PEDIATRIC & NEONATAL DOSAGE HANDBOOK

A Universal Resource for Clinicians
Treating Pediatric and Neonatal Patients

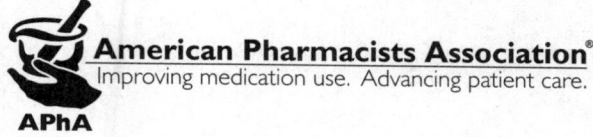

American Pharmacists Association®
Improving medication use. Advancing patient care.
APhA

Lexicomp is the official drug reference for the
American Pharmacists Association.

21st Edition

Carol K. Taketomo, PharmD
Jane H. Hodding, PharmD
Donna M. Kraus, PharmD, FAPhA, FCCP

Lexicomp®

PEDIATRIC & NEONATAL DOSAGE HANDBOOK

A Universal Resource for Clinicians
Treating Pediatric and Neonatal Patients

Carol K. Taketomo, PharmD
Director, Pharmacy and Nutritional Services
Children's Hospital Los Angeles
Los Angeles, California

Jane Hurlburt Hodding, PharmD
Executive Director, Pharmacy and Nutritional Services
Long Beach Memorial Medical Center and Miller Children's Hospital
Long Beach, California

Donna M. Kraus, PharmD, FAPhA, FPPAG, FCCP
Associate Professor of Pharmacy Practice
Departments of Pharmacy Practice and Pediatrics
Pediatric Clinical Pharmacist
University of Illinois at Chicago
Chicago, Illinois

Lexicomp®

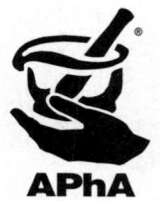

APhA

NOTICE

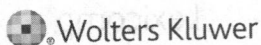

Lexicomp®

1100 Terex Road • Hudson, Ohio • 44236
(330) 650-6506

ISBN 978-1-59195-336-4 (Domestic Edition)

ISBN 978-1-59195-337-1 (International Edition)

Wolters Kluwer

TABLE OF CONTENTS

Preface... 2
Acknowledgments... 5
Neonatal Editorial Advisory Panel.. 5
Editorial Advisory Panel.. 6
About the Authors.. 7
Description of Sections and Fields Used in This Handbook.. 13
Definition of Age Group Terminology.. 14
Pregnancy Categories... 17
Abbreviations, Acronyms, and Symbols.. 18
Preventing Prescribing Errors... 19
FDA Name Differentiation Project: The Use of "Tall Man" Letters.. 29
Selected References.. 31

ALPHABETICAL LISTING OF DRUGS.. 34

APPENDIX 35
   Cardiology / Pulmonary.. 2189
   Comparative Drug Charts... 2191
   Conversion Tables.. 2219
   Cytochrome P450 Enzymes and Drug Metabolism.. 2244
   Dermatology.. 2247
   Endocrinology... 2255
   Gastroenterology and Nutrition.. 2266
   Growth and Development.. 2274
   Hematology / Oncology.. 2317
   Hepatology.. 2327
   Hotline Numbers... 2334
   Infectious Diseases / Immunology.. 2335
   Laboratory.. 2336
   Neonatology.. 2385
   Nephrology.. 2396
   Neurology... 2397
   Toxicology... 2402
   Miscellaneous... 2407
   2409

THERAPEUTIC CATEGORY & KEY WORD INDEX 2451

PREFACE

This twenty-first edition of the *Pediatric & Neonatal Dosage Handbook* is designed to be a practical and convenient guide to the dosing and usage of medications in neonates and children. The pediatric population is a dynamic group, with major changes in pharmacokinetics and pharmacodynamics taking place throughout infancy and childhood. Therefore, the need for the evaluation and establishment of medication dosing regimens in children of different ages is great.

Special considerations must be taken into account when dosing medications in pediatric and neonatal patients. Unfortunately, due to a lack of appropriate studies, most medications commonly used in neonates and children do not have FDA approved labeling for use in pediatric patients. Only 30% of drugs used in children in a 1988 survey carried FDA approval in their labeling. Seventy-five percent of medications listed in the *1990 Physicians' Desk Reference (PDR)* carried some type of precaution or disclaimer statement for use in children.[1] A more recent analysis of information in the 1998, 2002, and 2007 *PDR* found that although over 50% of prescription drug products carried FDA-approved labeling for use in pediatric patients, the percent of drugs with pediatric labeling actually **decreased** over time (1998: 55.9%; 2002: 54.3%; and 2007: 51.3%).[2] In addition, the number of drug entities with FDA-approved labeling for use in neonates decreased by 39% during this time frame. Another study found that 45% of parenteral medications used in the neonatal intensive care unit are not approved by the FDA for use in neonates.[3] Thus, further studies are needed to improve FDA drug labeling for pediatric patients, especially for neonates (and particularly preterm neonates).[4,5]

Investigations have also demonstrated the need for further improvement in FDA drug labeling for medications specifically used in critically ill children. One study found that 67% of medications used in a pediatric intensive care unit did not have FDA-approved labeling for use in pediatric patients or only had approval for use in limited age groups.[6] Of all drugs prescribed in a pediatric cardiac intensive care unit (CICU), 36% were prescribed "off-label" (ie, the drug did not have an FDA-approved labeled indication based on the patient's age); 94% of patients received one or more off-label medications; and the frequency of use of off-label drugs was higher in CICU patients who were younger, and in those with a higher severity of illness.[7] Considering the large number of medications without FDA-approved labeling that are used in critically ill neonates and children, further pediatric studies are clearly warranted to improve FDA drug labeling, and the safe and effective use of medications in these patients.

The FDA Modernization Act of 1997, the Children's Health Act of 2000, the Best Pharmaceuticals for Children Act of 2002, and the Pediatric Research Equity Act of 2003 have all helped to increase pediatric drug studies. The recent FDA Amendment Act of 2007, which was signed into law in September 2007, reauthorizes and amends the Pediatric Research Equity Act and the Best Pharmaceuticals for Children Act (Title IV and Title V, Public Law 110-85, 110th Congress). The Food and Drug Administration Safety and Innovation Act of 2012 renews and strengthens the Best Pharmaceuticals for Children Act and the Pediatric Research Equity Act by making these two laws permanent (and no longer subject to reauthorization every five years).

The FDA Modernization Act of 1997 (Section 111, Public Law 105-115, 105th Congress) **encouraged** pharmaceutical companies to conduct pediatric drug studies by allowing 6 months of market exclusivity to certain designated drugs. A list of drugs, for which additional pediatric information may produce pediatric healthcare benefits, was required by this law to be developed by the U.S. Department of Health and Human Services (HHS), with input from the American Academy of Pediatrics, the Pediatric Pharmacology Research Unit Network,[8] and the U.S. Pharmacopoeia. To date, the FDA has received 872 proposals from pharmaceutical companies to conduct pediatric drug studies under this Act (and subsequent acts) and has issued 449 written requests for studies. If these pediatric studies are completed as the FDA has specified, then these medications will qualify for the 6-month patent extension or additional market exclusivity. Two hundred two products have already had their marketing patents extended by this law and to date, 512 pediatric labeling changes have occurred.[9]

The pediatric section of the FDA Modernization Act was renewed by Congress and signed into law January 4, 2002. This new law, called the Best Pharmaceuticals for Children Act, reauthorized the use of the 6-month patent extension to **encourage** pharmaceutical companies to conduct pediatric drug research. This law called for the establishment of an Office of Pediatric Therapeutics within the FDA and established an FDA Pediatric Pharmacology Advisory Committee and a Pediatric Sub-committee of the Oncologic Drugs Advisory Committee. It also created a research fund for pediatric studies of drugs that are off patent, granted a special "priority status" to pediatric labeling changes, required the Department of Health and Human Services (along with the Institute of Medicine) to conduct a study to assess federally funded pediatric research, and called for the development of a Final Rule that required drug labeling to include a toll-free number to report adverse events.[10]

The Best Pharmaceuticals for Children Act was reauthorized, amended, and signed into law in September 2007, as part of the FDA Amendment Act of 2007.[9] This amended law establishes an internal review committee (the Pediatric Review Committee) within the FDA to review written requests that were issued and the submitted reports from drug manufacturers.[11] It also requires manufacturers who were granted a patent extension to revise pediatric labeling in a timely manner; reduces the patent extension from 6 months to 3 months for drugs with combined gross sales >1 billion dollars; prohibits the extension of market exclusivity for >9 months; requires manufacturers to explain why a pediatric formulation cannot be developed (when requested to perform pediatric studies); requires product labeling to include information about pediatric studies whether or not the studies demonstrate that the drug is safe and effective; requires the government to notify the public of pediatric drug formulations that were developed and studied and found to be safe and effective, but not introduced into the market within 1 year; and requires that a report be submitted to congress that assesses the use of patent extensions in making sure that medications used by pediatric patients are tested and properly labeled.[12]

The 1998 Pediatric Final Rule was an FDA regulation, titled "Regulations Requiring Manufacturers to Assess the Safety and Effectiveness of New Drugs and Biological Products in Pediatric Patients; Final Rule".[13] This important regulation **required** that manufacturers conduct pediatric studies for certain new and marketed drugs and biological products. This requirement was mandatory, and its scope included new drugs (ie, new chemical entities, new dosage forms, new indications, new routes of administration, and new dosing regimens) and certain marketed drugs (ie, where the drug product offered meaningful therapeutic benefit or had substantial use in pediatric patients, AND the absence of pediatric labeling posed a risk). This FDA regulation became effective April 1, 1999, but studies mandated under this rule were not required to be submitted to the FDA before ecember 2, 2000. The 1998 Pediatric Final Rule and the authority of the FDA to **require** manufacturers to conduct pediatric udies was challenged with a law suit. In March 2002, the FDA requested a 2-month stay on the lawsuit, so it could publish a otice and suspend the 1998 Pediatric Final Rule for 2 years. During the 2 year suspension of the Rule, the FDA planned to udy whether the Best Pharmaceuticals for Children Act of 2002 made the 1998 Final Rule unnecessary. After multiple rganizations lobbied Congress and the president, the Secretary of Health and Human Services announced in April 2002, that e FDA would continue to defend the Pediatric Final Rule of 1998 in court. However, on October 17, 2002, the U.S. District Court r the District of Columbia barred the FDA from enforcing the Pediatric Final Rule. Fortunately, Congress passed the Pediatric esearch Equity Act of 2003 (Public Law S.650, 108th Congress). This law essentially reinstates the Pediatric Final Rule and uthorizes the FDA to **require** pharmaceutical manufacturers to conduct pediatric studies of certain drugs and biological roducts. It also establishes an FDA Pediatric Advisory Committee. The Pediatric Research Equity Act was reauthorized, mended, and signed into law in September 2007, as part of the FDA Amendment Act of 2007.

he Children's Health Act of 2000 was signed into law on October 17, 2000. This important law establishes a Pediatric Research itiative (headed by the Director of the NIH) and provides funds to increase support for pediatric clinical research.

he Food and Drug Administration Safety and Innovation Act (FDASIA) was signed into law on July 9, 2012.[14] The pediatric rovisions of this law renew and strengthen the Best Pharmaceuticals for Children Act and the Pediatric Research Equity Act. DASIA makes both of these important Acts permanent and thus ensures that pediatric patients will have a permanent place in rug research and development. This new law requires a pediatric study plan to be submitted earlier by drug manufacturers ubject to the Pediatric Research Equity Act. It also gives the FDA new authority to help ensure that requirements of the Pediatric tesearch Equity Act are met in a more timely fashion. These requirements should help increase pediatric drug development and enerate pediatric drug information more quickly. FDASIA also addresses several neonatal concerns. It requires the Office of 'ediatric Therapeutics to include a member with expertise in a pediatric subgroup that is less likely to be studied under other aws, and specifies that for five years after enactment, this should include an individual with expertise in neonatology. The Act lso specifies that an FDA employee with expertise in neonatology should be a member of the Pediatric Review Committee. DASIA also requires Best Pharmaceuticals for Children Act requests for pediatric drug studies to include a rationale for not ncluding neonatal studies if none are requested. These requirements should help to increase neonatal drug information.

Vhile these important laws, plus other FDA regulations such as the FDA labeling changes[15] that required expanded information the Pediatric Use section of the package insert for all prescription drugs, will help to increase and disseminate pediatric and eonatal drug information; the practice of off-label prescribing in pediatric patients is a common occurrence.

urrently, however, most commonly used pharmacy references do not include information regarding pediatric and neonatal losing, drug administration, or special pediatric or neonatal concerns. It is, therefore, not surprising that in order to obtain ediatric and neonatal dosing information, oftentimes the pediatric clinician is faced with extensive literature searches to arrive at logical dose. This handbook serves as a compilation of recommended pediatric and neonatal doses found in the literature and rovides relevant clinical information regarding the use of drugs in neonates, children, and adolescents.[4]

New in This Edition

his new edition incorporates additions and revisions in a format that we hope the user will find beneficial.

s with each edition, drug monographs have been updated and revised, including updates to many monographs based on new uideline recommendations. Sixteen new monographs have been added: Adapalene and Benzoyl Peroxide, Anagrelide, Capreomycin, Cefditoren, Chenodiol, Dolutegravir, Entecavir, Etodolac, Hydrocodone and Chlorpheniramine, Hydrocodone nd Homatropine, Letrozole, Mitotane, Oxandrolone, Rifaxim, Tinidazole, and Vinorelbine. Three monographs have been leleted because the drugs are no longer available in the U.S.: Pemirolast; Piperacillin; and Sodium Nitrite, Sodium Thiosulfate, nd Amyl Nitrite. Also in this edition, the betamethasone monograph was split into two monographs based on the route: Betamethasone (Systemic) and Beatmethasone (Topical). This brings the total number of drug monographs to 997.

Eight appendix pieces were revised and updated: Carbohydrate Content of Medications; HIV appendices (Adult and Adolescent HIV, Pediatric HIV, Perinatal HIV); Immunization Guidelines; Oral Medications That Should Not Be Crushed or Altered; Pediatric Parenteral Nutrition; and Preprocedure Sedatives in Children.

Ve hope this edition continues to be a valuable and practical source of clinical drug information for the pediatric healthcare professional. We welcome comments to further improve future editions.

References

1. Food and Drug Letter, Washington Business Information, Inc. November 23, 1990.

2. Young L, Lawes F, Tordoff J, Norris P, Reith D. Access to prescribing information for paediatric medicines in the USA: post-modernization. *Br J Clin Pharmacol*. 2009;67(3):341-346.

3. Kumar P, Walker JK, Hurt KM, Bennett KM, Grosshans N, Fotis MA. Medication use in the neonatal intensive care unit: current patterns and off-label use of parenteral medications. *J Pediatr*. 2008;152:412.

4. American Academy of Pediatrics, Committee on Drugs. Off-label use of drugs in children. *Pediatrics*. 2014;133:563-567.

5. Milne CP, Davis J. The pediatric studies initiative: after 15 years have we reached the limits of the law? *Clinical Therapeutics*. 2014:36:156-162.

6. Yang CP, Veltri MA, Anton B, Taster M, Berkowitz ID. Food and Drug Administration approval for medications used in the pediatric intensive care unit: a continuing conundrum. *Pediatr Crit Care Med*. 2011;12:e195-e199.

7. Maltz LA, Klugman D, Spaeder MC, Wessel DL. Off-label drug use in a single-center pediatric cardiac intensive care unit. *World J Pediatr Congenital Heart Surg*. 2013;4:262-266.

8. NIH funds network of centers for pediatric drug research. *Am J Hosp Pharm*. 1994;51:2546.

9. http://www.fda.gov/Drugs/DevelopmentApprovalProcess/DevelopmentResources/ucm049867.htm

10. Birenbaum D. Pediatric initiatives: a regulatory perspective of the U.S. experience. 2002. Available at http://www.fda.gov/cder/pediatric/presentation/Ped_Init_2002_ DB/index.htm

11. Establishment of the Pediatric Review Committee, available at http://www.fda.gov/cder/pediatric/Pediatric_Review_Committee_Establishment%20_Memo.pdf

12. Ref B.S. 1156. The best pharmaceuticals for children amendments of 2007. Available at http://www.washingtonwatch.com/bills/show/110 SN 1156.html

13. "Department of Health and Human Services, Food and Drug Administration, 21CFR Parts 201, 312, 314, and 601 regulations requiring manufacturers to assess the safety and effectiveness of new drugs and biological products in pediatric patients; final rule. *Fed Regist.* 1998;63(231):66631-66672.

14. Food and Drug Administration Safety and Innovation Act (FDASIA), Title V - Pediatric Drugs and Devices, Public Law 112-144, 112th Congress, July 9, 2012. Available at http://www.gpo.gov/fdsys/pkg/PLAW-112publ144/pdf/PLAW-112publ144.pdf

15. "Pediatric use drug labeling NDA supplements due by December 1996 - FDA final rule; agency establishing pediatric subcommittee to track implementation. *F-D-C Reports - The Pink Sheet.* Wallace Werble Jr, Publisher; 1994.

ACKNOWLEDGMENTS

Special acknowledgement goes to all Lexicomp staff for their contributions to this handbook.

The authors wish to thank their families, friends, and colleagues who supported them in their efforts to complete this handbook.

Special thanks goes to Chris Lomax, PharmD, who played a significant role in bringing APhA and Lexicomp together.

In addition, Dr Taketomo would like to thank Robert Taketomo, PharmD, MBA for his professional guidance and continued support, and the pharmacy staff at Children's Hospital, Los Angeles, for their assistance.

Dr Kraus would like to especially thank Keith A. Rodvold, PharmD, for his ongoing professional and personal support, and the pediatric and neonatal clinical pharmacists at the Children's Hospital University of Illinois for their assistance.

Dr Hodding would like to thank Glenn Hodding, PharmD; Neepa Rai, PharmD; and the pediatric pharmacists at Miller Children's Hospital for their continued professional and personal support.

Some of the material contained in this book was a result of pediatric pharmacy contributors throughout the United States and Canada. Lexicomp has assisted many pediatric medical institutions to develop hospital-specific formulary manuals that contain clinical drug information as well as dosing. Working with these pediatric clinical pharmacists, pediatric hospital pharmacy and therapeutics committees, and hospital drug information centers, Lexicomp has developed an evolutionary drug database that reflects the practice of pediatric pharmacy in these major pediatric institutions.

Special thanks to Jenny Campbell of Campbell and Co. Cartooning, Chagrin Falls, Ohio, who makes our *Pediatric & Neonatal Dosage Handbook* come alive with her wonderful cover illustrations.

NEONATAL EDITORIAL ADVISORY PANEL

EDITORIAL ADVISORY PANEL

8

effrey P. Gonzales, PharmD, BCPS
ritical Care Clinical Pharmacy Specialist
niversity of Maryland Medical Center

ohn Grabenstein, RPh, PhD, FAPhA
harmacotherapy Contributor
Volters Kluwer Health

Roland Grad, MDCM, MSc, CCFP, FCFP
ssociate Professor
epartment of Family Medicine
IcGill University

arry D. Gray, PhD, ABMM
irector, Clinical Microbiology
riHealth Laboratories
ethesda and Good Samaritan Hospitals

racy Hagemann, PharmD
ssociate Professor
ollege of Pharmacy
he University of Oklahoma

IoEllen L. Hanigosky, PharmD
linical Coordinator
epartment of Hematology/Oncology/Bone Marrow Transplant
hildren's Hospital of Akron

Martin D. Higbee, PharmD
ssociate Professor
epartment of Pharmacy Practice and Science
he University of Arizona

lane Hurlburt Hodding, PharmD
xecutive Director, Inpatient Pharmacy Services and Clinical Nutrition Services
ong Beach Memorial Medical Center and Miller Children's Hospital

Mark T. Holdsworth, PharmD
Associate Professor of Pharmacy & Pediatrics
and *Pharmacy Practice Area Head*
ollege of Pharmacy
he University of New Mexico

Edward Horn, PharmD, BCPS
Clinical Specialist, Transplant Surgery
Allegheny General Hospital

Collin A. Hovinga, PharmD
Director of Research and *Associate Professor*
Dell Children's Medical Center
UT Austin School of Pharmacy

Darrell T. Hulisz, PharmD
Associate Professor
Department of Family Medicine
Case Western Reserve University

Douglas L. Jennings, PharmD, BCPS
Clinical Pharmacy Specialist, Cardiovascular Surgery
Jackson Memorial Hospital

Sallie Johnson, PharmD, BCPS, AQ Cardiology
Clinical Pharmacy Specialist, Cardiology
Penn State Milton S. Hershey Medical Center

Michael A. Kahn, DDS
Professor and Chairman
Department of Oral and Maxillofacial Pathology
Tufts University School of Dental Medicine

Jeannette Kaiser, MT, MBA
Medical Technologist
Akron General Medical Center

Julie J. Kelsey, PharmD
Clinical Specialist
Women's Health and Family Medicine
Department of Pharmacy Services
University of Virginia Health System

Patrick J. Kiel, PharmD, BCPS, BCOP
Clinical Pharmacy Specialist
Hematology and Stem Cell Transplant
Indiana University Simon Cancer Center

Polly E. Kintzel, PharmD, BCPS, BCOP
Clinical Pharmacy Specialist-Oncology
Spectrum Health

Michael Klepser, PharmD, FCCP
Professor of Pharmacy
Department of Pharmacy Practice
Ferris State University

Daren Knoell, PharmD
Associate Professor of Pharmacy Practice and Internal Medicine
Davis Heart and Lung Research Institute
The Ohio State University

David Knoppert, MScPhm, FCCP, MSc, FCSHP
Clinical Leader - Paediatrics
Pharmacy Services
London Health Sciences Centre
Children's Health Research Institute

Sandra Knowles, RPh, BScPhm
Drug Policy Research Specialist
Li Ka Shing Institute
St. Michael's Hospital

Jill M. Kolesar, PharmD, FCCP, BCPS
Associate Professor
School of Pharmacy
University of Wisconsin Paul P. Carbone Comprehensive Cancer Center

Susannah E. Koontz, PharmD, BCOP
Principal and Consultant
Pediatric Hematology/Oncology and Stem Cell Transplantation/Cellular Therapy
Koontz Oncology Consulting, LLC

Donna M. Kraus, PharmD, FAPhA, FPPAG, FCCP
Associate Professor of Pharmacy Practice
and *Pediatric Clinical Pharmacist*
Departments of Pharmacy Practice and Pediatrics
University of Illinois

Daniel L. Krinsky, RPh, MS
Manager, MTM Services
Giant Eagle Pharmacy
Assistant Professor
Department of Pharmacy Practice
Northeast Ohio Medical University (NEOMED)

Tim T.Y. Lau, PharmD, ACPR, FCSHP
Pharmacotherapeutic Specialist in Infectious Diseases
Pharmaceutical Sciences
Vancouver General Hospital

Mandy C. Leonard, PharmD, BCPS
Assistant Professor
Cleveland Clinic Lerner College of Medicine of Case Western University
Assistant Director, Drug Information Services
Cleveland Clinic

Jennifer L. Placencia, PharmD
Neonatal Clinical Pharmacy Specialist
Texas Children's Hospital

James A. Ponto, MS, RPh, BCNP
Chief Nuclear Pharmacist
Department of Radiology
University of Iowa, Hospitals and Clinics
Professor of Clinical Pharmacy
Department of Pharmacy Practice and Science
University of Iowa College of Pharmacy

Amy L. Potts, PharmD, BCPS
Assistant Director
Department of Pharmacy
PGY1 & PGY2 Residency Program Director
Monroe Carell Jr. Children's Hospital at Vanderbilt

Sally Rafie, PharmD, BCPS
Medical Safety Pharmacist
UC San Diego Health System

Esta Razavi, PharmD
Clinical Editor
Wolters Kluwer Health

James Reissig, PharmD
Assistant Director, Clinical Services
Akron General Medical Center

A.J. (Fred) Remillard, PharmD
Assistant Dean, Research and Graduate Affairs
College of Pharmacy and Nutrition
University of Saskatchewan

Elizabeth Rich, RN, BSN, BA
Registered Nurse – Critical Care
Hillcrest Hospital

Curtis M. Rimmermann, MD, MBA, FACC
Gus P. Karos Chair
Clinical Cardiovascular Medicine
Cleveland Clinic

Renee Rivard, PharmD
Consultant, Independent Medical Writer
Wolters Kluwer Health

P. David Rogers, PharmD, PhD, FCCP
Director, Clinical and Translational Therapeutics
University of Tennessee College of Pharmacy

James L. Rutkowski, DMD, PhD
Editor-in-Chief
Journal of Oral Implantology

Amy Rybarczyk, PharmD, BCPS
Pharmacotherapy Specialist, Internal Medicine
Akron General Medical Center

Jennifer K. Sekeres, PharmD, BCPS
Infectious Diseases Clinical Specialist
Cleveland Clinic

Todd P. Semla, MS, PharmD, BCPS, FCCP, AGSF
National PBM Clinical Program Manager – Mental Health & Geriatrics
Department of Veterans Affairs
Pharmacy Benefits Management Services
Associate Professor, Clinical
Department of Medicine, Psychiatry and Behavioral Health
Feinberg School of Medicine
Northwestern University

Chasity M. Shelton, PharmD, BCPS, BCNSP
Assistant Professor of Clinical Pharmacy
Department of Clinical Pharmacy
Neonatal Clinical Pharmacy Specialist
University of Tennessee Health Science Center

Vanessa Sherwood, BSc
Drug Information Pharmacist
IWK Pharmacy, Operations and Support Services

Pamela J. Sims, PharmD, PhD
Professor
Department of Pharmaceutical, Social, and Administrative Sciences
McWhorter School of Pharmacy
Samford University

Grant Sklar, PharmD, BCPS
Assistant Professor, Department of Pharmacy
and *Principal Clinical Pharmacist, General Medicine*
National University Hospital of Singapore

Joseph Snoke, RPh, BCPS
Manager
Core Pharmacology Group
Wolters Kluwer Health

Patricia L. Spenard, PharmD
Clinical Editor
Wolters Kluwer Health

Joni Lombardi Stahura, BS, PharmD, RPh
Pharmacotherapy Specialist
Wolters Kluwer Health

Kim Stevens, RN
Home Care
Samaritan Regional Health System

Stephen Marc Stout, PharmD, MS, BCPS
Pharmacotherapy Specialist
Wolters Kluwer Health

Dan Streetman, PharmD, RPh
Pharmacotherapy Specialist
Wolters Kluwer Health

Darcie-Ann Streetman, PharmD, RPh
Pharmacotherapy Specialist
Wolters Kluwer Health

Carol K. Taketomo, PharmD
Director of Pharmacy and Nutrition Services
Children's Hospital Los Angeles

Mary Temple-Cooper, PharmD
Pediatric Clinical Research Specialist
Hillcrest Hospital

Kelan Thomas, PharmD, MS, BCPS, BCPP
Assistant Professor of Pharmacy Practice
Touro University California, College of Pharmacy
Clinical Pharmacist
St. Helena Hospital Center for Behavioral Health Office

Elizabeth A. Tomsik, PharmD, BCPS
Senior Director
Content
Wolters Kluwer Health

Dana Travis, RPh
Pharmacotherapy Specialist
Wolters Kluwer Health

ABOUT THE AUTHORS

Carol K. Taketomo, PharmD

Dr Taketomo received her doctorate from the University of Southern California School of Pharmacy. Subsequently, she completed a clinical pharmacy residency at the University of California Medical Center in San Diego. With over 30 years of clinical experience at one of the largest pediatric teaching hospitals in the nation, she is an acknowledged expert in the practical aspects of pediatric drug distribution and clinical pharmacy practice. She currently holds the appointment of Adjunct Assistant Professor of Pharmacy Practice at the University of Southern California School of Pharmacy.

In her current capacity as Director of Pharmacy and Nutritional Services at Children's Hospital of Los Angeles, Dr Taketomo plays an active role in the education and training of the medical, pharmacy, and nursing staff. She coordinates the Pharmacy Department's quality assurance and drug use evaluation programs, maintains the hospital's strict formulary program, and is the editor of the house staff manual. Her particular interests are strategies to influence physician prescribing patterns, introducing LEAN concepts into clinical practice and transitions of care, and methods to decrease medication errors in the pediatric setting. She has been the author of numerous publications and is an active presenter at professional meetings.

Dr Taketomo is a member of the American Pharmacists Association (APhA), American Society of Health-System Pharmacists (ASHP), California Society of Hospital Pharmacists (CSHP), and Southern California Pediatric Pharmacy Group.

Jane Hurlburt Hodding, PharmD

Dr Hodding earned a doctorate and completed her pharmacy residency at the University of California School of Pharmacy (UCSF) in San Francisco. She has held teaching positions as Assistant Clinical Professor of Pharmacy at UCSF as well as Assistant Clinical Professor of Pharmacy Practice at the University of Southern California in Los Angeles and now holds the position of Assistant Dean at UCSF School of Pharmacy. Currently, Dr Hodding is the Executive Director, Pharmacy and Nutritional Services at Long Beach Memorial and Miller Children's Hospital in Long Beach, California.

Throughout her 34 years of pediatric pharmacy practice, Dr Hodding has actively pursued methods to improve the safety of medication use in neonates, children, and adolescents. She has actively practiced as a clinical pharmacy specialist in neonatal intensive care, pediatric intensive care, and pediatric hematology/oncology. Parenteral nutrition is another area of focus. She has published numerous articles covering neonatal medication administration and aminoglycoside and theophylline clearance in premature infants.

Dr Hodding is a member of the American Pharmacists Association (APhA), American Society of Health-System Pharmacists (ASHP), and California Society of Hospital Pharmacists (CSHP). She is frequently an invited speaker on the topics of Medication Safety in Children, A Multidisciplinary Approach; Monitoring Drug Therapy in the NICU; Fluid and Electrolyte Therapy in Children; Drug Therapy Considerations in Children; and Parenteral Nutrition in the Premature Infant.

Donna M. Kraus, PharmD, FAPhA, FPPAG, FCCP

Dr Kraus received her Bachelor of Science in Pharmacy from the University of Illinois at Chicago (UIC). She worked for several years as a hospital pediatric/obstetric satellite pharmacist before earning her doctorate degree at the UIC. Dr Kraus then completed a postdoctoral pediatric specialty residency at the University of Texas Health Science Center in San Antonio. She served as a pediatric intensive care clinical pharmacist for 15 years and for the past 16 years has been an ambulatory care pediatric clinical pharmacist, specializing in pediatric HIV pharmacotherapy and patient/parent medication adherence. Dr Kraus has also served as a clinical pharmacist consultant to a pediatric long-term care facility for over 21 years. She currently holds the appointment of Associate Professor of Pharmacy Practice in both the Departments of Pharmacy Practice and Pediatrics at the University of Illinois in Chicago.

In her 37 years of active pharmacy experience, Dr Kraus has dealt with pediatric pharmacy issues and pharmacotherapy problems. She is an active educator and has been a guest lecturer in China, Thailand, and Hong Kong. Dr Kraus has played a leading role in the advanced training of postgraduate pharmacists and has been the Director of the UIC (ASHP accredited) Pediatric Residency and Fellowship Program for 27 years. Dr Kraus' research areas include pediatric drug dosing and developmental pharmacokinetics and pharmacodynamics. She has published a number of articles on various issues of pediatric pharmacy and pharmacotherapy.

Dr Kraus has been an active member of numerous professional associations including the American Pharmacists Association (APhA), American Society of Health-System Pharmacists (ASHP), Illinois Pharmacists Association (IPhA), American College of Clinical Pharmacy (ACCP), and Illinois College of Clinical Pharmacy (ICCP). She has served as Chairperson of the ASHP Commission on Therapeutics; member of the Board of Directors of the Pediatric Pharmacy Advocacy Group (PPAG); Member-at-Large of the Academy of Pharmaceutical Research and Science (APhA); member of the ASHP, Commission on Credentialing, Design/Writing Group, Educational Outcomes, Goals and Objectives for Postgraduate Year Two (PGY2) Pediatric Pharmacy Residency Programs (2007); member of the Alliance for Pediatric Quality, Improve First Measures Task Force; and member of the PPAG Advisory Board. Dr Kraus also served as an Editorial Board member of the *American Journal of Health-System Pharmacy* and the *Journal of Pediatric Pharmacy Practice*. Currently, she serves as an Editorial Board member of *The Journal of Pediatric Pharmacology and Therapeutics*. Dr Kraus was recently named by PPAG as the 2013 recipient of the Richard A. Helms Award of Excellence in Pediatric Pharmacy Practice. This award recognizes sustained and meritorious contributions to PPAG and to pediatric pharmacy practice; and contributions of importance to education, new knowledge, and outreach. Dr Kraus has been awarded Fellow status by the American Pharmacists Association, the Pediatric Pharmacy Advocacy Group, and the American College of Clinical Pharmacy. She is the APhA designated author for this handbook.

DESCRIPTION OF SECTIONS AND FIELDS USED IN THIS HANDBOOK

The *Pediatric* & *Neonatal Dosage Handbook, 21st edition* is organized into a drug information section, an appendix, and a therapeutic category & key word index.

Drug information is presented in a consistent format and provides the following:

Generic Name	U.S. adopted name. "Tall Man" lettering appears for look-alike generic drug names as recommended by the FDA. See "FDA Differentiation Project: The Use of 'Tall Man' Letters" on page 31.
Pronunciation	Phonetic pronunciation guide
Medication Safety Issues	In an effort to promote the safe use of medications, this field is intended to highlight possible sources of medication errors such as sound-alike/look-alike drugs or highly concentrated formulations which require vigilance on the part of health care professionals. In addition, medications which have been associated with severe consequences in the event of a medication error are also identified in this field.
Related Information	Cross-reference to other pertinent drug information found in the Appendix.
Brand Names: U.S.	Trade names (manufacturer-specific) found in the United States. The symbol [DSC] appears after trade names that have been recently discontinued.
Brand Names: Canada	Trade names found in Canada
Therapeutic Category	Unique systematic classification of medications
Generic Availability (U.S.)	Indicates availability of generic products in the United States
Use	Information pertaining to appropriate indications or use of the drug. Labeled uses will be indicated in parentheses by "FDA-approved in", followed by the specific patient population. "FDA-approved in all ages" denotes ages day 0 through adult. This specific FDA approval information is currently being phased in to all monographs. Age-specific FDA approval may not be present in some monographs; product labeling should be consulted for additional detail. Uses mentioned at the end of the section without "FDA-approved" language are unique off-label pediatric uses.
Prescribing and Access Restrictions	Provides information on any special requirements regarding the prescribing, obtaining, or dispensing of drugs, including access restrictions pertaining to drugs with REMS elements and those drugs with access restrictions that are not REMS-related
Medication Guide Available	Identifies drugs that have an FDA-approved Medication Guide
Pregnancy Risk Factor	Five categories established by the FDA to indicate the potential of a systemically absorbed drug for causing risk to fetus
Pregnancy Considerations	A summary of human and/or animal information pertinent to or associated with the use of the drug as it relates to clinical effects on the fetus, newborn, or pregnant women
Breast-Feeding Considerations	A summary of available information pertinent to or associated with the human use of the drug as it relates to clinical effects on the nursing infant or postpartum woman
Contraindications	Information pertaining to disease states and patient populations in which the drug should not be used
Warnings	Hazardous conditions related to use of the drug; the notation **[U.S. Boxed Warning]** immediately follows information which has been adapted from the boxed warnings of the FDA-approved labeling. Consult the product labeling for the exact wording of black box warning through the manufacturer's or the FDA website.
Precautions	Disease states or patient populations in which the drug should be cautiously used
Adverse Reactions	Side effects are grouped by body system and include a listing of the more common and/or serious side effects. Due to space limitations, every reported side effect is not listed.
Drug Interactions	
Metabolism/Transport Effects	If a drug has demonstrated involvement with cytochrome P450 enzymes, or other metabolism or transport proteins, this field will identify the drug as an inhibitor, inducer, or substrate of the specific enzyme(s) (eg, CYP1A2 or UGT1A1). CYP450 isoenzymes are identified as substrates (minor or major), inhibitors (weak, moderate, or strong), and inducers (weak or strong).
Avoid Concomitant Use	Designates drug combinations which should not be used concomitantly, due to an unacceptable risk:benefit assessment. Frequently, the concurrent use of the agents is explicitly prohibited or contraindicated by the product labeling
Increased Effect/Toxicity	Drug combinations that result in a increased or toxic therapeutic effect between the drug listed in the monograph and other drugs or drug classes

Decreased Effect	Drug combinations that result in a decreased therapeutic effect between the drug listed in the monograph and other drugs or drug classes
Food Interactions	Possible important interactions between the drug listed in the monograph and food, alcohol, or other beverages
Stability	Storage, refrigeration, and compatibility information
Mechanism of Action	How the drug works in the body to elicit a response
Pharmacodynamics	Dose-response relationships including onset of action, time of peak action, and duration of action
Pharmacokinetics	Drug movement through the body over time. Pharmacokinetics deals with absorption, distribution, protein binding, metabolism, bioavailability, half-life, time to peak concentration, elimination, and clearance of drugs. Pharmacokinetic parameters help predict drug concentration and dosage requirements. Information is adult data unless noted.
Dosing: Neonatal	The amount of the drug to be typically given or taken during therapy; may also include dosing information for preterm neonates. Please note that doses for neonates may be listed by variable parameters: Postnatal age (PNA) (eg, PNA ≤7 days), gestational age (GA), postmenstrual age (PMA), and/or by body weight (eg, 1200 to 2000 g or 1.2 to 2 kg). Neonatal-specific dosing adjustment in renal impairment for select drugs will be provided in this field if available. For additional information, consult **Dosing: Usual** field for suggested renal impairment adjustment.
Dosing: Usual	The amount of the drug to be typically given or taken during therapy; may include dosing information for infants, children, adolescents, and adults. Dosing information not from product labeling will have a citation and supporting reference at the end of monograph.

When both fixed-milligram doses and weight-based, milligram per kilogram (mg/kg) doses are listed, the milligram per kilogram dosing method is preferred. When weight-based (mg/kg) and maximum doses are provided, use the weight-based (mg/kg) dose to calculate the milligram dose for the patient, but do **not** exceed the maximum dose listed. A *usual* maximum dose may be exceeded only if clinically indicated. Do **not** exceed adult maximum dosage unless otherwise noted. If using a fixed-milligram dosing guideline according to age, special care and lower doses should be used in children who have a low weight for their age. When ranges of doses are listed, initiate therapy at the lower end of the range and titrate the dose accordingly.

For select drugs, the dosing adjustment in renal impairment or dosing interval in renal impairment is given according to creatinine clearance (CrCl). Since most studies that recommend dosing guidelines in renal dysfunction are conducted in adult patients, CrCl is usually expressed in units of mL/minute. However, in order to extrapolate the adult information to the pediatric population, one must assume that the adults studied were of standard surface area (ie, 1.73 m^2). Therefore, although the value of CrCl listed for dosing adjustment in renal impairment or dosing interval in renal impairment may be expressed in mL/minute, it is assumed to be equal to the same value in mL/minute/1.73 m^2.

To calculate the dose in a pediatric patient with renal dysfunction, first calculate the normal dose (ie, the dose for a patient without renal dysfunction), then use the guidelines to adjust the dose. For example, the normal piperacillin dose for a 20 kg child is 200 to 300 mg/kg/day divided every 4 to 6 hours. If one selected 300 mg/kg/day divided every 6 hours, the dose would be 1.5 g every 6 hours in normal renal function. If CrCl was 20 to 40 mL/minute/1.73 m^2, the dose would be 1.5 g every 8 hours and if CrCl was <20 mL/minute/1.73 m^2, the dose would be 1.5 g every 12 hours. Dosing adjustments in renal impairment are adult data, unless otherwise indicated.

Usual Infusion Concentrations: Neonatal	Information describing the usual concentrations of drugs for continuous infusion administration in the neonatal population, as appropriate. Concentrations are derived from the literature, manufacturer recommendation, or organizational recommendations (eg, the Institute for Safe Medication Practices [ISMP]) and are universally established. Institution-specific standard concentrations may differ from those listed.
Usual Infusion Concentrations: Pediatric	Information describing the usual concentrations of drugs for continuous infusion administration in pediatric population, as appropriate. Concentrations are derived from the literature, manufacturer recommendation, or organizational recommendations (eg, the Institute for Safe Medication Practices [ISMP]) and are universally established. Institution-specific standard concentrations may differ from those listed.
Administration	Information regarding the recommended reconstitution, final concentration, and rate for administration of parenteral drugs are listed when appropriate, along with pertinent oral, ophthalmic, and topical administration information.
Vesicant/Extravasation Risk	Indicates whether the drug is considered to be a vesicant and likely to cause significant morbidity if the infusion infiltrates soft tissues
Monitoring Parameters	Laboratory tests and patient physical parameters that should be monitored for safety and efficacy of drug therapy are listed when appropriate.

Reference Range	Therapeutic drug concentrations, such as specific target concentrations, timing of serum samples, etc; toxic serum concentrations are listed when appropriate
Test Interactions	Listing of assay interferences when relevant; (S) = Serum; (U) = Urine; (B) = Blood
Additional Information	Other data and facts about the drug are offered when appropriate.
Product Availability	Provides availability information on products that have been approved by the FDA, but are not yet available for use. Estimates for when a product may be available are included, when this information is known. May also provide any unique or critical drug availability issues.
Controlled Substance	Contains controlled substance schedule information as assigned by the United States Drug Enforcement Administration (DEA) or Canadian Controlled Substance Act (CDSA). CDSA information is only provided for drugs available in Canada and not available in the U.S.
Dosage Forms Considerations	More specific information regarding product concentrations, ingredients, package sizes, amount of doses per container, and other important details pertaining to various formulations of medications
Dosage Forms	Information with regard to form, strength, and availability of the drug in the United States. **Note:** Additional formulation information (eg, excipients, preservatives) is included when available. Please consult labeling for further information.
Extemporaneous Preparations	Directions for preparing liquid formulations from solid drug products. May include stability information and references.
References	Bibliographic information referring to specific pediatric literature findings, especially doses

Appendix

The appendix offers a compilation of tables, guidelines, and conversion information which can often be helpful when considering patient care. This section is broken down into various sections for ease of use.

Therapeutic Category & Key Word Index

This index provides a useful listing of an easy-to-use therapeutic classification system. Also listed are controlled substances and preservative free, sugar free, dye free, and alcohol free medications.

DEFINITION OF AGE GROUP TERMINOLOGY

formation in this handbook is listed according to specific age or by age group. The following are definitions of age groups and e-related terminologies. These definitions should be used unless otherwise specified in the monograph.

Gestational age (GA)[1]	The time from conception until birth. More specifically, gestational age is defined as the number of weeks from the first day of the mother's last menstrual period (LMP) until the birth of the baby. Gestational age at birth is assessed by the date of the LMP and by physical exam (Dubowitz score).
Postnatal age (PNA)[1]	Chronological age since birth
Postmenstrual age (PMA)[1]	Postmenstrual age is calculated as gestational age plus postnatal age (PMA = GA + PNA).
Neonate	A full-term newborn 0 to 28 days postnatal age. Some experts may also apply this terminology to a premature neonate who is >28 days but whose postmenstrual age (PMA) is ≤42 to 46 weeks.
Premature neonate[2]	Neonate born at <37 weeks gestational age
Term neonate[2]	Neonate born at 37 weeks 0 days to 41 weeks 6 days (average ~40 weeks) gestational age
Infant	1 month (>28 days) to 12 months of age
Child/Children	1 to 12 years of age
Adolescent	13 to 18 years of age
Adult	>18 years of age

[1]Engle WA; American Academy of Pediatrics Committee on Fetus and Newborn. Age terminology during the perinatal period. *Pediatrics.* 2004;114 (5):1362-1364.
[2]Fleischman AR, Oinuma M, Clark SL. Rethinking the definition of 'term pregnancy'. *Obstet Gynecol.* 2010;116(1):136-139.

PREGNANCY CATEGORIES

Pregnancy Categories (sometimes referred to as pregnancy risk factors) are a letter system currently required under the *Teratogenic Effects* subsection of the product labeling. The system was initiated in 1979. The categories are required to be part of the package insert for prescription drugs that are systemically absorbed.

The categories are defined as follows:

A   Adequate and well-controlled studies in pregnant women have not shown that the drug increases the risk of fetal abnormalities.

B   Animal reproduction studies show no evidence of impaired fertility or harm to the fetus; however, no adequate and well-controlled studies have been conducted in pregnant women.
or
Animal reproduction studies have shown adverse events; however, studies in pregnant women have not shown that the drug increases the risk of abnormalities.

C   Animal reproduction studies have shown an adverse effect on the fetus. There are no adequate and well-controlled studies in humans and the benefits from the use of the drug in pregnant women may be acceptable, despite its potential risks.
or
Animal reproduction studies have not been conducted.

D   Based on human data, the drug can cause fetal harm when administered to pregnant women, but the potential benefits from the use of the drug may be acceptable, despite its potential risks.

X   Studies in animals or humans have demonstrated fetal abnormalities (or there is positive evidence of fetal risk based on reports and/or marketing experience) and the risk of using the drug in pregnant women clearly outweighs any possible benefit (for example, safer drugs or other forms of therapy are available).

The categories do not take into consideration nonteratogenic effects (that information is currently presented separately). In 2008, the Food and Drug Administration (FDA) proposed new labeling requirements which would eliminate the use of the pregnancy category system and replace it with scientific data and other information specific to the use of the drug in pregnant women. These proposed changes were suggested because the current category system may be misleading. For instance, some practitioners may believe that risk increases from category A to B to C to D to X, which is not the intent. In addition, practitioners may not be aware that some medications are categorized based on animal data, while others are based on human data. When the new labeling requirements are approved, product labeling will contain pregnancy and lactation subsections, each describing a risk summary, clinical considerations, and section for specific data.

For full descriptions of the current and proposed labeling requirements, refer to the following websites:

Labeling Requirements for Prescription Drugs and/or Insulin (Code of Federal Regulations, Title 21, Volume 4, Revised April 1, 2010). http://www.accessdata.fda.gov/scripts/cdrh/cfdocs/cfCFR/CFRSearch.cfm?fr=201.57

Content and Format of Labeling for Human Prescription Drug and Biological Products; Requirements for Pregnancy and Lactation Labeling (Federal Register, May 29, 2008). https://www.federalregister.gov/articles/2008/05/29/E8-11806/content-and-format-of-labeling-for-human-prescription-drug-and-biological-products-requirements-for

ABBREVIATIONS, ACRONYMS, AND SYMBOLS

Abbreviations Which May Be Used in This Reference

Abbreviation	Meaning
½NS	0.45% sodium chloride
5-HT	5-hydroxytryptamine
AACT	American Academy of Clinical Toxicology
AAP	American Academy of Pediatrics
AAPC	antibiotic-associated pseudomembranous colitis
ABG	arterial blood gases
ABMT	autologous bone marrow transplant
ABW	adjusted body weight
ACC	American College of Cardiology
ACE	angiotensin-converting enzyme
ACLS	advanced cardiac life support
ACOG	American College of Obstetricians and Gynecologists
ACTH	adrenocorticotrophic hormone
ADH	antidiuretic hormone
ADHD	attention-deficit/hyperactivity disorder
ADI	adequate daily intake
ADLs	activities of daily living
AED	antiepileptic drug
AHA	American Heart Association
AHCPR	Agency for Health Care Policy and Research
AIDS	acquired immunodeficiency syndrome
AIMS	Abnormal Involuntary Movement Scale
ALL	acute lymphoblastic leukemia
ALS	amyotrophic lateral sclerosis
ALT	alanine aminotransferase (formerly called SGPT)
AMA	American Medical Association
AML	acute myeloblastic leukemia
ANA	antinuclear antibodies
ANC	absolute neutrophil count
ANLL	acute nonlymphoblastic leukemia
aPTT	activated partial thromboplastin time
ARB	angiotensin receptor blocker
ARDS	acute respiratory distress syndrome
ASA-PS	American Society of Anesthesiologists – Physical Status P1: Normal, healthy patient P2: Patient having mild systemic disease P3: Patient having severe systemic disease P4: Patient having severe systemic disease which is a constant threat to life P5: Moribund patient; not expected to survive without the procedure P6: Patient declared brain-dead; organs being removed for donor purposes
AST	aspartate aminotransferase (formerly called SGOT)
ATP	adenosine triphosphate
AUC	area under the curve (area under the serum concentration-time curve)
A-V	atrial-ventricular
BDI	Beck Depression Inventory
BEC	blood ethanol concentration
BLS	basic life support
BMI	body mass index
BMT	bone marrow transplant
BP	blood pressure
BPD	bronchopulmonary disease or dysplasia

Abbreviations Which May Be Used in This Reference (continued)

Abbreviation	Meaning
BPH	benign prostatic hyperplasia
BPRS	Brief Psychiatric Rating Scale
BSA	body surface area
BUN	blood urea nitrogen
CABG	coronary artery bypass graft
CAD	coronary artery disease
CADD	computer ambulatory drug delivery
cAMP	cyclic adenosine monophosphate
CAN	Canadian
CAPD	continuous ambulatory peritoneal dialysis
CAS	chemical abstract service
CBC	complete blood count
CBT	cognitive behavioral therapy
CDC	Centers for Disease Control and Prevention
CF	cystic fibrosis
CFC	chlorofluorocarbons
CGI	Clinical Global Impression
CHD	coronary heart disease
CHF	congestive heart failure; chronic heart failure
CI	cardiac index
CIE	chemotherapy-induced emesis
C-II	schedule two controlled substance
C-III	schedule three controlled substance
C-IV	schedule four controlled substance
C-V	schedule five controlled substance
CIV	continuous I.V. infusion
CLL	chronic lymphocytic leukemia
C_{max}	maximum plasma concentration
C_{min}	minimum plasma concentration
CML	chronic myelogenous leukemia
CMV	cytomegalovirus
CNS	central nervous system or coagulase negative staphylococcus
COLD	chronic obstructive lung disease
COPD	chronic obstructive pulmonary disease
COX	cyclooxygenase
CPK	creatine phosphokinase
CPR	cardiopulmonary resuscitation
CrCl	creatinine clearance
CRF	chronic renal failure
CRP	C-reactive protein
CRRT	continuous renal replacement therapy
CSF	cerebrospinal fluid
CSII	continuous subcutaneous insulin infusion
CT	computed tomography
CVA	cerebrovascular accident
CVP	central venous pressure
CVVH	continuous venovenous hemofiltration
CVVHD	continuous venovenous hemodialysis
CVVHDF	continuous venovenous hemodiafiltration
CYP	cytochrome
$D_5\frac{1}{4}NS$	dextrose 5% in sodium chloride 0.2%
$D_5\frac{1}{2}NS$	dextrose 5% in sodium chloride 0.45%
D_5LR	dextrose 5% in lactated Ringer's

Abbreviations Which May Be Used in This Reference (continued)

Abbreviation	Meaning
D₅NS	dextrose 5% in sodium chloride 0.9%
D₅W	dextrose 5% in water
D₁₀W	dextrose 10% in water
DBP	diastolic blood pressure
DEHP	di(3-ethylhexyl)phthalate
DIC	disseminated intravascular coagulation
DL_co	pulmonary diffusion capacity for carbon monoxide
DM	diabetes mellitus
DMARD	disease modifying antirheumatic drug
DNA	deoxyribonucleic acid
DSC	discontinued
DSM-IV	Diagnostic and Statistical Manual
DVT	deep vein thrombosis
EBV	Epstein-Barr virus
ECG	electrocardiogram
ECHO	echocardiogram
ECMO	extracorporeal membrane oxygenation
ECT	electroconvulsive therapy
ED	emergency department
EEG	electroencephalogram
EF	ejection fraction
EG	ethylene glycol
EGA	estimated gestational age
eGFR	estimated glomerular filtration rate
EIA	enzyme immunoassay
ELBW	extremely low birth weight
ELISA	enzyme-linked immunosorbent assay
EPS	extrapyramidal side effects
ESA	erythropoiesis-stimulating agent
ESR	erythrocyte sedimentation rate
ESRD	end stage renal disease
E.T.	endotracheal
EtOH	alcohol
FDA	Food and Drug Administration (United States)
FEV₁	forced expiratory volume exhaled after 1 second
FSH	follicle-stimulating hormone
FTT	failure to thrive
FVC	forced vital capacity
G-6-PD	glucose-6-phosphate dehydrogenase
GA	gestational age
GABA	gamma-aminobutyric acid
GAD	generalized anxiety disorder
GE	gastroesophageal
GERD	gastroesophageal reflux disease
GFR	glomerular filtration rate
GGT	gamma-glutamyltransferase
GI	gastrointestinal
GU	genitourinary
GVHD	graft versus host disease
HAM-A	Hamilton Anxiety Scale
HAM-D	Hamilton Depression Scale
HARS	HIV-associated adipose redistribution syndrome
HCAHPS	Hospital Consumer Assessment of Healthcare Providers and Systems

Abbreviations Which May Be Used in This Reference *(continued)*

Abbreviation	Meaning
Hct	hematocrit
HDL-C	high density lipoprotein cholesterol
HF	heart failure
HFA	hydrofluoroalkane
HFSA	Heart Failure Society of America
Hgb	hemoglobin
HIV	human immunodeficiency virus
HMG-CoA	3-hydroxy-3-methylglutaryl-coenzyme A
HOCM	hypertrophic obstructive cardiomyopathy
HPA	hypothalamic-pituitary-adrenal
HPLC	high performance liquid chromatography
HSV	herpes simplex virus
HTN	hypertension
HUS	hemolytic uremic syndrome
IBD	inflammatory bowel disease
IBS	irritable bowel syndrome
IBW	ideal body weight
ICD	implantable cardioverter defibrillator
ICH	intracranial hemorrhage
ICP	intracranial pressure
IDDM	insulin-dependent diabetes mellitus
IDSA	Infectious Diseases Society of America
IgG	immune globulin G
IHSS	idiopathic hypertrophic subaortic stenosis
ILCOR	International Liaison Committee on Resuscitation
I.M.	intramuscular
INR	international normalized ration
Int. unit	international unit
I.O.	intraosseous
I & O	input and output
IOP	intraocular pressure
IQ	intelligence quotient
I.T.	intrathecal
ITP	idiopathic thrombocytopenic purpura
IUGR	intrauterine growth retardation
I.V.	intravenous
IVH	intraventricular hemorrhage
IVP	intravenous push
IVPB	intravenous piggyback
JIA	juvenile idiopathic arthritis
JNC	Joint National Committee
JRA	juvenile rheumatoid arthritis
kg	kilogram
KIU	kallikrein inhibitor unit
KOH	potassium hydroxide
LAMM	L-α-acetyl methadol
LDH	lactate dehydrogenase
LDL-C	low density lipoprotein cholesterol
LE	lupus erythematosus
LFT	liver function test
LGA	large for gestational age
LH	luteinizing hormone
LP	lumbar posture

Abbreviations Which May Be Used in This Reference (continued)

Abbreviation	Meaning
LR	lactated Ringer's
LV	left ventricular
LVEF	left ventricular ejection fraction
LVH	left ventricular hypertrophy
MAC	*Mycobacterium avium* complex
MADRS	Montgomery Asbery Depression Rating Scale
MAO	monoamine oxidase
MAOIs	monamine oxidase inhibitors
MAP	mean arterial pressure
MDD	major depressive disorder
MDRD	modification of diet in renal disease
MDRSP	multidrug resistant *streptococcus pneumoniae*
MI	myocardial infarction
MMSE	mini mental status examination
MOPP	mustargen (mechlorethamine), Oncovin® (vincristine), procarbazine, and prednisone
M/P	milk to plasma ratio
MPS I	mucopolysaccharidosis I
MRHD	maximum recommended human dose
MRI	magnetic resonance imaging
MRSA	methicillin-resistant *Staphylococcus aureus*
MUGA	multiple gated acquisition scan
NAEPP	National Asthma Education and Prevention Program
NAS	neonatal abstinence syndrome
NCI	National Cancer Institute
ND	nasoduodenal
NF	National Formulary
NFD	Nephrogenic fibrosing dermopathy
NG	nasogastric
NIDDM	noninsulin-dependent diabetes mellitus
NIH	National Institute of Health
NIOSH	National Institute for Occupational Safety and Health
NKA	no known allergies
NKDA	No known drug allergies
NMDA	n-methyl-d-aspartate
NMS	neuroleptic malignant syndrome
NNRTI	non-nucleoside reverse transcriptase inhibitor
NRTI	nucleoside reverse transcriptase inhibitor
NS	normal saline (0.9% sodium chloride)
NSAID	nonsteroidal anti-inflammatory drug
NSF	nephrogenic systemic fibrosis
NSTEMI	Non-ST-elevation myocardial infarction
NYHA	New York Heart Association
OA	osteoarthritis
OCD	obsessive-compulsive disorder
OHSS	ovarian hyperstimulation syndrome
O.R.	operating room
OTC	over-the-counter (nonprescription)
PABA	para-aminobenzoic acid
PACTG	Pediatric AIDS Clinical Trials Group
PALS	pediatric advanced life support
PAT	paroxysmal atrial tachycardia
PCA	patient-controlled analgesia
PCI	percutaneous coronary intervention

Abbreviation	Meaning
PCP	*Pneumocystis jiroveci* pneumonia (also called *Pneumocystis carinii* pneumonia)
PCWP	pulmonary capillary wedge pressure
PD	Parkinson's disease; peritoneal dialysis
PDA	patent ductus arteriosus
PDE-5	phosphodiesterase-5
PE	pulmonary embolism
PEG tube	percutaneous endoscopic gastrostomy tube
P-gp	P-glycoprotein
PHN	post-herpetic neuralgia
PICU	Pediatric Intensive Care Unit
PID	pelvic inflammatory disease
PIP	peak inspiratory pressure
PMA	postmenstrual age
PMDD	premenstrual dysphoric disorder
PNA	postnatal age
PONV	postoperative nausea and vomiting
PPHN	persistent pulmonary hypertension of the neonate
PPN	peripheral parenteral nutrition
PROM	premature rupture of membranes
PSVT	paroxysmal supraventricular tachycardia
PT	prothrombin time
PTH	parathyroid hormone
PTSD	post-traumatic stress disorder
PTT	partial thromboplastin time
PUD	peptic ulcer disease
PVC	premature ventricular contraction
PVD	peripheral vascular disease
PVR	peripheral vascular resistance
QT_c	corrected QT interval
QT_cF	corrected QT interval by Fredricia's formula
RA	rheumatoid arthritis
RAP	right arterial pressure
RDA	recommended daily allowance
REM	rapid eye movement
REMS	risk evaluation and mitigation strategies
RIA	radioimmunoassay
RNA	ribonucleic acid
RPLS	reversible posterior leukoencephalopathy syndrome
RSV	respiratory syncytial virus
SA	sinoatrial
SAD	seasonal affective disorder
SAH	subarachnoid hemorrhage
SBE	subacute bacterial endocarditis
SBP	systolic blood pressure
S_{cr}	serum creatinine
SERM	selective estrogen receptor modulator
SGA	small for gestational age
SGOT	serum glutamic oxaloacetic aminotransferase
SGPT	serum glutamic pyruvate transaminase
SI	International System of Units or Systeme international d'Unites
SIADH	syndrome of inappropriate antidiuretic hormone secretion
SIDS	sudden infant death syndrome
SLE	systemic lupus erythematosus

Abbreviations Which May Be Used in This Reference *(continued)*

Abbreviation	Meaning
SLEDD	sustained low-efficiency daily diafiltration
SNRI	serotonin norepinephrine reuptake inhibitor
SSKI	saturated solution of potassium iodide
SSRIs	selective serotonin reuptake inhibitors
STD	sexually transmitted disease
STEM I	ST-elevation myocardial infarction
SVR	systemic vascular resistance
SVT	supraventricular tachycardia
SWFI	sterile water for injection
SWI	sterile water for injection
$T_{1/2}$	half-life
T_3	triiodothyronine
T_4	thyroxine
TB	tuberculosis
TC	total cholesterol
TCA	tricyclic antidepressant
TD	tardive dyskinesia
TG	triglyceride
TIA	transient ischemic attack
TIBC	total iron binding capacity
TMA	thrombotic microangiopathy
T_{max}	time to maximum observed concentration, plasma
TNF	tumor necrosis factor
TPN	total parenteral nutrition
TSH	thyroid stimulating hormone
TT	thrombin time
TTP	thrombotic thrombocytopenic purpura
UA	urine analysis
UC	ulcerative colitis
ULN	upper limits of normal
URI	upper respiratory infection
USAN	United States Adopted Names
USP	United States Pharmacopeia
UTI	urinary tract infection
UV	ultraviolet
V_d	volume of distribution
V_{dss}	volume of distribution at steady-state
VEGF	vascular endothelial growth factor
VF	ventricular fibrillation
VLBW	very low birth weight
VMA	vanillylmandelic acid
VT	ventricular tachycardia
VTE	venous thromboembolism
vWD	von Willebrand disease
VZV	varicella zoster virus
WHO	World Health Organization
w/v	weight for volume
w/w	weight for weight
YBOC	Yale Brown Obsessive-Compulsive Scale
YMRS	Young Mania Rating Scale

Common Weights, Measures, or Apothecary Abbreviations

Abbreviation	Meaning
<[1]	less than
>[1]	greater than
≤	less than or equal to
≥	greater than or equal to
ac	before meals or food
ad	to, up to
ad lib	at pleasure
AM	morning
AMA	against medical advice
amp	ampul
amt	amount
aq	water
aq. dest.	distilled water
ASAP	as soon as possible
a.u.[1]	each ear
bid	twice daily
bm	bowel movement
C	Celsius, centigrade
cal	calorie
cap	capsule
cc[1]	cubic centimeter
cm	centimeter
comp	compound
cont	continue
d	day
d/c[1]	discharge
dil	dilute
disp	dispense
div	divide
dtd	give of such a dose
Dx	diagnosis
elix, el	elixir
emp	as directed
et	and
ex aq	in water
F	Fahrenheit
f, ft	make, let be made
g	gram
gr	grain
gtt	a drop
h	hour
hs[1]	at bedtime
kcal	kilocalorie
kg	kilogram
L	liter
liq	a liquor, solution
M	molar
mcg	microgram
m. dict	as directed
mEq	milliequivalent

Common Weights, Measures, or Apothecary Abbreviations *(continued)*

Abbreviation	Meaning
mg	milligram
microL	microliter
min	minute
mL	milliliter
mm	millimeter
mM	millimole
mm Hg	millimeters of mercury
mo	month
mOsm	milliosmoles
ng	nanogram
nmol	nanomole
no.	number
noc	in the night
non rep	do not repeat, no refills
NPO	nothing by mouth
NV	nausea and vomiting
O, Oct	a pint
o.d.[1]	right eye
o.l.	left eye
o.s.[1]	left eye
o.u.[1]	each eye
pc, post cib	after meals
PM	afternoon or evening
P.O.	by mouth
P.R.	rectally
prn	as needed
pulv	a powder
q	every
qad	every other day
qd[1,2]	every day, daily
qh	every hour
qid	four times a day
qod[1,2]	every other day
qs	a sufficient quantity
qs ad	a sufficient quantity to make
Rx	take, a recipe
S.L.	sublingual
stat	at once, immediately
SubQ	subcutaneous
supp	suppository
syr	syrup
tab	tablet
tal	such
tid	three times a day
tr, tinct	tincture
trit	triturate
tsp	teaspoon
u.d.	as directed
ung	ointment
v.o.	verbal order

Common Weights, Measures, or Apothecary Abbreviations *(continued)*

Abbreviation	Meaning
w.a.	while awake
x3	3 times
x4	4 times
y	year

[1]ISMP error-prone abbreviation

[2]JCAHO Do Not Use list

Additional abbreviations used and defined within a specific monograph or text piece may only apply to that text.

REFERENCES

The Institute for Safe Medication Practices (ISMP) list of Error-Prone Abbreviations, Symbols, and Dose Designations. Available at http://www.ismp.org/Tools/errorproneabbreviations.pdf

The Joint Commission Official "Do Not Use" list. Available at http://www.jointcommission.org/facts_about_the_official_/

PREVENTING PRESCRIBING ERRORS

Prescribing errors account for the majority of reported medication errors and have prompted healthcare professionals to focus on the development of steps to make the prescribing process safer. Prescription legibility has been attributed to a portion of these errors and legislation has been enacted in several states to address prescription legibility. However, eliminating handwritten prescriptions and ordering medications through the use of technology [eg, computerized prescriber order entry (CPOE)] has been the primary recommendation. Whether a prescription is electronic, typed, or hand-printed, additional safe practices should be considered for implementation to maximize the safety of the prescribing process. Listed below are suggestions for safer prescribing:

- Ensure correct patient by using at least 2 patient identifiers on the prescription (eg, full name, birth date, or address). Review prescription with the patient or patient's caregiver.

- If pediatric patient, document patient's birth date or age and most recent weight. If geriatric patient, document patient's birth date or age.

- Prevent drug name confusion: For more information, see http://www.ismp.org/tools/confuseddrugnames.pdf.

  - Use TALLman lettering (eg, buPROPion, busPIRone, predniSONE, prednisoLONE). For more information, see http://www.fda.gov/drugs/drugsafety/medicationerrors/default.htm.

  - Avoid abbreviated drug names (eg, MSO_4, $MgSO_4$, MS, HCT, 6MP, MTX), as they may be misinterpreted and cause error.

  - Avoid investigational names for drugs with FDA approval (eg, FK-506, CBDCA).

  - Avoid chemical names such as 6-mercaptopurine or 6-thioguanine, as sixfold overdoses have been given when these were not recognized as chemical names. The proper names of these drugs are mercaptopurine or thioguanine.

  - Use care when prescribing drugs that look or sound similar (eg, look-alike, sound-alike drugs). Common examples include: Celebrex vs Celexa, hydroxyzine vs hydralazine, Zyprexa vs Zyrtec.

- Avoid dangerous, error-prone abbreviations (eg, regardless of letter-case: U, IU, QD, QOD, μg, cc, @). Do not use apothecary system or symbols. Additionally, text messaging abbreviations (eg, "2Day") should never be used.

  - For more information, see http://www.ismp.org/tools/errorproneabbreviations.pdf.

- Always use a leading zero for numbers less than 1 (0.5 mg is correct and .5 mg is **incorrect**) and never use a trailing zero for whole numbers (2 mg is correct and 2.0 mg is **incorrect**).

- Always use a space between a number and its units as it is easier to read. There should be no periods after the abbreviations mg or mL (10 mg is correct and 10mg is **incorrect**).

- For doses that are greater than 1,000 dosing units, use properly placed commas to prevent 10-fold errors (100,000 units is correct and 100000 units is **incorrect**).

- Do not prescribe drug dosage by the type of container in which the drug is available (eg, do not prescribe "1 amp", "2 vials", etc).

- Do not write vague or ambiguous orders which have the potential for misinterpretation by other healthcare providers. Examples of vague orders to avoid: "Resume pre-op medications," "give drug per protocol," or "continue home medications."

- Review each prescription with patient (or patient's caregiver) including the medication name, indication, and directions for use.

- Take extra precautions when prescribing *high alert drugs* (drugs that can cause significant patient harm when prescribed in error). Common examples of these drugs include: Anticoagulants, chemotherapy, insulins, opioids, and sedatives.

  - For more information, see http://www.ismp.org/tools/institutionalhighalert.asp or http://www.ismp.org/communityRx/tools/ambulatoryhighalert.asp.

  To Err Is Human: Building a Safer Health System, Kohn LT, Corrigan JM, Donaldson MS, eds. Washington, D.C.: National Academy Press. 2000.

A Complete Outpatient Prescription[1]

A complete outpatient prescription can prevent the prescriber, the pharmacist, and/or the patient from making a mistake and can eliminate the need for further clarification. The complete outpatient prescription should contain:

- Patient's full name

- Medication indication

- Allergies

- Prescriber name and telephone or pager number

- For pediatric patients: Their birth date or age and current weight

- For geriatric patients: Their birth date or age

- Drug name, dosage form and strength

- For pediatric patients: Intended daily weight-based dose so that calculations can be checked by the pharmacist (ie, mg/kg/day or units/kg/day)
- Number or amount to be dispensed
- Complete instructions for the patient or caregiver, including the purpose of the medication, directions for use (including dose), dosing frequency, route of administration, duration of therapy, and number of refills.
- Dose should be expressed in convenient units of measure.
- When there are recognized contraindications for a prescribed drug, the prescriber should indicate knowledge of this fact to the pharmacist (ie, when prescribing a potassium salt for a patient receiving an ACE inhibitor, the prescriber should write "K serum leveling being monitored").

Upon dispensing of the final product, the pharmacist should ensure that the patient or caregiver can effectively demonstrate the appropriate administration technique. An appropriate measuring device should be provided or recommended. Household teaspoons and tablespoons should not be used to measure liquid medications due to their variability and inaccuracies in measurement; oral medication syringes are recommended.

For additional information, see http://www.ismp.org/Newsletters/acutecare/articles/20020601.asp

[1]Levine SR, Cohen MR, Blanchard NR, et al. Guidelines for preventing medication errors in pediatrics. *J Pediatr Pharmacol Ther.* 2001;6:426-442.

FDA NAME DIFFERENTIATION PROJECT: THE USE OF "TALL MAN" LETTERS

Confusion between similar drug names is an important cause of medication errors. For years, The Institute For Safe Medication Practices (ISMP), has urged generic manufacturers to use a combination of large and small letters as well as bolding (ie, chlorpro**MAZINE** and chlorpro**PAMIDE**) to help distinguish drugs with look-alike names, especially when they share similar strengths. Recently the FDA's Division of Generic Drugs began to issue recommendation letters to manufacturers suggesting this novel way to label their products to help reduce this drug name confusion. Although this project has had marginal success, the method has successfully eliminated problems with products such as diphenhydr**AMINE** and dimenhy**DRINATE**. Hospitals should also follow suit by making similar changes in their own labels, preprinted order forms, computer screens and printouts, and drug storage location labels.

Lexi-Comp, Inc. Medical Publishing will use "Tall-Man" letters for the drugs suggested by the FDA or recommended by ISMP.

The following is a list of generic and brand name product names and recommended revisions.

Drug Product	Recommended Revision
acetazolamide	aceta**ZOLAMIDE**
alprazolam	**ALPRAZ**olam
amiloride	a**MIL**oride
amlodipine	am**LODIP**ine
aripiprazole	**ARIP**iprazole
atomoxetine	ato**MOX**etine
atorvastatin	atorva**STAT**in
Avinza	**AVIN**za
azacitidine	aza**CITID**ine
azathioprine	aza**THIO**prine
bupropion	bu**PROP**ion
buspirone	bus**PIR**one
carbamazepine	car**BAM**azepine
carboplatin	**CARBO**platin
cefazolin	ce**FAZ**olin
cefotetan	cefo**TE**tan
cefoxitin	cef**OX**itin
ceftazidime	cef**TAZ**idime
ceftriaxone	cef**TRIAX**one
Celebrex	Cele**BREX**
Celexa	Cele**XA**
chlordiazepoxide	chlordiaze**POXIDE**
chlorpromazine	chlorpro**MAZINE**
chlorpropamide	chlorpro**PAMIDE**
cisplatin	**CIS**platin
clobazam	clo**BAZ**am
clomiphene	clomi**PHENE**
clomipramine	clomi**PRAMINE**
clonazepam	clonaze**PAM**
clonidine	clo**NID**ine
clozapine	clo**ZAP**ine
cycloserine	cyclo**SERINE**
cyclosporine	cyclo**SPORINE**
dactinomycin	**DACTIN**omycin
daptomycin	**DAPTO**mycin
daunorubicin	**DAUNO**rubicin
dimenhydrinate	dimenhy**DRINATE**
diphenhydramine	diphenhydr**AMINE**
dobutamine	**DOBUT**amine
docetaxel	**DOCE**taxel

Drug Product	Recommended Revision
dopamine	**DOP**amine
doxorubicin	**DOXO**rubicin
duloxetine	**DUL**oxetine
ephedrine	e**PHED**rine
epinephrine	**EPINEPH**rine
epirubicin	**EPI**rubicin
eribulin	eri**BUL**in
fentanyl	fenta**NYL**
flavoxate	flavox**ATE**
fluoxetine	**FLU**oxetine
fluphenazine	flu**PHENAZ**ine
fluvoxamine	fluvoxa**MINE**
glipizide	glipi**ZIDE**
glyburide	gly**BURIDE**
guaifenesin	guai**FEN**esin
guanfacine	guan**FACINE**
Humalog	Huma**LOG**
Humulin	Humu**LIN**
hydralazine	hydr**ALAZINE**
hydrocodone	**HYDRO**codone
hydromorphone	**HYDRO**morphone
hydroxyzine	hydr**OXY**zine
idarubicin	**IDA**rubicin
infliximab	in**FLIX**imab
Invanz	**INV**anz
isotretinoin	**ISO**tretinoin
Klonopin	Klono**PIN**
Lamictal	La**MIC**tal
Lamisil	Lam**ISIL**
lamivudine	lami**VUD**ine
lamotrigine	lamo**TRI**gine
levetiracetam	Lev**ETIRA**cetam
levocarnitine	lev**OCARN**itine
lorazepam	**LOR**azepam
medroxyprogesterone	medroxy**PROGESTER**one
metformin	met**FORMIN**
methylprednisolone	methyl**PREDNIS**olone
methyltestosterone	methyl**TESTOSTER**one
metronidazole	metro**NIDAZOLE**
mitomycin	mito**MY**cin
mitoxantrone	Mito**XAN**trone
Nexavar	Nex**AVAR**
Nexium	Nex**IUM**
nicardipine	ni**CAR**dipine
nifedipine	**NIFE**dipine
nimodipine	ni**MOD**ipine
Novolin	Novo**LIN**
Novolog	Novo**LOG**
olanzapine	**OLANZ**apine
oxcarbazepine	**OX**carbazepine
oxycodone	oxy**CODONE**
Oxycontin	Oxy**CONTIN**
paclitaxel	**PACL**itaxel
paroxetine	**PAR**oxetine

Drug Product	Recommended Revision
pazopanib	PAZOPanib
pemetrexed	PEMEtrexed
penicillamine	penicillAMINE
pentobarbital	PENTobarbital
phenobarbital	PHENobarbital
ponatinib	PONATinib
pralatrexate	PRALAtrexate
prednisolone	prednisoLONE
prednisone	predniSONE
Prilosec	PriLOSEC
Prozac	PROzac
quetiapine	QUEtiapine
quinidine	quiNIDine
quinine	quiNINE
rabeprazole	RABEprazole
Risperdal	RisperDAL
risperidone	risperiDONE
rituximab	riTUXimab
romidepsin	romiDEPsin
romiplostim	romiPLOStim
ropinirole	rOPINIRole
Sandimmune	sandIMMUNE
Sandostatin	SandoSTATIN
Seroquel	SEROquel
Sinequan	SINEquan
sitagliptin	sitaGLIPtin
Solu-Cortef	Solu-CORTEF
Solu-Medrol	Solu-MEDROL
sorafenib	SORAfenib
sufentanil	SUFentanil
sulfadiazine	sulfADIAZINE
sulfasalazine	sulfaSALAzine
sumatriptan	SUMAtriptan
sunitinib	SUNItinib
Tegretol	TEGretol
tiagabine	tiaGABine
tizanidine	tiZANidine
tolazamide	TOLAZamide
tolbutamide	TOLBUTamide
tramadol	traMADol
trazodone	traZODone
Trental	TRENtal
valacyclovir	valACYclovir
valganciclovir	valGANciclovir
vinblastine	vinBLAStine
vincristine	vinCRIStine
zolmitriptan	ZOLMitriptan
Zyprexa	ZyPREXA
Zyrtec	ZyrTEC

FDA and ISMP lists of look-alike drug names with recommended tall man letter. http://www.ismp.org/tools/tallmanletters.pdf. Accessed January 6, 2011. Name differentiation project. http://www.fda.gov/Drugs/DrugSafety/MedicationErrors/ucm164587.htm. Accessed January 6, 2011. U.S. Pharmacopeia. USP quality review: use caution – avoid confusion. March 2001, No. 76. http://www.usp.org

SELECTED REFERENCES

AHFS Drug Information. McEvoy GK, ed. Bethesda, MD: American Society of Health-System Pharmacists; 2013.

Applied Therapeutics: The Clinical Use of Drugs. 10th ed. Koda-Kimble MA, Young LY, Alldredge BK, et al, eds. Philadelphia, PA: Lippincott Williams & Wilkins; 2012.

Drug Facts and Comparisons. St Louis, MO: J.B. Facts and Comparisons (part of Wolters Kluwer Health Inc); 2013.

Drug Information Handbook. 22nd ed. Hudson, OH: Wolters Kluwer Health; 2013.

Drug Prescribing in Renal Failure: Dosing Guidelines for Adults and Children. 5th ed. Aronoff GR, Bennett WM, Berns JS, et al, eds. Philadelphia, PA: American College of Physicians; 2007.

Food Medication Interactions. 13th ed. Pronsky ZM, Redfern CM, Crowe J, et al, eds. Pottstown, PA: Food Medication Interactions; 2003.

Handbook of Injectable Drugs. 17th ed. Trissel LA, ed. Bethesda, MD: American Society of Health-System Pharmacists; 2012.

Handbook of Nonprescription Drugs: An Interactive Approach to Self-Care. 16th ed. Washington, DC: American Pharmacists Association; 2009.

Handbook on Extemporaneous Formulations for Pediatric, Geriatric, and Special Needs Patients. 2nd ed. Jew RK, Soo-Hoo W, Erush SC, eds. Bethesda, MD: American Society of Health-System Pharmacists; 2010.

Manual of Neonatal Care. 7th ed. Cloherty JP, Eichenwald EC, Stark AR, eds. Philadelphia, PA: Lippincott Williams & Wilkins; 2012.

Nathan and Oski's Hematology of Infancy and Childhood. 7th ed. Orkin S, Nathan D, Ginsburg D, et al, eds. Philadelphia, PA: Saunders Elsevier; 2009.

Nelson's Pocket Book of Pediatric Antimicrobial Therapy. 19th ed. Bradley JS, Nelson JD, Kimberlin DK, et al, eds. Philadelphia, PA: Lippincott Williams & Wilkins; 2012.

Nelson Textbook of Pediatrics. 19th ed. Kliegman RM, Stanton BF, St. Gemell JW, et al, eds. Philadelphia, PA: Saunders Elsevier; 2011.

Neonatal and Pediatric Pharmacology: Therapeutic Principles in Practice. 3rd ed. Yaffe SJ, Aranda JV, eds. Baltimore, MD: Lippincott Williams & Wilkins; 2004.

Pediatric Drug Formulations. 5th ed. Nahata MC, ed. Cincinnati, OH: Harvey Whitney Books Company; 2003.

Pediatric Endocrinology. 3rd ed. Sperling MA, ed. Philadelphia, PA: Saunders Elsevier; 2008.

Pediatric Pharmacology and Therapeutics. Radde IC, MacLead SM, eds. St. Louis, MO: Mosby; 1993.

Principles and Practice of Infectious Diseases. 7th ed. Mandell GL, Bennett JE, Dolin R, eds. Philadelphia, PA: Churchill Livingstone; 2010.

Principles and Practice of Pediatric Oncology. 6th ed. Pizzo PA, Poplack DG, eds. Philadelphia, PA: Lippincott Williams & Wilkins; 2011.

Red Book: 2012 Report of the Committee on Infectious Diseases. 29th ed. Pickering LK, ed. Elk Grove Village, IL: American Academy of Pediatrics; 2012.

Rogers' Textbook of Pediatric Intensive Care. 4th ed. Nichols DG, ed. Philadelphia, PA: Lippincott, Williams & Wilkins; 2008.

Rudolph's Pediatrics. 22nd ed. Rudolph C, Rudolph AM, Lister G, et al, eds. New York: McGraw-Hill Medical; 2011.

Teddy Bear Book: Pediatric Injectable Drugs. 9th ed. Phelps SJ, Hak EB, Crill CM, eds. Bethesda, MD: American Society of Health-System Pharmacists; 2010.

Textbook of Pediatric Infectious Diseases. 6th ed. Feigin RD, Cherry JD, Demmler-Harrison GJ, et al, eds. Philadelphia, PA: Saunders Elsevier; 2009.

Trissel's Stability of Compounded Formulations. 4th ed. Trissel LA, ed. Washington, DC: American Pharmaceutical Association; 2009.

ALPHABETICAL LISTING OF DRUGS

◆ **A-25 [OTC]** *see* Vitamin A *on page 2146*

Abacavir (a BAK a veer)

Related Information
Adult and Adolescent HIV *on page 2348*
Pediatric HIV *on page 2338*
Perinatal HIV *on page 2356*
Brand Names: U.S. Ziagen
Brand Names: Canada Ziagen®
Therapeutic Category Antiretroviral Agent; HIV Agents (Anti-HIV Agents); Nucleoside Reverse Transcriptase Inhibitor (NRTI)
Generic Availability (U.S.) May be product dependent
Use Treatment of HIV-1 infection in combination with other antiretroviral agents (FDA approved in ages ≥3 months and adults); **Note:** HIV regimens consisting of **three** antiretroviral agents are strongly recommended.
Medication Guide Available Yes
Pregnancy Risk Factor C
Pregnancy Considerations Adverse events have been observed in some animal reproduction studies. Abacavir has a high level of transfer across the human placenta. No increased risk of overall birth defects has been observed following first trimester exposure according to data collected by the antiretroviral pregnancy registry. Cases of lactic acidosis/hepatic steatosis syndrome related to mitochondrial toxicity have been reported in pregnant women with prolonged use of nucleoside analogues. It is not known if pregnancy itself potentiates this known side effect; however, women may be at increased risk of lactic acidosis and liver damage. In addition, these adverse events are similar to other rare but life-threatening syndromes which occur during pregnancy (eg, HELLP syndrome). Hepatic enzymes and electrolytes should be monitored in women receiving nucleoside analogues and clinicians should watch for early signs of the syndrome. In addition, mitochondrial dysfunction may develop in infants following in utero exposure. The pharmacokinetics of abacavir are not significantly changed by pregnancy and dose adjustment is not needed for pregnant women. The DHHS Perinatal HIV Guidelines consider abacavir in combination with lamivudine to be a preferred NRTI backbone for use in antiretroviral-naive pregnant women.

Regardless of CD4 count or HIV RNA copy number, all HIV-infected pregnant women should receive a combination antiretroviral (ARV) drug regimen. A combination of antepartum, intrapartum, and infant ARV prophylaxis is recommended. ARV therapy should be started as soon as possible in women with symptomatic infection. Although earlier initiation may be more effective in reducing the perinatal transmission of HIV, initiation may be delayed until after 12 weeks gestation in women who do not require immediate treatment after careful consideration of maternal conditions (eg, nausea and vomiting) and the potential risks of first trimester fetal exposure for specific agents. A scheduled cesarean delivery at 38 weeks gestation is recommended for all women with HIV RNA >1000 copies/mL or unknown concentrations near delivery in order to decrease transmission. If ARV therapy must be interrupted for <24 hours during the peripartum period, stop then restart all medications simultaneously in order to decrease the chance of developing resistance. Long-term follow-up is recommended for all infants exposed to ARV medications. In couples who want to conceive, the HIV-infected partner should attain maximum viral suppression prior to conception.

Healthcare providers are encouraged to enroll pregnant women exposed to antiretroviral medications in the Antiretroviral Pregnancy Registry (1-800-258-4263 or www.APRegistry.com). Healthcare providers caring for HIV-infected women and their infants may contact the National Perinatal HIV Hotline (888-448-8765) for clinical consultation (DHHS [perinatal], 2014).

Breast-Feeding Considerations Abacavir is excreted into breast milk. Maternal or infant antiretroviral therapy does not completely eliminate the risk of postnatal HIV transmission. In addition, multiclass-resistant virus has been detected in breast-feeding infants despite maternal therapy. Therefore, in the United States, where formula is accessible, affordable, safe, and sustainable, and the risk of infant mortality due to diarrhea and respiratory infections is low, complete avoidance of breast-feeding by HIV-infected women is recommended to decrease potential transmission of HIV (DHHS [perinatal], 2014).

Contraindications Hypersensitivity to abacavir or any component (**do not rechallenge** patients who have experienced hypersensitivity reactions to abacavir [regardless of *HLA-B*5701* status], potentially fatal hypersensitivity reactions may occur); moderate or severe hepatic dysfunction

Warnings Serious and sometimes fatal hypersensitivity reactions may occur **[U.S. Boxed Warning]**. Patients testing positive for the presence of the *HLA-B*5701* allele are at a significantly increased risk for hypersensitivity reactions **[U.S. Boxed Warning]**. Screening for *HLA-B*5701* allele status is recommended prior to initiating therapy or reinitiating therapy in patients of unknown genotype status, including patients who previously tolerated therapy. Patients who test positive for the *HLA-B*5701* allele should have an abacavir allergy recorded in their medical record and should **not** receive abacavir. If a suspected abacavir hypersensitivity reaction occurs during therapy, regardless of *HLA-B*5701* status, abacavir should be discontinued immediately and permanently. Hypersensitivity reactions may also occur in patients who test negative for the *HLA-B*5701* allele, but at a significantly lower rate.

Abacavir hypersensitivity is a multiorgan clinical syndrome **[U.S. Boxed Warning]**. Discontinue therapy immediately in patients who show signs or symptoms of 2 or more of the following: Fever, skin rash, respiratory symptoms (including cough, dyspnea, or pharyngitis), GI symptoms (including nausea, vomiting, diarrhea, or abdominal pain), and constitutional symptoms (including fatigue, malaise, or achiness). Carefully consider the diagnosis of hypersensitivity reaction in patients who present with acute onset respiratory symptoms, even if other diagnoses, such as bronchitis, flu-like illness, pharyngitis, or pneumonia, are possible. Permanently discontinue abacavir if hypersensitivity reaction cannot be ruled out, even when other diagnoses are possible (regardless of *HLA-B*5701* status) **[U.S. Boxed Warning]**. Skin rash may be maculopapular or urticarial, but can be variable in appearance; erythema multiforme has been reported; hypersensitivity reaction may occur without a rash. Other symptoms may include edema, lethargy, myolysis, paresthesia, shortness of breath, mouth ulcerations, conjunctivitis, lymphadenopathy, and abnormal findings on chest x-ray (ie, infiltrates that can be localized). Anaphylaxis, renal failure, hepatic failure, respiratory failure, ARDS, hypotension, and death may also occur in association with hypersensitivity reactions. Laboratory abnormalities include increases in liver function tests, elevated CPK or serum creatinine, and lymphopenia.

Do not restart abacavir or any other abacavir-containing product after a hypersensitivity reaction occurs **[U.S. Boxed Warning]**; more severe symptoms can recur within hours and may include life-threatening hypotension and death. Fatal hypersensitivity reactions have occurred following the reintroduction of abacavir in patients whose therapy was interrupted for other reasons [U.S. Boxed Warning]. These patients had no identified history or had unrecognized symptoms of abacavir hypersensitivity. Reactions occurred within hours. In some cases, signs of a hypersensitivity reaction may have been previously present, but attributed to other medical conditions (acute onset respiratory diseases, gastroenteritis, reactions to other medications). If abacavir or any other abacavir-containing product is to be restarted following an interruption in therapy, the patient must first be evaluated for previously unsuspected symptoms of hypersensitivity. Do not restart abacavir or any other abacavir-containing product, if hypersensitivity is suspected or cannot be ruled out (regardless of HLA-B*5701 status). Hypersensitivity reactions occur in 5% to 8% of adult and pediatric patients (actual incidence varies by race/ethnicity); most hypersensitivity reactions occur within the first 6 weeks of therapy, but can occur at any time; one study reported a higher incidence of severe hypersensitivity reactions with once daily dosing compared with twice daily dosing (see product information).

Cases of lactic acidosis, severe hepatomegaly with steatosis and death have been reported with the use of abacavir and other NRTIs [U.S. Boxed Warning]; most of these cases have been in women; prolonged nucleoside use, obesity, and prior liver disease may be risk factors; use with extreme caution in patients with other risk factors for liver disease; discontinue abacavir in patients who develop laboratory or clinical evidence of lactic acidosis or pronounced hepatotoxicity.

The oral solution contains propylene glycol; toxicities have been reported with use of products containing propylene glycol, including hyperosmolality, lactic acidosis, seizures, and respiratory depression; in neonates large amounts of propylene glycol delivered orally, intravenously (eg, >3000 mg/day), or topically have been associated with potentially fatal toxicities which can include metabolic acidosis, seizures, renal failure, and CNS depression; use oral solution containing propylene glycol with caution (AAP, 1997; Shehab, 2009).

Precautions Use with caution and decrease the dose in patients with mild hepatic dysfunction; use in moderate to severe hepatic dysfunction is contraindicated. Fat redistribution and accumulation [ie, central obesity, peripheral wasting, facial wasting, breast enlargement, dorsocervical fat enlargement (buffalo hump), and cushingoid appearance] have been observed in patients receiving antiretroviral agents (causal relationship not established). Always use abacavir in combination with other antiretroviral agents; do not add abacavir as a single agent to antiretroviral regimens that are failing; resistance to abacavir develops relatively slowly, but cross resistance between abacavir and other nucleoside reverse transcriptase inhibitors (NRTIs) may occur; limited response may be seen in patients with HIV isolates containing multiple mutations conferring resistance to NRTIs or in patients with a prolonged prior NRTI exposure. Use with caution in patients with plasma HIV RNA levels ≥100,000 copies/mL as earlier virologic failure has been observed in one study (DHHS [adult], 2014).

Immune reconstitution syndrome (an acute inflammatory response to residual or indolent opportunistic infections) may occur in HIV patients during initial treatment with combination antiretroviral agents, including abacavir; this syndrome may require further patient assessment and therapy. Autoimmune disorders (eg, Grave's disease, Guillain-Barré syndrome, and polymyositis) have been reported in patients experiencing immune reconstitution; time to onset is variable and may occur many months after antiretroviral treatment is initiated.

Use has been associated with an increased risk of myocardial infarction (MI) in observational studies; however, based on a meta-analysis of 26 randomized trials, the FDA has concluded there is not an increased risk. Consider using with caution in patients with risks for coronary heart disease and minimizing modifiable risk factors (eg, hypertension, hyperlipidemia, diabetes mellitus, and smoking) prior to use.

May cause mild hyperglycemia; more common in pediatric patients. May cause diarrhea; severe diarrhea may occur at a higher incidence in patients receiving once daily dosing.

Adverse Reactions Hypersensitivity reactions (which may be fatal) occur in ~5% of patients. Symptoms may include abdominal pain, anaphylaxis, arthralgia, conjunctivitis, diarrhea, edema, fatigue, fever, headache, hepatic failure, lethargy, lymphadenopathy, malaise, mouth ulcerations, myalgia, myolysis, nausea, paresthesia, rash (including erythema multiforme), renal failure, respiratory symptoms (eg, adult respiratory distress syndrome, cough, dyspnea, pharyngitis, respiratory failure), vomiting.

Note: Rates of adverse reactions were defined during combination therapy with other antiretrovirals (lamivudine and efavirenz or lamivudine and zidovudine). Only reactions which occurred at a higher frequency in adults (except where noted) than in the comparator group are noted. Adverse reaction rates attributable to abacavir alone are not available.

Central nervous system: Abnormal dreams, anxiety, depression, dizziness, fatigue, fever/chills, headache, malaise

Dermatologic: Rash

Gastrointestinal: Abdominal pain, diarrhea, nausea, vomiting

Hematologic: Thrombocytopenia

Hepatic: AST increased

Neuromuscular & skeletal: Musculoskeletal pain

Miscellaneous: Hypersensitivity reactions, infection

Rare but important or life-threatening: Erythema multiforme, hepatotoxicity, immune reconstitution syndrome, lactic acidosis, MI, pancreatitis, Stevens-Johnson syndrome, toxic epidermal necrolysis

Drug Interactions

Metabolism/Transport Effects None known.

Avoid Concomitant Use There are no known interactions where it is recommended to avoid concomitant use.

Increased Effect/Toxicity

The levels/effects of Abacavir may be increased by: Ganciclovir-Valganciclovir; Ribavirin

Decreased Effect

The levels/effects of Abacavir may be decreased by: Protease Inhibitors

Food Interactions Ethanol decreases the elimination of abacavir and may increase the risk of toxicity. Management: Monitor patients.

Stability Store tablets and oral solution at 20°C to 25°C (68°F to 77°F). Oral solution may be refrigerated; do not freeze.

Mechanism of Action Nucleoside reverse transcriptase inhibitor. Abacavir is a guanosine analogue which is phosphorylated to carbovir triphosphate which interferes with HIV viral RNA-dependent DNA polymerase resulting in inhibition of viral replication.

Pharmacokinetics (Adult data unless noted)

Absorption: Rapid and extensive

Distribution: Apparent V_d: 0.86 ± 0.15 L/kg

CSF to plasma AUC ratio: 27% to 33%

Protein binding: 50%

Metabolism: Hepatic via alcohol dehydrogenase and glucuronyl transferase to inactive carboxylate and glucuronide metabolites; not significantly metabolized by cytochrome P450 enzymes; intracellulary metabolized to carbovir triphosphate (active metabolite)

Bioavailability: Tablet: 83%; solution and tablet provide comparable AUCs

Half-life, elimination (serum):

Pediatric patients ≥3 months to ≤13 years: 1 to 1.5 hours (Hughes, 1999; Kline, 1999)

Adults: 1.54 ± 0.63 hours

Hepatic impairment (mild): Increases half-life by 58%

Half-life, intracellular: 12 to 26 hours

Time to peak serum concentration (Hughes, 1999):

Pediatric patients ≥3 months to ≤13 years: Within 1.5 hours

Adults: 1 to 1.7 hours

Elimination: Urine: ~83% (1.2% as unchanged drug, 30% as 5'-carboxylic acid metabolite, 36% as the glucuronide, and 15% as other metabolites); feces (16% total dose)

Clearance (apparent): Single dose 8 mg/kg (Hughes, 1999):

Pediatric patients ≥3 months to ≤13 years: 17.84 mL/minute/kg

Adults: 10.14 mL/minute/kg

Dosing: Usual

Pediatric: **HIV infection, treatment:** Oral: **Note:** Use in combination with other antiretroviral agents:

Infants <3 months: Not approved for use; safety, efficacy, and dosage not established

Infants ≥3 months, Children, and Adolescents <16 years: 8 mg/kg/dose twice daily; maximum dose: 300 mg/dose (DHHS [pediatric], 2014)

Alternate dosing:

Weight-based dosing for patients ≥14 kg who are able to swallow tablets (scored 300 mg tablets):

14 to 21 kg: 150 mg (½ tablet) twice daily

>21 to <30 kg: 150 mg (½ tablet) in the morning and 300 mg (1 tablet) in the evening

≥30 kg: 300 mg (1 tablet) twice daily

Once-daily dosing: Children and Adolescents <16 years: 16 to 20 mg/kg/dose once daily; maximum dose: 600 mg/dose. Not recommended as **initial** dosing in pediatric patients. May be used as a component of a once-daily regimen in clinically stable patients who have undetectable viral loads and stable CD4 counts for more than 6 months (DHHS [pediatric], 2014).

Adolescents ≥16 years: Oral: 300 mg twice daily or 600 mg once daily (DHHS [pediatric], 2014)

Adult: **HIV infection, treatment:** Oral: Use in combination with other antiretroviral agents: 300 mg twice daily or 600 mg once daily

Dosing adjustment in renal impairment: There are no dosage adjustments provided in the manufacturer's labeling; however, renal is a minor route of elimination.

Dosing adjustment in hepatic impairment:

Mild hepatic impairment (Child-Pugh score 5 to 6): Adults: 200 mg twice daily (using oral solution)

Moderate to severe hepatic impairment (Child-Pugh score >6): All patients: Use is contraindicated

Administration Oral: May be administered without regard to food

Monitoring Parameters HLA-B*5701 genotype status prior to initiating therapy or resuming therapy in patients of unknown HLA-B*5701 status (including patients previously tolerating therapy); signs and symptoms of hypersensitivity reaction (in all patients, but especially in those untested for the HLA-B*5701 allele)

Note: Monitor CD4 percentage (if <5 years of age) or CD4 count (if ≥5 years of age) at least every 3 to 4 months (DHHS [pediatric], 2014).

Prior to initiation of therapy: Genotypic resistance testing, CD4 and viral load (every 3 to 4 months), CBC with differential, LFTs, BUN, creatinine, electrolytes, glucose,

urinalysis (every 6 to 12 months), and assessment of readiness for adherence with medication regimen. At initiation and with any change in treatment regimen: CBC with differential, electrolytes, calcium, phosphate, glucose, LFTs, bilirubin, urinalysis (at initiation), BUN, creatinine, albumin, total protein, lipid panel (at initiation), CD4, and viral load. After 1 to 2 weeks of therapy: Signs of medication toxicity and adherence. After 2 to 4 weeks of therapy: CBC with differential, viral load, signs of medication toxicity, and adherence; then every 3-4 months: CBC with differential, electrolytes, glucose, LFTs, bilirubin, BUN, creatinine, CD4, viral load, signs of medication toxicity, and adherence. Lipid panel and urinalysis every 6 to 12 months. CD4 monitoring frequency may be decreased to every 6 to 12 months in children who are adherent to therapy if the value is well above the threshold for opportunistic infections, viral suppression is sustained, and the clinical status is stable for more than 2 to 3 years (DHHS [pediatric], 2014). Monitor for growth and development, signs of, HIV-specific physical conditions, HIV disease progression, opportunistic infections or lactic acidosis; serum creatine kinase.

Additional Information The patient Medication Guide, which includes written manufacturer information, should be dispensed to the patient with each new prescription and refill; the Warning Card describing the hypersensitivity reaction should be given to the patient to carry with them.

The development of the abacavir hypersensitivity reaction has been associated with certain HLA genotypes (eg, HLA-B*5701, HLA-DR7, HLA-DQ3) which may help predict which patients are at risk for developing the abacavir hypersensitivity reaction (Hetherington, 2002; Lucas, 2007; Mallal, 2002). Patients who test positive for the HLA-B*5701 allele should have an abacavir allergy recorded in their medical record and should **not** receive abacavir. All patients who receive abacavir (and their caregivers) should be educated about the risk of abacavir hypersensitivity reactions (including patients who test negative for the HLA-B*5701 allele, as the risk for the reaction is not completely eliminated). Approximately 4% of patients who test negative for the HLA-B*5701 allele will experience a clinically suspected abacavir hypersensitivity reaction compared to 61% of those who test positive for the HLA-B*5701 allele.

The prevalence of HLA-B*5701 in the United States has been estimated to be 8% in Caucasians, 2.5% in African-Americans, 2% in Hispanics, 1% in Asians; in the sub-Saharan Africa it is <1%. Pretherapy identification of HLA-B*5701-positive patients and subsequent avoidance of abacavir therapy in these patients has been shown to significantly reduce the occurrence of abacavir-associated hypersensitivity reactions. A skin patch test is in development for clinical screening purposes; however, only PCR-mediated genotyping methods are currently in clinical practice use for documentation of this susceptibility marker. A familial predisposition to the abacavir hypersensitivity reaction has also been reported; use abacavir with great caution in children of parents who experience a hypersensitivity reaction to abacavir (Peyriére, 2001).

Reverse transcriptase mutations of K65R, L74V, Y115F, and M184V have been associated with abacavir resistance; at least 2-3 mutations are needed to decrease HIV susceptibility by 10-fold. The presence of a multiple number of these abacavir resistance-associated mutations, may confer cross-resistance for other nucleoside or nucleotide reverse transcriptase inhibitors (eg, didanosine, emtricitabine, lamivudine, zalcitabine, or tenofovir). A progressive decrease in abacavir susceptibility is associated with an increasing number of thymidine analogue mutations (TAMs; M41L, D67N, K70R, L210W, T215Y/F, K219E/R/H/Q/N).

Dosage Forms Excipient information presented when available (limited, particularly for generics); consult specific product labeling.
Solution, Oral:
Ziagen: 20 mg/mL (240 mL) [contains methylparaben, propylene glycol, propylparaben, saccharin sodium; strawberry-banana flavor]
Tablet, Oral:
Ziagen: 300 mg [scored]
Generic: 300 mg

References

American Academy of Pediatrics Committee on Drugs. "Inactive" ingredients in pharmaceutical products: update (subject review). *Pediatrics.* 1997;99(2):268-278.

DHHS Panel on Antiretroviral Guidelines for Adults and Adolescents, "Guidelines for the Use of Antiretroviral Agents in HIV-Infected Adults and Adolescents," May 1, 2014. Available at http://www.aidsinfo.nih.gov

DHHS Panel on Antiretroviral Therapy and Medical Management of HIV-Infected Children, "Guidelines for the Use of Antiretroviral Agents in Pediatric HIV Infection," February 12, 2014. Available at http://aidsinfo.nih.gov

DHHS Panel on Treatment of HIV-Infected Pregnant Women and Prevention of Perinatal Transmission, "Recommendations for the Use of Antiretroviral Drugs in Pregnant HIV-1-Infected Women for Maternal Health and Interventions to Reduce Perinatal HIV-1 Transmission in the United States," March 28, 2014. Available at http://aidsinfo.nih.gov

Foster RH and Faulds D, "Abacavir," *Drugs*, 1998, 55(5):729-36.

Hetherington S, Hughes AR, Mosteller M, et al, "Genetic Variations in HLA-B Region and Hypersensitivity Reactions to Abacavir," *Lancet*, 2002, 359(9312):1121-2.

Hughes W, McDowell JA, Shenep J, et al, "Safety and Single-Dose Pharmacokinetics of Abacavir (1592U89) in Human Immunodeficiency Virus Type 1-Infected Children," *Antimicrob Agents Chemother*, 1999, 43(3):609-15.

Kline MW, Blanchard S, Fletcher CV, et al, "A Phase I Study of Abacavir (1592U89) Alone and in Combination With Other Antiretroviral Agents in Infants and Children With Human Immunodeficiency Virus Infection," *Pediatrics*, 1999, 103(4):e47. Available at http://www.pediatrics.org/cgi/content/full/103/4/e47

Lucas A, Nolan D, and Mallal S, "HLA-B*5701 Screening for Susceptibility to Abacavir Hypersensitivity," *J Antimicrob Chemother*, 2007, 59 (4):591-3.

Mallal S, Nolan D, Witt C, et al, "Association Between Presence of HLA-B*5701, HLA-DR7, and HLA-DQ3 and Hypersensitivity to HIV-1 Reverse-Transcriptase Inhibitor Abacavir," *Lancet*, 2002, 359 (9308):727-32.

Paediatric European Network for Treatment of AIDS (PENTA), "Comparison of Dual Nucleoside-Analogue Reverse-Transcriptase Inhibitor Regimens With and Without Nelfinavir in Children with HIV-1 Who Have Not Previously Been Treated: The PENTA 5 Randomised Trial," *Lancet*, 2002, 359(9308):733-40.

Peyriére H, Nicolas J, Siffert M, et al, "Hypersensitivity Related to Abacavir in Two Members of a Family," *Ann Pharmacother*, 2001, 35(10):1291-2.

Shehab N, Lewis CL, Streetman DD, Donn SM. Exposure to the pharmaceutical excipients benzyl alcohol and propylene glycol among critically ill neonates. *Pediatr Crit Care Med.* 2009;10 (2):256-259.

Abacavir and Lamivudine
(a BAK a veer & la MI vyoo deen)

Related Information
Adult and Adolescent HIV *on page 2348*
Pediatric HIV *on page 2338*
Perinatal HIV *on page 2356*

Brand Names: U.S. Epzicom®
Brand Names: Canada Kivexa™
Therapeutic Category Antiretroviral Agent; HIV Agents (Anti-HIV Agents); Nucleoside Analog Reverse Transcriptase Inhibitor (NRTI)
Generic Availability (U.S.) No
Use Treatment of HIV-1 infection in combination with other antiretroviral agents (FDA approved in ages ≥18 years and adults); **Note:** HIV regimens consisting of **three** antiretroviral agents are strongly recommended.
Medication Guide Available Yes
Pregnancy Risk Factor C

Pregnancy Considerations Animal reproduction studies have not been conducted with this combination. See individual agents. The DHHS Perinatal HIV Guidelines consider abacavir in combination with lamivudine to be a preferred NRTI backbone for use in antiretroviral-naive pregnant women (DHHS [perinatal], 2014).
Breast-Feeding Considerations Abacavir and lamivudine are excreted into breast milk. See individual agents.
Contraindications Hypersensitivity to abacavir, lamivudine, or any component; hepatic impairment. **Do not rechallenge** patients who have experienced hypersensitivity reactions to abacavir (regardless of *HLA-B*5701* status); potentially fatal hypersensitivity reactions may occur.

Warnings Serious and sometimes fatal hypersensitivity reactions to abacavir may occur **[U.S. Boxed Warning]**. Patients testing positive for the presence of the *HLA-B*5701* allele are at a significantly increased risk for hypersensitivity reactions **[U.S. Boxed Warning]**. Screening of *HLA-B*5701* allele status is recommended prior to initiating therapy or reinitiating therapy in patients of unknown genotype status, including patients who previously tolerated therapy. Patients who test positive for the *HLA-B*5701* allele should have an abacavir allergy recorded in their medical record and should **not** receive abacavir. If a suspected abacavir hypersensitivity reaction occurs during therapy, regardless of *HLA-B*5701* status, abacavir should be discontinued immediately and permanently. Hypersensitivity reactions may also occur in patients who test negative for the *HLA-B*5701* allele, but at a significantly lower rate.

Abacavir hypersensitivity is a multiorgan clinical syndrome **[U.S. Boxed Warning]**. Discontinue therapy immediately in patients who show signs or symptoms of 2 or more of the following: Fever, skin rash, respiratory symptoms (including cough, dyspnea, or pharyngitis), GI symptoms (including nausea, vomiting, diarrhea, or abdominal pain), and constitutional symptoms (including fatigue, malaise, or achiness). Carefully consider the diagnosis of hypersensitivity reaction in patients who present with acute onset respiratory symptoms, even if other diagnoses, such as bronchitis, flu-like illness, pharyngitis, or pneumonia, are possible. Permanently discontinue abacavir-containing medications if hypersensitivity reaction cannot be ruled out, even when other diagnoses are possible (regardless of *HLA-B*5701* status) **[U.S. Boxed Warning]**. Skin rash may be maculopapular or urticarial, but can be variable in appearance; erythema multiforme has been reported; hypersensitivity reaction may occur without a rash. Other symptoms may include edema, lethargy, myolysis, paresthesia, shortness of breath, mouth ulcerations, conjunctivitis, lymphadenopathy, and abnormal findings on chest x-ray (ie, infiltrates that can be localized). Anaphylaxis, renal failure, hepatic failure, respiratory failure, ARDS, hypotension, and death may also occur in association with hypersensitivity reactions. Laboratory abnormalities include increases in liver function tests, elevated CPK or serum creatinine, and lymphopenia.

Do not restart abacavir, Epzicom, or any other abacavir-containing product after a hypersensitivity reaction occurs **[U.S. Boxed Warning]**; more severe symptoms can recur within hours and may include life-threatening hypotension and death. Fatal hypersensitivity reactions have occurred following the reintroduction of abacavir in patients whose therapy was interrupted for other reasons **[U.S. Boxed Warning]**. These patients had no identified history or had unrecognized symptoms of abacavir hypersensitivity. Reactions occurred within hours. In some cases, signs of a hypersensitivity reaction may have been previously present, but attributed to other medical conditions (acute onset respiratory diseases, gastroenteritis, or reactions to other medications). If abacavir, Epzicom®, or any other abacavir-containing product is to be restarted following an interruption in therapy, the patient must first be evaluated for previously unsuspected symptoms of hypersensitivity. **Do not restart** abacavir, Epzicom®, or any other abacavir-containing product if hypersensitivity is suspected or cannot be ruled out (regardless of *HLA-B*5701* status). Hypersensitivity reactions occur in 5% to 8% of adult and pediatric patients (actual incidence varies by race/ethnicity); most hypersensitivity reactions occur within the first 6 weeks of therapy, but can occur at any time.

Cases of lactic acidosis, severe hepatomegaly with steatosis, and death have been reported in patients receiving nucleoside analogues **[U.S. Boxed Warning]**; most of these cases have been in women; prolonged nucleoside use, obesity, and prior liver disease may be risk factors; use with extreme caution in patients with other risk factors for liver disease; discontinue Epzicom® in patients who develop laboratory or clinical evidence of lactic acidosis or pronounced hepatotoxicity.

The major clinical toxicity of lamivudine in pediatric patients is pancreatitis; discontinue therapy if clinical signs, symptoms, or laboratory abnormalities suggestive of pancreatitis occur. HIV-infected patients who are coinfected with hepatitis B may experience severe acute exacerbations and clinical symptoms or laboratory evidence of hepatitis when a lamivudine-containing medication is discontinued **[U.S. Boxed Warning]**; most cases are self-limited, but fatalities have been reported; monitor patients closely for at least several months after discontinuation of abacavir and lamivudine; initiation of antihepatitis B therapy may be required. **Note:** HIV-infected patients should be screened for hepatitis B infection prior to starting lamivudine therapy. Concomitant use of combination antiretroviral therapy with interferon alfa (with or without ribavirin) has resulted in hepatic decompensation (with some fatalities) in patients coinfected with HIV and HCV; monitor patients closely, especially for hepatic decompensation; consider discontinuation of abacavir and lamivudine if needed; consider dose reduction or discontinuation of interferon alfa, ribavirin, or both if clinical toxicities, including hepatic decompensation, worsen.

Epzicom contains abacavir and lamivudine as a fixed-dose combination; do not use in patients with renal dysfunction (CrCl ≤50 mL/minute) who require lamivudine dosage adjustment or in patients with hepatic dysfunction. Abacavir is contraindicated in patients with moderate to severe hepatic dysfunction; patients with mild hepatic impairment require abacavir dosage reduction.

Precautions Fat redistribution and accumulation [ie, central obesity, peripheral wasting, facial wasting, breast enlargement, dorsocervical fat enlargement (buffalo hump), and cushingoid appearance] have been observed in patients receiving antiretroviral agents (causal relationship not established). Resistance to abacavir develops relatively slowly, but cross resistance between abacavir and other nucleoside reverse transcriptase inhibitors (NRTIs) may occur; limited response may be seen in patients with HIV isolates containing multiple mutations conferring resistance to NRTIs or in patients with a prolonged prior NRTI exposure.

Immune reconstitution syndrome (an acute inflammatory response to residual or indolent opportunistic infections) may occur in HIV patients during initial treatment with combination antiretroviral agents, including abacavir; this syndrome may require further patient assessment and therapy. Autoimmune disorders (eg, Grave's disease, Guillain-Barré syndrome, and polymyositis) have been reported in patients experiencing immune reconstitution; time to onset is variable and may occur many months after antiretroviral treatment is initiated.

Use of abacavir has been associated with an increased risk of myocardial infarction (MI) in observational studies; however, based on a meta-analysis of 26 randomized trials with abacavir therapy, the FDA has concluded there is not an increased risk. Consider using with caution in patients with risks for coronary heart disease and minimizing modifiable risk factors (eg, hypertension, hyperlipidemia, diabetes mellitus, and smoking) prior to use.

Do not administer Epzicom with abacavir- or lamivudine-containing products (eg, Epivir, Combivir, Trizivir, or Ziagen) or emtricitabine-containing products (eg, Atripla, Complera, Emtriva, Stribild, or Truvada).

Abacavir may cause mild hyperglycemia; more common in pediatric patients.

Adverse Reactions See individual agents.

Postmarketing and/or case reports: Alopecia, anaphylaxis, anemia, aplastic anemia, breath sounds abnormal, CPK increased, erythema multiforme, fat redistribution, hepatic steatosis, hepatitis B exacerbation, hyperglycemia, hypersensitivity reaction, immune reconstitution syndrome, lactic acidosis, lymphadenopathy, muscle weakness, pancreatitis, paresthesia, peripheral neuropathy, rhabdomyolysis, seizure, splenomegaly, Stevens-Johnson syndrome, stomatitis, urticaria, weakness, wheezing

Drug Interactions

Metabolism/Transport Effects None known.

Avoid Concomitant Use

Avoid concomitant use of Abacavir and Lamivudine with any of the following: Emtricitabine

Increased Effect/Toxicity

Abacavir and Lamivudine may increase the levels/effects of: Emtricitabine

The levels/effects of Abacavir and Lamivudine may be increased by: Ganciclovir-Valganciclovir; Ribavirin; Trimethoprim

Decreased Effect

The levels/effects of Abacavir and Lamivudine may be decreased by: Protease Inhibitors

Food Interactions Ethanol decreases the elimination of abacavir and may increase the risk of toxicity. Management: Monitor patients.

Stability Store at 25°C (77°F); excursions permitted to 15°C to 30°C (59°F to 86°F).

Mechanism of Action Nucleoside reverse transcriptase inhibitor combination.

Abacavir is a guanosine analogue which is phosphorylated to carbovir triphosphate which interferes with HIV viral RNA-dependent DNA polymerase resulting in inhibition of viral replication.

Lamivudine is a cytosine analog. After lamivudine is triphosphorylated, the principle mode of action is inhibition of HIV reverse transcription via viral DNA chain termination; inhibits RNA-dependent DNA polymerase activities of reverse transcriptase.

Pharmacokinetics (Adult data unless noted) One Epzicom tablet is bioequivalent, in the extent (AUC) of absorption and peak concentration, to two abacavir 300 mg tablets and two lamivudine 150 mg tablets; see individual agents

Dosing: Usual

Pediatric: **HIV infection, treatment:**

Children and Adolescents ≤50 kg: Not recommended; product is a fixed-dose combination.

Adolescents ≥16 years of age weighing >50 kg: Oral: 1 tablet daily (DHHS [pediatric], 2014)

Adult: **HIV infection, treatment:** Oral: 1 tablet daily

Dosing adjustment in renal impairment: CrCl ≤50 mL/minute: Use not recommended; use individual antiretroviral agents to reduce dosage

Dosing adjustment in hepatic impairment: Use is contraindicated; use individual antiretroviral agents to reduce dosage

Administration May be administered without regards to meals.

Monitoring Parameters HLA-B*5701 genotype status prior to initiating therapy or resuming therapy in patients of unknown HLA-B*5701 status (including patients previously tolerating therapy); signs and symptoms of abacavir hypersensitivity reaction (in all patients, but especially in those untested for the HLA-B*5701 allele)

Note: Monitor CD4 percentage (if <5 years of age) or CD4 count (if ≥5 years of age) at least every 3 to 4 months (DHHS [pediatric], 2014).

Prior to initiation of therapy: Genotypic resistance testing, CD4 and viral load (every 3 to 4 months), CBC with differential, LFTs, BUN, creatinine, electrolytes, glucose, urinalysis (every 6 to 12 months), and assessment of readiness for adherence with medication regimen. At initiation and with any change in treatment regimen: CBC with differential, electrolytes, calcium, phosphate, glucose, LFTs, bilirubin, urinalysis (at initiation), BUN, creatinine, albumin, total protein, lipid panel (at initiation), CD4, and viral load. After 1 or 2 weeks of therapy: Signs of medication toxicity and adherence. After 2 to 4 weeks of therapy: CBC with differential, viral load, signs of medication toxicity, and adherence; then every 3 to 4 months: CBC with differential, electrolytes, glucose, LFTs, bilirubin, BUN, creatinine, CD4, viral load, signs of medication toxicity, and adherence. Every 6 to 12 months: Lipid panel and urinalysis. CD4 monitoring frequency may be decreased to every 6 to 12 months in children who are adherent to therapy if the value is well above the threshold for opportunistic infections, viral suppression is sustained, and the clinical status is stable for more than 2 to 3 years (DHHS [pediatric], 2014). Monitor for growth and development, signs of HIV-specific physical conditions, HIV disease progression, opportunistic infections, pancreatitis, or lactic acidosis; serum creatinine kinase.

Additional Information The development of the abacavir hypersensitivity reaction has been associated with certain HLA genotypes (eg, HLA-B*5701, HLA-DR7, HLA-DQ3) which may help predict which patients are at risk for developing the abacavir hypersensitivity reaction (Hetherington, 2002; Lucas, 2007; Mallal, 2002). Patients who test positive for the HLA-B*5701 allele should have an abacavir allergy recorded in their medical record and should **not** receive abacavir. All patients who receive abacavir (and their caregivers) should be educated about the risk of abacavir hypersensitivity reactions (including patients who test negative for the HLA-B*5701 allele, as the risk for the reaction is not completely eliminated). Approximately 4% of patients who test negative for the HLA-B*5701 allele will experience a clinically suspected abacavir hypersensitivity reaction compared to 61% of those who test positive for the HLA-B*5701 allele.

The prevalence of HLA-B*5701 in the United States has been estimated to be 8% in Caucasians, 2.5% in African-Americans, 2% in Hispanics, <1% in Asians; in the sub-Saharan Africa it is 1%. Pretherapy identification of HLA-B*5701-positive patients and subsequent avoidance of abacavir therapy in these patients has been shown to significantly reduce the occurrence of abacavir-associated hypersensitivity reactions. A skin patch test is in development for clinical screening purposes; however, only PCR-mediated genotyping methods are currently in clinical practice for documentation of this susceptibility marker. A familial predisposition to the abacavir hypersensitivity reaction has been reported; use abacavir with great caution in children of parents who experience a hypersensitivity reaction to abacavir (Peyriére, 2001).

Reverse transcriptase mutations of K65R, L74V, Y115F, and M184V have been associated with abacavir resistance; at least 2 to 3 mutations are needed to decrease HIV susceptibility by 10-fold. The presence of a multiple number of these abacavir resistance-associated mutations, may confer cross-resistance for other nucleoside or nucleotide reverse transcriptase inhibitors (eg, didanosine, emtricitabine, lamivudine, zalcitabine, or tenofovir). A progressive decrease in abacavir susceptibility is associated with an increasing number of thymidine analogue mutations (TAMs; M41L, D67N, K70R, L210W, T215Y/F, K219E/R/H/Q/N).

Dosage Forms Excipient information presented when available (limited, particularly for generics); consult specific product labeling.

Tablet:

Epzicom®: Abacavir 600 mg and lamivudine 300 mg

References

DHHS Panel on Antiretroviral Therapy and Medical Management of HIV-Infected Children, "Guidelines for the Use of Antiretroviral Agents in Pediatric HIV Infection," February 12, 2014. Available at http://aidsinfo.nih.gov

Hetherington S, Hughes AR, Mosteller M, et al. Genetic variations in HLA-B region and hypersensitivity reactions to abacavir. Lancet. 2002;359(9312):1121-1122.

Lucas A, Nolan D, Mallal S. HLA-B*5701 screening for susceptibility to abacavir hypersensitivity. J Antimicrob Chemother. 2007;59(4):591-593.

Mallal S, Nolan D, Witt C, et al. Association between presence of HLA-B*5701, HLA-DR7, and HLA-DQ3 and hypersensitivity to HIV-1 reverse-transcriptase inhibitor abacavir. Lancet. 2002;359(9308):727-732.

Peyriére H, Nicolas J, Siffert M, et al. Hypersensitivity related to abacavir in two members of a family. Ann Pharmacother. 2001;35(10):1291-1292.

Abacavir, Lamivudine, and Zidovudine

(a BAK a veer, la MI vyoo deen, & zye DOE vyoo deen)

Related Information

Adult and Adolescent HIV on page 2348
Pediatric HIV on page 2338
Perinatal HIV on page 2356

Brand Names: U.S. Trizivir®

Brand Names: Canada Trizivir®

Therapeutic Category Antiretroviral Agent; HIV Agents (Anti-HIV Agents); Nucleoside Analog Reverse Transcriptase Inhibitor (NRTI)

Generic Availability (U.S.) Yes

Use Treatment of HIV-1 infection, either alone or in combination with other antiretroviral agents (FDA approved in adolescents ≥40 kg and adults); **Note:** HIV regimens consisting of **three** antiretroviral agents are strongly recommended; **Note:** Data on the use of this triple NRTI combination regimen in patients with baseline viral loads >100,000 copies/mL is limited.

Medication Guide Available Yes

Pregnancy Risk Factor C

Pregnancy Considerations Animal reproduction studies have not been conducted with this combination. The DHHS Perinatal HIV Guidelines generally do not recommend this combination in antiretroviral-naïve pregnant women due to inferior virologic activity (DHHS [Perinatal], 2014). See individual agents.

Breast-Feeding Considerations Abacavir, lamivudine, and zidovudine are excreted into breast milk. See individual agents.

Contraindications Hypersensitivity to abacavir, lamivudine, zidovudine, or any component; hepatic impairment. **Do not rechallenge** patients who have experienced hypersensitivity reactions to abacavir (regardless of HLA-B*5701 status), potentially fatal hypersensitivity reactions may occur

Warnings Serious and sometimes fatal hypersensitivity reactions to abacavir may occur **[U.S. Boxed Warning]**.

Patients testing positive for the presence of the *HLA-B*5701* allele are at a significantly increased risk for hypersensitivity reactions **[U.S. Boxed Warning]**. Screening for *HLA-B*5701* allele status is recommended prior to initiating therapy or reinitiating therapy in patients of unknown genotype status, including patients who previously tolerated therapy. Patients who test positive for the *HLA-B*5701* allele should have an abacavir allergy recorded in their medical record and should **not** receive abacavir. If a suspected abacavir hypersensitivity reaction occurs during therapy, regardless of *HLA-B*5701* status, abacavir should be discontinued immediately and permanently. Hypersensitivity reactions may also occur in patients who test negative for the *HLA-B*5701* allele, but at a significantly lower rate.

Abacavir hypersensitivity is a multiorgan clinical syndrome **[U.S. Boxed Warning]**. Discontinue therapy immediately in patients who show signs or symptoms of 2 or more of the following: Fever, skin rash, respiratory symptoms (including cough, dyspnea, or pharyngitis) and GI symptoms (including nausea, vomiting, diarrhea, or abdominal pain), and constitutional symptoms (including fatigue, malaise, or achiness). Carefully consider the diagnosis of hypersensitivity reaction in patients who present with acute onset respiratory symptoms, even if other diagnoses, such as bronchitis, flu-like illness, pharyngitis, or pneumonia, are possible. Permanently discontinue abacavir-containing medications if hypersensitivity reaction cannot be ruled out, even when other diagnoses are possible (regardless of *HLA-B*5701* status) **[U.S. Boxed Warning]**. Skin rash may be maculopapular or urticarial, but can be variable in appearance; erythema multiforme has been reported; hypersensitivity reaction may occur without a rash. Other symptoms may include edema, lethargy, myolysis, paresthesia, shortness of breath, mouth ulcerations, conjunctivitis, lymphadenopathy, and abnormal findings on chest x-ray (ie, infiltrates that can be localized). Anaphylaxis, renal failure, hepatic failure, respiratory failure, ARDS, hypotension, and death may also occur in association with hypersensitivity reactions. Laboratory abnormalities include increases in liver function tests, elevated CPK or serum creatinine, and lymphopenia.

Do not restart abacavir, Trizivir, or any other abacavir-containing product after a hypersensitivity reaction occurs **[U.S. Boxed Warning]**; more severe symptoms can recur within hours and may include life-threatening hypotension and death. Fatal hypersensitivity reactions have occurred following the reintroduction of abacavir in patients whose therapy was interrupted for other reasons **[U.S. Boxed Warning]**. These patients had no identified history or had unrecognized symptoms of abacavir hypersensitivity. Reactions occurred within hours. In some cases, signs of a hypersensitivity reaction may have been previously present, but attributed to other medical conditions (acute onset respiratory diseases, gastroenteritis, reactions to other medications). If abacavir, Trizivir, or any other abacavir-containing product is to be restarted following an interruption in therapy, the patient must first be evaluated for previously unsuspected symptoms of hypersensitivity. **Do not restart** abacavir, Trizivir, or any other abacavir-containing product if hypersensitivity is suspected or cannot be ruled out (regardless of *HLA-B*5701* status). Hypersensitivity reactions occur in 5% to 8% of adult and pediatric patients (actual incidence varies by race/ethnicity); most hypersensitivity reactions occur within the first 6 weeks of therapy, but can occur at any time.

Cases of lactic acidosis, severe hepatomegaly with steatosis, and death have been reported in patients receiving nucleoside analogues **[U.S. Boxed Warning]**; most of these cases have been in women; prolonged nucleoside use, obesity, and prior liver disease may be risk factors;

use with extreme caution in patients with other risk factors for liver disease; discontinue Trizivir in patients who develop laboratory or clinical evidence of lactic acidosis or pronounced hepatotoxicity.

The major clinical toxicity of lamivudine in pediatric patients is pancreatitis; discontinue therapy if clinical signs, symptoms, or laboratory abnormalities suggestive of pancreatitis occur. HIV-infected patients who are coinfected with hepatitis B may experience severe acute exacerbations and clinical symptoms or laboratory evidence of hepatitis when a lamivudine-containing medication is discontinued **[U.S. Boxed Warning]**; most cases are self-limited, but fatalities have been reported; monitor patients closely for at least several months after discontinuation of abacavir, lamivudine, and zidovudine; initiation of antihepatitis B therapy may be required. **Note:** HIV-infected patients should be screened for hepatitis B infection prior to starting lamivudine therapy. Concomitant use of combination antiretroviral therapy with interferon alfa (with or without ribavirin) has resulted in hepatic decompensation (with some fatalities) in patients coinfected with HIV and HCV; monitor patients closely, especially for hepatic decompensation, neutropenia, and anemia; consider discontinuation of abacavir, lamivudine, and zidovudine if needed; consider dose reduction or discontinuation of interferon alfa, ribavirin, or both if clinical toxicities, including hepatic decompensation, worsen.

Zidovudine is associated with hematologic toxicity including granulocytopenia and severe anemia requiring transfusions **[U.S. Boxed Warning]**; use with caution in patients with ANC <1000 cells/mm^3 or hemoglobin <9.5 g/dL; consider interruption of therapy for significant anemia (Hgb <7.5 g/dL or reduction >25% of baseline) or neutropenia (ANC <750 cells/mm^3 or reduction >50% from baseline); use of erythropoietin or filgrastim may be necessary in some patients. Prolonged use of zidovudine may cause myositis and myopathy **[U.S. Boxed Warning]**.

Trizivir contains abacavir, lamivudine, and zidovudine as a fixed-dose combination; do not use in patients weighing <40 kg, in patients with renal dysfunction (CrCl <50 mL/minute) who require lamivudine and zidovudine dosage adjustment, or in patients with hepatic dysfunction. Patients with mild to moderate hepatic dysfunction or liver cirrhosis require zidovudine dosage adjustment; abacavir is contraindicated in patients with moderate to severe hepatic dysfunction; patients with mild hepatic impairment require abacavir dosage reduction.

Precautions Use of abacavir has been associated with an increased risk of myocardial infarction (MI) in observational studies; however, based on a meta-analysis of 26 randomized trials with abacavir therapy, the FDA has concluded there is not an increased risk. Consider using with caution in patients with risks for coronary heart disease and minimizing modifiable risk factors (eg, hypertension, hyperlipidemia, diabetes mellitus, and smoking) prior to use. HIV therapy-experienced patients may have a lower response to the abacavir component.

Fat redistribution and accumulation [ie, central obesity, peripheral wasting, facial wasting, breast enlargement, dorsocervical fat enlargement (buffalo hump), and cushingoid appearance] have been observed in patients receiving antiretroviral agents (causal relationship not established). Resistance to abacavir develops relatively slowly, but cross resistance between abacavir and other nucleoside reverse transcriptase inhibitors (NRTIs) may occur; limited response may be seen in patients with HIV isolates containing multiple mutations conferring resistance to NRTIs or in patients with a prolonged prior NRTI exposure.

Immune reconstitution syndrome (an acute inflammatory response to residual or indolent opportunistic infections) may occur in HIV patients during initial treatment with combination antiretroviral agents; this syndrome may require further patient assessment and therapy. Autoimmune disorders (eg, Grave's disease, Guillain-Barré syndrome, and polymyositis) have been reported in patients experiencing immune reconstitution; time to onset is variable and may occur many months after antiretroviral treatment is initiated.

Do not administer Trizivir with abacavir, lamivudine, or zidovudine-containing products (eg, Epivir, Combivir, Epzicom, or Ziagen) or emtricitabine-containing products (eg, Atripla, Complera, Emtriva, Stribild, or Truvada).

Adverse Reactions Fatal hypersensitivity reactions have occurred in patients taking abacavir (in Trizivir®). If Trizivir® is to be restarted following an interruption in therapy, first evaluate the patient for previously unsuspected symptoms of hypersensitivity. Do not restart if hypersensitivity is suspected or if hypersensitivity cannot be ruled out.

The following information is based on CNA3005 study data concerning effects noted in patients receiving abacavir, lamivudine, and zidovudine. See individual agents for additional information.

Central nervous system: Anxiety, depression, fatigue, fever/chills, headache, malaise
Dermatologic: Rash
Endocrine & metabolic: Triglycerides increased
Gastrointestinal: Amylase increased, diarrhea, GGT increased, nausea, pancreatitis, vomiting
Hematologic: Neutropenia
Hepatic: ALT increased
Neuromuscular & skeletal: CPK increased
Otic: Ear infection
Respiratory: Nose/throat infection
Miscellaneous: Hypersensitivity, viral infection

Drug Interactions

Metabolism/Transport Effects Refer to individual components.

Avoid Concomitant Use

Avoid concomitant use of Abacavir, Lamivudine, and Zidovudine with any of the following: CloZAPine; Dipyrone; Emtricitabine; Stavudine

Increased Effect/Toxicity

Abacavir, Lamivudine, and Zidovudine may increase the levels/effects of: CloZAPine; Emtricitabine; Ribavirin

The levels/effects of Abacavir, Lamivudine, and Zidovudine may be increased by: Acyclovir-Valacyclovir; Clarithromycin; Dipyrone; DOXOrubicin (Conventional); DOXOrubicin (Liposomal); Fluconazole; Ganciclovir-Valganciclovir; Interferons; Methadone; Probenecid; Raltegravir; Trimethoprim; Valproic Acid and Derivatives

Decreased Effect

Abacavir, Lamivudine, and Zidovudine may decrease the levels/effects of: Stavudine

The levels/effects of Abacavir, Lamivudine, and Zidovudine may be decreased by: Clarithromycin; DOXOrubicin (Conventional); DOXOrubicin (Liposomal); Protease Inhibitors; Rifamycin Derivatives

Food Interactions Ethanol decreases the elimination of abacavir and may increase the risk of toxicity. Management: Monitor patients.

Stability Store at 25°C (77°F); excursions permitted to 15°C to 30°C (59°F to 86°F).

Mechanism of Action The combination of abacavir, lamivudine, and zidovudine is believed to act synergistically to inhibit reverse transcriptase via DNA chain termination after incorporation of the nucleoside analogue as well as to delay the emergence of mutations conferring resistance.

Pharmacokinetics (Adult data unless noted) One Trizivir tablet is bioequivalent, in the extent (AUC) and rate of absorption (peak concentration and time to peak concentration), to one abacavir 300 mg tablet, one lamivudine 150 mg tablet, plus one zidovudine 300 mg tablet; see individual agents

Dosing: Usual

Pediatric: **HIV infection, treatment:** May use alone or in combination with other antiretroviral agents:
Children and Adolescents <40 kg: Not recommended; product is a fixed-dose combination
Adolescents ≥40 kg: Oral: 1 tablet twice daily
Adult: **HIV infection, treatment:** Oral: 1 tablet twice daily
Dosing adjustment in renal impairment: CrCl <50 mL/minute: Use not recommended (use individual antiretroviral agents to reduce dosage).
Dosing adjustment in hepatic impairment: Use is contraindicated; use individual antiretroviral agents to reduce dosage.

Administration May be administered without regard to meals

Monitoring Parameters HLA-B*5701 genotype status prior to initiating therapy or resuming therapy in patients of unknown HLA-B*5701 status (including patients previously tolerating therapy); signs and symptoms of abacavir hypersensitivity reaction (in all patients, but especially in those untested for the HLA-B*5701 allele)
Note: Monitor CD4 percentage (if <5 years of age) or CD4 count (if ≥5 years of age) at least every 3 to 4 months (DHHS [pediatric], 2014)

Prior to initiation of therapy: Genotypic resistance testing, CD4 and viral load (every 3 to 4 months), CBC with differential, LFTs, BUN, creatinine, electrolytes, glucose, urinalysis (every 6 to 12 months), and assessment of readiness for adherence with medication regimen. At initiation and with any change in treatment regimen: CBC with differential, electrolytes, calcium, phosphate, glucose, LFTs, bilirubin, urinalysis (at initiation), BUN, creatinine, albumin, total protein, lipid panel (at initiation), CD4, and viral load. After 1 to 2 weeks of therapy: Signs of medication toxicity and adherence. After 2 to 4 weeks of therapy: CBC with differential, viral load, signs of medication toxicity and adherence; then every 3 to 4 months: CBC with differential, electrolytes, glucose, LFTs, bilirubin, BUN, creatinine, CD4, viral load, signs of medication toxicity, and adherence. Lipid panel and urinalysis every 6 to 12 months. CD4 monitoring frequency may be decreased to every 6 to 12 months in children who are adherent to therapy if the value is well above the threshold for opportunistic infections, viral suppression is sustained, and the clinical status is stable for more than 2 to 3 years (DHHS [pediatric], 2014). Monitor for growth and development, signs of HIV-specific physical conditions, HIV disease progression, opportunistic infections, hepatotoxicity, anemia, pancreatitis, or lactic acidosis; serum creatine kinase

Additional Information The development of the abacavir hypersensitivity reaction has been associated with certain HLA genotypes (eg, HLA-B*5701, HLA-DR7, HLA-DQ3) which may help predict which patients are at risk for developing the abacavir hypersensitivity reaction (Hetherington, 2002; Lucas, 2007; Mallal, 2002). Patients who test positive for the HLA-B*5701 allele should have an abacavir allergy recorded in their medical record and should **not** receive abacavir. All patients who receive abacavir (and their caregivers) should be educated about the risk of abacavir hypersensitivity reactions (including patients who test negative for the HLA-B*5701 allele, as the risk for the reaction is not completely eliminated). Approximately 4% of patients who test negative for the HLA-B*5701 allele will experience a clinically suspected abacavir hypersensitivity reaction compared to 61% of those who test positive for the *HLA-B*5701* allele.

The prevalence of *HLA-B*5701* in the United States has been estimated to be 8% in Caucasians, 2.5% in African-Americans, 2% in Hispanics, 1% in Asians; in the sub-Saharan Africa it is <1%. Pretherapy identification of *HLA-B*5701*-positive patients and subsequent avoidance of abacavir therapy in these patients has been shown to significantly reduce the occurrence of abacavir-associated hypersensitivity reactions. A skin patch test is in development for clinical screening purposes; however, only PCR-mediated genotyping methods are currently in clinical practice use for documentation of this susceptibility marker. A familial predisposition to the abacavir hypersensitivity reaction has been reported; use abacavir with great caution in children of parents who experience a hypersensitivity reaction to abacavir (Peyriére, 2001).

Reverse transcriptase mutations of K65R, L74V, Y115F, and M184V have been associated with abacavir resistance; at least 2 to 3 mutations are needed to decrease HIV susceptibility by 10-fold. The presence of a multiple number of these abacavir resistance-associated mutations may confer cross-resistance for other nucleoside or nucleotide reverse transcriptase inhibitors (eg, didanosine, emtricitabine, lamivudine, zalcitabine, or tenofovir). A progressive decrease in abacavir susceptibility is associated with an increasing number of thymidine analogue mutations (TAMs; M41L, D67N, K70R, L210W, T215Y/F, K219E/R/H/Q/N).

Dosage Forms Excipient information presented when available (limited, particularly for generics); consult specific product labeling.

Tablet, oral:

Trizivir®: Abacavir sulfate 300 mg, lamivudine 150 mg, and zidovudine 300 mg

Generic: Abacavir sulfate 300 mg, lamivudine 150 mg, and zidovudine 300 mg

References

DHHS Panel on Antiretroviral Guidelines for Adults and Adolescents, "Guidelines for the Use of Antiretroviral Agents in HIV-Infected Adults and Adolescents," May 1, 2014. Available at http://www.aidsinfo.nih.gov

DHHS Panel on Antiretroviral Therapy and Medical Management of HIV-Infected Children, "Guidelines for the Use of Antiretroviral Agents in Pediatric HIV Infection," February 12, 2014. Available at http://aidsinfo.nih.gov

Hetherington S, Hughes AR, Mosteller M, et al, "Genetic Variations in HLA-B Region and Hypersensitivity Reactions to Abacavir," *Lancet*, 2002, 359(9312):1121-2.

Lucas A, Nolan D, and Mallal S, "HLA-B*5701 Screening for Susceptibility to Abacavir Hypersensitivity," *J Antimicrob Chemother*, 2007, 59 (4):591-3.

Mallal S, Nolan D, Witt C, et al, "Association Between Presence of HLA-B*5701, HLA-DR7, and HLA-DQ3 and Hypersensitivity to HIV-1 Reverse-Transcriptase Inhibitor Abacavir," *Lancet*, 2002, 359 (9308):727-32.

Peyriére H, Nicolas J, Siffert M, et al, "Hypersensitivity Related to Abacavir in Two Members of a Family," *Ann Pharmacother*, 2001, 35(10):1291-2.

Saez-Llorens X, Nelson RP, Emmanuel P, et al, "A Randomized, Double-Blind Study of Triple Nucleoside Therapy of Abacavir, Lamivudine, and Zidovudine Versus Lamivudine and Zidovudine in Previously Treated Human Immunodeficiency Virus Type 1-Infected Children," *Pediatrics*, 2001, 107(1). Available at http://www.pediatrics.org/cgi/content/full/107/1/e4

Trizivir (abacavir, lamivudine, and zidovudine) [prescribing information]. Research Triangle Park, NC: ViiV Healthcare; May 2012.

◆ **Abacavir Sulfate** see Abacavir on page 36

◆ **Abacavir Sulfate and Lamivudine** see Abacavir and Lamivudine on page 39

Abatacept (ab a TA sept)

Medication Safety Issues

Sound-alike/look-alike issues:
Orencia may be confused with Oracea

Brand Names: U.S. Orencia

Brand Names: Canada Orencia

Therapeutic Category Antirheumatic, Disease Modifying

Generic Availability (U.S.) No

Use Treatment of moderately- to severely-active polyarticular juvenile idiopathic arthritis as monotherapy or concomitantly with methotrexate (I.V.: FDA approved in ages 6-17 years). Treatment of moderately- to severely-active rheumatoid arthritis as monotherapy or in combination with other DMARDs (I.V.; SubQ: FDA approved in adults). Note: Abatacept should not be used in combination with TNF antagonists or with other biologic rheumatoid arthritis drugs, such as anakinra.

Pregnancy Risk Factor C

Pregnancy Considerations Adverse effects were not observed in animal studies. Due to the potential risk for development of autoimmune disease in the fetus, use during pregnancy only if clearly needed. A pregnancy registry has been established to monitor outcomes of women exposed to abatacept during pregnancy (1-877-311-8972).

Breast-Feeding Considerations It is not known if abatacept is excreted into human milk. Due to the potential for serious adverse reactions in the nursing infant, a decision should be made to discontinue nursing or to discontinue the drug, taking into account the importance of treatment to the mother.

Contraindications Hypersensitivity to abatacept or any component

Warnings Serious and potentially fatal infections (including tuberculosis and sepsis) have been reported, particularly in patients receiving concomitant immunosuppressive therapy. Use caution when considering the use of abatacept in patients with a history of recurrent infections; with conditions that predispose them to infections; or with chronic, latent, or localized infections. Closely monitor patients who develop a new infection while undergoing treatment. If a patient develops a serious infection, discontinue abatacept. Patients receiving abatacept in combination with TNF antagonists had higher rates of infections than patients on TNF antagonists alone (concurrent use with TNF antagonists is not recommended); monitor for signs and symptoms of infection when transitioning from TNF-blocking agents to abatacept. Concurrent use with anakinra is not recommended due to insufficient experience. Reactivation of hepatitis B may occur in chronic carriers of the virus; evaluate prior to abatacept initiation and during treatment in patients at risk for hepatitis B infection.

Patients should be evaluated for latent tuberculosis with a tuberculin skin test prior to starting abatacept. Treatment of latent tuberculosis should be initiated before abatacept is used; safety in tuberculosis-positive patients has not been established. Use may affect defenses against malignancies (via T cell inhibition); impact on the development and course of malignancies is not fully defined. As compared to the general population, an increased risk of lymphoma and lung cancer has been noted in clinical trials; however, rheumatoid arthritis has been previously associated with an increased rate of lymphoma.

Rare cases of anaphylaxis or anaphylactoid reactions have been reported with intravenous administration; may occur with first infusion. Other reactions possibly associated with hypersensitivity including hypotension, urticaria, and dyspnea occurred within 24 hours of infusion; medications for the treatment of hypersensitivity reactions should be readily available during infusion. If anaphylaxis or other serious allergic reaction occurs, stop the infusion; institute appropriate therapy; abatacept therapy should be permanently discontinued.

Precautions Use with caution in patients with chronic obstructive pulmonary disease; higher incidences of adverse effects (COPD exacerbation, cough, rhonchi, dyspnea) have been observed; monitor closely. Patients should be brought up-to-date with all immunizations before initiating therapy. Live vaccines should not be given concurrently or within 3 months of discontinuation of therapy. Potentially significant interactions may exist, requiring dose or frequency adjustment, additional monitoring, and/ or selection of alternative therapy. Consult drug interactions database for more detailed information. Injectable formulation for I.V. infusion contains maltose which may result in falsely-elevated serum glucose readings on the day of infusion.

Adverse Reactions Note: COPD patients experienced a higher frequency of COPD-related adverse reactions (COPD exacerbation, cough, dyspnea, pneumonia, rhonchi)

Cardiovascular: Hypertension
Central nervous system: Dizziness, headache
Dermatologic: Skin rash
Gastrointestinal: Abdominal pain, diarrhea, dyspepsia, nausea
Genitourinary: Urinary tract infection
Immunologic: Immunogenicity
Infection: Herpes simplex infection, influenza
Local: Injection site reaction
Neuromuscular & skeletal: Back pain, limb pain
Respiratory: Bronchitis, cough, nasopharyngitis, pneumonia, rhinitis, sinusitis, upper respiratory tract infection
Miscellaneous: Antibody development, fever, infection, infusion-related reaction
Rare but important or life-threatening: Acute lymphocytic leukemia, anaphylactoid reaction, anaphylaxis, cellulitis, diverticulitis, dyspnea, exacerbation of arthritis, exacerbation of chronic obstructive pulmonary disease, hypersensitivity, hypotension, joint wear, malignant lymphoma, malignant neoplasm (including malignant melanoma, malignant neoplasm of the bile duct, malignant neoplasm of bladder, malignant neoplasm of breast, malignant neoplasm of cervix, malignant neoplasm of kidney, malignant neoplasm of prostate, malignant neoplasm of skin, malignant neoplasm of thyroid, myelodysplastic syndrome, and uterine neoplasm), malignant neoplasm of lung, ovarian cyst, pruritus, pyelonephritis, rhonchi, urticaria, varicella, vasculitis (including hypersensitivity angiitis [cutaneous vasculitis and leukocytoclastic vasculitis]), wheezing

Drug Interactions

Metabolism/Transport Effects None known.

Avoid Concomitant Use

Avoid concomitant use of Abatacept with any of the following: Anakinra; Anti-TNF Agents; BCG; Belimumab; Natalizumab; Pimecrolimus; RiTUXimab; Tacrolimus (Topical); Tocilizumab; Tofacitinib; Vaccines (Live)

Increased Effect/Toxicity

Abatacept may increase the levels/effects of: Belimumab; Leflunomide; Natalizumab; Tofacitinib; Vaccines (Live)

The levels/effects of Abatacept may be increased by: Anakinra; Anti-TNF Agents; Denosumab; Pimecrolimus; RiTUXimab; Roflumilast; Tacrolimus (Topical); Tocilizumab; Trastuzumab

Decreased Effect

Abatacept may decrease the levels/effects of: BCG; Coccidioidin Skin Test; Sipuleucel-T; Vaccines (Inactivated); Vaccines (Live)

The levels/effects of Abatacept may be decreased by: Echinacea

Stability

Prefilled syringe: Store at 2°C to 8°C (36°F to 46°F); do not freeze; protect from light.

Powder for injection: Store intact vial at 2°C to 8°C (36°F to 46°F); protect from light. Reconstitute vial with 10 mL SWI using a silicone-free disposable syringe (translucent particles may develop in solutions prepared with a siliconized syringe). After further dilution in NS, store for up to 24 hours at room temperature or refrigerate. Use within 24 hours of reconstitution.

Mechanism of Action Selective costimulation modulator; inhibits T-cell (T-lymphocyte) activation by binding to CD80 and CD86 on antigen presenting cells (APC), thus blocking the required CD28 interaction between APCs and T cells. Activated T lymphocytes are found in the synovium of rheumatoid arthritis patients.

Pharmacokinetics (Adult data unless noted)

Distribution: V_{dss}: 0.07 L/kg (range: 0.02 to 0.13 L/kg)
Bioavailability: SubQ: 78.6% (relative to I.V. administration)
Half-life elimination: RA: 13.1 days (range: 8 to 25 days)
Clearance: 0.22 to 0.23 mL/hour/kg
Children 6 to 17 years: JIA: 0.4 mL/hour/kg (increases with baseline body weight)

Dosing: Usual

Pediatric:

Juvenile idiopathic arthritis: Children and Adolescents 6 to 17 years: **Note:** Dose is based on body weight at each dose administration. I.V.: Following the initial I.V. infusion, repeat I.V. dose at 2 weeks and 4 weeks after the initial infusion, and every 4 weeks thereafter. Patient weight:
<75 kg: 10 mg/kg
75 to 100 kg: 750 mg
>100 kg: 1000 mg

Rheumatoid arthritis: Adolescents ≥18 years:
I.V.: Weight-based dosing: Following the initial I.V. infusion (using the weight-based dosing), repeat I.V. infusion (using the same weight-based dosing) at 2 weeks and 4 weeks after the initial infusion, and every 4 weeks thereafter.
<60 kg: 500 mg
60 to 100 kg: 750 mg
>100 kg: 1000 mg
SubQ: 125 mg once weekly. **Note:** SubQ dosing may be initiated with or without an I.V. loading dose.
If initiating with an I.V. loading dose: Administer the initial I.V. infusion (using the weight-based dosing), then administer 125 mg SubQ within 24 hours of the infusion, followed by 125 mg SubQ once weekly thereafter.
If transitioning from I.V. therapy to SubQ therapy: Administer the first SubQ dose instead of the next scheduled I.V. dose.

Adult: **Rheumatoid arthritis:**
I.V.: Dosing is according to body weight. Following the initial I.V. infusion (using the weight-based dosing), repeat I.V. infusion (using the same weight-based dosing) at 2 weeks and 4 weeks after the initial infusion, and every 4 weeks thereafter.
<60 kg: 500 mg
60 to 100 kg: 750 mg
>100 kg: 1000 mg
SubQ: 125 mg once weekly. **Note:** SubQ dosing may be initiated with or without an I.V. loading dose.
If initiating with an I.V. loading dose: Administer the initial I.V. infusion (using the weight-based dosing), then administer 125 mg SubQ within 24 hours of the infusion, followed by 125 mg SubQ once weekly thereafter.
If transitioning from I.V. therapy to SubQ therapy: Administer the first SubQ dose instead of the next scheduled I.V. dose.

Dosing adjustment for renal impairment: There are no dosage adjustments provided in the manufacturer's labeling; not studied.

Dosing adjustment for hepatic impairment: There are no dosage adjustments provided in the manufacturer's labeling; not studied.

Administration

I.V.: Prepare abatacept using only the silicone-free disposable syringe provided with each vial [for information on obtaining additional silicone-free disposable syringes contact Bristol-Myers Squibb at 1-800-ORENCIA]. Following reconstitution, remove an equal volume of solution from a 100 mL NS infusion bag before adding the abatacept dose to the bag with the silicone-free syringe. Mix gently; do not shake. Administer through a 0.2 to 1.2 micron low protein-binding filter. Infuse over 30 minutes at a final concentration not to exceed 10 mg/mL.

SubQ: Allow prefilled syringe to warm to room temperature for 30 to 60 minutes prior to administration. Inject into the front of the thigh (preferred), abdomen (except for 2-inch area around the navel), or the outer area of the upper arms (if administered by a caregiver). Rotate injection sites (≥1 inch apart); do not administer into tender, bruised, red, or hard skin.

Monitoring Parameters Monitor improvement of symptoms and physical function assessments (eg, joint swelling, pain, and tenderness; ESR or C-reactive protein level). Latent TB screening prior to initiating therapy; signs/symptoms of infection (prior to, during, and following therapy); CBC with differential; HBV screening prior to initiating signs and symptoms of hypersensitivity reaction; signs/symptoms of malignancy

Test Interactions Contains maltose; may result in falsely elevated blood glucose levels with dehydrogenase pyrroloquinolinequinone or glucose-dye-oxidoreductase testing methods on the day of infusion. Glucose monitoring methods which utilize glucose dehydrogenase nicotine adenine dinucleotide (GDH-NAD), glucose oxidase, or glucose hexokinase are recommended.

Dosage Forms Excipient information presented when available (limited, particularly for generics); consult specific product labeling.

Solution, Subcutaneous [preservative free]:
Orencia: 125 mg/mL (1 mL)
Solution Reconstituted, Intravenous [preservative free]:
Orencia: 250 mg (1 ea)

References

Bruce SP and Boyce EG, "Update on Abatacept: A Selective Costimulation Modulator for Rheumatoid Arthritis," *Ann Pharmacother*, 2007, 41(7):1153-62.

Orencia (abatacept) [prescribing information]. Princeton, NJ: Bristol-Myers Squibb; December 2013.

Ruperto N, Lovell DJ, Quartier P, et al, "Abatacept in Children With Juvenile Idiopathic Arthritis: A Randomised, Double-Blind, Placebo-Controlled Withdrawal Trial," *Lancet*, 2008, 372(9636):383-91.

◆ **Abbott-43818** see Leuprolide *on page 1215*

◆ **Abbott-Pantoprazole (Can)** see Pantoprazole *on page 1595*

◆ **ABC** see Abacavir *on page 36*

◆ **Abelcet** see Amphotericin B (Lipid Complex) *on page 152*

◆ **Abelcet® (Can)** see Amphotericin B (Lipid Complex) *on page 152*

◆ **Abenol (Can)** see Acetaminophen *on page 47*

◆ **Abilify** see ARIPiprazole *on page 196*

◆ **Abilify Discmelt** see ARIPiprazole *on page 196*

◆ **Abilify Maintena** see ARIPiprazole *on page 196*

◆ **ABLC** see Amphotericin B (Lipid Complex) *on page 152*

◆ **Absorica** see ISOtretinoin *on page 1161*

◆ **Abstral** see FentaNYL *on page 853*

◆ **Acanya** see Clindamycin and Benzoyl Peroxide *on page 502*

Acarbose (AY car bose)

Medication Safety Issues

Sound-alike/look-alike issues:
Precose® may be confused with PreCare®

High alert medication:
The Institute for Safe Medication Practices (ISMP) includes this medication among its list of drug classes which have a heightened risk of causing significant patient harm when used in error.

International issues:
Precose® [U.S., Malaysia] may be confused with Precosa brand name for *Saccharomyces boulardii* [Finland, Sweden]

Brand Names: U.S. Precose

Brand Names: Canada Glucobay™

Therapeutic Category Antidiabetic Agent, Alpha-glucosidase Inhibitor; Antidiabetic Agent, Oral

Generic Availability (U.S.) Yes

Use Management of type II diabetes mellitus (noninsulin-dependent, NIDDM) when hyperglycemia cannot be managed by diet alone; may be used concomitantly with metformin, a sulfonylurea, or insulin to improve glycemic control

Pregnancy Risk Factor B

Pregnancy Considerations Adverse events have not been reported in animal reproduction studies. Low amounts of acarbose are absorbed systemically which should limit fetal exposure. Limited information is available describing pregnancy outcomes following maternal use of acarbose.

For women with diabetes, maternal hyperglycemia can be associated with adverse effects in the fetus, neonate, and mother. To prevent adverse events, prior to conception and throughout pregnancy, the maternal HbA_{1c} should be kept close to normal but without causing significant hypoglycemia. The use of most oral antihyperglycemic agents in pregnant women is not recommended for routine management of GDM or type 2 diabetes mellitus in pregnant women; insulin is the drug of choice for the control of diabetes mellitus during pregnancy (ACOG, 2005; ADA, 2013; Kitzmiller, 2008; Metzger, 2007).

Breast-Feeding Considerations It is not known if acarbose is found in breast milk; however, low amounts of acarbose are absorbed systemically in adults, which may limit the amount that could distribute into breast milk. Although breast-feeding is encouraged for all women, including those with diabetes, the safety of acarbose during breast-feeding has not yet been established (Metzger, 2007). Breast-feeding is not recommended by the manufacturer.

Contraindications Hypersensitivity to acarbose or any component; diabetic ketoacidosis; cirrhosis; patients with inflammatory bowel disease, colonic ulceration, partial intestinal obstruction, or patients predisposed to intestinal obstruction; patients who have chronic intestinal diseases associated with marked disorders of digestion or absorption; patients who have conditions that may deteriorate as a result of increased gas formation in the intestine

Warnings Dose-related elevations in serum transaminases occurred in 15% of acarbose-treated patients in long-term studies; these elevations were asymptomatic, reversible, more common in females, and not associated with other evidence of liver dysfunction; acarbose serum levels are proportionately higher in patients with renal dysfunction (S_{cr} >2 mg/dL); until long term clinical studies are completed, use in renally-compromised patients is not recommended

Precautions Hypoglycemia may occur when used in combination with sulfonylureas or insulin; oral glucose (absorption is not affected by acarbose) should be used instead of sucrose (table sugar) for the treatment of mild to moderate hypoglycemia

Adverse Reactions

Gastrointestinal: Diarrhea and abdominal pain tend to return to pretreatment levels over time; frequency and intensity of flatulence tend to abate with time

Hepatic: Transaminases increased

Rare but important or life-threatening: Edema, erythema, exanthema, hepatitis, ileus/subileus, jaundice, liver damage, pneumatosis cystoides intestinalis, rash, thrombocytopenia, urticaria

Drug Interactions

Metabolism/Transport Effects None known.

Avoid Concomitant Use There are no known interactions where it is recommended to avoid concomitant use.

Increased Effect/Toxicity

Acarbose may increase the levels/effects of: Hypoglycemic Agents

The levels/effects of Acarbose may be increased by: Androgens; Herbs (Hypoglycemic Properties); MAO Inhibitors; Neomycin; Pegvisomant; Salicylates; Selective Serotonin Reuptake Inhibitors

Decreased Effect

Acarbose may decrease the levels/effects of: Digoxin

The levels/effects of Acarbose may be decreased by: Corticosteroids (Orally Inhaled); Corticosteroids (Systemic); Danazol; Loop Diuretics; Luteinizing Hormone-Releasing Hormone Analogs; Somatropin; Thiazide Diuretics

Mechanism of Action Competitive inhibitor of pancreatic α-amylase and intestinal brush border α-glucosidases, resulting in delayed hydrolysis of ingested complex carbohydrates and disaccharides and absorption of glucose; dose-dependent reduction in postprandial serum insulin and glucose peaks; inhibits the metabolism of sucrose to glucose and fructose

Pharmacodynamics Average decrease in fasting blood sugar: 20-30 mg/dL

Pharmacokinetics (Adult data unless noted)

Absorption: <2% absorbed as active drug

Metabolism: Metabolized exclusively within the GI tract, principally by intestinal bacteria and by digestive enzymes; 13 metabolites have been identified

Bioavailability: Low systemic bioavailability of parent compound

Elimination: Fraction absorbed as intact drug is almost completely excreted in urine

Dosing: Usual Oral:

Adolescents and Adults: Dosage must be individualized on the basis of effectiveness and tolerance; do not exceed the maximum recommended dose (use slow titration to prevent or minimize GI effects):

Initial: 25 mg 3 times/day; increase in 25 mg/day increments in 2-4 week intervals to maximum dose

Maximum dose:

Patients ≤60 kg: 50 mg 3 times/day

Patients >60 kg: 100 mg 3 times/day

Dosing adjustment in renal impairment:

Administration Oral: Administer with first bite of each main meal

Monitoring Parameters Fasting blood glucose; hemoglobin A₁c; liver enzymes every 3 months for the first year of therapy and periodically thereafter

Reference Range Target range:

Blood glucose: Fasting and preprandial: 80-120 mg/dL; bedtime: 100-140 mg/dL

Glycosylated hemoglobin (hemoglobin A_{1c}): <7%

Additional Information Acarbose has been used successfully to treat postprandial hypoglycemia in children with Nissen fundoplications. Six children (4-25 months) initially received 12.5 mg before each bolus feeding of formula containing complex carbohydrates. The dosage was increased in 12.5 mg increments (dosage range: 12.5-50 mg per dose) until postprandial serum glucose was stable ≥60 mg/dL. Most commonly reported side effects were flatulence, abdominal distension, and diarrhea (Ng, 2001).

Dosage Forms Excipient information presented when available (limited, particularly for generics); consult specific product labeling.

Tablet, Oral:

Precose: 25 mg, 50 mg, 100 mg

Generic: 25 mg, 50 mg, 100 mg

References

American College of Obstetricians and Gynecologists Committee on Practice Bulletins, "Clinical Management Guidelines for Obstetrician-Gynecologists. Number 60, March 2005. Progestational Diabetes Mellitus," *Obstet Gynecol*, 2005, 105(3):675-85.

American Diabetes Association, "Standards of Medical Care in Diabetes – 2013," *Diabetes Care*, 2013, 36(Suppl 1):S11-66.

DeFronzo RA, "Pharmacologic Therapy for Type 2 Diabetes Mellitus," *Ann Intern Med*, 1999, 131(4):281-303.

Kitzmiller JL, Block JM, Brown FM, et al, "Managing Preexisting Diabetes for Pregnancy: Summary of Evidence and Consensus Recommendations for Care," *Diabetes Care*, 2008, 31(5):1060-79.

Metzger BE, Buchanan TA, Coustan DR, et al, "Summary and Recommendations of the Fifth International Workshop-Conference on Gestational Diabetes Mellitus," *Diabetes Care*, 2007, 30(Suppl 2):S251-60.

Ng DD, Ferry RJ Jr, Kelly A, et al, "Acarbose Treatment of Postprandial Hypoglycemia in Children After Nissen Fundoplication," *J Pediatr*, 2001, 139(6):877-9.

◆ **Accel-Amlodipine (Can)** *see* AmLODIPine *on page 135*

◆ **Accel-Clarithromycin (Can)** *see* Clarithromycin *on page 490*

◆ **Accolate** *see* Zafirlukast *on page 2164*

◆ **Accolate® (Can)** *see* Zafirlukast *on page 2164*

◆ **AccuNeb [DSC]** *see* Albuterol *on page 84*

◆ **Accupril** *see* Quinapril *on page 1788*

◆ **Accutane** *see* ISOtretinoin *on page 1161*

◆ **Accutane® (Can)** *see* ISOtretinoin *on page 1161*

◆ **Acephen [OTC]** *see* Acetaminophen *on page 47*

◆ **Acerola C 500 [OTC]** *see* Ascorbic Acid *on page 206*

◆ **Acetadote** *see* Acetylcysteine *on page 60*

Acetaminophen (a seet a MIN oh fen)

Medication Safety Issues

Sound-alike/look-alike issues:

Acephen may be confused with AcipHex

FeverALL may be confused with Fiberall

Triaminic Children's Fever Reducer Pain Reliever may be confused with Triaminic cough and cold products

Tylenol may be confused with atenolol, timolol, Tylenol PM, Tylox

Other safety concerns:

Duplicate therapy issues: This product contains acetaminophen, which may be a component of combination products. Do not exceed the maximum recommended daily dose of acetaminophen.

Infant concentration change: All children's and infant acetaminophen products are available as 160 mg/ 5 mL. Some remaining infant concentrated solutions of 80 mg/0.8 mL and 100 mg/mL may still be available on pharmacy shelves or in patient homes. Check concentrations closely prior to administering or dispensing and verify concentration available to patients prior to recommending a dose (November 2011).

Injection: Reports of 10-fold overdose errors using the parenteral product have occurred in the U.S. and ▶

Europe; calculation of doses in "mg" and subsequent administration of the dose in "mL" using the commercially available concentration of 10 mg/mL contributed to these errors. Expressing doses as mg and mL, as well as pharmacy preparation of doses, may decrease error potential (Dart, 2012; ISMP, 2012).

International issues:

Depon [Greece] may be confused with Depen brand name for penicillamine [U.S.]; Depin brand name for nifedipine [India]; Dipen brand name for diltiazem [Greece]

Duorol [Spain] may be confused with Diuril brand name for chlorothiazide [U.S., Canada]

Paralen [Czech Republic] may be confused with Aralen brand name for chloroquine [U.S., Mexico]

Related Information

Acetaminophen Serum Level Nomogram *on page 2407*

Oral Medications That Should Not Be Crushed or Altered *on page 2438*

Brand Names: U.S. Acephen [OTC]; Aspirin Free Anacin Extra Strength [OTC]; Cetafen Extra [OTC]; Cetafen [OTC]; Excedrin Tension Headache [OTC]; Feverall [OTC]; Little Fevers [OTC]; Mapap Arthritis Pain [OTC]; Mapap Children's [OTC]; Mapap Extra Strength [OTC]; Mapap Infant's [OTC]; Mapap Junior Rapid Tabs [OTC]; Mapap [OTC]; Non-Aspirin Pain Reliever [OTC]; Nortemp Children's [OTC]; Ofirmev; Pain & Fever Children's [OTC]; Pain Eze [OTC]; Q-Pap Children's [OTC]; Q-Pap Extra Strength [OTC]; Q-Pap Infant's [OTC]; Q-Pap [OTC]; Rap-iMed Children's [OTC]; RapiMed Junior [OTC]; Silapap Children's [OTC]; Silapap Infant's [OTC]; Triaminic Children's Fever Reducer Pain Reliever [OTC]; Tylenol 8 Hour [OTC]; Tylenol Arthritis Pain Extended Relief [OTC]; Tylenol Children's Meltaways [OTC]; Tylenol Children's [OTC]; Tylenol Extra Strength [OTC]; Tylenol Jr. Meltaways [OTC]; Tylenol [OTC]; Valorin Extra [OTC]; Valorin [OTC]

Brand Names: Canada Abenol; Apo-Acetaminophen; Atasol; Novo-Gesic; Pediatrix; Tempra; Tylenol

Therapeutic Category Analgesic, Non-narcotic; Antipyretic

Generic Availability (U.S.) Yes: Excludes extended release products; injectable formulation

Use

Oral:

Immediate release:

Oral suspension, chewable tablets: Relief of minor aches and pains due to the common cold, flu, sore throat, headaches, and toothaches; reduction of fever (All indications: OTC products: FDA approved in infants and children <12 years; consult specific product formulations for appropriate age groups)

Caplet/tablet: Relief of minor aches and pains due to the common cold, headaches, minor pain of arthritis, backache, menstrual cramps, muscle aches, and toothaches (All indications: OTC products: FDA approved in ages ≥6 years and adults; consult specific product formulation for appropriate age group)

Extended release: Relief of minor aches and pains due to the common cold, headaches, backache, muscle aches, menstrual cramps, toothaches, and minor pain of arthritis; reduction of fever (All indications: OTC products: FDA approved in ages ≥12 or 18 years and adults; consult specific product formulations for appropriate age groups)

Parenteral: Treatment of mild to moderate pain and fever; treatment of moderate to severe pain when combined with opioid analgesia (All indications: FDA approved in ages ≥2 years and adults)

Rectal: Relief of minor aches, pains, and headaches; reduction of fever (All indications: OTC products: FDA approved in ages ≥6 months and adults; consult specific product formulation for appropriate age group)

Pregnancy Risk Factor C (intravenous)

Pregnancy Considerations Animal reproduction studies have not been conducted with intravenous acetaminophen, therefore, acetaminophen I.V. is classified as pregnancy category C. Acetaminophen crosses the placenta and can be detected in cord blood, newborn serum, and urine immediately after delivery. An increased risk of teratogenic effects has not been observed following maternal use of acetaminophen during pregnancy. Prenatal constriction of the ductus arteriosus has been noted in case reports following maternal use during the third trimester. The use of acetaminophen in normal doses during pregnancy is not associated with an increased risk of miscarriage or still birth; however, an increase in fetal death or spontaneous abortion may be seen following maternal overdose if treatment is delayed. Frequent maternal use of acetaminophen during pregnancy may be associated with wheezing and asthma in early childhood. The absorption may be delayed and the bioavailability of acetaminophen may be decreased in some women during pregnancy due to delayed gastric emptying.

Breast-Feeding Considerations Low concentrations of acetaminophen are excreted into breast milk and can be detected in the urine of nursing infants. Adverse reactions have generally not been observed; however, a rash caused by acetaminophen exposure was reported in one breast-feeding infant.

Contraindications Hypersensitivity to acetaminophen or any component

Additional product specific contraindication: Ofirmev: Severe hepatic impairment or severe active liver disease

OTC labeling: When used for self-medication, do not use with other drug products containing acetaminophen (prescription or nonprescription) or if allergic to acetaminophen or any of the inactive ingredients

Warnings Acetaminophen has been associated with acute liver failure, at times resulting in liver transplant and death. Hepatotoxicity is usually associated with excessive acetaminophen intake (>4 g/day in adults) and often involves more than one product that contains acetaminophen **[U.S. Boxed Warning]**. In addition, chronic daily dosing may also result in liver damage in some patients. Limit acetaminophen dose from all sources (prescription, OTC, combination products) and all routes of administration (I.V., oral, rectal) to maximum dose listed for specific age groups. Use with caution in patients with alcoholic liver disease; consuming ≥3 alcoholic drinks/day may increase the risk of liver damage. Use caution in patients with hepatic impairment or active liver disease; use of I.V. formulation is contraindicated in patients with severe hepatic impairment or severe active liver disease.

Take care to avoid dosing errors with acetaminophen injection which could result in accidental overdose and death; ensure that the dose in mg is not confused with mL, dosing in patients <50 kg is based on body weight, infusion pumps are properly programmed, and total daily dose of acetaminophen from all sources does not exceed the maximum daily limits **[U.S. Boxed Warning]**.

Hypersensitivity and anaphylactic reactions have been reported including life-threatening anaphylaxis; discontinue immediately if symptoms occur. Serious and potentially fatal skin reactions, including acute generalized exanthematous pustulosis (AGEP), Stevens-Johnson Syndrome (SJS), and toxic epidermal necrolysis (TEN), have occurred rarely with acetaminophen use. Discontinue therapy at the first appearance of skin rash.

Gelcap and geltab contain benzyl alcohol; some elixir preparations contain benzoic acid; liquid preparations (ie, elixir, liquid, suspension, and drops) may contain sodium benzoate; benzoic acid (benzoate) is a metabolite of benzyl alcohol; large amounts of benzyl alcohol (≥99 mg/kg/day) have been associated with a potentially fatal toxicity ("gasping syndrome") in neonates; the "gasping syndrome" consists of metabolic acidosis, respiratory distress, gasping respirations, CNS dysfunction (including convulsions, intracranial hemorrhage), hypotension and cardiovascular collapse; avoid use of acetaminophen products containing sodium benzoate in neonates; *in vitro* and animal studies have shown that benzoate displaces bilirubin from protein binding sites. Elixir, suspension, and some oral drops and liquids contain propylene glycol; toxicities have been reported with use of products containing propylene glycol, including hyperosmolality, lactic acidosis, seizures, and respiratory depression; in neonates large amounts of propylene glycol delivered orally, intravenously (eg, >3000 mg/day), or topically have been associated with potentially fatal toxicities which can include metabolic acidosis, seizures, renal failure, and CNS depression; use products containing propylene glycol with caution (AAP, 1997; Shehab, 2009).

Suppositories contain polysorbate 80 (Tween 80) which may cause allergic reactions in susceptible individuals. In premature neonates, thrombocytopenia, ascites, pulmonary deterioration, and renal and hepatic failure have been reported after receiving parenteral products containing polysorbate 80 (Alade, 1986; CDC, 1984).

When used for self-medication (OTC), patients should be instructed to stop use and contact health care provider if symptoms get worse or new symptoms appear, redness or swelling is present in the painful area, fever lasts >3 days (all ages), or pain (excluding sore throat) lasts longer than: Adults: 10 days, Children and Adolescents: 5 days, Infants: 3 days. When treating children with sore throat, if sore throat is severe, persists for >2 days, or is followed by fever, rash, headache, nausea, or vomiting, consult health care provider immediately. Do not give more than 5 doses in 24 hours or use with other drugs that contain acetaminophen; severe liver damage may occur.

Precautions Use with caution in patients with chronic malnutrition or severe renal impairment; use intravenous formulation with caution in patients with severe hypovolemia.

Although several case reports of acetaminophen-associated hemolytic anemia have been reported in patients with G-6-PD deficiency, a direct cause and effect relationship has not been well established (concurrent illnesses such as fever or infection may precipitate hemolytic anemia in patients with G-6-PD deficiency; therefore, acetaminophen is generally thought to be safe when given in therapeutic doses to patients with G-6-PD deficiency.

Some products (eg, chewable tablets) contain aspartame which is metabolized to phenylalanine and must be avoided (or used with caution) in patients with phenylketonuria.

Adverse Reactions Oral, Rectal:
Dermatologic: Skin rash

Endocrine & metabolic: Decreased serum bicarbonate, decreased serum calcium, decreased serum sodium, hyperchloremia, hyperuricemia, increased serum glucose

Genitourinary: Nephrotoxicity (with chronic overdose)

Hematologic & oncologic: Anemia, leukopenia, neutropenia, pancytopenia

Hepatic: Increased serum alkaline phosphatase, increased serum bilirubin

Hypersensitivity: Hypersensitivity reaction (rare)

Renal: Hyperammonemia, renal disease (analgesic)

I.V.:
Cardiovascular: Hypertension, hypotension, peripheral edema, tachycardia

Central nervous system: Agitation (children), anxiety, fatigue, headache (more common in adults), insomnia (more common in adults), trismus

Dermatologic: Pruritus (children), skin rash

Endocrine & metabolic: Hypervolemia, hypoalbuminemia, hypokalemia, hypomagnesemia, hypophosphatemia

Gastrointestinal: Abdominal pain, diarrhea, headache (more common in adults), insomnia (more common in adults), nausea (more common in adults), vomiting (more common in adults)

Genitourinary: Oliguria (children)

Hematologic & oncologic: Anemia

Hepatic: Increased serum transaminases

Local: Infusion site reaction (pain)

Neuromuscular & skeletal: Limb pain, muscle spasm

Ophthalmic: Periorbital edema

Respiratory: Abnormal breath sounds, atelectasis (children), dyspnea, hypoxia, pleural effusion, pulmonary edema, stridor, wheezing

Miscellaneous: Fever

Rare but important or life-threatening: Anaphylaxis, hepatic injury (dose-related), hypersensitivity reaction, severe dermatological reaction (acute generalized exanthematous pustulosis, Stevens-Johnson syndrome, toxic epidermal necrolysis)

Drug Interactions
Metabolism/Transport Effects Substrate of CYP1A2 (minor), CYP2A6 (minor), CYP2C9 (minor), CYP2D6 (minor), CYP2E1 (minor), CYP3A4 (minor); **Note:** Assignment of Major/Minor substrate status based on clinically relevant drug interaction potential; **Inhibits** CYP3A4 (weak)

Avoid Concomitant Use
Avoid concomitant use of Acetaminophen with any of the following: Pimozide

Increased Effect/Toxicity
Acetaminophen may increase the levels/effects of: ARIPiprazole; Busulfan; Dasatinib; Dofetilide; Imatinib; Lomitapide; Mipomersen; Phenylephrine (Systemic); Pimozide; Prilocaine; Sodium Nitrite; SORAfenib; Vitamin K Antagonists

The levels/effects of Acetaminophen may be increased by: Alcohol (Ethyl); Dasatinib; Isoniazid; Metyrapone; Nitric Oxide; Probenecid; SORAfenib

Decreased Effect
The levels/effects of Acetaminophen may be decreased by: Anticonvulsants (Hydantoin); Barbiturates; CarBAMazepine; Cholestyramine Resin; Peginterferon Alfa-2b

Food Interactions Rate of absorption may be decreased when given with food. Management: Administer without regard to food.

Stability Note: See individual product literature for detailed temperature information.

Injection: Store intact vials at 20°C to 25°C (68°F to 77°F); do not refrigerate or freeze. Use within 6 hours of opening vial or transferring to another container.

Oral formulations: Store at controlled room temperature.

Suppositories: Store at <27°C (80°F). Do not freeze.

Mechanism of Action Although not fully elucidated, believed to inhibit the synthesis of prostaglandins in the central nervous system and work peripherally to block pain impulse generation; produces antipyresis from inhibition of hypothalamic heat-regulating center

Pharmacodynamics
Onset of action:

Oral: <1 hour

I.V.: Analgesia: 5-10 minutes; Antipyretic: Within 30 minutes

Peak effect: I.V.: Analgesia: 1 hour

Duration:

I.V., Oral: Analgesia: 4-6 hours

I.V.: Antipyretic: ≥6 hours

Pharmacokinetics (Adult data unless noted) Note:

With the exception of half-life (see below), the pharmaco-kinetic profile in pediatric patients (0-18 years) is similar to adult patients.

Absorption: Primarily absorbed in small intestine (rate of absorption dependent upon gastric emptying); minimal absorption from stomach; varies by dosage form

Distribution: ~1 L/kg at therapeutic doses

Protein binding: 10% to 25% at therapeutic concentrations; 8% to 43% at toxic concentrations

Metabolism: At normal therapeutic dosages, primarily hepatic metabolism to sulfate and glucuronide conjugates, while a small amount is metabolized by CYP2E1 to a highly reactive intermediate N-acetyl-p-benzoquinone imine (NAPQI), which is conjugated rapidly with glutathione and inactivated to nontoxic cysteine and mercapturic acid conjugates. At toxic doses (as little as 4000 mg in a single day), glutathione conjugation becomes insufficient to meet the metabolic demand causing an increase in NAPQI concentrations, which may cause hepatic cell necrosis. Oral administration is subject to first-pass metabolism.

Half-life:

Neonates: ~7 hours

Infants: ~4 hours

Children and Adolescents: ~3 hours

Adults: ~2 hours; severe renal insufficiency (CrCl <30 mL/minute): 2-5.3 hours

Time to peak serum concentration:

Oral: Immediate release: 10-60 minutes (may be delayed in acute overdoses)

I.V.: 15 minutes

Elimination: Urine (<5% unchanged; 60% to 80% as glucuronide metabolites; 20% to 30% as sulfate metabolites; ~8% cysteine and mercapturic acid metabolites)

Dosing: Neonatal

Pain or fever:

Oral (Anand, 2001; Anand, 2002):

GA 28-32 weeks: 10-12 mg/kg/dose every 6-8 hours; maximum daily dose: 40 mg/kg/day

GA 33-37 weeks or term neonates <10 days: 10-15 mg/kg/dose every 6 hours; maximum daily dose: 60 mg/kg/day

Term neonates ≥10 days: 10-15 mg/kg/dose every 4-6 hours; maximum daily dose: 90 mg/kg/day

I.V.: Limited data available; dose not established; Note: Some experts do not recommend the [...] aminophen in premature neonates [...] until pharmacokinetic and pharmaco[...] have been conducted in this age grou[...] 2011).

Loading dose (Allegaert, 2007; [...] 20 mg/kg/dose

Maintenance dose (Allegaert, 2007; Bartocci, 2007):

PMA 28 to 32 weeks: 10 mg/kg/dos[...] some suggest 7.5 mg/kg/dose eve[...] imum daily dose: 22.5 mg/kg/day

PMA 33 to 36 weeks: 10 mg/kg/do[...] some suggest 7.5 to 10 mg/kg/do[...] maximum daily dose: 40 mg/kg/da[...]

PMA ≥37 weeks: 10 mg/kg/dose ev[...] imum daily dose: 40 mg/kg/day

Note: Manufacturer neonatal pha[...] suggests that 7.5 mg/kg/dose eve[...] ces a similar pharmacokinetic exp[...] dosing in children ≥2 years.

Rectal (Anand, 2001; Anand, 2002):

GA 28-32 weeks: 20 mg/kg/dose eve[...] imum daily dose: 40 mg/kg/day

GA 33-37 weeks or term neonates [...] dose: 30 mg/kg; then 15 mg/kg/do[...] maximum daily dose: 60 mg/kg/day

Term infants ≥10 days: Loading dose: 30 mg/kg; then 20 mg/kg/dose every 6-8 hours; maximum daily dose: 90 mg/kg/day

Dosing: Usual Note:

In 2011, McNeil Consumer Healthcare reduced the maximum daily doses and increased the dosing interval on the labeling of some of their acetaminophen OTC products used in older pediatric patients (usually children ≥12 years and adolescents) and adults in an attempt to protect consumers from inadvertent overdoses. For example, the maximum daily dose of Extra Strength Tylenol OTC and Regular Strength Tylenol OTC were decreased to 3000 mg/day and 3250 mg/day respectively, and the dosing interval for Extra Strength Tylenol OTC was increased. Health care professionals may still prescribe or recommend the 4 g adult daily maximum to patients ≥12 years of age (but are advised to use their own discretion and clinical judgment) (McNeil Consumer Healthcare, 2014).

Pediatric:

Pain or fever: Note: Limit acetaminophen dose from all sources (prescription and OTC); maximum daily dose of acetaminophen should be limited to ≤75 mg/kg/day in ≤5 divided doses and not to exceed 4000 mg/day for most products although some formulations suggest lower maximum daily dosing (see dosing information for further detail):

Oral: **Note:** With OTC use, should not exceed recommended treatment duration unless directed by health care provider; for fever: 3 days (all ages); pain (excluding sore throat): Children ≥12 years and adolescents: 10 days, children: 5 days, or infants: 3 days; sore throat in children: 2 days

Weight-directed dosing: Infants, Children, and Adolescents: 10 to 15 mg/kg/dose every 4 to 6 hours as needed (American Pain Society, 2008; Kleigman, 2011; Sullivan, 2011); do not exceed 5 doses in 24 hours; maximum daily dose: 75 mg/kg/**day** not to exceed 4000 mg/**day**

Fixed dosing:

Oral suspension, chewable tablets: Infants and Children <12 years: Consult specific product formulations for appropriate age groups. See table; use of weight to select dose is preferred; if weight is not available, then use age; doses may be repeated every 4 hours; maximum: 5 doses/day

(handwritten note)
max dose: 75 mg/kg/day ÷5
do not exceed 4000 mg/day

Recommended:
10-15 mg/kg/dose @ 4-6 HRS.

shake suspension
give w/ food

Children ≥12 years and Adolescents:

Regular strength: 650 mg every 4 to 6 hours; maximum daily dose: 3250 mg/**day** unless directed by a physician; under physician supervision daily doses ≤4000 mg may be used

Extra strength: 1000 mg every 6 hours; maximum daily dose: 3000 mg/**day** unless directed by a physician; under physician supervision daily doses ≤4000 mg may be used

Extended release: Children ≥12 years and Adolescents: 1300 mg every 8 hours; maximum daily dose: 3900 mg/**day**

I.V.:

Infants and Children <2 years: 7.5 to 15 mg/kg/dose every 6 hours; maximum daily dose: 60 mg/kg/**day** (Wilson-Smith, 2009)

Children ≥2 years and Adolescents:

<50 kg: 15 mg/kg/dose every 6 hours **or** 12.5 mg/kg/dose every 4 hours; maximum single dose: 15 mg/kg up to 750 mg; maximum daily dose: 75 mg/kg/**day** not to exceed 3750 mg

≥50 kg: 1000 mg every 6 hours **or** 650 mg every 4 hours; maximum single dose: 1000 mg; maximum daily dose: 4000 mg/**day**

Rectal:

Weight-directed dosing: Infants and Children <12 years: 10 to 20 mg/kg/dose every 4 to 6 hours as needed; do **not** exceed 5 doses in 24 hours. **Note:** Although the perioperative use of high-dose rectal acetaminophen (eg, 25-45 mg/kg/dose) has been investigated in several studies, its routine use remains controversial; optimal dosage and dosing frequency to ensure efficacy and safety have not yet been established (Buck, 2001).

Fixed dosing:

Infants 6 to 11 months: 80 mg every 6 hours; maximum daily dose: 320 mg/**day**

Infants and Children 12 to 36 months: 80 mg every 4 to 6 hours; maximum daily dose: 400 mg/**day**

Children >3 to 6 years: 120 mg every 4 to 6 hours; maximum daily dose: 600 mg/**day**

Children >6 up to 12 years: 325 mg every 4 to 6 hours; maximum daily dose: 1625 mg/**day**

Children ≥12 years and Adolescents: 650 mg every 4 to 6 hours; maximum daily dose: 3900 mg/**day**

Adult: **Note:** Limit acetaminophen dose from all sources (prescription and OTC) to <4 g/day. No dose adjustment required when converting between different acetaminophen formulations:

Pain or fever:

I.V.:

<50 kg: 15 mg/kg every 6 hours or 12.5 mg/kg every 4 hours; maximum single dose: 15 mg/kg up to 750 mg; maximum daily dose: 75 mg/kg/**day** (≤3750 mg/day)

≥50 kg: 1000 mg every 6 hours or 650 mg every 4 hours; maximum single dose: 1000 mg/dose; maximum daily dose: 4000 mg/**day**

Oral:

Immediate release: **Note:** Actual OTC dosing recommendations may vary by product and/or manufacturer: 325 to 650 mg every 4 to 6 hours or 1000 mg 3 to 4 times/day; maximum daily dose: 4000 mg/**day**

Extended release: 1300 mg every 8 hours; maximum daily dose: 3900 mg/**day**

Rectal: 325 to 650 mg every 4 to 6 hours or 1000 mg 3 to 4 times daily; maximum daily dose: 4000 mg/**day**

Dosing adjustment in renal impairment:

I.V.: Children ≥2 years, Adolescents, and Adults: CrCl ≤30 mL/minute: Use with caution; consider decreasing daily dose and extending dosing interval

Oral (Aronoff, 2007):

Infants, Children, and Adolescents:

GFR ≥10 mL/minute/1.73 m^2: No adjustment required

GFR <10 mL/minute/1.73 m^2: Administer every 8 hours

Intermittent hemodialysis or peritoneal dialysis: Administer every 8 hours

CRRT: No adjustments necessary

Adults:

CrCl 10-50 mL/minute: Administer every 6 hours

CrCl <10 mL/minute: Administer every 8 hours

Intermittent hemodialysis or peritoneal dialysis: No adjustment necessary

CRRT: Administer every 8 hours

Dosing adjustment in hepatic impairment: Use with caution. Limited, low-dose therapy is usually well-tolerated in hepatic disease/cirrhosis; however, cases of hepatotoxicity at daily acetaminophen dosages <4000 mg/day have been reported. Avoid chronic use in hepatic impairment.

Administration

Oral: Administer with food to decrease GI upset; shake drops and suspension well before use; do not crush or chew extended release products

Parenteral: For I.V. infusion only. May administer undiluted over 15 minutes. Use within 6 hours of opening vial or transferring to another container. Discard any unused portion; single-use vials only. pH: 5.5; osmolarity: 290 mOsmol/kg

For doses <1000 mg (<50 kg): Withdraw appropriate dose from vial and place into separate empty, sterile container prior to administration

For doses ≥1000 mg (≥50 kg): Insert vented I.V. set through vial stopper

Rectal: Remove wrapper; insert suppository well up into the rectum

Test Interactions Acetaminophen may cause false-positive urinary 5-hydroxyindoleacetic acid.

Additional Information 2 mg propacetamol (prodrug) = 1 mg paracetamol = 1 mg acetaminophen

Drops may contain saccharin.

Acetaminophen (15 mg/kg/dose given orally every 6 hours for 24 hours) did **not** relieve the intraoperative or the immediate postoperative pain associated with neonatal circumcision; some benefit was seen 6 hours after circumcision (Howard, 1994).

There is currently no scientific evidence to support alternating acetaminophen with ibuprofen in the treatment of fever (Mayoral, 2000).

Based on recommendations provided by the Food and Drug Administration (FDA), all over-the-counter (OTC) pediatric single-ingredient acetaminophen liquid products will transition to a single concentration of 160 mg/5 mL; the transition began in 2011 and will continue into 2012. The concentration of acetaminophen infant drops (previously 80 mg/0.8 mL) will now be the same as children's acetaminophen products (160 mg/5 mL) and as a result, new dosing on a volume-per-weight (or volume-per-age) basis will apply. The recommended mg/kg dose is unaffected.

Dosage Forms Excipient information presented when available (limited, particularly for generics); consult specific product labeling. [DSC] = Discontinued product

Caplet, oral: 500 mg

Cetafen Extra: 500 mg

Mapap Extra Strength: 500 mg

Mapap Extra Strength: 500 mg [scored]

Pain Eze: 650 mg

Tylenol: 325 mg

Tylenol Extra Strength: 500 mg

Caplet, extended release, oral:
Mapap Arthritis Pain: 650 mg
Tylenol 8 Hour: 650 mg
Tylenol Arthritis Pain Extended Relief: 650 mg
Capsule, oral:
Mapap Extra Strength: 500 mg
Captab, oral: 500 mg
Elixir, oral:
Mapap Children's: 160 mg/5 mL (118 mL, 480 mL) [ethanol free; contains benzoic acid, propylene glycol, sodium benzoate; cherry flavor]
Gelcap, oral: 500 mg
Mapap: 500 mg
Gelcap, rapid release, oral: 500 mg
Tylenol Extra Strength: 500 mg
Geltab, oral: 500 mg
Excedrin Tension Headache: 500 mg [contains caffeine 65 mg/geltab]
Injection, solution [preservative free]:
Ofirmev: 10 mg/mL (100 mL)
Liquid, oral: 160 mg/5 mL (120 mL, 473 mL); 500 mg/5 mL (240 mL)
Mapap Extra Strength: 500 mg/5 mL (237 mL) [contains propylene glycol, sodium 9 mg/15 mL, sodium benzoate; cherry flavor]
Q-Pap Children's: 160 mg/5 mL (118 mL, 473 mL) [ethanol free; contains propylene glycol, sodium 2 mg/5 mL, sodium benzoate; cherry flavor]
Q-Pap Children's: 160 mg/5 mL (118 mL) [ethanol free; contains propylene glycol, sodium 2 mg/5 mL, sodium benzoate; grape flavor]
Silapap Children's: 160 mg/5 mL (118 mL, 237 mL, 473 mL) [ethanol free, sugar free; contains propylene glycol, sodium benzoate; cherry flavor]
Tylenol Extra Strength: 500 mg/15 mL (240 mL) [ethanol free; contains propylene glycol, sodium benzoate; cherry flavor]
Solution, oral: 160 mg/5 mL (5 mL, 10 mL, 20 mL)
Pain & Fever Children's: 160 mg/5 mL (118 mL, 473 mL) [ethanol free, sugar free; contains propylene glycol, sodium 1 mg/5 mL, sodium benzoate; cherry flavor]
Solution, oral (drops): 80 mg/0.8 mL (15 mL [DSC])
Little Fevers: 80 mg/mL (30 mL) [dye free, ethanol free, gluten free; contains propylene glycol, sodium benzoate; berry flavor]
Q-Pap Infant's: 80 mg/0.8 mL (15 mL) [ethanol free; contains propylene glycol; fruit flavor]
Silapap Infant's: 80 mg/0.8 mL (15 mL, 30 mL) [ethanol free; contains propylene glycol, sodium benzoate; cherry flavor]
Suppository, rectal: 120 mg (12s); 325 mg (12s); 650 mg (12s)
Acephen: 120 mg (12s, 50s, 100s); 325 mg (6s, 12s, 50s, 100s); 650 mg (12s, 50s, 100s)
Feverall: 80 mg (6s, 50s); 120 mg (6s, 50s); 325 mg (6s, 50s); 650 mg (50s)
Suspension, oral: 160 mg/5 mL (5 mL, 10.15 mL, 20.3 mL)
Mapap Children's: 160 mg/5 mL (118 mL) [ethanol free; contains propylene glycol, sodium benzoate; cherry flavor]
Mapap Infant's: 160 mg/5 mL (59 mL) [dye free, ethanol free; contains propylene glycol, sodium benzoate; cherry flavor]
Nortemp Children's: 160 mg/5 mL (118 mL) [ethanol free; contains propylene glycol, sodium benzoate; cotton candy flavor]
Pain & Fever Children's: 160 mg/5 mL (60 mL) [ethanol free; contains propylene glycol, sodium benzoate; cherry flavor]
Q-Pap Children's: 160 mg/5 mL (118 mL) [ethanol free; contains sodium 2 mg/5 mL, sodium benzoate; bubblegum flavor]

Q-Pap Children's: 160 mg/5 mL (118 mL) [ethanol free; contains sodium 2 mg/5 mL, sodium benzoate; cherry flavor]
Q-Pap Children's: 160 mg/5 mL (118 mL) [ethanol free; contains sodium 2 mg/5 mL, sodium benzoate; grape flavor]
Tylenol Children's: 160 mg/5 mL (120 mL) [dye free, ethanol free; contains propylene glycol, sodium benzoate; cherry flavor]
Tylenol Children's: 160 mg/5 mL (120 mL) [ethanol free; contains propylene glycol, sodium 2 mg/5 mL, sodium benzoate; bubblegum flavor]
Tylenol Children's: 160 mg/5 mL (60 mL, 120 mL) [ethanol free; contains propylene glycol, sodium 2 mg/5 mL, sodium benzoate; cherry flavor]
Tylenol Children's: 160 mg/5 mL (120 mL) [ethanol free; contains propylene glycol, sodium 2 mg/5 mL, sodium benzoate; grape flavor]
Tylenol Children's: 160 mg/5 mL (120 mL) [ethanol free; contains propylene glycol, sodium 2 mg/5 mL, sodium benzoate; strawberry flavor]
Syrup, oral:
Triaminic Children's Fever Reducer Pain Reliever: 160 mg/5 mL (118 mL) [contains benzoic acid, sodium 6 mg/5 mL; bubblegum flavor]
Triaminic Children's Fever Reducer Pain Reliever: 160 mg/5 mL (118 mL) [contains sodium 5 mg/5 mL, sodium benzoate; grape flavor]
Tablet, oral: 325 mg, 500 mg
Aspirin Free Anacin Extra Strength: 500 mg
Cetafen: 325 mg
Mapap: 325 mg
Non-Aspirin Pain Reliever: 325 mg
Q-Pap: 325 mg [scored]
Q-Pap Extra Strength: 500 mg [scored]
Tylenol: 325 mg
Tylenol Extra Strength: 500 mg
Valorin: 325 mg [sugar free]
Valorin Extra: 500 mg [sugar free]
Tablet, chewable, oral: 80 mg
Mapap Children's: 80 mg [fruit flavor]
Tablet, orally disintegrating, oral: 80 mg, 160 mg
Mapap Children's: 80 mg [bubblegum flavor]
Mapap Children's: 80 mg [grape flavor]
Mapap Junior Rapid Tabs: 160 mg [bubblegum flavor]
RapiMed Children's: 80 mg [gluten free, sugar free; bubblegum flavor]
RapiMed Children's: 80 mg [gluten free, sugar free; wild grape flavor]
RapiMed Junior: 160 mg [gluten free, sugar free; bubblegum flavor]
RapiMed Junior: 160 mg [gluten free, sugar free; wild grape flavor]
Tylenol Children's Meltaways: 80 mg [scored; bubblegum flavor]
Tylenol Children's Meltaways: 80 mg [scored; grape flavor]
Tylenol Jr. Meltaways: 160 mg [bubblegum flavor]
Tylenol Jr. Meltaways: 160 mg [grape flavor]

References

Alade SL, Brown RE, Paquet A. Polysorbate 80 and e-ferol toxicity. Pediatrics. 1986;77(4):593-597.

Allegaert K, Murat I, and Anderson BJ, "Not All Intravenous Paracetamol Formulations Are Created Equal..." Paediatr Anaesth, 2007, 17(8):811-2.

Allegaert K, Palmer GM, and Anderson BJ, "The Pharmacokinetics of Intravenous Paracetamol in Neonates: Size Matters Most," Arch Dis Child, 2011, 96(6):575-80.

American Academy of Pediatrics: Committee on Drugs, "Acetaminophen Toxicity in Children," Pediatrics, 2001, 108(4):1020-4.

American Academy of Pediatrics Committee on Drugs. "Inactive" ingredients in pharmaceutical products: update (subject review). Pediatrics. 1997;99(2):268-278.

Anand KJ and International Evidence-Based Group for Neonatal Pain, "Consensus Statement for the Prevention and Management of Pain in the Newborn," *Arch Pediatr Adolesc Med*, 2001, 155(2):173-80.

Anand KJ, Chair, International Evidence-Based Group for Neonatal Pain, personal correspondence, April 2002.

Aronoff GR, Bennett WM, Berns JS, et al, *Drug Prescribing in Renal Failure: Dosing Guidelines for Adults and Children*, 5th ed. Philadelphia, PA: American College of Physicians; 2007.

Bartocci M and Lundeberg S, "Intravenous Paracetamol: The 'Stockholm Protocol' for Postoperative Analgesia of Term and Preterm Neonates," *Paediatr Anaesth*, 2007, 17(11):1120-1.

Birmingham PK, Tobin MJ, Fisher DM, et al, "Initial and Subsequent Dosing of Rectal Acetaminophen in Children: A 24-Hour Pharmacokinetic Study of New Dose Recommendations," *Anesthesiology*, 2001, 94(3):385-9.

Buck ML, "Perioperative Use of High-Dose Rectal Acetaminophen," *Pediatr Pharm*, 2001, 7(9), http://www.medscape.com/viewarticle/415082.

Centers for Disease Control and Prevention (CDC). Unusual syndrome with fatalities among premature infants: association with a new intravenous vitamin E product. *MMWR*. 1984;33(14):198-199.

Children's Tylenol meltaways chewable tablets (acetaminophen) [prescribing information]. Fort Washington, PA: McNeil-PPC, Inc; 2014.

Children's Tylenol oral suspension liquid (acetaminophen) [prescribing information]. Fort Washington, PA: McNeil-PPC, Inc; 2014.

Dart RC, Rumack BH. Intravenous acetaminophen in the United States: iatrogenic dosing errors. *Pediatrics*. 2012;129(2):349-353.

FeverAll suppositories (acetaminophen) [prescribing information]. Lincolnton, NC: Actavis; 2014.

Frequently Asked Questions About New Dosing for Extra Strength Tylenol Products. Fort Washington, PA: McNeil-PPC, Inc; 2014. Available at http://www.tylenolprofessional.com/assets/v4/faqs-new-dosing.pdf

Hahn TW, Henneberg SW, Holm-Knudsen RJ, et al, "Pharmacokinetics of Rectal Paracetamol After Repeated Dosing in Children," *Br J Anaesth*, 2000, 85(4):512-9.

Howard CR, Howard FM, and Weitzman ML, "Acetaminophen Analgesia in Neonatal Circumcision: The Effect on Pain," *Pediatrics*, 1994, 93(4):641-646.

Infants' Tylenol oral suspension (acetaminophen) [prescribing information]. Fort Washington, PA: McNeil-PPC, Inc; 2014.

Institute for Safe Medication Practices (ISMP). IV acetaminophen and overdoses in kids. *ISMP Medication Safety Alert*, April 19, 2012. Available at http://ismp.org/Newsletters/acutecare/issue.asp?dt=20120419

Jr. Tylenol meltaways chewable tablets (acetaminophen) [prescribing information]. Fort Washington, PA: McNeil-PPC, Inc; 2014.

Kliegman RM, Stanton BF, St. Gemell JW, et al, eds. *Nelson Textbook of Pediatrics*. 19th ed. Philadelphia, PA: Saunders Elsevier;2011.

Mayoral CE, Marino RV, Rosenfeld W, et al, "Alternating Antipyretics: Is This An Alternative?" *Pediatrics*, 2000, 105(5):1009-12.

Ofirmev (acetaminophen) [package insert]. San Diego, CA: Cadence Pharmaceuticals, Inc; 2013.

"Principles of Analgesic Use in the Treatment of Acute Pain and Cancer Pain," 6th ed, Glenview, IL: American Pain Society, 2008.

Shehab N, Lewis CL, Streetman DD, Donn SM. Exposure to the pharmaceutical excipients benzyl alcohol and propylene glycol among critically ill neonates. *Pediatr Crit Care Med*. 2009;10(2):256-259.

Sullivan JE, Farrar HC. Fever and antipyretic use in children. *Pediatrics*. 2011;127(3):580-587.

Tylenol arthritis pain extended release caplets (acetaminophen) [prescribing information]. Fort Washington, PA: McNeil-PPC, Inc; 2014.

Tylenol extra strength caplets (acetaminophen) [prescribing information]. Fort Washington, PA: McNeil-PPC, Inc; 2014.

Tylenol for Healthcare Professionals. Fort Washington, PA: McNeil-PPC, Inc; 2014. Available at http://www.tylenolprofessional.com/pediatrics.html

Tylenol 8 HR extended release caplets (acetaminophen) [prescribing information]. Fort Washington, PA: McNeil-PPC, Inc; 2014.

Tylenol regular strength tablets (acetaminophen) [prescribing information]. Fort Washington, PA: McNeil-PPC, Inc; 2014.

van den Anker JN and Tibboel D, "Pain Relief in Neonates: When to Use Intravenous Paracetamol," *Arch Dis Child*, 2011, 96(6):573-4.

van Lingen RA, Deinum HT, Quak CM, et al, "Multiple-Dose Pharmacokinetics of Rectally Administered Acetaminophen in Term Infants," *Clin Pharmacol Ther*, 1999, 66(5):509-15.

Wilson-Smith EM and Morton NS, "Survey of I.V. Paracetamol (Acetaminophen) Use in Neonates and Infants Under 1 Year of Age by UK Anesthetists," *Paediatr Anaesth*, 2009, 19(4):329-37.

Acetaminophen and Codeine
(a seet a MIN oh fen & KOE deen)

Medication Safety Issues
Sound-alike/look-alike issues:
Tylenol® may be confused with atenolol, timolol, Tylox®

High alert medication:
The Institute for Safe Medication Practices (ISMP) includes this medication among its list of drug classes which have a heightened risk of causing significant patient harm when used in error.

Other safety concerns:
Duplicate therapy issues: This product contains acetaminophen, which may be a component of other combination products. Do not exceed the maximum recommended daily dose of acetaminophen.

T3 is an error-prone abbreviation (mistaken as liothyronine)

International issues:
Codex: Brand name for acetaminophen/codeine [Brazil], but also the brand name for *saccharomyces boulardii* [Italy]

Codex [Brazil] may be confused with Cedax brand name for ceftibuten [U.S. and multiple international markets]

Brand Names: U.S. Capital® and Codeine; Tylenol® with Codeine No. 3; Tylenol® with Codeine No. 4

Brand Names: Canada ratio-Emtec-30; ratio-Lenoltec; Triatec-30; Triatec-8; Triatec-8 Strong; Tylenol Elixir with Codeine; Tylenol No. 1; Tylenol No. 1 Forte; Tylenol No. 2 with Codeine; Tylenol No. 3 with Codeine; Tylenol No. 4 with Codeine

Therapeutic Category Analgesic, Narcotic

Generic Availability (U.S.) Yes: excludes suspension

Use Relief of mild to moderate pain (FDA approved in ages ≥3 years and adults)

Pregnancy Risk Factor C

Pregnancy Considerations Animal reproduction studies have not been conducted with this combination. Refer to individual monographs.

Breast-Feeding Considerations Refer to individual monographs.

Contraindications Hypersensitivity to acetaminophen, codeine phosphate, or any component; postoperative pain management in pediatric patients who have undergone tonsillectomy and/or adenoidectomy

Warnings Acetaminophen may cause severe hepatotoxicity **[U.S. Boxed Warning]**, potentially requiring liver transplant or resulting in death; hepatotoxicity is usually associated with excessive acetaminophen intake (>4 g/day in adults). Risk is increased with alcohol use, preexisting liver disease, and intake of more than one source of acetaminophen-containing medications. Chronic daily dosing in adults has also resulted in liver damage in some patients. Do not exceed maximum daily doses; consider acetaminophen content of all products (prescription and OTC), including combination products when evaluating the total daily dose of acetaminophen; adults ingesting >4 g/day of acetaminophen should seek medical attention immediately.

Respiratory depression and death have occurred in children who received codeine following tonsillectomy and/or adenoidectomy and were found to have evidence of being ultrarapid metabolizers of codeine due to a CYP2D6 polymorphism **[U.S. Boxed Warning]**; patients with this phenotype may have extensive conversion of codeine to morphine with resultant increased serum morphine concentrations; this may result in increased opioid-mediated effects and possible life-threatening respiratory depression or signs of overdose (eg, extreme sleepiness, confusion, shallow breathing) at usual therapeutic doses of codeine; codeine is contraindicated in the postoperative pain management of children who have undergone tonsillectomy and/or adenoidectomy. Deaths have also occurred in nursing infants after being exposed to high concentrations of morphine because the mothers were ultrarapid metabolizers of codeine. Ultrarapid metabolizers of codeine [ie, patients with more than two copies of functional alleles (CYP2D6 genotype with gene duplications denoted as *1/*1xN or *1/*2xN)] are at increased risk of opioid toxicity; avoid the use of codeine in these patients; consider alternative analgesics such as morphine or a nonopioid agent (Crews, 2012). The observed occurrence of the CYP2D6 "ultrarapid" phenotype is: North Africans, Ethiopians, and Arabs: 16% to 28%; African-Americans: 3%; Caucasians: 1% to 10%; Hispanics: 0.5% to 1%; and Chinese and Japanese: 0.5% to 1%. Use with caution in patients with severe respiratory disease (COPD, sleep apnea); may lead to potentially fatal respiratory depression. Respiratory depression may occur at therapeutic dosages in any patient; use with extreme caution in patients with respiratory diseases including asthma, emphysema, COPD, cor pulmonale, hypoxia, hypercapnia, preexisting respiratory depression, significantly decreased respiratory reserve, other obstructive pulmonary disease, kyphoscoliosis, or other skeletal disorder which may alter respiratory function. Codeine should be prescribed in all patients in the lowest effective dose and for the shortest period of time; patients and caregivers should be informed about risks and signs of morphine overdose. Due to the incidence of serious side effects and fatalities associated with codeine use in children, Health Canada is no longer recommending codeine use in any child <12 years of age.

Hypersensitivity and anaphylactic reactions have been reported with acetaminophen and codeine; use with caution in patients with hypersensitivity reactions to other phenanthrene derivative opioid agonists (morphine, hydrocodone, hydromorphone, levorphanol, oxycodone, oxymorphone); discontinue immediately if symptoms of allergic or hypersensitivity reactions occur. Serious and potentially fatal skin reactions, including acute generalized exanthematous pustulosis (AGEP), Stevens-Johnson Syndrome (SJS), and toxic epidermal necrolysis (TEN), have occurred rarely with acetaminophen use. Discontinue therapy at the first appearance of skin rash.

Codeine may cause CNS depression which may impair physical or mental abilities; patients must be cautioned about performing tasks which require mental alertness (eg, operating machinery or driving). Use with caution in patients with CNS depression/coma. Use caution when combining with other CNS depressants (eg, centrally acting antiemetics, general anesthetics, phenothiazines, sedative-hypnotics) as there may be additive CNS effects. If combined therapy is needed, consider reducing the dose of one or both agents.

Use with extreme caution in patients with head injury, intracranial lesions, or elevated intracranial pressure; exaggerated elevation of ICP may occur. May cause hypotension; use with caution in patients with circulatory shock, hypovolemia, impaired myocardial function, or those receiving drugs which may exaggerate hypotensive effects (including phenothiazines or general anesthetics). Codeine may obscure diagnosis or clinical course of patients with acute abdominal conditions.

Physical and psychological dependence may occur; abrupt discontinuation after prolonged use may result in withdrawal symptoms or seizures. Warn patients of possible impairment of alertness or physical coordination. Concurrent use of agonist/antagonist analgesics (ie, pentazocine, nalbuphine, and butorphanol) may precipitate withdrawal symptoms and/or reduce analgesic efficacy in patients following prolonged therapy with mu opioid agonists. High potential for abuse; healthcare providers should be alert to problems of abuse, misuse, and diversion. Infants born to women physically dependent on opioids will also be physically dependent and may experience respiratory difficulties or opioid withdrawal symptoms [neonatal abstinence syndrome (NAS)]. Onset, duration and severity of NAS depend upon the drug used (maternal), duration of use, maternal dose, and rate of drug elimination by the newborn. Symptoms of opioid withdrawal may include excessive crying, diarrhea, fever, hyper-reflexia, irritability, tremors, vomiting, or failure to gain weight. Opioid withdrawal syndrome in the neonate may be life-threatening and should be promptly treated.

Some tablets contain metabisulfite which may cause allergic reactions in susceptible individuals. Oral solution contains alcohol (7%).

Suspension contains propylene glycol; toxicities have been reported with use of products containing propylene glycol, including hyperosmolality, lactic acidosis, seizures and respiratory depression; in neonates large amounts of propylene glycol delivered orally, intravenously (eg, >3000 mg/day), or topically have been associated with potentially fatal toxicities which can include metabolic acidosis, seizures, renal failure, and CNS depression; use suspension containing propylene glycol with caution (AAP, 1997; Shehab, 2009).

Suspension contains and other liquid products may contain sodium benzoate; benzoic acid (benzoate) is a metabolite of benzyl alcohol; large amounts of benzyl alcohol (≥99 mg/kg/day) have been associated with a potentially fatal toxicity ("gasping syndrome") in neonates; the "gasping syndrome" consists of metabolic acidosis, respiratory distress, gasping respirations, CNS dysfunction (including convulsions, intracranial hemorrhage), hypotension and cardiovascular collapse; avoid use of acetaminophen and codeine products containing sodium benzoate in neonates; in vitro and animal studies have shown that benzoate displaces bilirubin from protein binding sites.

Precautions Use with caution in patients with adrenal insufficiency (Addison's disease); prostatic hyperplasia; urinary stricture; thyroid dysfunction; or severe liver, pulmonary, or renal insufficiency. Use with caution in biliary tract disease or acute pancreatitis; may cause spasm of the sphincter of Oddi.

Although several case reports of acetaminophen-associated hemolytic anemia have been reported in patients with G-6-PD deficiency, a direct cause and effect relationship has not been well established (concurrent illnesses such as fever or infection may precipitate hemolytic anemia in patients with G-6-PD deficiency); therefore, acetaminophen is generally thought to be safe when given in therapeutic doses to patients with G-6-PD deficiency.

Adverse Reactions

Central nervous system: Dizziness, euphoria, sedation, voice disorder

Dermatologic: Pruritus

Gastrointestinal: Abdominal pain, constipation, nausea, vomiting

Hypersensitivity: Histamine release

Respiratory: Dyspnea

Rare but important or life-threatening: Antidiuretic hormone disease, biliary tract spasm, bradycardia, drug dependence, hypotension, increased intracranial pressure, miosis, palpitations, peripheral vasodilation, respiratory depression, urinary retention

Drug Interactions

Metabolism/Transport Effects Refer to individual components.

Avoid Concomitant Use

Avoid concomitant use of Acetaminophen and Codeine with any of the following: Azelastine (Nasal); Paraldehyde; Pimozide; Thalidomide

Increased Effect/Toxicity

Acetaminophen and Codeine may increase the levels/effects of: Alvimopan; ARIPiprazole; Azelastine (Nasal); Buprenorphine; Busulfan; CNS Depressants; Dasatinib; Desmopressin; Diuretics; Dofetilide; Hydrocodone; Imatinib; Lomitapide; Methotrimeprazine; Metyrosine; Mipomersen; Mirtazapine; Paraldehyde; Phenylephrine (Systemic); Pimozide; Pramipexole; Prilocaine; ROPINIRole; Rotigotine; Selective Serotonin Reuptake Inhibitors; Sodium Nitrite; SORAfenib; Thalidomide; Vitamin K Antagonists; Zolpidem

The levels/effects of Acetaminophen and Codeine may be increased by: Alcohol (Ethyl); Amphetamines; Anticholinergic Agents; Antipsychotic Agents (Phenothiazines); Brimonidine (Topical); Cannabis; Dasatinib; Doxylamine; Dronabinol; Droperidol; HydrOXYzine; Isoniazid; Kava Kava; Magnesium Sulfate; Methotrimeprazine; Metyrapone; Nabilone; Nitric Oxide; Perampanel; Probenecid; Rufinamide; Sodium Oxybate; Somatostatin Analogs; SORAfenib; Succinylcholine; Tapentadol; Tetrahydrocannabinol

Decreased Effect

Acetaminophen and Codeine may decrease the levels/effects of: Pegvisomant

The levels/effects of Acetaminophen and Codeine may be decreased by: Ammonium Chloride; Anticonvulsants (Hydantoin); Barbiturates; CarBAMazepine; Cholestyramine Resin; CYP2D6 Inhibitors (Moderate); CYP2D6 Inhibitors (Strong); Mixed Agonist / Antagonist Opioids; Naltrexone; Peginterferon Alfa-2b

Stability Store at 20°C to 25°C (68°F to 77°F); protect from light.

Mechanism of Action

Acetaminophen: Although not fully elucidated, believed to inhibit the synthesis of prostaglandins in the central nervous system and peripherally block pain impulse generation; produces antipyresis from inhibition of hypothalamic heat-regulating center.

Codeine: Binds to opiate receptors in the CNS, causing inhibition of ascending pain pathways, altering the perception of and response to pain; causes cough suppression by direct central action in the medulla; produces generalized CNS depression.

Caffeine (contained in some non-U.S. formulations) is a CNS stimulant; use with acetaminophen and codeine increases the level of analgesia provided by each agent.

Pharmacokinetics (Adult data unless noted) See individual agents.

Dosing: Usual Note: Doses should be titrated to appropriate analgesic effect:

Children and Adolescents: **Analgesia:** Oral:

Dosage for individual components:

Codeine: 0.5 to 1 mg/kg/dose every 4 to 6 hours; maximum dose: 60 mg/dose (APS, 2008); **Note:** Do not use for postoperative tonsillectomy and/or adenoidectomy pain management.

Acetaminophen: 10 to 15 mg/kg/dose every 4 to 6 hours; do **not** exceed 5 doses in 24 hours; maximum daily dose: 75 mg/kg/**day** not to exceed 4000 mg/**day**

Manufacturer's labeling: Oral solution: Dosage expressed as mL of formulation containing 120 mg acetaminophen and 12 mg codeine per 5 mL:

Children:

3 to 6 years: 5 mL 3 to 4 times daily as needed

7 to 12 years: 10 mL 3 to 4 times daily as needed

Adolescents: 15 mL every 4 hours as needed

Adults: **Analgesia:** Oral: 1 to 2 tablets every 4 hours; maximum total dose: 12 tablets/24 hours

Codeine: 30-60 mg/dose every 4-6 hours

Acetaminophen: Maximum total dose: 4000 mg/24 hours

Dosing adjustment in renal impairment: Children, Adolescents, and Adults: There are no specific dosage adjustments provided in the manufacturer's labeling; however, clearance may be reduced; active metabolites may accumulate. Use with caution; initiate at lower doses or longer dosing intervals followed by careful titration. See individual monographs for specific adjustments.

Dosing adjustment in hepatic impairment: Children, Adolescents, and Adults: There are no dosage adjustments provided in the manufacturer's labeling; however, product contains acetaminophen; use with caution. Cases of hepatotoxicity at daily acetaminophen dosages <4 g/day have been reported. See individual monographs.

Administration Oral: Administer with food to decrease GI upset; shake suspension well before use

Monitoring Parameters Pain relief, respiratory rate, mental status, blood pressure, bowel function; signs of misuse, abuse, and addiction

Test Interactions See individual agents.

Additional Information Tylenol® With Codeine elixir contains saccharin

Controlled Substance C-III; C-V

Dosage Forms Excipient information presented when available (limited, particularly for generics); consult specific product labeling.

Solution, oral [C-V]: Acetaminophen 120 mg and codeine phosphate 12 mg per 5 mL (5 mL, 10 mL, 12.5 mL, 15 mL, 120 mL, 480 mL)

Suspension, oral [C-V]:

Capital and Codeine: Acetaminophen 120 mg and codeine phosphate 12 mg per 5 mL (480 mL) [alcohol free; contains propylene glycol, sodium benzoate; fruit punch flavor]

Tablet, oral [C-III]: Acetaminophen 300 mg and codeine phosphate 15 mg; acetaminophen 300 mg and codeine phosphate 30 mg; acetaminophen 300 mg and codeine phosphate 60 mg

Tylenol with Codeine No. 3: Acetaminophen 300 mg and codeine phosphate 30 mg [contains sodium metabisulfite]

Tylenol with Codeine No. 4: Acetaminophen 300 mg and codeine phosphate 60 mg [contains sodium metabisulfite]

References

American Academy of Pediatrics Committee on Drugs. "Inactive" ingredients in pharmaceutical products: update (subject review). *Pediatrics.* 1997;99(2):268-278.

Crews KR, Gaedigk A, Dunnenberger HM, et al, "Clinical Pharmacogenetics Implementation Consortium (CPIC) Guidelines for Codeine Therapy in the Context of Cytochrome P450 2D6 (CYP2D6) Genotype," *Clin Pharmacol Ther,* 2012, 91(2):321-6.

Khan K and Chang J, "Neonatal Abstinence Syndrome Due to Codeine," *Arch Dis Child Fetal Neonatal Ed,* 1997, 76(1):F59-60.

Koren G, Cairns J, Chitayat D, et al, "Pharmacogenetics of Morphine Poisoning in a Breastfed Neonate of a Codeine-Prescribed Mother," *Lancet,* 2006, 368(9536):704.

"Principles of Analgesic Use in the Treatment of Acute Pain and Cancer Pain," 6th ed, Glenview, IL: American Pain Society, 2008.

Reynolds EW, Riel-Romero RM, and Bada HS, "Neonatal Abstinence Syndrome and Cerebral Infarction Following Maternal Codeine Use During Pregnancy," *Clin Pediatr (Phila),* 2007, 46(7):639-45.

Shehab N, Lewis CL, Streetman DD, Donn SM. Exposure to the pharmaceutical excipients benzyl alcohol and propylene glycol among critically ill neonates. *Pediatr Crit Care Med.* 2009;10 (2):256-259.

Spigset O and Hägg S, "Analgesics and Breast-Feeding: Safety Considerations," *Paediatr Drugs,* 2000, 2(3):223-38.

U.S. Food and Drug Administration Center for Drug Evaluation and Research, "FDA Public Health Advisory: Use of Codeine By Some Breastfeeding Mothers May Lead to Life-Threatening Side Effects in Nursing Babies," available at: http://www.fda.gov/cder/drug/advisory/codeine.htm.

◆ **Acetaminophen and Hydrocodone** *see* Hydrocodone and Acetaminophen *on page 1027*

◆ **Acetaminophen and Oxycodone** *see* Oxycodone and Acetaminophen *on page 1573*

◆ **Acetazolam (Can)** *see* AcetaZOLAMIDE *on page 56*

AcetaZOLAMIDE (a set a ZOLE a mide)

Medication Safety Issues
International issues:
Diamox [Canada and multiple international markets] may be confused with Diabinese brand name for chlorpropamide [Multiple international markets]; Dobutrex brand name for dobutamine [Multiple international markets]; Trimox brand name for amoxicillin [Brazil]; Zimox brand name for amoxicillin [Italy] and carbidopa/levodopa [Greece]

Related Information
Oral Medications That Should Not Be Crushed or Altered *on page 2438*

Brand Names: U.S. Diamox Sequels

Brand Names: Canada Acetazolam; Diamox®

Therapeutic Category Anticonvulsant, Miscellaneous; Carbonic Anhydrase Inhibitor; Diuretic, Carbonic Anhydrase Inhibitor

Generic Availability (U.S.) Yes

Use
Oral:
Immediate release tablets: Adjunct treatment of edema due to congestive heart failure, drug-induced edema, centrencephalic epilepsies, chronic simple (open-angle) glaucoma, secondary glaucoma, and preoperatively in acute angle-closure glaucoma where delay of surgery is desired (FDA approved in adults); prevention or amelioration of symptoms associated with acute mountain sickness (FDA approved in adults)
Extended release capsules: Adjunctive treatment of chronic simple (open-angle) glaucoma, secondary glaucoma, and preoperatively in acute angle-closure glaucoma where delay of surgery is desired (FDA approved in adults); prevention or amelioration of symptoms associated with acute mountain sickness (FDA approved in adults)
Parenteral: Adjunct treatment of edema due to congestive heart failure, drug-induced edema, centrencephalic epilepsies, chronic simple (open-angle) glaucoma, secondary glaucoma, and preoperatively in acute angle-closure glaucoma where delay of surgery is desired (FDA approved in adults)

Pregnancy Risk Factor C

Pregnancy Considerations Adverse events have been observed in animal reproduction studies. Limited data is available following the use of acetazolamide in pregnant women for the treatment of idiopathic intracranial hypertension (Falardeau, 2013; Kesler, 2013).

Pregnant women exposed to acetazolamide during pregnancy for the treatment of seizure disorders are encouraged to enroll themselves into the AED Pregnancy Registry by calling 1-888-233-2334. Additional information is available at aedpregnancyregistry.org

Breast-Feeding Considerations Acetazolamide is excreted into breast milk. In a case report, low concentrations of acetazolamide were detected in the breast milk and the infant serum following a maternal dose of acetazolamide 500 mg twice daily. Acetazolamide concentrations in the breast milk were 1.3-2.1 mcg/mL, 1-9 hours after the dose. Acetazolamide concentrations in the infant serum were 0.2-0.6 mcg/mL, 2-12 hours after nursing. Maternal plasma concentrations were 5.2-6.4 mcg/mL, 1-7 hours after the dose. All levels were obtained on days 4-5 of therapy, 10 days after delivery (Söderman, 1984).

Due to the potential for serious adverse reactions in the nursing infant, the manufacturer recommends a decision be made whether to discontinue nursing or to discontinue the drug, taking into account the importance of treatment to the mother.

Contraindications Hypersensitivity to acetazolamide, any component, or other sulfonamides; decreased serum sodium and/or potassium concentrations; suprarenal gland failure; hyperchloremic acidosis; cirrhosis; or severe hepatic or renal disease; long-term administration in patients with chronic noncongestive angle-closure glaucoma

Warnings Fatalities associated with sulfonamides, although rare, have occurred due to severe reactions including Stevens-Johnson syndrome, toxic epidermal necrolysis, hepatic necrosis, agranulocytosis, aplastic anemia, and other blood dyscrasias; discontinue use at first sign of rash or any sign of adverse reaction. Chemical similarities are present among sulfonamides, sulfonylureas, carbonic anhydrase inhibitors, thiazides, and loop diuretics (except ethacrynic acid). Use in patients with sulfonylurea allergy is specifically contraindicated in product labeling; however, a risk of cross reaction exists in patients with allergy to any of these compounds; avoid use when previous reaction has been severe. Discontinue if signs of hypersensitivity are noted. Anorexia, tachypnea, lethargy, metabolic acidosis, and death have been reported in patients receiving acetazolamide and high-dose aspirin concomitantly. Tolerance to antiepileptic effects may require dosage adjustment. Impairment of mental alertness and/or physical coordination may occur; incidence may be higher with dose increases.

Precautions Use with caution in patients with hepatic dysfunction; use is contraindicated in patients with cirrhosis or severe hepatic disease; avoid electrolyte and acid/base imbalances that might lead to hepatic encephalopathy. Use with caution in patients with respiratory acidosis; may worsen acidosis. Use with caution in patients with mild to moderate renal impairment; dosage adjustment may be necessary; use is contraindicated in patients with several renal disease. Use with caution in patients with prediabetes or diabetes mellitus; may see a change in glucose control. Increasing the dose does not increase diuresis and may increase the incidence of drowsiness and/or paresthesia; often results in a reduction of diuresis. Intramuscular administration is painful because of the alkaline pH of the drug; use by this route is not recommended. Growth retardation has been reported in children receiving chronic therapy (possibly due to chronic acidosis).

Adverse Reactions Frequency not defined.
Cardiovascular: Flushing
Central nervous system: Ataxia, confusion, convulsions, depression, dizziness, drowsiness, excitement, fatigue, flaccid paralysis, headache, malaise, paresthesia
Dermatologic: Allergic skin reaction, skin photosensitivity, Stevens-Johnson syndrome, toxic epidermal necrolysis, urticaria
Endocrine & metabolic: Electrolyte imbalance, growth retardation (children), hyperglycemia, hypoglycemia, hypokalemia, hyponatremia, metabolic acidosis
Gastrointestinal: Decreased appetite, diarrhea, dysgeusia, glycosuria, melena, nausea, vomiting
Genitourinary: Crystalluria, hematuria
Hematologic and oncologic: Agranulocytosis, aplastic anemia, leukopenia, thrombocytopenia, thrombocytopenic purpura
Hepatic: Abnormal hepatic function tests, cholestatic jaundice, fulminant hepatic necrosis, hepatic insufficiency
Hypersensitivity: Anaphylaxis
Local: Pain at injection site
Ophthalmic: Myopia

Otic: Auditory disturbance, tinnitus

Renal: Polyuria, renal failure

Miscellaneous: Fever

Drug Interactions

Metabolism/Transport Effects Inhibits CYP3A4 (weak)

Avoid Concomitant Use

Avoid concomitant use of AcetaZOLAMIDE with any of the following: Carbonic Anhydrase Inhibitors; Pimozide

Increased Effect/Toxicity

AcetaZOLAMIDE may increase the levels/effects of: Alpha-/Beta-Agonists (Indirect-Acting); Amifostine; Amphetamines; Anticonvulsants (Barbiturate); Anticonvulsants (Hydantoin); Antihypertensives; ARIPiprazole; CarBAMazepine; Carbonic Anhydrase Inhibitors; CycloSPORINE (Systemic); Dofetilide; DULoxetine; Flecainide; Hypotensive Agents; Lomitapide; Memantine; MetFORMIN; Obinutuzumab; Pimozide; Primidone; QuiNIDine; RiTUXimab; Sodium Bicarbonate; Sodium Phosphates

The levels/effects of AcetaZOLAMIDE may be increased by: Alfuzosin; Analgesics (Opioid); Barbiturates; Brimonidine (Topical); Diazoxide; Herbs (Hypotensive Properties); MAO Inhibitors; Pentoxifylline; Phosphodiesterase 5 Inhibitors; Prostacyclin Analogues; Salicylates

Decreased Effect

AcetaZOLAMIDE may decrease the levels/effects of: Lithium; Methenamine; Primidone; Trientine

The levels/effects of AcetaZOLAMIDE may be decreased by: Herbs (Hypertensive Properties); Ketorolac (Nasal); Ketorolac (Systemic); Mefloquine; Methylphenidate; Orlistat; Yohimbine

Stability

Oral:

Immediate release tablets: Store at 15°C to 30°C (59°F to 86°F); dispense in a well-closed container.

Extended release capsules: Store at 20°C to 25°C (68°F to 77°F); dispense in a well-closed container.

Parenteral: Store intact vials at 20°C to 25°C (68°F to 77°F); after reconstitution, acetazolamide injection is stable for 12 hours at room temperature and for 3 days when refrigerated.

Mechanism of Action Reversible inhibition of the enzyme carbonic anhydrase resulting in reduction of hydrogen ion secretion at renal tubule and an increased renal excretion of sodium, potassium, bicarbonate, and water. Decreases production of aqueous humor and inhibits carbonic anhydrase in central nervous system to retard abnormal and excessive discharge from CNS neurons.

Pharmacodynamics

Onset of action:

Capsule, extended release: 2 hours

Tablet: 1-1.5 hours

I.V.: 2 minutes

Maximum effect:

Capsule, extended release: 3-6 hours

Tablet: 1-4 hours

I.V.: 15 minutes

Duration:

Capsule, extended release: 18-24 hours

Tablet: 8-12 hours

I.V.: 4-5 hours

Pharmacokinetics (Adult data unless noted)

Absorption: Appears to be dose dependent; erratic with daily doses >10 mg/kg

Distribution: Into erythrocytes and kidneys; crosses the blood-brain barrier

Protein binding: 95%

Half-life: 2.4-5.8 hours

Time to peak serum concentration: Immediate release tablet: 1-4 hours; extended release capsules: 3-6 hours

Elimination: 70% to 100% of an I.V. or tablet dose and 47% of an extended release capsule excreted unchanged in urine within 24 hours

Dosing: Usual

Infants, Children, and Adolescents:

Altitude illness, acute: Limited data available: Oral:

Prevention: 2.5 mg/kg/dose every 12 hours started either the day before (preferred) or on the day of ascent and may be discontinued after staying at the same elevation for 2-3 days or if descent initiated; maximum dose: 125 mg/dose (Luks, 2010). **Note:** The International Society for Mountain Medicine does not recommend prophylaxis in children except in the rare circumstance of unavoidable rapid ascent or in children with known previous susceptibility to acute mountain sickness (Pollard, 2001).

Treatment: Acute mountain sickness (AMS); moderate: 2.5 mg/kg/dose every 8-12 hours; maximum single dose: 250 mg. **Note:** With high altitude cerebral edema, dexamethasone is the primary treatment; however, acetazolamide may be used adjunctively with the same treatment dose (Luks, 2010; Pollard, 2001).

Glaucoma: Limited data available: Oral:

Children <12 years: Immediate release: 10-30 mg/kg/day divided every 6-8 hours; maximum daily dose: 1000 mg/day (Portellos, 1998; Sabri, 2006)

Children ≥12 years and Adolescents: 15-30 mg/kg/day; maximum daily dose: 1000 mg/day; dosing interval determined by dosage form: Immediate release tablet: Divided doses every 6-8 hours; Extended release capsules: Divided doses twice daily (Pagliaro, 2002; Sabri, 2006)

Edema: Limited data available: Oral, I.V.: Immediate release: 5 mg/kg/dose every other day in the morning (Pagliaro, 2002)

Epilepsy, short-term management: Limited data available: Oral: Immediate release: Usual range: 4-16 mg/kg/day in 3-4 divided doses; may titrate; maximum daily dose: 30 mg/kg/day or 1000 mg/day (whichever is less) (Reiss, 1996); **Note:** Minimal additional benefit with doses >16 mg/kg/day; **extended release capsule is not recommended for treatment of epilepsy**

Pseudotumor cerebri: Limited data available: Oral:

Children: Usual reported dose: Initial: 15-25 mg/kg/day in 2-3 divided doses; may increase if needed to a maximum daily dose: 100 mg/kg/day or 2000 mg/day (whichever is less); therapy continued until resolution of headache, disc swelling, and visual field abnormalities; usually several months (eg, 3-9 months) (Distelmaier, 2006; Hacifazlioglu, 2012; Ko, 2010; Per, 2013; Rangwalla, 2007; Soler, 1998; Spennato, 2011; Standridge, 2010).

Adolescents: Initial: 500 mg twice daily; may increase if needed to a maximum daily dose: 4000 mg/day (Standridge, 2010)

Adults:

Glaucoma: Oral, I.V.:

Chronic simple (open-angle): 250 mg 1-4 times/day or 500 mg extended release capsule twice daily

Secondary or acute (closed-angle): 250-500 mg; maintenance: 125-250 mg every 4 hours (250 mg every 12 hours may be more effective in short-term treatment of some patients)

Edema: Oral, I.V.: 250-375 mg once daily

Epilepsy: Oral: 8-30 mg/kg/day in divided doses. A lower dosing range of 4-16 mg/kg/day in 1-4 divided doses has also been recommended; maximum daily dose: 30 mg/kg/day or 1000 mg/day (Oles, 1989; Reiss, 1996). **Note:** Minimal additional benefit with doses >16 mg/kg/day; **extended release capsule is not recommended for treatment of epilepsy**

Altitude sickness: Oral: 500-1000 mg daily in divided doses every 8-12 hours (immediate release tablets) or divided every 12-24 hours (extended release capsules). These doses are associated with more frequent and/or increased side effects. Alternative dosing has been recommended:

Prevention: 125 mg twice daily; beginning either the day before (preferred) or on the day of ascent; may be discontinued after staying at the same elevation for 2-3 days or if descent initiated (Basnyat, 2006; Luks, 2010). **Note:** In situations of rapid ascent (such as rescue or military operations), 1000 mg/day is recommended by the manufacturer. The Wilderness Medical Society recommends consideration of using dexamethasone in addition to acetazolamide in these situations (Luks, 2010).

Treatment: 250 mg twice daily. **Note:** With high altitude cerebral edema, dexamethasone is the primary treatment; however, acetazolamide may be used adjunctively with the same treatment dose (Luks, 2010).

Dosing interval in renal impairment: There are no dosage adjustments provided in the manufacturer's labeling; acetazolamide is contraindicated in severe renal impairment. The following adjustments have been recommended (Aronoff, 2007): Oral, I.V.: Adults: **Note:** Renally adjusted dose recommendations are based on doses of 250 mg every 6 hours:

CrCl >50 mL/minute: No dosage adjustment recommended

CrCl 10-50 mL/minute: Administer every 12 hours

CrCl <10 mL/minute: Avoid use; contraindicated

Hemodialysis: Moderately dialyzable (20% to 50%)

Peritoneal dialysis: Supplemental dose is not necessary (Schwenk, 1994)

Dosing adjustment in hepatic impairment: There are no dosage adjustments provided in the manufacturer's labeling; however, acetazolamide is contraindicated in patients with cirrhosis or severe liver impairment.

Administration

Oral: Administer with food to decrease GI upset; tablet may be crushed and suspended in cherry or chocolate syrup to disguise the bitter taste of the drug

Parenteral:

I.V.: Reconstitute with at least 5 mL SWI to provide a solution containing not more than 100 mg/mL; maximum concentration: 100 mg/mL; maximum rate of I.V. infusion: 500 mg/minute

I.M.: Not generally recommended as the drug's alkaline pH makes it very painful

Monitoring Parameters Serum electrolytes, CBC and platelet counts; intraocular pressure in glaucoma patients; monitor growth in pediatric patients

Test Interactions May cause false-positive results for urinary protein with Albustix®, Labstix®, Albutest®, Bumintest®; interferes with HPLC theophylline assay and serum uric acid levels

Additional Information Sodium content of 500 mg injection: 2.049 mEq

Dosage Forms Excipient information presented when available (limited, particularly for generics); consult specific product labeling.

Capsule Extended Release 12 Hour, Oral:

Diamox Sequels: 500 mg

Generic: 500 mg

Solution Reconstituted, Injection [preservative free]:

Generic: 500 mg (1 ea)

Tablet, Oral:

Generic: 125 mg, 250 mg

Extemporaneous Preparations A 25 mg/mL oral suspension may be made with tablets and either a 1:1 mixture of Ora-Sweet® and Ora-Plus® or a 1:1 mixture of Ora-Sweet® SF and Ora-Plus®. Crush twelve 250 mg tablets in a mortar and reduce to a fine powder. Add small portions of chosen vehicle and mix to a uniform paste; mix while adding the vehicle in incremental proportions to **almost** 120 mL; transfer to a calibrated bottle, rinse mortar with vehicle, and add quantity of vehicle sufficient to make 120 mL. Label "shake well" and "refrigerate". Stable for 60 days (Allen, 1996). When diluted in 120 mL solution of cherry syrup concentrate diluted 1:4 with simple syrup, NF, it is stable 60 days refrigerated (preferred) or at room temperature (Nahata, 2004).

Allen LV Jr and Erickson MA 3rd, "Stability of Acetazolamide, Allopurinol, Azathioprine, Clonazepam, and Flucytosine in Extemporaneously Compounded Oral Liquids," *Am J Health Syst Pharm,* 1996, 53(16):1944-9.

Nahata MC, Pai VB, and Hipple TF, *Pediatric Drug Formulations,* 5th ed, Cincinnati, OH: Harvey Whitney Books Co, 2004.

References

Aronoff GR, Bennett WM, Berns JS, et al, eds. *Drug Prescribing in Renal Failure: Dosing Guidelines for Adults and Children.* 5th ed. Philadelphia, PA: American College of Physicians; 2007.

Basnyat B, Gertsch JH, Holck PS, et al. Acetazolamide 125 mg BD is Not Significantly Different from 375 mg BD in the Prevention of Acute Mountain Sickness: The Prophylactic Acetazolamide Dosage Comparison for Efficacy (PACE) Trial. *High Alt Med Biol.* 2006;7(1):17-27.

Distelmaier F, Sengler U, Messing-Juenger M, et.al. *Pseudotumor cerebri* as an important differential diagnosis of papilledema in children. *Brain and Development.* 2006;28:190-195.

Falardeau J, Lobb BM, Golden S, et al, "The Use of Acetazolamide During Pregnancy in Intracranial Hypertension Patients," *J Neuroophthalmol,* 2013, 33(1):9-12.

Hacifazlioglu N, Yilmaz Y. *Pseudotumour cerebri* in children: etiological, clinical features and treatment modalities. *European Journal of Paediatric Neurology.* 2012;12:349-355.

Kennedy CR, Ayers S, Campbell MJ, et.al. Randomized, controlled trial of acetazolamide and furosemide in posthemorrhagic ventricular dialation in infancy: follow-up at 1 year. *Pediatrics.* 2001;108:597-607.

Kesler A and Kupferminc M, "Idiopathic Intracranial Hypertension and Pregnancy," *Clin Obstet Gynecol,* 2013, 56(2):389-96.

Ko MW,Liu GT. Pediatric idiopathic intracranial hypertension (*Pseudotumor cerebri*). *Horm Res Paediatr.* 2010;74:381-389.

Libenson MH, Kaye EM, Rosman NP, et al, "Acetazolamide and Furosemide for Posthemorrhagic Hydrocephalus of the Newborn," *Pediatr Neurol,* 1999, 20(3):185-91.

Luks AM, McIntosh SE, Grissom CK, et al. Wilderness Medical Society consensus guidelines for the prevention and treatment of acute altitude illness. *Wilderness Environ Med.* 2010;21(2):146-155.

Pagliaro LA and Pagliaro AM, eds.*Problems in Pediatric Drug Therapy.*4th ed. Washington, DC: American Pharmaceutical Association; 2002.

Per H, Canpolat M, Gumus H, et.al. Clinical spectrum of the *pseudotumor cerebri* in children: etiological, clinical features, treatment and prognosis. *Brain Dev.* 2013;35:561-568.

Rangwala LM, Liu GT. Pediatric idiopathic intracranial hypertension. *Survey of Ophthalmology.* 2007;52(6):597-617.

Reiss WG and Oles KS, "Acetazolamide in the Treatment of Seizures," *Ann Pharmacother,* 1996, 30(5):514-9.

Shinnar S, Gammon K, Bergman EW Jr, et al, "Management of Hydrocephalus in Infancy: Use of Acetazolamide and Furosemide to Avoid Cerebrospinal Fluid Shunts," *J Pediatr,* 1985, 107(1):31-7.

Söderman P, Hartvig P, and Fagerlund C, "Acetazolamide Excretion Into Human Breast Milk," *Br J Clin Pharmacol,* 1984, 17(5):599-600.

Soler D, Cox T, Bullock P, et.al. Diagnosis and management of benign intracranial hypertension. *Arch Dis Child.* 1998;78:89-94.

Schwenk MH, St. Peter WL, Meese MG, et al. Acetazolamide toxicity and pharmacokinetics in ratients receiving hemodialysis. *Pharmacotherapy.* 1995;15(4):522-527.

Spennato P, Ruggiero C, Parlato RS, et al. *Pseudotumor cerebri. Childs Nerv Syst.* 2011;27:215-235.

Standridge S. Idiopathic intracranial hypertension in children: a review and algorithm. *Pediatric Neurology.* 2010;43(6): 377-390.

Acetic Acid (a SEE tik AS id)

Medication Safety Issues

Sound-alike/look-alike issues:

Acetic acid for irrigation may be confused with glacial acetic acid

VoSol® may be confused with Vexol®,VoSol® HC

Therapeutic Category Otic Agent, Anti-infective; Topical Skin Product

Generic Availability (U.S.) Yes

Use

Otic solution: Treatment of superficial infections of the external auditory canal (FDA approved in ages ≥3 years and adults)

Irrigation solution: Irrigation of the bladder; periodic irrigation of indwelling catheters (FDA approved in adults)

Pregnancy Risk Factor C

Pregnancy Considerations Animal reproduction studies have not been conducted. Systemic absorption following bladder irrigation is not likely unless open lesions are present.

Breast-Feeding Considerations Use with caution in breast-feeding women.

Contraindications Hypersensitivity to acetic acid or any component

Irrigation: Use during transurethral procedures

Otic solution: Perforated tympanic membrane

Warnings Irrigation solution is not for internal intake or I.V. infusion; irrigation use only. Use of bladder irrigation in patients with mucosal lesions of urinary bladder may cause irritation. Open lesions of the bladder mucosa may result in systemic acidosis from absorption. Discontinue use if pain or hematuria occur during irrigation.

Otic solution is for external, topical use only; transient stinging and burning may occur with the initial use in an acutely inflamed ear; discontinue promptly if sensitization or irritation occur.

Adverse Reactions

Irrigation solution:

Endocrine & Metabolic: Systemic acidosis

Genitourinary: Urologic pain

Local: Irritation

Renal: Hematuria

Otic solution: Otic: Irritation, burning, stinging

Drug Interactions

Metabolism/Transport Effects None known.

Avoid Concomitant Use

Avoid concomitant use of Acetic Acid with any of the following: BCG

Increased Effect/Toxicity There are no known significant interactions involving an increase in effect.

Decreased Effect

Acetic Acid may decrease the levels/effects of: BCG; Sodium Picosulfate

Stability

Irrigation solution: Store at 20°C to 25°C (68°F to 77°F); do not exceed 66°C (150°F); do not freeze. Discard the unused portion as it does not contain preservatives.

Otic solution: Store at 20°C to 25°C (68°F to 77°F).

Dosing: Usual

Children ≥3 years and Adolescents: **Otitis externa:** Otic: Insert saturated wick of cotton; keep moist 24 hours by adding 3-5 drops every 4-6 hours; remove wick after 24 hours and instill 5 drops 3-4 times daily. **Note:** In children, 3-4 drops may be sufficient due to the smaller capacity of the ear canal.

Adults:

Irrigation, transurethral: Note: Dosage of an irrigating solution depends on the capacity or surface area of the structure being irrigated

Urinary bladder, continuous or intermittent irrigation: Transurethral: 0.25% irrigation solution: Usual volume: 500-1500 mL per 24 hours; the rate of administration will approximate the rate of urine flow

Indwelling urinary catheter, periodic irrigation to maintain patency: Transurethral: 0.25% irrigation solution: ~50 mL is required for each irrigation

Otitis externa: Otic: Insert saturated wick of cotton; keep moist 24 hours by adding 3-5 drops every 4-6 hours; remove wick after 24 hours and instill 5 drops 3-4 times daily

Administration Not for internal intake or I.V. infusion; topical use or irrigation use only

Bladder irrigation: Urine pH should be checked at least 4 times daily and the irrigation rate adjusted to maintain a pH of 4.5-5; increasing the rate decreases the pH and vice versa

Dosage Forms Excipient information presented when available (limited, particularly for generics); consult specific product labeling.

Solution, Irrigation:

Generic: 0.25% (250 mL, 500 mL, 1000 mL)

Solution, Otic:

Generic: 2% (15 mL, 60 mL)

◆ **Acetoxyl® (Can)** see Benzoyl Peroxide on page 275

◆ **Acetoxymethylprogesterone** see MedroxyPROGESTERone on page 1318

Acetylcholine (a se teel KOE leen)

Medication Safety Issues

Sound-alike/look-alike issues:

Acetylcholine may be confused with acetylcysteine

Brand Names: U.S. Miochol-E

Brand Names: Canada Miochol®-E

Therapeutic Category Cholinergic Agent, Ophthalmic; Ophthalmic Agent, Miotic

Generic Availability (U.S.) No

Use Produces complete miosis in cataract surgery, keratoplasty, iridectomy and other anterior segment surgery where rapid miosis is required (FDA approved in adults)

Contraindications Hypersensitivity to acetylcholine chloride or any component

Warnings Open under aseptic conditions only; do not gas sterilize

Precautions Systemic cholinergic effects rarely occur, but can cause problems for patients with acute CHF, bronchial asthma, peptic ulcer, GI spasm, and urinary tract obstruction. During cataract surgery, use only after lens is in place.

Adverse Reactions

Cardiovascular: Bradycardia, flushing, hypotension

Ocular: Clouding, corneal edema, decompensation

Respiratory: Dyspnea

Miscellaneous: Diaphoresis

Drug Interactions

Metabolism/Transport Effects None known.

Avoid Concomitant Use There are no known interactions where it is recommended to avoid concomitant use.

Increased Effect/Toxicity

The levels/effects of Acetylcholine may be increased by: Acetylcholinesterase Inhibitors; Beta-Blockers

Decreased Effect There are no known significant interactions involving a decrease in effect.

Stability Store at 4°C to 25°C (39°F to 77°F); do not freeze. Prepare solution immediately before use; do not use solution which is not clear and colorless.

Mechanism of Action Causes contraction of the sphincter muscles of the iris, resulting in miosis and contraction of the ciliary muscle, leading to accommodation spasm

Pharmacodynamics

Onset of action: Miosis occurs promptly

Duration: ~20 minutes (Kanski, 1968); duration as long as 6 hours has been reported (Roszkowska, 1998)

Dosing: Usual Miosis; intraoperative: Adults: Intraocular: 0.5-2 mL of 1% injection (5-20 mg) instilled into anterior chamber before or after securing one or more sutures

Dosing adjustment in renal impairment: There are no dosage adjustments provided in the manufacturer's labeling.

Dosing adjustment in hepatic impairment: There are no dosage adjustments provided in the manufacturer's labeling.

Administration Ophthalmic: Open under aseptic conditions only. Attach filter before irrigating eye. Instill into anterior chamber before or after securing one or more sutures; instillation should be gentle and parallel to the iris face and tangential to the pupil border; in cataract surgery, acetylcholine should be used only after delivery of the lens

Dosage Forms Excipient information presented when available (limited, particularly for generics); consult specific product labeling.

Solution Reconstituted, Intraocular, as chloride:
Miochol-E: 20 mg (1 ea) [contains mannitol]

References

Kanski JJ, "Miotics," *Br J Ophthalmol*, 1968, 52(12):936-7.
Roszkowska AM, Ferreri G, Squeri CA, et al, "Effect of Intraocular Acetylcholine and Carbachol on the Corneal Endothelium. *In vivo* Comparative Study," *Ophthalmologica*, 1998, 212(6):407-9.

◆ **Acetylcholine Chloride** see Acetylcholine on page 59

Acetylcysteine (a se teel SIS teen)

Medication Safety Issues

Sound-alike/look-alike issues:
Acetylcysteine may be confused with acetylcholine
Mucomyst® may be confused with Mucinex®

Related Information
Acetaminophen Serum Level Nomogram on page 2407

Brand Names: U.S. Acetadote

Brand Names: Canada Acetylcysteine Injection; Acetylcysteine Solution; Mucomyst®; Parvolex®

Therapeutic Category Antidote, Acetaminophen; Mucolytic Agent

Generic Availability (U.S.) Yes

Use
Inhalation: Adjunctive therapy in patients with abnormal or viscid mucous secretions in bronchopulmonary diseases, pulmonary complications of surgery, and cystic fibrosis; diagnostic bronchial studies [FDA approved in pediatric patients (age not specified) and adults]

Injection, Oral: Antidote for acute acetaminophen toxicity; prevention of radiocontrast-induced renal dysfunction [FDA approved in pediatric patients (age not specified) and adults]

Has also been used orally and rectally to treat distal intestinal obstruction syndrome (previously known as "meconium ileus or its equivalent")

Pregnancy Risk Factor B

Pregnancy Considerations Adverse events were not observed in animal reproduction studies. Based on limited reports using acetylcysteine to treat acetaminophen poisoning in pregnant women, acetylcysteine has been shown to cross the placenta and may provide protective levels in the fetus.

Acetylcysteine may be used to treat acetaminophen overdose in during pregnancy (Wilkes, 2005). In general, medications used as antidotes should take into consideration the health and prognosis of the mother; antidotes should be administered to pregnant women if there is a clear indication for use and should not be withheld because of fears of teratogenicity (Bailey, 2003).

Breast-Feeding Considerations It is not known if acetylcysteine is excreted in breast milk. The manufacturer recommends that caution be exercised when administering acetylcysteine to nursing women. Based on its pharmacokinetics, the drug should be nearly completely cleared 30 hours after administration; therefore, nursing women may consider resuming nursing 30 hours after dosing is complete.

Contraindications Hypersensitivity to acetylcysteine or any component

Warnings Acute flushing and erythema have been reported; usually occurs within 30-60 minutes and may

resolve spontaneously. Serious anaphylactoid reactions have also been reported and are more commonly associated with I.V. administration, but may also occur with oral administration (Mroz, 1997). When used for acetaminophen poisoning, the incidence is reduced when the initial intravenous loading dose is administered over 60 minutes. The acetylcysteine infusion may be interrupted until the treatment of allergic symptoms is initiated; the infusion can then be carefully restarted. Treatment for anaphylactoid reactions should be immediately available during administration. Use with caution in patients with asthma or history of bronchospasm as these patients may be at increased risk. Conversely, patients with high acetaminophen levels (>150 mg/dL) may be at a reduced risk for anaphylactoid reactions (Pakravan, 2008; Sandilands, 2009; Waring, 2008).

Acetylcysteine is indicated in patients with a serum acetaminophen concentration that indicates they are at "possible" risk or greater for hepatotoxicity when plotted on the Rumack-Matthew nomogram. There are several situations where the nomogram is of limited use. Serum acetaminophen concentrations obtained <4 hours postingestion are not interpretable; patients presenting late may have undetectable serum concentrations, despite having received a toxic dose. The nomogram is less predictive of hepatic injury following an acute overdose with an extended release acetaminophen product. The nomogram also does not take into account patients who may be at higher risk of acetaminophen toxicity (eg, alcoholics, malnourished patients). Nevertheless, acetylcysteine should be administered to any patient with signs of hepatotoxicity, even if serum acetaminophen concentration is low or undetectable. Patients who present >24 hours after an acute ingestion or patients who present following an acute ingestion at an unknown time may be candidates for acetylcysteine therapy; consultation with a poison control center or clinical toxicologist is highly recommended.

The Rumack-Matthew nomogram is not designed to be used following repeated supratherapeutic ingestions (RSTIs). In general, an accurate past medical history, including a comprehensive acetaminophen ingestion history, in conjunction with AST concentrations and serum acetaminophen concentrations, may give the clinician insight as to the patient's risk of acetaminophen toxicity. Some experts recommend that acetylcysteine be administered to any patient with "higher than expected" serum acetaminophen concentrations or serum acetaminophen concentration >10 mcg/mL, even in the absence of hepatic injury; others recommend treatment for patients with laboratory evidence and/or signs and symptoms of hepatotoxicity (Hendrickson, 2006; Jones, 2000). Consultation with a poison control center or a clinical toxicologist is highly recommended.

Precautions Use with caution in patients with asthma or previous history of bronchospasm. Since increased bronchial secretions may develop after inhalation, percussion, postural drainage, and suctioning should follow; if bronchospasm occurs, administer a bronchodilator; discontinue acetylcysteine if bronchospasm progresses.

Adverse Reactions

Inhalation:
Central nervous system: Chills, drowsiness, fever
Gastrointestinal: Nausea, stomatitis, vomiting
Local: Irritation, stickiness on face following nebulization
Respiratory: Bronchospasm, hemoptysis, rhinorrhea
Miscellaneous: Acquired sensitization (rare), clamminess, unpleasant odor during administration

Intravenous:
Cardiovascular: Edema, flushing, tachycardia
Dermatologic: Pruritus, rash, urticaria
Gastrointestinal: Nausea, vomiting

Respiratory: Pharyngitis, rhinorrhea, rhonchi, throat tightness

Miscellaneous: Anaphylactoid reaction

Rare but important or life-threatening: Anaphylaxis, angioedema, bronchospasm, chest tightness, cough, dizziness, dyspnea, headache, hypotension, respiratory distress, stridor, wheezing

Oral (Bebarta, 2010; Mroz, 1997):
Cardiovascular: Hypotension, tachycardia
Dermatologic: Angioedema, pruritus, urticaria
Gastrointestinal: Nausea, vomiting
Respiratory: Bronchospasm

Drug Interactions

Metabolism/Transport Effects None known.

Avoid Concomitant Use There are no known interactions where it is recommended to avoid concomitant use.

Increased Effect/Toxicity There are no known significant interactions involving an increase in effect.

Decreased Effect There are no known significant interactions involving a decrease in effect.

Stability

Solution for injection (Acetadote®): Store unopened vials at 20°C to 25°C (68°F to 77°F). Following reconstitution with D$_5$W, solution is stable for 24 hours at room temperature. A color change may occur in opened vials (light purple) and does not affect the safety or efficacy. Contact with rubber, copper, iron, and cork may inactivate the drug.

Solution for inhalation: Store unopened vials at 20°C to 25°C (68°F to 77°F); excursions permitted to 15°C to 30°C (59°F to 86°F); once opened, store under refrigeration and use within 96 hours. A color change may occur in opened vials (light purple) and does not affect the safety or efficacy. Contact with rubber, copper, iron, and cork may inactivate the drug.

Mechanism of Action Exerts mucolytic action through its free sulfhydryl group which opens up the disulfide bonds in the mucoproteins thus lowering mucous viscosity.

In patients with acetaminophen toxicity, acetylcysteine acts as a hepatoprotective agent by restoring hepatic glutathione, serving as a glutathione substitute, and enhancing the nontoxic sulfate conjugation of acetaminophen.

The presumed mechanism in preventing contrast-induced nephropathy is its ability to scavenge oxygen-derived free radicals and improve endothelium-dependent vasodilation.

Pharmacodynamics

Onset of action: Inhalation: Mucus liquefaction occurs maximally within 5-10 minutes

Duration: Inhalation: Mucus liquefaction: More than 1 hour

Pharmacokinetics (Adult data unless noted)

Distribution: V$_d$: 0.47 L/kg

Protein binding: 83%

Half-life:
Reduced acetylcysteine: 2 hours
Total acetylcysteine:
Newborns: 11 hours
Adults: 5.6 hours

Time to peak serum concentration: Oral: 1-2 hours

Elimination: Urine

Dosing: Usual

Infants, Children, and Adolescents:

Acetaminophen poisoning: Infants, Children, and Adolescents: Begin treatment within 8 hours of ingestion to optimize therapy in patients whose serum acetaminophen levels fall above the "possible" toxicity line on the Rumack-Matthew nomogram. Treatment is also indicated in patients with a history of known or suspected acute acetaminophen ingestion of >150 mg/kg (child) or >7.5 g (adolescent) total dose when plasma levels are not available within 8-10 hours of ingestion or in patients presenting >24 hours after acute ingestion who have a measurable acetaminophen level.

Oral: 72-hour regimen: Consists of 18 doses; total dose delivered: 1330 mg/kg

Loading dose: 140 mg/kg

Maintenance dose: 70 mg/kg every 4 hours for 17 doses; repeat dose if emesis occurs within 1 hour of administration; **Note:** Consultation with a poison control center or clinical toxicologist is highly recommended when considering the discontinuation of oral acetylcysteine prior to the conclusion of a full 18-dose course of therapy.

I.V. (Acetadote®): 21-hour regimen: Consists of 3 doses; total dose delivered: 300 mg/kg

Loading dose: 150 mg/kg (maximum: 15 g) infused over 60 minutes

Second dose: 50 mg/kg (maximum: 5000 mg) infused over 4 hours

Third dose: 100 mg/kg (maximum: 10 g) infused over 16 hours

Respiratory conditions, adjuvant therapy: Note: Patients should receive an aerosolized bronchodilator 10-15 minutes prior to acetylcysteine:

Nebulized inhalation:

Face mask, mouth piece, tracheostomy:
Infants: 1-2 mL of 20% solution (may be further diluted with sodium chloride or sterile water for inhalation) or 2-4 mL of 10% solution (undiluted); administer 3-4 times daily

Children: 3-5 mL of 20% solution (may be further diluted with sodium chloride or sterile water for inhalation) or 6-10 mL of 10% solution (undiluted); administer 3-4 times daily

Adolescents: 3-5 mL of 20% solution (may be further diluted with sodium chloride or sterile water for inhalation) or 6-10 mL of 10% solution (undiluted); administer 3-4 times daily; usual dosing range: 20% solution: 1-10 mL or 10% solution: 2-20 mL every 2-6 hours

Tent, croupette: 10% or 20% solution: Dose must be individualized; dose is volume of solution necessary to maintain a very heavy mist in tent or croupette; in some cases, may require up to 300 mL solution/treatment

Direct instillation: Children and Adolescents:
Endotracheal: 1-2 mL of 10% to 20% solution every 1-4 hours as needed

Percutaneous endotracheal catheter: 1-2 mL of 20% or 2-4 mL of 10% solution every 1-4 hours via syringe attached to catheter

Diagnostic bronchogram: Children and Adolescents: Nebulization or endotracheal: 1-2 mL of 20% solution or 2-4 mL of 10% solution administered 2-3 times prior to procedure

Distal intestinal obstruction syndrome (previously known as meconium ileus equivalent): Limited data available; dosing regimens variable (polyethylene glycol has become more widely used for this indication):

Oral:
Children <10 years: 30 mL of 10% solution diluted in 30 mL juice or soda 3 times/day for 24 hours

Children 10 years and Adolescents: 60 mL of 10% solution diluted in 60 mL juice or soda 3 times/day for 24 hours

Note: Prior to treatment, administer a phosphosoda enema. A clear liquid diet should be used during the 24-hour acetylcysteine treatment

Rectal enema: Children: Varying dosages; 100-300 mL of 4% to 6% solution 2-4 times/day; 50 mL of 20% solution 1-4 times/day and 5-30 mL of 10% to 20% solution 3-4 times/day have been used; rectal enemas appear to have less favorable results than oral administration (Mascarenhas, 2003)

Adults:

Acetaminophen poisoning: Only the 72-hour oral and 21-hour I.V. regimens are FDA approved. Ideally, in patients with an acute acetaminophen ingestion, treatment should begin within 8 hours of ingestion or as soon as possible after ingestion. In patients who present following RSTI and treatment is deemed appropriate, acetylcysteine should be initiated immediately.

Oral: 72-hour regimen: Consists of 18 doses; total dose delivered: 1330 mg/kg
  Loading dose: 140 mg/kg
  Maintenance dose: 70 mg/kg every 4 hours; repeat dose if emesis occurs within 1 hour of administration; **Note:** Consultation with a poison control center or clinical toxicologist is highly recommended when considering the discontinuation of oral acetylcysteine prior to the conclusion of a full 18-dose course of therapy.

I.V. (Acetadote®): 21-hour regimen: Consists of 3 doses; total dose delivered: 300 mg/kg
  Loading dose: 150 mg/kg (maximum: 15 g) infused over 60 minutes
  Second dose: 50 mg/kg (maximum: 5 g) infused over 4 hours
  Third dose: 100 mg/kg (maximum: 10 g) infused over 16 hours

Respiratory conditions; adjuvant therapy: Note: Patients should receive an aerosolized bronchodilator 10-15 minutes prior to dose.

Inhalation, nebulization (face mask, mouth piece, tracheostomy): Acetylcysteine 10% and 20% solution (dilute 20% solution with sodium chloride or sterile water for inhalation); 10% solution may be used undiluted: 3-5 mL of 20% solution or 6-10 mL of 10% solution until nebulized given 3-4 times/day; dosing range: 1-10 mL of 20% solution or 2-20 mL of 10% solution every 2-6 hours

Inhalation, nebulization (tent, croupette): Dose must be individualized; may require up to 300 mL solution/treatment

Direct instillation:
  Into tracheostomy: 1-2 mL of 10% to 20% solution every 1-4 hours
  Through percutaneous intratracheal catheter: 1-2 mL of 20% or 2-4 mL of 10% solution every 1-4 hours via syringe attached to catheter

Diagnostic bronchogram: Nebulization or intratracheal: 1-2 mL of 20% solution or 2-4 mL of 10% solution administered 2-3 times prior to procedure

Prevention of radiocontrast-induced renal dysfunction: Oral: 600 mg twice daily for 2 days (beginning the day before the procedure); hydrate patient concurrently

Administration

Oral: For treatment of acetaminophen overdosage, administer as a 5% solution; to prepare 5% solution, dilute the 20% solution (inhalation formulation) 1:3 with a cola, orange juice, or other soft drink; use within 1 hour of preparation. If patient vomits within 1 hour of dose, readminister. **Note:** The unpleasant odor (sulfur-like) becomes less noticeable as treatment progresses. It is helpful to put the acetylcysteine on ice, in a cup with a cover, and drink through a straw; alternatively, administer via an NG tube.

Inhalation solution: May be administered by nebulization either undiluted (both 10% and 20%) or diluted in NS

Rectal: Dilute the inhalation solution in NS to the desired final concentration and administer rectally

Parenteral: I.V.: Three infusions of different lengths: Dilute first dose (150 mg/kg) in 200 mL D$_5$W and infuse over 60 minutes; dilute second dose (50 mg/kg) in 500 mL D$_5$W and infuse over 4 hours; dilute third dose (100 mg/kg) in 1000 mL D$_5$W and infuse over 16 hours; for children <40 kg and patients who are fluid restricted, the manufacturer

recommends reducing the diluent to a "proportional" amount. See table for manufacturer's recommended infusion guideline for patients <40 kg. Or as an alternative to proportionally lower the diluent volume, a reasonable approach might be to utilize the concentrations resulting from using the recommended dilution for the dosage in a 50 kg patient. The calculated concentration would range between 5 mg/mL (maintenance infusion) to 37.5 mg/mL (loading dose).

Infusion Guide by Weight for Patients <40 kg

Body Weight (kg)	LOADING Dose 150 mg/kg over 60 min		SECOND Dose 50 mg/kg over 4 h		THIRD Dose 100 mg/kg over 16 h	
	Acetylcysteine Dose mg (mL)	5% Dextrose (mL)	Acetylcysteine Dose mg (mL)	5% Dextrose (mL)	Acetylcysteine Dose mg (mL)	5% Dextrose (mL)
10	1500 (7.5)	30	500 (2.5)	70	1000 (5)	140
15	2250 (11.25)	45	750 (3.75)	105	1500 (7.5)	210
20	3000 (15)	60	1000 (5)	140	2000 (10)	280
25	3750 (18.75)	100	1250 (6.25)	250	2500 (12.5)	500
30	4500 (22.5)	100	1500 (7.5)	250	3000 (15)	500

Monitoring Parameters When used in acetaminophen overdose, determine acetaminophen level as soon as possible, but no sooner than 4 hours after ingestion of immediate release formulations or 2 hours after ingestion of liquid formulations (to ensure peak levels have been obtained); coingestion of acetaminophen with other medications which may delay GI peristalsis eg, antihistamines, opioids, may require repeated serum levels to determine the peak serum level; liver function tests

Dosage Forms Excipient information presented when available (limited, particularly for generics); consult specific product labeling.

Injection, solution [preservative free]: 20% (30 mL)
  Acetadote: 20% [200 mg/mL] (30 mL)
Solution, for inhalation/oral: 10% [100 mg/mL] (10 mL, 30 mL); 20% [200 mg/mL] (10 mL, 30 mL)
Solution, for inhalation/oral [preservative free]: 10% [100 mg/mL] (4 mL, 10 mL); 20% [200 mg/mL] (4 mL, 10 mL, 30 mL)

References

Bailey B, "Are There Teratogenic Risks Associated With Antidotes Used in the Acute Management of Poisoned Pregnant Women?" *Birth Defects Res A Clin Mol Teratol*, 2003, 67(2):133-40.

Hanly JG and Fitzgerald MX, "Meconium Ileus Equivalent in Older Patients With Cystic Fibrosis," *Br Med J (Clin Res Ed)*, 1983, 286 (6375):1411-3.

Hendrickson RG and Bizovi KE, "Acetaminophen," *Goldfrank's Toxicologic Emergencies*, 8th edition, Flomenbaum NE, Goldfrank LR, Hoffman RS, et al, eds, New York: The McGraw-Hill Companies, Inc, 2006, 523-43.

Jones AL, "Mechanism of Action and Value of N-Acetylcysteine in the Treatment of Early and Late Acetaminophen Poisoning: A Critical Review," *J Toxicol Clin Toxicol*, 1998, 36(4):277-85.

Jones AL, "Recent Advances in the Management of Late Paracetamol Poisoning," *Emerg Med*, 2000, 12(1):14-21.

Mascarenhas MR, "Treatment of Gastrointestinal Problems in Cystic Fibrosis," *Curr Treat Options Gastroenterol*, 2003, 6(5):427-441.

Mroz L, Benitez JG, and Krenzelok E, "Angioedema With Oral Acetylcysteine," *Ann Emerg Med*, 1997, 30(2):240-1.

Pakravan N, Waring WS, Sharma S, et al, "Risk Factors and Mechanisms of Anaphylactoid Reactions to Acetylcysteine in Acetaminophen Overdose," *Clin Toxicol*, 2008, 46(8):697-702.

Rashid ST, Salman M, Myint F, et al, "Prevention of Contrast-Induced Nephropathy in Vascular Patients Undergoing Angiography: A Randomized Controlled Trial of Intravenous N-Acetylcysteine," *J Vasc Surg*, 2004, 40(6):1136-41.

Sandilands EA and Bateman DN, "Adverse Reactions Associated With Acetylcysteine," *Clin Toxicol (Phila)*, 2009, 47(2):81-8.

Tepel M, van der Giet M, Schwarzfeld C, et al, "Prevention of Radiographic-Contrast-Agent-Induced Reductions in Renal Function by Acetylcysteine," *N Engl J Med*, 2000, 343(3):180-4.

Walson PD and Groth JF Jr, "Acetaminophen Hepatotoxicity After Prolonged Ingestion," *Pediatrics*, 1993, 91(5):1021-2.

Waring WS, Stephen AF, Robinson OD, et al,"Lower Incidence of Anaphylactoid Reactions to N-Acetylcysteine in Patients With High Acetaminophen Concentrations After Overdose," *Clin Toxicol (Phila)*, 2008, 46(6):496-500.

Wilkes JM, Clark LE, and Herrera JL, "Acetaminophen Overdose in Pregnancy," *South Med J*, 2005, 98(11):1118-22.

◆ **Acetylcysteine Injection (Can)** *see* Acetylcysteine *on page 60*

◆ **Acetylcysteine Sodium** *see* Acetylcysteine *on page 60*

◆ **Acetylcysteine Solution (Can)** *see* Acetylcysteine *on page 60*

◆ **Acetylsalicylic Acid** *see* Aspirin *on page 212*

◆ **Achromycin** *see* Tetracycline *on page 1996*

◆ **Aciclovir** *see* Acyclovir (Systemic) *on page 63*

◆ **Aciclovir** *see* Acyclovir (Topical) *on page 68*

◆ **Acid Control (Can)** *see* Famotidine *on page 843*

◆ **Acid Reducer [OTC]** *see* Famotidine *on page 843*

◆ **Acid Reducer [OTC]** *see* Ranitidine *on page 1805*

◆ **Acid Reducer (Can)** *see* Ranitidine *on page 1805*

◆ **Acid Reducer Maximum Strength [OTC]** *see* Famotidine *on page 843*

◆ **Acid Reducer Maximum Strength [OTC] [DSC]** *see* Ranitidine *on page 1805*

◆ **Acidulated Phosphate Fluoride** *see* Fluoride *on page 894*

◆ **Acilac (Can)** *see* Lactulose *on page 1193*

◆ **Aciphex** *see* RABEprazole *on page 1797*

◆ **AcipHex Sprinkle** *see* RABEprazole *on page 1797*

◆ **Aclovate** *see* Alclometasone *on page 87*

◆ **Acne-Clear [OTC]** *see* Benzoyl Peroxide *on page 275*

◆ **Acne Medication [OTC]** *see* Benzoyl Peroxide *on page 275*

◆ **Acne Medication 5 [OTC]** *see* Benzoyl Peroxide *on page 275*

◆ **Acne Medication 10 [OTC]** *see* Benzoyl Peroxide *on page 275*

◆ **Act [OTC]** *see* Fluoride *on page 894*

◆ **ACT-D** *see* DACTINomycin *on page 580*

◆ **Actemra** *see* Tocilizumab *on page 2040*

◆ **ACTH** *see* Corticotropin *on page 545*

◆ **Acthar** *see* Corticotropin *on page 545*

◆ **Acthar HP** *see* Corticotropin *on page 545*

◆ **ActHIB** *see* Haemophilus b Conjugate Vaccine *on page 994*

◆ **Acticin** *see* Permethrin *on page 1647*

◆ **Actidose-Aqua [OTC]** *see* Charcoal, Activated *on page 432*

◆ **Actidose/Sorbitol [OTC]** *see* Charcoal, Activated *on page 432*

◆ **Actifed® (Can)** *see* Triprolidine and Pseudoephedrine *on page 2090*

◆ **Actigall** *see* Ursodiol *on page 2095*

◆ **Actinomycin** *see* DACTINomycin *on page 580*

◆ **Actinomycin D** *see* DACTINomycin *on page 580*

◆ **Actinomycin CI** *see* DACTINomycin *on page 580*

◆ **Actiq** *see* FentaNYL *on page 853*

◆ **Activase** *see* Alteplase *on page 104*

◆ **Activase rt-PA (Can)** *see* Alteplase *on page 104*

◆ **Activated Carbon** *see* Charcoal, Activated *on page 432*

◆ **Activated Charcoal** *see* Charcoal, Activated *on page 432*

◆ **Activated Dimethicone** *see* Simethicone *on page 1891*

◆ **Activated Ergosterol** *see* Ergocalciferol *on page 774*

◆ **Activated Methylpolysiloxane** *see* Simethicone *on page 1891*

◆ **Activated PCC** *see* Anti-inhibitor Coagulant Complex (Human) *on page 180*

◆ **Active-Cyclobenzaprine** *see* Cyclobenzaprine *on page 558*

◆ **Active-Tramadol** *see* TraMADol *on page 2060*

◆ **Act Kids [OTC]** *see* Fluoride *on page 894*

◆ **Act Restoring [OTC]** *see* Fluoride *on page 894*

◆ **Act Total Care [OTC]** *see* Fluoride *on page 894*

◆ **Acular** *see* Ketorolac (Ophthalmic) *on page 1184*

◆ **Acular® (Can)** *see* Ketorolac (Ophthalmic) *on page 1184*

◆ **Acular LS** *see* Ketorolac (Ophthalmic) *on page 1184*

◆ **Acular LS® (Can)** *see* Ketorolac (Ophthalmic) *on page 1184*

◆ **Acuvail** *see* Ketorolac (Ophthalmic) *on page 1184*

◆ **ACV** *see* Acyclovir (Systemic) *on page 63*

◆ **ACV** *see* Acyclovir (Topical) *on page 68*

◆ **Acycloguanosine** *see* Acyclovir (Systemic) *on page 63*

◆ **Acycloguanosine** *see* Acyclovir (Topical) *on page 68*

Acyclovir (Systemic) (ay SYE kloe veer)

Medication Safety Issues
Sound-alike/look-alike issues:
Acyclovir may be confused with ganciclovir, Retrovir, valacyclovir

Zovirax may be confused with Doribax, Valtrex, Zithromax, Zostrix, Zyloprim, Zyvox

Related Information
Management of Drug Extravasations *on page 2255*

Brand Names: U.S. Zovirax

Brand Names: Canada Apo-Acyclovir; Mylan-Acyclovir; Nu-Acyclovir; ratio-Acyclovir; Teva-Acyclovir; Zovirax

Therapeutic Category Antiviral Agent, Oral; Antiviral Agent, Parenteral

Generic Availability (U.S.) Yes

Use
Parenteral: Treatment of initial and prophylaxis of recurrent mucosal and cutaneous herpes simplex (HSV 1 and HSV 2) infections in immunocompromised patients (FDA approved in all ages); treatment of severe initial episodes of herpes genitalis in immunocompetent patients (FDA approved in ages ≥12 years and adults); treatment of herpes simplex encephalitis, including neonatal herpes simplex virus (FDA approved in all ages); treatment of varicella-zoster virus (VZV) infections in immunocompromised patients (FDA approved in all ages)

Oral: Treatment of chickenpox (varicella) in immunocompetent patients (FDA approved in ages ≥2 years and adults); treatment of initial episodes and prophylaxis of recurrent herpes simplex (HSV 2, genital herpes) and acute treatment of herpes zoster (shingles) (FDA approved in adults)

Has also been used for treatment of varicella-zoster infections in healthy, nonpregnant persons >13 years of age, children >12 months of age who have a chronic skin or lung disorder or are receiving long-term aspirin therapy, and immunocompromised patients; oral therapy has also been used for suppression following parenteral treatment of neonatal HSV infection

◀ **Pregnancy Risk Factor** B

Pregnancy Considerations Teratogenic effects were not observed in animal reproduction studies. Acyclovir has been shown to cross the human placenta (Henderson, 1992). Results from a pregnancy registry, established in 1984 and closed in 1999, did not find an increase in the number of birth defects with exposure to acyclovir when compared to those expected in the general population. However, due to the small size of the registry and lack of long-term data, the manufacturer recommends using during pregnancy with caution and only when clearly needed. Acyclovir may be appropriate for the treatment of genital herpes in pregnant women (CDC, 2010).

Breast-Feeding Considerations Acyclovir is excreted in breast milk. The manufacturer recommends that caution be exercised when administering acyclovir to nursing women. Limited data suggest exposure to the nursing infant of ~0.3 mg/kg/day following oral administration of acyclovir to the mother. Nursing mothers with herpetic lesions near or on the breast should avoid breast-feeding (Gartner, 2005).

Contraindications Hypersensitivity to acyclovir, valacyclovir, or any component

Warnings HSV and VZV with reduced susceptibility to acyclovir have been isolated from immunocompromised patients, especially patients with advanced HIV disease. Thrombocytopenic purpura/hemolytic uremic syndrome (TTP/HUS) has been reported in immunocompromised patients receiving acyclovir. Renal failure, in some cases resulting in death, has been reported with acyclovir use; dehydration, preexisting renal disease, and nephrotoxic drugs increase risk; use with caution in patients with renal disease, dehydration, or those receiving other nephrotoxic agents; dosage should be reduced in patients with renal impairment. Maintain adequate hydration; dilute I.V. product appropriately and infuse over 1 hour to prevent acyclovir crystal accumulation in renal tubules.

Precautions Use caution in patients with underlying neurologic disease, significant hypoxia, or hepatic or electrolyte abnormalities; with I.V. therapy, patients (~1%) can exhibit encephalopathic changes, including lethargy, obtundation, tremors, confusion, hallucinations, agitation, seizures, and coma.

Adverse Reactions

Oral:
Central nervous system: Headache, malaise
Gastrointestinal: Diarrhea, nausea, vomiting

Parenteral:
Dermatologic: Hives, itching, rash
Gastrointestinal: Nausea, vomiting
Hepatic: Liver function tests increased
Local: Inflammation at injection site, phlebitis
Renal: Acute renal failure, BUN increased, creatinine increased

All forms: Rare but important or life-threatening: Abdominal pain, aggression, agitation, anemia, anorexia, ataxia, coma, confusion, consciousness decreased, delirium, desquamation, disseminated intravascular coagulopathy (DIC), dizziness, dysarthria, encephalopathy, fatigue, fever, gastrointestinal distress, hallucinations, hematuria, hemolysis, hepatitis, hyperbilirubinemia, hypotension, insomnia, jaundice, leukocytoclastic vasculitis, leukocytosis, leukopenia, lymphadenopathy, mental depression, myalgia, neutrophilia, pain, psychosis, renal failure, renal pain, seizure, somnolence, sore throat, thrombocytopenia, thrombocytopenic purpura/hemolytic uremic syndrome (TTP/HUS), thrombocytosis, visual disturbances

Drug Interactions

Metabolism/Transport Effects None known.

Avoid Concomitant Use
Avoid concomitant use of Acyclovir (Systemic) with any of the following: Zoster Vaccine

Increased Effect/Toxicity
Acyclovir (Systemic) may increase the levels/effects of: Mycophenolate; Tenofovir; Zidovudine

The levels/effects of Acyclovir (Systemic) may be increased by: Mycophenolate

Decreased Effect
Acyclovir (Systemic) may decrease the levels/effects of: Zoster Vaccine

Food Interactions Food does not affect absorption of oral acyclovir.

Stability
Oral: Store capsules, tablets, and oral suspension at 15°C to 25°C (59°F to 77°F); protect capsules and tablets from moisture and dispense in a tightly closed container.
Parenteral: Store intact vials at 15°C to 25°C (59°F to 77°F). Reconstituted parenteral solutions remain stable for 12 hours at room temperature. Do not refrigerate reconstituted solutions or solutions diluted for infusion as they may precipitate. Once diluted for infusion, use within 24 hours. Incompatible with blood products and protein-containing solutions.

Mechanism of Action Acyclovir is converted to acyclovir monophosphate by virus-specific thymidine kinase then further converted to acyclovir triphosphate by other cellular enzymes. Acyclovir triphosphate inhibits DNA synthesis and viral replication by competing with deoxyguanosine triphosphate for viral DNA polymerase and being incorporated into viral DNA.

Pharmacokinetics (Adult data unless noted)
Absorption: Oral: 15% to 30%
Distribution: Widely distributed throughout the body including brain, kidney, lungs, liver, spleen, muscle, uterus, vagina, and the CSF; CSF acyclovir concentration is 50% of serum concentration
V_d:
Neonates to 3 months of age: 28.8 L/1.73 m^2
Children 1 to 2 years: 31.6 L/1.73 m^2
Children 2 to 7 years: 42 L/1.73 m^2
Protein binding: <9% to 33%
Metabolism: Converted by viral enzymes to acyclovir monophosphate, and further converted to diphosphate then triphosphate (active form) by cellular enzymes
Bioavailability: Oral: 10% to 20%; decreases with increasing dose
Half-life, terminal phase:
Neonates: 4 hours
Children 1 to 12 years: 2 to 3 hours
Adults: 2 to 3.5 hours (with normal renal function); hemodialysis: ~5 hours
Time to peak serum concentration: Oral: Within 1.5 to 2 hours
Elimination: Primary route is the kidney with 60% to 90% of a dose excreted unchanged in the urine
Dialysis: Hemodialysis removes ~60% of dose while removal by peritoneal dialysis is to a lesser extent

Dosing: Neonatal
HSV infection, treatment: I.V.: 20 mg/kg/dose every 8 hours for 14 to 21 days; CNS and disseminated infections: 21 day treatment duration; skin and mucous membrane infections: 14 day treatment duration (CDC, 2010; Kimberlin, 2013; *Red Book* [AAP], 2012)
HSV, chronic suppression following disseminated or CNS infection: Limited data available: Oral:
AAP Recommendation (low dose, 6-month-course): 300 mg/m^2/dose every 8 hours; begin after completion of a 14- to 21-day-course of I.V. therapy dependent upon type of infection; duration of therapy: 6 months (Kimberlin, 2011; Kimberlin, 2013)
Alternate dosing (high-dose, 2-year-course) (Tiffany, 2005): Begin after completion of a 21-day-course of I.V. therapy; dosing based on a prospective trial of 16 consecutive neonates (GA: Premature: n=4; term=12;

age at treatment: Neonate: n=14; PNA >30 days: n=1); pharmacokinetic data were used to determine dosing regimen to maintain serum acyclovir concentration above target of 2 mcg/mL; treatment was continued for 2 years in 14 of 16 patients; results showed normal neurodevelopmental outcomes in 69% and normal motor development in 70%; no untoward effects were reported during the study duration.

Initial dosing: Approximate dose: 1200 to 1600 mg/m²/dose twice daily

Preterm neonate: Proportional decrease of full-term initial dose

Full term or near term: 400 mg twice daily

Maintenance dosing: In the trial, serum acyclovir concentrations were evaluated to assess adequacy of dosing to maintain serum concentrations above the target of 2 to 3 mcg/mL. Samples were collected 1 hour after a witnessed dose; if the acyclovir serum concentration approached or was below the target; the dose was increased to the next greater 200 mg increment. Serum concentrations were evaluated every 3 months; in order to limit the phlebotomy losses, follow-up serum concentrations were not evaluated outside of routine monitoring.

Varicella zoster (chickenpox), treatment: I.V.: 10 to 15 mg/kg/dose every 8 hours for 5 to 10 days; continue for ≥48 hours after the last new lesions have appeared (Ogilvie, 1998; Sauerbrei, 2007; Smith, 2009)

Dosing adjustment in renal impairment:

Manufacturer's labeling: I.V.:

>50 mL/minute/1.73m²: No adjustments necessary

25 to 50 mL/minute/1.73m²: Administer every 12 hours

10 to 25mL/minute/1.73m²: Administer every 24 hours

0 to 10 mL/minute/1.73m²: Administer 50% of the dose every 24 hours

Alternate dosing: The following adjustments have been recommended (Englund, 1991): I.V.:

S_{cr} 0.8 to 1.1 mg/dL: Administer 20 mg/kg/dose every 12 hours

S_{cr} 1.2 to 1.5 mg/dL: Administer 20 mg/kg/dose every 24 hours

S_{cr} >1.5 mg/dL: Administer 10 mg/kg/dose every 24 hours

Dosing: Usual Note: Obese patients should be dosed using ideal body weight.

Pediatric:

HSV neonatal infection, treatment and suppressive therapy in very young infants (independent of HIV status):

Treatment (disseminated, CNS, or skin, eye, or mouth disease): Infants 1 to 3 months: I.V.: 20 mg/kg/dose every 8 hours; treatment duration: For cutaneous and mucous membrane infections (skin, eye, or mouth): 14 days; for CNS or disseminated infection: 21 days (CDC, 2010; Kimberlin, 2013; Red Book [AAP], 2012)

Chronic suppressive therapy: Limited data available: Oral:

AAP Recommendation (low dose, 6-month-course): Infants: 300 mg/m²/dose every 8 hours; begin after completion of a 14- to 21-day-course of I.V. therapy dependent upon type of infection; duration of therapy: 6 months (Kimberlin, 2011; Kimberlin, 2013)

Alternate dosing (high dose, 2-year-course) (Tiffany, 2005): Infants and Children <3 years: Begin after completion of a 21-day course of I.V. therapy; dosing based on a prospective trial of 16 consecutive neonates (GA: Premature: n=4; term= 12; age at treatment: Neonate: n=14; PNA >30 days: n=1); pharmacokinetic data were used to determine dosing regimen to maintain serum acyclovir concentration above target of 2 to 3 mcg/mL; treatment was continued for 2 years in 14 of 16 patients; results showed normal neurodevelopmental outcomes in

69% and normal motor development in 70%; no untoward effects were reported during the study duration.

Initial dosing: 400 mg twice daily; approximate dose: 1200 to 1600 mg/m²/dose twice daily

Maintenance dosing: **Note:** Approximate doses for patients born at term:

Infants 1 to <5 months: 400 mg twice daily

Infants 5 to <9 months: 600 mg twice daily

Infants and Children 9 to <15 months: 800 mg twice daily

Children 15 to 24 months: 1000 mg twice daily

Note: In the trial, serum acyclovir concentrations were evaluated to assess adequacy of dosing to maintain serum concentrations above the target of 2 to 3 mcg/mL. Samples were collected 1 hour after a witnessed dose; if the acyclovir serum concentration approached or was below the target; the dose was increased to the next greater 200 mg increment. Maximum dose: 1200 mg. Serum concentrations were evaluated every 3 months; in order to limit the phlebotomy losses, follow-up serum concentrations were not evaluated outside of routine monitoring.

HSV encephalitis, treatment: I.V.:

Infants and Children 3 months to <12 years:

Non-HIV-exposed/-positive: 10 to 15 mg/kg/dose every 8 hours for 14 to 21 days (Red Book [AAP], 2012)

HIV-exposed/-positive: 10 mg/kg/dose every 8 hours for 21 days; do not discontinue therapy until the repeat CSF HSV DNA PCR is negative (CDC, 2009)

Children ≥12 years and Adolescents (independent of HIV status): 10 mg/kg/dose every 8 hours for 14 to 21 days (Red Book [AAP], 2012)

HSV genital infection:

First infection, mild to moderate: Oral:

Non-HIV-exposed/-positive:

Children <12 years: 40 to 80 mg/kg/**day** divided in 3 to 4 doses per day for 5 to 10 days; maximum daily dose: 1000 mg/**day** (Red Book [AAP], 2012)

Children and Adolescents ≥12 years: 200 mg every 4 hours while awake (5 times daily) **or** 400 mg 3 times daily for 7 to 10 days; treatment can be extended beyond 10 days if healing is not complete (CDC, 2010; Red Book [AAP], 2012)

HIV-exposed/-positive:

Children <45 kg: 20 mg/kg/dose 3 times daily for 5 to 14 days; maximum dose: 400 mg (CDC, 2009)

Children ≥45 kg: 400 mg twice daily for 5 to 14 days (CDC, 2009)

Adolescents: 400 mg 3 times daily for 5 to 14 days (DHHS [adult], 2013)

First infection, severe (independent of HIV status): I.V.: Children and Adolescents ≥12 years: 5 mg/kg/dose every 8 hours for 5 to 7 days (Red Book [AAP], 2012)

Recurrent infection: Oral:

Children <12 years: 10 mg/kg/dose every 8 hours for up to 12 months; maximum daily dose: 1000 mg/**day**; re-evaluate after 12 months (Red Book [AAP], 2009)

Children and Adolescents ≥12 years:

Non-HIV-exposed/-positive: 200 mg every 4 hours while awake (5 times daily) for 5 days **or** 800 mg twice daily for 5 days **or** 800 mg 3 times daily for 2 days (CDC, 2010; Red Book [AAP], 2012)

HIV-exposed/-positive: Adolescents: 400 mg 3 times daily for 5 to 14 days (DHHS [adult], 2013)

Suppression, chronic: Oral:

Non-HIV-exposed/-positive:

Children <12 years: Limited data available: Oral: 20 to 25 mg/kg/dose twice daily; maximum dose: 400 mg (Bradley, 2011)

Children and Adolescents ≥12 years: 400 mg twice daily for up to 12 months (CDC, 2010; *Red Book* [AAP], 2012)

HIV-exposed/-positive:
Infants and Children: 20 mg/kg/dose twice daily; maximum dose: 400 mg (CDC, 2009)
Adolescents: 400 mg twice daily (DHHS [adult], 2013)

HSV gingivostomatitis (HIV-exposed/-positive) (CDC, 2009):
Mild, symptomatic: Oral: Infants and Children: 20 mg/kg/dose 3 times daily for 5 to 10 days; maximum dose: 400 mg
Moderate to severe, symptomatic: I.V.: Infants and Children: 5 to 10 mg/kg/dose every 8 hours; switch to oral therapy once lesions begin to regress

HSV, herpes labialis (cold sore) recurrent, chronic suppressive therapy: Oral: Children: 30 mg/kg/**day** in 3 divided doses for up to 12 months; maximum daily dose: 1000 mg/**day**; re-evaluate after 12 months (*Red Book* [AAP], 2012)

HSV mucosal or cutaneous infection (immunocompromised host):
Treatment:
I.V.: Infants, Children, and Adolescents: 10 mg/kg/dose every 8 hours for 7 to 14 days (*Red Book* [AAP], 2012)
Oral: Children ≥2 years and Adolescents: 1000 mg/**day** in 3 to 5 divided doses for 7 to 14 days; some suggest the maximum daily dose should not exceed 80 mg/kg/**day** (*Red Book*, 2009; *Red Book* [AAP], 2012)
Suppression, chronic (cutaneous, ocular) episodes: Oral:
Infants and Children (HIV-exposed/-positive): 20 mg/kg/dose twice daily for 5 to 14 days; maximum dose: 400 mg (CDC, 2009)
Children and Adolescents ≥12 years (independent of HIV status): 400 mg twice daily for up to 12 months (*Red Book* [AAP], 2012)

HSV orolabial (HIV-exposed/-positive): Adolescents: Oral: 400 mg 3 times daily for 5 to 10 days (DHHS [adult], 2013)

HSV progressive or disseminated infection, treatment (immunocompromised host) including HIV-exposed/-positive:
Non-HIV-exposed/-positive: Infants, Children, and Adolescents: I.V.: 10 mg/kg/dose every 8 hours for 7 to 21 days (*Red Book* [AAP], 2012)
HIV-exposed/-positive: Infants, Children, and Adolescents: I.V.: 10 mg/kg/dose every 8 hours for 21 days (CDC, 2009)

HSV prophylaxis; immunocompromised hosts, seropositive:
Hematopoietic stem cell transplant (HSCT) in seropositive recipient (Tomblyn, 2009):
Prevention of early reactivation: **Note:** Begin at conditioning and continue until engraftment or resolution of mucositis; whichever is longer (~30 days post-HSCT)
Infants, Children, and Adolescents <40 kg:
I.V.: 250 mg/m²/dose every 8 hours **or** 125 mg/m²/dose every 6 hours; maximum daily dose: 80 mg/**day**
Oral: 60 to 90 mg/kg/**day** in 2 to 3 divided doses
Children and Adolescents ≥40 kg:
I.V.: 250 mg/m²/dose every 12 hours
Oral: 400 to 800 mg twice daily
Prevention of late reactivation: **Note:** Treatment during first year after HSCT.
Infants, Children, and Adolescents <40 kg: Oral: 60 to 90 mg/kg/**day** in 2 to 3 divided doses; maximum daily dose: 800 mg twice daily

Children and Adolescents ≥40 kg: Oral: 800 mg twice daily

HIV-exposed/-positive, prevention of HSV reactivation:
Oral: Infants and Children: 20 mg/kg/dose twice daily, maximum dose: 400 mg (CDC, 2009)

Other immunocompromised hosts who are HSV seropositive:
I.V.: Infants, Children, and Adolescents: 5 mg/kg/dose every 8 hours during period of risk (*Red Book* [AAP], 2012)
Oral: Children ≥2 years and Adolescents: 200 mg every 4 hours while awake (5 doses daily) **or** 200 mg every 8 hours (*Red Book* [AAP], 2012)

Varicella zoster (chickenpox or shingles), prophylaxis (HIV-exposed/-positive): Oral: **Note:** Consider use if >96 hours postexposure or if VZV-immune globulin is not available; begin therapy 7 to 10 days after exposure
Infants and Children: 20 mg/kg/dose 4 times daily for 5 to 7 days; maximum dose: 800 mg (CDC, 2009)
Adolescents: 800 mg 5 times daily for 5 to 7 days (DHHS, 2013)

Varicella zoster (chickenpox), treatment:
Immunocompetent host:
Ambulatory therapy: Oral: Children ≥2 years and Adolescents: 20 mg/kg/dose 4 times daily for 5 days; maximum daily dose: 3200 mg/**day** (*Red Book* [AAP], 2012)
Hospitalized patient: I.V.: Children ≥2 years and Adolescents: 10 mg/kg/dose **or** 500 mg/m²/dose every 8 hours for 7 to 10 days (*Red Book* [AAP], 2012)

Immunocompromised host (non-HIV-exposed/-positive): I.V.:
Infants: 10 mg/kg/dose every 8 hours for 7 to 10 days (*Red Book* [AAP], 2012)
Children and Adolescents: 500 mg/m²/dose every 8 hours for 7 to 10 days; some experts recommend 10 mg/kg/dose every 8 hours (*Red Book* [AAP], 2012)

HIV-exposed/-positive:
Mild, uncomplicated disease and no or moderate immune suppression: Oral:
Infants and Children: 20 mg/kg/dose 4 times daily for 7 to 10 days or until no new lesions for 48 hours; maximum dose: 800 mg (CDC, 2009)
Adolescents: 800 mg 5 times daily for 5 to 7 days (DHHS [adult], 2013)
Severe, complicated disease or severe immune suppression: I.V.:
Infants: 10 mg/kg/dose every 8 hours for 7 to 10 days or until no new lesions for 48 hours (CDC, 2009)
Children: 10 mg/kg/dose **or** 500 mg/m²/dose every 8 hours for 7 to 10 days or until no new lesions for 48 hours (CDC, 2009)
Adolescents: 10 to 15 mg/kg/dose every 8 hours for 7 to 10 days; may convert to oral therapy after defervescence and if no evidence of visceral involvement is evident (DHHS [adult], 2013)

Varicella zoster (shingles; herpes zoster), treatment:
Immunocompetent host:
Ambulatory therapy: Oral: Children ≥12 years and Adolescents: 800 mg every 4 hours (5 doses per day) for 5 to 7 days (*Red Book* [AAP], 2012)
Hospitalized patient: I.V.:
Infants: 10 mg/kg/dose every 8 hours for 7 ti 10 days (*Red Book* [AAP], 2012)
Children and Adolescents: 500 mg/m²/dose every 8 hours for 7 to 10 days; some experts recommend 10 mg/kg/dose every 8 hours (*Red Book,* [AAP] 2012)

Immunocompromised host (non-HIV-exposed/-positive): I.V.: Infants, Children, and Adolescents: 10 mg/kg/dose every 8 hours for 7 to 10 days (*Red Book* [AAP], 2012)

HIV-exposed/-positive:

Mild, uncomplicated disease and no or moderate immune suppression: Oral:

Infants and Children: 20 mg/kg/dose 4 times daily for 7 to 10 days; maximum dose: 800 mg; consider longer course if resolution of lesions is slow (CDC, 2009)

Adolescents: 800 mg 5 times daily for 7 to 10 days, longer if lesions resolve slowly (DHHS [adult], 2013)

Severe immune suppression or complicated disease; trigeminal nerve involvement, extensive multidermatomal zoster or extensive cutaneous lesions or visceral involvement: I.V.:

Infants: 10 mg/kg/dose every 8 hours until resolution of cutaneous lesions and visceral disease clearly begins, then convert to oral therapy to complete a 10 to 14 day total course of therapy (CDC, 2009)

Children: 10 mg/kg/dose **or** 500 mg/m² every 8 hours until resolution of cutaneous lesions and visceral disease clearly begins, then convert to oral therapy to complete a 10 to 14 day total course of therapy (CDC, 2009)

Adolescents: 10 to 15 mg/kg/dose every 8 hours until clinical improvement is evident, then convert to oral therapy to complete a 10 to 14 day total course of therapy (DHHS [adult], 2013)

Varicella zoster, acute retinal necrosis, treatment (HIV-exposed/-positive):

Initial treatment: I.V.: **Note:** Follow up I.V. therapy with oral acyclovir or valacyclovir maintenance therapy.

Infants: 10 to 15 mg/kg/dose every 8 hours for 10 to 14 days (CDC, 2009)

Children: 10 to 15 mg/kg/dose **or** 500 mg/m²/dose every 8 hours for 10 to 14 days (CDC, 2009)

Adolescents: 10 to 15 mg/kg/dose every 8 hours for 10 to 14 days (DHHS [adult], 2013)

Maintenance treatment; begin after 10 to 14 day course of I.V. acyclovir: Oral: Infants and Children: 20 mg/kg/dose every 8 hours for a total duration of therapy of 4 to 6 weeks (CDC, 2009)

Adult:

HSV encephalitis: I.V.: 10 mg/kg/dose every 8 hours for 10 days; 10 to 15 mg/kg/dose every 8 hours for 14 to 21 days has also been reported

HSV genital infection:

I.V.: Immunocompetent: Initial episode, severe: 5 mg/kg/dose every 8 hours for 5 to 7 days **or** 5 to 10 mg/kg/dose every 8 hours for 2 to 7 days, follow with oral therapy to complete at least 10 days of therapy (CDC, 2010)

Oral:

Initial episode: 200 mg every 4 hours while awake (5 times/day) **or** 400 mg 3 times daily for 7 to 10 days (CDC, 2010)

Recurrence: 200 mg every 4 hours while awake (5 times/day) for 5 days; begin at earliest signs of disease

Alternatively, the following regimens are also recommended by the CDC: 400 mg 3 times daily for 5 days; 800 mg twice daily for 5 days; 800 mg 3 times daily for 2 days (CDC, 2010)

Chronic suppression: 400 mg twice daily (CDC 2010) or 200 mg 3 to 5 times daily, for up to 12 months followed by re-evaluation

HSV mucocutaneous: Immunocompromised: Treatment: I.V.: 5 mg/kg/dose every 8 hours for 7 days (Leflore, 2000); dosing for up to 14 days also reported

Varicella Zoster (chickenpox): Begin treatment within the first 24 hours of rash onset:

Oral: >40 kg (immunocompetent): 800 mg/dose 4 times daily for 5 days

I.V.:

Manufacturer's labeling (immunocompromised): 10 mg/kg/dose every 8 hours for 7 days

AIDS*info* guidelines (immunocompromised): 10 to 15 mg/kg/dose every 8 hours for 7 to 10 days (DHHS, 2013)

Herpes zoster (shingles):

Immunocompetent: Oral: 800 mg every 4 hours (5 times daily) for 7 to 10 days

Immunocompromised: I.V.: 10 mg/kg/dose **or** 500 mg/m²/dose every 8 hours for 7 days

Dosing adjustment in renal impairment:

Oral: Children, Adolescents, and Adults:

CrCl >25 mL/minute/1.73 m²: No adjustment required

CrCl 10 to 25 mL/minute/1.73 m²:

Normal dosing regimen 200 mg every 4 hours or 400 mg every 12 hours: No adjustment required

Normal dosing regimen 800 mg every 4 hours: Administer 800 mg every 8 hours

CrCl <10 mL/minute/1.73 m²:

Normal dosing regimen 200 mg every 4 hours or 400 mg every 12 hours: Administer 200 mg every 12 hours

Normal dosing regimen 800 mg every 4 hours: Administer 800 mg every 12 hours

Intermittent hemodialysis (IHD): Administer after hemodialysis on dialysis days

I.V.: Infants, Children, Adolescents, and Adults:

CrCl >50 mL/minute/1.73 m²: No adjustment required

CrCl 25 to 50 mL/minute/1.73 m²: Administer every 12 hours

CrCl 10 to 25 mL/minute/1.73 m²: Administer every 24 hours

CrCl <10 mL/minute/1.73 m²: Administer 50% of dose every 24 hours

Intermittent hemodialysis (IHD): Administer 50% of dose every 24 hours; administer after hemodialysis on dialysis days (Aronoff, 2007)

Peritoneal dialysis (PD): Administer 50% of normal dose every 24 hours; no supplemental dose needed (Aronoff, 2007)

Continuous renal replacement therapy (CRRT):

Infants, Children, and Adolescents: I.V.: 10 mg/kg/dose every 12 hours (Aronoff, 2007)

Adults: Drug clearance is highly dependent on the method of renal replacement, filter type, and flow rate. Appropriate dosing requires close monitoring of pharmacologic response, signs of adverse reactions due to drug accumulation, as well as drug concentrations in relation to target trough (if appropriate). The following are general recommendations only (based on dialysate flow/ultrafiltration rates of 1 to 2 L/hour and minimal residual renal function) and should not supersede clinical judgment (Heintz, 2009; Trotman, 2005):

CVVH: I.V.: 5 to 10 mg/kg every 24 hours

CVVHD/CVVHDF: I.V.: 5 to 10 mg/kg every 12 to 24 hours

Note: The higher end of dosage range (eg, 10 mg/kg every 12 hours for CVVHDF) is recommended for viral meningoencephalitis and varicella zoster virus infections.

Dosing adjustment in hepatic impairment: There are no dosage adjustments provided in the manufacturer's labeling.

Administration

Oral: May administer with or without food; shake suspension well before use

Parenteral: Reconstitute vial for injection with SWI; do not use SWI containing parabens or benzyl alcohol; further dilute to a final concentration ≤7 mg/mL and administer by slow I.V. infusion over at least 1 hour; rapid infusion is associated with nephrotoxicity due to crystalluria and renal tubular damage and should be avoided. In patients who require fluid restriction, a concentration of up to 10 mg/mL has been infused; concentration >10 mg/mL increases the risk of phlebitis. Avoid I.V. push, I.M., or SubQ administration.

Vesicant/Extravasation Risk Irritant at concentrations >7 mg/mL

Monitoring Parameters Urinalysis, BUN, serum creatinine, urine output; liver enzymes, CBC; neutrophil count at least twice weekly in neonates receiving acyclovir 60 mg/kg/day I.V.

Additional Information Sodium content of 1 g: 4.2 mEq

Dosage Forms Excipient information presented when available (limited, particularly for generics); consult specific product labeling.

Capsule, Oral:
Zovirax: 200 mg
Generic: 200 mg
Solution, Intravenous, as sodium [strength expressed as base]:
Generic: 50 mg/mL (10 mL, 20 mL)
Solution Reconstituted, Intravenous, as sodium [strength expressed as base]:
Generic: 500 mg (1 ea); 1000 mg (1 ea)
Suspension, Oral:
Zovirax: 200 mg/5 mL (473 mL) [banana flavor]
Generic: 200 mg/5 mL (473 mL)
Tablet, Oral:
Zovirax: 400 mg, 800 mg
Generic: 400 mg, 800 mg

References
American Academy of Pediatrics (AAP). In: Pickering LK, Baker CJ, Kimberlin DW, Long SS, eds. *Red Book: 2012 Report of the Committee on Infectious Diseases.* 29th ed. Elk Grove Village, IL: American Academy of Pediatrics; 2012.
American Academy of Pediatrics Committee on Infectious Diseases, "The Use of Oral Acyclovir in Otherwise Healthy Children With Varicella," *Pediatrics*, 1993, 91(3):674-6.
Aronoff GR, Bennett WM, Berns JS, et al, *Drug Prescribing in Renal Failure: Dosing Guidelines for Adults and Children*, 5th ed, Philadelphia, PA: American College of Physicians, 2007.
Bradley JS, Nelson JD, Kimberlin DK, et al, eds. *Nelson's Pocket Book of Pediatric Antimicrobial Therapy*. 19th ed. Philadelphia, PA: Lippincott Williams & Wilkins; 2012.
Centers for Disease Control and Prevention (CDC), "Guidelines for the Prevention and Treatment of Opportunistic Infections Among HIV-Exposed and HIV-Infected Children," *MMWR Recomm Rep*, 2009, 58(RR-11):1-166. Available at http://aidsinfo.nih.gov/contentfiles/Pediatric_OI.pdf
Centers for Disease Control and Prevention (CDC), "Sexually Transmitted Diseases Treatment Guidelines, 2010," *MMWR Recomm Rep*, 2010, 59(RR-12):1-110.
DHHS Panel on Opportunistic Infections (OI) in HIV-Infected Adults and Adolescents. Guidelines for prevention and treatment of opportunistic infections in HIV-infected adults and adolescents: recommendations from the Centers for Disease Control and Prevention (CDC), the National Institutes of Health (NIH), and the HIV Medicine Association (HIVMA) of the Infectious Diseases Society of America (IDSA). May 7, 2013. Available at http://aidsinfo.nih.gov/contentfiles/lvguidelines/adult_oi.pdf
Englund JA, Fletcher CV, and Balfour HH Jr, "Acyclovir Therapy in Neonates," *J Pediatr*, 1991, 119(1 Pt 1):129-35.
Gartner LM, Morton J, Lawrence RA, et al, "Breastfeeding and the Use of Human Milk," *Pediatrics*, 2005, 115(2):496-506.
Heintz BH, Matzke GR, and Dager WE, "Antimicrobial Dosing Concepts and Recommendations for Critically Ill Adult Patients Receiving Continuous Renal Replacement Therapy or Intermittent Hemodialysis," *Pharmacotherapy*, 2009, 29(5):562-77.
Henderson GI, Hu ZQ, Johnson RF, et al, "Acyclovir Transport by the Human Placenta," *J Lab Clin Med*, 1992, 120(6):885-92.
Kimberlin DW, Baley J, AAP Committee on Infectious Diseases, et al. "Guidance on management of asymptomatic neonates born to women with active genital herpes lesions. *Pediatrics.* 2013;131(2):e635-646.
Kimberlin DW, Lin CY, Jacobs RF, et al, "Safety and Efficacy of High-Dose Intravenous Acyclovir in the Management of Neonatal Herpes Simplex Virus Infections," *Pediatrics*, 2001, 108(2):230-8.
Kimberlin DW, Whitley RJ, Wan W, et al, "Oral Acyclovir Suppression and Neurodevelopment After Neonatal Herpes," *N Engl J Med*, 2011, 365(14):1284-92.
Ogilvie MM, "Antiviral Prophylaxis and Treatment in Chickenpox. A Review Prepared for the UK Advisory Group on Chickenpox on Behalf of the British Society for the Study of Infection," *J Infect*, 1998, 36 (Suppl 10):31-8.
Red Book: 2009 Report of the Committee on Infectious Diseases, 28th ed, Pickering LK, ed, Elk Grove Village, IL: American Academy of Pediatrics, 2009.
Sauerbrei A and Wutzler P, "Herpes Simplex and Varicella-Zoster Virus Infections During Pregnancy: Current Concepts of Prevention, Diagnosis and Therapy. Part 2: Varicella-Zoster Virus Infections," *Med Microbiol Immunol*, 2007, 196(2):95-102.
Smith CK and Arvin AM, "Varicella in the Fetus and Newborn," *Semin Fetal Neonatal Med*, 2009, 14(4):209-17.
Tiffany KF, Benjamin DK Jr, Palasanthiran P, et al, "Improved Neurodevelopmental Outcomes Following Long-Term High-Dose Oral Acyclovir Therapy in Infants With Central Nervous System and Disseminated Herpes Simplex Disease," *J Perinatol*, 2005, 25 (3):156-61.
Tomblyn M, Chiller T, Einsele H, et al, "Guidelines for Preventing Infectious Complications Among Hematopoietic Cell Transplantation Recipients: A Global Perspective," *Biol Blood Marrow Transplant*, 2009, 15(10):1143-238.
Trotman RL, Williamson JC, Shoemaker DM, et al, "Antibiotic Dosing in Critically Ill Adult Patients Receiving Continuous Renal Replacement Therapy," *Clin Infect Dis*, 2005, 41:1159-66.

Acyclovir (Topical) (ay SYE kloe veer)

Medication Safety Issues
Sound-alike/look-alike issues:
Acyclovir may be confused with ganciclovir, Retrovir, valacyclovir
Zovirax may be confused with Doribax, Valtrex Zithromax, Zostrix, Zyloprim, Zyvox
International issues:
Opthavir [Mexico] may be confused with Optivar brand name for azelastine [U.S.]

Brand Names: U.S. Sitavig; Zovirax

Brand Names: Canada Zovirax

Therapeutic Category Antiviral Agent, Topical

Generic Availability (U.S.) May be product dependent

Use
Topical (cream): Treatment of recurrent herpes labialis (cold sores) (FDA approved in ages ≥12 years and adults)
Topical (ointment): Management of initial genital herpes and in limited, nonlife-threatening mucocutaneous HSV infections in immunocompromised patients (FDA approved in adults)

Pregnancy Risk Factor B

Pregnancy Considerations Teratogenic effects were not observed in animal studies. When administered orally, acyclovir crosses the placenta. Refer to the Acyclovir, Systemic monograph for details. The amount of acyclovir available systemically following topical application of the cream or ointment is significantly less in comparison to oral doses.

Breast-Feeding Considerations When administered orally, acyclovir enters breast milk. Refer to the Acyclovir, Systemic monograph for details. The amount of acyclovir available systemically following topical application of the cream or ointment is significantly less in comparison to oral doses. Nursing mothers with herpetic lesions near or on the breast should avoid breast-feeding.

Contraindications Hypersensitivity to acyclovir, valacyclovir, or any component

Warnings Physical contact should be avoided when lesions are present; transmission may also occur in the absence of symptoms. Treatment should begin with the first signs or symptoms. Acyclovir ointment should not be used for prevention of recurrent HSV infections.

Precautions For external use only to the lips and face; do not apply to eye or inside the mouth or nose. Treatment should begin with the first signs or symptoms. Use with caution in immunocompromised patients.

Adverse Reactions

Central nervous system: Lethargy (buccal tablet)

Dermatologic: Erythema (buccal tablet), local pain (ointment; mild; includes transient burning and stinging), skin rash (buccal tablet)

Gastrointestinal: Aphthous stomatitis (buccal tablet), gingival pain (buccal tablet)

Local: Application site irritation (buccal tablet), application site reaction (cream; including dry lips, desquamation, dryness of skin, cracked lips, burning skin, pruritus, flakiness of skin, and stinging on skin)

Rare but important or life-threatening: Anaphylaxis, eczema

Drug Interactions

Metabolism/Transport Effects None known.

Avoid Concomitant Use There are no known interactions where it is recommended to avoid concomitant use.

Increased Effect/Toxicity There are no known significant interactions involving an increase in effect.

Decreased Effect There are no known significant interactions involving a decrease in effect.

Stability

Cream: Store at ≤25°C (77°F); excursions permitted to 15°C to 30°C (59°F to 86°F).

Ointment: Store at 15°C to 25°C (59°F to 77°F) in a dry place.

Mechanism of Action Acyclovir is converted to acyclovir monophosphate by virus-specific thymidine kinase then further converted to acyclovir triphosphate by other cellular enzymes. Acyclovir triphosphate inhibits DNA synthesis and viral replication by competing with deoxyguanosine triphosphate for viral DNA polymerase and being incorporated into viral DNA.

Pharmacokinetics (Adult data unless noted) Absorption: Poorly absorbed

Dosing: Usual

Topical:

Cream: Herpes labialis (cold sores): Children ≥12 years and Adults: Apply 5 times/day for 4 days

Ointment:

Genital HSV, immunocompromised: Adults: Initial episode: 1/2" ribbon of ointment for a 4" square surface area every 3 hours (6 times/day) for 7 days

Mucocutaneous HSV, nonlife-threatening, immunocompromised: Adults: Ointment: 1/2" ribbon of ointment for a 4" square surface area every 3 hours (6 times/day) for 7 days

Administration For topical use only; do not apply to eye, inside the mouth or nose, or on unaffected skin.

Cream: Apply layer of cream to cover only the cold sore or cover the area with symptoms; rub cream in until it disappears.

Ointment: Use a fingercot or rubber glove when applying ointment to prevent autoinoculation of other body sites or transmission of infection to other persons.

Product Availability

Sitavig: FDA approved April 2013; anticipated availability is currently unknown

Sitavig buccal tablets are indicated for the treatment of recurrent herpes labialis (cold sores) in immunocompetent adults.

Dosage Forms Excipient information presented when available (limited, particularly for generics); consult specific product labeling.

Cream, External:

Zovirax: 5% (5 g) [contains cetosteryl alcohol, propylene glycol]

Ointment, External:

Zovirax: 5% (30 g)

Generic: 5% (5 g, 15 g, 30 g)

Tablet, Buccal:

Sitavig: 50 mg [contains milk protein concentrate]

Acyclovir and Hydrocortisone
(ay SYE kloe veer & hye droe KOR ti sone)

Brand Names: U.S. Xerese™

Therapeutic Category Antiviral Agent, Topical; Corticosteroid, Topical

Generic Availability (U.S.) No

Use Early treatment of recurrent herpes labialis (cold sores) to shorten healing time and to reduce likelihood of ulceration (FDA approved in ages ≥12 years and adults)

Pregnancy Risk Factor B

Pregnancy Considerations Animal reproduction studies and studies in pregnant women have not been conducted with Xerese™. Systemic exposure of acyclovir and hydrocortisone after topical administration is minimal. See individual agents.

Breast-Feeding Considerations Systemic exposure of acyclovir and hydrocortisone after topical administration is minimal. See individual agents.

Contraindications Hypersensitivity to acyclovir, hydrocortisone, or any component

Warnings May cause local sensitization and irritation. For external use only to area around the mouth and lips; do not apply to mucosal membranes (inside of mouth or nose), eyes, or genital area. If healing fails after 2 weeks of therapy, patient should contact prescriber.

Precautions Use with caution in immunocompromised patients; safety and efficacy data are insufficient.

Adverse Reactions Rare but important or life-threatening: Dermatologic: Burning, contact dermatitis, dryness, erythema, flaking, pigmentation changes, sensitization, signs/symptoms of inflammation, tingling

Drug Interactions

Metabolism/Transport Effects Refer to individual components.

Avoid Concomitant Use

Avoid concomitant use of Acyclovir and Hydrocortisone with any of the following: Aldesleukin

Increased Effect/Toxicity

Acyclovir and Hydrocortisone may increase the levels/effects of: Ceritinib; Deferasirox

The levels/effects of Acyclovir and Hydrocortisone may be increased by: Telaprevir

Decreased Effect

Acyclovir and Hydrocortisone may decrease the levels/effects of: Aldesleukin; Corticorelin; Hyaluronidase; Telaprevir

Stability Store at 20°C to 25°C (68°F to 77°F); excursions permitted to 15°C to 30°C (59°F to 86°F); do not freeze.

Mechanism of Action See individual agents.

Pharmacokinetics (Adult data unless noted) See individual agents.

Dosing: Usual Children ≥12 years, Adolescents, and Adults: **Herpes labialis (cold sores):** Topical: Apply 5 times daily for 5 days; initiate therapy at first sign of infection (ie, during the prodrome or when lesions appear)

Administration Topical: For external use only. Wash hands before and after use. Apply to clean, dry area; use sufficient amount to cover the affected area(s), including the outer margin of cold sore; do not rub affected area nor cover area with a bandage. Do not bathe or shower for 30 minutes following application. Not for use in the eye, inside the mouth or nose, or on the genitals.

Dosage Forms Excipient information presented when available (limited, particularly for generics); consult specific product labeling.

Cream, topical:
   Xerese®: Acyclovir 5% and hydrocortisone 1% (5 g)

References
Strand A, Böttiger D, Gever LN, et al, "Safety and Tolerability of Combination Acyclovir 5% and Hydrocortisone 1% Cream in Adolescents With Recurrent Herpes Simplex Labialis," *Pediatr Dermatol*, 2012, 29(1):105-10.

◆ **ACZ885** *see* Canakinumab *on page 361*

◆ **Aczone** *see* Dapsone (Topical) *on page 589*

◆ **Aczone™ (Can)** *see* Dapsone (Topical) *on page 589*

◆ **Adacel** *see* Diphtheria and Tetanus Toxoids, and Acellular Pertussis Vaccine *on page 686*

◆ **Adacel®-Polio (Can)** *see* Diphtheria and Tetanus Toxoids, Acellular Pertussis, and Poliovirus Vaccine *on page 682*

◆ **Adalat XL (Can)** *see* NIFEdipine *on page 1497*

◆ **Adalat CC** *see* NIFEdipine *on page 1497*

Adalimumab (a da LIM yoo mab)

Medication Safety Issues
Sound-alike/look-alike issues:
   Humira may be confused with Humulin, Humalog
   Humira Pen may be confused with HumaPen Memoir
Brand Names: U.S. Humira; Humira Pen; Humira Pen-Crohns Starter; Humira Pen-Psoriasis Starter
Brand Names: Canada Humira
Therapeutic Category Antirheumatic, Disease Modifying; Gastrointestinal Agent, Miscellaneous; Monoclonal Antibody; Tumor Necrosis Factor (TNF) Blocking Agent
Generic Availability (U.S.) No
Use Treatment of moderately- to severely-active polyarticular juvenile idiopathic arthritis (JIA) alone or in combination with methotrexate (FDA approved in ages 4-17 years); moderately- to severely-active rheumatoid arthritis (RA) alone or in combination with methotrexate or other nonbiologic, disease-modifying antirheumatic drugs (DMARDs) (FDA approved in adults); active psoriatic arthritis alone or in combination with nonbiologic DMARDs (FDA approved in adults); ankylosing spondylitis (FDA approved in adults); treatment of moderately to severely active Crohn's disease in patients with inadequate response to conventional treatment or patients who have lost response to or are intolerant of infliximab (FDA approved in adults); treatment of moderate to severe chronic plaque psoriasis when systemic therapy is required and other agents are less appropriate (FDA approved in adults); and treatment of moderately to severely active ulcerative colitis in patients unresponsive to immunosuppressants (FDA approved in adults). **Note:** Efficacy in ulcerative colitis patients who are intolerant or no longer responsive to other TNF blockers has not been established. Has also been used in children with idiopathic or JIA-associated uveitis and chronic uveitis.
Medication Guide Available Yes
Pregnancy Risk Factor B
Pregnancy Considerations Adverse events were not observed in animal reproduction studies. Adalimumab crosses the placenta and can be detected in cord blood at birth at concentrations higher than those in the maternal serum. In one study of pregnant women with inflammatory bowel disease, adalimumab was found to be measurable in a newborn for up to 11 weeks following delivery. Maternal doses of adalimumab were 40 mg every other week (n=9) or 40 mg weekly (n=1) and the last dose was administered 0.14-8 weeks prior to delivery (median 5.5 weeks) (Mahadevan, 2013). If therapy for inflammatory bowel disease is needed during pregnancy, adalimumab should be discontinued before 30 weeks gestation in order to decrease exposure to the newborn. In addition, the administration of live vaccines should be postponed until anti-TNF concentrations in the infant are negative (Habal, 2012; Mahadeven, 2013; Zelinkova, 2013).

Women exposed to adalimumab during pregnancy for the treatment of an autoimmune disease (eg, inflammatory bowel disease) may contact the OTIS Autoimmune Diseases Study at 877-311-8972.
Breast-Feeding Considerations Low concentrations of adalimumab may be detected in breast milk but are unlikely to be absorbed by a nursing infant. The manufacturer recommends caution be used if administered to a nursing woman.
Contraindications Hypersensitivity to adalimumab or any component
Warnings Patients receiving adalimumab are at increased risk for serious infections which may result in hospitalization and/or fatality **[U.S. Boxed Warning]**; infections usually developed in patients >65 years, receiving concomitant immunosuppressive agents (eg, methotrexate or corticosteroids), and may present as disseminated (rather than local) disease. Active tuberculosis (or reactivation of latent tuberculosis); invasive fungal (including aspergillosis, blastomycosis, candidiasis, coccidioidomycosis, histoplasmosis, and pneumocystosis); and bacterial, viral, or other opportunistic infections (including legionellosis and listeriosis) have been reported in patients receiving TNF-blocking agents, including adalimumab. Monitor closely for signs/symptoms of infection; discontinue for serious infection or sepsis. Consider risks versus benefits prior to use in patients with a history of chronic or recurrent infection. Consider empiric antifungal therapy in patients who are at risk for invasive fungal infection and develop severe systemic illness. Caution should be exercised when considering use in the elderly or in patients with conditions that predispose them to infections (eg, diabetes) or residence/travel from areas of endemic mycoses (blastomycosis, coccidioidomycosis, histoplasmosis), or with latent or localized infections. Do not initiate adalimumab therapy with clinically important active infection. Patients who develop a new infection while undergoing treatment should be monitored closely. Avoid concomitant use with anakinra (interleukin-1 antagonist) or abatacept; neutropenia and serious infections have been reported with other TNF-blockers (etanercept) when used with anakinra and abatacept.

New onset tuberculosis and reactivation of tuberculosis (disseminated or extrapulmonary) has been reported while on adalimumab; most cases have been reported within the first 8 months of treatment. Patients should be evaluated for latent tuberculosis infection with a tuberculin skin test prior to therapy **[U.S. Boxed Warning]**. Patients with initial negative tuberculin skin tests should receive continued monitoring for tuberculosis throughout treatment; active tuberculosis has developed in this population during treatment. Use with caution in patients who have resided in regions where tuberculosis is endemic. If initial tuberculin skin test is positive (induration >5 mm, regardless if previously vaccinated with BCG), initiate treatment for latent TB prior to starting adalimumab; consider antituberculosis treatment for patients with history of latent or active TB in which complete course of therapy cannot be confirmed or those with risk factors for TB despite testing negative for latent TB.

In children and adolescents, lymphomas and other malignancies, some fatal, have been reported with use of TNF blockers **[U.S. Boxed Warning]**. Half the cases are lymphomas (Hodgkin's and non-Hodgkin's) and the other cases are varied, but include malignancies not typically observed in this population. Most patients were receiving concomitant immunosuppressants. Hepatosplenic T-cell lymphoma (HSTCL), a rare T-cell lymphoma, has also been reported **[U.S. Boxed Warning]**; postmarketing reports were primarily in patients with Crohn's disease or ulcerative colitis treated with adalimumab and who received concomitant azathioprine or mercaptopurine; reports occurred predominantly in adolescent and young adult males. Use of adalimumab may affect defenses against malignancies; impact on the development and course of malignancies is not fully defined. As compared to the general population, an increased risk of lymphoma has been noted in clinical trials; however, rheumatoid arthritis has been previously associated with an increased rate of lymphoma. A higher incidence of nonmelanoma skin cancers was noted in adalimumab-treated patients (0.7/100 patient years), when compared to the control group (0.2/100 patient years). In an analysis of children and adolescents who had received TNF-blockers (etanercept and infliximab), the FDA identified 48 cases of malignancy. Of the 48 cases, ~50% were lymphomas (eg, Hodgkin's and non-Hodgkin's lymphoma). Other malignancies such as leukemia, melanoma, and solid organ tumors were reported; malignancies rarely seen in children (eg, leiomyosarcoma, hepatic malignancies, and renal cell carcinoma) were also observed. Of note, most of these cases (88%) were receiving other immunosuppressive medications (eg, azathioprine and methotrexate). The role of TNF blockers in the development of malignancies in children cannot be excluded. The FDA also reviewed 147 postmarketing reports of leukemia (including acute myeloid leukemia, chronic lymphocytic leukemia, and chronic myeloid leukemia) in patients (children and adults) using TNF-blockers. Average onset time to development of leukemia was within the first 1-2 years of TNF blocker initiation. Although most patients were receiving other immunosuppressive agents, the role of TNF blockers in the development of leukemia could not be excluded. The FDA concluded that there is a possible association with the development of leukemia and the use of TNF blockers. Patients should be monitored closely for signs and symptoms suggestive of malignancy, evidence of which should result in prompt discontinuation of the medication and appropriate diagnostic evaluation. Healthcare professionals should report any malignancies in patients being treated with TNF-blockers to the FDA's MedWatch program.

May also cause new-onset psoriasis; improvement was seen when the TNF-blocker was discontinued; monitor closely for signs and symptoms suggestive of new-onset psoriasis, evidence of which should result in prompt discontinuation of the medication and appropriate diagnostic evaluation.

May rarely cause hypersensitivity reactions; anaphylaxis and angioneurotic edema have been reported. Therapy should be immediately discontinued and appropriate therapy initiated if anaphylactic or other serious allergic reaction occurs.

Rare reactivation of hepatitis B (HBV) has occurred in chronic carriers of the virus, usually in patients receiving concomitant immunosuppressants; evaluate for HBV prior to initiation in all patients. Monitor during and for several months following discontinuation of treatment in HBV carriers; interrupt therapy if reactivation occurs and treat appropriately with antiviral therapy; if resumption of therapy is deemed necessary, exercise caution and monitor patient closely.

Injection contains polysorbate 80 (Tween 80®) which may cause allergic reactions in susceptible individuals. The needle cover of syringe contains latex; patients with latex allergy should avoid contact.

Precautions Use with caution in patients with preexisting or recent onset central or peripheral nervous system demyelinating disorders; rare cases of new-onset or exacerbation of demyelinating disorders (eg, multiple sclerosis, optic neuritis, Guillain-Barré syndrome) have been reported; consider discontinuing use in patients who develop peripheral or central nervous system demyelinating disorders during treatment. Rare cases of pancytopenia (including aplastic anemia) have been reported with TNF-blocking agents; if significant hematologic abnormalities occur, consider discontinuing therapy. Use with caution in patients with congestive heart failure (CHF) or decreased left ventricular function; worsening or new onset CHF have been reported with TNF blockers. Patients should be brought up to date with all immunizations before initiating therapy; live vaccines should not be given concurrently. There are no data available concerning secondary transmission of infection from live vaccine in patients receiving adalimumab. Positive antinuclear antibody titers have been detected in patients (with negative baselines); rare cases of autoimmune disorder, including lupus-like syndrome, have been reported; monitor and discontinue if symptoms develop.

Adverse Reactions

Cardiovascular: Atrial fibrillation, cardiac arrest, cardiac arrhythmia, cardiac failure, chest pain, coronary artery disease, deep vein thrombosis, hypertension, hypertensive encephalopathy, myocardial infarction, palpitations, pericardial effusion, pericarditis, peripheral edema, subdural hematoma, syncope, tachycardia, vascular disease

Central nervous system: Confusion, headache, myasthenia, paresthesia

Dermatologic: Alopecia, cellulitis, erysipelas, skin rash

Endocrine & metabolic: Dehydration, hypercholesterolemia, hyperlipidemia, ketosis, menstrual disease, parathyroid disease

Gastrointestinal: Abdominal pain, diverticulitis, esophagitis, gastroenteritis, gastrointestinal hemorrhage, nausea, vomiting

Genitourinary: Cholecystitis, cholelithiasis, cystitis, hematuria, pelvic pain, urinary tract infection

Hematologic & oncologic: Adenoma, agranulocytosis, carcinoma (including breast, gastrointestinal, skin, urogenital), granulocytopenia, leukopenia, malignant lymphoma, malignant melanoma, pancytopenia, paraproteinemia, polycythemia, positive ANA titer

Hepatic: Hepatic necrosis, increased serum alkaline phosphatase

Hypersensitivity: Hypersensitivity reaction (more common in children)

Immunologic: Antibody development (significance unknown)

Infection: Herpes zoster, sepsis, serious infection (more common in adults [Burmester, 2012])

Local: Injection site reaction

Neuromuscular & skeletal: Arthralgia, arthritis, arthropathy, back pain, bone fracture, increased creatine phosphokinase, limb pain, multiple sclerosis, muscle cramps, myasthenia, osteonecrosis, septic arthritis, synovitis, systemic lupus erythematosus, tendon disease, tremor

Ophthalmic: Cataract

Renal: Nephrolithiasis, pyelonephritis

Respiratory: Asthma, bronchospasm, dyspnea, flu-like symptoms, pleural effusion, pneumonia, respiratory depression, sinusitis, tuberculosis (including reactivation of latent infection; disseminated, miliary, lymphatic, peritoneal and pulmonary); upper respiratory tract infection

Miscellaneous: Abnormal healing, accidental injury, fever, postoperative complication (infection)

Rare but important or life-threatening: Abscess (limb, perianal), anal fissure, anaphylactoid reaction, anaphylaxis, angioedema, aplastic anemia, appendicitis, bacterial infection, basal cell carcinoma, cerebrovascular accident, cervical dysplasia, circulatory shock, cytopenia, dermal ulcer, endometrial hyperplasia, erythema multiforme, fixed drug eruption, fulminant necrotizing fasciitis, fungal infection, Guillain-Barre syndrome, hepatic failure, hepatitis B (reactivation), hepatosplenic T-cell lymphomas (children, adolescents, and young adults), herpes simplex infection, histoplasmosis, hypersensitivity angiitis, increased serum transaminases, interstitial pulmonary disease (eg, pulmonary fibrosis), intestinal obstruction, intestinal perforation, leukemia, liver metastases, lupus-like syndrome, lymphadenopathy, lymphocytosis, malignant neoplasm of ovary, meningitis (viral), Merkel cell carcinoma, mycobacterium avium complex, myositis (children and adolescents), neutropenia, optic neuritis, pancreatitis, pharyngitis (children and adolescents), protozoal infection, psoriasis (including new onset, palmoplantar, pustular, or exacerbation), pulmonary embolism, respiratory failure, sarcoidosis, septic shock, skin granuloma (annulare; children and adolescents), Stevens-Johnson syndrome, streptococcal pharyngitis (children and adolescents), testicular neoplasm, thrombocytopenia, vasculitis (systemic), viral infection

Drug Interactions

Metabolism/Transport Effects None known.

Avoid Concomitant Use

Avoid concomitant use of Adalimumab with any of the following: Abatacept; Anakinra; BCG; Belimumab; Canakinumab; Certolizumab Pegol; InFLIXimab; Natalizumab; Pimecrolimus; Rilonacept; Tacrolimus (Topical); Tocilizumab; Tofacitinib; Vaccines (Live); Vedolizumab

Increased Effect/Toxicity

Adalimumab may increase the levels/effects of: Abatacept; Anakinra; Belimumab; Canakinumab; Certolizumab Pegol; InFLIXimab; Leflunomide; Natalizumab; Rilonacept; Tofacitinib; Vaccines (Live); Vedolizumab

The levels/effects of Adalimumab may be increased by: Abciximab; Denosumab; Pimecrolimus; Roflumilast; Tacrolimus (Topical); Tocilizumab; Trastuzumab

Decreased Effect

Adalimumab may decrease the levels/effects of: BCG; Coccidioidin Skin Test; CycloSPORINE (Systemic); Sipuleucel-T; Theophylline Derivatives; Vaccines (Inactivated); Vaccines (Live); Warfarin

The levels/effects of Adalimumab may be decreased by: Echinacea

Stability Store at 2°C to 8°C (36°F to 46°F); do not freeze; protect from light; store in original carton until administration

Mechanism of Action Adalimumab is a recombinant monoclonal antibody that binds to human tumor necrosis factor alpha (TNF-alpha), thereby interfering with binding to TNFα receptor sites and subsequent cytokine-driven inflammatory processes. Elevated TNF levels in the synovial fluid are involved in the pathologic pain and joint destruction in immune-mediated arthritis. Adalimumab decreases signs and symptoms of psoriatic arthritis, rheumatoid arthritis, and ankylosing spondylitis. It inhibits progression of structural damage of rheumatoid and psoriatic arthritis. Reduces signs and symptoms and maintains clinical remission in Crohn disease and ulcerative colitis; reduces epidermal thickness and inflammatory cell infiltration in plaque psoriasis.

Pharmacokinetics (Adult data unless noted)

Distribution: V_d: 4.7-6 L; synovial fluid concentrations: 31% to 96% of serum

Bioavailability: Absolute: 64%

Half-life: ~2 weeks (range: 10-20 days)

Time to peak serum concentration: SubQ: 131 ± 56 hours

Elimination: Clearance increased in the presence of anti-adalimumab antibodies; decreased in patients ≥40 years

Dosing: Usual

Children and Adolescents:

Juvenile idiopathic arthritis (JIA): SubQ: Children and Adolescents 4-17 years:
15 kg to <30 kg: 20 mg every other week
≥30 kg: 40 mg every other week

Crohn's disease; moderate to severe; refractory: Limited data available: SubQ: Children and Adolescents: 6-17 years: The largest clinical trial (n=188) to date reported a proportionally larger number of patients went into clinical remission or showed clinical response utilizing the higher end dosages shown below compared to the lower dosages; however, response rate differences were not statistically significant; may be less effective in patients with previous infliximab therapy (Hyams, 2012; Rosh, 2009):

Induction:
<40 kg: 80 mg on Week 0 followed by 40 mg on Week 2
≥40 kg: 160 mg on Week 0 followed by 80 mg on Week 2

Maintenance dose: Start on Week 4 (ie, 2 weeks after induction completed):
<40 kg: 10 mg or 20 mg every other week, if needed, dose may be increased by changing to weekly dosing
≥40 kg: 20 mg or 40 mg every other week; if needed, dose may be increased by changing to weekly dosing

Uveitis: Limited data available; SubQ: Children ≥3 years and Adolescents:
Body surface area-based dosing: 24 mg/m² every 2 weeks (Simonini, 2011)
Weight-based dosing (Biester, 2007; Sens, 2012; Tynjala, 2008):
<30 kg: 20 mg every other week
>30 kg: 40 mg every other week

Adults:

Ankylosing spondylitis: SubQ: 40 mg every other week

Crohn's disease: SubQ: Initial: 160 mg divided into 4 doses (ie, given as 4 injections on day 1 or as 2 injections per day over 2 consecutive days), then 80 mg 2 weeks later (day 15); maintenance: 40 mg every other week beginning day 29; **Note:** Some patients may require 40 mg every week as maintenance therapy (Lichtenstein, 2009).

Plaque psoriasis: SubQ: Initial: 80 mg as a single dose; maintenance: 40 mg every other week beginning 1 week after initial dose

Psoriatic arthritis: SubQ: 40 mg every other week

Rheumatoid arthritis: SubQ: 40 mg every other week; may be administered with other DMARDs; patients not taking methotrexate may increase dose to 40 mg every week

Ulcerative colitis: SubQ:
Initial: 160 mg (given as 4 injections on day 1 or as 2 injections daily over 2 consecutive days), then 80 mg 2 weeks later (day 15)
Maintenance: 40 mg every other week beginning day 29. **Note:** Only continue maintenance dose in patients demonstrating clinical remission by 8 weeks (day 57) of therapy.

Dosing adjustment in renal impairment: There are no dosage adjustments provided in the manufacturer's labeling.

Dosing adjustment in hepatic impairment: There are no dosage adjustments provided in the manufacturer's labeling.

Administration For SubQ injection into thigh or lower abdomen (avoid areas within 2 inches of navel); rotate injection sites. Do not use if solution is discolored or contains particulate matter. Do not administer to skin which is red, tender, bruised, or hard. To reduce pain of injection, some centers use 0.2 mL of 1% lidocaine and add adalimumab dose to the lidocaine syringe swirling gently to mix contents prior to administration (Ayala, 2008). Prefilled pens and syringes are available for use by patients (self-administration); the vial is intended for institutional use only. Vials do not contain a preservative; discard unused portion.

Monitoring Parameters Monitor improvement of symptoms and physical function assessments. Latent TB screening prior to initiating and during therapy; signs/symptoms of infection (prior to, during, and following therapy); CBC with differential; signs/symptoms/worsening of heart failure; HBV screening prior to initiating (all patients), HBV carriers (during and for several months following therapy); signs and symptoms of hypersensitivity reaction; symptoms of lupus-like syndrome; signs/symptoms of malignancy (eg, splenomegaly, hepatomegaly, abdominal pain, persistent fever, night sweats, weight loss).

Dosage Forms Excipient information presented when available (limited, particularly for generics); consult specific product labeling.

Kit, Subcutaneous [preservative free]:
Humira: 20 mg/0.4 mL, 40 mg/0.8 mL [contains polysorbate 80]
Humira Pen: 40 mg/0.8 mL [contains polysorbate 80]
Humira Pen-Crohns Starter: 40 mg/0.8 mL [contains polysorbate 80]
Humira Pen-Psoriasis Starter: 40 mg/0.8 mL [contains polysorbate 80]

References

Ayala RS, Groh BP, Robbins LM, et al, "The Addition of Injectable Lidocaine to Adalimumab Results in Decreased Injection Site Pain and Increased Acceptance of Therapy," 2008, American College of Rheumatology Annual Scientific Meeting, San Francisco, CA (poster).

Beukelman T, Patkar NM, Saag KG, et al, "2011 American College of Rheumatology Recommendations for the Treatment of Juvenile Idiopathic Arthritis: Initiation and Safety Monitoring of Therapeutic Agents for the Treatment of Arthritis and Systemic Features," *Arthritis Care Res (Hoboken)*, 2011, 63(4):465-82.

Biester S, Deuter C, Michels H, et al, "Adalimumab in the Therapy of Uveitis in Childhood," *Br J Ophthalmol*, 2007, 91(3):319-24.

Furst DE, Keystone EC, Kirkham B, et al, "Updated Consensus Statement on Biological Agents for the Treatment of Rheumatic Diseases, 2008," *Ann Rheum Dis*, 2008, 67 Suppl 3:iii2-25.

Habal FM and Huang VW, "Review Article: A Decision-Making Algorithm For the Management of Pregnancy in the Inflammatory Bowel Disease Patient," *Aliment Pharmacol Ther*, 2012, 35(5):501-15.

Hyams JS, Griffiths A, Markowitz J, et al, "Safety and Efficacy of Adalimumab for Moderate to Severe Crohn's Disease in Children," *Gastroenterology*, 2012, 143(2):365-74.

Lichtenstein GR, Hanauer SB, and Sandborn WJ, "Management of Crohn's Disease in Adults," *Am J Gastroenterol*, 2009, 104(2):465-83.

Lovell DJ, Ruperto N, Goodman S, et al, "Adalimumab With or Without Methotrexate in Juvenile Rheumatoid Arthritis," *N Engl J Med*, 2008, 359(8):810-20.

Mahadevan U, Wolf DC, Dubinsky M, et al, "Placental Transfer of Anti-Tumor Necrosis Factor Agents in Pregnant Patients With Inflammatory Bowel Disease," *Clin Gastroenterol Hepatol*, 2013, 11(3):286-92.

Rosh JR, Lerer T, Markowitz J, et al, "Retrospective Evaluation of the Safety and Effect of Adalimumab Therapy (RESEAT) in Pediatric Crohn's Disease," *Am J Gastroenterol*, 2009, 104(12):3042-9.

Sen ES, Sharma S, Hinchcliffe A, et al, "Use of Adalimumab in Refractory Non-infectious Childhood Chronic Uveitis: Efficacy in Ocular Disease - a Case Cohort Interventional Study," *Rheumatology (Oxford)*, 2012, 51(12):2199-203.

Simonini G, Taddio A, Cattalini M, et al, "Prevention of Flare Recurrences in Childhood-Refractory Chronic Uveitis: An Open-Label Comparative Study of Adalimumab Versus Infliximab," *Arthritis Care Res (Hoboken)*, 2011, 63(4):612-8.

Tynjälä P, Kotaniemi K, Lindahl P, et al, "Adalimumab in Juvenile Idiopathic Arthritis-Associated Chronic Anterior Uveitis," *Rheumatology (Oxford)*, 2008, 47(3):339-44.

Zelinkova Z, van der Ent C, Bruin KF, et al, "Effects of Discontinuing Anti-Tumor Necrosis Factor Therapy During Pregnancy on the Course of Inflammatory Bowel Disease and Neonatal Exposure," *Clin Gastroenterol Hepatol*, 2013, 11(3):318-21.

◆ **Adamantanamine Hydrochloride** *see* Amantadine on page 112

Adapalene (a DAP a leen)

Brand Names: U.S. Differin
Brand Names: Canada Differin®; Differin® XP
Therapeutic Category Acne Products
Generic Availability (U.S.) May be product dependent
Use Topical treatment of acne vulgaris (FDA approved in ages ≥12 years and adults)
Pregnancy Risk Factor C
Pregnancy Considerations Adverse effects were observed in animal reproduction studies. Retinoids may cause harm when administered during pregnancy. A case report described maternal use of adapalene 1 month prior to pregnancy and through 13 weeks gestation; cerebral and ocular malformations were reported in the exposed fetus which resulted in termination of pregnancy (Autret, 1997). In clinical trials, women of childbearing potential were required to have a negative pregnancy test prior to therapy.
Breast-Feeding Considerations It is not known if adapalene is excreted in breast milk. The manufacturer recommends that caution be exercised when administering adapalene to nursing women.
Contraindications Hypersensitivity to adapalene or any component
Warnings Use is associated with increased susceptibility/sensitivity to UV light; avoid exposure to sunlight and sunlamps; use sunscreen and protective apparel when exposure cannot be avoided. Weather extremes (wind or cold) may also be irritating. Certain cutaneous signs and symptoms such as erythema, dryness, scaling, burning, or pruritus may occur during treatment; these are most likely to occur during the first 2-4 weeks and will usually lessen with continued use. Depending on the severity of irritation, a moisturizer may be used or there may be a need to reduce the frequency or discontinue use. For external use only, avoid contact with abraded skin, mucous membranes, eyes, mouth, or angles of the nose. Wax depilation is not recommended.
Precautions Use with caution in patients with eczema; avoid application to abrasions, eczematous, or sunburned skin.

Adverse Reactions

Dermatologic: Burning/stinging, desquamation, dryness, erythema, pruritus, scaling, skin discomfort, skin irritation, sunburn

Rare but important or life-threatening: Acne flares, angioedema (gel), application site pain (gel), conjunctivitis, contact dermatitis, dermatitis, eczema, eyelid edema, facial edema (gel), lip swelling (gel), rash (cream/gel), skin discoloration

Drug Interactions

Metabolism/Transport Effects None known.

Avoid Concomitant Use
Avoid concomitant use of Adapalene with any of the following: Multivitamins/Fluoride (with ADE); Multivitamins/Minerals (with ADEK, Folate, Iron); Multivitamins/Minerals (with AE, No Iron)

Increased Effect/Toxicity
Adapalene may increase the levels/effects of: Porfimer

The levels/effects of Adapalene may be increased by: Multivitamins/Fluoride (with ADE); Multivitamins/Minerals (with ADEK, Folate, Iron); Multivitamins/Minerals (with AE, No Iron)

Decreased Effect
Adapalene may decrease the levels/effects of: Contraceptives (Progestins)

Stability

Cream: Store at 20°C to 25°C (68°F to 77°F); do not freeze.

Gel: Store at 20°C to 25°C (68°F to 77°F); excursions permitted to 15°C to 30°C (59°F to 86°F); do not freeze.

Lotion: Store at 20°C to 25°C (68°F to 77°F); excursions permitted to 15°C to 30°C (59°F to 86°F); do not refrigerate or freeze; protect from light.

Mechanism of Action Retinoid-like compound which is a modulator of cellular differentiation, keratinization, and inflammatory processes, all of which represent important features in the pathology of acne vulgaris

Pharmacodynamics Onset of action: 8-12 weeks

Pharmacokinetics (Adult data unless noted)

Absorption: Absorption through the skin is very low; only trace amounts have been measured in serum after chronic application

Elimination: Primarily in bile

Dosing: Usual Children ≥12 years, Adolescents, and Adults: **Acne, treatment:** Topical: Apply once daily in the evening

Dosing adjustment in renal impairment: There are no dosage adjustments provided in the manufacturer's labeling; however, dosage adjustment unlikely necessary due to low systemic absorption.

Dosing adjustment in hepatic impairment: There are no dosage adjustments provided in the manufacturer's labeling; however, dosage adjustment unlikely necessary due to low systemic absorption.

Administration Topical: For external use only. After cleansing the affected area with mild or soapless cleanser, apply a thin film of medication before retiring in the evening. Avoid contact with eyes, angles of the nose, lips and mucous membranes.

Monitoring Parameters Reduction in lesion size and/or inflammation; reduction in the number of lesions

Dosage Forms Excipient information presented when available (limited, particularly for generics); consult specific product labeling.

Cream, External:
Differin: 0.1% (45 g)
Generic: 0.1% (45 g)

Gel, External:
Differin: 0.1% (45 g)
Differin: 0.3% (45 g) [contains edetate disodium, methylparaben, propylene glycol]
Generic: 0.1% (45 g); 0.3% (45 g)

Lotion, External:
Differin: 0.1% (59 mL) [contains methylparaben, propylene glycol, propylparaben]

References

Autret E, Berjot M, Jonville-Béra AP, et al, "Anophthalmia and Agenesis of Optic Chiasma Associated With Adapalene Gel in Early Pregnancy," *Lancet*, 1997, 350(9074):339.

Eichenfield LF, Krakowski AC, Piggott C, et al, "Evidence-Based Recommendations for the Diagnosis and Treatment of Pediatric Acne," *Pediatrics*, 2013, (131 Suppl 3):S163-86.

Adapalene and Benzoyl Peroxide
(a DAP a leen & BEN zoe il peer OKS ide)

Brand Names: U.S. Epiduo®

Brand Names: Canada Tactuo™

Therapeutic Category Acne Products; Topical Skin Product; Topical Skin Product, Acne

Generic Availability (U.S.) No

Use Treatment of acne vulgaris (FDA approved in ages ≥9 years and adults)

Pregnancy Risk Factor C

Pregnancy Considerations There are no well-controlled studies in pregnant women. Use only if benefit outweighs the potential risk to fetus.

Contraindications Hypersensitivity to adapalene, benzoyl peroxide, benzoic acid, or any component

Warnings Use is associated with increased susceptibility/sensitivity to UV light; avoid exposure to sunlight and

sunlamps; use sunscreen and protective apparel when exposure cannot be avoided. Weather extremes, such as wind or cold, may be irritating to patients under treatment. Certain cutaneous signs and symptoms, such as erythema, dryness, scaling, burning, or pruritus, may occur during treatment; these are most likely to occur during the first 2-4 weeks and will usually lessen with continued use. May cause allergic contact or irritant dermatitis. Depending on the severity of irritation, a moisturizer may be used or there may be a need to reduce the frequency or discontinue use. For external use only; avoid contact with abraded skin, mucous membranes, eyes, mouth, or angles of the nose. Wax depilation is not recommended in areas being treated.

Precautions Avoid application to cuts, abrasions, eczematous or sunburned skin; use with caution in patients with eczema. Use concomitant topical acne therapy with caution; avoid concomitant topical products that may be irritating which may include medicated or abrasive soaps, products with skin-drying effects, and products with high concentration of alcohol, astringents, spices, or limes. May cause bleaching of hair or clothing.

Adverse Reactions

Dermatologic: Burning, contact dermatitis, dry skin, erythema, scaling, skin irritation, stinging

Rare but important or life-threatening: Blistering, conjunctivitis, eczema, eyelid edema, facial swelling, pain, photosensitivity, pruritus, rash, skin discoloration

Drug Interactions

Metabolism/Transport Effects None known.

Avoid Concomitant Use

Avoid concomitant use of Adapalene and Benzoyl Peroxide with any of the following: Multivitamins/Fluoride (with ADE); Multivitamins/Minerals (with ADEK, Folate, Iron); Multivitamins/Minerals (with AE, No Iron)

Increased Effect/Toxicity

Adapalene and Benzoyl Peroxide may increase the levels/effects of: Porfimer

The levels/effects of Adapalene and Benzoyl Peroxide may be increased by: Multivitamins/Fluoride (with ADE); Multivitamins/Minerals (with ADEK, Folate, Iron); Multivitamins/Minerals (with AE, No Iron)

Decreased Effect

Adapalene and Benzoyl Peroxide may decrease the levels/effects of: Contraceptives (Progestins)

Stability Store at 25°C; excursions permitted to 15°C to 30°C (59°F to 86°F); protect from light and heat.

Mechanism of Action

Benzoyl peroxide releases free-radical oxygen which oxidizes bacterial proteins in the sebaceous follicles decreasing the number of anaerobic bacteria and decreasing irritating-type free fatty acids.

Adapalene is a retinoid-like compound which is a modulator of cellular differentiation, keratinization, and inflammatory processes, all of which represent important features in the pathology of acne vulgaris.

Pharmacodynamics Onset of action: ≥4-8 weeks (Eichenfield, 2013)

Pharmacokinetics (Adult data unless noted)

Metabolism: Benzoyl peroxide: Converted to benzoic acid in skin

Elimination: Adapalene: Primarily through bile; Benzoyl peroxide: Urine

Dosing: Usual Note: Application of more than recommended amount or more frequent administration does not result in quicker onset of action and is associated with more irritant effects.

Pediatric: **Acne vulgaris:** Children ≥7 years and Adolescents; limited data in children <9 years: Topical: Apply a thin film once daily to affected areas of cleansed and dried skin (Eichenfield, 2013)

Adult: **Acne vulgaris:** Topical: Apply a thin film once daily to affected areas of cleansed and dried skin

Administration Apply a pea-sized amount for each affected area of the face (eg, forehead, chin, each cheek). Skin should be clean and dry before applying. For external use only; avoid applying to eyes and mucous membranes.

Dosage Forms Excipient information presented when available (limited, particularly for generics); consult specific product labeling.

Gel, topical:
Epiduo®: Adapalene 0.1% and benzoyl peroxide 2.5% (45 g)

References
Eichenfield LF, Krakowski AC, Piggott C, et al. Evidence-based recommendations for the diagnosis and treatment of pediatric acne. *Pediatrics.* 2013;(131 Suppl 3):S163-186.

◆ **ADD 234037** see Lacosamide on page 1189
◆ **Addamel N** see Trace Elements on page 2059
◆ **Addaprin [OTC]** see Ibuprofen on page 1059
◆ **Adderall** see Dextroamphetamine and Amphetamine on page 632
◆ **Adderall XR** see Dextroamphetamine and Amphetamine on page 632

Adefovir (a DEF o veer)

Brand Names: U.S. Hepsera
Brand Names: Canada Hepsera
Therapeutic Category Antiretroviral Agent, Reverse Transcriptase Inhibitor (Nucleotide)
Generic Availability (U.S.) Yes
Use Treatment of chronic hepatitis B with evidence of active viral replication and either persistent elevations of ALT or AST or histologically active disease (FDA approved in ages ≥12 years and adults)
Pregnancy Risk Factor C
Pregnancy Considerations Adverse events were observed in some animal reproduction studies. Pregnant women exposed to adefovir should be registered with the pregnancy registry (800-258-4263).
Breast-Feeding Considerations It is not known if adefovir is excreted in breast milk. Due to the potential for serious adverse reactions in the nursing infant, a decision should be made whether to discontinue nursing or to discontinue the drug, taking into account the importance of treatment to the mother.
Contraindications Hypersensitivity to adefovir or any component
Warnings Severe, acute exacerbation of hepatitis B may occur upon discontinuation **[U.S. Boxed Warning]**; exacerbations (ALT elevation ≥10 times ULN) may occur in up to 25% of patients and usually within 12 weeks; may be self-limited or resolve upon resuming treatment; risk may be increased with advanced liver disease or cirrhosis. Monitor liver function several months after stopping treatment; reinitiation of antihepatitis B therapy may be required.

Chronic administration may result in treatment-limiting nephrotoxicity in patients at risk for or with underlying renal dysfunction **[U.S. Boxed Warning]**; nephrotoxicity is characterized by gradual increase in serum creatinine and decrease in serum phosphorus; use with caution in patients with renal dysfunction or in patients at risk for development of nephrotoxicity including those on concurrent nephrotoxic agents (eg, cyclosporine, tacrolimus, aminoglycosides, vancomycin, or NSAIDs); dosage adjustment may be required in patients with preexisting renal dysfunction or in those who develop renal dysfunction during therapy. Calculate creatinine clearance before initiation of therapy.

May cause the development of HIV resistance in patients with unrecognized or untreated HIV infection **[U.S. Boxed Warning]**; determine HIV status prior to initiating treatment with adefovir.

Fatal cases of lactic acidosis and severe hepatomegaly with steatosis have been reported with the use of nucleoside analogues alone or in combination with other antiretrovirals **[U.S. Boxed Warning]**; use with caution in patients with risk factors for liver disease; risk may be increased with female gender, obesity, pregnancy, and prolonged treatment; suspend if clinical or laboratory findings suggestive of lactic acidosis or hepatotoxicity (transaminase elevation may or may not accompany hepatomegaly and steatosis).

Precautions Efficacy in pediatric patients <12 years has not been reported; in clinical trials of children 2-12 years, positive responses to adefovir therapy were observed (13% to 17% of subjects evaluated); however, findings did not reach statistical significance (Jonas, 2008). Use with caution in patients with decompensated liver function and prolonged use (>1 year) due to high rate of resistance accompanied by rebound increase viral load which may further decrease liver function (and possibly fatal outcome). Not recommended as first-line therapy of chronic HBV due to weak antiviral activity and high rate of resistance; may be more appropriate as second-line agent in treatment-naïve patients. Combination therapy with lamivudine in nucleoside-naïve patients has not been shown to provide synergistic antiviral effects. In patients with lamivudine-resistant HBV, switching to adefovir monotherapy was associated with a higher risk of adefovir resistance compared to adding adefovir to lamivudine therapy (Lok, 2009). Do not use concurrently with tenofovir (Viread®) or any product containing tenofovir (eg, Truvada®, Atripla®, Complera®).

Adverse Reactions
Central nervous system: Headache
Dermatologic: Pruritus, rash
Endocrine & metabolic: Hypophosphatemia
Gastrointestinal: Abdominal pain, diarrhea, dyspepsia, flatulence, nausea, vomiting
Hepatic: Hepatitis exacerbation
Neuromuscular & skeletal: Back pain, weakness
Renal: Hematuria, renal failure, serum creatinine increased
Respiratory: Cough, rhinitis
Postmarketing and/or case reports: Fanconi syndrome, hepatitis, myopathy, nephrotoxicity, osteomalacia, pancreatitis, proximal renal tubulopathy

Drug Interactions
Metabolism/Transport Effects None known.
Avoid Concomitant Use
Avoid concomitant use of Adefovir with any of the following: Tenofovir
Increased Effect/Toxicity
Adefovir may increase the levels/effects of: Tenofovir

The levels/effects of Adefovir may be increased by: Ganciclovir-Valganciclovir; Ribavirin; Tenofovir
Decreased Effect
Adefovir may decrease the levels/effects of: Tenofovir
Food Interactions Food does not have a significant effect on adefovir absorption. Management: Administer without regard to meals.
Stability Store at 25°C (77°F), excursions permitted to 15°C to 30°C (59°F to 86°F).
Mechanism of Action Acyclic nucleotide reverse transcriptase inhibitor (adenosine analog) which interferes with HBV viral RNA-dependent DNA polymerase resulting in inhibition of viral replication.

◀ **Pharmacokinetics (Adult data unless noted) Note:** Pharmacokinetic data reported in pediatric patients (12-18 years) similar to reported adult data.

Distribution: 0.35-0.39 L/kg

Protein binding: ≤4%

Metabolism: Prodrug; rapidly converted to adefovir (active metabolite) in intestine

Bioavailability: 59%

Half-life elimination: 7.5 hours; prolonged in renal impairment

Time to peak serum concentration: Median: 1.75 hours (range: 0.58-4 hours)

Elimination: Urine (45% as active metabolite within 24 hours)

Dialysis: ~35% of dose (10 mg) removed during 4 hours hemodialysis session

Dosing: Usual

Children ≥2 years and Adolescents: **Hepatitis B infection, chronic: Note:** Optimal duration of treatment not established, continuation of therapy for at least 6 months after seroconversion has been suggested (Jonas, 2010). Prolonged therapy (4 years) has been reported to be safe and well-tolerated in pediatric patients (2 to 18 years). Patients not achieving a <2 log decrease in serum HBV DNA after at least 6 months of therapy should either receive additional treatment or be switched to an alternative therapy (Jonas, 2012; Lok, 2009).

Children 2 to <7 years: Limited data available; efficacy results variable: Oral: 0.3 mg/kg/dose once daily; maximum dose: 10 mg (Jonas, 2008; Jonas, 2012)

Children ≥7 to <12 years: Limited data available; efficacy results variable: Oral: 0.25 mg/kg/dose once daily; maximum dose: 10 mg (Jonas, 2008; Jonas, 2012)

Children ≥12 years and Adolescents: Oral: 10 mg once daily

Adults: **Hepatitis B infection, chronic:** Oral: 10 mg once daily

Treatment duration (AASLD practice guidelines):

Hepatitis Be antigen (HBeAg) positive chronic hepatitis: Treat ≥1 year until HBeAg seroconversion and undetectable serum HBV DNA; continue therapy for ≥6 months after HBeAg seroconversion

HBeAg negative chronic hepatitis: Treat >1 year until hepatitis B surface antigen (HBsAg) clearance

Note: Patients not achieving a <2 log decrease in serum HBV DNA after at least 6 months of therapy should either receive additional treatment or be switched to an alternative therapy (Lok, 2009).

Dosage adjustment in renal impairment:

Children ≥12 years and Adolescents: There are no dosage adjustments provided in manufacturer's labeling; no data available; consider dosage reduction.

Adults:

Manufacturer's labeling: Oral:

CrCl ≥50 mL/minute: No dosage adjustment necessary

CrCl 30 to 49 mL/minute: 10 mg every 48 hours

CrCl 10 to 29 mL/minute: 10 mg every 72 hours

CrCl <10 mL/minute: There are no dosage adjustments provided in manufacturer's labeling; no data available in nonhemodialysis patients.

Hemodialysis: 10 mg every 7 days (following dialysis)

The following guidelines have been used by some clinicians (Aronoff, 2007): Oral:

CrCl ≥50 mL/minute: No dosage adjustment necessary

CrCl 30 to 49 mL/minute: 10 mg every 48 hours

CrCl ≤19 mL/minute: 10 mg every 72 hours

Administration Oral: May be administered without regard to food.

Monitoring Parameters HIV status (prior to initiation of therapy); serum creatinine (prior to initiation and during therapy); LFTs for several months following discontinuation of adefovir; HBV DNA (every 3 to 6 months during therapy); HBeAg and anti-HBe

Dosage Forms Excipient information presented when available (limited, particularly for generics); consult specific product labeling.

Tablet, Oral, as dipivoxil:

Hepsera: 10 mg

Generic: 10 mg

References

Aronoff GR, Bennett WM, Berns JS, et al, *Drug Prescribing in Renal Failure: Dosing Guidelines for Adults and Children*, 5th ed, Philadelphia, PA: American College of Physicians; 2007.

Haber BA, Block JM, Jonas MM, et al, "Recommendations for Screening, Monitoring, and Referral of Pediatric Chronic Hepatitis B," *Pediatrics*, 2009, 124(5):1007-13.

Jonas MM, Block JM, Haber BA, et al, "Treatment of Children With Chronic Hepatitis B Virus Infection in the United States: Patient Selection and Therapeutic Options," *Hepatology*, 2010, 52 (6):2192-205.

Jonas MM, Kelly D, Pollack H, et al, "Safety, Efficacy, and Pharmacokinetics of Adefovir Dipivoxil in Children and Adolescents (Age 2 to <18 Years) With Chronic Hepatitis B," *Hepatology*, 2008, 47 (6):1863-71.

Jonas MM, Kelly D, Pollack H, et al, "Efficacy and Safety of Long-Term Adefovir Dipivoxil Therapy in Children With Chronic Hepatitis B Infection," *Pediatr Infect Dis J*, 2012, 31(6):578-82.

Lok AS and McMahon BJ, "Chronic Hepatitis B: Update 2009," *Hepatology*, 2009, 50(3):661-2.

Sokal EM, Kelly D, Wirth S, et al, "The Pharmacokinetics and Safety of Adefovir Dipivoxil in Children and Adolescents With Chronic Hepatitis B Virus Infection," *J Clin Pharmacol*, 2008, 48(4):512-7.

◆ **Adefovir Dipivoxil** see Adefovir on page 75

◆ **Adenocard** see Adenosine on page 76

◆ **Adenoscan** see Adenosine on page 76

Adenosine (a DEN oh seen)

Medication Safety Issues

High alert medication:

This medication is in a class the Institute for Safe Medication Practices (ISMP) includes among its list of drug classes that have a heightened risk of causing significant patient harm when used in error.

Related Information

Adult ACLS Algorithms on page 2198

Pediatric ALS (PALS) Algorithms on page 2195

Brand Names: U.S. Adenocard; Adenoscan

Brand Names: Canada Adenocard; Adenosine Injection, USP; PMS-Adenosine

Therapeutic Category Antiarrhythmic Agent, Miscellaneous

Generic Availability (U.S.) Yes

Use Treatment of paroxysmal supraventricular tachycardia (PSVT), including that associated with accessory bypass tracts (eg, Wolff-Parkinson-White syndrome) (FDA approved in all ages); **Note:** When clinically advisable, appropriate vagal maneuvers should be attempted prior to adenosine administration; used in PALS algorithms for probable supraventricular tachycardia, stable regular monomorphic wide-complex tachycardia as a therapeutic (if arrhythmia supraventricular) and diagnostic maneuver; used in adult ACLS for stable narrow-complex regular tachycardias, unstable narrow-complex regular tachycardias while preparations are made for electrical cardioversion, stable regular monomorphic wide-complex tachycardia as a therapeutic (if arrhythmia supraventricular) and diagnostic maneuver; investigationally used as a continuous infusion for the treatment of primary pulmonary hypertension in adults and persistent pulmonary hypertension of the newborn (PPHN)

Pregnancy Risk Factor C

Pregnancy Considerations Animal reproduction studies have not been conducted. Adenosine is an endogenous substance and adverse fetal effects would not be anticipated. Case reports of administration during pregnancy have indicated no adverse effects on fetus or newborn attributable to adenosine (Blomström-Lundqvist, 2003). ACLS guidelines suggest use is safe and effective in pregnancy (Neumar, 2010).

Breast-Feeding Considerations Adenosine is endogenous in breast milk (Sugawara, 1995).

Contraindications Hypersensitivity to adenosine or any component; second and third degree A-V block or sick sinus syndrome unless pacemaker placed

Warnings Heart block, including transient or prolonged asystole may occur as well as other arrhythmias; episodes of asystole or other arrhythmias may be fatal; if arrhythmia is not due to re-entry pathway through A-V node or sinus node (ie, atrial fibrillation, flutter, or tachycardia or ventricular tachycardia), adenosine will not terminate the arrhythmia but can produce transient ventriculoatrial or A-V block; possible mutagenic effects

Precautions Bronchoconstriction may occur in asthmatics (avoid use in patients with bronchospasm or bronchoconstriction); use with caution in patients with underlying dysfunction of sinus or A-V node, obstructive lung disease, and those taking digoxin or verapamil; initial adenosine dose should be significantly decreased in patients receiving dipyridamole

Adverse Reactions

Cardiovascular: Atrioventricular block, cardiac arrhythmia (transient and new arrhythmia after cardioversion; eg, atrial fibrillation, atrial premature contractions, premature ventricular contractions), chest pain, chest pressure (and discomfort), depression of ST segment on ECG, hypotension, palpitations

Central nervous system: Apprehension, dizziness, headache, nervousness, numbness, paresthesia

Dermatologic: Diaphoresis, facial flushing

Gastrointestinal: Gastrointestinal distress, Nausea

Neuromuscular & skeletal: Neck discomfort (includes throat, jaw), upper extremity discomfort

Respiratory: Dyspnea, hyperventilation

Rare but important or life-threatening: Asystole (prolonged), atrial fibrillation, blurred vision, bradycardia, bronchospasm, burning sensation, cardiac arrest (fatal and nonfatal), increased intracranial pressure, injection site reaction, loss of consciousness, myocardial infarction, respiratory arrest, seizure, torsades de pointes, transient hypertension, ventricular arrhythmia, ventricular fibrillation, ventricular tachycardia

Drug Interactions

Metabolism/Transport Effects None known.

Avoid Concomitant Use There are no known interactions where it is recommended to avoid concomitant use.

Increased Effect/Toxicity
The levels/effects of Adenosine may be increased by: CarBAMazepine; Digoxin; Dipyridamole; Nicotine

Decreased Effect
The levels/effects of Adenosine may be decreased by: Caffeine and Caffeine Containing Products; Theophylline Derivatives

Stability Store at controlled room temperature 15°C to 30°C (59°F to 86°F); do **not** refrigerate, precipitation may occur (dissolve by warming to room temperature); contains no preservatives, discard unused portion

Mechanism of Action

Antiarrhythmic actions: Slows conduction time through the AV node, interrupting the re-entry pathways through the AV node, restoring normal sinus rhythm

Myocardial perfusion scintigraphy: Adenosine also causes coronary vasodilation and increases blood flow in normal coronary arteries with little to no increase in stenotic coronary arteries; thallium-201 uptake into the stenotic coronary arteries will be less than that of normal coronary arteries revealing areas of insufficient blood flow.

Pharmacodynamics

Onset of action: Rapid
Duration: Very brief

Pharmacokinetics (Adult data unless noted)

Metabolism: Removed from systemic circulation primarily by vascular endothelial cells and erythrocytes (by cellular uptake); rapidly metabolized intracellularly; phosphorylated by adenosine kinase to adenosine monophosphate (AMP) which is then incorporated into high-energy pool; intracellular adenosine is also deaminated by adenosine deaminase to inosine; inosine can be metabolized to hypoxanthine, then xanthine and finally to uric acid.

Half-life: <10 seconds

Dosing: Neonatal Paroxysmal supraventricular tachycardia: Rapid I.V.: Initial dose: 0.05-0.1 mg/kg; if not effective within 1-2 minutes, increase dose by 0.05-0.1 mg/kg increments every 1-2 minutes to a maximum single dose of 0.3 mg/kg or until termination of PSVT

Dosing: Usual Paroxysmal supraventricular tachycardia:
PALS Guidelines, 2010: Infants and Children: Rapid I.V.; I.O.: Initial: 0.1 mg/kg (maximum: 6 mg); if not effective, give 0.2 mg/kg (maximum: 12 mg) (PALS, 2010)

Manufacturer's recommendations: Rapid I.V.:
Infants, Children, and Adolescents <50 kg: Initial dose: 0.05-0.1 mg/kg; if not effective within 1-2 minutes, increase dose by 0.05-0.1 mg/kg increments every 1-2 minutes to a maximum single dose of 0.3 mg/kg or until termination of PSVT

Children and Adolescents ≥50 kg and Adults: 6 mg, if not effective within 1-2 minutes, 12 mg may be given; may repeat 12 mg bolus if needed. **Note:** Initial dose of adenosine should be reduced to 3 mg if patient is currently receiving carbamazepine or dipyridamole, has a transplanted heart, or if adenosine is administered via central line (ACLS, 2010).

Administration Parenteral: For rapid bolus I.V. use, administer over 1-2 seconds at peripheral I.V. site closest to patient's heart (I.V. administration into lower extremities may result in therapeutic failure or requirement of higher doses); follow each bolus with NS flush (infants and children: 5-10 mL; adults: 20 mL); **Note:** The use of two syringes (one with adenosine dose and the other with NS flush) connected to a T-connector or stopcock is recommended for I.V. and I.O. administration (PALS, 2010). If given I.V. peripherally in adults, elevate the extremity for 10-20 seconds after the NS flush. To administer doses <600 mcg (0.2 mL of commercial product), a dilution with NS (final concentration: 300 mcg/mL) may be made. **Note:** Preliminary results in adults suggest adenosine may be administered via a **central line** at lower doses (eg, Adults: Initial dose: 3 mg); FDA approved labeling for pediatric patients weighing <50 kg states that doses listed may be administered either peripherally or centrally (further studies are needed)

Monitoring Parameters Continuous ECG, heart rate, blood pressure, respirations

Additional Information Not effective in atrial flutter, atrial fibrillation, or ventricular tachycardia; short duration of action is an advantage as adverse effects are usually rapidly self-limiting; effects may be prolonged in patients with denervated transplanted hearts. Individualize treatment of prolonged adverse effects: Give I.V. fluids for hypotension, aminophylline/theophylline may antagonize effects.

Limited information is available regarding the use of adenosine for the treatment of persistent pulmonary hypertension of the newborn (PPHN); efficacy, optimal dose, and duration of therapy is not established; a randomized, masked, placebo-controlled pilot study of 18 term infants with PPHN used initial doses of 25 mcg/kg/minute (n=9);

after 30 minutes, doses were increased to 50 mcg/kg/minute if no improvement in PaO$_2$ was observed; all patients received study drug via central line into the right atrium (inserted via the umbilical vein); significant improvement in oxygenation was observed in 4 of 9 newborns receiving 50 mcg/kg/minute; hypotension or tachycardia were not observed; further studies are needed (Kondur, 1996).

Adenosine is also available as Adenoscan®, which is used in adults as an adjunct to thallium-201 myocardial perfusion scintigraphy; see package insert for further information on this use.

Dosage Forms Excipient information presented when available (limited, particularly for generics); consult specific product labeling.

Solution, Intravenous:
Adenocard: 6 mg/2 mL (2 mL); 12 mg/4 mL (4 mL)
Adenoscan: 3 mg/mL (20 mL, 30 mL)
Generic: 3 mg/mL (20 mL, 30 mL); 6 mg/2 mL (2 mL)
Solution, Intravenous [preservative free]:
Generic: 3 mg/mL (20 mL, 30 mL); 6 mg/2 mL (2 mL); 12 mg/4 mL (4 mL)

References

Blomström-Lundqvist C, Scheinman MM, Aliot EM, et al, "ACC/AHA/ESC Guidelines for the Management of Patients With Supraventricular Arrhythmias–Executive Summary. A Report of the American College of Cardiology/American Heart Association Task Force on Practice Guidelines and the European Society of Cardiology Committee for Practice Guidelines (Writing Committee to Develop Guidelines for the Management of Patients With Supraventricular Arrhythmias)," Circulation, 2003, 108(15):1871-909.

Eubanks AP and Artman M, "Administration of Adenosine to a Newborn of 26 Weeks' Gestation," Pediatr Cardiol, 1994, 15(3):157-8.

Field JM, Hazinski MF, Sayre MR, et al, "Part 1: Executive Summary: 2010 American Heart Association Guidelines for Cardiopulmonary Resuscitation and Emergency Cardiovascular Care," Circulation, 2010, 122(18 Suppl 3):640-56.

Kleinman ME, Chameides L, Schexnayder SM, et al, "Part 14: Pediatric Advanced Life Support: 2010 American Heart Association Guidelines for Cardiopulmonary Resuscitation and Emergency Cardiovascular Care," Circulation, 2010, 122(18 Suppl 3):876-908.

Konduri GG, Garcia DC, Kazzi NJ, et al, "Adenosine Infusion Improves Oxygenation in Term Infants With Respiratory Failure," Pediatrics, 1996, 97(3):295-300.

McIntosh-Yellin NL, Drew BJ, and Scheinman MM, "Safety and Efficacy of Central Intravenous Bolus Administration of Adenosine for Termination of Supraventricular Tachycardia," J Am Coll Cardiol, 1993, 22 (3):741-5.

Neumar RW, Otto CW, Link MS, et al, "Part 8: Adult Advanced Cardiovascular Life Support: 2010 American Heart Association Guidelines for Cardiopulmonary Resuscitation and Emergency Cardiovascular Care," Circulation, 2010, 122(18 Suppl 3):729-67.

Paul T and Pfammatter JP, "Adenosine: An Effective and Safe Antiarrhythmic Drug in Pediatrics," Pediatr Cardiol, 1997, 18(2):118-26.

Sherwood MC, Lau KC, and Sholler GF, "Adenosine in the Management of Supraventricular Tachycardia in Children," J Paediatr Child Health, 1998, 34(1):53-6.

Sugawara M, Sato N, Nakano T, et al, "Profile of Nucleotides and Nucleosides of Human Milk," J Nutr Sci Vitaminol (Tokyo), 1995, 41 (4):409-18.

Till J, Shinebourne EA, Rigby ML, et al, "Efficacy and Safety in the Treatment of Supraventricular Tachycardia in Infants and Children," Br Heart J, 1989, 62(3):204-11.

Zeigler V, "Adenosine in the Pediatric Population: Nursing Implications," Pediatr Nurs, 1991, 17(6):600-2.

◆ **Adenosine Injection, USP (Can)** see Adenosine on page 76

◆ **ADH** see Vasopressin on page 2121

◆ **Adoxa** see Doxycycline on page 721

◆ **Adoxa Pak 1/100** see Doxycycline on page 721

◆ **Adoxa Pak 1/150** see Doxycycline on page 721

◆ **Adoxa Pak 2/100** see Doxycycline on page 721

◆ **Adrenaclick** see EPINEPHrine (Systemic, Oral Inhalation) on page 761

◆ **Adrenalin** see EPINEPHrine (Nasal) on page 765

◆ **Adrenalin** see EPINEPHrine (Systemic, Oral Inhalation) on page 761

◆ **Adrenalin® (Can)** see EPINEPHrine (Nasal) on page 765

◆ **Adrenaline** see EPINEPHrine (Nasal) on page 765

◆ **Adrenaline** see EPINEPHrine (Systemic, Oral Inhalation) on page 761

◆ **Adrenocorticotropic Hormone** see Corticotropin on page 545

◆ **ADR (error-prone abbreviation)** see DOXOrubicin (Conventional) on page 718

◆ **Adria** see DOXOrubicin (Conventional) on page 718

◆ **Adriamycin** see DOXOrubicin (Conventional) on page 718

◆ **Adriamycin PFS (Can)** see DOXOrubicin (Conventional) on page 718

◆ **Adrucil** see Fluorouracil (Systemic) on page 897

◆ **Adsorbent Charcoal** see Charcoal, Activated on page 432

◆ **Advagraf (Can)** see Tacrolimus (Systemic) on page 1963

◆ **Advair (Can)** see Fluticasone and Salmeterol on page 916

◆ **Advair Diskus** see Fluticasone and Salmeterol on page 916

◆ **Advair HFA** see Fluticasone and Salmeterol on page 916

◆ **Advanced Eye Relief™ Dry Eye Environmental [OTC]** see Artificial Tears on page 205

◆ **Advanced Eye Relief™ Dry Eye Rejuvenation [OTC]** see Artificial Tears on page 205

◆ **Advate** see Antihemophilic Factor (Recombinant) on page 172

◆ **Advil [OTC]** see Ibuprofen on page 1059

◆ **Advil (Can)** see Ibuprofen on page 1059

◆ **Advil® Cold & Sinus [OTC]** see Pseudoephedrine and Ibuprofen on page 1772

◆ **Advil® Cold & Sinus (Can)** see Pseudoephedrine and Ibuprofen on page 1772

◆ **Advil® Cold & Sinus Daytime (Can)** see Pseudoephedrine and Ibuprofen on page 1772

◆ **Advil Junior Strength [OTC]** see Ibuprofen on page 1059

◆ **Advil Migraine [OTC]** see Ibuprofen on page 1059

◆ **Advil Pediatric Drops (Can)** see Ibuprofen on page 1059

◆ **Aerius® (Can)** see Desloratadine on page 611

◆ **Aerius® Kids (Can)** see Desloratadine on page 611

◆ **Afeditab CR** see NIFEdipine on page 1497

◆ **Afinitor** see Everolimus on page 821

◆ **Afinitor Disperz** see Everolimus on page 821

◆ **AFirm 1X [OTC]** see Vitamin A on page 2146

◆ **AFirm 2X [OTC]** see Vitamin A on page 2146

◆ **AFirm 3X [OTC]** see Vitamin A on page 2146

◆ **Afluria** see Influenza Virus Vaccine (Inactivated) on page 1103

◆ **Afluria Preservative Free** see Influenza Virus Vaccine (Inactivated) on page 1103

◆ **Afrezza** see Insulin Regular on page 1134

◆ **Afrin 12 Hour [OTC]** see Oxymetazoline (Nasal) on page 1577

◆ **Afrin Childrens [OTC]** see Phenylephrine (Nasal) on page 1660

- **Afrin Extra Moisturizing [OTC]** *see* Oxymetazoline (Nasal) *on page 1577*
- **Afrin Menthol Spray [OTC]** *see* Oxymetazoline (Nasal) *on page 1577*
- **Afrin Nasal Spray [OTC]** *see* Oxymetazoline (Nasal) *on page 1577*
- **Afrin NoDrip Original [OTC]** *see* Oxymetazoline (Nasal) *on page 1577*
- **Afrin NoDrip Sinus [OTC]** *see* Oxymetazoline (Nasal) *on page 1577*
- **Afrin Saline Nasal Mist [OTC]** *see* Sodium Chloride *on page 1902*
- **Afrin Sinus [OTC]** *see* Oxymetazoline (Nasal) *on page 1577*

Agalsidase Beta (aye GAL si days BAY ta)

Medication Safety Issues
Sound-alike/look-alike issues:
Agalsidase beta may be confused with agalsidase alfa, alglucerase, alglucosidase alfa

Brand Names: U.S. Fabrazyme

Brand Names: Canada Fabrazyme®

Therapeutic Category Enzyme, α-galactosidase A; Fabry's Disease, Treatment Agent

Generic Availability (U.S.) No

Use Treatment of Fabry's disease

Pregnancy Risk Factor B

Pregnancy Considerations Animal reproduction studies have not demonstrated adverse effects. There are no adequate and well-controlled studies in pregnant women. Women of childbearing potential are encouraged to enroll in Fabry registry (www.fabryregistry.com or 1-800-745-4447).

Breast-Feeding Considerations Nursing mothers are encouraged to enroll in Fabry registry.

Contraindications Hypersensitivity to agalsidase beta or any component

Warnings Infusion-related reactions (ranging from mild to severe) including fever, rigors, chest tightness, hypertension, hypotension, pruritus, myalgia, dyspnea, urticaria, abdominal pain, and headache have been reported; these reactions may be minimized by pretreatment with acetaminophen and an antihistamine; if an infusion related reaction occurs, regardless of pretreatment, decreasing the infusion rate, temporarily stopping the infusion, and/or additional administration of analgesics, antihistamines, or corticosteroids may ameliorate the reaction.

Precautions Use with caution in patients with compromised cardiac function (seen in advanced Fabry's disease) due to an increased potential for severe infusion related reactions; monitor these patients closely; patients may develop IgG antibodies to agalsidase beta

Adverse Reactions Note: The most common and serious adverse reactions are infusion reactions (symptoms may include fever, tachycardia, hyper-/hypotension, throat tightness, dyspnea, chills, abdominal pain, paresthesia, pruritus, urticaria, vomiting).

Cardiovascular: Bradycardia, chest pain/discomfort, facial edema, flushing, hyper-/hypotension, pallor, peripheral edema, tachycardia, ventricular wall thickening

Central nervous system: Anxiety, chills, depression, dizziness, fatigue, fever, headache, hypoesthesia, pain

Dermatologic: Bruising, excoriation, pruritus, rash, urticaria

Gastrointestinal: Abdominal pain, diarrhea, nausea, toothache, vomiting, xerostomia

Local: Infusion site reactions, postprocedural complication, procedural pain, thermal burn

Neuromuscular & skeletal: Back pain, burning sensation, fall, muscle spasms, myalgia, pain in extremity, paresthesia

Otic: Hearing impairment, tinnitus

Renal: Creatinine increased

Respiratory: Congestion, cough, dyspnea, lower respiratory infection, nasal congestion, pharyngitis, sinusitis, throat tightness, upper respiratory tract infection, wheezing,

Miscellaneous: Feeling cold, fungal infection, IgG antibody formation, viral infection

Other reported severe reactions: Anaphylaxis, allergic reactions, arrhythmia, ataxia, cardiac arrest, cardiac output decreased, nephrotic syndrome, stroke, vertigo

Rare but important or life-threatening: Anaphylactic shock, angioedema (including dysphagia, edema of ears, edema of eye, edema of lips, edema of tongue, pharyngeal edema), arthralgia, bronchospasm, cerebrovascular accident, erythema, heart failure, hypoxia, hyperhidrosis, lacrimation increased, leukocytoclastic vasculitis, lymphadenopathy, MI, oxygen saturation decreased, palpitation, pneumonia, renal failure, respiratory failure, rhinorrhea, sepsis, weakness

Drug Interactions

Metabolism/Transport Effects None known.

Avoid Concomitant Use
Avoid concomitant use of Agalsidase Beta with any of the following: Amiodarone; Chloroquine; Gentamicin (Systemic)

Increased Effect/Toxicity There are no known significant interactions involving an increase in effect.

Decreased Effect
The levels/effects of Agalsidase Beta may be decreased by: Amiodarone; Chloroquine; Gentamicin (Systemic)

Stability Store in refrigerator 2°C to 8°C (36°F to 46°F); reconstituted solution is stable for 24 hours refrigerated

Mechanism of Action Agalsidase beta is a recombinant form of the enzyme alpha-galactosidase-A, which is required for the hydrolysis of GL-3 and other glycosphingolipids. The compounds may accumulate (over many years) within the tissues of patients with Fabry disease, leading to renal and cardiovascular complications. In clinical trials of limited duration, agalsidase been noted to reduce tissue inclusions of a key sphingolipid (GL-3). It is believed that long-term enzyme replacement may reduce clinical manifestations of renal failure, cardiomyopathy, and stroke. However, the relationship to a reduction in clinical manifestations has not been established.

Pharmacokinetics (Adult data unless noted)
Distribution: V_d:
Children: 247-1097 mL/kg
Adults: 80-570 mL/kg
Half-life (dose dependent):
Children: 86-151 minutes
Adults: 45-102 minutes
Clearance:
Children: 1.1-5.8 mL/minute/kg
Adults: 0.8-4.9 mL/minute/kg

Dosing: Usual I.V.: Children and Adults: 1 mg/kg/dose every two weeks

Administration I.V.: Reconstitute each 35 mg vial with 7.2 mL SWI and each 5 mg vial with 1.1 mL SWI to result in 5 mg/mL concentrations; swirl to dissolve; do not shake; further dilute dosage in NS (see chart below for dilution volumes). Initial infusion not to exceed 15 mg/hour (0.25 mg/minute); after patient tolerance to initial infusion rate is established, the infusion rate may be increased in increments of 3-5 mg/hour (0.05-0.08 mg/minute) with subsequent infusions. Per the manufacturer's recommendation: For patients weighing <30 kg, the maximum infusion rate should remain at 0.25 mg/minute; for patients weighing >30 kg, the administration duration should not be less than 1.5 hours (based upon individual tolerability). An initial maximum infusion rate of 0.01 mg/minute should be used for rechallenge in patients with IgE antibodies; may increase infusion rate (doubling the infusion rate every 30 minutes) to a maximum rate of 0.25 mg/minute as tolerated. A 0.2 micron low protein-binding filter may be used during administration. Pretreatment with acetaminophen and an antihistamine is recommended to reduce infusion related side effects

Recommended Minimum Volumes for Dilution

Patient Weight (kg)	Minimum Total Volume (mL)
<35	50
35.1-70	100
70.1-100	250
>100	500

Monitoring Parameters Vital signs during infusion; infusion-related reactions; globotriasylceramide (GL3) plasma levels; improvement in disease symptomatology

Reference Range Normal endogenous activity of alpha-galactosidase A in plasma is approximately 170 nmol/hour/mL; in patients with Fabry's disease this activity is <1.5 nmol/hour/mL

Normal (goal) globotriasylceramide (GL3) <1.2 ng/micro-liter

Additional Information Agalsidase beta is an orphan drug; a Fabry Patient Support Group (800-745-4447) is available to assist patients in obtaining reimbursement from private insurers, Medicare, and Medicaid, and a Charitable Access Program sponsored by Genzyme provides the drug gratis to those patients in need. Detailed information regarding organizations and websites is also available in the Expert Panel Recommendations (Desnick, 2003)

Dosage Forms Excipient information presented when available (limited, particularly for generics); consult specific product labeling.

Solution Reconstituted, Intravenous:
  Fabrazyme: 5 mg (1 ea); 35 mg (1 ea) [contains mouse protein (murine) (hamster)]

References
Desnick RJ, Brady R, Barranger J, et al, "Fabry Disease, an Under-Recognized Multisystemic Disorder: Expert Recommendations for Diagnosis, Management, and Enzyme Replacement Therapy," *Ann Intern Med,* 2003, 138(4):338-46.

◆ **AgNO₃** *see* Silver Nitrate *on page 1889*

◆ **Agriflu (Can)** *see* Influenza Virus Vaccine (Inactivated) *on page 1103*

◆ **Agrylin** *see* Anagrelide *on page 166*

◆ **AHF (Human)** *see* Antihemophilic Factor (Human) *on page 170*

◆ **AHF (Human)** *see* Antihemophilic Factor/von Willebrand Factor Complex (Human) *on page 177*

◆ **AHF (Recombinant)** *see* Antihemophilic Factor (Recombinant) *on page 172*

◆ **Ahi-Temozolomide Capsules (Can)** *see* Temozolomide *on page 1972*

◆ **A-hydroCort** *see* Hydrocortisone (Systemic) *on page 1034*

◆ **A-Hydrocort** *see* Hydrocortisone (Systemic) *on page 1034*

◆ **A-hydroCort** *see* Hydrocortisone (Topical) *on page 1038*

◆ **AICC** *see* Anti-inhibitor Coagulant Complex (Human) *on page 180*

◆ **Airomir (Can)** *see* Albuterol *on page 84*

◆ **AJ-Cisplatin (Can)** *see* CISplatin *on page 481*

◆ **AJ-PIP/TAZ (Can)** *see* Piperacillin and Tazobactam *on page 1679*

◆ **Akne-Mycin** *see* Erythromycin (Topical) *on page 785*

◆ **AK Pentolate Oph Soln (Can)** *see* Cyclopentolate *on page 560*

◆ **AK-Poly-Bac™** *see* Bacitracin and Polymyxin B *on page 257*

◆ **AK Sulf Liq (Can)** *see* Sulfacetamide (Ophthalmic) *on page 1943*

◆ **Akten** *see* Lidocaine (Ophthalmic) *on page 1241*

◆ **Akwa Tears® [OTC]** *see* Ocular Lubricant *on page 1521*

◆ **Ala Cort** *see* Hydrocortisone (Topical) *on page 1038*

◆ **Alamag [OTC]** *see* Aluminum Hydroxide and Magnesium Hydroxide *on page 111*

◆ **Ala Scalp** *see* Hydrocortisone (Topical) *on page 1038*

◆ **ala seb [OTC]** *see* Sulfur and Salicylic Acid *on page 1956*

◆ **Alavert [OTC]** *see* Loratadine *on page 1278*

◆ **Alavert™ Allergy and Sinus [OTC]** *see* Loratadine and Pseudoephedrine *on page 1279*

◆ **Alaway [OTC]** *see* Ketotifen (Ophthalmic) *on page 1185*

◆ **Alaway Childrens Allergy [OTC]** *see* Ketotifen (Ophthalmic) *on page 1185*

Albendazole (al BEN da zole)

Medication Safety Issues
  Sound-alike/look-alike issues:
    Albenza® may be confused with Aplenzin™, Relenza®
  International issues:
    Albenza [U.S.] may be confused with Avanza brand name for mirtazapine [Australia]

Brand Names: U.S. Albenza

Therapeutic Category Anthelmintic

Generic Availability (U.S.) No

Use Treatment of parenchymal neurocysticercosis due to active lesions caused by larval forms of *Taenia solium* (pork tapeworm) and treatment of cystic hydatid disease of the liver, lung, and peritoneum caused by the larval form of *Echinococcus granulosus* (dog tapeworm) [FDA approved in pediatric patients (age not specified) and adults]. Is also active against and has been used in the treatment of *Ascaris lumbricoides* (roundworm), *Ancylostoma caninum, Ancylostoma duodenale, Necator americanus* (hookworm), *Enterobius vermicularis* (pinworm), cutaneous larva migrans, *Gnathostoma spinigerum, Gongylonema* sp; *Mansonella perstans* (filariasis), *Opisthorchis sinensis* (liver fluke), visceral larva migrans (toxocariasis), *Echinococcus multilocularis, Clonorchis sinensis* (Chinese liver fluke), *Giardia lamblia, Cysticecus cellulosae, Trichuris trichiura* (whipworm), microsporidiosis, *Capillaria philippinensis, Baylisascaris procyonis,* and *Strongyloides stercoralis.*

Pregnancy Risk Factor C

Pregnancy Considerations Adverse events were observed in animal reproduction studies. Albendazole should not be used during pregnancy, if at all possible. The manufacturer recommends a pregnancy test prior to therapy in women of reproductive potential. Women should be advised to avoid pregnancy for at least 1 month following therapy. Discontinue if pregnancy occurs during treatment.

Breast-Feeding Considerations Albendazole excretion into breast milk was studied following a single oral 400 mg dose in breast-feeding women 2 weeks to 6 months postpartum (n=33). Mean albendazole concentrations 6 hours after the dose were 63.7 ± 11.9 ng/mL (maternal serum) and 31.9 ± 9.2 ng/mL (milk). An active and inactive metabolite was also detected in breast milk (Abdel-tawab, 2009). The manufacturer recommends that caution be exercised when administering albendazole to nursing women.

Contraindications Hypersensitivity to albendazole, any component, or the benzimidazole class of compounds

Warnings Agranulocytosis, aplastic anemia, granulocytopenia, leukopenia, and pancytopenia have occurred leading to fatalities (rare). Patients with liver disease, including hepatic echinococcosis, appear to be at greater risk for bone marrow suppression. Monitor blood counts at the beginning of each 28-day cycle and every 2 weeks while on therapy. Discontinue therapy in all patients who develop clinically significant decreases in blood cell counts. Women of childbearing age should only begin treatment after a negative pregnancy test and should be cautioned against becoming pregnant during and for at least 1 month after treatment cessation with albendazole since it may cause fetal harm.

Precautions Use with caution in patients with abnormal liver function tests or decreased total leukocyte count (increased risk for hepatotoxicity and bone marrow suppression); discontinue albendazole if significant elevation of liver enzymes occur; may restart therapy when liver enzymes decrease to pretreatment values. During treatment, death of parasites within the brain may produce neurological symptoms (eg, seizures, increased ICP, focal signs) and an inflammatory response; corticosteroids should be used during the first week of treatment to prevent cerebral hypertensive episodes. In patients treated with albendazole for other conditions, preexisting neurocysticercosis may be uncovered and neurological symptoms (eg, seizures, increased ICP, and focal signs) may occur soon after treatment; appropriate steroid and anticonvulsant therapy should be started immediately. Albendazole may induce further retinal damage in patients having retinal lesions with neurocysticercosis.

Adverse Reactions

Central nervous system: Dizziness, fever, headache, intracranial pressure increased, meningeal signs, vertigo

Dermatologic: Alopecia

Gastrointestinal: Abdominal pain, nausea, vomiting

Hepatic: LFTs increased

Rare but important or life-threatening: Acute liver failure, acute renal failure, aplastic anemia, agranulocytosis, erythema multiforme, granulocytopenia, hepatitis, hypersensitivity reaction, leukopenia, neutropenia, pancytopenia, rash, Stevens-Johnson syndrome, thrombocytopenia, urticaria

Drug Interactions

Metabolism/Transport Effects Substrate of CYP1A2 (minor), CYP3A4 (minor); **Note:** Assignment of Major/Minor substrate status based on clinically relevant drug interaction potential

Avoid Concomitant Use There are no known interactions where it is recommended to avoid concomitant use.

Increased Effect/Toxicity

The levels/effects of Albendazole may be increased by: Grapefruit Juice

Decreased Effect

The levels/effects of Albendazole may be decreased by: Aminoquinolines (Antimalarial); CarBAMazepine; PHENobarbital; Phenytoin

Food Interactions Albendazole serum levels may be increased if taken with a fatty meal (increases the oral bioavailability by up to 5 times). Management: Should be administered with a high-fat meal (peanuts or ice cream).

Stability Store between 20°C and 25°C (68°F to 77°F)

Mechanism of Action Active metabolite, albendazole sulfoxide, causes selective degeneration of cytoplasmic microtubules in intestinal and tegmental cells of intestinal helminths and larvae; glycogen is depleted, glucose uptake and cholinesterase secretion are impaired, and desecratory substances accumulate intracellulary. ATP production decreases causing energy depletion, immobilization, and worm death.

Pharmacokinetics (Adult data unless noted) Note: In pediatric patients (6-13 years), pharmacokinetic values were reported to be similar to adult data.

Absorption: Poorly absorbed from the GI tract

Distribution: Widely distributed throughout the body including urine, bile, liver, cyst wall, cyst fluid, and CSF

Protein binding: 70%

Metabolism: Extensive first-pass metabolism; hepatic metabolism to albendazole sulfoxide, an active metabolite

Half-life: Albendazole sulfoxide: 8-12 hours

Time to peak serum concentration: 2-5 hours for the metabolite

Elimination: Biliary

Dosing: Usual Children and Adults: Oral:

Neurocysticercosis *(Taenia solium):* **Note:** Patients should receive concurrent corticosteroid for the first week of albendazole therapy and anticonvulsant therapy as required.

<60 kg: 15 mg/kg/day in 2 divided doses (maximum: 800 mg/day) for 8-30 days

≥60 kg: 400 mg twice daily for 8-30 days

Hydatid disease *(Echinococcus granulosus):*

<60 kg: 15 mg/kg/day in 2 divided doses (maximum: 800 mg/day); 28-day cycle followed by a 14-day albendazole-free interval, for a total of 3 cycles

≥60 kg: 400 mg twice daily; 28-day cycle followed by a 14-day albendazole-free interval, for a total of 3 cycles

Ancylostoma caninum, ascariasis (roundworm), hookworm, trichuriasis (whipworm): 400 mg as a single dose *(Red Book,* 2009)

Ascariasis: Children 12 months to 2 years: 200 mg as a single dose (World Health Organization Model Formulary for Children, 2010)

Baylisascaris procyonis: Children: 25 mg/kg/day for 20 days started as soon as possible (up to 3 days after possible infection) may prevent clinical disease and is recommended for children with known exposure (eg, ingestion of raccoon stool or contaminated soil). No drug has been demonstrated to be effective *(Red Book,* 2009).

Capillariasis: 400 mg once daily for 10 days *(Red Book,* 2009)

Clonorchis sinensis (Chinese liver fluke): 10 mg/kg/day once daily for 7 days *(Red Book,* 2009)

Cutaneous larva migrans: 400 mg once daily for 3 days *(Red Book,* 2009)

Enterobius vermicularis (pinworm): 400 mg as a single dose; repeat in 2 weeks *(Red Book,* 2009)

Filariasis *(Mansonella perstans):* 400 mg twice daily for 10 days *(Red Book,* 2009)

Filariasis *(Wuchereria Bancroft,* microfilaria reduction or suppression): 400 mg as a single dose (in combination with either ivermectin or diethylcarbamazine). **Note:** Albendazole/ivermectin combination does not kill all the adult worms *(Red Book,* 2009).

Giardiasis *(Giardia duodenalis) (Red Book,* 2009):

Children: 10 mg/kg/day once daily for 5 days

Adults: 400 mg once daily for 5 days

Gnathostoma spinigerum (Gnathostomiasis): 400 mg twice daily for 21 days *(Red Book,* 2009)

Gongylonema sp (Gongylonemiasis): 400 mg once daily for 3 days *(Red Book,* 2009)

Microsporidia infection (except *Enterocytozoon sp.* and *V. corneae*) in HIV-exposed/positive infants and children: 15 mg/kg/day in 2 divided doses (maximum: 800 mg/day) continued until immune reconstitution after HAART initiation

Microsporidiosis in non-HIV patients (*Red Book*, 2009):
Disseminated: 400 mg twice daily
Intestinal: 400 mg twice daily for 21 days
Ocular: 400 mg twice daily in combination with fumagillin
Strongyloidiasis (*Strongyloides stercoralis*): 400 mg twice daily for 7 days (*Red Book*, 2009)
Trichinellosis (*Trichinella spiralis*): 400 mg twice daily for 8-14 days (*Red Book*, 2009)
Visceral larva migrans (*Toxocariasis*): 400 mg twice daily for 5 days (*Red Book*, 2009)

Administration Oral: Administer with food. For children who have difficulty swallowing whole tablets, tablet may be crushed or chewed and swallowed with a drink of water.

Monitoring Parameters Monitor liver function tests, CBC at start of each cycle and every 2 weeks during therapy, fecal specimens for ova and parasites; pregnancy test

Dosage Forms Excipient information presented when available (limited, particularly for generics); consult specific product labeling.

Tablet, Oral:
Albenza: 200 mg [contains saccharin sodium]

References

Abdel-tawab AM, Bradley M, Ghazaly EA, et al, "Albendazole and its Metabolites in the Breast Milk of Lactating Women Following a Single Oral Dose of Albendazole," *Br J Clin Pharmacol*, 2009, 68(5):737-42.

Baranwal AK, Singhi PD, Khandelwal N, et al, "Albendazole Therapy in Children With Focal Seizures and Single Small Enhancing Computerized Tomographic Lesions: A Randomized, Placebo-Controlled, Double Blind Trial," *Pediatr Infect Dis J*, 1998, 17(8):696-700.

Centers for Disease Control and Prevention (CDC), "Guidelines for the Prevention and Treatment of Opportunistic Infections Among HIV-Exposed and HIV-Infected Children," *MMWR Recomm Rep*, 2009, 58(RR-11):1-166. Available at http://aidsinfo.nih.gov/contentfiles/Pediatric_OI.pdf

Jung H, Sanchez M, Gonzalez-Astiazaran A, et al, "Clinical Pharmacokinetics of Albendazole in Children With Neurocysticercosis," *Am J Ther*, 1997, 4(1):23-6.

Paul I, Gnanamani G, and Nallam NR, "Intestinal Helminth Infections Among School Children in Visakhapatnam," *Indian J Pediatr*, 1999, 66(5):669-73.

Pengsaa K, Sirivichayakul C, Pojjaroen-anant C, et al, "Albendazole Treatment for *Giardia intestinalis* Infections in School Children," *Southeast Asian J Trop Med Public Health*, 1999, 30(1):78-83.

Red Book: 2009 Report of the Committee on Infectious Diseases, 28th ed, Pickering LK, ed, Elk Grove Village, IL: American Academy of Pediatrics, 2009.

World Health Organization, "WHO Model Formulary for Children," 2010.

◆ **Albenza** *see* Albendazole *on page 80*

◆ **Albuked 5** *see* Albumin *on page 82*

◆ **Albuked 25** *see* Albumin *on page 82*

Albumin (al BYOO min)

Medication Safety Issues
Sound-alike/look-alike issues:
Albutein® may be confused with albuterol
Buminate® may be confused with bumetanide

Brand Names: U.S. Albuked 25; Albuked 5; Albumin-ZLB; Albuminar-25; Albuminar-5; AlbuRx; Albutein; Buminate; Flexbumin; Human Albumin Grifols; Kedbumin; Plasbumin-25; Plasbumin-5

Brand Names: Canada Alburex® 25; Alburex® 5; Albutein 25%; Albutein 5%; Buminate-25%; Buminate-5%; Plasbumin®-25; Plasbumin®-5

Therapeutic Category Blood Product Derivative; Plasma Volume Expander

Generic Availability (U.S.) Yes

Use Treatment of hypovolemia; plasma volume expansion and maintenance of cardiac output in the treatment of certain types of shock or impending shock;

hypoproteinemia resulting in generalized edema or decreased intravascular volume (eg, hypoproteinemia associated with acute nephrotic syndrome, premature neonates)

Note: PALS and Neonatal Resuscitation 2000 Guidelines recommend isotonic crystalloid solutions (eg, NS or LR) as initial volume expansion; albumin is used less frequently due to limited supply, potential risk of infections, and an association with an increase in mortality (identified by meta-analyses); few studies in these analyses included children, so no firm conclusions in pediatric patients can be made

Pregnancy Risk Factor C

Pregnancy Considerations Animal reproduction studies have not been conducted. Albumin is used for the treatment of ovarian hyperstimulation syndrome (ASRM, 2008). Use for other indications may be considered in pregnant women when contraindications to nonprotein colloids exist (Liumbruno, 2009).

Breast-Feeding Considerations Endogenous albumin is found in breast milk.

Contraindications Hypersensitivity to albumin or any component; patients with severe anemia or cardiac failure

Warnings Use 25% concentration with extreme caution and infuse slowly in preterm neonates, due to increased risk of IVH (from rapid expansion of intravascular volume). Some products (eg, Albuminar®, Buminate®) contain natural rubber latex (in certain components of the product packaging) which may cause allergic reactions in susceptible individuals; avoid use in patients with allergy to latex

Precautions Rapid infusion of albumin solutions may cause vascular overload. Do not administer albumin to burn patients for the first 24 hours after the burn (capillary exudation of albumin will occur); use with caution in patients with hepatic or renal failure (added protein load) and in patients who require sodium restriction; monitor for signs of hypervolemia

Due to the occasional shortage of 5% human albumin, 5% solutions may at times be prepared by diluting 25% human albumin with NS or with D₅W (if sodium load is a concern); however, **do not use sterile water** to dilute albumin solutions, as this may result in hypotonic-associated hemolysis which can be fatal

May contain aluminum; toxic aluminum concentrations may be seen with high doses, prolonged use, or renal dysfunction. Premature neonates are at higher risk due to immature renal function and aluminum intake from other parenteral sources. Parenteral aluminum exposure of >4-5 mcg/kg/day is associated with CNS and bone toxicity and tissue loading may occur at lower doses.

Adverse Reactions
Cardiovascular: Congestive heart failure (precipitation), edema, hypertension, hypotension, tachycardia
Central nervous system: Chills, headache
Dermatologic: Pruritus, skin rash, urticaria
Endocrine & metabolic: Hypervolemia
Gastrointestinal: Nausea, vomiting
Hypersensitivity: Anaphylaxis
Respiratory: Bronchospasm, pulmonary edema
Miscellaneous: Fever

Drug Interactions
Metabolism/Transport Effects None known.
Avoid Concomitant Use There are no known interactions where it is recommended to avoid concomitant use.
Increased Effect/Toxicity There are no known significant interactions involving an increase in effect.
Decreased Effect There are no known significant interactions involving a decrease in effect.

Stability Use within 4 hours after opening vial, do not use if turbid or contains a deposit; do not use SWI to dilute albumin

Mechanism of Action Provides increase in intravascular oncotic pressure and causes mobilization of fluids from interstitial into intravascular space

Pharmacodynamics Duration of volume expansion: ~24 hours

Pharmacokinetics (Adult data unless noted) Half-life: 21 days

Dosing: Neonatal I.V.: **Note:** Albumin **5%** should be used in hypovolemic or intravascularly depleted patients; albumin **25%** should be used in patients with fluid or sodium restrictions (eg, patients with hypoproteinemia and generalized edema, or nephrotic syndrome). Dose depends on condition of patient:

Hypoproteinemia: 0.5-1 g/kg/dose of 25% albumin; may repeat every 1-2 days

Hypovolemia, hypotension: Usual dose: 0.5 g/kg/dose of 5% albumin (10 mL/kg/dose); range: 0.25-0.5 g/kg/dose of 5% albumin (5-10 mL/kg/dose)

Dosing: Usual I.V.: **Note:** Albumin **5%** should be used in hypovolemic or intravascularly depleted patients; albumin **25%** should be used in patients with fluid or sodium restrictions (eg, patients with hypoproteinemia and generalized edema, or nephrotic syndrome). Dose depends on condition of patient:

Infants and Children:

Hypoproteinemia: 0.5-1 g/kg/dose of 25% albumin; may repeat every 1-2 days

Hypovolemia: 0.5-1 g/kg/dose (10-20 mL/kg/dose of 5% albumin); may repeat as needed; maximum dose: 6 g/kg/day (120 mL/kg/day of 5% albumin)

Nephrotic syndrome: 0.25-1 g/kg/dose of 25% albumin

Adults: 25 g; no more than 250 g should be administered within 48 hours

Nephrotic syndrome: 12.5-50 g/day in 3-4 divided doses

Administration Parenteral: I.V.: Too rapid infusion may result in vascular overload

Albuminar®: May administer via the administration set provided (in-line 60 micron filter) or via any administration set; use of filter is optional; size of filter may vary according to institutional policy. Method of filter sterilization used by manufacturer includes 0.2 micron filter; however, aggregates may form under storage, shipping, and handling. Administration via very small filter will not damage product, but will slow flow rate.

Albutein®: May administer via the administration set provided (in-line 50 micron filter) or via any administration set; use of filter is optional; size of filter may vary according to institutional policy. Method of production includes passage through 0.22 micron filter. May administer via filter as small as 0.22 microns.

Buminate®: Administer via the administration set provided (in-line 15 micron filter) or via any filtered administration set; use ≥5 micron filter to ensure adequate flow rate

Plasbumin®: May administer with or without an I.V. filter; filter as small as 0.22 microns may be used

Hypoproteinemia: Infuse over 2-4 hours; for neonates, dose may be added to hyperalimentation fluid and infused over 24 hours; **Note:** Hyperalimentation fluid containing >25 g/L of albumin is more likely to occlude 0.22 micron in-line filters; but hyperalimentation solutions containing albumin in concentrations as low as 10.8 g/L have also occluded 0.22 micron filters; use ≥5 micron filter to ensure adequate flow rate; addition of albumin to hyperalimentation solutions may increase potential for growth of bacteria or fungi.

Hypovolemia: Rate of infusion depends on severity of hypovolemia and patient's symptoms; usually infuse dose over 30-60 minutes (faster infusion rates may be clinically necessary)

Maximum rates of I.V. infusion after initial volume replacement:

5%: 2-4 mL/minute

25%: 1 mL/minute

To prepare 5% albumin from 25%, see Precautions.

Monitoring Parameters Observe for signs of hypervolemia, pulmonary edema, cardiac failure, vital signs, I & O, Hgb, Hct, urine specific gravity

Additional Information In certain conditions (eg, hypoproteinemia with generalized edema, nephrotic syndrome), doses of albumin may be followed with I.V. furosemide: 0.5-1 mg/kg/dose.

Both albumin 5% and 25% contain 130-160 mEq/L of sodium; albumin 5% is osmotically equivalent to an equal volume of plasma; albumin 25% is osmotically equivalent to 5 times its volume of plasma.

Dosage Forms Excipient information presented when available (limited, particularly for generics); consult specific product labeling.

Solution, Intravenous:

Albumin-ZLB: 5% (250 mL, 500 mL); 25% (50 mL, 100 mL)

Albuminar-5: 5% (250 mL, 500 mL)

Albuminar-25: 25% (50 mL, 100 mL)

AlbuRx: 5% (250 mL, 500 mL)

Albutein: 25% (50 mL, 100 mL)

Buminate: 5% (250 mL, 500 mL); 25% (20 mL)

Human Albumin Grifols: 25% (50 mL, 100 mL)

Plasbumin-5: 5% (50 mL, 250 mL)

Plasbumin-25: 25% (20 mL, 50 mL, 100 mL)

Generic: 5% (50 mL); 25% (50 mL, 100 mL)

Solution, Intravenous [preservative free]:

Albuked 5: 5% (250 mL)

Albuked 25: 25% (50 mL, 100 mL)

Albutein: 5% (250 mL, 500 mL); 25% (50 mL, 100 mL)

Flexbumin: 25% (50 mL, 100 mL)

Kedbumin: 25% (50 mL, 100 mL)

Plasbumin-25: 5% (50 mL, 250 mL)

Plasbumin-25: 25% (20 mL, 50 mL, 100 mL)

Generic: 5% (100 mL, 250 mL, 500 mL); 25% (50 mL, 100 mL)

References

Department Health and Human Services, Food Drug Administration, "Aluminum in Large and Small Volume Parenterals Used in Total Parenteral Nutrition," *Federal Register*, 2000, 65(17):4103-11.

"Guidelines 2000 for Cardiopulmonary Resuscitation and Emergency Cardiovascular Care, Part 10: Pediatric Advanced Life Support, The American Heart Association in Collaboration With the International Liaison Committee on Resuscitation," *Circulation*, 2000, 102(8 Suppl): I306.

"Guidelines 2000 for Cardiopulmonary Resuscitation and Emergency Cardiovascular Care, Part 11: Neonatal Resuscitation, The American Heart Association in Collaboration With the International Liaison Committee on Resuscitation," *Circulation*, 2000, 102(8 Suppl):I352.

"Hemolysis Associated With 25% Human Albumin Diluted With Sterile Water - United States, 1994-1998," *MMWR Morb Mortal Wkly Rep*, 1999, 48(8):157-9.

Lynch SK, Mullett MD, Graeber JE, et al, "A Comparison of Albumin-Bolus Therapy Versus Normal Saline-Bolus Therapy for Hypotension in Neonates," *J Perinatol*, 2008, 28(1):29-33.

◆ **Albuminar-5** *see Albumin on page 82*

◆ **Albuminar-25** *see Albumin on page 82*

◆ **Albumin (Human)** *see Albumin on page 82*

◆ **Albumin-ZLB** *see Albumin on page 82*

◆ **Alburex® 5 (Can)** *see Albumin on page 82*

◆ **Alburex® 25 (Can)** *see Albumin on page 82*

◆ **AlbuRx** *see Albumin on page 82*

◆ **Albutein** *see Albumin on page 82*

◆ **Albutein 5% (Can)** *see Albumin on page 82*

◆ **Albutein 25% (Can)** *see Albumin on page 82*

Albuterol (al BYOO ter ole)

Medication Safety Issues

Sound-alike/look-alike issues:

Albuterol may be confused with Albutein, atenolol

Proventil may be confused with Bentyl, PriLOSEC, Prinivil

Salbutamol may be confused with salmeterol

Ventolin may be confused with phentolamine, Benylin, Vantin

Related Information

Oral Medications That Should Not Be Crushed or Altered on page 2438

Brand Names: U.S. AccuNeb [DSC]; ProAir HFA; Proventil HFA; Ventolin HFA; VoSpire ER

Brand Names: Canada Airomir; Apo-Salvent; Apo-Salvent AEM; Apo-Salvent CFC Free; Apo-Salvent Sterules; Dom-Salbutamol; Novo-Salbutamol; PHL-Salbutamol; PMS-Salbutamol; ratio-Ipra-Sal; ratio-Salbutamol; Salbutamol HFA; Sandoz-Salbutamol; Teva-Salbutamol; Teva-Salbutamol Sterinebs P.F.; Ventolin Diskus; Ventolin HFA; Ventolin I.V. Infusion; Ventolin Nebules P.F.

Therapeutic Category Adrenergic Agonist Agent; Antiasthmatic; Beta$_2$-Adrenergic Agonist; Bronchodilator; Sympathomimetic

Generic Availability (U.S.) May be product dependent

Use

Oral: Treatment of bronchospasm in patients with reversible obstructive airway disease (Syrup: FDA approved in ages ≥2 years and adults; Immediate release and extended release tablets: FDA approved in ages ≥6 years and adults). **Note:** Although an FDA approved indication, the use of oral albuterol for management of acute asthma or long-term daily maintenance treatment is not recommended due to long onset of action and risk of side effects (GINA, 2008; GINA, 2012; NAEPP, 2007)

Oral inhalation:

Inhalation aerosol (metered dose inhaler): Treatment or prevention of bronchospasm in patients with reversible obstructive airway disease; prevention of exercise-induced bronchospasm (All indications: FDA approved in ages ≥4 years and adults)

Nebulization solution: Treatment of bronchospasm in patients with reversible obstructive airway disease (AccuNeb: FDA approved in ages 2-12 years; Proventil: FDA approved in ages ≥12 years and adults; treatment of acute attacks of bronchospasm (FDA approved in ages 2 years and adults; Proventil: FDA approved in ages ≥12 years and adults). **Note:** Approval ages for generics may vary; consult prescribing information for specific information.

Pregnancy Risk Factor C

Pregnancy Considerations Adverse events were observed in some animal reproduction studies. Albuterol crosses the placenta (Boulton, 1997). Congenital anomalies (cleft palate, limb defects) have rarely been reported following maternal use during pregnancy. Multiple medications were used in most cases, no specific pattern of defects has been reported, and no relationship to albuterol has been established. The amount of albuterol available systemically following inhalation is significantly less in comparison to oral doses.

Uncontrolled asthma is associated with adverse events on pregnancy (increased risk of perinatal mortality, preeclampsia, preterm birth, low birth weight infants). Albuterol is the preferred short acting beta agonist when treatment for asthma is needed during pregnancy (NAEPP, 2005; NAEPP, 2007).

Albuterol may affect uterine contractility. Maternal pulmonary edema and other adverse events have been reported when albuterol was used for tocolysis. Albuterol is not approved for use as a tocolytic; use caution when needed to treat bronchospasm in pregnant women. Use of the injection (Canadian product; not available in the U.S.) is specifically contraindicated in women during the first or second trimester who may be at risk of threatened abortion.

Breast-Feeding Considerations It is not known if albuterol is excreted into breast milk. The amount of albuterol available systemically following inhalation is significantly less in comparison to oral doses. According to the manufacturer, the decision to continue or discontinue breast-feeding during therapy should take into account the risk of exposure to the infant and the benefits of treatment to the mother. The use of beta-2-receptor agonists are not considered a contraindication to breast feeding (NAEPP, 2005).

Contraindications Hypersensitivity to albuterol or any component

Documentation of allergenic cross-reactivity for drugs in this class is limited; however, because of similarities in chemical structure and/or pharmacologic actions, the possibility of cross-sensitivity cannot be ruled out with certainty.

Warnings Inhaled albuterol can produce paradoxical bronchospasm that may be life-threatening; typically occurs with initial use of a new canister; discontinue therapy immediately if this occurs and distinguish from inadequate response or a hypersensitivity reaction. Excessive or prolonged use can lead to tolerance; excessive use has also been associated with deaths, possibly due to cardiac arrest. Increasing use (>2 days/week) for symptom relief (not prevention of exercise-induced bronchospasm) generally indicates inadequate control of asthma and the need for initiating or intensifying anti-inflammatory treatment. Optimize anti-inflammatory treatment before initiating maintenance treatment with albuterol. Generally, do not use as a component of chronic therapy without an anti-inflammatory agent; only the mildest forms of asthma (Step 1 and/or exercise-induced) would not require concurrent use of an anti-inflammatory agent based upon asthma guidelines. Regularly scheduled, daily, chronic use of short-acting beta agonists (eg, albuterol) is not recommended (NAEPP, 2007).

Immediate hypersensitivity reactions (urticaria, angioedema, rash, bronchospasm, anaphylaxis, and oropharyngeal edema) have been reported. In children receiving oral albuterol therapy, erythema multiforme and Stevens-Johnson syndrome have been reported (rare). Outbreaks of lower respiratory tract colonization and infection have been attributed to contaminated multidose albuterol bottles.

Precautions Use with caution in patients with cardiovascular disease (arrhythmia or hypertension or HF); beta-agonists may cause elevation in blood pressure, heart rate; beta$_2$-agonists may also increase risk of arrhythmias. Use with caution in patients with hypokalemia; beta$_2$-agonists may decrease serum potassium. Use with caution in patients with seizure disorders; beta-agonists may result in CNS stimulation/excitation. CNS stimulation, hyperactivity, and insomnia occur more frequently in younger children than in adults. Use with caution in patients with diabetes mellitus; beta$_2$-agonists may increase serum glucose. Use with caution in patients with glaucoma; may elevate intraocular pressure. Use with caution in hyperthyroidism; may stimulate thyroid activity. Patients must be instructed to seek medical attention in cases where acute symptoms are not relieved or a previous level of response is diminished. The need to increase frequency of use may indicate deterioration of asthma, and treatment must not be delayed. A spacer device or valved holding chamber is recommended when using a metered dose inhaler.

Adverse Reactions

Cardiovascular: Angina pectoris, atrial fibrillation, cardiac arrhythmia, chest discomfort, chest pain, extrasystoles, flushing, hypertension, hypotension, palpitations, supraventricular tachycardia, tachycardia

Central nervous system: Central nervous system stimulation, dizziness, drowsiness, headache, insomnia, irritability, migraine, nervousness, nightmares, restlessness, seizure, vertigo

Dermatologic: Diaphoresis, skin rash, urticaria

Endocrine & metabolic: Hyperglycemia, hypokalemia, lactic acidosis

Gastrointestinal: Diarrhea, dysgeusia, dyspepsia, gastroenteritis, nausea, vomiting, xerostomia

Genitourinary: Difficulty in micturition

Hematologic & oncologic: Lymphadenopathy

Hypersensitivity: Anaphylaxis, angioedema, hypersensitivity reaction

Local: Pain at injection site

Neuromuscular & skeletal: Muscle cramps, musculoskeletal pain, tremor, weakness

Otic: Otitis media

Respiratory: Bronchospasm, cough, epistaxis, exacerbation of asthma, laryngitis, oropharyngeal edema, oropharyngeal irritation, pharyngitis, rhinitis, upper respiratory tract inflammation, viral upper respiratory tract infection

Rare but important or life-threatening: Glossitis, hoarseness, ischemic heart disease, metabolic acidosis, pulmonary edema, throat irritation, tongue ulcer

Drug Interactions

Metabolism/Transport Effects None known.

Avoid Concomitant Use

Avoid concomitant use of Albuterol with any of the following: Beta-Blockers (Nonselective); Iobenguane I 123

Increased Effect/Toxicity

Albuterol may increase the levels/effects of: Atosiban; Loop Diuretics; Sympathomimetics; Thiazide Diuretics

The levels/effects of Albuterol may be increased by: AtoMOXetine; Cannabinoid-Containing Products; Linezolid; MAO Inhibitors; Tricyclic Antidepressants

Decreased Effect

Albuterol may decrease the levels/effects of: Iobenguane I 123

The levels/effects of Albuterol may be decreased by: Beta-Blockers (Beta1 Selective); Beta-Blockers (Nonselective); Betahistine

Stability

Oral:

Syrup: Store at 20°C to 25°C (68°F to 77°F).

Tablet: Store at 20°C to 25°C (68°F to 77°F).

Tablet, extended release: Store at 20°C to 25°C (68°F to 77°F).

Oral inhalations:

HFA aerosols: Store at 15°C to 25°C (59°F to 77°F).

Ventolin HFA: Discard when counter reads 000 or 12 months after removal from protective pouch, whichever comes first. Store with mouthpiece down.

Solution for nebulization (0.5%): Store at 2°C to 25°C (36°F to 77°F).

AccuNeb: Store at 2°C to 25°C (36°F to 77°F). Do not use if solution changes color or becomes cloudy. Use within 1 week of opening foil pouch.

Mechanism of Action
Relaxes bronchial smooth muscle by action on beta$_2$-receptors with little effect on heart rate

Pharmacodynamics

Nebulization/oral inhalation:

Maximum effect: Peak bronchodilation: 0.5-2 hours

Duration: 2-5 hours

Oral:

Maximum effect: Peak bronchodilatation: Immediate release: 2-3 hours

Duration: Immediate release: 4-6 hours; extended release tablets: Up to 12 hours

Pharmacokinetics (Adult data unless noted)

Metabolism: By the liver to an inactive sulfate

Half-life:

Oral: 2.7-5 hours

Inhalation: 3.8 hours

Elimination: 30% appears in urine as unchanged drug

Dosing: Neonatal

Bronchodilation: Limited data available: Oral inhalation:

Nebulization: Usual reported dose: 1.25-2.5 mg/dose (Ballard, 2002). In a retrospective report, 16 VLBW neonates (mean GA: 26.1 ± 1.2 weeks; mean birthweight: 817 ± 211 g) received 1.25 mg/dose every 8 hours for >2 weeks (Mhanna, 2009)

Inhalation, aerosol (metered dose inhaler); mechanically ventilated patients: 90 mcg/spray: 1-2 puffs administered into the ventilator circuit was the most frequently reported dose in a survey of 68 neonatal intensive care units (Ballard, 2002); typically used every 6 hours (Fok, 1998); may consider more frequent use if clinically indicated

Dosing: Usual

Pediatric:

Asthma, acute exacerbation: Oral inhalation:

Inhalation aerosol (metered dose inhaler): 90 mcg/puff:

Children: Limited data available in ages <4 years: 4-8 puffs every 20 minutes for 3 doses then every 1-4 hours

Adolescents: 4-8 puffs every 20 minutes for up to 4 hours then every 1-4 hours

Nebulization:

Infants and Children: Limited data in ages <2 years:

Intermittent: 0.15 mg/kg (minimum dose: 2.5 mg) every 20 minutes for 3 doses then 0.15-0.3 mg/kg not to exceed 10 mg every 1-4 hours (NAEPP, 2007)

Continuous: Dosing regimens variable; optimal dosage not established

NIH Guidelines: 0.5 mg/kg/hour (NAEPP, 2007)

Alternate dosing: Limited data available: 0.3 mg/kg/hour has also been used safely in the treatment of severe status asthmaticus in children (Papo, 1993); higher doses of 3 mg/kg/hour ± 2.2 mg/kg/hour in children (n=19, mean age: 20.7 months ± 38 months) resulted in no cardiotoxicity (Katz, 1993)

Adolescents:

Intermittent: 2.5-5 mg every 20 minutes for 3 doses then 2.5-10 mg every 1-4 hours as needed

Continuous: 10-15 mg/hour

Asthma, maintenance therapy (nonacute) (NAEPP, 2007): Oral inhalation:

Inhalation, aerosol (metered dose inhaler): Infants, Children, and Adolescents: Limited data available in ages <4 years: 90 mcg/puff: 2 puffs every 4-6 hours as needed. **Note:** Not recommended for long-term daily maintenance treatment; regular use exceeding 2 days/week for symptom control (not prevention of exercise-induced bronchospasm) indicates the need for additional long-term control therapy.

Nebulization: Limited data in ages <2 years:

Albuterol Nebulization Dosage

Age	Dose (mg)	0.5% Solution (mL)	0.083% Solution (mL)	Frequency
Infants and Children <5 y	0.63-2.5 mg	0.13-0.5 mL	0.76-3 mL	Every 4-6 h
Children ≥5 y and Adolescents	1.25-5 mg	0.25-1 mL	1.5-6 mL	Every 4-8 h

Bronchospasm, treatment:
Oral inhalation:
Inhalation, aerosol (metered dose inhaler):
Manufacturer's labeling: Children ≥4 years and Adolescents: 90 mcg/puff: 1-2 puffs every 4-6 hours
Alternate dosing: Limited data available: Infants, Children, and Adolescents: 90 mcg/puff: 4-8 puffs every 15-20 minutes for 3 doses; then every 1-4 hours (Hegenbarth, 2008)
Nebulization:
Manufacturer labeling: Children ≥2 years and Adolescents:
10-15 kg: 1.25 mg 3-4 times/day
>15 kg: 2.5 mg 3-4 times/day
Alternate dosing: Limited data available (Hegenbarth, 2008): Infants, Children, and Adolescents:
Intermittent: 0.5% (5 mg/mL) solution: 2.5 mg every 20 minutes for 3 doses, then 0.15-0.3 mg/kg up to 10 mg every 1-4 hours
Continuous (prolonged nebulization): 0.5 mg/kg/hour up to 10-15 mg/hour
Oral: **Note:** Not the preferred route for treatment of asthma; inhalation via nebulization or MDI is preferred (GINA, 2008; GINA, 2012; NAEPP, 2007)
Immediate release formulation (syrup, tablets):
Children 2-6 years: 0.1-0.2 mg/kg/dose 3 times daily; maximum dose: 4 mg
Children 6-12 years: 2 mg/dose 3-4 times daily
Adolescents: 2-4 mg/dose 3-4 times daily
Sustained release formulation (tablets):
Children ≥6 years: 0.3-0.6 mg/kg/**day** divided twice daily; maximum daily dose: 8 mg/**day**
Adolescents: 4 mg/dose twice daily; may increase to 8 mg/dose twice daily
Exercise-induced bronchospasm; prevention:
(NAEPP, 2007; Parsons, 2013): Oral inhalation:
Inhalation, aerosol (metered dose inhaler): Limited data available in ages <4 years: 90 mcg/puff:
Infants and Children <5 years: 1-2 puffs 5-20 minutes before exercising
Children ≥5 years and Adolescents: 2 puffs 5-20 minutes before exercising
Adult:
Bronchospasm:
Metered dose inhaler (90 mcg/puff): 2 puffs every 4-6 hours as needed (NAEPP, 2007):
Acute treatment: 1-2 puffs; additional puffs may be necessary if inadequate relief; however, patients should be advised to promptly consult health care provider or seek medical attention if no relief from acute treatment
Maintenance: 1-2 puffs 3-4 times daily (maximum: 8 puffs daily)
Nebulization: 2.5 mg 3-4 times daily as needed; Quick relief: 1.25-5 mg every 4-8 hours as needed (NAEPP, 2007)
Oral: **Note:** Oral is not the preferred route for treatment of asthma; inhalation via nebulization or MDI is preferred (NAEPP, 2007).
Regular release: 2-4 mg/dose 3-4 times daily; maximum dose not to exceed 32 mg daily (divided doses)

Extended release: 8 mg every 12 hours; maximum dose not to exceed 32 mg/day (divided doses). A 4 mg dose every 12 hours may be sufficient in some patients, such as adults of low body weight.
Exacerbation of asthma (acute, severe) (NAEPP, 2007):
Metered dose inhaler: 4-8 puffs every 20 minutes for up to 4 hours, then every 1-4 hours as needed
Nebulization solution: 2.5-5 mg every 20 minutes for 3 doses, then 2.5-10 mg every 1-4 hours as needed, or 10-15 mg/hour by continuous nebulization
Exercise-induced bronchospasm (prevention):
Metered dose inhaler (90 mcg/puff): 2 puffs 5-30 minutes prior to exercise
Dosing adjustment in renal impairment: All patients: Use with caution in patients with renal impairment. No dosage adjustment required, including patients on hemodialysis, peritoneal dialysis, or CRRT (Aronoff, 2007).
Dosing adjustment in hepatic impairment: There are no dosage adjustments provided in manufacturer's labeling.

Administration
Oral inhalation:
Inhalation, aerosol (metered dose inhaler): Prime the inhaler (before first use or if it has not been used for more than 2 weeks) by releasing 4 test sprays into the air away from the face (3 test sprays for ProAir HFA); shake well before use; use spacer for children <5 years of age and consider adding a face mask for infants and children <4 years of age. HFA inhalers should be cleaned with warm water at least once per week; allow to air dry completely prior to use.
Nebulization: Using 0.5% solution, dilute dosage in 1-2 mL NS (0.083% solution and AccuNeb do not require further dilution); adjust nebulizer flow to deliver dosage over 5-15 minutes; avoid contact of the dropper tip (multidose bottle) with any surface, including the nebulizer reservoir and associated ventilator equipment. For continuous nebulization, the total amount of fluid delivered is determined by nebulizer delivery device; usually 25-30 mL per 1 hours of nebulization, protocols may vary by institution (Hegenbarth, 2008).
Oral: Administer with food; do not crush or chew extended release tablets

Monitoring Parameters Serum potassium, oxygen saturation, heart rate, pulmonary function tests, respiratory rate, use of accessory muscles during respiration, suprasternal retractions; arterial or capillary blood gases (if patient's condition warrants)

Test Interactions Increased renin (S), increased aldosterone (S)

Dosage Forms Considerations
ProAir HFA 8.5 g canisters and Proventil HFA 6.7 g canisters contain 200 inhalations.
Ventolin HFA 18 g canisters contain 200 inhalations and the 8 g canisters contain 60 inhalations.

Dosage Forms Excipient information presented when available (limited, particularly for generics); consult specific product labeling. [DSC] = Discontinued product
Aerosol Solution, Inhalation:
ProAir HFA: 90 mcg/actuation (8.5 g)
Proventil HFA: 90 mcg/actuation (6.7 g)
Ventolin HFA: 90 mcg/actuation (8 g, 18 g)
Nebulization Solution, Inhalation:
Generic: 0.63 mg/3 mL (3 mL); 0.083% [2.5 mg/3 mL] (3 mL); 0.5% [2.5 mg/0.5 mL] (20 mL)
Nebulization Solution, Inhalation [preservative free]:
AccuNeb: 0.63 mg/3 mL (3 mL [DSC]); 1.25 mg/3 mL [DSC]
Generic: 0.63 mg/3 mL (3 mL); 1.25 mg/3 mL (3 mL); 0.083% [2.5 mg/3 mL] (3 mL); 0.5% [2.5 mg/0.5 mL] (1 ea)
Syrup, Oral:
Generic: 2 mg/5 mL (473 mL)

Tablet, Oral:
Generic: 2 mg, 4 mg
Tablet Extended Release 12 Hour, Oral:
VoSpire ER: 4 mg [contains fd&c blue #1 aluminum lake, fd&c yellow #10 aluminum lake]
VoSpire ER: 8 mg
Generic: 4 mg, 8 mg

References

Ballard J, Lugo RA, and Salyer JW, "A Survey of Albuterol Administration Practices in Intubated Patients in the Neonatal Intensive Care Unit," *Respir Care*, 2002, 47(1):31-8.

Boulton DW, Fawcett JP, and Fiddes TM, "Transplacental Distribution of Salbutamol Enantiomers at Caesarian Section," *Br J Clin Pharmacol*,1997, 44(6):587-90.

Fok TF, Lam K, Ng PC, et al, "Randomised Crossover Trial of Salbutamol Aerosol Delivered by Metered Dose Inhaler, Jet Nebuliser, and Ultrasonic Nebuliser in Chronic Lung Disease," *Arch Dis Child Fetal Neonatal Ed*, 1998, 79(2):F100-4.

Hegenbarth MA and American Academy of Pediatrics Committee on Drugs, "Preparing for Pediatric Emergencies: Drugs to Consider," *Pediatrics*, 2008, 121(2):433-43.

Katz RW, Kelly HW, Crowley MR, et al, "Safety of Continuous Nebulized Albuterol for Bronchospasm in Infants and Children," *Pediatrics*, 1993, 92(5):666-69.

Mhanna MJ, Patel JS, Patel S, et al, "The Effects of Racemic Albuterol Versus Levalbuterol in Very Low Birth Weight Infants," *Pediatr Pulmonol*, 2009, 44(8):778-83.

National Asthma Education and Prevention Program, "Expert Panel Report: Guidelines for the Diagnosis and Management of Asthma Update on Selected Topics–2002," *J Allergy Clin Immunol*, 2002, 110 (5 Suppl):S141-219.

National Asthma Education and Prevention Program (NAEPP), "Expert Panel Report 3 (EPR-3): Guidelines for the Diagnosis and Management of Asthma," *Clinical Practice Guidelines*, National Institutes of Health, National Heart, Lung, and Blood Institute, NIH Publication No. 08-4051, prepublication 2007; available at http://www.nhlbi.nih.gov/guidelines/asthma/asthgdln.htm.

National Asthma Education and Prevention Program (NAEPP) Working Group Report on "Managing Asthma During Pregnancy: Recommendations for Pharmacologic Treatment," National Institutes of Health, National Heart, Lung, and Blood Institute, NIH Publication No. 05-5236, March 2005. Available at http://www.nhlbi.nih.gov/health/prof/lung/asthma/astpreg/astpreg_full.pdf

O'Callaghan C, Milner AD, and Swarbrick A, "Nebulized Salbutamol Does Have a Protective Effect on Airways in Children Under One Year Old," *Arch Dis Child*, 1988, 63(5):479-83.

Papo MC, Frank J, and Thompson AE, "A Prospective, Randomized Study of Continuous Versus Intermittent Nebulized Albuterol for Severe Status Asthmaticus in Children," *Crit Care Med*, 1993, 21 (10):1479-86.

Parsons JP, Hallstrand TS, Mastronarde JG, et al. An official American Thoracic Society Clinical Practice Guideline: exercise-induced bronchoconstriction. *Am J Respir Crit Care Med*. 2013;187(9): 1016-1027.

Rachelefsky GS and Siegel SC, "Asthma in Infants and Children - Treatment of Childhood Asthma: Part II," *J Allergy Clin Immunol*, 1985, 76(3):409-25.

Schuh S, Parkin P, Rajan A, et al, "High- Versus Low-Dose, Frequently Administered, Nebulized Albuterol in Children With Severe, Acute Asthma," *Pediatrics*, 1989, 83(4):513-8.

Schuh S, Reider MJ, Canny G, et al, "Nebulized Albuterol in Acute Childhood Asthma: Comparison of Two Doses," *Pediatrics*, 1990, 86 (4):509-13.

◆ **Albuterol Sulfate** see Albuterol on page 84

◆ **Alcaine** see Proparacaine on page 1755

◆ **Alcaine® (Can)** see Proparacaine on page 1755

◆ **Alcalak [OTC]** see Calcium Carbonate on page 346

Alclometasone (al kloe MET a sone)

Medication Safety Issues
Sound-alike/look-alike issues:
Aclovate® may be confused with Accolate®
International issues:
Cloderm: Brand name for alclometasone [Indonesia], but also brand name for clobetasol [China, India, Malaysia, Singapore, Thailand]; clocortolone [U.S., Canada]; clotrimazole [Germany]

Related Information
Topical Corticosteroids on page 2224
Brand Names: U.S. Aclovate
Therapeutic Category Adrenal Corticosteroid; Anti-inflammatory Agent; Corticosteroid, Topical; Glucocorticoid
Generic Availability (U.S.) Yes
Use Treatment of inflammation and pruritic manifestations of corticosteroid-responsive dermatosis (low to medium potency topical corticosteroid) (FDA approved in ages ≥1 year and adults); **Note:** In pediatric patients, safety and efficacy ≥3 weeks have not been established.
Pregnancy Risk Factor C
Pregnancy Considerations Some corticosteroids were found to be teratogenic following topical application in animal reproduction studies. Topical products are not recommended for extensive use, in large quantities, or for long periods of time in pregnant women.
Breast-Feeding Considerations Systemic corticosteroids are excreted in human milk. It is not known if sufficient quantities of alclometasone are absorbed following topical administration to produce detectable amounts in breast milk.
Contraindications Hypersensitivity to alclometasone or any component
Warnings Hypothalamic-pituitary-adrenal (HPA) suppression may occur; acute adrenal insufficiency (adrenal crisis) may occur with abrupt withdrawal after long-term therapy or with stress; withdrawal and discontinuation of corticosteroids should be done carefully. Adverse systemic effects (eg, hyperglycemia, glycosuria, fluid and electrolyte changes) may occur when topical steroids are used in large areas of the body, denuded areas, for prolonged periods of time, with an occlusive dressing, and/or in infants and small children; infants and small children may be more susceptible to HPA axis suppression or other systemic toxicities due to larger skin surface area to body mass ratio, particularly if applying to >20% of BSA; use with caution in pediatric patients. If HPA suppression occurs, consider withdrawal of alclometasone, reduction in frequency of application, or substitution with a less potent corticosteroid. Cushing's syndrome and intracranial hypertension have also been reported in pediatric patients. May cause inhibition of bone growth in pediatric patients. Immunosuppression may occur; patients may be more susceptible to infections; avoid exposure to chickenpox and measles. Corticosteroids may activate latent opportunistic infections or exacerbate systemic fungal infections. Prolonged treatment with corticosteroids has been associated with the development of Kaposi's sarcoma (case reports); if noted, discontinuation of therapy should be considered. Allergic contact dermatitis can occur and is usually diagnosed by failure to heal rather than clinical exacerbation, diagnostic patch testing may corroborate observation.

Ointment and cream contain propylene glycol; toxicities have been reported with use of products containing propylene glycol, including hyperosmolality, lactic acidosis, seizures, and respiratory depression; in neonates large amounts of propylene glycol delivered orally, intravenously (eg, >3000 mg/day), or topically have been associated with potentially fatal toxicities which can include metabolic acidosis, seizures, renal failure, and CNS depression; use ointment and cream containing propylene glycol with caution (AAP, 1997; Shehab, 2009).

Precautions Do not use for diaper dermatitis. Avoid use with occlusive dressing or application to denuded skin or to large surface areas. Avoid using higher than recommended doses; suppression of HPA axis function may occur. Reduction in growth velocity may occur when corticosteroids are administered to pediatric patients by any route; monitor growth. Prolonged use may result in fungal ▶

or bacterial superinfection. Use may be associated with local sensitization.

Adverse Reactions

Dermatologic: Acne, allergic dermatitis, hypopigmentation, perioral dermatitis, skin atrophy, striae, miliaria

Endocrine & metabolic: HPA axis suppression, Cushing's syndrome, growth retardation

Local: Burning, erythema, itching, irritation, dryness, folliculitis, papular rash

Miscellaneous: Secondary infection

Drug Interactions

Metabolism/Transport Effects None known.

Avoid Concomitant Use

Avoid concomitant use of Alclometasone with any of the following: Aldesleukin

Increased Effect/Toxicity

Alclometasone may increase the levels/effects of: Ceritinib; Deferasirox

The levels/effects of Alclometasone may be increased by: Telaprevir

Decreased Effect

Alclometasone may decrease the levels/effects of: Aldesleukin; Corticorelin; Hyaluronidase; Telaprevir

Stability Store between 2°C and 30°C (36°F and 86°F)

Mechanism of Action Stimulates the synthesis of enzymes needed to decrease inflammation, suppress mitotic activity, and cause vasoconstriction

Pharmacodynamics

Initial response (Ruthven, 1988):

Eczema: 5.3 days

Psoriasis: 6.7 days

Peak response (Ruthven, 1988):

Eczema: 13.9 days

Psoriasis: 14.8 days

Pharmacokinetics (Adult data unless noted) Absorption: Topical: 3% (when left on intact skin without an occlusive dressing for 8 hours). Percutaneous absorption varies and depends on many factors including vehicle used, integrity of epidermis, dose, and use of occlusive dressing; absorption is increased by occlusive dressings or with decreased integrity of skin (eg, inflammation or skin disease). Absorption also depends upon the anatomical site: Forearm 1%; scalp 4%; scrotum 36%

Dosing: Usual Children, Adolescents, and Adults: Topical: Apply to affected area 2-3 times daily. Therapy should be discontinued when control is achieved; if no improvement is seen within 2 weeks, reassessment of diagnosis may be necessary. Safety and efficacy have not been established for long term use (>3 weeks) in children. In general, the treated skin should not be covered due to potential increased absorption; however, occlusive dressings may be used when treating refractory lesions of psoriasis and other deep-seated dermatoses such as localized neurodermatitis (lichen simplex chronicus); monitor closely for toxicity.

Administration Topical: Apply sparingly in a thin film; rub in lightly; for external use only; avoid contact with the eyes; generally not for routine use on the face, underarms, or groin area (including diapered area). Do not use on open wounds or weeping lesions. The treated skin area should not be bandaged or covered unless directed by the prescriber. Wash hands thoroughly before and after use.

Monitoring Parameters Clinical signs and symptoms of improvement in condition; assessment of HPA suppression (eg, ACTH stimulation test, morning plasma cortisol test, urinary free cortisol test) if treatment for prolonged periods or if HPA axis suppression is suspected; growth in pediatric patients

Dosage Forms Excipient information presented when available (limited, particularly for generics); consult specific product labeling.

Cream, External, as dipropionate:

Aclovate: 0.05% (15 g, 60 g) [contains cetearyl alcohol, propylene glycol]

Generic: 0.05% (15 g, 45 g, 60 g)

Ointment, External, as dipropionate:

Generic: 0.05% (15 g, 45 g, 60 g)

References

American Academy of Pediatrics Committee on Drugs. "Inactive" ingredients in pharmaceutical products: update (subject review). Pediatrics. 1997;99(2):268-278.

Goedert JJ, Vitale F, Lauria C, et al, "Risk Factors for Classical Kaposi's Sarcoma," J Natl Cancer Inst, 2002, 94(22):1712-8.

Ruthven K, Fortune S, Daniels VG, et al, "Surveillance Study of Aclometasone Dipropionate for the Treatment of Steroid-Responsive Dermatoses in General Practice," Curr Ther Res, 1988, 44:493-502.

Shehab N, Lewis CL, Streetman DD, Donn SM. Exposure to the pharmaceutical excipients benzyl alcohol and propylene glycol among critically ill neonates. Pediatr Crit Care Med. 2009;10 (2):256-259.

◆ **Alclometasone Dipropionate** see Alclometasone on page 87

◆ **Alcohol, Absolute** see Alcohol (Ethyl) on page 88

◆ **Alcohol, Dehydrated** see Alcohol (Ethyl) on page 88

Alcohol (Ethyl) (AL koe hol, ETH il)

Medication Safety Issues

Sound-alike/look-alike issues:

Ethanol may be confused with Ethyol®, Ethamolin®

Brand Names: U.S. Epi-Clenz™ [OTC]; Gel-Stat™ [OTC]; GelRite™ [OTC]; Isagel® [OTC]; Lavacol® [OTC]; Prevacare® [OTC]; Protection Plus® [OTC]; Purell® 2 in 1 [OTC]; Purell® Lasting Care [OTC]; Purell® Moisture Therapy [OTC]; Purell® with Aloe [OTC]; Purell® [OTC]

Brand Names: Canada Biobase-G™; Biobase™

Therapeutic Category Anti-infective Agent, Topical; Antidote, Ethylene Glycol Toxicity; Antidote, Methanol Toxicity; Fat Occlusion (Central Venous Catheter); Treatment Agent; Neurolytic

Generic Availability (U.S.) Yes

Use Antidote for the treatment of methanol and ethylene glycol intoxication; neurolysis of nerves or ganglia for the relief of intractable, chronic pain in such conditions as inoperable cancer and trigeminal neuralgia (dehydrated alcohol injection); topical anti-infective; treatment of occluded central venous catheters due to lipid deposition from fat emulsion infusion (particularly 3-in-1 admixture)

Pregnancy Risk Factor C (injection)

Pregnancy Considerations Reproduction studies have not been conducted with alcohol injection. Ethanol crosses the placenta, enters the fetal circulation, and has teratogenic effects in humans. The following withdrawal symptoms have been noted in the neonate following maternal ethanol consumption during pregnancy: Crying, hyperactivity, irritability, poor suck, tremors, seizures, poor sleeping pattern, hyperphagia, and diaphoresis. Fetal alcohol syndrome (FAS) is a term referring to a combination of physical, behavioral, and cognitive abnormalities resulting from ethanol exposure during fetal development. Since a "safe" amount of ethanol consumption during pregnancy has not been determined, the AAP recommends those women who are pregnant or planning a pregnancy refrain from all ethanol intake. When used as an antidote during the second or third trimester, FAS is not likely to occur due to the short treatment period; use during the first trimester is controversial.

Breast-Feeding Considerations Ethanol is found in breast milk. Drowsiness, diaphoresis, deep sleep, weakness, decreased linear growth, and abnormal weight gain have been reported in infants following large amounts of ethanol ingestion by the mother. Ingestion >1 g/kg/day decreases milk ejection reflex. The actual clearance of ethanol from breast milk is dependent upon the mother's weight and amount of ethanol consumed.

Contraindications Hypersensitivity to ethyl alcohol; seizure disorder and diabetic coma; subarachnoid injection of dehydrated alcohol in patients receiving anticoagulants

Warnings Ethyl alcohol is a flammable liquid and should be kept cool and away from any heat source; proper positioning of the patient for neurolytic administration is essential to control localization of the injection of dehydrated alcohol (which is hypobaric) into the subarachnoid space; avoid extravasation; not for SubQ administration; do not administer simultaneously with blood due to the possibility of pseudoagglutination or hemolysis; may potentiate severe hypoprothrombic bleeding; clinical evaluation and periodic lab determinations, including serum ethyl alcohol levels, are necessary to monitor effectiveness, changes in electrolyte concentrations, and acid-base balance (when used as an antidote)

Precautions Use with caution in diabetics (ethyl alcohol decreases blood sugar), hepatic impairment, patients with gout, shock, following cranial surgery, and in anticipated postpartum hemorrhage; monitor blood glucose closely, particularly in children as treatment of ingestions is associated with hypoglycemia; avoid extravasation during I.V. administration; ethyl alcohol passes freely into breast milk at a level approximately equivalent to maternal serum level; effects on the infant are insignificant until maternal blood level reaches 300 mg/dL; minimize dermal exposure of ethyl alcohol in infants as significant systemic absorption and toxicity can occur

Adverse Reactions
Cardiovascular: Flushing, hypotension
Central nervous system: Agitation, CNS depression, coma, disorientation, drowsiness, encephalopathy, headache, sedation, seizure (rare), vertigo
Endocrine & metabolic: Hypoglycemia
Gastrointestinal: Gastric irritation, nausea, vomiting
Genitourinary: Urinary retention
Local: Nerve and tissue destruction, phlebitis
Renal: Polyuria
Miscellaneous: Intoxication

Drug Interactions

Metabolism/Transport Effects None known.

Avoid Concomitant Use
Avoid concomitant use of Alcohol (Ethyl) with any of the following: Acitretin; Agomelatine; Amisulpride; Azelastine (Nasal); Bedaquiline; CycloSERINE; Didanosine; Disulfiram; Gabapentin Enacarbil; Hydrocodone; MAO Inhibitors; MetFORMIN; Methadone; Methylphenidate; MetroNIDAZOLE (Systemic); Mirtazapine; Paraldehyde; Perampanel; Pipamperone [INT]; Sodium Oxybate; Stiripentol; Sulpiride; Tapentadol; Tinidazole; Topiramate; Trabectedin

Increased Effect/Toxicity
Alcohol (Ethyl) may increase the levels/effects of: Acetaminophen; Acetohydroxamic Acid; Acitretin; Agomelatine; Amantadine; Aminophylline; Azelastine (Nasal); Bedaquiline; Bromocriptine; Buprenorphine; BuPROPion; CloBAZam; CycloSERINE; Didanosine; Diethylpropion; Doxylamine; Ethionamide; Ezogabine; Fesoterodine; Fosphenytoin; Gabapentin Enacarbil; Hydrocodone; ISOtretinoin; Levomilnacipran; Lomitapide; MAO Inhibitors; MetFORMIN; Methadone; Methylphenidate; Metyrosine; Mipomersen; Mirtazapine; Niacin; NIFEdipine; OXcarbazepine; Oxybutynin; Paraldehyde; Phendimetrazine; Phentermine; Phenytoin; Phosphodiesterase 5 Inhibitors; Pramipexole; Propranolol; ROPINIRole; Rotigotine; Rufinamide; Selective Serotonin Reuptake Inhibitors; Serotonin/Norepinephrine Reuptake Inhibitors; Sodium Oxybate; Sulpiride; Tacrolimus (Systemic); Tapentadol; Theophylline; Thiazide Diuretics; Topiramate; Trabectedin; TraZODone; Treprostinil; Trimethobenzamide; Trospium; Varenicline

The levels/effects of Alcohol (Ethyl) may be increased by: Amisulpride; Bromocriptine; BuPROPion; Cannabis; CefoTEtan; Chloramphenicol; Cisapride; CNS Depressants; Disulfiram; Dronabinol; Efavirenz; Griseofulvin; Ketoconazole (Systemic); MetroNIDAZOLE (Systemic); MetroNIDAZOLE (Topical); Nabilone; Perampanel; Pipamperone [INT]; Stiripentol; Sulfonylureas; Tacrolimus (Topical); Tetrahydrocannabinol; Tinidazole; Verapamil

Decreased Effect
Alcohol (Ethyl) may decrease the levels/effects of: Cyproterone; Fosphenytoin; Phenytoin; Propranolol; Vitamin K Antagonists

The levels/effects of Alcohol (Ethyl) may be decreased by: Efavirenz

Stability Store at room temperature; do not use unless solution is clear and container is intact

Mechanism of Action When used to treat ethylene glycol or methanol toxicity, ethyl alcohol competitively inhibits alcohol dehydrogenase, an enzyme which catalyzes the metabolism of ethylene glycol and methanol to their toxic metabolites.

Pharmacokinetics (Adult data unless noted)
Distribution: V_d: 0.6-0.7 L/kg
Metabolism: Hepatic to acetaldehyde or acetate by alcohol dehydrogenase
Clearance: Adults: 15-20 mg/dL/hour (range: 10-34 mg/dL/hour)
Dialysis: Hemodialysis clearance: 300-400 mL/minute with an ethanol removal rate of 280 mg/minute

Dosing: Usual

Absolute ethanol/ethyl alcohol (EtOH):
Treatment of methanol or ethylene glycol ingestion: Children, Adolescents, and Adults:
Loading dose (LD):
Oral: 0.8-1 mL/kg of 95% EtOH or 2 mL/kg of 40% EtOH (equivalent to 80 proof undiluted liquor) or 1.8 mL/kg of 43% EtOH (equivalent to 86 proof undiluted liquor)
I.V.: 8-10 mL/kg of 10% EtOH solution, not to exceed 200 mL
Modified loading dose (if ingestion consists of both EtOH **and** methanol or ethylene glycol): The loading dose is reduced in a proportional manner related to the measured EtOH blood level by multiplying the calculated loading dose described above by the following factor:

$$LD \times \left[\frac{100 - (\text{patient's serum ethanol level in mg/dL})}{100} \right]$$

Maintenance dose: See table

	Non-Drinker	Average Drinker	Chronic Drinker
EtOH dosage by weight	66 mg/kg/h	110 mg/kg/h	154 mg/kg/h
Oral: 43% EtOH (34 g EtOH/dL; 86 proof undiluted liquor)	0.2 mL/kg/h	0.3 mL/kg/h	0.46 mL/kg/h
Oral: 95% EtOH (75 g EtOH/dL)	0.1 mL/kg/h	0.15 mL/kg/h	0.2 mL/kg/h
I.V.: 10% EtOH (7.9 g EtOH/dL)	0.83 mL/kg/h	1.4 mL/kg/h	2 mL/kg/h

Note: Continue therapy until methanol or ethylene glycol blood level <10 mg/dL

Dosage adjustment for hemodialysis: See table

Maintenance Dose Adjustment of Dialysis[1]:

	Non-Drinker	Chronic Drinker
EtOH dosage by weight	169 mg/kg/h	257 mg/kg/h
Oral: 43% EtOH (34 g EtOH/dL)	0.5 mL/kg/h	0.77 mL/kg/h
I.V.: 10% EtOH (7.9 g EtOH/dL)	2.13 mL/kg/h	3.26 mL/kg/h

[1]Due to considerable variability of EtOH clearance between patients, adjust dosage as needed based upon serum EtOH levels.

Treatment of fat occlusion of central venous catheters: Children and Adults: I.V. (see institutional-based protocol for catheter clearance assessment, the following assessment is a general methodology): Up to 3 mL of 70% ethanol (maximum: 0.55 mL/kg); instill a volume equal to the internal volume of the catheter; may repeat if patency not restored after 30- minute dwell time; if dose repeated, reassess after 4-hour dwell time

Dehydrated alcohol injection: Therapeutic neurolysis (nerve or ganglion block): Adults: Intraneural: Dosage variable depending upon the site of injection, eg, trigeminal neuralgia: 0.05-0.5 mL as a single injection per interspace vs subarachnoid injection: 0.5-1 mL as a single injection per interspace; single doses >1.5 mL are seldom required

Liquid denatured alcohol: Topical: Children and Adults: Apply as needed

Administration
Oral: Dilute ethanol in 6 ounces orange juice and give over 30 minutes

Parenteral: Not for SubQ administration; I.V.: Dilute absolute alcohol for I.V. administration to a final concentration of 5% to 10% v/v in D_5W or $D_{10}W$; infuse loading dose plus 1 hour of maintenance dosage over 60 minutes; for treatment of occluded central venous catheter, a 70% dilution of ethanol may be made by adding 0.8 mL SWI to 2 mL 98% ethanol; instill with a volume equal to the internal volume of the catheter; assess patency at 30 minutes (or per institutional protocol); may repeat

Intraneural: Separate needles should be used for each of multiple injections or sites to prevent residual alcohol deposition at sites not intended for tissue destruction; inject slowly after determining proper placement of needle; since dehydrated alcohol is hypobaric when compared with spinal fluid, proper positioning of the patient is essential to control localization of injections into the subarachnoid space

Monitoring Parameters Antidotal therapy: Blood ethanol levels (at the end of the loading dose, every hour until stabilized, and then every 8-12 hours thereafter); blood glucose, electrolytes (including serum magnesium), arterial pH, blood gases, methanol or ethylene glycol blood levels, heart rate, blood pressure

Reference Range
Symptoms associated with serum ethanol levels:
Nausea and vomiting: Serum level >100 mg/dL
Coma: Serum level >300 mg/dL
Antidote for methanol/ethylene glycol: Goal range: Blood ethanol level: 100-150 mg/dL (22-32 mmol/liter)

Additional Information Eighty-proof spirits contain 40% ethanol; 86 proof spirits contain 43% ethanol

Dosage Forms Excipient information presented when available (limited, particularly for generics); consult specific product labeling.

Aerosol, foam, topical [instant hand sanitizer]:
Epi-Clenz™: 70% (240 mL) [contains aloe, vitamin E]

Gel, topical [foam/instant hand sanitizer]:
Epi-Clenz™: 70% (480 mL) [contains aloe, vitamin E]
Gel, topical [instant hand sanitizer]: 62% (1.5 mL, 118 mL, 354 mL, 473 mL)
Epi-Clenz™: 70% (45 mL, 120 mL, 480 mL) [contains aloe, vitamin E]
Gel-Stat™: 62% (120 mL, 480 mL) [contains aloe, vitamin E]
GelRite™: 67% (120 mL, 480 mL)
GelRite™: 67% (800 mL) [contains vitamin E]
Isagel®: 60% (59 mL, 118 mL, 621 mL, 800 mL)
Prevacare®: 60% (120 mL, 240 mL, 960 mL, 1200 mL, 1500 mL)
Purell®: 62% (60 mL, 360 mL, 1000 mL)
Purell®: 62% (15 mL, 30 mL, 59 mL, 60 mL, 120 mL, 236 mL, 240 mL, 250 mL, 360 mL, 500 mL, 800 mL, 1000 mL, 2000 mL) [contains moisturizers, vitamin E]
Purell®: 62% (15 mL, 60 mL, 360 mL, 800 mL, 1000 mL) [contains vitamin E]
Purell® Lasting Care: 62% (120 mL, 240 mL, 1000 mL) [contains moisturizers]
Purell® Moisture Therapy: 62% (75 mL)
Purell® with Aloe: 62% (60 mL, 120 mL, 354 mL, 800 mL, 1000 mL, 2000 mL) [contains aloe, moisturizers, tartrazine, vitamin E]
Purell® with Aloe: 62% (15 mL, 59 mL, 236 mL) [contains aloe, tartrazine, vitamin E]
Injection, solution [dehydrated, preservative free]: 98% (1 mL, 5 mL)
Liquid, topical [denatured]: 70% (480 mL, 3840 mL)
Liquid, topical [denatured/rubbing alcohol]:
Lavacol®: 70% (473 mL)
Lotion, topical [instant hand sanitizer]:
Purell® 2 in 1: 62% (60 mL, 360 mL, 1000 mL)
Pad, topical [instant hand sanitizer/towelette]:
Isagel®: 60% (50s, 300s)
Purell®: 62% (24s) [contains aloe, moisturizers, tartrazine, vitamin A, vitamin E]
Purell®: 62% (35s, 175s) [contains moisturizers, vitamin E]
Solution, topical [instant hand sanitizer]:
Protection Plus®: 62% (800 mL)

References
Barceloux DG, Bond GR, Krenzelok EP, et al, "American Academy of Clinical Toxicology Practice Guidelines on the Treatment of Methanol Poisoning," J Toxicol Clin Toxicol, 2002, 40(4):415-46.

Chernow B, ed, "Poisoning," Essentials of Critical Care Pharmacology, 2nd ed, Baltimore: Williams & Wilkins, 1994, 501-29.

Pennington CR and Pithie AD, "Ethanol Lock in the Management of Catheter Occlusion," JPEN J Parenter Enteral Nutr, 1987, 11 (5):507-8.

Poisoning and Drug Overdose, 2nd ed, Olson KR, ed, Norwalk, Connecticut: Appleton and Lange, 1994, 339-40.

Werlin SL, Lausten T, Jessens, et al, "Treatment of Central Venous Catheter Occlusions With Ethanol and Hydrochloric Acid," JPEN J Parenter Enteral Nutr, 1995, 19(5):416-8.

◆ **Aldactazide** see Hydrochlorothiazide and Spironolactone on page 1025

◆ **Aldactazide 25 (Can)** see Hydrochlorothiazide and Spironolactone on page 1025

◆ **Aldactazide 50 (Can)** see Hydrochlorothiazide and Spironolactone on page 1025

◆ **Aldactone** see Spironolactone on page 1930

Aldesleukin (al des LOO kin)

Medication Safety Issues
Sound-alike/look-alike issues:
Aldesleukin may be confused with oprelvekin
Proleukin® may be confused with oprelvekin

High alert medication:
The Institute for Safe Medication Practices (ISMP) includes this medication among its list of drug classes

which have a heightened risk of causing significant patient harm when used in error.

Related Information

Emetogenic Potential of Antineoplastic Agents in Children *on page 2327*

Safe Handling of Hazardous Drugs *on page 2419*

Brand Names: U.S. Proleukin

Brand Names: Canada Proleukin®

Therapeutic Category Antineoplastic Agent, Biologic Response Modulator; Antineoplastic Agent, Miscellaneous; Biological Response Modulator

Generic Availability (U.S.) No

Use Treatment of metastatic renal cell carcinoma and metastatic melanoma (FDA approved in adults); has been used in the treatment of acute myeloid leukemia (AML)

Pregnancy Risk Factor C

Pregnancy Considerations Maternal toxicity and embryocidal effects were noted in animal studies. There are no adequate and well-controlled studies in pregnant women; use during pregnancy only if benefits to the mother outweigh potential risk to the fetus. Contraception is recommended for fertile males or females using this medication.

Breast-Feeding Considerations Due to the potential for serious adverse reactions in the nursing infant, breast-feeding should be discontinued during treatment.

Contraindications Hypersensitivity to aldesleukin or any component; abnormal thallium stress test or pulmonary function tests; organ allografts (due to increased risk of rejection); **retreatment** in patients who have experienced sustained ventricular tachycardia (≥5 beats), cardiac rhythm disturbances not controlled or unresponsive to management, recurrent chest pain with ECG changes (consistent with angina or MI), intubation required >72 hours, cardiac tamponade; renal dysfunction requiring dialysis >72 hours, coma or toxic psychosis lasting >48 hours, repetitive or difficult to control seizures, bowel ischemia/perforation, and GI bleeding requiring surgery

Warnings Hazardous agent; use appropriate precautions for handling and disposal (NIOSH, 2012). High-dose aldesleukin therapy is associated with capillary leak syndrome (CLS), resulting in hypotension and reduced organ perfusion (occurring within 2-12 hours after start of treatment) which may be severe and fatal and is characterized by vascular tone loss and extravasation of plasma proteins and fluid into extravascular space **[U.S. Boxed Warning]**; CLS may be associated with cardiac arrhythmias, angina, MI, respiratory insufficiency requiring intubation, GI bleeding or infarction, renal insufficiency, edema, and mental status changes; therapy should be restricted to patients with normal cardiac and pulmonary functions as defined by thallium stress and formal pulmonary function testing. Monitor fluid status and organ perfusion status carefully; consider fluids and/or pressor agents to maintain organ perfusion. Withhold treatment for signs of organ failure (due to hypoperfusion), altered mental status, reduced urine output, systolic BP <90 mm Hg (in adults), or cardiac arrhythmia. Once blood pressure is normalized, may consider diuretics for excessive weight gain/edema. Recovery from CLS generally begins soon after treatment cessation. Hold aldesleukin administration in patients developing moderate to severe lethargy or somnolence as continued administration may result in coma **[U.S. Boxed Warning]**; may exacerbate disease symptoms in patients with clinically unrecognized or untreated CNS metastases thoroughly evaluate and treat all patients with CNS metastases prior to therapy

Precautions Use with extreme caution in patients with normal thallium stress tests and pulmonary functions tests who have a history of prior cardiac or pulmonary disease **[U.S. Boxed Warning]**; intensive aldesleukin treatment is associated with impaired neutrophil function (reduced chemotaxis) and with an increased risk of disseminated infection (particularly with *Staphylococcus aureus*) including sepsis and bacterial endocarditis **[U.S. Boxed Warning]**; patients with indwelling central lines are particularly at increased risk of infection; treat preexisting bacterial infections prior to initiation of aldesleukin therapy; standard supportive care during high-dose aldesleukin treatment includes acetaminophen to relieve fever and chills and an H_2 antagonist to reduce the risk of GI ulceration and/or bleeding; closely monitor for thyroid abnormalities; mental status changes (irritability, confusion, depression) can occur and may indicate bacteremia, sepsis, hypoperfusion, CNS malignancy, or CNS toxicity; use with caution in patients with known seizure disorders; use with caution in patients with autoimmune disease or inflammatory disorders; may exacerbate condition; exacerbation and/or new onset have been reported with aldesleukin and interferon alfa combination therapy; may impair hepatic function; concomitant hepatotoxic agents may increase the risk of hepatotoxicity; adults must have a serum creatinine ≤1.5 mg/dL prior to treatment; may impair renal function; concomitant nephrotoxic agents may increase the risk of renal toxicity; enhancement of cellular immune function may increase the risk of allograft rejection in transplant patients; an acute array of symptoms resembling aldesleukin adverse reactions (fever, chills, nausea, rash, pruritus, diarrhea, hypotension, edema and oliguria) were observed within 1-4 hours after iodinated contrast media administration, usually when given within 4 weeks after aldesleukin treatment, although has been reported several months after aldesleukin treatment. Should be administered under the supervision of an experienced cancer chemotherapy physician in a facility with cardiopulmonary or intensive specialists and intensive care facilities available **[U.S. Boxed Warning]**.

Adverse Reactions

Cardiovascular: Arrhythmia, cardiac arrest, cardiovascular disorder (includes blood pressure and HF and ECG changes), edema, hypotension, MI, peripheral edema, supraventricular tachycardia, tachycardia, vasodilation, ventricular tachycardia

Central nervous system: Anxiety, chills, coma, confusion, dizziness, fever, malaise, pain, psychosis, somnolence, stupor

Dermatologic: Exfoliative dermatitis, pruritus, rash

Endocrine & metabolic: Acidosis, hypocalcemia, hypomagnesemia

Gastrointestinal: Abdomen enlarged, abdominal pain, anorexia, diarrhea, nausea, stomatitis, vomiting, weight gain

Hematologic: Anemia, coagulation disorder (includes intravascular coagulopathy), leukopenia, thrombocytopenia

Hepatic: Alkaline phosphatase increased, AST increased, hyperbilirubinemia

Neuromuscular & skeletal: Weakness

Renal: Acute renal failure, anuria, creatinine increased, oliguria

Respiratory: Apnea, cough, dyspnea; lung disorder (includes pulmonary congestion, rales, and rhonchi); respiratory disorder (includes acute respiratory distress syndrome, infiltrates and pulmonary changes); rhinitis

Miscellaneous: Antibody formation, infection, sepsis

Rare but important or life-threatening: Allergic interstitial nephritis, anaphylaxis, angioedema, asthma, atrial arrhythmia, AV block, blindness (transient or permanent), bowel infarction/necrosis/perforation, bradycardia, bullous pemphigoid, capillary leak syndrome, cardiomyopathy, cellulitis, cerebral edema, cerebral lesions, cerebral vasculitis, cholecystitis, colitis, crescentic IgA glomerulonephritis, Crohn's disease exacerbation, delirium, depression (severe; leading to suicide), diabetes mellitus, duodenal ulcer, encephalopathy, endocarditis, extrapyramidal syndrome, hemorrhage (including cerebral, gastrointestinal, retroperitoneal, subarachnoid, subdural), hepatic failure, hepatitis, hepatosplenomegaly, hypertension, hyperuricemia, hypothermia, hyperthyroidism, inflammatory arthritis, injection site necrosis, insomnia, intestinal obstruction, intestinal perforation, leukocytosis, malignant hyperthermia, meningitis, myocardial ischemia, myocarditis, myopathy, myositis, neuralgia, neuritis, neuropathy, neutropenia, NPN increased, oculobulbar myasthenia gravis, optic neuritis, organ perfusion decreased, pancreatitis, pericardial effusion, pericarditis, peripheral gangrene, phlebitis, pneumonia, pneumothorax, pulmonary edema, pulmonary embolus, respiratory acidosis, respiratory arrest, respiratory failure, rhabdomyolysis, scleroderma, seizure, Stevens-Johnson syndrome, stroke, syncope, thrombosis, thyroiditis, tracheoesophageal fistula, transient ischemic attack, tubular necrosis, ventricular extrasystoles

Drug Interactions

Metabolism/Transport Effects None known.

Avoid Concomitant Use

Avoid concomitant use of Aldesleukin with any of the following: CloZAPine; Corticosteroids; Dipyrone

Increased Effect/Toxicity

Aldesleukin may increase the levels/effects of: CloZAPine; DULoxetine; Hypotensive Agents; Iodinated Contrast Agents

The levels/effects of Aldesleukin may be increased by: Barbiturates; Dipyrone; Interferons (Alfa)

Decreased Effect

The levels/effects of Aldesleukin may be decreased by: Corticosteroids

Stability Hazardous agent; use appropriate precautions for handling and disposal (NIOSH, 2012). Store in refrigerator; do not freeze; reconstituted solution is stable 48 hours in refrigerator or at room temperature; since aldesleukin contains no preservatives, refrigerated storage of the reconstituted solution is preferred; reconstituted solution packaged in tuberculin syringes for SubQ administration are stable 14 days refrigerated and 6 hours at room temperature; compatible **only** with D_5W; incompatible with sodium chloride solutions; do not mix with other medications; protect from light.

Mechanism of Action Aldesleukin is a human recombinant interleukin-2 product which promotes proliferation, differentiation, and recruitment of T and B cells, natural killer (NK) cells, and thymocytes; causes cytolytic activity in a subset of lymphocytes and subsequent interactions between the immune system and malignant cells; can stimulate lymphokine-activated killer (LAK) cells and tumor-infiltrating lymphocytes (TIL) cells.

Pharmacokinetics (Adult data unless noted)

Absorption: Oral: Not absorbed

Distribution: Primarily into plasma, lymphocytes, lungs, liver, kidney, and spleen

V_d: Adults: 4-7 L

Metabolism: Metabolized to amino acids in the cells lining the proximal convoluted tubules of the kidney

Half-life:

Children:

Distribution: 14 ± 6 minutes

Elimination: 51 ± 11 minutes

Adults:

Distribution: 6-27 minutes

Elimination: 85 minutes

Time to peak serum concentration: SubQ: 2-3 hours

Clearance: Adults: 7.2-16.1 L/hour

Dosing: Usual A wide variety of dosages have been or are currently under investigation (refer to individual protocols): Infants, Children, and Adolescents: **Acute Myeloid Leukemia (AML):** I.V.: 9 million units/m^2/day (9 x 10^6 units/m^2/day) continuous infusion over 24 hours daily for 4 days; followed in 4 days with 1.6 million units/m^2/day (1.6 x 10^6 units/m^2/day) continuous infusion over 24 hours daily for 10 days (Lange, 2008)

Adults: **Metastatic renal cell carcinoma and metastatic melanoma:** I.V.: Initial: 600,000 units/kg every 8 hours for a maximum of 14 doses; repeat after 9 days for a total of 28 doses per course; retreat if tumor shrinkage observed (and if no contraindications) at least 7 weeks after previous course

Dosage modification for toxicity (Adults): Hold or interrupt a dose, **do not dose reduce:**

Cardiovascular toxicity:

Withhold dose for atrial fibrillation, supraventricular tachycardia, or bradycardia that is persistent, recurrent, or requires treatment; may resume when asymptomatic with full recovery to normal sinus rhythm

Withhold dose for systolic BP <90 mm Hg (with increasing pressor requirements); may resume treatment when systolic BP ≥90 mm Hg and stable or pressor requirements improve

Withhold dose for any ECG change consistent with MI, ischemia, myocarditis (with or without chest pain), or suspected cardiac ischemia; may resume when asymptomatic, MI/myocarditis have been ruled out, suspicion of angina is low, or there is no evidence of ventricular hypokinesia

CNS toxicity: Withhold dose for mental status change, including moderate confusion or agitation; may resume when resolved completely

Dermatologic toxicity: Withhold dose for bullous dermatitis or marked worsening of preexisting skin condition; may treat with antihistamines or topical products (do not use topical steroids); may resume with resolution of all signs of bullous dermatitis

Gastrointestinal: Withhold dose for stool guaiac repeatedly >3-4+; may resume with negative stool guaiac

Hepatotoxicity: Withhold dose and discontinue treatment for balance of cycle for signs of hepatic failure, encephalopathy, increasing ascites, liver pain, hypoglycemia; may initiate a new course, if indicated, only after at least 7 weeks past resolution of all signs of hepatic failure (including hospital discharge)

Infection: Withhold dose for sepsis syndrome, clinically unstable; may resume when sepsis syndrome has resolved, patient is clinically stable, and infection is under treatment

Renal toxicity:

Withhold dose for serum creatinine >4.5 mg/dL (or ≥4 mg/dL with severe volume overload, acidosis, or hyperkalemia); may resume when <4 mg/dL and fluid/electrolyte status is stable

Withhold dose for persistent oliguria or urine output <10 mL/hour for 16-24 hours with rising serum creatinine; may resume when urine output >10 mL/hour with serum creatinine decrease of >1.5 mg/dL or normalization

Respiratory toxicity: Withhold dose for oxygen saturation <90%; may resume when >90%

Retreatment with aldesleukin is **contraindicated** with the following toxicities: Sustained ventricular tachycardia (≥5 beats), refractory uncontrolled or unresponsive cardiac arrhythmias, recurrent chest pain with ECG changes consistent with angina or MI, cardiac tamponade, intubation >72 hours, renal failure requiring dialysis for >72 hours, coma or toxic psychosis lasting >48 hours, repetitive or refractory seizures, bowel ischemia/perforation, or GI bleeding requiring surgery

Administration Hazardous agent; use appropriate precautions for handling and disposal (NIOSH, 2012).

I.V.: Reconstitute with 1.2 mL preservative-free SWI (swirl, do not shake); resulting concentration is 18 million (18 x 10^6) units/mL (1.1 mg/mL); further dilute dosage in D_5W [plastic (polyvinyl chloride) bags result in more consistent drug delivery and are recommended] to a final concentration between 0.49-1.1 million units/mL (30-70 mcg/mL) and infuse over 15 minutes; allow solution to reach room temperature prior to administration; for continuous infusions, dilute in D_5W maintaining the same final concentration; final dilutions <0.49 million units/mL (30 mcg/mL) or >1.1 million units/mL (70 mcg/mL) have shown increased variability in drug stability and bioactivity and should be avoided; addition of 0.1% albumin has been used to increase stability and decrease the extent of sorption if low final concentrations cannot be avoided; do not use in-line filter when administering; flush line before and after with D_5W

SubQ: Reconstituted solution may be administered subcutaneously without further dilution (**Note:** Subcutaneous administration is a non-FDA approved route)

Monitoring Parameters Baseline chest x-ray, pulmonary function tests and thallium stress study; CBC with differential, platelet counts, electrolytes, BUN, serum creatinine, hepatic enzymes, vital signs, weight, pulse oximetry, arterial blood gases (if pulmonary symptoms), fluid intake and output; cardiac monitoring (in a patient with a decreased blood pressure, especially systolic BP <90 mm Hg); ECG if an abnormal complex or rhythm is seen; monitor for change in mental status, and for signs of infection

Additional Information 18×10^6 int. units = 1.1 mg protein

Dosage Forms Excipient information presented when available (limited, particularly for generics); consult specific product labeling.

Solution Reconstituted, Intravenous [preservative free]:
  Proleukin: 22,000,000 units (1 ea)

References

Bergmann L, Heil G, Kolbe K, et al, "Interleukin-2 Bolus Infusion as Late Consolidation Therapy in 2nd Remission of Acute Myeloblastic Leukemia," *Leuk Lymphoma*, 1995, 16(3-4):271-9.

Lange BJ, Smith FO, Feusner J, et al, "Outcomes in CCG-2961, a Children's Oncology Group Phase 3 Trial for Untreated Pediatric Acute Myeloid Leukemia: A Report From the Children's Oncology Group," *Blood*, 2008, 111(3):1044-53.

National Institute for Occupational Safety and Health (NIOSH), "NIOSH List of Antineoplastic and Other Hazardous Drugs in Healthcare Settings 2012." Available at http://www.cdc.gov/niosh/docs/2012-150/pdfs/2012-150.pdf. Accessed January 21, 2013.

Sievers EL, Lange BJ, Sondel PM, et al, "Feasibility, Toxicity, and Biologic Response of Interleukin-2 After Consolidation Chemotherapy for Acute Myelogenous Leukemia: A Report From the Children's Cancer Group," *J Clin Oncol*, 1998, 16(3):914-9.

Whittington R and Faulds D, "Interleukin-2: A Review of Its Pharmacological Properties and Therapeutic Use in Patients With Cancer," *Drugs*, 1993, 46(3):446-514.

◆ **Aldomet** see Methyldopa on page 1376

◆ **Aldurazyme** see Laronidase on page 1210

◆ **Aldurazyme® (Can)** see Laronidase on page 1210

◆ **Aler-Dryl [OTC]** see DiphenhydrAMINE (Systemic) on page 673

◆ **Alertec® (Can)** see Modafinil on page 1429

◆ **Alevazol [OTC]** see Clotrimazole (Topical) on page 527

◆ **Aleve [OTC]** see Naproxen on page 1470

◆ **Aleve (Can)** see Naproxen on page 1470

◆ **Aleveer [OTC]** see Capsaicin on page 367

◆ **Alfenta** see Alfentanil on page 93

Alfentanil (al FEN ta nil)

Medication Safety Issues

Sound-alike/look-alike issues:
  Alfentanil may be confused with Anafranil, fentanyl, remifentanil, sufentanil
  Alfenta may be confused with Sufenta

High alert medication:
  The Institute for Safe Medication Practices (ISMP) includes this medication among its list of drug classes which have a heightened risk of causing significant patient harm when used in error.

Related Information
  Opioid Conversion Table on page 2242

Brand Names: U.S. Alfenta

Brand Names: Canada Alfenta; Alfentanil Injection, USP

Therapeutic Category Analgesic, Narcotic; General Anesthetic

Generic Availability (U.S.) Yes

Use Analgesia; analgesia adjunct; anesthetic agent

Pregnancy Risk Factor C

Pregnancy Considerations Adverse events were observed in some animal reproduction studies. Alfentanil is known to cross the placenta, which may result in severe respiratory depression in the newborn (Mattingly, 2003). When used for pain relief during labor, opioids may temporarily affect the heart rate of the fetus (ACOG, 2002). Use during labor and delivery is not recommended by the manufacturer.

Breast-Feeding Considerations Alfentanil is excreted into breast milk. Significant concentrations were observed in breast milk following administration of alfentanil 60 mcg/kg to nine women who underwent postpartum tubal ligation; concentrations were undetectable after 28 hours. The manufacturer recommends that caution be used if administered to nursing women. Parenteral opioids used during labor have the potential to interfere with a newborn's natural reflex to nurse within the first few hours after birth. Nursing infants exposed to large doses of opioids should be monitored for apnea and sedation (Montgomery, 2012).

Contraindications Hypersensitivity to alfentanil hydrochloride or any component; increased intracranial pressure; severe respiratory depression

Warnings Rapid I.V. infusion may result in skeletal muscle and chest wall rigidity → impaired ventilation → respiratory distress/arrest; inject slowly over 3-5 minutes; nondepolarizing skeletal muscle relaxant may be required. Due to the high incidence of apnea, hypotension, tachycardia, and muscle rigidity, alfentanil should be administered by individuals specifically trained in the use of anesthetic agents and should not be used in diagnostic or therapeutic procedures outside the monitored anesthesia setting; resuscitative and intubation equipment should be readily available.

Precautions Alfentanil shares the toxic potentials of opioid agonists and precautions of opioid agonist therapy should be observed. Use with caution in patients with bradycardia. Use with caution in patients with hypovolemia, cardiovascular disease (including acute MI), or drugs which may exaggerate hypotensive effects (including phenothiazines or general anesthetics); may cause hypotension. Use with caution in patients with preexisting respiratory compromise (hypoxia and/or hypercapnia), COPD or other obstructive pulmonary disease, and kyphoscoliosis or other skeletal disorder which may alter respiratory function. Use with extreme caution in patients with head injury, intracranial lesions, or elevated intracranial pressure; exaggerated elevation of ICP may occur. Use with caution in patients with a history of drug abuse or acute alcoholism; potential for drug dependency exists; tolerance and psychological and physical dependence may occur with prolonged use.

Adverse Reactions

Cardiovascular: Bradycardia, cardiac arrhythmia, orthostatic hypotension, peripheral vasodilation

Central nervous system: CNS depression, confusion, drowsiness, intracranial pressure increased, sedation

Endocrine & metabolic: Antidiuretic hormone release

Gastrointestinal: Constipation, nausea, vomiting

Ocular: Blurred vision

Rare but important or life-threatening: Convulsions, mental depression, paradoxical CNS excitation or delirium, dizziness, dysesthesia, rash, urticaria, itching, biliary tract spasm, urinary tract spasm, respiratory depression, ▶

bronchospasm, laryngospasm, physical and psychological dependence with prolonged use; cold, clammy skin

Drug Interactions

Metabolism/Transport Effects Substrate of CYP3A4 (major); **Note:** Assignment of Major/Minor substrate status based on clinically relevant drug interaction potential

Avoid Concomitant Use

Avoid concomitant use of Alfentanil with any of the following: Azelastine (Nasal); Conivaptan; Crizotinib; Enzalutamide; Fusidic Acid (Systemic); MAO Inhibitors; Paraldehyde; Thalidomide

Increased Effect/Toxicity

Alfentanil may increase the levels/effects of: Alcohol (Ethyl); Alvimopan; Azelastine (Nasal); Beta-Blockers; Buprenorphine; Calcium Channel Blockers (Nondihydropyridine); CNS Depressants; Desmopressin; Diuretics; Hydrocodone; MAO Inhibitors; Methotrimeprazine; Metyrosine; Mirtazapine; Paraldehyde; Pramipexole; Propofol; ROPINIRole; Rotigotine; Selective Serotonin Reuptake Inhibitors; Thalidomide; Zolpidem

The levels/effects of Alfentanil may be increased by: Amphetamines; Anticholinergic Agents; Antifungal Agents (Azole Derivatives, Systemic); Antipsychotic Agents (Phenothiazines); Brimonidine (Topical); Cannabis; Ceritinib; Cimetidine; Conivaptan; Crizotinib; CYP3A4 Inhibitors (Moderate); CYP3A4 Inhibitors (Strong); Dasatinib; Diazepam; Diltiazem; Doxylamine; Dronabinol; Droperidol; Fluconazole; Fusidic Acid (Systemic); HydrOXYzine; Ivacaftor; Kava Kava; Luliconazole; Macrolide Antibiotics; Magnesium Sulfate; Methotrimeprazine; Mifepristone; Nabilone; Perampanel; Rufinamide; Simeprevir; Sodium Oxybate; Stiripentol; Succinylcholine; Tapentadol; Tetrahydrocannabinol

Decreased Effect

Alfentanil may decrease the levels/effects of: Pegvisomant

The levels/effects of Alfentanil may be decreased by: Ammonium Chloride; Enzalutamide; Mixed Agonist / Antagonist Opioids; Naltrexone; Rifamycin Derivatives

Mechanism of Action Binds with stereospecific receptors at many sites within the CNS, increases pain threshold, alters pain perception, inhibits ascending pain pathways; is an ultra short-acting opioid

Pharmacodynamics

Onset of action: Within 5 minutes

Duration: <15-20 minutes

Pharmacokinetics (Adult data unless noted) An early study of continuous infusion suggested nonlinear pharmacokinetics in neonates (Wiest, 1991).

Distribution: V_d beta:

Newborns, premature: 1 L/kg

Children: 0.163-0.48 L/kg

Adults: 0.46 L/kg

Protein binding:

Neonates: 67%

Adults: 88% to 92%

Bound to alpha$_1$-acid glycoprotein

Metabolism: Hepatic

Half-life, elimination:

Newborns, premature: 320-525 minutes

Children: 40-60 minutes

Adults: 83-97 minutes

Dosing: Neonatal I.V.: Doses should be titrated to appropriate effects; wide range of doses is dependent upon desired degree of analgesia/anesthesia

Dose not established; reported range: 9-20 mcg/kg/dose; a high percentage of neonates (GA: 30-40 weeks; PNA <3 days) receiving alfentanil (prior to procedures) at doses of 9-15 mcg/kg (mean dose: 11.7 mcg/kg) developed chest wall rigidity; 9 out of 20 (45%) developed mild or moderate rigidity that did not affect ventilation, while 4 out of

20 (20%) had severe rigidity interfering with respiration for ~5-10 minutes (Pokela, 1992). In a separate study, severe muscle rigidity developed in 5 out of 8 (63%) neonates (GA: 29-36 weeks; PNA 2-6 days) following a dose of 20 mcg/kg (Saarenmaa, 1996); use of a skeletal muscle relaxant to prevent chest wall rigidity is recommended; however, smaller alfentanil doses may be required in newborns.

Dosing: Usual I.V.: Doses should be titrated to appropriate effects; wide range of doses is dependent upon desired degree of analgesia/anesthesia

Children:

Pre-induction, emergence agitation prevention, analgesia in tonsillectomy, or dental procedure patients undergoing general anesthesia: 10-20 mcg/kg/dose (Rahman Al-Refai, 2007; Annila, 1999; Bartolek, 2007; Kim, 2009; Kwak, 2010; Ng, 1999)

Procedural analgesia for LP or bone marrow aspiration (in addition to propofol): Intermittent doses of 2-3 mcg/kg/dose (total dose: mean: 1.4 mcg/kg ± 2.4; range: 1.8-9.6 mcg/kg) were administered to 20 patients ages 2-16 years old (von Heijne, 2004)

Adults: Use lean body weight for patients who weigh >20% over ideal body weight; see table.

Alfentanil: Adult Dosing

Indication	Approximate Duration of Anesthesia (minute)	Induction Period (Initial Dose) (mcg/kg)	Maintenance Period (Increments/ Infusion)	Total Dose (mcg/kg)	Effects
Incremental injection	≤30	8-20	3-5 mcg/kg or 0.5-1 mcg/kg/minute	8-40	Spontaneously breathing or assisted ventilation when required.
	30-60	20-50	5-15 mcg/kg	Up to 75	Assisted or controlled ventilation required. Attenuation of response to laryngoscopy and intubation.
Continuous infusion	>45	50-75	0.5-3 mcg/kg/minute; average infusion rate: 1-1.5 mcg/kg/minute	Dependent on duration of procedure	Assisted or controlled ventilation required. Some attenuation of response to intubation and incision, with intraoperative stability.
Anesthetic induction	>45	130-245	0.5-1.5 mcg/kg/minute or general anesthetic	Dependent on duration of procedure	Assisted or controlled ventilation required. Administer slowly (over 3 minutes). Concentration of inhalation agents reduced by 30% to 50% for initial hour.

Administration Parenteral: I.V.: Inject slowly over 3-5 minutes or by I.V. continuous infusion; maximum concentration: 80 mcg/mL

Monitoring Parameters Respiratory rate, blood pressure, heart rate, neurological status (for degree of analgesia/anesthesia)

Controlled Substance C-II

Dosage Forms Excipient information presented when available (limited, particularly for generics); consult specific product labeling.

Injectable, Injection [preservative free]:

Alfenta: 500 mcg/mL (2 mL, 5 mL)

Generic: 500 mcg/mL (2 mL, 5 mL)

References

ACOG Committee on Practice Bulletins-Obstetrics, "ACOG Practice Bulletin. Clinical Management Guidelines for Obstetrician-Gynecologists Number 36, July 2002. Obstetric Analgesia and Anesthesia," Obstet Gynecol, 2002, 100(1):177-91.

Annila P, Viitanen H, Reinikainen P, et al, "Induction Characteristics of Thiopentone/Suxamethonium, Propofol/Alfentanil or Halothane Alone in Children Aged 1-3 Years," *Eur J Anaesthesiol*, 1999, 16(6):359-66.

Bartolek D, Lajtman Z, Zdravcević-Sakić K, et al, "The Optimal Pediatric Induction Dose of Propofol in Combination With Reduced-Dose Rocuronium and Alfentanil for Day-Case Tonsillectomy in Children," *Int J Pediatr Otorhinolaryngol*, 2007, 71(12):1873-81.

Davis PJ, Killian A, Stiller RL, et al, "Pharmacokinetics of Alfentanil in Newborn Premature Infants and Older Children," *Dev Pharmacol Ther*, 1989, 13(1):21-7.

Kim JY, Chang YJ, Lee JY, et al, "Post-Induction Alfentanil Reduces Sevoflurane-Associated Emergence Agitation in Children Undergoing an Adenotonsillectomy," *Acta Anaesthesiol Scand*, 2009, 53 (5):678-81.

Kwak HJ, Kim JY, Min SK, et al, "Optimal Bolus Dose of Alfentanil for Successful Tracheal Intubation During Sevoflurane Induction With and Without Nitrous Oxide in Children," *Br J Anaesth*, 2010, 104 (5):628-32.

Marlow N, Weindling AM, Van Peer A, et al, "Alfentanil Pharmacokinetics in Preterm Infants," *Arch Dis Child*, 1990, 65(4 Spec No):349-51.

Mattingly JE, D'Alessio J, and Ramanathan J, "Effects of Obstetric Analgesics and Anesthetics on the Neonate: A Review," *Paediatr Drugs*, 2003, 5(9):615-27.

Meistelman C, Saint-Maurice C, Lepaul M, et al, "A Comparison of Alfentanil Pharmacokinetics in Children and Adults," *Anesthesiology*, 1987, 66(1):13-6.

Montgomery A, Hale TW, and Academy Of Breastfeeding Medicine, "ABM Clinical Protocol #15: Analgesia and Anesthesia For the Breastfeeding Mother, Revised 2012," *Breastfeed Med*, 2012, 7 (6):547-53.

Ng KP and Wang CY, "Alfentanil for Intubation Under Halothane Anaesthesia in Children," *Paediatr Anaesth*, 1999, 9(6):491-4.

Pokela ML, Ryhänen PT, Koivisto ME, et al, "Alfentanil-Induced Rigidity in Newborn Infants," *Anesth Analg*, 1992, 75(2):252-7.

Rahman Al-Refai A, Al-Mujadi H, Petrova Ivanova M, et al, "Prevention of Pain on Injection of Propofol: A Comparison of Remifentanil With Alfentanil in Children," *Minerva Anestesiol*, 2007, 73(4):219-23.

Saarenmaa E, Huttunen P, Leppäluoto J, et al, "Alfentanil as Procedural Pain Relief in Newborn Infants," *Arch Dis Child Fetal Neonatal Ed*, 1996, 75(2):F103-7.

Von Heijne M, Bredlöv B, Söderhäll S, et al, "Propofol or Propofol - Alfentanil Anesthesia for Painful Procedures in the Pediatric Oncology Ward," *Paediatr Anaesth*, 2004, 14(8):670-5.

Wiest DB, Ohning BL, and Garner SS, "The Disposition of Alfentanil in Neonates With Respiratory Distress," *Pharmacotherapy*, 1991, 11 (4):308-11.

♦ **Alfentanil Hydrochloride** see Alfentanil on page 93

♦ **Alfentanil Injection, USP (Can)** see Alfentanil on page 93

♦ **Alglucosidase** see Alglucosidase Alfa on page 95

Alglucosidase Alfa (al gloo KOSE i dase AL fa)

Medication Safety Issues
Sound-alike/look-alike issues:
Alglucosidase alfa may be confused with agalsidase alfa, agalsidase beta, alglucerase

Brand Names: U.S. Lumizyme; Myozyme

Brand Names: Canada Myozyme®

Therapeutic Category Enzyme

Generic Availability (U.S.) No

Use
Myozyme®: Replacement therapy of alpha-glucosidase (GAA) for infantile-onset Pompe disease [FDA approved in pediatric patients (age not specified)]

Lumizyme®: Replacement therapy of alpha-glucosidase (GAA) for late-onset (noninfantile) Pompe disease without evidence of cardiac hypertrophy (FDA approved in ages ≥8 years and adults)

Prescribing and Access Restrictions As a requirement of the REMS program, access to this medication is restricted. Lumizyme® is available only through Lumizyme® ACE (Alglucosidase Alfa Control and Education) program; only trained and certified prescribers and healthcare facilities enrolled in the program may prescribe, dispense, or administer Lumizyme®. Patients must be

enrolled in and meet all the conditions of the program to receive therapy. For enrollment, call 1-800-745-4447.

Access to Myozyme® is restricted by the manufacturer, and allowed only to patients <8 years of age with infantile-onset or late-onset Pompe disease (who are restricted from access to Lumizyme®) or to patients of any age with a diagnosis of infantile-onset Pompe disease or evidence of cardiac hypertrophy. To obtain Myozyme®, call 1-800-745-4447; no formal distribution program is established, but availability is controlled by Genzyme.

Pregnancy Risk Factor B

Pregnancy Considerations Animal reproduction studies have not demonstrated teratogenicity or fertility impairment. Limited information is available related to use of alglucosidase alfa in pregnant women (deVries 2011). A registry has been established for Pompe patients; women of childbearing potential are encouraged to enroll in the registry (www.pomperegistry.com or 1-800-745-4447).

Breast-Feeding Considerations Endogenous acid alfa-glucosidase can be detected in breast milk; concentrations are lower in women with Pompe disease. Following an infusion of alglucosidase alfa in one woman with Pompe disease, maximum enzyme activity was found in breast milk 2.5 hours after the dose and was ~0.3% of the maternal peak plasma value. Activity in breast milk returned to baseline values within 24 hours after the infusion (de Vries, 2011). A registry has been established for Pompe patients; women who are nursing are encouraged to enroll in the registry (www.pomperegistry.com or 1-800-745-4447)

Contraindications Hypersensitivity to alglucosidase alfa or any component

Warnings Life-threatening anaphylactic reactions have been observed in some patients during and within 3 hours after infusions. Therefore, appropriate medical support should be readily available when alglucosidase alfa is administered. **[U.S. Boxed Warning]** Reactions have included anaphylactic shock, cardiac arrest, respiratory distress, hypotension, bradycardia, hypoxia, bronchospasm, throat tightness, dyspnea, angioedema, and urticaria. Experience from clinical trials and expanded access programs has shown approximately 14% of patients treated with alglucosidase alfa develop allergic reaction involving at least 2 of the 3 following body systems: Cardiovascular, respiratory, or cutaneous. If anaphylactic or other severe allergic reaction occurs, immediately discontinue administration and provide appropriate medical treatment. Use extreme caution if readministration is attempted. Patients who develop IgE antibodies to alglucosidase alfa may be at a higher risk for occurrence of anaphylaxis and severe allergic reactions.

Patients with compromised cardiac or respiratory function may be at risk of serious acute exacerbation of their cardiac or respiratory compromise due to infusion reactions and may require additional monitoring. **[U.S. Boxed Warning]**; acute cardiorespiratory failure requiring intubation and inotropic support has been reported up to 72 hours postinfusion in patients with infantile-onset Pompe disease with underlying cardiac hypertrophy which may possibly be secondary to intravenous fluid overload from drug administration.

Infusion-related reactions are common; reactions may occur at any time during administration or for up to 2 hours postinfusion; discontinue immediately for severe hypersensitivity or anaphylactic reaction; mild-to-moderate reactions may be managed by reducing the infusion rate and/or administering antihistamines and/or antipyretics. Appropriate medical support for the management of infusion reactions should be readily available. Use caution with subsequent infusions; infusion reactions have occurred despite premedication with antihistamines, antipyretics, and/or steroids. Patients with acute underlying illness are at greater risk for infusion reactions. Although less common, delayed onset (within 48 hours after administration) infusion reactions have also occurred.

Cardiac arrhythmias (including ventricular fibrillation, ventricular tachycardia, and bradycardia) have been observed in patients with cardiac hypertrophy in patients undergoing general anesthesia during central venous catheter placement; relationship not well established; use caution.

Injection contains polysorbate 80 (Tween 80®) which may cause allergic reactions in susceptible individuals. In premature neonates, thrombocytopenia, ascites, pulmonary deterioration, and renal and hepatic failure have been reported after receiving parenteral products containing polysorbate 80 (Alade, 1986; CDC, 1984). Infusion of polysorbate 80-containing solutions through polyvinyl chloride tubing may cause DEHP to leach into the solution; in immature animals, exposure to DEHP may adversely affect the development of the male reproductive tract.

Lumizyme® is available only through a restricted distribution program due to the potential risk of rapid disease progression in patients <8 years of age **[U.S. Boxed Warning]**. Only health care providers enrolled in the program may prescribe, dispense, or administer Lumizyme® (Lumizyme ACE Program® 1-800-745-4447).

Precautions Systemic immune mediated and severe cutaneous reactions have been reported. Patients should be monitored for the development of systemic immune-complex mediated reactions involving the skin and other organs during therapy. Nephrotic syndrome secondary to membranous glomerulonephritis has also been observed.

Adverse Reactions

Cardiovascular: Bradycardia, chest pain, flushing, oxygen saturation decreased, peripheral edema, tachycardia

Central nervous system: Drowsiness, headache, malaise, pain, pain (postprocedural), vertigo

Dermatologic: Diaper rash, hyperhidrosis, pruritus, skin rash, urticaria

Endocrine & metabolic: Hypokalemia

Gastrointestinal: Abdominal pain, constipation, diarrhea, dyspepsia, gastroenteritis, gastroesophageal reflux disease, oral candidiasis, vomiting

Hematologic & oncologic: Anemia, lymphadenopathy

Hypersensitivity: Anaphylaxis

Immunologic: Development of IgG antibodies (may affect efficacy)

Local: Catheter infection, infusion site reaction

Neuromuscular & skeletal: Muscle twitching, musculoskeletal pain, myalgia, stiffness, tremor

Ophthalmic: Blurred vision

Otic: Auditory impairment, otalgia, otitis media

Renal: Nephrolithiasis

Respiratory: Bronchiolitis, cough, dyspnea, epistaxis, nasopharyngitis, pharyngitis, pneumonia, respiratory distress, respiratory failure, respiratory tract infection, rhinitis, rhinorrhea, tachypnea, upper respiratory tract infection

Miscellaneous: Fever, infusion related reaction

Rare but important or life-threatening: Acute cardiorespiratory failure, agitation, angioedema, aortic dissection, apnea, arthritis, bronchospasm, cardiac arrest, cardiac failure, cardiorespiratory arrest, cerebrovascular accident, chest discomfort, conjunctivitis, coronary artery disease, cyanosis, dehydration, dermal ulcer, edema, erythema, facial edema, facial erythema, fatigue, flu-like symptoms, hemothorax, herniated disk, hyperparathyroidism, hypersensitivity, hypertension, hypervolemia, hypotension, increased erythrocyte sedimentation rate, increased lacrimation, insomnia, irritability, livedo reticularis, muscle spasm, nausea, nephrotic syndrome (secondary to membranous glomerulonephritis), pallor,

periorbital edema, pharyngeal edema, pneumothorax, proteinuria, pulmonary infection, respiratory syncytial virus infection, restlessness, retching, rigors, sepsis, skin necrosis, stridor, wheezing

Drug Interactions

Metabolism/Transport Effects None known.

Avoid Concomitant Use There are no known interactions where it is recommended to avoid concomitant use.

Increased Effect/Toxicity There are no known significant interactions involving an increase in effect.

Decreased Effect There are no known significant interactions involving a decrease in effect.

Stability Store vials between 2°C and 8°C (36°F and 46°F); do not freeze. Protect from light. Allow vials to reach room temperature prior to reconstitution. Final solutions for infusion should be used immediately if possible, but may be stored for up to 24 hours between 2°C and 8°C (36°F and 46°F); do not freeze. Protect from light.

Mechanism of Action Alglucosidase alfa is a recombinant form of the enzyme acid alpha-glucosidase (GAA), which is required for glycogen cleavage. Due to an inherited GAA deficiency or absence, glycogen accumulates in the tissues of patients with Pompe disease, leading to progressive muscle weakness. In infantile-onset Pompe disease, glycogen accumulates in cardiac and skeletal muscles and hepatic tissue, leading to cardiomyopathy and respiratory failure. Juvenile- and adult-onset Pompe disease are limited to glycogen accumulation in skeletal muscle, leading to respiratory failure. Alglucosidase alfa binds to mannose-6-phosphate receptors on the cell surface, is internalized, and transported to lysosomes where it is activated for increased enzymatic glycogen cleavage.

Pharmacokinetics (Adult data unless noted)

Distribution: V_{ss}: Infants 1-7 months: 80-147 mL/kg

Half-life elimination: Infants 1-7 months and adults: 2-3 hours

Elimination: Clearance:
Infants 1-7 months: 24-25 mL/hour/kg
Adults: 601 mL/hour

Dosing: Usual Pompe disease:

Infantile-onset: Myozyme®: Infants ≥1 month, Children, and Adolescents: I.V.: 20 mg/kg over ~4 hours every 2 weeks

Late-onset (noninfantile): Lumizyme®: Children ≥8 years, Adolescents, and Adults: I.V.: 20 mg/kg over ~4 hours every 2 weeks

Administration Visually inspect the powder in the vial for particulate matter prior to reconstitution. After vial reaches room temperature, reconstitute each vial with 10.3 mL SWI. Inject slowly down internal side wall of vial (do not inject into powder; avoid foaming). Roll and tilt gently; do not invert, swirl, or shake. Resulting solution contains 5 mg/mL. Visually inspect the solution following reconstitution for particulate matter. To make final infusion, add the desired dose amount of reconstituted solution to 50-1000 mL NS (volume determined by patient's weight; see product labeling for complete details) to make a final concentration of 0.5-4 mg/mL. Do not use filter needle for preparation. Remove airspace from infusion bag prior to admixture to minimize particle formation due to sensitivity of drug to air-liquid interfaces. Do not shake. Final solutions for infusion should be used immediately if possible, but may be stored for up to 24 hours between 2°C and 8°C (36°F and 46°F); do not freeze. Protect from light.

Infuse over ~4 hours; initiate at 1 mg/kg/hour. If tolerated, increase by 2 mg/kg/hour every 30 minutes to a maximum rate of 7 mg/kg/hour. Decrease rate or temporarily hold for infusion reactions. Infuse through a low protein-binding, 0.2 micron in-line filter. Do not administer products with visualized particulate matter.

Monitoring Parameters Liver enzymes (baseline and periodically; elevation may be due to disease process);

vital signs during and following infusion; immune mediated reactions; volume overload; periodic urinalysis

The manufacturer recommends monitoring for IgG antibody formation every 3 months for 2 years, then annually. Consider testing if patient develops allergic or other suspected immune mediated reaction. No commercial tests are available; however, sampling kits can be obtained by contacting Genzyme Corporation at 1-800-745-4447.

Additional Information Patients with sustained positive IgG antibody titers (≥12,800) to alglucosidase alfa may have poorer clinical response. Most patients (89%) develop antibodies within the first 3 months of therapy; concern is with patients with sustained high (≥12,800) antibody titers. Patients developing a decreased motor function should be tested for neutralization of enzyme uptake or activity. Infusion reactions are more common in antibody-positive patients. Patients with moderate-to-severe or recurrent reactions with suspected mast-cell activation may be tested for alglucosidase alfa-specific IgE antibodies.

Dosage Forms Excipient information presented when available (limited, particularly for generics); consult specific product labeling.

Solution Reconstituted, Intravenous [preservative free]:
Lumizyme: 50 mg (1 ea) [contains polysorbate 80]
Myozyme: 50 mg (1 ea)

References

Alade SL, Brown RE, and Paquet A Jr, "Polysorbate 80 and E-Ferol Toxicity," *Pediatrics*, 1986, 77(4):593-7.

Centers for Disease Control (CDC), "Unusual Syndrome With Fatalities Among Premature Infants: Association With a New Intravenous Vitamin E Product," *MMWR Morb Mortal Wkly Rep*, 1984, 33 (14):198-9.

de Vries JM, Brugma JD, Ozkan L, et al, "First Experience With Enzyme Replacement Therapy During Pregnancy and Lactation in Pompe Disease," *Mol Genet Metab*, 2011, 104(4):552-5.

Kishnani PS, Corzo D, Nicolino M, et al, "Recombinant Human Acid [Alpha]-Glucosidase: Major Clinical Benefits in Infantile-Onset Pompe Disease," *Neurology*, 2007, 68(2):99-109.

Kishnani PS, Nicolino M, Voit T, et al, "Chinese Hamster Ovary Cell-Derived Recombinant Human Acid Alpha-Glucosidase in Infantile-Onset Pompe Disease," *J Pediatr*, 2006, 149(1):89-97.

Schoser B, Hill V, and Raben N, "Therapeutic Approaches in Glycogen Storage Disease Type II/Pompe Disease," *Neurotherapeutics*, 2008, 5(4):569-78.

◆ **Alinia** *see* Nitazoxanide *on page 1500*

◆ **Alkeran** *see* Melphalan *on page 1328*

◆ **Alkeran® (Can)** *see* Melphalan *on page 1328*

◆ **All Day Allergy [OTC]** *see* Cetirizine *on page 431*

◆ **All Day Allergy Childrens [OTC]** *see* Cetirizine *on page 431*

◆ **All Day Pain Relief [OTC]** *see* Naproxen *on page 1470*

◆ **All Day Relief [OTC]** *see* Naproxen *on page 1470*

◆ **Allegra® (Can)** *see* Fexofenadine *on page 870*

◆ **Allegra Allergy [OTC]** *see* Fexofenadine *on page 870*

◆ **Allegra Allergy Childrens [OTC]** *see* Fexofenadine *on page 870*

◆ **Aller-Chlor [OTC]** *see* Chlorpheniramine *on page 448*

◆ **Allerdryl® (Can)** *see* DiphenhydrAMINE (Systemic) *on page 673*

◆ **Allergy [OTC]** *see* Chlorpheniramine *on page 448*

◆ **Allergy [OTC]** *see* Loratadine *on page 1278*

◆ **Allergy 4 Hour [OTC] [DSC]** *see* Chlorpheniramine *on page 448*

◆ **Allergy Relief [OTC]** *see* Chlorpheniramine *on page 448*

◆ **Allergy Relief [OTC]** *see* DiphenhydrAMINE (Systemic) *on page 673*

◆ **Allergy Relief [OTC]** *see* Loratadine *on page 1278*

◆ **Allergy Relief Childrens [OTC]** *see* DiphenhydrAMINE (Systemic) *on page 673*

◆ **Allergy Relief For Kids [OTC]** *see* Loratadine *on page 1278*

◆ **Allergy-Time [OTC]** *see* Chlorpheniramine *on page 448*

◆ **Allernix (Can)** *see* DiphenhydrAMINE (Systemic) *on page 673*

◆ **Aller-Relief [OTC] (Can)** *see* Cetirizine *on page 431*

◆ **Allfen CD** *see* Guaifenesin and Codeine *on page 985*

◆ **Allfen CDX** *see* Guaifenesin and Codeine *on page 985*

◆ **Alloprin (Can)** *see* Allopurinol *on page 97*

Allopurinol (al oh PURE i nole)

Medication Safety Issues
Sound-alike/look-alike issues:
Allopurinol may be confused with Apresoline
Zyloprim may be confused with ZORprin, Zovirax

Brand Names: U.S. Aloprim; Zyloprim

Brand Names: Canada Alloprin; Apo-Allopurinol; JAMP-Allopurinol; Mar-Allopurinol; Novo-Purol; Zyloprim

Therapeutic Category Antigout Agent; Uric Acid Lowering Agent

Generic Availability (U.S.) May be product dependent

Use Prevention of attacks of gouty arthritis and nephropathy; also used in treatment of secondary hyperuricemia which may occur during treatment of tumors or leukemia; prevention of recurrent calcium oxalate calculi

Pregnancy Risk Factor C

Pregnancy Considerations Adverse events were observed in some animal reproduction studies. Allopurinol crosses the placenta (Torrance, 2009). An increased risk of adverse fetal events has not been observed (limited data) (Hoeltzenbein, 2013).

Breast-Feeding Considerations Allopurinol and its metabolite are excreted into breast milk; the metabolite was also detected in the serum of the nursing infant (Kamilli, 1993). The U.S. manufacturer recommends caution be used when administering allopurinol to nursing women. The Canadian labeling contraindicates use in nursing women except those with hyperuricemia secondary to malignancy.

Contraindications Hypersensitivity to allopurinol or any component

Warnings Do not use to treat asymptomatic hyperuricemia; monitor liver function and complete blood counts before initiating therapy and periodically

Precautions Reduce dosage in renal impairment; discontinue drug at the first sign of rash; risk of skin rash may be increased in patients receiving amoxicillin or ampicillin; risk of hypersensitivity may be increased in patients receiving thiazides and possibly ACE inhibitors

Adverse Reactions
Dermatologic: Skin rash
Endocrine & metabolic: Gout (acute)
Gastrointestinal: Diarrhea, nausea
Hepatic: Increased liver enzymes, increased serum alkaline phosphatase
Rare but important or life-threatening: Ageusia, agranulocytosis, alopecia, angioedema, aplastic anemia, cataract, cholestatic jaundice, ecchymoses, eczematoid dermatitis, eosinophilia, exfoliative dermatitis, hepatic necrosis, hepatitis, hepatomegaly, hyperbilirubinemia, hypersensitivity reaction, leukocytosis, leukopenia, lichen planus, macular retinitis, myopathy, necrotizing angiitis, nephritis, neuritis, neuropathy, onycholysis, pancreatitis, purpura, renal failure, skin granuloma (annulare), Stevens-Johnson syndrome, thrombocytopenia, toxic epidermal necrolysis, toxic pustuloderma, uremia, vasculitis, vesicobullous dermatitis

Drug Interactions
Metabolism/Transport Effects None known.
Avoid Concomitant Use
Avoid concomitant use of Allopurinol with any of the following: Didanosine; Pegloticase; Tegafur
Increased Effect/Toxicity
Allopurinol may increase the levels/effects of: Amoxicillin; Ampicillin; Anticonvulsants (Hydantoin); AzaTHIOprine; Bendamustine; CarBAMazepine; ChlorproPAMIDE; Cyclophosphamide; Didanosine; Mercaptopurine; Pegloticase; Theophylline Derivatives; Vitamin K Antagonists

The levels/effects of Allopurinol may be increased by: ACE Inhibitors; Loop Diuretics; Thiazide Diuretics
Decreased Effect
Allopurinol may decrease the levels/effects of: Tegafur

The levels/effects of Allopurinol may be decreased by: Antacids
Stability Reconstituted parenteral solution should be stored at room temperature; do not refrigerate; use within 10 hours of preparation; physically **incompatible** when mixed with or infused through the same line with the following: Amikacin, amphotericin B, carmustine, cefotaxime, chlorpromazine, cimetidine, clindamycin, cytarabine, dacarbazine, daunorubicin, diphenhydramine, doxorubicin, doxycycline, droperidol, floxuridine, gentamicin, haloperidol, hydroxyzine, idarubicin, imipenem-cilastatin, mechlorethamine, meperidine, metoclopramide, methylprednisolone sodium succinate, minocycline, nalbuphine, netilmicin, ondansetron, prochlorperazine, promethazine, sodium bicarbonate, streptozocin, tobramycin, vinorelbine
Mechanism of Action Allopurinol inhibits xanthine oxidase, the enzyme responsible for the conversion of hypoxanthine to xanthine to uric acid. Allopurinol is metabolized to oxypurinol which is also an inhibitor of xanthine oxidase; allopurinol acts on purine catabolism, reducing the production of uric acid without disrupting the biosynthesis of vital purines.
Pharmacodynamics Decrease in serum uric acid occurs in 1-2 days with a nadir achieved in 1-3 weeks
Pharmacokinetics (Adult data unless noted)
Absorption: Oral: ~80% from the GI tract
Distribution: Into breast milk; breast milk to plasma ratio: 0.9-1.4
Protein binding: <1%
Metabolism: ~75% of drug metabolized to active metabolites, chiefly oxypurinol
Half-life:
Parent: 1-3 hours
Oxypurinol metabolite: 18-30 hours in patients with normal renal function
Time to peak serum concentration: Within 2-6 hours
Dialysis: Allopurinol and oxypurinol are dialyzable
Dosing: Usual
Prevention of acute uric acid nephropathy in myeloproliferative neoplastic disorders (beginning 1-2 days before chemotherapy): Daily doses >300 mg should be administered in divided doses:
Children ≤10 years:
I.V.: 200 mg/m²/day in 1-3 divided doses; maximum dose: 600 mg/day
Oral: 10 mg/kg/day in 2-3 divided doses or 200-300 mg/m²/day in 2-4 divided doses; maximum dose: 800 mg/day
Alternative:
<6 years: 150 mg/day in 3 divided doses
6-10 years: 300 mg/day in 2-3 divided doses
Children >10 years and Adults:
I.V.: 200-400 mg/m²/day in 1-3 divided doses; maximum: 600 mg/day
Oral: 600-800 mg/day in 2-3 divided doses

Gout: Children >10 years and Adults: Oral:
Mild: 200-300 mg/day
Severe: 400-600 mg/day
Recurrent calcium oxalate stones: Children >10 years and Adults: Oral: 200-300 mg daily in divided or single daily dosage
Dosing adjustment in renal impairment:
CrCl >50 mL/minute: No dosage change
CrCl 10-50 mL/minute: Reduce dosage to 50% of recommended
CrCl <10 mL/minute: Reduce dosage to 30% of recommended
Administration
Oral: Administer after meals with plenty of fluid
Parenteral: Reconstitute 500 mg vial with 25 mL SWI; prior to administration, further dilute with D_5W or NS to a maximum concentration of 6 mg/mL; rate of infusion is dependent upon the volume of infusate (in research studies, 100-300 mg doses were infused over 30 minutes)
Monitoring Parameters CBC, liver function tests, renal function, serum uric acid; 24-hour urinary urate (when treating calcium oxalate stones)
Reference Range
Uric acid: Male: 3.0-7.0 mg/dL; Female: 2.0-6.0 mg/dL
Urinary urate excretion: Male: <800 mg/day; Female: <750 mg/day
Dosage Forms Excipient information presented when available (limited, particularly for generics); consult specific product labeling.
Solution Reconstituted, Intravenous, as sodium [preservative free]:
Aloprim: 500 mg (1 ea)
Tablet, Oral, as sodium:
Zyloprim: 100 mg, 300 mg [scored]
Generic: 100 mg, 300 mg
Extemporaneous Preparations A 20 mg/mL oral suspension may be made with tablets and either a 1:1 mixture of Ora-Sweet® and Ora-Plus® or a 1:1 mixture of Ora-Sweet® SF and Ora-Plus® or a 1:4 mixture of cherry syrup concentrate and simple syrup, NF. Crush eight 300 mg tablets in a mortar and reduce to a fine powder. Add small portions of chosen vehicle and mix to a uniform paste; mix while adding the vehicle in incremental proportions to **almost** 120 mL; transfer to a calibrated bottle, rinse mortar with vehicle, and add quantity of vehicle sufficient to make 120 mL. Label "shake well". Stable for 60 days refrigerated or at room temperature (Allen, 1996; Nahata, 2004).

Allen LV Jr and Erickson MA 3rd, "Stability of Acetazolamide, Allopurinol, Azathioprine, Clonazepam, and Flucytosine in Extemporaneously Compounded Oral Liquids," *Am J Health Syst Pharm*, 1996, 53(16):1944-9.
Nahata MC, Pai VB, and Hipple TF, *Pediatric Drug Formulations*, 5th ed, Cincinnati, OH: Harvey Whitney Books Co, 2004.

References
Bennett WM, Aronoff GR, Golper TA, et al, *Drug Prescribing in Renal Failure*, Philadelphia, PA: American College of Physicians, 1987.
Hoeltzenbein M, Stieler K, Panse M, et al, "Allopurinol Use During Pregnancy - Outcome of 31 Prospectively Ascertained Cases and a Phenotype Possibly Indicative for Teratogenicity," *PLoS One*, 2013, 8 (6):e66637.
Kamilli I and Gresser U, "Allopurinol and Oxypurinol in Human Breast Milk," *Clin Investig*, 1993, 71(2):161-4.
Krakoff IH and Murphy ML, "Hyperuricemia in Neoplastic Disease in Children: Prevention With Allopurinol, A Xanthine Oxidase Inhibitor" *Pediatrics*, 1968, 41(1):52-6.
Torrance HL, Benders MJ, Derks JB, et al, "Maternal Allopurinol During Fetal Hypoxia Lowers Cord Blood Levels of the Brain Injury Marker S-100B," *Pediatrics*, 2009, 124(1):350-7.

◆ **Allopurinol Sodium** *see* Allopurinol *on page 97*

◆ **All-*trans* Retinoic Acid** *see* Tretinoin (Systemic) *on page 2068*

◆ **All-*trans* Vitamin A Acid** *see* Tretinoin (Systemic) *on page 2068*

Almotriptan (al moh TRIP tan)

Medication Safety Issues
Sound-alike/look-alike issues:
Axert may be confused with Antivert
Brand Names: U.S. Axert
Brand Names: Canada Axert; Mylan-Almotriptan; Sandoz-Almotriptan
Therapeutic Category Antimigraine Agent; Serotonin 5-HT$_{1D}$ Receptor Agonist
Generic Availability (U.S.) No
Use Acute treatment of migraine with or without aura (FDA approved in ages 12-17 years and adults); **Note:** FDA labeled indication in adolescents is for patients with history of migraine lasting ≥4 hours when left untreated
Pregnancy Risk Factor C
Pregnancy Considerations Adverse events were observed in animal reproduction studies. Information related to almotriptan use in pregnancy is limited (Källén, 2011; Nezvalová-Henriksen, 2010; Nezvalová-Henriksen, 2012). Until additional information is available, other agents are preferred for the initial treatment of migraine in pregnancy (Da Silva, 2012; MacGregor, 2012; Williams, 2012).
Breast-Feeding Considerations It is not known if almotriptan is excreted in breast milk. The manufacturer recommends that caution be exercised when administering almotriptan to nursing women.
Contraindications Hypersensitivity to almotriptan or any component; known or suspected ischemic heart disease (eg, angina pectoris, MI, documented silent ischemia, coronary artery vasospasm, Prinzmetal's variant angina, other significant underlying cardiovascular disease); cerebrovascular syndromes (eg, stroke, TIA), peripheral vascular disease (eg, ischemic bowel disease), uncontrolled hypertension, concomitant use (within last 24 hours) of ergotamine derivatives and/or ergotamine-containing medications or other 5-HT$_1$ agonist (eg, triptans); management of hemiplegic or basilar migraine
Warnings Serious coronary events, including coronary artery vasospasm, transient ischemia, acute MI, life-threatening arrhythmias (eg, ventricular tachycardia/fibrillation), and death have been reported with 5-HT$_1$ agonist administration; avoid use in patients with risk factors for coronary artery disease, unless cardiovascular disease can be ruled out; consider administering first dose under close supervision to patients at high risk for coronary disease. Patients who experience sensations of chest pain/pressure/tightness or symptoms suggestive of angina following dosing should be evaluated for coronary artery disease or Prinzmetal's angina before receiving additional doses. If dosing resumed and symptoms recur, ECG monitoring is recommended. Periodically evaluate cardiovascular system in patients with risk factors for coronary artery disease. Cerebrovascular events (eg, cerebral hemorrhage, subarachnoid hemorrhage, stroke) have been reported with 5-HT$_1$ agonist (triptan) administration. Vasospasm-related events (eg, peripheral vascular ischemia, colonic ischemia with abdominal pain and bloody diarrhea) have been reported with 5-HT$_1$ agonists; transient and permanent blindness and significant partial vision loss have been very rarely reported; further evaluation is recommended in patients with signs and symptoms suggestive of reduced peripheral arterial blood flow following 5-HT$_1$ agonist (eg, triptan) use. Potentially fatal serotonin syndrome may occur when triptans are used in combination with SSRIs (eg, fluoxetine, sertraline) or SNRIs (eg, venlafaxine); monitor carefully if the two drugs are used concomitantly.
Precautions Use with caution in patients with controlled hypertension; temporary increases in peripheral vascular resistance and blood pressure may occur; significant elevation in blood pressure, including hypertensive crisis, has also been reported on rare occasions in patients with and without a history of hypertension; use is contraindicated in patients with uncontrolled hypertension. Use with caution and reduce the dose in patients with impaired hepatic or renal function. Use with caution in patients with sulfonamide hypersensitivity; almotriptan contains a sulfonyl group which is structurally different from a sulfonamide; however, cross-reactivity in patients with sulfonamide allergy has not been evaluated. In adolescent patients, almotriptan has not been shown to be effective at relieving migraine symptoms (eg, nausea, photophobia, phonophobia). Other potentially serious neurological conditions should be ruled out prior to acute migraine therapy. Almotriptan (given at >2.5 times the maximum oral daily dose) has caused corneal opacities in dogs; other animal studies suggest it may bind to the melanin of the eye; human studies are not available.

Adverse Reactions
Central nervous system: Dizziness, headache, somnolence
Gastrointestinal: Nausea, vomiting, xerostomia
Neuromuscular & skeletal: Paresthesia
Rare but important or life-threatening: Anaphylactic shock, angina, angioedema, breast pain, colitis, coronary artery vasospasm, hemiplegia, hypertension, myocardial ischemia, MI, neuropathy, rash, seizure, syncope, tachycardia, ventricular fibrillation, ventricular tachycardia, vertigo

Drug Interactions
Metabolism/Transport Effects Substrate of CYP2D6 (minor), CYP3A4 (minor); **Note:** Assignment of Major/Minor substrate status based on clinically relevant drug interaction potential
Avoid Concomitant Use
Avoid concomitant use of Almotriptan with any of the following: Ergot Derivatives; MAO Inhibitors
Increased Effect/Toxicity
Almotriptan may increase the levels/effects of: Antipsychotics; Droxidopa; Ergot Derivatives; Metoclopramide; Serotonin Modulators

The levels/effects of Almotriptan may be increased by: Antiemetics (5HT3 Antagonists); Antipsychotics; CYP3A4 Inhibitors (Strong); Ergot Derivatives; MAO Inhibitors
Decreased Effect
The levels/effects of Almotriptan may be decreased by: Peginterferon Alfa-2b
Stability Store at 25°C (77°F); excursions permitted to 15°C to 30°C (59°F to 86°F).
Mechanism of Action Selective agonist for serotonin (5-HT$_{1B}$ and 5-HT$_{1D}$ receptors) in cranial arteries; causes vasoconstriction and reduces sterile inflammation associated with antidromic neuronal transmission correlating with relief of migraine
Pharmacokinetics (Adult data unless noted) Note: Reported values are similar between adolescent and adult patients (Baldwin, 2004).
Absorption: Well absorbed
Distribution: Apparent V_d: ~180-200 L
Protein binding: ~35%
Metabolism: MAO type A oxidative deamination (~27% of dose); via CYP3A4 and 2D6 (~12% of dose) to inactive metabolites
Bioavailability: ~70%
Half-life: Mean: 3-5 hours (Baldwin, 2004; McEnroe, 2005)
Time to peak serum concentration: 1-3 hours
Elimination: Urine (~75%; ~40% of total dose as unchanged drug); feces (~13% of total dose as unchanged drug and metabolites)

Dosing: Usual Adolescents 12-17 years and Adults: Oral: Initial: 6.25-12.5 mg in a single dose; if headache returns, may repeat the dose after 2 hours; no more than 2 doses (maximum daily dose: 25 mg). In clinical trials, 12.5 mg dose tended to be more effective in adults; individualize dose based on patient response.

Dosage adjustment in hepatic impairment: Adolescents and Adults: Initial: 6.25 mg in a single dose; maximum daily dose: 12.5 mg

Dosage adjustment in renal impairment: Adolescents and Adults: Severe renal impairment (CrCl ≤30 mL/minute): Initial: 6.25 mg in a single dose; maximum daily dose: 12.5 mg

Administration May administer without regard to meals.

Additional Information Safety of treating >4 headaches per month is not established; almotriptan is not indicated for migraine prophylaxis; safety and efficacy for cluster headaches have not been established.

Dosage Forms Excipient information presented when available (limited, particularly for generics); consult specific product labeling.

Tablet, Oral, as maleate:
Axert: 6.25 mg
Axert: 12.5 mg [contains fd&c blue #2 (indigotine)]

References
Baldwin JR, Fleishaker JC, Azie NE, et al, "A Comparison of the Pharmacokinetics and Tolerability of the Anti-migraine Compound Almotriptan in Healthy Adolescents and Adults," *Cephalalgia*, 2004, 24(4):288-92.

Berenson F, Vasconcellos E, Pakalnis A, et al, "Long-Term, Open-Label Safety Study of Oral Almotriptan 12.5 mg for the Acute Treatment of Migraine in Adolescents," *Headache*, 2010, 50(5):795-807.

Da Silva AN and Tepper SJ, "Acute Treatment of Migraines," *CNS Drugs*, 2012, 26(10):823-39.

Källén B, Nilsson E, and Otterblad Olausson P, "Delivery Outcome After Maternal Use of Drugs for Migraine: A Register Study in Sweden," *Drug Saf*, 2011, 34(8):691-703.

Linder SL, Mathew NT, Cady RK, et al, "Efficacy and Tolerability of Almotriptan in Adolescents: A Randomized, Double-Blind, Placebo-Controlled Trial," *Headache*, 2008, 48(9):1326-36.

MacGregor EA, "Headache in Pregnancy," *Neurol Clin*, 2012, 30 (3):835-66.

McEnroe JD and Fleishaker JC, "Clinical Pharmacokinetics of Almotriptan, a Serotonin 5-HT(1B/1D) Receptor Agonist for the Treatment of Migraine," *Clin Pharmacokinet*, 2005, 44(3):237-46.

Nezvalová-Henriksen K, Spigset O, and Nordeng HM, "Errata in 'Triptan Exposure During Pregnancy and the Risk of Major Congenital Malformations and Adverse Pregnancy Outcomes: Results From the Norwegian Mother and Child Sohort Study,'" *Headache*, 2012, 52 (8):1319-20.

Nezvalová-Henriksen K, Spigset O, and Nordeng H, "Triptan Exposure During Pregnancy and the Risk of Major Congenital Malformations and Adverse Pregnancy Outcomes: Results From the Norwegian Mother and Child Cohort Study," *Headache*, 2010, 50(4):563-75.

Williams SH and Kehr HA, "An Update in the Treatment of Neurologic Disorders During Pregnancy-Focus on Migraines and Seizures," *J Pharm Pract*, 2012, 25(3):341-51.

◆ **Almotriptan Malate** see Almotriptan on page 99

◆ **Alocril** see Nedocromil on page 1474

◆ **Alocril® (Can)** see Nedocromil on page 1474

◆ **Alodox Convenience** see Doxycycline on page 721

◆ **Aloe Vesta Antifungal [OTC]** see Miconazole (Topical) on page 1410

◆ **Aloprim** see Allopurinol on page 97

◆ **Alora** see Estradiol (Systemic) on page 796

◆ **Aloxi** see Palonosetron on page 1586

◆ **Alpha-Galactosidase-A (Recombinant)** see Agalsidase Beta on page 79

◆ **Alphagan (Can)** see Brimonidine (Ophthalmic) on page 303

◆ **Alphagan P** see Brimonidine (Ophthalmic) on page 303

◆ **Alphanate®** see Antihemophilic Factor/von Willebrand Factor Complex (Human) on page 177

◆ **AlphaNine SD** see Factor IX (Human) on page 835

◆ **AlphaTrex** see Betamethasone (Topical) on page 285

◆ **Alph-E [OTC]** see Vitamin E on page 2148

◆ **Alph-E-Mixed [OTC]** see Vitamin E on page 2148

◆ **Alph-E-Mixed 1000 [OTC]** see Vitamin E on page 2148

ALPRAZolam (al PRAY zoe lam)

Medication Safety Issues
Sound-alike/look-alike issues:
ALPRAZolam may be confused with alprostadil, LORazepam, triazolam

Xanax® may be confused with Fanapt®, Lanoxin®, Tenex®, Tylox®, Xopenex®, Zantac®, ZyrTEC®

BEERS Criteria medication:
This drug may be potentially inappropriate for use in geriatric patients (Quality of evidence - high; Strength of recommendation - strong).

Related Information
Oral Medications That Should Not Be Crushed or Altered on page 2438

Brand Names: U.S. ALPRAZolam Intensol; ALPRAZolam XR; Niravam; Xanax; Xanax XR

Brand Names: Canada Apo-Alpraz®; Apo-Alpraz® TS; Mylan-Alprazolam; NTP-Alprazolam; Nu-Alpraz; Teva-Alprazolam; Xanax TS™; Xanax®

Therapeutic Category Antianxiety Agent; Benzodiazepine

Generic Availability (U.S.) May be product dependent

Use Treatment of generalized anxiety disorder (GAD); symptoms of anxiety (short-term treatment); anxiety associated with depression; management of panic disorder, with or without agoraphobia

Pregnancy Risk Factor D

Pregnancy Considerations Benzodiazepines have the potential to cause harm to the fetus. Alprazolam and its metabolites cross the human placenta. Teratogenic effects have been observed with some benzodiazepines; however, additional studies are needed. The incidence of premature birth and low birth weights may be increased following maternal use of benzodiazepines; hypoglycemia and respiratory problems in the neonate may occur following exposure late in pregnancy. Neonatal withdrawal symptoms may occur within days to weeks after birth and "floppy infant syndrome" (which also includes withdrawal symptoms) has been reported with some benzodiazepines (Bergman, 1992; Iqbal, 2002; Wikner, 2007).

Breast-Feeding Considerations Benzodiazepines are excreted into breast milk. In a study of eight postpartum women, peak concentrations of alprazolam were found in breast milk ~1 hour after the maternal dose and the half-life was ~14 hours. Samples were obtained over 36 hours following a single oral dose of alprazolam 0.5 mg. Metabolites were not detected in breast milk. In this study, the estimated exposure to the breast-feeding infant was ~3% of the weight-adjusted maternal dose (Oo, 1995). Drowsiness, lethargy, or weight loss in nursing infants have been observed in case reports following maternal use of some benzodiazepines (Iqbal, 2002). Breast-feeding is not recommended by the manufacturer.

Contraindications Hypersensitivity to alprazolam, any component, or other benzodiazepines; severe uncontrolled pain, narrow-angle glaucoma, severe respiratory depression, preexisting CNS depression; not to be used in pregnancy or lactation or in patients taking certain medications

Warnings Withdrawal symptoms including seizures have occurred 18 hours to 3 days after abrupt discontinuation; when discontinuing therapy, decrease daily dose by no more than 0.5 mg every 3 days; reduce dose in patients with significant hepatic disease. Concentrated oral solution contains propylene glycol; toxicities have been reported with use of products containing propylene glycol, including hyperosmolality, lactic acidosis, seizures, and respiratory depression; in neonates large amounts of propylene glycol delivered orally, intravenously (eg, >3000 mg/day), or topically have been associated with potentially fatal toxicities which can include metabolic acidosis, seizures, renal failure, and CNS depression; use oral solution containing propylene glycol with caution (AAP, 1997; Shehab, 2009).

Precautions Use with caution in patients with hepatic impairment. Use with caution in patients with renal impairment or predisposition to urate nephropathy; has weak uricosuric properties. Use with caution in patients with depression, particularly if suicidal risk may be present; episodes of mania or hypomania have occurred in depressed patients treated with alprazolam. Use with caution in patients with a history of drug abuse or acute alcoholism; potential for drug dependency exists. Tolerance and psychological and physical dependence may occur with prolonged use (generally >10 days). Use with caution in patients with respiratory disease. Use with caution in patients receiving other CNS depressants or psychoactive medication; effects with other sedative drugs or ethanol may be potentiated. Use with caution in patients taking strong CYP3A4 inhibitors, moderate or strong CYP3A4 inducers, and major CYP3A4 substrates (see Drug Interactions); consider alternative agents that avoid or lessen the potential for CYP-mediated interactions. Use with caution in debilitated patients. Use with extreme caution in patients who are at risk of falls; benzodiazepines have been associated with falls and traumatic injury. Use with caution in obese patients; may have prolonged action when discontinued.

Adverse Reactions

Central nervous system: Abnormal dreams, agitation, akathisia, altered mental status, ataxia, cognitive dysfunction, confusion, depersonalization, depression, derealization, disinhibition, disorientation, disturbance in attention, dizziness, drowsiness, dysarthria, dystonia, fatigue, fear, hallucination, headache, hypersomnia, hypoesthesia, insomnia, irritability, lethargy, malaise, memory impairment, nervousness, nightmares, paresthesia, restlessness, sedation, seizure, talkativeness, vertigo

Dermatologic: Dermatitis, diaphoresis, skin rash

Endocrine & metabolic: Decreased libido, Increased libido, menstrual disease, weight gain, weight loss

Gastrointestinal: Abdominal pain, anorexia, change in appetite, constipation, diarrhea, dyspepsia, nausea, sialorrhea, vomiting, xerostomia

Genitourinary: Difficulty in micturition, dysmenorrhea, sexual disorder, urinary incontinence

Hepatic: Increased liver enzymes, increased serum bilirubin, jaundice

Neuromuscular & skeletal: Arthralgia, back pain, dyskinesia, muscle cramps, muscle twitching, myalgia, tremor, weakness

Ophthalmic: Blurred vision

Respiratory: Allergic rhinitis, dyspnea, hyperventilation, nasal congestion, upper respiratory tract infection

Rare but important or life-threatening: Amnesia, angioedema, diplopia, falling, galactorrhea, gynecomastia, hepatic failure, hepatitis, homicidal ideation, hyperprolactinemia, hypomania, mania, peripheral edema, sleep apnea, Stevens-Johnson syndrome, suicidal ideation, tinnitus

Drug Interactions

Metabolism/Transport Effects Substrate of CYP3A4 (major); **Note:** Assignment of Major/Minor substrate status based on clinically relevant drug interaction potential

Avoid Concomitant Use

Avoid concomitant use of ALPRAZolam with any of the following: Azelastine (Nasal); Conivaptan; Fusidic Acid (Systemic); Indinavir; Itraconazole; Ketoconazole

(Systemic); Methadone; OLANZapine; Paraldehyde; Sodium Oxybate; Thalidomide

Increased Effect/Toxicity

ALPRAZolam may increase the levels/effects of: Alcohol (Ethyl); Azelastine (Nasal); Buprenorphine; CloZAPine; CNS Depressants; Hydrocodone; Methadone; Methotrimeprazine; Metyrosine; Mirtazapine; Paraldehyde; Pramipexole; ROPINIRole; Rotigotine; Selective Serotonin Reuptake Inhibitors; Sodium Oxybate; Thalidomide; Zolpidem

The levels/effects of ALPRAZolam may be increased by: Antifungal Agents (Azole Derivatives, Systemic); Aprepitant; Boceprevir; Brimonidine (Topical); Calcium Channel Blockers (Nondihydropyridine); Cannabis; Ceritinib; Cimetidine; Conivaptan; Contraceptives (Estrogens); Contraceptives (Progestins); CYP3A4 Inhibitors (Moderate); CYP3A4 Inhibitors (Strong); Dasatinib; Doxylamine; Dronabinol; Droperidol; Fosaprepitant; Fusidic Acid (Systemic); Grapefruit Juice; HydrOXYzine; Indinavir; Isoniazid; Itraconazole; Ivacaftor; Kava Kava; Ketoconazole (Systemic); Luliconazole; Macrolide Antibiotics; Magnesium Sulfate; Methotrimeprazine; Mifepristone; Nabilone; OLANZapine; Perampanel; Protease Inhibitors; Proton Pump Inhibitors; Rufinamide; Selective Serotonin Reuptake Inhibitors; Simeprevir; Stiripentol; Tapentadol; Telaprevir; Tetrahydrocannabinol

Decreased Effect

The levels/effects of ALPRAZolam may be decreased by: Bosentan; CarBAMazepine; CYP3A4 Inducers (Strong); Dabrafenib; Deferasirox; Mitotane; Rifamycin Derivatives; Siltuximab; St Johns Wort; Theophylline Derivatives; Tocilizumab; Yohimbine

Food Interactions Alprazolam serum concentration is unlikely to be increased by grapefruit juice because of alprazolam's high oral bioavailability. The C_{max} of the extended release formulation is increased by 25% when a high-fat meal is given 2 hours before dosing. T_{max} is decreased 33% when food is given immediately prior to dose and increased by 33% when food is given ≥1 hour after dose. Management: Administer without regard to food.

Stability Orally-disintegrating tablet: Store at room temperature of 20°C to 25°C (68°F to 77°F). Protect from moisture. Discard any cotton packaged inside bottle; reseal bottle tightly.

Mechanism of Action Binds to stereospecific benzodiazepine receptors on the postsynaptic GABA neuron at several sites within the central nervous system, including the limbic system, reticular formation. Enhancement of the inhibitory effect of GABA on neuronal excitability results by increased neuronal membrane permeability to chloride ions. This shift in chloride ions results in hyperpolarization (a less excitable state) and stabilization.

Pharmacokinetics (Adult data unless noted)

Absorption: Oral:

Immediate release tablet: Rapidly and well absorbed

Extended release tablet: Rate of absorption is increased following night time dosing (versus morning dosing)

Distribution: 0.9-1.2 L/kg; distributes into breast milk

Protein binding: 80%

Metabolism: Extensive in the liver, primarily via cytochrome P450 isoenzyme CYP3A; major metabolites: alpha-hydroxy-alprazolam (about half as active as alprazolam), 4-hydroxyalprazolam (active), and a benzophenone metabolite (inactive). **Note:** Active metabolites are not likely to contribute to pharmacologic effects due to low levels of activity and low concentrations.

Bioavailability: Similar for extended and immediate release tablets (~90%)

Half-life: Adults: 6.3-26.9 hours; mean: 11.2 hours; **Note:** Half-life may be 25% longer in Asians compared to Caucasians.

Time to peak serum concentration:
Immediate release tablet: Within 1-2 hours
Orally-disintegrating tablet: 1.5-2 hours (if given with or without water); **Note:** Time to peak serum concentration occurs ~15 minutes earlier when taken with water (versus without)
Elimination: Excretion of metabolites and parent compound in urine

Dosing: Usual Oral: **Note:** Titrate dose to effect; use lowest effective dose
Children <18 years: Immediate release: Dose not established; investigationally in children 7-16 years of age (n=13), initial doses of 0.005 mg/kg or 0.125 mg/dose were given 3 times/day for situational anxiety and increments of 0.125-0.25 mg/dose were used to increase doses to maximum of 0.02 mg/kg/dose or 0.06 mg/kg/day; a range of 0.375-3 mg/day was needed (Pfefferbaum, 1987). **Note:** A more recent study in 17 children (8-17 years of age) with overanxious disorder or avoidant disorders used initial daily doses of 0.25 mg for children <40 kg and 0.5 mg for those >40 kg. The dose was titrated at 2-day intervals to a maximum of 0.04 mg/kg/day. Required doses ranged from 0.5-3.5 mg/day with a mean of 1.6 mg/day. Based on clinical global ratings, alprazolam appeared to be better than placebo, however, this difference was **not** statistically significant (Simeon, 1992); further studies are needed.
Adults:
Anxiety: Immediate release: Initial: 0.25-0.5 mg 3 times/day; titrate dose upward as needed every 3-4 days; maximum dose: 4 mg/day given in divided doses
Panic disorder:
Immediate release: Initial: 0.5 mg 3 times/day; titrate dose upward as needed every 3-4 days in increments ≤1 mg/day; mean dose used in controlled trials: 5-6 mg/day; maximum dose: 10 mg/day (rarely required)
Extended release: Initial: 0.5-1 mg once daily; titrate dose upward as needed every 3-4 days in increments ≤1 mg/day; usual dose: 3-6 mg/day; maximum dose: 10 mg/day (rarely required)
Switching from immediate release to extended release: Administer the same total daily dose, but give once daily; if effect is not adequate, titrate dose as above

Administration Oral:
Immediate release tablet: Administer with food to decrease GI upset
Extended release tablet: Administer once daily, preferably in the morning; do not crush, chew, or break; swallow whole
Orally-disintegrating tablet: Do not remove tablets from bottle until right before dose; using dry hands, place tablet on top of tongue. If using one-half of tablet, immediately discard remaining half (half tablet may not remain stable). Administration with water is not necessary (water is not required to aid dissolution or swallowing)

Monitoring Parameters CNS status, respiratory rate
Additional Information If used for an extended period of time, long-term usefulness of alprazolam should be periodically re-evaluated for an individual patient.

Controlled Substance C-IV
Dosage Forms Excipient information presented when available (limited, particularly for generics); consult specific product labeling. [DSC] = Discontinued product
Concentrate, Oral:
ALPRAZolam Intensol: 1 mg/mL (30 mL) [unflavored flavor]
Tablet, Oral:
Xanax: 0.25 mg [scored]
Xanax: 0.5 mg [scored; contains fd&c yellow #6 (sunset yellow)]
Xanax: 1 mg [scored; contains fd&c blue #2 (indigotine)]

Xanax: 2 mg [scored]
Generic: 0.25 mg, 0.5 mg, 1 mg, 2 mg
Tablet Dispersible, Oral:
Niravam: 0.25 mg, 0.5 mg [DSC], 1 mg [DSC], 2 mg [DSC] [scored; orange flavor]
Generic: 0.25 mg, 0.5 mg, 1 mg, 2 mg
Tablet Extended Release 24 Hour, Oral:
ALPRAZolam XR: 0.5 mg
ALPRAZolam XR: 1 mg [contains fd&c yellow #10 (quinoline yellow)]
ALPRAZolam XR: 2 mg [contains fd&c blue #2 (indigotine)]
ALPRAZolam XR: 3 mg [contains fd&c blue #2 (indigotine), fd&c yellow #10 (quinoline yellow)]
Xanax XR: 0.5 mg
Xanax XR: 1 mg [contains fd&c yellow #10 (quinoline yellow)]
Xanax XR: 2 mg [contains fd&c blue #2 (indigotine)]
Xanax XR: 3 mg [contains fd&c blue #2 (indigotine), fd&c yellow #10 (quinoline yellow)]
Generic: 0.5 mg, 1 mg, 2 mg, 3 mg
Extemporaneous Preparations Note: Commercial oral solution is available (Alprazolam Intensol™: 1 mg/mL [dye free, ethanol free, sugar free; contains propylene glycol]

A 1 mg/mL oral suspension may be made with tablets and one of three different vehicles (a 1:1 mixture of Ora-Sweet® and Ora-Plus®, a 1:1 mixture of Ora-Sweet® SF and Ora-Plus®, or a 1:4 mixture of cherry syrup with Simple Syrup, NF). Crush sixty 2 mg tablets in a mortar and reduce to a fine powder. Add 40 mL of vehicle and mix to a uniform paste; mix while adding the vehicle in incremental proportions to **almost** 120 mL; transfer to a calibrated bottle, rinse mortar with vehicle, and add a quantity of vehicle sufficient to make 120 mL. Label "shake well" and "refrigerate". Stable for 60 days.
Nahata MC, Pai VB, and Hipple TF, *Pediatric Drug Formulations*, 5th ed, Cincinnati, OH: Harvey Whitney Books Co, 2004.

References

American Academy of Pediatrics Committee on Drugs. "Inactive" ingredients in pharmaceutical products: update (subject review). *Pediatrics.* 1997;99(2):268-278.
Bergman U, Rosa FW, Baum C, et al, "Effects of Exposure to Benzodiazepine During Fetal Life," *Lancet*, 1992, 340(8821):694-6.
Bernstein GA, Garfinkel BD, and Borchardt CM, "Comparative Studies of Pharmacotherapy for School Refusal," *J Am Acad Child Adolesc Psychiatry*, 1990, 29(5):773-81.
DeVane CL, Hill M, and Antal EJ, "Therapeutic Drug Monitoring of Alprazolam in Adolescents With Asthma," *Ther Drug Monit*, 1998, 20(3):257-60.
Iqbal MM, Sobhan T, Ryals T, et al, "Effects of Commonly Used Benzodiazepines on the Fetus, the Neonate, and the Nursing Infant," *Psychiatr Serv*, 2002, 53(1):39-49.
Oo CY, Kuhn RJ, Desai N, et al, "Pharmacokinetics in Lactating Women: Prediction of Alprazolam Transfer Into Milk," *Br J Clin Pharmacol*, 1995, 40(3):231-6.
Pfefferbaum B, Overall JE, Boren HA, et al, "Alprazolam in the Treatment of Anticipatory and Acute Situational Anxiety in Children With Cancer," *J Am Acad Child Adolesc Psychiatry*, 1987, 26(4):532-5.
Shehab N, Lewis CL, Streetman DD, Donn SM. Exposure to the pharmaceutical excipients benzyl alcohol and propylene glycol among critically ill neonates. *Pediatr Crit Care Med.* 2009;10 (2):256-259.
Simeon JG and Ferguson HB, "Alprazolam Effects in Children With Anxiety Disorders," *Can J Psychiatry*, 1987, 32(7):570-4.
Simeon JG, Ferguson HB, Knott V, et al, "Clinical, Cognitive, and Neurophysiological Effects of Alprazolam in Children and Adolescents With Overanxious and Avoidant Disorders," *J Am Acad Child Adolesc Psychiatry*, 1992, 31(1):29-33.
Wikner BN, Stiller CO, Bergman U, et al, "Use of Benzodiazepines and Benzodiazepine Receptor Agonists During Pregnancy: Neonatal Outcome and Congenital Malformations," *Pharmacoepidemiol Drug Saf*, 2007, 16(11):1203-10.

◆ **ALPRAZolam Intensol** see ALPRAZolam *on page 100*
◆ **ALPRAZolam XR** see ALPRAZolam *on page 100*
◆ **Alprolix** see Factor IX (Recombinant) *on page 838*

Alprostadil (al PROS ta dill)

Medication Safety Issues
Sound-alike/look-alike issues:
Alprostadil may be confused with alPRAZolam
Related Information
Emergency Drip Calculations *on page 2191*
Brand Names: U.S. Caverject; Caverject Impulse; Edex; Muse; Prostin VR
Brand Names: Canada Alprostadil Injection USP; Caverject; Muse Pellet; Prostin VR
Therapeutic Category Prostaglandin
Generic Availability (U.S.) May be product dependent
Use Temporary maintenance of patency of ductus arteriosus in neonates with ductal-dependent congenital heart disease until surgery can be performed. These defects include cyanotic (eg, pulmonary atresia, pulmonary stenosis, tricuspid atresia, Fallot's tetralogy, transposition of the great vessels) and acyanotic (eg, interruption of aortic arch, coarctation of aorta, hypoplastic left ventricle) heart disease.

Investigationally used for the treatment of pulmonary hypertension in infants and children with congenital heart defects with left-to-right shunts
Adult males: Diagnosis and treatment of erectile dysfunction
Pregnancy Risk Factor X/C (Muse)
Pregnancy Considerations Adverse events were observed in animal reproduction studies. Alprostadil is not indicated for use in women. The manufacturer of Muse recommends a condom barrier when being used during sexual intercourse with a pregnant women.
Breast-Feeding Considerations Alprostadil is not indicated for use in women.
Contraindications Hypersensitivity to alprostadil or any component; respiratory distress syndrome or persistent fetal circulation
Warnings Apnea occurs in 10% to 12% of neonates with congenital heart defects (especially in those weighing <2 kg at birth) and usually appears during the first hour of drug infusion **[U.S. Boxed Warnings]**. May cause gastric outlet obstruction in neonates secondary to antral hyperplasia; occurrence is related to duration of therapy and cumulative dose. Infuse alprostadil at lowest effective dose and for shortest period of time; weigh risks of long-term effects versus benefits.
Precautions Use cautiously in neonates with bleeding tendencies. If hypotension or pyrexia occurs, the infusion rate should be reduced until symptoms subside; severe hypotension, apnea, or bradycardia requires drug discontinuation with cautious reinstitution at a lower dose. Flushing of arm or face during infusion may indicate misplacement of intra-arterial catheter and drug infusing into subclavian or carotid artery; repositioning of catheter necessary. Tissue necrosis may occur with extravasation of concentrated solutions (due to high osmolality). Cortical proliferation (cortical hyperostosis) of long bones has been associated with long-term infusions of alprostadil; incidence and severity are related to duration of therapy and cumulative dose; **Note:** Cortical hyperostosis may present with clinical symptoms that mimic cellulitis or osteomyelitis (eg, symptomatic bone tenderness, soft tissue swelling).

Adverse Reactions
Intraurethral:
Central nervous system: Dizziness, headache, pain
Genitourinary: Penile pain, testicular pain, urethral bleeding (minor), urethral burning, vulvovaginal pruritus (female partner)
Rare but important or life-threatening: Tachycardia
Intracavernosal injection:
Cardiovascular: Hypertension

Central nervous system: Dizziness, headache
Genitourinary: Penile disease, penile pain, penile rash, penile swelling, prolonged erection (>4 hours), Peyronie's disease
Local: Bruising at injection site, hematoma at injection site
Rare but important or life-threatening: Balanitis, injection site hemorrhage, priapism
Intravenous:
Cardiovascular: Bradycardia, cardiac arrest, edema, flushing, hypertension, hypotension, tachycardia
Central nervous system: Dizziness, headache, seizure
Endocrine & metabolic: Hypokalemia
Gastrointestinal: Diarrhea
Hematologic & oncologic: Disseminated intravascular coagulation
Infection: Sepsis
Local: Local pain (in structures other than the injection site)
Neuromuscular & skeletal: Back pain
Respiratory: Apnea, cough, flu-like symptoms, nasal congestion, sinusitis, upper respiratory infection
Miscellaneous: Fever
Rare but important or life-threatening: Anemia, anuria, bradypnea, cardiac failure, cerebral hemorrhage, gastroesophageal reflux disease, hematuria, hemorrhage, hyperbilirubinemia, hyperemia, hyperirritability, hyperkalemia, hypoglycemia, hypothermia, neck hyperextension, peritonitis, second degree atrioventricular block, shock, supraventricular tachycardia, thrombocytopenia, ventricular fibrillation
Drug Interactions
Metabolism/Transport Effects None known.
Avoid Concomitant Use
Avoid concomitant use of Alprostadil with any of the following: Phosphodiesterase 5 Inhibitors
Increased Effect/Toxicity
The levels/effects of Alprostadil may be increased by: Phosphodiesterase 5 Inhibitors
Decreased Effect There are no known significant interactions involving a decrease in effect.
Stability Compatible in D_5W, $D_{10}W$, and saline solutions; refrigerate ampuls at 2°C to 8°C. Avoid direct contact of undiluted alprostadil with the plastic walls of volumetric infusion chambers because the drug will interact with the plastic and create a hazy solution; discard solution and volumetric chamber if this occurs.
Mechanism of Action Causes vasodilation by means of direct effect on vascular and ductus arteriosus smooth muscle; relaxes trabecular smooth muscle by dilation of cavernosal arteries when injected along the penile shaft, allowing blood flow to and entrapment in the lacunar spaces of the penis (ie, corporeal veno-occlusive mechanism)
Pharmacodynamics
Maximum effect:
Acyanotic congenital heart disease: Usual: 1.5-3 hours; range: 15 minutes to 11 hours
Cyanotic congenital heart disease: Usual: ~30 minutes
Duration: Ductus arteriosus will begin to close within 1-2 hours after drug is stopped
Pharmacokinetics (Adult data unless noted)
Metabolism: ~70% to 80% metabolized by oxidation during a single pass through the lungs; metabolite (13,14 dihydro-PGE_1) is active and has been identified in neonates
Half-life: 5-10 minutes; since the half-life is so short, the drug must be administered by continuous infusion
Elimination: Metabolites excreted in urine
Dosing: Neonatal Continuous I.V. infusion: 0.05-0.1 mcg/kg/minute; once therapeutic response is achieved, reduce rate to lowest effective dosage; with unsatisfactory response, increase rate gradually; maintenance: 0.01-0.4 mcg/kg/minute; higher doses may be required in patients receiving ECMO support (Stone, 2006); apnea may be

less likely to occur at doses <0.015 mcg/kg/minute (Browning Carmo, 2007). **Note:** PGE_1 is usually given at an infusion rate of 0.1 mcg/kg/minute, but it is often possible to reduce the dosage to $^1/_2$ or even $^1/_{10}$ without losing the therapeutic effect.

Dosing: Usual Continuous I.V. infusion: Infants: 0.05-0.1 mcg/kg/minute; once therapeutic response is achieved, reduce rate to lowest effective dosage; with unsatisfactory response, increase rate gradually; maintenance: 0.01-0.4 mcg/kg/minute. **Note:** PGE_1 is usually given at an infusion rate of 0.1 mcg/kg/minute, but it is often possible to reduce the dosage to $^1/_2$ or even $^1/_{10}$ without losing the therapeutic effect.

Usual Infusion Concentrations: Neonatal I.V. infusion: 10 mcg/mL

Usual Infusion Concentrations: Pediatric I.V. infusion: 10 mcg/mL **or** 20 mcg/mL

Administration Parenteral: I.V. continuous infusion into a large vein or alternatively through an umbilical artery catheter placed at the ductal opening; maximum concentration listed (per package insert) for I.V. infusion: 20 mcg/mL; has also been administered via continuous infusion into the right pulmonary artery for investigational treatment of pulmonary hypertension in infants and children with congenital heart defects with left-to-right shunts; rate of infusion (mL/hour) = dose (mcg/kg/minute) x weight (kg) x 60 minutes/hour divided by standard concentration (mcg/mL)

Monitoring Parameters Arterial pressure, respiratory rate, heart rate, temperature, pO_2; monitor for gastric obstruction in patients receiving PGE_1 for longer than 120 hours; x-rays may be needed to assess cortical hyperostosis in patients receiving prolonged PGE_1 therapy

Additional Information Therapeutic response is indicated by an increase in systemic blood pressure and pH in those with restricted systemic blood flow and acidosis, or by an increase in oxygenation (pO_2) in those with restricted pulmonary blood flow. Most cases of bone changes occurred 4-6 weeks after starting alprostadil, but it has occurred as early as 9 days; cortical hyperostosis usually resolves over 6-12 months after stopping PGE_1 therapy

Other dosage forms of alprostadil [Caverject® injection, Caverject® Impulse™ injection, Edex® injection, and Muse® Pellet (urethral)] are indicated for the diagnosis and treatment of erectile dysfunction in adult males; see package inserts for further information for this use.

Dosage Forms Excipient information presented when available (limited, particularly for generics); consult specific product labeling.

Kit, Intracavernosal:
Caverject Impulse: 10 mcg [contains benzyl alcohol]
Caverject Impulse: 20 mcg
Edex: 10 mcg, 20 mcg, 40 mcg
Pellet, Urethral:
Muse: 125 mcg (1 ea, 6 ea); 250 mcg (1 ea, 6 ea); 500 mcg (1 ea, 6 ea); 1000 mcg (1 ea, 6 ea)
Solution, Injection:
Prostin VR: 500 mcg/mL (1 mL) [contains benzyl alcohol]
Generic: 500 mcg/mL (1 mL)
Solution Reconstituted, Intracavernosal:
Caverject: 20 mcg (1 ea)
Caverject: 20 mcg (1 ea); 40 mcg (1 ea) [contains benzyl alcohol]

References

Browning Carmo KA, Barr P, West M, et al, "Transporting Newborn Infants With Suspected Duct Dependent Congenital Heart Disease on Low-Dose Prostaglandin E1 Without Routine Mechanical Ventilation," *Arch Dis Child Fetal Neonatal Ed*, 2007, 92(2):F117-9.

Institute for Safe Medication Practices (ISMP), "Standard Concentrations of Neonatal Drug Infusions," *ISMP*, 2011.

Kaufman MB and El-Chaar GM, "Bone and Tissue Changes Following Prostaglandin Therapy in Neonates," *Ann Pharmacother*, 1996, 30 (3):269-74, 277.

Lewis AB, Freed MD, Heymann MA, et al, "Side Effects of Therapy With Prostaglandin E₁ in Infants With Critical Congenital Heart Disease," *Circulation*, 1981, 64(5):893-8.

Peled N, Dagan O, Babyn P, et al, "Gastric-Outlet Obstruction Induced by Prostaglandin Therapy in Neonates," *N Engl J Med*, 1992, 327 (8):505-10.

Phillips MS, "Standardizing I.V. Infusion Concentrations: National Survey Results," *Am J Health Syst Pharm*, 2011, 68(22):2176-82.

Stone DM, Frattarelli DA, Karthikeyan S, et al, "Altered Prostaglandin E1 Dosage During Extracorporeal Membrane Oxygenation in a Newborn With Ductal-Dependent Congenital Heart Disease," *Pediatr Cardiol*, 2006, 27(3):360-3.

Weesner KM, "Hemodynamic Effects of Prostaglandin E₁ in Patients With Congenital Heart Disease and Pulmonary Hypertension," *Cathet Cardiovasc Diagn*, 1991, 24(1):10-5.

Woo K, Emery J, and Peabody J, "Cortical Hyperostosis: A Complication of Prolonged Prostaglandin Infusion in Infants Awaiting Cardiac Transplantation," *Pediatrics*, 1994, 93(3):417-20.

◆ **Alprostadil Injection USP (Can)** *see* Alprostadil *on page 103*

◆ **Alsuma** *see* SUMAtriptan *on page 1958*

◆ **Altacaine** *see* Tetracaine (Ophthalmic) *on page 1995*

◆ **Altachlore [OTC]** *see* Sodium Chloride *on page 1902*

◆ **Altafrin** *see* Phenylephrine (Ophthalmic) *on page 1661*

◆ **Altamist Spray [OTC]** *see* Sodium Chloride *on page 1902*

◆ **Altarussin [OTC]** *see* GuaiFENesin *on page 984*

◆ **Altaryl [OTC]** *see* DiphenhydrAMINE (Systemic) *on page 673*

Alteplase (AL te plase)

Medication Safety Issues
Sound-alike/look-alike issues:
Activase may be confused with Cathflo Activase, TNKase
Alteplase may be confused with Altace
"tPA" abbreviation should not be used when writing orders for this medication; has been misread as TNKase (tenecteplase)

High alert medication:
The Institute for Safe Medication Practices (ISMP) includes this medication (I.V.) among its list of drugs which have a heightened risk of causing significant patient harm when used in error.

Brand Names: U.S. Activase; Cathflo Activase

Brand Names: Canada Activase rt-PA; Cathflo Activase

Therapeutic Category Thrombolytic Agent; Thrombotic Occlusion (Central Venous Catheter), Treatment Agent

Generic Availability (U.S.) No

Use
Activase: Thrombolytic agent used in treatment of acute MI, acute ischemic stroke, and acute massive pulmonary embolism (All indications: FDA approved in adults)
CathFlo Activase: Treatment of occluded central venous access devices (catheters) to restore function (FDA approved in pediatric patients [age not specified] and adults)

Pregnancy Risk Factor C

Pregnancy Considerations Adverse events were observed in animal reproduction studies. The risk of bleeding may be increased in pregnant women. Information related to alteplase use in pregnancy is limited (Leonhardt, 2006; Li, 2012) and most guidelines consider pregnancy to be a relative contraindication for its use (Jaff, 2011; Jauch, 2013; O'Gara, 2013). Alteplase should not be withheld from pregnant women in life-threatening situations but should be avoided when safer alternatives are available (Bates, 2012; Li, 2012; Leonhardt, 2006; Vanden Hoek, 2010).

Breast-Feeding Considerations It is not known if alteplase is excreted in breast milk. The manufacturer recommends that caution be exercised when administering alteplase to nursing women.

Contraindications Hypersensitivity to alteplase or any component

Activase: Additional indication-specific contraindications:

Treatment of acute MI or pulmonary embolism: Active internal bleeding; known bleeding diathesis; history of CVA; intracranial neoplasm, arteriovenous malformation, or aneurysm; recent intracranial or intraspinal surgery or trauma; severe uncontrolled hypertension

Treatment of acute ischemic stroke: Active internal bleeding; known bleeding diathesis (including but not limited to: Current use of oral anticoagulants or an INR >1.7 or PT >15 seconds, administration of heparin within 48 hours before the onset of stroke and an elevated aPTT at presentation, platelet count <100,000/mm^3); evidence of intracranial hemorrhage on pretreatment evaluation; history of intracranial hemorrhage; suspicion of subarachnoid hemorrhage; recent (within 3 months) intracranial or intraspinal surgery, serious head trauma, or previous stroke; intracranial neoplasm, arteriovenous malformation, or aneurysm; seizure at the onset of stroke; uncontrolled hypertension at time of treatment (eg, adults with blood pressures of >185 mm Hg systolic or >110 mm Hg diastolic)

Warnings Systemic alteplase therapy may cause bleeding (internal, superficial, or surface bleeding); concurrent use of heparin anticoagulation may increase bleeding; monitor all potential bleeding sites. Avoid I.M. injections and nonessential handling of patient; carefully perform venipunctures and only when necessary. If an arterial puncture is required, use vessel in an upper extremity that can be manually compressed. Stop alteplase (and heparin) if serious bleeding occurs (effects of heparin can be reversed by protamine). Do not exceed recommended total doses (Adults: Acute ischemic stroke: 90 mg; acute myocardial infarction or pulmonary embolism: 100 mg); doses ≥150 mg are associated with an increase in intracranial hemorrhage compared to doses ≤100 mg. Significant bleeding complications including neonatal IVH and hemorrhage requiring PRBC transfusion have been reported in pediatric patients receiving systemic tPA therapy for thrombolysis (Monagle, 2012; Weiner, 1998).

Risks of bleeding from alteplase may be increased in the following conditions (risks vs benefits should be weighed carefully before use): Recent (within 10 days) major surgery (eg, CABG, obstetrical delivery, organ biopsy, previous puncture of noncompressible vessels), prolonged CPR with evidence of thoracic trauma, lumbar puncture within 1 week, cerebrovascular disease, recent GI or GU bleeding, recent trauma, hypertension (eg, adults with systolic BP ≥175 mm Hg and/or diastolic BP ≥110 mm Hg), patients with an increased risk of left heart thrombus (eg, mitral stenosis with atrial fibrillation), acute pericarditis, subacute bacterial endocarditis, hemostatic defects including ones caused by severe renal or hepatic dysfunction, significant hepatic dysfunction, diabetic hemorrhagic retinopathy or other hemorrhagic ophthalmic conditions, pregnancy, septic thrombophlebitis or occluded AV cannula at seriously infected site, advanced age (eg, >75 years old), current use of oral anticoagulants (eg, warfarin), and any other condition in which bleeding would be a significant risk or would be especially difficult to manage due to its location. For systemic use, pretreatment lab studies should include platelet count, PT/PTT, fibrinogen, fibrin degradation products, plasminogen, antithrombin III, protein S, protein C; blood pressure should be monitored during and after therapy.

Risk of bleeding is increased in patients receiving other anticoagulants. In the treatment of acute ischemic stroke, avoid aspirin for 24 hours following administration of alteplase; administration within 24 hours increases the risk of hemorrhagic transformation. Concurrent heparin anticoagulation may contribute to bleeding. In the treatment of acute ischemic stroke, concurrent use of anticoagulants was not permitted during the initial 24 hours of the <3-hour window trial (NINDS, 1995). The AHA/ASA does not recommend initiation of anticoagulant therapy within 24 hours of treatment with alteplase (Jauch, 2013). Initiation of SubQ heparin (≤10,000 units) or equivalent doses of low molecular weight heparin for prevention of DVT during the first 24 hours of the 3 to 4.5 hour window trial was permitted and did not increase the incidence of intracerebral hemorrhage (Hacke, 2008). For acute PE, withhold heparin during the 2-hour infusion period. Alteplase may be administered to patients with AIS having received direct thrombin inhibitors (eg, dabigatran) or direct factor Xa inhibitors (eg, rivaroxaban) when sensitive laboratory tests (eg, aPTT, INR, platelet count, ECT, TT, or appropriate direct factor Xa activity assays) are normal or the patient has not received a dose of these agents for >2 days (assuming normal renal function). When treating acute ischemic stroke 3 to 4.5 hours after symptom onset, the use of alteplase should be avoided with current use of any oral anticoagulant regardless of INR (Jauch, 2013). In the treatment of STEMI, adjunctive use of parenteral anticoagulants (eg, enoxaparin, heparin, or fondaparinux) is recommended to improve vessel patency and prevent reocclusion and may also contribute to bleeding; monitor for bleeding (ACCF/AHA; O'Gara, 2013).

For treatment of acute ischemic stroke, risks of alteplase therapy may be increased in patients with major early signs of infarct on CT and in those with severe neurological deficit at presentation (risks versus benefits should be weighed carefully). Patients who present **within 3 hours** of stroke symptom onset should be treated with alteplase unless contraindications exist. A longer time window (**3 to 4.5 hours** after symptom onset) has been shown to be safe and efficacious for select individuals (Hacke, 2008; Jauch, 2013).Treatment of patients with minor neurological deficit or with rapidly improving symptoms is not recommended.

Cholesterol embolism may occur (rare). Risk of stroke in acute MI patients who are at low risk for death from cardiac causes and who present with high blood pressure, may be greater than the survival benefit from thrombolytic therapy. Reperfusion arrhythmias may occur following coronary thrombolysis. In patients with pulmonary embolism, alteplase has not been proven to adequately treat underlying DVT; possible re-embolization from DVT may occur.

Injection contains polysorbate 80 (Tween 80) which may cause allergic reactions in susceptible individuals. In premature neonates, thrombocytopenia, ascites, pulmonary deterioration, and renal and hepatic failure have been reported after receiving parenteral products containing polysorbate 80 (Alade, 1986; CDC, 1984). Infusion of polysorbate 80-containing solutions through polyvinyl chloride tubing may cause DEHP to leach into the solution; in immature animals, exposure to DEHP may adversely affect the development of the male reproductive tract.

Precautions Use with caution if systemic alteplase is readministered; has not been studied; discontinue immediately if anaphylactoid reaction occurs.

Before instilling alteplase, consider other causes of central venous catheter occlusion (eg, mechanical failure, constriction by a suture, catheter malposition, and drug precipitates or lipid deposits within the lumen of the catheter) before use; do not use vigorous suction when determining catheter occlusion (vascular wall damage or collapse of soft-walled catheters may occur); avoid excessive pressure when instilling alteplase into an occluded catheter

(catheter may rupture or clot may become dislodged and enter the circulation). The use of alteplase has not been evaluated in patients who are at risk for bleeding; use with caution in patients with active internal bleeding or those who have had any of the following within 48 hours: Surgery, puncture of noncompressible vessels, obstetrical delivery, or percutaneous biopsy of viscera or deep tissues; use with caution in patients with thrombocytopenia, hemostatic defects including ones caused by severe renal or hepatic dysfunction, any condition in which bleeding would be a significant risk or would be especially difficult to manage due to its location, or those who are at a high risk for embolic complications (eg, venous thrombosis in the region of the catheter). Discontinue use and withdraw alteplase from catheter if serious bleeding in a critical location occurs. Use with caution in patients with known or suspected catheter infection (use of alteplase in these patients may release a localized infection in the catheter into the systemic circulation). Use of >2 doses of alteplase for line occlusion has not been studied.

Adverse Reactions As with all drugs which may affect hemostasis, bleeding is the major adverse effect associated with alteplase. Hemorrhage may occur at virtually any site. Risk is dependent on multiple variables, including the dosage administered, concurrent use of multiple agents which alter hemostasis, and patient predisposition. Rapid lysis of coronary artery thrombi by thrombolytic agents may be associated with reperfusion-related atrial and/or ventricular arrhythmia. **Note:** Lowest rate of bleeding complications expected with dose used to restore catheter function.

Cardiovascular: Hypotension

Central nervous system: Fever

Dermatologic: Bruising

Gastrointestinal: GI hemorrhage, nausea, vomiting

Genitourinary: GU hemorrhage

Hematologic: Bleeding

Local: Bleeding at catheter puncture site

Rare but important or life-threatening: Angioedema (orolingual), intracranial hemorrhage, retroperitoneal hemorrhage, pericardial hemorrhage, gingival hemorrhage, epistaxis, allergic reaction (anaphylaxis, anaphylactoid reactions, laryngeal edema, rash, and urticaria)

Additional cardiovascular events associated **with use in STEMI:** AV block, asystole, bradycardia, cardiac arrest, cardiac tamponade, cardiogenic shock, cholesterol crystal embolization, electromechanical dissociation, heart failure, hemorrhagic bursitis, mitral regurgitation, myocardial rupture, recurrent ischemia/infarction, pericardial effusion, pericarditis, pulmonary edema, ruptured intracranial AV malformation, seizure, thromboembolism, ventricular tachycardia

Additional events associated **with use in pulmonary embolism:** Pleural effusion, pulmonary re-embolization, pulmonary edema, thromboembolism

Additional events associated **with use in stroke:** Cerebral edema, cerebral herniation, new ischemic stroke, seizure

Drug Interactions

Metabolism/Transport Effects None known.

Avoid Concomitant Use There are no known interactions where it is recommended to avoid concomitant use.

Increased Effect/Toxicity

Alteplase may increase the levels/effects of: Anticoagulants; Dabigatran Etexilate

The levels/effects of Alteplase may be increased by: Agents with Antiplatelet Properties; Herbs (Anticoagulant/Antiplatelet Properties); Salicylates

Decreased Effect

The levels/effects of Alteplase may be decreased by: Aprotinin; Nitroglycerin

Stability

Activase: The lyophilized product may be stored at room temperature (not to exceed 30°C [86°F]), or under refrigeration (2°C to 8°C [36°F to 46°F]), protect from light. Once reconstituted, it should be used within 8 hours when stored between 2°C to 30°C (36°F to 86°F).

Cathflo Activase: Store lyophilized product under refrigeration (2°C to 8°C [36°F to 46°F]); protect from light. Once reconstituted, it should be used within 8 hours when stored between 2°C to 30°C (36°F to 86°F).

Solutions of 0.5 mg/mL, 1 mg/mL, and 2 mg/mL in SWI retained ≥94% of fibrinolytic activity at 48 hours when stored at 2°C in plastic syringes; these solutions retained ≥90% of fibrinolytic activity when stored in plastic syringes at -25°C or -70°C for 7 or 14 days, thawed at room temperature and then stored at 2°C for 48 hours (Davis, 2000). Solutions of 1 mg/mL in SWI were stable for 22 weeks in plastic syringes when stored at -30°C and for ~1 month in glass vials when stored at -20°C; bioactivity remained unchanged for 6 months in propylene containers when stored at -20°C and for 2 weeks in glass vials when stored at -70°C (Generali, 2001).

Mechanism of Action Initiates local fibrinolysis by binding to fibrin in a thrombus (clot) and converts entrapped plasminogen to plasmin

Pharmacodynamics Duration: >50% present in plasma cleared ~5 minutes after infusion terminated, ~80% cleared within 10 minutes; fibrinolytic activity persists for up to 1 hour after infusion terminated (Semba, 2000)

Pharmacokinetics (Adult data unless noted)

Distribution: V_d (initial): Approximates plasma volume

Half-life: Initial: 5 minutes

Elimination: Clearance: Rapidly from circulating plasma; 380 to 570 mL/minute; primarily hepatic; 80% of unbound drug is cleared within 10 minutes

Dosing: Neonatal

Occluded I.V. catheter: Intracatheter: **Dose listed is per lumen; for multilumen catheters, treat one lumen at a time; do not infuse into patient; dose should always be aspirated out of catheter after dwell.**

Manufacturer's labeling: Central venous catheter: Use a 1 mg/mL concentration; instill a volume equal to 110% of the internal lumen volume of the catheter; do not exceed 2 mg in 2 mL; leave in lumen for up to 2 hours, then aspirate out of catheter; may instill a second dose if catheter remains occluded after 2-hour dwell time

Alternate dosing:

Chest guidelines (Monagle, 2008): Limited data available: Central venous catheter: 0.5 mg diluted in NS to a volume equal to the internal volume of the lumen; instill in lumen over 1 to 2 minutes; leave in lumen for 1 to 2 hours, then aspirate out of catheter; flush catheter with NS. **Note:** The most recent guidelines (2012) continue to recommend alteplase as a treatment option but specific dosage recommendation is not provided (Monagle, 2012).

Soylu, 2010: Limited data available: Central venous catheter: 0.25 to 0.5 mg/mL solution; instill a volume to fill the catheter; leave in lumen for up to 2 hours, then aspirate out of catheter; dosing described in trial of 18 neonates including four patients with GA ≤32 weeks

Systemic thrombosis: Note: Dose must be titrated to effect. No pediatric studies have compared local to systemic thrombolytic therapy; therefore, there is no evidence to suggest that local infusions are superior. The pediatric patients' small vessel size may increase the chance of local damage to blood vessels and formation of a new thrombus; however, local infusion may be appropriate for catheter-related thrombosis if the catheter is already in place (Monagle, 2012). Various "low-dose" regimens have been used, both with local (or regional) and systemic administration.

Standard dose infusion: I.V.: **Note:** The optimal dose for various thrombotic conditions is not established; most published papers consist of case reports and series; few prospective neonatal studies have been conducted; dose must be titrated to effect (eg, fibrinogen >100 to 150 mg/dL). Administration of FFP may be considered prior to dose infusion. Current *Chest* guidelines recommend use only when major vessel occlusion is causing critical compromise of organs or limbs in the neonate (Monagle, 2012).

Chest guidelines (Monagle, 2012): Limited data available: Usual dose: 0.5 mg/kg/**hour** for 6 hours; reported range: 0.1 to 0.6 mg/kg/**hour**; some patients may require longer or shorter duration of therapy. Higher doses may be associated with an increased incidence of serious bleeding (Monagle, 2008; Monagle, 2012).

Additional reported standard dose regimens:

No loading dose regimens: Very limited data available: Seven neonates (GA: 24 to 38 weeks) with arterial thrombosis received a continuous I.V. infusion of 0.1 mg/kg/**hour** initially; infusion rate was titrated to maintain fibrinogen levels >100 mg/dL; dosage increases were made in 0.1 mg/kg/**hour** increments every 6 hours to a maximum of 0.4 mg/kg/**hour**; no heparin was used in these patients (Weiner, 1998). In case series of three neonates (GA: 26 to 36 weeks) with infective endocarditis and intracardiac thrombosis, a daily intermittent infusion of 0.2 mg/kg/**hour** over 6 hours for 5 days was used (Anderson, 2009).

Loading dose regimens: Limited data available; dosage reported varies widely: One trial of 16 neonates used a loading dose of 0.1 mg/kg over 10 minutes, followed by an intermittent infusion of 0.3 mg/kg/**hour** infusion for 3 hours every 12 to 24 hours as determined by response and monitoring parameters; a maximum of 4 additional intermittent doses were allowed; heparin was held during alteplase infusion (Farnoux, 1998). In another trial, a loading dose of 0.7 mg/kg bolus over 30 to 60 minutes was used followed by continuous I.V. infusion at an initial rate of 0.2 mg/kg/**hour** for 1 to 4 days in 13 neonates (GA: 27 to 42 weeks) with catheter-related thrombosis (used in conjunction with heparin infusion); reported effective range: 0.1 to 0.3 mg/kg/**hour** (Hartmann, 2001).

Low dose infusion: Very limited data available: Initial dose: I.V.: 0.02 to 0.03 mg/kg/**hour**, titrate dose based on patient response, range reported 0.01 to 0.06 mg/kg/**hour**; duration of therapy based on patient response. A trial comparing standard-dose and low-dose alteplase in pediatric patients included five neonates (four preterm; PNA 1 to 14 days) with acute thrombosis in low-dose group; dosing in neonates was initiated at 0.03 mg/kg/**hour**, in three neonates receiving systemic therapy, the effective dose was 0.03 mg/kg/**hour** in one patient and 0.06 mg/kg/**hour** in the other two patients; the remaining two neonates received local infusions and required a higher infusion rate (0.1 mg/kg/**hour** and 0.24 mg/kg/**hour**); duration of therapy ranged from 48 to 70 hours; complete clot resolution occurred in all patients. One preterm neonate with staphylococcal sepsis experienced a subdural bleed at the dose of 0.24 mg/kg/**hour** (Wang, 2003). One case series of four neonates and infants (PNA: 25 to 43 days, 2 preterm) with caval thrombosis due to central line reported using 0.02 to 0.1 mg/kg/**hour** with mixed results; resolution of clot occurred in only two patients (Anderson, 1991).

Dosing: Usual

Pediatric:

Occluded I.V. catheters: Infants, Children, Adolescents: Intracatheter: **Dose listed is per lumen; for multilumen catheters, treat one lumen at a time; do not infuse into patient; dose should always be aspirated out of catheter after dwell.**

Manufacturer's labeling: Central venous catheter:

Patients <30 kg: Use a 1 mg/mL concentration; instill a volume equal to 110% of the internal lumen volume of the catheter; do not exceed 2 mg in 2 mL; may instill a second dose if catheter remains occluded after 2-hour dwell time

Patients ≥30 kg: 2 mg in 2 mL; may instill second dose if catheter remains occluded after 2-hour dwell time

Chest guidelines (Monagle, 2008): **Note:** The most recent guidelines (2012) continue to recommend alteplase as a treatment option but specific dosage recommendation is not provided (Monagle, 2012)

Central venous catheter: **Note:** Some institutions use lower doses (eg, 0.25 mg/0.5 mL) in infants 1 to <3 months

Patients ≤10 kg: 0.5 mg diluted in NS to a volume equal to the internal volume of the lumen; instill in lumen over 1 to 2 minutes; leave in lumen for 1 to 2 hours, then **aspirate out of catheter, do not infuse into patient;** flush catheter with NS.

Patients >10 kg: 1 mg in 1 mL of NS; use a volume equal to the internal volume of the lumen; maximum: 2 mg in 2 mL per lumen; instill in each lumen over 1 to 2 minutes; leave in lumen for 1 to 2 hours; then **aspirate out of catheter, do not infuse into patient;** flush catheter with NS

SubQ port:

Patients ≤10 kg: 0.5 mg diluted with NS to 3 mL

Patients >10 kg: 2 mg diluted with NS to 3 mL

Systemic thrombosis: Note: Dose must be titrated to effect. No pediatric studies have compared local to systemic thrombolytic therapy; therefore, there is no evidence to suggest that local infusions are superior. The pediatric patients' small vessel size may increase the chance of local damage to blood vessels and formation of a new thrombus; however, local infusion may be appropriate for catheter-related thromboses if the catheter is already in place (Monagle, 2012).

Standard dose infusion: Limited data available; optimal dose not established; most published papers consist of case reports; few prospective pediatric studies have been conducted; several studies have used the following doses (Levy, 1991; Weiner, 1998): Infants, Children, and Adolescents: *Chest*, 2012 and AHA 2013 recommendations: I.V.: Usual dose: 0.5 mg/kg/**hour** for 6 hours; range: 0.1 to 0.6 mg/kg/**hour**; some patients may require longer or shorter duration of therapy; higher doses may be associated with an increased incidence of serious bleeding (Giglia, 2013; Monagle, 2008; Monagle 2012).

Low-dose infusion: Limited data available. Various "low-dose" regimens have been used: Infants, Children, and Adolescents:

AHA 2013 recommendations: I.V.: 0.03 to 0.06 mg/kg/**hour** for 12 to 48 hours; maximum hourly dose: 2 mg/hour (Giglia, 2013)

Additional reported regimens: I.V.:

Wang, 2003: Initial: 0.01 to 0.03 mg/kg/**hour**; usual effective range: 0.015 to 0.03 mg/kg/**hour**; duration of therapy based on clinical response; in this study of 17 pediatric patients (1.5 to 18 years) with acute and chronic thrombus, dosing was titrated to effect up to 0.06 mg/kg/**hour** in children and adolescents; final effective range: 0.007 to 0.06 mg/kg/**hour**; administration included systemic therapy as well as local infusions directly at site of thrombus (n=4); duration of therapy ranged from 4 to 96 hours. A similar dosing range has been reported in pediatric case reports (Doyle, 1992).

Leary, 2010: Initial: 0.03 to 0.06 mg/kg/**hour** for 12 to 48 hours; doses were titrated as necessary up to 0.12 mg/kg/**hour**; dosing from a retrospective study of 23 patients (median age: 12 years, range: 6 months to 21.5 years) diagnosed with DVT; eight patients required a dose increase to 0.12 mg/kg/**hour**; overall response rate: 59%, with complete clot resolution in 18% and partial resolution in 41%

Bratincsák, 2013: Initial: 0.05 mg/kg/**hour** for 30 minutes, if no signs of bleeding, rate increased to 0.1 mg/kg/**hour**; therapy used in 12 children with arterial or femoral vascular occlusions following cardiac catheterization

Catheter-directed infusion: Limited data available: Children and Adolescents: Intra-arterial, I.V. (administered through catheter or via catheter with tip placed at anatomic site of clot): 0.025 mg/kg/**hour** or 0.5 to 2 **mg/hour** for 12 to 24 hours (Giglia, 2013)

Parapneumonic effusion: Limited data available: Infants >3 months, Children, and Adolescents: Intrapleural:

Fixed dose: 4 mg in 40 mL NS, first dose at time of chest tube placement with 1-hour dwell time, repeat every 24 hours for 3 days (total of 3 doses) (Bradley, 2011; St. Peter, 2009)

Weight-directed: 0.1 mg/kg (maximum: 3 mg) in 10 to 30 mL NS, first dose after chest tube placement, 0.75- to 1-hour dwell time, repeat every 8 hours for 3 days (total of 9 doses) (Bradley, 2011; Hawkins, 2004)

Adult:

ST-elevation myocardial infarction (STEMI): I.V. (Activase): **Note:** Manufacturer's labeling recommends 3-hour infusion regimen; however, accelerated regimen preferred by the ACCF/AHA (O'Gara, 2013).

Accelerated regimen (weight-based):

Patients ≤67 kg: Infuse 15 mg I.V. bolus over 1 to 2 minutes followed by infusions of 0.75 mg/kg (not to exceed 50 mg) over 30 minutes then 0.5 mg/kg (not to exceed 35 mg) over 1 hour; maximum total dose: 100 mg

Patients >67 kg: Total dose: 100 mg over 1.5 hours; administered as a 15 mg I.V. bolus over 1 to 2 minutes followed by infusions of 50 mg over 30 minutes, then 35 mg over 1 hour; maximum total dose: 100 mg

Note: Thrombolytic should be administered within 30 minutes of hospital arrival. Administer concurrent aspirin, clopidogrel, and anticoagulant therapy (ie, unfractionated heparin, enoxaparin, or fondaparinux) with alteplase (O'Gara, 2013).

Acute massive or submassive pulmonary embolism (PE): I.V. (Activase): 100 mg over 2 hours; may be administered as a 10 mg bolus followed by 90 mg over 2 hours as was done in patients with submassive PE (Konstantinides, 2002). **Note:** Not recommended for submassive PE with minor RV dysfunction, minor myocardial necrosis, and no clinical worsening or low-risk PE (ie, normotensive, no RV dysfunction, normal biomarkers) (Jaff, 2011).

Acute ischemic stroke: I.V. (Activase): Within 3 hours of the onset of symptom onset **or** within 3 to 4.5 hours of symptom onset (Hacke, 2008; Jauch, 2013): **Note:** Perform noncontrast-enhanced CT or MRI prior to administration. Initiation of anticoagulants (eg, heparin) or antiplatelet agents (eg, aspirin) within 24 hours after starting alteplase is not recommended; however, initiation of aspirin within 24 to 48 hours after stroke onset is recommended (Jauch, 2013). Initiation of SubQ heparin (≤10,000 units) or equivalent doses of low molecular weight heparin for prevention of DVT during the first 24 hours of the 3 to 4.5 hour window trial did not increase incidence of intracerebral hemorrhage (Hacke, 2008).

Recommended total dose: 0.9 mg/kg (maximum total dose: 90 mg)

Patients ≤100 kg: Load with 0.09 mg/kg (10% of 0.9 mg/kg dose) as an I.V. bolus over 1 minute, followed by 0.81 mg/kg (90% of 0.9 mg/kg dose) as a continuous infusion over 60 minutes

Patients >100 kg: Load with 9 mg (10% of 90 mg) as an I.V. bolus over 1 minute, followed by 81 mg (90% of 90 mg) as a continuous infusion over 60 minutes

Central venous catheter clearance: Intracatheter (Cathflo Activase 1 mg/mL):

Patients <30 kg: 110% of the internal lumen volume of the catheter, not to exceed 2 mg/2 mL; retain in catheter for 0.5 to 2 hours; may instill a second dose if catheter remains occluded

Patients ≥30 kg: 2 mg (2 mL); retain in catheter for 0.5 to 2 hours; may instill a second dose if catheter remains occluded

Dosing adjustment in renal impairment: There are no dosage adjustments provided in manufacturer's labeling.

Dosing adjustment in hepatic impairment: There are no dosage adjustments provided in manufacturer's labeling.

Usual Infusion Concentrations: Pediatric I.V. infusion: 0.5 mg/mL or 1 mg/mL

Administration Parenteral:

I.V.: Activase: Reconstitute vials with supplied diluent (SWI); do not reconstitute with bacteriostatic water for injection; use large bore needle and syringe to reconstitute 50 mg vial (50 mg vial has a vacuum) and accompanying transfer device to reconstitute 100 mg vial (100 mg vial does not contain vacuum); swirl gently, do not shake; final concentration after reconstitution: 1 mg/mL. Reconstituted solution should be clear or pale yellow and transparent with a pH of 5 to 7.3. The 1 mg/mL solution may be administered or may be diluted further (immediately before use) with an equal volume of NS or D₅W to yield a final concentration of 0.5 mg/mL; swirl gently, do not shake; dilutions to concentrations <0.5 mg/mL are not recommended for routine clinical use; dilutions <0.5 mg/mL using D₅W or SWI may result in a precipitate (Frazin, 1990).

Prepare bolus dose using one of the following methods: 1) Remove bolus dose from reconstituted vial using syringe and needle; for 50 mg vial: do not prime syringe with air, insert needle into vial stopper; for 100 mg vial, insert needle away from puncture mark created by transfer device; 2) Remove bolus dose from a port on the infusion line after priming; 3) Program an infusion pump to deliver the bolus at the beginning of the infusion. Administer the remaining dose as follows: From 50 mg vial: Use polyvinyl chloride I.V. bag or glass vial and infusion set; from 100 mg vial: Use same puncture site made by transfer device to insert spike end of infusion set and infuse from vial.

Intracatheter: CathFlo Activase: Reconstitute vial with 2.2 mL of SWI; do not reconstitute with bacteriostatic water for injection; allow vial to stand undisturbed so large bubbles may dissipate; swirl gently, do not shake; complete dissolution occurs within 3 minutes; final concentration after reconstitution: 1 mg/mL. Discard any unused solution (solution does not contain preservatives).

Instill the appropriate dose into the occluded catheter; do not force solution into catheter; leave in lumen; evaluate catheter function (by attempting to aspirate blood) after 30 minutes; if catheter is functional, aspirate 4-5 mL of blood out of catheter in patients ≥10 kg or 3 mL in patients <10 kg to remove drug and residual clot, then gently flush catheter with NS; if catheter is still occluded, leave alteplase in lumen and evaluate catheter function after 120 minutes of dwell time; if catheter is functional, aspirate 4-5 mL of blood out of catheter in patients ≥10 kg or 3 mL in patients <10 kg and gently flush with NS; if catheter remains occluded after 120 minutes of dwell time, a second dose may be instilled by repeating the above administration procedure.

Intrapleural: Instill dose into chest tube at time of chest tube placement and clamp drain. Although the optimum dwell time has not been determined, clinical trials more often have used either a 45 minute (Hawkins, 2004) or 1 hour (Rahman, 2011; St. Peter, 2009) dwell time; after dwell period, release clamp and connect chest tube to continuous suction.

Monitoring Parameters

Systemic use: Blood pressure; CBC, reticulocyte, platelet count; fibrinogen level, plasminogen, fibrin/fibrinogen degradation products, PT, PTT, signs of bleeding

Intracatheter use: Catheter function (by attempting to aspirate blood); signs of sepsis, GI bleeding, bleeding at injection site, and venous thrombosis

Test Interactions Altered results of coagulation and fibrinolytic activity tests

Additional Information Activase and CathFlo Activase also contain L-arginine and phosphoric acid (for pH adjustment).

Advantages of alteplase include: Low immunogenicity, short half-life, direct activation of plasminogen, and a strong and specific affinity for fibrin. Failure of thrombolytic agents in newborns/neonates may occur due to the low plasminogen concentrations (~50% to 70% of adult levels); supplementing plasminogen (via administration of fresh frozen plasma) may possibly help. Osmolality of 1 mg/mL solution is ~215 mOsm/kg.

Dosage Forms Excipient information presented when available (limited, particularly for generics); consult specific product labeling.

Solution Reconstituted, Injection:
Cathflo Activase: 2 mg (1 ea)
Solution Reconstituted, Intravenous:
Activase: 50 mg (1 ea); 100 mg (1 ea)

References

Activase (alteplase) [prescribing information]. South San Francisco, CA: Genentech, Inc; December 2012.

Alade SL, Brown RE, and Paquet A Jr, "Polysorbate 80 and E-Ferol Toxicity," *Pediatrics*, 1986, 77(4):593-7.

Anderson BJ, Keeley SR, and Johnson ND, "Caval Thrombolysis in Neonates Using Low Doses of Recombinant Human Tissue-Type Plasminogen Activator," *Anaesth Intensive Care*, 1991, 19(1):22-7.

Anderson B, Urs P, Tudehope D, et al, "The Use of Recombinant Tissue Plasminogen Activator in the Management of Infective Intracardiac Thrombi in Pre-term Infants With Thrombocytopaenia," *J Paediatr Child Health*, 2009, 45(10):598-601.

Andrew M, Brooker L, Leaker M, et al, "Fibrin Clot Lysis by Thrombolytic Agents is Impaired in Newborns Due to a Low Plasminogen Concentration," *Thromb Haemost*, 1992, 68(3):325-30.

Bates SM, Greer IA, Middeldorp S, et al, "VTE, Thrombophilia, Antithrombotic Therapy, and Pregnancy: Antithrombotic Therapy and Prevention of Thrombosis, 9th ed: American College of Chest Physicians Evidence-Based Clinical Practice Guidelines," *Chest*, 2012, 141(2 Suppl):e691S-736S.

Bradley JS, Byington CL, Shah SS, et al. The management of community-acquired pneumonia in infants and children older than 3 months of age: clinical practice guidelines by the Pediatric Infectious Diseases Society and the Infectious Diseases Society of America. *Clin Infect Dis*. 2011;53(7):e25-76.

Bratincsák A, Moore JW, El-Said HG. Low dose tissue plasminogen activator treatment for vascular thrombosis following cardiac catheterization in children: a single center experience. *Catheter Cardiovasc Interv*. 2013;82(5):782-785.

Cada DJ, Levien T, and Baker DE, "Alteplase," *Hospital Pharmacy*, 2002, 37(2): 148-54.

Cathflo Activase (alteplase) [prescribing information]. South San Francisco, CA: Genentech, Inc; March 2010.

Centers for Disease Control (CDC), "Unusual Syndrome With Fatalities Among Premature Infants: Association With a New Intravenous Vitamin E Product," *MMWR Morb Mortal Wkly Rep*, 1984, 33 (14):198-9.

Choi M, Massicotte MP, Marzinotto V, et al, "The Use of Alteplase to Restore Patency of Central Venous Lines in Pediatric Patients: A Cohort Study," *J Pediatr*, 2001, 139(1):152-6.

Davis SN, Vermeulen L, Banton J, et al, "Activity and Dosage of Alteplase Dilution for Clearing Occlusions of Venous-Access Devices," *Am J Health Syst Pharm*, 2000, 57(11):1039-45.

Doyle E, Britto J, Freeman J, et al, "Thrombolysis With Low Dose Tissue Plasminogen Activator," *Arch Dis Child*, 1992, 67(12):1483-4.

Farnoux C, Camard O, Pinquier D, et al, "Recombinant Tissue-Type Plasminogen Activator Therapy of Thrombosis in 16 Neonates," *J Pediatr*, 1998, 133(1):137-40.

Frazin BS, "Maximal Dilution of Activase," *Am J Hosp Pharm*, 1990, 47 (5):1016.

Generali J and Cada DJ, "Alteplase (t-PA) Bolus: Occluded Catheters," *Hospital Pharmacy*, 2001, 36(1):93-103.

Giglia TM, Massicotte MP, Tweddell JS, et al. Prevention and treatment of thrombosis in pediatric and congenital heart disease: a scientific statement from the American Heart Association. *Circulation*. 2013;128 (24):2622-2703.

Hacke W, Kaste M, Bluhmki E, et al. Thrombolysis with alteplase 3 to 4.5 hours after acute ischemic stroke. *N Engl J Med*. 2008; 359 (13):1317-1329.

Hartmann J, Hussein A, Trowitzsch E, et al, "Treatment of Neonatal Thrombus Formation With Recombinant Tissue Plasminogen Activator: Six Years Experience and Review of the Literature," *Arch Dis Child Fetal Neonatal Ed*, 2001, 85(1):F18-22.

Hawkins JA, Scaife ES, Hillman ND, Feola GP. Current treatment of pediatric empyema. *Semin Thorac Cardiovasc Surg*. 2004;16 (3):196-200.

Jaff MR, McMurtry MS, Archer SL, et al, "Management of Massive and Submassive Pulmonary Embolism, Iliofemoral Deep Vein Thrombosis, and Chronic Thromboembolic Pulmonary Hypertension: A Scientific Statement from the American Heart Association," *Circulation*, 2011, 123(16):1788-830.

Jauch EC, Saver JL, Adams HP Jr, et al, "Guidelines for the Early Management of Patients With Acute Ischemic Stroke: A Guideline for Healthcare Professionals From the American Heart Association/ American Stroke Association," *Stroke*, 2013, 44(3):870-947.

Konstantinides S, Geibel A, Heusel G, et al. Heparin plus alteplase compared with heparin alone in patients with submassive pulmonary embolism. *N Engl J Med*. 2002;347(15):1143-1150.

Leary SE, Harrod VL, de Alarcon PA, Reiss UM. Low-dose systemic thrombolytic therapy for deep vein thrombosis in pediatric patients. *J Pediatr Hematol Oncol*. 2010;32(2):97-102.

Leonhardt G, Gaul C, Nietsch HH, et al, "Thrombolytic Therapy in Pregnancy," *J Thromb Thrombolysis*, 2006, 21(3):271-6.

Levy M, Benson LN, Burrows PE, et al, "Tissue Plasminogen Activator for the Treatment of Thromboembolism in Infants and Children," *J Pediatr*, 1991, 118(3):467-72.

Li Y, Margraf J, Kluck B, et al, "Thrombolytic Therapy For Ischemic Stroke Secondary to Paradoxical Embolism in Pregnancy: A Case Report and Literature Review," *Neurologist*, 2012, 18(1):44-8.

Monagle P, Chalmers E, Chan A, et al, "Antithrombotic Therapy in Neonates and Children: American College of Chest Physicians Evidence-Based Clinical Practice Guidelines (8th Edition)," *Chest*, 2008, 133(6 Suppl):887S-968S.

Monagle P, Chan A, Goldenberg NA, et al. Antithrombotic therapy in neonates and children: American College of Chest Physicians Evidence-Based Clinical Practice Guidelines, 9th Edition. *Chest*, 2012, 141(2 Suppl):e737-801.

Nowak-Gottl U, Auberger K, Halimeh S, et al, "Thrombolysis in Newborns and Infants," *Thromb Haemost*, 1999, 82 (Suppl 1):112-6.

O'Gara PT, Kushner FG, Ascheim DD, et al, "2013 ACCF/AHA Guideline for the Management of ST-Elevation Myocardial Infarction: A Report of the American College of Cardiology Foundation/American Heart Association Task Force on Practice Guidelines," *Circulation*, 2013, 127(4):e362-425.

Ponec D, Irwin D, Haire WD, et al, "Recombinant Tissue Plasminogen Activator (Alteplase) for Restoration of Flow in Occluded Central Venous Access Devices: A Double-Blind Placebo-Controlled Trial - The Cardiovascular Thrombolytic to Open Occluded Lines (COOL) Efficacy Trial," *J Vasc Intern Radiol*, 2001, 12(8):951-5.

Rahman NM, Maskell NA, West A, et al. Intrapleural use of tissue plasminogen activator and DNase in pleural infection. *N Engl J Med*. 2011;365(6):518-526.

Semba CP, Bakal CW, Calis KA, et al. Alteplase as an alternative to urokinase. Advisory Panel on Catheter-Directed Thrombolytic Therapy. *J Vasc Interv Radiol*. 2000;11(3):279-287.

Soylu H, Brandão LR, and Lee KS, "Efficacy of Local Instillation of Recombinant Tissue Plasminogen Activator for Restoring Occluded Central Venous Catheters in Neonates," *J Pediatr*, 2010, 156 (2):197-201.

St Peter SD, Tsao, K, Harrison C, et al. Thoracoscopic decortication vs tube thoracostomy with fibrinolysis for empyema in children: a prospective, randomized trial. *J Pediatr Surg*. 2009;44(1):106-111.

Tissue plasminogen activator for acute ischemic stroke. The National Institute of Neurological Disorders and Stroke rt-PA Stroke Study Group. *N Engl J Med*. 1995;333(24):1581-1587.

Vanden Hoek TL, Morrison LJ, Shuster M, et al, "Part 12: Cardiac Arrest in Special Situations: 2010 American Heart Association Guidelines for Cardiopulmonary Resuscitation and Emergency Cardiovascular Care," *Circulation*, 2010, 122(18 Suppl 3):829-61.

Wang M, Hays T, Balasa V, et al. Low-dose tissue plasminogen activator thrombolysis in children. *J Pediatr Hematol Oncol.* 2003;25 (5):379-386.

Weiner GM, Castle VP, DiPietro MA, et al, "Successful Treatment of Neonatal Arterial Thromboses With Recombinant Tissue Plasminogen Activator," *J Pediatr,* 1998, 133(1):133-6.

◆ **Alteplase, Recombinant** see Alteplase on page 104

◆ **Alteplase, Tissue Plasminogen Activator, Recombinant** see Alteplase on page 104

◆ **Alti-Flurbiprofen (Can)** see Flurbiprofen (Systemic) on page 908

◆ **Alti-Ipratropium (Can)** see Ipratropium (Nasal) on page 1146

◆ **Alti-MPA (Can)** see MedroxyPROGESTERone on page 1318

◆ **Altoprev** see Lovastatin on page 1286

Aluminum Acetate (a LOO mi num AS e tate)

Brand Names: U.S. Domeboro [OTC]; Gordon Boro-Packs [OTC]; Pedi-Boro [OTC]

Therapeutic Category Topical Skin Product

Generic Availability (U.S.) Yes, may be product dependent

Use Astringent wet dressing for relief of inflammatory conditions of the skin and to reduce weeping that may occur in dermatitis; relieve minor skin irritations due to poison ivy, poison oak, poison sumac, insect bites, athlete's foot, and rashes caused by soaps, detergents, cosmetics, or jewelry

Pregnancy Considerations Animal reproduction studies have not been conducted. The amount of aluminum acetate available systemically following topical application is unknown.

Breast-Feeding Considerations It is not known if topically administered aluminum acetate is excreted in breast milk.

Contraindications Use with topical collagenase

Precautions Do not use plastic or other impervious material to prevent evaporation

Drug Interactions

Metabolism/Transport Effects None known.

Avoid Concomitant Use

Avoid concomitant use of Aluminum Acetate with any of the following: BCG

Increased Effect/Toxicity There are no known significant interactions involving an increase in effect.

Decreased Effect

Aluminum Acetate may decrease the levels/effects of: BCG; Sodium Picosulfate

Dosing: Usual Children and Adults: Topical: Soak the affected area in the solution 2-4 times/day for 15-30 minutes or apply wet dressing soaked in the solution 2-4 times/day for 30-minute treatment periods; rewet dressing with solution every few minutes to keep it moist

Administration Topical: Keep away from eyes, external use only; one powder packet dissolved in 16 oz of water makes a modified Burow's solution equivalent to a 1:40 dilution, 2 packets: 1:20 dilution, 3 packets: 1:13 dilution. When used as a compress or wet dressing, soak a clean soft cloth in the solution. Apply cloth loosely to affected area for 15-30 minutes.

Dosage Forms Excipient information presented when available (limited, particularly for generics); consult specific product labeling.

Powder, for solution, topical: Aluminum sulfate 1191 mg and calcium acetate 839 mg per packet (12s)

Domeboro: Aluminum sulfate tetradecahydrate 1347 mg and calcium acetate monohydrate 952 mg per packet (12s, 100s)

Gordon Boro-Packs: Aluminum sulfate 49% and calcium acetate 51% per packet (100s)

Pedi-Boro: Aluminum sulfate tetradecahydrate 1191 mg and calcium acetate monohydrate 839 mg per packet (12s, 100s)

Aluminum Hydroxide
(a LOO mi num hye DROKS ide)

Brand Names: U.S. DermaMed [OTC]

Brand Names: Canada Amphojel®; Basaljel®

Therapeutic Category Antacid; Antidote; Gastrointestinal Agent, Gastric or Duodenal Ulcer Treatment; Protectant, Topical

Generic Availability (U.S.) May be product dependent

Use

Oral: Adjunct for the relief of peptic ulcer pain and to promote healing of peptic ulcers; relief of sour stomach or stomach upset associated with hyperacidity; relief of heartburn; treatment of gastritis, esophagitis, and gastroesophageal reflux disease; reduce phosphate absorption in hyperphosphatemia

Topical: Temporary protection of minor cuts, scrapes, burns, and other skin irritations

Pregnancy Considerations Most aluminum-containing antacids are considered low risk during pregnancy (Mahadevan, 2006).

Contraindications Hypersensitivity to aluminum salts or any component

Warnings

Oral: Hypophosphatemia may occur with prolonged aluminum hydroxide administration or with large doses; aluminum toxicity and osteomalacia may occur in patients with chronic kidney disease.

Topical: Not for application over deep wounds, puncture wounds, infected areas, or lacerations. When used for self medication (OTC use), consult with healthcare provider if needed for >7 days or for use in children <6 months of age.

Precautions Use oral aluminum hydroxide with caution in patients with decreased bowel motility and dehydration, gastric outlet obstruction, renal failure, CHF, edema, cirrhosis, and in patients who have an upper GI hemorrhage

Adverse Reactions

Gastrointestinal: Constipation, discoloration of feces (white speckles), fecal impaction, nausea, stomach cramps, vomiting

Endocrine & metabolic: Hypomagnesemia, hypophosphatemia

Drug Interactions

Metabolism/Transport Effects None known.

Avoid Concomitant Use

Avoid concomitant use of Aluminum Hydroxide with any of the following: Deferasirox; PONATinib; QuiNINE; Raltegravir; Vitamin D Analogs

Increased Effect/Toxicity

Aluminum Hydroxide may increase the levels/effects of: Amphetamines; Dexmethylphenidate; Methylphenidate

The levels/effects of Aluminum Hydroxide may be increased by: Ascorbic Acid; Calcium Polystyrene Sulfonate; Citric Acid Derivatives; Multivitamins/Fluoride (with ADE); Multivitamins/Minerals (with ADEK, Folate, Iron); Multivitamins/Minerals (with AE, No Iron); Sodium Polystyrene Sulfonate; Vitamin D Analogs

Decreased Effect

Aluminum Hydroxide may decrease the levels/effects of: ACE Inhibitors; Allopurinol; Anticonvulsants (Hydantoin); Antipsychotic Agents (Phenothiazines); Atazanavir; Bisacodyl; Bisphosphonate Derivatives; Bosutinib; Cefditoren; Cefpodoxime; Cefuroxime; Chenodiol; Chloroquine; Corticosteroids (Oral); Dabigatran Etexilate; Dabrafenib; Dasatinib; Deferasirox; Deferiprone; Delavirdine; Dolutegravir; Eltrombopag; Elvitegravir; Erlotinib; Ethambutol;

Fexofenadine; Gabapentin; HMG-CoA Reductase Inhibitors; Hyoscyamine; Iron Salts; Isoniazid; Itraconazole; Ketoconazole (Systemic); Levothyroxine; Mesalamine; Methenamine; Multivitamins/Fluoride (with ADE); Mycophenolate; Nilotinib; PAZOPanib; PenicillAMINE; Phosphate Supplements; PONATinib; Potassium Acid Phosphate; Protease Inhibitors; QuiNINE; Quinolone Antibiotics; Raltegravir; Rilpivirine; Riociguat; Strontium Ranelate; Sulpiride; Tetracycline Derivatives; Trientine; Ursodiol; Vismodegib

Stability Avoid freezing

Mechanism of Action Neutralizes hydrochloride in stomach to form Al $(Cl)_3$ salt + H_2O

Pharmacodynamics

Duration: Dependent on gastric emptying time

Fasting state: 20-60 minutes

One hour after meals: Up to 3 hours

Pharmacokinetics (Adult data unless noted) Elimination: Excreted by the kidneys (normal renal function): 17% to 30%; combines with dietary phosphate in the intestine and is excreted in the feces

Dosing: Usual

Oral:

Antacid:

Children: 300-900 mg between meals and at bedtime

Adolescents and Adults: 600-1200 mg between meals and at bedtime; or 600 mg 5-6 times/day between meals; maximum daily dose: 3600 mg/day; do not use maximum daily dose for more than 2 weeks without physician consultation

Hyperphosphatemia associated with chronic renal failure:

Children: 30 mg/kg/day in divided doses 3 or 4 times/day; maximum daily dose: 3000 mg/day; titrate to normal serum phosphorus level

Adolescents and Adults: 300-600 mg 3 or 4 times/day; maximum daily dose: 3000 mg/day

Topical: Apply to affected area as needed; reapply at least every 12 hours

Administration

Oral: Shake suspension well before use; dose should be followed with water

Antacid: Administer 1-3 hours after meals

To decrease phosphorus: Administer within 20 minutes of a meal

Topical: For external use only

Monitoring Parameters Monitor for GI complaints, stool frequency; serum phosphate and serum aluminum concentrations in patients with chronic kidney disease

Reference Range Baseline serum aluminum level <20 mcg/L

Test Interactions Decreased phosphorus, inorganic (S)

Additional Information Sodium content of ALternaGel®: <0.11 mEq per 5 mL

Dosage Forms Excipient information presented when available (limited, particularly for generics); consult specific product labeling.

Ointment, External:

DermaMed: (113 g)

Suspension, Oral:

Generic: 320 mg/5 mL (473 mL)

References

Avner ED, Harmon W, and Niaudet P, "Chronic Renal Disease," Pediatric Nephrology, 5th ed, Baltimore, MD: Lippincott Williams & Wilkins, 2003, 1363.

"K/DOQI Clinical Practice Guidelines for Bone Metabolism and Disease in Chronic Kidney Disease. Guideline 11. Aluminum Overload and Toxicity in CKD," 2002, available at www.kidney.org/professionals/kdoqi/guidelines_bone/guide11.htm.

Mahadevan U and Kane S, "American Gastroenterological Association Institute Medical Position Statement on the Use of Gastrointestinal Medications in Pregnancy," Gastroenterology, 2006, 131(1):278-82.

Aluminum Hydroxide and Magnesium Hydroxide

(a LOO mi num hye DROKS ide & mag NEE zhum hye DROK side)

Brand Names: U.S. Alamag [OTC]; Mag-Al Ultimate [OTC]; Mag-Al [OTC]

Brand Names: Canada Diovol®; Diovol® Ex; Gelusil® Extra Strength; Mylanta™

Therapeutic Category Antacid; Gastrointestinal Agent, Gastric or Duodenal Ulcer Treatment

Generic Availability (U.S.) No

Use Adjunct for the relief of heartburn, peptic ulcer pain, and to promote healing of peptic ulcers; relief of stomach upset associated with hyperacidity

Pregnancy Considerations See individual agents.

Breast-Feeding Considerations See individual agents.

Contraindications Hypersensitivity to aluminum hydroxide, magnesium hydroxide, or any component

Warnings Some liquids/suspensions contain propylene glycol; toxicities have been reported with use of products containing propylene glycol, including hyperosmolality, lactic acidosis, seizures, and respiratory depression; in neonates large amounts of propylene glycol delivered orally, intravenously (eg, >3000 mg/day), or topically have been associated with potentially fatal toxicities which can include metabolic acidosis, seizures, renal failure, and CNS depression; use liquids/suspensions containing propylene glycol with caution (AAP, 1997; Shehab, 2009).

Precautions Use with caution in patients with decreased bowel motility, dehydration, diarrhea, appendicitis, gastric outlet obstruction, and in patients who have an upper GI hemorrhage. There are reports of osteomalacia and osteoporosis due to aluminum toxicity associated with use. Prolonged antacid therapy may result in hypophosphatemia; aluminum in antacid may form insoluble complexes with phosphate leading to decreased phosphate absorption in the GI tract. Rarely, severe hypophosphatemia can lead to anorexia, muscle weakness, malaise, and osteomalacia. Use with caution in patients with renal impairment; avoid use in severe renal impairment; hypermagnesemia or aluminum intoxication may occur in severe renal impairment, particularly with prolonged use. Aluminum intoxication may lead to osteomalacia or dialysis encephalopathy. Some tablets may contain phenylalanine which must be avoided (or used with caution) in patients with phenylketonuria

Adverse Reactions

Gastrointestinal: Constipation, chalky taste, cramping, fecal discoloration (white speckles), fecal impaction, nausea, vomiting

Endocrine & metabolic: Hypophosphatemia (rare), hypermagnesemia (rare)

Drug Interactions

Metabolism/Transport Effects None known.

Avoid Concomitant Use

Avoid concomitant use of Aluminum Hydroxide and Magnesium Hydroxide with any of the following: Calcium Polystyrene Sulfonate; Deferasirox; PONATinib; QuiNINE; Raltegravir; Sodium Polystyrene Sulfonate; Vitamin D Analogs

Increased Effect/Toxicity

Aluminum Hydroxide and Magnesium Hydroxide may increase the levels/effects of: Amphetamines; Calcium Channel Blockers; Calcium Polystyrene Sulfonate; Dexmethylphenidate; Gabapentin; Methylphenidate; Misoprostol; Neuromuscular-Blocking Agents; QuiNIDine; Sodium Polystyrene Sulfonate

The levels/effects of Aluminum Hydroxide and Magnesium Hydroxide may be increased by: Ascorbic Acid; Calcium Channel Blockers; Citric Acid Derivatives; Multivitamins/Fluoride (with ADE); Multivitamins/Minerals (with ADEK, Folate, Iron); Multivitamins/Minerals (with AE, No Iron); Vitamin D Analogs

Decreased Effect

Aluminum Hydroxide and Magnesium Hydroxide may decrease the levels/effects of: ACE Inhibitors; Allopurinol; Anticonvulsants (Hydantoin); Antipsychotic Agents (Phenothiazines); Atazanavir; Bisacodyl; Bisphosphonate Derivatives; Bosutinib; Cefditoren; Cefpodoxime; Cefuroxime; Chenodiol; Chloroquine; Corticosteroids (Oral); Dabigatran Etexilate; Dabrafenib; Dasatinib; Deferasirox; Deferiprone; Delavirdine; Dolutegravir; Eltrombopag; Elvitegravir; Erlotinib; Ethambutol; Fexofenadine; Gabapentin; HMG-CoA Reductase Inhibitors; Hyoscyamine; Iron Salts; Isoniazid; Itraconazole; Ketoconazole (Systemic); Levothyroxine; Mesalamine; Methenamine; Multivitamins/Fluoride (with ADE); Mycophenolate; Nilotinib; PAZOPanib; PenicillAMINE; Phosphate Supplements; PONATinib; Potassium Acid Phosphate; Protease Inhibitors; QuiNINE; Quinolone Antibiotics; Raltegravir; Rilpivirine; Riociguat; Strontium Ranelate; Sulpiride; Tetracycline Derivatives; Trientine; Ursodiol; Vismodegib

The levels/effects of Aluminum Hydroxide and Magnesium Hydroxide may be decreased by: Trientine

Stability Store at room temperature; avoid freezing

Pharmacodynamics Duration: Dependent on gastric emptying time

Fasting state: 20-60 minutes

1 hour after meals: May be up to 3 hours

Dosing: Usual Note: Chronic administration is not recommended in children (Rudolph, 2001); dosing information for children is limited; very few published clinical trials are available. The following pediatric dosing represents suggestions from review articles (for children <12 years) or product labeling (children ≥12 years):

Liquid (aluminum hydroxide 200 mg and magnesium hydroxide 200 mg per 5 mL):

Children <12 years: 0.5-1 mL/kg/dose after meals and at bedtime (maximum dose: 15 mL) (Orenstein, 1988)

Children ≥12 years and Adults: 10-20 mL 4 times/day (maximum daily dose: 80 mL/day)

Suspension (aluminum hydroxide 500 mg and magnesium hydroxide 500 mg per 5 mL): Children ≥12 years and Adults: 10-20 mL 4 times/day, between meals and at bedtime (maximum daily dose: 45 mL/day)

Tablet (aluminum hydroxide 300 mg and magnesium hydroxide 150 mg):

Children 6-11 years: 1-2 tablets 4 times/day

Children ≥12 years and Adults: 1-2 tablets after meals and at bedtime, or as needed (maximum: 16 tablets/day)

Administration Oral:

Liquid, suspension: Shake suspensions well before use; administer 1-2 hours after meals when stomach acidity is highest

Tablet: Chew tablets thoroughly before swallowing or allow tablets to dissolve slowly in mouth; follow by a full glass of water

Monitoring Parameters GI complaints, stool frequency; serum phosphate concentrations in patients on hemodialysis receiving chronic aluminum-containing antacid therapy; serum electrolytes in patients with renal impairment receiving magnesium-containing antacids

Dosage Forms Excipient information presented when available (limited, particularly for generics); consult specific product labeling. [DSC] = Discontinued product

Liquid, oral:

Mag-Al: Aluminum hydroxide 200 mg and magnesium hydroxide 200 mg per 5 mL (30 mL) [dye free, ethanol free, sugar free; contains propylene glycol, sodium 4 mg/5 mL; peppermint flavor]

Suspension, oral:

Mag-Al Ultimate: Aluminum hydroxide 500 mg and magnesium hydroxide 500 mg per 5 mL (20 mL) [contains propylene glycol, sodium 4 mg/5 mL; peppermint flavor]

Tablet, chewable:

Alamag: Aluminum hydroxide 300 mg and magnesium hydroxide 150 mg [contains phenylalanine 2.63 mg; wild cherry flavor]

References

American Academy of Pediatrics Committee on Drugs. "Inactive" ingredients in pharmaceutical products: update (subject review). *Pediatrics.* 1997;99(2):268-278.

Nord KS, "Peptic Ulcer Disease in the Pediatric Population," *Pediatr Clin North Am,* 1988, 35(1):117-40.

Orenstein SR and Orenstein DM, "Gastroesophageal Reflux and Respiratory Disease in Children," *J Pediatr,* 1988, 112(6):847-58.

Rudolph CD, Mazur LJ, Liptak GS, et al, "Guidelines for Evaluation and Treatment of Gastroesophageal Reflux in Infants and Children: Recommendations of the North American Society for Pediatric Gastroenterology and Nutrition," *J Pediatr Gastroenterol Nutr,* 2001, 32 (Suppl 2):S1-31.

Shaffer SE and Levine S, "Gastroesophageal Reflux in Children," *Hosp Pharm,* 2003, 38(3):212-7.

Shapiro GG and Christie DL, "Gastroesophageal Reflux in Steroid-Dependent Asthmatic Youths," *Pediatrics,* 1979, 63(2):207-12.

Shehab N, Lewis CL, Streetman DD, Donn SM. Exposure to the pharmaceutical excipients benzyl alcohol and propylene glycol among critically ill neonates. *Pediatr Crit Care Med.* 2009;10 (2):256-259.

Sutphen JL, Dillard VL, and Pipan ME, "Antacid and Formula Effects on Gastric Acidity in Infants With Gastroesophageal Reflux," *Pediatrics,* 1986, 78(1):55-7.

◆ **Aluminum Sucrose Sulfate, Basic** *see* Sucralfate *on page 1940*

◆ **Aluminum Sulfate and Calcium Acetate** *see* Aluminum Acetate *on page 110*

◆ **Aluminum Sulfate Tetradecahydrate and Calcium Acetate** *see* Aluminum Acetate *on page 110*

◆ **Alupent** *see* Metaproterenol *on page 1352*

◆ **Alvesco** *see* Ciclesonide (Oral Inhalation) *on page 461*

◆ **Alvesco® (Can)** *see* Ciclesonide (Oral Inhalation) *on page 461*

Amantadine (a MAN ta deen)

Medication Safety Issues

Sound-alike/look-alike issues:

Amantadine may be confused with ranitidine, rimantadine

Symmetrel may be confused with Synthroid®

Brand Names: Canada Dom-Amantadine; Mylan-Amantadine; PHL-Amantadine; PMS-Amantadine

Therapeutic Category Anti-Parkinson's Agent (Dopamine Agonist); Antiviral Agent; Antiviral Agent, Adamantane

Generic Availability (U.S.) Yes

Use Prophylaxis and treatment of influenza A viral infection (FDA approved in ages ≥1 year and adults); **Note:** Due to high resistance rates, amantadine is no longer recommended by the CDC for the treatment or prophylaxis of influenza A (CDC, 2011); symptomatic and adjunct treatment of parkinsonism; treatment of drug-induced extrapyramidal reactions (FDA approved in adults); has also been used for attention-deficit/hyperactivity disorder (ADHD), autism, fatigue associated with multiple sclerosis, and in post-traumatic brain injury for behavior and cognition

Pregnancy Risk Factor C

Pregnancy Considerations Teratogenic effects were observed in animal studies and in case reports in humans.

Influenza infection may be more severe in pregnant women. Untreated influenza infection is associated with an increased risk of adverse events to the fetus and an increased risk of complications or death to the mother. Oseltamivir and zanamivir are currently recommended for the treatment or prophylaxis influenza in pregnant women and women up to 2 weeks postpartum. Antiviral agents are currently recommended as an adjunct to vaccination and should not be used as a substitute for vaccination in pregnant women (consult current CDC guidelines).

Healthcare providers are encouraged to refer women exposed to influenza vaccine, or who have taken an antiviral medication during pregnancy to the Vaccines and Medications in Pregnancy Surveillance System (VAMPSS) by contacting The Organization of Teratology Information Specialists (OTIS) at (877) 311-8972

Breast-Feeding Considerations The CDC recommends that women infected with the influenza virus follow general precautions (eg, frequent hand washing) to decrease viral transmission to the child. Mothers with influenza-like illnesses at delivery should consider avoiding close contact with the infant until they have received 48 hours of antiviral medication, fever has resolved, and cough and secretions can be controlled. These measures may help decrease (but not eliminate) the risk of transmitting influenza to the newborn during breast-feeding. During this time, breast milk can be expressed and bottle-fed to the infant by another person who is not infected. Protective measures, such as wearing a face mask, changing into a clean gown or clothing, and strict hand hygiene should be continued by the mother for ≥7 days after the onset of symptoms or until symptom-free for 24 hours. Infant care should be performed by a noninfected person when possible (consult current CDC guidelines).

Contraindications Hypersensitivity to amantadine hydrochloride or any component

Warnings Deaths due to amantadine overdose have been reported with the lowest lethal dose being 1 gram. Drug overdose has resulted in cardiac (ie, arrhythmia, tachycardia, hypertension), respiratory, renal, or central nervous system toxicity. Due to increased resistance, the ACIP has recommended that rimantadine and amantadine no longer be used for the treatment or prophylaxis of influenza A in the United States until susceptibility has been re-established; consult current guidelines.

May cause CNS depression, which may impair physical or mental abilities; patients must be cautioned about performing tasks which require mental alertness (eg, operating machinery or driving). Use has been associated with neuroleptic malignant syndrome (associated with dose reduction or abrupt discontinuation). Dopamine agonists used for Parkinson's disease or restless legs syndrome have been associated with compulsive behaviors and/or loss of impulse control, which has manifested as pathological gambling, libido increases (hypersexuality), and/or binge eating. Causality has not been established and controversy exists as to whether this phenomenon is related to the underlying disease, prior behaviors/addictions, and/or drug therapy. Dose reduction or discontinuation of therapy has been reported to reverse these behaviors in some, but not all cases. Risk for melanoma development is increased in Parkinson's disease patients; drug causation or factors contributing to risk have not been established. Patients should be monitored closely and periodic skin examinations should be performed. There have been reports of suicidal ideation/attempt in patients with and without a history of psychiatric illness. May exacerbate mental problems in patients with a history of mental illness; use with caution in patients with uncontrolled psychosis or severe psychoneurosis. May cause a withdrawal syndrome of agitation, anxiety, delirium, delusions, depression, hallucinations, paranoia, parkinsonian crisis, slurred speech, or stupor; gradually taper dose avoid abrupt discontinuation of therapy.

Oral solution contains propylene glycol; toxicities have been reported with use of products containing propylene glycol, including hyperosmolality, lactic acidosis, seizures,

and respiratory depression; in neonates large amounts of propylene glycol delivered orally, intravenously (eg, >3000 mg/day), or topically have been associated with potentially fatal toxicities which can include metabolic acidosis, seizures, renal failure, and CNS depression; use oral solution containing propylene glycol with caution (AAP, 1997; Shehab, 2009).

Precautions Use with caution in patients with renal impairment; dosage reduction recommended. Use with caution in patients with hepatic impairment; rarely, elevations in transaminases have been reported. Use with caution in patients with heart failure, peripheral edema, or orthostatic hypotension; dosage reduction may be required. Use with caution in patients with a history of recurrent and eczematoid dermatitis. Use with caution in patients with a history of seizure disorder or with concurrent CNS stimulant use; may increase seizure activity or EEG disturbances in patients with preexisting seizure disorder. Avoid in untreated angle closure glaucoma.

Adverse Reactions

Cardiovascular: Orthostatic hypotension, peripheral edema

Central nervous system: Agitation, anxiety, ataxia, confusion, delirium, depression, dizziness, dream abnormality, fatigue, hallucinations, headache, insomnia, irritability, lightheadedness, nervousness, somnolence

Dermatologic: Livedo reticularis

Gastrointestinal: Anorexia, constipation, diarrhea, nausea, xerostomia

Respiratory: Dry nose

Rare but important or life-threatening: Aggressive behavior, agranulocytosis, alkaline phosphatase increased, allergic reaction, ALT increased, AST increased, amnesia, anaphylaxis, arrhythmia, bilirubin increased, BUN increased, cardiac arrest, CHF, coma, CPK increased, creatinine increased, delusions, diaphoresis, dysphagia, dyspnea, eczematoid dermatitis, euphoria, GGT increased, heart failure, hyperkinesis, LDH increased, leukopenia, mania, neutropenia, neuroleptic malignant syndrome (NMS; associated with dose reduction or abrupt withdrawal of amantadine), oculogyric episodes, paresthesia, photosensitivity, psychosis, pulmonary edema, rash, respiratory failure (acute), seizures, suicidal ideation, suicide, urinary retention, withdrawal reactions (may include delirium, hallucinations, and psychosis), visual disturbances

Reported with dopamine agonists: Impulsive/compulsive behaviors (eg, pathological gambling, hypersexuality, binge eating)

Drug Interactions

Metabolism/Transport Effects None known.

Avoid Concomitant Use

Avoid concomitant use of Amantadine with any of the following: Amisulpride

Increased Effect/Toxicity

Amantadine may increase the levels/effects of: BuPROPion; Glycopyrrolate; Highest Risk QTc-Prolonging Agents; Moderate Risk QTc-Prolonging Agents; Trimethoprim

The levels/effects of Amantadine may be increased by: Alcohol (Ethyl); MAO Inhibitors; Methylphenidate; Mifepristone; Trimethoprim

Decreased Effect

Amantadine may decrease the levels/effects of: Amisulpride; Antipsychotics (Typical); Influenza Virus Vaccine (Live/Attenuated)

The levels/effects of Amantadine may be decreased by: Amisulpride; Antipsychotics (Atypical); Antipsychotics (Typical); Metoclopramide

Stability Store tablets and syrup at 25°C (77°F); excursions permitted to 15°C to 30°C (59°F to 86°F)

◄ **Mechanism of Action**

Antiviral:

The mechanism of amantadine's antiviral activity has not been fully elucidated. It appears to primarily prevent the release of infectious viral nucleic acid into the host cell by interfering with the transmembrane domain of the viral M2 protein. Amantadine is also known to prevent viral assembly during replication. Amantadine inhibits the replication of influenza A virus isolates from each of the subtypes (ie, H1N1, H2N2 and H3N2), but has very little or no activity against influenza B virus isolates.

Parkinson disease:

The exact mechanism of amantadine in the treatment of Parkinson disease and drug-induced extrapyramidal reactions is not known. Data from early animal studies suggest that amantadine may have direct and indirect effects on dopamine neurons; however, recent studies have demonstrated that amantadine is a weak, noncompetitive NMDA receptor antagonist. Although amantadine has not been shown to possess direct anticholinergic activity, clinically, it exhibits anticholinergic-like side effects (dry mouth, urinary retention, and constipation).

Pharmacokinetics (Adult data unless noted)

Absorption: Well absorbed

Distribution: V_d: Normal: 1.5-6.1 L/kg; Renal failure: 5.1 ± 0.2 L/kg; in saliva, tear film, and nasal secretions; in animals, tissue (especially lung) concentrations higher than serum concentrations; crosses blood-brain barrier

Protein binding: Normal renal function: ~67%; Hemodialysis: ~59%

Metabolism: Not appreciable; small amounts of an acetyl metabolite identified

Bioavailability: 86% to 90%

Half-life: Normal renal function: 16 ± 6 hours (9-31 hours); Healthy, older (≥60 years) males: 29 hours (range: 20-41 hours); End-stage renal disease: 7-10 days

Time to peak serum concentration: 2-4 hours

Elimination: Urine (80% to 90% unchanged) by glomerular filtration and tubular secretion

Dialysis: Negligible amounts removed

Dosing: Usual

Children and Adolescents:

Attention-deficit/hyperactivity disorder (ADHD): Limited data available: Oral: Children ≥5 years and Adolescents: Initial: 50 mg/**day**; titrate up at 4-7 day intervals in 50 mg increments to effect; reported range: 50-150 mg/**day** in divided doses 1-3 times daily (morning, noon, and 4 PM); maximum daily dose (weight-dependent): <30 kg: 100 mg/**day**; ≥30 kg: 150 mg/**day** (Donfrancesco, 2007; King, 2001; Mohammadi, 2010); dosing based on two small open-label trials (n=24, n=20; age range: 5-14 years) which suggested improvements in symptoms and ADHD outcome scores; a comparison trial with methylphenidate (n=40) did not detect differences in efficacy between the treatment groups (Mohammadi, 2010); further studies are needed.

Autism (hyperactivity, irritability): Limited data available: Oral: Children ≥5 years and Adolescents: Initial: 2.5 mg/kg/dose once daily for 1 week, then increase to 2.5 mg/kg/dose twice daily; maximum daily dose: 200 mg/**day**; dosing based on short-term (4-week) double-blind, placebo-controlled trial of 39 pediatric patients (treatment group, n=19) which showed improvement in clinician-rated behavioral and hyperactivity ratings (King, 2001a).

Influenza A treatment/prophylaxis: Oral: **Note:** Due to issues of resistance, amantadine is no longer recommended for the treatment or prophylaxis of influenza A. Please refer to the current ACIP recommendations. The following is based on the manufacturer's labeling and ACIP recommendations:

Influenza A treatment:

1-9 years: 5 mg/kg/**day** in 2 divided doses (manufacturer's labeling: 4.4-8.8 mg/kg/**day**); maximum daily dose: 150 mg/**day**

≥10 years and <40 kg: 5 mg/kg/**day** in 2 divided doses (CDC, 2011)

≥10 years and ≥40 kg: 100 mg twice daily (CDC, 2011)

Note: Initiate within 24-48 hours after onset of symptoms; continue for 24-48 hours after symptom resolution (duration of therapy is generally 3-5 days)

Influenza A prophylaxis: Refer to "Influenza A treatment" dosing

Note: Continue prophylaxis throughout the peak influenza activity in the community or throughout the entire influenza season in patients who cannot be vaccinated. Development of immunity following vaccination takes ~2 weeks; amantadine therapy should be considered for high-risk patients from the time of vaccination until immunity has developed. For ages <9 years receiving influenza vaccine for the first time, amantadine prophylaxis should continue for 6 weeks (4 weeks after the first dose and 2 weeks after the second dose).

Multiple-sclerosis associated lassitude (fatigue): Limited data available (Pohl, 2007): Oral:

<10 years or weight <40 kg: 2.5 mg/kg/dose twice daily; maximum daily dose: 150 mg/**day**

≥10 years and weight ≥40 kg: 100 mg twice daily, may titrate dose to clinical response; maximum daily dose: 400 mg/**day**

Traumatic brain injury (TBI): Limited data available: Oral:

Children ≥6 years and Adolescents <16 years: 4-6 mg/kg/**day** in 2 divided doses; maximum daily dose (age or weight dependent): If <10 years or <40 kg: 150 mg/**day**; if ≥10 years or ≥40 kg: 200 mg/**day** (Beers, 2005; McMahon, 2009). While total daily dose similar in trials, the reported dosing approaches and efficacy results are variable (eg, timing of therapy initiation, duration of study, outcome measures) (Williams, 2007). In an open-label, case-controlled trial of 27 pediatric patients with TBI within the last 24 months prior to enrollment (n=17 amantadine treatment, n=10 controls), patients received 5 mg/kg/**day** for entire study period of 12 weeks; results showed improvement in behavior (parental report) and a subset analysis suggested therapy more effective on cognition for those with more recent injury (Beers, 2005). In a double-blind, placebo-controlled crossover trial of seven pediatric patients (mean age: 12.7 years) with TBI within last 12 weeks prior to enrollment, therapy was initiated at 4 mg/kg/**day** up to 300 mg/**day** for 1 week, and increased to 6 mg/kg/**day** up to 400 mg/**day** for Weeks 2 and 3 of the study duration; improved consciousness observed during treatment period of study (McMahon, 2009; Vargus-Adams, 2010). Further studies are needed.

Adolescents ≥16 years: Initial: 100 mg twice daily for 14 days; on Week 3 increase to 150 mg twice daily; may further increase to 200 mg twice daily on Week 4 if needed; dosing based on a multicenter, double-blind, placebo-controlled trial of 184 patients (age range: 16-65 years; treatment group, n= 87) which showed 4 weeks of amantadine therapy initiated at 4-16 weeks postinjury increased the rate of functional recovery (Giacino, 2012). Further studies are needed.

Adults:

Drug-induced extrapyramidal symptoms: Oral: 100 mg twice daily; may increase to 300 mg/day in divided doses, if needed

Parkinson's disease: Oral: Usual dose: 100 mg twice daily as monotherapy; may increase to 400 mg/day in divided doses, if needed, with close monitoring

Note: Patients with a serious concomitant illness or those receiving high doses of other antiparkinson drugs should be started at 100 mg/day; may increase to 100 mg twice daily, if needed, after one to several weeks

Influenza A treatment/prophylaxis: Oral: **Note:** Due to issues of resistance, amantadine is no longer recommended for the treatment or prophylaxis of influenza A. Please refer to the current ACIP recommendations. The following is based on the manufacturer's labeling:

Influenza A treatment: 200 mg once daily **or** 100 mg twice daily (may be preferred to reduce CNS effects)

Note: Initiate within 24-48 hours after onset of symptoms; continue for 24-48 hours after symptom resolution (duration of therapy is generally 3-5 days)

Influenza A prophylaxis: 200 mg once daily **or** 100 mg twice daily (may be preferred to reduce CNS effects)

Note: Continue prophylaxis throughout the peak influenza activity in the community or throughout the entire influenza season in patients who cannot be vaccinated. Development of immunity following vaccination takes ~2 weeks; amantadine therapy should be considered for high-risk patients from the time of vaccination until immunity has developed.

Dosing interval in renal impairment: Adults:

CrCl 30-50 mL/minute: Administer 200 mg on day 1, then 100 mg/day

CrCl 15-29 mL/minute: Administer 200 mg on day 1, then 100 mg on alternate days

CrCl <15 mL/minute: Administer 200 mg every 7 days

Hemodialysis: Administer 200 mg every 7 days

Peritoneal dialysis: No supplemental dose is needed

Continuous arteriovenous or venous-venous hemofiltration: No supplemental dose is needed

Administration Oral: May be taken without regard to food. For regimens with multiple daily dosing, timing of doses may vary based upon patient tolerance (eg, if insomnia develops, administer evening dose several hours before bedtime) and use [for ADHD, administer morning and noon; if thrice daily dosing, last dose should be given around 4 PM (Mohammadi, 2010)].

Monitoring Parameters Renal function; mental status, monitor for signs of neurotoxicity; periodic skin exam for melanoma, blood pressure

Test Interactions May interfere with urine detection of amphetamines/methamphetamines (false-positive).

Dosage Forms Excipient information presented when available (limited, particularly for generics); consult specific product labeling.

Capsule, Oral, as hydrochloride:

Generic: 100 mg

Syrup, Oral, as hydrochloride:

Generic: 50 mg/5 mL (10 mL, 473 mL)

Tablet, Oral, as hydrochloride:

Generic: 100 mg

References

American Academy of Pediatrics Committee on Drugs. "Inactive" ingredients in pharmaceutical products: update (subject review). *Pediatrics.* 1997;99(2):268-278.

Aoki FY and Sitar DS, "Clinical Pharmacokinetics of Amantadine Hydrochloride," *Clin Pharmacokinet,* 1988, 14(1):35-51.

Beers SR, Skold A, Dixon CE, et al, "Neurobehavioral Effects of Amantadine After Pediatric Traumatic Brain Injury: A Preliminary Report," *J Head Trauma Rehabil,* 2005, 20(5):450-63.

Bradley JS, Byington CL, Shah SS, et al, "The Management of Community-Acquired Pneumonia in Infants and Children Older Than 3 Months of Age: Clinical Practice Guidelines by the Pediatric Infectious Diseases Society and the Infectious Diseases Society of America", *Clin Infect Dis,* 2011, 53(7):e25-76.

Centers for Disease Control and Prevention (CDC), "Influenza Division, National Center for Immunization and Respiratory Diseases. Antiviral Agents for the Treatment and Chemoprophylaxis of Influenza — Recommendations of the Advisory Committee on Immunization Practices (ACIP)," *MMWR Surveill Summ,* 2011, 60(1):1-28.

Centers for Disease Control and Prevention (CDC), "Interim Guidance: Considerations Regarding 2009 Novel H1N1 Flu Virus in Intrapartum and Postpartum Hospital Settings," Available at http://www.cdc.gov/h1n1flu/guidance/obstetric.htm

Centers for Disease Control and Prevention (CDC), "Prevention and Control of Influenza. Recommendations of the Advisory Committee on Immunization Practices (ACIP)," *MMWR Recomm Rep,* 2008, 56 (early release):1-60. Available at http://www.cdc.gov/mmwr/preview/mmwrhtml/rr57e717a1.htm

Chitnis T, Krupp L, Yeh A, et al, "Pediatric Multiple Sclerosis," *Neurol Clin,* 2011, 29(2):481-505.

Donfrancesco R, Calderoni D, and Vitiello B, "Open-Label Amantadine in Children With Attention-Deficit/Hyperactivity Disorder," *J Child Adolesc Psychopharmacol,* 2007, 17(5):657-64.

Giacino JT, Whyte J, Bagiella E, et al, "Placebo-Controlled Trial of Amantadine for Severe Traumatic Brain Injury," *N Engl J Med,* 2012, 366(9):819-26.

Green LB, Hornyak JE, and Hurvitz EA, "Amantadine in Pediatric Patients With Traumatic Brain Injury: A Retrospective, Case-Controlled Study," *Am J Phys Med Rehabil,* 2004, 83(12):893-7.

King BH, Wright DM, Handen BL, et al, "Double-Blind, Placebo-Controlled Study of Amantadine Hydrochloride in the Treatment of Children With Autistic Disorder," *J Am Acad Child Adolesc Psychiatry,* 2001a, 40(6):658-65.

King BH, Wright DM, Snape M, et al, "Case Series: Amantadine Open-Label Treatment of Impulsive and Aggressive Behavior in Hospitalized Children With Developmental Disabilities," *J Am Acad Child Adolesc Psychiatry,* 2001, 40(6):654-7.

McMahon MA, Vargus-Adams JN, Michaud LJ, et al, "Effects of Amantadine in Children With Impaired Consciousness Caused by Acquired Brain Injury: A Pilot Study," *Am J Phys Med Rehabil,* 2009, 88(7):525-32.

Mohammadi MR, Kazemi MR, Zia E, et al, "Amantadine Versus Methylphenidate in Children and Adolescents With Attention Deficit/Hyperactivity Disorder: A Randomized, Double-Blind Trial," *Hum Psychopharmacol,* 2010, 25(7-8):560-5.

Patrick PD, Blackman JA, Mabry JL, et al, "Dopamine Agonist Therapy in Low-Response Children Following Traumatic Brain Injury," *J Child Neurol,* 2006, 21(10):879-85.

Pohl D, Waubant E, Banwell B, et al, "Treatment of Pediatric Multiple Sclerosis and Variants," *Neurology,* 2007, 68(16 Suppl 2):54-65.

Shehab N, Lewis CL, Streetman DD, Donn SM. Exposure to the pharmaceutical excipients benzyl alcohol and propylene glycol among critically ill neonates. *Pediatr Crit Care Med.* 2009;10 (2):256-259.

Strong DK, Eisenstat DD, Bryson SM, et al, "Amantadine Neurotoxicity in a Pediatric Patient With Renal Insufficiency," *DICP,* 1991, 25 (11):1175-7.

Thompson AJ, Toosy AT, and Ciccarelli O, "Pharmacological Management of Symptoms in Multiple Sclerosis: Current Approaches and Future Directions," *Lancet Neurol,* 2010, 9(12):1182-99.

Vargus-Adams JN, McMahon MA, Michaud LJ, et al, "Pharmacokinetics of Amantadine in Children With Impaired Consciousness Due to Acquired Brain Injury: Preliminary Findings Using a Sparse-Sampling Technique," *PMR,* 2010, 2(1):37-42.

Williams SE, "Amantadine Treatment Following Traumatic Brain Injury in Children," *Brain Inj,* 2007, 21(9):885-9.

◆ **Amantadine Hydrochloride** *see* Amantadine *on page 112*

◆ **Ambien** *see* Zolpidem *on page 2182*

◆ **Ambien CR** *see* Zolpidem *on page 2182*

◆ **AmBisome** *see* Amphotericin B (Liposomal) *on page 155*

◆ **AmBisome® (Can)** *see* Amphotericin B (Liposomal) *on page 155*

◆ **A-Methapred** *see* MethylPREDNISolone *on page 1386*

◆ **Amethocaine Hydrochloride** *see* Tetracaine (Ophthalmic) *on page 1995*

◆ **Amethocaine Hydrochloride** *see* Tetracaine (Systemic) *on page 1994*

◆ **Amethocaine Hydrochloride** *see* Tetracaine (Topical) *on page 1995*

◆ **Amethopterin** *see* Methotrexate *on page 1367*

◆ **Ametop (Can)** *see* Tetracaine (Topical) *on page 1995*

◆ **Amicar** *see* Aminocaproic Acid *on page 122*

◆ **Amidate** *see* Etomidate *on page 814*

Amifostine (am i FOS teen)

Medication Safety Issues
Sound-alike/look-alike issues:
Ethyol® may be confused with ethanol
Brand Names: U.S. Ethyol
Brand Names: Canada Ethyol®
Therapeutic Category Antidote, Cisplatin; Cytoprotective Agent
Generic Availability (U.S.) Yes
Use Reduction of cumulative renal toxicity associated with repeated administration of cisplatin in patients with advanced ovarian cancer (FDA approved in adults); reduction of moderate to severe xerostomia from radiation treatment of the head and neck where the radiation port includes a substantial portion of the parotid glands (FDA approved in adults); has also been used as a cytoprotective agent to selectively protect normal tissues against toxicity due to cytotoxic chemotherapy
Pregnancy Risk Factor C
Pregnancy Considerations Animal studies have demonstrated embryotoxicity. There are no adequate and well-controlled studies in pregnant women.
Breast-Feeding Considerations Due to the potential for adverse reactions in the nursing infant, breast-feeding should be discontinued.
Contraindications Hypersensitivity to amifostine, aminothiol compounds, or any component
Warnings Due to limited experience and the possibility of amifostine interference with antineoplastic efficacy, amifostine should not be administered to patients receiving definitive radiation therapy or in settings in which chemotherapy (for malignancies other than ovarian cancer) can produce a significant survival benefit or cure, except in the context of a clinical trial.

Reports of clinically relevant hypocalcemia are rare, but serum calcium levels should be monitored in patients at risk of hypocalcemia (eg, those patients receiving multiple doses of amifostine, patients with nephrotic syndrome); may require calcium supplementation.

Hypotension may occur during or shortly after infusion; reported incidence is 62% and higher in patients with head and neck cancer, esophageal cancer, nonsmall cell lung cancer, prior neck radiation, or hypercalcemia; adequately hydrate prior to treatment (patients who are hypotensive or dehydrated should not receive amifostine) and keep in a supine position during the infusion. Monitor blood pressure every 5 minutes during the infusion. If hypotension requiring interruption of therapy occurs, patients should be placed in the Trendelenburg position and given an infusion of normal saline using a separate I.V. line; subsequent infusions may require a dose reduction. Interrupt antihypertensive therapy for 24 hours before treatment; according to the manufacturer, patients who cannot safely stop their antihypertensives 24 hours before should not receive amifostine. Infusions >15 minutes are associated with a higher incidence of adverse effects.

The incidence of nausea and vomiting is higher in patients receiving amifostine, compared to chemotherapy alone. Antiemetic medications, including dexamethasone I.V. and a serotonin 5-HT$_3$ receptor antagonist, should be administered prior to and in conjunction with amifostine. Use with caution in patients for whom the adverse effects of nausea/vomiting may have serious adverse events.

Rare hypersensitivity reactions, including anaphylaxis and allergic reaction, have been reported. Discontinue if allergic reaction occurs; do not rechallenge. Medications for the treatment of hypersensitivity reactions should be available. Serious cutaneous reactions, including erythema multiforme, Stevens-Johnson syndrome, toxic epidermal necrolysis, toxoderma, and exfoliative dermatitis have been reported with amifostine; may be delayed, developing up to weeks after treatment initiation. Cutaneous reactions have been reported more frequently when used as a radioprotectant. Discontinue treatment for severe/serious cutaneous reaction or with fever. Withhold treatment and obtain dermatologic consultation for rash involving lips or mucosa (of unknown etiology outside of radiation port) and for bullous, edematous, or erythematous lesions on hands, feet, or trunk; reinitiate only after careful evaluation.
Precautions Use with caution in patients with cardiovascular conditions such as ischemic heart diseases, arrhythmias, CHF, or in any patient who may be adversely affected by hypotension. Use with caution in patients with cerebrovascular disease such as history of stroke or TIA.

Adverse Reactions
Cardiovascular: Hypotension
Endocrine & metabolic: Hypocalcemia
Gastrointestinal: Nausea/vomiting
Rare but important or life-threatening: Apnea, anaphylactoid reactions, anaphylaxis, arrhythmia, atrial fibrillation, atrial flutter, back pain, bradycardia, cardiac arrest, chest pain, chest tightness, chills, cutaneous eruptions, dizziness, erythema multiforme, exfoliative dermatitis, extrasystoles, dyspnea, fever, flushing, hiccups, hypersensitivity reactions (fever, rash, hypoxia, dyspnea, laryngeal edema), hypertension (transient), hypoxia, malaise, MI, myocardial ischemia, pruritus, rash (mild), renal failure, respiratory arrest, rigors, seizure, sneezing, somnolence, Stevens-Johnson syndrome, supraventricular tachycardia, syncope, tachycardia, toxic epidermal necrolysis, toxoderma, urticaria

Drug Interactions
Metabolism/Transport Effects None known.
Avoid Concomitant Use There are no known interactions where it is recommended to avoid concomitant use.
Increased Effect/Toxicity
The levels/effects of Amifostine may be increased by: Antihypertensives
Decreased Effect There are no known significant interactions involving a decrease in effect.
Stability Store intact vial at 20°C to 25°C (68°F to 77°F). Reconstituted solution and solutions diluted to 5-40 mg/mL in NS are chemically stable for 5 hours at room temperature or 24 hours if refrigerated.
Mechanism of Action Prodrug that is dephosphorylated by alkaline phosphatase in tissues to a pharmacologically-active free thiol metabolite. The free thiol is available to bind to, and detoxify, reactive metabolites of cisplatin; and can also act as a scavenger of free radicals that may be generated (by cisplatin or radiation therapy) in tissues.

Pharmacokinetics (Adult data unless noted)
Distribution: V$_d$: 6.4 L; unmetabolized prodrug is largely confined to the intravascular compartment; active metabolite is distributed into normal tissues with high concentrations in bone marrow, GI mucosa, skin, liver, and salivary glands
Protein binding: 4%
Metabolism: Amifostine (phosphorylated prodrug) is hydrolyzed by alkaline phosphatase to an active free sulfhydryl compound (WR-1065)
Half-life:
Children: 9.3 minutes (Fouladi, 2001)
Adults: 8 minutes
Elimination: Metabolites excreted in urine

Dosing: Usual Refer to individual protocols.

Pediatric:

Cytoprotective agent against cisplatin or high-dose alkylating agents: Limited data available: Dose not established, variable efficacy results:

Gastrointestinal and hematologic toxicity reduction: Infants, Children, and Adolescents: I.V.: 740 mg/m^2/dose once daily prior to cytotoxic chemotherapy. In a study of patients (n=11, age range: 2.5 months to 17 years) receiving the same combination chemotherapy at the same doses (including cisplatin or high-dose alkylating agent) with or without amifostine, patients who received amifostine had significantly reduced incidences of mucositis and gastrointestinal toxicities and a significantly reduced requirement for erythrocyte transfusions. However, there was no difference in the number of platelet transfusions required (Cetingül, 2009). In another study in osteosarcoma patients treated with cisplatin or carboplatin as part of combination chemotherapy, there was a reduction in neutrophil and leukocyte toxicity in patients who received amifostine (n=17) compared to those who did not (n=19); however, amifostine did not protect against platelet effects (Petrilli, 2002). Other studies have not shown protection against myelosuppression (Adamson, 1995, Bernstein, 2006).

Nephrotoxicity reduction: Children and Adolescents: I.V.: 740 mg/m^2/dose given immediately prior to cisplatin. In a small study of intracavitary cisplatin therapy for solid tumors, three patients (ages: 2-6 years) received amifostine. Of these patients, only one experienced persistent renal dysfunction (Katzenstein, 2010).

Reduction of platinum-induced hearing loss: Children and Adolescents 3-20 years: I.V.: 600 mg/m^2/dose given immediately prior to and 3 hours into cisplatin administration has been shown to reduce cisplatin-induced hearing loss in patients with average-risk medulloblastoma. Amifostine did not protect against hearing loss in patients with high-risk medulloblastoma (Fouladi, 2008, Gurney, 2014). Other studies using a single dose of 740 mg/m^2 or 825 mg/m^2 immediately prior to cisplatin did not prevent ototoxicity (Katzenstein, 2009; Marina, 2005; Petrilli, 2002).

Xerostomia, moderate to severe from radiation of the head and neck, reduction: Limited data available: Children ≥7 years and Adolescents: SubQ: 200 mg once daily given 30 minutes prior to standard fraction radiation therapy. Dosing based on a small pilot study in pediatric patients who received subcutaneous amifostine (n=5, age range: 7-15 years) for a total of 129 injections. No grade 3 or 4 mucosal or skin reactions occurred (Anacak, 2007). Further studies are needed.

Adult: **Note:** Antiemetic medication, including dexamethasone 20 mg I.V. and a serotonin 5-HT$_3$ receptor antagonist, is recommended prior to and in conjunction with amifostine.

Cisplatin-induced renal toxicity, reduction: I.V.: 910 mg/m^2 once daily administered 30 minutes prior to cytotoxic chemotherapy

The infusion of amifostine should be interrupted if the systolic blood pressure decreases significantly from baseline, as defined below:

Decrease of 20 mm Hg if baseline systolic blood pressure <100

Decrease of 25 mm Hg if baseline systolic blood pressure 100-119

Decrease of 30 mm Hg if baseline systolic blood pressure 120-139

Decrease of 40 mm Hg if baseline systolic blood pressure 140-179

Decrease of 50 mm Hg if baseline systolic blood pressure ≥180

If blood pressure returns to normal within 5 minutes (assisted by fluid administration and postural management) and the patient is asymptomatic, the infusion may be restarted so that the full dose of amifostine may be administered. If the full dose of amifostine cannot be administered, the dose of amifostine for subsequent cycles should be 740 mg/m^2.

Xerostomia, moderate to severe from radiation of the head and neck, reduction: I.V.: 200 mg/m^2 once daily starting 15-30 minutes prior to standard fraction radiation therapy

Dosing adjustment in renal impairment: There are no dosage adjustments provided in the manufacturer's labeling.

Dosing adjustment in hepatic impairment: There are no dosage adjustments provided in the manufacturer's labeling.

Administration Parenteral: I.V.: Reconstitute 500 mg vial with 9.7 mL of NS to a concentration of 50 mg/mL; dose must be further diluted with NS to a final concentration of 5-40 mg/mL. Administer amifostine doses ≥600 mg/m^2 as an I.V. intermittent infusion over 15 minutes since the 15-minute infusion is better tolerated than a more prolonged infusion. Administer 200 mg/m^2 dose as a 3-minute infusion. Patients should be kept in supine position during infusion and amifostine should be interrupted if the blood pressure decreases significantly from baseline or if the patient develops symptoms related to decreased cerebral or cardiovascular perfusion. Patients experiencing decreased blood pressure should receive a rapid infusion of NS and be kept supine or placed in the Trendelenburg position. Amifostine can be restarted if the blood pressure returns to the baseline level.

Monitoring Parameters Baseline blood pressure followed by a blood pressure reading every 5 minutes during the infusion and after administration if clinically indicated; monitor electrolytes, urinalysis, serum calcium, serum magnesium; monitor I & O; evaluate for cutaneous reactions prior to each dose

Dosage Forms Excipient information presented when available (limited, particularly for generics); consult specific product labeling.

Solution Reconstituted, Intravenous:

Ethyol: 500 mg (1 ea)

Generic: 500 mg (1 ea)

Solution Reconstituted, Intravenous [preservative free]:

Generic: 500 mg (1 ea)

References

Adamson PC, Balis FM, Belasco JE, et al, "A Phase I Trial of Amifostine (WR-2721) and Melphalan in Children With Refractory Cancer," *Cancer Res*, 1995, 55(18): 4069-72.

Anacak Y, Kamer S, Haydaroglu A. Daily subcutaneous amifostine administration during irradiation of pediatric head and neck cancers. *Pediatr Blood Cancer* . 2007;48:579-581.

Bernstein MJ, Devidas M, Lafreniere D, et al. Intensive therapy with growth factor support for patients with Ewing tumor metastatic at diagnosis: pediatric oncology group/children's cancer group phase II study 9457 – a report from the children's oncology group. *Journal of Clinical Oncology*. 2006;24(1):152-159.

Cetingül N, Midyat L, Kantar M, Demirağ B, Aksoylar S, Kansoy S. Cytoprotective effects of amifostine in the treatment of childhood malignancies. *Pediatr Blood Cancer*. 2009;52:829-833.

Ethyol (amifostine) [prescribing information]. Bedford, OH: Ben Venue, Inc; January 2009.

Fouladi M, Chinagumpala M, Ashley D, et al. Amifostine protects against cisplatin-induced ototoxicity in children with average-risk medulloblastoma. *J Clin Oncol*. 2008;26(22):3749-3755.

Fouladi M, Stempak D, Gammon J, et al, "Phase I Trial of a Twice-Daily Regimen of Amifostine With Ifosfamide, Carboplatin, and Etoposide Chemotherapy in Children With Refractory Carcinoma," *Cancer*, 2001, 92(4):914-23.

Katzenstein HM, Chang KW, Krailo M, et.al. Amifostine does not prevent platinum-induced hearing loss associated with the treatment of children with hepatoblastoma. A report of the intergroup hepatoblastoma study P9645 as a part of the children's oncology group. *Cancer*. 2009;115(24):5828-5835.

Katzenstein HM, Petricca S, Ricketts R, et al. Intracavitary cisplatin therapy for pediatric malignancies. *Pediatr Blood Cancer* . 2010;55:452-456.

Marina N, Chang KW, Malogolowkin M, et al. Amifostine does not protect agains the ototoxicity of high-dose cisplatin combined with etoposide and bleomycin in pediatric germ-cell tumors. *Cancer.* 2005;104:841-847.

Petrilli AS, Oliveira DT, Ginani VC, et al. Use of amifostine in the therapy of osteosarcoma in children and adolescemts. *Journal of Pediatric Hematology/Oncology.* 2002;24(3):188-191.

Shaw LM, Bonner H, and Lieberman R, "Pharmacokinetic Profile of Amifostine," *Semin Oncol*, 1996, 23(4 Suppl 8):18-22.

Amikacin (am i KAY sin)

Medication Safety Issues
Sound-alike/look-alike issues:
Amikacin may be confused with Amicar, anakinra
Amikin may be confused with Amicar, Kineret

Brand Names: Canada Amikacin Sulfate Injection, USP; Amikin

Therapeutic Category Antibiotic, Aminoglycoside

Generic Availability (U.S.) Yes

Use Treatment of serious infections (bone and respiratory infections, endocarditis, and septicemia) due to organisms resistant to gentamicin and tobramycin, including *Pseudomonas*, *Klebsiella*, *Enterobacter*, *Serratia*, *Proteus*, and *Providencia* species, and *E. coli* (FDA approved in all ages); has also been used for documented infection of susceptible mycobacterial organisms

Pregnancy Risk Factor D

Pregnancy Considerations Adverse events were not observed in the initial animal reproduction studies; however, renal toxicity has been reported in additional studies. Amikacin crosses the placenta, produces detectable serum levels in the fetus, and concentrates in the fetal kidneys. Because of several reports of total irreversible bilateral congenital deafness in children whose mothers received another aminoglycoside (streptomycin) during pregnancy, the manufacturer classifies amikacin as pregnancy risk factor D. Although serious side effects to the fetus have not been reported following maternal use of amikacin, a potential for harm exists.

Due to pregnancy-induced physiologic changes, some pharmacokinetic parameters of amikacin may be altered. Pregnant women have an average-to-larger volume of distribution which may result in lower peak serum levels than for the same dose in nonpregnant women. Serum half-life may also be shorter.

Breast-Feeding Considerations Amikacin is excreted into breast milk in trace amounts; however, it is not absorbed when taken orally. This limited oral absorption may minimize exposure to the nursing infant. Nondose-related effects could include modification of bowel flora. Breast-feeding is not recommended by the manufacturer.

Contraindications Hypersensitivity to amikacin sulfate, any component, or other aminoglycosides

Warnings Aminoglycosides are associated with significant nephrotoxicity **[U.S. Boxed Warning]**. Vestibular and permanent bilateral auditory ototoxicity can occur **[U.S. Boxed Warning]**; tinnitus or vertigo are indications of vestibular injury and impending bilateral irreversible deafness. Risk of nephrotoxicity and ototoxicity is increased in patients with impaired renal function, dehydration, high-dose therapy, or prolonged therapy. Peak and trough serum concentrations should be monitored periodically during therapy to assure adequate concentrations are achieved and to avoid potentially toxic levels **[U.S. Boxed Warning]**. Ototoxicity is associated with high serum concentrations persisting for prolonged periods; nephrotoxicity is associated with high serum trough concentrations. Risk of nephrotoxicity increases when used concurrently with other potentially nephrotoxic drugs **[U.S. Boxed Warning]**; renal damage is usually reversible. Risk of ototoxicity increases with use of potent diuretics **[U.S. Boxed Warning]**; may cause neuromuscular blockade and respiratory paralysis **[U.S. Boxed Warning]**; risk increased with concomitant use of anesthesia or muscle relaxants. Prolonged use may result in fungal or bacterial superinfection, including *C. difficile*-associated diarrhea (CDAD) and pseudomembranous colitis; CDAD has been observed >2 months postantibiotic treatment. Not intended for long-term therapy due to toxic hazards associated with extended administration. Aminoglycosides can cause fetal harm when administered to a pregnant woman and have been associated with several reports of total irreversible bilateral congenital deafness in pediatric patients exposed *in utero*. Some products contain sulfites which may cause allergic reactions in susceptible individuals.

Precautions Use with caution in patients with preexisting renal impairment; modify dosage in patients with renal impairment; monitor renal and eighth nerve function in patients with known or suspected renal impairment **[U.S. Boxed Warning]**. Use with caution in patients with auditory or vestibular impairment. Use with caution in patients with myasthenia gravis, hypocalcemia, and in conditions which depress neuromuscular transmission; may cause neuromuscular blockade and respiratory paralysis; risk increased with concomitant use of anesthesia or muscle relaxants. Use with caution in pediatric patients on extracorporeal membrane oxygenation (ECMO); pharmacokinetics of aminoglycosides may be altered; dosage adjustment and close monitoring necessary.

Cross-allergenicity with other aminoglycosides has been observed. Avoid intramuscular administration in paralyzed patients, due to poor circulation in the atrophic muscles which may result in slower absorption and lower peak serum concentrations; use intravenous route.

Adverse Reactions
Central nervous system: Neurotoxicity
Genitourinary: Nephrotoxicity
Otic: Auditory ototoxicity, vestibular ototoxicity
Rare but important or life-threatening: Dyspnea, eosinophilia, hypersensitivity reaction

Drug Interactions
Metabolism/Transport Effects None known.

Avoid Concomitant Use
Avoid concomitant use of Amikacin with any of the following: BCG; Mannitol

Increased Effect/Toxicity
Amikacin may increase the levels/effects of: AbobotulinumtoxinA; Bisphosphonate Derivatives; CARBOplatin; Colistimethate; CycloSPORINE (Systemic); Neuromuscular-Blocking Agents; OnabotulinumtoxinA; RimabotulinumtoxinB; Tenofovir

The levels/effects of Amikacin may be increased by: Amphotericin B; Capreomycin; Cephalosporins (2nd Generation); Cephalosporins (3rd Generation); Cephalosporins (4th Generation); CISplatin; Loop Diuretics; Mannitol; Nonsteroidal Anti-Inflammatory Agents; Tenofovir; Vancomycin

Decreased Effect
Amikacin may decrease the levels/effects of: BCG; Sodium Picosulfate; Typhoid Vaccine

The levels/effects of Amikacin may be decreased by: Penicillins

Stability Store intact vials at 20°C to 25°C (68°F to 77°F); dilutions of 0.25 mg/mL and 5 mg/mL are stable for 24 hours at room temperature, 60 days under refrigeration, and 30 days frozen. Previous refrigerated or thawed frozen solutions are stable for 24 hours when stored at room temperature.

Mechanism of Action Inhibits protein synthesis in susceptible bacteria by binding to 30S ribosomal subunits

Pharmacodynamics Displays concentration-dependent killing; bacteriocidal

Pharmacokinetics (Adult data unless noted)

Absorption:
I.M.: Rapid
Oral: Poorly absorbed

Distribution: V_d: 0.25 L/kg; primarily into extracellular fluid (highly hydrophilic); 12% of serum concentration penetrates into bronchial secretions; poor penetration into the blood-brain barrier even when meninges are inflamed; V_d is increased in neonates and patients with edema, ascites, fluid overload; V_d is decreased in patients with dehydration

Protein-binding: ≤11%

Half-life:
Infants:
Low birth weight, 1-3 days of age: 7 hours
Full-term >7 days: 4-5 hours
Children: 1.6-2.5 hours
Adolescents: 1.5 ± 1 hour
Adults: Normal renal function: 1.4-2.3 hours
Anuria: 28-86 hours; half-life and clearance are dependent on renal function

Time to peak serum concentration:
I.M.: Within 45-120 minutes
I.V.: Within 30 minutes following a 30-minute infusion

Elimination: Urine (94% to 98%); excreted unchanged via glomerular filtration within 24 hours

Dialysis: Dialyzable (50% to 100%); supplemental dose recommended after hemodialysis or peritoneal dialysis

Dosing: Neonatal Note: Dose not well-defined in premature infants; monitor closely. Dosage should be based on actual weight unless the patient has hydrops fetalis. Consider single-dose administration with serum concentration monitoring in patients with urine output <1 mL/kg/hour or serum creatinine >1.3 mg/dL rather than scheduled dosing. Consider prolongation of dosing interval when coadministered with ibuprofen or indomethacin or in neonates with history of the following: Birth depression, birth hypoxia/asphyxia, or cyanotic congenital heart disease.

General dosing; susceptible infection: I.V.:
Age-directed dosing (Allegaert, 2006; Allegaert, 2008; Labaune, 2001; Sherwin, 2009): **Note:** Postmenstrual age is the sum of gestational age (weeks) and postnatal age (weeks) (Engle, 2004):
PMA ≤27 weeks: 15-20 mg/kg/dose every 48 hours
PMA 28-33 weeks: 15-20 mg/kg/dose every 36 hours
PMA ≥34 weeks: 15 mg/kg/dose every 24 hours
Weight-directed dosing (Red Book, 2012)
Body weight <1 kg:
PNA ≤14 days: 15 mg/kg/dose every 48 hours
PNA 15-28 days: 15 mg/kg/dose every 24-48 hours
Body weight 1-2 kg:
PNA ≤7 days: 15 mg/kg/dose every 48 hours
PNA 8-28 days: 15 mg/kg/dose every 24-48 hours
Body weight >2 kg:
PNA ≤7 days: 15 mg/kg/dose every 24 hours
PNA 8-28 days: 15 mg/kg/dose every 12-24 hours

Meningitis: I.V.: **Note:** Use smaller doses and longer intervals for neonates <2 kg (Tunkel, 2004):
PNA ≤7 days and ≥2 kg: 15-20 mg/kg/**day** divided every 12 hours
PNA >7 days and ≥2 kg: 30 mg/kg/**day** divided every 8 hours

Dosing: Usual Note: Dosage should be based on an estimate of ideal body weight. In morbidly obese children, adolescents, and adults, dosage requirement may best be estimated using a dosing weight of IBW + 0.4 (TBW - IBW). Dosage should be individualized based upon serum concentration monitoring.

Infants, Children, and Adolescents:

General dosing, severe, susceptible infections: I.M., I.V.: 15-22.5 mg/kg/**day** divided every 8 hours (Red Book, 2012); some consultants recommend initial doses of 30 mg/kg/**day** divided every 8 hours in patients who may require larger doses

CNS infections:
Meningitis (Tunkel, 2004):
Infants and Children: I.V.: 20-30 mg/kg/**day** divided every 8 hours
Adolescents: I.V.: 15 mg/kg/**day** divided every 8 hours
VP-shunt infection, ventriculitis: Limited data available: Intraventricular/intrathecal **(use a preservative free preparation)**: 5-50 mg/**day**; usual dose: 30 mg/**day**

Cystic fibrosis, pulmonary infection:
Traditional dosing: I.V., I.M.: 10 mg/kg/dose every 8 hours
Extended-interval dosing: I.V.: 30 mg/kg/dose every 24 hours (Flume, 2009); **Note:** The CF Foundation recommends extended-interval dosing as preferred over traditional dosing.

Intra-abdominal infection, complicated: I.V.: 15-22.5 mg/kg/day divided every 8-24 hours (Solomkin, 2010)

Mycobacterium, avium complex infection (MAC):
Infants and Children: I.V.: 15-30 mg/kg/**day** divided every 12-24 hours as part of a multiple drug regimen; maximum daily dose: 1500 mg/**day** (DHHS, [pediatric], 2013)
Adolescents: I.V.: 10-15 mg/kg/**day** every 24 hours as part of a multiple drug regimen; maximum daily dose: 1500 mg/**day** (DHHS [adult], 2013)

Tuberculosis, drug-resistant:
Infants, Children, and Adolescents ≤14 years: I.M., I.V.: 15-30 mg/kg/dose once daily as part of a multiple drug regimen; maximum daily dose: 1000 mg/**day** (ATS/CDC/IDSA, 2003; DHHS [pediatric], 2013)
Adolescents ≥15 years, HIV-exposed/-positive: I.M., I.V.: 15 mg/kg/dose once daily as part of a multiple drug regimen for the first 2-3 months; maximum daily dose: 1000 mg/**day** (ATS/CDC/IDSA, 2003; DHHS [adult], 2013)

Peritonitis (CAPD): Intraperitoneal: Continuous: Loading dose: 25 mg per liter of dialysate; maintenance dose: 12 mg per liter (Warady, 2012)

Adults: Individualization is critical because of the low therapeutic index

Initial and periodic peak and trough plasma drug levels should be determined, particularly in critically ill patients with serious infections or in disease states known to significantly alter aminoglycoside pharmacokinetics (eg, cystic fibrosis, burns, or major surgery). Manufacturer recommends a maximum daily dose of 15 mg/kg/**day** (or 1500 mg/**day** in heavier patients). Higher doses may be warranted based on therapeutic drug monitoring or susceptibility information.

Usual dosage range: I.M., I.V.: 5-7.5 mg/kg/dose every 8 hours; **Note:** Some clinicians suggest a daily dose of 15-20 mg/kg for all patients with normal renal function. This dose is at least as efficacious with similar, if not less, toxicity than conventional dosing.

Hospital-acquired pneumonia (HAP): I.V.: 20 mg/kg/day with antipseudomonal beta-lactam or carbapenem (ATS guidelines, 2005)

Meningitis (susceptible gram-negative organisms): I.V.: 5 mg/kg every 8 hours (administered with another bacteriocidal drug)

Mycobacterium fortuitum, M. chelonae, or M. abscessus: I.V.: 10-15 mg/kg daily for at least 2 weeks with high-dose cefoxitin

Dosing interval in renal impairment:
Infants, Children, and Adolescents: I.M., I.V.:
The following adjustments have been recommended (Aronoff, 2007); **Note:** Renally adjusted dose recommendations are based on doses of 5-7.5 mg/kg/dose every 8 hours:
GFR >50 mL/minute/1.73 m^2: No adjustment required
GFR 30-50 mL/minute/1.73 m^2: Administer every 12-18 hours
GFR 10-29 mL/minute/1.73 m^2: Administer every 18-24 hours
GFR <10 mL/minute/1.73 m^2: Administer every 48-72 hours
Intermittent hemodialysis: 5 mg/kg/dose; redose as indicated by serum concentrations
Peritoneal dialysis (PD): 5 mg/kg/dose; redose as indicated by serum concentrations
Continuous renal replacement therapy (CRRT): 7.5 mg/kg/dose every 12 hours, monitor serum concentrations
Adults: **Note:** Some patients may require larger or more frequent doses if serum levels document the need (ie, cystic fibrosis or febrile granulocytopenic patients):
CrCl ≥60 mL/minute: Administer every 8 hours
CrCl 40-60 mL/minute: Administer every 12 hours
CrCl 20-40 mL/minute: Administer every 24 hours
CrCl <20 mL/minute: Loading dose, then monitor levels
Intermittent hemodialysis (IHD) (administer after hemodialysis on dialysis days): Dializable (20%; variable; dependent on filter, duration, and type of HD): 5-7.5 mg/kg every 48-72 hours. Follow levels. Redose when pre-HD serum concentration <10 mg/L; redose when post-HD serum concentration <6-8 mcg/mL (Heintz, 2009). **Note:** Dosing dependent on the assumption of 3 times complete IHD sessions.
Peritoneal dialysis (PD): Dose as CrCl <20 mL/minute: Follow levels.
Continuous renal replacement therapy (CRRT) (Heintz, 2009; Trotman, 2005): Drug clearance is highly dependent on the method of renal replacement, filter type, and flow rate. Appropriate dosing requires close monitoring of pharmacologic response, signs of adverse reactions due to drug accumulation, as well as drug concentrations in relation to target trough (if appropriate). The following are general recommendations only (based on dialysate flow/ultrafiltration rates of 1-2 L/hour and minimal residual renal function) and should not supersede clinical judgment:
CVVH/CVVHD/CVVHDF: Loading dose of 10 mg/kg followed by maintenance dose of 7.5 mg/kg every 24-48 hours
Note: For severe gram-negative rod infections, target peak serum concentration of 15-30 mcg/mL; redose when serum concentration <10 mcg/mL (Heintz, 2009).

Administration

Parenteral: Administer other antibiotics, such as penicillins and cephalosporins, at least 1 hour before or after an amikacin dose; simultaneous administration may result in reduced antibacterial efficacy. Administer around-the-clock to promote less variation in peak and trough serum levels.
I.M.: Administer undiluted I.M into large muscle mass. Slower absorption and lower peak concentrations, probably due to poor circulation in the atrophic muscle, may occur following I.M. injection; in paralyzed patients, suggest I.V. route
I.V. intermittent infusion: Infuse over 30-60 minutes; in infants infusion over 1-2 hours is recommended by the manufacturer. Final concentration should not exceed 10 mg/mL.

Monitoring Parameters Urinalysis, urine output, BUN, serum creatinine, peak and trough serum amikacin concentrations; be alert to ototoxicity
With conventional dosing, typically obtain serum concentration after the third dose; exceptions for earlier monitoring may include neonates or patients with rapidly changing renal function. With extended-interval dosing, usually obtain serum concentration after first, second, or third dose.
Not all infants and children who receive aminoglycosides require monitoring of serum aminoglycoside concentrations. Indications for use of aminoglycoside serum concentration monitoring include:
• Treatment course >5 days
• Patients with decreased or changing renal function
• Patients with poor therapeutic response
• Neonates and Infants <3 months of age
• Atypical body constituency (obesity, expanded extracellular fluid volume)
• Clinical need for higher doses or shorter intervals (eg, cystic fibrosis, burns, endocarditis, meningitis, critically ill patients, relatively resistant organisms)
• Patients on hemodialysis or chronic ambulatory peritoneal dialysis
• Signs of nephrotoxicity or ototoxicity
• Concomitant use of other nephrotoxic agents

Reference Range Therapeutic levels:
Peak:
Life-threatening infections: 25-40 mcg/mL
Serious infections: 20-25 mcg/mL
Urinary tract infections: 15-20 mcg/mL
Trough: <8 mcg/mL; the American Thoracic Society (ATS) recommends trough levels of <4-5 mcg/mL for patients with hospital-acquired pneumonia
Timing of serum samples: Draw peak 30 minutes after completion of 30-minute infusion or at 1 hour following initiation of infusion or I.M. injection; draw trough within 30 minutes prior to next dose; aminoglycoside levels measured from blood taken from Silastic® central catheters can sometimes give falsely elevated readings

Test Interactions Some penicillin derivatives may accelerate the degradation of aminoglycosides *in vitro*, leading to a potential underestimation of aminoglycoside serum concentration.

Additional Information Some penicillins (eg, carbenicillin, ticarcillin, and piperacillin) have been shown to inactivate aminoglycosides *in vitro*. This has been observed to a greater extent with tobramycin and gentamicin, while amikacin has shown greater stability against inactivation. Concurrent use of these agents may pose a risk of reduced antibacterial efficacy *in vivo*, particularly in the setting of profound renal impairment; however, definitive clinical evidence is lacking. If combination penicillin/aminoglycoside therapy is desired in a patient with renal dysfunction, separation of doses (if feasible), and routine monitoring of aminoglycoside levels, CBC, and clinical response should be considered.

Dosage Forms Excipient information presented when available (limited, particularly for generics); consult specific product labeling.
Solution, Injection, as sulfate:
Generic: 500 mg/2 mL (2 mL); 1 g/4 mL (4 mL)
Solution, Injection, as sulfate [preservative free]:
Generic: 1 g/4 mL (4 mL)

References

Allegaert K, Anderson BJ, Cossey V, et al, "Limited Predictability of Amikacin Clearance in Extreme Premature Neonates at Birth," *Br J Clin Pharmacol*, 2006, 61(1):39-48.
Allegaert K, Scheers I, Cossey V, et al, "Covariates of Amikacin Clearance in Neonates: The Impact of Postnatal Age on Predictability," *Drug Metab Lett*, 2008, 2(4):286-9.
American Academy of Pediatrics (AAP). In: Pickering LK, Baker CJ, Kimberlin DW, Long SS, eds. *Red Book: 2012 Report of the*

Committee on Infectious Diseases. 29th ed. Elk Grove Village, IL: American Academy of Pediatrics; 2012.

American Thoracic Society and Infectious Diseases Society of America, "Guidelines for the Management of Adults With Hospital-Acquired, Ventilator-Associated, and Healthcare-Associated Pneumonia," *Am J Respir Crit Care Med*, 2005, 171(4):388-416.

American Thoracic Society, CDC, and Infectious Diseases Society of America, "Treatment of Tuberculosis," *MMWR Recomm Rep*, 2003, 52(RR-11):1-77.

Aronoff GR, Bennett WM, Berns JS, et al, *Drug Prescribing in Renal Failure: Dosing Guidelines for Adults and Children*, 5th ed, Philadelphia, PA: American College of Physicians, 2007.

DHHS. Guidelines for the prevention and treatment of opportunistic infections among HIV-exposed and HIV-infected children: recommendations from the National Institutes of Health, Centers for Disease Control and Prevention, the HIV Medicine Association of the Infectious Diseases Society of America, the Pediatric Infectious Diseases Society, and the American Academy of Pediatrics. November 6, 2013. Available at http://aidsinfo.nih.gov

DHHS Panel on Opportunistic Infections (OI) in HIV-Infected Adults and Adolescents, "Guidelines for Prevention and Treatment of Opportunistic Infections in HIV-Infected Adults and Adolescents: Recommendations From the Centers for Disease Control and Prevention (CDC), the National Institutes of Health (NIH), and the HIV Medicine Association (HIVMA) of the Infectious Diseases Society of America (IDSA)," May 7, 2013. Available at http://aidsinfo.nih.gov/contentfiles/lvguidelines/adult_oi.pdf

Engle WA and American Academy of Pediatrics Committee on Fetus and Newborn, "Age Terminology During the Perinatal Period," *Pediatrics*, 2004, 114(5):1362-4.

Flume PA, Mogayzel PJ Jr, Robinson KA, et al, "Cystic Fibrosis Pulmonary Guidelines: Treatment of Pulmonary Exacerbations," *Am J Respir Crit Care Med*, 2009, 180(9):802-8.

Gilbert VE, Beals JD Jr, Natelson SE, et al, "Treatment of Cerebrospinal Fluid Leaks and Gram-Negative Bacillary Meningitis With Large Doses of Intrathecal Amikacin and Systemic Antibiotics," *Neurosurgery*, 1986, 18(4):402-6.

Heintz BH, Matzke GR, and Dager WE, "Antimicrobial Dosing Concepts and Recommendations for Critically Ill Adult Patients Receiving Continuous Renal Replacement Therapy or Intermittent Hemodialysis," *Pharmacotherapy*, 2009, 29(5):562-77.

Kasiakou SK, Rafailidis PI, Liaropoulos K, et al, "Cure of Post-Traumatic Recurrent Multiresistant Gram-Negative Rod Meningitis With Intraventricular Colistin," *J Infect*, 2005, 50(4):348-52.

Kenyon CF, Knoppert DC, Lee SK, et al, "Amikacin Pharmacokinetics and Suggested Dosage Modifications for the Preterm Infant," *Antimicrob Agents Chemother*, 1990, 34(2):265-8.

Labaune JM, Bleyzac N, Maire P, et al, "Once-a-Day Individualized Amikacin Dosing for Suspected Infection at Birth Based on Population Pharmacokinetic Models," *Biol Neonate*, 2001, 80(2):142-7.

Public Health Service Task Force on Prophylaxis and Therapy for *Mycobacterium avium* Complex, "Recommendations on Prophylaxis and Therapy for Disseminated *Mycobacterium avium* Complex Disease in Patients Infected With the Human Immunodeficiency Virus," *N Engl J Med*, 1993, 329(12):898-904.

Rodríguez Guardado A, Blanco A, Asensi V, et al, "Multidrug-Resistant Acinetobacter Meningitis in Neurosurgical Patients With Intraventricular Catheters: Assessment of Different Treatments," *J Antimicrob Chemother*, 2008, 61(4):908-13.

Sherwin CM, Svahn S, Van der Linden A, et al, "Individualised Dosing of Amikacin in Neonates: A Pharmacokinetic/Pharmacodynamic Analysis," *Eur J Clin Pharmacol*, 2009, 65(7):705-13.

Solomkin JS, Mazuski JE, Bradley JS, et al, "Diagnosis and Management of Complicated Intra-Abdominal Infections in Adults and Children: Guidelines by the Surgical Infection Society and the Infectious Diseases Society of America," *Clin Infect Dis*, 2010, 50(2):133-64.

Starke JR and Correa AG, "Management of Mycobacterial Infection and Disease in Children," *Pediatr Infect Dis J*, 1995, 14(6):455-69.

Trotman RL, Williamson JC, Shoemaker DM, et al, "Antibiotic Dosing in Critically Ill Adult Patients Receiving Continuous Renal Replacement Therapy," *Clin Infect Dis*, 2005, 41(8):1159-66.

Tunkel AR, Hartman BJ, Kaplan SL, et al, "Practice Guidelines for the Management of Bacterial Meningitis," *Clin Infect Dis*, 2004, 39 (9):1267-84.

Vogelstein B, Kowarski A, and Lietman PS, "The Pharmacokinetics of Amikacin in Children," *J Pediatr*, 1977, 91(2):333-9.

Warady BA, Bakkaloglu S, Newland J, et al, "Consensus Guidelines for the Prevention and Treatment of Catheter-Related Infections and Peritonitis in Pediatric Patients Receiving Peritoneal Dialysis: 2012 Update," *Perit Dial Int*, 2012, (32 Suppl 2):S32-86.

♦ **Amikacin Sulfate** *see Amikacin on page 118*

♦ **Amikacin Sulfate Injection, USP (Can)** *see Amikacin on page 118*

♦ **Amikin (Can)** *see Amikacin on page 118*

AMILoride (a MIL oh ride)

Medication Safety Issues
Sound-alike/look-alike issues:
AMILoride may be confused with amiodarone, amLODIPine, inamrinone

Brand Names: Canada Apo-Amiloride®; Midamor

Therapeutic Category Antihypertensive Agent; Diuretic, Potassium Sparing

Generic Availability (U.S.) Yes

Use Management of edema associated with CHF, hepatic cirrhosis, and hyperaldosteronism; hypertension; primary hyperaldosteronism; hypokalemia induced by kaliuretic diuretics

Pregnancy Risk Factor B

Pregnancy Considerations Adverse events were not observed in animal reproduction studies.

Breast-Feeding Considerations It is not known if amiloride is excreted in breast milk. Due to the potential for serious adverse reactions in the nursing infant, a decision should be made whether to discontinue nursing or to discontinue the drug, taking into account the importance of treatment to the mother.

Contraindications Hypersensitivity to amiloride or any component; hyperkalemia; anuria; acute or chronic renal insufficiency; and evidence of diabetic nephropathy; concomitant use of potassium supplements (except in severe and/or refractory hypokalemia) or potassium-sparing diuretics

Warnings Severe hyperkalemia can occur **[U.S. Boxed Warning]**. Incidence is greater in patients with renal impairment, diabetes mellitus, and in elderly patients. Serum potassium levels must be monitored at frequent intervals especially when dosages are changed or with any illness that may cause renal dysfunction. Amiloride should be discontinued in diabetic patients for at least 3 days prior to glucose tolerance testing; discontinue if serum potassium >5.5 mEq/L; risk of hyperkalemia is reduced with concomitant use of thiazide diuretic.

Precautions Use with caution in patients with dehydration, electrolyte imbalance, metabolic or respiratory acidosis, diabetes (particularly those with nephropathy), hyponatremia, impaired renal function, or hepatic dysfunction; patients receiving potassium or other potassium-sparing diuretics; use with caution and modify dosage in patients with decreased renal function

Adverse Reactions
Central nervous system: Dizziness, fatigue, headache

Endocrine & metabolic: Dehydration, gynecomastia, hyperchloremic metabolic acidosis, hyperkalemia, hyponatremia

Gastrointestinal: Abdominal pain, change in appetite, constipation, diarrhea, gas pain, nausea, vomiting

Genitourinary: Impotence

Neuromuscular & skeletal: Muscle cramps, weakness

Respiratory: Cough, dyspnea

Rare but important or life-threatening: Bladder spasm, cardiac arrhythmia, chest pain, dysuria, gastrointestinal hemorrhage, increased intraocular pressure, jaundice, orthostatic hypotension, palpitations, polyuria

Drug Interactions
Metabolism/Transport Effects None known.

Avoid Concomitant Use
Avoid concomitant use of AMILoride with any of the following: CycloSPORINE (Systemic); Spironolactone; Tacrolimus (Systemic)

Increased Effect/Toxicity
AMILoride may increase the levels/effects of: ACE Inhibitors; Amifostine; Ammonium Chloride; Antihypertensives; Cardiac Glycosides; CycloSPORINE (Systemic); Dofetilide; DULoxetine; Hypotensive Agents;

Obinutuzumab; RiTUXimab; Sodium Phosphates; Spironolactone; Tacrolimus (Systemic)

The levels/effects of AMILoride may be increased by: Alfuzosin; Analgesics (Opioid); Angiotensin II Receptor Blockers; Barbiturates; Brimonidine (Topical); Canagliflozin; Diazoxide; Drospirenone; Eplerenone; Heparin; Heparin (Low Molecular Weight); Herbs (Hypotensive Properties); MAO Inhibitors; Nonsteroidal Anti-Inflammatory Agents; Pentoxifylline; Phosphodiesterase 5 Inhibitors; Potassium Salts; Prostacyclin Analogues; Tolvaptan

Decreased Effect

AMILoride may decrease the levels/effects of: Cardiac Glycosides; QuiNIDine

The levels/effects of AMILoride may be decreased by: Herbs (Hypertensive Properties); Methylphenidate; Nonsteroidal Anti-Inflammatory Agents; Yohimbine

Mechanism of Action Blocks epithelial sodium channels in the late distal convoluted tubule (DCT), and collecting duct which inhibits sodium reabsorption from the lumen. This effectively reduces intracellular sodium, decreasing the function of Na+/K+ATPase, leading to potassium retention and decreased calcium, magnesium, and hydrogen excretion. As sodium uptake capacity in the DCT/collecting duct is limited, the natriuretic, diuretic, and antihypertensive effects are generally considered weak.

Pharmacodynamics

Onset of action: 2 hours

Maximum effect: 6-10 hours

Duration: 24 hours

Pharmacokinetics (Adult data unless noted)

Absorption: 50%

Distribution: Adults: V_d: 350-380 L

Metabolism: No active metabolites

Half-life: Adults:

Normal renal function: 6-9 hours

End-stage renal disease: 21-144 hours

Elimination: Unchanged drug, equally in urine and feces

Dosing: Usual Oral:

Hypertension:

Children: 0.4-0.625 mg/kg/day; maximum dose: 20 mg/day

Adults: 5-10 mg/day in 1-2 divided doses (JNC 7)

Edema:

Children 6-20 kg: 0.625 mg/kg/day in 1-2 divided doses; maximum dose: 10 mg/day

Children >20 kg and Adults: 5-10 mg/day in 1-2 divided doses; maximum dose: 20 mg/day

Dosing adjustment in renal impairment:

CrCl 10-50 mL/minute: Administer at 50% of normal dose

CrCl <10 mL/minute: Avoid use

Administration Oral: Administer with food or milk

Monitoring Parameters Serum potassium, sodium, creatinine, BUN, blood pressure, fluid balance

Test Interactions May falsely elevate serum digoxin levels done by radioimmunoassay

Additional Information Studies utilizing aerosolized amiloride (5 mmol/L in 0.3% saline) in adult cystic fibrosis patients (Tomkiewcz, 1993) have suggested that inhaled amiloride is capable of improving the rheologic properties of the abnormally thickened mucus by increasing mucus sodium content

Dosage Forms Excipient information presented when available (limited, particularly for generics); consult specific product labeling.

Tablet, Oral, as hydrochloride:

Generic: 5 mg

Extemporaneous Preparations A 1 mg/mL oral suspension may be made with tablets. Crush ten 5 mg tablets in a mortar and reduce to a fine powder. Add small proportions up to 20 mL of Glycerin BP or Glycerin, USP and mix to uniform paste; mix while adding sterile water in incremental proportions to **almost** 50 mL; transfer to a calibrated bottle, rinse mortar with sterile water, and add quantity of sterile water sufficient to make 50 mL. Label "shake well" and "refrigerate". Stable for 21 days.

Nahata MC, Pai VB, and Hipple TF, *Pediatric Drug Formulations,* 5th ed, Cincinnati, OH: Harvey Whitney Books Co, 2004.

References

Chobanian AV, Bakris GL, Black HR, et al, "The Seventh Report of the Joint National Committee on Prevention, Detection, Evaluation, and Treatment of High Blood Pressure: The JNC 7 Report," *JAMA,* 2003, 289(19):2560-72.

National High Blood Pressure Education Program Working Group on High Blood Pressure in Children and Adolescents, "The Fourth Report on the Diagnosis, Evaluation, and Treatment of High Blood Pressure in Children and Adolescents," *Pediatrics,* 2004, 114(2 Suppl):555-76.

Tomkiewcz RP, App, EM, Zayas JG, et al, "Amiloride Inhalation Therapy in Cystic Fibrosis. Influence on Ion Content, Hydration, and Rheology of Sputum," *Am Rev Resp Dis,* 1993, 148:1002-7.

van der Vorst MM, Kist JE, van der Heijden AJ, et al, "Diuretics in Pediatrics: Current Knowledge and Future Prospects," *Paediatr Drugs,* 2006, 8(4):245-64.

◆ **Amiloride Hydrochloride** *see* AMILoride *on page 121*

◆ **2-Amino-6-Mercaptopurine** *see* Thioguanine *on page 2010*

◆ **2-Amino-6-Methoxypurine Arabinoside** *see* Nelarabine *on page 1477*

◆ **Aminobenzylpenicillin** *see* Ampicillin *on page 159*

Aminocaproic Acid (a mee noe ka PROE ik AS id)

Medication Safety Issues

Sound-alike/look-alike issues:

Amicar® may be confused with amikacin, Amikin®

International issues:

Amicar [U.S.] may be confused with Omacor brand name for Omega-3-Acid Ethyl Esters [multiple international markets]

Brand Names: U.S. Amicar

Therapeutic Category Hemostatic Agent

Generic Availability (U.S.) Yes

Use To enhance hemostasis when fibrinolysis contributes to bleeding (causes may include cardiac surgery, hematologic disorders, neoplastic disorders, abruptio placentae, hepatic cirrhosis, and urinary fibrinolysis) (FDA approved in adults); has also been used for traumatic hyphema, prevention of perioperative bleeding, refractory hematuria, and prevention of bleeding associated with ECMO in high-risk patients

Pregnancy Risk Factor C

Pregnancy Considerations Animal reproduction studies have not been conducted.

Breast-Feeding Considerations It is not known if aminocaproic acid is excreted in breast milk. The manufacturer recommends that caution be exercised when administering aminocaproic acid to nursing women

Contraindications Hypersensitivity to aminocaproic acid or any component; disseminated intravascular coagulation (without concomitant heparin); evidence of an intravascular clotting process

Warnings Avoid rapid I.V. administration; may induce hypotension, bradycardia, or arrhythmia; rapid injection of undiluted solution is not recommended. Intrarenal obstruction may occur secondary to glomerular capillary thrombosis or clots in the renal pelvis and ureters; consider risks versus benefits when using for hematuria. Do not use unless hyperfibrinolysis has been confirmed with laboratory studies; inhibition of fibrinolysis may promote clotting or thrombosis; more likely due to the presence of DIC. Do not administer with factor IX complex concentrates or anti-inhibitor coagulant complexes; may increase risk for thrombosis. Skeletal muscle weakness ranging from mild myalgias and fatigue to severe myopathy with rhabdomyolysis and acute renal failure has been reported with prolonged use; monitor CPK; discontinue treatment with a rise in CPK.

Injection contains benzyl alcohol which may cause allergic reactions in susceptible individuals; large amounts of benzyl alcohol (≥99 mg/kg/day) have been associated with a potentially fatal toxicity ("gasping syndrome") in neonates; the "gasping syndrome" consists of metabolic acidosis, respiratory distress, gasping respirations, CNS dysfunction (including convulsions, intracranial hemorrhage), hypotension and cardiovascular collapse; avoid use of injection in neonates; in vitro and animal studies have shown that benzoate, a metabolite of benzyl alcohol, displaces bilirubin from protein-binding sites

Precautions Use with caution in renal impairment; accumulation of aminocaproic acid may occur and dosage adjustment may be needed; may also increase serum potassium; monitor patients closely. Use with caution in hepatic impairment; monitor patients closely.

Adverse Reactions
Cardiovascular: Arrhythmia, bradycardia, edema, hypotension, intracranial hypertension, peripheral ischemia, syncope, thrombosis

Central nervous system: Confusion, delirium, dizziness, fatigue, hallucinations, headache, malaise, seizure, stroke

Dermatologic: Rash, pruritus

Gastrointestinal: Abdominal pain, anorexia, cramps, diarrhea, GI irritation, nausea, vomiting

Genitourinary: Dry ejaculation

Hematologic: Agranulocytosis, bleeding time increased, leukopenia, thrombocytopenia

Local: Injection site necrosis, injection site pain, injection site reactions

Neuromuscular & skeletal: CPK increased, myalgia, myositis, myopathy, rhabdomyolysis (rare), weakness

Ophthalmic: Vision decreased, watery eyes

Otic: Tinnitus

Renal: BUN increased, intrarenal obstruction (glomerular capillary thrombosis), myoglobinuria (rare), renal failure (rare)

Respiratory: Dyspnea, nasal congestion, pulmonary embolism

Miscellaneous: Allergic reaction, anaphylactoid reaction, anaphylaxis

Rare but important or life-threatening: Hepatic lesion, hyperkalemia, myocardial lesion

Drug Interactions
Metabolism/Transport Effects None known.

Avoid Concomitant Use
Avoid concomitant use of Aminocaproic Acid with any of the following: Anti-inhibitor Coagulant Complex (Human); Factor IX (Human); Factor IX (Recombinant); Factor IX Complex (Human) [(Factors II, IX, X)]

Increased Effect/Toxicity
Aminocaproic Acid may increase the levels/effects of: Anti-inhibitor Coagulant Complex (Human); Factor IX (Human); Factor IX (Recombinant); Factor IX Complex (Human) [(Factors II, IX, X)]; Fibrinogen Concentrate (Human)

The levels/effects of Aminocaproic Acid may be increased by: Fibrinogen Concentrate (Human); Tretinoin (Systemic)

Decreased Effect There are no known significant interactions involving a decrease in effect.

Stability
Oral (tablets and solution): Store at 15°C to 30°C (59°F to 86°F); dispense in a tightly closed container; do not freeze solution.

Parenteral: Store intact vials at 20°C to 25°C (68°F to 77°F); excursions permitted to 15°C to 30°C (59°F to 86°F). Further dilution in D_5W, NS, or LR is required before administration. Solutions diluted to 20 mg/mL or 100 mg/mL in D_5W or NS are stable for 7 days at 4°C or 23°C; dilutions in D_5W may develop a slight yellow color when stored at warmer temperatures [ie, 23°C (73°F)]; potency is not affected.

Mechanism of Action Binds competitively to plasminogen; blocking the binding of plasminogen to fibrin and the subsequent conversion to plasmin, resulting in inhibition of fibrin degradation (fibrinolysis).

Pharmacodynamics Onset of action: Inhibition of fibrinolysis: Within 1-72 hours; onset shortened substantially with loading dose

Pharmacokinetics (Adult data unless noted)
Distribution: Widely distributes through intravascular and extravascular compartments

Metabolism: Hepatic metabolism is minimal

Bioavailability: Oral: 100%

Half-life: 1-2 hours

Time to peak serum concentration: Oral: 1.2 ± 0.45 hours

Elimination: Urine (65% as unchanged drug, 11% as metabolite)

Dosing: Neonatal
Prevention of bleeding associated with extracorporeal membrane oxygenation (ECMO), high-bleeding risk patients: Limited data available: I.V.: 100 mg/kg prior to or immediately after cannulation, followed by 25-30 mg/kg/hour for up to 72 hours; target activated clotting time (ACT) range during therapy of 180-200 seconds has been used (Downard, 2003; Horwitz, 1998; Wilson, 1993); variable results; patients requiring surgery just prior to or while on ECMO seem to benefit most; further studies needed

Prevention of perioperative bleeding associated with cardiac surgery: Limited data available: I.V.: 75 mg/kg administered at the beginning and end of cardiopulmonary bypass, along with 75 mg/100 mL added to the priming fluid for cardiopulmonary bypass (Martin, 2011)

Dosing: Usual
Infants, Children, and Adolescents:

Control of hemorrhage (oral, epistaxis, menorrhagia) in hemophilic patients, adjunct treatment: Limited data available: Oral: 50-100 mg/kg/dose every 6 hours; maximum daily dose: 24 **g/day** (Acharya, 2011)

Control of mucosal bleeding in thrombocytopenia/ platelet dysfunction: Limited data available: Oral, I.V.: 50-100 mg/kg/dose every 6 hours; maximum daily dose: 24 **g/day** (Bussel, 2011; Lipton, 2011)

Hematuria (gross; upper tract), refractory: Limited data available: Children ≥11 years and Adolescents: Oral: 100 mg/kg/dose every 6 hours; continue for 2 days beyond resolution of hematuria; dosing based on case series (n=4) which showed hematuria resolution within 2-7 days; risks and benefits must be weighed prior to use; further studies needed (Kaye, 2010)

Prevention of bleeding associated with dental procedures in hemophilic patients: Limited data available: Oral: 50-100 mg/kg/dose every 6 hours; maximum daily dose: 24 **g/day**; used in conjunction with DDAVP or factor replacement therapy; continue for up to 7 days or until mucosal healing is complete (Acharya, 2011)

Prevention of bleeding associated with extracorporeal membrane oxygenation (ECMO), high-bleeding risk patients: Limited data available: I.V.: 100 mg/kg prior to or immediately after cannulation, followed by 25-30 mg/kg/hour for up to 72 hours; target activated clotting time (ACT) range during therapy of 180-200 seconds has been used (Downard, 2003; Horwitz, 1998; Wilson, 1993); variable results; patients requiring surgery just prior to or while on ECMO seem to benefit most; further studies needed

Prevention of perioperative bleeding associated with cardiac surgery: Limited data available:

Infants and Children <2 years: Dosing regimens variable: I.V.: In the largest trial (n=120, all patients <20 kg), a dose of 75 mg/kg was administered at the beginning and end of cardiopulmonary bypass (CPB), and 75 mg/100 mL was added to the CPB priming fluid (Martin, 2011a). Another study group in two separate trials (n=110, age range: 2 months to 14 years) used a 100 mg/kg dose after induction, during CPB pump priming, and when weaning CPB (over 3 hours) for a total of three doses (Chauhan, 2000; Chauhan, 2004).

Children ≥2 years and Adolescents: I.V.: 100 mg/kg after induction, during CPB pump priming, and when weaning CPB (over 3 hours) for a total of 3 doses; regimen used in two separate trials (n=110, age range: 2 months to 14 years) (Chauhan, 2000; Chauhan, 2004)

Prevention of perioperative bleeding associated with spinal surgery (eg, idiopathic scoliosis): Limited data available: Children ≥11 years and Adolescents: I.V.: 100 mg/kg (maximum dose: 5 **g**) administered over 15-20 minutes after induction, followed by a continuous I.V. infusion of 10 mg/kg/hour for the remainder of the surgery; discontinued at time of wound closure (Florentino-Pineda, 2001; Florentino-Pineda, 2004)

Traumatic hyphema: Oral: 50-100 mg/kg/dose every 4 hours for 5 days; maximum daily dose: 30 **g/day** (Brandt, 2001; Crouch, 1999; Teboul, 1995)

Adults: **Acute bleeding:** Oral, I.V.: Loading dose: 4-5 **g** during the first hour, followed by 1 **g**/hour for 8 hours (or 1.25 **g**/hour using oral solution) or until bleeding controlled (maximum daily dose: 30 **g**

Dosage adjustment in renal impairment: No dosage adjustments are provided in the manufacturer's labeling, but aminocaproic acid may accumulate in patients with decreased renal function; use with caution.

Dosage adjustment in hepatic impairment: No dosage adjustments are provided in the manufacturer's labeling (has not been studied).

Administration

Oral: May administer without regard to food

Parenteral: Further dilute in D_5W or NS to a maximum concentration of 20 mg/mL and administer I.V. over 15-60 minutes (rate dependent upon use); or a continuous I.V. infusion may be used. Do not administer undiluted; rapid I.V. injection (IVP) of undiluted solution is not recommended due to possible hypotension, bradycardia, and arrhythmia.

Monitoring Parameters Fibrinogen, fibrin split products, serum creatinine kinase (long-term therapy); serum potassium, BUN, creatinine

Reference Range Therapeutic concentration: >130 mcg/mL (concentration necessary for inhibition of fibrinolysis)

Dosage Forms Excipient information presented when available (limited, particularly for generics); consult specific product labeling.

Solution, Intravenous:
Generic: 250 mg/mL (20 mL)

Syrup, Oral:
Amicar: 25% (473 mL) [raspberry flavor]
Generic: 25% (237 mL, 473 mL)

Tablet, Oral:
Amicar: 500 mg, 1000 mg [scored]
Generic: 500 mg, 1000 mg

References

Acharya S, "Hemostatic Disorders," Manual of Pediatric Hematology and Oncology, 5th ed, Lanzkowsky P, ed, Burlington, MA: Academic Press, 2011, 402-3.

Brandt MT and Haug RH, "Traumatic Hyphema: A Comprehensive Review," J Oral Maxillofac Surg, 2001, 59(12):1462-70.

Bussel J and Renaud T, "Disorders of Platelets," Manual of Pediatric Hematology and Oncology, 5th ed, Lanzkowsky P, ed, Burlington, MA: Academic Press, 2011, 372.

Chauhan S, Das SN, Bisoi A, et al, "Comparison of Epsilon Aminocaproic Acid and Tranexamic Acid in Pediatric Cardiac Surgery," J Cardiothorac Vasc Anesth, 2004, 18(2):141-3.

Chauhan S, Kumar BA, Rao BH, et al, "Efficacy of Aprotinin, Epsilon Aminocaproic Acid, or Combination in Cyanotic Heart Disease," Ann Thorac Surg, 2000, 70(4):1308-12.

Crouch ER Jr and Crouch ER, "Management of Traumatic Hyphema: Therapeutic Options," J Pediatr Ophthalmol Strabismus, 1999, 36 (5):238-50.

Downard CD, Betit P, Chang RW, et al, "Impact of AMICAR on Hemorrhagic Complications of ECMO: A Ten-Year Review," J Pediatr Surg, 2003, 38(8):1212-6.

Florentino-Pineda I, Blakemore LC, Thompson GH, et al, "The Effect of Epsilon-Aminocaproic Acid on Perioperative Blood Loss in Patients With Idiopathic Scoliosis Undergoing Posterior Spinal Fusion: A Preliminary Prospective Study," Spine (Phila Pa 1976), 2001, 26 (10):1147-51.

Florentino-Pineda I, Thompson GH, Poe-Kochert C, et al, "The Effect of Amicar on Perioperative Blood Loss in Idiopathic Scoliosis: The Results of a Prospective, Randomized Double-Blind Study," Spine (Phila Pa 1976), 2004, 29(3):233-8.

Horwitz JR, Cofer BR, Warner BW, et al, "A Multicenter Trial of 6-Aminocaproic Acid (Amicar) in the Prevention of Bleeding in Infants on ECMO," J Pediatr Surg, 1998, 33(11):1610-3.

Kaye JD, Smith EA, Kirsch AJ, et al, "Preliminary Experience With Epsilon Aminocaproic Acid for Treatment of Intractable Upper Tract Hematuria in Children With Hematological Disorders," J Urol, 2010, 184(3):1152-7.

Lipton JM, "Bone Marrow Failure," Manual of Pediatric Hematology and Oncology, 5th ed, Lanzkowsky P, ed, Burlington, MA: Academic Press, 2011, 131.

Martin K, Breuer T, Gertler R, et al, "Tranexamic Acid Versus ε-Aminocaproic Acid: Efficacy and Safety in Paediatric Cardiac Surgery," Eur J Cardiothorac Surg, 2011a, 39(6):892-7.

Martin K, Gertler R, Liermann H, et al, "Switch From Aprotinin to ε-Aminocaproic Acid: Impact on Blood Loss, Transfusion, and Clinical Outcome in Neonates Undergoing Cardiac Surgery," Br J Anaesth, 2011, 107(6):934-9.

Teboul BK, Jacob JL, Barsoum-Homsy M, et al, "Clinical Evaluation of Aminocaproic Acid for Managing Traumatic Hyphema in Children," Ophthalmology, 1995, 102(11):1646-53.

Williams GD, Bratton SL, Riley EC, et al, "Efficacy of Epsilon-Aminocaproic Acid in Children Undergoing Cardiac Surgery," J Cardiothorac Vasc Anesth, 1999, 13(3):304-8.

Wilson JM, Bower LK, Fackler JC, et al, "Aminocaproic Acid Decreases the Incidence of Intracranial Hemorrhage and Other Hemorrhagic Complications of ECMO," J Pediatr Surg, 1993, 28(4):536-40.

Aminophylline (am in OFF i lin)

Medication Safety Issues

Sound-alike/look-alike issues:
Aminophylline may be confused with amitriptyline, ampicillin

Related Information
Management of Drug Extravasations on page 2255
Theophylline on page 2005

Brand Names: Canada Aminophylline Injection; JAA-Aminophylline

Therapeutic Category Antiasthmatic; Bronchodilator; Respiratory Stimulant; Theophylline Derivative

Generic Availability (U.S.) Yes

Use Treatment of symptoms and reversible airflow obstruction associated with asthma, COPD, or other chronic lung diseases [FDA approved in pediatric patients (age not specified) and adults]; has also been used for treatment of apnea of prematurity and to increase diaphragmatic contractility

Pregnancy Risk Factor C

Pregnancy Considerations Refer to Theophylline monograph.

Breast-Feeding Considerations Refer to Theophylline monograph.

Contraindications Hypersensitivity to aminophylline, theophylline, ethylenediamine, or any component

Warnings If a patient develops signs and symptoms of theophylline toxicity (eg, persistent, repetitive vomiting), serum concentrations should be measured and subsequent doses held. Theophylline clearance may be decreased in neonates, infants <3 months of age with decreased renal function, infants <1 year, elderly patients >60 years of age, in patients following cessation of smoking, in patients with certain disease states (ie, acute pulmonary edema, congestive heart failure, cor pulmonale, fever, hepatic disease, hypothyroidism, acute hepatitis, cirrhosis, sepsis with multiorgan failure, and shock), and when metabolic inhibitors (eg, cimetidine, erythromycin, tacrine) are administered or metabolic inducers (eg, carbamazepine, rifampin) are discontinued. Due to potential saturation of theophylline clearance at serum concentrations within (or in some patients less than) the therapeutic range, dosage adjustment should be made in small increments (maximum: 25% dose increase). Additional increases in dose due to an exacerbation of symptoms should not be made unless the steady state serum theophylline concentration is <10 mcg/mL.

Precautions

Prior to initiation of aminophylline therapy or dosage increase, various drug interactions and disease states that may alter theophylline clearance should be considered. Aminophylline and theophylline may exacerbate certain medical conditions [eg, acute peptic ulcer disease, seizure disorders, and cardiac arrhythmias (excluding bradyarrhythmias)]; use with extreme caution in these patients. Vesicant; ensure proper catheter or needle position prior to and during infusion. Avoid extravasation.

Adverse Reactions Adverse events observed at therapeutic serum levels:

Cardiovascular: Flutter, tachycardia

Central nervous system: Behavior alterations (children), headache, insomnia, irritability, restlessness, seizures

Dermatologic: Allergic skin reactions, exfoliative dermatitis

Gastrointestinal: Diarrhea, nausea, vomiting

Neuromuscular & skeletal: Tremor

Renal: Diuresis (transient)

Drug Interactions

Metabolism/Transport Effects Substrate of CYP1A2 (major), CYP2C9 (minor), CYP2D6 (minor), CYP2E1 (major), CYP3A4 (major); **Note:** Assignment of Major/Minor substrate status based on clinically relevant drug interaction potential; **Inhibits** CYP1A2 (weak)

Avoid Concomitant Use

Avoid concomitant use of Aminophylline with any of the following: Conivaptan; Fusidic Acid (Systemic); Iobenguane I 123; Riociguat

Increased Effect/Toxicity

Aminophylline may increase the levels/effects of: Formoterol; Indacaterol; Pancuronium; Riociguat; Sympathomimetics

The levels/effects of Aminophylline may be increased by: Abiraterone Acetate; Alcohol (Ethyl); Allopurinol; Antithyroid Agents; AtoMOXetine; Cannabinoid-Containing Products; Ceritinib; Cimetidine; Conivaptan; CYP1A2 Inhibitors (Moderate); CYP1A2 Inhibitors (Strong); CYP3A4 Inhibitors (Moderate); CYP3A4 Inhibitors (Strong); Dasatinib; Deferasirox; Disulfiram; Estrogen Derivatives; Febuxostat; FluvoxaMINE; Fusidic Acid (Systemic); Interferons; Isoniazid; Ivacaftor; Linezolid; Luliconazole; Macrolide Antibiotics; Methotrexate; Mexiletine; Mifepristone; Pentoxifylline; Propafenone; QuiNINE; Quinolone Antibiotics; Simeprevir; Stiripentol; Thiabendazole; Ticlopidine; Vemurafenib; Zafirlukast

Decreased Effect

Aminophylline may decrease the levels/effects of: Adenosine; Benzodiazepines; CarBAMazepine; Fosphenytoin; Iobenguane I 123; Lithium; Pancuronium; Phenytoin; Regadenoson; Thiopental; Zafirlukast

The levels/effects of Aminophylline may be decreased by: Adalimumab; Aminoglutethimide; Barbiturates; Beta-Blockers (Beta1 Selective); Beta-Blockers (Nonselective); Bosentan; Cannabis; CarBAMazepine; CYP1A2 Inducers (Strong); CYP3A4 Inducers (Strong); Cyproterone; Dabrafenib; Deferasirox; Fosphenytoin; Isoproterenol; Mitotane; Peginterferon Alfa-2b; Phenytoin; Protease Inhibitors; Siltuximab; St Johns Wort; Thyroid Products; Tocilizumab

Food Interactions

Ethanol: Ethanol may decrease theophylline clearance. Management: Avoid or limit ethanol.

Food: Food does not appreciably affect absorption. Changes in diet may affect the elimination of theophylline; charcoal-broiled foods may increase elimination, reducing half-life by 50%. Management: Avoid extremes of dietary protein and carbohydrate intake.

Stability Parenteral: Store at 20°C to 25°C (68°F to 77°F); protect from light. Do not use solutions if discolored or if crystals are present.

Mechanism of Action Causes bronchodilatation, diuresis, CNS and cardiac stimulation, and gastric acid secretion by blocking phosphodiesterase which increases tissue concentrations of cyclic adenine monophosphate (cAMP) which in turn promote catecholamine stimulation of lipolysis, glycogenolysis, and gluconeogenesis and induce release of epinephrine from adrenal medulla cells

Pharmacokinetics (Adult data unless noted) Aminophylline is the ethylenediamine salt of theophylline, pharmacokinetic parameters are those of **theophylline**; fraction available: 79% (eg, 100 mg aminophylline = 79 mg theophylline); refer to theophylline monograph.

Dosing: Neonatal Note: All dosages expressed as aminophylline; dose should be individualized based on serum concentrations. Due to longer half-life than older patients, the time to achieve steady-state serum concentration is prolonged in neonates (see theophylline half-life table); obtain serum theophylline concentration after 48 to 72 hours of therapy (usually 72 hours in neonates); repeat values should be obtained 3 days after each change in dosage or weekly if on a stabilized dosage. If renal function decreased, consider dose reduction and additional monitoring.

Apnea of prematurity: I.V.:

Manufacturer's labeling:

Loading dose: 5.7 mg/kg/dose

Maintenance:

PNA ≤24 days: 1.27 mg/kg/dose every 12 hours to achieve a target concentration of 7.5 mcg/mL

PNA >24 days: 1.9 mg/kg/dose every 12 hours to achieve a target concentration of 7.5 mcg/mL

Alternate dosing:

Loading dose: 5 to 8 mg/kg/dose; in a prospective randomized controlled trial of 61 neonates (birth weight: <1500 g), a loading dose of 8 mg/kg/dose achieved targeted theophylline serum concentrations in more patients compared to a loading dose of 6 mg/kg/dose (Hochwald, 2002)

Maintenance: Initial: 2 to 6 mg/kg/day divided every 8 to 12 hours (Bhatt-Mehta, 2003; Hochwald, 2002); increased dosages may be indicated as liver metabolism increases; monitor serum concentrations to determine appropriate dosages

Dosing adjustment in renal impairment: Dose reduction and frequent monitoring of serum theophylline concentrations are required in neonates with decreased renal function; 50% of dose is excreted unchanged in the urine of neonates.

Dosing: Usual All dosages expressed as **aminophylline**; use ideal body weight to calculate dose; adjust dose based on steady-state serum concentrations.

Pediatric:

Obstructive airway disease, acute symptoms: Infants, Children, and Adolescents: **Note:** Not recommended for the treatment of asthma exacerbations (NAEPP, 2007).

◄ *Loading dose:* I.V.:
Patients **not currently receiving** aminophylline or the-ophylline: 5.7 mg/kg/dose
Patients **currently receiving** aminophylline or theo-phylline: A loading dose is not recommended without first obtaining a serum theophylline concentration in patients who have received aminophylline or theophyl-line within the past 24 hours. The loading dose should be calculated as follows:

Dose = (C desired – C measured) (V_d)
C desired = desired serum theophylline concen-tration
C measured = measured serum theophylline con-centration

Maintenance dose: Continuous I.V. infusion: **Note:** Dos-ing presented is to achieve a target concentration of 10 mcg/mL. Lower initial doses may be required in patients with reduced theophylline clearance. Dosage should be adjusted according to serum concentration measure-ments during the first 12- to 24-hour period.
Infants 4 to 6 weeks: 1.9 mg/kg/dose every 12 hours
Infants 6 to 52 weeks: Dose (mg/kg/**hour**) = [(0.008 X age in weeks) + 0.21] divided by 0.79
Children 1 to <9 years: 1.01 mg/kg/**hour**
Children 9 to <12 years: 0.89 mg/kg/**hour**
Adolescents 12 to <16 years (otherwise healthy, non-smokers): 0.63 mg/kg/**hour**; maximum dose: 1139 mg/**day** unless serum concentrations indicate need for larger dose
Adolescents 12 to <16 years (cigarette or marijuana smokers): 0.89 mg/kg/**hour**
Adolescents ≥16 years (otherwise healthy, non-smokers): 0.51 mg/kg/**hour**; maximum dose: 1139 mg/**day** unless serum concentrations indicate need for larger dose
Cardiac decompensation, cor pulmonale, hepatic dys-function, sepsis with multiorgan failure, shock: Infants, Children, and Adolescents: Initial: 0.25 mg/kg/**hour**; maximum dose: 507 mg/**day** unless serum concen-trations indicate need for larger dose.

Adult: **Obstructive airway disease, acute symptoms:**
Loading dose: I.V.:
Patients **not currently receiving** aminophylline or the-ophylline: 5.7 mg/kg/dose
Patients **currently receiving** aminophylline or theo-phylline: A loading dose is not recommended without first obtaining a serum theophylline concentration in patients who have received aminophylline or theophyl-line within the past 24 hours. The loading dose should be calculated as follows:

Dose = (desired serum theophylline concentration - measured serum theophylline concentration) (V_d)

Maintenance dose: I.V.: **Note:** Dosing presented is to achieve a target theophylline concentration of 10 mcg/mL unless otherwise noted. Lower initial doses may be required in patients with reduced theophylline clearance. Dosage should be adjusted according to serum level measurements during the first 12- to 24-hour period.
Adults ≤60 years (otherwise healthy, nonsmokers): 0.51 mg/kg/**hour**; maximum: 1139 mg/**day** unless serum levels indicate need for larger dose
Adults >60 years: 0.38 mg/kg/**hour**; maximum dose: 507 mg/**day** unless serum concentrations indicate need for larger dose
Cardiac decompensation, cor pulmonale, hepatic dys-function, sepsis with multiorgan failure, shock: Initial: 0.25 mg/kg/**hour**; maximum dose: 507 mg/**day** unless serum concentrations indicate need for larger dose.

Dosage adjustment based on serum theophylline con-centrations:
Infants, Children, Adolescents, and Adults: **Note:** Recheck serum theophylline concentrations 12 hours (children) or 24 hours (adults) after I.V. dose
<9.9 mcg/mL: If tolerated, but symptoms remain, increase dose by ~25%. Recheck serum theophylline concentrations.
10 to 14.9 mcg/mL: Maintain dosage if tolerated. Recheck serum concentrations at 24-hour intervals.
15 to 19.9 mcg/mL: Consider 10% dose reduction to improve safety margin even if dose is tolerated.
20 to 24.9 mcg/mL: Decrease dose by ~25%. Recheck serum concentrations.
25 to 30 mcg/mL: Stop infusion for 12 hours (children) or 24 hours (adults) and decrease subsequent doses by at least 25%. Recheck serum concentrations.
>30 mcg/mL: Stop dosing and treat overdose; if resumed, decrease subsequent doses by at least 50%. Recheck serum concentrations.
Dosing adjustment in renal impairment:
Infants 1 to 3 months: Consider dose reduction and frequent monitoring of serum theophylline concentra-tions
Infants >3 months, Children, Adolescents, and Adults: No adjustment necessary
Dosing adjustment in hepatic impairment: Infants, Chil-dren, Adolescents, and Adults: Initial: 0.25 mg/kg/**hour**; maximum dose: 507 mg/**day** unless serum concentra-tions indicate need for larger dose
Usual Infusion Concentrations: Pediatric I.V. infu-sion: 1 mg/mL
Administration Parenteral: For I.V. administration only (I.M. use is not recommended; I.M. administration causes intense pain). Loading doses should be administered over 30 minutes; further dilute to a concentration of 1 mg/mL and infuse over 20 to 30 minutes; maximum concentration: 25 mg/mL; maximum rate of infusion: 0.36 mg/kg/minute, and not to exceed 25 mg/minute

Vesicant; ensure proper needle or catheter placement prior to and during I.V. infusion. Avoid extravasation. If extrav-asation occurs, stop infusion immediately and disconnect (leave needle/cannula in place); gently aspirate extrava-sated solution (do **NOT** flush the line); initiate hyaluroni-dase antidote (See Management of Drug Extravasations for more details); remove needle/cannula; apply dry cold compresses (Hurst, 2004); elevate extremity.
Vesicant/Extravasation Risk Vesicant
Monitoring Parameters Serum theophylline concentra-tions, heart rate, respiratory rate, number and severity of apnea spells (when used for apnea of prematurity); arterial or capillary blood gases (if applicable); pulmonary function tests
Reference Range Therapeutic concentrations:
Asthma: 5-15 mcg/mL
Apnea of prematurity: 6-12 mcg/mL; goal concentration is reduced due to decreased protein binding and higher free fraction

Guidelines for Drawing Theophylline Serum Concentrations

Dosage Form	When to Obtain Sample[A]
I.V. bolus	30 min after end of 30-min infusion
Continuous I.V. infusion	12-24 h after initiation of infusion

[A]The time to achieve steady-state serum concentration is prolonged in patients with longer half-lives (eg, infants and adults with cardiac or liver failure; see Theophylline half-life table). In these patients, serum theophylline concentrations should be drawn after 48-72 hours of therapy; may need to obtain concentrations prior to steady-state to assess the patient's current progress or evaluate potential toxicity.

Test Interactions Plasma glucose, uric acid, free fatty acids, total cholesterol, HDL, HDL/LDL ratio, and urinary free cortisol excretion may be increased by theophylline. Theophylline may decrease triiodothyronine.

Additional Information Theophylline dose is 79% of aminophylline dose.

Each mg/kg of theophylline administered as a bolus will increase the serum theophylline concentration by an average of 2 mcg/mL.

Dosage Forms Excipient information presented when available (limited, particularly for generics); consult specific product labeling.

Solution, Intravenous, as dihydrate:
Generic: 25 mg/mL (10 mL, 20 mL)

References

Aronson JK, Hardman M, and Reynolds DJ, "ABC of Monitoring Drug Therapy. Theophylline, "*BMJ,* 1992, 305(6865):1355-8.

Bhatt-Mehta V and Schumacher RE, "Treatment of Apnea of Prematurity," *Paediatr Drugs,* 2003, 5(3):195-210.

Hochwald C, Kennedy K, Chang J, et al, "A Randomized, Controlled, Double-Blind Trial Comparing Two Loading Doses of Aminophylline," *J Perinatol,* 2002, 22(4):275-8.

Hurst S, McMillan M. Innovative solutions in critical care units: extravasation guidelines. *Dimens Crit Care Nurs.* 2004;23(3):125-128.

National Asthma Education and Prevention Program (NAEPP), "Expert Panel Report 3 (EPR-3): Guidelines for the Diagnosis and Management of Asthma," Clinical Practice Guidelines, National Institutes of Health, National Heart, Lung, and Blood Institute, NIH Publication No. 08-4051, prepublication 2007. Available at http://www.nhlbi.nih.gov/guidelines/asthma/asthgdln.htm

◆ **Aminophylline Injection (Can)** *see* Aminophylline *on page 124*

◆ **5-Aminosalicylic Acid** *see* Mesalamine *on page 1347*

Amiodarone (a MEE oh da rone)

Medication Safety Issues

Sound-alike/look-alike issues:

Amiodarone may be confused with aMILoride, inamrinone

Cordarone may be confused with Cardura, Cordran

High alert medication:

The Institute for Safe Medication Practices (ISMP) includes this medication among its list of drugs which have a heightened risk of causing significant patient harm when used in error.

BEERS Criteria medication:

This drug may be potentially inappropriate for use in geriatric patients (Quality of evidence - high; Strength of recommendation - strong).

Related Information

Adult ACLS Algorithms *on page 2198*
Pediatric ALS (PALS) Algorithms *on page 2195*

Brand Names: U.S. Cordarone; Nexterone; Pacerone

Brand Names: Canada Amiodarone Hydrochloride Injection; Apo-Amiodarone; Ava-Amiodarone; Cordarone; Dom-Amiodarone; Mylan-Amiodarone; PHL-Amiodarone; PMS-Amiodarone; PRO-Amiodarone; ratio-Amiodarone; Riva-Amiodarone; Sandoz-Amiodarone; Teva-Amiodarone

Therapeutic Category Antiarrhythmic Agent, Class III

Generic Availability (U.S.) Yes

Use

Oral: Management of life-threatening recurrent ventricular arrhythmias [eg, recurrent ventricular fibrillation (VF) or recurrent hemodynamically unstable ventricular tachycardia (VT)] unresponsive to other therapy or in patients intolerant to other therapy (FDA approved in adults)

I.V.: Initiation of management and prophylaxis of frequently recurrent VF and hemodynamically unstable VT unresponsive to other therapy; VF and VT in patients requiring amiodarone who are not able to take oral therapy (All indications: FDA approved in adults)

Note: Also has been used to treat supraventricular arrhythmias unresponsive to other therapy. Amiodarone is recommended in the PALS guidelines for SVT (unresponsive to vagal maneuvers and adenosine). It is recommended in both the PALS and ACLS guidelines for cardiac arrest with pulseless VT or VF (unresponsive to defibrillation, CPR, and vasopressor administration) and control of hemodynamically-stable monomorphic VT or wide-complex tachycardia of uncertain origin. The drug is also recommended in the ACLS guidelines for re-entry SVT (unresponsive to vagal maneuvers and adenosine); control of rapid ventricular rate due to conduction via an accessory pathway in pre-excited atrial arrhythmias; control of stable narrow-complex tachycardia; and control of polymorphic VT with a normal QT interval.

Medication Guide Available Yes

Pregnancy Risk Factor D

Pregnancy Considerations Adverse events have been observed in some animal reproduction studies. Amiodarone crosses the placenta (~10% to 50%) and may cause fetal harm when administered to a pregnant woman, leading to congenital goiter and hypo- or hyperthyroidism. Growth retardation and premature birth have also been noted (ESG, 2011). Amiodarone should be used in pregnant women only to treat arrhythmias that are life-threatening or refractory to other treatments (Blomström-Lundqvist, 2003; ESG, 2011).

Breast-Feeding Considerations Amiodarone and its active metabolite are excreted into human milk. Breast-feeding may lead to significant infant exposure and potential toxicity. Due to the long half-life, amiodarone may be present in breast milk for several days following discontinuation of maternal therapy (Hall, 2003). The manufacturer recommends that breast-feeding be discontinued if treatment is needed.

Contraindications Hypersensitivity to amiodarone, iodine, or any component; severe sinus node dysfunction; marked sinus bradycardia, second or third degree A-V block; cardiogenic shock; bradycardia-induced syncope (except if pacemaker is placed)

Warnings Amiodarone is not considered a first-line antiarrhythmic due to high incidence of toxicity **[U.S. Boxed Warning]**; 75% of patients experience adverse effects with large doses; discontinuation is required in 5% to 20% of patients. Amiodarone has several potentially fatal toxicities **[U.S. Boxed Warning]**; the most noteworthy being pulmonary toxicity. Pulmonary toxicity from amiodarone can occur from indirect or direct toxicity and result in hypersensitivity pneumonitis (including eosinophilic pneumonia) or interstitial/alveolar pneumonitis, respectively. Early onset pulmonary toxicity (ie, occurring over days to weeks) has been reported with oral amiodarone (with or without initial I.V. use) and may progress to respiratory failure or death. Educate patients about monitoring for symptoms of pulmonary toxicity (eg, nonproductive cough, dyspnea, pleuritic pain, hemoptysis, wheezing, weight loss, fever, malaise). Evaluate new respiratory symptoms; preexisting pulmonary disease does not increase risk of developing pulmonary toxicity, but if pulmonary toxicity develops then the prognosis is worse. Lung damage (abnormal diffusion capacity) may occur without symptoms. Use of lower amiodarone doses (loading and maintenance) may be associated with a lower incidence of pulmonary toxicity. The lowest effective dose should be used to appropriately treat the arrhythmia. Reserve amiodarone for use in life-threatening arrhythmias refractory to other therapy.

Liver toxicity is also common, but is usually mild with evidence of increased liver enzymes; severe liver toxicity can occur and has been fatal in a few cases; discontinue or reduce dose of amiodarone if hepatic enzymes exceed 3 times normal or double in a patient with an elevated ▶

baseline. Use with caution in patients with hepatic impairment; monitor closely.

Amiodarone may worsen or precipitate arrhythmias **[U.S. Boxed Warning]**, including torsade de pointes; when possible, hypokalemia and hypomagnesemia should be corrected prior to amiodarone use due to increased risk for torsade de pointes. Amiodarone may prolong the QT interval and should not be used in patients with congenital long QT syndrome (Fishberger, 2009); use with caution when administering with other drugs that prolong the QT interval; obtain expert consultation. Amiodarone is a potent inhibitor of cytochrome P450 enzymes and p-glycoprotein; serious drug interactions may occur; prolongation of the QT interval, with or without torsade de pointes, has been reported in patients receiving amiodarone concomitantly with macrolide antibiotics, azoles, or fluoroquinolones. Hypotension with I.V. use occurs in about 16% of patients, may be associated with infusion rate, and may be fatal; hypotension with rapid administration has been attributed to the excipients (polysorbate 80 and benzyl alcohol); Nexterone® injection does not contain these excipients and may have a lower incidence of hypotension. In adults, I.V. daily doses >2100 mg are associated with greater risk of hypotension; hypotension may respond to slowing the infusion, volume expansion, or administration of calcium, vasopressor drugs, or positive inotropic agents. Bradycardia and AV block may occur; temporary pacemaker should be available when I.V. product is used in patients with known predisposition to bradycardia or AV block. Patients should be hospitalized for initiation of therapy and loading dose administration **[U.S. Boxed Warning]**.

Chronic administration of antiarrhythmic drugs may affect defibrillation or pacing thresholds in patients with implantable cardiac devices (eg, defibrillators, pacemakers); assess thresholds when initiating amiodarone and during therapy. In pediatric patients (n=61, age: 30 days to 15 years), dose-related cardiovascular adverse reactions were common (hypotension 36%, bradycardia 20%, and AV block 15%) and in some cases, severe or life-threatening. Optic neuropathy and/or optic neuritis resulting in visual impairment may occur at any time and can progress to permanent blindness; prompt ophthalmic exam is recommended if visual impairment occurs; re-evaluate amiodarone therapy if optic neuropathy or neuritis occurs. Corneal microdeposits occur in most adults receiving amiodarone, and may cause visual disturbances in some patients (blurred vision, halos); asymptomatic corneal deposits alone are not generally considered a reason to discontinue treatment. Corneal refractive laser surgery is generally contraindicated in patients receiving amiodarone (per manufacturers of the laser surgery devices). Chronic administration of oral amiodarone rarely leads to the peripheral neuropathy; may resolve when amiodarone is discontinued, but this resolution has been slow and incomplete.

Amiodarone partially inhibits the peripheral conversion of thyroxine (T_4) to triiodothyronine (T_3); serum T_4 and reverse triiodothyronine (RT_3) concentrations may be increased and serum T_3 concentrations may be decreased; most patients remain clinically euthyroid; however, clinical hypothyroidism or hyperthyroidism may occur. Hyperthyroidism may result in potentially fatal thyrotoxicosis and may aggravate or cause breakthrough arrhythmias (possibly fatal); consider the possibility of hyperthyroidism if any new signs of arrhythmia appear; use with caution and monitor thyroid function closely in patients with thyroid disease. Amiodarone HCl contains 37% iodine by weight and is a potential source of large amounts of iodine; ~3 mg of inorganic iodine per 100 mg of amiodarone is released into the systemic circulation (RDA for iodine in adults is 150 mcg); avoid use during pregnancy and while breast-feeding (fetal/neonatal goiters, hypothyroidism, and possible cerebral damage may occur). Oral amiodarone has caused dose-related thyroid tumors in rats; cases of thyroid nodules/thyroid cancer have been reported in patients treated with amiodarone; hyperthyroidism was also present in some of these patients.

Nexterone® injection does not contain polysorbate (Tween® 80) and benzyl alcohol; however, other injectable amiodarone products may; see product specific information. Polysorbate 80 or benzyl alcohol may cause allergic reactions in susceptible individuals; large amounts of benzyl alcohol (≥99 mg/kg/day) have been associated with a potentially fatal toxicity ("gasping syndrome") in neonates; the "gasping syndrome" consists of metabolic acidosis, respiratory distress, gasping respirations, CNS dysfunction (including convulsions, intracranial hemorrhage), hypotension, and cardiovascular collapse; use amiodarone products containing benzyl alcohol with caution in neonates; *in vitro* and animal studies have shown that benzoate, a metabolite of benzyl alcohol, displaces bilirubin from protein binding sites. In premature neonates, thrombocytopenia, ascites, pulmonary deterioration, and renal and hepatic failure have been reported after receiving parenteral products containing polysorbate 80 (Alade, 1986; CDC, 1984). Infusion of polysorbate 80-containing solutions through polyvinyl chloride tubing may cause DEHP to leach into the solution; in immature animals, exposure to DEHP may adversely affect the development of the male reproductive tract. In order to decrease the potential exposure of infants to plasticizers, consider the use of bolus dosing in 1 mg/kg aliquots (Perry, 1996).

Precautions Avoid excessive exposure to sunlight; may cause photosensitivity; patients should be counseled to avoid excessive exposure to sunlight and to use proper sun protection. This photosensitivity could manifest as a blue-grey discoloration of exposed skin; risk may be increased in patients with fair complexion and may be related to cumulative dose and duration of therapy. Amiodarone may enhance myocardial depressant and conduction effects of anesthetics; monitor surgical patients closely; also associated with increased risk of adult respiratory distress syndrome (ARDS) postoperatively.

Adverse Reactions In a recent meta-analysis, adult patients taking lower doses of amiodarone (152-330 mg daily for at least 12 months) were more likely to develop thyroid, neurologic, skin, ocular, and bradycardic abnormalities than those taking placebo (Vorperian, 1997). Pulmonary toxicity was similar in both the low-dose amiodarone group and in the placebo group but there was a trend towards increased toxicity in the amiodarone group. Gastrointestinal and hepatic events were seen to a similar extent in both the low-dose amiodarone group and placebo group.

Cardiovascular: AV block, bradycardia, cardiac arrhythmia, conduction abnormalities, CHF, edema, flushing, hypotension, SA node dysfunction; additional effects associated with I.V. administration include asystole, atrial fibrillation, cardiac arrest, electromechanical dissociation, pulseless electrical activity (PEA), ventricular tachycardia, and cardiogenic shock

Central nervous system: Abnormal gait/ataxia, dizziness, fatigue, headache, impaired memory, involuntary movement, insomnia, malaise, peripheral neuropathy, poor coordination, sleep disturbances, tremor

Dermatologic: Photosensitivity, slate blue skin discoloration

Endocrine & metabolic: Hyperthyroidism, hypothyroidism, libido decreased

Gastrointestinal: Abdominal pain, abnormal salivation, abnormal taste (oral), anorexia, constipation, diarrhea, nausea (I.V.), vomiting

Hematologic: Coagulation abnormalities

Hepatic: AST or ALT level >2x normal, hepatitis and cirrhosis

Local: Phlebitis (I.V., with concentrations >3 mg/mL)

Ocular: Corneal microdeposits, halo vision, optic neuritis, visual disturbances

Respiratory: Alveolar pneumonitis, ARDS, hypersensitivity pneumonitis, interstitial pneumonitis, pulmonary fibrosis (cough, fever, malaise), pulmonary inflammation

Miscellaneous: Abnormal smell (oral)

Rare but important or life-threatening: Acute intracranial hypertension (I.V.), acute renal failure, acute respiratory distress syndrome, agranulocytosis, alopecia, anaphylactic shock, angioedema, aplastic anemia, bone marrow granuloma, bronchiolitis obliterans organizing pneumonia (BOOP), bronchospasm, cholestatic hepatitis, confusion, delirium, demyelinating polyneuropathy, disorientation, drug rash with eosinophilia and systemic symptoms (DRESS), dyspnea, encephalopathy, eczema, eosinophilic pneumonia, epididymitis (noninfectious), erectile dysfunction, erythema multiforme, exfoliative dermatitis, fever, granuloma, hallucination, hemolytic anemia, hemoptysis, hyperglycemia, hypertriglyceridemia, hypotension (oral), hypoxia, impotence, injection site reactions, leukocytoclastic vasculitis, muscle weakness, myopathy, neutropenia, optic neuropathy, pancreatitis, pancytopenia, parkinsonian symptoms, photophobia, pleural effusion, pleuritis, proarrhythmia, pruritus, pseudotumor cerebri, pulmonary alveolar hemorrhage, pulmonary edema, pulmonary infiltrates, pulmonary mass, QT interval increased, rash, renal impairment, renal insufficiency, respiratory failure, rhabdomyolysis, SIADH, sinus arrest, skin cancer, spontaneous ecchymosis, Stevens-Johnson syndrome, thrombocytopenia, thyroid nodules, thyroid cancer, thyrotoxicosis, torsade de pointes (rare), toxic epidermal necrolysis, urticaria, vasculitis, ventricular fibrillation, wheezing

Drug Interactions

Metabolism/Transport Effects Substrate of CYP1A2 (minor), CYP2C19 (minor), CYP2C8 (major), CYP2D6 (minor), CYP3A4 (major), P-glycoprotein; **Note:** Assignment of Major/Minor substrate status based on clinically relevant drug interaction potential; **Inhibits** CYP1A2 (weak), CYP2A6 (moderate), CYP2B6 (weak), CYP2C9 (moderate), CYP2D6 (moderate), CYP3A4 (weak), P-glycoprotein

Avoid Concomitant Use

Avoid concomitant use of Amiodarone with any of the following: Agalsidase Alfa; Agalsidase Beta; Antiarrhythmic Agents (Class Ia); Azithromycin (Systemic); Bosutinib; Ceritinib; Conivaptan; Fingolimod; Fusidic Acid (Systemic); Grapefruit Juice; Highest Risk QTc-Prolonging Agents; Ivabradine; Mifepristone; Moderate Risk QTc-Prolonging Agents; PAZOPanib; Pimozide; Propafenone; Protease Inhibitors; Silodosin; Tegafur; Thioridazine; Topotecan; VinCRIStine (Liposomal)

Increased Effect/Toxicity

Amiodarone may increase the levels/effects of: Afatinib; Antiarrhythmic Agents (Class Ia); Beta-Blockers; Bosentan; Bosutinib; Bradycardia-Causing Agents; Brentuximab Vedotin; Cannabis; Cardiac Glycosides; Carvedilol; Ceritinib; Colchicine; CycloSPORINE (Systemic); CYP2A6 Substrates; CYP2C9 Substrates; CYP2D6 Substrates; Dabigatran Etexilate; DOXOrubicin (Conventional); Dronabinol; Everolimus; Fesoterodine; Flecainide; Fosphenytoin; Highest Risk QTc-Prolonging Agents; HMG-CoA Reductase Inhibitors; Lidocaine (Systemic); Lidocaine (Topical); Lomitapide; Loratadine; Metoprolol; Mipomersen; Nebivolol; PAZOPanib; P-glycoprotein/ABCB1 Substrates; Phenytoin; Pimozide; Porfimer; Propafenone; Prucalopride; Rifaximin; Rivaroxaban; Silodosin; Tetrahydrocannabinol; Thioridazine; Topotecan; VinCRIStine (Liposomal); Vitamin K Antagonists

The levels/effects of Amiodarone may be increased by: Azithromycin (Systemic); Boceprevir; Calcium Channel Blockers (Nondihydropyridine); Cimetidine; Conivaptan; Cyclophosphamide; CYP2C8 Inhibitors (Moderate); CYP2C8 Inhibitors (Strong); CYP3A4 Inhibitors (Moderate); CYP3A4 Inhibitors (Strong); Deferasirox; Fingolimod; Fosphenytoin; Fusidic Acid (Systemic); Grapefruit Juice; Ivabradine; Ivacaftor; Lidocaine (Topical); Luliconazole; Mifepristone; Moderate Risk QTc-Prolonging Agents; P-glycoprotein/ABCB1 Inhibitors; Protease Inhibitors; QTc-Prolonging Agents (Indeterminate Risk and Risk Modifying); Simeprevir; Stiripentol; Telaprevir

Decreased Effect

Amiodarone may decrease the levels/effects of: Agalsidase Alfa; Agalsidase Beta; Clopidogrel; Codeine; Sodium Iodide I131; Tamoxifen; Tegafur; TraMADol

The levels/effects of Amiodarone may be decreased by: Bile Acid Sequestrants; Bosentan; CYP2C8 Inducers (Strong); CYP3A4 Inducers (Strong); Dabrafenib; Deferasirox; Etravirine; Fosphenytoin; Grapefruit Juice; Mitotane; Orlistat; Peginterferon Alfa-2b; P-glycoprotein/ABCB1 Inducers; Phenytoin; Rifampin; Siltuximab; St Johns Wort; Tocilizumab

Food Interactions Food increases the rate and extent of absorption of amiodarone. Grapefruit juice increases bioavailability of oral amiodarone by 50% and decreases the conversion of amiodarone to N-DEA (active metabolite); altered effects are possible. Management: Take consistently with regard to meals; grapefruit juice should be avoided during therapy.

Stability

Tablets:

Cordarone®: Store at 20°C to 25°C (68°F to 77°F); protect from light; dispense in a light-resistant, tightly closed container.

Pacerone®: Store at 20°C to 25°C (68°F to 77°F); excursions permitted to 15°C to 30°C (59°F to 86°F); protect from light; dispense in a light-resistant, tightly closed container

Injection: Store at 20°C to 25°C (68°F to 77°F); protect from light during storage; protect from excessive heat. There is no need to protect diluted solutions from light during I.V. administration. When admixed in D₅W to a final concentration of 1-6 mg/mL, it is stable for 24 hours in glass or polyolefin bottles and for 2 hours in polyvinyl chloride bags; do not use evacuated glass containers; buffer may cause precipitation. Although amiodarone adsorbs to polyvinyl chloride tubing, all clinical studies used polyvinyl chloride tubing and the recommended doses take adsorption into account; therefore, in adults, polyvinyl chloride tubing is recommended.

Nexterone®: Store at 20°C to 25°C (68°F to 77°F); excursions permitted to 15°C to 30°C (59°F to 86°F); protect from light and excessive heat. May be diluted in D₅W or NS to a final concentration of 1-6 mg/mL and administered in polyvinyl chloride, polyolefin, or glass containers. Do not use evacuated glass containers; buffer may cause precipitation.

Mechanism of Action Class III antiarrhythmic agent which inhibits adrenergic stimulation (alpha- and beta-blocking properties), affects sodium, potassium, and calcium channels, prolongs the action potential and refractory period in myocardial tissue; decreases AV conduction and sinus node function

Pharmacodynamics

Onset of action: Oral: 2-3 days to 1-3 weeks after starting therapy; I.V.: (electrophysiologic effects) within hours; antiarrhythmic effects: 2-3 days to 1-3 weeks; mean onset of effect may be shorter in children vs adults and in patients receiving I.V. loading doses

◄ Maximum effect: Oral: 1 week to 5 months

Duration of effects after discontinuation of oral therapy: Variable, 2 weeks to months: Children: less than a few weeks; adults: several months

Pharmacokinetics (Adult data unless noted)

Absorption: Oral: Slow and incomplete

Distribution:

I.V.: Rapid redistribution with a decrease to 10% of peak values within 30-45 minutes after completion of infusion

V_{dss}: I.V. single dose: Mean range: 40-84 L/kg

Oral: V_d: 66 L/kg: Range: 18-148 L/kg

Protein binding: >96%

Metabolism: Hepatic via CYP3A4 and CYP2C8 to active metabolite, N-desethylamiodarone; possible enterohepatic recirculation

Bioavailability: Oral: ~50% (range: 35% to 65%)

Half-life:

Amiodarone:

Single dose: 58 days (range: 15-142 days)

Oral chronic therapy: Mean range: 40-55 days (range: 26-107 days)

I.V. single dose: Mean range: 9-36 days

Half-life is shortened in children vs adults

N-desethylamiodarone (active metabolite):

Single dose: 36 days (range 14-75 days)

Oral chronic therapy: 61 days

I.V. single dose: Mean range: 9-30 days

Time to peak serum concentration: Oral: 3-7 hours

Elimination: Via biliary excretion; <1% excreted unchanged in urine

Dosing: Neonatal

Supraventricular tachycardia: Limited data available:

Oral: Loading dose: 10-20 mg/kg/day in 2 divided doses for 7-10 days; dosage should then be reduced to 5-10 mg/kg/day once daily and continued for 2-7 months; dosing based on a study of 50 infants (<9 months of age) and neonates (as young as 1 day of life); **Note:** Patients who received a higher loading dose (20 mg/kg/day) were more likely to have a prolongation of the corrected QT interval (Etheridge, 2001); further studies are needed.

Tachyarrhythmia, including junctional ectopic tachycardia (JET), paroxysmal supraventricular tachycardia (PSVT): Limited data available; optimal dose not established; further studies are needed; the following dosing is based on studies that included neonates, infants, and children.

Loading dose: I.V.: 5 mg/kg given over 60 minutes; **Note:** Bolus infusion rates should generally not exceed 0.25 mg/kg/minute unless clinically indicated; most studies used bolus infusion time of 60 minutes to avoid hypotension; may repeat initial loading dose to a maximum total initial load: 10 mg/kg; do not exceed total daily bolus of 15 mg/kg/day (Etheridge, 2001; Figa, 1994; Haas, 2008; Raja, 1994; Soult, 1995).

Continuous I.V. infusion (if needed): **Note:** Reported dosing units for regimens are variable (mcg/kg/minute and mg/kg/day); use caution to ensure appropriate dose and dosing units are used; taper infusion as soon as clinically possible and switch to oral therapy if necessary.

Dosing based on **mcg/kg/minute**: Initial: 5 **mcg/kg/minute**; increase incrementally as clinically needed; usual required dose: 10 **mcg/kg/minute**; range: 5-15 **mcg/kg/minute** (Figa, 1994; Kovacikova, 2009; Lane, 2010)

Dosing based on **mg/kg/day**: Initial: 10 **mg/kg/day**; increase incrementally as clinically needed; range: 10-20 **mg/kg/day** (Haas, 2008; Lane, 2010; Raja, 1994; Soult, 1995)

Dosing: Usual

Infants, Children, and Adolescents:

Perfusing tachycardias: I.V., I.O.: Loading dose: 5 mg/kg (maximum: 300 mg/dose) over 20-60 minutes; may repeat twice up to maximum total dose of 15 mg/kg during acute treatment (PALS, 2010)

Pulseless VT or VF: I.V., I.O.: 5 mg/kg (maximum: 300 mg/dose) rapid bolus; may repeat twice up to a maximum total dose of 15 mg/kg during acute treatment (PALS, 2010)

Tachyarrhythmia, including junctional ectopic tachycardia (JET), paroxysmal supraventricular tachycardia (PSVT): Limited data available; further studies are needed

Oral: Loading dose: 10-15 mg/kg/day in 1-2 divided doses/day for 4-14 days or until adequate control of arrhythmia or prominent adverse effects occur; dosage should be reduced to 5 mg/kg/day given once daily for several weeks; if arrhythmia does not recur, reduce to lowest effective dosage possible; usual daily minimal dose: 2.5 mg/kg/day; maintenance doses may be given for 5 of 7 days/week

Note: For infants, some have suggested BSA-directed dosing: Loading dose: 600-800 mg/**1.73 m²/day** in 1-2 divided doses (equivalent to 347-462 mg/m²/day); maintenance dose: 200-400 mg/**1.73 m²/day** once daily (equivalent to 116-231 mg/m²/day) (Bucknall, 1986; Coumel, 1980; Coumel, 1983; Paul, 1994)

Note: Prolongation of the corrected QT interval was more likely in infants <9 months of age who received higher loading doses (20 mg/kg/day vs 10 mg/kg/day in 2 divided doses) (n=50; mean age: 1 ± 1.5 months) (Etheridge, 2001)

I.V.: Loading dose: 5 mg/kg (maximum: 300 mg/dose) given over 60 minutes; **Note:** Bolus infusion rates should generally not exceed 0.25 mg/kg/minute unless clinically indicated; most studies used bolus infusion time of 60 minutes to avoid hypotension; may repeat initial loading dose to a maximum total initial load: 10 mg/kg; do not exceed total daily bolus of 15 mg/kg/**day** (Etheridge, 2001; Figa, 1994; Haas, 2008; Raja, 1994; Soult, 1995)

Note: Dividing the 5 mg/kg loading dose into 1 mg/kg aliquots (each administered over 5-10 minutes) has been used; an additional 1-5 mg/kg loading dose was given in the same manner, if needed, after 30 minutes (Perry, 1996)

Continuous I.V. infusion (if needed); **Note:** Reported dosing units for regimens are variable (mcg/kg/minute and mg/kg/day); use caution to ensure appropriate dose and dosing units are used; taper infusion as soon as clinically possible and switch to oral therapy if necessary.

Dosing based on **mcg/kg/minute**: Initial: 5 **mcg/kg/minute**; increase incrementally as clinically needed; usual required dose: 10 **mcg/kg/minute**; range: 5-15 **mcg/kg/minute**; maximum daily dose: 2200 mg/**day** (Figa, 1994; Kovacikova, 2009; Lane, 2010)

Dosing based on **mg/kg/day**: Initial: 10 **mg/kg/day**; increase incrementally as clinically needed; range: 10-20 **mg/kg/day**; maximum daily dose: 2200 mg/**day** (Lane, 2010; Perry, 1996; Raja, 1994; Soult, 1995)

Adults: **Note:** Lower loading and maintenance doses are preferable in women and all patients with low body weight.

Pulseless VT or VF (ACLS, 2010): I.V. push, I.O.: Initial: 300 mg; if pulseless VT or VF continues after subsequent defibrillation attempt or recurs, administer supplemental dose of 150 mg. **Note:** In this setting, administering **undiluted** is preferred (Dager, 2006; Skrifvars, 2004). *The Handbook of Emergency*

Cardiovascular Care (Hazinski, 2010) and the 2010 ACLS guidelines (Neumar, 2010) do not make any specific recommendations regarding dilution of amiodarone in this setting. Experience is limited with I.O. administration of amiodarone (Neumar, 2010).

Upon return of spontaneous circulation, follow with an infusion of 1 mg/minute for 6 hours, then 0.5 mg/minute for 18 hours (mean daily doses >2100 mg/day have been associated with hypotension).

Perfusing tachycardias (ACLS, 2010): I.V.: Bolus doses for hemodynamically stable VT or wide QRS tachycardia of uncertain origin (regular rhythm): 150 mg given over 10 minutes; may repeat if necessary, followed by an infusion of 1 mg/minute for 6 hours, then 0.5 mg/minute; maximum daily dose: 2200 mg/**day** (Neumar, 2010)

Ventricular arrhythmias: Manufacturer's labeling:

Oral: Loading dose: 800-1600 mg/day in 1-2 divided doses for 1-3 weeks, then when adequate arrhythmia control is achieved, decrease to 600-800 mg/day in 1-2 divided doses for 1 month; maintenance: 400 mg daily; lower doses are recommended for supraventricular arrhythmias

I.V.: Loading dose: 1050 mg delivered over 24 hours as follows: 150 mg given over 10 minutes (at a rate of 15 mg/minute) followed by 360 mg given over 6 hours (at a rate of 1 mg/minute); follow with maintenance dose: 540 mg given over the next 18 hours (at a rate of 0.5 mg/minute); after the first 24 hours the maintenance dose is continued at 0.5 mg/minute; additional supplemental bolus doses of 150 mg infused over 10 minutes may be given for breakthrough VF or hemodynamically unstable VT; maintenance dose infusion may be increased to control arrhythmia; mean daily doses >2.1 g/day have been associated with hypotension

Atrial fibrillation: Pharmacologic cardioversion (ACC/AHA/ESC Practice Guidelines):

Oral:

Inpatient: 1200-1800 mg/day in divided doses until 10 **g** total, then 200-400 mg/day maintenance

Outpatient: 600-800 mg/day in divided doses until 10 **g** total, then 200-400 mg/day maintenance; although not supported by clinical evidence, a maintenance dose of 100 mg/day is commonly used especially for the elderly or patients with low body mass (Fuster, 2006; Zimetbaum, 2007). **Note:** Other regimens have been described and may be used clinically:

400 mg 3 times daily for 5-7 days, then 400 mg daily for 1 month, then 200 mg daily

or

10 mg/kg/day for 14 days, followed by 300 mg daily for 4 weeks, followed by maintenance dosage of 200 mg daily (Roy, 2000)

I.V.: 5-7 mg/kg over 30-60 minutes, then 1200-1800 mg/day continuous infusion until 10 **g** total; maintenance: See oral dosing.

Atrial fibrillation prophylaxis following open heart surgery: Note: A variety of regimens have been used in clinical trials, including oral and intravenous regimens:

Oral: Starting in postop recovery, 400 mg twice daily for up to 7 days. Alternative regimen of amiodarone: 600 mg/day for 7 days prior to surgery, followed by 200 mg/day until hospital discharge; has also been shown to decrease the risk of postoperative atrial fibrillation

I.V.: Starting at postop recovery, 1000 mg infused over 24 hours for 2 days has been shown to reduce the risk of postoperative atrial fibrillation

Atrial fibrillation, recurrent: No standard regimen defined; examples of regimens include: Oral: Initial: 10 mg/kg/day for 14 days; followed by 300 mg/day for 4 weeks, followed by maintenance dosage of 200 mg/day (Roy, 2000). Other regimens have been described and are used clinically (ie, 400 mg 3 times daily for 5-7 days, then 400 mg daily for 1 month, then 200 mg daily).

Transition from I.V. to oral therapy: Conversion from I.V. to oral therapy has not been formally evaluated. Some experts recommend a 1-2 day overlap when converting from I.V. to oral therapy especially when treating ventricular arrhythmias. Use the following as a guide assuming patient received 0.5 mg/minute for the listed duration of I.V. infusion:

<1 week infusion: 800-1600 mg/day

1-3 week infusion: 600-800 mg/day

>3 week infusion: 400 mg/day

Recommendations for conversion to intravenous amiodarone after oral administration: During long-term amiodarone therapy (ie, ≥4 months), the mean plasma-elimination half-life of the active metabolite of amiodarone in adults is 61 days. Replacement therapy may not be necessary in such patients if oral therapy is discontinued for a period <2 weeks, since any changes in serum amiodarone concentrations during this period may **not** be clinically significant.

Dosing adjustment in renal impairment: Adults: I.V., Oral: No adjustment necessary; nondialyzable (parent and metabolite)

Dosing adjustment in hepatic impairment: Adults; I.V., Oral: No dosage adjustments are recommended in the manufacturer labeling; however, dosage adjustment may be necessary in substantial hepatic impairment; use with caution. If hepatic enzymes exceed 3 times normal or double in a patient with an elevated baseline, consider decreasing the dose or discontinuing amiodarone.

Usual Infusion Concentrations: Pediatric Note: Premixed solutions available.

I.V. infusion: 1.8 mg/mL

Administration

Oral: Administer at same time in relation to meals; do not administer with grapefruit juice. In adults, may administer in divided doses with meals if GI upset occurs or if taking large daily dose.

I.V.: Adjust administration rate to patient's clinical condition and urgency: give slowly to patients who have a pulse (ie, perfusing arrhythmia). With perfusing arrhythmias (eg, atrial fibrillation, stable ventricular tachycardia), do not exceed recommended I.V. concentrations or rates of infusion listed below (severe hepatic toxicity may occur). Slow the infusion rate if hypotension or bradycardia develops.

Pulseless VT or VF:

Infants, Children, and Adolescents: Administer via rapid I.V. bolus. **Note:** PALS guidelines do not specify dilution of bolus dose. Adult data in this setting suggest administration of undiluted drug may be preferred (Dager, 2006; Skrifvars, 2004). *The Handbook of Emergency Cardiovascular Care* (Hazinski, 2010) and the 2010 ACLS guidelines (Neumar, 2010) do not make any specific recommendations regarding dilution of amiodarone in this setting.

Adults: May be administered rapidly and undiluted. **Note:** *The Handbook of Emergency Cardiovascular Care* (Hazinski, 2010) and the 2010 ACLS guidelines (Neumar, 2010) do not make any specific recommendations regarding dilution of amiodarone in this setting; however, in this setting, administering undiluted is preferred (Dager, 2006; Skrifvars, 2004).

Perfusing arrhythmias: Information based on adult data: Injection must be diluted before I.V. use. Administer via central venous catheter, if possible; increased phlebitis may occur with peripheral infusions >3 mg/mL in D_5W, but concentrations ≤2.5 mg/mL may be less irritating; the use of a central venous catheter with concentrations >2 mg/mL for infusions >1 hour is recommended. Maximum concentration for infusion: 6 mg/mL. An in-line filter has been recommended during administration for continuous infusions to reduce the incidence of phlebitis. The use of polyvinyl chloride tubing is recommended in adults. Must be infused via volumetric infusion device; drop size of I.V. solution may be reduced and underdosage may occur if drop counter-infusion sets are used.

Infants, Children, and Adolescents: Administer loading dose over 20-60 minutes; no data regarding concentration for infusion are available; take adult concentrations into consideration when diluting.

Adults: Usual dilutions: First loading infusion: 150 mg in 100 mL D_5W (1.5 mg/mL) for infusion over 10 minutes; then 900 mg in 500 mL D_5W (1.8 mg/mL) to deliver rest of dose

Monitoring Parameters Heart rate and rhythm, blood pressure, ECG, chest x-ray, pulmonary function tests, thyroid function tests; serum glucose, electrolytes (especially potassium and magnesium), triglycerides, liver enzymes; ophthalmologic exams including fundoscopy and slit-lamp examinations, physical signs and symptoms of thyroid dysfunction (lethargy, edema of hands and feet, weight gain or loss), and pulmonary toxicity (dyspnea, cough; oxygen saturation, blood gases). Monitor pacing or defibrillation thresholds in patients with implantable cardiac devices (eg, pacemakers, defibrillators) at initiation of therapy and periodically during treatment.

Reference Range Therapeutic: Chronic oral dosing: 1-2.5 mg/L (SI: 2-4 micromoles/L) (parent); desethyl metabolite (active) is present in equal concentration to parent drug; serum concentrations may not be of great value for predicting toxicity and efficacy; toxicity may occur even at therapeutic concentrations

Additional Information Intoxication with amiodarone necessitates ECG monitoring; bradycardia may be atropine resistant, I.V. isoproterenol or cardiac pacemaker may be required; hypotension, cardiogenic shock, heart block, QT prolongation and hepatotoxicity may also be seen; patients should be monitored for several days following overdose due to long half-life

I.V. product is used for acute treatment; the duration of I.V. treatment is usually 48-96 hours; however, in adults, infusions may be used cautiously for 2-3 weeks; there is limited experience with administering infusions for >3 weeks

Dosage Forms Excipient information presented when available (limited, particularly for generics); consult specific product labeling.

Solution, Intravenous, as hydrochloride:
Nexterone: 150 mg/100 mL (100 mL); 360 mg/200 mL (200 mL)
Generic: 150 mg/3 mL (3 mL); 450 mg/9 mL (9 mL); 900 mg/18 mL (18 mL)
Tablet, Oral, as hydrochloride:
Cordarone: 200 mg [scored]
Pacerone: 100 mg
Pacerone: 200 mg [scored; contains fd&c red #40, fd&c yellow #6 (sunset yellow)]
Pacerone: 400 mg [scored; contains fd&c yellow #10 aluminum lake]
Generic: 100 mg, 200 mg, 400 mg

Extemporaneous Preparations A 5 mg/mL oral suspension may be made with tablets and either a 1:1 mixture of Ora-Sweet® and Ora-Plus® or a 1:1 mixture of Ora-Sweet® SF and Ora-Plus® adjusted to a pH between 6-7 using a sodium bicarbonate solution (5 g/100 mL of distilled water). Crush five 200 mg tablets in a mortar and reduce to a fine powder. Add small portions of the chosen vehicle and mix to a uniform paste; mix while adding the vehicle in incremental proportions to **almost** 200 mL;

transfer to a calibrated bottle, rinse mortar with vehicle, and add quantity of vehicle sufficient to make 200 mL. Label "shake well" and "protect from light". Stable for 42 days at room temperature or 91 days refrigerated (preferred) (Nahata, 2004).

Nahata MC, Pai VB, and Hipple TF, *Pediatric Drug Formulations*, 5th ed, Cincinnati, OH: Harvey Whitney Books Co, 2004.

References

Alade SL, Brown RE, and Paquet A Jr, "Polysorbate 80 and E-Ferol Toxicity," *Pediatrics*, 1986, 77(4):593-7.

Blomström-Lundqvist C, Scheinman MM, Aliot EM, et al, "ACC/AHA/ESC Guidelines for the Management of Patients With Supraventricular Arrhythmias–Executive Summary. A Report of the American College of Cardiology/American Heart Association Task Force on Practice Guidelines and the European Society of Cardiology Committee for Practice Guidelines (Writing Committee to Develop Guidelines for the Management of Patients With Supraventricular Arrhythmias)," *Circulation*, 2003, 108(15):1871-909.

Bucknall CA, Keeton BR, Curry PV, et al, "Intravenous and Oral Amiodarone for Arrhythmias in Children," *Br Heart J*, 1986, 56(3):278-84.

Centers for Disease Control (CDC), "Unusual Syndrome With Fatalities Among Premature Infants: Association With a New Intravenous Vitamin E Product," *MMWR Morb Mortal Wkly Rep*, 1984, 33(14):198-9.

Chalmers JR, Bobek MB, and Militello MA, "Visual Compatibility of Amiodarone Hydrochloride Injection With Various Intravenous Drugs," *Am J Health Syst Pharm*, 2001, 58(6):504-6.

Coumel P and Fidelle J, "Amiodarone in the Treatment of Cardiac Arrhythmias in Children: One Hundred Thirty-Five Cases," *Am Heart J*, 1980, 100(6 Pt 2):1063-9.

Dager WE, Sanoski CA, Wiggins BS, et al, "Pharmacotherapy Considerations in Advanced Cardiac Life Support," *Pharmacotherapy*, 2006, 26(12):1703-29.

Etheridge SP, Craig JE, and Compton SJ, "Amiodarone is Safe and Highly Effective Therapy for Supraventricular Tachycardia in Infants," *Am Heart J*, 2001, 141(1):105-10.

European Society of Gynecology (ESG); Association for European Paediatric Cardiology (AEPC); German Society for Gender Medicine (DGesGM), et al, "ESC Guidelines on the Management of Cardiovascular Diseases During Pregnancy: The Task Force on the Management of Cardiovascular Diseases During Pregnancy of the European Society of Cardiology (ESC)," *Eur Heart J*, 2011, 32(24):3147-97.

Figa FH, Gow RM, Hamilton RM, et al, "Clinical Efficacy and Safety of Intravenous Amiodarone in Infants and Children," *Am J Cardiol*, 1994, 74(6):573-7.

Fishberger SB, Hannan RL, Welch EM, et al, "Amiodarone for Pediatric Resuscitation: A Word of Caution," *Pediatr Cardiol*, 2009, 30(7):1006-8.

Fuster V, Rydén LE, Cannom DS, et al, "ACC/AHA/ESC 2006 Guidelines for the Management of Patients With Atrial Fibrillation-Executive Summary: A Report of the American College of Cardiology/American Heart Association Task Force on Practice Guidelines and the European Society of Cardiology Committee for Practice Guidelines (Writing Committee to Revise the 2001 Guidelines for the Management of Patients With Atrial Fibrillation)," *J Am Coll Cardiol*, 2006, 48(4):854-906.

Haas NA and Camphausen CK, "Impact of Early and Standardized Treatment With Amiodarone on Therapeutic Success and Outcome in Pediatric Patients With Postoperative Tachyarrhythmia," *J Thorac Cardiovasc Surg*, 2008, 136(5):1215-22.

Hall CM and McCormick KP, "Amiodarone and Breast Feeding," *Arch Dis Child Fetal Neonatal Ed*, 2003, 88(3):F255-4.

Hazinski MF, Samson R, and Schexnayder S, *2010 Handbook of Emergency Cardiovascular Care for Healthcare Providers*, South Deerfield, MA: American Heart Association, 2010.

Kleinman ME, Chameides L, Schexnayder SM, et al, "Part 14: Pediatric Advanced Life Support: 2010 American Heart Association Guidelines for Cardiopulmonary Resuscitation and Emergency Cardiovascular Care," *Circulation*, 2010, 122(18 Suppl 3):876-908.

Kovacikova L, Hakacova N, Dobos D, et al, "Amiodarone as a First-Line Therapy for Postoperative Junctional Ectopic Tachycardia," *Ann Thorac Surg*, 2009, 88(2):616-22.

Lane RD, Nguyen KT, Niemann JT, et al, "Amiodarone for the Emergency Care of Children," *Pediatr Emerg Care*, 2010, 26(5):382-9.

Neumar RW, Otto CW, Link MS, et al, "Part 8: Adult Advanced Cardiovascular Life Support: 2010 American Heart Association Guidelines for Cardiopulmonary Resuscitation and Emergency Cardiovascular Care," *Circulation*, 2010, 122(18 Suppl 3):729-67.

Paul T and Guccione P, "New Antiarrhythmic Drugs in Pediatric Use: Amiodarone," *Pediatr Cardiol*, 1994, 15(3):132-8.

Perry JC, Fenrich AL, Hulse JE, et al, "Pediatric Use of Intravenous Amiodarone: Efficacy and Safety in Critically Ill Patients From a Multicenter Protocol," *J Am Coll Cardiol*, 1996, 27(5):1246-50.

Phillips MS, "Standardizing I.V. Infusion Concentrations: National Survey Results," *Am J Health Syst Pharm*, 2011, 68(22):2176-82.

Raja P, Hawker RE, Chaikitpinyo A, et al, "Amiodarone Management of Junctional Ectopic Tachycardia After Cardiac Surgery in Children," *Br Heart J*, 1994, 72(3):261-5.

Roy D, Talajic M, Dorian P, et al, "Amiodarone to Prevent Recurrence of Atrial Fibrillation. Canadian Trial of Atrial Fibrillation Investigators," *N Engl J Med*, 2000, 342(13):913-20.

Skrifvars MB, Kuisma M, Boyd J, et al, "The Use of Undiluted Amiodarone in the Management of Out-of-Hospital Cardiac Arrest," *Acta Anaesthesiol Scand*, 2004, 48(5):582-7.

Soult JA, Munoz M, Lopez JD, et al, "Efficacy and Safety of Intravenous Amiodarone for Short-Term Treatment of Paroxysmal Supraventricular Tachycardia in Children," *Pediatr Cardiol*, 1995, 16(1):16-9.

Vorperian VR, Havighurst TC, Miller S, et al, "Adverse Effects of Low Dose Amiodarone: A Meta-analysis," *J Am Coll Cardiol*, 1997, 30 (3):791-8.

Zimetbaum P, "Amiodarone for Atrial Fibrillation," *N Engl J Med*, 2007, 356(9):935-41.

◆ **Amiodarone Hydrochloride** *see* Amiodarone *on page 127*

◆ **Amiodarone Hydrochloride Injection (Can)** *see* Amiodarone *on page 127*

Amitriptyline (a mee TRIP ti leen)

Medication Safety Issues
Sound-alike/look-alike issues:
Amitriptyline may be confused with aminophylline, imipramine, nortriptyline

Elavil may be confused with Aldoril, Eldepryl, enalapril, Equanil, Plavix

BEERS Criteria medication:
This drug may be potentially inappropriate for use in geriatric patients (Quality of evidence - high [moderate for SIADH]; Strength of recommendation - strong).

Related Information
Antidepressant Agents *on page 2219*

Medications for Which a Single Dose May Be Fatal When Ingested by a Toddler *on page 2408*

Brand Names: Canada Apo-Amitriptyline; Bio-Amitriptyline; Elavil; Levate; Novo-Triptyn; PMS-Amitriptyline

Therapeutic Category Antidepressant, Tricyclic (Tertiary Amine); Antimigraine Agent

Generic Availability (U.S.) Yes

Use Treatment of various forms of depression, often in conjunction with psychotherapy; analgesic for certain chronic and neuropathic pain; migraine prophylaxis

Medication Guide Available Yes

Pregnancy Risk Factor C

Pregnancy Considerations Adverse events have been observed in some animal reproduction studies. Amitriptyline crosses the human placenta; CNS effects, limb deformities, and developmental delay have been noted in case reports (causal relationship not established). Tricyclic antidepressants may be associated with irritability, jitteriness, and convulsions (rare) in the neonate (Yonkers, 2009).

The ACOG recommends that therapy for depression during pregnancy be individualized; treatment should incorporate the clinical expertise of the mental health clinician, obstetrician, primary healthcare provider, and pediatrician (ACOG, 2008). According to the American Psychiatric Association (APA), the risks of medication treatment should be weighed against other treatment options and untreated depression. For women who discontinue antidepressant medications during pregnancy and who may be at high risk for postpartum depression, the medications can be restarted following delivery (APA, 2010). Treatment algorithms have been developed by the ACOG and the APA for the management of depression in women prior to conception and during pregnancy (Yonkers, 2009). Although not a first-line agent, amitriptyline may be used for the treatment of post-traumatic stress disorder in pregnant women (Bandelow, 2008). Migraine prophylaxis should be avoided during pregnancy; if needed, amitriptyline may be used if other agents are ineffective or contraindicated (Pringsheim, 2012).

Breast-Feeding Considerations Amitriptyline is excreted into breast milk. Based on information from six mother/infant pairs, following maternal use of amitriptyline 75-175 mg/day, the estimated exposure to the breast-feeding infant would be 0.2% to 1.9% of the weight-adjusted maternal dose. Adverse events have not been reported in nursing infants (four cases). Infants should be monitored for signs of adverse events; routine monitoring of infant serum concentrations is not recommended (Fortinguerra, 2009). Migraine prophylaxis should be avoided in women who are nursing; if needed, amitriptyline may be used if other agents are ineffective or contraindicated (Pringsheim, 2012). Due to the potential for serious adverse reactions in the nursing infant, the manufacturer recommends a decision be made whether to discontinue nursing or to discontinue the drug, taking into account the importance of treatment to the mother.

Contraindications Hypersensitivity to amitriptyline (cross-sensitivity with other tricyclics may occur) or any component; narrow-angle glaucoma; use of MAO inhibitors within 14 days (potentially fatal reactions may occur); concurrent use of cisapride; use during acute recovery phase after MI

Warnings Amitriptyline is not approved for use in pediatric patients. Clinical worsening of depression or suicidal ideation and behavior may occur in children and adults with major depressive disorder **[U.S. Boxed Warning]**. In clinical trials, antidepressants increased the risk of suicidal thinking and behavior (suicidality) in children, adolescents, and young adults (18-24 years of age) with major depressive disorder and other psychiatric disorders. This risk must be considered before prescribing antidepressants for any clinical use. Short-term studies did **not** show an increased risk of suicidality with antidepressant use in patients >24 years of age and showed a decreased risk in patients ≥65 years.

Patients of all ages who are treated with antidepressants for any indication require appropriate monitoring and close observation for clinical worsening of depression, suicidality, and unusual changes in behavior, especially during the first few months after antidepressant initiation or when the dose is adjusted. Family members and caregivers should be instructed to closely observe the patient (ie, daily) and communicate condition with healthcare provider. Patients should also be monitored for associated behaviors (eg, anxiety, agitation, panic attacks, insomnia, irritability, hostility, aggressiveness, impulsivity, akathisia, hypomania, mania) which may increase the risk for worsening depression or suicidality. Worsening depression or emergence of suicidality (or associated behaviors listed above) that is abrupt in onset, severe, or not part of the presenting symptoms, may require discontinuation or modification of drug therapy.

Do not discontinue abruptly in patients receiving high doses chronically (withdrawal symptoms may occur). To reduce risk of intentional overdose, write prescriptions for the smallest quantity consistent with good patient care. Screen individuals for bipolar disorder prior to treatment (using antidepressants alone may induce manic episodes in patients with this condition). May worsen psychosis in some patients.

Precautions Use with caution in patients with cardiac conduction disturbances, cardiovascular disease, seizure disorders, diabetes mellitus, narrow-angle glaucoma, increased intraocular pressure, history of urinary retention or bowel obstruction, hepatic or renal dysfunction, hyperthyroidism or those receiving thyroid hormone replacement; degree of sedation, anticholinergic effects, and risk of orthostatic hypotension are very high relative to other antidepressants; manufacturer does not recommend use in children <12 years of age

Adverse Reactions Anticholinergic effects may be pronounced; moderate to marked sedation can occur (tolerance to these effects usually occurs).

Frequency not defined.

Cardiovascular: Atrioventricular conduction disturbance, cardiac arrhythmia, cardiomyopathy (rare), cerebrovascular accident, ECG changes (nonspecific), edema, facial edema, heart block, hypertension, myocardial infarction, orthostatic hypotension, palpitations, syncope, tachycardia

Central nervous system: Anxiety, ataxia, cognitive dysfunction, coma, confusion, delusions, disorientation, dizziness, drowsiness, dysarthria, EEG pattern changes, excitement, extrapyramidal reaction (including abnormal involuntary movements and tardive dyskinesia), fatigue, hallucinations, headache, hyperpyrexia, insomnia, lack of concentration, nightmares, numbness, paresthesia, peripheral neuropathy, restlessness, sedation, seizure, tingling of extremities

Dermatologic: Allergic skin rash, alopecia, diaphoresis, skin photosensitivity, urticaria

Endocrine & metabolic: Altered serum glucose, decreased libido, galactorrhea, gynecomastia, increased libido, SIADH, weight gain, weight loss

Gastrointestinal: Ageusia, anorexia, constipation, diarrhea, melanoglossia, nausea, paralytic ileus, parotid gland enlargement, stomatitis, unpleasant taste, vomiting, xerostomia

Genitourinary: Breast hypertrophy, impotence, testicular swelling, urinary frequency, urinary retention, urinary tract dilation

Hematologic & oncologic: Bone marrow depression (including agranulocytosis, leukopenia, and thrombocytopenia), eosinophilia, purpura

Hepatic: Hepatic failure, hepatitis (rare; including altered liver function and jaundice)

Hypersensitivity: Tongue edema

Neuromuscular & skeletal: Lupus-like syndrome, tremor, weakness

Ophthalmic: Accommodation disturbance, blurred vision, increased intraocular pressure, mydriasis

Otic: Tinnitus

Miscellaneous: Diaphoresis, drug withdrawal (nausea, headache, malaise, irritability, restlessness, dream and sleep disturbance, mania [rare], and hypomania [rare])

Rare but important or life-threatening: Neuroleptic malignant syndrome (rare), serotonin syndrome (rare)

Drug Interactions

Metabolism/Transport Effects Substrate of CYP1A2 (minor), CYP2B6 (minor), CYP2C19 (minor), CYP2C9 (minor), CYP2D6 (major), CYP3A4 (minor); **Note:** Assignment of Major/Minor substrate status based on clinically relevant drug interaction potential; **Inhibits** CYP1A2 (weak), CYP2C19 (weak), CYP2C9 (weak), CYP2D6 (weak), CYP2E1 (weak)

Avoid Concomitant Use

Avoid concomitant use of Amitriptyline with any of the following: Aclidinium; Azelastine (Nasal); Cisapride; Iobenguane I 123; Ipratropium (Oral Inhalation); Linezolid; MAO Inhibitors; Methylene Blue; Moxonidine; Paraldehyde; Potassium Chloride; Thalidomide; Tiotropium; Umeclidinium

Increased Effect/Toxicity

Amitriptyline may increase the levels/effects of: Abobotulinumtoxin A; Alcohol (Ethyl); Alpha-/Beta-Agonists (Direct-Acting); Alpha1-Agonists; Amphetamines; Analgesics (Opioid); Anticholinergic Agents; Antipsychotics; ARIPiprazole; Aspirin; Azelastine (Nasal); Beta2-Agonists; Buprenorphine; Cannabinoid-Containing Products; Cisapride; Citalopram; CNS Depressants;

Desmopressin; Escitalopram; Highest Risk QTc-Prolonging Agents; Hydrocodone; Methotrimeprazine; Methylene Blue; Metyrosine; Mirabegron; Moderate Risk QTc-Prolonging Agents; NSAID (COX-2 Inhibitor); NSAID (Nonselective); OnabotulinumtoxinA; Paraldehyde; Potassium Chloride; Pramipexole; QuiNIDine; RimabotulinumtoxinB; ROPINIRole; Rotigotine; Serotonin Modulators; Sodium Phosphates; Sulfonylureas; Thalidomide; Thiazide Diuretics; Tiotropium; TraMADol; Vitamin K Antagonists; Yohimbine; Zolpidem

The levels/effects of Amitriptyline may be increased by: Abiraterone Acetate; Aclidinium; Altretamine; Antiemetics (5HT3 Antagonists); Antipsychotics; Brimonidine (Topical); BuPROPion; Cannabis; Cimetidine; Cinacalcet; Citalopram; Cobicistat; CYP2D6 Inhibitors (Moderate); CYP2D6 Inhibitors (Strong); Darunavir; Dexmethylphenidate; Doxylamine; Dronabinol; Droperidol; DULoxetine; Escitalopram; FLUoxetine; FluvoxaMINE; HydrOXYzine; Ipratropium (Oral Inhalation); Kava Kava; Linezolid; Lithium; Magnesium Sulfate; MAO Inhibitors; Methotrimeprazine; Methylphenidate; Metoclopramide; Metyrosine; Mifepristone; Nabilone; PARoxetine; Perampanel; Pramlintide; Protease Inhibitors; QuiNIDine; Rufinamide; Sertraline; Sodium Oxybate; Tapentadol; Terbinafine (Systemic); Tetrahydrocannabinol; Thyroid Products; Topiramate; TraMADol; Umeclidinium; Valproic Acid and Derivatives

Decreased Effect

Amitriptyline may decrease the levels/effects of: Acetylcholinesterase Inhibitors (Central); Alpha2-Agonists; Alpha2-Agonists (Ophthalmic); Iobenguane I 123; Moxonidine; Secretin

The levels/effects of Amitriptyline may be decreased by: Acetylcholinesterase Inhibitors (Central); Barbiturates; CarBAMazepine; Peginterferon Alfa-2b; St Johns Wort

Mechanism of Action Increases the synaptic concentration of serotonin and/or norepinephrine in the central nervous system by inhibition of their reuptake by the presynaptic neuronal membrane pump.

Pharmacodynamics Onset of action: Therapeutic antidepressant effects begin in 7-21 days; maximum effects may not occur for ≥2 weeks and as long as 4-6 weeks

Pharmacokinetics (Adult data unless noted)

Absorption: Oral: Rapid, well absorbed

Protein binding: >90%

Metabolism: In the liver to nortriptyline (active), hydroxy derivatives and conjugated derivatives

Half-life, adults: 9-25 hours (15-hour average)

Time to peak serum concentration: Within 4 hours

Elimination: Renal excretion of 18% as unchanged drug; small amounts eliminated in feces by bile

Dialysis: Nondialyzable

Dosing: Usual Oral:

Chronic pain management: Children: Initial: 0.1 mg/kg at bedtime, may advance as tolerated over 2-3 weeks to 0.5-2 mg/kg at bedtime

Depressive disorders: **Note:** Not FDA approved for use in pediatric patients; controlled clinical trials have not shown tricyclic antidepressants to be superior to placebo for the treatment of depression in children and adolescents (Dopheide, 2006; Wagner, 2005).

Children: Investigationally initial doses of 1 mg/kg/day given in 3 divided doses with increases to 1.5 mg/kg/day have been reported in a small number of children (n=9) 9-12 years of age; clinically, doses up to 3 mg/kg/day (5 mg/kg/day if monitored closely) have been proposed

Adolescents: Initial: 25-50 mg/day; may give in divided doses; increase gradually to 100 mg/day in divided doses; maximum dose: 200 mg/day

Migraine prophylaxis: Children: Limited studies exist; one small study (n=24; mean age: 8 years; range: 6-12 years)

used increasing doses over 5 days to reach a final dose of 1.5 mg/kg/day; effectiveness was seen in 19 of 24 patients, but 5 children dropped out of the trial due to adverse effects (Sorge, 1982). A recent large open-label trial in 192 children (mean age 12 ± 3 years) with >3 headaches/month (61% with migraine, 8% with migraine with aura, and 10% with tension-type headaches) used an initial dose of 0.25 mg/kg/day given before bedtime; doses were increased every 2 weeks by 0.25 mg/kg/day to a final dose of 1 mg/kg/day; patients also used appropriate abortive medications and lifestyle adjustments; at initial re-evaluation (mean: 67 days after initiation of therapy), the mean number of headaches per month significantly decreased from 17.1 to 9.2; the mean duration of headaches decreased from 11.5 to 6.3 hours; continued improvement was observed at follow-up visits; minimal adverse effects were reported. **Note:** Mean final dose was 0.99 ± 0.23 mg/kg; range: 0.16-1.7 mg/kg/day; ECGs were obtained on children receiving >1 mg/kg/day or in those describing a cardiac side effect (Hershey, 2000). Further studies are needed.

Depression: Adults: Initial: 50-100 mg/day single dose at bedtime or in divided doses; dose may be gradually increased up to 300 mg/day; once symptoms are controlled, decrease gradually to lowest effective dose

Administration Oral: May administer with food to decrease GI upset

Monitoring Parameters Heart rate, blood pressure, mental status, weight. Monitor patient periodically for symptom resolution; monitor for worsening depression, suicidality, and associated behaviors (especially at the beginning of therapy or when doses are increased or decreased).

Reference Range Note: Plasma levels do not always correlate with clinical effectiveness

Therapeutic:

Amitriptyline plus nortriptyline (active metabolite): 100-250 ng/mL (SI: 360-900 nmol/L)

Nortriptyline 50-150 ng/mL (SI: 190-570 nmol/L)

Toxic: >500 ng/mL (SI: >1800 nmol/L)

Additional Information Due to promotion of weight gain with amitriptyline, other antidepressants (ie, imipramine or desipramine) may be preferred in heavy or obese children and adolescents

Dosage Forms Excipient information presented when available (limited, particularly for generics); consult specific product labeling.

Tablet, Oral, as hydrochloride:

Generic: 10 mg, 25 mg, 50 mg, 75 mg, 100 mg, 150 mg

References

ACOG Committee on Practice Bulletins-Obstetrics, "ACOG Practice Bulletin: Clinical Management Guidelines for Obstetrician-Gynecologists Number 92, April 2008 (Replaces Practice Bulletin Number 87, November 2007). Use of Psychiatric Medications During Pregnancy and Lactation," *Obstet Gynecol*, 2008, 111(4):1001-20.

American Psychiatric Association (APA), "Treatment Recommendations for Patients With Major Depressive Disorder," 3rd ed, May 2010. Available at http://www.psychiatryonline.com/pracGuide/pracGuideTopic_7.aspx

Bandelow B, Zohar J, Hollander E, et al, "World Federation of Societies of Biological Psychiatry (WFSBP) Guidelines for the Pharmacological Treatment of Anxiety, Obsessive-Compulsive and Post-Traumatic Stress Disorders – First Revision," *World J Biol Psychiatry*, 2008, 9 (4): 248-312. Available at http://www.wfsbp.org/fileadmin/user_upload/Treatment_Guidelines/Guidelines_Anxiety_revision.pdf

Dopheide JA, "Recognizing and Treating Depression in Children and Adolescents," *Am J Health Syst Pharm*, 2006, 63(3):233-43.

Elser JM and Woody RC, "Migraine Headache in the Infant and Young Child," *Headache*, 1990, 30(6):366-8.

Fortinguerra F, Clavenna A, and Bonati M, "Psychotropic Drug Use During Breastfeeding: A Review of the Evidence," *Pediatrics*, 2009, 124(4):547-56.

Hershey AD, Powers SW, Bentti AL, et al, "Effectiveness of Amitriptyline in the Prophylactic Management of Childhood Headaches," *Headache*, 2000, 40(7):539-49.

Kashani JH, Shekim WO, and Reid JC, "Amitriptyline in Children With Major Depressive Disorder: A Double-Blind Crossover Pilot Study," *J Am Acad Child Psychiatry*, 1984, 23(3):348-51.

Levy HB, Harper CR, and Weinberg WA, "A Practical Approach to Children Failing in School," *Pediatr Clin North Am*, 1992, 39 (4):895-928.

Pringsheim T, Davenport W, Mackie G, et al, "Canadian Headache Society Guideline for Migraine Prophylaxis," *Can J Neurol Sci*, 2012, 39(2 Suppl 2):S1-59.

Sorge F, Barone P, Steardo L, et al, "Amitriptyline as a Prophylactic for Migraine in Children," *Acta Neurol (Napoli)*, 1982, 4(5):362-7.

Wagner KD, "Pharmacotherapy for Major Depression in Children and Adolescents," *Prog Neuropsychopharmacol Biol Psychiatry*, 2005, 29 (5):819-26.

Yonkers KA, Wisner KL, Stewart DE, et al, "The Management of Depression During Pregnancy: A Report From the American Psychiatric Association and the American College of Obstetricians and Gynecologists," *Obstet Gynecol*, 2009, 114(3):703-13.

◆ **Amitriptyline Hydrochloride** *see* Amitriptyline *on page 133*

◆ **AmLactin® [OTC]** *see* Lactic Acid and Ammonium Hydroxide *on page 1191*

AmLODIPine (am LOE di peen)

Medication Safety Issues

Sound-alike/look-alike issues:

AmLODIPine may be confused with aMILoride

Norvasc may be confused with Navane, Norvir, Vascor

International issues:

Norvasc [U.S., Canada, and multiple international markets] may be confused with Vascor brand name for imidapril [Philippines] and simvastatin [Malaysia, Singapore, and Thailand]

Brand Names: U.S. Norvasc

Brand Names: Canada Accel-Amlodipine; Amlodipine-Odan; Apo-Amlodipine; Auro-Amlodipine; Bio-Amlodipine; CO Amlodipine; Dom-Amlodipine; GD-Amlodipine; JAMP-Amlodipine; Mar-Amlodipine; Mint-Amlodipine; Mylan-Amlodipine; Norvasc; PHL-Amlodipine; PMS-Amlodipine; Q-Amlodipine; RAN-Amlodipine; ratio-Amlodipine; Riva-Amlodipine; Sandoz Amlodipine; Septa-Amlodipine; Teva-Amlodipine; ZYM-Amlodipine

Therapeutic Category Antianginal Agent; Antihypertensive Agent; Calcium Channel Blocker; Calcium Channel Blocker, Dihydropyridine

Generic Availability (U.S.) Yes

Use Treatment of hypertension (FDA approved in ages ≥6 years and adults); chronic stable angina (FDA approved in adults); vasospastic (Prinzmetal's) angina (FDA approved in adults); angiographically documented CAD [to decrease risk of hospitalization (due to angina) and coronary revascularization procedure] (FDA approved in adults)

Pregnancy Risk Factor C

Pregnancy Considerations Adverse events were observed in some animal reproduction studies. Untreated chronic maternal hypertension is associated with adverse events in the fetus, infant, and mother. If treatment for hypertension during pregnancy is needed, other agents are preferred (ACOG, 2013).

Breast-Feeding Considerations It is not known if amlodipine is excreted into breast milk. The manufacturer recommends nursing be discontinued during treatment.

Contraindications Hypersensitivity to amlodipine or any component

Warnings May increase frequency, duration, and severity of angina or precipitate acute MI during initiation of therapy or dosage increase (particularly in patients with severe obstructive coronary artery disease)

Precautions Use with caution and reduce the dose in patients with hepatic impairment; titrate dose slowly in patients with severe hepatic impairment. Symptomatic hypotension may occur; use with caution in patients with severe aortic stenosis; acute hypotension may rarely occur

Adverse Reactions

Cardiovascular: Flushing (more common in females), palpitations, peripheral edema (more common in females)

Central nervous system: Dizziness, drowsiness, fatigue, male sexual disorder

Dermatologic: Pruritus, skin rash

Gastrointestinal: Abdominal pain, nausea

Neuromuscular & skeletal: Muscle cramps, weakness

Respiratory: Dyspnea, pulmonary edema

Rare but important or life-threatening: Acute interstitial nephritis, angioedema, anorexia, atrial fibrillation, bradycardia, cardiac arrhythmia, cholestasis, conjunctivitis, depersonalization, depression, diarrhea, difficulty in micturition, diplopia, dysphagia, epistaxis, erythema multiforme, erythematous rash, exfoliative dermatitis, eye pain, female sexual disorder, gingival hyperplasia, gynecomastia, hepatitis, hot flash, hyperglycemia, hypersensitivity angiitis, hypersensitivity reaction, hypoesthesia, increased serum transaminases, increased thirst, insomnia, jaundice, leukopenia, maculopapular rash, myalgia, nocturia, nonthrombocytopenic purpura, orthostatic hypotension, osteoarthritis, pain, pancreatitis, paresthesia, peripheral ischemia, peripheral neuropathy, phototoxicity, purpura, rigors, Stevens-Johnson syndrome, syncope, tachycardia, thrombocytopenia, tremor, urinary frequency, vasculitis, ventricular tachycardia, weight gain, weight loss

Drug Interactions

Metabolism/Transport Effects **Substrate** of CYP3A4 (major); **Note:** Assignment of Major/Minor substrate status based on clinically relevant drug interaction potential; **Inhibits** CYP1A2 (weak), CYP2A6 (weak), CYP2B6 (weak), CYP2C8 (weak), CYP2C9 (weak), CYP2D6 (weak), CYP3A4 (weak)

Avoid Concomitant Use

Avoid concomitant use of AmLODIPine with any of the following: Conivaptan; Fusidic Acid (Systemic); Pimozide

Increased Effect/Toxicity

AmLODIPine may increase the levels/effects of: Amifostine; Antihypertensives; ARIPiprazole; Atosiban; Beta-Blockers; Calcium Channel Blockers (Nondihydropyridine); Dofetilide; DULoxetine; Fosphenytoin; Hypotensive Agents; Lomitapide; Magnesium Salts; Neuromuscular-Blocking Agents (Nondepolarizing); Nitroprusside; Obinutuzumab; Phenytoin; Pimozide; QuiNIDine; RiTUXimab; Simvastatin; Tacrolimus (Systemic)

The levels/effects of AmLODIPine may be increased by: Alfuzosin; Alpha1-Blockers; Antifungal Agents (Azole Derivatives, Systemic); Barbiturates; Brimonidine (Topical); Calcium Channel Blockers (Nondihydropyridine); Ceritinib; Conivaptan; CycloSPORINE (Systemic); CYP3A4 Inhibitors (Moderate); CYP3A4 Inhibitors (Strong); Dasatinib; Diazoxide; Fluconazole; Fusidic Acid (Systemic); Grapefruit Juice; Herbs (Hypotensive Properties); Ivacaftor; Luliconazole; Macrolide Antibiotics; Magnesium Salts; MAO Inhibitors; Mifepristone; Pentoxifylline; Phosphodiesterase 5 Inhibitors; Prostacyclin Analogues; Protease Inhibitors; QuiNIDine; Simeprevir; Stiripentol

Decreased Effect

AmLODIPine may decrease the levels/effects of: Clopidogrel; QuiNIDine

The levels/effects of AmLODIPine may be decreased by: Barbiturates; Bosentan; Calcium Salts; CarBAMazepine; CYP3A4 Inducers (Strong); Dabrafenib; Deferasirox; Efavirenz; Herbs (Hypotensive Properties); Melatonin; Methylphenidate; Mitotane; Nafcillin; Rifamycin Derivatives; Siltuximab; St Johns Wort; Tocilizumab; Yohimbine

Food Interactions Grapefruit juice may modestly increase amlodipine levels. Management: Monitor closely with concurrent use.

Stability Store at room temperature of 15°C to 30°C (59°F to 86°F); dispense in tightly-closed, light-resistant container

Mechanism of Action Inhibits calcium ion from entering the "slow channels" or select voltage-sensitive areas of vascular smooth muscle and myocardium during depolarization, producing a relaxation of coronary vascular smooth muscle and coronary vasodilation; increases myocardial oxygen delivery in patients with vasospastic angina. Amlodipine directly acts on vascular smooth muscle to produce peripheral arterial vasodilation reducing peripheral vascular resistance and blood pressure.

Pharmacodynamics Antihypertensive effects: Duration: ≥24 hours with chronic daily dosing

Pharmacokinetics (Adult data unless noted)

Absorption: Oral: Well absorbed

Distribution: Distribution into breast milk is unknown

Mean V_d:

Children >6 years: Similar to adults on a mg per kg basis; **Note:** Weight-adjusted V_d in younger children (<6 years of age) may be greater than in older children (Flynn, 2006)

Adults: 21 L/kg

Protein binding: 93%

Metabolism: In the liver with 90% metabolized to inactive metabolites

Bioavailability: Oral: 64% to 90%

Half-life: Terminal: 30-50 hours

Time to peak serum concentrations: 6-12 hours

Elimination: 10% of parent drug and 60% of metabolites are excreted in the urine

Clearance: May be decreased in patients with hepatic insufficiency or moderate to severe heart failure; weight-adjusted clearance in children >6 years of age is similar to adults; **Note:** Weight-adjusted clearance in younger children (<6 years of age) may be greater than in older children (Flynn, 2006)

Dialysis: Not dialyzable

Dosing: Usual Oral:

Children: Hypertension: **Note:** For a summary of other pediatric studies see Additional Information

Children 1-5 years: Limited information exists in the literature. One population pharmacokinetic study found that children <6 years of age had weight-adjusted clearance and V_d of amlodipine that were significantly greater than children ≥6 years of age. This may suggest the need for higher mg/kg/day doses in younger children (<6 years of age); however, the study included only a small number of younger children (n=11) (Flynn, 2006). One retrospective pediatric study (n=55) that included only eight patients 1-6 years of age used initial doses of 0.05-0.1 mg/kg/day; doses were titrated upwards as needed; mean required dose was significantly higher in patients 1-6 years of age (0.3 ± 0.16 mg/kg/day) compared to older children (6-12 years: 0.16 ± 0.12 mg/kg/day; 12-20 years: 0.14 ± 0.1 mg/kg/day) (Flynn, 2000a). Further studies are needed.

Children 6-17 years: Manufacturer recommendations: 2.5-5 mg once daily; doses >5 mg daily have not been fully studied.

Note: Limited data exists in the literature. In the only randomized, placebo-controlled trial of amlodipine in children (n=268; mean age: 12.1 years; range: 6-16 years), a significant reduction in systolic blood pressure (compared to placebo) was observed in both the 2.5 mg once daily and the 5 mg once daily amlodipine groups. The authors recommend an initial dose of 0.06 mg/kg/day with a maximum dose of 0.34 mg/kg/day (not to exceed 10 mg/day) (Flynn, 2004).

Adults:

Hypertension: Initial: 2.5-5 mg once daily; use initial dose of 2.5 mg once daily in patients who are small or fragile, and when adding amlodipine to other antihypertensive therapy; in general, titrate dose over 7-14 days to fully assess effects; usual dose: 5 mg once daily; maximum dose: 10 mg once daily; usual dosage range (JNC 7): 2.5-10 mg once daily

Angina or CAD: 5-10 mg once daily; use lower dose for patients with hepatic impairment; most patients with CAD require 10 mg once daily

Dosing adjustment in renal impairment: Not needed; patients may receive the usual initial dose

Dosing adjustment in hepatic impairment: Adults: Angina: Initial: 5 mg once daily; Hypertension: Initial: 2.5 mg once daily

Administration Oral: May be administered without regard to food; use caution if administered with grapefruit juice

Monitoring Parameters Blood pressure, liver enzymes

Additional Information Summary of additional pediatric studies:

In one prospective study, 21 hypertensive children (mean age: 13.1 years; range: 6-17 years) received the following initial daily doses of amlodipine based on weight groups: Children <50 kg: 0.05 mg/kg/day; children 50-70 kg: 2.5 mg daily; children >70 kg: 5 mg daily; mean initial dose: 0.07 ± 0.04 mg/kg/day; doses were increased by 25% to 50% (rounded to the nearest 2.5 mg) every 5-7 days to a maximum of 0.5 mg/kg/day, as needed to control blood pressure; the mean required dose was almost twice as high for children <13 years of age (0.29 ± 0.13 mg/kg/day) compared to children ≥13 years of age (0.16 ± 0.11 mg/kg/day) (Tallian, 1999).

In a small randomized crossover trial, amlodipine was compared to nifedipine or felodipine in 11 hypertensive children (mean age: 16 years; range: 9-17 years); amlodipine was administered once daily as a liquid preparation (tablets dissolved in water immediately prior to administration); an initial daily dose of 0.1 mg/kg/day (maximum: 5 mg daily) was increased by 50% to 100% after 1 week to a maximum of 10 mg/day, as needed for blood pressure control; mean initial dose: 0.09 ± 0.01 mg/kg/day; mean required dose: 0.12 mg/kg/day (Rogan, 2000). A third prospective study used fixed mg doses, rather than dosing on a mg/kg basis (Pfammatter, 1998).

A prospective study in 43 pediatric outpatients with chronic kidney disease (median age: 9 years; range: 1-19 years) used the following initial daily doses of amlodipine based on weight groups: Children 10-30 kg: 2.5 mg once daily; children ≥31 kg: 5 mg once daily. Doses were increased if needed to a maximum of 0.5 mg/kg/day (20 mg/day). Younger patients required significantly higher mg/kg/day doses of amlodipine compared to older children. This relationship was not observed when the dose was expressed as mg/m²/day. The authors recommend a dose of 7-10 mg/m² given once daily (von Vigier, 2001).

Five retrospective studies used a variety of initial amlodipine doses ranging from 0.05-0.13 mg/kg/day; mean required dose after dosage titration for all aged pediatric patients) ranged from 0.15-0.23 mg/kg/day (Andersen, 2006; Flynn, 2000a; Khattak, 1998; Parker 2002; Silverstein, 1999). Two of these studies noted a relationship between dose and age, with younger patients requiring higher mg/kg/day doses. Several retrospective studies used twice daily dosing in younger children, but it is unknown whether this reflects altered pharmacokinetics or physician prescribing habits. One population pharmacokinetic study suggests there is no justification for twice-daily dosing of amlodipine children (Flynn, 2006). Further pediatric studies are needed.

Dosage Forms Excipient information presented when available (limited, particularly for generics); consult specific product labeling.

Tablet, Oral:
Norvasc: 2.5 mg, 5 mg, 10 mg
Generic: 2.5 mg, 5 mg, 10 mg

Extemporaneous Preparations A 1 mg/mL oral suspension may be made with tablets and either a 1:1 mixture of simple syrup and 1% methylcellulose or a 1:1 mixture of Ora-Plus® and Ora-Sweet®. Crush fifty 5 mg tablets in a mortar and reduce to a fine powder. Add small portions of the chosen vehicle and mix to a uniform paste; mix while adding the vehicle in incremental proportions to **almost** 250 mL; transfer to a calibrated bottle, rinse mortar with vehicle, and add quantity of vehicle sufficient to make 250 mL. Label "shake well" and "refrigerate". Stable for 56 days at room temperature or 91 days refrigerated.

Nahata MC, Morosco RS, and Hipple TF, "Stability of Amlodipine Besylate in Two Liquid Dosage Forms," *J Am Pharm Assoc (Wash)*, 1999, 39(3):375-7.

References

American College of Obstetricians and Gynecologists (ACOG), "ACOG Practice Bulletin No. 125: Chronic Hypertension in Pregnancy," *Obstet Gynecol*, 2012, 119(2 Pt 1):396-407.

Andersen J, Groshong T, and Tobias JD, "Preliminary Experience With Amlodipine in the Pediatric Population," *Am J Ther*, 2006, 13 (3):198-204.

Chobanian AV, Bakris GL, Black HR, et al, "The Seventh Report of the Joint National Committee on Prevention, Detection, Evaluation, and Treatment of High Blood Pressure: The JNC 7 report," *JAMA*, 2003, 289(19):2560-72.

Flynn JT and Pasko DA, "Calcium Channel Blockers: Pharmacology and Place in Therapy of Pediatric Hypertension," *Pediatr Nephrol*, 2000, 15(3-4):302-16.

Flynn JT, Nahata MC, Mahan JD Jr, et al, "Population Pharmacokinetics of Amlodipine in Hypertensive Children and Adolescents," *J Clin Pharmacol*, 2006, 46(8):905-16.

Flynn JT, Newburger JW, Daniels SR, et al, "A Randomized, Placebo-Controlled Trial of Amlodipine in Children With Hypertension," *J Pediatr*, 2004, 145(3):353-9.

Flynn JT, Smoyer WE, and Bunchman TE, "Treatment of Hypertensive Children With Amlodipine," *Am J Hypertens*, 2000a, 13(10):1061-6.

Josefsson M, Zackrisson AL, and Ahlner J, "Effect of Grapefruit Juice on the Pharmacokinetics of Amlodipine in Healthy Volunteers," *Eur J Clin Pharmacol*, 1996, 51(2):189-93.

Khattak S, Rogan JW, Saunders EF, et al, "Efficacy of Amlodipine in Pediatric Bone Marrow Transplant Patients," *Clin Pediatr (Phila)*, 1998, 37(1):31-5.

Meredith PA and Elliott HL, "Clinical Pharmacokinetics of Amlodipine," *Clin Pharmacokinet*, 1992, 22(1):22-31.

National High Blood Pressure Education Program Working Group on High Blood Pressure in Children and Adolescents, "The Fourth Report on the Diagnosis, Evaluation, and Treatment of High Blood Pressure in Children and Adolescents," *Pediatrics*, 2004, 114(2 Suppl 4th Report):555-76.

Parker ML, Robinson RF, and Nahata MC, "Amlodipine Therapy in Pediatric Patients With Hypertension," *J Am Pharm Assoc*, 2002, 42 (1):114-7.

Pfammatter JP, Clericetti-Affolter C, Truttmann AC, et al, "Amlodipine Once-Daily in Systemic Hypertension," *Eur J Pediatr*, 1998, 157 (8):618-21.

Rogan JW, Lyszkiewicz DA, Blowey D, et al, "A Randomized Prospective Crossover Trial of Amlodipine in Pediatric Hypertension," *Pediatr Nephrol*, 2000, 14(12):1083-7.

Silverstein DM, Palmer J, Baluarte HJ, et al, "Use of Calcium-Channel Blockers in Pediatric Renal Transplant Recipients," *Pediatr Transplant*, 1999, 3(4):288-92.

Tallian KB, Nahata MC, Turman MA, et al, "Efficacy of Amlodipine in Pediatric Patients With Hypertension," *Pediatr Nephrol*, 1999, 13 (4):304-10.

Vincent J, Harris SI, Foulds G, et al, "Lack of Effect of Grapefruit Juice on the Pharmacokinetics and Pharmacodynamics of Amlodipine," *Br J Clin Pharmacol*, 2000, 50(5):455-63.

von Vigier RO, Franscini LM, Bianda ND, et al, "Antihypertensive Efficacy of Amlodipine in Children With Chronic Kidney Diseases," *J Hum Hypertens*, 2001, 15(6):387-91.

◆ **Amlodipine Besylate** see AmLODIPine *on page 135*

◆ **Amlodipine-Odan (Can)** see AmLODIPine *on page 135*

◆ **Ammens® Original Medicated [OTC]** see Zinc Oxide *on page 2176*

◆ **Ammens® Shower Fresh [OTC]** see Zinc Oxide *on page 2176*

◆ **Ammonapse** see Sodium Phenylbutyrate *on page 1912*

Ammonium Chloride (a MOE nee um KLOR ide)

Therapeutic Category Metabolic Alkalosis Agent; Urinary Acidifying Agent

Generic Availability (U.S.) Yes

Use Diuretic or systemic and urinary acidifying agent; treatment of hypochloremia

Pregnancy Risk Factor C

Pregnancy Considerations Reproduction studies have not been conducted.

Contraindications Hypersensitivity to ammonium chloride or any component; severe hepatic and renal dysfunction; patients with primary respiratory acidosis

Warnings Monitor closely for signs and symptoms of ammonia toxicity, including diaphoresis, altered breathing, bradycardia, arrhythmias, retching, twitching, and coma.

Precautions Use with caution in patients with primary respiratory acidosis or pulmonary insufficiency.

Adverse Reactions
Central nervous system: Coma, drowsiness, EEG abnormalities, headache, mental confusion, seizure
Dermatologic: Rash
Endocrine & metabolic: Calcium-deficient tetany, hyperchloremia, hypokalemia, metabolic acidosis, potassium may be decreased, sodium may be decreased
Gastrointestinal: Abdominal pain, gastric irritation, nausea, vomiting
Hepatic: Ammonia may be increased
Local: Pain at site of injection
Neuromuscular & skeletal: Twitching
Respiratory: Hyperventilation

Drug Interactions
Metabolism/Transport Effects None known.
Avoid Concomitant Use There are no known interactions where it is recommended to avoid concomitant use.
Increased Effect/Toxicity
Ammonium Chloride may increase the levels/effects of: Salicylates

The levels/effects of Ammonium Chloride may be increased by: Potassium-Sparing Diuretics
Decreased Effect
Ammonium Chloride may decrease the levels/effects of: Alpha-/Beta-Agonists (Indirect-Acting); Amphetamines; Analgesics (Opioid)

Stability Store intact vials at 20°C to 25°C (68°F to 77°F).

Mechanism of Action Increases acidity by increasing free hydrogen ion concentration

Pharmacokinetics (Adult data unless noted)
Metabolism: In the liver
Elimination: In urine

Dosing: Usual
Infants, Children, and Adolescents:
Metabolic alkalosis: I.V.: **Note:** Ammonium chloride is an alternative treatment and should be used only after sodium and potassium chloride supplementation has been optimized. The following equations represent different methods of chloride or alkalosis correction utilizing either the serum Cl⁻, the serum HCO₃⁻, or the base excess. These equations will yield different requirements of ammonium chloride. Initially, administer 1/2 to 2/3 of the calculated dose, and then re-evaluate.
Dosing of mEq NH₄Cl via the chloride-deficit method (hypochloremia):
$$mEq\ NH_4Cl = 0.2\ L/kg \times wt\ in\ kg \times [103 - serum\ Cl^-]\ mEq/L$$
Dosing of mEq NH₄Cl via the bicarbonate-excess method (refractory hypochloremic metabolic alkalosis):
$$mEq\ NH_4Cl = 0.5\ L/kg \times wt\ in\ kg \times [serum\ HCO_3^- - 24]\ mEq/L$$

Dosing of mEq NH₄Cl via the base excess method:
$$mEq\ NH_4Cl = 0.3\ L/kg \times wt\ in\ kg \times base\ excess\ (mEq/L)$$
Urinary acidification: I.V.: 75 mg/kg/day in 4 divided doses; maximum daily dose: 6 g

Adults: **Metabolic alkalosis:** The following equations represent different methods of correction utilizing either the serum HCO₃⁻, the serum chloride, or the base excess; administer 50% of dose over 12 hours, then re-evaluate:
Dosing of mEq NH₄Cl via the chloride-deficit method (hypochloremia):
Dose of mEq NH₄Cl = [0.2 L/kg × body weight (kg)] × [103 - observed serum chloride; **Note:** 0.2 L/kg is the estimated chloride volume of distribution and 103 is the average normal serum chloride concentration (mEq/L)
Dosing of mEq NH₄Cl via the bicarbonate-excess method (refractory hypochloremic metabolic alkalosis):
Dose of NH₄Cl = [0.5 L/kg × body weight (kg)] × (observed serum HCO₃⁻ - 24); **Note:** 0.5 L/kg is the estimated bicarbonate volume of distribution and 24 is the average normal serum bicarbonate concentration (mEq/L)
These equations will yield different requirements of ammonium chloride.

Administration
Parenteral: Dilute to 0.2 mEq/mL and infuse I.V. over 3 hours; maximum concentration: 0.4 mEq/mL; maximum rate of infusion: 1 mEq/kg/hour

Monitoring Parameters Serum electrolytes, serum ammonia

Dosage Forms Excipient information presented when available (limited, particularly for generics); consult specific product labeling.
Injection, solution: Ammonium 5 mEq/mL and chloride 5 mEq/mL (20 mL) [equivalent to ammonium chloride 267.5 mg/mL]

◆ **Ammonium Hydroxide and Lactic Acid** *see* Lactic Acid and Ammonium Hydroxide *on page 1191*

◆ **Ammonium Lactate** *see* Lactic Acid and Ammonium Hydroxide *on page 1191*

◆ **Ammonul®** *see* Sodium Phenylacetate and Sodium Benzoate *on page 1911*

◆ **Amnesteem** *see* ISOtretinoin *on page 1161*

Amobarbital (am oh BAR bi tal)

Medication Safety Issues
BEERS Criteria medication:
This drug may be potentially inappropriate for use in geriatric patients (Quality of evidence - high; Strength of recommendation - strong).

Brand Names: U.S. Amytal Sodium

Brand Names: Canada Amytal®

Therapeutic Category Anticonvulsant, Barbiturate; Barbiturate; General Anesthetic; Hypnotic; Sedative

Generic Availability (U.S.) No

Use Hypnotic in short-term treatment of insomnia; to reduce anxiety and provide sedation preoperatively. Has been used as an alternative agent for treatment of refractory tonic-clonic seizures. See Additional Information for special uses.

Pregnancy Risk Factor D

Pregnancy Considerations Barbiturates cross the placenta and distribute in fetal tissue. Teratogenic effects have been reported with 1st trimester exposure. Exposure during the 3rd trimester may lead to symptoms of acute withdrawal following delivery; symptoms may be delayed up to 14 days.

Breast-Feeding Considerations Small amounts of barbiturates are excreted in breast milk; information specific for amobarbital is not available.

Contraindications Hypersensitivity to barbiturates or any component; marked hepatic impairment; dyspnea or airway obstruction; porphyria

Warnings Tolerance and/or psychological and physical dependence may occur; abrupt discontinuation after prolonged use may result in withdrawal symptoms or seizures; withdraw gradually if used over extended periods of time; use with caution in patients with depression or suicidal tendencies, or in patients with a history of drug abuse. When used as a hypnotic for the treatment of insomnia, effectiveness is limited to ≤2 weeks. Rapid I.V. administration may cause respiratory depression, apnea, laryngospasm, or hypotension. Solution for injection is highly alkaline and extravasation may cause local tissue damage. Necrosis may occur; avoid inadvertent intra-arterial injection (various reactions ranging from transient pain to gangrene of the limb may occur); stop injection if patient complains of pain in limb. May cause CNS depression, which may impair physical or mental abilities; patients must be cautioned about performing tasks which require mental alertness (eg, operating machinery or driving). Effects with other sedative drugs or ethanol may be potentiated.

Precautions Use with caution in patients with acute or chronic pain (paradoxical excitement may occur or important symptoms may be masked), hepatic dysfunction (decreased dosage may be needed; avoid use in patients with premonitory signs of hepatic coma), hypoadrenalism (effects of exogenous or endogenous corticosteroids may be decreased), pregnancy (fetal abnormalities may occur; infants may experience withdrawal symptoms with chronic maternal use), CHF, renal impairment (decreased dosage may be needed), hypovolemic shock, or in children (barbiturates may produce paradoxical excitement). Safety and efficacy have not been established in children <6 years of age.

Adverse Reactions Reported as barbiturate use (not specifically amobarbital).

Cardiovascular: Bradycardia, hypotension, syncope

Central nervous system: Agitation, anxiety, ataxia, confusion, CNS depression, dizziness, fever, hallucinations, headache, insomnia, nightmares, nervousness, psychiatric disturbances, somnolence, thinking abnormal

Gastrointestinal: Constipation, nausea, vomiting

Hematologic: Megaloblastic anemia (following chronic phenobarbital use)

Hepatic: Liver damage

Local: Injection site reaction

Neuromuscular & skeletal: Hyperkinesia

Respiratory: Apnea, atelectasis (postoperative), hypoventilation

Miscellaneous: Hypersensitivity reaction (including angioedema, rash, and exfoliative dermatitis)

Drug Interactions

Metabolism/Transport Effects Induces CYP2A6 (strong)

Avoid Concomitant Use

Avoid concomitant use of Amobarbital with any of the following: Azelastine (Nasal); Paraldehyde; Somatostatin Acetate; Thalidomide; Voriconazole

Increased Effect/Toxicity

Amobarbital may increase the levels/effects of: Alcohol (Ethyl); Azelastine (Nasal); Buprenorphine; CNS Depressants; Hydrocodone; Hypotensive Agents; Meperidine; Methotrimeprazine; Metyrosine; Mirtazapine; Paraldehyde; Pramipexole; ROPINIRole; Rotigotine; Selective Serotonin Reuptake Inhibitors; Thalidomide; Thiazide Diuretics; Zolpidem

The levels/effects of Amobarbital may be increased by: Brimonidine (Topical); Cannabis; Chloramphenicol; Doxylamine; Dronabinol; Droperidol; Felbamate; HydrOXYzine; Kava Kava; Magnesium Sulfate; Methotrimeprazine; Nabilone; Perampanel; Primidone; Rufinamide; Sodium Oxybate; Somatostatin Acetate; Tapentadol; Tetrahydrocannabinol; Valproic Acid and Derivatives

Decreased Effect

Amobarbital may decrease the levels/effects of: Acetaminophen; Beta-Blockers; Calcium Channel Blockers; Chloramphenicol; Contraceptives (Estrogens); Contraceptives (Progestins); Corticosteroids (Systemic); CycloSPORINE (Systemic); CYP2A6 Substrates; Doxycycline; Etoposide; Etoposide Phosphate; Felbamate; Griseofulvin; LamoTRIgine; Propafenone; Teniposide; Theophylline Derivatives; Tricyclic Antidepressants; Valproic Acid and Derivatives; Vitamin K Antagonists; Voriconazole

The levels/effects of Amobarbital may be decreased by: Multivitamins/Minerals (with ADEK, Folate, Iron); Pyridoxine; Rifamycin Derivatives

Stability Powder should be stored at 15°C to 30°C (59°F to 86°F). Reconstitute with SWI to make a 10% I.V. solution; a 20% solution may be made for I.M. use. Rotate vial to dissolve, do not shake. Do not use unless a clear solution forms within 5 minutes. Following reconstitution, solution should be used within 30 minutes.

Mechanism of Action Interferes with transmission of impulses from the thalamus to the cortex of the brain resulting in an imbalance in central inhibitory and facilitatory mechanisms

Pharmacodynamics

Onset of action: Rapid, within minutes

Maximum effect: Hours

Duration: Variable

Pharmacokinetics (Adult data unless noted)

Distribution: Readily crosses placenta; small amounts enter breast milk

Metabolism: Primarily hepatic via microsomal enzymes

Half-life: Adults: 15-40 hours (mean: 25 hours)

Elimination: Metabolites are eliminated in the urine and feces; negligible amounts excreted unchanged in urine

Dosing: Usual Note: Dosage should be individualized with consideration of patient's age, weight, and medical condition.

Children:

Sedative: I.M., I.V.: 6-12 years: Manufacturer's dosing range: 65-500 mg

Hypnotic: I.M., I.V.: 2-3 mg/kg/dose given before bedtime (maximum: 500 mg)

Adults:

Hypnotic: I.M., I.V.: 65-200 mg at bedtime (mean range: I.M.: 65-500 mg; maximum single dose: 1000 mg)

Sedative: I.M., I.V.: 30-50 mg 2-3 times/day

Dosing adjustment in renal/hepatic impairment: Dosing should be reduced; specific recommendations not available; drug is contraindicated in patients with marked hepatic impairment; avoid use in patients with premonitory signs of hepatic coma

Administration

I.M.: Administer deeply into a large muscle. Do not use more than 5 mL at any single site (may cause tissue damage)

I.V.: Use only when I.M. administration is not feasible. Administer by slow I.V. injection (maximum: 50 mg/minute in adults)

Monitoring Parameters Vital signs should be monitored during injection and for several hours after administration. If using I.V., monitor patency of I.V. access; extravasation may cause local tissue damage. Monitor hematologic, renal, and hepatic function with prolonged therapy.

◀

Reference Range
Therapeutic: 1-5 mcg/mL (SI: 4-22 µmol/L)
Toxic: >10 mcg/mL (SI: >44 µmol/L)
Lethal: >50 mcg/mL

Additional Information Amobarbital has also been used for therapeutic or diagnostic "amobarbital interviewing" (Kavirajan, 1999) and the "Wada test" (ie, intracarotid amobarbital procedure) to lateralize speech and memory functions prior to brain surgery, in order to prevent or predict the degree of impact of the surgery (Breier, 2001; Grote, 2005; Hamer, 2000; Szabo, 1993).

Controlled Substance C-II

Dosage Forms Excipient information presented when available (limited, particularly for generics); consult specific product labeling.
Solution Reconstituted, Injection, as sodium:
Amytal Sodium: 500 mg (1 ea)

References
Bengner T, Haettig H, Merschhemke M, et al, "Memory Assessment During the Intracarotid Amobarbital Procedure: Influence of Injection Order," *Neurology*, 2003, 61(11):1582-7.

Breier JI, Simos PG, Wheless JW, et al, "Language Dominance in Children as Determined by Magnetic Source Imaging and the Intracarotid Amobarbital Procedure: A Comparison," *J Child Neurol*, 2001, 16(2):124-30.

Grote CL and Meador K, "Has Amobarbital Expired? Considering the Future of the Wada," *Neurology*, 2005, 65(11):1692-3.

Hamer HM, Wyllie E, Stanford L, et al, "Risk Factors for Unsuccessful Testing During the Intracarotid Amobarbital Procedure in Preadolescent Children," *Epilepsia*, 2000, 41(5):554-63.

Kavirajan H, "The Amobarbital Interview Revisited: A Review of the Literature Since 1966," *Harv Rev Psychiatry*, 1999, 7(3):153-65.

Kim HS, Wan X, Mathers DA, et al, "Selective GABA-Receptor Actions of Amobarbital on Thalamic Neurons," *Br J Pharmacol*, 2004, 143 (4):485-94.

Redmond GP, Bell JJ, and Perel JM, "Effect of Human Growth Hormone on Amobarbital Metabolism in Children," *Clin Pharmacol Ther*, 1978, 24(2):213-8.

Szabó CA and Wyllie E, "Intracarotid Amobarbital Testing for Language and Memory Dominance in Children," *Epilepsy Res*, 1993, 15 (3):239-46.

◆ **Amobarbital Sodium** see Amobarbital on page 138

◆ **Amoclan** see Amoxicillin and Clavulanate on page 144

Amoxicillin (a moks i SIL in)

Medication Safety Issues
Sound-alike/look-alike issues:
Amoxicillin may be confused with amoxapine, Augmentin®
Amoxil may be confused with amoxapine
International issues:
Fisamox [Australia] may be confused with Fosamax brand name for alendronate [U.S., Canada, and multiple international markets] and Vigamox brand name for moxifloxacin [U.S., Canada, and multiple international markets]
Limoxin [Mexico] may be confused with Lanoxin brand name for digoxin [U.S., Canada, and multiple international markets]; Lincocin brand name for lincomycin [U.S., Canada, and multiple international markets]
Zimox: Brand name for amoxicillin [Italy], but also the brand name for carbidopa/levodopa [Greece]
Zimox [Italy] may be confused with Diamox which is the brand name for acetazolamide [Canada and multiple international markets]

Related Information
H. pylori Treatment in Pediatric Patients on page 2311
Oral Medications That Should Not Be Crushed or Altered on page 2438
Prevention of Infective Endocarditis on page 2336
Brand Names: U.S. Moxatag
Brand Names: Canada Apo-Amoxi®; Mylan-Amoxicillin; Novamoxin®; NTP-Amoxicillin; Nu-Amoxi; PHL-Amoxicillin; PMS-Amoxicillin; Pro-Amox-250; Pro-Amox-500

Therapeutic Category Antibiotic, Penicillin
Generic Availability (U.S.) May be product dependent
Use
Immediate Release preparations (oral suspension, chewable tablets, tablets, and capsules): Treatment of infections of ear, nose, skin, and soft tissue, genitourinary tract, or upper or lower respiratory tract due to susceptible (beta-lactamase negative) organisms including *H. influenzae*, *N. gonorrhoeae*, *E. coli*, *P. mirabilis*, *E. faecalis*, streptococci, and nonpenicillinase-producing staphylococci (FDA approved in all ages); treatment of gonorrhea (FDA approved in ages ≥2 years and adults); combination therapy of *Helicobacter pylori* (FDA approved in adults); has also been used for the treatment of Lyme disease, prophylaxis of bacterial endocarditis, prophylaxis in sickle cell or asplenic patients, and postexposure prophylaxis and treatment of anthrax
Extended release tablet (Moxatag®): Treatment of tonsillitis and/or pharyngitis secondary to *Streptococcus pyogenes* (FDA approved in ages ≥12 years and adults)

Pregnancy Risk Factor B
Pregnancy Considerations Adverse events have not been observed in animal reproduction studies. Maternal use of amoxicillin has generally not resulted in an increased risk of adverse fetal effects; however, an increased risk of cleft lip with cleft palate has been observed in some studies. It is the drug of choice for the treatment of chlamydial infections in pregnancy and for anthrax prophylaxis when penicillin susceptibility is documented. Amoxicillin may be used in certain situations prior to vaginal delivery in women at high risk for endocarditis.

Due to pregnancy-induced physiologic changes, oral amoxicillin clearance is increased during pregnancy resulting in lower concentrations and smaller AUCs. Oral ampicillin-class antibiotics are poorly absorbed during labor.

Breast-Feeding Considerations Very small amounts of amoxicillin are excreted in breast milk. The manufacturer recommends that caution be exercised when administering amoxicillin to nursing women. Nondose-related effects could include modification of bowel flora and allergic sensitization of the infant.

Contraindications Hypersensitivity to amoxicillin, penicillin, other beta-lactams, or any component

Warnings Serious and occasionally severe or fatal hypersensitivity (anaphylactoid) reactions have been reported in patients on penicillin therapy, especially with a history of beta-lactam hypersensitivity, history of sensitivity to multiple allergens, or previous IgE-mediated reactions (eg, anaphylaxis, angioedema, urticaria). Administration to patients with confirmed penicillin allergies should be avoided; in patients with confirmed cephalosporin allergy, consider skin testing to rule out cross-sensitivity to penicillins.

Epstein-Barr virus infection (infectious mononucleosis), acute lymphocytic leukemia, or cytomegalovirus infection increases risk for amoxicillin-induced maculopapular rash. Appearance of a rash should be carefully evaluated to differentiate a nonallergic amoxicillin rash from a hypersensitivity reaction. Amoxicillin rash occurs in 5% to 10% of children receiving amoxicillin and is a generalized dull, red, maculopapular rash, generally appearing 3-14 days after the start of therapy. It normally begins on the trunk and spreads over most of the body. It may be most intense at pressure areas, elbows, and knees. A high percentage (43% to 100%) of patients with infectious mononucleosis have developed rash during therapy; amoxicillin-class antibiotics are not recommended in these patients. Prolonged use may result in fungal or bacterial superinfection including *C. difficile*-associated diarrhea (CDAD); CDAD has been observed >2 months postantibiotic treatment.

Immediate release preparations are not interchangeable on a mg:mg basis with the extended release tablet. Some oral suspensions may contain sodium benzoate; benzoic acid (benzoate) is a metabolite of benzyl alcohol; large amounts of benzyl alcohol (≥99 mg/kg/day) have been associated with a potentially fatal toxicity ("gasping syndrome") in neonates; the "gasping syndrome" consists of metabolic acidosis, respiratory distress, gasping respirations, CNS dysfunction (including convulsions, intracranial hemorrhage), hypotension and cardiovascular collapse; avoid use of amoxicillin products containing sodium benzoate in neonates; *in vitro* and animal studies have shown that benzoate displaces bilirubin from protein binding sites

Precautions Use caution in renal impairment, dosage adjustment is required; avoid use of extended release 775 mg tablet and immediate release 875 mg tablet in patients with CrCl <30 mL/minute or patients requiring hemodialysis. Use with caution in patients with a history of colitis, cephalosporin allergy, or asthma. Chewable tablets contain aspartame which is metabolized to phenylalanine and must be used with caution in patients with phenylketonuria.

Adverse Reactions
Cardiovascular: Hypersensitivity angiitis
Central nervous system: Agitation, anxiety, behavioral changes, confusion, dizziness, headache, hyperactivity (reversible), insomnia, seizure
Dermatologic: Acute generalized exanthematous pustulosis, erythematous maculopapular rash, erythema multiforme, exfoliative dermatitis, Stevens-Johnson syndrome, toxic epidermal necrolysis, urticaria
Gastrointestinal: Dental discoloration (brown, yellow, or gray; rare), diarrhea, hemorrhagic colitis, melanoglossia, mucocutaneous candidiasis, nausea, pseudomembranous colitis, vomiting
Genitourinary: Crystalluria
Hematologic & oncologic: Agranulocytosis, anemia, eosinophilia, hemolytic anemia, leukopenia,thrombocytopenia, thrombocytopenia purpura
Hepatic: Cholestatic hepatitis, cholestatic jaundice, hepatitis (acute cytolytic), increased serum ALT, increased serum AST
Hypersensitivity: Anaphylaxis
Immunologic: Serum sickness-like reaction

Drug Interactions
Metabolism/Transport Effects None known.
Avoid Concomitant Use
Avoid concomitant use of Amoxicillin with any of the following: BCG; Probenecid
Increased Effect/Toxicity
Amoxicillin may increase the levels/effects of: Methotrexate; Vitamin K Antagonists

The levels/effects of Amoxicillin may be increased by: Allopurinol; Probenecid
Decreased Effect
Amoxicillin may decrease the levels/effects of: BCG; Mycophenolate; Sodium Picosulfate; Typhoid Vaccine

The levels/effects of Amoxicillin may be decreased by: Tetracycline Derivatives

Stability
Immediate release formulations (oral suspension, chewable tablets, tablets, capsules): Store at 20°C to 25°C (68°F to 77°F); dispense in a tight, light-resistant container; reconstituted suspensions are stable for 14 days at room temperature or refrigerated; refrigeration is preferred
Extended release tablets: Store at 25°C (77°F); excursions permitted to 15°C to 30°C (59°F to 86°F).

Mechanism of Action Inhibits bacterial cell wall synthesis by binding to one or more of the penicillin-binding proteins (PBPs) which in turn inhibits the final transpeptidation step of peptidoglycan synthesis in bacterial cell walls, thus inhibiting cell wall biosynthesis. Bacteria eventually lyse due to ongoing activity of cell wall autolytic enzymes (autolysins and murein hydrolases) while cell wall assembly is arrested.

Pharmacokinetics (Adult data unless noted)
Absorption: Oral: Rapid and nearly complete (74% to 92% of a single dose is absorbed)
  Extended-release tablet: Rate of absorption is slower compared to immediate-release formulation
Distribution: Into liver, lungs, prostate, muscle, middle ear effusions, maxillary sinus secretions, bone, gallbladder, bile, and into ascitic and synovial fluids
Protein binding: 17% to 20%, lower in neonates
Metabolism: Partially hepatic
Half-life:
  Neonates, full-term: 3.7 hours
  Infants and children: 1-2 hours
  Adults: Normal renal function: 0.7-1.4 hours
  Patients with CrCl <10 mL/minute: 7-21 hours
Time to peak serum concentration:
  Capsule: Within 2 hours
  Extended release: 3.1 hours
  Suspension: Neonates: 3-4.5 hours; children: 1 hour
Elimination: Renal excretion (60% unchanged drug)

Dosing: Neonatal
Note: All neonatal dosing recommendations based on immediate release product formulations (ie, oral suspension).
General dosing, susceptible infection: Oral: 20 to 30 mg/kg/day in divided doses every 12 hours
Otitis media, acute (AOM): Oral: 30 to 40 mg/kg/day in divided doses every 8 hours (Bradley, 2014)
UTI, prophylaxis (hydronephrosis, vesicoureteral reflux): Oral: 10 to 15 mg/kg once daily (Belarmino, 2006; Greenbaum, 2006; Matoo, 2007)

Dosing: Usual
Pediatric: **Note:** Unless otherwise specified, all pediatric dosing recommendations based on immediate release product formulations (oral suspension, chewable tablet, tablet, and capsule).
General dosing, susceptible infection: Oral:
  Mild to moderate infection:
    Infants ≤3 months:
      AAP recommendations (*Red Book*, 2012): 25 to 50 mg/kg/day in divided doses every 8 hours
      Manufacturer labeling: 20 to 30 mg/kg/day in divided doses every 12 hours
    Infants >3 months, Children, and Adolescents:
      AAP recommendations (*Red Book*, 2012): 25 to 50 mg/kg/day in divided doses every 8 hours; maximum dose: 500 mg/dose
      Manufacturer's labeling: 20 to 40 mg/kg/day in divided doses every 8 hours (maximum dose: 500 mg/dose) **or** 25 to 45 mg/kg/day in divided doses every 12 hours (maximum dose: 875 mg/dose)
  Severe infection (as step-down therapy): Infants, Children, and Adolescents: Oral: 80 to 100 mg/kg/day in divided doses every 8 hours; maximum dose: 500 mg/dose for most indications (*Red Book*, 2012)
Anthrax: Oral:
  Cutaneous, community-acquired or bioterrorism-related (Stevens, 2005):
    Children <20 kg: 40 mg/kg/day in divided doses every 8 hours for 5 to 9 days
    Children ≥20 kg: 500 mg every 8 hours for 5 to 9 days
  Inhalational, postexposure prophylaxis (ACIP recommendations): **Note:** Use only if *B. anthracis* isolate is susceptible to amoxicillin (MIC ≤0.125 mcg/mL). Continue therapy for 30 to ≥60 days depending on

vaccination status and for 14 days after the third vaccine dose (CDC, 2010); see Additional Information
Children <40 kg: Oral:
CDC recommendations: 45 mg/kg/day in divided doses every 8 hours; maximum dose: 500 mg/dose
AAP recommendations: 80 mg/kg/day in divided doses every 8 hours; maximum dose: 500 mg/dose. This higher dose is recommended due to the lack of data on lower amoxicillin dosages for treating anthrax and the high mortality rate (*Red Book*, 2012)
Children ≥40 kg: 500 mg every 8 hours

Endocarditis, prophylaxis: Infants, Children, and Adolescents: Oral: 50 mg/kg 1 hour before procedure; maximum dose: 2000 mg/dose (Wilson, 2007)

Lyme disease: Infants, Children, and Adolescents: Oral: 50 mg/kg/day in divided doses every 8 hours; maximum dose: 500 mg/dose (Halperin, 2007; Wormser, 2006)

Otitis media, acute (AOM): Infants ≥2 months and Children: Oral: 80 to 90 mg/kg/day in divided doses every 12 hours; some experts recommend initiating with 90 mg/kg/day (Bradley, 2014; Lieberthal, 2013; *Red Book*, 2012)

Peritonitis, prophylaxis (for patients receiving peritoneal dialysis who require dental procedures): Infants, Children, and Adolescents: Oral: 50 mg/kg administered 30 to 60 minutes before dental procedure; maximum dose: 2000 mg/dose (Warady, 2012)

Pneumonia, community-acquired: Infants ≥3 months, Children, and Adolescents: Oral: **Note:** In pediatric patients 5 to 15 years of age, a macrolide antibiotic may be a more reasonable first choice since *M. pneumoniae* is the chief cause of pneumonia in this age group (Bradley, 2011)
Empiric therapy for presumed bacterial pneumonia: 90 mg/kg/day in divided doses every 12 hours; maximum daily dose: 4000 mg/day
Group A *Streptococcus*: 50 to 75 mg/kg/day in divided doses every 12 hours; maximum daily dose: 4000 mg/day
Haemophilus influenza: 75 to 100 mg/kg/day in divided doses every 8 hours; maximum daily dose: 4000 mg/day
Streptococcus pneumonia (penicillin MIC ≤2 mcg/mL); mild infection or step-down therapy: 90 mg/kg/day in divided doses every 12 hours **or** 45 mg/kg/day in divided doses every 8 hours; maximum daily dose: 4000 mg/day

Pneumococcal infection prophylaxis for anatomic or functional asplenia [eg, sickle cell disease (SCD)] (Price, 2007; *Red Book*, 2012;): Oral:
Before 2 months of age (or as soon as SCD is diagnosed or asplenia occurs) through 5 years of age: 20 mg/kg/day in divided doses every 12 hours; maximum dose: 250 mg/dose
≥6 years: 250 mg every 12 hours; **Note:** The decision to discontinue penicillin prophylaxis after 5 years of age in children who have not experienced invasive pneumococcal infection and have received recommended pneumococcal immunizations is patient and clinician dependent.

Rhinosinusitis, acute bacterial; uncomplicated: Note: AAP guidelines recommend amoxicillin as first-line empiric therapy for pediatric patients 1 to 18 years with uncomplicated cases and where resistance is not suspected; however, the IDSA guidelines consider amoxicillin/clavulanate as the preferred therapy (Chow, 2012; Wald, 2013): Children and Adolescents: Oral:
Low dose: 45 mg/kg/day in divided doses every 12 hours
High dose (use reserved for select patients; see **Note**): 80 to 90 mg/kg/day in divided doses every 12 hours; maximum dose: 1000 mg/dose; **Note:** Should only be

used in the following: Mild to moderate infections in communities with a high prevalence of nonsusceptible *S. pneumoniae* resistance

Tonsillopharyngitis; Group A streptococcal infection, treatment and primary prevention of rheumatic fever: Oral:
Immediate release (oral suspension, chewable tablets, tablets, capsules): Children and Adolescents 3 to 18 years: 50 mg/kg once daily **or** 25 mg/kg twice daily for 10 days; maximum daily dose: 1000 mg/day (Gerber, 2009; Shulman, 2012)
Extended release tablets: Children ≥12 years and Adolescents: 775 mg once daily for 10 days; **Note:** Patient must be able to swallow tablet whole.

UTI, prophylaxis (hydronephrosis, vesicoureteral reflux): Oral: Infants ≤2 months: 10 to 15 mg/kg once daily; some suggest administration in the evening (drug resides in bladder longer); **Note:** Due to resistance, amoxicillin should not be used for prophylaxis after 2 months of age (Belarmino, 2006; Greenbaum, 2006; Mattoo, 2007).

Adults:
General dosing, susceptible infection: Oral: Immediate release: 250 to 500 mg every 8 hours **or** 500 to 875 mg tablets twice daily **or** extended release tablet 775 mg once daily

Chlamydial infection during pregnancy: Oral: 500 mg 3 times daily for 7 days (CDC, 2010)

Endocarditis prophylaxis: Oral: 2000 mg 30 to 60 minutes before procedure

***H. pylori* eradication:** Oral: 1000 mg twice daily for 14 days in combination with a proton pump inhibitor and at least one other antibiotic (clarithromycin)

Tonsillitis and/or pharyngitis: Oral: Extended release tablets: 775 mg once daily for 10 days

Dosing adjustment in renal impairment:
Infants, Children, and Adolescents: There are no dosage adjustments provided in the manufacturer's labeling; however, the following guidelines have been used by some clinicians (Aronoff, 2007): Oral:
Immediate release: Infants, Children, and Adolescents:
Mild to moderate infection: Dosing based on 25 to 50 mg/kg/day divided every 8 hours:
GFR >30 mL/minute/1.73 m^2: No adjustment required
GFR 10 to 29 mL/minute/1.73 m^2: 8 to 20 mg/kg/dose every 12 hours
GFR <10 mL/minute/1.73 m^2: 8 to 20 mg/kg/dose every 24 hours
Hemodialysis: Moderately dialyzable (20% to 50%); ~30% removed by 3-hour hemodialysis: 8 to 20 mg/kg/dose every 24 hours; give after dialysis
Peritoneal dialysis: 8 to 20 mg/kg/dose every 24 hours
Severe infection: Dosing based on 80 to 90 mg/kg/day divided every 12 hours:
GFR >30 mL/minute/1.73 m^2: No adjustment required
GFR 10 to 29 mL/minute/1.73 m^2: 20 mg/kg/dose every 12 hours; do not use the 875 mg tablet
GFR <10 mL/minute/1.73 m^2: 20 mg/kg/dose every 24 hours; do not use the 875 mg tablet
Hemodialysis: Moderately dialyzable (20% to 50%); ~30% removed by 3-hour hemodialysis: 20 mg/kg/dose every 24 hours; give after dialysis
Peritoneal dialysis: 20 mg/kg/dose every 24 hours
Extended release: Children ≥12 years and Adolescents: CrCl <30mL/minute: Do not use the 775 mg tablet
Adults: **Note:** The immediate release 875 mg tablet and the extended release 775 mg tablet should not be used in patients with a CrCl <30 mL/minute. Oral:
CrCl >30 mL/minute: No adjustment required.

CrCl 10-30 mL/minute: 250 to 500 mg every 12 hours depending on severity of infection

CrCl <10 mL/minute: 250 to 500 mg every 24 hours depending on severity of infection

Hemodialysis: Moderately dialyzable (20% to 50%); ~30% removed by 3-hour hemodialysis: Give dose after dialysis (Aronoff, 2007)

Peritoneal dialysis: 250 mg every 12 hours

Dosing adjustment in hepatic impairment: There are no dosage adjustments provided in the manufacturer's labeling.

Administration Oral:

Immediate release: May be administered on an empty or full stomach; may be mixed with formula, milk, cold drink, or juice; administer dose immediately after mixing; shake suspension well before use.

Extended release: Take within 1 hour of finishing a meal; do not chew or crush tablet.

Monitoring Parameters With prolonged therapy, monitor renal, hepatic, and hematologic function periodically; observe for change in bowel frequency; monitor for signs of anaphylaxis during first dose

Test Interactions May interfere with urinary glucose tests using cupric sulfate (Benedict's solution, Clinitest®)

Some penicillin derivatives may accelerate the degradation of aminoglycosides *in vitro*, leading to a potential underestimation of aminoglycoside serum concentration.

Additional Information Some penicillins (eg, carbenicillin, ticarcillin, and piperacillin) have been shown to inactivate aminoglycosides *in vitro*. This has been observed to a greater extent with tobramycin and gentamicin, while amikacin has shown greater stability against inactivation. Concurrent use of these agents may pose a risk of reduced antibacterial efficacy *in vivo*, particularly in the setting of profound renal impairment; however, definitive clinical evidence is lacking. If combination penicillin/aminoglycoside therapy is desired in a patient with renal dysfunction, separation of doses (if feasible), and routine monitoring of aminoglycoside levels, CBC, and clinical response should be considered.

Only use amoxicillin for postexposure inhalational anthrax prophylaxis if isolates of the specific *B. anthracis* are susceptible to amoxicillin (MIC ≤0.125 mcg/mL). Duration of antibiotic postexposure prophylaxis (PEP) is ≥60 days in a previously unvaccinated exposed person. Antimicrobial therapy should continue for 14 days after the third dose of PEP vaccine. Those who are partially or fully vaccinated should receive at least a 30-day course of antimicrobial PEP and continue with licensed vaccination regimen. Unvaccinated workers, even those wearing personal protective equipment with adequate respiratory protection, should receive antimicrobial PEP. Antimicrobial PEP is not required for fully vaccinated people (5-dose I.M. vaccination series with a yearly booster) who enter an anthrax area clothed in personal protective equipment. If respiratory protection is disrupted, a 30-day course of antimicrobial therapy is recommended (CDC, 2010).

Dosage Forms Excipient information presented when available (limited, particularly for generics); consult specific product labeling.

Capsule, Oral:

Generic: 250 mg, 500 mg

Suspension Reconstituted, Oral:

Generic: 125 mg/5 mL (80 mL, 100 mL, 150 mL); 200 mg/5 mL (50 mL, 75 mL, 100 mL); 250 mg/5 mL (80 mL, 100 mL, 150 mL); 400 mg/5 mL (50 mL, 75 mL, 100 mL)

Tablet, Oral:

Generic: 500 mg, 875 mg

Tablet Chewable, Oral:

Generic: 125 mg, 250 mg

Tablet Extended Release 24 Hour, Oral:

Moxatag: 775 mg [contains cremophor el, fd&c blue #2 aluminum lake]

References

American Academy of Pediatrics (AAP). In: Pickering LK, Baker CJ, Kimberlin DW, Long SS, eds. *Red Book: 2012 Report of the Committee on Infectious Diseases.* 29th ed. Elk Grove Village, IL: American Academy of Pediatrics; 2012.

Aronoff GR, Bennett WM, Berns JS, et al, *Drug Prescribing in Renal Failure: Dosing Guidelines for Adults and Children,* 5th ed. Philadelphia, PA: American College of Physicians; 2007.

Belarmino JM and Kogan BA, "Management of Neonatal Hydronephrosis," *Early Hum Dev,* 2006, 82(1):9-14.

Boguniewicz M and Leung DY, "Hypersensitivity Reactions to Antibiotics Commonly Used in Children," *Pediatr Infect Dis J,* 1995, 14 (3):221-31.

Bradley JS, Byington CL, Shah SS, et al, "The Management of Community-Acquired Pneumonia in Infants and Children Older Than 3 Months of Age: Clinical Practice Guidelines by the Pediatric Infectious Diseases Society and the Infectious Diseases Society of America", *Clin Infect Dis,* 2011, 53(7):e25-76.

Bradley JS, Nelson JD, Kimberlin DK, et al, eds. *Nelson's Pocket Book of Pediatric Antimicrobial Therapy.* 20th ed. Philadelphia, PA: Lippincott Williams & Wilkins; 2014.

Canafax DM, Yuan Z, Chonmaitree T, et al, "Amoxicillin Middle Ear Fluid Penetration and Pharmacokinetics in Children with Acute Otitis Media," *Pediatr Infect Dis J,* 1998, 17(2):149-56.

CDC and Johns Hopkins Working Group on Civilian Biodefense, "Commentary on Non-Labeled Dosing of Oral Amoxicillin in Adults and Pediatrics for Post-Exposure Inhalational Anthrax," December 10, 2001, http://www.fda.gov/cder/drugprepare/amox-anthrax.htm.

Centers for Disease Control and Prevention (CDC), "Use of Anthrax Vaccine in the United States. Recommendations of the Advisory Committee on Immunization Practices," *MMWR Recomm Rep,* 2010, 59(RR-6):1-30.

Chow AW, Benninger MS, Brook I, et al, "IDSA Clinical Practice Guideline for Acute Bacterial Rhinosinusitis in Children and Adults," *Clin Infect Dis,* 2012, 54(8):e72-112.

Dajani AS, Taubert KA, Wilson WW, et al, "Prevention of Bacterial Endocarditis. Recommendations by the American Heart Association," *JAMA,* 1997, 277(22):1794-1801.

Gerber MA, Baltimore RS, Eaton CB, et al, "Prevention of Rheumatic Fever and Diagnosis and Treatment of Acute *Streptococcal pharyngitis*: A Scientific Statement from the American Heart Association Rheumatic Fever, Endocarditis, and Kawasaki Disease Committee of the Council on Cardiovascular Disease in the Young, the Interdisciplinary Council on Functional Genomics and Translational Biology, and the Interdisciplinary Council on Quality of Care and Outcomes Research: Endorsed by the American Academy of Pediatrics," *Circulation,* 2009, 119(11):1541-51.

Greenbaum LA and Mesrobian HG, "Vesicoureteral Reflux," *Pediatr Clin North Am,* 2006, 53(3):413-27.

Halperin JJ, Shapiro ED, Logigian E, et al, "Practice Parameter: Treatment of Nervous System Lyme Disease (an Evidence-Based Review): Report of the Quality Standards Subcommittee of the American Academy of Neurology," *Neurology,* 2007, 69(1):91-102.

Lieberthal AS, Carroll AE, Chonmaitree T, et al, "The Diagnosis and Management of Acute Otitis Media," *Pediatrics,* 2013, 131(3): e964-99.

Mattoo TK, "Medical Management of Vesicoureteral Reflux - Quiz Within the Article. Don't Overlook Placebos," *Pediatr Nephrol,* 2007, 22(8):1113-20.

McIntosh K, "Community-Acquired Pneumonia in Children," *N Engl J Med,* 2002, 346(6):429-37.

Shulman ST, Bisno AL, Clegg HW, et al, "Clinical Practice Guideline for the Diagnosis and Management of Group A Streptococcal Pharyngitis: 2012 Update by the Infectious Diseases Society of America," *Clin Infect Dis,* 2012. Available at http://aapredbook.aappublications.org/cgi/content/full

Stevens DL, Bisno AL, Chambers HF, et al, "Practice Guidelines for the Diagnosis and Management of Skin and Soft-Tissue Infections," *Clin Infect Dis,* 2005, 41(10):1373-406.

Wald ER, Applegate KE, Bordley C, et al. Clinical practice guideline for the diagnosis and management of acute bacterial sinusitis in children aged 1-18 years. *Pediatrics.* 2013;132:e262.

Warady BA, Bakkaloglu S, Newland J, et al "Consensus Guidelines for the Prevention and Treatment of Catheter-Related Infections and Peritonitis in Pediatric Patients Receiving Peritoneal Dialysis: 2012 Update," *Perit Dial Int,* 2012, 32(Suppl 2):S32-86.

Wilson W, Taubert KA, Gewitz M, et al, "Prevention of Infective Endocarditis: Guidelines From the American Heart Association: A Guideline From the American Heart Association Rheumatic Fever, Endocarditis, and Kawasaki Disease Committee, Council on Cardiovascular Disease in the Young, and the Council on Clinical Cardiology, Council on Cardiovascular Surgery and Anesthesia, and the

Quality of Care and Outcomes Research Interdisciplinary Working Group," *Circulation*, 2007, 116(15):1736-54.

Wormser GP, Dattwyler RJ, Shapiro ED, et al, "The Clinical Assessment, Treatment, and Prevention of Lyme Disease, Human Granulocytic Anaplasmosis, and Babesiosis: Clinical Practice Guidelines by the Infectious Diseases Society of America," *Clin Infect Dis*, 2006, 43 (9):1089-134.

Amoxicillin and Clavulanate
(a moks i SIL in & klav yoo LAN ate)

Medication Safety Issues
Sound-alike/look-alike issues:
Augmentin may be confused with amoxicillin, Azulfidine
Related Information
Oral Medications That Should Not Be Crushed or Altered on page 2438
Brand Names: U.S. Amoclan; Augmentin; Augmentin ES-600; Augmentin XR
Brand Names: Canada Amoxi-Clav; Apo-Amoxi-Clav; Clavulin; Novo-Clavamoxin; ratio-Aclavulanate
Therapeutic Category Antibiotic, Beta-lactam and Beta-lactamase Combination; Antibiotic, Penicillin
Generic Availability (U.S.) Yes
Use Infections caused by susceptible organisms involving the lower respiratory tract, otitis media, sinusitis, skin and skin structure, and urinary tract; spectrum same as amoxicillin in addition to beta-lactamase producing *M. catarrhalis*, *H. influenzae*, *N. gonorrhoeae*, and *S. aureus* (excluding MRSA) (FDA approved in all ages)
Pregnancy Risk Factor B
Pregnancy Considerations Adverse events have not been observed in animal reproduction studies. Both amoxicillin and clavulanic acid cross the placenta. Maternal use of amoxicillin/clavulanate has generally not resulted in an increased risk of birth defects. A possible increased risk of necrotizing enterocolitis in neonates or bowel disorders in children exposed to amoxicillin/clavulanate *in utero* has been observed. In women with acute infections during pregnancy, amoxicillin/clavulanate may be given if an antibiotic is required and appropriate based on bacterial sensitivity; however, use is not recommended in the management of preterm premature rupture of membranes. Oral ampicillin-class antibiotics are poorly absorbed during labor. When used during pregnancy, pharmacokinetic changes have been observed with amoxicillin alone (refer to the Amoxicillin monograph for details).
Breast-Feeding Considerations Amoxicillin is found in breast milk. The manufacturer recommends that caution be used if administered to breast-feeding women. The use of amoxicillin/clavulanate may be safe while breast-feeding. However, the risk of adverse events in the infant may be increased when compared to the use of amoxicillin alone and the risk may be related to maternal dose. Nondose-related effects could include modification of bowel flora and allergic sensitization of the infant.
Contraindications Hypersensitivity to amoxicillin, clavulanic acid, other beta-lactam antibacterials (eg, penicillins, cephalosporins), or any component; history of amoxicillin/clavulanic acid-associated cholestatic jaundice or hepatic dysfunction
Warnings Serious and occasionally severe or fatal hypersensitivity (anaphylactoid) reactions have been reported in patients on penicillin therapy, especially with a history of beta-lactam hypersensitivity, history of sensitivity to multiple allergens, or previous IgE-mediated reactions (eg, anaphylaxis, angioedema, urticaria). Administration to patients with confirmed penicillin or cephalosporin allergies should be avoided. Epstein-Barr virus infection (infectious mononucleosis), acute lymphocytic leukemia, or cytomegalovirus infection increase risk for penicillin-induced maculopapular rash. Appearance of a rash should be carefully evaluated to differentiate a nonallergic ampicillin rash from

a hypersensitivity reaction; rash occurs in 5% to 10% of children and is a generalized dull red, maculopapular rash, generally appearing 3-14 days after the start of therapy. It normally begins on the trunk and spreads over most of the body. It may be most intense at pressure areas, elbows, and knees. A high percentage (43% to 100%) of patients with infectious mononucleosis have developed rash during therapy; ampicillin-class antibiotics are not recommended in these patients. Prolonged use may result in fungal or bacterial superinfection, including *C. difficile*-associated diarrhea (CDAD) and pseudomembranous colitis; CDAD has been observed >2 months postantibiotic treatment. Seizures have been reported with rapid I.V. administration (over <3 minutes).
Precautions Use with caution in patients with renal dysfunction; doses and/or frequency of administration should be modified in response to the degree of renal impairment. The chewable tablets and oral suspensions contain aspartame, which is metabolized to phenylalanine and must be avoided (or used with caution) in patients with phenylketonuria. May cause diarrhea; reported incidence (≤14.5%) is higher than with amoxicillin alone. Due to amoxicillin-clavulanic acid ratios, not all products are interchangeable; use of an inappropriate product for a specific dosage could result in either diarrhea (which may be severe) or subtherapeutic clavulanic acid concentrations leading to decreased clinical efficacy.
Adverse Reactions
Dermatologic: Diaper rash, skin rash, urticaria
Gastrointestinal: Abdominal distress, diarrhea, loose stools, nausea, vomiting
Genitourinary: Vaginitis
Infection: Candidiasis, vaginal mycosis
Rare but important or life-threatening: Cholestatic jaundice, flatulence, headache, hepatic insufficiency, hepatitis, increased liver enzymes, increased serum alkaline phosphatase, prolonged prothrombin time, thrombocythemia, vasculitis (hypersensitivity)
Additional adverse reactions seen with **ampicillin-class antibiotics:** Acute generalized exanthematous pustulosis, agitation, agranulocytosis, anaphylaxis, anemia, angioedema, anxiety, behavioral changes, confusion, convulsions, crystalluria, dental discoloration, dizziness, dyspepsia, enterocolitis, eosinophilia, erythema multiforme, exfoliative dermatitis, gastritis, glossitis, hematuria, hemolytic anemia, hemorrhagic colitis, hyperactivity, immune thrombocytopenia, increased serum bilirubin, increased serum transaminases, insomnia, interstitial nephritis, leukopenia, melanoglossia, mucocutaneous candidiasis, pruritus, pseudomembranous colitis, serum sickness-like reaction, Stevens-Johnson syndrome, stomatitis, thrombocytopenia, toxic epidermal necrolysis
Drug Interactions
Metabolism/Transport Effects None known.
Avoid Concomitant Use
Avoid concomitant use of Amoxicillin and Clavulanate with any of the following: BCG; Probenecid
Increased Effect/Toxicity
Amoxicillin and Clavulanate may increase the levels/effects of: Methotrexate; Vitamin K Antagonists

The levels/effects of Amoxicillin and Clavulanate may be increased by: Allopurinol; Probenecid
Decreased Effect
Amoxicillin and Clavulanate may decrease the levels/effects of: BCG; Mycophenolate; Sodium Picosulfate; Typhoid Vaccine

The levels/effects of Amoxicillin and Clavulanate may be decreased by: Tetracycline Derivatives
Stability Store tablets and dry powder at or below 25°C (77°F). Reconstituted oral suspension should be refrigerated; discard unused suspension after 10 days.

Mechanism of Action Clavulanic acid binds and inhibits beta-lactamases that inactivate amoxicillin resulting in amoxicillin having an expanded spectrum of activity. Amoxicillin inhibits bacterial cell wall synthesis by binding to one or more of the penicillin-binding proteins (PBPs) which in turn inhibits the final transpeptidation step of peptidoglycan synthesis in bacterial cell walls, thus inhibiting cell wall biosynthesis. Bacteria eventually lyse due to ongoing activity of cell wall autolytic enzymes (autolysins and murein hydrolases) while cell wall assembly is arrested.

Pharmacokinetics (Adult data unless noted)
Absorption: Both amoxicillin and clavulanate are well absorbed
Distribution: Both widely distributed into lungs, pleural, peritoneal, synovial, and ascitic fluid as well as bone, gynecologic tissue, and middle ear fluid
Protein binding:
Amoxicillin: 17% to 20%
Clavulanate: 25%
Metabolism: Clavulanic acid: Hepatically metabolized
Half-life of both agents in adults with normal renal function: ~1 hour; amoxicillin pharmacokinetics are not affected by clavulanic acid
Time to peak serum concentration: Within 2 hours
Elimination: Urine (amoxicillin 50% to 70% unchanged drug; clavulanic acid 25% to 40% unchanged drug)

Dosing: Neonatal Note: Dosing based on amoxicillin component; dose and frequency are product specific; not all products are interchangeable, using a product with the incorrect amoxicillin:clavulanate ratio could result in subtherapeutic clavulanate concentrations or severe diarrhea:
Oral: 30 mg amoxicillin component/kg/day divided every 12 hours using the 125 mg/5 mL suspension **only**

Dosing: Usual Note: Dosing based on amoxicillin component; dose and frequency are product specific; not all products are interchangeable; using a product with the incorrect amoxicillin:clavulanic acid ratio could result in subtherapeutic clavulanic acid concentrations or severe diarrhea.

Infants <3 months: **General dosing, susceptible infection:** Oral: 30 mg amoxicillin/kg/day in divided doses every 12 hours using the 125 mg/5 mL oral suspension **only**
Infants ≥3 months, Children, and Adolescents:
  General dosing, susceptible infection: Oral:
    AAP recommendation: Mild to moderate infection (*Red Book*, 2012)
      Twice daily dosing:
        25-45 mg amoxicillin/kg/day in divided doses twice daily using the 200 mg/5 mL or 400 mg/5 mL oral suspension, or the 200 mg or 400 mg **chewable** tablet formulation; maximum single dose: 875 mg amoxicillin
        High dose: 90 mg amoxicillin/kg/day in divided doses twice daily using the 600 mg/5 mL formulation; **Note:** This formulation should only be used for patients weighing <40 kg; reserve for recurrent infection or previous treatment failure.
      Three times daily dosing: 20-40 mg amoxicillin/kg/day in divided doses 3 times daily using 125 mg/5 mL or 250 mg/5 mL oral suspension or 500 mg tablet formulations; maximum single dose: 500 mg amoxicillin
    Manufacturer's labeling:
      Infants, Children, and Adolescents ≥3 months and <40 kg:
        Less severe infection:
          Twice daily dosing: 25 mg amoxicillin/kg/day in divided doses twice daily using the 200 mg/5 mL or 400 mg/5 mL oral suspension or the 200 mg or 400 mg **chewable** tablets; maximum single dose: 875 mg amoxicillin

          Three times daily dosing: 20 mg amoxicillin/kg/day in divided doses 3 times daily using the 125 mg/5 mL or 250 mg/5 mL oral suspension; maximum single dose: 500 mg amoxicillin
        Severe infection:
          Twice daily dosing: 45 mg amoxicillin/kg/day in divided doses twice daily using the 200 mg/5 mL or 400 mg/5 mL oral suspension or the 200 mg or 400 mg **chewable** tablets; maximum single dose: 875 mg amoxicillin
          Three times daily dosing: 40 mg amoxicillin/kg/day in divided doses 3 times daily using the 125 mg/5 mL or 250 mg/5 mL oral suspension; maximum single dose: 500 mg amoxicillin

Otitis media, acute: Infants ≥6 months and Children: Oral: 90 mg amoxicillin/kg/day in divided doses every 12 hours for 10 days using the 600 mg/5 mL oral suspension **only** in children with severe illness, who have received amoxicillin in the past 30 days, who have treatment failure at 48-72 hours on first-line therapy, and when coverage for β-lactamase positive *H. influenzae* and *M. catarrhalis* is needed (Lieberthal, 2013). **Note:** Per the manufacturer, the 600 mg/5 mL formulation should only be used for patients weighing <40 kg.

Pneumonia, community-acquired: beta-lactamase positive *H. influenzae* strains: Oral:
  Standard dose: 45 mg amoxicillin/kg/day in divided doses 3 times daily using the 125 mg/5 mL or 250 mg/5 mL oral suspension formulation; maximum single dose: 500 mg amoxicillin (Bradley, 2011)
  High dose: 90 mg amoxicillin/kg/day in divided doses 2 times daily (Bradley, 2011) using the 600 mg/5 mL oral suspension formulation. A wider dosing range of 80-100 mg/kg/day divided every 8 hours has also been used (Bradley, 2002). **Note:** Per the manufacturer, the 600 mg/5 mL formulation should only be used for patients weighing <40 kg.

Rhinosinusitis, acute bacterial: Oral:
  AAP recommendations (Wald, 2013): Children and Adolescents: High-dose (use reserved for select patients; see **Note**): 80-90 mg amoxicillin/kg/day divided every 12 hours, using the 600 mg/5 mL oral suspension **only**; treatment duration variable: 10-28 days, some have suggested discontinuation of therapy 7 days after resolution of signs and symptoms of infection. **Note:** Recommended for patients with any of the following: Moderate to severe infection, age <2 years, childcare attendance, or recent antibiotic treatment. Per the manufacturer, the 600 mg/5 mL formulation should only be used for patients weighing <40 kg.
  IDSA recommendations (Chow, 2012):
    Infants ≥3 months, Children, and Adolescents <40 kg:
      First-line therapy:
        Low dose: 45 mg amoxicillin/kg/day divided every 12 hours for 10-14 days using the 200 mg/5 mL or 400 mg/5 mL oral suspension, or the 200 mg and 400 mg **chewable** tablets formulations **only**
        High dose (use reserved for select patients; see **Note**): 90 mg amoxicillin/kg/day divided every 12 hours, using the 600 mg/5 mL oral suspension **only**; **Note:** Should only be used in the following: Areas with high endemic rates of penicillin-nonsusceptible *S. pneumoniae*, patients with severe infections, daycare attendance, age <2 years, recent hospitalization, antibiotic use within the past month, or patients who are immunocompromised
      Second-line therapy; if initial therapy fails: 90 mg amoxicillin/kg/day divided every 12 hours for 10-14 days using the 600 mg/5 mL oral suspension **only**

Children and Adolescents ≥40 kg:
First-line therapy:
Low dose: 500 mg every 8 hours using the 500 mg tablet **only or** 875 mg every 12 hours using the 875 mg tablet **only** for 5-7 days
High dose (use reserved for select patients; see **Note**): 2000 mg (two 1000 mg extended release tablets) every 12 hours; **Note:** Should only be used in the following: Areas with high endemic rates of penicillin-nonsusceptible S. pneumoniae, patients with severe infections, recent hospitalization, antibiotic use within the past month, or patients who are immunocompromised.
Second-line therapy if initial therapy fails: 2000 mg (two 1000 mg tablets **only**) every 12 hours for 10 days

Skin and soft tissue infections, impetigo: Oral: 25 mg amoxicillin/kg/day in divided doses twice daily using the 200 mg/5 mL or 400 mg/5 mL oral suspension or the 200 mg or 400 mg **chewable** tablets; maximum single dose: 875 mg amoxicillin (Stevens, 2005)

Streptococci, group A; chronic carrier treatment: Oral: 40 mg amoxicillin/kg/day in divided doses every 8 hours for 10 days using the 125 mg/5 mL or 250 mg/5 mL oral suspension or 500 mg tablet; maximum single dose: 500 mg amoxicillin (Shulman, 2012)

Urinary tract infections: Oral: Infants and Children 2-24 months: 20-40 mg/kg/day in divided doses 3 times daily using the 125 mg/5 mL or 250 mg/5 mL oral suspension; maximum single dose: 500 mg amoxicillin (AAP, 2011)

Adults:
General dosing, susceptible infection: Oral:
Less severe infection: 250 mg every 8 hours using the 250 mg tablet **only**; **or** 500 mg every 12 hours using the 500 mg tablet, 125 mg/5 mL suspension, or 250 mg/5 mL suspension **only**
More severe infections and respiratory tract infections: 500 mg every 8 hours using the 500 mg tablet, 125 mg/5 mL suspension, or 250 mg/5 mL suspension **only**; **or** 875 mg every 12 hours using the 875 mg tablet, 200 mg/5 mL suspension, or 400 mg/5 mL suspension **only**

Rhinosinusitis, acute bacterial: Oral:
Immediate release tablet: 500 mg every 8 hours using the 500 mg tablet or 875 mg every 12 hours using the 875 mg tablet for 5-7 days
Extended release tablet: 2000 mg (two 1000 mg tablets) every 12 hours for 10 days
Note: May use high-dose therapy (extended release: 2000 mg every 12 hours) if initial therapy fails, in areas with high endemic rates of penicillin-nonsusceptible S. pneumoniae, those with severe infections, age >65 years, recent hospitalization, antibiotic use within the past month, or who are immunocompromised (Chow, 2012).

Bite wounds (animal/human) or erysipelas: Oral: 875 mg every 12 hours using the 875 mg tablet, 200 mg/5 mL suspension, or 400 mg/5 mL suspension **only**; **or** 500 mg every 8 hours using the 500 mg tablet, 125 mg/5 mL suspension, or 250 mg/5 mL suspension **only**

Diabetic foot: Oral: 2000 mg every 12 hours for 7-14 days using the 1000 mg extended release tablet **only**

Febrile neutropenia: Oral: 875 mg every 12 hours using the 875 mg tablet, 200 mg/5 mL suspension, or 400 mg/5 mL suspension **only**

Pneumonia: Oral:
Aspiration: 875 mg every 12 hours using the 875 mg tablet, 200 mg/5 mL suspension, or 400 mg/5 mL suspension **only**
Community-acquired: 2000 mg every 12 hours for 7-10 days using the 1000 mg extended release tablet **only**

Pyelonephritis (acute, uncomplicated): Oral: 875 mg every 12 hours **or** 500 mg every 8 hours

Skin abscess: Oral: 875 mg every 12 hours using the 875 mg tablet, 200 mg/5 mL suspension, or 400 mg/5 mL suspension **only**

Streptococci, **group A, chronic carrier treatment** (IDSA guidelines): Oral: 40 mg/kg/day divided every 8 hours (maximum daily dose: 2000 mg/**day**) for 10 days (Shulman, 2012)

Dosing adjustment in renal impairment:
Infants, Children, and Adolescents: There are no dosage adjustments provided in the manufacturer's labeling; however, the following guidelines have been used by some clinicians (Aronoff, 2007): Oral:
Mild to moderate infection: Dosing based on 25-50 mg amoxicillin/kg/day divided every 8 hours:
GFR >30 mL/minute/1.73 m^2: No adjustment required
GFR 10-29 mL/minute/1.73 m^2: 8-20 amoxicillin/kg/dose every 12 hours
GFR <10 mL/minute/1.73 m^2: 8-20 amoxicillin/kg/dose every 24 hours
Hemodialysis: 8-20 mg amoxicillin/kg/dose every 24 hours; give after dialysis
Peritoneal dialysis: 8-20 mg amoxicillin/kg/dose every 24 hours
Severe infection: Dosing based on 80-90 mg amoxicillin/kg/day divided every 12 hours:
CrCl >30 mL/minute/1.73 m^2: No adjustment required
CrCl 10-29 mL/minute/1.73 m^2: 20 mg amoxicillin/kg/dose every 12 hours; do not use the 875 mg tablet
CrCl <10 mL/minute/1.73 m^2: 20 mg amoxicillin/kg/dose every 24 hours; do not use the 875 mg tablet
Hemodialysis: 20 mg amoxicillin/kg/dose every 24 hours; give after dialysis; do not use the 875 mg tablet
Peritoneal dialysis: 20 mg amoxicillin/kg/dose every 24 hours; do not use the 875 mg tablet
Adults:
CrCl ≥30 mL/minute: No adjustment required
CrCl <30 mL/minute: Do not use 875 mg tablet or extended release tablets
CrCl 10-30 mL/minute: 250-500 mg every 12 hours
CrCl <10 mL/minute: 250-500 mg every 24 hours
Hemodialysis: Moderately dialyzable (30%): 250-500 mg every 24 hours; administer an additional dose during and after dialysis. Do not use extended release tablets.
Peritoneal dialysis: Moderately dialyzable (20% to 50%):
Amoxicillin: Administer 250 mg every 12 hours
Clavulanic acid: Dose for CrCl <10 mL/minute

Dosing adjustment in hepatic impairment: There are no dosage adjustments provided in the manufacturer's labeling; use with caution. Use contraindicated in patients with a history of amoxicillin and clavulanate-associated hepatic dysfunction.

Administration Oral: Can be given without regard to meals. Administer at the start of a meal to decrease the frequency or severity of GI side effects; may mix with milk, formula, or juice; shake suspension well before use

Monitoring Parameters With prolonged therapy, monitor renal, hepatic, and hematologic function periodically; monitor for signs of anaphylaxis during first dose

Test Interactions May interfere with urinary glucose tests using cupric sulfate (Benedict's solution, Clinitest®, Fehling's solution).
Some penicillin derivatives may accelerate the degradation of aminoglycosides *in vitro*, leading to a potential underestimation of aminoglycoside serum concentration.

Additional Information Products may not be interchangeable. Both the 250 mg and 500 mg tablets contain the same amount of clavulanic acid; two 250 mg tablets are not equivalent to one 500 mg tablet. Additionally, four 250 mg tablets or two 500 mg tablets are not equivalent to a single 1000 mg extended release tablet. Based upon usual dosing in pediatric patients <40 kg, typical "TID" regimens provide 5-10 mg/kg/day of clavulanate and "BID" regimens 3.4-6.4 mg/kg/day.

Some penicillins (eg, carbenicillin, ticarcillin, piperacillin) have been shown to inactivate aminoglycosides *in vitro*. This has been observed to a greater extent with tobramycin and gentamicin, while amikacin has shown greater stability against inactivation. Concurrent use of these agents may pose a risk of reduced antibacterial efficacy *in vivo*, particularly in the setting of profound renal impairment. However, definitive clinical evidence is lacking. If combination penicillin/aminoglycoside therapy is desired in a patient with renal dysfunction, separation of doses (if feasible), and routine monitoring of aminoglycoside levels, CBC, and clinical response should be considered.

Dosage Forms Excipient information presented when available (limited, particularly for generics); consult specific product labeling. [DSC] = Discontinued product

Powder for suspension, oral:

Generic: 200: Amoxicillin 200 mg and clavulanate potassium 28.5 mg per 5 mL (50 mL, 75 mL, 100 mL); 250: Amoxicillin 250 mg and clavulanate potassium 62.5 mg per 5 mL (75 mL, 100 mL, 150 mL); 400: Amoxicillin 400 mg and clavulanate potassium 57 mg per 5 mL (50 mL, 75 mL, 100 mL); 600: Amoxicillin 600 mg and clavulanate potassium 42.9 mg per 5 mL (75 mL, 125 mL, 200 mL)

Amoclan:

200: Amoxicillin 200 mg and clavulanate potassium 28.5 mg per 5 mL (50 mL, 75 mL, 100 mL) [contains phenylalanine 7 mg/5 mL and potassium 0.14 mEq/5 mL; fruit flavor]

400: Amoxicillin 400 mg and clavulanate potassium 57 mg per 5 mL (50 mL, 75 mL, 100 mL) [contains phenylalanine 7 mg/5 mL and potassium 0.29 mEq/5 mL; fruit flavor]

600: Amoxicillin 600 mg and clavulanate potassium 42.9 mg per 5 mL (75 mL, 125 mL, 200 mL) [contains phenylalanine 7 mg/5 mL, potassium 0.248 mEq/5 mL; orange flavor]

Augmentin:

125: Amoxicillin 125 mg and clavulanate potassium 31.25 mg per 5 mL (75 mL, 100 mL, 150 mL) [contains potassium 0.16 mEq/5 mL; banana flavor]

200: Amoxicillin 200 mg and clavulanate potassium 28.5 mg per 5 mL (50 mL, 75 mL, 100 mL) [contains phenylalanine 7 mg/5 mL and potassium 0.14 mEq/5 mL; orange flavor] [DSC]

250: Amoxicillin 250 mg and clavulanate potassium 62.5 mg per 5 mL (75 mL, 100 mL, 150 mL) [contains potassium 0.32 mEq/5 mL; orange flavor]

400: Amoxicillin 400 mg and clavulanate potassium 57 mg per 5 mL (50 mL, 75 mL, 100 mL) [contains phenylalanine 7 mg/5 mL and potassium 0.29 mEq/5 mL; orange flavor] [DSC]

Augmentin ES-600:

600: Amoxicillin 600 mg and clavulanate potassium 42.9 mg per 5 mL (75 mL, 125 mL, 200 mL) [contains phenylalanine 7 mg/5 mL, potassium 0.23 mEq/5 mL; strawberry cream flavor]

Tablet, oral:

Generic: 250: Amoxicillin 250 mg and clavulanate potassium 125 mg; 500: Amoxicillin 500 mg and clavulanate potassium 125 mg; 875: Amoxicillin 875 mg and clavulanate potassium 125 mg

Augmentin:

250: Amoxicillin 250 mg and clavulanate potassium 125 mg [contains potassium 0.63 mEq/tablet] [DSC]

500: Amoxicillin 500 mg and clavulanate potassium 125 mg [contains potassium 0.63 mEq/tablet]

875: Amoxicillin 875 mg and clavulanate potassium 125 mg [contains potassium 0.63 mEq/tablet]

Tablet, chewable, oral:

Generic: 200: Amoxicillin 200 mg and clavulanate potassium 28.5 mg [contains phenylalanine]; 400: Amoxicillin 400 mg and clavulanate potassium 57 mg [contains phenylalanine]

Tablet, extended release, oral:

Generic: Amoxicillin 1000 mg and clavulanate acid 62.5 mg

Augmentin XR: 1000: Amoxicillin 1000 mg and clavulanate acid 62.5 mg [contains potassium 12.6 mg (0.32 mEq) and sodium 29.3 mg (1.27 mEq) per tablet; packaged in either a 7-day or 10-day package]

References

American Academy of Pediatrics, Subcommittee on Urinary Tract Infection, Steering Committee on Quality Improvement and Management, and Roberts KB, "Urinary Tract Infection: Clinical Practice Guideline for the Diagnosis and Management of the Initial UTI in Febrile Infants and Children 2 to 24 Months," *Pediatrics*, 2011, 128 (3):595-610.

Bradley JS, Byington CL, Shah SS, et al, "The Management of Community-Acquired Pneumonia in Infants and Children Older Than 3 Months of Age: Clinical Practice Guidelines by the Pediatric Infectious Diseases Society and the Infectious Diseases Society of America", *Clin Infect Dis*, 2011, 53(7):e25-76.

Bradley JS, "Management of Community-Acquired Pediatric Pneumonia in an Era of Increasing Antibiotic Resistance and Conjugate Vaccines," *Pediatr Infect Dis J*, 2002, 21(6):592-8.

Chow AW, Benninger MS, Brook I, et al, "IDSA Clinical Practice Guideline for Acute Bacterial Rhinosinusitis in Children and Adults," *Clin Infect Dis*, 2012, 54(8):e72-e112.

Lieberthal AS, Carroll AE, Chonmaitree T, et al, "The Diagnosis and Management of Acute Otitis Media," *Pediatrics*, 2013, 131(3): e964-99.

Reed MD, "Clinical Pharmacokinetics of Amoxicillin and Clavulanate," *Pediatr Infect Dis J*, 1996, 15(10):949-54.

Shulman ST, Bisno AL, Clegg HW, et al, "Clinical Practice Guideline for the Diagnosis and Management of Group A Streptococcal Pharyngitis: 2012 Update by the Infectious Diseases Society of America," *Clin Infect Dis*, 2012.

Todd PA and Benfield P, "Amoxicillin/Clavulanic Acid. An Update of Its Antibacterial Activity, Pharmacokinetic Properties and Therapeutic Use," *Drugs*, 1990, 39(2):264-307.

Wald ER, Applegate KE, Bordley C, et al. Clinical practice guideline for the diagnosis and management of acute bacterial sinusitis in children aged 1-18 years. *Pediatrics*. 2013;132:e262.

◆ **Amoxicillin and Clavulanate Potassium** *see* Amoxicillin and Clavulanate *on page 144*

◆ **Amoxicillin and Clavulanic Acid** *see* Amoxicillin and Clavulanate *on page 144*

◆ **Amoxicillin Trihydrate** *see* Amoxicillin *on page 140*

◆ **Amoxi-Clav (Can)** *see* Amoxicillin and Clavulanate *on page 144*

◆ **Amoxil** *see* Amoxicillin *on page 140*

◆ **Amoxycillin** *see* Amoxicillin *on page 140*

◆ **Amoxycillin and Clavulanate Potassium** *see* Amoxicillin and Clavulanate *on page 144*

◆ **Amoxycillin and Clavulanic Acid** *see* Amoxicillin and Clavulanate *on page 144*

◆ **Amphadase** *see* Hyaluronidase *on page 1020*

◆ **Amphetamine and Dextroamphetamine** *see* Dextroamphetamine and Amphetamine *on page 632*

◆ **Amphojel® (Can)** *see* Aluminum Hydroxide *on page 110*

Amphotericin B (Conventional)

(am foe TER i sin bee con VEN sha nal)

Medication Safety Issues

High alert medication:

The Institute for Safe Medication Practices (ISMP) includes this medication (intrathecal administration) among its list of drugs which have a heightened risk of causing significant patient harm when used in error.

Other safety concerns:

Conventional amphotericin formulations (Amphocin, Fungizone) may be confused with lipid-based formulations (AmBisome, Abelcet, Amphotec).

Large overdoses have occurred when conventional formulations were dispensed inadvertently for lipid-based products. Single daily doses of conventional amphotericin formulation never exceed 1.5 mg/kg.

Brand Names: Canada Fungizone

Therapeutic Category Antifungal Agent, Systemic; Antifungal Agent, Topical

Generic Availability (U.S.) Yes

Use Treatment of severe systemic infections and central nervous system infections caused by susceptible fungi, such as *Candida* species, *Histoplasma capsulatum*, *Cryptococcus neoformans*, *Aspergillus* species, *Blastomyces dermatitidis*, *Torulopsis glabrata*, and *Coccidioides immitis* [FDA approved in pediatric patients (age not specified) and adults]; has also been used for fungal peritonitis; irrigant for bladder fungal infections; used in fungal infection in patients with bone marrow transplantation, amebic meningoencephalitis, ocular aspergillosis (intraocular injection), and chemoprophylaxis (low-dose I.V.)

Pregnancy Risk Factor B

Pregnancy Considerations Adverse events were not observed in animal reproduction studies. Amphotericin crosses the placenta and enters the fetal circulation. No teratogenic or undue systemic toxicity (electrolyte imbalance or renal dysfunction) has been reported in the mother or fetus. Toxic maternal effects are to be expected and must be monitored (Perfect, 2010). Amphotericin B is recommended for the treatment of serious systemic fungal diseases in pregnant women. Refer to current guidelines (King, 1998).

Breast-Feeding Considerations It is not known if amphotericin is excreted into breast milk. Due to its poor oral absorption, systemic exposure to the nursing infant is expected to be decreased; however, because of the potential for toxicity, breast-feeding is not recommended (Mactal-Haaf, 2001).

Contraindications Hypersensitivity to amphotericin B or any component

Warnings Amphotericin I.V. is used primarily for the treatment of patients with progressive and potentially fatal fungal infections **[U.S. Boxed Warning]**; do not use for noninvasive forms of fungal disease. Verify the product name and dosage if dose exceeds 1.5 mg/kg **[U.S. Boxed Warning]**; overdosage may result in cardiorespiratory arrest. Anaphylaxis has been reported with amphotericin B-containing drugs; facilities for cardiopulmonary resuscitation should be available during administration due to the possibility of anaphylactic reaction. If severe respiratory distress occurs during administration, the infusion should be immediately discontinued; during the initial dosing, the drug should be administered under close clinical observation. Acute reactions (eg, fever, shaking chills, hypotension, anorexia, nausea, vomiting, headache, tachypnea) may occur 1-3 hours after starting an intravenous infusion. These reactions are usually more common with the first few doses and generally diminish with subsequent doses. May premedicate patients who experience mild adverse reactions with acetaminophen and diphenhydramine 30 minutes prior to the amphotericin B infusion; meperidine and ibuprofen may help to reduce fevers and chills; hydrocortisone can be added to the infusion solution to reduce febrile and other systemic reactions. If therapy is stopped for >7 days, restart at the lowest dose recommended and increase gradually. In adults, amphotericin B administration of daily dose by continuous I.V. infusion over 24 hours has shown fewer adverse effects and reduced incidence of nephrotoxicity (Eriksson, 2001; Imhof, 2003; Peleg, 2004).

Precautions Due to the nephrotoxic potential of amphotericin B, other nephrotoxic drugs should be avoided; hydration and sodium repletion prior to administration may reduce the risk of developing nephrotoxicity (Branch, 1988); frequent monitoring of renal function is recommended; use with caution in patients with renal impairment. In adults, patients experiencing moderate to severe nephrotoxicity during conventional amphotericin B treatment had three or more risk factors which included body weight ≥90 kg, male sex, mean daily amphotericin B dosage ≥35 mg, chronic kidney disease, or concomitant use of amikacin or cyclosporine (Harbath,1991).

Acute pulmonary reactions have been reported in patients simultaneously receiving intravenous amphotericin B and leukocyte transfusions; separate these infusions temporally as much as possible and monitor pulmonary function. Administer by slow I.V. infusion; rapid infusion has been associated with hypotension, hypokalemia, arrhythmias, and shock. Avoid extravasation; may cause chemical irritation; monitor infusion site; heparin 1 unit/1 mL of infusion solution can be added to reduce phlebitis. Use caution with intraperitoneal administration; use associated with irritation to the peritoneum and abdominal pain; not routinely used unless intolerance to other therapies (Warady, 2000).

Adverse Reactions

Systemic:

Cardiovascular: Flushing, hypertension, hypotension

Central nervous system: Arachnoiditis, chills, delirium, headache (less frequent with I.T), malaise, neuralgia (lumbar; especially with I.T. therapy), pain (less frequent with I.T), paresthesia (especially with I.T. therapy)

Endocrine & metabolic: Hypokalemia, hypomagnesemia

Gastrointestinal: Anorexia, diarrhea, epigastric pain, heartburn, nausea (less frequent with I.T), stomach cramps, vomiting (less frequent with I.T)

Genitourinary: Urinary retention

Hematologic & oncologic: Anemia (normochromic-normocytic), leukocytosis

Local: Pain at injection site (with or without phlebitis or thrombophlebitis [incidence may increase with peripheral infusion of admixtures])

Renal: Renal function abnormality (including azotemia, renal tubular acidosis, nephrocalcinosis [>0.1 mg/mL]), renal insufficiency

Respiratory: Tachypnea

Miscellaneous: Fever

Rare but important or life-threatening: Acute hepatic failure, agranulocytosis, anuria, blood coagulation disorder, bone marrow depression, bronchospasm, cardiac arrest, cardiac arrhythmia, cardiac failure, convulsions, diplopia, dyspnea, eosinophilia, exfoliation of skin, hearing loss, hemorrhagic gastroenteritis, hepatitis, hypersensitivity pneumonitis, increased liver enzymes, jaundice, leukoencephalopathy, leukopenia, maculopapular rash, melena, nephrogenic diabetes insipidus, oliguria, peripheral neuropathy, pruritus, pulmonary edema, renal failure, renal tubular acidosis, shock, Stevens-Johnson syndrome, thrombocytopenia, tinnitus, toxic epidermal necrolysis, ventricular fibrillation, vertigo (transient), visual disturbance, wheezing

Drug Interactions

Metabolism/Transport Effects None known.

Avoid Concomitant Use

Avoid concomitant use of Amphotericin B (Conventional) with any of the following: Saccharomyces boulardii

Increased Effect/Toxicity

Amphotericin B (Conventional) may increase the levels/effects of: Aminoglycosides; Colistimethate; CycloSPORINE (Systemic); Flucytosine

The levels/effects of Amphotericin B (Conventional) may be increased by: Corticosteroids (Orally Inhaled); Corticosteroids (Systemic)

Decreased Effect

Amphotericin B (Conventional) may decrease the levels/effects of: Saccharomyces boulardii

The levels/effects of Amphotericin B (Conventional) may be decreased by: Antifungal Agents (Azole Derivatives, Systemic)

Stability Store intact vials at 2°C to 8°C (36°F to 46°F). Protect from light. Reconstitute only with SWI without preservatives; do not use bacteriostatic water; benzyl alcohol, sodium chloride, or other electrolyte solutions may cause precipitation; reconstituted vials are stable protected from light for 24 hours at room temperature and 1 week refrigerated. Can be further diluted in D_5W, $D_{10}W$, up to $D_{20}W$, and protected from light; parenteral admixtures are stable for 24 hours at room temperature and 2 days under refrigeration; irrigating solutions should be diluted in sterile water. Short-term exposure (<24 hours) to light during I.V. infusion does **not** appreciably affect potency

Mechanism of Action Binds to ergosterol altering cell membrane permeability in susceptible fungi and causing leakage of cell components with subsequent cell death. Proposed mechanism suggests that amphotericin causes an oxidation-dependent stimulation of macrophages (Lyman, 1992).

Pharmacokinetics (Adult data unless noted)

Absorption: Poor oral absorption

Distribution: Minimal amounts enter the aqueous humor, bile, pericardial fluid, pleural fluid, and synovial fluid

CNS penetration:

Preterm neonates (GA: 27.4 ± 5 weeks): High interpatient variability; 40% to 90% of serum concentrations (Baley, 1990)

Adults: Poor

V_d: Pediatric patients (0-18 years): Highly variable; reported range: 0.38-3.99 L/kg (Benson, 1989; Koren, 1988)

Protein binding: 90%

Half-life:

Premature neonates (GA: 27.4 ± 5 weeks): 14.8 hours (range: 5-82 hours) (Baley, 1990)

Infants and Children (4 months to 14 years): 18.1 ± 6.6 hours (range: 11.9-40.3 hours) (Benson, 1989)

Adult:

Initial: 15-48 hours

Terminal phase: 15 days

Elimination: Urine (2% to 5% unchanged); ~40% eliminated over 7-day period and may be detected in urine for up to 8 weeks after discontinued use

Clearance (Benson, 1989):

Infants and Children (8 months to 9 years): 0.57 ± 0.152 mL/minute/kg

Children and Adolescents (10-14 years): 0.24 ± 0.02 mL/minute/kg

Dialysis: Poorly dialyzed

Dosing: Neonatal Medication errors, including deaths, have resulted from confusion between lipid-based forms of amphotericin (Abelcet®, Amphotec®, AmBisome®) and conventional amphotericin B for injection; conventional amphotericin B for injection doses should not exceed 1.5 mg/kg/day

General dosing, susceptible infections:

I.V.: **Note:** Maintaining a sodium intake of >4 mEq/kg/day in premature neonates may reduce amphotericin B-associated nephrotoxicity (Turcu, 2009)

Initial: 0.5 mg/kg/dose once daily. The daily dose can then be gradually increased, usually in 0.25 mg/kg increments on each subsequent day until the desired daily dose is reached; maximum daily dose: 1.5 mg/kg/**day**; in critically ill patients, more rapid dosage acceleration (up to 0.5 mg/kg increments on each subsequent day) may be warranted

Maintenance dose: 0.25-1 mg/kg/dose once daily; infuse over 2-6 hours; rapidly progressing disease may require short-term use of doses up to 1.5 mg/kg/**day**; once therapy has been established, amphotericin B can be administered on an every-other-day basis at 1-1.5 mg/kg/dose

Irrigation, bladder: Limited data available: 50 **mcg**/mL solution, administered as either a continuous irrigation or as an intermittent irrigation 3 times per day with a dwell time of 60-90 minutes; dosing based on two case reports in neonates [PNA at treatment: 3 weeks; 3 months (PCA: 42 weeks)] (Ku, 2004; Martinez-Pajares, 2010)

Intrathecal, intraventricular, or intracisternal (preferably into the lateral ventricles through a cisternal Ommaya reservoir): Limited data available; some dosing based on experience in older pediatric patients: 25-100 **mcg** every 48-72 hours; increase to 500 **mcg** as tolerated (Chiou, 1994; Murphy; 2000; Red Book, 2012)

Blastomycosis, **treatment:** I.V.: 1 mg/kg/dose once daily (Chapman, 2008)

Candidiasis:

Invasive, treatment: I.V.: 1 mg/kg/dose once daily for at least 3 weeks (Pappas, 2009)

Urinary tract infections, asymptomatic (high-risk patients); treatment: I.V.: 1 mg/kg/dose once daily (Pappas, 2009)

Urologic procedures; prophylaxis: I.V.: 0.3-0.6 mg/kg/dose once daily for several days before and after procedure (Pappas, 2009)

Dosing: Usual Medication errors, including deaths, have resulted from confusion between lipid-based forms of amphotericin (Abelcet®, Amphotec®, AmBisome®) and conventional amphotericin B for injection; conventional amphotericin B for injection doses should not exceed 1.5 mg/kg/day

Note: Premedication: For patients who experience infusion-related immediate reactions, premedicate with the following drugs 30-60 minutes prior to drug administration: NSAID (with or without diphenhydramine) **or** acetaminophen with diphenhydramine **or** hydrocortisone. If the patient experiences rigors during the infusion, meperidine may be administered.

Infants and Children:

Test dose: I.V.: 0.1 mg/kg/dose to a maximum of 1 mg; infuse over 20-60 minutes; an alternative method to the 0.1 mg/kg test dose is to initiate therapy with 0.25 mg/kg amphotericin administered over 6 hours; frequent observation of the patient and assessment of vital signs during the first several hours of the infusion is recommended; many clinicians believe a test dose is unnecessary

General dosing, susceptible infections:

I.V.:

Initial: 0.25-0.5 mg/kg/dose once daily; gradually increase daily, usually in 0.25 mg/kg increments until the desired daily dose is reached (maximum daily dose: 1.5 mg/kg/**day**); in critically ill patients, more rapid dosage acceleration may be warranted [eg, ≥0.5 mg/kg daily dose increase; others have initiated at target dose for life-threatening infection (DHHS [pediatric], 2013)

Maintenance dose: 0.25-1 mg/kg/dose once daily; rapidly progressing disease may require short-term use of doses to 1.5 mg/kg/**day**; once therapy has been established, amphotericin B may be administered on an every-other-day basis at 1-1.5 mg/kg/dose in some cases

Intrathecal, intraventricular, or intracisternal (preferably into the lateral ventricles through a cisternal Ommaya reservoir): Limited data available: 25-100 mcg every 72 hours; increase to 500 mcg as tolerated (Chiou, 1994; Murphy, 2000; *Red Book*, 2012)

Irrigation, bladder: Limited data available: 50 mcg/mL solution, administered as either a continuous irrigation or as an intermittent irrigation 3 times per day with a dwell time of 60-90 minutes (Fisher, 2011; Gubbins, 1999)

Aspergillosis:

Prophylaxis, immunocompromised: Limited data available: Intranasal: 7 mg amphotericin B in 7 mL sterile water was placed in a De Vilbiss atomizer and the aerosolized solution was instilled intranasally to each nostril 4 times daily delivering an average of 5 mg amphotericin/day to reduce the frequency of invasive aspergillosis in neutropenic patients (Jeffery, 1991)

Treatment, HIV-exposed/-positive: I.V.: 1-1.5 mg/kg/dose once daily for ≥12 weeks; duration should be individualized based upon clinical response (CDC, 2009)

Blastomycosis (independent of HIV status), moderately severe to severe disease:
I.V.: 0.7-1 mg/kg/dose once daily as initial therapy for 1-2 weeks, followed with oral itraconazole for a total of 12 months (Chapman, 2008)

Candidiasis; treatment:

Non-HIV-exposed/-positive (Pappas, 2009): I.V.:

Invasive: 0.5-1 mg/kg/dose once daily; duration of therapy dependent upon severity and site of infection

Urinary tract infections:

Prophylaxis, urologic procedures: 0.3-0.6 mg/kg daily for several days before and after procedure

Treatment:

Asymptomatic (high-risk patients): 1 mg/kg/dose once daily

Symptomatic: 0.3-0.6 mg/kg/dose once daily; duration for 1-7 days for symptomatic cystitis, 14 days for pyelonephritis

HIV-exposed/-positive: I.V.:

Invasive: 0.5-1.5 mg/kg/dose once daily; after fever resolution and stabilization, may decrease dose to 1.5 mg/kg once every other day; for candidemia, continue treatment for 2-3 weeks after last positive blood culture (CDC, 2009)

Esophageal: 0.3-0.7 mg/kg/dose once daily (DHHS [pediatric], 2013)

Oropharyngeal: 0.3-0.5 mg/kg/dose once daily (DHHS [pediatric], 2013)

Coccidioidomycosis:

Non-HIV-exposed/-positive (Galgiani, 2005):

Disseminated (non-CNS) disease: I.V. 0.5-1.5 mg/kg/dose every day or every other day; with or without concomitant azole antifungal; duration determined by clinical response

CNS disease: Intrathecal: 0.1-1.5 mg/dose; frequency ranging from daily to weekly (with or without concomitant azole therapy); initiate at a low dose and increase until intolerance (eg, severe vomiting, exhaustion, or transient dose-related mental status changes); duration determined by clinical response

Pulmonary disease, diffuse: I.V. 0.5-1.5 mg/kg/dose every day or every other day for several weeks, followed by an oral azole antifungal for a total length of therapy ≥12 months

HIV-exposed/-positive: Disseminated (non-CNS) disease, diffuse pulmonary disease; severely ill: I.V.: 0.5-1 mg/kg/dose once daily until clinical improvement; minimum of several weeks of therapy (DHHS [pediatric], 2013)

Cryptococcal disease:

CNS disease:

Non-HIV-exposed/-positive: I.V.: 0.7-1 mg/kg/dose once daily plus flucytosine; **Note:** Minimum 2-4-week induction, followed by consolidation and chronic suppressive therapy; may increase amphotericin dose to 1.5 mg/kg/day if flucytosine is not tolerated (Perfect, 2010)

HIV-exposed/-positive: I.V.: 1 mg/kg/day plus flucytosine or fluconazole; **Note:** Minimum 2-week induction, followed by consolidation and chronic suppressive therapy; a longer duration of induction therapy may be necessary if CSF is not negative or lack of clinical improvement; may increase amphotericin dose to 1.5 mg/kg/day alone or in combination with fluconazole if flucytosine is not tolerated (DHHS [pediatric], 2013)

Disseminated (non-CNS disease) or severe pulmonary disease: *Independent of HIV status:* I.V.: 0.7-1 mg/kg/dose once daily with or without flucytosine; duration of therapy depends on the site and severity of the infection and clinical response

Histoplasmosis:

Non-HIV-exposed/-positive: Severe disseminated (non-CNS) or pulmonary disease: I.V.: 0.7-1 mg/kg/dose once daily; **Note:** Minimum 1-2-week induction, followed by consolidation therapy (Wheat, 2007)

HIV-exposed/-positive: CNS or severe disseminated disease: I.V.: 0.7-1 mg/kg/dose once daily; **Note:** Conventional amphotericin B is an alternative therapy, lipid formulations are preferred (DHHS [pediatric], 2013)

Duration of induction:

Severe or moderately severe pulmonary disease: 1-2 week minimum

Disseminated or clinical improvement delayed: ≥2 weeks

CNS involvement: 4-6 weeks

Peritonitis (CAPD):

Intraperitoneal, dialysate: Children: 0.5-2 mg per liter of dialysate; either with or without low-dose I.V. amphotericin B therapy (Manley, 2000; Raajimakers, 2007; Warady, 2000)

I.V.: 1 mg/kg dose once daily (Warady, 2000)

Adolescents:

Test dose: I.V.: 0.1 mg/kg/dose to a maximum of 1 mg; infuse over 20-60 minutes; an alternative method to the 0.1 mg/kg test dose is to initiate therapy with 0.25 mg/kg amphotericin administered over 6 hours; frequent observation of the patient and assessment of vital signs during the first several hours of the infusion is recommended; many clinicians believe a test dose is unnecessary

General dosing, susceptible infections:

I.V.:

Initial: 0.25-0.5 mg/kg/dose once daily; gradually increase daily, usually in 0.25 mg/kg increments until the desired daily dose is reached (maximum daily dose: 1.5 mg/kg/**day**); in critically ill patients, more rapid dosage acceleration may be warranted (eg, ≥0.5 mg/kg daily dose increase)

Maintenance dose: 0.25-1 mg/kg/dose once daily; rapidly progressing disease may require short-term use of doses to 1.5 mg/kg/**day**; once therapy has been established, amphotericin B may be administered on an every-other-day basis at 1-1.5 mg/kg/dose in some cases

Intrathecal, intraventricular, or intracisternal (preferably into the lateral ventricles through a central Ommaya reservoir): Limited data available; some dosing based on experience in older pediatric patients: 25-100 **mcg** every 48-72 hours; increase to 500 **mcg** as tolerated (*Red Book*, 2012)

Irrigation, bladder: Limited data available: 50 **mcg**/mL solution, administered as either a continuous irrigation or as an intermittent irrigation administered 3 times per day with a dwell time of 60-90 minutes (Fisher, 2011; Gubbins, 1999)

Aspergillosis:

Prophylaxis; immunocompromised: Limited data available: Intranasal: 7 mg amphotericin B in 7 mL sterile water was placed in a De Vilbiss atomizer and the aerosolized solution was instilled intranasally to each nostril 4 times daily delivering an average of 5 mg amphotericin/**day** to reduce the frequency of invasive aspergillosis in neutropenic patients (Jeffery, 1991)

Treatment; HIV-exposed/-positive: I.V.: 1 mg/kg/dose once daily until CD4 count is >200 cells/mm[3] and evidence of clinical response (DHHS [adult], 2013)

Blastomycosis **(independant of HIV status), moder-ately severe to severe disease:** I.V.: 0.7-1 mg/kg/dose once daily as initial therapy for 1-2 weeks, followed with oral itraconazole for a total of 12 months (Chap-man, 2008)

Candidiasis:

Non-HIV-exposed/-positive (Pappas 2009):

Invasive: I.V.: 0.5-1 mg/kg/dose once daily; duration of therapy dependent upon severity and site of infection

Urinary tract infections:

Prophylaxis, urologic procedures: I.V.: 0.3-0.6 mg/kg daily for several days before and after procedure

Treatment:

Asymptomatic (high-risk patients): I.V.: 1 mg/kg/dose once daily

Symptomatic: I.V.: 0.3-0.6 mg/kg/dose once daily; duration for 1-7 days for symptomatic cystitis, 14 days for pyelonephritis

HIV-exposed/-positive (DHHS [adult], 2013):

Esophageal: I.V.: 0.6 mg/kg/dose once daily for 14-21 days

Oropharyngeal, refractory: I.V.: 0.6 mg/kg/dose once daily for at least 7-14 days; depending upon response, a longer duration may be required

Coccidioidomycosis:

Non-HIV-exposed/-positive (Galgiani, 2005):

Disseminated (non-CNS) disease: I.V.: 0.5-1.5 mg/kg/dose every day or every other day; with or without concomitant azole antifungal; duration determined by clinical response

CNS disease: Intrathecal: 0.1-1.5 mg/dose; frequency ranging from daily to weekly (with or without con-comitant azole therapy); initiate at a low dose and increase until intolerance is noted (eg, severe vomit-ing, exhaustion, or transient dose-related mental status changes); duration determined by clinical response

Pulmonary disease, diffuse: I.V.: 0.5-1.5 mg/kg/dose every day or every other day for several weeks, followed by an oral azole antifungal for a total length of therapy ≥12 months

HIV-exposed/-positive: Non-CNS disease: I.V.: 0.7-1 mg/kg/dose once daily until clinical improvement (DHHS [adult], 2013)

Cryptococcal disease (independent of HIV status):

CNS disease: I.V.: 0.7-1 mg/kg/dose once daily plus flucytosine or fluconazole; **Note:** Minimum 2-week induction, followed by consolidation and chronic sup-pressive therapy (DHHS [adult], 2013; Perfect, 2010)

Disseminated (non-CNS disease) or severe pulmonary disease: I.V.: 0.7-1 mg/kg/dose once daily with or

without flucytosine; duration of therapy depends on the site and severity of infection and clinical response (Perfect, 2010)

Histoplasma: *Non-HIV-exposed/-positive:* Severe disse-minated (non-CNS) or pulmonary disease: I.V.: 0.7-1 mg/kg/dose once daily; **Note:** Minimum 1-2-week induction, followed by consolidation therapy (Wheat, 2007)

Leishmaniasis, visceral (HIV-exposed/-positive): I.V.: 0.5-1 mg/kg/dose once daily for a total cumulative dose of 1500-2000 mg (DHHS [adult], 2013)

Peritonitis (CAPD):

Intraperitoneal, dialysate: 0.5-2 mg per liter of dialysate, either with or without low-dose I.V. amphotericin B therapy (Manley, 2000; Raajimakers, 2007; Warady, 2000)

I.V.: 1 mg/kg once daily (Warady, 2000)

Adults:

Test dose: I.V.: 1 mg infused over 20-30 minutes. Many clinicians believe a test dose is unnecessary.

Susceptible fungal infections: I.V.: 0.3-1.5 mg/kg/dose once daily; 1-1.5 mg/kg over 4-6 hours every other day may be given once therapy is established; aspergillosis, rhinocerebral mucormycosis, often require 1-1.5 mg/kg/day; maximum daily dose: 1.5 mg/kg/**day**

Peritoneal dialysis (PD): Administration in dialysate: 1-2 mg per liter of dialysate, either with or without low-dose I.V. amphotericin B (a total dose of 2-10 mg/kg given over 7-14 days). Precipitate may form in ionic dialysate solutions.

Dosing adjustment in renal impairment: Infants, Chil-dren, Adolescents, and Adults:

If renal dysfunction is due to the drug, the daily total can be decreased by 50% or the dose can be given every other day. I.V. therapy may take several months.

Renal replacement therapy: Poorly dialyzed; no supple-mental dose or dosage adjustment necessary, including patients on intermittent hemodialysis or CRRT.

Dosing adjustment in hepatic impairment: There are no dosage adjustments provided in the manufacturer's labeling.

Administration

Intrathecal: Dilute dose in 0.5-2 mL of D$_5$W; use only preservative-free ingredients (Klaus, 1989)

Parenteral: Amphotericin B is administered by I.V. infusion over 2-6 hours; infuse at a final concentration not to exceed 0.1 mg/mL through a peripheral venous catheter; in patients unable to tolerate a large fluid volume, ampho-tericin B at a final concentration not to exceed 0.5 mg/mL in D$_5$W or D$_{10}$W may be administered through a central venous catheter; an in-line filter (>1 micron mean pore diameter) may be used for administration (Kintzel, 1992).

Monitoring Parameters Renal function (monitor fre-quently during therapy: Every other day during dose increases and at least weekly, thereafter), electrolytes (especially potassium and magnesium), liver function tests, temperature, PT/PTT, CBC; monitor input and out-put; monitor for signs of hypokalemia (muscle weakness, cramping, drowsiness, ECG changes, etc); blood pres-sure, temperature, pulse, respiration, I.V. site

Dosage Forms Excipient information presented when available (limited, particularly for generics); consult specific product labeling.

Solution Reconstituted, Injection, as desoxycholate:

Generic: 50 mg (1 ea)

References

American Academy of Pediatrics (AAP). In: Pickering LK, Baker CJ, Kimberlin DW, Long SS, eds. *Red Book: 2012 Report of the Commit-tee on Infectious Diseases.* 29th ed. Elk Grove Village, IL: American Academy of Pediatrics; 2012.

Baley JE, Meyers C, Kliegman RM, et al, "Pharmacokinetics, Outcome of Treatment, and Toxic Effects of Amphotericin B and 5-Fluorocyto-sine in Neonates," *J Pediatr,* 1990, 116(5):791-7.

Benson JM and Nahata MC, "Pharmacokinetics of Amphotericin B in Children," *Antimicrob Agents Chemother*, 1989, 33(11):1989-93.

Branch RA, "Prevention of Amphotericin B-Induced Renal Impairment. A Review on the Use of Sodium Supplementation," *Arch Intern Med*, 1988, 148(11):2389-94.

Centers for Disease Control and Prevention (CDC), "Guidelines for the Prevention and Treatment of Opportunistic Infections Among HIV-Exposed and HIV-Infected Children: Recommendations From CDC, the National Institutes of Health, the HIV Medicine Association of the Infectious Diseases Society of America, the Pediatric Infectious Diseases Society, and the American Academy of Pediatrics," *MMWR Recomm Rep*, 2009, 58(RR-11):1-166.

Chapman SW, Dismukes WE, Proia LA, et al, "Clinical Practice Guidelines for the Management of Blastomycosis: 2008 Update by the Infectious Diseases Society of America," *Clin Infect Dis*, 2008, 46 (12):1801-12.

Chiou CC, Wong TT, Lin HH, et al, "Fungal Infection of Ventriculoperitoneal Shunts in Children," *Clin Infect Dis*, 1994, 19(6):1049-53.

DHHS. Guidelines for the prevention and treatment of opportunistic infections among HIV-exposed and HIV-infected children: recommendations from the National Institutes of Health, Centers for Disease Control and Prevention, the HIV Medicine Association of the Infectious Diseases Society of America, the Pediatric Infectious Diseases Society, and the American Academy of Pediatrics. November 6, 2013. Available at http://aidsinfo.nih.gov

DHHS Panel on Opportunistic Infections (OI) in HIV-Infected Adults and Adolescents, "Guidelines for Prevention and Treatment of Opportunistic Infections in HIV-Infected Adults and Adolescents: Recommendations from the Centers for Disease Control and Prevention (CDC), the National Institutes of Health (NIH), and the HIV Medicine Association (HIVMA) of the Infectious Diseases Society of America (IDSA)," May 7, 2013. Available at http://aidsinfo.nih.gov/contentfiles/lvguidelines/adult_oi.pdf

Eriksson U, Seifert B, and Schaffner A, "Comparison of Effects of Amphotericin B Deoxycholate Infused Over 4 or 24 Hours: Randomised Controlled Trial," *BMJ*, 2001, 322(7286):579-82.

Fisher JF, Sobel JD, Kauffman CA, et al, "Candida Urinary Tract Infections-Treatment," *Clin Infect Dis*, 2011, 52(Suppl 6):S457-66.

Galgiani JN, Ampel NM, Blair JE, et al, "Coccidioidomycosis," *Clin Infect Dis*, 2005, 41(9):1217-23.

Gubbins PO, McConnell SA, and Penzak SR, "Current Management of Funguria," *Am J Health Syst Pharm*, 1999, 56(19):1929-35.

Harbarth S, Pestotnik SL, Lloyd JF, et al, "The Epidemiology of Nephrotoxicity Associated With Conventional Amphotericin B Therapy," *Am J Med*, 2001, 111(7):528-34.

Imhof A, Walter RB, and Schaffner A, "Continuous Infusion of Escalated Doses of Amphotericin B Deoxycholate: An Open-Label Observational Study," *Clin Infect Dis*, 2003, 36(8):943-51.

Jeffery GM, Beard ME, Ikram RB, et al, "Intranasal Amphotericin B Reduces the Frequency of Invasive Aspergillosis in Neutropenic Patients," *Am J Med*, 1991, 90(6):685-92.

King CT, Rogers PD, Cleary JD, et al, "Antifungal Therapy During Pregnancy," *Clin Infect Dis*, 1998, 27(5):1151-60.

Kintzel PE and Smith GH, "Practical Guidelines for Preparing and Administering Amphotericin B," *Am J Hosp Pharm*, 1992, 49 (5):1156-64.

Klaus JR, Knodel LC, and Kavanagh RE, "Administration Guidelines for Parenteral Drug Therapy. Part I: Pediatric Patients," *J Pharm Technol*, 1989, 5(3):101-28.

Koren G, Lau A, Klein J, et al, "Pharmacokinetics and Adverse Effects of Amphotericin B in Infants and Children," *J Pediatr*, 1988, 113 (3):559-63.

Ku JH, Kim ME, Jeon YS, et al, "Urinary Ascites and Anuria Caused by Bilateral Fungal Balls in a Premature Infant," *Arch Dis Child Fetal Neonatal Ed*, 2004, 89(1):F92-3.

Mactal-Haaf C, Hoffman M, and Kuchta A, "Use of Anti-infective Agents During Lactation, Part 3: Antivirals, Antifungals, and Urinary Antiseptics," *J Hum Lact*, 2001, 17(2):160-6.

Manley HJ, Grabe DW, Norcross M, et al, "Stability of Amphotericin B-Lipid Complex (Abelcet) in Peritoneal Dialysis Solutions," *Perit Dial Int*, 2000, 20(1):87-90.

Martinez-Pajares JD, Martinez-Ferriz MC, Moreno-Perez D, et al, "Management of Obstructive Renal Failure Caused by Bilateral Renal Aspergilloma in an Immunocompetent Newborn," *J Med Microbiol*, 2010, 59(Pt 3):367-9.

Murphy K, Bradley J, and James HE, "The Treatment of *Candida albicans* Shunt Infections," *Childs Nerv Syst*, 2000, 16(1):4-7.

Pappas PG, Kauffman CA, Andes D, et al, "Clinical Practice Guidelines for the Management of Candidiasis: 2009 Update by the Infectious Diseases Society of America," *Clin Infect Dis*, 2009, 48(5):503-35.

Pappas PG, Chetchotisakd P, Larsen RA, et al, "A Phase II Randomized Trial of Amphotericin B Alone or Combined With Fluconazole in the Treatment of HIV-Associated Cryptococcal Meningitis," *Clin Infect Dis*, 2009, 48(12):1775-83.

Peleg AY and Woods ML, "Continuous and 4 h Infusion of Amphotericin B: A Comparative Study Involving High-Risk Haematology Patients," *J Antimicrob Chemother*, 2004, 54(4):803-8.

Perfect JR, Dismukes WE, Dromer F, et al, "Clinical Practice Guidelines for the Management of Cryptococcal Disease: 2010 Update by the Infectious Diseases Society of America," *Clin Infect Dis*, 2010, 50 (3):291-322.

Raaijmakers R, Schröder C, Monnens L, et al, "Fungal Peritonitis in Children on Peritoneal Dialysis," *Pediatr Nephrol*, 2007, 22(2):288-93.

Turcu R, Patterson MJ, and Omar S, "Influence of Sodium Intake on Amphotericin B-Induced Nephrotoxicity Among Extremely Premature Infants," *Pediatr Nephrol*, 2009, 24(3):497-505.

Warady BA, Schaefer F, Holloway M, et al, "Consensus Guidelines for the Treatment of Peritonitis in Patients Receiving Peritoneal Dialysis," *Perit Dial Int*, 2000, 20(6):610-24.

Wheat LJ, Freifeld AG, Kleiman MB, et al, "Clinical Practice Guidelines for the Management of Patients With Histoplasmosis: 2007 Update by the Infectious Diseases Society of America," *Clin Infect Dis*, 2007, 45 (7):807-25.

◆ **Amphotericin B Deoxycholate** *see* Amphotericin B (Conventional) *on page 147*

◆ **Amphotericin B Desoxycholate** *see* Amphotericin B (Conventional) *on page 147*

Amphotericin B (Lipid Complex)
(am foe TER i sin bee LIP id KOM pleks)

Medication Safety Issues

High alert medication:

The Institute for Safe Medication Practices (ISMP) includes this medication among its list of drugs which have a heightened risk of causing significant patient harm when used in error.

Other safety concerns:

Lipid-based amphotericin formulations (Abelcet®) may be confused with conventional formulations (Fungizone®) or with other lipid-based amphotericin formulations (amphotericin B liposomal [AmBisome®]; amphotericin B cholesteryl sulfate complex [Amphotec®])

Large overdoses have occurred when conventional formulations were dispensed inadvertently for lipid-based products. Single daily doses of conventional amphotericin formulation never exceed 1.5 mg/kg.

Brand Names: U.S. Abelcet

Brand Names: Canada Abelcet®

Therapeutic Category Antifungal Agent, Systemic

Generic Availability (U.S.) No

Use Treatment of invasive fungal infections in patients who are refractory to or intolerant of conventional amphotericin B therapy (FDA approved in children and adults)

Pregnancy Risk Factor B

Pregnancy Considerations Adverse events were not observed in animal reproduction studies. Amphotericin crosses the placenta and enters the fetal circulation. Amphotericin B is recommended for the treatment of serious, systemic fungal diseases in pregnant women, refer to current guidelines (King, 1998).

Breast-Feeding Considerations It is not known if amphotericin is excreted into breast milk. Due to its poor oral absorption, systemic exposure to the nursing infant is expected to be decreased; however, because of the potential for toxicity, breast-feeding is not recommended (Mactal-Haaf, 2001).

Contraindications Hypersensitivity to amphotericin B or any component

Warnings Anaphylaxis has been reported with amphotericin B-containing drugs; if a severe anaphylactic reaction occurs, discontinue infusion immediately; patient should not receive further infusions of amphotericin B lipid complex; facilities for cardiopulmonary resuscitation should be available during administration due to the possibility of anaphylactic reaction

Precautions Acute reactions (including fever and chills) may occur 1-2 hours after starting an intravenous infusion; reactions are usually more common with the first few doses and generally diminish with subsequent doses.

Due to the nephrotoxic potential of amphotericin B, other nephrotoxic drugs should be avoided. Concurrent use with antineoplastic agents may enhance the potential for renal toxicity, bronchospasm, or hypotension. Acute pulmonary reactions have been reported in patients simultaneously receiving intravenous amphotericin B and leukocyte transfusions; separate these infusions temporally as much as possible and monitor pulmonary function.

Adverse Reactions Nephrotoxicity and infusion-related hyperpyrexia, rigor, and chilling are reduced relative to amphotericin deoxycholate.

Cardiovascular: Cardiac arrest, chest pain, hyper-/hypotension

Central nervous system: Chills, fever, headache, pain

Dermatologic: Rash

Endocrine & metabolic: Bilirubinemia, hypokalemia

Gastrointestinal: Abdominal pain, diarrhea, gastrointestinal hemorrhage, nausea, vomiting

Hematologic: Anemia, leukopenia, thrombocytopenia

Renal: Renal failure, serum creatinine increased

Respiratory: Dyspnea, respiratory disorder, respiratory failure

Miscellaneous: Infection, multiple organ failure, sepsis

Rare but important or life-threatening: Allergic reactions, anaphylactoid reactions, anuria, arrhythmias, asthma, blood dyscrasias, bronchospasm, BUN increased, cardiomyopathy, cerebral vascular accident, cholangitis, cholecystitis, coagulation abnormalities, deafness, dysuria, encephalopathy, eosinophilia, erythema multiforme, exfoliative dermatitis, extrapyramidal syndrome, hearing loss, hemoptysis, hepatic failure (acute), hepatitis, hepatomegaly, hepatotoxicity, hyper-/hypocalcemia, hyperkalemia, hypomagnesemia, injection site reaction, jaundice, leukocytosis, MI, myasthenia, oliguria, peripheral neuropathy, pleural effusion, pulmonary edema, pulmonary embolism, renal function decreased, renal tubular acidosis, seizures, shock, tachycardia, thrombophlebitis, transaminases increased, veno-occlusive liver disease, ventricular fibrillation, vertigo (transient), visual impairment

Drug Interactions

Metabolism/Transport Effects None known.

Avoid Concomitant Use

Avoid concomitant use of Amphotericin B (Lipid Complex) with any of the following: Saccharomyces boulardii

Increased Effect/Toxicity

Amphotericin B (Lipid Complex) may increase the levels/effects of: Aminoglycosides; Colistimethate; CycloSPORINE (Systemic); Flucytosine

The levels/effects of Amphotericin B (Lipid Complex) may be increased by: Corticosteroids (Orally Inhaled); Corticosteroids (Systemic)

Decreased Effect

Amphotericin B (Lipid Complex) may decrease the levels/effects of: Saccharomyces boulardii

The levels/effects of Amphotericin B (Lipid Complex) may be decreased by: Antifungal Agents (Azole Derivatives, Systemic)

Stability Store intact vials at 2°C to 8°C (36°F to 46°F); do not freeze; protect from light. Solutions for infusion are stable in D_5W for 48 hours at 2°C to 8°C (36°F to 46°F) and 6 hours at room temperature and should be protected from light. Do not dilute with saline solutions or mix with other drugs or electrolytes.

Mechanism of Action Binds to ergosterol altering cell membrane permeability in susceptible fungi and causing leakage of cell components with subsequent cell death. Proposed mechanism suggests that amphotericin causes an oxidation-dependent stimulation of macrophages.

Pharmacokinetics (Adult data unless noted) Exhibits nonlinear kinetics; volume of distribution and clearance from blood increases with increasing dose

Distribution: High tissue concentration found in the liver, spleen, and lung

Half-life, terminal: 173 hours

Elimination: 0.9% of dose excreted in urine over 24 hours; effects of hepatic and renal impairment on drug disposition are unknown

Dialysis: Not hemodialyzable

Dosing: Neonatal Candidiasis, invasive: Limited data available: I.V.: 2.5-5 mg/kg/dose once daily; dosing based on experience reported in 28 neonates [median GA: 27 weeks; median weight: 1.06 kg (range: 0.48-4.9 kg)] (Würthwein, 2005); IDSA guidelines suggest an initial dose of 3 mg/kg (Pappas, 2009). Another report describes therapy initiation using a dose escalation approach with an initial dose of 1 mg/kg on day 1, followed by a daily increase of 1 mg/kg/day to a goal of 5 mg/kg/day (n=10; mean GA: 30.7 ± 3.9 weeks) (Cetin, 2005)

Dosing: Usual

Infants and Children: **Note:** For patients who experience infusion-related immediate reactions, premedicate with the following drugs 30-60 minutes prior to drug administration: NSAID (with or without diphenhydramine) or acetaminophen with diphenhydramine or hydrocortisone. If the patient experiences rigors during the infusion, meperidine may be administered.

General dosing, susceptible infections: I.V.: 5 mg/kg/dose once daily

Aspergillosis, **invasive:**

Non-HIV-exposed/-infected: I.V.: 5 mg/kg/dose once daily; duration should be individualized based upon response (Walsh, 2008)

HIV-exposed/-infected: I.V.: 5 mg/kg/dose once daily for at least 12 weeks; duration should be individualized based on clinical response (CDC, 2009)

Blastomycosis, **invasive:** I.V.: 3-5 mg/kg/day for initial therapy usually for 1-2 weeks, if CNS infection 4-6 weeks may be needed; follow with oral itraconazole for a total of 12 months (Chapman, 2008)

Candidiasis, **invasive:**

Non-HIV-exposed/-infected: I.V.: 3-5 mg/kg/dose once daily; duration of therapy dependent upon severity and site of infection (Pappas, 2009)

HIV-exposed/-infected: I.V.: 5 mg/kg/dose once daily until 2-3 weeks after the last positive blood culture; may be used in combination with oral flucytosine for severe disease (eg, CNS involvement) (DHHS [pediatric], 2013)

Coccidioidomycosis, **invasive:**

Non-HIV-exposed/-infected:

Disseminated infection, nonpulmonary: I.V.: 2-5 mg/kg/day with or without concomitant azole antifungal therapy (Galgiani, 2005)

Pulmonary infection, diffuse: I.V.: 2-5 mg/kg/day for several weeks, followed by an oral azole antifungal for a total length of therapy ≥12 months (Galgiani, 2005)

HIV-exposed/-infected: *Non-CNS infection:* I.V.: 5 mg/kg/dose once daily until clinical improvement; dose may be increased to as high as 10 mg/kg/dose once daily for life-threatening infection (DHHS [pediatric], 2013)

Cryptococcosis:

Disseminated (non-CNS or severe pulmonary disease) (independent of HIV status): I.V.: 5 mg/kg/dose once daily; for severe infection in HIV-exposed/-infected patients, may consider the addition of flucytosine (DHHS [pediatric], 2013; Perfect, 2010)

Meningitis: I.V.:

Non-HIV-exposed/-positive: 5 mg/kg/dose once daily with or without oral flucytosine for a minimum 2-week induction; combination with flucytosine is the preferred treatment (Perfect, 2010)

HIV-exposed/-positive: 5 mg/kg/day plus flucytosine or fluconazole; **Note:** Minimum 2 week induction, followed by consolidation and chronic suppressive therapy; a longer duration of induction therapy may be necessary if CSF is not negative or lack of clinical improvement (DHHS [pediatric], 2013)

Histoplasmosis, acute pulmonary disease: I.V.: 3-5 mg/kg/day for 1-2 weeks followed by oral itraconazole for a total of 12 weeks; conventional amphotericin B typically preferred (Wheat, 2007)

Adolescents: **Note:** For patients who experience infusion-related immediate reactions, premedicate with the following drugs 30-60 minutes prior to drug administration: NSAID (with or without diphenhydramine) or acetaminophen with diphenhydramine or hydrocortisone 50-100 mg. If the patient experiences rigors during the infusion, meperidine may be administered.

General dosing, susceptible infection: I.V.: 5 mg/kg/dose once daily

Aspergillosis, **invasive:**

Non-HIV-exposed/-infected: I.V.: 5 mg/kg/day; duration of treatment depends on site of infection, extent of disease, and level of immunosuppression (Walsh, 2008)

HIV-exposed/-infected: I.V.: 5 mg/kg/day treat until CD4 count >200 cells/mm^3 and evidence of clinical response (DHHS [adult], 2013)

Blastomycosis, **invasive:** I.V.: 3-5 mg/kg/day for 1-2 weeks or until improvement, followed by oral itraconazole (Chapman, 2008)

Candida **infection:**

General invasive candidal disease: I.V.: 3-5 mg/kg/day; duration of therapy dependent upon severity and site of infection. **Note:** In chronic disseminated candidiasis, transition to fluconazole after several weeks in stable patients is preferred (Pappas, 2009)

CNS infection: I.V.: 3-5 mg/kg/day (with or without flucytosine) for several weeks, followed by fluconazole (Pappas, 2009)

Endocarditis: I.V.: 3-5 mg/kg/dose once daily (with or without flucytosine); continue to treat for 4-6 weeks after device removal unless device cannot be removed then chronic suppression with fluconazole is recommended (Pappas, 2009)

Esophageal: HIV-exposed/-positive: I.V.: 3-4 mg/kg/dose once daily for 14-21 days (DHHS [adult], 2013)

Oropharyngeal, refractory: HIV-exposed/-positive: I.V.: 3-4 mg/kg/dose once daily for at least 7-14 days; depending upon response a longer duration may be required (DHHS [adult], 2013)

Coccidioidomycosis, **invasive:**

Non-HIV-exposed/-infected:

Disseminated infection, nonpulmonary: I.V.: 2-5 mg/kg/day with or without concomitant azole antifungal therapy (Galgiani, 2005)

Pulmonary infection, diffuse: I.V.: 2-5 mg/kg/day for several weeks, followed by an oral azole antifungal for a total length of therapy ≥12 months (Galgiani, 2005)

HIV-exposed/-infected: *Non-CNS infection:* I.V.: 4-6 mg/kg/day until clinical improvement, then switch to fluconazole or itraconazole (DHHS [adult], 2013)

Cryptococcosis **infection:**

Non-HIV-exposed/-infected:

Disseminated infection: I.V.: 5 mg/kg/day (with flucytosine if possible) for ≥4 weeks may be used for severe pulmonary cryptococcosis or for cryptococcemia with evidence of high fungal burden, followed by

oral fluconazole. **Note:** If flucytosine is not given or treatment is interrupted, consider prolonging induction therapy for an additional 2 weeks (Perfect, 2010).

Meningitis, non-transplant patients: I.V.: Induction therapy: 5 mg/kg/day (with flucytosine if possible) for ≥4 weeks followed by oral fluconazole; should be used as an alternative to conventional amphotericin B in patients with renal concerns. **Note:** If flucytosine is not given or treatment is interrupted, consider prolonging induction therapy for an additional 2 weeks (Perfect, 2010).

Meningitis, transplant patients: I.V.: Induction therapy: 5 mg/kg/day (with flucytosine) for at least 2 weeks followed by oral fluconazole. **Note:** If flucytosine is not given, duration of therapy should be 4-6 weeks (Perfect, 2010).

HIV-exposed/-infected: *Cryptococcal meningitis or disseminated:* I.V.: Induction therapy: 5 mg/kg/day with flucytosine for at least 2 weeks, followed by oral fluconazole (DHHS [adult], 2013; Perfect, 2010); should be used as an alternative to conventional amphotericin B in patients with renal concerns. **Note:** If flucytosine is not given due to intolerance, duration of amphotericin B lipid complex therapy should be 4-6 weeks (Perfect, 2010).

Histoplasmosis:

Non-HIV-exposed/-positive: *Disseminated (non-CNS) or pulmonary disease:* I.V.: 5 mg/kg/dose once daily for 1-2 weeks followed by oral itraconazole (Wheat, 2007)

HIV-exposed/-positive: *Disseminated disease (moderately severe to severe):* Induction: I.V.: 3 mg/kg/dose once daily; **Note:** Minimum 2 week induction, longer if clinical improvement delayed; followed by oral itraconazole (DHHS [adult], 2013)

Leishmaniasis, visceral (HIV-exposed/-positive) (DHHS [adult], 2013):

Treatment: I.V.: 2-4 mg/kg/dose once daily **or** an interrupted schedule of 4 mg/kg/dose on days 1-5, and on days 10, 17, 24, 31, and 38 to achieve a total dose of 20-60 mg/kg

Chronic maintenance: I.V.: 3 mg/kg/dose every 21 days; **Note:** Use reserved for patients with visceral infection and CD4 count <200 cells/mm^3

Sporotrichosis **infection:** I.V.:

Meningeal: 5 mg/kg/day for 4-6 weeks, followed by oral itraconazole (Kauffman, 2007)

Pulmonary, osteoarticular, and disseminated: 3-5 mg/kg/day, followed by oral itraconazole after a favorable response is seen with amphotericin initial therapy (Kauffman, 2007)

Adults: **Note:** For patients who experience infusion-related immediate reactions, premedicate with the following drugs 30-60 minutes prior to drug administration: NSAID (with or without diphenhydramine) or acetaminophen with diphenhydramine or hydrocortisone 50-100 mg. If the patient experiences rigors during the infusion, meperidine may be administered. **General dosing, susceptible infection:** I.V.: 5 mg/kg/dose once daily

Dosing adjustment in renal impairment: Infants, Children, Adolescents, and Adults:

Manufacturer's recommendations: There are no dosage adjustments provided in manufacturer's labeling (has not been studied).

Alternate recommendations: The following adjustments have been recommended (Aronoff, 2007):

Hemodialysis: No supplemental dosage necessary

Peritoneal dialysis: No supplemental dosage necessary

Continuous renal replacement therapy (CRRT): No supplemental dosage necessary

Dosing adjustment in hepatic impairment: There are no dosage adjustments provided in manufacturer's labeling (has not been studied).

Administration Parenteral: I.V.: Prior to administration, amphotericin B lipid complex 5 mg/mL concentrated suspension must be diluted in D_5W by gently shaking the vial until solution contains no sediment; the appropriate dose is drawn into one or more sterile 20 mL syringes using an 18 gauge needle. The needle is removed and replaced with a 5 micrometer filter needle which can be used to filter the contents of up to 4 vials of drug. Contents of the syringe are injected via the filter needle into the I.V. container of D_5W diluting amphotericin B lipid complex to a final concentration of 1 mg/mL. Limited data suggests $D_{10}W$ and $D_{15}W$ may also be used for dilution (data on file [Sigma-Tau Pharmaceuticals, 2014]). A maximum concentration of 2 mg/mL may be used in fluid-restricted patients. Flush line with D_5W prior to infusion. Gently shake the I.V. container of diluted drug to insure that contents are thoroughly mixed then administer at a rate of 2.5 mg/kg/hour (over 2 hours). The manufacturer recommends that an in-line filter should NOT be used during administration of amphotericin B lipid complex. If infusion time exceeds 2 hours, mix the contents by gently rotating the infusion bag every 2 hours.

Monitoring Parameters BUN, serum creatinine, liver function tests, serum electrolytes, CBC; vital signs, I & O; monitor for signs of hypokalemia (muscle weakness, cramping, drowsiness, ECG changes, etc)

Additional Information The lipid portion of amphotericin B lipid complex formulation contains 0.045 kcal per 5 mg; for patients receiving parenteral nutrition, adjustment to the amount of lipids may be necessary (Sacks, 1997).

Dosage Forms Excipient information presented when available (limited, particularly for generics); consult specific product labeling.

Suspension, Intravenous:
Abelcet: 5 mg/mL (20 mL)

References

Adler-Shohet F, Waskin H, and Lieberman JM, "Amphotericin B Lipid Complex for Neonatal Invasive Candidiasis," *Arch Dis Child Fetal Neonatal Ed*, 2001, 84(2):F131-3.

Aronoff GR, Bennett WM, Berns JS, et al, *Drug Prescribing in Renal Failure: Dosing Guidelines for Adults and Children*, 5th ed, Philadelphia, PA: American College of Physicians, 2007, 97, 169.

Centers for Disease Control and Prevention (CDC). Guidelines for the prevention and treatment of opportunistic infections among HIV-exposed and HIV-infected children. *MMWR Recomm Rep*. 2009;58 (RR-11):1-166.

Cetin H, Yalaz M, Akisu M, et al, "The Efficacy of Two Different Lipid-Based Amphotericin B in Neonatal Candida Septicemia," *Pediatr Int*, 2005, 47(6):676-80.

Chapman SW, Dismukes WE, Proia LA, et al, "Clinical Practice Guidelines for the Management of Blastomycosis: 2008 Update by the Infectious Diseases Society of America," *Clin Infect Dis*, 2008, 46 (12):1801-12.

DHHS. Guidelines for the prevention and treatment of opportunistic infections among HIV-exposed and HIV-infected children: recommendations from the National Institutes of Health, Centers for Disease Control and Prevention, the HIV Medicine Association of the Infectious Diseases Society of America, the Pediatric Infectious Diseases Society, and the American Academy of Pediatrics. November 6, 2013. Available at http://aidsinfo.nih.gov

DHHS Panel on Opportunistic Infections (OI) in HIV-Infected Adults and Adolescents, "Guidelines for Prevention and Treatment of Opportunistic Infections in HIV-Infected Adults and Adolescents: Recommendations from the Centers for Disease Control and Prevention (CDC), the National Institutes of Health (NIH), and the HIV Medicine Association (HIVMA) of the Infectious Diseases Society of America (IDSA)," May 7, 2013. Available at http://aidsinfo.nih.gov/contentfiles/lvguidelines/adult_oi.pdf

Galgiani JN, Ampel NM, Blair JE, et al, "Coccidioidomycosis," *Clin Infect Dis*, 2005, 41(9):1217-23.

King CT, Rogers PD, Cleary JD, et al, "Antifungal Therapy During Pregnancy," *Clin Infect Dis*, 1998, 27(5):1151-60.

Mactal-Haaf C, Hoffman M, and Kuchta A, "Use of Anti-infective Agents During Lactation, Part 3: Antivirals, Antifungals, and Urinary Antiseptics," *J Hum Lact*, 2001, 17(2):160-6.

Pappas PG, Kauffman CA, Andes D, et al, "Clinical Practice Guidelines for the Management of Candidiasis: 2009 Update by the Infectious Diseases Society of America," *Clin Infect Dis*, 2009, 48(5):503-35.

Perfect JR, Dismukes WE, Dromer F, et al, "Clinical Practice Guidelines for the Management of Cryptococcal Disease: 2010 Update by the Infectious Diseases Society of America," *Clin Infect Dis*, 2010, 50 (3):291-322.

Sacks GS and Cleary JD, "Nutritional Impact of Lipid-Associated Amphotericin B Formulations," *Ann Pharmacother*, 1997, 31(1):121-2.

Tunkel AR, Glaser CA, Bloch KC, et al, "The Management of Encephalitis: Clinical Practice Guidelines from the Infectious Diseases Society of America," *Clin Infect Dis*, 2008, 47(3):303-27.

Walsh TJ, Anaissie EJ, Denning DW, et al, "Treatment of Aspergillosis: Clinical Practice Guidelines of the Infectious Diseases Society of America," *Clin Infect Dis*, 2008, 46(3):327-60.

Wheat LJ, Freifeld AG, Kleiman MB, et al, "Clinical Practice Guidelines for the Management of Patients With Histoplasmosis: 2007 Update by the Infectious Diseases Society of America," *Clin Infect Dis*, 2007, 45 (7):807-25.

Würthwein G, Groll AH, Hempel G, et al, "Population Pharmacokinetics of Amphotericin B Lipid Complex in Neonates," *Antimicrob Agents Chemother*, 2005, 49(12):5092-8.

Amphotericin B (Liposomal)
(am foe TER i sin bee lye po SO mal)

Medication Safety Issues
High alert medication:
The Institute for Safe Medication Practices (ISMP) includes this medication among its list of drugs which have a heightened risk of causing significant patient harm when used in error.

Other safety concerns:
Lipid-based amphotericin formulations (AmBisome®) may be confused with conventional formulations (Amphocin®, Fungizone®) or with other lipid-based amphotericin formulations (Abelcet®, Amphotec®)

Large overdoses have occurred when conventional formulations were dispensed inadvertently for lipid-based products. Single daily doses of conventional amphotericin formulation never exceed 1.5 mg/kg.

Brand Names: U.S. AmBisome

Brand Names: Canada AmBisome®

Therapeutic Category Antifungal Agent, Systemic

Generic Availability (U.S.) No

Use Empirical therapy for presumed fungal infection in febrile, neutropenic patients; treatment of patients with *Aspergillus* species, *Candida* species, and/or *Cryptococcus* species infections refractory to amphotericin B desoxycholate (conventional amphotericin), or in patients where renal impairment or unacceptable toxicity precludes the use of amphotericin B desoxycholate; treatment of cryptococcal meningitis in HIV-infected patients; treatment of visceral leishmaniasis (all indications: FDA approved in ages ≥1 month and adults). Has also been used for treatment of systemic *Histoplasmosis* infection, blastomycosis, coccidioidomycosis, and mucormycosis

Pregnancy Risk Factor B

Pregnancy Considerations Adverse events were not observed in animal reproduction studies. Amphotericin crosses the placenta and enters the fetal circulation. Amphotericin B is recommended for the treatment of serious systemic fungal diseases in pregnant women; refer to current guidelines (King, 1998).

Breast-Feeding Considerations It is not known if amphotericin is excreted into breast milk. Due to its poor oral absorption, systemic exposure to the nursing infant is expected to be decreased; however, because of the potential for toxicity, breast-feeding is not recommended (Mactal-Haaf, 2001).

Contraindications Hypersensitivity to amphotericin B desoxycholate or any component

Warnings Anaphylaxis has been reported with amphotericin B-containing drugs; if a severe anaphylactic reaction occurs, discontinue infusion immediately; patient should not receive further infusions of amphotericin B liposome;

facilities for cardiopulmonary resuscitation should be available during administration due to the possibility of anaphylactic reaction

Precautions Due to the nephrotoxic potential of amphotericin B, other nephrotoxic drugs should be avoided. Acute infusion reactions (including fever and chills) may occur 1-2 hours after starting infusions; reactions are more common with the first few doses and generally diminish with subsequent doses administered at a slower infusion rate. Acute pulmonary reactions have been reported in patients simultaneously receiving intravenous amphotericin B and leukocyte transfusions; separate these infusions temporally as much as possible and monitor pulmonary function. Concurrent use with antineoplastic agents may enhance the potential for renal toxicity, bronchospasm, or hypotension.

Adverse Reactions Nephrotoxicity and infusion-related hyperpyrexia, rigor, and chilling are reduced relative to amphotericin deoxycholate.

Cardiovascular: Atrial fibrillation, bradycardia, cardiac arrest, cardiac arrhythmia, cardiomegaly, chest pain, edema, facial edema, flushing, heart valve disease, hypertension, hypotension, localized phlebitis, orthostatic hypotension, peripheral edema, tachycardia, vascular disorder, vasodilatation

Central nervous system: Abnormality in thinking, agitation, anxiety, chills, coma, confusion, depression, dizziness, drowsiness, dysesthesia, dystonia, hallucination, headache, insomnia, malaise, nervousness, pain, paresthesia, rigors, seizure

Dermatologic: Alopecia, cellulitis, dermal ulcer, dermatological reaction, diaphoresis, maculopapular rash, pruritus, skin discoloration, skin rash, urticaria, vesiculobullous dermatitis, xeroderma

Endocrine & metabolic: Acidosis, hyperchloremia, hyperglycemia, hyperkalemia, hypermagnesemia, hypernatremia, hyperphosphatemia, hypervolemia, hypocalcemia, hypokalemia, hypomagnesemia, hyponatremia, hypophosphatemia, increased lactate dehydrogenase, increased nonprotein nitrogen

Gastrointestinal: Abdominal pain, anorexia, aphthous stomatitis, constipation, diarrhea, dyspepsia, dysphagia, enlargement of abdomen, eructation, fecal incontinence, flatulence, gastrointestinal hemorrhage, gingival hemorrhage, hematemesis, hemorrhoids, hiccups, increased serum amylase, intestinal obstruction, mucositis, nausea, rectal disease, stomatitis, vomiting, xerostomia

Genitourinary: Dysuria, hematuria, nephrotoxicity, toxic nephrosis, urinary incontence, vaginal hemorrhage

Hematologic & oncologic: Anemia, blood coagulation disorder, bruise, decreased prothrombin time, hemophthalmos, hemorrhage, hypoproteinemia, increased prothrombin time, leukopenia, oral hemorrhage, petechia, purpura, thrombocytopenia

Hepatic: Abnormal hepatic function tests (not specified), hepatic injury, hepatic veno-occlusive disease, hepatomegaly, hyperbilirubinemia, increased serum alkaline phosphatase, increased serum ALT, increased serum AST

Hypersensitivity: Delayed hypersensitivity, hypersensitivity reaction, transfusion reaction

Immunologic: Graft versus host disease

Infection: Infection, herpes simplex infection, sepsis

Local: Inflammation at injection site

Neuromuscular & skeletal: Arthralgia, back pain, myalgia, neck pain, osteallgia, tremor, weakness

Ophthalmic: Conjunctivitis, dry eyes

Renal: Acute renal failure, increased blood urea nitrogen, increased serum creatinine, renal failure, renal function abnormality

Respiratory: Asthma, atelectasis, cough, dry nose, dyspnea, epistaxis, flu-like symptoms, hemoptysis, hyperventilation, hypoxia, pharyngitis, pleural effusion, pneumonia, pulmonary disease, pulmonary edema, respiratory alkalosis, respiratory failure, respiratory insufficiency, rhinitis, sinusitis

Miscellaneous: Infusion related reactions (fever, chills, vomiting, nausea, dyspnea, tachycardia, hypertension, vasodilation, hypotension, hyperventilation, hypoxia), procedural complication

Rare but important or life-threatening: Agranulocytosis, angioedema, cyanosis, hemorrhagic cystitis, hypoventilation, rhabdomyolysis

Drug Interactions

Metabolism/Transport Effects None known.

Avoid Concomitant Use

Avoid concomitant use of Amphotericin B (Liposomal) with any of the following: Saccharomyces boulardii

Increased Effect/Toxicity

Amphotericin B (Liposomal) may increase the levels/effects of: Aminoglycosides; Colistimethate; CycloSPORINE (Systemic); Flucytosine

The levels/effects of Amphotericin B (Liposomal) may be increased by: Corticosteroids (Orally Inhaled); Corticosteroids (Systemic)

Decreased Effect

Amphotericin B (Liposomal) may decrease the levels/effects of: Saccharomyces boulardii

The levels/effects of Amphotericin B (Liposomal) may be decreased by: Antifungal Agents (Azole Derivatives, Systemic)

Stability Store unopened vials at temperatures ≤25°C (≤77°F); reconstituted drug is stable for 24 hours under refrigeration at 2°C to 8°C (36°F to 46°F); do not freeze. Do not dilute with saline solutions or mix with other drugs or electrolytes; may cause precipitant formation. Manufacturer's labeling states infusion should begin within 6 hours of dilution with D_5W; data on file with Astellas Pharma shows extended formulation stability (see table) when admixed at 0.2-2 mg/mL (in polyolefin or polyvinyl chloride bags) in various dextrose solutions. For infants and small children, dilutions of 0.2-0.5 mg/mL may be used.

AmBisome® Stability

Solution		Temperature	Stability
D_5W	2 mg/mL	2°C to 8°C	14 days
	0.2 mg/mL	2°C to 8°C	11 days
	0.2-2 mg/mL	23°C to 27°C	24 hours
$D_{10}W$	0.2-2 mg/mL	2°C to 8°C	48 hours
$D_{20}W$	2 mg/mL	2°C to 8°C	48 hours
$D_{25}W$	2 mg/mL	2°C to 8°C	48 hours

Mechanism of Action Binds to ergosterol altering cell membrane permeability in susceptible fungi and causing leakage of cell components with subsequent cell death. Proposed mechanism suggests that amphotericin causes an oxidation-dependent stimulation of macrophages (Lyman, 1992).

Pharmacokinetics (Adult data unless noted) Exhibits nonlinear kinetics (greater than proportional increase in serum concentration with an increase in dose)

Distribution: V_d: 0.1-0.16 L/kg

Half-life (terminal): 100-153 hours

Dosing: Neonatal Candidiasis, invasive: Limited data available: I.V.: 3-5 mg/kg/dose once daily for ≥3 weeks (Cetin, 2005; Juster-Reicher, 2003; Pappas, 2009; Queiroz-Telles, 2008); doses as high as 7 mg/kg/dose once daily have been used (Juster-Reicher, 2003); another report describes a dose escalation approach with dosing initiated with 1 mg/kg/dose on day 1 and increased by 1 mg/kg/dose once daily to a maximum of 5 mg/kg/dose once daily (preterm neonate: n=40; term neonate: n=4) (Scarcella, 1998)

Dosing: Usual

Infants and Children: Note: Premedication: For patients who experience infusion-related immediate reactions, premedicate with the following drugs 30-60 minutes prior to drug administration: NSAID (with or without diphenhydramine) **or** acetaminophen with diphenhydramine **or** hydrocortisone. If the patient experiences rigors during the infusion, meperidine may be administered.

General dosing:

Empiric therapy: I.V.: 3 mg/kg/dose once daily

Treatment, susceptible systemic infection: I.V.: 3-5 mg/kg/dose once daily

Aspergillosis, invasive:

Non-HIV-exposed/-positive: I.V.: 3-5 mg/kg/dose once daily (Walsh, 2008)

HIV-exposed/-positive: I.V.: 5 mg/kg/dose once daily for at least 12 weeks; durations should be individualized based on clinical response (CDC, 2009); doses as high as 10 mg/kg/dose have been used in patients with documented *Aspergillus* infection

Blastomycosis, invasive: I.V.: 3-5 mg/kg/day for initial therapy, if CNS infection 4-6 weeks may be needed; followed by oral itraconazole for a total of 12 months (Chapman, 2008)

Candidiasis, invasive:

Non-HIV-exposed/-positive: I.V.: 3-5 mg/kg/dose once daily; duration of therapy dependent upon severity and site of infection (Filioti, 2007; Pappas, 2009)

HIV-exposed/-positive: I.V.: 5 mg/kg/dose once daily until 2-3 weeks after the last positive blood culture; may be used in combination with oral flucytosine for severe disease (eg, CNS involvement) (DHHS [pediatric], 2013)

Coccidioidomycosis, invasive:

Non-HIV-exposed/-positive:

Disseminated infection, nonpulmonary: I.V.: 2-5 mg/kg/day with or without concomitant azole antifungal (Galgiani, 2005)

Pulmonary infection, diffuse: I.V.: 2-5 mg/kg/day for several weeks, followed by an oral azole antifungal for a total length of therapy ≥12 months (Galgiani, 2005)

HIV-exposed/-positive: *Non-CNS infection:* I.V.: 5 mg/kg/dose once daily until clinical improvement (minimum of several weeks of therapy); may be increased to as high as 10 mg/kg/dose once daily for life-threatening infection (DHHS [pediatric], 2013)

Cryptococcosis, invasive:

Disseminated cryptococcosis (non-CNS or severe pulmonary disease) (independent of HIV status): I.V.: 3-5 mg/kg/dose once daily; may consider addition of oral flucytosine (DHHS [pediatric], 2013; Perfect, 2010)

Meningitis (HIV-exposed/-positive): I.V.: 6 mg/kg/dose once daily with or without oral flucytosine or fluconazole for a minimum 2-week induction; **Note:** Minimum 2 week induction, followed by consolidation and chronic suppressive therapy; a longer duration of induction therapy may be necessary if CSF is not negative or lack of clinical improvement (DHHS [pediatric], 2013)

Histoplasmosis:

Non-HIV-exposed/-positive: *Acute pulmonary disease:* I.V.: 3-5 mg/kg/day for 1-2 weeks followed by oral itraconazole for a total of 12 weeks; conventional amphotericin B typically preferred (Wheat, 2007)

HIV-exposed/-positive:

Disseminated infection (non-CNS disease): Treatment: I.V.: 3-5 mg/kg/dose once daily for at least 2 weeks for induction; if itraconazole not tolerated for consolidation therapy, may continue for 4-6 weeks (DHHS [pediatric], 2013)

CNS disease: Acute therapy: I.V.: 5 mg/kg/dose once daily for 4-6 weeks, followed by consolidation therapy (DHHS [pediatric], 2013)

Visceral leishmaniasis:

Immunocompetent patients: I.V.: Initial: 3 mg/kg/dose once daily on days 1-5; then repeat dose (3 mg/kg) on days 14 and 21. **Note:** Repeat course may be given to patients who do not achieve parasitic clearance.

Immunocompromised patients: I.V.: Initial: 4 mg/kg/dose once daily on days 1-5; then repeat dose (4 mg/kg) on days 10, 17, 24, 31, 38

Adolescents: Note: Premedication: For patients who experience nonanaphylactic infusion-related immediate reactions, premedicate with the following drugs 30-60 minutes prior to drug administration: NSAID (with or without diphenhydramine) **or** acetaminophen with diphenhydramine **or** hydrocortisone. If the patient experiences rigors during the infusion, meperidine may be administered.

General dosing: I.V.: 3-6 mg/kg/dose once daily; **Note:** Higher doses (15 mg/kg/day) have been used clinically (Walsh, 2001)

Aspergillosis, invasive:

Non-HIV-exposed/-positive: I.V.: 3-5 mg/kg/dose once daily (Walsh, 2008)

HIV-exposed/-positive: I.V.: 5 mg/kg/dose once daily until CD4 count >200 cells/mm^3 and evidence of clinical response (DHHS [adult], 2013); doses as high as 10 mg/kg/dose have been used in patients with documented *Aspergillus* infection

Blastomycosis, invasive: I.V.: 3-5 mg/kg/day for initial therapy, if CNS infection 4-6 weeks may be needed; followed by oral itraconazole for a total of 12 months (Chapman, 2008)

Candidiasis:

Empiric therapy: I.V.: 3-5 mg/kg/dose once daily (Pappas, 2009)

Treatment:

General invasive Candidal disease (Independent of HIV status): I.V.: 3-5 mg/kg/dose once daily (Filioti, 2007; Pappas, 2009); **Note:** In HIV-exposed/-positive patients, doses at the higher end of the range may be considered (5 mg/kg/day); combination therapy with flucytosine may also be appropriate in some situations (DHHS [adult], 2013).

Endocarditis (Non-HIV-exposed/-positive): I.V.: 3-5 mg/kg/dose once daily (with or without flucytosine) for 6 weeks after valve replacement (Pappas, 2009)

Esophageal (HIV-exposed/-positive): I.V.: 3-4 mg/kg/dose once daily for 14-21 days (DHHS [adult], 2013)

Oropharyngeal, refractory (HIV-exposed/-positive): I.V.: 3-4 mg/kg/dose once daily for at least 7-14 days; depending upon response a longer duration may be required (DHHS [adult], 2013)

Coccidioidomycosis, invasive:

Non-HIV-exposed/-positive:

Disseminated infection, nonpulmonary: I.V.: 2-5 mg/kg/day with or without concomitant azole antifungal (Galgiani, 2005)

Pulmonary infection, diffuse: I.V.: 2-5 mg/kg/day for several weeks, followed by an oral azole antifungal for a total length of therapy ≥12 months (Galgiani, 2005)

HIV-exposed/-positive: *Non-CNS infection:* I.V.: 4-6 mg/kg/dose once daily until clinical improvement (minimum of several weeks of therapy) (DHHS [adult], 2013)

Cryptococcosis, **invasive:**

Disseminated cryptococcosis (non-CNS or severe pulmonary disease)

Non-HIV-exposed: I.V.: 3-4 mg/kg/dose once daily for at least 14 days; may consider addition of oral flucytosine (Perfect, 2010)

HIV-exposed/-positive: I.V.: 3-4 mg/kg/dose once daily with or without fluconazole (DHHS [adult], 2013)

Meningitis (HIV-exposed/-positive): I.V.: 3-4 mg/kg/dose once daily with or without fluconazole (DHHS [adult], 2013); doses up to 6 mg/kg/dose have been reported for treatment of meningoencephalitis and may be considered for treatment failure or high fungal burden disease (Perfect, 2010)

Histoplasmosis:

Non-HIV-exposed/-positive: I.V.: 3-5 mg/kg/day for 1-2 weeks followed by itraconazole (Wheat, 2007)

HIV-exposed/-positive (DHHS [adult], 2013): I.V.:

Non-CNS infection: 3 mg/kg/dose once daily

CNS infection: 5 mg/kg/dose once daily

Leishmaniasis:

Immunocompetent: Visceral infection: I.V.: 3 mg/kg/dose on days 1-5, and 3 mg/kg/dose on days 14 and 21; a repeat course may be given in patients who do not achieve parasitic clearance

HIV-exposed/-positive (DHHS [adult], 2013): I.V.:

Cutaneous or visceral infection, treatment:: I.V.: 2-4 mg/kg/dose once daily **or** an interrupted schedule of 4 mg/kg/dose on days 1-5, and on days 10, 17, 24, 31, and 38 to achieve a total dose of 20-60 mg/kg

Chronic maintenance therapy: I.V.: 4 mg/kg/dose every 2-4 weeks; **Note:** Use reserved for patients with visceral infection and CD4 count <200 cells/mm^3:

Sporotrichosis **infection:**

Disseminated, pulmonary, or osteoarticular disease: I.V.: 3-5 mg/kg/day, followed by oral itraconazole after a favorable response is seen with amphotericin initial therapy (Kauffman, 2007)

Meningeal: I.V.: 5 mg/kg/day for 4-6 weeks, followed by oral itraconazole (Kauffman, 2007)

Adults: **Note:** Premedication: For patients who experience nonanaphylactic infusion-related immediate reactions, premedicate with the following drugs 30-60 minutes prior to drug administration: NSAID (with or without diphenhydramine) **or** acetaminophen with diphenhydramine **or** hydrocortisone. If the patient experiences rigors during the infusion, meperidine may be administered. **General dosing, susceptible infection:** I.V.: 3-6 mg/kg/day; **Note:** Higher doses (15 mg/kg/day) have been used clinically (Walsh, 2001)

Dosing adjustment in renal impairment: Infants, Children, Adolescents, and Adults: No dosage adjustment provided in manufacturer's labeling (has not been studied).

Dosing adjustment in hepatic impairment: Infants, Children, Adolescents, and Adults: No dosage adjustment provided in manufacturer's labeling (has not been studied).

Administration Parenteral: I.V.: Reconstitute with 12 mL SWI to a concentration of 4 mg/mL; shake vigorously for at least 30 seconds, until dispersed into a translucent yellow suspension; a 5-micron filter should be on the syringe used to inject the reconstituted product from the vial into the diluent. AmBisome® may be diluted with D$_5$W, D$_{10}$W, D$_{20}$W, or D$_{25}$W to a final concentration of 1-2 mg/mL; in infants and small children, a lower concentration of 0.2-0.5 mg/mL may be used to provide sufficient volume for infusion. Do not use in-line filter less than 1 micron to administer AmBisome®. Flush line with D$_5$W prior to

infusion; infusion of diluted AmBisome® should start within 6 hours of preparation; infuse over 2 hours; infusion time may be reduced to 1 hour in patients who tolerate the treatment

Monitoring Parameters BUN, serum creatinine, liver function tests, serum electrolytes (particularly magnesium and potassium), CBC, vital signs, I & O; monitor for signs of hypokalemia (muscle weakness, cramping, drowsiness, ECG changes); monitor cardiac function if used concurrently with corticosteroids

Test Interactions Falsely-elevated serum phosphate may occur when using the PHOSm assay.

Additional Information The lipid portion of amphotericin B (liposomal) formulation contains 0.27 kcal per 5 mg; for patients receiving parenteral nutrition, adjustment to the amount of lipids may be necessary (Sacks, 1997).

Dosage Forms Excipient information presented when available (limited, particularly for generics); consult specific product labeling.

Suspension Reconstituted, Intravenous:

AmBisome: 50 mg (1 ea) [contains cholesterol, distearoyl phosphatidylglycerol, hydrogenated soy phosphatidylcholine, sodium succinate hexahydrate, sucrose, tocopherol, dl-alpha]

References

Centers for Disease Control and Prevention (CDC). Guidelines for the prevention and treatment of opportunistic infections among HIV-exposed and HIV-infected children. *MMWR Recomm Rep.* 2009;58 (RR-11):1-166. Available at http://aidsinfo.nih.gov/contentfiles/Pediatric_OI.pdf

Cetin H, Yalaz M, Akisu M, et al, "The Efficacy of Two Different Lipid-Based Amphotericin B in Neonatal Candida Septicemia," *Pediatr Int,* 2005, 47(6):676-80.

Chapman SW, Dismukes WE, Proia LA, et al, "Clinical Practice Guidelines for the Management of Blastomycosis: 2008 Update by the Infectious Diseases Society of America," *Clin Infect Dis,* 2008, 46 (12):1801-12.

DHHS. Guidelines for the prevention and treatment of opportunistic infections among HIV-exposed and HIV-infected children: recommendations from the National Institutes of Health, Centers for Disease Control and Prevention, the HIV Medicine Association of the Infectious Diseases Society of America, the Pediatric Infectious Diseases Society, and the American Academy of Pediatrics. November 6, 2013. Available at http://aidsinfo.nih.gov

DHHS Panel on Opportunistic Infections (OI) in HIV-Infected Adults and Adolescents, "Guidelines for Prevention and Treatment of Opportunistic Infections in HIV-Infected Adults and Adolescents: Recommendations from the Centers for Disease Control and Prevention (CDC), the National Institutes of Health (NIH), and the HIV Medicine Association (HIVMA) of the Infectious Diseases Society of America (IDSA)," May 7, 2013. Available at http://aidsinfo.nih.gov/contentfiles/lvguidelines/adult_oi.pdf

Emminger W, Graninger W, Emminger-Schmidmeir W, et al, "Tolerance of High Doses of Amphotericin B by Infusion of a Liposomal Formulation in Children With Cancer," *Ann Hematol,* 1994, 68:27-31.

Filioti J, Spiroglou K, Panteliadis CP, et al, "Invasive Candidiasis in Pediatric Intensive Care Patients: Epidemiology, Risk Factors, Management, and Outcome," *Intensive Care Med,* 2007, 33(7):1272-83.

Galgiani JN, Ampel NM, Blair JE, et al, "Coccidioidomycosis," *Clin Infect Dis,* 2005, 41(9):1217-23.

Juster-Reicher A, Flidel-Rimon O, Amitay M, "High-Dose Liposomal Amphotericin B in the Therapy of Systemic Candidiasis in Neonates," *Eur J Clin Microbiol Infect Dis,* 2003, 22(10):603-7.

Kauffman CA, Bustamante B, Chapman SW, et al, "Clinical Practice Guidelines for the Management of Sporotrichosis: 2007 Update by the Infectious Diseases Society of America," *Clin Infect Dis,* 2007, 45 (10):1255-65.

King CT, Rogers PD, Cleary JD, et al, "Antifungal Therapy During Pregnancy," *Clin Infect Dis,* 1998, 27(5):1151-60.

Mactal-Haaf C, Hoffman M, and Kuchta A, "Use of Anti-infective Agents During Lactation, Part 3: Antivirals, Antifungals, and Urinary Antiseptics," *J Hum Lact,* 2001, 17(2):160-6.

Pappas PG, Kauffman CA, Andes D, et al, "Clinical Practice Guidelines for the Management of *Candidiasis*: 2009 Update by the Infectious Diseases Society of America," *Clin Infect Dis,* 2009, 48(5):503-35.

Perfect JR, Dismukes WE, Dromer F, et al, "Clinical Practice Guidelines for the Management of Cryptococcal Disease: 2010 Update by the Infectious Diseases Society of America," *Clin Infect Dis,* 2010, 50 (3):291-322.

Queiroz-Telles F, Berezin E, Leverger G, et al, "Micafungin Versus Liposomal Amphotericin B for Pediatric Patients With Invasive

Candidiasis: Substudy of a Randomized Double-Blind Trial," *Pediatr Infect Dis J*, 2008, 27(9):820-6.

Sacks GS and Cleary JD, "Nutritional Impact of Lipid-Associated Amphotericin B Formulations," *Ann Pharmacother*, 1997, 31(1):121-2.

Scarcella A, Pasquariello MB, Giugliano B, et al, "Liposomal Amphotericin B Treatment for Neonatal Fungal Infections," *Pediatr Infect Dis J*, 1998, 17(2):146-8.

Tunkel AR, Glaser CA, Bloch KC, et al, "The Management of Encephalitis: Clinical Practice Guidelines by the Infectious Diseases Society of America," *Clin Infect Dis*, 2008, 47(3):303-27.

Walsh TJ, Anaissie EJ, Denning DW, et al, "Treatment of Aspergillosis: Clinical Practice Guidelines of the Infectious Diseases Society of America," *Clin Infect Dis*, 2008, 46(3):327-60.

Walsh TJ, Finberg RW, Arndt C, et al, "Liposomal Amphotericin B for Empirical Therapy in Patients With Persistent Fever and Neutropenia," *N Engl J Med*, 1999, 340:764-71.

Walsh TJ, Goodman JL, Pappas P, et al, "Safety, Tolerance, and Pharmacokinetics of High-Dose Liposomal Amphotericin B (AmBisome®) in Patients Infected With Aspergillus Species and Other Filamentous Fungi: Maximum Tolerated Dose Study," *Antimicrob Agents Chemother*, 2001, 45(12):3487-96.

Wheat LJ, Freifeld AG, Kleiman MB, et al, "Clinical Practice Guidelines for the Management of Patients With Histoplasmosis: 2007 Update by the Infectious Diseases Society of America," *Clin Infect Dis*, 2007, 45 (7):807-25.

◆ **Amphotericin B Liposome** *see* Amphotericin B (Liposomal) *on page 155*

Ampicillin (am pi SIL in)

Medication Safety Issues
Sound-alike/look-alike issues:
Ampicillin may be confused with aminophylline
Related Information
Prevention of Infective Endocarditis *on page 2336*
Brand Names: Canada Ampicillin for Injection; Apo-Ampi®; Novo-Ampicillin; Nu-Ampi
Therapeutic Category Antibiotic, Penicillin
Generic Availability (U.S.) Yes
Use Treatment of susceptible respiratory, gastrointestinal, and urinary tract infections; bacterial meningitis, septicemia, and endocarditis [FDA approved in pediatric patients (age not specified) and adults]; susceptible organisms may include streptococci, pneumococci, enterococci, nonpenicillinase-producing staphylococci, *Listeria*, meningococci; some strains of *H. influenzae*, *P. mirabilis*, *Salmonella*, *Shigella*, *E. coli*, *Enterobacter*, and *Klebsiella*; has also been used as empiric therapy for neonatal sepsis or meningitis and endocarditis prophylaxis
Pregnancy Risk Factor B
Pregnancy Considerations Adverse events have not been observed in animal reproduction studies. Ampicillin crosses the placenta, providing detectable concentrations in the cord serum and amniotic fluid (Bolognese, 1968; Fisher, 1967; MacAulay, 1966). Maternal use of ampicillin has generally not resulted in an increased risk of birth defects (Aselton, 1985; Czeizel, 2001b; Heinonen, 1977; Jick, 1981; Puhó, 2007). Ampicillin is recommended for use in pregnant women for the management of preterm premature rupture of membranes (PPROM) and for the prevention of early-onset group B streptococcal (GBS) disease in newborns. Ampicillin may also be used in certain situations prior to vaginal delivery in women at high risk for endocarditis (ACOG, 2013; ACOG No. 120, 2011; ACOG No. 485, 2011; CDC [RR-10], 2010).

The volume of distribution of ampicillin is increased during pregnancy and the half-life is decreased. As a result, serum concentrations in pregnant patients are approximately 50% of those in nonpregnant patients receiving the same dose. Higher doses may be needed during pregnancy. Although oral absorption is not altered during pregnancy, oral ampicillin is poorly absorbed during labor (Philipson, 1977; Philipson, 1978; Wasz-Höckert, 1970).

Breast-Feeding Considerations Ampicillin is excreted in breast milk. The manufacturer recommends that caution be exercised when administering ampicillin to nursing women. Due to the low concentrations in human milk, minimal toxicity would be expected in the nursing infant. Nondose-related effects could include modification of bowel flora and allergic sensitization.

Contraindications Hypersensitivity to ampicillin, any penicillin, or any component

Warnings Serious and occasionally severe or fatal hypersensitivity (anaphylactoid) reactions have been reported in patients on penicillin therapy, especially with a history of beta-lactam hypersensitivity, history of sensitivity to multiple allergens, or previous IgE-mediated reactions (eg, anaphylaxis, angioedema, urticaria). Administration to patients with confirmed penicillin allergies should be avoided; in patients with confirmed cephalosporin allergy, consider skin testing to rule out cross-sensitivity to penicillins. Epstein-Barr virus infection (infectious mononucleosis), acute lymphocytic leukemia, or cytomegalovirus infection increase risk for ampicillin-induced maculopapular rash. Appearance of a rash should be carefully evaluated to differentiate a nonallergic ampicillin rash from a hypersensitivity reaction; rash occurs in 5% to 10% of children and is a generalized dull red, maculopapular rash, generally appearing 3-14 days after the start of therapy. It normally begins on the trunk and spreads over most of the body. It may be most intense at pressure areas, elbows, and knees. A high percentage (43% to 100%) of patients with infectious mononucleosis have developed rash during therapy; ampicillin-class antibiotics are not recommended in these patients. Prolonged use may result in fungal or bacterial superinfection, including *C. difficile*-associated diarrhea (CDAD) and pseudomembranous colitis; CDAD has been observed >2 months postantibiotic treatment. Seizures have been reported with rapid I.V. administration (over <3 minutes).

Precautions Use with caution in patients with renal impairment; dosage adjustment recommended; use with caution in patients allergic to cephalosporins and asthmatic patients.

Adverse Reactions
Central nervous system: Brain disease (penicillin-induced), glossalgia, seizure, sore mouth
Dermatologic: Erythema multiforme, exfoliative dermatitis, skin rash, urticaria
  Note: Appearance of a rash should be carefully evaluated to differentiate (if possible) nonallergic ampicillin rash from hypersensitivity reaction. Incidence is higher in patients with viral infection, *Salmonella* infection, lymphocytic leukemia, or patients that have hyperuricemia.
Gastrointestinal: Diarrhea, enterocolitis, glossitis, melanoglossia, nausea, oral candidiasis, pseudomembranous colitis, stomatitis, vomiting
Hematologic & oncologic: Agranulocytosis, anemia, eosinophilia, hemolytic anemia, immune thrombocytopenia, leukopenia
Hepatic: Increased serum AST
Hypersensitivity: Anaphylaxis
Immunologic: Serum sickness-like reaction
Renal: Interstitial nephritis (rare)
Respiratory: Stridor
Miscellaneous: Fever

Drug Interactions
Metabolism/Transport Effects None known.
Avoid Concomitant Use
  Avoid concomitant use of Ampicillin with any of the following: BCG; Probenecid
Increased Effect/Toxicity
  Ampicillin may increase the levels/effects of: Methotrexate; Vitamin K Antagonists

  The levels/effects of Ampicillin may be increased by: Allopurinol; Probenecid

▶

◀ **Decreased Effect**

Ampicillin may decrease the levels/effects of: Atenolol; BCG; Mycophenolate; Sodium Picosulfate; Typhoid Vaccine

The levels/effects of Ampicillin may be decreased by: Chloroquine; Lanthanum; Tetracycline Derivatives

Food Interactions Food decreases ampicillin absorption rate; may decrease ampicillin serum concentration. Management: Take at equal intervals around-the-clock, preferably on an empty stomach (1 hour before or 2 hours after meals). Maintain adequate hydration, unless instructed to restrict fluid intake.

Stability

Oral: Store capsules and powder for suspension at 20°C to 25°C (68°F to 77°F); after reconstitution, suspension is stable for 14 days under refrigeration.

Parenteral: Store intact vials 20°C to 25°C (68°F to 77°F); excursions permitted to 15°C to 30°C (59°F to 86°F); after reconstitution, solutions for I.M. or direct I.V. should be used within 1 hour. Solutions for I.V. infusion in NS are stable for 8 hours at room temperature (25°C) or 2 days under refrigeration (4°C); solutions mixed in D_5W are only stable for 2 hours due to inactivation by dextrose at room temperature.

Mechanism of Action Inhibits bacterial cell wall synthesis by binding to one or more of the penicillin-binding proteins (PBPs) which in turn inhibits the final transpeptidation step of peptidoglycan synthesis in bacterial cell walls, thus inhibiting cell wall biosynthesis. Bacteria eventually lyse due to ongoing activity of cell wall autolytic enzymes (autolysins and murein hydrolases) while cell wall assembly is arrested.

Pharmacokinetics (Adult data unless noted)

Absorption: Oral: 50%

Distribution: Into bile; penetration into CSF occurs with inflamed meninges only; low excretion into breast milk

Protein binding:

Neonates: 10%

Adults: 15% to 18%

Half-life:

Neonates:

PNA 2-7 days: 4 hours

PNA 8-14 days: 2.8 hours

PNA 15-30 days: 1.7 hours

Children and Adults: 1-1.8 hours

Anuric patients: 8-20 hours

Time to peak serum concentration: Oral: Within 1-2 hours

Elimination: ~90% of drug excreted unchanged in urine within 24 hours; excreted in bile

Dosing: Neonatal

General dosing, susceptible infection (*Red Book*, 2012): I.M., I.V.:

Body weight <1 kg:

PNA ≤14 days: 50 mg/kg/dose every 12 hours

PNA 15-28 days: 50 mg/kg/dose every 8 hours

Body weight 1-2 kg:

PNA ≤7 days: 50 mg/kg/dose every 12 hours

PNA 8-28 days: 50 mg/kg/dose every 8 hours

Body weight >2 kg:

PNA ≤7 days: 50 mg/kg/dose every 8 hours

PNA 8-28 days: 50 mg/kg/dose every 6 hours

Bacteremia, Group B streptococcal (presumed or proven) (*Red Book*, 2012): **Note:** Treatment of bacteremia without a defined focus should be for at least 10 days: I.M., I.V.:

Body weight ≤2 kg:

PNA ≤7 days: 100 mg/kg/dose every 12 hours

PNA 8-28 days: 50 mg/kg/dose every 8 hours

Body weight >2 kg:

PNA ≤7 days: 100 mg/kg/dose every 12 hours

PNA 8-28 days: 50 mg/kg/dose every 6 hours

Meningitis, Group B streptococcal: I.V.:

PNA ≤7 days: 50-100 mg/kg/dose every 8 hours for at least 14 days if uncomplicated; some experts have also recommended 75 mg/kg/dose every 6 hours (*Red Book*, 2012; Tunkel, 2004)

PNA >7 days: 50-75 mg/kg/dose every 6 hours for at least 14 days if uncomplicated; some experts have also recommended 75 mg/kg/dose every 6 hours (*Red Book*, 2012; Tunkel, 2004)

Surgical prophylaxis: I.V.: 50 mg/kg as a single dose (*Red Book*, 2012)

Dosing: Usual

Infants, Children, and Adolescents:

General dosing, susceptible infection (*Red Book*, 2012):

Mild to moderate infection:

Oral: 50-100 mg/kg/day divided every 6 hours; maximum daily dose: 4000 mg/**day**

I.M., I.V.: 100-150 mg/kg/day divided every 6 hours; maximum daily dose: 4000 mg/**day**

Severe infection: I.M., I.V.: 200-400 mg/kg/day divided every 6 hours; maximum daily dose: 12 g/**day**

Community-acquired pneumonia (CAP) (IDSA/PIDS, 2011): Infants >3 months, Children, and Adolescents:

Note: May consider addition of vancomycin or clindamycin to empiric therapy if community-acquired MRSA suspected. In children ≥5 years, a macrolide antibiotic should be added if atypical pneumonia cannot be ruled out.

Empiric treatment or *S. pneumoniae* (MICs for penicillin ≤2 mcg/mL) or *H. influenzae* (beta-lactamase negative) in fully immunized patients: I.V.: 150-200 mg/kg/day divided every 6 hours

Group A *Streptococcus*: I.V.: 200 mg/kg/day divided every 6 hours

S. pneumoniae (MICs for penicillin ≥4 mcg/mL): I.V.: 300-400 mg/kg/day divided every 6 hours

Endocarditis (Baddour, 2005):

Treatment: I.V.: 300 mg/kg/day divided every 4-6 hours in combination with other antibiotics for at least 4-6 weeks; some organisms may require longer duration (Baddour, 2005)

Prophylaxis:

Dental procedure or respiratory tract procedures (eg, tonsillectomy, adenoidectomy): I.V., I.M.: 50 mg/kg within 30-60 minutes before procedure; maximum single dose: 2000 mg (Wilson, 2007)

Genitourinary and gastrointestinal tract procedures (high-risk patients): I.V., I.M.: 50 mg/kg within 30 minutes prior to procedure; maximum dose: 2000 mg; followed by ampicillin 25 mg/kg (or amoxicillin 25 mg/kg orally) 6 hours later; must be used in combination with gentamicin. **Note:** As of April 2007, the American Heart Association guidelines now recommend prophylaxis only in patients undergoing invasive procedures and in whom underlying cardiac conditions may predispose to a higher risk of adverse outcomes should infection occur. Routine prophylaxis for GI/GU procedures is no longer recommended.

Intra-abdominal infection, complicated: I.V.: 200 mg/kg/**day** divided every 6 hours; maximum single dose: 2000 mg; maximize doses if undrained abdominal abscesses (Solomkin, 2010)

Meningitis: I.V.: 200-400 mg/kg/**day** divided every 6 hours; maximum daily dose: 12 g/**day** (*Red Book*, 2012; Tunkel, 2004)

Peritonitis (CAPD): Intraperitoneal: 125 mg per liter of dialysate for 2 weeks (Warady, 2012)

Surgical prophylaxis: I.V.: 50 mg/kg 30-60 minutes prior to procedure; may repeat in 2 hours; maximum single dose: 2000 mg (Bratzler, 2013; *Red Book*, 2012)

Adults:

Usual dosage range:
Oral: 250-500 mg every 6 hours
I.M., I.V.: 1000-2000 mg every 4-6 hours or 50-250 mg/kg/**day** in divided doses (maximum daily dose: 12 **g/day**)

Cholangitis (acute): I.V.: 2000 mg every 4 hours with gentamicin

Diverticulitis: I.M., I.V.: 2000 mg every 6 hours with metronidazole

Endocarditis:
Infective: I.V.: 12 **g/day** via continuous infusion or divided every 4 hours
Prophylaxis: Dental, oral, or respiratory tract procedures: I.M., I.V.: 2000 mg within 30-60 minutes prior to procedure in patients not allergic to penicillin and unable to take oral amoxicillin. Intramuscular injections should be avoided in patients who are receiving anticoagulant therapy. In these circumstances, orally administered regimens should be given whenever possible. Intravenously administered antibiotics should be used for patients who are unable to tolerate or absorb oral medications. **Note:** American Heart Association (AHA) guidelines now recommend prophylaxis only in patients undergoing invasive procedures and in whom underlying cardiac conditions may predispose to a higher risk of adverse outcomes should infection occur.
Prophylaxis in total joint replacement patient: I.M., I.V.: 2000 mg 1 hour prior to the procedure
Genitourinary and gastrointestinal tract procedures: I.M., I.V.:
High-risk patients: 2000 mg within 30 minutes prior to procedure, followed by ampicillin 1000 mg (or amoxicillin 1000 mg orally) 6 hours later; must be used in combination with gentamicin. **Note:** As of April 2007, routine prophylaxis for GI/GU procedures is no longer recommended by the AHA.
Moderate-risk patients: 2000 mg within 30 minutes prior to procedure

Group B strep prophylaxis (intrapartum): I.V.: 2000 mg initial dose, then 1000 mg every 4 hours until delivery

***Listeria* infections:** I.V.: 2000 mg every 4 hours (consider addition of aminoglycoside)

Mild to moderate infections: Oral: 250-500 mg every 6 hours

Prosthetic joint infection, *Enterococcus* spp (penicillin-susceptible): I.V.: 12 **g** continuous infusion every 24 hours **or** 2000 mg every 4 hours for 4-6 weeks; consider addition of aminoglycoside (Osmon, 2013)

Sepsis/meningitis: I.V.: 150-250 mg/kg/**day** divided every 3-4 hours (range: 6-12 **g/day**)

Urinary tract infections (*Enterococcus* suspected): I.V.: 1000-2000 mg every 6 hours with gentamicin

Dosing adjustment in renal impairment:
Infants, Children, and Adolescents: The following adjustments have been recommended (Aronoff, 2007). **Note:** Renally adjusted dose recommendations are based on doses of 100-200 mg/kg/day divided every 6 hours: I.M., I.V.:
GFR 30-50 mL/minute/1.73 m^2: 35-50 mg/kg/dose every 6 hours
GFR 10-29 mL/minute/1.73 m^2: 35-50 mg/kg/dose every 8-12 hours
GFR <10 mL/minute/1.73 m^2: 35-50 mg/kg/dose every 12 hours
Intermittent hemodialysis: 35-50 mg/kg/dose every 12 hours
Peritoneal dialysis (PD): 35-50 mg/kg/dose every 12 hours
Continuous renal replacement therapy (CRRT): 35-50 mg/kg/dose every 6 hours

Adults:
CrCl >50 mL/minute: Administer every 6 hours
CrCl 10-50 mL/minute: Administer every 6-12 hours
CrCl <10 mL/minute: Administer every 12-24 hours
Intermittent hemodialysis (IHD) (administer after hemodialysis on dialysis days): Dialyzable (20% to 50%): I.V.: 1-2 g every 12-24 hours (Heintz, 2009). **Note:** Dosing dependent on the assumption of 3 times/week, complete IHD sessions.
Peritoneal dialysis (PD): 250 mg every 12 hours
Continuous renal replacement therapy (CRRT) (Heintz, 2009): Drug clearance is highly dependent on the method of renal replacement, filter type, and flow rate. Appropriate dosing requires close monitoring of pharmacologic response, signs of adverse reactions due to drug accumulation, as well as drug concentrations in relation to target trough (if appropriate). The following are general recommendations only (based on dialysate flow/ultrafiltration rates of 1-2 L/hour and minimal residual renal function) and should not supersede clinical judgment:
CVVH: Loading dose of 2000 mg followed by 1000-2000 mg every 8-12 hours
CVVHD: Loading dose of 2000 mg followed by 1000-2000 mg every 8 hours
CVVHDF: Loading dose of 2000 mg followed by 1000-2000 mg every 6-8 hours

Administration
Oral: Administer around-the-clock to promote less variation in peak and trough serum levels. Administer on an empty stomach (ie, 1 hour prior to or 2 hours after meals) to increase total absorption; shake suspension well before using
Parenteral:
I.M.: Reconstitute vial with SWI to a final concentration of 125-250 mg/mL; administer intramuscularly
I.V.:
I.V. push: Reconstitute vial with SWI (see manufacturer labeling for specific details). Doses ≤500 mg should be administered over 3-5 minutes; doses >500 mg should be administered over 10-15 minutes; rapid administration has been associated with seizures.
Intermittent I.V. infusion: Infuse over 10-15 minutes at a concentration not to exceed 30 mg/mL

Monitoring Parameters With prolonged therapy monitor renal, hepatic, and hematologic function periodically; observe for change in bowel frequency; observe for signs of anaphylaxis with first dose

Test Interactions May interfere with urinary glucose tests using cupric sulfate (Benedict's solution, Clinitest®)

Some penicillin derivatives may accelerate the degradation of aminoglycosides *in vitro*, leading to a potential underestimation of aminoglycoside serum concentration.

Additional Information Sodium content: Oral suspension (250 mg/5 mL, 5 mL): 10 mg (0.4 mEq); parenteral (1 g): 66.7 mg (3 mEq)

Some penicillins (eg, carbenicillin, ticarcillin, and piperacillin) have been shown to inactivate aminoglycosides *in vitro*. This has been observed to a greater extent with tobramycin and gentamicin, while amikacin has shown greater stability against inactivation. Concurrent use of these agents may pose a risk of reduced antibacterial efficacy *in vivo*, particularly in the setting of profound renal impairment; however, definitive clinical evidence is lacking. If combination penicillin/aminoglycoside therapy is desired in a patient with renal dysfunction, separation of doses (if feasible), and routine monitoring of aminoglycoside levels, CBC, and clinical response should be considered.

Dosage Forms Excipient information presented when available (limited, particularly for generics); consult specific product labeling.

Capsule, Oral:
Generic: 250 mg, 500 mg
Solution Reconstituted, Injection, as sodium [strength expressed as base]:
Generic: 125 mg (1 ea); 250 mg (1 ea); 500 mg (1 ea); 1 g (1 ea); 2 g (1 ea); 10 g (1 ea)
Solution Reconstituted, Injection, as sodium [strength expressed as base, preservative free]:
Generic: 250 mg (1 ea); 500 mg (1 ea)
Solution Reconstituted, Intravenous, as sodium [strength expressed as base]:
Generic: 1 g (1 ea); 2 g (1 ea); 10 g (1 ea)
Solution Reconstituted, Intravenous, as sodium [strength expressed as base, preservative free]:
Generic: 10 g (1 ea)
Suspension Reconstituted, Oral:
Generic: 125 mg/5 mL (100 mL, 200 mL); 250 mg/5 mL (100 mL, 200 mL)

References

American Academy of Pediatrics (AAP). In: Pickering LK, Baker CJ, Kimberlin DW, Long SS, eds. Red Book: 2012 Report of the Committee on Infectious Diseases. 29th ed. Elk Grove Village, IL: American Academy of Pediatrics; 2012.

American College of Obstetricians and Gynecologists (ACOG). Practice bulletins no. 139: premature rupture of membranes. Obstet Gynecol. 2013;122(4):918-930.

American College of Obstetricians and Gynecologists, "ACOG Practice Bulletin No. 120: Use of Prophylactic Antibiotics in Labor and Delivery," Obstet Gynecol, 2011, 117(6):1472-83.

American College of Obstetricians and Gynecologists Committee on Obstetric Practice, "ACOG Committee Opinion No. 485: Prevention of Early-Onset Group B Streptococcal Disease in Newborns," Obstet Gynecol, 2011, 117(4):1019-27.

Aronoff GR, Bennett WM, Berns JS, et al, Drug Prescribing in Renal Failure: Dosing Guidelines for Adults and Children, 5th ed, Philadelphia, PA: American College of Physicians, 2007, 55, 149.

Aselton P, Jick H, Milunsky A, et al, "First-Trimester Drug Use and Congenital Disorders," Obstet Gynecol, 1985, 65(4):451-5.

Baddour LM, Wilson WR, Bayer AS, et al, "Infective Endocarditis. Diagnosis, Antimicrobial Therapy, and Management of Complications: A Statement for Healthcare Professionals From the Committee on Rheumatic Fever, Endocarditis, and Kawasaki Disease, Council on Cardiovascular Disease in the Young, and the Councils on Clinical Cardiology, Stroke, and Cardiovascular Surgery and Anesthesia, American Heart Association - Executive Summary: Endorsed by the Infectious Diseases Society of America," Circulation, 2005, 111 (23):3167-184.

Boguniewicz M and Leung DY, "Hypersensitivity Reactions to Antibiotics Commonly Used in Children," Pediatr Infect Dis J, 1995, 14 (3):221-31.

Bolognese RJ, "Ampicillin: Transfer Into Fetus and Amniotic Fluid," Rocky Mt Med J, 1968, 65(8):72-4.

Bradley JS, Byington CL, Shah SS, et al, "The Management of Community-Acquired Pneumonia in Infants and Children Older Than 3 Months of Age: Clinical Practice Guidelines by the Pediatric Infectious Diseases Society and the Infectious Diseases Society of America", Clin Infect Dis, 2011, 53(7):e25-76.

Bratzler DW, Dellinger EP, Olsen KM, et al, "Clinical Practice Guidelines for Antimicrobial Prophylaxis in Surgery," Am J Health Syst Pharm, 2013, 70(3):195-283.

Brown RD, Campoli-Richards DM, "Antimicrobial Therapy in Neonates, Infants, and Children," Clin Pharmacokinet, 1989, 17(Suppl 1):105-15.

Centers for Disease Control and Prevention (CDC), "Prevention of Perinatal Group B Streptococcal Disease-Revised Guidelines From CDC, 2010," MMWR Recomm Rep, 2010, 59(RR-10):1-36.

Chow MS, Quintiliani R, and Nightingale CH, "In Vivo Inactivation of Tobramycin by Ticarcillin. A Case Report," JAMA, 1982, 247(5):658-9.

Czeizel AE, Rockenbauer M, Sørensen HT, et al, "A Population-Based Case-Control Teratologic Study of Ampicillin Treatment During Pregnancy," Am J Obstet Gynecol, 2001b, 185(1):140-7.

Daly JS, Dodge RA, Glew RH, et al, "Effect of Time and Temperature on Inactivation of Aminoglycosides by Ampicillin at Neonatal Dosages," J Perinatol, 1997, 17(1):42-5.

Farchione LA, "Inactivation of Aminoglycosides by Penicillins," J Antimicrob Chemother, 1982, 8(Suppl A):27-36.

Fisher AM and Smith MR, "The Prophylactic Use of Ampicillin and Its Trans-Placental Passage After Amniotomy," J Obstet Gynaecol Br Commonw, 1967, 74(6):855-61.

Heinonen OP, Slone D, and Shapiro S, "Birth Defects and Drugs in Pregnancy," Publishing Sciences Group, Inc, Littleton, MA, 1977.

Heintz BH, Matzke GR, and Dager WE, "Antimicrobial Dosing Concepts and Recommendations for Critically Ill Adult Patients Receiving

Continuous Renal Replacement Therapy or Intermittent Hemodialysis," Pharmacotherapy, 2009, 29(5):562-77.

Jick H, Holmes LB, Hunter JR, et al, "First-Trimester Drug Use and Congenital Disorders," JAMA, 1981, 246(4):343-6.

MacAulay MA, Abou-Sabe M, and Charles D, "Placental Transfer of Ampicillin," Am J Obstet Gynecol, 1966, 96(7):943-50.

Osmon DR, Berbari EF, Berendt AR, et al, "Diagnosis and Management of Prosthetic Joint Infection: Clinical Practice Guideline by the Infectious Diseases Society of America," Clin Infect Dis, 2013, 56(1):e1-25.

Philipson A, "Pharmacokinetics of Ampicillin During Pregnancy," J Infect Dis, 1977, 136(3):370-6.

Puhó EH, Szunyogh M, Métneki J, et al, "Drug Treatment During Pregnancy and Isolated Orofacial Clefts in Hungary," Cleft Palate Craniofac J, 2007, 44(2):194-202.

Shaffer CL, Davey AM, Ransom JL, et al, "Ampicillin-Induced Neurotoxicity in Very-Low-Birth-Weight Neonates," Ann Pharmacother, 1998, 32(4):482-4.

Solomkin JS, Mazuski JE, Bradley JS, et al, "Diagnosis and Management of Complicated Intra-abdominal Infection in Adults and Children: Guidelines by the Surgical Infection Society and the Infectious Diseases Society of America," Clin Infect Dis, 2010, 50(2):133-64.

Tunkel AR, Hartman BJ, Kaplan SL, et al, "Practice Guidelines for the Management of Bacterial Meningitis," Clin Infect Dis, 2004, 39 (9):1267-84.

Warady BA, Bakkaloglu S, Newland J, et al, "Consensus Guidelines for the Prevention and Treatment of Catheter-Related Infections and Peritonitis in Pediatric Patients Receiving Peritoneal Dialysis: 2012 Update," Perit Dial Int, 2012, (32 Suppl 2):S32-86.

Wasz-Höckert O, Nummi S, Vuopala S, et al, "Transplacental Passage of Azidocillin, Ampicillin and Penicillin G During Early and Late Pregnancy," Acta Paediatr Scand Suppl, 1970, 206(Suppl 206):109.

Wilson W, Taubert KA, Gewitz M, et al, "Prevention of Infective Endocarditis. Guidelines From the American Heart Association. A Guideline From the American Heart Association Rheumatic Fever, Endocarditis, and Kawasaki Disease Committee, Council on Cardiovascular Disease in the Young, and the Council on Clinical Cardiology, Council on Cardiovascular Surgery and Anesthesia, and the Quality of Care and Outcomes Research Interdisciplinary Working Group," Circulation, 2007, 115.

Ampicillin and Sulbactam
(am pi SIL in & SUL bak tam)

Brand Names: U.S. Unasyn®
Brand Names: Canada Unasyn®
Therapeutic Category Antibiotic, Beta-lactam and Beta-lactamase Combination; Antibiotic, Penicillin
Generic Availability (U.S.) Yes
Use Treatment of susceptible bacterial infections involved with skin and skin structure (FDA approved in ages ≥1 year and adults); treatment of susceptible bacterial intra-abdominal infections and gynecological infections (FDA approved in adults); spectrum is that of ampicillin plus organisms producing beta-lactamases such as Staphylococcus sp, Streptococcus sp, H. influenzae, E. coli, K. pneumonia, Proteus sp (including P. mirabilis), Acinetobacter calcoaceticus, Providencia rettgeri, Providencia stuartii, Morganella morganii, Neisseria gonorrhoeae, Enterobacter sp, and anaerobes (including B. fragilis, P. multocida)
Pregnancy Risk Factor B
Pregnancy Considerations Adverse events have not been observed in animal reproduction studies. Both ampicillin and sulbactam cross the placenta. Maternal use of penicillins has generally not resulted in an increased risk of birth defects. When used during pregnancy, pharmacokinetic changes have been observed with ampicillin alone (refer to the Ampicillin monograph for details). Ampicillin/sulbactam may be considered for prophylactic use prior to cesarean delivery (consult current guidelines).
Breast-Feeding Considerations Ampicillin and sulbactam are both excreted into breast milk in low concentrations. The manufacturer recommends that caution be used if administering to lactating women. Nondose-related effects could include modification of bowel flora and allergic sensitization of the infant. The maternal dose of sulbactam does not need altered in the postpartum period. Also refer to the Ampicillin monograph.

Contraindications Hypersensitivity to ampicillin, sulbactam, any component, or penicillins

Warnings Serious and occasionally fatal hypersensitivity (anaphylactoid) reactions have been reported in patients on penicillin therapy, especially with a history of beta-lactam hypersensitivity, history of sensitivity to multiple allergens, or previous IgE-mediated reactions (eg, anaphylaxis, angioedema, urticaria). Administration to patients with confirmed penicillin allergies should be avoided; in patients with confirmed cephalosporin allergy, consider skin testing to rule out cross-sensitivity to penicillins. Epstein-Barr virus infection (infectious mononucleosis), acute lymphocytic leukemia, or cytomegalovirus infection increase risk for ampicillin-induced maculopapular rash. Appearance of a rash should be carefully evaluated to differentiate a nonallergic ampicillin rash from a hypersensitivity reaction; rash occurs in 5% to 10% of children and is a generalized dull red, maculopapular rash, generally appearing 3-14 days after the start of therapy. It normally begins on the trunk and spreads over most of the body. It may be most intense at pressure areas, elbows, and knees. A high percentage (43% to 100%) of patients with infectious mononucleosis have developed rash during ampicillin therapy; ampicillin-class antibiotics are not recommended in these patients. Prolonged use may result in fungal or bacterial superinfection, including *C. difficile*-associated diarrhea (CDAD) and pseudomembranous colitis; CDAD has been observed >2 months postantibiotic treatment. Seizures have been reported with rapid I.V. administration (over <3 minutes) of ampicillin.

Precautions Use with caution in patients with renal impairment; dosage adjustment recommended; use with caution in patients allergic to cephalosporins and asthmatic patients.

Adverse Reactions Also see Ampicillin.

Cardiovascular: Thrombophlebitis

Dermatologic: Skin rash

Gastrointestinal: Diarrhea

Hypersensitivity: Hypersensitivity reaction (may include serum sickness, urticaria, bronchospasm, hypotension, etc)

Local: Pain at injection site (I.M./I.V.)

Rare but important or life-threatening: Abdominal distention, agranulocytosis, anemia, candidiasis, chest pain, chills, constriction of the pharynx, dysuria, edema, eosinophilia, epistaxis, erythema, facial swelling, fatigue, flatulence, gastritis, glossitis, hairy tongue, headache, increased liver enzymes, interstitial nephritis, leukopenia, lymphocytosis (abnormal), malaise, mucous membrane bleeding, nausea, pruritus, pseudomembranous colitis, seizure, stomatitis, substernal pain, thrombocytopenia, urinary retention, vomiting

Drug Interactions

Metabolism/Transport Effects None known.

Avoid Concomitant Use

Avoid concomitant use of Ampicillin and Sulbactam with any of the following: BCG; Probenecid

Increased Effect/Toxicity

Ampicillin and Sulbactam may increase the levels/effects of: Methotrexate; Vitamin K Antagonists

The levels/effects of Ampicillin and Sulbactam may be increased by: Allopurinol; Probenecid

Decreased Effect

Ampicillin and Sulbactam may decrease the levels/effects of: Atenolol; BCG; Mycophenolate; Sodium Picosulfate; Typhoid Vaccine

The levels/effects of Ampicillin and Sulbactam may be decreased by: Chloroquine; Lanthanum; Tetracycline Derivatives

Stability Store intact vials at 20°C to 25°C (68°F to 77°F).

I.M.: Concentration of 250 mg ampicillin/mL should be used within 1 hour after preparation with SWI or lidocaine (0.5% or 2%)

Intermittent I.V. infusion: Solutions further diluted in NS are stable up to 72 hours (20 mg ampicillin/mL) under refrigeration (4°C) compared to dextrose solutions (at same concentrations) which are stable for only 4 hours

Mechanism of Action Inhibits bacterial cell wall synthesis by binding to one or more of the penicillin-binding proteins (PBPs) which in turn inhibits the final transpeptidation step of peptidoglycan synthesis in bacterial cell walls, thus inhibiting cell wall biosynthesis. Bacteria eventually lyse due to ongoing activity of cell wall autolytic enzymes (autolysins and murein hydrolases) while cell wall assembly is arrested. The addition of sulbactam, a beta-lactamase inhibitor, to ampicillin extends the spectrum of ampicillin to include some beta-lactamase-producing organisms.

Pharmacokinetics (Adult data unless noted)

Ampicillin: See Ampicillin monograph

Sulbactam:

Distribution: Into bile, blister and tissue fluids; poor penetration into CSF with uninflamed meninges; higher concentrations attained with inflamed meninges; V_d (Nahata, 1999):

Children 1-12 years: ~0.35 L/kg

Adults: 0.25 L/kg

Protein binding: 38%

Half-life:

Children 1-12 years: Mean range: ~0.7-0.9 hours with normal renal function (Nahata, 1999)

Adults: 1-1.3 hours with normal renal function

Elimination: Urine (~75% to 85% as unchanged drug) within 8 hours

Dosing: Neonatal Note: Unasyn® (ampicillin/sulbactam) is a combination product formulated in a 2:1 ratio (eg, each 3 g vial contains 2 g of ampicillin and 1 g of sulbactam); review dosing units carefully. Dosage recommendations are expressed as mg of the **ampicillin** component.

Susceptible infection (non-CNS), treatment: I.V.:

Premature neonate: 100 mg/kg/day divided every 12 hours; dosing based on a pharmacokinetic analysis of 15 premature neonates using a 1:1 formulation of ampicillin to sulbactam (GA ≤28 weeks: n=6; GA >28 weeks: n=9) (Sutton, 1986)

Full-term neonate: 100 mg/kg/day divided every 8 hours for ≤8 days was used in 108 neonates (GA ≥37 weeks) (Manzoni, 2009)

Dosing: Usual Note: Unasyn® (ampicillin/sulbactam) is a combination product formulated in a 2:1 ratio (eg, each 3 g vial contains 2 g of ampicillin and 1 g of sulbactam); review dosing units carefully.

Infants, Children, and Adolescents <40 kg: **Note:** Dosage recommendations are expressed as mg of the **ampicillin** component.

General dosing, susceptible infection:

AAP dosing:

Mild to moderate infection: I.V.: 100-200 mg ampicillin/kg/day divided every 6 hours; maximum dose: 1000 mg ampicillin (*Red Book*, 2012); may also be administered I.M. (Bradley, 2012)

Severe infection: I.V.: 200 mg ampicillin/kg/day divided every 6 hours; maximum dose: 2000 mg (*Red Book*, 2012); higher doses up to 400 mg ampicillin/kg/day may be required for some infections (ie, meningitis)

Manufacturer's labeling: Children ≥1 year and Adolescents <40 kg: I.V.: 200 mg ampicillin/kg/day divided every 6 hours; maximum dose: 2000 mg ampicillin

Endocarditis, treatment: I.V.: 200 mg ampicillin/kg/day divided every 4-6 hours with gentamicin (optional; dependent upon organism) for at least 4-6 weeks; some organisms may require longer duration (Baddour, 2005) ▶

163

Intra-abdominal infection: I.V.: 200 mg ampicillin/kg/day divided every 6 hours; **Note:** Due to high rates of *E. coli* resistance, not recommended for the treatment of community-acquired intra-abdominal infections (Solomkin, 2010)

Meningitis: I.V.: 200-400 mg ampicillin/kg/day divided every 6 hours (*Red Book*, 2009)

Rhinosinusitis, severe infection requiring hospitalization: Children and Adolescents: I.V.: 200-400 mg ampicillin/kg/day divided every 6 hours for 10-14 days; maximum dose: 2000 mg ampicillin (Chow, 2012)

Skin, soft tissue infection: I.V.: 200 mg ampicillin/kg/day divided every 6 hours

Children ≥40 kg and Adolescents ≥40 kg: **Note:** Doses expressed as total grams of the **ampicillin/sulbactam combination**.

General dosing, susceptible infection: I.M., I.V.: 1.5-3 **g** every 6 hours (maximum daily dose: Unasyn® 12 g/day)

Amnionitis, cholangitis, diverticulitis, endometritis (with doxycycline), endophthalmitis, epididymitis/orchitis, liver abscess (with metronidazole), peritonitis: I.V.: 3 **g** every 6 hours; **Note:** Due to high rates of *E. coli* resistance, not recommended for the treatment of community-acquired intra-abdominal infections (Solomkin, 2010)

Bite (human, canine/feline): *Pasteurella multocida:* I.V.: 1.5-3 **g** every 6 hours (Stevens, 2005)

Endocarditis: I.V.: 3 **g** every 6 hours with gentamicin (optional; dependent upon organism) for 4-6 weeks (Baddour, 2005)

Pelvic inflammatory disease: I.V.: 3 **g** every 6 hours with doxycycline (CDC, 2010)

Rhinosinusitis, severe infection requiring hospitalization: I.V.: 1.5-3 **g** every 6 hours for 5-7 days (Chow, 2012)

Urinary tract infections, pyelonephritis: I.V.: 3 **g** every 6 hours for 14 days

Adults: **Note:** Doses expressed as total grams of the **ampicillin/sulbactam combination. General dosing, susceptible infection:** I.M., I.V.: 1.5-3 **g** every 6 hours (maximum daily dose: Unasyn® 12 **g**/day)

Dosing interval in renal impairment: Children and Adults: **Note:** Doses expressed as **ampicillin/sulbactam combination**. I.V.:

CrCl ≥30 mL/minute/1.73 m^2: No dosage adjustment required.

CrCl 15-29 mL/minute/1.73 m^2: Administer every 12 hours.

CrCl 5-14 mL/minute/1.73 m^2: Administer every 24 hours.

Intermittent hemodialysis (IHD): Adults: 1.5-3 **g** every 12-24 hours (administer after hemodialysis on dialysis days) (Heintz, 2009). **Note:** Dosing dependent on the assumption of 3 times/week, complete IHD sessions.

Peritoneal dialysis (PD): Adults: 3 **g** every 24 hours

Continuous renal replacement therapy (CRRT): Adults: Drug clearance is highly dependent on the method of renal replacement, filter type, and flow rate. Appropriate dosing requires close monitoring of pharmacologic response, signs of adverse reactions due to drug accumulation, as well as drug concentrations in relation to target trough (if appropriate). The following are general recommendations only (based on dialysate flow/ultrafiltration rates of 1-2 L/hour and minimal residual renal function) and should not supersede clinical judgment (Heintz, 2009; Trotman, 2005):

CVVH: Initial: 3 **g**; maintenance: 1.5-3 **g** every 8-12 hours

CVVHD: Initial: 3 **g**; maintenance: 1.5-3 **g** every 8 hours

CVVHDF: Initial: 3 **g**; maintenance: 1.5-3 **g** every 6-8 hours

Administration Parenteral:

I.M.: Reconstitute with SWI or lidocaine (0.5% or 2%) to a final concentration of 375 mg/mL of Unasyn® (ie, 250 mg/mL of ampicillin and 125 mg/mL of sulbactam); administer by deep I.M. injection

I.V.: Administered by slow I.V. injection over 10-15 minutes or by intermittent I.V. infusion over 15-30 minutes; final concentration should not exceed 45 mg/mL Unasyn® (30 mg/mL of ampicillin and 15 mg/mL of sulbactam)

Monitoring Parameters With prolonged therapy monitor hematologic, renal, and hepatic function; observe for change in bowel frequency; monitor for signs of anaphylaxis during first dose

Test Interactions May interfere with urinary glucose tests using cupric sulfate (Benedict's solution, Clinitest®).

Some penicillin derivatives may accelerate the degradation of aminoglycosides *in vitro*, leading to a potential underestimation of aminoglycoside serum concentration.

Additional Information Some penicillins (eg, carbenicillin, ticarcillin, and piperacillin) have been shown to inactivate aminoglycosides *in vitro*. This has been observed to a greater extent with tobramycin and gentamicin, while amikacin has shown greater stability against inactivation. Concomitant use of these agents may pose a risk of reduced antibacterial efficacy *in vivo*, particularly in the setting of profound renal impairment; however, definitive clinical evidence is lacking. If combination penicillin/aminoglycoside therapy is desired in a patient with renal dysfunction, separation of doses (if feasible), and routine monitoring of aminoglycoside concentrations, CBC, and clinical response should be considered.

Dosage Forms Excipient information presented when available (limited, particularly for generics); consult specific product labeling.

Injection, powder for reconstitution: 1.5 g: Ampicillin 1 g and sulbactam 0.5 g; 3 g: Ampicillin 2 g and sulbactam 1 g; 15 g: Ampicillin 10 g and sulbactam 5 g

Unasyn®:

1.5 g: Ampicillin 1 g and sulbactam 0.5 g [contains sodium 115 mg (5 mEq)/1.5 g)]

3 g: Ampicillin 2 g and sulbactam 1 g [contains sodium 115 mg (5 mEq)/1.5 g)]

15 g: Ampicillin 10 g and sulbactam 5 g [bulk package; contains sodium 115 mg (5 mEq)/1.5 g)]

References

American Academy of Pediatrics (AAP). In: Pickering LK, Baker CJ, Kimberlin DW, Long SS, eds. *Red Book: 2012 Report of the Committee on Infectious Diseases.* 29th ed. Elk Grove Village, IL: American Academy of Pediatrics; 2012.

Baddour LM, Wilson WR, Bayer AS, et al, "Infective Endocarditis: Diagnosis, Antimicrobial Therapy, and Management of Complications: A Statement for Healthcare Professionals From the Committee on Rheumatic Fever, Endocarditis, and Kawasaki Disease, Council on Cardiovascular Disease in the Young, and the Councils on Clinical Cardiology, Stroke, and Cardiovascular Surgery and Anesthesia, American Heart Association: Endorsed by the Infectious Diseases Society of America," *Circulation,* 2005, 111(23):e394-434.

Bradley JS, Nelson JD, Kimberlin DK, et al, eds. *Nelson's Pocket Book of Pediatric Antimicrobial Therapy.* 19th ed. Philadelphia, PA: Lippincott Williams & Wilkins; 2012.

Chow AW, Benninger MS, Brook I, et al, "IDSA Clinical Practice Guideline for Acute Bacterial Rhinosinusitis in Children and Adults," *Clin Infect Dis,* 2012, 54(8):e72-112.

Heintz BH, Matzke GR, Dager WE, "Antimicrobial Dosing Concepts and Recommendations for Critically Ill Adult Patients Receiving Continuous Renal Replacement Therapy or Intermittent Hemodialysis," *Pharmacotherapy,* 2009, 29(5):562-77.

Li PK, Szeto CC, Piraino B, et al, "Peritoneal Dialysis-Related Infections Recommendations: 2010 Update," *Perit Dial Int,* 2010, 30(4):393-423.

Lipsky BA, Berendt AR, Cornia PB, et al, "2012 Infectious Diseases Society of America Clinical Practice Guideline for the Diagnosis and Treatment of Diabetic Foot Infections," *Clin Infect Dis,* 2012, 54(12):e132-73.

Manzoni P, Esposito S, Gallo E, et al, "Switch Therapy in Full-Term Neonates With Presumed or Proven Bacterial Infection," *J Chemother,* 2009, 21(1):68-73.

Mermel LA, Allon M, Bouza E, et al, "Clinical Practice Guidelines for the Diagnosis and Management of Intravascular Catheter-Related Infection: 2009 Update by the Infectious Diseases Society of America," *Clin Infect Dis*, 2009, 49(1):1-45.

Nahata MC, Vashi VI, Swanson RN, et al, "Pharmacokinetics of Ampicillin and Sulbactam in Pediatric Patients," *Antimicrob Agents Chemother*, 1999, 43(5):1225-9.

Red Book: 2009 Report of the Committee on Infectious Diseases, "Amebiasis," 28th ed, Pickering LK, ed, Elk Grove Village, IL: American Academy of Pediatrics, 2009. Available at http://aapredbook.-aappublications.org/cgi/content/full/2009/1/3.3

Solomkin JS, Mazuski JE, Bradley JS, et al, "Diagnosis and Management of Complicated Intra-Abdominal Infections in Adults and Children: Guidelines by the Surgical Infection Society and the Infectious Diseases Society of America," *Clin Infect Dis*, 2010, 50(2):133-64.

Stevens DL, Bisno AL, Chambers HF, et al, "Practice Guidelines for the Diagnosis and Management of Skin and Soft-Tissue Infections," *Clin Infect Dis*, 2005, 41(10):1373-406.

Sutton AM, Turner TL, Cockburn F, et al, "Pharmacokinetic Study of Sulbactam and Ampicillin Administered Concomitantly by Intraarterial or Intravenous Infusion in the Newborn," *Rev Infect Dis*, 1986, 8 (Suppl 5):518-22.

Trotman RL, Williamson JC, Shoemaker DM, et al, "Antibiotic Dosing in Critically Ill Adult Patients Receiving Continuous Renal Replacement Therapy," *Clin Infect Dis*, 2005, 41(8):1159-66.

Workowski KA, Berman S, and Centers for Disease Control and Prevention (CDC), "Sexually Transmitted Diseases Treatment Guidelines, 2010," *MMWR Recomm Rep*, 2010, 59(RR-12):1-110.

◆ **Ampicillin for Injection (Can)** *see* Ampicillin *on page 159*

◆ **Ampicillin Sodium** *see* Ampicillin *on page 159*

◆ **Ampicillin Trihydrate** *see* Ampicillin *on page 159*

◆ **Amrix** *see* Cyclobenzaprine *on page 558*

◆ **Amylase, Lipase, and Protease** *see* Pancrelipase *on page 1591*

Amyl Nitrite (AM il NYE trite)

Therapeutic Category Antidote, Cyanide; Vasodilator, Coronary

Generic Availability (U.S.) Yes

Use Treatment of angina pectoris (FDA approved in adults); has also been used as an adjunct treatment of cyanide poisoning

Note: Given the widespread use of newer nitrate compounds, the use of amyl nitrite for patients experiencing angina pectoris has fallen out of favor.

Pregnancy Risk Factor C

Pregnancy Considerations Animal reproduction studies have not been conducted. Because amyl nitrate significantly decreases systemic blood pressure and therefore blood flow to the fetus, use is contraindicated in pregnancy (per manufacturer). In addition, fetal hemoglobin may be more susceptible methemoglobin conversion (Valenzuela, 1986).

Breast-Feeding Considerations It is not known if amyl nitrite is excreted in breast milk. The manufacturer recommends that caution be exercised when administering amyl nitrite to nursing women.

Contraindications Hypersensitivity to nitrates or any component; recent head trauma or cerebral hemorrhage; glaucoma; pregnancy

Warnings Amyl nitrite may cause methemoglobin formation and severe hypotension resulting in diminished oxygen-carrying capacity; serious adverse effects may occur at doses less than twice the recommended therapeutic dose. Monitor for adequate perfusion and oxygenation; ensure patient is euvolemic. Use with caution in patients with preexisting diminished oxygen or cardiovascular reserve (eg, smoke inhalation victims, anemia, substantial blood loss, and cardiac or respiratory compromise), in patients at greater risk for developing methemoglobinemia (eg, infants or patients with congenital methemoglobin reductase deficiency) and in patients who may be susceptible to injury from vasodilation; the use of hydroxocobalamin is recommended in these patients. Amyl nitrite may cause harm to the fetus if administered to a pregnant woman; may significantly decrease systemic blood pressure and blood flow.

Due to the risk for serious adverse effects, use with caution in patients in whom the diagnosis of cyanide poisoning is uncertain; however, if clinical suspicion of cyanide poisoning is high, treatment should not be delayed. Treatment of cyanide poisoning should include decontamination and supportive therapy. Collection of pretreatment blood cyanide concentrations does not preclude administration and should not delay administration in the emergency management of highly suspected or confirmed cyanide toxicity. Pretreatment levels may be useful as postinfusion levels may be inaccurate. Monitor patients for return of symptoms for 24-48 hours; repeat treatment should be administered if symptoms return. Consider consultation with a poison control center at 1-800-222-1222.

Fire victims may present with both cyanide and carbon monoxide poisoning. Carbon monoxide poisoning leads to carboxyhemoglobinemia which decreases the oxygen-carrying capacity; use of amyl nitrite which induces methemoglobinemia may worsen oxygen-carrying capacity. In this scenario, sodium thiosulfate may be used alone to promote the clearance of cyanide. Due to the slow onset of action of sodium thiosulfate, may consider using hydroxocobalamin alone or in combination with sodium thiosulfate (Howland, 2011).

Precautions Use with caution in patients with coronary artery disease and patients with hypotension; transient episodes of dizziness, weakness, syncope, and cerebral ischemia secondary to postural hypotension may occur. Use with caution in patients with increased intracranial pressure; use is contraindicated in patients with recent head trauma or cerebral hemorrhage. Use with extreme caution or avoid in patients with severe aortic stenosis; may reduce coronary perfusion resulting in ischemia; considered by some to be a contraindication (Reagan, 2005).

Adverse Reactions

Cardiovascular: Cerebral ischemia, facial flushing, hypotension, orthostatic hypotension, pallor, shock, syncope, tachycardia, vasodilation

Central nervous system: Dizziness, headache, intracranial pressure increased, restlessness

Dermatologic: Dermatitis, irritation

Gastrointestinal: Fecal incontinence, nausea, vomiting

Genitourinary: Urinary incontinence

Hematologic: Hemolytic anemia, methemoglobinemia

Neuromuscular & skeletal: Weakness

Ocular: Intraocular pressure increased, irritation

Miscellaneous: Diaphoresis

Drug Interactions

Metabolism/Transport Effects None known.

Avoid Concomitant Use

Avoid concomitant use of Amyl Nitrite with any of the following: Phosphodiesterase 5 Inhibitors; Riociguat

Increased Effect/Toxicity

Amyl Nitrite may increase the levels/effects of: DULoxetine; Hypotensive Agents; Prilocaine; Riociguat; Sodium Nitrite

The levels/effects of Amyl Nitrite may be increased by: Barbiturates; Nitric Oxide; Phosphodiesterase 5 Inhibitors

Decreased Effect There are no known significant interactions involving a decrease in effect.

Stability Store at 2°C to 8°C (36°F to 46°F), protect from light; flammable, avoid exposure to heat or flame

Mechanism of Action Relaxes vascular smooth muscle; decreases venous ratios and arterial blood pressure; ▶

reduces left ventricular work; decreases myocardial O_2 consumption. When used for cyanide poisoning, amyl nitrite promotes the formation of methemoglobin which competes with cytochrome oxidase for the cyanide ion. Cyanide combines with methemoglobin to form cyanomethemoglobin, thereby freeing the cytochrome oxidase and allowing aerobic metabolism to continue.

Pharmacodynamics

Onset of action: Angina: Within 30 seconds
Duration: Angina: 3-5 minutes

Pharmacokinetics (Adult data unless noted)

Absorption: Inhalation: Readily absorbed through respiratory tract
Metabolism: In the liver to form inorganic nitrates (less potent)
Half-life:
Amyl nitrite: <1 hour
Methemoglobin: 1 hour
Elimination: Renal; ~33%

Dosing: Usual

Infants, Children and Adolescents:
Cyanide poisoning: Inhalation: 0.3 mL ampul crushed into a gauze pad and placed in front of the patient's mouth (or endotracheal tube if patient is intubated) to inhale over 15-30 seconds; repeat every minute until sodium nitrite can be administered. **Note:** Must separate administrations by at least 30 seconds to allow for adequate oxygenation; each ampul will last for ~3 minutes. Amyl nitrite is a temporary intervention that should only be used until I.V. sodium nitrite infusion is ready for administration.

Adults:
Cyanide poisoning: Inhalation: 0.3 mL ampul crushed into a gauze pad and placed in front of the patient's mouth (or endotracheal tube if patient is intubated) to inhale over 15-30 seconds; repeat every minute until sodium nitrite can be administered. **Note:** Must separate administrations by at least 30 seconds to allow for adequate oxygenation; each ampul will last for ~3 minutes. Amyl nitrite is a temporary intervention that should only be used until I.V. sodium nitrite infusion is ready for administration.

Angina: Inhalation: 2-6 nasal inhalations from 1 crushed ampul; may repeat in 3-5 minutes

Administration Administer nasally via inhalation. The patient should be lying down during administration. Crush the ampul in a gauze pad and place in front of patient's mouth (or endotracheal tube if intubated) and allow patient to inhale for 15-30 seconds; repeat every minute until sodium nitrite can be administered. One ampul lasts for ~3 minutes.

Monitoring Parameters Monitor blood pressure and heart rate during therapy
Cyanide poisoning: Monitor for at least 24-48 hours after administration; hemoglobin/hematocrit; co-oximetry; serum lactate levels; venous-arterial PO_2 gradient; serum methemoglobin and oxyhemoglobin. Pretreatment cyanide levels may be useful diagnostically.

Reference Range Symptoms associated with blood cyanide levels:
Flushing and tachycardia: 0.5-1 mcg/mL
Obtundation: 1-2.5 mcg/mL
Coma and respiratory depression: >2.5 mcg/mL
Death: >3 mcg/mL

Dosage Forms Excipient information presented when available (limited, particularly for generics); consult specific product labeling.
Liquid, for inhalation: USP: 85% to 103% (0.3 mL)

References

Agency for Toxic Substances and Disease Registry (ATSDR), "Medical Management Guidelines for Hydrogen Cyanide (HCN)," 2001. Available at http://www.atsdr.cdc.gov/MHMI/mmg8.pdf

Berlin CM Jr, "The Treatment of Cyanide Poisoning in Children," Pediatrics, 1970, 46(5):793-6.
Geller RJ, Barthold C, Saiers JA, et al, "Pediatric Cyanide Poisoning: Causes, Manifestations, Management, and Unmet Needs," Pediatrics, 2006, 118(5):2146-58.
Gracia R and Shepherd G, "Cyanide Poisoning and Its Treatment," Pharmacotherapy, 2004, 24(10):1358-65.
Hall AH, Dart R, and Bogdan G, "Sodium Thiosulfate or Hydroxocobalamin for the Empiric Treatment of Cyanide Poisoning?" Ann Emerg Med, 2007, 49(6):806-13.
Howland MA, "Antidotes in Depth: Sodium and Amyl Nitrite," Goldfrank's Toxicologic Emergencies, 9th ed, Nelson LS, Hoffman RS, Lewin NA, et al, eds, New York, NY: McGraw-Hill Companies, Inc, 2011, 1519-22.
Lavon O and Bentur Y, "Does Amyl Nitrite Have a Role in the Management of Pre-Hospital Mass Casualty Cyanide Poisoning?" Clin Toxicol (Phila), 2010, 48(6):477-84.
Mokhlesi B, Leikin JB, Murray P, et al, "Adult Toxicology in Critical Care: Part II: Specific Poisonings," Chest, 2003, 123(3):897-922.
Nichol LM, Mills NL, and Starkey IR, "Amyl Nitrite Induced Cerebral and Coronary Vasospasm," QJM, 2011, 104(1):83-4.
Reagan BW, Helmcke F, and Kerut EK, "Commonly Used Respiratory and Pharmacologic Interventions in the Echocardiography Laboratory," Echocardiography, 2005, 22(5):455-60.
Valenzuela A, Guerra R, Lazcano L, et al, "Differential Prooxidative Effect of Adult and Fetal Hemoglobin," FEBS Lett, 1986, 196 (2):353-6.

◆ **Amylobarbitone** see Amobarbital on page 138

◆ **Amytal® (Can)** see Amobarbital on page 138

◆ **Amytal Sodium** see Amobarbital on page 138

◆ **Anacaine** see Benzocaine on page 273

◆ **Anafranil** see ClomiPRAMINE on page 510

◆ **Anafranil® (Can)** see ClomiPRAMINE on page 510

Anagrelide (an AG gre lide)

Medication Safety Issues
Sound-alike/look-alike issues:
Anagrelide may be confused with anastrozole

Brand Names: U.S. Agrylin

Brand Names: Canada Agrylin; Dom-Anagrelide; Mylan-Anagrelide; PMS-Anagrelide; Sandoz-Anagrelide

Therapeutic Category Antiplatelet Agent; Phosphodiesterase Enzyme Inhibitor; Phosphodiestrerase-3 Enzyme Inhibitor

Generic Availability (U.S.) Yes

Use Treatment of thrombocythemia secondary to myeloproliferative disorders to decrease elevated platelet count and the associated risk of thrombosis and ameliorate symptoms including thrombo-hemorrhagic events (FDA approved in ages >6 years and adults)

Pregnancy Risk Factor C

Pregnancy Considerations Adverse events were observed in some animal reproduction studies. Data regarding use of anagrelide during pregnancy is limited. The manufacturer recommends effective contraception in women of childbearing potential.

Breast-Feeding Considerations It is not known if anagrelide is excreted in breast milk. Due to the potential for serious adverse reactions in the nursing infant, a decision should be made whether to discontinue nursing or to discontinue the drug, taking into account the importance of treatment to the mother.

Contraindications Hypersensitivity to anagrelide or any component; severe hepatic impairment

Warnings Ventricular tachycardia and torsade de pointes have been reported with anagrelide therapy. In a clinical trial of adult patients, dose-related increases in heart rate and mean QT_c interval have been observed; the maximum change in mean heart rate was ~8 beats per minute (bpm) at a dose of 0.5 mg and ~29 bpm with a 2.5 mg dose; the maximum mean change in QT_c I (individual subject correlation) from placebo was 7 ms and 13 ms with doses of 0.5 mg and 2.5 mg, respectively. Prior to initiating therapy, obtain a baseline EKG and cardiovascular examination and monitor periodically during therapy. Do not use in patients with hypokalemia, congenital long QT syndrome, a known history of acquired QT_c prolongation, or with concomitant drugs which may prolong the QT_c interval.

As with other phosphodiesterase 3 (PDE3) inhibitors, anagrelide may cause vasodilation, tachycardia, palpitations, and heart failure; PDE3 inhibitors are associated with decreased survival (compared to placebo) in patients with class III or IV heart failure. Hypotension accompanied by dizziness may occur, particularly with higher doses. Use with caution in patients with known or suspected cardiovascular disease (eg, heart failure, bradyarrhythmias, electrolyte abnormalities); benefits should outweigh risks; pretreatment cardiovascular evaluation (including ECG) and careful monitoring during treatment is recommended.

Interstitial lung disease including allergic alveolitis, eosinophilic pneumonia, and interstitial pneumonitis has been associated with use; onset is from 1 week to several years, usually presenting with progressive dyspnea with lung infiltrations; symptoms usually improve after discontinuation. Renal abnormalities including renal failure have been observed with anagrelide use; may be associated with preexisting renal impairment, although dosage adjustment due to renal insufficiency not required; monitor closely in patients with renal insufficiency.

Precautions Use with caution in patients with mild to moderate hepatic impairment; in patients with moderate impairment, anagrelide exposure was increased eightfold; dosage reduction is required; monitor patients for cardiovascular effect and QT_c prolongation; use is contraindicated in severe hepatic impairment. Hepatotoxicity (elevated ALT and AST) may occur; monitor liver function prior to and during treatment. Use caution with concomitant aspirin therapy; major hemorrhagic events have been reported; other potentially significant interactions may exist, requiring dose or frequency adjustment, additional monitoring, and/or selection of alternative therapy. Consult drug interactions database for more detailed information.

Adverse Reactions
Cardiovascular: Angina pectoris, cardiac arrhythmia, cardiac failure, chest pain, edema, hypertension, orthostatic hypotension, palpitations, peripheral edema, syncope, tachycardia, thrombosis, vasodilatation
Central nervous system: Amnesia, chills, confusion, depression, dizziness, drowsiness, headache, insomnia, malaise, migraine, nervousness, pain, paresthesia
Dermatologic: Alopecia, pruritus, skin rash, skin photosensitivity
Endocrine & skeletal: Dehydration
Gastrointestinal: Abdominal pain, anorexia, aphthous stomatitis, constipation, diarrhea, dyspepsia, eructation, flatulence, gastritis, gastrointestinal distress, gastrointestinal hemorrhage, melena, nausea, vomiting
Genitourinary: Dysuria
Hematologic & oncologic: Anemia, bruise, hemorrhage, lymphadenopathy, thrombocytopenia
Neuromuscular & skeletal: Arthralgia, back pain, leg cramps, myalgia, weakness
Ophthalmic: Amblyopia, diplopia, visual field defect
Otic: Tinnitus
Renal: Hematuria, renal function abnormality, renal failure
Respiratory: Asthma, bronchitis, cough, dyspnea, epistaxis, flu-like symptoms, pharyngitis, pneumonia, rhinitis, sinusitis
Miscellaneous: Fever
Rare but important or life-threatening: Atrial fibrillation, cardiomegaly, cardiomyopathy, cerebrovascular accident, complete atrioventricular block, duodenal ulcer, eosinophilic pneumonia, gastric ulcer, hepatotoxicity, hypersensitivity pneumonitis, increased serum ALT, increased serum AST, interstitial nephritis, interstitial

pneumonitis, leukocytosis, myocardial infarction, pancreatitis, pericardial effusion, pericarditis, pleural effusion, prolonged Q-T interval on ECG, pulmonary fibrosis, pulmonary hypertension, pulmonary infiltrates, seizure, torsades de pointes, ventricular tachycardia

Drug Interactions
Metabolism/Transport Effects Substrate of CYP1A2 (minor)
Avoid Concomitant Use
Avoid concomitant use of Anagrelide with any of the following: Highest Risk QTc-Prolonging Agents; Ivabradine; Mifepristone; Moderate Risk QTc-Prolonging Agents; Riociguat; Urokinase
Increased Effect/Toxicity Antiplatelet agents may enhance the adverse/toxic effects of drotrecogin alfa. Concurrent use of NSAIDs, salicylates, or treprostinil may enhance the adverse/toxic effects of antiplatelet agents.
Decreased Effect
The levels/effects of Anagrelide may be decreased by: Nonsteroidal Anti-Inflammatory Agents
Food Interactions Food has no clinically significant effect on absorption. Management: Administer without regard to meals.
Stability Store at 25°C (77°F); excursions permitted to 15°C to 30°C (59°F to 86°F); protect from light.
Mechanism of Action Anagrelide appears to inhibit cyclic nucleotide phosphodiesterase and the release of arachidonic acid from phospholipase, possibly by inhibiting phospholipase A_2. It also causes a dose-related reduction in platelet production, which results from decreased megakaryocyte hypermaturation (disrupts the postmitotic phase of maturation).
Pharmacodynamics
Onset of action: Initial: Within 7-14 days
Maximum effect: Complete response (platelets ≤600,000/mm³): 4-12 weeks
Duration: 6-24 hours; upon discontinuation, platelet count begins to rise within 4 days
Pharmacokinetics (Adult data unless noted) Note: In pediatric patients 7-14 years; data has shown a decreased maximum serum concentration (48%) and AUC (55%) compared to adults when normalized to dose and bodyweight.
Metabolism: Hepatic, partially via CYP1A2; to two major metabolites, RL603 and 3-hydroxy anagrelide
Bioavailability: Food has no clinically significant effect
Half-life, elimination: 1.3 hours; similar data reported in pediatric patients 7-14 years
Time to peak, serum concentration: 1 hour; similar data reported in pediatric patients 7-14 years.
Elimination: Urine (<1% as unchanged drug)
Dosing: Usual
Pediatric:
Essential thrombocythemia: Very limited data available; several small case series: Children ≥6 years and Adolescents: Oral: Initial: 0.5 mg 2-3 times daily; increase at weekly intervals in 0.5 mg increments until platelet count begins to decrease; usual reported maintenance dose range: 1-2.5 mg/day; maximum daily dose: 10 mg/**day** (per manufacturer) although the maximum reported dose for essential thrombocythemia: 4 mg/**day**; once platelet count normalizes, further adjust dose to lowest effective dose; in some cases, discontinuation of therapy has been accomplished (Chintagumpala, 1995; Lackner, 1998; Lackner, 2006); **Note:** Essential thrombocytopenia is also considered a type myeloproliferative disorder.

Secondary thrombocythemia (associated with myeloproliferative disorders): Children >6 years and Adolescents: Oral: Initial: 0.5 mg once daily; usual range: 0.5 mg 1-4 times daily; median maintenance daily dose: Patient age 7-11 years: 1.75 mg/day; patient age: 11-14 years: 2 mg; **Note:** Maintain initial dose for ≥1 week, then adjust to the lowest effective dose to reduce and maintain platelet count <600,000/mm^3 ideally to the normal range; the dose must not be increased by >0.5 mg per day in any 1 week; maximum single dose: 2.5 mg; maximum daily dose: 10 mg/**day**

Adult: **Thrombocythemia:** Oral: Initial: 0.5 mg 4 times daily or 1 mg twice daily (most patients will experience adequate response at dose ranges of 1.5-3 mg/day); **Note:** Maintain initial dose for ≥1 week, then adjust to the lowest effective dose to reduce and maintain platelet count <600,000/mm^3 ideally to the normal range; the dose must not be increased by >0.5 mg per day in any 1 week; maximum single dose: 2.5 mg; maximum daily dose: 10 mg

Dosing adjustment in renal impairment: Children, Adolescents, and Adults: No adjustment required in renal insufficiency; monitor closely.

Dosing adjustment in hepatic impairment: Adults: Moderate impairment: Initial: 0.5 mg once daily; maintain for at least 1 week with careful monitoring of cardiovascular status; the dose must not be increased by >0.5 mg/day in any 1 week

Severe impairment: Use is contraindicated

Administration May be administered without regard to food.

Monitoring Parameters Platelet count (every 2 days during the first week of treatment and at least weekly until the maintenance dose is reached; continue to monitor after cessation of treatment); CBC with differential (monitor closely during first 2 weeks of treatment), liver function (ALT and AST; baseline and during treatment), BUN, and serum creatinine (monitor closely during first weeks of treatment); serum electrolytes; blood pressure; heart rate; cardiovascular exam including ECG (pretreatment; monitor during therapy), signs/symptoms of interstitial lung disease. Monitor for thrombosis or bleeding.

Dosage Forms Excipient information presented when available (limited, particularly for generics); consult specific product labeling.

Capsule, Oral:
Agrylin: 0.5 mg
Generic: 0.5 mg, 1 mg

References

Agrylin (anagrelide) [prescribing information]. Wayne, PA: Shire US Inc; February 2014.

Chintagumpala MM, Kennedy LL, Steuber CP. Treatment of essential thrombocythemia with anagrelide. *J Pediatr.* 1995;127:495-198.

Doubek M, Brychtova Y, Doubek R, et al. Anagrelide therapy in pregnancy: report of a case of essential thrombocythemia. *Ann Hematol.* 2004;83(11):726-727.

Giona F, Teofili L, Moleti ML, et al. Thrombocythemia and polycythemia in patients younger than 20 years at diagnosis: clinical and biologic features, treatment, and long-term outcome. *Blood.* 2012;119(10): 2219-2227.

Lackner H, Urban C, Benesch M, et al. Long-term use of anagrelide in the treatment of children with essential thrombocythemia. *Eur J Haematol.* 2006;77:358-359.

Lackner H, Urban C, Beham-Schmid C, et al. Treatment of children with anagrelide for thrombocythemia. *J Pediatr Hematol/Oncol.* 1998;20 (5): 469-473.

Mazzucconi MG, Redi R, Bernasconi S, et al. A long-term study of young patients with essential thrombocythemia treated with anagrelide. *Hematologica.* 2004;89:1306-13.

◆ **Anagrelide Hydrochloride** *see* Anagrelide *on page 166*

Anakinra (an a KIN ra)

Medication Safety Issues
Sound-alike/look-alike issues:
Anakinra may be confused with amikacin, Ampyra™
Kineret® may be confused with Amikin®

Brand Names: U.S. Kineret

Brand Names: Canada Kineret®

Therapeutic Category Antirheumatic, Disease Modifying; Interleukin-1 Receptor Antagonist

Generic Availability (U.S.) No

Use Treatment of neonatal-onset multisystem inflammatory disease (NOMID), also known as chronic infantile neurological cutaneous and articular syndrome (CINCA), which is a cryopyrin-associated periodic syndrome (CAPS) [FDA approved in pediatric patients (age not specified) and adults]; treatment of moderately to severely active rheumatoid arthritis in patients who have failed one or more disease-modifying antirheumatic drugs (DMARDs); may be used alone or in combination with DMARDs that are not tumor necrosis factor (TNF)-blocking agents (eg, etanercept, adalimumab) (FDA approved in ages ≥18 years and adults); has also been used for reducing signs and symptoms of systemic onset juvenile idiopathic arthritic (SOJIA) and polyarticular-course juvenile idiopathic arthritis (JIA)

Pregnancy Risk Factor B

Pregnancy Considerations Animal reproduction studies have not revealed any evidence of impaired fertility or harm to fetus. Women exposed to anakinra during pregnancy may contact the Organization of Teratology Information Services (OTIS), Rheumatoid Arthritis and Pregnancy Study at 1-877-311-8972.

Breast-Feeding Considerations Endogenous interleukin-1 receptor antagonist can be found in breast milk; although specific excretion of anakinra is not known. Use caution if administering to a nursing woman.

Contraindications Hypersensitivity to *E. coli*-derived proteins, anakinra, or any component

Warnings Use associated with increased risk of developing serious infections; risk is higher if used concurrently with etanercept or if patient has asthma. Patients who develop a new infection while undergoing treatment should be monitored closely. If a patient receiving anakinra for rheumatoid arthritis develops a serious infection, therapy should be discontinued; if a patient receiving anakinra for NOMID develops a serious infection, the risk of a NOMID flare should be weighed against the risk associated with continued treatment. Do not initiate therapy in patients with active infection, including chronic or local infections. Safety and efficacy have not been evaluated in immunosuppressed patients or patients with chronic infection; the impact on active or chronic infections has not been determined. Immunosuppressive therapy (including anakinra) may lead to reactivation of latent tuberculosis or other atypical or opportunistic infections; test patients for latent TB prior to initiation, and treat latent TB infection prior to use. Use is not recommended in combination with tumor necrosis factor antagonists.

Injection contains polysorbate 80 (Tween 80®) which may cause allergic reactions in susceptible individuals. Infusion of polysorbate 80-containing solutions through polyvinyl chloride tubing may cause DEHP to leach into the solution; in immature animals, exposure to DEHP may adversely affect the development of the male reproductive tract. May cause angioedema, hypersensitivity, anaphylaxis, or anaphylactoid reactions; discontinue use if severe hypersensitivity occurs; medications for the treatment of hypersensitivity reactions should be available for immediate use.

Precautions Injection site reactions commonly occur and are generally mild with a duration of 14-28 days. Use may affect defenses against malignancies; impact on the development and course of malignancies is not fully defined. As compared to the general population, an increased risk of lymphoma has been noted in clinical trials; however, rheumatoid arthritis has been previously associated with an increased rate of lymphoma. Use with caution in patients with a history of significant hematologic abnormalities; therapy is associated with uncommon but significant decreases in hematologic parameters (particularly neutrophil counts). Assess neutrophil count at baseline, monthly for 3 months, then every 3 months for up to 1 year. In a limited number of patients with NOMID, neutropenia resolved over time with continued anakinra administration. Patients should be brought up-to-date with all immunizations before initiating therapy; live vaccines should not be given concurrently. There is no data available concerning the effects of therapy on vaccination or secondary transmission of live vaccines in patients receiving therapy. Patients with latex allergy should not handle the needle cover of the diluent syringe since it contains latex. Use with caution in patients with renal impairment; consider extended dosing intervals for severe renal dysfunction (CrCl <30 mL/minute) and end stage renal disease. Potentially significant interactions may exist, requiring dose or frequency adjustment, additional monitoring, and/or selection of alternative therapy. Consult drug interactions database for more detailed information.

Adverse Reactions
Central nervous system: Fever, headache
Gastrointestinal: Diarrhea, nausea
Hematologic: Neutropenia
Local: Injection site reaction
Neuromuscular & skeletal: Arthralgia
Respiratory: Nasopharyngitis
Miscellaneous: Infection (including serious)
Rare but important or life-threatening: Cellulitis, hepatitis (noninfectious), hypersensitivity reactions (including anaphylaxis, angioedema, pruritus, rash, urticaria), increased serum transaminases, leukopenia, opportunistic infection, pneumonia (bacterial), pulmonary fibrosis, secondary malignancies (including lymphoma, melanoma), thrombocytopenia

Drug Interactions
Metabolism/Transport Effects None known.
Avoid Concomitant Use
Avoid concomitant use of Anakinra with any of the following: Abatacept; Anti-TNF Agents; BCG; Canakinumab; Natalizumab; Pimecrolimus; Tacrolimus (Topical); Tofacitinib; Vaccines (Live)
Increased Effect/Toxicity
Anakinra may increase the levels/effects of: Abatacept; Canakinumab; Leflunomide; Natalizumab; Tofacitinib; Vaccines (Live)

The levels/effects of Anakinra may be increased by: Anti-TNF Agents; Denosumab; Pimecrolimus; Roflumilast; Tacrolimus (Topical); Trastuzumab
Decreased Effect
Anakinra may decrease the levels/effects of: BCG; Coccidioidin Skin Test; Sipuleucel-T; Vaccines (Inactivated); Vaccines (Live)

The levels/effects of Anakinra may be decreased by: Echinacea
Stability Store at 2°C to 8°C (36°F to 46°F); do not freeze. Do not shake. Protect from light.
Mechanism of Action Antagonist of the interleukin-1 (IL-1) receptor. Endogenous IL-1 is induced by inflammatory stimuli and mediates a variety of immunological responses, including degradation of cartilage (loss of proteoglycans) and stimulation of bone resorption.

Pharmacokinetics (Adult data unless noted)
Bioavailability: SubQ: 95%
Half-life elimination: Terminal: 4-6 hours; severe renal impairment (CrCl <30 mL/minute): ~7 hours; ESRD: 9.7 hours (Yang, 2003)
Time to peak serum concentration: SubQ: 3-7 hours
Dosing: Usual
Pediatric:
Neonatal-onset multisystem inflammatory disease (NOMID) or chronic infantile neurological, cutaneous, and articular syndrome (CINCA) [cryopyrin-associated periodic syndromes (CAPS)]: Infants, Children, and Adolescents: SubQ: Initial: 1-2 mg/kg/day in 1-2 divided doses; adjust dose in 0.5-1 mg/kg increments as needed to control inflammation; usual maintenance dose: 3-4 mg/kg/day; maximum daily dose: 8 mg/kg/**day. Note:** Once-daily administration is preferred; however, the dose may also be divided and administered twice daily.
Juvenile idiopathic arthritis (JIA): Limited data available: SubQ:
Systemic-onset JIA (SOJIA): Children and Adolescents: Initial: 1-2 mg/kg/dose once daily; maximum initial dose: 100 mg; if no response, may titrate typically at 2-week intervals by doubling dose up to 4 mg/kg/dose once daily; maximum dose: 200 mg (Dewitt, 2012; Gattorno, 2006; Hedrich, 2012; Irigoyen, 2006; Lequerré, 2008; Nigrovi, 2011; Quartier, 2011)
Polyarticular course JIA: Children ≥2 years and Adolescents: 1 mg/kg once daily; maximum dose: 100 mg (Ilowite, 2009; Reiff, 2005)
Rheumatoid arthritis: Adolescents ≥18 years: SubQ: 100 mg once daily; administer at approximately the same time each day
Adult:
Neonatal-onset multisystem inflammatory disease (NOMID) or chronic infantile neurological, cutaneous, and articular syndrome (CINCA) [cryopyrin-associated periodic syndromes (CAPS)]: SubQ: Initial: 1-2 mg/kg daily in 1-2 divided doses; adjust dose in 0.5-1 mg/kg increments as needed; usual maintenance dose: 3-4 mg/kg daily; maximum daily dose: 8 mg/kg/**day. Note:** The prefilled syringe does not allow doses lower than 20 mg to be administered.
Rheumatoid arthritis: SubQ: 100 mg once daily; administer at approximately the same time each day
Dosing adjustment in renal impairment:
CrCl ≥30 mL/minute: No dosage adjustment necessary
CrCl <30 mL/minute:
NOMID: Infants, Children, Adolescents, and Adults: Decrease frequency of administration to every other day
Rheumatoid arthritis: Adolescents ≥18 years and Adults: Consider 100 mg every other day
ESRD: <2.5% of the dose is removed by hemodialysis or CAPD:
NOMID: Infants, Children, Adolescents, and Adults: Decrease frequency of administration to every other day
Rheumatoid arthritis: Adolescents ≥18 years and Adults: 100 mg every other day
Dosing adjustment in hepatic impairment: There are no dosage adjustments provided in the manufacturer's labeling (has not been studied).
Administration SubQ: Rotate injection sites: Outer area of upper arms, abdomen (do not use within 2 inches of belly button), front of middle thighs, or upper outer buttocks; injection should be given at least 1 inch away from previous injection site. Allow solution to warm to room temperature prior to use (30 minutes). Do not shake. Provided in single-use, preservative-free syringes with 27-gauge needles; discard any unused portion.

Monitoring Parameters CBC with differential (baseline, then monthly for 3 months, then every 3 months for a period up to 1 year); serum creatinine

Juvenile idiopathic arthritis: PPD screening (baseline and annually); CBC with differential and platelets, C-reactive protein, ESR, ferritin, and LDH [baseline, at follow-up visits (1-2 weeks, 1, 2, 6, and 9 months)] and with any treatment change (DeWitt, 2012)

Additional Information Anakinra is produced by recombinant DNA/*E. coli* technology.

Dosage Forms Excipient information presented when available (limited, particularly for generics); consult specific product labeling.

Solution, Subcutaneous [preservative free]:
   Kineret: 100 mg/0.67 mL (0.67 mL) [contains disodium edta, polysorbate 80]

References

Callejas JL, Oliver J, Martín J, et al, "Anakinra in Mutation-Negative CINCA Syndrome," *Clin Rheumatol*, 2007, 26(4):576-7.

Dewitt EM, Kimura Y, Beukelman T, et al. Consensus treatment plans for new-onset systemic juvenile idiopathic arthritis. *Arthritis Care Res (Hoboken)*. 2012;64(7):1001-1010.

Gattorno M, Piccini A, Lasiglié D, et al, "The Pattern of Response to Anti-Interleukin-1 Treatment Distinguishes Two Subsets of Patients With Systemic-Onset Juvenile Idiopathic Arthritis," *Arthritis Rheum*, 2008, 58(5):1505-15.

Goldbach-Mansky R, Dailey NJ, Canna SW, et al, "Neonatal-Onset Multisystem Inflammatory Disease Responsive to Interleukin-1Beta Inhibition," *N Engl J Med*, 2006, 355(6):581-92.

Hedrich CM, Bruck N, Fiebig B, Gahr M. Anakinra: a safe and effective first-line treatment in systemic onset juvenile idiopathic arthritis (SoJIA). *Rheumatol Int.* 2012;32(11):3525-3530.

Ilowite N, Porras O, Reiff A, et al, "Anakinra in the Treatment of Polyarticular-Course Juvenile Rheumatoid Arthritis: Safety and Preliminary Efficacy Results of a Randomized Multicenter Study," *Clin Rheumatol*, 2009, 28(2):129-37.

Irigoyen P, Olson J, Horn C, et al, "Treatement of Systemic Onset Juvenile Idiopathic Arthritis With Anakinra," *Ped Rheumatol Online J*, 2006, 4(2):123-34

Kashiwagi Y, Kawashima H, Nishimata S, et al, "Extreme Efficiency of Anti-Interleukin 1 Agent (Anakinra) in a Japanese Case of CINCA Syndrome," *Clin Rheumatol*, 2008, 27(2):277-9.

Lequerré T, Quartier P, Rosellini D, et al, "Interleukin-1 Receptor Antagonist (Anakinra) Treatment in Patients With Systemic-Onset Juvenile Idiopathic Arthritis or Adult Onset Still Disease: Preliminary Experience in France," *Ann Rheum Dis*, 2008, 67(3):302-8.

Lovell DJ, Bowyer SL, and Solinger AM, "Interleukin-1 Blockade by Anakinra Improves Clinical Symptoms in Patients With Neonatal-Onset Multisystem Inflammatory Disease," *Arthritis Rheum*, 2005, 52(4):1283-6.

Matsubayashi T, Sugiura H, Arai T, et al, "Anakinra Therapy for CINCA Syndrome With a Novel Mutation in Exon 4 of the CIAS1 Gene," *Acta Paediatr*, 2006, 95(2):246-9.

Neven B, Marvillet I, Terrada C, et al. Long-term efficacy of the interleukin-1 receptor antagonist anakinra in ten patients with neonatal-onset multisystem inflammatory disease/chronic infantile neurologic, cutaneous, articular syndrome. *Arthritis and Rheumatism*. 2010;62(1): 258-267.

Nigrovic PA, Mannion M, Prince FH, et al. Anakinra as first-line disease-modifying therapy in systemic juvenile idiopathic arthritis: report of forty-six patients from an international multicenter series. *Arthritis Rheum*. 2011;63(2):545-555.

Ohlsson V, Baildam E, Foster H, et al, "Anakinra Treatment for Systemic Onset Juvenile Idiopathic Arthritis (SOJIA)," *Rheumatology (Oxford)*, 2008, 47(4):555-6.

Pascual V, Allantaz F, Arce E, et al, "Role of Interleukin-1 (IL-1) in the Pathogenesis of Systemic Onset Juvenile Idiopathic Arthritis and Clinical Response to IL-1 Blockade," *J Exp Med*, 2005, 201 (9):1479-86.

Quartier P, Allantaz F, Cimaz R, et al. A multicentre, randomised, double-blind, placebo-controlled trial with the interleukin-1 receptor antagonist anakinra in patients with systemic-onset juvenile idiopathic arthritis (ANAJIS trial). *Ann Rheum Dis*. 2011;70(5):747-754.

Reiff A, "The Use of Anakinra in Juvenile Arthritis," *Curr Rheumatol Rep*, 2005, 7(6):434-40.

Rigante D, Ansuini V, Caldarelli M, et al, "Hydrocephalus in CINCA Syndrome Treated With Anakinra," *Childs Nerv Syst*, 2006, 22 (4):334-7.

Yang BB, Baughman S, and Sullivan JT, "Pharmacokinetics of Anakinra in Subjects With Different Levels of Renal Function," *Clin Pharmacol Ther*, 2003, 74(1):85-94.

◆ **Anaprox** *see* Naproxen *on page 1470*

◆ **Anaprox DS** *see* Naproxen *on page 1470*

◆ **Anascorp** *see* Centruroides Immune F(ab')$_2$ (Equine) *on page 428*

◆ **Anaspaz** *see* Hyoscyamine *on page 1056*

◆ **Anbesol [OTC]** *see* Benzocaine *on page 273*

◆ **Anbesol® Baby (Can)** *see* Benzocaine *on page 273*

◆ **Anbesol Cold Sore Therapy [OTC]** *see* Benzocaine *on page 273*

◆ **Anbesol JR [OTC]** *see* Benzocaine *on page 273*

◆ **Anbesol Maximum Strength [OTC]** *see* Benzocaine *on page 273*

◆ **Ancef** *see* CeFAZolin *on page 393*

◆ **Anchoic Acid** *see* Azelaic Acid *on page 244*

◆ **Ancobon** *see* Flucytosine *on page 882*

◆ **Andriol (Can)** *see* Testosterone *on page 1986*

◆ **Androderm** *see* Testosterone *on page 1986*

◆ **AndroGel** *see* Testosterone *on page 1986*

◆ **AndroGel Pump** *see* Testosterone *on page 1986*

◆ **Andropository (Can)** *see* Testosterone *on page 1986*

◆ **Androxy** *see* Fluoxymesterone *on page 906*

◆ **AneCream [OTC]** *see* Lidocaine (Topical) *on page 1242*

◆ **AneCream5 [OTC]** *see* Lidocaine (Topical) *on page 1242*

◆ **Anectine** *see* Succinylcholine *on page 1938*

◆ **Aneurine Hydrochloride** *see* Thiamine *on page 2009*

◆ **Anexate (Can)** *see* Flumazenil *on page 888*

◆ **Anhydrous Glucose** *see* Dextrose *on page 637*

◆ **Ansaid (Can)** *see* Flurbiprofen (Systemic) *on page 908*

◆ **Ansamycin** *see* Rifabutin *on page 1822*

◆ **Antacid [OTC]** *see* Calcium Carbonate *on page 346*

◆ **Antacid Extra Strength [OTC]** *see* Calcium Carbonate *on page 346*

◆ **Anti-D Immunoglobulin** *see* Rh$_o$(D) Immune Globulin *on page 1815*

◆ **Anti-CD20 Monoclonal Antibody** *see* RiTUXimab *on page 1841*

◆ **Anti-Dandruff [OTC]** *see* Selenium Sulfide *on page 1877*

◆ **Anti-Diarrheal [OTC]** *see* Loperamide *on page 1270*

◆ **Antidigoxin Fab Fragments, Ovine** *see* Digoxin Immune Fab *on page 663*

◆ **Antidiuretic Hormone** *see* Vasopressin *on page 2121*

◆ **Antifungal [OTC]** *see* Miconazole (Topical) *on page 1410*

◆ **Anti-Fungal [OTC]** *see* Tolnaftate *on page 2044*

Antihemophilic Factor (Human)
(an tee hee moe FIL ik FAK tor HYU man)

Medication Safety Issues
Sound-alike/look-alike issues:
   Factor VIII may be confused with Factor XIII
Other safety concerns:
   Confusion may occur due to the omitting of "Factor VIII" from some product labeling. Review product contents carefully prior to dispensing any antihemophilic factor.

Brand Names: U.S. Hemofil M; Koāte®-DVI; Monoclate-P®

Brand Names: Canada Hemofil M

Therapeutic Category Antihemophilic Agent; Blood Product Derivative

Generic Availability (U.S.) Yes

Use Prevention and treatment of hemorrhagic episodes in patients with hemophilia A (classical hemophilia);

perioperative management of patients with hemophilia A; can provide therapeutic effects in patients with acquired factor VIII inhibitors <10 Bethesda units/mL

Pregnancy Risk Factor C

Pregnancy Considerations Animal reproduction studies have not been conducted. Parvovirus B19 or hepatitis A, which may be present in plasma-derived products, may affect a pregnant woman more seriously than nonpregnant women.

Breast-Feeding Considerations It is not known if this product is excreted into breast milk.

Contraindications

All products: Hypersensitivity to any component (see table) Antihemophilic factor, human (Method M, monoclonal purified); Hemofil M; Monoclate-P®: Hypersensitivity to mouse protein

Antihemophilic Factor (Human) [Factor VIII (Human)] Products

Product	Preparation and Purification Methods	Viral Inactivation	Stabilizers and Excipients
Hemofil M	• Method M process • Immunoaffinity chromatography using murine monoclonal antibody • Ion exchange chromatography	• Organic solvent/detergent treatment	• Albumin (human)[1] • Polyethylene glycol[1] • Histidine[1] • Glycine[1] • Mouse protein • Tri-n-butyl phosphate • Octoxynol 9
Koāte®-DVI	• Purified from cold insoluble fraction of fresh-frozen plasma • Gel permeation chromatography	• Organic solvent/detergent treatment • Heat treatment (dry; in lyophilized form in final container; 80°C x 72 hours)	• Albumin (human) • Polyethylene glycol • Glycine • Polysorbate 80 • Tri-n-butyl phosphate • Calcium • Aluminum • Histidine
Monoclate-P®	• Immunoaffinity chromatography using murine monoclonal antibody	• Heat treatment in aqueous solution (pasteurization; 60°C x 10 hours)	• Albumin (human)[1] • Sodium (300-450 millimoles/L) • Calcium chloride • Mannitol • Histidine • Hydrochloric acid and/or sodium hydroxide (pH adjustment) • Mouse protein

Note: Source of all products is pooled human plasma.

[1]Listed as a stabilizer in the product's package insert.

Warnings Hemofil M contains natural rubber latex (in certain components of the product packaging) which may cause allergic reactions in susceptible individuals; avoid use in patients with allergy to latex. Koāte®-DVI contains polysorbate 80 (Tween 80®) which may cause allergic reactions in susceptible individuals. In premature neonates, thrombocytopenia, ascites, pulmonary deterioration, and renal and hepatic failure have been reported after receiving parenteral products containing polysorbate 80 (Alade, 1986; CDC, 1984). Infusion of polysorbate 80-containing solutions through polyvinyl chloride tubing may cause DEHP to leach into the solution; in immature animals, exposure to DEHP may adversely affect the development of the male reproductive tract.

Precautions Clinical response to recommended doses may vary; dosage must be individualized based on coagulation studies (performed prior to treatment and at regular intervals during treatment) and clinical response. Human antihemophilic factor is prepared from pooled plasma and even with heat treated or other viral attenuated processes, the risk of viral transmission (ie, viral hepatitis, HIV, parvovirus B19, and theoretically, Creutzfeldt-Jacob disease agent) is not totally eradicated. Hepatitis B vaccination is recommended for all patients receiving human antihemophilic factor and hepatitis A vaccination is recommended for seronegative patients. [**Note:** The use of recombinant antihemophilic factor products (such as Advate, Helixate® FS, Kogenate® FS, Recombinate™, or ReFacto®) substantially decreases the risk of viral transmission because these products are biosynthetically prepared]. Progressive anemia and hemolysis may occur in individuals with blood groups A, B, and AB who receive large or frequent doses of human antihemophilic factor due to trace amounts of blood group A and B isohemagglutinins.

Formation of factor VIII inhibitors (neutralizing antibodies to AHF human) may occur; reported incidence is 3% to 52%; an increase of inhibitor antibody concentration is seen at 2-7 days, with peak concentrations at 1-3 weeks after therapy; children <5 years of age are at greatest risk; higher doses of AHF may be needed if antibody is present; if antibody concentration is >10 Bethesda units/mL, patients may not respond to larger doses and alternative treatment modalities may be needed; monitor patients appropriately. Allergic-type hypersensitivity reactions including anaphylaxis may occur; discontinue therapy immediately if urticaria, hives, hypotension, tightness of the chest, wheezing, dyspnea, faintness, or anaphylaxis develop; emergency treatment and resuscitative measures (eg, epinephrine, oxygen) may be needed. Products vary by preparation method (see table); final formulations contain human albumin.

Adverse Reactions Rare but important or life-threatening: Acute hemolytic anemia, AHF inhibitor development, allergic reactions (rare), anaphylaxis (rare), bleeding tendency increased, blurred vision, chest tightness, chills, fever, headache, hyperfibrinogenemia, jittery feeling, lethargy, nausea, somnolence, stinging at the infusion site, stomach discomfort, tingling, urticaria, vasomotor reactions with rapid infusion, vomiting

Drug Interactions

Metabolism/Transport Effects None known.

Avoid Concomitant Use There are no known interactions where it is recommended to avoid concomitant use.

Increased Effect/Toxicity There are no known significant interactions involving an increase in effect.

Decreased Effect There are no known significant interactions involving a decrease in effect.

Stability

Storage: Store unopened vials under refrigeration 2°C to 8°C (36°F to 46°F); avoid freezing (to prevent damage to diluent vial)

Hemofil M: May also be stored at room temperature (≤30°C or 86°F)

Koāte®-DVI: May also be stored at room temperature (≤25°C or 77°F) for up to 6 months

Monoclate-P®: May also be stored at room temperature (≤30°C or 86°F) for up to 6 months

Reconstitution: If refrigerated, the dried concentrate and diluent should be warmed to room temperature before reconstitution; see individual product labeling for specific reconstitution guidelines; gently agitate or rotate vial after adding diluent, do not shake vigorously (**Note:** For Koāte®-DVI: Swirl vigorously without creating excessive foaming); use filter needle provided by manufacturer to draw product into syringe; use one filter needle per vial; do **not** refrigerate after reconstitution (precipitation may occur); administer within 3 hours after reconstitution; **Note:** Use plastic syringes, since AHF may stick to the surface of glass syringes

Mechanism of Action Protein (factor VIII) in normal plasma which is necessary for clot formation and maintenance of hemostasis; activates factor X in conjunction with activated factor IX; activated factor X converts prothrombin to thrombin, which converts fibrinogen to fibrin, and with factor XIII forms a stable clot

Pharmacodynamics Maximum effect: 1-2 hours

Pharmacokinetics (Adult data unless noted)
Distribution: Does not readily cross the placenta
Half-life: 4-24 hours; mean = 12 hours (biphasic)

Dosing: Usual Children and Adults: I.V.: Individualize dosage based on coagulation studies performed prior to and during treatment at regular intervals:

Hemophilia A: For every 1 international unit per kg body weight of AHF (human) administered, factor VIII level should increase by 2%; calculated dosage should be adjusted to the actual vial size

Formula to calculate dosage required, based on desired increase in factor VIII (% of normal) (**Note:** This formula assumes that the patient's baseline AHF level is <1%):
Units required = Body weight (kg) x 0.5 x desired increase in factor VIII (units/dL or % of normal)

Hospitalized patients: 20-50 units/kg/dose; may be higher for special circumstances. Dose can be given every 12-24 hours and more frequently in special circumstances.

Hemophilia A with high titer of inhibitor antibody: 50-75 units/kg/hour has been given

General dosing guidelines (consult individual product labeling for specific dosage recommendations):

Minor hemorrhage (required peak postinfusion AHF level: 20% to 40%): 10-20 units/kg; repeat every 12-24 hours for 1-3 days until bleeding is resolved or healing achieved; mild superficial or early hemorrhages may respond to a single dose

Moderate hemorrhage (required peak postinfusion AHF level: 30% to 60%): 15-30 units/kg; repeat every 12-24 hours for ≥3 days until pain and disability are resolved
Alternatively (to achieve peak postinfusion AHF level: 50%) Initial: 25 units/kg; maintenance: 10-15 units/kg every 8-12 hours

Severe/life-threatening hemorrhage (required peak postinfusion AHF level: 60% to 100%): 30-50 units/kg; repeat every 8-24 hours until threat is resolved
Alternatively (to achieve peak postinfusion AHF level: 80% to 100%): 40-50 units/kg; maintenance: 20-25 units/kg every 8-12 hours

Minor surgery (required peak postinfusion AHF level: Range 30% to 80%): 15-40 units/kg; dose is highly dependent upon procedure and specific product recommendations; for some procedures, a single dose plus oral antifibrinolytic therapy within 1 hour is sufficient; in other procedures, may repeat dose every 12-24 hours as needed

Major surgery (required peak pre- and postsurgery AHF level: 80% to 100%): 40-50 units/kg; repeat every 8-24 hours depending on state of healing

Prophylaxis: May also be given on a regular schedule to prevent bleeding

Administration Parenteral: I.V. administration only; see Stability for reconstitution and dosage preparation; administer through a separate line, do not mix with drugs or other I.V. fluids

Maximum rate of administration is product dependent:
Hemofil® M: 10 mL/minute
Monoclate-P®: 2 mL/minute
Koate®-DVI: Total dose may be given over 5-10 minutes; adjust administration rate based on patient response

Monitoring Parameters Bleeding; heart rate and blood pressure (before and during I.V. administration); AHF levels prior to and during treatment; monitor for development of inhibitor antibodies by clinical observation (eg, inadequate control of bleeding with adequate doses) and laboratory tests (eg, inhibitor level, Bethesda assay). In patients with blood groups A, B, or AB who receive large or frequent doses, monitor Hct, direct Coombs' test, and signs of intravascular hemolysis

Reference Range
Plasma antihemophilic factor level:
Normal range: 50% to 150%
Level to prevent spontaneous hemorrhage: 5%
Required peak postinfusion AHF activity in blood (as % of normal or units/dL plasma):
Early hemarthrosis, muscle bleed, or oral bleed: 20% to 40%
More extensive hemarthrosis, muscle bleed, or hematoma: 30% to 60%
Life-threatening bleeds (such as head injury, throat bleed, severe abdominal pain): 80% to 100%
Minor surgery, including tooth extraction: 60% to 80%
Major surgery: 80% to 100% (pre- and postoperative)

Additional Information One unit of AHF is equal to the factor VIII activity present in 1 mL of normal human plasma. If bleeding is not controlled with adequate dose, test for the presence of factor VIII inhibitor; larger doses of AHF may be therapeutic with inhibitor titers <10 Bethesda units/mL; it may not be possible or practical to control bleeding if inhibitor titers >10 Bethesda units/mL (due to the very large AHF doses required); other treatments [eg, antihemophilic factor (porcine), factor IX complex concentrates, recombinant factor VIIa, or anti-inhibitor coagulant complex] may be needed in patients with inhibitor titers >10 Bethesda units/mL.

Dosage Forms Excipient information presented when available (limited, particularly for generics); consult specific product labeling. [DSC] = Discontinued product
Injection, powder for reconstitution:
Hemofil M: ~250 units, ~500 units, ~1000 units, ~1700 units [contains albumin (human), mouse protein; packaging may contain natural rubber latex]. Supplied with diluent.
Koāte®-DVI: ~250 units, ~500 units, ~1000 units [contains albumin (human), aluminum, polysorbate 80]. Supplied with diluent.
Monoclate-P®: ~250 units, ~500 units, ~1000 units, ~1500 units [contains albumin (human), mouse protein]. Supplied with diluent.

References
Alade SL, Brown RE, and Paquet A Jr, "Polysorbate 80 and E-Ferol Toxicity," *Pediatrics*, 1986, 77(4):593-7.
Centers for Disease Control (CDC), "Unusual Syndrome With Fatalities Among Premature Infants: Association With a New Intravenous Vitamin E Product," *MMWR Morb Mortal Wkly Rep*, 1984, 33 (14):198-9.
Liesner RJ, "Prophylaxis in Haemophilic Children," *Blood Coagul Fibrinolysis*, 1997, 8(Suppl 1):S7-10.
Scharrer I, Bray GL, and Neutzling O, "Incidence of Inhibitors in Haemophilia A Patients–A Review of Recent Studies of Recombinant and Plasma-Derived Factor VIII Concentrates," *Haemophilia*, 1999, 5 (3):145-54.
Shord SS and Lindley CM, "Coagulation Products and Their Uses," *Am J Health Syst Pharm*, 2000, 57(15):1403-20.

Antihemophilic Factor (Recombinant)
(an tee hee moe FIL ik FAK tor ree KOM be nant)

Medication Safety Issues
Sound-alike/look-alike issues:
Factor VIII may be confused with Factor XIII
Other safety concerns:
Confusion may occur due to the omitting of "Factor VIII" from some product labeling. Review product contents carefully prior to dispensing any antihemophilic factor.

Brand Names: U.S. Advate; Helixate FS; Kogenate FS; Kogenate FS Bio-Set; Recombinate; Xyntha; Xyntha Solofuse

Brand Names: Canada Advate; Helixate FS; Kogenate FS; Xyntha

Therapeutic Category Antihemophilic Agent
Generic Availability (U.S.) No
Use Note: Antihemophilic Factor (Recombinant) is not indicated for the treatment of von Willebrand disease.

Advate: Prevention and control of hemorrhagic episodes in patients with hemophilia A; perioperative management of patients with hemophilia A; routine prophylaxis to prevent or reduce the frequency of bleeding episodes in patients with hemophilia A (All indications: FDA approved in ages 0-16 years and adults)

Helixate FS, Kogenate FS: Prevention and control of hemorrhagic episodes in patients with hemophilia A; perioperative management of patients with hemophilia A; routine prophylaxis to reduce the frequency of bleeding episodes and reduce the risk of joint damage in children with hemophilia A with no preexisting joint damage (All indications: FDA approved in ages 0-16 years)

Recombinate: Prevention and control of hemorrhagic episodes in patients with hemophilia A (FDA approved in all ages); perioperative management of patients with hemophilia A (FDA approved in all ages)

Xyntha: Prevention and control of hemorrhagic episodes in patients with hemophilia A (FDA approved in ages ≥12 years and adults); perioperative management of patients with hemophilia A (FDA approved in ages ≥12 years and adults)

Has also been used in patients with acquired factor VIII inhibitors <10 Bethesda units/mL
Pregnancy Risk Factor C
Pregnancy Considerations Animal reproduction studies have not been conducted. Safety and efficacy in pregnant women has not been established. Use during pregnancy only if clearly needed.
Breast-Feeding Considerations It is not known if antihemophilic factor (recombinant) is excreted in breast milk. The manufacturer recommends that caution be exercised when administering antihemophilic factor (recombinant) to nursing women.
Contraindications

All products: Hypersensitivity or intolerance to any component

Advate; Helixate FS; Kogenate FS: Hypersensitivity to mouse or hamster protein

Recombinate: Hypersensitivity to mouse, hamster, or bovine protein

Xyntha: Hypersensitivity to hamster protein

Warnings Allergic-type hypersensitivity reactions including anaphylaxis may occur; discontinue therapy immediately if urticaria, hives, hypotension, tightness of the chest, wheezing, or anaphylaxis develop; emergency treatment and resuscitative measures (eg, epinephrine, oxygen) may be needed. Clinical response to antihemophilic factor administration may vary; dosage must be individualized based on coagulation studies (performed prior to treatment and at regular intervals during treatment) and clinical response. If bleeding is not controlled with the recommended dose, determine plasma level of factor VIII and follow with a sufficient dose to achieve satisfactory clinical response. If plasma levels of factor VIII fail to increase as expected or bleeding continues, suspect the presence of an inhibitor; test as appropriate. Formation of factor VIII inhibitors (neutralizing antibodies to AHF recombinant) may occur at any time, but is more common in young children with severe hemophilia during the first years of therapy, or in patients at any age who received little prior therapy with factor VIII; monitor patients appropriately. Some products may contain polysorbate 80 (Tween 80) which may cause allergic reactions in susceptible individuals. In premature neonates, thrombocytopenia, ascites, pulmonary deterioration, and renal and hepatic failure

have been reported after receiving parenteral products containing polysorbate 80 (Alade, 1986; CDC, 1984). Infusion of polysorbate 80-containing solutions through polyvinyl chloride tubing may cause DEHP to leach into the solution; in immature animals, exposure to DEHP may adversely affect the development of the male reproductive tract. Consult product specific labeling for further detail on excipients.
Precautions Recombinate contains natural rubber latex (in certain components of the product packaging) which may cause allergic reactions in susceptible individuals; avoid use in patients with allergy to latex. Recombinate may contain bovine protein; Advate, Helixate FS, Kogenate FS, Recombinate, and Xyntha may contain trace amounts of mouse or hamster protein; formation of antibodies to mouse, hamster, or bovine protein may occur. Products vary by preparation method. Recombinate formulation is stabilized using human albumin; Helixate FS, Kogenate FS, and Xyntha formulations are stabilized using sucrose.
Adverse Reactions

Central nervous system: Chills, dizziness, fever, headache, pain

Dermatologic: Pruritus, rash, urticaria

Gastrointestinal: Constipation, diarrhea, nausea, taste perversion, vomiting

Local: Injection site reactions

Neuromuscular & skeletal: Arthralgia, joint swelling, pain in extremity, weakness

Otic: Ear infection, ear pain

Respiratory: Cough, dyspnea, nasopharyngitis, pharyngolaryngeal pain

Miscellaneous: Catheter thrombosis, catheter infection, factor VIII inhibitor formation, flu-like syndrome, influenza

Rare but important or life-threatening: Abdominal pain, adenopathy, allergic reactions, anaphylaxis, anemia, angioedema, anorexia, arthralgia, AST increased, chest discomfort, chest pain, cyanosis, depersonalization, diaphoresis, dyspnea, edema, epistaxis, erythema, facial edema, facial flushing, factor VIII decreased, fatigue, GI hemorrhage, hematoma, hives, hot flashes, hyperhidrosis, hypersensitivity reaction, hyper-/hypotension (slight), infection, laryngeal edema, lethargy, malaise, pallor, paresthesia, restlessness, rhinitis, rigors, shortness of breath, somnolence, tachycardia, tremor, urinary tract infection, vasodilation, venous catheter access complications

Drug Interactions
Metabolism/Transport Effects None known.
Avoid Concomitant Use There are no known interactions where it is recommended to avoid concomitant use.
Increased Effect/Toxicity There are no known significant interactions involving an increase in effect.
Decreased Effect There are no known significant interactions involving a decrease in effect.
Stability Prior to reconstitution, store refrigerated at 2°C to 8°C (36°F to 46°F); avoid freezing. Use within 3 hours of reconstitution. Do not refrigerate after reconstitution.

Advate: May also be stored at room temperature [not to exceed 30°C (86°F)] for up to 6 months; do not return to refrigerator.

Helixate FS, Kogenate FS: May also be stored at room temperature [not to exceed 25°C (77°F)] up to 12 months; do not return to refrigerator. Avoid prolonged exposure to light during storage; store in carton prior to use.

Recombinate: May also be stored at room temperature, not to exceed 30°C (86°F).

Xyntha: May also be stored at room temperature [not to exceed 25°C (77°F)] up to 3 months; after room temperature storage, product may be returned to the refrigerator until the expiration date; however, do not store at room temperature and return to refrigerator temperature more than once. Avoid prolonged exposure to light during storage.

Xyntha Solofuse: May also be stored at room temperature [not to exceed 25°C (77°F)] up to 3 months; do not return to refrigerator. Avoid prolonged exposure to light during storage.

Mechanism of Action Factor VIII replacement, necessary for clot formation and maintenance of hemostasis. It activates factor X in conjunction with activated factor IX; activated factor X converts prothrombin to thrombin, which converts fibrinogen to fibrin, and with factor XIII forms a stable clot.

Pharmacokinetics (Adult data unless noted) Half-life: Children 4-18 years of age (mean age: 12 years): 10.7 hours (range: 7.8-15.3)
Adults: 11-15 hours

Dosing: Neonatal

Individualize dosage based on coagulation studies performed prior to treatment and at regular intervals during treatment; for every 1 international unit per kg body weight of rAHF administered, factor VIII level should increase by 2% (or 2 units/dL); calculated dosage should be adjusted to the actual vial size

Control or prevention of bleeding in patients with factor VIII deficiency (hemophilia A): I.V.: Dosage is expressed in units of factor VIII activity (ie, international units) and must be individualized based on formulation, severity of factor VIII deficiency, extent and location of bleed, and clinical situation of patient.

Formula for units required to raise blood level:
Number of Factor VIII Units required = body weight (in kg) x 0.5 units/kg per units/dL x desired factor VIII level increase (units/dL or%)
For example, for a desired 100% level in a 3 kg patient who has an actual level of 20%: Number of Factor VIII Units needed = 3 kg x 80% x 0.5 units/kg per units/dL = 120 units

Manufacturer's labeling: Advate, Helixate FS, Kogenate FS, Recombinate: Desired Factor VIII level, dosing interval, and duration based on hemorrhage type: I.V.:
Minor hemorrhage (early joint hemorrhage, mild muscle or oral bleed): 10-20 units/kg/dose
Desired factor VIII levels (% or units/dL): 20-40
Frequency of dosing: Every 8-24 hours
Duration of treatment: 1-3 days until bleeding is resolved or healing achieved; mild, superficial, or early hemorrhages may respond to a single dose
Moderate hemorrhage (intramuscular bleed, hematoma, moderate bleeding into oral cavity, definite joint bleed, and known trauma): 15-30 units/kg/dose
Desired factor VIII levels (% or units/dL): 30-60
Frequency of dosing: Every 8-24 hours
Duration of treatment: ≥3 days until bleeding, pain, and disability are resolved or healing is achieved
Severe/life-threatening hemorrhage (GI, intracranial, intra-abdominal, intrathoracic bleeding, retroperitoneal, retropharyngeal, illiopsoas, CNS bleeding or head trauma, fractures):
Helixate FS, Kogenate FS: Initial: 40-50 units/kg; maintenance: 20-25 units/kg/dose
Desired factor VIII levels (% or units/dL): 80-100
Frequency of dosing: Every 8-12 hours
Duration of treatment: Until bleeding is resolved (duration not specified)
Advate, Recombinate: 30-50 units/kg/dose
Desired factor VIII levels (% or units/dL): 60-100
Frequency of dosing: Every 6-12 hours (Advate) or every 8-24 hours (Recombinate)
Duration of treatment: Until bleeding is resolved (duration not specified)

Perioperative management: I.V.:
Minor surgery (including dental extractions):
Advate: 30-50 units/kg as bolus infusion beginning within 1 hour prior to surgery; for dental procedures, adjunctive therapy may be considered

Desired factor VIII levels (% or units/dL): 60-100
Frequency of dosing: Every 12-24 hours as needed to control bleeding
Duration of treatment: Until bleeding is resolved (duration not specified)
Helixate FS, Kogenate FS: 15-30 units/kg/dose
Desired factor VIII levels (% or units/dL): 30-60
Frequency of dosing: Every 12-24 hours
Duration of treatment: Until bleeding is resolved (duration not specified)
Recombinate:
Desired factor VIII levels (% or units/dL): 60-80
Frequency of dosing: Single dose plus oral antifibrinolytic therapy within 1 hour is sufficient for most cases
Major surgery (tonsillectomy, hernia repair, intracranial, intra-abdominal, or intrathoracic surgery; joint replacement, trauma):
Advate: 40-60 units/kg/dose
Desired factor VIII levels (% or units/dL): Pre- and postoperative levels: 80-120; verify 100% activity has been achieved prior to surgery
Frequency of dosing: Every 6-24 hours as needed
Duration of treatment: Based on desired level and state of healing
Helixate FS, Kogenate FS: 50 units/kg/dose
Desired factor VIII levels (% or units/dL): Pre- and postoperative levels: 100; verify 100% activity has been achieved prior to surgery
Frequency of dosing: Every 6-12 hours as needed
Duration of treatment: Until healing is complete (~10-14 days)
Recombinate:
Desired factor VIII levels (% or units/dL): Pre- and postoerative: 80-100
Frequency of dosing: Every 8-24 hours depending on state of healing

Routine prophylaxis: I.V.:
Advate: 20-40 units/kg/dose every other day (3-4 times weekly). Alternatively, an every-third-day dosing regimen may be used to target factor VIII trough levels of ≥1%
Helixate FS, Kogenate FS: **Note:** For use in patients with no preexisting joint damage: 25 units/kg/dose given every other day.

Dosing: Usual
Pediatric:

Individualize dosage based on coagulation studies performed prior to treatment and at regular intervals during treatment; for every 1 international unit per kg body weight of rAHF administered, factor VIII level should increase by 2% (or 2 units/dL); calculated dosage should be adjusted to the actual vial size

Control or prevention of bleeding in patients with factor VIII deficiency (hemophilia A): I.V.: Infants, Children, and Adolescents: Dosage is expressed in units of factor VIII activity (ie, international units) and must be individualized based on formulation, severity of factor VIII deficiency, extent and location of bleed, and clinical situation of patient.

Formula for units required to raise blood level:
Number of Factor VIII Units required = body weight (in kg) x 0.5 units/kg per units/dL x desired VIII level increase (units/dL or%)
For example, for a desired 100% level in a 25 kg patient who has an actual level of 20%: Number of Factor VIII Units needed = 25 kg x 80% x 0.5 units/kg per units/dL = 1000 units

Manufacturer's labeling: Advate, Helixate FS, Kogenate FS, Recombinate, Xyntha: Desired factor VIII level, dosing interval, and duration based on hemorrhage type: I.V.:
Minor hemorrhage (early joint hemorrhage, mild muscle or oral bleed): 10-20 units/kg/dose

Desired factor VIII levels (% or units/dL): 20-40

Frequency of dosing: Every 8-24 hours (Advate: <6 years old) **or** every 12-24 hours (Advate: ≥6 years old; Helixate FS; Kogentae FS; Xyntha)

Duration of treatment: 1-3 days until bleeding is resolved or healing achieved; mild, superficial, or early hemorrhages may respond to a single dose

Moderate hemorrhage (intramuscular bleed, hematoma, moderate bleeding into oral cavity, definite joint bleed, and known trauma): 15-30 units/kg/dose

Desired factor VIII levels (% or units/dL): 30-60

Frequency of dosing: Every 8-24 hours (Advate: <6 years old) **or** every 12-24 hours (Advate: ≥6 years old; Helixate FS; Kogenate FS; Xyntha)

Duration of treatment: ≥3 days until bleeding, pain, and disability are resolved or healing is achieved

Severe/life-threatening hemorrhage (GI, intracranial, intra-abdominal, intrathoracic bleeding, retroperitoneal, retropharyngeal, illiopsoas, CNS bleeding or head trauma, fractures):

Helixate FS, Kogenate FS: Initial: 40-50 units/kg; maintenance: 20-25 units/kg/dose

Desired factor VIII levels (% or units/dL): 80-100

Frequency of dosing: Every 8-12 hours

Duration of treatment: Until bleeding is resolved (duration not specified)

Advate, Recombinate, Xyntha: 30-50 units/kg/dose

Desired factor VIII levels (% or units/dL): 60-100

Frequency of dosing: Every 6-12 hours (Advate: <6 years old) **or** 8-24 hours (Advate: ≥6 years old; Recombinate; Xyntha)

Duration of treatment: Until bleeding is resolved (duration not specified)

Alternative dosing: **Note:** The following recommendations reflect guideline recommendations for general dosing requirements; may vary from those found within prescribing information or practitioner preference:

I.V.: Infants, Children, and Adolescents: Desired factor VIII level to maintain and duration based on site of hemorrhage/clinical situation (when no significant resource constraints exist) [WFH guidelines (Srivastava, 2013)]. **Note:** Factor VIII level may either be expressed as units/dL or as%. Dosing frequency most commonly corresponds to the half-life of factor VIII but should be determined based on an assessment of factor VIII levels before the next dose.

Joint: 40-60 units/dL for 1-2 days; may be longer if response is inadequate

Superficial muscle (no neurovascular compromise): 40-60 units/dL for 2-3 days, sometimes longer if response is inadequate

Iliopsoas and deep muscle with neurovascular injury, or substantial blood loss: Initial: 80-100 units/dL for 1-2 days; Maintenance: 30-60 units/dL for 3-5 days, sometimes longer as secondary prophylaxis during physiotherapy

CNS/head: Initial: 80-100 units/dL for 1-7 days; Maintenance: 50 units/dL for 8-21 days

Throat and neck: Initial: 80-100 units/dL for 1-7 days; Maintenance: 50 units/dL for 8-14 days

Gastrointestinal: Initial: 80-100 units/dL for 7-14 days; Maintenance: 50 units/dL (duration not specified)

Renal: 50 units/dL for 3-5 days

Deep laceration: 50 units/dL for 5-7 days

Continuous I.V. infusion: Infants, Children, and Adolescents: Limited data available: **Note:** For patients who require prolonged periods of treatment (eg, intracranial hemorrhage or surgery) to avoid peaks and troughs associated with intermittent infusions [Batorova, 2002; Poon, 2012; WFH guidelines (Srivastava, 2013)]:

Following initial bolus to achieve the desired factor VIII level: Initial dosing: 2-4 units/kg/hour; adjust dose based on frequent factor VIII assays and calculation of factor VIII clearance at steady-state using the following equations:

Factor VIII clearance (mL/kg/hour) = (current infusion rate in units/kg/hour) / (plasma Factor level in units/**mL**)

New infusion rate (units/kg/hour) = (factor VIII clearance in mL/kg/hour) x (desired plasma level in units/**mL**)

Perioperative management: I.V.: Infants, Children, and Adolescents:

Manufacturer's labeling: Desired factor VIII level, dosing interval, and duration based on surgery type:

Minor surgery (including dental extractions):

Advate: 30-50 units/kg as bolus infusion beginning within 1 hour prior to surgery; for dental procedures, adjunctive therapy may be considered

Desired factor VIII levels (% or units/dL): 60-100

Frequency of dosing: Every 12-24 hours as needed to control bleeding

Duration of treatment: Until bleeding is resolved (duration not specified)

Helixate FS, Kogenate FS, Xyntha: 15-30 units/kg/dose; for dental procedures, a single dose plus oral antifibrinolytic therapy within 1 hour may be sufficient

Desired factor VIII levels (% or units/dL): 30-60

Frequency of dosing: Every 12-24 hours

Duration of treatment: 3-4 days or until bleeding is resolved

Recombinate:

Desired factor VIII levels (% or units/dL): 60-80

Frequency of dosing: Single dose plus oral antifibrinolytic therapy within 1 hour is sufficient for most cases

Major surgery (tonsillectomy, hernia repair, intracranial, intra-abdominal or intrathoracic surgery; joint replacement, trauma):

Advate: 40-60 units/kg/dose

Desired factor VIII levels (% or units/dL): Pre- and postoperative levels: 80-120; verify 100% activity has been achieved prior to surgery

Frequency of dosing: Every 6-24 hours (<6 years old) **or** every 8-24 hours (≥6 years old) as needed

Duration of treatment: Based on desired level and state of healing

Helixate FS, Kogenate FS: 50 units/kg/dose

Desired factor VIII levels (% or units/dL): Pre- and postoperative levels: 100; verify 100% activity has been achieved prior to surgery

Frequency of dosing: Every 6-12 hours as needed

Duration of treatment: Until healing is complete (~10-14 days)

Recombinate: 40-50 units/kg/dose

Desired factor VIII levels (% or units/dL): Pre- and postoperative: 80-100

Frequency of dosing: Every 8-24 hours

Duration of treatment: Based on state of healing

Xyntha: Children ≥12 years and Adolescents:

Desired factor VIII levels (% or units/dL): 60-100

Frequency of dosing: Every 8-24 hours

Duration of treatment: Until bleeding is resolved and wound healing is achieved

Alternative dosing: **Note:** The following recommendations reflect guideline recommendations for general dosing requirements; may vary from those found within prescribing information or practitioner preference:

I.V.: Desired factor VIII level to maintain and duration based on site of hemorrhage/clinical situation (when no significant resource constraints exist) [WFH guidelines (Srivastava, 2013)]. **Note:** Factor VIII level may either be expressed as units/dL or as%. Dosing frequency most commonly corresponds to the half-life of factor VIII but should be determined based on an assessment of factor VIII levels before the next dose.

Surgery (major):

Preop: 80-100 units/dL

Postop: 60-80 units/dL for 1-3 days; then 40-60 units/dL for 4-6 days; then 30-50 units/dL for 7-14 days

Surgery (minor):

Preop: 50-80 units/dL

Postop: 30-80 units/dL for 1-5 days depending on procedure type

Continuous I.V. infusion: Infants, Children, and Adolescents: Limited data available: Initial: 25-50 units/kg prior to surgery, followed by continuous infusion at a rate of 3-5 units/kg/hour; regimen based on two studies evaluating use in pediatric surgery patients (age range: 0.9-17 years); rate was adjusted and additional boluses given as needed to maintain desired factor VIII level (Batorova, 2012; Dingli, 2002)

Routine prophylaxis: I.V.: Infants, Children, and Adolescents:

Manufacturer's labeling:

Advate: 20-40 units/kg/dose every other day (3-4 times weekly). Alternatively, an every-third-day dosing regimen may be used to target factor VIII trough levels of ≥1%

Helixate FS, Kogenate FS: **Note:** For use in patients with no preexisting joint damage: 25 units/kg/dose given every other day

Alternative dosing: 15-30 units/kg/dose 3 times weekly (WFH guidelines [Srivastava, 2013] [Utrecht protocol]) **or** 25-40 units/kg/dose 3 times weekly (WFH guidelines [Srivastava, 2013] [Malmö protocol]) **or** 25-50 units/kg/dose administered 3 times weekly **or** every other day (National Hemophilia Foundation, MASAC recommendation, 2007); optimum regimen has yet to be defined.

Adults:

Hemophilia: I.V.: **Individualize dosage based on coagulation studies performed prior to treatment and at regular intervals during treatment.** In general, administration of factor VIII 1 unit/kg will increase circulating factor VIII levels by ~2 units/dL (or 2%). (General guidelines presented; consult individual product labeling for specific dosing recommendations.)

Dosage based on desired factor VIII increase (%):

To calculate dosage needed based on desired factor VIII increase (%):

Body weight (kg) x 0.5 units/kg x desired factor VIII increase (%) = units factor VIII required

For example: 50 kg x 0.5 units/kg x 30 (% increase) = 750 units factor VIII

Dosage based on expected factor VIII increase (%):

It is also possible to calculate the **expected**% factor VIII increase:

(# units administered x 2%/units/kg) divided by body weight (kg) = expected% factor VIII increase

For example: (1400 units x 2%/units/kg) divided by 70 kg = 40%

General guidelines (consult individual product labeling for specific dosage recommendations):

Minor hemorrhage: 10-20 units/kg as a single dose to achieve FVIII plasma level ~20% to 40% of normal. Mild superficial or early hemorrhages may respond to a single dose; may repeat dose every 12-24 hours for 1-3 days until bleeding is resolved or healing achieved.

Moderate hemorrhage/minor surgery: 15-30 units/kg to achieve FVIII plasma level 30% to 60% of normal. May repeat 1 dose at 12-24 hours if needed. Some products suggest continuing for ≥3 days until pain and disability are resolved.

Major to life-threatening hemorrhage: Initial dose 30-50 units/kg followed by a maintenance dose of 20-50 units/kg every 8-24 hours until threat is resolved, to achieve FVIII plasma level 60% to 100% of normal.

Minor surgery (including tooth extraction): 15-50 units/kg to raise factor VIII level to ~30% to 100% before procedure/surgery. May repeat every 12-24 hours until bleeding is resolved.

Major surgery: 40-60 units/kg given preoperatively to raise factor VIII level to ~60% to 120% before surgery begins. May repeat as necessary after 6-24 hours until wound healing. Intensity of therapy may depend on type of surgery and postoperative regimen.

If bleeding is not controlled with adequate dose, test for presence of inhibitor. It may not be possible or practical to control bleeding if inhibitor titers >10 Bethesda units/mL.

Administration

Reconstitution: If refrigerated, the dried concentrate and diluent should be warmed to room temperature before reconstitution; see individual product labeling for specific reconstitution guidelines; gently agitate or rotate vial after adding diluent, do not shake vigorously. Use filter needle provided by manufacturer to draw product into syringe (all products except Xyntha); do **not** refrigerate after reconstitution; administer within 3 hours after reconstitution; **Note:** Use plastic syringes, since rAHF may stick to the surface of glass syringes.

Parenteral: I.V. administration only; adjust administration rate based on patient response

Advate: Infuse over ≤5 minutes; maximum infusion rate: 10 mL/minute

Helixate FS, Kogenate FS: Infuse over 1-15 minutes; based on patient tolerability; use sterile administration set provided by manufacturer.

Recombinate:

Reconstitution with 5 mL of SWFI: Infuse at a maximum rate of 5 mL/minute

Reconstitution with 10 mL of SWFI: Infuse at a maximum rate of 10 mL/minute

Xyntha, Xyntha Solufuse: Infuse over several minutes; adjust based on patient comfort. Do not admix or administer in same tubing as other medications.

WFH recommendations: Infuse slowly with maximum rate determined by age: Young children: 100 **units/**minute; Adults: 3 mL/minute; may also administer as a continuous infusion in select patients (WFH guidelines [Srivastava, 2013]).

Monitoring Parameters Bleeding; heart rate and blood pressure (before and during I.V. administration); factor VIII levels prior to and during treatment; monitor for the development of inhibitor antibodies by clinical observations (eg, inadequate control of bleeding with adequate doses) and laboratory tests (eg, inhibitor level, Bethesda assay)

Reference Range

Classification of hemophilia; normal is defined as 1 unit/mL of factor VIII

Severe: Factor level <1% of normal

Moderate: Factor level 1% to 5% of normal

Mild: Factor level >5% to <40% of normal

Additional Information One unit of rAHF is equal to the factor VIII activity present in 1 mL of fresh pooled human plasma. If bleeding is not controlled with adequate dose, test for the presence of factor VIII inhibitor; larger doses of rAHF may be therapeutic with inhibitor titers <10 Bethesda units/mL; it may not be possible or practical to control bleeding if inhibitor titers >10 Bethesda units/mL (due to the very large rAHF doses required); other treatments [eg, antihemophilic factor (porcine), factor IX complex concentrates, recombinant factor VIIa, or anti-inhibitor coagulant complex] may be needed in patients with inhibitor titers >10 Bethesda units/mL

Product Availability

Novoeight: FDA approved October 2013; availability anticipated in the second quarter of 2015.

Novoeight is indicated for use in children and adults with hemophilia A (congenital factor VIII deficiency or classic hemophilia) for control and prevention of bleeding episodes, perioperative management, and routine prophylaxis to prevent or reduce the frequency of bleeding episodes.

Eloctate: FDA approved June 2014; anticipated availability is mid-2014.

Eloctate, Antihemophilic Factor (Recombinant), Fc fusion protein, is indicated for use in adults and children with Hemophilia A.

Dosage Forms Excipient information presented when available (limited, particularly for generics); consult specific product labeling.

Kit, Intravenous:

Kogenate FS: 250 units, 500 units, 1000 units [contains mouse protein (murine) (hamster)]

Kit, Intravenous [preservative free]:

Helixate FS: 250 units, 500 units, 1000 units, 2000 units, 3000 units [contains polysorbate 80]

Kogenate FS: 2000 units, 3000 units [contains mouse protein (murine) (hamster)]

Kogenate FS Bio-Set: 250 units, 500 units, 1000 units, 2000 units, 3000 units

Xyntha: 250 units, 500 units, 1000 units, 2000 units [albumin free; contains mouse protein (murine) (hamster), polysorbate 80]

Xyntha Solofuse: 250 units, 500 units, 1000 units, 2000 units, 3000 units [albumin free; contains mouse protein (murine) (hamster), polysorbate 80]

Solution Reconstituted, Intravenous [preservative free]:

Advate: 250 units (1 ea); 500 units (1 ea); 1000 units (1 ea); 1500 units (1 ea); 2000 units (1 ea); 3000 units (1 ea); 4000 units (1 ea) [albumin free; contains polysorbate 80]

Recombinate: 220-400 units (1 ea); 401-800 units (1 ea); 801-1240 units (1 ea); 1241-1800 units (1 ea); 1801-2400 units (1 ea) [contains albumin human, polyethylene glycol, polysorbate 80]

References

Alade SL, Brown RE, and Paquet A Jr, "Polysorbate 80 and E-Ferol Toxicity," *Pediatrics*, 1986, 77(4):593-7.

Abshire TC, Brackmann HH, Scharrer I, et al, "Sucrose Formulated Recombinant Human Antihemophilic Factor VIII is Safe and Efficacious for Treatment of Hemophilia A in Home Therapy. International Kogenate-FS Study Group," *Thromb Haemost*, 2000, 83(6):811-6.

Batorova A, Holme P, Gringeri A, et al. Continuous infusion in haemophilia: current practice in Europe. *Haemophilia*. 2012;18(5):753-759.

Batorova A, Martinowitz U. Continuous infusion of coagulation factors. *Haemophilia*. 2002;8(3):170-177.

Bray GL, Gomperts ED, Courter S, et al, "A Multicenter Study of Recombinant Factor VIII (Recombinate): Safety, Efficacy, and Inhibitor Risk in Previously Untreated Patients With Hemophilia A. The Recombinate Study Group," *Blood*, 1994, 83(9):2428-35.

Centers for Disease Control (CDC), "Unusual Syndrome With Fatalities Among Premature Infants: Association With a New Intravenous Vitamin E Product," *MMWR Morb Mortal Wkly Rep*, 1984, 33 (14):198-9.

Dingli D, Gastineau DA, Gilchrist GS, Nichols WL, Wilke JL. Continuous factor VIII infusion therapy in patients with haemophilia A undergoing surgical procedures with plasma-derived or recombinant factor VIII concentrates. *Haemophilia*. 2002;8(5):629-634.

Kelly KM, Butler RB, Farace L, et al, "Superior In Vivo Response of Recombinant Factor VIII Concentrate in Children With Haemophilia A," *J Pediatr*, 1997, 130(4):537-40.

Liesner RJ, "Prophylaxis in Haemophilic Children," *Blood Coagul Fibrinolysis*, 1997, 8(Suppl 1):S7-10.

National Hemophilia Foundation. MASAC recommendations concerning prophylaxis (regular administration of clotting factor concentrate to prevent bleeding). 2007. Available at http://www.hemophilia.org/NHFWeb/Resource/StaticPages/menu0/menu5/menu57/masac179.pdf

Poon MC, Card R. Hemophilia management in transfusion medicine. *Transfus Apher Sci.* 2012;46(3):299-307.

Scharrer I, Bray GL, and Neutzling O, "Incidence of Inhibitors in Haemophilia A Patients - A Review of Recent Studies of Recombinant and Plasma-Derived Factor VIII Concentrates," *Haemophilia*, 1999, 5 (3):145-54.

Shord SS and Lindley CM, "Coagulation Products and Their Uses," *Am J Health Syst Pharm*, 2000, 57(15):1403-20.

Schwartz RS, Abildgaard CF, Aledort LM, et al, "Human Recombinant DNA-Derived Antihemophilic Factor (Factor VIII) in the Treatment of Hemophilia A. Recombinant Factor VIII Study Group," *N Engl J Med*, 1990, 323(26):1800-5.

Srivastava A, Brewer AK, Mauser-Bunschoten EP, et al. Guidelines for the management of hemophilia. *Haemophilia*. 2013;19(1):e1-47.

Antihemophilic Factor/von Willebrand Factor Complex (Human)

(an tee hee moe FIL ik FAK tor von WILL le brand FAK tor KOM plex HYU man)

Medication Safety Issues

Sound-alike/look-alike issues:

Factor VIII may be confused with Factor XIII

Brand Names: U.S. Alphanate®; Humate-P®; Wilate®

Brand Names: Canada Humate-P®

Therapeutic Category Antihemophilic Agent; Blood Product Derivative

Generic Availability (U.S.) No

Use

Hemophilia A (Factor VIII deficiency): Alphanate®, Humate-P®: Prevention and treatment of hemorrhage episodes in hemophilia A (classic hemophilia) (Alphanate®: FDA approved in ages >16 years and adults; Humate-P®: FDA approved in adults); prevention and treatment of hemorrhagic episodes with acquired factor VIII deficiency (Alphanate®: FDA approved in ages >16 years and adults)

von Willebrand disease (VWD):

Alphanate®: Prophylaxis for surgical and/or invasive procedures in patients with VWD when desmopressin is either ineffective or contraindicated [FDA approved in pediatric patients (age not specified) and adults]. **Note:** Not indicated for patients with severe VWD undergoing major surgery.

Humante-P®: Treatment of spontaneous and trauma-induced hemorrhagic episodes and prevention of excessive perioperative bleeding in patients with mild to moderate and severe VWD where the use of desmopressin is suspected or known to be inadequate (FDA approved in ages ≥1 month and adults). **Note:** Not indicated for the prophylaxis of spontaneous bleeding episodes.

Wilate®: Treatment of spontaneous and trauma-induced bleeding in patients with severe VWD, including mild or moderate disease when use of desmopressin is known or suspected to be inadequate or contraindicated (FDA approved in ages ≥5 years and adults). **Note:** Not indicated for prophylaxis of spontaneous bleeding or prevention of excessive bleeding during and after surgery.

Pregnancy Risk Factor C

Pregnancy Considerations Animal reproduction studies have not been conducted. Parvovirus B19 or hepatitis A, which may be present in plasma-derived products, may affect a pregnant woman more seriously than nonpregnant women.

Breast-Feeding Considerations No human or animal data is available. Breast-feeding is not recommended by the manufacturer.

Contraindications History of anaphylactic or severe systemic response to antihemophilic factor (AHF) or von Willebrand factor products; hypersensitivity to any component

Warnings Thromboembolic events in patients with von Willebrand disease receiving antihemophilic factor/von Willebrand factor complex have been reported; risk of these events may be increased with ongoing use; monitor concentrations of von Willebrand factor and factor VIII closely; avoid excessive increases in factor VIII activity. Incidence of thrombosis may be increased in patients with other risk factors for thrombosis and females. Allergic reactions, including anaphylaxis, has been observed; monitor patients closely during infusion; patients experiencing anaphylactic reactions should be evaluated for the presence of inhibitors; discontinue therapy immediately if urticaria, hives, hypotension, tightness of the chest, wheezing, dyspnea, faintness, or anaphylaxis develop.

Alphanate® and Wilate® contain polysorbate 80 (Tween 80®) which may cause allergic reactions in susceptible individuals. In premature neonates, thrombocytopenia, ascites, pulmonary deterioration, and renal and hepatic failure have been reported after receiving parenteral products containing polysorbate 80 (Alade, 1986; CDC, 1984). Infusion of polysorbate 80-containing solutions through polyvinyl chloride tubing may cause DEHP to leach into the solution; in immature animals, exposure to DEHP may adversely affect the development of the male reproductive tract.

Precautions Human antihemophilic factor/von Willebrand factor complex is prepared from pooled plasma; even with heat treated or other viral attenuated processes, the risk of viral transmission (ie, viral hepatitis, HIV, parvovirus B19, and theoretically, Creutzfeldt-Jakob disease agent) is not totally eradicated. Hepatitis B vaccination is recommended for all patients receiving human antihemophilic factor/von Willebrand factor complex and hepatitis A vaccination is recommended for seronegative patients.

Alphanate®, Humate-P® contain trace amounts of blood groups A and B isohemagglutinins; progressive anemia and hemolysis may occur in individuals with blood groups A, B, and AB who receive large or frequent doses of human antihemophilic factor/von Willebrand factor complex due to trace amounts of blood group A and B isohemagglutinins; use with caution in these patients.

Formation of factor VIII inhibitors (neutralizing antibodies to AHF human) may occur, particularly in patients with Type 3 (severe) von Willebrand factor; reported overall incidence is 3% to 52%; an increase of inhibitor antibody concentration is seen at 2-7 days, with peak concentrations at 1-3 weeks after therapy; children <5 years of age may also be at greatest risk. Patients who develop antibodies (usually antibody concentration >10 Bethesda units/mL) against von Willebrand factor will not have an effective clinical response to therapy and infusions may result in anaphylactic reactions; these patients should be managed by an experienced physician and alternatives to therapy should be considered. Any patient who has an inadequate response to therapy or a severe adverse reaction should be evaluated for the presence of inhibitors. The dosage requirement will vary in patients with factor VIII inhibitors; optimal treatment should be determined by clinical response. In patients with Hemophilia A, the dosage requirement will vary in patients with factor VIII inhibitors; optimal treatment should be determined by clinical response.

Adverse Reactions

Cardiovascular: Cardiorespiratory arrest, chest tightness, edema, femoral venous thrombosis, flushing, hypervolemia, orthostatic hypotension, shock, thromboembolic events, vasodilation

Central nervous system: Chills, dizziness, fever, headache, lethargy, pain, seizure, somnolence

Dermatologic: Itching, pruritus, rash, urticaria

Endocrine & metabolic: Parotid gland swelling

Gastrointestinal: Nausea, vomiting

Hematologic: Hematocrit decreased (moderate), hemorrhage, hemolysis, pseudothrombocytopenia (severe)

Hepatic: ALT increased

Local: Injection site stinging, phlebitis

Neuromuscular & skeletal: Extremity pain, joint pain, paresthesia, rigors

Respiratory: Cough, dyspnea, pharyngitis, pulmonary embolus (large doses)

Miscellaneous: Allergic reactions, anaphylactic reactions, factor VIII inhibitor formation, hypersensitivity reactions, von Willebrand factor inhibitor formation

Drug Interactions

Metabolism/Transport Effects None known.

Avoid Concomitant Use There are no known interactions where it is recommended to avoid concomitant use.

Increased Effect/Toxicity There are no known significant interactions involving an increase in effect.

Decreased Effect There are no known significant interactions involving a decrease in effect.

Stability

Alphanate®: Store intact vials at ≤25°C (77°F); do not freeze. Use within 3 hours of reconstitution; do not refrigerate after reconstitution.

Humate-P®: Store intact vials at ≤25°C (≤77°F); avoid freezing. Use within 3 hours of reconstitution. Do not refrigerate after reconstitution, precipitation may occur.

Wilate®: Store intact vials at 2°C to 8°C (36°F to 46°F); do not freeze. Protect from light. Intact vials may also be stored at room temperature [not to exceed 25°C (77°F)] for ≤6 months. Once stored at room temperature, do not return to the refrigerator. Following reconstitution, use solution immediately.

Mechanism of Action Factor VIII and von Willebrand factor (VWF), obtained from pooled human plasma, are used to replace endogenous factor VIII and VWF in patients with hemophilia or VWD. Factor VIII in conjunction with activated factor IX, activates factor X which converts prothrombin to thrombin and fibrinogen to fibrin. VWF promotes platelet aggregation and adhesion to damaged vascular endothelium and acts as a stabilizing carrier protein for factor VIII. (Circulating levels of functional VWF are measured as ristocetin cofactor activity [VWF:RCo].)

Pharmacodynamics

Onset: Shortening of bleeding time: Immediate

Maximum effect: 1-2 hours

Duration: VWD: Shortening of bleeding time: <6 hours postinfusion; VWF multimers detected in the plasma: 24 hours after infusion

Pharmacokinetics (Adult data unless noted)

Distribution: V_{dss}: VWF:RCo: 53-72 mL/kg

Half-life, elimination:

FVIII coagulant activity (FVIII:C 8-28 hours in patients with hemophilia A

VWF:RCo: 3-34 hours in patients with VWD

Dosing: Usual Note: Individualize dosage based on coagulation studies performed prior to and during treatment at regular intervals:

Hemophilia A; Factor VIII deficiency: Alphanate®, Humate-P®: General guidelines provided (consult specific product labeling for Alphanate® or Humate-P®):

Infants, Children, Adolescents, and Adults: Limited data in pediatric patients <16 years: I.V.: In general, administration of 1 unit/kg of factor VIII will increase circulating factor VIII levels by ~2 units/dL (or 2%); calculated dosage should be adjusted to the actual vial size.

The formula to calculate required dosage based on desired increase in factor VIII (% of normal); **Note:** This formula assumes that the patient's baseline AHF level is <1%:

Units required = Body weight (kg) x 0.5 x desired increase in factor VIII (units or% of normal)

Minor hemorrhage: Loading dose: FVIII:C 15 units/kg to achieve FVIII:C plasma level ~30% of normal. One infusion may be adequate. If second infusion is needed, half the loading dose may be given once or twice daily for 1-2 days.

Moderate hemorrhage: Loading dose: FVIII:C 25 units/kg to achieve FVIII:C plasma level ~50% of normal. Maintenance: FVIII:C 15 units/kg every 8-12 hours for 1-2 days in order to maintain FVIII:C plasma levels at 30% of normal. Repeat the same dose once or twice daily for up to 7 days or until adequate wound healing.

Life-threatening hemorrhage: Loading dose: FVIII:C 40-50 units/kg. Maintenance: FVIII:C 20-25 units/kg every 8 hours to maintain FVIII:C plasma levels at 80% to 100% of normal for 7 days. Continue same dose once or twice daily for another 7 days in order to maintain FVIII:C levels at 30% to 50% of normal.

von Willebrand disease (VWD); treatment: Dosage is expressed in international units of von Willebrand factor: Ristocetin cofactor (VWF:RCo): Dose must be individualized based on type of VWD, extent and location of bleeding, clinical status of patient, and coagulation studies performed prior to and at regular intervals during treatment. Products are not identical and should not be used interchangeably (NHLBI, 2007).

Hemorrhage:

Humate P: Infants, Children, Adolescents, and Adults: I.V.: **Note:** In general, administration of 1 unit/kg of factor VIII would be expected to raise circulating VWF:RCo ~5 units/dL

Type 1, mild VWD: Major hemorrhage or minor hemorrhage (if desmopressin is not appropriate):
Loading dose: 40-60 units/kg
Maintenance dose: 40-50 units/kg/dose every 8-12 hours for 3 days, maintain VWF:RCo nadir >50%; follow with 40-50 units/kg once daily for up to 7 days

Type 1, moderate or severe VWD:
Minor hemorrhage: 40-50 units/kg/dose for 1-2 doses
Major hemorrhage:
Loading dose: 50-75 units/kg
Maintenance dose: 40-60 units/kg/dose every 8-12 hours for 3 days; maintain VWF:RCo nadir >50%; follow with 40-60 units/kg/dose once daily for up to 7 days

Types 2 and 3 VWD:
Minor hemorrhage: 40-50 units/kg/dose for 1-2 doses
Major hemorrhage:
Loading dose: 60-80 units/kg
Maintenance dose: 40-60 units/kg/dose every 8-12 hours for 3 days, maintain VWF:RCo nadir >50%; follow with 40-60 units/kg/dose once daily for up to 7 days

Wilate: Children ≥5 years, Adolescents, and Adults: I.V.:
Minor hemorrhage:
Loading dose: 20-40 units/kg
Maintenance dose: 20-30 units/kg/dose every 12-24 hours for ≤3 days, keeping the VWF:RCo nadir >30%
Major hemorrhage:
Loading dose: 40-60 units/kg
Maintenance dose: 20-40 units/kg/dose every 12-24 hours for 5-7 days, keeping the VWF:RCo nadir >50%

von Willebrand disease (VWD); surgical/procedural prophylaxis: Note: Not for patients with type 3 VWD undergoing major surgery

Alphanate:

Infants, Children, and Adolescents: I.V.:
Preoperative dose: 75 units/kg as a single dose 1 hour prior to surgery
Maintenance dose: 50-75 units/kg/dose every 8-12 hours as clinically needed. May reduce dose after third postoperative day; continue treatment until healing is complete. Goal is to keep the VWF:RCo nadir >50 units/dL at least for the first 3 days (NHLBI, 2007)

Adults (except patients with type 3 undergoing major surgery): I.V.:
Preoperative dose: 60 units/kg 1 hour prior to surgery
Maintenance dose: 40-60 units/kg/dose every 8-12 hours as clinically needed. May reduce dose after third postoperative day; continue treatment until healing is complete. For minor procedures, maintain VWF of 40% to 50% during postoperative days 1-3; for major procedures maintain VWF of 40% to 50% for ≥3-7 days postoperative.

Humate-P®: Infants, Children, Adolescents, and Adults: I.V.:
Emergency surgery: 50-60 units/kg; monitor trough coagulation factor levels for subsequent doses
Surgical management (nonemergency): **Note:** Whenever possible, the *in vivo* recovery (IVR) should be measured and baseline plasma VWF:RCo and FVIII activity should be assessed in all patients prior to surgery. The formula to calculate the IVR is as follows: Measure baseline plasma VWF:RCo; then infuse VWF:RCo 60 units/kg I.V. at time zero; measure VWF:RCo at 30 minutes after infusion. IVR = (plasma VWF:RCo at 30 minutes minus plasma VWF:RCof at baseline) divided by 60 units/kg.
Loading dose: Loading dose calculation based on baseline target VWF:RCo: (Target peak VWF:RCo - Baseline VWF:RCo) x weight (in kg) / IVR = units VWF:RCo required. Administer loading dose 1-2 hours prior to surgery. **Note:** If *in vivo* recovery (IVR) is not available, assume IVR of 2 units/dL for every one VWF:RCo unit/kg administered.
Target peak VWF:RCo concentrations following loading dose:
Major surgery/emergency: 100 units/dL
Minor/oral surgery: 50-60 units/dL
Note: Oral surgery is <2 extractions of nonmolars without bony involvement; extractions of ≥2 teeth or >1 impacted wisdom tooth is considered major surgery.
Maintenance dose: Initial: One-half loading dose followed by subsequent dosing determined by target trough concentrations, generally administered every 8-12 hours; patients with shorter half-lives may require dosing every 6 hours

Target maintenance trough VWF:RCo concentrations and minimum duration of treatment:

Major surgery: >50 units/dL for up to 3 days, followed by >30 units/dL; minimum duration of treatment: 72 hours

Minor surgery: ≥30 units/dL; minimum duration of treatment: 48 hours

Oral surgery: ≥30 units/dL; minimum duration of treatment: 8-12 hours

Administration Reconstitution: If refrigerated, the dried concentrate and diluent should be warmed to room temperature before reconstitution; see product labeling for specific reconstitution guidelines; gently swirl or rotate vial after adding diluent, do not shake vigorously. Use provided filter transfer set to withdraw solution from vial of Alphanate® or Humate-P®; remove filter spike prior to administration. Use provided transfer device to reconstitute Wilate®. **Note:** Use plastic syringes; AHF may stick to the surface of glass syringes. Discard unused contents and administration equipment after use.

Parenteral: I.V.: Administer through a separate line, do not mix with drugs or other I.V. fluids

Alphanate®: Infuse slowly; maximum rate: 10 mL/minute

Humate-P®: Infuse slowly; maximum rate: 4 mL/minute

Wilate®: Infuse slowly at a rate of 2-4 mL/minute

Monitoring Parameters Signs and symptoms of intravascular hemolysis or bleeding; heart rate and blood pressure (before and during I.V. administration). AHF levels prior to and during treatment; in patients with circulating inhibitors, the inhibitor level should be monitored; hematocrit; VWF activity (circulating levels of functional VWF are measured as ristocetin cofactor activity [VWF: RCo]). In surgical patients, monitor VWF:RCo at baseline and after surgery, trough VWF:RCo and FVIII:C at least daily.

Reference Range Hemophilia: Classification of hemophilia; normal is defined as 1 unit/mL of factor VIII:C

Severe: Factor level <1% of normal

Moderate: Factor level 1% to 5% of normal

Mild: Factor level >5% to 30% of normal

Additional Information One unit of AHF is equal to the factor VIII activity present in 1 mL of normal human plasma. If bleeding is not controlled with adequate dose, test for the presence of factor VIII inhibitor; larger doses of AHF may be therapeutic with inhibitor titers <10 Bethesda units/mL; it may not be possible or practical to control bleeding if inhibitor titers >10 Bethesda units/mL (due to the very large AHF doses required); other treatments [eg, antihemophilic factor (porcine), factor IX complex concentrates, recombinant factor VIIa, or anti-inhibitor coagulant complex] may be needed in patients with inhibitor titers >10 Bethesda units/mL.

Exact potency varies among products and between lots of the same product; each vial contains the exact labeled amount of VWF activity, as measured with the Ristocetin cofactor activity (VWF:RCo), and factor VIII (FVIII) activity and should be consulted prior to use. However, the average ratio between VWF:RCo and FVIII among available products is:

Alphanate®: Average ratio not provided by manufacturer or in available literature

Humate-P®: Average ratio of VWF:RCo to FVIII is 2.4:1

Wilate®: Average ratio of VWF:RCo to FVIII is ~1:1

Dosage Forms Excipient information presented when available (limited, particularly for generics); consult specific product labeling. [DSC] = Discontinued product

Injection, powder for reconstitution [human derived]:

Alphanate®:

250 units [Factor VIII and VWF:RCo ratio varies by lot; contains sodium ≥10 mEq/vial, albumin and polysorbate 80; packaged with diluent]

500 units [Factor VIII and VWF:RCo ratio varies by lot; contains sodium ≥10 mEq/vial, albumin and polysorbate 80; packaged with diluent]

1000 units [Factor VIII and VWF:RCo ratio varies by lot; contains sodium ≥10 mEq/vial, albumin and polysorbate 80; packaged with diluent]

1500 units [Factor VIII and VWF:RCo ratio varies by lot; contains sodium ≥10 mEq/vial, albumin and polysorbate 80; packaged with diluent]

Humate-P®:

FVIII 250 units and VWF:RCo 600 units [contains albumin; packaged with diluent]

FVIII 500 units and VWF:RCo 1200 units [contains albumin; packaged with diluent]

FVIII 1000 units and VWF:RCo 2400 units [contains albumin; packaged with diluent]

Wilate®:

FVIII 450 units and VWF:RCo 450 units [contains polysorbate 80 (in diluent); packaged with diluent] [DSC]

FVIII 500 units and VWF:RCo 500 units [contains polysorbate 80 (in diluent); packaged with diluent]

FVIII 900 units and VWF:RCo 900 units [contains polysorbate 80 (in diluent); packaged with diluent] [DSC]

FVIII 1000 units and VWF:RCo 1000 units [contains polysorbate 80 (in diluent); packaged with diluent]

References

Alade SL, Brown RE, and Paquet A Jr, "Polysorbate 80 and E-Ferol Toxicity," *Pediatrics,* 1986, 77(4):593-7.

Centers for Disease Control (CDC), "Unusual Syndrome With Fatalities Among Premature Infants: Association With a New Intravenous Vitamin E Product," *MMWR Morb Mortal Wkly Rep,* 1984, 33 (14):198-9.

NHLBI VWD Expert Panel, "The Diagnosis, Evaluation, and Management of von Willebrand Disease. US Department of Health and Human Services, National Institutes of Health, National Heart Lung and Blood Institute, 2007, NIH No. 08-5832.

World Federation of Hemophilia, "Guidelines for the Management of Hemophilia," 2005. Available at http://www.wfh.org/2/docs/Publications/Diagnosis_and_Treatment/Guidelines_Mng_Hemophilia.pdf

◆ **Anti-Hist Allergy [OTC]** *see* DiphenhydrAMINE (Systemic) *on page 673*

Anti-inhibitor Coagulant Complex (Human)

(an TEE in HI bi tor coe AG yoo lant KOM pleks HYU man)

Brand Names: U.S. Feiba NF

Brand Names: Canada FEIBA NF

Therapeutic Category Antihemophilic Agent; Blood Product Derivative

Generic Availability (U.S.) No

Use Control of spontaneous bleeding episodes or to cover surgical interventions in hemophilia A and hemophilia B patients [FDA approved in infants (>28 days of life), children, and adults]

Pregnancy Risk Factor C

Pregnancy Considerations Animal reproduction studies have not been conducted.

Breast-Feeding Considerations It is not known if this product is excreted in breast milk. The manufacturer recommends that caution be exercised when administering anti-inhibitor coagulant complex to nursing women.

Contraindications Hypersensitivity to anti-inhibitor coagulant complex or any component; patients with a normal coagulation mechanism; significant signs of disseminated intravascular coagulation (DIC); treatment of bleeding due to coagulation factor deficiencies in the absence of inhibitors to coagulation factors VIII or IX; acute thromboembolism (including myocardial infarction)

Warnings Not for use in patients with bleeding episodes resulting from coagulation factor deficiencies without circulating inhibitors. Product is prepared from pooled human plasma; may contain infectious agents that can transmit disease; screening of donors, as well as testing and/or inactivation or removal of certain viruses, reduces the risk (rare). WBCT, aPTT, and TEG tests do not correlate with clinical efficacy; dosing to normalize these values may result in DIC. Discontinue immediately if symptoms of DIC occur. Thrombotic and thromboembolic events (including venous thrombosis, pulmonary embolism, DIC, MI, and stroke) may occur, particularly following administration of high doses and/or in patients with thrombotic risk factors **[U.S. Boxed Warning]**. Single doses of 100 units/kg or a daily dose of 200 units/kg should not be exceeded; patients receiving maximum single or daily doses must be monitored for the development of DIC and/or symptoms of acute coronary ischemia. High doses should be used for the shortest time necessary to control bleeding. Thromboembolic events may be increased with concurrent use of an antifibrinolytic (tranexamic acid, aminocaproic acid); avoid or delay use of antifibrinolytic for at least 12 hours. Anamnestic rises in inhibitor (antibody) levels have been observed in 20% of the patients which may result in prolonged refractoriness to subsequent therapy.

Allergic reactions (including severe anaphylactoid reactions) have been observed following administration. Discontinue immediately with signs/symptoms of hypersensitivity. Appropriate medication including epinephrine should be readily available.

Precautions Use with extreme caution in patients with thrombotic risk factors (eg, history of CHD, liver disease, DIC, postoperative immobilization, neonates, elderly patients); systemic antifibrinolytics (eg, tranexamic acid, aminocaproic acid) should not be used within 12 hours of Feiba NF dose; if signs of DIC occur (eg, chest pain, heart rate changes, blood pressure changes, or cough), discontinue infusion and initiate appropriate therapeutic measures

Adverse Reactions

Cardiovascular: Blood pressure decreased, chest discomfort/pain, flushing, hyper-/hypotension, MI, tachycardia, thromboembolism

Central nervous system: Chills, dizziness, fever, headache, hypoesthesia (including facial), malaise, paresthesia, somnolence

Dermatologic: Angioedema, pruritus, rash, urticaria

Gastrointestinal: Abdominal discomfort, diarrhea, dysgeusia, nausea, vomiting

Hematologic: DIC, stroke (embolic/thrombotic), thrombosis (arterial/venous)

Local: Injection site pain

Respiratory: Bronchospasm, cough, dyspnea, pulmonary embolism, wheezing

Miscellaneous: Allergic reaction (including anaphylaxis), anamnestic response, hypersensitivity

Drug Interactions

Metabolism/Transport Effects None known.

Avoid Concomitant Use

Avoid concomitant use of Anti-inhibitor Coagulant Complex (Human) with any of the following: Antifibrinolytic Agents

Increased Effect/Toxicity

The levels/effects of Anti-inhibitor Coagulant Complex (Human) may be increased by: Antifibrinolytic Agents

Decreased Effect There are no known significant interactions involving a decrease in effect.

Stability Prior to reconstitution, store at room temperature [maximum of 25°C (77°F)]; store in original package to protect from light. Do **not** refrigerate after reconstitution.

Mechanism of Action Multiple interactions of the components in anti-inhibitor coagulant complex restore the impaired thrombin generation of hemophilia patients with inhibitors. *In vitro*, anti-inhibitor coagulant complex shortens the activated partial thromboplastin time of plasma containing factor VIII inhibitor.

Dosing: Usual Dosage is dependent upon the severity and location of bleeding, type and level of inhibitors, and whether the patient has a history of an anamnestic increase in antihemophilic inhibitor levels following use of preparations containing antihemophilic factor. Maximum dose should only be exceeded if bleeding severity warrants; monitor closely for DIC and/or coronary ischemia.

Infants, Children, and Adults: I.V.: **Note:** Considered a first-line treatment when factor VIII inhibitor titer is >5 Bethesda units (BU) (antihemophilic factor may be preferred when titer <5 BU)

General dosing: 50-100 units/kg (maximum: 200 units/kg/**day**); dosage may vary with the bleeding site and severity

Joint hemorrhage: 50 units/kg every 12 hours; may increase to 100 units/kg every 12 hours; (maximum: 200 units/kg/**day**)

Mucous membrane bleeding: 50 units/kg every 6 hours; may increase to 100 units/kg every 6 hours for up to two doses (maximum: 200 units/kg/**day**)

Soft tissue hemorrhage: 100 units/kg every 12 hours (maximum: 200 units/kg/**day**)

Other severe hemorrhages: 100 units/kg every 12 hours; may be given every 6 hours if needed (maximum: 200 units/kg/**day**)

Administration I.V.: Reconstitute with provided diluent; swirl gently; do not shake; do **not** refrigerate after reconstitution; use within 3 hours of reconstitution; administer without further dilution. Maximum rate of infusion: 2 units/kg/minute

Monitoring Parameters Monitor for control of bleeding; signs and symptoms of DIC (blood pressure changes, pulse rate changes, chest pain/cough, fibrinogen decreased, platelet count decreased, fibrin-fibrinogen degradation products, significantly-prolonged thrombin time, PT, or partial thromboplastin time); hemoglobin and hematocrit; hypotension; have epinephrine ready to treat hypersensitivity reactions. **Note:** Tests used to control efficacy such as aPTT, WBCT, and TEG do not correlate with clinical improvement. Dosing to normalize these values may result in DIC.

Additional Information Note: Dosage is expressed in units of factor VIII inhibitor bypassing activity. One unit of activity is defined as that amount of anti-inhibitor coagulant complex that shortens the activated partial thromboplastin time (aPTT) of a high titer factor VIII inhibitor reference plasma to 50% of the blank value.

Dosage Forms Excipient information presented when available (limited, particularly for generics); consult specific product labeling.

Solution Reconstituted, Intravenous:

Feiba NF: (1 ea)

Solution Reconstituted, Intravenous [preservative free]:

Feiba NF: 500 units (1 ea); 1000 units (1 ea); 2500 units (1 ea)

◆ **Anti-Itch [OTC]** *see* DiphenhydrAMINE (Topical) *on page 677*

◆ **Anti-Itch Maximum Strength [OTC]** *see* DiphenhydrAMINE (Topical) *on page 677*

◆ **Anti-Itch Maximum Strength [OTC]** *see* Hydrocortisone (Topical) *on page 1038*

Antipyrine and Benzocaine

(an tee PYE reen & BEN zoe kane)

Brand Names: U.S. Aurodex®

Brand Names: Canada Auralgan®

Therapeutic Category Otic Agent, Analgesic; Otic Agent, Cerumenolytic

Generic Availability (U.S.) Yes

Use Temporary relief of pain and reduction of inflammation associated with acute otitis media (congestive and serous stages); facilitates ear wax removal

Pregnancy Risk Factor C

Pregnancy Considerations Animal reproduction studies have not been conducted with this combination.

Contraindications Hypersensitivity to antipyrine, benzocaine, or any component; perforated tympanic membrane; ear discharge

Warnings Methemoglobinemia has been reported with benzocaine topical products containing higher concentrations (14% to 20%) of benzocaine but is rare with combination products (concentration: 1.4%) (Rodriguez, 1994). Fatal methemoglobinemia was reported in a 4 month old infant who received 3 times the prescribed dose of ear drops containing benzocaine 0.25% and antipyrine 5.4%; causality was not proven (Logan, 2005). Use of otic anesthetics may mask symptoms of a fulminating middle ear infection (acute otitis media); not intended for prolonged use. Discontinue if sensitization or irritation occur.

Precautions For use in ears only, do not apply to eyes.

Adverse Reactions No adverse reactions are reported in the manufacturer's labeling. Refer to Benzocaine monograph.

Drug Interactions

Metabolism/Transport Effects None known.

Avoid Concomitant Use There are no known interactions where it is recommended to avoid concomitant use.

Increased Effect/Toxicity

Antipyrine and Benzocaine may increase the levels/effects of: Prilocaine; Sodium Nitrite

The levels/effects of Antipyrine and Benzocaine may be increased by: Nitric Oxide

Decreased Effect There are no known significant interactions involving a decrease in effect.

Stability Store at 20°C to 25°C (68°F to 77°F); excursions permitted to 15°C to 30°C (59°F to 86°F); protect from light, heat, and freezing. Do not use if brown or contains a precipitate. Discard 6 months after opening

Mechanism of Action Antipyrine has analgesic properties; benzocaine is a local anesthetic; the glycerin base provides decreased middle ear pressure by osmosis.

Pharmacodynamics Onset of action: Pain relief: ~30 minutes (Hoberman, 1997)

Dosing: Usual Infants, Children, Adolescents, and Adults:

Acute otitis media, adjunct for associated pain and swelling: Otic: Fill ear canal, then moisten cotton pledget, place in external ear; repeat every 1-2 hours until pain and congestion are relieved

Ear wax removal; adjunct to loosen cerumen and to dry the ear canal or minimize associated discomfort: Otic: Instill drops 3 times daily for 2-3 days; moisten cotton pledget with antipyrine and benzocaine solution and place in external ear after solution instillation

Dosing adjustment in renal impairment: There are no dosage adjustments provided in the manufacturer's labeling.

Dosing adjustment in hepatic impairment: There are no dosage adjustments provided in the manufacturer's labeling.

Administration Otic: Patient should lie down with affected ear upward and medication instilled; remain in the position to allow penetration of solution. Avoid touching dropper to ears or fingers. Do not rinse dropper after use.

Acute otitis media: Fill ear canal with solution, then moisten cotton pledget with antipyrine and benzocaine solution and place in external ear

Ear wax removal: Moisten cotton pledget with antipyrine and benzocaine solution and place in external ear after solution instillation

Additional Information Product availability variable, some products previously on market (eg, Auralgan) are no longer available due to FDA regulations; see website for additional information at http://www.fda.gov/Drugs/GuidanceComplianceRegulatoryInformation/EnforcementActivitiesbyFDA/SelectedEnforcementActionsonUnapprovedDrugs/ucm238675.htm#ophthalmic

Dosage Forms Excipient information presented when available (limited, particularly for generics); consult specific product labeling.

Solution, otic [drops]: Antipyrine 5.4% and benzocaine 1.4% (10 mL, 15 mL)

Aurodex™: Antipyrine 5.4% and benzocaine 1.4% (10 mL)

References
Hoberman A, Paradise JL, Reynolds EA, et al, "Efficacy of Auralgan for Treating Ear Pain in Children With Acute Otitis Media," *Arch Pediatr Adolesc Med*, 1997, 151(7):675-8.
Logan BK and Gordon AM, "Death of an Infant Involving Benzocaine," *J Forensic Sci*, 2005, 50(6):1486-8.
Rodriguez LF, Smolik LM, and Zbehlik AJ, "Benzocaine-Induced Methemoglobinemia: Report of a Severe Reaction and Review of the Literature," *Ann Pharmacother*, 1994, 28(5):643-9.

Antithymocyte Globulin (Equine)
(an te THY moe site GLOB yu lin, E kwine)

Medication Safety Issues
Sound-alike/look-alike issues:
Antithymocyte globulin equine (Atgam®) may be confused with antithymocyte globulin rabbit (Thymoglobulin®)
Atgam® may be confused with Ativan®

Brand Names: U.S. Atgam

Brand Names: Canada Atgam®

Therapeutic Category Immunosuppressant Agent; Polyclonal Antibody

Generic Availability (U.S.) No

Use Prevention and/or treatment of acute renal allograft rejection [FDA approved in pediatrics (age not specified) and adults]; treatment of moderate to severe aplastic anemia in patients not considered suitable candidates for bone marrow transplantation; [FDA approved in pediatrics (age not specified) and adults]; has also been used in prevention or treatment of graft-vs-host disease following allogenic stem cell transplantation; prevention and treatment of other solid organ (other than renal) allograft rejection; treatment of myelodysplastic syndrome (MDS)

Pregnancy Risk Factor C

Pregnancy Considerations Animal reproduction studies have not been conducted. Women exposed to Atgam® during pregnancy may be enrolled in the National Transplantation Pregnancy Registry (877-955-6877).

Breast-Feeding Considerations It is not known if antithymocyte globulin (equine) is excreted into breast milk. The manufacturer recommends caution be used if administered to a nursing woman.

Contraindications Hypersensitivity to ATG (history of severe systemic reaction with prior administration), any component, or other equine gamma globulins

Warnings Should only be used by physicians experienced in immunosuppressive therapy or management of renal transplant patients **[U.S. Boxed Warning]**; adequate laboratory and supportive medical resources must be readily available in the facility for patient management **[U.S. Boxed Warning]**. Anaphylaxis (symptoms can include hypotension, respiratory distress, pain in the chest, rash, and tachycardia) may occur at any time during ATG therapy. Epinephrine and oxygen should be readily available to treat anaphylaxis.

Therapy should be discontinued in patients who experience any symptoms of anaphylaxis (rash, tachycardia, dyspnea, hypotension); severe unremitting hemolysis, or in transplant patients who experience severe, unremitting leukopenia or thrombocytopenia

Precautions Product potency may vary from lot to lot. Product of equine and human plasma; may have a risk of transmitting disease, including a theoretical risk of Creutzfeldt-Jakob disease (CJD). Monitor closely for signs of infection; the incidence of cytomegalovirus (CMV) infection may be increased.

Adverse Reactions

Cardiovascular: Bradycardia, cardiac irregularity, chest pain, edema, heart failure, hyper-/hypotension, myocarditis

Central nervous system: Agitation, chills, fever, headache, lethargy, lightheadedness, listlessness, seizure, viral encephalopathy

Dermatologic: Pruritus, rash, urticaria

Gastrointestinal: Diarrhea, nausea, stomatitis, vomiting

Hematologic: Leukopenia, thrombocytopenia

Hepatic: Hepatosplenomegaly, liver function tests abnormal

Local: Burning soles/palms, injection site reactions (pain, redness, swelling), phlebitis, thrombophlebitis,

Neuromuscular & skeletal: Aches, arthralgia, back pain, joint stiffness, myalgia

Ocular: Periorbital edema

Renal: Proteinuria, renal function tests abnormal

Respiratory: Dyspnea, pleural effusion, respiratory distress

Miscellaneous: Anaphylactic reaction, diaphoresis, lymphadenopathy, night sweats, serum sickness, viral infection

Rare but important or life-threatening: Abdominal pain, acute renal failure, anaphylactoid reaction, anemia, aplasia, apnea, confusion, cough, deep vein thrombosis, disorientation, dizziness, eosinophilia, epigastric pain, epistaxis, erythema, faintness, flank pain, GI bleeding, GI perforation, granulocytopenia, hemolysis, hemolytic anemia, herpes simplex reactivation, hiccups, hyperglycemia, iliac vein obstruction, infection, involuntary movement, kidney enlarged/ruptured, laryngospasm, malaise, neutropenia, pancytopenia, paresthesia, pulmonary edema, renal artery thrombosis, rigidity, sore mouth/throat, tachycardia, toxic epidermal necrosis, tremor, vasculitis, viral hepatitis, weakness, wound dehiscence

Drug Interactions

Metabolism/Transport Effects None known.

Avoid Concomitant Use

Avoid concomitant use of Antithymocyte Globulin (Equine) with any of the following: BCG; Natalizumab; Pimecrolimus; Tacrolimus (Topical); Tofacitinib; Vaccines (Live)

Increased Effect/Toxicity

Antithymocyte Globulin (Equine) may increase the levels/effects of: Leflunomide; Natalizumab; Tofacitinib; Vaccines (Live)

The levels/effects of Antithymocyte Globulin (Equine) may be increased by: Denosumab; Pimecrolimus; Roflumilast; Tacrolimus (Topical); Trastuzumab

Decreased Effect

Antithymocyte Globulin (Equine) may decrease the levels/effects of: BCG; Coccidioidin Skin Test; Sipuleucel-T; Vaccines (Inactivated); Vaccines (Live)

The levels/effects of Antithymocyte Globulin (Equine) may be decreased by: Echinacea

Stability Store ampuls at 2°C to 8°C (36°F to 46°F); do not freeze. Dilute in ½NS or NS; when diluted to concentrations up to 4 mg/mL, ATG infusion solution is stable for 24 hours if refrigerated; use of dextrose solutions is not recommended; precipitation can occur in solutions with a low salt concentration (ie, D_5W)

Mechanism of Action Immunosuppressant involved in the elimination of antigen-reactive T lymphocytes (killer cells) in peripheral blood or alteration in the function of T-lymphocytes, which are involved in humoral immunity and partly in cell-mediated immunity; induces complete or partial hematologic response in aplastic anemia

Pharmacokinetics (Adult data unless noted)

Distribution: Poor into lymphoid tissues; binds to circulating lymphocytes, granulocytes, platelets, bone marrow cells

Half-life, plasma: 1.5-12 days

Elimination: ~1% of dose excreted in urine

Dosing: Usual Intradermal skin test is recommended prior to administration of the initial dose of ATG; use 0.1 mL of a fresh 1:1000 dilution of ATG in NS; observe the skin test every 15 minutes for 1 hour; a local reaction ≥10 mm diameter with a wheal or erythema or both should be considered a positive skin test; if a positive skin test occurs, the first infusion should be administered in a controlled environment with intensive life support immediately available. A systemic reaction precludes further administration of the drug. The absence of a reaction does **not** preclude the possibility of an immediate sensitivity reaction.

I.V.: Children and Adults:

Aplastic anemia protocol: 10-20 mg/kg/day for 8-14 days; additional every other day therapy can be administered up to a total of 21 doses in 28 days. One study (Rosenfeld, 1995) used a dose of 40 mg/kg/day once daily over 4 hours for 4 days.

Renal allograft: Dosage range: Children: 5-25 mg/kg/day; Adults: 10-30 mg/kg/day

Induction dose (delaying the onset of allograft rejection): 15 mg/kg/day for 14 days, then every other day for 14 days for a total of 21 doses in 28 days. Initial dose should be administered within 24 hours before or after transplantation.

Treatment of rejection: 10-15 mg/kg/day for 14 days; additional every other day therapy can be administered up to a total of 21 doses

Acute GVHD treatment (unlabeled use): 30 mg/kg/dose every other day for 6 doses (MacMillan, 2007) or 15 mg/kg/dose twice daily for 10 doses (MacMillan, 2002)

Dosage adjustment for toxicity:

Anaphylaxis: Stop infusion immediately; administer epinephrine. May require corticosteroids, respiration assistance, and/or other resuscitative measures. Do not resume infusion.

Hemolysis (severe and unremitting): May require discontinuation of treatment

Administration Parenteral: Do not shake diluted or undiluted ATG solution to prevent excessive foaming and denaturation of the product. ATG should be added to an inverted bottle of sterile diluent so that undiluted drug does not contact air inside the bottle. Allow diluted ATG to reach room temperature before infusion. Administer via central line; use of high flow central vein will minimize the occurrence of phlebitis and thrombosis; administer by slow I.V. infusion through a 0.2-1 micron in-line filter over 4-8 hours at a final concentration not to exceed 4 mg ATG/mL

Monitoring Parameters Lymphocyte profile; CBC with differential and platelet count, vital signs during administration, renal function test

Dosage Forms Excipient information presented when available (limited, particularly for generics); consult specific product labeling.

Injectable, Intravenous:

Atgam: 50 mg/mL (5 mL) [thimerosal free]

References

Macmillan ML, Couriel D, Weisdorf DJ, et al, "A Phase 2/3 Multicenter Randomized Clinical Trial of ABX-CBL Versus ATG as Secondary

Therapy for Steroid-Resistant Acute Graft-Versus-Host Disease," *Blood*, 2007, 109(6):2657-62.

MacMillan ML, Weisdorf DJ, Davies SM, et al, "Early Antithymocyte Globulin Therapy Improves Survival in Patients With Steroid-Resistant Acute Graft-Versus-Host Disease," *Biol Blood Marrow Transplant*, 2002, 8(1):40-6.

Rosenfeld SJ, Kimball J, Vining D, et al, "Intensive Immunosuppression With Antithymocyte Globulin and Cyclosporine as Treatment for Severe Acquired Aplastic Anemia," *Blood*, 1995, 85(11):3058-65.

Taylor DO, Edwards LB, Aurora P, et al, "Registry of the International Society for Heart and Lung Transplantation: Twenty-Fifth Official Adult Heart Transplant Report–2008," *J Heart Lung Transplant*, 2008, 27 (9):943-56.

Webster A, Chapman JR, Craig JC, et al. "Polyclonal and Monoclonal Antibodies for Preventing Acute Rejection Episodes in Kidney Transplant Recipients," *Cochrane Database of Systematic Reviews*, 2006, Issue 2.

Whitehead B, James I, Helms P, et al, "Intensive Care Management of Children Following Heart and Heart-Lung Transplantation," *Intensive Care Med*, 1990, 16(7):426-30.

Antithymocyte Globulin (Rabbit)

(an te THY moe site GLOB yu lin RAB bit)

Medication Safety Issues
Sound-alike/look-alike issues:
Antithymocyte globulin rabbit (Thymoglobulin®) may be confused with antithymocyte globulin equine (Atgam®)

Brand Names: U.S. Thymoglobulin

Brand Names: Canada Thymoglobulin

Therapeutic Category Immunosuppressant Agent

Generic Availability (U.S.) No

Use Treatment of acute rejection of renal transplant; used in conjunction with concomitant immunosuppression (FDA approved in adults); has also been used as induction therapy in renal transplant; treatment of myelodysplastic syndrome (MDS); prevention and/or treatment of acute rejection after bone marrow, heart/lung, liver, intestinal, or multivisceral transplantation in conjunction with other immunosuppressive agents

Pregnancy Risk Factor C

Pregnancy Considerations Animal reproduction studies have not been conducted. Women exposed to thymoglobulin during pregnancy may be enrolled in the National Transplantation Pregnancy Registry (877-955-6877).

Breast-Feeding Considerations This product has not been evaluated in nursing women; the manufacturer recommends that breast-feeding be discontinued if therapy is needed.

Contraindications Hypersensitivity to antithymocyte globulin, rabbit proteins, or any component; acute or chronic infection

Warnings Adequate laboratory and supportive medical resources must be readily available in the facility for patient management. Anaphylaxis has been reported with the use of antithymocyte globulin (rabbit). Epinephrine, oxygen, and resuscitative equipment should be readily available to treat anaphylaxis. Release of cytokines by activated monocytes and lymphocytes may cause fatal cytokine release syndrome (CRS) during administration of antithymocyte globulin. Rapid infusion rates have been associated with CRS in case reports. Severe or life-threatening symptoms include hypotension, acute respiratory distress syndrome, pulmonary edema, myocardial infarction, and tachycardia; symptoms range from a mild, self-limiting "flu-like" reaction to severe, life-threatening reactions.

Thrombocytopenia or neutropenia may result from cross-reactive antibodies and is reversible following dose reduction or discontinuation. Risk of post-transplant lymphoproliferative disease or other malignancies may be increased with prolonged use or overdosage of antithymocyte globulin (rabbit) in association with other immunosuppressants.

Precautions Infusion may cause fever and chills. Infuse first dose slowly over a minimum of 6 hours into a high flow vein; 1 hour prior to infusion, premedicate with corticosteroids, acetaminophen, and/or an antihistamine to reduce incidence of side effects during infusion. Reduce dose in patients with WBC between 2000-3000 cells/mm^3 or if the platelet count is between 50,000-75,000 cells/ mm^3. Consider discontinuing antithymocyte globulin (rabbit) if WBC <2000 cells/mm^3 or platelets <50,000 cells/ mm^3. Patients should not be immunized with attenuated live virus vaccines during or shortly after treatment; safety of immunization following therapy has not been studied. Should only be used by physicians experienced in immunosuppressive therapy for the treatment of renal transplant patients **[U.S. Boxed Warning]**.

Adverse Reactions
Cardiovascular: Hypertension, peripheral edema, tachycardia

Central nervous system: Chills, dizziness, fever, headache, malaise, pain

Endocrine & metabolic: Hyperkalemia

Gastrointestinal: Abdominal pain, diarrhea, gastritis, gastrointestinal moniliasis, nausea

Genitourinary: Urinary tract infection

Hematologic: Leukopenia, thrombocytopenia

Neuromuscular & skeletal: Weakness

Respiratory: Dyspnea

Miscellaneous: Antirabbit antibody development, cytomegalovirus infection, herpes simplex infection, oral moniliasis, sepsis, systemic infection

Rare but important or life-threatening: Anaphylaxis, cytokine release syndrome, PTLD, neutropenia, serum sickness (delayed)

Drug Interactions
Metabolism/Transport Effects None known.

Avoid Concomitant Use
Avoid concomitant use of Antithymocyte Globulin (Rabbit) with any of the following: BCG; Natalizumab; Pimecrolimus; Tacrolimus (Topical); Tofacitinib; Vaccines (Live)

Increased Effect/Toxicity
Antithymocyte Globulin (Rabbit) may increase the levels/ effects of: Leflunomide; Natalizumab; Tofacitinib; Vaccines (Live)

The levels/effects of Antithymocyte Globulin (Rabbit) may be increased by: Denosumab; Pimecrolimus; Roflumilast; Tacrolimus (Topical); Trastuzumab

Decreased Effect
Antithymocyte Globulin (Rabbit) may decrease the levels/ effects of: BCG; Coccidioidin Skin Test; Sipuleucel-T; Vaccines (Inactivated); Vaccines (Live)

The levels/effects of Antithymocyte Globulin (Rabbit) may be decreased by: Echinacea

Stability Store intact vial in refrigerator; protect from light; do not freeze. Allow diluent and contents of vial to reach room temperature prior to reconstitution; reconstituted product is stable for up to 24 hours at room temperature; however, since it contains no preservatives, it should be used immediately following reconstitution; compatible with D$_5$W or NS; Y-site injection compatible with hydrocortisone sodium succinate and heparin 100 units/mL in D$_5$W or NS; incompatible with heparin 2 units/mL in D$_5$W

Mechanism of Action Polyclonal antibody which appears to cause immunosuppression by acting on T-cell surface antigens and depleting CD4 lymphocytes

Pharmacodynamics Onset of action (T-cell depletion): Within one day

Pharmacokinetics (Adult data unless noted) Half-life: 2-3 days

Dosing: Usual IV: (refer to individual protocols):
Children:
Bone marrow transplantation: 1.5-3 mg/kg/day once daily for 4 consecutive days before transplantation

Treatment of graft-versus-host disease: 1.5 mg/kg/dose once daily or every other day

Renal transplantation:

Induction: 1-2 mg/kg/day once daily for 4-5 days initiated at time of transplant

Acute rejection: 1.5mg/kg/day once daily for 7-14 days

Heart/lung transplantation:

Induction: 1-2 mg/kg/day depending on baseline platelet count once daily for 5 days

Rejection: 2 mg/kg/day once daily for 5 days

Liver, intestinal, or multivisceral transplant:

Preconditioning/induction: Pretransplant: 2 mg/kg; postop day 1: 3 mg/kg

Rejection: 1.5 mg/kg/day once daily for 7-14 days based upon biopsy results; maximum dose: 2 mg/kg/dose

Adults: Acute renal transplant rejection: 1.5 mg/kg/day once daily for 7-14 days

Administration Parenteral: Administer by slow I.V. infusion over 6-12 hours for the preconditioning/induction dose or over 6 hours for the initial acute rejection treatment dose; infuse over 4 hours for subsequent doses if first dose tolerated. Administer through an in-line filter with pore size of 0.22 microns via central line or high flow vein at a final concentration of 0.5 mg/mL in NS or D$_5$W.

Monitoring Parameters Platelet count, CBC with differential, lymphocyte count, vital signs during infusion

Test Interactions Potential interference with rabbit antibody-based immunoassays

Additional Information Antiviral therapy should be given prophylactically during antithymocyte globulin (rabbit) use.

Dosage Forms Excipient information presented when available (limited, particularly for generics); consult specific product labeling.

Solution Reconstituted, Intravenous:

Thymoglobulin: 25 mg (1 ea) [contains glycine, mannitol, sodium chloride]

References

Di Filippo S, Boissonnat P, Sassolas F, et al, "Rabbit Antithymocyte Globulin as Induction Immunotherapy in Pediatric Heart Transplantation," *Transplantation*, 2003, 75(3):354-8.

Horan JT, Liesveld JL, Fenton P, et al, "Hematopoietic Stem Cell Transplantation for Multiply Transfused Patients With Sickle Cell Disease and Thalassemia After Low-Dose Total Body Irradiation, Fludarabine, and Rabbit Anti-thymocyte Globulin," *Bone Marrow Transplant*, 2005, 35(2):171-7.

Starzl TE, Murase N, Abu-Elmagd K, et al, "Tolerogenic Immunosuppression for Organ Transplantation," *Lancet*, 2003, 361 (9368):1502-10.

Thymoglobulin [package insert], Cambridge, MA:Genzyme Corp; 2005.

Trissel LA and Saenz CA, "Physical Compatibility of Antithymocyte Globulin (Rabbit) With Heparin Sodium and Hydrocortisone Sodium Succinate," *Am J Health Syst Pharm*, 2003, 60(16):1650-2.

◆ **Antithymocyte Immunoglobulin** *see* Antithymocyte Globulin (Equine) *on page 182*

◆ **Antithymocyte Immunoglobulin** *see* Antithymocyte Globulin (Rabbit) *on page 184*

◆ **Antitumor Necrosis Factor Alpha (Human)** *see* Adalimumab *on page 70*

◆ **Anti-VEGF Monoclonal Antibody** *see* Bevacizumab *on page 288*

◆ **Anti-VEGF rhuMAb** *see* Bevacizumab *on page 288*

◆ **Antivenin (*Centruroides*) Immune F(ab')$_2$ (Equine)** *see* Centruroides Immune F(ab')$_2$ (Equine) *on page 428*

◆ **Antivenin (Crotalidae) Polyvalent, FAB (Ovine)** *see* Crotalidae Polyvalent Immune Fab (Ovine) *on page 553*

Antivenin (*Latrodectus mactans*)

(an tee VEN in lak tro DUK tus MAK tans)

Therapeutic Category Antivenin
Generic Availability (U.S.) Yes

Use Treatment of patients with symptoms (eg, cramping, intractable pain, hypertension) refractory to supportive measures due to *Latrodectus mactans* (black widow spider) envenomation (FDA approved in children and adults); has also been used for treatment of patients with symptoms (eg, cramping, intractable pain, hypertension) refractory to supportive measures due to other *Latrodectus* spp (including *L. bishopi*, *L. geometricus*, *L. hesperus*, and *L. variolus*) envenomation

Pregnancy Risk Factor C

Pregnancy Considerations Animal reproduction studies have not been conducted. Use during pregnancy (second and third trimester) has been described in case reports; all patients delivered healthy infants (Handel, 1994; Russell, 1979; Sherman, 2000). In general, medications used as antidotes should take into consideration the health and prognosis of the mother; antidotes should be administered to pregnant women if there is a clear indication for use and should not be withheld because of fears of teratogenicity (Bailey, 2003).

Breast-Feeding Considerations It is not known if antivenin (*Latrodectus mactans*) is excreted in breast milk. The manufacturer recommends that caution be exercised when administering antivenin (*Latrodectus mactans*) to nursing women.

Warnings Anaphylaxis and serum sickness have been reported in patients who received *Latrodectus mactans* antivenin. Allergic reactions may be less frequent than described in initial studies (Clark, 2001; Offerman, 2011). One retrospective study reviewed 163 cases of black widow spider envenomation; 58 patients received antivenin therapy and only one case of anaphylaxis occurred (Clark, 1992). The risk of reaction appears to be greatest with bolus administration of undiluted antivenin (Clark, 2001). Delayed serum sickness, albeit uncommon, may occur 1-2 weeks following administration, especially when large doses are used (Clark, 2001). Patients with atopic sensitivity to horses may have an increased risk of experiencing an immediate sensitivity reaction to the antivenin; carefully review allergies and history of exposure to products containing horse serum; use with caution in patients with asthma, hay fever, or urticaria; fatal anaphylaxis has been reported in patients with a history of asthma. All patients require close monitoring in a setting where resuscitation can be performed.

A skin or conjunctival test may be performed prior to use; however, the utility of skin and conjunctival tests to accurately identify patients at risk of early (anaphylactic) or late (serum sickness) hypersensitivity reactions to horse-derived antivenins has been questioned (WHO, 2005). One mL of normal horse serum (1:10 dilution) is included for sensitivity testing. The absence of a skin or conjunctival hypersensitivity reaction does not exclude anaphylaxis or hypersensitivity following antivenin administration. False-negative rate for skin testing is 10% with similar agents. Conversely, hypersensitivity is not an absolute contraindication in a significantly envenomated patient.

A desensitization protocol is available if sensitivity tests are mildly or questionably positive to reduce risk of immediate severe hypersensitivity reaction. According to the manufacturer, desensitization should be performed when antivenin administration would be lifesaving; however, the risk of anaphylaxis should be weighed against the risks associated with delayed antivenin administration (Rojnuckarin, 2009). Some products may contain thimerosal.

Adverse Reactions

Dermatologic: Rash (rare; associated with hypersensitivity reaction)

Neuromuscular & skeletal: Muscle cramps

Miscellaneous: Anaphylaxis, hypersensitivity reactions, serum sickness

Drug Interactions

Metabolism/Transport Effects None known.

Avoid Concomitant Use There are no known interactions where it is recommended to avoid concomitant use.

Increased Effect/Toxicity There are no known significant interactions involving an increase in effect.

Decreased Effect There are no known significant interactions involving a decrease in effect.

Stability Store at 2°C to 8°C (36°F to 46°F); do not freeze. After reconstitution, appearance may be opalescent and color may be light (straw) to very dark (iced tea); potency is not affected.

Mechanism of Action Neutralizes the venom of *Latrodectus mactans* (black widow spiders), but may also be effective following envenomation by other *Latrodectus* species (including *L. bishopi, L. geometricus, L. hesperus,* and *L. variolus*) (Clark, 2001; Isbister, 2003).

Pharmacodynamics Onset of action: Within 30 minutes with envenomation symptoms subsiding after 1-3 hours

Dosing: Usual

Infants, Children, and Adolescents: **Note:** Limited data in infants (Monte 2011; Nordt, 2012). The initial dose of antivenin should be administered as soon as possible for prompt relief of symptoms. Delayed antivenin administration may still be effective in treating patients with prolonged or refractory symptoms resulting from black widow spider bites; a case report describes use of antivenin administration up to 90 hours after bite (O'Malley, 1999); however, delayed administration may decrease effectiveness (Edberg, 2009).

Sensitivity testing: Intradermal skin test or conjunctival test may be performed prior to antivenin administration:

Skin test: Intradermal: Up to 0.02 mL of a 1:10 dilution of normal horse serum (provided in kit) in NS; evaluate after 10 minutes against a control test (intradermal injection of 0.02 mL NS). **Note:** Positive reaction consists of an urticarial wheal surrounded by a zone of erythema.

Conjunctival test: Instill 1 drop of 1:100 dilution of normal horse serum into conjunctival sac; a positive reaction is indicated by itching of the eye and/or reddening of conjunctiva, usually occurring within 10 minutes

Desensitization: In separate vials or syringes, prepare 1:10 and 1:100 dilutions of antivenin in NS:

SubQ: Inject 0.1 mL, followed by 0.2 mL and 0.5 mL of a 1:100 dilution at 15- to 30-minute intervals. During desensitization procedure, proceed with the next dose only if a reaction has **not** occurred following the previous dose. Repeat procedure with a 1:10 dilution of antivenin; and then with undiluted antivenin. If no reaction has occurred following administration of 0.5 mL of undiluted antivenin, continue the dose at 15-minute intervals until the entire dose has been administered.

If a reaction occurs, apply a tourniquet proximal to the injection site and administer epinephrine (1:1000) SubQ or I.V. proximal to the tourniquet or into another extremity. Wait at least 30 minutes, then administer another antivenin injection at the previous dilution which did not evoke a reaction.

Latrodectus mactans **(black widow spider) envenomation; other *Latrodectus* spp envenomation** (Clark, 2001): Limited data available for some types of envenomations. **Note:** If a positive reaction to a skin or conjunctival test occurs and antivenin therapy is necessary, pretreat the patient with intravenous diphenhydramine and an H_2-blocker while having a syringe of epinephrine (1:1000) at the bedside:

Infants and Children <12 years: I.M.; I.V. (preferred): One vial (2.5 mL); a second dose may be needed in some cases; more than 1 to 2 vials are rarely required

Children ≥12 years and Adolescents: I.M., I.V.: One vial (2.5 mL); a second dose may be needed in some cases; more than 1 to 2 vials are rarely required

Adults: The initial dose of antivenin should be administered as soon as possible for prompt relief of symptoms. Delayed antivenin administration may still be effective in treating patients with prolonged or refractory symptoms resulting from black widow spider bites; case report of antivenin administration up to 90 hours after bite (O'Malley, 1999); however, delayed administration may decrease effectiveness (Edberg, 2009).

Sensitivity testing: Intradermal skin test or conjunctival test may be performed prior to antivenin administration:

Skin test: Intradermal: Up to 0.02 mL of a 1:10 dilution of normal horse serum in NS; evaluate after 10 minutes against a control test (intradermal injection of NS). **Note:** A positive reaction is an urticarial wheal surrounded by a zone of erythema.

Conjunctival test: Ophthalmic: Instill 1 drop of a 1:10 dilution of normal horse serum into the conjunctival sac; **Note:** Itching of the eye and/or reddening of conjunctiva indicates a positive reaction, usually occurring within 10 minutes.

Desensitization: In separate vials or syringes, prepare 1:10 and 1:100 dilutions of antivenin in NS.

SubQ: Inject 0.1 mL, 0.2 mL, and 0.5 mL of the 1:100 dilution at 15- to 30-minute intervals. During this procedure, proceed with the next dose only if a reaction has **not** occurred following the previous dose. Repeat procedure using the 1:10 dilution and then undiluted antivenin. If no reaction has occurred following administration of 0.5 mL of undiluted antivenin, continue the dose at 15-minute intervals until the entire dose has been administered.

If a reaction occurs, apply a tourniquet proximal to the injection site and administer epinephrine (1:1000) SubQ or I.V. proximal to the tourniquet or into another extremity. Wait at least 30 minutes; then administer another antivenin injection at the previous dilution which did not evoke a reaction.

Dosing adjustment for renal impairment: There are no dosage adjustments provided in the manufacturer's labeling.

Dosing adjustment for hepatic impairment: There are no dosage adjustments provided in the manufacturer's labeling.

Administration

Parenteral: Reconstitute vial containing 6000 units of antivenin with 2.5 mL provided diluent or SWI; gently shake vial (with the needle still in the rubber stopper) to dissolve powder. Excessive agitation or shaking of the reconstituted vial may cause foaming, which may lead to denaturation of the antivenin. When reconstituted, solution can range from a light straw to a dark tea color.

I.M.: Administer the anterolateral thigh. Apply tourniquet if an adverse reaction occurs.

I.V.: Preferred in severe cases, with shock, or in children <12 years of age. There appears to be no clinical difference in efficacy between the I.M. and I.V. route of administration (Isbister, 2008). Dilute reconstituted antivenin with 10 to 50 mL of NS; infuse over 15 to 30 minutes (Clark, 2001). If an immediate hypersensitivity reaction occurs, immediately interrupt antivenin infusion and provide appropriate supportive therapy. If administration of antivenin can be resumed after control of the reaction, reinitiate at a slower infusion rate.

Monitoring Parameters Vital signs; hypersensitivity reactions; serum sickness (for 8-12 days following administration); worsening of symptoms due to envenomation

Additional Information The venom of the black widow spider is a neurotoxin that causes release of a presynaptic neurotransmitter. Within 1 hour of the bite, the clinical effects of black widow spider envenomation (BWSE)

include sharp pain, muscle spasm, weakness, tremor, severe abdominal pain with rigidity, hypertension, respiratory distress, diaphoresis, and facial swelling. Priapism has been reported in pediatric patients following BWSE (Hoover, 2004; Quan, 2009).

Dosage Forms Excipient information presented when available (limited, particularly for generics); consult specific product labeling.

Kit, Injection:

Generic: 6000 Antivenin units

References

Antivenin (*Latrodectus mactans*) (black widow spider antivenin) [prescribing information]. Whitehouse Station, NJ: Merck & Co; February 2014.

Bailey B, "Are There Teratogenic Risks Associated With Antidotes Used in the Acute Management of Poisoned Pregnant Women?" *Birth Defects Res A Clin Mol Teratol*, 2003, 67(2):133-40.

Clark RF, "The Safety and Efficacy of Antivenin *Latrodectus mactans*," *J Toxicol Clin Toxicol*, 2001, 39(2):125-7.

Clark RF, Wethern-Kestner S, Vance MV, et al, "Clinical Presentation and Treatment of Black Widow Spider Envenomation: A Review of 163 Cases," *Ann Emerg Med*, 1992, 21(7):782-7.

Diaz JH, "The Global Epidemiology, Syndromic Classification, Management, and Prevention of Spider Bites," *Am J Trop Med Hyg*, 2004, 71 (2):239-50.

Edberg AL, Lanphear JR, Riley BD, et al, "Toxic Traveler? Latrodectus Species Envenomation in Michigan With Refractory Symptoms After Antivenin Administration," *Clin Toxicol (Phila)*, 2009, 47(4):356-7.

Handel CC, Izquierdo LA, and Curet LB, "Black Widow Spider (*Latrodectus mactans*) Bite During Pregnancy," *West J Med*, 1994, 160 (3):261-2.

Hoover NG and Fortenberry JD, "Use of Antivenin to Treat Priapism After a Black Widow Spider Bite," *Pediatrics*, 2004, 114(1):e128-9.

Isbister GK and Fan HW, "Spider Bite," *Lancet*, 2011, 378 (9808):2039-47.

Isbister GK, Brown SG, Miller M, et al, "A Randomised Controlled Trial of Intramuscular vs Intravenous Antivenom for latrodectism-the RAVE Study," *QJM*, 2008, 101(7):557-65.

Isbister GK, Graudins A, White J, et al, "Antivenom Treatment in Arachnidism," *J Toxicol Clin Toxicol*, 2003, 41(3):291-300.

Monte AA, Bucher-Bartelson B, and Heard KJ, "A US Perspective of Symptomatic *Latrodectus spp.* Envenomation and Treatment: A National Poison Data System Review," *Ann Pharmacother*, 2011, 45 (12):1491-8.

Nordt SP, Clark RF, Lee A, et al, "Examination of Adverse Events Following Black Widow Antivenom Use in California," *Clin Toxicol (Phila)*, 2012, 50(1):70-3.

Offerman SR, Daubert GP, and Clark RF, "The Treatment of Black Widow Spider Envenomation With Antivenin *Latrodectus Mactans*: A Case Series," *Permanente J*, 2011, 15(3):76-81.

O'Malley GF, Dart RC, and Kuffner EF, "Successful Treatment of Latrodectism With Antivenin After 90 Hours," *N Engl J Med*, 1999, 340(8):657.

Quan D and Ruha AM, "Priapism Associated With *Latrodectus mactans* Envenomation," *Am J Emerg Med*, 2009, 27(6):759, e1-2.

Rojnuckarin P, "Antivenom Skin Test: Theory Versus Practice," *Acta Tropica*, 2009, 109(1):86.

Russel FE, Marcus P, and Streng JA, "Black Widow Spider Envenomation During Pregnancy: Report of a Case," *Toxicon*, 1979, 17 (2):188-9.

Saucier JR, "Arachnid Envenomation," *Emerg Med Clin North Am*, 2004, 22(2):405-22.

Sherman RP, Groll JM, Gonzalez DI, et al, "Black Widow Spider (*Latrodectus mactans*) Envenomation in a Term Pregnancy," *Curr Surg*, 2000, 57(4):346-8.

World Health Organization, "Guidelines for the Clinical Management of Snake Bites in the South-East Asia Region," 2005, World Health Organization, Geneva. Available at http://www.searo.who.int/Link-Files/SDE_mgmt_snake-bite.pdf

◆ **Antivenin Scorpion** *see Centruroides* Immune F(ab')₂ (Equine) *on page 428*

◆ **Antivenom (*Centruroides*) Immune F(ab')₂ (Equine)** *see Centruroides* Immune F(ab')₂ (Equine) *on page 428*

◆ **Antivenom (Crotalidae) Polyvalent, FAB (Ovine)** *see Crotalidae* Polyvalent Immune Fab (Ovine) *on page 553*

◆ **Antivenom Scorpion** *see Centruroides* Immune F(ab')₂ (Equine) *on page 428*

◆ **Antivert** *see* Meclizine *on page 1317*

◆ **Antizol** *see* Fomepizole *on page 927*

◆ **Anucort-HC** *see* Hydrocortisone (Topical) *on page 1038*

◆ **Anu-Med [OTC]** *see* Phenylephrine (Topical) *on page 1662*

◆ **Anusol-HC** *see* Hydrocortisone (Topical) *on page 1038*

◆ **Anuzinc (Can)** *see* Zinc Sulfate *on page 2176*

◆ **Anzemet** *see* Dolasetron *on page 703*

◆ **APAP (abbreviation is not recommended)** *see* Acetaminophen *on page 47*

◆ **aPCC** *see* Anti-inhibitor Coagulant Complex (Human) *on page 180*

◆ **Apidra** *see* Insulin Glulisine *on page 1123*

◆ **Apidra® (Can)** *see* Insulin Glulisine *on page 1123*

◆ **Apidra SoloStar** *see* Insulin Glulisine *on page 1123*

◆ **Aplenzin** *see* BuPROPion *on page 327*

◆ **Apo-Acetaminophen (Can)** *see* Acetaminophen *on page 47*

◆ **Apo-Acyclovir (Can)** *see* Acyclovir (Systemic) *on page 63*

◆ **Apo-Allopurinol (Can)** *see* Allopurinol *on page 97*

◆ **Apo-Alpraz® (Can)** *see* ALPRAZolam *on page 100*

◆ **Apo-Alpraz® TS (Can)** *see* ALPRAZolam *on page 100*

◆ **Apo-Amiloride® (Can)** *see* AMILoride *on page 121*

◆ **Apo-Amiodarone (Can)** *see* Amiodarone *on page 127*

◆ **Apo-Amitriptyline (Can)** *see* Amitriptyline *on page 133*

◆ **Apo-Amlodipine (Can)** *see* AmLODIPine *on page 135*

◆ **Apo-Amoxi® (Can)** *see* Amoxicillin *on page 140*

◆ **Apo-Amoxi-Clav (Can)** *see* Amoxicillin and Clavulanate *on page 144*

◆ **Apo-Ampi® (Can)** *see* Ampicillin *on page 159*

◆ **Apo-Atenol (Can)** *see* Atenolol *on page 222*

◆ **Apo-Atomoxetine (Can)** *see* AtoMOXetine *on page 224*

◆ **Apo-Atorvastatin (Can)** *see* AtorvaSTATin *on page 227*

◆ **Apo-Azathioprine (Can)** *see* AzaTHIOprine *on page 241*

◆ **Apo-Azithromycin® (Can)** *see* Azithromycin (Systemic) *on page 247*

◆ **Apo-Baclofen® (Can)** *see* Baclofen *on page 259*

◆ **Apo-Beclomethasone (Can)** *see* Beclomethasone (Nasal) *on page 267*

◆ **Apo-Benztropine® (Can)** *see* Benztropine *on page 276*

◆ **Apo-Bisacodyl [OTC] (Can)** *see* Bisacodyl *on page 293*

◆ **Apo-Brimonidine (Can)** *see* Brimonidine (Ophthalmic) *on page 303*

◆ **Apo-Brimonidine P (Can)** *see* Brimonidine (Ophthalmic) *on page 303*

◆ **Apo-Buspirone® (Can)** *see* BusPIRone *on page 332*

◆ **Apo-Cal (Can)** *see* Calcium Carbonate *on page 346*

◆ **Apo-Candesartan (Can)** *see* Candesartan *on page 363*

◆ **Apo-Capto (Can)** *see* Captopril *on page 368*

◆ **Apo-Carbamazepine (Can)** *see* CarBAMazepine *on page 372*

◆ **Apo-Carvedilol (Can)** *see* Carvedilol *on page 385*

◆ **Apo-Cefaclor® (Can)** *see* Cefaclor *on page 391*

◆ **Apo-Cefadroxil (Can)** *see* Cefadroxil *on page 392*

◆ **Apo-Cefprozil® (Can)** *see* Cefprozil *on page 412*

◆ **Apo-Cefuroxime (Can)** *see* Cefuroxime *on page 422*

◆ **Apo-Cephalex (Can)** *see* Cephalexin *on page 429*

◆ **Apo-Cetirizine® [OTC] (Can)** *see* Cetirizine *on page 431*

◆ **Apo-Chlorthalidone (Can)** *see* Chlorthalidone *on page 453*

◆ **Apo-Ciclopirox (Can)** *see* Ciclopirox *on page 465*

◆ **Apo-Cimetidine® (Can)** *see* Cimetidine *on page 469*

◆ **Apo-Ciproflox (Can)** *see* Ciprofloxacin (Systemic) *on page 471*

◆ **Apo-Citalopram® (Can)** *see* Citalopram *on page 484*

◆ **Apo-Clarithromycin (Can)** *see* Clarithromycin *on page 490*

◆ **Apo-Clindamycin (Can)** *see* Clindamycin (Systemic) *on page 495*

◆ **Apo-Clobazam (Can)** *see* CloBAZam *on page 504*

◆ **Apo-Clomipramine® (Can)** *see* ClomiPRAMINE *on page 510*

◆ **Apo-Clonazepam (Can)** *see* ClonazePAM *on page 514*

◆ **Apo-Clonidine® (Can)** *see* CloNIDine *on page 516*

◆ **Apo-Clopidogrel (Can)** *see* Clopidogrel *on page 521*

◆ **Apo-Clorazepate® (Can)** *see* Clorazepate *on page 524*

◆ **Apo-Clozapine (Can)** *see* CloZAPine *on page 527*

◆ **Apo-Cromolyn Nasal Spray [OTC] (Can)** *see* Cromolyn (Nasal) *on page 553*

◆ **Apo-Cyclobenzaprine (Can)** *see* Cyclobenzaprine *on page 558*

◆ **Apo-Cyclosporine (Can)** *see* CycloSPORINE (Systemic) *on page 564*

◆ **Apo-Desmopressin® (Can)** *see* Desmopressin *on page 612*

◆ **Apo-Dexamethasone (Can)** *see* Dexamethasone (Systemic) *on page 615*

◆ **Apo-Diazepam® (Can)** *see* Diazepam *on page 640*

◆ **Apo-Diclo (Can)** *see* Diclofenac (Systemic) *on page 645*

◆ **Apo-Diclo Rapide (Can)** *see* Diclofenac (Systemic) *on page 645*

◆ **Apo-Diclo SR (Can)** *see* Diclofenac (Systemic) *on page 645*

◆ **Apo-Digoxin (Can)** *see* Digoxin *on page 658*

◆ **Apo-Diltiaz (Can)** *see* Diltiazem *on page 667*

◆ **Apo-Diltiaz CD (Can)** *see* Diltiazem *on page 667*

◆ **Apo-Diltiaz Injectable (Can)** *see* Diltiazem *on page 667*

◆ **Apo-Diltiaz SR (Can)** *see* Diltiazem *on page 667*

◆ **Apo-Diltiaz TZ (Can)** *see* Diltiazem *on page 667*

◆ **Apo-Dimenhydrinate® [OTC] (Can)** *see* DimenhyDRINATE *on page 670*

◆ **Apo-Dipyridamole FC® (Can)** *see* Dipyridamole *on page 693*

◆ **Apo-Divalproex (Can)** *see* Valproic Acid and Derivatives *on page 2102*

◆ **Apo-Docusate Calcium [OTC] (Can)** *see* Docusate *on page 701*

◆ **Apo-Docusate Sodium [OTC] (Can)** *see* Docusate *on page 701*

◆ **Apo-Doxazosin (Can)** *see* Doxazosin *on page 712*

◆ **Apo-Doxepin (Can)** *see* Doxepin (Systemic) *on page 715*

◆ **Apo-Doxy (Can)** *see* Doxycycline *on page 721*

◆ **Apo-Doxy Tabs (Can)** *see* Doxycycline *on page 721*

◆ **Apo-Enalapril (Can)** *see* Enalapril *on page 744*

◆ **Apo-Erythro Base (Can)** *see* Erythromycin (Systemic) *on page 780*

◆ **Apo-Erythro E-C (Can)** *see* Erythromycin (Systemic) *on page 780*

◆ **Apo-Erythro-ES (Can)** *see* Erythromycin (Systemic) *on page 780*

◆ **Apo-Erythro-S (Can)** *see* Erythromycin (Systemic) *on page 780*

◆ **Apo-Esomeprazole (Can)** *see* Esomeprazole *on page 793*

◆ **Apo-Etodolac (Can)** *see* Etodolac *on page 812*

◆ **Apo-Famciclovir® (Can)** *see* Famciclovir *on page 842*

◆ **Apo-Famotidine® (Can)** *see* Famotidine *on page 843*

◆ **Apo-Famotidine® Injectable (Can)** *see* Famotidine *on page 843*

◆ **Apo-Fentanyl Matrix (Can)** *see* FentaNYL *on page 853*

◆ **Apo-Ferrous Gluconate® (Can)** *see* Ferrous Gluconate *on page 866*

◆ **Apo-Ferrous Sulfate® (Can)** *see* Ferrous Sulfate *on page 868*

◆ **Apo-Flecainide® (Can)** *see* Flecainide *on page 874*

◆ **Apo-Fluconazole (Can)** *see* Fluconazole *on page 877*

◆ **Apo-Flunisolide® (Can)** *see* Flunisolide (Nasal) *on page 890*

◆ **Apo-Fluoxetine (Can)** *see* FLUoxetine *on page 901*

◆ **Apo-Flurazepam® (Can)** *see* Flurazepam *on page 907*

◆ **Apo-Flurbiprofen (Can)** *see* Flurbiprofen (Systemic) *on page 908*

◆ **Apo-Fluticasone® (Can)** *see* Fluticasone (Nasal) *on page 913*

◆ **Apo-Fluvoxamine (Can)** *see* FluvoxaMINE *on page 922*

◆ **Apo-Folic® (Can)** *see* Folic Acid *on page 925*

◆ **Apo-Fosinopril (Can)** *see* Fosinopril *on page 938*

◆ **Apo-Furosemide (Can)** *see* Furosemide *on page 948*

◆ **Apo-Gabapentin (Can)** *see* Gabapentin *on page 950*

◆ **Apo-Glyburide (Can)** *see* GlyBURIDE *on page 974*

◆ **Apo-Haloperidol (Can)** *see* Haloperidol *on page 998*

◆ **Apo-Haloperidol LA (Can)** *see* Haloperidol *on page 998*

◆ **Apo-Hydralazine® (Can)** *see* HydrALAZINE *on page 1022*

◆ **Apo-Hydro (Can)** *see* Hydrochlorothiazide *on page 1023*

◆ **Apo-Hydroxyquine (Can)** *see* Hydroxychloroquine *on page 1048*

◆ **Apo-Hydroxyurea (Can)** *see* Hydroxyurea *on page 1051*

◆ **Apo-Hydroxyzine (Can)** *see* HydrOXYzine *on page 1054*

◆ **Apo-Ibuprofen (Can)** *see* Ibuprofen *on page 1059*

◆ **Apo-Imatinib (Can)** *see* Imatinib *on page 1072*

◆ **Apo-Indomethacin (Can)** *see* Indomethacin *on page 1096*

◆ **Apo-Ipravent® (Can)** *see* Ipratropium (Nasal) *on page 1146*

◆ **Apo-Irbesartan (Can)** *see* Irbesartan *on page 1147*

◆ **Apo-K (Can)** *see* Potassium Chloride *on page 1708*

◆ **Apo-Ketoconazole (Can)** *see* Ketoconazole (Systemic) *on page 1177*

◆ **Apo-Ketorolac® (Can)** *see* Ketorolac (Systemic) *on page 1180*

◆ **Apo-Ketorolac Injectable® (Can)** *see* Ketorolac (Systemic) *on page 1180*

◆ **Apo-Ketorolac® Ophthalmic (Can)** *see* Ketorolac (Ophthalmic) *on page 1184*

◆ **Apo-Labetalol (Can)** *see* Labetalol *on page 1186*

◆ **Apo-Lactulose® (Can)** *see* Lactulose *on page 1193*

◆ **Apo-Lamivudine (Can)** *see* LamiVUDine *on page 1194*

◆ **Apo-Lamivudine HBV (Can)** *see* LamiVUDine *on page 1194*

♦ **Apo-Lamotrigine® (Can)** see LamoTRIgine on page 1199

♦ **Apo-Lansoprazole® (Can)** see Lansoprazole on page 1206

♦ **Apo-Letrozole (Can)** see Letrozole on page 1211

♦ **Apo-Levetiracetam (Can)** see LevETIRAcetam on page 1219

♦ **Apo-Levobunolol® (Can)** see Levobunolol on page 1223

♦ **APO-Levofloxacin (Can)** see Levofloxacin (Systemic) on page 1228

♦ **Apo-Lisinopril (Can)** see Lisinopril on page 1262

♦ **Apo-Lithium® Carbonate (Can)** see Lithium on page 1266

♦ **Apo-Lithium® Carbonate SR (Can)** see Lithium on page 1266

♦ **Apo-Loperamide® (Can)** see Loperamide on page 1270

♦ **Apo-Loratadine (Can)** see Loratadine on page 1278

♦ **Apo-Lorazepam (Can)** see LORazepam on page 1280

♦ **Apo-Losartan (Can)** see Losartan on page 1283

♦ **Apo-Lovastatin (Can)** see Lovastatin on page 1286

♦ **Apo-Medroxy® (Can)** see MedroxyPROGESTERone on page 1318

♦ **Apo-Meloxicam (Can)** see Meloxicam on page 1325

♦ **Apo-Metformin® (Can)** see MetFORMIN on page 1353

♦ **Apo-Methotrexate (Can)** see Methotrexate on page 1367

♦ **Apo-Methylphenidate (Can)** see Methylphenidate on page 1379

♦ **Apo-Methylphenidate SR (Can)** see Methylphenidate on page 1379

♦ **Apo-Metoclop (Can)** see Metoclopramide on page 1391

♦ **Apo-Metoprolol (Can)** see Metoprolol on page 1396

♦ **Apo-Metoprolol SR (Can)** see Metoprolol on page 1396

♦ **Apo-Metoprolol (Type L) (Can)** see Metoprolol on page 1396

♦ **Apo-Minocycline® (Can)** see Minocycline on page 1420

♦ **Apo-Mometasone® (Can)** see Mometasone (Nasal) on page 1433

♦ **Apo-Montelukast (Can)** see Montelukast on page 1438

♦ **Apo-Mycophenolate (Can)** see Mycophenolate on page 1453

♦ **Apo-Nadol (Can)** see Nadolol on page 1460

♦ **Apo-Napro-Na (Can)** see Naproxen on page 1470

♦ **Apo-Napro-Na DS (Can)** see Naproxen on page 1470

♦ **Apo-Naproxen (Can)** see Naproxen on page 1470

♦ **Apo-Naproxen EC (Can)** see Naproxen on page 1470

♦ **Apo-Naproxen SR (Can)** see Naproxen on page 1470

♦ **Apo-Nifed PA (Can)** see NIFEdipine on page 1497

♦ **Apo-Nitrofurantoin (Can)** see Nitrofurantoin on page 1502

♦ **Apo-Nizatidine (Can)** see Nizatidine on page 1508

♦ **Apo-Nortriptyline® (Can)** see Nortriptyline on page 1512

♦ **Apo-Oflox® (Can)** see Ofloxacin (Systemic) on page 1521

♦ **Apo-Olanzapine (Can)** see OLANZapine on page 1525

♦ **Apo-Olanzapine ODT (Can)** see OLANZapine on page 1525

♦ **Apo-Omeprazole (Can)** see Omeprazole on page 1535

♦ **Apo-Ondansetron® (Can)** see Ondansetron on page 1544

♦ **Apo-Orciprenaline® (Can)** see Metaproterenol on page 1352

♦ **Apo-Oxaprozin (Can)** see Oxaprozin on page 1562

♦ **Apo-Oxcarbazepine® (Can)** see OXcarbazepine on page 1564

♦ **Apo-Oxybutynin (Can)** see Oxybutynin on page 1568

♦ **Apo-Oxycodone/Acet (Can)** see Oxycodone and Acetaminophen on page 1573

♦ **Apo-Oxycodone CR (Can)** see OxyCODONE on page 1569

♦ **Apo-Paclitaxel® (Can)** see PACLitaxel on page 1579

♦ **Apo-Pantoprazole (Can)** see Pantoprazole on page 1595

♦ **Apo-Paroxetine (Can)** see PARoxetine on page 1609

♦ **Apo-Pen VK (Can)** see Penicillin V Potassium on page 1635

♦ **Apo-Perphenazine® (Can)** see Perphenazine on page 1648

♦ **Apo-Pimozide® (Can)** see Pimozide on page 1677

♦ **Apo-Piroxicam (Can)** see Piroxicam on page 1683

♦ **Apo-Pravastatin® (Can)** see Pravastatin on page 1720

♦ **Apo-Prazo (Can)** see Prazosin on page 1724

♦ **Apo-Prednisone (Can)** see PredniSONE on page 1732

♦ **Apo-Primidone® (Can)** see Primidone on page 1737

♦ **Apo-Procainamide® (Can)** see Procainamide on page 1740

♦ **Apo-Prochlorperazine (Can)** see Prochlorperazine on page 1745

♦ **Apo-Propranolol (Can)** see Propranolol on page 1759

♦ **Apo-Quetiapine (Can)** see QUEtiapine on page 1783

♦ **Apo-Quinapril (Can)** see Quinapril on page 1788

♦ **Apo-Quinidine® (Can)** see QuiNIDine on page 1791

♦ **Apo-Quinine® (Can)** see QuiNINE on page 1794

♦ **Apo-Rabeprazole (Can)** see RABEprazole on page 1797

♦ **Apo-Ranitidine (Can)** see Ranitidine on page 1805

♦ **Apo-Risperidone (Can)** see RisperiDONE on page 1831

♦ **Apo-Rizatriptan® (Can)** see Rizatriptan on page 1845

♦ **Apo-Rosuvastatin (Can)** see Rosuvastatin on page 1853

♦ **Apo-Salvent (Can)** see Albuterol on page 84

♦ **Apo-Salvent AEM (Can)** see Albuterol on page 84

♦ **Apo-Salvent CFC Free (Can)** see Albuterol on page 84

♦ **Apo-Salvent Sterules (Can)** see Albuterol on page 84

♦ **Apo-Sertraline (Can)** see Sertraline on page 1879

♦ **Apo-Sildenafil (Can)** see Sildenafil on page 1884

♦ **Apo-Simvastatin (Can)** see Simvastatin on page 1892

♦ **Apo-Sotalol (Can)** see Sotalol on page 1925

♦ **Apo-Sucralfate (Can)** see Sucralfate on page 1940

♦ **Apo-Sulfasalazine (Can)** see SulfaSALAzine on page 1954

♦ **Apo-Sulfatrim (Can)** see Sulfamethoxazole and Trimethoprim on page 1948

♦ **Apo-Sulfatrim DS (Can)** see Sulfamethoxazole and Trimethoprim on page 1948

♦ **Apo-Sulfatrim Pediatric (Can)** see Sulfamethoxazole and Trimethoprim on page 1948

♦ **Apo-Sulin (Can)** see Sulindac on page 1957

♦ **Apo-Sumatriptan (Can)** see SUMAtriptan on page 1958

◆ **Apo-Tamox® (Can)** *see* Tamoxifen *on page 1968*

◆ **Apo-Terazosin® (Can)** *see* Terazosin *on page 1981*

◆ **Apo-Terbinafine (Can)** *see* Terbinafine (Systemic) *on page 1982*

◆ **Apo-Tetra (Can)** *see* Tetracycline *on page 1996*

◆ **Apo-Theo LA® (Can)** *see* Theophylline *on page 2005*

◆ **Apo-Timol® (Can)** *see* Timolol (Systemic) *on page 2026*

◆ **Apo-Timop® (Can)** *see* Timolol (Ophthalmic) *on page 2028*

◆ **Apo-Tobramycin (Can)** *see* Tobramycin (Systemic, Oral Inhalation) *on page 2034*

◆ **Apo-Topiramate (Can)** *see* Topiramate *on page 2046*

◆ **Apo-Trazodone (Can)** *see* TraZODone *on page 2065*

◆ **Apo-Trazodone D (Can)** *see* TraZODone *on page 2065*

◆ **Apo-Triazo® (Can)** *see* Triazolam *on page 2080*

◆ **Apo-Trifluoperazine® (Can)** *see* Trifluoperazine *on page 2082*

◆ **Apo-Trimethoprim® (Can)** *see* Trimethoprim *on page 2087*

◆ **Apo-Valacyclovir® (Can)** *see* ValACYclovir *on page 2097*

◆ **Apo-Valganciclovir® (Can)** *see* ValGANciclovir *on page 2099*

◆ **Apo-Valproic (Can)** *see* Valproic Acid and Derivatives *on page 2102*

◆ **Apo-Valsartan (Can)** *see* Valsartan *on page 2108*

◆ **Apo-Venlafaxine XR (Can)** *see* Venlafaxine *on page 2125*

◆ **Apo-Verap (Can)** *see* Verapamil *on page 2129*

◆ **Apo-Verap SR (Can)** *see* Verapamil *on page 2129*

◆ **Apo-Warfarin® (Can)** *see* Warfarin *on page 2156*

◆ **Apo-Zidovudine® (Can)** *see* Zidovudine *on page 2168*

◆ **APPG** *see* Penicillin G Procaine *on page 1634*

◆ **Apprilon (Can)** *see* Doxycycline *on page 721*

Aprepitant (ap RE pi tant)

Medication Safety Issues
Sound-alike/look-alike issues:
Aprepitant may be confused with fosaprepitant
Emend® (aprepitant) oral capsule formulation may be confused with Emend® for injection (fosaprepitant)

Brand Names: U.S. Emend

Brand Names: Canada Emend®

Therapeutic Category Antiemetic; Substance P/Neurokinin 1 Receptor Antagonist

Generic Availability (U.S.) No

Use Prevention of acute and delayed nausea and vomiting associated with initial and repeat courses of moderate and highly emetogenic cancer chemotherapy (MEC & HEC) (in combination with other antiemetic agents); prevention of postoperative nausea and vomiting (PONV) (FDA approved in ages ≥18 years and adults).

Pregnancy Risk Factor B

Pregnancy Considerations Teratogenic effects were not observed in animal reproduction studies. Use during pregnancy only if clearly needed. Efficacy of hormonal contraceptive may be reduced; alternative or additional methods of contraception should be used both during treatment with fosaprepitant or aprepitant and for at least 1 month following the last fosaprepitant/aprepitant dose.

Breast-Feeding Considerations It is not known if aprepitant is excreted in breast milk. Due to the potential for adverse reactions in the nursing infant, the decision to discontinue aprepitant or to discontinue breast-feeding should take into account the benefits of treatment to the mother.

Contraindications Hypersensitivity to aprepitant or any component; concurrent use with pimozide, terfenadine, astemizole, or cisapride

Warnings Aprepitant has the potential to significantly interact with many medications; increased serum concentrations of pimozide, terfenadine, astemizole, or cisapride could result in serious or life-threatening adverse effects. Concomitant use with warfarin may result in clinically significant decrease in INR; patients on warfarin should have INR monitored closely, particularly at 7-10 days following initiation of 3-day aprepitant therapy or a single 40 mg aprepitant oral dose in an adult for prevention of postoperative nausea and vomiting.

Efficacy of oral contraceptives may be reduced during treatment with aprepitant; alternative or additional methods of birth control should be used both during treatment with aprepitant and for at least 1 month following the last aprepitant dose.

Precautions Use with caution in patients with severe hepatic impairment (Child-Pugh class C); use has not been studied. Use with caution in patients receiving medications metabolized by CYP3A4 as decreased metabolism and subsequent elevation of serum concentration may occur; the effect of aprepitant on orally administered CYP3A4 substrates may be greater than that seen with intravenously administered CYP3A4 substrates. A single 40 mg aprepitant oral dose in an adult is not likely to alter serum concentrations of CYP3A4 substrates. Use with caution and monitor closely in patients receiving docetaxel, paclitaxel, etoposide, irinotecan, ifosfamide, imatinib, vinorelbine, vinblastine, and vincristine as they are known to be metabolized by CYP3A4 isoenzymes. Other potentially significant interactions may exist requiring dose or frequency adjustment, additional monitoring, and/or selection of alternative therapy. Consult drug interactions database for more detailed information.

Chronic continuous use for prevention of nausea and vomiting is not recommended because it has not been studied. Aprepitant has not been studied for the treatment of established nausea and vomiting.

Adverse Reactions Note: Adverse reactions reported as part of a combination chemotherapy regimen or with general anesthesia.

Cardiovascular: Bradycardia, hypotension
Central nervous system: Dizziness, fatigue
Endocrine & metabolic: Dehydration
Gastrointestinal: Abdominal pain, constipation, diarrhea, dyspepsia, epigastric distress, gastritis, hiccups, nausea, stomatitis
Genitourinary Proteinuria
Hepatic: Increased serum ALT, increased serum AST
Neuromuscular & skeletal: Weakness
Renal: Increased blood urea nitrogen
Rare but important or life-threatening: Acid regurgitation, acne vulgaris, anaphylaxis, anemia, angioedema, anxiety, arthralgia, back pain, candidiasis, confusion, conjunctivitis, cough, decreased appetite, decreased serum albumin, decreased visual acuity, deep vein thrombosis, depression, diabetes mellitus, diaphoresis, disorientation, dysarthria, dysgeusia, dysphagia, dyspnea, dysuria, edema, enterocolitis, eructation, erythrocyturia, febrile neutropenia, flatulence, flushing, glycosuria, herpes simplex infection, hyperglycemia, hypersensitivity reaction, hypertension, hypoesthesia, hypokalemia, hyponatremia, hypothermia, hypovolemia, hypoxia, increased serum alkaline phosphatase, increased serum bilirubin, leukocytosis, leukocyturia, malaise, miosis, musculoskeletal pain, myalgia, myasthenia, myocardial infarction, neutropenic sepsis, obstipation, pain, palpitations, pelvic pain,

perforated duodenal ulcer, peripheral neuropathy, peripheral sensory neuropathy, pharyngitis, pharyngolaryngeal pain, pneumonia, pneumonitis, pruritus, pulmonary embolism, renal insufficiency, respiratory insufficiency, respiratory tract infection, rhinorrhea, rigors, sensory disturbance, septic shock, sialorrhea, skin rash, Stevens-Johnson syndrome, syncope, tachycardia, thrombocytopenia, toxic epidermal necrolysis, tremor, urinary tract infection, urticaria, voice disorder, weight loss, wheezing, xerostomia

Drug Interactions

Metabolism/Transport Effects Substrate of CYP1A2 (minor), CYP2C19 (minor), CYP3A4 (major); **Note:** Assignment of Major/Minor substrate status based on clinically relevant drug interaction potential; **Inhibits** CYP2C19 (weak), CYP2C9 (weak), CYP3A4 (moderate); **Induces** CYP2C9 (strong), CYP3A4 (weak/moderate)

Avoid Concomitant Use

Avoid concomitant use of Aprepitant with any of the following: Axitinib; Bosutinib; Cisapride; Conivaptan; Fusidic Acid (Systemic); Ibrutinib; Ivabradine; Lomitapide; Pimozide; Simeprevir; Tolvaptan; Ulipristal

Increased Effect/Toxicity

Aprepitant may increase the levels/effects of: Avanafil; Benzodiazepines (metabolized by oxidation); Bosentan; Bosutinib; Budesonide (Systemic, Oral Inhalation); Cannabis; Cisapride; Colchicine; Corticosteroids (Systemic); CYP3A4 Substrates; Diltiazem; Dofetilide; DOXOrubicin (Conventional); Dronabinol; Eplerenone; Everolimus; FentaNYL; Halofantrine; Ibrutinib; Imatinib; Ivabradine; Ivacaftor; Lomitapide; Lurasidone; OxyCODONE; Pimecrolimus; Pimozide; Propafenone; Ranolazine; Rivaroxaban; Salmeterol; Saxagliptin; Simeprevir; Tetrahydrocannabinol; Tolvaptan; Ulipristal; Vilazodone; Zuclopenthixol

The levels/effects of Aprepitant may be increased by: Ceritinib; Conivaptan; CYP3A4 Inhibitors (Moderate); CYP3A4 Inhibitors (Strong); Dasatinib; Diltiazem; Fusidic Acid (Systemic); Luliconazole; Mifepristone; Stiripentol

Decreased Effect

Aprepitant may decrease the levels/effects of: ARIPiprazole; Axitinib; Contraceptives (Estrogens); Contraceptives (Progestins); CYP2C9 Substrates; Diclofenac (Systemic); Ifosfamide; PARoxetine; Saxagliptin; Simeprevir; TOLBUTamide; Warfarin

The levels/effects of Aprepitant may be decreased by: Bosentan; CYP3A4 Inducers (Strong); Dabrafenib; Deferasirox; Mitotane; PARoxetine; Rifampin; Siltuximab; St Johns Wort; Tocilizumab

Food Interactions Aprepitant serum concentration may be increased when taken with grapefruit juice. Management: Avoid concurrent use.

Stability Store at room temperature of 20°C to 25°C (68°F to 77°F).

Mechanism of Action Prevents acute and delayed vomiting by inhibiting the substance P/neurokinin 1 (NK$_1$) receptor; augments the antiemetic activity of 5-HT$_3$ receptor antagonists and corticosteroids to inhibit acute and delayed phases of chemotherapy-induced emesis.

Pharmacokinetics (Adult data unless noted)

Distribution: V$_d$: ~70 L; crosses the blood-brain barrier

Protein binding: >95%

Metabolism: Extensively hepatic via CYP3A4 (major); CYP1A2 and CYP2C19 (minor); forms 7 metabolites (weakly active)

Bioavailability: 60% to 65%

Half-life: ~9-13 hours

Time to peak serum concentration: 3-4 hours

Elimination: Primarily via metabolism

Clearance: 62-90 mL/minute

Dosing: Usual Pediatric:

Prevention of chemotherapy-induced nausea and vomiting: Children ≥11 years and Adolescents (>40 kg): Oral: 125 mg 1 hour prior to chemotherapy on day 1, followed by 80 mg once daily on days 2 and 3 (in combination with a corticosteroid and 5-HT$_3$ antagonist antiemetic) (Gore, 2009; Smith, 2005)

Adult:

Prevention of chemotherapy-induced nausea and vomiting: Oral:

Highly emetogenic chemotherapy: 125 mg 1 hour prior to chemotherapy on day 1, followed by 80 mg once daily on days 2 and 3 (in combination with a 5-HT$_3$ antagonist antiemetic on day 1 and dexamethasone on days 1-4)

Moderately emetogenic chemotherapy: 125 mg 1 hour prior to chemotherapy on day 1, followed by 80 mg once daily on days 2 and 3 (in combination with a 5-HT$_3$ antagonist antiemetic and dexamethasone on day 1)

Prevention of PONV: Oral: 40 mg within 3 hours prior to induction

Dosage adjustment in renal impairment:

Mild, moderate, or severe impairment: No dosage adjustment necessary.

Dialysis-dependent end-stage renal disease (ESRD): No dosage adjustment necessary.

Dosage adjustment in hepatic impairment:

Mild to moderate impairment (Child-Pugh class A or B): No dosage adjustment necessary.

Severe impairment (Child-Pugh class C): Use with caution; no data available

Administration Oral: May be administered without regard to food, 1 hour prior to chemotherapy on day 1 of treatment and in the morning on the subsequent next 2 days or within 3 hours prior to induction of anesthesia.

Dosage Forms Excipient information presented when available (limited, particularly for generics); consult specific product labeling.

Capsule, Oral:

Emend: 40 mg, 80 mg, 125 mg, 80 mg & 125 mg

Extemporaneous Preparations A 20 mg/mL oral aprepitant suspension may be prepared with capsules and a 1:1 combination of Ora-Sweet® and Ora-Plus® (or Ora-Blend®). Empty the contents of four 125 mg capsules into a mortar and reduce to a fine powder (process will take 10-15 minutes). Add small portions of vehicle and mix to a uniform paste. Add sufficient vehicle to form a liquid; transfer to a graduated cylinder, rinse mortar with vehicle, and add quantity of vehicle sufficient to make 25 mL. Label "shake well" and "refrigerate". Stable for 90 days refrigerated.

Dupuis LL, Lingertat-Walsh K, and Walker SE, "Stability of an Extemporaneous Oral Liquid Aprepitant Formulation," *Support Care Cancer,* 2009, 17(6):701-6.

References

American Society of Clinical Oncology, Kris MG, Hesketh PJ, et al, "American Society of Clinical Oncology Guideline for Antiemetics in Oncology: Update 2006," *J Clin Oncol,* 2006, 24(18):2932-47.

Choi MR, Jiles C, and Seibel NL, "Aprepitant Use in Children, Adolescents, and Young Adults for the Control of Chemotherapy-Induced Nausea and Vomiting (CINV)," *J Pediatr Hematol Oncol,* 2010, 32 (7):268-71.

Gore L, Chawla S, Petrilli A, et al, "Aprepitant in Adolescent Patients for Prevention of Chemotherapy-Induced Nausea and Vomiting: A Randomized, Double-Blind, Placebo-Controlled Study of Efficacy and Tolerability," *Pediatr Blood Cancer,* 2009, 52(2):242-7.

National Comprehensive Cancer Network® (NCCN), "Clinical Practice Guidelines in Oncology™: Antiemesis," Version 1.2011. Available at http://www.nccn.org/professionals/physician_gls/PDF/antiemesis.pdf

Smith AR, Repka TL, and Weigel BJ, "Aprepitant for the Control of Chemotherapy Induced Nausea and Vomiting in Adolescents," *Pediatr Blood Cancer,* 2005, 45(6):857-60.

◆ **Aprepitant Injection** *see* Fosaprepitant *on page 934*

◆ **Apresoline** *see* HydrALAZINE *on page 1022*

◆ **Apresoline® (Can)** *see* HydrALAZINE *on page 1022*

◆ **Apriso** *see* Mesalamine *on page 1347*

◆ **Aprodine [OTC]** *see* Triprolidine and Pseudoephedrine *on page 2090*

◆ **Aptivus** *see* Tipranavir *on page 2031*

◆ **Aptivus® (Can)** *see* Tipranavir *on page 2031*

◆ **Aquacort® (Can)** *see* Hydrocortisone (Topical) *on page 1038*

◆ **AquaMEPHYTON® (Can)** *see* Phytonadione *on page 1671*

◆ **Aquanil HC [OTC]** *see* Hydrocortisone (Topical) *on page 1038*

◆ **Aquasol A** *see* Vitamin A *on page 2146*

◆ **Aquasol E [OTC]** *see* Vitamin E *on page 2148*

◆ **Aquavit-E [OTC]** *see* Vitamin E *on page 2148*

◆ **Aqueous Procaine Penicillin G** *see* Penicillin G Procaine *on page 1634*

◆ **Aqueous Vitamin D [OTC]** *see* Cholecalciferol *on page 455*

◆ **Aqueous Vitamin E [OTC]** *see* Vitamin E *on page 2148*

◆ **Ara-C** *see* Cytarabine (Conventional) *on page 573*

◆ **Arabinosylcytosine** *see* Cytarabine (Conventional) *on page 573*

◆ **Aralen** *see* Chloroquine *on page 444*

◆ **Aranesp (Can)** *see* Darbepoetin Alfa *on page 592*

◆ **Aranesp (Albumin Free)** *see* Darbepoetin Alfa *on page 592*

◆ **Arbinoxa** *see* Carbinoxamine *on page 377*

◆ **Arcalyst** *see* Rilonacept *on page 1828*

◆ **Aredia (Can)** *see* Pamidronate *on page 1587*

◆ **Arestin Microspheres (Can)** *see* Minocycline *on page 1420*

Argatroban (ar GA troh ban)

Medication Safety Issues
Sound-alike/look-alike issues:
Argatroban may be confused with Aggrastat, Orgaran
High alert medication:
The Institute for Safe Medication Practices (ISMP) includes this medication among its list of drugs which have a heightened risk of causing significant patient harm when used in error.

Therapeutic Category Anticoagulant, Thrombin Inhibitor
Generic Availability (U.S.) Yes
Use Prophylaxis or treatment of thrombosis in patients with heparin-induced thrombocytopenia (HIT) (FDA approved in adults); anticoagulant for percutaneous coronary intervention (PCI) in patients who have or are at risk for thrombosis associated HIT (FDA approved in adults). Has also been studied in children with HIT for procedural anticoagulation including cardiac catheterization, extracorporeal membrane oxygenation (ECMO), and hemodialysis/hemofiltration

Pregnancy Risk Factor B
Pregnancy Considerations Adverse events were not observed in animal studies. Information related to argatroban in pregnancy is limited. Use of parenteral direct thrombin inhibitors in pregnancy should be limited to those women who have severe allergic reactions to heparin, including heparin-induced thrombocytopenia, and who cannot receive danaparoid (Guyatt, 2012).

Breast-Feeding Considerations It is not known if argatroban is excreted in human milk. Because of the serious potential of adverse effects to the nursing infant, a decision to discontinue nursing or discontinue argatroban should be considered.

Contraindications Hypersensitivity to argatroban or any component; overt major bleeding

Warnings Prior to initiation of argatroban therapy, all other parenteral anticoagulants should be discontinued and adequate time lapsed. Hemorrhage is the most frequent complication of argatroban; bleeding can occur at any site in the body. Use with extreme caution in patients with increased risk of hemorrhage. Risk factors for hemorrhage include intensity of anticoagulation; bacterial endocarditis; congenital or acquired bleeding disorders; recent puncture of large vessels or organ biopsy; recent CVA, stroke, or intracerebral surgery; severe hypertension; renal impairment; recent major surgery, especially of the brain, spinal cord, or eye; recent major bleeding (intracranial, GI, intraocular, or pulmonary); GI lesions (eg, ulcerations); immediately after lumbar puncture; spinal anesthesia. Monitor for signs and symptoms of bleeding including unexplained decrease in hematocrit or blood pressure. Argatroban is for I.V. use only.

Precautions Use with caution and reduce dose in patients with hepatic impairment; may require >4 hours to achieve full reversal of argatroban anticoagulant effect following treatment in patients with hepatic impairment. Avoid use during PCI in patients with elevations of ALT/AST (≥3 times the upper limit of normal); use in these patients has not been evaluated. Use with caution and reduce the dose in critically ill patients, patients with multiple organ dysfunction, heart failure, severe anasarca, or postcardiac surgery; clearance is reduced in these patients. Limited pediatric pharmacokinetic and dosing information is available; the appropriate goals of anticoagulation and duration of treatment in pediatric patients have not been established. In pediatric trials, hypokalemia and abdominal pain were reported (Young, 2007).

Argatroban prolongs the PT/INR. Concomitant use with warfarin will cause increased prolongation of the PT and INR greater than that of warfarin alone. If warfarin is initiated concurrently with argatroban, initial PT/INR goals while on argatroban may require modification; alternative guidelines for monitoring therapy should be followed. Safety and efficacy for use with thrombolytic agents have not been established.

Adverse Reactions As with all anticoagulants, bleeding is the major adverse effect of argatroban. Hemorrhage may occur at virtually any site. Risk is dependent on multiple variables, including the intensity of anticoagulation and patient susceptibility.

Cardiovascular: Atrial fibrillation, bradycardia, CABG-related bleeding (minor), cardiac arrest, cerebrovascular disorder, chest pain, hypotension, MI, myocardial ischemia, thrombosis, vasodilation, ventricular tachycardia

Central nervous system: Fever, headache, intracranial bleeding, pain

Dermatologic: Skin reactions (bullous eruption, rash)

Gastrointestinal: Abdominal pain, diarrhea, GI bleed, nausea, vomiting

Genitourinary: Genitourinary bleed and hematuria, urinary tract infection

Hematologic: Hematocrit decreased, hemoglobin decreased (<2 g/dL)

Local: Bleeding at injection or access site

Neuromuscular & skeletal: Back pain

Renal: Abnormal renal function

Respiratory: Cough, dyspnea, hemoptysis, pneumonia

Miscellaneous: Infection, sepsis

Rare but important or life-threatening: Allergic reactions, constipation (infants and children), GERD, hypokalemia (infants and children), limb and below-the-knee stump bleed, multisystem hemorrhage and DIC, pulmonary edema, retroperitoneal bleeding

Drug Interactions

Metabolism/Transport Effects None known.

Avoid Concomitant Use

Avoid concomitant use of Argatroban with any of the following: Apixaban; Dabigatran Etexilate; Omacetaxine; Rivaroxaban; Urokinase; Vorapaxar

Increased Effect/Toxicity

Argatroban may increase the levels/effects of: Anticoagulants; Collagenase (Systemic); Deferasirox; Ibritumomab; Omacetaxine; Rivaroxaban; Tositumomab and Iodine I 131 Tositumomab

The levels/effects of Argatroban may be increased by: Agents with Antiplatelet Properties; Apixaban; Dabigatran Etexilate; Dasatinib; Herbs (Anticoagulant/Antiplatelet Properties); Ibrutinib; Nonsteroidal Anti-Inflammatory Agents; Omega-3 Fatty Acids; Pentosan Polysulfate Sodium; Prostacyclin Analogues; Salicylates; Sugammadex; Thrombolytic Agents; Tibolone; Tipranavir; Urokinase; Vitamin E; Vorapaxar

Decreased Effect

The levels/effects of Argatroban may be decreased by: Estrogen Derivatives; Progestins

Stability Store unused vials at 25°C (77°F) with excursions permitted to 15°C to 30°C (59°F to 86°F) in original carton (to protect from light); do not freeze. Prepared solution is stable for 24 hours at 25°C (77°F) with excursions permitted to 15°C to 30°C (59°F to 86°F) in ambient indoor light. Do not expose to direct sunlight. Prepared solution that is protected from light and kept at controlled room temperature of 20°C to 25°C (68°F to 77°F) or under refrigeration at 2°C to 8°C (36°F to 46°F) is stable for up to 96 hours. Additional light resistant measures (eg, foil protection for I.V. lines) are not needed.

Mechanism of Action A direct, highly-selective thrombin inhibitor. Reversibly binds to the active thrombin site of free and clot-associated thrombin. Inhibits fibrin formation; activation of coagulation factors V, VIII, and XIII; activation of protein C; and platelet aggregation.

Pharmacodynamics Onset of action: Immediate

Pharmacokinetics (Adult data unless noted)

Distribution: Distributes primarily to intracellular fluid
V_d: 174 mL/kg

Protein binding: Total: 54%; Albumin: 20%; α_1-acid glycoprotein: 34%

Metabolism: Hepatic via hydroxylation and aromatization. Metabolism via CYP3A4/5 to four known metabolites plays a minor role. Unchanged argatroban is the major plasma component. Plasma concentration of primary metabolite (M1) is 0% to 20% of the parent drug; M1 is three- to fivefold weaker.

Half-life, terminal: 39-51 minutes; hepatic impairment: 181 minutes

Elimination: Feces via biliary secretion (65%; 14% unchanged); urine (22%; 16% unchanged)

Clearance:
Pediatric patients (seriously ill): 0.16 L/kg/hour; 50% lower than healthy adults
Pediatric patients (seriously ill with elevated bilirubin due to hepatic impairment or cardiac complications; n=4): 0.03 L/kg/hour; 80% lower than pediatric patients with normal bilirubin
Adult: 0.31 L/kg/hour (5.1 mL/kg/minute); hepatic impairment: 1.9 mL/kg/minute

Dialysis: Hemodialysis: 20% dialyzed

Dosing: Usual I.V.

Infants and Children ≤16 years: Note: Limited data available; dosing regimens not established. Titration of maintenance dose must consider multiple factors including current argatroban dose, current aPTT, target aPTT, and clinical status of the patient. For specific uses, required maintenance dose is highly variable between patients. Additionally, during the course of treatment,

patient's dosing requirements may change as clinical status changes (eg, sicker patients require lower dose); frequent dosage adjustments may be required to maintain desired anticoagulant activity (Alsoufi, 2004; Boshkov 2006). If argatroban therapy is used concurrently with or following FFP or a thrombolytic, some centers decrease dose by half (Alsoufi, 2004).

Heparin-induced thrombocytopenia: I.V. continuous infusion: (manufacturer's recommendations):

Initial dose: 0.75 mcg/kg/minute

Maintenance dose: Measure aPTT after 2 hours; adjust dose until the steady-state aPTT is 1.5-3 times the initial baseline value, not exceeding 100 seconds; adjust in increments of 0.1-0.25 mcg/kg/minute for normal hepatic function; reduce dose in hepatic impairment.

Note: A lower initial infusion rate may be needed in other pediatric patients with reduced clearance of argatroban (eg, patients with heart failure, multiple organ system failure, severe anasarca, or postcardiac surgery). This precaution is based on adult studies of patients with these disease states who had reduced argatroban clearance.

Conversion to oral anticoagulant: Because there may be a combined effect on the INR when argatroban is combined with warfarin, loading doses of warfarin should not be used. Warfarin therapy should be started at the expected daily dose. Once combined INR on warfarin and argatroban is >4, stop argatroban. Repeat INR measurement in 4-6 hours; if INR is below therapeutic level, argatroban therapy may be restarted. Repeat procedure daily until desired INR on warfarin alone is obtained. Another option is to use factor X levels to monitor the effect of warfarin anticoagulation. When factor X level is <0.3, warfarin is considered therapeutic and at which time argatroban can be discontinued (Alsoufi, 2004; Boshkov, 2006).

Adults: Heparin-induced thrombocytopenia: I.V. continuous infusion:

Initial dose: 2 mcg/kg/minute; use actual body weight up to 130 kg (BMI up to 51 kg/m²) (Rice, 2007)

Maintenance dose: Patient may not be at steady state but measure aPTT after 2 hours; adjust dose until the steady-state aPTT is 1.5-3.0 times the initial baseline value, not exceeding 100 seconds; dosage should not exceed 10 mcg/kg/minute

Note: Critically-ill patients with normal hepatic function became excessively anticoagulated with FDA approved or lower starting doses of argatroban. Doses between 0.15-1.3 mcg/kg/minute were required to maintain aPTTs in the target range (Reichert, 2003). In a prospective observational study of critically-ill patients with multiple organ dysfunction (MODS) and suspected or proven HIT, an initial infusion dose of 0.2 mcg/kg/minute was found to be sufficient and safe in this population (Beiderlinden, 2007). Consider reducing starting dose to 0.2 mcg/kg/minute in critically-ill patients with MODS defined as a minimum number of two organ failures. Another report of a cardiac patient with anasarca secondary to acute renal failure had a reduction in argatroban clearance similar to patients with hepatic dysfunction. Reduced clearance may have been due to reduced liver perfusion (de Denus, 2003). The American College of Chest Physicians has recommended an initial infusion rate of 0.5-1.2 mcg/kg/minute for patients with heart failure, MODS, severe anasarca, or postcardiac surgery (Hirsch, 2008).

Conversion to oral anticoagulant: Because there may be a combined effect on the INR when argatroban is combined with warfarin, loading doses of warfarin should not be used. Warfarin therapy should be started at the expected daily dose.

◄ Patients receiving ≤2 mcg/kg/minute of argatroban: Argatroban therapy can be stopped when the combined INR on warfarin and argatroban is >4; repeat INR measurement in 4-6 hours; if INR is below therapeutic level, argatroban therapy may be restarted. Repeat procedure daily until desired INR on warfarin alone is obtained.

Patients receiving >2 mcg/kg/minute of argatroban: In order to predict the INR on warfarin alone, reduce dose of argatroban to 2 mcg/kg/minute; measure INR for argatroban and warfarin 4-6 hours after dose reduction; argatroban therapy can be stopped when the combined INR on warfarin and argatroban is >4. Repeat INR measurement in 4-6 hours; if INR is below therapeutic level, argatroban therapy may be restarted. Repeat procedure daily until desired INR on warfarin alone is obtained.

Note: The American College of Chest Physicians recommends monitoring chromogenic factor X assay when transitioning from argatroban to warfarin (Hirsh, 2008). Factor X levels <45% have been associated with INR values >2 after the effects of argatroban have been eliminated (Arpino, 2005).

Dosing adjustment in renal impairment: Dosage adjustment is not required.

Dosing adjustment in hepatic impairment: Decreased clearance is seen with hepatic impairment; dose should be reduced.

Infants and Children ≤16 years: Heparin-induced thrombocytopenia; I.V. continuous infusion:
Initial dose: 0.2 mcg/kg/minute
Maintenance dose: Measure aPTT after 2 hours; adjust dose until the steady-state aPTT is 1.5-3 times the initial baseline value, not exceeding 100 seconds; adjust in increments of ≤0.05 mcg/kg/minute.

Adults: Moderate hepatic impairment: I.V. continuous infusion: Initial dose: 0.5 mcg/kg/minute; monitor aPTT closely; adjust dose as clinically needed. **Note:** During PCI, avoid use in patients with elevations of ALT/AST (>3 times ULN); the use of argatroban in these patients has not been evaluated.

Usual Infusion Concentrations: Pediatric Note: Premixed solutions available.

I.V. infusion: 1000 mcg/mL

Administration For I.V. use only. Solution must be diluted prior to administration; dilute each 250 mg vial with 250 mL of diluent; final concentration: 1 mg/mL. May be mixed with NS, D₅W, or LR. Mix by repeated inversion for 1 minute. A slight but brief haziness may occur prior to mixing. Do not mix with other medications.

Monitoring Parameters HIT: Obtain baseline aPTT prior to start of therapy. Check aPTT 2 hours after start of therapy and any dosage adjustment. Monitor hemoglobin, hematocrit, platelets, signs and symptoms of bleeding.

Test Interactions Argatroban may elevate PT/INR levels in the absence of warfarin. If warfarin is started, initial PT/INR goals while on argatroban may require modification. The American College of Chest Physicians suggests monitoring chromogenic factor X assay when transitioning from argatroban to warfarin (Garcia, 2012) or overlapping administration of warfarin for a minimum of 5 days until INR is within target range; recheck INR after anticoagulant effect of argatroban has dissipated (Guyatt, 2012). Factor Xa levels <45% have been associated with INR values >2 after the effects of argatroban have been eliminated (Arpino, 2005).

Additional Information Molecular weight: 526.66; argatroban is a synthetic anticoagulant (direct thrombin inhibitor) derived from L-arginine. Increases in aPTT, ACT, PT, INR, and TT occur in a dose-dependent fashion with increasing doses of argatroban. Adult studies have established the use of aPTT for patients with HIT and ACT for

patients with PCI procedures. Therapeutic ranges for PT, INR, and TT have not been identified.

A reversal agent to argatroban is not available. Should life-threatening bleeding occur, discontinue argatroban immediately, obtain an aPTT and other coagulation tests, and provide symptomatic and supportive care.

Infants and Children ≤16 years: Doses reported in the literature for infants and children with HIT for procedural anticoagulation:

Cardiac Catheterization: Dose not established; the following doses have been used in limited reports: Initial I.V. bolus dose: 150-250 mcg/kg, followed by continuous I.V. infusion at an initial rate 5-15 mcg/kg/minute; one case series adjusted the continuous infusion dose to maintain target ACT >300 seconds (n=4). **Note:** Data is limited to an open-labeled study of a mixed population that included six pediatric cardiac catheterization patients and case reports/series (n=4 patients) [Alsoufi, 2004; GlaxoSmithKline Result Summary, 2007 (manufacturer unpublished data); Young, 2007]. Further studies are required before these doses can be recommended.

ECMO: Dose not established; data is limited to an open-labeled study of a mixed population that included one infant on ECMO, published and submitted abstracts, and case reports/series (n=16 patients) [Alsoufi, 2004; GlaxoSmithKline Result Summary, 2007 (manufacturer unpublished data); Hursting, 2006; Potter, 2007; Tcheng, 2004]. Further studies are required before these doses can be recommended.

The reported argatroban doses used to prime the ECMO circuit have varied widely; more recent reports utilize an ECMO priming dose between 30-50 mcg based upon patient's clinical status and ACT, followed by a continuous I.V. infusion at an initial rate of 0.5-2 mcg/kg/minute; continuous infusion doses were adjusted to maintain target ACT of at least 200 seconds; reported ACT target ranges varied from 160-300 seconds or aPTT 2 times initial baseline value. Dosing requirements ranging from 0.1-24 mcg/kg/minute have been reported. If patient not previously anticoagulated on heparin prior to starting argatroban, an initial bolus dose may be required.

Hemodialysis/Hemofiltration: Dose not established; clinical data limited to case series/reports (Alsoufi, 2004; Hursting, 2006; Young, 2007). Further studies are required before these doses can be recommended. The following doses have been used in limited reports: I.V. continuous infusion: Initial dose: 0.5-2 mcg/kg/minute; infusions were adjusted to maintain target ACT at least >160 seconds or aPTT >50 seconds; when reported, ACT target ranges were 160-200 seconds and aPTT 50-75 seconds. Reported dosing requirements were 0.1-2 mcg/kg/minute. If patient not previously anticoagulated on heparin prior to starting argatroban, an initial bolus dose may be required; initial bolus doses of 65 mcg/kg and 250 mcg/kg have each been reported.

Dosage Forms Excipient information presented when available (limited, particularly for generics); consult specific product labeling.
Solution, Intravenous:
Generic: 125 mg/125 mL (125 mL); 100 mg/mL (2.5 mL)
Solution, Intravenous [preservative free]:
Generic: 50 mg/50 mL (50 mL)

References

Alsoufi B, Boshkov LK, Kirby A, et al, "Heparin-Induced Thrombocytopenia (HIT) in Pediatric Cardiac Surgery: An Emerging Cause of Morbidity and Mortality," *Semin Thorac Cardiovasc Surg Pediatr Card Surg Annu*, 2004, 7:155-71.

Arpino PA, Demirjian Z, and Van Cott EM, "Use of the Chromogenic Factor X Assay to Predict the International Normalized Ratio in

Patients Transitioning From Argatroban to Warfarin," *Pharmacotherapy*, 2005, 25(2):157-64.

Beiderlinden M, Treschan TA, Gorlinger K, et al, "Argatroban Anticoagulation in Critically Ill Patients," *Ann Pharmacother*, 2007, 41(5):749-54.

Boshkov LK, Kirby A, Shen I, et al, "Recognition and Management of Heparin-Induced Thrombocytopenia in Pediatric Cardiopulmonary Bypass Patients," *Ann Thorac Surg*, 2006, 81(6):S2355-9.

de Denus S and Spinler SA, "Decreased Argatroban Clearance Unaffected by Hemodialysis in Anasarca," *Ann Pharmacother*, 2003, 37(9):1237-40.

GlaxoSmithKline Result Summary, Study No: SKF105043/013, "An Open-Label Study of Argatroban Injection to Evaluate the Safety and Effectiveness in Pediatric Patients Requiring Anticoagulation Alternatives to Heparin," July 2, 2007. Available at: http://www.gsk-clinicalstudyregister.com/files/pdf/22691.pdf.

Guyatt GH, Akl EA, Crowther M, et al, "Executive Summary: Antithrombotic Therapy and Prevention of Thrombosis, 9th ed: American College of Chest Physicians Evidence-Based Clinical Practice Guidelines," *Chest*, 2012, 141(2 Suppl):7-47.

Hirsh J, Guyatt G, Albers GW, et al, "Executive Summary: American College of Chest Physicians Evidence-Based Clinical Practice Guidelines (8th Edition)," *Chest*, 2008, 133(6 Suppl):71-109.

Hursting MJ, Dubb J, and Verme-Gibboney CN, "Argatroban Anticoagulation in Pediatric Patients: A Literature Analysis," *J Pediatr Hematol Oncol*, 2006, 28(1):4-10.

Potter KE, Raj A, and Sullivan JE, "Argatroban for Anticoagulation in Pediatric Patients With Heparin-Induced Thrombocytopenia Requiring Extracorporeal Life Support," *J Pediatr Hematol Oncol*, 2007, 29(4):265-8.

Reichert MG, MacGregor DA, Kincaid EH, et al, "Excessive Argatroban Anticoagulation for Heparin-Induced Thrombocytopenia," *Ann Pharmacother*, 2003, 37(5):652-4.

Rice L, Hursting MJ, Baillie GM, et al, "Argatroban Anticoagulation in Obese Versus Nonobese Patients: Implications for Treating Heparin-Induced Thrombocytopenia," *J Clin Pharmacol*, 2007, 47(8):1028-34.

Scott LK, Grier LR, and Conrad SA, "Heparin-Induced Thrombocytopenia in a Pediatric Patient Receiving Extracorporeal Membrane Oxygenation Managed With Argatroban," *Pediatr Crit Care Med*, 2006, 7(5):473-5.

Tcheng WY and Wong W, "Successful Use of Argatroban in Pediatric Patients Requiring Anticoagulant Alternatives to Heparin," *Blood*, 2004,104:107b-108b.

Young G and Boshkov L, "Prospective Study of Direct Thrombin Inhibition With Argatroban in Pediatric Patients Requiring Non-Heparin Anticoagulation," *Blood*, 2007, 110.

Young G, "New Anticoagulants in Children," *Hematology Am Soc Hematol Educ Program*, 2008, 245-50.

Arginine (AR ji neen)

Medication Safety Issues
Administration issues:
The Food and Drug Administration (FDA) has identified several cases of fatal arginine overdose in children and has recommended that healthcare professionals always recheck dosing calculations prior to administration of arginine. Doses used in children should not exceed usual adult doses.

Brand Names: U.S. R-Gene 10

Therapeutic Category Diagnostic Agent, Growth Hormone Function; Metabolic Alkalosis Agent; Urea Cycle Disorder (UCD) Treatment Agent

Generic Availability (U.S.) No

Use Pituitary function test (stimulant for the release of growth hormone); management of severe, uncompensated, metabolic alkalosis (pH ≥7.55) **after** optimizing therapy with sodium or potassium chloride supplements; treatment agent for urea cycle disorders (FDA approved in children and adults)

Pregnancy Risk Factor B

Pregnancy Considerations Teratogenic effects were not observed in animal studies; however, the manufacturer does not recommend use of arginine during pregnancy.

Breast-Feeding Considerations Amino acids are excreted in breast milk, the amount following arginine administration is not known.

Contraindications Hypersensitivity to arginine or any component

Warnings Use extreme caution when administering to neonates and children as overdosage has resulted in hyperchloremic metabolic acidosis, cerebral edema, or possibly death. Use with caution in renal or hepatic failure. For I.V. administration only; avoid extravasation; may cause local tissue damage.

Precautions Arginine hydrochloride is metabolized to nitrogen-containing products for excretion; the temporary effect of a high nitrogen load on the kidneys should be evaluated; accumulation of excess arginine may result in an overproduction of nitric oxide, leading to vasodilation and hypotension; each 1 mEq chloride delivers 1 mEq hydrogen; monitor acid base balance closely, particularly in neonates

Adverse Reactions
Cardiovascular: Flushing (with rapid I.V. infusion)
Central nervous system: Headache
Gastrointestinal: Nausea, vomiting
Local: Venous irritation
Neuromuscular & skeletal: Numbness
Rare but important or life-threatening: Anaphylaxis, cerebral edema, hematuria, hyperkalemia, hypersensitivity reaction, injection site reaction, skin burn/necrosis (due to extravasation), lethargy, loss of consciousness, perioral tingling

Drug Interactions
Metabolism/Transport Effects None known.
Avoid Concomitant Use There are no known interactions where it is recommended to avoid concomitant use.
Increased Effect/Toxicity There are no known significant interactions involving an increase in effect.
Decreased Effect There are no known significant interactions involving a decrease in effect.

Mechanism of Action Stimulates pituitary release of growth hormone and prolactin through origins in the hypothalamus; patients with impaired pituitary function have lower or no increase in plasma concentrations of growth hormone after administration of arginine. Arginine hydrochloride has been used for severe metabolic alkalosis due to its high chloride content. Arginine hydrochloride has been used investigationally to treat metabolic alkalosis. Arginine contains 475 mEq of hydrogen ions and 475 mEq of chloride ions/L. Arginine is metabolized by the liver to produce hydrogen ions. It may be used in patients with relative hepatic insufficiency because arginine combines with ammonia in the body to produce urea. Arginine is a precursor to nitric oxide and can produce vasodilation and inhibition of platelet aggregation.

Pharmacokinetics (Adult data unless noted)
Absorption: Oral: Well absorbed
Bioavailability: ~68%
Time to peak serum concentration:
Oral: 1.5-2 hours
I.V.: 30 minutes
Half-life: 0.7-1.3 hours
V_d: 33-100 L/kg

Dosing: Neonatal
I.V.:
Treatment of urea cycle disorders (in combination with sodium phenylacetate and sodium benzoate):
Argininosuccinic acid lyase (ASL) or argininosuccinic acid synthetase (ASS) disorders or pending definitive diagnosis: 600 mg/kg as a loading dose followed by 600 mg/kg/day as a continuous infusion.
Carbamyl phosphate synthetase (CPS) or ornithine transcarbamylase (OTC) disorder: 200 mg/kg as a loading dose followed by 200 mg/kg/day as a continuous infusion.
Intermittent hyperammonemic crisis in patients with urea cycle disorders:
ASL or ASS: 0.6 g/kg or 12 g/m² loading dose followed by 0.6 g/kg/day or 12 g/m²/day continuous infusion

CPS or OTC: 0.2 g/kg or 4 g/m^2 loading dose followed by 0.2 g/kg/day or 4 g/m^2/day continuous infusion

I.V., Oral: Necrotizing enterocolitis (NEC), prevention: 261 mg/kg/day added to enteral or parenteral nutrition beginning on day of life 2-5 and continued for 28 consecutive days. In a single-center, prospective, double-blind, randomized, placebo-controlled trial of 75 neonates (GA: <32 weeks; birth weight: <1250 g) in Canada, arginine supplementation decreased the NEC incidence when compared to placebo (6.7% vs 27%) (Amin, 2002; Shah, 2007). **Note:** The only commercial product available in the U.S. is arginine HCl injection and it is not known whether the hydrochloride salt was used in the Canadian study. Increased administration of HCl in this patient population could result in hyperchloremic metabolic acidosis.

Dosing: Usual I.V.: (**Note:** Each 1 g provides 4.75 mEq chloride)

Growth hormone reserve test:
Children: 0.5 g/kg over 30 minutes
Adults: 30 g (300 mL) over 30 minutes

Treatment of urea cycle disorders: Infants, Children, and Adults (in combination with sodium phenylacetate and sodium benzoate):
Argininosuccinic acid lyase (ASL) or argininosuccinic acid synthetase (ASS) disorders or pending definitive diagnosis: 600 mg/kg as a loading dose followed by 600 mg/kg/day as a continuous infusion
Carbamyl phosphate synthetase (CPS) or ornithine transcarbamylase (OTC) disorder: 200 mg/kg as a loading dose followed by 200 mg/kg/day as a continuous infusion. A single case using 60 mg/kg/hour for 12 hours has been reported (Kodama, 1996).

Intermittent hyperammonemic crisis in patients with urea cycle disorders: Infants, Children, and Adults:
ASL or ASS: 0.6 g/kg or 12 g/m^2 loading dose followed by 0.6 g/kg/day or 12 g/m^2/day continuous infusion
CPS or OTC: 0.2 g/kg or 4 g/m^2 loading dose followed by 0.2 g/kg/day or 4 g/m^2/day continuous infusion

Metabolic alkalosis: Infants, Children, and Adults: **Note:** Arginine hydrochloride is an alternative treatment for uncompensated metabolic alkalosis after sodium chloride and potassium chloride supplementation have been optimized; it should not be used as initial therapy for chloride supplementation.
Arginine hydrochloride dose (mEq) = 0.5 x weight (kg) x [HCO_3^- - 24] where HCO_3^- = the patient's serum bicarbonate concentration in mEq/L (Adrogué, 1998; Martin, 1982); give $^1/_2$ to $^2/_3$ of calculated dose and re-evaluate
To correct hypochloremia: Infants, Children, and Adults: Arginine hydrochloride dose (mEq) = 0.2 x weight (kg) x [103 - Cl$^-$] where Cl$^-$ = the patient's serum chloride concentration in mEq/L (Martin, 1982); give $^1/_2$ to $^2/_3$ of calculated dose and re-evaluate

Administration Parenteral: May be infused without further dilution (however, very irritating to tissues, dilution is recommended); administration through a central line is recommended; maximum rate of I.V. infusion: 1 g/kg/hour (4.75 mEq/kg/hour) (maximum dose: 60 g/hour = 285 mEq over 1 hour); infuse loading doses for urea cycle disorders over 90 minutes

Monitoring Parameters Acid-base status (arterial or capillary blood gases), serum electrolytes, BUN, glucose, plasma growth hormone concentrations (when evaluating growth hormone reserve), plasma ammonia and amino acids (when treating urea cycle disorders)

Reference Range If intact pituitary function, human growth hormone levels should rise after arginine administration to 10-30 ng/mL (control range: 0-6 ng/mL)

Additional Information When treating urea cycle disorders, sodium bicarbonate use may be necessary to neutralize the acidifying effects of arginine HCl.

Dosage Forms Excipient information presented when available (limited, particularly for generics); consult specific product labeling.
Solution, Intravenous, as hydrochloride [preservative free]: R-Gene 10: 10% (300 mL)

References

Adrogué HJ and Madias NE, "Management of Life-Threatening Acid-Base Disorders. Second of Two Parts," *N Engl J Med*, 1998, 338 (2):107-11.

Amin HJ, Zamora SA, McMillan DD, et al, "Arginine Supplementation Prevents Necrotizing Enterocolitis in the Premature Infant," *J Pediatr*, 2002, 140(4):425-31.

Batshaw ML, MacArthur RB, and Tuchman M, "Alternative Pathway Therapy for Urea Cycle Disorders: Twenty Years Later," *J Pediatr*, 2001, 138(1 Suppl):S46-54.

Bode-Böger SM, Böger RH, Galland A, et al, "L-Arginine-Induced Vasodilation in Healthy Humans: Pharmacokinetic-Pharmacodynamic Relationship," *Br J Clin Pharmacol*, 1998, 46(5):489-97.

Bushinsky DA and Gennari FJ, "Life-Threatening Hyperkalemia Induced by Arginine," *Ann Intern Med*, 1978, 89(5 Pt 1):632-4.

Kodama H, Mori Y, Kubota K, et al, "Intravenous Arginine Dramatically Improved Hyperammonemia in a Patient With Late-Onset Ornithine Transcarbamylase Deficiency," *Tohoku J Exp Med*, 1996, 180 (1):83-6.

Martin WJ and Matzke GR, "Treating Severe Metabolic Alkalosis," *Clin Pharm*, 1982, 1(1):42-8.

Shah P and Shah V, "Arginine Supplementation for Prevention of Necrotising Enterocolitis in Preterm Infants," *Cochrane Database Syst Rev*, 2007, (3):CD004339.

Summar M, "Current Strategies for the Management of Neonatal Urea Cycle Disorders," *J Pediatr*, 2001, 138(1 Suppl):S30-9.

◆ **Arginine HCl** see Arginine on page 195
◆ **Arginine Hydrochloride** see Arginine on page 195
◆ **8-Arginine Vasopressin** see Vasopressin on page 2121
◆ **Aridol** see Mannitol on page 1301

ARIPiprazole (ay ri PIP ray zole)

Medication Safety Issues
Sound-alike/look-alike issues:
Abilify may be confused with Ambien
ARIPiprazole may be confused with proton pump inhibitors (dexlansoprazole, esomeprazole, lansoprazole, omeprazole, pantoprazole, RABEprazole)

BEERS Criteria medication:
This drug may be potentially inappropriate for use in geriatric patients (Quality of evidence - moderate; Strength of recommendation - strong).

Other safety issues:
There are two formulations available for intramuscular administration: Abilify is an immediate release short-acting formulation and Abilify Maintena is an extended-release formulation. These products are **not** interchangeable.

Brand Names: U.S. Abilify; Abilify Discmelt; Abilify Maintena

Brand Names: Canada Abilify; Abilify Maintena

Therapeutic Category Antipsychotic Agent, Atypical

Generic Availability (U.S.) No

Use
Oral: Acute and maintenance treatment of schizophrenia (FDA approved in ages ≥13 years and adults); acute and maintenance treatment of bipolar disorder (with acute manic or mixed episodes) (FDA approved in ages ≥10 years and adults); adjunctive therapy (to lithium or valproate) for acute treatment of bipolar disorder (with acute manic or mixed episodes) (FDA approved in ages ≥10 years and adults); treatment of irritability associated with autistic disorder (including symptoms of aggression, deliberate self-injurious behavior, temper tantrums, quickly changing moods) (FDA approved in ages 6-17 years); adjunctive treatment (to antidepressants) of major depressive disorder (FDA approved in adults). Has also been used in children and adolescents for treatment of ADHD, conduct disorders, Tourette's syndrome, and

irritability associated with other pervasive developmental disorders.

Injection: Acute treatment of agitation associated with schizophrenia or bipolar disorder (manic or mixed) (FDA approved in adults)

Medication Guide Available Yes

Pregnancy Risk Factor C

Pregnancy Considerations Adverse events were observed in animal reproduction studies. Aripiprazole crosses the placenta; aripiprazole and dehydro-aripiprazole can be detected in the cord blood at delivery (Nguyen, 2011; Wantanabe, 2011). Antipsychotic use during the third trimester of pregnancy has a risk for abnormal muscle movements (extrapyramidal symptoms [EPS]) and/or withdrawal symptoms in newborns following delivery. Symptoms in the newborn may include agitation, feeding disorder, hypertonia, hypotonia, respiratory distress, somnolence, and tremor; these effects may be self-limiting or require hospitalization.

Treatment algorithms have been developed by the ACOG and the APA for the management of depression in women prior to conception and during pregnancy (Yonkers, 2009). The ACOG recommends that therapy during pregnancy be individualized; treatment with psychiatric medications during pregnancy should incorporate the clinical expertise of the mental health clinician, obstetrician, primary healthcare provider, and pediatrician. Safety data related to atypical antipsychotics during pregnancy is limited and routine use is not recommended. However, if a woman is inadvertently exposed to an atypical antipsychotic while pregnant, continuing therapy may be preferable to switching to a typical antipsychotic that the fetus has not yet been exposed to; consider risk:benefit (ACOG, 2008).

Healthcare providers are encouraged to enroll women 18-45 years of age exposed to aripiprazole during pregnancy in the Atypical Antipsychotics Pregnancy Registry (866-961-2388 or http://www.womensmentalhealth.org/ pregnancyregistry).

Breast-Feeding Considerations Aripiprazole is excreted in breast milk (Schlotterbeck, 2007; Watanabe, 2011). In one case report, milk concentrations were ~20% of the maternal plasma concentration (maternal dose: 15 mg/day; ~6 months postpartum) (Schlotterbeck, 2007); however, aripiprazole was not detected in the breast milk in a second case (limit of detection 10 ng/mL; maternal dose: 15 mg/day; ~1 month postpartum) (Lutz, 2010). Aripiprazole was also detected in the neonatal blood 6 days after delivery in a breast-fed infant also exposed during pregnancy. In this case report, the authors suggest *in utero* exposure could have contributed to the findings due to the long elimination half-life of aripiprazole (Watanabe, 2011). In one report, lactation was not able to be established, possibly due to changes in maternal prolactin potentially caused by aripiprazole (Mendhekar, 2006). The manufacturer recommends a decision be made whether to discontinue nursing or to discontinue the drug, taking into account the importance of treatment to the mother.

Contraindications Hypersensitivity to aripiprazole or any component

Warnings Aripiprazole is **not** FDA approved for the (adjunctive) treatment of depression in pediatric patients. Clinical worsening of depression or suicidal ideation and behavior may occur in children and adults with major depressive disorder **[U.S. Boxed Warning]**. In clinical trials, antidepressants increased the risk of suicidal thinking and behavior (suicidality) in children, adolescents, and young adults (18-24 years of age) with major depressive disorder and other psychiatric disorders. This risk must be considered before prescribing antidepressants for any clinical use. Short-term studies did **not** show an increased risk of suicidality with antidepressant use in patients

>24 years of age and showed a decreased risk in patients ≥65 years.

Patients of all ages who are treated with antidepressants for any indication require appropriate monitoring and close observation for clinical worsening of depression, suicidality, and unusual changes in behavior, especially during the first few months after antidepressant initiation or when the dose is adjusted. Family members and caregivers should be instructed to closely observe the patient (ie, daily) and communicate condition with healthcare provider. Patients should also be monitored for associated behaviors (eg, anxiety, agitation, panic attacks, insomnia, irritability, hostility, aggressiveness, impulsivity, akathisia, hypomania, mania) which may increase the risk for worsening depression or suicidality. Worsening depression or emergence of suicidality (or associated behaviors listed above) that is abrupt in onset, severe, or not part of the presenting symptoms, may require discontinuation or modification of drug therapy. To reduce risk of intentional overdose, write prescriptions for the smallest quantity consistent with good patient care. Screen individuals for bipolar disorder prior to treatment of depression (using antidepressants alone may induce manic episodes in patients with this condition).

May cause neuroleptic malignant syndrome (symptoms include hyperpyrexia, altered mental status, muscle rigidity, autonomic instability, acute renal failure, rhabdomyolysis, and elevated CPK). May cause extrapyramidal reactions, including pseudoparkinsonism, acute dystonic reactions, akathisia, and tardive dyskinesia (risk of these reactions is low relative to other neuroleptics, and is dose-dependent; to decrease risk of tardive dyskinesia: Use smallest dose and shortest duration possible; evaluate continued need periodically; risk of dystonia is increased with the use of high potency and higher doses of conventional antipsychotics and in males and younger patients).

Hyperglycemia has been reported with atypical antipsychotics, which may be severe and include potentially fatal ketoacidosis or hyperosmolar coma; reports of hyperglycemia with aripiprazole therapy have been few and specific risk associated with this agent is not known. Use with caution and monitor glucose closely in patients with diabetes mellitus (or with risk factors such as family history or obesity); measure fasting blood glucose at the beginning of therapy and periodically during therapy in these patients; monitor for symptoms of hyperglycemia in all patients treated with aripiprazole; measure fasting blood glucose in patients who develop symptoms. Leukopenia, neutropenia, and agranulocytosis (sometimes fatal) have been reported in clinical trials and postmarketing reports with antipsychotic use; presence of risk factors (eg, preexisting low WBC or history of drug-induced leuko/neutropenia) should prompt periodic blood count assessment. Discontinue therapy at first signs of blood dyscrasias or if absolute neutrophil count <1000/mm³.

Pediatric psychiatric disorders are frequently serious mental disorders which present with variable symptoms that do not always match adult diagnostic criteria. Conduct a thorough diagnostic evaluation and carefully consider risks of psychotropic medication before initiation in pediatric patients with schizophrenia, bipolar disorder, or irritability associated with autistic disorder. Medication therapy for pediatric patients with these disorders is indicated as part of a total treatment program that frequently includes educational, psychological, and social interventions.

An increased risk of death has been reported with the use of antipsychotics in elderly patients with dementia-related psychosis **[U.S. Boxed Warning]**; most deaths seemed to be cardiovascular (eg, sudden death, heart failure) or infectious (eg, pneumonia) in nature. An increased incidence of cerebrovascular adverse events (eg, transient

▶

◄ ischemic attack, stroke), including fatalities, has been reported with the use of aripiprazole in elderly patients with dementia-related psychosis. Aripiprazole is not approved for the treatment of patients with dementia-related psychosis.

Precautions Use with caution in patients with seizure disorders (seizures have been rarely reported), in suicidal patients, patients with concomitant systemic illnesses, patients with unstable heart disease or a recent history of MI (these patients not adequately studied), and in those at risk of aspiration pneumonia (esophageal dysmotility and aspiration have been associated with antipsychotic agents). May cause orthostatic hypotension; use with caution in patients at risk for this effect or in those who would not tolerate transient hypotensive episodes (eg, cerebrovascular disease, cardiovascular disease, hypovolemia, or concurrent medication use which may predispose to hypotension). May cause somnolence (dose-related). May cause alteration of temperature regulation (use with caution in patients exposed to temperature extremes).

Aripiprazole may cause a higher than normal weight gain in children and adolescents; monitor growth (including weight, height, BMI, and waist circumference) in pediatric patients receiving aripiprazole; compare weight gain to standard growth curves. **Note:** A prospective, nonrandomized cohort study followed 338 antipsychotic naïve pediatric patients (age: 4-19 years) for a median of 10.8 weeks (range: 10.5-11.2 weeks) and reported the following significant mean increases in weight in kg (and% change from baseline): Olanzapine: 8.5 kg (15.2%), quetiapine: 6.1 kg (10.4%), risperidone: 5.3 kg (10.4%), and aripiprazole: 4.4 kg (8.1%) compared to the control cohort: 0.2 kg (0.65%). Increases in metabolic indices (eg, serum cholesterol, triglycerides, glucose) were also reported; however, these changes were not significant in patients receiving aripiprazole (Correll, 2009); additionally, in clinical trials, lipid changes observed with aripiprazole monotherapy in pediatric patients were similar to those observed with placebo. Biannual monitoring of cardiometabolic indices after the first 3 months of therapy is suggested (Correll, 2009).

Children and adolescents may experience a higher frequency of some adverse effects than adults, including EPS (20% vs 5%), fatigue (17% vs 8%), and somnolence (23% vs 6%).

Oral solution contains 400 mg fructose and 200 mg sucrose per mL. Orally disintegrating tablets contain aspartame which is metabolized to phenylalanine and must be avoided (or used with caution) in patients with phenylketonuria.

Adverse Reactions

Cardiovascular: Chest pain, hypertension, orthostatic hypotension, peripheral edema, tachycardia

Central nervous system: Agitation, akathisia (dose-related; more common in adults), anxiety, ataxia, cognitive dizziness, drooling (children), drowsiness (more common in children), dysfunction (more common in children), dystonia (children), extrapyramidal reaction (dose-related), fatigue (dose-related; more common in children), headache (more common in adults), hypersomnia (children), insomnia, lethargy (children), nervousness, pain, restlessness, sedation (dose-related; more common in children)

Dermatologic: Skin rash (children)

Endocrine & metabolic: Increased thirst (children), weight gain (≥7% body weight), weight loss

Gastrointestinal: Abdominal distress, constipation (more common in adults), decreased appetite (children), diarrhea (children), dyspepsia, gastric distress, increased appetite (children), nausea, sialorrhea (dose-related), toothache, upper abdominal pain (children), vomiting, xerostomia (more common in adults)

Genitourinary: Dysmenorrhea (children)

Local: Injection site reaction (injection)

Neuromuscular & skeletal: Arthralgia (more common in adults), dyskinesia (children), increased creatine phosphokinase, limb pain, muscle cramps, muscle spasm, myalgia, stiffness (more common in adults), tremor (dose-related), weakness

Ophthalmic: Accommodation disturbance, blurred vision

Respiratory: Aspiration pneumonia, cough, dyspnea, nasal congestion, nasopharyngitis (children), pharyngolaryngeal pain, rhinorrhea (children), upper respiratory tract infection

Miscellaneous: Fever (children)

Rare but important or life-threatening: Abnormal bilirubin levels, agranulocytosis, akinesia, alopecia, amenorrhea, anaphylaxis, angina pectoris, angioedema, anorexia, anorgasmia, atrial fibrillation, atrial flutter, atrioventricular block, bradycardia, cardiorespiratory arrest, catatonia, cerebrovascular accident, choreoathetosis, cogwheel rigidity, delirium, depression, diabetes mellitus, diabetic ketoacidosis, diplopia, disruption of body temperature regulation, edema, erectile dysfunction, esophagitis, extrasystoles, gynecomastia, hepatitis, homicidal ideation, hostility, hyperglycemia, hyperlipidemia, hypersensitivity, hypertonia, hypoglycemia, hypokalemia, hypokinesia, hyponatremia, hypotension, hypothermia, hypotonia, increased blood urea nitrogen, increased creatinine clearance, increased gamma-glutamyl transferase, increased lactate dehydrogenase, increased serum prolactin, intentional injury, ischemic heart disease, jaundice, leukopenia, mastalgia, memory impairment, myocardial infarction, myoclonus, neuroleptic malignant syndrome, neutropenia, nocturia, pancreatitis, Parkinson's disease, priapism, prolonged Q-T interval on ECG, rhabdomyolysis, seizure (including injection), suicidal ideation, suicidal tendencies, supraventricular tachycardia, syncope, tardive dyskinesia, thrombocytopenia, tics, tonic-clonic seizures, uncontrolled diabetes mellitus, urinary retention, ventricular tachycardia

Drug Interactions

Metabolism/Transport Effects Substrate of CYP2D6 (major), CYP3A4 (major); **Note:** Assignment of Major/Minor substrate status based on clinically relevant drug interaction potential

Avoid Concomitant Use

Avoid concomitant use of ARIPiprazole with any of the following: Amisulpride; Azelastine (Nasal); Conivaptan; Fusidic Acid (Systemic); Metoclopramide; Paraldehyde; Sulpiride; Thalidomide

Increased Effect/Toxicity

ARIPiprazole may increase the levels/effects of: Alcohol (Ethyl); Amisulpride; Azelastine (Nasal); Buprenorphine; CNS Depressants; DULoxetine; FLUoxetine; Haloperidol; Highest Risk QTc-Prolonging Agents; Hydrocodone; Methotrimeprazine; Methylphenidate; Metyrosine; Mirtazapine; Moderate Risk QTc-Prolonging Agents; Paraldehyde; PARoxetine; Ritonavir; Selective Serotonin Reuptake Inhibitors; Serotonin Modulators; Sulpiride; Thalidomide; Zolpidem

The levels/effects of ARIPiprazole may be increased by: Abiraterone Acetate; Acetylcholinesterase Inhibitors (Central); Brimonidine (Topical); Cannabis; Ceritinib; Conivaptan; CYP2D6 Inhibitors (Moderate); CYP2D6 Inhibitors (Strong); CYP2D6 Inhibitors (Weak); CYP3A4 Inhibitors (Moderate); CYP3A4 Inhibitors (Strong); CYP3A4 Inhibitors (Weak); Dasatinib; Doxylamine; Dronabinol; Droperidol; DULoxetine; FLUoxetine; Fusidic Acid (Systemic); Haloperidol; HydrOXYzine; Ivacaftor; Kava Kava; Lithium; Luliconazole; Magnesium Sulfate; Methotrimeprazine; Methylphenidate; Metoclopramide; Metyrosine; Mifepristone; Nabilone; PARoxetine; Perampanel; Ritonavir; Serotonin Modulators; Sertraline;

Simeprevir; Sodium Oxybate; Stiripentol; Tapentadol; Tetrahydrocannabinol

Decreased Effect

ARIPiprazole may decrease the levels/effects of: Amphetamines; Anti-Parkinson's Agents (Dopamine Agonist); Haloperidol; Quinagolide

The levels/effects of ARIPiprazole may be decreased by: CYP3A4 Inducers; Dabrafenib; Lithium; Mitotane; Peginterferon Alfa-2b; Siltuximab; St Johns Wort; Tocilizumab

Food Interactions Ingestion with a high-fat meal delays time to peak plasma level. Management: Administer without regard to meals.

Stability Store at 25°C (77°F); excursions permitted to 15°C to 30°C (59°F to 86°F). Protect injection from light; store in original container; keep in carton until ready to use. Use oral solution within 6 months after opening, but not beyond the manufacturer expiration date.

Mechanism of Action Aripiprazole is a quinolinone antipsychotic which exhibits high affinity for D_2, D_3, $5-HT_{1A}$, and $5-HT_{2A}$ receptors; moderate affinity for D_4, $5-HT_{2C}$, $5-HT_7$, alpha$_1$ adrenergic, and H_1 receptors. It also possesses moderate affinity for the serotonin reuptake transporter; has no affinity for muscarinic (cholinergic) receptors. Aripiprazole functions as a partial agonist at the D_2 and $5-HT_{1A}$ receptors, and as an antagonist at the $5-HT_{2A}$ receptor.

Pharmacodynamics

Onset: Initial: 1-3 weeks

Pharmacokinetics (Adult data unless noted) Note: In pediatric patients 10-17 years of age, the pharmacokinetic parameters of aripiprazole and dehydro-aripiprazole have been shown to be similar to adult values when adjusted for weight.

Absorption: Well absorbed

Distribution: V_{dss}: 4.9 L/kg

Protein binding: ≥99%, primarily to albumin

Metabolism: Hepatic, via CYP2D6 and CYP3A4; the dehydro-aripiprazole metabolite has affinity for D_2 receptors similar to the parent drug and represents 40% of the parent drug exposure in plasma

Bioavailability: I.M.: 100%; Oral: Tablet: 87%; **Note:** Orally disintegrating tablets are bioequivalent to tablets; oral solution to tablet ratio of geometric mean for peak concentration is 122% and for AUC is 114%.

Half-life elimination: Aripiprazole: 75 hours; dehydro-aripiprazole: 94 hours

CYP2D6 poor metabolizers: Aripiprazole: 146 hours

Time to peak serum concentration: I.M.: 1-3 hours; tablet: 3-5 hours

Elimination: Feces (55%, ~18% of dose as unchanged drug); urine (25%, <1% unchanged drug)

Dosing: Usual Note: Oral solution may be substituted for the oral tablet on a mg-per-mg basis, up to 25 mg. Patients receiving 30 mg tablets should be given 25 mg oral solution. Orally disintegrating tablets (Abilify Discmelt®) are bioequivalent to the immediate release tablets (Abilify®).

Children and Adolescents:

Attention-Deficit/Hyperactivity Disorder (ADHD): Limited data available: Children ≥8 years and Adolescents: Oral: Initial: 2.5 mg/day; may increase on a weekly basis by 2.5 mg/day increments as tolerated; maximum daily dose: 10 mg/day; dosing based on an open-label, pilot study (n=23, age: 8-12 years) which reported significant improvement in ADHD outcome scores without an impact on cognitive measures (positive or negative); mean final dose: 6.7 ± 2.4 mg/day (Findling, 2008). Other aripiprazole published reports in pediatric and adolescent patients in which ADHD is a comorbid diagnosis within the study population exist; however, effectiveness in ADHD was not a reported primary outcome measure (Bastiaens, 2009; Budman, 2008;

Findling, 2009; Murphy, 2009; Valicenti-McDermott, 2006).

Autism; treatment of associated irritability (including aggression, deliberate self-injurious behavior, temper tantrums, and quickly changing moods): Children and Adolescents 6-17 years: Oral: Initial: 2 mg daily for 7 days, followed by 5 mg daily; subsequent dose increases may be made in 5 mg increments every ≥7 days, up to a maximum daily dose of 15 mg/**day**

Bipolar I disorder (acute manic or mixed episodes): Children and Adolescents 10-17 years: Oral: Initial: 2 mg daily for 2 days, followed by 5 mg daily for 2 days with a further increase to target dose of 10 mg daily; subsequent dose increases may be made in 5 mg increments, up to a maximum daily dose of 30 mg/**day. Note:** The safety of doses >30 mg/day has not been evaluated.

Conduct disorder (CD); aggression: Limited data available: Children ≥6 years and Adolescents: Oral: Patient weight <25 kg: 1 mg/day; 25-50 kg: 2 mg/day; 51-70 kg: 5 mg/day; >70 kg: 10 mg/day; may titrate after 2 weeks to clinical effectiveness; maximum daily dose: 15 mg/**day**. Dosing based on an open-label, prospective study (n=23; age: 6-17 years) which evaluated pharmacokinetics and effectiveness in patients with a primary diagnosis of CD (with or without comorbid ADHD); results showed improvement in CD symptom scores with only minor improvements in cognition (Findling, 2009).

Pervasive Developmental Disorder Not Otherwise Specified (PDD-NOS) or Asperger's Disorder; treatment of associated irritability (aggression, self-injury, tantrums): Limited data available: Children ≥4 years and Adolescents: Oral:

Preschool age: Initial dose: 1.25 mg/day with titration every ≥5 days in 1.25 mg/day increments as tolerated or clinically indicated (Masi, 2009)

Prepubertal children: Initial dose: 1.25-2.5 mg/day with titration every 3-5 days in 1.25-2.5 mg/day increments as tolerated or clinically indicated; maximum daily dose: 15 mg/**day** (Masi, 2009; Stigler, 2009)

Adolescents: Initial dose: 2.5-5 mg/day with titration every 5 days in 2.5-5 mg/day increments as tolerated or clinically indicated; doses >5 mg/day were divided twice daily; if sleep disorder was reported, the dose was given in morning and/or at lunchtime (Masi, 2009); maximum daily dose: 15 mg/**day** (Stigler, 2009)

An open-labeled, pilot study (n=25; mean age: 8.6 years; range: 5-17 years) reported an 88% response with a mean final dose of 7.8 mg/day (range: 2.5-15 mg/day) (Stigler, 2009). A retrospective, non-controlled, open-label study of 34 PDD patients (mean age: 10.2 years; range: 4-15 years) included 10 patients with autistic disorder and 24 patients with PDD-NOS reported a mean final dose: 8.1 ± 4.9 mg/day and an overall response rate of 32.4% (29.2% in patients with PDD-NOS) (Masi, 2009). In a retrospective chart review of children and adolescents with developmental disability and a wide range of psychiatric disorders (n=32; age: 5-19 years), a mean starting dose of aripiprazole of 7.1 ± 0.32 mg/day and a mean maintenance dose of 10.55 ± 6.9 mg/day was used; a response rate of 56% was reported for the overall population. However, a study population subset analysis in patients with mental retardation (n=18) showed a lower response rate in patients with mental retardation with PDD-NOS (38%) than in patients with mental retardation without PDD-NOS (100%) (Valicenti-McDermott, 2006).

Schizophrenia: Adolescents 13-17 years: Oral: Initial: 2 mg daily for 2 days, followed by 5 mg daily for 2 days with a further increase to target dose of 10 mg daily; subsequent dose increases may be made in 5 mg

increments up to a maximum daily dose of 30 mg/**day**.
Note: 30 mg/day was **not** found to be more effective than the 10 mg/day dose.

Tourette's syndrome, tic disorders: Limited data available: Children ≥7 years and Adolescents: Oral: Initial: 1.25-5 mg/day; daily doses were increased by 1.25-2.5 mg weekly or by 5 mg every 2 weeks; maximum daily dose: 20 mg/day. Dosing based on several open-label trials and a retrospective case series; reported mean required doses ranged from 3.3-11.7 mg/day (Budman, 2008; Murphy, 2009; Seo, 2008; Yoo, 2007; Yoo, 2011). Further studies are needed.

Adults:

Acute agitation (schizophrenia/bipolar mania): I.M.: 9.75 mg as a single dose (range: 5.25-15 mg); may repeat at ≥2-hour intervals to a maximum daily dose of 30 mg/**day**); **Note:** A dose of 15 mg was **not** shown to be more effective than 9.75 mg dose.

Bipolar disorder (acute manic or mixed episodes): Oral: Initial: 15 mg once daily (as monotherapy or as adjunctive therapy with lithium or valproate); usual: 15 mg once daily; may be increased to a maximum daily dose of 30 mg/**day**; doses >30 mg/day have not been evaluated. Continue for up to 6 weeks; efficacy of continued treatment >6 weeks has not been established

Depression (adjunctive with antidepressants): Oral: Initial: 2-5 mg/day; dosage adjustments of up to 5 mg/day may be made in intervals of ≥1 week; usual dose: 2-15 mg/day

Schizophrenia: Oral: Initial: 10-15 mg once daily; usual: 10-15 mg once daily; may be increased to a maximum daily dose of 30 mg/**day**. Dosage titration should not be more frequent than every 2 weeks. **Note:** Doses higher than 10-15 mg once daily were **not** found to be more effective.

Dosage adjustment with concurrent CYP450 inducer or inhibitor therapy: Children, Adolescents, and Adults: Oral:

CYP3A4 inducers (eg, carbamazepine): Aripiprazole dose should be doubled; dose should be subsequently reduced if concurrent inducer agent discontinued.

Strong CYP3A4 inhibitors (eg, ketoconazole): Aripiprazole dose should be reduced to 50% of the usual dose, and proportionally increased upon discontinuation of the inhibitor agent.

CYP2D6 inhibitors (eg, fluoxetine, paroxetine): Aripiprazole dose should be reduced to 50% of the usual dose, and proportionally increased upon discontinuation of the inhibitor agent. **Note:** When aripiprazole is administered as adjunctive therapy to patients with MDD, the dose should **not** be adjusted, follow usual dosing recommendations.

CYP3A4 and CYP2D6 inhibitors: Aripiprazole dose should be reduced to 25% of the usual dose. In patients receiving inhibitors of differing (eg, moderate 3A4/strong 2D6) or same (eg, moderate 3A4/moderate 2D6) potencies (excluding concurrent strong inhibitors), further dosage adjustments can be made to achieve the desired clinical response. In patients receiving strong CYP3A4 and 2D6 inhibitors, aripiprazole dose is proportionally increased upon discontinuation of one or both inhibitor agents.

Dosage adjustment based on CYP2D6 metabolizer status: Children, Adolescents, and Adults: Oral: Aripiprazole dose should be reduced to 50% of the usual dose in CYP2D6 poor metabolizers and to 25% of the usual dose in poor metabolizers receiving a concurrent strong CYP3A4 inhibitor; subsequently adjust dose for favorable clinical response.

Dosage adjustment in renal impairment: No dosage adjustment required.

Dosage adjustment in hepatic impairment: No dosage adjustment required.

Administration

Oral (all dosage forms): May be administered with or without food.

Orally-disintegrating tablet: Do not remove tablet from blister pack until ready to administer; do not push tablet through foil (tablet may become damaged); peel back foil to expose tablet; use dry hands to remove tablet and place immediately on tongue. Tablet dissolves rapidly in saliva and may be swallowed without liquid; if needed, tablet can be taken with liquid. Do not split tablet.

Injection: For I.M. use only; do not administer SubQ or I.V.; inject slowly into deep muscle mass

Monitoring Parameters Vital signs; CBC with differential; fasting lipid profile and fasting blood glucose/Hb A_{1c} (prior to treatment, at 3 months, then annually); weight, growth, BMI, and waist circumference (especially in children), personal/family history of diabetes, blood pressure, mental status, abnormal involuntary movement scale (AIMS), extrapyramidal symptoms (EPS). Weight should be assessed prior to treatment, at 4 weeks, 8 weeks, 12 weeks, and then at quarterly intervals. Consider titrating to a different antipsychotic agent for a weight gain ≥5% of the initial weight. Monitor patient periodically for symptom resolution; monitor for worsening depression, suicidality, and associated behaviors (especially at the beginning of therapy or when doses are increased or decreased)

Additional Information Long-term usefulness of aripiprazole should be periodically re-evaluated in patients receiving the drug for extended periods of time.

Dosage Forms Excipient information presented when available (limited, particularly for generics); consult specific product labeling.

Solution, Intramuscular:
Abilify: 9.75 mg/1.3 mL (1.3 mL)

Solution, Oral:
Abilify: 1 mg/mL (150 mL) [contains methylparaben, propylene glycol, propylparaben; orange cream flavor]

Suspension Reconstituted, Intramuscular:
Abilify Maintena: 300 mg (1 ea); 400 mg (1 ea)

Tablet, Oral:
Abilify: 2 mg, 5 mg, 10 mg, 15 mg, 20 mg, 30 mg

Tablet Dispersible, Oral:
Abilify Discmelt: 10 mg, 15 mg [contains aspartame, fd&c blue #2 aluminum lake]

References

ACOG Committee on Practice Bulletins-Obstetrics, "ACOG Practice Bulletin: Clinical Management Guidelines for Obstetrician-Gynecologists Number 92, April 2008 (Replaces Practice Bulletin Number 87, November 2007). Use of Psychiatric Medications During Pregnancy and Lactation," *Obstet Gynecol*, 2008, 111(4):1001-20.

American Diabetes Association, American Psychiatric Association, American Association of Clinical Endocrinologists, et al, "Consensus Development Conference on Antipsychotic Drugs and Obesity and Diabetes," *Diabetes Care*, 2004, 27(2):596-601.

Bastiaens L, "A Non-Randomized, Open Study With Aripiprazole and Ziprasidone for the Treatment of Aggressive Behavior in Youth in a Community Clinic," *Community Ment Health J*, 2009, 45(1):73-7.

Budman C, Coffey BJ, Shechter R, et al, "Aripiprazole in Children and Adolescents With Tourette Disorder With and Without Explosive Outbursts," *J Child Adolesc Psychopharmacol*, 2008, 18(5):509-15.

Correll CU, Manu P, Olshanskiy V, et al, "Cardiometabolic Risk of Second-Generation Antipsychotic Medications During First-Time Use in Children and Adolescents," *JAMA*, 2009, 302(16):1765-73.

Findling RL, Kauffman R, Sallee FR, et al, "An Open-Label Study of Aripiprazole: Pharmacokinetics, Tolerability, and Effectiveness in Children and Adolescents With Conduct Disorder," *J Child Adolesc Psychopharmacol*, 2009, 19(4):431-9.

Findling RL, Short EJ, Leskovec T, et al, "Aripiprazole in Children With Attention-Deficit/Hyperactivity Disorder," *J Child Adolesc Psychopharmacol*, 2008, 18(4):347-54.

Lutz UC, Hiemke C, Wiatr G, et al, "Aripiprazole in Pregnancy and Lactation: A Case Report," *J Clin Psychopharmacol*, 2010. 30 (2):204-5.

Marcus RN, Owen R, Kamen L, et al, "A Placebo-Controlled, Fixed-Dose Study of Aripiprazole in Children and Adolescents With

Irritability Associated With Autistic Disorder," *J Am Acad Child Adolesc Psychiatry*, 2009, 48(11):1110-9.

Masi G, Cosenza A, Millepiedi S, et al, "Aripiprazole Monotherapy in Children and Young Adolescents With Pervasive Developmental Disorders: A Retrospective Study," *CNS Drugs*, 2009, 23(6):511-21.

Mendhekar DN, Sunder KR, and Andrade C, "Aripiprazole Use in a Pregnant Schizoaffective Woman," *Bipolar Disord*, 2006, 8 (3):299-300.

Murphy TK, Mutch PJ, Reid JM, et al, "Open Label Aripiprazole in the Treatment of Youth With Tic Disorders," *J Child Adolesc Psychopharmacol*, 2009, 19(4):441-7.

Nguyen T, Teoh S, Hackett LP, et al, "Placental Transfer of Aripiprazole," *Aust N Z J Psychiatry*, 2011, 45(6):500-1.

Owen R, Sikich L, Marcus RN, et al, "Aripiprazole in the Treatment of Irritability in Children and Adolescents With Autistic Disorder," *Pediatrics*, 2009, 124(6):1533-40.

Schlotterbeck P, Leube D, Kircher T, et al, "Aripiprazole in Human Milk," *Int J Neuropsychopharmacol*, 2007, 10(3):433.

Seo WS, Sung HM, Sea HS, et al, "Aripiprazole Treatment of Children and Adolescents With Tourette Disorder or Chronic Tic Disorder," *J Child Adolesc Psychopharmacol*, 2008, 18(2):197-205.

Stigler KA, Diener JT, Kohn AE, et al, "Aripiprazole in Pervasive Developmental Disorder Not Otherwise Specified and Asperger's Disorder: A 14-Week, Prospective, Open-Label Study," *J Child Adolesc Psychopharmacol*, 2009, 19(3):265-74.

Valicenti-McDermott MR and Demb H, "Clinical Effects and Adverse Reactions of Off-Label Use of Aripiprazole in Children and Adolescents With Developmental Disabilities," *J Child Adolesc Psychopharmacol*, 2006, 16(5):549-60.

Watanabe N, Kasahara M, Sugibayashi R, et al, "Perinatal Use of Aripiprazole: A Case Report," *J Clin Psychopharmacol*, 2011, 31 (3):377-9.

Yonkers KA, Wisner KL, Stewart DE, et al, "The Management of Depression During Pregnancy: A Report From the American Psychiatric Association and the American College of Obstetricians and Gynecologists," *Obstet Gynecol*, 2009, 114(3):703-13.

Yoo HK, Choi SH, Park S, et al, "An Open-Label Study of the Efficacy and Tolerability of Aripiprazole for Children and Adolescents With Tic Disorders," *J Clin Psychiatry*, 2007, 68(7):1088-93.

Yoo HK, Lee JS, Paik KW, et al, "Open-Label Study Comparing the Efficacy and Tolerability of Aripiprazole and Haloperidol in the Treatment of Pediatric Tic Disorders," *Eur Child Adolesc Psychiatry*, 2011, 20(3):127-35.

◆ **Aristospan® (Can)** *see* Triamcinolone (Systemic) *on page 2072*

◆ **Aristospan Intra-Articular** *see* Triamcinolone (Systemic) *on page 2072*

◆ **Aristospan Intralesional** *see* Triamcinolone (Systemic) *on page 2072*

◆ **Armour Thyroid** *see* Thyroid, Desiccated *on page 2018*

◆ **Arranon** *see* Nelarabine *on page 1477*

Arsenic Trioxide (AR se nik tri OKS id)

Medication Safety Issues

High alert medication:

This medication is in a class the Institute for Safe Medication Practices (ISMP) includes among its list of drugs which have a heightened risk of causing significant patient harm when used in error.

Related Information

Emetogenic Potential of Antineoplastic Agents in Children *on page 2327*

Management of Drug Extravasations *on page 2255*

Safe Handling of Hazardous Drugs *on page 2419*

Brand Names: U.S. Trisenox

Brand Names: Canada Trisenox

Therapeutic Category Antineoplastic Agent, Miscellaneous

Generic Availability (U.S.) No

Use Remission induction and consolidation in patients with relapsed or refractory acute promyelocytic leukemia (APL) characterized by t(15;17) translocation or PML/RAR-alpha gene expression (FDA approved in ages ≥4 years and adults); has also been used in the initial treatment of APL and the treatment of myelodysplastic syndrome (MDS)

Pregnancy Risk Factor D

Pregnancy Considerations Increased resorptions, neural-tube defects, and ophthalmic abnormalities have been observed in animal studies. Arsenic crosses the human placenta. In studies of women exposed to high levels of arsenic from drinking water, cord blood levels were similar to maternal serum levels. Dimethylarsinic acid (DMA) was the form of arsenic found in the fetus. An increased risk of low birth weight and still births were observed in women who ingested high levels of dietary arsenic. Women of childbearing potential should avoid pregnancy. The Canadian labeling contraindicates use in pregnant women. It also recommends that women of childbearing potential avoid pregnancy, and male patients wear condoms during intercourse with women who are pregnant or of childbearing potential during therapy and for 3 months following therapy discontinuation.

Breast-Feeding Considerations Arsenic is naturally found in breast milk; concentrations range from 0.2-6 mcg/kg. In studies of women exposed to high levels of arsenic from drinking water, breast milk concentrations were low (~3.1 mcg/kg) and did not correlate with maternal serum levels. The possible effect of maternal arsenic trioxide therapy on breast milk concentrations is not known. Due to the potential for serious adverse reactions in a nursing infant, breast-feeding during therapy is not recommended. The Canadian labeling contraindicates use in nursing women and recommends avoiding nursing for 3 months after therapy discontinuation.

Contraindications Hypersensitivity to arsenic or any component

Warnings Hazardous agent; use appropriate precautions for handling and disposal (NIOSH, 2012). May prolong the QT interval. May lead to torsade de pointes or complete AV block **[U.S. Boxed Warnings]**. Risk factors for torsade de pointes include extent of prolongation, HF, a history of torsade de pointes, preexisting QT interval prolongation, patients taking medications known to prolong the QT interval or potassium-wasting diuretics, and conditions which cause hypokalemia or hypomagnesemia. If possible, discontinue all medications known to prolong the QT interval. A baseline 12-lead ECG, serum electrolytes (potassium, calcium, magnesium), and creatinine should be obtained prior to treatment **[U.S. Boxed Warning]**. Correct electrolyte abnormalities prior to treatment and monitor potassium and magnesium levels during therapy (maintain potassium >4 mEq/dL and magnesium >1.8 mg/dL). If baseline QT_c >500 msec, correct prior to treatment. If QT_c >500 during treatment, reassess, correct contributing factors, and consider temporarily withholding treatment. If syncope or irregular heartbeat develops during therapy, hospitalize patient and do not reinitiate therapy until QT_c <460 msec, electrolytes abnormalities are corrected, and syncope or irregular heartbeat has resolved. Monitor ECG weekly; more frequently if clinically indicated.

May cause retinoic-acid-acute promyelocytic leukemia (RA-APL) syndrome or APL differentiation syndrome (dyspnea, fever, weight gain, pulmonary infiltrates, and pleural or pericardial effusions) in patients with APL **[U.S. Boxed Warning]**; may be fatal. High-dose steroids (dexamethasone 10 mg I.V. twice daily for ≥3 days; begin at initial presentation and taper over 2 weeks) have been used for treatment; in general, most patients may continue arsenic trioxide during treatment of APL differentiation syndrome. May lead to the development of hyperleukocytosis (leukocytes ≥10,000/mm³); did not correlate with baseline WBC counts and generally were not as high during consolidation as observed during induction treatment.

Precautions Use with caution in patients with hepatic impairment; in patients with severe hepatic impairment, monitor closely for toxicity. Use with caution in patients with severe renal impairment; systemic exposure to metabolites may be higher; has not been studied in dialysis patients. Monitor electrolytes, CBC with differential, and coagulation parameters at least twice a week during induction and weekly during consolidation; more frequently if clinically indicated. Should be administered under the supervision of a physician experienced in acute leukemia management **[U.S. Boxed Warning]**.

Adverse Reactions

Cardiovascular: Abnormal ECG (not QT prolongation), atrial dysrhythmia, chest pain, edema, facial edema, flushing, hyper-/hypotension, pallor, palpitation, QT interval >500 msec, tachycardia, torsade de pointes

Central nervous system: Agitation, anxiety, coma, confusion, depression, dizziness, fatigue, fever, headache, insomnia, pain, seizure, somnolence

Dermatologic: Bruising, dermatitis, dry skin, erythema, hyperpigmentation, local exfoliation, petechia, pruritus, skin lesions, urticaria

Endocrine & metabolic: Acidosis, hyperglycemia, hyperkalemia, hypocalcemia, hypoglycemia, hypokalemia, hypomagnesemia, intermenstrual bleeding

Gastrointestinal: Abdominal distension, abdominal pain, abdominal tenderness, anorexia, appetite decreased, caecitis, constipation, diarrhea, dyspepsia, fecal incontinence, gastrointestinal hemorrhage, hemorrhagic diarrhea, loose stools, nausea, oral blistering, oral candidiasis, sore throat, vomiting, weight gain/loss, xerostomia

Genitourinary: Incontinence, vaginal hemorrhage

Hematologic: Anemia, APL differentiation syndrome, DIC, febrile neutropenia, hemorrhage, leukocytosis, neutropenia, thrombocytopenia

Hepatic: ALT increased, AST increased

Local: Injection site: Edema, erythema, pain

Neuromuscular & skeletal: Arthralgia, back pain, bone pain, limb pain, myalgia, neck pain, neuropathy, paresthesia, rigors, tremor, weakness

Ocular: Blurred vision, dry eye, eye irritation, eyelid edema, painful red eye

Otic: Earache, tinnitus

Renal: Renal failure, renal impairment, oliguria

Respiratory: Breath sounds decreased, cough, crepitations, dyspnea, epistaxis, hemoptysis, hypoxia, nasopharyngitis, pleural effusion, postnasal drip, pulmonary edema, rales, rhonchi, sinusitis, tachypnea, upper respiratory tract infection, wheezing

Miscellaneous: Bacterial infection, diaphoresis increased, herpes simplex, injection site edema, herpes zoster, hypersensitivity, lymphadenopathy, night sweats, sepsis

Rare but important or life-threatening: Acute respiratory distress syndrome, AV block, capillary leak syndrome, CHF, heart block, hypoalbuminemia, hyponatremia, hypophosphatemia, lipase increased, mitochondrial myopathy, pancytopenia, peripheral neuropathy, pneumonitis, pulmonary infiltrate, respiratory distress, stomatitis, ventricular extrasystoles, ventricular tachycardia

Drug Interactions

Metabolism/Transport Effects None known.

Avoid Concomitant Use

Avoid concomitant use of Arsenic Trioxide with any of the following: CloZAPine; Dipyrone; Highest Risk QTc-Prolonging Agents; Ivabradine; Mifepristone; Moderate Risk QTc-Prolonging Agents

Increased Effect/Toxicity

Arsenic Trioxide may increase the levels/effects of: CloZAPine; Highest Risk QTc-Prolonging Agents; Hypoglycemic Agents

The levels/effects of Arsenic Trioxide may be increased by: Dipyrone; Herbs (Hypoglycemic Properties); Ivabradine; MAO Inhibitors; Mifepristone; Moderate Risk QTc-Prolonging Agents; QTc-Prolonging Agents

(Indeterminate Risk and Risk Modifying); Salicylates; Selective Serotonin Reuptake Inhibitors

Decreased Effect

The levels/effects of Arsenic Trioxide may be decreased by: Loop Diuretics

Stability Hazardous agent; use appropriate precautions for handling and disposal (NIOSH, 2012). Store at 25°C (77°F); excursions permitted to 15°C to 30°C (59°F to 86°F); do not freeze. Following dilution in D_5W or NS; stable for 24 hours at room temperature or 48 hours when refrigerated.

Mechanism of Action Induces apoptosis in APL cells via morphological changes and DNA fragmentation; also damages or degrades the fusion protein PML-RAR alpha

Pharmacokinetics (Adult data unless noted)

Distribution: V_d: As^{III}: 562 L; widely distributed throughout body tissues; orally administered arsenic trioxide distributes into the CNS

Metabolism: Arsenic trioxide is immediately hydrolyzed to the active form, arsenious acid (As^{III}) which is methylated (hepatically) to the less active pentavalent metabolites, monomethylarsonic acid (MMA^V) and dimethylarsinic acid (DMA^V) by methyltransferases; As^{III} is also oxidized to the minor metabolite, arsenic acid (As^V)

Half-life elimination: AS^{III}: 10-14 hours; MMA^V: ~32 hours; DMA^V: ~72 hours

Time to peak serum concentrations: As^{III}: At the end of infusion; MMA^V and DMA^V: ~10-24 hours

Elimination: Urine (MMA^V, DMA^V, and 15% of a dose as unchanged As^{III})

Dosing: Usual I.V.:

Children and Adolescents:

Acute promyelocytic leukemia (APL), relapsed or refractory: Children ≥4 years and Adolescents:

Induction: 0.15 mg/kg/day; administer daily until bone marrow remission; maximum induction: 60 doses

Consolidation: 0.15 mg/kg/day starting 3-6 weeks after completion of induction therapy; maximum consolidation: 25 doses over a period of up to 5 weeks

APL initial treatment: Limited data available

Induction, consolidation, and maintenance (Mathews, 2006): Dosing based on experience available for children ≥3 years; however, age was not an exclusion criteria in clinical trial

Induction: 0.15 mg/kg/day (maximum dose: 10 mg); administer daily until bone marrow remission; maximum induction: 60 doses

Consolidation: 0.15 mg/kg/day (maximum dose: 10 mg) for 4 weeks, starting 4 weeks after completion of induction therapy

Maintenance: 0.15 mg/kg/dose (maximum dose: 10 mg) administered 10 days per month for 6 months, starting 4 weeks after completion of consolidation therapy

In combination with tretinoin (Ravandi, 2009): Dosing based on experience available for adolescents ≥14 years; however, age was not an exclusion criteria in clinical trial

Induction (beginning 10 days after initiation of tretinoin): 0.15 mg/kg/day until bone marrow remission; maximum induction: 75 doses

Consolidation: 0.15 mg/kg/day Monday through Friday for 4 weeks every 8 weeks for 4 cycles (weeks 1 to 4, 9 to 12, 17 to 20, and 25 to 28)

Adults:

APL, relapsed or refractory:

Induction: 0.15 mg/kg/day; administer daily until bone marrow remission; maximum induction: 60 doses

Consolidation: 0.15 mg/kg/day starting 3-6 weeks after completion of induction therapy; maximum consolidation: 25 doses over a period of up to 5 weeks

ARTEMETHER AND LUMEFANTRINE

Dosage adjustment in renal impairment:
Severe renal impairment (CrCl <30 mL/minute): Use with caution (systemic exposure to metabolites may be higher); may require dosage reduction; monitor closely for toxicity
Dialysis patients: Has not been studied

Dosage adjustment in hepatic impairment: Use with caution; severe hepatic impairment (Child-Pugh class C): Monitor closely for toxicity

Administration Hazardous agent; use appropriate precautions for handling and disposal (NIOSH, 2012). Dilute in 100-250 mL D₅W or NS. Does not contain a preservative; properly discard unused portion. Do not mix with other medications. Infuse over 1-2 hours. If acute vasomotor reactions occur, may infuse over a maximum of 4 hours. Does not require administration via a central venous catheter; pH: 7.5-8.5

Vesicant/Extravasation Risk May be an irritant

Monitoring Parameters Baseline then weekly 12-lead ECG; monitor electrolytes, CBC with differential, and coagulation at baseline then at least twice weekly during induction and at least weekly during consolidation; more frequent monitoring may be necessary in unstable patients

Dosage Forms Excipient information presented when available (limited, particularly for generics); consult specific product labeling.
Solution, Intravenous:
Trisenox: 10 mg/10 mL (10 mL)

References

Au WY, Tam S, Fong BM, et al, "Determinants of Cerebrospinal Fluid Arsenic Concentration in Patients With Acute Promyelocytic Leukemia on Oral Arsenic Trioxide Therapy," *Blood*, 2008, 112(9):3587-90.

Concha G, Vogler G, Lezcano D, et al, "Exposure to Inorganic Arsenic Metabolites During Early Human Development," *Toxicol Sci*, 1998, 44 (2):185-90.

"Dietary Reference Intakes for Vitamin A, Vitamin K, Arsenic, Boron, Chromium, Copper, Iodine, Iron, Manganese, Molybdenum, Nickel, Silicon, Vanadium, and Zinc," Food and Nutrition Board, Institute of Medicine. National Academy of Sciences, Washington, DC: National Academy Press, 2001, 162-84.

Fox E, Razzouk BI, Widemann BC, et al, "Phase 1 Trial and Pharmacokinetic Study of Arsenic Trioxide in Children and Adolescents With Refractory or Relapsed Acute Leukemia, Including Acute Promyelocytic Leukemia or Lymphoma," *Blood*, 2008, 111(2):566-73.

Gore SD, Gojo I, Sekeres MA, et al, "Single Cycle of Arsenic Trioxide-Based Consolidation Chemotherapy Spares Anthracycline Exposure in the Primary Management of Acute Promyelocytic Leukemia," *J Clin Oncol*, 2010, 28(6):1047-53.

Mathews V, George B, Chendamarai E, et al, "Single-Agent Arsenic Trioxide in the Treatment of Newly Diagnosed Acute Promyelocytic Leukemia: Long-Term Follow-Up Data," *J Clin Oncol*, 2010, 28 (24):3866-71.

Mathews V, George B, Lakshmi KM, et al, "Single-Agent Arsenic Trioxide in the Treatment of Newly Diagnosed Acute Promyelocytic Leukemia: Durable Remissions With Minimal Toxicity," *Blood*, 2006, 107(7):2627-32.

National Comprehensive Cancer Network® (NCCN), "Practice Guidelines in Oncology: Acute Myeloid Leukemia, Version 3, 2010." Available at http://www.nccn.org/professionals/physician_gls/PDF/aml.pdf

National Institute for Occupational Safety and Health (NIOSH), "NIOSH List of Antineoplastic and Other Hazardous Drugs in Healthcare Settings 2012." Available at http://www.cdc.gov/niosh/docs/2012-150/pdfs/2012-150.pdf. Accessed January 21, 2013.

Powell BL, Moser B, Stock W, et al, "Arsenic Trioxide Improves Event-Free and Over-All Survival for Adults With Acute Promyelocytic Leukemia: North American Leukemia Intergroup Study C9710," *Blood*, 2010, 116(19):3751-7.

Powell BL, Moser B, Stock W, et al, "Effect of Consolidation With Arsenic Trioxide (As2O3) on Event-Free Survival (EFS) and Overall Survival (OS) Among Patients With Newly Diagnosed Acute Promyelocytic Leukemia (APL): North American Intergroup Protocol C9710," *J Clin Oncol*, 2007, 25(18s):2 [abstract 2 from 2007 ASCO Annual Meeting].

Ravandi F, Estey E, Jones D, et al, "Effective Treatment of Acute Promyelocytic Leukemia With All-Trans-Retinoic Acid, Arsenic Trioxide, and Gemtuzumab Ozogamicin," *J Clin Oncol*, 2009, 27 (4):504-10.

Von Ehrenstein OS, Guha Mazumder DN, Hira-Smith M, et al, "Pregnancy Outcomes, Infant Mortality, and Arsenic in Drinking Water in West Bengal, India," *Am J Epidemiol*, 2006,163(7):662-9.

Yang CY, Chang CC, Tsai SS, et al, "Arsenic in Drinking Water and Adverse Pregnancy Outcome in an Arseniasis-Endemic Area in Northeastern Taiwan," *Environ Res*, 2003, 91(1):29-34.

◆ **Artane** see Trihexyphenidyl *on page 2085*

◆ **Artemether and Benflumetol** see Artemether and Lumefantrine *on page 203*

Artemether and Lumefantrine
(ar TEM e ther & loo me FAN treen)

Brand Names: U.S. Coartem
Therapeutic Category Antimalarial Agent
Generic Availability (U.S.) No
Use Treatment of acute, uncomplicated malaria infections due to *Plasmodium falciparum*, including malaria in geographical regions where chloroquine resistance has been reported [FDA approved in children ≥2 months (and at least 5 kg) and adults]
Note: Not approved for treatment of severe or complicated *Plasmodium falciparum* malaria or prevention of malaria
Pregnancy Risk Factor C
Pregnancy Considerations Animal studies have demonstrated increased fetal resorption and postimplantation loss during the period of organogenesis. Safety data from an observational pregnancy study included 500 pregnant women exposed to artemether/lumefantrine and did not show an increased in adverse outcomes or teratogenic effects over background rate. Approximately one-third of these patients were in the third trimester. Efficacy has not been established in pregnant patients. Treatment failures with standard doses have been reported in pregnant women in areas where drug resistant parasites are prevalent. This may be attributed to lower serum concentration of both artemether and lumefantrine in this population (McGready, 2008). Use during pregnancy only if potential benefit justifies potential risk to the fetus.
Breast-Feeding Considerations The benefits of breast-feeding to mother and infants should be weighed against the potential risk from infant exposure to artemether and lumefantrine.
Contraindications Hypersensitivity to artemether, lumefantrine, or any component; concurrent use with strong CYP3A4 inducers (eg, rifampin, carbamazepine, phenytoin, St John's wort)
Warnings QT interval prolongation has been reported in patients taking artemether/lumefantrine; avoid use in patients at risk for QT prolongation, including patients with a history of long QT syndrome, family history of congenital QT prolongation or sudden death, symptomatic arrhythmias, clinically-relevant bradycardia, severe heart disease, known hypokalemia, hypomagnesemia, or concurrent administration of antiarrhythmics (eg, Class Ia or III), drugs metabolized by CYP2D6 known to have cardiac effects (eg, flecainide, tricyclic antidepressants), or other drugs known to prolong the QT interval (eg, antipsychotics, antidepressants, macrolides, fluoroquinolones, triazole antifungals, or cisapride). Concomitant use of agents that promote hypokalemia or hypomagnesemia should be avoided.
Precautions Use with caution in patients receiving CYP3A4 inhibitors, substrates, or inducers as loss of concomitant drug efficacy or QT prolongation may occur. Use contraindicated in patients receiving strong CYP3A4 inducers. Avoid use in patients receiving medications metabolized by CYP2D6 as plasma concentrations of these coadministered medications may increase. Do not use within 1 month of halofantrine (not available in the U.S.) due to the potential additive effects on the QT interval. Drugs that prolong the QT interval (including quinidine and quinine) should be used with caution following treatment with artemether/lumefantrine due to lumefantrine's long half-life and potential for additive effects on the

QT interval. If mefloquine is administered prior to lumefantrine, decreased lumefantrine exposure may occur due to mefloquine-induced decreased bile production; encourage food consumption and monitor efficacy.

In the event of disease reappearance after treatment with artemether/lumefantrine, patients should be treated with a different antimalarial drug. Use caution in patients with severe hepatic or renal impairment as it has not been studied in these populations.

Adverse Reactions

Cardiovascular: Palpitation

Central nervous system: Chills, dizziness, fatigue, fever, headache, insomnia, malaise, sleep disturbances, vertigo

Dermatologic: Pruritus, rash

Gastrointestinal: Abdominal pain, anorexia, diarrhea, nausea, splenomegaly, vomiting

Hematologic: Anemia

Hepatic: AST increased, hepatomegaly

Neuromuscular & skeletal: Arthralgia, myalgia, weakness

Respiratory: Cough, nasopharyngitis, rhinitis

Rare but important or life-threatening: Acrodermatitis, angioedema, agitation, ALT increased, asthma, ataxia, back pain, bronchitis, bullous skin eruption, conjunctivitis, constipation, clonus, dyspepsia, dysphagia, eosinophilia, fine motor delay, gait disturbance, hearing loss, hematocrit decreased, hematuria, hyper-reflexia, hypersensitivity reactions, hypoesthesia, hypokalemia, impetigo, infection (viral/bacterial/parasitic), leukocytosis, leukopenia, lymphocyte morphology abnormal, mood swings, nystagmus, peptic ulcer, pharyngolaryngeal pain, proteinuria, QT prolongation, tinnitus, thrombocytopenia, thrombocytosis, tremor, urticaria

Drug Interactions

Metabolism/Transport Effects Refer to individual components.

Avoid Concomitant Use

Avoid concomitant use of Artemether and Lumefantrine with any of the following: Antimalarial Agents; Artemether; Axitinib; CYP3A4 Inducers (Strong); Halofantrine; Highest Risk QTc-Prolonging Agents; Ivabradine; Lumefantrine; Mifepristone; Moderate Risk QTc-Prolonging Agents; Simeprevir; St Johns Wort; Thioridazine

Increased Effect/Toxicity

Artemether and Lumefantrine may increase the levels/ effects of: Antimalarial Agents; Antipsychotic Agents (Phenothiazines); CYP2D6 Substrates; Dapsone (Systemic); Dapsone (Topical); DOXOrubicin (Conventional); Etravirine; Fesoterodine; Halofantrine; Highest Risk QTc-Prolonging Agents; Lumefantrine; Metoprolol; Nebivolol; Thioridazine

The levels/effects of Artemether and Lumefantrine may be increased by: Antimalarial Agents; Artemether; CYP3A4 Inhibitors (Strong); Dapsone (Systemic); Etravirine; Grapefruit Juice; Ivabradine; Mifepristone; Moderate Risk QTc-Prolonging Agents; QTc-Prolonging Agents (Indeterminate Risk and Risk Modifying)

Decreased Effect

Artemether and Lumefantrine may decrease the levels/ effects of: ARIPiprazole; Axitinib; Codeine; Contraceptives (Estrogens); Contraceptives (Progestins); Ibrutinib; Saxagliptin; Simeprevir; Tamoxifen; TraMADol

The levels/effects of Artemether and Lumefantrine may be decreased by: Bosentan; CYP3A4 Inducers (Strong); Dabrafenib; Deferasirox; Efavirenz; Etravirine; Siltuximab; St Johns Wort; Tocilizumab

Food Interactions Absorption of artemether and lumefantrine is increased in the presence of food. The bioavailability of artemether increases two- to threefold and lumefantrine increases 16-fold (particularly a high-fat meal). Administration with grapefruit juice may result in increased concentrations of artemether and/or lumefantrine and potentiate QT prolongation. Management: Administer with a full meal for maximal absorption. Avoid grapefruit juice.

Stability Store at 25°C (77°F); excursions permitted to 15°C to 30°C (59°F to 86°F).

Mechanism of Action A coformulation of artemether and lumefantrine with activity against *Plasmodium falciparum*. Artemether and major metabolite dihydroartemisinin (DHA) are rapid schizontocides with activity attributed to the endoperoxide moiety common to each substance. Artemether inhibits an essential calcium adenosine triphosphatase. The exact mechanism of lumefantrine is unknown, but it may inhibit the formation of β-hematin by complexing with hemin. Both artemether and lumefantrine inhibit nucleic acid and protein synthesis. Artemether rapidly reduces parasite biomass and lumefantrine eliminates residual parasites.

Pharmacokinetics (Adult data unless noted)

Absorption:

Artemether: Rapid; enhanced with food

Lumefantrine: Initial absorption at 2 hours; enhanced with food

Protein binding:

Artemether: 95%

Dihydroartemisinin (DHA): 47% to 76%

Lumefantrine: 99.7%

Metabolism: Artemether is hepatically metabolized to an active metabolite, dihydroartemisinin (DHA) catalyzed predominately by CYP3A4/5 and to a lesser extent by CYP2B6, CYP2C9, and CYP2C19. The artemether/DHA AUC ratio is 1.2 after one dose and 0.3 after six doses which may indicate autoinduction. Lumefantrine is hepatically metabolized to desbutyl-lumefantrine by CYP3A4.

Bioavailability: Absorption is increased in the presence of food. The bioavailability of artemether increases two- to threefold and lumefantrine increases 16-fold (particularly a high-fat meal)

Half-life:

Artemether: 1-2 hours

DHA: 2 hours

Lumefantrine: 72-144 hours

Time to peak serum concentration:

Artemether: ~2 hours

Lumefantrine: ~6-8 hours

Elimination: No excretion data exist for humans

Dosing: Usual Malaria, uncomplicated (due to *P. falciparum*, including chloroquine resistant *P. falciparum*):

Note: Not for treatment of severe or complicated *Plasmodium falciparum* malaria or prevention of malaria

Infants ≥2 months, Children, and Adolescents ≤16 years: Oral:

5 kg to <15 kg: One tablet at hour 0 and at hour 8 on the first day and then one tablet twice daily (in the morning and evening) on days 2 and 3 (total of 6 tablets per treatment course)

15 kg to <25 kg: Two tablets at hour 0 and at hour 8 on the first day and then two tablets twice daily (in the morning and evening) on days 2 and 3 (total of 12 tablets per treatment course)

25 kg to <35 kg: Three tablets at hour 0 and at hour 8 on the first day and then three tablets twice daily (in the morning and evening) on day 2 and 3 (total of 18 tablets per treatment course)

≥35 kg: Four tablets at hour 0 and at hour 8 on the first day and then four tablets twice daily (in the morning and evening) on days 2 and 3 (total of 24 tablets per treatment course)

Adolescents >16 years and Adults (≥35 kg): Oral: Four tablets at hour 0 and at hour 8 on the first day and then four tablets twice daily (in the morning and evening) on days 2 and 3 (total of 24 tablets per treatment course). If patient is <35 kg, refer to dosing in children.

Administration Administer with a full meal for best absorption. For infants, children, and patients unable to swallow tablets: Crush tablet and mix with 5-10 mL of water in a clean container; administer; rinse container with water and administer remaining contents. The crushed mixture should be followed with food/milk, infant formula, pudding, porridge, or broth if possible. Repeat dose if vomiting occurs within 2 hours of administration; for persistent vomiting, explore alternative therapy.

Monitoring Parameters Monitor for adequate food consumption and efficacy.

Dosage Forms Excipient information presented when available (limited, particularly for generics); consult specific product labeling.

Tablet:
Coartem: Artemether 20 mg and lumefantrine 120 mg

References

Alecrim MG, Lacerda MV, Mourão MP, et al, "Successful Treatment of *Plasmodium falciparum* Malaria With a Six-Dose Regimen of Artemether-Lumefantrine Versus Quinine-Doxycycline in the Western Amazon Region of Brazil," *Am J Trop Med Hyg*, 2006, 74(1):20-5.

Centers for Disease Control and Prevention (CDC), "Guidelines for Treatment of Malaria in the United States," Treatment Table Update, September 23, 2011. Available at http://www.cdc.gov/malaria/resources/pdf/treatmenttable.pdf

Centers for Disease Control and Prevention (CDC), "Treatment of Malaria (Guidelines for Clinicians)." Available at http://www.cdc.gov/malaria/pdf/clinicalguidance.pdf

Makanga M, Premji Z, Falade C, et al, "Efficacy and Safety of the Six-Dose Regimen of Artemether-Lumefantrine in Pediatrics With Uncomplicated *Plasmodium falciparum* Malaria: a Pooled Analysis of Individual Patient Data," *Am J Trop Med Hyg*, 2006, 74(6):991-8.

McGready R, Tan SO, Ashley EA, et al, "A Randomised Controlled Trial of Artemether-Lumefantrine Versus Artesunate for Uncomplicated *Plasmodium falciparum* Treatment in Pregnancy," *PLoS Med*, 2008, 5(12):e253.

Omari AA, Gamble C, and Garner P, "Artemether-Lumefantrine (Six-Dose Regimen) for Treating Uncomplicated *Falciparum* Malaria," *Cochrane Database Syst Rev*, 2005, Issue 4, Art. No.: CD005564.

Toovey S and Jamieson A, "Audiometric Changes Associated With the Treatment of Uncomplicated *Falciparum* malaria With Co-Artemether," *Trans R Soc Trop Med Hyg*, 2004, 98(5):261-7.

"World Health Organization Guidelines for the Treatment of Malaria Second Edition," Available at http://www.cdc.gov/malaria/diagnosis_-treatment/treatment.html

---

Artificial Tears (ar ti FISH il tears)

Medication Safety Issues

Sound-alike/look-alike issues:
Isopto® Tears may be confused with Isoptin®

Brand Names: U.S. Advanced Eye Relief™ Dry Eye Environmental [OTC]; Advanced Eye Relief™ Dry Eye Rejuvenation [OTC]; Bion® Tears [OTC]; HypoTears [OTC]; Murine Tears® [OTC]; Soothe® Hydration [OTC]; Soothe® [OTC]; Systane® Ultra [OTC]; Systane® [OTC]; Tears Again® [OTC]; Tears Naturale® Forte [OTC]; Tears Naturale® Free [OTC]; Tears Naturale® II [OTC]; Viva-Drops® [OTC]

Brand Names: Canada Teardrops®

Therapeutic Category Ophthalmic Agent, Miscellaneous

Generic Availability (U.S.) Yes

Use Ophthalmic lubricant; for relief of dry eyes and eye irritation; protectant against further irritation (OTC: FDA approved in adults; refer to product-specific information regarding FDA approval in pediatric patients); has also been used for symptomatic treatment of dry eye associated with conjunctivitis, blepharitis, and keratitis

Contraindications Hypersensitivity to any component (consult product-specific information)

Warnings Individual product formulations may include (as an active ingredient) polyvinyl alcohol, povidone, carboxymethylcellulose, hydroxymethylcellulose, hydroxypropyl methylcellulose, or dextran 70; refer to product labeling for specific ingredients. Additionally, some formulations contain propylene glycol; toxicities have been reported with use of products containing propylene glycol, including hyperosmolality, lactic acidosis, seizures and respiratory depression; in neonates large amounts of propylene glycol delivered orally, intravenously (eg, >3000 mg/day), or topically have been associated with potentially fatal toxicities which can include metabolic acidosis, seizures, renal failure, and CNS depression; use products containing propylene glycol with caution (AAP, 1997; Shehab, 2009). Some formulations may contain polysorbate 80 (Tween 80®) which may cause allergic reactions in susceptible individuals. In premature neonates, thrombocytopenia, ascites, pulmonary deterioration, and renal and hepatic failure have been reported after receiving parenteral products containing polysorbate 80 (Alade, 1986; *MMWR*, 1984).

Precautions Ophthalmic solutions may contain benzalkonium chloride which may be absorbed by contact lenses; remove contact lenses before use. Preservative-free formulations are single-use containers; once opened they should be discarded; do not reuse. When used for self-medication (OTC), use should be discontinued and healthcare provider contacted if changes in vision, eye pain, continued redness, or irritation occur, or if the condition worsens or persists for more than 72 hours. Use in neonates or infants should be directed by a prescriber. To avoid contamination, do not touch tip of container to any surface. Replace cap after using. Do not use if solution is cloudy or changes color.

Adverse Reactions Ocular: blurred vision, crusting of eyelids, mild stinging

Drug Interactions

Metabolism/Transport Effects None known.

Avoid Concomitant Use There are no known interactions where it is recommended to avoid concomitant use.

Increased Effect/Toxicity There are no known significant interactions involving an increase in effect.

Decreased Effect There are no known significant interactions involving a decrease in effect.

Stability Store at room temperature; see product-specific labeling for any additional storage requirements.

Mechanism of Action Products contain demulcents (ie, cellulose derivatives, dextran 70, gelatin, polyols, polyvinal alcohol, or povidone); usually a water-soluble polymer, applied topically to the eye to protect and lubricate mucous membrane surfaces and relieve dryness and irritation

Dosing: Neonatal Ophthalmic: **Ocular dryness/irritation:** 1 drop into eye(s) as needed to relieve symptoms; **Note:** Neonatal data are unavailable; dosage extrapolated from older pediatric patients.

Dosing: Usual Ophthalmic:

Infants, Children, and Adolescents:
Ocular dryness/irritation: 1-2 drops into eye(s) as needed to relieve symptoms

Dry eye associated with ocular inflammation (eg, blepharitis, conjunctivitis, keratitis): 1-2 drops into eye(s) at least twice daily or as needed to relieve symptoms (Sethuraman, 2009)

Adults: **Ocular dryness/irritation:** 1-2 drops into eye(s) as needed to relieve symptoms

Administration Wash hands thoroughly before administration; do not touch tip of container to the eye or any surface; replace cap after use. Some products should not be used with contact lenses; consult specific product information.

Dosage Forms Excipient information presented when available (limited, particularly for generics); consult specific product labeling.

Solution, ophthalmic:
Advanced Eye Relief™ Dry Eye Environmental: Glycerin 1% (15 mL) [contains benzalkonium chloride]

Advanced Eye Relief™ Dry Eye Rejuvenation: Glycerin 0.3% and propylene glycol 1% (30 mL) [contains benzalkonium chloride]

HypoTears: Polyvinyl alcohol 1% and polyethylene glycol 400 1% (30 mL) [contains benzalkonium chloride]

Murine Tears®: Polyvinyl alcohol 0.5% and povidone 0.6% (15 mL) [contains benzalkonium chloride]

Soothe® Hydration: Povidone 1.25% (15 mL)

Systane® Ultra: Polyethylene glycol 400 0.4% and propylene glycol 0.3% (5 mL, 10 mL)

Systane®: Polyethylene glycol 400 0.4% and propylene glycol 0.3% (5 mL, 15 mL, 30 mL)

Tears Again®: Polyvinyl alcohol 1.4% (30 mL) [contains benzalkonium chloride]

Tears Naturale® II: Dextran 70 0.1% and hydroxypropyl methylcellulose 2910 0.3% (30 mL)

Tears Naturale® Forte: Dextran 70 1%, glycerin 0.2%, and hydroxypropyl methylcellulose 2910 0.3% (30 mL)

Solution, ophthalmic [preservative free]:

Bion® Tears: Dextran 70 0.1% and hydroxypropyl methylcellulose 2910 0.3% per 0.4 mL (28s)

Soothe®: Glycerin 0.6% and propylene glycol 0.6% per 0.6 mL (28s)

Systane® Ultra: Polyethylene glycol 400 0.4% and propylene glycol 0.3% per 0.4 mL (24s)

Tears Naturale® Free: Dextran 70 0.1% and hydroxypropyl methylcellulose 2910 0.3% per 0.5 mL (36s, 60s)

Viva-Drops®: Polysorbate 80 1% (0.5 mL, 10 mL)

References

Alade SL, Brown RE, and Paquet A Jr, "Polysorbate 80 and E-Ferol Toxicity," *Pediatrics*, 1986, 77(4):593-7.

American Academy of Pediatrics Committee on Drugs. "Inactive" ingredients in pharmaceutical products: update (subject review). *Pediatrics*. 1997;99(2):268-278.

Centers for Disease Control (CDC), "Unusual Syndrome With Fatalities Among Premature Infants: Association With a New Intravenous Vitamin E Product," *MMWR Morb Mortal Wkly Rep*, 1984, 33 (14):198-9.

Sethuraman U and Kamat D, "The Red Eye: Evaluation and Management," *Clin Pediatr (Phila)*, 2009, 48(6):588-600.

Shehab N, Lewis CL, Streetman DD, Donn SM. Exposure to the pharmaceutical excipients benzyl alcohol and propylene glycol among critically ill neonates. *Pediatr Crit Care Med*. 2009;10 (2):256-259.

◆ **As₂O₃** *see* Arsenic Trioxide *on page* 201

◆ **ASA** *see* Aspirin *on page* 212

◆ **5-ASA** *see* Mesalamine *on page* 1347

◆ **Asacol (Can)** *see* Mesalamine *on page* 1347

◆ **Asacol 800 (Can)** *see* Mesalamine *on page* 1347

◆ **Asacol HD** *see* Mesalamine *on page* 1347

◆ **Asaphen (Can)** *see* Aspirin *on page* 212

◆ **Asaphen E.C. (Can)** *see* Aspirin *on page* 212

◆ **Ascocid [OTC]** *see* Ascorbic Acid *on page* 206

◆ **Ascocid-ISO-pH [OTC]** *see* Ascorbic Acid *on page* 206

◆ **Ascor L 500** *see* Ascorbic Acid *on page* 206

◆ **Ascor L NC** *see* Ascorbic Acid *on page* 206

Ascorbic Acid (a SKOR bik AS id)

Medication Safety Issues

International issues:

Rubex [Ireland] may be confused with Brivex brand name for brivudine [Switzerland]

Rubex: Brand name for ascorbic acid [Ireland], but also the brand name for doxorubicin [Brazil]

Brand Names: U.S. Acerola C 500 [OTC]; Asco-Tabs-1000 [OTC]; Ascocid [OTC]; Ascocid-ISO-pH [OTC]; Ascor L 500; Ascor L NC; BProtected Vitamin C [OTC]; C Complex [OTC]; C-500 [OTC]; C-Time [OTC]; Cemill SR [OTC]; Cemill [OTC]; Chew-C [OTC]; Ester-C [OTC]; Fruit C 500 [OTC]; Fruit C [OTC]; Fruity C [OTC]; Mega-C/A Plus; Ortho-CS 250; Vita-C [OTC]

Brand Names: Canada Proflavanol C™; Revitalose C-1000®

Therapeutic Category Nutritional Supplement; Urinary Acidifying Agent; Vitamin, Water Soluble

Generic Availability (U.S.) May be product dependent

Use

Oral: Dietary supplement of Vitamin C (OTC: FDA approved in adults); has also been used for urinary acidification

Parenteral: Prevention and treatment of scurvy (All indications: FDA approved in adults)

Pregnancy Risk Factor C

Pregnancy Considerations Animal reproduction studies have not been conducted. Maternal plasma concentrations of ascorbic acid decrease as pregnancy progresses due to hemodilution and increased transfer to the fetus. Some pregnant women (eg, smokers) may require supplementation greater than the RDA (IOM, 2000).

Breast-Feeding Considerations Ascorbic acid is found in breast milk; regulatory mechanisms prevent concentrations from exceeding a required amount (IOM, 2000).

Contraindications Hypersensitivity to ascorbic acid or any component

Warnings Liquid may contain sodium benzoate; benzoic acid (benzoate) is a metabolite of benzyl alcohol; large amounts of benzyl alcohol (≥99 mg/kg/day) have been associated with a potentially fatal toxicity ("gasping syndrome") in neonates; the "gasping syndrome" consists of metabolic acidosis, respiratory distress, gasping respirations, CNS dysfunction (including convulsions, intracranial hemorrhage), hypotension, and cardiovascular collapse; use liquid-containing sodium benzoate with caution in neonates; *in vitro* and animal studies have shown that benzoate displaces bilirubin from protein binding sites

Precautions Use with caution in patients with concurrent anticoagulant therapy, sodium-restricted diet, diabetes, or patients prone to recurrent renal calculi (eg, dialysis patients); these patients should not take excessive doses for extended periods of time. High doses (>RDA) should be avoided during pregnancy; ascorbic acid actively crosses the placenta; fetal effects of high doses of vitamin C are not known.

Some products contain sulfites which may cause allergic reactions in susceptible individuals. Some oral products contain aspartame which is metabolized to phenylalanine and must be avoided (or used with caution) in patients with phenylketonuria. The parenteral product may contain aluminum; toxic aluminum concentrations may be seen with high doses, prolonged use, or renal dysfunction. Premature neonates are at higher risk due to immature renal function and aluminum intake from other parenteral sources. Parenteral aluminum exposure of >4-5 mcg/kg/day is associated with CNS and bone toxicity and tissue loading may occur at lower doses.

Adverse Reactions

Endocrine & metabolic: Hyperoxaluria (with large doses)

Rare but important or life-threatening: Dizziness, fatigue, flank pain, headache

Drug Interactions

Metabolism/Transport Effects None known.

Avoid Concomitant Use There are no known interactions where it is recommended to avoid concomitant use.

Increased Effect/Toxicity

Ascorbic Acid may increase the levels/effects of: Aluminum Hydroxide; Deferoxamine; Estrogen Derivatives

Decreased Effect

Ascorbic Acid may decrease the levels/effects of: Amphetamines; Bortezomib; CycloSPORINE (Systemic)

The levels/effects of Ascorbic Acid may be decreased by: Copper

Stability Parenteral: Store at <23°C (<73°F); protect from light. Use within 4 hours of vial entry; discard remaining portion; protect oral dosage forms from light; ascorbic acid solution is rapidly oxidized.

Mechanism of Action Not fully understood; necessary for collagen formation and tissue repair; involved in some oxidation-reduction reactions as well as other metabolic pathways, such as synthesis of carnitine, steroids, and catecholamines and conversion of folic acid to folinic acid

Pharmacodynamics Onset of action: Reversal of scurvy symptoms: 2 days to 3 weeks

Pharmacokinetics (Adult data unless noted)

Absorption: Oral: Readily absorbed; absorption is an active process and is thought to be dose-dependent

Distribution: Widely distributed

Protein binding: 25%

Metabolism: Hepatic, by oxidation and sulfation

Elimination: In urine; there is an individual specific renal threshold for ascorbic acid; when blood levels are high, ascorbic acid is excreted in urine, whereas when the levels are subthreshold (doses up to 80 mg/day) very little if any ascorbic acid is excreted into urine

Dosing: Neonatal

Adequate Intake (AI): Oral: 40 mg daily (~6 mg/kg/day)

Parenteral nutrition, maintenance requirement (Vanek, 2012): I.V.:

Preterm: 15-25 mg/kg/day

Term: 80 mg daily

Dosing: Usual

Infants, Children, and Adolescents:

Adequate Intake (AI): Oral:

1-6 months: 40 mg daily (~6 mg/kg/day)

7-12 months: 50 mg daily (~6 mg/kg/day)

Recommended daily allowance (RDA): Oral:

1-3 years: 15 mg daily

4-8 years: 25 mg daily

9-13 years: 45 mg daily

14-18 years: Males: 75 mg daily, females: 65 mg daily

Dietary supplement: Oral: 35-100 mg daily

Parenteral nutrition, maintenance requirement (Vanek, 2012): I.V.:

Infants: 15-25 mg/kg/day; maximum daily dose: 80 mg/**day**

Children and Adolescents: 80 mg daily

Scurvy: Oral, I.M., I.V., SubQ: Initial: 100 mg/dose 3 times daily for 1 week (300 mg/day) followed by 100 mg once daily until normalization of tissue saturation, usually 1-3 months (AAP, 2009; Weinstein, 2001)

Urinary acidification: Oral: 500 mg every 6-8 hours

Adults:

Recommended daily allowance (RDA): Oral: **Note:** Upper limit of intake should not exceed 2000 mg/day

Males: 90 mg daily

Females: 75 mg daily

Pregnant females:

≤18 years: 80 mg daily; upper limit of intake should not exceed 1800 mg/day

19-50 years: 85 mg daily; upper limit of intake should not exceed 2000 mg/day

Lactating females:

≤18 years: 115 mg daily; upper limit of intake should not exceed 1800 mg/day

19-50 years: 120 mg daily; upper limit of intake should not exceed 2000 mg/day

Adult smoker: Add an additional 35 mg daily

Dietary supplement (variable): Oral: 50-200 mg daily

Parenteral nutrition, maintenance requirement: I.V.: ASPEN Recommendations: 200 mg/day (Vanek, 2012)

Scurvy: Oral, I.V., I.M., SubQ: 100-250 mg 1-2 times daily for at least 2 weeks

Urinary acidification: Oral: 4-12 **grams** daily in 3-4 divided doses

Wound healing: I.V.: 300-500 mg daily for 7-10 days

Severe burns: I.V.: 1000-2000 mg daily

Administration

Oral: May be administered without regard to meals

Parenteral: Use only in circumstances when the oral route is not possible; I.M. preferred parenteral route due to improved utilization; for I.V. use dilute in equal volume D_5W or NS, and infuse over at least 10 minutes; rapid infusion may cause dizziness

Reference Range

Normal levels: 10-20 mcg/mL

Scurvy: <1-1.5 mcg/mL

Test Interactions False-positive urinary glucose with cupric sulfate reagent, false-negative urinary glucose with glucose oxidase method; false-negative stool occult blood 48-72 hours after ascorbic acid ingestion

Additional Information Sodium content of 1 g: ~5 mEq

Dosage Forms Excipient information presented when available (limited, particularly for generics); consult specific product labeling. [DSC] = Discontinued product

Capsule Extended Release, Oral:

C-Time: 500 mg

Generic: 500 mg

Capsule Extended Release, Oral [preservative free]:

Generic: 500 mg

Crystals, Oral:

Vita-C: (120 g, 480 g) [animal products free, gelatin free, gluten free, lactose free, no artificial color(s), no artificial flavor(s), starch free, sugar free, yeast free]

Granules, Oral:

Generic: (100 g, 500 g, 1000 g)

Liquid, Oral:

BProtected Vitamin C: 500 mg/5 mL (236 mL) [contains propylene glycol, saccharin sodium, sodium benzoate; citrus flavor]

Generic: 500 mg/5 mL (473 mL)

Powder, Oral:

Ascocid: (227 g)

Generic: (113 g, 120 g, 480 g)

Powder Effervescent, Oral:

Ascocid-ISO-pH: (150 g) [corn free, rye free, wheat free]

Solution, Injection:

Generic: 500 mg/mL (50 mL)

Solution, Injection [preservative free]:

Ascor L 500: 500 mg/mL (50 mL)

Ascor L NC: 500 mg/mL (50 mL) [corn free]

Mega-C/A Plus: 500 mg/mL (50 mL)

Solution, Injection, as sodium ascorbate [preservative free]:

Ortho-CS 250: 250 mg/mL (100 mL) [contains edetate disodium, water, sterile]

Generic: 250 mg/mL (30 mL)

Syrup, Oral:

Generic: 500 mg/5 mL (118 mL, 473 mL)

Tablet, Oral:

Asco-Tabs-1000: 1000 mg [color free, starch free, sugar free]

Ester-C:

Generic: 100 mg, 250 mg, 500 mg, 1000 mg, 1000 mg

Tablet, Oral [preservative free]:

Generic: 250 mg, 500 mg

Tablet Chewable, Oral:

Chew-C: 500 mg

Fruit C 500: 500 mg [animal products free, gelatin free, gluten free, kosher certified, lactose free, no artificial color(s), no artificial flavor(s), starch free, sugar free, yeast free]

Fruit C: 100 mg [animal products free, gelatin free, gluten free, lactose free, no artificial color(s), no artificial flavor(s), starch free, sugar free, yeast free]

Fruity C: 250 mg

Generic: 100 mg, 250 mg, 500 mg

Tablet Chewable, Oral [preservative free]:
C-500: 500 mg [animal products free, gluten free, soy free, starch free, yeast free; orange flavor]
Generic: 500 mg,
Tablet Extended Release, Oral:
C Complex: [contains rose hips]
Cemill: 500 mg
Cemill SR: 1000 mg
Generic: 500 mg, 1000 mg, 1500 mg
Tablet Extended Release, Oral [preservative free]:
C Complex: [corn free, no artificial color(s), no artificial flavor(s), starch free, sugar free, wheat free, yeast free]
Generic: 1000 mg [DSC]
Wafer, Oral [preservative free]:
Acerola C 500: 500 mg (50 ea) [corn free, no artificial color(s), no artificial flavor(s), wheat free, yeast free; contains acerola (malpighia glabra)]

References

American Academy of Pediatrics Committee on Nutrition, "Micronutrients: Vitamin K," *Pediatric Nutrition Handbook*, 6th ed, Kleinman RE, ed, Elk Grove Village, IL: American Academy of Pediatrics, 2009, 484.

Department Health and Human Services, Food Drug Administration, "Aluminum in Large and Small Volume Parenterals Used in Total Parenteral Nutrition," *Federal Register*, 2000, 65(17):4103-11.

"Dietary Reference Intakes for Vitamin C, Vitamin E, Selenium, and Carotenoids. A Report of the Panel on Dietary Antioxidants and Related Compounds Food and Nutrition Board, Institute of Medicine," National Academy of Sciences, Washington, DC: National Academy Press, 2000.

Ellis CN, Vanderveen EE, and Rasmussen JE, "Scurvy. A Case Caused by Peculiar Dietary Habits," *Arch Dermatol*, 1984, 120(9):1212-4.

Institute of Medicine (IOM), *Dietary Reference Intakes for Vitamin C, Vitamin E, Selenium, and Carotenoids*, Washington, DC: National Academy Press, 2000.

Vanek VW, Borum P, Buchman A, et al, "A.S.P.E.N. Position Paper: Recommendations for Changes in Commercially Available Parenteral Multivitamin and Multi-trace Element Products," *Nutr Clin Pract*, 2012, 27(4):440-91.

Weinstein M, Babyn P, and Zlotkin S, "An Orange a Day Keeps the Doctor Away: Scurvy in the Year 2000," *Pediatrics*, 2001, 108(3):E55.

◆ **Asco-Tabs-1000 [OTC]** *see* Ascorbic Acid *on page 206*

◆ **Ascriptin Maximum Strength [OTC]** *see* Aspirin *on page 212*

◆ **Ascriptin Regular Strength [OTC]** *see* Aspirin *on page 212*

◆ **Asmanex 7 Metered Doses** *see* Mometasone (Oral Inhalation) *on page 1432*

◆ **Asmanex 14 Metered Doses** *see* Mometasone (Oral Inhalation) *on page 1432*

◆ **Asmanex 30 Metered Doses** *see* Mometasone (Oral Inhalation) *on page 1432*

◆ **Asmanex 60 Metered Doses** *see* Mometasone (Oral Inhalation) *on page 1432*

◆ **Asmanex 120 Metered Doses** *see* Mometasone (Oral Inhalation) *on page 1432*

◆ **Asmanex HFA** *see* Mometasone (Oral Inhalation) *on page 1432*

◆ **Asmanex Twisthaler (Can)** *see* Mometasone (Oral Inhalation) *on page 1432*

◆ **ASNase** *see* Asparaginase (E. coli) *on page 208*

◆ **Asparaginase** *see* Asparaginase (E. coli) *on page 208*

Asparaginase (E. coli) (a SPEAR a ji nase e ko lye)

Medication Safety Issues
Sound-alike/look-alike issues:
Asparaginase (E. coli) may be confused with asparaginase (Erwinia), pegaspargase

Elspar may be confused with Elaprase, Erwinaze, Oncaspar

High alert medication:
This medication is in a class the Institute for Safe Medication Practices (ISMP) includes among its list of drug classes which have a heightened risk of causing significant patient harm when used in error.

Related Information
Emetogenic Potential of Antineoplastic Agents in Children *on page 2327*
Safe Handling of Hazardous Drugs *on page 2419*

Brand Names: U.S. Elspar [DSC]
Brand Names: Canada Kidrolase
Therapeutic Category Antineoplastic Agent, Enzyme; Antineoplastic Agent, Miscellaneous
Generic Availability (U.S.) No
Use Treatment (in combination with other chemotherapy agents) of acute lymphoblastic leukemia (ALL) (FDA approved in all ages); has also been used for treatment of non-Hodgkin's lymphoma and acute myeloid leukemia
Pregnancy Risk Factor C
Pregnancy Considerations Adverse events were observed in animal reproduction studies. Use during pregnancy only if clearly needed.
Breast-Feeding Considerations It is not known if asparaginase is excreted in human milk. Due to the potential for serious adverse reactions in the nursing infant, the decision to discontinue asparaginase or to discontinue breast-feeding should take into account the importance of treatment to the mother.
Contraindications Hypersensitivity to asparaginase (E. coli-derived), or any component; history of serious thrombosis, pancreatitis, or serious hemorrhagic events with prior L-asparaginase treatment
Warnings Hazardous agent; use appropriate precautions for handling and disposal (NIOSH, 2012). Asparaginase should be administered under the supervision of a physician experienced in the use of cancer chemotherapy agents. Severe allergic reactions may occur; incidence of hypersensitivity reactions in children is 20% with E. coli asparaginase and <5% with Erwinia asparaginase; monitor for 1 hour after administration (although reactions may also occur beyond 1 hour after administration); immediate treatment for hypersensitivity reactions should be available during administration (diphenhydramine, epinephrine, steroid, and oxygen). Discontinue asparaginase if serious allergic reaction occurs. Prior exposure to asparaginase is a risk factor for allergic reactions; I.V. administration (compared to I.M. or SubQ administration) and younger age also may be associated with hypersensitivity reactions (Stock, 2011; Woo, 2000). There is a potential for patients to develop asparaginase antibodies which may result in hypersensitivity reactions or lead to faster clearance of asparaginase.

Increased prothrombin time, partial thromboplastin time, and hypofibrinogenemia may occur; cerebrovascular hemorrhage has been reported; monitor coagulation parameters at baseline and periodically during and after therapy. Fresh frozen plasma may be used to replace coagulation factors in patients with severe coagulopathy. Use with caution in patients with an underlying coagulopathy; use is contraindicated with a history of serious hemorrhagic event with prior asparaginase treatment. Serious thrombosis, including sagittal sinus thrombosis, may occur; discontinue with serious thrombotic events. Anticoagulation prophylaxis during therapy may be considered in some patients (Farge, 2013). The risk for thrombosis may be higher in adult patients (Stock, 2011). Use is contraindicated with a history of serious thrombosis with prior asparaginase treatment.

May cause serious and possibly fulminant or fatal pancreatitis; promptly evaluate patients with abdominal pain; the manufacturer recommends to discontinue if pancreatitis develops; however, may consider continuing therapy for asymptomatic chemical pancreatitis (amylase or lipase >3 times ULN) or only radiologic abnormalities in older adolescents and adults; monitor closely for rising amylase and/or lipase levels (Stock, 2011). Discontinue permanently for clinical pancreatitis (eg, vomiting, severe abdominal pain) with amylase/lipase elevation >3 times ULN for >3 days and/or development of a pancreatic pseudocyst (Stock, 2011). Use is contraindicated with a history of pancreatitis with prior asparaginase treatment.

Posterior reversible encephalopathy syndrome (PRES) has been observed in patients treated with asparaginase (in combination with other chemotherapy agents). Monitor for signs/symptoms of PRES (eg, altered mental status, headache, hypertension, seizures, visual disturbances); interrupt therapy for suspected PRES. Control blood pressure and closely monitor for seizure activity.

Altered liver function tests (eg, increased AST, ALT, alkaline phosphatase, bilirubin, and decreased serum albumin, plasma fibrinogen) may occur with therapy; fulminant hepatic failure has also occurred. Fatty liver may be observed on biopsy. Use with caution in patients with preexisting hepatic impairment; may alter function. Monitor liver function tests at baseline and periodically during treatment. May cause hyperglycemia/glucose intolerance (some cases may be irreversible); cases of diabetic ketoacidosis have been observed; monitor blood glucose.

Precautions Do not interchange *E. coli* asparaginase for *Erwinia* asparaginase or pegaspargase; ensure the proper formulation, route of administration, and dose prior to administration. Appropriate measures should be taken to prevent tumor lysis syndrome and subsequent hyperuricemia and uric acid nephropathy; consider antihyperuricemic therapy, hydration, and urinary alkalinization.

Adverse Reactions

Central nervous system: Agitation, chills, coma, confusion, depression, disorientation, fatigue, fever, hallucinations, seizure, somnolence, stupor

Endocrine & metabolic: Hyperglycemia/glucose intolerance, hyperuricemia

Gastrointestinal: Abdominal cramps, acute pancreatitis, anorexia, nausea, stomatitis, vomiting

Hematologic: Hypofibrinogenemia and depression of clotting factors V and VIII, variable decrease in factors VII and IX, severe protein C deficiency and decrease in antithrombin III (may be dose limiting or fatal)

Hepatic: Alkaline phosphatase, bilirubin, and transaminases increased (transient)

Hypersensitivity: Acute allergic reactions (anaphylaxis, angioedema, arthralgia, bronchospasm, fever, hypotension, rash, urticaria; may be dose limiting in some patients, may be fatal)

Renal: Azotemia

Miscellaneous: Allergic reaction (including anaphylaxis), antibody formation/immunogenicity

Rare but important or life-threatening: Acute renal failure, albumin decreased, cerebrovascular hemorrhage, diabetic ketoacidosis, disorientation, fatty liver, glucosuria, hallucinations, hemorrhagic pancreatitis, hepatic failure, hepatoxicity (may be fatal), hyperammonemia, hyper-/hypolipidemia, hyperthermia, hypocholesterolemia, hypotension, insulin-dependent diabetes, intracranial hemorrhage, irritability, ketoacidosis, malabsorption syndrome, myelosuppression (mild–to-moderate anemia, leukopenia, and thrombocytopenia; onset: 7 days; nadir: 14 days; recovery: 21 days), pancreatic pseudocyst, Parkinsonian symptoms (including tremor and increased muscle tone), partial thromboplastin time increased, peripheral edema, proteinuria, prothrombin time increased, renal

insufficiency, reversible posterior leukoencephalopathy syndrome, serum ammonia increased, serum cholesterol decreased, stroke (hemorrhagic and thrombotic), thrombosis (including cerebrovascular, sagittal sinus, venous)

Drug Interactions

Metabolism/Transport Effects None known.

Avoid Concomitant Use There are no known interactions where it is recommended to avoid concomitant use.

Increased Effect/Toxicity

Asparaginase (E. coli) may increase the levels/effects of: Dexamethasone (Systemic)

Decreased Effect There are no known significant interactions involving a decrease in effect.

Stability Store intact vials at 2°C to 8°C (36°F to 46°F). Reconstituted solutions are stable for 1 week refrigerated at 8°C (Stecher, 1999); however, the manufacturer recommends that reconstituted solutions should be discarded after 8 hours since there is no preservative. Discard immediately if solution becomes cloudy. Solutions for I.V. infusion are stable for 8 hours at room temperature or under refrigeration. A 5 micron filter may be used to remove fiber-like particles without loss of potency; use of a 0.2 micron filter may result in loss of potency.

Mechanism of Action In leukemic cells, asparaginase hydrolyzes L-asparagine to ammonia and L-aspartic acid, leading to depletion of asparagine. Leukemia cells, especially lymphoblasts, require exogenous asparagine; normal cells can synthesize asparagine. Asparagine depletion in leukemic cells leads to inhibition of protein synthesis and apoptosis. Asparaginase is cycle-specific for the G_1 phase.

Pharmacokinetics (Adult data unless noted)

Distribution: Slightly higher than plasma volume; <1% CSF penetration

Metabolism: Systemically degraded

Half-life: I.M.: 34 to 49 hours; I.V.: 8 to 30 hours

Time to peak serum concentrations: I.M.: 14 to 24 hours

Elimination: In patients who have experienced hypersensitivity reactions, increased clearance has been observed.

Dosing: Usual Note: Dose, frequency, number of doses, and start date may vary by protocol and treatment phase. Refer to individual protocols.

Pediatric:

Acute lymphoblastic leukemia (ALL):

Manufacturer's labeling: Infants, Children, and Adolescents: I.V., I.M.: 6000 units/m²/dose 3 times weekly for 9 doses in combination with other chemotherapy agents

Alternate dosing: Limited data available:

CCG 1922 protocol (Bostrom, 2003): Children 1 to 10 years: I.M.:

Induction: 6000 units/m²/dose 3 times weekly for 9 doses beginning either on day 2, 3, or 4

Delayed intensification: 6000 units/m²/dose on Monday, Wednesday, and Friday for 6 doses beginning day 3

DFCI-ALL Consortium protocol 00-01 (Vrooman, 2013): Children and Adolescents: I.M.:

Induction: 25,000 units/m² for 1 dose (in combination with other chemotherapy agents)

Intensification:

Fixed dose: 25,000 units/m²/dose weekly (in combination with other chemotherapy agents) for 30 weeks

Individualized dose: I.M.: Initial dose: 12,500 units/m^2/dose weekly (in combination with other chemotherapy agents); doses were adjusted based on nadir serum asparaginase activity (NSAA) determinations; NSAA was obtained prior to the second and fourth doses and then every 3 weeks thereafter; asparaginase was administered for 30 weeks; minimum dose: 6000 units/m^2; maximum dose: 25,000 units/m^2 (Vrooman, 2013). Doses were adjusted as follows based on most recent dose:

NSAA <0.025 units/mL: Increase dose by 80%, immediately assess for *E. coli* asparaginase antibody

NSAA 0.025 to <0.05 units/mL: Increase dose by 60%

NSAA 0.05 to <0.08 units/mL: Increase dose by 40%

NSAA 0.08 to <0.1 units/mL: Increase dose by 20%

NSAA 0.1 to <0.14 units/mL: No change; continue current dose

NSAA 0.14 to <0.2 units/mL: Decrease dose by 20%

NSAA >0.2 units/mL: Decrease dose by 40%

DFCI-ALL Consortium protocol 95-01 (Moghrabi, 2007): Infants, Children, and Adolescents: I.M.:

Induction: 25,000 units/m^2 for 1 dose on day 4 (in combination with other chemotherapy agents)

Intensification: 25,000 units/m^2/dose weekly (in combination with other chemotherapy agents) for 20 weeks

POG Study 8704 (T-3) (Amylon, 1999): Children and Adolescents: I.M.:

Induction: 10,000 units/m^2/dose on days 27, 29, and 31 for 3 doses (in combination with other chemotherapy agents)

Continuation: I.M.: 25,000/units/m^2/dose weekly for 20 weeks beginning on day 99 (in combination with other chemotherapy agents)

POG Study 9411: Children and Adolescents: Induction: I.M.: 10,000 units/m^2/dose on days 1, 3, 5, 8, 10, 12, 15, 17, 19, 22, 24, and 26 (in combination with other chemotherapy agents) (Kelly, 2013)

Lymphoblastic lymphoma: Limited data available:

EORTC CLG 58881: Infants, Children, and Adolescents: I.V.: 10,000 units/m^2/dose twice weekly (on days 12, 15, 18, 22, 25, 29, 32, and 35) in combination with other chemotherapy agents; for reinduction, similar dosing has been used for 4 doses on days 8, 11, 15, and 18 (Uyttebroeck, 2008)

POG Study 8704 (T-3) (Amylon, 1999): Children and Adolescents: I.M.:

Induction: 10,000 units/m^2/dose on days 27, 29, and 31 for 3 doses (in combination with other chemotherapy agents)

Continuation: I.M.: 25,000/units/m^2/dose weekly for 20 weeks beginning on day 99 (in combination with other chemotherapy agents)

St. Jude NHL 13 (Sandlund, 2009): Children and Adolescents: I.M.: Induction: 10,000 units/m^2/dose on days 2, 4, 6, 8, 10, and 12 (in combination with other chemotherapy agents)

Adult: **Note:** Utilize patient's actual body weight (full weight) for calculation of body surface area- or weight-based dosing, particularly when the intent of therapy is curative; manage regimen-related toxicities in the same manner as for nonobese patients; if a dose reduction is utilized due to toxicity, consider resumption of full weight-based dosing with subsequent cycles, especially if cause of toxicity (eg, hepatic or renal impairment) is resolved (Griggs, 2012).

Acute lymphoblastic leukemia (ALL):

Manufacturer's labeling: I.V., I.M.: 6000 units/m^2/dose 3 times weekly

Alternate dosing: Hyper-CVAD regimen: I.V. 20,000 units weekly for 4 doses (starting on day 2) during either months 7 and 19 or months 7 and 11 of intensification phase (Thomas, 2010)

Lymphoblastic lymphoma: Hyper-CVAD regimen: I.V.: 20,000 units weekly for 4 doses (starting on day 2) for 2 cycles (months 7 and 11) during maintenance phase (Thomas, 2004)

Dosing adjustment for toxicity: Infants, Children, Adolescents, and Adults: I.V., I.M.:

Allergic reaction/hypersensitivity: Discontinue for severe reactions.

Neurotoxicity (posterior reversible encephalopathy syndrome; PRES): Interrupt therapy for suspected PRES; control blood pressure and closely monitor for seizure activity.

Pancreatitis: Discontinue permanently (per manufacturer.)

Thrombotic event: Discontinue for serious reactions.

Dosing adjustment in renal impairment: Infants, Children, Adolescents, and Adults: I.V., I.M.: There are no dosage adjustments provided in the manufacturer's labeling.

Dosing adjustment in renal impairment: Infants, Children, Adolescents, and Adults: I.V., I.M.: There are no dosage adjustments provided in the manufacturer's labeling.

Administration Hazardous agent; use appropriate precautions for handling and disposal (NIOSH, 2012). Observe patients for 1 hour after administration; have epinephrine, diphenhydramine, and hydrocortisone at the bedside. A physician should be readily accessible.

I.M.: The manufacturer recommends reconstitution of the lyophilized powder with 2 mL NS to a concentration of 5000 units/mL; however, some institutions reconstitute with 1 mL NS for I.M. use, resulting in a concentration of 10,000 units/mL. Shake well, but not too vigorously. Maximum 2 mL volume is recommended for I.M. injections; if the volume to be administered is >2 mL, use multiple injection sites

I.V.: Reconstitute vial with 5 mL SWI or NS to a final concentration of 2000 units/mL; must be infused over a minimum of 30 minutes. Gelatinous fiber-like particles may develop on standing; filtration through a 5-micron filter during administration will remove the particles with no loss of potency.

Monitoring Parameters CBC with differential, coagulation parameters (baseline and periodic), urinalysis, amylase, liver enzymes, and bilirubin (baseline and periodic), renal function tests, urine glucose, blood glucose, uric acid. Monitor vital signs during administration and for allergic reaction, be prepared to treat anaphylaxis at each administration; monitor for onset of abdominal pain, seizure activity, and mental status changes.

Test Interactions Decreased thyroxine and thyroxine-binding globulin

Product Availability Elspar: Manufacturing of asparaginase *(E. coli)* was discontinued by Lundbeck at the end of 2012. Elspar was acquired by Recordati Rare Diseases; availability information is currently unavailable.

Dosage Forms Excipient information presented when available (limited, particularly for generics); consult specific product labeling. [DSC] = Discontinued product

Solution Reconstituted, Injection:

Elspar: 10,000 units (1 ea [DSC])

References

Amylon MD, Shuster J, Pullen J, et al, "Intensive High-Dose Asparaginase Consolidation Improves Survival for Pediatric Patients With T Cell Acute Lymphoblastic Leukemia and Advanced Stage

Lymphoblastic Lymphoma: A Pediatric Oncology Group Study," *Leukemia*, 1999, 13(3):335–42.

Asselin BL, Whitin JC, Coppola DJ, et al, "Comparative Pharmacokinetic Studies of Three Asparaginase Preparations," *J Clin Oncol*, 1993, 11(9):1780-6.

Avramis VI, Sencer S, Periclou AP, et al, "A Randomized Comparison of Native *Escherichia coli* Asparaginase and Polyethylene Glycol Conjugated Asparaginase for Treatment of Children With Newly Diagnosed Standard-Risk Acute Lymphoblastic Leukemia: A Children's Cancer Group Study," *Blood*, 2002, 99(6):1986-94.

Bostrom BC, Sensel MR, Sather HN, et al. Dexamethasone versus prednisone and daily oral versus weekly intravenous mercaptopurine for patients with standard-risk acute lymphoblastic leukemia: a report from the children's cancer group. *Blood*. 2003;101(10):3809-3817.

Clavell LA, Gelber RD, Cohen HJ, et al, "Four-Agent Induction and Intensive Asparaginase Therapy for Treatment of Childhood Acute Lymphoblastic Leukemia," *N Engl J Med*, 1986, 315(11):657-63.

Elspar (asparaginase) [prescribing information]. Deerfield, IL: Lundbeck; July 2013.

Farge D, Debourdeau P, Beckers M, et al. International clinical practice guidelines for the treatment of and prophylaxis of venous thromboembolism in patients with cancer. *J Thromb Haemost*. 2013;1(1):56-70.

Griggs JJ, Mangu PB, Anderson H, et al. Appropriate chemotherapy dosing for obese adult patients with cancer: American Society of Clinical Oncology Clinical Practice Guideline. *J Clin Oncol*. 2012;30(13):1553-1561.

Kelly ME, Lu X, Devidas M, et al. Treatment of relapsed precursor-B acute lymphoblastic leukemia with intensive chemotherapy: POG (Pediatric Oncology Group) study 9411 (SIMAL 9). *J Pediatr Hematol Oncol*. 2013;35(7):509-513.

Moghrabi A, Levy DE, Asselin B, et al. Results of the Dana-Farber Cancer Institute ALL Consortium Protocol 95-01 for children with acute lymphoblastic leukemia. *Blood*. 2007;109(3):896-904.

National Institute for Occupational Safety and Health (NIOSH), "NIOSH List of Antineoplastic and Other Hazardous Drugs in Healthcare Settings 2012." Available at http://www.cdc.gov/niosh/docs/2012-150/pdfs/2012-150.pdf. Accessed January 21, 2013.

Sandlund JT, Pui CH, Zhou Y, et al. Effective treatment of advanced-stage childhood lymphoblastic lymphoma without prophylactic cranial irradiation: results of St Jude NHL13 study. *Leukemia*. 2009;23(6):1127-1130.

Stecher AL, de Deus PM, Polikarpov I, et al, "Stability of L-Asparaginase: An Enzyme Used in Leukemia Treatment," *Pharm Acta Helv*, 1999, 74(1):1-9.

Stock W, Douer D, DeAngelo DJ, et al. Prevention and management of asparaginase/pegasparaginase-associated toxicities in adults and older adolescents: recommendations of an expert panel. *Leuk Lymphoma*. 2011;52(12):2237-2253.

Thomas DA, O'Brien S, Cortes J, et al. Outcome with the Hyper-CVAD regimens in lymphoblastic lymphoma. *Blood*. 2004;104(6):1624-1630.

Thomas DA, O'Brien S, Faderl S, et al. Chemoimmunotherapy with a modified Hyper-CVAD and rituximab regimen improves outcome in *de novo* Philadelphia Chromosome-Negative Precursor B-Lineage Acute Lymphoblastic Leukemia. *J Clin Oncol*. 2010;28(24):3880-3889.

Uyttebroeck A, Suciu S, Laureys G, et al. Treatment of childhood T-cell lymphoblastic lymphoma according to the strategy for acute lymphoblastic leukaemia, without radiotherapy: long term results of the EORTC CLG 58881 trial. *Eur J Cancer*. 2008;44(6):840-846.

Vrooman LM, Stevenson KE, Supko JG, et al. Postinduction dexamethasone and individualized dosing of *Escherichia Coli* L-asparaginase each improve outcome of children and adolescents with newly diagnosed acute lymphoblastic leukemia: results from a randomized study–Dana-Farber Cancer Institute ALL Consortium Protocol 00-01. *J Clin Onco*. 2013;31(9):1202-1210.

Woo MH, Hak LJ, Storm MC, et al. Hypersensitivity or development of antibodies to asparaginase does not impact treatment outcome of childhood acute lymphoblastic leukemia. *J Clin Onco*. 2000;18(7):1525-1532.

Asparaginase (*Erwinia*)
(a SPEAR a ji nase er WIN i ah)

Medication Safety Issues
Sound-alike/look-alike issues:
Asparaginase (*Erwinia*) may be confused with asparaginase (*E. coli*), pegaspargase

Erwinaze may be confused with Elaprase, Elspar, Oncaspar

High alert medication:
This medication is in a class the Institute for Safe Medication Practices (ISMP) includes among its list of drug classes which have a heightened risk of causing significant patient harm when used in error.

Related Information
Safe Handling of Hazardous Drugs *on page 2419*

Brand Names: U.S. Erwinaze

Brand Names: Canada Erwinase

Therapeutic Category Antineoplastic Agent, Enzyme; Antineoplastic Agent, Miscellaneous

Generic Availability (U.S.) No

Use Treatment (in combination with other chemotherapy agents) of acute lymphoblastic leukemia (ALL) in patients with hypersensitivity to *E. coli*-derived asparaginase (FDA approved in ages ≥2 years and adults)

Prescribing and Access Restrictions Erwinaze is distributed through Accredo Health Group, Inc. (1-877-900-9223).

Pregnancy Risk Factor C

Pregnancy Considerations Adverse events were observed in animal reproduction studies. Use during pregnancy only if clearly needed.

Breast-Feeding Considerations It is not known if asparaginase *Erwinia chrysanthemi* is excreted in breast milk. Due to the potential for serious adverse reactions in the nursing infant, the manufacturer recommends a decision be made whether to discontinue nursing or to discontinue the drug, taking into account the importance of treatment to the mother.

Contraindications Hypersensitivity reactions, including anaphylaxis to asparaginase (*Erwinia*) or any component; history of serious pancreatitis, serious thrombosis, or serious hemorrhagic event with prior asparaginase treatment

Warnings Hazardous agent; use appropriate precautions for handling and disposal (NIOSH, 2012). Severe hypersensitivity reactions, including anaphylaxis, have occurred in 5% of patients in clinical trials. Immediate treatment for anaphylactic reactions should be available during administration; discontinue for serious hypersensitivity reactions and administer appropriate treatment as necessary.

Pancreatitis has been reported in 4% of patients in clinical trials; promptly evaluate with symptoms suggestive of pancreatitis. For mild pancreatitis, withhold treatment until signs and symptoms subside and amylase returns to normal; may resume after resolution. Discontinue for severe or hemorrhagic pancreatitis characterized by abdominal pain >72 hours and amylase ≥2 x ULN. Further use is contraindicated if severe pancreatitis is diagnosed.

Serious thrombotic events, including sagittal sinus thrombosis, have been reported with asparaginase formulations. Decreases in fibrinogen, protein C activity, protein S activity, and antithrombin III have been noted following a 2-week treatment course; use with caution in patients with an underlying coagulopathy. Discontinue for hemorrhagic or thrombotic events; may resume treatment after resolution; contraindicated with history of serious thrombosis or hemorrhagic event with prior asparaginase treatment.

Glucose intolerance occurred in 2% of patients in the clinical trials; may be irreversible; monitor glucose levels (baseline and periodic) during treatment; may require insulin administration.

Adverse Reactions
Hypersensitivity: Hypersensitivity reaction (includes anaphylaxis, urticaria)

Cardiovascular: Thrombosis

Endocrine & metabolic: Decreased glucose tolerance, hyperglycemia

Gastrointestinal: Abdominal pain, diarrhea, nausea, pancreatitis, vomiting

Hepatic: Abnormal transaminase, hyperbilirubinemia

Local: Injection site reaction

Miscellaneous: Fever

Rare but important or life-threatening: Acute renal failure, anorexia, bone marrow depression (rare), changes in serum lipids, disseminated intravascular coagulation, hemorrhage, hepatomegaly, hyperammonemia, increased alkaline phosphatase, malabsorption syndrome, seizure, transient ischemic attacks, weight loss

Drug Interactions

Metabolism/Transport Effects None known.

Avoid Concomitant Use There are no known interactions where it is recommended to avoid concomitant use.

Increased Effect/Toxicity

Asparaginase (Erwinia) may increase the levels/effects of: Dexamethasone (Systemic)

Decreased Effect There are no known significant interactions involving a decrease in effect.

Stability Hazardous agent; use appropriate precautions for handling and disposal (NIOSH, 2012). Store intact vials at 2°C to 8°C (36°F to 48°F). Protect from light. Within 15 minutes of reconstitution, withdraw appropriate volume for dose into a polypropylene syringe. Do not freeze or refrigerate reconstituted solution; discard if not administered within 4 hours.

Mechanism of Action Asparaginase catalyzes the deamidation of asparagine to aspartic acid and ammonia, reducing circulating levels of asparagine. Leukemia cells lack asparagine synthetase and are unable to synthesize asparagine. Asparaginase reduces the exogenous asparagine source for the leukemic cells, resulting in cytotoxicity specific to leukemic cells.

Pharmacokinetics (Adult data unless noted) Half-life elimination: I.M.: ~16 hours (Asselin, 1993; Avramis, 2005)

Dosing: Usual

Acute lymphoblastic leukemia (ALL): I.M.: Children ≥1 year, Adolescents, and Adults:

As a substitute for pegaspargase: 25,000 units/m²/dose 3 times weekly (Mon, Wed, Fri) for 6 doses for each planned pegaspargase dose

As a substitute for asparaginase (E. coli): 25,000 units/m²/dose for each planned asparaginase (E. coli) dose

Dosage adjustment for toxicity:

Hemorrhagic or thrombotic event: Discontinue treatment; may resume treatment upon symptom resolution.

Pancreatitis:

Mild pancreatitis: Withhold treatment until signs and symptoms subside and amylase returns to normal; may resume after resolution.

Severe or hemorrhagic pancreatitis (abdominal pain >72 hours and amylase ≥2 x ULN): Discontinue treatment; further use is contraindicated.

Serious hypersensitivity: Discontinue treatment.

Dosing adjustment in renal impairment: There are no dosage adjustments provided in the manufacturer's labeling.

Dosing adjustment in hepatic impairment: There are no dosage adjustments provided in the manufacturer's labeling.

Administration Hazardous agent; use appropriate precautions for handling and disposal (NIOSH, 2012). Reconstitute each vial with 1 mL of preservative-free sodium chloride 0.9% (NS) to obtain a concentration of 10,000 units/mL, or with 2 mL preservative-free NS to obtain a concentration of 5,000 units/mL. Gently direct the NS down the wall of the vial (do not inject forcefully into or onto the powder). Dissolve by gently swirling or mixing; do not shake or invert the vial. Resulting reconstituted solution should be clear and colorless and free of visible particles or protein aggregates. Administer I.M.; volume of each single injection site should be limited to 2 mL; use multiple injection sites for volumes >2 mL. Following administration observe patient for hypersensitivity reactions; have resuscitation equipment and medication available for treatment of anaphylaxis.

Monitoring Parameters CBC with differential, amylase, liver enzymes, blood glucose (baseline and periodically during treatment), coagulation parameters, symptoms of hypersensitivity; symptoms of pancreatitis, thrombosis, or hemorrhage

Dosage Forms Excipient information presented when available (limited, particularly for generics); consult specific product labeling.

Solution Reconstituted, Intramuscular:

Erwinaze: 10,000 units (1 ea)

References

Asselin BL, Whitin JC, Cappola DJ, et al, "Comparative Pharmacokinetic Studies of Three Asparaginase Preparations," *J Clin Oncol*, 1993, 11(9):1780-6.

Avramis VI and Panosyan EH, "Pharmacokinetic/Pharmacodynamic Relationships of Asparaginase Formulations: The Past, the Present and Recommendations for the Future," *Clin Pharmacokinet*, 2005, 44 (4):367-93.

Cheung KC, van den Bemt PM, Torringa ML, et al, "Erroneous Exchange of Asparaginase Forms in the Treatment of Acute Lymphoblastic Leukemia," *J Pediatr Hematol Oncol*, 2011, 33(3):e109-13.

Duval M, Suciu S, Ferster A, et al, "Comparison of *Escherichia Coli* -Asparaginase With *Erwinia*-Asparaginase in the Treatment of Childhood Lymphoid Malignancies: Results of a Randomized European Organisation for Research and Treatment of Cancer – Children's Leukemia Group Phase 3 Trial," *Blood*, 2002, 99(8):2734-9.

Grace RF, Dahlberg SE, Neuberg D, et al, "The Frequency and Management of Asparaginase-Related Thrombosis in Paediatric and Adult Patients With Acute Lymphoblastic Leukaemia Treated on Dana-Farber Cancer Institute Consortium Protocols," *Br J Haematol*, 2011, 152(4):452-9.

National Institute for Occupational Safety and Health (NIOSH), "NIOSH List of Antineoplastic and Other Hazardous Drugs in Healthcare Settings 2012." Available at http://www.cdc.gov/niosh/docs/ 2012-150/pdfs/2012-150.pdf. Accessed January 21, 2013.

Salzer W, Asselin B, Supko JG, et al, "Administration of Erwinia Asparaginase (Erwinase®) Following Allergy to PEG-Asparaginase In Children and Young Adults With Acute Lymphoblastic Leukemia Treated on AALL07P2 Achieves Therapeutic Nadir Serum Asparaginase Activity: A Report From the Children's Oncology Group (COG)," *Blood*, 2010, 116(21):2134 [abstract 2134 from 2010 ASH Annual Meeting].

Schrey D, Speitel K, Lanvers-Kaminsky C, et al, "Five-Year Single-Center Study of Asparaginase Therapy Within the ALL-BFM 2000 Trial," *Pediatr Blood Cancer*, 2011, 57(3):378-84.

Vrooman LM, Supko JG, Neuberg DS, et al, "*Erwinia* Asparaginase After Allergy to E. coli Asparaginase in Children With Acute Lymphoblastic Leukemia," Pediatr Blood Cancer, 2010, 54(2):199-205.

Zalewska-Szewczyk B, Gach A, Wyka K, et al, "The Cross-Reactivity of Anti-Asparaginase Antibodies Against Different L-Asparaginase Preparations," *Clin Exp Med*, 2009, 9(2):113-6.

◆ **Asparaginase Erwinia chrysanthemi** *see* Asparaginase (Erwinia) *on page 211*

◆ **Aspart Insulin** *see* Insulin Aspart *on page 1114*

◆ **Aspercin [OTC]** *see* Aspirin *on page 212*

◆ **Aspergum [OTC]** *see* Aspirin *on page 212*

Aspirin (AS pir in)

Medication Safety Issues

Sound-alike/look-alike issues:

Aspirin may be confused with Afrin

Ascriptin may be confused with Aricept

Ecotrin may be confused with Edecrin, Epogen

Halfprin may be confused with Haltran

ZORprin may be confused with Zyloprim

International issues:

Cartia [multiple international markets] may be confused with Cartia XT brand name for diltiazem [U.S.]

BEERS Criteria medication:

This drug may be potentially inappropriate for use in geriatric patients (Quality of evidence - moderate; Strength of recommendation - strong).

Related Information

Oral Medications That Should Not Be Crushed or Altered *on page 2438*

Brand Names: U.S. Ascriptin Maximum Strength [OTC]; Ascriptin Regular Strength [OTC]; Aspercin [OTC]; Aspergum [OTC]; Aspir-low [OTC]; Aspirtab [OTC]; Bayer

Aspirin Extra Strength [OTC]; Bayer Aspirin Regimen Adult Low Strength [OTC]; Bayer Aspirin Regimen Children's [OTC]; Bayer Aspirin Regimen Regular Strength [OTC]; Bayer Genuine Aspirin [OTC]; Bayer Plus Extra Strength [OTC]; Bayer Women's Low Dose Aspirin [OTC]; Buffasal [OTC]; Bufferin Extra Strength [OTC]; Bufferin [OTC]; Buffinol [OTC]; Ecotrin Arthritis Strength [OTC]; Ecotrin Low Strength [OTC]; Ecotrin [OTC]; Halfprin [OTC]; St Joseph Adult Aspirin [OTC]; Tri-Buffered Aspirin [OTC]

Brand Names: Canada Asaphen; Asaphen E.C.; Entrophen; Novasen; Praxis ASA EC 81 Mg Daily Dose; Pro-AAS EC-80

Therapeutic Category Analgesic, Non-narcotic; Anti-inflammatory Agent; Antiplatelet Agent; Antipyretic; Non-steroidal Anti-inflammatory Drug (NSAID), Oral; Salicylate

Generic Availability (U.S.) Yes: Excludes gum

Use Treatment of mild to moderate pain, inflammation, and fever (OTC: All products: FDA approved in adults; refer to product-specific information regarding FDA approval in pediatric patients, most products FDA approved in ages ≥12 years), has also been used for adjunctive treatment of Kawasaki disease; prevention of vascular mortality during suspected acute MI; prevention of recurrent MI; prevention of MI in patients with angina; prevention of recurrent stroke and mortality following TIA or stroke; management of rheumatoid arthritis, and rheumatic fever; adjunctive therapy in revascularization procedures (coronary artery bypass graft, percutaneous transluminal coronary angioplasty, carotid endarterectomy)

Pregnancy Considerations Salicylates have been noted to cross the placenta and enter fetal circulation. Adverse effects reported in the fetus include mortality, intrauterine growth retardation, salicylate intoxication, bleeding abnormalities, and neonatal acidosis. Use of aspirin close to delivery may cause premature closure of the ductus arteriosus. Adverse effects reported in the mother include anemia, hemorrhage, prolonged gestation, and prolonged labor (Østensen, 1998). Low-dose aspirin may be used to prevent preeclampsia in women with a history of early-onset preeclampsia and preterm delivery (<34 0/7 weeks), or preeclampsia in ≥1 prior pregnancy (ACOG, 2013). Low-dose aspirin is used to treat complications resulting from antiphospholipid syndrome in pregnancy (either primary or secondary to SLE) (Carp, 2004; Guyatt, 2012; Tincani, 2003). In general, low doses during pregnancy needed for the treatment of certain medical conditions have not been shown to cause fetal harm, however, discontinuing therapy prior to delivery is recommended (Østensen, 2006). Use of safer agents for routine management of pain or headache should be considered.

Breast-Feeding Considerations Low amounts of aspirin can be found in breast milk. Milk/plasma ratios ranging from 0.03-0.3 have been reported. Peak levels in breast milk are reported to be at ~9 hours after a dose. Metabolic acidosis was reported in one infant following an aspirin dose of 3.9 g/day in the mother. The WHO considers occasional doses of aspirin to be compatible with breast-feeding, but to avoid long-term therapy and consider monitoring the infant for adverse effects (WHO, 2002). Other sources suggest avoiding aspirin while breast-feeding due to the theoretical risk of Reye's syndrome (Bar-Oz, 2003; Spigset, 2000). When used for vascular indications, breast-feeding may be continued during low-dose aspirin therapy (Guyatt, 2012).

Contraindications Hypersensitivity to salicylates or any component; history of asthma, urticaria, or allergic-type reaction to aspirin, or other NSAIDs; patients with the "aspirin triad" [asthma, rhinitis (with or without nasal polyps), and aspirin intolerance] (fatal asthmatic and anaphylactoid reactions may occur in these patients); inherited or acquired bleeding disorders (including factor VII and factor IX deficiency)

Warnings Do not use aspirin in children <12 years (APS, 2008) and adolescents (per manufacturer) who have or who are recovering from chickenpox or flu symptoms (due to the association with Reye's syndrome); when using aspirin, changes in behavior (along with nausea and vomiting) may be an early sign of Reye's syndrome; instruct patients and caregivers to contact their healthcare provider if these symptoms occur. Use with caution in patients with erosive gastritis or peptic ulcer disease.

Low-dose aspirin for cardioprotective effects is associated with a two- to fourfold increase in upper GI events (eg, symptomatic or complicated ulcers); the risks of these events increase with increasing aspirin dose; during the chronic phase of aspirin dosing, doses >81 mg are not recommended unless indicated (Bhatt, 2008). When NSAIDS/COX-2 inhibitors are used concomitantly with ≤325 mg of aspirin, the risk of gastrointestinal complications (eg, ulcer) substantially increased; concomitant gastroprotective therapy (eg, proton pump inhibitors) is recommended (Bhatt, 2008).

In the treatment of acute ischemic stroke, avoid aspirin for 24 hours following administration of alteplase; administration within 24 hours increases the risk of hemorrhagic transformation (Jauch, 2013). Concurrent use of aspirin and clopidogrel is not recommended for secondary prevention of ischemic stroke or TIA in patients unable to take oral anticoagulants due to hemorrhagic risk (Furie, 2011).

When self-medicating (OTC use) for pain, fever, and/or inflammation, notify healthcare provider if pain or inflammation does not improve within 10 days or fever lasts >3 days. Discontinue and contact healthcare provider if tinnitus or hearing impairment occurs. Some products may contain tartrazine which may cause allergic reactions in susceptible individuals. Some tablets contain polysorbate 80 (Tween 80®) which may cause allergic reactions in susceptible individuals.

Precautions Use with caution in patients with mild to moderate renal impairment (high dosages); avoid use in severe renal impairment. Use with caution in patients with platelet and bleeding disorders or hepatic impairment; avoid use in severe hepatic impairment; heavy ethanol use (>3 drinks/day) can also increase bleeding risks. Use with caution in patients with dehydration. In general, low doses during pregnancy needed for the treatment of certain medical conditions have not been shown to cause fetal harm; however, discontinuing therapy prior to delivery is recommended and if possible, avoid use during the third trimester of pregnancy. Use of safer agents for routine management of pain or headache throughout pregnancy should be considered. In surgical patients, aspirin should be avoided (if possible) for 1-2 weeks prior to surgery, to reduce the risk of excessive bleeding [except in patients with cardiac stents that have not completed their full course of dual antiplatelet therapy (aspirin, clopidogrel); patient-specific situations need to be discussed with cardiologist; AHA/ACC/SCAI/ACS/ADA Science Advisory provides recommendations].

Adverse Reactions As with all drugs which may affect hemostasis, bleeding is associated with aspirin. Hemorrhage may occur at virtually any site. Risk is dependent on multiple variables including dosage, concurrent use of multiple agents which alter hemostasis, and patient susceptibility. Many adverse effects of aspirin are dose related, and are extremely rare at low dosages. Other serious reactions are idiosyncratic, related to allergy or individual sensitivity.

Cardiovascular: Dysrhythmias, edema, hypotension, tachycardia

Central nervous system: Agitation, cerebral edema, coma, confusion, dizziness, fatigue, headache, hyperthermia, insomnia, lethargy, nervousness

Dermatologic: Angioedema, rash, urticaria

Endocrine & metabolic: Acidosis, dehydration, hyperglycemia, hyperkalemia, hypernatremia (buffered forms), hypoglycemia (children)

Gastrointestinal: Duodenal ulcers, dyspepsia, epigastric discomfort, gastrointestinal ulceration, gastric erosions, gastric erythema, heartburn, nausea, stomach pain, vomiting

Hematologic: Anemia, bleeding, coagulopathy, disseminated intravascular coagulation (DIC), hemolytic anemia, iron-deficiency anemia, prothrombin times prolonged, thrombocytopenia

Hepatic: Hepatitis (reversible), hepatotoxicity, transaminases increased

Neuromuscular & skeletal: Acetabular bone destruction (OA), rhabdomyolysis, weakness

Otic: Hearing loss, tinnitus

Renal: BUN increased, interstitial nephritis, papillary necrosis, proteinuria, renal failure (including cases caused by rhabdomyolysis), serum creatinine increased

Respiratory: Asthma, bronchospasm, dyspnea, hyperpnea, laryngeal edema, noncardiogenic pulmonary edema, respiratory alkalosis, tachypnea

Miscellaneous: Anaphylaxis, low birth weight, peripartum bleeding, prolonged pregnancy and labor, Reye's syndrome, stillbirths

Postmarketing and/or case reports: Cholestatic jaundice, colitis, colonic ulceration, conduction defect and atrial fibrillation (toxicity), coronary artery spasm, delirium, esophageal stricture, esophagitis with esophageal ulcer, esophageal hematoma, ischemic brain infarction, oral mucosal ulcers (aspirin-containing chewing gum), periorbital edema, rectal stenosis (suppository), rhinosinusitis

Drug Interactions

Metabolism/Transport Effects Substrate of CYP2C9 (minor); **Note:** Assignment of Major/Minor substrate status based on clinically relevant drug interaction potential; **Induces** CYP2C19 (weak/moderate)

Avoid Concomitant Use

Avoid concomitant use of Aspirin with any of the following: Floctafenine; Influenza Virus Vaccine (Live/Attenuated); Ketorolac (Nasal); Ketorolac (Systemic); Omacetaxine; Urokinase

Increased Effect/Toxicity

Aspirin may increase the levels/effects of: Agents with Antiplatelet Properties; Alendronate; Anticoagulants; Apixaban; Carbonic Anhydrase Inhibitors; Carisoprodol; Collagenase (Systemic); Corticosteroids (Systemic); Dabigatran Etexilate; Heparin; Hypoglycemic Agents; Ibritumomab; Methotrexate; NSAID (COX-2 Inhibitor); Omacetaxine; PRALAtrexate; Rivaroxaban; Salicylates; Thrombolytic Agents; Ticagrelor; Tositumomab and Iodine I 131 Tositumomab; Urokinase; Valproic Acid and Derivatives; Varicella Virus-Containing Vaccines; Vitamin K Antagonists

The levels/effects of Aspirin may be increased by: Agents with Antiplatelet Properties; Ammonium Chloride; Antidepressants (Tricyclic, Tertiary Amine); Calcium Channel Blockers (Nondihydropyridine); Dasatinib; Floctafenine; Ginkgo Biloba; Glucosamine; Herbs (Anticoagulant/Antiplatelet Properties); Ibrutinib; Influenza Virus Vaccine (Live/Attenuated); Ketorolac (Nasal); Ketorolac (Systemic); Loop Diuretics; Multivitamins/Fluoride (with ADE); Multivitamins/Minerals (with ADEK, Folate, Iron); Multivitamins/Minerals (with AE, No Iron); NSAID (Nonselective); Omega-3 Fatty Acids; Pentosan Polysulfate Sodium; Pentoxifylline; Potassium Acid Phosphate; Prostacyclin Analogues; Selective Serotonin Reuptake Inhibitors; Serotonin/Norepinephrine Reuptake Inhibitors; Tipranavir; Treprostinil; Vitamin E

Decreased Effect

Aspirin may decrease the levels/effects of: ACE Inhibitors; Carisoprodol; Hyaluronidase; Loop Diuretics; Multivitamins/Fluoride (with ADE); Multivitamins/Minerals (with ADEK, Folate, Iron); Multivitamins/Minerals (with AE, No Iron); NSAID (Nonselective); Probenecid; Ticagrelor; Tiludronate

The levels/effects of Aspirin may be decreased by: Corticosteroids (Systemic); Floctafenine; Ketorolac (Nasal); Ketorolac (Systemic); NSAID (Nonselective)

Food Interactions Food may decrease the rate but not the extent of oral absorption. Benedictine liqueur, prunes, raisins, tea, and gherkins have a potential to cause salicylate accumulation. Fresh fruits containing vitamin C may displace drug from binding sites, resulting in increased urinary excretion of aspirin. Curry powder, paprika, licorice; may cause salicylate accumulation. These foods contain 6 mg salicylate/100 g. An ordinary American diet contains 10-200 mg/day of salicylate. Management: Administer with food or large volume of water or milk to minimize GI upset. Limit curry powder, paprika, licorice.

Stability Store oral dosage forms (caplets, tablets) at room temperature; protect from moisture; see product-specific labeling for details. Keep suppositories in refrigerator, do not freeze; hydrolysis of aspirin occurs upon exposure to water or moist air, resulting in salicylate and acetate; acetate possesses a vinegar-like odor; do not use if a strong odor is present

Mechanism of Action Irreversibly inhibits cyclooxygenase-1 and 2 (COX-1 and 2) enzymes, via acetylation, which results in decreased formation of prostaglandin precursors; irreversibly inhibits formation of prostaglandin derivative, thromboxane A_2, via acetylation of platelet cyclooxygenase, thus inhibiting platelet aggregation; has antipyretic, analgesic, and anti-inflammatory properties

Pharmacokinetics (Adult data unless noted)

Absorption: From the stomach and small intestine

Distribution: Readily distributes into most body fluids and tissues; hydrolyzed to salicylate (active) by esterases in the GI mucosa, red blood cells, synovial fluid and blood

Metabolism: Primarily by hepatic microsomal enzymes

Half-life: 15-20 minutes; metabolic pathways are saturable such that salicylate half-life is dose-dependent ranging from 3 hours at lower doses (300-600 mg), 5-6 hours (after 1 g) and 10 hours with higher doses

Time to peak serum concentration: Salicylate: ~1-2 hours

Elimination: Renal as salicylate and conjugated metabolites

Dosing: Neonatal Full-term neonate: **Antiplatelet effects:** Postoperative congenital heart repair or recurrent arterial ischemic stroke: Oral: Adequate neonatal studies have not been performed; neonatal dosage is derived from clinical experience and is not well established; suggested doses: 1-5 mg/kg/dose once daily (Monagle, 2012). Doses are typically rounded to a convenient amount (eg, 1/4 of 81 mg tablet)

Dosing: Usual

Infants, Children, and Adolescents: **Note:** Doses are typically rounded to a convenient amount (eg, 1/4 of 81 mg tablet):

Analgesic: Oral, rectal: **Note:** Do not use aspirin in children <12 years (APS, 2008) and adolescents (per manufacturer) who have or who are recovering from chickenpox or flu symptoms due to the association with Reye's syndrome (APS, 2008):

Infants, Children, and Adolescents weighing <50 kg: 10-15 mg/kg/dose every 4-6 hours; maximum daily dose: The lesser value of either 120 mg/kg/**day** or 4000 mg/**day** (APS, 2008)

Children ≥12 years and Adolescents weighing ≥50 kg: 325-650 mg every 4-6 hours; maximum daily dose: 4000 mg/**day**

Anti-inflammatory: Oral: Initial: 60-90 mg/kg/**day** in divided doses; usual maintenance: 80-100 mg/kg/**day** divided every 6-8 hours; monitor serum concentrations (Levy, 1978)

Antiplatelet effects: Limited data available: Oral: Adequate pediatric studies have not been performed; pediatric dosage is derived from adult studies and clinical experience and is not well established; suggested doses have ranged from 1-5 mg/kg/dose once daily (Monagle, 2012) to 5-10 mg/kg/dose once daily. Doses are typically rounded to a convenient amount (eg, 1/2 of 81 mg tablet).

Acute ischemic stroke (AIS):
Noncardioembolic: 1-5 mg/kg/dose once daily for ≥2 years; patients with recurrent AIS or TIAs should be transitioned to clopidogrel, LMWH, or warfarin (Monagle, 2012)
Secondary to Moyamoya and non-Moyamoya vasculopathy: 1-5 mg/kg/dose once daily; **Note:** In non-Moyamoya vasculopathy, continue aspirin for 3 months, with subsequent use guided by repeat cerebrovascular imaging (Monagle, 2012).

Prosthetic heart valve:
Bioprosthetic aortic valve (with normal sinus rhythm): 1-5 mg/kg/dose once daily for 3 months (Guyatt, 2012; Monagle, 2012)
Mechanical aortic and/or mitral valve: 1-5 mg/kg/dose once daily combined with vitamin K antagonist (eg, warfarin) is recommended as first-line antithrombotic therapy (Guyatt, 2012; Monagle, 2012). Alternative regimens: 6-20 mg/kg/dose once daily in combination with dipyridamole (Bradley, 1985; El Makhlouf, 1987; LeBlanc, 1993; Serra, 1987; Solymar, 1991)

Blalock-Taussig shunts; postoperative; primary prophylaxis: 1-5 mg/kg/dose once daily (Monagle, 2012)

Fontan surgery, postoperative; primary prophylaxis: 1-5 mg/kg/dose once daily (Monagle, 2012)

Ventricular assist device (VAD) placement: 1-5 mg/kg/dose once daily initiated within 72 hours of VAD placement; should be used with heparin (initiated between 8-48 hours following implantation) and with or without dipyridamole (Monagle, 2012)

Kawasaki disease: Limited data available: Oral: 80-100 mg/kg/**day** divided every 6 hours for up to 14 days until fever resolves for at least 48 hours; then decrease dose to 1-5 mg/kg/**day** once daily. In patients without coronary artery abnormalities, give lower dose (eg, 1-5 mg/kg/**day**; AHA suggests 3-5 mg/kg/**day**) for 6-8 weeks. In patients with coronary artery abnormalities, low-dose aspirin should be continued indefinitely (in addition to therapy with warfarin) (Monagle, 2012; Newburger, 2004; *Red Book*, 2012)

Rheumatic fever: Limited data available: Oral: Initial: 100 mg/kg/**day** divided into 4-5 doses; if response inadequate, may increase dose to 125 mg/kg/**day**; continue for 2 weeks; then decrease dose to 60-70 mg/kg/**day** in divided doses for an additional 3-6 weeks (WHO Guidelines, 2001)

Migratory polyarthritis, with carditis without cardiomegaly or congestive heart failure: Initial: 100 mg/kg/**day** in 4 divided doses for 3-5 days, followed by 75 mg/kg/**day** in 4 divided doses for 4 weeks

Carditis and cardiomegaly or congestive heart failure: At the beginning of the tapering of the prednisone dose, aspirin should be started at 75 mg/kg/**day** in 4 divided doses for 6 weeks

Adults:
Acute coronary syndrome (ST-segment elevation myocardial infarction [STEMI], unstable angina (UA)/non-ST-segment elevation myocardial infarction [NSTEMI]): Oral: Initial: 162-325 mg given on presentation (patient should chew nonenteric-coated aspirin especially if not taking before presentation); for patients unable to take oral, may use rectal suppository [300-600 mg (Antman, 2004; Maalouf, 2009)]. Maintenance (secondary prevention): 75-162 mg once daily indefinitely (Anderson, 2007) or 81-325 mg once daily; 81 mg once daily preferred (O'Gara, 2013). **Note:** When aspirin is used with ticagrelor, the recommended maintenance dose of aspirin is 81 mg/day (Jneid, 2012; O'Gara, 2013).

UA/NSTEMI: Concomitant antiplatelet therapy (Jneid, 2012):
If invasive strategy chosen: Aspirin is recommended in combination with either clopidogrel, ticagrelor (or prasugrel if at the time of PCI) or an I.V. GP IIb/IIIa inhibitor (if given before PCI, eptifibatide and tirofiban are preferred agents).
If noninvasive strategy chosen: Aspirin is recommended in combination with clopidogrel or ticagrelor.

Analgesic and antipyretic:
Oral: 325-650 mg every 4-6 hours; maximum daily dose: 4000 mg/**day**
Rectal: 300-600 mg every 4-6 hours; maximum daily dose: 4000 mg/**day**

Anti-inflammatory: Oral: Initial: 2400-3600 mg/day in divided doses; usual maintenance: 3600-5400 mg/day; monitor serum concentrations

CABG: Oral: 100-325 mg once daily initiated either preoperatively or within 6 hours postoperatively; continue indefinitely (Hillis, 2011)

Coronary artery disease (CAD), established: Oral: 75-100 mg once daily (Guyatt, 2012)

PCI: Oral:
Nonemergent PCI: Preprocedure: 81-325 mg [325 mg (nonenteric coated) in aspirin-naive patients] starting at least 2 hours (preferably 24 hours) before procedure. Postprocedure: 81 mg once daily continued indefinitely [in combination with a P2Y$_{12}$ inhibitor (eg, clopidogrel, prasugrel, ticagrelor) up to 12 months] (Levine, 2011)
Primary PCI: Preprocedure: 162-325 mg as early as possible prior to procedure; 325 mg preferred followed by a maintenance dose of 81 mg once daily even when a stent is deployed (O'Gara, 2013)
Alternatively, in patients who have undergone elective PCI with either bare metal or drug-eluting stent placement: The American College of Chest Physicians recommends the use of 75-325 mg once daily (in combination with clopidogrel) for 1 month (BMS) or 3-6 months (dependent upon DES type) followed by 75-100 mg once daily (in combination with clopidogrel) for up to12 months. For patients who underwent PCI but did not have stent placement, 75-325 mg once daily (in combination with clopidogrel) for 1 month is recommended. In either case, single antiplatelet therapy (either aspirin or clopidogrel) is recommended indefinitely (Guyatt, 2012).

Primary prevention: Oral:
American College of Cardiology/American Heart Association: Prevention of myocardial infarction: 75-162 mg once daily. **Note:** Patients are most likely to benefit if their 10-year coronary heart disease risk is ≥6% (Antman, 2004).

American College of Chest Physicians: Prevention of myocardial infarction and stroke: Select individuals ≥50 years of age (without symptomatic cardiovascular disease): 75-100 mg once daily (Guyatt, 2012; Grade 2B, weak recommendation)

Stroke/TIA: Oral:

Acute ischemic stroke/TIA: Initial: 160-325 mg within 48 hours of stroke/TIA onset, followed by 75-100 mg once daily (Guyatt, 2012). The AHA/ASA recommends an initial dose of 325 mg within 24-48 hours after stroke; do not administer aspirin within 24 hours after administration of alteplase (Jauch, 2013).

Cardioembolic, secondary prevention (oral anticoagulation unsuitable): 75-100 mg once daily (in combination with clopidogrel) (Guyatt, 2012)

Cryptogenic with patent foramen ovale (PFO) or atrial septal aneurysm: 50-100 mg once daily (Guyatt, 2012)

Noncardioembolic, secondary prevention: 75-325 mg once daily (Smith, 2011) **or** 75-100 mg once daily (Guyatt, 2012). **Note:** Combination aspirin/extended release dipyridamole or clopidogrel is preferred over aspirin alone (The ACTIVE Investigators, 2009; Guyatt, 2012).

Women at high risk, primary prevention: 81 mg once daily **or** 100 mg every other day (Goldstein, 2010)

Dosing adjustment in renal impairment:

Infants, Children, and Adolescents: The following the adjustments have been recommended (Aronoff, 2007):

GFR ≥10 mL/minute/1.73 m^2: No dosage adjustment necessary.

GFR <10 mL/minute/1.73 m^2: Avoid use.

Intermittent hemodialysis: Dialyzable: 50% to 100%; administer daily dose after dialysis session

Peritoneal dialysis: Avoid use

CRRT: No dosage adjustment necessary; monitor serum concentrations

Adults:

CrCl <10 mL/minute: Avoid use.

Dialyzable (50% to 100%)

Administration Oral: Administer with water, food, or milk to decrease GI upset. Do not crush or chew enteric coated tablets; these preparations should be swallowed whole. For acute myocardial infarction, have patient chew immediate release tablet.

Monitoring Parameters Serum salicylate concentration with chronic use; may not be necessary in Kawasaki disease; **Note:** Decreased aspirin absorption and increased salicylate clearance has been observed in children with acute Kawasaki disease; these patients rarely achieve therapeutic serum salicylate concentrations; thus, monitoring of serum salicylate concentrations is not necessary in most of these children.

Reference Range

Timing of serum samples: Peak concentrations usually occur 2 hours after normal doses but may occur 6-24 hours after acute toxic ingestion.

Salicylate serum concentrations correlate with the pharmacological actions and adverse effects observed. See table.

Serum Salicylate: Clinical Correlations

Serum Salicylate Concentration (mcg/mL)	Desired Effects	Adverse Effects / Intoxication
~100	Antiplatelet Antipyresis Analgesia	GI intolerance and bleeding, hypersensitivity, hemostatic defects
150-300	Anti-inflammatory	Mild salicylism
250-400	Treatment of rheumatic fever	Nausea/vomiting, hyperventilation, salicylism, flushing, sweating, thirst, headache, diarrhea, and tachycardia
>400-500		Respiratory alkalosis, hemorrhage, excitement, confusion, asterixis, pulmonary edema, convulsions, tetany, metabolic acidosis, fever, coma, cardiovascular collapse, renal and respiratory failure

Test Interactions False-negative results for glucose oxidase urinary glucose tests (Clinistix®); false-positives using the cupric sulfate method (Clinitest®); also, interferes with Gerhardt test, VMA determination; 5-HIAA, xylose tolerance test and T_3 and T_4

Dosage Forms Excipient information presented when available (limited, particularly for generics); consult specific product labeling.

Caplet, oral: 500 mg

Bayer® Aspirin Extra Strength: 500 mg

Bayer® Genuine Aspirin: 325 mg

Bayer® Women's Low Dose Aspirin: 81 mg [contains elemental calcium 300 mg]

Caplet, oral [buffered]:

Ascriptin® Maximum Strength: 500 mg [contains aluminum hydroxide, calcium carbonate, magnesium hydroxide]

Bayer® Plus Extra Strength: 500 mg [contains calcium carbonate]

Caplet, enteric coated, oral:

Bayer® Aspirin Regimen Regular Strength: 325 mg

Gum, chewing, oral:

Aspergum®: 227 mg (12s) [cherry flavor]

Aspergum®: 227 mg (12s) [orange flavor]

Suppository, rectal: 300 mg (12s); 600 mg (12s)

Tablet, oral: 325 mg

Aspercin: 325 mg

Aspirtab: 325 mg

Bayer® Genuine Aspirin: 325 mg

Tablet, oral [buffered]: 325 mg

Ascriptin® Regular Strength: 325 mg [contains aluminum hydroxide, calcium carbonate, magnesium hydroxide]

Buffasal: 325 mg [contains magnesium oxide]

Bufferin®: 325 mg [contains calcium carbonate, magnesium carbonate, magnesium oxide]

Bufferin® Extra Strength: 500 mg [contains calcium carbonate, magnesium carbonate, magnesium oxide]

Buffinol: 324 mg [sugar free; contains magnesium oxide]

Tri-Buffered Aspirin: 325 mg [contains calcium carbonate, magnesium carbonate, magnesium oxide]

Tablet, chewable, oral: 81 mg

Bayer® Aspirin Regimen Children's: 81 mg [cherry flavor]

Bayer® Aspirin Regimen Children's: 81 mg [orange flavor]

St Joseph® Adult Aspirin: 81 mg

Tablet, enteric coated, oral: 81 mg, 325 mg, 650 mg
Aspir-low: 81 mg
Bayer® Aspirin Regimen Adult Low Strength: 81 mg
Ecotrin®: 325 mg
Ecotrin® Arthritis Strength: 500 mg
Ecotrin® Low Strength: 81 mg
Halfprin®: 81 mg
St Joseph® Adult Aspirin: 81 mg

References

ACOG Committee on Obstetric Practice, "ACOG Practice Bulletin. Diagnosis and Management of Preeclampsia and Eclampsia. Number 33, January 2002. American College of Obstetricians and Gynecologists," *Int J Gynaecol Obstet*, 2002, 77(1):67-75.

The ACTIVE Investigators. Effect of clopidogrel added to aspirin in patients with atrial fibrillation. *N Engl J Med*. 2009;360:2066-2078.

Antman EM, Anbe DT, Armstrong PW, et al, "ACC/AHA Guidelines for the Management of Patients With ST-Elevation Myocardial Infarction: A Report of the American College of Cardiology/American Heart Association Task Force on Practice Guidelines (Committee to Revise the 1999 Guidelines for the Management of Patients with Acute Myocardial Infarction)," *Circulation*, 2004, 110(9):e82-292.

Aronoff GR, Bennett WM, Berns JS, et al, *Drug Prescribing in Renal Failure: Dosing Guidelines for Adults and Children*, 5th ed. Philadelphia, PA: American College of Physicians; 2007.

Bar-Oz B, Bulkowstein M, Benyamini L, et al, "Use of Antibiotic and Analgesic Drugs During Lactation," *Drug Saf*, 2003, 26(13):925-35.

Bhatt DL, Scheiman J, Abraham NS, et al, "ACCF/ACG/AHA 2008 Expert Consensus Document on Reducing the Gastrointestinal Risks of Antiplatelet Therapy and NSAID Use: A Report of the American College of Cardiology Foundation Task Force on Clinical Expert Consensus Documents," *J Am Coll Cardiol*, 2008, 52(18):1502-17.

Bradley LM, Midgley FM, Watson DC, et al, "Anticoagulation Therapy in Children With Mechanical Prosthetic Cardiac Valves," *Am J Cardiol*, 1985, 56(8):533-5.

Capone ML, Sciulli MG, Tacconelli S, et al, "Pharmacodynamic Interaction of Naproxen With Low-Dose Aspirin in Healthy Subjects," *J Am Coll Cardiol*, 2005, 45(8):1295-1301.

Carp HJ, "Antiphospholipid Syndrome in Pregnancy," *Curr Opin Obstet Gynecol*, 2004, 16(2):129-35.

Catella-Lawson F, Reilly MP, Kapoor SC, et al, "Cyclooxygenase Inhibitors and the Antiplatelet Effects of Aspirin," *N Engl J Med*, 2001, 345(25):1809-17.

Cryer B, Verlin RG, Cooper SA, et al, "Double-Blind, Randomized, Parallel, Placebo-Controlled Study Of Ibuprofen Effects On Thromboxane B2 Concentrations In Aspirin-Treated Healthy Adult Volunteers," *Clin Ther*, 2005, 27 (2):185-191.

el Makhlouf A, Friedli B, Oberhänsli I, et al, "Prosthetic Heart Valve Replacement in Children. Results and Follow-Up of 273 Patients," *J Thorac Cardiovasc Surg*, 1987, 93(1):80-5.

Furie KL, Kasner SE, Adams RJ, et al, "Guidelines for the Prevention of Stroke in Patients With Stroke or Transient Ischemic Attack: A Guideline for Healthcare Professionals From the American Heart Association/American Stroke Association," *Stroke*, 2011, 42(1):227-76.

Goldstein LB, Bushnell CD, Adams RJ, et al, "Guidelines for the Primary Prevention of Stroke: A Guideline for Healthcare Professionals From the American Heart Association/American Stroke Association," *Stroke*, 2011, 42(2):517-84.

Guyatt GH, Akl EA, Crowther M, et al, "Executive Summary: Antithrombotic Therapy and Prevention of Thrombosis, 9th ed: American College of Chest Physicians Evidence-Based Clinical Practice Guidelines," *Chest*, 2012, 141(2 Suppl):7-47.

Hathaway WE, "Use of Antiplatelet Agents in Pediatric Hypercoagulable States," *Am J Dis Child*, 1984, 138(3):301-4.

Hillis LD, Smith PK, Anderson JL, et al, "2011 ACCF/AHA Guideline for Coronary Artery Bypass Graft Surgery: Executive Summary: A Report of the American College of Cardiology Foundation/American Heart Association Task Force on Practice Guidelines," *Circulation*, 2011, 124(23):2610-42.

Jauch EC, Saver JL, Adams HP Jr, et al, "Guidelines for the Early Management of Patients With Acute Ischemic Stroke: A Guideline for Healthcare Professionals From the American Heart Association/American Stroke Association," *Stroke*, 2013, 44(3):870-947.

Jneid H, Anderson JL, Wright RS, et al, "2012 ACCF/AHA Focused Update of the Guideline for the Management of Patients With Unstable Angina/Non-ST-Elevation Myocardial Infarction (Updating the 2007 Guideline and Replacing the 2011 Focused Update): A Report of the American College of Cardiology Foundation/American Heart Association Task Force on Practice Guidelines," *Circulation*, 2012, 126(7):875-910.

LeBlanc JG, Sett SS, and Vince DJ, "Antiplatelet Therapy in Children With Left-Sided Mechanical Prostheses," *Eur J Cardiothorac Surg*, 1993, 7(4):211-5.

Levine GN, Bates ER, Blankenship JC, et al, "2011 ACCF/AHA/SCAI Guideline for Percutaneous Coronary Intervention: A Report of the American College of Cardiology Foundation/American Heart

Association Task Force on Practice Guidelines and the Society for Cardiovascular Angiography and Interventions," *Circulation*, 2011, 124(23):e574-651.

Levy G, "Clinical Pharmacokinetics of Aspirin," *Pediatrics*, 1978, 62(5 Pt 2 Suppl):867-72.

Maalouf R, Mosley M, James Kallail K, et al, "A Comparison of Salicylic Acid Levels in Normal Subjects After Rectal Versus Oral Dosing," *Acad Emerg Med*, 2009, 16(2):157-61.

Monagle P, Chan A, Goldenberg NA, et al, "Antithrombotic Therapy in Neonates and Children: American College of Chest Physicians Evidence-Based Clinical Practice Guidelines (9th Edition)," *Chest*, 2012, 141(2 Suppl):e737-801.

Newburger JW, Takahashi M, Gerber MA, et al, "Diagnosis, Treatment, and Long-Term Management of Kawasaki Disease: A Statement for Health Professionals From the Committee on Rheumatic Fever, Endocarditis, and Kawasaki Disease, Council on Cardiovascular Disease in the Young, American Heart Association," *Pediatrics*, 2004, 114(6):1708-33.

O'Gara PT, Kushner FG, Ascheim DD, et al, "2013 ACCF/AHA Guideline for the Management of ST-Elevation Myocardial Infarction: A Report of the American College of Cardiology Foundation/American Heart Association Task Force on Practice Guidelines," *Circulation*, 2013, 127(4):e362-425.

Østensen M, Khamashta M, Lockshin M, "Anti-inflammatory and Immunosuppressive Drugs and Reproduction," *Arthritis Res Ther*, 2006, 8 (3):209.

Østensen M, "Nonsteroidal Anti-inflammatory Drugs During Pregnancy," *Scand J Rheumatol Suppl*, 1998, 107:128-32.

Red Book: 2012 Report of the Committee on Infectious Diseases, "Antibacterial Drugs Dosage Tables," 29th ed, Pickering LK, ed, Elk Grove Village, IL: American Academy of Pediatrics, 2012, 808-16.

Serra AJ, McNicholas KW, Olivier HF Jr, et al, "The Choice of Anticoagulation in Pediatric Patients With the St. Jude Medical Valve Prostheses," *J Cardiovasc Surg (Torino)*, 1987, 28(5):588-91.

Smith SC Jr, Benjamin EJ, Bonow RO, et al, "AHA/ACCF Secondary Prevention and Risk Reduction Therapy for Patients With Coronary and Other Atherosclerotic Vascular Disease: 2011 Update: A Guideline From the American Heart Association and American College of Cardiology Foundation," *Circulation*, 2011, 124(22):2458-73.

Solymar L, Rao PS, Mardini MK, et al, "Prosthetic Valves in Children and Adolescents," *Am Heart J*, 1991, 121(2 Pt 1):557-68.

Spigset O and Hagg S, "Analgesics and Breast-Feeding: Safety Considerations," *Paediatr Drugs*, 2000, 2(3):223-38.

Tincani A, Branch W, Levy RA, et al, "Treatment of Pregnant Patients With Antiphospholipid Syndrome," *Lupus*, 2003, 12(7):524-9.

World Health Organization (WHO), "Breastfeeding and Maternal Medication, Recommendations for Drugs in the Eleventh WHO Model List of Essential Drugs," 2013. Available at http://www.who.int/maternal_-child_adolescent/documents/55732/en/index.html

World Health Organization (WHO), "Rheumatic Fever and Rheumatic Heart Disease," 2004. Available at http://www.who.int/cardiovascular_diseases/resources/trs923/en/

◆ **Aspirin and Oxycodone** *see* Oxycodone and Aspirin *on page 1575*

◆ **Aspirin Free Anacin Extra Strength [OTC]** *see* Acetaminophen *on page 47*

◆ **Aspir-low [OTC]** *see* Aspirin *on page 212*

◆ **Aspirtab [OTC]** *see* Aspirin *on page 212*

◆ **Astagraf XL** *see* Tacrolimus (Systemic) *on page 1963*

◆ **Astelin [DSC]** *see* Azelastine (Nasal) *on page 245*

◆ **Astelin (Can)** *see* Azelastine (Nasal) *on page 245*

◆ **Astepro** *see* Azelastine (Nasal) *on page 245*

◆ **Asthmanefrin Refill [OTC]** *see* EPINEPHrine (Systemic, Oral Inhalation) *on page 761*

◆ **Asthmanefrin Starter Kit [OTC]** *see* EPINEPHrine (Systemic, Oral Inhalation) *on page 761*

◆ **Astramorph** *see* Morphine (Systemic) *on page 1440*

◆ **Atacand** *see* Candesartan *on page 363*

◆ **Atarax (Can)** *see* HydrOXYzine *on page 1054*

◆ **Atasol (Can)** *see* Acetaminophen *on page 47*

Atazanavir (at a za NA veer)

Related Information
Adult and Adolescent HIV *on page 2348*
Pediatric HIV *on page 2338*
Perinatal HIV *on page 2356*
Brand Names: U.S. Reyataz
Brand Names: Canada Reyataz
Therapeutic Category Antiretroviral Agent; HIV Agents (Anti-HIV Agents); Protease Inhibitor
Generic Availability (U.S.) No
Use Treatment of HIV infection in combination with other antiretroviral agents (FDA approved in ages ≥3 months weighing ≥10 kg and adults). **Note:** HIV regimens consisting of **three** antiretroviral agents are strongly recommended; low-dose ritonavir (booster dose) is recommended in combination with atazanavir in antiretroviral-experienced patients with prior virologic failure.

Pregnancy Risk Factor B
Pregnancy Considerations Adverse events were not observed in animal reproduction studies. Atazanavir has a low level of transfer across the human placenta with cord blood concentrations reported as 13% to 21% of maternal serum concentrations at delivery. An increased risk of teratogenic effects has not been observed based on information collected by the antiretroviral pregnancy registry. A small increased risk of preterm birth has been associated with maternal use of protease inhibitor-based combination antiretroviral (ARV) therapy during pregnancy; however, the benefits of use generally outweigh this risk and protease inhibitors (PIs) should not be withheld if otherwise recommended. Hyperglycemia, new onset of diabetes mellitus, or diabetic ketoacidosis have been reported with PIs; it is not clear if pregnancy increases this risk. Hyperbilirubinemia or hypoglycemia may occur in neonates following *in utero* exposure to atazanavir, although data are conflicting.

The DHHS Perinatal HIV Guidelines recommend atazanavir as a preferred PI in antiretroviral-naive pregnant women when combined with low-dose ritonavir boosting. Pharmacokinetic studies suggest that standard dosing during pregnancy may provide decreased plasma concentrations and some experts recommend increased doses during the second and third trimesters. However, the manufacturer notes that dose adjustment is not required unless using concomitant H₂-receptor blockers or tenofovir or for ARV-naive pregnant women taking efavirenz. May give as once-daily dosing.

Regardless of CD4 count or HIV RNA copy number, all HIV-infected pregnant women should receive a combination antiretroviral (ARV) drug regimen. A combination of antepartum, intrapartum, and infant ARV prophylaxis is recommended. ARV therapy should be started as soon as possible in women with symptomatic infection. Although earlier initiation may be more effective in reducing the perinatal transmission of HIV, initiation may be delayed until after 12 weeks gestation in women who do not require immediate treatment after careful consideration of maternal conditions (eg, nausea and vomiting) and the potential risks of first trimester fetal exposure for specific agents. A scheduled cesarean delivery at 38 weeks gestation is recommended for all women with HIV RNA >1000 copies/mL or unknown concentrations near delivery in order to decrease transmission. If ARV therapy must be interrupted for <24 hours during the peripartum period, stop then restart all medications simultaneously in order to decrease the chance of developing resistance. Long-term follow-up is recommended for all infants exposed to ARV medications. In couples who want to conceive, the HIV-infected partner should attain maximum viral suppression prior to conception.

Healthcare providers are encouraged to enroll pregnant women exposed to antiretroviral medications in the Antiretroviral Pregnancy Registry (1-800-258-4263 or www.APRegistry.com). Healthcare providers caring for HIV-infected women and their infants may contact the National Perinatal HIV Hotline (888-448-8765) for clinical consultation (DHHS [perinatal], 2014).

Breast-Feeding Considerations Atazanavir is excreted into breast milk. Maternal or infant antiretroviral therapy does not completely eliminate the risk of postnatal HIV transmission. In addition, multiclass-resistant virus has been detected in breast-feeding infants despite maternal therapy. Therefore, in the United States, where formula is accessible, affordable, safe, and sustainable, and the risk of infant mortality due to diarrhea and respiratory infections is low, complete avoidance of breast-feeding by HIV-infected women is recommended to decrease potential transmission of HIV (DHHS [perinatal], 2014).

Contraindications Hypersensitivity (eg, Stevens-Johnson syndrome, erythema multiforme, or toxic skin eruptions) to atazanavir or any component; concurrent therapy with medications that largely rely on cytochrome P450 isoenzyme CYP3A or UGT1A1 for clearance and that have an association between increased plasma concentrations and serious or life-threatening effects including the following: Alfuzosin, cisapride, dihydroergotamine, ergotamine, ergonovine, irinotecan, lovastatin, methylergonovine, midazolam (oral), pimozide, sildenafil [when used for pulmonary artery hypertension (eg, Revatio)], simvastatin, triazolam; concurrent therapy with indinavir, nevirapine, rifampin, or the herbal medicine St John's wort (*Hypericum perforatum*)

Warnings Atazanavir is an inhibitor of cytochrome P450 isoenzyme CYP3A and uridine diphosphate glucuronosyl transferase (UGT1A1; a glucuronidation enzyme). Administration of atazanavir with drugs that are primarily metabolized by CYP3A or UGT1A1 may result in increased serum concentrations of the other drug and lead to an increase or prolongation of adverse effects. Due to potential serious and/or life-threatening drug interactions, some drugs are contraindicated or not recommended for concurrent use; other drug interactions require dosage or regimen adjustment or monitoring of serum concentrations of drugs coadministered with atazanavir.

Asymptomatic elevations in unconjugated (indirect) bilirubin occur commonly (in approximately 50% of patients) during therapy with atazanavir; this reversible hyperbilirubinemia is related to inhibition of uridine diphosphate glucuronosyl transferase; consider alternative therapy if bilirubin is >5 times upper limits of normal (long-term safety data is not available for such patients) or if jaundice or scleral icterus become a cosmetic concern for the patient; evaluate alternative etiologies if elevated transaminase also occur. Do not use atazanavir in infants <3 months of age due to potential risk of kernicterus.

Skin rash may occur with atazanavir use, usually mild to moderate; maculopapular; reported incidence: Pediatric patients: 14% (Grade 2 to 4); adults: 21% (all grades); median onset: 7.3 weeks; treatment may be continued if rash is mild to moderate (rash may resolve; median duration: 1.4 weeks); discontinue therapy in cases of severe rash. Protease inhibitors have been associated with a variety of hypersensitivity reactions (some severe), including rash, erythema multiforme, Stevens-Johnson syndrome (rare), and/or toxic skin eruptions [including DRESS (drug rash, eosinophilia and systemic symptoms) syndrome]. It is generally recommended to discontinue treatment if severe rash or moderate symptoms accompanied by other systemic symptoms occur.

Postmarketing cases of nephrolithiasis and/or cholelithiasis have been reported; consider temporary interruption of therapy or discontinuation if signs or symptoms of nephrolithiasis and/or cholethiasis occur.

The oral powder contains phenylalanine which must be avoided (or used with caution) in patients with phenylketonuria.

Precautions Atazanavir may prolong the P-R interval; rare cases of second-degree AV block and other conduction abnormalities have also been reported; ECG monitoring should be considered in patients with preexisting conduction abnormalities or with medications which prolong A-V conduction (dosage adjustment is required with some agents). Concomitant use of salmeterol is not recommended due to increased risk of cardiovascular adverse events, including QT_c prolongation. Hyperglycemia, changes in glucose tolerance, exacerbation of diabetes, DKA, and new-onset diabetes mellitus have been reported in patients receiving protease inhibitors; use with caution in patients with diabetes mellitus.

Use atazanavir with caution in patients with mild to moderate hepatic impairment; consider dosage adjustment in patients with moderate hepatic dysfunction; atazanavir is **not** recommended for use in patients with severe hepatic impairment; the use of atazanavir **plus** ritonavir is not recommended in patients with hepatic impairment. Do not use concurrently with colchicine in patients with renal or hepatic impairment. Atazanavir may exacerbate preexisting hepatic dysfunction; use with caution in patients with hepatitis B or C or in patients with marked elevations in hepatic transaminases. Use with caution and adjust dose (and add ritonavir) in antiretroviral-naïve patients with end-stage renal disease managed with hemodialysis; do not use atazanavir in antiretroviral-experienced patients with end-stage renal disease managed with hemodialysis. Use with caution in patients with hemophilia; spontaneous bleeding episodes have been reported in patients with hemophilia type A and B receiving protease inhibitors.

Fat redistribution and accumulation [ie, central obesity, peripheral wasting, facial wasting, breast enlargement, dorsocervical fat enlargement (buffalo hump), and cushingoid appearance] have been observed in patients receiving antiretroviral agents (causal relationship not established); less common with atazanavir than other protease inhibitors. May cause hypercholesterolemia less frequently than with other protease inhibitors.

Immune reconstitution syndrome (an acute inflammatory response to residual or indolent opportunistic infections) may occur in HIV patients during initial treatment with combination antiretroviral agents, including atazanavir; this syndrome may require further patient assessment and therapy. Autoimmune disorders (eg, Graves' disease, Guillain-Barré syndrome, and polymyositis) have been reported in patients experiencing immune reconstitution; time to onset is variable and may occur many months after antiretroviral treatment is initiated. May cause cough; reported incidence in children 21%. May cause fever; higher incidence observed in children compared to adults (19% vs 2%).

Adverse Reactions Includes data from both treatment-naive and treatment-experienced patients; listed for adults unless otherwise specified.

Cardiovascular: First degree atrioventricular block, second degree atrioventricular block, peripheral edema

Central nervous system: Depression, dizziness, headache (more common in children), insomnia, peripheral neuropathy

Dermatologic: Skin rash (more common in adults)

Endocrine & metabolic: Hyperglycemia, hypoglycemia (children), increased amylase (children and adults), increased serum cholesterol (≥240 mg/dL), increased serum triglycerides

Gastrointestinal: Abdominal pain, diarrhea (more common in children), increased serum lipase (children and adults), nausea, vomiting (more common in children)

Hematologic & oncologic: Decreased hemoglobin (children and adults), neutropenia (more common in children), thrombocytopenia

Hepatic: Increased serum ALT (children and adults; more common in patients seropositive for hepatitis B and/or C), increased serum AST (more common in patients seropositive for hepatitis B and/or C), increased serum bilirubin (children and adults), jaundice

Neuromuscular & skeletal: Increased creatine phosphokinase, limb pain (children), myalgia

Respiratory: Cough (children), nasal congestion (children), oropharyngeal pain (children), rhinorrhea (children), wheezing (children)

Miscellaneous: Fever (more common in children)

Rare but important or life-threatening: Cholecystitis, cholelithiasis, cholestasis, complete atrioventricular block (rare), diabetes mellitus, DRESS syndrome, edema, erythema multiforme, immune reconstitution syndrome, interstitial nephritis, left bundle branch block, maculopapular rash, nephrolithiasis, pancreatitis, prolongation P-R interval on ECG, prolonged Q-T interval on ECG, Stevens-Johnson syndrome, torsades de pointes

Drug Interactions

Metabolism/Transport Effects Substrate of CYP3A4 (major); **Note:** Assignment of Major/Minor substrate status based on clinically relevant drug interaction potential; **Inhibits** CYP1A2 (weak), CYP2C8 (weak), CYP2C9 (weak), CYP3A4 (strong), UGT1A1

Avoid Concomitant Use

Avoid concomitant use of Atazanavir with any of the following: Ado-Trastuzumab Emtansine; Alfuzosin; Amiodarone; Apixaban; Avanafil; Axitinib; Bosutinib; Buprenorphine; Cabozantinib; Ceritinib; Cisapride; Conivaptan; Crizotinib; Dronedarone; Eplerenone; Ergot Derivatives; Etravirine; Everolimus; Fusidic Acid (Systemic); Halofantrine; Ibrutinib; Indinavir; Irinotecan; Ivabradine; Lapatinib; Lomitapide; Lovastatin; Lurasidone; Macitentan; Midazolam; Nevirapine; Nilotinib; Nisoldipine; Pimozide; QuiNIDine; Ranolazine; Red Yeast Rice; Regorafenib; Rifampin; Rivaroxaban; Salmeterol; Silodosin; Simeprevir; Simvastatin; St Johns Wort; Tamsulosin; Ticagrelor; Tipranavir; Tolvaptan; Toremifene; Triazolam; Ulipristal; Vemurafenib; VinCRIStine (Liposomal); Vorapaxar; Voriconazole

Increased Effect/Toxicity

Atazanavir may increase the levels/effects of: Ado-Trastuzumab Emtansine; Alfuzosin; Almotriptan; Alosetron; ALPRAZolam; Amiodarone; Apixaban; ARIPiprazole; AtorvaSTATin; Avanafil; Axitinib; Bedaquiline; Bortezomib; Bosentan; Bosutinib; Brentuximab Vedotin; Brinzolamide; Budesonide (Nasal); Budesonide (Systemic, Oral Inhalation); Buprenorphine; Cabozantinib; Calcium Channel Blockers (Dihydropyridine); Calcium Channel Blockers (Nondihydropyridine); Cannabis; CarBAMazepine; Ceritinib; Cisapride; Clarithromycin; Colchicine; Conivaptan; Contraceptives (Progestins); Corticosteroids (Orally Inhaled); Crizotinib; Cyclophosphamide; CycloSPORINE (Systemic); CYP3A4 Substrates; Digoxin; DOXOrubicin (Conventional); Dronabinol; Dronedarone; Dutasteride; Enfuvirtide; Eplerenone; Ergot Derivatives; Etravirine; Everolimus; FentaNYL; Fesoterodine; Fluticasone (Nasal); Fluticasone (Oral Inhalation); GuanFACINE; Halofantrine; Highest Risk QTc-Prolonging Agents; Ibrutinib; Iloperidone; Imatinib; Indinavir; Irinotecan; Ivabradine; Ivacaftor; Ixabepilone; Lacosamide; Lapatinib; Levomilnacipran; Lomitapide; Lovastatin; Lurasidone; Macitentan; Maraviroc; Meperidine; MethylPREDNISolone; Midazolam; Mifepristone; Moderate Risk QTc-Prolonging Agents; Nefazodone; Nevirapine; Nilotinib; Nisoldipine; Ospemifene; OxyCODONE;

Paricalcitol; PAZOPanib; Pimecrolimus; Pimozide; Pitavastatin; PONATinib; Propafenone; Protease Inhibitors; QUEtiapine; QuiNIDine; Ranolazine; Red Yeast Rice; Regorafenib; Repaglinide; Rifabutin; Rilpivirine; Riociguat; Rivaroxaban; RomiDEPsin; Rosuvastatin; Ruxolitinib; Salmeterol; Saxagliptin; Sildenafil; Silodosin; Simeprevir; Simvastatin; SORAfenib; Tacrolimus (Systemic); Tacrolimus (Topical); Tadalafil; Tamsulosin; Temsirolimus; Tenofovir; Tetrahydrocannabinol; Ticagrelor; Tofacitinib; Tolterodine; Tolvaptan; Toremifene; TraZODone; Triazolam; Tricyclic Antidepressants; Ulipristal; Vardenafil; Vemurafenib; Vilazodone; VinCRIStine (Liposomal); Vorapaxar; Voriconazole; Warfarin; Zuclopenthixol

The levels/effects of Atazanavir may be increased by: Clarithromycin; Conivaptan; CycloSPORINE (Systemic); CYP3A4 Inhibitors (Moderate); CYP3A4 Inhibitors (Strong); Enfuvirtide; Fusidic Acid (Systemic); Indinavir; Luliconazole; Mifepristone; Posaconazole; Simeprevir; Stiripentol; Telaprevir

Decreased Effect
Atazanavir may decrease the levels/effects of: Abacavir; Boceprevir; Clarithromycin; Contraceptives (Estrogens); Delavirdine; Didanosine; Ifosfamide; Meperidine; Prasugrel; Telaprevir; Ticagrelor; Valproic Acid and Derivatives; Voriconazole; Zidovudine

The levels/effects of Atazanavir may be decreased by: Antacids; Boceprevir; Bosentan; Buprenorphine; CarBAMazepine; CYP3A4 Inducers (Strong); Dabrafenib; Deferasirox; Didanosine; Efavirenz; Etravirine; Garlic; H2-Antagonists; Minocycline; Mitotane; Nevirapine; Proton Pump Inhibitors; Rifampin; Siltuximab; St Johns Wort; Tenofovir; Tipranavir; Tocilizumab; Voriconazole

Food Interactions Bioavailability of atazanavir increased when taken with food. Management: Administer with food.

Stability
Capsules: Store at 25°C (77°F); excursions permitted to 15°C to 30°C (59°F to 86°F).

Oral powder: Store below 30°C (86°F) in original packet; do not open until ready to use. Mixture of oral powder and food or beverage may be kept at room temperature of 20°C to 30°C (68°F to 86°F) for up to 1 hour prior to administration.

Mechanism of Action Binds to the site of HIV-1 protease activity and inhibits cleavage of viral Gag-Pol polyprotein precursors into individual functional proteins required for infectious HIV. This results in the formation of immature, noninfectious viral particles.

Pharmacokinetics (Adult data unless noted)
Absorption: Rapid; enhanced with food

Distribution: CSF: Plasma concentration ratio (range): 0.0021 to 0.0226

Protein binding: 86%; binds to both alpha$_1$-acid glycoprotein and albumin (similar affinity)

Metabolism: Hepatic, primarily by cytochrome P450 isoenzyme CYP3A; also undergoes biliary elimination; major biotransformation pathways include mono-oxygenation and deoxygenation; minor pathways for parent drug or metabolites include glucuronidation, N-dealkylation, hydrolysis and oxygenation with dehydrogenation; 3 minor inactive metabolites have been identified

Half-life:
Adults: Unboosted: 7 to 8 hours, Boosted with ritonavir: 9 to 18 hours

Adults with hepatic impairment: 12 hours

Time to peak serum concentration: 2 hours

Elimination: 13% of the dose is excreted in the urine (7% as unchanged drug); 79% of the dose is excreted in feces (20% as unchanged drug)

Dosing: Neonatal Not recommended due to risk of kernicterus

Dosing: Usual Pediatric: **HIV infection, treatment:** Use in combination with other antiretroviral agents. Oral:

Infants 1 to <3 months: Not recommended due to risk of kernicterus

Infants ≥3 months, Children, and Adolescents <18 years: **Note:** Pediatric patients <13 years of age must receive atazanavir **plus** ritonavir taken together once daily with food. Dosing recommendations do not exist for patients <40 kg who receive concomitant tenofovir. For all pediatric patients, follow the adult recommendations about timing of concomitant H$_2$-receptor blockers and proton pump inhibitors; do not exceed recommended adult maximum doses of these concurrent agents. Pediatric patients ≥13 years and ≥40 kg who receive concomitant tenofovir, H$_2$-receptor blockers, or proton pump inhibitors must take atazanavir **plus** ritonavir.

Ritonavir unboosted regimen: Antiretroviral-naïve patients ≥13 years and ≥40 kg who are not able to tolerate ritonavir: Atazanavir 400 mg once daily (without ritonavir). **Note:** Ritonavir boosted atazanavir dosing regimen is preferred; data indicates that higher atazanavir dosing (ie, higher on a mg/kg or mg/m^2 basis than predicted by adult dosing guidelines) may be needed when atazanavir is used without ritonavir boosting in children and adolescents (DHHS [pediatric], 2014).

Ritonavir boosted regimen: Antiretroviral-naïve and experienced patients:

Oral powder: Infants and Children weighing 10 to <25 kg:
10 to <15 kg: 200 mg (4 packets) **plus** ritonavir 80 mg once daily
15 to <25 kg: 250 mg (5 packets) **plus** ritonavir 80 mg once daily

Oral capsule: Children and Adolescents 6 to <18 years:
15 kg to <20 kg: Atazanavir 150 mg **plus** ritonavir 100 mg once daily
20 kg to <40 kg: Atazanavir 200 mg **plus** ritonavir 100 mg once daily; some experts would increase to 300 mg atazanavir for patients ≥35 kg, especially when given with tenofovir (DHHS [pediatric], 2014)
≥40 kg: Atazanavir 300 mg **plus** ritonavir 100 mg once daily

Adolescents ≥18 years and Adults: **HIV infection, treatment:** Oral:

Antiretroviral-naïve patients: Atazanavir 300 mg once daily **plus** ritonavir 100 mg once daily **or** atazanavir 400 mg once daily in patients unable to tolerate ritonavir.

Antiretroviral-experienced patients: Atazanavir 300 mg once daily **plus** ritonavir 100 mg once daily. **Note:** Atazanavir without ritonavir is not recommended in antiretroviral-experienced patients with prior virologic failure.

Pregnant patients (antiretroviral-naïve): Atazanavir 300 mg once daily **plus** ritonavir 100 mg once daily. **Note:** Preferred regimen for pregnant patients who are antiretroviral-naïve. Postpartum dosage adjustment not needed. Observe patient for adverse events, especially within 2 months after delivery. Dose adjustments required for concomitant tenofovir **or** H$_2$ antagonist use (insufficient information for dose adjustment if **both** tenofovir and an H$_2$ antagonist are used). Some experts recommend atazanavir 400 mg plus ritonavir 100 mg in all pregnant women during the second and third trimesters due to decreased plasma concentrations (DHHS [perinatal], 2014).

Dosing adjustments for concomitant therapy:

Coadministration with efavirenz:

Antiretroviral-naïve patients: Adults: Atazanavir 400 mg **plus** ritonavir 100 mg once daily (as a single dose, administered with food); give with efavirenz 600 mg (administered on an empty stomach, preferably at bedtime); do **not** use efavirenz and atazanavir without booster doses of ritonavir.

Antiretroviral-experienced patients: Concurrent use not recommended due to decreased atazanavir exposure

Coadministration with H₂-receptor antagonists:

Antiretroviral-naïve patients: Daily dose of atazanavir **plus** ritonavir given simultaneously with, or at least 10 hours after, the H₂-receptor antagonist; dosage of H₂-receptor antagonist must be limited to the equivalent of 40 mg dose of famotidine twice daily in adults; administer with food

Patients unable to tolerate ritonavir: Adults: Atazanavir 400 mg once daily given at least 2 hours before or at least 10 hours after an H₂ antagonist; dosage of H₂-receptor antagonist must be limited to the equivalent daily dose of ≤40 mg famotidine (single dose: ≤20 mg)

Antiretroviral-experienced patients: Daily dose of atazanavir **plus** ritonavir given simultaneously with, or at least 10 hours after, the H₂-receptor antagonist; dosage of H₂-receptor antagonist must be limited to the equivalent of a 20 mg dose of famotidine twice daily in adults; administer with food

Antiretroviral-experienced pregnant patients in the second or third trimester: Adults: Atazanavir 400 mg plus ritonavir 100 mg simultaneously with, or at least 10 hours after an H₂ antagonist. **Note:** Insufficient information for dose adjustment if tenofovir **and** an H₂-antagonist are used.

Coadministration with proton pump inhibitor:

Antiretroviral-naïve patients: Daily dose of atazanavir **plus** ritonavir given 12 hours after the proton pump inhibitor; dosage of proton pump inhibitor must be limited to the equivalent of a 20 mg dose of omeprazole/day in adults; administer with food

Antiretroviral-experienced patients: Concurrent use **not** recommended

Coadministration with didanosine buffered or enteric-coated formulations: All patients: Administer atazanavir 2 hours before or 1 hour after didanosine buffered or enteric-coated formulations

Coadministration with tenofovir: Adults:

Antiretroviral-naïve patients: Atazanavir 300 mg **plus** ritonavir 100 mg given with tenofovir 300 mg (all as a single daily dose); administer with food; do **not** use tenofovir and atazanavir without booster doses of ritonavir; if H₂-receptor antagonist is coadministered, increase atazanavir to 400 mg **plus** ritonavir 100 mg once daily (see Coadministration with H₂-receptor antagonist)

Antiretroviral-experienced patients: Atazanavir 300 mg plus ritonavir 100 mg given with tenofovir 300 mg (all as a single daily dose); if H₂ antagonist coadministered (not to exceed equivalent daily dose of ≤40 mg famotidine), increase atazanavir to 400 mg (plus ritonavir 100 mg) once daily

Antiretroviral-experienced pregnant patients in the second or third trimester: Atazanavir 400 mg plus ritonavir 100 mg. **Note:** Insufficient information for dose adjustment if tenofovir **and** an H₂ antagonist are used.

Dosing adjustment in renal impairment:

Patients with renal impairment, including severe renal impairment who are not managed with hemodialysis: No dosage adjustment required

Patients with end-stage renal disease managed with hemodialysis: Not appreciably removed during hemodialysis. Only 2.1% of the dose was removed during a 4-hour dialysis session; however, mean AUC, peak, and trough serum concentrations were 25% to 43% lower (versus adults with normal renal function) when atazanavir was administered either prior to, or after hemodialysis; mechanism of the decrease is not currently known.

Antiretroviral-naïve patients: Adults: Atazanavir 300 mg **plus** ritonavir 100 mg once daily

Antiretroviral-experienced patients: Do not use atazanavir; dosage is not known

Dosing adjustment in hepatic impairment:

Mild to moderate hepatic insufficiency: Adults: Use with caution; if moderate hepatic impairment (Child-Pugh class B) and no prior virologic failure, consider dose reduction of atazanavir to 300 mg once daily

Severe hepatic impairment (Child-Pugh Class C): Do not use

Note: Patients with underlying hepatitis B or C or those with marked elevations in transaminases prior to treatment may be at increased risk of hepatic decompensation or further increases in transaminases with atazanavir therapy (monitor patients closely). Combination therapy with ritonavir in patients with hepatic impairment is **not** recommended.

Administration Administer with food to enhance absorption. Administer atazanavir 2 hours before or 1 hour after didanosine buffered formulations, didanosine enteric-coated capsules, other buffered medications, or antacids. Administer atazanavir (with ritonavir) simultaneously with, or at least 10 hours after, H₂-receptor antagonists; administer atazanavir (without ritonavir) at least 2 hours before or at least 10 hours after H₂-receptor antagonist. Administer atazanavir (with ritonavir) 12 hours after proton pump inhibitor.

Additional formulation specific information:

Oral capsules: Swallow capsules whole, do not open.

Oral powder: It is preferable to mix oral powder with food such as applesauce or yogurt. Mixing oral powder with a beverage (eg milk, infant formula, or water) may be used for infants who can drink from a cup. For young infants (<6 months) who cannot eat solid food or drink from a cup, oral powder should be mixed with infant formula and given using an oral dosing syringe. Administration of atazanavir and infant formula using an infant bottle is not recommended because full dose may not be delivered. Determine the number of packets (4 or 5 packets) needed. Mix with a small amount (one tablespoon) of soft food (preferred, eg, applesauce, yogurt) or beverage (milk, formula, water). After administration, add an additional small amount of soft food or beverage to the container, mix, and feed the residual amount to insure that the entire dose has been consumed. Administer oral powder within 1 hour of mixing with food or beverage.

Monitoring Parameters Note: Monitor CD4 percentage (if <5 years of age) or CD4 count (if ≥5 years of age) at least every 3 to 4 months (DHHS [pediatric], 2014).

Prior to initiation of therapy: Genotypic resistance testing, CD4 and viral load (every 3 to 4 months), CBC with differential, LFTs, BUN, creatinine, electrolytes, glucose, urinalysis (every 6 to 12 months), and assessment of readiness for adherence with medication regimen. At initiation and with any change in treatment regimen: CBC with differential, electrolytes, calcium, phosphate, glucose, LFTs, bilirubin, urinalysis (at initiation), BUN, creatinine, albumin, total protein, lipid panel (at initiation), CD4, and viral load. After 1 to 2 weeks of therapy: Signs of medication toxicity and adherence. After 2 to 4 weeks of therapy: CBC with differential, viral load, signs of medication toxicity, and adherence; then every 3 to 4 months: CBC with differential, electrolytes, glucose, LFTs, bilirubin, BUN, creatinine, CD4, viral load, signs of medication toxicity, and adherence. Every 6 to 12 months: Lipid panel and urinalysis. CD4 monitoring frequency may be decreased to every 6 to 12 months in children who are adherent to therapy if the value is well above the threshold for opportunistic infections, viral suppression is sustained, and the clinical status is stable for more than 2 to 3 years (DHHS [pediatric], 2014). Monitor for growth and development, signs of HIV-specific physical conditions, HIV disease progression, opportunistic infections or pancreatitis.

Reference Range Plasma trough concentration ≥150 ng/mL (DHHS [adult, pediatric], 2014)

Additional Information Preliminary studies have shown that appropriate atazanavir serum concentrations are difficult to achieve in pediatric patients even with higher doses (on a mg/kg or m^2 basis). Optimal dosing in children <6 years of age is under investigation; the addition of low-dose ritonavir (booster doses) to increase atazanavir serum concentrations may be required and is currently being evaluated. Results of a pediatric Phase II clinical trial suggest that when used **without** ritonavir boosting, children ≥6 and <13 years of age require atazanavir 520 mg/m^2/day and adolescents ≥13 years of age require atazanavir 620 mg/m^2/day (once daily doses of 600 to 900 mg/day). When used in combination **with** ritonavir, the study used atazanavir 205 mg/m^2/day (once daily doses of 250 to 375 mg/day) (DHHS [pediatric], 2014).

Product Availability Reyataz oral powder: FDA approved June 2014; anticipated availability is currently unknown.

Dosage Forms Excipient information presented when available (limited, particularly for generics); consult specific product labeling.

Capsule, Oral, as sulfate:
Reyataz: 150 mg, 200 mg, 300 mg [contains fd&c blue #2 (indigotine)]

References

DHHS Panel on Antiretroviral Guidelines for Adults and Adolescents. Guidelines for the use of antiretroviral agents in HIV-1-infected adults and adolescents, Department of Health and Human Services. May 1, 2014. Available at http://www.aidsinfo.nih.gov/ContentFiles/AdultandAdolescentGL.pdf

DHHS Panel on Antiretroviral Therapy and Medical Management of HIV-Infected Children. Guidelines for the use of antiretroviral agents in pediatric HIV infection. February 12, 2014. Available at http://aidsinfo.nih.gov

DHHS Panel on Treatment of HIV-Infected Pregnant Women and Prevention of Perinatal Transmission. Recommendations for the use of antiretroviral drugs in pregnant HIV-1-infected women for maternal health and interventions to reduce perinatal HIV-1 transmission in the United States. March 28, 2014. Available at http://aidsinfo.nih.gov

Goldsmith DR, Perry CM. Atazanavir. *Drugs*. 2003;63(16):1679-1693.

Musial BL, Chojnacki JK, Coleman CI. Atazanavir: a new protease inhibitor to treat HIV infection. *Am J Health Syst Pharm*. 2004;61 (13):1365-1374.

Reyataz (atazanavir) [prescribing information]. Princeton, NJ: Bristol-Myers Squibb Company; June 2014.

◆ **Atazanavir Sulfate** see Atazanavir on page 218

Atenolol (a TEN oh lole)

Medication Safety Issues
Sound-alike/look-alike issues:
Atenolol may be confused with albuterol, Altenol, timolol, Tylenol

Tenormin may be confused with Imuran, Norpramin, thiamine, Trovan

Brand Names: U.S. Tenormin

Brand Names: Canada Apo-Atenolol; Ava-Atenolol; CO Atenolol; Dom-Atenolol; JAMP-Atenolol; Mint-Atenolol; Mylan-Atenolol; Nu-Atenol; PMS-Atenolol; RAN-Atenolol; ratio-Atenolol; Riva-Atenolol; Sandoz-Atenolol; Septa-Atenolol; Tenormin; Teva-Atenolol

Therapeutic Category Antianginal Agent; Antihypertensive Agent; Beta-Adrenergic Blocker

Generic Availability (U.S.) Yes

Use Treatment of hypertension, alone or in combination with other agents (FDA approved in adults); management of angina pectoris (FDA approved in adults); post-MI patients (to reduce cardiovascular mortality) (FDA approved in adults); acute alcohol withdrawal; supraventricular and ventricular arrhythmias; migraine headache prophylaxis

Pregnancy Risk Factor D

Pregnancy Considerations Studies in pregnant women have demonstrated a risk to the fetus; therefore, the manufacturer classifies atenolol as pregnancy category D. Atenolol crosses the placenta and is found in cord blood. In a cohort study, an increased risk of cardiovascular defects was observed following maternal use of beta-blockers during pregnancy. Intrauterine growth restriction (IUGR), small placentas, as well as fetal/neonatal bradycardia, hypoglycemia, and/or respiratory depression have been observed following *in utero* exposure to beta-blockers as a class. Adequate facilities for monitoring infants at birth should be available. Untreated chronic maternal hypertension and pre-eclampsia are also associated with adverse events in the fetus, infant, and mother. The maternal pharmacokinetic parameters of atenolol during the second and third trimesters are within the ranges reported in nonpregnant patients. Although atenolol has shown efficacy in the treatment of hypertension in pregnancy, it is not the drug of choice due to potential IUGR in the infant.

Breast-Feeding Considerations Atenolol is excreted in breast milk and has been detected in the serum and urine of nursing infants. Peak concentrations in breast milk have been reported to occur between 2 to 8 hours after the maternal dose and in some cases are higher than the peak maternal serum concentration. Although most studies have not reported adverse events in nursing infants, avoiding maternal use while nursing infants with renal dysfunction or infants <44 weeks postconceptual age has been suggested. Beta-blockers with less distribution into breast milk may be preferred. The manufacturer recommends that caution be exercised when administering atenolol to nursing women.

Contraindications Hypersensitivity to atenolol or any component; pulmonary edema, cardiogenic shock, bradycardia, heart block, or uncompensated CHF

Warnings Exacerbation of angina, arrhythmias, and, in some cases, MI may occur following abrupt discontinuation of beta-blockers **[U.S. Boxed Warning]**; avoid abrupt discontinuation, wean slowly, and monitor for signs and symptoms of ischemia. Atenolol should not be administered to patients with untreated pheochromocytoma. Atenolol may mask clinical signs of hyperthyroidism (exacerbation of symptoms of hyperthyroidism, including thyroid storm, may occur following abrupt discontinuation). Atenolol decreases the ability of the heart to respond to reflex adrenergic stimuli and may increase the risk of general anesthesia and surgical procedures; use caution with anesthetic agents that decrease myocardial function. Beta-blocker use has been associated with induction or exacerbation of psoriasis, but cause and effect have not been firmly established.

Precautions Use with caution and modify dosage in patients with renal impairment; use with caution in patients with CHF, bronchospastic disease, diabetes mellitus, and hyperthyroidism. Use with caution in nursing women; clinically significant bradycardia may occur in breast-fed infants; infants with renal dysfunction and premature infants may be at higher risk for adverse effects; breast-fed infants and neonates born to mothers receiving atenolol may be at increased risk for hypoglycemia. Patients who have a history of anaphylactic hypersensitivity reactions to various substances may be more reactive while receiving beta-blockers; these patients may not be responsive to the normal doses of epinephrine used to treat hypersensitivity reactions.

Adverse Reactions

Cardiovascular: Chest pain, edema, heart failure, hypotension, persistent bradycardia, Raynaud's phenomenon, second- or third-degree AV block

Central nervous system: Confusion, depression, dizziness, fatigue, headache, insomnia, lethargy, mental impairment, nightmares

Gastrointestinal: Constipation, diarrhea, nausea

Genitourinary: Impotence

Miscellaneous: Cold extremities

Rare but important or life-threatening: Alopecia, dyspnea (especially with large doses), hallucinations, impotence, liver enzymes increased, lupus syndrome, Peyronie's disease, positive ANA, psoriasiform rash, psychosis, thrombocytopenia, wheezing

Drug Interactions

Metabolism/Transport Effects None known.

Avoid Concomitant Use

Avoid concomitant use of Atenolol with any of the following: Ceritinib; Floctafenine; Methacholine

Increased Effect/Toxicity

Atenolol may increase the levels/effects of: Alpha-/Beta-Agonists (Direct-Acting); Alpha1-Blockers; Alpha2-Agonists; Amifostine; Antihypertensives; Bradycardia-Causing Agents; Bupivacaine; Cardiac Glycosides; Ceritinib; Cholinergic Agonists; DULoxetine; Ergot Derivatives; Fingolimod; Grass Pollen Allergen Extract (5 Grass Extract); Hypotensive Agents; Insulin; Lidocaine (Systemic); Lidocaine (Topical); Mepivacaine; Methacholine; Midodrine; Obinutuzumab; RiTUXimab; Sulfonylureas

The levels/effects of Atenolol may be increased by: Acetylcholinesterase Inhibitors; Alpha2-Agonists; Amiodarone; Anilidopiperidine Opioids; Barbiturates; Brimonidine (Topical); Calcium Channel Blockers (Dihydropyridine); Calcium Channel Blockers (Nondihydropyridine); Diazoxide; Dipyridamole; Disopyramide; Dronedarone; Floctafenine; Glycopyrrolate; Herbs (Hypotensive Properties); MAO Inhibitors; Pentoxifylline; Phosphodiesterase 5 Inhibitors; Prostacyclin Analogues; Regorafenib; Reserpine

Decreased Effect

Atenolol may decrease the levels/effects of: Beta2-Agonists; Theophylline Derivatives

The levels/effects of Atenolol may be decreased by: Ampicillin; Herbs (Hypertensive Properties); Methylphenidate; Nonsteroidal Anti-Inflammatory Agents; Yohimbine

Food Interactions Atenolol serum concentrations may be decreased if taken with food. Management: Administer without regard to meals.

Mechanism of Action Competitively blocks response to beta-adrenergic stimulation, selectively blocks beta$_1$-receptors with little or no effect on beta$_2$-receptors except at high doses

Pharmacodynamics

Beta-blocking effect:

Onset of action: Oral: ≤1 hour

Maximum effect: Oral: 2-4 hours

Duration: Oral: ≥24 hours

Antihypertensive effect:

Duration: Oral: 24 hours

Pharmacokinetics (Adult data unless noted)

Absorption: Incomplete from the GI tract; ~50% absorbed

Distribution: Does not cross the blood-brain barrier; low lipophilicity; distributes into breast milk at a concentration 1.5-6.8 times the maternal plasma concentration

Protein binding: Low (6% to 16%)

Half-life, beta:

Neonates: Mean: 16 hours, up to 35 hours

Children 5-16 years of age: Mean: 4.6 hours; range: 3.5-7 hours; children >10 years of age may have longer half-life (>5 hours) compared to children 5-10 years of age (<5 hours)

Adults: 6-7 hours

Prolonged half-life with renal dysfunction

Time to peak serum concentration: Oral: Within 2-4 hours

Elimination: 40% as unchanged drug in urine, 50% in feces

Dialysis: Moderately dialyzable (20% to 50%)

Dosing: Usual Oral: Hypertension:

Children: Initial: 0.5-1 mg/kg/day given once daily or divided in 2 doses per day; titrate dose to effect; usual range: 0.5-1.5 mg/kg/day; maximum dose: 2 mg/kg/day; do not exceed adult maximum dose of 100 mg/day (National High Blood Pressure Education Program Working Group on High Blood Pressure in Children and Adolescents, 2004)

Adults: Initial: 25-50 mg once daily; titrate dose to effect; usual dose: 50-100 mg once daily; usual dosage range (JNC 7): 25-100 mg once daily; maximum dose: 100 mg once daily

See table for oral dosing interval in renal impairment.

Creatinine Clearance	Maximum Oral Dose	Frequency of Administration
15-35 mL/min	50 mg or 1 mg/kg/dose	Daily
<15 mL/min	50 mg or 1 mg/kg/dose	Every other day

Administration Oral: May be administered without regard to food

Monitoring Parameters Blood pressure, heart rate, ECG, fluid intake and output, daily weight, respiratory rate

Test Interactions Increased glucose; decreased HDL

Additional Information In diabetic patients, atenolol may potentiate hypoglycemia and mask signs and symptoms of hypoglycemia; limited data suggests that atenolol may have a shorter half-life and faster clearance in patients with Marfan syndrome. Higher doses (2 mg/kg/day divided every 12 hours) have been used in patients with Marfan syndrome (6-22 years of age) to decrease aortic root growth rate and prevent aortic dissection or rupture; further studies are needed.

Dosage Forms Excipient information presented when available (limited, particularly for generics); consult specific product labeling.

Tablet, Oral:

Tenormin: 25 mg

Tenormin: 50 mg [scored]

Tenormin: 100 mg

Generic: 25 mg, 50 mg, 100 mg

Extemporaneous Preparations A 2 mg/mL oral suspension may be made with tablets. Crush four 50 mg tablets in a mortar and reduce to a fine powder. Add a small amount of glycerin and mix to a uniform paste. Mix while adding Ora-Sweet® SF vehicle in incremental proportions to almost 100 mL; transfer to a calibrated bottle, rinse mortar with vehicle, and add quantity of vehicle sufficient to make 100 mL. Label "shake well" and "refrigerate". Stable for 90 days.

Nahata MC, Pai VB, and Hipple TF, *Pediatric Drug Formulations*, 5th ed, Cincinnati, OH: Harvey Whitney Books Co, 2004.

References

Brauchli YB, Jick SS, Curtin F, et al, "Association Between Beta-Blockers, Other Antihypertensive Drugs and Psoriasis: Population-Based Case-Control Study," *Br J Dermatol*, 2008, 158(6):1299-307.

Buck ML, Wiest D, Gillette PC, et al, "Pharmacokinetics and Pharmacodynamics of Atenolol in Children," *Clin Pharmacol Ther*, 1989, 46 (6):629-33.

Case CL, Trippel DL, and Gillette PC, "New Antiarrhythmic Agents in Pediatrics," *Pediatr Clin North Am*, 1989, 36(5):1293-320.

Chobanian AV, Bakris GL, Black HR, et al, "The Seventh Report of the Joint National Committee on Prevention, Detection, Evaluation, and Treatment of High Blood Pressure: The JNC 7 report," *JAMA*, 2003, 289(19):2560-72.

Gold MH, Holy AK, and Roenigk HH Jr, "Beta-Blocking Drugs and Psoriasis. A Review of Cutaneous Side Effects and Retrospective Analysis of Their Effects on Psoriasis," *J Am Acad Dermatol*, 1988, 19 (5 Pt 1):837-41.

National High Blood Pressure Education Program Working Group on High Blood Pressure in Children and Adolescents, "The Fourth Report on the Diagnosis, Evaluation, and Treatment of High Blood Pressure in Children and Adolescents," *Pediatrics*, 2004, 114(2 Suppl 4th Report):555-76.

Schön MP and Boehncke WH, "Psoriasis," *N Engl J Med*, 2005, 352 (18):1899-912.

Trippel DL and Gillette PC, "Atenolol in Children With Supraventricular Tachycardia," *Am J Cardiol*, 1989, 64(3):233-6.

Trippel DL and Gillette PC, "Atenolol in Children With Ventricular Arrhythmias," *Am Heart J*, 1990, 119(6):1312-6.

◆ **ATG** *see* Antithymocyte Globulin (Equine) *on page 182*

◆ **Atgam** *see* Antithymocyte Globulin (Equine) *on page 182*

◆ **Atgam® (Can)** *see* Antithymocyte Globulin (Equine) *on page 182*

◆ **Athletes Foot Spray [OTC]** *see* Tolnaftate *on page 2044*

◆ **Ativan** *see* LORazepam *on page 1280*

◆ **Atlizumab** *see* Tocilizumab *on page 2040*

AtoMOXetine (AT oh mox e teen)

Medication Safety Issues
Sound-alike/look-alike issues:
AtoMOXetine may be confused with atorvaSTATin
Related Information
Oral Medications That Should Not Be Crushed or Altered *on page 2438*
Brand Names: U.S. Strattera
Brand Names: Canada Apo-Atomoxetine; DOM-Atomoxetine; Mylan-Atomoxetine; PMS-Atomoxetine; RIVA-Atomoxetine; Sandoz-Atomoxetine; Strattera; Teva-Atomoxetine
Therapeutic Category Norepinephrine Reuptake Inhibitor, Selective
Generic Availability (U.S.) No
Use Treatment of attention-deficit/hyperactivity disorder (ADHD) (FDA approved in ages ≥6 years and adults)
Medication Guide Available Yes
Pregnancy Risk Factor C
Pregnancy Considerations Adverse events have been observed in animal reproduction studies. Information related to atomoxetine use in pregnancy is limited; appropriate contraception is recommended for sexually active women of childbearing potential (Heiligenstein, 2003).
Breast-Feeding Considerations It is not known if atomoxetine is excreted in breast milk. The manufacturer recommends that caution be exercised when administering atomoxetine to nursing women.
Contraindications Hypersensitivity to atomoxetine or any component; concurrent use or use within 14 days of MAO inhibitors; narrow-angle glaucoma; current or past history of pheochromocytoma; severe cardiovascular disorders in which the condition would be expected to deteriorate with clinically relevant blood pressure or heart rate increases.
Warnings Atomoxetine has been associated with an increased risk of suicidal thinking in children and adolescents with ADHD **[U.S. Boxed Warning]**. This risk must be considered before prescribing atomoxetine in pediatric patients. Children and adolescents who start treatment with atomoxetine require close monitoring for suicidal thinking and behavior, or clinical worsening, especially during the first few months after initiation of a course of therapy or when the dosage is changed. Family members and caregivers should be instructed to closely observe the patient and communicate their condition with the healthcare provider. Recommended monitoring includes daily observation by family members and caregivers. Patients should also be

monitored for associated behaviors (eg, agitation, irritability, anxiety, akathisia, aggressiveness, insomnia, hostility, impulsivity, panic attacks, hypomania, mania) which may be precursors to emerging suicidality. Emergence of suicidality or associated behaviors listed above, that is abrupt in onset, severe, or not part of the presenting symptoms, may require discontinuation or modification of drug therapy.

Psychiatric adverse events may occur. Atomoxetine may exacerbate symptoms of behavior disturbance and thought disorder in patients with preexisting psychosis. New-onset psychosis or mania may occur in patients without a prior history of psychotic illness or mania, even at standard doses. Atomoxetine may induce mixed/manic episodes in patients with bipolar disorder; patients should be screened for bipolar disorder prior to treatment; consider discontinuation if such symptoms (eg, delusional thinking, hallucinations, or mania) occur. New or worsening symptoms of hostility or aggressive behaviors have been associated with atomoxetine (causal relationship not established) particularly with the initiation of therapy; monitor for development or worsening of these behaviors.

Rare, severe liver injury has been reported with atomoxetine including liver failure (requiring transplantation) and death; the majority of cases occurred within 120 days of initiation of therapy; discontinue atomoxetine and do not restart if signs or symptoms of hepatotoxic reaction (eg, jaundice, pruritus, flu-like symptoms) or laboratory evidence of liver injury are observed. Use with caution in patients with hepatic impairment; dosage adjustments may be necessary.

Serious cardiovascular events including sudden death may occur in patients with preexisting structural cardiac abnormalities or other serious heart problems. Sudden death has been reported in children and adolescents; sudden death, stroke, and MI have been reported in adults. Avoid the use of atomoxetine in patients with known serious structural cardiac abnormalities, cardiomyopathy, serious heart rhythm abnormalities, coronary artery disease, or other serious cardiac problems that could place patients at an increased risk to the noradrenergic effects of atomoxetine. Patients should be carefully evaluated for cardiac disease prior to initiation of therapy. The American Heart Association recommends that all children diagnosed with ADHD who may be candidates for medication, such as atomoxetine, should have a thorough cardiovascular assessment prior to initiation of therapy. This assessment should include a combination of medical history, family history, and physical examination focusing on cardiovascular disease risk factors. An ECG is not mandatory but should be considered. If a child displays symptoms of cardiovascular disease, including chest pain, dyspnea, or fainting, parents should seek immediate medical care for the child. In a recent retrospective study on the possible association between stimulant medication use and sudden death in children, 564 previously healthy children who died suddenly in motor vehicle accidents were compared to a group of 564 previously healthy children who died suddenly. Two of the 564 (0.4%) children in motor vehicle accidents were taking stimulant medications compared to 10 of 564 (1.8%) children who died suddenly. While the authors of this study conclude there may be an association between stimulant use and sudden death in children, there were a number of limitations to the study and the FDA cannot conclude this information impacts the overall risk:benefit profile of these medications (Gould, 2009). In a large retrospective cohort study involving 1,200,438 children and young adults (aged 2-24 years), none of the currently available stimulant medications or atomoxetine were shown to increase the risk of serious cardiovascular events (ie, acute MI, sudden cardiac death, or stroke) in current (adjusted hazard ratio: 0.75; 95% CI: 0.31-1.85) or former (adjusted hazard ratio: 1.03; 95% CI: 0.57-1.89) users compared to nonusers. It should be noted that due to the upper limit of the 95% CI, the study could not rule out a doubling of the risk, albeit low (Cooper, 2011).

May cause significant increases in blood pressure and heart rate; in pediatric clinical trials, incidences of maximum increases in SBP, DBP, and HR compared to placebo were as follows: SBP (≥20 mm Hg): 12.5% vs 8.7%; DBP (≥15 mm Hg): 21.5% vs 14.1%; and HR (≥20 bpm): 23.4% vs 11.5%; monitor blood pressure and pulse at baseline, with dosage increases, and periodically during therapy. Use caution in patients with underlying medical conditions which may be exacerbated by increases in blood pressure and/or heart rate, including hypertension, tachycardia, or other cardiovascular or cerebrovascular conditions; use is contraindicated in patients with severe cardiovascular disorders who may experience clinical deterioration of condition with clinical increases in blood pressure or heart rate.

Allergic reactions (including anaphylaxis, rash, urticaria, and angioneurotic edema) may occur (rare).

In pediatric patients, suppression of growth (height and weight) has been reported during the initial 9-12 months of therapy and has been shown to recover to normative values by 3 years of therapy; this growth pattern has been observed to be independent of pubertal status and patient's metabolic profile (ie, poor or extensive metabolizer); growth should be monitored during treatment.

Precautions May cause orthostatic hypotension or syncope; use with caution in patients with conditions that predispose to hypotension or with conditions associated with abrupt heart rate or blood pressure changes. May cause new onset or exacerbation of Raynaud's phenomenon. May cause urinary retention or hesitancy; use with caution in patients with a history of urinary retention or bladder outlet obstruction. May rarely cause priapism; prompt medical attention may be required.

Use with caution in patients who are cytochrome P450 CYP2D6 poor metabolizers; bioavailability and drug exposure may be increased; dosage adjustments are recommended; the incidence of some adverse reactions are reported to be increased in poor metabolizers of CYP2D6 substrates including decreased appetite, increases in blood pressure or heart rate, insomnia, sedation, depression, tremor, early morning awakening, pruritus, and mydriasis. Use caution with concurrent use of strong CYP2D6 inhibitors (eg, paroxetine, fluoxetine, and quinidine); modification of atomoxetine dose may be required.

Adverse Reactions

Cardiovascular: Cold extremities, flushing, increased diastolic blood pressure, orthostatic hypotension, palpitations, syncope, systolic hypertension, tachycardia

Central nervous system: Abnormal dreams, agitation, anxiety, chills, depression, disturbed sleep, dizziness, drowsiness, emotional lability, fatigue, headache, insomnia, irritability, jitteriness, paresthesia (higher in adults; postmarketing observation in children), restlessness

Dermatologic: Excoriation, hyperhidrosis, skin rash

Endocrine & metabolic: Decreased libido, hot flash, increased thirst, menstrual disease, weight loss

Gastrointestinal: Abdominal pain, anorexia, constipation, decreased appetite, diarrhea, dysgeusia, dyspepsia, flatulence, nausea, vomiting, xerostomia

Genitourinary: Dysmenorrhea, dysuria, ejaculatory disorder, erectile dysfunction, orgasm abnormal, pollakiuria, prostatitis, urinary frequency, urinary retention

Neuromuscular & skeletal: Back pain, muscle spasm, tremor, weakness

Ophthalmic: Blurred vision, conjunctivitis, mydriasis

Respiratory: Oropharyngeal pain, pharyngolaryngeal pain, sinus headache

Miscellaneous: Therapeutic response unexpected

Rare but important or life-threatening: Aggressive behavior, allergy disorder, anaphylaxis, angioedema, cerebrovascular accident, delusions, growth suppression (children), hallucination, hepatotoxicity, hostility, hypersensitivity reaction, hypomania, impulsivity, jaundice, mania, myocardial infarction, panic attack, pelvic pain, peripheral vascular disease, priapism, prolonged Q-T interval on ECG, Raynaud's phenomenon, seizure (including patients with no prior history or known risk factors for seizure), severe hepatic disease, suicidal ideation, testicular pain, tics

Drug Interactions

Metabolism/Transport Effects Substrate of CYP2C19 (minor), CYP2D6 (major); **Note:** Assignment of Major/Minor substrate status based on clinically relevant drug interaction potential; **Inhibits** CYP2D6 (weak), CYP3A4 (weak)

Avoid Concomitant Use

Avoid concomitant use of AtoMOXetine with any of the following: Iobenguane I 123; MAO Inhibitors; Pimozide

Increased Effect/Toxicity

AtoMOXetine may increase the levels/effects of: ARIPiprazole; Beta2-Agonists; Dofetilide; Lomitapide; Pimozide; Sympathomimetics

The levels/effects of AtoMOXetine may be increased by: Abiraterone Acetate; CYP2D6 Inhibitors (Moderate); CYP2D6 Inhibitors (Strong); Darunavir; MAO Inhibitors

Decreased Effect

AtoMOXetine may decrease the levels/effects of: Iobenguane I 123

The levels/effects of AtoMOXetine may be decreased by: Peginterferon Alfa-2b

Stability Store at 25°C (77°F); excursions permitted to 15°C to 30°C (59°F to 86°F).

Mechanism of Action Selectively inhibits the reuptake of norepinephrine (Ki 4.5 nM) with little to no activity at the other neuronal reuptake pumps or receptor sites.

Pharmacokinetics (Adult data unless noted) The pharmacokinetics in pediatric patients ≥6 years of age have been shown to be similar to those of adult patients.

Absorption: Oral: Rapid

Distribution: V_d: I.V.: 0.85 L/kg

Protein binding: 98%, primarily albumin

Metabolism: Hepatic, primarily by oxidative metabolism via CYP2D6 to 4-hydroxyatomoxetine (major metabolite regardless of CYP2D6 status, active, equipotent to atomoxetine) with subsequent glucuronidation; also metabolized via CYP2C19 to N-desmethylatomoxetine (active, minimal activity). **Note:** CYP2D6 poor metabolizers have atomoxetine AUCs that are ~10-fold higher and peak concentrations that are ~fivefold greater than extensive metabolizers; 4-hyroxyatomoxetine plasma concentrations are very low (extensive metabolizers: 1% of atomoxetine concentrations; poor metabolizers: 0.1% of atomoxetine concentrations

Bioavailability: Extensive metabolizers: 63%; poor metabolizers: 94%

Half-life:

Atomoxetine: Extensive metabolizers: 5.2 hours; poor metabolizers: 21.6 hours

4-hydroxyatomoxetine: Extensive metabolizers: 6-8 hours

N-desmethylatomoxetine: Extensive metabolizers: 6-8 hours; poor metabolizers: 34-40 hours

Time to peak serum concentration: 1-2 hours; delayed 3 hours by high-fat meal

Elimination: Urine: <3% is excreted unchanged; 80% excreted as 4-hydroxyatomoxetine glucuronide; feces: <17%

Dosing: Usual Attention-deficit/hyperactivity disorder:
Children ≥6 years and Adolescents, weighing ≤70 kg: Oral: Initial: 0.5 mg/kg/day; increase after a minimum of 3 days to ~1.2 mg/kg/day; may administer once daily in the morning or divide into 2 doses and administer in the morning and late afternoon/early evening; maximum daily dose: 1.4 mg/kg/**day** or 100 mg/**day**, whichever is less. **Note:** Doses >1.2 mg/kg/day have not been shown to provide additional benefit.

Dosage adjustment with concurrent strong CYP2D6 inhibitors (eg, paroxetine, fluoxetine, quinidine) use or patients known to be CYP2D6 poor metabolizers: Oral: Initial: 0.5 mg/kg/day for 4 weeks; increase dose to 1.2 mg/kg/day only if clinically needed and the initial dose is well tolerated; do not exceed 1.2 mg/kg/**day**

Children ≥6 years and Adolescents, weighing >70 kg and Adults: Oral: Initial: 40 mg daily; increase after a minimum of 3 days to ~80 mg daily; may administer once daily in the morning or divide into 2 doses and administer in morning and late afternoon/early evening. After an additional 2-4 weeks, may increase (if needed) to maximum daily dose: 100 mg/**day**.

Dosage adjustment with concurrent strong CYP2D6 inhibitors (eg, paroxetine, fluoxetine, quinidine) use or patients known to be CYP2D6 poor metabolizers: Oral: Initial: 40 mg daily for 4 weeks; increase dose to 80 mg daily only if clinically needed and the initial dose is well tolerated; do not exceed 80 mg daily

Dosage adjustment in renal impairment: Children ≥6 years, Adolescents, and Adults: No dosage adjustments are recommended.

Dosage adjustment in hepatic impairment: Children ≥6 years, Adolescents, and Adults:
Moderate hepatic impairment (Child-Pugh class B): Administer 50% of normal dose
Severe hepatic impairment (Child-Pugh class C): Administer 25% of normal dose

Administration Oral: May be administered without regard to food. Do not crush, chew, or open capsule; swallow whole with water or other liquids. **Note:** Atomoxetine is an ocular irritant; if capsule is opened accidently and contents come into contact with eye, flush eye immediately with water and obtain medical advice; wash hands and any potentially contaminated surface as soon as possible.

Monitoring Parameters Family members and caregivers need to monitor patient daily for emergence of irritability, agitation, unusual changes in behavior, and suicide ideation. Pediatric patients should be monitored closely for suicidality, clinical worsening, or unusual changes in behavior, especially during the initial few months of therapy or at times of dose changes. Appearance of symptoms needs to be immediately reported to healthcare provider.

Evaluate for cardiac disease prior to initiation of therapy with thorough medical history, family history, and physical exam; consider ECG; perform ECG and echocardiogram if findings suggest cardiac disease; promptly conduct cardiac evaluation in patients who develop chest pain, unexplained syncope, or any other symptom of cardiac disease during treatment. Monitor body weight, BMI, height and growth rate (in children); CNS activity; blood pressure and heart rate and rhythm (baseline, following dose increases, and periodically during treatment); liver enzymes in patients with symptoms of liver dysfunction; sleep, appetite, abnormal movements. Patients should be re-evaluated at appropriate intervals to assess continued need of the medication. Monitor for new psychotic symptoms, appearance or worsening of aggressive behavior, or hostility.

Additional Information Atomoxetine hydrochloride is the R(-) isomer. Therapy may be discontinued without being tapered. Total daily doses >150 mg/day and single doses >120 mg/dose have not been systematically evaluated. Medications used to treat ADHD should be part of a total treatment program that may include other components such as psychological, educational, and social measures. If used for an extended period of time, long-term usefulness of atomoxetine should be periodically re-evaluated for the individual patient.

Dosage Forms Excipient information presented when available (limited, particularly for generics); consult specific product labeling.
Capsule, Oral:
Strattera: 10 mg, 18 mg, 25 mg, 40 mg, 60 mg
Strattera: 80 mg, 100 mg [contains fd&c blue #2 (indigotine)]

References

American Academy of Pediatrics, "ADHD: Clinical Practice Guideline for the Diagnosis, Evaluation, and Treatment of Attention-Deficit/Hyperactivity Disorder in Children and Adolescents," *Pediatrics*, 2011, 128(5):1007-22.

American Academy of Pediatrics/American Heart Association Clarification of Statement on Cardiovascular Evaluation and Monitoring of Children and Adolescents With Heart Disease Receiving Medications for ADHD; available at: http://americanheart.mediaroom.com/index.php?s=43&item=422.

Biderman J, Heiligenstein JH, Faries DE, at al, "Efficacy of Atomoxetine Versus Placebo in School-Age Girls With Attention-Deficit/Hyperactivity Disorder," *Pediatrics*, 2002, 110(6), http://www.pediatrics.org/cgi/content/full/110/6/e75.

Cooper WO, Habel LA, Sox CM, et al, "ADHD Drugs and Serious Cardiovascular Events in Children and Young Adults," *N Engl J Med*, 2011, 365(20):1896-904.

Dopheide JA and Pliszka SR, "Attention-Deficit-Hyperactivity Disorder: An Update," *Pharmacotherapy*, 2009, 29(6):656-79.

Gould MS, Walsh BT, Munfakh JL, et al, "Sudden Death and Use of Stimulant Medications in Youths," *Am J Psychiatry*, 2009, 166 (9):992-1001.

Heiligenstein J, Michelson D, Wernicke J, et al, "Atomoxetine and Pregnancy; Author Reply," *J Am Acad Child Adolesc Psychiatry*, 2003, 42(8): 884-5.

Kratochvil CJ, Heiligenstein JH, Dittmann R, et al, "Atomoxetine and Methylphenidate Treatment in Children With ADHD: A Prospective, Randomized, Open-Label trial," *J Am Acad Child Adolesc Psychiatry*, 2002, 41(7):776-84.

Michelson D, Allen AJ, Busner J, et al, "Once-Daily Atomoxetine Treatment for Children and Adolescents With Attention Deficit Hyperactivity Disorder: A Randomized, Placebo-Controlled Study," *Am J Psychiatry*, 2002, 159(11):1896-901.

Michelson D, Faries D, Wernicke J, et al, "Atomoxetine in the Treatment of Children and Adolescents With Attention-Deficit/Hyperactivity Disorder: A Ramdomized, Placebo-Controlled, Dose-Response Study," *Pediatrics*, 2001, 108(5), http://www.pediatrics.org/cgi/content/full/108/5/e83.

Newcorn JH, Michelson D, Kratochvil CJ, et al, "Low-Dose Atomoxetine for Maintenance Treatment of Attention-Deficit/Hyperactivity Disorder," *Pediatrics*, 2006, 118(6):e1701-6.

Pliszka S and AACAP Work Group on Quality Issues, "Practice Parameter for the Assessment and Treatment of Children and Adolescents With Attention-Deficit/Hyperactivity Disorder," *J Am Acad Child Adolesc Psychiatry*, 2007, 46(7):894-921.

Spencer T, Heiligenstein JH, Biederman J, et al, "Results From 2 Proof-of-Concept, Placebo-Controlled Studies of Atomoxetine in Children With Attention-Deficit/Hyperactivity Disorder," *J Clin Psychiatry*, 2002, 63(12):1140-7.

Vetter VL, Elia J, Erickson C, et al, "Cardiovascular Monitoring of Children and Adolescents With Heart Disease Receiving Stimulant Drugs: A Scientific Statement From the American Heart Association Council on Cardiovascular Disease in the Young Congenital Cardiac Defects Committee and the Council on Cardiovascular Nursing," *Circulation*, 2008, 117(18):2407-23.

Wernicke JF and Kratochvil CJ, "Safety Profile of Atomoxetine in the Treatment of Children and Adolescents With ADHD," *J Clin Psychiatry*, 2002, 63(Suppl 12):50-5.

◆ **Atomoxetine Hydrochloride** see AtoMOXetine on page 224

AtorvaSTATin (a TORE va sta tin)

Medication Safety Issues

Sound-alike/look-alike issues:

AtorvaSTATin may be confused with atoMOXetine, lovastatin, nystatin, pitavastatin, pravastatin, rosuvastatin, simvastatin

Lipitor may be confused with labetalol, Levatol, lisinopril, Loniten, Lopid, Mevacor, Zocor, ZyrTEC

Brand Names: U.S. Lipitor

Brand Names: Canada Apo-Atorvastatin; Ava-Atorvastatin; CO Atorvastatin; Dom-Atorvastatin; GD-Atorvastatin; Lipitor; Mylan-Atorvastatin; Novo-Atorvastatin; PMS-Atorvastatin; RAN-Atorvastatin; ratio-Atorvastatin; Sandoz-Atorvastatin

Therapeutic Category Antilipemic Agent; HMG-CoA Reductase Inhibitor

Generic Availability (U.S.) Yes

Use Hyperlipidemia: Adjunct to dietary therapy in pediatric patients with heterozygous familial hypercholesterolemia if LDL-C remains ≥190 mg/dL, if ≥160 mg/dL with family history of premature CHD or presence of ≥2 cardiovascular risk factors (FDA approved in boys and postmenarchal girls 10-17 years). Adjunct to dietary therapy to decrease elevated serum total and low density lipoprotein cholesterol (LDL-C), apolipoprotein B (apo-B), and triglyceride levels, and to increase high density lipoprotein cholesterol (HDL-C) in patients with primary hypercholesterolemia (heterozygous, familial and nonfamilial) and mixed dyslipidemia (Fredrickson types IIa and IIb) (FDA approved in adults); treatment of homozygous familial hypercholesterolemia (FDA approved in adults); treatment of isolated hypertriglyceridemia (Fredrickson type IV); treatment of primary dysbetalipoproteinemia (Fredrickson Type III) (FDA approved in adults)

Primary prevention of cardiovascular disease in high risk patients (FDA approved in adults); risk factors include: Age ≥55 years, smoking, hypertension, low HDL-C, or family history of early coronary heart disease; secondary prevention of cardiovascular disease to reduce the risk of MI, stroke, revascularization procedures, and angina in patients with evidence of coronary heart disease and to reduce the risk of hospitalization for heart failure. Has also been used in prevention of graft coronary artery disease in heart transplant patients.

Pregnancy Risk Factor X

Pregnancy Considerations Adverse events were observed in animal reproductions studies. There are reports of congenital anomalies following maternal use of HMG-CoA reductase inhibitors in pregnancy; however, maternal disease, differences in specific agents used, and the low rates of exposure limit the interpretation of the available data (Godfrey, 2012; Lecarpentier, 2012). Cholesterol biosynthesis may be important in fetal development; serum cholesterol and triglycerides increase normally during pregnancy. The discontinuation of lipid lowering medications temporarily during pregnancy is not expected to have significant impact on the long term outcomes of primary hypercholesterolemia treatment.

Use of atorvastatin is contraindicated in pregnancy or those who may become pregnant. HMG-CoA reductase inhibitors should be discontinued prior to pregnancy (ADA, 2013). If treatment of dyslipidemias is needed in pregnant women or in women of reproductive age, other agents are preferred (Berglund, 2012; Stone, 2013). The manufacturer recommends administration to women of childbearing potential only when conception is highly unlikely and patients have been informed of potential hazards.

Breast-Feeding Considerations It is not known if atorvastatin is excreted into breast milk. Due to the potential for serious adverse reactions in a nursing infant, use while breast-feeding is contraindicated by the manufacturer.

Contraindications Hypersensitivity to atorvastatin or any component; active liver disease; unexplained persistent elevations of serum transaminases; pregnancy; breast-feeding

Warnings Patients receiving HMG-CoA reductase inhibitors have developed rhabdomyolysis with or without acute renal failure and/or myopathy; patients should be monitored closely; risk is dose-related and is increased with concurrent use of other lipid-lowering medications (eg, fibric acid derivatives or niacin at doses >1 g/day) or during concurrent use with potent CYP3A4 inhibitor or large quantities of grapefruit juice (>1 quart/day). With concurrent use of erythromycin, clarithromycin, itraconazole, and protease inhibitors (eg, lopinavir, ritonavir); dosage reductions of atorvastatin recommended. Avoid use with cyclosporine, tipranivir plus ritonavir, or telaprevir. Ensure patient is on the lowest effective atorvastatin dose in all circumstances. Discontinue in any patient in which CPK levels are markedly elevated (>10 times ULN) or if myopathy is suspected/diagnosed; monitoring of CPK may be warranted, but may not prevent severe myopathy. The manufacturer recommends temporary discontinuation for elective major surgery, acute medical or surgical conditions, or in any patient experiencing an acute or serious condition predisposing to renal failure (eg, sepsis, hypotension, trauma, uncontrolled seizures). However, based upon current evidence, HMG-CoA reductase inhibitor therapy should be continued in the perioperative period unless risk outweighs cardioprotective benefit. Use caution in patients with renal impairment, inadequately treated hypothyroidism, and those taking other drugs associated with myopathy (eg, colchicine); these patients are predisposed to myopathy. Patients should be instructed to report unexplained muscle pain, tenderness, weakness, or brown urine.

An autoimmune-mediated myopathy (IMNM), has been reported (rarely) with HMG-CoA reductase inhibitor therapy; presents as proximal muscle weakness with elevated CPK levels, which persists despite discontinuation of HMG-CoA reductase inhibitor therapy; additionally, muscle biopsy may show necrotizing myopathy with limited inflammation; immunosuppressive therapy (eg, corticosteroids, azathioprine) may be used for treatment. Patients with a history of hemorrhagic stroke may be at increased risk for another when taking atorvastatin. Tablets contain polysorbate 80 (Tween 80®) which may cause allergic reactions in susceptible individuals.

Postmarketing reports of fatal and nonfatal hepatic failure are rare; if serious hepatotoxicity with clinical symptoms and/or hyperbilirubinemia or jaundice occurs during treatment, interrupt therapy. If an alternate etiology is not identified, do not restart atorvastatin. Liver enzyme tests should be obtained at baseline and as clinically indicated; routine periodic monitoring of liver enzymes is not necessary. Use with caution in patients with history of heavy alcohol use or a previous history of liver disease.

Precautions Increases in Hb A_{1c} and fasting blood glucose have been reported with HMG-CoA reductase inhibitors; however, the benefits of statin therapy far outweigh the risk of dysglycemia. Secondary causes of hyperlipidemia should be ruled out prior to therapy; has not been studied when the primary lipid abnormality is chylomicron elevation (Fredrickson types I and V).

Although rare, reversible cognitive impairment (including confusion, forgetfulness, amnesia, and memory loss) can occur with HMG-CoA reductase inhibitors. These cognitive symptoms have been reported at variable times during therapy (1 day to years after initiation) and are reversible with discontinuation; resolution usually occurs within ~3 weeks. Cases have not been associated with fixed or progressive dementia; nor have they been associated with age, specific HMG-CoA reductase inhibitor, dose, or concomitant medication use.

Adverse Reactions

Central nervous system: Insomnia

Gastrointestinal: Dyspepsia, nausea

Gastrointestinal: Diarrhea

Genitourinary: Urinary tract infection

Respiratory: Nasopharyngitis

Hepatic: Transaminases increased (with 80 mg/day dosing)

Neuromuscular & skeletal: Arthralgia, limb pain, muscle spasms, musculoskeletal pain, myalgia

Respiratory: Pharyngolaryngeal pain

Rare but important or life-threatening: Alkaline phosphatase increased, alopecia, amnesia (reversible), anaphylaxis, anemia, angioneurotic edema, anorexia, biliary pain, blood glucose increased, blurred vision, bullous rash, bullous rash, bursitis, cholestasis, cholestatic jaundice, cognitive impairment (reversible), colitis, confusion (reversible), CPK increased, depression, diabetes mellitus (new onset), dizziness, duodenal ulcer, dysphagia, ecchymosis, emotional lability, epistaxis, eructation, erythema multiforme, esophagitis, fatigue, flatulence, gastritis, gastroenteritis, gingival hemorrhage, glossitis, glycosylated hemoglobin (Hb A_{1c}) increased, hematuria, hepatic failure, hepatitis, hyper-/hypoglycemia, incoordination, jaundice, joint swelling, leg cramps, malaise, melena, memory disturbance (reversible), memory impairment (reversible), metrorrhagia, migraine, muscle fatigue, myasthenia, myopathy, myositis, neck pain, neck rigidity, nephritis, nightmare, pancreatitis, paresthesia, parosmia, peripheral neuropathy, petechiae, photosensitivity, pruritus, rectal hemorrhage, rhabdomyolysis, Stevens-Johnson syndrome, stomatitis, syncope, taste loss, taste perversion, tendinous contracture, tendon rupture, tenesmus, thrombocytopenia, tinnitus, torticollis, toxic epidermal necrolysis, urticaria, vaginal hemorrhage, vomiting

Additional class-related events or case reports (not necessarily reported with atorvastatin therapy): Cataracts, cirrhosis, dermatomyositis, eosinophilia, erectile dysfunction, extraocular muscle movement impaired, fulminant hepatic necrosis, gynecomastia, hemolytic anemia, immune-mediated necrotizing myopathy (IMNM), interstitial lung disease, ophthalmoplegia, peripheral nerve palsy, polymyalgia rheumatica, positive ANA, renal failure (secondary to rhabdomyolysis), systemic lupus erythematosus-like syndrome, thyroid dysfunction, tremor, vasculitis, vertigo

Drug Interactions

Metabolism/Transport Effects Substrate of CYP3A4 (major), P-glycoprotein, SLCO1B1; **Note:** Assignment of Major/Minor substrate status based on clinically relevant drug interaction potential; **Inhibits** CYP3A4 (weak), P-glycoprotein

Avoid Concomitant Use

Avoid concomitant use of AtorvaSTATin with any of the following: Bosutinib; Conivaptan; CycloSPORINE (Systemic); Fusidic Acid (Systemic); Gemfibrozil; PAZOPanib; Pimozide; Posaconazole; Red Yeast Rice; Silodosin; Telaprevir; Tipranavir; Topotecan; VinCRIStine (Liposomal)

Increased Effect/Toxicity

AtorvaSTATin may increase the levels/effects of: Afatinib; Aliskiren; ARIPiprazole; Bosutinib; Brentuximab Vedotin; Cimetidine; Colchicine; DAPTOmycin; Digoxin; Diltiazem; Dofetilide; DOXOrubicin (Conventional); Everolimus; Ketoconazole (Systemic); Lomitapide; Midazolam; PAZOPanib; P-glycoprotein/ABCB1 Substrates; Pimozide; Prucalopride; Rifaximin; Rivaroxaban; Silodosin; Spironolactone; Topotecan; Trabectedin; Verapamil; VinCRIStine (Liposomal)

The levels/effects of AtorvaSTATin may be increased by: Amiodarone; Azithromycin (Systemic); Bezafibrate; Boceprevir; Ceritinib; Clarithromycin; Cobicistat; Colchicine; Conivaptan; CycloSPORINE (Systemic); CYP3A4 Inhibitors (Moderate); CYP3A4 Inhibitors (Strong); Cyproterone; Danazol; Dasatinib; Diltiazem; Dronedarone; Eltrombopag; Erythromycin (Systemic); Fenofibrate and Derivatives; Fluconazole; Fusidic Acid (Systemic); Gemfibrozil; Grapefruit Juice; Itraconazole; Ivacaftor; Ketoconazole (Systemic); Luliconazole; Mifepristone; Niacin; Niacinamide; P-glycoprotein/ABCB1 Inhibitors; Posaconazole; Protease Inhibitors; QuiNINE; Raltegravir; Ranolazine; Red Yeast Rice; Sildenafil; Simeprevir; Stiripentol; Telaprevir; Telithromycin; Tipranavir; Voriconazole

Decreased Effect

AtorvaSTATin may decrease the levels/effects of: Dabigatran Etexilate; Lanthanum

The levels/effects of AtorvaSTATin may be decreased by: Antacids; Bexarotene (Systemic); Bile Acid Sequestrants; Bosentan; CYP3A4 Inducers (Strong); Dabrafenib; Deferasirox; Efavirenz; Etravirine; Fosphenytoin; Mitotane; P-glycoprotein/ABCB1 Inducers; Phenytoin; Rifamycin Derivatives; Siltuximab; St Johns Wort; Tocilizumab

Food Interactions Atorvastatin serum concentrations may be increased by grapefruit juice. Management: Avoid concurrent intake of large quantities of grapefruit juice (>1 quart/day).

Stability Store at 20°C to 25°C (68°F to 77°F); dispense in a tightly closed container.

Mechanism of Action Inhibitor of 3-hydroxy-3-methylglutaryl coenzyme A (HMG-CoA) reductase, the rate-limiting enzyme in cholesterol synthesis (reduces the production of mevalonic acid from HMG-CoA); this then results in a compensatory increase in the expression of LDL receptors on hepatocyte membranes and a stimulation of LDL catabolism

Pharmacodynamics

Onset of action: Within 2 weeks

Maximum effect: After 4 weeks

LDL reduction: 10 mg/day: 39% (for each doubling of this dose, LDL is lowered approximately 6%)

Pharmacokinetics (Adult data unless noted)

Absorption: Oral: Rapidly absorbed; extensive first-pass metabolism in GI mucosa and liver

Distribution: V_d: ~381 L

Protein binding: >98%

Metabolism: Extensive metabolism to ortho- and parahydroxylated derivatives and various beta-oxidation products with equivalent *in vitro* activity to atorvastatin; plasma concentrations are elevated in patients with chronic alcoholic liver disease and Childs-Pugh class A and B liver disease

Bioavailability: Absolute: 14%

Half-life: 14 hours (half-life of inhibitory activity due to active metabolites is 20-30 hours)

Time to peak serum concentration: 1-2 hours

Elimination: Primarily in bile following hepatic and/or extrahepatic metabolism; does not appear to undergo enterohepatic recirculation; <2% excreted in urine

Dialysis: Due to the high protein binding, atorvastatin is not expected to be cleared by dialysis (not studied)

Dosing: Usual Dosage should be individualized according to the baseline LDL-C level, the recommended goal of therapy, and patient response; adjustments should be made at intervals of 4 weeks (adults: 2-4 weeks).

Children and Adolescents:

Heterozygous familial and nonfamilial hypercholesterolemia: Oral: **Note:** Begin treatment if after adequate trial of diet, the following are present: LDL-C ≥190 mg/dL or LDL-C remains ≥160 mg/dL and positive family history of premature cardiovascular disease or meets NCEP classification (NHLBI 2011). Therapy may be considered for children 8-9 years of age meeting the above criteria or for children with diabetes mellitus and LDL-C ≥130 mg/dL (Daniels, 2008).

Children 6-10 years of age (Tanner stage I): Limited data available: Initial: 5 mg once daily; if LDL-C target not achieved after 4 weeks may increase to maximum daily dose: 10 mg/**day**; dosing based on trial which included 13 patients as part of a larger study population (n=45); efficacy and tolerability were similar to a group of children age 10-17 years receiving 10-20 mg/day (Gandelman, 2011)

Children and Adolescents 10-17 years: Initial: 10 mg once daily; if LDL-C target not achieved after 4 weeks may increase to a maximum daily dose: 20 mg/**day**; doses >20 mg have not been studied

Hyperlipidemia: Oral: Children and Adolescents 10-17 years (males and postmenarchal females): Initial: 10 mg once daily; if LDL-C target not achieved after 1-3 months, may increase to a maximum daily dose: 20 mg/**day**; doses >20 mg have not been studied (McCrindle, 2007; NHLBI, 2011)

Prevention of graft coronary artery disease: Limited data available: Oral: Children and Adolescents: 0.2 mg/kg/day rounded to nearest 2.5 mg increment; not to exceed age-appropriate doses (Chin, 2002; Chin, 2008)

Adults:

Hypercholesterolemia (heterozygous familial and nonfamilial) and mixed hyperlipidemia (Fredrickson types IIa and IIb): Oral: Initial: 10-20 mg once daily; patients requiring >45% reduction in LDL-C may be started at 40 mg once daily; range: 10-80 mg once daily

Homozygous familial hypercholesterolemia: Oral: 10-80 mg once daily

Dosage adjustment for atorvastatin with concomitant medications: Adults:

Boceprevir, nelfinavir: Use lowest effective atorvastatin dose (not to exceed 40 mg daily)

Clarithromycin, itraconazole, fosamprenavir, ritonavir (plus darunavir, fosamprenavir, or saquinavir): Use lowest effective atorvastatin dose (not to exceed 20 mg daily)

Dosing adjustment in renal impairment: Children ≥10 years, Adolescents, and Adults: Because atorvastatin does not undergo significant renal excretion, dose modification is not necessary.

Dosing adjustment in hepatic impairment: There are no dosage adjustments provided in the manufacturer labeling; contraindicated in active liver disease or in patients with unexplained persistent elevations of serum transaminases.

Administration Oral: May be taken without regard to meals or time of day

Monitoring Parameters

Pediatric patients: Baseline: ALT, AST, and creatine phosphokinase levels (CPK); fasting lipid panel (FLP) and repeat ALT and AST should be checked after 4 weeks of therapy; if no myopathy symptoms or laboratory abnormalities, then monitor FLP, ALT, and AST every 3-4 months during the first year and then every 6 months thereafter (NHLBI, 2011)

Adults: Baseline CPK (recheck CPK in any patient with symptoms suggestive of myopathy; discontinue therapy if markedly elevated); baseline liver function tests (LFTs) and repeat when clinically indicated thereafter. Patients with elevated transaminase levels should have a second (confirmatory) test and frequent monitoring until values normalize; discontinue if increase in ALT/AST is persistently >3 times ULN (NCEP, 2002)

Lipid panel (total cholesterol, HDL, LDL, triglycerides):

ATP III recommendations (NCEP, 2002): Baseline; 6-8 weeks after initiation of drug therapy; if dose increased, then at 6-8 weeks until final dose determined. Once treatment goal achieved, follow-up intervals may be reduced to every 4-6 months. Lipid panel should be assessed at least annually, and preferably at each clinic visit.

Manufacturer recommendation: Analyze lipid panel at initiation and 2-4 weeks after each titration.

Dosage Forms Excipient information presented when available (limited, particularly for generics); consult specific product labeling.

Tablet, Oral:

Lipitor: 10 mg, 20 mg, 40 mg, 80 mg

Generic: 10 mg, 20 mg, 40 mg, 80 mg

References

American Diabetes Association, "Standards of Medical Care in Diabetes-2013," *Diabetes Care*, 2013, 36(Suppl 1):S11-66.

Belay B, Belamarich PF, and Tom-Revzon C, "The Use of Statins in Pediatrics: Knowledge Base, Limitations, and Future Directions," *Pediatrics*, 2007, 119(2):370-80.

Berglund L, Brunzell JD, Goldberg AC, et al, "Evaluation and Treatment of Hypertriglyceridemia: An Endocrine Society Clinical Practice Guideline," *J Clin Endocrinol Metab*, 2012, 97(9):2969-89.

Chin C, Gamberg P, Miller J, et al, "Efficacy and Safety of Atorvastatin After Pediatric Heart Transplantation," *J Heart Lung Transplant*, 2002, 21(11):1213-7.

Chin C, Lukito SS, Shek J, et al, "Prevention of Pediatric Graft Coronary Artery Disease: Atorvastatin," *Pediatr Transplant*, 2008, 12(4):442-6.

Daniels SR, Greer FR, and Committee on Nutrition, "Lipid Screening and Cardiovascular Health in Childhood," *Pediatrics*, 2008, 122 (1):198-208.

"Executive Summary of The Third Report of The National Cholesterol Education Program (NCEP) Expert Panel on Detection, Evaluation, and Treatment of High Blood Cholesterol in Adults (Adult Treatment Panel III)," *JAMA*, 2001, 285(19):2486-97.

Godfrey LM, Erramouspe J, and Cleveland KW, "Teratogenic Risk of Statins in Pregnancy," *Ann Pharmacother*, 2012, 46(10):1419-24.

Lecarpentier E, Morel O, Fournier T, et al, "Statins and Pregnancy: Between Supposed Risks and Theoretical Benefits," *Drugs*, 2012, 72 (6):773-88.

McCrindle BW, Ose L, and Marais AD, "Efficacy and Safety of Atorvastatin in Children and Adolescents With Familial Hypercholesterolemia or Severe Hyperlipidemia: A Multicenter, Randomized, Placebo-Controlled Trial," *J Pediatr*, 2003, 143(1):74-80.

McCrindle BW, Urbina EM, Dennison BA, et al, "Drug Therapy of High-Risk Lipid Abnormalities in Children and Adolescents: A Scientific Statement From the American Heart Association Atherosclerosis, Hypertension, and Obesity in Youth Committee, Council of Cardiovascular Disease in the Young, With the Council on Cardiovascular Nursing," *Circulation*, 2007, 115(14):1948-67.

National Heart, Lung, and Blood Institute, "Expert Panel on Integrated Guidelines for Cardiovascular Health and Risk Reduction in Children and Adolescents," Clinical Practice Guidelines, 2011, National Institutes of Health. Available at http://www.nhlbi.nih.gov/guidelines/cvd_ped/peds_guidelines_full.pdf

"Third Report of the National Cholesterol Education Program Expert Panel on Detection, Evaluation, and Treatment of High Blood Cholesterol in Adults (Adult Treatment Panel III)," May 2001, www.nhlbi.nih.gov/guidelines/cholesterol.

◆ **Atorvastatin Calcium** see AtorvaSTATin on page 227

Atovaquone (a TOE va kwone)

Brand Names: U.S. Mepron
Brand Names: Canada Mepron®
Therapeutic Category Antiprotozoal
Generic Availability (U.S.) Yes

Use Prevention of *Pneumocystis jirovecii* pneumonia (PCP) and second-line treatment of mild to moderate PCP in patients intolerant of trimethoprim/sulfamethoxazole (TMP/SMX) (FDA approved in ages ≥13 years and adults); mild to moderate PCP is defined as an alveolar-arterial oxygen diffusion gradient ≤45 mm Hg and PaO_2 ≥60 mm Hg on room air; patients intolerant of TMP/SMX are defined as having a significant rash (ie, Stevens-Johnson-like syndrome), neutropenia, or hemolysis; has also been used for the treatment of babesiosis and the prevention of first episode of toxoplasmosis in HIV-infected children and adults

Pregnancy Risk Factor C

Pregnancy Considerations Adverse events were observed in animal reproduction studies. Diagnosis and treatment of *Pneumocystis jirovecii* pneumonia (PCP) in pregnant women is the same as in nonpregnant women; however, information specific to the use of atovaquone in pregnancy is limited (DHHS [OI], 2013).

Breast-Feeding Considerations It is not known if atovaquone is excreted in breast milk. The manufacturer recommends that caution be exercised when administering atovaquone to nursing women.

Contraindications Hypersensitivity to atovaquone or any component

Warnings Clinical experience with atovaquone has been limited to patients with mild to moderate PCP; treatment of more severe episodes of PCP has not been systematically studied

Suspension contains benzyl alcohol which may cause allergic reactions in susceptible individuals; large amounts of benzyl alcohol (≥99 mg/kg/day) have been associated with a potentially fatal toxicity ("gasping syndrome") in neonates; the "gasping syndrome" consists of metabolic acidosis, respiratory distress, gasping respirations, CNS dysfunction (including convulsions, intracranial hemorrhage), hypotension and cardiovascular collapse; avoid use in neonates; *in vitro* and animal studies have shown that benzoate, a metabolite of benzyl alcohol, displaces bilirubin from protein binding sites

Precautions For patients who have difficulty taking atovaquone with food or who have chronic diarrhea, stomach or intestinal problems which may result in drug malabsorption, parenteral therapy with other agents should be considered since a low serum atovaquone concentration could lead to treatment failure

Adverse Reactions

Cardiovascular: Hypotension

Central nervous system: Anxiety, depression, dizziness, fever, headache, insomnia, pain

Dermatologic: Pruritus, rash

Endocrine & metabolic: Hyper-/hypoglycemia, hyponatremia

Gastrointestinal: Abdominal pain, amylase increased, anorexia, constipation, diarrhea, heartburn, nausea, taste perversion, vomiting

Hematologic: Anemia, neutropenia

Hepatic: Liver enzymes increased

Neuromuscular & skeletal: Weakness

Renal: BUN increased, creatinine increased

Respiratory: Bronchospasm, cough, dyspnea, rhinitis, sinusitis

Miscellaneous: Oral moniliasis

Rare but important or life-threatening: Acute renal failure, allergic reaction, angioedema, erythema multiforme, hepatitis (rare), hypersensitivity reactions, liver failure (rare), methemoglobinemia, pancreatitis, skin desquamation, Stevens-Johnson syndrome, throat tightness, thrombocytopenia, urticaria, vortex keratopathy

Drug Interactions

Metabolism/Transport Effects None known.

Avoid Concomitant Use

Avoid concomitant use of Atovaquone with any of the following: Efavirenz; Rifamycin Derivatives; Ritonavir

Increased Effect/Toxicity

Atovaquone may increase the levels/effects of: Etoposide

Decreased Effect

Atovaquone may decrease the levels/effects of: Indinavir

The levels/effects of Atovaquone may be decreased by: Efavirenz; Metoclopramide; Rifamycin Derivatives; Ritonavir; Tetracycline

Food Interactions Ingestion with a fatty meal increases absorption. Management: Administer with food, preferably high-fat meals (peanuts or ice cream).

Stability Store at 15°C to 25°C (59°F to 77°F). Do not freeze.

Mechanism of Action Inhibits electron transport in mitochondria resulting in the inhibition of key metabolic enzymes responsible for the synthesis of nucleic acids and ATP

Pharmacokinetics (Adult data unless noted)

Absorption: Oral:

Infants and Children <2 years of age: Decreased absorption

Adults: Oral suspension: Absorption is enhanced 1.4-fold with food; decreased absorption with single doses exceeding 750 mg

Distribution: V_{dss}: 0.6 L/kg; CSF concentration is <1% of the plasma concentration

Protein binding: >99%

Bioavailability: Suspension (administered with food): 47%

Half-life, elimination:

Children (4 months to 12 years): 60 hours (range: 31-163 hours)

Adults: 2.9 days

Adults with AIDS: 2.2 days

Time to peak serum concentration: Dual peak serum concentrations at 1 to 8 hours and at 24 to 96 hours after dose due to enterohepatic cycling

Elimination: ~94% is recovered as unchanged drug in feces; 0.6% excreted in urine

Dosing: Neonatal Oral: *Pneumocystis jirovecii* pneumonia (PCP) (CDC, 2009): Treatment: 30-40 mg/kg/day divided twice daily

Dosing: Usual Oral:

Infants and Children:

Pneumocystis jirovecii pneumonia (PCP) (CDC, 2009):

Treatment:

1 to <3 months: 30-40 mg/kg/day divided twice daily (maximum dose: 1500 mg/day)

3-23 months: 45 mg/kg/day divided twice daily (maximum dose: 1500 mg/day)

≥24 months: 30-40 mg/kg/day divided twice daily (maximum dose: 1500 mg/day)

Prophylaxis:

1-3 months: 30 mg/kg/day once daily (maximum dose: 1500 mg/day)

4-24 months: 45 mg/kg/day once daily (maximum dose: 1500 mg/day)

>24 months: 30 mg/kg/day once daily (maximum dose: 1500 mg/day)

Toxoplasma gondii, prophylaxis (CDC, 2009):

1-3 months: 30 mg/kg once daily (maximum dose: 1500 mg/day)

4-24 months: 45 mg/kg once daily (maximum dose: 1500 mg/day)

>24 months: 30 mg/kg once daily (maximum dose: 1500 mg/day)

Babesiosis: 40 mg/kg/day divided twice daily (maximum dose: 1500 mg/day) with azithromycin 12 mg/kg/day once daily for 7-10 days

Adolescents 13-16 years and Adults:
Pneumocystis jirovecii pneumonia (PCP):
Treatment: 750 mg/dose twice daily for 21 days
Prophylaxis: 1500 mg once daily
Toxoplasma gondii encephalitis (CDC, 2009):
Prophylaxis: 1500 mg once daily
Treatment: 750 mg 4 times daily or 1500 mg twice daily for at least 6 weeks after resolution of signs and symptoms
Suppression after treatment: 750 mg 2-4 times/day
Babesiosis: 750 mg/dose twice daily for 7-10 days with azithromycin; 600 mg once daily for 7-10 days (*Red Book*, 2009)

Administration Oral: Administer with food or a high-fat meal; gently shake suspension before using

Monitoring Parameters CBC with differential, liver enzymes, serum chemistries, serum amylase

Additional Information The suspension contains the inactive ingredient poloxamer 188

Dosage Forms Excipient information presented when available (limited, particularly for generics); consult specific product labeling.
Suspension, Oral:
Mepron: 750 mg/5 mL (5 mL, 210 mL) [contains benzyl alcohol; citrus flavor]
Generic: 750 mg/5 mL (210 mL)

References

Centers for Disease Control and Prevention (CDC), "Guidelines for the Prevention and Treatment of Opportunistic Infections Among HIV-Exposed and HIV-Infected Children," *MMWR Recomm Rep*, 2009, 58(RR-11):1-166. Available at http://aidsinfo.nih.gov/contentfiles/Pediatric_OI.pdf

DHHS Panel on Opportunistic Infections (OI) in HIV-Infected Adults and Adolescents, "Guidelines for Prevention and Treatment of Opportunistic Infections in HIV-Infected Adults and Adolescents: Recommendations from the Centers for Disease Control and Prevention (CDC), the National Institutes of Health (NIH), and the HIV Medicine Association (HIVMA) of the Infectious Diseases Society of America (IDSA)," May 7, 2013. Available at http://aidsinfo.nih.gov/contentfiles/lvguidelines/adult_oi.pdf

"Guidelines for Prevention and Treatment of Opportunistic Infections in HIV-Infected Adults and Adolescents. Panel on Clinical Practices for Treatment of HIV Infection," June 18, 2008, *MMWR Recomm Rep*, 2009, 58(RR-4). Available at: http://www.aidsinfo.nih.gov.

Haile LG and Flaherty JF, "Atovaquone: A Review," *Ann Pharmacother*, 1993, 27(12):1488-94.

Hughes W, Dorenbaum A, Yogev R, et al, "Phase I Safety and Pharmacokinetics Study of Micronized Atovaquone Human Immunodeficiency Virus-Infected Infants and Children. Pediatric AIDS Clinical Trials Group," *Antimicrob Agents Chemother*, 1998, 42(6):1315-8.

Hughes W, Leoung G, Kramer F, et al, "Comparison of Atovaquone (566C80) With Trimethoprim-Sulfamethoxazole to Treat *Pneumocystis carinii* Pneumonia in Patients With AIDS," *N Engl J Med*, 1993, 328 (21):1521-7.

Red Book: 2009 Report of the Committee on Infectious Diseases, 28th ed, Pickering LK, ed, Elk Grove Village, IL: American Academy of Pediatrics, 2009.

Atovaquone and Proguanil
(a TOE va kwone & pro GWA nil)

Brand Names: U.S. Malarone®
Brand Names: Canada Malarone®; Malarone® Pediatric
Therapeutic Category Antimalarial Agent
Generic Availability (U.S.) Yes: Excludes pediatric strength tablet
Use Prevention (FDA approved in pediatric patients >11 kg and adults) or treatment (FDA approved in pediatric patients >5 kg and adults) of acute, uncomplicated *P. falciparum* malaria, including chloroquine-resistant *P. falciparum*

Pregnancy Risk Factor C

Pregnancy Considerations Teratogenic effects were not observed with the combination of atovaquone/proguanil in animal reproduction studies using concentrations similar to the estimated human exposure. The pharmacokinetics of atovaquone and proguanil are changed during pregnancy.

Malaria infection in pregnant women may be more severe than in nonpregnant women. Because *P. falciparum* malaria can cause maternal death and fetal loss, pregnant women traveling to malaria-endemic areas must use personal protection against mosquito bites. Atovaquone/proguanil may be used as an alternative treatment of malaria in pregnant women; consult current CDC guidelines.

Breast-Feeding Considerations Small quantities of proguanil are found in breast milk. This combination is not recommended if nursing infants <5 kg (safety data is limited concerning therapeutic use in infants <5 kg)

Contraindications Hypersensitivity to atovaquone, proguanil, or any component of the formulation; prophylactic use in severe renal impairment (CrCl <30 mL/minute)

Warnings Liver function test abnormalities and hepatitis have been reported with use. One case of hepatic failure has been reported. Not indicated for severe or complicated malaria.

Precautions Absorption of atovaquone may be decreased in patients who have diarrhea or vomiting; monitor closely and consider use of an antiemetic. If severe, consider use of an alternative antimalarial. Delayed cases of *P. falciparum* malaria may occur after stopping prophylaxis; travelers returning from endemic areas who develop febrile illnesses should be evaluated for malaria. Recrudescent infections or infections following prophylaxis with this agent should be treated with alternative agent(s). Use with caution in patients with preexisting renal disease. Parasite relapse is common when used to treat *P. vivax*.

Adverse Reactions The following adverse reactions were reported in patients being treated for malaria. When used for prophylaxis, reactions are similar to those seen with placebo.

Central nervous system: Dizziness, headache
Dermatologic: Pruritus
Gastrointestinal: Abdominal pain, anorexia, diarrhea, nausea, vomiting
Hepatic: Transaminase increases (increased LFT values typically normalized after ~4 weeks)
Neuromuscular & skeletal: Weakness
Rare but important or life-threatening: Anaphylaxis (rare), anemia (rare), angioedema, cholestasis, erythema multiforme (rare), hallucinations, hepatitis (rare), hepatic failure (case report), neutropenia, pancytopenia (with severe renal impairment), photosensitivity, psychotic episodes (rare), rash, seizure (rare), Stevens-Johnson syndrome (rare), stomatitis, urticaria, vasculitis (rare)

Drug Interactions
Metabolism/Transport Effects None known.
Avoid Concomitant Use
Avoid concomitant use of Atovaquone and Proguanil with any of the following: Artemether; Efavirenz; Lumefantrine; Rifamycin Derivatives; Ritonavir

Increased Effect/Toxicity
Atovaquone and Proguanil may increase the levels/effects of: Antipsychotic Agents (Phenothiazines); Dapsone (Systemic); Dapsone (Topical); Etoposide; Lumefantrine; Warfarin

The levels/effects of Atovaquone and Proguanil may be increased by: Artemether; Dapsone (Systemic)

Decreased Effect
Atovaquone and Proguanil may decrease the levels/effects of: Indinavir

The levels/effects of Atovaquone and Proguanil may be decreased by: Efavirenz; Metoclopramide; Rifamycin Derivatives; Ritonavir; Tetracycline

Food Interactions Atovaquone taken with dietary fat significantly increases the rate and extent of absorption; AUC is increased 2-3 times and C_{max} is increased 5 times as compared to administration during a fasted state.

Management: Administer with food or milk-based drink at the same time each day.

Stability Store tablets at 25°C (77°F)

Mechanism of Action

Atovaquone: Selectively inhibits parasite mitochondrial electron transport.

Proguanil: The metabolite cycloguanil inhibits dihydrofolate reductase, disrupting deoxythymidylate synthesis. Together, atovaquone/cycloguanil affect the erythrocytic and exoerythrocytic stages of development.

Pharmacokinetics (Adult data unless noted)

Atovaquone: See Atovaquone monograph.

Proguanil:

Absorption: Extensive

Distribution: V_d: Pediatric patients: 42 L/kg

Protein binding: 75%

Metabolism: Hepatic to active metabolites, cycloguanil (via CYP2C19) and 4-chlorophenylbiguanide

Half-life elimination: 12-21 hours

Elimination: Urine (40% to 60%)

Dosing: Usual Oral:

Children (dosage based on body weight):

Prevention of malaria: Start 1-2 days prior to entering a malaria-endemic area, continue throughout the stay and for 7 days after leaving area. Take as a single dose, once daily. **Note:** AAP (*Red Book*, 2009) states that atovaquone and proguanil can be used for prevention in a child ≥5 kg if travel cannot be avoided to areas where chloroquine-resistant *P. falciparum* exists.

5-8 kg: Atovaquone/proguanil: 31.25 mg/12.5 mg

9-10 kg: Atovaquone/proguanil: 46.88 mg/18.75 mg

Manufacturer's dosing:

11-20 kg: Atovaquone/proguanil 62.5 mg/25 mg

21-30 kg: Atovaquone/proguanil 125 mg/50 mg

31-40 kg: Atovaquone/proguanil 187.5 mg/75 mg

>40 kg: Atovaquone/proguanil 250 mg/100 mg

Treatment of acute malaria: Take as a single dose, once daily for 3 consecutive days.

5-8 kg: Atovaquone/proguanil 125 mg/50 mg

9-10 kg: Atovaquone/proguanil 187.5 mg/75 mg

11-20 kg: Atovaquone/proguanil 250 mg/100 mg

21-30 kg: Atovaquone/proguanil 500 mg/200 mg

31-40 kg: Atovaquone/proguanil 750 mg/300 mg

>40 kg: Atovaquone/proguanil 1 g/400 mg

Adults:

Prevention of malaria: Atovaquone/proguanil 250 mg/100 mg once daily; start 1-2 days prior to entering a malaria-endemic area, continue throughout the stay and for 7 days after leaving area

Treatment of acute malaria: Atovaquone/proguanil 1 g/400 mg as a single dose, once daily for 3 consecutive days. **Note:** Consultants recommend dividing the daily dose in 2 to decrease nausea and vomiting.

Dosage adjustment in renal impairment: Should not be used as prophylaxis in severe renal impairment (CrCl <30 mL/minute). For treatment of malaria, alternative regimens should be used in patients with CrCl <30 mL/minute unless benefits outweigh the risks. No dosage adjustment required in mild to moderate renal impairment.

Dosage adjustment in hepatic impairment: No dosage adjustment required in mild to moderate hepatic impairment. No data available for use in severe hepatic impairment.

Administration Administer with food or milk at the same time each day. If vomiting occurs within 1 hour of administration, repeat the dose. Tablets are not palatable if chewed due to bitter taste. For children who have difficulty swallowing tablets, tablets may be crushed and mixed with condensed milk just prior to administration.

Dosage Forms Excipient information presented when available (limited, particularly for generics); consult specific product labeling.

Tablet, oral: Atovaquone 250 mg and proguanil hydrochloride 100 mg

Malarone®: Atovaquone 250 mg and proguanil hydrochloride 100 mg

Tablet, oral [pediatric]:

Malarone®: Atovaquone 62.5 mg and proguanil hydrochloride 25 mg

References

Centers for Disease Control and Prevention (CDC), "Guidelines for the Prevention and Treatment of Opportunistic Infections Among HIV-Exposed and HIV-Infected Children," *MMWR Recomm Rep*, 2009, 58(RR-11):1-166. Available at http://aidsinfo.nih.gov/contentfiles/Pediatric_OI.pdf

Red Book: 2009 Report of the Committee on Infectious Diseases, 28th ed, Pickering LK, ed, Elk Grove Village, IL: American Academy of Pediatrics, 2009, 98-104.

♦ **Atovaquone and Proguanil Hydrochloride** see Atovaquone and Proguanil *on page 231*

♦ **ATRA** see Tretinoin (Systemic) *on page 2068*

Atracurium (a tra KYOO ree um)

Medication Safety Issues

High alert medication:

The Institute for Safe Medication Practices (ISMP) includes this medication among its list of drugs which have a heightened risk of causing significant patient harm when used in error.

Other safety concerns:

United States Pharmacopeia (USP) 2006: The Interdisciplinary Safe Medication Use Expert Committee of the USP has recommended the following:

- Hospitals, clinics, and other practice sites should institute special safeguards in the storage, labeling, and use of these agents and should include these safeguards in staff orientation and competency training.

- Healthcare professionals should be on **high alert** (especially vigilant) whenever a neuromuscular-blocking agent (NMBA) is stocked, ordered, prepared, or administered.

Brand Names: Canada Atracurium Besylate Injection

Therapeutic Category Neuromuscular Blocker Agent, Nondepolarizing; Skeletal Muscle Relaxant, Paralytic

Generic Availability (U.S.) Yes

Use Adjunct to general anesthesia, to facilitate endotracheal intubation, and to provide skeletal muscle relaxation during surgery or mechanical ventilation (FDA approved in ages ≥1 month and adults)

Pregnancy Risk Factor C

Pregnancy Considerations Adverse events were observed in animal reproduction studies. Small amounts of atracurium have been shown to cross the placenta when given to women during cesarean section.

Breast-Feeding Considerations It is not known if atracurium is excreted in breast milk. The manufacturer recommends that caution be exercised when administering atracurium to nursing women.

Contraindications Hypersensitivity to atracurium besylate or any component

Warnings Ventilation must be supported during neuromuscular blockade; atracurium should only be administered by individuals who are experienced in the maintenance of an adequate airway and respiratory support. Atracurium does not alter consciousness; use in conjunction with adequate sedation or anesthesia. Severe allergic reactions have been reported with neuromuscular-blocking agents including atracurium; cross-sensitivity with other neuromuscular-blocking agents may occur; use extreme caution in patients with previous anaphylactic reactions. Reduce initial dosage and inject slowly (over 1-2 minutes) in patients in whom substantial histamine release would be potentially hazardous (eg, patients with clinically important cardiovascular disease); maintenance of an adequate airway and respiratory support is critical.

Some formulations may contain benzyl alcohol which may cause allergic reactions in susceptible individuals; large amounts of benzyl alcohol (≥99 mg/kg/day) have been associated with a potentially fatal toxicity ("gasping syndrome") in neonates; the "gasping syndrome" consists of metabolic acidosis, respiratory distress, gasping respirations, CNS dysfunction (including convulsions, intracranial hemorrhage), hypotension and cardiovascular collapse; avoid use of atracurium products containing benzyl alcohol in neonates; use preservative free product; *in vitro* and animal studies have shown that benzoate, a metabolite of benzyl alcohol, displaces bilirubin from protein binding sites; avoid use of preservative-containing formulation in neonates.

Precautions Certain clinical conditions may result in potentiation or antagonism of neuromuscular blockade, see table. Increased sensitivity in patients with myasthenia gravis, Eaton-Lambert syndrome; resistance to neuromuscular blockade in burn patients (>30% of body) for period of 5-70 days postinjury; resistance in patients with muscle trauma, denervation, immobilization, infection, and prolonged treatment with atracurium. When used in conjunction with anesthetics, bradycardia may be more common with atracurium than with other neuromuscular blocking agents; it has no clinically significant effects on heart rate to counteract the bradycardia produced by anesthetics.

Clinical Conditions Affecting Neuromuscular Blockade

Potentiation	Antagonism
Acidosis	Alkalosis
Acute intermittent porphyria	Demyelinating lesions
Electrolyte abnormalities	Diabetes mellitus
Hypermagnesemia	Hypercalcemia
Severe hyponatremia	Peripheral neuropathies
Severe hypocalcemia	
Severe hypokalemia	
Hepatic failure	
Neuromuscular diseases	
Renal failure	

Adverse Reactions Mild, rare, and generally suggestive of histamine release

Cardiovascular: Flushing

Rare but important or life-threatening: Bronchial secretions, erythema, hives, itching, wheezing

Postmarketing and/or case reports: Acute quadriplegic myopathy syndrome (prolonged use), allergic reaction, bradycardia, bronchospasm, dyspnea, hypotension, injection site reaction, laryngospasm, myositis ossificans (prolonged use), seizure, tachycardia, urticaria

Causes of prolonged neuromuscular blockade: Accumulation of active metabolites; cumulative drug effect; metabolism/excretion decreased (hepatic and/or renal impairment); electrolyte imbalance (hypokalemia, hypocalcemia, hypermagnesemia, hypernatremia); excessive drug administration; hypothermia

Drug Interactions

Metabolism/Transport Effects None known.

Avoid Concomitant Use

Avoid concomitant use of Atracurium with any of the following: QuiNINE

Increased Effect/Toxicity

Atracurium may increase the levels/effects of: Cardiac Glycosides; Corticosteroids (Systemic); OnabotulinumtoxinA; RimabotulinumtoxinB

The levels/effects of Atracurium may be increased by: AbobotulinumtoxinA; Aminoglycosides; Calcium Channel Blockers; Capreomycin; Clindamycin (Topical); Colistimethate; CycloSPORINE (Systemic); Fosphenytoin-Phenytoin; Inhalational Anesthetics; Ketorolac (Nasal); Ketorolac (Systemic); Lincosamide Antibiotics; Lithium; Loop Diuretics; Magnesium Salts; Polymyxin B; Procainamide; QuiNIDine; QuiNINE; Spironolactone; Tetracycline Derivatives; Vancomycin

Decreased Effect

The levels/effects of Atracurium may be decreased by: Acetylcholinesterase Inhibitors; Fosphenytoin-Phenytoin; Loop Diuretics

Stability Store intact vials at 2°C to 8°C (36°F to 46°F); protect from freezing; use vials within 14 days upon removal from the refrigerator to room temperature of 25°C (77°F). Unstable in alkaline solutions; compatible with D_5W, D_5NS, and NS; dilutions of 0.2 mg/mL or 0.5 mg/mL are stable for up to 24 hours at room temperature or under refrigeration; do not dilute in LR.

Mechanism of Action Blocks neural transmission at the myoneural junction by binding with cholinergic receptor sites

Pharmacodynamics

Onset of action: I.V.: 1-4 minutes

Maximum effect: Within 3-5 minutes

Duration: Recovery begins in 20-35 minutes when anesthesia is balanced

Pharmacokinetics (Adult data unless noted)

Distribution: V_d:

Infants: 0.21 L/kg

Children: 0.13 L/kg

Adults: 0.1 L/kg

Metabolism: Some metabolites are active; undergoes rapid nonenzymatic degradation (Hofmann elimination) in the bloodstream; additional metabolism occurs via ester hydrolysis

Half-life: Elimination:

Infants: 20 minutes

Children: 17 minutes

Adults: 16 minutes

Elimination: Clearance:

Infants: 7.9 mL/kg/minute

Children: 6.8 mL/kg/minute

Adults: 5.3 mL/kg/minute

Dosing: Neonatal Paralysis/skeletal muscle relaxation: I.V.: 0.25-0.4 mg/kg initially followed by maintenance doses of 0.25 mg/kg as needed to maintain neuromuscular blockade **or** a continuous I.V. infusion 0.4 mg/kg/**hour** (Clarkson, 2001; Kalli, 1988); **Note:** Higher intermittent doses (eg, 0.5 mg/kg) have been associated with toxicity and fatal outcomes in premature neonates (Clarkson, 2001)

Dosing: Usual Paralysis/skeletal muscle relaxation:

Infants and Children ≤2 years:

I.V.: 0.3-0.4 mg/kg initially followed by maintenance doses of 0.3-0.4 mg/kg as needed to maintain neuromuscular blockade

Continuous I.V. infusion: 0.6-1.2 mg/kg/**hour** or 10-20 **mcg**/kg/minute

Children >2 years to Adults:

I.V.: 0.4-0.5 mg/kg then 0.08-0.1 mg/kg 20-45 minutes after initial dose to maintain neuromuscular block; repeat dose at 15- to 25-minute intervals

Continuous I.V. infusion: Initial: 0.54-0.6 mg/kg/**hour** or 9-10 **mcg**/kg/minute at initial signs of recovery from bolus dose; block is usually maintained by a rate of 0.3-0.54 mg/kg/**hour** or 5-9 **mcg**/kg/minute (range: 0.1-0.9 mg/kg/**hour** or 2-15 **mcg**/kg/minute).

Dosage adjustment in hepatic or renal impairment: Not necessary

Dosage adjustment with enflurane or isoflurane: Reduce dosage by 33%

Dosage adjustment with induced hypothermia (cardiobypass surgery): Reduce dosage by 50%

Administration Parenteral: May be administered without further dilution by rapid I.V. injection; for continuous I.V. infusions, dilute to a maximum concentration of 0.5 mg/mL (more concentrated solutions have reduced stability, ie, <24 hours at room temperature); not for I.M. injection due to tissue irritation

Monitoring Parameters Muscle twitch response to peripheral nerve stimulation, heart rate, blood pressure, assisted ventilation status

Additional Information Neuromuscular blockade may be reversed with neostigmine; atropine or glycopyrrolate should be available to treat excessive cholinergic effects from neostigmine

Dosage Forms Excipient information presented when available (limited, particularly for generics); consult specific product labeling.

Solution, Intravenous, as besylate:
Generic: 50 mg/5 mL (5 mL); 100 mg/10 mL (10 mL)
Solution, Intravenous, as besylate [preservative free]:
Generic: 50 mg/5 mL (5 mL)

References

Clarkson A, Choonara I, and Martin P, "Suspected Toxicity of Atracurium in the Neonate," *Paediatr Anaesth*, 2001, 11(5):631-2.

Kalli I and Meretoja OA, "Infusion of Atracurium in Neonates, Infants and Children. A Study of Dose Requirements," *Br J Anaesth*, 1988, 60 (6):651-4.

Martin LD, Bratton SL, and O'Rourke PP, "Clinical Uses and Controversies of Neuromuscular Blocking Agents in Infants and Children," *Crit Care Med*, 1999, 27(7):1358-68.

◆ **Atracurium Besylate** see Atracurium on page 232

◆ **Atracurium Besylate Injection (Can)** see Atracurium on page 232

◆ **Atralin** see Tretinoin (Topical) on page 2071

◆ **Atriance™ (Can)** see Nelarabine on page 1477

◆ **Atripla** see Efavirenz, Emtricitabine, and Tenofovir on page 735

◆ **AtroPen** see Atropine on page 234

Atropine (A troe peen)

Medication Safety Issues

BEERS Criteria medication:
This drug may be potentially inappropriate for use in geriatric patients (Quality of evidence - varies based on comorbidity; Strength of recommendation - varies based on comorbidity)

Related Information

Adult ACLS Algorithms on page 2198
Pediatric ALS (PALS) Algorithms on page 2195

Brand Names: U.S. AtroPen; Atropine-Care; Isopto Atropine

Brand Names: Canada Dioptic's Atropine Solution; Isopto® Atropine

Therapeutic Category Antiasthmatic; Anticholinergic Agent; Anticholinergic Agent, Ophthalmic; Antidote; Organophosphate Poisoning; Antispasmodic Agent, Gastrointestinal; Bronchodilator; Ophthalmic Agent, Mydriatic

Generic Availability (U.S.) May be product dependent

Use

Parenteral:
Auto-injector: Antidote for anticholinesterase poisoning (carbamate insecticides, nerve agents, organophosphate insecticides, muscarinic poisoning) (FDA approved in all ages)
Injection: Preoperative medication to inhibit salivation and secretions; treatment of symptomatic sinus bradycardia, AV block (nodal level) adjuvant use with anticholinesterases (eg, edrophonium, neostigmine) to decrease their side effects during reversal of

neuromuscular blockade [All indications: FDA approved in pediatric patients (age not specified) and adults];
Note: Use is no longer recommended in the management of asystole or pulseless electrical activity (PEA) (ACLS, 2010)

Ophthalmic: Produce mydriasis and cycloplegia for examination of the retina and optic disc and accurate measurement of refractive errors; produce papillary dilation in inflammatory conditions (eg, uveitis) (All indications: FDA approved in adults; refer to product-specific information regarding FDA approval in pediatric patients)

Prescribing and Access Restrictions The AtroPen® formulation is available for use primarily by the Department of Defense.

Pregnancy Risk Factor B/C (manufacturer specific)

Pregnancy Considerations Animal reproduction studies have not been conducted. Atropine has been found to cross the human placenta.

Breast-Feeding Considerations Trace amounts of atropine are excreted into breast milk. Anticholinergic agents may suppress lactation.

Contraindications Hypersensitivity to atropine sulfate or any component; narrow-angle glaucoma
Additional contraindications:
Injection: Pyloric stenosis, prostatic hypertrophy; asthma (I.V. use for treatment); pediatric patients who have previously had a severe systemic reaction to atropine; **Note:** For the treatment of life-threatening organophosphate or carbamate insecticide or nerve agent poisoning, there are no contraindications
Ophthalmic: Predisposition to glaucoma, adhesions between the iris and lens

Warnings The AtroPen formulation is available for use primarily by the Department of Defense as an initial treatment of the muscarinic symptoms of insecticide or nerve agent poisoning; its use should be reserved for individuals who have had adequate training in the recognition and treatment of this type of intoxication. Atropine reverses the muscarinic but not the nicotinic effects associated with anticholinesterase toxicity. Clinical symptoms consistent with highly suspected organophosphate or carbamate insecticides or nerve agent poisoning should be treated with antidote immediately; administration should not be delayed for confirmatory laboratory tests. Signs of atropinization include flushing, mydriasis, tachycardia, and dryness of the mouth or nose. Monitor effects closely when administering subsequent injections as necessary. The presence of these effects is not indicative of the success of therapy; inappropriate use of mydriasis as an indicator of successful treatment has resulted in atropine toxicity. Reversal of bronchial secretions is the preferred indicator of success. Adjunct treatment with a cholinesterase reactivator (eg, pralidoxime) may be required in patients with toxicity secondary to organophosphorus insecticides or nerve agents. Treatment should always include proper evacuation and decontamination procedures; medical personnel should protect themselves from inadvertent contamination. Antidotal administration is intended only for initial management; definitive and more extensive medical care is required following administration. Individuals should not rely solely on antidote for treatment, as other supportive measures (eg, artificial respiration) may still be required.

Parenteral atropine (I.V.) should not be used to treat asthma; the high doses required to treat asthma may cause excessive drying of bronchiolar mucous plugs. Avoid relying on atropine for effective treatment of type II second- or third-degree AV block (with or without a new wide QRS complex). Although no evidence exists for significant detrimental effects, routine use of atropine for asystole or bradycardic PEA is unlikely to have a therapeutic benefit and is no longer recommended (ACLS, 2010).

Pediatric patients are more susceptible to toxic effects of anticholinergic agents than adults; care should be taken to prevent overexposure. Avoid use if possible in patients with obstructive uropathy or in other conditions resulting in urinary retention; use is contraindicated in patients with prostatic hypertrophy. In patients with myasthenia gravis, use atropine with extreme caution when used to treat side effects of acetylcholinesterase inhibition or avoid; may precipitate a myasthenic crisis.

Precautions Use with caution in patients with hepatic or renal impairment; effects of atropine may be prolonged in severe hepatic or renal impairment. Use with caution in presence of high environmental temperature; heat prostration can occur. Use with caution in children with spastic paralysis or brain damage; children are at increased risk for rapid rise in body temperature due to suppression of sweat gland activity. Paradoxical hyperexcitability may occur in children given large doses. Infants with Down's syndrome have both increased sensitivity to cardiac effects and mydriasis. Use with caution in patients with pyloric stenosis or hiatal hernia associated with reflux esophagitis; avoid use in patients with paralytic ileus, intestinal atony of the elderly or debilitated patient, severe ulcerative colitis, and toxic megacolon complicating ulcerative colitis. Use with caution in cardiovascular disease (myocardial ischemia, heart failure, tachyarrhythmias, and/ or hypertension); treatment-related blood pressure increases and tachycardia may lead to ischemia, precipitate an MI, or increase arrhythmogenic potential. In sensitive individuals, psychosis may occur. Use with caution in patients with autonomic neuropathy. Use with caution in patients with hyperthyroidism.

In heart transplant recipients, atropine will likely be ineffective in treatment of bradycardia due to lack of vagal innervation of the transplanted heart. Cholinergic reinnervation may occur over time (years), so atropine may be used cautiously; however, some may experience paradoxical slowing of the heart rate and high-degree AV block upon administration (ACLS, 2010; Bernheim, 2004).

Adverse Reactions Severity and frequency of adverse reactions are dose related and vary greatly; listed reactions are limited to significant and/or life-threatening.

Cardiovascular: Cardiac arrhythmia, flushing, hypotension, palpitations, tachycardia
Central nervous system: Ataxia, coma, delirium, disorientation, dizziness, drowsiness, excitement, hallucination, headache, insomnia, nervousness
Dermatologic: Anhidrosis, scarlatiniform rash, skin rash, urticaria
Gastrointestinal: Ageusia, bloating, constipation, delayed gastric emptying, nausea, paralytic ileus, vomiting, xerostomia
Genitourinary: Urinary hesitancy, urinary retention
Hypersensitivity: Anaphylaxis
Neuromuscular & skeletal: Laryngospasm, weakness
Ocular: Angle-closure glaucoma, blurred vision, cycloplegia, dry eye syndrome, increased intraocular pressure, mydriasis
Respiratory: Dry nose, dry throat, dyspnea, pulmonary edema
Miscellaneous: Fever

Drug Interactions
Metabolism/Transport Effects None known.
Avoid Concomitant Use
Avoid concomitant use of Atropine with any of the following: Aclidinium; Ipratropium (Oral Inhalation); Potassium Chloride; Tiotropium; Umeclidinium

Increased Effect/Toxicity
Atropine may increase the levels/effects of: AbobotulinumtoxinA; Analgesics (Opioid); Anticholinergic Agents; Cannabinoid-Containing Products; Mirabegron; OnabotulinumtoxinA; Potassium Chloride; RimabotulinumtoxinB; Thiazide Diuretics; Tiotropium; Topiramate

The levels/effects of Atropine may be increased by: Aclidinium; Ipratropium (Oral Inhalation); Pramlintide; Umeclidinium
Decreased Effect
Atropine may decrease the levels/effects of: Acetylcholinesterase Inhibitors (Central); Secretin

The levels/effects of Atropine may be decreased by: Acetylcholinesterase Inhibitors (Central)
Stability
Ophthalmic: Store at 20°C to 25°C (68°F to 77°F); keep tightly closed.
Parenteral:
Auto-injector (AtroPen): Store at 25°C (77°F), excursions permitted to 15°C to 30°C (59°F to 86°F); do not freeze; protect from light.
Injection: Store at 20°C to 25°C (68°F to 77°F). Preparation of bulk atropine solution for mass chemical terrorism at a concentration of 1 mg/mL is stable for 72 hours at 4°C to 8°C (39°F to 46°F); 20°C to 25°C (68°F to 77°F); 32°C to 36°C (90°F to 97°F) (Dix, 2003).
Mechanism of Action Blocks the action of acetylcholine at parasympathetic sites in smooth muscle, secretory glands, and the CNS; increases cardiac output, dries secretions. Atropine reverses the muscarinic effects of cholinergic poisoning due to agents with acetylcholinesterase inhibitor activity by acting as a competitive antagonist of acetylcholine at muscarinic receptors. The primary goal in cholinergic poisonings is reversal of bronchorrhea and bronchoconstriction. Atropine has no effect on the nicotinic receptors responsible for muscle weakness, fasciculations, and paralysis.
Pharmacodynamics
Inhibition of salivation:
Onset of action: I.M.: 30 minutes
Maximum effect: I.M.: 1-1.6 hours
Duration: I.M.: Up to 4 hours
Increased heart rate:
Onset of action: I.M.: 5-40 minutes
Maximum effect:
I.M.: 20 minutes to 1 hour
I.V.: 2-4 minutes
Pharmacokinetics (Adult data unless noted)
Absorption: Well absorbed from all dosage forms
Distribution: Widely distributes throughout the body; crosses the blood-brain barrier
Protein binding: 14% to 22%
Metabolism: Hepatic via enzymatic hydrolysis
Half-life:
Children <2 years: 6.9 ± 3 hours
Children >2 years: 2.5 ± 1.2 hours
Adults: 3 ± 0.9 hours
Time to peak serum concentration: I.M.: Auto-injector: 3 minutes
Elimination: Urine (30% to 50% as unchanged drug and metabolites)
Dosing: Neonatal
Bradycardia: Note: Not part of neonatal resuscitation algorithm; some institutions have used the following:
I.V., I.O.: 0.02 mg/kg/dose; use of a minimum dosage of 0.1 mg will result in dosages >0.02 mg/kg and is not recommended (Barrington, 2011); there is no documented minimum dosage in this age group; may repeat once in 3 to 5 minutes; reserve use for those patients unresponsive to improved oxygenation and epinephrine

Endotracheal: 0.04 to 0.06 mg/kg/dose; may repeat once if needed

Inhibit salivation and secretions (preanesthesia): I.M., I.V., SubQ: Patient weight <5 kg: 0.02 mg/kg/dose 30 to 60 minutes preoperatively then every 4 to 6 hours as needed; use of a minimum dosage of 0.1 mg will result in dosages >0.02 mg/kg and is not recommended (Barrington, 2011); there is no documented minimum dosage in this age group

Intubation, nonemergent (preferred vagolytic): I.M., I.V.: 0.02 mg/kg/dose (Kumar, 2010)

Organophosphate or carbamate insecticide or nerve agent poisoning: Note: The dose of atropine required varies considerably with the severity of poisoning. The total amount of atropine used for carbamate poisoning is usually less than with organophosphate insecticide or nerve agent poisoning. Severely poisoned patients may exhibit significant tolerance to atropine; ≥2 times the suggested doses may be needed. Titrate to pulmonary status (decreased bronchial secretions); consider administration of atropine via continuous I.V. infusion in patients requiring large doses of atropine. Once patient is stable for a period of time, the dose/dosing frequency may be decreased. Pralidoxime is a component of the management of organophosphate insecticide and nerve agent toxicity; refer to pralidoxime for the specific route and dose.

I.V., I.M.: Initial: 0.05 to 0.1 mg/kg; repeat every 5 to 10 minutes as needed, doubling the dose if previous dose did not induce atropinization (Hegenbarth, 2008; Reigart, 1999; Rotenberg, 2003). Maintain atropinization by administering repeat doses as needed for ≥2 to 12 hours based on recurrence of symptoms (Reigart, 1999).

Continuous I.V. infusion: Following atropinization (see above), administer 10% to 20% of the total loading dose required to induce atropinization as a continuous I.V. infusion per hour; adjust as needed to maintain adequate atropinization without atropine toxicity (Eddleston, 2004; Roberts, 2007)

I.M.: AtroPen: 0.25 mg (yellow pen):

Mild symptoms (≥2 mild symptoms): Administer one 0.25 mg (yellow pen) dose as soon as an exposure is known or strongly suspected. If severe symptoms develop after the first dose, 2 additional doses should be repeated in rapid succession 10 minutes after the first dose; do not administer more than 3 doses. If profound anticholinergic effects occur in the absence of excessive bronchial secretions, further doses of atropine should be withheld. Mild symptoms of insecticide or nerve agent poisoning, as provided by manufacturer in the AtroPen product labeling to guide therapy, include: Blurred vision, bradycardia, breathing difficulties, chest tightness, coughing, drooling, miosis, muscular twitching, nausea, runny nose, salivation increased, stomach cramps, tachycardia, teary eyes, tremor, vomiting, or wheezing.

Severe symptoms (≥1 severe symptom): Immediately administer **three** 0.25 mg (yellow pen) doses. Severe symptoms of insecticide or nerve agent poisoning, as provided by manufacturer in the AtroPen product labeling to guide therapy, include: Breathing difficulties (severe), confused/strange behavior, defecation (involuntary), muscular twitching/generalized weakness (severe), respiratory secretions (severe), seizure, unconsciousness, urination (involuntary); **Note:** Neonates and infants may become drowsy or unconscious with muscle floppiness as opposed to muscle twitching.

Endotracheal: Increase the dose by 2 to 3 times the usual I.V. dose. Mix with 3 to 5 mL of normal saline and administer. Flush with 3 to 5 mL of NS and follow with 5 assisted manual ventilations (Rotenberg, 2003)

Refraction: Ophthalmic: Instill 1 drop of 0.25% solution 3 times/day for 3 days before the procedure

Uveitis: Ophthalmic: Instill 1 drop of 0.5% solution 1 to 3 times daily

Dosing: Usual
Pediatric:

Bradycardia: Infants, Children, and Adolescents:

I.V., I.O.: 0.02 mg/kg/dose; minimum dose recommended by PALS: 0.1 mg; however, use of a minimum dosage of 0.1 mg in patients <5 kg will result in dosages >0.02 mg/kg and is not recommended (Barrington, 2011); there is no documented minimum dosage in this age group; maximum single dose: 0.5 mg; may repeat once in 3 to 5 minutes; maximum total dose: 1 mg (PALS, 2010).

Endotracheal: 0.04 to 0.06 mg/kg/dose; may repeat once if needed (PALS, 2010)

Inhibit salivation and secretions (preanesthesia): Infants, Children, and Adolescents: I.M., I.V., SubQ: Administer dose 30 to 60 minutes preoperatively then every 4 to 6 hours as needed:

Weight-directed dosing (Nelson, 1996):

Infants weighing <5 kg: 0.02 mg/kg/dose; use of a fixed minimum dosage of 0.1 mg will result in dosages >0.02 mg/kg; there is no documented minimum dosage in this age group

Infants and Children weighing ≥5 kg: 0.01 to 0.02 mg/kg/dose; maximum single dose: 0.4 mg; minimum dose: 0.1 mg

Fixed dosing:

3 to 7 kg (7 to 16 lb): 0.1 mg
8 to 11 kg (17 to 24 lb): 0.15 mg
11 to 18 kg (24 to 40 lb): 0.2 mg
18 to 29 kg (40 to 65 lb): 0.3 mg
≥30 kg (≥65 lb): 0.4 mg

Organophosphate or carbamate insecticide or nerve agent poisoning: Infants, Children, and Adolescents: **Note:** The dose of atropine required varies considerably with the severity of poisoning. The total amount of atropine used for carbamate poisoning is usually less than with organophosphate insecticide or nerve agent poisoning. Severely poisoned patients may exhibit significant tolerance to atropine; ≥2 times the suggested doses may be needed. Titrate to pulmonary status (decreased bronchial secretions); consider administration of atropine via continuous I.V. infusion in patients requiring large doses of atropine. Once patient is stable for a period of time, the dose/dosing frequency may be decreased. Pralidoxime is a component of the management of organophosphate insecticide and nerve agent toxicity; refer to pralidoxime for the specific route and dose.

I.V., I.M.: Initial: 0.05 to 0.1 mg/kg; repeat every 5 to 10 minutes as needed, doubling the dose if previous dose does not induce atropinization (Hegenbarth, 2008; Reigart, 1999; Rotenberg, 2003). Maintain atropinization by administering repeat doses as needed for ≥2 to 12 hours based on recurrence of symptoms (Reigart, 1999).

Continuous I.V. infusion: Following atropinization, administer 10% to 20% of the total loading dose required to induce atropinization as a continuous I.V. infusion per hour; adjust as needed to maintain adequate atropinization without atropine toxicity (Eddleston, 2004; Roberts, 2007)

I.M. (AtroPen): Number of doses dependent upon symptom severity:

Weight-directed dosing:
<6.8 kg (15 lb): 0.25 mg/dose (yellow pen)
6.8 to 18 kg (15 to 40 lb): 0.5 mg/dose (blue pen)
18 to 41 kg (40 to 90 lb): 1 mg/dose (dark red pen)
>41 kg (>90 lb): 2 mg/dose (green pen)

Mild symptoms (≥2 mild symptoms): Administer the weight-based dose listed above as soon as an exposure is known or strongly suspected. If severe symptoms develop after the first dose, 2 additional doses should be repeated in rapid succession 10 minutes after the first dose; do not administer more than 3 doses. If profound anticholinergic effects occur in the absence of excessive bronchial secretions, further doses of atropine should be withheld. Mild symptoms of insecticide or nerve agent poisoning, as provided by manufacturer in the AtroPen product labeling to guide therapy, include: Blurred vision, bradycardia, breathing difficulties, chest tightness, coughing, drooling, miosis, muscular twitching, nausea, runny nose, salivation increased, stomach cramps, tachycardia, teary eyes, tremor, vomiting, or wheezing.

Severe symptoms (≥1 severe symptom): Immediately administer **three** weight-based doses in rapid succession. Symptoms of insecticide or nerve agent poisoning, as provided by manufacturer in the AtroPen product labeling to guide therapy, include: Breathing difficulties (severe), confused/strange behavior, defecation (involuntary), muscular twitching/generalized weakness (severe), respiratory secretions (severe), seizure, unconsciousness, urination (involuntary); **Note:** Infants may become drowsy or unconscious with muscle floppiness as opposed to muscle twitching.

Endotracheal: Increase the dose by 2 to 3 times the usual I.V. dose. Mix with 3 to 5 mL of normal saline and administer. Flush with 3 to 5 mL of NS and follow with 5 assisted manual ventilations (Rotenberg, 2003).

Refraction: Ophthalmic:

Infants: Instill 1 drop of 0.25% solution 3 times/day for 3 days before the procedure

Children: 1 to 5 years: Instill 1 drop of 0.5% solution 3 times/day for 3 days before the procedure

Children and Adolescents >5 years or Children with dark irides: Instill 1 drop of 1% solution 3 times/day for 3 days before the procedure

Uveitis: Infants, Children, and Adolescents: Ophthalmic: Instill 1 drop of 0.5% solution 1 to 3 times daily

Adult: **Note:** Doses <0.5 mg have been associated with paradoxical bradycardia.

Bradycardia: I.V.: 0.5 mg every 3 to 5 minutes, not to exceed a total of 3 mg or 0.04 mg/kg (ACLS, 2010)

Neuromuscular blockade reversal: I.V.: 25 to 30 mcg/kg 30-60 seconds before neostigmine or 7 to 10 mcg/kg 30 to 60 seconds before edrophonium

Organophosphate or carbamate insecticide or nerve agent poisoning: Note: The dose of atropine required varies considerably with the severity of poisoning. The total amount of atropine used for carbamate poisoning is usually less than with organophosphate insecticide or nerve agent poisoning. Severely poisoned patients may exhibit significant tolerance to atropine; ≥2 times the suggested doses may be needed. Titrate to pulmonary status (decreased bronchial secretions); consider administration of atropine via continuous I.V. infusion in patients requiring large doses of atropine. Once patient is stable for a period of time, the dose/dosing frequency may be decreased. If atropinization occurs after 1 to 2 mg of atropine then re-evaluate working diagnosis (Reigart, 1999). Pralidoxime is a component of the management of organophosphate insecticide and nerve agent toxicity; refer to Pralidoxime monograph for the specific route and dose.

I.M. (AtroPen):

Mild symptoms (≥2 mild symptoms): Administer 2 mg as soon as an exposure is known or strongly suspected. If severe symptoms develop after the first

dose, 2 additional doses should be repeated in rapid succession 10 minutes after the first dose; do not administer more than 3 doses. If profound anticholinergic effects occur in the absence of excessive bronchial secretions, further doses of atropine should be withheld. Mild symptoms of insecticide or nerve agent poisoning, as provided by manufacturer in the AtroPen® product labeling to guide therapy, include: Blurred vision, bradycardia, breathing difficulties, chest tightness, coughing, drooling, miosis, muscular twitching, nausea, runny nose, salivation increased, stomach cramps, tachycardia, teary eyes, tremor, vomiting, or wheezing.

Severe symptoms (≥1 severe symptom): Immediately administer **three** 2 mg doses in rapid succession. Severe symptoms of insecticide or nerve agent poisoning, as provided by manufacturer in the AtroPen product labeling to guide therapy include: Breathing difficulties (severe), confused/strange behavior, defecation (involuntary), muscular twitching/generalized weakness (severe), respiratory secretions (severe), seizure, unconsciousness, urination (involuntary)

Inhibit salivation and secretions (preanesthesia): I.M., I.V., SubQ: 0.4 to 0.6 mg 30 to 60 minutes preop and repeat every 4 to 6 hours as needed

Mydriasis, cycloplegia (preprocedure): Ophthalmic: Solution (1%): Instill 1 to 2 drops 1 hour before the procedure

Uveitis: Ophthalmic:

Solution (1%): Instill 1 to 2 drops up to 4 times/day

Ointment: Apply a small amount in the conjunctival sac up to 3 times/day. Compress the lacrimal sac by digital pressure for 1 to 3 minutes after instillation

Dosing adjustment in renal impairment: There are no dosage adjustments provided in the manufacturer's labeling.

Dosing adjustment in hepatic impairment: There are no dosage adjustments provided in the manufacturer's labeling.

Administration

Endotracheal: Administer and flush with 1 to 5 mL NS or SWI based on patient size, followed by 5 manual ventilations. Absorption may be greater with sterile water. Stop compressions (if using for cardiac arrest), spray the drug quickly down the tube. Follow immediately with several quick insufflations and continue chest compressions.

Parenteral:

I.V.: Administer undiluted by rapid I.V. injection; slow injection may result in paradoxical bradycardia

I.M.: AtroPen: Administer to the outer thigh. Firmly grasp the autoinjector with the green tip (0.5 mg, 1 mg, and 2 mg autoinjector) or black tip (0.25 mg autoinjector) pointed down; remove the yellow safety release (0.5 mg, 1 mg, and 2 mg autoinjector) or gray safety release (0.25 autoinjector). Firmly jab the green tip at a 90°angle against the outer thigh; may be administered through clothing as long as pockets at the injection site are empty. In thin patients or patients <6.8 kg (15 lb), bunch up the thigh prior to injection. Hold the autoinjector in place for 10 seconds following the injection; remove the autoinjector and massage the injection site. After administration, the needle will be visible; if the needle is not visible, repeat the above steps with more pressure. After use, bend the needle against a hard surface (needle does not retract) to avoid accidental injury.

Preparation of bulk atropine solution for mass chemical terrorism: Add atropine sulfate powder to 100 mL NS in polyvinyl chloride bags to yield a final concentration of 1 mg/mL (Dix, 2003)

Ophthalmic: Instill solution into conjunctival sac of affected eye(s); compress lacrimal sac with digital pressure for 2-3 minutes after instillation; avoid contact of bottle tip with eye or skin

Monitoring Parameters Heart rate, blood pressure, pulse, mental status; intravenous administration requires a cardiac monitor

Organophosphate or carbamate insecticide or nerve agent poisoning: Heart rate, blood pressure, respiratory status, oxygenation secretions. Maintain atropinization with repeated dosing as indicated by clinical status. Crackles in lung bases, or continuation of cholinergic signs, may be signs of inadequate dosing. Pulmonary improvement may not parallel other signs of atropinization. Monitor for signs and symptoms of atropine toxicity (eg, fever, muscle fasciculations, delirium); if toxicity occurs, discontinue atropine and monitor closely.

Additional Information Due to the discontinuance of 0.5% ophthalmic solutions commercially, 0.5% and 0.25% solutions may be prepared under sterile conditions by dilution of 1% atropine ophthalmic solution with artificial tears; 0.5%: An equal part dilution (equal volume of 1% atropine with artificial tears) and 0.25%: Dilute 2.5 mL 1% atropine with 7.5 mL artificial tears

Dosage Forms Excipient information presented when available (limited, particularly for generics); consult specific product labeling.

Device, Intramuscular, as sulfate:
AtroPen: 0.25 mg/0.3 mL (0.3 mL) [pyrogen free]
AtroPen: 0.5 mg/0.7 mL (0.7 mL); 1 mg/0.7 mL (0.7 mL); 2 mg/0.7 mL (0.7 mL) [pyrogen free; contains phenol]
Ointment, Ophthalmic, as sulfate:
Generic: 1% (3.5 g)
Solution, Injection, as sulfate:
Generic: 0.05 mg/mL (5 mL); 0.1 mg/mL (5 mL, 10 mL); 0.4 mg/mL (1 mL, 20 mL); 1 mg/mL (1 mL)
Solution, Injection, as sulfate [preservative free]:
Generic: 0.4 mg/mL (1 mL); 0.8 mg/mL (0.5 mL); 1 mg/mL (1 mL)
Solution, Ophthalmic, as sulfate:
Atropine-Care: 1% (2 mL, 5 mL, 15 mL) [contains benzalkonium chloride, edetate disodium]
Isopto Atropine: 1% (5 mL, 15 mL)
Generic: 1% (5 mL, 15 mL)

References

Andriessen P, Janssen BJ, Berendsen RC, et al, "Cardiovascular Autonomic Regulation in Preterm Infants: The Effect of Atropine," *Pediatr Res*, 2004, 56(6):939-46.
Atropine sulfate [prescribing information]. Eatontown, NJ: West-Ward Pharmaceuticals; July 2011.
Atropine sulfate [prescribing information]. El Monte, CA: International Medication Systems, Limited; August 2010.
Atropine sulfate [prescribing information]. Lake Forest, IL: Hospira, Inc; November 2004.
Barrington KJ, "The Myth of a Minimum Dose for Atropine," *Pediatrics*, 2011, 127(4):783-4.
Bernheim A, Fatio R, Kiowski W, et al, "Atropine Often Results in Complete Atrioventricular Block or Sinus Arrest After Cardiac Transplantation: An Unpredictable and Dose-Independent Phenomenon," *Transplantation*, 2004, 77(8):1181-5.
Dempsey EM, Al Hazzani F, Faucher D, et al, "Facilitation of Neonatal Endotracheal Intubation With Mivacurium and Fentanyl in the Neonatal Intensive Care Unit," *Arch Dis Child Fetal Neonatal Ed*, 2006, 91 (4):F279-82.
Dix J, Weber RJ, Frye RF, et al, "Stability of Atropine Sulfate Prepared for Mass Chemical Terrorism," *J Toxicol Clin Toxicol*, 2003, 41 (6):771-5.
Eddleston M, Dawson A, Karalliedde L, et al, "Early Management After Self-Poisoning with an Organophosphorus or Carbamate Pesticide – A Treatment Protocol for Junior Doctors," *Crit Care*, 2004, 8(6): R391-7.
Field JM, Hazinski MF, Sayre MR, et al, "Part 1: Executive Summary: 2010 American Heart Association Guidelines for Cardiopulmonary Resuscitation and Emergency Cardiovascular Care," *Circulation*, 2010, 122(18 Suppl 3):S640-56.
Hegenbarth MA, "Preparing for Pediatric Emergencies: Drugs to Consider," *Pediatrics*, 2008, 121(2):433-43.
Kleinman ME, Chameides L, Schexnayder SM, et al, "Part 14: Pediatric Advanced Life Support (PALS): 2010 American Heart Association Guidelines for Cardiopulmonary Resuscitation and Emergency Cardiovascular Care," *Circulation*, 2010, 122(18 Suppl 3):S876-908.
Kumar P, Denson SE, Mancuso TJ, et al, "Premedication for Nonemergency Endotracheal Intubation in the Neonate," *Pediatrics*, 2010, 125(3):608-15.
Nelson WE, Behrman RE, Kliegman RM, et al, eds. *Nelson Textbook of Pediatrics*. 15th ed. Philadelphia, PA: WB Saunders Company; 1996.
Neumar RW, Otto CW, Link MS, et al, "Part 8: Adult Advanced Cardiovascular Life Support (ACLS): 2010 American Heart Association Guidelines for Cardiopulmonary Resuscitation and Emergency Cardiovascular Care," *Circulation*, 2010, 122(18 Suppl 3):S729-67.
Oei J, Hari R, Butha T, et al, "Facilitation of Neonatal Nasotracheal Intubation With Premedication: A Randomized Controlled Trial," *J Paediatr Child Health*, 2002, 38(2):146-50.
Reigart JR and Roberts JR, "Recognition and Management of Pesticide Poisonings," U.S. Environmental Protection Agency, Washington, DC, 5th ed, 1999: 34-47. Available at http://www.epa.gov/oppfead1/safety/healthcare/handbook/handbook.htm
Roberts DM and Aaron CK, "Management of Acute Organophosphorus Pesticide Poisoning," *BMJ*, 2007, 334(7594):629-34.
Roberts KD, Leone TA, Edwards WH, et al, "Premedication for Nonemergent Neonatal Intubations: A Randomized, Controlled Trial Comparing Atropine and Fentanyl to Atropine, Fentanyl, and Mivacurium," *Pediatrics*, 2006, 118(4):1583-91.
Rotenberg JS and Newmark J, "Nerve Agent Attacks on Children: Diagnosis and Management," *Pediatrics*, 2003, 112(3 Pt 1):648-58.

◆ **Atropine and Diphenoxylate** see Diphenoxylate and Atropine *on page 678*

◆ **Atropine-Care** see Atropine *on page 234*

◆ **Atropine, Hyoscyamine, Phenobarbital, and Scopolamine** see Hyoscyamine, Atropine, Scopolamine, and Phenobarbital *on page 1058*

◆ **Atropine Sulfate** see Atropine *on page 234*

◆ **Atrovent** see Ipratropium (Nasal) *on page 1146*

◆ **Atrovent® (Can)** see Ipratropium (Nasal) *on page 1146*

◆ **Atrovent HFA** see Ipratropium (Oral Inhalation) *on page 1144*

Attapulgite (at a PULL gite)

Medication Safety Issues
Sound-alike/look-alike issues:
Kaopectate® may be confused with Kayexalate®
Note: Attapulgite preparations have been discontinued in the U.S.; refer to Bismuth monograph for newly-reformulated Kaopectate® products.

Brand Names: Canada Kaopectate® Children's [OTC]; Kaopectate® Extra Strength [OTC]; Kaopectate® [OTC]

Therapeutic Category Antidiarrheal

Use Treatment of uncomplicated diarrhea

Contraindications Hypersensitivity to attapulgite or any component

Warnings Not to be used for self-medication for diarrhea >48 hours or in the presence of high fever in infants and children <3 years of age; do not use for diarrhea associated with pseudomembranous enterocolitis or in diarrhea caused by toxigenic bacteria

Drug Interactions
Metabolism/Transport Effects None known.
Avoid Concomitant Use There are no known interactions where it is recommended to avoid concomitant use.
Increased Effect/Toxicity There are no known significant interactions involving an increase in effect.
Decreased Effect There are no known significant interactions involving a decrease in effect.

Mechanism of Action Nonselectively absorbs excess intestinal fluid, thereby reducing stool liquidity. May interfere with absorption of nutrients and other drugs as well.

Dosing: Usual Adequate controlled clinical studies documenting the efficacy of attapulgite are lacking; its usage and dosage has been primarily empiric; the following are manufacturer's recommended dosages

Oral: Give after each bowel movement

Children:

3-6 years: 300-750 mg/dose; maximum dose: 7 doses/day or 2250 mg/day

6-12 years: 600-1500 mg/dose; maximum dose: 7 doses/day or 4500 mg/day

Children >12 years and Adults: 1200-3000 mg/dose; maximum dose: 8 doses/day or 9000 mg/day

Administration May be administered without regard to meals; shake liquid preparation well before use

Additional Information Kaopectate®, Kaopectate® Advanced Formula, Children's Kaopectate®, and Kaopectate® Maximum Strength have been reformulated. Previously, Kaopectate® contained attapulgite. The new formulation contains only bismuth subsalicylate. Bismuth salicylate has significant contraindications, particularly in children with influenza and chickenpox. Please refer to bismuth monograph for product information. During the transition period, the older formulation may still be available, read product label closely.

Product Availability Not available in U.S.

◆ **ATV** see Atazanavir on page 218

◆ **Augmentin** see Amoxicillin and Clavulanate on page 144

◆ **Augmentin ES-600** see Amoxicillin and Clavulanate on page 144

◆ **Augmentin XR** see Amoxicillin and Clavulanate on page 144

◆ **Auralgan® (Can)** see Antipyrine and Benzocaine on page 181

Auranofin (au RANE oh fin)

Medication Safety Issues
Sound-alike/look-alike issues:
Ridaura® may be confused with Cardura®

Brand Names: U.S. Ridaura

Brand Names: Canada Ridaura®

Therapeutic Category Gold Compound

Generic Availability (U.S.) No

Use Management of active stage of classic or definite rheumatoid arthritis in patients who do not respond to or tolerate other agents (FDA approved in adults)

Pregnancy Risk Factor C

Pregnancy Considerations Adverse events were observed in animal reproduction studies.

Breast-Feeding Considerations Injectable gold salts have been detected in breast milk.

Contraindications Any history of gold-induced disorders including anaphylactoid reactions, necrotizing enterocolitis, exfoliative dermatitis, pulmonary fibrosis, bone marrow aplasia, or other severe hematologic disorders

Warnings May be associated with significant toxicity involving dermatologic, gastrointestinal, hematologic, pulmonary, renal, and hepatic systems **[U.S. Boxed Warning]**; patient education is required. In patients with a history of abnormalities of these organ systems, risk of toxicity is increased and symptoms of gold toxicity may be difficult to detect; consider alternative therapy. Hematologic signs of gold toxicity include decrease in hemoglobin, leukocytes, granulocytes, and platelets; avoid use in patients with a history of blood dyscrasias (anemia, agranulocytosis), hemorrhagic diathesis, or drug induced granulocytopenia. Therapy should be discontinued if platelet count falls to <100,000/mm^3, WBC <4000, granulocytes <1500/mm^3. Dermatitis and lesions of the mucous membranes are common and may be serious; pruritus may precede the early development of a skin reaction; consider alternative therapy in patient with dermatitis; exfoliative dermatitis is a contraindication. Gold dermatitis may be aggravated by sun exposure; avoid exposure to sunlight and artificial light sources (sunlamps, tanning booth/bed). Signs of GI toxicity include persistent diarrhea, stomatitis, and enterocolitis; avoid use in patients with prior inflammatory bowel disease; use is contraindicated in patients with necrotizing enterocolitis. In pediatric trials, diarrhea was the most common adverse effect (Giannini, 1990). May be associated with the development of cholestatic jaundice; consider alternative therapy in patients with hepatic impairment. May be associated with interstitial fibrosis; monitor closely. Renal toxicity ranges from mild proteinuria to nephrotic syndrome; perform urinalysis regularly and discontinue treatment if proteinuria or hematuria develop.

Auranofin capsules contain benzyl alcohol which may cause allergic reactions in susceptible individuals; large amounts of benzyl alcohol (≥99 mg/kg/day) have been associated with a potentially fatal toxicity ("gasping syndrome") in neonates; in vitro and animal studies have shown that benzoate displaces bilirubin from protein binding sites; avoid use of auranofin in neonates.

Precautions Use with caution and modify dose in patients with renal impairment; consider alternative therapy

Adverse Reactions
Dermatologic: Alopecia, pruritus, rash, urticaria
Gastrointestinal: Abdominal pain, anorexia, constipation, diarrhea/loose stools, dysgeusia, dyspepsia, flatulence, glossitis, nausea, stomatitis, vomiting
Hematologic: Eosinophilia, leukopenia, thrombocytopenia
Hepatic: Transaminases increased
Ocular: Conjunctivitis
Renal: Hematuria, proteinuria
Rare but important or life-threatening: Agranulocytosis, aplastic anemia, angioedema, corneal deposits, dysphagia, enterocolitis (ulcerative), fever, GI hemorrhage, gingivitis, gold bronchitis, hepatotoxicity, interstitial pneumonitis, jaundice, metallic taste, melena, neutropenia, pancytopenia, peripheral neuropathy, pure red cell aplasia. **Note:** Exfoliative dermatitis has been reported with other gold compounds.

Drug Interactions
Metabolism/Transport Effects None known.
Avoid Concomitant Use There are no known interactions where it is recommended to avoid concomitant use.
Increased Effect/Toxicity There are no known significant interactions involving an increase in effect.
Decreased Effect There are no known significant interactions involving a decrease in effect.

Stability Store at 15°C to 30°C (59°F to 86°F); dispense in a tight, light-resistant container.

Mechanism of Action The exact mechanism of action of gold is unknown; gold is taken up by macrophages which results in inhibition of phagocytosis and lysosomal membrane stabilization; other actions observed are decreased serum rheumatoid factor and alterations in immunoglobulins. Additionally, complement activation is decreased, prostaglandin synthesis is inhibited, and lysosomal enzyme activity is decreased.

Pharmacodynamics Onset of action: Therapeutic response may not be seen for 3-4 months after start of therapy, as long as 6 months in some patients

Pharmacokinetics (Adult data unless noted) Note: Due to rapid metabolism, the pharmacokinetics of auranofin are based on gold concentrations, not auranofin.
Absorption: Oral: 25%
Protein binding: 60%
Metabolism: Rapid; intact auranofin not detectable in the blood

Half-life: 21-31 days (half-life dependent upon single or multiple dosing)

Time to peak serum concentration: Within 2 hours

Elimination: 60% of absorbed gold is eliminated in urine while the remainder is eliminated in feces

Dosing: Usual

Children ≥18 months and Adolescents ≤17 years: **Juvenile idiopathic arthritis (rheumatoid):** Limited data available: Oral: Initial: 0.1-0.15 mg/kg/day in 1-2 divided doses; usual maintenance: 0.15 mg/kg/day in 1-2 divided doses; maximum daily dose: 0.2 mg/kg/**day** or 9 mg/**day.** **Note:** With current market availability, may not be able to replicate the exact dosing used in trials; in trials, doses were rounded to nearest whole mg using 1 mg tablet (no longer available) (Brewer, 1983; Giannini, 1990; Marcolongo, 1988)

Adults: **Rheumatoid arthritis:** Oral: 6 mg/day in 1-2 divided doses; after 6 months may be increased to 9 mg/day in 3 divided doses; if still no response after 3 months at 9 mg/day, discontinue drug

Dosage adjustment in renal impairment: Adults: There are no dosage adjustments provided in the manufacturer's labeling. The following guidelines have been used by some clinicians (Aronoff, 2007):

CrCl 50-80 mL/minute: Reduce dose to 50%

CrCl <50 mL/minute: Avoid use

Dosage adjustment in hepatic impairment: There are no dosage adjustments provided in the manufacturer's labeling.

Administration Take with or without food; some centers have recommended to administer with food if it causes GI upset.

Monitoring Parameters Baseline and periodic (at least monthly): CBC with differential, platelet count, urinalysis for protein; baseline renal and liver function tests; skin and oral mucosa examinations; specific questioning for symptoms of pruritus, rash, stomatitis, or metallic taste

Reference Range Gold: Normal: 0-0.1 mcg/mL (SI: 0-0.0064 micromoles/L); Therapeutic: 1-3 mcg/mL (SI: 0.06-0.18 micromoles/L); Urine <0.1 mcg/24 hours

Test Interactions May enhance the response to a tuberculin skin test

Additional Information Metallic taste may indicate stomatitis

Dosage Forms Excipient information presented when available (limited, particularly for generics); consult specific product labeling.

Capsule, Oral:

Ridaura: 3 mg [contains benzyl alcohol]

References

Aronoff GR, Bennett WM, Berns JS, et al. *Drug Prescribing in Renal Failure: Dosing Guidelines for Adults and Children.* 5th ed. Philadelphia, PA: American College of Physicians; 2007.

Brewer EJ, Giannini EH, Person DA. Early experiences with auranofin in juvenile rheumatoid arthritis. *Am J Med.* 1983;75(6A):152-156.

Giannini EH, Brewer EJ, Kuzmina N, et.al. Auranofin in the treatment of juvenile rheumatoid arthritis. *Arthritis Rheum.* 1990;33(4):466-476.

Marcolongo R, Mathieu A, Pala R, et al. The efficacy and safety of auranofin in the treatment of juvenile rheumatoid arthritis. *Arthritis Rheum.* 1988;31(8):981-983.

◆ **Auraphene-B [OTC]** *see* Carbamide Peroxide on page 377

◆ **Auro-Amlodipine (Can)** *see* AmLODIPine on page 135

◆ **Auro-Cefprozil (Can)** *see* Cefprozil on page 412

◆ **Auro-Cefuroxime (Can)** *see* Cefuroxime on page 422

◆ **Auro-Ciprofloxacin (Can)** *see* Ciprofloxacin (Systemic) on page 471

◆ **Auro-Citalopram (Can)** *see* Citalopram on page 484

◆ **Auro-Cyclobenzaprine (Can)** *see* Cyclobenzaprine on page 558

◆ **Aurodex®** *see* Antipyrine and Benzocaine on page 181

◆ **Auro-Gabapentin (Can)** *see* Gabapentin on page 950

◆ **Auro-Irbesartan (Can)** *see* Irbesartan on page 1147

◆ **Auro-Lamotrigine (Can)** *see* LamoTRIgine on page 1199

◆ **Auro-Letrozole (Can)** *see* Letrozole on page 1211

◆ **Auro-Levetiracetam (Can)** *see* LevETIRAcetam on page 1219

◆ **Auro-Lisinopril (Can)** *see* Lisinopril on page 1262

◆ **Auro-Losartan (Can)** *see* Losartan on page 1283

◆ **Auro-Meloxicam (Can)** *see* Meloxicam on page 1325

◆ **Auro-Montelukast (Can)** *see* Montelukast on page 1438

◆ **Auro-Montelukast Chewable Tablets (Can)** *see* Montelukast on page 1438

◆ **Auro-Nevirapine (Can)** *see* Nevirapine on page 1487

◆ **Auro-Omeprazole (Can)** *see* Omeprazole on page 1535

◆ **Auro-Paroxetine (Can)** *see* PARoxetine on page 1609

◆ **Auro-Quetiapine (Can)** *see* QUEtiapine on page 1783

◆ **Auro-Sertraline (Can)** *see* Sertraline on page 1879

◆ **Auro-Simvastatin (Can)** *see* Simvastatin on page 1892

◆ **Auro-Terbinafine (Can)** *see* Terbinafine (Systemic) on page 1982

◆ **AURO-Topiramate (Can)** *see* Topiramate on page 2046

◆ **Auvi-Q** *see* EPINEPHrine (Systemic, Oral Inhalation) on page 761

◆ **Ava-Amiodarone (Can)** *see* Amiodarone on page 127

◆ **Ava-Atenolol (Can)** *see* Atenolol on page 222

◆ **Ava-Atorvastatin (Can)** *see* AtorvaSTATin on page 227

◆ **Ava-Azithromycin (Can)** *see* Azithromycin (Systemic) on page 247

◆ **Ava-Baclofen (Can)** *see* Baclofen on page 259

◆ **Ava-Bupropion SR (Can)** *see* BuPROPion on page 327

◆ **Ava-Carvedilol (Can)** *see* Carvedilol on page 385

◆ **Ava-Cefprozil (Can)** *see* Cefprozil on page 412

◆ **Ava-Citalopram (Can)** *see* Citalopram on page 484

◆ **Ava-Clarithromycin (Can)** *see* Clarithromycin on page 490

◆ **Ava-Clindamycin (Can)** *see* Clindamycin (Systemic) on page 495

◆ **Ava-Cyclobenzaprine (Can)** *see* Cyclobenzaprine on page 558

◆ **Ava-Diclofenac (Can)** *see* Diclofenac (Systemic) on page 645

◆ **Ava-Diclofenac SR (Can)** *see* Diclofenac (Systemic) on page 645

◆ **Ava-Diltiazem (Can)** *see* Diltiazem on page 667

◆ **Ava-Enalapril (Can)** *see* Enalapril on page 744

◆ **Ava-Famciclovir (Can)** *see* Famciclovir on page 842

◆ **Ava-Fluoxetine (Can)** *see* FLUoxetine on page 901

◆ **Ava-Fluvoxamine (Can)** *see* FluvoxaMINE on page 922

◆ **Ava-Fosinopril (Can)** *see* Fosinopril on page 938

◆ **AVA-Furosemide (Can)** *see* Furosemide on page 948

◆ **Avage** *see* Tazarotene on page 1971

◆ **Ava-Glyburide (Can)** *see* GlyBURIDE on page 974

◆ **Ava-Hydrochlorothiazide (Can)** *see* Hydrochlorothiazide on page 1023

◆ **Ava-Irbesartan (Can)** *see* Irbesartan on page 1147

◆ **Avakine** *see* InFLIXimab on page 1099

◆ **Ava-Levetiracetam (Can)** *see* LevETIRAcetam on page 1219

- ◆ **AVA-Levofloxacin (Can)** *see* Levofloxacin (Systemic) *on page 1228*
- ◆ **Ava-Lovastatin (Can)** *see* Lovastatin *on page 1286*
- ◆ **Ava-Meloxicam (Can)** *see* Meloxicam *on page 1325*
- ◆ **Ava-Metformin (Can)** *see* MetFORMIN *on page 1353*
- ◆ **Ava-Metoprolol (Can)** *see* Metoprolol *on page 1396*
- ◆ **Ava-Metoprolol (Type L) (Can)** *see* Metoprolol *on page 1396*
- ◆ **Avamys® (Can)** *see* Fluticasone (Nasal) *on page 913*
- ◆ **Ava-Naproxen EC (Can)** *see* Naproxen *on page 1470*
- ◆ **Avandia** *see* Rosiglitazone *on page 1850*
- ◆ **Ava-Nortriptyline (Can)** *see* Nortriptyline *on page 1512*
- ◆ **Ava-Olanzapine (Can)** *see* OLANZapine *on page 1525*
- ◆ **Ava-Omeprazole (Can)** *see* Omeprazole *on page 1535*
- ◆ **Ava-Pantoprazole (Can)** *see* Pantoprazole *on page 1595*
- ◆ **Avapro** *see* Irbesartan *on page 1147*
- ◆ **Ava-Quetiapine (Can)** *see* QUEtiapine *on page 1783*
- ◆ **Ava-Risperidone (Can)** *see* RisperiDONE *on page 1831*
- ◆ **Ava-Simvastatin (Can)** *see* Simvastatin *on page 1892*
- ◆ **Avastin** *see* Bevacizumab *on page 288*
- ◆ **Ava-Sumatriptan (Can)** *see* SUMAtriptan *on page 1958*
- ◆ **AVA-Topiramate (Can)** *see* Topiramate *on page 2046*
- ◆ **Ava-Valsartan (Can)** *see* Valsartan *on page 2108*
- ◆ **Avaxim (Can)** *see* Hepatitis A Vaccine *on page 1005*
- ◆ **Avaxim-Pediatric (Can)** *see* Hepatitis A Vaccine *on page 1005*
- ◆ **Aveed** *see* Testosterone *on page 1986*
- ◆ **Aventyl® (Can)** *see* Nortriptyline *on page 1512*
- ◆ **Avidoxy** *see* Doxycycline *on page 721*
- ◆ **AVINza** *see* Morphine (Systemic) *on page 1440*
- ◆ **Avita** *see* Tretinoin (Topical) *on page 2071*
- ◆ **AVP** *see* Vasopressin *on page 2121*
- ◆ **Axert** *see* Almotriptan *on page 99*
- ◆ **Axid** *see* Nizatidine *on page 1508*
- ◆ **Axid AR [OTC]** *see* Nizatidine *on page 1508*
- ◆ **Axiron** *see* Testosterone *on page 1986*
- ◆ **Aygestin** *see* Norethindrone *on page 1511*
- ◆ **Ayr [OTC]** *see* Sodium Chloride *on page 1902*
- ◆ **Ayr Nasal Mist Allergy/Sinus [OTC]** *see* Sodium Chloride *on page 1902*
- ◆ **Ayr Saline Nasal [OTC]** *see* Sodium Chloride *on page 1902*
- ◆ **Ayr Saline Nasal Drops [OTC]** *see* Sodium Chloride *on page 1902*
- ◆ **Ayr Saline Nasal Gel [OTC]** *see* Sodium Chloride *on page 1902*
- ◆ **Ayr Saline Nasal No-Drip [OTC]** *see* Sodium Chloride *on page 1902*
- ◆ **AYR Saline Nasal Rinse [OTC]** *see* Sodium Chloride *on page 1902*
- ◆ **Azactam** *see* Aztreonam *on page 254*
- ◆ **Azactam in Dextrose** *see* Aztreonam *on page 254*
- ◆ **Azasan** *see* AzaTHIOprine *on page 241*
- ◆ **AzaSite** *see* Azithromycin (Ophthalmic) *on page 253*

AzaTHIOprine (ay za THYE oh preen)

Medication Safety Issues
Sound-alike/look-alike issues:
AzaTHIOprine may be confused with azaCITIDine, azidothymidine, azithromycin, Azulfidine
Imuran may be confused with Elmiron, Enduron, Imdur, Inderal, Tenormin
Other safety concerns:
Azathioprine is metabolized to mercaptopurine; concurrent use of these commercially-available products has resulted in profound myelosuppression.

Related Information
Safe Handling of Hazardous Drugs *on page 2419*
Brand Names: U.S. Azasan; Imuran
Brand Names: Canada Apo-Azathioprine; Imuran; Mylan-Azathioprine; Teva-Azathioprine
Therapeutic Category Immunosuppressant Agent
Generic Availability (U.S.) Yes
Use Adjunct with other agents in prevention of kidney transplant rejection (FDA approved in adults); management of active rheumatoid arthritis (FDA approved in adults); has also been used as an immunosuppressant in a variety of autoimmune diseases such as SLE, juvenile idiopathic arthritis (JIA), JIA-associated uveitis, myasthenia gravis, and autoimmune hepatitis, and as a steroid-sparing agent for inflammatory bowel disease
Pregnancy Risk Factor D
Pregnancy Considerations Adverse events have been observed in animal reproduction studies. Azathioprine crosses the placenta in humans; congenital anomalies, immunosuppression, hematologic toxicities (lymphopenia, pancytopenia), and intrauterine growth retardation have been reported. Azathioprine should not be used to treat rheumatoid arthritis during pregnancy. Women of childbearing potential should avoid becoming pregnant during treatment.

The National Transplantation Pregnancy Registry (NTPR, Temple University) is a registry for pregnant women taking immunosuppressants following any solid organ transplant. The NTPR encourages reporting of all immunosuppressant exposures during pregnancy in transplant recipients at 877-955-6877.
Breast-Feeding Considerations Azathioprine is excreted in breast milk. Due to potential for serious adverse reactions in the nursing infant, breast-feeding is not recommended by the manufacturer.
Contraindications Hypersensitivity to azathioprine or any component; pregnancy (patients with rheumatoid arthritis); patients with rheumatoid arthritis previously treated with alkylating agents (eg, cyclophosphamide, chlorambucil, melphalan) may have a prohibitive risk of neoplasia with azathioprine treatment
Warnings Hazardous agent: Use appropriate precautions for handling and disposal (NIOSH, 2012). Immunosuppressive agents, including azathioprine, increase the risk of development of malignancy; lymphoma (in post-transplant patients) and hepatosplenic T-cell lymphoma (HSTCL) (in patients with inflammatory bowel disease) have been reported **[U.S. Boxed Warning]**. Patients should be informed of the risk for malignancy development. Hepatosplenic T-cell lymphoma (HSTCL) is a rare white blood cell cancer that is usually fatal and has predominantly occurred in adolescents and young adults treated for Crohn disease or ulcerative colitis and receiving TNF blockers (eg, adalimumab, certolizumab pegol, etanercept, golimumab), azathioprine, and/or mercaptopurine. Most cases of HSTCL have occurred in patients treated with a combination of immunosuppressant agents, although there have been reports of HSTCL in patients receiving azathioprine or mercaptopurine monotherapy.

Renal transplant patients are also at increased risk for malignancy (eg, skin cancer, lymphoma); limit sun and ultraviolet light exposure and use appropriate sun protection.

Dose-related hematologic toxicities (leukopenia, thrombocytopenia, anemias, including macrocytic anemia or pancytopenia) may occur; may be severe and/or delayed. Patients with intermediate thiopurine methyltransferase (TPMT) activity may be at risk for increased hematologic toxicity at conventional azathioprine doses; those with low or absent TPMT activity are at risk for severe, life-threatening myelotoxicity. TPMT genotyping or phenotyping may assist in identifying patients at risk for developing toxicity; consider TPMT testing in patients with abnormally low CBC unresponsive to dose reduction. TPMT testing does not substitute for CBC monitoring. Myelosuppression may be more severe with renal transplants experiencing rejection. Monitor CBC with differential and platelets weekly during the first month, then twice a month for 2 months, then monthly (or more frequently if clinically indicated). May require treatment interruption or dose reduction. Patients on concurrent therapy with drugs which may inhibit TPMT (eg, olsalazine) or xanthine oxidase (eg, allopurinol) may be at higher risk for myelosuppressive effects. Dose adjustment of azathioprine may be recommended when used concurrently with allopurinol; patients with low or absent TPMT activity may require further dose reductions or discontinuation. Azathioprine is metabolized to mercaptopurine; concomitant use may result in profound myelosuppression and should be avoided. Potentially significant interactions may exist, requiring dose or frequency adjustment, additional monitoring, and/or selection of alternative therapy. Consult drug interactions database for more detailed information.

Chronic immunosuppression increases the risk of serious, sometimes fatal, infections (bacterial, viral, fungal, protozoal, and opportunistic). Progressive multifocal leukoencephalopathy (PML), an opportunistic CNS infection caused by reactivation of the JC virus, has been reported in patients receiving immunosuppressive therapy, including azathioprine; promptly evaluate any patient presenting with neurological changes. Consider decreasing the degree of immunosuppression with consideration to the risk of organ rejection in transplant patients. Immune response to vaccines may be diminished.

The development of secondary hemophagocytic lymphohistiocytosis (HLH), a rare and frequently fatal activation of macrophages which causes phagocytosis of all bone marrow blood cell lines, is increased (100-fold) in pediatric patients diagnosed with inflammatory bowel disease due to chronic inflammation; this risk is further increased with concomitant thiopurine (ie, azathioprine or mercaptopurine) therapy, Epstein-Barr virus or possibly other infections; if patient on thiopurine therapy presents with fever for at least 5 days, cervical lymphadenopathy and lymphopenia, discontinue immunosuppressive therapy and further diagnostic evaluation for HLH should be performed; delay in diagnosis has been associated with increased mortality (Biank, 2011).

Severe nausea, vomiting, diarrhea, rash, fever, malaise, myalgia, hypotension, and liver enzyme abnormalities may occur within the first several weeks of treatment and are generally reversible upon discontinuation.

Precautions Use with caution in renal impairment; dosage reductions may be necessary.

Use with caution in patients with hepatic impairment. Hepatotoxicity (transaminase, bilirubin, and alkaline phosphatase elevations) may occur, usually in renal transplant patients and generally within 6 months of transplant; normally reversible with discontinuation; monitor liver function periodically. Rarely, hepatic sinusoidal obstruction syndrome (SOS; formerly called veno-occlusive disease [VOD]) has been reported; discontinue azathioprine if hepatic SOS is suspected. Should be prescribed by physicians familiar with the risks, including hematologic toxicities and mutagenic potential **[U.S. Boxed Warning]**.

Adverse Reactions

Central nervous system: Malaise

Gastrointestinal: Diarrhea, nausea and vomiting (rheumatoid arthritis)

Hematologic and oncologic: Leukopenia (more common in renal transplant), neoplasia (renal transplant), thrombocytopenia

Hepatic: Hepatotoxicity, increased serum alkaline phosphatase, increased serum bilirubin, increased serum transaminases

Infection: Increased susceptibility to infection (more common in renal transplant; includes bacterial, fungal, protozoal, viral, opportunistic, and reactivation of latent infections)

Neuromuscular & skeletal: Myalgia

Miscellaneous: Fever

Rare but important or life-threatening: Abdominal pain, acute myelocytic leukemia, alopecia, anemia, arthralgia, bone marrow depression, hemorrhage, hepatic veno-occlusive disease, hepatosplenic T-cell lymphomas, hypersensitivity, hypotension, interstitial pneumonitis (reversible), JC virus infection, macrocytic anemia, malignant lymphoma, malignant neoplasm of skin, negative nitrogen balance, pancreatitis, pancytopenia, progressive multifocal leukoencephalopathy, skin rash, steatorrhea, Sweet's syndrome (acute febrile neutrophilic dermatosis)

Drug Interactions

Metabolism/Transport Effects None known.

Avoid Concomitant Use

Avoid concomitant use of AzaTHIOprine with any of the following: BCG; Febuxostat; Mercaptopurine; Natalizumab; Pimecrolimus; Tacrolimus (Topical); Tofacitinib; Vaccines (Live)

Increased Effect/Toxicity

AzaTHIOprine may increase the levels/effects of: Cyclophosphamide; Leflunomide; Mercaptopurine; Natalizumab; Tofacitinib; Vaccines (Live)

The levels/effects of AzaTHIOprine may be increased by: 5-ASA Derivatives; ACE Inhibitors; Allopurinol; Denosumab; Febuxostat; Pimecrolimus; Ribavirin; Roflumilast; Sulfamethoxazole; Tacrolimus (Topical); Trastuzumab; Trimethoprim

Decreased Effect

AzaTHIOprine may decrease the levels/effects of: BCG; Coccidioidin Skin Test; Sipuleucel-T; Vaccines (Inactivated); Vaccines (Live); Vitamin K Antagonists

The levels/effects of AzaTHIOprine may be decreased by: Echinacea

Stability

Tablet:

Azasan: Store at 20°C to 25°C (68°F to 77°F); protect from light.

Imuran: Store at 15°C to 25°C (59°F to 77°F); protect from light.

Mechanism of Action Azathioprine is an imidazolyl derivative of mercaptopurine; metabolites are incorporated into replicating DNA and halt replication; also block the pathway for purine synthesis (Taylor, 2005). The 6-thioguanine nucleotide metabolites appear to mediate the majority of azathioprine's immunosuppressive and toxic effects.

Pharmacokinetics (Adult data unless noted)

Absorption: Oral: Well absorbed

Protein binding: ~30%

Metabolism: Hepatic; metabolized to 6-mercaptopurine via glutathione S-transferase (GST). Further metabolism in the liver and GI tract, via three major pathways: Hypoxanthine guanine phosphoribosyltransferase (to active metabolites: 6-thioguanine-nucleotides, or 6-TGNs), xanthine oxidase (to inactive metabolite: 6-thiouric acid), and thiopurine methyltransferase (TPMT) (to inactive metabolite: 6-methylmercaptopurine)

Time to peak serum concentration: Oral: 1 to 2 hours (including metabolites)

Half-life, elimination: Azathioprine and mercaptopurine: Variable: ~2 hours (Taylor, 2005)

Elimination: Urine (primarily as metabolites)

Dosing: Usual Note: Patients with intermediate TPMT activity may be at risk for increased myelosuppression; those with low or absent TPMT activity receiving conventional azathioprine doses are at risk for developing severe, life-threatening myelotoxicity. Dosage reductions are recommended for patients with reduced TPMT activity. **Note:** I.V. dose is equivalent to oral dose (dosing should be transitioned from I.V. to oral as soon as tolerated).

Pediatric:

Hepatitis, autoimmune: Limited data available: Children and Adolescents: Oral: Initial: 0.5 mg/kg/dose once daily; titrate as needed up to 2 mg/kg/dose once daily; for long-term therapy, a low-dose of 1 to 1.5 mg/kg/day may be effective in some patients (Della Corte, 2012; Vitfell-Pedersen, 2012)

Inflammatory bowel disease: Limited data available: Infants, Children, and Adolescents: Oral: 2 to 2.5 mg/kg/dose once daily; titrate to effect; usual reported range: 1 to 3 mg/kg/dose once daily; reported maximum daily dose: 4 mg/kg/day or 200 mg/day; may takes several weeks of therapy to be fully effective (Fuentes, 2003; Punati, 2011; Riello, 2011; Sandhu, 2010). Some data suggest that pediatric patients ≤6 years may require higher doses to achieve remission; a median dose of 3.51 mg/kg/day (maximum daily dose: 5 mg/kg/day) was reported to induce remission in 62% of patients ≤6 years of age vs 17% of those receiving lower doses (ie, <2 to 3 mg/kg/day study group; median dose: 2.46 mg/kg/day) (Grossman, 2008).

Immune thrombocytopenia (ITP), chronic refractory: Limited data available: Children ≥2 years and Adolescents: Oral: Maintenance: 2 to 2.5 mg/kg/day, rounded to the nearest 50 mg (Boruchov, 2007)

Juvenile-idiopathic arthritis (rheumatoid arthritis): Limited data available: Children and Adolescents: Oral: 2 to 2.5 mg/kg/dose once daily; data limited to single double-blind, placebo-controlled trial of pediatric patients (n=17 treatment group); efficacy results were not statistically significant (response rate: Treatment: 41% vs placebo: 27%); data suggested a minimum trial of 12 weeks to fully assess therapeutic response (AHRQ, 2011; Hashkes, 2005; Kvien, 1986)

Lupus nephritis, mild: Limited data available: Children and Adolescents: Oral: 2 to 2.5 mg/kg/dose once daily (Bertsias, 2012; Marks, 2010); **Note:** Some data suggest less effective in non-Caucasian pediatric patients; some centers recommend use for primary induction in Caucasian patients with less severe disease (Adams, 2006; Marks, 2010).

Myasthenia gravis, juvenile: Limited data available: Children and Adolescents: Oral: 1 to 3 mg/kg/dose once daily (Ashraf, 2006; Lindner, 1997)

Transplantation, solid organ: Limited data available: Infants, Children, and Adolescents: Oral: Initial: 3 to 5 mg/kg/dose once daily, beginning at the time of transplant; maintenance: 1 to 3 mg/kg/dose once daily (Denfield, 2010; Ford, 2006)

Uveitis, JIA-associated: Limited data available: Children and Adolescents: Oral: Initial mean dose: 2.4 mg/kg/dose once daily; reported range: 1.4 to 3.2 mg/kg/dose once daily; in a retrospective review of 41 children, a mean maintenance 2.1 mg/kg/dose (range: 1 to 2.8 mg/kg/dose) once daily was reported as monotherapy and/or in combination with other immunosuppressive agents; infectious etiology was excluded; the authors recommend doses of <3 mg/kg/day (Goebel, 2011)

Adult:

Renal transplantation (treatment usually started the day of transplant; however, has been initiated [rarely] 1 to 3 days prior to transplant): Oral: Initial: 3 to 5 mg/kg/day usually given as a single daily dose, then maintenance 1 to 3 mg/kg/day

Rheumatoid arthritis: Oral:

Initial: 1 mg/kg/day (50 to 100 mg) given once daily or divided twice daily for 6 to 8 weeks; may increase by 0.5 mg/kg every 4 weeks until response or up to a maximum daily dose of 2.5 mg/**day**; an adequate trial should be a minimum of 12 weeks

Maintenance dose: Reduce dose by 0.5 mg/kg (~25 mg daily) every 4 weeks until lowest effective dose is reached; optimum duration of therapy not specified; may be discontinued abruptly

Dosage adjustment for concomitant use with allopurinol:

Infants, Children, and Adolescents: Limited data available

Adults: Reduce azathioprine dose to one-third or one-fourth the usual dose when used concurrently with allopurinol. Patients with low or absent TPMT activity may require further dose reductions or discontinuation.

Dosage adjustment for toxicity:

Infants, Children, and Adolescents: Limited data available

Adults:

Rapid WBC count decrease, persistently low WBC count, or serious infection: Reduce dose or temporarily withhold treatment.

Severe toxicity in renal transplantation: May require discontinuation.

Hepatic sinusoidal obstruction syndrome (SOS; venoocclusive disease): Permanently discontinue.

Dosing adjustment in renal impairment:

Infants, Children, and Adolescents (Aronoff, 2007):

GFR >50 mL/minute/1.73 m^2: No adjustment required.

GFR 10 to 50 mL/minute/1.73 m^2: Administer 75% of dose once daily.

GFR <10 mL/minute/1.73 m^2: Administer 50% of dose once daily.

Hemodialysis (dialyzable; ~45% removed in 8 hours): Administer 50% of normal dose once daily.

CAPD: Administer 50% of normal dose once daily.

CRRT: Administer 75% of normal dose once daily.

Adults: There are no specific dosage adjustments provided in manufacturer's labeling; however, oliguric patients, particularly those with tubular necrosis in the immediate post-transplant period (cadaveric transplant) may have delayed clearance and typically receive lower doses. The following adjustments have been recommended (Aronoff, 2007):

CrCl >50 mL/minute: No adjustment required.

CrCl 10 to 50 mL/minute: Administer 75% of normal dose.

CrCl <10 mL/minute: Administer 50% of normal dose.

Hemodialysis (dialyzable; ~45% removed in 8 hours): Administer 50% of normal dose; supplement: 0.25 mg/kg

CRRT: Administer 75% of normal dose.

Dosing adjustment in hepatic impairment: There are no dosage adjustments provided in the manufacturer's labeling.

Administration Hazardous agent; use appropriate precautions for handling and disposal (NIOSH, 2012). Oral: Administer with food or may administer in divided doses to decrease GI upset.

Monitoring Parameters CBC with differential and platelets (weekly during first month, twice monthly for months 2 and 3, then monthly; monitor more frequently with dosage modifications), total bilirubin, liver function tests, creatinine clearance, TPMT genotyping or phenotyping (consider TPMT testing in patients with abnormally low CBC unresponsive to dose reduction); monitor for symptoms of infection

For use as immunomodulatory therapy in inflammatory bowel disease (Crohn disease or ulcerative colitis), monitor CBC with differential weekly for 1 month, then biweekly for 1 month, followed by monitoring every 1-2 months throughout the course of therapy; monitor more frequently if symptomatic. LFTs should be assessed every 3 months. Monitor for signs/symptoms of malignancy (eg, splenomegaly, hepatomegaly, abdominal pain, persistent fever, night sweats, weight loss).

Test Interactions TPMT phenotyping results will not be accurate following recent blood transfusions.

Dosage Forms Excipient information presented when available (limited, particularly for generics); consult specific product labeling.

Tablet, Oral:
Azasan: 75 mg, 100 mg [scored]
Imuran: 50 mg [scored]
Generic: 50 mg

Extemporaneous Preparations Hazardous agent: Use appropriate precautions for handling and disposal.

A 50 mg/mL oral suspension may be prepared with tablets. Crush one-hundred-twenty 50 mg tablets in a mortar and reduce to a fine powder. Add 40 mL of either cherry syrup (diluted 1:4 with Simple Syrup, USP); a 1:1 mixture of Ora-Sweet® and Ora-Plus®; or a 1:1 mixture of Ora-Sweet® SF and Ora-Plus®, and mix to a uniform paste. Mix while adding the vehicle in incremental proportions to almost 120 mL; transfer to a calibrated bottle, rinse mortar with vehicle, and add quantity of vehicle sufficient to make 120 mL. Label "shake well", "refrigerate", and "protect from light". Stable for 60 days refrigerated.

Allen LV Jr and Erickson MA 3rd, "Stability of Acetazolamide, Allopurinol, Azathioprine, Clonazepam, and Flucytosine in Extemporaneously Compounded Oral Liquids," Am J Health Syst Pharm, 1996, 53(16):1944-9.

References

Adams A, MacDermott EJ, and Lehman TJ, "Pharmacotherapy of Lupus Nephritis in Children: A Recommended Treatment Approach," Drugs, 2006, 66(9):1191-207.

Aronoff GR, Bennett WM, Berns JS, et al, Drug Prescribing in Renal Failure: Dosing Guidelines for Adults and Children, 5th ed. Philadelphia, PA: American College of Physicians, 2007, p. 97, 177.

Ashraf VV, Taly AB, Veerendrakumar M, et al, "Myasthenia Gravis in Children: A Longitudinal Study," Acta Neurol Scand, 2006, 114 (2):119-23.

Bertsias GK, Tektonidou M, Amoura Z, et al, "Joint European League Against Rheumatism and European Renal Association-European Dialysis and Transplant Association (EULAR/ERA-EDTA) Recommendations for the Management of Adult and Paediatric Lupus Nephritis," Ann Rheum Dis, 2012, 71(11):1771-82.

Biank VF, Sheth MK, Talano J, et al, "Association of Crohn's Disease, Thiopurines, and Primary Epstein-Barr Virus Infection With Hemophagocytic Lymphohistiocytosis," J Pediatr, 2011, 159(5):808-12.

Boruchov DM, Gururangan S, Driscoll MC, et al, "Multiagent Induction and Maintenance Therapy for Patients With Refractory Immune Thrombocytopenic Purpura (ITP)," Blood, 2007, 110(10):3526-31.

Della Corte C, Sartorelli MR, Sindoni CD, et al, "Autoimmune Hepatitis in Children: An Overview of the Disease Focusing on Current Therapies," Eur J Gastroenterol Hepatol, 2012, 24(7):739-46.

Denfield SW, "Strategies to Prevent Cellular Rejection in Pediatric Heart Transplant Recipients," Paediatr Drugs, 2010, 12(6):391-403.

Ford KA, "Paediatric Immunosuppression Following Solid Organ Transplantation," Arch Dis Child Educ Pract, 2006, 91:ep87-ep91.

Fuentes D, Torrente F, Keady S, et al, "High-Dose Azathioprine in Children With Inflammatory Bowel Disease," Aliment Pharmacol Ther, 2003, 17(7):913-21.

Goebel JC, Roesel M, Heinz C, et al, "Azathioprine as a Treatment Option for Uveitis in Patients With Juvenile Idiopathic Arthritis," Br J Ophthalmol, 2011, 95(2):209-13.

Grossman AB, Noble AJ, Mamula P, et al, "Increased Dosing Requirements for 6-Mercaptopurine and Azathioprine in Inflammatory Bowel Disease Patients Six Years and Younger," Inflamm Bowel Dis, 2008, 14(6):750-5.

Hashkes PJ and Laxer RM, "Medical Treatment of Juvenile Idiopathic Arthritis," JAMA, 2005, 294(13):1671-84.

Imuran (azathioprine) [prescribing information]. San Diego, CA: Prometheus Laboratories Inc: February 2014.

Kemper AR, Coeytaux R, Sanders GD, et al, "Disease-Modifying Antirheumatic Drugs (DMARDs) in Children With Juvenile Idiopathic Arthritis (JIA)," Agency for Healthcare Research and Quality, AHRQ Comparative Effectiveness Reviews, 2011.

Kvien TK, Hoyeraal HM, and Sandstad B, "Azathioprine Versus Placebo in Patients With Juvenile Rheumatoid Arthritis: A Single Center Double Blind Comparative Study," J Rheumatol, 1986, 13(1):118-23.

Leichter HE, Sheth KJ, Gerlach MJ, et al, "Outcome of Renal Transplantation in Children Aged 1-5 and 6-18 Years," Child Nephrol Urol, 1992, 12(1):1-5.

Lindner A, Schalke B, and Toyka KV, "Outcome in Juvenile-Onset Myasthenia Gravis: A Retrospective Study With Long-Term Follow-Up of 79 Patients," J Neurol, 1997, 244(8):515-20.

Marks SD and Tullus K, "Modern Therapeutic Strategies for Paediatric Systemic Lupus Erythematosus and Lupus Nephritis," Acta Paediatr, 2010, 99(7):967-74.

National Institute for Occupational Safety and Health (NIOSH), "NIOSH List of Antineoplastic and Other Hazardous Drugs in Healthcare Settings 2012." Available at http://www.cdc.gov/niosh/docs/2012-150/pdfs/2012-150.pdf. Accessed January 21, 2013.

Palace J, Newsom-Davis J, and Lecky B, "A Randomized Double-Blind Trial of Prednisolone Alone or With Azathioprine in Myasthenia Gravis. Myasthenia Gravis Study Group," Neurology, 1998, 50 (6):1778-83.

Punati J, Markowitz J, Lerer T, et al, "Effect of Early Immunomodulator Use in Moderate to Severe Pediatric Crohn Disease," Inflamm Bowel Dis, 2008, 14(7):949-54.

Riello L, Talbotec C, Garnier-Lengliné H, et al, "Tolerance and Efficacy of Azathioprine in Pediatric Crohn's Disease," Inflamm Bowel Dis, 2011, 17(10):2138-43.

Sandhu BK, Fell JME, Beattie RM, et al, "Guidelines for the Management of Inflammatory Bowel Disease in Children in the United Kingdom," JPGN, 2010, 50:S1-S13.

Sathasivam S, "Steroids and Immunosuppressant Drugs in myasthenia Gravis," Nat Clin Pract Neurol, 2008, 4(6):317-27.

Taylor AL, Watson CJ, Bradley JA. Immunosuppressive agents in solid organ transplantation: mechanisms of action and therapeutic efficacy. Crit Rev Oncol Hematol. 2005;56(1):23-46.

Vitfell-Pedersen J, Jorgensen MH, Müller K, et al, "Autoimmune Hepatitis in Children in Eastern Denmark," J Pediatr Gastroenterol Nutr, 2012, 55(4):376-9.

◆ **Azathioprine Sodium** see AzaTHIOprine on page 241

Azelaic Acid (a zeh LAY ik AS id)

Brand Names: U.S. Azelex; Finacea
Brand Names: Canada Finacea®
Therapeutic Category Acne Products
Generic Availability (U.S.) No
Use Topical:
Cream: Azelex: Treatment of mild to moderate inflammatory acne vulgaris (FDA approved in ages ≥12 years and adults)
Gel: Finacea: Treatment of inflammatory papules and pustules of mild to moderate rosacea (FDA approved in adults)

Pregnancy Risk Factor B

Pregnancy Considerations Adverse events were observed in animal reproduction studies following oral administration. Minimal systemic absorption (<4%) occurs following topical administration.

Breast-Feeding Considerations The manufacturer recommends that caution be exercised when administering azelaic acid to nursing women. Minimal systemic absorption (<4%) occurs following topical administration; a significant change from baseline azelaic acid levels in the milk is not expected.

Contraindications Hypersensitivity to azelaic acid, propylene glycol, or any component

Warnings May cause skin irritation; discontinue use if severe skin irritation or sensitivity occurs. Cream and gel contain benzoic acid; benzoic acid (benzoate) is a metabolite of benzyl alcohol which may cause allergic reactions in susceptible individuals; large amounts of benzyl alcohol (≥99 mg/kg/day) have been associated with a potentially fatal toxicity ("gasping syndrome") in neonates; do not use in neonates; *in vitro* and animal studies have shown that benzoate displaces bilirubin from protein binding. Cream and gel formulations contain propylene glycol; toxicities have been reported with use of products containing propylene glycol, including hyperosmolality, lactic acidosis, seizures, and respiratory depression; in neonates large amounts of propylene glycol delivered orally, intravenously (eg, >3000 mg/day), or topically have been associated with potentially fatal toxicities which can include metabolic acidosis, seizures, renal failure, and CNS depression; use cream and gel formulations containing propylene glycol with caution (AAP, 1997; Shehab, 2009). Gel also contains polysorbate 80 (Tween 80) which may cause allergic reactions in susceptible individuals.

Precautions Due to isolated reports of hypopigmentation, use cautiously in patients with dark complexions; monitor for changes in skin color. Avoid foods that may cause erythema (spicy foods, thermally hot foods and drinks, and alcoholic beverages) when applying gel for treatment of rosacea. For topical use only; avoid contact with eyes, mouth, mucous membranes, or open wounds.

Adverse Reactions
Dermatologic: Acne (gel), burning/stinging/tingling, contact dermatitis, dry skin/peeling/scaling/xerosis, edema (gel), erythema, irritation, pruritus (gel)

Rare but important or life-threatening: Asthma exacerbation, allergic reaction, dermatitis, herpes labialis exacerbation, hypertrichosis, iridocyclitis, rash, reddening, small depigmented spots, vitiligo depigmentation

Drug Interactions
Metabolism/Transport Effects None known.

Avoid Concomitant Use There are no known interactions where it is recommended to avoid concomitant use.

Increased Effect/Toxicity There are no known significant interactions involving an increase in effect.

Decreased Effect There are no known significant interactions involving a decrease in effect.

Stability
Azelex: Store at 15°C to 30°C (59°F to 86°F); do not freeze. Store product on its side.

Finacea: Store at 25°C (77°F); excursions permitted to 15°C to 30°C (59°F to 86°F).

Mechanism of Action Azelaic acid is a dietary constituent normally found in whole grain cereals; can be formed endogenously. Exact mechanism is not known. *In vitro*, azelaic acid possesses antimicrobial activity against *Propionibacterium acnes* and *Staphylococcus epidermidis*. May decrease microcomedo formation.

Pharmacodynamics Onset of action (cream): Within 4 weeks

Pharmacokinetics (Adult data unless noted)
Absorption (cream): ~3% to 5% penetrates stratum corneum; up to 10% found in epidermis and dermis; 4% systemic absorption

Half-life (elimination): Topical: 12 hours

Elimination: Primarily unchanged in the urine

Dosing: Usual Topical:
Children ≥12 years and Adolescents: **Acne vulgaris:** Cream (Azelex 20%): Apply twice daily in the morning and evening; may reduce to once daily if persistent skin irritation occurs.

Adults:
  Acne vulgaris: Cream (Azelex 20%): Apply twice daily in the morning and evening; may reduce to once daily if persistent skin irritation occurs.
  Rosacea: Gel (Finacea 15%): Apply to affected areas of the face twice daily in the morning and evening; reassess if no improvement after 12 weeks of therapy.

Administration Topical: Apply a thin film and gently massage into to clean, dry skin; wash hands following application. Avoid the use of occlusive dressings or wrappings. For gel formulation, cosmetics may be applied after the gel has dried. Use only mild soaps or soapless cleansing lotion for facial cleansing. Not intended for intravaginal, ophthalmic, or oral use.

Monitoring Parameters Reduction in lesion size and/or inflammation; reduction in the number of lesions

Dosage Forms Excipient information presented when available (limited, particularly for generics); consult specific product labeling.
Cream, External:
  Azelex: 20% (30 g, 50 g)
Gel, External:
  Finacea: 15% (50 g) [contains benzoic acid, disodium edta, polysorbate 80, propylene glycol]

References
American Academy of Pediatrics Committee on Drugs. "Inactive" ingredients in pharmaceutical products: update (subject review). *Pediatrics.* 1997;99(2):268-278.

Shehab N, Lewis CL, Streetman DD, Donn SM. Exposure to the pharmaceutical excipients benzyl alcohol and propylene glycol among critically ill neonates. *Pediatr Crit Care Med.* 2009;10 (2):256-259.

Azelastine (Nasal) (a ZEL as teen)

Medication Safety Issues
Sound-alike/look-alike issues:
  Astelin may be confused with Astepro
Brand Names: U.S. Astelin [DSC]; Astepro
Brand Names: Canada Astelin
Therapeutic Category Antihistamine, Nasal
Generic Availability (U.S.) Yes
Use
Astelin: Treatment of the symptoms of seasonal allergic rhinitis (FDA approved in ages ≥5 years and adults) and vasomotor rhinitis (FDA approved in ages ≥12 years and adults)

Astepro: Treatment of the symptoms of seasonal allergic rhinitis and perennial allergic rhinitis (FDA approved in ages ≥6 years and adults)

Pregnancy Risk Factor C

Pregnancy Considerations Adverse events were observed in some animal reproduction studies. Azelastine is systemically absorbed following nasal inhalation and may have side effects similar to other antihistamines. However, data related to the use of azelastine in pregnancy is limited; if treatment for rhinitis in a pregnant woman is needed, other agents are preferred (Wallace, 2008).

Breast-Feeding Considerations It is not known if azelastine (nasal) is excreted in breast milk. The manufacturer recommends that caution be exercised when administering azelastine (nasal) to nursing women.

Contraindications Hypersensitivity to azelastine or any component

Precautions May cause CNS depression, which may impair physical or mental abilities; patients must be cautioned about performing tasks which require mental alertness (eg, operating machinery or driving). Effects may be potentiated when used with other sedative drugs or ethanol.

Adverse Reactions Note: Adverse reactions may be dose-, indication-, or product-dependent:

Cardiovascular: Flushing, hypertension, tachycardia

Central nervous system: Abnormality in thinking, anxiety, bitter taste, depersonalization, depression, dizziness, drowsiness, dysesthesia, fatigue, headache, hypoesthesia, malaise, nervousness, sleep disorder, vertigo

Dermatologic: Contact dermatitis, eczema, furunculosis, folliculitis

Endocrine & metabolic: Albuminuria, amenorrhea, weight gain

Gastrointestinal: Abdominal pain, ageusia, aphthous stomatitis, constipation, diarrhea, dysgeusia (children 6-11 years), gastroenteritis, glossitis, increased appetite, nausea, toothache, vomiting, xerostomia

Genitourinary: Hematuria, mastalgia

Hepatic: Increased serum ALT

Hypersensitivity: Hypersensitivity reaction

Infection: Cold symptoms, herpes simplex infection, upper respiratory tract infections (children 6-11 years), viral infection

Neuromuscular & skeletal: Back pain, dislocation of temporomandibular joint, hyperkinesia, limb pain, myalgia, rheumatoid arthritis

Ophthalmic: Conjunctivitis, eye pain, watery eyes

Renal: Polyuria

Respiratory: Asthma, bronchitis, bronchospasm, burning sensation of the nose, cough, epistaxis, laryngitis, nasal congestion, nasal discomfort, nasal mucosa ulcer, paranasal sinus hypersecretion, paroxysmal nocturnal dyspnea, pharyngitis, pharyngolaryngeal pain, postnasal drip, sinusitis, sneezing, sore throat

Miscellaneous: Fever, laceration

Rare but important or life-threatening: Altered sense of smell, anaphylactoid reaction, anosmia, atrial fibrillation, chest pain, confusion, drug tolerance, increased serum transaminases, muscle spasm, urinary retention, xerophthalmia

Drug Interactions

Metabolism/Transport Effects Substrate of CYP1A2 (minor), CYP2C19 (minor), CYP2D6 (minor), CYP3A4 (minor); **Note:** Assignment of Major/Minor substrate status based on clinically relevant drug interaction potential; **Inhibits** CYP2B6 (weak), CYP2C19 (weak), CYP2C9 (weak), CYP2D6 (weak), CYP3A4 (weak)

Avoid Concomitant Use

Avoid concomitant use of Azelastine (Nasal) with any of the following: Aclidinium; Alcohol (Ethyl); CNS Depressants; Ipratropium (Oral Inhalation); Paraldehyde; Pimozide; Potassium Chloride; Thalidomide; Tiotropium; Umeclidinium

Increased Effect/Toxicity

Azelastine (Nasal) may increase the levels/effects of: AbobotulinumtoxinA; Anticholinergic Agents; Cannabinoid-Containing Products; Dofetilide; Lomitapide; Metyrosine; Mirabegron; OnabotulinumtoxinA; Paraldehyde; Pimozide; Potassium Chloride; Pramipexole; RimabotulinumtoxinB; ROPINIRole; Rotigotine; Selective Serotonin Reuptake Inhibitors; Thalidomide; Thiazide Diuretics; Tiotropium

The levels/effects of Azelastine (Nasal) may be increased by: Aclidinium; Alcohol (Ethyl); Brimonidine (Topical); Cannabis; CNS Depressants; Dronabinol; Ipratropium (Oral Inhalation); Kava Kava; Magnesium Sulfate; Nabilone; Pramlintide; Rufinamide; Tetrahydrocannabinol; Umeclidinium

Decreased Effect

Azelastine (Nasal) may decrease the levels/effects of: Acetylcholinesterase Inhibitors (Central); Benzylpenicilloyl Polylysine; Betahistine; Hyaluronidase; Secretin

The levels/effects of Azelastine (Nasal) may be decreased by: Acetylcholinesterase Inhibitors (Central); Amphetamines; Peginterferon Alfa-2b

Stability

Astelin®: Store at 20°C to 25°C (68°F to 77°F); protect from freezing.

Astepro®: Store in the upright position at 20°C to 25°C (68°F to 77°F); protect from light; protect from freezing.

Mechanism of Action Competes with histamine for H_1-receptor sites on effector cells and inhibits the release of histamine and other mediators involved in the allergic response; when used intranasally, reduces hyper-reactivity of the airways; increases the motility of bronchial epithelial cilia, improving mucociliary transport

Pharmacodynamics

Onset of action: 30 minutes to 1 hour

Maximum effect: 3 hours

Duration: 12 hours

Pharmacokinetics (Adult data unless noted)

Protein binding: 88%; desmethylazelastine: 97%

Metabolism: Metabolized by cytochrome P450 enzyme system; active metabolite desmethylazelastine

Bioavailability: 40%

Half-life, elimination: Azelastine: 22-25 hours; desmethylazelastine: 52-57 hours

Time to peak serum concentration: 2-4 hours

Elimination: Clearance: 0.5 L/hour/kg

Dosing: Usual Note: Astepro and Astelin are not interchangeable; Astelin delivers 137 mcg/spray; Astepro 0.1% delivers 137 mcg/spray; Astepro 0.15% delivers 205.5 mcg/spray

Children and Adolescents:

Perennial allergic rhinitis: Intranasal:

Astepro 0.1%: Children 6-11 years: 1 spray **per nostril** twice daily

Astepro 0.15%:

Children 6-11 years: 1 spray **per nostril** twice daily

Children ≥12 years and Adolescents: 2 sprays **per nostril** twice daily

Seasonal allergic rhinitis: Intranasal:

Astelin:

Children 5-11 years: 1 spray **per nostril** twice daily

Children ≥12 years and Adolescents: 1-2 sprays **per nostril** twice daily

Astepro 0.1%:

Children 6-11 years: 1 spray **per nostril** twice daily

Children ≥12 years and Adolescents: 1-2 sprays **per nostril** twice daily

Astepro 0.15%: Children ≥12 years and Adolescents: 1-2 sprays **per nostril** twice daily **or** 2 sprays **per nostril** once daily

Vasomotor rhinitis: Intranasal: Astelin: Children ≥12 years and Adolescents: 2 sprays **per nostril** twice daily

Adults:

Perennial allergic rhinitis: (Astepro 0.15%): Intranasal: 2 sprays **per nostril** twice daily

Seasonal allergic rhinitis: Intranasal:

Astelin, Astepro 0.1%: 1-2 sprays **per nostril** twice daily

Astepro 0.15%: 1-2 sprays **per nostril** twice daily or 2 sprays **per nostril** once daily

Vasomotor rhinitis (Astelin): Intranasal: 2 sprays **per nostril** twice daily

Dosing adjustment in renal impairment: There are no dosage adjustments provided in the manufacturer's labeling.

Dosing adjustment in hepatic impairment: There are no dosage adjustments provided in the manufacturer's labeling.

Administration Before use, the delivery system should be primed with 4 sprays (Astelin), 6 sprays (Astepro), or until a fine mist appears; when 3 or more days have elapsed since the last use, the pump should be reprimed with 2 sprays or until a fine mist appears. Blow nose to clear nostrils. Remove the dust cover. Keep head tilted downward when spraying. Insert applicator into nostril, keeping bottle upright, and close off the other nostril. Breathe in through nose. While inhaling, press pump to release spray. Alternate sprays between nostrils. After each use, wipe the spray tip with a clean tissue or cloth. Avoid spraying in eyes or mouth.

Dosage Forms Considerations Astelin and Astepro 30 mL bottles contain 200 sprays each.

Dosage Forms Excipient information presented when available (limited, particularly for generics); consult specific product labeling. [DSC] = Discontinued product
Solution, Nasal, as hydrochloride:
Astelin: 137 mcg/spray (30 mL [DSC]) [contains benzalkonium chloride, edetate disodium]
Astepro: 0.15% (30 mL) [contains benzalkonium chloride, edetate disodium]
Generic: 137 mcg/spray (30 mL); 0.15% (30 mL)

References
Wallace DV, Dykewicz MS, Bernstein DI, et al, "The Diagnosis and Management of Rhinitis: An Updated Practice Parameter," *J Allergy Clin Immunol*, 2008, 122(2 Suppl):1-84.

Azelastine (Ophthalmic) (a ZEL as teen)

Medication Safety Issues
Sound-alike/look-alike issues:
Optivar® may be confused with Optiray®, Optive™
International issues:
Optivar [U.S.] may be confused with Opthavir brand name for acyclovir [Mexico]
Brand Names: U.S. Optivar
Therapeutic Category Antiallergic, Ophthalmic
Generic Availability (U.S.) Yes
Use Treatment of itching of the eye associated with allergic conjunctivitis
Pregnancy Risk Factor C
Pregnancy Considerations Animal reproduction studies have shown toxic effects to the fetus at maternally toxic doses.
Breast-Feeding Considerations It is not known if azelastine (ophthalmic) is excreted in breast milk. The manufacturer recommends that caution be exercised when administering azelastine (ophthalmic) to nursing women.
Contraindications Hypersensitivity to azelastine or any component
Warnings Ophthalmic solution not for use in contact lens-related irritation; preservative in ophthalmic solution may be absorbed by soft contact lenses; wait at least 10 minutes after instillation before inserting soft contact lenses
Adverse Reactions
Central nervous system: Fatigue, headache
Dermatologic: Pruritus
Gastrointestinal: Bitter taste
Ocular: Blurred vision (temporary), conjunctivitis, eye pain, transient burning/stinging
Respiratory: Asthma, dyspnea, pharyngitis, rhinitis
Miscellaneous: Flu-like syndrome
Drug Interactions
Metabolism/Transport Effects None known.
Avoid Concomitant Use There are no known interactions where it is recommended to avoid concomitant use.
Increased Effect/Toxicity There are no known significant interactions involving an increase in effect.
Decreased Effect There are no known significant interactions involving a decrease in effect.

Mechanism of Action Competes with histamine for H_1-receptor sites on effector cells and inhibits the release of histamine and other mediators involved in the allergic response

Dosing: Usual Ophthalmic: Children ≥3 years and Adults: Instill 1 drop into each affected eye twice daily

Administration Apply finger pressure to lacrimal sac during and for 1-2 minutes after instillation to decrease risk of systemic effects; avoid contact of bottle tip with skin or eye.

Dosage Forms Excipient information presented when available (limited, particularly for generics); consult specific product labeling.
Solution, Ophthalmic, as hydrochloride:
Optivar: 0.05% (6 mL) [contains benzalkonium chloride]
Generic: 0.05% (6 mL)

◆ **Azelastine Hydrochloride** see Azelastine (Nasal) on page 245
◆ **Azelastine Hydrochloride** see Azelastine (Ophthalmic) on page 247
◆ **Azelex** see Azelaic Acid on page 244
◆ **Azidothymidine** see Zidovudine on page 2168
◆ **Azidothymidine, Abacavir, and Lamivudine** see Abacavir, Lamivudine, and Zidovudine on page 41

Azithromycin (Systemic) (az ith roe MYE sin)

Medication Safety Issues
Sound-alike/look-alike issues:
Azithromycin may be confused with azathioprine, erythromycin
Zithromax® may be confused with Fosamax®, Zinacef®, Zovirax®
Related Information
Prevention of Infective Endocarditis on page 2336
Brand Names: U.S. Zithromax; Zithromax Tri-Pak; Zithromax Z-Pak; Zmax
Brand Names: Canada Apo-Azithromycin®; Ava-Azithromycin; Azithromycin for Injection; CO Azithromycin; Dom-Azithromycin; GD-Azithromycin; Mylan-Azithromycin; Novo-Azithromycin; PHL-Azithromycin; PMS-Azithromycin; PRO-Azithromycin; ratio-Azithromycin; Riva-Azithromycin; Sandoz-Azithromycin; Zithromax®; Zithromax® For Intravenous Injection; Zmax SR™
Therapeutic Category Antibiotic, Macrolide
Generic Availability (U.S.) Yes
Use
Oral:
Immediate release; oral suspension, tablets: Treatment of acute otitis media due to *H. influenzae, M. catarrhalis,* or *S. pneumoniae* (FDA approved in pediatric patient ages >6 months); treatment of pharyngitis/tonsillitis due to *S. pyogenes* (FDA approved in ages ≥2 years and adults); treatment of community-acquired pneumonia due to susceptible organisms, including *C. pneumoniae, M. pneumoniae, H. influenzae, S. pneumoniae* (FDA approved in ages ≥6 months and adults). [Oral azithromycin is not indicated for use in patients with pneumonia who have moderate to severe disease and judged to be inappropriate for oral therapy or have any risk factors such as cystic fibrosis, nosocomial infection, known or suspected bacteremia, hospitalization, elderly or debilitated patients, or patients with significant underlying health problems that may compromise their ability to respond to their illness (including immunodeficiency or functional asplenia)]; treatment of sinusitis or COPD exacerbation due to *H. influenzae, M. catarrhalis,* or *S. pneumoniae* (FDA approved in adults); treatment of infections of the skin and skin structure, acute pelvic inflammatory disease, chancroid, and urethritis and cervicitis due to susceptible strains of *C. trachomatis,*

N. gonorrhoeae, M. catarrhalis, H. influenzae, S. aureus, S. pyogenes, S. pneumoniae, Mycoplasma pneumoniae, M. avium complex, *C. psittaci,* and *C. pneumoniae* (FDA approved in adults). Has also been used for treatment of babesiosis, pertussis, endocarditis prophylaxis in penicillin allergic patients, and cystic fibrosis lung disease

Extended release (Zmax®); oral suspension: Treatment of community-acquired pneumonia due to *C. pneumoniae, M. pneumoniae, H. influenzae, S. pneumonia* (FDA approved in ages ≥6 months and adults); treatment of acute bacterial sinusitis due to *H. influenzae, M. catarrhalis,* or *S. pneumoniae* (FDA approved in adults)

Parenteral: Treatment of community-acquired pneumonia due to susceptible *C. pneumoniae, L. pneumophilia, M. pneumoniae, H. influenzae, S. aureus, S. pneumoniae*; treatment of pelvic inflammatory disease due to susceptible *C. pneumonia, N. gonorrhoeae,* or *M. hominis* (FDA approved in adults)

Pregnancy Risk Factor B

Pregnancy Considerations Adverse events were not observed in animal reproduction studies. Azithromycin crosses the placenta (Ramsey, 2003). The maternal serum half-life of azithromycin is unchanged in early pregnancy and decreased at term; however, high concentrations of azithromycin are sustained in the myometrium and adipose tissue (Fischer, 2012; Ramsey, 2003). Azithromycin is recommended for the treatment of several infections, including chlamydia, gonococcal infections, and *Mycobacterium avium* complex (MAC) in pregnant patients (consult current guidelines) (CDC, 2010; DHHS, 2013).

Breast-Feeding Considerations Azithromycin is excreted in low amounts into breast milk (Kelsey, 1994). Decreased appetite, diarrhea, rash, and somnolence have been reported in nursing infants exposed to macrolide antibiotics (Goldstein, 2009). The manufacturer recommends that caution be exercised when administering azithromycin to breast-feeding women.

Contraindications Hypersensitivity to azithromycin or any component, erythromycin, other macrolide, or ketolide antibiotics; concurrent use of pimozide due to potential cardiotoxicity; history of cholestatic jaundice/hepatic dysfunction association with prior azithromycin use

Warnings Macrolides have been associated with rare QT$_c$ prolongation and ventricular arrhythmias, including torsade de pointes; consider avoiding use in patients with prolonged QT interval, congenital long QT syndrome, history of torsade de pointes, bradyarrhythmias, uncorrected hypokalemia or hypomagnesemia, clinically significant bradycardia, uncompensated heart failure, or concurrent use of Class IA (eg, quinidine, procainamide) or Class III (eg, amiodarone, dofetilide, sotalol) antiarrhythmic agents or other drugs known to prolong the QT interval; use with caution in patients at risk for prolonged cardiac repolarization. A recent retrospective cohort study done in Tennessee Medicaid patients demonstrated an increased cardiac risk with azithromycin relative to amoxicillin or ciprofloxacin, and similar risk compared to levofloxacin; notably, increased cardiac mortality (an estimated 47 additional deaths per 1 million 5-day courses of treatment compared to amoxicillin) was associated with higher baseline cardiovascular risk (Ray, 2012); however, this data may not be generalizable to the population as a whole (Ray, 1989). Another nationwide historical cohort study done involving young to middle-aged adults in Denmark did not demonstrate an increased risk of cardiovascular death when compared to the use of penicillin V nor did azithromycin demonstrate an increased risk of cardiovascular death when compared to amoxicillin in a *post hoc* analysis of the same study (Svanstrom, 2013).

Oral azithromycin should not be used to treat pneumonia that is considered inappropriate for outpatient oral therapy.

May mask or delay symptoms of incubating gonorrhea or syphilis so appropriate culture and susceptibility tests should be performed prior to initiating azithromycin. Pseudomembranous colitis, including *Clostridium difficile*-associated diarrhea (CDAD) ranging from mild diarrhea to fatal colitis has been reported with use of antibiotics, including azithromycin; CDAD has been observed >2 months postantibiotic treatment. If CDAD is suspected or confirmed, azithromycin may need to be discontinued and CDAD treatment and supportive care initiated. Serious allergic reactions, including anaphylaxis, angioedema, Stevens-Johnson syndrome, and toxic epidermal necrolysis, have been reported; reappearance of allergic reaction may occur shortly after discontinuation of symptomatic treatment even without further azithromycin exposure. Patients who experience allergic reactions may require prolonged periods of observation and symptomatic treatment, possibly due to the drug's long tissue half-life.

Hepatic impairment, including hepatocellular and/or cholestatic hepatitis, with or without jaundice, hepatic necrosis, failure, and death have been reported in older children and adults; it may be accompanied by malaise, nausea, vomiting, abdominal colic, and fever; discontinue use immediately if signs/symptoms of hepatic impairment occur.

Formulations of azithromycin (immediate release vs extended release) are not interchangeable on a mg per mg basis due to different pharmacokinetic profiles.

Precautions Use with caution in patients with impaired hepatic function and patients with severe renal impairment (GFR <10 mL/minute). Use with caution in patients with myasthenia gravis; exacerbation and new onset of symptoms have occurred.

Adverse Reactions

Dermatologic: Pruritus, skin rash

Gastrointestinal: Abdominal pain, anorexia, diarrhea, nausea, stomach cramps, vomiting

Genitourinary: Vaginitis

Local: (with I.V. administration): Local inflammation, pain at injection site

Rare but important or life-threatening: Acute renal failure, ageusia, aggressive behavior, anaphylaxis, anemia, angioedema, anosmia, auditory disturbance, candidiasis, cardiac arrhythmia (including ventricular tachycardia), chest pain, cholestatic jaundice, conjunctivitis (pediatric patients), deafness, DRESS syndrome, eczema, edema, enteritis, erythema multiforme (rare), fungal dermatitis, fungal infection, gastritis, hearing loss, hepatic failure, hepatic necrosis, hepatitis, hyperactivity, hyperkinesia, hypotension, increased liver enzymes, insomnia, interstitial nephritis, jaundice, leukopenia, melena, mucositis, nephritis, neutropenia (mild), oral candidiasis, pancreatitis, pharyngitis, pleural effusion, prolonged Q-T interval on ECG (rare), pseudomembranous colitis, pyloric stenosis, seizure, skin photosensitivity, Stevens-Johnson syndrome (rare), syncope, taste perversion, thrombocytopenia, tongue discoloration (rare), torsades de pointes (rare), toxic epidermal necrolysis (rare), vesiculobullous rash

Drug Interactions

Metabolism/Transport Effects Substrate of CYP3A4 (minor); **Note:** Assignment of Major/Minor substrate status based on clinically relevant drug interaction potential; **Inhibits** CYP1A2 (weak), P-glycoprotein

Avoid Concomitant Use

Avoid concomitant use of Azithromycin (Systemic) with any of the following: Amiodarone; BCG; Highest Risk QTc-Prolonging Agents; Ivabradine; Mifepristone; Pimozide; QuiNINE; Terfenadine

Increased Effect/Toxicity

Azithromycin (Systemic) may increase the levels/effects of: Amiodarone; AtorvaSTATin; Cardiac Glycosides;

CycloSPORINE (Systemic); Highest Risk QTc-Prolonging Agents; Ivermectin (Systemic); Lovastatin; Moderate Risk QTc-Prolonging Agents; Pimozide; QuiNINE; Rilpivirine; Rivaroxaban; Simvastatin; Tacrolimus (Systemic); Tacrolimus (Topical); Terfenadine; Vitamin K Antagonists

The levels/effects of Azithromycin (Systemic) may be increased by: Ivabradine; Mifepristone; Nelfinavir; QTc-Prolonging Agents (Indeterminate Risk and Risk Modifying)

Decreased Effect

Azithromycin (Systemic) may decrease the levels/effects of: BCG; Sodium Picosulfate; Typhoid Vaccine

Food Interactions Rate and extent of GI absorption may be altered depending upon the formulation. Azithromycin suspension, not tablet form, has significantly increased absorption (46%) with food. Management: Immediate release suspension and tablet may be taken without regard to food; extended release suspension should be taken on an empty stomach (at least 1 hour before or 2 hours following a meal).

Stability

Oral:

Tablets: Store at or below 30°C (86°F).

Oral suspension:

Immediate release single dose packets: Store at 5°C to 30°C (41°F to 86°F).

Immediate release bottle: Store dry powder at or below 30°C (86°F). After reconstitution, may be stored for 10 days at room temperature or in the refrigerator.

Extended release microspheres (Zmax): Store dry powder at or below 30°C (86°F). After reconstitution, store at room temperature; do not refrigerate or freeze; must be consumed within 12 hours following reconstitution. Any suspension remaining after dosing must be discarded.

Parenteral: Store intact vials at or below 30°C (86°F). After reconstitution, 100 mg/mL solution is stable for 24 hours at room temperature. When further diluted to a concentration of 1-2 mg/mL, this solution is stable for 24 hours at room temperature or 7 days if refrigerated.

Mechanism of Action Inhibits RNA-dependent protein synthesis at the chain elongation step; binds to the 50S ribosomal subunit resulting in blockage of transpeptidation

Pharmacokinetics (Adult data unless noted)

Absorption: Oral: Rapid from the GI tract

Distribution: Extensive tissue distribution into skin, lungs, tonsils, bone, prostate, cervix; CSF concentrations are low

V_d: 31-33 L/kg

Protein binding: 7% to 51% (concentration-dependent and dependent on alpha$_1$-acid glycoprotein concentrations)

Metabolism: Hepatic to inactive metabolites

Bioavailability: Tablet, immediate release oral suspension: 34% to 52%; extended release oral suspension: 28% to 43%

Half-life, terminal:

Infants and Children 4 months to 15 years: 54.5 hours

Adults: Immediate release: 68-72 hours; Extended release: 59 hours

Time to peak serum concentration: Oral:

Immediate release: 2-3 hours

Extended release oral suspension: 3-5 hours

Elimination: 50% of dose is excreted unchanged in bile; 6% to 14% of dose is excreted unchanged in urine

Dosing: Neonatal Note: Extended release suspension (Zmax) is not interchangeable with immediate-release formulations. All oral doses are expressed as immediate release azithromycin unless otherwise specified.

General dosing, susceptible infection (*Red Book* [AAP], 2012):

Oral: 10-20 mg/kg once daily

I.V.: 10 mg/kg once daily

Bronchopulmonary dysplasia, prevention: Limited data available: Oral, I.V.: 10 mg/kg once daily for 7 days, followed by 5 mg/kg once daily for 5 weeks was used in 19 mechanically ventilated premature neonates (mean GA: 25.6 weeks; PNA: <72 hours; birth weight ≤1000 g) and decreased corticosteroid use and duration of mechanical ventilation compared to placebo (Ballard, 2007)

Chlamydial conjunctivitis or chlamydial pneumonia: Oral, I.V.: 20 mg/kg once daily for 3 days (*Red Book* [AAP], 2012)

Pertussis, treatment and postexposure prophylaxis: Oral, I.V.: 10 mg/kg once daily for 5 days (*Red Book* [AAP], 2012)

Dosing: Usual Note: Extended release suspension (Zmax) is not interchangeable with immediate-release formulations. All doses are expressed as immediate release azithromycin unless otherwise specified.

Pediatric:

General dosing, susceptible infection (*Red Book* [AAP], 2012): Infants, Children, and Adolescents:

Mild to moderate infection: Oral: 5 -12 mg/kg/dose; typically administered as 10-12 mg/kg/dose on day 1 followed by 5-6 mg/kg once daily for remainder of treatment duration; usual maximum dose for the total course: 1500-2000 mg

Serious infection: I.V.: 10 mg/kg once daily; maximum dose: 500 mg

Acute otitis media (AOM): Infants, Children, and Adolescents: Oral: **Note:** Due to increased *S pneumonia* and *H. influenzae* resistance, azithromycin is not routinely recommended as a treatment option (Lieberthal, 2013)

Single dose regimen: 30 mg/kg as a single dose; maximum dose: 1500 mg; if patient vomits within 30 minutes of dose, repeat dosing has been administered although limited data available on safety

Three-day regimen: 10 mg/kg once daily for 3 days; maximum dose: 500 mg

Five-day regimen: 10 mg/kg once on day 1 (maximum dose: 500 mg), followed by 5 mg/kg (maximum dose: 250 mg) once daily on days 2-5

Babesiosis: Infants, Children, and Adolescents: Oral: 10 mg/kg once on day 1 (maximum dose: 500 mg), then 5 mg/kg once daily on days 2-10 (maximum dose: 250 mg) in combination with atovaquone; longer duration of therapy may be necessary in some cases; in immunocompromised patients, higher doses (eg, adults: 600-1000 mg daily) may be required (*Red Book*, 2012; Wormser, 2006)

Bartonellosis: Oral:

Cat scratch disease (*B. henselae*) with extensive lymphadenopathy: *Non-HIV-exposed/-positive:*

Infants, Children, and Adolescents ≤45.5 kg: 10 mg/kg once on day 1 (maximum dose: 500 mg), followed by 5 mg/kg once daily on days 2-5 (maximum dose: 250 mg) (Rolain, 2004)

Children and Adolescents >45.5 kg: 500 mg as a single dose on day 1, then 250 mg once daily for 4 additional days (Bass, 1998; Stevens, 2005)

Cutaneous bacillary angiomatosis (*B. henselae* or *B. quintana*): *HIV- exposed/-positive:* Infants, Children, and Adolescents: 5-12 mg/kg once daily; maximum dose: 600 mg; usual treatment duration: 3 months (CDC, 2009)

Chancroid (CDC, 2010; *Red Book*, 2012): Oral:

<45 kg: 20 mg/kg as a single dose; maximum dose: 1000 mg

≥45 kg: 1000 mg as a single dose

Chlamydial infections:

Cervicitis, urethritis (*C. trachomatis*): Children and Adolescents ≥45 kg: Oral: 1000 mg as a single dose (CDC, 2010; *Red Book* [AAP], 2012)

Conjunctivitis: Infants: Oral, I.V.: 20 mg/kg once daily for 3 days (Red Book [AAP], 2012)

Pneumonia, community-acquired (Bradley, 2011): Infants >3 months, Children, and Adolescents:

Mild infection or step-down therapy: Oral: 10 mg/kg once on day 1 (maximum dose: 500 mg) followed by 5 mg/kg once daily on days 2-5 (maximum dose: 250 mg)

Severe infection: I.V.: 10 mg/ kg once daily for at least 2 days, then transition to oral route with a single daily dose of 5 mg/kg to complete course of therapy; maximum dose: 500 mg

Cystic fibrosis; improve lung function, reduce exacerbation frequency: Limited data available; dosing regimen variable (Flume, 2007; Saiman, 2003; Saiman; 2010): Children ≥6 years and ≥18 kg and Adolescents: Oral:

18-35.9 kg: 250 mg three times weekly (Monday, Wednesday, Friday)

≥36 kg: 500 mg three times weekly (Monday, Wednesday, Friday)

Diarrhea, infectious:

Campylobacter: Infants, Children, and Adolescents: Oral: 10 mg/kg once daily for 3 days; maximum dose: 500 mg (Red Book [AAP], 2012)

Shigellosis: Infants, Children, and Adolescents: Oral:

AAP Recommendation: 12 mg/kg once on day 1 (maximum dose: 500 mg), followed by 6 mg/kg once daily on days 2-5 (maximum dose: 250 mg) (Red Book [AAP], 2012)

Alternate dosing: 10 mg/kg once daily for 3 days (Dupont, 2009; Mackell, 2005); WHO Guidelines recommend up to 20 mg/kg/dose and in some cases, a wider range of duration of therapy (eg, 1-5 days) (WHO, 2005)

Endocarditis; prophylaxis: Infants, Children, and Adolescents: Oral: 15 mg/kg/dose 30-60 minutes before procedure; maximum dose: 500 mg (Wilson, 2007)

Gonococcal infection; uncomplicated (cervicitis, urethritis, anorectal): Oral:

Children <45 kg: 20 mg/kg as a single dose; maximum dose: 1000 mg (Red Book [AAP], 2012)

Children >8 years and ≥45 kg and Adolescents: 1000 mg as a single dose (CDC, 2012; Red Book, 2012)

Group A streptococcal infection; treatment of streptococcal tonsillopharyngitis:

Manufacturer's labeling and AHA guidelines: Infants, Children, and Adolescents: Limited data in infants and children <2 years: Oral: 12 mg/kg/dose once daily for 5 days; maximum single dose: 500 mg; total dose for course: 60 mg/kg (Gerber, 2009)

Alternate dosing:

IDSA guidelines: Infants, Children, and Adolescents: Oral: 12 mg/kg (maximum: 500 mg) on day 1 followed by 6 mg/kg/dose (maximum: 250 mg) once daily on days 2 through 5 (Red Book [AAP] 2012; Shulman, 2012); **Note:** Recommended by the Infectious Disease Society of America (IDSA) as an alternative agent for group A streptococcal pharyngitis in penicillin-allergic patients (Shulman, 2012).

Three-day regimen: Limited data available: Children and Adolescents: Oral: 20 mg/kg/dose once daily for 3 days; maximum single dose: 1000 mg (Cohen, 2004; O'Doherty, 1996)

Meningococcal disease, chemoprophylaxis of high-risk contacts: Infants, Children, and Adolescents: Oral: 10 mg/kg as a single dose; maximum dose: 500 mg; **Note:** Not routinely recommended; may consider if fluoroquinolone resistance detected (Red Book [AAP], 2012)

Mycobacterium avium complex (MAC) infection:

HIV-exposed/-positive:

Infants and Children (DHHS [pediatric], 2013): Oral:

Treatment: 10-12 mg/kg once daily (maximum dose: 500 mg) in combination with ethambutol, with or without rifabutin; treatment duration at least 12 months; dependent upon clinical response

Primary prevention of first episode: Preferred: 20 mg/kg once weekly (maximum dose: 1200 mg) **or** alternatively, 5 mg/kg/day once daily (maximum dose: 250 mg/day)

Secondary prevention of recurring episodes: 5 mg/kg once daily (maximum dose: 250 mg) in combination with ethambutol, with or without rifabutin

Adolescents (DHHS [adult], 2013): Oral:

Treatment: 500-600 mg daily in combination with ethambutol

Primary prophylaxis: 1200 mg once weekly **or** alternatively, 600 mg twice weekly

Secondary prophylaxis: 500-600 mg daily in combination with ethambutol

Non-HIV-exposed/-positive (Bradley, 2011): Infants >3 months, Children, and Adolescents:

Mild infection or step-down therapy: Oral: 10 mg/kg once on day 1 (maximum dose: 500 mg) followed by 5 mg/kg once daily on days 2-5 (maximum dose: 250 mg)

Severe infection: I.V.: 10 mg/kg once daily for at least 2 days (maximum dose: 500 mg), then transition to oral route with a single daily dose of 5 mg/kg to complete course of therapy (maximum dose: 250 mg)

Peritonitis, prophylaxis for patients receiving peritoneal dialysis who require dental procedures: Infants, Children, and Adolescents: Oral: 15 mg/kg administered 30-60 minutes before dental procedure; maximum dose: 500 mg (Warady, 2012)

Pertussis (CDC, 2005, Red Book, 2012): Oral, I.V.:

Infants 1-5 months: 10 mg/kg/dose once daily for 5 days

Infants ≥6 months, Children, and Adolescents: 10 mg/kg once on day 1 (maximum dose: 500 mg), followed by 5 mg/kg once daily on days 2-5 (maximum dose: 250 mg)

Pneumonia, community-acquired (excluding mycobacterial and chlamydial):

Oral:

Immediate release: Infants >3 months, Children, and Adolescents: 10 mg/kg once on day 1 (maximum dose: 500 mg), followed by 5 mg/kg (maximum dose: 250 mg/day) once daily on days 2-5 (Bradley, 2011)

Extended release oral suspension (Zmax): Infants ≥6 months, Children, and Adolescents: 60 mg/kg as a single dose; maximum dose: 2000 mg

I.V.: Infants >3 months, Children, and Adolescents: 10 mg/kg once daily for at least 2 days, follow I.V. therapy by the oral route with a single daily dose of 5 mg/kg to complete a 5-day course of therapy; maximum dose: 500 mg (Bradley, 2011)

Rhinosinusitis, bacterial: Oral: Infants ≥6 months, Children, and Adolescents: 10 mg/kg once daily for 3 days; maximum dose: 500 mg. **Note:** Although FDA approved, macrolides are not recommended for empiric therapy due to high rates of resistance (Chow, 2012)

Sexual victimization, prophylaxis: Oral: **Note:** Use in combination with cefixime or ceftriaxone and completion of hepatitis B virus immunization; also consider prophylaxis for trichomoniasis and bacterial vaginosis (CDC, 2010; Red Book [AAP], 2012).

Children <45 kg: 20 mg/kg as a single dose

Children ≥45 kg and Adolescents: 1000 mg as a single dose

***Toxoplasma gondii*, encephalitis (HIV-exposed/-positive); treatment and prevention:** Oral: Adolescents: 900-1200 mg once daily in combination with pyrimethamine/leucovorin; treatment duration: 6 weeks or longer if extensive disease or incomplete response at 6 weeks (DHHS [adult], 2013)

Adult:

Rhinosinusitis, bacterial: Oral: 500 mg once daily for 3 days. **Note:** Although FDA approved, macrolides are not recommended for empiric therapy due to high rates of resistance (Chow, 2012).

Alternate regimen: Extended release suspension (Zmax): 2000 mg as a single dose

Chancroid due to *H. ducreyi*: Oral: 1000 mg as a single dose (CDC, 2010)

Cervicitis, urethritis: Nongonococcal *Chlamydia trachomatis*: Oral: 1000 mg as a single dose

Gonococcal infection, uncomplicated (cervix, rectum, urethra): Oral: 1000 mg as a single dose in combination with ceftriaxone (preferred) or cefixime (only if ceftriaxone unavailable); if cefixime is used, test-of-cure in 7 days is recommended (CDC, 2012). **Note:** Monotherapy with azithromycin single dose of 2000 mg has been associated with resistance and/or treatment failure; however, may be appropriate for treatment of a gonococcal infection in pregnant women who cannot tolerate a cephalosporin (CDC, 2010).

Patients with severe cephalosporin allergy: 2000 mg as a single dose and test-of-cure in 7 days (CDC, 2012)

Gonococcal infection, uncomplicated (pharynx): Oral: 1000 mg as a single dose in combination with ceftriaxone (CDC, 2012)

Gonococcal infection, expedited partner therapy: Oral: 1000 mg as a single dose in combination with cefixime (CDC, 2012). **Note:** Only used if a heterosexual partner cannot be linked to evaluation and treatment in a timely manner; dose delivered to partner by patient, collaborating pharmacy, or disease investigation specialist.

Granuloma inguinale (donovanosis): Oral: 1000 mg once a week for at least 3 weeks and until lesions have healed (CDC, 2010)

Endocarditis prophylaxis: Oral: 500 mg 30-60 minutes before procedure. **Note:** American Heart Association (AHA) guidelines now recommend prophylaxis only in patients undergoing invasive procedures and in whom underlying cardiac conditions may predispose to a higher risk of adverse outcomes should infection occur. As of April 2007, routine prophylaxis for GI/GU procedures is no longer recommended by the AHA (Wilson, 2007).

Mild to moderate respiratory tract, skin, and soft tissue infections: Oral: 500 mg in a single loading dose on day 1 followed by 250 mg daily as a single dose on days 2-5

Alternative regimen: Bacterial exacerbation of COPD: 500 mg daily for a total of 3 days

***Mycobacterium avium* complex disease, disseminated, in patients with advanced HIV infection:** Oral: Treatment: 600 mg daily in combination with ethambutol

Primary prophylaxis: 1200 mg once weekly (preferred), with **or** without rifabutin or alternatively, 600 mg twice weekly (DHHS [adult], 2013)

Secondary prophylaxis: 500-600 mg daily in combination with ethambutol (DHHS [adult], 2013)

Pelvic inflammatory disease: I.V.: 500 mg as a single dose for 1-2 days, follow I.V. therapy by the oral route with a single daily dose of 250 mg to complete a 7-day course of therapy

Pharyngitis/tonsillitis, group A streptococci:
Manufacturer labeling: Oral: 500 mg on day 1 followed by 250 mg once daily on days 2-5

IDSA guidelines: Oral: 12 mg/kg (maximum: 500 mg) on day 1 followed by 6 mg/kg/dose (maximum: 250 mg) once daily days 2 to 5. **Note:** Recommended by the Infectious Disease Society of America (IDSA) as an alternative agent for group A streptococcal pharyngitis in penicillin-allergic patients (Shulman, 2012).

Pneumonia, community-acquired:
Oral: 500 mg on day 1 followed by 250 mg once daily on days 2-5

Alternate regimen: Extended release suspension (Zmax®): 2000 mg as a single dose

I.V.: 500 mg as a single dose for at least 2 days; follow I.V. therapy by the oral route with a single daily dose of 500 mg to complete a 7- to 10-day course of therapy

Pertussis: Oral: 500 mg on day 1 followed by 250 mg once daily on days 2-5 (CDC, 2005)

Prophylaxis against sexually transmitted diseases following sexual assault: Oral: 1000 mg as a single dose (in combination with a cephalosporin and metronidazole) (CDC, 2010)

Dosing adjustment in renal impairment: Infants ≥6 months, Children, Adolescents, and Adults:

Use with caution in patients with GFR <10 mL/minute (AUC increased by 35% compared to patients with normal renal function); however, no dosage adjustment is provided in the manufacturer's labeling.

No supplemental dose or dosage adjustment necessary, including patients on intermittent hemodialysis, peritoneal dialysis, or continuous renal replacement therapy (eg, CVVHD) (Aronoff, 2007; Heintz, 2009).

Dosing adjustment in hepatic impairment: Azithromycin is predominantly hepatically eliminated; however, there is no dosage adjustment provided in the manufacturer's labeling. Use with caution due to potential for hepatotoxicity (rare); discontinue immediately for signs or symptoms of hepatitis.

Administration

Oral:

Immediate release: May administer without regard to food; do not administer with antacids that contain aluminum or magnesium.

Oral suspension, multiple doses: Shake well before use.

Oral suspension 1000 mg packet for a single dose: Prepare by mixing contents of 1 packet with approximately 60 mL of water; administer the entire contents immediately; add an additional 60 mL of water, mix, and drink. Do not use to administer any other dose except 1000 mg or 2000 mg.

Extended release oral suspension: Prepare 2000 mg azithromycin suspension by reconstituting with 60 mL of water (final concentration: 27 mg/mL). Shake suspension well before use; administer on an empty stomach 1 hour before or 2 hours after a meal. May be administered without regard to antacids containing aluminum or magnesium.

Parenteral: **Do not give I.M. or by direct I.V. injection.** Administer I.V. infusion at a final concentration of 1 mg/mL over 3 hours; for a 2 mg/mL concentration, infuse over 1 hour; do not infuse over a period of less than 60 minutes.

Monitoring Parameters Liver function tests, WBC with differential; number and type of stools/day for diarrhea; monitor patients receiving azithromycin and drugs known to interact with erythromycin (ie, theophylline, digoxin, anticoagulants, triazolam) since there are still very few studies examining drug-drug interactions with azithromycin. When used as part of alternative treatment for gonococcal infection, test-of-cure 7 days after dose (CDC, 2012).

Dosage Forms Excipient information presented when available (limited, particularly for generics); consult specific product labeling.

Packet, Oral, as dihydrate [strength expressed as base]:
Zithromax: 1 g (3 ea, 10 ea) [cherry-banana flavor]
Generic: 1 g (3 ea, 10 ea)

Solution Reconstituted, Intravenous, as dihydrate [strength expressed as base]:
Zithromax: 500 mg (1 ea)

Solution Reconstituted, Intravenous, as hydrogencitrate [strength expressed as base]:
Generic: 2.5 g (1 ea)

Solution Reconstituted, Intravenous, as monohydrate [strength expressed as base]:
Generic: 500 mg (1 ea)

Solution Reconstituted, Intravenous, as monohydrate [strength expressed as base, preservative free]:
Generic: 500 mg (1 ea)

Suspension Reconstituted, Oral, as dihydrate [strength expressed as base]:
Zithromax: 100 mg/5 mL (15 mL) [cherry-vanilla-banana flavor]
Zithromax: 200 mg/5 mL (15 mL, 22.5 mL, 30 mL) [cherry flavor]
Zmax: 2 g (1 ea) [cherry-banana flavor]
Generic: 100 mg/5 mL (15 mL); 200 mg/5 mL (15 mL, 22.5 mL, 30 mL)

Suspension Reconstituted, Oral, as monohydrate [strength expressed as base]:
Generic: 100 mg/5 mL (15 mL); 200 mg/5 mL (15 mL, 22.5 mL, 30 mL)

Tablet, Oral, as anhydrous:
Generic: 250 mg, 500 mg, 600 mg

Tablet, Oral, as dihydrate [strength expressed as base]:
Zithromax: 250 mg, 500 mg, 600 mg
Zithromax Tri-Pak: 500 mg
Zithromax Z-Pak: 250 mg
Generic: 250 mg, 500 mg, 600 mg

Tablet, Oral, as monohydrate [strength expressed as base]:
Generic: 250 mg, 500 mg, 600 mg

References

American Academy of Pediatrics (AAP). In: Pickering LK, Baker CJ, Kimberlin DW, Long SS, eds. *Red Book: 2012 Report of the Committee on Infectious Diseases.* 29th ed. Elk Grove Village, IL: American Academy of Pediatrics; 2012.

American College of Obstetricians and Gynecologists, "ACOG Practice Bulletin No. 120: Use of Prophylactic Antibiotics in Labor and Delivery," *Obstet Gynecol,* 2011, 117(6):1472-83.

Aronoff GR, Bennett WM, Berns JS, et al, *Drug Prescribing in Renal Failure: Dosing Guidelines for Adults and Children,* 5th ed, Philadelphia, PA: American College of Physicians, 2007.

Ballard HO, Anstead MI, and Shook LA, "Azithromycin in the Extremely Low Birth Weight Infant for the Prevention of Bronchopulmonary Dysplasia: A Pilot Study," *Respir Res,* 2007, 8:41.

Bass JW, Freitas BC, Freitas AD, et al, "Prospective Randomized Double Blind Placebo-Controlled Evaluation of Azithromycin for Treatment of Cat-Scratch Disease," *Pediatr Infect Dis J,* 1998, 17 (6):447-52.

Bradley JS, Byington CL, Shah SS, et al, "The Management of Community-Acquired Pneumonia in Infants and Children Older Than 3 Months of Age: Clinical Practice Guidelines by the Pediatric Infectious Diseases Society and the Infectious Diseases Society of America", *Clin Infect Dis,* 2011, 53(7):e25-76.

Bryant KA, Humbaugh K, Brothers K, et al, "Measures to Control an Outbreak of Pertussis in a Neonatal Intermediate Care Nursery After Exposure to a Healthcare Worker," *Infect Control Hosp Epidemiol,* 2006, 27(6):541-5.

Centers for Disease Control and Prevention (CDC), "Guidelines for the Prevention and Treatment of Opportunistic Infections Among HIV-Exposed and HIV-Infected Children," *MMWR Recomm Rep,* 2009, 58(RR-11):1-166. Available at http://aidsinfo.nih.gov/contentfiles/Pediatric_OI.pdf

Centers for Disease Control and Prevention (CDC), "Recommended Antimicrobial Agents for the Treatment and Postexposure Prophylaxis of Pertussis: 2005 CDC Guidelines," *MMWR Recomm Rep,* 2005, 54 (RR-14):1-16.

Centers for Disease Control and Prevention (CDC), "Sexually Transmitted Diseases Treatment Guidelines, 2010," *MMWR Recomm Rep,* 2010, 59(RR-12):1-110.

Centers for Disease Control and Prevention (CDC), "Update to CDC's Sexually Transmitted Diseases Treatment Guidelines, 2010: Oral Cephalosporins No Longer a Recommended Treatment for Gonococcal Infections," *MMWR Morb Mortal Wkly Rep,* 2012, 61(31):590-4.

Chow AW, Benninger MS, Brook I, et al, "IDSA Clinical Practice Guideline for Acute Bacterial Rhinosinusitis in Children and Adults," *Clin Infect Dis,* 2012 54(8):e72-e112.

Cohen R. Defining the optimum treatment regimen for azithromycin in acute tonsillopharyngitis. *Pediatr Infect Dis J.* 2004;23(2 Suppl): S129-134.

DHHS. Guidelines for the prevention and treatment of opportunistic infections among HIV-exposed and HIV-infected children: recommendations from the National Institutes of Health, Centers for Disease Control and Prevention, the HIV Medicine Association of the Infectious Diseases Society of America, the Pediatric Infectious Diseases Society, and the American Academy of Pediatrics. November 6, 2013. Available at http://aidsinfo.nih.gov

DHHS Panel on Opportunistic Infections (OI) in HIV-Infected Adults and Adolescents, "Guidelines for Prevention and Treatment of Opportunistic Infections in HIV-Infected Adults and Adolescents: Recommendations from the Centers for Disease Control and Prevention (CDC), the National Institutes of Health (NIH), and the HIV Medicine Association (HIVMA) of the Infectious Diseases Society of America (IDSA)," May 7, 2013. Available at http://aidsinfo.nih.gov/contentfiles/lvguidelines/adult_oi.pdf

Drew RH and Gallis HA, "Azithromycin-Spectrum of Activity, Pharmacokinetics, and Clinical Applications," *Pharmacotherapy,* 1992, 12 (3):161-73.

DuPont HL, "Clinical Practice. Bacterial Diarrhea," *N Engl J Med,* 2009, 361(16):1560-9.

Fischer JH, Sarto GE, Habibi M, et al, "Influence of Body Weight, Ethnicity, Oral Contraceptives, and Pregnancy on the Pharmacokinetics of Azithromycin in Women of Childbearing Age," *Antimicrob Agents Chemother,* 2012, 56(2):715-24.

Flume PA, O'Sullivan BP, Robinson KA, et al, "Cystic Fibrosis Pulmonary Guidelines: Chronic Medications for Maintenance of Lung Health," *Am J Respir Crit Care Med,* 2007, 176(10):957-69.

Foulds G, Shepard RM, and Johnson RB, "The Pharmacokinetics of Azithromycin in Human Serum and Tissues," *J Antimicrob Chemother,* 1990, 25(Suppl A):73-82.

Gerber MA, Baltimore RS, Eaton CB, et al, "Prevention of Rheumatic Fever and Diagnosis and Treatment of Acute Streptococcal Pharyngitis: A Scientific Statement From the American Heart Association Rheumatic Fever, Endocarditis, and Kawasaki Disease Committee of the Council on Cardiovascular Disease in the Young, the Interdisciplinary Council on Functional Genomics and Translational Biology, and the Interdisciplinary Council on Quality of Care and Outcomes Research: Endorsed by the American Academy of Pediatrics," *Circulation,* 2009, 119(11):1541-51.

Goldstein LH, Berlin M, Tsur L, et al, "The Safety of Macrolides During Lactation," *Breastfeed Med,* 2009, 4(4):197-200.

Heintz BH, Matzke GR, and Dager WE, "Antimicrobial Dosing Concepts and Recommendations for Critically Ill Adult Patients Receiving Continuous Renal Replacement Therapy or Intermittent Hemodialysis," *Pharmacotherapy,* 2009, 29(5):562-77.

Jacobs RF, Maples HD, Aranda JV, et al, "Pharmacokinetics of Intravenously Administered Azithromycin in Pediatric Patients," *Pediatr Infect Dis J,* 2005, 24(1):34-9.

Kelsey JJ, Moser LR, Jennings JC, et al, "Presence of Azithromycin Breast Milk Concentrations: A Case Peport," *Am J Obstet Gynecol,* 1994, 170(5 Pt 1):1375-6.

Lieberthal AS, Carroll AE, Chonmaitree T, et al, "The Diagnosis and Management of Acute Otitis Media," *Pediatrics,* 2013, 131(3): e964-99.

Lockwood AM, Cole S, and Rabinovich M, "Azithromycin-Induced Liver Injury," *Am J Health Syst Pharm,* 2010, 67(10):810-4.

Mackell S, "Traveler's Diarrhea in the Pediatric Population: Etiology and Impact," *Clin Infect Dis,* 2005, 41(Suppl 80):S547-52.

Nahata MC, Koranyi KI, Gadgil SD, et al, "Pharmacokinetics of Azithromycin After Oral Administration of Multiple Doses of Suspension," *Antimicrob Agents Chemother,* 1993, 37(2):314-16.

O'Doherty B. Azithromycin versus penicillin V in the treatment of paediatric patients with acute streptococcal pharyngitis/tonsillitis. Paediatric Azithromycin Study Group. *Eur J Clin Microbiol Infect Dis.* 1996;15(9):718-724.

Ramsey PS, Vaules MB, Vasdev GM, et al, "Maternal and Transplacental Pharmacokinetics of Azithromycin," *Am J Obstet Gynecol,* 2003, 188(3):714-8.

Ray WA, Griffin MR. Use of Medicaid data for pharmacoepidemiology. *American Journal of Epidemiology.* 1989;129(4):837-849.

Ray WA, Murray KT, Hall K, et al, "Azithromycin and the Risk of Cardiovascular Death," *N Engl J Med,* 2012, 366(20):1881-90.

Rolain JM, Brouqui P, Koehler JE, et al, "Recommendations for Treatment of Human Infections Caused by Bartonella Species," *Antimicrob Agents Chemother*, 2004, 48(6):1921-33.

Saiman L, Anstead M, Mayer-Hamblett N, et al, "Effect of Azithromycin on Pulmonary Function in Patients With Cystic Fibrosis Uninfected With *Pseudomonas aeruginosa*: A Randomized Controlled Trial," *JAMA*, 2010, 303(17):1707-15.

Saiman L, Marshall BC, Mayer-Hamblett N, et al, "Azithromycin in Patients With Cystic Fibrosis Chronically Infected With *Pseudomonas aeruginosa*: A Randomized Controlled Trial," *JAMA*, 2003, 290 (13):1749-56.

Shulman ST, Bisno AL, Clegg HW, et al, "Clinical Practice Guideline for the Diagnosis and Management of Group A Streptococcal Pharyngitis: 2012 Update by the Infectious Diseases Society of America," *Clin Infect Dis*, 2012.

Starke JR and Correa AG, "Management of Mycobacterial Infection and Disease in Children," *Pediatr Infect Dis J*, 1995, 14(6):455-69.

Svanström H, Pasternak B, Hviid A. Use of azithromycin and death from cardiovascular causes. *N Engl J Med*. 2013;368(18):1704-1712.

Warady BA, Bakkaloglu S, Newland J, et al, "Consensus Guidelines for the Prevention and Treatment of Catheter-Related Infections and Peritonitis in Pediatric Patients Receiving Peritoneal Dialysis: 2012 Update," *Perit Dial Int*, 2012, 32(Suppl 2):S32-86.

Wilson W, Taubert KA, Gewitz M, et al, "Prevention of Infective Endocarditis: Guidelines From the American Heart Association: A Guideline From the American Heart Association Rheumatic Fever, Endocarditis, and Kawasaki Disease Committee, Council on Cardiovascular Disease in the Young, and the Council on Clinical Cardiology, Council on Cardiovascular Surgery and Anesthesia, and the Quality of Care and Outcomes Research Interdisciplinary Working Group," *Circulation*, 2007, 116(15):1736-54.

World Health Organization (WHO), "Guidelines for the Control of Shigellosis, Including Epidemics Due to Shigella dysenteriae Type 1," 2005. Available at http://whqlibdoc.who.int/publications/2005/9241592330.pdf

Azithromycin (Ophthalmic) (az ith roe MYE sin)

Medication Safety Issues
Sound-alike/look-alike issues:
Azithromycin may be confused with azathioprine, erythromycin

Brand Names: U.S. AzaSite

Therapeutic Category Antibiotic, Ophthalmic

Generic Availability (U.S.) No

Use Treatment of bacterial conjunctivitis due to susceptible CDC coryneform group G, *H. influenzae*, *S. aureus*, *S. mitis* group, or *S. pneumoniae* (FDA approved in ages ≥1 year and adults); has also been used for *Ophthalmia neonatorum* prophylaxis

Pregnancy Risk Factor B

Pregnancy Considerations Adverse events were not observed in animal reproduction studies. The amount of azithromycin available systemically following topical application of the ophthalmic drops is estimated to be below quantifiable limits. Systemic absorption would be required in order for azithromycin to cross the placenta and reach the fetus. When administered orally or I.V., azithromycin crosses the placenta. Refer to the Azithromycin (Systemic) monograph for details.

Breast-Feeding Considerations It is not known if azithromycin is excreted into breast milk following ophthalmic administration. The amount of azithromycin available systemically following topical application of the ophthalmic drops is estimated to be below quantifiable limits. Systemic absorption would be required in order for azithromycin to enter breast milk. The manufacturer recommends that caution be exercised when administering azithromycin eye drops to nursing women. When administered orally or I.V., azithromycin enters breast milk. Refer to the Azithromycin (Systemic) monograph for details.

Contraindications Hypersensitivity to azithromycin or any component, erythromycin, other macrolide, or ketolide antibiotics

Warnings Severe hypersensitivity reactions, including anaphylaxis, angioedema, and dermatologic reactions, have been reported with systemic use of azithromycin. Prolonged use may lead to overgrowth of nonsusceptible organisms, including fungi. Discontinue use and institute alternative therapy if superinfection is suspected. Contains benzalkonium chloride which may be absorbed by contact lenses; contact lens should not be worn during treatment.

Precautions For topical ophthalmic use only; do not inject subconjunctivally or introduce directly into the anterior chamber of the eye.

Adverse Reactions
Ocular: Eye irritation
Rare but important or life-threatening: Abnormal taste, blurred vision, contact dermatitis, corneal erosion, dry eyes, eye pain, facial edema, hives, nasal congestion, ocular reactions (burning, discharge, irritation, itching, stinging), periocular swelling, punctate keratitis, rash, sinusitis, urticaria, visual acuity decreased

Drug Interactions
Metabolism/Transport Effects None known.

Avoid Concomitant Use There are no known interactions where it is recommended to avoid concomitant use.

Increased Effect/Toxicity There are no known significant interactions involving an increase in effect.

Decreased Effect There are no known significant interactions involving a decrease in effect.

Stability Store sealed bottle at 2°C to 8°C (36°F to 46°F). Once bottle is opened, store in refrigerator for ≤14 days; discard any remaining solution after 14 days.

Mechanism of Action Inhibits RNA-dependent protein synthesis at the chain elongation step; binds to the 50S ribosomal subunit resulting in blockage of transpeptidation

Dosing: Neonatal Gonococcal ophthalmia or chlamydial ophthalmia, prophylaxis (*Ophthalmia neonatorum*): Limited data available: 1-2 drops in each conjunctival sac; efficacy studies are lacking; however, may consider use during shortages of erythromycin ophthalmic ointment (CDC, 2006)

Dosing: Usual Bacterial conjunctivitis: Children ≥1 year and Adults: Instill 1 drop in the affected eye(s) twice daily (8-12 hours apart) for 2 days, then 1 drop once daily for 5 days.

Administration For topical ophthalmic use only. Avoid contacting tip with skin or eye. Invert closed bottle and shake once before each use. Remove cap with bottle inverted. Tilt head back and gently squeeze inverted bottle to instill drop.

Dosage Forms Excipient information presented when available (limited, particularly for generics); consult specific product labeling.
Solution, Ophthalmic:
AzaSite: 1% (2.5 mL) [contains benzalkonium chloride, disodium edta]

References
Center for Disease Control and Prevention (CDC), "CDC Guidance on Shortage of Erythromycin (0.5%) Ophthalmic Ointment," Available at http://www.cdc.gov/std/treatment/2006/erythromycinOintmentShortage.htm. Date accessed: May 13, 2011.

◆ **Azithromycin Dihydrate** see Azithromycin (Systemic) on page 247

◆ **Azithromycin for Injection (Can)** see Azithromycin (Systemic) on page 247

◆ **Azithromycin Monohydrate** see Azithromycin (Systemic) on page 247

◆ **Azo-Gesic [OTC]** see Phenazopyridine on page 1651

◆ **Azolen Tincture [OTC]** see Miconazole (Topical) on page 1410

◆ **AZT™ (Can)** see Zidovudine on page 2168

◆ **AZT + 3TC (error-prone abbreviation)** see Lamivudine and Zidovudine on page 1198

◆ **AZT, Abacavir, and Lamivudine** see Abacavir, Lamivudine, and Zidovudine on page 41

◆ **AZT (error-prone abbreviation)** *see* Zidovudine on page 2168

◆ **Azthreonam** *see* Aztreonam *on page 254*

Aztreonam (AZ tree oh nam)

Medication Safety Issues
Sound-alike/look-alike issues:
Aztreonam may be confused with azidothymidine

Brand Names: U.S. Azactam; Azactam in Dextrose; Cayston

Brand Names: Canada Cayston

Therapeutic Category Antibiotic, Miscellaneous

Generic Availability (U.S.) May be product dependent

Use
Injection: Treatment of patients with documented multidrug resistant aerobic gram-negative infection in which beta-lactam therapy is contraindicated; used for UTI, lower respiratory tract infections, intra-abdominal infections, and gynecological infections caused by susceptible organisms (FDA approved in ages ≥9 months and adults); treatment of susceptible skin and skin-structure infections and septicemia (FDA approved in adults)

Inhalation (nebulized, Cayston®): Improve respiratory symptoms in cystic fibrosis patients with *Pseudomonas aeruginosa* in the lungs (FDA approved in ages ≥7 years and adults)

Prescribing and Access Restrictions Cayston (aztreonam inhalation solution) is only available through a select group of specialty pharmacies and cannot be obtained through a retail pharmacy. Because Cayston® may only be used with the Altera Nebulizer System, it can only be obtained from the following specialty pharmacies: Cystic Fibrosis Services, Inc; IV Solutions; Foundation Care; and Pharmaceutical Specialties, Inc. This network of specialty pharmacies ensures proper access to both the drug and device. To obtain the medication and proper nebulizer, contact the Cayston Access Program at 1-877-7CAYSTON (1-877-722-9786) or at www.cayston.com.

Pregnancy Risk Factor B

Pregnancy Considerations Adverse events have not been observed in animal reproduction studies; therefore, the manufacturer classifies aztreonam as pregnancy category B. Aztreonam crosses the placenta and enters cord blood during middle and late pregnancy. Distribution to the fetus is minimal in early pregnancy. The amount of aztreonam available systemically following inhalation is significantly less in comparison to doses given by injection.

Breast-Feeding Considerations Very small amounts of aztreonam are excreted in breast milk. The poor oral absorption of aztreonam (<1%) may limit adverse effects to the infant. Nondose-related effects could include modification of bowel flora. Maternal use of aztreonam inhalation is not likely to pose a risk to breast-feeding infants.

Contraindications Hypersensitivity to aztreonam or any component

Warnings May cause hypersensitivity reaction; patients with history of hypersensitivity reactions to cephalosporins or pencillins may experience cross-sensitivity; use with caution in patients with a history of cephalosporin or penicillin allergy, especially IgE-mediated reactions (eg, anaphylaxis, angioedema, urticaria). Prolonged use may result in fungal or bacterial superinfection, including *C. difficile*-associated diarrhea (CDAD) and pseudomembranous colitis; CDAD has been observed >2 months post-antibiotic treatment; use with caution in patients with a history of colitis. Bronchospasm may occur following nebulization; administer a short-acting bronchodilator 15 minutes to 4 hours prior to each dose of Cayston® or a long-acting bronchodilator 30 minutes to 12 hours prior to each dose of Cayston®. Safety and efficacy have not been established for nebulized inhalation patients colonized with *Burkholderia cepacia* or in patients with FEV1 <25% or >75% predicted. To reduce the development of resistant bacteria and maintain efficacy, reserve use of inhalation solution for CF patients with known *Pseudomonas aeruginosa*.

Precautions Use with caution and reduce injectable dose in patients with renal impairment; no dosing adjustment is necessary in patients receiving the inhalation formulation.

Adverse Reactions
Inhalation:
Cardiovascular: Chest discomfort

Dermatologic: Skin rash

Gastrointestinal: Abdominal pain, vomiting

Respiratory: Bronchospasm, cough, nasal congestion, sore throat, wheezing

Miscellaneous: Fever (more common in children)

Rare but important or life-threatening: Arthralgia, facial edema, hypersensitivity reaction, joint swelling, tightness in chest and throat

Injection:
Dermatologic: Rash (more common in children)

Gastrointestinal: Diarrhea, nausea, vomiting

Hematologic & oncologic: Eosinophilia (more common in children), neutropenia (more common in children), thrombocythemia (more common in children)

Hepatic: Increased serum transaminases (ALT/AST; children)

Local: Inflammation at injection site, injection site reaction (erythema, induration; more common in children), pain at injection site (more common in children)

Renal: Increased serum creatinine (children)

Miscellaneous: Fever

Rare but important or life-threatening: Anaphylaxis, anemia, angioedema, aphthous stomatitis, *Clostridium difficile* associated diarrhea, erythema multiforme, exfoliative dermatitis, gastrointestinal hemorrhage, hepatitis, leukocytosis, leukopenia, oral mucosa ulcer, pancytopenia, positive direct Coombs test, prolonged partial thromboplastin time, prolonged prothrombin time, pseudomembranous colitis, seizure, thrombocytopenia, toxic epidermal necrolysis, vaginitis, ventricular bigeminy (transient), ventricular premature contractions (transient), vulvovaginal candidiasis

Drug Interactions
Metabolism/Transport Effects None known.

Avoid Concomitant Use
Avoid concomitant use of Aztreonam with any of the following: BCG

Increased Effect/Toxicity There are no known significant interactions involving an increase in effect.

Decreased Effect
Aztreonam may decrease the levels/effects of: BCG; Sodium Picosulfate; Typhoid Vaccine

Stability
Inhalation: Store intact vials and diluent ampules at 2°C to 8°C (36°F to 46°F). May be stored at 25°C (77°F) for up to 28 days; protect from light. Reconstituted solution must be used immediately.

Parenteral:
I.M.: Store intact vials at room temperature. Reconstituted solution is stable for 48 hours at room temperature or 7 days refrigerated. Do **not** mix with any local anesthetic agent. Reconstitute vial with at least 3 mL SWFI, sterile bacteriostatic water for injection, NS, or bacteriostatic sodium chloride per gram of aztreonam; immediately shake vigorously.

Premixed GALAXY containers for I.V.: Store frozen at -20°C or less (-4°F or less). Thaw at room temperature or in a refrigerator; do not force thaw. Thawed solution should be used within 48 hours if stored at room temperature or within 14 days if stored under refrigeration. **Do not refreeze.**

Vials for I.V.: Store intact vials at room temperature; avoid excessive heat. Reconstituted solution (≤20 mg/mL, or >20 mg/mL in NS or SWFI **only**) is stable 48 hours at room temperature and 7 days when refrigerated.

Mechanism of Action Inhibits bacterial cell wall synthesis by binding to one or more of the penicillin-binding proteins (PBPs) which in turn inhibits the final transpeptidation step of peptidoglycan synthesis in bacterial cell walls, thus inhibiting cell wall biosynthesis. Bacteria eventually lyse due to ongoing activity of cell wall autolytic enzymes (autolysins and murein hydrolases) while cell wall assembly is arrested. Monobactam structure makes cross-allergenicity with beta-lactams unlikely.

Pharmacokinetics (Adult data unless noted)

Absorption: I.M.: Well absorbed; Oral inhalation: Poorly absorbed

Distribution: Injection: Widely distributed into body tissues, cerebrospinal fluid, bronchial secretions, peritoneal fluid, bile, and bone

V_d:

Neonates: 0.26-0.36 L/kg

Children: 0.2-0.29 L/kg

Adults: 0.2 L/kg

Protein binding: 56%

Half-life: Injection:

Neonates:

<7 days, ≤2.5 kg: 5.5-9.9 hours

<7 days, >2.5 kg: 2.6 hours

1 week to 1 month: 2.4 hours

Children 2 months to 12 years: 1.7 hours

Children with cystic fibrosis: 1.3 hours

Adults: 1.3-2.2 hours (half-life prolonged in renal failure)

Time to peak serum concentration: Within 60 minutes after an I.M. dose

Elimination:

Injection: 60% to 70% excreted unchanged in the urine by active tubular secretion and glomerular filtration; 12% excreted in feces

Inhalation: Urine (10% of the total dose)

Dialysis: Moderately dialyzable

Hemodialysis: 27% to 58% in 4 hours

Peritoneal dialysis: 10% with a 6-hour dwell time

Dosing: Neonatal General dosing, susceptible infection: I.M., I.V. (*Red Book*, 2012):

Body weight <1 kg:

PNA ≤14 days: 30 mg/kg/dose every 12 hours

PNA 15-28 days: 30 mg/kg/dose every 8-12 hours

Body weight 1-2 kg:

PNA ≤7 days: 30 mg/kg/dose every 12 hours

PNA 8-28 days: 30 mg/kg/dose every 8-12 hours

Body weight >2 kg:

PNA ≤7 days: 30 mg/kg/dose every 8 hours

PNA 8-28 days: 30 mg/kg/dose every 6 hours

Dosing: Usual

Infants, Children, and Adolescents:

General dosing, susceptible infection: I.M., I.V. (*Red Book*, 2012):

Mild to moderate infection: 30 mg/kg every 8 hours; maximum daily dose: 3000 mg/**day**

Severe infection: 30 mg/kg every 6-8 hours; maximum daily dose: 8 g/**day**

Cystic fibrosis (*Pseudomonas aeruginosa*):

Inhalation (nebulizer): Children ≥7 years and Adolescents: 75 mg via nebulization 3 times daily (at least 4 hours apart) for 28 days; administer in repeated cycles of 28 days on drug, followed by 28 days off drug

I.V.: 150-200 mg/kg/day in divided doses every 6-8 hours; higher doses have been used: 200-300 mg/kg/day divided every 6 hours; maximum daily dose: 12 **g/day** (Zobell, 2012)

Intra-abdominal infections, complicated: I.V.: 90-120 mg/kg/day divided every 6-8 hours; maximum dose: 2000 mg (Solomkin, 2010)

Peritonitis (CAPD): Intraperitoneal: Continuous: Loading dose: 1000 mg per liter of dialysate; maintenance dose: 250 mg per liter (Warady, 2000)

Surgical prophylaxis: Children and Adolescents: I.V.: 30 mg/kg as a single dose; may repeat in 4 hours; maximum dose: 2000 mg (Bratzler, 2013)

Adults:

General dosing, susceptible infection:

Moderately severe systemic infections:

I.M.: 1000 mg every 8-12 hours

I.V.: 1000-2000 mg every 8-12 hours

Severe systemic or life-threatening infections (especially if caused by *Pseudomonas aeruginosa*): I.V.: 2000 mg every 6-8 hours; maximum daily dose: 8 **g/day**

Cystic fibrosis (*Pseudomonas aeruginosa*): Inhalation (nebulizer): 75 mg via nebulization 3 times daily (at least 4 hours apart) for 28 days; administer in repeated cycles of 28 days on drug, followed by 28 days off drug

Meningitis (gram-negative): I.V.: 2000 mg every 6-8 hours

Urinary tract infection: I.M., I.V.: 500-1000 mg every 8-12 hours

Dosing adjustment in renal impairment:

Infants, Children, and Adolescents: I.M., I.V.: The following adjustments have been recommended (Aronoff, 2007). **Note:** Renally adjusted dose recommendations are based on doses of 90-120 mg/kg/**day** divided every 8 hours.

GFR ≥30 mL/minute/1.73 m²: No adjustment required

GFR 10-29 mL/minute/1.73 m²: 15-20 mg/kg every 8 hours

GFR <10 mL/minute/1.73 m²: 7.5-10 mg/kg every 12 hours

Intermittent hemodialysis: 7.5-10 mg/kg every 12 hours

Peritoneal dialysis (PD): 7.5-10 mg/kg every 12 hours

Continuous renal replacement therapy (CRRT): No adjustment required.

Inhalation (nebulized): No adjustment required.

Adults:

I.M., I.V.:

CrCl 10-30 mL/minute: Give 50% of the usual dose at the usual interval

CrCl <10 mL/minute: Give a full first dose, then give 25% of the dose at the usual interval

Hemodialysis: Give a full first dose, then give 25% of the dose at the usual interval; for serious infections give 12.5% of the initial dose after each dialysis session. Alternatively, may administer 500 mg every 12 hours (Heintz, 2009). **Note:** Dosing dependent on the assumption of 3 times weekly, complete IHD sessions.

Peritoneal dialysis: Give a full first dose, then give 25% of the dose at the usual interval

Continuous renal replacement therapy (CRRT) (Heintz, 2009; Trotman, 2005): Drug clearance is highly dependent on the method of renal replacement, filter type, and flow rate. Appropriate dosing requires close monitoring of pharmacologic response, signs of adverse reactions due to drug accumulation, as well as drug concentrations in relation to target trough (if appropriate). The following are general recommendations only (based on dialysate flow/ultrafiltration rates of 1-2 L/hour and minimal residual renal function) and should not supersede clinical judgment:

CVVH: Loading dose of 2000 mg followed by 1000-2000 mg every 12 hours

CVVHD/CVVHDF: Loading dose of 2000 mg followed by either 1000 mg every 8 hours **or** 2000 mg every 12 hours (Heintz, 2009)

Inhalation (nebulized): No adjustment required.

Dosing adjustment in hepatic impairment: There are no dosage adjustments provided in the manufacturer's labeling; however, minor hepatic elimination of aztreonam does occur. Use with caution in patients with impaired hepatic function; appropriate monitoring is recommended.

Administration Parenteral:

I.V.: Administer by IVP over 3-5 minutes at a maximum concentration of 66 mg/mL or by intermittent infusion over 20-60 minutes at a final concentration not to exceed 20 mg/mL.

I.M.: Deep I.M. injection at a concentration of ≤333 mg/mL into a large muscle mass such as the upper outer quadrant of the gluteus maximus or lateral part of the thigh. Doses >1000 mg should be administered I.V.

Inhalation: Administer only using an Altera® nebulizer system; dose can be nebulized over 2-3 minutes. Do not mix with other inhaled nebulizer medications. Administer a bronchodilator before administration of aztreonam (short-acting 15 minutes to 4 hours before; long-acting: 30 minutes to 12 hours before). Administer doses ≥4 hours apart.

Monitoring Parameters

Injection: Periodic renal and hepatic function tests; monitor for stool frequency; monitor for signs of anaphylaxis during first dose

Inhalation: FEV₁

Test Interactions May interfere with urine glucose tests containing cupric sulfate (Benedict's solution, Clinitest); positive Coombs' test

Dosage Forms Excipient information presented when available (limited, particularly for generics); consult specific product labeling.

Solution, Intravenous:

Azactam in Dextrose: 1 g (50 mL); 2 g (50 mL) [sodium free]

Solution Reconstituted, Inhalation [preservative free]:

Cayston: 75 mg (84 mL) [arginine free]

Solution Reconstituted, Injection:

Azactam: 1 g (1 ea); 2 g (1 ea) [sodium free]

Generic: 1 g (1 ea); 2 g (1 ea)

References

American Academy of Pediatrics (AAP). In: Pickering LK, Baker CJ, Kimberlin DW, Long SS, eds. *Red Book: 2012 Report of the Committee on Infectious Diseases.* 29th ed. Elk Grove Village, IL: American Academy of Pediatrics; 2012.

Aronoff GR, Bennett WM, Berns JS, et al, *Drug Prescribing in Renal Failure: Dosing Guidelines for Adults and Children,* 5th ed, Philadelphia, PA: American College of Physicians, 2007.

Bosso JA and Black PG, "The Use of Aztreonam in Pediatric Patients: A Review," *Pharmacotherapy,* 1991, 11(1):20-5.

Bratzler DW, Dellinger EP, Olsen KM, et al, "Clinical Practice Guidelines for Antimicrobial Prophylaxis in Surgery," *Am J Health Syst Pharm,* 2013, 70(3):195-283.

Heintz BH, Matzke GR, and Dager WE, "Antimicrobial Dosing Concepts and Recommendations for Critically Ill Adult Patients Receiving Continuous Renal Replacement Therapy or Intermittent Hemodialysis," *Pharmacotherapy,* 2009, 29(5):562-77.

Le J, Ashley ED, Neuhauser MM, et al, "Consensus Summary of Aerosolized Antimicrobial Agents: Application of Guideline Criteria," *Pharmacotherapy,* 2010, 30(6):562-84.

Retsch-Bogart GZ, Quittner AL, Gibson RL, et al, "Efficacy and Safety of Inhaled Aztreonam Lysine for Airway Pseudomonas in Cystic Fibrosis," *Chest,* 2009, 135(5):1223-32.

Solomkin JS, Mazuski JE, Bradley JS, et al, "Diagnosis and Management of Complicated Intra-abdominal Infections in Adults and Children: Guidelines by the Surgical Infection Society and the Infectious Diseases Society of America," *Clin Infect Dis,* 2010, 50(2):133-64.

Stutman HR, Chartrand SA, Tolentino T, et al, "Aztreonam Therapy for Serious Gram-Negative Infections in Children," *Am J Dis Child,* 1986, 140(11):1147-51.

Tunkel AR, Hartman BJ, Kaplan SL, et al, "Practice Guidelines for the Management of Bacterial Meningitis," *Clin Infect Dis,* 2004, 39 (9):1267-84.

Warady BA, Schaefer F, Holloway M, et al, "Consensus Guidelines for the Treatment of Peritonitis in Pediatric Patients Receiving Peritoneal Dialysis," *Perit Dial Int,* 2000, 20(6):610-24.

Zobell JT, Young DC, Waters CD, et al, "Optimization of Anti-pseudomonal Antibiotics for Cystic Fibrosis Pulmonary Exacerbations: I. Aztreonam and Carbapenems," *Pediatr Pulmonol,* 2012, 47 (12):1147-58.

◆ **Azulfidine** see SulfaSALAzine on page 1954
◆ **Azulfidine EN-tabs** see SulfaSALAzine on page 1954
◆ **B-2-400 [OTC]** see Riboflavin on page 1821
◆ **B6** see Pyridoxine on page 1778
◆ **Baby Anbesol [OTC]** see Benzocaine on page 273
◆ **Baby Aspirin** see Aspirin on page 212
◆ **Baby Ayr Saline [OTC]** see Sodium Chloride on page 1902
◆ **BabyBIG®** see Botulism Immune Globulin (Intravenous-Human) on page 301
◆ **Bacid® [OTC]** see Lactobacillus on page 1191
◆ **Bacid® (Can)** see Lactobacillus on page 1191
◆ **Baciguent (Can)** see Bacitracin on page 256
◆ **BACiiM** see Bacitracin on page 256
◆ **Baciject (Can)** see Bacitracin on page 256

Bacitracin (bas i TRAY sin)

Medication Safety Issues

Sound-alike/look-alike issues:

Bacitracin may be confused with Bactrim, Bactroban

Brand Names: U.S. BACiiM

Brand Names: Canada Baciguent; Baciject

Therapeutic Category Antibiotic, Miscellaneous; Antibiotic, Topical

Generic Availability (U.S.) Yes

Use Treatment of pneumonia and empyema caused by susceptible staphylococci; prevention or treatment of superficial skin infections; due to its toxicity, use of bacitracin systemically or as an irrigant should be limited to situations where less toxic alternatives would not be effective; treatment of antibiotic-associated colitis

Pregnancy Considerations It is unknown if bacitracin crosses the placenta. The minimal absorption after topical use should limit the amount of medication available for transfer to the fetus. If ophthalmic agents are needed during pregnancy, the minimum effective dose should be used in combination with punctual occlusion to decrease potential exposure to the fetus.

Breast-Feeding Considerations It is unknown if bacitracin is distributed in human milk. The minimal absorption after topical use should limit the amount of medication available for transfer.

Contraindications Hypersensitivity to bacitracin or any component; I.M. use is not recommended in patients with renal impairment

Warnings I.M. use may cause renal failure due to tubular and glomerular necrosis **[U.S. Boxed Warning]**; avoid concurrent use with other nephrotoxic drugs; discontinue use if toxicity occurs; monitor renal function prior to therapy and daily during therapy **[U.S. Boxed Warning]**; ensure adequate fluid intake and urinary output; should only be used where adequate laboratory facilities are available and when constant supervision is possible; avoid concomitant use with other nephrotoxic drugs if possible; do not administer intravenously because severe thrombophlebitis occurs; bacitracin may be absorbed from denuded areas and irrigation sites

Precautions Prolonged use may result in overgrowth of nonsusceptible organisms

Adverse Reactions

Cardiovascular: Chest tightness, edema of face/lips, hypotension

Central nervous system: Pain

Dermatologic: Itching, rash

Gastrointestinal: Anorexia, diarrhea, nausea, rectal itching, vomiting

Hematologic: Blood dyscrasias

Renal: Nephrotoxicity (with systemic administration)

Miscellaneous: Anaphylaxis, diaphoresis

Drug Interactions

Metabolism/Transport Effects None known.

Avoid Concomitant Use

Avoid concomitant use of Bacitracin with any of the following: BCG

Increased Effect/Toxicity There are no known significant interactions involving an increase in effect.

Decreased Effect

Bacitracin may decrease the levels/effects of: BCG; Sodium Picosulfate

Stability Sterile powder should be stored in the refrigerator; once reconstituted, bacitracin is stable for 1 week under refrigeration (2°C to 8°C); incompatible with diluents containing parabens

Mechanism of Action Inhibits bacterial cell wall synthesis by preventing transfer of mucopeptides into the growing cell wall

Pharmacokinetics (Adult data unless noted)

Absorption: Poor from mucous membranes and intact skin; rapid following I.M. administration

Protein binding: Minimally bound to plasma proteins

Time to peak serum concentration: I.M.: Within 1-2 hours

Elimination: Slow elimination into the urine with 10% to 40% of a dose excreted within 24 hours

Dosing: Usual

I.M. (not recommended):

Infants:

≤2.5 kg: 900 units/kg/day in 2-3 divided doses

>2.5 kg: 1000 units/kg/day in 2-3 divided doses

Children: 800-1200 units/kg/day divided every 8 hours

Adults: 10,000-25,000 units/dose every 6 hours; not to exceed 100,000 units/day

Children and Adults:

Topical: Apply 1-5 times/day

Irrigation, solution: 50-100 units/mL in NS, LR, or sterile water for irrigation; soak sponges in solution for topical compresses 1-5 times/day or as needed during surgical procedures

Antibiotic-associated colitis: Adults: Oral: 25,000 units every 6 hours for 7-10 days

Administration

Parenteral: For I.M. administration, pH of urine should be kept above 6 by using sodium bicarbonate; bacitracin sterile powder should be dissolved in NS injection containing 2% procaine hydrochloride; administer I.M. injection into the upper outer quadrant of the buttocks; alternate injection sites

Topical: Apply thin layer to the cleansed affected area. May cover with a sterile bandage. For external use only. Do not use topical ointment in the eyes.

Monitoring Parameters I.M.: Urinalysis, renal function tests

Dosage Forms Excipient information presented when available (limited, particularly for generics); consult specific product labeling. [DSC] = Discontinued product

Ointment, Ophthalmic:

Generic: 500 units/g (1 g, 3.5 g)

Ointment, External, as zinc [strength expressed as base]:

Generic: 500 units/g (1 ea, 14 g, 14.2 g, 15 g, 28 g, 28.35 g, 28.4 g, 30 g [DSC], 120 g, 454 g)

Solution Reconstituted, Intramuscular:

BACiiM: 50,000 units (1 ea)

Generic: 50,000 units (1 ea)

Solution Reconstituted, Intramuscular [preservative free]:

Generic: 50,000 units (1 ea)

References

Kelly CP, Pothoulakis C, and LaMont JT, "*Clostridium difficile* Colitis," *N Engl J Med*, 1994, 330(4):257-62.

Bacitracin and Polymyxin B

(bas i TRAY sin & pol i MIKS in bee)

Medication Safety Issues

Sound-alike/look-alike issues:

Betadine® may be confused with Betagan®, betaine

Brand Names: U.S. AK-Poly-Bac™; Polycin™; Polysporin® [OTC]

Brand Names: Canada LID-Pack®; Optimyxin®

Therapeutic Category Antibiotic, Ophthalmic; Antibiotic, Topical

Generic Availability (U.S.) Yes

Use Treatment of superficial infections involving the conjunctiva and/or cornea caused by susceptible organisms; prevent infection in minor cuts, scrapes and burns

Pregnancy Risk Factor C

Pregnancy Considerations Animal reproduction studies have not been conducted with this combination. See individual agents.

Breast-Feeding Considerations It is not known if bacitracin or polymyxin B are excreted into breast milk. The manufacturer recommends that caution be exercised when administering to nursing women. See individual agents.

Contraindications Hypersensitivity to polymyxin, bacitracin, or any component

Precautions Prolonged use may result in overgrowth of nonsusceptible organisms

Adverse Reactions Local: Anaphylactoid reactions, burning, conjunctival erythema, itching, rash, swelling

Drug Interactions

Metabolism/Transport Effects None known.

Avoid Concomitant Use

Avoid concomitant use of Bacitracin and Polymyxin B with any of the following: BCG

Increased Effect/Toxicity

Bacitracin and Polymyxin B may increase the levels/effects of: Colistimethate; Neuromuscular-Blocking Agents

The levels/effects of Bacitracin and Polymyxin B may be increased by: Capreomycin

Decreased Effect

Bacitracin and Polymyxin B may decrease the levels/effects of: BCG; Sodium Picosulfate

Mechanism of Action See individual agents.

Pharmacokinetics (Adult data unless noted) Absorption: Insignificant from intact skin or mucous membrane

Dosing: Usual Children and Adults:

Ophthalmic: Instill ¼" to ½" directly into conjunctival sac(s) every 3-4 hours depending on severity of the infection

Topical: Apply a small amount of ointment or dusting of powder to the affected area 1-3 times/day

Administration Ophthalmic: Do not use topical ointment in the eyes; avoid contact of tube tip with skin or eye

Dosage Forms Excipient information presented when available (limited, particularly for generics); consult specific product labeling.

Ointment, ophthalmic: Bacitracin 500 units and polymyxin B 10,000 units per g (3.5 g)

AK-Poly-Bac™: Bacitracin 500 units and polymyxin B 10,000 units per g (3.5 g)

Polycin™: Bacitracin 500 units and polymyxin B 10,000 units per g (3.5 g)

Ointment, topical: Bacitracin 500 units and polymyxin B 10,000 units per g (15 g, 30 g)

Polysporin®: Bacitracin 500 units and polymyxin B 10,000 units per g (0.9 g, 15 g, 30 g)

Powder, topical:

Polysporin®: Bacitracin 500 units and polymyxin B 10,000 units per g (10 g)

Bacitracin, Neomycin, and Polymyxin B
(bas i TRAY sin, nee oh MYE sin, & pol i MIKS in bee)

Brand Names: U.S. Neo-Polycin™; Neosporin® Neo To Go® [OTC]; Neosporin® Topical [OTC]
Therapeutic Category Antibiotic, Ophthalmic; Antibiotic, Topical
Generic Availability (U.S.) Yes
Use Help prevent infection in minor cuts, scrapes and burns; short-term treatment of superficial external ocular infections caused by susceptible organisms
Pregnancy Risk Factor C
Pregnancy Considerations Animal reproduction studies have not been conducted with this combination. See individual agents.
Breast-Feeding Considerations It is not known if bacitracin, neomycin, or polymyxin B is excreted into breast milk. The manufacturer recommends that caution be exercised when administering to nursing women. See individual agents.
Contraindications Hypersensitivity to neomycin, polymyxin B, zinc bacitracin, or any component
Warnings Symptoms of neomycin sensitization include itching, reddening, edema, failure to heal; ophthalmic ointments may retard corneal healing
Precautions Prolonged use may result in overgrowth of nonsusceptible organisms
Adverse Reactions
Dermatologic: Allergic contact dermatitis, reddening
Local: Failure to heal, irritation, itching, swelling
Ophthalmic: Conjunctival edema
Miscellaneous: Anaphylaxis
Drug Interactions
Metabolism/Transport Effects None known.
Avoid Concomitant Use
Avoid concomitant use of Bacitracin, Neomycin, and Polymyxin B with any of the following: BCG; Mannitol
Increased Effect/Toxicity
Bacitracin, Neomycin, and Polymyxin B may increase the levels/effects of: AbobotulinumtoxinA; Acarbose; Bisphosphonate Derivatives; CARBOplatin; Colistimethate; CycloSPORINE (Systemic); Neuromuscular-Blocking Agents; OnabotulinumtoxinA; RimabotulinumtoxinB; Tenofovir; Vitamin K Antagonists

The levels/effects of Bacitracin, Neomycin, and Polymyxin B may be increased by: Amphotericin B; Capreomycin; Cephalosporins (2nd Generation); Cephalosporins (3rd Generation); Cephalosporins (4th Generation); CISplatin; Loop Diuretics; Mannitol; Nonsteroidal Anti-Inflammatory Agents; Tenofovir; Vancomycin
Decreased Effect
Bacitracin, Neomycin, and Polymyxin B may decrease the levels/effects of: BCG; Cardiac Glycosides; Sodium Picosulfate; SORAfenib

The levels/effects of Bacitracin, Neomycin, and Polymyxin B may be decreased by: Penicillins
Mechanism of Action See individual agents.
Dosing: Usual Children and Adults:
Ophthalmic ointment: Instill into the conjunctival sac 1 or more times daily every 3-4 hours for 7-10 days
Topical: Apply 1-3 times/day
Administration
Ophthalmic: Avoid contamination of the tip of the ointment tube
Topical: Apply a thin layer to the cleansed affected area; may cover with a sterile bandage
Dosage Forms Excipient information presented when available (limited, particularly for generics); consult specific product labeling.

Ointment, ophthalmic: Bacitracin 400 units, neomycin 3.5 mg, and polymyxin B 10,000 units per g (3.5 g)
Neo-Polycin™: Bacitracin 400 units, neomycin 3.5 mg, and polymyxin B 10,000 units per g (3.5 g)
Ointment, topical: Bacitracin 400 units, neomycin 3.5 mg, and polymyxin B 5000 units per g (0.9 g, 15 g, 30 g, 454 g)
Neosporin®: Bacitracin 400 units, neomycin 3.5 mg, and polymyxin B 5000 units per g (15 g, 30 g)
Neosporin® Neo To Go®: Bacitracin 400 units, neomycin 3.5 mg, and polymyxin B 5000 units per g (0.9 g)

Bacitracin, Neomycin, Polymyxin B, and Hydrocortisone
(bas i TRAY sin, nee oh MYE sin, pol i MIKS in bee, & hye droe KOR ti sone)

Brand Names: U.S. Cortisporin® Ointment; Neo-Polycin™ HC
Brand Names: Canada Cortisporin® Topical Ointment
Therapeutic Category Antibiotic, Ophthalmic; Antibiotic, Otic; Antibiotic, Topical; Corticosteroid, Ophthalmic; Corticosteroid, Otic; Corticosteroid, Topical
Generic Availability (U.S.) Yes: Ophthalmic ointment
Use
Ophthalmic: Prevention and treatment of susceptible inflammatory conditions where bacterial infection (or risk of infection) is present (FDA approved in adults)
Topical: Treatment of corticosteroid-responsive dermatoses with secondary infection (FDA approved in adults)
Pregnancy Risk Factor C
Pregnancy Considerations Adverse events have been observed with topical corticosteroids in animal reproduction studies. See individual agents.
Breast-Feeding Considerations It is not known if systemic absorption following topical administration results in detectable quantities in human milk. Breast-feeding is not recommended by the manufacturer. See individual agents.
Contraindications Hypersensitivity to bacitracin, neomycin, polymyxin B, hydrocortisone, or any component; not for use in viral infections, fungal diseases, mycobacterial infections, or if eardrum is perforated (topical)
Warnings Neomycin may cause cutaneous and conjunctival sensitization presenting as itching, reddening, edema, and failure to heal. Neomycin may cause permanent hearing loss; risk of ototoxicity is increased in patients with longstanding otitis media or tympanic perforation. Systemic absorption of hydrocortisone may cause hyperglycemia, glycosuria, fluid and electrolyte changes and HPA axis suppression which can lead to adrenal crisis; risk is increased when used over large surface areas, for prolonged periods, or with occlusive dressings; children are more susceptible to topical corticosteroid-induced HPA axis suppression and Cushing's syndrome; prolonged use of corticosteroids may also increase the incidence of secondary infection, mask acute infection (including fungal infections), prolong or exacerbate viral infections, or limit response to vaccines; prolonged treatment with corticosteroids has been associated with the development of Kaposi's sarcoma (case reports); if noted, discontinuation of therapy should be considered.
Ophthalmic ointment: Should never be directly introduced into the anterior chamber; may delay corneal healing. Prolonged use may result in ocular hypertension/glaucoma, corneal and scleral thinning, potentially resulting in perforation.
Precautions Use with caution in glaucoma; avoid use following ocular cataract surgery; inadvertent contamination of multiple-dose ophthalmic products has caused bacterial keratitis
Adverse Reactions For additional information, see individual agents.

Ophthalmic ointment:
Dermatologic: Delayed wound healing, rash
Ocular: Cataracts, corneal thinning, glaucoma, irritation, keratitis (bacterial), intraocular pressure increase, optic nerve damage, scleral thinning
Miscellaneous: Hypersensitivity (including anaphylaxis), secondary infection, sensitization to kanamycin, paromomycin, streptomycin, and gentamicin

Topical ointment:
Dermatologic: Acneiform eruptions, allergic contact dermatitis, burning skin, dryness, folliculitis, hypertrichosis, hypopigmentation, irritation, maceration of skin, miliaria, ocular hypertension, perioral dermatitis, pruritus, skin atrophy, striae
Otic: Ototoxicity
Renal: Nephrotoxicity
Miscellaneous: Hypersensitivity (including anaphylaxis), secondary infection, sensitization to karamycin, paromycin, streptomycin, and gentamicin

Drug Interactions
Metabolism/Transport Effects Refer to individual components.

Avoid Concomitant Use
Avoid concomitant use of Bacitracin, Neomycin, Polymyxin B, and Hydrocortisone with any of the following: Aldesleukin; BCG; Mannitol

Increased Effect/Toxicity
Bacitracin, Neomycin, Polymyxin B, and Hydrocortisone may increase the levels/effects of: AbobotulinumtoxinA; Acarbose; Bisphosphonate Derivatives; CARBOplatin; Ceritinib; Colistimethate; CycloSPORINE (Systemic); Deferasirox; Neuromuscular-Blocking Agents; OnabotulinumtoxinA; RimabotulinumtoxinB; Tenofovir; Vitamin K Antagonists

The levels/effects of Bacitracin, Neomycin, Polymyxin B, and Hydrocortisone may be increased by: Amphotericin B; Capreomycin; Cephalosporins (2nd Generation); Cephalosporins (3rd Generation); Cephalosporins (4th Generation); CISplatin; Loop Diuretics; Mannitol; Nonsteroidal Anti-Inflammatory Agents; Telaprevir; Tenofovir; Vancomycin

Decreased Effect
Bacitracin, Neomycin, Polymyxin B, and Hydrocortisone may decrease the levels/effects of: Aldesleukin; BCG; Cardiac Glycosides; Corticorelin; Hyaluronidase; Sodium Picosulfate; SORAfenib; Telaprevir

The levels/effects of Bacitracin, Neomycin, Polymyxin B, and Hydrocortisone may be decreased by: Penicillins

Stability
Ointment: Store at controlled room temperature of 15°C to 25°C (59°F to 77°F).
Ophthalmic ointment: Store at controlled room temperature of 15°C to 30°C (59°F to 86°F).

Mechanism of Action See individual agents.
Pharmacokinetics (Adult data unless noted) See individual agents.

Dosing: Usual Children and Adults:
Ophthalmic: Ointment: Instill 1/2" ribbon to inside of lower lid every 3-4 hours until improvement occurs
Topical: Apply thin film sparingly 2-4 times/day for up to 7 days. Therapy should be discontinued when control is achieved or after a week; if no improvement is seen, reassessment of diagnosis may be necessary.

Monitoring Parameters If ophthalmic ointment is used >10 days or in patients with glaucoma, monitor intraocular pressure (IOP).

Dosage Forms Excipient information presented when available (limited, particularly for generics); consult specific product labeling.

Ointment, ophthalmic: Bacitracin 400 units, neomycin 3.5 mg, polymyxin B 10,000 units, and hydrocortisone 10 mg per g (3.5 g)
Neo-Polycin™ HC: Bacitracin 400 units, neomycin 3.5 mg, polymyxin B 10,000 units, and hydrocortisone 10 mg per g (3.5 g)
Ointment, topical:
Cortisporin®: Bacitracin 400 units, neomycin 3.5 mg, polymyxin B 5000 units, and hydrocortisone 10 mg per g (15 g)

Baclofen (BAK loe fen)

Medication Safety Issues
Sound-alike/look-alike issues:
Baclofen may be confused with Bactroban®
Lioresal® may be confused with lisinopril, Lotensin®
High alert medication:
The Institute for Safe Medication Practices (ISMP) includes this medication (intrathecal administration) among its list of drugs which have a heightened risk of causing significant patient harm when used in error.

Brand Names: U.S. EnovaRX-Baclofen; Gablofen; Lioresal

Brand Names: Canada Apo-Baclofen®; Ava-Baclofen; Dom-Baclofen; Lioresal®; Lioresal® D.S.; Lioresal® Intrathecal; Med-Baclofen; Mylan-Baclofen; Novo-Baclofen; Nu-Baclo; PHL-Baclofen; PMS-Baclofen; ratio-Baclofen; Riva-Baclofen

Therapeutic Category Skeletal Muscle Relaxant, Nonparalytic

Generic Availability (U.S.) May be product dependent

Use Treatment of cerebral spasticity, reversible spasticity associated with multiple sclerosis or spinal cord lesions; intrathecal use for the management of spasticity in patients who are unresponsive to oral baclofen or experience intolerable CNS side effects; treatment of trigeminal neuralgia; adjunctive treatment of tardive dyskinesia

Pregnancy Risk Factor C

Pregnancy Considerations Adverse events were observed in animal reproduction studies. Withdrawal symptoms in the neonate were noted in a case report following the maternal use of oral baclofen 20 mg 4 times/day throughout pregnancy (Ratnayaka, 2001). Plasma concentrations following administration of intrathecal baclofen are significantly less than those with oral doses; exposure to the fetus is expected to be limited (Morton, 2009).

Breast-Feeding Considerations Baclofen is excreted into breast milk. Very small amounts were found in the breast milk of a woman 14 days postpartum after oral use. Following a single oral dose of baclofen 20 mg, the total amount of baclofen excreted in breast milk within 26 hours was 22 mcg (Eriksson, 1981). Adverse events were not observed in a nursing infant following maternal use of intrathecal baclofen 200 mcg/day throughout pregnancy and while nursing (Morton, 2009). Due to the potential for adverse events in the nursing infant, breast-feeding is not recommended by the manufacturer.

Contraindications Hypersensitivity to baclofen or any component; injection for intrathecal use is not recommended or intended for I.V., I.M., SubQ, or epidural administration

Warnings Should not be used when spasticity is used to maintain posture or balance; due to the life-threatening complications of intrathecal use, physicians must be adequately trained in its use; abrupt withdrawal of oral baclofen has been reported to precipitate hallucinations and/or seizures. Abrupt discontinuation of intrathecal baclofen regardless of the cause, has resulted in sequelae that include high fever, altered mental status, exaggerated rebound spasticity, and muscle rigidity, that in rare cases, has advanced to rhabdomyolysis, multiple organ system failure, and death **[U.S. Boxed Warning]**. Early symptoms of withdrawal include: Return of baseline spasticity, pruritus, hypotension, and paresthesias. Clinical characteristics of advanced withdrawal may resemble autonomic dysreflexia, sepsis, malignant hyperthermia, neuroleptic-malignant syndrome, and other conditions associated with hypermetabolic state or widespread rhabdomyolysis. Patients at increased risk those include spinal cord injuries at T-6 or above, those with communication difficulties, and those history of withdrawal symptoms from oral baclofen. If restoration of intrathecal baclofen is delayed, oral baclofen or benzodiazepine treatment may be used as a temporary measure.

Precautions Use with caution in patients with seizure disorder, impaired renal function, peptic ulcer disease, stroke, ovarian cysts, psychotic disorders, autonomic dysreflexia (intrathecal therapy); careful attention to programming and monitoring of intrathecal baclofen is recommended to prevent abrupt discontinuation

Adverse Reactions
Cardiovascular: Hypotension
Central nervous system: Ataxia, confusion, drowsiness, fatigue, headache, hypotonia, insomnia, psychiatric disturbance, slurred speech, vertigo
Dermatologic: Skin rash
Gastrointestinal: Constipation, nausea
Genitourinary: Polyuria
Neuromuscular & skeletal: Weakness
Rare but important or life-threatening: Chest pain, dyspnea, dysuria, hematuria, impotence, inhibited ejaculation, nocturia, palpitations, syncope, urinary incontinence, urinary retention
Withdrawal reactions have occurred with abrupt discontinuation (particularly severe with intrathecal use).

Drug Interactions
Metabolism/Transport Effects None known.
Avoid Concomitant Use
Avoid concomitant use of Baclofen with any of the following: Azelastine (Nasal); Paraldehyde; Thalidomide
Increased Effect/Toxicity
Baclofen may increase the levels/effects of: Alcohol (Ethyl); Azelastine (Nasal); Buprenorphine; CNS Depressants; Hydrocodone; Methotrimeprazine; Metyrosine; Mirtazapine; Paraldehyde; Pramipexole; ROPINIRole; Rotigotine; Selective Serotonin Reuptake Inhibitors; Thalidomide; Zolpidem

The levels/effects of Baclofen may be increased by: Brimonidine (Topical); Cannabis; Doxylamine; Dronabinol; Droperidol; HydrOXYzine; Kava Kava; Magnesium Sulfate; Methotrimeprazine; Nabilone; Perampanel; Rufinamide; Sodium Oxybate; Tapentadol; Tetrahydrocannabinol
Decreased Effect There are no known significant interactions involving a decrease in effect.

Mechanism of Action Inhibits the transmission of both monosynaptic and polysynaptic reflexes at the spinal cord level, possibly by hyperpolarization of primary afferent fiber terminals, with resultant relief of muscle spasticity

Pharmacodynamics
Oral: Muscle relaxation effects require 3-4 days and maximal clinical effects are not seen for 5-10 days
Intrathecal:
Bolus:
Onset of action: 30 minutes to 1 hour
Maximum effect: 4 hours
Duration: 4-8 hours
Continuous intrathecal infusion:
Onset of action: 6-8 hours
Maximum activity: 24-48 hours

Pharmacokinetics (Adult data unless noted)
Oral:
Absorption: Rapid; absorption from the GI tract is thought to be dose dependent
Protein binding: 30%
Metabolism: Minimal in the liver (15%)
Half-life: 2.5-4 hours
Time to peak serum concentration: Oral: Within 2-3 hours
Elimination: 85% of dose excreted in urine and feces as unchanged drug
Intrathecal:
Half-life, CSF elimination: 1.5 hours
Clearance, CSF: 30 mL/hour

Dosing: Usual
Oral: Dose-related side effects (eg, sedation) may be minimized by slow titration; lower initial doses than described below (2.5-5 mg **daily**) may be used with subsequent titration to 8 hourly doses.
Children: Limited published data in children; the following is a compilation of small prospective studies (Albright, 1996; Milla, 1977; Scheinberg, 2006) and one large retrospective analysis of baclofen use in children (Lubsch, 2006):
<2 years: 10-20 mg **daily** divided every 8 hours; titrate dose every 3 days in increments of 5-15 mg/day to a maximum of 40 mg **daily**
2-7 years: 20-30 mg **daily** divided every 8 hours; titrate dose every 3 days in increments of 5-15 mg/day to a maximum of 60 mg **daily**
≥8 years: 30-40 mg **daily** divided every 8 hours; titrate dosage as above to a maximum of 120 mg **daily**
Note: Lubsch retrospective analysis noted that higher daily dosages of baclofen were needed as the time increased from injury onset, as age increased, and as the number of concomitant antispasticity medications increased. Each of these variables may represent drug tolerance or progressive spasticity. In this review, doses as high as 200 mg **daily** were used.
Adults: 5 mg 3 times/day, may increase 5 mg/dose every 3 days to a maximum of 80 mg/day
Intrathecal: Children and Adults:
Screening dosage: 50 mcg for 1 dose and observe for 4-8 hours; very small children may receive 25 mcg; if ineffective, a repeat dosage increased by 50% (eg, 75 mcg) may be repeated in 24 hours; if still suboptimal, a third dose increased by 33% (eg, 100 mcg) may be repeated in 24 hours; patients who do not respond to 100 mcg intrathecally should not be considered for continuous chronic administration via an implantable pump
Maintenance dose: Continuous infusion: Initial: Depending upon the screening dosage and its duration:
If the screening dose duration >8 hours: Daily dose = effective screening dose
If the screening dose duration <8 hours: Daily dose = **twice** effective screening dose
Continuous infusion dose mcg/hour = daily dose divided by 24 hours
Note: Further adjustments in infusion rate may be done every 24 hours as needed; for spinal cord-related spasticity, increase in 10% to 30% increments/24 hours; for spasticity of cerebral origin, increase in 5% to 10% increments/24 hours
Average daily dose:
Children ≤12 years: 100-300 mcg/day (4.2-12.5 mcg/hour); doses as high as 1000 mcg/day have been used
Children >12 years and Adults: 300-800 mcg/day (12.5-33 mcg/hour); doses as high as 2000 mcg/day have been used

Administration
Oral: Administer with food or milk

Parenteral: Intrathecal: Test dosage: Use dilute concentration (50 mcg/mL) and inject over at least 1 minute; for maintenance infusion via implantable infusion pump, concentrations of 500-2000 mcg/mL may be used; do not abruptly discontinue intrathecal baclofen administration

Monitoring Parameters Muscle rigidity, spasticity (decrease in number and severity of spasms), modified Ashworth score

Test Interactions Increased alkaline phosphatase, AST, glucose, ammonia (B); decreased bilirubin (S)

Dosage Forms Considerations EnovaRX-Baclofen is a compounding kit. Refer to manufacturer's package insert for compounding instructions.

Dosage Forms Excipient information presented when available (limited, particularly for generics); consult specific product labeling.
Cream, External:
EnovaRX-Baclofen: 1% (60 g, 120 g) [contains cetyl alcohol]
Solution, Intrathecal [preservative free]:
Gablofen: 50 mcg/mL (1 mL); 10,000 mcg/20 mL (20 mL); 20,000 mcg/20 mL (20 mL); 40,000 mcg/20 mL (20 mL) [antioxidant free]
Lioresal: 0.05 mg/mL (1 mL); 10 mg/20 mL (20 mL); 10 mg/5 mL (5 mL); 40 mg/20 mL (20 mL) [antioxidant free]
Tablet, Oral:
Generic: 10 mg, 20 mg

Extemporaneous Preparations A 5 mg/mL oral suspension may be made with tablets. Crush thirty 20 mg tablets in a mortar and reduce to a fine powder. Add a small amount of glycerin and mix to a uniform paste. Mix while adding Simple Syrup, NF in incremental proportions to **almost** 120 mL; transfer to a calibrated bottle, rinse mortar with vehicle, and add a sufficient quantity of vehicle to make 120 mL. Label "shake well" and "refrigerate". Stable for 35 days (Johnson, 1993).

A 10 mg/mL oral suspension may be made with tablets. Crush one-hundred-twenty 10 mg tablets in a mortar and reduce to a fine powder. Add small portions (60 mL) of a 1:1 mixture of Ora-Sweet® and Ora-Plus® and mix to a uniform paste; mix while adding the vehicle in incremental proportions to **almost** 120 mL; transfer to a calibrated bottle, rinse mortar with vehicle, and add quantity of vehicle sufficient to make 120 mL. Label "shake well" and "refrigerate". Stable for 60 days (Allen, 1996).

Allen LV Jr and Erickson MA 3rd, "Stability of Baclofen, Captopril, Diltiazem Hydrochloride, Dipyridamole, and Flecainide Acetate in Extemporaneously Compounded Oral Liquids," *Am J Health Syst Pharm*, 1996, 53(18):2179-84.
Johnson CE and Hart SM, "Stability of an Extemporaneously Compounded Baclofen Oral Liquid," *Am J Hosp Pharm*, 1993, 50 (11):2353-5.

References
Albright AL, "Baclofen in the Treatment of Cerebral Palsy," *J Child Neurol*, 1996, 11(2):77-83.
Eriksson G and Swahn CG, "Concentrations of Baclofen in Serum and Breast Milk From a Lactating Woman," *Scand J Clin Lab Invest*, 1981, 41(2):185-7.
Lubsch L, Habersang R, Haase M, et al, "Oral Baclofen and Clonidine for Treatment of Spasticity in Children," *J Child Neurol*, 2006, 21 (12):1090-2.
Milla PJ and Jackson AD, "A Controlled Trial of Baclofen in Children With Cerebral Palsy," *J Int Med Res*, 1977, 5(6):398-404.
Morton CM, Rosenow J, Wong C, et al, "Intrathecal Baclofen Administration During Pregnancy: A Case Series and Focused Clinical Review," *PM R*, 2009, 1(11):1025-9.
Ratnayaka BD, Dhaliwal H, and Watkin S, "Drug Points: Neonatal Convulsions After Withdrawal of Baclofen," *BMJ*, 2001, 323(7304):85.
Scheinberg A, Hall K, Lam LT, et al, "Oral Baclofen in Children With Cerebral Palsy: A Double-Blind Cross-Over Pilot Study," *J Paediatr Child Health*, 2006, 42(11):715-20.

◆ **Bactocill in Dextrose** *see* Oxacillin *on page 1555*

◆ **Bactrim** *see* Sulfamethoxazole and Trimethoprim *on page 1948*

◆ **Bactrim DS** *see* Sulfamethoxazole and Trimethoprim *on page 1948*

◆ **Bactroban** *see* Mupirocin *on page 1452*

◆ **Bactroban Nasal** *see* Mupirocin *on page 1452*

◆ **Baking Soda** *see* Sodium Bicarbonate *on page 1901*

◆ **BAL** *see* Dimercaprol *on page 672*

◆ **Bal in Oil** *see* Dimercaprol *on page 672*

◆ **Balmex® [OTC]** *see* Zinc Oxide *on page 2176*

◆ **Balminil Decongestant (Can)** *see* Pseudoephedrine *on page 1770*

◆ **Balminil DM E (Can)** *see* Guaifenesin and Dextromethorphan *on page 987*

◆ **Balminil Expectorant (Can)** *see* GuaiFENesin *on page 984*

◆ **Balnetar [OTC]** *see* Coal Tar *on page 532*

Balsalazide (bal SAL a zide)

Medication Safety Issues
Sound-alike/look-alike issues:
Colazal® may be confused with Clozaril®

Brand Names: U.S. Colazal; Giazo

Therapeutic Category 5-Aminosalicylic Acid Derivative; Anti-inflammatory Agent

Generic Availability (U.S.) May be product dependent

Use
Capsules: Short-term treatment of mildly to moderately active ulcerative colitis (FDA approved in ages ≥5 years and adults); Pediatric patients (5-17 years): 8 weeks of therapy; Adult patients: 12 weeks of therapy
Tablets (Giazo™): Short-term treatment (8 weeks) of mildly to moderately active ulcerative colitis (FDA approved in males ≥18 years and adults)

Pregnancy Risk Factor B

Pregnancy Considerations Teratogenic effects were not observed in animal reproduction studies. Mesalamine (5-aminosalicylic acid) is the active metabolite of balsalazide; mesalamine is known to cross the placenta.

Breast-Feeding Considerations Mesalamine, 5-aminosalicylic acid, is the active metabolite of balsalazide. Low levels of mesalamine enter breast milk; a case of bloody diarrhea in a breast-fed infant has been reported.

Contraindications Hypersensitivity to balsalazide or metabolites, salicylates, or any component

Warnings May exacerbate symptoms of ulcerative colitis; reported incidence higher in children than adults (6% vs 1%). May cause an acute intolerance syndrome (cramping, acute abdominal pain, bloody diarrhea; sometimes fever, headache, rash); discontinue if this occurs. Hepatoxicity (some cases fatal) including increased liver function tests, jaundice, cholestatic jaundice, cirrhosis, and hepatocellular damage, including liver necrosis and failure, has been reported with products that contain mesalamine or are metabolized to mesalamine, including balsalazide. Giazo™ oral tablets were not found effective in adult female patients.

Precautions Use with caution in patients with renal impairment; renal toxicity has been observed with other mesalamine (5-aminosalicylic acid) products. Patients with pyloric stenosis may have prolonged gastric retention, delaying release of drug in the colon. May cause staining of teeth or tongue if capsule is opened and sprinkled on food. Children may experience a higher frequency of some adverse effects than adults, including: Headache (15% vs 8%), abdominal pain (~13% vs 6%), and vomiting (10% vs ≤4%)

Adverse Reactions

Central nervous system: Fatigue, fever, headache (more common in children than adults), insomnia

Endocrine & metabolic: Dysmenorrhea

Gastrointestinal: Abdominal pain (more common in children than adults), anorexia, cramps, constipation, diarrhea, dyspepsia, flatulence, hematochezia, nausea, stomatitis, ulcerative colitis exacerbation, vomiting, xerostomia

Genitourinary: Urinary tract infection

Hematologic: Anemia

Neuromuscular & skeletal: Arthralgia, musculoskeletal pain, myalgia

Respiratory: Cough, pharyngolaryngeal pain, pharyngitis, respiratory infection, rhinitis

Miscellaneous: Flu-like syndrome

Rare but important or life-threatening: Alopecia, alveolitis, AST increased, back pain, blood pressure increased, cholestatic jaundice, cirrhosis, defecation urgency, dizziness, dyspnea, edema, erythema nodosum, facial edema, fever, gastroenteritis, gastroesophageal reflux, hard stool, heart rate increased, hepatocellular damage, hepatotoxicity, hyperbilirubinemia, hypersensitivity, interstitial nephritis, jaundice, Kawasaki-like syndrome, lethargy, liver failure, liver necrosis, liver function tests increased, malaise, myocarditis, pain, pancreatitis, pericarditis, pleural effusion, pneumonia (with and without eosinophilia), pruritus, rash, renal failure, vasculitis

Drug Interactions

Metabolism/Transport Effects None known.

Avoid Concomitant Use There are no known interactions where it is recommended to avoid concomitant use.

Increased Effect/Toxicity

Balsalazide may increase the levels/effects of: Heparin; Heparin (Low Molecular Weight); Thiopurine Analogs; Varicella Virus-Containing Vaccines

The levels/effects of Balsalazide may be increased by: Nonsteroidal Anti-Inflammatory Agents

Decreased Effect

Balsalazide may decrease the levels/effects of: Cardiac Glycosides

Stability Store at 20°C to 25°C (68°F to 77°F); excursions permitted between 15°C to 30°C (59°F to 86°F)

Mechanism of Action Balsalazide is a prodrug, converted by bacterial azoreduction to 5-aminosalicylic acid (mesalamine, active), 4-aminobenzoyl-β-alanine (inert), and their metabolites. 5-aminosalicylic acid may decrease inflammation by blocking the production of arachidonic acid metabolites topically in the colon mucosa.

Pharmacodynamics Onset of action: Delayed; may require several days to weeks (2 weeks); similar in adults and children

Pharmacokinetics (Adult data unless noted)

Absorption: Very low and variable; in children, reported systemic absorption of 5-ASA (active) lower than adults (C_{max}: 67% lower, AUC: 64% lower)

Protein binding: ≥99%

Metabolism: Azoreduced in the colon to 5-aminosalicylic acid (active), 4-aminobenzoyl-β-alanine (inert), and N-acetylated metabolites

Half-life: Primary effect is topical (colonic mucosa); therapeutic effect appears not to be influenced by the systemic half-life of balsalazide (1.9 hours) or its metabolites (5-ASA [9.5 hours], N-Ac-5-ASA [10.4 hours])

Time to peak serum concentration: Capsule: 1-2 hours; Tablet: 0.5 hours

Elimination: Feces (65% as 5-aminosalicylic acid, 4-aminobenzoyl-β-alanine, and N-acetylated metabolites); urine (11.3% as N-acetylated metabolites); Parent drug: Urine or feces (<1%)

Dosing: Usual

Children ≥5 years and Adolescents ≤17 years: **Ulcerative colitis:** Oral: Capsules: 2.25 g/day or 6.75 g/day for up to 8 weeks administered as either:

2.25 g (three 750 mg capsules) 3 times daily (total daily dose: 6.75 g/day)

or

750 mg (one capsule) 3 times daily (total daily dose: 2.25 g/day)

Note: Limited blinded clinical trial in children did not demonstrate significant improvement between total daily doses of 6.75 g or 2.25 g (Quiros, 2009).

Adolescents ≥18 years and Adults: **Ulcerative colitis:**

Capsule: 2.25 g (three 750 mg capsules) 3 times daily for up to 8-12 weeks

Tablet (Giazo™): Males: 3.3 g (three 1.1 g tablets) twice daily for up to 8 weeks

Dosing adjustment in renal impairment: There are no dosage adjustments provided in manufacturer's labeling. Renal toxicity has been observed with other 5-aminosalicylic acid products; use with caution.

Dosing adjustment in hepatic impairment: There are no dosage adjustments provided in manufacturer's labeling.

Administration

Capsules: Should be swallowed whole or may be opened and sprinkled on applesauce. Applesauce mixture may be chewed; swallow immediately, do not store mixture for later use. When sprinkled on food, may cause staining of teeth or tongue. Color variation of powder inside capsule (ranging from orange to yellow) is expected.

Tablets: Administer with or without food.

Monitoring Parameters Improvement or worsening of symptoms; renal function (prior to initiation, then periodically); liver function tests

Additional Information Balsalazide 750 mg is equivalent to mesalamine 267 mg.

Dosage Forms Excipient information presented when available (limited, particularly for generics); consult specific product labeling.

Capsule, Oral, as disodium:

Colazal: 750 mg

Generic: 750 mg

Tablet, Oral:

Giazo: 1.1 g

References

Connell W and Miller A, "Treating Inflammatory Bowel Disease During Pregnancy: Risks and Safety of Drug Therapy," *Drug Safety*, 1999, 21 (4):311-23.

Diav-Citrin O, Park YH, Veerasuntharam G, et al, "The Safety of Mesalamine in Human Pregnancy: A Prospective Controlled Cohort Study," *Gastroenterology*, 1998, 114(1):23-8.

Dubinsky M, Abraham B, and Mahadevan U, "Management of the Pregnant IBD Patient," *Inflamm Bowel Dis*, 2008, 14(12):1736-50.

Quiros JA, Heyman MB, Pohl JF, et al, "Safety, Efficacy, and Pharmacokinetics of Balsalazide in Pediatric Patients With Mild-to-Moderate Active Ulcerative Colitis: Results of a Randomized, Double-Blind Study," *J Pediatr Gastroenterol Nutr*, 2009, 49(5):571-9.

Scherl EJ, Pruitt R, Gordon GL, et al, "Safety and Efficacy of a New 3.3 g b.i.d. Tablet Formulation in Patients With Mild-to-Moderately-Active Ulcerative Colitis: A Multicenter, Randomized, Double-Blind, Placebo-Controlled Study," *Am J Gastroenterol*, 2009, 104(6):1452-9.

◆ **Balsalazide Disodium** *see* Balsalazide *on page 261*

◆ **Banophen [OTC]** *see* DiphenhydrAMINE (Systemic) *on page 673*

◆ **Banophen [OTC]** *see* DiphenhydrAMINE (Topical) *on page 677*

◆ **Banzel** *see* Rufinamide *on page 1858*

◆ **Banzel™ (Can)** *see* Rufinamide *on page 1858*

◆ **Baraclude** *see* Entecavir *on page 757*

◆ **Baridium [OTC]** *see* Phenazopyridine *on page 1651*

◆ **Basaljel® (Can)** *see* Aluminum Hydroxide *on page 110*

◆ **Base Ointment** *see* Zinc Oxide *on page 2176*

Basiliximab (ba si LIK si mab)

Brand Names: U.S. Simulect
Brand Names: Canada Simulect®
Therapeutic Category Monoclonal Antibody
Generic Availability (U.S.) No

Use In combination with an immunosuppressive regimen (cyclosporine and corticosteroids), induction therapy for the prophylaxis of acute organ rejection in patients receiving renal transplants (FDA approved in pediatric patients [age not specified] and adults); basiliximab has also been used in liver and heart transplant patients

Pregnancy Risk Factor B

Pregnancy Considerations Teratogenic effects were not observed in animal studies. IL-2 receptors play an important role in the development of the immune system. Use in pregnant women only when benefit exceeds potential risk to the fetus. Women of childbearing potential should use effective contraceptive measures before beginning treatment and for 4 months after completion of therapy with this agent. The National Transplantation Pregnancy Registry (NTPR, Temple University) is a registry for pregnant women taking immunosuppressants following any solid organ transplant. The NTPR encourages reporting of all immunosuppressant exposures during pregnancy in transplant recipients at 877-955-6877.

Breast-Feeding Considerations It is not known whether basiliximab is excreted in human milk. Because many immunoglobulins are secreted in milk and the potential for serious adverse reactions exists, a decision should be made whether to discontinue nursing or discontinue the drug, taking into account the importance of the drug to the mother.

Contraindications Hypersensitivity to basiliximab, murine proteins, or any component of the formulation

Warnings Severe, acute hypersensitivity reactions, including anaphylaxis, have been reported following initial exposure or re-exposure to basiliximab. Patients in whom concomitant immunosuppression was prematurely discontinued (eg, abandoned transplantation or early loss of graft) are at particular risk of developing a severe hypersensitivity reaction upon readministration. If a severe hypersensitivity reaction occurs, basiliximab should be permanently discontinued. Medications for the management of severe allergic reactions should be available for immediate use.

Precautions May result in an increased susceptibility to infection or an increased risk for developing lymphoproliferative disorders. Treatment with basiliximab may result in the development of human antimurine antibodies (HAMA); however, limited evidence suggesting the use of muromonab-CD3 or other murine products is not precluded. Basiliximab should only be prescribed by physicians experienced in immunosuppression therapy and management of organ transplant patients **[U.S. Boxed Warning]**. Patients receiving basiliximab should be treated at facilities specially equipped and staffed to manage organ transplant patients. In renal transplant patients receiving basiliximab plus prednisone, cyclosporine, and mycophenolate, new-onset diabetes, glucose intolerance, and impaired fasting glucose were observed at rates significantly higher than observed in patients receiving prednisone, cyclosporine, and mycophenolate without basiliximab (Aasebo, 2010).

Adverse Reactions

Cardiovascular: Abnormal heart sounds, angina, arrhythmia, atrial fibrillation, chest pain, generalized edema, heart failure, hyper-/hypotension, peripheral edema, tachycardia

Central nervous system: Agitation, anxiety, depression, dizziness, fatigue, fever, headache, hypoesthesia, insomnia, malaise, pain

Dermatologic: Acne, cyst, hypertrichosis, pruritus, rash, skin disorder, skin ulceration, wound complications

Endocrine & metabolic: Acidosis, dehydration, diabetes mellitus, fluid overload, glucocorticoids increased, hyper-/hypocalcemia, hypercholesterolemia, hyperglycemia, hyper-/hypokalemia, hyperlipemia, hypertriglyceridemia, hyperuricemia, hypoglycemia, hypomagnesemia, hyponatremia, hypophosphatemia, hypoproteinemia

Gastrointestinal: Abdomen enlarged, abdominal pain, constipation, diarrhea, dyspepsia esophagitis, flatulence, gastroenteritis, GI hemorrhage, gingival hyperplasia, melena, moniliasis, nausea, stomatitis (including ulcerative), vomiting, weight gain

Genitourinary: Bladder disorder, dysuria, genital edema (male), impotence, ureteral disorder, urinary frequency, urinary retention, urinary tract infection

Hematologic: Anemia, hematoma, hemorrhage, leukopenia, polycythemia, purpura, thrombocytopenia, thrombosis

Neuromuscular & skeletal: Arthralgia, arthropathy, back pain, cramps, fracture, hernia, leg pain, myalgia, neuropathy, paresthesia, rigors, tremor, weakness

Ocular: Abnormal vision, cataract, conjunctivitis

Renal: Albuminuria, hematuria, nonprotein nitrogen increased, oliguria, renal function abnormal, renal tubular necrosis

Respiratory: Bronchitis, bronchospasm, cough, dyspnea, infection (upper respiratory), pharyngitis, pneumonia, pulmonary edema, rhinitis, sinusitis

Miscellaneous: Accidental trauma, cytomegalovirus (CMV) infection, herpes infection (simplex and zoster), infection, sepsis

Rare but important or life-threatening: Anaphylaxis, capillary leak syndrome, cytokine release syndrome, diabetes (new onset), fasting glucose impaired, glucose intolerance, hypersensitivity reaction (including heart failure, hypotension, tachycardia, bronchospasm, dyspnea, pulmonary edema, respiratory failure, sneezing, pruritus, rash, urticaria), lymphoproliferative disease

Drug Interactions

Metabolism/Transport Effects None known.

Avoid Concomitant Use

Avoid concomitant use of Basiliximab with any of the following: BCG; Belimumab; Natalizumab; Pimecrolimus; Tacrolimus (Topical); Tofacitinib; Vaccines (Live)

Increased Effect/Toxicity

Basiliximab may increase the levels/effects of: Belimumab; Hypoglycemic Agents; Leflunomide; Natalizumab; Tofacitinib; Vaccines (Live)

The levels/effects of Basiliximab may be increased by: Abciximab; Denosumab; Herbs (Hypoglycemic Properties); MAO Inhibitors; Pimecrolimus; Roflumilast; Salicylates; Selective Serotonin Reuptake Inhibitors; Tacrolimus (Topical); Trastuzumab

Decreased Effect

Basiliximab may decrease the levels/effects of: BCG; Coccidioidin Skin Test; Sipuleucel-T; Vaccines (Inactivated); Vaccines (Live)

The levels/effects of Basiliximab may be decreased by: Echinacea; Loop Diuretics

Stability Store intact vials under refrigeration 2°C to 8°C (36°F to 46°F). Reconstituted solution should be used immediately after reconstitution; however, may be stored at 2°C to 8°C for up to 24 hours or at room temperature for up to 4 hours. Discard the reconstituted solution within 24 hours. Do not shake.

Mechanism of Action Chimeric (murine/human) immunosuppressant monoclonal antibody which blocks the alpha-chain of the interleukin-2 (IL-2) receptor complex; this receptor is expressed on activated T lymphocytes and is a critical pathway for activating cell-mediated allograft rejection

▶

Pharmacodynamics Duration: 36 days ± 14 days (determined by IL-2R alpha saturation in patients also on cyclosporine and corticosteroids)

Pharmacokinetics (Adult data unless noted) Note:
Values based on data from renal transplant patients
Distribution: V_{dss}:
Children 1-11 years: 4.8 ± 2.1 L
Adolescents 12-16 years: 7.8 ± 5.1 L
Adults: 8.6 ± 4.1 L
Half-life:
Children 1-11 years: 9.5 ± 4.5 days
Adolescents 12-16 years: 9.1 ± 3.9 days
Adults: 7.2 ± 3.2 days
Elimination: Clearance:
Children 1-11 years: 17 ± 6 mL/hour; in pediatric liver transplant patients, significant basiliximab loss through ascites fluid can increase total body clearance and reduce IL-2R (CD25) saturation duration; dosage adjustments may be necessary (Cintorino, 2006; Kovarik, 2002; Spada, 2006)
Adolescents 12-16 years: 31 ±19 mL/hour
Adults: 41 ± 19 mL/hour

Dosing: Usual Note: Patients previously administered basiliximab should only be re-exposed to a subsequent course of therapy with extreme caution.
Infants, Children, and Adolescents:
Renal transplantation: I.V.:
Patient weight <35 kg:
Initial dose: 10 mg administered within 2 hours prior to renal transplant surgery
Second dose: 10 mg administered 4 days after transplantation; hold second dose if complications occur (including severe hypersensitivity reactions or graft loss)
Patient weight ≥35 kg:
Initial dose: 20 mg administered within 2 hours prior to renal transplant surgery
Second dose: 20 mg administered 4 days after transplantation; hold second dose if complications occur (including severe hypersensitivity reactions or graft loss)
Liver transplantation: I.V.: Limited data available (Cintorino, 2006; Kovarik, 2002; Spada, 2006):
Patient weight <35 kg:
Initial dose: 10 mg administered within 6 hours of organ perfusion
Second dose: 10 mg administered 4 days after transplantation; hold second dose if complications occur (including severe hypersensitivity reactions or graft loss)
Third dose: 10 mg has been repeated on postoperative days 8-10 if ascites fluid loss exceeds 70 mL/kg or >5 L
Patient weight ≥35 kg:
Initial dose: 20 mg administered within 6 hours of organ perfusion
Second dose: 20 mg administered 4 days after transplantation; hold second dose if complications occur (including severe hypersensitivity reactions or graft loss)
Third dose: 20 mg has been repeated on postoperative days 8-10 if ascites fluid loss exceeds 70 mL/kg or if total ascites volume ≥5 L
Heart transplantation: I.V.: Limited data available (Ford, 2005; Grundy, 2009):
Patient weight <35 kg:
Initial dose: 10 mg administered immediately before cardiopulmonary by-pass started or within 6 hours of organ perfusion
Second dose: 10 mg administered 4 days after transplantation; hold second dose if complications occur (including severe hypersensitivity reactions or graft loss)

Patient weight ≥35 kg:
Initial dose: 20 mg administered immediately before cardiopulmonary by-pass started or within 6 hours of organ perfusion
Second dose: 20 mg administered 4 days after transplantation; hold second dose if complications occur (including severe hypersensitivity reactions or graft loss)
Adults: **Renal transplantation:** I.V.:
Initial dose: 20 mg administered within 2 hours prior to renal transplant surgery
Second dose: 20 mg administered 4 days after transplantation; hold second dose if complications occur (including severe hypersensitivity reactions or graft loss)
Dosing adjustment in renal impairment: There are no dosage adjustments provided in manufacturer's labeling.
Dosing adjustment in hepatic impairment: There are no dosage adjustments provided in manufacturer's labeling.
Administration For I.V. administration only. Administer only after assurance that patient will receive renal graft and immunosuppression. Reconstitute with preservative free SWI (reconstitute 10 mg vial with 2.5 mL, 20 mg vial with 5 mL). Shake the vial gently to dissolve. Reconstituted basiliximab solution may be administered without further dilution as a bolus injection over 10 minutes or further dilute in NS or D_5W to a final concentration of 0.4 mg/mL and infuse over 20-30 minutes. When mixing the solution, gently invert the bag to avoid foaming. Do not shake the bag. Bolus injection is associated with nausea, vomiting, and local pain at the injection site.
Monitoring Parameters CBC with differential, vital signs, immunologic monitoring of T cells, renal function, serum glucose, signs or symptoms of hypersensitivity, infection
Reference Range Serum concentration >0.2 mcg/mL
Dosage Forms Excipient information presented when available (limited, particularly for generics); consult specific product labeling.
Solution Reconstituted, Intravenous [preservative free]:
Simulect: 10 mg (1 ea); 20 mg (1 ea)

References

Aasebø W, Midtvedt K, Valderhaug TG, et al, "Impaired Glucose Homeostasis in Renal Transplant Recipients Receiving Basiliximab," *Nephrol Dial Transplant*, 2010, 25(4):1289-93.

Bamgbola FO, Del Rio M, Kaskel FJ, et al, "Non-Cardiogenic Pulmonary Edema During Basiliximab Induction in Three Adolescent Renal Transplant Patients," *Pediatr Transplant*, 2003, 7(4):315-20.

Cintorino D, Riva S, Spada M, et al, "Corticosteroid-Free Immunosuppression in Pediatric Liver Transplantation: Safety and Efficacy After a Short-Term Follow-Up," *Transplant Proc*, 2006, 38(4):1099-100.

Dolan N, Waldron M, O'Connell M, et al, "Basiliximab Induced Non-Cardiogenic Pulmonary Edema in Two Pediatric Renal Transplant Recipients," *Pediatr Nephrol*, 2009, 24(11):2261-5.

Ford KA, Cale CM, Rees PG, et al, "Initial Data on Basiliximab in Critically Ill Children Undergoing Heart Transplantation," *J Heart Lung Transplant*, 2005, 24(9):1284-8.

Goulet O, Sauvat F, Ruemmele F, et al, "Results of the Paris Program: Ten Years of Pediatric Intestinal Transplantation," *Transplant Proc*, 2005, 37(4):1667-70.

Grundy N, Simmonds J, Dawkins H, et al, "Pre-Implantation Basiliximab Reduces Incidence of Early Acute Rejection in Pediatric Heart Transplantation," *J Heart Lung Transplant*, 2009, 28(12):1279-84.

Ji SQ, Chen HR, Yan HM, et al, "Anti-CD25 Monoclonal Antibody (Basiliximab) for Prevention of Graft-Versus-Host Disease After Haploidentical Bone Marrow Transplantation for Hematological Malignancies," *Bone Marrow Transplant*, 2005, 36(4):349-54.

Kovarik JM, Gridelli BG, Martin S, et al, "Basiliximab in Pediatric Liver Transplantation: A Pharmacokinetic-Derived Dosing Algorithm," *Pediatr Transplant*, 2002, 6(3):224-30.

Spada M, Petz W, Bertani A, et al, "Randomized Trial of Basiliximab Induction Versus Steroid Therapy in Pediatric Liver Allograft Recipients Under Tacrolimus Immunosuppression," *Am J Transplant*, 2006, 6(8):1913-21.

◆ **Baycadron** see Dexamethasone (Systemic) on page 615
◆ **Bayer Aspirin Extra Strength [OTC]** see Aspirin on page 212

- ◆ **Bayer Aspirin Regimen Adult Low Strength [OTC]** *see* Aspirin *on page 212*
- ◆ **Bayer Aspirin Regimen Children's [OTC]** *see* Aspirin *on page 212*
- ◆ **Bayer Aspirin Regimen Regular Strength [OTC]** *see* Aspirin *on page 212*
- ◆ **Bayer Genuine Aspirin [OTC]** *see* Aspirin *on page 212*
- ◆ **Bayer Plus Extra Strength [OTC]** *see* Aspirin *on page 212*
- ◆ **Bayer Women's Low Dose Aspirin [OTC]** *see* Aspirin *on page 212*
- ◆ **Baza Antifungal [OTC]** *see* Miconazole (Topical) *on page 1410*
- ◆ **BCNU** *see* Carmustine *on page 382*
- ◆ **Bebulin VH** *see* Factor IX Complex (Human) [(Factors II, IX, X)] *on page 833*

Beclomethasone (Oral Inhalation)
(be kloe METH a sone)

Related Information
Inhaled Corticosteroids *on page 2223*
Brand Names: U.S. Qvar
Brand Names: Canada QVAR
Therapeutic Category Adrenal Corticosteroid; Anti-inflammatory Agent; Antiasthmatic; Corticosteroid, Inhalant (Oral); Glucocorticoid
Generic Availability (U.S.) No
Use Long-term (chronic) control of persistent bronchial asthma (FDA approved in ages ≥5 years and adults); **not** indicated for the relief of acute bronchospasm. Also used to help reduce or discontinue oral corticosteroid therapy for asthma.
Pregnancy Risk Factor C
Pregnancy Considerations Adverse events were observed in some animal reproduction studies. Hypoadrenalism may occur in newborns following maternal use of corticosteroids in pregnancy. Based on available data, an overall increased risk of congenital malformations or a decrease in fetal growth has not been associated with maternal use of inhaled corticosteroids during pregnancy (Bakhireva, 2005; NAEPP, 2005; Namazy, 2004). Uncontrolled asthma is associated with adverse events in pregnancy (increased risk of perinatal mortality, pre-eclampsia, preterm birth, low birth weight infants). Inhaled corticosteroids are recommended for the treatment of asthma during pregnancy (most information available using budesonide) (ACOG, 2008; NAEPP, 2005).
Breast-Feeding Considerations Other corticosteroids have been found in breast milk; however, information for beclomethasone is not available. Due to the potential for serious adverse reactions in the nursing infant, the manufacturer recommends a decision be made whether to discontinue nursing or to discontinue the drug, taking into account the importance of treatment to the mother. Use of inhaled corticosteroids is not a contraindication to breast-feeding (NAEPP, 2005).
Contraindications Hypersensitivity to beclomethasone or any component; primary treatment of status asthmaticus or other acute episodes of bronchial asthma where intensive treatment is needed
Warnings Fatalities have occurred due to adrenal insufficiency in asthmatic patients during and after switching from systemic corticosteroids to aerosol steroids; several months may be required for full recovery of hypothalamic-pituitary-adrenal (HPA) function; patients receiving higher doses of systemic corticosteroids (eg, adults receiving ≥20 mg of prednisone per day) may be at greater risk; during this period of HPA suppression, aerosol steroids do not provide the systemic glucocorticoid or

mineralocorticoid activity needed to treat patients requiring stress doses (ie, patients with major stress such as trauma, surgery, or infections, or other conditions associated with severe electrolyte loss). When used at high doses or for a prolonged time, hypercorticism and HPA suppression (including adrenal crisis) may occur; use with inhaled or systemic corticosteroids (even alternate-day dosing) may increase risk of HPA suppression. Acute adrenal insufficiency may occur with abrupt withdrawal after long-term use or with stress; withdrawal and discontinuation of corticosteroids should be done carefully; patients with HPA axis suppression may require doses of systemic glucocorticosteroids prior to, during, and after unusual stress (eg, surgery). Immunosuppression may occur; patients may be more susceptible to infections; avoid exposure to chickenpox and measles. Switching from systemic corticosteroids to inhalation may unmask allergic conditions (such as eczema, conjunctivitis, and rhinitis) that were previously suppressed by systemic steroids. Bronchospasm may occur after use of inhaled asthma medications; if bronchospasm with wheezing occurs after use, a fast-acting bronchodilator may be used; discontinue orally inhaled corticosteroid and initiate alternative chronic therapy.

C. albicans infections of the mouth and pharynx may occur with orally inhaled corticosteroid use, mostly mild to moderate in nature; interruption of therapy may be necessary at times while antifungal therapy is employed; advise patients to rinse mouth after use. Hypersensitivity reactions with angioedema and swelling of the lips, tongue, and pharynx have been reported rarely.

Precautions Avoid using higher than recommended dosages; suppression of HPA function, reduced bone mineral density, hypercorticism (Cushing's syndrome) may occur; titrate to lowest effective dose. Reduction in growth velocity may occur when corticosteroids are administered to pediatric patients, even at recommended doses via inhaled route; reduction in growth velocity is related to dose and duration of exposure; monitor growth. With beclomethasone-HFA (Qvar) the mean reduction in growth velocity was 0.5 cm/year less than that with the previous beclomethasone CFC inhaler formulation. Use with extreme caution in patients with respiratory tuberculosis, untreated systemic infections, or ocular herpes simplex. Use with caution and monitor patients closely with hepatic dysfunction. Rare cases of increased IOP, glaucoma, or cataracts have been reported with inhaled corticosteroids. Use of Qvar with a spacer device is not recommended in children <5 years of age due to the decreased amount of medication that is delivered with increasing wait times; patients should be instructed to inhale immediately if using a spacer device.

Adverse Reactions
Central nervous system: Headache, pain, voice disorder
Gastrointestinal: Nausea
Genitourinary: Dysmenorrhea
Neuromuscular & skeletal: Back pain
Respiratory: Cough, pharyngitis, rhinitis, sinusitis, upper respiratory tract infection
Rare but important or life-threatening: Anaphylactoid reaction, anaphylaxis, behavioral changes (such as aggressiveness, depression, sleep disturbances, psychomotor hyperactivity, suicidal ideation; more common in children/adolescents), decreased linear skeletal growth rate (in children/adolescents), hypersensitivity reaction (immediate and delayed; including angioedema, bronchospasm, rash, urticaria), HPA-axis suppression; rarely glaucoma, increased intraocular pressure, and cataracts have been reported with inhaled corticosteroids

Drug Interactions
Metabolism/Transport Effects None known.

Avoid Concomitant Use

Avoid concomitant use of Beclomethasone (Oral Inhalation) with any of the following: Aldesleukin; BCG; Natalizumab; Pimecrolimus; Tacrolimus (Topical); Tofacitinib

Increased Effect/Toxicity

Beclomethasone (Oral Inhalation) may increase the levels/effects of: Amphotericin B; Ceritinib; Deferasirox; Leflunomide; Loop Diuretics; Natalizumab; Thiazide Diuretics; Tofacitinib

The levels/effects of Beclomethasone (Oral Inhalation) may be increased by: Denosumab; Pimecrolimus; Tacrolimus (Topical); Telaprevir; Trastuzumab

Decreased Effect

Beclomethasone (Oral Inhalation) may decrease the levels/effects of: Aldesleukin; Antidiabetic Agents; BCG; Coccidioidin Skin Test; Corticorelin; Hyaluronidase; Sipuleucel-T; Telaprevir; Vaccines (Inactivated)

The levels/effects of Beclomethasone (Oral Inhalation) may be decreased by: Echinacea

Stability Store at 25°C (77°F); excursions permitted between 15°C to 30°C (59°F to 86°F). Do not store near heat or open flame; do not puncture canister, or throw into fire or incinerator; exposure to temperatures >49°C (120°F) may cause bursting. Store Qvar so inhaler rests on concave end of canister (with plastic actuator on top).

Mechanism of Action Controls the rate of protein synthesis; depresses the migration of polymorphonuclear leukocytes, fibroblasts; reverses capillary permeability and lysosomal stabilization at the cellular level to prevent or control inflammation

Pharmacodynamics Onset of action: Within 1-2 days in some patients; usually within 1-2 weeks; Maximum effect: 3-4 weeks

Pharmacokinetics (Adult data unless noted)

Absorption: Readily absorbed; quickly hydrolyzed by pulmonary esterases to active metabolite, beclomethasone-17-monoproprionate (17-BMP), prior to absorption

Distribution: V_d: Beclomethasone dipropionate (BDP): 20 L; 17-BMP: 424 L

Protein binding: BDP 87%; 17-BMP: 94% to 96%

Metabolism: BDP is a prodrug (inactive) which undergoes rapid hydrolysis to 17-BMP (active monoester) during absorption; BDP is also metabolized in the liver via cytochrome P450 isoenzyme CYP3A4 to 17-BMP and two other less active metabolites: Beclomethasone-21-monopropionate (21-BMP) and beclomethasone (BOH)

Half-life, elimination: BDP: 0.5 hours; 17-BMP: 2.7 hours

Time to peak serum concentration: BDP: 0.5 hours; 17-BMP: 0.7 hours

Elimination: Primary route of excretion is via feces (~60%); <10% to 12% of oral dose excreted in urine as metabolites

Dosing: Usual

Pediatric: **Note:** Doses should be titrated to the lowest effective dose once asthma is controlled: **Asthma, maintenance therapy:** Children ≥5 years and Adolescents: Inhalation, oral:

Manufacturer's labeling (Qvar):

Children 5-11 years: Initial: 40 mcg twice daily; maximum dose: 80 mcg twice daily

Children ≥12 years and Adolescents:

No previous inhaled corticosteroids: Initial: 40-80 mcg twice daily; maximum dose: 320 mcg twice daily

Previous inhaled corticosteroid use: Initial: 40-160 mcg twice daily; maximum dose: 320 mcg twice daily

Note: Therapeutic ratio between Qvar and other beclomethasone inhalers (eg, CFC formulations; however, none are currently available in U.S.) has not been established.

Alternate dosing: NIH Asthma Guidelines (NAEPP, 2007): HFA formulation (Qvar):

Children 5-11 years: Administer in divided doses:

"Low" dose: 80-160 mcg/day (40 mcg/puff: 2-4 puffs/day or 80 mcg/puff: 1-2 puffs/day)

"Medium" dose: >160-320 mcg/day (40 mcg/puff: 4-8 puffs/day or 80 mcg/puff: 2-4 puffs/day)

"High" dose: >320 mcg/day (40 mcg/puff: >8 puffs/day or 80 mcg/puff: >4 puff/day)

Children ≥12 years and Adolescents:

"Low" dose: 80-240 mcg/day (40 mcg/puff: 2-6 puffs/day or 80 mcg/puff: 1-3 puffs/day)

"Medium" dose: >240-480 mcg/day (40 mcg/puff: 6-12 puffs/day or 80 mcg/puff: 3-6 puffs/day)

"High" dose: >480 mcg/day (40 mcg/puff: >12 puffs/day or 80 mcg/puff: 6 puffs/day)

Conversion from oral systemic corticosteroid to orally inhaled corticosteroid: Initiation of oral inhalation therapy should begin in patients whose asthma is reasonably stabilized on oral corticosteroids (OCS). A gradual dose reduction of OCS should begin ~7 days after starting inhaled therapy. U.S. labeling recommends reducing prednisone dose no more rapidly than ≤2.5 mg/day (or equivalent of other OCS) every 1-2 weeks in adolescents or adults. If adrenal insufficiency occurs, temporarily increase the OCS dose and follow with a more gradual withdrawal. **Note:** When transitioning from systemic to inhaled corticosteroids, supplemental systemic corticosteroid therapy may be necessary during periods of stress or during severe asthma attacks.

Adult: **Asthma:** Inhalation, oral (doses should be titrated to the lowest effective dose once asthma is controlled):

Patients previously on bronchodilators only: Initial dose 40-80 mcg twice daily; maximum dose: 320 mcg twice day

Patients previously on inhaled corticosteroids: Initial dose 40-160 mcg twice daily; maximum dose: 320 mcg twice daily

NIH Asthma Guidelines (NIH, 2007):

"Low" dose: 80-240 mcg/day

"Medium" dose: >240-480 mcg/day

"High" dose: >480 mcg/day

Conversion from oral systemic corticosteroid to orally inhaled corticosteroid: Initiation of oral inhalation therapy should begin in patients whose asthma is reasonably stabilized on oral corticosteroids (OCS). A gradual dose reduction of OCS should begin ~7 days after starting inhaled therapy. U.S. labeling recommends reducing prednisone dose no more rapidly than ≤2.5 mg/day (or equivalent of other OCS) every 1-2 weeks. If adrenal insufficiency occurs, temporarily increase the OCS dose and follow with a more gradual withdrawal. **Note:** When transitioning from systemic to inhaled corticosteroids, supplemental systemic corticosteroid therapy may be necessary during periods of stress or during severe asthma attacks.

Administration Qvar, metered dose inhaler: Canister does not need to be shaken prior to use. Prime canister by spraying twice into the air prior to initial use or if not in use for >10 days. Avoid spraying in face or eyes. Exhale fully prior to bringing inhaler to mouth. Place inhaler in mouth, close lips around mouthpiece, and inhale slowly and deeply while pressing down on the canister with your finger. Remove inhaler and hold breath for approximately 5-10 seconds. Rinse mouth and throat after use to prevent *Candida* infection. Do not wash or put inhaler in water; mouth piece may be cleaned with a dry tissue or cloth. Discard after the "discard by" date or after labeled number of doses has been used, even if container is not completely empty. Patients using a spacer should inhale immediately due to decreased amount of medication that is delivered with a delayed inspiration. **Note:** Use of Qvar with a spacer device is not recommended in children <5 years of age due to the decreased amount of medication that is delivered with increasing wait times; patients should be instructed to inhale immediately if using a spacer device.

Monitoring Parameters Check mucous membranes for signs of fungal infection; monitor growth in pediatric patients; monitor IOP with therapy >6 weeks. Monitor for symptoms of asthma, FEV_1, peak flow, and/or other pulmonary function tests

Additional Information Qvar: Does not contain chlorofluorocarbons (CFCs), uses hydrofluoroalkane (HFA) as the propellant; is a solution formulation; uses smaller-size particles which results in a higher percent of drug delivered to the respiratory tract and lower recommended doses than other products. An open-label, randomized, multicenter, 12-month study in 300 asthmatic children 5-11 years of age indicated that QVAR provided long-term control of asthma at approximately half the dose compared with a CFC propelled beclomethasone MDI and spacer (Pedersen, 2002).

Dosage Forms Considerations QVAR 8.7 g canisters contain 120 inhalations.

Dosage Forms Excipient information presented when available (limited, particularly for generics); consult specific product labeling.

Aerosol Solution, Inhalation, as dipropionate:

Qvar: 40 mcg/actuation (8.7 g); 80 mcg/actuation (8.7 g)

References

ACOG Committee on Practice Bulletins-Obstetrics, "ACOG Practice Bulletin: Clinical Management Guidelines for Obstetrician-Gynecologists Number 90, February 2008: Asthma in Pregnancy," *Obstet Gynecol*, 2008, 111(2 Pt 1):457-64.

Bakhireva LN, Jones KL, Schatz M, et al, "Asthma Medication Use in Pregnancy and Fetal Growth," *J Allergy Clin Immunol*, 2005, 116 (3):503-9.

Namazy J, Schatz M, Long L, et al, "Use of Inhaled Steroids by Pregnant Asthmatic Women Does Not Reduce Intrauterine Growth," *J Allergy Clin Immunol*, 2004, 113(3):427-32.

National Asthma Education and Prevention Program (NAEPP), "Expert Panel Report 3 (EPR-3): Guidelines for the Diagnosis and Management of Asthma," *Clinical Practice Guidelines*, National Institutes of Health, National Heart, Lung, and Blood Institute, NIH Publication No. 08-4051, prepublication 2007; available at http://www.nhlbi.nih.gov/guidelines/asthma/asthgdln.htm.

National Asthma Education and Prevention Program (NAEPP) Working Group Report on "Managing Asthma During Pregnancy: Recommendations for Pharmacologic Treatment," National Institutes of Health, National Heart, Lung, and Blood Institute, NIH Publication No. 05-5236, March 2005. Available at http://www.nhlbi.nih.gov/health/prof/lung/asthma/astpreg/astpreg_full.pdf

QVAR [package insert], Horsham, PA:Teva Respiratory, LLC: 2012.

Pedersen S, Warner J, Wahn U, et al, "Growth, Systemic Safety, and Efficacy During 1 Year of Asthma Treatment With Different Beclomethasone Dipropionate Formulations: An Open-Label, Randomized Comparison of Extra Fine and Conventional Aerosols in Children," *Pediatrics*, 2002, 109(6), http://www.pediatrics.org/cgi/content/full/109/6/e92.

Tinkelman DG, Reed CE, Nelson HS, et al, "Aerosol Beclomethasone Dipropionate Compared With Theophylline as Primary Treatment of Chronic, Mild-to-Moderately Severe Asthma in Children," *Pediatrics*, 1993, 92(1):64-77.

Wyatt R, Waschek J, Weinberger M, et al, "Effects of Inhaled Beclomethasone Dipropionate and Alternate-Day Prednisone on Pituitary-Adrenal Function in Children With Chronic Asthma," *N Engl J Med*, 1978, 299(25):1387-92.

Beclomethasone (Nasal) (be kloe METH a sone)

Brand Names: U.S. Beconase AQ; Qnasl

Brand Names: Canada Apo-Beclomethasone; Mylan-Beclo AQ; Rivanase AQ

Therapeutic Category Corticosteroid, Intranasal

Generic Availability (U.S.) No

Use

Beconase® AQ: Management of nasal symptoms associated with seasonal or perennial allergic and non-allergic (vasomotor) rhinitis and prevention of recurrence of nasal polyps following surgical removal (FDA approved in ages ≥6 years and adults)

Qnasl™: Management of nasal symptoms associated with seasonal and perennial allergic rhinitis (FDA approved in ages ≥12 years and adults)

Intranasal corticosteroids have also been used as an adjunct to antibiotics in empiric treatment of acute bacterial rhinosinusitis primarily in patients with history of allergic rhinitis (Chow, 2012), in pediatric patients with mild obstructive sleep apnea syndrome who cannot undergo adenotonsillectomy or who still have symptoms after surgery (Marcus, 2012), and for children with nasal obstruction caused by adenoidal hypertrophy.

Pregnancy Risk Factor C

Pregnancy Considerations Adverse events were observed in some animal reproduction studies. Hypoadrenalism may occur in newborns following maternal use of corticosteroids in pregnancy; monitor. Intranasal corticosteroids are recommended for the treatment of rhinitis during pregnancy; the lowest effective dose should be used (NAEPP, 2005; Wallace, 2008).

Breast-Feeding Considerations Other corticosteroids have been found in breast milk; however, information for beclomethasone is not available. The manufacturer recommends caution be used if administered to a nursing woman. Use of inhaled corticosteroids is not a contraindication to breast-feeding (NAEPP, 2005).

Contraindications Hypersensitivity to beclomethasone or any component

Warnings HPA suppression or hypercorticism (Cushing's syndrome) may occur with use of higher than recommended doses or at typical doses in susceptible patients. Acute adrenal insufficiency may occur with abrupt withdrawal after long-term use, with stress, or when converting from systemic to topical corticosteroid therapy; withdrawal or discontinuation of corticosteroids should be done carefully; patients with HPA axis suppression may require doses of systemic glucocorticosteroids prior to, during, and after unusual stress (eg, surgery). Immunosuppression may occur; patients may be more susceptible to infections; avoid exposure to chickenpox and measles.

Precautions Avoid using higher than recommended dosages; suppression of HPA function, suppression of linear growth (ie, reduction of growth velocity), reduced bone mineral density, or hypercorticism (Cushing's syndrome) may occur; titrate to lowest effective dose. Reduction in growth velocity may occur when corticosteroids are administered to pediatric patients, even at recommended doses via intranasal route (monitor growth). Use beclomethasone with extreme caution in patients with respiratory tuberculosis; untreated bacterial, fungal, systemic viral or parasitic infections; or ocular herpes simplex. Localized *Candida* infections of the nose and pharynx have been reported rarely; interruption of therapy may be necessary while antifungal therapy is employed. Corticosteroids impair wound healing; avoid use in patients with recent nasal ulcers, nasal surgery, or nasal trauma; allow healing to occur before use. Glaucoma, increased intraocular pressure, and cataracts have been reported following the intranasal application of corticosteroids; monitor patients who have change in vision and in patients with a history of increased ocular pressure, glaucoma, or cataracts. Use of nasal beclomethasone in place of systemic corticosteroids may unmask allergies (eg, eczema, rhinitis) that were previously controlled by the systemic corticosteroids. Rare cases of immediate hypersensitivity reactions or nasal septum perforation may occur with intranasal corticosteroids.

Adverse Reactions

Central nervous system: Headache, lightheadedness

Dermatologic: Angioedema, rash, urticaria

Endocrine & metabolic: Growth velocity reduction in children and adolescents, HPA function suppression (dose related), weight gain

Gastrointestinal: Dry/irritated nose, throat and mouth, hoarseness, localized *Candida* or *Aspergillus* infection, loss of smell, loss of taste, nausea, unpleasant smell, unpleasant taste, vomiting

Local: Burning, epistaxis, localized *Candida* infection, nasal septum perforation (rare), nasal stuffiness, nosebleeds, rhinorrhea, sneezing, transient irritation, ulceration of nasal mucosa (rare)

Ocular: Cataracts (rare), glaucoma (rare), intraocular pressure increased (rare), tearing

Respiratory: Cough, paradoxical bronchospasm (rare), pharyngitis, sinusitis, wheezing

Miscellaneous: Anaphylactic/anaphylactoid reactions, immediate and delayed hypersensitivity reactions

Drug Interactions

Metabolism/Transport Effects None known.

Avoid Concomitant Use There are no known interactions where it is recommended to avoid concomitant use.

Increased Effect/Toxicity

Beclomethasone (Nasal) may increase the levels/effects of: Ceritinib

Decreased Effect There are no known significant interactions involving a decrease in effect.

Stability

Beconase® AQ: Store between 15°C to 30°C (59°F to 86°F).

Qnasl™: Store at 25°C (77°F), excursions permitted to 15°C to 30°C (59°F to 86°F). Do not puncture. Do not store near heat or open flame. Do not expose to temperatures higher than 49°C (120°F).

Mechanism of Action Controls the rate of protein synthesis; depresses the migration of polymorphonuclear leukocytes, fibroblasts; reverses capillary permeability and lysosomal stabilization at the cellular level to prevent or control inflammation

Pharmacodynamics Onset of action: Within a few days up to 2 weeks

Pharmacokinetics (Adult data unless noted)

Distribution: V_d: Beclomethasone dipropionate (BDP): 20 L; 17-BMP: 424 L

Protein binding: BDP 87%; 17-BMP: 94% to 96%

Metabolism: BDP is a prodrug (inactive) which undergoes rapid hydrolysis to 17-BMP (active monoester) during absorption; BDP is also metabolized in the liver via cytochrome P450 isoenzyme CYP3A4 to 17-BMP and two other less active metabolites: Beclomethasone-21-monopropionate (21-BMP) and beclomethasone (BOH)

Bioavailability: Beconase AQ®: 17-BMP: 44% (43% from swallowed portion)

Half-life, elimination: BDP: 0.5 hours; 17-BMP: 2.7 hours

Elimination: Feces (60%), urine (12%; as free and conjugated metabolites)

Dosing: Usual Note: Product formulations are not interchangeable: Beconase® AQ: One spray delivers 42 mcg; Qnasl®: One spray delivers 80 mcg

Children and Adolescents:

Nasal airway obstruction/adenoidal hypertrophy: Limited data available; dosing regimens variable: Intranasal: Beconase AQ®: Children 5-12 years: Initial: 168 mcg twice daily delivered as 84 mcg (2 sprays) **per nostril** twice daily for 4 weeks, followed by 84 mcg twice daily delivered as 42 mcg (1 spray) **per nostril** twice daily. Dosing based on a double-blind, placebo-controlled crossover study (n=17, age range: 5-11 years); results showed significant reduction in adenoid hypertrophy and related obstructive nasal symptoms following 4 weeks of beclomethasone therapy vs placebo (Demain, 1995). Positive efficacy findings were also observed in a single-blind, placebo-controlled

crossover study of 53 children (mean age: 3.8 ± 1.3 years) using a total daily dose of 400 mcg/day [200 mcg twice daily (using 50 mcg/spray formulation, not available in U.S.)] delivered as 100 mcg (2 sprays) **per nostril** twice daily (Criscuoli, 2003). Lower daily dosage (200 mcg/day) have not been found effective (Lepcha, 2002).

Allergic rhinitis: Intranasal:

Beconase® AQ:

Children 6-12 years: Initial: 84 mcg twice daily delivered as 42 mcg (1 spray) **per nostril** twice daily; may increase if needed to 168 mcg twice daily delivered as 84 mcg (2 sprays) **per nostril** twice daily; once symptoms are adequately controlled, decrease dose to 84 mcg twice daily delivered as 42 mcg (1 spray) **per nostril** twice daily.

Children and Adolescents ≥12 years: 84 or 168 mcg twice daily delivered as 42 mcg (1 spray) or 84 mcg (2 sprays) **per nostril** twice daily.

Qnasl™: Children and Adolescents ≥12 years: 320 mcg once daily delivered as 160 mcg (2 sprays) **per nostril** once daily

Nasal polyps (postsurgical prophylaxis), vasomotor rhinitis: Intranasal: Beconase® AQ:

Children 6-12 years: Initial: 84 mcg twice daily delivered as 42 mcg (1 spray) **per nostril** twice daily; may increase if needed to 168 mcg twice daily delivered as 84 mcg (2 sprays) **per nostril** twice daily; once symptoms are adequately controlled, decrease dose to 84 mcg twice daily delivered as 42 mcg (1 spray) **per nostril** twice daily

Children and Adolescents ≥12 years: 84 or 168 mcg twice daily delivered as 42 mcg (1 spray) or 84 mcg (2 sprays) **per nostril** twice daily

Adults:

Allergic rhinitis: Intranasal:

Beconase® AQ: 84 or 168 mcg twice daily delivered as 42 mcg (1 spray) or 84 mcg (2 sprays) **per nostril** twice daily

Qnasl™: 320 mcg once daily delivered as 160 mcg (2 sprays) **per nostril** once daily

Nasal polyps (postsurgical prophylaxis), vasomotor rhinitis: Intranasal: Beconase AQ®: 84 or 168 mcg twice daily delivered as 42 mcg (1 spray) or 84 mcg (2 sprays) **per nostril** twice daily

Dosing adjustment in renal impairment: There are no dosage adjustments provided in the manufacturer's labeling.

Dosing adjustment in hepatic impairment: There are no dosage adjustments provided in the manufacturer's labeling.

Administration Shake well prior to each use. Blow nose to clear nostrils. Insert applicator into nostril, keeping bottle upright, and close off the other nostril. Breathe in through nose. While inhaling, press pump to release spray. Avoid spraying directly onto the nasal septum or into eyes. Discard after the "discard by" date or after labeled number of doses has been used, even if bottle is not completely empty.

Beconase® AQ: Prior to initial use, prime pump 6 times (or until fine spray appears); repeat priming if product not used for ≥7 days. Nasal applicator and dust cap may be washed in warm water and dry thoroughly.

Qnasl™: Prior to initial use, prime pump 4 times. If product not used for ≥7 days, prime pump 2 times.

Monitoring Parameters Mucous membranes for signs of fungal infection, growth (pediatric patients), signs/symptoms of HPA axis suppression/adrenal insufficiency; ocular changes

Additional Information When used short term as adjunctive therapy in acute bacterial rhinosinusitis (ABRS), intranasal steroids show modest symptomatic improvement and few adverse effects; improvement is primarily due to increased sinus drainage. Use should be considered optional in ABRS; however, intranasal corticosteroids should be routinely prescribed to ABRS patients who have a history of or concurrent allergic rhinitis (Chow, 2012).

Dosage Forms Considerations
Beconase AQ 25 g bottles contain 180 sprays.
Qnasl 8.7 g bottles contain 120 actuations.

Dosage Forms Excipient information presented when available (limited, particularly for generics); consult specific product labeling.
Aerosol Solution, Nasal, as dipropionate:
Qnasl: 80 mcg/actuation (8.7 g)
Suspension, Nasal, as dipropionate:
Beconase AQ: 42 mcg/spray (25 g) [contains benzalkonium chloride]

References

Chow AW, Benninger MS, Brook I, et al, "IDSA Clinical Practice Guideline For Acute Bacterial Rhinosinusitis in Children and Adults," *Clin Infect Dis*, 2012, 54(8):e72-e112.

Criscuoli G, D'Amora S, Ripa G, et al, "Frequency of Surgery Among Children Who Have Adenotonsillar Hypertrophy and Improve After Treatment With Nasal Beclomethasone," *Pediatrics*, 2003, 111(3):e236-8.

Demain JG and Goetz DW, "Pediatric Adenoidal Hypertrophy and Nasal Airway Obstruction: Reduction With Aqueous Nasal Beclomethasone," *Pediatrics*, 1995, 95(3):355-64.

Lepcha A, Kurien M, Job A, et al, "Chronic Adenoid Hypertrophy in Children - Is Steroid Nasal Spray Beneficial?" *Indian J Otolaryngol Head Neck Surg*, 2002, 54(4):280-4.

Marcus CL, Brooks LJ, Draper KA, et al, "Diagnosis and Management of Childhood Obstructive Sleep Apnea Syndrome," *Pediatrics*, 2012, 130(3):576-84.

National Asthma Education and Prevention Program (NAEPP) Working Group Report on "Managing Asthma During Pregnancy: Recommendations for Pharmacologic Treatment," National Institutes of Health, National Heart, Lung, and Blood Institute, NIH Publication No. 05-5236, March 2005. Available at http://www.nhlbi.nih.gov/health/prof/lung/asthma/astpreg/astpreg_full.pdf

Wallace DV, Dykewicz MS, Bernstein DI, et al, "The Diagnosis and Management of Rhinitis: An Updated Practice Parameter," *J Allergy Clin Immunol*, 2008, 122(2 Suppl):S1-84.

◆ **Beclomethasone Dipropionate** see Beclomethasone (Nasal) *on page 267*

◆ **Beconase AQ** see Beclomethasone (Nasal) *on page 267*

◆ **Belladonna Alkaloids With Phenobarbital** see Hyoscyamine, Atropine, Scopolamine, and Phenobarbital *on page 1058*

Belladonna and Opium (bel a DON a & OH pee um)

Medication Safety Issues
Sound-alike/look-alike issues:
B&O may be confused with beano
High alert medication:
The Institute for Safe Medication Practices (ISMP) includes this medication among its list of drug classes which have a heightened risk of causing significant patient harm when used in error.
BEERS Criteria medication:
This drug may be potentially inappropriate for use in geriatric patients (Quality of evidence - moderate; Strength of recommendation - strong).

Therapeutic Category Analgesic, Narcotic; Antispasmodic Agent, Urinary

Generic Availability (U.S.) Yes

Use Relief of moderate to severe pain associated with rectal or bladder tenesmus that may occur in postoperative states and neoplastic situations; relief of pain associated with ureteral spasms not responsive to nonopioid analgesics and to space intervals between injections of opioids

Pregnancy Risk Factor C

Pregnancy Considerations Reproduction studies have not been conducted with this product. Refer to Atropine and Morphine (Systemic) monographs for additional information.

Breast-Feeding Considerations It is not known if/how much morphine or atropine may be found in breast milk following rectal administration of this product. Refer to Atropine and Morphine (Systemic) monographs for additional information.

Contraindications Hypersensitivity to belladonna, atropine, opium alkaloids, morphine, or any component; glaucoma; severe renal or hepatic disease; obstructive uropathy; obstructive disease of the GI tract; severe respiratory depression; convulsive disorders; acute alcoholism; premature labor

Warnings Opium shares the toxic potential of opioid agonists; usual precautions of opioid agonist therapy should be observed; not recommended for use in children <12 years

Precautions Use with caution in patients with cardiac, respiratory, hepatic, or renal dysfunction, severe prostatic hypertrophy, or history of opioid abuse; use with caution in patients with increased intracranial pressure

Adverse Reactions
Cardiovascular: Palpitation
Central nervous system: Dizziness, drowsiness
Dermatologic: Pruritus, urticaria
Gastrointestinal: Constipation, nausea, vomiting, xerostomia
Genitourinary: Urinary retention
Ocular: Blurred vision, photophobia

Drug Interactions
Metabolism/Transport Effects None known.
Avoid Concomitant Use
Avoid concomitant use of Belladonna and Opium with any of the following: Aclidinium; Azelastine (Nasal); Ipratropium (Oral Inhalation); Paraldehyde; Potassium Chloride; Thalidomide; Tiotropium; Umeclidinium

Increased Effect/Toxicity
Belladonna and Opium may increase the levels/effects of: AbobotulinumtoxinA; Alcohol (Ethyl); Alvimopan; Analgesics (Opioid); Anticholinergic Agents; Azelastine (Nasal); Buprenorphine; Cannabinoid-Containing Products; CNS Depressants; Desmopressin; Diuretics; Hydrocodone; Methotrimeprazine; Metyrosine; Mirabegron; Mirtazapine; OnabotulinumtoxinA; Paraldehyde; Potassium Chloride; Pramipexole; RimabotulinumtoxinB; ROPINIRole; Rotigotine; Selective Serotonin Reuptake Inhibitors; Thalidomide; Thiazide Diuretics; Tiotropium; Topiramate; Zolpidem

The levels/effects of Belladonna and Opium may be increased by: Aclidinium; Amphetamines; Anticholinergic Agents; Antipsychotic Agents (Phenothiazines); Brimonidine (Topical); Cannabis; Doxylamine; Dronabinol; Droperidol; HydrOXYzine; Ipratropium (Oral Inhalation); Kava Kava; Magnesium Sulfate; MAO Inhibitors; Methotrimeprazine; Nabilone; Perampanel; Pramlintide; Rufinamide; Sodium Oxybate; Succinylcholine; Tapentadol; Tetrahydrocannabinol; Umeclidinium

Decreased Effect
Belladonna and Opium may decrease the levels/effects of: Acetylcholinesterase Inhibitors (Central); Pegvisomant; Secretin

The levels/effects of Belladonna and Opium may be decreased by: Acetylcholinesterase Inhibitors (Central); Ammonium Chloride; Mixed Agonist / Antagonist Opioids; Naltrexone

Stability Store at room temperature; avoid freezing

Mechanism of Action The pharmacologically active agents present in the belladonna component are atropine and scopolamine. Atropine blocks the action of acetylcholine at parasympathetic sites in smooth muscle, secretory glands, and the CNS causing a relaxation of smooth muscle and drying of secretions. The principle agent in opium is morphine. Morphine binds to opiate receptors in the CNS, causing inhibition of ascending pain pathways, altering the perception of and response to pain.

Pharmacodynamics Opium: Onset of action: Within 30 minutes

Pharmacokinetics (Adult data unless noted) Metabolism: Hepatic

Dosing: Usual Rectal: Adults: 1 suppository 1-2 times/day, up to 4 doses/day

Administration Rectal: Remove from foil; moisten finger and suppository; insert rectally

Controlled Substance C-II

Dosage Forms Excipient information presented when available (limited, particularly for generics); consult specific product labeling.

Suppository: Belladonna extract 16.2 mg and opium 30 mg; belladonna extract 16.2 mg and opium 60 mg

◆ **Benadryl [OTC]** see DiphenhydrAMINE (Systemic) on page 673

◆ **Benadryl® (Can)** see DiphenhydrAMINE (Systemic) on page 673

◆ **Benadryl Allergy [OTC]** see DiphenhydrAMINE (Systemic) on page 673

◆ **Benadryl Allergy Childrens [OTC]** see DiphenhydrAMINE (Systemic) on page 673

◆ **Benadryl® Cream (Can)** see DiphenhydrAMINE (Topical) on page 677

◆ **Benadryl Dye-Free Allergy [OTC]** see DiphenhydrAMINE (Systemic) on page 673

◆ **Benadryl Itch Relief [OTC]** see DiphenhydrAMINE (Topical) on page 677

◆ **Benadryl® Itch Relief Stick (Can)** see DiphenhydrAMINE (Topical) on page 677

◆ **Benadryl Itch Stopping [OTC]** see DiphenhydrAMINE (Topical) on page 677

◆ **Benadryl Maximum Strength [OTC]** see DiphenhydrAMINE (Topical) on page 677

◆ **Benadryl® Spray (Can)** see DiphenhydrAMINE (Topical) on page 677

Benazepril (ben AY ze pril)

Medication Safety Issues
Sound-alike/look-alike issues:
Benazepril may be confused with Benadryl
Lotensin may be confused with Lioresal, lorcaserin, lovastatin

Brand Names: U.S. Lotensin

Brand Names: Canada Lotensin

Therapeutic Category Angiotensin-Converting Enzyme (ACE) Inhibitor; Antihypertensive Agent

Generic Availability (U.S.) Yes

Use Treatment of hypertension, either alone or in combination with a thiazide diuretic (FDA approved in ages ≥6 years and adults)

Pregnancy Risk Factor D

Pregnancy Considerations [U.S. Boxed Warning]: Drugs that act on the renin-angiotensin system can cause injury and death to the developing fetus. Discontinue as soon as possible once pregnancy is detected. Benazepril crosses the placenta; teratogenic effects may occur following maternal use during pregnancy. Drugs that act on the renin-angiotensin system are associated with oligohydramnios. Oligohydramnios, due to decreased fetal renal function, may lead to fetal lung hypoplasia and skeletal malformations. Their use in pregnancy is also associated with anuria, hypotension, renal failure, skull hypoplasia, and death in the fetus/neonate. Chronic maternal hypertension itself is also associated with adverse events in the fetus/infant. ACE inhibitors

are not recommended during pregnancy to treat maternal hypertension or heart failure. Use of an ACE inhibitor should also be avoided in any woman of reproductive age. Women who are planning a pregnancy should be considered for other medication options if an ACE inhibitor is currently prescribed or the ACE inhibitor should be discontinued as soon as possible once pregnancy is detected. The exposed fetus should be monitored for fetal growth, amniotic fluid volume, and organ formation. Infants exposed to an ACE inhibitor in utero should be monitored for hyperkalemia, hypotension, and oliguria (exchange transfusions or dialysis may be needed). These adverse events are generally associated with maternal use in the second and third trimesters.

Untreated chronic maternal hypertension is also associated with adverse events in the fetus, infant, and mother. The use of ACE inhibitors is not recommended to treat chronic uncomplicated hypertension in pregnant women and should generally be avoided in women of reproductive potential (ACOG, 2013).

Breast-Feeding Considerations Small amounts of benazepril and benazeprilat are found in breast milk.

Contraindications Hypersensitivity to benazepril, any component, or other ACE inhibitors; patients with a history of angioedema (with or without prior ACE inhibitor therapy)

Warnings Angioedema can occur at any time during treatment (especially following first dose). Angioedema may occur in the head, neck, extremities, or intestines; patients with angioedema of the intestines may present with abdominal pain (with or without nausea or vomiting); angioedema of the larynx, glottis, or tongue may cause airway obstruction, especially in patients with a history of airway surgery. Prolonged monitoring may be required, even in patients with swelling of only the tongue (ie, without respiratory distress) because treatment with corticosteroids and antihistamines may not be sufficient; very rare fatalities have occurred with angioedema of the larynx or tongue; appropriate treatment (eg, establishing patent airway and/or SubQ epinephrine) should be readily available for patients with angioedema of larynx, glottis, or tongue, in whom airway obstruction is likely to occur.

Anaphylactic/anaphylactoid reactions can occur with ACE inhibitors. Life-threatening anaphylactoid reactions may be seen during hemodialysis (eg, CVVHD) with high-flux dialysis membranes (eg, AN69), and rarely, during low density lipoprotein apheresis with dextran sulfate cellulose. Rare cases of anaphylactoid reactions have been reported in patients undergoing sensitization treatment with hymenoptera (bee, wasp) venom while receiving ACE inhibitors.

Benazepril has been associated with rare but potentially fatal cases of agranulocytosis, neutropenia, or leukopenia with myeloid hypoplasia; higher risk for development of neutropenia is associated with renal impairment; risk is further increased in patients with both renal impairment and collagen vascular disease (eg, systemic lupus erythematosus); onset of neutropenia is usually within 3 months of ACE inhibitor initiation; closely monitor CBC with differential for the first 3 months of therapy and periodically thereafter in these patients; neutrophil count generally returns to baseline within 2 weeks of discontinuation.

ACE inhibitor use has been associated with deterioration of renal function and/or increases in serum creatinine, particularly in patients with low renal blood flow (eg, renal artery stenosis, heart failure) whose glomerular filtration rate (GFR) is dependent on efferent arteriolar vasoconstriction by angiotensin II; deterioration may result in oliguria, acute renal failure, and progressive azotemia. Small increases in serum creatinine may occur following initiation; consider discontinuation only in patients with progressive and/or significant deterioration in renal function.

A rare toxicity associated with ACE inhibitors includes cholestatic jaundice, which may progress to fulminant hepatic necrosis; discontinue if marked elevation of hepatic transaminases or jaundice occurs and initiate appropriate medical treatment.

Drugs that act on the renin-angiotensin system can cause injury and death to the developing fetus. Discontinue as soon as possible once pregnancy is detected **[U.S. Boxed Warning]**. Concomitant use of an ARB or renin inhibitor (eg, aliskiren) is associated with an increased risk of hypotension, hyperkalemia, and renal dysfunction. Concomitant use with aliskiren should be avoided in patients with GFR <60 mL/minute and is contraindicated in patients with diabetes mellitus (regardless of GFR).

Precautions Use with caution in patients with renal impairment; dosage reduction may be necessary; avoid rapid dosage escalation which may lead to further renal impairment. Use with caution in patients with unstented unilateral/bilateral renal artery stenosis. When unstented bilateral renal artery stenosis is present, use is generally avoided due to the elevated risk of deterioration in renal function unless possible benefits outweigh risks.

Use with caution when initiating therapy and in volume-depleted patients; may cause symptomatic hypotension with or without syncope, usually with the first several doses; correct volume depletion prior to initiation; initiate lower doses in patients with sodium or volume depletion; close monitoring of patient is required especially with initial dosing and dosing increases; blood pressure must be lowered at a rate appropriate for the patient's clinical condition. Although dose reduction may be necessary, hypotension alone is not a reason for discontinuation of future ACE inhibitor use especially in patients with heart failure where a reduction in systolic blood pressure is a desirable observation. Use caution in patients with ischemic heart disease or cerebrovascular disease during therapy initiation; observe closely due to the potential consequences posed by falling blood pressure (eg, MI, stroke); fluid replacement may be required to restore blood pressure; therapy may then be resumed; discontinue therapy in patients whose hypotension recurs. Use with caution in patients with severe aortic stenosis; may reduce coronary perfusion resulting in ischemia. Use with caution in patients with hypertrophic cardiomyopathy (HCM) and outflow tract obstruction since reduction in afterload may worsen symptoms associated with this condition.

May cause hyperkalemia; risk factors include renal dysfunction, diabetes mellitus, concomitant use of potassium-sparing diuretics, potassium supplements, and/or potassium-containing salts; use with caution, if at all, with these agents, and monitor potassium closely.

Use with caution before, during, or immediately after major surgery; cardiopulmonary bypass, intraoperative blood loss or vasodilating anesthesia increases endogenous renin release; use of ACE inhibitors perioperatively will blunt angiotensin II formation and may result in hypotension.

An ACE inhibitor cough is a dry, hacking, nonproductive one that usually occurs within the first few months of treatment and should generally resolve within 1-4 weeks after discontinuation of the ACE inhibitor. In pediatric patients, an isolated dry hacking cough lasting >3 weeks was reported in seven of 42 pediatric patients (17%) receiving ACE inhibitors (von Vigier, 2000); a review of pediatric randomized-controlled ACE inhibitor trials reported a lower incidence of 3.2%; a higher incidence of cough has been reported in pediatric patients receiving benazepril (15.2%); however, this may have resulted from differences in study methodology (Baker-Smith, 2010). Other causes of cough should be considered (eg, pulmonary congestion in patients with heart failure) and excluded prior to discontinuation.

Adverse Reactions

Central nervous system: Dizziness, drowsiness, headache, orthostatic dizziness

Renal: Increased serum creatinine, renal insufficiency (may occur in patients with bilateral renal artery stenosis or hypovolemia)

Respiratory: Cough

Rare but important or life-threatening: Agranulocytosis, alopecia, anaphylactoid reaction, angina pectoris, angioedema (includes head, neck, and intestinal angioedema), arthralgia, arthritis, asthma, dermatitis, dyspnea, ECG changes, eosinophilia, flushing, gastritis, hemolytic anemia, hyperbilirubinemia, hyperglycemia, hyperkalemia, hypersensitivity, hypertonia, hyponatremia, hypotension, impotence, increased blood urea nitrogen (transient), increased serum transaminases, increased uric acid, insomnia, leukopenia, myalgia, neutropenia, orthostatic hypotension, palpitations, pancreatitis, paresthesia, pemphigus, peripheral edema, proteinuria, pruritus, shock, skin photosensitivity, skin rash, Stevens-Johnson syndrome, syncope, thrombocytopenia, vomiting

Anaphylaxis, eosinophilic pneumonitis, neutropenia, agranulocytosis, renal failure, and renal insufficiency have been reported with other ACE inhibitors. In addition, a syndrome including arthralgia, elevated ESR, eosinophilia, fever, interstitial nephritis, myalgia, rash, and vasculitis has been reported to be associated with ACE inhibitors.

Drug Interactions

Metabolism/Transport Effects None known.

Avoid Concomitant Use There are no known interactions where it is recommended to avoid concomitant use.

Increased Effect/Toxicity

Benazepril may increase the levels/effects of: Allopurinol; Amifostine; Antihypertensives; AzaTHIOprine; CycloSPORINE (Systemic); DULoxetine; Ferric Gluconate; Gold Sodium Thiomalate; Grass Pollen Allergen Extract (5 Grass Extract); Hypotensive Agents; Iron Dextran Complex; Lithium; Nonsteroidal Anti-Inflammatory Agents; Obinutuzumab; RiTUXimab; Sodium Phosphates

The levels/effects of Benazepril may be increased by: Alfuzosin; Aliskiren; Angiotensin II Receptor Blockers; Barbiturates; Brimonidine (Topical); Canagliflozin; Diazoxide; DPP-IV Inhibitors; Eplerenone; Everolimus; Heparin; Heparin (Low Molecular Weight); Herbs (Hypotensive Properties); Hydrochlorothiazide; Loop Diuretics; MAO Inhibitors; Pentoxifylline; Phosphodiesterase 5 Inhibitors; Potassium Salts; Potassium-Sparing Diuretics; Prostacyclin Analogues; Sirolimus; Temsirolimus; Thiazide Diuretics; TiZANidine; Tolvaptan; Trimethoprim

Decreased Effect

Benazepril may decrease the levels/effects of: Hydrochlorothiazide

The levels/effects of Benazepril may be decreased by: Antacids; Aprotinin; Herbs (Hypertensive Properties); Icatibant; Lanthanum; Methylphenidate; Nonsteroidal Anti-Inflammatory Agents; Salicylates; Yohimbine

Stability Store at temperatures ≤30°C (86°F); protect from moisture; dispense in tight container

Mechanism of Action Competitive inhibition of angiotensin I being converted to angiotensin II, a potent vasoconstrictor, through the angiotensin I-converting enzyme (ACE) activity, with resultant lower levels of angiotensin II which causes an increase in plasma renin activity and a reduction in aldosterone secretion

◀ **Pharmacodynamics** Adults:

Maximum effect:

Reduction in plasma angiotensin-converting enzyme (ACE) activity: 1-2 hours after 2-20 mg dose

Reduction in blood pressure: Single dose: 2-4 hours; Continuous therapy: 2 weeks

Duration: Reduction in plasma angiotensin-converting enzyme (ACE) activity: >90% inhibition for 24 hours after 5-20 mg dose

Pharmacokinetics (Adult data unless noted)

Absorption: Oral: 37%; rapidly absorbed; **Note:** Metabolite (benazeprilat) is unsuitable for oral administration due to poor absorption

Distribution: V_d: ~8.7 L

Protein binding: Benazepril: 97%; benazeprilat: 95%

Metabolism: Rapidly and extensively metabolized (primarily in the liver) to benazeprilat (active metabolite), via cleavage of ester group; extensive first-pass effect. Benazeprilat is about 200 times more potent than benazepril. Parent and active metabolite undergo glucuronide conjugation

Half-life: Benazeprilat: Terminal:

Children and Adolescents 6-16 years: 5 hours

Adults: 22 hours

Time to peak serum concentration: Oral:

Parent drug: 0.5-1 hour

Active metabolite (benazeprilat):

Fasting: 1-2 hours

Nonfasting: 2-4 hours

Elimination: Hepatic clearance is the main elimination route of unchanged benazepril. Only trace amounts of unchanged benazepril appear in the urine; 20% of dose is excreted in urine as benazeprilat, 8% as benazeprilat glucuronide, and 4% as benazepril glucuronide

Clearance: Nonrenal excretion (ie, biliary) appears to contribute to the elimination of benazeprilat (11% to 12% in healthy adults); biliary clearance may be increased in patients with severe renal impairment

Dialysis: ~6% of metabolite removed within 4 hours of dialysis following 10 mg of benazepril administered 2 hours prior to procedure; parent compound not found in dialysate

Dosing: Usual Hypertension: Note: Dosage must be titrated according to patient's response; use lowest effective dose

Children ≥6 years and Adolescents: Oral: Initial: 0.2 mg/kg/dose once daily as monotherapy; maximum initial dose: 10 mg/**day**; maintenance: 0.1-0.6 mg/kg/dose once daily; maximum daily dose: 40 mg/**day**

Adults: Oral: Initial: 10 mg once daily in patients not receiving a diuretic; maintenance: 20-80 mg/day as a single dose or 2 divided doses; the need for twice daily dosing should be assessed by monitoring peak (2-6 hours after dosing) and trough blood pressure responses

Note: To decrease the risk of hypotension, patients taking diuretics should have diuretics discontinued 2-3 days prior to starting benazepril; diuretic may be resumed if blood pressure is not controlled with benazepril monotherapy. If diuretics cannot be discontinued prior to starting benazepril, then an initial dose of benazepril of 5 mg once daily should be used.

Dosing adjustment in renal impairment:

Children and Adolescents: CrCl <30 mL/minute/1.73 m²: Use is not recommended (insufficient data exists; dose not established)

Adults: CrCl <30 mL/minute/1.73 m²: Initial: 5 mg once daily, then increase as required to a maximum of 40 mg/day

Administration Oral: May be administered without regard to food.

Monitoring Parameters Blood pressure (supervise for at least 2 hours after the initial dose or any dosage increase for significant orthostasis); renal function, WBC, serum potassium; monitor for angioedema and anaphylactoid reactions

Dosage Forms Excipient information presented when available (limited, particularly for generics); consult specific product labeling.

Tablet, Oral, as hydrochloride:

Lotensin: 10 mg, 20 mg, 40 mg

Generic: 5 mg, 10 mg, 20 mg, 40 mg

Extemporaneous Preparations A 2 mg/mL oral suspension may be made with tablets. Mix fifteen benazepril 20 mg tablets in an amber polyethylene terephthalate bottle with Ora-Plus® 75 mL. Shake for 2 minutes, allow suspension to stand for ≥1 hour, then shake again for at least 1 additional minute. Add Ora-Sweet® 75 mL to suspension and shake to disperse. Will make 150 mL of a 2 mg/mL suspension. Label "shake well" and "refrigerate". Stable for 30 days.

Lotensin® prescribing information, Novartis Pharmaceuticals Corporation, Suffern, NY, 2009.

References

ALLHAT Officers and Coordinators for the ALLHAT Collaborative Research Group, "Major Outcomes in High-Risk Hypertensive Patients Randomized to Angiotensin-Converting Enzyme Inhibitor or Calcium Channel Blocker vs Diuretic: The Antihypertensive and Lipid-Lowering Treatment to Prevent Heart Attack Trial (ALLHAT)," *JAMA*, 2002, 288(23):2981-97.

Antman EM, Anbe DT, Armstrong PW, et al, "ACC/AHA Guidelines for the Management of Patients With ST-Elevation Myocardial Infarction - Executive Summary: A Report of the American College of Cardiology/American Heart Association Task Force on Practice Guidelines (Writing Committee to Revise the 1999 Guidelines for the Management of Patients With Acute Myocardial Infarction)," *Circulation*, 2004, 110:588-636.

Baker-Smith CM, Benjamin DK Jr, Califf RM, et al, "Cough in Pediatric Patients Receiving Angiotensin-Converting Enzyme Inhibitor Therapy or Angiotensin Receptor Blocker Therapy in Randomized Controlled Trials," *Clin Pharmacol Ther*, 2010, 87(6):668-71.

Brown NJ, Ray WA, Snowden M, et al, "Black Americans Have an Increased Rate of Angiotensin-Converting Enzyme Inhibitor-Associated Angioedema," *Clin Pharmacol Ther*, 1996, 60(1):8-13.

Chase MP, Fiarman GS, Scholz FJ, et al, "Angioedema of the Small Bowel Due to an Angiotensin-Converting Enzyme Inhibitor," *J Clin Gastroenterol*, 2000, 31(3):254-7.

Chobanian AV, Bakris GL, Black HR, et al, "The Seventh Report of the Joint National Committee on Prevention, Detection, Evaluation, and Treatment of High Blood Pressure: The JNC 7 Report," *JAMA*, 2003, 289(19):2560-72.

Conlin PR, Moore TJ, Swartz SL, et al, "Effect of Indomethacin on Blood Pressure Lowering by Captopril and Losartan in Hypertensive Patients," *Hypertension*, 2000, 36(3):461-5.

"Consensus Recommendations for the Management of Chronic Heart Failure. On Behalf of the Membership of the Advisory Council to Improve Outcomes Nationwide in Heart Failure," *Am J Cardiol*, 1999, 83(2A):1A-38A.

Cooper WO, Hernandez-Diaz S, Arbogast PG, et al, "Major Congenital Malformations After First-Trimester Exposure to ACE Inhibitors," *N Engl J Med*, 2006, 354(23):2443-51.

"Guidelines for the Evaluation and Management of Heart Failure. Report of the American College of Cardiology/American Heart Association Task Force on Practice Guidelines (Committee on Evaluation and Management of Heart Failure)," *Circulation*, 1995, 92(9):2764-84.

Kaiser G, Ackermann R, Brechbühler S, et al, "Pharmacokinetics of the Angiotensin Converting Enzyme Inhibitor Benazepril.HCl (CGS 14 824 A) in Healthy Volunteers After Single and Repeated Administration)," *Biopharm Drug Dispos*, 1989, 10(4):365-76.

"K/DOQI Clinical Practice Guidelines for Chronic Kidney Disease: Evaluation, Classification, and Stratification. Kidney Disease Outcome Quality Initiative," *Am J Kidney Dis*, 2002, 39(2 Suppl 2):1-246.

Konstam MA, Dracup K, Baker, DW, et al, "Heart Failure Evaluation and Care of Patients With Left-Ventricular Systolic Dysfunction," *J Card Fail*, 1995, 1(2):183-7.

Mastrobattista JM, "Angiotensin Converting Enzyme Inhibitors in Pregnancy," *Semin Perinatol*, 1997, 21(2):124-34.

National High Blood Pressure Education Program Working Group on High Blood Pressure in Children and Adolescents, "The Fourth Report on the Diagnosis, Evaluation, and Treatment of High Blood Pressure in Children and Adolescents," *Pediatrics*, 2004, 114(2 Suppl):555-76.

Packer M, Poole-Wilson PA, Armstrong PW, et al, "Comparative Effects of Low and High Doses of the Angiotensin-Converting Enzyme Inhibitor, Lisinopril, on Morbidity and Mortality in Chronic Heart Failure," *Circulation*, 1999, 100(23):2312-8.

Cepacol Sore Throat + Coating: 15 mg (16 ea) [sugar free; contains brilliant blue fcf (fd&c blue #1), fd&c yellow #10 (quinoline yellow); lemon-lime flavor]

Cepacol Sore Throat Max Numb: 15 mg (16 ea) [sugar free; contains fd&c red #40; cherry flavor]

Sore Throat Relief: 10 mg (2 ea) [wild cherry flavor]

Trocaine Throat: 10 mg (1 ea)

Ointment, External:
Anacaine: 10% (30 g)
Anbesol Cold Sore Therapy: 20% (9 g) [contains aloe, vitamin e]
Chiggerex: 2% (52.5 g)
Foille: 5% (28 g)

Solution, Mouth/Throat:
Benz-O-Sthetic: 20% (30 mL) [contains polyethylene glycol, saccharin]
Benzocaine Oral Anesthetic: 20% (59.7 g) [contains alcohol, usp, polyethylene glycol, saccharin sodium]
Hurricaine: 20% (57 g) [contains polyethylene glycol, saccharin sodium]
Hurricaine: 20% (30 mL) [contains polyethylene glycol, saccharin sodium; pina colada flavor]
Hurricaine: 20% (57 g, 30 mL) [contains polyethylene glycol, saccharin sodium; wild cherry flavor]
HurriCaine One: 20% (2 ea, 25 ea) [contains polyethylene glycol, saccharin sodium]
Kank-A Mouth Pain: 20% (9.75 mL) [contains benzyl alcohol, propylene glycol, saccharin sodium]
Topex Topical Anesthetic: 20% (57 g) [cherry flavor]

Solution, Otic:
Pinnacaine Otic: 20% (15 mL)

Strip, Mouth/Throat:
Ora-film: 6% (12 ea) [contains brilliant blue fcf (fd&c blue #1), menthol, methylparaben, propylparaben, tartrazine (fd&c yellow #5)]

Swab, Mouth/Throat:
Benz-O-Sthetic: 20% (2 ea) [contains benzyl alcohol, polyethylene glycol, saccharin sodium]
Benz-O-Sthetic: 20% (2 ea) [contains benzyl alcohol, polyethylene glycol, saccharin sodium; cherry flavor]
Hurricaine: 20% (72 ea) [contains polyethylene glycol, saccharin sodium; wild cherry flavor]

◆ Benzocaine and Antipyrine see Antipyrine and Benzocaine on page 181

◆ Benzocaine Oral Anesthetic [OTC] see Benzocaine on page 273

◆ Benz-O-Sthetic [OTC] see Benzocaine on page 273

Benzoyl Peroxide (BEN zoe il peer OKS ide)

Medication Safety Issues
Sound-alike/look-alike issues:
Benzoyl peroxide may be confused with benzyl alcohol
Benoxyl® may be confused with Brevoxyl®, Peroxyl®
Benzac® may be confused with Benza®
Brevoxyl® may be confused with Benoxyl®
Fostex® may be confused with pHisoHex®

Brand Names: U.S. Acne Medication 10 [OTC]; Acne Medication 5 [OTC]; Acne Medication [OTC]; Acne-Clear [OTC]; Benzac AC Wash; Benzac W Wash; BenzEFoam; BenzEFoamUltra; BenzePrO; BenzePrO Short Contact; Benziq; Benziq LS; Benziq Wash; Benzoyl Peroxide Cleanser [OTC]; Benzoyl Peroxide Wash; Benzoyl Peroxide Wash [OTC]; BP Cleansing [OTC]; BP Foam; BP Gel [OTC]; BP Wash; BP Wash [OTC]; BPO; BPO Creamy Wash; BPO Creamy Wash [OTC]; BPO Foaming Cloths; BPO-10 Wash [OTC]; BPO-5 Wash [OTC]; Clearplex V [OTC]; Clearplex X; Clearskin [OTC]; Desquam-X Wash [OTC]; Inova; Lavoclen-4 Acne Wash; Lavoclen-4 Creamy Wash; Lavoclen-8 Acne Wash; Lavoclen-8 Creamy Wash; Neutrogena Clear Pore [OTC]; OC8 [OTC]; Oscion

Cleanser; PanOxyl Wash [OTC]; PanOxyl [OTC]; Pan-Oxyl-4 Creamy Wash [OTC]; PanOxyl-8 Creamy Wash [OTC]; PR Benzoyl Peroxide Wash; Riax; SE BPO Wash; Zaclir Cleansing

Brand Names: Canada Acetoxyl®; Benoxyl®; Benzac AC®; Benzac W® Gel; Benzac W® Wash; Desquam-X®; Oxyderm™; PanOxyl®; Solugel®

Therapeutic Category Acne Products; Topical Skin Product

Generic Availability (U.S.) May be product dependent

Use Treatment of mild to moderate acne vulgaris (FDA approved in ages ≥12 years and adults)

Pregnancy Risk Factor C

Pregnancy Considerations Animal reproduction studies have not been conducted; ~2% of the applied dose is expected to be absorbed systemically (Akhavan, 2003).

Breast-Feeding Considerations It is not known if benzoyl peroxide is excreted in breast milk. The manufacturer recommends that caution be exercised when administering benzoyl peroxide to nursing women.

Contraindications Hypersensitivity to benzoyl peroxide, benzoic acid, or any component

Warnings Discontinue if burning, swelling, irritation, or undue dryness occurs.

Precautions For external use only; may bleach hair, carpeting, or colored fabrics; avoid contact with eyes, eyelids, lips, mucous membranes, open wounds, and highly inflamed or denuded skin; use a sunscreen and minimize exposure to sunlight or artificial light sources

Adverse Reactions Dermatologic: Contact dermatitis, dryness, erythema, irritation, peeling, stinging

Drug Interactions
Metabolism/Transport Effects None known.
Avoid Concomitant Use There are no known interactions where it is recommended to avoid concomitant use.
Increased Effect/Toxicity There are no known significant interactions involving an increase in effect.
Decreased Effect There are no known significant interactions involving a decrease in effect.

Mechanism of Action Releases free-radical oxygen which oxidizes bacterial proteins in the sebaceous follicles decreasing the number of anaerobic bacteria and decreasing irritating-type free fatty acids

Pharmacokinetics (Adult data unless noted)
Absorption: ~5% through the skin
Metabolism: Major metabolite is benzoic acid
Elimination: In the urine as benzoate

Dosing: Usual Children ≥12 years, Adolescents, and Adults: Topical:
Topical formulations: Apply sparingly once daily; gradually increase to 2-3 times/day if needed. If excessive dryness or peeling occurs, reduce dose frequency or concentration. If excessive stinging or burning occurs, remove with mild soap and water; resume use the next day
Topical cleansers: Wash once or twice daily; control amount of drying or peeling by modifying dose frequency or concentration

Administration Topical: Shake lotion before using; cleanse skin before applying; for external use only. Avoid contact with eyes, eyelids, lips, and mucous membranes; rinse with water if accidental contact occurs

Additional Information Granulation may indicate effectiveness; gels are more penetrating than creams and last longer than creams or lotions

Dosage Forms Excipient information presented when available (limited, particularly for generics); consult specific product labeling.
Bar, External:
PanOxyl: 10% (1 ea)
Cream, External:
Clearskin: 10% (30 g)

Foam, External:
BenzEFoam: 5.3% (60 g, 100 g) [contains cetearyl alcohol, disodium edta, methylparaben, propylene glycol, propylparaben]
BenzEFoamUltra: 9.8% (100 g) [contains cetearyl alcohol, disodium edta, methylparaben, propylene glycol, propylparaben]
BenzePrO: 5.3% (60 g, 100 g) [contains cetearyl alcohol, disodium edta, methylparaben, propylene glycol, propylparaben, trolamine (triethanolamine)]
BenzePrO Short Contact: 9.8% (100 g) [contains cetearyl alcohol, disodium edta, methylparaben, propylene glycol, propylparaben]
BP Foam: 5.3% (60 g, 100 g); 9.8% (100 g) [contains methylparaben, propylparaben]
Riax: 5.5% (100 g); 9.5% (100 g) [contains methylparaben, propylparaben]
Generic: 5.3% (60 g, 100 g); 9.8% (100 g)
Gel, External:
Acne Medication 5: 5% (42.5 g) [contains edetate disodium]
Acne Medication 10: 10% (42.5 g) [contains edetate disodium]
Acne-Clear: 10% (42.5 g)
Benziq: 5.25% (50 g) [contains benzyl alcohol, disodium edta, trolamine (triethanolamine)]
Benziq LS: 2.75% (50 g) [contains trolamine (triethanolamine)]
BP Gel: 5% (60 g) [contains benzyl alcohol, edetate disodium, trolamine (triethanolamine)]
BP Gel: 10% (60 g) [contains benzyl alcohol, disodium edta, trolamine (triethanolamine)]
BPO: 4% (42.5 g); 8% (42.5 g) [contains benzyl alcohol, cetyl alcohol]
Clearplex V: 5% (45 g)
Clearplex X: 10% (45 g)
OC8: 7% (45 g) [contains disodium edta, propylene glycol]
Generic: 2.5% (60 g); 5% (60 g, 90 g); 10% (60 g, 90 g)
Kit, External:
Benzoyl Peroxide Wash: 8 & 5%, Liquid wash 4% (170.1 g) and bar soap 5% (2 x 21 g) [contains cetearyl alcohol, methylparaben]
BPO Creamy Wash: 4 & 5%, 8 & 5% [contains disodium edta, methylparaben]
Inova: 4 & 5%, 8 & 5% [contains disodium edta, methylparaben]
Lavoclen-4 Acne Wash: 4% [soap free; contains butylparaben, cetearyl alcohol, methylparaben, propylparaben]
Lavoclen-4 Acne Wash: 4% [soap free; contains butylparaben, methylparaben, propylparaben]
Lavoclen-8 Acne Wash: 8% [soap free; contains butylparaben, cetearyl alcohol, methylparaben, propylparaben]
Lavoclen-8 Acne Wash: 8% [soap free; contains butylparaben, methylparaben, propylparaben]
Liquid, External:
Benzac AC Wash: 5% (226 g)
Benzac W Wash: 5% (226 g)
Benziq Wash: 5.25% (175 g) [contains benzyl alcohol, cetyl alcohol, disodium edta, propylene glycol]
Benzoyl Peroxide Wash: 5% (148 g, 237 g) [contains cetyl alcohol, edetate disodium, propylene glycol]
Benzoyl Peroxide Wash: 5% (142 g, 227 g) [contains edetate disodium]
Benzoyl Peroxide Wash: 10% (148 g, 237 g) [contains cetyl alcohol, edetate disodium, propylene glycol]
Benzoyl Peroxide Wash: 10% (142 g, 227 g) [contains edetate disodium]
BP Wash: 2.5% (227 g); 5% (113 g, 142 g, 227 g) [contains cetearyl alcohol, methylparaben]
BP Wash: 5.25% (175 g); 7% (473 mL) [contains benzyl alcohol, cetyl alcohol, propylene glycol, trolamine (triethanolamine)]

BP Wash: 10% (142 g, 227 g) [contains cetearyl alcohol, methylparaben]
BPO-10 Wash: 10% (227 g) [contains methylparaben, propylene glycol, propylparaben]
BPO-5 Wash: 5% (227 g) [contains methylparaben, propylene glycol, propylparaben]
Desquam-X Wash: 5% (140 g); 10% (140 g) [contains edetate disodium]
Lavoclen-4 Creamy Wash: 4% (170.1 g) [contains cetearyl alcohol, methylparaben]
Lavoclen-8 Creamy Wash: 8% (170.1 g) [contains cetearyl alcohol, methylparaben]
Neutrogena Clear Pore: 3.5% (125 mL) [contains disodium edta, menthol]
PanOxyl: 2.5% (156 g) [soap free; contains cetearyl alcohol]
PanOxyl Wash: 10% (156 g) [contains alcohol, usp, methylparaben]
PanOxyl-4 Creamy Wash: 4% (170.1 g) [contains cetearyl alcohol, methylparaben]
PanOxyl-8 Creamy Wash: 8% (170.1 g) [contains cetearyl alcohol, methylparaben]
PR Benzoyl Peroxide Wash: 7% (473 mL) [contains cetyl alcohol, edetate disodium, propylene glycol]
SE BPO Wash: 7% (180 g) [contains edetate disodium, methylparaben]
Lotion, External:
Acne Medication 5: 5% (30 mL) [odorless; contains disodium edta]
Acne Medication: 10% (30 mL) [odorless; contains edetate disodium]
Benzoyl Peroxide Cleanser: 6% (170.3 g, 340.2 g) [contains cetyl alcohol, edetate disodium, propylene glycol]
BP Cleansing: 4% (297 g) [contains cetyl alcohol, propylene glycol]
Oscion Cleanser: 6% (170.3 g, 340.2 g)
Zaclir Cleansing: 8% (297 g)
Miscellaneous, External:
BPO Foaming Cloths: 3% (60 ea); 6% (60 ea); 9% (60 ea) [contains methylparaben]

References
Akhavan A and Bershad S, "Topical Acne Drugs: Review of Clinical Properties, Systemic Exposure, and Safety," *Am J Clin Dermatol*, 2003, 4(7):473-92.
Winston MH and Shalita AR, "Acne Vulgaris: Pathogenesis and Treatment," *Pediatr Clin North Am*, 1991, 38(4):889-903.

◆ **Benzoyl Peroxide and Adapalene** *see* Adapalene and Benzoyl Peroxide *on page 74*
◆ **Benzoyl Peroxide and Clindamycin** *see* Clindamycin and Benzoyl Peroxide *on page 502*
◆ **Benzoyl Peroxide Cleanser [OTC]** *see* Benzoyl Peroxide *on page 275*
◆ **Benzoyl Peroxide Wash** *see* Benzoyl Peroxide *on page 275*

Benztropine (BENZ troe peen)

Medication Safety Issues
Sound-alike/look-alike issues:
Benztropine may be confused with bromocriptine
BEERS Criteria medication:
This drug may be potentially inappropriate for use in geriatric patients (Parkinson's disease: Quality of evidence - moderate; Strength of recommendation - strong).
Brand Names: U.S. Cogentin
Brand Names: Canada Apo-Benztropine®; Benztropine Omega; PMS-Benztropine
Therapeutic Category Anti-Parkinson's Agent; Anticholinergic Agent; Antidote, Drug-induced Dystonic Reactions
Generic Availability (U.S.) Yes

Use Adjunctive treatment of parkinsonism (FDA approved in adults); treatment of drug-induced extrapyramidal effects (except tardive dyskinesia) (FDA approved in adults)

Pregnancy Considerations Animal reproduction studies have not been conducted. Paralytic ileus (which resolved rapidly) was reported in two newborns exposed to a combination of benztropine and chlorpromazine during the second and third trimesters and the last 6 weeks of pregnancy, respectively (Falterman, 1980).

Breast-Feeding Considerations It is not known if benztropine is excreted in breast milk. Anticholinergic agents may suppress lactation.

Contraindications Hypersensitivity to benztropine mesylate or any component; pediatric patients <3 years of age

Warnings Severe anhidrosis and fatal hyperthermia have occurred; risk increased with hot environments, prolonged outdoor exposure, or concomitant use of phenothiazines, haloperidol, or other drugs with anticholinergic or antidopaminergic activity; alcoholic patients, elderly patients or patients with CNS disease; use with caution in hot weather or during exercise. The anticholinergic effects may be of concern in children; contraindicated in children <3 years of age due to atropine-like adverse effects.

May be associated with confusion, visual hallucinations, or excitement (generally at higher dosages); intensification of symptoms or toxic psychosis may occur in patients with mental disorders; use with caution and monitor closely. May cause CNS depression, which may impair physical or mental abilities; patients must be cautioned about performing tasks which require mental alertness (eg, operating machinery or driving). When given in large doses or to susceptible patients, may cause weakness and inability to move particular muscle groups. Avoid use in patients with myasthenia gravis; may precipitate myasthenic crisis. Not recommended for use in patients with tardive dyskinesia; benztropine does not relieve symptoms of tardive dyskinesia and may potentially exacerbate symptoms.

Precautions Use with caution in patients with tachycardia, cardiac arrhythmias, hypertension, or hypotension. Use with caution in patients with obstructive disease of the GI tract (eg, pyloric or duodenal obstruction). Use with caution in patients with glaucoma; avoid use in angle-closure glaucoma. Use with caution in patients with hepatic or renal impairment. Use with caution in patients with prostatic hyperplasia and/or urinary stricture or retention. Potentially significant interactions may exist, requiring dose or frequency adjustment, additional monitoring, and/ or selection of alternative therapy. Consult drug interactions database for more detailed information.

Adverse Reactions

Cardiovascular: Tachycardia

Central nervous system: Confusion, depression, disorientation, heatstroke, hyperthermia, lethargy, memory impairment, nervousness, numbness of fingers, psychotic symptoms (exacerbation of preexisting symptoms), toxic psychosis, visual hallucination

Dermatologic: Skin rash

Gastrointestinal: Constipation, nausea, paralytic ileus, vomiting, xerostomia

Genitourinary: Dysuria, urinary retention

Ophthalmic: Blurred vision, mydriasis

Drug Interactions

Metabolism/Transport Effects Substrate of CYP2D6 (minor); **Note:** Assignment of Major/Minor substrate status based on clinically relevant drug interaction potential

Avoid Concomitant Use

Avoid concomitant use of Benztropine with any of the following: Aclidinium; Ipratropium (Oral Inhalation); Potassium Chloride; Tiotropium; Umeclidinium

Increased Effect/Toxicity

Benztropine may increase the levels/effects of: AbobotulinumtoxinA; Analgesics (Opioid); Anticholinergic Agents; Cannabinoid-Containing Products; Mirabegron; OnabotulinumtoxinA; Potassium Chloride; RimabotulinumtoxinB; Thiazide Diuretics; Tiotropium; Topiramate

The levels/effects of Benztropine may be increased by: Aclidinium; Ipratropium (Oral Inhalation); Pramlintide; Umeclidinium

Decreased Effect

Benztropine may decrease the levels/effects of: Acetylcholinesterase Inhibitors (Central); Ioflupane I 123; Secretin

The levels/effects of Benztropine may be decreased by: Acetylcholinesterase Inhibitors (Central); Peginterferon Alfa-2b

Stability Store at 20°C to 25°C (68°F to 77°F).

Mechanism of Action Possesses both anticholinergic and antihistaminic effects. *In vitro* anticholinergic activity approximates that of atropine; *in vivo* it is only about half as active as atropine. Animal data suggest its antihistaminic activity and duration of action approach that of pyrilamine maleate. May also inhibit the reuptake and storage of dopamine, thereby prolonging the action of dopamine.

Pharmacodynamics

Onset of action:

Oral: Within 1 hour

Parenteral: Within 15 minutes

Duration: 6-48 hours

Dosing: Usual Note: I.V. route should be reserved for situations when oral or I.M. are not appropriate.

Children and Adolescents: **Drug-induced extrapyramidal reaction:** Oral, I.M., I.V.:

Children ≥3 years: 0.02-0.05 mg/kg/dose 1-2 times daily; use in children <3 years should be reserved for life-threatening emergencies (Bellman, 1974; Habre, 1999; Joseph, 1995; Teoh, 2002)

Adolescents: 1-4 mg every 12-24 hours (Nelson, 1996)

Adults:

Acute dystonia: I.M., I.V.: 1-2 mg as a single dose

Drug-induced extrapyramidal symptom: Oral, I.M., I.V.: 1-4 mg 1-2 times daily or 1-2 mg 2-3 times daily for reactions developing soon after initiation of antipsychotic medication; usually provides relief within 1-2 days, but may continue for up to 1-2 weeks; withdraw after 1-2 weeks to reassess continued need for therapy. May reinitiate benztropine if symptoms recur.

Parkinsonism, idiopathic or postencephalitic: Oral, I.M., I.V.: Usual dose: 1-2 mg daily; range: 0.5-6 mg/day in a single dose at bedtime or divided in 2-4 doses; titrate dose in 0.5 mg increments at 5- to 6-day intervals to achieve the desired effect; maximum daily dose: 6 mg/**day**

Note: Dosing should be individualized based on patient age, weight, and type of parkinsonism being treated. Lower initial doses may be appropriate for older and thinner patients. Low initial doses (0.5-1 mg) may also be appropriate for idiopathic parkinsonism and may be adequate for maintenance. Higher initial doses (2 mg daily) may be required for postencephalitic parkinsonism. Dosing schedule should also be individualized; patients may respond more favorably to either once-daily bedtime dosing or 2-4 divided doses throughout the day; however, once-daily bedtime dosing is often effective.

Dosing adjustment in renal impairment: There are no dosage adjustments provided in the manufacturer's labeling.

Dosing adjustment in hepatic impairment: There are no dosage adjustments provided in the manufacturer's labeling.

Administration

Oral: May be given with or without food; administration with food may decrease GI upset.

Parenteral: I.V. route should be reserved for situations when oral or I.M. are not appropriate. Manufacturer's labeling states there is no difference in onset of effect after I.V. or I.M. injection and therefore there is usually no need to use the I.V. route. No specific instructions on administering benztropine I.V. are provided in the labeling. The I.V. route has been reported in the literature in adults (slow I.V. push when reported), although specific instructions are lacking (Sachdev, 1993; Schramm, 2002).

Dosage Forms Excipient information presented when available (limited, particularly for generics); consult specific product labeling.

Solution, Injection, as mesylate:
Cogentin: 1 mg/mL (2 mL)
Generic: 1 mg/mL (2 mL)
Tablet, Oral, as mesylate:
Generic: 0.5 mg, 1 mg, 2 mg

References

Bellman MH.Treatment of phenothiazine drug intoxication with bentropine. *Arch Dis Child.*1974;49(8):664-665.

Falterman CG and Richardson CJ, "Small Left Colon Syndrome Associated With Maternal Ingestion of Psychotropic Drugs," *J Pediatr*, 1980, 97(2):308-10.

Habre W, Wilson D, Johnson CM. Extrapyrimidal side-effects from droperidol mixed with morphine for patient-controlled analgesia in two children. *Paediatric Anaesthesia.* 1999;9:362-364.

Joseph MM, King WD. Dystonic reaction following recommended use of a cold syrup. *Annals of Emergency Medicine.* 1995;26(6):749-751.

Nelson WE, Behrman RE, Kliegman RM, et al, eds. *Nelson Textbook of Pediatrics.* 15th ed. Philadelphia, PA: WB Saunders Company; 1996.

Sachdev P, Loneragan C. Intravenous benztropine and propranolol challenges in tardive akathisia. *Psychopharmacology (Berl).* 1993;113(1):119-122.

Schramm BM, Orser BA. Dystonic reaction to propofol attenuated by benztropine (Cogentin). *Anesth Analg,* 2002;94(5):1237-1240.

Teoh L, Allen H, Kowalenko N. Drug-induced extrapyramidal reactions. *J Paediatr Child Health.* 2002;38:95-97.

◆ **Benztropine Mesylate** see Benztropine on page 276

◆ **Benztropine Omega (Can)** see Benztropine on page 276

Benzyl Alcohol (BEN zill AL koe hol)

Medication Safety Issues
Sound-alike/look-alike issues:
Benzyl alcohol may be confused with benzoyl peroxide

Brand Names: U.S. Ulesfia; Zilactin [OTC]

Therapeutic Category Analgesic, Topical; Antiparasitic Agent, Topical; Pediculocide; Topical Skin Product

Generic Availability (U.S.) No

Use

Lotion: Treatment of head lice infestation (FDA approved in ages ≥6 months and adults)

Liquid (topical): Temporary relief of pain caused by cold sores/fever blisters (FDA approved in ages ≥2 years and adults)

Pregnancy Risk Factor B

Pregnancy Considerations Teratogenic effects were not observed in animal studies. There are no well-controlled human studies with topical benzyl alcohol in pregnancy. Use only if clearly needed.

Breast-Feeding Considerations It is unknown if benzyl alcohol is distributed in human milk. Use with caution.

Contraindications Hypersensitivity to benzyl alcohol or any component

Warnings Large amounts of benzyl alcohol (≥99 mg/kg/day) have been associated with a potentially fatal toxicity ("gasping syndrome") in neonates; the "gasping syndrome" consists of metabolic acidosis, respiratory distress, gasping respirations, CNS dysfunction (including convulsions, intracranial hemorrhage), hypotension, and cardiovascular collapse; avoid use in neonates

Precautions For external use only; if contact with eyes occurs, flush immediately with water; allergic or irritant dermatitis may occur

Adverse Reactions

Dermatologic: Erythema, pruritus
Local: Anesthesia, hypoesthesia, irritation, pain
Ocular: Ocular irritation
Rare but important or life-threatening: Dandruff, dermatitis, dryness, excoriation, exfoliation, paresthesia, rash, thermal burn

Drug Interactions

Metabolism/Transport Effects None known.

Avoid Concomitant Use There are no known interactions where it is recommended to avoid concomitant use.

Increased Effect/Toxicity There are no known significant interactions involving an increase in effect.

Decreased Effect There are no known significant interactions involving a decrease in effect.

Stability

Lotion: Store at 20°C to 25°C (68°F to 77°F); excursions permitted to 15°C to 30°C (59°F to 86°F); do not freeze.

Liquid (topical): Store at 15°C to 20°C (59°F to 86°F). Flammable; keep away from fire or flame.

Mechanism of Action Inhibits respiration of lice by obstructing respiratory spiracles causing lice asphyxiation. No ovicidal activity.

Pharmacokinetics (Adult data unless noted) Absorption: Quantifiable serum plasma concentrations reported following prolonged exposure (30 minutes) in patients 6 months to 11 years of age

Dosing: Usual

Lotion (Ulesfia™): Treatment of head lice infestation: Children ≥6 months of age and adults: Apply appropriate volume for hair length to dry hair, saturate the scalp completely, leave on for 10 minutes, rinse thoroughly with water; repeat in 7 days.

Hair length 0-2 inches: 4-6 ounces
Hair length 2-4 inches: 6-8 ounces
Hair length 4-8 inches: 8-12 ounces
Hair length 8-16 inches: 12-24 ounces
Hair length 16-22 inches: 24-32 ounces
Hair length >22 inches: 32-48 ounces

Liquid (topical) [Zilactin®-L (OTC)]: Cold sores/fever blisters: Children ≥2 years of age and adults: Moisten cotton swab with several drops of liquid; apply to affected area up to 4 times/day; do not use for more than 7 days

Administration For topical use only. Do not swallow liquid or lotion.

Lotion (Ulesfia™): Apply under adult supervision to dry hair, until entire scalp and hair are saturated. Leave on for 10 minutes then rinse thoroughly. Avoid contact with eyes. Wash hands after application. A lice comb may be used to remove dead lice after both treatments.

Liquid (topical) [Zilactin®-L (OTC)]: Apply to affected area only with moistened cotton swab. Allow to dry for 15 seconds. Avoid contact with eyes.

Dosage Forms Excipient information presented when available (limited, particularly for generics); consult specific product labeling.

Gel, Mouth/Throat:
Zilactin: 10% (7.1 g) [contains propylene glycol, sd alcohol]
Lotion, External:
Ulesfia: 5% (227 g) [contains polysorbate 80, trolamine (triethanolamine)]

◆ **Benzylpenicillin Benzathine** see Penicillin G Benzathine on page 1629

◆ **Benzylpenicillin Potassium** see Penicillin G (Parenteral/Aqueous) on page 1631

◆ **Benzylpenicillin Sodium** *see* Penicillin G (Parenteral/Aqueous) *on page 1631*

Benzylpenicilloyl Polylysine
(BEN zil pen i SIL oyl pol i LIE seen)

Brand Names: U.S. Pre-Pen®
Therapeutic Category Diagnostic Agent
Generic Availability (U.S.) No
Use Adjunct in assessing the risk of administering penicillin (penicillin G or benzylpenicillin) in patients suspected of a clinical penicillin hypersensitivity [FDA approved in pediatric patients (age not specified) and adults]. Has also been used as an adjunct in assessment of hypersensitivity to other beta-lactam antibiotics (penicillins and cephalosporins) to determine the safety of penicillin administration in patients with a history of reaction to cephalosporins
Pregnancy Risk Factor C
Pregnancy Considerations Animal reproduction studies have not been conducted with benzylpenicilloyl polylysine. The Centers for Disease Control and Prevention (CDC) states that penicillin skin testing may be useful in assessing suspected penicillin hypersensitivity in pregnant women diagnosed with syphilis (of any stage) due to a lack of proven alternatives to the use of penicillin in this population (CDC, 2006).
Contraindications Systemic or marked local reaction to a previous administration of benzylpenicilloyl polylysine skin test; patients with a known severe hypersensitivity to penicillin should not be tested.
Warnings Rare systemic allergic reactions, including anaphylaxis, have been associated with penicillin skin testing. Penicillin skin testing should only be performed by skilled medical personnel under direct supervision of a physician, and testing should be performed only in an appropriate healthcare setting prepared for the immediate treatment with epinephrine. To decrease the risk of a systemic allergic reaction, the manufacturer recommends puncture skin testing prior to intradermal testing. Patients with a reliable history of a severe life-threatening penicillin allergy, including Stevens-Johnson syndrome or TEN, should **not** receive penicillin skin testing. Responses to skin testing may be attenuated by concurrent administration of antihistamines. Consider delaying testing until these medications can be withheld to allow time for their effects to dissipate; hydroxyzine and diphenhydramine should be discontinued for at least 4 days before skin testing (Boguniewicz, 1995).

According to the manufacturer, a negative skin test is associated with an incidence of immediate allergic reactions of <5% after penicillin administration and a positive skin test may indicate >50% incidence of allergic reaction occurring after penicillin administration. Adequate penicillin skin testing should ideally involve reagents of both the major antigenic determinant (penicilloyl-polylysine) and minor determinants (penicilloate or penilloate). Benzylpenicilloyl polylysine alone does not identify those patients who react to a minor antigenic determinant. The minor determinant mixture (MDM) is not commercially available in the U.S.; however, diluted penicillin G (concentration: 10,000 U/mL) has been used as a minor determinant for skin testing purposes (Bernstein, 2008). Penicillin skin testing does not predict the occurrence of late reactions (eg, Type II, III, IV, or idiopathic reactions).
Adverse Reactions
Cardiovascular: Hypotension
Dermatologic: Angioneurotic edema, pruritus, erythema, urticaria
Local: Inflammation (intense; at skin test site), wheal (locally)
Respiratory: Dyspnea
Miscellaneous: Systemic allergic reactions (including anaphylaxis; rare)

Drug Interactions
Metabolism/Transport Effects None known.
Avoid Concomitant Use There are no known interactions where it is recommended to avoid concomitant use.
Increased Effect/Toxicity There are no known significant interactions involving an increase in effect.
Decreased Effect
The levels/effects of Benzylpenicilloyl Polylysine may be decreased by: Alpha-/Beta-Agonists; Alpha1-Agonists; Antihistamines
Stability Refrigerate at 2°C to 8°C (36°F to 46°F); discard if left at room temperature for longer than 1 day.
Mechanism of Action Benzylpenicilloyl polylysine, a conjugate of the benzylpenicilloyl structural group (hapten) and the poly-l-lysine carrier (protein), is an antigen which reacts with benzylpenicilloyl IgE antibodies to elicit the release of chemical mediators, thereby producing type I (immediate or accelerated) urticarial reactions in patients hypersensitive to penicillins.
Dosing: Usual Children and Adults: **Note:** Benzylpenicilloyl polylysine should always be applied first via the puncture technique. **Do not administer intradermally to patients who have positive reactions to a puncture test.**
Puncture scratch test: Apply a small drop of the skin test solution using a 22-28 gauge needle and to make a single shallow puncture of the epidermis through the drop of solution. A positive reaction consists of a pale wheal surrounding the puncture site which develops within 10 minutes and ranges from 5-15 mm or more in diameter (wheal may be surrounded by erythema and variable degrees of itching). If a positive response is evident, the solution should be wiped off immediately. If the puncture test is negative or equivocal (<5 mm wheal, with little or no erythema and no itching) 15 minutes following the puncture test, an intradermal test may be performed.
Intradermal test: Using a 0.5 to 1 mL tuberculin syringe with a 3/8 to 5/8 inch, 26- to 30-gauge short bevel needle; inject a volume of skin test solution sufficient to raise a small intradermal bleb ~3 mm in diameter intradermally and duplicate at least 2 cm apart. A control of 0.9% sodium chloride or allergen-diluting solution should be injected at least 5 cm from the antigen test site. Most skin responses to the intradermal test will develop within 5-15 minutes. A response to the skin test is read at 20 minutes.
Interpretation of intradermal test:
(-) Negative: No increase in size of original bleb or no greater reaction compared to the control site.
(±) Ambiguous: Wheal only slightly larger than original bleb with or without erythematous flare and slightly larger than control site; **or** discordance between duplicate test sites.
(+) Positive: Itching and marked increase in size of original bleb to ≥5 mm. Wheal may exhibit pseudopods and be >20 mm in diameter.
Control site should be reactionless. If wheal >2-3 mm develops at control site, repeat the test. If same reaction occurs, consultation is necessary.
Administration
Puncture test: Administer initially by puncture technique on the inner volvar aspect of the forearm; observe 15 minutes for reaction. If negative reaction, follow with an intradermal injection.
Intradermal test: Do **not** administer intradermally to patients with a positive reaction to a puncture test (wheal of 5-15 mm or more in diameter). Administer the intradermal test on the upper, outer arm, below the deltoid muscle in the event a severe hypersensitivity reaction occurs and a tourniquet needs to be applied. During the skin test, immediate treatment with epinephrine should also be available. Observe 20 minutes for reaction.

▶

Monitoring Parameters Observe 15 minutes (puncture) or 20 minutes (intradermal) for reaction.

Additional Information Penicillin skin testing is the preferred method of evaluating patients with possible penicillin specific IgE-mediated (Type I) immediate hypersensitivity reactions, when performed using the appropriate major and minor determinant reagents. Testing detects the presence or absence of penicillin-specific IgE antibodies; therefore, it is not useful to detect non-IgE mediated reactions. Patients testing positive to benzylpenicilloyl polylysine possess IgE antibodies against the benzylpenicilloyl structural group (B-lactam ring). The possibility exists for patients to have selective IgE antibodies directed against the R-group side chain structure of certain penicillins, rather than the core beta-lactam structure. Therefore, these patients may test negative to the penicillin major and minor determinants, but be allergic to semisynthetic penicillins (eg, amoxicillin, ampicillin) only and tolerate other penicillin compounds (Bernstein, 2008). Skin testing has also been used in some centers to determine safety of penicillin administration in patients with prior reactions to cephalosporins.

Dosage Forms Excipient information presented when available (limited, particularly for generics); consult specific product labeling.

Injection, solution:
  Pre-Pen®: 6 x 10^-5 M (0.25 mL)

References

Bernstein IL, Li JT, Bernstein DI, et al, "Allergy Diagnostic Testing: An Updated Practice Parameter," *Ann Allergy Asthma Immunol*, 2008, 100(3 Suppl 3):1-148.

Boguniewicz M and Leung DYM, "Hypersensitivity Reactions to Antibiotics Commonly Used in Children," *Pediatr Infect Dis J*, 1995, 14 (3):221-31.

Centers for Disease Control and Prevention, "Sexually Transmitted Diseases Treatment Guidelines, 2006," *MMWR Recomm Rep*, 2009, 55(RR-11):1-94. Available at http://www.cdc.gov/std/treatment/2006/rr5511.pdf.

Macy E, Mangat R, and Burchette RJ, "Penicillin Skin Testing in Advance of Need: Multiyear Follow-Up in 568 Test Result-Negative Subjects Exposed to Oral Penicillins," *J Allergy Clin Immunol*, 2003, 111(5):1111-5.

Salkind AR, Cuddy PG, and Foxworth JW, "The Rational Clinical Examination. Is This Patient Allergic to Penicillin? An Evidence-Based Analysis of the Likelihood of Penicillin Allergy," *JAMA*, 2001, 285 (19):2498-505.

Wendel GD Jr, Stark BJ, Jamison RB, et al, "Penicillin Allergy and Desensitization in Serious Infections During Pregnancy," *N Engl J Med*, 1985, 312(19):1229-32.

◆ **Benzylpenicilloyl-polylysine** see Benzylpenicilloyl Polylysine on page 279

Beractant (ber AKT ant)

Medication Safety Issues
Sound-alike/look-alike issues:
  Survanta® may be confused with Sufenta®
Brand Names: U.S. Survanta
Brand Names: Canada Survanta®
Therapeutic Category Lung Surfactant
Generic Availability (U.S.) No
Use Prevention and treatment of respiratory distress syndrome (RDS) in premature infants

Prophylactic therapy: Infants with body weight <1250 g who are at risk for developing or with evidence of surfactant deficiency

Rescue therapy: Treatment of infants with RDS confirmed by x-ray and requiring mechanical ventilation

Pregnancy Considerations Beractant is only indicated for use in premature infants.

Warnings Rapidly affects oxygenation and lung compliance and should be restricted to a highly supervised use in a clinical setting with immediate availability of clinicians experienced with intubation and ventilatory management

of premature infants. If transient episodes of bradycardia and decreased oxygen saturation occur, discontinue the dosing procedure and initiate measures to alleviate the condition; produces rapid improvements in lung oxygenation and compliance that may require immediate reductions in ventilator settings and FiO$_2$.

Precautions Use of beractant in infants <600 g birth weight or >1750 g birth weight has not been evaluated

Adverse Reactions During the dosing procedure:
Cardiovascular: Transient bradycardia
Respiratory: Oxygen desaturation
Rare but important or life-threatening: Apnea, endotracheal tube blockage, hypercarbia, hyper-/hypotension, post-treatment nosocomial sepsis probability increased, pulmonary air leaks, pulmonary interstitial emphysema, vasoconstriction

Drug Interactions
Metabolism/Transport Effects None known.
Avoid Concomitant Use
  Avoid concomitant use of Beractant with any of the following: Ceritinib
Increased Effect/Toxicity
  Beractant may increase the levels/effects of: Bradycardia-Causing Agents; Ceritinib
Decreased Effect There are no known significant interactions involving a decrease in effect.

Stability Refrigerate; protect from light; prior to administration warm by standing at room temperature for 20 minutes or hold in hand for 8 minutes; artificial warming methods should **not** be used; unused, unopened vials warmed to room temperature may be returned to the refrigerator within 24 hours of warming only once

Mechanism of Action Replaces deficient or ineffective endogenous lung surfactant in neonates with respiratory distress syndrome (RDS) or in neonates at risk of developing RDS. Surfactant prevents the alveoli from collapsing during expiration by lowering surface tension between air and alveolar surfaces.

Dosing: Neonatal Endotracheal:
Prophylactic treatment: 4 mL/kg (100 mg phospholipids/kg) as soon as possible; as many as 4 doses may be administered during the first 48 hours of life, no more frequently than 6 hours apart. The need for additional doses is determined by evidence of continuing respiratory distress or if the infant is still intubated and requiring at least 30% inspired oxygen to maintain a PaO$_2$ ≤80 torr.
Rescue treatment: 4 mL/kg (100 mg phospholipids/kg) as soon as the diagnosis of RDS is made; may repeat if needed, no more frequently than every 6 hours to a maximum of 4 doses

Administration Endotracheal: For endotracheal administration only. Do not shake; if settling occurs during storage, gently swirl. Suction infant prior to administration; inspect solution to verify complete mixing of the suspension. Administer endotracheally by instillation through a 5-French end-hole catheter inserted into the infant's endotracheal tube. Administer the dose in four 1 mL/kg aliquots. Each quarter-dose is instilled over 2-3 seconds; each quarter-dose is administered with the infant in a different position; slightly downward inclination with head turned to the right, then repeat with head turned to the left; then slightly upward inclination with head turned to the right, then repeat with head turned to the left.

Monitoring Parameters Continuous heart rate and transcutaneous O$_2$ saturation should be monitored during administration; frequent ABG sampling is necessary to prevent postdosing hyperoxia and hypocarbia.

Dosage Forms Excipient information presented when available (limited, particularly for generics); consult specific product labeling.
Suspension, Inhalation:
  Survanta: Phospholipids 25 mg/mL (4 mL, 8 mL)

◆ **Berinert** *see* C1 Inhibitor (Human) *on page 337*

Besifloxacin (be si FLOX a sin)

Brand Names: U.S. Besivance
Brand Names: Canada Besivance™
Therapeutic Category Antibiotic, Fluoroquinolone; Antibiotic, Ophthalmic; Ophthalmic Agent
Generic Availability (U.S.) No
Use Treatment of bacterial conjunctivitis (FDA approved in ages ≥1 year and adults)
Pregnancy Risk Factor C
Pregnancy Considerations Oral besifloxacin has been shown to be fetotoxic in animal studies at doses that were also maternally toxic. Quinolone exposure during human pregnancy has been reported with other agents (refer to Ciprofloxacin and Ofloxacin monographs). The low plasma concentrations of besifloxacin following ophthalmic use (<1.3 ng/mL in nonpregnant patients) should limit fetal exposure.
Breast-Feeding Considerations Other quinolones are known to be excreted in breast milk. The manufacturer recommends using caution if besifloxacin is administered while nursing.
Contraindications Hypersensitivity to besifloxacin or any component
Warnings Do not inject ophthalmic solution subconjunctivally or introduce directly into the anterior chamber of the eye. Prolonged use may result in fungal or bacterial superinfection; discontinue use and initiate alternative therapy if superinfection occurs. Severe hypersensitivity reactions, including anaphylaxis, have occurred with systemic quinolone therapy. Prompt discontinuation of drug should occur if skin rash or other symptoms arise.
Precautions Contact lenses should not be worn during treatment of ophthalmic infections.
Adverse Reactions
Central nervous system: Headache
Ocular: Blurred vision, conjunctival redness, irritation, pain, pruritus
Drug Interactions
Metabolism/Transport Effects None known.
Avoid Concomitant Use There are no known interactions where it is recommended to avoid concomitant use.
Increased Effect/Toxicity There are no known significant interactions involving an increase in effect.
Decreased Effect There are no known significant interactions involving a decrease in effect.
Stability Store between 15°C to 25°C (59°F to 77°F); protect from light.
Mechanism of Action Inhibits both DNA gyrase and topoisomerase IV. DNA gyrase is an essential bacterial enzyme required for DNA replication, transcription, and repair. Topoisomerase IV is an essential bacterial enzyme required for decatenation during cell division. Inhibition effect is bactericidal.
Pharmacokinetics (Adult data unless noted) Half-life elimination: ~7 hours
Dosing: Usual Ophthalmic: Children ≥1 year and Adults: Bacterial conjunctivitis: Instill 1 drop into affected eye(s) 3 times/day (4-12 hours apart) for 7 days
Administration Ophthalmic: Wash hands before and after instillation. Shake bottle once prior to each administration. Avoid contaminating the applicator tip with affected eye(s).
Monitoring Parameters Signs and symptoms of infection or hypersensitivity reaction
Dosage Forms Excipient information presented when available (limited, particularly for generics); consult specific product labeling.

Suspension, Ophthalmic:
Besivance: 0.6% (5 mL) [contains benzalkonium chloride, edetate disodium dihydrate]

References
Cambau E, Matrat S, Pan XS, et al, "Target Specificity of the New Fluoroquinolone Besifloxacin in *Streptococcus pneumoniae, Staphylococcus aureus* and *Escherichia coli*," *J Antimicrob Chemother,* 2009, 63(3):443-50.
Karpecki P, DePaolis M, Hunter JA, et al, "Besifloxacin Ophthalmic Suspension 0.6% in Patients With Bacterial Conjunctivitis: A Multicenter, Prospective, Randomized, Double-Masked, Vehicle-Controlled, 5-Day Efficacy and Safety Study," *Clin Ther,* 2009, 31 (3):514-26.

◆ **Besifloxacin Hydrochloride** *see* Besifloxacin *on page 281*
◆ **Besivance** *see* Besifloxacin *on page 281*
◆ **Besivance™ (Can)** *see* Besifloxacin *on page 281*
◆ **β,β-Dimethylcysteine** *see* PenicillAMINE *on page 1627*
◆ **9-Beta-D-Ribofuranosyladenine** *see* Adenosine *on page 76*
◆ **Betacaine (Can)** *see* Lidocaine (Topical) *on page 1242*
◆ **Beta Care Betatar Gel [OTC]** *see* Coal Tar *on page 532*
◆ **Betaderm (Can)** *see* Betamethasone (Topical) *on page 285*
◆ **Betagan** *see* Levobunolol *on page 1223*
◆ **Betagan® (Can)** *see* Levobunolol *on page 1223*
◆ **Beta HC [OTC]** *see* Hydrocortisone (Topical) *on page 1038*

Betaine (BAY ta een)

Medication Safety Issues
Sound-alike/look-alike issues:
Betaine may be confused with Betadine®
Cystadane® may be confused with cysteamine, cysteine
Brand Names: U.S. Cystadane
Brand Names: Canada Cystadane®
Therapeutic Category Homocystinuria, Treatment Agent
Generic Availability (U.S.) May be product dependent
Use Treatment of homocystinuria to reduce elevated homocysteine blood concentrations (FDA approved in ages 24 days to 17 years and adults); homocystinuria includes deficiencies or defects in cystathionine beta-synthase (CBS), 5,10-methylenetetrahydrofolate reductase (MTHFR), and cobalamin cofactor metabolism (cbl)
Prescribing and Access Restrictions Cystadane® may be obtained by contacting Accredo Health Group Inc at 1-888-454-8860.
Pregnancy Risk Factor C
Pregnancy Considerations Animal reproduction studies have not been conducted with betaine. It is not known whether betaine can cause fetal harm when administered to a pregnant woman or can affect reproductive capacity. Betaine should be given to a pregnant woman only if needed.
Breast-Feeding Considerations Betaine is found naturally in human breast milk. The influence from betaine therapy is unknown.
Contraindications Hypersensitivity to betaine or any component
Warnings Cerebral edema has been reported in patients with hypermethioninemia, including a few patients treated with betaine. Treatment of CBS with betaine may further increase methionine serum concentrations (due to remethylation of homocysteine to methionine); monitor methionine serum concentrations in patients with CBS deficiency; maintain methionine concentrations <1,000 micromol/L. Therapy should be directed by a physician with expertise managing homocystinuria patients.

Adverse Reactions

Gastrointestinal: Diarrhea, dysgeusia, GI distress, nausea

Rare but important or life-threatening: Alopecia, anorexia, agitation, cerebral edema (associated with hypermethioninemia), dental disorders, depression, hives, glossitis, irritability, personality disorder, sleep disturbances, skin odor abnormalities, urinary incontinence, vomiting

Drug Interactions

Metabolism/Transport Effects None known.

Avoid Concomitant Use There are no known interactions where it is recommended to avoid concomitant use.

Increased Effect/Toxicity There are no known significant interactions involving an increase in effect.

Decreased Effect There are no known significant interactions involving a decrease in effect.

Stability Store at 15°C to 30°C (59°F to 86°F); protect from moisture

Mechanism of Action Betaine acts as a methyl group donor in the remethylation of homocysteine to methionine. Homocystinuria is an inborn error of metabolism in which elevated plasma homocysteine levels can lead to mental retardation, ocular abnormalities, osteoporosis, premature atherosclerosis and thromboembolic disease. Remethylation is one of the two divergent pathways in the metabolism of homocysteine. The second pathway involves transulfuration of homocysteine to produce cysteine. A number of enzymes and cofactors are also involved in these pathways.

Dosing: Neonatal Oral: PNA ≥24 days (PMA not specified): 100 mg/kg/day divided into 2 doses; increase at weekly intervals in 50 mg/kg/day increments; minimal benefit has been shown in patients treated with >150 mg/kg/day or exceeding a twice daily dosing schedule

Dosing: Usual Oral: **Note:** Minimal benefit has been seen with dosages >150 mg/kg/day or >20 g/day or exceeding a twice daily dosing schedule.

Infants and Children <3 years: 100 mg/kg/day divided in 2 doses; increase at weekly intervals in 50 mg/kg/day increments

Children ≥3 years, Adolescents, and Adults: 3 g twice daily; doses up to 20 g/day have been needed to control homocysteine plasma concentrations in some patients

Administration Oral: Shake bottle lightly before opening; measure prescribed amount with provided measuring scoop and dissolve in 4-6 ounces of water, juice, milk, or formula; may also mix with food; administer immediately; do not use if powder does not completely dissolve or gives a colored solution

Monitoring Parameters Plasma homocysteine concentration (should be low or undetectable); plasma methionine (CBS patients)

Additional Information Vitamin B$_6$, vitamin B$_{12}$, and folate have been helpful in the management of homocystinuria and are often used in conjunction.

Dosage Forms Excipient information presented when available (limited, particularly for generics); consult specific product labeling.

Powder, Oral, as anhydrous:

Cystadane: 1 g/scoop (180 g)

Tablet, Oral, as anhydrous:

Generic: 300 mg

References

Burns SP, Iles RA, Ryalls M, et al "Methylgenesis From Betaine in Cystathionine-Beta-Synthase Deficiency," *Biochem Soc Trans*, 1993, 21:455S.

Devlin AM, Hajipour L, Gholkar A, "Cerebral Edema Associated With Betaine Treatment in Classical Homocystinuria," *J Pediatr*, 2001,144 (4):545-8.

Kishi T, Kawamura I, Harada Y, et al, "Effect of Betaine on S-Adenosylmethionine Levels in the Cerebrospinal Fluid in a Patient With Methylenetetrahydrofolate Reductase Deficiency and Peripheral Neuropathy," *J Inherit Metab Dis*, 1994, 17(5):560-5.

Lawson-Yuen A and Levy, HL, "The Use of Betaine in the Treatment of Elevated Homocysteine," *Mol Genet Metab*, 2006, 88(3):201-7.

Matthews A, Johnson TN, Rostami-Hodjegan A, et al, "An Indirect Response Model of Homocysteine Suppression by Betaine: Optimising the Dosage Regimen of Betaine in Homocystinuria," *Br J Clin Pharmacol*, 2002, 54(2):140-6.

Smolin LA, Benevenga NJ, and Berlow S, "The Use of Betaine for the Treatment of Homocystinuria," *J Pediatr*, 1981, 99:467-72.

◆ **Betaine Anhydrous** *see* Betaine *on page 281*

◆ **Betaject (Can)** *see* Betamethasone (Systemic) *on page 282*

◆ **Betaloc (Can)** *see* Metoprolol *on page 1396*

Betamethasone (Systemic) (bay ta METH a sone)

Related Information

Corticosteroids Systemic Equivalencies *on page 2222*

Brand Names: U.S. Celestone; Celestone Soluspan

Brand Names: Canada Betaject; Celestone Soluspan

Therapeutic Category Corticosteroid, Systemic

Generic Availability (U.S.) May be product dependent

Use

I.M.: Anti-inflammatory or immunosuppressant agent in the treatment of a variety of diseases when oral therapy not feasible including those of allergic, hematologic, dermatologic, endocrine, gastrointestinal, ophthalmic, neoplastic, rheumatic, autoimmune, nervous system, renal, and respiratory origin (FDA approved in pediatric patients [age not specified] and adults)

Intra-articular or soft tissue administration: Adjunctive therapy for short-term administration (to tide the patient over an acute episode or exacerbation) in acute gouty arthritis, acute and subacute bursitis, acute nonspecific tenosynovitis, epicondylitis, rheumatoid arthritis, synovitis of osteoarthritis (FDA approved in pediatric patients [age not specified] and adults)

Intralesional: Treatment of alopecia areata; discoid lupus erythematosus; keloids; localized hypertrophic, infiltrated, inflammatory lesions of granuloma annulare, lichen planus, lichen simplex chronicus (neurodermatitis), and psoriatic plaques; necrobiosis lipoidica diabeticorum (FDA approved in pediatric patients [age not specified] and adults); has also been used for treatment of infantile hemangioma

Pregnancy Risk Factor C

Pregnancy Considerations Adverse events have been observed with corticosteroids in animal reproduction studies. Betamethasone crosses the placenta (Brownfoot, 2013); and is partially metabolized by placental enzymes to an inactive metabolite (Murphy, 2007). Some studies have shown an association between first trimester systemic corticosteroid use and oral clefts (Park-Wyllie, 2000; Pradat, 2003). Systemic corticosteroids may have an effect on fetal growth (decreased birth weight); however, information is conflicting (Lunghi, 2010). Hypoadrenalism may occur in newborns following maternal use of corticosteroids during pregnancy; monitor.

Because antenatal corticosteroid administration may reduce the incidence of intraventricular hemorrhage, necrotizing enterocolitis, neonatal mortality, and respiratory distress syndrome, the injection is often used in patients with preterm premature rupture of membranes (membrane rupture between 24 0/7 weeks and 34 0/7 weeks of gestation) who are at risk of preterm delivery (ACOG, 2013). When systemic corticosteroids are needed in pregnancy, it is generally recommended to use the lowest effective dose for the shortest duration of time, avoiding high doses during the first trimester (Leachman, 2006; Lunghi, 2010; Makol, 2011; Østensen, 2009).

Women exposed to betamethasone during pregnancy for the treatment of an autoimmune disease may contact the OTIS Autoimmune Diseases Study at 877-311-8972.

Breast-Feeding Considerations Corticosteroids are excreted in human milk. The onset of milk secretion after birth may be delayed and the volume of milk produced may be decreased by antenatal betamethasone therapy; this affect was seen when delivery occurred 3-9 days after the betamethasone dose in women between 28 and 34 weeks gestation. Antenatal betamethasone therapy did not affect milk production when birth occurred <3 days or >10 days of treatment (Henderson, 2008).

The manufacturer notes that when used systemically, maternal use of corticosteroids have the potential to cause adverse events in a nursing infant (eg, growth suppression, interfere with endogenous corticosteroid production) and therefore recommends that caution be exercised when administering betamethasone to nursing women. If there is concern about exposure to the infant, some guidelines recommend waiting 4 hours after the maternal dose of an oral systemic corticosteroid before breast-feeding in order to decrease potential exposure to the infant (based on a study using prednisolone) (Bae, 2011; Leachman, 2006; Makol, 2011; Ost, 1985).

Contraindications Hypersensitivity to betamethasone, or any component

Additional dose- or route-specific contraindications:
Immunosuppressive doses: Immunization with live or live-attenuated vaccines
I.M.: Idiopathic thrombocytopenia (ITP)

Documentation of allergenic cross-reactivity for drugs in this class is limited. However, because of similarities in chemical structure and/or pharmacologic actions, the possibility of cross-sensitivity cannot be ruled out with certainty.

Warnings Hypothalamic-pituitary-adrenal (HPA) suppression or Cushing's syndrome may occur, particularly in younger children or in patients receiving high doses for prolonged periods; acute adrenal insufficiency (adrenal crisis) may occur with abrupt withdrawal after long-term therapy or with stress; withdrawal and discontinuation of corticosteroids should be tapered slowly and carefully; patients with HPA axis suppression may require doses of systemic glucocorticosteroids prior to, during, and after unusual stress (eg, surgery). **Note:** Adrenal suppression with failure to thrive has been reported in infants after receiving intralesional corticosteroid injections for treatment of hemangioma (Goyal, 2004).

Immunosuppression may occur; patients may be more susceptible to infections; prolonged use of corticosteroids may also increase the incidence of secondary infection, mask acute infection (including fungal infections), prolong or exacerbate viral or fungal infections, activate latent opportunistic infections, or limit response to vaccines. Exposure to chickenpox should be avoided; corticosteroids should not be used to treat ocular herpes simplex; use caution in patients with a history of ocular herpes simplex. Corticosteroids should not be used for cerebral malaria or viral hepatitis. Close observation is required in patients with latent tuberculosis and/or TB reactivity; restrict use in active TB (only in conjunction with antituberculosis treatment). Avoid injection into an infected site; injection into a previously infected joint is not recommended. If infection is suspected, joint fluid examination is recommended. If septic arthritis occurs after injection, initiate appropriate antimicrobial therapy.

May cause osteoporosis (at any age) or inhibition of bone growth in pediatric patients. Use with caution in patients with osteoporosis. In a population-based study of children, risk of fracture was shown to be increased with >4 courses of corticosteroids; underlying clinical condition may also impact bone health and osteoporotic effect of corticosteroids (Leonard, 2006).

Corticosteroid use may cause psychiatric disturbances, including depression, euphoria, insomnia, mood swings, and personality changes. preexisting psychiatric conditions may be exacerbated by corticosteroid use. Acute myopathy may occur with high doses, usually in patients with neuromuscular transmission disorders; myopathy may involve ocular and/or respiratory muscles; monitor creatine kinase; recovery may be delayed. Increased IOP, open-angle glaucoma, and cataracts may occur, especially with prolonged use; monitor IOP in patients on prolonged therapy. Rare cases of anaphylactoid reactions have been reported with corticosteroids.

Administer products only via recommended route; suspension for injection (betamethasone acetate) is for intramuscular, intra-articular, or intralesional use only, do not administer intravenously. Intra-articular injection may be systemically absorbed. Intra-articular injection may result in joint tissue damage. Injection of corticosteroids into unstable joints is not recommended.

Precautions Avoid using higher than recommended doses; suppression of HPA function, suppression of linear growth (ie, reduction of growth velocity), reduced bone mineral density, hypercorticism (Cushing's syndrome), hyperglycemia, or glucosuria may occur; titrate to lowest effective dose. Reduction in growth velocity may occur when corticosteroids are administered to pediatric patients by any route; monitor growth. Use with extreme caution in patients with respiratory tuberculosis or untreated systemic infections. Use with caution in patients with hypertension, heart failure, or renal impairment; long-term use has been associated with fluid retention and hypertension. Use with caution in patients with GI diseases (diverticulitis, fresh intestinal anastomoses, peptic ulcer, ulcerative colitis) due to risk of GI bleeding and perforation. Avoid ethanol; may enhance gastric mucosal irritation. High-dose corticosteroids should not be used for management of head injury; increased mortality was observed in patients receiving high-dose I.V. methylprednisolone. Use with caution in patients with myasthenia gravis; exacerbation of symptoms has occurred, especially during initial treatment with corticosteroids. Use with caution in patients with hepatic impairment, including cirrhosis; enhanced pharmacologic effect due to decreased metabolism and long-term use has been associated with fluid retention. Use with caution following acute MI; corticosteroids have been associated with myocardial rupture.

Use with caution in patients with diabetes; corticosteroids may alter glucose regulation, leading to hyperglycemia. Use with caution in patients with cataracts and/or glaucoma; increased intraocular pressure, open-angle glaucoma, and cataracts have occurred with prolonged use; consider routine eye exams in chronic users. Use with caution in patients with a history of seizure disorder; seizures have been reported with adrenal crisis. Use with caution in patients with thyroid dysfunction; changes in thyroid status may necessitate dosage adjustments; metabolic clearance of corticosteroids increases in hyperthyroid patients and decreases in hypothyroid patients. Prolonged treatment with corticosteroids has been associated with the development of Kaposi's sarcoma (case reports); if noted, discontinuation of therapy should be considered.

Potentially significant drug-drug interactions may exist, requiring dose or frequency adjustment, additional monitoring, and/or selection of alternative therapy. Consult drug interactions database for more detailed information.

Adverse Reactions

Cardiovascular: Congestive heart failure, edema, hyper-/hypotension

Central nervous system: Dizziness, headache, insomnia, intracranial pressure increased, lightheadedness, nervousness, pseudotumor cerebri, seizure, vertigo

Dermatologic: Ecchymoses, facial erythema, fragile skin, hirsutism, hyper-/hypopigmentation, perioral dermatitis (oral), petechiae, striae, wound healing impaired

Endocrine & metabolic: Amenorrhea, Cushing's syndrome, diabetes mellitus, growth suppression, hyperglycemia, hypokalemia, menstrual irregularities, pituitary-adrenal axis suppression, protein catabolism, sodium retention, water retention

Local: Injection site reactions (intra-articular use), sterile abscess

Neuromuscular & skeletal: Arthralgia, muscle atrophy, fractures, muscle weakness, myopathy, osteoporosis, necrosis (femoral and humeral heads)

Ocular: Cataracts, glaucoma, intraocular pressure increased

Miscellaneous: Anaphylactoid reaction, diaphoresis, hypersensitivity, secondary infection

Drug Interactions

Metabolism/Transport Effects None known.

Avoid Concomitant Use

Avoid concomitant use of Betamethasone (Systemic) with any of the following: Aldesleukin; BCG; Indium 111 Capromab Pendetide; Mifepristone; Natalizumab; Pimecrolimus; Tacrolimus (Topical); Tofacitinib

Increased Effect/Toxicity

Betamethasone (Systemic) may increase the levels/ effects of: Acetylcholinesterase Inhibitors; Amphotericin B; Androgens; Ceritinib; Deferasirox; Leflunomide; Loop Diuretics; Natalizumab; NSAID (COX-2 Inhibitor); NSAID (Nonselective); Thiazide Diuretics; Tofacitinib; Vaccines (Live); Warfarin

The levels/effects of Betamethasone (Systemic) may be increased by: Antifungal Agents (Azole Derivatives, Systemic); Aprepitant; Calcium Channel Blockers (Nondihydropyridine); Denosumab; Estrogen Derivatives; Fluconazole; Fosaprepitant; Indacaterol; Macrolide Antibiotics; Mifepristone; Neuromuscular-Blocking Agents (Nondepolarizing); Pimecrolimus; Quinolone Antibiotics; Roflumilast; Salicylates; Tacrolimus (Topical); Telaprevir; Trastuzumab

Decreased Effect

Betamethasone (Systemic) may decrease the levels/ effects of: Aldesleukin; Antidiabetic Agents; BCG; Calcitriol; Coccidioidin Skin Test; Corticorelin; Hyaluronidase; Indium 111 Capromab Pendetide; Isoniazid; Salicylates; Sipuleucel-T; Telaprevir; Urea Cycle Disorder Agents; Vaccines (Inactivated)

The levels/effects of Betamethasone (Systemic) may be decreased by: Aminoglutethimide; Barbiturates; Echinacea; Mifepristone; Mitotane; Primidone; Rifamycin Derivatives

Stability Store at 25°C (77°F); excursions are permitted between 15°C and 30°C (59°F and 86°F). Protect from light.

Mechanism of Action Controls the rate of protein synthesis; depresses the migration of polymorphonuclear leukocytes, fibroblasts; reverses capillary permeability and lysosomal stabilization at the cellular level to prevent or control inflammation

Dosing: Usual Note: Dosages expressed as combined amount of betamethasone sodium phosphate and betamethasone acetate; 1 mg is equivalent to betamethasone sodium phosphate 0.5 mg and betamethasone acetate 0.5 mg. Dosage should be based on severity of disease and patient response; use lowest effective dose for shortest period of time to avoid HPA axis suppression

Pediatric:

General dosing, treatment of inflammatory and allergic conditions: Infants, Children, and Adolescents: I.M.: Initial: 0.02 to 0.3 mg/kg/day (0.6 to 9 mg/m^2/ day) in 3 or 4 divided doses

Infantile hemangioma, severe: Limited data available: Infants and Children: Intralesional: Dosage dependent upon size of lesion: Commonly reported: 6 mg administered as a 6 mg/mL (in combination with triamcinolone injection) divided into multiple injections along the lesion perimeter; reported range: 1.5 to 18 mg/dose; doses usually administered every 8 to 14 weeks; reported range: 6 to 25 weeks (Buckmiller, 2008; Chowdri, 1994; Kushner, 1985; Praseyono, 2011). Dosing based on small trials and case-series, mostly reported in infants and children ≤4 years of age. The largest experience (n=70, age range: 2 months to 12 years) prospectively used a betamethasone/triamcinolone combination injection (1.5 to 18 mg betamethasone acetate) and showed that 89.23% of lesions with an initial volume <20 cc^3 regressed by more than 50%, but only 22.2% of lesions with an initial volume >20 cc^3 displayed a good or excellent response (Chowdri, 1994). Another trial (n=25, age range: 7 weeks to 2 years) used lower doses of 3 to 12 mg (in combination with triamcinolone); 16 patients experienced a marked response (Kushner, 1985).

Adult: **Note:** Dosages expressed as combined amount of betamethasone sodium phosphate and betamethasone acetate; 1 mg is equivalent to betamethasone sodium phosphate 0.5 mg and betamethasone acetate 0.5 mg. Base dosage on severity of disease and patient response

General dosing: I.M.: Initial: 0.25 to 9 mg/day

Antenatal fetal maturation: I.M.: In women with preterm premature rupture of membranes (membrane rupture between 24 0/7 weeks and 34 0/7 weeks of gestation), a single course of corticosteroids is recommended if there is a risk of preterm delivery (ACOG, 2013). Although the optimal corticosteroid and dose have not been determined, betamethasone 12 mg every 24 hours for a total of 2 doses has been used in most studies (Brownfoot, 2013).

Bursitis (other than of the foot), tenosynovitis, peritendinitis: Intrabursal: 3 to 6 mg (0.5 to1 mL) for 1 dose; several injections may be required for acute exacerbations or chronic conditions; reduced doses may be warranted for repeat injections

Dermatologic: Intralesional: 1.2 mg/cm^2 (0.2 mL/cm^2) for 1 dose (maximum: 6 mg [1 mL] weekly)

Foot disorders: Intra-articular: 1.5 mg to 6 mg (0.25 to1 mL) per dose at 3- to 7-day intervals. Dose is based upon condition:

Bursitis: 1.5 mg to 3 mg (0.25 to 0.5 mL)

Tenosynovitis: 3 mg (0.5 mL)

Acute gouty arthritis: 3 mg to 6 mg (0.5 to1 mL)

Multiple sclerosis: I.M.: 30 mg daily for 1 week, followed by 12 mg every other day for 4 weeks

Rheumatoid and osteoarthritis: Intra-articular: 3 mg to 12 mg (0.5 to 2 mL) for 1 dose. Dose is based upon the joint size:

Very large (eg, hip): 6 to 12 mg (1 to 2 mL)

Large (eg, knee, ankle, shoulder): 6 mg (1 mL)

Medium (eg, elbow, wrist): 3 to 6 mg (0.5 to 1 mL)

Small (eg, inter- or metacarpophalangeal, sternoclavicular): 1.5 mg to 3 mg (0.25 to 0.5 mL)

Dosing adjustment in renal impairment: There are no dosage adjustments provided in the manufacturer's labeling.

Dosing adjustment in hepatic impairment: There are no dosage adjustments provided in the manufacturer's labeling.

Administration If suspension is coadministered with a local anesthetic, it may be mixed in syringe with 1% or 2% lidocaine HCl (without parabens). Withdraw the dose of betamethasone suspension from the vial into the syringe, then draw up the local anesthetic into the syringe, and shake the syringe briefly. Do not inject the local anesthetic directly into the suspension vial.

I.M.: Do **not** give injectable suspension I.V.

Intrabursal: Tendinitis, tenosynovitis: Inject into affected tendon sheaths (not directly into tendons)

Intralesional: Using a 25-gauge tuberculin syringe with ½-inch needle inject a uniform depot; for infantile hemangioma, 26- and 27-gauge needles have been used for administration. Should be injected directly into the lesion area. Do **not** inject subcutaneously.

Monitoring Parameters Intraocular pressure (if therapy >6 weeks); weight, height, and linear growth (with chronic use); assess HPA suppression. Monitor blood pressure, serum glucose, potassium, calcium, hemoglobin, occult blood loss, and clinical presence of adverse effects.

Test Interactions May suppress the wheal and flare reactions to skin test antigens

Dosage Forms Excipient information presented when available (limited, particularly for generics); consult specific product labeling.

Solution, Oral, as base:

Celestone: 0.6 mg/5 mL (118 mL) [cherry-orange flavor] [DSC]

Suspension, Injection:

Celestone Soluspan: Betamethasone sodium phosphate 3 mg and betamethasone acetate 3 mg per 1 mL (5 mL) [contains benzalkonium chloride, edetate disodium]

Generic: Betamethasone sodium phosphate 3 mg and betamethasone acetate 3 mg per 1 mL (5 mL)

References

ACOG practice bulletins no. 139: premature rupture of membranes. *Obstet Gynecol.* 2013;122(4):918-930.

Betamethasone sodium phosphate and betamethasone acetate injectable suspension [prescribing information]. Shirley, NY: American Regent, Inc; December 2009.

Boot AM, Nauta J, Hokken-Koelega AC, Pols HA, de Ridder MA, de Muinck Keizer-Schrama SM. Renal transplantation and osteoporosis. *Arch Dis Child.* 1995;72(6):502-506.

Bowman H, Lennard TW. Immunosuppressive drugs. *Br J Hosp Med.* 1992;48(9):570-573.

Brownfoot FC, Gagliardi DI, Bain E, Middleton P, Crowther CA. Different corticosteroids and regimens for accelerating fetal lung maturation for women at risk of preterm birth. *Cochrane Database Syst Rev.* 2013;29;8:CD006764.

Buckmiller LM, Francis CL, Glade RS. Intralesional steroid injection for proliferative parotid hemangiomas. *Int J Pediatr Otorhinolaryngo.* 2008;72:81-87.

Celestone soluspan (betamethasone sodium phosphate and betamethasone acetate injectable suspension) [prescribing information]. Whitehouse Station, NY: Merck & Co, Inc; May 2012.

Chowdri NA, Darzi MA, Fazili Z, Iqbal S. Intralesional corticosteroid therapy for childhood cutaneous hemangiomas. *Ann Plast Surg.* 1994;33(1):46-51.

Cooper MS, Stewart PM. Corticosteroid insufficiency in acutely ill patients. *N Engl J Med.* 2003;348(8):727-734.

Coursin DB, Wood KE. Corticosteroid supplementation for adrenal onsufficiency. *JAMA.* 2002;287(2):236-240.

Gamsu HR, Mullinger BM, Donnai P, Dash CH. Antenatal administration of betamethasone to prevent respiratory distress syndrome in preterm infants: report of a UK Multicentre Trial. *Br J Obstet Gynaecol.* 1989;96(4):401-410.

Goedert JJ, Vitale F, Lauria C, et al. Risk factors for classical Kaposi's Sarcoma. *J Natl Cancer Inst.* 2002;94(22):1712-1718.

Grotz WH, Mundinger FA, Gugel B, Exner VM, Kirste G, Schollmeyer PJ. Bone mineral density after kidney transplantation: a cross-sectional study in 190-graft recipients up to 20 years after transplantation. *Transplantation.* 1995;59(7):982-986.

Gutin PH. Corticosteroid therapy in patients with brain tumors. *Natl Cancer Inst Monogr.* 1977;46:151-156.

Henderson JJ, Hartmann PE, Newnham JP, Simmer K. Effect of preterm birth and antenatal corticosteroid treatment on lactogenesis II in women. *Pediatrics.* 2008;121(1):e92-100.

Hochberg MC, Altman RD, April KT, et al. American College of Rheumatology 2012 recommendations for the use of nonpharmacologic and pharmacologic therapies in osteoarthritis of the hand, hip, and knee. *Arthritis Care Res (Hoboken).* 2012;64(4):465-474.

Kimberly RP. Glucocorticoids. *Curr Opin Rheumatol.* 1994;6 (3):273-280.

Koutroulis I, Papoutsis J, Kroumpouzos G. Atopic dermatitis in pregnancy: current status and challenges. *Obstet Gynecol Surv.* 2011;66 (10):654-663.

Kushner BJ. The treatment of periorbital infantile hemangioma with intralesional corticosteroid. *Plast Reconstruc Surg.* 1985;76 (4):517-524.

Lam DS, Fan DS, Ng JS, Yu CB, Wong CY, Cheung AY. Ocular hypertensive and anti-inflammatory responses to different dosages of topical dexamethasone in children: a randomized trial. *Clin Experiment Ophthalmol.* 2005;33(3):252-258.

Leachman SA, Reed BR. The use of dermatologic drugs in pregnancy and lactation. *Dermatol Clin.* 2006;24(2):167-197.

Leonard MB. Glucocorticoid-induced osteoporosis in children: impact of the underlying disease. *Pediatrics.* 2007;119 (Suppl 2):S166-174.

Liggins GC, Howie RN. A controlled trial of antepartum glucocorticoid treatment of respiratory distress syndrome in premature infants. *Pediatrics.* 1972;50(4):515-525.

Lowenthal RM, Jestrimski KW. Corticosteroid drugs: their role in oncological practice. *Med J Aust.* 1986;144(2):81-85.

Lunghi L, Pavan B, Biondi C, et al. Use of glucocorticoids in pregnancy. *Curr Pharm Des.* 2010;16(32):3616-3637.

Makol A, Wright K, Amin S. Rheumatoid arthritis and pregnancy: safety considerations in pharmacological management. *Drugs.* 2011;71 (15):1973-1987.

McGee S, Hirschmann J. Use of corticosteroids in treating infectious diseases. *Arch Intern Med.* 2008;168(10):1034-1046.

Murphy VE, Fittock RJ, Zarzycki PK, Delahunty MM, Smith R, Clifton VL. Metabolism of synthetic steroids by the human placenta. *Placenta.* 2007;28(1):39-46.

Østensen M, Forger F. Management of RA medications in pregnant patients. *Nat Rev Rheumatol.* 2009;5(7):382-390.

Ost L, Wettrell G, Björkhem I, Rane A, Prednisolone excretion in human milk. *J Pediatr.* 1985;106(6):1008-1011.

Park-Wyllie L, Mazzotta P, Pastuszak A, et al. Birth defects after maternal exposure to corticosteroids: prospective cohort study and meta-analysis of epidemiological studies. *Teratology.* 2000;62 (6):385-392.

Pradat P, Robert-Gnansia E, Di Tanna GL, et al. First trimester exposure to corticosteroids and oral clefts. *Birth Defects Res A Clin Mol Teratol.* 2003;67(12):968-970.

Prasetyono TO, Djoenaedi I. Efficacy of intralesional steroid injection in head and neck hemangioma: a systematic review. *Ann Plast Surg.* 2011;66(1):98-106.

Report of a Workshop by the British Association for Paediatric Nephrology and Research Unit, Royal College of Physicians. Consensus statement on management and audit potential for steroid responsive nephrotic syndrome, *Arch Dis Child.* 1994;70(2):151-157.

Betamethasone (Topical) (bay ta METH a sone)

Medication Safety Issues

Sound-alike/look-alike issues:

Luxiq may be confused with Lasix

Related Information

Topical Corticosteroids *on page 2224*

Brand Names: U.S. AlphaTrex; Diprolene; Diprolene AF; Luxiq

Brand Names: Canada Betaderm; Betnesol; Celestoderm V; Celestoderm V/2; Diprolene; Diprosone; Luxiq; Prevex B; ratio-Ectosone; Ratio-Topilene; Ratio-Topisone; Rivasone; Rolene; Rosone; Taro-Sone; Valisone Scalp Lotion

Therapeutic Category Corticosteroid, Topical

Generic Availability (U.S.) Yes

Use

Betamethasone dipropionate (augmented): Treatment of inflammation and pruritus associated with corticosteroid-responsive dermatoses of the skin (Cream, lotion, and ointment: FDA approved in ages ≥13 years and adults; Gel: FDA approved in ages ≥12 years and adults)

Betamethasone valerate:

Cream, lotion, and ointment: Treatment of inflammation and pruritus associated with corticosteroid-responsive dermatoses of the skin (FDA approved in pediatric patients [age not specified] and adults)

Foam: Treatment of inflammation and pruritus associated with corticosteroid-responsive dermatoses of the scalp including psoriasis (FDA approved in adults)

Pregnancy Risk Factor C

Pregnancy Considerations Adverse events have been observed with corticosteroids in animal reproduction studies. Topical corticosteroids are preferred over systemic for treating conditions, such as psoriasis or atopic dermatitis in pregnant women; high potency corticosteroids are not recommended during the first trimester. Topical products are not recommended for extensive use, in large quantities, or for long periods of time in pregnant women (Bae, 2011; Koutroulis, 2011; Leachman, 2006). Refer to the Betamethasone Systemic monograph for additional information.

Breast-Feeding Considerations Corticosteroids are excreted in human milk. It is not known if systemic absorption following topical administration results in detectable quantities in human milk. Do not apply topical corticosteroids to nipples; hypertension was noted in a nursing infant exposed to a topical corticosteroid while nursing (Leachman, 2006).

The manufacturer notes that when used systemically, maternal use of corticosteroids have the potential to cause adverse events in a nursing infant (eg, growth suppression, interfere with endogenous corticosteroid production) and therefore recommends that caution be exercised when administering betamethasone to nursing women.

Contraindications Hypersensitivity to betamethasone, other corticosteroids, or any component

Warnings Topical corticosteroids may be absorbed percutaneously. The extent of absorption is dependent on several factors, including epidermal integrity (intact vs abraded skin), formulation, age of the patient, prolonged duration of use, and the use of occlusive dressings. Percutaneous absorption of topical steroids is increased in neonates (especially preterm neonates), infants, and young children.

Hypothalamic-pituitary-adrenal (HPA) suppression may occur, particularly in younger children or in patients receiving high doses for prolonged periods; acute adrenal insufficiency (adrenal crisis) may occur with abrupt withdrawal after long-term therapy or with stress. Patients receiving large doses of potent topical steroids should be periodically evaluated for HPA axis suppression using urinary free cortisol and ACTH stimulation tests. HPA axis suppression was observed in 32% of infants and children (age range: 3 months to 12 years) being treated with betamethasone dipropionate cream (0.05%) for atopic dermatitis in an open-label trial (n=60); the incidence was greater in younger patients vs older children (mean reported incidence for age ranges: ≤1 year: 50%; 2 to 8 years: 32% to 38%; 9 to 12 years: 17%). If HPA suppression occurs, consider withdrawal of betamethasone, reduction in frequency of application or substitution with a less potent steroid. Recovery is usually prompt and complete upon drug discontinuation, but may require supplemental systemic corticosteroids if signs and symptoms of steroid withdrawal occur. In stressful situations, HPA axis-suppressed patients may require doses of systemic glucocorticoids prior to, during, and after unusual stress (eg, surgery). Infants and small children may be more susceptible to HPA axis suppression, intracranial hypertension, Cushing syndrome, or other systemic toxicities due to larger skin surface area to body mass ratio. Prolonged use may also affect growth velocity; growth should be routinely monitored in pediatric patients; use with caution in pediatric patients. Use lowest dose possible for shortest period of time to avoid HPA axis suppression. Use should be limited to small areas and for a period of ≤2 weeks to minimize adverse effects. Avoid concurrent use of other corticosteroids.

Betamethasone valerate foam products contains propylene glycol; toxicities have been reported with use of products containing propylene glycol, including hyperosmolality, lactic acidosis, seizures and respiratory depression; in neonates large amounts of propylene glycol delivered orally, intravenously (eg, >3000 mg/day), or topically have been associated with potentially fatal toxicities which can include metabolic acidosis, seizures, renal failure, and CNS depression; use foam products containing propylene glycol with caution (AAP, 1997; Shehab, 2009).

Precautions Do not use for diaper dermatitis. Avoid use with occlusive dressing or application to denuded skin or to large surface areas. Avoid using higher than recommended doses; suppression of HPA axis function may occur. Reduction in growth velocity may occur when corticosteroids are administered to pediatric patients by any route; monitor growth. Prolonged use may result in fungal or bacterial superinfection. Use may be associated with local sensitization. Augmented gel, lotion, or ointment should not be used for the treatment of rosacea or perioral dermatitis and should not be applied to the face, groin, or in the axillae.

Foam: Formulation contains alcohol and propane/butane; do not expose to open flame or smoking during or immediately after application. Do not puncture or incinerate container.

Adverse Reactions

Dermatologic: Acneiform eruptions, allergic dermatitis, burning, dry skin, erythema, folliculitis, hypertrichosis, irritation, miliaria, pruritus, skin atrophy, striae, vesiculation

Endocrine and metabolic effects have occasionally been reported with topical use.

Drug Interactions

Metabolism/Transport Effects None known.

Avoid Concomitant Use

Avoid concomitant use of Betamethasone (Topical) with any of the following: Aldesleukin

Increased Effect/Toxicity

Betamethasone (Topical) may increase the levels/effects of: Ceritinib; Deferasirox

The levels/effects of Betamethasone (Topical) may be increased by: Telaprevir

Decreased Effect

Betamethasone (Topical) may decrease the levels/ effects of: Aldesleukin; Corticorelin; Hyaluronidase; Telaprevir

Stability

Betamethasone dipropionate (augmented formulations):
Cream/lotion/ointment: Store at 25°C (77°F); excursions permitted to 15°C to 30°C (59°F to 86°F).
Gel: Store between 2°C and 25°C (36°F and 77°F).
Betamethasone valerate:
Cream/lotion/ointment: Store at 15°C to 30°C (59°F to 86°F).
Foam: Store at 20°C to 25°C (68°F to 77°F). Do not expose to heat and/or store at ≥49°C (120°F). Do not store in direct sunlight. Contents are flammable.

Mechanism of Action Controls the rate of protein synthesis; depresses the migration of polymorphonuclear leukocytes, fibroblasts; reverses capillary permeability and lysosomal stabilization at the cellular level to prevent or control inflammation

Pharmacokinetics (Adult data unless noted)

Absorption: Topical corticosteroids are absorbed percutaneously. The extent of absorption is dependent on several factors, including epidermal integrity (intact vs abraded skin), formulation, age of the patient, prolonged duration of use, and the use of occlusive dressings. Percutaneous absorption of topical steroids is increased in neonates (especially preterm neonates), infants, and young children.

Metabolism: Hepatic

Elimination: Urine and bile

Dosing: Usual Dosage should be based on severity of disease and patient response; use smallest amount for shortest period of time to avoid HPA axis suppression.

Note: Therapy should be discontinued when control is achieved.

Pediatric: **Dermatoses (corticosteroid-responsive):** Topical:

Betamethasone valerate:

Cream/ointment: Children and Adolescents: Apply a thin film to the affected area once to 3 times daily; usually once or twice daily application is effective.

Lotion: Children and Adolescents: Apply a few drops to the affected area twice daily; in some cases, more frequent application may be necessary; following improvement reduce to once daily application

Betamethasone dipropionate (augmented formulation):

Cream/ointment: Adolescents: Apply a thin film to affected area once or twice daily; maximum dose: 50 g/week; evaluate continuation of therapy if no improvement within 2 weeks of treatment.

Gel: Children and Adolescents ≥12 years: Apply a thin layer to the affected area once or twice daily; rub in gently; maximum dose: 50 g/week; not recommended for use longer than 2 weeks

Lotion: Adolescents: Apply a few drops to the affected area once or twice daily; rub in gently; maximum dose: 50 mL/week; not recommended for use for longer than 2 weeks.

Adult:

Dermatoses (corticosteroid-responsive): Topical:

Cream: Apply 1 to 3 times daily; **Note**: Twice daily application is usually effective.

Cream, augmented formulation: Apply once or twice daily (maximum dose: 45 g week). **Note:** Reassess if no improvement after 2 weeks of treatment.

Gel, augmented formulation: Apply once or twice daily; rub in gently (maximum: 50 g/week); **Note:** Reassess if no improvement after 2 weeks of treatment.

Lotion: Apply a few drops twice daily

Lotion, augmented formulation: Apply a few drops once or twice daily; rub in gently (maximum dose: 50 mL/week). **Note**: Reassess if no improvement after 2 weeks of treatment.

Ointment: Apply 1 to 3 times daily; **Note:** Twice daily application is usually effective.

Ointment, augmented formulation: Apply once or twice daily (maximum dose: 50 g/week); **Note:** Reassess if no improvement after 2 weeks of treatment.

Psoriasis: Foam: Apply to the scalp twice daily, once in the morning and once at night; **Note:** Therapy should be discontinued when control is achieved; reassess if no improvement after 2 weeks of treatment.

Dosing adjustment in renal impairment: There are no dosage adjustments provided in the manufacturer's labeling.

Dosing adjustment in hepatic impairment: There are no dosage adjustments provided in the manufacturer's labeling.

Administration Topical: For external use only. Apply sparingly to affected areas. Not for use on broken skin or in areas of infection. Do not apply to wet skin unless directed; do not cover with occlusive dressing. Do not apply very high potency agents to face, groin, axillae, or diaper area.

Betamethasone valerate:

Foam: Invert can and dispense a small amount onto a saucer or other cool surface. Do not dispense directly into hands as foam will begin to melt immediately upon contact with warm skin. Pick up small amounts of foam and gently massage into affected areas until foam disappears. Repeat until entire affected scalp area is treated. Avoid fire, flame, and/or smoking during and immediately following application.

Lotion: Shake well prior to use.

Monitoring Parameters Growth in pediatric patients; assess HPA axis suppression (eg, ACTH stimulation test, morning plasma cortisol test, urinary free cortisol test)

Test Interactions May suppress the wheal and flare reactions to skin test antigens

Additional Information

Very high potency (super high potency): Augmented betamethasone dipropionate ointment, lotion

High potency: Augmented betamethasone dipropionate cream, betamethasone dipropionate cream and ointment

Intermediate potency: Betamethasone dipropionate lotion, betamethasone valerate cream

Dosage Forms Excipient information presented when available (limited, particularly for generics); consult specific product labeling.

Cream, External, as dipropionate [strength expressed as base]:

Diprolene AF: 0.05% (15 g, 50 g)

Generic: 0.05% (15 g, 45 g, 50 g)

Cream, External, as valerate [strength expressed as base]:

Generic: 0.1% (15 g, 45 g)

Foam, External, as valerate:

Luxiq: 0.12% (50 g, 100 g) [contains alcohol, usp, cetyl alcohol, propylene glycol]

Foam, External, as valerate [strength expressed as base]:

Generic: 0.12% (50 g, 100 g)

Gel, External, as dipropionate [strength expressed as base]:

AlphaTrex: 0.05% (15 g, 50 g)

Generic: 0.05% (15 g, 50 g)

Lotion, External, as dipropionate [strength expressed as base]:

Diprolene: 0.05% (30 mL, 60 mL) [contains isopropyl alcohol, propylene glycol]

Generic: 0.05% (30 mL, 60 mL)

Lotion, External, as valerate [strength expressed as base]:

Generic: 0.1% (60 mL)

Ointment, External, as dipropionate [strength expressed as base]:

Diprolene: 0.05% (15 g, 50 g)

Generic: 0.05% (15 g, 45 g, 50 g)

Ointment, External, as valerate [strength expressed as base]:

Generic: 0.1% (15 g, 45 g)

References

American Academy of Pediatrics Committee on Drugs. "Inactive" ingredients in pharmaceutical products: update (subject review). *Pediatrics.* 1997;99(2):268-278.

Bae YS, Van Voorhees AS, Hsu S, et al, "Review of Treatment Options For Psoriasis in Pregnant or Lactating Women: From the Medical Board of the National Psoriasis Foundation," *J Am Acad Dermatol,* 2012, 67(3):459-77.

Betamethasone dipropionate [prescribing information]. Melville, NY: Fougera Pharmaceuticals, Inc; May 2012.

Betamethasone valerate (augmented cream, ointment, and lotion formulations) [prescribing information]. Melville, NY: Fougera; March 2013.

Diprolene AF (augmented betamethasone dipropionate) [prescribing information]. Whitehouse Station, NJ: Merck & Co, Inc; May 2012.

Diprolene (augmented betamethasone dipropionate) [prescribing information]. Whitehouse Station, NJ: Merck & Co, Inc; October 2012.

Koutroulis I, Papoutsis J, and Kroumpouzos G, "Atopic Dermatitis in Pregnancy: Current Status and Challenges," *Obstet Gynecol Surv,* 2011, 66(10):654-63.

Leachman SA and Reed BR, "The Use of Dermatologic Drugs in Pregnancy and Lactation," *Dermatol Clin,* 2006, 24(2):167-97, vi.

Luxiq (betamethasone valerate) [prescribing information]. Research Triangle Park, NC: Stiefel Laboratories, Inc; June 2011.

Shehab N, Lewis CL, Streetman DD, Donn SM. Exposure to the pharmaceutical excipients benzyl alcohol and propylene glycol among critically ill neonates. *Pediatr Crit Care Med.* 2009;10 (2):256-259.

◆ **Betamethasone Acetate** *see* Betamethasone (Systemic) *on page 282*

◆ **Betamethasone Dipropionate** *see* Betamethasone (Topical) *on page 285*

◆ **Betamethasone Dipropionate, Augmented** *see* Betamethasone (Topical) *on page 285*

◆ **Betamethasone Sodium Phosphate** *see* Betamethasone (Systemic) *on page 282*

◆ **Betamethasone Valerate** *see* Betamethasone (Topical) *on page 285*

◆ **Betapace** *see* Sotalol *on page 1925*

◆ **Betapace AF** *see* Sotalol *on page 1925*

◆ **Betasal [OTC]** *see* Salicylic Acid *on page 1860*

◆ **Betasept Surgical Scrub [OTC]** *see* Chlorhexidine Gluconate *on page 441*

◆ **Betaxin (Can)** *see* Thiamine *on page 2009*

Bethanechol (be THAN e kole)

Medication Safety Issues
Sound-alike/look-alike issues:
Bethanechol may be confused with betaxolol
Brand Names: U.S. Urecholine
Brand Names: Canada Duvoid®; PHL-Bethanechol; PMS-Bethanechol
Therapeutic Category Cholinergic Agent
Generic Availability (U.S.) Yes
Use Treatment of nonobstructive urinary retention and retention due to neurogenic bladder; gastroesophageal reflux
Pregnancy Risk Factor C
Pregnancy Considerations Reproduction studies have not been conducted.
Breast-Feeding Considerations It is not known if bethanechol is excreted in breast milk. Due to the potential for serious adverse reactions in the nursing infant, a decision should be made whether to discontinue nursing or to discontinue the drug, taking into account the importance of treatment to the mother.
Contraindications Hypersensitivity to bethanechol chloride or any component; do not use in patients with mechanical obstruction of the GI or GU tract; do not use in patients with hyperthyroidism, peptic ulcer, bronchial asthma, or cardiac disease

Adverse Reactions
Cardiovascular: Flushing, hypotension, tachycardia
Central nervous system: Colic, headache, malaise, seizure
Dermatologic: Diaphoresis
Gastrointestinal: Abdominal cramps, borborygmi, diarrhea, eructation, nausea, salivation, vomiting
Genitourinary: Urinary urgency
Ophthalmic: Lacrimation, miosis
Respiratory: Asthma, bronchoconstriction

Drug Interactions
Metabolism/Transport Effects None known.
Avoid Concomitant Use There are no known interactions where it is recommended to avoid concomitant use.
Increased Effect/Toxicity
The levels/effects of bethanechol may be increased by: Acetylcholinesterase Inhibitors; Beta-Blockers
Decreased Effect There are no known significant interactions involving a decrease in effect.
Mechanism of Action Due to stimulation of the parasympathetic nervous system, bethanechol increases bladder muscle tone causing contractions which initiate urination. Bethanechol also stimulates gastric motility, increases gastric tone and may restore peristalsis.

Pharmacodynamics
Onset of action: Oral: 30-90 minutes
Duration: Oral: Up to 6 hours

Pharmacokinetics (Adult data unless noted)
Absorption: Oral: Variable
Metabolic fate and excretion have not been determined

Dosing: Usual Oral:
Children:
Abdominal distention or urinary retention: 0.6 mg/kg/day divided 3-4 times/day
Gastroesophageal reflux: 0.1-0.2 mg/kg/dose or 3 mg/m²/dose given 30 minutes to 1 hour before each meal to a maximum of 4 times/day
Adults: 10-50 mg 2-4 times/day
Administration Oral: Administer on an empty stomach to reduce nausea and vomiting
Test Interactions Increased lipase, amylase (S), bilirubin, aminotransferase [ALT/AST] (S)
Dosage Forms Excipient information presented when available (limited, particularly for generics); consult specific product labeling.
Tablet, Oral, as chloride:
Urecholine: 5 mg, 10 mg [scored]
Urecholine: 25 mg, 50 mg [scored; contains fd&c yellow #10 (quinoline yellow), fd&c yellow #6 (sunset yellow)]
Generic: 5 mg, 10 mg, 25 mg, 50 mg
Extemporaneous Preparations A 1 mg/mL solution may be made with tablets. Crush twelve 10 mg tablets in a mortar and reduce to a fine powder. Add small portions of sterile water and mix to a uniform paste; mix while adding sterile water in incremental proportions to **almost** 120 mL; transfer to a calibrated bottle, rinse mortar with sterile water, and add quantity of sterile water sufficient to make 120 mL. Label "shake well" and "refrigerate". Stable for 30 days (Schlatter, 1997).

A 5 mg/mL suspension may be made with tablets and either a 1:1 mixture of Ora-Plus® and Ora-Sweet® or Ora-Plus® and Ora-Sweet® SF or 1:4 concentrated cherry syrup and simple syrup, NF mixture. Crush twelve 50 mg tablets in a mortar and reduce to a fine powder. Add small portions of chosen vehicle and mix to a uniform paste; mix while adding the vehicle in incremental proportions to **almost** 120 mL; transfer to a calibrated bottle, rinse mortar with vehicle, and add quantity of vehicle sufficient to make 120 mL. Label "shake well" and "refrigerate". Stable for 60 days refrigerated (preferred) or at room temperature (Allen, 1998; Nahata, 2004).

Allen LV Jr and Erickson MA, "Stability of Bethanechol Chloride, Pyrazinamide, Quinidine Sulfate, Rifampin, and Tetracycline Hydrochloride in Extemporaneously Compounded Oral Liquids," *Am J Health Syst Pharm*, 1998, 55(17):1804-9.

Nahata MC, Pai VB, and Hipple TF, *Pediatric Drug Formulations*, 5th ed, Cincinnati, OH: Harvey Whitney Books Co, 2004.

Schlatter JL and Saulnier JL, "Bethanechol Chloride Oral Solutions: Stability and Use in Infants," *Ann Pharmacother*, 1997, 31(3):294-6.

◆ **Bethanechol Chloride** *see* Bethanechol *on page 288*

◆ **Bethkis** *see* Tobramycin (Systemic, Oral Inhalation) *on page 2034*

◆ **Betimol** *see* Timolol (Ophthalmic) *on page 2028*

◆ **Betnesol (Can)** *see* Betamethasone (Topical) *on page 285*

Bevacizumab (be vuh SIZ uh mab)

Medication Safety Issues
Sound-alike/look-alike issues:
Avastin may be confused with Astelin
Bevacizumab may be confused with brentuximab, cetuximab, ranibizumab, riTUXimab
High alert medication:
This medication is in a class the Institute for Safe Medication Practices (ISMP) includes among its list of drug classes which have a heightened risk of causing significant patient harm when used in error.
International issues:
Avastin [U.S., Canada, and multiple international markets] may be confused with Avaxim, a brand name for

hepatitis A vaccine [Canada and multiple international markets]

Related Information

Emetogenic Potential of Antineoplastic Agents in Children *on page 2327*

Brand Names: U.S. Avastin

Brand Names: Canada Avastin

Therapeutic Category Antineoplastic Agent, Monoclonal Antibody; Antineoplastic Agent, Vascular Endothelial Growth Factor (VEGF) Inhibitor; Vascular Endothelial Growth Factor (VEGF) Inhibitor

Generic Availability (U.S.) No

Use Treatment of metastatic colorectal cancer (FDA approved in adults); treatment of unresectable, locally advanced recurrent or metastatic nonsquamous, nonsmall cell lung cancer (FDA approved in adults); glioblastoma with progressive disease following prior therapy as single agent (FDA approved in adults); and metastatic renal cell cancer (FDA approved in adults). Has also been used in the treatment of pediatric refractory solid tumors and primary CNS tumors; has been used intravitreally for retinopathy of prematurity (Stage 3+).

Pregnancy Risk Factor C

Pregnancy Considerations Teratogenic effects have been observed in animal reproduction studies. Angiogenesis is of critical importance to human fetal development, and bevacizumab inhibits angiogenesis. Adequate contraception during therapy is recommended (and for ≥6 months following last dose of bevacizumab). Patients should also be counseled regarding prolonged exposure following discontinuation of therapy due to the long half-life of bevacizumab.

Based on animal studies, bevacizumab may disrupt normal menstrual cycles and impair fertility by several effects, including reduced endometrial proliferation and follicular developmental arrest. Some parameters do not recover completely, or recover very slowly following discontinuation.

Breast-Feeding Considerations It is not known if bevacizumab is excreted in breast milk. Immunoglobulins are excreted in breast milk, and it is assumed that bevacizumab may appear in breast milk. Because of the potential for serious adverse reactions in the nursing infant, the decision to discontinue bevacizumab or to discontinue breast-feeding during therapy should take into account the benefits of treatment to the mother. The half-life of bevacizumab is up to 50 days (average 20 days), and this should be considered when decisions are made concerning breast-feeding resumption.

Note: Canadian labeling recommends to discontinue breast-feeding during treatment and to avoid breast-feeding a minimum of 6 months following discontinuation of treatment.

Contraindications Hypersensitivity to bevacizumab, murine proteins, or any component.

Warnings Surgical and wound healing complications have been reported and were sometimes fatal (not related to treatment duration) **[U.S. Boxed Warning]**; monitor patients for signs/symptoms of improper wound healing. Permanently discontinue in patients who develop these complications. The appropriate intervals between administration of bevacizumab and surgical procedures to avoid impairment in wound healing has not been established. Do not initiate therapy within 28 days of major surgery and only following complete healing of the incision. Bevacizumab should be discontinued at least 28 days prior to elective surgery and the estimated half-life (20 days) should be considered. In a retrospective review of central venous access device placements, a greater risk of wound dehiscence was observed when port placement and

bevacizumab administration were separated by <14 days (Erinjeri, 2011).

Severe or fatal hemorrhage, including hemoptysis, gastrointestinal bleeding, central nervous system hemorrhage, epistaxis, and vaginal bleeding, have been reported up to 5 times more frequently if receiving bevacizumab; avoid use in patients with recent hemoptysis (>2.5 mL blood) **[U.S. Boxed Warning]**; significant pulmonary bleeding (primarily in patients with nonsmall cell lung cancer with squamous cell histology) has also been reported; discontinuation of treatment is recommended in all patients with serious hemorrhage. Use with caution in patients with CNS metastases; one case of CNS hemorrhage was observed in a study of NSCLC patients with CNS metastases. Use with caution in patients at risk for thrombocytopenia.

Infection with resultant permanent vision loss has been reported following intravitreal injection of repackaged bevacizumab; use proper aseptic technique when manipulating commercially available dosage forms. Some experts recommend caution regarding use in premature neonates for ROP outside of controlled, clinical trials (Quinn, 2011); systemic absorption after intravitreal administration with decreases in VEGF serum concentration (as low as 9% of baseline systemic concentration) have been reported in a case series of 11 neonates (Sato, 2012); short- and long-term implications of systemic exposure are unknown; monitoring is recommended.

May cause CHF and/or potentiate cardiotoxic effects of anthracyclines. CHF is more common with prior anthracycline exposure and/or left chest wall irradiation. Among approved and nonapproved uses evaluated thus far, the incidence of heart failure (HF) and/or left ventricular dysfunction (including LVEF decline) is higher in patients receiving bevacizumab plus chemotherapy when compared to chemotherapy alone; use with caution in patients with cardiovascular disease; the safety of therapy resumption or continuation in patients with cardiac dysfunction has not been studied. In studies of patients with metastatic breast cancer, the incidence of grades 3 or 4 HF was increased in patients receiving bevacizumab plus paclitaxel when compared to the control arm; patients with metastatic breast cancer who received prior anthracycline therapy had a higher rate of HF compared to those receiving paclitaxel alone (3.8% vs 0.6%, respectively). Bevacizumab is no longer FDA approved for the treatment of breast cancer.

Bevacizumab may cause and/or worsen hypertension significantly; use with caution in patients with preexisting hypertension and monitor BP closely (every 2-3 weeks during treatment; regularly after discontinuation if bevacizumab-induced hypertension occurs or worsens). Permanent discontinuation is recommended in patients who experience hypertensive crisis or encephalopathy. Temporarily discontinue in patients who develop uncontrolled hypertension. Proteinuria and/or nephrotic syndrome have been associated with bevacizumab; risk is increased in patients with a history of hypertension; interrupt therapy for moderate to severe proteinuria pending further evaluation; in adults, withhold treatment for ≥2 g proteinuria/24 hours and resume when proteinuria is <2 g/24 hours; discontinue in patients with nephrotic syndrome.

Cases of reversible posterior leukoencephalopathy syndrome (RPLS) have been reported; discontinue therapy if RPLS occurs. Symptoms such as headache, seizure, confusion, lethargy, blindness, or other vision or neurologic disturbances may occur from 16 hours to 1 year after treatment initiation. Resolution of symptoms usually occurs within days after discontinuation; however, neurologic sequelae may remain. RPLS may be associated with hypertension; discontinue bevacizumab and begin ▶

management of hypertension if present. Bevacizumab is associated with hypersensitivity reactions and/or infusion-related reactions. Interrupt therapy if patient experiences severe hypersensitivity reaction or infusion reaction which includes hypertension, hypertensive crises associated with neurologic manifestations, wheezing, oxygen desaturation, chest pain, headaches, rigors, and diaphoresis. Micro-angiopathic hemolytic anemia (MAHA) has been reported when bevacizumab has been used in combination with sunitinib.

Bevacizumab may impair fertility and have adverse effects on fetal development; adequate contraception during therapy and following discontinuation is recommended. In premenopausal women receiving bevacizumab in combination with mFOLFOX (fluorouracil/oxaliplatin based chemotherapy) the incidence of ovarian failure (amenorrhea ≥3 months) was higher (34%) compared to women who received mFOLFOX alone (2%). Ovarian function recovered in some patients after treatment was discontinued. Premenopausal women should be informed of the potential risk of ovarian failure.

Bevacizumab, in combination with chemotherapy (or biologic therapy), is associated with an increased risk of treatment-related mortality; a higher risk of fatal adverse events was identified in a meta-analysis of 16 trials in which bevacizumab was used for the treatment of various cancers (breast cancer, colorectal cancer, nonsmall cell lung cancer, pancreatic cancer, prostate cancer, and renal cell cancer) and compared to chemotherapy alone (Ranpura, 2011).

An increased risk for arterial thromboembolic events (eg, stroke, MI, TIA, angina) is associated with bevacizumab use in combination with chemotherapy. History of arterial thromboembolism or ≥65 years of age may present an even greater risk; permanently discontinue if serious arterial thromboembolic event occurs. Although patients with cancer are at risk for venous thromboembolism, a meta-analysis of 15 controlled trials has demonstrated an increased risk for venous thromboembolism in patients who received bevacizumab (Nalluri, 2008).

Gastrointestinal perforation, sometimes fatal, has been reported **[U.S. Boxed Warning]**; most cases occur within 50 days of treatment initiation; monitor for signs/symptoms (eg, fever, abdominal pain with constipation and/or nausea/vomiting). Severe and sometimes fatal fistula formation (including enterocutaneous, esophageal, duodenal, and rectal fistulas) and nongastrointestinal fistulas (including tracheoesophageal, bronchopleural, biliary, vaginal, and bladder fistulas) most commonly within the first 6 months of treatment; discontinue therapy in patients who develop these complications.

When used in combination with myelosuppressive chemotherapy, increased rates of severe or febrile neutropenia and neutropenic infection were reported. The incidence of hand-foot syndrome is increased in patients treated with bevacizumab plus sorafenib in comparison to those treated with sorafenib monotherapy. Osteonecrosis of the jaw has been associated with bevacizumab use alone or in combination with other chemotherapies, steroids, and bisphosphonates. A report of three pediatric patients (ages: 10 years, 13 years, and 17 years) has also described cases of osteonecrosis of the wrist and knee (Fangusaro, 2013).

Precautions Use with caution in patients with cardiovascular disease or acquired coagulopathy. Ocular inflammation has been reported with repeated intravitreal use; monitor patients for signs or symptoms. Use with caution in patients with renal or hepatic impairment; safety and efficacy have not been established. An increase in diastolic and systolic blood pressures was noted in a retrospective review of patients with renal insufficiency (CrCl ≤60 mL/minute) who received bevacizumab for renal cell cancer (Gupta, 2011).

Adverse Reactions Reported monotherapy and as part of combination chemotherapy regimens.

Cardiovascular: Arterial thrombosis (including cardio-/cerebrovascular), cardiac failure, deep vein thrombosis, hyper-/hypotension, intra-abdominal thrombosis (venous), pulmonary embolism, syncope, thromboembolism, venous thromboembolism, ventricular dysfunction (left)

Central nervous system: Dizziness, fatigue, headache, pain, neuropathy, taste disorder, voice disorder

Dermatologic: Acne vulgaris, alopecia, dermal ulcer, exfoliative dermatitis, skin discoloration, xeroderma

Endocrine & metabolic: Dehydration, hyponatremia, weight loss

Gastrointestinal: Abdominal pain, anorexia, colitis, constipation, diarrhea, dry mouth, dyspepsia, fistula, flatulence, gastritis, gastrointestinal hemorrhage, gastrointestinal perforation, gastroesophageal reflux disease, gingival hemorrhage (minor), gingival pain, gingivitis, intestinal obstruction, nausea, oral mucosa ulcer, stomatitis, vomiting, xerostomia

Genitourinary: Proteinuria (median onset: 5.6 months; median time to resolution: 6.1 months), vaginal hemorrhage

Hematologic & oncologic: Febrile neutropenia, hemorrhage (including CNS), leukopenia, neutropenia, neutropenic infection, thrombocytopenia

Infection: Abscess (tooth; intra-abdominal), infection (pneumonia, catheter infection, or wound infection)

Neuromuscular & skeletal: Back pain, myalgia, weakness

Ophthalmic: Blurred vision

Otic: Deafness, tinnitus

Respiratory: Dyspnea, epistaxis, hemoptysis (nonsquamous histology), pneumonitis, rhinitis, upper respiratory tract infection

Miscellaneous: Infusion related reaction, postoperative wound complication (including dehiscence)

Rare but important or life-threatening: Anaphylaxis, anastomotic ulcer, angina pectoris, antibody development (anti-bevacizumab and neutralizing), bladder fistula, bronchopleural fistula, cerebral infarction, conjunctival hemorrhage, endophthalmitis (infectious and sterile), enterocutaneous fistula, fistula of bile duct, fulminant necrotizing fasciitis, gastrointestinal fistula (including duodenal and esophageal), gastrointestinal ulcer, hemolytic anemia (microangiopathic; when used in combination with sunitinib), hemorrhagic stroke, hypersensitivity, hypertensive crisis, hypertensive encephalopathy, increased intraocular pressure, inflammation of anterior segment of eye (toxic anterior segment syndrome), intestinal necrosis, intraocular inflammation (iritis, vitritis), mesenteric thrombosis, myocardial infarction, nasal septum perforation, nephrotic syndrome, ocular hyperemia, osteonecrosis (jaw), ovarian failure, pancytopenia, permanent vision loss, polyserositis, pulmonary hemorrhage, pulmonary hypertension, rectal fistula, renal failure, renal fistula, renal thrombotic microangiopathy, retinal detachment, retinal hemorrhage, reversible posterior leukoencephalopathy syndrome (RPLS), sepsis, subarachnoid hemorrhage, tracheoesophageal fistula, transient ischemic attacks, ureteral spasm, vaginal fistula, vitreous hemorrhage, vitreous opacity

Drug Interactions

Metabolism/Transport Effects None known.

Avoid Concomitant Use

Avoid concomitant use of Bevacizumab with any of the following: Belimumab; CloZAPine; Dipyrone; SUNItinib

Increased Effect/Toxicity

Bevacizumab may increase the levels/effects of: Antineoplastic Agents (Anthracycline, Systemic); Belimumab;

Bisphosphonate Derivatives; CloZAPine; Irinotecan; SORAfenib; SUNItinib

The levels/effects of Bevacizumab may be increased by: Abciximab; Dipyrone; SUNItinib

Decreased Effect There are no known significant interactions involving a decrease in effect.

Stability Store vials at 2°C to 8°C (36°F to 46°F); protect from light; do not freeze or shake. **Do not mix** with dextrose-containing solutions (concentration-dependent degradation may occur). Diluted solution is stable for up to 8 hours under refrigeration.

Mechanism of Action Bevacizumab is a recombinant, humanized monoclonal antibody which binds to, and neutralizes, vascular endothelial growth factor (VEGF), preventing its association with endothelial receptors, Flt-1 and KDR. VEGF binding initiates angiogenesis (endothelial proliferation and the formation of new blood vessels). The inhibition of microvascular growth is believed to retard the growth of all tissues (including metastatic tissue).

Pharmacokinetics (Adult data unless noted)
Half-life:
I.V.:
Pediatric patients (age: 1-21 years): Median: 11.8 days (range: 4.4-14.6 days) (Glade-Bender, 2008)
Adults: 20 days (range: 11-50 days)
Intravitreal: ~5-10 days (Bakri, 2007; Krohne, 2008)

Dosing: Neonatal Retinopathy of prematurity (ROP): Limited data available; dosing regimens variable; optimal dose not established: PMA ≥31 weeks and PNA ≥28 days: Intravitreal injection: Usual dosing: 0.625 mg (0.025 mL) as a single dose in the affected eye; dosing was used in 70 premature neonates (140 eyes) with Stage 3+ ROP in a prospective, randomized comparative trial with laser therapy; the primary outcome studied was recurrence of ROP, which was lower in the treatment group (6%) compared to conventional laser therapy (26%) (Mintz-Hittner, 2011). This same dose was used in a larger retrospective trial of 85 preterm neonates (162 eyes) with Stage 3 ROP as either primary therapy or salvage therapy after laser treatment; ROP regression occurred in 83% of treated eyes (Wu, 2013). Other doses reported range from 0.37-1.25 mg in the affected eye (Harder, 2013, Micieli, 2009; Spandau, 2013). Some experts recommend caution regarding use outside of a clinical trial (Quinn, 2011); systemic absorption with decreases in VEGF serum concentration have been reported in a case series of 11 neonates after intravitreal administration of doses consistent with those in reported in the literature (Sato, 2012); further studies are needed.

Dosing: Usual Refer to individual protocols; details concerning dosing in combination regimens should also be consulted.

Children and Adolescents:
Refractory solid tumor: Limited data available: I.V.: 5-15 mg/kg/dose every 2 weeks in a 28-day course (Glade-Bender, 2008) **or** 5-10 mg/kg every 2-3 weeks (Benesch, 2008)
Primary CNS tumor; recurrent/refractory (high/low grade gliomas, medulloblastoma): Limited data available; efficacy results variable: I.V.: 10 mg/kg/dose every 2 weeks (Aguilera, 2011; Aguilera, 2013; Packer, 2009; Parekh, 2011; Reismüller, 2010) or days 1 and 15 of each 28 day cycle (Kang, 2008); mostly used in combination with irinotecan with/without temozolmide **or** 15 mg/kg/dose every 3 weeks has also been used (Parekh, 2011; Reismüller, 2010). In general, when treating high-grade glioma, patients with contrast-enhancing disease showed greater response or remained stable, while patients with noncontrast-enhancing disease had disease progression (Parekh, 2011); others have observed only minimal efficacy in patients with high grade glioma (Narayana, 2010)

Adults:
Colorectal cancer, metastatic, in combination with fluorouracil-based chemotherapy: I.V.: 5 mg/kg every 2 weeks in combination with bolus IFL **or** 10 mg/kg every 2 weeks in combination with FOLFOX4
Colorectal cancer, metastatic, following first-line therapy containing bevacizumab: I.V.: 5 mg/kg every 2 weeks **or** 7.5 mg/kg every 3 weeks in combination with fluoropyrimidine-irinotecan or fluoropyrimidine-oxaliplatin based regimen
Non-small cell lung cancer (nonsquamous): I.V.: 15 mg/kg every 3 weeks in combination with carboplatin and paclitaxel
Glioblastoma: I.V.: 10 mg/kg every 2 weeks as monotherapy
Renal cell cancer, metastatic: I.V.: 10 mg/kg every 2 weeks in combination with interferon alfa
Dosing adjustment for renal impairment: There are no dosage adjustments provided in manufacturer's labeling.
Dosing adjustment for hepatic impairment: There are no dosage adjustments provided in manufacturer's labeling.

Administration
Parenteral: I.V. infusion: Dilute prescribed dose of bevacizumab in 100 mL NS; infuse the initial dose over 90 minutes; second infusion may be shortened to 60 minutes if the initial infusion is well-tolerated. Third and subsequent infusions may be shortened to 30 minutes if the 60-minute infusion is well-tolerated. Do **not** administer via I.V. push.
Intravitreal injection: Inject undiluted bevacizumab solution. The major clinical trial for ROP used an insulin syringe (0.3 mL syringe with a 31 gauge, 5/16 inch needle) to accurately deliver the dose; each 1 unit on an insulin syringe is equivalent to 0.01 mL; typical bevacizumab dose of 0.625 mg would equate to 2.5 units on an insulin syringe using a 25 mg/mL solution. In this ROP trial, the injection site was anesthetized with a drop of tetracaine hydrochloride 0.5% ophthalmic solution or proparacaine hydrochloride 0.5% ophthalmic solution prior to bevacizumab administration and sterilized before and after administration with a drop of povidone-iodine 5% ophthalmic solution. Following the procedure, a topical ophthalmic antibiotic drop was also administered every 6 hours for 7 days (Mintz-Hittner, 2011).
pH: 6.2

Monitoring Parameters
I.V. administration: Monitor for signs of an infusion reaction during infusion; blood pressure (continue to monitor blood pressure during and after bevacizumab has been discontinued). Monitor CBC with differential; signs/symptoms of GI perforation or abscess (abdominal pain, constipation, vomiting, fever); signs/symptoms of bleeding including hemoptysis, GI bleeding, CNS bleeding, epistaxis. Signs of wound dehiscence or healing complications. Urinalysis for proteinuria, nephrotic syndrome
Intravitreal administration: Monitor blood pressure, heart rate, respiratory rate, and oxygen saturation prior to, during, and after the procedure; monitor for signs and symptoms of infection or ocular inflammation; consider short- and long-term monitoring for sequelae of systemic absorption when used in neonates (Sato, 2012)

Dosage Forms Excipient information presented when available (limited, particularly for generics); consult specific product labeling.
Solution, Intravenous [preservative free]:
Avastin: 100 mg/4 mL (4 mL); 400 mg/16 mL (16 mL)

References
Aguilera DG, Goldman S, Fangusaro J. Bevacizumab and irinotecan in the treatment of children with recurrent/refractory medulloblastoma. *Pediatr Blood Cancer.* 2011;56:491-494.
Aguilera D, Mazewskli C, Fangusaro J, et al. Response to bevacizumab, irinotecan, and temozolomide in children with relapsed

medulloblastoma: a multi-institutional experience. *Childs Nerv Syst*. 2013;29:589-596.

Bakri SJ, Snyder MR, Reid JM, et al, "Pharmacokinetics of Intravitreal Bevacizumab (Avastin)," *Ophthalmology*, 2007, 114(5):855-9.

Benesch M, Windelberg M, Sauseng W, et al, "Compassionate Use of Bevacizumab (Avastin®) in Children and Young Adults With Refractory or Recurrent Solid Tumors," *Ann Oncol*, 2008, 19(4):807-13.

Choueiri TK, Mayer EL, Je Y, et al, "Congestive Heart Failure Risk in Patients With Breast Cancer Treated With Bevacizumab," *J Clin Oncol*, 2011, 29(6):632-8.

Erinjeri JP, Fong AJ, Kemeny NE, et al, "Timing of Administration of Bevacizumab Chemotherapy Affects Wound Healing After Chest Wall Port Placement," *Cancer*, 2011, 117(6):1296-301.

Fangusaro J, Gururangan S, Jakacki RI, et al. Bevacizumab-associated osteonecrosis of the wrist and knee in three pediatric patients with recurrent CNS tumors. *Journal of Clincial Oncology*. 2013;31(2): e24-27.

Glade Bender JL, Adamson PC, Reid JM, et al, "Phase I Trial and Pharmacokinetic Study of Bevacizumab in Pediatric Patients With Refractory Solid Tumors: A Children's Oncology Group Study," *J Clin Oncol*, 2008, 26(3):399-405.

Gupta S, Parsa VB, Heilbrun LK, et al, "Safety and Efficacy of Molecularly Targeted Agents in Patients With Metastatic Kidney Cancer With Renal Dysfunction," *Anticancer Drugs*, 2011, 22 (8):794-800.

Harder BC, von Baltz S, Jonas JB, Schlichtenbrede FC. Intravitreal low-dosage bevacizumab for retinopathy of prematurity. *Acta Ophthalmol*. 2013. [Epub ahead of print].

Kang TY, Jin T, Elinzano H, et al. Irinotecan and bevacizumab in progressive primary brain tumors, an evaluation of efficacy and safety. *J Neurooncol*. 2008;89:113-118.

Krohne TU, Eter N, Holz FG, et al, "Intraocular Pharmacokinetics of Bevacizumab After a Single Intravitreal Injection in Humans," *Am J Ophthalmol*, 2008, 146(4):508-12.

Micieli JA, Surkont M, and Smith AF, "A Systematic Analysis of the Off-Label Use of Bevacizumab for Severe Retinopathy of Prematurity," *Am J Ophthalmol*, 2009, 148(4):536-543.e2.

Mintz-Hittner HA, Kennedy KA, Chuang AZ, et al, "Efficacy of Intravitreal Bevacizumab for Stage 3+ Retinopathy of Prematurity," *N Engl J Med*, 2011, 364(7):603-15.

Mintz-Hittner HA, personal communication, August 2011.

Nalluri SR, Chu D, Keresztes R, et al, "Risk of Venous Thromboembolism With the Angiogenesis Inhibitor Bevacizumab in Cancer Patients: A Meta-Analysis," *JAMA*, 2008, 300(19):2277-85.

Narayana A, Kunnakkat S, Chacko-Mathew J, et al. Bevacizumab in recurrent high-grade pediatric gliomas. *Neuro Oncology*. 2010;12 (9):985-990.

Packer RJ, Jakacki R, Horn M, et al. Objective response of multiply recurrent low-grade gliomas to bevacizumab and irinotecan. *Pediatr Blood Cancer*. 2009;52:791-795.

Parekh C, Jubran R, Erdreich-Epstein A, et al. Treatment of children with recurrent high grade gliomas with a bevacizumab containing regimen. *J Neurooncol*. 2011;103: 673-680.

Quinn GE and Rubin SE, "Caution Urged in Using Bevacizumab Outside Clinical Trials, " *AAP News*, 2011, 32;46.

Ranpura V, Hapani S, and Wu S, "Treatment-Related Mortality With Bevacizumab in Cancer Patients," *JAMA*, 2011, 305(5):487-94.

Reismüller B, Azizi AA, Peyrl A, et al, "Feasibility and Tolerability of Bevacizumab in Children With Primary CNS Tumors," *Pediatr Blood Cancer*, 2010, 54(5):681-6.

Sato T, Wada K, Arahori H, et al, "Serum Concentrations of Bevacizumab (Avastin) and Vascular Endothelial Growth Factor in Infants With Retinopathy of Prematurity," *Am J Ophthalmol*, 2012, 153(2):327-333.

Spandau U, Tomic Z, Ewald U, et.al. Time to consider a new treatment protocol for aggressive posterior retinopathy of prematurity? *Acta Ophthalmologica*. 2013;170-175.

Wu W, Kuo H, Yeh P, et.al. An updated study of the use of bevacizumab in the treatment of patients with prethreshold retinopathy of prematurity in Taiwan. *Am J Ophthalmol*. 2013;155:150-158.

◆ **Biaxin** *see* Clarithromycin *on page 490*

◆ **Biaxin XL** *see* Clarithromycin *on page 490*

◆ **Biaxin XL Pac** *see* Clarithromycin *on page 490*

◆ **Biaxin BID (Can)** *see* Clarithromycin *on page 490*

◆ **Bicillin L-A** *see* Penicillin G Benzathine *on page 1629*

◆ **Bicillin® L-A (Can)** *see* Penicillin G Benzathine *on page 1629*

◆ **Bicitra** *see* Sodium Citrate and Citric Acid *on page 1906*

◆ **BiCNU** *see* Carmustine *on page 382*

◆ **BiCNU® (Can)** *see* Carmustine *on page 382*

◆ **Bidex [OTC]** *see* GuaiFENesin *on page 984*

◆ **BIG-IV** *see* Botulism Immune Globulin (Intravenous-Human) *on page 301*

◆ **Biltricide** *see* Praziquantel *on page 1723*

◆ **Bio-D-Mulsion [OTC]** *see* Cholecalciferol *on page 455*

◆ **Bio-D-Mulsion Forte [OTC]** *see* Cholecalciferol *on page 455*

◆ **Bio-Amitriptyline (Can)** *see* Amitriptyline *on page 133*

◆ **Bio-Amlodipine (Can)** *see* AmLODIPine *on page 135*

◆ **Biobase™ (Can)** *see* Alcohol (Ethyl) *on page 88*

◆ **Biobase-G™ (Can)** *see* Alcohol (Ethyl) *on page 88*

◆ **Bio-Diazepam (Can)** *see* Diazepam *on page 640*

◆ **Bio-Furosemide (Can)** *see* Furosemide *on page 948*

◆ **Bio-Hydrochlorothiazide (Can)** *see* Hydrochlorothiazide *on page 1023*

◆ **Bio-Letrozole (Can)** *see* Letrozole *on page 1211*

◆ **Bioniche Promethazine (Can)** *see* Promethazine *on page 1748*

◆ **Bion® Tears [OTC]** *see* Artificial Tears *on page 205*

◆ **BioQuin® Durules™ (Can)** *see* QuiNIDine *on page 1791*

◆ **Bio-Statin** *see* Nystatin (Oral) *on page 1516*

Biotin (BYE oh tin)

Therapeutic Category Biotinidase Deficiency, Treatment Agent; Nutritional Supplement; Vitamin, Water Soluble

Use Treatment of primary biotinidase deficiency; nutritional biotin deficiency; component of the vitamin B complex

Contraindications Hypersensitivity to biotin or any component

Mechanism of Action Functions as a coenzyme; involved in carboxylation, transcarboxylation, and decarboxylation reactions of gluconeogenesis, lipogenesis, fatty acid synthesis, propionate metabolism, and the catabolism of leucine

Dosing: Neonatal Oral:
Adequate intake (AI): 5 mcg/day (~0.7 mcg/kg/day)
Biotinidase deficiency: 5-10 mg once daily

Dosing: Usual Oral:
Adequate intake (AI): Infants, Children, and Adults: There is no official RDA.
Infants:
1 to <6 months: 5 mcg/day (~0.7 mcg/kg/day)
6-12 months: 6 mcg/day (~0.7 mcg/kg/day)
Children:
1-3 years: 8 mcg/day
4-8 years: 12 mcg/day
9-13 years: 20 mcg/day
14-18 years: 25 mcg/day
Adults: 30 mcg/day
Biotinidase deficiency: Infants, Children, and Adults: 5-10 mg once daily
Biotin deficiency: Children and Adults: 5-20 mg once daily

Administration Oral: May be administered without regard to meals

Reference Range Serum biotinidase activity

Dosage Forms Capsule: 1 mg

References
McVoy JR, Levy HL, Lawler M, et al, "Partial Biotinidase Deficiency: Clinical and Biochemical Features," *J Pediatr*, 1990, 116(1):78-83.

Salbert BA, Pellock JM, and Wolf B, "Characterization of Seizures Associated With Biotinidase Deficiency," *Neurology*, 1993, 43 (7):1351-5.

Standing Committee on the Scientific Evaluation of Dietary Reference Intakes, Food and Nutrition Board, Institute of Medicine, "Dietary Reference Intakes for Thiamin, Riboflavin, Niacin, Vitamin B6, Folate, Vitamin B12, Pantothenic Acid, Biotin and Choline," *National Academy of Sciences*, Washington, DC: National Academy Press, 1999. Available at http://www.nap.edu

Wastell HJ, Bartlett K, Dale G, et al, "Biotinidase Deficiency: A Survey of 10 Cases," *Arch Dis Child*, 1988, 63(10):1244-9.

◆ **Biphentin (Can)** *see* Methylphenidate *on page 1379*
◆ **Bisac-Evac [OTC]** *see* Bisacodyl *on page 293*

Bisacodyl (bis a KOE dil)

Medication Safety Issues
Sound-alike/look-alike issues:
Doxidan may be confused with doxepin
Dulcolax (bisacodyl) may be confused with Dulcolax (docusate)

Related Information
Oral Medications That Should Not Be Crushed or Altered *on page 2438*

Brand Names: U.S. Bisac-Evac [OTC]; Bisacodyl EC [OTC]; Bisacodyl Laxative [OTC]; Biscolax [OTC]; Correct [OTC]; Ducodyl [OTC]; Dulcolax [OTC]; Ex-Lax Ultra [OTC]; Fleet Bisacodyl [OTC]; Fleet Laxative [OTC]; Gentle Laxative [OTC]; Laxative [OTC]; Magic Bullets [OTC]; Stimulant Laxative [OTC]; Womens Laxative [OTC]

Brand Names: Canada Apo-Bisacodyl [OTC]; Bisacodyl-Odan [OTC]; Bisacolax [OTC]; Carter's Little Pills [OTC]; Codulax [OTC]; Dulcolax For Women [OTC]; Dulcolax [OTC]; PMS-Bisacodyl [OTC]; ratio-Bisacodyl [OTC]; Silver Bullet Suppository [OTC]; Soflax EX [OTC]; The Magic Bullett [OTC]; Woman's Laxative [OTC]

Therapeutic Category Laxative, Stimulant

Generic Availability (U.S.) May be product dependent

Use Treatment of constipation; colonic evacuation prior to procedures or examination

Pregnancy Considerations Plasma concentrations of BHPM (the active metabolite of bisacodyl) are low (median: 61 ng/mL; range: 21-194 ng/mL) following doses of 10 mg/day for 7 days (Friedrich, 2011). Although not first choice for the treatment of constipation in pregnant women, short-term use of stimulant laxatives is generally considered safe in pregnancy; long-term use should be avoided (Cullen, 2007; Prather, 2004; Wald, 2003).

Breast-Feeding Considerations Neither bisacodyl nor its active metabolite (BHPM) were detectable in breast milk following administration of bisacodyl 10 mg once daily for 7 days to eight lactating women (limit of detection: 1 ng/mL) (Friedrich, 2011).

Contraindications Hypersensitivity to bisacodyl or any component; do not use in patients with abdominal pain, appendicitis, obstruction, nausea or vomiting; not to be used during pregnancy or lactation

Warnings Stimulant laxatives are habit-forming; long-term use may result in laxative dependence and loss of normal bowel function.

Precautions Bisacodyl tannex powder for preparation as a rectal solution should be used with caution in patients with ulceration of the colon

Adverse Reactions Rare but important or life-threatening: Electrolyte and fluid imbalance (metabolic acidosis or alkalosis, hypocalcemia), mild abdominal cramps, nausea, rectal burning, vertigo, vomiting

Drug Interactions
Metabolism/Transport Effects None known.
Avoid Concomitant Use There are no known interactions where it is recommended to avoid concomitant use.
Increased Effect/Toxicity There are no known significant interactions involving an increase in effect.
Decreased Effect
The levels/effects of Bisacodyl may be decreased by: Antacids

Stability Store enteric-coated tablets and rectal suppositories at <30°C.

Mechanism of Action Stimulates peristalsis by directly irritating the smooth muscle of the intestine, possibly the colonic intramural plexus; alters water and electrolyte secretion producing net intestinal fluid accumulation and laxation

Pharmacodynamics Onset of action:
Oral: Within 6-10 hours
Rectal: 15-60 minutes

Pharmacokinetics (Adult data unless noted)
Absorption: Oral, rectal: <5% absorbed systemically
Metabolism: In the liver
Elimination: Conjugated metabolites excreted in breast milk, bile, and urine

Dosing: Usual
Bisacodyl (Dulcolax®) tablet: Oral:
Children 3-12 years: 5-10 mg or 0.3 mg/kg/day as a single dose
Children ≥12 years and Adults: 5-15 mg/day as a single dose; maximum dose: 30 mg
Bisacodyl (Dulcolax®) suppository: Rectal:
Children:
<2 years: 5 mg/day as a single dose
2-11 years: 5-10 mg/day as a single dose
Children ≥12 years and Adults: 10 mg/day as a single dose

Administration Oral: Administer on an empty stomach with water; patient should swallow tablet whole; do not break or chew enteric-coated tablet; do not administer within 1 hour of ingesting antacids, alkaline material, milk, or dairy products

Additional Information In a randomized prospective study of 70 patients, bisacodyl tablets were given orally once daily in the morning for 2 days before colonoscopy to 19 patients (dose for children <5 years: 5 mg; 5-12 years: 10 mg; >12 years: 15 mg) with a Fleet® enema given on the morning of the procedure without any dietary restriction. Results showed that bisacodyl without dietary restriction provided unsatisfactory colon cleansing.

Dosage Forms Excipient information presented when available (limited, particularly for generics); consult specific product labeling.
Enema, Rectal:
Fleet Bisacodyl: 10 mg/30 mL (37 mL)
Suppository, Rectal:
Bisac-Evac: 10 mg (1 ea, 8 ea, 12 ea, 50 ea, 100 ea, 500 ea, 1000 ea)
Bisacodyl Laxative: 10 mg (12 ea)
Biscolax: 10 mg (12 ea, 100 ea)
Dulcolax: 10 mg (4 ea, 8 ea, 16 ea, 28 ea, 50 ea)
Gentle Laxative: 10 mg (4 ea, 8 ea, 12 ea)
Laxative: 10 mg (12 ea, 100 ea)
Magic Bullets: 10 mg (12 ea, 100 ea)
Generic: 10 mg (12 ea, 50 ea, 100 ea)
Tablet Delayed Release, Oral:
Bisacodyl EC: 5 mg
Bisacodyl EC: 5 mg [contains fd&c yellow #10 (quinoline yellow), fd&c yellow #6 (sunset yellow)]
Bisacodyl EC: 5 mg [contains fd&c yellow #10 aluminum lake, fd&c yellow #6 aluminum lake]
Correct: 5 mg
Ducodyl: 5 mg
Dulcolax: 5 mg [contains fd&c yellow #10 (quinoline yellow), methylparaben, propylparaben, sodium benzoate]
Ex-Lax Ultra: 5 mg [contains fd&c yellow #6 (sunset yellow), methylparaben]
Fleet Laxative: 5 mg
Gentle Laxative: 5 mg
Stimulant Laxative: 5 mg
Stimulant Laxative: 5 mg [contains fd&c yellow #10 aluminum lake, fd&c yellow #6 aluminum lake]
Womens Laxative: 5 mg
Womens Laxative: 5 mg [contains fd&c blue #1 aluminum lake, sodium benzoate, tartrazine (fd&c yellow #5)]

References

BaKer SS, Liptak GS, Colletti RB, et al, "Constipation in Infants and Children: Evaluation and Treatment," 2000, www.naspgn.org/constipation.

Cullen G and O'Donoghue D, "Constipation and Pregnancy," *Best Pract Res Clin Gastroenterol*, 2007, 21(5):807-18.

Dahshan A, Lin CH, Peters J, et al, "A Randomized, Prospective Study to Evaluate the Efficacy and Acceptance of Three Bowel Preparations for Colonoscopy in Children," *Am J Gastroenterol*, 1999, 94 (12):3497-501.

Friedrich C, Richter E, Trommeshauser D, et al, "Absence of Excretion of the Active Moiety of Bisacodyl and Sodium Picosulfate Into Human Breast Milk: An Open-Label, Parallel-Group, Multiple-Dose Study in Healthy Lactating Women," *Drug Metab Pharmacokinet*, 2011, 26 (5):458-64.

Prather CM, "Pregnancy-Related Constipation," *Curr Gastroenterol Rep*, 2004, 6(5):402-4.

Wald A, "Constipation, Diarrhea, and Symptomatic Hemorrhoids During Pregnancy," *Gastroenterol Clin North Am*, 2003, 32(1):309-22.

◆ **Bisacodyl EC [OTC]** *see* Bisacodyl *on page 293*

◆ **Bisacodyl Laxative [OTC]** *see* Bisacodyl *on page 293*

◆ **Bisacodyl-Odan [OTC] (Can)** *see* Bisacodyl *on page 293*

◆ **Bisacolax [OTC] (Can)** *see* Bisacodyl *on page 293*

◆ **bis(chloroethyl) nitrosourea** *see* Carmustine *on page 382*

◆ **bis-chloronitrosourea** *see* Carmustine *on page 382*

◆ **Biscolax [OTC]** *see* Bisacodyl *on page 293*

◆ **Bismatrol [OTC]** *see* Bismuth *on page 294*

◆ **Bismatrol [OTC]** *see* Bismuth *on page 294*

◆ **Bismatrol Maximum Strength [OTC]** *see* Bismuth *on page 294*

Bismuth (BIZ muth)

Medication Safety Issues
Sound-alike/look-alike issues:
Kaopectate® may be confused with Kayexalate®
Other safety concerns:
Maalox® Total Relief® is a different formulation than other Maalox® liquid antacid products which contain aluminum hydroxide, magnesium hydroxide, and simethicone.
Canadian formulation of Kaopectate® does not contain bismuth; the active ingredient in the Canadian formulation is attapulgite.

Related Information
H. pylori Treatment in Pediatric Patients *on page 2311*

Brand Names: U.S. Bismatrol Maximum Strength [OTC]; Bismatrol [OTC]; Diotame [OTC]; Kao-Tin [OTC]; Peptic Relief [OTC]; Pepto-Bismol To-Go [OTC]; Pepto-Bismol [OTC]; Pink Bismuth [OTC]; Stomach Relief Max St [OTC]; Stomach Relief Plus [OTC]; Stomach Relief [OTC]

Therapeutic Category Antidiarrheal; Gastrointestinal Agent, Gastric or Duodenal Ulcer Treatment

Generic Availability (U.S.) Yes

Use
Subsalicylate formulation: Symptomatic treatment of mild, nonspecific diarrhea including traveler's diarrhea; chronic infantile diarrhea; adjunctive treatment of *Helicobacter pylori*-associated antral gastritis

Subgallate formulation: An aid to reduce fecal odors from a colostomy or ileostomy

Pregnancy Considerations Following oral administration, bismuth and salicylates cross the placenta. The use of salicylates in pregnancy may adversely affect the newborn (Lione, 1988). Use during pregnancy is not recommended (Mahadevan, 2007).

Breast-Feeding Considerations Low amounts of salicylates enter breast milk; refer to the aspirin monograph for additional information (Bar-Oz, 2004). A case report describes bowel obstruction in a breast-fed infant whose mother applied a bismuth-containing ointment to her nipples prior to breast-feeding (Anonymous, 1974).

Contraindications Hypersensitivity to bismuth, salicylates, or any component; history of severe GI bleeding or coagulopathy

Warnings Kaopectate® has been reformulated to contain **only** bismuth subsalicylate; follow dosage recommendations closely. Do not use subsalicylate in patients with a viral infection, such as influenza or chickenpox, because of the risk of Reye's syndrome; when using bismuth subsalicylate, changes in behavior (along with nausea and vomiting) may be an early sign of Reye's syndrome; instruct patients and caregivers to contact their healthcare provider if these symptoms occur; subsalicylate should be used with caution if patient is taking aspirin, due to additive toxicity; use with caution in children <3 years of age; be aware of salicylate content when prescribing for use in children. May cause bleeding.

Precautions May interfere with radiologic examinations of GI tract as bismuth is radiopaque; should not be used in patients with a history of bleeding disorder, gastrointestinal ulcer disease, or those taking anticoagulants, clopidogrel, NSAIDS, and/or oral antidiabetic agents.

Adverse Reactions Subsalicylate formulation:
Central nervous system: Anxiety, confusion, headache, mental depression, slurred speech
Gastrointestinal: Discoloration of the tongue (darkening), grayish black stools, impaction may occur in infants and debilitated patients
Neuromuscular & skeletal: Muscle spasms, weakness
Otic: Hearing loss, tinnitus

Drug Interactions
Metabolism/Transport Effects None known.

Avoid Concomitant Use There are no known interactions where it is recommended to avoid concomitant use.

Increased Effect/Toxicity There are no known significant interactions involving an increase in effect.

Decreased Effect
Bismuth may decrease the levels/effects of: Tetracycline Derivatives

Mechanism of Action Bismuth subsalicylate exhibits both antisecretory and antimicrobial action. This agent may provide some anti-inflammatory action as well. The salicylate moiety provides antisecretory effect and the bismuth exhibits antimicrobial directly against bacterial and viral gastrointestinal pathogens.

Pharmacokinetics (Adult data unless noted)
Absorption: Bismuth is minimally absorbed (<1%) across the GI tract while salicylate salt is readily absorbed (80%)
Distribution: Salicylate: V_d: 170 mL/kg
Protein binding, plasma: Bismuth and salicylate: >90%
Metabolism: Bismuth salts undergo chemical dissociation after oral administration; salicylate is extensively metabolized in the liver
Half-life:
Bismuth: Terminal: 21-72 days
Salicylate: Terminal: 2-5 hours
Elimination:
Bismuth: Renal, biliary
Salicylate: Only 10% excreted unchanged in urine

Dosing: Usual Oral: Bismuth subsalicylate: **(bismuth subsalicylate liquid dosages expressed in mL of 262 mg/15 mL concentration):**
Nonspecific diarrhea: Children: 100 mg/kg/day divided into 5 equal doses for 5 days (maximum: 4.19 g/day) **or**
Children: Up to 8 doses/24 hours:
3-6 years: 1/3 tablet or 5 mL (87 mg) every 30 minutes to 1 hour as needed
6-9 years: 2/3 tablet or 10 mL (175 mg) every 30 minutes to 1 hour as needed
9-12 years: 1 tablet or 15 mL (262 mg) every 30 minutes to 1 hour as needed

Adults: 2 tablets or 30 mL (524 mg) every 30 minutes to 1 hour as needed up to 8 doses/24 hours

Chronic infantile diarrhea:

2-24 months: 2.5 mL (44 mg) every 4 hours

24-48 months: 5 mL (87 mg) every 4 hours

48-70 months: 10 mL (175 mg) every 4 hours

Prevention of traveler's diarrhea: Adults: 2.1 g/day or 2 tablets 4 times/day before meals and at bedtime

Helicobacter pylori-associated antral gastritis: Dosage in children is not well established, the following dosages have been used [in conjunction with ampicillin and metronidazole or (in adults) tetracycline and metronidazole]:

Children ≤10 years: 15 mL (262 mg) 4 times/day for 6 weeks

Children >10 years and Adults: 30 mL (524 mg) solution or two 262 mg tablets 4 times/day for 6 weeks

Dosing adjustment in renal impairment: Avoid use in patients with renal failure

Administration Oral: Shake liquid well before using; chew tablets or allow to dissolve in mouth before swallowing

Test Interactions Increased uric acid, increased AST; bismuth absorbs x-rays and may interfere with diagnostic procedures of GI tract

Additional Information Bismuth subsalicylate: 262 mg = 130 mg nonaspirin salicylate; 525 mg = 236 mg nonaspirin salicylate

Dosage Forms Excipient information presented when available (limited, particularly for generics); consult specific product labeling.

Suspension, Oral, as subsalicylate:

Bismatrol: 262 mg/15 mL (236 mL) [contains benzoic acid, d&c red #22 (eosine), saccharin sodium; wintergreen flavor]

Bismatrol Maximum Strength: 525 mg/15 mL (236 mL) [contains benzoic acid, d&c red #22 (eosine), saccharin sodium; wintergreen flavor]

Kao-Tin: 262 mg/15 mL (236 mL, 473 mL) [contains fd&c red #40, saccharin sodium, sodium benzoate]

Peptic Relief: 262 mg/15 mL (237 mL) [sugar free; contains benzoic acid, d&c red #22 (eosine), saccharin sodium; mint flavor]

Pepto-Bismol: 262 mg/15 mL (473 mL) [contains benzoic acid, d&c red #22 (eosine), saccharin sodium]

Pink Bismuth: 262 mg/15 mL (236 mL)

Pink Bismuth: 262 mg/15 mL (237 mL) [contains benzoic acid, d&c red #22 (eosine), saccharin sodium]

Stomach Relief: 262 mg/15 mL (237 mL, 355 mL) [contains d&c red #22 (eosine), saccharin sodium]

Stomach Relief: 527 mg/30 mL (240 mL, 480 mL)

Stomach Relief Max St: 525 mg/15 mL (237 mL) [contains d&c red #22 (eosine), saccharin sodium]

Stomach Relief Plus: 525 mg/15 mL (240 mL, 480 mL)

Tablet Chewable, Oral, as subsalicylate:

Bismatrol: 262 mg [contains aspartame]

Diotame: 262 mg

Peptic Relief: 262 mg

Pepto-Bismol To-Go: 262 mg [sugar free; contains fd&c red #40 aluminum lake, saccharin sodium; cherry flavor]

Pink Bismuth: 262 mg

Pink Bismuth: 262 mg [contains saccharin sodium]

Stomach Relief: 262 mg [contains aspartame]

Generic: 262 mg

References

Bar-Oz B, Bulkowstein M, Benyamini L, et al, "Use of Antibiotic and Analgesic Drugs During Lactation," *Drug Saf*, 2003, 26(13):925-35.

Drumm B, Sherman P, Karmali M, et al, "Treatment of *Campylobacter pylori*-associated Antral Gastritis in Children With Bismuth Subsalicylate and Ampicillin," *J Pediatr*, 1988, 113(5):908-12.

Lione A, "Nonprescription Drugs as a Source of Aluminum, Bismuth, and Iodine During Pregnancy," *Reprod Toxicol*, 1987-8, 1(4):243-52.

Mahadevan U, "Gastrointestinal Medications in Pregnancy," *Best Pract Res Clin Gastroenterol*, 2007, 21(5):849-77.

Soriano-Brucher HE, Avendano P, O'Ryan M, et al, "Use of Bismuth Subsalicylate in Acute Diarrhea in Children," *Rev Infect Dis*, 1990, 12 (Suppl 1):S51-5.

Walsh JH and Peterson WL, "The Treatment of *Helicobacter pylori* Infection in the Management of Peptic Ulcer Disease," *N Engl J Med*, 1995, 333(15):984-91.

◆ **Bismuth Subsalicylate** *see* Bismuth *on page 294*

◆ **Bis-POM PMEA** *see* Adefovir *on page 75*

◆ **Bistropamide** *see* Tropicamide *on page 2092*

◆ **Bivalent Human Papillomavirus Vaccine** *see* Papillomavirus (Types 16, 18) Vaccine (Human, Recombinant) *on page 1603*

◆ **Bivigam** *see* Immune Globulin *on page 1084*

◆ **Bi-Zets/Benzotroches [OTC]** *see* Benzocaine *on page 273*

◆ **BL4162A** *see* Anagrelide *on page 166*

◆ **Black Widow Spider Species Antivenin** *see* Antivenin (*Latrodectus mactans*) *on page 185*

◆ **Black Widow Spider Species Antivenom** *see* Antivenin (*Latrodectus mactans*) *on page 185*

◆ **Blenoxane** *see* Bleomycin *on page 295*

◆ **Blenoxane® (Can)** *see* Bleomycin *on page 295*

◆ **Bleo** *see* Bleomycin *on page 295*

Bleomycin (blee oh MYE sin)

Medication Safety Issues

Sound-alike/look-alike issues:

Bleomycin may be confused with Cleocin

High alert medication:

This medication is in a class the Institute for Safe Medication Practices (ISMP) includes among its list of drugs which have a heightened risk of causing significant patient harm when used in error.

International issues:

Some products available internationally may have vial strength and dosing expressed as international units or milligrams (instead of units or USP units). Refer to prescribing information for specific strength and dosing information.

Related Information

Emetogenic Potential of Antineoplastic Agents in Children *on page 2327*

Management of Drug Extravasations *on page 2255*

Safe Handling of Hazardous Drugs *on page 2419*

Brand Names: Canada Blenoxane®; Bleomycin Injection, USP

Therapeutic Category Antineoplastic Agent, Antibiotic

Generic Availability (U.S.) Yes

Use Palliative treatment of squamous cell carcinoma (of the head and neck, penis, cervix, or vulva), testicular carcinoma, Hodgkin's lymphoma, and non-Hodgkin's lymphoma; sclerosing agent to control malignant effusions (FDA approved in adults); has also been used in the treatment of germ cell tumors and pediatric Hodgkin's lymphoma

Pregnancy Risk Factor D

Pregnancy Considerations Adverse effects were observed in animal reproduction studies. Women of childbearing potential should avoid becoming pregnant during treatment.

Breast-Feeding Considerations It is not known if bleomycin is excreted in breast milk. Due to the potential for serious adverse reactions in the nursing infant, the manufacturer recommends against breast-feeding during treatment.

Contraindications Hypersensitivity to bleomycin sulfate or any component

Warnings Hazardous agent; use appropriate precautions for handling and disposal (NIOSH, 2012). Occurrence of pulmonary fibrosis (commonly presenting as pneumonitis; occasionally progressing to pulmonary fibrosis) is the most severe toxicity; risk is higher in elderly patients and patients receiving >400 units total lifetime dose **[U.S. Boxed Warning]**; but has also been reported in younger patients on low doses. Other possible risk factors include smoking and patients with prior radiation therapy or receiving concurrent oxygen (especially high-inspired oxygen doses). A review of patients receiving bleomycin for the treatment of germ cell tumors suggests risk for pulmonary toxicity is increased in patients >40 years of age, with glomerular filtration rate <80 mL/minute, advanced disease, and cumulative doses >300 units (O'Sullivan, 2003). Pulmonary toxicity may include bronchiolitis obliterans and organizing pneumonia (BOOP), eosinophilic hypersensitivity, and interstitial pneumonitis, progressing to pulmonary fibrosis (Sleijfer, 2001); pulmonary toxicity may be due to a lack of the enzyme which inactivates bleomycin (bleomycin hydrolase) in the lungs (Morgan, 2011; Sleijfer, 2001). If pulmonary changes occur, withhold treatment and investigate if drug-related. In children a younger age at treatment, cumulative dose ≥400 units/m^2 (combined with chest irradiation) and renal impairment are associated with a higher incidence of pulmonary toxicity (Huang, 2011).

A severe idiosyncratic reaction consisting of hypotension, mental confusion, fever, chills, and wheezing (similar to anaphylaxis) has been reported in 1% of lymphoma patients treated with bleomycin **[U.S. Boxed Warning]**. Since these reactions usually occur after the first or second dose, careful monitoring is essential after these doses.

Precautions Use caution when administering O$_2$ during surgery to patients who have received bleomycin; the risk of bleomycin-related pulmonary toxicity is increased. Use caution with renal impairment (CrCl <50 mL/minute); may require dose adjustment; may cause renal or hepatic toxicity. Should be administered under the supervision of an experienced cancer chemotherapy physician **[U.S. Boxed Warning]**. Some products available internationally may have vial strength and dosing expressed as international units or milligrams (instead of units or USP units). Refer to prescribing information for specific dosing information. Potentially significant interactions may exist, requiring dose or frequency adjustment, additional monitoring, and/or selection of alternative therapy. Consult drug interactions database for more detailed information.

Adverse Reactions

Dermatologic: Diffuse scleroderma, erythema, hyperkeratosis, induration, onycholysis, pain at the tumor site, phlebitis, pruritus, rash, skin thickening, striae, vesiculation; peeling of the skin (particularly on the palmar and plantar surfaces of the hands and feet); hyperpigmentation, alopecia, nailbed changes may also occur (appear dose related and reversible with discontinuation)

Gastrointestinal: Anorexia, stomatitis and mucositis, weight loss

Respiratory: Death, hypoxia, Interstitial pneumonitis (acute or chronic), pulmonary fibrosis, rales, tachypnea; symptoms include cough, dyspnea, and bilateral pulmonary infiltrates. The pathogenesis is not certain, but may be due to damage of pulmonary, vascular, or connective tissue. Response to steroid therapy is variable and somewhat controversial.

Miscellaneous: Acute febrile reactions; anaphylactoid-like reactions (characterized by hypotension, confusion, fever, chills, and wheezing; onset may be immediate or delayed for several hours); idiosyncratic reactions

Rare but important or life-threatening: Angioedema, cerebrovascular accident, cerebral arteritis, chest pain, coronary artery disease, flagellate hyperpigmentation, hepatotoxicity, malaise, MI, myelosuppression (rare), myocardial ischemia, nausea, pericarditis, Raynaud's phenomenon, renal toxicity, scleroderma-like skin changes, Stevens-Johnson syndrome, thrombotic microangiopathy, toxic epidermal necrolysis, vomiting

Drug Interactions

Metabolism/Transport Effects None known.

Avoid Concomitant Use

Avoid concomitant use of Bleomycin with any of the following: BCG; Brentuximab Vedotin; Natalizumab; Pimecrolimus; Tacrolimus (Topical); Tofacitinib; Vaccines (Live)

Increased Effect/Toxicity

Bleomycin may increase the levels/effects of: Leflunomide; Natalizumab; Tofacitinib; Vaccines (Live)

The levels/effects of Bleomycin may be increased by: Brentuximab Vedotin; Denosumab; Filgrastim; Gemcitabine; Pimecrolimus; Roflumilast; Sargramostim; Tacrolimus (Topical); Trastuzumab

Decreased Effect

Bleomycin may decrease the levels/effects of: BCG; Cardiac Glycosides; Coccidioidin Skin Test; Phenytoin; Sipuleucel-T; Vaccines (Inactivated); Vaccines (Live)

The levels/effects of Bleomycin may be decreased by: Echinacea

Stability Hazardous agent; use appropriate precautions for handling and disposal (NIOSH, 2012). Store under refrigeration at 2°C to 8°C (36°F to 46°F); intact vials are stable 4 weeks at room temperature; solutions reconstituted in NS are stable for up to 28 days refrigerated and 14 days at room temperature; however, the manufacturer recommends stability of 24 hours in NS at room temperature. Incompatible when admixed with aminophylline, ascorbic acid, cefazolin, diazepam, hydrocortisone, mitomycin, nafcillin, penicillin G; dilution in dextrose solutions may result in a 10% loss of activity within 24 hours.

Mechanism of Action Inhibits synthesis of DNA; binds to DNA leading to single- and double-strand breaks; also inhibits (to a lesser degree) RNA and protein synthesis

Pharmacokinetics (Adult data unless noted)

Absorption: I.M. and intrapleural administration: 30% to 50% of I.V. serum concentrations; intraperitoneal and SubQ routes produce serum concentrations equal to those of I.V.

Distribution: V$_d$: 22 L/m^2; highest concentrations in skin, kidney, lung, and heart tissues; lowest in testes and GI tract; does not cross blood-brain

Protein binding: 1%

Metabolism: Via several tissues, including hepatic, GI tract, skin, pulmonary, renal, and serum

Half-life elimination: Biphasic (renal function dependent):
Children: 2.1 to 3.5 hours
Adults:
  Normal renal function: Initial: 1.3 hours; Terminal: 9 hours
  End-stage renal disease: Initial: 2 hours; Terminal: 30 hours

Time to peak serum concentration: I.M.: Within 30 minutes

Elimination: Urine (50% to 70% as active drug)

Dosing: Usual Note: An international consideration with use is that dosages below are expressed as USP units; 1 USP unit = 1 mg (by potency) = 1000 international units (Stefanou, 2001). The risk for pulmonary toxicity increases with cumulative lifetime dose >400 units. Refer to individual protocols for specific dosage and interval information.

Pediatric:

Test dose for lymphoma patients: Children and Adolescents: I.M., I.V., SubQ: Because of the possibility of an anaphylactoid reaction, the manufacturer recommends administering 1 to 2 units of bleomycin before the first 1 to 2 doses; monitor vital signs every 15 minutes; wait a minimum of 1 hour before administering remainder of dose; if no acute reaction occurs, then the regular dosage schedule may be followed. **Note:** Test doses may not be predictive of a reaction (Lam, 2005) and/or may produce false-negative results.

Hodgkin lymphoma (combination regimen):

ABVD regimen: Children and Adolescents: I.V.: 10 units/m^2 on days 1 and 15 of a 28-day treatment cycle in combination with doxorubicin, vinblastine, dacarbazine (Hutchinson, 1998)

BEACOPP regimen: Children and Adolescents: I.V. 10 units/m^2 on day 7 of a 21-day treatment cycle in combination with etoposide, doxorubicin, cyclophosphamide, vincristine, procarbazine, and prednisone (Kelly, 2002)

Stanford V: Adolescent ≥16 years: 5 units/m^2/dose in weeks 2, 4, 6, 8, 10, and 12 in combination with mechlorethamine, vinblastine, vincristine, doxorubicin, etoposide, and prednisone (Horning, 2000; Horning, 2002)

Malignant germ cell cancer (combination therapy) (Cushing, 2004): I.V.:

Infants: 0.5 **mg**/kg/dose day 1 of a 21-day treatment cycle for 4 cycles

Children and Adolescents: 15 units/m^2 day 1 of a 21-day treatment cycle for 4 cycles

Adults:

Test dose for lymphoma patients: I.M., I.V., SubQ: Because of the possibility of an anaphylactoid reaction, the manufacturer recommends administering 1 to 2 units of bleomycin before the first 1 to 2 doses; monitor vital signs every 15 minutes; wait a minimum of 1 hour before administering remainder of dose; if no acute reaction occurs, then the regular dosage schedule may be followed. **Note:** Test doses may not be predictive of a reaction (Lam, 2005) and/or may produce false-negative results.

Hodgkin's lymphoma (combination regimens): I.V.:

ABVD: 10 units/m^2 days 1 and 15 of a 28-day treatment cycle (Straus, 2004)

BEACOPP: 10 units/m^2 day 8 of a 21-day treatment cycle (Dann, 2007; Diehl, 2003)

Stanford V: 5 units/m^2/dose in weeks 2, 4, 6, 8, 10, and 12 (Horning, 2000; Horning, 2002)

Malignant pleural effusion: Intrapleural: 60 units as a single instillation; mix in 50-100 mL of NS and instill into the pleural cavity via a thoracostomy tube

Dosing adjustment in obesity: Adults: Fixed doses (dosing which is independent of body weight or BSA) are used in some protocols (eg, testicular cancer); due to toxicity concerns, the same fixed dose should also be considered for obese patients (Griggs, 2012).

Dosing adjustment in renal impairment: Adults:

Manufacturer's labeling: **Note:** Creatinine clearance should be estimated using the Cockcroft-Gault formula:

CrCl >50 mL/minute: No dosage adjustment necessary

CrCl 40 to 50 mL/minute: Administer 70% of normal dose

CrCl 30 to 40 mL/minute: Administer 60% of normal dose

CrCl 20 to 30 mL/minute: Administer 55% of normal dose

CrCl 10 to 20 mL/minute: Administer 45% of normal dose

CrCl 5 to 10 mL/minute: Administer 40% of normal dose

The following guidelines have been used by some clinicians:

Aronoff, 2007: Continuous renal replacement therapy (CRRT): Administer 75% of dose

Kintzel, 1995:

CrCl 46 to 60 mL/minute: Administer 70% of dose

CrCl 31 to 45 mL/minute: Administer 60% of dose

CrCl <30 mL/minute: Consider use of alternative drug

Dosing adjustment in hepatic impairment: There are no dosage adjustments provided in the manufacturer's

labeling (has not been studied); however, adjustment for hepatic impairment is not necessary (King, 2001).

Dosing adjustment for toxicity:

Pulmonary changes: Discontinue until determined not to be drug-related.

Pulmonary diffusion capacity for carbon monoxide (DL$_{CO}$) <30% to 35% of baseline: Discontinue treatment.

Administration Hazardous agent; use appropriate precautions for handling and disposal (NIOSH, 2012).

Parenteral:

I.M.: May cause pain at injection site.

I.V.: Reconstitute 15-unit vial with 5 mL NS and the 30-unit vial with 10 mL NS. Administer I.V. slowly over at least 10 minutes at a concentration not to exceed 3 units/mL; bleomycin for continuous I.V. infusion can be further diluted in NS; administration by continuous infusion may produce less severe pulmonary toxicity.

SubQ: Reconstitute 15-unit vial with NS or sterile or bacteriostatic water for injection; 15 units/mL concentration may be used for administration; may cause pain at injection site

Intrapleural: Adults: 60 units in 50 to 100 mL NS; use of topical anesthetics or opioid analgesia is usually not necessary. Use appropriate precautions for handling and disposal.

Vesicant/Extravasation Risk May be an irritant

Monitoring Parameters Pulmonary function tests, including total lung volume, forced vital capacity, diffusion capacity for carbon monoxide; vital capacity, total lung capacity, and pulmonary capillary blood volume may be better indicators of changes induced by bleomycin (Sleijfer, 2001), chest x-ray; renal function, hepatic function, vital signs, and temperature initially; CBC with differential and platelet count; check body weight at regular intervals

Dosage Forms Excipient information presented when available (limited, particularly for generics); consult specific product labeling.

Solution Reconstituted, Injection:

Generic: 15 units (1 ea); 30 units (1 ea)

Solution Reconstituted, Injection [preservative free]:

Generic: 15 units (1 ea); 30 units (1 ea)

References

Aronoff GR, Bennett WM, Berns JS, et al, *Drug Prescribing in Renal Failure: Dosing Guidelines for Adults and Children*, 5th ed, Philadelphia, PA: American College of Physicians, 2007, 97.

Bleomycin [prescribing information]. Schaumburg, IL: APP Pharmaceuticals, LLC; October 2008.

Carver JR, Shapiro CL, Ng A, et al, "American Society of Clinical Oncology Clinical Evidence Review on the Ongoing Care of Adult Cancer Survivors: Cardiac and Pulmonary Late Effects," *J Clin Oncol*, 2007, 25(25):3991-4008.

Cushing B, Giller R, Cullen JW, et al, "Randomized Comparison of Combination Chemotherapy With Etoposide, Bleomycin, and Either High-Dose or Standard-Dose Cisplatin in Children and Adolescents With High-Risk Malignant Germ Cell Tumors: A Pediatric Intergroup Study – Pediatric Oncology Group 9049 and Children's Cancer Group 8882," *J Clin Oncol*, 2004, 22(13):2691-700.

Dann EJ, Bar-Shalom R, Tamir A, et al, "Risk-Adapted BEACOPP Regimen Can Reduce the Cumulative Dose of Chemotherapy for Standard and High-Risk Hodgkin Lymphoma With No Impairment of Outcome," *Blood*, 2007, 109(3):905-9.

Diehl V, Franklin J, Pfreundschuh M, et al, "Standard and Increased-Dose BEACOPP Chemotherapy Compared With COPP-ABVD for Advanced Hodgkin's Disease," *N Engl J Med*, 2003, 348(24):2386-95.

Engert A, Franklin J, Eich HT, et al, "Two Cycles of Doxorubicin, Bleomycin, Vinblastine, and Dacarbazine Plus Extended-Field Radiotherapy Is Superior to Radiotherapy Alone in Early Favorable Hodgkin's Lymphoma: Final Results of the GHSG HD7 Trial," *J Clin Oncol*, 2007, 25(23):3495-502.

Griggs JJ, Mangu PB, Anderson H, et al, "Appropriate Chemotherapy Dosing For Obese Adult Patients With Cancer: American Society of Clinical Oncology Clinical Practice Guideline," *J Clin Oncol*, 2012, 30 (13):1553-61.

Horning SJ, Hoppe RT, Breslin S, et al, "Stanford V and Radiotherapy for Locally Extensive and Advanced Hodgkin's Disease: Mature Results of a Prospective Clinical Trial," *J Clin Oncol*, 2002, 20 (3):630-7.

Horning SJ, Williams J, Bartlett NL, et al, "Assessment of the Stanford V Regimen and Consolidative Radiotherapy for Bulky and Advanced Hodgkin's Disease: Eastern Cooperative Oncology Group Pilot Study E1492," *J Clin Oncol*, 2000, 18(5):972-80.

Hoskin PJ, Lowry L, Horwich A, et al, "Randomized Comparison of the Stanford V Regimen and ABVD in the Treatment of Advanced Hodgkin's Lymphoma: United Kingdom National Cancer Research Institute Lymphoma Group Study ISRCTN 64141244," *J Clin Oncol*, 2009, 27(32):5390-6.

Huang TT, Hudson MM, Stokes DC, et al, "Pulmonary Outcomes in Survivors of Childhood Cancer: A Systematic Review," *Chest*, 2011, 140(4): 881-901.

Hutchinson RJ, Fryer CJ, Davis PC, et al, "MOPP or Radiation in Addition to ABVD in the Treatment of Pathologically Staged Advanced Hodgkin's Disease in Children: Results of the Children's Cancer Group Phase III Trial," *J Clin Oncol*, 1998, 16(3):897-906.

Ibrahimi OA and Anderson RR, "Images in Clinical Medicine. Bleomycin-Induced Flagellate Hyperpigmentation," *N Engl J Med*, 2010, 363 (24):e36.

Johnson PW, Radford JA, Cullen MH, et al, "Comparison of ABVD and Alternating or Hybrid Multidrug Regimens for the Treatment of Advanced Hodgkin's Lymphoma: Results of the United Kingdom Lymphoma Group LY09 Trial (ISRCTN97144519)," *J Clin Oncol*, 2005, 23(36):9208-18.

Kelly KM, Sposto R, Hutchinson R, et al. BEACOPP chemotherapy is a highly effective regimen in children and adolescents with high-risk Hodgkin lymphoma: a report from the Children's Oncology Group. *Blood*. 2011;117(9):2596-2603.

King PD and Perry MC, "Hepatotoxicity of Chemotherapy," *Oncologist*, 2001, 6(2):162-76.

Kintzel PE and Dorr RT, "Anticancer Drug Renal Toxicity and Elimination: Dosing Guidelines for Altered Renal Function," *Cancer Treat Rev*, 1995, 21(1):33-64.

Kung FH, Schwartz CL, Ferree CR, et al, "POG 8625: A Randomized Trial Comparing Chemotherapy With Chemoradiotherapy for Children and Adolescents With Stages I, IIA, IIIA1 Hodgkin Disease: A Report From the Children's Oncology Group," *J Pediatr Hematol Oncol*, 2006, 28(6):362-8.

Lam MS, "The Need for Routine Bleomycin Test Dosing in the 21st Century," *Ann Pharmacother*, 2005, 39(11):1897-902.

National Comprehensive Cancer Network® (NCCN), "Clinical Practice Guidelines in Oncology™: Head and Neck Cancers," Version 1.2011. Available at http://www.nccn.org/professionals/physician_gls/PDF/head-and-neck.pdf

National Institute for Occupational Safety and Health (NIOSH), "NIOSH List of Antineoplastic and Other Hazardous Drugs in Healthcare Settings 2012." Available at http://www.cdc.gov/niosh/docs/2012-150/pdfs/2012-150.pdf. Accessed January 21, 2013.

Stefanou A, Siderov J, Society of Hospital Pharmacists of Australia Committee of Specialty Practice in Oncology. Medical errors. Dosage nomenclature of bleomycin needs to be standardised to avoid errors. *BMJ*. 2001;322(7299):1423-1424.

Straus DJ, Portlock CS, Qin J, et al, "Results of a Prospective Randomized Clinical Trial of Doxorubicin, Bleomycin, Vinblastine, and Dacarbazine (ABVD) Followed by Radiation Therapy (RT) Versus ABVD Alone for Stages I, II, and IIIA Nonbulky Hodgkin Disease," *Blood*, 2004, 104(12):3483-9.

◆ **Bleomycin Injection, USP (Can)** *see* Bleomycin *on page 295*

◆ **Bleomycin Sulfate** *see* Bleomycin *on page 295*

◆ **Bleph-10** *see* Sulfacetamide (Ophthalmic) *on page 1943*

◆ **Bleph 10 DPS (Can)** *see* Sulfacetamide (Ophthalmic) *on page 1943*

◆ **BLM** *see* Bleomycin *on page 295*

◆ **Bloxiverz** *see* Neostigmine *on page 1486*

◆ **BMS-188667** *see* Abatacept *on page 44*

◆ **BMS-232632** *see* Atazanavir *on page 218*

◆ **BMS 337039** *see* ARIPiprazole *on page 196*

◆ **B&O** *see* Belladonna and Opium *on page 269*

◆ **BOL-303224-A** *see* Besifloxacin *on page 281*

◆ **Boostrix** *see* Diphtheria and Tetanus Toxoids, and Acellular Pertussis Vaccine *on page 686*

Bosentan (boe SEN tan)

Medication Safety Issues
Sound-alike/look-alike issues:
Tracleer® may be confused with TriCor®

Related Information
Oral Medications That Should Not Be Crushed or Altered *on page 2438*
Safe Handling of Hazardous Drugs *on page 2419*
Brand Names: U.S. Tracleer
Brand Names: Canada CO Bosentan; Mylan-Bosentan; PMS-Bosentan; Sandoz-Bosentan; Tracleer®
Therapeutic Category Endothelin Receptor Antagonist
Generic Availability (U.S.) No
Use Treatment of pulmonary arterial hypertension (PAH) [WHO Group I] in patients with NYHA Class II, III, or IV symptoms to improve exercise capacity and decrease the rate of clinical deterioration (FDA approved in ages >12 years and adults); **Note:** Clinical trials establishing effectiveness included primarily patients with NYHA Functional Class II-IV symptoms.

Prescribing and Access Restrictions As a requirement of the REMS program, access to this medication is restricted. Bosentan (Tracleer®) is only available through Tracleer® Access Program (T.A.P.). Only prescribers and pharmacies registered with T.A.P. may prescribe and dispense bosentan. Further information may be obtained from the manufacturer, Actelion Pharmaceuticals (1-866-228-3546 or http://www.tracleer.com/hcp/prescribing-tracleer.asp).

Medication Guide Available Yes
Pregnancy Risk Factor X
Pregnancy Considerations [U.S. Boxed Warning]: May cause birth defects; use in pregnancy is contraindicated. Exclude pregnancy prior to initiation of therapy and obtain pregnancy tests monthly during treatment. Reliable contraception must be used during therapy and for 1 month after stopping treatment. Hormonal contraceptives (oral, injectable, transdermal, or implantable) may not be effective and a second method of contraception (nonhormonal) is required. Patients with tubal ligation or an implanted IUD (Copper T 380A or LNg 20) do not need additional contraceptive measures. When a hormonal or barrier contraceptive is used, one additional method of contraception is still needed if a male partner has had a vasectomy. When initiating treatment for women of reproductive potential, a negative pregnancy test should be documented within the first 5 days of a normal menstrual period and ≥11 days after the last unprotected intercourse. A missed menses or suspected pregnancy should be reported to a healthcare provider and prompt immediate pregnancy testing. Sperm counts may be reduced in men during treatment. Women of childbearing potential should avoid splitting, crushing, or handling broken tablets and exposure to the generated dust (tablet splitting is currently outside of product labeling).

Breast-Feeding Considerations Due to the potential risk of adverse events in a nursing infant, a decision should be made to discontinue nursing or discontinue therapy.

Contraindications Hypersensitivity to bosentan or any component; pregnancy; concurrent use of cyclosporine or glyburide

Warnings Hazardous agent; use appropriate precautions for handling and disposal (NIOSH, 2012). Women of childbearing potential should avoid splitting, crushing, or handling broken tablets and exposure to the generated dust (should be dissolved in water if necessary).

Serious hepatic injury, including rare reports of cirrhosis and liver failure may occur **[U.S. Boxed Warning]**. Dose-dependent elevations in liver aminotransferases (ALT and AST) of at least 3 times the ULN may occur at any time during therapy in up to 11% of patients; elevations in bilirubin may occur in some cases; progression of liver enzyme elevation is generally slow and asymptomatic and usually reversible after drug interruption or discontinuation of therapy. Rare cases of hepatic cirrhosis have been reported after prolonged use (>12 months) and in patients receiving multiple medications. Monitor liver enzymes at baseline and monthly thereafter. Use with caution in patients with mildly impaired liver function; avoid use in moderate to severe hepatic impairment. Avoid use in patients with elevated serum transaminases (>3 times ULN) at baseline; adjust dosage if elevations in liver enzymes occur during therapy. Treatment should be discontinued in patients who develop elevated transaminases (ALT or AST) in combination with symptoms of hepatic injury (unusual fatigue, jaundice, nausea, vomiting, abdominal pain, and/or fever) or elevated serum bilirubin ≥2 times ULN. Consider the benefits of treatment versus the risk of hepatotoxicity when initiating therapy in patients with WHO Class II symptoms. Patients with WHO Class II symptoms who received bosentan demonstrated a decrease in the rate of clinical deterioration; however, only a trend for improved exercise capacity was observed. The risk of serious hepatic injury should be weighed against these benefits in this group of patients, as serious hepatic injury may preclude future use of bosentan as the disease progresses.

May cause birth defects; use in pregnancy contraindicated **[U.S. Boxed Warning]**. Exclude pregnancy prior to initiation of therapy; obtain monthly pregnancy tests during treatment. Reliable contraception must be used during therapy and for 1 month after stopping treatment. Hormonal contraceptives (oral, injectable, transdermal, or implantable) may not be effective and a second method of contraception (nonhormonal) is required. Patients with tubal ligation or an implanted IUD (Copper T 380A or LNg 20) do not need additional contraceptive measures.

Because of the risks of hepatic impairment and the high likelihood of teratogenic effects, bosentan is only available through the Tracleer® Access Program (T.A.P.) **[U.S. Boxed Warning]**. Patients, prescribers, and pharmacies must be registered with and meet conditions of T.A.P. Call 1-866-228-3546 or visit http://www.tracleer.com/hcp/prescribing-tracleer.asp for more information.

Bosentan may interact with many medications and may result in potentially serious and/or life-threatening adverse events; concurrent use with some medications is contraindicated (ie, cyclosporine, glyburide) and other medications may require dosage adjustments. Consult drug interactions database for more detailed information.

Precautions Use with caution in patients with low hemoglobin levels or ischemic cardiovascular disease; may cause dose-related decreases in hematocrit and hemoglobin (≥1 g/dL in up to 57% of patients, typically in first 6 weeks of therapy; markedly decreased hemoglobin may occur in up to 6% of patients); measure hemoglobin prior to initiating therapy, at 1 and 3 months, and every 3 months thereafter. Significant decreases in hemoglobin in the absence of other causes may warrant the discontinuation of therapy. May cause fluid retention, worsening of CHF, weight gain, and leg edema; **Note:** PAH itself may cause fluid retention and edema; if significant fluid retention occurs, further evaluation may be necessary to determine the cause and appropriate treatment or discontinuation of bosentan therapy. If pulmonary edema occurs, consider the possibility of pulmonary veno-occlusive disease (PVOD) and discontinue bosentan. Sperm count may be reduced in men during treatment; no changes in sperm function or hormone levels have been noted; fertility issues may require discussion with patient.

Adverse Reactions

Cardiovascular: Chest pain, edema, flushing, hypotension, palpitation, syncope

Central nervous system: Headache

Dermatologic: Pruritus

Endocrine & metabolic: Spermatogenesis inhibition

Hematologic: Anemia, decreased hemoglobin

Hepatic: Abnormal hepatic function, transaminases increased

Neuromuscular & skeletal: Arthralgia

Respiratory: Respiratory tract infection, sinusitis

Rare but important or life-threatening: Anaphylaxis, angioneurotic edema, heart failure (exacerbation), cirrhosis (prolonged therapy), hyperbilirubinemia, hypersensitivity, jaundice, leukocytoclastic vasculitis, leukopenia, liver failure (rare), neutropenia, peripheral edema, rash, thrombocytopenia, weight gain

Drug Interactions

Metabolism/Transport Effects Substrate of CYP2C9 (minor), CYP3A4 (minor), SLCO1B1; **Note:** Assignment of Major/Minor substrate status based on clinically relevant drug interaction potential; **Induces** CYP2C9 (weak/moderate), CYP3A4 (weak/moderate)

Avoid Concomitant Use

Avoid concomitant use of Bosentan with any of the following: Axitinib; CycloSPORINE (Systemic); GlyBURIDE; Simeprevir

Increased Effect/Toxicity

The levels/effects of Bosentan may be increased by: Atazanavir; Boceprevir; Cobicistat; CycloSPORINE (Systemic); CYP2C9 Inhibitors (Moderate); CYP2C9 Inhibitors (Strong); CYP3A4 Inhibitors (Moderate); CYP3A4 Inhibitors (Strong); Darunavir; Eltrombopag; Fosamprenavir; GlyBURIDE; Indinavir; Lopinavir; Nelfinavir; Phosphodiesterase 5 Inhibitors; Rifampin; Ritonavir; Saquinavir; Telaprevir; Tipranavir

Decreased Effect

Bosentan may decrease the levels/effects of: ARIPiprazole; Atazanavir; Axitinib; Boceprevir; Contraceptives (Estrogens); Contraceptives (Progestins); CycloSPORINE (Systemic); CYP3A4 Substrates; Darunavir; Fosamprenavir; GlyBURIDE; HMG-CoA Reductase Inhibitors; Ibrutinib; Indinavir; Lopinavir; Nelfinavir; Phosphodiesterase 5 Inhibitors; Saquinavir; Saxagliptin; Simeprevir; Telaprevir; Tipranavir; Vitamin K Antagonists

The levels/effects of Bosentan may be decreased by: GlyBURIDE; Rifampin

Food Interactions Bioavailability of bosentan is not affected by food. Bosentan serum concentrations may be increased by grapefruit juice. Management: Avoid grapefruit/grapefruit juice.

Stability Hazardous agent; use appropriate precautions for handling and disposal (NIOSH, 2012). Store at controlled room temperature of 20°C to 25°C (68°F to 77°F); excursions permitted to 15°C to 30°C (59°F to 86°F).

Mechanism of Action Blocks endothelin receptors on vascular endothelium and smooth muscle. Stimulation of these receptors is associated with vasoconstriction. Although bosentan blocks both ET_A and ET_B receptors, the affinity is higher for the A subtype.

Pharmacokinetics (Adult data unless noted)

Distribution: Does not distribute into RBCs; V_d: ~18 L

Protein binding: >98% to plasma proteins (primarily albumin)

Metabolism: Extensive in the liver via cytochrome P450 isoenzymes CYP2C9 and CYP3A4 to three metabolites (one has pharmacologic activity and may account for 10% to 20% of drug effect); steady-state plasma concentrations are 50% to 65% of those attained after single dose (most likely due to autoinduction of liver enzymes); steady-state is attained within 3-5 days

Bioavailability: ~50%

Half-life: Healthy subjects: 5 hours; half-life may be prolonged in PAH, as AUC is 2-fold greater in adults with PAH versus healthy subjects

Time to peak serum concentration: Oral: Within 3-5 hours

Elimination: Biliary excretion; urine (<3% as unchanged drug)

Dialysis: Not likely to be removed (due to extensive protein binding and high molecular weight)

Dosing: Neonatal Note: Very limited information exists; further studies are needed

Full-Term Neonate: Oral: 1 mg/kg/dose twice daily short-term use (2-16 days) in three full-term neonates has been reported. In the initial report, two full-term neonates (8 days and 14 days old) with persistent pulmonary hypertension of the newborn (PPHN) and transposition of the great arteries received bosentan prior to cardiac surgery; patients also received other therapies (Goissen, 2008). A case report describes the use of bosentan monotherapy for PPHN in a full-term neonate as primary course of treatment initiated at 29 hours of life; therapy was weaned after 72 hours through the following dose reductions: 0.5 mg/kg/dose twice daily followed by 0.5 mg/kg once daily and subsequent discontinuation at 96 hours of treatment (Nakwan, 2009).

Dosing: Usual

Infants, Children, and Adolescents: **Pulmonary arterial hypertension:**

Infants ≥7 months and Children: Limited data exist; further studies needed (Barst, 2003; Ivy, 2004; Maiya, 2006; Rosenzweig, 2005):

Fixed dosing:

5 to <10 kg: Initial: 15.6 mg daily for 4 weeks; increase to maintenance dose of 15.6 mg twice daily

10-20 kg: Initial: 31.25 mg daily for 4 weeks; increase to maintenance dose of 31.25 mg twice daily

>20-40 kg: Initial: 31.25 mg twice daily for 4 weeks; increase to maintenance dose of 62.5 mg twice daily

>40 kg: Initial: 62.5 mg twice daily for 4 weeks; increase to maintenance dose of 125 mg twice daily

Weight-based dosing: Children ≥2 years: Initial: 0.75-1 mg/kg/dose twice daily for 4 weeks (maximum dose: 62.5 mg); then increase to maintenance dose of 2 mg/kg/dose twice daily (maximum dose: ≤40 kg: 62.5 mg; maximum dose: >40 kg: 125 mg); a higher daily dose of 4 mg/kg/dose twice daily has been studied but has not been shown to produce higher serum concentrations than 2 mg/kg/dose and is not recommended by authors of the trial (Beghetti, 2009; Beghetti, 2009a, Villanueva, 2006)

Adolescents <40 kg: Initial and maintenance: 62.5 mg twice daily

Adolescents ≥40 kg: Initial: 62.5 mg twice daily for 4 weeks; increase to maintenance dose of 125 mg twice daily; **Note:** Doses >125 mg twice daily do not provide additional benefit sufficient to offset the increased risk of hepatic injury. When discontinuing treatment, consider a reduction in dosage to 62.5 mg twice daily for 3-7 days to avoid clinical deterioration.

Adults: **Pulmonary arterial hypertension:** Initial: 62.5 mg twice daily for 4 weeks; increase to maintenance dose of 125 mg twice daily; adults <40 kg should be maintained at 62.5 mg twice daily. **Note:** Doses >125 mg twice daily do not provide additional benefit sufficient to offset the increased risk of hepatic injury. When discontinuing treatment, consider a reduction in dosage to 62.5 mg twice daily for 3-7 days (to avoid clinical deterioration).

Coadministration with protease inhibitor regimen: Adults:

Dosage adjustment for concurrent use with atazanavir/ritonavir, darunavir/ritonavir, fosamprenavir, lopinavir/ritonavir, ritonavir, saquinavir/ritonavir, tipranavir/ritonavir:

Coadministration of bosentan in patients currently receiving one of these protease inhibitor regimens for at least 10 days: Begin with bosentan 62.5 mg once daily or every other day based on tolerability

Coadministration of one of these protease inhibitor regimens in patients currently receiving bosentan: Discontinue bosentan at least 36 hours prior to the initiation of an above protease inhibitor regimen. After at least 10 days of the protease inhibitor regimen, resume bosentan 62.5 mg once daily or every other day based on tolerability

Dosage adjustment for concurrent use with indinavir or nelfinavir:

Coadministration of bosentan in patients currently receiving indinavir or nelfinavir: Begin with bosentan 62.5 mg once daily or every other day based on tolerability

Coadministration of indinavir or nelfinavir in patients currently receiving bosentan: Adjust bosentan to 62.5 mg once daily or every other day based on tolerability

Dosing adjustment in renal impairment: No dosage adjustment required.

Dosing adjustment in hepatic impairment: Adolescents and Adults:

Mild impairment (Child-Pugh class A): No dosage adjustment necessary.

Moderate to severe impairment (Child-Pugh class B and C) and/or baseline transaminase >3 times ULN: Use not recommended; systemic exposure significantly increased in patients with moderate impairment (not studied in patients with severe impairment).

Dosing adjustment based on serum transaminase elevation: Adults: If any elevation, regardless of degree, is accompanied by clinical symptoms of hepatic injury (unusual fatigue, nausea, vomiting, abdominal pain, fever, or jaundice) or a serum bilirubin ≥2 times ULN, treatment should be stopped.

AST/ALT >3 times but ≤5 times ULN: Confirm elevation with additional test; if confirmed, reduce dose to 62.5 mg or interrupt treatment. Monitor transaminase levels at least every 2 weeks. May continue or reintroduce treatment, as appropriate, following return to pretreatment aminotransferase values. When reintroducing treatment, begin with starting dose and recheck transaminases within 3 days and at least every 2 weeks thereafter.

AST/ALT >5 times but ≤8 times upper limit of normal: Confirm elevation with additional test; if confirmed, stop treatment. Monitor transaminase levels at least every 2 weeks. May reintroduce treatment, as appropriate, following return to pretreatment aminotransferase values. When reintroducing treatment, begin with starting dose and recheck transaminases within 3 days and at least every 2 weeks thereafter.

AST/ALT >8 times upper limit of normal: Stop treatment and do not reintroduce.

Administration Hazardous agent; use appropriate precautions for handling and disposal (NIOSH, 2012).

Oral: May be administered without regard to meals. Avoid grapefruit and grapefruit juice. Women of childbearing potential should avoid splitting, crushing, or handling broken tablets and exposure to the generated dust (tablets should be dissolved in water if necessary).

Monitoring Parameters Serum transaminase (AST and ALT) and bilirubin should be determined prior to the initiation of therapy and at monthly intervals thereafter. Monitor for clinical signs and symptoms of liver injury (eg, abdominal pain, fatigue, fever, jaundice, nausea, vomiting). Hemoglobin and hematocrit should be measured at baseline, after 1 and 3 months of treatment, and every 3 months thereafter.

A woman of childbearing potential must have a negative pregnancy test prior to the initiation of therapy, monthly thereafter, and 1 month after stopping therapy.

Additional Information The addition of bosentan to epoprostenol therapy in 8 children (8-18 years of age) with idiopathic PAH allowed for a reduction in the epoprostenol dose (and its associated side effects) in 7 of the 8 children.

Epoprostenol was able to be discontinued in 3 of the 8 children (Ivy, 2004). The results from the European post-marketing surveillance program in children 2-11 years of age confirm the need for monthly measurement of liver aminotransferases in pediatric patients for the duration of bosentan treatment (Beghetti, 2008).

Clinical studies in adults have shown that bosentan was **not** effective in the treatment of CHF in patients with left ventricular dysfunction; hospitalizations for CHF were more common during the first 1-2 months after initiation of the drug.

Dosage Forms Excipient information presented when available (limited, particularly for generics); consult specific product labeling.

Tablet, Oral:

Tracleer: 62.5 mg, 125 mg

Extemporaneous Preparations Hazardous agent: Use appropriate precautions for handling and disposal.

Note: Tablets are not scored; a commercial pill cutter should be used to prepare a 31.25 mg dose from the 62.5 mg tablet; the half-cut 62.5 mg tablets are stable for up to 4 weeks when stored at room temperature in the high-density polyethylene plastic bottle provided by the manufacturer. Since bosentan is classified as a teratogen (Pregnancy Risk Factor X), individuals should avoid exposure to bosentan powder (dust) by taking appropriate measures (eg, using gloves and mask); women of child-bearing potential should avoid exposure to dust generated from broken or split tablets.

Crushing of the tablets is not recommended; bosentan tablets will disintegrate rapidly (within 5 minutes) in 5-25 mL of water to create a suspension. An appropriate aliquot of the suspension can be used to deliver the prescribed dose. Any remaining suspension should be discarded. Bosentan should not be mixed or dissolved in liquids with a low (acidic) pH (eg, fruit juices) due to poor solubility; the drug is most soluble in solutions with a pH >8.5.

References

Adatia I, "Improving the Outcome of Childhood Pulmonary Arterial Hypertension: The Effect of Bosentan in the Setting of a Dedicated Pulmonary Hypertension Clinic," *J Am Coll Cardiol*, 2005, 46 (4):705-6.

Apostolopoulou SC, Manginas A, Cokkinos DV, et al, "Long-Term Oral Bosentan Treatment in Patients With Pulmonary Arterial Hypertension Related to Congenital Heart Disease: A 2-Year Study," *Heart*, 2007, 93(3):350-4.

Barst RJ, Ivy D, Dingemanse J, et al, "Pharmacokinetics, Safety, and Efficacy of Bosentan in Pediatric Patients With Pulmonary Arterial Hypertension," *Clin Pharmacol Ther*, 2003, 73(4):372-82.

Beghetti M, "Bosentan in Pediatric Patients With Pulmonary Arterial Hypertension," *Curr Vasc Pharmacol*, 2009, 7(2):225-33.

Beghetti M, "Current Treatment Options in Children With Pulmonary Arterial Hypertension and Experiences With Oral Bosentan," *Eur J Clin Invest*, 2006, 36(Suppl 3):16-24.

Beghetti M, Haworth SG, Bonnet D, et al, "Pharmacokinetic and Clinical Profile of a Novel Formulation of Bosentan in Children With Pulmonary Arterial Hypertension: The FUTURE-1 Study," *Br J Clin Pharmacol*, 2009a, 68(6):948-55.

Beghetti M, Hoeper MM, Kiely DG, et al, "Safety Experience With Bosentan in 146 Children 2-11 Years Old With Pulmonary Arterial Hypertension: Results From the European Postmarketing Surveillance Program," *Pediatr Res*, 2008, 64(2):200-4.

Carter NJ and Keating GM, "Bosentan: In Pediatric Patients With Pulmonary Arterial Hypertension," *Paediatr Drugs*, 2010, 12(1):63-73.

Gilbert N, Luther YC, Miera O, et al, "Initial Experience With Bosentan (Tracleer®) as Treatment for Pulmonary Arterial Hypertension (PAH) Due to Congenital Heart Disease in Infants and Young Children," *Z Kardiol*, 2005, 94(9):570-4.

Goissen C, Ghyselen L, Tourneux P, et al, "Persistent Pulmonary Hypertension of the Newborn With Transposition of the Great Arteries: Successful Treatment With Bosentan," *Eur J Pediatr*, 2008, 167 (4):437-40.

Ivy DD, Doran A, Claussen L, et al, "Weaning and Discontinuation of Epoprostenol in Children With Idiopathic Pulmonary Arterial Hypertension Receiving Concomitant Bosentan," *Am J Cardiol*, 2004, 93 (7):943-6.

Ivy DD, Rosenzweig EB, Lemarié JC, et al, "Long-Term Outcomes in Chidren With Pulmonary Arterial Hypertension Treated With Bosentan in Real-World Clinical Settings," *Am J Cardiol*, 2010, 106(9):1332-8.

Lunze K, Gilbert N, Mebus S, et al, "First Experience With an Oral Combination Therapy Using Bosentan and Sildenafil for Pulmonary Arterial Hypertension," *Eur J Clin Invest*, 2006, 36 Suppl 3:32-8.

Maiya S, Hislop AA, Flynn Y, et al, "Response to Bosentan in Children With Pulmonary Hypertension," *Heart*, 2006, 92(5):664-70.

Nakwan N, Choksuchat D, Saksawad R, et al, "Successful Treatment of Persistent Pulmonary Hypertension of the Newborn With Bosentan," *Acta Paediatr*, 2009, 98(10):1683-5.

National Institute for Occupational Safety and Health (NIOSH), "NIOSH List of Antineoplastic and Other Hazardous Drugs in Healthcare Settings 2012." Available at http://www.cdc.gov/niosh/docs/2012-150/pdfs/2012-150.pdf. Accessed January 21, 2013.

Rosenzweig EB, Ivy DD, Widlitz A, et al, "Effects of Long-Term Bosentan in Children With Pulmonary Arterial Hypertension," *J Am Coll Cardiol*, 2005, 46(4):697-704.

Sitbon O, Beghetti M, Petit J, et al, "Bosentan for the Treatment of Pulmonary Arterial Hypertension Associated With Congenital Heart Defects," *Eur J Clin Invest*, 2006, 36(Suppl 3):25-31.

Villanueva D. Medical Information Manager, Actelion, personal correspondence, March 2006.

◆ **Botox** *see* OnabotulinumtoxinA *on page 1541*

◆ **Botox Cosmetic** *see* OnabotulinumtoxinA *on page 1541*

◆ **Botulinum Toxin Type A** *see* OnabotulinumtoxinA *on page 1541*

◆ **Botulinum Toxin Type B** *see* RimabotulinumtoxinB *on page 1829*

Botulism Immune Globulin (Intravenous-Human)

(BOT yoo lism i MYUN GLOB you lin, in tra VEE nus, YU man)

Medication Safety Issues

Sound-alike/look-alike issues:

BabyBIG® may be confused with HBIG

Brand Names: U.S. BabyBIG®

Therapeutic Category Immune Globulin

Generic Availability (U.S.) No

Use Treatment of infant botulism caused by toxin type A or B (FDA approved in ages <1 year)

Prescribing and Access Restrictions Access to botulism immune globulin is restricted through the Infant Botulism Treatment and Prevention Program (IBTPP). Healthcare providers must contact the IBTPP on-call physician at (510) 231-7600 to review treatment indications and to obtain the medication. For more information, refer to http://www.infantbotulism.org or contact IBTPP@infantbotulism.org.

Pregnancy Considerations Botulism immune globulin is only indicated for use in neonates.

Contraindications Hypersensitivity to immune globulin or any component; IgA deficiency (BabyBIG® contains trace amounts of immunoglobulin A)

Warnings Renal dysfunction and/or acute renal failure has been reported with the administration of immune globulin intravenous (IGIV); 88% of the cases were associated with the administration of sucrose-containing IGIV products at doses of 400 mg/kg or greater. BabyBIG® contains sucrose as a stabilizer. BabyBIG® is made from human plasma which carries the risk of blood-borne virus transmission, including the disease-causing agent for Creutzfeldt-Jakob disease. Like any other blood product, the risks and benefits of this agent should be discussed between the patient's legal guardian and the attending physician.

An aseptic meningitis syndrome has been reported to occur with high total doses of other I.V. immune globulin products (eg, 2 g/kg of IGIV). Symptoms usually present within hours to days of treatment. Signs and symptoms may include severe headache, nuchal rigidity, photophobia, nausea, vomiting, painful eye movement, and fever. Cerebrospinal fluid may be positive with pleocytosis and increased protein concentrations. IGIV has been associated with antiglobulin hemolysis; monitor for signs of hemolytic anemia.

Hyperproteinemia, increased serum viscosity, and hyponatremia may occur following administration of IGIV products; distinguish hyponatremia from pseudohyponatremia to prevent volume depletion, a further increase in serum viscosity, and a higher risk of thrombotic events. These adverse events have not been reported with botulism immune globulin. Thrombotic events have been reported with administration of IGIV; use with caution in patients with a history of atherosclerosis or cardiovascular and/or thrombotic risk factors or patients with known/suspected hyperviscosity. Consider a baseline assessment of blood viscosity in patients at risk for hyperviscosity. Infuse at lowest practical rate in patients at risk for thrombotic events. Noncardiogenic pulmonary edema has been reported with IGIV use. Monitor for transfusion-related acute lung injury (TRALI). TRALI is characterized by severe respiratory distress, pulmonary edema, hypoxemia, and fever in the presence of normal left ventricular function and usually occurs within 1-6 hours after infusion.

Precautions Use with caution in patients at increased risk for developing acute renal failure (patients with preexisting renal insufficiency, diabetes mellitus, volume depletion, sepsis, paraproteinemia, and concomitant nephrotoxic drugs). Assure that patients are not volume depleted prior to the initiation of BabyBIG®. If a minor reaction occurs during infusion (eg, flushing), decrease infusion rate; if anaphylaxis or significant hypotension occurs, discontinue infusion.

Adverse Reactions

Cardiovascular: Blood pressure increased/decreased, cardiac murmur, edema, pallor, peripheral coldness, tachycardia

Central nervous system: Agitation, body temperature decreased, irritability, pyrexia

Dermatologic: Contact dermatitis, erythematous rash

Endocrine & metabolic: Dehydration, hyponatremia, metabolic acidosis

Gastrointestinal: Abdominal distension, dysphagia, loose stools, vomiting

Hematologic: Anemia, hemoglobin decreased

Local: Injection site erythema, injection site reaction

Otic: Otitis media

Renal: Neurogenic bladder

Respiratory: Atelectasis, breath sounds decreased cough, dyspnea, lower respiratory tract infection, nasal congestion, oxygen saturation decreased, rales, rhonchi, stridor, tachypnea

Miscellaneous: Infusion rate reactions (includes back pain, chills, fever, muscle cramps, nausea, vomiting, wheezing), oral candidiasis, intubation

Drug Interactions

Metabolism/Transport Effects None known.

Avoid Concomitant Use There are no known interactions where it is recommended to avoid concomitant use.

Increased Effect/Toxicity There are no known significant interactions involving an increase in effect.

Decreased Effect

Botulism Immune Globulin (Intravenous-Human) may decrease the levels/effects of: Vaccines (Live)

Stability Store between 2°C to 8°C (35.6°F to 46.4°F). Since BabyBIG® does not contain a preservative, reconstituted vials should be used within 2 hours. Do not mix with other drugs.

Mechanism of Action BIG-IV is purified immunoglobulin derived from the plasma of adults immunized with botulinum toxoid types A and B. BIG-IV provides antibodies to neutralize circulating toxins.

Pharmacodynamics Duration: ~6 months with a single infusion

Pharmacokinetics (Adult data unless noted) Half-life: Infants: ~28 days

Dosing: Neonatal I.V.: Dosage is specific to the manufactured lot, as of March 2012 (Lot 4 production): Total dose is 75 mg/kg as a single I.V. infusion. Start as soon as diagnosis of infant botulism is made; refer to product specific information.

Dosing: Usual I.V.: Infants: Dosage is specific to the manufactured lot, as of March 2012 (Lot 4 production): Total dose is 75 mg/kg as a single I.V. infusion. Start as soon as diagnosis of infant botulism is made; refer to product specific information.

Administration Do not administer I.M. or SubQ

I.V. infusion: Add 2 mL SWI to 100 mg vial, resulting in 50 mg/mL solution; rotate vial gently to wet all the powder and avoid foaming. Do not shake vial. Allow solution to stand 30 minutes until it clears. Infusion should be started within 2 hours of reconstitution and be completed within 4 hours of reconstitution. Use low volume tubing for administration via a separate line. If this is not possible, piggyback BabyBIG® into a preexisting line containing either NS or a dextrose solution ($D_{2.5}W$, D_5W, $D_{10}W$, or $D_{20}W$) with or without added NaCl. Do not dilute more than 1:2 with any of the above solutions. Drug concentration should be no less than 25 mg/mL. Administer via an in-line 18 micron filter.

Initial: Administer slowly at 25 mg/kg/hour (0.5 mL/kg/hour using the 50 mg/mL concentration) for the first 15 minutes; after 15 minutes, rate may be increased to the maximum infusion rate of 50 mg/kg/hour (1 mL/kg/hour using the 50 mg/mL concentration) to the end of the infusion (infusion should conclude within 4 hours of reconstitution unless infusion rate is decreased due to an adverse reaction).

Monitoring Parameters Vital signs and blood pressure monitored continuously during the infusion. BUN and serum creatinine should be monitored prior to initial infusion. Periodic monitoring of renal function tests and urine output in patients at risk for developing renal failure.

Additional Information Once the patient is approved and purchase agreement is faxed, the original copy of the purchase agreement must be returned to the IBTPP via overnight courier, and payment must be wired within 5 business days. Arrange for courier pick-up of BabyBIG® from FFF Enterprises in Temecula, CA.

Prior to March 2012, dosing recommendations were for **Lot 3** for a total dose of 100 mg/kg/dose.

Dosage Forms Excipient information presented when available (limited, particularly for generics); consult specific product labeling.

Injection, powder for reconstitution [preservative free]:
BabyBIG®: ~100 mg [contains albumin (human), sucrose; supplied with diluent]

References

Arnon SS, Schechter R, Maslanka SE, et al, "Human Botulism Immune Globulin for the Treatment of Infant Botulism," N Engl J Med, 2006, 354(5):462-71.

Infant Botulism Treatment and Prevention Program, Department of Communicable Disease Control, California Department of Health Services, http://infantbotulism.org

Underwood K, Rubin S, Deakers T, et al, "Infant Botulism: A 30-Year Experience Spanning the Introduction of Botulism Immune Globulin Intravenous in the Intensive Care Unit at Childrens Hospital Los Angeles," Pediatrics, 2007, 120(6):e1380-5.

◆ **Boudreaux's® Butt Paste [OTC]** see Zinc Oxide on page 2176

◆ **Bovine Lung Surfactant** see Beractant on page 280

◆ **Bovine Lung Surfactant** see Calfactant on page 360

◆ **BP Cleansing [OTC]** see Benzoyl Peroxide on page 275

◆ **BP Foam** see Benzoyl Peroxide on page 275

◆ **BP Gel [OTC]** see Benzoyl Peroxide on page 275

◆ **BPO** *see* Benzoyl Peroxide *on page 275*

◆ **BPO-5 Wash [OTC]** *see* Benzoyl Peroxide *on page 275*

◆ **BPO-10 Wash [OTC]** *see* Benzoyl Peroxide *on page 275*

◆ **BPO Creamy Wash** *see* Benzoyl Peroxide *on page 275*

◆ **BPO Foaming Cloths** *see* Benzoyl Peroxide *on page 275*

◆ **BProtected Pedia D-Vite [OTC]** *see* Cholecalciferol *on page 455*

◆ **BProtected Pedia Iron [OTC]** *see* Ferrous Sulfate *on page 868*

◆ **BProtected Vitamin C [OTC]** *see* Ascorbic Acid *on page 206*

◆ **BP Wash** *see* Benzoyl Peroxide *on page 275*

◆ **Brethaire** *see* Terbutaline *on page 1984*

◆ **Brethine** *see* Terbutaline *on page 1984*

◆ **Brevibloc** *see* Esmolol *on page 791*

◆ **Brevibloc® (Can)** *see* Esmolol *on page 791*

◆ **Brevibloc in NaCl** *see* Esmolol *on page 791*

◆ **Brevibloc® Premixed (Can)** *see* Esmolol *on page 791*

◆ **Brevital® (Can)** *see* Methohexital *on page 1365*

◆ **Brevital Sodium** *see* Methohexital *on page 1365*

◆ **Bricanyl** *see* Terbutaline *on page 1984*

◆ **Bricanyl® Turbuhaler® (Can)** *see* Terbutaline *on page 1984*

Brimonidine (Ophthalmic) (bri MOE ni deen)

Medication Safety Issues
Sound-alike/look-alike issues:
Brimonidine may be confused with bromocriptine

Brand Names: U.S. Alphagan P

Brand Names: Canada Alphagan; Apo-Brimonidine; Apo-Brimonidine P; PMS-Brimonidine Tartrate; ratio-Brimonidine; Sandoz-Brimonidine

Therapeutic Category Alpha-Adrenergic Agonist, Ophthalmic; Glaucoma, Treatment Agent

Generic Availability (U.S.) Yes

Use Lowering of IOP in patients with open-angle glaucoma or ocular hypertension (FDA approved in ages ≥2 years and adults)

Pregnancy Risk Factor B

Pregnancy Considerations Teratogenic effects were not observed in animal reproduction studies.

Breast-Feeding Considerations It is not known if brimonidine is excreted in breast milk. Due to the potential for serious adverse reactions in the nursing infant, a decision should be made whether to discontinue nursing or to discontinue the drug, taking into account the importance of treatment to the mother.

Contraindications Hypersensitivity to brimonidine or any component; use in neonates, infants, and children <2 years

Warnings May cause CNS depression, particularly in young children; the most common adverse effect reported in a study of pediatric glaucoma patients was somnolence and decreased alertness (50% to 83% in children 2-6 years of age); these effects resulted in a 16% discontinuation of treatment rate; children >7 years (>20 kg) had a much lower rate of somnolence (25%); apnea, bradycardia, hypotension, hypothermia, hypotonia, and somnolence have been reported in infants receiving brimonidine

Precautions Use with caution in patients receiving concomitant MAO inhibitor therapy or with severe cardiovascular disease, hepatic or renal impairment (not studied), depression, cerebral or coronary insufficiency, Raynaud's phenomenon, orthostatic hypotension, or thromboangiitis. Some formulations may contain benzalkonium chloride which may be adsorbed by soft contact lenses; remove contacts prior to administration and wait 15 minutes before reinserting.

Adverse Reactions
Cardiovascular: Hyper-/hypotension
Central nervous system: Alertness decreased (children), dizziness, fatigue, headache, insomnia, somnolence
Dermatologic: Rash
Endocrine & metabolic: Hypercholesterolemia
Gastrointestinal: Dyspepsia, xerostomia
Neuromuscular & skeletal: Weakness
Ocular: Allergic conjunctivitis, blepharitis, blepharoconjunctivitis, blurred vision, burning sensation, cataract, conjunctival edema, conjunctival folliculosis, conjunctival hemorrhage, conjunctival hyperemia, conjunctivitis, dry eye, epiphora, eye discharge, eye pruritus, eyelid disorder, eyelid edema, eyelid erythema, follicular conjunctivitis, foreign body sensation, irritation, keratitis, ocular allergic reaction, pain, photophobia, stinging, superficial punctate keratopathy, visual disturbance, visual acuity worsened, visual field defect, vitreous detachment, vitreous floaters, watery eyes
Respiratory: Bronchitis, cough, dyspnea, pharyngitis, rhinitis, sinus infection, sinusitis
Miscellaneous: Allergic reaction, flu-like syndrome, infection
Rare but important or life-threatening: Anterior uveitis, bradycardia, depression, hypersensitivity, iritis, keratoconjunctivitis sicca, miosis, nausea, skin reactions (erythema, eyelid pruritus, vasodilation), tachycardia; apnea, bradycardia, hypothermia, and hypotonia have been reported in infants

Drug Interactions
Metabolism/Transport Effects None known.

Avoid Concomitant Use
Avoid concomitant use of Brimonidine (Ophthalmic) with any of the following: Azelastine (Nasal); Iobenguane I 123; Paraldehyde; Thalidomide

Increased Effect/Toxicity
Brimonidine (Ophthalmic) may increase the levels/effects of: Alcohol (Ethyl); Azelastine (Nasal); Beta-Blockers; Buprenorphine; CNS Depressants; DULoxetine; Hydrocodone; Hypotensive Agents; Methotrimeprazine; Metyrosine; Paraldehyde; Pramipexole; ROPINIRole; Rotigotine; Selective Serotonin Reuptake Inhibitors; Thalidomide; Zolpidem

The levels/effects of Brimonidine (Ophthalmic) may be increased by: Barbiturates; Beta-Blockers; Brimonidine (Topical); Cannabis; Doxylamine; Dronabinol; Droperidol; HydrOXYzine; Kava Kava; Magnesium Sulfate; MAO Inhibitors; Methotrimeprazine; Nabilone; Perampanel; Rufinamide; Sodium Oxybate; Tapentadol; Tetrahydrocannabinol

Decreased Effect
Brimonidine (Ophthalmic) may decrease the levels/effects of: Iobenguane I 123

The levels/effects of Brimonidine (Ophthalmic) may be decreased by: Mirtazapine; Serotonin/Norepinephrine Reuptake Inhibitors; Tricyclic Antidepressants

Stability Store at 15°C to 25°C (59°F to 77°F).

Mechanism of Action Selective agonism for alpha$_2$-receptors; causes reduction of aqueous humor formation and increased uveoscleral outflow

Pharmacodynamics Maximum effect: 2 hours

Pharmacokinetics (Adult data unless noted)
Metabolism: Extensive in liver
Half-life: 2 hours
Time to peak serum concentration: Ophthalmic: Within 0.5-2.5 hours

◀ **Dosing: Usual Glaucoma, ocular hypertension:** Children ≥2 years, Adolescents, and Adults: Ophthalmic: Instill 1 drop into lower conjunctival sac of affected eye(s) 3 times daily (approximately every 8 hours)

Administration Ophthalmic: Instill into conjunctival sac avoiding contact of bottle tip with skin or eye; apply finger pressure to lacrimal sac during and for 1-2 minutes after instillation to decrease risk of absorption and systemic effects. Administer other topical ophthalmic medications at least 5 minutes apart; generic formulation contains benzalkonium chloride which may be absorbed by soft contact lenses; wait at least 15 minutes after administration to insert soft contact lenses.

Monitoring Parameters IOP

Dosage Forms Excipient information presented when available (limited, particularly for generics); consult specific product labeling.

Solution, Ophthalmic, as tartrate:
Alphagan P: 0.1% (5 mL, 10 mL, 15 mL); 0.15% (5 mL, 10 mL, 15 mL) [contains carboxymethylcellulose sodium]
Generic: 0.15% (5 mL, 10 mL, 15 mL); 0.2% (5 mL, 10 mL, 15 mL)

References
Berlin RJ, Lee UT, Samples JR, et al, "Ophthalmic Drops Causing Coma in an Infant," *J Pediatr*, 2001, 138(3):441-3.
Carlsen JO, Zabriskie NA, Kwon YH, et al, "Apparent Central Nervous System Depression in Infants After the Use of Topical Brimonidine," *Am J Ophthalmol*, 1999, 128(2):255-6.
Enyedi LB and Freedman SF, "Safety and Efficacy of Brimonidine in Children With Glaucoma," *J AAPOS*, 2001, 5(5):281-4.

◆ **Brimonidine Tartrate** *see* Brimonidine (Ophthalmic) *on page 303*

◆ **Brisdelle** *see* PARoxetine *on page 1609*

◆ **British Anti-Lewisite** *see* Dimercaprol *on page 672*

◆ **BRL 43694** *see* Granisetron *on page 980*

Bromocriptine (broe moe KRIP teen)

Medication Safety Issues
Sound-alike/look-alike issues:
Bromocriptine may be confused with benztropine, brimonidine
Cycloset® may be confused with Glyset®
Parlodel® may be confused with pindolol, Provera®

Related Information
Serotonin Syndrome *on page 2405*

Brand Names: U.S. Cycloset; Parlodel

Brand Names: Canada Dom-Bromocriptine; PMS-Bromocriptine

Therapeutic Category Anti-Parkinson's Agent, Dopamine Agonist; Antidiabetic Agent, Dopamine Agonist; Antidiabetic Agent, Oral; Ergot Derivative

Generic Availability (U.S.) Yes

Use Treatment of dysfunctions associated with hyperprolactinemia, including amenorrhea with or without galactorrhea, infertility, or hypogonadism (FDA approved in adults); treatment of prolactin-secreting adenomas (FDA approved in ages ≥11 years and adults); treatment of acromegaly (FDA approved in adults); treatment of Parkinson's disease (FDA approved in adults); treatment of type 2 diabetes mellitus as an adjunct to diet and exercise (Cycloset®: FDA approved in adults); has also been used for neuroleptic malignant syndrome

Pregnancy Risk Factor B

Pregnancy Considerations No evidence of teratogenicity or fetal toxicity in animal studies. Bromocriptine is used for ovulation induction in women with hyperprolactinemia. In general, therapy should be discontinued if pregnancy is confirmed unless needed for treatment of macroprolactinoma. Data collected from women taking bromocriptine during pregnancy suggest the incidence of birth defects is not increased with use. However, the majority of women discontinued use within 8 weeks of pregnancy. Women not seeking pregnancy should be advised to use appropriate contraception.

Breast-Feeding Considerations A previous indication for prevention of postpartum lactation was withdrawn voluntarily by the manufacturer following reports of serious adverse reactions, including stroke, MI, seizures, and severe hypertension. Use during breast-feeding is specifically contraindicated in the product labeling for Cycloset®. Use in postpartum women with a history of coronary artery disease or other severe cardiovascular conditions is specifically contraindicated in the product labeling for Parlodel® (unless withdrawal of medication is medically contraindicated). Based on the risk/benefit assessment, other treatments should be considered for lactation suppression.

Contraindications Hypersensitivity to bromocriptine, ergot alkaloids, or any component

Parlodel®: Uncontrolled hypertension; pregnancy (risk:benefit evaluation must be performed in women who become pregnant during treatment for acromegaly, prolactinoma, or Parkinson's disease; hypertension during treatment should generally result in efforts to withdraw therapy); postpartum women with a history of coronary artery disease or other severe cardiovascular conditions (unless withdrawal of medication is medically contraindicated)

Cycloset®: Syncopal migraine; breast-feeding

Warnings Complete evaluation of pituitary function should be completed prior to initiation of treatment for any hyperprolactinemia-associated dysfunction. Patients not seeking pregnancy or those with large adenomas should be advised to use contraception other than oral contraceptives during treatment with bromocriptine. Pregnancy testing is recommended at least every 4 weeks during the amenorrheic period and, once menses are reinitiated, every time a patient misses a menstrual period.

Symptomatic hypotension may occur in a significant number of patients (up to 30%) especially during the first days of treatment. Ergot alkaloids and derivatives have been associated with fibrotic valve thickening (eg, aortic, mitral, tricuspid) and is usually associated with long-term, chronic use. Hypertension, seizures, MI, and stroke have been rarely associated with therapy. Severe headache or visual changes may precede events. The onset of reactions may be immediate or delayed (often may occur in the second week of therapy). Patients who receive bromocriptine during and immediately following pregnancy as a continuation of previous therapy (eg, acromegaly) should be closely monitored for cardiovascular effects. Prolactin-secreting adenomas may expand and compress the optic or other cranial nerves. Monitoring and careful evaluation of visual changes during the treatment of hyperprolactinemia is recommended to differentiate between tumor shrinkage and traction on the optic chiasm. Rapidly progressing visual field loss requires neurosurgical consultation. In most cases, compression resolves following delivery.

Rare cases of pleural and pericardial effusions as well as pleural and pulmonary fibrosis and constrictive pericarditis have been reported, particularly with long term and high-dose treatment. Retroperitoneal fibrosis has also been reported.

In the treatment of acromegaly, discontinuation is recommended if tumor expansion occurs during therapy. Cold sensitive digital vasospasm may occur in some patients with acromegaly and may be reversed with dosage reduction. Discontinuation of therapy in patients with macroadenomas has been associated with rapid regrowth of tumor and increased prolactin serum levels. Patients treated with pituitary radiation should have an annual 4-8 week withdrawal from bromocriptine to assess both the clinical effects of radiation on the disease process as well as the effects of bromocriptine. Recurrence of signs and symptoms or increases in growth hormone indicate the need to resume treatment.

Safety has not been established for therapy duration >2 years in patients with Parkinson's disease. Concurrent use with levodopa has been associated with an increased risk of hallucinations; consider dosage reduction and/or discontinuation in patients with hallucinations. Hallucinations may require weeks to months before resolution. Dopamine agonists used to treat Parkinson's have been associated with compulsive behaviors and/or loss of impulse control, which has manifested as pathological gambling/spending, libido increases (hypersexuality), and/or binge eating. Causality has not been established, and controversy exists as to whether this phenomenon is related to the underlying disease, prior behaviors/addictions, and/or drug therapy. Dose reduction or discontinuation of therapy has been reported to reverse these behaviors in some, but not all cases. Risk for melanoma development is increased in Parkinson's disease patients; drug causation or factors contributing to risk have not been established. Patients should be monitored closely and periodic skin examinations should be performed. Bromocriptine has been associated with sudden onset of sleep during daily activities, in some cases without awareness or warning signs primarily in patients with Parkinson's disease. A reduction in dosage or termination of therapy may be necessary. Patients must be cautioned about performing tasks which require mental alertness. Dopaminergic agents have been associated with a syndrome resembling neuroleptic malignant syndrome on abrupt withdrawal or significant dosage reduction after long-term use; gradual dosage reduction is recommended when discontinuing therapy.

In the management of type 2 diabetes mellitus, Cycloset® ("quick-release" tablet) should not be interchanged with any other bromocriptine product due to formulation differences and resulting pharmacokinetic profile. Therapy is not appropriate in patients with diabetic ketoacidosis (DKA) or type 1 diabetes mellitus due to lack of efficacy in these patient populations. There is limited efficacy information regarding use in combination with thiazolidinediones or in combination with insulin. Combination therapy with other hypoglycemic agents may increase risk for hypoglycemic events; dose reduction of concomitant hypoglycemics may be warranted. Concomitant use with dopamine receptor antagonists, including neuroleptic agents with dopamine receptor antagonist properties (clozapine, olanzapine, ziprasidone), is not recommended; efficacy may be reduced. Concomitant use of dopamine agonists is not recommended.

Precautions Use with caution in patients with cardiovascular disease (myocardial infarction, arrhythmia), peptic ulcer, dementia, hepatic and/or renal impairment, and psychosis. Not recommended for use to control or prevent lactation or in patients with uncontrolled hypertension. Concurrent antihypertensives or drugs which may alter blood pressure should be used with caution. Avoid use in patients with rare hereditary galactose intolerance, severe lactase deficiency, or glucose-galactose malabsorption.

Adverse Reactions

Cardiovascular: Hypotension (including postural/orthostatic), Raynaud's phenomenon, syncope, vasospasm (digital)

Central nervous system: Dizziness, drowsiness, fatigue, headache, lightheadedness

Endocrine & metabolic: Hypoglycemia

Gastrointestinal: Abdominal cramps, anorexia, constipation, diarrhea, dyspepsia, gastrointestinal hemorrhage, nausea, vomiting, xerostomia

Infection: Increased susceptibility to infection

Neuromuscular & skeletal: Weakness

Ophthalmic: Amblyopia

Respiratory: Flu-like symptoms, nasal congestion, rhinitis, sinusitis

Rare but important or life-threatening: Acquired valvular heart disease, alopecia, bradycardia, cardiac arrhythmia, cerebrovascular accident (postpartum), confusion, constrictive pericarditis, depression, dysphagia, epileptiform seizures, ergot alkaloids toxicity, erythromelalgia, gastrointestinal ulcer, hallucination, hypertension (postpartum), increased cerebrospinal fluid pressure, insomnia, myocardial infarction (postpartum), narcolepsy, paresthesia, pericardial effusion, peripheral edema, pleural effusion, pleurisy, psychomotor agitation, pulmonary fibrosis, retroperitoneal fibrosis, seizure (postpartum), status epilepticus (postpartum), tachycardia, transient blindness, urinary incontinence, urinary retention, vasodepressor syncope, ventricular tachycardia

Drug Interactions

Metabolism/Transport Effects Substrate of CYP3A4 (major); **Note:** Assignment of Major/Minor substrate status based on clinically relevant drug interaction potential; **Inhibits** CYP1A2 (weak), CYP3A4 (weak)

Avoid Concomitant Use

Avoid concomitant use of Bromocriptine with any of the following: Alpha-/Beta-Agonists; Alpha1-Agonists; Amisulpride; Conivaptan; Fusidic Acid (Systemic); Lorcaserin; Nitroglycerin; Pimozide; Protease Inhibitors; Serotonin 5-HT1D Receptor Agonists

Increased Effect/Toxicity

Bromocriptine may increase the levels/effects of: Alcohol (Ethyl); Alpha-/Beta-Agonists; Alpha1-Agonists; BuPROPion; CycloSPORINE (Systemic); Dofetilide; Lomitapide; Metoclopramide; Pimozide; Serotonin 5-HT1D Receptor Agonists; Serotonin Modulators

The levels/effects of Bromocriptine may be increased by: Alcohol (Ethyl); Antiemetics (5HT3 Antagonists); Beta-Blockers; Ceritinib; Conivaptan; CYP3A4 Inhibitors (Moderate); CYP3A4 Inhibitors (Strong); Dasatinib; Fusidic Acid (Systemic); Ivacaftor; Lorcaserin; Luliconazole; Macrolide Antibiotics; MAO Inhibitors; Methylphenidate; Mifepristone; Nitroglycerin; Protease Inhibitors; Serotonin 5-HT1D Receptor Agonists; Simeprevir; Stiripentol

Decreased Effect

Bromocriptine may decrease the levels/effects of: Amisulpride; Antipsychotics (Typical); Nitroglycerin

The levels/effects of Bromocriptine may be decreased by: Amisulpride; Antipsychotics (Atypical); Antipsychotics (Typical); Metoclopramide

Stability Store at or below 25°C (77°F); protect from light.

Mechanism of Action Semisynthetic ergot alkaloid derivative and a dopamine receptor agonist which activates postsynaptic dopamine receptors in the tuberoinfundibular (inhibiting pituitary prolactin secretion) and nigrostriatal pathways (enhancing coordinated motor control).

In the treatment of type 2 diabetes mellitus, the mechanism of action is unknown; however, bromocriptine is believed to affect circadian rhythms which are mediated, in part, by dopaminergic activity, and are believed to play a role in obesity and insulin resistance. It is postulated that bromocriptine (when administered during the morning and released into the systemic circulation in a rapid, 'pulse-like' dose) may reset hypothalamic circadian activities which have been altered by obesity, thereby resulting in the reversal of insulin resistance and decreases in glucose production, without increasing serum insulin concentrations.

Pharmacodynamics Reduction of prolactin concentrations (Parlodel®):
Onset of action: 1-2 hours
Maximum effect: 5-10 hours
Duration: 8-12 hours

Pharmacokinetics (Adult data unless noted)
Bioavailability: Parlodel®: 28%; Cycloset®: 65% to 95%
Distribution: V_d: ~61L
Protein binding: 90% to 96%
Metabolism: Primarily hepatic via CYP3A4; extensive first-pass biotransformation (93%)
Half-life: Parlodel®: ~5 hours; Cycloset®: 6 hours
Time to peak serum concentration:
Parlodel®: 2.5 ± 2 hours
Cycloset®: 53 minutes (fasted); 90-120 minutes (high-fat meal)
Elimination: Feces (82%); urine (2% to 6% as unchanged drug)

Dosing: Usual
Children and Adolescents: **Hyperprolactinemia:**
Children and Adolescents 11-15 years (based on limited information): Oral: Initial: 1.25-2.5 mg daily; dosage may be increased as tolerated to achieve a therapeutic response; usual dosage range: 2.5-10 mg daily
Adolescents ≥16 years: Oral: Initial: 1.25-2.5 mg daily; may be increased by 2.5 mg/day as tolerated every 2-7 days until optimal response; usual dosage range: 2.5-15 mg daily
Adults:
Acromegaly: Oral: Initial: 1.25-2.5 mg daily increasing by 1.25-2.5 mg daily as necessary every 3-7 days; usual dose: 20-30 mg/day (maximum: 100 mg/day)
Hyperprolactinemia: Oral: Initial: 1.25-2.5 mg daily; may be increased by 2.5 mg daily as tolerated every 2-7 days until optimal response; usual dosage range: 2.5-15 mg daily
Neuroleptic malignant syndrome (NMS): Oral: 2.5 mg (orally or via gastric tube) every 8-12 hours, increased to a maximum of 45 mg daily, if needed; continue therapy until NMS is controlled, then taper slowly (Gortney, 2009; Strawn, 2007)
Parkinsonism: Oral: 1.25 mg twice daily, increased by 2.5 mg/day in 2- to 4-week intervals as needed (maximum daily dose: 100 mg/day)
Type 2 diabetes mellitus (Cycloset®): Oral: Initial: 0.8 mg once daily; may increase at weekly intervals in 0.8 mg increments as tolerated; usual dose: 1.6-4.8 mg daily (maximum: 4.8 mg daily)
Dosing adjustment in hepatic impairment: No guidelines are available; however, may be necessary due to extensive metabolism

Administration Oral: May be taken with food to decrease GI distress
Cycloset®: Administer within 2 hours of waking in the morning

Monitoring Parameters Monitor blood pressure closely as well as hepatic, hematopoietic, and cardiovascular function; visual field monitoring is recommended (prolactinoma); pregnancy testing during amenorrheic period; growth hormone and prolactin levels; Hb A_{1c} and serum glucose (type 2 diabetes mellitus)

Additional Information Usually used with levodopa or levodopa/carbidopa to treat Parkinson's disease. When adding bromocriptine, the dose of levodopa/carbidopa can usually be decreased.

Dosage Forms Excipient information presented when available (limited, particularly for generics); consult specific product labeling.
Capsule, Oral:
Parlodel: 5 mg
Generic: 5 mg
Tablet, Oral:
Cycloset: 0.8 mg

Parlodel: 2.5 mg [scored]
Generic: 2.5 mg

References
de Groot AN, van Dongen PW, Vree TB, et al, "Ergot Alkaloids. Current Status and Review of Clinical Pharmacology and Therapeutic Use Compared With Other Oxytocics in Obstetrics and Gynaecology," *Drugs*, 1998, 56(4):523-35.
Gillam MP, Fideleff H, Boquete HR, et al, "Prolactin Excess: Treatment and Toxicity," *Pediatr Endocrinol Rev*, 2004, 2(suppl)1:108-14.
Gortney JS, Fagan A, and Kissack JC, "Neuroleptic Malignant Syndrome Secondary to Quetiapine," *Ann Pharmacother*, 2009, 43 (4):785-91.
Lejoyeux M, et al, "Serotonin Syndrome: Incidence, Symptoms, and Treatment," *CNS Drugs*, 1994, 2:132-43.
Melmed S and Braunstein GD, "Bromocriptine and Pleuropulmonary Disease," *Arch Intern Med*, 1989, 149(2):258-9.
Molitch ME, "Management of Prolactinomas During Pregnancy," *J Reprod Med*, 1999, 44(12 Suppl):1121-6.
Morgans D, "Re: Parlodel," *Aust N Z J Obstet Gynaecol*, 1995, 35 (2):228-9.
Mueller PS, Vester JW, and Fermaglich J, "Neuroleptic Malignant Syndrome. Successful Treatment With Bromocriptine," *JAMA*, 1983, 249(3):386-8.
Parkes D, "Drug Therapy: Bromocriptine," *N Engl J Med*, 1979, 301 (16):873-8.
Strawn JR, Keck PE Jr, and Caroff SN, "Neuroleptic Malignant Syndrome," *Am J Psychiatry*, 2007, 164(6):870-6.

◆ **Bromocriptine Mesylate** see Bromocriptine on page 304

Brompheniramine and Pseudoephedrine
(brome fen IR a meen & soo doe e FED rin)

Brand Names: U.S. Brotapp [OTC]; BroveX PSB [OTC]; J-Tan D PD [OTC]; Lodrane D [OTC]; LoHist PSB [OTC] [DSC]; Q-Tapp Cold & Allergy [OTC]

Therapeutic Category Antihistamine/Decongestant Combination

Generic Availability (U.S.) Yes

Use Temporary relief of symptoms associated with allergic rhinitis including rhinorrhea, sneezing, itchy watery eyes, and itching of the nose and throat and temporary relief of nasal congestion associated with common cold, hay fever, or upper respiratory allergies (promotes nasal and/or sinus drainage). FDA approved ages and OTC availability varies with dosage form and generic market; consult product specific labeling.
Oral:
Capsules (Lodrane-D): FDA approved in ages >12 years and adults
Drops (J-Tan D PD): FDA approved in ages 2-12 years
Elixir (Q-Tapp): FDA approved in ages ≥6 years and adults
Liquid:
Brotapp: FDA approved in ages ≥6 years and adults
Rynex PSE: FDA approved in ages ≥2 years and adults

Contraindications Hypersensitivity to brompheniramine, pseudoephedrine, or any component; MAO inhibitor therapy (or 2 weeks following MAO inhibitor use)

Warnings Safety and efficacy for the use of cough and cold products in children <2 years of age is limited. Serious adverse effects including death have been reported (in some cases, high blood concentrations of pseudoephedrine were found). The FDA notes that there are no approved OTC uses for these products in children <2 years of age. Healthcare providers are reminded to ask caregivers about the use of OTC cough and cold products in order to avoid exposure to multiple medications containing the same ingredient. Antihistamines may cause excitation in young children.

When used for self-medication (OTC), notify healthcare provider if symptoms do not improve within 7 days or are accompanied by fever or onset of new symptoms. Discontinue and contact healthcare provider if nervousness, dizziness, or sleeplessness occur.

Brompheniramine may cause drowsiness; alcohol, sedatives, and tranquilizers may increase this effect; patients must be cautioned about performing tasks which require mental alertness (eg, operating machinery or driving). Antihistamines may cause paradoxical excitation in young children.

Multiple concentrations of oral liquid formulations (drops, elixir, and liquid) exist; close attention must be paid to the concentration when ordering or administering. Some products may contain sodium benzoate; benzoic acid (benzoate) is a metabolite of benzyl alcohol; large amounts of benzyl alcohol (≥99 mg/kg/day) have been associated with a potentially fatal toxicity ("gasping syndrome") in neonates; avoid use in neonates; in vitro and animal studies have shown that benzoate displaces bilirubin from protein binding sites.

Precautions Use with caution in patients with concurrent sedative use, mild-moderate hypertension, heart disease, arrhythmias, diabetes mellitus, thyroid disease, asthma, emphysema, chronic bronchitis, glaucoma, and prostatic hypertrophy; consult physician prior to use

Adverse Reactions

Cardiovascular: Arrhythmias, flushing, hypertension, pallor, palpitation, tachycardia

Central nervous system: Convulsions, CNS stimulation, dizziness, excitability (children; rare), giddiness, hallucinations, headache, insomnia, irritability, lassitude, nervousness, sedation

Gastrointestinal: Anorexia, diarrhea, dyspepsia, nausea, vomiting, xerostomia

Genitourinary: Dysuria, urinary retention (with BPH)

Neuromuscular skeletal: Tremors, weakness

Ocular: Diplopia

Renal: Polyuria

Respiratory: Respiratory difficulty

Drug Interactions

Metabolism/Transport Effects None known.

Avoid Concomitant Use

Avoid concomitant use of Brompheniramine and Pseudoephedrine with any of the following: Aclidinium; Azelastine (Nasal); Ergot Derivatives; Iobenguane I 123; Ipratropium (Oral Inhalation); MAO Inhibitors; Paraldehyde; Potassium Chloride; Thalidomide; Tiotropium; Umeclidinium

Increased Effect/Toxicity

Brompheniramine and Pseudoephedrine may increase the levels/effects of: AbobotulinumtoxinA; Alcohol (Ethyl); Analgesics (Opioid); Anticholinergic Agents; Azelastine (Nasal); Buprenorphine; Cannabinoid-Containing Products; CNS Depressants; Hydrocodone; Methotrimeprazine; Metyrosine; Mirabegron; Mirtazapine; OnabotulinumtoxinA; Paraldehyde; Potassium Chloride; Pramipexole; RimabotulinumtoxinB; ROPINIRole; Rotigotine; Selective Serotonin Reuptake Inhibitors; Sympathomimetics; Thalidomide; Thiazide Diuretics; Tiotropium; Topiramate; Zolpidem

The levels/effects of Brompheniramine and Pseudoephedrine may be increased by: Aclidinium; Alkalinizing Agents; AtoMOXetine; Brimonidine (Topical); Cannabinoid-Containing Products; Cannabis; Carbonic Anhydrase Inhibitors; Doxylamine; Dronabinol; Droperidol; Ergot Derivatives; HydrOXYzine; Ipratropium (Oral Inhalation); Kava Kava; Linezolid; Magnesium Sulfate; MAO Inhibitors; Methotrimeprazine; Nabilone; Perampanel; Pramlintide; Rufinamide; Serotonin/Norepinephrine Reuptake Inhibitors; Sodium Oxybate; Tapentadol; Tetrahydrocannabinol; Umeclidinium

Decreased Effect

Brompheniramine and Pseudoephedrine may decrease the levels/effects of: Acetylcholinesterase Inhibitors (Central); Benzylpenicilloyl Polylysine; Betahistine; FentaNYL; Hyaluronidase; Iobenguane I 123; Secretin

The levels/effects of Brompheniramine and Pseudoephedrine may be decreased by: Acetylcholinesterase Inhibitors (Central); Alpha1-Blockers; Amphetamines; Spironolactone; Urinary Acidifying Agents

Stability

Oral: Store at room temperatature.

Brotapp liquid: Store at 20°C to 25°C (68°F to 77°F).

J-Tan D PD drops: Store at 15°C to 30°C (59°F to 86°F); dispense in a tight, light-resistant container.

Q-Tapp elixir: Store at 15°C to 30°C (59°F to 86°F).

Rynex PSE: Store at 15°C to 30°C (59°F to 86°F); dispense in a tight container.

Mechanism of Action Brompheniramine maleate is an antihistamine with H_1-receptor activity; pseudoephedrine, a sympathomimetic amine and isomer of ephedrine, acts as a decongestant in respiratory tract mucous membranes with less vasoconstrictor action than ephedrine in normotensive individuals.

Pharmacodynamics See individual monograph for Pseudoephedrine.

Brompheniramine component only:

Maximum effect: Within 3-9 hours

Duration: 4-6 hours

Pharmacokinetics (Adult data unless noted) See individual monograph for Pseudoephedrine.

Brompheniramine component only:

Distribution: V_d: Children 6-12 years: ~20 L/kg (Simons, 1999), Adults: ~12 L/kg (Simons, 1982)

Metabolism: Hepatic, extensive (Simons, 2004)

Half-life: Children 6-12 years: 12.4 hours (Simons, 1999), Adults: ~25 hours (Simons, 1982)

Time to peak serum concentration: Oral: ~3 hours; similar data reported in children 6-12 years (Simons, 1982; Simons, 1999)

Elimination: Urine (50%, as inactive metabolites) (Bruce, 1968)

Dosing: Usual Note: Multiple concentrations of oral liquid formulations (drops, elixir, and liquid) exist; close attention must be paid to the concentration when ordering or administering

Children: **Allergic rhinitis and nasal congestion:** Oral:

Children 2 to <6 years:

Oral drops (J-Tan D PD, brompheniramine 1 mg and pseudoephedrine 7.5 mg per 1 mL dropper): 1 mL (1 dropperful) every 4-6 hours; maximum daily dose: 6 mL/24 hours

Oral liquid: Rynex PSE (brompheniramine 1 mg and pseudoephedrine 15 mg per 5 mL): 5 mL every 4-6 hours; maximum daily dose: 20 mL/24 hours

Children 6 to <12 years:

Oral drops: J-Tan D PD (brompheniramine 1 mg and pseudoephedrine 7.5 mg per 1 mL dropper): 2 mL (2 dropperfuls) every 4-6 hours; maximum daily dose: 12 mL/24 hours

Oral liquid: Brotapp, Q-Tapp, Rynex PSE (brompheniramine 1 mg and pseudoephedrine 15 mg per 5 mL): 10 mL every 4-6 hours; maximum daily dose: 40 mL/24 hours

Children 12 years of age:

Oral drops: J-Tan D PD (brompheniramine 1 mg and pseudoephedrine 7.5 mg per 1 mL dropper): 2 mL (2 dropperfuls) every 4-6 hours; maximum daily dose: 12 mL/24 hours

Oral liquid: Brotapp, Q-Tapp, Rynex PSE (brompheniramine 1 mg and pseudoephedrine 15 mg per 5 mL): 20 mL every 4-6 hours; maximum daily dose: 80 mL/24 hours

Adolescents: **Allergic rhinitis and nasal congestion:** Oral:

Oral capsules (Lodrane D, brompheniramine 4 mg and pseudoephedrine 60 mg): 1 capsule every 4-6 hours; maximum daily dose: 4 capsules/24 hours

Oral liquid (brompheniramine 1 mg and pseudoephedrine 15 mg per 5 mL): 20 mL every 4-6 hours; maximum daily dose: 80 mL/24 hours

Adults: **Rhinitis and nasal congestion:** Oral:

Oral capsules (brompheniramine 4 mg and pseudoephedrine 60 mg): 1 capsule every 4-6 hours; maximum daily dose: 4 capsules/24 hours

Oral liquid (brompheniramine 1 mg and pseudoephedrine 15 mg per 5 mL): 20 mL every 4-6 hours; maximum daily dose: 80 mL/24 hours

Test Interactions See individual agents.

Dosage Forms Excipient information presented when available (limited, particularly for generics); consult specific product labeling. [DSC] = Discontinued product

Capsule, oral:

Lodrane D: Brompheniramine maleate 4 mg and pseudoephedrine hydrochloride 60 mg

Liquid, oral:

Brotapp: Brompheniramine maleate 1 mg and pseudoephedrine hydrochloride 15 mg per 5 mL (120 mL, 240 mL, 480 mL) [ethanol free, sugar free; contains propylene glycol, sodium benzoate; grape flavor]

BroveX PSB: Brompheniramine maleate 4 mg and pseudoephedrine hydrochloride 20 mg per 5 mL (473 mL) [dye free, ethanol free, sugar free; contains propylene glycol; cotton candy flavor]

LoHist PSB: Brompheniramine maleate 4 mg and pseudoephedrine hydrochloride 20 mg per 5 mL (473 mL) [dye free, ethanol free, sugar free; cherry flavor] [DSC]

Q-Tapp Cold & Allergy: Brompheniramine maleate 1 mg and pseudoephedrine hydrochloride 15 mg per 5 mL (118 mL, 237 mL) [ethanol free; contains propylene glycol, sodium 2 mg/5 mL, sodium benzoate; grape flavor]

Liquid, oral [drops]:

J-Tan D PD: Brompheniramine maleate 1 mg and pseudoephedrine hydrochloride 7.5 mg per 1 mL (30 mL) [dye free, ethanol free, sugar free; contains propylene glycol; cotton candy flavor]

References
Bruce RB, Turnbull LB, Newman JH, et al. Metabolism of brompheniramine. J Med Chem. 1968;11(5):1031-1034.

Gentile DA, Friday GA, and Skoner DP, "Management of Allergic Rhinitis: Antihistamines and Decongestants," Immunol Allergy Clin NA, 2000, 20(2):355-68.

Simons FE. Advances in H1-antihistamines. N Engl J Med. 2004;351 (21):2203-2217.

Simons FE, Frith EM, Simons KJ. The pharmacokinetics and antihistaminic effects of brompheniramine. J Allergy Clin Immunol. 1982;70 (6):458-464.

Simons FE, Roberts JR, Gu X, et al. The clinical pharmacology of brompheniramine in children. J Allergy Clin Immunol. 1999; 103(2 Pt 1):223-226.

◆ **Brompheniramine Maleate and Pseudoephedrine Hydrochloride** see Brompheniramine and Pseudoephedrine on page 306

◆ **Brompheniramine Maleate and Pseudoephedrine Sulfate** see Brompheniramine and Pseudoephedrine on page 306

◆ **Broncho Saline [OTC]** see Sodium Chloride on page 1902

◆ **Brotapp [OTC]** see Brompheniramine and Pseudoephedrine on page 306

◆ **BroveX PSB [OTC]** see Brompheniramine and Pseudoephedrine on page 306

◆ **BTX-A** see OnabotulinumtoxinA on page 1541

◆ **Buckleys Chest Congestion [OTC]** see GuaiFENesin on page 984

◆ **Budeprion SR [DSC]** see BuPROPion on page 327

Budesonide (Systemic, Oral Inhalation)
(byoo DES oh nide)

Related Information
Inhaled Corticosteroids on page 2223
Oral Medications That Should Not Be Crushed or Altered on page 2438

Brand Names: U.S. Entocort EC; Pulmicort; Pulmicort Flexhaler; Uceris

Brand Names: Canada Entocort; Pulmicort Turbuhaler

Therapeutic Category Adrenal Corticosteroid; Anti-inflammatory Agent; Antiasthmatic; Corticosteroid, Inhalant (Oral); Glucocorticoid

Generic Availability (U.S.) May be product dependent

Use
Inhalation:

Nebulization: Maintenance therapy and prophylaxis of bronchial asthma (FDA approved in ages 1-8 years); **not** indicated for the relief of acute bronchospasm

Oral inhalation: Maintenance therapy and prophylaxis of bronchial asthma with or without oral corticosteroids (FDA approved in ages ≥6 years and adults); **not** indicated for the relief of acute bronchospasm

Oral:

Entocort® EC: Treatment of mild to moderate active Crohn's disease of the ileum and/or ascending colon and maintenance of remission for up to 3 months (FDA approved in adults); has also been used for treatment of protein-losing enteropathy in patients after Fontan procedure

Uceris™ ER: Induction of remission from active, mild to moderate ulcerative colitis (FDA approved in adults)

Pregnancy Risk Factor C (capsule, tablet)/B (inhalation)

Pregnancy Considerations Adverse events have been observed with corticosteroids in animal reproduction studies. Some studies have shown an association between first trimester systemic corticosteroid use and oral clefts (Park-Wyllie, 2000; Pradat, 2003). Systemic corticosteroids may also influence fetal growth (decreased birth weight); however, information is conflicting (Lunghi, 2010). Hypoadrenalism may occur in newborns following maternal use of corticosteroids in pregnancy; monitor. When systemic corticosteroids are needed in pregnancy, it is generally recommended to use the lowest effective dose for the shortest duration of time, avoiding high doses during the first trimester (Leachman, 2006; Lunghi, 2010). Budesonide may be used for the induction of remission in pregnant women with inflammatory bowel disease (Habal, 2012).

Based on available data, an overall increased risk of congenital malformations or a decrease in fetal growth has not been associated with maternal use of inhaled corticosteroids during pregnancy (Bakhireva, 2005; NAEPP, 2005; Namazy, 2004). In addition, studies of pregnant women specifically using inhaled budesonide have not demonstrated an increased risk of congenital abnormalities. Uncontrolled asthma is associated with adverse events on pregnancy (increased risk of perinatal mortality, pre-eclampsia, preterm birth, low birth weight infants). Inhaled corticosteroids are recommended for the treatment of asthma during pregnancy; budesonide is preferred (ACOG, 2008; NAEPP, 2005).

Breast-Feeding Considerations Following use of the powder for oral inhalation, ~0.3% to 1% of the maternal dose was found in breast milk. The maximum concentration appeared within 45 minutes of dosing. Plasma budesonide levels obtained from infants ~90 minutes after breast-feeding (~140 minutes after maternal dose) were below the limit of quantification. Concentrations of budesonide in breast milk are expected to be higher following administration of oral capsules/tablets than after an inhaled dose.

Due to the potential for serious adverse reactions in the nursing infant, the manufacturers of the oral tablets and capsules recommend a decision be made whether to discontinue nursing or to discontinue the drug, taking into account the importance of treatment to the mother. If there is concern about exposure to the infant, some guidelines recommend waiting 4 hours after the maternal dose of an oral systemic corticosteroid before breast-feeding in order to decrease potential exposure to the nursing infant (based on a study using prednisolone) (Habal, 2012; Ost, 1985).

According to the manufacturer of the product for inhalation, the decision to continue or discontinue breast-feeding during therapy should take into account the risk of minimal exposure to the infant and the benefits of breast-feeding to the mother. The use of inhaled corticosteroids is not considered a contraindication to breast-feeding (NAEPP, 2005).

Contraindications Hypersensitivity to budesonide or any component

Additional product specific contraindications:

Oral inhalation: Severe hypersensitivity to milk proteins; primary treatment of status asthmaticus or other acute episodes of bronchial asthma when intensive treatment is needed

Nebulization: Primary treatment of status asthmaticus or other acute episodes of bronchial asthma when intensive treatment is needed

Warnings Fatalities have occurred due to adrenal insufficiency in asthmatic patients during and after switching from systemic corticosteroids to aerosol or oral steroids with poor bioavailability; several months may be required for full recovery of hypothalamic-pituitary-adrenal (HPA) function; patients receiving higher doses of systemic corticosteroids (eg, adults receiving ≥20 mg of prednisone per day may be at greater risk; during this period of HPA suppression, aerosol steroids do **not** provide the systemic glucocorticoid or mineral corticoid activity needed to treat patients requiring stress doses (ie, patients with major stress, such as trauma, surgery, infections, or other conditions associated with severe electrolyte loss). When used at high doses, HPA suppression may occur; use with inhaled or systemic corticosteroids (even alternate-day dosing) or when switching patients from systemic corticosteroids to oral budesonide (due to lower bioavailability) may increase risk of HPA suppression. Acute adrenal insufficiency may occur with abrupt withdrawal after long-term use or with stress; withdrawal and discontinuation of corticosteroids should be done carefully; patients with HPA axis suppression may require doses of systemic glucocorticosteroids prior to, during, and after unusual stress (eg, surgery). Use of oral, inhaled, or nebulized budesonide in place of systemic corticosteroids may unmask allergies (eg, eczema, rhinitis) that were previously controlled by the systemic corticosteroids.

Immunosuppression may occur; patients may be more susceptible to infections; prolonged use of corticosteroids may also increase the incidence of secondary infection, mask acute infection (including fungal infections), prolong or exacerbate viral or fungal infections, activate latent opportunistic infections, or limit response to vaccines. Exposure to chickenpox should be avoided; corticosteroids should not be used to treat ocular herpes simplex; use caution in patients with a history of ocular herpes simplex. Corticosteroids should not be used for cerebral malaria or viral hepatitis. Close observation is required in patients with latent tuberculosis and/or TB reactivity; restrict use in active TB (only in conjunction with antituberculosis treatment). Amebiasis should be ruled out in any patient with recent travel to tropical climates or unexplained diarrhea prior to initiation of corticosteroids. Use with great caution in patients with known or suspected *Strongyloides* infection. *C. albicans* infections of the mouth and pharynx may occur with orally inhaled corticosteroid use, mostly mild to moderate; interruption of therapy may be necessary at times while antifungal therapy is employed; advise patients to rinse mouth after use.

Budesonide is not meant to relieve acute asthma or bronchospasm, rapidly deteriorating, or potentially life-threatening episodes of asthma; acute episodes should be treated with short-acting beta$_2$-agonist. Bronchospasm may occur after use of inhaled asthma medications; if this occurs, a fast-acting bronchodilator may be used; discontinue orally inhaled corticosteroid and initiate alternative chronic therapy.

Powder for oral inhalation (Pulmicort Flexhaler®) contains lactose (milk proteins) which may cause allergic reactions in patients with severe milk protein allergy.

Precautions Avoid using higher than recommended dosages; suppression of HPA function, suppression of linear growth (ie, reduction of growth velocity), reduced bone mineral density, or hypercorticism (Cushing's syndrome) may occur; titrate to lowest effective dose. Reduction in growth velocity [mean: 1 cm/year (range: 0.3-1.8 cm)] may occur when corticosteroids are administered to pediatric patients, even at recommended doses via oral, inhaled, or nebulized routes; reduction in growth velocity is related to dose and duration of exposure; monitor growth. Use with caution in patients with osteoporosis; decreases in bone mineral density have occurred with long term administration. A 12-week study in infants (n=141; 6-12 months of age) receiving budesonide nebulizations (0.5 mg or 1 mg once daily) vs placebo demonstrated a budesonide dose-dependent suppression of linear growth; in addition, although mean changes from baseline did not indicate budesonide-induced adrenal suppression, six infants who received budesonide had subnormal stimulated cortisol levels at week 12. Children and adolescents (n=18; 6-15 years) receiving budesonide nebulizations of 1 and 2 mg twice daily showed a significant reduction in urinary cortisol excretion; this reduction was not seen when patients were dosed at 1 mg/day (maximum recommended dose). Long-term effects of chronic use of budesonide nebulization on immunological or developmental processes of upper airways, mouth, and lung are unknown.

Use with caution with potent inhibitors of cytochrome P450 isoenzyme CYP3A4 (eg, ketoconazole, ritonavir, atazanavir, clarithromycin, indinavir, itraconazole, nefazodone, nelfinavir, saquinavir, telithromycin); may increase budesonide serum concentrations and result in systemic corticosteroid effects. Use oral budesonide with caution in patients with hypertension or heart failure; long-term use has been associated with fluid retention. Use oral budesonide with caution in patients with peptic ulcer disease; increased risk for perforation. Use oral budesonide with caution in patients with diabetes mellitus or a family history of diabetes mellitus; may alter glucose production/regulation, leading to hyperglycemia. Use oral budesonide with caution and consider dosage reduction in patients with hepatic cirrhosis. Eosinophilic conditions (eosinophilia, vasculitic rash, cardiac complications, worsening pulmonary symptoms, and/or neuropathy) may occur and are usually associated with withdrawal or decrease of oral corticosteroids after the initiation of inhaled corticosteroids; a causal relationship to budesonide has not been established. Rare cases of increased IOP, glaucoma, or cataracts may occur with inhaled corticosteroids.

Adverse Reactions

Oral capsules:

Cardiovascular: Chest pain, edema, facial edema, flushing, hypertension, palpitation, tachycardia

Central nervous system: Agitation, amnesia, confusion, dizziness, fever, headache, insomnia, malaise, nervousness, sleep disorder, somnolence, vertigo

Dermatologic: Acne, alopecia, bruising, dermatitis, eczema, hirsutism, purpura, skin disorder, striae

Endocrine & metabolic: Adrenal insufficiency, hypokalemia, intermenstrual bleeding, menstrual disorder

Gastrointestinal: Anus disorder, appetite increased, Crohn's disease exacerbation, diarrhea, dyspepsia, enteritis, epigastric pain, gastrointestinal fistula, glossitis, hemorrhoids, intestinal obstruction, nausea, oral candidiasis, tongue edema, tooth disorder, weight gain

Genitourinary: Dysuria, hematuria, micturition frequency, nocturia, pyuria, urinary tract infection

Hematologic: Anemia, leukocytosis, neutrophils abnormal

Hepatic: Alkaline phosphatase increased

Neuromuscular & skeletal: Arthralgia, arthritis, hyperkinesia, muscle cramping, myalgia, paresthesia, tremor, weakness

Ocular: Eye abnormality, vision abnormal

Otic: Ear infection

Respiratory: Bronchitis, dyspnea, pharynx disorder, respiratory infection, rhinitis, sinusitis

Miscellaneous: Abscess, C-reactive protein increased, diaphoresis, fat redistribution (moon face, buffalo hump), flu-like syndrome, erythrocyte sedimentation rate increased, viral infection

Rare but important or life-threatening: Anaphylaxis, intracranial hypertension (benign), mood swings

Oral inhaler (Pulmicort Flexhaler®):

Cardiovascular: Syncope

Central nervous system: Fever, headache, insomnia, pain

Dermatologic: Bruising

Gastrointestinal: Abdominal pain, dyspepsia, gastroenteritis (viral), nausea, oral candidiasis, taste perversion, vomiting, weight gain, xerostomia

Neuromuscular & skeletal: Arthralgia, back pain, fracture, hypertonia, myalgia, neck pain, weakness

Otic: Otitis media

Respiratory: Allergic rhinitis, cough, nasal congestion, nasopharyngitis, pharyngitis, respiratory infection, rhinitis, sinusitis, upper respiratory tract infection (viral)

Miscellaneous: Infection, voice alteration

Rare but important or life-threatening: Aggressiveness, anxiety, cataracts, depression, glaucoma, hypercorticism, hypersensitivity reactions (immediate and delayed [includes rash, contact dermatitis, angioedema, bronchospasm, urticaria]), hypocorticism, intraocular pressure increased, irritability, nervousness, psychosis, restlessness, throat irritation, wheezing (patients with severe milk allergy)

Oral tablets:

Central nervous system: Fatigue, headache, mood swings

Dermatologic: Acne, hirsutism

Endocrine & metabolic: Cortisol decreased

Gastrointestinal: Abdominal distension, constipation, flatulence, nausea, upper abdominal pain

Genitourinary: Urinary tract infection

Neuromuscular & skeletal: Arthralgia

Rare but important or life-threatening: Anaphylaxis, intracranial hypertension (benign)

Suspension for nebulization:

Cardiovascular: Chest pain

Central nervous system: Dysphonia, fatigue, mood swings

Dermatologic: Contact dermatitis, eczema, pruritus, purpura, pustular rash, rash

Gastrointestinal: Abdominal pain, anorexia, diarrhea, gastroenteritis, vomiting

Hematologic: Cervical lymphadenopathy

Neuromuscular & skeletal: Fracture, hyperkinesia, myalgia

Ocular: Conjunctivitis, eye infection

Otic: Earache, ear infection, otitis externa, otitis media

Respiratory: Cough, epistaxis, respiratory infection, rhinitis, stridor

Miscellaneous: Allergic reaction, flu-like syndrome, herpes simplex, infection, moniliasis, viral infection

Rare but important or life-threatening: Aggressiveness, anxiety, avascular necrosis of the femoral head, bronchitis, bruising, cataracts, depression, facial skin irritation, fever, glaucoma, growth suppression, headache, hypercorticism, hypersensitivity reactions (immediate and delayed [includes angioedema, bronchospasm, urticaria]), hypocorticism, intraocular pressure increased, irritability, nervousness, osteoporosis, pain, pharyngitis, psychosis, restlessness, sinusitis, throat irritation

Drug Interactions

Metabolism/Transport Effects Substrate of CYP3A4 (major); **Note:** Assignment of Major/Minor substrate status based on clinically relevant drug interaction potential

Avoid Concomitant Use

Avoid concomitant use of Budesonide (Systemic, Oral Inhalation) with any of the following: Aldesleukin; BCG; Conivaptan; Fusidic Acid (Systemic); Grapefruit Juice; Natalizumab; Pimecrolimus; Tacrolimus (Topical); Tofacitinib

Increased Effect/Toxicity

Budesonide (Systemic, Oral Inhalation) may increase the levels/effects of: Amphotericin B; Deferasirox; Leflunomide; Loop Diuretics; Natalizumab; Thiazide Diuretics; Tofacitinib

The levels/effects of Budesonide (Systemic, Oral Inhalation) may be increased by: Conivaptan; CYP3A4 Inhibitors (Moderate); CYP3A4 Inhibitors (Strong); Dasatinib; Denosumab; Fusidic Acid (Systemic); Grapefruit Juice; Ivacaftor; Luliconazole; Mifepristone; Pimecrolimus; Simeprevir; Stiripentol; Tacrolimus (Topical); Telaprevir; Trastuzumab

Decreased Effect

Budesonide (Systemic, Oral Inhalation) may decrease the levels/effects of: Aldesleukin; Antidiabetic Agents; BCG; Coccidioidin Skin Test; Corticorelin; Hyaluronidase; Sipuleucel-T; Vaccines (Inactivated)

The levels/effects of Budesonide (Systemic, Oral Inhalation) may be decreased by: Antacids; Bile Acid Sequestrants; Echinacea

Food Interactions Grapefruit juice may double systemic exposure of orally administered budesonide. Administration of capsules with a high-fat meal delays peak concentration, but does not alter the extent of absorption; administration of tablets with a high-fat meal decreases peak concentration (~27%). Management: Avoid grapefruit juice when using oral capsules or tablets.

Stability

Oral:

Entocort® EC capsules: Store at 15°C to 30°C (59°F to 86°F)

Ulceris™ ER tablets: Store at 25°C (77°F); excursions permitted to 15°C to 30°C (59°F to 86°F). Protect from light and moisture.

Inhalation:

Nebulization (Pulmicort Respules®): Store Respules® upright at 20°C to 25°C (68°F to 77°F); protect from light; do not refrigerate or freeze; do not mix with other medications; after foil packet has been opened, Respules® are stable for 2 weeks when protected from light; return unused Respules® to foil packet to protect from light; use opened Respules® promptly

Oral inhaler (Pulmicort Flexhaler®): Keep clean and dry; store at 20°C to 25°C (68°F to 77°F)

Mechanism of Action Controls the rate of protein synthesis; depresses the migration of polymorphonuclear leukocytes, fibroblasts; reverses capillary permeability

310

and lysosomal stabilization at the cellular level to prevent or control inflammation. Has potent glucocorticoid activity and weak mineralocorticoid activity.

Pharmacodynamics Clinical effects are due to direct local effect, rather than systemic absorption.

Onset of action:

Nebulization (control of asthma symptoms): Within 2-8 days

Oral inhalation: Within 24 hours

Maximum effect:

Nebulization: 4-6 weeks

Oral inhalation: ≥1-2 weeks

Pharmacokinetics (Adult data unless noted)

Distribution: V_d:

Children 4-6 years: 3 L/kg

Adults: 2.2-3.9 L/kg

Protein binding: 85% to 90%

Metabolism: Extensive hepatic metabolism via cytochrome P450 CYP3A isoenzyme to 2 major metabolites: 16α-hydroxyprednisolone and 6β-hydroxybudesonide; both are <1% as active as parent

Bioavailability:

Nebulization: Children 4-6 years: 6%

Oral inhalation: 39% of an inhaled metered dose is available systemically

Oral: 9% in healthy volunteers and 21% in patients with Crohn's disease (large first pass effect); **Note:** Oral bioavailability is 2.5-fold higher in patients with hepatic cirrhosis

Half-life:

Children 4-6 years: 2.3 hours (after nebulization)

Children 10-14 years: 1.5 hours

Adults: 2-3.6 hours

Time to peak serum concentration:

Nebulization: 20 minutes

Oral inhalation (Pulmicort Flexhaler®): 10 minutes

Oral capsules (Entocort® EC): 0.5-10 hours

Oral tablets, extended release (Uceris™): ~13 hours

Elimination: Urine (60% as metabolites; no unchanged drug) and feces (metabolites)

Clearance:

Children 4-6 years: 0.5 L/minute (~50% greater than healthy adults after weight adjustment)

Adults: 0.9-1.8 L/minute

Dosing: Usual

Infants, Children, and Adolescents

Asthma: Note: Doses should be titrated to the lowest effective dose once asthma is controlled:

Nebulization: Pulmicort Respules®:

Infants: Limited data available: Initial: 0.25 mg twice daily or 0.5 mg once daily; maximum daily dose: 1 mg/day (Baker, 1999; GINA, 2009)

Children and Adolescents:

Manufacturer's labeling: Children ≤8 years or Children >8 years and Adolescents unable to effectively use metered-dose inhalers:

Previously treated with bronchodilators alone: Initial: 0.25 mg twice daily or 0.5 mg once daily; maximum daily dose: 0.5 mg/**day**

Previously treated with inhaled corticosteroids: Initial: 0.25 mg twice daily or 0.5 mg once daily; maximum daily dose: 1 mg/**day**

Previously treated with oral corticosteroids: Initial: 0.5 mg twice daily or 1 mg once daily; maximum daily dose: 1 mg/**day**

Symptomatic children not responding to nonsteroidal asthma medications: Initial: 0.25 mg once daily may be considered

NIH Asthma Guidelines (NAEPP, 2007): Administer once daily or in divided doses twice daily

Children ≤4 years:

"Low" dose: 0.25-0.5 mg/**day**

"Medium" dose: >0.5-1 mg/**day**

"High" dose: >1 mg/**day**

Children 5-11 years:

"Low" dose: 0.5 mg/**day**

"Medium" dose: 1 mg/**day**

"High" dose: 2 mg/**day**

Oral inhalation: Pulmicort Flexhaler®:

Manufacturer's labeling:

Children and Adolescents age 6-17 years: Initial: 180 mcg twice daily (some patients may be initiated at 360 mcg twice daily); maximum single dose: 360 mcg

Adolescents ≥18 years: Initial: 360 mcg twice daily (some patients may be initiated at 180 mcg twice daily); maximum single dose: 720 mcg

Alternate dosing: NIH Asthma Guidelines (NAEPP, 2007): Administer in divided doses twice daily

Children 5-11 years:

"Low" dose: 180-400 mcg/**day** (90 mcg/inhalation, 2-4 inhalations per day or 180 mcg/inhalation, 1-2 inhalations per day)

"Medium" dose: >400-800 mcg/**day** (180 mcg/inhalation, 2-4 inhalations per day)

"High" dose: >800 mcg/**day** (180 mcg/inhalation, >4 inhalations per day)

Children ≥12 years and Adolescents:

"Low" dose: 180-600 mcg/**day** (90 mcg/inhalation, 2-6 inhalations per day or 180 mcg/inhalation, 1-3 inhalations per day)

"Medium" dose: >600-1200 mcg/**day** (180 mcg/inhalation, 3-6 inhalations per day)

"High" dose: >1200 mcg/**day** (180 mcg/inhalation, >6 inhalations per day)

Conversion from oral systemic corticosteroid to orally inhaled corticosteroid: Initiation of oral inhalation therapy should begin in patients whose asthma is reasonably stabilized on oral corticosteroids (OCS). A gradual dose reduction of OCS should begin ~7-10 days after starting inhaled therapy. Manufacturer's labeling recommends reducing prednisone dose by 2.5 mg/day (or equivalent of other OCS) on a weekly basis (patients using oral inhaler) or by ≤25% every 1-2 weeks (patients using respules). When transitioning from systemic to inhaled corticosteroids, supplemental systemic corticosteroid therapy may be necessary during periods of stress or during severe asthma attacks.

Crohn's disease; treatment, mild to moderate: Children ≥6 years and Adolescents: Limited data available: Oral capsule (Entocort® EC): Induction: 9 mg once daily or in divided doses every 8 hours for 7-8 weeks, followed by a maintenance dose of 6 mg daily for 3-4 weeks; therapy was discontinued after a total duration of 10-12 weeks (Escher, 2004; Levine, 2003; Levine, 2009). In another study of patients 10-19 years of age, a trend for higher remission rates using an initial dose of 12 mg daily for 4 weeks, followed by 9 mg daily for 3 weeks, followed by 6 mg daily for 3 weeks was observed (Levine, 2009). A retrospective study used doses of 0.45 mg/kg/day up to a maximum daily dose of 9 mg/day (n= 62; age range: 9.5-18 years; final dose in all patients: 9 mg/day) (Levine, 2002)

Protein-losing enteropathy (PLE) following Fontan: Limited data available: Children ≥7 years and Adolescents: Oral capsule (Entocort® EC): Initial: 9 mg once daily or in divided doses every 8 hours; after clinical improvement and albumin >3 g/dL may then wean dose over several weeks to 3 mg once daily or every other day; if during the weaning process the serum albumin decreases to <2.5 g/dL, do not further reduce dose, consider dosage increase. Dosing based on several case series describing institutional experiences, the majority of pediatric patients described were ≥7 years of age (n=17) (John, 2011; Schumacher, 2011; Thacker,

2010; Turner, 2012). Reported experience in children <7 years is very limited (n=1); in one report, an initial dose of 6 mg once daily was recommended for children <4 years; further studies are needed (Thacker, 2010).

Adults:

Asthma: Oral inhalation:

Manufacturer's labeling: Pulmicort Flexhaler®: Initial: 360 mcg twice daily (selected patients may be initiated at 180 mcg twice daily); may increase dose after 1-2 weeks of therapy in patients who are not adequately controlled; maximum: 720 mcg twice daily; **Note:** Doses should be titrated to the lowest effective dose once asthma is controlled.

NIH Asthma Guidelines (NAEPP, 2007):

"Low" dose: 180-600 mcg/**day** (180 mcg/inhalation, 1-3 inhalations per day)

"Medium" dose: >600-1200 mcg/**day** (180 mcg/inhalation, 3-6 inhalations per day)

"High" dose: >1200 mcg/**day** (180 mcg/inhalation, >6 inhalations per day)

Conversion from oral systemic corticosteroid to orally inhaled corticosteroid: Initiation of oral inhalation therapy should begin in patients whose asthma is reasonably stabilized on oral corticosteroids (OCS). A gradual dose reduction of OCS should begin ~7-10 days after starting inhaled therapy. Manufacturer's labeling recommends reducing prednisone dose by 2.5 mg/day (or equivalent of other OCS) on a weekly basis (patients using oral inhaler) or by ≤25% every 1-2 weeks (patients using respules). When transitioning from systemic to inhaled corticosteroids, supplemental systemic corticosteroid therapy may be necessary during periods of stress or during severe asthma attacks.

Crohn's Disease, active: Oral: Capsule (Entocort® EC): Treatment: 9 mg once daily in the morning for ≤8 weeks; may repeat the 8-week course for recurring episodes of active Crohn's disease; **Note:** When switching patients from oral prednisolone to oral budesonide, do not stop prednisolone abruptly; prednisolone taper should begin at the same time that budesonide is started.

Maintenance of remission: Following treatment of active disease and control of symptoms (Crohn's Disease Activity Index <150), use 6 mg once daily for up to 3 months; if symptoms are still controlled at 3 months, taper the dose to complete cessation; continuing remission dose >3 months has not been demonstrated to result in substantial benefit

Ulcerative colitis, active: Oral: Tablet (Ulceris™): 9 mg once daily in the morning for ≤8 weeks

Dosing adjustment in renal impairment: Inhalation, Nebulization, Oral: There are no dosage adjustments provided in the manufacturer's labeling (has not been studied).

Dosing adjustment in hepatic impairment:

Inhalation, Nebulization, Oral: There are no dosage adjustments provided in the manufacturer's labeling (has not been studied). However, budesonide undergoes hepatic metabolism; drug may accumulate with hepatic impairment; use with caution; monitor closely.

Oral: There are no specific dosage adjustments provided in the manufacturer's labeling. Budesonide undergoes hepatic metabolism; bioavailability is increased in cirrhosis; monitor closely for signs and symptoms of hypercorticism.

Moderate to severe liver disease:

Capsule (Entocort® EC): Manufacturer's labeling: Consider dosage reduction

Tablet (Ulceris™): Manufacturer's labeling: Consider discontinuing use

Administration

Inhalation:

Nebulization: Shake gently with a circular motion before use. Administer only with a compressed air driven jet nebulizer; do not use an ultrasonic nebulizer; use adequate flow rates and administer via appropriate size face mask or mouthpiece. Avoid exposure of nebulized medication to eyes. Rinse mouth following treatments to decrease risk of oral candidiasis (wash face if using face mask).

Oral inhaler: Pulmicort Flexhaler®: Hold inhaler in upright position (mouthpiece up) to load dose. Do not shake prior to use. Unit should be primed prior to first use. It will not need to be primed again, even if not used for a long time. Place mouthpiece between lips and inhale forcefully and deeply. Do not exhale through inhaler; do not use a spacer. Dose indicator does not move with every dose, usually only after 5 doses. Discard when dose indicator reads "0". Rinse mouth with water after use to reduce incidence of candidiasis.

Oral: May be administered without regard to meals.

Capsule: Manufacturer's labeling: Swallow whole; do not break, chew, or crush. Opening the capsule and sprinkling over applesauce has been evaluated *in vitro* and no change in the release properties of budesonide was found (Espmarker, 2002); this method of administration has also been used in patients unable to swallow the capsules in a study evaluating budesonide use in Crohn's disease (Thacker, 2010).

Tablet: Swallow whole; do not break, chew, or crush.

Monitoring Parameters Monitor growth in pediatric patients; inhalation: Check mucous membranes for signs of fungal infection; Asthma: FEV_1, peak flow, and/or other pulmonary function tests; Long-term use: Regular eye examinations and IOP, blood pressure, glucose, signs and symptoms of hypercorticism, or adrenal suppression.

Additional Information Budesonide capsules (Entocort™ EC) contain granules in a methylcellulose matrix; the granules are coated with a methacrylic acid polymer to protect from dissolution in the stomach; the coating dissolves at a pH >5.5 (duodenal pH); the methylcellulose matrix controls the release of drug in a time-dependent manner (until the drug reaches the ileum and ascending colon).

Dosage Forms Considerations Pulmicort Flexhaler 180 mcg/actuation canisters contain 120 actuations and the 90 mcg/actuation canisters contain 60 inhalations.

Dosage Forms Excipient information presented when available (limited, particularly for generics); consult specific product labeling.

Aerosol Powder Breath Activated, Inhalation:

Pulmicort Flexhaler: 90 mcg/actuation (1 ea); 180 mcg/actuation (1 ea) [contains milk protein]

Capsule Extended Release 24 Hour, Oral:

Entocort EC: 3 mg

Generic: 3 mg

Suspension, Inhalation:

Pulmicort: 0.25 mg/2 mL (2 mL); 0.5 mg/2 mL (2 mL); 1 mg/2 mL (2 mL) [contains disodium edta, polysorbate 80]

Generic: 0.25 mg/2 mL (2 mL); 0.5 mg/2 mL (2 mL)

Tablet Extended Release 24 Hour, Oral:

Uceris: 9 mg

References

"Asthma In Pregnancy," ACOG Practice Bulletin No. 90. American College of Obstetricians and Gynecologists, *Obstet Gynecol*, 2008, 111(2 Pt 1):457-64.

Baker JW, Mellon M, Wald J, et al, "A Multiple-Dosing, Placebo-Controlled Study of Budesonide Inhalation Suspension Given Once or Twice Daily for Treatment of Persistent Asthma in Young Children and Infants," *Pediatrics*, 1999, 103(2):414-21.

Bakhireva LN, Jones KL, Schatz M, et al, "Asthma Medication Use in Pregnancy and Fetal Growth," *J Allergy Clin Immunol*, 2005, 116 (3):503-9.

Escher JC and the European Collaborative Research Group on Budesonide in Paediatric IBD, "Budesonide Versus Prednisolone for the
Treatment of Active Crohn's Disease in Children: A Randomized,
Double-Blind, Controlled, Multicenter Trial," *Eur J Gastroenterol Hepatol*, 2004, 16(1):47-54.

Espmarker U, Kristensson M, and Langkilde F, "*In Vitro* Study of
Budesonide Capsultes (Entocort® EC) 3 mg After Exposure of the
Granules to Applesauce," *American Journal of Gastoenterology*,
2002, 97(9): s259-60.

From the Global Strategy for the Diagnosis and Management of Asthma
in Children 5 Years and Younger, Global Initiative for Asthma (GINA)
2009. Available at http://www.ginasthma.org/

Habal FM and Huang VW, "Review Article: A Decision-Making Algorithm For the Management of Pregnancy in the Inflammatory Bowel
Disease Patient," *Aliment Pharmacol Ther*, 2012, 35(5):501-15.

John AS, Driscoll DJ, Warnes CA, et al, "The Use of Oral Budesonide in
Adolescents and Adults With Protein-Losing Enteropathy After the
Fontan Operation," *Ann Thorac Surg*, 2011, 92(4):1451-6.

Leachman SA and Reed BR, "The Use of Dermatologic Drugs in
Pregnancy and Lactation," *Dermatol Clin*, 2006, 24(2):167-97, vi.

Levine A, Broide E, Stein M, et al, "Evaluation of Oral Budesonide for
Treatment of Mild and Moderate Exacerbations of Crohn's Disease in
Children," *J Pediatr*, 2002, 140(1):75-80.

Levine A, Kori M, Dinari G, et al, "Comparison of Two Dosing Methods
for Induction of Response and Remission With Oral Budesonide in
Active Pediatric Crohn's Disease: A Randomized Placebo-Controlled
Trial," *Inflamm Bowel Dis*, 2009, 15(7):1055-61.

Levine A, Weizman Z, Broide E, et al, "A Comparison of Budesonide
and Prednisone for the Treatment of Active Pediatric Crohn Disease,"
J Pediatr Gastroenterol Nutr, 2003, 36(2):248-52.

Lunghi L, Pavan B, Biondi C, et al, "Use of Glucocorticoids in Pregnancy," *Curr Pharm Des*, 2010, 16(32):3616-37.

National Asthma Education and Prevention Program (NAEPP), "Expert
Panel Report 3 (EPR-3): Guidelines for the Diagnosis and Management of Asthma," Clinical Practice Guidelines, National Institutes of
Health, National Heart, Lung, and Blood Institute, NIH Publication No.
08-4051, prepublication 2007. Available at http://www.nhlbi.nih.gov/
guidelines/asthma/asthgdln.htm

NAEPP Working Group Report on "Managing Asthma During Pregnancy: Recommendations for Pharmacologic Treatment," National
Institutes of Health, National Heart, Lung, and Blood Institute, NIH
Publication No. 05-5236, March 2005. Available at http://www.nhlbi.
nih.gov/health/prof/lung/asthma/astpreg_full.pdf

Namazy J, Schatz M, Long L, et al, "Use of Inhaled Steroids by
Pregnant Asthmatic Women Does Not Reduce Intrauterine Growth,"
J Allergy Clin Immunol, 2004, 113(3):427-32.

Park-Wyllie L, Mazzotta P, Pastuszak A, et al, "Birth defects After
Maternal Exposure to Corticosteroids: Prospective Cohort Study
and Meta-Analysis of Epidemiological Studies," *Teratology*, 2000, 62
(6):385-92.

Pradat P, Robert-Gnansia E, Di Tanna GL, et al, "First Trimester
Exposure to Corticosteroids and Oral Clefts," *Birth Defects Res A
Clin Mol Teratol*, 2003, 67(12):968-70.

Schumacher KR, Cools M, Goldstein BH, et al, "Oral Budesonide
Treatment for Protein-Losing Enteropathy in Fontan-Palliated
Patients," *Pediatr Cardiol*, 2011, 32(7):966-71.

Szefler SJ, "A Review of Budesonide Inhalation Suspension in the
Treatment of Pediatric Asthma," *Pharmacotherapy*, 2001, 21
(2):195-206.

Thacker D, Patel A, Dodds K, et al, "Use of Oral Budesonide in the
Management of Protein-Losing Enteropathy After the Fontan Operation," *Ann Thorac Surg*, 2010, 89(3):837-42.

Turner Z, Lanford L, and Webber S, "Oral Budesonide as a Therapy for
Protein-Losing Enteropathy in Patients Having Undergone Fontan
Palliation," *Congenit Heart Dis*, 2012, 7(1):24-30.

Budesonide (Nasal) (byoo DES oh nide)

Brand Names: U.S. Rhinocort Aqua

Brand Names: Canada Mylan-Budesonide AQ; Rhino-
cort® Aqua®; Rhinocort® Turbuhaler®

Therapeutic Category Adrenal Corticosteroid; Anti-
inflammatory Agent; Corticosteroid, Intranasal; Glucocorticoid

Generic Availability (U.S.) Yes

Use Management of nasal symptoms associated with seasonal or perennial allergic rhinitis (FDA approved in ages
≥6 years and adults)

Intranasal corticosteroids have also been used as an
adjunct to antibiotics in empiric treatment of acute bacterial
rhinosinusitis primarily in patients with history of allergic
rhinitis (Chow, 2012) and in pediatric patients with mild

obstructive sleep apnea syndrome who cannot undergo
adenotonsillectomy or who still have symptoms after surgery (Marcus, 2012).

Pregnancy Risk Factor B

Pregnancy Considerations Adverse events have been
observed with corticosteroids in animal reproduction studies. Hypoadrenalism may occur in newborns following
maternal use of corticosteroids in pregnancy; monitor.
Studies of pregnant women using intranasal budesonide
have not demonstrated an increased risk of abnormalities.
Intranasal corticosteroids are recommended for the treatment of rhinitis during pregnancy; the lowest effective dose
should be used (NAEPP, 2005; Wallace, 2008); budesonide is preferred (Wallace, 2008).

Breast-Feeding Considerations Following use of budesonide powder for oral inhalation, ~0.3% to 1% of the
maternal dose was found in breast milk. The maximum
concentration appeared within 45 minutes of dosing.
Plasma budesonide levels obtained from infants ~90
minutes after breast-feeding (~140 minutes after maternal
dose) were below the limit of quantification. Milk concentrations following the use of the nasal inhaler are expected
to be similar. The use of inhaled corticosteroids is not
considered a contraindication to breast feeding (NAEPP,
2005). The manufacturer recommends using only when
clinically appropriate, at the lowest effective dose, and
administering the dose following a feeding in order to
minimize potential exposure to the nursing infant.

Contraindications Hypersensitivity to budesonide or any
component

Warnings HPA suppression or hypercorticism (Cushing's
syndrome) may occur with use of higher than recommended doses or at typical doses in susceptible patients.
Acute adrenal insufficiency may occur with abrupt withdrawal after long-term use, with stress, or when converting
from systemic to topical corticosteroid therapy; withdrawal
or discontinuation of corticosteroids should be done carefully; patients with HPA axis suppression may require
doses of systemic glucocorticosteroids prior to, during,
and after unusual stress (eg, surgery). Immunosuppression may occur; patients may be more susceptible to
infections; avoid exposure to chickenpox and measles.
Epistaxis may occur.

Potent inhibitors of cytochrome P450 isoenzyme CYP3A4
(eg, atazanavir, clarithromycin, indinavir, itraconazole,
ketoconazole, nefazodone, nelfinavir, ritonavir, saquinavir,
telithromycin) may significantly increase budesonide
serum concentrations and result in systemic corticosteroid
effects.

Precautions Avoid using higher than recommended dosages; suppression of HPA function, suppression of linear
growth (ie, reduction of growth velocity), reduced bone
mineral density, or hypercorticism (Cushing's syndrome)
may occur; titrate to lowest effective dose. Reduction in
growth velocity may occur when corticosteroids are administered to pediatric patients, even at recommended doses
via intranasal route (monitor growth). Use budesonide with
extreme caution in patients with respiratory tuberculosis;
untreated bacterial, fungal, systemic viral or parasitic infections; or ocular herpes simplex. Localized *Candida* infections of the nose and pharynx have been reported rarely;
interruption of therapy may be necessary while antifungal
therapy is employed. Corticosteroids impair wound healing; avoid use in patients with recent nasal ulcers, nasal
surgery, or nasal trauma; allow healing to occur before
use. Glaucoma, increased intraocular pressure and cataracts have been reported following the intranasal application of corticosteroids; monitor patients who have change
in vision and in patients with a history of increased ocular
pressure, glaucoma, or cataracts. Use of nasal budesonide in place of systemic corticosteroids may unmask
allergies (eg, eczema, rhinitis) that were previously

controlled by the systemic corticosteroids. Rare cases of immediate hypersensitivity reactions or nasal septum perforation may occur with intranasal corticosteroids.

Adverse Reactions Reaction severity varies by dose and duration; not all adverse reactions have been reported with each dosage form.

Respiratory: Bronchospasm, cough, epistaxis, nasal congestion, nasal irritation, pharyngitis, throat irritation

Rare but important or life-threatening: Anosmia, growth suppression, hypersensitivity reactions (immediate and delayed [includes rash, contact dermatitis, angioedema, bronchospasm]), nasal septum perforation, pharyngeal disorders (irritation, throat pain, itchy throat)

Drug Interactions

Metabolism/Transport Effects Substrate of CYP3A4 (minor); **Note:** Assignment of Major/Minor substrate status based on clinically relevant drug interaction potential

Avoid Concomitant Use There are no known interactions where it is recommended to avoid concomitant use.

Increased Effect/Toxicity

Budesonide (Nasal) may increase the levels/effects of: Ceritinib

The levels/effects of Budesonide (Nasal) may be increased by: CYP3A4 Inhibitors (Strong); Telaprevir

Decreased Effect There are no known significant interactions involving a decrease in effect.

Stability Store with valve up at 20°C to 25°C (68°F to 77°F). Protect from light; do not freeze.

Mechanism of Action Controls the rate of protein synthesis; depresses the migration of polymorphonuclear leukocytes, fibroblasts; reverses capillary permeability and lysosomal stabilization at the cellular level to prevent or control inflammation. Has potent glucocorticoid activity and weak mineralocorticoid activity.

Pharmacodynamics Clinical effects are due to direct local effect, rather than systemic absorption.

Onset of action: Within 10 hours

Maximum effect: 2 weeks

Duration after discontinuation: Several days

Pharmacokinetics (Adult data unless noted)

Distribution: V_d: 2-3 L/kg

Protein binding: 85% to 90%

Metabolism: Extensively metabolized by the liver via cytochrome P450 CYP3A isoenzyme to 2 major metabolites: 16α-hydroxyprednisolone and 6β-hydroxybudesonide; both are <1% as active as parent

Bioavailability: Intranasal 34%, Oral ~10%

Half-life: 2-3 hours

Time to peak serum concentration: 30 minutes

Elimination: 60% to 66% of dose renally excreted as metabolites; no unchanged drug found in urine; remainder via feces as metabolites

Dosing: Usual

Children ≥6 years and Adolescents: **Seasonal or perennial rhinitis:** Intranasal (Rhinocort® Aqua®): Initial: 64 mcg once daily delivered as 32 mcg (1 spray) **per nostril** once daily; dose may be increased if needed

Maximum daily dose:

Children <12 years: 128 mcg once daily delivered as 64 mcg (2 sprays) **per nostril** once daily

Children and Adolescents ≥12 years: 256 mcg once daily delivered as 128 mcg (4 sprays) **per nostril** once daily

Adults: **Seasonal or perennial rhinitis:** Intranasal (Rhinocort® Aqua®): Initial: 64 mcg once daily delivered as 32 mcg (1 spray) **per nostril** once daily; dose may be increased if needed; maximum daily dose: 256 mcg once daily delivered as 128 mcg (4 sprays) **per nostril** once daily

Dosing adjustment in renal impairment: There are no dosage adjustments provided in the manufacturer's labeling (not studied).

Dosing adjustment in hepatic impairment: There are no dosage adjustments provided in the manufacturer's labeling. Systemic availability of budesonide may be increased in patients with hepatic impairment; monitor closely for signs and symptoms of hypercorticism; dosage reduction may be required.

Administration Shake gently prior to each use. Before first use, prime by pressing pump 8 times or until a fine spray appears. If ≥2 days between use, repeat priming with 1 spray or until a fine spray appears. If >14 days between use, rinse applicator and repeat priming with 2 sprays or until a fine spray appears. Blow nose to clear nostrils before each use. Insert applicator into nostril, keeping bottle upright, and close off the other nostril. Breathe in through nose. While inhaling, press pump to release spray. After administration lean head backward for a few seconds; avoid blowing nose for 15 minutes after use. Do not spray into eyes or mouth. Discard after labeled number of doses has been used, even if bottle is not completely empty.

Monitoring Parameters Mucous membranes for signs of fungal infection, growth (pediatric patients), signs/symptoms of HPA axis suppression/adrenal insufficiency; ocular changes

Additional Information When used short term as adjunctive therapy in acute bacterial rhinosinusitis (ABRS), intranasal steroids show modest symptomatic improvement and few adverse effects; improvement is primarily due to increased sinus drainage. Use should be considered optional in ABRS; however, intranasal corticosteroids should be routinely prescribed to ABRS patients who have a history of or concurrent allergic rhinitis (Chow, 2012).

Dosage Forms Considerations

Rhinocort Aqua 8.6 g bottles contain 120 sprays.

Dosage Forms Excipient information presented when available (limited, particularly for generics); consult specific product labeling.

Suspension, Nasal:

Rhinocort Aqua: 32 mcg/actuation (8.6 g) [contains disodium edta, polysorbate 80]

Generic: 32 mcg/actuation (8.6 g)

References

Chow AW, Benninger MS, Brook I, et al, "IDSA Clinical Practice Guideline For Acute Bacterial Rhinosinusitis in Children and Adults," *Clin Infect Dis,* 2012, 54(8):e72-e112.

Marcus CL, Brooks LJ, Draper KA, et al, "Diagnosis and Management of Childhood Obstructive Sleep Apnea Syndrome," *Pediatrics,* 2012, 130(3):576-84.

NAEPP Working Group Report on "Managing Asthma During Pregnancy: Recommendations for Pharmacologic Treatment," National Institutes of Health, National Heart, Lung, and Blood Institute, NIH Publication No. 05-5236, March 2005. Available at http://www.nhlbi. nih.gov/health/prof/lung/asthma/astpreg/astpreg_full.pdf

Wallace DV, Dykewicz MS, Bernstein DI, et al, "The Diagnosis and Management of Rhinitis: An Updated Practice Parameter," *J Allergy Clin Immunol,* 2008, 122(2 Suppl):1-84.

◆ **Budesonide and Eformoterol** *see* Budesonide and Formoterol *on page 314*

Budesonide and Formoterol

(byoo DES oh nide & for MOH te rol)

Brand Names: U.S. Symbicort

Brand Names: Canada Symbicort

Therapeutic Category Adrenal Corticosteroid; Adrenergic Agonist Agent; Anti-inflammatory Agent; Antiasthmatic; Beta₂-Adrenergic Agonist; Bronchodilator; Corticosteroid, Inhalant (Oral); Glucocorticoid

Use Maintenance treatment of asthma (FDA approved in ages ≥12 years and adults); maintenance treatment of airflow obstruction associated with chronic obstructive pulmonary disease (COPD), including chronic bronchitis and emphysema (FDA approved in adults); **NOT** indicated for the relief of acute bronchospasm

Medication Guide Available Yes

Pregnancy Risk Factor C

Pregnancy Considerations Adverse events were observed in animal reproduction studies using this combination. Refer to individual agents.

Breast-Feeding Considerations It is not known if formoterol is excreted into breast milk; budesonide is excreted in small amounts. The manufacturer does not recommend use of this combination product in breast-feeding women. Refer to individual agents.

Contraindications Hypersensitivity to adrenergic amines, formoterol, budesonide, or any component; treatment of acute asthma or status asthmaticus

Warnings Long-acting beta$_2$-agonists (LABAs), including formoterol, increase the risk of asthma-related deaths **[U.S. Boxed Warning]**. Budesonide and formoterol should only be prescribed in patients not adequately controlled on asthma-controller medications (ie, inhaled corticosteroid) or whose disease severity requires initiation of two maintenance therapies. In a large clinical trial, LABA (salmeterol) use was associated with an increase in asthma-related deaths compared to placebo (when added to usual asthma therapy); risk is considered a class effect among all LABAs. Data are not available to determine if the addition of an inhaled corticosteroid lessens this increased risk of death associated with LABA use or if LABA use also increases the risk of death in patients with COPD. Assess patients at regular intervals once asthma control is maintained on combination therapy to determine if step-down therapy is appropriate (without loss of asthma control), and if the patient can be maintained on an inhaled corticosteroid alone. LABAs are not appropriate in patients whose asthma is adequately controlled on low- or medium-dose inhaled corticosteroids. LABAs may increase the risk of asthma-related hospitalization in pediatric and adolescent patients **[U.S. Boxed Warning]**; when addition of a LABA is clinically indicated in patients <18 years of age, a combination product containing a LABA and an inhaled corticosteroid is preferred to ensure compliance.

Budesonide and formoterol is not meant to relieve acute asthmatic or COPD symptoms, rapidly deteriorating, or potentially life-threatening episodes of asthma or COPD; acute episodes should be treated with short-acting beta$_2$-agonist. Routine use of inhaled, short-acting beta$_2$-agonists should be discontinued prior to initiation of budesonide and formoterol. Budesonide and formoterol should not be used more frequently than recommended (twice daily), at higher doses, or with any additional long-acting beta$_2$-adrenergic agonist; adverse cardiovascular effects (possibly fatal) have been reported with excessive beta$_2$-adrenergic overstimulation. Paroxysmal bronchospasm (which can be fatal) has been reported with formoterol and other inhaled beta$_2$-agonist agents; if this occurs, discontinue treatment; most commonly occurs with first use of a new canister or vial. Symptoms of laryngeal spasm, irritation, or swelling, such as stridor and choking, have been reported; if this occurs, discontinue treatment.

Fatalities have occurred due to adrenal insufficiency in asthmatic patients during and after switching from systemic corticosteroids to inhaled steroids; several months may be required for full recovery of hypothalamic-pituitary-adrenal (HPA) function; patients receiving higher doses of systemic corticosteroids (eg, adults receiving ≥20 mg/day of prednisone) may be at greater risk; during this period of adrenal suppression, inhaled steroids do not provide the systemic glucocorticoid or mineralocorticoid activity needed to treat patients requiring stress doses (ie, patients with major stress such as trauma, surgery, infections, or other conditions associated with severe electrolyte loss). When used at high doses, HPA suppression may occur; use of inhaled or systemic corticosteroids (even alternate day dosing) may increase risk of HPA suppression. Acute adrenal insufficiency may occur with abrupt withdrawal after long-term use or with stress; withdrawal or discontinuation of corticosteroid therapy should be done carefully; patients with HPA axis suppression may require doses of systemic glucocorticosteroids prior to, during, and after unusual stress (eg, surgery). Switching patients from systemic corticosteroids to inhaled steroids may unmask allergic conditions (eg, rhinitis, conjunctivitis, eczema, arthritis, eosinophilic conditions) previously suppressed by the systemic steroid. Immunosuppression may occur; patients may be more susceptible to infections; avoid exposure to chickenpox and measles.

C. albicans infections of the mouth and pharynx may occur with orally inhaled corticosteroid use, mostly mild to moderate; interruption of therapy may be necessary at times while antifungal therapy is employed; advise patients to rinse mouth after use. Hypersensitivity reactions with angioedema and swelling of the lips, tongue, and pharynx have been reported rarely.

Not recommended for use with strong CYP3A4 inhibitors (eg, ketoconazole, ritonavir, atazanavir, clarithromycin, indinavir, itraconazole, nefazodone, nelfinavir, saquinavir, telithromycin) due to potential for an increased risk of cardiovascular events and may also increase budesonide serum concentrations and result in systemic corticosteroid effects.

Precautions Use with caution in patients with cardiovascular disorders (especially coronary insufficiency, arrhythmias, hypertension, heart failure), although uncommon at recommended doses, beta-agonists may cause elevation in BP and HR and result in CNS stimulation and excitation. Caution should also be used in patients with thyrotoxicosis, seizure disorders, or conditions that are unusually sensitive to sympathomimetic amines. Transient hypokalemia from intracellular shunting may occur and produce adverse cardiovascular effects. Use with caution in patients with diabetes mellitus (DM); beta$_2$-agonists can increase serum glucose aggravating preexisting DM and ketoacidosis. Use caution in patients with hepatic impairment. Immediate hypersensitivity reactions (urticaria, angioedema, rash, bronchospasm) have been reported.

Suppression of HPA function, suppression of linear growth (ie, reduction of growth velocity), reduced bone mineral density or hypercorticism (Cushing's syndrome) may occur; titrate to lowest effective dose. Reduction in growth velocity [mean: 1 cm/year (range: 0.3-1.8 cm)] may occur when corticosteroids are administered to pediatric patients, even at recommended doses via inhaled route; related to dose and duration of exposure; monitor growth. Use with extreme caution in patients with respiratory tuberculosis, untreated systemic infections, or ocular herpes simplex. Rare cases of increased IOP, glaucoma, or cataracts have been reported with inhaled corticosteroids, including budesonide. Pneumonia and other lower respiratory tract infections have been reported in patients with COPD following the use of inhaled corticosteroids; monitor COPD patients closely since pneumonia symptoms may overlap symptoms of exacerbations.

Adverse Reactions Note: Adverse events may be dose related; causation not established. Also see individual agents.

Central nervous system: Dizziness, headache

Gastrointestinal: Oral candidiasis, stomach discomfort, vomiting

Neuromuscular & skeletal: Back pain

Respiratory: Bronchitis, lower respiratory tract infection, nasal congestion, nasopharyngitis, pharyngolaryngeal pain, sinusitis, upper respiratory tract infections

Miscellaneous: Influenza

Rare but important or life-threatening): Agitation, anaphylaxis, angina, angioedema, anxiety, atrial arrhythmia,

◀

behavioral disturbances, bronchospasm, bruising, cataract, cough, depression, dermatitis, dysphonia, exanthema, extrasystoles, glaucoma, growth velocity decreased (pediatric patients), hypercorticism symptoms, hyper-/hypotension, hyperglycemia, hypersensitivity reactions, hypokalemia, immunosuppression, intraocular pressure increased, muscle cramps, nausea, nervousness, palpitation, pruritus, rash, restlessness, sleep disturbances, tachycardia, throat irritation, tremor, urticaria, ventricular arrhythmia

Drug Interactions

Metabolism/Transport Effects Refer to individual components.

Avoid Concomitant Use

Avoid concomitant use of Budesonide and Formoterol with any of the following: Aldesleukin; BCG; Beta-Blockers (Nonselective); Conivaptan; Fusidic Acid (Systemic); Grapefruit Juice; Highest Risk QTc-Prolonging Agents; Iobenguane I 123; Ivabradine; Long-Acting Beta2-Agonists; Mifepristone; Natalizumab; Pimecrolimus; Tacrolimus (Topical); Tofacitinib

Increased Effect/Toxicity

Budesonide and Formoterol may increase the levels/ effects of: Amphotericin B; Atosiban; Deferasirox; Highest Risk QTc-Prolonging Agents; Leflunomide; Long-Acting Beta2-Agonists; Loop Diuretics; Moderate Risk QTc-Prolonging Agents; Natalizumab; Sympathomimetics; Thiazide Diuretics; Tofacitinib

The levels/effects of Budesonide and Formoterol may be increased by: AtoMOXetine; Caffeine and Caffeine Containing Products; Cannabinoid-Containing Products; Conivaptan; CYP3A4 Inhibitors (Moderate); CYP3A4 Inhibitors (Strong); Dasatinib; Denosumab; Fusidic Acid (Systemic); Grapefruit Juice; Inhalational Anesthetics; Ivabradine; Ivacaftor; Linezolid; Luliconazole; MAO Inhibitors; Mifepristone; Pimecrolimus; QTc-Prolonging Agents (Indeterminate Risk and Risk Modifying); Simeprevir; Stiripentol; Tacrolimus (Topical); Telaprevir; Theophylline Derivatives; Trastuzumab; Tricyclic Antidepressants

Decreased Effect

Budesonide and Formoterol may decrease the levels/ effects of: Aldesleukin; Antidiabetic Agents; BCG; Coccidioidin Skin Test; Corticorelin; Hyaluronidase; Iobenguane I 123; Sipuleucel-T; Vaccines (Inactivated)

The levels/effects of Budesonide and Formoterol may be decreased by: Antacids; Beta-Blockers (Beta1 Selective); Beta-Blockers (Nonselective); Betahistine; Bile Acid Sequestrants; Echinacea

Stability Store at controlled room temperature of 20°C to 25°C (68°F to 77°F) with mouthpiece down; do not expose to temperatures >120°F; do not puncture or incinerate.

Mechanism of Action Formoterol relaxes bronchial smooth muscle by selective action on beta₂ receptors with little effect on heart rate. Formoterol has a long-acting effect. Budesonide is a corticosteroid which controls the rate of protein synthesis, depresses the migration of polymorphonuclear leukocytes/fibroblasts, and reverses capillary permeability and lysosomal stabilization at the cellular level to prevent or control inflammation.

Pharmacodynamics See individual agents.

Pharmacokinetics (Adult data unless noted) See individual agents.

Dosing: Usual

Pediatric: Asthma; maintenance treatment: Oral inhalation:

Children 5 to 11 years: Budesonide 80 mcg/formoterol 4.5 mcg (Symbicort 80/4.5): 2 inhalations twice daily. Do not exceed 4 inhalations/day (Morice, 2008; NAEPP, 2007)

Children and Adolescents ≥12 years not controlled on low-medium dose inhaled corticosteroids: Budesonide

80 mcg/formoterol 4.5 mcg (Symbicort 80/4.5): 2 inhalations twice daily. Do not exceed 4 inhalations/day. In patients not adequately controlled following 2 weeks of therapy, consider the higher dose combination.

Children and Adolescents ≥12 years not controlled on medium-high dose inhaled corticosteroids: Budesonide 160 mcg/formoterol 4.5 mcg (Symbicort 160/4.5): 2 inhalations twice daily. Do not exceed 4 inhalations/day.

Adult:

Asthma: Oral inhalation: Symbicort 80/4.5, Symbicort 160/4.5: 2 inhalations twice daily. Do not exceed 4 inhalations/day. Recommended starting dose combination is determined according to asthma severity. In patients not adequately controlled on the lower combination dose following 1 to 2 weeks of therapy, consider the higher dose combination.

COPD: Oral inhalation: Symbicort 160/4.5: 2 inhalations twice daily. Do not exceed 4 inhalations/day.

Administration Prior to first use, inhaler must be primed by releasing 2 test sprays into the air (away from the face); shake well for 5 seconds before each use. Inhaler must be reprimed if inhaler has not been used for >7 days or has been dropped. Discard after labeled number of inhalations has been used or within 3 months after foil wrap has been removed; do not use immerse in water or use "float test" to determine number of inhalations left.

Monitoring Parameters Pulmonary function tests, vital signs, CNS stimulation, serum glucose, serum potassium; check mucous membranes for signs of fungal infection; monitor growth in pediatric patients

Dosage Forms Excipient information presented when available (limited, particularly for generics); consult specific product labeling.

Aerosol for oral inhalation:

Symbicort 80/4.5: Budesonide 80 mcg and formoterol fumarate dihydrate 4.5 mcg per actuation (6.9 g) [60 metered inhalations]; budesonide 80 mcg and formoterol fumarate dihydrate 4.5 mcg per actuation (10.2 g) [120 metered inhalations]

Symbicort 160/4.5: Budesonide 160 mcg and formoterol fumarate dihydrate 4.5 mcg per actuation (6 g) [60 metered inhalations]; budesonide 160 mcg and formoterol fumarate dihydrate 4.5 mcg per actuation (10.2 g) [120 metered inhalations]

References

Morice AH, Peterson S, Beckman O, Osmanliev D. Therapeutic comparison of a new budesonide/formoterol pMDI with budesonide pMDI and budesonide/formoterol DPI in asthma. *Int J Clin Pract.* 2007;61 (11):1874-1883.

National Asthma Education and Prevention Program (NAEPP), "Expert Panel Report 3 (EPR-3): Guidelines for the Diagnosis and Management of Asthma," *Clinical Practice Guidelines,* National Institutes of Health, National Heart, Lung, and Blood Institute, NIH Publication No. 08-4051, prepublication 2007. Available at http://www.nhlbi.nih.gov/ guidelines/asthma/asthgdln.htm

Pohunek P, Kuna P, Jorup C, et al, "Budesonide/Formoterol Improves Lung Function Compared With Budesonide Alone in Children With Asthma," *Pediatr Allergy Immunol,* 2006, 17(6):458-65.

◆ **Buffasal [OTC]** *see* Aspirin *on page* 212

◆ **Bufferin [OTC]** *see* Aspirin *on page* 212

◆ **Bufferin Extra Strength [OTC]** *see* Aspirin *on page* 212

◆ **Buffinol [OTC]** *see* Aspirin *on page* 212

Bumetanide (byoo MET a nide)

Medication Safety Issues

Sound-alike/look-alike issues:

Bumetanide may be confused with Buminate

Bumex may be confused with Brevibloc, Buprenex

International issues:

Bumex [U.S.] may be confused with Permax brand name for pergolide [multiple international markets]

Brand Names: Canada Burinex

Therapeutic Category Antihypertensive Agent; Diuretic, Loop

Generic Availability (U.S.) Yes

Use Management of edema secondary to heart failure or hepatic or renal disease, including nephrotic syndrome (FDA approved in adults); has also been used to reverse oliguria in preterm neonates and for the treatment of hypertension alone or in combination with other antihypertensive agents

Pregnancy Risk Factor C

Pregnancy Considerations Adverse events have been observed in some animal reproduction studies.

Breast-Feeding Considerations It is not known if bumetanide is excreted in breast milk. Breast-feeding is not recommended by the manufacturer. Diuretics have the potential to decrease milk volume and suppress lactation.

Contraindications Hypersensitivity to bumetanide or any component; anuria or increasing azotemia; hepatic coma; severe electrolyte depletion (until condition is improved or corrected)

Warnings Loop diuretics are potent diuretics; excess amounts can lead to profound diuresis with fluid and electrolyte loss **[U.S. Boxed Warning]**; close medical supervision and dose evaluation is required. Potassium supplementation and/or use of potassium-sparing diuretics may be necessary to prevent hypokalemia. Monitor fluid status and renal function in an attempt to prevent oliguria, azotemia, and reversible increases in BUN and creatinine; close medical supervision of aggressive diuresis required. Coadministration of antihypertensives may increase the risk of hypotension.

Ototoxicity has been demonstrated following oral administration of torsemide and following rapid I.V. administration of other loop diuretics. Other possible risk factors may include use in renal impairment, excessive doses, and concurrent use of other ototoxins (eg, aminoglycosides).

Although rare, thrombocytopenia has been reported; routinely monitor for possible occurrence.

Parenteral formulation contains benzyl alcohol; large amounts of benzyl alcohol (≥99 mg/kg/day) have been associated with a potentially fatal toxicity ("gasping syndrome") in neonates; the "gasping syndrome" consists of metabolic acidosis, respiratory distress, gasping respirations, CNS dysfunction (including convulsions, intracranial hemorrhage), hypotension and cardiovascular collapse; avoid use of parenteral formulations containing benzyl alcohol in neonates; *in vitro* and animal studies have shown that benzoate displaces bilirubin from protein binding sites. *In vitro* studies using pooled sera from critically ill neonates have shown bumetanide to be a potent displacer of bilirubin; use with caution in neonates at risk for kernicterus.

Precautions Use with caution in patients with cirrhosis; avoid sudden changes in fluid and electrolyte balance and acid/base status which may lead to hepatic encephalopathy. Administration with an aldosterone antagonist or potassium-sparing diuretic may provide additional diuretic efficacy and maintain normokalemia.

Chemical similarities are present among sulfonamides, sulfonylureas, carbonic anhydrase inhibitors, thiazides, and loop diuretics (except ethacrynic acid); the manufacturer's labeling states that bumetanide may be used in patients allergic to furosemide. Use in patients with sulfonylurea allergy is not specifically contraindicated in product labeling; however, a risk of cross-reaction exists in patients with allergy to any of these compounds; avoid use when previous reaction has been severe. Discontinue if signs of hypersensitivity are noted.

Bumetanide increases urinary excretion of calcium and magnesium and may lead to hypocalcemia and hypomagnesemia; asymptomatic hyperuricemia has also been reported. Glucose alterations may occur with bumetanide use; serum glucose should be monitored during therapy especially in patients with or suspected to have diabetes.

Adverse Reactions

Central nervous system: Dizziness

Endocrine & metabolic: Bicarbonate altered, calcium altered, CO_2 content altered, hyperglycemia, hyperuricemia, hypochloremia, hypokalemia, hyponatremia, phosphorus altered

Neuromuscular & skeletal: Muscle cramps

Renal: Azotemia, serum creatinine increased

Miscellaneous: LDH altered

Rare but important or life-threatening: Abdominal pain, alkaline phosphatase altered, arthritic pain, asterixis, bilirubin altered, chest pain, cholesterol altered, creatinine clearance altered, dehydration, diaphoresis, diarrhea, ear discomfort, ECG changes, encephalopathy (in patients with preexisting liver disease), erectile dysfunction, fatigue, headache, hearing impaired, hemoglobin/hematocrit altered, hives, hyperventilation, hypotension, musculoskeletal pain, nausea, nipple tenderness, orthostatic hypotension, ototoxicity, premature ejaculation, prothrombin time altered, pruritus, rash, renal failure, Stevens-Johnson syndrome, thrombocytopenia, toxic epidermal necrolysis, transaminase altered, upset stomach, urine glucose increased, urine protein increased, vertigo, vomiting, WBC altered, weakness, xerostomia

Drug Interactions

Metabolism/Transport Effects None known.

Avoid Concomitant Use There are no known interactions where it is recommended to avoid concomitant use.

Increased Effect/Toxicity

Bumetanide may increase the levels/effects of: ACE Inhibitors; Allopurinol; Amifostine; Aminoglycosides; Antihypertensives; Cardiac Glycosides; CISplatin; Dofetilide; DULoxetine; Hypotensive Agents; Ivabradine; Lithium; Methotrexate; Neuromuscular-Blocking Agents; Obinutuzumab; RisperiDONE; RiTUXimab; Salicylates; Sodium Phosphates; Topiramate

The levels/effects of Bumetanide may be increased by: Alfuzosin; Analgesics (Opioid); Barbiturates; Beta2-Agonists; Brimonidine (Topical); Canagliflozin; Corticosteroids (Orally Inhaled); Corticosteroids (Systemic); CycloSPORINE (Systemic); Diazoxide; Herbs (Hypotensive Properties); Licorice; MAO Inhibitors; Methotrexate; Pentoxifylline; Phosphodiesterase 5 Inhibitors; Probenecid; Prostacyclin Analogues

Decreased Effect

Bumetanide may decrease the levels/effects of: Hypoglycemic Agents; Lithium; Neuromuscular-Blocking Agents

The levels/effects of Bumetanide may be decreased by: Bile Acid Sequestrants; Fosphenytoin; Herbs (Hypertensive Properties); Methotrexate; Methylphenidate; Nonsteroidal Anti-Inflammatory Agents; Phenytoin; Probenecid; Salicylates; Yohimbine

Food Interactions Bumetanide serum levels may be decreased if taken with food. Management: It has been recommended that bumetanide be administered without food (Bard, 2004).

Stability

Oral: Store at 15°C to 30°C (59°F to 86°F); protect from light

Parenteral: Store at 20°C to 25°C (68°F to 77°F); protect from light; may discolor when exposed to light

Mechanism of Action Inhibits reabsorption of sodium and chloride in the ascending loop of Henle and proximal renal tubule, interfering with the chloride-binding cotransport system, thus causing increased excretion of water, ▶

sodium, chloride, magnesium, phosphate, and calcium; it does not appear to act on the distal tubule

Pharmacodynamics
Onset of action:
Oral, I.M.: Within 30-60 minutes
I.V.: Within a few minutes
Maximum effect:
Oral, I.M.: 1-2 hours
I.V.: 15-30 minutes
Duration:
Oral: 4-6 hours
I.V.: 2-3 hours

Pharmacokinetics (Adult data unless noted)
Distribution: V_d: Neonates and infants: 0.26-0.39 L/kg
Protein binding: 95%
Neonates: 97%
Metabolism: Partial metabolism occurs in the liver
Bioavailability: 59% to 89% (median: 80%)
Half-life:
Premature and full term neonates: 6 hours (range up to 15 hours)
Infants <2 months: 2.5 hours
Infants 2-6 months: 1.5 hours
Adults: 1-1.5 hours
Time to peak serum concentration: 0.5-2 hours
Elimination: Unchanged drug excreted in urine (45%); biliary/fecal (2%)
Clearance:
Preterm and full term neonates: 0.2-1.1 mL/minute/kg
Infants <2 months: 2.17 mL/minute/kg
Infants 2-6 months: 3.8 mL/minute/kg
Adults: 2.9 ± 0.2 mL/minute/kg

Dosing: Neonatal Oral, I.M., I.V.: **Note:** Doses in the higher end of the range may be required for patients with heart failure:
Preterm neonates: 0.01-0.05 mg/kg/dose every 24-48 hours (Lopez-Samplas, 1997; Shankaran, 1995); a retrospective trial reported a mean dose of 0.03 mg/kg/dose every 12-24 hours for oliguric acute renal failure (n=35; PMA: 24-36 weeks) (maximum reported dose: 0.06 mg/kg/dose) (Oliveros, 2011)
Term neonates: 0.01-0.05 mg/kg/dose every 12-24 hours (Sullivan, 1996; Ward, 1977)

Dosing: Usual
Infants and Children: Oral, I.M., I.V.: 0.015-0.1 mg/kg/dose every 6-24 hours (maximum dose: 10 mg/day); a prospective, open-label dose-range study in infants (mean age: 2 months; range: 0-6 months) reported a maximal diuretic response at doses 0.035-0.04 mg/kg/dose every 6-8 hours, and no additional clinical benefit (ie, urine output) at doses >0.05 mg/kg/dose (Sullivan, 1996)
Adults:
Edema:
Oral: 0.5-2 mg/dose 1-2 times/day; if diuretic response to initial dose is not adequate, may repeat in 4-5 hours for up to 2 doses (maximum daily dose: 10 mg/**day**)
I.M., I.V.: 0.5-1 mg/dose; may repeat in 2-3 hours for up to 2 doses if needed (maximum daily dose: 10 mg/**day**)
Hypertension: Oral: 0.5 mg daily (maximum daily dose: 5 mg/**day**); usual dosage range (JNC 7): 0.5-2 mg divided twice daily (Chobanian, 2003)

Administration
Oral: Administer with food to decrease GI irritation
Parenteral: Administer without additional dilution by direct I.V. injection over 1-2 minutes; for intermittent I.V. infusion, dilute in D_5W, LR, or NS and infuse over 5 minutes (Rudy, 1991); pH: 6.8-7.8

Monitoring Parameters Blood pressure, serum electrolytes, renal function, urine output

Additional Information Patients with impaired hepatic function must be monitored carefully, often requiring reduced doses; larger doses may be necessary in patients with impaired renal function to obtain the same therapeutic response; 1 mg bumetanide approximately equivalent in potency to 40 mg furosemide

Dosage Forms Excipient information presented when available (limited, particularly for generics); consult specific product labeling.
Solution, Injection:
Generic: 0.25 mg/mL (2 mL, 4 mL, 10 mL)
Tablet, Oral:
Generic: 0.5 mg, 1 mg, 2 mg

References
Brater DC, "Clinical Pharmacology of Loop Diuretics," *Drugs*, 1991, 41 Suppl 3:14-22.
Chobanian AV, Bakris GL, Black HR, et al, "The Seventh Report of the Joint National Committee on Prevention, Detection, Evaluation, and Treatment of High Blood Pressure: The JNC 7 Report," *JAMA*, 2003, 289(19):2560-72.
Cook JA, Smith DE, Cornish LA, et al, "Kinetics, Dynamics, and Bioavailability of Bumetanide in Healthy Subjects and Patients With Congestive Heart Failure," *Clin Pharmacol Ther*, 1988, 44(5):487-500.
Lopez-Samblas AM, Adams JA, Goldberg RN, et al, "The Pharmacokinetics of Bumetanide in the Newborn Infant," *Biol Neonate*, 1997, 72 (5):265-72.
Oliveros M, Pham JT, John E, et al, "The Use of Bumetanide for Oliguric Acute Renal Failure in Preterm Infants," *Pediatr Crit Care Med*, 2011, 12(2):210-4.
Rudy DW, Voelker JR, Greene PK, et al, "Loop Diuretics for Chronic Renal Insufficiency: A Continuous Infusion Is More Efficacious Than Bolus Therapy," *Ann Intern Med*, 1991, 115(5):360-6.
Shankaran S, Liang KC, Ilagan N, et al, "Mineral Excretion Following Furosemide Compared With Bumetanide Therapy in Premature Infants," *Pediatr Nephrol*, 1995, 9(2):159-62.
Sullivan JE, Witte MK, Yamashita TS, et al, "Analysis of the Variability in the Pharmacokinetics and Pharmacodynamics of Bumetanide in Critically Ill Infants," *Clin Pharmacol Ther*, 1996, 60(4):414-23.
Sullivan JE, Witte MK, Yamashita TS, et al, "Dose-Ranging Evaluation of Bumetanide Pharmacodynamics in Critically Ill Infants," *Clin Pharmacol Ther*, 1996, 60(4):424-34.
Ward OC and Lam LK, "Bumetanide in Heart Failure in Infancy," *Arch Dis Child*, 1977, 52(11):877-82.
Wells TG, "The Pharmacology and Therapeutics of Diuretics in the Pediatric Patient," *Pediatr Clin North Am*, 1990, 37(2):463-504.

◆ **Bumex** *see* Bumetanide *on page 316*

◆ **Buminate** *see* Albumin *on page 82*

◆ **Buminate-5% (Can)** *see* Albumin *on page 82*

◆ **Buminate-25% (Can)** *see* Albumin *on page 82*

◆ **Bunavail** *see* Buprenorphine and Naloxone *on page 324*

◆ **Buphenyl** *see* Sodium Phenylbutyrate *on page 1912*

Bupivacaine (byoo PIV a kane)

Medication Safety Issues
Sound-alike/look-alike issues:
Bupivacaine may be confused with mepivacaine, ropivacaine
Marcaine® may be confused with Narcan®
High alert medication:
The Institute for Safe Medication Practices (ISMP) includes this medication (epidural administration) among its list of drug classes which have a heightened risk of causing significant patient harm when used in error.

Brand Names: U.S. Bupivacaine Spinal; Marcaine; Marcaine Preservative Free; Marcaine Spinal; Sensorcaine; Sensorcaine-MPF; Sensorcaine-MPF Spinal

Brand Names: Canada Marcaine®; Sensorcaine®

Therapeutic Category Local Anesthetic, Injectable

Generic Availability (U.S.) Yes

Use Local anesthetic (injectable) for peripheral nerve block, infiltration, sympathetic block, caudal or epidural block, retrobulbar block

Pregnancy Risk Factor C

Pregnancy Considerations Adverse events were observed in animal reproduction studies. Bupivacaine crosses the placenta. Bupivacaine is approved for use at term in obstetrical anesthesia or analgesia. **[U.S. Boxed Warning]: The 0.75% is not recommended for obstetrical anesthesia.** Bupivacaine 0.75% solutions have been associated with cardiac arrest following epidural anesthesia in obstetrical patients and use of this concentration is not recommended for this purpose. Use in obstetrical paracervical block anesthesia is contraindicated.

Breast-Feeding Considerations Bupivacaine is excreted in breast milk. Due to the potential for serious adverse reactions in the nursing infant, a decision should be made whether to discontinue nursing or to discontinue the drug, taking into account the importance of treatment to the mother.

Contraindications Hypersensitivity to bupivacaine hydrochloride, other amide-type anesthetics, or any component; not recommended for I.V. regional anesthesia (Bier block); obstetrical paracervical block anesthesia (use is associated with fetal bradycardia and death); 0.75% concentration in obstetrical anesthesia

Warnings Convulsions due to systemic toxicity leading to cardiac arrest have been reported, presumably following unintentional I.V. injection; some products contain sulfites which may cause allergic reactions in susceptible individuals; **do not use solutions containing preservatives for caudal or epidural block.** Infants may be at greater risk for bupivacaine toxicity because α_1-acid-glycoprotein, the major serum protein to which bupivacaine is bound, is lower in infants compared with older children; use epidural infusions with caution in infants and monitor closely; increased toxicity may be minimized by limiting the duration of infusion to ≤48 hours (McCloskey, 1992). Reduce epidural infusion dosage in patients with seizure disorders or at increased risk for seizures (eg, electrolyte imbalance) (Berde, 1992). Chondrolysis has been reported following continuous intra-articular infusion; intra-articular administration of local anesthetics is not an FDA-approved route of administration.

Precautions Use with caution in patients with liver disease and impaired cardiovascular function; when used for epidural anesthesia, a smaller test dose is recommended to evaluate the patient's response

Adverse Reactions Note: Most effects are dose related, and are often due to accelerated absorption from the injection site, unintentional intravascular injection, or slow metabolic degradation. The development of any central nervous system symptoms may be an early indication of more significant toxicity (seizure).

Cardiovascular: Bradycardia, cardiac arrest, heart block, hypotension, palpitation, ventricular arrhythmia

Central nervous system: Anxiety, dizziness, restlessness, seizure; rare symptoms (usually associated with unintentional subarachnoid injection during high spinal anesthesia) include cranial nerve palsies, headache, paralysis, paresthesia, persistent anesthesia, and septic meningitis

Gastrointestinal: Nausea, vomiting; rare symptoms (usually associated with unintentional subarachnoid injection during high spinal anesthesia) include fecal incontinence and loss of sphincter control

Genitourinary: Rare symptoms (usually associated with unintentional subarachnoid injection during high spinal anesthesia) include loss of perineal sensation, loss of sexual function, and urinary incontinence

Neuromuscular & skeletal: Chondrolysis (continuous intra-articular administration), weakness

Ocular: Blurred vision, pupillary constriction

Otic: Tinnitus

Respiratory: Apnea, hypoventilation (usually associated with unintentional subarachnoid injection during high spinal anesthesia)

Miscellaneous: Allergic reactions (angioedema, pruritus, urticaria), anaphylactoid reactions

Drug Interactions

Metabolism/Transport Effects Substrate of CYP1A2 (minor), CYP2C19 (minor), CYP2D6 (minor), CYP3A4 (minor); **Note:** Assignment of Major/Minor substrate status based on clinically relevant drug interaction potential

Avoid Concomitant Use There are no known interactions where it is recommended to avoid concomitant use.

Increased Effect/Toxicity

The levels/effects of Bupivacaine may be increased by: Beta-Blockers; Hyaluronidase

Decreased Effect

Bupivacaine may decrease the levels/effects of: Technetium Tc 99m Tilmanocept

The levels/effects of Bupivacaine may be decreased by: Peginterferon Alfa-2b

Stability Store at room temperature; solutions containing epinephrine should be protected from light; bupivacaine 0.4375 mg/mL when mixed with epinephrine 0.6875 mcg/mL and fentanyl 1.25 mcg/mL is stable refrigerated for 20 days and at room temperature for 48 hours; bupivacaine 625 mcg/mL or 1250 mcg/mL mixed with morphine sulfate 100 mcg/mL or 500 mcg/mL in NS is stable for 72 hours at room temperature

Mechanism of Action Blocks both the initiation and conduction of nerve impulses by decreasing the neuronal membrane's permeability to sodium ions, which results in inhibition of depolarization with resultant blockade of conduction

Pharmacodynamics

Onset of anesthetic action: Dependent on total dose, concentration, and route administered, but generally occurs within 4-10 minutes

Duration: 1.5-8.5 hours (depending upon route of administration)

Pharmacokinetics (Adult data unless noted)

Distribution: V_d:

Infants: 3.9 ± 2 L/kg

Children: 2.7 ± 0.2 L/kg

Protein binding: 84% to 95%

Metabolism: In the liver

Half-life (age-dependent):

Neonates: 8.1 hours

Adults: 2.7 hours

Time to peak serum concentration: Caudal, epidural, or peripheral nerve block: 30-45 minutes

Elimination: Small amounts (~6%) excreted in urine unchanged

Clearance:

Infants: 7.1 ± 3.2 mL/kg/minute

Children: 10 ± 0.7 mL/kg/minute

Dosing: Neonatal Dose varies with procedure, depth of anesthesia, vascularity of tissues, duration of anesthesia, and condition of patient. Continuous epidural (caudal or lumbar) infusion: Limited data available (Berde, 1992): Loading dose: 2-2.5 mg/kg (0.8-1 mL/kg of 0.25% bupivacaine)

Infusion dose:

Dose: 0.2-0.25 mg/kg/**hour**

Dose (using 0.25% solution): 0.08-0.1 mL/kg/**hour**

Dose (using 0.125% solution): 0.16-0.2 mL/kg/**hour**

Dose (using 0.05% solution): 0.4-0.5 mL/kg/**hour**

Dosing: Usual Dose varies with procedure, depth of anesthesia, vascularity of tissues, duration of anesthesia, and condition of patient.

Caudal block (with or without epinephrine, **preservative free**):

Children: 1-3.7 mg/kg

Adults: 15-30 mL of 0.25% or 0.5%

Epidural block, **preservative free** (other than caudal block):
Children: 1.25 mg/kg/dose
Adults: 10-20 mL of 0.25%, 0.5%, or 0.75%
Peripheral nerve block: 5 mL dose of 0.25% or 0.5% (12.5-25 mg); maximum dose: 400 mg/day
Sympathetic nerve block: 20-50 mL of 0.25% (no epinephrine) solution
Continuous epidural (caudal or lumbar) infusion: Limited information in infants and children:
Loading dose: 2-2.5 mg/kg (0.8-1 mL/kg of 0.25% bupivacaine)
Infusion dose: See table

Bupivacaine Infusion Dose

Age	Dose	Dose (using 0.25% solution)	Dose (using 0.125% solution)	Dose (using 0.05% solution)
Infants ≤4 mo	0.2-0.25 mg/kg/h	0.08-0.1 mL/kg/h	0.16-0.2 mL/kg/h	0.4-0.5 mL/kg/h
Infants >4 mo and children	0.4-0.5 mg/kg/h	0.16-0.2 mL/kg/h	0.32-0.4 mL/kg/h	0.8-1 mL/kg/h
Adults	5-20 mg/h	2-8 mL/h	4-16 mL/h	10-40 mL/h

Administration Solutions containing preservatives should not be used for epidural or caudal blocks; for epidural infusion, may use undiluted or diluted with preservative free NS

Reference Range Toxicity: 2-4 mcg/mL (however, some experts have suggested that the rate of rise of the serum level is more predictive of toxicity than the actual value; Scott, 1975)

Additional Information For epidural infusion, lower dosages of bupivacaine may be effective when used in combination with opioid analgesics

Dosage Forms Excipient information presented when available (limited, particularly for generics); consult specific product labeling.
Solution, Injection, as hydrochloride:
Marcaine: 0.25% (50 mL); 0.5% (50 mL) [contains methylparaben]
Sensorcaine: 0.25% (50 mL); 0.5% (50 mL) [contains methylparaben]
Sensorcaine-MPF: 0.25% (10 mL, 30 mL); 0.5% (10 mL, 30 mL); 0.75% (10 mL, 30 mL) [methylparaben free]
Generic: 0.25% (10 mL, 30 mL, 50 mL); 0.5% (10 mL, 30 mL, 50 mL); 0.75% (10 mL, 30 mL)
Solution, Injection, as hydrochloride [preservative free]:
Marcaine: 0.75% (10 mL, 30 mL)
Marcaine Preservative Free: 0.25% (10 mL, 30 mL); 0.5% (10 mL, 30 mL)
Generic: 0.25% (10 mL, 20 mL, 30 mL); 0.5% (10 mL, 20 mL, 30 mL); 0.75% (10 mL, 20 mL, 30 mL)
Solution, Intrathecal, as hydrochloride [preservative free]:
Bupivacaine Spinal: 0.75% [7.5 mg/mL] (2 mL)
Marcaine Spinal: 0.75% [7.5 mg/mL] (2 mL)
Sensorcaine-MPF Spinal: 0.75% [7.5 mg/mL] (2 mL)

References

Berde CB, "Convulsions Associated With Pediatric Regional Anesthesia," *Anesth Analg*, 1992, 75(2):164-6.
Desparmet J, Meistelman C, Barre J, et al, "Continuous Epidural Infusion of Bupivacaine for Postoperative Pain Relief in Children," *Anesthesiology*, 1987, 67(1):108-10.
Luz G, Innerhofer P, Bachmann B, et al, "Bupivacaine Plasma Concentrations During Continuous Epidural Anesthesia in Infants and Children," *Anesth Analg*, 1996, 82(2):231-4.
McCloskey JJ, Haun SE, and Deshpande JK, "Bupivacaine Toxicity Secondary to Continuous Caudal Epidural Infusion in Children," *Anesth Analg*, 1992, 75(2):287-90.
Scott DB, "Evaluation of Clinical Tolerance of Local Anaesthetic Agents," *Br J Anaesth*, 1975, 47:328-31.

◆ **Bupivacaine Hydrochloride** *see* Bupivacaine *on page 318*

◆ **Bupivacaine Spinal** *see* Bupivacaine *on page 318*
◆ **Buprenex** *see* Buprenorphine *on page 320*

Buprenorphine (byoo pre NOR feen)

Medication Safety Issues
Sound-alike/look-alike issues:
Buprenex may be confused with Brevibloc, Bumex
High alert medication:
The Institute for Safe Medication Practices (ISMP) includes this medication among its list of drug classes which have a heightened risk of causing significant harm when used in error.

Brand Names: U.S. Buprenex; Butrans
Brand Names: Canada Butrans
Therapeutic Category Analgesic, Narcotic; Opioid Partial Agonist
Generic Availability (U.S.) May be product dependent
Use
Oral: Sublingual tablet: Treatment of opioid dependence (FDA approved in ages ≥16 years and adults)
Parenteral: Management of moderate to severe pain (FDA approved in ages ≥2 years and adults)
Transdermal: Management of moderate to severe chronic pain in patients requiring an around-the-clock opioid analgesic for an extended period of time (FDA approved in adults)

Prescribing and Access Restrictions Prescribing of tablets for opioid dependence is limited to physicians who have met the qualification criteria and have received a DEA number specific to prescribing this product. Tablets will be available through pharmacies and wholesalers which normally provide controlled substances.
Medication Guide Available Yes
Pregnancy Risk Factor C
Pregnancy Considerations Adverse effects have been observed in some animal reproduction studies. Buprenorphine crosses the placenta; buprenorphine and norbuprenorphine can be detected in newborn serum, urine, and meconium following in utero exposure (CSAT, 2004). Following chronic opioid therapy in pregnancy, adverse events in the newborn (including withdrawal) may occur; monitoring of the neonate is recommended. The minimum effective dose should be used if opioids are needed (Chou, 2009). The onset of withdrawal in infants of women receiving buprenorphine during pregnancy ranged from day 1 to day 8 of life, most occurring on day 1. Symptoms of withdrawal may include agitation, apnea, bradycardia, convulsions, hypertonia, myoclonus, respiratory depression, and tremor.

Buprenorphine is currently considered an alternate treatment for pregnant women who need therapy for opioid addiction (CSAT, 2004; Dow, 2012); however, use in pregnancy for this purpose is increasing (ACOG, 2012; Soyka, 2013). Buprenorphine should not be used to treat pain during labor. Women receiving buprenorphine for the treatment of addiction should be maintained on their daily dose of buprenorphine in addition to receiving the same pain management options during labor and delivery as opioid-naïve women; maintenance doses of buprenorphine will not provide adequate pain relief. Narcotic agonist-antagonists should be avoided for the treatment of labor pain in women maintained on buprenorphine due to the risk of precipitating acute withdrawal. In addition, buprenorphine should not be given to women in labor taking methadone (ACOG, 2012).

Amenorrhea may develop secondary to substance abuse; pregnancy may occur following the initiation of buprenorphine maintenance treatment. Contraception counseling is recommended to prevent unplanned pregnancies (Dow, 2012).

Breast-Feeding Considerations Buprenorphine is excreted in breast milk. Breast-feeding is not recommended by the manufacturer. Nursing infants exposed to large doses of opioids should be monitored for apnea and sedation (Montgomery, 2012).

When buprenorphine is used to treat opioid addiction in nursing women, most guidelines do not contraindicate breast-feeding as long as the infant is tolerant to the dose and other contraindications do not exist; caution should be used when nursing infants not previously exposed (ACOG, 2012; CSAT, 2004; Montgomery, 2012). If additional illicit substances are being abused, women treated with buprenorphine should pump and discard breast milk until sobriety is established (ACOG, 2012; Dow, 2012).

Contraindications Hypersensitivity to buprenorphine or any component. Additional contraindications for transdermal patch: Significant respiratory depression; acute or severe bronchial asthma; known or suspected paralytic ileus.

Warnings Respiratory depression may occur; use with caution and in reduced doses in patients with preexisting respiratory depression, decreased respiratory reserve, hypoxia, hypercapnia, significant COPD, or cor pulmonale, and in those receiving medications with CNS or respiratory depressant effects; respiratory depression may not be reversible with naloxone; mechanical ventilation may be required. Patients who are cachectic or debilitated may be at higher risk for respiratory depression; monitor closely.

May cause CNS depression which may impair physical or mental abilities; patients must be cautioned about performing tasks which require mental alertness (eg, operating machinery or driving); use caution when combining with other CNS depressants (eg, centrally acting antiemetics, general anesthetics, phenothiazines, sedative-hypnotics) due to additive CNS effects. If combination therapy is needed, consider dosage reduction of one or both agents. Physical and psychological dependence may occur; abrupt discontinuation after prolonged use may result in withdrawal symptoms; compared to full-opioid agonists, withdrawal from buprenorphine may be milder and may be delayed in onset; opioid antagonist activity of buprenorphine may precipitate acute opioid withdrawal in opioid-dependent individuals. Infants born to women physically dependent on opioids, including buprenorphine, will also be physically dependent and may experience respiratory difficulties or opioid withdrawal symptoms [neonatal abstinence syndrome (NAS)]. Onset, duration, and severity of NAS depend upon the drug used (maternal), duration of use, maternal dose, and rate of drug elimination by the newborn. Symptoms of newborn opioid withdrawal may include excessive crying, diarrhea, fever, hyper-reflexia, irritability, tremors, vomiting, or failure to gain weight. Opioid withdrawal syndrome in the neonate, unlike in adults, may be life-threatening and should be promptly treated. Onset of symptoms ranged from day 1 to day 8 of life, most occurring on day 1 of life in infants of women receiving buprenorphine sublingual tablets during pregnancy; rare cases of convulsions (with one case of apnea and bradycardia) have also been reported.

Hepatitis and other hepatic events have been reported in patients receiving buprenorphine for the treatment of opioid dependence; infection with viral hepatitis, concomitant use of potentially hepatotoxic drugs, preexisting liver enzyme abnormalities, and ongoing drug use may have contributed to liver abnormalities. Monitor liver function tests in all patients prior to and during therapy. Hypersensitivity reactions, including bronchospasm, angioneurotic edema, and anaphylactic shock have also been reported. Acute and chronic hypersensitivity reactions have also been reported. Orthostatic hypotension may occur in ambulatory patients.

Dosage form specific warnings:

Transdermal patch: May cause potentially life-threatening respiratory depression even with therapeutic use **[U.S. Boxed Warning]**. Ensure proper dosing and titration; monitor for respiratory depression, especially within the first 24-72 hours of initiation or dose escalation. Use is contraindicated in patients with respiratory depression or acute or severe bronchial asthma. May cause QT prolongation; do not exceed one 20 **mcg**/hour transdermal patch; avoid using in patients with history of long QT syndrome or in patients with predisposing factors increasing the risk of QT abnormalities (eg, concurrent medications such as antiarrhythmics, hypokalemia, unstable heart failure, unstable atrial fibrillation). Potential for abuse **[U.S. Boxed Warning]**; healthcare providers should be alert to problems of abuse, misuse, and diversion. Risk of opioid abuse is increased in patients with a history or family history of alcohol or drug abuse or mental illness. Buprenorphine transdermal patches should only be prescribed by healthcare professionals familiar with the use of potent opioids for chronic pain. Proper storage, handling, and disposal of used patches is essential to prevent accidental exposure and potentially fatal overdose, especially in children **[U.S. Boxed Warning]**; to properly dispose of Butrans® patch, fold it over on itself and flush down the toilet; alternatively, seal the used patch in the provided Patch-Disposal Unit and dispose of in the trash. Misuse of the patch by chewing, snorting, or injecting the contents within the transdermal patch may result in uncontrolled delivery of buprenorphine may result in overdose; fatalities have been reported. Avoid exposure of application site and surrounding area to direct external heat sources. Buprenorphine release from the patch is temperature-dependent and may result in overdose. Patients who experience fever or increase in core temperature should be monitored closely. Application site reactions, including rare cases of severe reactions (eg, vesicles, discharge, "burns"), have been observed with use; onset varies from days to months after initiation; patients should be instructed to report severe reactions promptly.

Precautions Use with extreme caution in patients with head injury or increased intracranial pressure; exaggerated elevation of ICP may occur. Avoid use of buprenorphine in patients with CNS depression or coma as these patients are susceptible to intracranial effects of CO_2 retention. Use with caution in patients with hepatic insufficiency or severe renal impairment; dosage adjustments may be needed. Parenteral use may cause hypotension; use with caution in patients with hypovolemia, cardiovascular disease (including acute MI), or drugs which may exaggerate hypotensive effects (including phenothiazines or general anesthetics). Use with caution in patients with biliary tract disease or pancreatitis; may cause spasm of the sphincter of Oddi. Use with caution in patients with seizure disorders; may induce or aggravate seizures. May obscure diagnosis or clinical course of patients with acute abdominal conditions. Caution is also advised when used in patients with toxic psychosis, hypothyroidism, Addison's disease, urethral stricture, prostatic hypertrophy; acute alcoholism, delirium tremens, or kyphoscoliosis.

Adverse Reactions

Injection:

Cardiovascular: Hypotension

Central nervous system: Dizziness/vertigo, headache, sedation

Gastrointestinal: Nausea, vomiting

Ocular: Miosis

Respiratory: Respiratory depression

Miscellaneous: Diaphoresis

Rare but important or life-threatening: Amblyopia, anaphylactic shock, apnea, bradycardia, conjunctivitis, coma, cyanosis, depersonalization, depression, diplopia, euphoria, hallucinations, hypersensitivity reactions, hypertension, injection site reaction, psychosis, seizures, slurred speech, tachycardia, urinary retention, Wenckebach block

Tablet:
Central nervous system: Anxiety, chills, depression, dizziness, fever, headache, insomnia, nervousness, pain, somnolence
Gastrointestinal: Abdominal pain, constipation, diarrhea, dyspepsia, nausea, vomiting
Local: Abscess formation
Neuromuscular & skeletal: Back pain, weakness
Ocular: Lacrimation
Respiratory: Cough, pharyngitis, rhinitis
Miscellaneous: Diaphoresis, flu-like syndrome, infection, withdrawal syndrome
Rare but important or life-threatening: Anaphylactic shock, angioedema, hepatic encephalopathy, hepatic failure, hepatic necrosis, hepatitis (including cytolytic), hepatorenal syndrome, hypersensitivity reactions, transaminases increased

Transdermal patch:
Cardiovascular: Chest pain, hypertension, peripheral edema
Central nervous system: Anxiety, depression, dizziness, fatigue, fever, headache, hypoesthesia, insomnia, migraine, somnolence
Dermatologic: Hyperhydrosis, pruritus, rash
Gastrointestinal: Abdominal discomfort, anorexia, constipation, diarrhea, dyspepsia, nausea, upper abdominal pain, vomiting, xerostomia
Genitourinary: Urinary tract infection
Local: Application site erythema, application site irritation, application site pruritus, application site rash
Neuromuscular & skeletal: Arthralgia, back pain, joint swelling, muscle spasms, musculoskeletal pain, myalgia, neck pain, pain in extremity, paresthesia, tremor, weakness
Respiratory: Bronchitis, cough, dyspnea, nasopharyngitis, pharyngolaryngeal pain, sinusitis, upper respiratory tract infection
Miscellaneous: Flu-like syndrome
Rare but important or life-threatening: ALT increased, angina, angioedema, application site dermatitis, asthma exacerbation, bradycardia, contact dermatitis, diverticulitis, hallucinations, hyper/hypoventilation, hypersensitivity reactions, hypotension, ileus, loss of consciousness, memory impairment, mental impairment, mental status changes, miosis (dose-related), orthostatic hypotension, psychoses, respiratory depression, respiratory distress, respiratory failure, syncope, tachycardia, urinary incontinence, urinary retention, vasodilatation, visual disturbances, withdrawal syndrome

Drug Interactions
Metabolism/Transport Effects Substrate of CYP3A4 (major); **Note:** Assignment of Major/Minor substrate status based on clinically relevant drug interaction potential; **Inhibits** CYP1A2 (weak), CYP2A6 (weak), CYP2C19 (weak), CYP2D6 (weak)

Avoid Concomitant Use
Avoid concomitant use of Buprenorphine with any of the following: Atazanavir; Azelastine (Nasal); Conivaptan; Fusidic Acid (Systemic); MAO Inhibitors; Paraldehyde; Thalidomide

Increased Effect/Toxicity
Buprenorphine may increase the levels/effects of: Alvimopan; Azelastine (Nasal); Desmopressin; Diuretics; Hydrocodone; MAO Inhibitors; Methotrimeprazine; Metyrosine; Paraldehyde; Pramipexole; ROPINIRole; Rotigotine; Selective Serotonin Reuptake Inhibitors; Thalidomide; Zolpidem

The levels/effects of Buprenorphine may be increased by: Alcohol (Ethyl); Amphetamines; Anticholinergic Agents; Atazanavir; Boceprevir; Brimonidine (Topical); Cannabis; Ceritinib; CNS Depressants; Conivaptan; CYP3A4 Inhibitors (Moderate); CYP3A4 Inhibitors (Strong); Dasatinib; Dronabinol; Droperidol; Fusidic Acid (Systemic); Ivacaftor; Kava Kava; Luliconazole; Magnesium Sulfate; Methotrimeprazine; Mifepristone; Nabilone; Perampanel; Rufinamide; Simeprevir; Sodium Oxybate; Stiripentol; Succinylcholine; Tapentadol; Tetrahydrocannabinol

Decreased Effect
Buprenorphine may decrease the levels/effects of: Atazanavir; Pegvisomant

The levels/effects of Buprenorphine may be decreased by: Ammonium Chloride; Boceprevir; Bosentan; CYP3A4 Inducers (Strong); Dabrafenib; Deferasirox; Efavirenz; Etravirine; Mitotane; Naltrexone; Siltuximab; St Johns Wort; Tocilizumab

Stability
Injection: Protect from exposure to excessive heat of >40°C (>104°F) or prolonged exposure to light.
Sublingual tablet: Store at 25°C (77°F); excursions permitted to 15°C to 30°C (59°F to 86°F).
Transdermal patch: Store at 25°C (77°F); excursions permitted to 15°C to 30°C (59°F to 86°F).

Mechanism of Action Buprenorphine exerts its analgesic effect via high affinity binding to μ opiate receptors in the CNS; displays partial mu agonist and weak kappa antagonist activity

Pharmacodynamics I.M.:
Onset of action: 15 minutes
Maximum effect: 1 hour
Duration: ≥6 hours

Pharmacokinetics (Adult data unless noted)
Absorption: I.M., SubQ: 30% to 40%
Distribution: CSF concentrations are ~15% to 25% of plasma concentrations
V_d:
Premature neonates (GA: 27-32 weeks): 6.2 ± 2.1 L/kg (Barrett, 1993)
Children 4-7 years: 3.2 ± 2 L/kg (Olkkola, 1989)
Adults: 430 L
Protein binding: 96%, primarily to alpha and beta globulin
Metabolism: Hepatic, via both N-dealkylation (to an active metabolite, norbuprenorphine) and glucuronidation; norbuprenorphine also undergoes glucuronidation; extensive first-pass effect
Bioavailability: Relative to I.V. administration:
I.M.: 70%
Sublingual tablet: 29%
Transdermal patch: 15%
Half-life:
I.V.:
Premature neonates (GA: 27-32 weeks): 20 ± 8 hours (Barrett, 1993)
Children 4-7 years: ~1 hour (Olkkola, 1989)
Adults: 2.2 hours
Sublingual: 37 hours
Transdermal patch (apparent half-life): ~26 hours
Time to peak serum concentration:
Sublingual: 30 minutes to 1 hour (Kuhlman, 1996)
Transdermal patch: Steady state achieved by day 3
Elimination: 30% of the dose is excreted in the urine (1% as unchanged drug; 9.4% as conjugated drug; 2.7% as norbuprenorphine; and 11% as conjugated norbuprenorphine) and 69% in feces (33% as unchanged drug; 5% as conjugated drug; 21% as norbuprenorphine; and 2% as conjugated norbuprenorphine)
Clearance: Related to hepatic blood flow
Premature neonates (GA: 27-32 weeks): 0.23 ± 0.07 L/hour/kg (Barrett, 1993)

Children 4-7 years: 3.6 ± 1.1 L/hour/kg (Olkkola, 1989)
Adults: 0.78-1.32 L/hour/kg

Dosing: Neonatal Neonatal abstinence syndrome (NAS):
Very limited data available: Full-term neonates: Sublingual solution (0.075 mg/mL): Initial: 5.3 mcg/kg/dose every 8 hours; dosing based on birth weight; may increase dose in 25% increments based on targeted NAS scores; a rescue dose of 50% of the previous dose may be used for inadequate control between scheduled doses; once a maximum daily dose of 60 mcg/kg/day reached, pheno-barbital therapy may be added. After 3 days of dose stabilization, buprenorphine may be weaned based on NAS scores using 10% daily dose reductions. Dosing based on an open-label comparative trial with morphine (each treatment group, n= 12); in the clinical trial, doses were increased if a single NAS score was ≥12 or NAS scale scores ≥24 total on three measures; neonates with maternal concomitant benzodiazepine or chronic alcohol abuse were excluded from the trial; results showed a significant decrease in length of NAS treatment and hos-pital stay compared to morphine treatment arm (Kraft, 2011). In the pilot trial, a lower initial dose of sublingual buprenorphine (4.4 mcg/kg/dose every 8 hours) was used; clinically the majority of patients had NAS symptoms controlled; no differences in outcome variables (length of treatment and hospital) were detected and pharmacoki-netic analysis showed >98% of serum concentrations were less than the target concentration needed to control absti-nence symptoms in adults (Kraft, 2008).

Dosing: Usual Note: Dose should be titrated to appro-priate effect.
Use 1/2 of the dose listed in patients with preexisting respiratory depression, decreased respiratory reserve, hypoxia, hypercapnia, significant COPD, or cor pulmonale, and in those receiving medications with CNS or respiratory depressant effects.

Children and Adolescents:

Moderate to severe pain:

Children 2-12 years: I.M., slow I.V. injection: 2-6 **mcg**/kg every 4-6 hours; **Note:** 3 mcg/kg/dose has been most commonly studied; not all children have faster clear-ance rates than adults; some children may require dosing intervals of every 6-8 hours; observe clinical effects to establish the proper dosing interval

Adolescents: I.M., slow I.V. injection: Initial: Opioid-naive: 0.3 mg every 6-8 hours as needed; initial dose may be repeated once in 30-60 minutes if clinically needed

Opioid dependence: Note: Do not start induction with buprenorphine until objective and clear signs of with-drawal are apparent (otherwise withdrawal may be precipitated). Adolescents ≥16 years: Sublingual:

Induction: Target range: 12-16 mg/day (doses during one induction study used 8 mg on day 1, followed by 16 mg on day 2; other studies accomplished induction over 3-4 days). Treatment should begin at least 4 hours after last use of heroin or short-acting opioid, preferably when first signs of withdrawal appear. Titrat-ing dose to clinical effect should be done as rapidly as possible to prevent undue withdrawal symptoms and patient drop-out during the induction period. There is little controlled experience with induction in patients on methadone or other long-acting opioids; consult expert physician experienced with this procedure.

Maintenance: **Note:** Patients should be switched to the buprenorphine/naloxone combination product for maintenance and for unsupervised therapy; initial target dose: 12-16 mg/day; then adjust dose in 2-4 mg increments/decrements to a dose that adequately suppresses opioid withdrawal; usual range: 4-24 mg/day

Adults:

Moderate to severe pain: I.M., slow I.V. injection: Initial: Opioid-naive: 0.3 mg every 6-8 hours as needed; initial

dose may be repeated once in 30-60 minutes if clinically needed; **Note:** In adults, single doses of up to 0.6 mg administered I.M. may occasionally be required; usual dosage range: 0.15-0.6 mg every 4-8 hours as needed

Opioid dependence: Note: Do not start induction with buprenorphine until objective and clear signs of with-drawal are apparent (otherwise withdrawal may be precipitated). Sublingual:

Induction: Target range: 12-16 mg/day (doses during one induction study used 8 mg on day 1, followed by 16 mg on day 2; other studies accomplished induction over 3-4 days). Treatment should begin at least 4 hours after last use of heroin or short-acting opioid, preferably when first signs of withdrawal appear. Titrat-ing dose to clinical effect should be done as rapidly as possible to prevent undue withdrawal symptoms and patient drop-out during the induction period. There is little controlled experience with induction in patients on methadone or other long-acting opioids; consult expert physician experienced with this procedure.

Maintenance: **Note:** Patients should be switched to the buprenorphine/naloxone combination product for maintenance and for unsupervised therapy; initial target dose: 12-16 mg/day; then adjust dose in 2-4 mg increments/decrements to a dose that adequately suppresses opioid withdrawal; usual range: 4-24 mg/day

Chronic pain (moderate to severe):

Transdermal patch:

Opioid-naive patients: Initial: 5 **mcg**/hour applied once every 7 days

Opioid-experienced patients (conversion from other opioids to buprenorphine): Taper the current around-the-clock opioid for up to 7 days to ≤30 mg/day of oral morphine or equivalent before initiating therapy. Short-acting analgesics as needed may be continued until analgesia with transdermal buprenorphine is attained. There is a potential for buprenorphine to precipitate withdrawal in patients already receiving opioids.

Patients who were receiving daily dose of <30 mg of oral morphine equivalents: Initial: 5 **mcg**/hour applied once every 7 days

Patients who were receiving daily dose of 30-80 mg of oral morphine equivalents: Initial: 10 **mcg**/hour applied once every 7 days

Patient who were receiving daily dose of >80 mg of oral morphine equivalents: Buprenorphine trans-dermal patch, even at the maximum dose of 20 **mcg**/hour applied once every 7 days, may **not** provide adequate analgesia; **consider the use of an alternate analgesic.**

Dose titration (opioid-naive or opioid-experienced patients): May increase dose, based on patient's supplemental short-acting analgesic requirements, with a minimum titration interval of 72 hours. Max-imum dose: 20 **mcg**/hour applied once every 7 days; risk for QT_c prolongation increases with doses ≥20 **mcg**/hour patch

Discontinuation of therapy: Taper dose gradually every 7 days to prevent withdrawal; consider initiat-ing immediate-release opioids, if needed.

Dosing adjustment in renal impairment:
There are no dosage adjustments provided in manufacturer's labeling (has not been studied).

Dosing adjustment in hepatic impairment:
Injection, sublingual tablet: Children, Adolescents, and Adults: Use caution due to extensive hepatic metabo-lism; dosage adjustments recommended although no specific recommendations are provided by the manu-facturer.

Transdermal patch: Adults:

Mild to moderate impairment: Initial: No dosage adjustment needed; peak plasma levels (C_{max}) and exposure (AUC) were not increased in patients with mild to moderate hepatic impairment following intravenous administration.

Severe impairment: Not studied; consider alternative therapy with more flexibility for dosing adjustments.

Administration

Oral:

Sublingual solution: In neonates, place dose under tongue; insert pacifier to help reduce swallowing of dose (Kraft, 2008; Kraft, 2011)

Sublingual tablet: Place tablet under the tongue until dissolved; do not swallow. If 2 or more tablets are needed per dose, all tablets may be placed under the tongue at once, or 2 tablets may be placed under the tongue at a time; to ensure consistent bioavailability, subsequent doses should always be taken the same way.

Parenteral:

I.M.: Administer via deep I.M. injection

I.V.: Administer slowly, over at least 2 minutes

Topical: Transdermal patch: Apply patch to intact, non-irritated skin only. Apply to a hairless or nearly hairless skin site. If hairless site is not available, do not shave skin (as absorption from patch can be increased); hair at application site should be clipped. Prior to application, if the site must be cleaned, clean with clear water and allow to dry completely; do not use soaps, alcohol, lotions, or abrasives due to potential for increased skin absorption. Do not use any patch that has been damaged, cut, or manipulated in any way. Remove patch from protective pouch immediately before application. Remove the protective backing, and apply the sticky side of the patch to one of eight possible application sites (upper outer arm, upper chest, upper back, or the side of the chest [each site on either side of the body]). Firmly press patch in place and hold for ~10 seconds. Change patch every 7 days. Rotate patch application sites; wait ≥21 days before reapplying another patch to the same skin site. Avoid exposing application site to external heat sources (eg, heating pad, electric blanket, heat lamp, hot tub). If there is difficulty with patch adhesion, the edges of the system may be taped in place with first-aid tape. If the patch falls off during the 7-day dosing interval, dispose of the patch and apply a new patch to a different skin site. To properly dispose of Butrans® patch, fold it over on itself and flush down the toilet; alternatively, seal the used patch in the provided Patch-Disposal Unit and dispose of in the trash.

Monitoring Parameters Pain relief, respiratory rate, mental status, blood pressure; liver enzymes (baseline and periodic), symptoms of withdrawal, CNS depression, application site reactions (transdermal patch)

Additional Information Equianalgesic doses (parenteral): Buprenorphine 0.3 mg = morphine 10 mg; buprenorphine has a longer duration of action than morphine

Symptoms of overdose include CNS and respiratory depression, pinpoint pupils, hypotension, and bradycardia; treatment is supportive; naloxone may have limited effects in reversing respiratory depression; doxapram has also been used as a respiratory stimulant.

Controlled Substance C-III

Dosage Forms Excipient information presented when available (limited, particularly for generics); consult specific product labeling.

Patch Weekly, Transdermal:

Butrans: 5 mcg/hr (4 ea); 10 mcg/hr (4 ea); 15 mcg/hr (4 ea); 20 mcg/hr (4 ea)

Solution, Injection:

Buprenex: 0.3 mg/mL (1 mL)

Generic: 0.3 mg/mL (1 mL)

Tablet Sublingual, Sublingual:

Generic: 2 mg, 8 mg

Extemporaneous Preparations A 0.075 mg/mL solution can be made using the 0.3 mg/mL injection, 95% ethanol, and simple syrup. Add 1.26 mL of 95% ethanol to 0.3 mg buprenorphine obtained from an 0.3 mg/1 mL ampule, mix well, and add quantity of simple syrup sufficient to obtain 4 mL (final volume). Solution is stable under refrigeration and at room temperature for 30 days when stored in amber glass bottles and for 7 days when stored in oral syringes (Anagnostis, 2011; Anagnostis, 2013).

Anagnostis EA, Sadaka RE, Sailor LA, et al, "Formulation of Buprenorphine for Sublingual Use in Neonates," *J Pediatr Pharmacol Ther*, 2011, 16(4):281-4.

Anagnostis EA, personal communication, March 2013.

References

ACOG Committee on Health Care for Underserved Women and American Society of Addiction Medicine, "ACOG Committee Opinion No. 524: Opioid Abuse, Dependence, and Addiction in Pregnancy," *Obstet Gynecol*, 2012, 119(5):1070-6.

Barrett DA, Simpson J, Rutter N, et al, "The Pharmacokinetics and Physiological Effects of Buprenorphine Infusion in Premature Neonates," *Br J Clin Pharmacol*, 1993, 36(3):215-9.

Center for Substance Abuse Treatment (CSAT), *Clinical Guidelines for the Use of Buprenorphine in the Treatment of Opioid Addiction*, Treatment Improvement Protocol (TIP) Series 40. DHHS Publication No. (SMA) 04-3939. Rockville, MD: Substance Abuse and Mental Health Services Administration, 2004

Chou R, Fanciullo GJ, Fine PG, et al, "Clinical Guidelines For the Use of Chronic Opioid Therapy in Chronic Noncancer Pain," *J Pain*, 2009, 10 (2):113-30.

Dow K, Ordean A, Murphy-Oikonen J, et al, "Neonatal Abstinence Syndrome Clinical Practice Guidelines For Ontario," *J Popul Ther Clin Pharmacol*, 2012, 19(3):e488-506.

Hamunen K, Olkkola KT, and Maunuksela EL, "Comparison of the Ventilatory Effects of Morphine and Buprenorphine in Children," *Acta Anaesthesiol Scand*, 1993, 37(5):449-53.

Kraft WK, Dysart K, Greenspan JS, et al, "Revised Dose Schema of Sublingual Buprenorphine in the Treatment of the Neonatal Opioid Abstinence Syndrome," *Addiction*, 2011, 106(3):574-80.

Kraft WK, Gibson E, Dysart K, et al, "Sublingual Buprenorphine for Treatment of Neonatal Abstinence Syndrome: A Randomized Trial," *Pediatrics*, 2008, 122(3):e601-7.

Kuhlman JJ Jr, Lalani S, Magliulo J Jr, et al, "Human Pharmacokinetics of Intravenous, Sublingual, and Buccal Buprenorphine," *J Anal Toxicol*, 1996, 20(6):369-78.

Maunuksela EL, Korpela R, and Olkkola KT, "Comparison of Buprenorphine With Morphine in the Treatment of Postoperative Pain in Children," *Anesth Analg*, 1988, 67(3):233-9.

Maunuksela EL, Korpela R, and Olkkola KT, "Double-Blind, Multiple-Dose Comparison of Buprenorphine and Morphine in Postoperative Pain of Children," *Br J Anaesth*, 1988, 60(1):48-55.

Montgomery A, Hale TW, and Academy Of Breastfeeding Medicine, "ABM Cinical Protocol #15: Analgesia and Anesthesia For the Breastfeeding Mother, Revised 2012," *Breastfeed Med*, 2012, 7(6):547-53.

Olkkola KT, Leijala MA, and Maunuksela EL, "Paediatric Ventilatory Effects of Morphine and Buprenorphine Revisited," *Paediatr Anaesth*, 1995, 5(5):303-5.

Olkkola KT, Maunuksela EL, and Korpela R, "Pharmacokinetics of Intravenous Buprenorphine in Children," *Br J Clin Pharmacol*, 1989, 28(2):202-4.

Soyka M, "Buprenorphine Use in Pregnant Opioid Users: A Critical Review," *CNS Drugs*, 2013, 27(8):653-62.

US Department of Health and Human Services, Substance Abuse and Mental Health Services Administration, and Center for Substance Abuse Treatment (CSAT), "Clinical Guidelines for the Use of Buprenorphine in the Treatment of Opioid Addiction," 2005. Available at http://kap.samhsa.gov/products/tools/keys/pdfs/KK_40.pdf

Welsh CJ, Suman M, Cohen A, et al, "The Use of Intravenous Buprenorphine for the Treatment of Opioid Withdrawal in Medically Ill Hospitalized Patients," *Am J Addict*, 2002, 11(2): 135-40.

Buprenorphine and Naloxone

(byoo pre NOR feen & nal OKS one)

Medication Safety Issues

High alert medication:

The Institute for Safe Medication Practices (ISMP) includes this medication among its list of drug classes

which have a heightened risk of causing significant patient harm when used in error.

Other safety concerns:

Potential for over- or underdosing when switching among various formulations and between strengths of the sublingual films: **Not all strengths of sublingual tablets and films are bioequivalent to one another.** In addition, systemic exposure between the various strengths of sublingual films may be different; pharmacists should not substitute one or more film strengths for another (eg, dispense three 4 mg films for one 12 mg film, or vice-versa) without physician approval. Any patient switching between sublingual tablet and sublingual film formulation or between one or more strengths of the sublingual films should be monitored for over- or underdosing.

Brand Names: U.S. Suboxone; Zubsolv

Brand Names: Canada Suboxone

Therapeutic Category Analgesic, Narcotic; Opioid Partial Agonist

Generic Availability (U.S.) Yes: Sublingual tablet

Use Maintenance treatment of opioid dependence as part of a complete plan that includes counseling and psychosocial support (Sublingual tablet: FDA approved in ages ≥16 years and adults; Sublingual film: FDA approved in adults)

Prescribing and Access Restrictions Prescribing of tablets for opioid dependence is limited to physicians who have met the qualification criteria and have received a DEA number specific to prescribing this product. Tablets will be available through pharmacies and wholesalers which normally provide controlled substances.

Medication Guide Available Yes

Pregnancy Risk Factor C

Pregnancy Considerations Adverse effects have been observed in some animal reproduction studies. See individual agents.

Breast-Feeding Considerations Buprenorphine and its active metabolite, norbuprenorphine, are excreted in breast milk. It is not known if naloxone is excreted into breast milk, however, systemic absorption following oral administration is low (Smith, 2012) and any exposure of naloxone to a nursing infant would therefore be limited.

In general, breast-feeding is not recommended by the manufacturers of buprenorphine-containing products; the manufacturer of Zubsolv buprenorphine and naloxone sublingual tablets recommends that caution be exercised when administering this specific combination product to nursing women. See individual agents.

Contraindications Hypersensitivity to buprenorphine, naloxone, or any component

Warnings Buprenorphine may cause CNS depression which may impair physical or mental abilities; patients must be cautioned about performing tasks which require mental alertness (eg, operating machinery or driving); use caution when combining with other CNS depressants (eg, centrally acting antiemetics, general anesthetics, phenothiazines, sedative-hypnotics) due to additive CNS effects. If combination therapy is needed, consider dosage reduction of one or both agents.

Respiratory depression may occur; use with extreme caution in patients with respiratory diseases including asthma, emphysema, COPD, cor pulmonale, hypoxia, hypercapnia, preexisting respiratory depression, significantly decreased respiratory reserve, other obstructive pulmonary disease, kyphoscoliosis, or other skeletal disorder which may alter respiratory function. Patients who are cachectic or debilitated may be at higher risk for respiratory depression; monitor closely. Naloxone may be used in the management of respiratory depression, but higher doses and repeated administration may be

necessary; mechanical ventilation may be required. Coma and death resulting from respiratory depression have been reported; many reports are associated with misuse by self-injection in combination with benzodiazepines and other CNS depressants including alcohol.

May increase ICP; use with extreme caution in patients with head injury, intracranial lesions, or elevated intracranial pressure. May cause hypotension; use with caution in patients with circulatory shock, hypovolemia, impaired myocardial function, or those receiving drugs which may exaggerate hypotensive effects (including phenothiazines or general anesthetics). Buprenorphine may obscure diagnosis or clinical course of patients with acute abdominal conditions.

Physical and psychological dependence may occur; abrupt discontinuation after prolonged use may result in withdrawal symptoms; compared to full-opioid agonists, withdrawal from buprenorphine may be milder and may be delayed in onset; opioid antagonist activity of buprenorphine may precipitate acute opioid withdrawal in opioid-dependent individuals. Naloxone may precipitate intense withdrawal symptoms in patients addicted to opioids when administered before the opioid effects have subsided, or if misused parenterally in opioid-dependent individuals. Infants born to women physically dependent on opioids, including buprenorphine, will also be physically dependent and may experience respiratory difficulties or opioid withdrawal symptoms [neonatal abstinence syndrome (NAS)]. Onset, duration, and severity of NAS depend upon the drug used (maternal), duration of use, maternal dose, and rate of drug elimination by the newborn. Symptoms of newborn opioid withdrawal may include excessive crying, diarrhea, fever, hyper-reflexia, irritability, tremors, vomiting, or failure to gain weight. Opioid withdrawal syndrome in the neonate, unlike in adults, may be life-threatening and should be promptly treated. Onset of symptoms ranged from day 1 to day 8 of life, most occurring on day 1 of life in infants of women receiving buprenorphine sublingual tablets during pregnancy; rare cases of convulsions (with one case of apnea and bradycardia) have also been reported.

High potential for abuse; healthcare providers should be alert to problems of abuse, misuse, and diversion. Oral buprenorphine is not approved for management of pain; deaths have been reported in opioid-naive patients receiving oral buprenorphine for analgesia.

Hepatitis and other hepatic events have been reported in patients receiving buprenorphine for the treatment of opioid dependence; infection with viral hepatitis, concomitant use of potentially hepatotoxic drugs, preexisting liver enzyme abnormalities, and ongoing drug use may have contributed to liver abnormalities. Monitor liver function tests in all patients prior to and during therapy. Hypersensitivity reactions, including bronchospasm, angioneurotic edema, and anaphylactic shock have also been reported.

Use caution when changing between tablet and sublingual film; potential for greater bioavailability with certain sublingual film strengths compared to the same strength of the sublingual tablet strength exists; monitor closely for either over- or underdosing when switching patients from one formulation to another. Size and compositions of the various strengths of sublingual films are different; various combinations of these strengths may result in different systemic exposure; pharmacists should not substitute one or more film strengths for another (eg, three 4 mg films compared to one 12 mg film, or vice-versa) without physician approval; patients should be monitored for over- or underdosing when various film strengths are switched. **Keep out of the reach of children and discard any open units**

properly; contains an amount of medication that can be fatal to children.

Precautions Use with caution in patients with hepatic insufficiency or severe renal impairment; dosage adjustments may be needed. Use with caution in patients with biliary tract disease or pancreatitis; may cause spasm of the sphincter of Oddi. Use with caution in patients with seizure disorders; may induce or aggravate seizures. Caution is also advised when used in patients with coma, toxic psychosis, hypothyroidism, Addison's disease, urethral stricture, prostatic hypertrophy, acute alcoholism, and delirium tremens.

Adverse Reactions Also see individual agents.

Cardiovascular: Vasodilation

Central nervous system: Headache, pain

Gastrointestinal: Abdominal pain, constipation, erythema (oral mucosa; film), glossodynia (film), oral hypoesthesia (film), nausea, vomiting

Miscellaneous: Diaphoresis, withdrawal syndrome

Drug Interactions

Metabolism/Transport Effects Refer to individual components.

Avoid Concomitant Use

Avoid concomitant use of Buprenorphine and Naloxone with any of the following: Atazanavir; Azelastine (Nasal); Conivaptan; Fusidic Acid (Systemic); MAO Inhibitors; Paraldehyde; Thalidomide

Increased Effect/Toxicity

Buprenorphine and Naloxone may increase the levels/ effects of: Alvimopan; Azelastine (Nasal); Desmopressin; Diuretics; Hydrocodone; MAO Inhibitors; Methotrimeprazine; Metyrosine; Paraldehyde; Pramipexole; ROPINIRole; Rotigotine; Selective Serotonin Reuptake Inhibitors; Thalidomide; Zolpidem

The levels/effects of Buprenorphine and Naloxone may be increased by: Alcohol (Ethyl); Amphetamines; Anticholinergic Agents; Atazanavir; Boceprevir; Brimonidine (Topical); Cannabis; Ceritinib; CNS Depressants; Conivaptan; CYP3A4 Inhibitors (Moderate); CYP3A4 Inhibitors (Strong); Dasatinib; Dronabinol; Droperidol; Fusidic Acid (Systemic); Ivacaftor; Kava Kava; Luliconazole; Magnesium Sulfate; Methotrimeprazine; Mifepristone; Nabilone; Perampanel; Rufinamide; Simeprevir; Sodium Oxybate; Stiripentol; Succinylcholine; Tapentadol; Tetrahydrocannabinol

Decreased Effect

Buprenorphine and Naloxone may decrease the levels/ effects of: Atazanavir; Pegvisomant

The levels/effects of Buprenorphine and Naloxone may be decreased by: Ammonium Chloride; Boceprevir; Bosentan; CYP3A4 Inducers (Strong); Dabrafenib; Deferasirox; Efavirenz; Etravirine; Mitotane; Naltrexone; Siltuximab; St Johns Wort; Tocilizumab

Stability Store at 25°C (77°F); excursions permitted to 15°C to 30°C (59°F to 86°F).

Mechanism of Action See individual agents.

Pharmacodynamics Maximum effect: Buprenorphine: 100 minutes; Naloxone: No clinically significant effect when administered sublingually

Pharmacokinetics (Adult data unless noted) Also see individual agents.

Absorption: High variability among patients, but low variability within each individual patient.

Protein binding: Buprenorphine: ~96%; Naloxone: ~45%

Bioavailability: Potential for greater bioavailability with certain strengths of the sublingual film compared to the same strength of the sublingual tablet exists. Although pharmacokinetics were similar between the sublingual formulations, bioequivalence is variable. In addition, the sizes and compositions between the sublingual film

strengths are different which may result in different systemic exposures.

Half-life: Film: Buprenorphine: 24-42 hours; Naloxone: 2-12 hours

Dosing: Usual Note: Sublingual tablets and film contain a free-base ratio of buprenorphine:naloxone of 4:1. Doses based on buprenorphine content; titrate to appropriate effect.

Opioid dependence, maintenance treatment: Sublingual: Adolescents ≥16 years (sublingual tablets) and Adults (sublingual film or sublingual tablets):

Manufacturer's labeling:

Induction: Not recommended; initial treatment should begin using buprenorphine sublingual tablets (see Buprenorphine monograph)

Maintenance: Target dose: 16 mg/day as a single daily dose; dosage should be adjusted in increments of 2 mg or 4 mg to a dose that adequately suppresses opioid withdrawal; usual range: 4-24 mg/day; **Note:** Combination product for maintenance and for unsupervised therapy (if patient's clinical stability permits)

Alternate dosing [Center for Substance Abuse Treatment Guidelines (CSAT), 2004]:

Induction (for patients dependent on **short-acting** opioids and whose last dose of opioids was >12-24 hours prior to induction):

Day 1: Initial: 4 mg; may repeat dose after >2 hours if withdrawal symptoms not relieved; Day 1 maximum daily dose: 8 mg/**day**

Day 2:

- If no withdrawal symptoms, repeat total daily dose from Day 1
- If withdrawal symptoms are present, increase Day 1 dose by 4 mg; if withdrawal symptoms not relieved after >2 hours, may administer an additional 4 mg; Day 2 maximum daily dose: 16 mg/**day**

Subsequent induction days:

- If withdrawal symptoms are not present, daily dose is established (stabilization dose).
- If withdrawal symptoms are present, increase dose in increments of 2 mg or 4 mg each day as needed for symptom relief. Target daily dose by the end of the first week: 12 mg or 16 mg/day; maximum daily dose: 32 mg/**day**

Stabilization: Usual dose: 16-24 mg/day; maximum dose: 32 mg/**day**

Switching between sublingual tablets and sublingual film: Same dosage should be used as the previous administered product. **Note:** Potential for greater bioavailability with the sublingual film compared to the sublingual tablet exists; monitor closely for either over- or underdosing when switching patients from one formulation to another.

Switching between different strengths of sublingual films: Systemic exposure may be different with various combinations of sublingual film strengths; pharmacists should not substitute one or more film strengths for another (eg, switching from three 4 mg films to a single 12 mg film, or vice-versa) without physician approval and patients should be monitored closely for either over- or underdosing when switching between film strengths.

Dosing adjustment in renal impairment: There are no dosage adjustments are provided in manufacturer's labeling.

Dosing adjustment in hepatic impairment: Moderate to severe impairment: Dosage adjustments recommended; however, no specific dosage adjustment recommendations provided by manufacturer; monitor patients closely.

Administration

Sublingual film: Film should be placed under the tongue. Keep under the tongue until film dissolves completely; film should not be chewed, swallowed, or moved after placement. If more than 1 film is needed, the additional film should be placed under the tongue on the opposite side from the first film to minimize overlapping as much as possible.

Sublingual tablets: Place tablet under the tongue until dissolved; do not swallow. If 2 or more tablets are needed per dose, all tablets may be placed under the tongue at once, or 2 tablets may be placed under the tongue at a time; to ensure consistent bioavailability, subsequent doses should always be taken the same way.

Monitoring Parameters Symptoms of withdrawal, respiratory rate, mental status, blood pressure; liver function tests (baseline and periodically during therapy)

Additional Information Naloxone has been added to the formulation to decrease the abuse potential of dissolving tablets or film in water and using as an injection (precipitation of severe withdrawal would occur in opioid dependent patients if the tablets or film were misused in this manner).

Product Availability Bunavail: FDA approved June 2014; anticipated availability in third quarter 2014.

Bunavail is a buccal film indicated for the maintenance treatment of opioid dependence, as part of a complete treatment plan (eg, counseling, psychosocial support).

Controlled Substance C-III

Dosage Forms Excipient information presented when available (limited, particularly for generics); consult specific product labeling.

Film, sublingual:

Suboxone: Buprenorphine 2 mg and naloxone 0.5 mg (30s); buprenorphine 4 mg and naloxone 1 mg (30s); buprenorphine 8 mg and naloxone 2 mg (30s); buprenorphine 12 mg and naloxone 3 mg (30s) [lime flavor]

Tablet, sublingual: Buprenorphine 2 mg and naloxone 0.5 mg; buprenorphine 8 mg and naloxone 2 mg

Zubsolv: Buprenorphine 1.4 mg and naloxone 0.36 mg; buprenorphine 5.7 mg and naloxone 1.4 mg [menthol flavor]

References

Center for Substance Abuse Treatment, "Clinical Guidelines for the Use of Buprenorphine in the Treatment of Opioid Addiction. Treatment Improvement Protocol (TIP) Series 40. DHHS Publication No. (SMA) 04-3939," Rockville, MD: Substance Abuse and Mental Health Services Administration, 2004.

Smith K, Hopp M, Mundin G, et al, "Low Absolute Bioavailability of Oral Naloxone in Healthy Subjects," *Int J Clin Pharmacol Ther*, 2012, 50 (5):360-7.

◆ **Buprenorphine Hydrochloride** see Buprenorphine on page 320

◆ **Buprenorphine Hydrochloride and Naloxone Hydrochloride Dihydrate** see Buprenorphine and Naloxone on page 324

◆ **Buproban** see BuPROPion on page 327

BuPROPion (byoo PROE pee on)

Medication Safety Issues

Sound-alike/look-alike issues:

Aplenzin may be confused with Albenza, Relenza

BuPROPion may be confused with busPIRone

Forfivo XL may be confused with Forteo

Wellbutrin XL may be confused with Wellbutrin SR

Zyban may be confused with Diovan

Related Information

Antidepressant Agents on page 2219

Oral Medications That Should Not Be Crushed or Altered on page 2438

Brand Names: U.S. Aplenzin; Budeprion SR [DSC]; Buproban; Forfivo XL; Wellbutrin; Wellbutrin SR; Wellbutrin XL; Zyban

Brand Names: Canada Ava-Bupropion SR; Bupropion SR; Mylan-Bupropion XL; Novo-Bupropion SR; PMS-Bupropion SR; ratio-Bupropion SR; Sandoz-Bupropion SR; Wellbutrin SR; Wellbutrin XL; Zyban

Therapeutic Category Antidepressant, Dopamine-Reuptake Inhibitor; Smoking Cessation Aid

Generic Availability (U.S.) Yes

Use Treatment of major depressive disorder (Aplenzin™, Forfivo™ XL, Wellbutrin®, Wellbutrin SR®, Wellbutrin XL®: FDA approved in adults), seasonal affective disorder (SAD) (Aplenzin™, Wellbutrin XL®: FDA approved in adults); adjunct in smoking cessation (Buproban®, Zyban®: FDA approved in adults); has also been used to treat ADHD

Medication Guide Available Yes

Pregnancy Risk Factor C

Pregnancy Considerations Adverse events have been observed in some animal reproduction studies. Bupropion and its metabolites were found to cross the placenta in *in vitro* studies (Earhart, 2012). An increased risk of congenital malformations has not been observed following maternal use of bupropion during pregnancy; however, data specific to cardiovascular malformations is inconsistent. The long-term effects on development and behavior have not been studied. The ACOG recommends that antidepressant therapy during pregnancy be individualized; treatment of depression during pregnancy should incorporate the clinical expertise of the mental health clinician, obstetrician, primary healthcare provider, and pediatrician. According to the American Psychiatric Association (APA), the risks of medication treatment should be weighed against other treatment options and untreated depression. For women who discontinue antidepressant medications during pregnancy and who may be at high risk for postpartum depression, the medications can be restarted following delivery. Treatment algorithms have been developed by the ACOG and the APA for the management of depression in women prior to conception and during pregnancy (ACOG, 2008; APA, 2010; Yonkers, 2009). There is insufficient information related to the use of bupropion to recommend use in pregnancy (ACOG, 2010).

Breast-Feeding Considerations Bupropion and its metabolites are excreted into breast milk. The estimated dose to a nursing infant varies by study and has been reported as ~2% of the weight-adjusted maternal dose (range: 1.4% to 10.6%) (Davis, 2009; Haas, 2004). Adverse events have been reported with some antidepressants and a seizure was noted in one 6-month old nursing infant exposed to bupropion (a causal effect could not be confirmed) (Chaudron, 2004; Hale, 2010). Recommendations for use in nursing women vary by manufacturer labeling.

Contraindications Hypersensitivity to bupropion or any component; seizure disorder; anorexia/bulimia; use of MAO inhibitors or MAO inhibitors intended to treat psychiatric disorders (concurrently or within 14 days of discontinuing either bupropion or the MAO inhibitor); initiation of bupropion in a patient receiving linezolid or intravenous methylene blue; patients undergoing abrupt discontinuation of ethanol or sedatives (including benzodiazepines); patients receiving other dosage forms of bupropion

Aplenzin™: Additional contraindications: Other conditions that increase seizure risk, including arteriovenous malformation, severe head injury, severe stroke, CNS tumor, or CNS infection or abrupt discontinuation of barbiturates or antiepileptics

Warnings Clinical worsening of depression or suicidal ideation and behavior may occur in children and adults with major depressive disorder **[U.S. Boxed Warning]**. In clinical trials, antidepressants increased the risk of suicidal thinking and behavior (suicidality) in children, adolescents, and young adults (18-24 years of age) with major depressive disorder and other psychiatric disorders. This risk must be considered before prescribing antidepressants for any clinical use. Short-term studies did **not** show an increased risk of suicidality with antidepressant use in patients >24 years of age and showed a decreased risk in patients ≥65 years.

Patients of all ages who are treated with antidepressants for any indication require appropriate monitoring and close observation for clinical worsening of depression, suicidality, and unusual changes in behavior, especially during the first few months after antidepressant initiation or when the dose is adjusted. Family members and caregivers should be instructed to closely observe the patient (ie, daily) and communicate condition with healthcare provider. Patients should also be monitored for associated behaviors (eg, anxiety, agitation, panic attacks, insomnia, irritability, hostility, aggressiveness, impulsivity, akathisia, hypomania, mania) which may increase the risk for worsening depression or suicidality. Worsening depression or emergence of suicidality (or associated behaviors listed above) that is abrupt in onset, severe, or not part of the presenting symptoms, may require discontinuation or modification of drug therapy.

Do not discontinue abruptly in patients receiving high doses chronically; withdrawal symptoms may occur (Dopheide, 2006). To reduce risk of intentional overdose, write prescriptions for the smallest quantity consistent with good patient care. May worsen psychosis in some patients or precipitate a shift to mania or hypomania in patients with bipolar disorder. Antidepressant monotherapy in patients with bipolar disorder should be avoided. Patients presenting with depressive symptoms should be screened for bipolar disorder. Bupropion is not FDA approved for the treatment of bipolar depression.

Serious neuropsychiatric events, including depression, suicidal thoughts, suicide attempt, and suicide, have been reported with use for smoking cessation **[U.S. Boxed Warning]**; neuropsychiatric symptoms including psychosis, hallucinations, paranoia, delusions, hostility, agitation, aggression, anxiety, panic, and homicidal ideation have also been reported; some cases may have been complicated by symptoms of nicotine withdrawal following smoking cessation. Smoking cessation (with or without treatment) is associated with nicotine withdrawal symptoms (including depression or agitation), or the exacerbation of underlying psychiatric illness; however, some of the behavioral disturbances reported occurred in treated patients who continued to smoke. These neuropsychiatric symptoms (eg, mood disturbances, psychosis, hostility) have occurred in patients with and without preexisting psychiatric disease; many cases resolved following therapy discontinuation although in some cases, symptoms persisted. Monitor all patients for behavioral changes and psychiatric symptoms (eg, agitation, depression, suicidal behavior, suicidal ideation); inform patients to discontinue treatment and contact their healthcare provider immediately if they experience any behavioral and/or mood changes.

The American Heart Association recommends that all children diagnosed with ADHD who may be candidates for medication, such as bupropion, should have a thorough cardiovascular assessment prior to initiation of therapy. These recommendations are based upon reports of serious cardiovascular adverse events (including sudden death) in patients (both children and adults) taking usual doses of stimulant medications. Most of these patients were found to have underlying structural heart disease (eg, hypertrophic obstructive cardiomyopathy). This assessment should include a combination of thorough medical history, family history, and physical examination. An ECG is not mandatory but should be considered.

Anaphylactoid/anaphylactic reactions have occurred, with symptoms of pruritus, urticaria, angioedema, and dyspnea. Serious reactions have been (rarely) reported, including Stevens-Johnson syndrome, erythema multiforme, and anaphylactic shock. Arthralgia, myalgia, and fever with rash and other symptoms suggestive of delayed hypersensitivity resembling serum sickness may occur.

Bupropion may cause a dose-related risk of seizures. Use is contraindicated in patients with a history of seizures or certain conditions with high-seizure risk (eg, arteriovenous malformation, severe head injury, CNS tumor, CNS infection, history of anorexia/bulimia, or patients undergoing abrupt discontinuation of ethanol, benzodiazepines, barbiturates, or antiepileptic drugs). Use caution with concurrent use of antipsychotics, antidepressants, theophylline, systemic corticosteroids, stimulants (including cocaine), anorectants, other medications that may lower seizure threshold, hypoglycemic agents, or with excessive use of ethanol, benzodiazepines, sedative/hypnotics, or opioids. Use with caution in seizure-potentiating metabolic disorders (eg, hypoglycemia, hyponatremia, severe hepatic impairment, and hypoxia). The dose-dependent risk of seizures may be reduced by gradual dose increases and limiting the daily dose to bupropion hydrochloride ≤450 mg or bupropion hydrobromide ≤522 mg in adults. Use of multiple bupropion formulations is contraindicated. Permanently discontinue if seizure occurs during therapy. Chewing, crushing, or dividing long-acting products may increase seizure risk.

Concurrent use of MOA inhibitors including reversible MAO inhibitors (eg, linezolid, methylene blue) is contraindicated; however, if urgent treatment with linezolid or I.V. methylene blue is required in a patient already receiving bupropion and potential benefits outweigh potential risks, discontinue bupropion promptly and administer linezolid or I.V. methylene blue. Monitor for increased risk of hypertensive reactions for 2 weeks or until 24 hours after the last dose of linezolid or I.V. methylene blue, whichever comes first. May resume bupropion 24 hours after the last dose of linezolid or I.V. methylene blue.

Bupropion is available as hydrochloride and hydrobromide (Aplenzin™) salt formulations which are not interchangeable due to differences in the amount of bupropion supplied. Budeprion SR® 100 mg tablets contain tartrazine which may cause allergic reactions in susceptible individuals.

Precautions May cause CNS stimulation (restlessness, anxiety, agitation, insomnia) or anorexia. Use in patients with depression may be associated with neuropsychiatric symptoms such as delusions, hallucinations, psychosis, confusion, paranoia, and concentrations disturbance. May increase the risks associated with electroconvulsive therapy (ECT). Consider discontinuing, when possible, prior to ECT. May cause weight loss; use caution in patients where weight loss is not desirable.

Use with caution in patients with cardiovascular disease, history of hypertension, recent MI, or coronary artery disease; treatment-emergent hypertension (including some severe cases) has been reported, both with bupropion alone and in combination with nicotine transdermal systems. Use with caution and decrease the dose and/or frequency in patients with hepatic or renal dysfunction. May cause motor or cognitive impairment in some patients, which may impair physical or mental abilities; patients must be cautioned about performing tasks which require mental alertness (eg, operating machinery or driving).

Extended release tablet: Insoluble tablet shell may remain intact and be visible in the stool.

Adverse Reactions

Cardiovascular: Cardiac arrhythmia, chest pain, flushing, hypertension, hypotension, palpitations, tachycardia

Central nervous system: Abnormal dreams, agitation, akathisia, anxiety, central nervous system stimulation, confusion, depression, dizziness, drowsiness, headache, hostility, insomnia, irritability, memory impairment, migraine, nervousness, pain, paresthesia, sensory disturbance, sleep disorder, twitching

Dermatologic: Diaphoresis, pruritus, skin rash, urticaria

Endocrine & metabolic: Decreased libido, hot flash, menstrual disease, weight gain, weight loss

Gastrointestinal: Abdominal pain, anorexia, increased appetite, constipation, diarrhea, dysgeusia, dyspepsia, dysphagia, flatulence, nausea, vomiting, xerostomia

Genitourinary: Urinary tract infection, urinary urgency, vaginal hemorrhage

Hypersensitivity: Hypersensitivity reaction (including anaphylaxis, pruritus, urticaria)

Infection: Infection

Neuromuscular & skeletal: Arthralgia, arthritis, myalgia, neck pain, tremor, weakness

Ophthalmic: Amblyopia, blurred vision

Otic: Auditory disturbance, tinnitus

Renal: Polyuria

Respiratory: Cough, pharyngitis, sinusitis, upper respiratory infection

Miscellaneous: Fever

Rare but important or life-threatening:Abnormal accommodation, akinesia, alopecia, amnesia, anaphylactic shock, anaphylactoid reaction, anemia, angioedema, aphasia, ataxia, atrioventricular block, cerebrovascular accident, colitis, coma, cystitis, deafness, delayed hypersensitivity, delirium, delusions, depersonalization, derealization, diplopia, dysarthria, dyskinesia, dyspareunia, dysphoria, dystonia, dysuria, edema, EEG pattern changes, erythema multiforme, esophagitis, euphoria, exfoliative dermatitis, extrapyramidal reaction, extrasystoles, facial edema, gastric ulcer, gastroesophageal reflux disease, gastrointestinal hemorrhage, gingival hemorrhage, glossitis, glycosuria, gynecomastia, hallucination, hepatic injury, hepatic insufficiency, hepatitis, hirsutism, hyperglycemia, hyperkinesia, hypertonia, hypoglycemia, hypokinesia, hypomania, impotence, increased intraocular pressure, increased libido, intestinal perforation, jaundice, leukocytosis, leukopenia, lymphadenopathy, manic behavior, myasthenia, mydriasis, myocardial infarction, myoclonus, neuralgia, neuropathy, orthostatic hypotension, painful erection, pancreatitis, pancytopenia, paranoia, pneumonia, psychiatric signs and symptoms, pulmonary embolism, rhabdomyolysis, salpingitis, sciatica, seizure (dose-related), SIADH, skin photosensitivity, Stevens-Johnson syndrome, stomatitis, suicidal ideation, syncope, tardive dyskinesia, thrombocytopenia, tongue edema, urinary incontinence, urinary retention, vasodilatation

Drug Interactions

Metabolism/Transport Effects Substrate of CYP1A2 (minor), CYP2A6 (minor), CYP2B6 (major), CYP2C9 (minor), CYP2D6 (minor), CYP2E1 (minor), CYP3A4 (minor); Note: Assignment of Major/Minor substrate status based on clinically relevant drug interaction potential; Inhibits CYP2D6 (strong)

Avoid Concomitant Use

Avoid concomitant use of BuPROPion with any of the following: MAO Inhibitors; Pimozide; Tamoxifen; Thioridazine

Increased Effect/Toxicity

BuPROPion may increase the levels/effects of: Alcohol (Ethyl); ARIPiprazole; AtoMOXetine; CYP2D6 Substrates; DOXOrubicin (Conventional); Fesoterodine; FLUoxetine; FluvoxaMINE; Iloperidone; Lorcaserin; Metoprolol; Nebivolol; PARoxetine; Pimozide; Propafenone; Tetrabenazine; Thioridazine; Tricyclic Antidepressants; Vortioxetine

The levels/effects of BuPROPion may be increased by: Alcohol (Ethyl); Anti-Parkinson's Agents (Dopamine Agonist); CYP2B6 Inhibitors (Moderate); CYP2B6 Inhibitors (Strong); MAO Inhibitors; Mifepristone; Quazepam

Decreased Effect

BuPROPion may decrease the levels/effects of: Codeine; Iloperidone; Ioflupane I 123; Tamoxifen; TraMADol

The levels/effects of BuPROPion may be decreased by: CYP2B6 Inducers (Strong); Dabrafenib; Efavirenz; Lopinavir; Peginterferon Alfa-2b; Ritonavir

Stability

Extended release tablets:

Aplenzin™, Wellbutrin XL®: Store at 25°C (77°F); excursions permitted to 15°C to 30°C (59°F to 86°F).

Forfivo™ XL: Store at 20°C to 25°C (68°F to 77°F).

Immediate release tablets: Store at 15°C to 25°C (59°F to 77°F). Protect from light and moisture.

Sustained release tablets: Wellbutrin SR®, Zyban®: Store at 20°C to 25°C (68°F to 77°F). Dispense in tight, light-resistant container.

Mechanism of Action

Aminoketone antidepressant structurally different from all other marketed antidepressants; like other antidepressants the mechanism of bupropion's activity is not fully understood. Bupropion is a relatively weak inhibitor of the neuronal uptake of norepinephrine and dopamine, and does not inhibit monoamine oxidase or the reuptake of serotonin. Metabolite inhibits the reuptake of norepinephrine. The primary mechanism of action is thought to be dopaminergic and/or noradrenergic.

Pharmacodynamics

Onset of action: 1-2 weeks

Maximum effect: 8-12 weeks

Duration: 1-2 days

Pharmacokinetics (Adult data unless noted)

Absorption: Rapid

Distribution: V_d: ~20-47 L/kg (Laizure, 1985)

Protein binding: 84%

Metabolism: Extensively hepatic via CYP2B6 to hydroxybupropion; non-CYP-mediated metabolism to erythrohydrobupropion and threohydrobupropion; these 3 metabolites are active. Preliminary studies suggest hydroxybupropion is 50% and erythrohydrobupropion and threohydrobupropion are 20% as active as parent drug. Bupropion also undergoes oxidation to form the glycine conjugate of meta-chlorobenzoic acid, the major urinary metabolite.

Half-life:

Distribution: 3-4 hours

Elimination: ~14 hours (range: 8-24 hours); Metabolites: Hydroxybupropion: 20 ± 5 hours; Erythrohydrobupropion: 33 ± 10 hours; Threohydrobupropion: 37 ± 13 hours

Extended release (Aplenzin™): 21 ± 7 hours; Metabolites: Hydroxybupropion: 24 ± 5 hours; Erythrohydrobupropion: 31 ± 8 hours; Threohydrobupropion: 51 ± 9 hours

Time to peak serum concentration: Bupropion: Immediate release: ~2 hours; sustained release: ~3 hours; extended release: ~5 hours [Forfivo™ XL: 5 hours (fasting); 12 hours (fed)]

Metabolites: Hydroxybupropion, erythrohydrobupropion, threohydrobupropion: ~7 hours

Elimination: Urine (87%); feces (10%); only 0.5% of the dose is excreted as unchanged drug

Dosing: Usual

Note: Bupropion is available as either hydrochloride or hydrobromide (Aplenzin™) salt formulations which are not interchangeable on a mg per mg basis; dosage expressed in terms of the salt formulation.

▶

Children and Adolescents:

Attention-deficit/hyperactivity disorder: Limited data available: Children and Adolescents: Oral:

Immediate release, hydrochloride salts: Initial: 3 mg/kg/**day** in 2-3 divided doses; maximum initial dose: 150 mg/**day**; titrate dose as needed to a maximum daily dose of 6 mg/kg/**day** or 300 mg/**day** with no single dose >150 mg (Dopheide, 2009; Pliszka, 2007).

Sustained release (Wellbutrin SR®) and extended release (Wellbutrin XL®), hydrochloride salts: May be used in place of regular tablets, once the daily dose is titrated using the immediate release product and the titrated 12-hour dosage corresponds to a sustained release tablet (Wellbutrin SR®) or the 24-hour dosage range corresponds to an extended release tablet size (Wellbutrin XL®)

Depression, refractory to SSRIs: Limited data available, further studies needed. **Note:** May be most beneficial in patients with comorbid ADHD, conduct disorder, substance abuse problems or who want to quit smoking (Dopheide, 2006). Treatment should be periodically evaluated at appropriate intervals to ensure lowest effective dose is used.

Immediate release, hydrochloride salt: Children ≤11 years: Oral: Initial: 37.5 mg twice daily; titrate to response; usual dosage range: 100-400 mg/**day** (Dopheide, 2006)

Sustained release, hydrochloride salt (Wellbutrin SR®): Children ≥11 years and Adolescents: Oral: Initial: 2 mg/kg up to 100 mg administered as a morning dose; may titrate as needed every 2-3 weeks using the following titration schedule: Step 2: Increase up to 3 mg/kg every morning; Step 3: Increase up to 3 mg/kg every morning and 2 mg/kg at 5 pm; Step 4: Increase up to 3 mg/kg/dose twice daily; maximum dose: 150 mg; reported mean effective dose: Morning: 2.2 mg/kg and afternoon: 1.7 mg/kg (Daviss, 2001)

Extended release, hydrochloride salt (Wellbutrin XL®): Children ≥12 years and Adolescents: Oral: Initial: 150 mg once daily; may titrate after 2 weeks to 300 mg once daily if adequate response not achieved; dosing based on a pharmacokinetic study in eight patients with depression (Daviss, 2006); doses as high as 400 mg/**day** have been reported (Dopheide, 2006); may also be used once the daily dose is titrated using the immediate release product and the 24-hour dosage range corresponds to an extended release tablet size (Wellbutrin XL).

Smoking cessation: Limited data available; further studies needed: Adolescents ≥14 years and ≥40.5 kg: Sustained release, hydrochloride salt (Buproban®, Zyban®): Oral: Initial: 150 mg once daily for 3 days; increase to 150 mg twice daily; treatment should start while the patient is still smoking in order to allow drug to reach steady-state levels prior to smoking cessation; generally, patients should stop smoking during the second week of treatment; maximum daily dose: 300 mg/**day**; short-term efficacy was demonstrated in 104 adolescents who received therapy for 7 weeks with cessation counseling (Muramoto, 2007).

Adults:

Depression: Note: Treatment should be periodically evaluated at appropriate intervals to ensure lowest effective dose is used.

Immediate release, hydrochloride salt: Initial: 100 mg twice daily; after 3 days may increase to the usual dose of 100 mg 3 times daily; if no clinical improvement after several weeks, may increase to a maximum dose of 150 mg 3 times daily

Sustained release, hydrochloride salt: Initial: 150 mg daily in the morning; if tolerated, as early as day 4, may increase to a target dose of 150 mg twice daily; if no clinical improvement after several weeks, may increase to a maximum dose of 200 mg twice daily; **Note:** Interval between successive doses should be at least 8 hours.

Extended release:

Hydrochloride salt: Initial: 150 mg once daily in the morning; if tolerated, as early as day 4, may increase to 300 mg once daily; if no clinical improvement after several weeks, may increase to maximum dose of 450 mg once daily; **Note:** Forfivo™ XL may only be used after initial dose titration with other bupropion products.

Hydrochloride salt (Forfivo™ XL): Switching from Wellbutrin® immediate release, SR®, or XL® to Forfivo™ XL: Patients receiving 300 mg daily of bupropion hydrochloride for at least 2 weeks and requiring a dose increase or patients already taking 450 mg daily of bupropion hydrochloride may switch to Forfivo™ XL 450 mg once daily.

Hydrobromide salt (Aplenzin™): Initial: 174 mg once daily in the morning; may increase as early as day 4 of dosing to 348 mg once daily (target); maximum dose: 522 mg daily (if no improvement seen after several weeks on 348 mg); **Note:** In patients receiving 348 mg once daily, taper dose down to 174 mg once daily prior to discontinuing.

Switching from hydrochloride salt formulation (eg, Wellbutrin® immediate release, SR®, XL®, or Forfivo™ XL) to hydrobromide salt formulation (Aplenzin™):

Bupropion hydrochloride 150 mg daily is equivalent to bupropion hydrobromide 174 mg once daily

Bupropion hydrochloride 300 mg daily is equivalent to bupropion hydrobromide 348 mg once daily

Bupropion hydrochloride 450 mg daily is equivalent to bupropion hydrobromide 522 mg once daily

Seasonal affective disorder (SAD): Initial: 150 mg once daily (Wellbutrin XL®) or 174 mg once daily (Aplenzin™) in the morning; if tolerated, may increase after 1 week to 300 mg once daily (Wellbutrin XL®) or 348 mg once daily (Aplenzin™) in the morning.

Note: Prophylactic treatment should be reserved for those patients with frequent depressive episodes and/or significant impairment. Initiate treatment in the autumn prior to symptom onset, and discontinue in early spring with dose tapering to 150 mg once daily for 2 weeks (Wellbutrin XL®) or 174 mg once daily (Aplenzin™), then discontinue. Doses >300 mg daily (Wellbutrin XL®) or >348 mg daily (Aplenzin™) have not been studied in SAD.

Smoking cessation (Zyban®, Buproban®): Initial: 150 mg once daily for 3 days; increase to 150 mg twice daily; treatment should continue for 7-12 weeks

Note: Therapy should begin at least 1 week before target quit date. Target quit dates are generally in the second week of treatment. If patient successfully quits smoking after 7-12 weeks, may consider ongoing maintenance therapy based on individual patient risk: benefit. Efficacy of maintenance therapy (300 mg daily) has been demonstrated for up to 6 months. Conversely, if significant progress has not been made by the seventh week of therapy, success is unlikely and treatment discontinuation should be considered.

Dosing conversion between hydrochloride salt immediate (Wellbutrin®), sustained (Wellbutrin SR®), and extended release (Wellbutrin XL®, Forfivo™ XL) products: Convert using same total daily dose (up to the maximum recommended dose for a given dosage form), but adjust frequency as indicated for sustained (twice daily) or extended (once daily) release products.

Dosing adjustment in renal impairment: Adults: Immediate release, sustained release, and extended release formulations: There are no dosage adjustments provided in the manufacturer's labeling; however, limited pharmacokinetic information suggests elimination of bupropion and/or the active metabolites may be reduced. Use with caution and consider a reduction in dose and/or dosing frequency; closely monitor for adverse effects.

Forfivo™ XL: Use is not recommended.

Dosage adjustment in hepatic impairment: Adults:

Mild to moderate hepatic impairment: Immediate release, sustained release, and extended release formulations: Use with caution; consider reduced dosage and/or frequency.

Forfivo™ XL: Use is not recommended.

Severe hepatic cirrhosis: Use with extreme caution; maximum dose:

Aplenzin™: 174 mg every other day

Forfivo™ XL: Use is not recommended.

Wellbutrin®: 75 mg once daily

Wellbutrin SR®: 100 mg once daily or 150 mg every other day

Wellbutrin XL®: 150 mg every other day

Zyban®: 150 mg every other day

Administration Oral: May be taken without regard to meals. Do not crush, chew, or divide sustained or extended release tablets (hydrochloride and hydrobromide salt formulations); swallow whole. The insoluble shell of the extended-release tablet may remain intact during GI transit and is eliminated in the feces.

Monitoring Parameters Heart rate, blood pressure, mental status, weight. Monitor patient periodically for symptom resolution; monitor for worsening depression, suicidality, and associated behaviors (especially at the beginning of therapy or when doses are increased or decreased), anxiety, social functioning, mania, panic attacks, tics.

ADHD: Evaluate patients for cardiac disease prior to initiation of therapy for ADHD with thorough medical history, family history, and physical exam; consider ECG; perform ECG and echocardiogram if findings suggest cardiac disease; promptly conduct cardiac evaluation in patients who develop chest pain, unexplained syncope, or any other symptom of cardiac disease during treatment.

Reference Range Therapeutic levels (trough, 12 hours after last dose): 50-100 ng/mL

Test Interactions May interfere with urine detection of amphetamine/methamphetamine (false-positive). Decreased prolactin levels.

Dosage Forms Excipient information presented when available (limited, particularly for generics); consult specific product labeling. [DSC] = Discontinued product

Tablet, Oral, as hydrochloride:

Wellbutrin: 75 mg, 100 mg

Generic: 75 mg, 100 mg

Tablet Extended Release 12 Hour, Oral:

Generic: 150 mg

Tablet Extended Release 12 Hour, Oral, as hydrochloride:

Budeprion SR: 100 mg [DSC] [contains tartrazine (fd&c yellow #5)]

Budeprion SR: 150 mg [DSC]

Buproban: 150 mg

Wellbutrin SR: 100 mg, 150 mg, 200 mg

Zyban: 150 mg

Generic: 100 mg, 150 mg, 200 mg

Tablet Extended Release 24 Hour, Oral, as hydrobromide:

Aplenzin: 174 mg, 348 mg, 522 mg

Tablet Extended Release 24 Hour, Oral, as hydrochloride:

Forfivo XL: 450 mg

Wellbutrin XL: 150 mg, 300 mg

Generic: 150 mg, 300 mg

Tablet Extended Release 24 Hour, Oral, as hydrochloride [strength expressed as base]:

Generic: 300 mg

References

ACOG Committee on Practice Bulletins–Obstetrics, "ACOG Practice Bulletin: Clinical Management Guidelines for Obstetrician-Gynecologists Number 92, April 2008 (Replaces Practice Bulletin Number 87, November 2007). Use of Psychiatric Medications During Pregnancy and Lactation," *Obstet Gynecol*, 2008, 111(4):1001-20.

ACOG, "Committee Opinion No. 471: Smoking Cessation During Pregnancy," *Obstet Gynecol*, 2010, 116(5):1241-4.

American Academy of Pediatrics/American Heart Association Clarification of Statement on Cardiovascular Evaluation and Monitoring of Children and Adolescents With Heart Disease Receiving Medications for ADHD; available at: http://americanheart.mediaroon.com/index.php?s=43&item=422.

American Psychiatric Association, "Treatment Recommendations for Patients With Major Depressive Disorder," 3rd ed, May 2010. Available at http://www.psychiatryonline.com/pracGuide/pracGuideTopic_7.aspx

Chaudron LH and Schoenecker CJ, "Bupropion and Breastfeeding: A Case of a Possible Infant Seizure," *J Clin Psychiatry*, 2004, 65 (6):881-2.

Davidson J, "Seizures and Bupropion: A Review," *J Clin Psychiatry*, 1989, 50(7):256-61.

Davis MF, Miller HS, and Nolan PE Jr, "Bupropion Levels in Breast Milk for 4 Mother-Infant Pairs: More Answers to Lingering Questions," *J Clin Psychiatry*, 2009, 70(2):297-8.

Daviss WB, Bentivoglio P, Racusin R, et al, "Bupropion Sustained Release in Adolescents With Comorbid Attention-Deficit/Hyperactivity Disorder and Depression," *J Am Acad Child Adolesc Psychiatry*, 2001, 40(3):307-14.

Daviss WB, Perel JM, Birmaher B, et al, "Steady-State Clinical Pharmacokinetics of Bupropion Extended-Release in Youths," *J Am Acad Child Adolesc Psychiatry*, 2006, 45(12):1503-9.

Dopheide JA, "Recognizing and Treating Depression in Children and Adolescents," *Am J Health Syst Pharm*, 2006, 63(3):233-43.

Earhart AD, Patrikeeva S, Wang X, et al, "Transplacental Transfer and Metabolism of Bupropion," *J Matern Fetal Neonatal Med*, 2010, 23 (5):409-16.

Haas JS, Kaplan CP, Barenboim D, et al, "Bupropion in Breast Milk: An Exposure Assessment for Potential Treatment to Prevent Post-Partum Tobacco Use," *Tob Control*, 2004, 13(1):52-6.

Hack S, "Pediatric Bupropion-Induced Serum Sickness Like Reaction," *J Child Adolesc Psychopharmacol*, 2004, 14(3):478-80.

Hale TW, Kendall-Tackett K, Cong Z, et al, "Discontinuation Syndrome in Newborns Whose Mothers Took Antidepressants While Pregnant or Breastfeeding," *Breastfeed Med*, 2010, 5(6):283-8.

Jennison TA, Brown P, Crossett J, et al, "A High-Performance Liquid Chromatographic Method for Quantitating Bupropion in Human Plasma or Serum," *J Anal Toxicol*, 1995, 19(2):69-72.

Leverich GS, Altshuler LL, Frye MA, et al, "Risk of Switch in Mood Polarity to Hypomania or Mania in Patients with Bipolar Depression During Acute and Continuation Trials of Venlafaxine, Sertraline, and Bupropion as Adjuncts to Mood Stabilizers," *Am J Psychiatry*, 2006, 163(2):232-9.

McIntyre RS, Mancini DA, McCann S, et al, "Topiramate Versus Bupropion SR When Added to Mood Stabilizer Therapy for the Depressive Phase of Bipolar Disorder: A Preliminary Single-Blind Study," *Bipolar Disord*, 2002, 4(3):207-13.

Muramoto ML, Leischow SJ, Sherrill D, et al, "Randomized, Double-Blind, Placebo-Controlled Trial of 2 Dosages of Sustained-Release Bupropion for Adolescent Smoking Cessation," *Arch Pediatr Adolesc Med*, 2007, 161(11):1068-74.

Pass SE and Simpson RW, "Discontinuation and Reinstitution of Medications During the Perioperative Period," *Am J Health Syst Pharm*, 2004, 61(9):899-912.

Pliszka S, AACAP Work Group on Quality Issues. Practice parameter for the assessment and treatment of children and adolescents with attention-deficit/hyperactivity disorder. *J Am Acad Child Adolesc Psychiatry*. 2007 Jul;46(7):894-921.

Pliszka SR, Crismon ML, Hughes CW, et al, "The Texas Children's Medication Algorithm Project: Revision of the Algorithm for Pharmacotherapy of ADHD," *J Am Acad Child Adolesc Psychiatry*, 2006, 45 (6):642-57.

Riggs PD, Leon SL, Mikulich SK, et al, "An Open Trial of Bupropion for ADHD in Adolescents With Substance Use Disorders and Conduct Disorder," *J Am Acad Child Adolesc Psychiatry*, 1998, 37(12):1271-8.

Turpeinen M, Koivuviita N, Tolonen A, et al, "Effect of Renal Impairment on the Pharmacokinetics of Bupropion and Its Metabolites," *Br J Clin Pharmacol*, 2007, 64(2):165-73.

Van Wyck FJ, Manberg PJ, Miller LL, et al, "Overview of Clinically Significant Adverse Reactions to Bupropion," *J Clin Psychiatry*, 1983, 44(5 Pt 2):191-6.

Vetter VL, Elia J, Erickson C, et al, "Cardiovascular Monitoring of Children and Adolescents With Heart Disease Receiving Stimulant Drugs: A Scientific Statement From the American Heart Association Council on Cardiovascular Disease in the Young Congenital Cardiac

Defects Committee and the Council on Cardiovascular Nursing," *Circulation*, 2008, 117(18):2407-23.

Wagner KD, "Pharmacotherapy for Major Depression in Children and Adolescents," *Prog Neuropsychopharmacol Biol Psychiatry*, 2005, 29 (5):819-26.

Yonkers KA, Wisner KL, Stewart DE, et al, "The Management of Depression During Pregnancy: A Report From the American Psychiatric Association and the American College of Obstetricians and Gynecologists," *Obstet Gynecol*, 2009, 114(3):703-13.

◆ **Bupropion Hydrobromide** *see* BuPROPion on page 327

◆ **Bupropion Hydrochloride** *see* BuPROPion on page 327

◆ **Bupropion SR (Can)** *see* BuPROPion on page 327

◆ **Burinex (Can)** *see* Bumetanide on page 316

◆ **Burow's Solution** *see* Aluminum Acetate on page 110

◆ **Buscopan® (Can)** *see* Scopolamine (Systemic) on page 1872

◆ **BuSpar** *see* BusPIRone on page 332

BusPIRone (byoo SPYE rone)

Medication Safety Issues
Sound-alike/look-alike issues:
BusPIRone may be confused with buPROPion
Brand Names: Canada Apo-Buspirone®; Bustab®; Dom-Buspirone; Novo-Buspirone; PMS-Buspirone; Riva-Buspirone

Therapeutic Category Antianxiety Agent
Generic Availability (U.S.) Yes
Use Management of anxiety disorders
Pregnancy Risk Factor B
Pregnancy Considerations Adverse events have not been observed in animal reproduction studies.
Breast-Feeding Considerations It is not known if buspirone is excreted in breast milk. Breast-feeding is not recommended by the manufacturer.
Contraindications Hypersensitivity to buspirone or any component
Warnings Do not use concurrently with MAO inhibitors or within 10 days of MAO inhibitors as significant increases in blood pressure may occur. Buspirone does not possess antipsychotic activity and should not be used in place of appropriate antipsychotic treatment; two pediatric cases of possible psychotic deterioration have been reported (Soni, 1992).
Precautions Use with caution in patients with hepatic or renal dysfunction; use in severe hepatic or renal impairment is not recommended. Buspirone does not prevent or treat withdrawal from benzodiazepines or sedative/hypnotic drugs; if substituting buspirone for these agents, gradually withdraw the other drug(s) prior to initiating buspirone. Buspirone possesses a low potential for cognitive or motor impairment; however, until effects on an individual patient are known, patients should be warned to use caution when performing tasks which require mental alertness (eg, operating machinery or driving); effects may be potentiated when used with other sedative drugs or ethanol. Restlessness syndrome has been reported in a small number of patients; may be attributable to buspirone's antagonism of central dopamine receptors. Monitor for signs of any dopamine-related movement disorders (eg, dystonia, akathisia, pseudo-parkinsonism).

Adverse Reactions
Cardiovascular: Chest pain
Central nervous system: Anger, confusion, dizziness, dream disturbance, drowsiness, excitement, headache, hostility, lightheadedness, nervousness
Dermatologic: Rash
Gastrointestinal: Diarrhea, nausea
Neuromuscular & skeletal: Incoordination, musculoskeletal pain, numbness, paresthesia, tremor. weakness
Ocular: Blurred vision
Otic: Tinnitus
Respiratory: Nasal congestion, sore throat
Miscellaneous: Diaphoresis
Rare but important or life-threatening: Akathisia, alcohol abuse, allergic reaction, alopecia, ALT increased, amenorrhea, angioedema, anorexia, AST increased, ataxia, bleeding disorder, bradycardia, bruising, cardiomyopathy, claustrophobia, cogwheel rigidity, conjunctivitis, CVA, dyskinesia, dystonia, edema, enuresis, eosinophilia, epistaxis, EPS, galactorrhea, hallucination, heart failure, hyper-/hypotension, hyperventilation, irritable colon, leukopenia, memory impairment, menstrual irregularity, MI, ocular pressure increased, parkinsonism, personality disorders, photophobia, PID, psychosis, rectal bleeding, restless leg syndrome, seizure, serotonin syndrome, slow reaction time, slurred speech, suicidal ideation, syncope, thrombocytopenia, thyroid abnormality, transaminase increases, visual disturbances (tunnel vision)

Drug Interactions
Metabolism/Transport Effects Substrate of CYP2D6 (minor), CYP3A4 (major); **Note:** Assignment of Major/Minor substrate status based on clinically relevant drug interaction potential
Avoid Concomitant Use
Avoid concomitant use of BusPIRone with any of the following: Azelastine (Nasal); Conivaptan; Fusidic Acid (Systemic); MAO Inhibitors; Methylene Blue; Paraldehyde; Thalidomide
Increased Effect/Toxicity
BusPIRone may increase the levels/effects of: Alcohol (Ethyl); Antidepressants (Serotonin Reuptake Inhibitor/Antagonist); Antipsychotics; Azelastine (Nasal); Buprenorphine; CNS Depressants; Hydrocodone; MAO Inhibitors; Methotrimeprazine; Methylene Blue; Metoclopramide; Metyrosine; Paraldehyde; Pramipexole; ROPINIRole; Rotigotine; Selective Serotonin Reuptake Inhibitors; Serotonin Modulators; Thalidomide; Zolpidem

The levels/effects of BusPIRone may be increased by: Antiemetics (5HT3 Antagonists); Antifungal Agents (Azole Derivatives, Systemic); Antipsychotics; Brimonidine (Topical); Calcium Channel Blockers (Nondihydropyridine); Cannabis; Ceritinib; Conivaptan; CYP3A4 Inhibitors (Moderate); CYP3A4 Inhibitors (Strong); Dasatinib; Doxylamine; Dronabinol; Droperidol; Fusidic Acid (Systemic); Grapefruit Juice; HydrOXYzine; Ivacaftor; Kava Kava; Luliconazole; Macrolide Antibiotics; Magnesium Sulfate; Methotrimeprazine; Mifepristone; Nabilone; Perampanel; Rufinamide; Selective Serotonin Reuptake Inhibitors; Simeprevir; Sodium Oxybate; Stiripentol; Tapentadol; Tetrahydrocannabinol

Decreased Effect
BusPIRone may decrease the levels/effects of: Ioflupane I 123

The levels/effects of BusPIRone may be decreased by: Bosentan; CYP3A4 Inducers (Strong); Dabrafenib; Deferasirox; Mitotane; Peginterferon Alfa-2b; Rifamycin Derivatives; Siltuximab; St Johns Wort; Tocilizumab; Yohimbine

Food Interactions Food may decrease the absorption of buspirone, but it may also decrease the first-pass metabolism, thereby increasing the bioavailability of buspirone. Grapefruit juice may cause increased buspirone concentrations. Management: Administer with or without food, but must be consistent. Avoid intake of large quantities of grapefruit juice.

Stability Store at 25°C (77°F); excursions permitted between 15°C to 30°C (59°F to 86°F); protect from light.

Mechanism of Action The mechanism of action of buspirone is unknown. Buspirone has a high affinity for serotonin 5-HT$_{1A}$ and 5-HT$_2$ receptors, without affecting benzodiazepine-GABA receptors. Buspirone has moderate affinity for dopamine D$_2$ receptors.

Pharmacodynamics

Onset of action: Within 2 weeks

Maximum effect: 3-4 weeks, up to 4-6 weeks

Pharmacokinetics (Adult data unless noted)

Absorption: Rapid and complete, but bioavailability is limited by extensive first-pass effect; only 1.5% to 13% (mean 4%) of the oral dose reaches the systemic circulation unchanged

Protein binding: 86%

Distribution: V$_d$: Adults: 5.3 L/kg

Metabolism: In the liver by oxidation (by cytochrome P450 isoenzyme CYP3A4) to several metabolites including 1-pyrimidinyl piperazine (about 1/4 as active as buspirone)

Half-life: Adults: Mean: 2-3 hours; increased with renal or liver dysfunction

Time to peak serum concentration: 40-90 minutes

Elimination: 29% to 63% excreted in urine (primarily as metabolites)

Dosing: Usual

Pediatric: **Anxiety disorders:** Children and Adolescents: Oral: Limited information is available; dose is not well established. One pilot study of 15 children, 6-14 years of age (mean 10 years), with mixed anxiety disorders, used initial doses of 5 mg daily; doses were individualized with increases in increments of 5 mg/day every week as needed to a maximum dose of 20 mg/day divided into 2 doses; the mean dose required: 18.6 mg/day (Simeon, 1994). Some authors (Carrey, 1996 and Kutcher, 1992), based on their clinical experience, recommend higher doses (eg, 15-30 mg/day in 2 divided doses). An open-label study in 25 prepubertal inpatients (mean age: 8 ± 1.8 years; range: 5-11 years) with anxiety symptoms and moderately aggressive behavior used initial doses of 5 mg daily; doses were titrated upwards (over 3 weeks) by 5-10 mg every 3 days to a maximum dose of 50 mg/day; doses >5 mg/day were administered in 2 divided doses/day; buspirone was discontinued in 25% of the children due to increased aggression and agitation or euphoric mania; mean optimal dose (n=19): 28 mg/day; range: 10-50 mg/day; median: 30 mg/day (Pfeffer, 1997). Two placebo-controlled 6-week trials in children and adolescents (n=559; age: 6-17 years) with generalized anxiety disorder studied doses of 7.5-30 mg twice daily (15-60 mg/day); no significant differences between buspirone and placebo with respect to generalized anxiety disorder symptoms were observed (see package insert).

Adult: **Generalized anxiety disorders:** Oral: Initial: 7.5 mg twice daily; may increase every 2-3 days in increments of 2.5 mg twice daily to a maximum of 30 mg twice daily; a dose of 10-15 mg twice daily was most often used in clinical trials that allowed for dose titration

Dosing adjustment in renal impairment: Patients with impaired renal function demonstrated increased plasma levels and a prolonged half-life of buspirone. Use in patients with severe renal impairment not recommended.

Dosing adjustment in hepatic impairment: Patients with impaired hepatic function demonstrated increased plasma levels and a prolonged half-life of buspirone. Use in patients with severe hepatic impairment not recommended.

Administration Oral: Administer in a consistent manner in relation to food (ie, either always with food or always without food); may administer with food to decrease GI upset

Monitoring Parameters Mental status, signs and symptoms of anxiety, liver and renal function; signs of dopamine-related movement disorders (eg, dystonia, akathisia, pseudo-parkinsonism).

Test Interactions The presence of buspirone may result in a false positive on a urinary assay for metanephrine/catecholamine; discontinue buspirone ≥48 hours prior to collection of urine sample for catecholamines

Additional Information Not appropriate for "as needed" (prn) use or for brief, situational anxiety; buspirone is equipotent to diazepam on a milligram to milligram basis in the treatment of anxiety; however, unlike diazepam, the onset of buspirone is delayed

Dosage Forms Excipient information presented when available (limited, particularly for generics); consult specific product labeling.

Tablet, Oral, as hydrochloride:

Generic: 5 mg, 7.5 mg, 10 mg, 15 mg, 30 mg

References

Carrey NJ, Wiggins DM, and Milin RP, "Pharmacological Treatment of Psychiatric Disorders in Children and Adolescents," *Drugs*, 1996, 51 (5):750-9.

Gammans RE, Mayol RF, and LaBudde JA, "Metabolism and Disposition of Buspirone," *Am J Med*, 1986, 80(3B):41-51.

Hanna GL, Feibusch EL, and Albright KJ, "Buspirone Treatment of Anxiety, Associated With Pharyngeal Dysphagia in a Four-Year Old," *J Child Adolesc Psychopharmacol*, 1997, 7(2):137-43.

Kutcher SP, Reiter S, Gardner DM, et al, "The Pharmacotherapy of Anxiety Disorders in Children and Adolescents," *Psychiatr Clin North Am*, 1992, 15(1):41-67.

Pfeffer CR, Jiang H, and Domeshek LJ, "Buspirone Treatment of Psychiatrically Hospitalized Prepubertal Children With Symptoms of Anxiety and Moderately Severe Aggression," *J Child Adolesc Psychopharmacol*, 1997, 7(3):145-55.

Simeon JG, Knott VJ, DuBois C, et al, "Buspirone Therapy of Mixed Anxiety Disorders in Childhood and Adolescence: A Pilot Study," *J Child Adolesc Psychopharmacol*, 1994, 4(3):159-70.

Soni P and Weintraub AL, "Buspirone-Associated Mental Status Changes," *J Am Acad Child Adolesc Psychiatry*, 1992, 31(6):1098-9.

◆ **Buspirone Hydrochloride** see BusPIRone on page 332

◆ **Bussulfam** see Busulfan on page 333

◆ **Bustab® (Can)** see BusPIRone on page 332

Busulfan (byoo SUL fan)

Medication Safety Issues

Sound-alike/look-alike issues:

Myleran® may be confused with Alkeran®, Leukeran®, melphalan, Mylicon®

High alert medication:

This medication is in a class the Institute for Safe Medication Practices (ISMP) includes among its list of drug classes which have a heightened risk of causing significant patient harm when used in error.

Related Information

Emetogenic Potential of Antineoplastic Agents in Children on page 2327

Management of Drug Extravasations on page 2255

Safe Handling of Hazardous Drugs on page 2419

Brand Names: U.S. Busulfex; Myleran

Brand Names: Canada Busulfex®; Myleran®

Therapeutic Category Antineoplastic Agent, Alkylating Agent

Generic Availability (U.S.) No

Use

Oral: Palliative treatment of chronic myelogenous leukemia (CML) [FDA approved in pediatric patients (age not specified) and adults]; has also been used as a conditioning regimen prior to hemapoietic stem cell transplant

Parenteral: Conditioning regimen prior to allogeneic hematopoietic progenitor cell transplantation for CML in combination with cyclophosphamide [FDA approved in adults]

Pregnancy Risk Factor D

◀ **Pregnancy Considerations** Animal studies have demonstrated teratogenic effects. There are no adequate and well-controlled studies in pregnant women. May cause fetal harm if administered during pregnancy. The solvent in I.V. busulfan, DMA, is also associated with teratogenic effects and may impair fertility. Women of childbearing potential should avoid pregnancy while receiving busulfan treatment.

Breast-Feeding Considerations According to the manufacturer, the decision to continue or discontinue breast-feeding during therapy should take into account the risk of exposure to the infant and the benefits of treatment to the mother.

Contraindications Hypersensitivity to busulfan or any component

Additional route specific contraindication: Oral: Patients without a definitive diagnosis of CML

Warnings Hazardous agent; use appropriate precautions for handling and disposal (NIOSH, 2012). Bronchopulmonary dysplasia with pulmonary fibrosis ("busulfan lung") is associated with busulfan; onset is delayed with symptoms occurring at an average of 4 years (range: 4 months to 10 years) after treatment; may be fatal. Symptoms generally include a slow onset of cough, dyspnea and fever (low-grade), although acute symptomatic onset may also occur. Diminished diffusion capacity and decreased pulmonary compliance have been noted with pulmonary function testing. Differential diagnosis should rule out opportunistic pulmonary infection or leukemic pulmonary infiltrates; may require lung biopsy. Discontinue busulfan if toxicity develops. Pulmonary toxicity may be additive if administered with other cytotoxic agents also associated with pulmonary toxicity. Busulfan is potentially carcinogenic; malignant tumors and acute leukemias have been reported; chromosomal alterations may also occur.

Cellular dysplasia in many organs has been observed (in addition to lung dysplasia); giant hyperchromatic nuclei have been noted in adrenal glands, liver, lymph nodes, pancreas, thyroid, and bone marrow; may obscure routine diagnostic cytologic exams (eg, cervical smear). Busulfan use has also been associated with ovarian failure including failure to achieve puberty and amenorrhea in females

Severe bone marrow suppression is common even with recommended dosages **[U.S. Boxed Warning]**; may result in severe neutropenia, thrombocytopenia, anemia, bone marrow failure, and/or severe pancytopenia; pancytopenia may be prolonged (1 month up to 2 years) and may be reversible. Use with caution in patients with compromised bone marrow reserve (due to prior treatment or radiation therapy); reduce dosage in patients with bone marrow suppression; may require bone marrow biopsy. Monitor closely for signs of infection (due to neutropenia) or bleeding (due to thrombocytopenia).

High busulfan AUC values (>1500 micromolar/minute) may be associated with an increased risk of developing hepatic sinusoidal obstruction syndrome [SOS; formerly called veno-occlusive disease (VOD)]; reported incidence 7.7% to 12% with high-dose busulfan; patients who have received prior radiation therapy, ≥3 cycles of chemotherapy, or prior progenitor cell transplant are also at increased risk for developing SOS at recommended dosage regimens. Oral busulfan doses above 16 mg/kg (based on IBW) and concurrent use with alkylating agents may also increase the risk for hepatic SOS. Of the patients who developed SOS, it was fatal in 40% of the cases; monitor liver function tests periodically. Cardiac tamponade has been reported in pediatric patients with thalassemia treated with high-dose oral busulfan in combination with cyclophosphamide.

Seizures have been reported with busulfan; use with caution in patients predisposed to seizures, with a history of seizures, or head trauma. When using as a conditioning regimen for transplant, initiate prophylactic anticonvulsant therapy (eg, phenytoin) prior to treatment. Phenytoin increases busulfan clearance by ≥15%; busulfan pharmacokinetics and dosing recommendations for high-dose HSCT conditioning were studied with concomitant phenytoin therapy; if alternate anticonvulsants are used, busulfan clearance may be decreased and dosing should be monitored accordingly.

The solvent in busulfan injection is dimethylacetamide (DMA); DMA may impair fertility and may also be associated with hepatotoxicity, hallucinations, somnolence, lethargy, and confusion.

Precautions Should be administered under the supervision of an experienced cancer chemotherapy physician **[U.S. Boxed Warning]**. For the I.V. formulation, the physician should be experienced in management of hematopoietic stem cell transplantation and management of patients with severe pancytopenia. "Juvenile type" chronic myelogenous leukemia which typically occurs in young children and is associated with the absence of Philadelphia chromosome responds poorly to busulfan. Potentially significant interactions may exist, requiring dose or frequency adjustment, additional monitoring, and/or selection of alternative therapy. Consult drug interactions database for more detailed information.

Adverse Reactions

I.V.:

Cardiovascular: Arrhythmia, atrial fibrillation, cardiomegaly, chest pain, ECG abnormal, edema, heart block, heart failure, hyper-/hypotension, hypervolemia, pericardial effusion, tachycardia, tamponade, thrombosis, vasodilation, ventricular extrasystoles

Central nervous system: Agitation, anxiety, cerebral hemorrhage, chills, confusion, delirium, depression, dizziness, encephalopathy, fever, hallucination, headache, insomnia, lethargy, pain, seizure, somnolence

Dermatologic: Acne, alopecia, erythema nodosum, exfoliative dermatitis, maculopapular rash, pruritus, rash, skin discoloration, vesicular rash, vesiculobullous rash

Endocrine & metabolic: Hyperglycemia, hypocalcemia, hypokalemia, hypomagnesemia, hyponatremia, hypophosphatemia

Gastrointestinal: Abdominal fullness, abdominal pain, anorexia, constipation, diarrhea, dyspepsia, esophagitis, hematemesis, ileus, mucositis/stomatitis, nausea, pancreatitis, rectal disorder, vomiting, weight gain, xerostomia,

Hematologic: Anemia, lymphopenia, myelosuppression, neutropenia (median recovery: 13 days), prothrombin time increased, thrombocytopenia (median onset: 5-6 days)

Hepatic: Alkaline phosphatase increased, ALT increased, hepatic sinusoidal obstruction syndrome (SOS; veno-occlusive disease), hepatomegaly, hyperbilirubinemia, jaundice

Local: Injection site inflammation/pain

Neuromuscular & skeletal: Arthralgia, back pain, myalgia, weakness

Renal: BUN/creatinine increased, dysuria, hematuria, hemorrhagic cystitis, oliguria

Respiratory: Alveolar hemorrhage, asthma, atelectasis, cough, dyspnea, epistaxis, hemoptysis, hiccup, hyperventilation, hypoxia, lung disorder, pharyngitis, pleural effusion, pneumonia, rhinitis, sinusitis

Miscellaneous: Allergic reaction, infection (includes severe bacterial, viral [CMV], and fungal infections)

Oral:

Dermatologic: Hyperpigmentation of skin, rash

Endocrine & metabolic: Amenorrhea, ovarian suppression

Gastrointestinal: Xerostomia

Hematologic: Myelosuppression (anemia, leukopenia, thrombocytopenia)

I.V. and/or Oral: Rare but important or life-threatening: Acute leukemias, adrenal insufficiency, alopecia (permanent), aplastic anemia (may be irreversible), azoospermia, bronchopulmonary dysplasia, capillary leak syndrome, cataracts (rare), cheilosis, cholestatic jaundice, corneal thinning, dry skin, endocardial fibrosis, erythema multiforme, esophageal varices, gynecomastia, hepatic dysfunction, hepatocellular atrophy, hyperuricemia, hyperuricosuria, interstitial pulmonary fibrosis, malignant tumors, myasthenia gravis, neutropenic fever, ocular (lens) changes, ovarian failure, pancytopenia, porphyria cutanea tarda, pulmonary fibrosis, radiation myelopathy, radiation recall (skin rash), sepsis, sterility, testicular atrophy, thrombotic microangiopathy (TMA), tumor lysis syndrome, urticaria

Drug Interactions

Metabolism/Transport Effects None known.

Avoid Concomitant Use

Avoid concomitant use of Busulfan with any of the following: BCG; CloZAPine; Dipyrone; Natalizumab; Pimecrolimus; Tacrolimus (Topical); Tofacitinib; Vaccines (Live)

Increased Effect/Toxicity

Busulfan may increase the levels/effects of: CloZAPine; Ifosfamide; Leflunomide; Natalizumab; Tofacitinib; Vaccines (Live); Vitamin K Antagonists

The levels/effects of Busulfan may be increased by: Acetaminophen; Antifungal Agents (Azole Derivatives, Systemic); Denosumab; Dipyrone; MetroNIDAZOLE (Systemic); Pimecrolimus; Roflumilast; Tacrolimus (Topical); Trastuzumab

Decreased Effect

Busulfan may decrease the levels/effects of: BCG; Coccidioidin Skin Test; Sipuleucel-T; Vaccines (Inactivated); Vaccines (Live); Vitamin K Antagonists

The levels/effects of Busulfan may be decreased by: Echinacea; Fosphenytoin; Phenytoin

Stability

Oral: Store at 25°C (77°F); excursions permitted to 15°C to 30°C (59°F to 86°F).

Parenteral: Store intact ampuls and vials at 2°C to 8°C (36°F to 46°F); diluted busulfan solution is stable for up to 8 hours at room temperature; infusion must be completed within that 8 hour time frame. If diluted in NS, the solution is stable for 12 hours if refrigerated, but the infusion must be completed within that 12-hour time frame.

Mechanism of Action Busulfan is an alkylating agent which reacts with the N-7 position of guanosine and interferes with DNA replication and transcription of RNA. Busulfan has a more marked effect on myeloid cells than on lymphoid cells and is also very toxic to hematopoietic stem cells. Busulfan exhibits little immunosuppressive activity. Interferes with the normal function of DNA by alkylation and cross-linking the strands of DNA.

Pharmacokinetics (Adult data unless noted)

Absorption: Oral: Rapid and complete

Distribution: V_d: ~1 L/kg; distributes into CSF with levels equal to plasma

Protein binding: 32% plasma proteins; 47% to red blood cells

Metabolism: Extensively hepatic (may increase with multiple doses); glutathione conjugation followed by oxidation

Bioavailability: Oral: Highly variable: Children 1.5-6 years: 68% (range: 22% to 120%); adolescents and adults: 80% (range: 47% to 103%)

Half-life: Mean: 2.69 hours (± 0.49)

Time to peak serum concentration: Oral: Within 1-2 hours; I.V.: Within 5 minutes

Elimination: Urine (25% to 60% predominantly as metabolites; <2% as unchanged drug)

Clearance:
Children: 3.37 mL/minute/kg
Adults: 2.52 mL/minute/kg (range: 1.49-4.31 mL/minute/kg)

Dosing: Usual Dose, frequency, number of doses, and/or start date may vary by protocol and treatment phase. Refer to individual protocols. **Note:** Premedicate with prophylactic anticonvulsant therapy (eg, phenytoin) prior to high-dose busulfan treatment. Prophylactic antiemetics may be necessary for high-dose (HSCT) regimens.

Pediatric:

Chronic myelogenous leukemia (CML), palliation: Infants, Children, and Adolescents: Oral:

Remission induction: 0.06 mg/kg/dose once daily **or** 1.8 mg/m²/day once daily; titrate dose (or withhold) to maintain a leukocyte count >15,000/mm³; doses >4 mg/day should be reserved for patients with the most compelling symptoms

Maintenance: When leukocyte count ≥50,000/mm³: Resume induction dose **or** (if remission <3 months) 1-3 mg/day (to control hematologic status and prevent relapse)

Hematopoietic stem cell transplant (HSCT) conditioning regimen: Limited data available:

I.V.: Infants, Children, and Adolescents: **Note:** Dosing based on actual body weight:

≤12 kg: 1.1 mg/kg/dose every 6 hours for 16 doses
>12 kg: 0.8 mg/kg/dose every 6 hours for 16 doses

Adjust dose to desired AUC (1125 micromolar•minute) using the following formula:

Adjusted dose (mg) = Actual dose (mg) x [target AUC (micromolar•minute) / actual AUC (micromolar•minute)]

Reduced intensity conditioning regimen: Infants, Children, and Adolescents: 0.8 mg/kg/dose for one dose on either day -7 (related donor) or day -10 (unrelated donor or cord recipient) prior to transplant, followed by 7 additional doses of ~0.8 mg/kg/dose every 6 hours (actual dose based on pharmacokinetic analysis after initial dose) beginning days -3 and -2 (related donor) or days -6 and -5 (unrelated donor or cord recipient) prior to transplant; used in combination with fludarabine and antithymocyte globulin (rabbit). In clinical trials, there was no minimum age for inclusion; the youngest patient treated was 2 years (Pulsipher, 2009).

Oral:

Infants and Children <3 years:

Ewing sarcoma: 1 mg/kg/dose every 6 hours for 16 doses on days -6 to -3 prior to transplant in combination with melphalan (Drabco, 2012)

Thalessemia major: 1.25 mg/kg every 6 hours for 16 doses on day -9 to day -6 prior to transplant in combination with cyclophosphamide and antithymocyte globulin (horse); data is from patients who were considered Class 1 or Class 2 (ie, low risk for GVHD or transplant mortality) (Hussein, 2013)

Children ≥3 years and Adolescents: 1 mg/kg/dose every 6 hours for 16 doses prior to transplant; days of administration and combination therapy varied by disease: In Ewing sarcoma, on days -6 to -3 prior to transplant in combination with melphalan (Drabco, 2012); in thalassemia major, on days -9 to -6 in combination with cyclophosphamide and antithymocyte globulin (horse) (in this trial, patients were considered Class 1 or Class 2; ie, low risk for GVHD or transplant mortality) (Hussein, 2013) and in acute myeloid leukemia (AML), on days -9 to -6 in combination with cyclophosphamide (in this trial, patients were ≥16 years) (Cassileth, 1998).

Reduced intensity conditioning regimen: Children ≥10 years and Adolescents: 2 mg/kg/dose every 12 hours for 4 doses on days -8 and -7 in combination with fludarabine and antithymocyte globulin (horse); data is from patients with thalessmia major who were considered Class 3 (all risk factors with extensive liver damage and iron overload) (Hussein, 2013)

Adults:

Chronic myelogenous leukemia (CML), palliation:
Oral:
Remission induction: 0.06 mg/kg/dose once daily or 1.8 mg/m²/dose once daily; usual range: 4-8 mg/day; titrate dose (or withhold) to maintain leukocyte counts ≥15,000/mm³; doses >4 mg/day should be reserved for patients with the most compelling symptoms
Maintenance: When leukocyte count ≥50,000/mm³: Resume induction dose **or** (if remission <3 months) 1-3 mg/day (to control hematologic status and prevent relapse)

Hematopoietic stem cell (HSCT) conditioning regimen: I.V.: 0.8 mg/kg/dose every 6 hours for 4 days (a total of 16 doses); **Note:** Use ideal body weight or actual body weight, (whichever is lower) for dosing.
Obesity: For obese or severely-obese patients, use of an adjusted body weight [IBW + 0.25 x (actual − IBW)] is recommended.
Reduced intensity conditioning regimen: 0.8 mg/kg/day for 4 days starting 5 days prior to transplant (in combinations with fludarabine) (Ho, 2009)

Dosing adjustment in renal impairment:
I.V.: There are no dosage adjustment provided in the manufacturer's labeling (has not been studied).
Oral: There are no dosage adjustments are provided in the manufacturer's labeling; elimination appears to be independent of renal function; some clinicians suggest adjustment is not necessary (Aronoff, 2007).

Dosing adjustment in hepatic impairment:
I.V.: There are no dosage adjustments provided in the manufacturer's labeling (has not been studied).
Oral: There are no dosage adjustments provided in the manufacturer's labeling.

Administration Hazardous agent; use appropriate precautions for handling and disposal (NIOSH, 2012).
Oral: May be administered without regard to meals. To facilitate ingestion of high doses (for HSCT), may insert multiple tablets into clear gelatin capsules for administration.
Parenteral: Filter busulfan using 5 micron syringe filter provided, using one filter per ampul. If using the syringe filter in the forward flow direction, allow for ~0.16 mL of residual busulfan to remain in the filter. Dilute busulfan injection with either NS or D_5W to a final concentration of ≥0.5 mg/mL (diluent volume should be 10 times the volume of busulfan injection); infuse over 2 hours through a central venous catheter; flush line before and after each infusion with D_5W or NS. Do **not** use polycarbonate syringes or filter needles for preparation or administration.

Vesicant/Extravasation Risk May be an irritant

Monitoring Parameters CBC with differential and platelet count (weekly for palliative treatment; daily until engraftment for HSCT); liver function tests, bilirubin, and alkaline phosphatase daily thru BMT day +28.

If conducting therapeutic drug monitoring for AUC calculations in HSCT, monitor busulfan plasma concentrations at appropriate collection times (record collection times); for I.V. infusion: For calculating AUC:
After first dose, collect at 2 hours (end of infusion), 4 hours, and 6 hours (immediately prior to the next dose).
Any other dose, collect a pre-infusion concentration, then at 2 hours (end of infusion), 4 hours, and 6 hours (immediately prior to the next dose).

Dosage Forms Excipient information presented when available (limited, particularly for generics); consult specific product labeling.
Solution, Intravenous:
Busulfex: 6 mg/mL (10 mL)
Tablet, Oral:
Myleran: 2 mg

Extemporaneous Preparations Hazardous agent: Use appropriate precautions for handling and disposal.

A 2 mg/mL oral suspension can be prepared in a vertical flow hood with tablets and simple syrup. Crush one-hundred-twenty 2 mg tablets in a mortar and reduce to a fine powder. Add small portions of simple syrup and mix to a uniform paste; mix while adding the simple syrup in incremental proportions to **almost** 120 mL; transfer to a graduated cylinder, rinse mortar and pestle with simple syrup, and add quantity of vehicle sufficient to make 120 mL. Transfer contents of the graduated cylinder into an amber prescription bottle. Label "shake well", "refrigerate", and "caution chemotherapy". Stable for 30 days.
Allen LV, "Busulfan Oral Suspension," *US Pharm*, 1990, 15:94-5.

References

Aronoff GR, Bennett WM, Berns JS, et al, *Drug Prescribing in Renal Failure: Dosing Guidelines for Adults and Children.* 5th ed. Philadelphia, PA: American College of Physicians; 2007.

Cassileth PA, Harrington DP, Appelbaum FR, et al. Chemotherapy compared with autologous or allogeneic bone marrow transplantation in the management of acute myeloid leukemia in first remission. *NEJM.* 1998;339(23):1649-1656.

Drabco K, Raciborska A, Bilska K, et al. Consolidation of first-line therapy with busulphan and melphalan, and autologous stem cell rescue in children with Ewing's sarcoma. *Bone Marrow Transplantation.* 2012;47:1530-1534.

Ho VT, Aldridge J, Kim HT, et al, Comparison of tacrolimus and sirolimus (Tac/Sir) versus tacrolimus, sirolimus, and mini-methotrexate (Tac/Sir/MTX) as acute graft-versus-host disease prophylaxis after reduced-intensity conditioning allogeneic peripheral blood stem cell transplantation. *Biol Blood Marrow Transplant*, 2009;15(7):844-850.

Hussein AA, Al-Zaben A, Ghatasheh L, et al. Risk adopted allogeneic hematopoietic stem cell transplantation using a reduced intensity regimen for children with thalassemia major. *Pediatr Blood Cancer.* 2013;60:1345-1349.

Le Gall JB, Milone MC, Waxman IM, et al. The pharmacokinetics and safety of twice daily I.V. BU during conditioning in pediatric allo-SCT recipients. *Bone Marrow Transplantation.* 2013;48:19-25.

Liu H, Zhai X, Song Z, et al. Busulfan plus fludarabine as a myeloablative conditioning regimen compared with busulfan plus cyclophosphamide for acute myeloid leukemia in first complete remission undergoing allogeneic hematopoietic stem cell transplantation: a prospective and multicenter study. *J Hematol Oncol.* 2013;6:15-23.

National Institute for Occupational Safety and Health (NIOSH), "NIOSH List of Antineoplastic and Other Hazardous Drugs in Healthcare Settings 2012." Available at http://www.cdc.gov/niosh/docs/2012-150/pdfs/2012-150.pdf. Accessed January 21, 2013.

Ozkaynak MF, Weinberg K, Kohn D, et al, "Hepatic Veno-Occlusive Disease Post-Bone Marrow Transplantation in Children Conditioned With Busulfan and Cyclophosphamide: Incidence, Risk Factors, and Clinical Outcome," *Bone Marrow Transplant*, 1991, 7(6):467-74.

Pulsipher MA, Boucher KM, Wall D, et al. Reduced-intensity allogeneic transplantation in pediatric patients ineligible for myeloablative therapy: results of the Pediatric Blood and Marrow Transplant Consortium Study ONC0313. *Blood.* 2009;114:1429-1436.

Regazzi MB, Locatelli F, Buggia I, et al. Disposition of High Dose Busulfan in Pediatric Patients Undergoing Bone Marrow Transplantation," *Clin Pharmacol Ther*, 1993, 54(1):45-52.

Vassal G, Gouyette A, Hartmann O, et al, "Pharmacokinetics of High-Dose Busulfan in Children," *Cancer Chemother Pharmacol*, 1989, 24 (6):386-90.

◆ **Busulfanum** *see* Busulfan *on page 333*
◆ **Busulfex** *see* Busulfan *on page 333*
◆ **Busulfex® (Can)** *see* Busulfan *on page 333*
◆ **Busulphan** *see* Busulfan *on page 333*
◆ **Butrans** *see* Buprenorphine *on page 320*
◆ **BW-430C** *see* LamoTRIgine *on page 1199*
◆ **BW524W91** *see* Emtricitabine *on page 738*
◆ **C1 Esterase Inhibitor** *see* C1 Inhibitor (Human) *on page 337*

◆ **C1-INH** *see* C1 Inhibitor (Human) *on page 337*
◆ **C1-Inhibitor** *see* C1 Inhibitor (Human) *on page 337*
◆ **C1INHRP** *see* C1 Inhibitor (Human) *on page 337*
◆ **C2B8 Monoclonal Antibody** *see* RiTUXimab *on page 1841*
◆ **C-500 [OTC]** *see* Ascorbic Acid *on page 206*

C1 Inhibitor (Human) (cee won in HIB i ter HYU man)

Brand Names: U.S. Berinert; Cinryze
Brand Names: Canada Berinert
Therapeutic Category Blood Product Derivative
Generic Availability (U.S.) No
Use
Berinert: Treatment of acute abdominal, facial, or laryngeal attacks of hereditary angioedema (HAE) (FDA approved in adolescents and adults)
Cinryze: Routine prophylaxis against angioedema attacks in patients with HAE (FDA approved in adolescents and adults); has also been used for treatment of acute abdominal, facial, and laryngeal attacks of HAE
Prescribing and Access Restrictions Assistance with procurement and reimbursement of Cinryze is available for healthcare providers and patients through the CINRYZE-*Solutions* program (telephone: 1-877-945-1000) or at http://www.cinryze.com/Cinryze_Solutions/Default.aspx
Pregnancy Risk Factor C
Pregnancy Considerations Animal reproduction studies have not been conducted. Although information related to use during pregnancy is limited, plasma-derived human C1 inhibitor concentrate is the preferred treatment for HAE during pregnancy (Baker, 2013; Caballero, 2012). Women with HAE should be monitored closely during pregnancy and for at least 72 hours after delivery (Caballero, 2012).
Breast-Feeding Considerations It is not known if these products are excreted into breast milk. The manufacturers recommend caution be used if needed in a nursing woman. Lactation may increase the frequency of attacks and women should be monitored closely. Plasma-derived human C1 inhibitor concentrate is the preferred treatment for HAE during lactation (Caballero, 2012).
Contraindications Hypersensitivity or history of anaphylactic reactions to human C1 esterase inhibitor (C1-INH) preparations or any component
Warnings Severe hypersensitivity reactions (eg, urticaria, hives, wheezing, tightness of the chest, hypotension, anaphylaxis) may occur rarely during or after administration. Signs and symptoms of hypersensitivity reactions may be similar to the attacks associated with hereditary angioedema; therefore, consideration should be given to treatment methods. In the event of acute hypersensitivity reactions to C1-INH therapy, treatment should be discontinued and epinephrine should be available. Due to the potential for airway obstruction, patients suffering from an acute laryngeal HAE attack and self-administering should be informed to immediately seek medical attention following treatment.

Serious arterial and venous thromboembolic events have been reported at recommended doses and when used off-label at doses higher than recommended. Risk factors may include the presence of an indwelling venous catheter/access device, prior history of thrombosis, underlying atherosclerosis, use of oral contraceptives or certain androgens, morbid obesity, and immobility. Consider potential risk of thrombosis with use; closely monitor patients with preexisting risks for thrombotic events.
Precautions Product of human plasma; may potentially contain infectious agents which could transmit disease. Screening of donors reduces the risk, as does testing and/or inactivation or removal of certain viruses. Infections

thought to be transmitted by this product should be reported to the manufacturer. Products are not interchangeable; one unit of Cinryze is **NOT** equivalent to 1 international unit of Berinert.
Adverse Reactions
Central nervous system: Dizziness, fever, headache
Dermatologic: Erythema, pruritus, rash
Gastrointestinal: Abdominal pain/discomfort, abnormal taste, nausea, vomiting, xerostomia
Genitourinary: Vulvovaginal fungal infection
Local: Infusion-related reactions
Respiratory: Nasopharyngitis,upper respiratory tract infection
Miscellaneous: Flu-like syndrome, hereditary angioedema attack symptoms exacerbated, viral infection
Rare but important or life-threatening: Anaphylactic reaction, chills, hypersensitivity reaction, injection site erythema, injection site pain, shock, stroke, thrombotic events, transient ischemic attack
Drug Interactions
Metabolism/Transport Effects None known.
Avoid Concomitant Use There are no known interactions where it is recommended to avoid concomitant use.
Increased Effect/Toxicity There are no known significant interactions involving an increase in effect.
Decreased Effect There are no known significant interactions involving a decrease in effect.
Stability Store intact vials at 2°C to 25°C (36°F to 77°F); do not freeze. **Protect from light** prior to reconstitution. Once reconstituted, product should be clear and colorless or slightly blue (Cinryze); do not use if turbid, discolored, or contains particles; use within 3 hours (Cinryze) or 8 hours (Berinert) of reconstitution; do not refrigerate or freeze reconstituted solution.
Mechanism of Action C1 inhibitor, one of the serine proteinase inhibitors found in human blood, plays a role in regulating the complement and intrinsic coagulation (contact system) pathway, and is also involved in the fibrinolytic and kinin pathways. C1 inhibitor therapy in patients with C1 inhibitor deficiency, such as HAE, is believed to suppress contact system activation via inactivation of plasma kallikrein and factor XIIa, thus preventing bradykinin production. Unregulated bradykinin production is thought to contribute to the increased vascular permeability and angioedema observed in HAE.
Pharmacodynamics Onset of action:
C1-INH plasma concentration increase: Cinryze: 1 hour or less
Symptom relief; laryngeal:
Berinert: Median: 15 minutes per attack
Cinryze: Pediatric patients 6-17 years: Median: 30 minutes per attack; for the majority of patient unequivocal symptom relief reported within 1 hour (range: 15-135 minutes) (Lumry, 2013)
Duration of Action: Time to complete resolution of HAE symptoms: Berinert: Median: 8.4 hours
Pharmacokinetics (Adult data unless noted)
Distribution: V_{ss}: Berinert:
Children and Adolescents: (6-13 years, n=5): 0.02 L/kg (range: 0.017-0.026 L/kg)
Adults: 0.018 L/kg (range: 0.011-0.028 L/kg)
Half-life elimination:
Berinert:
Children 3 to <12 years: 16.7 hours
Adults: 22 hours (range: 17-24 hours)
Cinryze: 56 hours (range: 11-108 hours)
Time to peak serum concentration: Cinryze: ~4 hours

◄ **Dosing: Usual Note:** Products are not interchangeable; one unit of Cinryze is **NOT** equivalent to 1 unit of Berinert.

Pediatric:

Hereditary angioedema (HAE) attacks; routine prophylaxis: Cinryze: Children ≥6 years (Limited data available) and Adolescents: I.V.: 1000 units every 3-4 days (ie, twice weekly) (Lumry, 2013)

Hereditary angioedema (HAE) attacks (abdominal, facial or laryngeal); treatment:

Berinert: Children ≥6 years (Limited data available) and Adolescents: I.V.: 20 units/kg (Farkas, 2013; Wahn, 2012)

Cinryze: Limited data available: Children ≥6 years and Adolescents: I.V.: 1000 units; may repeat dose in 1 hour if needed (Lumry, 2013)

Adult:

Hereditary angioedema (HAE) attacks; routine prophylaxis: Cinryze: I.V.: 1000 units every 3-4 days

Hereditary angioedema (HAE) attacks (abdominal, facial, or laryngeal); treatment: Berinert: I.V.: 20 units/kg

Administration Parenteral:

Berinert: Allow vials to come to room temperature. Reconstitute each vial with 10 mL of SWI using the provided transfer set; final concentration: 50 units/mL. After combining with diluent, gently swirl (do not shake) vial to completely dissolve powder. Do not use if turbid, discolored, or contains particles. Administer I.V. at recommended infusion rate: 4 mL/minute (200 units/minute); discard any unused product.

Cinryze: Allow vials to come to room temperature. Do not use product if there is no vacuum in the vial. Reconstitute each vial with 5 mL of SWI using the provided transfer set; final concentration 100 units/mL. After combining with diluent, gently swirl (do not shake) vial to completely dissolve powder. Reconstituted product should be clear and colorless or slightly blue; do not use if turbid, discolored, or contains particles. A silicone-free syringe is recommended for reconstitution and administration. Administer I.V. at recommended infusion rate: 1 mL/minute (over 10 minutes; 100 units/minute); discard any unused product.

Self-administration: Following patient or caregiver training and instructions on self-administration, patient or caregiver may self-administer treatment (Berinert) or prophylaxis (Cinryze) therapy. Epinephrine should be available during self-administration in the event of an acute, severe hypersensitivity reaction. Patient suffering from an acute laryngeal HAE attack and self-administering should be informed to seek immediate medical attention following treatment (potential for airway obstruction to occur).

Monitoring Parameters Monitor patient closely for hypersensitivity reaction and thrombotic events during or after administration.

Additional Information

Cinryze: 1 unit corresponds to C1 inhibitor present in 1 mL of normal fresh plasma

Berinert: A single 500 unit vial contains 400-625 units of C1 inhibitor

Dosage Forms Excipient information presented when available (limited, particularly for generics); consult specific product labeling.

Kit, Intravenous:

Berinert: 500 units

Solution Reconstituted, Intravenous [preservative free]:

Cinryze: 500 units (1 ea)

References

Baker JW, Craig TJ, Riedl MA, et al, "Nanofiltered C1 Esterase Inhibitor (Human) for Hereditary Angioedema Attacks in Pregnant Women," *Allergy Asthma Proc,* 2013, 34(2):162-9.

Berinert (C1 esterase inhibitor [human]) [prescribing information]. Kankakee, IL: CSL Behring LLC; February 2014.

Caballero T, Farkas H, Bouillet L, et al, "International Consensus and Practical Guidelines on the Gynecologic and Obstetric Management

of Female Patients With Hereditary Angioedema Caused by C1 Inhibitor Deficiency," *J Allergy Clin Immunol,* 2012, 129(2):308-20.

Cinryze (C1 esterase inhibitor [human]) [prescribing information]. Exton, PA: ViroPharma Biologics, Inc; February 2014

Farkas H, Csuka D, Zotter Z, et al, "Treatment of Attacks With Plasma-Derived C1-Inhibitor Concentrate in Pediatric Hereditary Angioedema Patients," *J Allergy Clin Immunol,* 2013, 131(3):909-11.

Hermans C, "Successful Management With C1-Inhibitor Concentrate of Hereditary Angioedema Attacks During Two Successive Pregnancies: A Case Report," *Arch Gynecol Obstet,* 2007, 276(3):271-6.

Lumry W, Manning ME, Hurewitz DS, et al, "Nanofiltered C1-Esterase Inhibitor for the Acute Management and Prevention of Hereditary Angioedema Attacks Due to C1-Inhibitor Deficiency in Children," *J Pediatr,* 2013, 162(5):1017-22.

Wahn V, Aberer W, Eberl W, et al, "Hereditary Angioedema (HAE) in Children and Adolescents - A Consensus on Therapeutic Strategies," *Eur J Pediatr,* 2012, 171(9):1339-48.

Wasserman RL, Levy RJ, Bewtra AK, et al, "Prospective Study of C1 Esterase Inhibitor in the Treatment of Successive Acute Abdominal and Facial Hereditary Angioedema Attacks," *Ann Allergy Asthma Immunol,* 2011, 106(1):62-8.

♦ **CaEDTA** *see* Edetate CALCIUM Disodium *on page* 729

♦ **Cafcit®** *see* Caffeine *on page* 338

♦ **CAFdA** *see* Clofarabine *on page* 508

♦ **Cafergor (Can)** *see* Ergotamine and Caffeine *on page* 777

♦ **Cafergot** *see* Ergotamine and Caffeine *on page* 777

Caffeine (KAF een)

Brand Names: U.S. Cafcit®; Enerjets [OTC]; No Doz® Maximum Strength [OTC]; Vivarin® [OTC]

Therapeutic Category Central Nervous System Stimulant; Diuretic; Respiratory Stimulant

Generic Availability (U.S.) Yes: Tablet, caffeine and sodium benzoate injection, injection, oral solution

Use

Treatment of idiopathic apnea of prematurity **(caffeine citrate)**

Emergency stimulant in acute circulatory failure; diuretic; treatment of spinal puncture headaches **(caffeine sodium benzoate)**

Pregnancy Risk Factor C

Pregnancy Considerations Adverse events were observed in animal reproduction studies. Caffeine crosses the placenta; serum concentrations in the fetus are similar to those in the mother (Grosso, 2005). Based on current studies, usual dietary exposure to caffeine is unlikely to cause congenital malformations (Brent, 2011). However, available data shows conflicting results related to maternal caffeine use and the risk of other adverse events, such as spontaneous abortion or growth retardation (Brent, 2011; Jahanfar, 2013). The half-life of caffeine is prolonged during the second and third trimesters of pregnancy and maternal and fetal exposure is also influenced by maternal smoking or drinking (Brent, 2011; Koren, 2000). Current guidelines recommend limiting caffeine intake from all sources to ≤200 mg/day (ACOG, 2010).

Breast-Feeding Considerations Caffeine is detected in breast milk (Berlin, 1981; Hildebrant, 1983; Ryu, 1985a); concentrations may be dependent upon maternal consumption and her ability to metabolize (eg, smoker versus nonsmoker) (Brent, 2011). The ability of the breast-feeding child to metabolize caffeine is age-dependent (Hildebrant, 1983). Irritability and jitteriness have been reported in the nursing infant exposed to high concentrations of caffeine in breast milk (Martin, 2007). Infant heart rates and sleep patterns were not found to be affected in normal, full-term infants exposed to lesser amounts of caffeine (Ryu, 1985b).

Contraindications Hypersensitivity to caffeine or any component; sodium benzoate salt form in neonates

Warnings Do not interchange the caffeine citrate salt formulation with the caffeine sodium benzoate formulation; sodium benzoate has been associated with a potentially fatal toxicity ("gasping syndrome") in neonates; the "gasping syndrome" consists of metabolic acidosis, respiratory distress, gasping respirations, CNS dysfunction (including convulsions, intracranial hemorrhage), hypotension and cardiovascular collapse; *in vitro* and animal studies have shown that benzoate also displaces bilirubin from protein-binding sites; avoid use of products containing sodium benzoate in neonates. During a Cafcit® double-blind, placebo-controlled study, 6 of 85 patients developed necrotizing enterocolitis (NEC); 5 of these 6 patients had received caffeine citrate; although no causal relationship has been established, neonates who receive caffeine citrate should be closely monitored for the development of NEC. Caffeine serum levels should be closely monitored to optimize therapy and prevent serious toxicity.

Precautions Use with caution in patients with a history of peptic ulcer, impaired renal or hepatic function, seizure disorders, or cardiovascular disease; avoid in patients with symptomatic cardiac arrhythmias

Adverse Reactions Primarily serum-concentration related.

Cardiovascular: Angina, arrhythmia (ventricular), chest pain, flushing, palpitation, sinus tachycardia, tachycardia (supraventricular), vasodilation

Central nervous system: Agitation, delirium, dizziness, hallucinations, headache, insomnia, irritability, psychosis, restlessness

Dermatologic: Urticaria

Gastrointestinal: Esophageal sphincter tone decreased, gastritis

Neuromuscular & skeletal: Fasciculations

Ocular: Intraocular pressure increased (>180 mg caffeine), miosis

Renal: Diuresis

Drug Interactions

Metabolism/Transport Effects Substrate of CYP1A2 (major), CYP2C9 (minor), CYP2D6 (minor), CYP2E1 (minor), CYP3A4 (minor); **Note:** Assignment of Major/Minor substrate status based on clinically relevant drug interaction potential; **Inhibits** CYP1A2 (weak)

Avoid Concomitant Use

Avoid concomitant use of Caffeine with any of the following: Iobenguane I 123; Stiripentol

Increased Effect/Toxicity

Caffeine may increase the levels/effects of: Formoterol; Indacaterol; Sympathomimetics

The levels/effects of Caffeine may be increased by: Abiraterone Acetate; AtoMOXetine; Cannabinoid-Containing Products; CYP1A2 Inhibitors (Moderate); CYP1A2 Inhibitors (Strong); Deferasirox; Linezolid; Norfloxacin; Stiripentol; Vemurafenib

Decreased Effect

Caffeine may decrease the levels/effects of: Adenosine; Iobenguane I 123; Regadenoson

The levels/effects of Caffeine may be decreased by: Peginterferon Alfa-2b; Teriflunomide

Stability Caffeine citrate: Injection and oral solution contain no preservatives; injection is chemically stable for at least 24 hours at room temperature when diluted to 10 mg/mL (as caffeine citrate) with D_5W, $D_{50}W$, Intralipid® 20%, and Aminosyn® 8.5%; also compatible with dopamine (600 mcg/mL), calcium gluconate 10%, heparin (1 unit/mL), and fentanyl (10 mcg/mL) at room temperature for 24 hours

Mechanism of Action Increases levels of 3'5' cyclic AMP by inhibiting phosphodiesterase; CNS stimulant which increases medullary respiratory center sensitivity to carbon dioxide, stimulates central inspiratory drive, and improves skeletal muscle contraction (diaphragmatic contractility); prevention of apnea may occur by competitive inhibition of adenosine

Pharmacokinetics (Adult data unless noted)

Distribution: V_d:

Neonates: 0.8-0.9 L/kg

Children >9 months to Adults: 0.6 L/kg

Protein binding: 17%

Metabolism: Interconversion between caffeine and theophylline has been reported in preterm neonates (caffeine levels are ~25% of measured theophylline after theophylline administration and ~3% to 8% of caffeine would be expected to be converted to theophylline)

Half-life:

Neonates: 72-96 hours (range: 40-230 hours)

Infants >9 months, Children, and Adults: 5 hours

Time to peak serum concentration: Oral: Within 30 minutes to 2 hours

Elimination:

Neonates ≤1 month: 86% excreted unchanged in urine

Infants >1 month and Adults: Extensively liver metabolized to a series of partially demethylated xanthines and methyluric acids

Clearance:

Neonates: 8.9 mL/hour/kg (range: 2.5-17)

Adults: 94 mL/hour/kg

Dosing: Neonatal Oral, I.V.: Apnea of prematurity: **Caffeine citrate: Note:** Dose expressed as caffeine citrate; caffeine base is 1/2 the dose of the caffeine citrate:

Loading dose: Minimum dose: 20 mg/kg caffeine citrate; loading doses as high as 80 mg/kg of caffeine citrate have been reported (Steer, 2004); some centers repeat a load of 20 mg/kg as caffeine citrate to a maximum cumulative dose load of 80 mg/kg as caffeine citrate in refractory patients (Schmidt, 2006; Schmidt, 2007; Steer, 2004)

Maintenance dose: 5-10 mg/kg/day caffeine citrate once daily starting 24 hours after the loading dose; some centers increase maintenance dose in 5 mg/kg/day increments of caffeine citrate to a maximum of 20 mg/kg/day in refractory patients based on clinical response ± serum caffeine concentrations (Schmidt, 2006; Schmidt, 2007; Steer, 2004)

Dosing: Usual

Stimulant/diuretic: **Caffeine sodium benzoate:** Adults: I.M., I.V.: 500 mg as a single dose

Treatment of spinal puncture headache: **Caffeine sodium benzoate:** Adults: I.V.: 500 mg as a single dose; may repeat in 4 hours if headache unrelieved

Administration

Oral: May be administered without regard to feedings or meals; may administer injectable formulation (caffeine citrate) orally

Parenteral:

Caffeine citrate: Infuse loading dose over at least 30 minutes; maintenance dose may be infused over at least 10 minutes; may administer without dilution or diluted with D_5W to 10 mg caffeine citrate/mL

Caffeine sodium benzoate: I.V. as slow direct injection; for spinal headaches, dilute in 1000 mL NS and infuse over 1 hour; follow with 1000 mL NS, infuse over 1 hour; administer I.M. undiluted

Monitoring Parameters Heart rate, number and severity of apnea spells, serum caffeine levels

Reference Range

Therapeutic: Apnea of prematurity: 8-20 mcg/mL

Potentially toxic: >20 mcg/mL

Toxic: >50 mcg/mL

Dosage Forms Excipient information presented when available (limited, particularly for generics); consult specific product labeling. [DSC] = Discontinued product

Caplet:

NoDoz® Maximum Strength: 200 mg

◄ Injection, solution, as citrate [preservative free]: 20 mg/mL (3 mL) [equivalent to 10 mg/mL caffeine base]

Cafcit®: 20 mg/mL (3 mL) [equivalent to 10 mg/mL caffeine base]

Injection, solution [with sodium benzoate]: Caffeine 125 mg/mL and sodium benzoate 125 mg/mL (2 mL)

Lozenge:

Enerjets®: 75 mg (12s) [classic coffee, hazelnut cream, or mochamint flavor]

Solution, oral, as citrate [preservative free]: 20 mg/mL (3 mL) [equivalent to 10 mg/mL caffeine base]

Cafcit®: 20 mg/mL (3 mL) [equivalent to 10 mg/mL caffeine base]

Tablet: 200 mg

Vivarin®: 200 mg

Extemporaneous Preparations A 10 mg/mL oral solution of caffeine (as citrate) may be prepared from 10 g caffeine (anhydrous) combined with 10 g citric acid USP and dissolved in 1000 mL sterile water. Label "shake well" and "refrigerate". Stable for 3 months (Nahata, 2004).

A 20 mg/mL oral solution of caffeine (as citrate) may be made from 5 g caffeine (anhydrous) combined with 5 g citric acid USP and dissolved in 250 mL sterile water. Stir solution until completely clear, then add a 2:1 mixture of simple syrup and cherry syrup in sufficient quantity to make 500 mL. Label "shake well" and "refrigerate". Stable for 90 days (Eisenberg, 1984).

Eisenberg MG and Kang N, "Stability of Citrated Caffeine Solutions for Injectable and Enteral Use," *Am J Hosp Pharm*, 1984, 41(11):2405-6.

Nahata MC, Pai VB, and Hipple TF, *Pediatric Drug Formulations*, 5th ed, Cincinnati, OH: Harvey Whitney Books Co, 2004.

References

American College of Obstetricians and Gynecologists, "ACOG Committee Opinion No. 462: Moderate Caffeine Consumption During Pregnancy," *Obstet Gynecol*, 2010, 116(2 Pt 1):467-8.

Berlin CM Jr, "Excretion of Methylxanthines in Human Milk," *Semin Perinatol*, 1981, 5(4):389-94.

Bhatt-Mehta V and Schumacher RE, "Treatment of Apnea of Prematurity," *Paediatr Drugs*, 2003, 5(3):195-210.

Brent RL, Christian MS, Diener RM. Evaluation of the reproductive and developmental risks of caffeine. *Birth Defects Res B Dev Reprod Toxicol*. 2011;92(2):152-87.

Erenberg A, Leff RD, Haack DG, et al, "Caffeine Citrate for the Treatment of Apnea of Prematurity: A Double-Blind, Placebo-Controlled Study," *Pharmacotherapy*, 2000, 20(6):644-52.

Grosso LM, Bracken MB. Caffeine metabolism, genetics, and perinatal outcomes: a review of exposure assessment considerations during pregnancy. *Ann Epidemiol*. 2005;15(6):460-6.

Hildebrandt R and Gundert-Remy U, "Lack of Pharmacological Active Saliva Levels of Caffeine in Breast-Fed Infants," *Pediatr Pharmacol*, 1983, 3(3-4):237-44.

Jahanfar S, Jaafar SH. Effects of restricted caffeine intake by mother on fetal, neonatal and pregnancy outcome. *Cochrane Database Syst Rev*. 2013;2:CD006965.

Koren G, "Caffeine During Pregnancy? In Moderation," *Can Fam Physician*, 2000, 46(4):801-3.

Kriter KE and Blanchard J, "Management of Apnea in Infants," *Clin Pharm*, 1989, 8(8):577-87.

Martín I, López-Vílchez MA, Mur A, et al, "Neonatal Withdrawal Syndrome After Chronic Maternal Drinking of Mate," *Ther Drug Monit*, 2007, 29(1):127-9.

Ryu JE, "Caffeine in Human Milk and in Serum of Breast-Fed Infants," *Dev Pharmacol Ther*, 1985a, 8(6):329-37.

Ryu JE, "Effect of Maternal Caffeine Consumption on Heart Rate and Sleep Time of Breast-Fed Infants," *Dev Pharmacol Ther*, 1985b, 8 (6):355-63.

Schmidt B, Roberts RS, Davis P, et al, "Caffeine Therapy for Apnea of Prematurity," *N Engl J Med*, 2006, 354(20):2112-21.

Schmidt B, Roberts RS, Davis P, et al, "Long-Term Effects of Caffeine Therapy for Apnea of Prematurity," *N Engl J Med*, 2007, 357 (19):1893-902.

Steer P, Flenady V, Shearman A, et al, "High Dose Caffeine Citrate for Extubation of Preterm Infants: A Randomised Controlled Trial," *Arch Dis Child Fetal Neonatal Ed*, 2004, 89(6):F499-503.

◆ **Caffeine and Ergotamine** *see* Ergotamine and Caffeine *on page 777*

◆ **Caffeine and Sodium Benzoate** *see* Caffeine *on page 338*

◆ **Caffeine Citrate** *see* Caffeine *on page 338*

◆ **Caffeine Sodium Benzoate** *see* Caffeine *on page 338*

Calamine (KAL a meen)

Therapeutic Category Topical Skin Product

Generic Availability (U.S.) Yes

Use Employed primarily as an astringent, protectant, and soothing agent to relieve itching, pain, and discomfort for conditions such as poison ivy, poison oak, poison sumac, sunburn, insect bites, or minor skin irritations (FDA approved in ages ≥6 months and adults)

Contraindications Hypersensitivity to calamine or any component

Precautions For external use only; avoid contact with eyes and mucous membranes. When using for self-medication (OTC use), discontinue use and contact healthcare provider if needed for >7 days or if condition worsens.

Drug Interactions

Metabolism/Transport Effects None known.

Avoid Concomitant Use There are no known interactions where it is recommended to avoid concomitant use.

Increased Effect/Toxicity There are no known significant interactions involving an increase in effect.

Decreased Effect There are no known significant interactions involving a decrease in effect.

Stability Store at 15°C to 30°C (59°F to 86°F).

Dosing: Usual Skin protectant: Infants, Children, Adolescents, and Adults: Topical: Apply to affected area as often as needed; **Note:** For patients <6 months, consult a physician prior to use.

Administration Topical: Shake well before using. Apply to clean, dry skin; may apply using cotton or a soft cloth. Avoid contact with the eyes and mucous membranes; do not use on open wounds or burns.

Additional Information Active ingredients: Calamine, zinc oxide

Dosage Forms Excipient information presented when available (limited, particularly for generics); consult specific product labeling.

Lotion, External:

Generic: 8% (120 mL, 177 mL, 180 mL, 240 mL)

◆ **Calamine Lotion** *see* Calamine *on page 340*

◆ **Calan** *see* Verapamil *on page 2129*

◆ **Calan SR** *see* Verapamil *on page 2129*

◆ **Calax [OTC] (Can)** *see* Docusate *on page 701*

◆ **Calcarb 600 [OTC]** *see* Calcium Carbonate *on page 346*

◆ **Cal-Carb Forte [OTC]** *see* Calcium Carbonate *on page 346*

◆ **Calci-Chew [OTC]** *see* Calcium Carbonate *on page 346*

◆ **Calcidol [OTC]** *see* Ergocalciferol *on page 774*

◆ **Calciferol [OTC]** *see* Ergocalciferol *on page 774*

◆ **Calcijex (Can)** *see* Calcitriol *on page 342*

◆ **Calcimar (Can)** *see* Calcitonin *on page 340*

◆ **Calci-Mix [OTC]** *see* Calcium Carbonate *on page 346*

◆ **Calcionate [OTC]** *see* Calcium Glubionate *on page 353*

◆ **Calcite-500 (Can)** *see* Calcium Carbonate *on page 346*

Calcitonin (kal si TOE nin)

Medication Safety Issues

Sound-alike/look-alike issues:

Calcitonin may be confused with calcitriol

Miacalcin may be confused with Micatin

Administration issues:

Calcitonin nasal spray is administered as a single spray into **one** nostril daily, using alternate nostrils each day.

Brand Names: U.S. Fortical; Miacalcin
Brand Names: Canada Calcimar
Therapeutic Category Antidote, Hypercalcemia
Generic Availability (U.S.) Yes
Use

Parenteral: Treatment of Paget's disease of bone; adjunctive therapy for hypercalcemia; postmenopausal osteoporosis (FDA approved in adults); has also been used for osteogenesis imperfecta

Intranasal: Postmenopausal osteoporosis in women >5 years postmenopause with low bone mass (FDA approved in adults)

Pregnancy Risk Factor C
Pregnancy Considerations Decreased birth weight was observed in animal reproduction studies. Calcitonin does not cross the placenta. The nasal spray formulations are not indicated for use in pregnancy.

Breast-Feeding Considerations It is not known if calcitonin is excreted in human breast milk. Calcitonin has been shown to decrease milk production in animals. Breast-feeding is not recommended by the manufacturer.

Contraindications Hypersensitivity to calcitonin, salmon protein, or any component

Warnings Analyses of randomized controlled trials (in osteoporosis and osteoarthritis) have demonstrated a statistically significant increase in the risk of the development of cancer in calcitonin-treated patients (compared to placebo). The risk for malignancies is associated with long-term use of calcitonin. Definitive efficacy of calcitonin-salmon in decreasing fractures is lacking compared to other agents approved for osteoporosis treatment. Consider potential benefits of therapy against risks, including the potential risk for malignancy with long-term use.

Precautions Due to potential hypersensitivity reactions, a skin test is recommended prior to initiating parenteral therapy; the skin test is 0.1 mL of 10 unit/mL calcitonin injection in NS (must be prepared) injected intradermally; observe injection site for 15 minutes for wheal or significant erythema; when using intranasal formulation, periodic nasal examinations are recommended. Discontinue for nasal ulcerations >1.5 mm or those that penetrate below the mucosa.

Adverse Reactions

Cardiovascular: Angina pectoris, flushing, hypertension

Central nervous system: Depression, dizziness, fatigue

Dermatologic: Erythematous rash

Gastrointestinal: Abdominal pain, constipation, diarrhea, dyspepsia, nausea

Genitourinary: Cystitis

Hematologic & oncologic: Lymphadenopathy

Infection: Increased susceptibility to infection

Local: Injection site reaction

Neuromuscular & skeletal: Back pain, myalgia, osteoarthritis, paresthesia

Ophthalmic: Abnormal lacrimation, conjunctivitis

Respiratory: Bronchospasm, flu-like symptoms, nasal mucosa ulcer, rhinitis (including ulcerative), sinusitis, upper respiratory tract infection

Rare but important or life-threatening): Alopecia, altered sense of smell, anaphylactic shock, anaphylactoid reaction, anaphylaxis, anemia, anorexia, arthritis, bronchitis, bundle branch block, cerebrovascular accident, cholelithiasis, dermal ulcer, eczema, edema, gastritis, goiter, hearing loss, hematuria, hepatitis, hypersensitivity reaction, hyperthyroidism, malignant neoplasm, migraine, myocardial infarction, nephrolithiasis, neuralgia, nocturia, palpitations, parosmia, periorbital edema, pneumonia, polymyalgia rheumatica, polyuria, pyelonephritis, tachycardia, thrombophlebitis, tissue damage (nasal mucosal excoriation), vitreous opacity, weight gain

Drug Interactions

Metabolism/Transport Effects None known.

Avoid Concomitant Use There are no known interactions where it is recommended to avoid concomitant use.

Increased Effect/Toxicity There are no known significant interactions involving an increase in effect.

Decreased Effect
Calcitonin may decrease the levels/effects of: Lithium

Stability

Injection: Store under refrigeration at 2°C to 8°C (36°F to 46°F); protect from freezing.

Nasal: Store unopened bottle under refrigeration at 2°C to 8°C (36°F to 46°F); do not freeze.

Fortical®: After opening, store for up to 30 days at 20°C to 25°C (68°F to 77°F); excursions permitted to 15°C to 30°C (59°F to 86°F). Store in upright position.

Miacalcin®: After opening, store for up to 35 days at room temperature of 15°C to 30°C (59°F to 86°F). Store in upright position.

Mechanism of Action Peptide sequence similar to human calcitonin; functionally antagonizes the effects of parathyroid hormone. Directly inhibits osteoclastic bone resorption; promotes the renal excretion of calcium, phosphate, sodium, magnesium, and potassium by decreasing tubular reabsorption; increases the jejunal secretion of water, sodium, potassium, and chloride

Pharmacodynamics

Onset of action:

Hypercalcemia: I.M., SubQ: ~2 hours

Paget's disease: Within a few months; may take up to 1 year for neurologic symptom improvement

Duration: Hypercalcemia: I.M., SubQ: 6-8 hours

Pharmacokinetics (Adult data unless noted)

Absorption: Intranasal: Rapidly but highly variable and lower than I.M. administration

Metabolism: Rapidly in the kidneys, blood, and peripheral tissues

Bioavailability: I.M. 66%; SubQ: 71%

Half-life, elimination (terminal): I.M.: 58 minutes; SubQ: 59-64 minutes

Time to peak serum concentration: SubQ ~23 minutes

Elimination: As inactive metabolites in urine

Clearance: Salmon calcitonin: 3.1 mL/kg/minute

Dosing: Usual

Pediatric: **Osteogenesis imperfecta:** Infants >6 months, Children, and Adolescents: I.M., SubQ: 2 units/kg/dose 3 times/week (Castells, 1979)

Adult:

Paget's disease: Miacalcin: I.M., SubQ: Initial: 100 units/day; maintenance dose: 50 units/day or 50-100 units every 1-2 days; may be preferable to maintain doses of 100 units daily for serious deformity or neurologic involvement

Hypercalcemia: Miacalcin: Initial: I.M., SubQ: 4 units/kg every 12 hours for 1-2 days; may increase up to 8 units/kg every 12 hours; if the response remains unsatisfactory after 2 additional days, a further increase up to a maximum of 8 units/kg every 6 hours may be considered

Postmenopausal osteoporosis:

Miacalcin: I.M., SubQ: 100 units every other day

Fortical, Miacalcin: Intranasal: 200 units (1 spray) into **one** nostril daily

Administration

Intranasal: Spray into **one** nostril daily; alternate nostrils to reduce irritation. Before priming a new pump, allow it to reach room temperature first.

Parenteral: Do not exceed 2 mL volume per injection site; may be administered SubQ or I.M. SubQ is preferred for outpatient self administration; I.M. is preferred for larger injection volumes.

Monitoring Parameters Serum electrolytes and calcium; alkaline phosphatase and 24-hour urine collection for hydroxyproline excretion (Paget's disease); urinalysis ▶

(urine sediment); serum calcium; periodic nasal exams (intranasal use only)

Dosage Forms Excipient information presented when available (limited, particularly for generics); consult specific product labeling.

Solution, Injection:
Miacalcin: 200 units/mL (2 mL)

Solution, Nasal:
Fortical: 200 units/actuation (3.7 mL)
Miacalcin: 200 units/actuation (3.7 mL)
Generic: 200 units/actuation (3.7 mL)

References
Castells S, Colbert C, Chakrabarti C, et al, "Therapy of Osteogenesis Imperfecta With Synthetic Salmon Calcitonin," *J Pediatr,* 1979, 95(5 Pt 1):807-11.

◆ **Calcitonin (Salmon)** see Calcitonin on page 340
◆ **Cal-Citrate [OTC]** see Calcium Citrate on page 351

Calcitriol (kal si TRYE ole)

Medication Safety Issues
Sound-alike/look-alike issues:
Calcitriol may be confused with alfacalcidol, Calciferol, calcitonin, calcium carbonate, captopril, colestipol, paricalcitol, ropinirole

Administration issues:
Dosage is expressed in mcg (micrograms), **not** mg (milligrams); rare cases of acute overdose have been reported

Brand Names: U.S. Rocaltrol; Vectical
Brand Names: Canada Calcijex; Rocaltrol; Silkis
Therapeutic Category Rickets, Treatment Agent; Vitamin D Analog; Vitamin, Fat Soluble
Generic Availability (U.S.) Yes

Use
Oral/Injection: Management of secondary hyperparathyroidism and resultant metabolic bone disease in patients with moderate-to-severe chronic renal failure not yet on dialysis (FDA approved in ages ≥3 years and adults); management of hypocalcemia and resultant metabolic bone disease in patients on chronic renal dialysis (FDA approved in ages ≥18 years); management of hypocalcemia in patients with hypoparathyroidism (FDA approved in ages ≥1 year and adults) and pseudohypoparathyroidism (FDA approved in ages ≥6 years and adults)

Topical: Management of mild-to-moderate plaque psoriasis (FDA approved in ages ≥18 years)

Pregnancy Risk Factor C
Pregnancy Considerations Teratogenic effects have been observed in some animal reproduction studies. Mild hypercalcemia has been reported in a newborn following maternal use of calcitriol during pregnancy. Adverse effects on fetal development were not observed with use of calcitriol during pregnancy in women (N=9) with pseudovitamin D-dependent rickets. Doses were adjusted every 4 weeks to keep calcium concentrations within normal limits (Edouard, 2011). If calcitriol is used for the management of hypoparathyroidism in pregnancy, dose adjustments may be needed as pregnancy progresses and again following delivery. Vitamin D and calcium levels should be monitored closely and kept in the lower normal range.

Breast-Feeding Considerations Low levels are found in breast milk (~2 pg/mL).

Contraindications Hypersensitivity to calcitriol or any component; hypercalcemia; vitamin D toxicity; abnormal sensitivity to the effects of vitamin D

Warnings Excessive administration may lead to over suppression of PTH, hypercalcemia, hypercalciuria, hyperphosphatemia, and adynamic bone disease. Acute hypercalcemia may increase risk of cardiac arrhythmias and seizures. Chronic hypercalcemia may lead to generalized vascular and other soft-tissue calcification. Phosphate and vitamin D (and its derivatives) should be withheld during therapy to avoid hypercalcemia. Monitor serum calcium levels closely; the calcitriol dosage should be adjusted accordingly; serum calcium times phosphorus product (Ca x P) should not exceed 65 mg^2/dL^2 for infants and children <12 years of age and 55 mg^2/dL^2 for adolescents and adults. Not indicated for use in patients with rapidly worsening kidney function or those who are non-compliant with medications or follow-up (K/DOQI Guidelines, 2003).

Topical: May cause hypercalcemia; if alterations in calcium occur, discontinue treatment until levels return to normal.

Precautions Hypercalcemia potentiates digoxin toxicity; use concomitantly with caution

Topical: For external use only; not for ophthalmic, oral, or intravaginal use. Do not apply to facial skin, eyes, or lips. Absorption may be increased with occlusive dressings. Avoid or limit excessive exposure to natural or artificial sunlight or phototherapy. The safety and effectiveness have not been evaluated in patients with erythrodermic, exfoliative, or pustular psoriasis.

The parenteral product contains aluminum; toxic aluminum concentrations may be seen with high doses, prolonged use, or renal dysfunction. Premature neonates are at higher risk due to immature renal function and aluminum intake from other parenteral sources. Parenteral aluminum exposure of >4-5 mcg/kg/day is associated with CNS and bone toxicity and tissue loading may occur at lower doses.

Adverse Reactions
Oral, I.V.:
Cardiovascular: Cardiac arrhythmia, hypertension
Central nervous system: Apathy, headache, hyperthermia, psychosis, sensory disturbances, somnolence
Dermatologic: Erythema multiforme, erythematous skin disorders, pruritus, rash, urticaria
Endocrine & metabolic: Dehydration, growth suppression, hypercalcemia, hypercholesterolemia, libido decreased, polydipsia
Gastrointestinal: Abdominal pain, anorexia, constipation, metallic taste, nausea, pancreatitis, stomach ache, vomiting, weight loss, xerostomia
Genitourinary: Nocturia, urinary tract infection
Hepatic: ALT increased, AST increased
Local: Injection site pain (mild)
Neuromuscular & skeletal: Bone pain, myalgia, dystrophy, soft tissue calcification, weakness
Ocular: Conjunctivitis, photophobia
Renal: Albuminuria, BUN increased, creatinine increased, hypercalciuria, nephrocalcinosis, polyuria
Respiratory: Rhinorrhea
Miscellaneous: Allergic reaction, hypersensitivity reactions
Rare but important or life-threatening: Anaphylaxis

Topical:
Dermatologic: Pruritus, psoriasis, skin discomfort
Endocrine: Hypercalcemia
Genitourinary: Urine abnormality
Renal: Hypercalciuria
Rare but important or life-threatening: Kidney stones

Drug Interactions
Metabolism/Transport Effects Substrate of CYP3A4 (major); **Note:** Assignment of Major/Minor substrate status based on clinically relevant drug interaction potential; **Induces** CYP3A4 (weak/moderate)

Avoid Concomitant Use
Avoid concomitant use of Calcitriol with any of the following: Aluminum Hydroxide; Axitinib; Conivaptan; Fusidic Acid (Systemic); Multivitamins/Fluoride (with ADE);

Multivitamins/Minerals (with ADEK, Folate, Iron); Simeprevir; Sucralfate; Sucroferric Oxyhydroxide; Vitamin D Analogs

Increased Effect/Toxicity
Calcitriol may increase the levels/effects of: Aluminum Hydroxide; Cardiac Glycosides; Magnesium Salts; Sucralfate; Vitamin D Analogs

The levels/effects of Calcitriol may be increased by: Calcium Salts; Ceritinib; Conivaptan; CYP3A4 Inhibitors (Moderate); CYP3A4 Inhibitors (Strong); Danazol; Dasatinib; Fusidic Acid (Systemic); Ivacaftor; Luliconazole; Mifepristone; Multivitamins/Fluoride (with ADE); Multivitamins/Minerals (with ADEK, Folate, Iron); Stiripentol; Thiazide Diuretics

Decreased Effect
Calcitriol may decrease the levels/effects of: ARIPiprazole; Axitinib; Ibrutinib; Saxagliptin; Simeprevir

The levels/effects of Calcitriol may be decreased by: Bile Acid Sequestrants; Bosentan; Corticosteroids (Systemic); CYP3A4 Inducers (Strong); Dabrafenib; Deferasirox; Mineral Oil; Mitotane; Orlistat; Sevelamer; Siltuximab; St Johns Wort; Sucroferric Oxyhydroxide; Tocilizumab

Stability Store at room temperature; protect oral and I.V. formulations from light and heat. Do not refrigerate or freeze topical ointment.

Mechanism of Action Calcitriol, the active form of vitamin D (1,25 hydroxyvitamin D_3), binds to and activates the vitamin D receptor in kidney, parathyroid gland, intestine, and bone, stimulating intestinal calcium transport and absorption. It reduces PTH levels and improves calcium and phosphate homeostasis by stimulating bone resorption of calcium and increasing renal tubular reabsorption of calcium. Decreased renal conversion of vitamin D to its primary active metabolite (1,25 hydroxyvitamin D) in chronic renal failure leads to reduced activation of vitamin D receptor, which subsequently removes inhibitory suppression of parathyroid hormone (PTH) release; increased serum PTH (secondary hyperparathyroidism) reduces calcium excretion and enhances bone resorption.

The mechanism by which calcitriol is beneficial in the treatment of psoriasis has not been established.

Pharmacodynamics Oral:
Onset of action: 2 hours
Maximum effect: 10 hours
Duration: 3-5 days

Pharmacokinetics (Adult data unless noted)
Distribution: Breast milk: Very low (levels 2.2 ± 0.1 pg/mL)
Protein binding: 99.9%
Metabolism: Primarily to 1,24,25-trihydroxycholecalciferol and 1,24,25-trihydroxy ergocalciferol
Half-life:
Children 1.8-16 years undergoing peritoneal dialysis: 27.4 hours
Adults without renal dysfunction: 5-8 hours
Adults with CRF: 16.2-21.9 hours
Time to peak serum concentration: Oral: 3-6 hours
Elimination: Feces 27% and urine 7% excreted unchanged in 24 hours
Clearance: Children 1.8-16 years undergoing peritoneal dialysis: 15.3 mL/hour/kg

Dosing: Neonatal
Hypocalcemia secondary to hypoparathyroidism: Oral: 1 mcg once daily for the first 5 days of life
Alternate regimen: Oral: 0.02-0.06 mcg/kg/day; similar dosage has also been described in neonates with DiGeorge syndrome (Miller, 1983)
Hypocalcemic tetany:
I.V.: 0.05 mcg/kg once daily for 5-12 days

Oral: Initial: 0.25 mcg/dose once daily, followed by 0.01-0.10 mcg/kg/day divided in 2 doses (maximum daily dose: 2 mcg)

Dosing: Usual
Management of hypocalcemia in patients with chronic kidney disease (CKD): Indicated for therapy when serum levels of 25(OH)D are >30 ng/mL (75 nmol/L) and serum levels of intact parathyroid hormone (iPTH) are above the target range for the stage of CKD; serum levels of corrected total calcium are <9.5-10 mg/dL (2.37 mmol/L) and serum levels of phosphorus in children are less than age-appropriate upper limits of normal or in adults <4.6 mg/dL (1.49 mmol/L) (K/DOQI Guidelines, 2005):
Children and Adolescents: CKD Stages 2-4: Oral:
<10 kg: 0.05 mcg every other day
10-20 kg: 0.1-0.15 mcg daily
>20 kg: 0.25 mcg daily
Dosage adjustment:
If iPTH decrease is <30% after 3 months of therapy and serum levels of calcium and phosphorus are within the target ranges based upon the CKD Stage, increase dosage by 50%
If iPTH decrease <target range for CKD stage hold calcitriol therapy until iPTH increases to above target range; resume therapy at half the previous dosage (if dosage <0.25 mcg capsule or 0.05 mcg liquid, use every other day therapy)
If serum levels of total corrected calcium exceed 10.2 mg/dL (2.37 mmol/L) hold calcitriol therapy until serum calcium decreased to <9.8 mg/dL (2.37 mmol/L); resume therapy at half the previous dosage (if dosage <0.25 mcg capsule or 0.05 mcg liquid, use every other day therapy)
If serum levels of phosphorus increase to >age-appropriate upper limits, hold calcitriol therapy (initiate or increase phosphate binders until the levels of serum phosphorus decrease to age-appropriate limits); resume therapy at half the previous dosage
Children and Adolescents: CKD Stage 5: Oral, I.V.: Serum calcium times phosphorus product (Ca x P) should not exceed 65 mg^2/dL^2 for infants and children <12 years of age and 55 mg^2/dL^2 for adolescents, serum phosphorus should be within target, serum calcium <10 mg/dL (2.37 mmol/L):
iPTH 300-500 pg/mL: 0.0075 mcg/kg per dialysis session (3 times/week); not to exceed 0.25 mcg daily
iPTH >500-1000 pg/mL: 0.015 mcg/kg per dialysis session (3 times/week); not to exceed 0.5 mcg daily
iPTH >1000 pg/mL: 0.025 mcg/kg per dialysis session (3 times/week); not to exceed 1 mcg daily
Dosage adjustment: If iPTH decrease is <30% after 3 months of therapy and serum levels of calcium and phosphorus are within the target ranges based upon the CKD Stage 5, increase dosage by 50%
Adult CKD Stages 3 or 4: Serum calcium <9.5 mg/dL (2.37 mmol/L), serum phosphorus <5.5 mg/dL (1.77 mmol/L), serum calcium times phosphorus product (Ca x P) <55 mg^2/dL^2:
iPTH 300-600 pg/mL: Oral, I.V.: 0.5-1.5 mcg per dialysis session (3 times/week)
iPTH 600-1000 pg/mL: I.V.: 1-3 mcg per dialysis session (3 times/week); Oral: 1-4 mcg per dialysis session (3 times/week)
iPTH >1000 pg/mL: I.V. 3-5 mcg per dialysis session (3 times/week); Oral: 3-7 mcg per dialysis session (3 times/week)
Dosage adjustment:
If iPTH decrease <target range for CKD stage 5 hold calcitriol therapy until iPTH increases to above target range; resume therapy at half the previous dosage (if dosage <0.25 mcg capsule or 0.05 mcg liquid, use every other day therapy)

If serum levels of total corrected calcium exceed 9.5 mg/dL (2.37 mmol/L) hold calcitriol therapy until serum calcium decreased to <9.5 mg/dL (2.37 mmol/L); resume therapy at half the previous dosage (if dosage <0.25 mcg capsule or 0.05 mcg liquid, use every other day therapy)

If serum levels of phosphorus increase to >4.6 mg/dL (1.49 mmol/L), hold calcitriol therapy (initiate or increase phosphate binders until the levels of serum phosphorus decrease to 4.6 mg/dL (1.49 mmol/L); resume therapy at prior dosage

Note: Intermittent administration of calcitriol by I.V. or oral routes is more effective than daily oral calcitriol in lowering iPTH levels.

Hypoparathyroidism/pseudohypoparathyroidism: Oral (evaluate dosage at 2- to 4-week intervals):
Infants <1 year: 0.04-0.08 mcg/kg once daily
Children 1-5 years: 0.25-0.75 mcg once daily
Children >6 years and Adults: 0.5-2 mcg once daily

Vitamin D-dependent rickets: Children and Adults: Oral: 1 mcg once daily

Vitamin D-resistant rickets (familial hypophosphatemia): Children and Adults: Oral: Initial: 0.015-0.02 mcg/kg once daily; maintenance: 0.03-0.06 mcg/kg once daily; maximum dose: 2 mcg once daily

Psoriasis: Adults: Topical: Apply twice daily to affected areas (maximum: 200 g/week)

Administration
Oral: May be administered with or without meals; when administering small doses from the liquid-filled capsules, consider the following concentration for Rocaltrol®:
0.25 mcg capsule = 0.25 mcg per 0.17 mL
0.5 mcg capsule = 0.5 mcg per 0.17 mL
Parenteral: May be administered undiluted as a bolus dose I.V. through the catheter at the end of hemodialysis
Topical: Apply externally; not for ophthalmic, oral, or intra-vaginal use

Monitoring Parameters Signs and symptoms of vitamin D intoxication
Serum calcium and phosphorus:
I.V.: Twice weekly during initial phase, then at least monthly once dose established
Oral: At least every 2 weeks for 3 months or following dose adjustment, then monthly for 3 months, then every 3 months
Serum or plasma intact parathyroid hormone (iPTH): At least every 2 weeks for 3 months or following dose adjustment, then monthly for 3 months, then as per K/DOQI Guidelines below.
Per Kidney Disease Outcome Quality Initiative Practice Guidelines: Children (K/DOQI, 2005):
Stage 3 CKD: iPTH every 6 months
Stage 4 CKD: iPTH every 3 months
Stage 5 CKD: iPTH every 3 months
Per Kidney Disease Outcome Quality Initiative Practice Guidelines: Adults (K/DOQI, 2003):
Stage 3 CKD: iPTH every 12 months
Stage 4 CKD: iPTH every 3 months
Stage 5 CKD: iPTH every 3 months

Reference Range
Chronic kidney disease (CKD) is defined either as kidney damage or GFR <60 mL/minute/1.73 m² for ≥3 months); stages of CKD are described below:
CKD Stage 1: Kidney damage with normal or increased GFR; GFR >90 mL/minute/1.73m²
CKD Stage 2: Kidney damage with mild decrease in GFR; GFR 60-89 mL/minute/1.73 m²
CKD Stage 3: Moderate decrease in GFR; GFR 30-59 mL/minute/1.73 m²
CKD Stage 4: Severe decrease in GFR; GFR 15-29 mL/minute/1.73 m²
CKD Stage 5: Kidney failure; GFR <15 mL/minute/1.73 m² or dialysis

Target range for iPTH:
Stage 2 CKD: Children: 35-70 pg/mL (3.85-7.7 pmol/L)
Stage 3 CKD: Children and Adults: 35-70 pg/mL (3.85-7.7 pmol/L)
Stage 4 CKD: Children and Adults: 70-110 pg/mL (7.7-12.1 pmol/L)
Stage 5 CKD:
Children: 200-300 pg/mL (22-33 pmol/L)
Adults: 150-300 pg/mL (16.5-33 pmol/L)
Serum phosphorous:
Stages 1-4 CKD: Children: At or above the age-appropriate lower limits and no higher than age-appropriate upper limits
Stage 3 and 4 CKD: Adults: ≥2.7 to <4.6 mg/dL (≥0.87 to <1.49 mmol/L)
Stage 5 CKD:
Children 1-12 years: 4-6 mg/dL (1.29-1.94 mmol/L)
Children >12 years and Adults: 3.5-5.5 mg/dL (1.13-1.78 mmol/L)

Dosage Forms Excipient information presented when available (limited, particularly for generics); consult specific product labeling.
Capsule, Oral:
Rocaltrol: 0.25 mcg, 0.5 mcg [contains fd&c yellow #6 (sunset yellow), methylparaben, propylparaben]
Generic: 0.25 mcg, 0.5 mcg
Ointment, External:
Vectical: 3 mcg/g (100 g)
Generic: 3 mcg/g (100 g)
Solution, Intravenous:
Generic: 1 mcg/mL (1 mL)
Solution, Oral:
Rocaltrol: 1 mcg/mL (15 mL)
Generic: 1 mcg/mL (15 mL)

References
Department Health and Human Services, Food Drug Administration, "Aluminum in Large and Small Volume Parenterals Used in Total Parenteral Nutrition," *Federal Register*, 2000, 65(17):4103-11.
Edouard T, Alos N, Chabot G, et al, "Short- and Long-Term Outcome of Patients with Pseudo-Vitamin D Deficiency Rickets Treated with Calcitriol," *J Clin Endocrinol Metab*, 2011, 96(1):82-9.
"K/DOQI Clinical Practice Guidelines for Bone Metabolism and Disease in Children With Chronic Kidney Disease," *Am J Kidney Dis*, 2005, 46 (4 Suppl 1):S1-121.
"K/DOQI Clinical Practice Guidelines for Bone Metabolism and Disease in Chronic Kidney Disease. Guideline 1. Evaluation of Calcium and Phosphorus Metabolism," *Am J Kidney Dis*, 2003, 42(4 Suppl 3):52-7.
"K/DOQI Clinical Practice Guidelines for Bone Metabolism and Disease in Chronic Kidney Disease. Guideline 3. Evaluation of Serum Phosphorus Levels," *Am J Kidney Dis*, 2003, 42(4 Suppl 3):62-3.
"K/DOQI Clinical Practice Guidelines for Chronic Kidney Disease: Evaluation, Classification, and Stratification, Part 4. Definition and Classification of Stages of Chronic Kidney Disease," *Am J Kidney Dis*, 2002, 39(2 Suppl 1):46-75.
Sanchez CP, "Secondary Hyperparathyroidism in Children With Chronic Renal Failure: Pathogenesis and Treatment," *Paediatr Drugs*, 2003, 5 (11): 763-76.
Ziolkowska H, "Minimizing Bone Abnormalities in Children With Renal Failure," *Paediatr Drugs*, 2006, 8(4):205-22.

◆ **Calcium 600 [OTC]** *see* Calcium Carbonate *on page 346*

Calcium Acetate (KAL see um AS e tate)

Medication Safety Issues
Sound-alike/look-alike issues:
PhosLo® may be confused with Phos-Flur®, ProSom
Brand Names: U.S. Calphron [OTC]; Eliphos; PhosLo; Phoslyra
Brand Names: Canada PhosLo®
Therapeutic Category Calcium Salt; Electrolyte Supplement, Parenteral
Generic Availability (U.S.) May be product dependent
Use Treatment of hyperphosphatemia in end-stage renal failure (FDA approved in adults)
Pregnancy Risk Factor C

Pregnancy Considerations Animal reproduction studies have not been conducted. Calcium crosses the placenta. The amount of calcium reaching the fetus is determined by maternal physiological changes. Intestinal absorption of calcium increases during pregnancy. If use is required in pregnant patients with end stage renal disease, fetal harm is not expected if maternal calcium concentrations are monitored and maintained within normal limits as recommended (IOM, 2011).

Breast-Feeding Considerations Calcium is excreted in breast milk. The amount of calcium in breast milk is homeostatically regulated and not altered by maternal calcium intake (IOM, 2011).

Contraindications Hypersensitivity to calcium formulation; hypercalcemia, renal calculi, ventricular fibrillation

Warnings Multiple salt forms of calcium exist; close attention must be paid to the salt form when ordering and administering calcium; incorrect selection or substitution of one salt for another without proper dosage adjustment may result in serious over- or under-dosing. Some products may contain tartrazine which may cause allergic reactions in susceptible individuals. Avoid use of calcium-containing phosphate binders (calcium acetate or phosphate) in dialysis patients with hypercalcemia or whose plasma PTH concentrations are <150 pg/mL on two consecutive measurements. Mild to severe hypercalcemia may occur; decrease calcium acetate dose or temporarily discontinue, depending on severity of hypercalcemia; in addition, decrease or discontinue any concomitant vitamin D therapy. Chronic hypercalcemia may result in vascular calcification and other soft tissue calcification.

Precautions Use with caution in patients with sarcoidosis, respiratory failure, acidosis, renal or cardiac disease, and in patients who may be at risk of cardiac arrhythmias, including digitalized patients. Hypercalcemia and hypercalciuria are most likely to occur in hypoparathyroid patients receiving high doses of vitamin D. Calcium administration interferes with absorption of some minerals and drugs; use with caution. Some products may contain aspartame which is metabolized to phenylalanine and must be avoided in patients with phenylketonuria.

Adverse Reactions
Endocrine & metabolic: Hypercalcemia
Gastrointestinal: Diarrhea (oral solution), nausea, vomiting
Rare but important or life-threatening: Dizziness, edema, pruritus, weakness

Drug Interactions

Metabolism/Transport Effects None known.

Avoid Concomitant Use
Avoid concomitant use of Calcium Acetate with any of the following: Calcium Salts

Increased Effect/Toxicity
Calcium Acetate may increase the levels/effects of: CefTRIAXone; Vitamin D Analogs

The levels/effects of Calcium Acetate may be increased by: Calcium Salts; Multivitamins/Fluoride (with ADE); Multivitamins/Minerals (with ADEK, Folate, Iron); Thiazide Diuretics

Decreased Effect
Calcium Acetate may decrease the levels/effects of: Bisphosphonate Derivatives; Calcium Channel Blockers; Deferiprone; DOBUTamine; Dolutegravir; Eltrombopag; Estramustine; Multivitamins/Fluoride (with ADE); Phosphate Supplements; Quinolone Antibiotics; Strontium Ranelate; Tetracycline Derivatives; Thyroid Products; Trientine

The levels/effects of Calcium Acetate may be decreased by: Trientine

Food Interactions Foods that contain maltitol may have an additive laxative effect with the oral solution formulation (contains maltitol).

Mechanism of Action Combines with dietary phosphate to form insoluble calcium phosphate which is excreted in feces

Pharmacokinetics (Adult data unless noted)
Absorption: 25% to 35%; varies with age (infants 60%, prepubertal children 28%, pubertal children 34%, young adults 25%); decreased absorption occurs in patients with achlorhydria, renal osteodystrophy, steatorrhea, or uremia
Protein binding: 45%
Elimination: Primarily in the feces as unabsorbed calcium

Dosing: Usual Treatment of hyperphosphatemia in end-stage renal failure: Oral: Adults: Dose expressed in mg of **calcium acetate** (PhosLo®): 1334 mg (two 667 mg capsules) with each meal; may increase up to 2668 mg (four 667 mg capsules) with each meal; can be increased gradually to bring the serum phosphate value <6 mg/dL as long as hypercalcemia does not develop (usual dose: 2001-2668 mg calcium acetate with each meal); do not give additional calcium supplements

Administration Oral: Administer with plenty of fluids with meals to optimize effectiveness

Monitoring Parameters Serum calcium (twice weekly during initial dose adjustments), serum phosphorus; serum calcium-phosphorus product; intact parathyroid hormone (iPTH)

Reference Range
Calcium: Serum calcium: 8.5-10.5 mg/dL
Newborns: 7-12 mg/dL
0-2 years: 8.8-11.2 mg/dL
Serum phosphorus:
Stage 3 and 4 CKD: ≥2.7 to <4.6 mg/dL (adults); within age-appropriate limits (children)
Stage 5 CKD: 3.5-5.5 mg/dL (children >12 years and adults); 4-6 mg/dL (children 1-12 years)
Serum calcium-phosphorus product: Stage 3-5 CKD: <55 mg^2/dL^2 (children >12 years and adults); <65 mg^2/dL^2 (children ≤12 years)

Additional Information 1 g calcium acetate = 250 mg elemental calcium = 12.7 mEq calcium.

Elemental Calcium Content of Calcium Salts

Calcium Salt	Elemental Calcium (mg/1 g of salt form)	Calcium (mEq/g)
Calcium acetate	253	12.7
Calcium carbonate	400	20
Calcium chloride	273	13.6
Calcium citrate	211	10.5
Calcium glubionate	63.8	3.2
Calcium gluconate	93	4.65
Calcium lactate	130	6.5
Calcium phosphate (tribasic)	390	19.3

Dosage Forms Considerations
Calcium acetate is approximately 25% elemental calcium
Calcium acetate 667 mg = elemental calcium 169 mg = calcium 8.45 mEq = calcium 4.23 mmol

Dosage Forms Excipient information presented when available (limited, particularly for generics); consult specific product labeling.
Capsule, Oral:
PhosLo: 667 mg

Generic: 667 mg
Solution, Oral:
Phoslyra: 667 mg/5 mL (473 mL) [contains methylparaben, propylene glycol]
Tablet, Oral:
Calphron: 667 mg
Eliphos: 667 mg
Generic: 667 mg, 668 mg

References

Dietary Reference Intakes for Calcium and Vitamin D, Institute of Medicine (US) Committee to Review Dietary Reference Intakes for Vitamin D and Calcium, Ross AC, Taylor CL, et al, eds, Washington, DC: National Academies Press (US), 2011. Available at http://www.nap.edu/catalog.php?record_id=13050

◆ **Calcium Acetate and Aluminum Sulfate** *see* Aluminum Acetate *on page 110*

◆ **Calcium Antacid [OTC]** *see* Calcium Carbonate *on page 346*

◆ **Calcium Antacid Extra Strength [OTC]** *see* Calcium Carbonate *on page 346*

◆ **Calcium Antacid Ultra Max St [OTC]** *see* Calcium Carbonate *on page 346*

Calcium Carbonate (KAL see um KAR bun ate)

Medication Safety Issues
Sound-alike/look-alike issues:
Calcium carbonate may be confused with calcitriol
Children's Pepto may be confused with Pepto-Bismol products
Maalox and Children's Maalox may be confused with other Maalox products
Mylanta may be confused with Mynatal
International issues:
Remegel [Hungary, Great Britain, and Ireland] may be confused with Renagel brand name for sevelamer [U.S., Canada, and multiple international markets]
Remegel: Brand name for calcium carbonate [Hungary, Great Britain, and Ireland], but also the brand name for aluminum hydroxide and magnesium carbonate [Netherlands]

Brand Names: U.S. Alcalak [OTC]; Antacid Extra Strength [OTC]; Antacid [OTC]; Cal-Carb Forte [OTC]; Cal-Gest Antacid [OTC]; Cal-Mint [OTC]; Calcarb 600 [OTC]; Calci-Chew [OTC]; Calci-Mix [OTC]; Calcium 600 [OTC]; Calcium Antacid Extra Strength [OTC]; Calcium Antacid Ultra Max St [OTC]; Calcium Antacid [OTC]; Calcium High Potency [OTC]; Caltrate 600 [OTC]; Florical [OTC]; Maalox Childrens [OTC]; Maalox [OTC]; Os-Cal [OTC] [DSC]; Oysco 500 [OTC]; Titralac [OTC]; Tums E-X 750 [OTC]; Tums Freshers [OTC]; Tums Kids [OTC]; Tums Lasting Effects [OTC]; Tums Smoothies [OTC]; Tums Ultra 1000 [OTC]; Tums [OTC]

Brand Names: Canada Apo-Cal; Calcite-500; Caltrate; Caltrate Select; Os-Cal; Tums Chews Extra Strength; Tums Extra Strength; Tums Regular Strength; Tums Smoothies; Tums Ultra Strength

Therapeutic Category Antacid; Calcium Salt; Electrolyte Supplement, Oral

Generic Availability (U.S.) May be product dependent

Use Symptomatic relief of hyperacidity associated with peptic ulcer, gastritis, esophagitis, and hiatal hernia; treatment of hyperphosphatemia in end-stage renal failure; dietary supplement; prevention and treatment of calcium deficiency; topical treatment of hydrofluoric acid burns; adjunctive prevention and treatment of osteoporosis

Pregnancy Considerations Calcium crosses the placenta. Intestinal absorption of calcium increases during pregnancy. The amount of calcium reaching the fetus is determined by maternal physiological changes. Calcium requirements are the same in pregnant and nonpregnant females (IOM, 2011). Calcium-based antacids are considered low risk during pregnancy; excessive use should be avoided (Mahadevan, 2006).

Breast-Feeding Considerations Calcium is excreted in breast milk. The amount of calcium in breast milk is homeostatically regulated and not altered by maternal calcium intake. Calcium requirements are the same in lactating and nonlactating females (IOM 2011). Calcium-based antacids are probably compatible with breast-feeding (Mahadevan, 2006).

Contraindications Hypersensitivity to calcium formulation; hypercalcemia, renal calculi, ventricular fibrillation

Warnings Multiple salt forms of calcium exist; close attention must be paid to the salt form when ordering and administering calcium; incorrect selection or substitution of one salt for another without proper dosage adjustment may result in serious over- or under-dosing. Some products may contain tartrazine which may cause allergic reactions in susceptible individuals.

Precautions Use cautiously in patients with sarcoidosis, respiratory failure, acidosis, renal or cardiac disease; some chewable tablets contain phenylalanine which must be avoided in patients with phenylketonuria; some products may contain aspartame which is metabolized to phenylalanine and must be avoided in patients with phenylketonuria

Adverse Reactions Well tolerated
Central nervous system: Headache
Endocrine & metabolic: Hypercalcemia, hypophosphatemia
Gastrointestinal: Abdominal pain, acid rebound, anorexia, constipation, flatulence, laxative effect, nausea, vomiting, xerostomia
Miscellaneous: Milk-alkali syndrome with very high, chronic dosing and/or renal failure (or alkalosis, headache, hypercalcemia, irritability, nausea, renal impairment, weakness)

Drug Interactions
Metabolism/Transport Effects None known.
Avoid Concomitant Use
Avoid concomitant use of Calcium Carbonate with any of the following: Calcium Acetate; PONATinib
Increased Effect/Toxicity
Calcium Carbonate may increase the levels/effects of: Amphetamines; Calcium Acetate; Calcium Polystyrene Sulfonate; Dexmethylphenidate; Methylphenidate; QuiNIDine; Sodium Polystyrene Sulfonate; Vitamin D Analogs

The levels/effects of Calcium Carbonate may be increased by: Multivitamins/Fluoride (with ADE); Thiazide Diuretics
Decreased Effect
Calcium Carbonate may decrease the levels/effects of: ACE Inhibitors; Allopurinol; Anticonvulsants (Hydantoin); Antipsychotic Agents (Phenothiazines); Atazanavir; Bisacodyl; Bisphosphonate Derivatives; Bosutinib; Calcium Channel Blockers; Cefditoren; Cefpodoxime; Cefuroxime; Chloroquine; Corticosteroids (Oral); Dabigatran Etexilate; Dabrafenib; Dasatinib; Deferiprone; Delavirdine; DOBUTamine; Dolutegravir; Eltrombopag; Elvitegravir; Erlotinib; Estramustine; Gabapentin; HMG-CoA Reductase Inhibitors; Hyoscyamine; Iron Salts; Isoniazid; Itraconazole; Ketoconazole (Systemic); Mesalamine; Methenamine; Multivitamins/Fluoride (with ADE); Multivitamins/Minerals (with ADEK, Folate, Iron); Mycophenolate; Nilotinib; PAZOPanib; PenicillAMINE; Phosphate Supplements; PONATinib; Potassium Acid Phosphate; Protease Inhibitors; Quinolone Antibiotics; Rilpivirine; Riociguat; Strontium Ranelate; Sulpiride; Tetracycline Derivatives; Thyroid Products; Trientine; Vismodegib

The levels/effects of Calcium Carbonate may be decreased by: Trientine

Food Interactions Food may increase calcium absorption. Calcium may decrease iron absorption. Bran, foods high in oxalates, or whole grain cereals may decrease calcium absorption. Management: Administer preferably with food.

Stability Store at room temperature.

Mechanism of Action As dietary supplement, used to prevent or treat negative calcium balance; in osteoporosis, it helps to prevent or decrease the rate of bone loss. Calcium is an integral component of the skeleton and also moderates nerve and muscle performance and allows normal cardiac function. Also used to treat hyperphosphatemia in patients with chronic kidney disease by combining with dietary phosphate to form insoluble calcium phosphate, which is excreted in feces. Calcium salts as antacids neutralize gastric acidity resulting in increased gastric and duodenal bulk pH; they additionally inhibit proteolytic activity of pepsin if the pH is increased >4 and increase lower esophageal sphincter tone (IOM, 2011).

Pharmacodynamics Acid neutralizing capacity: Tums® 500 mg: 10 mEq, Tums® E-X 750 mg: 15mEq; Tums® Ultra 1000 mg: 20 mEq

Pharmacokinetics (Adult data unless noted)

Absorption: 25% to 35%; varies with age (infants 60%, prepubertal children 28%, pubertal children 34%, young adults 25%); decreased absorption occurs in patients with achlorhydria, renal osteodystrophy, steatorrhea, or uremia

Protein binding: 45%

Elimination: Primarily in the feces as unabsorbed calcium

Dosing: Neonatal Oral:

Adequate intake (AI): 200 mg/day of **elemental calcium**; requirements may vary on prematurity, postnatal age, and other clinical factors; serum calcium concentrations should be monitored closely to determine patient-specific needs

Hypocalcemia: Dose depends on clinical condition and serum calcium concentration: Dose expressed in mg of **elemental calcium**: 50-150 mg/kg/day in 4-6 divided doses; not to exceed 1000 mg/day (Avery, 1994; Riga, 2007; Thomas, 2012)

Dosing: Usual Oral:

Adequate intake (AI): Dosage expressed in terms of **elemental calcium**:
1-6 months: 200 mg/day
7-12 months: 260 mg/day

Recommended daily allowance (RDA): Dosage expressed in terms of **elemental calcium**; during pregnancy and lactation, requirements may change:
1-3 years: 700 mg/day
4-8 years: 1000 mg/day
9-18 years: 1300 mg/day
Females 19-50 years, males 19-70 years: 1000 mg/day
Females ≥51 years, males ≥71 years: 1200 mg/day

Antacid:

Children 2-5 years: Children's Pepto: 1 tablet (400 mg calcium carbonate) as symptoms occur; not to exceed 3 tablets/day

Children >5-11 years: Children's Pepto: 2 tablets (800 mg calcium carbonate) as symptoms occur; not to exceed 6 tablets/day

Children >11 years and Adults:

Tums®, Tums® E-X: Chew 2-4 tablets as symptoms occur; not to exceed 15 tablets (Tums®) or 10 tablets (Tums® E-X) per day

Tums® Ultra: Chew 2-3 tablets as symptoms occur; not to exceed 7 tablets per day

Hypocalcemia: Dose depends on clinical condition and serum calcium concentration: Dose expressed as **elemental calcium**:

Infants and Children: 45-65 mg/kg/day in 4 divided doses (Nelson, 1996)

Adults: 1-2 g or more per day in 3-4 divided doses

Treatment of hyperphosphatemia in end-stage renal failure: Children and Adults: Dose expressed as **calcium carbonate**: 1 g with each meal; increase as needed; range: 4-7 g/day

Adjunctive prevention and treatment of osteoporosis: Adults: 500 mg **elemental calcium** 2-3 times/day; recommended dosage includes dietary intake and should be adjusted depending upon the patient's diet; to improve absorption do not administer more than 500 mg **elemental calcium**/dose

Hydrofluoric acid (HF) burns (HF concentration <20%): Topical: Various topical calcium preparations have been used anecdotally for treatment of dermal exposure to HF solutions; calcium carbonate at concentrations ranging from 2.5% to 33% has been used; a topical calcium carbonate preparation must be compounded; apply topically as needed

Dosage adjustment in renal impairment: CrCl <25 mL/minute may require dosage adjustment depending upon serum calcium level

Administration

Oral: Administer with plenty of fluids with or immediately following meals; if using for phosphate-binding, administer with meals

Suspension: Shake well before administration

Chewable tablets: Thoroughly chew tablets before swallowing

Topical: Massage calcium carbonate slurry into exposed area for 15 minutes

Monitoring Parameters Serum calcium (ionized calcium preferred if available), phosphate, magnesium, heart rate, ECG

Reference Range

Calcium: Newborns: 7-12 mg/dL; 0-2 years: 8.8-11.2 mg/dL; 2 years to adults: 9-11 mg/dL

Calcium, ionized, whole blood: 4.4-5.4 mg/dL

Additional Information 1 g calcium carbonate = 400 mg elemental calcium = 20 mEq calcium. Due to a poor correlation between the serum ionized calcium (free) and total serum calcium, particularly in states of low albumin or acid/base imbalances, direct measurement of ionized calcium is recommended. If ionized calcium is unavailable, in low albumin states, the corrected **total** serum calcium may be estimated by this equation (assuming a normal albumin of 4 g/dL); [(4 − patient's albumin) x 0.8] + patient's measured total calcium

Elemental Calcium Content of Calcium Salts

Calcium Salt	Elemental Calcium (mg/1 g of salt form)	Calcium (mEq/g)
Calcium acetate	253	12.7
Calcium carbonate	400	20
Calcium chloride	273	13.6
Calcium citrate	211	10.5
Calcium glubionate	63.8	3.2
Calcium gluconate	93	4.65
Calcium lactate	130	6.5
Calcium phosphate (tribasic)	390	19.3

Dosage Forms Considerations

1 g calcium carbonate = elemental calcium 400 mg = calcium 20 mEq = calcium 10 mmol

Dosage Forms Excipient information presented when available (limited, particularly for generics); consult specific product labeling. [DSC] = Discontinued product

Capsule, Oral:
Calci-Mix: 1250 mg
Florical: 364 mg
Powder, Oral:
Generic: 800 mg/2 g (480 g)
Suspension, Oral:
Generic: 1250 mg/5 mL (5 mL, 473 mL, 500 mL)
Tablet, Oral:
Cal-Carb Forte: 1250 mg
Calcarb 600: 1500 mg [scored]
Calcium 600: 600 mg [scored]
Calcium 600: 600 mg [contains fd&c yellow #6 aluminum lake, soy polysaccharides]
Calcium High Potency: 600 mg
Caltrate 600: 1500 mg [scored]
Florical: 364 mg
Oysco 500: 500 mg [contains brilliant blue fcf (fd&c blue #1), tartrazine (fd&c yellow #5)]
Generic: 500 mg, 600 mg, 648 mg [DSC], 1250 mg
Tablet, Oral [preservative free]:
Calcium 600: 600 mg [lactose free, salt free, sugar free]
Generic: 500 mg, 600 mg, 1250 mg
Tablet Chewable, Oral:
Alcalak: 420 mg [mint flavor]
Antacid: 420 mg [mint flavor]
Antacid: 500 mg
Antacid: 500 mg [assorted fruit flavor]
Antacid: 500 mg [peppermint flavor]
Antacid: 500 mg [contains brilliant blue fcf (fd&c blue #1), fd&c yellow #10 (quinoline yellow), fd&c yellow #6 (sunset yellow)]
Antacid: 500 mg [contains fd&c blue #1 aluminum lake, fd&c red #40 aluminum lake, fd&c yellow #5 aluminum lake, fd&c yellow #6 aluminum lake]
Antacid Extra Strength: 750 mg [contains brilliant blue fcf (fd&c blue #1), fd&c red #40]
Antacid Extra Strength: 750 mg [contains fd&c red #40, fd&c yellow #6 (sunset yellow), tartrazine (fd&c yellow #5)]
Cal-Gest Antacid: 500 mg [contains fd&c blue #1 aluminum lake, fd&c yellow #10 aluminum lake, fd&c yellow #6 aluminum lake]
Cal-Mint: 260 mg [animal products free, gelatin free, gluten free, lactose free, no artificial color(s), no artificial flavor(s), starch free, sugar free, yeast free]
Calci-Chew: 1250 mg [cherry flavor]
Calcium Antacid: 500 mg
Calcium Antacid: 500 mg [contains brilliant blue fcf (fd&c blue #1), fd&c red #40, fd&c yellow #6 (sunset yellow), soybeans (glycine max), tartrazine (fd&c yellow #5); assorted flavor]
Calcium Antacid: 500 mg [contains fd&c blue #1 aluminum lake]
Calcium Antacid Extra Strength: 750 mg [assorted fruit flavor]
Calcium Antacid Extra Strength: 750 mg [contains brilliant blue fcf (fd&c blue #1), fd&c red #40, fd&c yellow #6 (sunset yellow), tartrazine (fd&c yellow #5); assorted flavor]
Calcium Antacid Extra Strength: 750 mg [contains fd&c blue #1 aluminum lake, fd&c red #40 aluminum lake]
Calcium Antacid Ultra Max St: 1000 mg [contains brilliant blue fcf (fd&c blue #1), fd&c red #40, fd&c yellow #6 (sunset yellow), soybeans (glycine max), tartrazine (fd&c yellow #5)]
Maalox: 600 mg [contains aspartame; wild berry flavor]
Maalox Childrens: 400 mg [contains aspartame; wild berry flavor]
Os-Cal: 1250 mg [DSC]
Titralac: 420 mg [low sodium, sugar free; contains saccharin]
Tums: 500 mg [gluten free]
Tums: 500 mg [gluten free; contains fd&c blue #1 aluminum lake, fd&c red #40 aluminum lake, fd&c yellow #6 aluminum lake, tartrazine (fd&c yellow #5)]
Tums E-X 750: 750 mg
Tums E-X 750: 750 mg [assorted flavor]
Tums E-X 750: 750 mg [gluten free; contains fd&c blue #1 aluminum lake, fd&c red #40 aluminum lake; assorted berries flavor]
Tums E-X 750: 750 mg [gluten free; contains fd&c blue #1 aluminum lake, fd&c red #40 aluminum lake, fd&c yellow #5 aluminum lake, fd&c yellow #6 aluminum lake; assorted fruit flavor]
Tums E-X 750: 750 mg [sugar free]
Tums Freshers: 500 mg [gluten free; contains brilliant blue fcf (fd&c blue #1); mint flavor]
Tums Kids: 750 mg [scored; contains fd&c blue #1 aluminum lake, fd&c red #40 aluminum lake; cherry flavor]
Tums Lasting Effects: 500 mg [contains fd&c red #40 aluminum lake, fd&c yellow #6 aluminum lake, tartrazine (fd&c yellow #5)]
Tums Smoothies: 750 mg [peppermint flavor]
Tums Smoothies: 750 mg [contains fd&c blue #1 aluminum lake, fd&c red #40 aluminum lake, fd&c yellow #6 aluminum lake, soybeans (glycine max); assorted tropical fruit flavor]
Tums Smoothies: 750 mg [contains fd&c blue #1 aluminum lake, fd&c red #40 aluminum lake, soybeans (glycine max); berry flavor]
Tums Smoothies: 750 mg [gluten free; contains fd&c blue #1 aluminum lake, fd&c red #40 aluminum lake, fd&c yellow #5 aluminum lake, fd&c yellow #6 aluminum lake, milk (cow)]
Tums Ultra 1000: 1000 mg [peppermint flavor]
Tums Ultra 1000: 1000 mg [contains fd&c blue #1 aluminum lake, fd&c red #40 aluminum lake, fd&c yellow #5 aluminum lake, fd&c yellow #6 aluminum lake; assorted berries flavor]
Tums Ultra 1000: 1000 mg [contains fd&c red #40 aluminum lake, fd&c yellow #6 aluminum lake, tartrazine (fd&c yellow #5); assorted tropical fruit flavor]
Tums Ultra 1000: 1000 mg [DSC] [gluten free]
Tums Ultra 1000: 1000 mg [gluten free; contains fd&c blue #1 aluminum lake, fd&c red #40 aluminum lake, fd&c yellow #6 aluminum lake, tartrazine (fd&c yellow #5)]
Generic: 260 mg, 500 mg
Tablet Chewable, Oral [preservative free]:
Generic: 500 mg

References

Avery GB, Fletcher MA, MacDonald MG, eds. Neonatology - Pathophysiology and Management of the Newborn. 4th ed. J.B. Philadelphia, PA: Lippincott Company; 1993.

Dietary Reference Intakes for Calcium and Vitamin D, Institute of Medicine (US) Committee to Review Dietary Reference Intakes for Vitamin D and Calcium, Ross AC, Taylor CL, et al, eds, Washington, DC: National Academies Press (US), 2011. Available at http://www.nap.edu/catalog.php?record_id=13050

Mahadevan U and Kane S, "American Gastroenterological Association Institute Medical Position Statement on the Use of Gastrointestinal Medications in Pregnancy," Gastroenterology, 2006, 131(1):278-82.

Nelson WE, Behrman RE, Kliegman RM, Arvin AM, eds. Nelson Textbook of Pediatrics. 15th ed. Philadelphia, PA: WR Saunders Company; 2004.

Rigo J, Pieltain C, Salle B, Senterre J. Enteral calcium, phosphate and vitamin D requirements and bone mineralization in preterm infants. Acta Paediatr. 2007;96(7):969-974.

Thomas TC, Smith JM, White PC, Adhikari S. Transient neonatal hypocalcemia: presentation and outcomes. Pediatrics. 2012;129(6):e1461-1467.

Calcium Chloride (KAL see um KLOR ide)

Medication Safety Issues

Sound-alike/look-alike issues:

Calcium chloride may be confused with calcium gluconate

Administration issues:

Calcium chloride may be confused with calcium gluconate.

Confusion with the different intravenous salt forms of calcium has occurred. There is a threefold difference in the primary cation concentration between calcium chloride (in which 1 g = 14 mEq [270 mg] of elemental Ca++) and calcium gluconate (in which 1 g = 4.65 mEq [90 mg] of elemental Ca++).

Prescribers should specify which salt form is desired. Dosages should be expressed either as mEq, mg, or grams of the salt form.

Related Information

Management of Drug Extravasations *on page 2255*

Therapeutic Category Calcium Salt; Electrolyte Supplement, Parenteral

Generic Availability (U.S.) Yes

Use Treatment of hypocalcemia and conditions secondary to hypocalcemia (eg, tetany, seizures, arrhythmias); treatment of cardiac disturbances secondary to hyperkalemia; adjunctive treatment of magnesium sulfate overdose [All indications: FDA approved in pediatric patients (age not specified) and adults]; has also been used for calcium channel blocker toxicity, or beta-blocker toxicity refractory to glucagon and vasopressors

Pregnancy Risk Factor C

Pregnancy Considerations Animal reproduction studies have not been conducted. Calcium crosses the placenta. The amount of calcium reaching the fetus is determined by maternal physiological changes. Calcium requirements are the same in pregnant and nonpregnant females (IOM, 2011). Information related to use as an antidote in pregnancy is limited. In general, medications used as antidotes should take into consideration the health and prognosis of the mother; antidotes should be administered to pregnant women if there is a clear indication for use and should not be withheld because of fears of teratogenicity (Bailey, 2003).

Breast-Feeding Considerations Calcium is excreted in breast milk. The amount of calcium in breast milk is homeostatically regulated and not altered by maternal calcium intake. Calcium requirements are the same in lactating and nonlactating females (IOM, 2011).

Contraindications Hypersensitivity to calcium formulation; hypercalcemia; known or suspected digoxin toxicity, ventricular fibrillation; not recommended as routine treatment in cardiac arrest (includes asystole, pulseless ventricular tachycardia, or pulseless electrical activity); in neonates: Concurrent intravenous use with ceftriaxone

Warnings Multiple salt forms of calcium exist; close attention must be paid to the salt form when ordering and administering calcium; incorrect selection or substitution of one salt for another without proper dosage adjustment may result in serious over- or underdosing. For I.V. use only; do not inject SubQ or I.M.; avoid rapid I.V. administration (do not exceed 100 mg/minute except in emergency situations). Avoid extravasation; adverse events from extravasation can be devastating (eg, profound tissue necrosis); monitor the I.V. site closely.

The parenteral product contains aluminum; toxic aluminum concentrations may be seen with high doses, prolonged use, or renal dysfunction. Premature neonates are at higher risk due to immature renal function and aluminum intake from other parenteral sources. Parenteral aluminum exposure of >4-5 mcg/kg/day is associated with CNS and bone toxicity and tissue loading may occur at lower doses.

Ceftriaxone may complex with calcium causing precipitation. Fatal lung and kidney damage associated with calcium-ceftriaxone precipitates has been observed in premature and term neonates. Due to reports of precipitation reaction in neonates, do not coadminister ceftriaxone with calcium-containing solutions, even via separate infusion lines/sites or at different times in any neonate. Ceftriaxone should not be administered simultaneously with any calcium-containing solution via a Y-site in any patient. However, ceftriaxone and calcium-containing solutions may be administered sequentially of one another for use in patients other than neonates if infusion lines are thoroughly flushed (with a compatible fluid) between infusions.

Precautions Use cautiously in patients with respiratory failure, acidosis, or renal impairment; acidifying effect of calcium chloride may potentiate acidosis. Use with caution in patients with chronic renal failure to avoid hypercalcemia; frequent monitoring of serum calcium and phosphorus is necessary. Use with caution in patients with severe hyperphosphatemia as elevated levels of phosphorus and calcium may result in soft tissue and pulmonary arterial calcium-phosphate precipitation. Use with caution in patients with severe hypokalemia as acute rises in serum calcium levels may result in life-threatening cardiac arrhythmias. Hypomagnesemia is a common cause of hypocalcemia; therefore, correction of hypocalcemia may be difficult in patients with concomitant hypomagnesemia. Evaluate serum magnesium and correct hypomagnesemia (if necessary), particularly if initial treatment of hypocalcemia is refractory. Use with caution in digitalized patients; hypercalcemia may precipitate cardiac arrhythmias; use is contraindicated with known or suspected digoxin toxicity.

Adverse Reactions

Cardiovascular (following rapid I.V. injection): Arrhythmia, bradycardia, cardiac arrest, hypotension, syncope, vasodilation

Central nervous system: Sense of oppression (with rapid I.V. injection)

Endocrine & metabolic: Hypercalcemia

Gastrointestinal: Irritation, chalky taste

Hepatic: Serum amylase increased

Local (following extravasation): Tissue necrosis

Neuromuscular & skeletal: Tingling sensation (with rapid I.V. injection)

Renal: Renal calculi

Miscellaneous: Hot flashes (with rapid I.V. injection)

Postmarketing and/or case reports: Calcinosis cutis

Drug Interactions

Metabolism/Transport Effects None known.

Avoid Concomitant Use

Avoid concomitant use of Calcium Chloride with any of the following: Calcium Acetate

Increased Effect/Toxicity

Calcium Chloride may increase the levels/effects of: Calcium Acetate; CefTRIAXone; Vitamin D Analogs

The levels/effects of Calcium Chloride may be increased by: Multivitamins/Fluoride (with ADE); Multivitamins/Minerals (with ADEK, Folate, Iron); Thiazide Diuretics

▶

Decreased Effect

Calcium Chloride may decrease the levels/effects of: Bisphosphonate Derivatives; Calcium Channel Blockers; Deferiprone; DOBUTamine; Dolutegravir; Eltrombopag; Multivitamins/Fluoride (with ADE); Phosphate Supplements; Tetracycline Derivatives; Thyroid Products; Trientine

The levels/effects of Calcium Chloride may be decreased by: Trientine

Stability Store intact vials at 20°C to 25°C (68°F to 77°F); excursions permitted to 15°C to 30°C (59°F to 86°F). Although calcium chloride is not routinely used in the preparation of parenteral nutrition, it is important to note that calcium-phosphate stability in parenteral nutrition solutions is dependent upon the pH of the solution, temperature, and relative concentration of each ion. The pH of the solution is primarily dependent upon the amino acid concentration. The higher the percentage amino acids, the lower the pH and the more soluble the calcium and phosphate. Individual commercially available amino acid solutions vary significantly with respect to pH lowering potential and consequent calcium phosphate compatibility.

Mechanism of Action Moderates nerve and muscle performance via action potential excitation threshold regulation

Pharmacokinetics (Adult data unless noted)

Protein binding: 40%, primarily to albumin (Wills, 1971)

Elimination: Primarily feces (80% as insoluble calcium salts); urine (20%)

Dosing: Neonatal

Daily maintenance calcium: I.V.: Dosage expressed in terms of **elemental calcium**: 3-4 **mEq**/kg/**day**

Parenteral nutrition, maintenance requirement (Mirtallo, 2004): I.V.: Dosage expressed in terms of **elemental calcium**: 2-4 **mEq**/kg/**day**

Hypocalcemia: I.V.: Dosage expressed in mg of **calcium chloride**: 10-20 mg/kg/dose, repeat every 4-6 hours if needed

Cardiac arrest in the presence of hyperkalemia or hypocalcemia, hypermagnesemia, or calcium channel blocker toxicity: I.V., I.O.: Dosage expressed in mg of **calcium chloride**: 20 mg/kg; may repeat in 10 minutes if necessary; if effective, consider I.V. infusion of 20-50 mg/kg/**hour**

Tetany: I.V.: Dosage expressed in mg of **calcium chloride**: 10 mg/kg over 5-10 minutes; may repeat after 6 hours or follow with an infusion with a maximum dose of 200 mg/kg/**day**

Dosing: Usual Infants, Children and Adolescents: **Note:** One gram of calcium chloride salt is equal to 270 mg of elemental calcium.

Daily maintenance calcium: I.V.: Dosage expressed in terms of **elemental calcium**

Infants and Children <25 kg: 1-2 **mEq**/kg/**day**

Children 25-45 kg: 0.5-1.5 **mEq**/kg/**day**

Children >45 kg and Adolescents: 0.2-0.3 **mEq**/kg/**day** or 10-20 **mEq**/**day**

Parenteral nutrition, maintenance requirement (Mirtallo, 2004): I.V.: **Note:** Dosage expressed in terms of **elemental calcium**

Infants and Children ≤50 kg: 0.5-4 **mEq**/kg/**day**

Children >50 kg and Adolescents: 10-20 **mEq**/kg/**day**

Hypocalcemia: Note: In general, I.V. calcium gluconate is preferred over I.V. calcium chloride in nonemergency settings due to the potential for extravasation with calcium chloride. Dosage expressed in mg of **calcium chloride**

Manufacturer's recommendations: I.V.: 2.7-5 mg/kg/dose every 4-6 hours; maximum dose: 1000 mg

Alternative dosing: I.V.: 10-20 mg/kg/dose; maximum dose: 1000 mg; repeat every 4-6 hours if needed

Cardiac arrest in the presence of hyperkalemia or hypocalcemia, hypermagnesemia, or calcium channel antagonist toxicity (PALS recommendations):

I.V., I.O.: Dosage expressed in mg of **calcium chloride:** 20 mg/kg/dose (maximum dose: 2000 mg); may repeat in 10 minutes if necessary; if effective, consider I.V. infusion of 20-50 mg/kg/**hour; Note:** Routine use in cardiac arrest is not recommended due to the lack of improved survival (Hegenbarth, 2008; Kleinman, 2010)

Calcium channel blocker toxicity: I.V.: Dosage expressed in mg of **calcium chloride**: 20 mg/kg/dose infused over 5-10 minutes; if effective, consider I.V. infusion of 20-50 mg/kg/**hour**

Hypocalcemia secondary to citrated blood infusion: I.V.: 0.45 mEq **elemental** calcium for each 100 mL citrated blood infused

Tetany:

I.V.: Dosage expressed in mg of **calcium chloride**: 10 mg/kg over 5-10 minutes; may repeat after 6 hours or follow with an infusion with a maximum dose of 200 mg/kg/**day**

Adults: **Dosages are expressed in terms of the calcium chloride salt based on a solution concentration of 100 mg/mL (10%) containing 1.4 mEq (27 mg)/mL elemental calcium.**

Hypocalcemia: I.V.:

Acute, symptomatic: Manufacturer's recommendations: 200-1000 mg every 1-3 days

Severe, symptomatic (eg, seizure, tetany): 1000 mg over 10 minutes; may repeat every 60 minutes until symptoms resolve (French, 2012)

Cardiac arrest or cardiotoxicity in the presence of hyperkalemia, hypocalcemia, or hypermagnesemia (ACLS recommendations): I.V.: 500-1000 mg over 2-5 minutes; may repeat as necessary (Vanden Hoek, 2010). **Note:** Routine use in cardiac arrest is not recommended due to the lack of improved survival (Neumar, 2010).

Dosing adjustment in renal impairment: No initial dosage adjustment necessary; however, accumulation may occur with renal impairment and subsequent doses may require adjustment based on serum calcium concentrations

Dosing adjustment in hepatic impairment: No initial dosage adjustment necessary; subsequent doses should be guided by serum calcium concentrations.

Administration Parenteral: Do not use scalp vein or small hand or foot veins for I.V. administration; central-line administration is the preferred route. Not for endotracheal administration. Do not inject calcium salts I.M. or administer SubQ since severe necrosis and sloughing may occur; extravasation of calcium can result in severe necrosis and tissue sloughing. Stop the infusion if the patient complains of pain or discomfort. Warm solution to body temperature prior to administration. Do not infuse calcium chloride in the same I.V. line as phosphate-containing solutions.

I.V.: For direct I.V. injection infuse slow IVP over 3-5 minutes or at a maximum rate of 50-100 mg calcium chloride/minute; in situations of cardiac arrest, calcium chloride may be administered over 10-20 seconds

I.V. infusion: Dilute to a final concentration of 20 mg/mL; administer 45-90 mg calcium chloride/kg over 1 hour; 0.6-1.2 mEq calcium/kg over 1 hour

Vesicant/Extravasation Risk Vesicant

Monitoring Parameters Serum calcium (ionized calcium preferred if available), phosphate, magnesium, heart rate, ECG

Reference Range

Age		Normal Values Serum Concentration
Calcium, total	Cord blood	9-11.5 mg/dL
	Newborn 3-24 hours	9-10.6 mg/dL
	Newborn 24-48 hours	7-12 mg/dL
	4-7 days	9-10.9 mg/dL
	Child	8.8-10.8 mg/dL
	Adolescent to Adult	8.4-10.2 mg/dL
Calcium, ionized, whole blood	Cord blood	5-6 mg/dL
	Newborn 3-24 hours	4.3-5.1 mg/dL
	Newborn 24-48 hours	4-4.7 mg/dL
	≥2 days	4.8-4.92 mg/dL (2.24-2.46 mEq/L)

Additional Information 1 g calcium chloride = 270 mg elemental calcium = 13.5 mEq calcium. Due to a poor correlation between the serum ionized calcium (free) and total serum calcium, particularly in states of low albumin or acid/base imbalances, direct measurement of ionized calcium is recommended. If ionized calcium is unavailable, in low albumin states, the corrected **total** serum calcium may be estimated by this equation (assuming a normal albumin of 4 g/dL); [(4 − patient's albumin) x 0.8] + patient's measured total calcium

Elemental Calcium Content of Calcium Salts

Calcium Salt	Elemental Calcium (mg/1 g of salt form)	Calcium (mEq/g)
Calcium acetate	253	12.7
Calcium carbonate	400	20
Calcium chloride	273	13.6
Calcium citrate	211	10.5
Calcium glubionate	63.8	3.2
Calcium gluconate	93	4.65
Calcium lactate	130	6.5
Calcium phosphate (tribasic)	390	19.3

Dosage Forms Considerations
1 g calcium chloride = elemental calcium 273 mg = calcium 13.6 mEq = calcium 6.8 mmol

Dosage Forms Excipient information presented when available (limited, particularly for generics); consult specific product labeling.
Solution, Intravenous:
 Generic: 10% (10 mL)
Solution, Intravenous [preservative free]:
 Generic: 10% (10 mL)

References
Bailey B, "Are There Teratogenic Risks Associated With Antidotes Used in the Acute Management of Poisoned Pregnant Women?" *Birth Defects Res A Clin Mol Teratol*, 2003, 67(2):133-40.

Department Health & Human Services, Food Drug Administration, "Aluminum in Large and Small Volume Parenterals Used in Total Parenteral Nutrition," *Federal Register*, 2000, 65(17):4103-11.

Field JM, Hazinski MF, Sayre MR, et al, "Part 1: Executive Summary: 2010 American Heart Association Guidelines for Cardiopulmonary Resuscitation and Emergency Cardiovascular Care," *Circulation*, 2010, 122(18 Suppl 3):640-56.

French S, Subauste J, and Geraci S, "Calcium Abnormalities in Hospitalized Patients," *South Med J*, 2012, 105(4):231-7.

Hegenbarth MA and American Academy of Pediatrics Committee on Drugs, "Preparing for Pediatric Emergencies: Drugs to Consider," *Pediatrics*, 2008, 121(2):433-43.

IOM (Institute of Medicine), Dietary Reference Intakes for Calcium and Vitamin D. Washington, DC: The National Academies Press, 2011.

Kleinman ME, Chameides L, Schexnayder SM, et al, "Part 14: Pediatric Advanced Life Support: 2010 American Heart Association Guidelines for Cardiopulmonary Resuscitation and Emergency Cardiovascular Care," *Circulation*, 2010, 122(18 Suppl 3):876-908.

Mirtallo J, Canada T, Johnson D, et al, "Safe Practices for Parenteral Nutrition," *JPEN J Parenter Enteral Nutr*, 2004, 28(6):S39-70.

Neumar RW, Otto CW, Link MS, et al, "Part 8: Adult Advanced Cardiovascular Life Support: 2010 American Heart Association Guidelines for Cardiopulmonary Resuscitation and Emergency Cardiovascular Care," *Circulation*, 2010, 122(18 Suppl 3):729-67.

Vanden Hoek TL, Morrison LJ, Shuster M, et al, "Part 12: Cardiac Arrest in Special Situations: 2010 American Heart Association Guidelines for Cardiopulmonary Resuscitation and Emergency Cardiovascular Care," *Circulation*, 2010, 122(18 Suppl 3):829-61.

Calcium Citrate (KAL see um SIT rate)

Medication Safety Issues
Sound-alike/look-alike issues:
 Citracal® may be confused with Citrucel®
Brand Names: U.S. Cal-Citrate [OTC]; Calcitrate [OTC]
Brand Names: Canada Osteocit®
Therapeutic Category Calcium Salt; Electrolyte Supplement, Oral
Generic Availability (U.S.) Yes
Use Treatment of hyperphosphatemia in end-stage renal failure; dietary supplement; prevention and treatment of calcium deficiency; adjunctive prevention and treatment of osteoporosis
Pregnancy Considerations Calcium crosses the placenta. Intestinal absorption of calcium increases during pregnancy. The amount of calcium reaching the fetus is determined by maternal physiological changes. Calcium requirements are the same in pregnant and nonpregnant females (IOM, 2011).
Breast-Feeding Considerations Calcium is excreted in breast milk. The amount of calcium in breast milk is homeostatically regulated and not altered by maternal calcium intake. Calcium requirements are the same in lactating and nonlactating females (IOM, 2011).
Contraindications Hypersensitivity to calcium formulation; hypercalcemia, renal calculi, ventricular fibrillation
Warnings Multiple salt forms of calcium exist; close attention must be paid to the salt form when ordering and administering calcium; incorrect selection or substitution of one salt for another without proper dosage adjustment may result in serious over- or under-dosing. Some products may contain tartrazine which may cause allergic reactions in susceptible individuals.
Precautions Use cautiously in patients with sarcoidosis, respiratory failure, acidosis, renal or cardiac disease; some products may contain aspartame which is metabolized to phenylalanine and must be avoided in patients with phenylketonuria
Adverse Reactions
Central nervous system: Headache
Endocrine & metabolic: Hypercalcemia, hypophosphatemia
Gastrointestinal: Abdominal pain, anorexia, constipation, nausea, vomiting
Mild hypercalcemia (calcium: >10.5 mg/dL) may be asymptomatic or manifest itself as anorexia, constipation, nausea, and vomiting

◄ More severe hypercalcemia (calcium: >12 mg/dL) is associated with coma confusion, delirium, and stupor
Miscellaneous: Thirst

Drug Interactions

Metabolism/Transport Effects None known.

Avoid Concomitant Use

Avoid concomitant use of Calcium Citrate with any of the following: Calcium Acetate

Increased Effect/Toxicity

Calcium Citrate may increase the levels/effects of: Aluminum Hydroxide; Calcium Acetate; Vitamin D Analogs

The levels/effects of Calcium Citrate may be increased by: Multivitamins/Fluoride (with ADE); Multivitamins/Minerals (with ADEK, Folate, Iron); Thiazide Diuretics

Decreased Effect

Calcium Citrate may decrease the levels/effects of: Bisphosphonate Derivatives; Calcium Channel Blockers; Deferiprone; DOBUTamine; Dolutegravir; Eltrombopag; Estramustine; Multivitamins/Fluoride (with ADE); Phosphate Supplements; Quinolone Antibiotics; Strontium Ranelate; Tetracycline Derivatives; Thyroid Products; Trientine

The levels/effects of Calcium Citrate may be decreased by: Trientine

Stability Store at room temperature.

Mechanism of Action Moderates nerve and muscle performance via action potential excitation threshold regulation

Pharmacokinetics (Adult data unless noted)

Absorption: 25% to 35%; varies with age (infants 60%, prepubertal children 28%, pubertal children 34%, young adults 25%); decreased absorption occurs in patients with achlorhydria, renal osteodystrophy, steatorrhea, or uremia

Protein binding: 45%

Elimination: Primarily in the feces as unabsorbed calcium

Dosing: Neonatal Oral:

Adequate intake (AI): 200 mg/day of **elemental calcium**; requirements may vary on prematurity, postnatal age, and other clinical factors; serum calcium concentrations should be monitored closely to determine patient-specific needs

Hypocalcemia: Dose depends on clinical condition and serum calcium concentration: Dose expressed in mg of **elemental calcium:** 50-150 mg/kg/day in 4-6 divided doses; not to exceed 1000 mg/day

Dosing: Usual Oral:

Adequate intake (AI): Dosage expressed in terms of **elemental calcium:**

1-6 months: 200 mg/day

7-12 months: 260 mg/day

Recommended daily allowance (RDA): Dosage expressed in terms of **elemental calcium;** during pregnancy and lactation, requirements may change:

1-3 years: 700 mg/day

4-8 years: 1000 mg/day

9-18 years: 1300 mg/day

Females 19-50 years, males 19-70 years: 1000 mg/day

Females ≥51 years, males ≥71 years: 1200 mg/day

Hypocalcemia: Dose depends on clinical condition and serum calcium concentration: Dose expressed as **elemental calcium:**

Children: 45-65 mg/kg/day in 4 divided doses

Adults: 1-2 g or more per day in 3-4 divided doses

Dietary supplement: Adults: 500 mg to 2 g divided 2-4 times/day

Adjunctive prevention and treatment of osteoporosis: Adults: 500 mg **elemental calcium** 2-3 times/day; recommended dosage includes dietary intake and should be adjusted depending upon the patient's diet; to improve

absorption do not administer more than 500 mg **elemental calcium**/dose

Dosage adjustment in renal impairment: CrCl <25 mL/minute may require dosage adjustment depending upon serum calcium level

Administration Oral: Administer with plenty of fluids; may administer without regard to food when using to treat/prevent deficiency conditions; administer with food when treating hyperphosphatemia or when administering granule formulation

Monitoring Parameters Serum calcium (ionized calcium preferred if available), phosphate, magnesium, heart rate, ECG

Reference Range

Calcium: Newborns: 7-12 mg/dL; 0-2 years: 8.8-11.2 mg/dL; 2 years to adults: 9-11 mg/dL

Calcium, ionized, whole blood: 4.4-5.4 mg/dL

Additional Information 1 g calcium citrate = 211 mg elemental calcium = 10.6 mEq calcium. Due to a poor correlation between the serum ionized calcium (free) and total serum calcium, particularly in states of low albumin or acid/base imbalances, direct measurement of ionized calcium is recommended. If ionized calcium is unavailable, in low albumin states, the corrected **total** serum calcium may be estimated by this equation (assuming a normal albumin of 4 g/dL); [(4 − patient's albumin) x 0.8] + patient's measured total calcium

Elemental Calcium Content of Calcium Salts

Calcium Salt	Elemental Calcium (mg/1 g of salt form)	Calcium (mEq/g)
Calcium acetate	253	12.7
Calcium carbonate	400	20
Calcium chloride	273	13.6
Calcium citrate	211	10.5
Calcium glubionate	63.8	3.2
Calcium gluconate	93	4.65
Calcium lactate	130	6.5
Calcium phosphate (tribasic)	390	19.3

Dosage Forms Considerations

1 g calcium citrate = elemental calcium 211 mg = calcium 10.5 mEq = calcium 5.25 mmol

Dosage Forms Excipient information presented when available (limited, particularly for generics); consult specific product labeling.

Capsule, Oral [preservative free]:

Cal-Citrate: 150 mg [dye free]

Granules, Oral:

Generic: 760 mg/3.5 g (480 g)

Tablet, Oral:

Generic: 250 mg, 950 mg, 1040 mg

Tablet, Oral [preservative free]:

Calcitrate: 950 mg [lactose free, milk derivatives/products, no artificial color(s), no artificial flavor(s), sodium free, soy free, sugar free, wheat free, yeast free]

References

Dietary Reference Intakes for Calcium and Vitamin D, Institute of Medicine (US) Committee to Review Dietary Reference Intakes for Vitamin D and Calcium, Ross AC, Taylor CL, et al, eds, Washington, DC: National Academies Press (US), 2011. Available at http://www.-nap.edu/catalog.php?record_id=13050

◆ **Calcium Disodium Edetate** *see* Edetate CALCIUM Disodium *on page 729*

♦ **Calcium Disodiumethylenediaminetetraacetic Acid** *see* Edetate CALCIUM Disodium *on page 729*

♦ **Calcium Folinate** *see* Leucovorin Calcium *on page 1213*

Calcium Glubionate (KAL see um gloo BYE oh nate)

Medication Safety Issues
Sound-alike/look-alike issues:
Calcium glubionate may be confused with calcium gluconate

Brand Names: U.S. Calcionate [OTC]

Therapeutic Category Calcium Salt; Electrolyte Supplement, Oral

Generic Availability (U.S.) Yes

Use Treatment and replacement of calcium deficiency; dietary supplement; adjunctive prevention and treatment of osteoporosis

Pregnancy Considerations Calcium crosses the placenta. Intestinal absorption of calcium increases during pregnancy. The amount of calcium reaching the fetus is determined by maternal physiological changes. Calcium requirements are the same in pregnant and nonpregnant females (IOM, 2011).

Breast-Feeding Considerations Calcium is excreted in breast milk. The amount of calcium in breast milk is homeostatically regulated and not altered by maternal calcium intake. Calcium requirements are the same in lactating and nonlactating females (IOM, 2011).

Contraindications Hypersensitivity to calcium formulation; hypercalcemia, renal calculi, ventricular fibrillation

Warnings Multiple salt forms of calcium exist; close attention must be paid to the salt form when ordering and administering calcium; incorrect selection or substitution of one salt for another without proper dosage adjustment may result in serious over- or under-dosing. Some products may contain tartrazine which may cause allergic reactions in susceptible individuals.

Precautions Use cautiously in patients with sarcoidosis, respiratory failure, acidosis, renal or cardiac disease; some products may contain aspartame which is metabolized to phenylalanine and must be avoided in patients with phenylketonuria

Adverse Reactions Symptoms reported with hypercalcemia:
Gastrointestinal: Abdominal pain, anorexia, constipation, nausea, thirst, vomiting, xerostomia
Genitourinary: Polyuria

Drug Interactions
Metabolism/Transport Effects None known.

Avoid Concomitant Use
Avoid concomitant use of Calcium Glubionate with any of the following: Calcium Acetate

Increased Effect/Toxicity
Calcium Glubionate may increase the levels/effects of: Calcium Acetate; Vitamin D Analogs

The levels/effects of Calcium Glubionate may be increased by: Multivitamins/Fluoride (with ADE); Multivitamins/Minerals (with ADEK, Folate, Iron); Thiazide Diuretics

Decreased Effect
Calcium Glubionate may decrease the levels/effects of: Bisphosphonate Derivatives; Calcium Channel Blockers; Deferiprone; DOBUTamine; Dolutegravir; Eltrombopag; Estramustine; Multivitamins/Fluoride (with ADE); Phosphate Supplements; Quinolone Antibiotics; Strontium Ranelate; Tetracycline Derivatives; Thyroid Products; Trientine

The levels/effects of Calcium Glubionate may be decreased by: Trientine

Food Interactions Food may increase calcium absorption. Calcium may decrease iron absorption. Bran, foods high in oxalates, or whole grain cereals may decrease calcium absorption. Management: Administer preferably with food.

Stability Store at room temperature.

Mechanism of Action As dietary supplement, used to prevent or treat negative calcium balance. The calcium in calcium salts moderates nerve and muscle performance and allows normal cardiac function.

Pharmacokinetics (Adult data unless noted)
Absorption: 25% to 35%; varies with age (infants 60%, prepubertal children 28%, pubertal children 34%, young adults 25%); decreased absorption occurs in patients with achlorhydria, renal osteodystrophy, steatorrhea, or uremia
Protein binding: 45%
Elimination: Primarily in the feces as unabsorbed calcium

Dosing: Neonatal Oral:
Adequate intake (AI): 200 mg/day of **elemental calcium**; requirements may vary on prematurity, postnatal age, and other clinical factors; serum calcium concentrations should be monitored closely to determine patient-specific needs
Hypocalcemia: Dose depends on clinical condition and serum calcium concentration:
Dose expressed in mg of **elemental calcium**: 50-150 mg/kg/day in 4-6 divided doses; not to exceed 1000 mg/day
Dose expressed in mg of **calcium glubionate**: 1200 mg/kg/day in 4-6 divided doses

Dosing: Usual Oral:
Adequate intake (AI): Dosage expressed in terms of **elemental calcium**:
1-6 months: 200 mg/day
7-12 months: 260 mg/day
Recommended daily allowance (RDA): Dosage expressed in terms of **elemental calcium**; during pregnancy and lactation, requirements may change:
1-3 years: 700 mg/day
4-8 years: 1000 mg/day
9-18 years: 1300 mg/day
Females ≥19-50 years, males 19-70 years: 1000 mg/day
Females ≥51 years, males ≥71 years: 1200 mg/day
Dietary supplement: Dosage below based on product containing: 1.8 g calcium glubionate/5 mL (115 mg **elemental calcium**/5 mL)
Infants <12 months: 5 mL/dose 5 times a day; may mix with juice or formula
Children <4 years: 10 mL/dose 3 times a day
Children ≥4 years and Adolescents: 15 mL/dose 3 times a day
Adults: 15 mL/dose 3 times a day
Pregnant or lactating women: 15 mL/dose 4 times a day
Hypocalcemia: Dose depends on clinical condition and serum calcium concentration:
Dose expressed as **elemental calcium**:
Children: 45-65 mg/kg/day in 4 divided doses
Adults: 1-2 g or more per day in 3-4 divided doses
Dose expressed as **calcium glubionate**:
Infants and Children: 600-2000 mg/kg/day in 4 divided doses up to a maximum of 9 g/day
Adults: 6-18 g/day in divided doses
Adjunctive prevention and treatment of osteoporosis: Adults: 500 mg **elemental calcium** 2-3 times/day; recommended dosage includes dietary intake and should be adjusted depending upon the patient's diet; to improve absorption do not administer more than 500 mg **elemental calcium**/dose
Dosage adjustment in renal impairment: CrCl <25 mL/ minute may require dosage adjustment depending upon serum calcium level

Administration Oral: Administer with plenty of fluids with or following meals; for phosphate binding, administer on an empty stomach before meals to optimize effectiveness

Monitoring Parameters Serum calcium (ionized calcium preferred if available), phosphate, magnesium, heart rate, ECG

Reference Range

Calcium: Newborns: 7-12 mg/dL; 0-2 years: 8.8-11.2 mg/dL; 2 years to adults: 9-11 mg/dL
Calcium, ionized, whole blood: 4.4-5.4 mg/dL

Test Interactions Decreased magnesium

Additional Information 1 g calcium glubionate = 64 mg elemental calcium = 3.2 mEq calcium. Due to a poor correlation between the serum ionized calcium (free) and total serum calcium, particularly in states of low albumin or acid/base imbalances, direct measurement of ionized calcium is recommended. If ionized calcium is unavailable, in low albumin states, the corrected **total** serum calcium may be estimated by this equation (assuming a normal albumin of 4 g/dL): [(4 − patient's albumin) x 0.8] + patient's measured total calcium

Elemental Calcium Content of Calcium Salts

Calcium Salt	Elemental Calcium (mg/1 g of salt form)	Calcium (mEq/g)
Calcium acetate	253	12.7
Calcium carbonate	400	20
Calcium chloride	273	13.6
Calcium citrate	211	10.5
Calcium glubionate	63.8	3.2
Calcium gluconate	93	4.65
Calcium lactate	130	6.5
Calcium phosphate (tribasic)	390	19.3

Dosage Forms Considerations

1 g calcium glubionate = elemental calcium 63.8 mg = calcium 3.2 mEq = calcium 1.6 mmol

Dosage Forms Excipient information presented when available (limited, particularly for generics); consult specific product labeling.

Syrup, Oral:
Calcionate: 1.8 g/5 mL (473 mL) [fruit flavor]

References

Dietary Reference Intakes for Calcium and Vitamin D, Institute of Medicine (US) Committee to Review Dietary Reference Intakes for Vitamin D and Calcium, Ross AC, Taylor CL, et al, eds, Washington, DC: National Academies Press (US), 2011. Available at http://www.-nap.edu/catalog.php?record_id=13050

Calcium Gluconate (KAL see um GLOO koe nate)

Medication Safety Issues

Sound-alike/look-alike issues:
Calcium gluconate may be confused with calcium glubionate, cupric sulfate

Administration issues:
Calcium gluconate may be confused with calcium chloride.

Confusion with the different intravenous salt forms of calcium has occurred. There is a threefold difference in the primary cation concentration between calcium gluconate (in which 1 g = 4.65 mEq [90 mg] of elemental Ca++) and calcium chloride (in which 1 g = 14 mEq [270 mg] of elemental Ca++).

Prescribers should specify which salt form is desired. Dosages should be expressed either as mEq, mg, or grams of the salt form.

Related Information

Management of Drug Extravasations *on page 2255*

Brand Names: U.S. Cal-Glu [OTC]

Therapeutic Category Antidote, Hydrofluoric Acid; Calcium Salt; Electrolyte Supplement, Oral; Electrolyte Supplement, Parenteral

Generic Availability (U.S.) Yes

Use

Parenteral: Treatment of hypocalcemia and conditions secondary to hypocalcemia (eg, tetany, seizures, arrhythmias); treatment of cardiac disturbances secondary to hyperkalemia; adjunctive treatment of rickets, osteomalacia, and magnesium sulfate overdose; decrease capillary permeability in allergic conditions, nonthrombocytopenic purpura, and exudative dermatoses (eg, dermatitis herpetiformis, pruritus secondary to certain drugs) (All indications: FDA approved in all ages); has also been used for calcium channel blocker toxicity and as a supplement in total parenteral nutrition admixtures

Oral: Dietary supplementation of calcium (OTC: FDA approved in adults)

Pregnancy Risk Factor C

Pregnancy Considerations Animal reproduction studies have not been conducted. Calcium crosses the placenta. The amount of calcium reaching the fetus is determined by maternal physiological changes. Calcium requirements are the same in pregnant and nonpregnant females (IOM, 2011). Information related to use as an antidote in pregnancy is limited. In general, medications used as antidotes should take into consideration the health and prognosis of the mother; antidotes should be administered to pregnant women if there is a clear indication for use and should not be withheld because of fears of teratogenicity (Bailey, 2003).

Breast-Feeding Considerations Calcium is excreted in breast milk. The amount of calcium in breast milk is homeostatically regulated and not altered by maternal calcium intake. Calcium requirements are the same in lactating and nonlactating females (IOM, 2011).

Contraindications Hypersensitivity to calcium formulation; hypercalcemia, ventricular fibrillation; in neonates: Concurrent intravenous use with ceftriaxone

Warnings Ceftriaxone may complex with calcium causing precipitation. Fatal lung and kidney damage associated with calcium-ceftriaxone precipitates has been observed in premature and term neonates. Due to reports of precipitation reaction in neonates, do not coadminister ceftriaxone with calcium-containing solutions, even via separate infusion lines/sites or at different times in any neonate. Ceftriaxone should not be administered simultaneously with any calcium-containing solution via a Y-site in any patient. However, ceftriaxone and calcium-containing solutions may be administered sequentially of one another for use in patients **other than neonates** if infusion lines are thoroughly flushed (with a compatible fluid) between infusions.

Avoid too rapid I.V. administration; do not exceed 200 mg/minute except in emergency situations; rapid I.V. administration may result in vasodilation, hypotension, bradycardia, arrhythmias, and cardiac arrest. Parenteral calcium is a vesicant; ensure proper catheter or needle position prior to and during infusion. Avoid extravasation; adverse events from extravasation can be devastating (eg, profound tissue necrosis); monitor the I.V. site closely.

Multiple salt forms of calcium exist; close attention must be paid to the salt form when ordering and administering calcium; incorrect selection or substitution of one salt for another without proper dosage adjustment may result in serious over- or under-dosing. Some products may contain tartrazine which may cause allergic reactions in susceptible individuals.

The parenteral product contains aluminum; toxic aluminum concentrations may be seen with high doses, prolonged use, or renal dysfunction. Premature neonates are at higher risk due to immature renal function and aluminum intake from other parenteral sources. Parenteral aluminum exposure of >4-5 mcg/kg/day is associated with CNS and bone toxicity and tissue loading may occur at lower doses.

Precautions Use with caution in patients with chronic renal failure to avoid hypercalcemia; frequent monitoring of serum calcium and phosphorus is necessary. Use with caution in patients with severe hyperphosphatemia as elevated levels of phosphorus and calcium may result in soft tissue and pulmonary arterial calcium-phosphate precipitation. Use with caution in patients with severe hypokalemia as acute rises in serum calcium levels may result in life-threatening cardiac arrhythmias. Hypomagnesemia is a common cause of hypocalcemia; therefore, correction of hypocalcemia may be difficult in patients with concomitant hypomagnesemia. Evaluate serum magnesium and correct hypomagnesemia (if necessary), particularly if initial treatment of hypocalcemia is refractory. Use with caution in digitalized patients; hypercalcemia may precipitate cardiac arrhythmias. Use caution when administering calcium supplements to patients with a history of kidney stones.

Oral calcium administration interferes with absorption of some minerals and drugs; use caution with concomitant administration times; concomitant administration of oral vitamin D and food will optimize calcium absorption.

Adverse Reactions
I.V.:
Cardiovascular (with rapid I.V. injection): Arrhythmia, bradycardia, cardiac arrest, hypotension, syncope, vasodilation
Central nervous system: Sense of oppression (with rapid I.V. injection)
Endocrine & metabolic: Hypercalcemia
Gastrointestinal: Chalky taste
Neuromuscular & skeletal: Tingling sensation (with rapid I.V. injection)
Miscellaneous: Heat waves (with rapid I.V. injection)
Postmarketing and/or case reports: Calcinosis cutis
Oral: Gastrointestinal: Constipation

Drug Interactions
Metabolism/Transport Effects None known.

Avoid Concomitant Use
Avoid concomitant use of Calcium Gluconate with any of the following: Calcium Acetate

Increased Effect/Toxicity
Calcium Gluconate may increase the levels/effects of: Calcium Acetate; CefTRIAXone; Vitamin D Analogs

The levels/effects of Calcium Gluconate may be increased by: Multivitamins/Fluoride (with ADE); Multivitamins/Minerals (with ADEK, Folate, Iron); Thiazide Diuretics

Decreased Effect
Calcium Gluconate may decrease the levels/effects of: Bisphosphonate Derivatives; Calcium Channel Blockers; Deferiprone; DOBUTamine; Dolutegravir; Eltrombopag; Estramustine; Multivitamins/Fluoride (with ADE); Phosphate Supplements; Quinolone Antibiotics; Strontium Ranelate; Tetracycline Derivatives; Thyroid Products; Trientine

The levels/effects of Calcium Gluconate may be decreased by: Trientine

Stability
Oral: Store at room temperature; consult product labeling for specific requirements.
Parenteral: Store intact vials at 20°C to 25°C (68°F to 77°F); excursions permitted to 15°C to 30°C (59°F to 86°F).
Calcium-phosphate stability in parenteral nutrition solutions is dependent upon the pH of the solution, temperature, and relative concentration of each ion. The pH of the solution is primarily dependent upon the amino acid concentration. The higher the percentage amino acids the lower the pH, the more soluble the calcium and phosphate. Individual commercially available amino acid solutions vary significantly with respect to pH lowering potential and consequent calcium phosphate compatibility.

Mechanism of Action Moderates nerve and muscle performance via action potential threshold regulation.
In hydrogen fluoride exposures, calcium gluconate provides a source of calcium ions to complex free fluoride ions and prevent or reduce toxicity; administration also helps to correct fluoride-induced hypocalcemia.

Pharmacokinetics (Adult data unless noted)
Absorption: Requires vitamin D; varies with age: Infants 60%, prepubertal children 28%, pubertal children 34%, young adults 25%; calcium is absorbed in soluble, ionized form; absorption increased in an acidic environment; decreased absorption occurs in patients with achlorhydria, renal osteodystrophy, steatorrhea, or uremia
Protein binding: ~40%, primarily to albumin (Wills, 1971)
Elimination: Primarily feces (as unabsorbed calcium salts); urine (20%)

Dosing: Neonatal
Adequate intake (AI): Oral: 200 mg/day of **elemental calcium**; requirements may vary on prematurity, postnatal age, and other clinical factors; serum calcium concentrations should be monitored closely to determine patient-specific needs (IOM, 2011)
Enteral nutrition, maintenance requirement (dietary intake; formula, breastmilk): Preterm neonates, birth weight <2000 g: Oral: 150 to 220 mg/kg/day of **elemental calcium** (Abrams, 2013)
Cardiac arrest in the presence of hyperkalemia or hypocalcemia, hypermagnesemia, or calcium channel blocker toxicity: Dose expressed as calcium gluconate: I.V., I.O.: 60 to 100 mg/kg/**dose**; may repeat in 10 minutes if necessary; if effective, consider I.V. infusion (Avery, 1994; Hegenbarth, 2008)
Hypocalcemia: Dose depends on clinical condition and serum calcium concentration; monitor closely:
General dosing:
Dose expressed as **calcium gluconate**: I.V.: 200 mg/kg every 6 to 12 hours or 400 mg/kg/day as a continuous infusion (Avery, 1994; Scott, 1984)
Dose expressed as **elemental calcium**:
I.V.: Usual range: 40 to 50 mg/kg/day as a continuous infusion; for asymptomatic hypocalcemia tapering regimen has been suggested: Initial: 80 mg/kg/day as a continuous infusion for 48 hours then reduce to 40 mg/kg/day continuous infusion typically for 24 hours (once normal serum calcium concentration documented) (Cloherty, 2012; Jain, 2010)
Oral: 50 to 150 mg/kg/day in 4 to 6 divided doses; not to exceed 1000 mg/**day** (Avery, 1994; Rigo, 2007).
Note: In general, other calcium salts may be more preferable oral dosage forms in neonatal patients; however, the 10% calcium gluconate injection may be given orally (Mimouni, 1994).
Symptomatic (ie, seizures, tetany): Dose expressed as **calcium gluconate**: I.V.: 100 to 200 mg/kg/**dose** over 5 to 10 minutes; followed by a continuous infusion 500 to 800 mg/kg/day (Cloherty, 2012; Jain, 2010; Mimouni, 1994; Nelson, 1996; Root, 1976; Zhou, 2009)

Parenteral nutrition, maintenance requirement: Dose expressed as **elemental calcium:** I.V.: 2 to 4 **mEq**/kg/day (Mirtallo, 2004)

Rickets (radiographic evidence), treatment: Dose expressed as **elemental calcium:** Oral: Initial: 20 mg/kg/day in 2 to 4 divided doses, increased as tolerated to usual range of 60 to 70 mg/kg/day in 2 to 4 divided doses; maximum daily dose of 80 mg/kg/day (Abrams, 2013; Avery, 1994)

Dosing: Usual

Pediatric:

Adequate intake (AI) (IOM, 2011): Dose expressed as **elemental calcium:** Oral:
1 to 6 months: 200 mg/day
7 to 12 months: 260 mg/day

Recommended daily allowance (RDA) (IOM, 2011): Dose expressed as **elemental calcium;** during pregnancy and lactation, requirements may change: Oral:
1 to 3 years: 700 mg/day
4 to 8 years: 1000 mg/day
9 to 18 years: 1300 mg/day

Parenteral nutrition, maintenance requirement (Mirtallo, 2004): **Note:** Dose expressed as **elemental calcium:** I.V.:
Infants and Children ≤50 kg: 0.5 to 4 **mEq**/kg/day
Children >50 kg and Adolescents: 10 to 20 **mEq**/day

Hypocalcemia: Dose depends on clinical condition and serum calcium concentration:
General dosing: Infants, Children, and Adolescents: Dose expressed as **calcium gluconate:** I.V.: 200 to 500 mg/kg/day as a continuous infusion or in 4 divided doses; usual adult maximum dose: 2000 mg/dose (Edmondson, 1990; Zhou, 2009)

Symptomatic (ie, seizures, tetany): Infants, Children, and Adolescents: Dose expressed as **calcium gluconate:** I.V.: 100 to 200 mg/kg/dose over 5 to 10 minutes; usual adult maximum dose: 2000 mg/dose; may repeat after 6 hours or follow with a continuous infusion of 200 to 800 mg/kg/day (Edmondson, 1990; Kelly, 2013; Misra, 2008; Nelson, 1996; Zhou, 2009)

Chronic therapy in asymptomatic patient: Infants and Children: Dose expressed as **calcium gluconate:** Oral: 500 mg/kg/day in divided doses every 4 to 8 hours (Nelson, 1996); usual maximum adult dose: 2000 mg/dose. **Note:** In general, other oral calcium salts (eg, carbonate, glubionate) are a more preferable oral dosage form option in young pediatric patients; however, the 10% calcium gluconate injection may be given orally (Mimouni, 1994).

Rickets (due to vitamin D deficiency); treatment: Infants and Children: Dose expressed as **elemental calcium:** Oral: 30 to 75 mg/kg/day in 3 divided doses; begin at higher end of range and titrate downward over 2 to 4 weeks (Misra, 2008). **Note:** In general, other oral calcium salts (eg, carbonate, glubionate) are a more preferable oral dosage formulation option in young pediatric patients; however, the 10% calcium gluconate injection may be given orally (Mimouni, 1994).

Cardiac arrest in the presence of hyperkalemia or hypocalcemia, hypermagnesemia, or calcium channel blocker toxicity: Infants, Children, and Adolescents: Dose expressed as **calcium gluconate:** I.V., I.O.: 60 to 100 mg/kg/**dose** (maximum dose: 3000 mg); may repeat in 10 minutes if necessary; if effective, consider I.V. infusion (Hegenbarth, 2008). **Note:** Routine use in cardiac arrest is not recommended due to the lack of improved survival (PALS [Kleinman], 2010).

Calcium channel blocker toxicity; hypotension/conduction disturbances: Infants, Children, and Adolescents: Dose expressed in mg of **calcium gluconate:** I.V., I.O.: 60 mg/kg/**dose** administered over 30 to 60 minutes (Hegenbarth, 2008). **Note:** Calcium chloride

may provide a more rapid increase of ionized calcium in critically ill children. Calcium gluconate may be substituted if calcium chloride is not available.

Adult: **Note:** Dose expressed in terms of the **calcium gluconate salt** (unless otherwise specified as elemental calcium). Doses expressed in terms of the **calcium gluconate salt** are based on a solution concentration of 100 mg/mL (10%) containing 0.465 mEq (9.3 mg)/mL elemental calcium, except where noted.

Recommended daily allowance (RDA) (IOM, 2011): **Note:** Expressed in terms of elemental calcium: Oral: Females/Males:
19 to 50 years: 1000 mg elemental calcium daily
≥51 years, females: 1200 mg elemental calcium daily
51 to 70 years, males: 1000 mg elemental calcium daily
Females, pregnant/lactating: Requirements are the same as in nonpregnant or nonlactating females

Hypocalcemia:

Intermittent I.V.:
Mild [ionized calcium: 4 to 5 mg/dL (1 to 1.2 mmol/L)]: 1000-2000 mg over 2 hours; asymptomatic patients may be given oral calcium (Ariyan, 2004; French, 2012)
Moderate to severe [without seizure or tetany; ionized calcium: <4 mg/dL (<1 mmol/L)]: 4000 mg over 4 hours (French, 2012)
Severe symptomatic (eg, seizure, tetany): 1000 to 2000 mg over 10 minutes; repeat every 60 minutes until symptoms resolve (French, 2012)
Note: Repeat ionized calcium measurement 6 to 10 hours after completion of administration. Check for hypomagnesemia and correct if present. Consider continuous infusion if hypocalcemia is likely to recur due to ongoing losses (French, 2012).
Continuous I.V. infusion: 5 to 20 mg/kg/hour (Pai, 2011)

Cardiac arrest or cardiotoxicity in the presence of hyperkalemia, hypocalcemia, or hypermagnesemia: I.V.: 1500 to 3000 mg over 2 to 5 minutes (Vanden Hoek, 2010); **Note:** Routine use in cardiac arrest is not recommended due to the lack of improved survival (Neumar, 2010).

Maintenance electrolyte requirements for parenteral nutrition: I.V. (Mirtallo, 2004): **Note:** Expressed in terms of elemental calcium: 10-20 mEq daily

Dosing adjustment in renal impairment: Infants, Children, Adolescents, and Adults: No initial dosage adjustment necessary; however, accumulation may occur with renal impairment and subsequent doses may require adjustment based on serum calcium concentrations.

Dosing adjustment in hepatic impairment: Infants, Children, Adolescents, and Adults: No initial dosage adjustment necessary; subsequent doses should be guided by serum calcium concentrations. In adult patients in the anhepatic stage of liver transplantation, equal rapid increases in ionized concentrations occur suggesting that calcium gluconate does not require hepatic metabolism for release of ionized calcium (Martin, 1990).

Administration

Oral: Administer with plenty of fluids with or following meals. The 10% calcium gluconate injection may be administered orally in young pediatric patients (Mimouni, 1994)

Parenteral: Observe the vial for the presence of particulates. If particulates are observed, place vial in a 60°C to 80°C water bath for 15 to 30 minutes (or until solution is clear); and occasionally shake to dissolve; cool to body/room temperature before use. Do not use vial if particulates do not dissolve. **Note:** Due to the potential presence of particulates, American Regent, Inc recommends the use of a 5 micron filter when preparing calcium gluconate containing I.V. solutions (Important Drug

Administration Information, American Regent, 2013); a similar recommendation has not been noted by other manufacturers. Do not inject calcium salts I.M. or administer SubQ since severe necrosis and sloughing may occur; extravasation of calcium can result in severe necrosis and tissue sloughing. Do not use scalp vein or small hand or foot veins for I.V. administration. Not for endotracheal administration.

I.V.: Administer slowly (~1.5 mL calcium gluconate 10% per minute; not to exceed 200 mg/minute except in emergency situations; requires cardiac monitoring) through a small needle into a large vein in order to avoid too rapid increases in the serum calcium and extravasation. In acute situations of symptomatic hypocalcemia, infusions over 5 to 10 minutes have been described in pediatric patients (Kelly, 2013; Misra, 2008)

I.V. infusion: May further dilute in D$_5$W or NS; a maximum concentration of 50 mg/mL has been used by some centers; infuse at a rate not to exceed 200 mg/minute.

Note: Due to the potential presence of particulates, American Regent, Inc recommends the use of a 0.22 micron in-line filter for I.V. administration of admixture (1.2 micron filter if admixture contains lipids) (Important Drug Administration Information, American Regent, 2013); a similar recommendation has not been noted by other manufacturers.

Vesicant; ensure proper needle or catheter placement prior to and during I.V. infusion. Avoid extravasation. If extravasation occurs, stop infusion immediately and disconnect (leave needle/cannula in place); gently aspirate extravasated solution (do NOT flush the line); initiate hyaluronidase antidote (See Management of Drug Extravasations for more details); remove needle/cannula; apply dry cold compresses (Hurst, 2004); elevate extremity.

Vesicant/Extravasation Risk Vesicant

Monitoring Parameters Serum calcium (ionized calcium preferred if available), phosphate, magnesium, heart rate, ECG

Reference Range

	Age	Normal Values Serum Concentration
Calcium, total	Cord blood	9 to 11.5 mg/dL
	Newborn 3 to 24 hours	9 to 10.6 mg/dL
	Newborn 24 to 48 hours	7 to 12 mg/dL
	4 to 7 days	9 to 10.9 mg/dL
	Child	8.8 to 10.8 mg/dL
	Adolescent to Adult	8.4 to 10.2 mg/dL
Calcium, ionized, whole blood	Cord blood	5 to 6 mg/dL
	Newborn 3 to 24 hours	4.3 to 5.1 mg/dL
	Newborn 24 to 48 hours	4 to 4.7 mg/dL
	≥2 days	4.8 to 4.92 mg/dL (2.24 to 2.46 mEq/L)

Test Interactions I.V. administration may produce falsely decreased serum and urine magnesium concentrations

Additional Information Due to a poor correlation between the serum ionized calcium (free) and total serum calcium, particularly in states of low albumin or acid/base imbalances, direct measurement of ionized calcium is recommended. If ionized calcium is unavailable, in low albumin states, the corrected **total** serum calcium may be estimated by this equation (assuming a normal albumin of 4 g/dL); [(4 − patient's albumin) x 0.8] + patient's measured total calcium

Elemental Calcium Content of Calcium Salts

Calcium Salt	Elemental Calcium (mg/1 g of salt form)	Calcium (mEq/g)
Calcium acetate	253	12.7
Calcium carbonate	400	20
Calcium chloride	273	13.6
Calcium citrate	211	10.5
Calcium glubionate	63.8	3.2
Calcium gluconate	93	4.65
Calcium lactate	130	6.5
Calcium phosphate (tribasic)	390	19.3

Dosage Forms Considerations
1 g calcium gluconate = elemental calcium 93 mg = calcium 4.65 mEq = calcium 2.33 mmol

Dosage Forms Excipient information presented when available (limited, particularly for generics); consult specific product labeling. [DSC] = Discontinued product

Capsule, Oral [preservative free]:
Cal-Glu: 500 mg [dye free]

Solution, Intravenous:
Generic: 10% (10 mL, 50 mL, 100 mL)

Solution, Intravenous [preservative free]:
Generic: 10% (100 mL)

Tablet, Oral:
Generic: 50 mg, 500 mg, 648 (60 Ca) mg [DSC]

References

Abrams SA, Committee on Nutrition. Calcium and vitamin D requirements of enterally fed preterm infants. *Pediatrics.* 2013;131(5):e1676-1683.

Ariyan CE, Sosa JA. Assessment and management of patients with abnormal calcium. *Crit Care Med.* 2004; 32(4 Suppl):146-154.

Avery GB, Fletcher MA, MacDonald MG, eds. *Neonatology - Pathophysiology and Management of the Newborn.* 4th ed. Philadelphia, PA: Lippincott Company; 1994.

Bailey B, "Are There Teratogenic Risks Associated With Antidotes Used in the Acute Management of Poisoned Pregnant Women?" *Birth Defects Res A Clin Mol Teratol*, 2003, 67(2):133-40.

Calcium gluconate [prescribing information]. Schaumberg, IL: APP Pharmaceuticals, LLC; February 2009.

Cloherty JP, Eichenwald EC, Hansen AR, Stark AR, eds. *Manual of Neonatal Care.* Philadelphia, PA: Lippincott Williams & Wilkins; 2011.

Department Health & Human Services, Food Drug Administration, "Aluminum in Large and Small Volume Parenterals Used in Total Parenteral Nutrition," *Federal Register*, 2000, 65(17):4103-11.

Edmondson S, Almquist TD. Iatrogenic hypocalcemic tetany. *Ann Emerg Med.* 1990;19(8):938-940.

French S, Subauste J, and Geraci S, "Calcium Abnormalities in Hospitalized Patients," *South Med J*, 2012, 105(4):231-7.

Hegenbarth MA and American Academy of Pediatrics Committee on Drugs, "Preparing for Pediatric Emergencies: Drugs to Consider," *Pediatrics*, 2008, 121(2):433-43.

Hurst S, McMillan M. Innovative solutions in critical care units: extravasation guidelines. *Dimens Crit Care Nurs.* 2004;23(3):125-128.

IOM (Institute of Medicine), *Dietary Reference Intakes for Calcium and Vitamin D*, Washington, DC: The National Academies Press, 2011. Available at http://www.nap.edu/catalog.php?record_id=13050

Jain A, Agarwal R, Sankar MJ, Deorari A, Paul VK. Hypocalcemia in the newborn. *Indian J Pediatr.* 2010;77(10):1123-1128.

Kelly A, Levine MA. Hypocalcemia in the critically ill patient. *J Intensive Care Med.* 2013;28(3):166-177.

Kleinman ME, Chameides L, Schexnayder SM, et al, "Part 14: Pediatric Advanced Life Support: 2010 American Heart Association Guidelines for Cardiopulmonary Resuscitation and Emergency Cardiovascular Care," *Circulation*, 2010, 122 (18 Suppl 3):876-908.

Martin TJ, Kang Y, Robertson KM, et al. Ionization and hemodynamic effects of calcium chloride and calcium gluconate in the absence of hepatic function. *Anesthesiology.* 1990; 71(1):62-65.

Mimouni F, Tsang RC. Neonatal hypocalcemia: to treat or not to treat? (A review). *J Am Coll Nutr.* 1994;13(5):408-415.

Mirtallo J, Canada T, Johnson D, et al, "Safe Practices for Parenteral Nutrition," *JPEN J Parenter Enteral Nutr*, 2004, 28(6):S39-70.

Misra M, Pacaud D, Petryk A, Collett-Solberg PF, Kappy M, Drug and Therapeutics Committee of the Lawson Wilkins Pediatric Endocrine Society. Vitamin D deficiency in children and its management: review of current knowledge and recommendations. *Pediatrics.* 2008;122 (2):398-417.

Nelson WE, Behrman RE, Kliegman RM, Arvin AM, eds. *Nelson Textbook of Pediatrics.* 15th ed. Philadelphia, PA: WR Saunders Company; 1996.

Neumar RW, Otto CW, Link MS, et al, "Part 8: Adult Advanced Cardiovascular Life Support: 2010 American Heart Association Guidelines for Cardiopulmonary Resuscitation and Emergency Cardiovascular Care," *Circulation,* 2010, 122(18 Suppl 3):729-67.

Pai AB. Chapter 59: disorders of calcium and phosphorus homeostasis. *Pharmacotherapy: A Pathophysiologic Approach.* 8th ed. Talbert RL, DiPiro JT, Matzke GR, et al, eds, New York, NY:McGraw-Hill, 2011.

Rigo J, Pieltain C, Salle B, Senterre J. Enteral calcium, phosphate and vitamin D requirements and bone mineralization in preterm infants. *Acta Paediatrica.* 2007;96:969-974.

Root AW, Harrison HE. Recent advances in calcium metabolism. II. Disorders of calcium homeostasis. *J Pediatr.* 1976;88(2):177-199.

Scott SM, Ladenson JH, Aguanna JJ, Walgate J, Hillman LS. Effect of calcium therapy in the sick premature infant with early neonatal hypocalcemia. *J Pediatr.* 1984;104(5):747-751.

Vanden Hoek TL, Morrison LJ, Shuster M, et al, "Part 12: Cardiac Arrest in Special Situations: 2010 American Heart Association Guidelines for Cardiopulmonary Resuscitation and Emergency Cardiovascular Care," *Circulation,* 2010, 122(18 Suppl 3):829-61.

Wills MR and Lewin MR, "Plasma Calcium Fractions and the Protein-Binding of Calcium in Normal Subjects and in Patients With Hypercalcaemia and Hypocalcaemia," *J Clin Pathol,* 1971, 24(9):856-66.

Worthley LI and Phillips PJ, "Intravenous Calcium Salts," *Lancet,* 1980, 2(8186):149.

Zhou P, Markowitz M. Hypocalcemia in infants and children. *Pediatr Rev.* 2009;30(5):190-192.

◆ **Calcium High Potency [OTC]** *see* Calcium Carbonate on page 346

Calcium Lactate (KAL see um LAK tate)

Brand Names: U.S. Cal-Lac [OTC]

Therapeutic Category Calcium Salt; Electrolyte Supplement, Oral

Generic Availability (U.S.) Yes

Use Prevention and treatment of calcium deficiency; dietary supplement; adjunctive prevention and treatment of osteoporosis

Pregnancy Considerations Calcium crosses the placenta. Intestinal absorption of calcium increases during pregnancy. The amount of calcium reaching the fetus is determined by maternal physiological changes. Calcium requirements are the same in pregnant and nonpregnant females (IOM, 2011).

Breast-Feeding Considerations Calcium is excreted in breast milk. The amount of calcium in breast milk is homeostatically regulated and not altered by maternal calcium intake. Calcium requirements are the same in lactating and nonlactating females (IOM, 2011).

Contraindications Hypersensitivity to calcium formulation; hypercalcemia, renal calculi, ventricular fibrillation

Warnings Multiple salt forms of calcium exist; close attention must be paid to the salt form when ordering and administering calcium; incorrect selection or substitution of one salt for another without proper dosage adjustment may result in serious over- or under-dosing. Some products may contain tartrazine which may cause allergic reactions in susceptible individuals.

Precautions Use cautiously in patients with sarcoidosis, respiratory failure, acidosis, renal or cardiac disease; some products may contain aspartame which is metabolized to phenylalanine and must be avoided in patients with phenylketonuria

Adverse Reactions Rare but important or life-threatening: Constipation, dizziness, dry mouth, headache, hypercalcemia, hypercalciuria, hypomagnesemia, hypophosphatemia, mental confusion, milk-alkali syndrome, nausea, vomiting

Drug Interactions

Metabolism/Transport Effects None known.

Avoid Concomitant Use

Avoid concomitant use of Calcium Lactate with any of the following: Calcium Acetate

Increased Effect/Toxicity

Calcium Lactate may increase the levels/effects of: Calcium Acetate; Vitamin D Analogs

The levels/effects of Calcium Lactate may be increased by: Multivitamins/Fluoride (with ADE); Multivitamins/Minerals (with ADEK, Folate, Iron); Thiazide Diuretics

Decreased Effect

Calcium Lactate may decrease the levels/effects of: Bisphosphonate Derivatives; Calcium Channel Blockers; Deferiprone; DOBUTamine; Dolutegravir; Eltrombopag; Estramustine; Multivitamins/Fluoride (with ADE); Phosphate Supplements; Quinolone Antibiotics; Strontium Ranelate; Tetracycline Derivatives; Thyroid Products; Trientine

The levels/effects of Calcium Lactate may be decreased by: Trientine

Stability Store at room temperature.

Mechanism of Action As dietary supplement, used to prevent or treat negative calcium balance; in osteoporosis, it helps to prevent or decrease the rate of bone loss. The calcium in calcium salts moderates nerve and muscle performance and allows normal cardiac function.

Pharmacokinetics (Adult data unless noted)

Absorption: 25% to 35%; varies with age (infants 60%, prepubertal children 28%, pubertal children 34%, young adults 25%); decreased absorption occurs in patients with achlorhydria, renal osteodystrophy, steatorrhea, or uremia

Protein binding: 45%

Elimination: Primarily in the feces as unabsorbed calcium

Dosing: Neonatal Oral:

Adequate intake (AI): 200 mg/day of **elemental calcium**; requirements may vary on prematurity, postnatal age, and other clinical factors; serum calcium concentrations should be monitored closely to determine patient-specific needs

Hypocalcemia: Dose depends on clinical condition and serum calcium concentration:

Dose expressed in mg of **elemental calcium**: 50-150 mg/kg/day in 4-6 divided doses; not to exceed 1000 mg/day

Dose expressed in mg of **calcium lactate**: 400-500 mg/kg/day divided every 4-6 hours

Dosing: Usual Oral:

Adequate intake (AI): Dosage expressed in terms of **elemental calcium:**

1-6 months: 200 mg/day

7-12 months: 260 mg/day

Recommended daily allowance (RDA): Dosage expressed in terms of **elemental calcium;** during pregnancy and lactation, requirements may change:

1-3 years: 700 mg/day

4-8 years: 1000 mg/day

9-18 years: 1300 mg/day

Females 19-50 years, males 19-70 years: 1000 mg/day

Females ≥51 years, males ≥71 years: 1200 mg/day

Hypocalcemia: Dose depends on clinical condition and serum calcium concentration:

Dose expressed as **elemental calcium**:

Children: 45-65 mg/kg/day in 4 divided doses

Adults: 1-2 g or more per day in 3-4 divided doses

Dose expressed as **calcium lactate**:

Infants: 400-500 mg/kg/day divided every 4-6 hours

Children: 500 mg/kg/day divided every 6-8 hours; maximum daily dose: 9 g

Adults: 1.5-3 g/day divided every 8 hours; maximum daily dose: 9 g

Adjunctive prevention and treatment of osteoporosis: Adults: 500 mg **elemental calcium** 2-3 times/day; recommended dosage includes dietary intake and should be adjusted depending upon the patient's diet; to improve absorption do not administer more than 500 mg **elemental calcium**/dose

Dosage adjustment in renal impairment: CrCl <25 mL/minute may require dosage adjustment depending upon serum calcium level

Administration Oral: Administer with plenty of fluids with or following meals

Monitoring Parameters Serum calcium (ionized calcium preferred if available), phosphate, magnesium, heart rate, ECG

Reference Range
Calcium: Newborns: 7-12 mg/dL; 0-2 years: 8.8-11.2 mg/dL; 2 years to adults: 9-11 mg/dL
Calcium, ionized, whole blood: 4.4-5.4 mg/dL

Additional Information 1 g calcium lactate = 130 mg elemental calcium = 6.5 mEq calcium. Due to a poor correlation between the serum ionized calcium (free) and total serum calcium, particularly in states of low albumin or acid/base imbalances, direct measurement of ionized calcium is recommended. If ionized calcium is unavailable, in low albumin states, the corrected **total** serum calcium may be estimated by this equation (assuming a normal albumin of 4 g/dL); [(4 − patient's albumin) x 0.8] + patient's measured total calcium

Elemental Calcium Content of Calcium Salts

Calcium Salt	Elemental Calcium (mg/1 g of salt form)	Calcium (mEq/g)
Calcium acetate	253	12.7
Calcium carbonate	400	20
Calcium chloride	273	13.6
Calcium citrate	211	10.5
Calcium glubionate	63.8	3.2
Calcium gluconate	93	4.65
Calcium lactate	130	6.5
Calcium phosphate (tribasic)	390	19.3

Dosage Forms Considerations
648 mg calcium lactate = elemental calcium 84 mg = calcium 4.2 mEq = calcium 2.1 mmol

Dosage Forms Excipient information presented when available (limited, particularly for generics); consult specific product labeling.
Capsule, Oral [preservative free]:
Cal-Lac: 500 mg [dye free]
Tablet, Oral:
Generic: 100 mg
Tablet, Oral [preservative free]:
Generic: 648 mg

References
Dietary Reference Intakes for Calcium and Vitamin D, Institute of Medicine (US) Committee to Review Dietary Reference Intakes for Vitamin D and Calcium, Ross AC, Taylor CL, et al, eds, Washington, DC: National Academies Press (US), 2011. Available at http://www.nap.edu/catalog.php?record_id=13050

◆ **Calcium Leucovorin** *see* Leucovorin Calcium
on page 1213

Calcium Phosphate (Tribasic)
(KAL see um FOS fate tri BAY sik)

Brand Names: U.S. Posture® [OTC]
Therapeutic Category Calcium Salt; Electrolyte Supplement, Oral
Generic Availability (U.S.) No
Use Prevention and treatment of calcium deficiency; dietary supplement; adjunctive prevention and treatment of osteoporosis
Pregnancy Considerations Calcium crosses the placenta. Intestinal absorption of calcium increases during pregnancy. The amount of calcium reaching the fetus is determined by maternal physiological changes. Calcium requirements are the same in pregnant and nonpregnant females (IOM, 2011).
Breast-Feeding Considerations Calcium is excreted in breast milk. The amount of calcium in breast milk is homeostatically regulated and not altered by maternal calcium intake. Calcium requirements are the same in lactating and nonlactating females (IOM, 2011).
Contraindications Hypersensitivity to calcium formulation; hypercalcemia, renal calculi, ventricular fibrillation
Warnings Multiple salt forms of calcium exist; close attention must be paid to the salt form when ordering and administering calcium; incorrect selection or substitution of one salt for another without proper dosage adjustment may result in serious over- or under-dosing. Some products may contain tartrazine which may cause allergic reactions in susceptible individuals.
Precautions Use cautiously in patients with sarcoidosis, respiratory failure, acidosis, renal or cardiac disease; some products may contain aspartame which is metabolized to phenylalanine and must be avoided in patients with phenylketonuria
Adverse Reactions Rare but important or life-threatening: Constipation, dry mouth, hypercalcemia, hypophosphatemia, milk-alkali syndrome, nausea
Drug Interactions
Metabolism/Transport Effects None known.
Avoid Concomitant Use
Avoid concomitant use of Calcium Phosphate (Tribasic) with any of the following: Calcium Acetate
Increased Effect/Toxicity
Calcium Phosphate (Tribasic) may increase the levels/effects of: Calcium Acetate; Vitamin D Analogs

The levels/effects of Calcium Phosphate (Tribasic) may be increased by: Bisphosphonate Derivatives; Multivitamins/Fluoride (with ADE); Thiazide Diuretics
Decreased Effect
Calcium Phosphate (Tribasic) may decrease the levels/effects of: Bisphosphonate Derivatives; Calcium Channel Blockers; Deferiprone; DOBUTamine; Dolutegravir; Eltrombopag; Estramustine; Multivitamins/Fluoride (with ADE); Phosphate Supplements; Quinolone Antibiotics; Strontium Ranelate; Tetracycline Derivatives; Thyroid Products; Trientine

The levels/effects of Calcium Phosphate (Tribasic) may be decreased by: Antacids; Calcium Salts; Iron Salts; Magnesium Salts; Multivitamins/Minerals (with ADEK, Folate, Iron); Sucralfate; Trientine
Stability Store at room temperature.
Mechanism of Action As dietary supplement, used to prevent or treat negative calcium balance; in osteoporosis, it helps to prevent or decrease the rate of bone loss. The calcium in calcium salts moderates nerve and muscle performance and allows normal cardiac function.
Pharmacokinetics (Adult data unless noted)
Absorption: 25% to 35%; varies with age (infants 60%, prepubertal children 28%, pubertal children 34%, young

adults 25%); decreased absorption occurs in patients with achlorhydria, renal osteodystrophy, steatorrhea, or uremia

Protein binding: 45%

Elimination: Primarily in the feces as unabsorbed calcium

Dosing: Usual Oral:

Adequate intake (AI): Dosage expressed in terms of **elemental calcium:**

1-6 months: 200 mg/day

7-12 months: 260 mg/day

Recommended daily allowance (RDA): Dosage expressed in terms of **elemental calcium;** during pregnancy and lactation, requirements may change:

1-3 years: 700 mg/day

4-8 years: 1000 mg/day

9-18 years: 1300 mg/day

Females 19-50 years, males 19-70 years: 1000 mg/day

Females ≥51 years, males ≥71 years: 1200 mg/day

Hypocalcemia: Dose depends on clinical condition and serum calcium concentration: Dose expressed as **elemental calcium:**

Children: 45-65 mg/kg/day in 4 divided doses

Adults: 1-2 g or more per day in 3-4 divided doses

Adjunctive prevention and treatment of osteoporosis: Adults: 500 mg **elemental calcium** 2-3 times/day; recommended dosage includes dietary intake and should be adjusted depending upon the patient's diet; to improve absorption do not administer more than 500 mg **elemental calcium**/dose

Dosage adjustment in renal impairment: CrCl <25 mL/minute may require dosage adjustment depending upon serum calcium level

Monitoring Parameters Serum calcium (ionized calcium preferred if available), phosphate, magnesium, heart rate, ECG

Reference Range

Calcium: Newborns: 7-12 mg/dL; 0-2 years: 8.8-11.2 mg/dL; 2 years to adults: 9-11 mg/dL

Calcium, ionized, whole blood: 4.4-5.4 mg/dL

Additional Information 1 g calcium phosphate, tribasic = 390 mg elemental calcium = 19.3 mEq calcium. Due to a poor correlation between the serum ionized calcium (free) and total serum calcium, particularly in states of low albumin or acid/base imbalances, direct measurement of ionized calcium is recommended. If ionized calcium is unavailable, in low albumin states, the corrected **total** serum calcium may be estimated by this equation (assuming a normal albumin of 4 g/dL); [(4 − patient's albumin) x 0.8] + patient's measured total calcium

Elemental Calcium Content of Calcium Salts

Calcium Salt	Elemental Calcium (mg/1 g of salt form)	Calcium (mEq/g)
Calcium acetate	253	12.7
Calcium carbonate	400	20
Calcium chloride	273	13.6
Calcium citrate	211	10.5
Calcium glubionate	63.8	3.2
Calcium gluconate	93	4.65
Calcium lactate	130	6.5
Calcium phosphate (tribasic)	390	19.3

Dosage Forms Excipient information presented when available (limited, particularly for generics); consult specific product labeling.

Caplet:

Posture®: Calcium 600 mg and phosphorus 280 mg [as tricalcium phosphate]

References

Dietary Reference Intakes for Calcium and Vitamin D, Institute of Medicine (US) Committee to Review Dietary Reference Intakes for Vitamin D and Calcium, Ross AC, Taylor CL, et al, eds, Washington, DC: National Academies Press (US), 2011. Available at http://www.nap.edu/catalog.php?record_id=13050

◆ **Caldolor** see Ibuprofen *on page 1059*

Calfactant (kaf AKT ant)

Brand Names: U.S. Infasurf

Therapeutic Category Lung Surfactant

Generic Availability (U.S.) No

Use Prevention and treatment of respiratory distress syndrome (RDS) in premature infants

Prophylactic therapy: Infants <29 weeks at significant risk for RDS

Treatment: Infants ≤72 hours of age with RDS (confirmed by clinical and radiologic findings and requiring endotracheal intubation)

Warnings Rapidly affects oxygenation and lung compliance and should be restricted to a highly supervised use in a clinical setting with immediate availability of clinicians experienced with intubation and ventilatory management of premature infants; if transient episodes of bradycardia and decreased oxygen saturation occur, discontinue the dosing procedure and initiate measures to alleviate the condition; produces rapid improvement in lung oxygenation and compliance that may require immediate reductions in ventilator settings and FiO$_2$; for intratracheal administration only

Precautions Transient episodes of reflux of calfactant into the endotracheal tube, cyanosis, bradycardia, or airway obstruction have occurred during dosing procedures; such episodes may require stopping administration and taking appropriate measures to alleviate the condition before resuming therapy

Adverse Reactions

Cardiovascular: Bradycardia, cyanosis

Respiratory: Airway obstruction, reflux, reintubation, requirement for manual ventilation

Drug Interactions

Metabolism/Transport Effects None known.

Avoid Concomitant Use

Avoid concomitant use of Calfactant with any of the following: Ceritinib

Increased Effect/Toxicity

Calfactant may increase the levels/effects of: Bradycardia-Causing Agents; Ceritinib

Decreased Effect There are no known significant interactions involving a decrease in effect.

Stability Refrigerate; protect from light; unopened, unused warmed vials of calfactant may be returned to refrigerator within 24 hours for future use; repeated warming to room temperature should be avoided

Mechanism of Action Endogenous lung surfactant is essential for effective ventilation because it modifies alveolar surface tension, thereby stabilizing the alveoli. Lung surfactant deficiency is the cause of respiratory distress syndrome (RDS) in premature infants and lung surfactant restores surface activity to the lungs of these infants.

Dosing: Neonatal Endotracheal: 3 mL/kg every 12 hours up to a total of 3 doses in the first 96 hours of life; repeat doses have been administered as frequently as every 6 hours for a total of up to 4 doses (if the neonate was still intubated and required at least 30% inspired oxygen to maintain arterial oxygen saturations >90% or with a PaO$_2$ ≤80 torr on >30% inspired oxygen) (Bloom, 2005; Kattwinkel, 2000)

Administration Intratracheal: Gently swirl to redisperse suspension; do not shake; administer dosage divided into two aliquots of 1.5 mL/kg each into the endotracheal tube; after each instillation, reposition the infant with either the right or left side dependent; administration is made while ventilation is continued over 20-30 breaths for each aliquot, with small bursts timed only during the inspiratory cycles; a pause followed by evaluation of the respiratory status and repositioning should separate the two aliquots; calfactant dosage has also been divided into four equal aliquots and administered with repositioning in four different positions (prone, supine, right and left lateral)

Monitoring Parameters Continuous heart rate and transcutaneous O_2 saturation should be monitored during administration; frequent ABG sampling is necessary to prevent postdosing hyperoxia and hypocarbia

Dosage Forms Excipient information presented when available (limited, particularly for generics); consult specific product labeling.

Suspension, Inhalation:
Infasurf: 35 mg phospholipids and 0.7 mg protein per mL (3 mL, 6 mL)

References

Bloom BT, Clark RH, and Infasurf Survanta Clinical Trial Group, "Comparison of Infasurf (Calfactant) and Survanta (Beractant) in the Prevention and Treatment of Respiratory Distress Syndrome," *Pediatrics*, 2005, 116(2):392-9.

Bloom BT, Kattwinkel J, Hall RT, et al, "Comparison of Infasurf® (Calf Lung Surfactant Extract) to Survanta® (Beractant) in the Treatment and Prevention of Respiratory Distress Syndrome," *Pediatrics*, 1997, 100(1):31-8.

Hudak ML, Martin DJ, Egan EA, et al, "A Multicenter Randomized Masked Comparison Trial of Synthetic Surfactant Versus Calf Lung Surfactant Extract in the Prevention of Neonatal Respiratory Distress Syndrome," *Pediatrics*, 1997, 100(1):39-50.

Kattwinkel J, Bloom BT, Delmore P, et al, "High- Versus Low-Threshold Surfactant Retreatment for Neonatal Respiratory Distress Syndrome," *Pediatrics*, 2000, 106(2 Pt 1):282-8.

◆ **Cal-Gest Antacid [OTC]** *see* Calcium Carbonate *on page 346*

◆ **Cal-Glu [OTC]** *see* Calcium Gluconate *on page 354*

◆ **Calicylic [OTC]** *see* Salicylic Acid *on page 1860*

◆ **Cal-Lac [OTC]** *see* Calcium Lactate *on page 358*

◆ **Cal-Mint [OTC]** *see* Calcium Carbonate *on page 346*

◆ **Calphron [OTC]** *see* Calcium Acetate *on page 344*

◆ **Caltrate (Can)** *see* Calcium Carbonate *on page 346*

◆ **Caltrate 600 [OTC]** *see* Calcium Carbonate *on page 346*

◆ **Caltrate Select (Can)** *see* Calcium Carbonate *on page 346*

◆ **Cambia** *see* Diclofenac (Systemic) *on page 645*

◆ **Camila** *see* Norethindrone *on page 1511*

◆ **Camphorated Tincture of Opium (error-prone synonym)** *see* Paregoric *on page 1605*

◆ **Camptosar** *see* Irinotecan *on page 1149*

◆ **Camptothecin-11** *see* Irinotecan *on page 1149*

Canakinumab (can a KIN ue mab)

Brand Names: U.S. Ilaris
Brand Names: Canada Ilaris
Therapeutic Category Interleukin-1 Receptor Antagonist; Monoclonal Antibody
Generic Availability (U.S.) No
Use Treatment of cryopyrin-associated periodic syndromes (CAPS), including familial cold autoinflammatory syndrome (FCAS) and Muckle-Wells syndrome (MWS) (FDA approved in ages ≥4 years and adults); treatment of active systemic for juvenile idiopathic arthritis (SJIA) (FDA approved in ages ≥2 years weighing at least 7.5 kg)
Medication Guide Available Yes

Pregnancy Risk Factor C
Pregnancy Considerations Adverse events were observed in animal reproduction studies. The Canadian product labeling recommends women of reproductive potential use effective contraception during treatment and for 3 months after the last dose.
Breast-Feeding Considerations It is not known if canakinumab is excreted into breast milk. The U.S. manufacturer labeling recommends caution be used if administered to nursing women. The Canadian labeling recommends avoiding use in nursing women.
Contraindications Hypersensitivity to canakinumab or any component
Warnings Hypersensitivity reactions, excluding anaphylactic reactions, have been reported with use; symptoms may be similar to those that are disease related; use is contraindicated in patients with known hypersensitivity to canakinumab. May decrease immune response to infection due to interleukin-1 (IL-1) blockade; serious infections have been reported during canakinumab therapy. Exercise caution when considering use in patients with a history of new or recurrent infections, conditions that predispose them to infections, latent infections [eg, tuberculoisis (TB)] or opportunistic infections. Patients who develop a new infection while undergoing treatment should be monitored closely; discontinue therapy if serious infection develops. Risk of serious infection increased with concurrent tumor necrosis factor (TNF)-blocker (eg, etanercept) use; manufacturer recommends avoiding concurrent therapy with TNF-blockers and other IL-1 blocking agents (eg, rilonacept). Avoid use in patients with active TB; patients should be evaluated for latent tuberculosis infection with a tuberculin skin test prior to starting therapy. Latent TB infections should be treated prior to initiating canakinumab therapy; monitor for signs/symptoms of active TB during therapy. Canakinumab contains polysorbate 80 (Tween 80®) which may cause allergic reactions in susceptible individuals; infusion of polysorbate 80-containing solutions through polyvinyl chloride tubing may cause DEHP to leach into the solution; in immature animals, exposure to DEHP may adversely affect the development of the male reproductive tract. Macrophage activation syndrome (MAS), which can be life-threatening, may develop in patients with SJIA and should be treated aggressively. Infection or worsening SJIA may be triggers for MAS.
Precautions Use may affect defenses against malignancies; impact on the development and course of malignancies is not fully defined. Patients should be brought up-to-date with all immunizations, including pneumococcal and influenza, before initiating therapy; live vaccines should not be given concurrently. Influenza reported in 17% of patients during clinical trials. No data are available concerning the effects of therapy on vaccine effectiveness or secondary transmission of live vaccines in patients receiving therapy. Vertigo has been reported exclusively in patients with MWS (9% to 14%); events appear self-resolving with continued therapy. May cause diarrhea (20%), nasopharyngitis (34%), and rhinitis (17%).
Adverse Reactions
Adverse events reported in treatment of CAPS unless otherwise noted.
Central nervous system: Headache, vertigo
Endocrine & metabolic: Calcium decreased
Gastrointestinal: Diarrhea, gastroenteritis, nausea, upper abdominal pain (SJIA), weight gain
Hematologic & oncologic: Decreased platelet count (mild, transient; SJIA), decreased white blood cell count (SJIA), eosinophils increased
Hepatic: Bilirubin increased, increased ALT, increased AST, increased serum transaminases (SJIA)
Immunologic: Antibody development (CAPS, SJIA)
Infection: Increased susceptibility to infection (SJIA)
Local: Injection site reaction (CAPS, SJIA)

Neuromuscular and skeletal: Musculoskeletal pain
Renal: Creatinine clearance decreased, proteinuria
Respiratory: Bronchitis, nasopharyngitis, pharyngitis, rhinitis
Miscellaneous: Influenza
Rare but important or life-threatening: Hypersensitivity reactions, neutropenia (SJIA)

Drug Interactions

Metabolism/Transport Effects None known.

Avoid Concomitant Use

Avoid concomitant use of Canakinumab with any of the following: Anti-TNF Agents; BCG; Belimumab; Interleukin-1 Inhibitors; Interleukin-1 Receptor Antagonist; Natalizumab; Pimecrolimus; Tacrolimus (Topical); Tofacitinib; Vaccines (Live)

Increased Effect/Toxicity

Canakinumab may increase the levels/effects of: Belimumab; Leflunomide; Natalizumab; Tofacitinib; Vaccines (Live)

The levels/effects of Canakinumab may be increased by: Abciximab; Anti-TNF Agents; Denosumab; Interleukin-1 Inhibitors; Interleukin-1 Receptor Antagonist; Pimecrolimus; Roflumilast; Tacrolimus (Topical); Trastuzumab

Decreased Effect

Canakinumab may decrease the levels/effects of: BCG; Coccidioidin Skin Test; Sipuleucel-T; Vaccines (Inactivated); Vaccines (Live)

The levels/effects of Canakinumab may be decreased by: Echinacea

Stability Store intact vial at 2°C to 8°C (36°F to 46°F); do not freeze; protect from light; avoid shaking product. After reconstitution, protect from light; stable for 1 hour at controlled room temperature or 4 hours under refrigeration at 2°C to 8°C (36°F to 46°F).

Mechanism of Action Canakinumab reduces inflammation by binding to interleukin-1 beta (IL-1β) (no binding to IL-1 alpha or IL-1 receptor antagonist) and preventing interaction with cell surface receptors. Cryopyrin-associated periodic syndromes (CAPS) refers to rare genetic syndromes caused by mutations in the nucleotide-binding domain, leucine rich family (NLR), pyrin domain containing 3 (NLRP-3) gene or the cold-induced autoinflammatory syndrome-1 (CIAS1) gene. Cryopyrin, a protein encoded by this gene, regulates IL-1β activation. Deficiency of cryopyrin results in excessive inflammation.

Pharmacodynamics Maximum effect: Within 8 days CRP and serum amyloid normalization

Pharmacokinetics (Adult data unless noted)

Distribution: Varies according to body weight: V_{dss}: Children: 0.097 L/kg (3.2 L in 33 kg); Adults: 0.086 L/kg (6 L in 70 kg)

Protein binding: Binds to serum IL-1β

Bioavailability: SubQ: 66%

Half-life elimination: Pediatric patients ≥4 years: 23-26 days; Adults: 26 days

Time to peak serum concentration: Pediatric patients ≥4 years: 2-7 days; Adults: ~7 days

Elimination: Clearance: Varies according to body weight (NCT 00685373, 2011):
Pediatric patients ≤40 kg: 0.083 L/day
Pediatric patients >40 kg and Adults: 0.18 L/day

Dosing: Usual

Children and Adolescents:

Cryopyrin-associated periodic syndromes (CAPS):
Children ≥3 years and Adolescents:
15-40 kg: SubQ: Initial: 2 mg/kg/dose every 8 weeks; may increase to 3 mg/kg/dose if response inadequate; if residual symptoms continue, higher doses ≤8 mg/kg/dose and/or an increased frequency have been used (Kuemmerle-Deschner, 2011)

>40 kg: SubQ: 150 mg/dose every 8 weeks; if residual symptoms continue, higher doses ≤600 mg/dose and/or an increased frequency have been used (Kuemmerle-Deschner, 2011)

Juvenile idiopathic arthritis; systemic: Children ≥2 years weighing at least 7.5 kg and Adolescents: SubQ: 4 mg/kg/dose every 4 weeks; maximum dose: 300 mg

Adults: **Cryopyrin-associated periodic syndromes (CAPS):** Patient weight >40 kg: SubQ: 150 mg/dose every 8 weeks

Dosing adjustment in renal impairment: Children ≥2 years, Adolescents, and Adults: There are no dosage adjustments provided in the manufacturer's labeling; has not been studied.

Dosing adjustment in hepatic impairment: Children ≥2 years, Adolescents, and Adults: There are no dosage adjustments provided in the manufacturer's labeling; has not been studied.

Administration SubQ: Reconstitute vial with 1 mL preservative-free SWI; swirl the vial at a 45°angle for ~1 minute, then allow solution to sit for 5 minutes. Continue product dissolution by gently turning vial (without touching rubber stopper) upside down and back 10 times; do not shake. Allow to sit at room temperature for ~15 minutes until solution is clear. Solution may have a slight brownish-yellow tint; do not use if distinctly brown in color or if particulate matter is present in solution. Final concentration is 150 mg/mL; no further dilution required prior to administration. Administer subcutaneously by a healthcare provider; avoid sites with scar tissue.

Monitoring Parameters CBC with differential, C-reactive protein (CRP), serum amyloid A; signs or symptoms of infection; latent TB screening (prior to initiating therapy), body weight. Eye examinations for patients with CAPS (Caorsi, 2013) and symptoms of disease for patients with CAPS or SJIA (Caorsi, 2013; Lachmann, 2009; Ruperto, 2012) were also monitored in clinical trials.

Dosage Forms Excipient information presented when available (limited, particularly for generics); consult specific product labeling.
Solution Reconstituted, Subcutaneous [preservative free]:
Ilaris: 180 mg (1 ea) [contains polysorbate 80]

References

Caorsi R, Lepore L, Zulian F, et al. The schedule of administration of canakinumab in cryopyrin associated periodic syndrome is driven by the phenotype severity rather than the age. *Arthritis Res Ther.* 2013;15(1):R33.

Furst DE, Keystone EC, Braun J, et al, "Updated Consensus Statement on Biological Agents for the Treatment of Rheumatic Diseases, 2010," *Ann Rheum Dis*, 2011, 70(Suppl 1)2-36.

Kuemmerle-Deschner JB, Hachulla E, Cartwright R, et al, "Two-Year Results From an Open-Label, Multicentre, Phase III Study Evaluating the Safety and Efficacy of Canakinumab in Patients With Cryopyrin-Associated Periodic Syndrome Across Different Severity Phenotypes," *Ann Rheum Dis*, 2011, Aug 21.

Lachmann HJ, Kone-Paut I, Kuemmerle-Deschner JB, et al, "Use of Canakinumab in the Cryopyrin-Associated Periodic Syndrome," *N Engl J Med*, 2009, 360(23):2416-25.

NCT 00685373, "Efficacy and Safety of ACZ885 in Patients With the Following Cryopyrin-Associated Periodic Syndromes: Familial Cold Autoinflammatory Syndrome, Muckle-Wells Syndrome, or Neonatal Onset Multisystem Inflammatory Disease", Unpublished data. Available at http://clinicaltrials.gov/ct2/show/NCT00685373?term=NCT+00685373&rank=1. Date Accessed: October 29, 2011

Ruperto N, Brunner H, Horneff G, et al, "Efficacy and Safety of Canakinumab, a Longacting Fully Human Anti-Interleukin-1ß Antibody, in Systemic Juvenile Idiopathic Arthritis With Active Systemic Features: Results From a Phase III Study," *Pediatric Rheumatology*, 2011, 9(Suppl 1):021.

Ruperto N, Brunner HI, Quartier P, et al. Two randomized trials of canakinumab in systemic juvenile idiopathic arthritis. *N Engl J Med.* 2012;367(25):2396-406.

Ruperto N, Quartier P, Wulffraat N, et al, "A Phase II, Multicenter, Open-Label Study Evaluating Dosing and Preliminary Safety and Efficacy of Canakinumab in Systemic Juvenile Idiopathic Arthritis With Active Systemic Features," *Arthritis Rheum*, 2012, 64(2):557-67.

◆ **Canasa** see Mesalamine on page 1347

◆ **Cancidas** *see* Caspofungin *on page 388*

◆ **Cancidas® (Can)** *see* Caspofungin *on page 388*

Candesartan (kan de SAR tan)

Medication Safety Issues
Sound-alike/look-alike issues:
Atacand may be confused with antacid
Brand Names: U.S. Atacand
Brand Names: Canada Apo-Candesartan; Atacand; CO Candesartan; DOM-Candesartan; JAMP-Candesartan; Mylan-Candesartan; PMS-Candesartan; Ran-Candesartan; Sandoz-Candesartan; Teva-Candesartan
Therapeutic Category Angiotensin II Receptor Blocker; Antihypertensive Agent
Generic Availability (U.S.) Yes
Use Treatment of hypertension alone or in combination with other antihypertensive agents (FDA approved in ages ≥1 year and adults); treatment of heart failure (NYHA class II-IV) (FDA approved in adults)
Pregnancy Risk Factor D
Pregnancy Considerations [U.S. Boxed Warning]: Drugs that act on the renin-angiotensin system can cause injury and death to the developing fetus. Discontinue as soon as possible once pregnancy is detected. The use of drugs which act on the renin-angiotensin system are associated with oligohydramnios. Oligohydramnios, due to decreased fetal renal function, may lead to fetal lung hypoplasia and skeletal malformations. Use is also associated with anuria, hypotension, renal failure, skull hypoplasia, and death in the fetus/neonate. The exposed fetus should be monitored for fetal growth, amniotic fluid volume, and organ formation. Infants exposed *in utero* should be monitored for hyperkalemia, hypotension, and oliguria (exchange transfusions or dialysis may be needed). These adverse events are generally associated with maternal use in the second and third trimesters.

Untreated chronic maternal hypertension is also associated with adverse events in the fetus, infant, and mother. The use of angiotensin II receptor blockers is not recommended to treat chronic uncomplicated hypertension in pregnant women and should generally be avoided in women of reproductive potential (ACOG, 2013).

Breast-Feeding Considerations It is not known if candesartan is excreted into breast milk. Due to the potential for serious adverse reactions in the nursing infant, the manufacturer recommends a decision be made whether to discontinue nursing or to discontinue the drug, taking into account the importance of treatment to the mother.

Contraindications Hypersensitivity to candesartan, any component, or other angiotensin II receptor blockers; concomitant use with aliskiren in patients with diabetes mellitus

Warnings Drugs that act on the renin-angiotensin system can cause injury and death to the developing fetus. Discontinue as soon as possible once pregnancy is detected **[U.S. Boxed Warning]**. Symptomatic hypotension may occur, especially in patients with an activated renin-angiotensin system (eg, volume- or salt-depleted patients receiving high doses of diuretic agents); use with caution in these patients; correct depletion before starting therapy or initiate therapy at a lower dose. Concomitant use of an ACE inhibitor or renin inhibitor (eg, aliskiren) is associated with an increased risk of hypotension, hyperkalemia, and renal dysfunction.

Angioedema has been reported rarely with some angiotensin II receptor antagonists (ARBs) and may occur at any time during treatment (especially following first dose); it may involve the head and neck (potentially compromising airway) or the intestine (presenting with abdominal pain). Patients with idiopathic or hereditary angioedema or previous angioedema associated with ACE-inhibitor therapy may be at an increased risk. Prolonged frequent monitoring may be required, especially if tongue, glottis, or larynx are involved, as they are associated with airway obstruction. Patients with a history of airway surgery may have a higher risk of airway obstruction. Discontinue therapy immediately if angioedema occurs. Aggressive early management is critical. Intramuscular (I.M.) administration of epinephrine may be necessary. Do not readminister to patients who have had angioedema with ARBs.

Precautions Use with caution in patients with hepatic impairment; systemic exposure increases in hepatic impairment; dosage adjustment is recommended in patients with moderate hepatic impairment. Pharmacokinetics have not been studied in severe hepatic impairment. Use with caution in patients with impaired renal function; use is associated with deterioration of renal function, precipitation of azotemia, and/or increases in serum creatinine, particularly in patients with low renal blood flow (eg, renal artery stenosis, heart failure); deterioration may result in oliguria, or acute renal failure. Small increases in serum creatinine may occur following initiation; consider discontinuation in patients with progressive and/or significant deterioration in renal function. Hyperkalemia may occur; risk factors include renal dysfunction, diabetes mellitus, concomitant use of potassium-sparing diuretics, potassium supplements, and/or potassium-containing salts; use with caution with these agents; monitor potassium closely. Use caution when initiating in heart failure; may need to adjust dose and/or concurrent diuretic therapy because of candesartan-induced hypotension. Not recommended for use in children <1 year due to possible effects on developing kidneys; has not been studied in children with GFR <30 mL/minute/1.73 m^2; use not recommended.

Adverse Reactions
Cardiovascular: Angina pectoris, hypotension, myocardial infarction, palpitations, tachycardia
Central nervous system: Anxiety, depression, dizziness, drowsiness, headache, paresthesia, vertigo
Dermatologic: Diaphoresis, skin rash
Endocrine & metabolic: Hyperglycemia, hyperkalemia, hypertriglyceridemia, hyperuricemia
Gastrointestinal: Dyspepsia, gastroenteritis
Genitourinary: Hematuria
Neuromuscular & skeletal: Back pain, increased creatine phosphokinase, myalgia, weakness
Renal: Increased serum creatinine
Respiratory: Dyspnea, epistaxis, pharyngitis, rhinitis, upper respiratory tract infection
Miscellaneous: Fever
Rare but important or life-threatening: Agranulocytosis, anemia, angioedema, hepatic insufficiency, hepatitis, hyponatremia, leukopenia, neutropenia, thrombocytopenia

Drug Interactions
Metabolism/Transport Effects Substrate of CYP2C9 (minor); **Note:** Assignment of Major/Minor substrate status based on clinically relevant drug interaction potential; **Inhibits** CYP2C8 (weak), CYP2C9 (weak)
Avoid Concomitant Use There are no known interactions where it is recommended to avoid concomitant use.
Increased Effect/Toxicity
Candesartan may increase the levels/effects of: ACE Inhibitors; Amifostine; Antihypertensives; CycloSPORINE (Systemic); DULoxetine; Hypotensive Agents; Lithium; Nonsteroidal Anti-Inflammatory Agents; Obinutuzumab; Potassium-Sparing Diuretics; RiTUXimab; Sodium Phosphates

The levels/effects of Candesartan may be increased by: Alfuzosin; Aliskiren; Barbiturates; Brimonidine (Topical); Canagliflozin; Diazoxide; Eplerenone; Heparin; Heparin ▶

(Low Molecular Weight); Herbs (Hypotensive Properties); MAO Inhibitors; Pentoxifylline; Phosphodiesterase 5 Inhibitors; Potassium Salts; Prostacyclin Analogues; Tolvaptan; Trimethoprim

Decreased Effect

The levels/effects of Candesartan may be decreased by: Herbs (Hypertensive Properties); Methylphenidate; Nonsteroidal Anti-Inflammatory Agents; Yohimbine

Stability Store at 25°C (77°F); excursions permitted to 15°C to 30°C (59°F to 86°F)

Mechanism of Action Candesartan is an angiotensin receptor antagonist. Angiotensin II acts as a vasoconstrictor. In addition to causing direct vasoconstriction, angiotensin II also stimulates the release of aldosterone. Once aldosterone is released, sodium as well as water are reabsorbed. The end result is an elevation in blood pressure. Candesartan binds to the AT1 angiotensin II receptor. This binding prevents angiotensin II from binding to the receptor thereby blocking the vasoconstriction and the aldosterone secreting effects of angiotensin II.

Pharmacodynamics

Antihypertensive effect:
Onset of action: Within 2 weeks
Maximum effect: 4-6 weeks

Pharmacokinetics (Adult data unless noted)

Absorption: Candesartan: Rapid and complete following conversion from candesartan cilexetil by GI esterases

Distribution: V_d: 0.13 L/kg

Protein binding: >99%

Metabolism: Converted to active candesartan, via ester hydrolysis during absorption from GI tract; hepatic (minor) via O-deethylation to inactive metabolite

Bioavailability, absolute: Candesartan: 15%

Half-life elimination: 9 hours; dose-dependent

Time to peak serum concentration: Pediatric patients (1-17 years), adults: 3-4 hours

Elimination: Excreted via biliary and renal routes; feces: 67%; urine: 33% (26% as unchanged drug). The AUC and C_{max} increased 30% and 56% in mild hepatic impairment and 145% and 73% in moderate hepatic impairment, respectively. The pharmacokinetics after candesartan administration have not been investigated in patients with severe hepatic impairment.

Clearance: Total body: 0.37 mL/minute/kg; Renal: 0.19 mL/minute/kg; decreased with severe renal impairment. In hypertensive patients with CrCl <30 mL/min/1.73 m^2, the AUC and C_{max} are approximately doubled. In heart failure patients with renal impairment, AUC is 36% and 65% higher and C_{max} is 15% and 55% higher in patients with mild and moderate renal impairment, respectively.

Dosing: Usual Note: Use of a lower initial dose is recommended in volume- and salt-depleted patients; dosage must be individualized

Children and Adolescents:

Hypertension:
Children 1 to <6 years: Oral: Initial: 0.2 mg/kg/**day** divided once or twice daily; titrate to response (within 2 weeks, antihypertensive effect usually observed); usual range: 0.05-0.4 mg/kg/**day** divided once or twice daily; maximum daily dose: 0.4 mg/kg/**day**; higher doses have not been studied.

Children and Adolescents 6 to <17 years: Oral:
<50 kg: Initial: 4-8 mg/**day** divided once or twice daily; titrate to response (within 2 weeks, antihypertensive effect usually observed); usual range: 2-16 mg/**day** divided once or twice daily; maximum daily dose: 32 mg/**day**; higher doses have not been studied.

>50 kg: Initial: 8-16 mg/**day** divided once or twice daily; titrate to response (within 2 weeks, antihypertensive effect usually observed); usual range: 4-32 mg/**day** divided once or twice daily; maximum daily dose: 32 mg/**day**; higher doses have not been studied.

Adolescents ≥17 years: Oral: Initial: 16 mg once daily (monotherapy); usual range: 8-32 mg/day divided once or twice daily; blood pressure response is dose-related over the range of 2-32 mg; larger doses do not appear to have a greater effect and there is relatively little experience with such doses

Adults:
Hypertension: Oral: Initial: 16 mg once daily (monotherapy); usual range: 8-32 mg/day divided once or twice daily; blood pressure response is dose-related over the range of 2-32 mg; larger doses do not appear to have a greater effect and there is relatively little experience with such doses

Congestive heart failure: Oral: Initial: 4 mg once daily; double the dose at 2-week intervals, as tolerated; target dose: 32 mg/day; **Note:** In selected cases, concurrent therapy with an ACE inhibitor may provide additional benefit.

Dosing adjustment in renal impairment:
Children and Adolescents 1 to <17 years:
CrCl ≥30 mL/minute/1.73 m^2: There are no dosage adjustments provided in the manufacturer's labeling; has not been studied in pediatric patients with renal impairment.

CrCl <30 mL/minute/1.73 m^2: Use is not recommended.

Adults: No initial dosage adjustment necessary; however, in patients with severe renal impairment (CrCl <30 mL/minute/1.73m^2) AUC and C_{max} were approximately doubled after repeated dosing.

Not removed by dialysis.

Dosing adjustment in hepatic impairment:
Mild hepatic impairment (Child-Pugh Class A): No initial dosage adjustment required

Moderate hepatic impairment (Child-Pugh Class B): Adults: Initial: 8 mg daily: AUC increased by 145%

Severe hepatic impairment (Child-Pugh Class C): There are no dosage adjustments provided in manufacturer's labeling (has not been studied); however, systemic exposure increases significantly in moderate impairment.

Administration Oral: May be administered without regard to meals.

Monitoring Parameters Blood pressure, serum creatinine, BUN, baseline and periodic electrolytes

Dosage Forms Excipient information presented when available (limited, particularly for generics); consult specific product labeling.

Tablet, Oral, as cilexetil:
Atacand: 4 mg, 8 mg, 16 mg, 32 mg [scored]
Generic: 4 mg, 8 mg, 16 mg, 32 mg

Extemporaneous Preparations Oral suspension may be made in concentrations ranging from 0.1 to 2 mg/mL; typically 1 mg/mL oral suspension suitable for majority of prescribed doses; any strength tablet may be used. A 1 mg/mL (total volume: 160 mL) oral suspension may be made with tablets and a 1:1 mixture of Ora-Plus® and Ora-Sweet SF®. Prepare the vehicle by adding 80 mL of Ora-Plus® and 80 mL of Ora-Sweet SF® or, alternatively, use 160 mL of Ora-Blend SF®. Add a small amount of vehicle to five 32 mg tablets and grind into a smooth paste using a mortar and pestle. Transfer the paste to a calibrated amber PET bottle, rinse the mortar and pestle clean using the vehicle, add this to the bottle, and then add a quantity of vehicle sufficient to make 160 mL. The suspension is stable at room temperature for 100 days unopened or 30 days after the first opening; do not freeze; label "shake well before use." (Atacand® prescribing information, 2013).

Atacand® prescribing information, AstraZeneca LP, Wilmington, DE, 2013.

References
American College of Obstetricians and Gynecologists (ACOG), "ACOG Practice Bulletin No. 125: Chronic Hypertension in Pregnancy," Obstet Gynecol, 2012, 119(2 Pt 1):396-407.

Chobanian AV, Bakris GL, Black HR, et al, "The Seventh Report of the Joint National Committee on Prevention, Detection, Evaluation, and Treatment of High Blood Pressure: The JNC 7 Report," *JAMA*, 2003, 289(19):2560-71.

Franks AM, O'Brien CE, Stowe CD, et al, "Candesartan Cilexetil Effectively Reduces Blood Pressure in Hypertensive Children," *Ann Pharmacother*, 2008, 42(10):1388-95.

Hoy SM and Keating GM, "Candesartan Cilexetil: In Children and Adolescents Aged 1 to <17 Years With Hypertension," *Am J Cardiovasc Drugs*, 2010, 10(5):335-42.

Schaefer F, van de Walle J, Zurowska A, et al, "Efficacy, Safety and Pharmacokinetics of Candesartan Cilexetil in Hypertensive Children From 1 to Less Than 6 Years of Age," *J Hypertens*, 2010, 28 (5):1083-90.

Trachtman H, Hainer JW, Sugg J, et al, "Efficacy, Safety, and Pharmacokinetics of Candesartan Cilexetil in Hypertensive Children Aged 6 to 17 Years," *J Clin Hypertens (Greenwich)*, 2008, 10(10):743-50.

◆ **Candesartan Cilexetil** *see* Candesartan *on page* 363

◆ **Candistatin (Can)** *see* Nystatin (Topical) *on page* 1517

◆ **CanesOral (Can)** *see* Fluconazole *on page* 877

◆ **Canesten® Topical (Can)** *see* Clotrimazole (Topical) *on page* 527

◆ **Canesten® Vaginal (Can)** *see* Clotrimazole (Topical) *on page* 527

◆ **Capastat Sulfate** *see* Capreomycin *on page* 365

◆ **Capex** *see* Fluocinolone (Topical) *on page* 892

◆ **Capex® (Can)** *see* Fluocinolone (Topical) *on page* 892

◆ **Capital® and Codeine** *see* Acetaminophen and Codeine *on page* 53

◆ **Capoten** *see* Captopril *on page* 368

Capreomycin (kap ree oh MYE sin)

Medication Safety Issues
Sound-alike/look-alike issues:
Capastat® may be confused with Cepastat®
Brand Names: U.S. Capastat Sulfate
Therapeutic Category Antibiotic, Miscellaneous; Antitubercular Agent
Generic Availability (U.S.) No
Use Treatment of pulmonary tuberculosis (TB) in conjunction with at least one other antituberculosis agent when primary anti-TB agents are ineffective (drug-resistant) or patient does not tolerate or resistant tubercle bacilli present (FDA approved in adults)
Pregnancy Risk Factor C
Pregnancy Considerations Capreomycin has been shown to be teratogenic in animal studies. **[U.S. Boxed Warning]: Safety has not been established in pregnant women**; use during pregnancy only if the potential benefit to the mother outweighs the possible risk to the fetus.
Breast-Feeding Considerations It is not known if capreomycin is excreted in breast milk. The manufacturer recommends that caution be exercised when administering capreomycin to nursing women.
Contraindications Hypersensitivity to capreomycin sulfate or any component
Warnings May cause renal injury including tubular necrosis, elevated BUN or serum creatinine, and abnormal urinary sediment; BUN elevation and abnormal urinary sediment are associated with prolonged therapy and the clinical significance of these findings is not fully established. Proteinuria frequently reported; electrolyte disturbances (hypokalemia, hypomagnesemia, and hypocalcemia) may result from renal injury (CDC, 2003). Use in patients with renal impairment must be undertaken with great caution, and the risk of additional renal injury should be weighed against the benefits of therapy **[U.S. Boxed Warning]**; monitor patients closely during therapy; if BUN >30 mg/dL occurs or other evidence of decreased renal function, consider capreomycin dosage reduction or discontinuation of therapy; discontinuation of therapy due

to renal toxicity has been reported in 20% to 25% of patients (CDC, 2003). Monitor renal function; urinalysis and electrolytes at baseline and periodically (monthly) throughout therapy (CDC, 2003; Seddon, 2012). May cause hearing loss; some cases may be irreversible. Tinnitus and vertigo have also been reported; more common in elderly patients and patients with preexisting renal impairment. In pediatric patients treated for multidrug-resistant TB, the reported incidence of hearing loss is variable (7% to 24%) with regimens that included either capreomycin or an aminoglycoside; the majority of children received amikacin compared to capreomycin; specific incidence with capreomycin not determined (Drobac, 2006; Seddon, 2013). Use in patients with preexisting auditory impairment must be undertaken with great caution, and the risk of additional eighth nerve impairment should be weighed against the benefits to be derived from therapy **[U.S. Boxed Warnings]**; audiometric measurements and vestibular function assessment should be completed at baseline and during therapy. Since other parenteral antituberculous agents (eg, streptomycin) also have similar and sometimes irreversible toxic effects, particularly on eighth cranial nerve and renal function, simultaneous administration of these agents with capreomycin is not recommended **[U.S. Boxed Warning]**. Use with nonantituberculous drugs (eg, aminoglycosides, vancomycin) having ototoxic or nephrotoxic potential should be undertaken only with great caution **[U.S. Boxed Warning]**. Prolonged use may result in fungal or bacterial superinfection, including *C. difficile*-associated diarrhea and pseudomembranous colitis. Safety and effectiveness in pediatric patients has not been established **[U.S. Boxed Warning]**.
Precautions May cause neuromuscular blockade after large intravenous doses; use with caution in patients with in conditions which depress neuromuscular transmission; risk increased with concomitant use of anesthesia (eg, ether)
Adverse Reactions
Hematologic: Eosinophilia (dose related, mild)
Otic: Ototoxicity
Renal: Nephrotoxicity (increased BUN)
Rare but important or life-threatening: Acute tubular necrosis, Bartter's syndrome, creatinine increased, hypersensitivity (maculopapular rash, urticaria and/or fever), hypocalcemia, hypokalemia, hypomagnesemia, injection site reactions (abscess, bleeding, induration and pain), leukocytosis, leukopenia, liver function decreased (BSP excretion decreased), renal injury, thrombocytopenia (rare), tinnitus, toxic nephritis, urinary sediment abnormal, vertigo
Drug Interactions
Metabolism/Transport Effects None known.
Avoid Concomitant Use
Avoid concomitant use of Capreomycin with any of the following: BCG
Increased Effect/Toxicity May increase effect/duration of nondepolarizing neuromuscular blocking agents. Additive toxicity (nephrotoxicity and ototoxicity), respiratory paralysis may occur with aminoglycosides (eg, streptomycin).
Decreased Effect
Capreomycin may decrease the levels/effects of: BCG; Sodium Picosulfate
Stability Store intact vial at 15°C to 30°C (59°F to 86°F); following reconstitution, may store under refrigeration for up to 24 hours; may develop a pale straw color and darken; not associated with loss of potency or toxicity.
Mechanism of Action Capreomycin is a cyclic polypeptide antimicrobial. It is administered as a mixture of capreomycin IA and capreomycin IB. The mechanism of action of capreomycin is not well understood. Mycobacterial species that have become resistant to other agents are

usually still sensitive to the action of capreomycin. However, significant cross-resistance with viomycin, kanamycin, and neomycin occurs.

Pharmacokinetics (Adult data unless noted)
Absorption: Oral: Not absorbed
Half-life elimination:
Normal renal function: 4-6 hours
Renal impairment:
CrCl 50-80 mL/minute: 7-10 hours
CrCl 20-40 mL/minute: 12-20 hours
CrCl 10 mL/minute: 29 hours
CrCl 0 mL/minute: 55 hours
Time to peak serum concentration: I.M.: 1-2 hours
Elimination: Urine (within 12 hours: 52% as unchanged drug)

Dosing: Usual
Infants, Children, Adolescents: **Tuberculosis; multidrug resistant (MDR):** Limited data available: **Note:** Usual duration of therapy is 4-6 months although older children may require up to 8 months of therapy; use in combination with at least 2-3 additional anti-TB agents (overall multidrug regimen dependent upon susceptibility profile/ patterns); regimens with less frequent dosing (ie, twice or three times weekly) have less clinical experience supporting efficacy (CDC, 2003; Seddon, 2012): I.M., I.V.:
Infants and Children weighing ≤40 kg: 15-30 mg/kg once daily; maximum daily dose: 1000 mg/**day** (CDC, 2003; DHHS [pediatric], 2013; Seddon, 2012)
Children weighing >40 kg and Adolescents: 15 mg/kg once daily; maximum daily dose: 1000 mg/**day** (CDC, 2003; DHHS [adult], 2013; Seddon, 2012)
Adults: **Tuberculosis:** I.M., I.V.: 1000 mg once daily (maximum dose: 20 mg/kg/dose) for 60-120 days, followed by 1000 mg 2-3 times/week **or** 15 mg/kg/day (maximum: 1000 mg/dose) for 2-4 months, followed by 15 mg/kg (maximum: 1000 mg/dose) 2-3 times/week (CDC, 2003)

Dosing interval in renal impairment: Adults: I.M., I.V.:
Manufacturer's labeling: Maximum single dose: 1000 mg
CrCl 110 mL/minute: Administer 13.9 mg/kg every 24 hours
CrCl 100 mL/minute: Administer 12.7 mg/kg every 24 hours
CrCl 80 mL/minute: Administer 10.4 mg/kg every 24 hours
CrCl 60 mL/minute: Administer 8.2 mg/kg every 24 hours
CrCl 50 mL/minute: Administer 7 mg/kg every 24 hours **or** 14 mg/kg every 48 hours
CrCl 40 mL/minute: Administer 5.9 mg/kg every 24 hours **or** 11.7 mg/kg every 48 hours
CrCl 30 mL/minute: Administer 4.7 mg/kg every 24 hours **or** 9.5 mg/kg every 48 hours **or** 14.2 mg/kg every 72 hours
CrCl 20 mL/minute: Administer 3.6 mg/kg every 24 hours **or** 7.2 mg/kg every 48 hours **or** 10.7 mg/kg every 72 hours
CrCl 10 mL/minute: Administer 2.4 mg/kg every 24 hours **or** 4.9 mg/kg every 48 hours **or** 7.3 mg/kg every 72 hours
CrCl 0 mL/minute: Administer 1.3 mg/kg every 24 hours **or** 2.6 mg/kg every 48 hours **or** 3.9 mg/kg every 72 hours
The following guidelines may also be used:
CDC, 2003:
CrCl ≥30 mL/minute: No adjustment required
CrCl <30 mL/minute and/or hemodialysis: 12-15 mg/kg (maximum dose: 1000 mg/dose) 2-3 days per week (**NOT** daily)
Aronoff, 2007:
CrCl ≥10 mL/minute: No adjustment required
CrCl <10 mL/minute: 1000 mg every 48 hours
Hemodialysis: Administer dose after hemodialysis only

Continuous renal replacement therapy (CRRT): 5 mg/kg every 24 hours
Dosing adjustment in hepatic impairment: There are no dosage adjustments provided in the manufacturer's labeling; some suggest that no extra precautions are needed (CDC, 2003).

Administration Parenteral:
I.V.: Reconstitute powder (1000 mg vial) with 2 mL of NS or SWI; allow 2-3 minutes for dissolution. Further dilute in NS 100 mL and infuse over 60 minutes.
I.M.: Administer by deep I.M. injection into large muscle mass; concentration for administration dependent upon dose:
1000 mg dose: Administer contents of vial reconstituted with NS or SWI
<1000 mg dose: Reconstitute 1000 mg vial to final concentration 210-370 mg/mL (see table):

Capreomycin Dilution for Doses <1000 mg (I.M. Administration)

Diluent Volume for 1000 mg Vial (mL)	Final Capreomycin Solution Volume (mL)	Final Concentration (approximate)*
2.15	2.85	370 mg/mL
2.63	3.33	315 mg/mL
3.3	4	260 mg/mL
4.3	5	210 mg/mL

* Retention volume taken into account for approximation of final concentration.

Monitoring Parameters
Pediatric patients: Audiometric measurements and vestibular function (baseline, monthly while on therapy, and at 6 months following discontinuation of therapy); renal function (baseline, weekly during therapy or monthly for first 6 months of therapy, then every 3 months and at 6 months following discontinuation of therapy); baseline and frequent assessment of serum electrolytes (including calcium, magnesium, and potassium), liver function tests, growth parameters (CDC, 2003; Seddon, 2012).
Adults: Audiometric measurements and vestibular function at baseline and during therapy; renal function at baseline and weekly during therapy; frequent assessment of serum electrolytes (including calcium, magnesium, and potassium), liver function tests

Additional Information Recommended dosages are designed to achieve a mean serum concentration of 10 mcg/mL which corresponds to the recommended concentration for susceptibility testing (CDC, 2003).

Dosage Forms Excipient information presented when available (limited, particularly for generics); consult specific product labeling.
Solution Reconstituted, Injection, as sulfate:
Capastat Sulfate: 1 g (1 ea)

References
Aronoff GR, Bennett WM, Berns JS, et al, *Drug Prescribing in Renal Failure: Dosing Guidelines for Adults and Children*, 5th ed. Philadelphia, PA: American College of Physicians, 2007.
Centers for Disease Control and Prevention (CDC), "Treatment of Tuberculosis," *MMWR Recomm Rep*, 2003, 52(RR-11):1-77. Available at http://www.cdc.gov/mmwr/preview/mmwrhtml/rr5211a1.htm
DHHS. Guidelines for the prevention and treatment of opportunistic infections among HIV-exposed and HIV-infected children: recommendations from the National Institutes of Health, Centers for Disease Control and Prevention, the HIV Medicine Association of the Infectious Diseases Society of America, the Pediatric Infectious Diseases Society, and the American Academy of Pediatrics. November 6, 2013. Available at http://aidsinfo.nih.gov
DHHS Panel on Opportunistic Infections (OI) in HIV-Infected Adults and Adolescents. Guidelines for prevention and treatment of opportunistic infections in HIV-infected adults and adolescents: recommendations from the Centers for Disease Control and Prevention (CDC), the

National Institutes of Health (NIH), and the HIV Medicine Association (HIVMA) of the Infectious Diseases Society of America (IDSA). May 7, 2013. Available at http://aidsinfo.nih.gov/contentfiles/lvguidelines/adult_oi.pdf

Drobac PC, Mukherjee JS, Joseph JK, et al. Community-based therapy for children with multidrug-resistant tuberculosis. *Pediatrics*. 2006;117 (6): 2022-2029.

Seddon JA, Furin JJ, Gale M, et al. Caring for children with drug-resistant tuberculosis- practice-based recommendations. *Am J Respir Crit Care Med*. 2012;186:953-964.

Seddon JA, Thee S, Jacobs K, et al. Hearing loss in children treated for multi-drug resistant tuberculosis. *J Infect*. 2013;66:320-3299.

◆ **Capreomycin Sulfate** see Capreomycin on page 365

Capsaicin (kap SAY sin)

Medication Safety Issues
Sound-alike/look-alike issues:
Zostrix® may be confused with Zestril®, Zovirax®

Brand Names: U.S. Aleveer [OTC]; Capzasin-HP® [OTC]; Capzasin-P® [OTC]; DiabetAid® Pain and Tingling Relief [OTC]; Qutenza™; Salonpas® Gel-Patch Hot [OTC]; Salonpas® Hot [OTC] [DSC]; Trixaicin HP [OTC]; Trixaicin [OTC]; Zostrix® Diabetic Foot Pain [OTC]; Zostrix® [OTC]; Zostrix®-HP [OTC]

Brand Names: Canada Zostrix®; Zostrix® H.P.

Therapeutic Category Analgesic, Topical; Topical Skin Product; Transient Receptor Potential Vanilloid 1 (TRPV1) Agonist

Generic Availability (U.S.) Yes: Cream

Use Topical treatment of pain associated with postherpetic neuralgia (FDA approved in adults); temporary treatment of minor pain associated with muscles and joints due to backache, strains, sprains, bruises, cramps, or arthritis; temporary relief of pain associated with diabetic neuropathy (FDA approved in adults; DiabetAid Pain and Tingling Relief: FDA approved in ages ≥2 years and adults; Salonpas® Hot: FDA approved in ages ≥12 years and adults); has also been used for postsurgical pain, pain associated with psoriasis, chronic neuralgias unresponsive to other forms of therapy, and intractable pruritus

Pregnancy Risk Factor B

Pregnancy Considerations Adverse events have not been observed in animal reproduction studies with capsaicin patch or liquid. Systemic absorption is limited following topical administration of the patch; plasma concentrations are below the limit of detection 3-6 hours after the patch is removed.

Breast-Feeding Considerations Systemic absorption is limited following topical administration of the patch. When using the topical high concentration (capsaicin 8%) patch, Qutenza™, the manufacturer recommends not breast-feeding on the day of treatment after the patch has been applied to reduce any potential infant exposure.

Contraindications Hypersensitivity to capsaicin or any component

Warnings When using the high concentration topical patch (Qutenza™), do not apply to face, scalp, or allow contact with eyes or mucous membranes; do not apply on skin not being treated. If an unintended area of skin is inadvertently exposed, the cleansing gel should be used. Postapplication pain should be treated with local cooling methods and/or analgesics (opioids may be necessary). Rapid removal of patches may lead to aerosolization of capsaicin; remove patches gently and slowly to decrease risk of aerosolization; inhalation of airborne capsaicin may result in coughing or sneezing; if shortness of breath occurs, medical care is required.

May cause serious burns (eg, first- to third-degree chemical burns) at the application site. In some cases, hospitalization has been required. Discontinue use and seek medical attention if signs of skin injury (eg, pain, swelling, or blistering) occur following application (FDA Drug Safety

Communication, 2012). Transient burning sensation (without skin damage) may occur and generally disappears after several days; discontinue use if severe burning develops. Stop use and consult a healthcare provider if redness or irritation develops, symptoms get worse, or symptoms resolve and then recur.

Precautions When using OTC topical products, apply externally; avoid contact with eyes or mucous membranes. Should not be applied to wounds or broken or irritated skin. Treated area should not be exposed to heat or direct sunlight. Affected area should not be tightly bandaged.

Use caution in patients with uncontrolled hypertension or a history of cardiovascular or cerebrovascular events when using the high concentration topical patch (Qutenza™); transient increases in blood pressure due to treatment-related pain have occurred during and after application of patch.

Adverse Reactions Topical patch (Qutenza™, capsaicin 8%):
Local: Erythema, pain
Cardiovascular: Hypertension (transient)
Dermatologic: Pruritus
Gastrointestinal: Nausea, vomiting
Local: Dryness, edema, erythema, papules, pruritus, swelling
Respiratory: Bronchitis, nasopharyngitis, sinusitis
Rare but important or life-threatening): Application site reactions (bruising, dermatitis, excoriation, exfoliation, hyperesthesia, inflammation, paresthesia, urticaria), burning sensation, cough, dizziness, dysgeusia, headache, hypoesthesia, peripheral edema, peripheral sensory neuropathy, skin odor (abnormal), throat irritation

Drug Interactions
Metabolism/Transport Effects Substrate of CYP2E1 (minor); **Note:** Assignment of Major/Minor substrate status based on clinically relevant drug interaction potential
Avoid Concomitant Use There are no known interactions where it is recommended to avoid concomitant use.
Increased Effect/Toxicity There are no known significant interactions involving an increase in effect.
Decreased Effect There are no known significant interactions involving a decrease in effect.

Stability
DiabetAid Pain and Tingling Relief, Zostrix®, Zostrix®-HP: Store at 15°C to 30°C (59°F to 86°F)
Qutenza™: Store at room temperature between 20°C to 25°C (68°F to 77°F). Excursions between 15°C to 30°C (59°F to 86°F) are permitted.

Mechanism of Action Capsaicin, a transient receptor potential vanilloid 1 receptor (TRPV1) agonist, activates TRPV1 ligand-gated cation channels on nociceptive nerve fibers, resulting in depolarization, initiation of action potential, and pain signal transmission to the spinal cord; capsaicin exposure results in subsequent desensitization of the sensory axons and inhibition of pain transmission initiation. In arthritis, capsaicin induces release of substance P, the principal chemomediator of pain impulses from the periphery to the CNS, from peripheral sensory neurons; after repeated application, capsaicin depletes the neuron of substance P and prevents reaccumulation. The functional link between substance P and the capsaicin receptor, TRPV1, is not well understood.

Pharmacodynamics Onset of action:
OTC products (capsaicin 0.025% to 0.1%): 2-4 weeks of continuous therapy
Qutenza™ patch: 1 week after application

Pharmacokinetics (Adult data unless noted)
Absorption: Topical patch (capsaicin 8%): Systemic absorption is transient and low (<5 ng/mL) in approximately one-third of patients when measured following 60-minute application. In patients with quantifiable

▶

concentrations, most fell below the limit of quantitation at 3-6 hours postapplication.

Half-life: Topical patch (capsaicin 8%): 1.64 hours (Babbar, 2009)

Dosing: Usual Topical:

Pain relief:

Lotion: Children >2 years, Adolescents, and Adults: OTC labeling (DiabetAid Tingling and Pain Relief): Apply to affected area 3-4 times/day

Patch: Adolescents ≥12 years and Adults: OTC labeling (Salonpas®-Hot): Apply patch to affected area up to 3-4 times/day for 7 days. Patch may remain in place for up to 8 hours

Cream, gel, liquid: Adults: Apply to affected area 3-4 times/day; efficacy may be decreased if used less than 3 times/day; best results seen after 2-4 weeks of continuous use

Postherpetic neuralgia: Patch [Qutenza™ (capsaicin 8%)]: Adults: Apply patch to most painful area for 60 minutes. Up to 4 patches may be applied in a single application. Treatment may be repeated ≥3 months as needed for return of pain (do not apply more frequently than every 3 months). Area should be pretreated with a topical anesthetic prior to patch application.

Administration

Topical products (cream, gel, liquid, lotion): Wear gloves to apply; apply thin film to the affected areas and gently rub in until absorbed; wash hands with soap and water after applying to avoid spreading to eyes or other sensitive areas of the body.

Topical patch (Salonpas®-Hot): Apply patch externally to clean and dry affected area. Backing film should be removed prior to application. Do not use within 1 hour prior to a bath or immediately after bathing. Do not use with a heating pad.

Topical patch [Qutenza™ (capsaicin 8%)]: Patch should only be applied by physician or by a healthcare professional under the close supervision of a physician. The treatment area must be identified and marked by a physician. The patch can be cut to match size/shape of treatment area. If necessary, excessive hair present on and surrounding the treatment area may be clipped (not shaved) to promote adherence. Prior to application, the treatment area should be cleansed with mild soap and water and dried thoroughly. The treatment area should be anesthetized with a topical anesthetic prior to patch application. Anesthetic should be removed with a dry wipe and area should be cleansed again with soap/water, and dried. Patch may then be applied to dry, intact skin within 2 hours of opening the sealed patch; apply patch using nitrile gloves (latex gloves should **NOT** be used). During application, slowly peel back the release liner under the patch. Patch should remain in place for 60 minutes. Do not touch the patch while it is on the skin. Remove patches gently and slowly. Following patch removal, apply cleansing gel to the treatment area and leave in place for at least 1 minute. All treatment materials should be disposed of according to biomedical waste procedures.

Monitoring Parameters Qutenza™: Blood pressure

Additional Information In patients with severe and persistent local discomfort, pretreatment with topical lidocaine 5% ointment or concurrent oral analgesics for the first 2 weeks of therapy have been effective in alleviating the initial burning sensation and enabling continuation of topical capsaicin

Dosage Forms Excipient information presented when available (limited, particularly for generics); consult specific product labeling. [DSC] = Discontinued product

Cream, topical: 0.025% (60 g)

Capzasin-HP®: 0.1% (42.5 g) [contains benzyl alcohol]

Capzasin-P®: 0.035% (42.5 g) [contains benzyl alcohol]

Trixaicin: 0.025% (60 g) [contains benzyl alcohol]

Trixaicin HP: 0.075% (60 g) [contains benzyl alcohol]

Zostrix®: 0.025% (60 g) [contains benzyl alcohol]

Zostrix® Diabetic Foot Pain: 0.075% (60 g) [contains benzyl alcohol]

Zostrix®-HP: 0.075% (60 g) [contains benzyl alcohol]

Gel, topical:

Capzasin-P®: 0.025% (42.5 g) [contains menthol]

Liquid, topical:

Capzasin-P®: 0.15% (29.5 mL)

Lotion, topical:

DiabetAid® Pain and Tingling Relief: 0.025% (120 mL)

Patch, topical:

Aleveer: 0.0375% (15s) [contains menthol 5%, and aloe]

Qutenza™: 8% (1s, 2s) [contains metal; supplied with cleansing gel]

Salonpas® Gel-Patch Hot: 0.025% (3s, 6s) [contains menthol]

Salonpas® Hot: 0.025% (1s [DSC]) [contains natural rubber/natural latex in packaging]

References

Babbar S, Marier JF, Mouksassi MS, et al, "Pharmacokinetic Analysis of Capsaicin After Topical Administration of a High-Concentration Capsaicin Patch to Patients With Peripheral Neuropathic Pain," Ther Drug Monit, 2009, 31(4):502-10.

Backonja M, Wallace MS, Blonsky ER, et al, "NGX-4010, a High-Concentration Capsaicin Patch, for the Treatment of Postherpetic Neuralgia: A Randomised, Double-Blind Study," Lancet Neurol, 2008, 7(12):1106-12.

Bernstein JE, Korman NJ, Bickers DR, et al, "Topical Capsaicin Treatment of Chronic Postherpetic Neuralgia," J Am Acad Dermatol, 1989, 21(2 Pt 1):265-70.

FDA Drug Safety Communication. Rare cases of serious burns with the use of over-the-counter topical muscle and joint pain relievers. 2012. Available at http://www.fda.gov/Drugs/DrugSafety/ucm318858.htm

Willcockson HH, Chen Y, Han JE, et al, "Effect of Genetic Deletion of the Vanilloid Receptor TRPV1 on the Expression of Substance P in Sensory Neurons of Mice With Adjuvant-Induced Arthritis," Neuropeptides, 2010, 44(4):293-7.

Captopril (KAP toe pril)

Medication Safety Issues

Sound-alike/look-alike issues:

Captopril may be confused with calcitriol, Capitrol, carvedilol

International issues:

Acepril [Great Britain] may be confused with Accupril which is a brand name for quinapril in the U.S.

Acepril: Brand name for captopril [Great Britain], but also the brand name for enalapril [Hungary, Switzerland]; lisinopril [Malaysia]

Brand Names: Canada Apo-Capto; Dom-Captopril; Mylan-Captopril; PMS-Captopril

Therapeutic Category Angiotensin-Converting Enzyme (ACE) Inhibitor; Antihypertensive Agent

Generic Availability (U.S.) Yes

Use Treatment of hypertension, heart failure, left ventricular dysfunction after myocardial infarction, and diabetic nephropathy (FDA approved in adults)

Pregnancy Risk Factor D

Pregnancy Considerations [U.S. Boxed Warning]: Drugs that act on the renin-angiotensin system can cause injury and death to the developing fetus. Discontinue as soon as possible once pregnancy is detected. Captopril crosses the placenta; teratogenic effects may occur following maternal use during pregnancy. Drugs that act on the renin-angiotensin system are associated with oligohydramnios. Oligohydramnios, due to decreased fetal renal function, may lead to fetal lung hypoplasia and skeletal malformations. Their use in pregnancy is also associated with anuria, hypotension, renal failure, skull hypoplasia, and death in the fetus/neonate. Chronic maternal hypertension itself is also associated with adverse events in the fetus/infant. ACE inhibitors are not recommended during pregnancy to treat maternal hypertension or heart failure. Use of an ACE inhibitor should also be avoided in any woman of reproductive age. Women who are planning a pregnancy should be considered for other medication options if an ACE inhibitor is currently prescribed or the ACE inhibitor should be discontinued as soon as possible once pregnancy is detected. The exposed fetus should be monitored for fetal growth, amniotic fluid volume, and organ formation. Infants exposed to an ACE inhibitor *in utero* should be monitored for hyperkalemia, hypotension, and oliguria (exchange transfusions or dialysis may be needed). These adverse events are generally associated with maternal use in the second and third trimesters.

Untreated chronic maternal hypertension is also associated with adverse events in the fetus, infant, and mother. The use of ACE inhibitors is not recommended to treat chronic uncomplicated hypertension in pregnant women and should generally be avoided in women of reproductive potential (ACOG, 2013).

Breast-Feeding Considerations Captopril is excreted in breast milk. Breast-feeding is not recommended by the manufacturer.

Contraindications Hypersensitivity to captopril, any component, or other ACE inhibitors; patients with idiopathic or hereditary angioedema or a history of angioedema with previous ACE inhibitor use

Warnings Angioedema can occur at any time during treatment (especially following first dose). The relative risk of angioedema with ACE inhibitors is higher within the first 30 days of use (compared to >1 year of use), for Black Americans (compared to Whites), for lisinopril or enalapril (compared to captopril), and for patients previously hospitalized within 30 days (Brown, 1996). Angioedema may occur in the head, neck, extremities, or intestines; patients with angioedema of the intestines may present with abdominal pain (with or without nausea or vomiting); angioedema of the larynx, glottis, or tongue may cause airway obstruction, especially in patients with a history of airway surgery. Prolonged monitoring may be required, even in patients with swelling of only the tongue (ie, without respiratory distress) because treatment with corticosteroids and antihistamines may not be sufficient; very rare fatalities have occurred with angioedema of the larynx or tongue; appropriate treatment (eg, establishing patent airway and/or SubQ epinephrine) should be readily available for patients with angioedema of larynx, glottis, or tongue, in whom airway obstruction is likely to occur.

Anaphylactic/anaphylactoid reactions can occur with ACE inhibitors. Life-threatening anaphylactoid reactions may be seen during hemodialysis (eg, CVVHD) with high-flux dialysis membranes (eg, AN69), and rarely, during low density lipoprotein apheresis with dextran sulfate cellulose. Rare cases of anaphylactoid reactions have been reported in patients undergoing sensitization treatment with hymenoptera (bee, wasp) venom while receiving ACE inhibitors.

Captopril has been associated with rare but potentially fatal cases of agranulocytosis, neutropenia, or leukopenia with myeloid hypoplasia; higher risk for development of neutropenia is associated with renal impairment; risk is further increased in patients with both renal impairment and collagen vascular disease (eg, systemic lupus erythematosus). Onset of neutropenia is usually within 3 months of captopril initiation; closely monitor CBC with differential for the first 3 months of therapy and periodically thereafter in these patients; neutrophil count generally returns to baseline within 2 weeks of discontinuation.

ACE inhibitor use has been associated with deterioration of renal function and/or increases in serum creatinine, particularly in patients with low renal blood flow (eg, renal artery stenosis, heart failure) whose glomerular filtration rate (GFR) is dependent on efferent arteriolar

vasoconstriction by angiotensin II; deterioration may result in oliguria, acute renal failure, and progressive azotemia. Small increases in serum creatinine may occur following initiation; consider discontinuation only in patients with progressive and/or significant deterioration in renal function.

A rare toxicity associated with ACE inhibitors includes cholestatic jaundice, which may progress to fulminant hepatic necrosis; discontinue if marked elevation of hepatic transaminases or jaundice occurs and initiate appropriate medical treatment.

Drugs that act on the renin-angiotensin system can cause injury and death to the developing fetus. Discontinue as soon as possible once pregnancy is detected **[U.S. Boxed Warning]**.

Concomitant use of an ARB or renin inhibitor (eg, aliskiren) is associated with an increased risk of hypotension, hyperkalemia, and renal dysfunction. Concomitant use with aliskiren should be avoided in patients with GFR <60 mL/minute and is contraindicated in patients with diabetes mellitus (regardless of GFR).

Precautions Use with caution in patients with renal impairment; dosage reduction may be necessary; avoid rapid dosage escalation which may lead to further renal impairment. Use with caution in patients with unstented unilateral/bilateral renal artery stenosis. When unstented bilateral renal artery stenosis is present, use is generally avoided due to the elevated risk of deterioration in renal function unless possible benefits outweigh risks.

Use with caution when initiating therapy and in volume-depleted patients; may cause symptomatic hypotension with or without syncope, usually with the first several doses; correct volume depletion prior to initiation; initiate lower doses in patients with sodium or volume depletion; close monitoring of patient is required, especially with initial dosing and dosing increases; blood pressure must be lowered at a rate appropriate for the patient's clinical condition. Although dose reduction may be necessary, hypotension alone is not a reason for discontinuation of future ACE inhibitor use, especially in patients with heart failure when a reduction in systolic blood pressure is a desirable observation. An observational study of 66 pediatric patients with heart failure reported hypotension in 15% of patients during therapy initiation at typical starting doses; close monitoring in an inpatient setting and low starting doses has been suggested in these patients (Momma, 2006; Orchard, 2010). Use with caution in patients with ischemic heart disease or cerebrovascular disease during therapy initiation; observe closely due to the potential consequences posed by falling blood pressure (eg, MI, stroke); fluid replacement may be required to restore blood pressure; therapy may then be resumed; discontinue therapy in patients whose hypotension recurs. Use with caution in patients with severe aortic stenosis; may reduce coronary perfusion resulting in ischemia. Use with caution in patients with hypertrophic cardiomyopathy (HCM) and outflow tract obstruction since reduction in afterload may worsen symptoms associated with this condition.

May cause hyperkalemia; risk factors include renal dysfunction, diabetes mellitus, concomitant use of potassium-sparing diuretics, potassium supplements, and/or potassium-containing salts; use with caution, if at all, with these agents and monitor potassium closely. Concurrent use of angiotensin receptor blockers (ARBs) may increase the risk of clinically significant adverse events (eg, renal dysfunction, hyperkalemia).

Extemporaneous preparations of liquid formulations may vary; this may affect the rate and extent of absorption causing intrapatient variability regarding dosing and safety profile for the patient; use with caution and monitor closely if dosage formulations are changed (Bhatt, 2011; Mulla, 2007).

Use with caution before, during, or immediately after major surgery; cardiopulmonary bypass, intraoperative blood loss, or vasodilating anesthesia increases endogenous renin release; use of ACE inhibitors perioperatively will blunt angiotensin II formation and may result in hypotension.

An ACE inhibitor cough is a dry, hacking, nonproductive one that usually occurs within the first few months of treatment and should generally resolve within 1-4 weeks after discontinuation of the ACE inhibitor; in pediatric patients, an isolated dry hacking cough lasting >3 weeks was reported in 7 of 42 pediatric patients (17%) receiving ACE inhibitors (von Vigier, 2000); a review of pediatric randomized-controlled ACE inhibitor trials reported a lower incidence of 3.2% (Baker-Smith, 2010). Other causes of cough should be considered (eg, pulmonary congestion in patients with heart failure) and excluded prior to discontinuation.

Adverse Reactions

Cardiovascular: Angina, angioedema, cardiac arrest, cerebrovascular insufficiency, chest pain, CHF, flushing, hypotension, MI, orthostatic hypotension, pallor, palpitation, Raynaud's syndrome, rhythm disturbances, syncope, tachycardia

Central nervous system: Ataxia, confusion, depression, nervousness, somnolence

Dermatologic: Bullous pemphigus, erythema multiforme, exfoliative dermatitis, pruritus, rash (maculopapular or urticarial), Stevens-Johnson syndrome

Endocrine & metabolic: Gynecomastia, hyperkalemia, alkaline phosphatase increased, bilirubin increased

Gastrointestinal: Dyspepsia, glossitis, pancreatitis

Genitourinary: Impotence, urinary frequency

Hematologic: Agranulocytosis, anemia, neutropenia pancytopenia, thrombocytopenia

Hepatic: Cholestasis, hepatic necrosis (rare), hepatitis, jaundice, hyponatremia (symptomatic), transaminases increased

Neuromuscular & skeletal: Asthenia, myalgia, myasthenia

Ocular: Blurred vision

Renal: Nephrotic syndrome, oliguria, polyuria, proteinuria, renal failure, renal insufficiency, serum creatinine increased, worsening of renal function (may occur in patients with bilateral renal artery stenosis or hypovolemia)

Respiratory: Bronchospasm, cough, eosinophilic pneumonitis, rhinitis

Miscellaneous: Anaphylactoid reactions, dysgeusia - loss of taste or diminished perception, hypersensitivity reactions (arthralgia, eosinophilia, fever, pruritus, rash)

Rare but important or life-threatening: Alopecia, angina, anorexia, aphthous ulcers, aplastic anemia, cholestatic jaundice, eosinophilia, erythrocyte sedimentation rate increased, exacerbations of Huntington's disease, glomerulonephritis, Guillain-Barré syndrome, hemolytic anemia, hyperthermia, insomnia, interstitial nephritis, Kaposi's sarcoma, peptic ulcer, pericarditis, psoriasis, seizure (in premature infants), systemic lupus erythematosus, vasculitis, visual hallucinations (Doane, 2013)

Drug Interactions

Metabolism/Transport Effects Substrate of CYP2D6 (major); **Note:** Assignment of Major/Minor substrate status based on clinically relevant drug interaction potential

Avoid Concomitant Use There are no known interactions where it is recommended to avoid concomitant use.

Increased Effect/Toxicity

Captopril may increase the levels/effects of: Allopurinol; Amifostine; Antihypertensives; AzaTHIOprine; CycloSPORINE (Systemic); DULoxetine; Ferric Gluconate;

Gold Sodium Thiomalate; Grass Pollen Allergen Extract (5 Grass Extract); Hypotensive Agents; Iron Dextran Complex; Lithium; Nonsteroidal Anti-Inflammatory Agents; Obinutuzumab; RiTUXimab; Sodium Phosphates

The levels/effects of Captopril may be increased by: Abiraterone Acetate; Alfuzosin; Aliskiren; Angiotensin II Receptor Blockers; Barbiturates; Brimonidine (Topical); Canagliflozin; CYP2D6 Inhibitors (Moderate); CYP2D6 Inhibitors (Strong); Darunavir; Diazoxide; DPP-IV Inhibitors; Eplerenone; Everolimus; Heparin; Heparin (Low Molecular Weight); Herbs (Hypotensive Properties); Loop Diuretics; MAO Inhibitors; Pentoxifylline; Phosphodiesterase 5 Inhibitors; Potassium Salts; Potassium-Sparing Diuretics; Prostacyclin Analogues; Sirolimus; Temsirolimus; Thiazide Diuretics; TiZANidine; Tolvaptan; Trimethoprim

Decreased Effect

The levels/effects of Captopril may be decreased by: Antacids; Aprotinin; Herbs (Hypertensive Properties); Icatibant; Lanthanum; Methylphenidate; Nonsteroidal Anti-Inflammatory Agents; Peginterferon Alfa-2b; Salicylates; Yohimbine

Food Interactions Captopril serum concentrations may be decreased if taken with food. Long-term use of captopril may lead to a zinc deficiency which can result in altered taste perception. Management: Take on an empty stomach 1 hour before or 2 hours after meals.

Stability Store at ≤30°C (86°F); protect from moisture and light.

Mechanism of Action Competitive inhibitor of angiotensin-converting enzyme (ACE); prevents conversion of angiotensin I to angiotensin II, a potent vasoconstrictor; results in lower levels of angiotensin II which causes an increase in plasma renin activity and a reduction in aldosterone secretion

Pharmacodynamics

Onset of action: Antihypertensive: Within 15 minutes

Maximum effect: Antihypertensive: 60-90 minutes; may require several weeks of therapy before full hypotensive effect is seen

Duration: Dose-related

Pharmacokinetics (Adult data unless noted)

Absorption: 60% to 75%

Distribution: 7 L/kg

Bioavailability: 75%

Protein binding: 25% to 30%

Metabolism: 50% metabolized

Half-life:

Infants with CHF: 3.3 hours; range: 1.2-12.4 hours (Pereira, 1991)

Children: 1.5 hours; range: 0.98-2.3 hours (Levy, 1991)

Normal adults (dependent upon renal and cardiac function): 1.9 hours

Adults with CHF: 2.1 hours

Anuria: 20-40 hours

Time to peak serum concentration: Within 1-2 hours

Elimination: 95% excreted in urine in 24 hours

Dosing: Neonatal Heart failure (afterload reduction); hypertension: Limited data available: **Note:** Dosage must be titrated according to patient's response; use lowest effective dose; lower doses (~1/2 of those listed) should be used in patients who are sodium and water depleted due to diuretic therapy

Premature neonates: Oral: Initial: 0.01 mg/kg/dose every 8-12 hours; titrate dose

Term neonates, PNA ≤7 days: Oral: Initial: 0.01 mg/kg/dose every 8-12 hours; titrate dose

Term neonates, PNA >7 days: Oral: Initial: 0.05-0.1 mg/kg/dose every 8-24 hours; titrate dose upward to maximum of 0.5 mg/kg/dose given every 6-24 hours

Dosing: Usual

Infants, Children and Adolescents:

Heart failure (afterload reduction): Limited data available: **Note:** Initiate therapy at lower end of range and titrate upward to prevent symptomatic hypotension (Momma, 2006):

Infants: Oral: 0.3-2.5 mg/kg/day divided every 8-12 hours; one study of infants (age: 1-7 months) with left-right shunt reported a mean dose of 1.3 mg/kg/day

Children and Adolescents: Oral: 0.3-6 mg/kg/day divided every 8-12 hours; maximum daily dose: 150 mg/day; in clinical trials, usual reported dosage range was 0.9-3.9 mg/kg/day

Hypertension: Limited data available: **Note:** Dosage must be titrated according to patient's response; use lowest effective dose; lower doses (~1/2 of those listed) should be used in patients who are sodium- and water-depleted due to diuretic therapy

Weight-based dosing:

Infants: Oral: Initial: 0.15-0.3 mg/kg/dose; titrate dose upward to maximum of 6 mg/kg/day in 1-4 divided doses; usual required dose: 2.5-6 mg/kg/day

Children and Adolescents: Oral: Initial: 0.3-0.5 mg/kg/dose every 8 hours; may titrate as needed up to maximum daily dose: 6 mg/kg/day in 3 divided doses (NHBPEP, 2004; NHLBI, 2011); maximum daily dose: 450 mg/day

Fixed dosing:

Older Children: Oral: Initial: 6.25-12.5 mg/dose every 12-24 hours; titrate as needed; maximum daily dose: 6 mg/kg/day in 2-4 divided doses; maximum daily dose: 450 mg/day

Adolescents: Oral: Initial: 12.5-25 mg/dose given every 8-12 hours; increase by 25 mg/dose at 1-2 week intervals based on patient response; maximum daily dose: 450 mg/day; usual dosage range for hypertension (JNC 7): Adolescents ≥18 years: 25-100 mg/day in 2 divided doses

Adults: **Note:** Titrate dose according to patient's response; use lowest effective dose.

Acute hypertension (urgency/emergency): Oral: 12.5-25 mg, may repeat as needed (may be given sublingually, but no therapeutic advantage demonstrated)

Heart failure: Oral:

Initial dose: 6.25-12.5 mg 3 times daily in conjunction with cardiac glycoside and diuretic therapy; initial dose depends upon patient's fluid/electrolyte status

Target dose: 50 mg 3 times daily

Hypertension: Oral: Initial dose: 25 mg 2-3 times daily [a lower initial dose of 12.5 mg 3 times daily may also be considered (VA Cooperative Study Group, 1984)]; may increase by 12.5-25 mg/dose at 1- to 2-week intervals up to 50 mg 3 times daily; add thiazide diuretic, unless severe renal impairment coexists then consider loop diuretic before further dosage increases or consider other treatment options; maximum dose: 150 mg 3 times daily

Usual dose range (JNC 7): 25-100 mg/day in 2 divided doses

LV dysfunction following MI: Oral: Initial: 6.25 mg; if tolerated, follow with 12.5 mg 3 times daily; then increase to 25 mg 3 times daily during next several days and then gradually increase over next several weeks to target dose of 50 mg 3 times daily (some dose schedules are more aggressive to achieve an increased goal dose within the first few days of initiation)

Diabetic nephropathy: Oral: Initial: 25 mg 3 times daily; may be taken with other antihypertensive therapy if required to further lower blood pressure

Dosing adjustment in renal impairment:

Infants, Children and Adolescents: The following adjustments have been recommended (Aronoff, 2007). **Note:** Renally adjusted dose recommendations are based on doses of 0.1-0.5 mg/kg/dose every 6-8 hours; maximum daily dose: 6 mg/kg/**day**.

GFR 10-50 mL/minute/1.73 m^2: Administer 75% of dose

GFR <10 mL/minute/1.73 m^2: Administer 50% of dose

Intermittent hemodialysis: Administer 50% of dose

Peritoneal dialysis (PD): Administer 50% of dose

Continuous renal replacement therapy (CRRT): Administer 75% of dose

Adults:

Manufacturer's labeling: Reduce initial daily dose and titrate slowly (1- to 2-week intervals) with smaller increments. Slowly back titrate to determine the minimum effective dose once the desired therapeutic effect has been reached.

The following adjustments have been recommended (Aronoff, 2007):

CrCl >50 mL/minute: Administer 100% of normal dose every 8-12 hours

CrCl 10-50 mL/minute: Administer 75% of normal dose every 12-18 hours

CrCl <10 mL/minute: Administer 50% of normal dose every 24 hours

Intermittent hemodialysis (IHD): Administer after hemodialysis on dialysis days

Peritoneal dialysis: Administer 75% of normal dose every 12-18 hours; supplemental dose is not necessary

Administration Oral: Administer on an empty stomach 1 hour before meals or 2 hours after meals; if crushing tablet and dissolving in water, allow adequate time for complete dissolution (>10 minutes) (Bhatt, 2011)

Monitoring Parameters Blood pressure, BUN, serum creatinine, renal function, urine dipstick for protein, serum potassium, WBC with differential, especially during first 3 months of therapy for patients with renal impairment and/or collagen vascular disease; monitor for angioedema and anaphylactoid reactions; hypovolemia and postural hypotension when beginning therapy, adjusting dosage, and on a regular basis throughout

Test Interactions Positive Coombs' [direct]; may cause false-positive results in urine acetone determinations using sodium nitroprusside reagent

Dosage Forms Excipient information presented when available (limited, particularly for generics); consult specific product labeling.

Tablet, Oral:

Generic: 12.5 mg, 25 mg, 50 mg, 100 mg

Extemporaneous Preparations A 1 mg/mL oral solution may be made by allowing two 50 mg tablets to dissolve in 50 mL of distilled water. Add the contents of one 500 mg sodium ascorbate injection ampul or one 500 mg ascorbic acid tablet and allow to dissolve. Add quantity of distilled water sufficient to make 100 mL. Label "shake well" and "refrigerate". Stable for 56 days refrigerated.

Nahata MC, Pai VB, and Hipple TF, *Pediatric Drug Formulations*, 5th ed, Cincinnati, OH: Harvey Whitney Books Co, 2004.

References

Aronoff GR, Bennett WM, Berns JS, et al, *Drug Prescribing in Renal Failure: Dosing Guidelines for Adults and Children*, 5th ed, Philadelphia, PA: American College of Physicians, 2007.

Baker-Smith CM, Benjamin DK Jr, Califf RM, et al, "Cough in Pediatric Patients Receiving Angiotensin-Converting Enzyme Inhibitor Therapy or Angiotensin Receptor Blocker Therapy in Randomized Controlled Trials," *Clin Pharmacol Ther*, 2010, 87(6):668-71.

Bhatt MD, Thomas JE, and Mondal TK, "Variation in Captopril Formulations in Pharmacies Across Canada," *Paediatr Child Health*, 2011, 16(4):e30-2.

Brown NJ, Ray WA, Snowden M, et al, "Black Americans Have an Increased Rate of Angiotensin-Converting Enzyme Inhibitor-Associated Angioedema," *Clin Pharmacol Ther*, 1996, 60(1):8-13.

Chobanian AV, Bakris GL, Black HR, et al, "The Seventh Report of the Joint National Committee on Prevention, Detection, Evaluation, and Treatment of High Blood Pressure: The JNC 7 Report," *JAMA*, 2003, 289(19):2560-72.

Levy M, Koren G, Klein J, et al, "Captopril Pharmacokinetics, Blood Pressure Response and Plasma Renin Activity in Normotensive Children With Renal Scarring," *Dev Pharmacol Ther*, 1991, 16 (4):185-93.

Mirkin BL and Newman TJ, "Efficacy and Safety of Captopril in the Treatment of Severe Childhood Hypertension: Report of the International Collaborative Study Group," *Pediatrics*, 1985, 75(6):1091-100.

Momma K, "ACE Inhibitors in Pediatric Patients With Heart Failure," *Paediatr Drugs*, 2006, 8(1):55-69.

Mulla H, Tofeig M, Bu'Lock F, et al, "Variations in Captopril Formulations Used to Treat Children With Heart Failure: A Survey in the United Kingdom," *Arch Dis Child*, 2007, 92(5):409-11.

National High Blood Pressure Education Program Working Group on High Blood Pressure in Children and Adolescents, "The Fourth Report on the Diagnosis, Evaluation, and Treatment of High Blood Pressure in Children and Adolescents," *Pediatrics*, 2004, 114(2 Suppl):555-76.

Orchard EA, Apps A, and Wilson N, "Use of Captopril in Paediatric Congestive Cardiac Failure: Early Effects on Blood Pressure and Renal Function," *Arch Dis Child*, 2010, 95(7):566-7.

Pereira CM, Tam YK, Collins-Nakai RL, "The Pharmacokinetics of Captopril in Infants With Congestive Heart Failure," *Ther Drug Monit*, 1991, 13(3):209-14.

Veterans Administration Cooperative Study Group on Antihypertensive Agents, "Low-Dose Captopril for the Treatment of Mild to Moderate Hypertension. I. Results of a 14-Week Trial," *Arch Intern Med*, 1984, 144(10):1947-53.

von Vigier RO, Mozzettini S, Truttmann AC, et al, "Cough is Common in Children Prescribed Converting Enzyme Inhibitors," *Nephron*, 2000, 84(1):98.

◆ **Capzasin-HP® [OTC]** *see Capsaicin on page 367*

◆ **Capzasin-P® [OTC]** *see Capsaicin on page 367*

◆ **Carac** *see Fluorouracil (Topical) on page 900*

◆ **Carafate** *see Sucralfate on page 1940*

◆ **Carbaglu** *see Carglumic Acid on page 381*

CarBAMazepine (kar ba MAZ e peen)

Medication Safety Issues

Sound-alike/look-alike issues:

CarBAMazepine may be confused with OXcarbazepine

Epitol may be confused with Epinal

TEGretol, TEGretol-XR may be confused with Mebaral, Toprol-XL, Toradol, TRENtal

BEERS Criteria medication:

This drug may be potentially inappropriate for use in geriatric patients (Quality of evidence - moderate; Strength of recommendation - strong).

Related Information

Oral Medications That Should Not Be Crushed or Altered *on page 2438*

Safe Handling of Hazardous Drugs *on page 2419*

Brand Names: U.S. Carbatrol; Epitol; Equetro; TEGretol; TEGretol-XR

Brand Names: Canada Apo-Carbamazepine; Dom-Carbamazepine; Mapezine; Mylan-Carbamazepine CR; Nu-Carbamazepine; PMS-Carbamazepine; Sandoz-Carbamazepine; Taro-Carbamazepine Chewable; Tegretol; Teva-Carbamazepine

Therapeutic Category Anticonvulsant, Miscellaneous

Generic Availability (U.S.) Yes

Use

Carbatrol, Epitol, Tegretol, Tegretol-XR: Treatment of generalized tonic-clonic, partial (especially complex partial), and mixed partial or generalized seizure disorder (Carbatrol,Tegretol: FDA approved in pediatric patients [age not specified] and adults; Tegretol-XR: FDA approved in ages ≥6 years and adults); relief of pain in trigeminal neuralgia or glossopharyngeal neuralgia (Carbatrol, Epitol, Tegretol, Tegretol XR: FDA approved in adults)

Equetro: Treatment of acute manic and mixed episodes associated with bipolar I disorders (FDA approved in adults)

Medication Guide Available Yes

Pregnancy Risk Factor D

Pregnancy Considerations Studies in pregnant women have demonstrated a risk to the fetus. Carbamazepine and its metabolites can be found in the fetus and may be associated with teratogenic effects, including spina bifida, craniofacial defects, cardiovascular malformations, and hypospadias. The risk of teratogenic effects is higher with anticonvulsant polytherapy than monotherapy.

Developmental delays have also been observed following *in utero* exposure to carbamazepine (per manufacturer); however, socioeconomic factors, maternal and paternal IQ, and polytherapy may contribute to these findings. Pregnancy may cause small decreases of carbamazepine plasma concentrations in the second and third trimesters; monitoring should be considered. When used for the treatment of bipolar disorder, use of carbamazepine should be avoided during the first trimester of pregnancy if possible. The use of a single medication for the treatment of bipolar disorder or epilepsy in pregnancy is preferred. Carbamazepine may decrease plasma concentrations of hormonal contraceptives; breakthrough bleeding or unintended pregnancy may occur and alternate or back-up methods of contraception should be considered.

Patients exposed to carbamazepine during pregnancy are encouraged to enroll themselves into the AED Pregnancy Registry by calling 1-888-233-2334. Additional information is available at www.aedpregnancyregistry.org.

Breast-Feeding Considerations Carbamazepine and its active epoxide metabolite are found in breast milk. Carbamazepine can also be detected in the serum of nursing infants. Transient hepatic dysfunction has been observed in some case reports. Nursing should be discontinued if adverse events are observed. According to the manufacturer, the decision to continue or discontinue breast-feeding during therapy should take into account the risk of exposure to the infant and the benefits of treatment to the mother. Respiratory depression, seizures, nausea, vomiting, diarrhea, and/or decreased feeding have been observed in neonates exposed to carbamazepine *in utero* and may represent a neonatal withdrawal syndrome.

Contraindications Hypersensitivity to carbamazepine, tricyclic antidepressants, or any component; patients with a history of bone marrow suppression; concomitant use or use within 14 days of MAO inhibitors; concurrent use with nefazodone; concomitant use of delavirdine or other nonnucleoside reverse transcriptase inhibitors

Warnings Hazardous agent; use appropriate precautions for handling and disposal (NIOSH, 2012).

The risk of developing aplastic anemia or agranulocytosis is increased during treatment **[U.S. Boxed Warning]**; a spectrum of hematologic effects has been reported with use (eg, agranulocytosis, aplastic anemia, neutropenia, leukopenia, thrombocytopenia, pancytopenia, and anemias); patients with a previous history of adverse hematologic reaction to any drug may be at increased risk; use with caution and assess risks and benefits of therapy. Monitor CBC, platelets, and differential at baseline and periodically during therapy; advise patients of early signs and symptoms which are fever, sore throat, mouth ulcers, infections, easy bruising, petechial or purpuric hemorrhage; discontinue carbamazepine if evidence of significant bone marrow depression occurs.

Potentially fatal, severe dermatologic reactions including Stevens-Johnson syndrome (SJS) and toxic epidermal necrolysis (TEN) may occur **[U.S. Boxed Warning]**; over 90% of patients who experience these reactions do so within the first few months of treatment; the risk is increased in patients with the variant *HLA-B*1502* allele, found almost exclusively in patients of Asian ancestry. The presence of this genetic variant exists in up to 15% of people of Asian descent, varying from <1% in Japanese and Koreans, to 2% to 4% of South Asians and Indians, to 10% to 15% of populations from China, Taiwan, Malaysia, and the Philippines. This variant is virtually absent in those of Caucasian, African-American, Hispanic, Native American, or European ancestry. Risk assessments have suggested that incidence of SJS/TEN in Asians could be ~60 cases/10,000 new users depending on the country of origin (a nearly 10-fold higher incidence than in predominantly Caucasian populations). Patients of Asian ancestry should be screened for the variant *HLA-B*1502* allele (genetic marker) prior to initiating therapy [U.S. Boxed Warning]. Avoid use in patients testing positive for the allele, unless the benefit clearly outweighs the risk; toxic dermatologic reactions can still occur infrequently in patients of any ethnicity who test negative for *HLA-B*1502*; discontinue therapy in patients who have a serious dermatologic reaction. The risk of SJS or TENS may also be increased if carbamazepine is used in combination with other antiepileptic drugs associated with these reactions. Presence of the *HLA-B*1502* allele has not been found to predict the risk of less serious dermatologic reactions such as anticonvulsant hypersensitivity syndrome or nonserious rash.

The risk of developing a hypersensitivity reaction may be increased in patients with the variant *HLA-A*3101* allele. These hypersensitivity reactions include SJS/TEN, maculopapular eruptions, and drug reaction with eosinophilia and systemic symptoms (DRESS/multiorgan hypersensitivity). The *HLA-A*3101* allele may occur more frequently in patients of African-American, Asian, European, Indian, Latin American, and Native American ancestry. Hypersensitivity has also been reported in patients experiencing reactions to other anticonvulsants; the history of hypersensitivity reactions in the patient or their immediate family members should be reviewed; use with caution and assess risks and benefits of therapy. Approximately 25% to 30% of patients allergic to carbamazepine will also have reactions with oxcarbazepine.

Potentially serious, sometimes fatal multiorgan hypersensitivity reactions [also known as drug reaction with eosinophilia and systemic symptoms (DRESS)] have been reported with some antiepileptic drugs including carbamazepine; monitor for signs and symptoms of possible disparate manifestations associated with lymphatic, hepatic, renal, and/or hematologic organ systems; rash and eosinophilia may also be present; discontinuation of carbamazepine and conversion to alternate therapy may be required.

Carbamazepine may activate latent psychosis and/or cause confusion or agitation; elderly patients may be at an increased risk for psychiatric effects. Avoid the use of carbamazepine in patients with hepatic porphyria (eg, variegate porphyria, acute intermittent porphyria, porphyria cutanea tarda); acute attacks of porphyria may occur. Use with caution in patients with hepatic impairment; dosage reduction may be needed. Rare cases of a hepatic failure and vanishing bile duct syndrome involving destruction and disappearance of the intrahepatic bile ducts have been reported. Clinical courses of vanishing bile duct syndrome have been variable ranging from fulminant to indolent. Some cases have also had features associated with other immunoallergic syndromes such as multiorgan hypersensitivity (DRESS syndrome) and serious dermatologic reactions including Stevens-Johnson syndrome.

Substitution of Tegretol with generic carbamazepine has resulted in decreased carbamazepine levels and increased seizure activity, as well as increased carbamazepine levels and toxicity. Monitoring of carbamazepine serum concentrations is mandatory when patients are switched from any product to another. Anticonvulsants should not be discontinued abruptly because of the possibility of increasing seizure frequency or precipitating status epilepticus; therapy should be withdrawn gradually, unless safety concerns require a more rapid withdrawal.

Hyponatremia caused by the syndrome of inappropriate antidiuretic hormone secretion (SIADH) may occur during therapy. Risk may be increased in the elderly or in patients also taking diuretics and may be dose-dependent. Consider discontinuation of carbamazepine in patients with symptomatic hyponatremia.

Antiepileptic drugs (AEDs) increase the risk of suicidal behavior and ideation in patients receiving these medications for any indication. Pooled analyses of placebo-controlled trials involving 11 different AEDs (regardless of indication) showed a twofold increased risk of suicidal thoughts or behavior (estimated incidence rate: 0.43% in AED treated patients compared to 0.24% of patients receiving placebo); increased risk was observed as early as 1 week after initiation of AED and continued through duration of trials (most trials ≤24 weeks); risk did not vary significantly by age (age range: 5-100 years). Consider risks and benefits of AEDs before prescribing. Monitor all patients receiving an AED for emergence of suicidal thoughts or behavior, thoughts of self-harm, any unusual changes in behavior or mood, or the emergence or worsening of depressive symptoms; notify healthcare provider immediately if symptoms or concerning behavior occur. Note: The FDA requires a Medication Guide for all antiepileptic drugs informing patients of this risk.

May cause CNS depression or impairment in judgment, cognition, and motor function, which may impair physical or mental abilities; patients must be cautioned about performing tasks which require mental alertness (eg, operating machinery or driving). Effects with other sedative drugs or ethanol may be potentiated.

The suspension may contain sorbitol; avoid use in patents with hereditary fructose intolerance.

Precautions Use with caution in renal impairment. Use caution in patients with underlying ECG abnormalities, preexisting cardiac damage, or patients who are at risk for conduction abnormalities; may cause conduction abnormalities.

Use with caution in patients with sensitivity to anticholinergic effects (urinary retention, increased IOP, constipation); carbamazepine has mild anticholinergic activity. Use with caution in patients taking strong CYP3A4 inducers or inhibitors; carbamazepine may significantly induce many CYP450 enzymes, including 1A2, 2B6, 2C8, 2C9, 2C19, and 3A4; use with caution with medications significantly metabolized through these pathways. Potentially significant interactions may exist, requiring dose or frequency adjustment, additional monitoring, and/or selection of alternative therapy. Consult drug interactions database for more detailed information.

Use with caution when treating patients with a mixed seizure disorder that includes atypical absence seizures (carbamazepine may increase frequency of generalized convulsions in these patients). Administration of the suspension will yield higher peak and lower trough serum levels than an equal dose of the tablet form (Tegretol); consider a lower starting dose given more frequently (same total daily dose) when using the suspension.

For bipolar disorder, use the smallest effective dose to reduce the risk of overdose/suicide; high-risk patients should be monitored for suicidal ideations; to reduce risk of intentional overdose, write prescriptions for the smallest quantity consistent with good patient care.

Adverse Reactions

Cardiovascular: Aggravation of coronary artery disease, atrioventricular block, cardiac arrhythmia, cardiac failure, edema, hypertension, hypotension, syncope, thromboembolism, thrombophlebitis

Central nervous system: Abnormality in thinking, agitation, amnesia, ataxia, chills, confusion, depression, dizziness, drowsiness, fatigue, hallucinations, headache, hyperacusis, neuroleptic malignant syndrome (NMS), paresthesia, peripheral neuritis, slurred speech, speech disturbance, talkativeness, twitching, vertigo

Dermatologic: Acute generalized exanthematous pustulosis, alopecia, diaphoresis, dyschromia, erythema multiforme, erythema nodosum, exfoliative dermatitis, onychomadesis, pruritus, skin photosensitivity, skin rash, Stevens-Johnson syndrome, toxic epidermal necrolysis, urticaria

Endocrine & metabolic: Abnormal thyroid function test, albuminuria, glycosuria, hypocalcemia, hyponatremia, porphyria, SIADH

Gastrointestinal: Abdominal pain, anorexia, constipation, diarrhea, gastric distress, glossitis, nausea, pancreatitis, stomatitis, vanishing bile duct syndrome, vomiting, xerostomia

Genitourinary: Azotemia, impotence, oliguria, urinary frequency, urinary retention

Hematologic & oncologic: Agranulocytosis, anemia, aplastic anemia, bone marrow depression, eosinophilia, leukocytosis, leukopenia, lymphadenopathy, pancytopenia, purpura, thrombocytopenia

Hepatic: Abnormal hepatic function tests, hepatic failure, hepatitis, jaundice

Hypersensitivity: Hypersensitivity reaction, multi-organ hypersensitivity

Neuromuscular & skeletal: Arthralgia, exacerbation of systemic lupus erythematosus, leg cramps, myalgia, osteoporosis, tremor, weakness

Ophthalmic: Blurred vision, cataract, conjunctivitis, diplopia, increased intraocular pressure, nystagmus, oculomotor disturbances

Otic: Tinnitus

Renal: Increased blood urea nitrogen, renal failure

Respiratory: Dry throat, pneumonia

Miscellaneous: Fever

Rare but important or life-threatening: Aseptic meningitis, defective spermatogenesis, hirsutism, lupus-like syndrome, maculopapular rash, paralysis, reduced fertility (male), suicidal ideation

Drug Interactions

Metabolism/Transport Effects Substrate of CYP2C8 (minor), CYP3A4 (major); **Note:** Assignment of Major/Minor substrate status based on clinically relevant drug interaction potential; **Induces** CYP1A2 (strong), CYP2B6 (strong), CYP2C19 (strong), CYP2C8 (strong), CYP2C9 (strong), CYP3A4 (strong), P-glycoprotein

Avoid Concomitant Use

Avoid concomitant use of CarBAMazepine with any of the following: Abiraterone Acetate; Apixaban; Apremilast; Artemether; Axitinib; Azelastine (Nasal); Bedaquiline; Boceprevir; Bortezomib; Bosutinib; Cabozantinib; Ceritinib; CloZAPine; Conivaptan; Crizotinib; Dabigatran Etexilate; Dienogest; Dipyrone; Dolutegravir; Dronedarone; Enzalutamide; Everolimus; Fusidic Acid (Systemic); Ibrutinib; Itraconazole; Ivacaftor; Lapatinib; Lumefantrine; Lurasidone; Macitentan; MAO Inhibitors; Mifepristone; Nefazodone; NIFEdipine; Nilotinib; Nisoldipine; Paraldehyde; PAZOPanib; Pirfenidone; Pomalidomide; PONATinib; Praziquantel; Ranolazine; Regorafenib; Reverse Transcriptase Inhibitors (Non-Nucleoside); Rivaroxaban; Roflumilast; RomiDEPsin; Simeprevir; Sofosbuvir; SORAfenib; Stiripentol; Tasimelteon; Telaprevir; Thalidomide; Ticagrelor; Tofacitinib; Tolvaptan; Toremifene; TraMADol;

Ulipristal; Vandetanib; Vemurafenib; VinCRIStine (Liposomal); Vorapaxar; Voriconazole

Increased Effect/Toxicity

CarBAMazepine may increase the levels/effects of: Adenosine; Alcohol (Ethyl); Azelastine (Nasal); Buprenorphine; Clarithromycin; ClomiPRAMINE; CloZAPine; CNS Depressants; Desmopressin; Eslicarbazepine; Fosphenytoin; Hydrocodone; Lithium; MAO Inhibitors; Methotrimeprazine; Metyrosine; Paraldehyde; Phenytoin; Pramipexole; Rotigotine; Thalidomide

The levels/effects of CarBAMazepine may be increased by: Allopurinol; Brimonidine (Topical); Calcium Channel Blockers (Nondihydropyridine); Cannabis; Carbonic Anhydrase Inhibitors; Cimetidine; Clarithromycin; Conivaptan; CYP3A4 Inhibitors (Moderate); CYP3A4 Inhibitors (Strong); Danazol; Darunavir; Dipyrone; Doxylamine; Dronabinol; Droperidol; Fluconazole; Fusidic Acid (Systemic); Grapefruit Juice; HydrOXYzine; Isoniazid; Kava Kava; LamoTRIgine; Luliconazole; Macrolide Antibiotics; Magnesium Sulfate; Methotrimeprazine; Nabilone; Nefazodone; Protease Inhibitors; QuiNINE; Selective Serotonin Reuptake Inhibitors; Sodium Oxybate; Stiripentol; Tapentadol; Telaprevir; Tetrahydrocannabinol; Thiazide Diuretics; TraMADol; Zolpidem

Decreased Effect

CarBAMazepine may decrease the levels/effects of: Abiraterone Acetate; Acetaminophen; Afatinib; Albendazole; Apixaban; Apremilast; ARIPiprazole; Artemether; Axitinib; Bazedoxifene; Bedaquiline; Bendamustine; Benzodiazepines (metabolized by oxidation); Boceprevir; Bortezomib; Bosutinib; Brentuximab Vedotin; Cabozantinib; Calcium Channel Blockers (Dihydropyridine); Calcium Channel Blockers (Nondihydropyridine); Canagliflozin; Cannabidiol; Cannabis; Caspofungin; Ceritinib; Clarithromycin; CloZAPine; Cobicistat; Contraceptives (Estrogens); Contraceptives (Progestins); Crizotinib; CycloSPORINE (Systemic); CYP1A2 Substrates; CYP2B6 Substrates; CYP2C19 Substrates; CYP2C8 Substrates; CYP2C9 Substrates; CYP3A4 Substrates; Dabigatran Etexilate; Dasatinib; Diclofenac (Systemic); Dienogest; Dolutegravir; DOXOrubicin (Conventional); Doxycycline; Dronabinol; Dronedarone; Elvitegravir; Enzalutamide; Eslicarbazepine; Everolimus; Exemestane; Ezogabine; Felbamate; FentaNYL; Fingolimod; Flunarizine; Fosphenytoin; Gefitinib; GuanFACINE; Haloperidol; Ibrutinib; Imatinib; Irinotecan; Itraconazole; Ivacaftor; Ixabepilone; Lacosamide; LamoTRIgine; Lapatinib; Linagliptin; Lopinavir; Lumefantrine; Lurasidone; Macitentan; Maraviroc; Mebendazole; Methadone; MethylPREDNISolone; Mifepristone; Nefazodone; NIFEdipine; Nilotinib; Nisoldipine; OXcarbazepine; Paliperidone; PAZOPanib; Perampanel; P-glycoprotein/ABCB1 Substrates; Phenytoin; Pirfenidone; Pomalidomide; PONATinib; Praziquantel; Protease Inhibitors; QUEtiapine; QuiNINE; Ranolazine; Regorafenib; Reverse Transcriptase Inhibitors (Non-Nucleoside); RisperiDONE; Rivaroxaban; Roflumilast; RomiDEPsin; Rufinamide; Saxagliptin; Selective Serotonin Reuptake Inhibitors; Simeprevir; Sofosbuvir; SORAfenib; SUNItinib; Tadalafil; Tasimelteon; Telaprevir; Temsirolimus; Tetrahydrocannabinol; Theophylline Derivatives; Thyroid Products; Ticagrelor; Tofacitinib; Tolvaptan; Topiramate; Toremifene; TraMADol; Treprostinil; Tricyclic Antidepressants; Ulipristal; Valproic Acid and Derivatives; Vandetanib; Vecuronium; Vemurafenib; Vilazodone; VinCRIStine (Liposomal); Vitamin K Antagonists; Vorapaxar; Voriconazole; Vortioxetine; Ziprasidone; Zolpidem; Zuclopenthixol

The levels/effects of CarBAMazepine may be decreased by: Bosentan; CYP3A4 Inducers (Strong); Dabrafenib; Deferasirox; Felbamate; Fosphenytoin; Ketorolac (Nasal); Ketorolac (Systemic); Mefloquine; Methylfolate;

Mitotane; Orlistat; Phenytoin; Reverse Transcriptase Inhibitors (Non-Nucleoside); Rufinamide; Siltuximab; St Johns Wort; Theophylline Derivatives; Tocilizumab; TraMADol; Valproic Acid and Derivatives

Food Interactions Carbamazepine serum levels may be increased if taken with food and/or grapefruit juice. Management: Avoid concurrent ingestion of grapefruit juice. Maintain adequate hydration, unless instructed to restrict fluid intake.

Stability Hazardous agent; use appropriate precautions for handling and disposal (NIOSH, 2012).

Carbatrol, Equetro: Store at 25°C (77°F); excursions permitted to 15°C to 30°C (59°F to 86°F); protect from light and moisture.

Epitol: Store at 20°C to 25°C (68°F to 77°F); protect from moisture; dispense in tightly closed container.

Tegretol-XR: Store at 15°C to 30°C (59°F to 86°F); protect from moisture; dispense in tightly closed container.

Tegretol tablets and chewable tablets: Store at ≤30°C (86°F); protect from light and moisture; dispense in tight, light-resistant container.

Tegretol suspension: Store at ≤30°C (86°F); dispense in tight, light-resistant container.

Mechanism of Action In addition to anticonvulsant effects, carbamazepine has anticholinergic, antineuralgic, antidiuretic, muscle relaxant, antimanic, antidepressive, and antiarrhythmic properties; may depress activity in the nucleus ventralis of the thalamus or decrease synaptic transmission or decrease summation of temporal stimulation leading to neural discharge by limiting influx of sodium ions across cell membrane or other unknown mechanisms; stimulates the release of ADH and potentiates its action in promoting reabsorption of water; chemically related to tricyclic antidepressants

Pharmacokinetics (Adult data unless noted)

Absorption: Slowly from the GI tract

Distribution: Carbamazepine and its active epoxide metabolite distribute into breast milk

V_d:

Neonates: 1.5 L/kg

Children: 1.9 L/kg

Adults: 0.59 to 2 L/kg

Protein binding: Carbamazepine: 75% to 90%, bound to alpha$_1$-acid glycoprotein and nonspecific binding sites on albumin; protein binding may be decreased in newborns Epoxide metabolite: 50% protein bound

Metabolism: Induces liver enzymes to increase metabolism and shorten half-life over time; metabolized in the liver by cytochrome P450 3A4 to active epoxide metabolite; epoxide metabolite is metabolized by epoxide hydrolase to the trans-diol metabolite; ratio of serum epoxide to carbamazepine concentrations may be higher in patients receiving polytherapy (vs monotherapy) and in infants (vs older children); boys may have faster carbamazepine clearances and may, therefore, require higher mg/kg/day doses of carbamazepine compared to girls of similar age and weight

Bioavailability, oral: 75% to 85%; relative bioavailability of extended release tablet to suspension: 89%

Half-life:

Carbamazepine:

Initial: 25 to 65 hours

Multiple dosing:

Children: 8 to 14 hours

Adults: 12 to 17 hours

Epoxide metabolite: 34 ± 9 hours

Time to peak serum concentration: Unpredictable

Immediate release: Multiple doses: Suspension: 1.5 hours; Tablet: 4 to 5 hours

Extended release: Carbatrol, Equetro: 19 hours (single dose), ~6 hours (multiple doses); Tegretol-XR: 3 to 12 hours

Elimination: Urine 72% (1% to 3% as unchanged drug); feces 28%

Dosing: Usual Dosage must be adjusted according to patient's response and serum concentrations.

Pediatric: **Epilepsy:** Oral: To convert from tablets (immediate release or extended release) or capsules to oral suspension, use the same total mg daily dose and divided into 4 daily doses; monitor serum concentrations. **Note:** Carbamazepine suspension may be administered rectally as maintenance doses, if oral therapy is not possible; when using carbamazepine suspension rectally, administer the same total daily dose, but give in small, diluted, multiple doses; dilute the oral suspension with an equal volume of water; if defecation occurs within the first 2 hours, repeat the dose (Graves, 1987).

Infants and Children:

<6 years: Initial: 10 to 20 mg/kg/day divided twice or 3 times daily as immediate release tablets or 4 times daily as suspension; increase dose every week until optimal response and therapeutic levels are achieved; maintenance dose: Divide into 3-4 doses daily (immediate release tablets or suspension); maximum recommended daily dose: 35 mg/kg/**day**

6 to 12 years: Initial: 100 mg twice daily [immediate release tablets or extended release tablets (Tegretol-XR)] or 50 mg of suspension 4 times daily (200 mg/day); increase by up to 100 mg/day at weekly intervals using a twice daily regimen of extended release tablets or 3 to 4 times daily regimen of other formulations until optimal response and therapeutic levels are achieved; usual maintenance: 400 to 800 mg/day; maximum recommended daily dose: 1000 mg/**day**

Adolescents: Initial: 200 mg twice daily (immediate release tablets, extended release tablets [Tegretol-XR], or extended release capsules [Carbatrol]) or 100 mg of suspension 4 times daily (400 mg daily); increase by up to 200 mg/day at weekly intervals using a twice daily regimen of extended release tablets or capsules, or a 3 to 4 times/day regimen of other formulations until optimal response and therapeutic levels are achieved; usual dose: 800 to 1200 mg/day

Maximum recommended daily doses:

Adolescents ≤15 years: 1000 mg/**day**

Adolescents >15 years: 1200 mg/**day**

Adult:

Epilepsy: Oral: Initial: 400 mg/day in 2 divided doses (tablets or extended release tablets or extended release capsules) or 4 divided doses (oral suspension); increase by up to 200 mg/day at weekly intervals using a twice daily regimen of extended release tablets or capsules, or a 3 to 4 times daily regimen of other formulations until optimal response and therapeutic levels are achieved; usual dose: 800 to 1200 mg/day

Maximum recommended daily dose: 1600 mg/**day**; however, some patients have required up to 2400 mg/**day**

Trigeminal or glossopharyngeal neuralgia: Oral:

Initial: 200 mg/day in 2 divided doses (tablets, extended release tablets, or extended release capsules) or 4 divided doses (oral suspension) with food, gradually increasing in increments of 200 mg/day as needed

Maintenance: Usual: 400 to 800 mg daily in 2 divided doses (tablets, extended release tablets, or extended release capsules) or 4 divided doses (oral suspension); maximum daily dose: 1200 mg/**day**

Bipolar disorder: Oral: Initial: 400 mg/day in 2 divided doses (tablets, extended release tablets, or extended release capsules) or 4 divided doses (oral suspension); may adjust by 200 mg/day increments; maximum daily dose: 1600 mg/**day**. **Note:** Equetro is the only formulation specifically approved by the FDA for the management of bipolar disorder.

◀ **Dosing adjustment in renal impairment:** Dosage adjustments are not required nor recommended in the manufacturer's labeling; however, the following guidelines have been used by some clinicians (Aronoff, 2007):

Infants, Children, and Adolescents: **Note:** Renally adjusted dose recommendations are based on doses of 10 to 20 mg/kg/**day** divided every 8 to 12 hours.

GFR ≥10 mL/minute/1.73 m²: No dosage adjustment required

GFR <10 mL/minute/1.73 m²: Administer 75% of normal dose

Intermittent hemodialysis: Administer 75% of normal dose; on dialysis days give dose **after** hemodialysis

Peritoneal dialysis (PD): Administer 75% of normal dose

Continuous renal replacement therapy (CRRT): Administer 75% of normal dose; monitor serum concentrations

Adults:

GFR ≥10 mL/minute: No dosage adjustment required

GFR <10 mL/minute: Administer 75% of dose

Intermittent hemodialysis: Administer 75% of normal dose; on dialysis days give dose **after** hemodialysis

Peritoneal dialysis (PD): Administer 75% of normal dose

Continuous renal replacement therapy (CRRT): No dosage adjustment recommended

Dosing adjustment in hepatic impairment: Infants, Children, Adolescents, and Adults: Use with caution in hepatic impairment; metabolized primarily in the liver.

Administration Hazardous agent; use appropriate precautions for handling and disposal (NIOSH, 2012).

Oral: Administer with food to decrease GI upset

Immediate release:

Chewable and conventional tablets: Administer with meals; may be given 2 to 3 times daily.

Oral suspension: Shake well before use; administer with meals; must be given on a 3 to 4 times daily schedule. When carbamazepine suspension has been combined with chlorpromazine or thioridazine solutions, a precipitate forms which may result in loss of effect. Therefore, it is recommended that the carbamazepine suspension dosage form not be administered at the same time with other liquid medicinal agents or diluents.

Extended release:

Capsules (Carbatrol, Equetro): Consists of three different types of beads: Immediate release, extended release, and enteric release. The bead types are combined in a ratio to allow twice daily dosing. Capsules may be opened and contents sprinkled over food such as a teaspoon of applesauce; do not store medication/food mixture for later use; drink fluids after dose to make sure mixture is completely swallowed; may be administered with or without food; do not crush or chew.

Tablet (Tegretol-XR): Administer with meals; should be dosed twice daily; examine XR tablets for cracks or chips or other damage; do not use damaged extended release tablets without release portal. Swallow tablet whole; do not crush or chew.

Monitoring Parameters *HLA-B*1502* genotype screening prior to therapy initiation in patients of Asian descent; CBC with platelet count, reticulocytes, serum iron, liver function tests, ophthalmic examinations (including slit-lamp, fundoscopy, and tonometry), urinalysis, BUN, lipid panel, serum drug concentrations, thyroid function tests, serum sodium; pregnancy test; observe patient for excessive sedation especially when instituting or increasing therapy; signs of edema, skin rash, and hypersensitivity reactions; signs and symptoms of suicidality (eg, anxiety, depression, behavior changes).

Reference Range Timing of serum samples: Absorption is slow; peak levels occur 8 to 65 hours after ingestion of the first dose; the half-life ranges from 8 to 60 hours; therefore, steady-state is achieved in 2 to 5 days

Epilepsy: Therapeutic concentrations: 4 to 12 mcg/mL (SI: 17 to 51 micromoles/L). Patients who require higher levels (8 to 12 mcg/mL [SI: 34 to 51 micromoles/L]) should be carefully monitored. Side effects (especially CNS) occur commonly at higher levels. If other anticonvulsants (enzyme inducers) are given, therapeutic range is 4 to 8 mcg/mL (SI: 17 to 34 micromoles/L) due to increase in unmeasured active epoxide metabolite.

Test Interactions May cause false-positive serum TCA screen; may interact with some pregnancy tests

Additional Information Carbamazepine is not effective in absence, myoclonic, akinetic, or febrile seizures; exacerbation of certain seizure types have been seen after initiation of carbamazepine therapy in children with mixed seizure disorders. Rectally administered carbamazepine is not useful in status epilepticus due to its slow absorption.

Investigationally, loading doses of the suspension (10 mg/kg for children <12 years of age and 8 mg/kg for children >12 years) were given (via NG or ND tubes followed by 5 to 10 mL of water to flush through tube) to PICU patients with frequent seizures/status; 5 of 6 patients attained mean plasma concentrations of 4.3 mcg/mL and 7.3 mcg/mL at 1 and 2 hours postload; concurrent enteral feeding or ileus may delay absorption of loading dose (Miles, 1990).

A recent study (Relling, 2000) demonstrated that enzyme-inducing antiepileptic drugs (AEDs) (carbamazepine, phenobarbital, and phenytoin) increased systemic clearance of antileukemic drugs (teniposide and methotrexate) and were associated with a worse event-free survival, CNS relapse, and hematologic relapse, (ie, lower efficacy), in B-lineage ALL children receiving chemotherapy; the authors recommend using nonenzyme-inducing AEDs in patients receiving chemotherapy for ALL.

Dosage Forms Excipient information presented when available (limited, particularly for generics); consult specific product labeling.

Capsule Extended Release 12 Hour, Oral:

Carbatrol: 100 mg [contains fd&c blue #2 (indigotine)]

Carbatrol: 200 mg, 300 mg

Equetro: 100 mg, 200 mg, 300 mg [contains fd&c blue #2 (indigotine)]

Generic: 100 mg, 200 mg, 300 mg

Suspension, Oral:

TEGretol: 100 mg/5 mL (450 mL) [contains fd&c yellow #6 (sunset yellow), propylene glycol; citrus-vanilla flavor]

Generic: 100 mg/5 mL (450 mL)

Tablet, Oral:

Epitol: 200 mg [scored]

TEGretol: 200 mg [scored; contains fd&c red #40]

Generic: 200 mg

Tablet Chewable, Oral:

Generic: 100 mg

Tablet Extended Release 12 Hour, Oral:

TEGretol-XR: 100 mg, 200 mg, 400 mg

Generic: 200 mg, 400 mg

Extemporaneous Preparations Hazardous agent: Use appropriate precautions for handling and disposal.

Note: Commercial oral suspension is available (20 mg/mL)

A 40 mg/mL oral suspension may be made with tablets. Crush twenty 200 mg tablets in a mortar and reduce to a fine powder. Add small portions of Simple Syrup, NF and mix to a uniform paste; mix while adding the vehicle in incremental proportions to **almost** 100 mL; transfer to a calibrated bottle, rinse mortar with vehicle, and add sufficient quantity of vehicle to make 100 mL. Label "shake well" and "refrigerate". Stable for 90 days.

Nahata MC, Pai VB, and Hipple TF, *Pediatric Drug Formulations*, 5th ed, Cincinnati, OH: Harvey Whitney Books Co, 2004.

References

Aronoff GR, Bennett WM, Berns JS, et al, *Drug Prescribing in Renal Failure: Dosing Guidelines for Adults and Children*, 5th ed, Philadelphia, PA: American College of Physicians, 2007.

Gilman JT, "Carbamazepine Dosing for Pediatric Seizure Disorders: The Highs and Lows," *DICP*, 1991, 25(10):1109-12.

Graves NM and Kriel RL, "Rectal Administration of Antiepileptic Drugs in Children," *Pediatr Neurol*, 1987, 3(6):321-6.

Korinthenberg R, Haug C, and Hannak D, "The Metabolization of Carbamazepine to CBZ-10,11 Epoxide in Children From the Newborn Age to Adolescence," *Neuropediatrics*, 1994, 25(4):214-6.

Liu H and Delgado MR, "Influence of Sex, Age, Weight, and Carbamazepine Dose on Serum Concentrations, Concentration Ratios, and Level/Dose Ratios of Carbamazepine and Its Metabolites," *Ther Drug Monit*, 1994, 16(5):469-76.

Matos ME, Burns MM, and Shannon MW, "False-Positive Tricyclic Antidepressant Drug Screen Results Leading to the Diagnosis of Carbamazepine Intoxication," *Pediatrics*, 2000, 105(5), http://www.pediatrics.org/cgi/content/full/105/5/e66.

Miles MV, Lawless ST, Tennison MB, et al, "Rapid Loading of Critically Ill Patients With Carbamazepine Suspension," *Pediatrics*, 1990, 86 (2):263-6.

National Institute for Occupational Safety and Health (NIOSH), "NIOSH List of Antineoplastic and Other Hazardous Drugs in Healthcare Settings 2012," National Institute for Occupational Safety and Health (NIOSH), at http://www.cdc.gov/niosh/docs/2012-150/pdfs/2012-150.pdf. Accessed January 21, 2013.

Relling MV, Pui CH, Sandlund JT, et al, "Adverse Effect of Anticonvulsants on Efficacy of Chemotherapy for Acute Lymphoblastic Leukaemia," *Lancet*, 2000, 356(9226):285-90.

Carbamide Peroxide (KAR ba mide per OKS ide)

Brand Names: U.S. Auraphene-B [OTC]; Debrox [OTC]; E-R-O Ear Drops [OTC]; E-R-O Ear Wax Removal System [OTC]; Ear Drops Earwax Aid [OTC]; Ear Wax Remover [OTC]; Earwax Treatment Drops [OTC]; Gly-Oxide [OTC]; Thera-Ear [OTC]

Therapeutic Category Otic Agent, Cerumenolytic

Generic Availability (U.S.) Yes

Use

Oral: Relief of minor inflammation of gums, oral mucosal surfaces and lips including canker sores and dental irritation; adjunct in oral hygiene

Otic: Emulsify and disperse ear wax

Contraindications Hypersensitivity to carbamide peroxide or any component; otic preparation should not be used in patients with a perforated tympanic membrane or following otic surgery; ear drainage, ear pain, or rash in the ear; dizziness; oral preparation should not be used for self medication in children <3 years of age

Warnings With prolonged use of oral carbamide peroxide, there is a potential for overgrowth of opportunistic organisms, damage to periodontal tissues, delayed wound healing

Adverse Reactions

Dermatologic: Rash

Local: Irritation, redness

Miscellaneous: Superinfection

Drug Interactions

Metabolism/Transport Effects None known.

Avoid Concomitant Use There are no known interactions where it is recommended to avoid concomitant use.

Increased Effect/Toxicity There are no known significant interactions involving an increase in effect.

Decreased Effect There are no known significant interactions involving a decrease in effect.

Stability Protect from heat and direct light

Mechanism of Action Carbamide peroxide releases hydrogen peroxide which serves as a source of nascent oxygen upon contact with catalase; deodorant action is probably due to inhibition of odor-causing bacteria; softens impacted cerumen due to its foaming action

Pharmacodynamics Onset of action: Otic: Slight disintegration of hard ear wax in 24 hours

Dosing: Usual

Oral: Children and Adults: Solution: Apply several drops undiluted to affected area of the mouth 4 times/day after meals and at bedtime for up to 7 days, expectorate after 2-3 minutes; as an adjunct to oral hygiene after brushing, swish 10 drops for 2-3 minutes, then expectorate

Otic: Solution:

Children <12 years: Individualize the dose according to patient size; 3 drops (range: 1-5 drops) twice daily for up to 4 days

Children ≥12 years and Adults: Instill 5-10 drops twice daily for up to 4 days

Administration

Oral: Apply undiluted solution with an applicator or cotton swab to the affected area after meals and at bedtime; or place drops on the tongue, mix with saliva, swish in the mouth for several minutes, then expectorate. Patient should not rinse mouth or drink fluids for 5 minutes after oral administration.

Otic: Instill drops into the external ear canal; keep drops in ear for several minutes by keeping head tilted or placing cotton in ear. Gently irrigate ear canal with warm water to remove loosened cerumen.

Dosage Forms Excipient information presented when available (limited, particularly for generics); consult specific product labeling.

Solution, Mouth/Throat:

Gly-Oxide: 10% (15 mL, 60 mL) [contains propylene glycol]

Solution, Otic:

Auraphene-B: 6.5% (15 mL)

Debrox: 6.5% (15 mL) [contains propylene glycol]

E-R-O Ear Drops: 6.5% (15 mL) [contains glycerin]

E-R-O Ear Wax Removal System: 6.5% (15 mL)

Ear Drops Earwax Aid: 6.5% (15 mL) [contains propylene glycol, trolamine (triethanolamine)]

Ear Wax Remover: 6.5% (15 mL) [contains propylene glycol]

Earwax Treatment Drops: 6.5% (15 mL)

Thera-Ear: 6.5% (15 mL)

◆ **Carbatrol** see CarBAMazepine on page 372

Carbinoxamine (kar bi NOKS a meen)

Medication Safety Issues

BEERS Criteria medication:

This drug may be potentially inappropriate for use in geriatric patients (Quality of evidence - moderate; Strength of recommendation - strong).

Brand Names: U.S. Arbinoxa; Karbinal ER; Palgic [DSC]

Therapeutic Category Antihistamine

Generic Availability (U.S.) May be product dependent

Use Symptomatic treatment of seasonal and perennial allergic rhinitis; vasomotor rhinitis; allergic conjunctivitis; mild manifestations of urticaria and angioedema; dermatographism; adjunct therapy for anaphylactic reactions (after acute manifestations controlled); amelioration of blood and plasma allergic reactions (All indications: FDA approved in ages ≥2 years and adults)

Pregnancy Risk Factor C

Pregnancy Considerations Animal reproduction studies have not been conducted. Maternal antihistamine use has generally not resulted in an increased risk of birth defects; however, information specific for the use of carbinoxamine during pregnancy has not been located. Although antihistamines are recommended for some indications in pregnant women, the use of other agents with specific pregnancy data may be preferred.

Breast-Feeding Considerations It is not known if carbinoxamine is excreted in breast milk. Premature infants and newborns have a higher risk of intolerance to antihistamines. Use while breast-feeding is contraindicated by the manufacturer. Antihistamines may decrease maternal serum prolactin concentrations when administered prior to the establishment of nursing.

Contraindications Hypersensitivity to carbinoxamine or any component; use with or within 14 days of MAO inhibitor therapy; infants and children <2 years of age, nursing mothers

Warnings Safety and efficacy for the use of cough and cold products in children <2 years of age is limited. Serious adverse effects including death have been reported in pediatric patients exposed to antihistamines, including carbinoxamine; use in contraindicated in pediatric patients <2 years.

Precautions Use with caution in patients with mild to moderate hypertension, cardiovascular disease, asthma, hyperthyroidism, increased intraocular pressure, GU or GI obstruction, or symptomatic prostatic hypertrophy. May cause paradoxical excitation in young children. May cause CNS depression, which may impair physical or mental abilities; patients must be cautioned about performing tasks which require mental alertness (eg, operating machinery or driving). Effects may be potentiated when used with other sedative drugs or ethanol.

Adverse Reactions Frequency not defined.

Cardiovascular: Chest tightness, extrasystoles, hypotension, palpitations, tachycardia

Central nervous system: Ataxia (most frequent), chills, confusion, dizziness (most frequent), drowsiness (most frequent), euphoria, excitability, fatigue, headache, hysteria, insomnia, irritability, nervousness, neuritis, paresthesia, restlessness, sedation (most frequent), seizure, vertigo

Dermatologic: Diaphoresis, skin photosensitivity, skin rash, urticaria

Endocrine & metabolic: Increased uric acid

Gastrointestinal: Anorexia, constipation, diarrhea, epigastric distress (most frequent), nausea, vomiting, xerostomia

Genitourinary: Difficulty in micturition, early menses, urinary frequency, urinary retention

Hematologic & oncologic: Agranulocytosis, hemolytic anemia, thrombocytopenia

Hypersensitivity: Anaphylactic shock, hypersensitivity reaction

Neuromuscular & skeletal: Tremor

Ophthalmic: Blurred vision, diplopia

Otic: Labyrinthitis, tinnitus

Respiratory: Dry nose, dry throat, nasal congestion, thickening of bronchial secretions (most frequent), wheezing

Drug Interactions

Metabolism/Transport Effects None known.

Avoid Concomitant Use

Avoid concomitant use of Carbinoxamine with any of the following: Aclidinium; Azelastine (Nasal); Ipratropium (Oral Inhalation); Paraldehyde; Potassium Chloride; Thalidomide; Tiotropium; Umeclidinium

Increased Effect/Toxicity

Carbinoxamine may increase the levels/effects of: AbobotulinumtoxinA; Alcohol (Ethyl); Analgesics (Opioid); Anticholinergic Agents; Azelastine (Nasal); Buprenorphine; Cannabinoid-Containing Products; CNS Depressants; Hydrocodone; Methotrimeprazine; Metyrosine; Mirabegron; Mirtazapine; OnabotulinumtoxinA; Paraldehyde; Potassium Chloride; Pramipexole; RimabotulinumtoxinB; ROPINIRole; Rotigotine; Selective Serotonin Reuptake Inhibitors; Thalidomide; Thiazide Diuretics; Tiotropium; Topiramate; Zolpidem

The levels/effects of Carbinoxamine may be increased by: Aclidinium; Brimonidine (Topical); Cannabis; Doxylamine; Dronabinol; Droperidol; HydrOXYzine; Ipratropium (Oral Inhalation); Kava Kava; Magnesium Sulfate; Methotrimeprazine; Nabilone; Perampanel; Pramlintide; Rufinamide; Sodium Oxybate; Tapentadol; Tetrahydrocannabinol; Umeclidinium

Decreased Effect

Carbinoxamine may decrease the levels/effects of: Acetylcholinesterase Inhibitors (Central); Benzylpenicilloyl Polylysine; Betahistine; Hyaluronidase; Secretin

The levels/effects of Carbinoxamine may be decreased by: Acetylcholinesterase Inhibitors (Central); Amphetamines

Stability Protect from light; store in a tightly closed, child-resistant container.

Arbinoxa™: Store at 20°C to 25°C (68°F to 77°F).

Palgic®: Store at 15°C to 30°C (59°F to 86°F).

Mechanism of Action Carbinoxamine competes with histamine for H_1-receptor sites on effector cells in the gastrointestinal tract, blood vessels, and respiratory tract.

Pharmacodynamics Duration: 4 hours

Pharmacokinetics (Adult data unless noted)

Absorption: Well absorbed from the GI tract

Metdabolism: Extensively hepatic

Half-life: 10-20 hours

Time to peak serum concentration: 1.5-5 hours

Elimination: Urine (as metabolites)

Dosing: Usual

Children and Adolescents: **Allergic rhinitis/urticaria:** Oral:

Children 2-5 years:

Weight directed (preferred): 0.2-0.4 mg/kg/day in divided doses 3-4 times daily

Fixed dose: 1-2 mg/dose 3-4 times daily; maximum daily dose: 0.4 mg/kg/**day**

Children 6-11 years: 2-4 mg/dose 3-4 times daily

Children ≥12 years and Adolescents: 4-6 mg/dose 3-4 times daily; maximum daily dose: 24 mg/**day**

Adults: **Allergic rhinitis/urticaria:** Oral: 4-8 mg/dose 3-4 times daily; maximum daily dose: 24 mg/**day**

Dosing adjustment in renal impairment: There are no dosage adjustments provided in manufacturer's labeling.

Dosing adjustment in hepatic impairment: There are no dosage adjustments provided in manufacturer's labeling.

Administration Oral: Administer on an empty stomach with water.

Product Availability Karbinal™ ER (extended release) oral suspension: FDA approved March 2013; anticipated availability is unknown. Consult the prescribing information for additional information.

Dosage Forms Excipient information presented when available (limited, particularly for generics); consult specific product labeling. [DSC] = Discontinued product

Liquid Extended Release, Oral, as maleate:

Karbinal ER: 4 mg/5 mL (480 mL) [contains methylparaben, polysorbate 80, propylparaben, sodium metabisulfite; strawberry-banana flavor]

Solution, Oral, as maleate:

Arbinoxa: 4 mg/5 mL (473 mL) [contains methylparaben, propylene glycol, propylparaben; bubble-gum flavor]

Palgic: 4 mg/5 mL (480 mL [DSC]) [contains methylparaben, propylene glycol, propylparaben; bubble-gum flavor]

Generic: 4 mg/5 mL (118 mL, 473 mL)

Tablet, Oral, as maleate:

Arbinoxa: 4 mg [scored]

Palgic: 4 mg [DSC] [scored]

Generic: 4 mg

◆ **Carbinoxamine Maleate** see Carbinoxamine on page 377

◆ **Carbocaine** *see* Mepivacaine *on page 1341*

◆ **Carbocaine® (Can)** *see* Mepivacaine *on page 1341*

◆ **Carbocaine Preservative-Free** *see* Mepivacaine *on page 1341*

◆ **Carbolith™ (Can)** *see* Lithium *on page 1266*

CARBOplatin (KAR boe pla tin)

Medication Safety Issues
Sound-alike/look-alike issues:
CARBOplatin may be confused with CISplatin, oxaliplatin
Paraplatin® may be confused with Platinol®
High alert medication:
This medication is in a class the Institute for Safe Medication Practices (ISMP) includes among its list of drug classes which have a heightened risk of causing significant patient harm when used in error.
BEERS Criteria medication:
This drug may be potentially inappropriate for use in geriatric patients (Quality of evidence - moderate; Strength of recommendation - strong).

Related Information
Emetogenic Potential of Antineoplastic Agents in Children *on page 2327*
Management of Drug Extravasations *on page 2255*
Safe Handling of Hazardous Drugs *on page 2419*

Brand Names: Canada Carboplatin Injection; Carboplatin Injection - LIQ IV

Therapeutic Category Antineoplastic Agent, Alkylating Agent; Antineoplastic Agent, Platinum Analog

Generic Availability (U.S.) Yes

Use Treatment of advanced ovarian carcinoma (FDA approved in adults); has also been used in the treatment of bladder cancer, breast cancer (metastatic), central nervous system tumors, cervical cancer (recurrent or metastatic), endometrial cancer, esophageal cancer, head and neck cancer, Hodgkin lymphoma (relapsed or refractory), malignant pleural mesothelioma, melanoma (advanced or metastatic), Merkel cell carcinoma, neuroendocrine tumors (adrenal gland and carcinoid tumors), non-Hodgkin lymphomas (relapsed or refractory), non-small cell lung cancer, prostate cancer, sarcomas (Ewing's sarcoma, osteosarcoma), small cell lung cancer, testicular cancer, thymic malignancies, unknown primary adenocarcinoma, Wilm's tumor, and as a conditioning regimen prior to hematopoietic stem cell transplantation

Pregnancy Risk Factor D

Pregnancy Considerations Embryotoxicity and teratogenicity have been observed in animal reproduction studies. May cause fetal harm if administered during pregnancy. Women of childbearing potential should avoid becoming pregnant during treatment.

Breast-Feeding Considerations Due to the potential for toxicity in nursing infants, breast-feeding is not recommended.

Contraindications Hypersensitivity to carboplatin, cisplatin, any component, other platinum-containing compounds, or mannitol; severe bone marrow suppression or excessive bleeding

Warnings Hazardous agent; use appropriate precautions for handling and disposal (NIOSH, 2012). When carboplatin is dosed using AUC as the endpoint, note that the calculated dose is the dose administered, not the dose based on body surface area; anaphylactic-like reactions can occur within minutes of administration **[U.S. Boxed Warning]**; risk for reaction increased in patients previously exposed to platinum therapy. Epinephrine, corticosteroids, and antihistamines have been used to treat symptoms. The risk of allergic reactions (including anaphylaxis) is increased in patients previously exposed to platinum therapy. Skin testing and desensitization protocols have been

reported (Confina-Cohen, 2005; Lee, 2004; Markman, 2003).

Precautions May cause severe, dose-limiting, dose-related bone marrow suppression **[U.S. Boxed Warning]**; patients who have received prior myelosuppressive therapy and patients with renal dysfunction are at increased risk for bone marrow suppression; anemia may be cumulative and require transfusion; reduce dosage in patients with bone marrow suppression; cycles should be delayed until WBC and platelet counts have recovered. May cause severe vomiting **[U.S. Boxed Warning]**; vomiting is dose-related and can be more severe in patients who previously received emetogenic therapy. High doses have resulted in severe abnormalities of liver function tests; reduce dosage in patients with impaired renal function (creatinine clearance values <60 mL/minute). Clinically significant hearing loss has been reported to occur in pediatric patients when carboplatin was administered at higher than recommended doses in combination with other ototoxic agents (eg, aminoglycosides). Loss of vision (reversible) has been reported with higher than recommended doses. Peripheral neuropathy occurs infrequently; the incidence of peripheral neuropathy is increased in patients who have previously received cisplatin treatment. When administered as sequential infusions, taxane derivatives (docetaxel, paclitaxel) should be administered before the platinum derivatives (carboplatin, cisplatin) to limit myelosuppression and to enhance efficacy.

When calculating the carboplatin dose using the Calvert formula and an estimated glomerular filtration rate (GFR), the laboratory method used to measure serum creatinine may impact dosing. Compared to other methods, standardized Isotope Dilution Mass Spectrometry (IDMS) may underestimate serum creatinine values in patients with low creatinine values (eg, ≤0.7 mg/dL) and therefore may overestimate GFR in patients with normal renal function. This may result in higher calculated carboplatin doses and increased toxicities. If using IDMS, the Food and Drug Administration (FDA) recommends that clinicians consider capping estimated GFR at a maximum of 125 mL/minute to avoid potential toxicity.

Should be administered under the supervision of an experienced cancer chemotherapy physician **[U.S. Boxed Warning]**.

Adverse Reactions
Central nervous system: Neurotoxicity, pain
Dermatologic: Alopecia
Endocrine & metabolic: Hypocalcemia, hypokalemia, hypomagnesemia, hyponatremia
Gastrointestinal: Abdominal pain, constipation, diarrhea, stomatitis/mucositis, nausea, taste dysgeusia, vomiting
Hematologic: Anemia, bleeding, hemorrhagic complications, leukopenia, myelosuppression (dose related and dose limiting; nadir at ~21 days with single-agent therapy), neutropenia, thrombocytopenia
Hepatic: Alkaline phosphatase increased, AST increased, bilirubin increased
Neuromuscular & skeletal: Peripheral neuropathy, weakness
Ocular: Visual disturbance
Otic: Ototoxicity
Renal: BUN increased, creatinine clearance decreased, creatinine increased
Miscellaneous: Hypersensitivity/allergic reaction, infection
Rare but important or life-threatening: Anaphylactic reaction, bronchospasm, cardiac failure, cerebrovascular accident, dehydration, embolism, erythema, hemolytic anemia (acute), hemolytic uremic syndrome (HUS), hyper-/hypotension, injection site reactions (pain, redness, swelling), limb ischemia (acute), necrosis (associated with extravasation), neutropenic fever, pruritus, rash, secondary malignancies, urticaria, vision loss

◀ **Drug Interactions**
Metabolism/Transport Effects None known.
Avoid Concomitant Use

Avoid concomitant use of CARBOplatin with any of the following: BCG; CloZAPine; Dipyrone; Natalizumab; Pimecrolimus; SORAfenib; Tacrolimus (Topical); Tofacitinib; Vaccines (Live)

Increased Effect/Toxicity

CARBOplatin may increase the levels/effects of: Bexarotene (Systemic); CloZAPine; Leflunomide; Natalizumab; Taxane Derivatives; Tofacitinib; Topotecan; Vaccines (Live)

The levels/effects of CARBOplatin may be increased by: Aminoglycosides; Denosumab; Dipyrone; Pimecrolimus; Roflumilast; SORAfenib; Tacrolimus (Topical); Trastuzumab

Decreased Effect

CARBOplatin may decrease the levels/effects of: BCG; Coccidioidin Skin Test; Fosphenytoin-Phenytoin; Sipuleucel-T; Vaccines (Inactivated); Vaccines (Live)

The levels/effects of CARBOplatin may be decreased by: Echinacea

Stability Hazardous agent; use appropriate precautions for handling and disposal (NIOSH, 2012). Store intact vials at room temperature of 25°C (77°F); excursions permitted to 15°C to 30°C (59°F to 86°F). Protect from light. Further dilution to a concentration as low as 0.5 mg/mL is stable at room temperature (25°C) for 8 hours in NS; stable at room temperature or under refrigeration for at least 9 days in D₅W, although the manufacturer states to use within 8 hours due to lack of preservative.

Powder for reconstitution: Reconstituted to a final concentration of 10 mg/mL is stable for 5 days at room temperature (25°C).

Solution for injection: Multidose vials are stable for up to 14 days after opening when stored at room temperature.

Mechanism of Action Carboplatin is a platinum compound alkylating agent which covalently binds to DNA; interferes with the function of DNA by producing inter-strand DNA cross-links

Pharmacokinetics (Adult data unless noted)
Distribution: V_d: 16 L (based on a dose of 300-500 mg/m²)
Protein binding: 0%; however, platinum (from carboplatin) is 30% protein bound
Half-life: Terminal: CrCl >60 mL/minute: Carboplatin: 2.5-5.9 hours (based on a dose of 300-500 mg/m²); platinum (from carboplatin): ≥5 days
Elimination: Urine (~70% as carboplatin within 24 hours; 3% to 5% as platinum within 1-4 days)

Dosing: Usual I.V. (refer to individual protocols):
Infants, Children, and Adolescents: **Note:** Some protocols calculate dose on the basis of body weight rather than body surface area in infants and young children (<3 years or ≤12 kg):
BSA-directed dosing:
Bone marrow transplant preparative regimen: Children: 500 mg/m²/day for 3 days (Gilheeney, 2010)
Glioma (Packer, 1997): Infants ≥3 months, Children, and Adolescents:
Induction: 175 mg/m² once weekly for 4 weeks every 6 weeks (2-week recovery period between courses) in combination with vincristine for 2 cycles
Maintenance: 175 mg/m² weekly for 4 weeks, with a 3-week recovery period between courses in combination with vincristine for ≤12 cycles
Sarcomas: Ewing's sarcoma, osteosarcoma: Children and Adolescents: 400 mg/m²/day for 2 days every 21 days (in combination with ifosfamide and etoposide) (Van Winkle, 2005)
Alternative carboplatin dosing: Some investigators calculate pediatric carboplatin doses using a modified

Calvert formula: Dosing based on target AUC (modified Calvert formula for use in children): Total dose (mg) = [Target AUC (mg/mL/minute)] x [GFR (mL/minute) + (0.36 x body weight in kilograms)]; **Note:** GFR in this equation is an exact measured value (eg, "raw" in mL/minute) **not** corrected for BSA (ie, **not** mL/minute/1.73 m²).
Note: Calvert formula was based on using chromic edetate (⁵¹Cr-EDTA) plasma clearance to establish GFR. Some clinicians have recommended that methods for estimating CrCl not be substituted for GFR since carboplatin dosing based on such estimates may not be predictive.
Note: The dose of carboplatin calculated is TOTAL mg DOSE not mg/m².
Adults:
Note: Doses for adults are commonly calculated by the target AUC using the Calvert formula, where **Total dose (mg) = Target AUC x (GFR + 25).** If estimating glomerular filtration rate (GFR) instead of measuring GFR, the Food and Drug Administration (FDA) recommends considering capping estimated GFR at a maximum of 125 mL/minute to avoid potential toxicity.
Ovarian cancer, advanced: I.V.: 360 mg/m² every 4 weeks (as a single agent) **or** 300 mg/m² every 4 weeks (in combination with cyclophosphamide) **or** target AUC 4-6 (in previously treated patients)
Dosage adjustment for toxicity: Platelets <50,000 cells/mm³ or ANC <500 cells/mm³: Administer 75% of dose
Dosage adjustment in renal impairment: Adults: **Note:** Dose determination with Calvert formula uses GFR and, therefore, inherently adjusts for renal dysfunction.
The manufacturer's labeling recommends the following dosage adjustment guidelines for single-agent therapy:
Baseline CrCl 41-59 mL/minute: Initiate at 250 mg/m² and adjust subsequent doses based on bone marrow toxicity
Baseline CrCl 16-40 mL/minute: Initiate at 200 mg/m² and adjust subsequent doses based on bone marrow toxicity
Baseline CrCl ≤15 mL/minute: No guidelines are available.
The following dosage adjustments have been used by some clinicians (for dosing based on mg/m²) (Aronoff, 2007):
Hemodialysis: Administer 50% of dose
Continuous ambulatory peritoneal dialysis (CAPD): Administer 25% of dose
Continuous renal replacement therapy (CRRT): 200 mg/m²
Dosage adjustment in hepatic impairment: Dosage adjustments are not provided in manufacturer's labeling.
Administration Hazardous agent; use appropriate precautions for handling and disposal (NIOSH, 2012).
Parenteral: Administer by I.V. intermittent infusion over 15-60 minutes although some protocols may require infusions up to 24 hours; reconstituted carboplatin 10 mg/mL should be further diluted to a final concentration of 0.5-2 mg/mL with D₅W or NS for administration. When administered as sequential infusions, taxane derivatives (docetaxel, paclitaxel) should be administered before platinum derivatives to limit myelosuppression and to enhance efficacy. Needles or I.V. administration sets that contain aluminum should not be used in the preparation or administration of carboplatin; aluminum can react with carboplatin resulting in precipitate formation and loss of potency.
Vesicant/Extravasation Risk May be an irritant
Monitoring Parameters CBC with differential and platelet count, serum electrolytes, urinalysis, serum creatinine and BUN, creatinine clearance, liver function tests

Dosage Forms Excipient information presented when available (limited, particularly for generics); consult specific product labeling.

Solution, Intravenous:
Generic: 50 mg/5 mL (5 mL); 150 mg/15 mL (15 mL); 450 mg/45 mL (45 mL); 600 mg/60 mL (60 mL)

Solution, Intravenous [preservative free]:
Generic: 50 mg/5 mL (5 mL); 150 mg/15 mL (15 mL); 450 mg/45 mL (45 mL); 600 mg/60 mL (60 mL)

Solution Reconstituted, Intravenous:
Generic: 150 mg (1 ea)

References

Abramson DH, Frank CM, and Dunkel IJ, "A Phase I/II Study of Subconjunctival Carboplatin for Intraocular Retinoblastoma," *Ophthalmology*, 1999, 106(10):1947-50.

Cairo MS, "The Use of Ifosfamide, Carboplatin, and Etoposide in Children With Solid Tumors," *Semin Oncol*, 1995, 22(3 Suppl 7):23-7.

Calvert AH, Newell DR, Grumbell LA, et al, "Carboplatin Dosage: Prospective Evaluation of a Simple Formula Based on Renal Function," *J Clin Oncol*, 1989, 7(11):1748-56.

Cheung Y-W, Cradock JC, Vishnuvajjala BR, et al, "Stability of Cisplatin, Iproplatin, Carboplatin, and Tetraplatin in Commonly Used Intravenous Solutions," *Am J Hosp Pharm*, 1987, 44:124-30.

Confino-Cohen R, Fishman A, Altaras M, et al, "Successful Carboplatin Desensitization in Patients With Proven Carboplatin Allergy," *Cancer*, 2005, 104(3):640-3.

Gilheeney SW, Khakoo Y, Souweidane M, et al, "Thiotepa/Topotecan/Carboplatin With Autologous Stem Cell Rescue in Recurrent/Refractory/Poor Prognosis Pediatric Malignancies of the Central Nervous System," *Pediatr Blood Cancer*, 2010, 54(4):591-5.

Lee CW, Matulonis UA, and Castells MC, "Carboplatin Hypersensitivity: A 6-h 12-Step Protocol Effective in 35 Desensitizations in Patients With Gynecological Malignancies and Mast Cell/IgE-Mediated Reactions," *Gynecol Oncol*, 2004, 95(2):370-6.

Lovett D, Kelsen D, Eisenberger M, et al, "A Phase II Trial of Carboplatin and Vinblastine in the Treatment of Advanced Squamous Cell Carcinoma of the Esophagus," *Cancer*, 1991, 67(2):354-6.

Markman M, Zanotti K, Peterson G, et al, "Expanded Experience With an Intradermal Skin Test to Predict for the Presence or Absence of Carboplatin Hypersensitivity," *J Clin Oncol*, 2003, 21(24):4611-4.

National Institute for Occupational Safety and Health (NIOSH), "NIOSH List of Antineoplastic and Other Hazardous Drugs in Healthcare Settings 2012." Available at http://www.cdc.gov/niosh/docs/2012-150/pdfs/2012-150.pdf. Accessed January 21, 2013.

Newell DR, Pearson AD, Balmanno K, et al, "Carboplatin Pharmacokinetics in Children: The Development of a Pediatric Dosing Formula. The United Kingdom Children's Cancer Study Group," *J Clin Oncol*, 1993, 11(12):2314-23.

Packer RJ, Ater J, Allen J, et al, "Carboplatin and Vincristine Chemotherapy for Children With Newly Diagnosed Progressive Low-Grade Gliomas," *J Neurosurg*, 1997, 86(5):747-54.

Pearson AD, Pinkerton CR, Lewis IJ, et al, "High-Dose Rapid and Standard Induction Chemotherapy for Patients Aged Over 1 Year With Stage 4 Neuroblastoma: A Randomised Trial," *Lancet Oncol*, 2008, 9(3):247-56.

van Winkle P, Angiolillo A, Krailo M, et al, "Ifosfamide, Carboplatin, and Etoposide (ICE) Reinduction Chemotherapy in a Large Cohort of Children and Adolescents With Recurrent/Refractory Sarcoma: The Children's Cancer Group (CCG) Experience," *Pediatr Blood Cancer*, 2005, 44(4):338-47.

Zeltzer PM, Epport K, Nelson MD Jr, et al, "Prolonged Response to Carboplatin in an Infant With Brain Stem Glioma," *Cancer*, 1991, 67(1):43-7.

◆ **Carboplatin Injection (Can)** see CARBOplatin on page 379

◆ **Carboplatin Injection - LIQ IV (Can)** see CARBOplatin on page 379

◆ **Carboxypeptidase-G2** see Glucarpidase on page 972

◆ **Cardene IV** see NiCARdipine on page 1493

◆ **Cardene SR** see NiCARdipine on page 1493

◆ **Cardizem** see Diltiazem on page 667

◆ **Cardizem CD** see Diltiazem on page 667

◆ **Cardizem LA** see Diltiazem on page 667

◆ **Cardura** see Doxazosin on page 712

◆ **Cardura-1 (Can)** see Doxazosin on page 712

◆ **Cardura-2 (Can)** see Doxazosin on page 712

◆ **Cardura-4 (Can)** see Doxazosin on page 712

◆ **Cardura XL** see Doxazosin on page 712

Carglumic Acid (kar GLU mik AS id)

Brand Names: U.S. Carbaglu

Therapeutic Category Antidote; Metabolic Alkalosis Agent; Urea Cycle Disorder (UCD) Treatment Agent

Generic Availability (U.S.) No

Use Adjunctive therapy for treatment of acute hyperammonemia due to N-acetylglutamate synthase (NAGS) deficiency (FDA approved in all ages); maintenance therapy for chronic hyperammonemia due to NAGS deficiency (FDA approved in all ages)

Prescribing and Access Restrictions Carbaglu is not available through pharmaceutical wholesalers or retail pharmacies, but only through direct shipping from the Accredo specialty pharmacy. Prescribers must contact Accredo Health Group at 888-454-8860 or refer to www.accredo.com to initiate patients on this product.

Pregnancy Risk Factor C

Pregnancy Considerations Teratogenic effects were reported in some animal reproduction studies. There are no adequate and well-controlled studies in pregnant women. However, due to the potential for irreversible fetal neurologic damage for untreated NAGS deficiency, women with this condition must remain on treatment throughout pregnancy.

Breast-Feeding Considerations It is not known if carglumic acid is excreted in breast milk. Breast-feeding is not recommended by the manufacturer.

Contraindications Hypersensitivity to carglumic acid or any component

Warnings Acute, uncontrolled hyperammonemia is a life-threatening emergency and may rapidly cause brain injury or death; carglumic acid in addition to other therapies, including dialysis (preferably hemodialysis), may be necessary until ammonia levels normalize. Since hyperammonemia is the result of protein catabolism, complete protein restriction is recommended to be maintained for 24 to 48 hours and caloric supplementation should be maximized to reverse catabolism and nitrogen turnover; monitor plasma ammonia concentrations and neurologic status.

Precautions Should be administered under the supervision of a medical personnel experienced in metabolic disorders. May cause vomiting, reported in ~25% of patients.

Adverse Reactions
Central nervous system: Fever, headache, somnolence
Dermatologic: Hyperhidrosis, rash
Gastrointestinal: Abdominal pain, anorexia, diarrhea, dysgeusia, vomiting, weight loss
Hematologic: Anemia
Neuromuscular & skeletal: Weakness
Otic: Ear infection
Respiratory: Nasopharyngitis, pneumonia, tonsillitis
Miscellaneous: Infections, influenza

Drug Interactions

Metabolism/Transport Effects None known.

Avoid Concomitant Use There are no known interactions where it is recommended to avoid concomitant use.

Increased Effect/Toxicity There are no known significant interactions involving an increase in effect.

Decreased Effect There are no known significant interactions involving a decrease in effect.

Stability Store at 2°C to 8°C (36°F to 46°F). After opening, do not refrigerate or store above 30°C (86°F); protect from moisture (keep container tightly closed). Discard 1 month after opening.

Mechanism of Action N-acetylglutamate synthase (NAGS) is a mitochondrial enzyme which produces N-acetylglutamate (NAG). NAG is a required allosteric activator of the hepatic mitochondrial enzyme, carbamoyl phosphate synthetase 1 (CPS 1), which converts ammonia into urea in the first step of the urea cycle. In NAGS-deficient patients, carglumic acid serves as a replacement for NAG.

Pharmacodynamics Onset of action: Within 24 hours

Pharmacokinetics (Adult data unless noted)

Distribution: V_d: ~2657 L

Metabolism: Via intestinal flora to carbon dioxide

Half-life, elimination: Median: 5.6 hours (range: 4.3-9.5 hours)

Time to peak serum concentration: Median: 3 hours

Elimination: Feces (60% as unchanged drug); urine (9% as unchanged drug)

Dosing: Neonatal

Acute hyperammonemia; adjunct therapy: Oral: 100-250 mg/kg/day given in 2 or 4 divided doses; titrate to age-appropriate plasma ammonia concentrations; concomitant ammonia-lowering therapy recommended.

Chronic hyperammonemia: Oral: Usual dose: <100 mg/kg/day given in 2 or 4 divided doses; titrate to age-appropriate plasma ammonia concentrations

Dosing: Usual

Pediatric:

Acute hyperammonemia: Infants, Children, and Adolescents: Oral: 100 to 250 mg/kg/day given in 2 or 4 divided doses; titrate to age-appropriate plasma ammonia concentrations; concomitant ammonia-lowering therapy recommended

Chronic hyperammonemia: Infants, Children, and Adolescents: Oral: Usual dose: <100 mg/kg/day given in 2 or 4 divided doses; titrate to age-appropriate plasma ammonia concentrations

Adult: **Note:** Dose should be rounded to the nearest 100 mg (1/2 tablet).

Acute hyperammonemia; adjunct therapy: Oral: 100 to 250 mg/kg/day given in 2 or 4 divided doses; titrate to age-appropriate plasma ammonia concentrations; concomitant ammonia-lowering therapy recommended

Chronic hyperammonemia: Oral: Usual dose: <100 mg/kg/day given in 2 or 4 divided doses; titrate to age-appropriate plasma ammonia concentrations

Administration Oral: Administer immediately before meals.

Preparation for administration: Disperse each 200 mg tablet in 2.5 mL of water and swallow; container should be rinsed and contents swallowed immediately; no other food or liquid should be used. Tablets do not dissolve completely and some particles may remain. For partial doses, gently shake the container, draw up the appropriate volume (80 mg/mL) of dispersion into an oral syringe, administer immediately, and discard unused portion. Oral syringe should be refilled with a minimum of 1-2 mL of water and administered immediately. This same dispersion may also be used for nasogastric tube administration, followed by flush with additional water to clear the tube.

Monitoring Parameters Plasma ammonia concentrations; physical signs/symptoms of hyperammonemia (eg, lethargy, ataxia, confusion, vomiting, seizures, memory impairment)

Dosage Forms Excipient information presented when available (limited, particularly for generics); consult specific product labeling.

Tablet, Oral:

Carbaglu: 200 mg [scored]

◆ **Carimune NF** see Immune Globulin on page 1084

◆ **Caripul (Can)** see Epoprostenol on page 770

Carmustine (kar MUS teen)

Medication Safety Issues

Sound-alike/look-alike issues:

Carmustine may be confused with bendamustine, lomustine

High alert medication:

This medication is in a class the Institute for Safe Medication Practices (ISMP) includes among its list of drug classes which have a heightened risk of causing significant patient harm when used in error.

Related Information

Emetogenic Potential of Antineoplastic Agents in Children on page 2327

Management of Drug Extravasations on page 2255

Safe Handling of Hazardous Drugs on page 2419

Brand Names: U.S. BiCNU; Gliadel Wafer

Brand Names: Canada BiCNU®; Gliadel Wafer®

Therapeutic Category Antineoplastic Agent, Alkylating Agent; Antineoplastic Agent, Alkylating Agent (Nitrosourea)

Generic Availability (U.S.) No

Use

Injection: Treatment of brain tumors (glioblastoma, brainstem glioma, medulloblastoma, astrocytoma, ependymoma, and metastatic brain tumor); multiple myeloma, Hodgkin's lymphoma, and non-Hodgkin's lymphomas (relapsed or refractory) (FDA approved in adults)

Wafer (implant): Adjunct to surgery in patients with recurrent glioblastoma multiforme; adjunct to surgery and radiation in patients with newly diagnosed high grade malignant glioma (FDA approved in adults)

Pregnancy Risk Factor D

Pregnancy Considerations Teratogenicity and embryotoxicity have been demonstrated in animal studies. Carmustine can cause fetal harm if administered to a pregnant woman. There are no adequate and well-controlled studies in pregnant women. Women of childbearing potential should avoid becoming pregnant while on treatment.

Breast-Feeding Considerations Due to the potential for serious adverse reactions in the nursing infant, breast-feeding should be discontinued.

Contraindications Hypersensitivity to carmustine or any component

Warnings Hazardous agent; use appropriate precautions for handling and disposal (NIOSH, 2012). Bone marrow suppression (may be delayed), notably thrombocytopenia and leukopenia, may lead to bleeding and overwhelming infection in an already compromised patient **[Injection: U.S. Boxed Warning]**; monitor blood counts weekly for at least 6 weeks after administration. Myelosuppression is cumulative. When given at the FDA-approved doses, treatment should not be administered less than 6 weeks apart. Consider nadir blood counts from prior dose for dosage adjustment. May cause bleeding (due to thrombocytopenia) or infections (due to neutropenia); monitor closely. Patients must have platelet counts >100,000/mm^3 and leukocytes >4000/mm^3 for a repeat dose. Anemia may occur (less common and less severe than leukopenia or thrombocytopenia). Long-term use is associated with the development of secondary malignancies (acute leukemias and bone marrow dysplasias).

Dose-related pulmonary fibrosis (sometimes fatal) may occur; patients receiving cumulative doses >1400 mg/m^2 are at higher risk; delayed onset of pulmonary fibrosis has occurred in children up to 17 years after carmustine treatment **[Injection: U.S. Boxed Warning]**; this occurred in patients aged 1-16 years using carmustine for the treatment of intracranial tumors; cumulative doses ranged from 770-1800 mg/m^2 (in combination with cranial radiotherapy). Pulmonary toxicity is characterized by pulmonary infiltrates and/or fibrosis and has been reported from 9 days to 43 months after nitrosourea treatment (including carmustine). Although pulmonary toxicity generally occurs in patients who have received prolonged treatment, pulmonary fibrosis has been reported with cumulative doses <1400 mg/m². In addition to high cumulative doses, other risk factors for pulmonary toxicity include history of lung disease and baseline predicted forced vital capacity (FVC) or carbon monoxide diffusing capacity (DLCO) <70%. Baseline and periodic pulmonary function tests are recommended. For high-dose treatment (transplant), acute lung injury may occur ~1-3 months post-transplant; advise patients to contact their transplant physician for dyspnea, cough, or fever; interstitial pneumonia may be managed with a course of corticosteroids.

Potentially significant interactions may exist, requiring dose or frequency adjustment, additional monitoring, and/or selection of alternative therapy. Consult drug interactions database for more detailed information.

Wafer: Monitor closely for known craniotomy-related complications (seizure, intracranial infection, abnormal wound healing, brain edema). Intracerebral mass effect (unresponsive to corticosteroids) has been reported; may lead to brain herniation. Avoid communication between the resection cavity and the ventricular system to prevent wafer migration; communications larger than the wafer should be closed prior to implantation; wafer migration may cause obstructive hydrocephalus.

Injection: Carmustine injection diluent contains absolute alcohol which can cause an "alcohol flushing syndrome" in susceptible patients; use with caution in patients with aldehyde dehydrogenase-2 deficiency.

Precautions Monitor infusion site closely for infiltration or injection site reactions; injection site burning and local tissue reactions, including swelling, pain, erythema, and necrosis have been reported. Use with caution in patients with hepatic impairment; reversible increases in transaminases, bilirubin, and alkaline phosphatase have been reported (rare); monitor liver function tests periodically during treatment. Use with caution in patients with renal impairment; renal failure, progressive azotemia, and decreased kidney size have been reported in patients who have received large cumulative dose or prolonged treatment; renal toxicity has also been reported in patients who have received lower cumulative doses; monitor renal function tests periodically during treatment. Ocular toxicity has been associates with intra-aterial intracarotid administration (unlabeled administration). Should be administered under the supervision of an experienced cancer chemotherapy physician **[Injection: U.S. Boxed Warning]**.

Adverse Reactions

I.V.:
Cardiovascular: Arrhythmia (with high doses), chest pain, flushing (with rapid infusion), hypotension, tachycardia
Central nervous system: Ataxia, dizziness
Central nervous system: Ethanol intoxication (with high doses), headache
Dermatologic: Hyperpigmentation/skin burning (after skin contact)
Gastrointestinal: Nausea (common; dose related), vomiting (common; dose related), mucositis (with high doses), toxic enterocolitis (with high doses)
Hematologic: Leukopenia (common; onset: 5-6 weeks; recovery: after 1-2 weeks), thrombocytopenia (common: onset: ~4 weeks; recovery: after 1-2 weeks), anemia, neutropenic fever, secondary malignancies (acute leukemia, bone marrow dysplasias)
Hepatic: Alkaline phosphatase increased, bilirubin increased, hepatic sinusoidal obstruction syndrome

(SOS; veno-occlusive disease; with high doses), transaminases increased
Local: Injection site reactions (burning, erythema, necrosis, pain, swelling)
Ocular: Conjunctival suffusion (with rapid infusion), neuroretinitis
Renal: Kidney size decreased, progressive azotemia, renal failure
Respiratory: Interstitial pneumonitis (with high doses), pulmonary fibrosis, pulmonary hypoplasia, pulmonary infiltrates
Miscellaneous: Allergic reaction, infection (with high doses)

Wafer:
Cardiovascular: Chest pain, deep thrombophlebitis, facial edema
Central nervous system: Anxiety, ataxia, brain edema, confusion, depression, facial paralysis, fever, hallucination, headache, hypesthesia, intracranial hypertension, meningitis, pain, seizure (grand mal), somnolence, speech disorder
Dermatologic: Abnormal wound healing, rash
Endocrine: Diabetes
Gastrointestinal: Abdominal pain, constipation, diarrhea, nausea, vomiting
Genitourinary: Urinary tract infection
Hematologic: Hemorrhage
Local: Abscess
Neuromuscular & skeletal: Back pain, weakness
Rare but important or life-threatening: Abnormal thinking, allergic reaction, amnesia, aspiration pneumonia, cerebral hemorrhage, cerebral infarction, coma, cyst formation, diplopia, dizziness, dysphagia, eye pain, fecal incontinence, gastrointestinal hemorrhage, hydrocephalus, hyperglycemia, hyper-/hypotension, hypokalemia, hyponatremia, insomnia, leukocytosis, monoplegia, neck pain, paranoia, peripheral edema, sepsis, thrombocytopenia, urinary incontinence, visual field defect

Drug Interactions

Metabolism/Transport Effects None known.

Avoid Concomitant Use
Avoid concomitant use of Carmustine with any of the following: BCG; CloZAPine; Dipyrone; Natalizumab; Pimecrolimus; Tacrolimus (Topical); Tofacitinib; Vaccines (Live)

Increased Effect/Toxicity
Carmustine may increase the levels/effects of: CloZAPine; Leflunomide; Natalizumab; Tofacitinib; Vaccines (Live)

The levels/effects of Carmustine may be increased by: Cimetidine; Denosumab; Dipyrone; Melphalan; Pimecrolimus; Roflumilast; Tacrolimus (Topical); Trastuzumab

Decreased Effect
Carmustine may decrease the levels/effects of: BCG; Cardiac Glycosides; Coccidioidin Skin Test; Sipuleucel-T; Vaccines (Inactivated); Vaccines (Live)

The levels/effects of Carmustine may be decreased by: Echinacea

Stability

Injection: Store intact vials and provided diluent under refrigeration at 2°C to 8°C (36°F to 46°F).
Reconstituted solutions are stable for 24 hours refrigerated (2°C to 8°C) and protected from light. Examine reconstituted vials for crystal formation prior to use. If crystals are observed, they may be redissolved by warming the vial to room temperature with agitation.
Solutions diluted to a concentration of 0.2 mg/mL in D_5W are stable for 8 hours at room temperature (25°C) in glass or polyolefin containers and protected from light.

Wafer: Store at or below -20°C (-4°F). Unopened foil pouches may be kept at room temperature for up to 6 hours

Mechanism of Action Interferes with the normal function of DNA and RNA by alkylation and cross-linking the strands of DNA and RNA, and by possible protein modification; may also inhibit enzyme processes by carbamylation of amino acids in protein

Pharmacokinetics (Adult data unless noted)

Distribution: 3.3 L/kg; readily crosses the blood-brain barrier since it is highly lipid soluble; CSF:plasma ratio >50%

Metabolism: Hepatic; rapid; forms active metabolites

Half-life: Biphasic: Initial: 1.4 minutes; Secondary: 20 minutes (active metabolites: plasma half-life of 67 hours)

Elimination: ~60% to 70% excreted as metabolites in the urine within 96 hours and 6% to 10% excreted as CO_2 by the lungs

Dosing: Usual

Infants, Children, and Adolescents: **Note:** Children are at increased risk for pulmonary toxicity due to carmustine, weigh risk vs benefit before use. Refer to individual protocols; dosing and frequency may vary.

Brain tumors, Myeloablative therapy prior to autologous stem cell rescue: Very limited data available; dose not established: I.V.: 100 mg/m^2/dose twice daily for 3 days (total: 600 mg/m^2) as part of a high dose combination chemotherapy regimen is most commonly reported in trials with mixed results (Dunkel, 1998, Finlay, 2008); however, a phase I trial identified a lower dose of 100 mg/m^2 once daily for 3 days (total: 300 mg/m^2) in combination with thiotepa as the maximum tolerated regimen with a high degree of pulmonary toxicity observed (Gilman, 2011). Further studies are needed.

Adults: **Note:** Utilize patient's actual body weight (full weight) for calculation of body surface area- or weight-based dosing, particularly when the intent of therapy is curative; manage regimen-related toxicities in the same manner as for nonobese patients; if a dose reduction is utilized due to toxicity, consider resumption of full weight-based dosing with subsequent cycles, especially if cause of toxicity (eg, hepatic or renal impairment) is resolved (Griggs, 2012).

Brain tumors, Hodgkin's lymphoma, multiple myeloma, non-Hodgkin's lymphoma: I.V.: 150-200 mg/m^2 every 6 weeks or 75-100 mg/m^2/day for 2 days every 6 weeks

Glioblastoma multiforme (recurrent), newly-diagnosed high-grade malignant glioma: Implantation (wafer): 8 wafers placed in the resection cavity (total dose: 61.6 mg); should the size and shape not accommodate 8 wafers, the maximum number of wafers allowed (up to 8) should be placed

Dosing adjustment in renal impairment: Adults: I.V.: The FDA-approved labeling does not contain renal dosing adjustment guidelines. The following dosage adjustments have been used by some clinicians (Kintzel, 1995):
CrCl 46-60 mL/minute: Administer 80% of dose
CrCl 31-45 mL/minute: Administer 75% of dose
CrCl ≤30 mL/minute: Consider use of alternative drug

Dosing adjustment in hepatic impairment: Dosage adjustment may be necessary; however, no specific guidelines are available.

Administration Hazardous agent; use appropriate precautions for handling and disposal (NIOSH, 2012).

Parenteral: Reconstitute initially with 3 mL of supplied diluent (dehydrated alcohol injection, USP); then further dilute with SWFI (27 mL), this provides a concentration of 3.3 mg/mL in ethanol 10%; protect from light; further dilute for infusion with D_5W using a non-PVC container; should be prepared in either glass or polyolefin containers due to significant absorption to PVC containers.

Infuse over 2 hours (infusions <2 hours may lead to injection site pain or burning); infuse through a free-flowing saline or dextrose infusion, or administer through a central catheter to alleviate venous pain/irritation.

High-dose carmustine (transplant dose): Infuse over a least 2 hours to avoid excessive flushing, agitation, and hypotension; was infused over 1 hour in some trials (Chopra, 1993). High-dose carmustine may be fatal if not followed by stem cell rescue. Monitor vital signs frequently during infusion; patients should be supine during infusion and may require the Trendelenburg position, fluid support, and vasopressor support.

Wafer: Double glove before handling; outer gloves should be discarded as chemotherapy waste after handling wafers. Any wafer or remnant that is removed upon repeat surgery should be discarded as chemotherapy waste. The outer surface of the external foil pouch is not sterile. Open pouch gently; avoid pressure on the wafers to prevent breakage. Wafer that are broken in half may be used, however, wafers broken into more than 2 pieces should be discarded in a biohazard container. Oxidized regenerated cellulose (Surgicel) may be placed over the wafer to secure; irrigate cavity prior to closure.

Vesicant/Extravasation Risk Irritant; infiltration may result in local pain, erythema, swelling, burning and skin necrosis; the alcohol-based diluent may be an irritant, especially with high doses.

Monitoring Parameters CBC with differential and platelet count (weekly for at least 6 weeks after a dose), pulmonary function tests (FVC, DLCO; at baseline and frequently during treatment), liver function (periodically), renal function tests (periodically); monitor blood pressure and vital signs during administration; monitor infusion site for possible infiltration

Wafer: Complications of craniotomy (seizures, intracranial infection, brain edema)

Dosage Forms Excipient information presented when available (limited, particularly for generics); consult specific product labeling.

Solution Reconstituted, Intravenous:
BiCNU: 100 mg (1 ea) [contains alcohol, usp]
Wafer, Implant:
Gliadel Wafer: 7.7 mg (8 ea) [contains polifeprosan 20]

References

Aronin PA, Mahaley MS Jr, Rudnick SA, et al, "Prediction of BCNU Pulmonary Toxicity in Patients With Malignant Gliomas," *N Engl J Med*, 1980, 303(4):183-8.

Chopra R, McMillan AK, Linch DC, et al. The place of high-dose BEAM therapy and autologous bone marrow transplantation in poor-risk Hodgkin's disease. A single-center eight-year study of 155 patients. *Blood*. 1993;81(5):1137-1145

Colvin M, Hartner J, and Summerfield M, "Stability of Carmustine in the Presence of Sodium Bicarbonate," *Am J Hosp Pharm*, 1980, 37 (5):677-8.

Dunkel IJ, Garvin JH Jr, Goldman S, et al, "High Dose Chemotherapy With Autologous Bone Marrow Rescue for Children With Diffuse Pontine Brain Stem Tumors. Children's Cancer Group," *J Neurooncol*, 1998, 37(1):67-73.

Favier M, De Cazanove F, Coste A, et al, "Stability of Carmustine in Polyvinyl Chloride Bags and Polyethylene-Lined Trilayer Plastic Containers," *Am J Health Syst Pharm*, 2001, 58(3):238-41.

Finlay JL, DHall G, Boyett JM, Dunkel IJ, Gardner SL, Goldman S, et al. Myeloablative chemotherapy with autologous bone marrow rescue in children and adolescents with recurrent malignant astrocytoma: outcome compared with conventional chemotherapy: a report from the Children's Oncology Group. *Pediatr Blood Cancer*. 2008;51:806-811.

Gilman AL, Jacobsen C, Bunin N, Levine J, Goldman F, Bendel A, et al. Phase I study of tandem high-dose chemotherapy with autologous peripheral blood stem cell rescue for children with recurrent brain tumors: a pediatric blood and marrow transplant consortium study. *Pediatr Blood Cancer*. 2011;57:506-513.

Griggs JJ, Mangu PB, Anderson H, et al. Appropriate Chemotherapy dosing for obese adult patients with cancer: American Society of Clinical Oncology Clinical Practice Guideline. *J Clin Oncol*. 2012;30 (13):1553-1561.

Kintzel PE, Dorr RT. Anticancer drug renal toxicity and elimination: dosing guidelines for altered renal function. *Cancer Treat Rev*. 1995;21(1):33-64.

National Institute for Occupational Safety and Health (NIOSH), "NIOSH List of Antineoplastic and Other Hazardous Drugs in Healthcare Settings 2012." Available at http://www.cdc.gov/niosh/docs/2012-150/pdfs/2012-150.pdf. Accessed January 21, 2013.

O'Driscoll BR, Hasleton PS, Taylor PM, et al, "Active Lung Fibrosis Up to 17 Years After Chemotherapy With Carmustine (BCNU) in Childhood," *N Engl J Med*, 1990, 323(6):378-82.

Papadakis V, Dunkel IJ, Cramer LD, et al, "High-Dose Carmustine, Thiotepa and Etoposide Followed by Autologous Bone Marrow Rescue for the Treatment of High Risk Central Nervous System Tumors," *Bone Marrow Transplant*, 2000, 26(2):153-60.

◆ **Carmustine Polymer Wafer** *see* Carmustine *on page 382*

◆ **Carmustinum** *see* Carmustine *on page 382*

◆ **Carnitine** *see* LevOCARNitine *on page 1224*

◆ **Carnitor** *see* LevOCARNitine *on page 1224*

◆ **Carnitor SF** *see* LevOCARNitine *on page 1224*

◆ **Carrington Antifungal [OTC]** *see* Miconazole (Topical) *on page 1410*

◆ **Carter's Little Pills [OTC] (Can)** *see* Bisacodyl *on page 293*

◆ **Cartia XT** *see* Diltiazem *on page 667*

Carvedilol (KAR ve dil ole)

Medication Safety Issues
Sound-alike/look-alike issues:
Carvedilol may be confused with atenolol, captopril, carbidopa, carteolol

Coreg may be confused with Corgard, Cortef, Cozaar

Related Information
Oral Medications That Should Not Be Crushed or Altered *on page 2438*

Brand Names: U.S. Coreg; Coreg CR

Brand Names: Canada Apo-Carvedilol; Ava-Carvedilol; Dom-Carvedilol; JAMP-Carvedilol; Mylan-Carvedilol; Novo-Carvedilol; PMS-Carvedilol; RAN-Carvedilol; ratio-Carvedilol; ZYM-Carvedilol

Therapeutic Category Antihypertensive Agent; Beta-Adrenergic Blocker, Nonselective With Alpha-Blocking Activity

Generic Availability (U.S.) May be product dependent

Use Treatment of mild to severe chronic heart failure of cardiomyopathic or ischemic origin (usually in addition to standard therapy) (FDA approved in ages ≥18 years and adults); management of hypertension, alone or in combination with other agents (FDA approved in ages ≥18 years and adults); reduction of cardiovascular mortality in patients with left ventricular dysfunction following MI (FDA approved in ages ≥18 years and adults)

Pregnancy Risk Factor C

Pregnancy Considerations Because adverse events were not observed in animal reproduction studies, carvedilol is classified as pregnancy category C. In a cohort study, an increased risk of cardiovascular defects was observed following maternal use of beta-blockers during pregnancy. Intrauterine growth restriction (IUGR), small placentas, as well as fetal/neonatal bradycardia, hypoglycemia, and/or respiratory depression have been observed following *in utero* exposure to beta-blockers as a class. Adequate facilities for monitoring infants at birth should be available. Untreated chronic maternal hypertension and pre-eclampsia are also associated with adverse events in the fetus, infant, and mother. Carvedilol is not currently recommended for the initial treatment of maternal hypertension during pregnancy.

Breast-Feeding Considerations It is not known if carvedilol is excreted into human milk. The manufacturer suggests that a decision should be made to either discontinue nursing or discontinue the medication.

Contraindications Hypersensitivity to carvedilol or any component; bronchial asthma or related bronchospastic conditions; sick sinus syndrome, second or third degree AV block, or severe bradycardia (except in patients with a functioning artificial pacemaker); cardiogenic shock; decompensated cardiac failure requiring intravenous inotropic therapy; severe hepatic impairment

Warnings Symptomatic hypotension with or without syncope may occur with carvedilol (usually within the first 30 days of therapy); close monitoring is required especially with initial dosing and dosing increases; blood pressure must be lowered at a rate appropriate for patient's clinical condition. Initiate carvedilol cautiously at a low dose with gradual up-titration, administer with food (to slow the rate of absorption), and monitor closely. Due to risk of syncope, avoid driving or hazardous tasks during initiation of therapy. Significant bradycardia may occur requiring dosage reduction. Cytochrome P450 isoenzyme CYP2D6 poor metabolizers may have a higher rate of dizziness during initiation and upwards titration of carvedilol, perhaps due to the higher serum concentrations of the alpha-blocking R(+) enantiomer and resulting vasodilation. Exacerbation of angina, arrhythmias, and in some cases MI may occur following abrupt discontinuation of beta-blockers; avoid abrupt discontinuation, wean carvedilol slowly over 1-2 weeks, monitor for signs and symptoms of ischemia.

Heart failure patients receiving carvedilol may experience a deterioration of renal function (rare); risk factors include underlying renal dysfunction, diffuse vascular disease, ischemic heart disease or low blood pressure (eg, adults with SBP <100 mm Hg); deterioration of renal function is reversible upon drug discontinuation. In the severe chronic heart failure trials, adult patients were excluded if they had a baseline serum creatinine >2.8 mg/dL or increasing serum creatinine. Initiate cautiously and monitor for possible deterioration in patient status (eg, symptoms of HF). Monitor renal function closely in these patients; decrease carvedilol dose or discontinue drug if renal function worsens. Worsening heart failure or fluid retention may occur during upward titration; dose reduction or temporary discontinuation may be necessary; adjustment of other medications (ACE inhibitors and/or diuretics) may also be required.

Generally, patients with bronchospastic disease should not receive beta-blockers; if used at all, therapy should be with the lowest possible dose with close monitoring. Beta-blocker use has been associated with induction or exacerbation of psoriasis, but cause and effect have not been firmly established.

Intraoperative floppy iris syndrome has been observed in cataract surgery patients who were on or were previously treated with alpha$_1$-blockers; causality has not been established and there appears to be no benefit in discontinuing alpha-blocker therapy prior to surgery. Instruct patients to inform ophthalmologist of carvedilol use when considering eye surgery.

Immediate release and extended release products are not interchangeable on a mg:mg basis due to pharmacokinetic differences. Some immediate release tablets contain polysorbate 80 (Tween 80) which may cause allergic reactions in susceptible individuals.

Precautions Use with caution in mild to moderate hepatic impairment; use is contraindicated in patients with severe hepatic impairment; manufacturer recommends discontinuation of therapy if liver injury occurs (confirmed by laboratory testing). Use with caution in patients with pheochromocytoma (untreated); adequate alpha-blockade is required prior to use of any beta-blocker. Use with caution in patients with history of severe anaphylaxis to allergens; patients who have a history of severe anaphylactic hypersensitivity reactions to various substances may be more reactive while receiving beta-blockers; these patients may not be responsive to the normal doses of epinephrine used to treat hypersensitivity reactions. Use with caution in diabetes mellitus; beta-blockers may block hypoglycemia-induced tachycardia and blood pressure changes and possibly mask the signs and symptoms of hypoglycemia (eg, sweating, anxiety); nonselective beta-blockers may augment the insulin-induced hypoglycemia and delay the recovery of serum glucose concentrations; monitor serum glucose closely. In patients with heart failure and diabetes, use of carvedilol may worsen hyperglycemia; may require adjustment of antidiabetic agents. Use with caution in patients with peripheral vascular disease; may aggravate arterial insufficiency; may precipitate or aggravate symptoms of arterial insufficiency in patients with PVD and Raynaud's disease; monitor for arterial obstruction. Use with caution in Prinzmetal's variant angina; beta-blockers may provoke chest pain. Use with caution in thyroid disease; may mask signs of hyperthyroidism (eg, tachycardia); if hyperthyroidism is suspected, carefully manage and monitor; abrupt withdrawal may exacerbate symptoms of hyperthyroidism or precipitate thyroid storm. Chronic beta-blocker therapy should not be routinely withdrawn prior to major surgery; use caution with anesthetic agents that decrease myocardial function. Use with caution with concurrent use of verapamil, diltiazem, or digoxin; bradycardia or heart block can occur.

Adverse Reactions

Cardiovascular: Angina, AV block, bradycardia, cerebrovascular accident, edema (including generalized, dependent, and peripheral), hyper-/hypotension, hyper-/hypovolemia, orthostatic hypotension, palpitation, syncope

Central nervous system: Depression, dizziness, fatigue, fever, headache, hypoesthesia, hypotonia, insomnia, malaise, somnolence, vertigo, weakness

Endocrine & metabolic: Diabetes mellitus, gout, hypercholesterolemia, hyper-/hypoglycemia, hyponatremia, hyperkalemia, hypertriglyceridemia, hyperuricemia

Gastrointestinal: Abdominal pain, diarrhea, melena, nausea, periodontitis, vomiting, weight gain/loss

Genitourinary: Impotence

Hematologic: Anemia, prothrombin decreased, purpura, thrombocytopenia

Hepatic: Alkaline phosphatase increased, GGT increased, transaminases increased

Neuromuscular & skeletal: Arthralgia, arthritis, back pain, muscle cramps, paresthesia

Ocular: Blurred vision

Renal: Albuminuria, BUN increased, creatinine increased, glycosuria, hematuria, nonprotein nitrogen increased, renal insufficiency

Respiratory: Cough, dyspnea, nasopharyngitis, dyspnea, nasal congestion, pulmonary edema, rales, rhinitis, sinus congestion

Miscellaneous: Allergy, flu-like syndrome, injury, sudden death

Rare but important or life-threatening: Anaphylactoid reaction, alopecia, angioedema, aplastic anemia, amnesia, asthma, bronchospasm, bundle branch block, cholestatic jaundice, concentration decreased, diaphoresis, erythema multiforme, exfoliative dermatitis, GI hemorrhage, HDL decreased, hearing decreased, hyperbilirubinemia, hypersensitivity reaction, hypokalemia, hypokinesia, interstitial pneumonitis, leukopenia, libido decreased, migraine, myocardial ischemia, nervousness, neuralgia, nightmares, pancytopenia, paresis, peripheral ischemia, photosensitivity, pruritus, rash (erythematous, maculopapular, and psoriaform), respiratory alkalosis, seizure, Stevens-Johnson syndrome, tachycardia, tinnitus, toxic epidermal necrolysis, urinary incontinence, urticaria, xerostomia

Drug Interactions

Metabolism/Transport Effects Substrate of CYP1A2 (minor), CYP2C9 (minor), CYP2D6 (major), CYP2E1 (minor), CYP3A4 (minor), P-glycoprotein; **Note:** Assignment of Major/Minor substrate status based on clinically relevant drug interaction potential; **Inhibits** P-glycoprotein

Avoid Concomitant Use

Avoid concomitant use of Carvedilol with any of the following: Beta2-Agonists; Bosutinib; Ceritinib; Floctafenine; Methacholine; PAZOPanib; Silodosin; Topotecan; VinCRIStine (Liposomal)

Increased Effect/Toxicity

Carvedilol may increase the levels/effects of: Afatinib; Alpha-/Beta-Agonists (Direct-Acting); Alpha1-Blockers; Alpha2-Agonists; Amifostine; Antihypertensives; Antipsychotic Agents (Phenothiazines); Bosutinib; Bradycardia-Causing Agents; Brentuximab Vedotin; Bupivacaine; Cardiac Glycosides; Ceritinib; Cholinergic Agonists; Colchicine; CycloSPORINE (Systemic); Dabigatran Etexilate; Digoxin; DOXOrubicin (Conventional); DULoxetine; Ergot Derivatives; Everolimus; Fingolimod; Grass Pollen Allergen Extract (5 Grass Extract); Hypotensive Agents; Insulin; Lidocaine (Systemic); Lidocaine (Topical); Mepivacaine; Methacholine; Midodrine; Obinutuzumab; PAZOPanib; P-glycoprotein/ABCB1 Substrates; Prucalopride; Rifaximin; RiTUXimab; Rivaroxaban; Silodosin; Sulfonylureas; Topotecan; VinCRIStine (Liposomal)

The levels/effects of Carvedilol may be increased by: Abiraterone Acetate; Acetylcholinesterase Inhibitors; Alpha2-Agonists; Aminoquinolines (Antimalarial); Amiodarone; Anilidopiperidine Opioids; Antipsychotic Agents (Phenothiazines); Barbiturates; Brimonidine (Topical); Calcium Channel Blockers (Dihydropyridine); Calcium Channel Blockers (Nondihydropyridine); Cimetidine; CYP2C9 Inhibitors (Moderate); CYP2C9 Inhibitors (Strong); CYP2D6 Inhibitors (Moderate); CYP2D6 Inhibitors (Strong); Darunavir; Diazoxide; Digoxin; Dipyridamole; Disopyramide; Dronedarone; Floctafenine; Herbs (Hypotensive Properties); MAO Inhibitors; NiCARdipine; Pentoxifylline; P-glycoprotein/ABCB1 Inhibitors; Phosphodiesterase 5 Inhibitors; Propafenone; Prostacyclin Analogues; Regorafenib; Reserpine; Selective Serotonin Reuptake Inhibitors

Decreased Effect

Carvedilol may decrease the levels/effects of: Beta2-Agonists; Theophylline Derivatives

The levels/effects of Carvedilol may be decreased by: Barbiturates; Herbs (Hypertensive Properties); Methylphenidate; Nonsteroidal Anti-Inflammatory Agents; Peginterferon Alfa-2b; P-glycoprotein/ABCB1 Inducers; Rifamycin Derivatives; Yohimbine

Food Interactions Food decreases rate but not extent of absorption. Management: Administration with food minimizes risks of orthostatic hypotension.

Stability

Immediate release tablet (Coreg®): Store below 30°C (86°F); protect from moisture; dispense in tightly closed, light resistant container

Extended release capsule (Coreg CR®): Store at 25°C (77°F); excursions permitted to 15°C to 30°C (59°F to 86°F); dispense in tightly closed, light-resistant container

Mechanism of Action As a racemic mixture, carvedilol has nonselective beta-adrenoreceptor and alpha-adrenergic blocking activity. No intrinsic sympathomimetic activity has been documented. Associated effects in hypertensive patients include reduction of cardiac output, exercise- or beta-agonist-induced tachycardia, reduction of reflex orthostatic tachycardia, vasodilation, decreased peripheral vascular resistance (especially in standing position), decreased renal vascular resistance, reduced plasma renin activity, and increased levels of atrial natriuretic peptide. In CHF, associated effects include decreased pulmonary capillary wedge pressure, decreased pulmonary artery pressure, decreased heart rate, decreased systemic vascular resistance, increased stroke volume index, and decreased right arterial pressure (RAP).

Pharmacodynamics Oral:

Onset of action:
  Alpha-blockade: Within 30 minutes
  Beta-blockade: Within 1 hour
  Maximum effect: Antihypertensive effect: ~1-2 hours

Pharmacokinetics (Adult data unless noted)

Absorption: Oral: Rapid and extensive, but with large first pass effect; first pass effect is stereoselective with R(+) enantiomer achieving plasma concentrations 2-3 times higher than S(-) enantiomer

Distribution: V_d: 115 L; distributes into extravascular tissues

Protein binding: >98%, primarily to albumin

Metabolism: Extensively (98%) hepatic primarily via CYP2D6 and 2C9 and to a lesser extent CYP3A4, 2C19, and 2E1; metabolized predominantly by aromatic ring oxidation and glucuronidation; oxidative metabolites undergo conjugation via glucuronidation and sulfation; three active metabolites (4'-hydroxyphenyl metabolite is 13 times more potent than parent drug for beta-blockade; however, active metabolites achieve plasma concentrations of only 1/10 of those for carvedilol). Metabolism is subject to genetic polymorphism; CYP2D6 poor metabolizers have a 2-3 fold higher plasma concentration of the R(+) enantiomer and a 20% to 25% increase in the S(-) enantiomer compared to extensive metabolizers.

Bioavailability: Immediate release tablets: 25% to 35%; extended release capsules: 85% of immediate release; bioavailability is increased in patients with CHF

Half-life:
  Infants and Children 6 weeks to 3.5 years (n=8): 2.2 hours (Laer, 2002)
  Children and Adolescents 5.5-19 years (n=7): 3.6 hours (Laer, 2002)
  Adults 7-10 hours; some have reported lower values:
  Adults 24-37 years (n=9): 5.2 hours (Laer, 2002)
  R(+)-carvedilol: 5-9 hours
  S(-)-carvedilol: 7-11 hours

Time to peak serum concentration: Extended release capsules: 5 hours

Elimination: <2% excreted unchanged in urine; metabolites are excreted via bile, into the feces

Dialysis: Hemodialysis does not significantly clear carvedilol

Dosing: Usual Note: Individualize dosage for each patient; monitor patients closely during initiation and upwards titration of dose; reduce dosage if bradycardia or hypotension occurs

Infants, Children, and Adolescents: **Note:** Pharmacokinetic data suggests a faster carvedilol elimination in young pediatric patients (<3.5 years) which may require more frequent dosing (3 times daily) and a higher target dose per kg (Laer, 2002; Shaddy, 2007).

  Heart Failure: Limited data available, efficacy results variable; optimal dose not established: Oral: Immediate release tablets: Initial: Reported mean: 0.075-0.08 mg/kg/dose twice daily; titrate as tolerated; may increase dose by typically 50% every 2 weeks; usual reported maintenance (target) dose range: 0.3-0.75 mg/kg/dose twice daily; the usual titration time to reach target dose was 11-14 weeks (Bruns, 2001; Rusconi, 2004); maximum daily dose: 50 mg/**day**. Dosing based on two retrospective analyses of a total 70 pediatric patients (age range: 3 months to 19 years) which showed improvement in left ventricular function and heart failure symptoms (67% to 68% of patients showed improvement in NYHA class). However, in a

large, a multicenter, double-blind, placebo-controlled, dose-finding trial in 161 pediatric patients (treatment group: n=103, median age range: 33-43 months), a lower target dose range of 0.2-0.4 mg/kg/dose twice daily did not result in a statistical difference in composite clinical end point scores compared to placebo; the authors suggested multiple factors for negative efficacy findings including that the study may have been underpowered due to unexpected, high improvement of the placebo-arm; a subset analysis suggests ventricular morphology may play a role in efficacy (Shaddy, 2007). Further studies are needed.

Adolescents ≥18 years and Adults: **Note:** Reduce dosage if heart rate drops to <55 beats/minute.

  Heart Failure: Note: Prior to initiating therapy, other CHF medications should be stabilized and fluid retention minimized.

  Immediate release tablets: Oral: Initial: 3.125 mg twice daily for 2 weeks; if tolerated, may increase to 6.25 mg twice daily. May double the dose every 2 weeks to the highest dose tolerated by patient.

  Maximum recommended dose:
    Mild to moderate heart failure:
      <85 kg: 25 mg twice daily
      >85 kg: 50 mg twice daily
    Severe heart failure: 25 mg twice daily

  Extended release capsules: Oral: Initial: 10 mg once daily for 2 weeks; if tolerated, may double the dose (eg, 20 mg, 40 mg) every 2 weeks up to 80 mg once daily; maintain on lower dose if higher dose is not tolerated

Hypertension:

  Immediate release tablets: Oral: Initial: 6.25 mg twice daily; if tolerated, dose should be maintained for 1-2 weeks, then increased to 12.5 mg twice daily; maximum daily dose: 50 mg/**day**

  Extended release capsules: Oral: Initial: 20 mg once daily; if tolerated, dose should be maintained for 1-2 weeks, then increased to 40 mg once daily if necessary; maximum daily dose: 80 mg/**day**

Left ventricular dysfunction following MI: Note: Initiate only after patient is hemodynamically stable and fluid retention has been minimized.

  Immediate release tablets: Oral: Initial: 3.125-6.25 mg twice daily; increase dosage incrementally (eg, from 6.25 to 12.5 mg twice daily) at intervals of 3-10 days, as tolerated, to a target dose of 25 mg twice daily

  Extended release capsules: Oral: Initial: 10-20 mg once daily; increase dosage incrementally at intervals of 3-10 days, as tolerated, to a target dose of 80 mg once daily

Conversion from immediate release to extended release (Coreg CR®):

  Current dose immediate release tablets 3.125 mg twice daily: Convert to extended release capsules 10 mg once daily

  Current dose immediate release tablets 6.25 mg twice daily: Convert to extended release capsules 20 mg once daily

  Current dose immediate release tablets 12.5 mg twice daily: Convert to extended release capsules 40 mg once daily

  Current dose immediate release tablets 25 mg twice daily: Convert to extended release capsules 80 mg once daily

Dosing adjustment in renal impairment: No adjustment required. **Note:** Mean AUCs were 40% to 50% higher in patients with moderate to severe renal dysfunction who received immediate release carvedilol, but the ranges of AUCs were similar to patients with normal renal function

Dosing adjustment in hepatic impairment:

  Mild to moderate impairment (Child-Pugh class A or B): There are no dosage adjustments provided in manufacturer's labeling; use with caution; monitor for symptoms of drug-induced toxicity.

Severe impairment (Child-Pugh class C): Use is contraindicated as drug is extensively metabolized by the liver. **Note:** Patients with severe cirrhotic liver disease achieved carvedilol serum concentrations four- to sevenfold higher than normal patients following a single dose of immediate release carvedilol

Administration

Immediate release tablets: Administer with food to decrease the risk of orthostatic hypotension.

Extended release capsules: Administer with food, preferably in the morning; do not crush or chew capsule; swallow whole; do not take in divided doses. Capsule may be opened and contents sprinkled on a spoonful of applesauce; swallow applesauce/medication mixture immediately; do not chew; do not store for later use; do not use warm applesauce; do not sprinkle capsule contents on food other than applesauce; drink fluids after dose to make sure mixture is completely swallowed.

Monitoring Parameters Heart rate, blood pressure (determine need for dosage increase based on trough blood pressure measurements and tolerance on standing systolic pressure 1 hour after dosing), weight; S_{Cr}, BUN, liver function; in patient with increased risk for developing renal dysfunction, monitor renal function during dosage titration

Additional Information CHF: Carvedilol is a nonselective beta blocker with alpha-blocking and antioxidant properties. It is the only beta blocker approved in adults for the treatment of heart failure. Beta blocker therapy, without intrinsic sympathomimetic activity, should be initiated in adult patients with **stable** CHF (NYHA Class II-IV). To date, carvedilol, sustained release metoprolol, and bisoprolol have demonstrated a beneficial effect on morbidity and mortality. It is important that beta blocker therapy be instituted initially at very low doses with gradual and very careful titration. Because carvedilol has alpha-adrenergic blocking effects, it may lower blood pressure to a greater extent. The definitive clinical benefits of the antioxidant property are not known at this time.

Coreg CR® extended release capsules are hard gelatin capsules filled with immediate-release and controlled-release microparticles containing carvedilol phosphate; the microparticles are drug-layered and coated with methacrylic acid copolymers.

Dosage Forms Excipient information presented when available (limited, particularly for generics); consult specific product labeling.

Capsule Extended Release 24 Hour, Oral, as phosphate:
Coreg CR: 10 mg, 20 mg, 40 mg, 80 mg
Tablet, Oral:
Coreg: 3.125 mg, 6.25 mg, 12.5 mg, 25 mg
Generic: 3.125 mg, 6.25 mg, 12.5 mg, 25 mg

Extemporaneous Preparations A 1.25 mg/mL carvedilol oral suspension may be made with tablets and one of two different vehicles (Ora-Blend™ or 1:1 mixture of Ora-Sweet® and Ora-Plus®). Crush five 25 mg tablets in a mortar and reduce to a fine powder; add 15 mL of purified water and mix to a uniform paste. Mix while adding chosen vehicle in incremental proportions to almost 100 mL; transfer to a calibrated amber bottle, rinse mortar with vehicle, and add quantity of vehicle sufficient to make 100 mL. Label "shake well". Stable for 84 days when stored in amber prescription bottles at room temperature (Loyd, 2006).

Carvedilol oral liquid suspensions (0.1 mg/mL and 1.67 mg/mL) made from tablets, water, Ora-Plus®, and Ora-Sweet® were stable for 12 weeks when stored in glass amber bottles at room temperature (25°C). Use one 3.125 mg tablet for the 0.1 mg/mL suspension or two 25 mg tablets for the 1.67 mg/mL suspension; grind

the tablet(s) and compound a mixture with 5 mL of water, 15 mL Ora-Plus®, and 10 mL Ora-Sweet®. Final volume of each suspension: 30 mL; label "shake well" (data on file, GlaxoSmithKline, Philadelphia, PA: DOF #132 [**Note:** Manufacturer no longer disseminates this document]).
Loyd A Jr, "Carvedilol 1.25 mg/mL Oral Suspension," *Int J Pharm Compounding*, 2006, 10(3):220.

References

Azeka E, Franchini Ramires JA, Valler C, et al, "Delisting of Infants and Children From the Heart Transplantation Waiting List After Carvedilol Treatment," *J Am Coll Cardiol*, 2002, 40(11):2034-8.

Brauchli YB, Jick SS, Curtin F, et al, "Association Between Beta-Blockers, Other Antihypertensive Drugs and Psoriasis: Population-Based Case-Control Study," *Br J Dermatol*, 2008, 158(6):1299-307.

Bruns LA and Canter CE, "Should Beta-Blockers be Used for the Treatment of Pediatric Patients With Chronic Heart Failure?" *Paediatr Drugs*, 2002, 4(12):771-8.

Bruns LA, Chrisant MK, Lamour JM, et al, "Carvedilol as Therapy in Pediatric Heart Failure: An Initial Multicenter Experience," *J Pediatr*, 2001, 138(4):505-11.

Gachara N, Prabhakaran S, Srinivas S, et al, "Efficacy and Safety of Carvedilol in Infants With Dilated Cardiomyopathy: A Preliminary Report," *Indian Heart J*, 2001, 53(1):74-8.

Giardini A, Formigari R, Bronzetti G, et al, "Modulation of Neurohormonal Activity After Treatment of Children in Heart Failure With Carvedilol," *Cardiol Young*, 2003, 13(4):333-6.

Gold MH, Holy AK, and Roenigk HH Jr, "Beta-Blocking Drugs and Psoriasis. A Review of Cutaneous Side Effects and Retrospective Analysis of Their Effects on Psoriasis," *J Am Acad Dermatol*, 1988, 19 (5 Pt 1):837-41.

Hsu DT and Pearson GD, "Heart Failure in Children: Part II: Diagnosis, Treatment, and Future Directions," *Circ Heart Fail*, 2009, 2(5):490-8.

Laer S, Mir TS, Behn F, et al, "Carvedilol Therapy in Pediatric Patients With Congestive Heart Failure: A Study Investigating Clinical and Pharmacokinetic Parameters," *Am Heart J*, 2002, 143(5):916-22.

Ratnapalan S, Griffiths K, Costei AM, et al, "Digoxin-Carvedilol Interactions in Children," *J Pediatr*, 2003, 142(5):572-4.

Rusconi P, Gomez-Marin O, Rossique-Gonzalez M, et al, "Carvedilol in Children With Cardiomyopathy: 3-Year Experience at a Single Institution," *J Heart Lung Transplant*, 2004, 23(7):832-8.

Schön MP and Boehncke WH, "Psoriasis," *N Engl J Med*, 2005, 352 (18):1899-912.

Shaddy RE, Boucek MM, Hsu DT, et al, "Carvedilol for Children and Adolescents With Heart Failure: A Randomized Controlled Trial," *JAMA*, 2007, 298(10):1171-9.

Shaddy RE, Curtin EL, Sower B, et al, "The Pediatric Randomized Carvedilol Trial in Children With Heart Failure: Rationale and Design," *Am Heart J*, 2002, 144(3):383-9.

Caspofungin (kas poe FUN jin)

Brand Names: U.S. Cancidas
Brand Names: Canada Cancidas®
Therapeutic Category Antifungal Agent, Echinocandin; Antifungal Agent, Systemic
Generic Availability (U.S.) No
Use Treatment of invasive aspergillosis in patients who are refractory to or intolerant of other therapies (ie, amphotericin B, lipid formulations of amphotericin B, and/or itraconazole); candidemia, intra-abdominal abscess, peritonitis, and pleural space infection caused by susceptible *Candida* species; esophageal candidiasis; empiric therapy of presumed fungal infection in febrile neutropenic patients (FDA approved in ages ≥3 months and adults)
Pregnancy Risk Factor C
Pregnancy Considerations Adverse events have been observed in animal reproduction studies. Caspofungin should be used during pregnancy only if potential benefit justifies the potential risk to the fetus.
Breast-Feeding Considerations It is not known if caspofungin is excreted in breast milk. The manufacturer recommends that caution be exercised when administering caspofungin to nursing women.
Contraindications Hypersensitivity to caspofungin or any component
Warnings Transient increases of alanine transaminase (ALT) and aspartate transaminase (AST) have been reported both with and without concomitant use of

cyclosporine; limit use in patients receiving cyclosporine to those in whom the potential benefit outweighs the risk

Precautions Use with caution and modify dose in patients with moderate hepatic impairment; safety and efficacy have not been established in children with any degree of hepatic impairment and adults with severe hepatic impairment; use with caution and modify dose in patients on concurrent drugs which induce drug clearance such as efavirenz, nevirapine, phenytoin, dexamethasone, carbamazepine, or rifampin

Adverse Reactions

Cardiovascular: Hypertension, hypotension, peripheral edema, tachycardia

Central nervous system: Chills, headache

Dermatologic: Erythema, pruritus, skin rash

Endocrine & metabolic: Hyperglycemia, hypokalemia, hypomagnesemia

Gastrointestinal: Abdominal pain, diarrhea, gastric irritation, nausea, vomiting

Hematologic & oncologic: Anemia, decreased hemoglobin, decreased hematocrit, decreased white blood cell count

Hepatic: Decreased serum albumin, increased serum alkaline phosphatase increased, increased serum ALT, increased serum AST, increased serum bilirubin

Immunologic: Graft versus host disease (infants, children, and adolescents)

Infection: Sepsis

Local: Catheter infection, localized phlebitis

Renal: Hematuria, increased blood urea nitrogen, increased serum creatinine

Respiratory: Cough, dyspnea, pleural effusion, pneumonia, respiratory distress, respiratory failure, rales

Miscellaneous: Fever, infusion related reaction, septic shock

Rare but important or life-threatening: Abdominal distention, adult respiratory distress syndrome, anaphylaxis, anorexia, anxiety, arthralgia, atrial fibrillation, back pain, bacteremia, blood coagulation disorder, bradycardia, cardiac arrest, cardiac arrhythmia, confusion, constipation, decreased appetite, decubitus ulcer, depression, dizziness, drowsiness, dyspepsia, dystonia, edema, epistaxis, erythema multiforme, exfoliation of skin, fatigue, febrile neutropenia, flushing, hematuria, hepatic failure, hepatic necrosis, hepatitis, hepatomegaly, hepatotoxicity, histamine release (including facial swelling, bronchospasm, sensation of warmth), hypercalcemia, hyperkalemia, hypervolemia, hypoxia, infusion site reaction (pain/pruritus/swelling), insomnia, jaundice, limb pain, myocardial infarction, nephrotoxicity (serum creatinine ≥2 x baseline value or ≥1 mg/dL in patients with serum creatinine above ULN range), pancreatitis, petechia, pulmonary edema, pulmonary infiltrates, renal failure, renal insufficiency, seizure, skin lesion, stridor, Stevens-Johnson syndrome, tachypnea, thrombocytopenia, tremor, urinary tract infection, urticaria, weakness

Drug Interactions

Metabolism/Transport Effects None known.

Avoid Concomitant Use

Avoid concomitant use of Caspofungin with any of the following: Saccharomyces boulardii

Increased Effect/Toxicity

The levels/effects of Caspofungin may be increased by: CycloSPORINE (Systemic)

Decreased Effect

Caspofungin may decrease the levels/effects of: Saccharomyces boulardii; Tacrolimus (Systemic)

The levels/effects of Caspofungin may be decreased by: Inducers of Drug Clearance; Rifampin

Stability Store lyophilized vial in refrigerator at 2°C to 8°C (36°F to 46°F); reconstitute 50 mg or 70 mg vial with 10.8 mL of NS (consult manufacturer's prescribing information for details); reconstituted solution may be stored at room temperature (≤25°C or ≤77°F) for 1 hour prior to preparation of the infusion solution; final infusion solution may be stored at room temperature (≤25°C or ≤77°F) for 24 hours or for 48 hours in the refrigerator; caspofungin is not stable in dextrose-containing solutions

Mechanism of Action Inhibits synthesis of β(1,3)-D-glucan, an essential component of the cell wall of susceptible fungi. Highest activity is in regions of active cell growth. Mammalian cells do not require β(1,3)-D-glucan, limiting potential toxicity.

Pharmacokinetics (Adult data unless noted)

Distribution: CSF concentrations: Nondetectable [<10 ng/mL (n=1)] (Sáez-Llorens, 2009)

Protein binding: 97% to albumin

Metabolism: Via hydrolysis and N-acetylation in the liver; undergoes spontaneous chemical degradation to an open-ring peptide and hydrolysis to amino acids

Half-life: Beta (distribution): 9-11 hours (~8 hours in children <12 years); terminal: 40-50 hours; beta phase half-life is 32% to 43% lower in pediatric patients than in adult patients

Elimination: 35% of dose excreted in feces primarily as metabolites; 41% of dose excreted in urine primarily as metabolites; 1.4% of dose excreted unchanged in urine

Dialysis: Not dialyzable

Dosing: Neonatal Note: Caspofungin treatment duration should be based on patient status and clinical response. Empiric therapy should be given until neutropenia resolves. In neutropenic patients, continue treatment for at least 7 days after both signs and symptoms of infection and neutropenia resolve. In patients with positive cultures, continue treatment for at least 14 days after the last positive culture.

I.V.: 25 mg/m^2/dose once daily; dosing based on a pharmacokinetic study of 18 neonates including preterm neonates that showed similar serum concentrations to standard adult doses. Reported trough concentrations were slightly elevated and not correlated with increased adverse events (Sáez-Llorens, 2009). Limited data available, further studies needed.

Dosing: Usual I.V.: Note: Caspofungin treatment duration should be based on patient status and clinical response. Empiric therapy should be given until neutropenia resolves. In neutropenic patients, continue treatment for at least 7 days after both signs and symptoms of infection and neutropenia resolve. In patients with positive cultures, continue treatment for at least 14 days after the last positive culture.

Infants 1 to <3 months: 25 mg/m^2/dose once daily; dosing based on a pharmacokinetic study of 18 infants that showed similar serum concentrations to standard adult doses (50 mg/day). Reported trough concentrations were slightly elevated and not correlated with increased adverse events (Sáez-Llorens, 2009)

Infants and Children 3 months to 17 years: Initial dose: 70 mg/m^2/dose on day 1, subsequent dosing: 50 mg/m^2/dose once daily; may increase to 70 mg/m^2/dose once daily if clinical response inadequate (maximum dose: 70 mg). Patients receiving carbamazepine, dexamethasone, efavirenz, nevirapine, phenytoin, or rifampin (and possibly other enzyme inducers): Consider 70 mg/m^2/dose once daily (maximum: 70 mg/day).

Adults: Loading dose: 70 mg on day 1, followed by 50 mg once daily thereafter; 70 mg daily dose has been administered and well tolerated in patients not clinically responding to the daily 50 mg dose; may need to adjust dose in patients receiving a concomitant enzyme inducer. Doses greater than the standard adult dosing regimen (ie, 150 mg once daily) have not demonstrated increased benefit or toxicity in patients with invasive candidiasis (Betts, 2009).

Esophageal candidiasis: 50 mg once daily with no loading dose

Patients receiving concomitant enzyme inducer:
Patients receiving rifampin: 70 mg caspofungin once daily
Patients receiving carbamazepine, dexamethasone, phenytoin, nevirapine, or efavirenz: May require an increase in caspofungin dose to 70 mg once daily
Dosing adjustment in renal impairment: No adjustment needed
Dosing adjustment in hepatic impairment (based on adult data):
Mild hepatic impairment (Child-Pugh score 5 to 6): No dosage adjustment necessary
Moderate hepatic impairment (Child-Pugh score 7 to 9): Decrease daily dose by 30%
Administration Administer by slow I.V. infusion over 1 hour (manufacturer); higher doses (eg, 150 mg) have been infused over ~2 hours (Betts, 2009); maximum concentration of 0.5 mg/mL diluted in NS, LR, 0.45% sodium chloride. Do not mix or coinfuse with other medications. Do not use diluents containing dextrose.
Monitoring Parameters Periodic liver function tests, serum potassium, CBC, hemoglobin
Dosage Forms Excipient information presented when available (limited, particularly for generics); consult specific product labeling.
Solution Reconstituted, Intravenous, as acetate:
Cancidas: 50 mg (1 ea); 70 mg (1 ea)
References
Betts RF, Nucci M, Talwar D, et al, "A Multicenter, Double-Blind Trial of a High-Dose Caspofungin Treatment Regimen Versus a Standard Caspofungin Treatment Regimen for Adult Patients With Invasive Candidiasis," *Clin Infect Dis*, 2009, 48(12):1676-84.
Centers for Disease Control and Prevention (CDC), "Guidelines for the Prevention and Treatment of Opportunistic Infections Among HIV-Exposed and HIV-Infected Children," *MMWR Recomm Rep*, 2009, 58(RR-11):1-166. Available at http://aidsinfo.nih.gov/contentfiles/Pediatric_OI.pdf
Pappas PG, Kauffman CA, Andes D, et al, "Clinical Practice Guidelines for the Management of Candidiasis: 2009 Update by the Infectious Diseases Society of America," *Clin Infect Dis*, 2009, 48(5):503-35.
Sáez-Llorens X, Macias M, Maiya P, et al, "Pharmacokinetics and Safety of Caspofungin in Neonates and Infants Less Than 3 Months of Age," *Antimicrob Agents Chemother*, 2009, 53(3):869-75.
Walsh TJ, Adamson PC, Seibel NL, et al, "Pharmacokinetics (PK) of Caspofungin (CAS) in Pediatric Patients (#M-896)," 42nd Interscience Conference on Antimicrobial Agents and Chemotherapy, San Diego, CA, Sept 27-30, 2002.
Walsh TJ, Adamson PC, Seibel NL, et al, "Pharmacokinetics, Safety, and Tolerability of Caspofungin in Children and Adolescents," *Antimicrob Agents Chemother*, 2005, 49(11):4536-45.
Walsh TJ, Teppler H, Donowitz GR, et al, "Caspofungin Versus Liposomal Amphotericin B for Empirical Antifungal Therapy in Patients With Persistent Fever and Neutropenia," *N Engl J Med*, 2004, 351 (14):1391-402.

◆ **Caspofungin Acetate** see Caspofungin on page 388

Castor Oil (KAS tor oyl)

Therapeutic Category Laxative, Stimulant
Generic Availability (U.S.) No
Use Preparation for rectal or bowel examination or surgery; rarely used to relieve constipation; also applied to skin as emollient and protectant
Pregnancy Considerations Ingestion of castor oil may be associated with induction of labor. Use of castor oil as a laxative during pregnancy should be avoided (Cullen, 2007; Hall, 2011; Wald, 2003).
Contraindications Hypersensitivity to castor oil; nausea, vomiting, abdominal pain, fecal impaction, GI bleeding, appendicitis, CHF, menstruation, dehydration
Warnings Long-term use may result in laxative dependence
Adverse Reactions
Cardiovascular: Hypotension
Central nervous system: Dizziness
Endocrine & metabolic: Electrolyte disturbance
Gastrointestinal: Abdominal cramps, diarrhea, nausea
Genitourinary: Pelvic congestion
Drug Interactions
Metabolism/Transport Effects None known.
Avoid Concomitant Use There are no known interactions where it is recommended to avoid concomitant use.
Increased Effect/Toxicity There are no known significant interactions involving an increase in effect.
Decreased Effect There are no known significant interactions involving a decrease in effect.
Stability Protect from heat (emulsion should be protected from freezing)
Mechanism of Action Acts primarily in the small intestine; hydrolyzed to ricinoleic acid which reduces net absorption of fluid and electrolytes and stimulates peristalsis
Pharmacodynamics Onset of action: Oral: Within 2-6 hours
Dosing: Usual Oral:
Castor oil:
Infants <2 years: 1-5 mL or 15 mL/m²/dose as a single dose
Children 2-11 years: 5-15 mL as a single dose
Children ≥12 years and Adults: 15-60 mL as a single dose
Emulsified castor oil:
Infants: 2.5-7.5 mL/dose
Children:
<2 years: 5-15 mL/dose
2-11 years: 7.5-30 mL/dose
Children ≥12 years and Adults: 30-60 mL/dose
Administration Oral: Do not administer at bedtime because of rapid onset of action; chill or administer with milk, juice, or carbonated beverage to improve palatability; administer on an empty stomach; castor oil emulsions should be shaken well before use
Monitoring Parameters I & O, serum electrolytes, stool frequency
References
Cullen G and O'Donoghue D, "Constipation and Pregnancy," *Best Pract Res Clin Gastroenterol*, 2007, 21(5):807-18.
Hall HG, McKenna LG, and Griffiths DL, "Complementary and Alternative Medicine for Induction of Labour," *Women Birth*, 2011.
Wald A, "Constipation, Diarrhea, and Symptomatic Hemorrhoids During Pregnancy," *Gastroenterol Clin North Am*, 2003, 32(1):309-22.

◆ **Cataflam** see Diclofenac (Systemic) on page 645
◆ **Catapres** see CloNIDine on page 516
◆ **Catapres® (Can)** see CloNIDine on page 516
◆ **Catapres-TTS-1** see CloNIDine on page 516
◆ **Catapres-TTS-2** see CloNIDine on page 516
◆ **Catapres-TTS-3** see CloNIDine on page 516
◆ **Cathflo Activase** see Alteplase on page 104
◆ **Caverject** see Alprostadil on page 103
◆ **Caverject Impulse** see Alprostadil on page 103
◆ **CaviRinse** see Fluoride on page 894
◆ **Cayston** see Aztreonam on page 254
◆ **CB-1348** see Chlorambucil on page 437
◆ **CBDCA** see CARBOplatin on page 379
◆ **CBZ** see CarBAMazepine on page 372
◆ **ccIIV3 [Flucelvax]** see Influenza Virus Vaccine (Inactivated) on page 1103
◆ **CCNU** see Lomustine on page 1268
◆ **C Complex [OTC]** see Ascorbic Acid on page 206
◆ **2-CdA** see Cladribine on page 488
◆ **CDCA** see Chenodiol on page 434
◆ **CDDP** see CISplatin on page 481
◆ **CE** see Estrogens (Conjugated/Equine, Systemic) on page 799

◆ **CE** *see* Estrogens (Conjugated/Equine, Topical) *on page 801*

◆ **Ceclor® (Can)** *see* Cefaclor *on page 391*

◆ **Cedax** *see* Ceftibuten *on page 416*

◆ **CEE** *see* Estrogens (Conjugated/Equine, Systemic) *on page 799*

◆ **CEE** *see* Estrogens (Conjugated/Equine, Topical) *on page 801*

◆ **CeeNU** *see* Lomustine *on page 1268*

Cefaclor (SEF a klor)

Medication Safety Issues
Sound-alike/look-alike issues:
Cefaclor may be confused with cephalexin

Related Information
Oral Medications That Should Not Be Crushed or Altered *on page 2438*

Brand Names: Canada Apo-Cefaclor®; Ceclor®; Novo-Cefaclor; Nu-Cefaclor; PMS-Cefaclor

Therapeutic Category Antibiotic, Cephalosporin (Second Generation)

Generic Availability (U.S.) Yes

Use Infections caused by susceptible bacteria including *Staph aureus*, *S. pneumoniae*, *S. pyogenes*, and *H. influenzae* (excluding β-lactamase negative, ampicillin-resistant strains); treatment of otitis media, sinusitis, and infections involving the respiratory tract, skin and skin structure, bone and joint; treatment of urinary tract infections caused by *E. coli*, *Klebsiella*, and *Proteus mirabilis*

Pregnancy Risk Factor B

Pregnancy Considerations Adverse events were not observed in animal reproduction studies. An increased risk of teratogenic effects has not been observed following maternal use of cefaclor.

Breast-Feeding Considerations Small amounts of cefaclor are excreted in breast milk. The manufacturer recommends that caution be exercised when administering cefaclor to nursing women. Nondose-related effects could include modification of bowel flora.

Contraindications Hypersensitivity to cefaclor, any component, or cephalosporins

Warnings Prolonged use may result in fungal or bacterial superinfection, including *C. difficile*-associated diarrhea (CDAD) and pseudomembranous colitis; CDAD has been observed >2 months postantibiotic treatment; use with caution in patients with a history of colitis; pseudomembranous colitis reported with cefaclor.

Oral suspension contains sodium benzoate; benzoic acid (benzoate) is a metabolite of benzyl alcohol; large amounts of benzyl alcohol (≥99 mg/kg/day) have been associated with a potentially fatal toxicity ("gasping syndrome") in neonates; the "gasping syndrome" consists of metabolic acidosis, respiratory distress, gasping respirations, CNS dysfunction (including convulsions, intracranial hemorrhage), hypotension, and cardiovascular collapse; use suspension containing sodium benzoate with caution in neonates; *in vitro* and animal studies have shown that benzoate displaces bilirubin from protein binding sites.

Precautions Use with caution in patients with impaired renal function; adjust dose in patients with severe renal impairment. Use with caution in patients with a history of penicillin hypersensitivity, especially IgE-mediated reactions (eg, anaphylaxis, angioedema, urticaria); cross-hypersensitivity among beta-lactam antibiotics may occur in up to 10% of patients with penicillin allergy history; may cause serum sickness-like reaction (estimated incidence ranges from 0.024% to 0.2% per drug course); majority of reactions have occurred in children <5 years of age with

symptoms of fever, rash, erythema multiforme, and arthralgia, often occurring during the second or third exposure.

Adverse Reactions
Dermatologic: Rash (maculopapular, erythematous, or morbilliform)
Gastrointestinal: Diarrhea
Genitourinary: Vaginitis
Hematologic: Eosinophilia
Hepatic: Increased transaminases
Miscellaneous: Moniliasis
Rare but important or life-threatening: Agitation, agranulocytosis, anaphylaxis, angioedema, aplastic anemia, arthralgia, cholestatic jaundice, CNS irritability, confusion, dizziness, hallucinations, hemolytic anemia, hepatitis, hyperactivity, insomnia, interstitial nephritis, nausea, nervousness, neutropenia, paresthesia, PT prolonged, pruritus, pseudomembranous colitis, seizure, serum-sickness, somnolence, Stevens-Johnson syndrome, thrombocytopenia, toxic epidermal necrolysis, urticaria, vomiting
Reactions reported with other cephalosporins: Abdominal pain, cholestasis, fever, hemorrhage, renal dysfunction, superinfection, toxic nephropathy

Drug Interactions
Metabolism/Transport Effects None known.
Avoid Concomitant Use
Avoid concomitant use of Cefaclor with any of the following: BCG
Increased Effect/Toxicity
Cefaclor may increase the levels/effects of: Aminoglycosides; Vitamin K Antagonists

The levels/effects of Cefaclor may be increased by: Probenecid
Decreased Effect
Cefaclor may decrease the levels/effects of: BCG; Sodium Picosulfate; Typhoid Vaccine

Food Interactions Cefaclor serum levels may be decreased slightly if taken with food. The bioavailability of cefaclor extended release tablets is decreased 23% and the maximum concentration is decreased 67% when taken on an empty stomach. Management: Administer without regard to food.

Stability Store capsule and unreconstituted powder for oral suspension at room temperature. Refrigerate suspension after reconstitution; discard after 14 days.

Mechanism of Action Inhibits bacterial cell wall synthesis by binding to one or more of the penicillin-binding proteins (PBPs) which in turn inhibits the final transpeptidation step of peptidoglycan synthesis in bacterial cell walls, thus inhibiting cell wall biosynthesis. Bacteria eventually lyse due to ongoing activity of cell wall autolytic enzymes (autolysins and murein hydrolases) while cell wall assembly is arrested.

Pharmacokinetics (Adult data unless noted)
Absorption: Oral: Well absorbed; acid stable
Distribution: Distributes into tissues and fluids including bone, pleural and synovial fluid; crosses the placenta; appears in breast milk
Protein binding: 25%
Half-life: 30-60 minutes (prolonged with renal impairment)
Time to peak serum concentration:
Capsule: 60 minutes
Suspension: 45-60 minutes
Elimination: Most of dose (80%) excreted unchanged in urine by glomerular filtration and tubular secretion
Dialysis: Moderately dialyzable (20% to 50%)

Dosing: Usual Oral:
Infants >1 month and Children: 20-40 mg/kg/day divided every 8-12 hours; maximum dose: 2 g/day (twice daily option is for treatment of otitis media or pharyngitis)
Otitis media: 40 mg/kg/day divided every 12 hours
Pharyngitis: 20 mg/kg/day divided every 12 hours

Adults: 250-500 mg every 8 hours

Dosing adjustment in renal impairment: CrCl <10 mL/minute: Administer 50% of dose

Administration Oral: Capsule, suspension: Administer 1 hour before or 2 hours after a meal; shake suspension well before use

Monitoring Parameters With prolonged therapy, monitor CBC and stool frequency periodically

Test Interactions Positive direct Coombs', false-positive urinary glucose test using cupric sulfate (Benedict's solution, Clinitest®, Fehling's solution), false-positive serum or urine creatinine with Jaffé reaction

Dosage Forms Excipient information presented when available (limited, particularly for generics); consult specific product labeling.

Capsule, Oral:
Generic: 250 mg, 500 mg
Suspension Reconstituted, Oral:
Generic: 125 mg/5 mL (150 mL); 250 mg/5 mL (150 mL); 375 mg/5 mL (100 mL)
Tablet Extended Release 12 Hour, Oral:
Generic: 500 mg

References

Boguniewicz M and Leung DYM, "Hypersensitivity Reactions to Antibiotics Commonly Used in Children," *Pediatr Infect Dis J*, 1995, 14 (3):221-31.

Hyslop DL, "Cefaclor Safety Profile: A Ten Year Review," *Clin Ther*, 1988, 11(Suppl A):83-94.

Levine LR, "Quantitative Comparison of Adverse Reactions to Cefaclor vs Amoxicillin in a Surveillance Study," *Pediatr Infect Dis*, 1985, 4 (4):358-61.

Cefadroxil (sef a DROKS il)

Brand Names: Canada Apo-Cefadroxil; PRO-Cefadroxil; Teva-Cefadroxil

Therapeutic Category Antibiotic, Cephalosporin (First Generation)

Generic Availability (U.S.) Yes

Use Treatment of susceptible bacterial infections including group A beta-hemolytic streptococcal pharyngitis or tonsillitis; skin and soft tissue infections caused by streptococci or staphylococci; urinary tract infections caused by *Klebsiella*, *E. coli*, and *Proteus mirabilis*

Pregnancy Risk Factor B

Pregnancy Considerations Adverse events have not been observed in animal reproduction studies. Cefadroxil crosses the placenta. Limited data is available concerning the use of cefadroxil in pregnancy; however, adverse fetal effects were not noted in a small clinical trial.

Breast-Feeding Considerations Very small amounts of cefadroxil are excreted in breast milk. The manufacturer recommends that caution be exercised when administering cefadroxil to nursing women. Nondose-related effects could include modification of bowel flora.

Contraindications Hypersensitivity to cefadroxil, any component, or cephalosporins

Warnings Prolonged use may result in superinfection; do not use in patients with immediate-type hypersensitivity reaction to penicillin

Oral suspension contains sodium benzoate; benzoic acid (benzoate) is a metabolite of benzyl alcohol; large amounts of benzyl alcohol (≥99 mg/kg/day) have been associated with a potentially fatal toxicity ("gasping syndrome") in neonates; the "gasping syndrome" consists of metabolic acidosis, respiratory distress, gasping respirations, CNS dysfunction (including convulsions, intracranial hemorrhage), hypotension and cardiovascular collapse; use cefadroxil oral suspensions containing sodium benzoate with caution in neonates; *in vitro* and animal studies have shown that benzoate displaces bilirubin from protein binding sites

Precautions Use with caution in patients who are hypersensitive to penicillin; modify dosage in patients with renal impairment

Adverse Reactions

Gastrointestinal: Diarrhea

Rare but important or life-threatening: Agranulocytosis, anaphylaxis, angioedema, cholestasis, *Clostridium difficile* associated diarrhea, dyspepsia, erythema multiforme, erythematous rash, genital candidiasis, hepatic failure, increased serum transaminases, maculopapular rash, neutropenia, pseudomembranous colitis, serum sickness, Stevens-Johnson syndrome, thrombocytopenia, vaginitis

Drug Interactions

Metabolism/Transport Effects None known.

Avoid Concomitant Use

Avoid concomitant use of Cefadroxil with any of the following: BCG

Increased Effect/Toxicity

Cefadroxil may increase the levels/effects of: Vitamin K Antagonists

The levels/effects of Cefadroxil may be increased by: Probenecid

Decreased Effect

Cefadroxil may decrease the levels/effects of: BCG; Sodium Picosulfate; Typhoid Vaccine

Food Interactions Concomitant administration with food, infant formula, or cow's milk does **not** significantly affect absorption.

Stability Refrigerate suspension after reconstitution; discard after 14 days

Mechanism of Action Inhibits bacterial cell wall synthesis by binding to one or more of the penicillin-binding proteins (PBPs) which in turn inhibits the final transpeptidation step of peptidoglycan synthesis in bacterial cell walls, thus inhibiting cell wall biosynthesis. Bacteria eventually lyse due to ongoing activity of cell wall autolytic enzymes (autolysins and murein hydrolases) while cell wall assembly is arrested.

Pharmacokinetics (Adult data unless noted)

Absorption: Oral: Rapid; well absorbed from GI tract

Distribution: V_d: 0.31 L/kg; crosses the placenta; appears in breast milk

Protein binding: 20%

Half-life: 1-2 hours; 20-24 hours in renal failure

Time to peak serum concentration: Within 70-90 minutes

Elimination: >90% of dose excreted unchanged in urine within 24 hours

Dosing: Usual Oral:

Infants and Children: 30 mg/kg/day divided twice daily up to a maximum of 2 g/day

Adolescents and Adults: 1-2 g/day in 1-2 divided doses; maximum dose for adults: 4 g/day

Dosing interval in renal impairment:

CrCl 10-25 mL/minute: Administer every 24 hours
CrCl <10 mL/minute: Administer every 36 hours

Administration Oral: May be administered without regard to food; administration with food may decrease nausea or vomiting; shake suspension well before use

Monitoring Parameters Stool frequency, resolution of infection

Test Interactions Positive direct Coombs', false-positive urinary glucose test using cupric sulfate (Benedict's solution, Clinitest®, Fehling's solution), false-positive serum or urine creatinine with Jaffé reaction

Dosage Forms Excipient information presented when available (limited, particularly for generics); consult specific product labeling.

Capsule, Oral, as monohydrate [strength expressed as base]:
Generic: 500 mg

Suspension Reconstituted, Oral, as monohydrate [strength expressed as base]:
Generic: 250 mg/5 mL (100 mL); 500 mg/5 mL (75 mL, 100 mL)
Tablet, Oral, as monohydrate [strength expressed as base]:
Generic: 1 g

References

Shulman ST, Bisno AL, Clegg HW, et al, "Clinical Practice Guideline for the Diagnosis and Management of Group A Streptococcal Pharyngitis: 2012 Update by the Infectious Diseases Society of America," *Clin Infect Dis*, 2012.

◆ **Cefadroxil Monohydrate** *see* Cefadroxil *on page 392*

CeFAZolin (sef A zoe lin)

Medication Safety Issues
Sound-alike/look-alike issues:
CeFAZolin may be confused with cefoTEtan, cefOXitin, cefprozil, cefTAZidime, cefTRIAXone, cephalexin

Related Information
Prevention of Infective Endocarditis *on page 2336*

Brand Names: Canada Cefazolin For Injection; Cefazolin For Injection, USP

Therapeutic Category Antibiotic, Cephalosporin (First Generation)

Generic Availability (U.S.) Yes

Use Treatment of susceptible infections involving the respiratory tract, skin and skin structure, urinary tract, biliary tract, bone and joint, genitals, and septicemia (FDA approved in ages ≥1 month and adults); perioperative prophylaxis (FDA approved in adults); treatment of bacterial endocarditis (FDA approved in adults); has also been used for bacterial endocarditis prophylaxis for dental and upper respiratory procedures

Pregnancy Risk Factor B

Pregnancy Considerations Adverse effects were not observed in animal reproduction studies. Cefazolin crosses the placenta. Adverse events have not been reported in the fetus following administration of cefazolin prior to cesarean section. Cefazolin is recommended for group B streptococcus prophylaxis in pregnant patients with a nonanaphylactic penicillin allergy. It is also one of the antibiotics recommended for prophylactic use prior to cesarean delivery and may be used in certain situations prior to vaginal delivery in women at high risk for endocarditis.

Due to pregnancy-induced physiologic changes, the pharmacokinetics of cefazolin are altered. The half-life is shorter, the AUC is smaller, and the clearance and volume of distribution are increased.

Breast-Feeding Considerations Small amounts of cefazolin are excreted in breast milk. The manufacturer recommends that caution be exercised when administering cefazolin to nursing women. Nondose-related effects could include modification of bowel flora.

Contraindications Hypersensitivity to cefazolin sodium, any component, or cephalosporins. Additional contraindications: Premix formulations in dextrose: Hypersensitivity to corn or corn products

Warnings Prolonged use may result in fungal or bacterial superinfection, including *C. difficile*-associated diarrhea (CDAD) and pseudomembranous colitis; CDAD has been observed >2 months postantibiotic treatment; use with caution in patients with a history of colitis. May cause hypersensitivity reaction; patients with history of hypersensitivity reactions to other cephalosporins or penicillins may experience cross-sensitivity; use with caution in patients with a history of penicillin allergy, especially IgE-mediated reactions (eg, anaphylaxis, angioedema, urticaria).

Precautions Use with caution in patients with impaired renal function; dosage adjustment may be needed. Use with caution in patients previously stabilized on anticoagulant therapy; may cause alteration in prothrombin activity; risk increased in renal or hepatic impairment, poor nutritional state, or prolonged course of therapy; monitor prothrombin times as necessary. Use with caution in patients with a history of seizure disorder; high levels, particularly in the presence of renal impairment, may increase risk of seizures.

Adverse Reactions
Cardiovascular: Localized phlebitis
Central nervous system: Seizure
Dermatologic: Pruritus, skin rash, Stevens-Johnson syndrome
Gastrointestinal: Abdominal cramps, anorexia, diarrhea, nausea, oral candidiasis, pseudomembranous colitis, vomiting
Genitourinary: Vaginitis
Hepatic: Hepatitis, increased serum transaminases
Hematologic: Eosinophilia, leukopenia, neutropenia, thrombocythemia, thrombocytopenia
Hypersensitivity: Anaphylaxis
Local: Pain at injection site
Renal: Increased blood urea nitrogen, increased serum creatinine, renal failure
Miscellaneous: Fever

Drug Interactions
Metabolism/Transport Effects None known.

Avoid Concomitant Use
Avoid concomitant use of CeFAZolin with any of the following: BCG

Increased Effect/Toxicity
CeFAZolin may increase the levels/effects of: Fosphenytoin; Phenytoin; Vitamin K Antagonists

The levels/effects of CeFAZolin may be increased by: Probenecid

Decreased Effect
CeFAZolin may decrease the levels/effects of: BCG; Sodium Picosulfate; Typhoid Vaccine

Stability
Vials: Store intact vials at 20°C to 25°C (68°F to 77°F); protect from light. Reconstituted solution is stable for 24 hours at room temperature or 10 days when refrigerated.
Duplex infusion bags: Prior to activation, store at 20°C to 25°C (68°F to 77°F); excursions permitted to 15°C to 30°C (59°F to 86°F). After activation, stable for 24 hours at room temperature or 7 days refrigerated.
Premixed Galaxy infusion bags: Store frozen at -20°C (-4°F); thaw at room temperature or under refrigeration; do not force thaw. Thawed solution is stable for 48 hours at room temperature and 30 days refrigerated; do not refreeze.

Mechanism of Action Inhibits bacterial cell wall synthesis by binding to one or more of the penicillin-binding proteins (PBPs) which in turn inhibits the final transpeptidation step of peptidoglycan synthesis in bacterial cell walls, thus inhibiting cell wall biosynthesis. Bacteria eventually lyse due to ongoing activity of cell wall autolytic enzymes (autolysins and murein hydrolases) while cell wall assembly is arrested.

Pharmacokinetics (Adult data unless noted)
Distribution: CSF penetration is poor; penetrates bone and synovial fluid well; distributes into bile
Protein binding: 74% to 86%
Metabolism: Minimally hepatic
Half-life:
Neonates: 3-5 hours
Adults: 90-150 minutes (prolonged with renal impairment) ▶

Time to peak serum concentration:
I.M.: Within 0.5-2 hours
I.V.: Within 5 minutes
Elimination: 80% to 100% excreted unchanged in urine

Dosing: Neonatal General dosing, susceptible infection (*Red Book*, 2012): I.M., I.V.:
Body weight <2 kg: 25 mg/kg/dose every 12 hours
Body weight >2 kg:
PNA ≤7 days: 25 mg/kg/dose every 12 hours
PNA 8-28 days: 25 mg/kg/dose every 8 hours

Dosing: Usual

Infants, Children, and Adolescents:

General dosing, susceptible infection (*Red Book*, 2012): I.M., I.V.:
Mild to moderate infections: 25-50 mg/kg/day divided every 8 hours; maximum dose: 1000 mg
Severe infections: 100-150 mg/kg/day divided every 8 hours; maximum dose: 2000 mg

Endocarditis, bacterial:
Prophylaxis for dental and upper respiratory procedures: I.M., I.V.: 50 mg/kg 30-60 minutes before procedure; maximum dose: 1000 mg (Wilson, 2007)
Treatment: I.V.: 100 mg/kg/day in divided doses every 8 hours for at least 6 weeks; with or without gentamicin; if prosthetic valve, also use in combination with rifampin; maximum dose: 2000 mg (Baddour, 2005)

Peritonitis (CAPD) (Warady, 2012):
Prophylaxis:
Touch contamination of PD line: Intraperitoneal: 125 mg per liter
Invasive dental procedures: I.V.: 25 mg/kg administered 30-60 minutes before procedure; maximum dose: 1000 mg
Gastrointestinal or genitourinary procedures: I.V.: 25 mg/kg administered 60 minutes before procedure; maximum dose: 2000 mg
Treatment: Intraperitoneal:
Intermittent: 20 mg/kg every 24 hours in the long dwell
Continuous: Loading dose: 500 mg per liter of dialysate; maintenance: 125 mg per liter of dialysate

Pneumonia, community-acquired pneumonia (CAP), S. aureus, methicillin susceptible: Infants ≥3 months, Children, and Adolescents: I.V.: 50 mg/kg/dose every 8 hours; maximum dose: 2000 mg (Bradley, 2011)

Skin and soft tissue infections, S. aureus, methicillin susceptible (mild to moderate): I.V.: 50 mg/kg/day in divided doses 3 times daily; maximum dose: 1000 mg (Stevens, 2005); higher doses may be required in severe cases

Surgical prophylaxis: Children and Adolescents: I.V.: 25-30 mg/kg 30-60 minutes before procedure, may repeat in 4 hours; maximum dose dependent upon patient weight: Weight <120 kg: 2000 mg; weight ≥120 kg: 3000 mg (Bratzler, 2013; *Red Book*, 2012)

Adults:

General dosing, susceptible infection:
Mild infection with gram-positive cocci: I.V.: 250-500 mg every 8 hours
Moderate to severe infections: I.V.: 500-1000 mg every 6-8 hours

Group B streptococcus (neonatal prophylaxis): I.V.: 2000 mg once, then 1000 mg every 8 hours until delivery (CDC, 2010)

Perioperative prophylaxis: I.M., I.V.: 1000 mg 30-60 minutes prior to surgery (may repeat in 2-5 hours intraoperatively); followed by 500-1000 mg every 6-8 hours for 24 hours postoperatively

Pneumonia, pneumococcal: I.V.: 500 mg every 12 hours

Urinary tract infection; uncomplicated: I.M., I.V.: 1000 mg every 12 hours

Dosing interval in renal impairment: I.M., I.V.:
Infants >1 month, Children, and Adolescents: After initial loading dose is administered, modify dose based on the degree of renal impairment:
CrCl >70 mL/minute: No dosage adjustment required
CrCl 40-70 mL/minute: Administer 60% of the usual daily dose divided every 12 hours
CrCl 20-40 mL/minute: Administer 25% of the usual daily dose divided every 12 hours
CrCl 5-20 mL/minute: Administer 10% of the usual daily dose given every 24 hours
Hemodialysis: 25 mg/kg/dose every 24 hours (Aronoff, 2007)
Peritoneal dialysis: 25 mg/kg/dose every 24 hours (Aronoff, 2007)
Continuous renal replacement therapy: 25 mg/kg/dose every 8 hours (Aronoff, 2007)

Adults: After initial loading dose is administered, modify dose based on the degree of renal impairment:
CrCl ≥55 mL/minute: No dosage adjustment required
CrCl 35-54 mL/minute: Administer full dose ≥every 8 hours
CrCl 11-34 mL/minute: Administer 50% of usual dose every 12 hours
CrCl ≤10 mL/minute: Administer 50% of usual dose every 18-24 hours
Intermittent hemodialysis (IHD) (administer after hemodialysis on dialysis days): Dialyzable (20% to 50%): 500-1000 mg every 24 hours **or** use 1000-2000 mg every 48-72 hours (Heintz, 2009); **Note:** Dosing dependent on the assumption of 3 times/week, complete IHD sessions. Alternatively, may administer 15-20 mg/kg (maximum dose: 2000 mg) after dialysis without regularly scheduled dosing (Ahern, 2003; Sowinski, 2001).
Peritoneal dialysis (PD): 500 mg every 12 hours
Continuous renal replacement therapy (CRRT) (Heintz, 2009; Trotman, 2005): Drug clearance is highly dependent on the method of renal replacement, filter type, and flow rate. Appropriate dosing requires close monitoring of pharmacologic response, signs of adverse reactions due to drug accumulation, as well as drug concentrations in relation to target trough (if appropriate). The following are general recommendations only (based on dialysate flow/ultrafiltration rates of 1-2 L/hour and minimal residual renal function) and should not supersede clinical judgment:
CVVH: Loading dose of 2000 mg, followed by 1000-2000 mg every 12 hours
CVVHD/CVVHDF: Loading dose of 2000 mg, followed by either 1000 mg every 8 hours **or** 2000 mg every 12 hours. **Note:** Dosage of 1000 mg every 8 hours results in similar steady-state concentrations as 2000 mg every 12 hours and is more cost effective (Heintz, 2009).

Dosing adjustment in hepatic impairment: There are no dosage adjustments provided in the manufacturer's labeling.

Administration Parenteral:
I.V.: Cefazolin may be administered IVP over 3-5 minutes at a maximum concentration of 100 mg/mL or I.V. intermittent infusion over 10-60 minutes at a final concentration of 20 mg/mL. In fluid-restricted patients, a concentration of 138 mg/mL has been administered IVP.
I.M.: Deep I.M. injection into a large muscle mass. May dilute vial using SWI to a final concentration between 225-330 mg/mL.

Monitoring Parameters Renal function periodically when used in combination with other nephrotoxic drugs, hepatic function tests, and CBC; prothrombin time in patients at risk; number and type of stools/day for diarrhea; monitor for signs of anaphylaxis during first dose

Test Interactions Positive direct Coombs', false-positive urinary glucose test using cupric sulfate (Benedict's solution, Clinitest, Fehling's solution), false-positive serum or urine creatinine with Jaffé reaction.

Some penicillin derivatives may accelerate the degradation of aminoglycosides *in vitro*, leading to a potential underestimation of aminoglycoside serum concentration.

Dosage Forms Excipient information presented when available (limited, particularly for generics); consult specific product labeling.

Solution, Intravenous:
Generic: 1 g (50 mL)
Solution Reconstituted, Injection:
Generic: 500 mg (1 ea); 1 g (1 ea); 10 g (1 ea); 20 g (1 ea); 100 g (1 ea); 300 g (1 ea)
Solution Reconstituted, Injection [preservative free]:
Generic: 500 mg (1 ea); 1 g (1 ea); 10 g (1 ea); 20 g (1 ea)
Solution Reconstituted, Intravenous:
Generic: 1 g (1 ea); 2 g (1 ea)

References

Ahern JW, Possidente CJ, Hood V, et al, "Cefazolin Dosing Protocol for Patients Receiving Long-Term Hemodialysis," *Am J Health Syst Pharm*, 2003, 60(2):178-81.

American Academy of Pediatrics (AAP). In: Pickering LK, Baker CJ, Kimberlin DW, Long SS, eds. *Red Book: 2012 Report of the Committee on Infectious Diseases*. 29th ed. Elk Grove Village, IL: American Academy of Pediatrics; 2012.

Aronoff GR, Bennett WM, Berns JS, et al, *Drug Prescribing in Renal Failure: Dosing Guidelines for Adults and Children*, 5th ed, Philadelphia, PA: American College of Physiciansm, 2007.

Baddour LM, Wilson WR, Bayer AS, et al, "Infective Endocarditis: Diagnosis, Antimicrobial Therapy, and Management of Complications: A Statement for Healthcare Professionals From the Committee on Rheumatic Fever, Endocarditis, and Kawasaki Disease, Council on Cardiovascular Disease in the Young, and the Councils on Clinical Cardiology, Stroke, and Cardiovascular Surgery and Anesthesia, American Heart Association: Endorsed by the Infectious Diseases Society of America", *Circulation*, 2005, 111(23):e394-434.

Bradley JS, Byington CL, Shah SS, et al, "The Management of Community-Acquired Pneumonia in Infants and Children Older Than 3 Months of Age: Clinical Practice Guidelines by the Pediatric Infectious Diseases Society and the Infectious Diseases Society of America", *Clin Infect Dis*, 2011, 53(7):e25-76.

Bratzler DW, Dellinger EP, Olsen KM, et al, "Clinical Practice Guidelines for Antimicrobial Prophylaxis in Surgery," *Am J Health Syst Pharm*, 2013, 70(3):195-283.

Centers for Disease Control and Prevention (CDC), "Prevention of Perinatal Group B Streptococcal Disease-Revised Guidelines From CDC, 2010," *MMWR Recomm Rep*, 2010, 59(RR-10):1-36.

Engelman R, Shahian D, Shemin R, et al, "The Society of Thoracic Surgeons Practice Guideline Series: Antibiotic Prophylaxis in Cardiac Surgery, Part II: Antibiotic Choice," *Ann Thorac Surg*, 2007, 83 (4):1569-76.

Heintz BH, Matzke GR, Dager WE, et al, "Antimicrobial Dosing Concepts and Recommendations for Critically Ill Adult Patients Receiving Continuous Renal Replacement Therapy or Intermittent Hemodialysis," *Pharmacotherapy*, 2009, 29(5):562-77.

Pickering LK, O'Connor DM, Anderson D, et al, "Clinical and Pharmacologic Evaluation of Cefazolin in Children," *J Infect Dis* 1973, 128 (Suppl):S407-1.

Robinson DC, Cookson TL, and Grisafe JA, "Concentration Guidelines for Parenteral Antibiotics in Fluid-Restricted Patients," *Drug Intell Clin Pharm*, 1987, 21(12):985-9.

Sowinski KM, Mueller BA, Grabe DW, et al, "Cefazolin Dialytic Clearance by High-Efficiency and High-Flux Hemodialyzers," *Am J Kidney Dis*, 2001, 37(4):766-76.

Stevens DL, Bisno AL, Chambers HF, et al, "Practice Guidelines for the Diagnosis and Management of Skin and Soft-Tissue Infections," *Clin Infect Dis*, 2005, 41(10):1373-406.

Trotman RL, Williamson JC, Shoemaker DM, et al, "Antibiotic Dosing in Critically Ill Adult Patients Receiving Continuous Renal Replacement Therapy," *Clin Infect Dis*, 2005, 41(8):1159-66.

Warady BA, Bakkaloglu S, Newland J, et al, "Consensus Guidelines for the Prevention and Treatment of Catheter-Related Infections and Peritonitis in Pediatric Patients Receiving Peritoneal Dialysis: 2012 Update," *Perit Dial Int*, 2012, (32 Suppl 2):S32-86.

Wilson W, Taubert KA, Gewitz M, et al, "Prevention of Infective Endocarditis: Guidelines from the American Heart Association: A Guideline from the American Heart Association Rheumatic Fever, Endocarditis, and Kawasaki Disease Committee, Council on Cardiovascular Disease in the Young, and the Council on Clinical Cardiology, Council on Cardiovascular Surgery and Anesthesia, and the Quality of Care and Outcomes Research Interdisciplinary Working Group," *Circulation*, 2007, 116(15):1736-54.

◆ **Cefazolin For Injection (Can)** *see* CeFAZolin on page 393
on page 393

◆ **Cefazolin For Injection, USP (Can)** *see* CeFAZolin on page 393

◆ **Cefazolin Sodium** *see* CeFAZolin on page 393

Cefdinir (SEF di ner)

Therapeutic Category Antibiotic, Cephalosporin (Third Generation)

Generic Availability (U.S.) Yes

Use Treatment of susceptible acute bacterial otitis media (FDA approved in ages 6 months to 12 years); treatment of susceptible acute maxillary sinusitis, pharyngitis/tonsillitis, and uncomplicated skin and skin structure infections (FDA approved in ages ≥6 months and adults); treatment of susceptible acute exacerbations of chronic bronchitis and community-acquired pneumonia (FDA approved in adolescents and adults)

Pregnancy Risk Factor B

Pregnancy Considerations Teratogenic events have not been observed in animal reproduction studies. An increase in most types of birth defects was not found following first trimester exposure to cephalosporins.

Breast-Feeding Considerations Cefdinir is not detectable in breast milk following a single cefdinir 600 mg dose. If present in breast milk, nondose-related effects could include modification of bowel flora.

Contraindications Hypersensitivity to cefdinir, any component, or cephalosporins

Warnings Prolonged use may result in fungal or bacterial superinfection, including *C. difficile*-associated diarrhea (CDAD) and pseudomembranous colitis; CDAD has been observed >2 months postantibiotic treatment; use with caution in patients with a history of colitis. Serum sickness-like reactions have been reported with signs and symptoms occurring after a few days of therapy and resolving a few days after drug discontinuation. May cause hypersensitivity reaction; patients with history of hypersensitivity reactions to other cephalosporins or penicillins may experience cross-sensitivity; use with caution in patients with a history of penicillin allergy, especially IgE-mediated reactions (eg, anaphylaxis, angioedema, urticaria). If an allergic reaction occurs, discontinue cefdinir.

Precautions Use with caution in patients with impaired renal function (CrCl <30 mL/minute); dosage adjustment is recommended.

Adverse Reactions

Central nervous system: Headache

Dermatologic: Rash

Endocrine & metabolic: Bicarbonate decreased, hyperglycemia, hyperphosphatemia

Gastrointestinal: Abdominal pain, diarrhea, nausea, vomiting

Genitourinary: Urine leukocytes increased, urine pH increased, urine specific gravity increased, vaginal moniliasis, vaginitis

Hematologic: Eosinophils increased, lymphocytes decreased/increased, platelets increased, PMN changes, WBC decreased/increased

Hepatic: Alkaline phosphatase increased, ALT increased

Renal: Glycosuria, microhematuria, proteinuria

Miscellaneous: GGT increased, lactate dehydrogenase increased

Rare but important or life-threatening: Allergic vasculitis, amylase increased, anaphylaxis, anorexia, asthma, AST increased, bilirubin increased, bleeding tendency, bloody diarrhea, BUN increased, cardiac failure, chest pain, ►

cholestasis, coagulation disorder, conjunctivitis, constipation, cutaneous moniliasis, disseminated intravascular coagulation (DIC), dizziness, dyspepsia, enterocolitis (acute), eosinophilic pneumonia, erythema multiforme, erythema nodosum, exfoliative dermatitis, facial edema, fever, flatulence, fulminant hepatitis, granulocytopenia, hemoglobin decreased, hemolytic anemia, hemorrhagic colitis, hepatic failure, hepatitis (acute), hyperkalemia, hyperkinesia, hypertension, hypocalcemia, hypophosphatemia, idiopathic thrombocytopenia purpura, ileus, insomnia, interstitial pneumonia (idiopathic), involuntary movement, jaundice, laryngeal edema, leukopenia, leukorrhea, loss of consciousness, maculopapular rash, melena, moniliasis, monocytes increased, myocardial infarction, nephropathy, pancytopenia, peptic ulcer, pneumonia (drug-induced), pruritus, pseudomembranous colitis, renal failure (acute), respiratory failure (acute), rhabdomyolysis, serum sickness, shock, somnolence, Stevens-Johnson syndrome, stomatitis, stools abnormal, thrombocytopenia, toxic epidermal necrolysis, upper GI bleed, urine specific gravity decreased, weakness, xerostomia

Additional reactions reported with other cephalosporins: Agranulocytosis, angioedema, aplastic anemia, asterixis, encephalopathy, hemorrhage, interstitial nephritis, neuromuscular excitability, PT prolonged, seizure, superinfection, and toxic nephropathy

Drug Interactions

Metabolism/Transport Effects None known.

Avoid Concomitant Use

Avoid concomitant use of Cefdinir with any of the following: BCG

Increased Effect/Toxicity

Cefdinir may increase the levels/effects of: Aminoglycosides; Vitamin K Antagonists

The levels/effects of Cefdinir may be increased by: Probenecid

Decreased Effect

Cefdinir may decrease the levels/effects of: BCG; Sodium Picosulfate; Typhoid Vaccine

The levels/effects of Cefdinir may be decreased by: Iron Salts; Multivitamins/Minerals (with ADEK, Folate, Iron)

Stability Capsules, powder for suspension: Store at 20°C to 25°C (68°F to 77°F), excursions permitted to 15°C to 30°C (59°F to 86°F). Once reconstituted, store suspension at room temperature; stable for 10 days.

Mechanism of Action Inhibits bacterial cell wall synthesis by binding to one or more of the penicillin-binding proteins (PBPs) which in turn inhibits the final transpeptidation step of peptidoglycan synthesis in bacterial cell walls, thus inhibiting cell wall biosynthesis. Bacteria eventually lyse due to ongoing activity of cell wall autolytic enzymes (autolysins and murein hydrolases) while cell wall assembly is arrested.

Pharmacokinetics (Adult data unless noted)

Distribution: Penetrates into blister fluid, middle ear fluid, tonsils, sinus, and lung tissues

V_d:

Children 6 months to 12 years: 0.67 ± 0.38 L/kg

Adults: 0.35 ± 0.29 L/kg

Protein binding: 60% to 70%

Metabolism: Minimal

Bioavailability:

Capsules: 16% to 21%

Suspension: 25%

Half-life, elimination: 1.7 (± 0.6) hours with normal renal function

Time to peak serum concentration: 2-4 hours

Elimination: 11.6% to 18.4% of a dose is excreted unchanged in urine

Dialysis: ~63% is removed by hemodialysis (4 hours duration)

Dosing: Usual

Infants, Children, and Adolescents: Oral:

General dosing, susceptible infection (*Red Book*, 2012): Mild to moderate infections: 14 mg/kg/day in divided doses 1-2 times daily; maximum daily dose: 600 mg/**day**

Bronchitis, acute exacerbation: Adolescents: 300 mg every 12 hours for 5-10 days **or** 600 mg every 24 hours for 10 days

Otitis media, acute (AOM): Infants ≥6 months and Children: 14 mg/kg/day in divided doses every 12-24 hours for 5-10 days; maximum daily dose: 600 mg/**day. Note:** Recommended by the AAP as an alternative agent for initial treatment in penicillin allergic patients (Lieberthal, 2013).

Pharyngitis/Tonsillitis: Note: Although FDA approved at twice daily dosing, duration <10 days is not recommended (Shulman, 2012).

Infants ≥6 months and Children: 7 mg/kg/dose every 12 hours for 5-10 days **or** 14 mg/kg/dose every 24 hours for 10 days; maximum daily dose: 600 mg/**day**

Adolescents: 300 mg every 12 hours for 5-10 days **or** 600 mg every 24 hours for 10 days

Pneumonia, community-acquired: Adolescents: 300 mg every 12 hours for 10 days

Skin and skin structure infection, uncomplicated:

Infants ≥6 months and Children: 14 mg/kg/day in divided doses twice daily for 10 days; maximum daily dose: 600 mg/**day**

Adolescents: 300 mg every 12 hours for 10 days

Sinusitis, acute maxillary: Note: Due to decreased *S. pneumonia* sensitivity, cefdinir is no longer recommended as monotherapy for the initial empiric treatment of sinusitis (Chow, 2012)

Infants ≥6 months and Children: 14 mg/kg/day in divided doses every 12-24 hours for 10 days; maximum daily dose: 600 mg/**day**

Adolescents: 300 mg every 12 hours **or** 600 mg every 24 hours for 10 days

Adults: Oral:

Bronchitis, acute exacerbation: 300 mg every 12 hours for 5-10 days **or** 600 mg once daily for 10 days

Pharyngitis/tonsillitis: 300 mg every 12 hours for 5-10 days **or** 600 mg once daily for 10 days. **Note:** Although FDA approved at twice daily dosing, duration <10 days is not recommended (Shulman, 2012).

Pneumonia, community-acquired: 300 mg every 12 hours for 10 days

Sinusitis, acute maxillary: 300 mg every 12 hours **or** 600 mg once daily for 10 days. **Note:** Due to decreased *S. pneumonia* sensitivity, cefdinir is no longer recommended as monotherapy for the initial empiric treatment of sinusitis (Chow, 2012).

Skin and skin structure infection (uncomplicated): 300 mg every 12 hours for 10 days

Dosing adjustment in renal impairment:

Infants, Children, Adolescents, and Adults: CrCl ≥30 mL/minute: No adjustment required

Infants and Children ≥6 months to 12 years: CrCl <30 mL/minute/1.73 m²: 7 mg/kg/dose once daily; maximum daily dose: 300 mg/**day**

Adolescents and Adults: CrCl <30 mL/minute: 300 mg once daily

Hemodialysis: Infants, Children, Adolescents, and Adults: Initial dose: 7 mg/kg/dose (maximum dose: 300 mg) every other day. At the conclusion of each hemodialysis session, an additional dose (7 mg/kg/dose up to 300 mg) should be given. Subsequent doses should be administered every other day.

Dosing adjustment in hepatic impairment: No dosage adjustments are recommended.

Administration Oral: May administer with or without food; administer with food if stomach upset occurs; administer cefdinir at least 2 hours before or after antacids or iron supplements; shake suspension well before use

Monitoring Parameters Evaluate renal function before and during therapy; with prolonged therapy, monitor coagulation tests, CBC, liver function test periodically, and number and type of stools/day for diarrhea. Observe for signs and symptoms of anaphylaxis during first dose.

Test Interactions False-positive reaction for urinary ketones may occur with nitroprusside- but not nitroferricyanide-based tests. False-positive urine glucose results may occur when using Clinitest®, Benedict's solution, or Fehling's solution; glucose-oxidase-based reaction systems (eg, Clinistix®, Tes-Tape®) are recommended. May cause positive direct Coombs' test.

Additional Information Oral suspension contains 2.82-2.94 g of sucrose per 5 mL.

Dosage Forms Excipient information presented when available (limited, particularly for generics); consult specific product labeling.

Capsule, Oral:
 Generic: 300 mg
Suspension Reconstituted, Oral:
 Generic: 125 mg/5 mL (60 mL, 100 mL); 250 mg/5 mL (60 mL, 100 mL)

References

American Academy of Pediatrics (AAP). In: Pickering LK, Baker CJ, Kimberlin DW, Long SS, eds. *Red Book: 2012 Report of the Committee on Infectious Diseases.* 29th ed. Elk Grove Village, IL: American Academy of Pediatrics; 2012.

Bradley JS, Byington CL, Shah SS, et al, "The Management of Community-Acquired Pneumonia in Infants and Children Older Than 3 Months of Age: Clinical Practice Guidelines by the Pediatric Infectious Diseases Society and the Infectious Diseases Society of America", *Clin Infect Dis,* 2011, 53(7):e25-76.

Chow AW, Benninger MS, Brook I, et al, "IDSA Clinical Practice Guideline for Acute Bacterial Rhinosinusitis in Children and Adults," *Clin Infect Dis,* 2012, 54(8):e72-e112.

Klein JO and McCracken GH Jr, "Summary: Role of a New Oral Cephalosporin, Cefdinir, for Therapy of Infections of Infants and Children," *Pediatr Infect Dis J,* 2000, 19(12 Suppl):S181-3.

Lieberthal AS, Carroll AE, Chonmaitree T, et al, "The Diagnosis and Management of Acute Otitis Media," *Pediatrics,* 2013, 131(3):e964-99.

Perry CM and Scott LJ, "Cefdinir: A Review of Its Use in the Management of Mild-to-Moderate Bacterial Infections," *Drugs,* 2004, 64 (13):1433-64.

Shulman ST, Bisno AL, Clegg HW, et al, "Clinical Practice Guideline for the Diagnosis and Management of Group A Streptococcal Pharyngitis: 2012 Update by the Infectious Diseases Society of America," *Clin Infect Dis,* 2012. Available at http://aapredbook.aappublications.org/cgi/content/full

Cefditoren (sef de TOR en)

Medication Safety Issues

International issues:
 Spectracef [U.S., Great Britain, Mexico, Portugal, Spain] may be confused with Spectrocef brand name for cefotaxime [Italy]

Brand Names: U.S. Spectracef

Therapeutic Category Antibiotic, Cephalosporin

Generic Availability (U.S.) Yes

Use Treatment of mild to moderate infections caused by susceptible bacteria including acute bacterial exacerbation of chronic bronchitis, community-acquired pneumonia, pharyngitis or tonsillitis, and uncomplicated skin and skin-structure infections (FDA approved in ages ≥12 years and adults)

Pregnancy Risk Factor B

Pregnancy Considerations Adverse events have not been observed in animal reproduction studies. An increase in most types of birth defects was not found following first trimester exposure to cephalosporins.

Breast-Feeding Considerations It is not known whether cefditoren is excreted in human milk. The manufacturer recommends caution when using cefditoren during breast-feeding. If cefditoren reaches the breast milk, the limited oral absorption may minimize the effect on the nursing infant. Nondose-related effects could include modification of bowel flora.

Contraindications Hypersensitivity to cefditoren, any component, other cephalosporins, milk protein; carnitine deficiency or inborn errors of metabolism that may result in clinically significant carnitine deficiency

Warnings May cause hypersensitivity reaction; patients with history of hypersensitivity reactions to other cephalosporins or penicillins may experience cross-sensitivity; use is contraindicated in patients with a history of cephalosporin allergy; use with caution in patients with a history of penicillin allergy, especially IgE-mediated reactions (eg, anaphylaxis, angioedema, urticaria). If an allergic reaction occurs, discontinue cefditoren. Tablets contain sodium caseinate which may cause hypersensitivity reactions in patients with milk protein hypersensitivity; use in patients with milk protein allergy is contraindicated; this does not affect patients with lactose intolerance.

Carnitine deficiency may result from prolonged use; cefditoren causes renal excretion of carnitine; plasma carnitine concentrations usually return to normal range within 7 to 10 days after discontinuation of therapy; contraindicated in patients with carnitine deficiency or inborn errors of metabolism that may result in clinically significant carnitine deficiency. May be associated with increased INR, especially in nutritionally deficient patients, prolonged treatment, hepatic or renal disease. Prolonged use may result in fungal or bacterial superinfection, including *C. difficile*-associated diarrhea (CDAD) and pseudomembranous colitis; CDAD has been observed >2 months postantibiotic treatment; use with caution in patients with a history of colitis.

Precautions Use with caution in patients with renal impairment; dosage adjustment may be needed for moderate to severe renal impairment. Use with caution in patients with severe hepatic impairment; use has not been studied. In patients with mild to moderate hepatic impairment, only slight changes in the AUC were observed. Use with caution in patients with a history of seizure disorder; high serum concentrations, particularly in the presence of renal impairment, may increase risk of seizures.

Adverse Reactions
Central nervous system: Headache
Endocrine & metabolic: Glucose increased
Gastrointestinal: Abdominal pain, diarrhea, dyspepsia, nausea, vomiting
Genitourinary: Vaginal moniliasis
Hematologic: Hematocrit decreased
Renal: Hematuria, urinary white blood cells increased
Rare but important or life-threatening: Acute renal failure, albumin decreased, allergic reaction, arthralgia, asthma, BUN increased, calcium decreased, coagulation time increased, eosinophilic pneumonia, erythema multiforme, fungal infection, hyperglycemia, interstitial pneumonia, leukopenia, leukorrhea, positive direct Coombs' test, potassium increased, pseudomembranous colitis, rash, sodium decreased, Stevens-Johnson syndrome, thrombocythemia, thrombocytopenia, toxic epidermal necrolysis, white blood cells increased/decreased
Reactions reported with other cephalosporins: Anaphylaxis, aplastic anemia, cholestasis, hemorrhage, hemolytic anemia, renal dysfunction, reversible hyperactivity, serum sickness-like reaction, toxic nephropathy

Drug Interactions

Metabolism/Transport Effects None known.

Avoid Concomitant Use There are no known interactions where it is recommended to avoid concomitant use. ▸

Increased Effect/Toxicity Increased levels of cefditoren with probenecid.

Decreased Effect Antacids and H_2 receptor antagonists decrease cefditoren levels.

Food Interactions Moderate- to high-fat meals increase bioavailability and maximum plasma concentration. Management: Take with meals. Maintain adequate hydration, unless instructed to restrict fluid intake.

Stability Store at 25°C (77°F); excursions permitted to 15°C to 30°C (59°F to 86°F); protect from light and moisture.

Mechanism of Action Inhibits bacterial cell wall synthesis by binding to one or more of the penicillin-binding proteins (PBPs) which in turn inhibits the final transpeptidation step of peptidoglycan synthesis in bacterial cell walls, thus inhibiting cell wall biosynthesis. Bacteria eventually lyse due to ongoing activity of cell wall autolytic enzymes (autolysins and murein hydrolases) while cell wall assembly is arrested.

Pharmacokinetics (Adult data unless noted)
Distribution: V_d: 9.3 ± 1.6 L
Protein binding: 88% (in vitro), primarily to albumin
Metabolism: Cefditoren pivoxil is hydrolyzed by esterases to cefditoren (active) and pivalate; cefditoren is not appreciable metabolized
Bioavailability: ~14% to 16%, increased by moderate to high-fat meal (mean AUC by 70%; maximum plasma concentration by 50%)
Half-life elimination: 1.6 ± 0.4 hours; increased with moderate (2.7 hours) and severe (4.7 hours) renal impairment
Time to peak serum concentration: 1.5 to 3 hours
Elimination: Urine (as cefditoren and pivaloylcarnitine)

Dosing: Usual
Pediatric:
General dosing, susceptible infection; mild to moderate infection: Children ≥12 years and Adolescents: Oral: 200 to 400 mg twice daily (Red Book [AAP, 2012])
Bronchitis, chronic; acute bacterial exacerbation: Children ≥12 years and Adolescents: Oral: 400 mg twice daily for 10 days
Pneumonia, community-acquired: Children ≥12 years and Adolescents: Oral: 400 mg twice daily for 14 days
Pharyngitis, tonsillitis:
Manufacturer's labeling: Children ≥12 years and Adolescents: Oral: 200 mg twice daily for 10 days
Alternate dosing: Infants ≥8 months and Children: Limited data available: Oral: 3 mg/kg/dose 3 times daily for 5 days; dosing based on a prospective study comparing 5 days of cefditoren (n=103, age range: 0.7 to 12.4 years) to 10 days of amoxicillin (n=155); efficacy and tolerability were similar for both groups; cefditoren was administered as a granule formulation that is not available in the U.S. (Ozaki, 2008)
Skin and skin structure infections, uncomplicated: Children ≥12 years and Adolescents: Oral: 200 mg twice daily for 10 days
Adult:
Bronchitis, chronic; acute bacterial exacerbation: Oral: 400 mg twice daily for 10 days
Pneumonia, community-acquired: Oral: 400 mg twice daily for 14 days
Pharyngitis, tonsillitis: Oral: 200 mg twice daily for 10 days
Skin and skin structure infections, uncomplicated: Oral: 200 mg twice daily for 10 days
Dosing adjustment in renal impairment: Children ≥12 years, Adolescents, and Adults:
CrCl ≥50 mL/minute/1.73 m²: No dosage adjustment necessary
CrCl 30-49 mL/minute/1.73 m²: Maximum dose: 200 mg twice daily
CrCl <30 mL/minute/1.73 m²: Maximum dose: 200 mg once daily

End stage renal disease: Appropriate dose has not been determined
Dosing adjustment in hepatic impairment: Children ≥12 years, Adolescents, and Adults:
Mild to moderate impairment (Child-Pugh Class A or B): No dosage adjustment necessary.
Severe impairment (Child-Pugh Class C): There are no dosage adjustment guidelines provided in the manufacturer's labeling (not studied).

Administration Oral: Administer with meals.

Monitoring Parameters Assess patient at beginning and throughout therapy for infection; observe for changes in bowel frequency, monitor for signs of anaphylaxis during first dose

Test Interactions May induce a positive direct Coomb's test. May cause a false-negative ferricyanide test. Glucose oxidase or hexokinase methods recommended for blood/plasma glucose determinations. False-positive urine glucose test when using copper reduction based assays (eg, Clinitest®).

Dosage Forms Excipient information presented when available (limited, particularly for generics); consult specific product labeling.
Tablet, Oral:
Spectracef: 200 mg, 400 mg [contains sodium caseinate]
Generic: 200 mg, 400 mg

References

American Academy of Pediatrics (AAP). In: Pickering LK, Baker CJ, Kimberlin DW, Long SS, eds. Red Book: 2012 Report of the Committee on Infectious Diseases. 29th ed. Elk Grove Village, IL: American Academy of Pediatrics; 2012.

Ozaki T, Nishimura N, Suzuki M, et.al. Five-day oral cefditoren pivoxil versus 10-day oral amoxicillin for pediatric group A streptococcal pharyngotonsillitis. J Infect Chemother. 2008;14:213-218.

Spectracef (cefditoren) [prescribing information]. Cary, NC: Cornerstone therapeutics Inc; 2001.

◆ **Cefditoren Pivoxil** see Cefditoren on page 397

Cefepime (SEF e pim)

Medication Safety Issues
Sound-alike/look-alike issues:
Cefepime may be confused with cefixime, cefTAZidime
Brand Names: U.S. Maxipime
Brand Names: Canada Maxipime
Therapeutic Category Antibiotic, Cephalosporin (Fourth Generation)
Generic Availability (U.S.) Yes
Use Treatment of pneumonia, uncomplicated skin and soft tissue infections, and complicated and uncomplicated urinary tract infections (including pyelonephritis) caused by susceptible organisms, and as empiric therapy for febrile neutropenic patients (FDA approved in ages ≥2 months and adults); used in combination with metronidazole for complicated intra-abdominal infections (FDA approved in adults). Cefepime is a fourth generation cephalosporin with activity against gram-negative bacteria, including Pseudomonas aeruginosa, E. coli, H. influenzae, M. catarrhalis, M morganii, P. mirabilis, and strains of Acinetobacter, Citrobacter, Enterobacter, Klebsiella, Providencia, and Serratia; active against gram-positive bacteria, such as Staphylococcus aureus, S. pyogenes, and S. pneumoniae
Pregnancy Risk Factor B
Pregnancy Considerations Adverse events were not observed in animal reproduction studies. Cefepime crosses the placenta.
Breast-Feeding Considerations Small amounts of cefepime are excreted in breast milk. The manufacturer recommends that caution be exercised when administering cefepime to nursing women. Nondose-related effects could include modification of bowel flora.

Contraindications Hypersensitivity to cefepime, any component, or other cephalosporins, penicillins, or beta-lactam antibiotics

Warnings Severe neurological reactions (some fatal) have been reported, including encephalopathy, myoclonus, seizures, and nonconvulsive status epilepticus; risk may be increased with high serum concentrations in the presence of renal impairment; adjust dose for renal dysfunction (CrCl ≤60 mL/minute); discontinue therapy if patient develops neurotoxicity; effects are often reversible upon discontinuation of cefepime. Use with caution in patients with a history of seizure disorders and in patients with renal impairment.

Prolonged use may result in fungal or bacterial superinfection, including *C. difficile*-associated diarrhea (CDAD) and pseudomembranous colitis; CDAD has been observed >2 months postantibiotic treatment; use with caution in patients with a history of colitis. May cause hypersensitivity reaction; patients with history of hypersensitivity reactions to other cephalosporins or penicillins may experience cross-sensitivity; use of cefepime in these patients is contraindicated.

Precautions The manufacturer does not recommend the use of cefepime in pediatric patients for the treatment of serious infections due to *Haemophilus influenzae* type b, for suspected meningitis, or for meningeal seeding from a distant infection site. However, limited data suggest that cefepime may be a valuable alternative for treating bacterial meningitis in children in conjunction with other agents like vancomycin in areas with a high incidence of cephalosporin nonsusceptible pneumococci (Haase, 2004). Use with caution in patients previously stabilized on anticoagulant therapy; may cause alteration in prothrombin activity; risk increased in renal or hepatic impairment, poor nutritional state, or prolonged course of therapy; monitor prothrombin times as necessary.

Adverse Reactions

Cardiovascular: Localized phlebitis

Central nervous system: Headache

Dermatologic: Pruritus, skin rash

Endocrine & metabolic: Hypophosphatemia

Gastrointestinal: Diarrhea, nausea, vomiting

Hematologic & oncologic: Eosinophilia, positive direct Coombs test (without hemolysis)

Hepatic: Abnormal partial thromboplastin time, abnormal prothrombin time, increased serum ALT, increased serum AST

Local: Local pain

Miscellaneous: Fever

Rare but important or life-threatening: Agranulocytosis, anaphylactic shock, anaphylaxis, brain disease, colitis, coma, confusion, decreased hematocrit, hallucination, hypercalcemia, hyperkalemia, hyperphosphatemia, hypocalcemia, increased blood urea nitrogen, increased serum alkaline phosphatase, increased serum bilirubin, increased serum creatinine, leukopenia, neutropenia, oral candidiasis, pseudomembranous colitis, seizure, status epilepticus (nonconvulsive), stupor, thrombocytopenia, urticaria, vaginitis

Drug Interactions

Metabolism/Transport Effects None known.

Avoid Concomitant Use

Avoid concomitant use of Cefepime with any of the following: BCG

Increased Effect/Toxicity

Cefepime may increase the levels/effects of: Aminoglycosides; Vitamin K Antagonists

The levels/effects of Cefepime may be increased by: Probenecid

Decreased Effect

Cefepime may decrease the levels/effects of: BCG; Sodium Picosulfate; Typhoid Vaccine

Stability

Vials: Store intact vial at 20°C to 25°C (68°F to 77°F); protect from light. Cefepime diluted with NS, D_5W, $D_{10}W$, and D_5NS is stable for 24 hours at 20°C to 25°C (68°F to 77°F) or for 7 days at 2°C to 8°C (36°F to 46°F).

Premixed solution: Store frozen at -20°C (-4°F). Thawed solution is stable for 24 hours at room temperature or 7 days under refrigeration; do not refreeze.

Mechanism of Action Inhibits bacterial cell wall synthesis by binding to one or more of the penicillin-binding proteins (PBPs) which in turn inhibits the final transpeptidation step of peptidoglycan synthesis in bacterial cell walls, thus inhibiting cell wall biosynthesis. Bacteria eventually lyse due to ongoing activity of cell wall autolytic enzymes (autolysis and murein hydrolases) while cell wall assembly is arrested.

Pharmacokinetics (Adult data unless noted)

Absorption: I.M.: Rapid and complete

Distribution: V_d:

Neonates (Capparelli, 2005):

PMA <30 weeks: 0.51 L/kg

PMA >30 weeks: 0.39 L/kg

Infants and Children 2 months to 11 years: 0.3 L/kg

Adults: 18 L, 0.26 L/kg; penetrates into inflammatory fluid at concentrations ~80% of serum concentrations and into bronchial mucosa at concentrations ~60% of plasma concentrations; crosses the blood-brain barrier

Protein binding: ~20%

Metabolism: Very little

Half-life:

Neonates: 4-5 hours (Lima-Rogel, 2008)

Children 2 months to 6 years: 1.77-1.96 hours

Adults: 2 hours

Hemodialysis: 13.5 hours

Continuous peritoneal dialysis: 19 hours

Elimination: At least 85% eliminated as unchanged drug in urine

Dosing: Neonatal

General dosing, susceptible infection (*Red Book*, 2012): I.M., I.V.: 30 mg/kg/dose every 12 hours

Meningitis: I.V.:

Body weight <1 kg:

PNA 0-14 days: 50 mg/kg/dose every 12 hours

PNA ≥14 days: 50 mg/kg/dose every 8 hours

Body weight 1-2 kg:

PNA 0-7 days: 50 mg/kg/dose every 12 hours

PNA ≥8 days: 50 mg/kg/dose every 8 hours

Body weight >2 kg: 50 mg/kg/dose every 8 hours

Pseudomonal infection: I.M., I.V.:

Body weight <1 kg:

PNA 0-14 days: 50 mg/kg/dose every 12 hours

PNA ≥14 days: 50 mg/kg/dose every 8 hours

Body weight 1-2 kg:

PNA 0-7 days: 50 mg/kg/dose every 12 hours

PNA ≥8 days: 50 mg/kg/dose every 8 hours

Body weight >2 kg: 50 mg/kg/dose every 8 hours

Dosing: Usual

Infants, Children, and Adolescents:

General dosing, susceptible infection (*Red Book*, 2012): I.M., I.V.:

Mild to moderate infection: 50 mg/kg/dose every 12 hours; maximum single dose: 2000 mg

Severe infection: 50 mg/kg/dose every 8-12 hours; maximum single dose: 2000 mg

Cystic fibrosis, acute pulmonary exacerbation: I.V: 50 mg/kg/dose every 8 hours; maximum dose: 2000 mg; patients with more resistant pseudomonal isolates (MIC ≥16 mg/L) may require 50 mg/kg/dose every 6 hours (Zobell, 2013)

Endocarditis, prosthetic valve, treatment within 1 year of replacement: I.V.: 50 mg/kg/dose every 8 hours in combination with vancomycin and rifampin for 6 weeks plus gentamicin for the first 2 weeks; maximum single dose: 2000 mg (Baddour, 2005)

Febrile neutropenia, empiric therapy: I.V.: 50 mg/kg/dose every 8 hours; maximum single dose: 2000 mg (*Red Book*, 2012); duration of therapy dependent upon febrile neutropenia risk-status; in high-risk patients, may discontinue empiric antibiotics if all of the following criteria met: Negative blood cultures at 48 hours; afebrile for at least 24 hours, and evidence of marrow recovery. In low-risk patients, may discontinue empiric antibiotics after 72 hours duration in patients with a negative blood culture and who have been afebrile for 24 hours regardless of marrow recovery status; follow-up closely (Lehrnbecher, 2012).

Intra-abdominal infection, complicated: I.V.: 50 mg/kg/dose every 12 hours in combination with metronidazole; maximum single dose: 2000 mg (Solomkin, 2010)

Meningitis: I.V.: 50 mg/kg/dose every 8 hours; maximum single dose: 2000 mg (Tunkel, 2004)

Pneumonia, moderate to severe: Infants ≥2 months, Children, and Adolescents: I.V.: 50 mg/kg/dose every 12 hours for 10 days; maximum single dose: 2000 mg

Skin and skin structure infections, uncomplicated: Infants ≥2 months, Children, and Adolescents: I.V.: 50 mg/kg/dose every 12 hours for 10 days; maximum single dose: 2000 mg

Urinary tract infection, complicated and uncomplicated: Infants ≥2 months, Children, and Adolescents: I.M., I.V.: 50 mg/kg/dose every 12 hours for 7-10 days; maximum single dose: 2000 mg; duration based on severity of infection: Mild to moderate: 7-10 days; severe/pyelonephritis: 10 days; **Note:** I.M. may be considered for mild to moderate infection only.

Adults:

Febrile neutropenia, monotherapy: I.V: 2000 mg every 8 hours for 7 days or until the neutropenia resolves

Intra-abdominal infections, complicated, severe (in combination with metronidazole): I.V.: 2000 mg every 12 hours for 7-10 days. **Note:** 2010 IDSA guidelines recommend 2000 mg every 8-12 hours for 4-7 days (provided source controlled). Not recommended for hospital-acquired intra-abdominal infections (IAI) associated with multidrug-resistant gram-negative organisms or in mild to moderate community-acquired IAIs due to risk of toxicity and the development of resistant organisms (Solomkin [IDSA], 2010).

Pneumonia: I.V.:

Nosocomial (HAP/VAP): 1000-2000 mg every 8-12 hours; **Note:** Duration of therapy may vary considerably (7-21 days); usually longer courses are required if *Pseudomonas*. In absence of *Pseudomonas*, and if appropriate empiric treatment used and patient responsive, it may be clinically appropriate to reduce duration of therapy to 7-10 days (American Thoracic Society Guidelines, 2005).

Community-acquired (including pseudomonal): 1000-2000 mg every 12 hours for 10 days

Skin and skin structure infections, uncomplicated: I.V.: 2000 mg every 12 hours for 10 days

Urinary tract infections, complicated and uncomplicated:

Mild to moderate: I.M., I.V.: 500-1000 mg every 12 hours for 7-10 days

Severe: I.V.: 2000 mg every 12 hours for 10 days

Dosing adjustment in renal impairment:

Infants, Children, and Adolescents:

Manufacturer's labeling: Infants ≥2 months, Children, and Adolescents: There are no dosage adjustments provided in the manufacturer's labeling; however,

similar dosage adjustments to adults would be anticipated based on comparable pharmacokinetics between children and adults.

Alternative dosing recommendations (Aronoff, 2007): **Note:** Renally adjusted dose recommendations are based on doses of 50 mg/kg/dose every 8-12 hours.

GFR >50 mL/minute/1.73 m^2: No adjustment needed

GFR 10-50 mL/minute/1.73 m^2: 50 mg/kg/dose every 24 hours

GFR <10 mL/minute/1.73 m^2: 50 mg/kg/dose every 48 hours

Intermittent hemodialysis: 50 mg/kg/dose every 24 hours

Peritoneal dialysis (PD): 50 mg/kg/dose every 24 hours

Continuous renal replacement therapy (CRRT): 50 mg/kg/dose every 12 hours

Adults: Recommended maintenance schedule based on creatinine clearance (may be estimated using the Cockcroft-Gault formula), compared to normal dosing schedule: See table.

Cefepime Hydrochloride

Creatinine Clearance (mL/minute)	Recommended Maintenance Schedule			
>60 (normal recommended dosing schedule)	500 mg every 12 hours	1000 mg every 12 hours	2000 mg every 12 hours	2000 mg every 8 hours
30-60	500 mg every 24 hours	1000 mg every 24 hours	2000 mg every 24 hours	2000 mg every 12 hours
11-29	500 mg every 24 hours	500 mg every 24 hours	1000 mg every 24 hours	2000 mg every 24 hours
<11	250 mg every 24 hours	250 mg every 24 hours	500 mg every 24 hours	1000 mg every 24 hours

Continuous ambulatory peritoneal dialysis (CAPD): Removed to a lesser extent than hemodialysis; administer normal recommended dose every 48 hours

Hemodialysis: 68% removed by hemodialysis: Initial: 1000 mg (single dose) on day 1. Maintenance: 500 mg once daily (1000 mg once daily in febrile neutropenic patients)

Continuous renal replacement therapy (CRRT) (Heintz, 2009; Trotman, 2005): Drug clearance is highly dependent on the method of renal replacement, filter type, and flow rate. Appropriate dosing requires close monitoring of pharmacologic response, signs of adverse reactions due to drug accumulation, as well as drug concentrations in relation to target trough (if appropriate). The following are general recommendations only (based on dialysate flow/ultrafiltration rates of 1-2 L/hour and minimal residual renal function) and should not supersede clinical judgment:

CVVH: Loading dose of 2000 mg followed by 1000-2000 mg every 12 hours

CVVHD/CVVHDF: Loading dose of 2000 mg followed by either 1000 mg every 8 hours **or** 2000 g every 12 hours. **Note:** Dosage of 1000 mg every 8 hours results in similar steady-state concentrations as 2000 mg every 12 hours and is more cost-effective (Heintz, 2009).

Note: Consider higher dosage of 4000 mg/day if treating *Pseudomonas* or life-threatening infections in order to maximize time above MIC (Trotman, 2005). Dosage of 2000 mg every 8 hours may be needed for gram-negative rods with MIC ≥4 mg/L (Heintz, 2009).

Dosing adjustment in hepatic impairment: No dosage adjustments are recommended.

Administration Parenteral:

I.V.: May dilute dose in D₅W, NS, D₁₀W, D₅NS, or D₅LR; final concentration should not exceed 40 mg/mL; administer as an intermittent I.V. infusion over 20-30 minutes; in adult clinical trials, cefepime has been administered by direct I.V. injection over 3-5 minutes at final concentrations of 40 mg/mL (Garretts, 1999) and 100 mg/mL (Jaruratanasirikul, 2002; Lipman, 1999) for severe infections

I.M.: May dilute vial using SWI, NS, D₅W, or 0.5% or 1% lidocaine to a final concentration of 280 mg/mL; administer by deep I.M. injection into large muscle mass

Monitoring Parameters With prolonged therapy, monitor renal and hepatic function periodically; number and type of stools/day for diarrhea; CBC with differential. Observe for signs and symptoms of anaphylaxis during first dose.

Test Interactions Positive direct Coombs', false-positive urinary glucose test using cupric sulfate (Benedict's solution, Clinitest®, Fehling's solution), false-positive serum or urine creatinine with Jaffé reaction, false-positive urinary proteins and steroids

Dosage Forms Excipient information presented when available (limited, particularly for generics); consult specific product labeling.

Solution, Intravenous, as hydrochloride:
Generic: 1 g/50 mL (50 mL); 2% (100 mL)
Solution Reconstituted, Injection, as hydrochloride:
Maxipime: 1 g (1 ea); 2 g (1 ea)
Generic: 1 g (1 ea); 2 g (1 ea)
Solution Reconstituted, Intravenous, as hydrochloride:
Maxipime: 1 g (1 ea); 2 g (1 ea)
Generic: 1 g/50 mL (1 ea); 2 g/50 mL (1 ea)

References

American Academy of Pediatrics (AAP). In: Pickering LK, Baker CJ, Kimberlin DW, Long SS, eds. *Red Book: 2012 Report of the Committee on Infectious Diseases.* 29th ed. Elk Grove Village, IL: American Academy of Pediatrics; 2012.

American Thoracic Society and Infectious Diseases Society of America, "Guidelines for the Management of Adults With Hospital-Acquired, Ventilator-Associated, and Healthcare-Associated Pneumonia," *Am J Respir Crit Care Med,* 2005, 171(4):388-416.

Arguedas AG, Stutman HR, Zaleska M, et al, "Cefepime. Pharmacokinetics and Clinical Response in Patients With Cystic Fibrosis," *Am J Dis Child,* 1992, 146(7):797-802.

Capparelli E, Hochwald C, Rasmussen M, et al, "Population Pharmacokinetics of Cefepime in the Neonate," *Antimicrob Agents Chemother,* 2005, 49(7):2760-6.

Garretts JC and Wagner DJ, "The Pharmacokinetics, Safety, and Tolerance of Cefepime Administered as an Intravenous Bolus or as a Rapid Infusion," *Ann Pharmacother,* 1999, 33(12):1258-61.

Haase MR, "Acute Bacterial Meningitis in Children," *J Pharm Pract,* 2004, 17:392.

Heintz BH, Matzke GR, and Dager WE, "Antimicrobial Dosing Concepts and Recommendations for Critically Ill Adult Patients Receiving Continuous Renal Replacement Therapy or Intermittent Hemodialysis," *Pharmacotherapy,* 2009, 29(5):562-77.

Jaruratanasirikul S, Sriwiriyajan S, and Ingviya N, "Continuous Infusion Versus Intermittent Administration of Cefepime in Patients With Gram-Negative Bacilli Bacteraemia," *J Pharm Pharmacol,* 2002, 54 (12):1693-6.

Lehrnbecher T, Phillips R, Alexander S, et al, "Guideline for the Management of Fever and Neutropenia in Children With Cancer and/or Undergoing Hematopoietic Stem-Cell Transplantation," *J Clin Oncol,* 2012, 30(35):4427-38.

Lima-Rogel V, Medina-Rojas EL, Del Carmen Milán-Segovia R, et al, "Population Pharmacokinetics of Cefepime in Neonates With Severe Nosocomial Infections," *J Clin Pharm Ther,* 2008, 33(3):295-306.

Lipman J, Wallis SC, and Rickard C, "Low Plasma Cefepime Levels in Critically Ill Septic Patients: Pharmacokinetic Modeling Indicates Improved Troughs With Revised Dosing," *Antimicrob Agents Chemother,* 1999, 43(10):2559-61.

Solomkin JS, Mazuski JE, Bradley JS, et al, "Diagnosis and Management of Complicated Intra-Abdominal Infections in Adults and Children: Guidelines by the Surgical Infection Society and the Infectious Diseases Society of America," *Clin Infect Dis,* 2010, 50(2):133-64.

Trotman RL, Williamson JC, Shoemaker DM, et al, "Antibiotic Dosing in Critically Ill Adult Patients Receiving Continuous Renal Replacement Therapy," *Clin Infect Dis,* 2005, 41(8):1159-66.

Tunkel AR, Hartman BJ, Kaplan SL, et al, "Practice Guidelines for the Management of Bacterial Meningitis," *Clin Infect Dis,* 2004, 39 (9):1267-84.

Wynd MA and Paladino JA, "Cefepime: A Fourth-Generation Parenteral Cephalosporin," *Ann Pharmacother,* 1996, 30(12):1414-24.

Zobell JT, Waters CD, Young DC, et al, "Optimization of Anti-Pseudomonal Antibiotics for Cystic Fibrosis Pulmonary Exacerbations: II. Cephalosporins and Penicillins," *Pediatr Pulmonol,* 2013, 48 (2):107-22.

◆ **Cefepime Hydrochloride** *see* Cefepime *on page 398*

Cefixime (sef IKS eem)

Medication Safety Issues
Sound-alike/look-alike issues:
Cefixime may be confused with cefepime
Suprax® may be confused with Sporanox®
International issues:
Cefiton: Brand name for cefixime [Portugal] may be confused with Ceftim brand name for ceftazidime [Portugal]; Ceftime brand name for ceftazidime [Thailand]; Ceftin brand name for cefuroxime [U.S., Canada]

Brand Names: U.S. Suprax

Brand Names: Canada Suprax®

Therapeutic Category Antibiotic, Cephalosporin (Third Generation)

Generic Availability (U.S.) No

Use Treatment of urinary tract infections, otitis media, acute exacerbations of chronic bronchitis due to susceptible organisms which may include *S. pneumoniae* and *pyogenes, H. influenzae, M. catarrhalis, E. coli,* and *P mirabilis*; treatment of pharyngitis and tonsillitis due to *S. pyogenes*; treatment of uncomplicated cervical/urethral gonorrhea due to *N. gonorrhoeae* (All indications: FDA approved in ages ≥6 months and adults); has also been used for management of irinotecan-associated diarrhea, prophylaxis for sexual victimization, and management of low risk febrile neutropenia

Pregnancy Risk Factor B

Pregnancy Considerations Teratogenic effects were not observed in animal reproduction studies. Cefixime crosses the placenta and can be detected in the amniotic fluid. An increase in most types of birth defects was not found following first trimester exposure to cephalosporins. Cefixime may be used for the treatment of gonococcal infections in pregnant women in certain situations (refer to current guidelines).

Breast-Feeding Considerations It is not known if cefixime is excreted in breast milk. The manufacturer recommends that consideration be given to discontinuing nursing temporarily during treatment. If present in breast milk, nondose-related effects could include modification of bowel flora.

Contraindications Hypersensitivity to cefixime, any component, or cephalosporins

Warnings Prolonged use may result in fungal or bacterial superinfection, including *C. difficile*-associated diarrhea (CDAD) and pseudomembranous colitis; CDAD has been observed >2 months postantibiotic treatment; use with caution in patients with a history of colitis. May cause hypersensitivity reaction; patients with history of hypersensitivity reactions to other cephalosporins or pencillins may experience cross-sensitivity; use with caution in patients with a history of penicillin allergy, especially IgE-mediated reactions (eg, anaphylaxis, angioedema, urticaria).

Suspension contains sodium benzoate; benzoic acid (benzoate) is a metabolite of benzyl alcohol; large amounts of benzyl alcohol (≥99 mg/kg/day) have been associated with a potentially fatal toxicity ("gasping syndrome") in neonates; the "gasping syndrome" consists of metabolic acidosis, respiratory distress, gasping respirations, CNS dysfunction (including convulsions, intracranial hemorrhage), hypotension and cardiovascular collapse; use suspension containing sodium benzoate with caution in ▶

neonates; *in vitro* and animal studies have shown that benzoate displaces bilirubin from protein binding sites

Precautions Use with caution in patients with impaired renal function; dosage adjustment required. Use with caution in patients previously stabilized on anticoagulant therapy; may cause alteration in prothrombin activity; risk increased in renal or hepatic impairment, poor nutritional state or prolonged course of therapy; monitor prothrombin times as necessary. May cause diarrhea; reported incidence (~16%) similar in children receiving oral suspension and adults receiving tablet dosage form. Use caution when interchanging product formulations; oral suspension and chewable tablets are bioequivalent but oral immediate release tablets are not bioequivalent; for some infections (eg, otitis media), dosing recommendations are product specific. Chewable tablets contain aspartame which is metabolized to phenylalanine; use with caution in phenylketonuric patients.

Adverse Reactions

Gastrointestinal: Abdominal pain, diarrhea, dyspepsia, flatulence, loose stools, nausea

Rare but important or life-threatening: Acute renal failure, anaphylactic/anaphylactoid reactions, angioedema, BUN increased, candidiasis, creatinine increased, dizziness, drug fever, eosinophilia, erythema multiforme, facial edema, fever, headache, hepatitis, hyperbilirubinemia, jaundice, leukopenia, neutropenia, pruritus, pseudomembranous colitis, PT prolonged, rash, seizure, serum sickness-like reaction, Stevens-Johnson syndrome, thrombocytopenia, toxic epidermal necrolysis, transaminases increased, urticaria, vaginitis, vomiting

Reactions reported with other cephalosporins: Agranulocytosis, aplastic anemia, colitis, hemolytic anemia, hemorrhage, interstitial nephritis, pancytopenia, superinfection

Drug Interactions

Metabolism/Transport Effects None known.

Avoid Concomitant Use

Avoid concomitant use of Cefixime with any of the following: BCG

Increased Effect/Toxicity

Cefixime may increase the levels/effects of: Aminoglycosides; Vitamin K Antagonists

The levels/effects of Cefixime may be increased by: Probenecid

Decreased Effect

Cefixime may decrease the levels/effects of: BCG; Sodium Picosulfate; Typhoid Vaccine

Food Interactions Food delays cefixime absorption. Management: May administer with or without food.

Stability Oral:

Capsule, chewable tablet, tablet: Store at 20°C to 25°C (68°F to 77°F).

Suspension: Store at 20°C to 25°C (68°F to 77°F). After reconstitution, oral suspension may be stored for 14 days at room temperature or under refrigeration; keep tightly closed.

Mechanism of Action Inhibits bacterial cell wall synthesis by binding to one or more of the penicillin-binding proteins (PBPs); which in turn inhibits the final transpeptidation step of peptidoglycan synthesis in bacterial cell walls, thus inhibiting cell wall biosynthesis. Bacteria eventually lyse due to ongoing activity of cell wall autolytic enzymes (autolysins and murein hydrolases) while cell wall assembly is arrested.

Pharmacokinetics (Adult data unless noted) Note: Chewable tablets and oral suspension are bioequivalent. However, oral suspension and tablet (nonchewable)/capsule formulations are **not** considered bioequivalent (in normal adult volunteers, oral suspension AUC ~10% to 25% greater compared with tablet after doses of 100-400 mg).

Absorption: Oral: 40% to 50%; capsule AUC reduced by ~15% and C_{max} by ~25% when taken with food

Distribution: Widely distributed throughout the body and reaches therapeutic concentration in most tissues and body fluids, including synovial, pericardial, pleural, peritoneal; bile, sputum, and urine; bone, myocardium, gallbladder, and skin and soft tissue

Protein binding: 65%

Half-life:

Normal renal function: 3-4 hours

Renal impairment: Up to 11.5 hours

Time to peak serum concentration: Tablet/suspension: 2-6 hours; capsules: 3-8 hours (delayed with food)

Elimination: Urine (50% of absorbed dose as active drug); feces (10%)

Dosing: Usual

Infants, Children, and Adolescents: **Note:** Unless otherwise specified, any dosage form may be used.

General dosing; susceptible infection (mild-moderate): Oral:

Weight-based:

Infants and Children weighing ≤45 kg: 8 mg/kg/day divided every 12-24 hours; maximum daily dose: 400 mg/**day** (*Red Book*, 2012)

Children weighing >45 kg and Adolescents: 400 mg daily

Fixed dosing: Infants ≥6 months and Children weighing ≤45 kg:

5 to <7.6 kg: 50 mg daily

7.6 to <10.1 kg: 80 mg daily

10.1 to <12.6 kg: 100 mg daily

12.6 to <20.6 kg: 150 mg daily

20.6 to <28.1 kg: 200 mg daily

28.1 to <33.1 kg: 250 mg daily

33.1 to <40.1 kg: 300 mg daily

40.1 to ≤45 kg: 350 mg daily

Febrile neutropenia (low-risk): Limited data available: Oral: Oral suspension: 8 mg/kg/day in divided doses every 12-24 hours; in most trials, cefixime therapy was initiated as step-down therapy after 48-72 hours of empiric parenteral antibiotic therapy with first cefixime dose administered at the end of the last I.V. infusion (Klassen, 2000; Lehrnbecher, 2012; Paganini, 2000; Shenep, 2001). **Note:** In clinical trials, doses were repeated if patient vomited within 2 hours.

Gonococcal infection, uncomplicated: Children ≥45 kg and Adolescents: 400 mg as a single dose in combination with oral azithromycin (preferred) or oral doxycycline (CDC, 2010). **Note:** CDC no longer recommends cefixime as a first-line agent, only use as an alternative agent with test-of-cure follow up in 7 days (CDC, 2012). In Canada, due to increased antimicrobial resistance, the recommended dose is 800 mg as a single dose for treatment of uncomplicated gonococcal infections in pediatric patients ≥9 years of age (Public Health Agency of Canada, 2012).

Irinotecan-associated diarrhea, prophylaxis: Limited data available: Oral: 8 mg/kg once daily; begin 5 days before oral irinotecan therapy and continue throughout course (Wagner, 2008)

Otitis media, acute: Oral: Oral suspension or chewable tablets:

Infants and Children weighing ≤45 kg: 8 mg/kg/day divided every 12-24 hours; maximum daily dose: 400 mg/**day**

Children >45 kg or Adolescents: 400 mg daily in divided doses every 12-24 hours

Pharyngitis or tonsillitis; *S. pyogenes*: Oral: **Note:** Not preferred for treatment in IDSA Guidelines due to unnecessary broad spectrum, and lack of selectivity for antibiotic resistant flora (Schulman, 2012)

Infants and Children weighing ≤45 kg: 8 mg/kg/day in divided doses every 12-24 hours for ≥10 days; maximum daily dose: 400 mg/day

Children weighing >45 kg and Adolescents: 400 mg daily in divided doses every 12-24 hours

Pneumonia, community-acquired (CAP); *haemophilus influenza* **types A-F or nontypeable; mild infection or step-down therapy:** Infants ≥3 months, Children, and Adolescents: Oral: 8 mg/kg/day in divided doses every 12-24 hours; maximum daily dose: 400 mg/day (IDSA/PIDS [Bradley, 2011]) *Red Book,* 2012)

Rhinosinusitis, acute bacterial: Oral: 4 mg/kg/dose every 12 hours with concomitant clindamycin for 10-14 days; maximum daily dose: 400 mg/day. **Note:** Recommended in patients with non-type I penicillin allergy, after failure of initial therapy or in patients at risk for antibiotic resistance (eg, daycare attendance, age <2 years, recent hospitalization, antibiotic use within the past month) (Chow, 2012).

Sexual victimization, prophylaxis: Children weighing ≥45 kg and Adolescents: Oral: 400 mg **plus** azithromycin or doxycycline and completion of hepatitis B virus immunization and consider prophylaxis for trichomoniasis and bacterial vaginosis (*Red Book,* 2012)

Typhoid fever (*Salmonella typhi*): Limited data available; efficacy results variable: Oral: 7.5-10 mg/kg/dose every 12 hours for 7-14 days (Girgis, 1995; Cao, 1999; Stephens, 2002)

Urinary tract infection; acute: Oral:

Manufacturer 's labeling:

Infants ≥6 months and Children weighing ≤45 kg: 8 mg/kg/day in divided doses every 12-24 hours

Children weighing >45 kg and Adolescents: 400 mg daily in divided doses every 12-24 hours

Alternate dosing: Infants and Children ≤2 years: Initial: 8 mg/kg/day every 24 hours for 7-14 days; in patients <24 months, shorter courses (1-3 days) have been shown to be inferior to longer durations of therapy (AAP, 2011)

Adults:

General dosing; susceptible infections: Oral: 400 mg daily in divided doses every 12-24 hours

Gonococcal infection, uncomplicated cervical/urethral/rectal gonorrhea due to *N. gonorrhoeae*: Oral: 400 mg as a single dose in combination with oral azithromycin (preferred) or oral doxycycline (CDC, 2010). **Note:** CDC no longer recommends cefixime as a first-line agent (ceftriaxone is the preferred cephalosporin), if cefixime is used as an alternative agent, test-of-cure follow up in 7 days is recommended; in addition, cefixime is **not** an option for the treatment of uncomplicated gonorrhea of the pharynx (CDC, 2012). In Canada, due to increased antimicrobial resistance, the Public Health Agency of Canada recommends 800 mg as a single dose for treatment of uncomplicated gonococcal infections.

Gonococcal infection, expedited partner therapy: Oral: 400 mg as a single dose in combination with oral azithromycin (CDC, 2012). **Note:** Only used if a heterosexual partner cannot be linked to evaluation and treatment in a timely manner; dose delivered to partner by patient, collaborating pharmacy, or disease investigation specialist.

***S. pyogenes* infections:** Oral: 400 mg daily in divided doses every 12-24 hours for 10 days

Dosing adjustment in renal impairment:

Infants ≥6 months, Children, and Adolescents: Very limited data available; some clinicians have suggested the following (Daschner, 2005; Dhib, 1991; Guay, 1986):

Mild to moderate impairment: No adjustment recommended

Severe impairment (GFR ≤10-20 mL/minute/1.73 m^2): Reduce dose by 50%

Anuric: Reduce dose by 50%

Hemodialysis, peritoneal dialysis: Not significantly removed

Adults: Manufacturer's labeling:

CrCl ≥60 mL/minute: No adjustment required

CrCl 21-59 mL/minute: 260 mg once daily

CrCl <20 mL/minute:

Chewable tablet, tablet: 200 mg once daily

100 mg/5 mL suspension: 172 mg once daily

200 mg/5 mL suspension: 176 mg once daily

500 mg/5 mL suspension: 180 mg once daily

Intermittent hemodialysis: Not significantly removed: 260 mg once daily

CAPD: Not significantly removed by peritoneal dialysis

Chewable tablet, tablet: 200 mg once daily

100 mg/5 mL suspension: 172 mg once daily

200 mg/5 mL suspension: 176 mg once daily

500 mg/5 mL suspension: 180 mg once daily

Dosing adjustment in hepatic impairment: There are no dosage adjustments provided in the manufacturer's labeling.

Administration Oral: May be administered with or without food; administer with food to decrease GI distress; shake suspension well before use; chewable tablets must be chewed or crushed before swallowing

Monitoring Parameters With prolonged therapy, monitor renal and hepatic function periodically; number and type of stools/day for diarrhea. Observe for signs and symptoms of anaphylaxis during first dose. When used as part of alternative treatment for gonococcal infection, test-of-cure 7 days after dose (CDC, 2012).

Test Interactions Positive direct Coombs', false-positive urinary glucose test using cupric sulfate (Benedict's solution, Clinitest®, Fehling's solution), may cause false-positive serum or urine creatinine with the alkaline picrate-based Jaffé reaction for measuring creatinine; false-positive urine ketones using tests with nitroprusside (but not those using nitroferricyanide).

Dosage Forms Excipient information presented when available (limited, particularly for generics); consult specific product labeling. [DSC] = Discontinued product

Capsule, Oral, as trihydrate:

Suprax: 400 mg

Suspension Reconstituted, Oral, as trihydrate:

Suprax: 100 mg/5 mL (50 mL) [strawberry flavor]

Suprax: 200 mg/5 mL (50 mL, 75 mL); 500 mg/5 mL (10 mL, 20 mL) [contains sodium benzoate; strawberry flavor]

Tablet, Oral, as trihydrate:

Suprax: 400 mg [DSC] [scored]

Tablet Chewable, Oral, as trihydrate:

Suprax: 100 mg, 200 mg [contains aspartame, fd&c red #40 aluminum lake; tutti-frutti flavor]

References

American Academy of Pediatrics Subcommittee on Urinary Tract Infection. Urinary tract infection: clinical practice guideline for the diagnosis and management of the initial UTI in febrile infants and children 2 to 24 months. *Pediatrics.* 2011;128(3):595-610.

Bradley JS, Byington CL, Shah SS, et al, "The Management of Community-Acquired Pneumonia in Infants and Children Older Than 3 Months of Age: Clinical Practice Guidelines by the Pediatric Infectious Diseases Society and the Infectious Diseases Society of America", *Clin Infect Dis*, 2011, 53(7):e25-76.

Cao XT, Kneen R, Nguyen TA, et al, "A Comparative Study of Ofloxacin and Cefixime for Treatment of Typhoid Fever in Children. The Dong Nai Pediatric Center Typhoid Study Group," *Pediatr Infect Dis J*, 1999, 18(3):245-8.

Centers for Disease Control and Prevention (CDC), "Sexually Transmitted Diseases Treatment Guidelines, 2010," *MMWR Recomm Rep*, 2010, 59(RR-12):1-110.

Centers for Disease Control and Prevention (CDC), "Update to CDC's Sexually Transmitted Diseases Treatment Guidelines, 2010: Oral Cephalosporins No Longer a Recommended Treatment for Gonococcal Infections", *MMWR Morb Mortal Wkly Rep*, 2012, 61(31):590-4.

Chow AW, Benninger MS, Brook I, et al, "IDSA Clinical Practice Guideline for Acute Bacterial Rhinosinusitis in Children and Adults," *Clin Infect Dis*, 2012, 54(8):e72-112.

Daschner M. Drug dosage in children with reduced renal function. *Pediatr Nephrol*. 2005;20:1675-1686.

Dhib M, Moulin B, Leroy A, et al. Relationship between renal function and disposition of oral cefixime. *Eur J Clin Pharmacol*. 1991;41:579-583.

Girgis NI, Sultan Y, Hammad O, et al, "Comparison of the Efficacy, Safety and Cost of Cefixime, Ceftriaxone and Aztreonam in the Treatment of Multidrug-Resistant *Salmonella typhi* Septicemia in Children," *Pediatr Infect Dis J*, 1995, 14(7):603-5.

Guay DRP, Meatherall RC, Harding GK, et al. Pharmacokinetics of cefixime (CL 284,635; FK 027) in healthy subjects and patients with renal insufficiency. *Antimicrob Agents Chemother*. 1986;30 (3):485-490.

Klaassen RJ, Allen U, and Doyle JJ, "Randomized Placebo-Controlled Trial of Oral Antibiotics in Pediatric Oncology Patients at Low-Risk With Fever and Neutropenia," *J Pediatr Hematol Oncol*, 2000, 22 (5):405-11.

Lehrnbecher T, Phillips R, Alexander S, et al, "Guideline for the Management of Fever and Neutropenia in Children With Cancer and/or Undergoing Hematopoietic Stem-Cell Transplantation," *J Clin Oncol*, 2012, 30(35):4427-38.

Paganini HR, Sarkis CM, De Martino MG, et al, "Oral Administration of Cefixime to Lower Risk Febrile Neutropenic Children With Cancer," *Cancer*, 2000, 88(12):2848-52.

Public Health Agency of Canada, "Canadian Guidelines on Sexually Transmitted Infections." Available at http://www.phac-aspc.gc.ca/std-mts/sti-its/alert/2011/alert-gono-eng.php. Accessed January 4, 2012.

Shenep JL, Flynn PM, Baker DK, et al, "Oral Cefixime Is Similar to Continued Intravenous Antibiotics in the Empirical Treatment of Febrile Neutropenic Children With Cancer," *Clin Infect Dis*, 2001, 32 (1):36-43.

Stephens I and Levine MM, "Management of Typhoid Fever in Children," *Pediatr Infect Dis J*, 2002, 21(2):157-8.

Wagner LM, Crews KR, Stewart CF, et al, "Reducing Irinotecan-Associated Diarrhea in Children," *Pediatr Blood Cancer*, 2008, 50 (2):201-7.

◆ **Cefixime Trihydrate** see Cefixime on page 401

◆ **Cefotan** see CefoTEtan on page 407

Cefotaxime (sef oh TAKS eem)

Medication Safety Issues

Sound-alike/look-alike issues:

Cefotaxime may be confused with cefOXitin, cefuroxime

International issues:

Spectracef [Italy] may be confused with Spectracef brand name for cefditoren [U.S., Great Britain, Mexico, Portugal, Spain]

Brand Names: U.S. Claforan; Claforan in D$_5$W

Brand Names: Canada Cefotaxime Sodium For Injection; Claforan

Therapeutic Category Antibiotic, Cephalosporin (Third Generation)

Generic Availability (U.S.) May be product dependent

Use Treatment of susceptible lower respiratory tract, skin and skin structure, bone and joint, intra-abdominal, genitourinary tract, and gynecologic infections, bacteremia/septicemia and documented or suspected central nervous system infections (eg, meningitis, ventriculitis) (FDA approved in all ages); prevention of postoperative surgical site infection in contaminated or potentially contaminated surgical procedures [eg, gastrointestinal and genitourinary tract surgeries and hysterectomy (abdominal or vaginal)] and caesarian section (FDA approved in all ages)

Pregnancy Risk Factor B

Pregnancy Considerations Adverse events have not been observed in animal reproduction studies. Cefotaxime crosses the human placenta and can be found in fetal tissue. An increase in most types of birth defects was not found following first trimester exposure to cephalosporins. During pregnancy, peak cefotaxime serum concentrations are decreased and the serum half-life is shorter. Cefotaxime is approved for use in women undergoing cesarean section (consult current guidelines for appropriate use).

Breast-Feeding Considerations Low concentrations of cefotaxime are found in breast milk. The manufacturer recommends that caution be exercised when administering cefotaxime to nursing women. Nondose-related effects could include modification of bowel flora. The pregnancy-related changes in cefotaxime pharmacokinetics continue into the early postpartum period.

Contraindications Hypersensitivity to cefotaxime, any component, or cephalosporins

Warnings Prolonged use may result in fungal or bacterial superinfection, including *C. difficile*-associated diarrhea (CDAD) and pseudomembranous colitis; CDAD has been observed >2 months postantibiotic treatment; use with caution in patients with a history of colitis. May cause hypersensitivity reaction; patients with history of hypersensitivity reactions to other cephalosporins or pencillins may experience cross-sensitivity; use with caution in patients with a history of penicillin allergy, especially IgE-mediated reactions (eg, anaphylaxis, angioedema, urticaria). Rapid bolus injection of cefotaxime (over <1 minute through a central venous catheter) has been associated with potentially life-threatening arrhythmias.

Precautions Use with caution in patients with impaired renal function. Granulocytopenia and more rarely agranulocytosis may develop during prolonged treatment (>10 days).

Adverse Reactions

Dermatologic: Pruritus, rash

Gastrointestinal: Colitis, diarrhea, nausea, vomiting

Local: Pain at injection site

Rare but important or life-threatening: Agranulocytosis, alkaline phosphatase increased, ALT increased, anaphylaxis, arrhythmia (after rapid I.V. injection via central catheter), AST increased, bilirubin increased, BUN increased, candidiasis, cholestasis, Coombs test (direct) positive, creatinine increased, encephalopathy, eosinophilia, erythema multiforme, fever, GGT increased, headache, hemolytic anemia, hepatitis, interstitial nephritis, jaundice, LDH increased, leukopenia, moniliasis, neutropenia, phlebitis, pseudomembranous colitis, Stevens-Johnson syndrome, thrombocytopenia, toxic epidermal necrolysis, transaminases increased, urticaria, vaginitis

Reactions reported with other cephalosporins: Aplastic anemia, hemorrhage, pancytopenia, renal dysfunction, seizure, superinfection, toxic nephropathy

Drug Interactions

Metabolism/Transport Effects None known.

Avoid Concomitant Use

Avoid concomitant use of Cefotaxime with any of the following: BCG

Increased Effect/Toxicity

Cefotaxime may increase the levels/effects of: Aminoglycosides; Vitamin K Antagonists

The levels/effects of Cefotaxime may be increased by: Probenecid

Decreased Effect

Cefotaxime may decrease the levels/effects of: BCG; Sodium Picosulfate; Typhoid Vaccine

Stability

Powder for injection: Store intact vial at 20°C to 25°C (68°F to 77°F); excursions permitted 15°C to 30°C (59°F to 86°F); protect from light and high temperatures. Reconstituted solution is stable for 12-24 hours at room temperature, 7-10 days when refrigerated and for 13 weeks when frozen; duration is dependent upon concentration; see manufacturer's labeling for specific information. Upon further dilution with NS or D$_5$W for I.V. infusion, solution is stable for 24 hours at room temperature, 5 days when refrigerated, or 13 weeks when frozen in Viaflex® plastic containers.

Premixed solution (manufacturer premixed): Store at -20°C (-4°F); once thawed, solutions are stable for 24 hours at room temperature or for 10 days refrigerated. Do not refreeze.

Mechanism of Action Inhibits bacterial cell wall synthesis by binding to one or more of the penicillin-binding proteins (PBPs) which in turn inhibits the final transpeptidation step of peptidoglycan synthesis in bacterial cell walls, thus inhibiting cell wall biosynthesis. Bacteria eventually lyse due to ongoing activity of cell wall autolytic enzymes (autolysins and murein hydrolases) while cell wall assembly is arrested. Cefotaxime has activity in the presence of some beta-lactamases, both penicillinases and cephaolsporinases, of gram-negative and gram-positive bacteria. *Enterococcus* species may be intrinsically resistant to cefotaxime. Most extended-spectrum beta-lactamase (ESBL)-producing and carbapenemase-producing isolates are resistant to cefotaxime.

Pharmacokinetics (Adult data unless noted)

Distribution: Into bronchial secretions, middle ear effusions, bone, bile; penetration into CSF when meninges are inflamed

Protein binding: 31% to 50%

Metabolism: Partially metabolized in the liver to active metabolite, desacetylcefotaxime

Half-life:

Cefotaxime:

Neonates, birth weight ≤1500 g: 4.6 hours

Neonates, birth weight >1500 g: 3.4 hours

Children: 1.5 hours

Adults: 1-1.5 hours (prolonged with renal and/or hepatic impairment)

Desacetylcefotaxime: 1.5-1.9 hours (prolonged with renal impairment)

Time to peak serum concentration: I.M.: Within 30 minutes

Elimination: Urine (~60% as unchanged drug and metabolites in urine)

Dialysis: Moderately dialyzable (20% to 50%)

Dosing: Neonatal

General dosing, susceptible infection: I.M., I.V. (*Red Book*, 2012):

Body weight <1 kg:

PNA ≤14 days: 50 mg/kg/dose every 12 hours

PNA 15-28 days: 50 mg/kg/dose every 8-12 hours

Body weight 1-2 kg:

PNA ≤7 days: 50 mg/kg/dose every 12 hours

PNA 8-28 days: 50 mg/kg/dose every 8-12 hours

Body weight >2 kg:

PNA ≤7 days: 50 mg/kg/dose every 12 hours

PNA 8-28 days: 50 mg/kg/dose every 8 hours; in some cases, every 6 hours dosing has been used

Gonococcal infection:

Disseminated or scalp abscess: I.M., I.V.: 25 mg/kg/dose every 12 hours for 7 days; therapy should be extended to 10-14 days if meningitis is documented (CDC, 2010)

Ophthalmia neonatorum: I.M., I.V.: 100 mg/kg as a single dose (*Red Book*, 2012)

Meningitis (Tunkel, 2004): I.V.: **Note:** Treat for a minimum of 21 days; use smaller doses and longer intervals for neonates <2 kg.

PNA ≤7 days and ≥2 kg: 100-150 mg/kg/**day** divided every 8-12 hours

PNA >7 days and ≥2 kg: 150-200 mg/kg/**day** divided every 6-8 hours

Dosing: Usual

Infants, Children, and Adolescents:

General dosing, susceptible infection: Infants, Children and Adolescents: I.M., I.V.:

AAP recommendations (*Red Book*, 2012):

Mild to moderate infection: 50-180 mg/kg/**day** in divided doses every 6-8 hours; maximum daily dose: 6 **g/day**

Severe infection: 200-225 mg/kg/day in divided doses every 4-6 hours; up to 300 mg/kg/**day** has been used for meningitis; maximum daily dose: 12 **g/day**

Manufacturer labeling:

<50 kg: 50-180 mg/kg/**day** divided every 4-6 hours

≥50 kg:

Uncomplicated infections: I.M., I.V.: 1000 mg every 12 hours

Moderate to severe infections: I.M., I.V.: 1000-2000 mg every 8 hours

Life-threatening infections: I.V.: 2000 mg every 4 hours, maximum dose: 12 **g/day**

Acute bacterial rhinosinusitis, severe infection requiring hospitalization: Children and Adolescents: I.V.: 100-200 mg/kg/**day** divided every 6 hours for 10-14 days; maximum dose: 2000 mg (Chow, 2012)

Enteric bacterial infections, empiric treatment (HIV-exposed/-positive): Adolescents: I.V.: 1000 mg every 8 hours (DHHS [adult], 2013)

Gonorrhea (as an alternative to ceftriaxone) (CDC, 2010; CDC, 2012): Children weighing ≥45 kg and Adolescents:

Uncomplicated gonorrhea of the cervix, urethra, or rectum: I.M.: 500 mg as a single dose in combination with oral azithromycin or oral doxycycline

Disseminated: I.V.: 1 g every 8 hours for a total duration of at least 7 days

Intra-abdominal infection, complicated: Infants, Children, and Adolescents: I.V.: 150-200 mg/kg/**day** divided every 6-8 hours; maximum dose: 2000 mg; use in combination with metronidazole (Solomkin, 2010)

Lyme disease, cardiac or CNS manifestations or recurrent arthritis: Infants, Children, and Adolescents: I.V.: 150-200 mg/kg/**day** in divided doses every 6-8 hours for 14-28 days; maximum daily dose: 6 **g/day** (Halperin, 2007; *Red Book*, 2012; Wormser, 2006)

Meningitis: Infants, Children, and Adolescents: I.V.: 225-300 mg/kg/**day** divided every 6-8 hours; maximum dose: 2000 mg; use in combination with vancomycin for empiric coverage (*Red Book*, 2012; Tunkel, 2004)

Peritonitis (CAPD) (Warady, 2012): Infants, Children, and Adolescents: Intraperitoneal:

Intermittent: 30 mg/kg/dose every 24 hours

Continuous: Loading dose: 500 mg per liter of dialysate; maintenance dose: 250 mg per liter; **Note:** 125 mg/liter has also been recommended as a maintenance dose (Aronoff, 2007)

Pneumonia:

Bacterial pneumonia (HIV-exposed/-positive): I.V.: 150-200 mg/kg/**day** divided every 6-8 hours; maximum single dose: 2000 mg (DHHS, 2013; DHHS [adult and pediatric], 2013); consider more frequent dosing for severe or life-threatening infections (every 4-6 hours) (*Red Book*, 2012)

Community-acquired pneumonia (CAP): Infants >3 months, Children, and Adolescents: I.V.: 50 mg/kg/dose every 8 hours; maximum dose: 2000 mg; **Note:** May consider addition of vancomycin or clindamycin to empiric therapy if community-acquired MRSA suspected. In children ≥5 years, a macrolide antibiotic should be added if atypical pneumonia cannot be ruled out (Bradley, 2011).

Salmonellosis (HIV-exposed/-positive): Adolescents: I.V.: 1000 mg every 8 hours (DHHS [adult], 2013)

Surgical prophylaxis: Children and Adolescents: I.V.: 50 mg/kg 30-60 minutes prior to the procedure; may repeat in 3 hours; maximum dose: 1000 mg (Bratzler, 2013)

Urinary tract infection: Infants and Children 2-24 months: I.M., I.V.: 150 mg/kg/day divided every 6-8 hours (AAP, 2011)

Adults:

Usual dosage range: I.M., I.V.: 1000-2000 mg every 4-12 hours

Uncomplicated infections: I.M., I.V.: 1000 mg every 12 hours

Moderate to severe infections: I.M., I.V.: 1000-2000 mg every 8 hours

Life-threatening infections: I.V.: 2000 mg every 4 hours

Caesarean section: I.M., I.V.: 1000 mg as soon as the umbilical cord is clamped, then 1000 mg at 6- and 12-hour intervals

Gonorrhea (CDC, 2010):

Uncomplicated gonorrhea of the cervix, urethra, or rectum: I.M.: 500 mg as a single dose in combination with oral azithromycin or oral doxycycline; may also administer 1000 mg as a single dose for rectal gonorrhea in males (per manufacturer labeling)

Disseminated: I.V.: 1000 mg every 8 hours for a total duration of at least 7 days

Sepsis: I.V.: 2000 mg every 6-8 hours

Dosing adjustment in renal impairment:

Infants, Children, and Adolescents: The following adjustments have been recommended (Aronoff, 2007). **Note:** Renally adjusted dose recommendations are based on doses of 100-200 mg/**kg/day** divided every 8 hours.

GFR 30-50 mL/minute/1.73 m^2: 35-70 mg/kg/dose every 8-12 hours

GFR 10-29 mL/minute/1.73 m^2: 35-70 mg/kg/dose every 12 hours

GFR <10 mL/minute/1.73 m^2: 35-70 mg/kg/dose every 24 hours

Intermittent hemodialysis: 35-70 mg/kg/dose every 24 hours

Peritoneal dialysis (PD): 35-70 mg/kg/dose every 24 hours

Continuous renal replacement therapy (CRRT): 35-70 mg/kg/dose every 12 hours

Adults:

Manufacturer's labeling: **Note:** Renal function may be estimated using Cockcroft-Gault formula for dosage adjustment purposes.

CrCl <20 mL/minute/1.73 m^2: Dose should be decreased by 50%.

Alternate Dosing: The following dosage adjustments have been recommended:

GFR >50 mL/minute: Administer every 6 hours (Aronoff, 2007)

GFR 10-50 mL/minute: Administer every 6-12 hours (Aronoff, 2007)

GFR <10 mL/minute: Administer every 24 hours **or** decrease the dose by 50% (and administer at usual intervals) (Aronoff, 2007)

Intermittent hemodialysis (IHD): 1-2 g every 24 hours (on dialysis days, administer after hemodialysis). **Note:** Dosing dependent on the assumption of 3 times/week, complete IHD sessions (Heintz, 2009).

Peritoneal dialysis (PD): 1 g every 24 hours (Aronoff, 2007)

Continuous renal replacement therapy (CRRT) (Heintz, 2009; Trotman, 2005): Drug clearance is highly dependent on the method of renal replacement, filter type, and flow rate. Appropriate dosing requires close monitoring of pharmacologic response, signs of adverse reactions due to drug accumulation, as well as drug concentrations in relation to target trough (if appropriate). The following are general recommendations only (based on dialysate flow/ultrafiltration rates of 1-2 L/hour and minimal residual renal function) and should not supersede clinical judgment:

CVVH: 1-2 g every 8-12 hours

CVVHD: 1-2 g every 8 hours

CVVHDF: 1-2 g every 6-8 hours

Administration Parenteral:

I.V.: May be administered I.V. push over 3-5 minutes at a maximum concentration of 200 mg/mL or as an intermittent I.V. infusion over 15-30 minutes at a final concentration of 20-60 mg/mL; avoid rapid injection (<1 minute) due to association with arrhythmias

I.M.: Reconstitute powder for injection with SWI to a final concentration between 230-330 mg/mL (see manufacturer labeling for specific details). Administer by deep I.M. injection into a large muscle mass such as the upper outer quadrant of the gluteus maximus. Doses of 2000 mg should be divided and administered at two different sites.

Monitoring Parameters Observe for signs and symptoms of anaphylaxis during first dose; monitor infusion site for extravasation; with prolonged therapy, monitor renal, hepatic, and hematologic function periodically; number and type of stools/day for diarrhea

Test Interactions Positive direct Coombs', false-positive urinary glucose test using cupric sulfate (Benedict's solution, Clinitest®, Fehling's solution), false-positive serum or urine creatinine with Jaffé reaction

Dosage Forms Excipient information presented when available (limited, particularly for generics); consult specific product labeling.

Solution, Intravenous:

Claforan in D$_5$W: 1 g/50 mL (50 mL); 2 g/50 mL (50 mL)

Solution Reconstituted, Injection:

Claforan: 500 mg (1 ea); 1 g (1 ea); 2 g (1 ea); 10 g (1 ea)

Generic: 500 mg (1 ea); 1 g (1 ea); 2 g (1 ea); 10 g (1 ea)

Solution Reconstituted, Intravenous:

Claforan: 1 g (1 ea); 2 g (1 ea)

References

American Academy of Pediatrics. Urinary tract infection: clinical practice guideline for the diagnosis and management of the initial UTI in febrile infants and children 2 to 24 months. *Pediatrics.* 2011;128 (3):595-610.

Aronoff GR, Bennett WM, Berns JS, et al, *Drug Prescribing in Renal Failure: Dosing Guidelines for Adults and Children,* 5th ed. Philadelphia, PA: American College of Physicians; 2007, p 55, 149.

Bradley JS, Byington CL, Shah SS, et al, "The Management of Community-Acquired Pneumonia in Infants and Children Older Than 3 Months of Age: Clinical Practice Guidelines by the Pediatric Infectious Diseases Society and the Infectious Diseases Society of America," *Clin Infect Dis,* 2011, 53(7):e25-76.

Bratzler DW, Dellinger EP, Olsen KM, et al, "Clinical Practice Guidelines for Antimicrobial Prophylaxis in Surgery," *Am J Health Syst Pharm,* 2013, 70(3):195-283.

Centers for Disease Control and Prevention (CDC), "Sexually Transmitted Diseases Treatment Guidelines, 2010," *MMWR Recomm Rep,* 2010, 59(RR-12):1-110.

Centers for Disease Control and Prevention (CDC), "Update to CDC's Sexually Transmitted Diseases Treatment Guidelines, 2010: Oral Cephalosporins No Longer a Recommended Treatment for Gonococcal Infections," *MMWR Morb Mortal Wkly Rep,* 2012, 61(31):590-4.

Chow AW, Benninger MS, Brook I, et al, "IDSA Clinical Practice Guideline for Acute Bacterial Rhinosinusitis in Children and Adults," *Clin Infect Dis,* 2012, 54(8):e72-112.

DHHS. Guidelines for the prevention and treatment of opportunistic infections among HIV-exposed and HIV-infected children: recommendations from the National Institutes of Health, Centers for Disease Control and Prevention, the HIV Medicine Association of the Infectious Diseases Society of America, the Pediatric Infectious Diseases Society, and the American Academy of Pediatrics. November 6, 2013. Available at http://aidsinfo.nih.gov

DHHS Panel on Opportunistic Infections (OI) in HIV-Infected Adults and Adolescents. Guidelines for prevention and treatment of opportunistic infections in HIV-infected adults and adolescents: recommendations from the Centers for Disease Control and Prevention (CDC), the National Institutes of Health (NIH), and the HIV Medicine Association (HIVMA) of the Infectious Diseases Society of America (IDSA). May 7, 2013. Available at http://aidsinfo.nih.gov/contentfiles/lvguidelines/adult_oi.pdf

Halperin JJ, Shapiro ED, Logigian E, et al, "Practice Parameter: Treatment of Nervous System Lyme Disease (an Evidence-Based Review): Report of the Quality Standards Subcommittee of the American Academy of Neurology," *Neurology,* 2007, 69(1):91-102.

Heintz BH, Matzke GR, Dager WE, "Antimicrobial Dosing Concepts and Recommendations for Critically Ill Adult Patients Receiving Continuous Renal Replacement Therapy or Intermittent Hemodialysis," *Pharmacotherapy,* 2009, 29(5):562-77.

Solomkin JS, Mazuski JE, Bradley JS, et al, "Diagnosis and Management of Complicated Intra-Abdominal Infections in Adults and

Children: Guidelines by the Surgical Infection Society and the Infectious Diseases Society of America," *Clin Infect Dis*, 2010, 50 (2):133-64.

Spritzer R, Kamp HJ, Dzoljic G, et al, "Five Years of Cefotaxime Use in a Neonatal Intensive Care Unit," *Pediatr Infect Dis J*, 1990, 9(2):92-6.

Trotman RL, Williamson JC, Shoemaker DM, et al, "Antibiotic Dosing in Critically Ill Adult Patients Receiving Continuous Renal Replacement Therapy," *Clin Infect Dis*, 2005, 41(8):1159-66.

Tunkel AR, Hartman BJ, Kaplan SL, et al, "Practice Guidelines for the Management of Bacterial Meningitis," *Clin Infect Dis*, 2004, 39 (9):1267-84.

Warady BA, Bakkaloglu S, Newland J, et al, "Consensus Guidelines for the Prevention and Treatment of Catheter-Related Infections and Peritonitis in Pediatric Patients Receiving Peritoneal Dialysis: 2012 Update," *Perit Dial Int*, 2012, (32 Suppl 2):S32-86.

Wormser GP, Dattwyler RJ, Shapiro ED, et al, "The Clinical Assessment, Treatment, and Prevention of Lyme Disease, Human Granulocytic Anaplasmosis, and Babesiosis: Clinical Practice Guidelines by the Infectious Diseases Society of America," *Clin Infect Dis*, 2006, 43 (9):1089-134.

◆ **Cefotaxime Sodium** *see* Cefotaxime *on page 404*

◆ **Cefotaxime Sodium For Injection (Can)** *see* Cefotaxime *on page 404*

CefoTEtan (SEF oh tee tan)

Medication Safety Issues
Sound-alike/look-alike issues:
CefoTEtan may be confused with ceFAZolin, cefOXitin, cefTAZidime, Ceftin®, cefTRIAXone

Therapeutic Category Antibiotic, Cephalosporin (Second Generation)

Generic Availability (U.S.) Yes

Use Treatment of susceptible lower respiratory tract, skin and skin structure, bone and joint, urinary tract, gynecologic, and intra-abdominal infections (FDA approved in adults); surgical prophylaxis (FDA approved in adults)

Pregnancy Risk Factor B

Pregnancy Considerations Adverse events have not been observed in animal reproduction studies. Cefotetan crosses the placenta and produces therapeutic concentrations in the amniotic fluid and cord serum. Cefotetan is one of the antibiotics recommended for prophylactic use prior to cesarean delivery.

Breast-Feeding Considerations Very small amounts of cefotetan are excreted in human milk. The manufacturer recommends caution when giving cefotetan to a breast-feeding mother. Nondose-related effects could include modification of bowel flora.

Contraindications Hypersensitivity to cefotetan, cephalosporins, any component, or patients who have experienced a cephalosporin-associated hemolytic anemia

Warnings Prolonged use may result in fungal or bacterial superinfection, including *C. difficile*-associated diarrhea (CDAD) and pseudomembranous colitis; CDAD has been observed >2 months postantibiotic treatment; use with caution in patients with a history of colitis. May cause hypersensitivity reaction; patients with history of hypersensitivity reactions to other cephalosporins or pencillins may experience cross-sensitivity; use with caution in patients with a history of penicillin allergy, especially IgE-mediated reactions (eg, anaphylaxis, angioedema, urticaria).

Severe and sometimes fatal cases of immune mediated hemolytic anemia have been reported with cefotetan administration. Risk of developing cefotetan-induced hemolytic anemia is 3-fold higher relative to other cephalosporins. Monitor hematologic parameters carefully during use; blood transfusion may be needed; consider cephalosporin-associated immune anemia in patients who have received cefotetan within 2-3 weeks (either as treatment or prophylaxis). May be associated with increased INR, especially in nutritionally deficient patients, prolonged treatment, hepatic or renal disease.

Precautions Use with caution in patients with renal impairment; modify dosing interval in severe impairment.

Adverse Reactions
Gastrointestinal: Diarrhea

Hepatic: Transaminases increased

Miscellaneous: Hypersensitivity reactions

Rare but important or life-threatening: Agranulocytosis, anaphylaxis, bleeding, BUN increased, creatinine increased, eosinophilia, fever, hemolytic anemia, leukopenia, nausea, nephrotoxicity, phlebitis, prolonged PT, pruritus, pseudomembranous colitis, rash, thrombocytopenia, thrombocytosis, urticaria, vomiting

Reactions reported with other cephalosporins: Agranulocytosis, aplastic anemia, cholestasis, colitis, hemolytic anemia, hemorrhage, pancytopenia, renal dysfunction, seizure, Stevens-Johnson syndrome, superinfection, toxic epidermal necrolysis, toxic nephropathy

Drug Interactions
Metabolism/Transport Effects None known.

Avoid Concomitant Use
Avoid concomitant use of CefoTEtan with any of the following: BCG

Increased Effect/Toxicity
CefoTEtan may increase the levels/effects of: Alcohol (Ethyl); Aminoglycosides; Carbocisteine; Vitamin K Antagonists

The levels/effects of CefoTEtan may be increased by: Probenecid

Decreased Effect
CefoTEtan may decrease the levels/effects of: BCG; Sodium Picosulfate; Typhoid Vaccine

Food Interactions Concurrent use with ethanol may cause a disulfiram-like reaction. Management: Monitor patients.

Stability
Parenteral:
Bulk vials: Store intact vials at 20°C to 25°C (68°F to 77°F); protect from light. Reconstituted vial should be used within 4 hours; upon further dilution, solution is stable for 24 hours at room temperature, 96 hours refrigerated.

Individual vials: Store intact vials at ≤22°C (≤72°F); protect from light. Reconstituted solution is stable for 24 hours at room temperature and for 96 hours when refrigerated when stored in the original container or packaged in glass or plastic syringes; solution is also stable for 1 week if frozen. Thawed solution should be used within 24 hours if stored at room temperature or 96 hours if stored under refrigeration. Do not refreeze.

DUPLEX Drug Delivery System: Store unactivated unit at 20°C to 25°C (68°F to 77°F); excursions permitted to 15°C to 30°C (59°F to 86°F). After activated, stable for 12 hours at room temperature or 5 days refrigerated. Do not freeze.

Mechanism of Action Inhibits bacterial cell wall synthesis by binding to one or more of the penicillin-binding proteins (PBPs) which in turn inhibits the final transpeptidation step of peptidoglycan synthesis in bacterial cell walls, thus inhibiting cell wall biosynthesis. Bacteria eventually lyse due to ongoing activity of cell wall autolytic enzymes (autolysins and murein hydrolases) while cell wall assembly is arrested.

Pharmacokinetics (Adult data unless noted)
Absorption: I.M.: Completely absorbed

Distribution: Distributes into tissues and fluids including gallbladder, kidney, skin, tonsils, uterus, sputum, prostatic and peritoneal fluids; poor penetration into CSF

Protein binding: 88%

Half-life: 3-4.6 hours, prolonged in patients with moderately impaired renal function (up to 10 hours)

Time to peak serum concentration: I.M.: Within 1.5-3 hours ▶

Elimination: 51% to 81% excreted as unchanged drug in urine, 20% of dose is excreted in bile

Dosing: Usual

Infants, Children, and Adolescents:

General dosing, susceptible infection (*Red Book*, 2012): I.M., I.V.:

Mild to moderate infection: 30 mg/kg/dose every 12 hours, maximum single dose: 2000 mg

Severe infection: 50 mg/kg/dose every 12 hours; usual maximum single dose: 2000 mg; for life-threatening infections doses as high as 3000 mg every 12 hours have been used

Intra-abdominal infection, complicated: I.V.: 20-40 mg/kg/dose every 12 hours. **Note:** Due to high rates of *B. fragilis* group resistance, not recommended for the treatment of community-acquired intra-abdominal infections (Solomkin, 2010).

Pelvic inflammatory disease: Adolescents: I.V.: 2000 mg every 12 hours; used in combination with doxycycline (CDC, 2010)

Surgical prophylaxis: Children and Adolescents: I.V.: 40 mg/kg 60 minutes prior to procedure; may redose in 6 hours; maximum dose: 2000 mg (Bratzler, 2013)

Adults:

General dosing, susceptible infection: I.M., I.V.: Usual dose: 1000-2000 mg every 12 hours for 5-10 days; 1000-2000 mg may be given every 24 hours for urinary tract infection; maximum single dose: 3000 mg. **Note:** Due to high rates of *B. fragilis* group resistance, not recommended for the treatment of community-acquired intra-abdominal infections (Solomkin, 2010).

Pelvic inflammatory disease: I.V.: 2000 mg every 12 hours; used in combination with doxycycline (CDC, 2010)

Surgical (perioperative) prophylaxis: I.V.: 1000-2000 mg 30-60 minutes prior to surgery; when used for cesarean section, dose should be given as soon as umbilical cord is clamped

Urinary tract infection: I.M., I.V.: 500 mg every 12 hours or 1000-2000 mg every 12-24 hours

Dosage adjustment in renal impairment:

Infants, Children, and Adolescents: Dosage adjustments are not provided in the manufacturer's labeling; however, the following guidelines have been used by some clinicians (Aronoff, 2007); **Note:** Renally adjusted dose recommendations are based on doses of 20-40 mg/kg/dose every 12 hours:

GFR ≥30 mL/minute/1.73 m^2: No adjustment required.

GFR 10-29 mL/minute/1.73 m^2: 20-40 mg/kg/dose every 24 hours

GFR <10 mL/minute/1.73 m^2: 20-40 mg/kg/dose every 48 hours

Intermittent hemodialysis: 20-40 mg/kg/dose every 48 hours; give after dialysis on dialysis days

Peritoneal dialysis (PD): 20-40 mg/kg/dose every 48 hours

Continuous renal replacement therapy (CRRT): 20-40 mg/kg/dose every 12 hours

Adults:

CrCl >30 mL/minute: No adjustment required

CrCl 10-30 mL/minute: Administer every 24 hours

CrCl <10 mL/minute: Administer every 48 hours

Hemodialysis: Dialyzable (5% to 20%); administer 1/4 the usual dose every 24 hours on days between dialysis; administer 1/2 the usual dose on the day of dialysis

Dosage adjustment for hepatic impairment: There are no dosage adjustments provided in the manufacturer's labeling.

Administration

Parenteral:

I.M.: Inject deep I.M. into large muscle mass at a concentration ≤500 mg/mL

I.V. intermittent: Infuse over 20-60 minutes at a concentration of 10-40 mg/mL

I.V. push: Inject direct I.V. over 3-5 minutes at a concentration ≤182 mg/mL

Monitoring Parameters CBC, prothrombin time, renal function tests; number and type of stools/day for diarrhea; signs and symptoms of hemolytic anemia; monitor for signs of anaphylaxis during first dose

Test Interactions Positive direct Coombs', false-positive urinary glucose test using cupric sulfate (Benedict's solution, Clinitest®, Fehling's solution), false-positive serum or urine creatinine with Jaffé reaction

Additional Information Sodium content of 1000 mg: 3.5 mEq. Chemical structure contains a methyltetrazolethiol side chain which may be responsible for the disulfiram-like reaction with alcohol and increased risk of bleeding

Dosage Forms Excipient information presented when available (limited, particularly for generics); consult specific product labeling.

Solution Reconstituted, Injection:

Generic: 1 g (1 ea); 2 g (1 ea); 10 g (1 ea)

Solution Reconstituted, Intravenous:

Generic: 1 g (1 ea); 2 g (1 ea)

References

Bratzler DW, Dellinger EP, Olsen KM, et al, "Clinical Practice Guidelines for Antimicrobial Prophylaxis in Surgery," *Am J Health Syst Pharm*, 2013, 70(3):195-283.

Centers for Disease Control and Prevention (CDC), "Sexually Transmitted Diseases Treatment Guidelines, 2010," *MMWR Recomm Rep*, 2010, 59(RR-12):1-110.

Martin C, Thomachot L, and Albanese J, "Clinical Pharmacokinetics of Cefotetan," *Clin Pharmacokinet*, 1994, 26(4):248-58.

Solomkin JS, Mazuski JE, Bradley JS, et al. Diagnosis and management of complicated intra-abdominal infections in adults and children: guidelines by the Surgical Infection Society and the Infectious Diseases Society of America. *Clin Infect Dis*. 2010;50(2):133-164.

◆ **Cefotetan Disodium** see CefoTEtan *on page 407*

CefOXitin (se FOKS i tin)

Medication Safety Issues

Sound-alike/look-alike issues:

CefOXitin may be confused with ceFAZolin, cefotaxime, cefoTEtan, cefTAZidime, cefTRIAXone, Cytoxan

Mefoxin may be confused with Lanoxin

Brand Names: U.S. Mefoxin

Brand Names: Canada Cefoxitin For Injection

Therapeutic Category Antibiotic, Cephalosporin (Second Generation)

Generic Availability (U.S.) May be product dependent

Use Treatment of susceptible lower respiratory tract, skin and skin structure, bone and joint, genitourinary tract, sepsis, gynecologic, and intra-abdominal infections and surgical prophylaxis (FDA approved in ages ≥3 months and adults)

Pregnancy Risk Factor B

Pregnancy Considerations Adverse events have not been observed in animal reproduction studies. Cefoxitin crosses the placenta and reaches the cord serum and amniotic fluid.

Peak serum concentrations of cefoxitin during pregnancy may be similar to or decreased compared to nonpregnant values. Maternal half-life may be shorter at term. Pregnancy-induced hypertension increases trough concentrations in the immediate postpartum period. Cefoxitin is one of the antibiotics recommended for prophylactic use prior to cesarean delivery.

Breast-Feeding Considerations Very small amounts of cefoxitin are excreted in breast milk. The manufacturer recommends that caution be exercised when administering cefoxitin to nursing women. Nondose-related effects could include modification of bowel flora. Cefoxitin pharmacokinetics may be altered immediately postpartum.

Contraindications Hypersensitivity to cefoxitin, any component, or cephalosporins; solutions containing dextrose may be contraindicated in patients with hypersensitivity to corn

Warnings High doses in children have been associated with an increased incidence of eosinophilia and elevation of serum AST. Prolonged use may result in fungal or bacterial superinfection, including *C. difficile*-associated diarrhea (CDAD) and pseudomembranous colitis; CDAD has been observed >2 months postantibiotic treatment; use with caution in patients with a history of colitis. May cause hypersensitivity reaction; patients with history of hypersensitivity reactions to other cephalosporins or penicillins may experience cross-sensitivity; use with caution in patients with a history of penicillin allergy, especially IgE-mediated reactions (eg, anaphylaxis, angioedema, urticaria).

Precautions Use with caution and modify dosage in patients with renal impairment

Adverse Reactions

Gastrointestinal: Diarrhea

Rare but important or life-threatening: Anaphylaxis, angioedema, bone marrow suppression, BUN increased, creatinine increased, dyspnea, eosinophilia, exacerbation of myasthenia gravis, exfoliative dermatitis, fever, hemolytic anemia, hypotension, interstitial nephritis, jaundice, leukopenia, nausea, nephrotoxicity (with aminoglycosides), phlebitis, prolonged PT, pruritus, pseudomembranous colitis, rash, thrombocytopenia, thrombophlebitis, toxic epidermal necrolysis, transaminases increased, urticaria, vomiting

Reactions reported with other cephalosporins: Agranulocytosis, aplastic anemia, cholestasis, colitis, erythema multiforme, hemolytic anemia, hemorrhage, pancytopenia, renal dysfunction, seizure, serum-sickness reactions, Stevens-Johnson syndrome, superinfection, toxic nephropathy, vaginitis

Drug Interactions

Metabolism/Transport Effects None known.

Avoid Concomitant Use

Avoid concomitant use of CefOXitin with any of the following: BCG

Increased Effect/Toxicity

CefOXitin may increase the levels/effects of: Aminoglycosides; Vitamin K Antagonists

The levels/effects of CefOXitin may be increased by: Probenecid

Decreased Effect

CefOXitin may decrease the levels/effects of: BCG; Sodium Picosulfate; Typhoid Vaccine

Stability Parenteral:

Vials: Store intact vials at 2°C to 25°C (36°F to 77°F); avoid exposures above 50°C. Reconstituted solution is stable for 6 hours at room temperature and for 7 days under refrigeration. When further diluted, it is stable for 24 hours at room temperature and 48 hours refrigerated.

DUPLEX container: Store unactivated container at 20°C to 25°C (68°F to 77°F); excursions permitted to 15°C to 30°C (59°F to 86°F); do not freeze. Following activation, solution is stable for 12 hours at room temperature and 7 days refrigerated.

GALAXY container (Mefoxin®): Store at or below -20°C (-4°F). Thaw at room temperature or under refrigeration; do not force thaw. Thawed solutions are stable for 24 hours at room temperature or 21 days when refrigerated; do not refreeze.

Mechanism of Action Inhibits bacterial cell wall synthesis by binding to one or more of the penicillin-binding proteins (PBPs) which in turn inhibits the final transpeptidation step of peptidoglycan synthesis in bacterial cell walls, thus inhibiting cell wall biosynthesis. Bacteria eventually lyse due to ongoing activity of cell wall autolytic enzymes (autolysins and murein hydrolases) while cell wall assembly is arrested.

Pharmacokinetics (Adult data unless noted)

Distribution: Distributes into tissues and fluids including ascitic, pleural, bile, and synovial fluids; poor penetration into CSF even with inflamed meninges

Protein binding: 65% to 79%

Half-life:

Neonates and Infants (PNA: 10-53 days): 1.4 hours (Regazzi, 1983)

Adults: 45-60 minutes, increases significantly with renal insufficiency

Time to peak serum concentration: I.M.: Within 20-30 minutes

Elimination: Urine (85% as unchanged drug)

Dosing: Neonatal General dosing; susceptible infection: Limited data available: I.V.: 90-100 mg/kg/day divided every 8 hours (Regazzi, 1983; Roos, 1980)

Dosing: Usual

Infants, Children, and Adolescents: Limited data available for infants <3 months:

General dosing, susceptible infection (*Red Book*, 2012): I.M., I.V.:

Mild-moderate infection: 80 mg/kg/day divided every 6-8 hours; maximum daily dose: 4000 mg/**day**

Severe infection: 160 mg/kg/day divided every 6 hours; maximum daily dose: 12 **g/day**

Manufacturer's labeling: Infants ≥3 months, Children, and Adolescents: 80-160 mg/kg/day divided every 4-6 hours; maximum daily dose: 12 **g/day**

Intra-abdominal infections, complicated: I.V.: 160 mg/kg/day divided every 4-6 hours; maximum daily dose: 8 **g/day** (Solomkin, 2010)

Surgical prophylaxis: I.V.:

Manufacturer's labeling: Infants ≥3 months, Children, and Adolescents: 30-40 mg/kg 30-60 minutes prior to initial incision, followed by 30-40 mg/kg every 6 hours for up to 24 hours; maximum single dose: 2000 mg

Alternate dosing (ASHP guidelines, endorsed by IDSA): Children and Adolescents: 40 mg/kg 30-60 minutes prior to surgery; may repeat in 2 hours; maximum single dose: 2000 mg [Bratzler, 2013; *Red Book* (AAP, 2012)]

Adults:

General dosing, susceptible infection: I.M., I.V.: 1000-2000 mg every 6-8 hours; maximum daily dose: 12 **g/day**; **Note:** I.M. injection is painful.

Uncomplicated infections: 1000 mg every 6-8 hours

Moderately severe to severe infections: 1000 mg every 4 hours **or** 2000 mg every 6-8 hours

Infection needing higher dosages (eg, gas gangrene): 2000 mg every 4 hours or 3000 mg every 6 hours

Pelvic inflammatory disease (Workowski, 2010; *Red Book*, 2012):

Inpatients: I.V.: 2000 mg every 6 hours **plus** doxycycline 100 mg orally every 12 hours until improved, followed by doxycycline to complete 14 days

Outpatients: I.M.: 2000 mg **plus** probenecid as a single dose, followed by doxycycline for 14 days

Surgical prophylaxis: I.M., I.V.: 2000 mg 30-60 minutes prior to surgery; may repeat in 2 hours intraoperatively (Bratzler, 2013), followed by 2000 mg every 6 hours for no more than 24 hours after surgery depending on the procedure.

Cesarean section: 2000 mg as a single dose administered as soon as the umbilical cord is clamped; may give an additional two doses at 4 and 8 hours after the initial dose.

Dosing adjustment in renal impairment:

Infants, Children, and Adolescents: The manufacturer's labeling suggests dosing modification consistent with the adult recommendations. Some clinicians have used the following guidelines (Aronoff, 2007): **Note:** Renally adjusted dose recommendations are based on doses of 20-40 mg/kg/dose every 6 hours.

GFR >50 mL/minute/1.73 m^2: No adjustment required.

GFR 30-50 mL/minute/1.73 m^2: 20-40 mg/kg/dose every 8 hours

GFR 10-29 mL/minute/1.73 m^2: 20-40 mg/kg/dose every 12 hours

GFR <10 mL/minute/1.73 m^2: 20-40 mg/kg/dose every 24 hours

Intermittent hemodialysis: Moderately dialyzable (20% to 50%): 20-40 mg/kg/dose every 24 hours

Peritoneal dialysis (PD): 20-40 mg/kg/dose every 24 hours

Continuous renal replacement therapy (CRRT): 20-40 mg/kg/dose every 8 hours

Adults: Initial loading dose of 1000-2000 mg, then:

CrCl >50 mL/minute: No adjustment required

CrCl 30-50 mL/minute: 1000-2000 mg every 8-12 hours

CrCl 10-29 mL/minute: 1000-2000 mg every 12-24 hours

CrCl 5-9 mL/minute: 500-1000 mg every 12-24 hours

CrCl <5 mL/minute: 500-1000 mg every 24-48 hours

Hemodialysis: Moderately dialyzable (20% to 50%): Loading dose of 1000-2000 mg after each hemodialysis; maintenance dose as noted above based on CrCl

Continuous arteriovenous or venovenous hemodiafiltration effects: 1000-2000 mg every 8-24 hours

Dosing adjustment in hepatic impairment: There are no dosage adjustments provided in the manufacturer's labeling.

Administration Parenteral:

IVP: Administer over 3-5 minutes at a maximum concentration of 200 mg/mL

I.V. intermittent infusion: Administer over 10-60 minutes at a final concentration not to exceed 40 mg/mL

I.M.: Deep I.M. injection into a large muscle mass such as the upper outer quadrant of the gluteus maximus. May dilute vial using SWI or 0.5% or 1% lidocaine to a final concentration of 400 mg/mL

Monitoring Parameters Renal function periodically when used in combination with other nephrotoxic drugs; liver function and hematologic function tests; number and type of stools/day for diarrhea. Observe for signs and symptoms of anaphylaxis during first dose.

Test Interactions Positive direct Coombs', false-positive urinary glucose test using cupric sulfate (Benedict's solution, Clinitest®, Fehling's solution), false-positive serum or urine creatinine with Jaffé reaction

Dosage Forms Excipient information presented when available (limited, particularly for generics); consult specific product labeling.

Solution, Intravenous:

Mefoxin: 1 g (50 mL); 2 g (50 mL)

Solution Reconstituted, Injection:

Generic: 10 g (1 ea)

Solution Reconstituted, Injection [preservative free]:

Generic: 10 g (1 ea)

Solution Reconstituted, Intravenous:

Generic: 1 g (1 ea); 2 g (1 ea)

Solution Reconstituted, Intravenous [preservative free]:

Generic: 1 g (1 ea); 2 g (1 ea)

References

American Academy of Pediatrics (AAP). In: Pickering LK, Baker CJ, Kimberlin DW, Long SS, eds. *Red Book: 2012 Report of the Committee on Infectious Diseases.* 29th ed. Elk Grove Village, IL: American Academy of Pediatrics; 2012.

Aronoff GR, Bennett WM, Berns JS, et al, *Drug Prescribing in Renal Failure: Dosing Guidelines for Adults and Children,* 5th ed, Philadelphia, PA: American College of Physicians, 2007.

Bratzler DW, Dellinger EP, Olsen KM, et al, "Clinical Practice Guidelines for Antimicrobial Prophylaxis in Surgery," *Am J Health Syst Pharm,* 2013, 70(3):195-283.

Feldman WE, Moffitt S, and Sprow N, "Clinical and Pharmacokinetic Evaluation of Parenteral Cefoxitin in Infants and Children," *Antimicrob Agents Chemother,* 1980, 17(4):669-74.

Regazzi MB, Chirico G, Cristiani D, et al, "Cefoxitin in Newborn Infants. A Clinical and Pharmacokinetic Study," *Eur J Clin Pharmacol,* 1983, 25(4):507-9.

Roos R, von Hattingberg HM, Belohradsky BH, et al. Pharmacokinetics of cefoxitin in premature and newborn infants studied by continuous serum level monitoring during combination therapy with penicillin and amikacin. *Infection.* 1980;8(6):301-306.

Solomkin JS, Mazuski JE, Bradley JS, et al, "Diagnosis and Management of Complicated Intra-Abdominal Infection in Adults and Children: Guidelines by the Surgical Infection Society and the Infectious Diseases Society of America," *Clin Infect Dis,* 2010, 50(2):133-64.

Workowski KA, Berman S, and Centers for Disease Control and Prevention (CDC), "Sexually Transmitted Diseases Treatment Guidelines, 2010," *MMWR Recomm Rep,* 2010, 59(RR-12):1-110.

◆ **Cefoxitin For Injection (Can)** see CefOXitin on page 408

◆ **Cefoxitin Sodium** see CefOXitin on page 408

Cefpodoxime (sef pode OKS eem)

Medication Safety Issues

Sound-alike/look-alike issues:

Vantin may be confused with Ventolin®

Therapeutic Category Antibiotic, Cephalosporin (Third Generation)

Generic Availability (U.S.) Yes

Use Treatment of susceptible acute, community-acquired pneumonia caused by *S. pneumoniae* or nonbeta-lactamase producing *H. influenzae* (FDA approved in ages ≥12 years and adults); alternative regimen for acute uncomplicated gonorrhea caused by *N. gonorrhoeae* (FDA approved in ages ≥12 years and adults); uncomplicated skin and skin structure infections caused by *S. aureus* or *S. pyogenes* (FDA approved in ages ≥12 years and adults); acute otitis media caused by *S. pneumoniae*, *S. pyogenes*, *H. influenzae*, or *M. catarrhalis* (FDA approved in ≥2 months to 12 years); pharyngitis or tonsillitis caused by *S. pyogenes* (FDA approved in ages ≥2 months and adults); acute maxillary sinusitis caused by *H. influenzae*, *S. pneumoniae*, and *M. catarrhalis* (FDA approved in ages ≥2 months and adults);and uncomplicated urinary tract infections caused by *E. coli*, *Klebsiella*, and *Proteus* spp. inactive against *Pseudomonas* and *Enterobacter* spp. (FDA approved in ages ≥12 years and adults)

Pregnancy Risk Factor B

Pregnancy Considerations Teratogenic events were not observed in animal reproduction studies. An increase in most types of birth defects was not found following first trimester exposure to cephalosporins.

Breast-Feeding Considerations Cefpodoxime is excreted in breast milk. The manufacturer recommends discontinuing nursing or discontinuing the medication in breast-feeding women. Nondose-related effects could include modification of bowel flora.

Contraindications Hypersensitivity to cefpodoxime, any component, or cephalosporins

Warnings Prolonged use may result in fungal or bacterial superinfection, including *C. difficile*-associated diarrhea (CDAD) and pseudomembranous colitis; CDAD has been observed >2 months postantibiotic treatment. Do not use in patients with immediate-type hypersensitivity reactions to penicillin

Suspension contains sodium benzoate; benzoic acid (benzoate) is a metabolite of benzyl alcohol; large amounts of benzyl alcohol (≥99 mg/kg/day) have been associated with a potentially fatal toxicity ("gasping syndrome") in neonates; the "gasping syndrome" consists of metabolic acidosis, respiratory distress, gasping respirations, CNS dysfunction (including convulsions, intracranial hemorrhage), hypotension and cardiovascular collapse; use suspension containing sodium benzoate with caution in neonates; *in vitro* and animal studies have shown that benzoate displaces bilirubin from protein binding sites

Precautions Use with caution in patients with history of penicillin hypersensitivity, impaired renal function, and patients with a history of colitis; modify dosage in patients with renal impairment. Some formulations contain phenylalanine and must be avoided or used with caution in patients with phenylketonuria.

Adverse Reactions

Central nervous system: Headache

Dermatologic: Diaper rash, rash

Gastrointestinal: Abdominal pain, diarrhea, nausea, vomiting

Genitourinary: Vaginal infection

Rare but important or life-threatening: Anaphylaxis, anxiety, appetite decreased, chest pain, cough, dizziness, epistaxis, eye itching, fatigue, fever, flatulence, flushing, fungal skin infection, hypotension, insomnia, malaise, nightmares, pruritus, pseudomembranous colitis, purpuric nephritis, salivation decreased, taste alteration, tinnitus, vaginal candidiasis, weakness

Reactions reported with other cephalosporins: Agranulocytosis, aplastic anemia, cholestasis, colitis, erythema multiforme, hemolytic anemia, hemorrhage, interstitial nephritis, toxic nephropathy, pancytopenia, renal dysfunction, seizure, serum-sickness reactions, Stevens-Johnson syndrome, superinfection, toxic epidermal necrolysis, urticaria, vaginitis

Drug Interactions

Metabolism/Transport Effects None known.

Avoid Concomitant Use

Avoid concomitant use of Cefpodoxime with any of the following: BCG

Increased Effect/Toxicity

Cefpodoxime may increase the levels/effects of: Aminoglycosides; Vitamin K Antagonists

The levels/effects of Cefpodoxime may be increased by: Probenecid

Decreased Effect

Cefpodoxime may decrease the levels/effects of: BCG; Sodium Picosulfate; Typhoid Vaccine

The levels/effects of Cefpodoxime may be decreased by: Antacids; H2-Antagonists

Food Interactions Food and/or low gastric pH delays absorption and may increase serum levels. Management: Take with or without food at regular intervals on an around-the-clock schedule to promote less variation in peak and trough serum levels.

Stability

Granules for suspension: Store at 20°C to 25°C (68°F to 77°F); after reconstitution, suspension may be stored in refrigerator for 14 days.

Tablet: Store at 20°C to 25°C (68°F to 77°F); protect from light.

Mechanism of Action Inhibits bacterial cell wall synthesis by binding to one or more of the penicillin-binding proteins (PBPs) which in turn inhibits the final transpeptidation step of peptidoglycan synthesis in bacterial cell walls, thus inhibiting cell wall biosynthesis. Bacteria eventually lyse due to ongoing activity of cell wall autolytic enzymes (autolysins and murein hydrolases) while cell wall assembly is arrested.

Pharmacokinetics (Adult data unless noted)

Absorption: Tablet: Enhanced in the presence of food or low gastric pH

Distribution: Good tissue penetration, including lung and tonsils; penetrates into pleural fluid; poor penetration into CSF; small amounts appear in breast milk

Protein binding: 22% to 33% (serum)

Metabolism: Following oral administration, cefpodoxime proxetil is de-esterified in the GI tract to the active metabolite, cefpodoxime

Bioavailability: Oral: 50%

Half-life: 2.2 hours (prolonged with renal impairment)

Time to peak serum concentration: Within 2-3 hours

Elimination: Primarily by the kidney with 29% to 33% of administered dose excreted unchanged in urine in 12 hours

Dosing: Usual Oral:

Infants ≥2 months and Children:

Acute otitis media: 5 mg/kg/dose every 12 hours for 5 days; maximum dose: 200 mg

Acute maxillary sinusitis: 5 mg/kg/dose every 12 hours for 10 days; maximum dose: 200 mg

Pharyngitis/tonsillitis: 5 mg/kg/dose every 12 hours for 5-10 days; maximum dose: 100 mg

Adolescents and Adults:

Acute community-acquired pneumonia and bacterial exacerbations of chronic bronchitis: 200 mg every 12 hours for 14 days and 10 days, respectively

Acute maxillary sinusitis: 200 mg every 12 hours for 10 days

Pharyngitis/tonsillitis: 100 mg every 12 hours for 5-10 days

Skin and skin structure: 400 mg every 12 hours for 7-14 days

Uncomplicated gonorrhea (male and female) and rectal gonococcal infections (female): 200 mg as a single dose

Uncomplicated urinary tract infection: 100 mg every 12 hours for 7 days

Dosing adjustment in renal impairment: CrCl <30 mL/minute: Administer every 24 hours

Hemodialysis: Administer dose 3 times/week after hemodialysis

Dosing adjustment in hepatic impairment: Not necessary in patient with cirrhosis

Administration Oral:

Tablet: Administer with food

Suspension: May administer with or without food; shake suspension well before use

Monitoring Parameters Observe patient for diarrhea; with prolonged therapy, monitor renal function periodically

Test Interactions Positive direct Coombs', false-positive urinary glucose test using cupric sulfate (Benedict's solution, Clinitest®, Fehling's solution), false-positive serum or urine creatinine with Jaffé reaction

Dosage Forms Excipient information presented when available (limited, particularly for generics); consult specific product labeling.

Suspension Reconstituted, Oral:

Generic: 50 mg/5 mL (50 mL, 100 mL); 100 mg/5 mL (50 mL, 100 mL)

Tablet, Oral:

Generic: 100 mg, 200 mg

References

Borin MT, "A Review of the Pharmacokinetics of Cefpodoxime Proxetil," *Drugs*, 1991, 42(Suppl 3):13-21.

Bradley JS, Byington CL, Shah SS, et al, "The Management of Community-Acquired Pneumonia in Infants and Children Older Than 3 Months of Age: Clinical Practice Guidelines by the Pediatric Infectious Diseases Society and the Infectious Diseases Society of America", *Clin Infect Dis*, 2011, 53(7):e25-76.

Fujii R, "Clinical Trials of Cefpodoxime Proxetil Suspension in Pediatrics," *Drugs*, 1991, 42(Suppl 3):57-60.

Mendelman PM, Del-Beccaro MA, McLinn SE, et al, "Cefpodoxime Proxetil Compared With Amoxicillin-Clavulanate for the Treatment of Otitis Media," *J Pediatr*, 1992, 121(3):459-65.

◆ **Cefpodoxime Proxetil** see Cefpodoxime on page 410

Cefprozil (sef PROE zil)

Medication Safety Issues

Sound-alike/look-alike issues:

Cefprozil may be confused with ceFAZolin, cefuroxime

Cefzil may be confused with Ceftin®

Brand Names: Canada Apo-Cefprozil®; Auro-Cefprozil; Ava-Cefprozil; Cefzil®; RAN™-Cefprozil; Sandoz-Cefprozil

Therapeutic Category Antibiotic, Cephalosporin (Second Generation)

Generic Availability (U.S.) Yes

Use Treatment of mild to moderate infections caused by susceptible organisms involving the upper respiratory tract and skin and skin structure (FDA approved in ages ≥2 years and adults); treatment of mild to moderate acute sinusitis and otitis media (FDA approved in ages ≥6 months and adults)

Pregnancy Risk Factor B

Pregnancy Considerations Adverse events were not observed in animal reproduction studies.

Breast-Feeding Considerations Small amounts of cefprozil are excreted in breast milk. The manufacturer recommends that caution be exercised when administering cefprozil to nursing women. Nondose-related effects could include modification of bowel flora.

Contraindications Hypersensitivity to cefprozil, any component, or cephalosporins

Warnings Prolonged use may result in fungal or bacterial superinfection, including C. difficile-associated diarrhea (CDAD) and pseudomembranous colitis; CDAD has been observed >2 months postantibiotic treatment; use with caution in patients with a history of colitis or gastrointestinal disease. May cause hypersensitivity reaction; patients with history of hypersensitivity reactions to other cephalosporins or pencillins may experience cross-sensitivity; use with caution in patients with a history of penicillin allergy, especially IgE-mediated reactions (eg, anaphylaxis, angioedema, urticaria). Immediate treatment for anaphylactic reaction should be available during administration.

Tablets and suspension contain polysorbate 80 (Tween 80®) which may cause allergic reactions in susceptible individuals. Oral suspension contains sodium benzoate; benzoic acid (benzoate) is a metabolite of benzyl alcohol; large amounts of benzyl alcohol (≥99 mg/kg/day) have been associated with a potentially fatal toxicity ("gasping syndrome") in neonates; use oral suspension containing sodium benzoate with caution in neonates; in vitro and animal studies have shown that benzoate displaces bilirubin from protein binding sites

Precautions Use with caution in patients with impaired renal function and in patients receiving concurrent therapy with potent diuretics; modify dosage in patients with severe renal impairment. Some products (eg, oral suspension) contain aspartame which is metabolized to phenylalanine and must be used with caution in patients with phenylketonuria.

Adverse Reactions

Central nervous system: Dizziness

Dermatologic: Diaper rash

Gastrointestinal: Abdominal pain, diarrhea, nausea, vomiting

Genitourinary: Genital pruritus, vaginitis

Hepatic: Transaminases increased

Miscellaneous: Superinfection

Rare but important or life-threatening: Anaphylaxis, angioedema, arthralgia, BUN increased, cholestatic jaundice, confusion, creatinine increased, eosinophilia, erythema multiforme, fever, headache, hyperactivity, insomnia, leukopenia, pseudomembranous colitis, rash, serum sickness, somnolence, Stevens-Johnson syndrome, thrombocytopenia, urticaria

Reactions reported with other cephalosporins: Agranulocytosis, aplastic anemia, colitis, hemolytic anemia, hemorrhage, interstitial nephritis, pancytopenia, renal dysfunction, seizure, superinfection, toxic epidermal necrolysis, toxic nephropathy, vaginitis

Drug Interactions

Metabolism/Transport Effects None known.

Avoid Concomitant Use

Avoid concomitant use of Cefprozil with any of the following: BCG

Increased Effect/Toxicity

Cefprozil may increase the levels/effects of: Aminoglycosides; Vitamin K Antagonists

The levels/effects of Cefprozil may be increased by: Probenecid

Decreased Effect

Cefprozil may decrease the levels/effects of: BCG; Sodium Picosulfate; Typhoid Vaccine

Food Interactions Food delays cefprozil absorption. Management: May administer with food.

Stability Store at 20°C to 25°C (68°F to 77°F); excursions permitted to 15°C to 30°C (59°F to 86°F). Refrigerate suspension after reconstitution; discard after 14 days.

Mechanism of Action Inhibits bacterial cell wall synthesis by binding to one or more of the penicillin-binding proteins (PBPs) which in turn inhibits the final transpeptidation step of peptidoglycan synthesis in bacterial cell walls, thus inhibiting cell wall biosynthesis. Bacteria eventually lyse due to ongoing activity of cell wall autolytic enzymes (autolysins and murein hydrolases) while cell wall assembly is arrested.

Pharmacokinetics (Adult data unless noted)

Absorption: Oral: Well absorbed

Distribution: 0.23 L/kg

Protein binding: 36%

Bioavailability: 95%

Half-life, elimination:

Infants and Children (6 months to 12 years): 1.5 hours

Adults:

Normal renal and hepatic function: 1.3 hours

Renal impairment: 5.2 hours

Renal failure: 5.9 hours

Hepatic impairment: 2 hours

Time to peak serum concentration: 1.5 hours (fasting state)

Elimination: 61% excreted unchanged in urine

Dosing: Usual

Infants, Children, and Adolescents:

General dosing, susceptible infection (*Red Book*, 2012): Oral: Mild to moderate infection: 7.5-15 mg/kg/dose twice daily; maximum single dose: 500 mg

Bronchitis, acute bacterial exacerbation or secondary bacterial infection: Adolescents: Oral: 500 mg every 12 hours for 10 days

Otitis media, acute: Infants ≥6 months and Children: Oral: 15 mg/kg/dose every 12 hours for 10 days; maximum single dose: 500 mg

Pharyngitis/tonsillitis: Oral:

Children ≥2 years: 7.5 mg/kg/dose every 12 hours for 10 days; maximum single dose: 500 mg

Adolescents: 500 mg every 24 hours for 10 days

Rhinosinusitis: Oral:

Infants ≥6 months and Children: 7.5-15 mg/kg/dose every 12 hours for 10 days; maximum single dose: 500 mg

Adolescents: 250-500 mg every 12 hours for 10 days

Skin and skin structure infection: Oral:

Children ≥2 years: 20 mg/kg/dose once daily for 10 days; maximum single dose: 500 mg

Adolescents: 250 mg every 12 hours **or** 500 mg every 12-24 hours for 10 days

Urinary tract infection: Oral: Infants and Children 2-24 months: 15 mg/kg/dose twice daily for 7-14 days (AAP, 2011)

Adults:

Bronchitis, acute bacterial exacerbation or secondary bacterial infection: Oral: 500 mg every 12 hours for 10 days

Pharyngitis/tonsillitis: Oral: 500 mg every 24 hours for 10 days

Rhinosinusitis: Oral: 250-500 mg every 12 hours for 10 days

Skin and skin structure infection, uncomplicated: Oral: 250 mg every 12 hours **or** 500 mg every 12-24 hours for 10 days

Dosing adjustment in renal impairment: All patients:
CrCl ≥30 mL/minute: No adjustment required.
CrCl <30 mL/minute: Reduce dose by 50%.

Intermittent hemodialysis: Administer after dialysis; ~55% is removed by hemodialysis. The following guidelines have been used by some clinicians (Aronoff, 2007):
Pediatric patients: Reduce dose by 50%
Adult patients: 250 mg after dialysis

Peritoneal dialysis (Aronoff, 2007): Reduce dose by 50%

Administration Oral: May administer with or without food; administer with food if stomach upset occurs; chilling improves flavor of suspension (do not freeze); shake suspension well before use

Monitoring Parameters Evaluate renal function before and during therapy; with prolonged therapy, monitor coagulation tests, CBC, and liver function tests periodically; monitor for signs of anaphylaxis during first dose.

Test Interactions Positive direct Coombs', false-positive urinary glucose test using cupric sulfate (Benedict's solution, Clinitest®, Fehling's solution), false-positive serum or urine creatinine with Jaffé reaction

Dosage Forms Excipient information presented when available (limited, particularly for generics); consult specific product labeling.

Suspension Reconstituted, Oral:
Generic: 125 mg/5 mL (50 mL, 75 mL, 100 mL); 250 mg/ 5 mL (50 mL, 75 mL, 100 mL)

Tablet, Oral:
Generic: 250 mg, 500 mg

References

American Academy of Pediatrics Subcommittee on Urinary Tract Infection, "Urinary Tract Infection: Clinical Practice Guideline for the Diagnosis and Management of the Initial UTI in Febrile Infants and Children 2 to 24 Months," *Pediatrics*, 2011, 128(3):595-610.

Arguedas AG, Zaleska M, Stutman HR, et al, "Comparative Trial of Cefprozil vs Amoxicillin Clavulanate Potassium in the Treatment of Children With Acute Otitis Media With Effusion," *Pediatr Infect Dis J*, 1991, 10(5):375-80.

Aronoff GR, Bennett WM, Berns JS, et al, *Drug Prescribing in Renal Failure: Dosing Guidelines for Adults and Children*, 5th ed. Philadelphia, PA: American College of Physicians, 2007.

Barriere SL, "Review of *In Vitro* Activity, Pharmacokinetic Characteristics, Safety, and Clinical Efficacy of Cefprozil, a New Oral Cephalosporin," *Ann Pharmacother*, 1993, 27(9):1082-9.

Bradley JS, Byington CL, Shah SS, et al, "The Management of Community-Acquired Pneumonia in Infants and Children Older Than 3 Months of Age: Clinical Practice Guidelines by the Pediatric Infectious Diseases Society and the Infectious Diseases Society of America", *Clin Infect Dis*, 2011, 53(7):e25-76.

Lowery N, Kearns GL, Young RA, et al, "Serum Sickness-Like Reactions Associated With Cefprozil Therapy," *J Pediatr*, 1994, 125 (2):325-8.

CefTAZidime (SEF tay zi deem)

Medication Safety Issues
Sound-alike/look-alike issues:
CefTAZidime may be confused with ceFAZolin, cefepime, cefoTEtan, cefOXitin, cefTRIAXone
Ceptaz may be confused with Septra

Tazicef may be confused with Tazidime

International issues:
Ceftim [Portugal] and Ceftime [Thailand] brand names for ceftazidime may be confused with Ceftin brand name for cefuroxime [U.S., Canada]; Cefiton brand name for cefixime [Portugal]

Brand Names: U.S. Fortaz; Fortaz in D_5W; Tazicef

Brand Names: Canada Ceftazidime For Injection; Fortaz

Therapeutic Category Antibiotic, Cephalosporin (Third Generation)

Generic Availability (U.S.) May be product dependent

Use Treatment of susceptible infections of the respiratory tract, urinary tract, gynecologic, skin and skin structure, intra-abdominal, osteomyelitis, sepsis, and meningitis (FDA approved in all ages); has also been used in management of febrile neutropenia and empiric therapy for febrile, granulocytopenic patients

Pregnancy Risk Factor B

Pregnancy Considerations Adverse events have not been observed in animal reproduction studies. Ceftazidime crosses the placenta and reaches the cord serum and amniotic fluid. An increase in most types of birth defects was not found following first trimester exposure to cephalosporins. Maternal peak serum concentration is unchanged in the first trimester. After the first trimester, serum concentrations decrease by approximately 50% of those in nonpregnant patients. Renal clearance is increased during pregnancy.

Breast-Feeding Considerations Very small amounts of ceftazidime are excreted in breast milk. The manufacturer recommends that caution be exercised when administering ceftazidime to nursing women. Ceftazidime in not absorbed when given orally; therefore, any medication that is distributed to human milk should not result in systemic concentrations in the nursing infant. Nondose-related effects could include modification of bowel flora.

Contraindications Hypersensitivity to ceftazidime, any component, or cephalosporins

Warnings Use with caution in patients with a history of penicillin allergy, especially IgE-mediated reactions (eg, anaphylaxis, angioedema, urticaria). Prolonged use may result in fungal or bacterial superinfection, including *C. difficile*-associated diarrhea (CDAD) and pseudomembranous colitis; CDAD has been observed >2 months postantibiotic treatment.

Elevated serum concentrations in renal insufficiency may lead to seizures, encephalopathy, coma, asterixis, neuromuscular excitability, and myoclonia; use with caution in patients with renal impairment; dose modification may be needed.

Precautions Intra-arterial administration may result in distal necrosis. Use with caution in patients previously stabilized on anticoagulant therapy; may cause alteration in prothrombin activity; risk increased in renal or hepatic impairment, poor nutritional state or prolonged course of therapy; monitor prothrombin times as necessary.

Adverse Reactions
Cardiovascular: Phlebitis

Endocrine & metabolic: Increased gamma-glutamyl transferase, increased lactate dehydrogenase

Gastrointestinal: Diarrhea

Hematologic & oncologic: Eosinophilia, positive direct Coombs test (without hemolysis), thrombocythemia

Hepatic: Increased serum alkaline phosphatase, increased serum ALT, increased serum AST

Hypersensitivity: Hypersensitivity reactions

Local: Inflammation at injection site, pain at injection site

Rare but important or life-threatening: Agranulocytosis, anaphylaxis, angioedema, asterixis, brain disease, candidiasis, *Clostridium difficile* associated diarrhea, erythema multiforme, hemolytic anemia, hyperbilirubinemia, increased lactate dehydrogenase, leukopenia, lymphocytosis, myoclonus, nausea, neuromuscular excitability, neutropenia, paresthesia, pseudomembranous colitis, renal disease (may be severe, including renal failure), renal insufficiency, seizure, skin rash, Stevens-Johnson syndrome, thrombocytopenia, toxic epidermal necrolysis, vaginitis

Drug Interactions

Metabolism/Transport Effects None known.

Avoid Concomitant Use

Avoid concomitant use of CefTAZidime with any of the following: BCG

Increased Effect/Toxicity

CefTAZidime may increase the levels/effects of: Aminoglycosides; Vitamin K Antagonists

The levels/effects of CefTAZidime may be increased by: Probenecid

Decreased Effect

CefTAZidime may decrease the levels/effects of: BCG; Sodium Picosulfate; Typhoid Vaccine

Stability

Fortaz® vials, powder for injection: Store intact vials at 15°C to 30°C (59°F to 86°F); protect from light. Reconstituted solution and solution further diluted for I.V. infusion are stable for 12 hours at room temperature, for 3 days when refrigerated, or for 12 weeks when frozen at -20°C (-4°F). After freezing, thawed solution in SWI for I.M. administration is stable for 3 hours at room temperature or 3 days when refrigerated; thawed solution in NS in a Viaflex® small volume container for I.V. administration is stable for 12 hours at room temperature or for 3 days when refrigerated; and thawed solution in SWI in the original container is stable for 8 hours at room temperature or for 3 days when refrigerated.

Fortaz® premixed solution: Store frozen below -20°C (below -4°F); once thawed, may remain at room temperature for up to 8 hours or refrigerated for up to 3 days.

Fortaz®, Tazicef®: ADD-Vantage® vials: Following dilution, may be stored for up to 12 hours at room temperature or 3 days under refrigeration. Freezing solutions in the ADD-Vantage® system is not recommended. Joined vials that have not been activated must be used within 14 days.

Tazicef® vials: Store intact vials at 20°C to 25°C (68°F to 77°F); protect from light. Reconstituted vials and solution further diluted for I.V. infusion are stable for 24 hours at room temperature, for 7 days when refrigerated, or for 12 weeks when frozen at -20°C (-4°F). When thawed, solution is stable for 8 hours at room temperature or 4 days when refrigerated.

Mechanism of Action Inhibits bacterial cell wall synthesis by binding to one or more of the penicillin-binding proteins (PBPs) which in turn inhibits the final transpeptidation step of peptidoglycan synthesis in bacterial cell walls, thus inhibiting cell wall biosynthesis. Bacteria eventually lyse due to ongoing activity of cell wall autolytic enzymes (autolysins and murein hydrolases) while cell wall assembly is arrested.

Pharmacokinetics (Adult data unless noted)

Distribution: Widely distributed throughout the body including bone, bile, skin, CSF (diffuses into CSF at higher concentrations when the meninges are inflamed), endometrium, heart, pleural and lymphatic fluids

Protein binding: <10%

Half-life:

Neonates <23 days: 2.2-4.7 hours

Adults: 1.9 hours (prolonged with renal impairment)

Time to peak serum concentration: I.M.: Within 60 minutes

Elimination: By glomerular filtration with 80% to 90% of the dose excreted as unchanged drug in urine within 24 hours

Dosing: Neonatal

General dosing, susceptible infection:

Manufacturer's labeling: I.V.: 30 mg/kg/dose every 12 hours

Alternate dosing (Red Book, 2012): I.M., I.V.:

Body weight <1 kg:

PNA ≤14 days: 50 mg/kg/dose every 12 hours; some reports use 25 mg/kg/dose every 24 hours with adequate serum concentrations in premature neonates (Low, 1985; Mulhall, 1985; van den Anker, 1995a; van den Anker, 1995)

PNA 15-28 days: 50 mg/kg/dose every 8-12 hours

Body weight 1-2 kg:

PNA ≤7 days: 50 mg/kg/dose every 12 hours

PNA 8-28 days: 50 mg/kg/dose every 8-12 hours

Body weight >2 kg:

PNA ≤7 days: 50 mg/kg/dose every 12 hours

PNA 8-28 days: 50 mg/kg/dose every 8 hours

Meningitis (Tunkel, 2004): I.V.:

PNA ≤7 days: 100-150 mg/kg/day divided every 8-12 hours

PNA >7 days: 150 mg/kg/day divided every 8 hours

Dosing: Usual

Infants, Children, and Adolescents:

General dosing, susceptible infection: I.M., I.V.:

Manufacturer's labeling: Infants and Children 1 month to 12 years: 30-50 mg/kg/dose every 8 hours; maximum daily dose: 6 g/**day**

Alternate dosing (Red Book, 2012):

Mild to moderate infections: 90-150 mg/kg/day divided every 8 hours; maximum daily dose: 3000 mg/**day**

Severe infections: 200-300 mg/kg/day divided every 8 hours; maximum daily dose: 6 g/**day**

Cystic fibrosis, lung infection caused by Pseudomonas spp: I.V.: 150-200 mg/kg/day divided every 6-8 hours, maximum daily dose: 6 g/**day**; higher doses have been used: 200-400 mg/kg/day divided every 6-8 hours; maximum daily dose: 12 g/**day** (Zobell, 2012)

Febrile neutropenia; empiric: I.V.: 50-100 mg/kg/dose every 8 hours; maximum daily dose: 6 g/**day** (Hughes, 2002); **Note:** Due to emerging resistance patterns, some centers have found empiric monotherapy is no longer reliable (Freifeld, 2011; Lehrnbecher, 2012).

Intra-abdominal infections, complicated: I.V.: 50 mg/kg/dose every 8 hours; maximum daily dose: 6 g/**day** (Solomkin, 2010)

Meningitis: I.V.: 150 mg/kg/day divided every 8 hours; maximum daily dose: 6 g/**day** (Tunkel, 2004)

Peritonitis (CAPD) (Warady, 2012): Intraperitoneal:

Intermittent: 20 mg/kg/dose every 24 hours in the long dwell

Continuous: Loading dose: 500 mg per liter of dialysate; maintenance dose: 125 mg per liter

Urinary tract infection: Infants and Children 2-24 months: I.V.: 100-150 mg/kg/day divided every 8 hours (AAP, 2011)

Adults:

Bacterial arthritis (gram-negative bacilli): I.V.: 1000-2000 mg every 8 hours

Bone and joint infections: I.V.: 2000 mg every 12 hours

Intra-abdominal infection, severe (in combination with metronidazole): I.V.: 2000 mg every 8 hours for 4-7 days (provided source controlled). Not recommended for hospital-acquired intra-abdominal infections (IAI) associated with multidrug-resistant gram-negative organisms or in mild to moderate community-acquired IAIs due to risk of toxicity and the development of resistant organisms (Solomkin, 2010).

Melioidosis: I.V.: 40 mg/kg/dose every 8 hours for 10 days, followed by oral therapy with doxycycline or TMP/SMX

Otitis externa: I.V.: 2000 mg every 8 hours

Peritonitis (CAPD):
Anuric, intermittent: 1000-1500 mg daily
Anuric, continuous (per liter exchange): Loading dose: 250 mg; maintenance dose: 125 mg

Pneumonia: I.V.:
Uncomplicated: 500-1000 mg every 8 hours
Complicated or severe: 2000 mg every 8 hours

Prosthetic joint infection, *Pseudomonas aeruginosa* **(alternative to cefepime or meropenem):** I.V.: 2000 mg every 8 hours for 4-6 weeks (consider addition of an aminoglycoside) (Osmon, 2013)

Skin and soft tissue infections: I.V., I.M.: 500-1000 mg every 8 hours

Severe infections, including meningitis, complicated pneumonia, endophthalmitis, CNS infection, osteomyelitis, gynecological, skin and soft tissue: I.V.: 2000 mg every 8 hours

Urinary tract infections: I.V., I.M.:
Uncomplicated: 250 mg every 12 hours
Complicated: 500 mg every 8-12 hours

Dosing adjustment in renal impairment:
Infants, Children, and Adolescents: The manufacturer recommends decreasing dosing frequency based on the calculated BSA adjusted creatinine clearance. The following guidelines have been used by some clinicians (Aronoff, 2007): **Note:** Renally adjusted dose recommendations are based on a usual dose of 25-50 mg/kg/dose every 8 hours:
GFR >50 mL/minute: No adjustment required
GFR 30-50 mL/minute: 50 mg/kg/dose every 12 hours
GFR 10-29 mL/minute: 50 mg/kg/dose every 24 hours
GFR ≤10 mL/minute: 50 mg/kg/dose every 48 hours
Hemodialysis: Dialyzable (50% to 100%): 50 mg/kg/dose every 48 hours, give after dialysis on dialysis days
Peritoneal dialysis: 50 mg/kg/dose every 48 hours
Continuous renal replacement therapy (CRRT): 50 mg/kg/dose every 12 hours

Adults:
CrCl >50 mL/minute: No adjustment required
CrCl 31-50 mL/minute: Administer 1000 mg every 12 hours
CrCl 16-30 mL/minute: Administer 1000 mg every 24 hours
CrCl 6-15 mL/minute: Loading dose 1000 mg, then 500 mg every 24 hours
CrCl ≤5 mL/minute: Loading dose 1000 mg, then 500 mg every 48 hours
Hemodialysis: Dialyzable (50% to 100%): Loading dose 1000 mg, then an additional 1000 mg after each dialysis period
Alternate dosing: 500-1000 mg every 24 hours **or** 1000-2000 mg every 48-72 hours (Heintz, 2009). **Note:** Dosing dependent on the assumption of 3 times per week, complete IHD sessions. Administer after hemodialysis on dialysis days.
Peritoneal dialysis: Loading dose 1000 mg, then 500 mg every 24 hours
Continuous renal replacement therapy (CRRT) (Heintz, 2009; Trotman, 2005): Drug clearance is highly dependent on the method of renal replacement, filter type, and flow rate. Appropriate dosing requires close monitoring of pharmacologic response, signs of adverse reactions due to drug accumulation, as well as drug concentrations in relation to target trough (if appropriate). The following are general recommendations only (based on dialysate flow/ultrafiltration rates of 1-2 L/hour and minimal residual renal function) and should not supersede clinical judgment:
CVVH: Loading dose of 2000 mg followed by 1000-2000 mg every 12 hours

CVVHD/CVVHDF: Loading dose of 2000 mg followed by either 1000 mg every 8 hours **or** 2000 mg every 12 hours. **Note:** Dosage of 1000 mg every 8 hours results in similar steady-state concentrations as 2000 mg every 12 hours and is more cost effective. Dosage of 2000 mg every 8 hours may be needed for gram-negative rods with MIC ≥4 mg/L (Heintz, 2009).
Note: For patients receiving CVVHDF, some recommend giving a loading dose of 2000 mg followed by 3000 mg over 24 hours as a continuous I.V. infusion to maintain concentrations ≥4 times the MIC for susceptible pathogens (Heintz, 2009).

Dosing adjustment in hepatic impairment: No adjustment required.

Administration Parenteral: Any carbon dioxide bubbles that may be present in the withdrawn solution should be expelled prior to injection
IVP: Administer over 3-5 minutes at a maximum concentration of 180 mg/mL
I.V. intermittent infusion: Administer over 15-30 minutes at a final concentration ≤40 mg/mL
I.M.: Deep I.M. injection into a large muscle mass such as the upper outer quadrant of the gluteus maximus or lateral part of the thigh. May dilute vial using SWI or 0.5% or 1% lidocaine to a final concentration of 280 mg/mL

Monitoring Parameters Renal function periodically when used in combination with aminoglycosides; with prolonged therapy also monitor hepatic and hematologic function periodically; number and type of stools/day for diarrhea. Observe for signs and symptoms of anaphylaxis during first dose. Monitor prothrombin time in patients at risk for increased INR (nutritionally deficient patients, prolonged treatment, hepatic or renal disease)

Test Interactions Positive direct Coombs', false-positive urinary glucose test using cupric sulfate (Benedict's solution, Clinitest®, Fehling's solution), false-positive serum or urine creatinine with Jaffé reaction

Dosage Forms Excipient information presented when available (limited, particularly for generics); consult specific product labeling.
Solution, Intravenous, as sodium [strength expressed as base]:
Fortaz in D₅W: 1 g (50 mL); 2 g (50 mL)
Tazicef: 1 g/50 mL (50 mL)
Solution Reconstituted, Injection:
Fortaz: 500 mg (1 ea); 1 g (1 ea); 2 g (1 ea); 6 g (1 ea)
Tazicef: 1 g (1 ea); 2 g (1 ea); 6 g (1 ea)
Generic: 1 g (1 ea); 2 g (1 ea); 6 g (1 ea); 100 g (1 ea)
Solution Reconstituted, Injection [preservative free]:
Generic: 1 g (1 ea); 2 g (1 ea); 6 g (1 ea)
Solution Reconstituted, Intravenous:
Fortaz: 1 g (1 ea); 2 g (1 ea)
Tazicef: 1 g (1 ea); 2 g (1 ea)
Generic: 1 g/50 mL (1 ea); 2 g/50 mL (1 ea)

References
American Academy of Pediatrics (AAP). In: Pickering LK, Baker CJ, Kimberlin DW, Long SS, eds. *Red Book: 2012 Report of the Committee on Infectious Diseases.* 29th ed. Elk Grove Village, IL: American Academy of Pediatrics; 2012.
American Academy of Pediatrics, "Urinary Tract Infection: Clinical Practice Guideline for the Diagnosis and Management of the Initial UTI in Febrile Infants and Children 2 to 24 Months," *Pediatrics,* 2011, 128(3):595-610.
Aronoff GR, Bennett WM, Berns JS, et al, *Drug Prescribing in Renal Failure: Dosing Guidelines for Adults and Children,* 5th ed. Philadelphia, PA: American College of Physicians; 2007.
Boccazzi A, Rizzo M, Caccamo ML, et al, "Comparison of the Concentrations of Ceftazidime in the Serum of Newborn Infants After Intravenous and Intramuscular Administration," *Antimicrob Agents Chemother,* 1980, 24(6):955-6.
Freifeld AG, Bow EJ, Sepkowitz KA, et al, "Clinical Practice Guideline for the Use of Antimicrobial Agents in Neutropenic Patients With Cancer: 2010 Update by the Infectious Diseases Society of America," *Clin Infect Dis,* 2011, 52(4):e56-93.

Heintz BH, Matzke GR, Dager WE, "Antimicrobial Dosing Concepts and Recommendations for Critically Ill Adult Patients Receiving Continuous Renal Replacement Therapy or Intermittent Hemodialysis," *Pharmacotherapy*, 2009, 29(5):562-77.

Hughes WT, Armstrong D, Bodey GP, et al, "2002 Guidelines for the Use of Antimicrobial Agents in Neutropenic Patients With Cancer," *Clin Infect Dis*, 2002, 34(6):730-51.

Lehrnbecher T, Phillips R, Alexander S, et al, "Guideline for the Management of Fever and Neutropenia in Children With Cancer and/or Undergoing Hematopoietic Stem-Cell Transplantation," *J Clin Oncol*, 2012, 30(35):4427-38.

Low DC, Bissenden JG, and Wise R, "Ceftazidime in Neonatal Infections," *Arch Dis Child*, 1985, 60(4):360-4.

McCracken GH Jr, Threlkeld N, and Thomas ML, "Pharmacokinetics of Ceftazidime in Newborn Infants," *Antimicrob Agents Chemother*, 1984, 26(4):583-4.

Mulhall A and de Louvois J, "The Pharmacokinetics and Safety of Ceftazidime in the Neonate," *J Antimicrob Chemother*, 1985, 15(1):97-103.

Osmon DR, Berbari EF, Berendt AR, et al, "Diagnosis and Management of Prosthetic Joint Infection: Clinical Practice Guideline by the Infectious Diseases Society of America," *Clin Infect Dis*, 2013, 56(1):e1-25.

Robinson DC, Cookson TL, and Grisafe JA, "Concentration Guidelines for Parenteral Antibiotics in Fluid-Restricted Patients," *Drug Intell Clin Pharm*, 1987, 21(12):985-9.

Solomkin JS, Mazuski JE, Bradley JS, et al, "Diagnosis and Management of Complicated Intra-Abdominal Infections in Adults and Children: Guidelines by the Surgical Infection Society and the Infectious Diseases Society of America," *Clin Infect Dis*, 2010, 50(2):133-64.

Tessin I, Trollfors B, Thiringer K, et al, "Concentrations of Ceftazidime, Tobramycin and Ampicillin in the Cerebrospinal Fluid of Newborn Infants," *Eur J Pediatr*, 1989, 148(7):679-81.

Trotman RL, Williamson JC, Shoemaker DM, et al, "Antibiotic Dosing in Critically Ill Adult Patients Receiving Continuous Renal Replacement Therapy," *Clin Infect Dis*, 2005, 41(8):1159-66.

van den Anker JN, Hop WC, Schoemaker RC, et al, "Ceftazidime Pharmacokinetics in Preterm Infants: Effect of Postnatal Age and Postnatal Exposure to Indomethacin," *Br J Clin Pharmacol*, 1995, 40(5):439-43.

van den Anker JN, Schoemaker RC, van der Heijden BJ, et al, "Once-Daily Versus Twice-Daily Administration of Ceftazidime in the Preterm Infant," *Antimicrob Agents Chemother*, 1995a, 39(9):2048-50.

Warady BA, Bakkaloglu S, Newland J, et al, "Consensus Guidelines for the Prevention and Treatment of Catheter-Related Infections and Peritonitis in Pediatric Patients Receiving Peritoneal Dialysis: 2012 Update," *Perit Dial Int*, 2012, 32(Suppl 2):S32-86.

Zobell JT, Waters CD, Young DC, et al, "Optimization of Anti-Pseudomonal Antibiotics for Cystic Fibrosis Pulmonary Exacerbations: II. Cephalosporins and Penicillins," *Pediatr Pulmonol*, 2013, 48(2):107-22.

◆ **Ceftazidime For Injection (Can)** *see* CefTAZidime on page 413

Ceftibuten (sef TYE byoo ten)

Medication Safety Issues
Sound-alike/look-alike issues:
Cedax® may be confused with Cidex®
International issues:
Cedax [U.S. and multiple international markets] may be confused with Codex brand name for acetaminophen/codeine [Brazil] and *Saccharomyces boulardii* [Italy]

Brand Names: U.S. Cedax

Therapeutic Category Antibiotic, Cephalosporin (Third Generation)

Generic Availability (U.S.) Yes

Use Treatment of acute exacerbations of chronic bronchitis, acute bacterial otitis media, pharyngitis/tonsillitis due to *H. influenzae* and *M. catarrhalis* (both beta-lactamase-producing and nonproducing strains), *S. pneumoniae* (penicillin-susceptible strains only), and *S. pyogenes*

Pregnancy Risk Factor B

Pregnancy Considerations Teratogenic effects were not observed in animal reproduction studies. An increase in most types of birth defects was not found following first trimester exposure to cephalosporins.

Breast-Feeding Considerations Ceftibuten was not detectable in milk after a single 200 mg dose (limit of detection: 1 mcg/mL). It is not known if it would be detectable after a 400 mg dose or multiple doses. The manufacturer recommends that caution be exercised when administering ceftibuten to nursing women. If ceftibuten does reach the human milk, nondose-related effects could include modification of bowel flora.

Contraindications Hypersensitivity to ceftibuten, any component, or cephalosporins

Warnings Prolonged use may result in superinfection. Pseudomembranous colitis has been reported with ceftibuten. Do not use in patients with immediate-type hypersensitivity reactions to penicillin. Cross hypersensitivity among beta-lactam antibiotics may occur in up to 10% of patients with penicillin allergy history.

Suspension contains sodium benzoate; benzoic acid (benzoate) is a metabolite of benzyl alcohol; large amounts of benzyl alcohol (≥99 mg/kg/day) have been associated with a potentially fatal toxicity ("gasping syndrome") in neonates; the "gasping syndrome" consists of metabolic acidosis, respiratory distress, gasping respirations, CNS dysfunction (including convulsions, intracranial hemorrhage), hypotension and cardiovascular collapse; use suspension containing sodium benzoate with caution in neonates; *in vitro* and animal studies have shown that benzoate displaces bilirubin from protein binding sites

Precautions Use with caution in patients with renal impairment, history of colitis, or in penicillin-sensitive patients; modify dosage in patients with moderate-to-severe renal impairment. May cause diarrhea, incidence is higher in younger patients (8% in patients ≤2 years; 2% in patients >2 years).

Adverse Reactions

Central nervous system: Dizziness, headache

Gastrointestinal: Abdominal pain, diarrhea, dyspepsia, loose stools, nausea, vomiting

Hematologic: Eosinophils increased, hemoglobin decreased, platelets increased

Hepatic: ALT increased, bilirubin increased

Renal: BUN increased

Rare but important or life-threatening: Agitation, alkaline phosphatase increased, anorexia, aphasia, AST increased, constipation, creatinine increased, dehydration, diaper rash, dyspnea, dysuria, eructation, fatigue, fever, flatulence, hematuria, hyperkinesia, insomnia, irritability, jaundice, leukopenia, melena, moniliasis, nasal congestion, paresthesia, platelets increased, pruritus, pseudomembranous colitis, psychosis, rash, rigors, serum-sickness reactions, somnolence, Stevens-Johnson syndrome, stridor, taste perversion, thrombocytopenia, toxic epidermal necrolysis, urticaria, vaginitis, xerostomia

Additional reactions reported with other cephalosporins: Allergic reaction, agranulocytosis, angioedema, aplastic anemia, anaphylaxis, asterixis, cholestasis, drug fever, encephalopathy, erythema multiforme, hemolytic anemia, hemorrhage, interstitial nephritis, neuromuscular excitability, neutropenia, pancytopenia, prolonged PT, renal dysfunction, seizure, superinfection, toxic nephropathy

Drug Interactions

Metabolism/Transport Effects None known.

Avoid Concomitant Use
Avoid concomitant use of Ceftibuten with any of the following: BCG

Increased Effect/Toxicity
Ceftibuten may increase the levels/effects of: Aminoglycosides; Vitamin K Antagonists

The levels/effects of Ceftibuten may be increased by: Probenecid

Decreased Effect
Ceftibuten may decrease the levels/effects of: BCG; Sodium Picosulfate; Typhoid Vaccine

The levels/effects of Ceftibuten may be decreased by: Multivitamins/Minerals (with ADEK, Folate, Iron); Multivitamins/Minerals (with AE, No Iron); Zinc Salts

Stability Store capsules and powder for oral suspension at room temperature; reconstituted suspension is stable for 14 days if refrigerated

Mechanism of Action Inhibits bacterial cell wall synthesis by binding to one or more of the penicillin-binding proteins (PBPs) which in turn inhibits the final transpeptidation step of peptidoglycan synthesis in bacterial cell walls, thus inhibiting cell wall biosynthesis. Bacteria eventually lyse due to ongoing activity of cell wall autolytic enzymes (autolysins and murein hydrolases) while cell wall assembly is arrested.

Pharmacokinetics (Adult data unless noted)
Absorption: Rapid; food decreases peak concentration and lowers AUC

Distribution: Distributes into middle ear fluid, bronchial secretions, sputum, tonsillar tissue, and blister fluid:
V_d:
Children: 0.5 L/kg
Adults: 0.21 L/kg
Protein binding: 65%
Bioavailability: 75% to 90%
Half-life:
Children: 1.9-2.5 hours
Adults: 2-3 hours; CrCl 30-49 mL/minute: 7 hours; CrCl 5-29 mL/minute: 13 hours; CrCl <5 mL/minute: 22 hours
Time to peak serum concentration: 2-3 hours
Elimination: 60% to 70% excreted unchanged in urine
Dialysis: 39% to 65% removed by a 2-4 hour hemodialysis

Dosing: Usual Oral:
Children <12 years: 9 mg/kg/day once daily for 10 days (maximum dose: 400 mg)
Children ≥12 years, Adolescents, and Adults: 400 mg once daily for 10 days

Dosing adjustment in renal impairment:
CrCl ≥50 mL/minute: No adjustment needed
CrCl 30-49 mL/minute: 4.5 mg/kg or 200 mg every 24 hours
CrCl 5-29 mL/minute: 2.25 mg/kg or 100 mg every 24 hours
Hemodialysis: Administer 9 mg/kg (maximum dose: 400 mg) after hemodialysis

Administration
Capsule: Administer without regard to food
Suspension: Shake suspension well before use. Administer 2 hours before or 1 hour after meals.

Monitoring Parameters Observe for signs and symptoms of anaphylaxis during first dose; with prolonged therapy, monitor renal, hepatic, and hematologic function periodically; number and type of stools/day for diarrhea

Test Interactions Positive direct Coombs', false-positive urinary glucose test using cupric sulfate (Benedict's solution, Clinitest®, Fehling's solution), false-positive serum or urine creatinine with Jaffé reaction

Dosage Forms Excipient information presented when available (limited, particularly for generics); consult specific product labeling.
Capsule, Oral:
Cedax: 400 mg [contains butylparaben, edetate calcium disodium, methylparaben, propylparaben]
Generic: 400 mg
Suspension Reconstituted, Oral:
Cedax: 90 mg/5 mL (60 mL, 90 mL, 120 mL) [contains polysorbate 80, sodium benzoate; cherry flavor]
Cedax: 180 mg/5 mL (30 mL, 60 mL) [contains sodium benzoate; cherry flavor]
Generic: 180 mg/5 mL (60 mL)

References

Barr WH, Affrime M, Lin CC, et al, "Pharmacokinetics of Ceftibuten in Children," *Pediatr Infect Dis J*, 1995, 14(7 Suppl):S93-101.

Bradley JS, Byington CL, Shah SS, et al, "The Management of Community-Acquired Pneumonia in Infants and Children Older Than 3 Months of Age: Clinical Practice Guidelines by the Pediatric Infectious Diseases Society and the Infectious Diseases Society of America", *Clin Infect Dis*, 2011, 53(7):e25-76.

Guay DR, "Ceftibuten: A New Expanded-Spectrum Oral Cephalosporin," *Ann Pharmacother*, 1997, 31(9):1022-33.

◆ **Ceftin** see Cefuroxime on page 422

CefTRIAXone (sef trye AKS one)

Medication Safety Issues
Sound-alike/look-alike issues:
CefTRIAXone may be confused with CeFAZolin, cefoTEtan, cefOXitin, cefTAZidime, Cetraxal
Rocephin may be confused with Roferon

Related Information
Prevention of Infective Endocarditis on page 2336

Brand Names: U.S. Rocephin

Brand Names: Canada Ceftriaxone for Injection USP; Ceftriaxone Sodium for Injection; Ceftriaxone Sodium for Injection BP

Therapeutic Category Antibiotic, Cephalosporin (Third Generation)

Generic Availability (U.S.) Yes

Use Treatment of sepsis, meningitis, infections of the lower respiratory tract, acute bacterial otitis media, skin and skin structure, bone and joint, intra-abdominal and urinary tract due to susceptible organisms (FDA approved in infants, children, adolescents, and adults); surgical prophylaxis (FDA approved in adults); documented or suspected uncomplicated gonococcal infection or pelvic inflammatory disease (FDA approved for adults)

Pregnancy Risk Factor B

Pregnancy Considerations Teratogenic effects have not been observed in animal reproduction studies. Ceftriaxone crosses the placenta and distributes to amniotic fluid. An increase in most types of birth defects was not found following first trimester exposure to cephalosporins. Pregnancy was found to influence the single dose pharmacokinetics of ceftriaxone when administered prior to delivery. The pharmacokinetics of ceftriaxone following multiple doses in the third trimester are similar to those of nonpregnant patients. Ceftriaxone is recommended for use in pregnant women for the treatment of gonococcal infections, Lyme disease, and may be used in certain situations prior to vaginal delivery in women at high risk for endocarditis (consult current guidelines).

Breast-Feeding Considerations Low concentrations of ceftriaxone are excreted in breast milk. The manufacturer recommends that caution be exercised when administering ceftriaxone to nursing women. Nondose-related effects could include modification of bowel flora.

Contraindications Hypersensitivity to ceftriaxone sodium, any component, or cephalosporins; do not use in hyperbilirubinemic neonates, particularly those who are premature since ceftriaxone is reported to displace bilirubin from albumin binding sites increasing the risk for kernicterus; do not use in neonates if they require or may require calcium-containing I.V. solutions (including parenteral nutrition solution)

Warnings Fatal reactions involving calcium-ceftriaxone precipitates in the lungs and kidneys of neonates have been reported, even when calcium-containing solutions were administered through separate sites and/or at different times. Ceftriaxone is incompatible with calcium and should not be reconstituted, admixed, or infused simultaneously with any calcium-containing solution (eg, LR, Hartmann's solution, parenteral nutrition) via a Y-site in any patient. Ceftriaxone and calcium-containing solutions may be administered sequentially in non-neonatal patients if the line is flushed thoroughly between infusions with a compatible solution.

Prolonged use may result in fungal or bacterial super-infection, including *C. difficile*-associated diarrhea (CDAD) and pseudomembranous colitis; CDAD has been observed >2 months postantibiotic treatment. Do not use in patients with immediate-type hypersensitivity reactions to penicillin. Severe cases (including some fatalities) of immune-related hemolytic anemia have been reported in patients receiving cephalosporins, including ceftriaxone; if hemolytic anemia develops, ceftriaxone should be discontinued until the etiology is identified. May be associated with increased INR (rarely), especially in nutritionally-deficient patients, prolonged treatment, and hepatic or renal disease. Secondary to biliary obstruction, pancreatitis has been reported rarely.

Precautions Use with caution in patients with gallbladder, biliary tract, liver, or pancreatic disease, or in patients with history of colitis or penicillin hypersensitivity. Abnormal gallbladder sonograms have been reported, possibly due to ceftriaxone-calcium precipitates; discontinue in patients who develop signs and symptoms of gallbladder disease. Use with caution in patients with concurrent hepatic dysfunction and significant renal disease; dosage should not exceed 2000 mg/day.

Adverse Reactions

Dermatologic: Rash

Gastrointestinal: Diarrhea

Hematologic: Eosinophilia, leukopenia, thrombocytosis

Hepatic: Transaminases increased

Local: Induration, pain, tenderness at injection site (I.V.); warmth, tightness, induration following I.M. injection; pain

Renal: BUN increased

Rare but important or life-threatening: Abdominal pain, agranulocytosis, alkaline phosphatase increased, allergic dermatitis, allergic pneumonitis, anaphylaxis, anemia, basophilia, biliary lithiasis, bilirubin increased, bronchospasm, chills, colitis, creatinine increased, diaphoresis, dizziness, dysgeusia, dyspepsia, edema, epistaxis, erythema multiforme, exanthema, fever, flatulence, flushing, gallbladder sludge, gallstones, glossitis, glycosuria, headache, hematuria, hemolytic anemia, jaundice, leukocytosis, Lyell's syndrome, lymphocytosis, lymphopenia, moniliasis, monocytosis, nausea, nephrolithiasis, neutropenia, oliguria, palpitation, pancreatitis, phlebitis, prolonged or decreased PT, pruritus, pseudomembranous colitis, renal and pulmonary ceftriaxone-calcium precipitations (neonates including some fatalities), seizure, serum sickness Stevens-Johnson syndrome, stomatitis, thrombocytopenia, toxic epidermal necrolysis, urinary casts, urticaria, vaginitis, vomiting

Reactions reported with other cephalosporins: Angioedema, allergic reaction, aplastic anemia, asterixis, cholestasis, encephalopathy, hemorrhage, hepatic dysfunction, hyperactivity (reversible), hypertonia, interstitial nephritis, LDH increased, neuromuscular excitability, pancytopenia, paresthesia, renal dysfunction, superinfection, toxic nephropathy

Drug Interactions

Metabolism/Transport Effects None known.

Avoid Concomitant Use

Avoid concomitant use of CefTRIAXone with any of the following: BCG

Increased Effect/Toxicity

CefTRIAXone may increase the levels/effects of: Aminoglycosides; Vitamin K Antagonists

The levels/effects of CefTRIAXone may be increased by: Calcium Salts (Intravenous); Probenecid; Ringer's Injection (Lactated)

Decreased Effect

CefTRIAXone may decrease the levels/effects of: BCG; Sodium Picosulfate; Typhoid Vaccine

Stability

Powder for injection: Store intact vial at ≤25°C (≤77°F). Protect from light.

Premixed solution (manufacturer premixed): Store at -20°C (-4°F); once thawed, solutions are stable for 3 days at room temperature of 25°C (77°F) or for 21 days refrigerated at 5°C (41°F). Do not refreeze.

Stability of reconstituted solutions:

10-40 mg/mL: Reconstituted in D_5W, $D_{10}W$, NS, or SWI: Stable for 2 days at room temperature of 25°C (77°F) or for 10 days when refrigerated at 4°C (39°F). Stable for 26 weeks when frozen at -20°C (-4°F) when reconstituted with D_5W or NS. Once thawed (at room temperature), solutions are stable for 2 days at room temperature of 25°C (77°F) or for 10 days when refrigerated at 4°C (39°F); does not apply to manufacturer's premixed bags. Do not refreeze.

100 mg/mL: Reconstituted in D_5W, SWI, or NS: Stable for 2 days at room temperature of 25°C (77°F) or for 10 days when refrigerated at 4°C (39°F). Reconstituted in lidocaine 1% solution or bacteriostatic water: Stable for 24 hours at room temperature of 25°C (77°F) or for 10 days when refrigerated at 4°C (39°F).

250-350 mg/mL: Reconstituted in D_5W, NS, lidocaine 1% solution, bacteriostatic water, or SWI: Stable for 24 hours at room temperature of 25°C (77°F) or for 3 days when refrigerated at 4°C (39°F).

Incompatible with calcium-containing solutions (including LR, Hartmann's solution, or parenteral nutrition); do not mix or administer ceftriaxone simultaneously with calcium-containing solutions via a Y-site.

Mechanism of Action Inhibits bacterial cell wall synthesis by binding to one or more of the penicillin-binding proteins (PBPs) which in turn inhibits the final transpeptidation step of peptidoglycan synthesis in bacterial cell walls, thus inhibiting cell wall biosynthesis. Bacteria eventually lyse due to ongoing activity of cell wall autolytic enzymes (autolysins and murein hydrolases) while cell wall assembly is arrested.

Pharmacokinetics (Adult data unless noted)

Absorption: I.M.: Complete

Distribution: Widely distributed throughout the body including gallbladder, lungs, bone, bile, CSF (diffuses into the CSF at higher concentrations when the meninges are inflamed)

V_d:

Neonates: 0.34-0.55 L/kg (Richards, 1984)

Infants and Children: 0.3-0.4 L/kg (Richards, 1984)

Adults: 6-14 L

Protein binding: 85% to 95%

Half-life:

Neonates (Martin, 1984):

1-4 days: 16 hours

9-30 days: 9 hours

Pediatric patients (age not specified): 4.1-6.6 hours (Richards, 1984)

Adults: Normal renal and hepatic function: 5-9 hours; renal impairment (mild to severe): 12-16 hours

Time to peak serum concentration: I.M.: 2-3 hours

Elimination: Unchanged in the urine (33% to 67%) by glomerular filtration and in feces via bile

Dosing: Neonatal Note: Use cefotaxime in place of ceftriaxone if hyperbilirubinemia is present or if patient is receiving calcium-containing intravenous solutions

General dosing, susceptible infection (*Red Book*, 2012): I.M., I.V.: 50 mg/kg/dose every 24 hours

Gonococcal infections (including CNS) (CDC, 2010): I.M., I.V.:
Prophylaxis: 25-50 mg/kg as a single dose; maximum single dose: 125 mg
Treatment: 25-50 mg/kg every 24 hours for 7 days, up to 10-14 days if meningitis is documented; maximum single dose: 125 mg

Meningitis, non-gonoccocal: Limited data available, dose not established: **Note:** In neonates, current IDSA guidelines suggest cefotaxime as the preferred nonpseudomonal third-generation cephalosporin; no ceftriaxone dosing is provided in the guidelines (Tunkel, 2004). Dosing based on an open-label prospective trial of 71 patients (age range: PNA 14 days to 15 years) which included 26 patients diagnosed with meningitis and a pharmacokinetic analysis of 20 neonates and infants (n=12 neonates; including six with PNA <14 days) with sepsis or meningitis; both trials reported adequate CSF penetration and favorable response (Martin, 1984; Yogev, 1986). I.V.:
PNA <14 days: 50 mg/kg/dose once daily
PNA ≥14 days: 100 mg/kg for one dose, followed by 80-100 mg/kg/dose once daily

Ophthalmia neonatorum, treatment: I.M., I.V.: 25-50 mg/kg as a single dose; maximum single dose: 125 mg (CDC, 2010; Red Book, 2012)

Dosing: Usual
Infants, Children, and Adolescents:
General dosing, susceptible infection: I.M., I.V.:
Mild to moderate infection: 50-75 mg/kg/dose once daily; maximum single dose: 1000 mg (Red Book, 2012)
Severe infection:
AAP recommendation (Red Book, 2012): 100 mg/kg/day divided every 12-24 hours
Manufacturer labeling (non-CNS): 50-75 mg/kg/day divided every 12 hours; maximum daily dose: 2000 mg/**day**
Chancroid: I.M.: 50 mg/kg as a single dose; maximum single dose: 250 mg (Red Book, 2012)
Endocarditis, bacterial: I.M., I.V.:
Prophylaxis: 50 mg/kg as a single dose; maximum single dose: 1000 mg (Red Book, 2012; Wilson, 2007)
Treatment (Baddour, 2005):
Enterococcal endocarditis (native or prosthetic valve): 100 mg/kg/day divided every 12 hours plus ampicillin for at least 8 weeks
HACEK microorganisms: 100 mg/kg once daily for 4 weeks
Viridans group streptococci and Streptococcus bovis (highly penicillin susceptible):
Native valve: 100 mg/kg once daily for 4 weeks or 2 weeks if given with gentamicin
Prosthetic valve: 100 mg/kg once daily for 6 weeks with 2 weeks of gentamicin
Viridans group streptococci and Streptococcus bovis (relatively resistant): Native valve: 100 mg/kg once daily for 4 weeks with 2 weeks of gentamicin
Note: American Heart Association (AHA) guidelines now recommend prophylaxis only in patients undergoing invasive procedures and in whom underlying cardiac conditions may predispose to a higher risk of adverse outcomes should infection occur. As of April 2007, routine prophylaxis for GI/GU procedures is no longer recommended by the AHA.
Enteric infection, bacteria, empiric therapy pending diagnostic studies (HIV-exposed/-positive): Adolescents: I.V.: 1000 mg every 24 hours (DHHS [adult], 2013)
Gonococcal infections:
Epididymitis, acute: I.M.: 250 mg in a single dose

Uncomplicated cervicitis, pharyngitis, proctitis, urethritis, and vulvovaginitis: Treatment and prophylaxis: **Note:** Due to increasing resistance, coadminister with azithromycin, erythromycin, or doxycycline (if ≥8 years) (Red Book, 2012): I.M.:
<45 kg: 125 mg as a single dose (CDC, 2010)
≥45 kg: 250 mg as a single dose (CDC, 2010; CDC, 2012)
Complicated: I.M., I.V.:
<45 kg (Red Book, 2012):
Disseminated infection: 50 mg/kg once daily for 7 days; maximum single dose: 1000 mg
Conjunctivitis: 50 mg/kg as a single dose; maximum single dose: 1000 mg
Meningitis or endocarditis: 50 mg/kg/day divided every 12 hours for 10-14 days (meningitis) or for 28 days (endocarditis); maximum daily dose: 2000 mg/**day**
≥45 kg (CDC, 2010):
Disseminated infection: 1000 mg once daily for 7 days
Meningitis: 1000-2000 mg every 12 hours for 10-14 days
Endocarditis: 1000-2000 mg every 12 hours for 28 days
Conjunctivitis: I.M.: 1000 mg in a single dose

Intra-abdominal infection, complicated: I.M., I.V.: 50-75 mg/kg/day divided every 12-24 hours; maximum daily dose: 2000 mg/**day** (Solomkin, 2010)

Lyme disease, neurologic involvement, persistent/ recurrent arthritis, heart block, or carditis: I.M., I.V.: 50-75 mg/kg once daily; maximum single dose: 2000 mg; duration dependent on symptoms and response (Halperin, 2007; Red Book, 2012; Wormser, 2006)

Meningitis: I.M., I.V.: Loading dose of 100 mg/kg may be administered at the start of therapy
Manufacturer labeling: 100 mg/kg/day divided every 12-24 hours for 7-14 days; maximum daily dose: 4000 mg/**day**
IDSA guidelines (Tunkel, 2004): 80-100 mg/kg/day divided every 12-24 hours; maximum daily dose: 4000 mg/**day**

Meningococcal infection, chemoprophylaxis for high-risk contacts (close exposure to patients with invasive meningococcal disease) (Red Book, 2012):
<15 years: I.M.: 125 mg in a single dose
≥15 years: I.M.: 250 mg in a single dose

Otitis media (AAP guidelines; Lieberthal, 2013):
Acute bacterial: I.M.: 50 mg/kg in a single dose; maximum single dose: 1000 mg
Persistent or relapsing: I.M., I.V.: 50 mg/kg once daily for 3 days; maximum single dose: 1000 mg

Peritonitis, prophylaxis for patients receiving peritoneal dialysis who require dental procedures: I.M., I.V.: 50 mg/kg administered 30-60 minutes before dental procedure; maximum dose: 1000 mg (Warady, 2012)

Pneumonia:
Bacterial pneumonia (HIV-exposed/-positive): I.V.: 50-100 mg/kg/day divided every 12-24 hours; maximum daily dose: 4000 mg/**day** (DHHS [adult and pediatric], 2013)
Community-acquired (CAP): (IDSA/PIDS [Bradley, 2011]): Infants >3 months, Children, and Adolescents: I.V.: 50-100 mg/kg/day divided every 12-24 hours; maximum daily dose 2000 mg/**day**. **Note:** May consider addition of vancomycin or clindamycin to empiric therapy if community-acquired MRSA suspected. Use the higher end of the range for penicillin-resistant S. pneumoniae; in children ≥5 years, a macrolide antibiotic should be added if atypical pneumonia cannot be ruled out; preferred in patients not fully immunized for H. influenzae type b and S. pneumoniae, or

significant local resistance to penicillin in invasive pneumococcal strains

Prophylaxis against sexually transmitted diseases following sexual assault (CDC, 2010):

≤45 kg: I.M.: 125 mg in a single dose (in combination with azithromycin and metronidazole)

>45 kg: I.M., I.V.: 250 mg in a single dose (in combination with azithromycin and metronidazole)

Rhinosinusitis, acute bacterial:

Ambulatory patients: Children and Adolescents: I.M., I.V.: 50 mg/kg as a single dose; maximum dose: 1000 mg; use for patients who are unable to tolerate oral medication, or unlikely to be adherent to the initial doses of antibiotic (Wald, 2013)

Severe infection requiring hospitalization: I.M., I.V.: 50 mg/kg/day divided every 12 hours for 10-14 days; maximum daily dose: 2000 mg/**day** (Chow, 2012)

Salmonellosis: Note: Salmonella in healthy patients typically does not require antibiotic treatment as it generally resolves in 5-7 days (CDC, 2013)

Infants <6 months of age or who have severe infection, prostheses, valvular heart disease, severe atherosclerosis, malignancy, or uremia: Non-*typhi* species diarrhea: I.M., I.V.: 100 mg/kg/day divided every 12-24 hours for 14 days; or longer if relapsing. **Note:** Not recommended for routine use (Guerrant, 2001).

HIV-exposed/-positive: Adolescents: I.V.: 1000 mg every 24 hours; duration dependent upon CD4 counts and presence of bacteremia (DHHS [adult], 2013)

If CD4 count ≥200 cells/mm^3: 7-14 days; if bacteremia present: At least 14 days or longer for complicated cases

If CD4 count <200 cells/mm^3: 2-6 weeks

Shigellosis: I.M., I.V.: 50-100 mg/kg once daily; usual duration 5 days; may shorten duration to 2 days if clinical response good and no extraintestinal involvement (*Red Book*, 2012; WHO, 2005)

Skin/skin structure infections: I.M., I.V.: 50-75 mg/kg/day in 1-2 divided doses; maximum daily dose: 2000 mg/**day**

***S. pneumoniae* infection, invasive** (*Red Book*, 2012): I.V.:

CNS infection: 100 mg/kg/day divided every 12-24 hours

Non-CNS infection: 50-75 mg/kg/day divided every 12-24 hours

Surgical prophylaxis: Children and Adolescents: I.V.: 50-75 mg/kg as a single dose; maximum single dose: 2000 mg (Bratzler, 2013)

Syphilis: Note: Not considered first-line therapy and use should be reserved for special circumstances with close monitoring and follow-up: I.M., I.V.:

Congenital syphilis; treatment: Infants >30 days: 75-100 mg/kg once daily for 10-14 days (CDC, 2010); **Note:** There is insufficient data regarding the use of ceftriaxone for treatment of congenital syphilis (penicillin is recommended); use should be reserved for situations of penicillin shortage

Postexposure prophylaxis (HIV-exposed/-positive): Adolescents: 1000 mg once daily for 8-10 days (DHHS [adult], 2013)

Treatment:

Early syphilis (independent of HIV status): Adolescents: 1000 mg once daily for 10-14 days; optimal dose and duration have not been defined (CDC, 2010)

Neurosyphillis, otic, ocular disease (HIV-exposed/-positive; penicillin-allergic): Adolescents: 2000 mg once daily for 10-14 days. **Note:** Penicillin desensitization is the preferred approach; use should be reserved when desensitization is not feasible (DHHS [adult], 2013).

Typhoid fever: I.V.: 80 mg/kg once daily for 14 days (Stephens, 2002)

Urinary tract infections: I.M., I.V.:

Infants and Children 2-24 months: 50-75 mg/kg once daily (AAP, 2011; Bradley, 2012)

Children >24 months and Adolescents: 50 mg/kg once daily; maximum single dose: 2000 mg (Bradley, 2012)

Adults:

General dosage, susceptible infection: I.M., I.V.: 1000-2000 mg every 12-24 hours, depending on the type and severity of infection; maximum daily dose: 4000 mg/**day**

Chancroid: I.M.: 250 mg as single dose (CDC, 2010)

Cholecystitis, mild to moderate: I.M., I.V.: 1000-2000 mg every 12-24 hours for 4-7 days (provided source controlled)

Gonococcal infections (CDC, 2010; CDC, 2012):

Conjunctivitis, complicated: I.M., I.V.: 1000 mg in a single dose

Disseminated: I.M., I.V.: 1000 mg once daily for 24-48 hours; may switch to cefixime (after improvement noted) to complete a total of 7 days of therapy

Endocarditis: I.M., I.V.: 1000-2000 mg every 12 hours for at least 28 days

Epididymitis, acute: I.M.: 250 mg in a single dose with doxycycline

Meningitis: I.M., I.V.: 1000-2000 mg every 12 hours for 10-14 days

Uncomplicated cervicitis, pharyngitis, urethritis: I.M.: 250 mg in a single dose with azithromycin (preferred) or doxycycline

Infective endocarditis: I.M., I.V.:

Native valve: 2000 mg once daily for 2-4 weeks; **Note:** If using 2-week regimen, concurrent gentamicin is recommended

Prosthetic valve: 2000 mg once daily for 6 weeks [with or without 2 weeks of gentamicin (dependent on penicillin MIC)]; **Note:** For HACEK organisms, duration of therapy is 4 weeks

Enterococcus faecalis (resistant to penicillin, aminoglycoside, and vancomycin), native or prosthetic valve: 2000 mg twice daily for ≥8 weeks administered concurrently with ampicillin

Prophylaxis: 1000 mg 30-60 minutes before procedure. Intramuscular injections should be avoided in patients who are receiving anticoagulant therapy. In these circumstances, orally administered regimens should be given whenever possible. Intravenously administered antibiotics should be used for patients who are unable to tolerate or absorb oral medications.

Note: American Heart Association (AHA) guidelines now recommend prophylaxis only in patients undergoing invasive procedures and in whom underlying cardiac conditions may predispose to a higher risk of adverse outcomes should infection occur. As of April 2007, routine prophylaxis for GI/GU procedures is no longer recommended by the AHA.

Intra-abdominal infection, complicated, community-acquired, mild to moderate (in combination with metronidazole): I.M., I.V.: 1000-2000 mg every 12-24 hours for 4-7 days (provided source controlled)

Lyme disease: I.V.: 2000 mg once daily for 14-28 days

Meningitis: I.V.: 2000 mg every 12 hours for 7-14 days (longer courses may be necessary for selected organisms)

Meningococcal infection, chemoprophylaxis for high-risk contacts (close exposure to patients with invasive meningococcal disease): I.M.: 250 mg in a single dose

Pelvic inflammatory disease: I.M.: 250 mg in a single dose plus doxycycline (with or without metronidazole) (CDC, 2010)

Pneumonia, community-acquired: I.V.: 1000 mg once daily, usually in combination with a macrolide; consider 2000 mg/day for patients at risk for more severe infection and/or resistant organisms (ICU status, age >65 years, disseminated infection)

Prophylaxis against sexually transmitted diseases following sexual assault: I.M.: 250 mg as a single dose (in combination with azithromycin and metronidazole) (CDC, 2010)

Pyelonephritis (acute, uncomplicated): Females: I.V.: 1000-2000 mg once daily (Stamm, 1993). Many physicians administer a single parenteral dose before initiating oral therapy (Warren, 1999).

Rhinosinusitis, acute bacterial, severe infection requiring hospitalization: I.V.: 1000-2000 mg every 12-24 hours for 5-7 days (Chow, 2012)

Surgical prophylaxis: I.V.: 1000 mg 30 minutes to 2 hours before surgery

Cholecystectomy: 1000-2000 mg every 12-24 hours, discontinue within 24 hours unless infection outside gallbladder suspected

Syphilis: I.M., I.V.: 1000 mg once daily for 10-14 days; **Note:** Alternative treatment for early syphilis, optimal dose, and duration have not been defined (CDC, 2010)

Dosage adjustment in renal impairment: No dosage adjustment is generally necessary in renal impairment; **Note:** Concurrent renal and hepatic dysfunction: Adult maximum daily dose: ≤2000 mg/day

Poorly dialyzed; no supplemental dose or dosage adjustment necessary, including patients on intermittent hemodialysis, peritoneal dialysis, or continuous renal replacement therapy (eg, CVVHD).

Dosage adjustment in hepatic impairment: No adjustment is generally necessary in hepatic impairment; **Note:** Concurrent renal and hepatic dysfunction: Adult maximum daily dose: ≤2000 mg/day

Administration Parenteral: Do not reconstitute or coadminister with calcium-containing solutions.

IVP: Administration over 2-4 minutes at a maximum concentration of 40-100 mg/mL has been reported in pediatric patients >11 years and adults primarily in the outpatient setting (Baumgartner, 1983; Garrelts, 1988; Poole, 1999) and over 5 minutes in pediatric patients ages newborn to 15 years with meningitis (Grubbauer, 1990; Martin, 1984). Rapid IVP injection over 5 minutes of a 2000 mg dose resulted in tachycardia, restlessness, diaphoresis, and palpitations in an adult patient (Lossos, 1994). I.V. push administration in young infants may also have been a contributing factor in risk of cardiopulmonary events occurring from interactions between ceftriaxone and calcium (Bradley, 2009).

I.V. intermittent infusion: Administer over 30 minutes; shorter infusion times (15 minutes) have been reported (Yogev, 1986); final concentration for I.V. infusion administration should not exceed 40 mg/mL

I.M. injection: May be diluted with SWI or 1% lidocaine to a final concentration of 250-350 mg/mL; administer I.M. injections deep into a large muscle mass

Monitoring Parameters CBC with differential, platelet count, PT, renal and hepatic function tests periodically; number and type of stools/day for diarrhea; observe for signs and symptoms of anaphylaxis

Test Interactions Positive direct Coombs', false-positive urinary glucose test using cupric sulfate (Benedict's solution, Clinitest®, Fehling's solution), false-positive serum or urine creatinine with Jaffé reaction

Additional Information Rocephin® contains 3.6 mEq sodium per gram of ceftriaxone.

Dosage Forms Excipient information presented when available (limited, particularly for generics); consult specific product labeling.

Solution, Intravenous:
Generic: 20 mg/mL (50 mL); 40 mg/mL (50 mL)

Solution Reconstituted, Injection:
Rocephin: 500 mg (1 ea); 1 g (1 ea)
Generic: 250 mg (1 ea); 500 mg (1 ea); 1 g (1 ea); 2 g (1 ea)

Solution Reconstituted, Intravenous:
Generic: 1 g (1 ea); 2 g (1 ea); 10 g (1 ea)

References

American Academy of Pediatrics (AAP). In: Pickering LK, Baker CJ, Kimberlin DW, Long SS, eds. Red Book: 2012 Report of the Committee on Infectious Diseases. 29th ed. Elk Grove Village, IL: American Academy of Pediatrics; 2012.

American Academy of Pediatrics, "Urinary Tract Infection: Clinical Practice Guideline for the Diagnosis and Management of the Initial UTI in Febrile Infants and Children 2 to 24 Months," Pediatrics, 2011, 128(3):595-610.

Baddour LM, Wilson WR, Bayer AS, et al, "Infective Endocarditis. Diagnosis, Antimicrobial Therapy, and Management of Complications: A Statement for Healthcare Professionals From the Committee on Rheumatic Fever, Endocarditis, and Kawasaki Disease, Council on Cardiovascular Disease in the Young, and the Councils on Clinical Cardiology, Stroke, and Cardiovascular Surgery and Anesthesia, American Heart Association - Executive Summary: Endorsed by the Infectious Diseases Society of America," Circulation, 2005, 111:3167-184.

Bradley JS, Byington CL, Shah SS, et al, "The Management of Community-Acquired Pneumonia in Infants and Children Older Than 3 Months of Age: Clinical Practice Guidelines by the Pediatric Infectious Diseases Society and the Infectious Diseases Society of America", Clin Infect Dis, 2011, 53(7):e25-76.

Bradley JS, Compogiannis LS, Murray WE, et al, "Pharmacokinetics and Safety of Intramuscular Injection of Concentrated Ceftriaxone in Children," Clin Pharm, 1992, 11(11):961-4.

Bradley JS, Nelson JD, Kimberlin DK, et al, eds. Nelson's Pocket Book of Pediatric Antimicrobial Therapy. 19th ed. Philadelphia, PA: Lippincott Williams & Wilkins; 2012.

Bradley JS, Wassel RT, Lee L, et al, "Intravenous Ceftriaxone and Calcium in the Neonate: Assessing the Risk for Cardiopulmonary Adverse Events," Pediatrics, 2009, 123(4):e609-13.

Bratzler DW, Dellinger EP, Olsen KM, et al, "Clinical Practice Guidelines for Antimicrobial Prophylaxis in Surgery," Am J Health Syst Pharm, 2013, 70(3):195-283.

Centers for Disease Control and Prevention (CDC). Salmonella, diagnosis and treatment. Availabel at http://www.cdc.gov/salmonella/general/diagnosis.html

Centers for Disease Control and Prevention (CDC), "Sexually Transmitted Diseases Treatment Guidelines, 2010, Gonococcal Infections," 2010.

Centers for Disease Control and Prevention (CDC), "Update to CDC's Sexually Transmitted Diseases Treatment Guidelines, 2010: Oral Cephalosporins No Longer a Recommended Treatment for Gonococcal Infections", MMWR Morb Mortal Wkly Rep, 2012, 61(31):590-4.

Chow AW, Benninger MS, Brook I, et al, "IDSA Clinical Practice Guideline for Acute Bacterial Rhinosinusitis in Children and Adults," Clin Infect Dis, 2012, 54(8):e72-112.

DHHS. Guidelines for the prevention and treatment of opportunistic infections among HIV-exposed and HIV-infected children: recommendations from the National Institutes of Health, Centers for Disease Control and Prevention, the HIV Medicine Association of the Infectious Diseases Society of America, the Pediatric Infectious Diseases Society, and the American Academy of Pediatrics. November 6, 2013. Available at http://aidsinfo.nih.gov

DHHS Panel on Opportunistic Infections (OI) in HIV-Infected Adults and Adolescents, "Guidelines for Prevention and Treatment of Opportunistic Infections in HIV-Infected Adults and Adolescents: Recommendations from the Centers for Disease Control and Prevention (CDC), the National Institutes of Health (NIH), and the HIV Medicine Association (HIVMA) of the Infectious Diseases Society of America (IDSA)," May 7, 2013. Available at http://aidsinfo.nih.gov/contentfiles/lvguidelines/adult_oi.pdf

Frenck RW Jr, Nakhla I, Sultan Y, et al, "Azithromycin Versus Ceftriaxone for the Treatment of Uncomplicated Typhoid Fever in Children," Clin Infect Dis, 2000, 31(5):1134-8.

Garrelts JC, Ast D, LaRocca J, et al, "Postinfusion Phlebitis After Intravenous Push Versus Intravenous Piggyback Administration of Antimicrobial Agents," Clin Pharm, 1988, 7(10):760-5.

Grubbauer HM, Dornbusch HJ, Dittrich P, et al, "Ceftriaxone Monotherapy for Bacterial Meningitis in Children," Chemotherapy, 1990, 36 (6):441-7.

Guerrant RL, Van Gilder T, Steiner TS, et al, "Practice Guidelines for the Management of Infectious Diarrhea," Clin Infect Dis, 2001, 32 (3):331-51.

Halperin JJ, Shapiro ED, Logigian E, et al, "Practice Parameter: Treatment of Nervous System Lyme Disease (an Evidence-Based Review): Report of the Quality Standards Subcommittee of the American Academy of Neurology," Neurology, 2007, 69(1):91-102.

Lieberthal AS, Carroll AE, Chonmaitree T, et al, "The Diagnosis and Management of Acute Otitis Media," *Pediatrics*, 2013, 131(3): e964-99.

Lossos IS and Lossos A, "Hazards of Rapid Administration of Ceftriaxone," *Ann Pharmacother*, 1994, 28(6):807-8.

Martin E, Koup JR, Paravicini U, et al, "Pharmacokinetics of Ceftriaxone in Neonates and Infants With Meningitis," *J Pediatr*, 1984, 105 (3):475-81.

Poole SM, Nowobilski-Vasilios A, and Free F, "Intravenous Push Medications in the Home," *J Intraven Nurs*, 1999, 22(4):209-15.

Richards DM, Heel RC, Brogden RN, et al, "Ceftriaxone: A Review of Its Antibacterial Activity, Pharmacological Properties and Therapeutic Use," *Drugs*, 1984, 27(6):469-527.

Solomkin JS, Mazuski JE, Bradley JS, et al, "Diagnosis and Management of Complicated Intra-Abdominal Infections in Adults and Children: Guidelines by the Surgical Infection Society and the Infectious Diseases Society of America," *Clin Infect Dis*, 2010, 15;50(2):133-64.

Stamm WE, Hooton TM, "Management of Urinary Tract Infections in Adults," *N Engl J Med*, 1993, 329(18):1328-34.

Stephens I and Levine MM, "Management of Typhoid Fever in Children," *Pediatr Infect Dis J*, 2002, 21(2):157-8.

Tunkel AR, Hartman BJ, Kaplan SL, et al, "Practice Guidelines for the Management of Bacterial Meningitis," *Clin Infect Dis*, 2004, 39 (9):1267-84.

Wald ER, Applegate KE, Bordley C, et.al. Clinical practice guideline for the diagnosis and management of acute bacterial sinusitis in children aged 1-18 years. *Pediatrics*. 2013;132:e262-280.

Warady BA, Bakkaloglu S, Newland J, et al, "Consensus Guidelines for the Prevention and Treatment of Catheter-Related Infections and Peritonitis in Pediatric Patients Receiving Peritoneal Dialysis: 2012 Update," *Perit Dial Int*, 2012, 32(Suppl 2):S32-86.

Warren JW, Abrutyn E, Hebel JR, et al, "Guidelines for Antimicrobial Treatment of Uncomplicated Acute Bacterial Cystitis and Acute Pyelonephritis in Women," *Clin Infect Dis*, 1999, 29(4):745-58.

Wilson W, Taubert KA, Gewitz M, et al, "Prevention of Infective Endocarditis. Guidelines From the American Heart Association. A Guideline From the American Heart Association Rheumatic Fever, Endocarditis, and Kawasaki Disease Committee, Council on Cardiovascular Disease in the Young, and the Council on Clinical Cardiology, Council on Cardiovascular Surgery and Anesthesia, and the Quality of Care and Outcomes Research Interdisciplinary Working Group," *Circulation*, 2007, 115.

World Health Organization (WHO), "Guidelines for the Control of Shigellosis, Including Epidemics Due to *Shigella dysenteriae* Type 1," 2005. Available at http://whqlibdoc.who.int/publications/2005/9241592330.pdf

Wormser GP, Dattwyler RJ, Shapiro ED, et al, "The Clinical Assessment, Treatment, and Prevention of Lyme Disease, Human Granulocytic Anaplasmosis, and Babesiosis: Clinical Practice Guidelines by the Infectious Diseases Society of America," *Clin Infect Dis*, 2006, 43 (9):1089-134.

Yogev R, Shulman ST, Chadwick EG, et al, "Once Daily Ceftriaxone for Central Nervous System Infections and Other Serious Pediatric Infections," *Pediatr Infect Dis*, 1986, 5(3):298-303.

◆ **Ceftriaxone for Injection USP (Can)** *see* CefTRIAXone *on page 417*

◆ **Ceftriaxone Sodium** *see* CefTRIAXone *on page 417*

◆ **Ceftriaxone Sodium for Injection (Can)** *see* CefTRIAXone *on page 417*

◆ **Ceftriaxone Sodium for Injection BP (Can)** *see* CefTRIAXone *on page 417*

Cefuroxime (se fyoor OKS eem)

Medication Safety Issues

Sound-alike/look-alike issues:
Cefuroxime may be confused with cefotaxime, cefprozil, deferoxamine

Ceftin may be confused with Cefzil, Cipro

Zinacef may be confused with Zithromax

International issues:
Ceftin [U.S., Canada] may be confused with Cefiton brand name for cefixime [Portugal]; Ceftim brand name for ceftazidime [Portugal]; Ceftime brand name for ceftazidime [Thailand]

Related Information
Oral Medications That Should Not Be Crushed or Altered *on page 2438*

Brand Names: U.S. Ceftin; Zinacef; Zinacef in Sterile Water

Brand Names: Canada Apo-Cefuroxime; Auro-Cefuroxime; Ceftin; Cefuroxime For Injection; Cefuroxime For Injection, USP; PRO-Cefuroxime; ratio-Cefuroxime

Therapeutic Category Antibiotic, Cephalosporin (Second Generation)

Generic Availability (U.S.) May be product dependent

Use
Oral suspension: Treatment of mild to moderate susceptible infections including pharyngitis/tonsillitis, acute bacterial maxillary sinusitis, acute bacterial otitis media, and impetigo (FDA approved in ages 3 months to 12 years)

Oral tablet: Treatment of mild to moderate susceptible infections involving the upper and lower respiratory tract, otitis media, acute bacterial maxillary sinusitis, urinary tract (uncomplicated), skin and soft tissue (uncomplicated), urethral and endocervical gonorrhea (uncomplicated), and early Lyme disease [FDA approved in pediatric patients (age not specified) and adults]

Parenteral: Treatment susceptible infections involving the upper and lower respiratory tract, urinary tract, skin and skin structure, sepsis, uncomplicated and disseminated gonorrhea, and bone and joints (FDA approved in ages ≥3 months and adults); surgical prophylaxis (FDA approved in adults)

Pregnancy Risk Factor B

Pregnancy Considerations Adverse events were not observed in animal reproduction studies. Cefuroxime crosses the placenta and reaches the cord serum and amniotic fluid. Placental transfer is decreased in the presence of oligohydramnios. Several studies have failed to identify an increased teratogenic risk to the fetus following maternal cefuroxime use.

During pregnancy, mean plasma concentrations of cefuroxime are 50% lower, the AUC is 25% lower, and the plasma half-life is shorter than nonpregnant values. At term, plasma half-life is similar to nonpregnant values and peak maternal concentrations after I.M. administration are slightly decreased. Pregnancy does not alter the volume of distribution. Cefuroxime is one of the antibiotics recommended for prophylactic use prior to cesarean delivery.

Breast-Feeding Considerations Cefuroxime is excreted in breast milk. Manufacturer recommendations vary; caution is recommended if cefuroxime I.V. is given to a nursing woman and it is recommended to consider discontinuing nursing temporarily during treatment following oral cefuroxime. Nondose-related effects could include modification of bowel flora.

Contraindications Hypersensitivity to cefuroxime, any component, or cephalosporins

Warnings Prolonged use may result in fungal or bacterial superinfection, including *C. difficile*-associated diarrhea (CDAD) and pseudomembranous colitis; CDAD has been observed >2 months postantibiotic treatment; use with caution in patients with a history of colitis. May cause hypersensitivity reaction; patients with history of hypersensitivity reactions to other cephalosporins or penicillins may experience cross-sensitivity; use with caution in patients with a history of penicillin allergy, especially IgE-mediated reactions (eg, anaphylaxis, angioedema, urticaria). Patients with renal or hepatic impairment, poor nutritional state, patients previously stabilized on anticoagulant therapy, or who have received a prolonged course of antimicrobial therapy are at risk for developing a fall in prothrombin activity. Monitor prothrombin time and consider administering vitamin K if indicated. Safety and efficacy in infants <3 months of age have not been established. Cefuroxime tablets and oral suspension are not bioequivalent; do not substitute. Cefuroxime tablets contain sodium benzoate; benzoic acid (benzoate) is a metabolite of benzyl alcohol; which may cause allergic reactions in susceptible individuals.

Precautions Use with caution and modify dosage in patients with renal impairment; use with caution in patients receiving concurrent treatment with potent diuretics; may adversely affect renal function. The oral suspension contains aspartame which is metabolized to phenylalanine and must be avoided (or used with caution) in patients with phenylketonuria.

Adverse Reactions
Dermatologic: Diaper rash

Endocrine & metabolic: Alkaline phosphatase increased, lactate dehydrogenase increased

Gastrointestinal: Diarrhea (duration-dependent), nausea/vomiting

Genitourinary: Vaginitis

Hematologic: Eosinophilia, hemoglobin and hematocrit decreased

Hepatic: Transaminases increased

Local: Thrombophlebitis

Rare but important or life-threatening: Anaphylaxis, angioedema, BUN increased, chest pain, cholestasis, colitis, creatinine increased, dyspnea, erythema multiforme, fever, GI bleeding, hemolytic anemia, hepatitis, hives, hyperbilirubinemia, hypersensitivity, interstitial nephritis, jaundice, leukopenia, neutropenia, pain at injection site, pancytopenia, positive Coombs test, prolonged PT/INR, pseudomembranous colitis, rash, renal dysfunction, seizure, Stevens-Johnson syndrome, stomach cramps, tachycardia, thrombocytopenia (rare), tongue swelling, toxic epidermal necrolysis, urticaria

Reactions reported with other cephalosporins: Agranulocytosis, aplastic anemia, asterixis, colitis, encephalopathy, hemorrhage, neuromuscular excitability, serumsickness reactions, superinfection, toxic nephropathy

Drug Interactions
Metabolism/Transport Effects None known.

Avoid Concomitant Use

Avoid concomitant use of Cefuroxime with any of the following: BCG

Increased Effect/Toxicity

Cefuroxime may increase the levels/effects of: Aminoglycosides; Vitamin K Antagonists

The levels/effects of Cefuroxime may be increased by: Probenecid

Decreased Effect

Cefuroxime may decrease the levels/effects of: BCG; Sodium Picosulfate; Typhoid Vaccine

The levels/effects of Cefuroxime may be decreased by: Antacids; H2-Antagonists

Food Interactions Bioavailability is increased with food; cefuroxime serum levels may be increased if taken with food or dairy products. Management: Administer tablet without regard to meals; suspension may be administered with food.

Stability
Oral suspension: Before reconstitution, store dry powder at 2°C to 30°C (36°F to 86°F). Reconstituted oral suspension should be stored in the refrigerator; discard after 10 days.

Oral tablets: Store at 15°C to 30°C (59°F to 86°F).

Parenteral: Store intact vials at 15°C to 30°C (59°F to 86°F); protect from light. Reconstituted injectable solution (100 mg/mL) or injectable suspension (200-220 mg/mL) is stable for 24 hours at room temperature or 48 hours when refrigerated. Diluted solutions are stable for 24 hours at room temperature and 7 days refrigerated. May be frozen for up to 6 months; once thawed, stable

for 24 hours at room temperature and 7 days refrigerated; do not refreeze.

ADD-Vantage vials: Joined, but not activated, vials are stable for 14 days. Once activated, stable for 24 hours at room temperature and 7 days refrigerated. Do not freeze.

Premix Galaxy® plastic containers: Store frozen at -20°C. Thaw container at room temperature or under refrigeration; do not force thaw. Thawed solution is stable for 24 hours at room temperature and 28 days refrigerated; do not refreeze.

Mechanism of Action Inhibits bacterial cell wall synthesis by binding to one or more of the penicillin-binding proteins (PBPs) which in turn inhibits the final transpeptidation step of peptidoglycan synthesis in bacterial cell walls, thus inhibiting cell wall biosynthesis. Bacteria eventually lyse due to ongoing activity of cell wall autolytic enzymes (autolysins and murein hydrolases) while cell wall assembly is arrested.

Pharmacokinetics (Adult data unless noted)
Distribution: Into bronchial secretions, synovial and pericardial fluid, kidneys, heart, liver, bone and bile; penetrates into CSF with inflamed meninges

Protein binding: 33% to 50%

Metabolism: Cefuroxime axetil (oral) is hydrolyzed in the intestinal mucosa and blood to cefuroxime

Bioavailability: Oral tablet: Fasting: 37%; following food: 52%; cefuroxime axetil suspension is less bioavailable than the tablet (91% of the AUC for tablets)

Half-life:

Premature neonates:

PNA ≤3 days: Median: 5.8 hours (de Louvois, 1982)

PNA ≥8 days: Median: 1.6-3.8 hours (de Louvois, 1982)

Children and Adolescents: 1.4-1.9 hours

Adults: 1-2 hours (prolonged in renal impairment)

Time to peak serum concentration:

Oral: Children: 3-4 hours; Adults: 2-3 hours

I.M.: Within 15-60 minutes

Elimination: Primarily 66% to 100% as unchanged drug in urine by both glomerular filtration and tubular secretion

Dosing: Neonatal
General dosing, susceptible infection: I.M., I.V. (*Red Book* [AAP], 2012):

Body weight <1 kg:

PNA ≤14 days: 50 mg/kg/dose every 12 hours

PNA 15 to 28 days: 50 mg/kg/dose every 8 to 12 hours

Body weight 1 to 2 kg:

PNA ≤7 days: 50 mg/kg/dose every 12 hours

PNA 8 to 28 days: 50 mg/kg/dose every 8 to 12 hours

Body weight >2 kg:

PNA ≤7 days: 50 mg/kg/dose every 12 hours

PNA 8 to 28 days: 50 mg/kg/dose every 8 hours

Dosing: Usual Note: Cefuroxime axetil film-coated tablets and oral suspension are not bioequivalent and are not substitutable on a mg/mg basis.

Pediatric:

General dosing, susceptible infection (*Red Book* [AAP], 2012): Infants, Children, and Adolescents:

Mild to moderate infection:

Oral: 20 to 30 mg/kg/day divided twice daily; maximum single dose: 500 mg

I.M., I.V.: 75 to 100 mg/kg/day divided in 3 doses; maximum single dose: 1500 mg

Severe infection: I.M., I.V.: 100 to 200 mg/kg/day divided in 3 to 4 doses; maximum single dose: 1500 mg

Bone and joint infection: Infants ≥3 months, Children, and Adolescents: I.M., I.V.: 50 mg/kg/dose every 8 hours; maximum single dose: 1500 mg

Bronchitis, acute (and exacerbations of chronic bronchitis): Adolescents: Oral tablets: 250 to 500 mg every 12 hours for 10 days

Gonorrhea, uncomplicated: Note: Due to increasing antimicrobial resistance, oral cephalosporins are no longer recommended for treatment of gonococcal infections (CDC, 2012). Adolescents: Oral tablet: 1000 mg as a single dose

Intra-abdominal infection complicated, community-acquired: Infants, Children, and Adolescents: I.M., I.V.: 150 mg/kg/day in divided doses every 6 to 8 hours; maximum single dose: 1500 mg (Solomkin, 2010)

Lyme disease: Infants, Children, and Adolescents:

Acrodermatitis chronica atrophicans: Oral: 15 mg/kg/dose every 12 hours for 21 days; maximum single dose: 500 mg (Wormser, 2006)

Early localized disease: Oral: 15 mg/kg/dose every 12 hours for 14 to 21 days; maximum single dose: 500 mg (*Red Book* [AAP], 2012; Wormser, 2006)

Late disease (arthritis): Oral: 15 mg/kg/dose every 12 hours for 28 days; maximum single dose: 500 mg (Wormser, 2006)

Nervous system disease: **Note:** Use only when doxycycline is contraindicated; doxycycline is the preferred treatment; Oral: 15 mg/kg/dose every 12 hours for 14 days; maximum single dose: 500 mg (Halperin, 2007)

Otitis media, acute: Infants ≥3 months and Children: Oral suspension: 15 mg/kg/dose twice daily for 10 days; maximum single dose: 500 mg (Lieberthal, 2013)

Alternate dosing for patients who can swallow a tablet whole: Oral tablet: 250 mg twice daily for 10 days

Pharyngitis/tonsillitis:

Infants ≥3 months and Children: Oral suspension: 10 mg/kg/dose twice daily for 10 days; maximum single dose: 250 mg

Adolescents: Oral tablets: 250 mg twice daily for 10 days

Pneumonia, bacterial (HIV-exposed/-positive): Infants and Children: I.V.: 35 to 50 mg/kg/dose 3 times daily; maximum single dose: 2000 mg (DHHS [pediatric], 2013)

Sinusitis:

Infants ≥3 months and Children:

Oral suspension: 15 mg/kg/dose twice daily for 10 days; maximum single dose: 500 mg

Alternate dosing for patients who can swallow a tablet whole: Oral tablet: 250 mg twice daily for 10 days

Adolescents: Oral tablet: 250 mg twice daily for 10 days

Skin and skin structure infection:

Animal or human bites (Stevens, 2005): Adolescents:

Oral: 500 mg twice daily

Parenteral: I.M., I.V.: 1000 mg once daily

Impetigo: Infants ≥3 months and Children: Oral suspension: 15 mg/kg/dose twice daily for 10 days; maximum single dose: 500 mg

Uncomplicated skin and skin structure infections: Adolescents: Oral tablets: 250 to 500 mg twice daily for 10 days

Surgical prophylaxis: Children and Adolescents: I.V.: 50 mg/kg 30 to 60 minutes prior to procedure; may repeat dose in 4 hours; maximum single dose: 1500 mg (Bratzler, 2013)

Urinary tract infection, uncomplicated:

Infants and Children 2 to 24 months: Oral: 10 to 15 mg/kg/dose twice daily (AAP, 2011)

Children >24 months: Moderate to severe disease (possible pyelonephritis): Oral: 20 to 30 mg/kg/day divided twice daily; maximum single dose: 500 mg (Bradley, 2012)

Adolescents: Oral tablets: 250 mg twice daily for 7 to 10 days

Adult:

Bronchitis, acute (and exacerbations of chronic bronchitis):

Oral: 250 to 500 mg every 12 hours for 10 days

I.V.: 500 to 750 mg every 8 hours (complete therapy with oral dosing)

Cellulitis, orbital: I.V.: 1500 mg every 8 hours

Cholecystitis, mild to moderate: I.V.: 1500 mg every 8 hours for 4 to 7 days (provided source controlled)

Gonorrhea:

Disseminated: I.M., I.V.: 750 mg every 8 hours

Uncomplicated:

Oral: 1000 mg as a single dose

I.M.: 1500 mg as single dose (administer in two different sites with oral probenecid)

Intra-abdominal infection, complicated, community-acquired, mild to moderate (in combination with metronidazole): I.V.: 1500 mg every 8 hours for 4 to 7 days (provided source controlled) (Solomkin, 2010)

Lyme disease (early): Oral: 500 mg twice daily for 20 days

Pharyngitis/tonsillitis and sinusitis: Oral: 250 mg twice daily for 10 days

Pneumonia, uncomplicated: I.M., I.V.: 750 mg every 8 hours

Severe or complicated infections: I.M., I.V.: 1500 mg every 8 hours (up to 1500 mg every 6 hours in life-threatening infections)

Skin/skin structure infection, uncomplicated:

Oral: 250 to 500 mg every 12 hours for 10 days

I.M., I.V.: 750 mg every 8 hours

Surgical prophylaxis:

Manufacturer's recommendation: I.V.: 1500 mg 30 minutes to 1 hour prior to procedure (if procedure is prolonged can give 750 mg every 8 hours I.V. or I.M.)

Open heart: I.V.: 1500 mg every 12 hours for a total of 4 doses starting at anesthesia induction

Alternative recommendation: I.V.: 1500 mg within 60 minutes prior to surgical incision. Doses may be repeated in 4 hours if procedure is lengthy or if there is excessive blood loss (Bratzler, 2013).

Urinary tract infection, uncomplicated:

Oral: 125 to 250 mg twice daily for 7 to 10 days

I.V., I.M.: 750 mg every 8 hours

Dosing interval in renal impairment:

Infants, Children, and Adolescents: The manufacturer's labeling recommends decreasing the frequency similar to adult recommendations. The following guidelines have been used by some clinicians (Aronoff, 2007). **Note:** Renally adjusted dose recommendations are based on doses of 30 mg/kg/day divided every 12 hours (oral) or 75 to 150 mg/kg/day divided every 8 hours (I.M., I.V.). Oral, Parenteral:

GFR ≥30 mL/minute/1.73 m^2: No adjustment required

GFR 10 to 29 mL/minute/1.73 m^2: Administer every 12 hours

GFR <10 mL/minute/1.73 m^2: Administer every 24 hours

Intermittent hemodialysis: Administer every 24 hours

Peritoneal dialysis: Administer every 24 hours

Adults:

Oral: No dosage adjustment required. Dose after dialysis on dialysis days (Aronoff, 2007).

Parenteral:

CrCl >20 mL/minute: No adjustment required

CrCl 10 to 20 mL/minute: 750 mg every 12 hours

CrCl <10 mL/minute: 750 mg every 24 hours

Peritoneal dialysis: Administer every 24 hours

Continuous renal replacement therapy (CRRT): 1000 mg every 12 hours

Dosing adjustment in hepatic impairment: There are no dosage adjustments provided in the manufacturer's labeling.

Administration

Oral: Cefuroxime axetil suspension must be administered with food; shake suspension well before use; tablets may be administered with or without food; administer with food to decrease GI upset; avoid crushing the tablet due to its bitter taste

Parenteral:
IVP: Administer over 3-5 minutes at a maximum concentration of 100 mg/mL
I.V. intermittent infusion: Administer over 15-30 minutes at a final concentration for administration ≤30 mg/mL; in fluid restricted patients, a concentration of 137 mg/mL may be administered
I.M.: Inject deep I.M. into large muscle mass at a concentration of 220 mg/mL; less painful when administered as an injectable suspension rather than a solution, and is less painful when administered into the buttock rather than the thigh

Monitoring Parameters With prolonged therapy, monitor renal, hepatic, and hematologic function periodically; number and type of stools/day for diarrhea; and prothrombin time. Observe for signs and symptoms of anaphylaxis during first dose.

Test Interactions Positive direct Coombs', false-positive urinary glucose test using cupric sulfate (Benedict's solution, Clinitest®, Fehling's solution); false-negative may occur with ferricyanide test. Glucose oxidase or hexokinase-based methods should be used.

Dosage Forms Excipient information presented when available (limited, particularly for generics); consult specific product labeling.
Solution, Intravenous, as sodium [strength expressed as base]:
Zinacef in Sterile Water: 1.5 g (50 mL)
Solution Reconstituted, Injection, as sodium [strength expressed as base]:
Zinacef: 750 mg (1 ea); 1.5 g (1 ea); 7.5 g (1 ea)
Generic: 750 mg (1 ea); 1.5 g (1 ea); 7.5 g (1 ea); 75 g (1 ea); 225 g (1 ea)
Solution Reconstituted, Intravenous, as sodium [strength expressed as base]:
Zinacef: 750 mg (1 ea); 1.5 g (1 ea)
Generic: 750 mg (1 ea); 1.5 g (1 ea); 7.5 g (1 ea)
Suspension Reconstituted, Oral, as axetil [strength expressed as base]:
Ceftin: 125 mg/5 mL (100 mL); 250 mg/5 mL (50 mL, 100 mL) [contains aspartame; tutti-frutti flavor]
Generic: 125 mg/5 mL (100 mL)
Tablet, Oral, as axetil [strength expressed as base]:
Ceftin: 250 mg, 500 mg
Generic: 250 mg, 500 mg

References

American Academy of Pediatrics, "Urinary Tract Infection: Clinical Practice Guideline for the Diagnosis and Management of the Initial UTI in Febrile Infants and Children 2 to 24 Months," *Pediatrics*, 2011, 128(3):595-610.
Aronoff GR, Bennett WM, Berns JS, et al, *Drug Prescribing in Renal Failure: Dosing Guidelines for Adults and Children*, 5th ed. Philadelphia, PA: American College of Physicians; 2007.
Bradley JS, Byington CL, Shah SS, et al, "The Management of Community-Acquired Pneumonia in Infants and Children Older Than 3 Months of Age: Clinical Practice Guidelines by the Pediatric Infectious Diseases Society and the Infectious Diseases Society of America", *Clin Infect Dis*, 2011, 53(7):e25-76.
Bradley JS, Nelson JD, Kimberlin DK, et al, eds. *Nelson's Pocket Book of Pediatric Antimicrobial Therapy*. 19th ed. Philadelphia, PA: Lippincott Williams & Wilkins; 2012.
Bratzler DW, Dellinger EP, Olsen KM, Perl TM, Auwaerter PG, Bolon MK, et al. Clinical practice guidelines for antimicrobial prophylaxis in surgery. *Am J Health Syst Pharm*. 2013;70(3):195-283.
Center for Disease Control (CDC), "Update to CDC's Sexually Transmitted Diseases Treatment Guidelines, 2010: Oral Cephalosporins No Longer a Recommended Treatment for Gonococcal Infections," *MMWR*, 2012, 61(31): 581-604.
de Louvois J, Mulhall A, and Hurley R, "Cefuroxime in the Treatment of Neonates," *Arch Dis Child*, 1982, 57(1):59-62.
DHHS. Guidelines for the prevention and treatment of opportunistic infections among HIV-exposed and HIV-infected children: recommendations from the National Institutes of Health, Centers for Disease Control and Prevention, the HIV Medicine Association of the Infectious Diseases Society of America, the Pediatric Infectious Diseases Society, and the American Academy of Pediatrics. November 6, 2013. Available at http://aidsinfo.nih.gov
DHHS Panel on Opportunistic Infections (OI) in HIV-Infected Adults and Adolescents. Guidelines for prevention and treatment of opportunistic infections in HIV-infected adults and adolescents: recommendations from the Centers for Disease Control and Prevention (CDC), the National Institutes of Health (NIH), and the HIV Medicine Association (HIVMA) of the Infectious Diseases Society of America (IDSA). May 7, 2013. Available at http://aidsinfo.nih.gov/contentfiles/lvguidelines/adult_oi.pdf
Halperin JJ, Shapiro ED, Logigian E, et al, "Practice Parameter: Treatment of Nervous System Lyme Disease (an Evidence-Based Review): Report of the Quality Standards Subcommittee of the American Academy of Neurology," *Neurology*, 2007, 69(1):91-102.
Lieberthal AS, Carroll AE, Chonmaitree T, et al, "The Diagnosis and Management of Acute Otitis Media," *Pediatrics*, 2013, 131(3):e964-99.
Nelson JD, "Cefuroxime: A Cephalosporin With Unique Applicability to Pediatric Practice," *Pediatr Infect Dis*, 1983, 2(5):394-6.
Solomkin JS, Mazuski JE, Bradley JS, et al, "Diagnosis and Management of Complicated Intra-Abdominal Infections in Adults and Children: Guidelines by the Surgical Infection Society and the Infectious Diseases Society of America," *Clin Infect Dis*, 2010, 50(2):133-64.
Stevens DL, Bisno AL, Chambers HF, et al, "Practice Guidelines for the Diagnosis and Management of Skin and Soft-Tissue Infections," *Clin Infect Dis*, 2005, 41(10):1373-406.
Tunkel AR, Hartman BJ, Kaplan SL, et al, "Practice Guidelines for the Management of Bacterial Meningitis," *Clin Infect Dis*, 2004, 39 (9):1267-84.
Wormser GP, Dattwyler RJ, Shapiro ED, et al, "The Clinical Assessment, Treatment, and Prevention of Lyme Disease, Human Granulocytic Anaplasmosis, and Babesiosis: Clinical Practice Guidelines by the Infectious Diseases Society of America," *Clin Infect Dis*, 2006, 43 (9):1089-134.

◆ **Cefuroxime Axetil** see Cefuroxime on page 422
◆ **Cefuroxime For Injection (Can)** see Cefuroxime on page 422
◆ **Cefuroxime For Injection, USP (Can)** see Cefuroxime on page 422
◆ **Cefuroxime Sodium** see Cefuroxime on page 422
◆ **Cefzil** see Cefprozil on page 412
◆ **Cefzil® (Can)** see Cefprozil on page 412
◆ **CeleBREX** see Celecoxib on page 425
◆ **Celebrex (Can)** see Celecoxib on page 425

Celecoxib (se le KOKS ib)

Medication Safety Issues
Sound-alike/look-alike issues:
CeleBREX may be confused with CeleXA, Cerebyx, Cervarix, Clarinex

Brand Names: U.S. CeleBREX

Brand Names: Canada Celebrex

Therapeutic Category Nonsteroidal Anti-inflammatory Drug (NSAID), COX-2 Selective

Generic Availability (U.S.) No

Use Relief of signs and symptoms of juvenile idiopathic arthritis (JIA) (FDA approved in ages ≥2 years weighing ≥10 kg); relief of sign and symptoms of osteoarthritis, adult rheumatoid arthritis, and ankylosing spondylitis (FDA approved in adults); management of acute pain (FDA approved in adults); treatment of primary dysmenorrhea (FDA approved in adults)

Medication Guide Available Yes

Pregnancy Risk Factor C (prior to 30 weeks gestation)/D (≥30 weeks gestation)

Pregnancy Considerations Teratogenic effects have been observed in some animal studies; therefore, celecoxib is classified as pregnancy category C. Celecoxib is a NSAID that primarily inhibits COX-2 whereas other currently available NSAIDs are nonselective for COX-1 and COX-2. The effects of this selective inhibition to the fetus have not been well studied and limited information is available specific to celecoxib. NSAID exposure during the first trimester is not strongly associated with congenital malformations; however, cardiovascular anomalies and cleft palate have been observed following NSAID exposure in some studies. The use of a NSAID close to conception may be associated with an increased risk of miscarriage. Nonteratogenic effects have been observed following NSAID administration during the third trimester including: Myocardial degenerative changes, prenatal constriction of the ductus arteriosus, fetal tricuspid regurgitation, failure of the ductus arteriosus to close postnatally; renal dysfunction or failure, oligohydramnios; gastrointestinal bleeding or perforation, increased risk of necrotizing enterocolitis; intracranial bleeding (including intraventricular hemorrhage), platelet dysfunction with resultant bleeding; pulmonary hypertension. Because it may cause premature closure of the ductus arteriosus, the use of celecoxib is not recommended ≥30 weeks gestation. The chronic use of NSAIDs in women of reproductive age may be associated with infertility that is reversible upon discontinuation of the medication. A registry is available for pregnant women exposed to autoimmune medications including celecoxib. For additional information contact the Organization of Teratology Information Specialists, OTIS Autoimmune Diseases Study, at 877-311-8972.

Breast-Feeding Considerations Small amounts of celecoxib are found in breast milk. The manufacturer recommends that caution be exercised when administering celecoxib to nursing women.

Contraindications Hypersensitivity to celecoxib, any component, sulfonamides (celecoxib is a sulfonamide), aspirin, or other NSAIDs; patients with the "aspirin triad" [asthma, rhinitis (with or without nasal polyps) and aspirin intolerance] (fatal asthmatic and anaphylactoid reactions may occur in these patients); perioperative pain in the setting of coronary artery bypass surgery (CABG); active GI bleed

Warnings NSAIDs are associated with an increased risk of serious adverse cardiovascular thrombotic events, including potentially fatal MI and stroke **[U.S. Boxed Warning]**; risk may be increased with duration of use or preexisting cardiovascular risk factors or disease; carefully evaluate cardiovascular risk profile prior to prescribing; use the lowest effective dose for the shortest duration of time, taking into consideration individual patient treatment goals; alternate therapies should be considered for patients at high risk. Use is contraindicated for treatment of perioperative pain in the setting of CABG surgery **[U.S. Boxed Warning]**; an increased incidence of MI and stroke was found in patients receiving COX-2 selective NSAIDs for the treatment of pain within the first 10-14 days after CABG surgery. NSAIDs may cause fluid retention, edema, and new onset or worsening of preexisting hypertension; use with caution in patients with hypertension, CHF, or fluid retention.

NSAIDs may increase the risk of gastrointestinal inflammation, ulceration, bleeding, and perforation **[U.S. Boxed Warning]**. These events, which can be potentially fatal, may occur at any time during therapy, and without warning. Use of celecoxib in patients with active GI bleeding is contraindicated. Use NSAIDs with extreme caution in patients with a history of GI bleeding or ulcers (these patients have a 10-fold increased risk for developing a GI bleed). Use NSAIDs with caution in patients with other risk factors which may increase GI bleeding (eg, concurrent therapy with aspirin, anticoagulants, and/or corticosteroids, longer duration of NSAID use, smoking, use of alcohol, and poor general health). Use the lowest effective dose for the shortest duration of time, taking into consideration individual patient treatment goals; alternate therapies should be considered for patients at high risk.

NSAIDs may compromise existing renal function; dose-dependent decreases in prostaglandin synthesis may result from NSAID use, reducing renal blood flow which may cause renal decompensation. Patients with impaired renal function, dehydration, heart failure, liver dysfunction,

those taking diuretics and ACE inhibitors are at greater risk of renal toxicity; use with caution in these patients; monitor renal function closely. NSAIDs are not recommended for use in patients with advanced renal disease. Long-term use of NSAIDs may cause renal papillary necrosis and other renal injury.

Even in patients without prior exposure, anaphylactoid reactions may occur; patients with "aspirin triad" [bronchial asthma, aspirin intolerance, and rhinitis (with or without nasal polyps)] are at increased risk; use is contraindicated in these patients. Do not use in patients who experience bronchospasm, asthma, rhinitis, or urticaria with NSAID or aspirin therapy. NSAIDs may cause serious and potentially fatal dermatologic adverse reactions including exfoliative dermatitis, Stevens-Johnson syndrome, and toxic epidermal necrolysis; discontinue use at first sign of skin rash or any other sign of hypersensitivity reaction. Avoid use of NSAIDs in late pregnancy (≥30 weeks gestation) as they may cause premature closure of the ductus arteriosus.

Precautions Use with caution in patients with moderate hepatic impairment; dose reduction is recommended; not recommended for use in patients with severe hepatic impairment (Child-Pugh Class C). Closely monitor patients with abnormal LFTs; severe hepatic reactions (eg, fulminant hepatitis, hepatic necrosis, jaundice, liver failure) have occurred with NSAID use, rarely; discontinue if signs or symptoms of liver disease develop, or if systemic manifestations occur.

Use with caution in patients with asthma; asthmatic patients may have aspirin-sensitive asthma which may be associated with severe and potentially fatal bronchospasm when aspirin or NSAIDs are administered. Anemia may sometimes occur; monitor hemoglobin and hematocrit in patients receiving long term therapy. Use with caution in pediatric patients with systemic-onset JIA; serious adverse reactions, including disseminated intravascular coagulation, may occur.

Use with caution and consider dosage reduction in patients who are known or suspected poor metabolizers of cytochrome P450 isoenzyme 2C9 substrates; these patients may have unusually high plasma levels due to reduced clearance. Consider alternate therapy in JIA patients who are identified to be CYP2C9 poor metabolizers. In a small pediatric study (n=4), the AUC of celecoxib was ~10 times higher in a child who was homozygous for CYP2C9*3, compared to children who were homozygous for the *1 allele (n=2) or who had the CYP2C9*1/*2 genotype; further studies are needed to determine if carriers of the CYP2C9*3 allele are at increased risk for cardiovascular toxicity or dose-related adverse effects of celecoxib, especially with long-term, high-dose use of the drug (Stempak, 2005). Adult subjects who were homozygous for CYP2C9*3/*3 displayed celecoxib serum concentrations 3-7 times higher than subjects with CYP2C9*1/*1 or CYP2C9*1/*3 genotypes. The frequency of CYP2C9*3/*3 genotype is estimated to be 0.3% to 1% in various ethnic groups. Long-term (>6 months) cardiovascular toxicity in children and adolescents has not been studied. Celecoxib should not be used as a substitute for corticosteroid therapy or to treat corticosteroid insufficiency. Avoid concomitant use of celecoxib and other NSAIDs.

Adverse Reactions

Cardiovascular: Angina, aortic valve incompetence, chest pain, coronary artery disorder, edema, facial edema, hypertension (aggravated), MI, palpitation, peripheral edema, sinus bradycardia, tachycardia, ventricular hypertrophy

Central nervous system: Anxiety, depression, dizziness, fatigue, fever, headache, hypoesthesia, insomnia, migraine, nervousness, pain, somnolence, vertigo

Dermatologic: Alopecia, bruising, cellulitis, dermatitis, dry skin, photosensitivity, pruritus, rash (erythematous), rash (including maculopapular), urticaria

Endocrine & metabolic: Hot flashes, hypercholesterolemia, hyperglycemia, hypokalemia, ovarian cyst, testosterone decreased

Gastrointestinal: Abdominal pain, anorexia, appetite increased, constipation, diarrhea, diverticulitis, dyspepsia, dysphagia, eructation, esophagitis, flatulence, gastritis, gastroenteritis, gastroesophageal reflux, gastrointestinal ulcer, hemorrhoids, hiatal hernia, melena, nausea, stomatitis, tenesmus, vomiting, weight gain, xerostomia

Genitourinary: Cystitis, dysuria, urinary frequency

Hematologic: Anemia, thrombocythemia

Hepatic: Alkaline phosphatase increased, transaminases increased

Neuromuscular & skeletal: Arthralgia, arthrosis, back pain, CPK increased, hypertonia, leg cramps, myalgia, paresthesia, synovitis, tendonitis

Ocular: Conjunctival hemorrhage, vitreous floaters

Otic: Deafness, labyrinthitis, tinnitus

Renal: Albuminuria, BUN increased, creatinine increased, hematuria, nonprotein nitrogen increased, renal calculi

Respiratory: Bronchitis, bronchospasm, cough, dyspnea, epistaxis, laryngitis, nasopharyngitis, pharyngitis, pneumonia, rhinitis, sinusitis, upper respiratory tract infection

Miscellaneous: Allergic reactions, allergy aggravated, cyst, diaphoresis, flu-like syndrome

Rare but important or life-threatening: Acute renal failure, agranulocytosis, anaphylactoid reactions, angioedema, anosmia, aplastic anemia, aseptic meningitis, cerebrovascular accident, CHF, cholelithiasis, colitis, DVT, erythema multiforme, esophageal perforation, exfoliative dermatitis, gangrene, gastrointestinal bleeding, hepatic failure, hepatic necrosis, hepatitis (including fulminant), hypoglycemia, hyponatremia, ileus, interstitial nephritis, intestinal obstruction, intestinal perforation, intracranial hemorrhage, jaundice, leukopenia, pancreatitis, pancytopenia, pulmonary embolism, renal papillary necrosis, sepsis, Stevens-Johnson syndrome, sudden death, suicide, syncope, thrombocytopenia, thrombophlebitis, toxic epidermal necrolysis, vasculitis, ventricular fibrillation

Drug Interactions

Metabolism/Transport Effects Substrate of CYP2C9 (major), CYP3A4 (minor); **Note:** Assignment of Major/Minor substrate status based on clinically relevant drug interaction potential; **Inhibits** CYP2C8 (moderate), CYP2D6 (moderate)

Avoid Concomitant Use

Avoid concomitant use of Celecoxib with any of the following: Floctafenine; Ketorolac (Nasal); Ketorolac (Systemic); Nonsteroidal Anti-Inflammatory Agents; NSAID (COX-2 Inhibitor); Omacetaxine; Thioridazine

Increased Effect/Toxicity

Celecoxib may increase the levels/effects of: 5-ASA Derivatives; Agents with Antiplatelet Properties; Aliskiren; Aminoglycosides; Anticoagulants; ARIPiprazole; Bisphosphonate Derivatives; CycloSPORINE (Systemic); CYP2C8 Substrates; CYP2D6 Substrates; Deferasirox; Desmopressin; Digoxin; DOXOrubicin (Conventional); Eplerenone; Estrogen Derivatives; Fesoterodine; Haloperidol; Lithium; Methotrexate; Metoprolol; Nebivolol; NSAID (COX-2 Inhibitor); Omacetaxine; Porfimer; Potassium-Sparing Diuretics; PRALAtrexate; Prilocaine; Quinolone Antibiotics; Sodium Nitrite; Tenofovir; Thioridazine; Vancomycin; Vitamin K Antagonists

The levels/effects of Celecoxib may be increased by: ACE Inhibitors; Angiotensin II Receptor Blockers; Antidepressants (Tricyclic, Tertiary Amine); Aspirin; Ceritinib; Corticosteroids (Systemic); CycloSPORINE (Systemic); CYP2C9 Inhibitors (Moderate); CYP2C9 Inhibitors (Strong); Floctafenine; Herbs (Anticoagulant/Antiplatelet Properties); Ketorolac (Nasal); Ketorolac (Systemic); Mifepristone; Nitric Oxide; Nonsteroidal Anti-Inflammatory Agents; Probenecid; Propafenone; Selective Serotonin Reuptake Inhibitors; Sodium Phosphates; Treprostinil

Decreased Effect

Celecoxib may decrease the levels/effects of: ACE Inhibitors; Agents with Antiplatelet Properties; Aliskiren; Angiotensin II Receptor Blockers; Beta-Blockers; Codeine; Eplerenone; HydrALAZINE; Loop Diuretics; Potassium-Sparing Diuretics; Prostaglandins (Ophthalmic); Selective Serotonin Reuptake Inhibitors; Tamoxifen; Thiazide Diuretics; TraMADol

The levels/effects of Celecoxib may be decreased by: Bile Acid Sequestrants; CYP2C9 Inducers (Strong); Dabrafenib; Peginterferon Alfa-2b

Food Interactions Peak concentrations are delayed and AUC is increased by 10% to 20% when taken with a high-fat meal. Management: Administer without regard to meals.

Stability Store at 25°C (77°F); excursions permitted to 15°C to 30°C (59°F to 86°F).

Mechanism of Action Inhibits prostaglandin synthesis by decreasing the activity of the enzyme, cyclooxygenase-2 (COX-2), which results in decreased formation of prostaglandin precursors; has antipyretic, analgesic, and anti-inflammatory properties. Celecoxib does not inhibit cyclooxygenase-1 (COX-1) at therapeutic concentrations.

Pharmacokinetics (Adult data unless noted)

Absorption: Prolonged due to low solubility

Distribution: V_d (apparent):

Children and Adolescents ~7-16 years (steady-state): 8.3 ± 5.8 L/kg (Stempak, 2002)

Adults: ~400 L

Protein binding: ~97%; primarily to albumin; binds to alpha 1-acid glycoprotein to a lesser extent

Metabolism: Hepatic via CYP2C9; forms 3 inactive metabolites (a primary alcohol, corresponding carboxylic acid, and its glucuronide conjugate)

Bioavailability: Absolute: Unknown. AUC was increased by 40% and 180% with mild and moderate hepatic impairment, respectively. **Note:** Meta-analysis suggests the AUC is 40% higher in Blacks compared to Caucasians (clinical significance unknown).

Half-life elimination:

Children and Adolescents ~7-16 years (steady-state): 6 ± 2.7 hours (range: 3-10 hours) (Stempak, 2002)

Adults: ~11 hours (fasted)

Time to peak serum concentration:

Children: Median: 3 hours (range: 1-5.8 hours) (Stempak, 2002)

Adults: ~3 hours

Elimination: Feces (57% as metabolites, <3% as unchanged drug); urine (27% as metabolites, <3% as unchanged drug); primary metabolites in feces and urine: Carboxylic acid metabolite (73% of dose); low amounts of glucuronide metabolite appear in urine

Dosing: Usual Note: Use the lowest effective dose for the shortest duration of time, consistent with individual patient goals.

Children ≥2 years and Adolescents: **Juvenile idiopathic arthritis (JIA):** Oral:

≥10 kg to ≤25 kg: 50 mg twice daily

>25 kg: 100 mg twice daily

Adults:

Acute pain or primary dysmenorrhea: Oral: Initial dose: 400 mg, followed by an additional 200 mg if needed on day 1; maintenance dose: 200 mg twice daily as needed

Ankylosing spondylitis: Oral: 200 mg/day as a single dose or in divided doses twice daily; if no effect after 6 weeks, may increase to 400 mg/day. If no response following 6 weeks of treatment with 400 mg/day, consider discontinuation and alternative treatment.

Osteoarthritis: Oral: 200 mg/day as a single dose or in divided doses twice daily

Rheumatoid arthritis: Oral: 100-200 mg twice daily

Dosing adjustment in poor metabolizers of CYP2C9 substrates: Use with caution in patients who are known or suspected poor metabolizers of cytochrome P450 isoenzyme 2C9 substrates.

Children ≥2 years and Adolescents: Consider alternate therapy in JIA patients who are poor metabolizers.

Adults: Consider initiation at 50% of the lowest recommended dose.

Dosing adjustment in renal impairment: Children ≥2 years, Adolescents, and Adults: Use is not recommended in patients with severe renal dysfunction.

Dosing adjustment in hepatic impairment: Children ≥2 years, Adolescents, and Adults:

Moderate hepatic impatient (Child-Pugh Class B): Reduce dose by 50%; monitor closely

Severe hepatic impairment (Child-Pugh Class C): Use is not recommended; has not been studied

Administration Lower doses (up to 200 mg twice daily) may be administered without regard to meals (may administer with food to reduce GI upset); larger doses should be administered with food to improve absorption. Do not administer with antacids. Capsules may be swallowed whole or the entire contents emptied onto a teaspoon of cool or room temperature applesauce; the contents of the capsule sprinkled onto applesauce may be stored under refrigeration for up to 6 hours.

Monitoring Parameters CBC; blood chemistry profile; occult blood loss; periodic liver function tests; renal function (urine output, serum BUN and creatinine); monitor efficacy (eg, in arthritic conditions: Pain, range of motion, grip strength, mobility), inflammation; observe for weight gain, edema; observe for bleeding, bruising; evaluate GI effects (abdominal pain, bleeding, dyspepsia); blood pressure (baseline and throughout therapy)

JIA: Monitor for development of abnormal coagulation tests in patients with systemic-onset JIA

Dosage Forms Excipient information presented when available (limited, particularly for generics); consult specific product labeling.

Capsule, Oral:

CeleBREX: 50 mg, 100 mg, 200 mg, 400 mg

References

Stempak D, Bukaveckas BL, Linder M, et al, "Cytochrome P450 2C9 Genotype: Impact on Celecoxib Safety and Pharmacokinetics in a Pediatric Patient," *Clin Pharmacol Ther*, 2005, 78(3):309-10.

Stempak D, Gammon J, Halton J, et al, "Modulation of Celecoxib Pharmacokinetics by Food in Pediatric Patients," *Clin Pharmacol Ther*, 2005a, 77(3):226-8.

Stempak D, Gammon J, Klein J, et al, "Single-Dose and Steady-State Pharmacokinetics of Celecoxib in Children," *Clin Pharmacol Ther*, 2002, 72(5):490-7.

◆ **Celestoderm V (Can)** *see* Betamethasone (Topical) *on page 285*

◆ **Celestoderm V/2 (Can)** *see* Betamethasone (Topical) *on page 285*

◆ **Celestone** *see* Betamethasone (Systemic) *on page 282*

◆ **Celestone Soluspan** *see* Betamethasone (Systemic) *on page 282*

◆ **CeleXA** *see* Citalopram *on page 484*

◆ **Celexa® (Can)** *see* Citalopram *on page 484*

◆ **CellCept** *see* Mycophenolate *on page 1453*

◆ **CellCept Intravenous** *see* Mycophenolate *on page 1453*

◆ **Cell Culture Inactivated Influenza Vaccine, Trivalent [Flucelvax]** *see* Influenza Virus Vaccine (Inactivated) *on page 1103*

◆ **Celontin** *see* Methsuximide *on page 1375*

◆ **Celontin® (Can)** *see* Methsuximide *on page 1375*

◆ **Celsentri (Can)** *see* Maraviroc *on page 1304*

◆ **Cemill [OTC]** *see* Ascorbic Acid *on page 206*

◆ **Cemill SR [OTC]** *see* Ascorbic Acid *on page 206*

◆ **Centany** *see* Mupirocin *on page 1452*

◆ **Centany AT** *see* Mupirocin *on page 1452*

◆ ***Centruroides* Immune FAB2 (Equine)** *see Centruroides* Immune F(ab')₂ (Equine) *on page 428*

Centruroides Immune F(ab')₂ (Equine)
(sen tra ROY dez i MYUN fab too E kwine)

Brand Names: U.S. Anascorp

Therapeutic Category Antivenin

Generic Availability (U.S.) No

Use Treatment of scorpion envenomation in patients with clinical signs of envenomation including, but not limited to, loss of muscle control, roving or abnormal eye movements, slurred speech, respiratory distress, excessive salivation, frothing at mouth, and vomiting (FDA approved in ages of neonates through adults)

Pregnancy Risk Factor C

Pregnancy Considerations Animal reproduction studies have not been conducted. In general, medications used as antidotes should take into consideration the health and prognosis of the mother; antidotes should be administered to pregnant women if there is a clear indication for use and should not be withheld because of fears of teratogenicity (Bailey, 2003).

Breast-Feeding Considerations It is not known if this product is excreted into breast milk. The manufacturer recommends caution be used if administered to a nursing woman.

Contraindications Hypersensitivity to *Centruroides* Immune F(ab')₂ (Equine) or any component

Warnings Product derived from equine (horse) immune globulin F(ab')2 fragments; anaphylaxis and anaphylactoid reactions are possible, especially in patients with known allergies to horse protein. Patients who have had previous treatment with *Centruroides* immune F(ab')2 or other equine-derived antivenom/antitoxin may be at a higher risk for hypersensitivity reactions. In patients who develop an anaphylactic reaction, discontinue the infusion and administer emergency care. Immediate treatment (eg, epinephrine 1:1000, corticosteroids, diphenhydramine) should be available. Delayed serum sickness may occur, usually within 2 weeks; monitor patients with follow-up visits for signs and symptoms (eg, arthralgia, fever, myalgia, rash). Product of equine (horse) plasma; may potentially contain infectious agents (eg, viruses) which could transmit disease. May contain small amounts of cresol resulting from the manufacturing process; local reactions and myalgias may occur.

Adverse Reactions

Central nervous system: Fatigue, fever, headache, lethargy

Dermatologic: Pruritus, rash

Gastrointestinal: Diarrhea, nausea, vomiting

Neuromuscular & skeletal: Myalgia

Respiratory: Cough, rhinorrhea

Rare but important or life-threatening: Aspiration, ataxia, chest tightness, eye edema, hypersensitivity, hypoxia, palpitation, pneumonia, respiratory distress, serum sickness (delayed)

Drug Interactions

Metabolism/Transport Effects None known.

Avoid Concomitant Use There are no known interactions where it is recommended to avoid concomitant use.

Increased Effect/Toxicity There are no known significant interactions involving an increase in effect.

Decreased Effect There are no known significant interactions involving a decrease in effect.

Stability Store unused vials at room temperature of 25°C (77°F); excursions permitted up to 40°C (104°F); do not freeze. Discard partially used vials. May further dilute in NS.

Mechanism of Action Contains venom-specific F(ab')$_2$ fragments of IgG which bind and neutralize venom toxins; thereby helping to remove the toxin from the target tissue and eliminate it from the body.

Pharmacodynamics Onset: Time to resolution of symptoms: Children: 1.28 ± 0.8 hours; Adults: 1.91 ± 1.4 hours; >95% of all patients will experience resolution of symptoms within 4 hours

Pharmacokinetics (Adult data unless noted)
Distribution: V$_{dss}$: 13.6 L ± 5.4 L
Half-life: 159 ± 57 hours

Dosing: Neonatal Scorpion envenomation: I.V.: Initial: 3 vials (~≤360 mg total protein and ≥450 LD50 [mouse] neutralizing units) initiated as soon as possible after scorpion sting; may administer additional vials in 1-vial increments every 30-60 minutes as needed

Dosing: Usual Scorpion envenomation: Infants, Children, Adolescents, and Adults: I.V.: Initial: 3 vials (~≤360 mg total protein and ≥450 LD50 [mouse] neutralizing units) initiated as soon as possible after scorpion sting; may administer additional vials in 1-vial increments every 30-60 minutes as needed.

Dosing adjustment in renal impairment: There are no dosage adjustments provided in manufacturer's labeling.

Dosing adjustment in hepatic impairment: There are no dosage adjustments provided in manufacturer's labeling.

Administration I.V.: Reconstitute each vial with 5 mL of NS; gently swirl to mix. Dilute dose (eg, 1-3 vials) with NS to a total volume of 50 mL. Administer over 10 minutes; others have reported beginning infusion slower at 25-50 mL/hour and then double the rate every 5 minutes as tolerated (Turri, 2011); monitor for return of symptoms of envenomation and repeat as needed. Medications (eg, epinephrine, corticosteroids, diphenhydramine) and equipment for resuscitation should be readily available in case of hypersensitivity reactions. I.M. administration should generally be avoided since the time to peak blood concentration may be prolonged with this route of administration (Turri, 2011; Vasquez, 2010). If unable to obtain intravenous access, intraosseous (full dose) and intramuscular (single vial dose) administration have been reported in a neonate and a 16 month old child (Hiller, 2010).

Monitoring Parameters Signs and symptoms of envenomation (eg, opsoclonus, involuntary muscle movement, slurred speech, paresthesias, respiratory distress, salivation, frothy sputum, vomiting); signs and symptoms of hypersensitivity reactions; follow-up visits for signs and symptoms of serum sickness (eg, arthralgia, fever, myalgia, rash)

Additional Information Each vial of *Centruroides* immune F(ab')$_2$ (equine) contains ≤120 mg total protein and ≥150 LD50 (mouse) neutralizing units.

Dosage Forms Excipient information presented when available (limited, particularly for generics); consult specific product labeling.
Solution Reconstituted, Intravenous [preservative free]:
Anascorp: (1 ea)

References
Bailey B, "Are There Teratogenic Risks Associated With Antidotes Used in the Acute Management of Poisoned Pregnant Women?" *Birth Defects Res A Clin Mol Teratol*, 2003, 67(2):133-40.
Boyer LV, Theodorou AA, Berg RA, et al, "Antivenom for Critically Ill Children With Neurotoxicity From Scorpion Stings," *N Engl J Med*, 2009, 360(20):2090-8.
Hiller K, Jarrod MM, Franke HA, et al, "Scorpion Antivenom Administered by Alternative Infusions," *Ann Emerg Med*, 2010, 56(3):309-10.
Tuuri RE and Reynolds S, "Scorpion Envenomation and Antivenom Therapy," *Pediatr Emerg Care*, 2011, 27(7):667-675.
Vasquez H, Chavez-Haro A, Garcia-Ubbelohde W, et al, "Pharmacokinetics of a F(ab')2 Scorpion Antivenom Administered Intramuscularly in Healthy Human Volunteers," *Int Immunopharmacol*, 2010, 10 (11):1318-24.

◆ **Cepacol Dual Relief [OTC]** *see* Benzocaine *on page 273*

◆ **Cepacol Sensations Hydra [OTC]** *see* Benzocaine *on page 273*

◆ **Cepacol Sensations Warming [OTC]** *see* Benzocaine *on page 273*

◆ **Cepacol Sore Throat [OTC]** *see* Benzocaine *on page 273*

◆ **Cepacol Sore Throat + Coating [OTC]** *see* Benzocaine *on page 273*

◆ **Cepacol Sore Throat Max Numb [OTC]** *see* Benzocaine *on page 273*

Cephalexin (sef a LEKS in)

Medication Safety Issues
Sound-alike/look-alike issues:
Cephalexin may be confused with cefaclor, ceFAZolin, ciprofloxacin
Keflex may be confused with Keppra, Valtrex

Related Information
Prevention of Infective Endocarditis *on page 2336*

Brand Names: U.S. Keflex

Brand Names: Canada Apo-Cephalex; Dom-Cephalexin; Keflex; Novo-Lexin; Nu-Cephalex; PMS-Cephalexin

Therapeutic Category Antibiotic, Cephalosporin (First Generation)

Generic Availability (U.S.) Yes

Use Treatment of susceptible bacterial infections, including those caused by group A beta-hemolytic *Streptococcus*, *Staphylococcus*, *Klebsiella pneumoniae*, *E. coli*, and *Proteus mirabilis*; not active against enterococci or methicillin-resistant staphylococci; used to treat susceptible infections of the respiratory tract, skin and skin structure, bone, genitourinary tract, and otitis media; alternative therapy for endocarditis prophylaxis

Pregnancy Risk Factor B

Pregnancy Considerations Adverse events were not observed in animal reproduction studies. Cephalexin crosses the placenta and produces therapeutic concentrations in the fetal circulation and amniotic fluid. An increased risk of teratogenic effects has not been observed following maternal use of cephalexin. Peak concentrations in pregnant patients are similar to those in nonpregnant patients. Prolonged labor may decrease oral absorption.

Breast-Feeding Considerations Small amounts of cephalexin are excreted in breast milk. The manufacturer recommends that caution be exercised when administering cephalexin to nursing women. Maximum milk concentration occurs ~4 hours after a single oral dose and gradually disappears by 8 hours after administration. Non-dose-related effects could include modification of bowel flora.

Contraindications Hypersensitivity to cephalexin, any component, or cephalosporins

Warnings Prolonged use may result in GI or genitourinary superinfection; do not use in patients with immediate-type hypersensitivity reactions to penicillin

Precautions Use with caution and modify dosage in patients with renal impairment; use with caution in patients with history of colitis or history of penicillin hypersensitivity. Tablets for oral suspension contain aspartame which is metabolized to phenylalanine and must be avoided (or used with caution) in patients with phenylketonuria.

Adverse Reactions

Central nervous system: Agitation, confusion, dizziness, fatigue, hallucinations, headache

Dermatologic: Angioedema, erythema multiforme (rare), rash, Stevens-Johnson syndrome (rare), toxic epidermal necrolysis (rare), urticaria

Gastrointestinal: Abdominal pain, diarrhea, dyspepsia, gastritis, nausea (rare), pseudomembranous colitis, vomiting (rare)

Genitourinary: Genital pruritus, genital moniliasis, vaginitis, vaginal discharge

Hematologic: Eosinophilia, hemolytic anemia, neutropenia, thrombocytopenia

Hepatic: ALT increased, AST increased, cholestatic jaundice (rare), transient hepatitis (rare)

Neuromuscular & skeletal: Arthralgia, arthritis, joint disorder

Renal: Interstitial nephritis (rare)

Miscellaneous: Allergic reactions, anaphylaxis

Drug Interactions

Metabolism/Transport Effects None known.

Avoid Concomitant Use

Avoid concomitant use of Cephalexin with any of the following: BCG

Increased Effect/Toxicity

Cephalexin may increase the levels/effects of: MetFORMIN; Vitamin K Antagonists

The levels/effects of Cephalexin may be increased by: Probenecid

Decreased Effect

Cephalexin may decrease the levels/effects of: BCG; Sodium Picosulfate; Typhoid Vaccine

The levels/effects of Cephalexin may be decreased by: Multivitamins/Minerals (with ADEK, Folate, Iron); Multivitamins/Minerals (with AE, No Iron); Zinc Salts

Food Interactions Peak antibiotic serum concentration is lowered and delayed, but total drug absorbed is not affected. Cephalexin serum levels may be decreased if taken with food. Management: Administer without regard to food.

Stability Refrigerate suspension after reconstitution; discard after 14 days; tablets for oral suspension should be used immediately after dissolving

Mechanism of Action Inhibits bacterial cell wall synthesis by binding to one or more of the penicillin-binding proteins (PBPs) which in turn inhibits the final transpeptidation step of peptidoglycan synthesis in bacterial cell walls, thus inhibiting cell wall biosynthesis. Bacteria eventually lyse due to ongoing activity of cell wall autolytic enzymes (autolysins and murein hydrolases) while cell wall assembly is arrested.

Pharmacokinetics (Adult data unless noted)

Absorption: Rapid (90%); delayed in young children and may be decreased up to 50% in neonates

Distribution: Into tissues and fluids including bone, pleural and synovial fluid; crosses the placenta; appears in breast milk

Protein binding: 6% to 15%

Half-life:

Neonates: 5 hours

Children 3-12 months: 2.5 hours

Adults: 0.5-1.2 hours (prolonged with renal impairment)

Time to peak serum concentration: Oral: Within 60 minutes

Elimination: 80% to 100% of dose excreted as unchanged drug in urine within 8 hours

Dialysis: Moderately dialyzable (20% to 50%)

Dosing: Usual Oral:

Children: 25-50 mg/kg/day divided every 6-8 hours; severe infections: 50-100 mg/kg/day divided every 6-8 hours; maximum dose: 4 g/day

Otitis media: 75-100 mg/kg/day divided every 6 hours

Streptococcal pharyngitis, skin and skin structure infections: 25-50 mg/kg/day divided every 12 hours

Endocarditis prophylaxis: 50 mg/kg 1 hour prior to procedure (maximum: 2 g)

Uncomplicated cystitis: Children >15 years: 500 mg every 12 hours for 7-14 days

Adults: 250-500 mg every 6 hours; maximum dose: 4 g/day

Streptococcal pharyngitis, skin and skin structure infections: 500 mg every 12 hours

Endocarditis prophylaxis: 2 g 1 hour prior to procedure

Uncomplicated cystitis: 500 mg every 12 hours for 7-14 days

Dosing interval in renal impairment:

CrCl 10-40 mL/minute: Administer every 8-12 hours

CrCl <10 mL/minute: Administer every 12-24 hours

Administration Oral: Administer on an empty stomach (ie, 1 hour prior to, or 2 hours after meals); administer with food if GI upset occurs; shake suspension well before use

Tablet for oral suspension: Mix tablet in a small amount of water (~10 mL); stir until thoroughly mixed; entire mixture should be administered immediately after mixing; rinse container with an additional small amount of water and drink contents to assure the whole dose is taken. **Do not** chew or swallow tablets. **Do not** mix with liquids other than water.

Monitoring Parameters With prolonged therapy, monitor renal, hepatic, and hematologic function periodically; number and type of stools/day for diarrhea

Test Interactions Positive direct Coombs', false-positive urinary glucose test using cupric sulfate (Benedict's solution, Clinitest®, Fehling's solution), false-positive serum or urine creatinine with Jaffé reaction, false-positive urinary proteins and steroids

Dosage Forms Excipient information presented when available (limited, particularly for generics); consult specific product labeling.

Capsule, Oral:

Keflex: 250 mg, 500 mg, 750 mg [contains brilliant blue fcf (fd&c blue #1), fd&c yellow #10 (quinoline yellow), fd&c yellow #6 (sunset yellow)]

Generic: 250 mg, 500 mg, 750 mg

Suspension Reconstituted, Oral:

Generic: 125 mg/5 mL (100 mL, 200 mL); 250 mg/5 mL (100 mL, 200 mL)

Tablet, Oral:

Generic: 250 mg, 500 mg

References

Bergan T, "Pharmacokinetic Properties of Cephalosporins," Drugs, 1987, 34 (Suppl 2):89-104.

Bradley JS, Byington CL, Shah SS, et al, "The Management of Community-Acquired Pneumonia in Infants and Children Older Than 3 Months of Age: Clinical Practice Guidelines by the Pediatric Infectious Diseases Society and the Infectious Diseases Society of America", Clin Infect Dis, 2011, 53(7):e25-76.

Shulman ST, Bisno AL, Clegg HW, et al, "Clinical Practice Guideline for the Diagnosis and Management of Group A Streptococcal Pharyngitis: 2012 Update by the Infectious Diseases Society of America," Clin Infect Dis, 2012.

◆ **Cephalexin Monohydrate** see Cephalexin on page 429

◆ **Ceprotin** see Protein C Concentrate (Human) on page 1766

◆ **Cerebyx** see Fosphenytoin on page 941

◆ **Cerebyx® (Can)** see Fosphenytoin on page 941

◆ **Cerezyme** see Imiglucerase on page 1076

◆ **Cerubidine (Can)** see DAUNOrubicin (Conventional) on page 599

◆ **Cervarix** see Papillomavirus (Types 16, 18) Vaccine (Human, Recombinant) on page 1603

◆ **C.E.S.** see Estrogens (Conjugated/Equine, Systemic) on page 799

◆ **C.E.S.** *see* Estrogens (Conjugated/Equine, Topical) *on page 801*

◆ **C.E.S.® (Can)** *see* Estrogens (Conjugated/Equine, Systemic) *on page 799*

◆ **Cesamet** *see* Nabilone *on page 1459*

◆ **Cesamet® (Can)** *see* Nabilone *on page 1459*

◆ **Cetafen [OTC]** *see* Acetaminophen *on page 47*

◆ **Cetafen Extra [OTC]** *see* Acetaminophen *on page 47*

Cetirizine (se TI ra zeen)

Medication Safety Issues
Sound-alike/look-alike issues:
Cetirizine may be confusd with sertraline
ZyrTEC may be confused with Lipitor, Serax, Xanax, Zantac, Zerit, Zocor, ZyPREXA, ZyrTEC-D
ZyrTEC (cetirizine) may be confused with ZyrTEC Itchy Eye (ketotifen)
International issues:
Benadryl international brand name for cetirizine [Great Britain, Phillipines], but also the brand name for acrivastine and pseudoephedrine [Great Britain] and several products containing diphenhydramine [U.S., Canada]

Brand Names: U.S. All Day Allergy Childrens [OTC]; All Day Allergy [OTC]; Cetirizine HCl Allergy Child [OTC]; Cetirizine HCl Childrens Alrgy [OTC]; Cetirizine HCl Childrens [OTC]; Cetirizine HCl Hives Relief [OTC]; ZyrTEC Allergy Childrens [OTC]; ZyrTEC Allergy [OTC]; ZyrTEC Childrens Allergy [OTC]; ZyrTEC Childrens Hives Relief [OTC]; ZyrTEC Hives Relief [OTC]

Brand Names: Canada Aller-Relief [OTC]; Apo-Cetirizine® [OTC]; Extra Strength Allergy Relief [OTC]; PMS-Cetirizine; Reactine [OTC]; Reactine™

Therapeutic Category Antihistamine

Generic Availability (U.S.) May be product dependent

Use Relief of symptoms associated with perennial and seasonal allergic rhinitis; treatment of the uncomplicated skin manifestations of chronic idiopathic urticaria

Pregnancy Considerations Maternal use of cetirizine has not been associated with an increased risk of major malformations. The use of antihistamines for the treatment of rhinitis during pregnancy is generally considered to be safe at recommended doses. Although safety data is limited, cetirizine may be a preferred second generation antihistamine for the treatment of rhinitis during pregnancy.

Breast-Feeding Considerations Cetirizine is excreted into breast milk.

Contraindications Hypersensitivity to cetirizine, hydroxyzine, or any component

Warnings Safety and efficacy for the use of cough and cold products in children <2 years of age is limited. Serious adverse effects including death have been reported. The FDA notes that there are no approved OTC uses for these products in children <2 years of age. Healthcare providers are reminded to ask caregivers about the use of OTC cough and cold products in order to avoid exposure to multiple medications containing the same ingredient. Doses >10 mg/day may cause significant drowsiness.

Precautions Use with caution in patients with hepatic or renal dysfunction

Adverse Reactions
Central nervous system: Dizziness, headache, fatigue, insomnia, malaise, somnolence
Gastrointestinal: Abdominal pain, diarrhea, dry mouth, nausea, vomiting
Respiratory: Bronchospasm, epistaxis, pharyngitis
Rare but important or life-threatening: Aggressive reaction, anaphylaxis, angioedema, ataxia, chest pain, confusion, convulsions, depersonalization, depression, edema, fussiness, hallucinations, hemolytic anemia, hepatitis, hypertension, hypotension (severe), irritability, liver function abnormal, nervousness, ototoxicity, palpitation, paralysis, paresthesia, photosensitivity, rash, suicidal ideation, suicide, taste perversion, tongue discoloration, tongue edema, tremor, visual field defect, weakness

Drug Interactions
Metabolism/Transport Effects Substrate of CYP3A4 (minor), P-glycoprotein; **Note:** Assignment of Major/Minor substrate status based on clinically relevant drug interaction potential

Avoid Concomitant Use
Avoid concomitant use of Cetirizine with any of the following: Aclidinium; Azelastine (Nasal); Ipratropium (Oral Inhalation); Paraldehyde; Potassium Chloride; Thalidomide; Tiotropium; Umeclidinium

Increased Effect/Toxicity
Cetirizine may increase the levels/effects of: AbobotulinumtoxinA; Alcohol (Ethyl); Analgesics (Opioid); Anticholinergic Agents; Azelastine (Nasal); Buprenorphine; Cannabinoid-Containing Products; CNS Depressants; Hydrocodone; Methotrimeprazine; Metyrosine; Mirabegron; Mirtazapine; OnabotulinumtoxinA; Paraldehyde; Potassium Chloride; Pramipexole; RimabotulinumtoxinB; ROPINIRole; Rotigotine; Selective Serotonin Reuptake Inhibitors; Thalidomide; Thiazide Diuretics; Tiotropium; Topiramate; Zolpidem

The levels/effects of Cetirizine may be increased by: Aclidinium; Brimonidine (Topical); Cannabis; Doxylamine; Dronabinol; Droperidol; HydrOXYzine; Ipratropium (Oral Inhalation); Kava Kava; Magnesium Sulfate; Methotrimeprazine; Nabilone; Perampanel; P-glycoprotein/ABCB1 Inhibitors; Pramlintide; Rufinamide; Sodium Oxybate; Tapentadol; Tetrahydrocannabinol; Umeclidinium

Decreased Effect
Cetirizine may decrease the levels/effects of: Acetylcholinesterase Inhibitors (Central); Benzylpenicilloyl Polylysine; Betahistine; Hyaluronidase; Secretin

The levels/effects of Cetirizine may be decreased by: Acetylcholinesterase Inhibitors (Central); Amphetamines; P-glycoprotein/ABCB1 Inducers

Food Interactions Cetirizine's absorption and maximal concentration are reduced when taken with food. Management: May be taken without regard to meals.

Stability Store at room temperature; protect syrup from light

Mechanism of Action Competes with histamine for H_1-receptor sites on effector cells in the gastrointestinal tract, blood vessels, and respiratory tract

Pharmacodynamics
Onset of action: 20-60 minutes
Duration: 24 hours

Pharmacokinetics (Adult data unless noted)
Absorption: Well absorbed from the GI tract
Distribution: V_d:
Children: 0.7 L/kg
Adults: 0.5-0.8 L/kg
Protein binding: 93%
Metabolism: Exact fate is unknown, limited hepatic metabolism
Half-life:
Children: 6.2 hours
Adults: 7.4-9 hours
Adults with mild-moderate renal failure: 19-21 hours
Time to peak serum concentration: 1 hour
Elimination: 60% to 70% excreted unchanged in urine
Dialysis: <10% removed during hemodialysis

Dosing: Usual Oral:
Children 6-12 months: 2.5 mg once daily
Children 12-23 months: Initial: 2.5 mg once daily; dosage may be increased to 2.5 mg twice daily

Children 2-5 years: 2.5 mg/day; may be increased to a maximum of 5 mg/day given either as a single dose or divided into 2 doses

Children ≥6 years to Adults: 5-10 mg/day as a single dose or divided into 2 doses

Dosage adjustment in renal or hepatic impairment:
Children <6 years: Cetirizine use not recommended
Children 6-11 years: <2.5 mg once daily
Children ≥12 and Adults:
CrCl 11-31 mL/minute, hemodialysis, or hepatic impairment: 5 mg once daily
CrCl <11 mL/minute, not on dialysis: Cetirizine use not recommended

Administration Oral: Administer without regard to food

Test Interactions May cause false-positive serum TCA screen. May suppress the wheal and flare reactions to skin test antigens.

Dosage Forms Excipient information presented when available (limited, particularly for generics); consult specific product labeling. [DSC] = Discontinued product
Capsule, Oral, as hydrochloride:
ZyrTEC Allergy: 10 mg
Solution, Oral, as hydrochloride:
All Day Allergy Childrens: 5 mg/5 mL (118 mL) [contains methylparaben, propylene glycol, propylparaben]
All Day Allergy Childrens: 5 mg/5 mL (118 mL) [dye free, gluten free; contains methylparaben, propylene glycol, propylparaben; grape flavor]
All Day Allergy Childrens: 1 mg/mL (118 mL [DSC]) [dye free, gluten free, sugar free; contains propylene glycol, sodium benzoate; grape flavor]
Cetirizine HCl Allergy Child: 5 mg/5 mL (120 mL) [alcohol free, dye free, gluten free, sugar free; contains methylparaben, propylene glycol, propylparaben; grape flavor]
Cetirizine HCl Allergy Child: 5 mg/5 mL (120 mL) [alcohol free, sugar free; contains methylparaben, propylene glycol, propylparaben]
Cetirizine HCl Childrens: 1 mg/mL (118 mL) [contains methylparaben, propylene glycol, propylparaben]
Cetirizine HCl Hives Relief: 5 mg/5 mL (120 mL) [alcohol free, sugar free; contains methylparaben, propylene glycol, propylparaben; grape flavor]
Generic: 1 mg/mL (473 mL)
Syrup, Oral, as hydrochloride:
Cetirizine HCl Childrens Alrgy: 1 mg/mL (118 mL, 120 mL) [contains methylparaben, propylene glycol, propylparaben; grape flavor]
ZyrTEC Childrens Allergy: 1 mg/mL (118 mL) [contains methylparaben, propylene glycol, propylparaben; banana-grape flavor]
ZyrTEC Childrens Allergy: 1 mg/mL (118 mL) [dye free, sugar free; contains propylene glycol, sodium benzoate]
ZyrTEC Childrens Allergy: 1 mg/mL (118 mL) [dye free, sugar free; contains propylene glycol, sodium benzoate; bubble-gum flavor]
ZyrTEC Childrens Allergy: 5 mg/5 mL (5 mL, 118 mL) [dye free, sugar free; contains propylene glycol, sodium benzoate; grape flavor]
ZyrTEC Childrens Hives Relief: 1 mg/mL (118 mL) [grape flavor]
Generic: 1 mg/mL (120 mL, 473 mL [DSC], 480 mL); 5 mg/5 mL (5 mL, 120 mL [DSC])
Tablet, Oral, as hydrochloride:
All Day Allergy: 10 mg
All Day Allergy: 10 mg [contains brilliant blue fcf (fd&c blue #1)]
ZyrTEC Allergy: 10 mg
ZyrTEC Hives Relief: 10 mg
Generic: 5 mg, 10 mg
Tablet Chewable, Oral, as hydrochloride:
All Day Allergy Childrens: 5 mg, 10 mg [tutti-frutti flavor]
ZyrTEC Childrens Allergy: 5 mg [grape flavor]

ZyrTEC Childrens Allergy: 10 mg [contains fd&c blue #2 aluminum lake; grape flavor]
Generic: 5 mg, 10 mg
Tablet Dispersible, Oral, as hydrochloride:
ZyrTEC Allergy Childrens: 10 mg [citrus flavor]

◆ **Cetirizine HCl Allergy Child [OTC]** *see* Cetirizine *on page 431*
◆ **Cetirizine HCl Childrens [OTC]** *see* Cetirizine *on page 431*
◆ **Cetirizine HCl Childrens Alrgy [OTC]** *see* Cetirizine *on page 431*
◆ **Cetirizine HCl Hives Relief [OTC]** *see* Cetirizine *on page 431*
◆ **Cetirizine Hydrochloride** *see* Cetirizine *on page 431*
◆ **Cetraxal** *see* Ciprofloxacin (Otic) *on page 476*
◆ **CFDN** *see* Cefdinir *on page 395*
◆ **CG** *see* Chorionic Gonadotropin (Human) *on page 460*
◆ **CGP 33101** *see* Rufinamide *on page 1858*
◆ **CGP-57148B** *see* Imatinib *on page 1072*
◆ **CGS-20267** *see* Letrozole *on page 1211*
◆ **Charac-25 [OTC] (Can)** *see* Charcoal, Activated *on page 432*
◆ **Charac-50 [OTC] (Can)** *see* Charcoal, Activated *on page 432*
◆ **Charactol-25 [OTC] (Can)** *see* Charcoal, Activated *on page 432*
◆ **Charactol-50 [OTC] (Can)** *see* Charcoal, Activated *on page 432*

Charcoal, Activated (CHAR kole AK tiv ay ted)

Medication Safety Issues
Sound-alike/look-alike issues:
Actidose® may be confused with Actos®
Related Information
Oral Medications That Should Not Be Crushed or Altered *on page 2438*
Brand Names: U.S. Actidose-Aqua [OTC]; Actidose/Sorbitol [OTC]; Char-Flo with Sorbitol [OTC]; EZ Char [OTC]; Kerr Insta-Char in Sorbitol [OTC]; Kerr Insta-Char [OTC]
Brand Names: Canada Charac-25 [OTC]; Charac-50 [OTC]; Charactol-25 [OTC]; Charactol-50 [OTC]; Charcodote Susp [OTC]; Charcodote TFS [OTC]; Charcodote-Aqueous Sus; Premium Activated Charcoal [OTC]
Therapeutic Category Antidiarrheal; Antidote, Adsorbent; Antiflatulent
Generic Availability (U.S.) May be product dependent
Use Emergency treatment in poisoning by drugs and chemicals (FDA approved in all ages); repetitive doses for GI dialysis in drug overdose to enhance the elimination of certain drugs (eg, theophylline, phenobarbital, carbamazepine, dapsone, quinine) (FDA approved in all ages); has also been used in uremia to adsorb various waste products; dietary supplement (digestive aid)
Pregnancy Considerations Activated charcoal is not absorbed systemically following oral administration. Systemic absorption would be required in order for activated charcoal to cross the placenta and reach the fetus. In general, medications used as antidotes should take into consideration the health and prognosis of the mother; antidotes should be administered to pregnant women if there is a clear indication for use and should not be withheld because of fears of teratogenicity (Bailey, 2003).
Breast-Feeding Considerations Activated charcoal is not absorbed systemically following oral administration.
Contraindications Patients with an unprotected airway (eg, depressed CNS state without endotracheal

intubation); patients at increased risk and severity of aspiration (eg, ingestion of hydrocarbon with a high potential for aspiration); patients at risk of GI perforation or hemorrhage due to medical conditions, recent surgery, or other pathology; **Note**: Ingestion of a corrosive (caustic) substance is **not** a contraindication if charcoal is used for coingested systemic toxin. Charcoal is not effective for cyanide, mineral acids, caustic alkalis, organic solvents, iron, ethanol, methanol, or lithium poisonings; do not use charcoal with sorbitol in patients with fructose intolerance; charcoal with sorbitol is not recommended in children <1 year of age

Warnings If charcoal in sorbitol is administered, doses should be limited to prevent excessive fluid and electrolyte losses. Excessive amounts of activated charcoal with sorbitol may cause hypernatremic dehydration in pediatric patients. Aspiration may cause tracheal obstruction in infants but usually not a major problem in adults; aspiration pneumonitis, bronchiolitis obliterans, and ARDS have been reported following aspiration of charcoal; however, these problems may be due to the aspiration of gastric contents and not charcoal per se.

Some suspensions (eg, Kerr Insta-Char®) contain sodium benzoate; benzoic acid (benzoate) is a metabolite of benzyl alcohol; large amounts of benzyl alcohol (≥99 mg/kg/day) have been associated with a potentially fatal toxicity ("gasping syndrome") in neonates; the "gasping syndrome" consists of metabolic acidosis, respiratory distress, gasping respirations, CNS dysfunction (including convulsions, intracranial hemorrhage), hypotension, and cardiovascular collapse; use activated charcoal products containing sodium benzoate with caution in neonates; *in vitro* and animal studies have shown that benzoate displaces bilirubin from protein binding sites.

Precautions When using ipecac with charcoal, induce vomiting with ipecac before administering activated charcoal since charcoal adsorbs ipecac syrup. Charcoal may cause vomiting; rate is higher with sorbitol; vomiting is hazardous in petroleum distillate and caustic ingestions. Charcoal (especially in multiple doses) may adsorb maintenance medications and place the patient at risk for exacerbation of concomitant disorders.

Adverse Reactions
Gastrointestinal: Abdominal distention, appendicitis, bowel obstruction, constipation, vomiting
Ocular: Corneal abrasion (with direct contact)
Respiratory: Aspiration, respiratory failure
Miscellaneous: Fecal discoloration (black)

Drug Interactions
Metabolism/Transport Effects None known.
Avoid Concomitant Use There are no known interactions where it is recommended to avoid concomitant use.
Increased Effect/Toxicity There are no known significant interactions involving an increase in effect.
Decreased Effect
Charcoal, Activated may decrease the levels/effects of: Leflunomide; Teriflunomide

Food Interactions The addition of some flavoring agents (eg, milk, ice cream, sherbet, marmalade) are known to reduce the adsorptive capacity, and therefore the efficacy, of activated charcoal and should be avoided in preference to activated charcoal-water slurries; nevertheless, these flavoring agents do not completely compromise the effectiveness of activated charcoal and may be necessary in some circumstances (eg, administration in pediatric patients) to enhance compliance (Cooney, 1995; Dagnone, 2002).

Stability Adsorbs gases from air; store in closed container
Mechanism of Action Adsorbs toxic substances, thus inhibiting GI absorption

Pharmacodynamics In studies using adult human volunteers: Mean **reduction** in drug absorption following a single dose of activated charcoal:
All size doses of activated charcoal:
    Given within 30 minutes after ingestion: 69.1% reduction
    Given at 60 minutes after ingestion: 34.4% reduction
50 g activated charcoal:
    Given within 30 minutes after ingestion: 88.6% reduction
    Given at 60 minutes after ingestion: 37.3% reduction

Pharmacokinetics (Adult data unless noted)
Absorption: Not absorbed from the GI tract
Metabolism: Not metabolized
Elimination: Excreted as charcoal in feces

Dosing: Usual Oral:
Acute poisoning:
    Single dose: Charcoal with sorbitol (**Note:** The use of repeated oral charcoal with sorbitol doses is not recommended):
        Infants <1 year: Not recommended
        Children 1-12 years: 1-2 g/kg or 25-50 g or approximately 5-10 times the weight of the ingested poison on a gram-to-gram basis; 1 g adsorbs 100-1000 mg of poison; in young children sorbitol should be repeated **no more** than 1-2 times/day
        Adolescents and Adults: 30-100 g
    Single dose: Charcoal in water (a cathartic such as sorbitol should be added in appropriate doses):
        Infants <1 year: 1 g/kg
        Children 1-12 years: 1-2 g/kg or 25-50 g
        Adolescents and Adults: 30-100 g or 1-2 g/kg
    Multiple dose: Charcoal in water (doses are repeated until clinical observations of toxicity subside and serum drug concentrations have returned to a subtherapeutic range or until the development of absent bowel sounds or ileus; use only one dose of cathartic daily):
        Infants <1 year: 1 g/kg every 4-6 hours
        Children 1-12 years: 1-2 g/kg or 15-30 g every 2-6 hours
        Adolescents and Adults: 25-60 g or 1-2 g/kg every 2-6 hours
Gastric dialysis: Adults: 20-50 g every 6 hours for 1-2 days

Administration Oral: Administer as soon as possible after ingestion, preferably within 1 hour for greatest effect. Shake well before use; do not mix with milk, ice cream, sherbet, or marmalade; may be mixed with chocolate or fruit syrup to increase palatability. Instruct patient to drink slowly, rapid administration may increase frequency of vomiting; if patient has persistent vomiting, multiple doses may be administered as a continuous enteral infusion

Monitoring Parameters Fluid status, sorbitol intake, number of stools, electrolytes if increase in stools or diarrhea occurs; continually assess for active bowel sounds in patients receiving multiple dose activated charcoal

Additional Information 5-6 tablespoonfuls of activated charcoal powder is approximately equal to 30 g; minimum dilution of 240 mL water per 20-30 g activated charcoal should be mixed as an aqueous slurry; multiple dose activated charcoal has been shown to be effective in increasing the elimination of certain drugs (carbamazepine, theophylline, phenobarbital) even after these drugs have been absorbed

The Position Paper on single dose activated charcoal by The American Academy of Clinical Toxicology and The European Association of Poisons Centres and Clinical Toxicologists (Chyka, 2005) does not advocate **routine** use of single dose activated charcoal in the treatment of poisoned patients. Scientific literature supports the use of activated charcoal within 1 hour of toxin ingestion, when it will be more likely to produce benefit. Studies in volunteers demonstrate that the effectiveness of activated charcoal decreases as the time of administration after toxin ingestion increases. Therefore, this publication states that activated charcoal may be considered up to 1 hour following ingestion of a potentially toxic amount of poison. In addition, the use of activated charcoal may be considered greater than 1 hour following ingestion, since the potential benefit cannot be excluded. Furthermore, based on current literature, the routine administration of a cathartic with activated charcoal is not recommended; when cathartics are used, only a single dose should be administered so as to decrease adverse effects (Position Paper: Cathartics, 2004).

A policy statement by the American Academy of Pediatrics states that it is currently premature to recommend the **routine** administration of activated charcoal as a home treatment strategy for poisonings (AAP, 2003).

Dosage Forms Excipient information presented when available (limited, particularly for generics); consult specific product labeling.

Liquid, Oral:

Actidose-Aqua: 15 g/72 mL (72 mL); 25 g/120 mL (120 mL); 50 g/240 mL (240 mL) [sweet flavor]

Actidose/Sorbitol: 25 g/120 mL (120 mL); 50 g/240 mL (240 mL) [sweet flavor]

Kerr Insta-Char: 25 g/120 mL (120 mL); 50 g/240 mL (240 mL) [contains fd&c red #40, methylparaben sodium, propylene glycol, propylparaben sodium, sodium benzoate; cherry flavor]

Kerr Insta-Char: 50 g/240 mL (240 mL) [contains propylene glycol]

Kerr Insta-Char in Sorbitol: 25 g/120 mL (120 mL); 50 g/240 mL (240 mL) [contains fd&c red #40, methylparaben sodium, propylene glycol, propylparaben sodium, sodium benzoate; cherry flavor]

Suspension, Oral:

Char-Flo with Sorbitol: 25 g (120 mL)

Suspension Reconstituted, Oral:

EZ Char: 25 g (1 ea) [contains bentonite]

References

American Academy of Pediatrics Committee on Injury, Violence, and Poison Prevention, "Poison Treatment in the Home," *Pediatrics*, 2003, 112(5):1182-5.

Bailey B, "Are There Teratogenic Risks Associated With Antidotes Used in the Acute Management of Poisoned Pregnant Women?" *Birth Defects Res A Clin Mol Teratol*, 2003, 67(2):133-40.

Burns MM, "Activated Charcoal as the Sole Intervention for Treatment After Childhood Poisoning," *Curr Opin Pediatr*, 2000, 12(2):166-71.

Chyka PA, Seger D, Krenzelok EP, et al, "Position Paper: Single-Dose Activated Charcoal," *Clin Toxicol (Phila)*, 2005, 43(2):61-87.

Cooney DO, *Development of Palatable Formulations, Activated Charcoal in Medical Applications*, Cooney DO, ed, New York, NY: Marcel Dekker, Inc, 1995, 397-417.

Dagnone D, Matsui D, and Rieder MJ, "Assessment of the Palatability of Vehicles for Activated Charcoal in Pediatric Volunteers," *Pediatr Emerg Care*, 2002, 18(1):19-21.

Farley TA, "Severe Hypernatremic Dehydration After Use of an Activated Charcoal-Sorbitol Suspension," *J Pediatr*, 1986, 109(4):719-22.

"Position Statement and Practice Guidelines on the Use of Multi-dose Activated Charcoal in the Treatment of Acute Poisoning. American Academy of Clinical Toxicology; European Association of Poisons Centres and Clinical Toxicologists," *J Toxicol Clin Toxicol*, 1999, 37 (6):731-51.

"Position Paper: Cathartics," *J Toxicol Clin Toxicol*, 2004, 42(3):243-53.

Shannon M, "Ingestion of Toxic Substances by Children," *N Engl J Med*, 2000, 342(3):186-91.

◆ **Charcodote-Aqueous Sus (Can)** *see* Charcoal, Activated *on page 432*

◆ **Charcodote Susp [OTC] (Can)** *see* Charcoal, Activated *on page 432*

◆ **Charcodote TFS [OTC] (Can)** *see* Charcoal, Activated *on page 432*

◆ **Char-Flo with Sorbitol [OTC]** *see* Charcoal, Activated *on page 432*

◆ **Chemet** *see* Succimer *on page 1937*

◆ **Chenodal** *see* Chenodiol *on page 434*

◆ **Chenodeoxycholic Acid** *see* Chenodiol *on page 434*

Chenodiol (kee noe DYE ole)

Brand Names: U.S. Chenodal
Therapeutic Category Bile Acid
Generic Availability (U.S.) No
Use Oral dissolution of radiolucent cholesterol gallstones in well-opacifying gallbladders in patients who are not candidates for surgery due to systemic disease or age (FDA approved in adults); has also been used for lipid storage diseases, including cerebrotendinous xanthomatosis, Zellweger syndrome, and other susceptible bile acid biosynthesis defects which result in low chenodeoxycholic acid concentrations

Prescribing and Access Restrictions Prescriptions are only dispensed by a specialty pharmacy, Centric Health Resources, which may be contacted at 866-758-7068.

Pregnancy Risk Factor X

Pregnancy Considerations Hepatic, renal, and adrenal lesions were observed in some animal reproduction studies. Use during pregnancy is contraindicated.

Breast-Feeding Considerations It is not known if chenodiol is excreted in breast milk. The manufacturer recommends that caution be exercised when administering chenodiol to nursing women.

Contraindications Hypersensitivity to chenodiol or any component; presence of known hepatocyte dysfunction or bile ductal abnormalities (eg, intrahepatic cholestasis, primary biliary cirrhosis, sclerosing cholangitis); a gallbladder confirmed as nonvisualizing after two consecutive single doses of dye; radiopaque stones; gallstone complications or compelling reasons for gallbladder surgery (eg, unremitting acute cholecystitis, cholangitis, biliary obstruction, gallstone pancreatitis, or biliary gastrointestinal fistula); pregnancy or patients who may become pregnant

Warnings Drug-induced liver toxicity may occur (dose-related); avoid or use with extreme caution in patients with hepatic impairment or elevated liver enzymes; use contraindicated in patients with known hepatocyte dysfunction or bile ductal abnormalities. Minor (≤3 X ULN), dose-related elevation of serum aminotransferases has been reported frequently (incidence: 30%); aminotransferase elevations >3 X ULN have also been reported less often (incidence: 2% to 3%); close monitoring of serum aminotransferase levels recommended during therapy; prompt discontinuation of therapy recommended if significant elevation of serum aminotransferase levels (>3 X ULN) or signs of hepatic impairment occur.

Precautions Dose-related diarrhea commonly occurs (up to 40% of patients). Diarrhea is usually mild, most frequently observed during therapy initiation, and does not interfere with therapy; however, diarrhea may be severe and a temporary dosage reduction or discontinuation may be required. Epidemiologic studies have suggested that bile acids may increase the risk of colon cancer. Evidence is weak and conflicting; however, a potential link between bile acids and colon cancer cannot be ruled out.

Careful selection of appropriate patients is necessary prior to therapy; studies have shown gallstone dissolution rates are higher in patients with small (<15 mm in diameter), radiolucent, and/or floatable stones. Radiopaque (calcified or partially calcified) stones and bile pigment stones do not respond to bile acid dissolution therapy. Response to therapy should be monitored with oral cholecystograms or ultrasonograms. Complete dissolution should be confirmed by one repeat test 1-3 months after continued therapy. If partial dissolution is not observed by 9-12 months, complete dissolution is unlikely. If no response is observed by 18 months, therapy should be discontinued; safety beyond 24 months of use has not been established.

Adverse Reactions

Endocrine & metabolic: LDL cholesterol increased, total cholesterol increased

Gastrointestinal: Abdominal cramps, abdominal pain, anorexia, biliary pain, constipation, diarrhea (including severe diarrhea requiring dose reduction), dyspepsia, flatulence, heartburn, nausea, vomiting

Hematologic: Leukopenia

Hepatic: Aminotransferase increased

Drug Interactions

Metabolism/Transport Effects None known.

Avoid Concomitant Use There are no known interactions where it is recommended to avoid concomitant use.

Increased Effect/Toxicity There are no known significant interactions involving an increase in effect.

Decreased Effect

The levels/effects of Chenodiol may be decreased by: Aluminum Hydroxide; Bile Acid Sequestrants; Estrogen Derivatives; Fibric Acid Derivatives

Stability Store at 20°C to 25°C (68°F to 77°F).

Mechanism of Action Chenodiol (chenodeoxycholic acid) is a naturally occurring human bile acid, normally constituting one-third of the total bile acid pool. Synthesis of chenodiol is regulated by the relative composition and flux of cholesterol and bile acids through the hepatocyte by a negative feedback effect on the rate-limiting enzymes for synthesis of cholesterol (HMG-CoA reductase) and bile acids (cholesterol 7 alpha-hydroxyl). In patients with cholesterol gallstones, chenodiol is believed to suppress hepatic synthesis of cholesterol and cholic acid, and inhibit biliary cholesterol secretion, which leads to increased production of cholesterol unsaturated bile thereby allowing for dissolution of gallstones.

Pharmacokinetics (Adult data unless noted)

Absorption: Rapid, almost completely absorbed in proximal small intestine (Crosignani, 1996)

Distribution: V_d: 1600 L (Crosignani, 1996)

Metabolism: Converted hepatically to taurine and glycine conjugates and secreted in bile; extensive first-pass hepatic clearance (60% to 80%); undergoes enterohepatic circulation; further metabolized in colon by bacteria to lithocholic acid; small portion of lithocholate is absorbed and converted to sulfolithocholyl conjugates in the liver

Half-life: 45 hours (Crosignani, 1996)

Elimination: Feces (80%, as lithocholate)

Dosing: Usual

Infants, Children, and Adolescents:

Gallstone dissolution: Limited data available: Oral: Children ≥12 years and Adolescents: 15 mg/kg/day divided 3 times daily with meals; dosing based on reported experience in three obese pediatric patients (age range: 12-13 years); **Note:** Not first-line therapy due to frequent side effect (increased LFT, diarrhea) and other therapeutic options available (Podda, 1982)

Inborn errors of bile acid biosynthesis: Limited data available: **Note:** Due to the rarity of the disease states, data is limited to very small case series and case reports; further studies are needed. Adjust dose based upon targeted bile acid or biosynthesis intermediate compound concentrations. Combination therapy with ursodeoxycholic acid (urosdiol) dependent on specific deficiency, and phenotypic presentation of syndrome.

Cerebrotendinous xanthomatosis: Oral: Initial: 10-15 mg/kg/day divided 1-3 times daily; in adolescents, a fixed dose of 750 mg/day has also been reported (Beringer, 2010; Kaufman, 2012; Setchell, 2006; van Heijst, 1998)

Steroid dehydrogenase or reductase deficiencies (susceptible): Oral: Usual initial range: 5-10 mg/kg/day divided once or twice daily; higher initial doses of 11-18 mg/kg/day have also been reported; a maintenance dose of 5 mg/kg/day was the most frequently reported and initiated once targeted bile acid normalized or stabilized (depending upon the syndrome) (Clayton, 1996; Clayton, 2011; Ichimiya, 1990; Riello, 2010)

Peroxisome deficiency, including Zellweger syndrome: Oral: 100-250 mg/day or 5 mg/kg/day have been used (Maeda, 2002; Setchell, 1992)

Adults: **Gallstone dissolution (monotherapy):** Oral: Initial: 250 mg twice daily for the first 2 weeks and increasing by 250 mg/day each week thereafter until the recommended or maximum tolerated dose is achieved; maintenance: 13-16 mg/kg/day in 2 divided doses. **Note:** Dosages <10 mg/kg are usually ineffective and may increase the risk of cholecystectomy.

Dosing adjustment in renal impairment: There are no dosage adjustments provided in manufacturer's labeling.

Dosing adjustment in hepatic impairment: Use extreme caution; contraindicated for use in presence of known hepatocyte dysfunction or bile duct abnormalities.

Administration May be taken without regard to meals.

Monitoring Parameters Serum aminotransferase levels (monthly for first 3 months, then every 3 months during therapy); serum cholesterol (every 6 months); for gallstone dissolution: Oral cholecystograms and/or ultrasonograms (6-9 month intervals for response to therapy); dissolutions of stones should be confirmed 1-3 months later; for bile acid biosynthesis defects: Targeted bile acids or intermediate product concentrations from either serum or blood should be measured (as appropriate) (Clatyon 2011; Setchell, 2006)

Dosage Forms Excipient information presented when available (limited, particularly for generics); consult specific product labeling.

Tablet, Oral:

Chenodal: 250 mg

References

Beringer VM, Gross B, Morad K, etal. Chronic diarrhea and juvenile cataracts: think cerebrotendinous xanthomatosis and treat. *Pediatrics.* 2010;123:143-147.

Clayton PT. Disorders of bile acid synthesis. *J Inherit Meab Dis.* 2011;34 593-604.

Clayton PT, Mills KA, Johnson AW, et al. Delta 4-3-oxosteroid 5ß-reductase deficiency: failure of ursodeoxycholic acid treatment and response to chenodeoxycholic acid plus cholic acid. *Gut.* 1996;38:623-628.

Crosignani A, Setchell KDR, Invernizzi P, etal. Clinical pharmacokinetics of therapeutic bile acids. *Clin Pharmacokineti.* 1996;30(5):333-358.

Ichimiya H, Nazer H, Gunasekaran T, et al. Treatment of chronic liver disease caused by 3ß-hydroxy-Δ5-C27-steroid dehydrogenase deficiency with chenodeoxycholic acid. *Archives of Disease in Childhood.* 1990;65:1121-1124.

Kaufman MA, Gonzalez-Moron D, Consalvo D, et al. Cerebrotendinous xanthomatosis revealed in drug-resistant epilepsy diagnostic workup. *Am J Med Sci.* 2012;343(4):332-333.

Maeda K, Kimura A, Yamoto Y, et al. Oral bile acid treatment in two Japanese patients with Zellweger syndrome. *Journal of Pediatric Gastroenterology and Nutrition.* 2002;35:227-230.

Podda M, Zuin M, Dioguardi ML, et al. Successful treatment of gallstones with bile acids in obese adolescents. *Arch Dis Child.* 1982;57(12):956-958.

Riello L, Antiga LD, Guido M, et al. Titration of bile acid supplements in 3ß-hydroxy-Δ5-C27-steroid dehydrogenase/isomerase deficiency. *JPGN.* 2010;50:655-660.

Setchell KD, Bragetti P, Zimmer-Nechemias L, et al. Oral bile acid treatment and the patient with Zellweger syndrome. *Hepatology.* 1992;15(2):198-207.

Setchell KDR, Heubi JE. Defects in bile acid biosynthesis – diagnosis and treatment. *Journal of Pediatric Gastroenterology and Nutrition.* 2006;43:17-22.

Van Heijst AJ, Verrips A, Wevers RA, et al. Treatment and follow-up of children with cerebrotendinous xanthomatosis. *Eur J Pediatr.* 1998;157(4):313-316.

◆ **Cheracol D [OTC]** see Guaifenesin and Dextromethorphan on page 987

◆ **Cheracol Plus [OTC]** see Guaifenesin and Dextromethorphan on page 987

- **Cheratussin** *see* GuaiFENesin *on page 984*
- **Chew-C [OTC]** *see* Ascorbic Acid *on page 206*
- **CHG** *see* Chlorhexidine Gluconate *on page 441*
- **Chickenpox Vaccine** *see* Varicella Virus Vaccine *on page 2116*
- **Chiggerex [OTC]** *see* Benzocaine *on page 273*
- **Chiggertox [OTC]** *see* Benzocaine *on page 273*
- **Childrens Advil [OTC]** *see* Ibuprofen *on page 1059*
- **Children's Advil® Cold (Can)** *see* Pseudoephedrine and Ibuprofen *on page 1772*
- **Childrens Ibuprofen [OTC]** *see* Ibuprofen *on page 1059*
- **Childrens Loratadine [OTC]** *see* Loratadine *on page 1278*
- **Childrens Motrin [OTC]** *see* Ibuprofen *on page 1059*
- **Childrens Motrin Jr Strength [OTC]** *see* Ibuprofen *on page 1059*
- **Childrens Silfedrine [OTC]** *see* Pseudoephedrine *on page 1770*
- **Children's Advil (Can)** *see* Ibuprofen *on page 1059*
- **Children's Europrofen (Can)** *see* Ibuprofen *on page 1059*
- **Children's Motion Sickness Liquid [OTC] (Can)** *see* DimenhyDRINATE *on page 670*
- **ChiRhoStim** *see* Secretin *on page 1876*
- **Chloditan** *see* Mitotane *on page 1425*
- **Chlodithane** *see* Mitotane *on page 1425*
- **Chloral** *see* Chloral Hydrate *on page 436*

Chloral Hydrate (KLOR al HYE drate)

Medication Safety Issues
High alert medication:
The Institute for Safe Medication Practices (ISMP) includes this medication among its list of drugs which have a heightened risk of causing significant patient harm when used in error.

Related Information
Oral Medications That Should Not Be Crushed or Altered *on page 2438*
Preprocedure Sedatives in Children *on page 2402*
Safe Handling of Hazardous Drugs *on page 2419*

Brand Names: Canada PMS-Chloral Hydrate

Therapeutic Category Hypnotic; Sedative

Use Short-term sedative and hypnotic (<2 weeks), sedative/hypnotic prior to nonpainful therapeutic or diagnostic procedures (eg, EEG, CT scan, MRI, ophthalmic exam, dental procedure)

Pregnancy Considerations Animal reproduction studies have not been conducted. Chloral hydrate crosses the placenta, and long-term use may lead to withdrawal symptoms in the neonate.

Breast-Feeding Considerations Chloral hydrate is excreted in breast milk; use by breast-feeding women may cause sedation in the infant.

Contraindications Hypersensitivity to chloral hydrate or any component; hepatic or renal impairment; severe cardiac disease. Oral forms are also contraindicated in patients with gastritis, esophagitis, or gastric or duodenal ulcers.

Warnings Hazardous agent; use appropriate precautions for handling and disposal; exposure may irritate skin and mucous membranes. Deaths and permanent neurologic injury from respiratory compromise have been reported in children sedated with chloral hydrate; respiratory obstruction may occur in children with tonsillar and adenoidal hypertrophy, obstructive sleep apnea, and Leigh's encephalopathy, and in ASA class III children; depressed levels of consciousness may occur; chloral hydrate should **not** be administered for sedation by nonmedical personnel or in a nonsupervised medical environment; sedation with chloral hydrate requires careful patient monitoring (Cote, 2000); animal studies suggest that chloral hydrate may depress the genioglossus muscle and other airway-maintaining muscles in patients who are already at risk for life-threatening airway obstruction (eg, obstructive sleep apnea); alternative sedative agents should be considered for these patients (Hershenson, 1984).

Trichloroethanol (TCE), an active metabolite of chloral hydrate, is a carcinogen in mice; there is no data in humans. Syrup may contain sodium benzoate; benzoic acid (benzoate) is a metabolite of benzyl alcohol; large amounts of benzyl alcohol (≥99 mg/kg/day) have been associated with a potentially fatal toxicity ("gasping syndrome") in neonates; the "gasping syndrome" consists of metabolic acidosis, respiratory distress, gasping respirations, CNS dysfunction (including convulsions, intracranial hemorrhage), hypotension and cardiovascular collapse; use chloral hydrate products containing sodium benzoate with caution in neonates; *in vitro* and animal studies have shown that benzoate displaces bilirubin from protein binding sites

Precautions Use with caution in neonates, drug and metabolites may accumulate with repeated use; prolonged use in neonates is associated with direct hyperbilirubinemia [active metabolite (TCE) competes with bilirubin for glucuronide conjugation in the liver]; use with caution in patients with porphyria. Tolerance to hypnotic effect develops, therefore, not recommended for use >2 weeks; taper dosage to avoid withdrawal with prolonged use. Avoid use in patients with moderate to severe renal failure (CrCl <50 mL/minute).

Adverse Reactions
Cardiovascular: Atrial arrhythmia, depression of myocardial contractility, hypotension, shortening of refractory periods, torsades de pointes, ventricular arrhythmia
Central nervous system: Abnormal gait, ataxia, confusion, delirium, dizziness, drowsiness, drug dependence (physical and psychological; with prolonged use or large doses), hallucinations, hangover effect, malaise, nightmares, paradoxical excitation, somnambulism, vertigo
Dermatologic: Skin rash (including erythema, eczematoid dermatitis, urticaria, scarlatiniform exanthems)
Endocrine & metabolic: Acute porphyria, ketonuria
Gastrointestinal: Diarrhea, flatulence, gastric irritation, nausea, vomiting
Hematologic & oncologic: Acute porphyria, eosinophilia, leukopenia
Ophthalmic: Allergic conjunctivitis, blepharoptosis, keratoconjunctivitis
Otic: Increased middle ear pressure (infants and children)
Respiratory: Airway obstruction (young children), laryngeal edema (children)
Miscellaneous: Drug tolerance

Drug Interactions
Metabolism/Transport Effects None known.
Avoid Concomitant Use
Avoid concomitant use of Chloral Hydrate with any of the following: Azelastine (Nasal); Furosemide; Paraldehyde; Sodium Oxybate; Thalidomide
Increased Effect/Toxicity
Chloral Hydrate may increase the levels/effects of: Alcohol (Ethyl); Azelastine (Nasal); Buprenorphine; CNS Depressants; Highest Risk QTc-Prolonging Agents; Hydrocodone; Methotrimeprazine; Metyrosine; Mirtazapine; Moderate Risk QTc-Prolonging Agents; Paraldehyde; Pramipexole; ROPINIRole; Rotigotine; Selective Serotonin Reuptake Inhibitors; Sodium Oxybate; Thalidomide; Vitamin K Antagonists; Zolpidem

The levels/effects of Chloral Hydrate may be increased by: Brimonidine (Topical); Cannabis; Doxylamine; Dronabinol; Droperidol; Furosemide; HydrOXYzine; Kava Kava; Magnesium Sulfate; Methotrimeprazine; Mifepristone; Nabilone; Perampanel; Rufinamide; Tapentadol; Tetrahydrocannabinol

Decreased Effect

The levels/effects of Chloral Hydrate may be decreased by: Flumazenil

Stability Sensitive to light; exposure to air causes volatilization; store in light-resistant, airtight container at room temperature; do not refrigerate

Mechanism of Action Central nervous system depressant effects are due to its active metabolite trichloroethanol, mechanism unknown

Pharmacodynamics

Onset of action: 10-20 minutes
Maximum effect: Within 30-60 minutes
Duration: 4-8 hours

Pharmacokinetics (Adult data unless noted)

Absorption: Oral, rectal: Well absorbed
Distribution: Crosses the placenta; distributes to breast milk
Protein binding: Trichloroethanol: 35% to 40%; trichloroacetic acid: ~94% (may compete with bilirubin for albumin binding sites)
Metabolism: Rapidly metabolized by alcohol dehydrogenase to trichloroethanol (active metabolite); trichloroethanol undergoes glucuronidation in the liver; variable amounts of chloral hydrate and trichloroethanol are metabolized in liver and kidney to trichloroacetic acid (inactive)
Half-life:
Chloral hydrate: Infants: 1 hour
Trichloroethanol (active metabolite):
Neonates: Range: 8.5-66 hours
Half-life decreases with increasing postmenstrual age (PMA):
Preterm infants (PMA 31-37 weeks): Mean half-life: 40 hours
Term infants (PMA 38-42 weeks): Mean half-life: 28 hours
Older children (PMA 57-708 weeks): Mean half-life: 10 hours
Adults: 8-11 hours
Trichloroacetic acid: Adults: 67.2 hours
Elimination: Metabolites excreted in urine; small amounts excreted in feces via bile
Dialysis: Dialyzable (50% to 100%)

Dosing: Neonatal Oral, rectal: 25 mg/kg/dose for sedation prior to a procedure; **Note:** Repeat doses should be used with great caution as drug and metabolites accumulate with repeated use; toxicity has been reported after 3 days in a preterm neonate and after 7 days in a term neonate receiving chloral hydrate 40-50 mg/kg every 6 hours

Dosing: Usual Oral, rectal:
Infants and Children:
Sedation, anxiety: 25-50 mg/kg/day divided every 6-8 hours, maximum dose: 500 mg/dose
Prior to EEG: 25-50 mg/kg/dose 30-60 minutes prior to EEG; may repeat in 30 minutes to a total maximum of 100 mg/kg or 1 g total for infants and 2 g total for children
Sedation, nonpainful procedure: 50-75 mg/kg/dose 30-60 minutes prior to procedure; may repeat 30 minutes after initial dose if needed, to a total maximum dose of 120 mg/kg or 1 g total for infants and 2 g total for children
Hypnotic: 50 mg/kg/dose at bedtime; maximum dose: 1 g/dose; total maximum: 1 g/day for infants and 2 g/day for children
Adults:
Sedation, anxiety: 250 mg 3 times/day

Hypnotic: 500-1000 mg at bedtime or 30 minutes prior to procedure, not to exceed 2 g/24 hours
Dosing adjustment in renal impairment:
CrCl ≥50 mL/minute: No dosage adjustment needed
CrCl <50 mL/minute: Avoid use

Administration

Oral: Minimize unpleasant taste and gastric irritation by administering with water, infant formula, fruit juice, or ginger ale; do not crush capsule, contains drug in liquid form with unpleasant taste
Rectal administration: May administer chloral hydrate syrup rectally

Monitoring Parameters Level of sedation; vital signs and O₂ saturation with doses used for sedation prior to procedure

Test Interactions May interfere with copper sulfate tests for glycosuria or with fluorometric urine catecholamine and urinary 17-hydroxycorticosteroid tests.

Additional Information Not an analgesic; osmolality of 500 mg/5 mL syrup is approximately 3500 mOsm/kg

References

American Academy of Pediatrics, Committee on Drugs and Committee on Environmental Health, "Use of Chloral Hydrate for Sedation in Children," *Pediatrics*, 1993, 92(3):471-3.

Buck ML, "Chloral Hydrate Use During Infancy," *Neonatal Pharmacology Quarterly*, 1992, 1(1):31-7.

Cote CJ, Karl HW, Notterman DA, et al, "Adverse Sedation Events in Pediatrics: Analysis of Medications Used for Sedation," *Pediatrics*, 2000, 106(4):633-44.

Hershenson M, Brouillette RT, Olsen E, et al, "The Effect of Chloral Hydrate on Genioglossus and Diaphragmatic Activity," *Pediatr Res*, 1984, 18(6):516-9.

Mayers DJ, Hindmarsh KW, Gorecki DK, et al, "Sedative/Hypnotic Effects of Chloral Hydrate in the Neonate: Trichloroethanol or Parent Drug?" *Dev Pharmacol Ther*, 1992, 19(2-3):141-6.

Mayers DJ, Hindmarsh KW, Sankaran K, et al, "Chloral Hydrate Disposition Following Single-Dose Administration to Critically Ill Neonates and Children," *Dev Pharmacol Ther*, 1991, 16(2):71-7.

Steinberg AD, "Should Chloral Hydrate be Banned?" *Pediatrics*, 1993, 92(3):442-6.

Chlorambucil (klor AM byoo sil)

Medication Safety Issues

Sound-alike/look-alike issues:
Chlorambucil may be confused with Chloromycetin®
Leukeran® may be confused with Alkeran®, leucovorin, Leukine®, Myleran®

High alert medication:
This medication is in a class the Institute for Safe Medication Practices (ISMP) includes among its list of drug classes which have a heightened risk of causing significant patient harm when used in error.

Related Information

Emetogenic Potential of Antineoplastic Agents in Children *on page 2327*
Oral Medications That Should Not Be Crushed or Altered *on page 2438*
Safe Handling of Hazardous Drugs *on page 2419*

Brand Names: U.S. Leukeran

Brand Names: Canada Leukeran®

Therapeutic Category Antineoplastic Agent, Alkylating Agent; Antineoplastic Agent, Alkylating Agent (Nitrogen Mustard)

Generic Availability (U.S.) No

Use Treatment of chronic lymphocytic leukemia (CLL), Hodgkin's and non-Hodgkin's lymphoma (FDA approved in adults); has also been used in the treatment of nephrotic syndrome (unresponsive to conventional therapy) and Waldenström's macroglobulinemia

Pregnancy Risk Factor D

Pregnancy Considerations Animal reproduction studies have demonstrated teratogenicity. Chlorambucil crosses the human placenta. Following exposure during the first trimester, case reports have noted adverse renal effects ▶

(unilateral agenesis). Women of childbearing potential should avoid becoming pregnant while receiving treatment. **[U.S. Boxed Warning]: Affects human fertility; probably mutagenic and teratogenic as well**; chromosomal damage has been documented. Reversible and irreversible sterility (when administered to prepubertal and pubertal males), azoospermia (in adult males) and amenorrhea (in females) have been observed. Fibrosis, vasculitis and depletion of primordial follicles have been noted on autopsy of the ovaries.

Breast-Feeding Considerations It is not known if chlorambucil is excreted in breast milk. Due to the potential for serious adverse reactions in the nursing infant, the decision to discontinue chlorambucil or to discontinue breast-feeding should take into account the benefits of treatment to the mother.

Contraindications Hypersensitivity to chlorambucil or any component; cross hypersensitivity (skin rash) may occur with other alkylating agents; previous resistance

Warnings Hazardous agent; use appropriate precautions for handling and disposal (NIOSH, 2012). Chlorambucil can severely suppress bone marrow function **[U.S. Boxed Warning]**; neutropenia may be severe. Reduce initial dosage if patient has received myelosuppressive or radiation therapy within the previous 4 weeks, or has a depressed baseline leukocyte or platelet count; chlorambucil dose should not exceed 0.1 mg/kg/day if bone marrow is hypoplastic. Irreversible bone marrow damage may occur with total doses approaching 6.5 mg/kg. Progressive lymphopenia may develop (recovery is generally rapid after discontinuation). Adversely affects human fertility **[U.S. Boxed Warning]**; chromosomal damage has been documented. Reversible and irreversible sterility (when administered to prepubertal and pubertal males), azoospermia (in adult males) and amenorrhea (in females) have been observed. Possibly mutagenic and teratogenic **[U.S. Boxed Warning]**; carcinogenic in humans **[U.S. Boxed Warning]**; acute myelocytic leukemia and secondary malignancies may be associated with chronic therapy. Duration of treatment and higher cumulative doses are associated with a higher risk for development of leukemia. Convulsions and severe skin reactions (eg, erythema multiforme, Stevens-Johnson syndrome and toxic epidermal necrolysis) have been reported.

Precautions Use with caution in patients with seizure disorder, head trauma, patients receiving epileptogenic drugs, and in patients with bone marrow suppression; avoid administration of live vaccines to immunocompromised patients; children with nephrotic syndrome may have an increased risk of seizures.

Adverse Reactions
Central nervous system: Agitation (rare), ataxia (rare), confusion (rare), drug fever, fever, focal/generalized seizure (rare), hallucinations (rare)
Dermatologic: Angioneurotic edema, erythema multiforme (rare), rash, skin hypersensitivity, Stevens-Johnson syndrome (rare), toxic epidermal necrolysis (rare), urticaria
Endocrine & metabolic: Amenorrhea, infertility, SIADH (rare)
Gastrointestinal: Diarrhea (infrequent), nausea (infrequent), oral ulceration (infrequent), vomiting (infrequent)
Genitourinary: Azoospermia, cystitis (sterile)
Hematologic: Neutropenia (onset: 3 weeks; recovery: 10 days after last dose), bone marrow failure (irreversible), bone marrow suppression, anemia, leukemia (secondary), leukopenia, lymphopenia, pancytopenia, thrombocytopenia
Hepatic: Hepatotoxicity, jaundice
Neuromuscular & skeletal: Flaccid paresis (rare), muscular twitching (rare), myoclonia (rare), peripheral neuropathy, tremor (rare)
Respiratory: Interstitial pneumonia, pulmonary fibrosis

Miscellaneous: Allergic reactions, malignancies (secondary)

Drug Interactions
Metabolism/Transport Effects None known.
Avoid Concomitant Use
Avoid concomitant use of Chlorambucil with any of the following: BCG; CloZAPine; Dipyrone; Natalizumab; Pimecrolimus; Tacrolimus (Topical); Tofacitinib; Vaccines (Live)
Increased Effect/Toxicity
Chlorambucil may increase the levels/effects of: CloZAPine; Leflunomide; Natalizumab; Tofacitinib; Vaccines (Live)

The levels/effects of Chlorambucil may be increased by: Denosumab; Dipyrone; Pimecrolimus; Roflumilast; Tacrolimus (Topical); Trastuzumab
Decreased Effect
Chlorambucil may decrease the levels/effects of: BCG; Coccidioidin Skin Test; Sipuleucel-T; Vaccines (Inactivated); Vaccines (Live)

The levels/effects of Chlorambucil may be decreased by: Echinacea
Food Interactions Absorption is decreased when administered with food. Management: Administer preferably on an empty stomach.
Stability Hazardous agent; use appropriate precautions for handling and disposal (NIOSH, 2012). Store in refrigerator; protect from light.
Mechanism of Action Alkylating agent; interferes with DNA replication and RNA transcription by alkylation and cross-linking the strands of DNA
Pharmacokinetics (Adult data unless noted)
Absorption: Oral: Rapid and almost completely absorbed from GI tract
Distribution: To liver, ascitic fluid, fat; extensively bound to plasma and tissue proteins; crosses the placenta
Protein binding: ~99%
Metabolism: In the liver to an active metabolite, phenylacetic acid mustard
Bioavailability: 56% to 100%
Half-life: Chlorambucil: 1.5 hours; phenylacetic acid mustard: 2.5 hours
Time to peak serum concentration: Chlorambucil: Within 1 hour; phenylacetic acid mustard: Within 2-4 hours
Elimination: 60% excreted in urine within 24 hours principally as metabolites; <1% excreted as unchanged drug or phenylacetic acid mustard in urine
Dialysis: Probably not dialyzable
Dosing: Usual Oral (refer to individual protocols):
Children:
General short courses: 0.1-0.2 mg/kg/day or 4.5 mg/m^2/day once daily for 3-6 weeks for remission induction (usual: 4-10 mg/day); maintenance therapy: 0.03-0.1 mg/kg/day (usual: 2-4 mg/day)
Relapsing steroid-sensitive nephrotic syndrome: 0.2 mg/kg/day once daily for 8 weeks
CLL:
Biweekly regimen: Initial: 0.4 mg/kg/dose every 2 weeks; increase dose by 0.1 mg/kg every 2 weeks until a response occurs and/or myelosuppression occurs
Monthly regimen: Initial: 0.4 mg/kg every 4 weeks, increase dose by 0.2 mg/kg every 4 weeks until a response occurs and/or myelosuppression occurs
Malignant lymphomas:
Non-Hodgkin's lymphoma: 0.1 mg/kg/day
Hodgkin's: 0.2 mg/kg/day
Adults: 0.1-0.2 mg/kg/day or 3-6 mg/m^2/day once daily for 3-6 weeks, then adjust dose on basis of blood counts
Administration Hazardous agent; use appropriate precautions for handling and disposal (NIOSH, 2012).

Oral: Administer 30-60 minutes before food; do not administer with acidic foods, hot foods, and spices

Monitoring Parameters Liver function tests, CBC with differential, hemoglobin, leukocyte and platelet counts, serum uric acid

Additional Information Myelosuppressive effects:
WBC: Moderate
Platelets: Moderate
Onset (days): 7
Nadir (days): 14-21

Dosage Forms Excipient information presented when available (limited, particularly for generics); consult specific product labeling.
Tablet, Oral:
Leukeran: 2 mg

Extemporaneous Preparations Hazardous agent: Use appropriate precautions for handling and disposal.

A 2 mg/mL oral suspension may be prepared with tablets. Crush sixty 2 mg tablets in a mortar and reduce to a fine powder. Add small portions of methylcellulose 1% and mix to a uniform paste (total methylcellulose: 30 mL); mix while adding simple syrup in incremental proportions to **almost** 60 mL; transfer to a graduated cylinder, rinse mortar and pestle with simple syrup, and add quantity of vehicle sufficient to make 60 mL. Transfer contents of graduated cylinder to an amber prescription bottle. Label "shake well", "refrigerate", and "protect from light". Stable for 7 days refrigerated.

Dressman JB and Poust RI, "Stability of Allopurinol and of Five Antineoplastics in Suspension," *Am J Hosp Pharm*, 1983, 40(4):616-8.

Nahata MC, Pai VB, and Hipple TF, *Pediatric Drug Formulations*, 5th ed, Cincinnati, OH: Harvey Whitney Books Co, 2004.

References

Baluarte HJ, Hiner L, and Gruskin AB, "Chlorambucil Dosage in Frequently Relapsing Nephrotic Syndrome: A Controlled Clinical Trial," *J Pediatr*, 1978, 92(2):295-8.

Durkan A, Hodson EM, Willis NS, et al, "Non-corticosteroid Treatment for Nephrotic Syndrome in Children," *Cochrane Database Syst Rev*, 2005, 18(2):CD002290.

National Institute for Occupational Safety and Health (NIOSH), "NIOSH List of Antineoplastic and Other Hazardous Drugs in Healthcare Settings 2012." Available at http://www.cdc.gov/niosh/docs/2012-150/pdfs/2012-150.pdf. Accessed January 21, 2013.

Singh BN and Malhotra BK, "Effects of Food on the Clinical Pharmacokinetics of Anticancer Agents: Underlying Mechanisms and Implications for Oral Chemotherapy," *Clin Pharmacokinet*, 2004, 43 (15):1127-56.

Williams SA, Makker SP, and Grupe WE, "Seizures: A Significant Side Effect of Chlorambucil Therapy in Children," *J Pediatr*, 1978, 93 (3):516-8.

◆ **Chlorambucilum** *see* Chlorambucil *on page 437*

◆ **Chloraminophene** *see* Chlorambucil *on page 437*

Chloramphenicol (klor am FEN i kole)

Medication Safety Issues
Sound-alike/look-alike issues:
Chloromycetin® may be confused with chlorambucil, Chlor-Trimeton®

Related Information
Safe Handling of Hazardous Drugs *on page 2419*

Brand Names: Canada Chloromycetin®; Chloromycetin® Succinate; Diochloram®; Pentamycetin®

Therapeutic Category Antibiotic, Miscellaneous

Generic Availability (U.S.) Yes

Use Treatment of serious infections caused by susceptible organisms [eg, Salmonella, rickettsia, *H. influenza* (meningitis), or cystic fibrosis pathogens] when less toxic drugs are ineffective (ie, resistance) or contraindicated (FDA approved in all ages)

Pregnancy Considerations Chloramphenicol crosses the placenta producing cord concentrations approaching maternal serum concentrations. An increased risk of teratogenic effects has not been associated with the use of chloramphenicol in pregnancy (Czeizel, 2000; Heinonen, 1977). "Gray Syndrome" has occurred in premature infants and newborns receiving chloramphenicol. The manufacturer recommends caution if used in a pregnant patient near term or during labor. Chloramphenicol may be used for the treatment of Rocky Mountain spotted fever in pregnant women although caution should be used when administration occurs during the third trimester (CDC, 2006).

Breast-Feeding Considerations Chloramphenicol and its inactive metabolites are excreted in breast milk. Chloramphenicol is well absorbed following oral administration; however, metabolism and excretion are highly variable in infants and children. The half-life is also significantly prolonged in low birth weight infants (Powell, 1982). Due to the potential for serious adverse reactions in the nursing infant, the manufacturer recommends that caution be exercised when administering chloramphenicol to nursing women. Other sources recommended avoiding use while breast-feeding, especially infants <34 weeks postconceptual age or when unusually large doses are needed (Atkinson, 1988; Matsuda, 1984; Plomp, 1983). Non-dose-related effects could include modification of bowel flora.

Contraindications Hypersensitivity to chloramphenicol or any component; previous toxic reaction to chloramphenicol; treatment of trivial or viral infections; bacterial prophylaxis

Warnings Hazardous agent; use appropriate precautions for handling and disposal (NIOSH, 2012). Serious and fatal blood dyscrasias (aplastic anemia, hypoplastic anemia, thrombocytopenia, and granulocytopenia) have occurred after short-term and prolonged therapy **[U.S. Boxed Warning]**; monitor CBC with platelets frequently in all patients **[U.S. Boxed Warning]**; discontinue if evidence of myelosuppression. Irreversible bone marrow suppression may occur weeks or months after therapy. Avoid repeated courses of treatment; avoid concurrent therapy with drugs that may also cause bone marrow depression. Should not be used when less potentially toxic agents are effective. Prolonged use may result in fungal or bacterial superinfection, including *C. difficile*-associated diarrhea (CDAD) and pseudomembranous colitis; CDAD has been observed >2 months postantibiotic treatment. Use in neonates (including premature) has resulted in "gray-baby syndrome" characterized by circulatory collapse, cyanosis, acidosis, abdominal distention (with or without emesis), myocardial depression, coma, and death; progression of symptoms is rapid; prompt termination of therapy required. Reaction appears to be associated with serum levels ≥50 mcg/mL and may be due to drug accumulation possibly caused by the impaired neonatal hepatic or renal function.

Precautions Use with caution in patients with G-6-PD deficiency. Use with caution in patients with impaired renal or hepatic function; may reduce ability to metabolize and excrete chloramphenicol; dosage adjustment may be necessary.

Adverse Reactions
Central nervous system: Confusion, delirium, depression, fever, headache
Dermatologic: Angioedema, rash, urticaria
Gastrointestinal: Diarrhea, enterocolitis, glossitis, nausea, stomatitis, vomiting
Hematologic: Aplastic anemia, bone marrow suppression, granulocytopenia, hypoplastic anemia, pancytopenia, thrombocytopenia
Ocular: Optic neuritis
Miscellaneous: Anaphylaxis, hypersensitivity reactions, Gray syndrome

Drug Interactions
Metabolism/Transport Effects Inhibits CYP2C19 (strong), CYP2C9 (weak), CYP3A4 (strong)

Avoid Concomitant Use

Avoid concomitant use of Chloramphenicol with any of the following: Ado-Trastuzumab Emtansine; Alfuzosin; Apixaban; Avanafil; Axitinib; BCG; Bosutinib; Cabozantinib; Ceritinib; CloZAPine; Conivaptan; Crizotinib; Dipyrone; Dronedarone; Eplerenone; Everolimus; Halofantrine; Ibrutinib; Ivabradine; Lapatinib; Lomitapide; Lovastatin; Lurasidone; Macitentan; Nilotinib; Nisoldipine; Pimozide; Ranolazine; Red Yeast Rice; Regorafenib; Rivaroxaban; Salmeterol; Silodosin; Simeprevir; Simvastatin; Tamsulosin; Ticagrelor; Tolvaptan; Toremifene; Ulipristal; Vemurafenib; VinCRIStine (Liposomal); Vorapaxar

Increased Effect/Toxicity

Chloramphenicol may increase the levels/effects of: Ado-Trastuzumab Emtansine; Alcohol (Ethyl); Alfuzosin; Almotriptan; Alosetron; Anticonvulsants (Hydantoin); Apixaban; ARIPiprazole; Avanafil; Axitinib; Barbiturates; Bedaquiline; Bortezomib; Bosentan; Bosutinib; Brentuximab Vedotin; Brinzolamide; Budesonide (Nasal); Budesonide (Systemic, Oral Inhalation); Cabozantinib; Cannabis; Carbocisteine; Ceritinib; Citalopram; CloZAPine; Colchicine; Conivaptan; Corticosteroids (Orally Inhaled); Crizotinib; CycloSPORINE (Systemic); CYP2C19 Substrates; CYP3A4 Substrates; Dienogest; Dofetilide; DOXOrubicin (Conventional); Dronabinol; Dronedarone; Dutasteride; Enzalutamide; Eplerenone; Everolimus; FentaNYL; Fesoterodine; Fluticasone (Nasal); Fluticasone (Oral Inhalation); GuanFACINE; Halofantrine; Ibrutinib; Iloperidone; Imatinib; Ivabradine; Ivacaftor; Ixabepilone; Lacosamide; Lapatinib; Levomilnacipran; Lomitapide; Lovastatin; Lumefantrine; Lurasidone; Macitentan; Maraviroc; MethylPREDNISolone; Mifepristone; Nilotinib; Nisoldipine; Ospemifene; OxyCODONE; Paricalcitol; PAZOPanib; Pimecrolimus; Pimozide; PONATinib; Propafenone; QUEtiapine; Ranolazine; Red Yeast Rice; Regorafenib; Repaglinide; Rilpivirine; Rivaroxaban; RomiDEPsin; Ruxolitinib; Salmeterol; Saxagliptin; Sildenafil; Silodosin; Simeprevir; Simvastatin; SORAfenib; Sulfonylureas; Tacrolimus (Systemic); Tadalafil; Tamsulosin; Tetrahydrocannabinol; Ticagrelor; Tofacitinib; Tolterodine; Tolvaptan; Toremifene; Ulipristal; Vardenafil; Vemurafenib; Vilazodone; VinCRIStine (Liposomal); Vitamin K Antagonists; Vorapaxar; Voriconazole; Zuclopenthixol

The levels/effects of Chloramphenicol may be increased by: Dipyrone

Decreased Effect

Chloramphenicol may decrease the levels/effects of: BCG; Clopidogrel; Cyanocobalamin; Prasugrel; Sodium Picosulfate; Ticagrelor; Typhoid Vaccine

The levels/effects of Chloramphenicol may be decreased by: Anticonvulsants (Hydantoin); Barbiturates; Rifampin

Stability Hazardous agent; use appropriate precautions for handling and disposal (NIOSH, 2012).
Store intact vials at 20°C to 25°C (68°F to 77°F). Reconstituted solutions (100 mg/mL) remain stable for 30 days. Use only clear solutions. Frozen solutions remain stable for 6 months.

Mechanism of Action Reversibly binds to 50S ribosomal subunits of susceptible organisms preventing amino acids from being transferred to growing peptide chains thus inhibiting protein synthesis

Pharmacokinetics (Adult data unless noted)

Distribution: Distributes to most tissues and body fluids; good CSF and brain penetration
  CSF concentration with uninflamed meninges: 21% to 50% of plasma concentration
  CSF concentration with inflamed meninges: 45% to 89% of plasma concentration
  V_d:
    Chloramphenicol: 0.5-1 L/kg

Chloramphenicol succinate: 0.2-3.1 L/kg; decreased with hepatic or renal dysfunction
Protein binding: Chloramphenicol: 60% decreased with hepatic or renal dysfunction and 30% to 40% in newborn infants
Metabolism:
  Chloramphenicol succinate: Hydrolized in the liver, kidney, and lungs to chloramphenicol (active)
  Chloramphenicol succinate: Hepatic to metabolites (inactive)
Bioavailability:
  Chloramphenicol: Oral: ~80%
  Chloramphenicol succinate: I.V.: ~70%; highly variable, dependant upon rate and extent of metabolism to chloramphenicol
Half-life:
  Neonates:
    1-2 days: 24 hours
    10-16 days: 10 hours
  Children: 4-6 hours
  Adults:
    Normal renal function: ~4 hours
    Chloramphenicol succinate: ~3 hours
    End-stage renal disease: 3-7 hours
    Hepatic disease: Prolonged
Elimination: ~30% as unchanged chloramphenicol succinate in urine; in infants and young children, 6% to 80% of the dose may be excreted unchanged in urine; 5% to 15% as chloramphenicol

Dosing: Neonatal Note: Follow serum concentrations closely to monitor for toxicity and efficacy in neonates due to variability in metabolism; use should be restricted to treatment of serious infections caused by susceptible organisms when less toxic drugs are ineffective (ie, resistance) or contraindicated.

Meningitis (Tunkel, 2004): I.V.: **Note:** Treat for a minimum of 21 days; use smaller doses and longer intervals for neonates <2 kg:
  PNA ≤7 days: 25 mg/kg/dose every 24 hours
  PNA 8-28 days: 25 mg/kg/dose every 12 hours or 50 mg/kg/dose every 24 hours

Severe infection: I.V.:
  Weight-based dosing: Limited data available (Prober, 1990):
    Patient weight:
      <1200 g: 22 mg/kg/dose every 24 hours
      1200-2000 g: 25 mg/kg/dose every 24 hours
  Age-based dosing: Limited data available:
    Premature neonate or term neonate with PNA ≤7 days: Dosing regimens variable: 25 mg/kg/dose every 24 hours or initiation with a loading dose of 20 mg/kg followed in 12 hours by a maintenance regimen of 12.5 mg/kg/dose every 12 hours (Rajchgot, 1982; Rajchgot, 1983; Weiss, 1960)
    Term neonate with PNA >7 days: Dosing regimens variable: 25 mg/kg/dose every 12 hours or 12.5 mg/kg/dose every 6 hours (Rajchgot, 1983; Weiss, 1960)
  Manufacturer's labeling: **Note:** Frequency recommended by the manufacturer for this age group is higher than other expert recommendations, which generally recommend no more frequent than every 12 hours; monitor serum concentrations closely.
    Preterm infants: 6.25 mg/kg/dose every 6 hours
    Term infants:
      PNA <14 days: 6.25 mg/kg/dose every 6 hours
      PNA ≥14 days: 12.5 mg/kg/dose every 6 hours

Dosing: Usual

Infants, Children, and Adolescents: **Note:** Follow serum concentrations closely to monitor for toxicity. Use should be restricted to treatment of serious infections when less toxic drugs are ineffective (ie, resistance) or contraindicated.

Meningitis: I.V.: 18.75-25 mg/kg/dose every 6 hours (Bradley, 2012; Kliegman, 2011; Tunkel, 2004)

Severe infections: I.V.:

Manufacturer's labeling: 12.5 mg/kg/dose every 6 hours; in some cases higher doses up to 25 mg/kg/dose every 6 hours may be required; higher doses should be promptly decreased when able

Alternate dosing: 12.5-25 mg/kg/dose every 6 hours; maximum daily dose: 4000 mg/**day** (AAP, 2012)

Adults: **Systemic infections:** I.V.: 50-100 mg/kg/day in divided doses every 6 hours

Dosing adjustment in renal impairment: Use with caution; monitor serum concentrations.

Dosing adjustment in hepatic impairment: Use with caution; monitor serum concentrations.

Administration Hazardous agent; use appropriate precautions for handling and disposal (NIOSH, 2012).

Parenteral: Should not be administered I.M.; has been shown to be ineffective. May administer I.V. push over at least 1 minute at a maximum concentration of 100 mg/mL, or I.V. intermittent infusion over 15-60 minutes at a final concentration for administration ≤25 mg/mL (Phelps, 2013). In neonates, some centers have administered as an intermittent I.V. infusion over 15-30 minutes at a concentration of 25 mg/mL (Prober, 1990; Rajchgot, 1983).

Monitoring Parameters CBC with differential and platelet counts (baseline and every 2 days during therapy), serum iron level, iron-binding capacity, periodic liver and renal function tests, serum drug concentration

Reference Range

Therapeutic concentrations:

Meningitis:

Peak: 15-25 mcg/mL

Trough: 5-15 mcg/mL

Other infections:

Peak: 10-20 mcg/mL

Trough: 5-10 mcg/mL

Timing of serum samples: Draw peak concentrations 0.5-1.5 hours after completion of I.V. dose; and trough immediately before next dose

Test Interactions May cause false-positive results in urine glucose tests when using cupric sulfate (Benedict's solution, Clinitest®).

Additional Information Sodium content of 1 g injection: 2.25 mEq

Dosage Forms Excipient information presented when available (limited, particularly for generics); consult specific product labeling.

Solution Reconstituted, Intravenous:

Generic: 1 g (1 ea)

References

Ambrose PJ, "Clinical Pharmacokinetics of Chloramphenicol and Chloramphenicol Succinate," *Clin Pharmacokinet*, 1984, 9(3):222-38.

American Academy of Pediatrics (AAP). In: Pickering LK, Baker CJ, Kimberlin DW, Long SS, eds. *Red Book: 2012 Report of the Committee on Infectious Diseases.* 29th ed. Elk Grove Village, IL: American Academy of Pediatrics; 2012.

Atkinson HC, Begg EJ, and Darlow BA, "Drugs in Human Milk. Clinical Pharmacokinetic Considerations," *Clin Pharmacokinet*, 1988, 14 (4):217-40

Bradley JS, Nelson JD, Kimberlin DK, et al, eds. *Nelson's Pocket Book of Pediatric Antimicrobial Therapy.* 19th ed. Philadelphia, PA: Lippincott Williams & Wilkins; 2012.

Center for Disease Control and Prevention (CDC), "Diagnosis and Management of Tickborne Rickettsial Diseases: Rocky Mountain Spotted Fever, Ehrlichioses, and Anaplasmosis - United States: A Practical Guide for Physicians and Other Health-Care and Public Health Professionals," *MMWR Recomm Rep,* 2006, 55(RR-4):1-29.

Czeizel AE, Rockenbauer M, and Sørensen HT, "A Population-Based Case-Control Teratologic Study of Oral Chloramphenicol Treatment During Pregnancy," *Eur J Epidemiol,* 2000, 16(4):323-7.

Heinonen OP, Slone D, and Shapiro S, *Birth Defects and Drugs in Pregnancy,* Littleton, MA: Publishing Sciences Group, Inc, 1977.

Kliegman RM, Stanton BF, St. Gemell JW, et al, eds. *Nelson Textbook of Pediatrics.* 19th ed. Philadelphia, PA: Saunders Elsevier;2011.

Matsuda S, "Transfer of Antibiotics Into Maternal Milk," *Biol Res Pregnancy Perinatol*, 1984, 5(2):57-60.

National Institute for Occupational Safety and Health (NIOSH), "NIOSH List of Antineoplastic and Other Hazardous Drugs in Healthcare Settings 2012." Available at http://www.cdc.gov/niosh/docs/2012-150/pdfs/2012-150.pdf. Accessed January 21, 2013.

Phelps SJ, Hak EB, Crill CM, eds. *Teddy Bear Book: Pediatric Injectable Drugs.* 10th ed. Bethesda, MD: American Society of Health-System Pharmacists;2013.

Plomp TA, Thiery M, and Maes RA, "The Passage of Thiamphenicol and Chloramphenicol Into Human Milk After Single and Repeated Oral Administration," *Vet Hum Toxicol*, 1983, 25(3):167-72.

Powell DA and Nahata MC, "Chloramphenicol: New Perspectives on an Old Drug," *Drug Intell Clin Pharm,* 1982, 16(4):295-300.

Prober CG, Stevenson DK, Benitz WE. The use of antibiotics in neonates weighing less than 1200 grams. *Pediatr Infect Dis J.* 1990; 9:111-121.

Rajchgot P, Prober CG, Soldin S, et al. Initiation of chloramphenicol therapy in the newborn infant. *J Pediatr.* 1982; 101:1018-1021.

Rajchgot P, Prober CG, Soldin SJ, et.al. Toward optimization of therapy in the neonate. *Clinical Pharmacology and Therapeutics.* 1983;33 (5):551-555.

Tunkel AR, Hartman BJ, Kaplan SL, et al, "Practice Guidelines for the Management of Bacterial Meningitis," *Clin Infect Dis,* 2004, 39 (9):1267-84.

Vozeh S, Schmidlin O, and Taeschner W, "Pharmacokinetic Drug Data," *Clin Pharmacokinet,* 1988, 15(4):254-82.

Weiss CF, Glazko AJ, Weston JK. Chloramphenicol in the newborn infant. *New Engl J Med.* 1960;262(16):787-794.

◆ **ChloraPrep One Step [OTC]** *see* Chlorhexidine Gluconate *on page 441*

◆ **Chlorbutinum** *see* Chlorambucil *on page 437*

◆ **Chlorethazine** *see* Mechlorethamine (Systemic) *on page 1315*

◆ **Chlorethazine Mustard** *see* Mechlorethamine (Systemic) *on page 1315*

Chlorhexidine Gluconate
(klor HEKS i deen GLOO koe nate)

Medication Safety Issues

Sound-alike/look-alike issues:

Peridex may be confused with Precedex

Brand Names: U.S. Betasept Surgical Scrub [OTC]; ChloraPrep One Step [OTC]; Hibiclens [OTC]; Hibistat [OTC]; Paroex; Peridex; Periogard; Tegaderm CHG Dressing [OTC]

Brand Names: Canada Hibidil 1:2000; ORO-Clense; Peridex Oral Rinse

Therapeutic Category Antibacterial, Topical; Antibiotic, Oral Rinse

Generic Availability (U.S.) May be product dependent

Use Skin cleanser for surgical scrub; cleanser for skin wounds; germicidal hand rinse; antibacterial dental rinse to reduce plaque formation and control gingivitis; prophylactic dental rinse to prevent oral infections in immunocompromised patients, particularly bone marrow transplant patients receiving cytotoxic therapy; and short-term substitute for toothbrushing in situations where the patient is unable to tolerate mechanical stimulation of the gums

Pregnancy Risk Factor B/C (manufacturer specific)

Pregnancy Considerations Adverse events have not been observed in animal reproduction studies following use of the oral rinse; use of periodontal chip has not been studied. Chlorhexidine gluconate oral rinse is poorly absorbed from the gastrointestinal tract.

Breast-Feeding Considerations It is not known if chlorhexidine gluconate is excreted in breast milk. The manufacturer recommends that caution be exercised when administering chlorhexidine gluconate oral rinse to nursing women. However, oral rinse is not intended for ingestion; patient should expectorate after rinsing.

Contraindications Hypersensitivity to chlorhexidine gluconate or any component; do not use as a preoperative skin preparation of the face or head (except Hibiclens® liquid)

as serious, permanent eye injury has occurred when chlorhexidine gluconate enters and remains in the eye during surgery.

Warnings For topical use only; there have been several case reports of anaphylaxis following disinfection with chlorhexidine; a case of bradycardic episodes after breast-feeding in a 2 day old infant whose mother used chlorhexidine gluconate topically on her breasts to prevent mastitis has been reported

Precautions Staining of oral surfaces, teeth, restorations, and dorsum of tongue may occur and may be visible as soon as 1 week after therapy begins; staining is more pronounced when there is a heavy accumulation of unremoved plaque and when teeth fillings have rough surfaces; stain does not have a clinically adverse effect, but because removal may not be possible, patients with frontal restoration should be advised of the potential permanency of the stain; avoid contact with meninges; corneal injury has been associated with direct eye contact; deafness has been associated with direct instillation into the middle ear through a perforated eardrum

Adverse Reactions

Oral:

Tartar on teeth increased, taste changes. Staining of oral surfaces (mucosa, teeth, dorsum of tongue) may be visible as soon as 1 week after therapy begins and is more pronounced when there is a heavy accumulation of unremoved plaque and when teeth fillings have rough surfaces. Stain does not have a clinically adverse effect but because removal may not be possible, patient with frontal restoration should be advised of the potential permanency of the stain.

Gastrointestinal: Oral irritation, tongue irritation

Rare but important or life-threatening: Dyspnea, facial edema, nasal congestion

Topical: Allergic reactions, dryness, sensitization, skin erythema and roughness

Drug Interactions

Metabolism/Transport Effects None known.

Avoid Concomitant Use There are no known interactions where it is recommended to avoid concomitant use.

Increased Effect/Toxicity There are no known significant interactions involving an increase in effect.

Decreased Effect There are no known significant interactions involving a decrease in effect.

Stability Store away from heat and direct light; do not freeze

Mechanism of Action Chlorhexidine has activity against gram-positive and gram-negative organisms, facultative anaerobes, aerobes, and yeast; it is both bacteriostatic and bactericidal, depending on its concentration. The bactericidal effect of chlorhexidine is a result of the binding of this cationic molecule to negatively charged bacterial cell walls and extramicrobial complexes. At low concentrations, this causes an alteration of bacterial cell osmotic equilibrium and leakage of potassium and phosphorous resulting in a bacteriostatic effect. At high concentrations of chlorhexidine, the cytoplasmic contents of the bacterial cell precipitate and result in cell death.

Pharmacokinetics (Adult data unless noted)

Absorption: ~30% of chlorhexidine is retained in the oral cavity following rinsing and is slowly released into the oral fluids; chlorhexidine is poorly absorbed from the GI tract and is not absorbed topically through intact skin

Serum concentrations: Detectable levels are not present in the plasma 12 hours after administration

Elimination: Primarily through the feces (~90%); <1% excreted in the urine

Dosing: Usual

Oral rinse (Peridex® or PerioGard®):

Children and Adults: 15 mL twice daily

Immunocompromised patient: 10-15 mL, 2-3 times/day

Cleanser: Children and Adults: Apply 5 mL per scrub or hand wash; apply 25 mL per body wash or hair wash

Administration

Oral rinse: Precede use of solution by flossing and brushing teeth, completely rinse toothpaste from mouth; swish undiluted oral rinse around in mouth for 30 seconds, then expectorate; caution patient not to swallow the medicine; avoid eating for 2-3 hours after treatment.

Topical:

Surgical scrub: Scrub 3 minutes and rinse thoroughly, wash for an additional 3 minutes

Hand wash: Wash for 15 seconds and rinse

Hand rinse: Rub vigorously for 15 seconds

Body wash: Wet body and/or hair, apply, rinse thoroughly, repeat.

Monitoring Parameters Improvement in gingival inflammation and bleeding; development of teeth or denture discoloration; dental prophylaxis to remove stains at regular intervals of no greater than 6 months.

Test Interactions If chlorhexidine is used as a disinfectant before midstream urine collection, a false-positive urine protein may result (when using dipstick method based upon a pH indicator color change).

Dosage Forms Excipient information presented when available (limited, particularly for generics); consult specific product labeling.

Liquid, External:

Betasept Surgical Scrub: 4% (118 mL, 237 mL, 473 mL, 946 mL, 3780 mL)

Hibiclens: 4% (15 mL, 118 mL, 236 mL, 473 mL, 946 mL, 3790 mL) [contains fd&c red #40, isopropyl alcohol]

Generic: 2% (118 mL); 4% (118 mL, 237 mL, 473 mL, 946 mL, 3800 mL)

Miscellaneous, External:

Hibistat: 0.5% (50 ea) [contains isopropyl alcohol]

Tegaderm CHG Dressing: (Dressing) (1 ea)

Pad, External:

Generic: 2% (2 ea, 6 ea)

Solution, External:

ChloraPrep One Step: 2% (3 mL, 10.5 mL) [latex free]

Solution, Mouth/Throat:

Paroex: 0.12% (473 mL) [alcohol free; contains fd&c red #40, propylene glycol]

Peridex: 0.12% (118 mL, 473 mL) [contains alcohol, usp, brilliant blue fcf (fd&c blue #1), saccharin sodium]

Periogard: 0.12% (473 mL) [mint flavor]

Generic: 0.12% (15 mL, 473 mL)

References

Quinn MW and Bini RM, "Bradycardia Associated With Chlorhexidine Spray," *Arch Dis Child*, 1989, 64(6):892-3.

Yong D, Parker FC, and Foran SM, "Severe Allergic Reactions and Intra-Urethral Chlorhexidine Gluconate," *Med J Aust*, 1995, 162 (5):257-8.

◆ **Chlormeprazine** see Prochlorperazine on page 1745

◆ **2-Chlorodeoxyadenosine** see Cladribine on page 488

◆ **Chloromag** see Magnesium Chloride on page 1291

◆ **Chloromycetin® (Can)** see Chloramphenicol on page 439

◆ **Chloromycetin® Succinate (Can)** see Chloramphenicol on page 439

Chloroprocaine (klor oh PROE kane)

Medication Safety Issues

Sound-alike/look-alike issues:

Nesacaine® may be confused with Neptazane™

High alert medication:

The Institute for Safe Medication Practices (ISMP) includes this medication (epidural administration) among its list of drug classes which have a heightened risk of causing significant patient harm when used in error.

Brand Names: U.S. Nesacaine; Nesacaine-MPF

Brand Names: Canada Nesacaine®-CE

Therapeutic Category Local Anesthetic, Injectable

Generic Availability (U.S.) Yes

Use Production of local or regional analgesia and anesthesia by local infiltration and peripheral nerve block techniques

Pregnancy Risk Factor C

Pregnancy Considerations Animal reproduction studies have not been conducted. Local anesthetics rapidly cross the placenta and may cause varying degrees of maternal, fetal, and neonatal toxicity. Close maternal and fetal monitoring (heart rate and electronic fetal monitoring advised) are required during obstetrical use. Maternal hypotension has resulted from regional anesthesia. Positioning the patient on her left side and elevating the legs may help. Epidural, paracervical, or pudendal anesthesia may alter the forces of parturition through changes in uterine contractility or maternal expulsive efforts. The use of some local anesthetic drugs during labor and delivery may diminish muscle strength and tone for the first day or two of life. Administration as a paracervical block is not recommended with toxemia of pregnancy, fetal distress, or prematurity. Administration of a paracervical block early in pregnancy has resulted in maternal seizures and cardiovascular collapse. Fetal bradycardia and acidosis also have been reported. Fetal depression has occurred following unintended fetal intracranial injection while administering a paracervical and/or pudendal block.

Breast-Feeding Considerations It is not known if chloroprocaine is excreted in breast milk. The manufacturer recommends that caution be exercised when administering chloroprocaine to nursing women.

Contraindications Hypersensitivity to chloroprocaine, PABA, any anesthetic of the ester type, or any component of the formulation; cerebrospinal diseases such as meningitis or syphilis, and septicemia (spinal anesthetic use)

Warnings Convulsions and cardiac arrhythmias resulting in cardiac arrest have been reported, presumably due to systemic toxicity following unintentional I.V. injection; should be administered in small incremental doses. Chloroprocaine solutions containing preservatives (methylparaben) are not to be used for lumbar or caudal anesthesia. When using for obstetrical anesthesia, 5% to 10% of cases where initial total doses of 120-400 mg were administered, have been associated with fetal bradycardia. Chondrolysis has been reported following continuous intra-articular infusion; intra-articular administration of local anesthetics is not an FDA-approved route of administration.

Precautions Use with extreme caution as lumbar or caudal anesthesia in patients with existing neurologic disease, spinal deformities, or severe hypertension; use with caution in patients with hypotension, cardiac disease, and hepatic or renal disease. Use caution in debilitated, elderly, or acutely-ill patients; dose reduction may be required. Adverse effects in the CNS and cardiovascular system are directly related to the blood level of procaine, route of administration, and physical status of the patient and more likely to occur after systemic administration rather than infiltration.

Adverse Reactions

Cardiovascular: Bradycardia, cardiac arrest, hypotension, ventricular arrhythmia

Central nervous system: Anxiety, dizziness, restlessness, seizure, tinnitus, unconsciousness

Dermatologic: Angioneurotic edema, erythema, pruritus, urticaria

Neuromuscular & skeletal: Chondrolysis (continuous intra-articular administration)

Ocular: Blurred vision

Respiratory: Respiratory arrest

Miscellaneous: Allergic reactions, anaphylactoid reactions

Drug Interactions

Metabolism/Transport Effects None known.

Avoid Concomitant Use There are no known interactions where it is recommended to avoid concomitant use.

Increased Effect/Toxicity

The levels/effects of Chloroprocaine may be increased by: Hyaluronidase

Decreased Effect

Chloroprocaine may decrease the levels/effects of: Technetium Tc 99m Tilmanocept

Stability Store at controlled room temperature of 15°C to 30°C (59°F to 86°F); protect from light. Solutions may not be resterilized by autoclaving.

Mechanism of Action Chloroprocaine HCl is benzoic acid, 4-amino-2-chloro-2-(diethylamino) ethyl ester monohydrochloride. Chloroprocaine is an ester-type local anesthetic, which stabilizes the neuronal membranes and prevents initiation and transmission of nerve impulses thereby affecting local anesthetic actions. Local anesthetics including chloroprocaine, reversibly prevent generation and conduction of electrical impulses in neurons by decreasing the transient increase in permeability to sodium. The differential sensitivity generally depends on the size of the fiber; small fibers are more sensitive than larger fibers and require a longer period for recovery. Sensory pain fibers are usually blocked first, followed by fibers that transmit sensations of temperature, touch, and deep pressure. High concentrations block sympathetic somatic sensory and somatic motor fibers. The spread of anesthesia depends upon the distribution of the solution. This is primarily dependent on the volume of drug injected.

Pharmacodynamics

Onset of action: 6-12 minutes

Duration (patient, type of block, concentration, and method of anesthesia dependent): Up to 1 hour

Pharmacokinetics (Adult data unless noted)

Metabolism: Rapidly hydrolyzed by plasma enzymes to 2-chloro-4-aminobenzoic acid and 8-diethylaminoethanol (80% conjugated before elimination)

Half-life (*in vitro*):

Neonates: 43 ± 2 seconds

Adult males: 21 ± 2 seconds

Adult females: 25 ± 1 second

Elimination: Very little excreted as unchanged drug in urine; metabolites: Cloro-aminobenzoic acid and diethylaminoethanol primarily excreted unchanged in urine

Dosing: Usual Dose varies with procedure, desired depth, and duration of anesthesia, desired muscle relaxation, vascularity of tissues, physical condition, and age of patient. The smallest dose and concentration required to produce the desired effect should be used.

Children >3 years: Maximum dose without epinephrine: 11 mg/kg

Adults: Maximum dose: 11 mg/kg; not to exceed 800 mg per treatment; with epinephrine: 14 mg/kg; not to exceed 1000 mg per treatment

Infiltration and peripheral nerve block:

Mandibular: 2-3 mL (40-60 mg) using 2%

Infraorbital: 0.5-1 mL (10-20 mg) using 2%

Brachial plexus: 30-40 mL (600-800 mg) using 2%

Digital (without epinephrine): 3-4 mL (30-40 mg) using 1%

Pudendal: 10 mL (200 mg) into each side (2 sites) using 2%

Paracervical: 3 mL (30 mg) per each of four sites using 1%

Caudal and lumbar epidural block:

Caudal: 15-25 mL using 2% to 3% solution; may repeat dose at 40- to 60-minute intervals

Lumbar: 2-2.5 mL per segment using 2% to 3% solution; usual total volume 15-25 mL; repeated doses 2-6 mL less than the original dose may be given at 40- to 50-minutes intervals

Administration Parenteral: Administer in small incremental doses; when using continuous intermittent catheter techniques, use frequent aspirations before and during the injection to avoid intravascular injection

Monitoring Parameters Blood pressure, heart rate, respiration, signs of CNS toxicity (lightheadedness, dizziness, tinnitus, restlessness, tremors, twitching, drowsiness, circumoral paresthesia)

Dosage Forms Excipient information presented when available (limited, particularly for generics); consult specific product labeling.

Solution, Injection, as hydrochloride:
Nesacaine: 1% (30 mL); 2% (30 mL) [contains disodium edta, methylparaben]
Solution, Injection, as hydrochloride [preservative free]:
Nesacaine-MPF: 2% (20 mL); 3% (20 mL) [methylparaben free]
Generic: 2% (20 mL); 3% (20 mL)

◆ **Chloroprocaine Hydrochloride** see Chloroprocaine on page 442

Chloroquine (KLOR oh kwin)

Medication Safety Issues

International issues:
Aralen [U.S., Mexico] may be confused with Paralen brand name for acetaminophen [Czech Republic]

Related Information
Medications for Which a Single Dose May Be Fatal When Ingested by a Toddler on page 2408

Brand Names: U.S. Aralen

Brand Names: Canada Aralen; Novo-Chloroquine

Therapeutic Category Amebicide; Antimalarial Agent

Generic Availability (U.S.) Yes

Use Suppression or chemoprophylaxis of malaria in chloroquine-sensitive areas [FDA approved in pediatric patients (age not specified) and adults]; treatment of uncomplicated acute attacks of malaria due to susceptible *Plasmodium* species, except chloroquine-resistant *Plasmodium falciparum* [FDA approved in pediatric patients (age not specified) and adults]; extraintestinal amebiasis (FDA approved in adults); has been used for treatment of rheumatoid arthritis, discoid lupus erythematosus, scleroderma, pemphigus

Pregnancy Considerations In animal reproduction studies, drug accumulated in fetal ocular tissues and remained for several months following drug elimination from the rest of the body. Chloroquine and its metabolites cross the placenta and can be detected in the cord blood and urine of the newborn infant (Akintonwa, 1988; Essien, 1982; Law, 2008). In one study, chloroquine and its metabolites were measurable in the cord blood 89 days (mean) after the last maternal dose (Law, 2008).

Malaria infection in pregnant women may be more severe than in nonpregnant women and has a high risk of maternal and perinatal morbidity and mortality. Therefore, pregnant women and women who are likely to become pregnant are advised to avoid travel to malaria-risk areas. Chloroquine is recommended for the treatment of pregnant women for uncomplicated malaria in chloroquine-sensitive regions; when caused by chloroquine-sensitive *P. vivax* or *P. ovale*, pregnant women should be maintained on chloroquine prophylaxis for the duration of their pregnancy (refer to current guidelines) (CDC, 2011; CDC, 2012).

Breast-Feeding Considerations Chloroquine and its metabolite can be detected in breast milk. Per product labeling, 11 lactating women with malaria were given a single oral dose of chloroquine 600 mg. The maximum daily dose to the breast-feeding infant was calculated to be 0.7% of the maternal dose. Additional information has been published and results are variable. In one study, the relative dose to the nursing infant was calculated to be 2.3% (chloroquine) and 1% (metabolite) of the weight-adjusted maternal dose with the samples obtained a median of 17 days after the last dose. Women in this study received chloroquine phosphate 750 mg daily for 3 days. This report also provides data from other studies, listing relative infant doses of chloroquine ranging from 0.9% to 9.5% of the maternal dose (Law, 2008). Due to the potential for serious adverse reactions in the nursing infant, the manufacturer recommends a decision be made whether to discontinue nursing or to discontinue the drug, taking into account the importance of treatment to the mother. Other sources consider the amount of chloroquine exposure to the nursing infant to be safe when normal maternal doses for malaria are used. However, the amount of chloroquine obtained by a nursing infant from breast milk would not provide adequate protection if therapy for malaria in the infant is needed (CDC, 2012).

Contraindications Hypersensitivity to 4-aminoquinoline compounds (eg, chloroquine, hydroxychloroquine) or any component; retinal or visual field changes

Warnings Physicians should be familiar with chloroquine before prescribing **[U.S. Boxed Warning]**. Resistance of *Plasmodium falciparum* to chloroquine is widespread, including everywhere that *P. falciparum* malaria is transmitted, except for areas of Central America (northwest of the Panama Canal), Haiti, the Dominican Republic, and most areas of the Middle East; cases of *Plasmodium vivax* resistance have been reported. Irreversible retinal damage has been reported in patients who received long-term or high-dose therapy; baseline and periodic ophthalmic exams should be performed. Periodically examine patients for evidence of muscular weakness; discontinue chloroquine if weakness occurs. Chloroquine may precipitate a severe attack of psoriasis in patients with psoriasis; may exacerbate porphyria in patients with porphyria.

Precautions Use with caution in patients with liver disease, G-6-PD deficiency, severe blood disorders, seizure disorders, preexisting auditory damage, or in conjunction with hepatotoxic drugs; use in pregnancy should be avoided, except for the suppression or treatment of malaria when, in the judgement of the prescriber, the potential benefit outweighs the potential risks to the fetus.

Adverse Reactions

Cardiovascular: Cardiomyopathy, ECG changes (rare; including prolonged QRS and QT_c intervals, T wave inversion or depression), hypotension (rare), torsades de pointes (rare)

Central nervous system: Agitation, anxiety, confusion, decreased deep tendon reflex, delirium, depression, extrapyramidal reaction (dystonia, dyskinesia, protrusion of the tongue, torticollis), hallucination, headache, insomnia, personality changes, polyneuropathy, psychosis, seizure

Dermatologic: Alopecia, bleaching of hair, blue gray skin pigmentation, erythema multiforme (rare), exacerbation of psoriasis, exfoliative dermatitis (rare), lichen planus, pleomorphic rash, pruritus, skin photosensitivity, Stevens-Johnson syndrome (rare), toxic epidermal necrolysis (rare), urticaria

Gastrointestinal: Abdominal cramps, anorexia, diarrhea, nausea, vomiting

Hematologic & oncologic: Agranulocytosis (rare; reversible), aplastic anemia, neutropenia, pancytopenia, thrombocytopenia

Hepatic: Hepatitis, increased liver enzymes

Hypersensitivity: Anaphylactoid reaction, anaphylaxis, angioedema

Immunologic: DRESS syndrome

Neuromuscular & skeletal: Myopathy, neuromuscular disease, proximal myopathy

Ophthalmic: Accommodation disturbances, blurred vision, corneal opacity (reversible), macular degeneration (may be irreversible), maculopathy (may be irreversible), nocturnal amblyopia, retinopathy (including irreversible changes in some patients long-term or high-dose therapy), visual field defects

Otic: Deafness (nerve), hearing loss (risk increased in patients with preexisting auditory damage), tinnitus

Drug Interactions

Metabolism/Transport Effects Substrate of CYP2D6 (major), CYP3A4 (major); **Note:** Assignment of Major/Minor substrate status based on clinically relevant drug interaction potential; **Inhibits** CYP2D6 (moderate)

Avoid Concomitant Use

Avoid concomitant use of Chloroquine with any of the following: Agalsidase Alfa; Agalsidase Beta; Artemether; Conivaptan; Fusidic Acid (Systemic); Highest Risk QTc-Prolonging Agents; Ivabradine; Lumefantrine; Mefloquine; Mifepristone; Thioridazine

Increased Effect/Toxicity

Chloroquine may increase the levels/effects of: Antipsychotic Agents (Phenothiazines); ARIPiprazole; Beta-Blockers; Cardiac Glycosides; CYP2D6 Substrates; Dapsone (Systemic); Dapsone (Topical); DOXOrubicin (Conventional); Fesoterodine; Highest Risk QTc-Prolonging Agents; Lumefantrine; Mefloquine; Metoprolol; Moderate Risk QTc-Prolonging Agents; Nebivolol; Prilocaine; Sodium Nitrite; Thioridazine

The levels/effects of Chloroquine may be increased by: Abiraterone Acetate; Artemether; Conivaptan; CYP2D6 Inhibitors (Moderate); CYP2D6 Inhibitors (Strong); CYP3A4 Inhibitors (Moderate); CYP3A4 Inhibitors (Strong); Dapsone (Systemic); Dasatinib; Fusidic Acid (Systemic); Ivabradine; Ivacaftor; Luliconazole; Mefloquine; Mifepristone; Nitric Oxide; QTc-Prolonging Agents (Indeterminate Risk and Risk Modifying); Simeprevir; Stiripentol

Decreased Effect

Chloroquine may decrease the levels/effects of: Agalsidase Alfa; Agalsidase Beta; Ampicillin; Anthelmintics; Codeine; Rabies Vaccine; Tamoxifen; TraMADol

The levels/effects of Chloroquine may be decreased by: Antacids; Bosentan; CYP3A4 Inducers (Strong); Dabrafenib; Deferasirox; Kaolin; Lanthanum; Mitotane; Peginterferon Alfa-2b; Siltuximab; St Johns Wort; Tocilizumab

Stability Protect from light. Store tablets at 25°C (77°F); excursions permitted to 15°C to 30°C (59°F to 86°F).

Mechanism of Action Binds to and inhibits DNA and RNA polymerase; interferes with metabolism and hemoglobin utilization by parasites; inhibits prostaglandin effects; chloroquine concentrates within parasite acid vesicles and raises internal pH resulting in inhibition of parasite growth; may involve aggregates of ferriprotoporphyrin IX acting as chloroquine receptors causing membrane damage; may also interfere with nucleoprotein synthesis

Pharmacokinetics (Adult data unless noted)

Absorption: Oral: Rapid

Distribution: Widely distributed in body tissues including eyes, heart, kidneys, liver, leukocytes, and lungs where retention is prolonged; crosses the placenta; appears in breast milk

Protein binding: 50% to 65%

Metabolism: Partially hepatic; main metabolite is desethylchloroquine

Half-life: 3-5 days

Time to peak serum concentration: Oral: Within 1-2 hours

Elimination: ~70% of dose excreted in urine (~35% unchanged); acidification of the urine increases elimination of drug; small amounts of drug may be present in urine months following discontinuation of therapy

Dialysis: Minimally removed by hemodialysis

Dosing: Usual Oral: **Note:** Dosage expressed in terms of base (10 mg base = 16.6 mg chloroquine phosphate):

Malaria:

Suppression or prophylaxis:

Infants and Children: Administer 5 mg base/kg/week on the same day each week (not to exceed 300 mg base/dose); begin 1-2 weeks prior to exposure; continue for 4 weeks after leaving endemic area; if suppressive therapy is not begun prior to exposure, double the initial loading dose to 10 mg base/kg and give in 2 divided doses 6 hours apart, followed by the usual dosage regimen

Adults: 300 mg base on the same day each week; begin 1-2 weeks prior to exposure; continue for 4 weeks after leaving endemic area; if suppressive therapy is not begun prior to exposure, double the initial loading dose to 600 mg base and give in 2 divided doses 6 hours apart, followed by the usual dosage regimen

Acute attack:

Infants and Children: 10 mg base/kg immediately (maximum: 600 mg base/dose), followed by 5 mg base/kg (maximum: 300 mg base/dose) administered at 6, 24, and 48 hours after first dose for a total of 4 doses (CDC, 2009)

Adults: 600 mg base/dose immediately, then 300 mg base/dose at 6, 24, and 48 hours after the first dose

Extraintestinal amebiasis:

Children: 10 mg base/kg once daily for 21 days (up to 600 mg base/day) (Seidel, 1984)

Adults: 600 mg base/day for 2 days followed by 300 mg base/day for at least 2-3 weeks

Rheumatoid arthritis, lupus erythematosus: Adults: 150 mg base once daily

Dosing adjustment in renal impairment: CrCl <10 mL/minute: Administer 50% of dose (Arnoff, 2007)

Administration Oral: Administer with meals to decrease GI upset; chloroquine phosphate tablets have also been mixed with chocolate syrup or enclosed in gelatin capsules to mask the bitter taste

Monitoring Parameters Periodic CBC, examination for muscular weakness, and ophthalmologic examination (visual acuity, slit-lamp, fundoscopic, and visual field tests) in patients receiving prolonged therapy

Additional Information *P. vivax* and *P. ovale* infections treated with chloroquine only can relapse due to hypnozoites; add primaquine to eradicate hypnozoites

Dosage Forms Excipient information presented when available (limited, particularly for generics); consult specific product labeling.

Tablet, Oral, as phosphate:

Aralen: 500 mg [equivalent to chloroquine base 300 mg]

Generic: 250 mg [equivalent to chloroquine base 150 mg], 500 mg [equivalent to chloroquine base 300 mg]

Extemporaneous Preparations A 15 mg chloroquine phosphate/mL oral suspension (equivalent to 9 mg chloroquine base/mL) may be made from tablets and a 1:1 mixture of Ora-Sweet® and Ora-Plus®. Crush three 500 mg chloroquine phosphate tablets (equivalent to 300 mg base/tablet) in a mortar and reduce to a fine powder. Add 15 mL of the vehicle and mix to a uniform paste; mix while adding the vehicle in incremental proportions to **almost** 100 mL; transfer to a calibrated bottle, rinse mortar with vehicle, and add quantity of vehicle sufficient to make 100 mL. Label "shake well before using" and "protect from light". Stable for up to 60 days when stored in the dark at room temperature or refrigerated (preferred).

Allen LV Jr and Erickson MA 3rd, "Stability of Alprazolam, Chloroquine Phosphate, Cisapride, Enalapril Maleate, and Hydralazine Hydrochloride in Extemporaneously Compounded Oral Liquids," *Am J Health Syst Pharm*, 1998, 55(18):1915-20.

References

Akintonwa A, Gbajumo SA, and Mabadeje AF, "Placental and Milk Transfer of Chloroquine in Humans," *Ther Drug Monit*, 1988, 10 (2):147-9.

Aronoff GR, Bennett WM, Berns JS, et al, *Drug Prescribing in Renal Failure: Dosing Guidelines for Adults and Children*, 5th ed, Philadelphia, PA: American College of Physicians, 2007, 73.

Centers for Disease Control and Prevention (CDC), "CDC Health Information for International Travel 2012," New York: Oxford University Press, 2012.

Centers for Disease Control and Prevention (CDC), "Guidelines for the Prevention and Treatment of Opportunistic Infections Among HIV-Exposed and HIV-Infected Children," *MMWR Recomm Rep*, 2009, 58(RR-11):1-166. Available at http://aidsinfo.nih.gov/contentfiles/Pediatric_OI.pdf

Centers for Disease Control and Prevention, "Guidelines for Treatment of Malaria in the United States." Available at http://www.cdc.gov/malaria/resources/pdf/treatmenttable.pdf.

Centers for Disease Control and Prevention, "Malaria Prescription Drug Information for Healthcare Providers." Available at http://www.cdc.gov/malaria/travel/drugs_hcp.htm.

Centers for Disease Control and Prevention, "Treatment of Malaria (Guidelines for Clinicians)." Available at http://www.cdc.gov/malaria/pdf/clinicalguidance.pdf.

Essien EE and Afamefuna GC, "Chloroquine and Its Metabolites in Human Cord Blood, Neonatal Blood, and Urine After Maternal Medication," *Clin Chem*, 1982, 28(5):1148-52.

Law I, Ilett KF, Hackett LP, et al, "Transfer of Chloroquine and Desethylchloroquine Across the Placenta and Into Milk in Melanesian Mothers," *Br J Clin Pharmacol*, 2008, 65(5):674-9.

Red Book: 2009 Report of the Committee on Infectious Diseases, "Amebiasis," 28th ed, Pickering LK, ed, Elk Grove Village, IL: American Academy of Pediatrics, 2009, 206-8.

Seidel J, "Diagnosis and Management of Amebic Liver Abscess in Children," *West J Med*, 1984, 140(6):932-3.

Wyler DJ, "Malaria Chemoprophylaxis for the Traveler," *N Engl J Med*, 1993, 329(1):31-7.

◆ **Chloroquine Phosphate** see Chloroquine on page 444

Chlorothiazide (klor oh THYE a zide)

Medication Safety Issues
International issues:
Diuril [U.S.] may be confused with Duorol brand name for acetaminophen [Spain]

Brand Names: U.S. Diuril; Sodium Diuril

Therapeutic Category Antihypertensive Agent; Diuretic, Thiazide

Generic Availability (U.S.) May be product dependent

Use
Oral: Suspension, tablets: Treatment of edema due to heart failure, hepatic cirrhosis, and estrogen or corticosteroid therapy (FDA approved in infants, children, and adults); treatment of various forms of renal dysfunction, including nephrotic syndrome, acute glomerulonephritis, and chronic renal failure (FDA approved in infants, children, and adults); management of hypertension either alone or in combination with other antihypertensive agents (FDA approved in infants, children, and adults); has also been used for bronchopulmonary dysplasia (BPD) and central diabetes insipidus of infancy; **Note:** Use in pregnancy should be reserved for those cases causing extreme discomfort and unrelieved by rest; should not be routinely used during pregnancy

Parenteral: Treatment of edema due to heart failure, hepatic cirrhosis, and estrogen or corticosteroid therapy (FDA approved in adults); treatment of various forms of renal dysfunction including nephrotic syndrome, acute glomerulonephritis, and chronic renal failure (FDA approved in adults); has also been used for bronchopulmonary dysplasia (BPD); **Note:** Use in pregnancy should be reserved for those cases causing extreme discomfort

and unrelieved by rest; should not be routinely used during pregnancy

Pregnancy Risk Factor C

Pregnancy Considerations Adverse events were not observed in animal reproduction studies; however, studies were not complete. Chlorothiazide crosses the placenta and is found in cord blood. Maternal use may cause may cause fetal or neonatal jaundice, thrombocytopenia, or other adverse events observed in adults. Use of thiazide diuretics to treat edema during normal pregnancies is not appropriate; use may be considered when edema is due to pathologic causes (as in the nonpregnant patient); monitor. Untreated chronic maternal hypertension is associated with adverse events in the fetus, infant, and mother (ACOG, 2013). Women who required thiazide diuretics for the treatment of hypertension prior to pregnancy may continue their use (ACOG, 2013).

Breast-Feeding Considerations Chlorothiazide is excreted into breast milk. Due to the potential for serious adverse reactions in the nursing infant, the manufacturer recommends a decision be made whether to discontinue nursing or to discontinue the drug, taking into account the importance of treatment to the mother. Diuretics have the potential to decrease milk volume and suppress lactation.

Contraindications Hypersensitivity to chlorothiazide or any component; cross-sensitivity with other thiazides or sulfonamides; anuria

Warnings Hypersensitivity reactions may occur with chlorothiazide; risk is increased in patients with a history of allergy or bronchial asthma. Chemical similarities are present among sulfonamides, sulfonylureas, carbonic anhydrase inhibitors, thiazides, and loop diuretics (except ethacrynic acid). Use in patients with sulfonamide allergy is specifically contraindicated in product labeling; however, a risk of cross-reaction exists in patients with allergy to any of these compounds; avoid use when previous reaction has been severe. Discontinue if signs of hypersensitivity are noted.

May cause hypokalemia; increased risk associated with aggressive diuresis, severe cirrhosis, or after prolonged therapy; alterations in adequate oral potassium intake may also increase risk; monitor serum potassium concentrations at baseline and periodically; correct hypokalemia prior to initiating therapy. Other electrolyte disorders may occur, including hyponatremia, hypomagnesemia, and hypochloremic metabolic alkalosis; monitor electrolytes. May cause SLE exacerbation or activation. Photosensitization may occur; patients should be counseled.

Oral suspension contains benzoic acid; benzoic acid is a metabolite of benzyl alcohol; large amounts of benzyl alcohol (≥99 mg/kg/day) have been associated with a potentially fatal toxicity ("gasping syndrome") in neonates; the "gasping syndrome" consists of metabolic acidosis, respiratory distress, gasping respirations, CNS dysfunction (including convulsions, intracranial hemorrhage), hypotension, and cardiovascular collapse; use the oral suspension containing benzyl alcohol with caution in neonates; *in vitro* and animal studies have shown that benzoate, a metabolite of benzyl alcohol, displaces bilirubin from protein binding sites.

Precautions Use with caution in patients with severe renal disease due to decreased efficacy; may precipitate azotemia. Use with caution in patients with severe hepatic dysfunction; in cirrhosis, avoid electrolyte and acid/base imbalances that might lead to hepatic encephalopathy. Use with caution in patients with prediabetes or diabetes mellitus; may alter glucose control. Use with caution in patients with a history of gout; may cause hyperuricemia and in certain patients with a history of gout, a familial predisposition to gout, or chronic renal failure, gout can be precipitated. Use with caution in patients with moderate or high cholesterol concentrations.

Use with caution in patients with hypercalcemia or parathyroid disease; thiazide diuretics may decrease renal calcium excretion; pathologic changes in the parathyroid glands with hypercalcemia and hypophosphatemia have been observed with prolonged use.

Adverse Reactions

Cardiovascular: Hypotension, orthostatic hypotension, necrotizing angiitis

Central nervous system: Dizziness, fever, headache, restlessness, vertigo

Dermatologic: Alopecia, erythema multiforme, exfoliative dermatitis, photosensitivity, purpura, rash, Stevens-Johnson syndrome, toxic epidermal necrolysis, urticaria

Endocrine & metabolic: Cholesterol increased, hypercalcemia, hyperglycemia, hyperuricemia, hypochloremic alkalosis, hypokalemia, hyponatremia, hypomagnesemia, triglycerides increased

Gastrointestinal: Abdominal cramping, anorexia, constipation, diarrhea, gastric irritation, nausea, pancreatitis, sialadenitis, vomiting

Genitourinary: Impotence

Hematologic: Agranulocytosis, aplastic anemia, hemolytic anemia, leukopenia, thrombocytopenia

Hepatic: Jaundice

Neuromuscular & skeletal: Muscle spasm, paresthesia, weakness

Ocular: Blurred vision, xanthopsia

Renal: Glycosuria, hematuria (I.V.), interstitial nephritis, renal failure, renal dysfunction

Respiratory: Pneumonitis, pulmonary edema, respiratory distress

Miscellaneous: Anaphylactic reactions, systemic lupus erythematosus

Drug Interactions

Metabolism/Transport Effects None known.

Avoid Concomitant Use

Avoid concomitant use of Chlorothiazide with any of the following: Dofetilide

Increased Effect/Toxicity

Chlorothiazide may increase the levels/effects of: ACE Inhibitors; Allopurinol; Amifostine; Antihypertensives; Calcium Salts; CarBAMazepine; Cyclophosphamide; Diazoxide; Dofetilide; DULoxetine; Hypotensive Agents; Ivabradine; Lithium; Multivitamins/Minerals (with ADEK, Folate, Iron); Multivitamins/Minerals (with AE, No Iron); Obinutuzumab; OXcarbazepine; Porfimer; RiTUXimab; Sodium Phosphates; Topiramate; Toremifene; Vitamin D Analogs

The levels/effects of Chlorothiazide may be increased by: Alcohol (Ethyl); Alfuzosin; Analgesics (Opioid); Anticholinergic Agents; Barbiturates; Beta2-Agonists; Brimonidine (Topical); Corticosteroids (Orally Inhaled); Corticosteroids (Systemic); Diazoxide; Herbs (Hypotensive Properties); Licorice; MAO Inhibitors; Multivitamins/Fluoride (with ADE); Pentoxifylline; Phosphodiesterase 5 Inhibitors; Prostacyclin Analogues; Selective Serotonin Reuptake Inhibitors

Decreased Effect

Chlorothiazide may decrease the levels/effects of: Antidiabetic Agents

The levels/effects of Chlorothiazide may be decreased by: Bile Acid Sequestrants; Herbs (Hypertensive Properties); Methylphenidate; Nonsteroidal Anti-Inflammatory Agents; Yohimbine

Food Interactions Chlorothiazide serum levels may be increased if taken with food. Management: Administer without regard to food.

Stability

Oral:

Suspension: Store at 15°C to 30°C (59°F to 86°F) in tightly closed container; protect from freezing

Tablets: Store at 20°C to 25°C (68°F to 77°F) in tightly closed container; protect from light and moisture

Parenteral: Store intact vial at 2°C to 25°C (36°F to 77°F); reconstituted solution is stable for 24 hours at room temperature

Mechanism of Action Inhibits sodium and chloride reabsorption in the distal tubules causing increased excretion of sodium, chloride, and water resulting in diuresis. Loss of potassium, hydrogen ions, magnesium, phosphate, and bicarbonate also occurs.

Pharmacodynamics

Onset of action: Diuresis: Oral: Within 2 hours; I.V.: Within 15 minutes

Maximum effect: Diuresis: Oral: 4 hours; I.V.: 30 minutes

Duration: Diuresis: Oral: ~6-12 hours; I.V.: 2 hours

Pharmacokinetics (Adult data unless noted)

Absorption: Oral: Poor

Bioavailability: 9% to 56%; dose-dependent

Half-life: 45-120 minutes

Time to peak serum concentration: Oral: Within 4 hours; I.V.: 30 minutes

Elimination: Urine (Oral: 10% to 15% excreted unchanged; I.V.: 96% excreted unchanged)

Dosing: Neonatal

Edema, heart failure, bronchopulmonary dysplasia: Limited data available; **Note:** The manufacturer states that I.V. and oral dosing are equivalent; however, some clinicians use lower I.V. doses due to poor oral absorption.

Oral: 20-40 mg/kg/day in 2 divided doses

I.V.: 5-10 mg/kg/day in 2 divided doses (Costello, 2007); doses up to 20 mg/kg/day have been used

Hyperinsulinemia hypoglycemia, congenital hyperinsulinism (adjunct therapy): Limited data available: Oral: 7-10 mg/kg/day in 2 divided doses in combination with diazoxide (Aynsley-Green, 2000; Hussain, 2004; Kapoor, 2009)

Diabetes insipidus (central): Limited data available: Oral: 10 mg/kg/day in 2 divided doses; may need to titrate dose to target urine osmolality: 100-150 mOsm/L (Rivkees, 2008)

Dosing: Usual

Infants, Children, and Adolescents: **Note:** The manufacturer states that I.V. and oral dosing are equivalent; however, some clinicians use lower I.V. doses due to the poor oral absorption.

Edema (diuresis), heart failure, hypertension:

Manufacturer labeling:

Infants <6 months: Oral: 10-30 mg/kg/day in divided doses once or twice daily

Infants ≥6 months, Children, and Adolescents: Oral: 10-20 mg/kg/day in divided doses once or twice daily

Maximum daily doses:

Infants and Children <2 years: 375 mg/**day**

Children 2-12 years: 1000 mg/**day**

Adolescents: 2000 mg/**day**

Alternate dosing:

Oral: 10-40 mg/kg/day in 2 divided doses

Maximum daily doses:

Infants and Children <2 years: 375 mg/**day**

Children ≥2 years and Adolescents: 1000 mg/**day**

I.V.: Limited data available: 5-10 mg/kg/day in divided doses once or twice daily (Costello, 2007); in some cases, doses up to 20 mg/kg/day have been used; maximum dose: 500 mg

Diabetes insipidus (central): Infants [breast milk-fed or formula (Similac PM 60/40)-fed]: Limited data available: Oral: 10 mg/kg/day in 2 divided doses; may need to titrate dose to target urine osmolality: 100-150 mOsm/L (Rivkees, 2008)

Adults: **Note:** The manufacturer states that I.V. and oral dosing are equivalent; however, some clinicians use lower I.V. doses due to the poor oral absorption.

Hypertension: Oral: 500-2000 mg/day divided in 1-2 doses (manufacturer labeling); doses of 125-500 mg/day have also been recommended (JNC 7)

Edema: Oral, I.V.: 500-1000 mg once or twice daily; intermittent treatment (eg, therapy on alternative days) may be appropriate for some patients

ACC/AHA 2009 Heart Failure Guidelines:

Oral: 250-500 mg once or twice daily (maximum daily dose: 1000 mg)

I.V.: 500-1000 mg once or twice daily plus a loop diuretic

Dosage adjustment in renal impairment: Infants, Children, Adolescents, and Adults: CrCl <10 mL/minute: Avoid use. Ineffective with CrCl <30 mL/minute unless in combination with a loop diuretic (Aronoff, 2007).

Note: ACC/AHA 2005 Heart Failure guidelines suggest that thiazides lose their efficacy when CrCl <40 mL/minute.

Administration

Oral: Administer with food; administer early in day to avoid nocturia; if multiple daily dosing, the last dose should not be administered later than 6:00 pm unless instructed otherwise. Shake suspension well before use.

Parenteral: Reconstitute 500 mg vial with 18 mL SWI (resulting in 28 mg/mL concentration); may administer by direct I.V. infusion over 3-5 minutes or further dilute in D_5W or NS and infuse over 30 minutes. Avoid extravasation of parenteral solution since it is extremely irritating to tissues; pH: 9.2-10. Do **not** administer via I.M. or SubQ route.

Monitoring Parameters Serum electrolytes, BUN, creatinine, blood pressure, fluid balance, body weight

Test Interactions May interfere with tests for parathyroid function

Dosage Forms Excipient information presented when available (limited, particularly for generics); consult specific product labeling.

Solution Reconstituted, Intravenous, as sodium [strength expressed as base]:
Sodium Diuril: 500 mg (1 ea)
Generic: 500 mg (1 ea)

Suspension, Oral:
Diuril: 250 mg/5 mL (237 mL) [contains alcohol, usp, benzoic acid, fd&c yellow #10 (quinoline yellow), methylparaben, propylparaben, saccharin sodium]

Tablet, Oral:
Generic: 250 mg, 500 mg

Extemporaneous Preparations A 50 mg/mL oral suspension may be made with tablets. Crush ten 500 mg chlorothiazide tablets in a mortar and reduce to a fine powder; mix with a small amount of glycerin to form a uniform paste. Add 2 g carboxymethylcellulose gel (mix 2 g carboxymethylcellulose with 5 to 10 mL water to form a paste; add 40 mL water and heat to 60°C with moderate stirring until dissolution occurs; cool and allow to stand for 1 to 2 hours to form a clear gel). Dissolve 500 mg citric acid in 5 mL water and add to chlorothiazide carboxymethylcellulose mixture with 0.1% parabens. Add a quantity of purified water sufficient to make 100 mL (Nahata, 2004). Label "shake well" and "refrigerate". Stable for 30 days.

Nahata MC, Pai VB, and Hipple TF, *Pediatric Drug Formulations*, 5th ed, Cincinnati, OH: Harvey Whitney Books Co, 2004.

References

American College of Obstetricians and Gynecologists (ACOG), "ACOG Practice Bulletin No. 125: Chronic Hypertension in Pregnancy," *Obstet Gynecol*, 2012, 119(2 Pt 1):396-407.

Aronoff GR, Bennett WM, Berns JS, et al, *Drug Prescribing in Renal Failure: Dosing Guidelines for Adults and Children*, 5th ed. Philadelphia, PA: American College of Physicians, 2007.

Aynsley-Green A, Hussain K, Hall J, et al, "Practical Management of Hyperinsulinism in Infancy," *Arch Dis Child Fetal Neonatal Ed*, 2000, 82(2):F98-107.

Chobanian AV, Bakris GL, Black HR, et al, "The Seventh Report of the Joint National Committee on Prevention, Detection, Evaluation, and Treatment of High Blood Pressure: The JNC 7 Report," *JAMA*, 2003, 289(19):2560-72.

Costello JM and Almodovar MC, "Emergency Care for Infants and Children With Acute Cardiac Disease," *Clin Pediatr Emerg Med*, 2007, 8:145-55.

Hunt SA, Abraham WT, Chin MH, et al, "ACC/AHA 2005 Guideline Update for the Diagnosis and Management of Chronic Heart Failure in the Adult: A Report of the American College of Cardiology/American Heart Association Task Force on Practice Guidelines (Writing Committee to Update the 2001 Guidelines for the Evaluation and Management of Heart Failure): Developed in Collaboration With the American College of Chest Physicians and the International Society for Heart and Lung Transplantation: Endorsed by the Heart Rhythm Society," *Circulation*, 2005, 112(12):e154-235.

Hussain K and Aynsley-Green A, "Hyperinsulinaemic Hypoglycaemia in Preterm Neonates," *Arch Dis Child Fetal Neonatal Ed*, 2004, 89(1):F65-7.

Kapoor RR, Flanagan SE, James C, et al, "Hyperinsulinaemic Hypoglycaemia," *Arch Dis Child*, 2009, 94(6):450-7.

Rivkees SA, "The Management of Central Diabetes Insipidus in Infancy," *US Pediatrics*, 2008, 66-8.

◆ **Chlorphen [OTC]** *see* Chlorpheniramine *on page 448*

Chlorpheniramine (klor fen IR a meen)

Medication Safety Issues

Sound-alike/look-alike issues:
Chlor-Trimeton® may be confused with Chloromycetin®

BEERS Criteria medication:
This drug may be potentially inappropriate for use in geriatric patients (Quality of evidence - moderate; Strength of recommendation - strong).

Related Information

Oral Medications That Should Not Be Crushed or Altered *on page 2438*

Brand Names: U.S. Aller-Chlor [OTC]; Allergy 4 Hour [OTC] [DSC]; Allergy Relief [OTC]; Allergy [OTC]; Allergy-Time [OTC]; Chlor-Trimeton Allergy [OTC]; Chlor-Trimeton [OTC]; Chlorphen [OTC]; Ed ChlorPed; Ed Chlorped Jr [OTC]; Ed ChlorPed [OTC]; Ed-Chlor-Tan; Ed-Chlortan [OTC]; Pharbechlor [OTC]

Brand Names: Canada Chlor-Tripolon®; Novo-Pheniram

Therapeutic Category Antihistamine

Generic Availability (U.S.) May be product dependent

Use Perennial and seasonal allergic rhinitis and other allergic symptoms including urticaria

Pregnancy Considerations Maternal chlorpheniramine use has generally not resulted in an increased risk of birth defects (Aselton, 1985; Gilboa, 2009; Heinonen, 1977; Jick, 1981). Antihistamines are recommended for the treatment of rhinitis, urticaria, and pruritus with rash in pregnant women (although second generation antihistamines may be preferred) (Angier, 2010; Wallace, 2008; Zuberbier, 2009). Antihistamines are not recommended for treatment of pruritus associated with intrahepatic cholestasis in pregnancy (Ambros-Rudolph, 2011; Kremer, 2011).

Breast-Feeding Considerations Chlorpheniramine is excreted into breast milk. Antihistamines may decrease maternal serum prolactin concentrations when administered prior to the establishment of nursing (Messinis, 1985).

Contraindications Hypersensitivity to chlorpheniramine maleate or any component; narrow-angle glaucoma, bladder neck obstruction, symptomatic prostatic hypertrophy, stenosing peptic ulcer, pyloroduodenal obstruction

Warnings Safety and efficacy for the use of cough and cold products in children <2 years of age is limited. Serious adverse effects including death have been reported. The FDA notes that there are no approved OTC uses for these products in children <2 years of age. Healthcare providers are reminded to ask caregivers about the use of OTC cough and cold products in order to avoid exposure to multiple medications containing the same ingredient. Children may be at increased risk for developing CNS stimulation

Precautions Use with caution in patients with asthma; young children may be more susceptible to side effects and CNS stimulation

Adverse Reactions

Central nervous system: Dizziness, excitability, fatigue, headache, nervousness, slight to moderate drowsiness

Gastrointestinal: Abdominal pain, diarrhea, increased appetite, nausea, weight gain, xerostomia

Genitourinary: Urinary retention

Neuromuscular & skeletal: Arthralgia, weakness

Ocular: Diplopia

Renal: Polyuria

Respiratory: Pharyngitis, thickening of bronchial secretions

Drug Interactions

Metabolism/Transport Effects Substrate of CYP2D6 (major), CYP3A4 (minor); **Note:** Assignment of Major/Minor substrate status based on clinically relevant drug interaction potential; **Inhibits** CYP2D6 (weak)

Avoid Concomitant Use

Avoid concomitant use of Chlorpheniramine with any of the following: Aclidinium; Azelastine (Nasal); Ipratropium (Oral Inhalation); Paraldehyde; Potassium Chloride; Thalidomide; Tiotropium; Umeclidinium

Increased Effect/Toxicity

Chlorpheniramine may increase the levels/effects of: AbobotulinumtoxinA; Alcohol (Ethyl); Analgesics (Opioid); Anticholinergic Agents; ARIPiprazole; Azelastine (Nasal); Buprenorphine; Cannabinoid-Containing Products; CNS Depressants; Hydrocodone; Methotrimeprazine; Metyrosine; Mirabegron; Mirtazapine; OnabotulinumtoxinA; Paraldehyde; Potassium Chloride; Pramipexole; RimabotulinumtoxinB; ROPINIRole; Rotigotine; Selective Serotonin Reuptake Inhibitors; Thalidomide; Thiazide Diuretics; Thioridazine; Tiotropium; Topiramate; Zolpidem

The levels/effects of Chlorpheniramine may be increased by: Abiraterone Acetate; Aclidinium; Brimonidine (Topical); Cannabis; CYP2D6 Inhibitors (Moderate); CYP2D6 Inhibitors (Strong); Darunavir; Doxylamine; Dronabinol; Droperidol; HydrOXYzine; Ipratropium (Oral Inhalation); Kava Kava; Magnesium Sulfate; Methotrimeprazine; Nabilone; Perampanel; Pramlintide; Rufinamide; Sodium Oxybate; Tapentadol; Tetrahydrocannabinol; Thioridazine; Umeclidinium

Decreased Effect

Chlorpheniramine may decrease the levels/effects of: Acetylcholinesterase Inhibitors (Central); Benzylpenicilloyl Polylysine; Betahistine; Hyaluronidase; Secretin

The levels/effects of Chlorpheniramine may be decreased by: Acetylcholinesterase Inhibitors (Central); Amphetamines; Peginterferon Alfa-2b

Mechanism of Action Competes with histamine for H_1-receptor sites on effector cells in the gastrointestinal tract, blood vessels, and respiratory tract

Pharmacodynamics

Onset of action: Oral: 6 hours

Duration: Oral: 24 hours

Pharmacokinetics (Adult data unless noted) (Data from chlorpheniramine maleate)

Distribution: V_d:

Children: 3.8 L/kg

Adults: 2.5-3.2 L/kg

Protein binding: 69% to 72%

Metabolism: Substantial metabolism in GI mucosa and on first pass through liver

Bioavailability: Chlorpheniramine:

Solution: 35% to 60%

Tablet: 25% to 45%

Half-life:

Children: Average: 9.6-13.1 hours (range: 5.2-23.1 hours)

Adults: 12-43 hours

Time to peak serum concentration: Oral (solution and conventional tablets): 2-6 hours

Elimination: 35% excreted in 48 hours

Dosing: Usual Oral:

Chlorpheniramine maleate:

Children <12 years: 0.35 mg/kg/day in divided doses every 4-6 hours or as an alternative

2-5 years: 1 mg every 4-6 hours

6-11 years: 2 mg every 4-6 hours, not to exceed 12 mg/day or timed release 8 mg every 12 hours

Children ≥12 years and Adults: 4 mg every 4-6 hours, not to exceed 24 mg/day or timed release 8-12 mg every 12 hours

Chlorpheniramine tannate:

Children 2 to <6 years: 2 mg (1.25 mL) twice daily; not to exceed 8 mg (5 mL) in a 24-hour period

Children 6 to <12 years: 4-8 mg (2.5-5 mL) twice daily; not to exceed 16 mg (10 mL) in a 24-hour period

Children ≥12 years and Adults: 8-16 mg (5-10 mL) twice daily; not to exceed 32 mg (20 mL) in a 24-hour period

Dexchlorpheniramine maleate:

Children 2-5 years: 0.5 mg every 4-6 hours, not to exceed 3 mg/day

Children 6-11 years: 1 mg every 4-6 hours, not to exceed 6 mg/day

Children ≥12 years and Adults: 2 mg every 4-6 hours; not to exceed 12 mg/day

Administration Oral: Administer with food to decrease GI distress; do not crush or chew timed release tablets; shake suspension well before use

Test Interactions May suppress the wheal and flare reactions to skin test antigens.

Dosage Forms Excipient information presented when available (limited, particularly for generics); consult specific product labeling. [DSC] = Discontinued product

Liquid, Oral, as maleate:

Ed ChlorPed: 2 mg/mL (60 mL) [contains fd&c red #40, propylene glycol, saccharin sodium, sodium benzoate; cotton candy flavor]

Suspension, Oral, as tannate:

Ed ChlorPed: 2 mg/mL (60 mL) [contains aspartame, methylparaben, propylene glycol, propylparaben; cotton candy flavor]

Syrup, Oral, as maleate:

Aller-Chlor: 2 mg/5 mL (118 mL [DSC]) [contains alcohol, usp, fd&c yellow #6 (sunset yellow), menthol, methylparaben, propylene glycol, propylparaben; fruit flavor]

Chlor-Trimeton: 2 mg/5 mL (120 mL) [contains alcohol, usp]

Ed Chlorped Jr: 2 mg/5 mL (118 mL, 473 mL) [alcohol free, sugar free; contains fd&c red #40, methylparaben, propylene glycol, propylparaben; cherry flavor]

Tablet, Oral, as maleate:

Aller-Chlor: 4 mg [scored; contains fd&c yellow #10 aluminum lake]

Allergy: 4 mg [contains fd&c yellow #10 (quinoline yellow)]

Allergy: 4 mg [contains fd&c yellow #10 aluminum lake]

Allergy: 4 mg [scored; contains fd&c yellow #10 aluminum lake]

Allergy 4 Hour: 4 mg [DSC] [contains fd&c yellow #10 (quinoline yellow)]

Allergy Relief: 4 mg [contains fd&c yellow #10 aluminum lake]

Allergy-Time: 4 mg [contains fd&c yellow #10 aluminum lake]

Chlor-Trimeton: 4 mg [scored]

Chlorphen: 4 mg [scored; contains fd&c yellow #10 (quinoline yellow)]

Ed-Chlortan: 4 mg [scored; contains fd&c yellow #10 aluminum lake]

Pharbechlor: 4 mg

◀ Generic: 4 mg
Tablet, Oral, as tannate:
Ed-Chlor-Tan: 8 mg [scored]
Tablet Extended Release, Oral, as maleate:
Chlor-Trimeton Allergy: 12 mg [contains fd&c blue #2 aluminum lake, fd&c yellow #10 aluminum lake, fd&c yellow #6 aluminum lake]
Chlor-Trimeton Allergy: 12 mg [contains fd&c yellow #6 (sunset yellow), fd&c yellow #6 aluminum lake]
Generic: 12 mg

◆ **Chlorpheniramine Maleate** see Chlorpheniramine on page 448

◆ **Chlorpheniramine Maleate and Hydrocodone Bitartrate** see Hydrocodone and Chlorpheniramine on page 1030

ChlorproMAZINE (klor PROE ma zeen)

Medication Safety Issues
Sound-alike/look-alike issues:
ChlorproMAZINE may be confused with chlordiazePOX-IDE, chlorproPAMIDE, clomiPRAMINE, prochlorperazine, promethazine
Thorazine may be confused with thiamine, thioridazine
BEERS Criteria medication:
This drug may be potentially inappropriate for use in geriatric patients (Quality of evidence - moderate; Strength of recommendation - strong).

Related Information
Medications for Which a Single Dose May Be Fatal When Ingested by a Toddler on page 2408
Prochlorperazine on page 1745
Serotonin Syndrome on page 2405

Brand Names: Canada Chlorpromazine Hydrochloride Inj; Teva-Chlorpromazine

Therapeutic Category Antiemetic; Antipsychotic Agent, Typical, Phenothiazine; Phenothiazine Derivative

Generic Availability (U.S.) Yes

Use Treatment of nausea and vomiting (FDA approved in ages 6 months to 12 years and adults), restlessness and apprehension prior to surgery (FDA approved in ages 6 months to 12 years and adults), severe behavioral problems in children displayed by combativeness and/or explosive hyperexcitable behavior and in short-term treatment of hyperactive children (FDA approved in ages 1-12 years); adjunct in the treatment of tetanus (Parenteral only: FDA approved in ages 6 months to 12 years and adults); schizophrenia (FDA approved in adults), psychotic disorders (FDA approved in adults), mania (FDA approved in adults), acute intermittent porphyria (FDA approved in adults), intractable hiccups (FDA approved in adults); has also been used in management of Tourette's syndrome, neonatal abstinence syndrome, and cyclic vomiting syndrome (prevention); management of chemotherapy-induced nausea and vomiting (CINV); treatment of delirium

Pregnancy Considerations Embryotoxicity was observed in animal reproduction studies. Jaundice or hyper-/hyporeflexia have been reported in newborn infants following maternal use of phenothiazines. Antipsychotic use during the third trimester of pregnancy has a risk for abnormal muscle movements (extrapyramidal symptoms [EPS]) and withdrawal symptoms in newborns following delivery. Symptoms in the newborn may include agitation, feeding disorder, hypertonia, hypotonia, respiratory distress, somnolence, and tremor; these effects may be self-limiting or require hospitalization.

Breast-Feeding Considerations Chlorpromazine and its metabolites have been detected in breast milk; concentrations in the milk do not correlate with those in the mother and may be higher than what is in the maternal plasma.

Contraindications Hypersensitivity to chlorpromazine hydrochloride, other phenothiazines, or any component; comatose states; presence or concurrent use of large doses (amounts) of CNS depressants (ethanol, narcotics, barbiturates)

Warnings May alter cardiac conduction; life-threatening arrhythmias have occurred with therapeutic doses of neuroleptics; may cause QT prolongation and subsequent torsade de pointes; avoid use in patients with diagnosed or suspected congenital long QT syndrome; avoid concurrent use with other drugs known to prolong QT_c interval. May be sedating; use with caution in disorders in which CNS depression is a feature; patients must be cautioned about performing tasks which require mental alertness (eg, operating machinery or driving); effects may be potentiated when used with other sedative drugs or ethanol; use is contraindicated with high doses of other sedative drugs (ethanol, barbiturates, narcotics).

Impaired core body temperature regulation may occur; use with caution with strenuous exercise, heat exposure, dehydration, and concomitant medication possessing anticholinergic effects. Relative to other neuroleptics, chlorpromazine has a moderate potency of cholinergic blockade. May mask toxicity of other drugs or conditions (eg, intestinal obstruction, Reye's syndrome, brain tumor) due to antiemetic effects.

May cause extrapyramidal symptoms (EPS), including pseudoparkinsonism, acute dystonic reactions, akathisia, and tardive dyskinesia (risk of these reactions is low-moderate relative to other neuroleptics, and is dose-dependent; to decrease risk of tardive dyskinesia: Use smallest dose and shortest duration possible; evaluate continued need periodically; risk of dystonia is increased with the use of high potency and higher doses of conventional antipsychotics and in males and younger patients). EPS occurring with chlorpromazine should be differentiated from possible CNS syndromes which may also cause vomiting (eg, Reye's syndrome, encephalopathy); avoid use in pediatric patients whose clinical presentation is suggestive of Reye's syndrome. Use may be associated with neuroleptic malignant syndrome (NMS); monitor for mental status changes, fever, muscle rigidity, and/or autonomic instability; risk may be increased in patients with Parkinson's disease or Lewy body dementia. Avoid abrupt discontinuation after prolonged use; abrupt discontinuation in patients receiving maintenance treatment may result in transient dyskinetic signs in some patients; these dyskinetic movements may not be distinguishable from tardive dyskinesia (except for duration). May cause pigmentary retinopathy and lenticular and corneal deposits, particularly with prolonged therapy.

Leukopenia, neutropenia, and agranulocytosis (sometimes fatal) have been reported in clinical trials and postmarketing reports with antipsychotic use; in the presence of risk factors (eg, preexisting low WBC or history of drug-induced leuko/neutropenia), evaluate risk versus benefit; if therapy initiated, periodic blood count assessment should be performed; discontinue therapy at first signs of blood dyscrasias or if absolute neutrophil count <1000/mm³.

An increased risk of death has been reported with the use of antipsychotics in elderly patients with dementia-related psychosis **[U.S. Boxed Warning]**; most deaths seemed to be cardiovascular (eg, sudden death, heart failure) or infectious (eg, pneumonia) in nature; chlorpromazine is not approved for this indication.

Tablets may contain benzoic acid; benzoic acid (benzoate) is a metabolite of benzyl alcohol; large amounts of benzyl alcohol (≥99 mg/kg/day) have been associated with a potentially fatal toxicity ("gasping syndrome") in neonates; the "gasping syndrome" consists of metabolic acidosis, respiratory distress, gasping respirations, CNS dysfunction (including convulsions, intracranial hemorrhage), hypotension, and cardiovascular collapse; use chlorpromazine products containing benzoic acid with caution in neonates; *in vitro* and animal studies have shown that benzoate displaces bilirubin from protein binding sites. Injection contains sulfites which may cause allergic reactions in susceptible individuals.

Precautions Use with caution in patients with hepatic or renal impairment or severe cardiovascular disease. Chlorpromazine may cause orthostatic hypotension; use with caution in patients at risk of this effect or in those who would not tolerate transient hypotensive episodes (cerebrovascular disease, cardiovascular disease, hypovolemia, or concurrent medication use which may predispose to hypotension/bradycardia); significant hypotension may occur, particularly with parenteral administration. Use with caution in patients with narrow-angle glaucoma; condition may be exacerbated by cholinergic blockade. Use with caution in patients with myasthenia gravis; condition may be exacerbated by cholinergic blockade. Use with caution in patients with Parkinson's disease; these patients may be more sensitive to adverse effects. Use with caution in patients with respiratory disease (eg, severe asthma, emphysema), particularly children, due to potential for CNS effects. Use with caution in patients at risk of seizures, including those with a history of seizures, head trauma, brain damage, alcoholism, or concurrent therapy with medications which may lower seizure threshold; antipsychotics may lower seizures threshold. Antipsychotics are associated with increased prolactin levels; clinical significance of hyperprolactinemia in patients with breast cancer or other prolactin-dependent tumors is unknown. Antipsychotic use has been associated with esophageal dysmotility and aspiration; use with caution in patients at risk of pneumonia (ie, Alzheimer's disease).

Adverse Reactions
Cardiovascular: Dizziness, nonspecific QT changes, orthostatic hypotension, tachycardia
Central nervous system: Akathisia, drowsiness, dystonias, neuroleptic malignant syndrome, pseudoparkinsonism, seizure, tardive dyskinesia
Dermatologic: Dermatitis, photosensitivity, skin pigmentation (slate gray)
Endocrine & metabolic: Amenorrhea, breast engorgement, false-positive pregnancy test, gynecomastia, hyper- or hypoglycemia, lactation
Gastrointestinal: Constipation, nausea, xerostomia
Genitourinary: Ejaculatory disorder, impotence, urinary retention
Hematologic: Agranulocytosis, aplastic anemia, eosinophilia, hemolytic anemia, leukopenia, thrombocytopenic purpura
Hepatic: Jaundice
Ocular: Blurred vision, corneal and lenticular changes, epithelial keratopathy, pigmentary retinopathy

Drug Interactions
Metabolism/Transport Effects Substrate of CYP1A2 (minor), CYP2D6 (major), CYP3A4 (minor); **Note:** Assignment of Major/Minor substrate status based on clinically relevant drug interaction potential; **Inhibits** CYP2D6 (moderate), CYP2E1 (weak)

Avoid Concomitant Use
Avoid concomitant use of ChlorproMAZINE with any of the following: Aclidinium; Amisulpride; Azelastine (Nasal); Highest Risk QTc-Prolonging Agents; Ipratropium (Oral Inhalation); Ivabradine; Metoclopramide; Mifepristone; Paraldehyde; Potassium Chloride; Sulpiride; Thalidomide; Thioridazine; Tiotropium; Umeclidinium

Increased Effect/Toxicity
ChlorproMAZINE may increase the levels/effects of: Abobotulinumtoxin A; Alcohol (Ethyl); Amisulpride; Analgesics (Opioid); Anticholinergic Agents; Antidepressants

(Serotonin Reuptake Inhibitor/Antagonist); ARIPiprazole; Azelastine (Nasal); Beta-Blockers; Buprenorphine; Cannabinoid-Containing Products; CNS Depressants; CYP2D6 Substrates; Desmopressin; DOXOrubicin (Conventional); Fesoterodine; Haloperidol; Highest Risk QTc-Prolonging Agents; Hydrocodone; Methotrimeprazine; Methylphenidate; Metoprolol; Metyrosine; Mirabegron; Mirtazapine; Moderate Risk QTc-Prolonging Agents; Nebivolol; Onabotulinumtoxin A; Paraldehyde; Porfimer; Potassium Chloride; Rimabotulinumtoxin B; Selective Serotonin Reuptake Inhibitors; Serotonin Modulators; Sulpiride; Thalidomide; Thiazide Diuretics; Thiopental; Thioridazine; Tiotropium; Topiramate; Valproic Acid and Derivatives; Zolpidem

The levels/effects of ChlorproMAZINE may be increased by: Abiraterone Acetate; Acetylcholinesterase Inhibitors (Central); Aclidinium; Antidepressants (Serotonin Reuptake Inhibitor/Antagonist); Antimalarial Agents; Beta-Blockers; Brimonidine (Topical); Cannabis; CYP2D6 Inhibitors (Moderate); CYP2D6 Inhibitors (Strong); Darunavir; Doxylamine; Dronabinol; Droperidol; Haloperidol; HydrOXYzine; Ipratropium (Oral Inhalation); Ivabradine; Kava Kava; Lithium; Magnesium Sulfate; Methotrimeprazine; Methylphenidate; Metoclopramide; Metyrosine; Mifepristone; Nabilone; Perampanel; Pramlintide; QTc-Prolonging Agents (Indeterminate Risk and Risk Modifying); Rufinamide; Serotonin Modulators; Sodium Oxybate; Tapentadol; Tetrahydrocannabinol; Umeclidinium

Decreased Effect
ChlorproMAZINE may decrease the levels/effects of: Acetylcholinesterase Inhibitors (Central); Amphetamines; Anti-Parkinson's Agents (Dopamine Agonist); Codeine; Quinagolide; Secretin; Tamoxifen; TraMADol

The levels/effects of ChlorproMAZINE may be decreased by: Acetylcholinesterase Inhibitors (Central); Antacids; Anti-Parkinson's Agents (Dopamine Agonist); Lithium; Peginterferon Alfa-2b

Stability
Oral: Store at 20°C to 25°C (68°F to 77°F); protect from light and moisture.
Parenteral: Store at 20°C to 25°C (68°F to 77°F), excursions permitted to 15°C to 30°C (59°F to 86°F); protect from freezing and light. A slightly yellowed solution does not indicate potency loss, but a markedly discolored solution should be discarded. Solution diluted with NS (1 mg/mL) and stored in 5 mL vials remains stable for 30 days.

Mechanism of Action Chlorpromazine is an aliphatic phenothiazine antipsychotic which blocks postsynaptic mesolimbic dopaminergic receptors in the brain; exhibits a strong alpha-adrenergic blocking effect and depresses the release of hypothalamic and hypophyseal hormones; believed to depress the reticular activating system, thus affecting basal metabolism, body temperature, wakefulness, vasomotor tone, and emesis

Pharmacodynamics
Onset of action:
Oral: 30-60 minutes
Antipsychotic effects: Gradual, may take up to several weeks
Maximum antipsychotic effect: 6 weeks to 6 months
Duration: Oral: 4-6 hours

Pharmacokinetics (Adult data unless noted)
Absorption: Oral: Rapid and virtually complete; large first-pass effect due to metabolism during absorption in the GI mucosa
Distribution: Widely distributed into most body tissues and fluids; crosses blood-brain barrier; V_d: 8-160 L/kg
Protein binding: 90% to 99%
Metabolism: Extensively in the liver by demethylation (followed by glucuronide conjugation) and amine oxidation

Bioavailability: Oral: ~32%

Half-life, biphasic:

Initial:

Children: 1.1 hours

Adults: ~2 hours

Terminal:

Children: 7.7 hours

Adults: ~30 hours

Elimination: Urine (<1% as unchanged drug) within 24 hours

Dosing: Neonatal Neonatal abstinence syndrome (withdrawal from maternal opioid use; controls CNS and gastrointestinal symptoms): Limited data available:

I.M.: Initial: 0.55 mg/kg/dose given every 6 hours; change to oral after ~4 days, decrease dose gradually over 2-3 weeks. **Note:** Chlorpromazine is rarely used for neonatal abstinence syndrome due to adverse effects such as hypothermia, cerebellar dysfunction, decreased seizure threshold, and eosinophilia; other agents are preferred (AAP Committee on Drugs, 1998; Hudak, 2012).

Dosing: Usual

Infants ≥6 months, Children, and Adolescents:

Behavior problems; severe: Note: Begin with low doses and gradually titrate as needed to lowest effective dose; route of administration should be determined by severity of symptoms.

Infants ≥6 months, Children, and Adolescents weighing ≤45.5 kg:

Oral: Initial: 0.55 mg/kg/dose every 4-6 hours as needed; may titrate as required; in severe cases, higher doses may be required (50-100 mg/**day**); in older children, higher daily doses (200 mg/**day** or higher) may be necessary; maximum daily dose: 500 mg/**day**; daily doses >500 mg have not been shown to further improve behavior in pediatric patients with severe mental impairment

I.M., I.V.: Initial: 0.55 mg/kg/dose every 6-8 hours as needed; may titrate as required in severe cases

Maximum recommended daily doses:

Children <5 years or weighing <22.7 kg: 40 mg/**day**

Children ≥5 years and Adolescents or weighing 22.7-45.5 kg: 75 mg/**day**

Adolescents weighing >45.5 kg:

Oral: Range: 30-800 mg/**day** in 2-4 divided doses, initiate at lower doses and titrate as needed; usual dose is 200 mg/**day**

I.M., I.V.: 25 mg initially, may repeat (25-50 mg) in 1-4 hours, gradually increase to a maximum of 400 mg/ dose every 4-6 hours until patient controlled; usual dose 200-800 mg/**day**

Nausea and vomiting, treatment (non-CINV):

Infants ≥6 months, Children, and Adolescents weighing ≤45.5 kg: Oral, I.M., I.V.: 0.55 mg/kg/dose every 6-8 hours as needed; in severe cases, higher doses may be needed; usual maximum daily dose: I.M., I.V.:

Children <5 years or weighing <22.7 kg: 40 mg/**day**

Children ≥5 years and Adolescents or weighing 22.7-45.5 kg: 75 mg/**day**

Adolescents weighing >45.5 kg:

Oral: 10-25 mg every 4-6 hours as needed

I.M., I.V.: Initial: 25 mg; if tolerated (no hypotension), then may give 25-50 mg every 4-6 hours as needed

Chemotherapy-induced nausea and vomiting (CINV); prevention: I.V.: Initial: 0.5 mg/kg/dose every 6 hours; if not controlled, may increase up to 1 mg/kg/dose; monitor for sedation, maximum dose: 50 mg; recommended in situations where corticosteroids are contraindicated (Dupuis, 2013)

Cyclic vomiting syndrome; abortive therapy: I.V.: 0.5-1 mg/kg/dose every 6 hours; maximum dose: 50 mg; in combination with diphenhydramine (for possible dystonic reactions) (Li, 2008)

Delirium, ICU associated: Limited data available (Silver, 2010):

Oral: 2.5-6 mg/kg/**day** divided every 4-6 hours

Maximum daily dose:

Children ≤5 years: 50 mg/**day**

Children >5 years and Adolescents: 200 mg/**day**

I.M.: 2.5-4 mg/kg/**day** divided every 6-8 hours; maximum daily dose: 40 mg/**day**

Preoperative sedation, anxiety:

Oral: 0.55 mg/kg/dose once 2-3 hours before surgery; maximum dose: 50 mg

I.M.: 0.55 mg/kg/dose once 1-2 hours before surgery; maximum dose: 25 mg

Tetanus:

Infants ≥6 months, Children, and Adolescents weighing ≤45.5 kg: I.M., I.V.: 0.55 mg/kg/dose every 6-8 hours; in severe cases higher doses may be needed

Usual maximum daily dose:

Children <5 years or weighing <22.7 kg: 40 mg/**day**

Children ≥5 years and Adolescents or weighing 22.7-45.5 kg: 75 mg/**day**

Adolescents weighing ≥45.5 kg: I.M., I.V.: 25-50 mg every 6-8 hours; begin with low dose and increase gradually based upon patient response

Adults:

Intractable hiccups:

Oral, I.M.: 25-50 mg 3-4 times daily

I.V. (refractory to oral or I.M. treatment): 25-50 mg via slow I.V. infusion

Nausea and vomiting:

Oral: 10-25 mg every 4-6 hours

I.M., I.V.: 25-50 mg every 4-6 hours

Schizophrenia/psychoses:

Oral: Range: 30-800 mg/day in 1-4 divided doses, initiate at lower doses and titrate as needed; usual dose is 200 mg/day; some patients may require 1-2 g/**day**

I.M., I.V.: 25 mg initially, may repeat (25-50 mg) in 1-4 hours, gradually increase to a maximum of 400 mg/ dose every 4-6 hours until patient controlled; usual dose 300-800 mg/**day**

Administration

Oral: Administer with water, food, or milk to decrease GI upset; brown precipitate may occur when chlorpromazine is mixed with caffeine-containing liquids

Parenteral: Do not administer SubQ (tissue damage and irritation may occur); for direct I.V. injection, dilute with NS to a maximum concentration of 1 mg/mL, administer slow I.V. at a rate not to exceed 0.5 mg/minute in children and 1 mg/minute in adults. To reduce the risk of hypotension, patients receiving I.V. chlorpromazine must remain lying down during and for 30 minutes after the injection. **Note:** Avoid skin contact with solution; may cause contact dermatitis.

Monitoring Parameters
Vital signs (especially with parenteral use); lipid profile, fasting blood glucose/Hgb A_{1c}; BMI; mental status; abnormal involuntary movement scale (AIMS); extrapyramidal symptoms (EPS); CBC in patients with risk factors for leukopenia/neutropenia; periodic eye exam with prolonged therapy

Reference Range
Relationship of plasma concentration to clinical response is not well established

Therapeutic: 50-300 ng/mL (SI: 157-942 nmol/L)

Toxic: >750 ng/mL (SI: >2355 nmol/L)

Test Interactions
False-positives for phenylketonuria, amylase, uroporphyrins, urobilinogen. May cause false-positive pregnancy test. May interfere with urine detection of amphetamine/methamphetamine and methadone (false-positives).

Additional Information
Although chlorpromazine has been used in combination with meperidine and promethazine as a premedication ("lytic cocktail"), this combination may have a higher rate of adverse effects compared to

alternative sedatives/analgesics (AAP, 1995). Use decreased doses in elderly or debilitated patients; dystonic reactions may be more common in patients with hypocalcemia; extrapyramidal reactions may be more common in pediatric patients, especially those with dehydration or acute illnesses (viral or CNS infections).

Dosage Forms Excipient information presented when available (limited, particularly for generics); consult specific product labeling.

Solution, Injection, as hydrochloride:
Generic: 25 mg/mL (1 mL, 2 mL)
Tablet, Oral, as hydrochloride:
Generic: 10 mg, 25 mg, 50 mg, 100 mg, 200 mg

References

American Academy of Pediatrics Committee on Drugs, "Neonatal Drug Withdrawal," *Pediatrics*, 1998, 101(6):1079-88.

American Academy of Pediatrics Committee on Drugs, "Reappraisal of Lytic Cocktail/Demerol®, Phenergan®, and Thorazine® (DPT) for the Sedation of Children," *Pediatrics*, 1995, 95(4):598-602.

Dupuis LL, Boodhan S, Holdsworth M, et al, "Guideline for the Prevention of Acute Nausea and Vomiting Due to Antineoplastic Medication in Pediatric Cancer Patients," *Pediatr Blood Cancer*, March 19, 2013.

Furlanut M, Benetello P, Baraldo M, et al, "Chlorpromazine Disposition in Relation to Age in Children," *Clin Pharmacokinet*, 1990, 18 (4):329-31.

Hudak ML and Tan RC, "Neonatal Drug Withdrawal," *Pediatrics*, 2012, 129(2):e540-60.

Li BU, Lefevre F, Chelimsky GG, et al, "North American Society for Pediatric Gastroenterology, Hepatology, and Nutrition Consensus Statement on the Diagnosis and Management of Cyclic Vomiting Syndrome," *J Pediatr Gastroenterol Nutr*, 2008, 47(3):379-93.

Mazurier E, Cambonie G, Barbotte E, et al, "Comparison of Chlorpromazine Versus Morphine Hydrochloride for Treatment of Neonatal Abstinence Syndrome," *Acta Paediatr*, 2008, 97(10):1358-61.

Silver GH, Kearney JA, Kutko MC, et al, "Infant Delirium in Pediatric Critical Care Settings," *Am J Psychiatry*, 2010, 167(10):1172-7.

◆ **Chlorpromazine Hydrochloride** see ChlorproMAZINE on page 450

◆ **Chlorpromazine Hydrochloride Inj (Can)** see ChlorproMAZINE on page 450

Chlorthalidone (klor THAL i done)

Brand Names: Canada Apo-Chlorthalidone
Therapeutic Category Diuretic, Thiazide
Generic Availability (U.S.) Yes
Use Treatment of edema due to heart failure; hepatic cirrhosis; estrogen or corticosteroid therapy; various forms of renal dysfunction, including nephrotic syndrome, acute glomerulonephritis, and chronic renal failure (FDA approved in adults); management of hypertension either alone or in combination with other antihypertensive agents (FDA approved in adults); **Note:** Use in pregnancy should be reserved for those cases causing extreme discomfort and unrelieved by rest; should not be routinely used during pregnancy.
Pregnancy Risk Factor B
Pregnancy Considerations Adverse events were not observed in animal reproduction studies. Chlorthalidone crosses the placenta and can be detected in cord blood. Maternal use may cause fetal or neonatal jaundice, thrombocytopenia, or other adverse events observed in adults. Use of thiazide diuretics to treat edema during normal pregnancies is not appropriate; use may be considered when edema is due to pathologic causes (as in the nonpregnant patient); monitor. Untreated chronic maternal hypertension is associated with adverse events in the fetus, infant, and mother. Women who require thiazide diuretics for the treatment of hypertension prior to pregnancy may continue their use (ACOG, 2013).
Breast-Feeding Considerations Thiazides are excreted into breast milk. Due to the potential for serious adverse reactions in the nursing infant, the manufacturer recommends a decision be made whether to discontinue nursing or to discontinue the drug, taking into account the importance of treatment to the mother. Diuretics have the potential to decrease milk volume and suppress lactation.

Contraindications Hypersensitivity to chlorthalidone or any component; cross-sensitivity with other thiazides or sulfonamides; anuria

Warnings Hypersensitivity reactions may occur with chlorthalidone and other thiazide diuretics; risk is increased in patients with a history of allergy or bronchial asthma. Chemical similarities are present among sulfonamides, sulfonylureas, carbonic anhydrase inhibitors, thiazides, and loop diuretics (except ethacrynic acid). Use in patients with sulfonamide allergy is specifically contraindicated in product labeling; a risk of crossreaction exists in patients with allergy to any of these compounds; avoid use when previous reaction has been severe. Discontinue if signs of hypersensitivity are noted.

May cause hypokalemia; increased risk associated with aggressive diuresis, severe cirrhosis, or after prolonged therapy; alterations in adequate oral potassium intake may also increase risk; monitor serum potassium concentrations at baseline and periodically; correct hypokalemia prior to initiating therapy. Other electrolyte disorders including hyponatremia, hypomagnesemia, and hypochloremic metabolic alkalosis may occur; monitor electrolytes. SLE exacerbation or activation has been reported with other thiazide-type diuretics. Photosensitization may occur; patients should be counseled.

Precautions Use with caution in patients with severe renal disease due to decreased efficacy and may precipitate azotemia. Use with caution in patients with severe hepatic dysfunction; in cirrhosis, avoid electrolyte and acid/base imbalances that might lead to hepatic encephalopathy or coma. Use with caution in patients with prediabetes or diabetes mellitus; may alter glucose control. Use with caution in patients a history of gout; may cause hyperuricemia and in certain patients with a history of gout, a familial predisposition to gout, or chronic renal failure, gout can be precipitated. Use with caution in patients with hypercalcemia or parathyroid disease; thiazide diuretics may decrease renal calcium excretion; pathologic changes in the parathyroid glands with hypercalcemia and hypophosphatemia have been observed with prolonged use.

Adverse Reactions

Dermatologic: Photosensitivity
Endocrine & metabolic: Hypokalemia
Gastrointestinal: Anorexia, dyspepsia
Rare but important or life-threatening: Agranulocytosis, aplastic anemia, cholecystitis, diabetes mellitus, gout, hypercalcemia, hyperglycemia, hypersensitivity reactions, hypochloremic alkalosis, hyponatremia, leukopenia, necrotizing angiitis, orthostatic hypotension, pancreatitis, renal impairment, thrombocytopenia, toxic epidermal necrolysis, vasculitis, xanthopsia

Drug Interactions

Metabolism/Transport Effects None known.

Avoid Concomitant Use

Avoid concomitant use of Chlorthalidone with any of the following: Dofetilide

Increased Effect/Toxicity

Chlorthalidone may increase the levels/effects of: ACE Inhibitors; Allopurinol; Amifostine; Antihypertensives; Calcium Salts; CarBAMazepine; Cyclophosphamide; Diazoxide; Dofetilide; DULoxetine; Hypotensive Agents; Ivabradine; Lithium; Multivitamins/Minerals (with ADEK, Folate, Iron); Multivitamins/Minerals (with AE, No Iron); Obinutuzumab; OXcarbazepine; Porfimer; RiTUXimab; Sodium Phosphates; Topiramate; Toremifene; Vitamin D Analogs

The levels/effects of Chlorthalidone may be increased by: Alcohol (Ethyl); Alfuzosin; Analgesics (Opioid); ▶

Anticholinergic Agents; Barbiturates; Beta2-Agonists; Brimonidine (Topical); Corticosteroids (Orally Inhaled); Corticosteroids (Systemic); Diazoxide; Herbs (Hypotensive Properties); Licorice; MAO Inhibitors; Multivitamins/Fluoride (with ADE); Pentoxifylline; Phosphodiesterase 5 Inhibitors; Prostacyclin Analogues; Selective Serotonin Reuptake Inhibitors

Decreased Effect
Chlorthalidone may decrease the levels/effects of: Antidiabetic Agents

The levels/effects of Chlorthalidone may be decreased by: Bile Acid Sequestrants; Herbs (Hypertensive Properties); Methylphenidate; Nonsteroidal Anti-Inflammatory Agents; Yohimbine

Stability Store 20°C to 25°C (68°F to 77°F); protect from light.

Mechanism of Action Sulfonamide-derived diuretic that inhibits sodium and chloride reabsorption in the cortical-diluting segment of the ascending loop of Henle

Pharmacodynamics
Onset of action: Diuresis: ~2 hours
Duration: Diuresis: 24-72 hours

Pharmacokinetics (Adult data unless noted)
Distribution: 0.14 L/kg; sequesters in erythrocytes
Protein binding: ~75%
Bioavailability: Chlorthalidone: ~65%; Thalitone®: 104% to 116% relative to an oral solution
Metabolism: Hepatic
Half-life: 40-60 hours; may be prolonged with renal impairment; Anuria: 81 hours
Time to peak serum concentration: 13.8 hours
Elimination: Urine (~50% to 65% as unchanged drug)

Dosing: Usual
Children and Adolescents: **Hypertension:** Oral: Initial: 0.3 mg/kg once daily; may titrate up to a maximum daily dose: 2 mg/kg/**day** or 50 mg/**day** (NHBPEP, 2004; NHLBI, 2011)
Adults:
Hypertension: Oral: 25-100 mg/day or 100 mg 3 times/week; usual dosage range (JNC 7): 12.5-25 mg/day
Edema: Initial: 50-100 mg/day or 100 mg on alternate days; maximum dose: 200 mg/day
Heart failure-associated edema: 12.5-25 mg once daily; maximum daily dose: 100 mg (ACC/AHA 2009 Heart Failure Guidelines)
Dosing adjustments in renal impairment: Adults: CrCl <10 mL/minute: Avoid use. Ineffective with low GFR (Aronoff, 2007)
Note: ACC/AHA 2009 Heart Failure Guidelines suggest that thiazides lose their efficacy when CrCl <40 mL/minute.

Administration Oral: Administer in the morning with food

Monitoring Parameters Serum electrolytes, BUN, creatinine, blood pressure, fluid balance, body weight

Dosage Forms Excipient information presented when available (limited, particularly for generics); consult specific product labeling.
Tablet, Oral:
Generic: 25 mg, 50 mg, 100 mg

References
American College of Obstetricians and Gynecologists (ACOG), "ACOG Practice Bulletin No. 125: Chronic Hypertension in Pregnancy," *Obstet Gynecol*, 2012, 119(2 Pt 1):396-407.
Aronoff GR, Bennett WM, Berns JS, et al, *Drug Prescribing in Renal Failure: Dosing Guidelines for Adults and Children*, 5th ed, Philadelphia, PA: American College of Physicians, 2007.
Chobanian AV, Bakris GL, Black HR, et al, "The Seventh Report of the Joint National Committee on Prevention, Detection, Evaluation, and Treatment of High Blood Pressure: The JNC 7 Report," *JAMA*, 2003, 289(19):2560-72.
Hunt SA, Abraham WT, Chin MH, et al, "2009 Focused Update Incorporated Into the ACC/AHA 2005 Guidelines for the Diagnosis and Management of Heart Failure in Adults: A Report of the American College of Cardiology Foundation/American Heart Association Task Force on Practice Guidelines Developed in Collaboration With the International Society for Heart and Lung Transplantation," *J Am Coll Cardiol*, 2009, 53(15):1-90.
National Heart, Lung, and Blood Institute, "Expert Panel on Integrated Guidelines for Cardiovascular Health and Risk Reduction in Children and Adolescents, Clinical Practice Guidelines, 2011," National Institutes of Health. Available at http://www.nhlbi.nih.gov/guidelines/cvd_ped/peds_guidelines_full.pdf. Date accessed: June 11, 2012.
National High Blood Pressure Education Program Working Group on High Blood Pressure in Children and Adolescents, "The Fourth Report on the Diagnosis, Evaluation, and Treatment of High Blood Pressure in Children and Adolescents," *Pediatrics*, 2004, 114(2 Suppl):555-76.

◆ **Chlor-Trimeton [OTC]** *see* Chlorpheniramine *on page 448*

◆ **Chlor-Trimeton Allergy [OTC]** *see* Chlorpheniramine *on page 448*

◆ **Chlor-Tripolon® (Can)** *see* Chlorpheniramine *on page 448*

◆ **Chlor-Tripolon ND® (Can)** *see* Loratadine and Pseudoephedrine *on page 1279*

Chlorzoxazone (klor ZOKS a zone)

Medication Safety Issues
BEERS Criteria medication:
This drug may be potentially inappropriate for use in geriatric patients (Quality of evidence - moderate; Strength of recommendation - strong).

Brand Names: U.S. Lorzone; Parafon Forte DSC

Therapeutic Category Skeletal Muscle Relaxant, Nonparalytic

Generic Availability (U.S.) Yes

Use Symptomatic treatment of muscle spasm and pain associated with acute musculoskeletal conditions

Pregnancy Considerations Animal reproduction studies have not been conducted.

Contraindications Hypersensitivity to chlorzoxazone or any component; impaired liver function

Warnings Serious (including fatal) hepatocellular toxicity has been reported rarely

Adverse Reactions
Central nervous system: Dizziness, drowsiness, lightheadedness, paradoxical stimulation, malaise
Dermatologic: Rash (rare), petechiae (rare), ecchymoses (rare), angioedema (very rare)
Gastrointestinal: Diarrhea, GI bleeding (rare), nausea, vomiting
Genitourinary: Urine discoloration
Hepatic: Liver dysfunction
Miscellaneous: Anaphylaxis (very rare)

Drug Interactions
Metabolism/Transport Effects Substrate of CYP1A2 (minor), CYP2A6 (minor), CYP2D6 (minor), CYP2E1 (minor), CYP3A4 (minor); **Note:** Assignment of Major/Minor substrate status based on clinically relevant drug interaction potential; **Inhibits** CYP2E1 (weak), CYP3A4 (weak)

Avoid Concomitant Use
Avoid concomitant use of Chlorzoxazone with any of the following: Azelastine (Nasal); Paraldehyde; Pimozide; Thalidomide

Increased Effect/Toxicity
Chlorzoxazone may increase the levels/effects of: Alcohol (Ethyl); ARIPiprazole; Azelastine (Nasal); Buprenorphine; CNS Depressants; Dofetilide; Hydrocodone; Lomitapide; Methotrimeprazine; Metyrosine; Mirtazapine; Paraldehyde; Pimozide; Pramipexole; ROPINIRole; Rotigotine; Selective Serotonin Reuptake Inhibitors; Thalidomide; Zolpidem

The levels/effects of Chlorzoxazone may be increased by: Brimonidine (Topical); Cannabis; Disulfiram; Doxylamine; Dronabinol; Droperidol; HydrOXYzine; Isoniazid;

Kava Kava; Magnesium Sulfate; Methotrimeprazine; Nabilone; Perampanel; Rufinamide; Sodium Oxybate; Tapentadol; Tetrahydrocannabinol

Decreased Effect

The levels/effects of Chlorzoxazone may be decreased by: Peginterferon Alfa-2b

Mechanism of Action Acts on the spinal cord and subcortical areas of the brain to inhibit polysynaptic reflex arcs involved in causing and maintaining skeletal muscle spasms

Pharmacodynamics

Onset of action: Within 60 minutes

Duration: 3-4 hours

Pharmacokinetics (Adult data unless noted)

Absorption: Oral: Readily

Metabolism: Extensive in the liver by glucuronidation

Half-life: ~60 minutes

Time to peak serum concentration: Adults: 1-2 hours

Elimination: In urine as conjugates; <1% excreted unchanged in urine

Dosing: Usual Oral:

Children: 20 mg/kg/day or 600 mg/m^2/day in 3-4 divided doses

Adults: 250-750 mg 3-4 times/day

Administration Oral: Administer with food

Monitoring Parameters Periodic liver function tests

Dosage Forms Excipient information presented when available (limited, particularly for generics); consult specific product labeling.

Tablet, Oral:

Lorzone: 375 mg [contains sodium benzoate]

Lorzone: 750 mg [scored; contains sodium benzoate]

Parafon Forte DSC: 500 mg [scored; contains brilliant blue fcf (fd&c blue #1), fd&c yellow #10 (quinoline yellow), sodium benzoate]

Generic: 500 mg

Cholecalciferol (kole e kal SI fer ole)

Medication Safety Issues

Sound-alike/look-alike issues:

Cholecalciferol may be confused with alfacalcidol, ergocalciferol

Administration issues:

Liquid vitamin D preparations have the potential for dosing errors when administered to infants. Droppers should be clearly marked to easily provide 400 international units. For products intended for infants, the FDA recommends that accompanying droppers deliver no more than 400 international units per dose.

Brand Names: U.S. Aqueous Vitamin D [OTC]; Bio-D-Mulsion Forte [OTC]; Bio-D-Mulsion [OTC]; BProtected Pedia D-Vite [OTC]; D-3-5 [OTC]; D-Vi-Sol [OTC]; D-Vita [OTC]; D3-50 [OTC]; Decara; Decara [OTC]; Delta D3 [OTC]; Dialyvite Vitamin D 5000 [OTC]; Dialyvite Vitamin D3 Max [OTC]; Pronutrients Vitamin D3 [OTC]; Vitamin D3 Super Strength [OTC]

Brand Names: Canada D-Vi-Sol®

Therapeutic Category Nutritional Supplement; Vitamin D Analog; Vitamin, Fat Soluble

Generic Availability (U.S.) Yes

Use Prevention and treatment of vitamin D deficiency and/or rickets; dietary supplement (FDA approved in all ages)

Pregnancy Considerations Adverse events were observed in animals when high maternal doses of vitamin D were administered during pregnancy. Vitamin D crosses the placenta but the transfer to the fetus from the mother is low. Maternal supplementation has not been shown to affect pregnancy outcomes. Vitamin D requirements are the same in pregnant and nonpregnant females (IOM, 2011).

Breast-Feeding Considerations Small quantities of vitamin D are found in breast milk following normal maternal exposure via sunlight and diet. The amount in breast milk does not correlate with serum levels in the infant. Therefore, vitamin D supplementation is recommended in all infants who are partially or exclusively breast fed. Hypercalcemia has been noted in a breast-feeding infant following maternal use of large doses of ergocalciferol; high doses should be avoided in lactating women (IOM, 2011).

Contraindications Hypersensitivity to cholecalciferol or any component; hypercalcemia

Precautions Adequate calcium intake is necessary for clinical response to cholecalciferol therapy; maintain adequate fluid intake

Adverse Reactions Endocrine & metabolic: Hypervitaminosis D (signs and symptoms include hypercalcemia, resulting in headache, nausea, vomiting, lethargy, confusion, sluggishness, abdominal pain, bone pain, polyuria, polydipsia, weakness, cardiac arrhythmias [eg, QT shortening, sinus tachycardia], soft tissue calcification, calciuria, and nephrocalcinosis)

Drug Interactions

Metabolism/Transport Effects Inhibits CYP2C19 (weak), CYP2C9 (weak), CYP2D6 (weak)

Avoid Concomitant Use

Avoid concomitant use of Cholecalciferol with any of the following: Aluminum Hydroxide; Multivitamins/Fluoride (with ADE); Multivitamins/Minerals (with ADEK, Folate, Iron); Sucralfate; Sucroferric Oxyhydroxide; Vitamin D Analogs

Increased Effect/Toxicity

Cholecalciferol may increase the levels/effects of: Aluminum Hydroxide; ARIPiprazole; Cardiac Glycosides; Sucralfate; Vitamin D Analogs

The levels/effects of Cholecalciferol may be increased by: Calcium Salts; Danazol; Multivitamins/Fluoride (with ADE); Multivitamins/Minerals (with ADEK, Folate, Iron); Thiazide Diuretics

Decreased Effect

The levels/effects of Cholecalciferol may be decreased by: Bile Acid Sequestrants; Mineral Oil; Orlistat; Sucroferric Oxyhydroxide

Stability Store at room temperature; protect from light

Pharmacokinetics (Adult data unless noted)

Protein binding: Extensively to vitamin D-binding protein

Metabolism: Hydroxylated in liver to calcidiol (25-OH-D3) then in kidney to the active form, calcitriol (1α,2-[OH]2 vitamin D$_3$)

Half-life: 19-25 hours

Elimination: As metabolites, urine and feces

Dosing: Neonatal

Adequate intake (AI): Oral: 400 units/day

Prevention of Vitamin D deficiency (Greer, 2000; Wagner, 2008): Oral:

Premature neonates: 400-800 units/day or 150-400 units/kg/day

Breast-fed neonates (fully or partially): 400 units/day beginning in the first few days of life. Continue supplementation until infant is weaned to ≥1000 mL/day or 1 qt/day of vitamin D-fortified formula or whole milk (after 12 months of age)

Formula-fed neonates ingesting <1000 mL of vitamin D-fortified formula: 400 units/day

Treatment of Vitamin D deficiency and/or rickets: Oral:

Note: In addition to calcium and phosphorus supplementation (Gordon, 2008; Misra, 2008): 1000 units/day for 2-3 months; once radiologic evidence of healing is observed, dose should be decreased to 400 units/day

Dosing: Usual

Infants, Children, and Adolescents:

Adequate intake (AI): Oral: Infants: 400 units/day

Recommended Daily Allowance (RDA): Oral: Children and Adolescents: 600 units/day

Prevention of Vitamin D deficiency: (Greer, 2000; Wagner, 2008): Oral:

Breast-fed infants (fully or partially): 400 units/day beginning in the first few days of life. Continue supplementation until infant is weaned to ≥1000 mL/day or 1 qt/day of vitamin D-fortified formula or whole milk (after 12 months of age)

Formula-fed infants ingesting <1000 mL of vitamin D-fortified formula: 400 units/day

Children ingesting <1000 mL of vitamin D-fortified milk: 400 units/day

Children with increased risk of vitamin D deficiency (chronic fat malabsorption, maintained on chronic antiseizure medications): Higher doses may be required; use laboratory testing [25(OH)D, PTH, bone mineral status] to evaluate

Adolescents without adequate intake: 400 units/day

Treatment Vitamin D deficiency and/or rickets: Oral:

Note: In addition to calcium and phosphorus supplementation (Gordon, 2008; Misra, 2008):

Infants 1-12 months: 1000-5000 units/day for 2-3 months; once radiologic evidence of healing is observed, dose should be decreased to 400 units/day

Children >12 months: 5000-10,000 units/day for 2-3 months; once radiologic evidence of healing is observed, dose should be decreased to 400 units/day

Children with increased risk of vitamin D deficiency (chronic fat malabsorption, maintained on chronic antiseizure medications): Higher doses may be required; use laboratory testing [25(OH)D, PTH, bone mineral status] to evaluate

Note: If poor compliance, single high dose may be used or repeated periodically

Treatment of Vitamin D insufficiency or deficiency associated with CKD (stages 2-5, 5D); serum 25 hydroxyvitamin D [25(OH)D] level ≤30 ng/mL (KDOQI Guidelines, 2009): Oral:

Serum 25(OH)D level 16-30 ng/mL: Children: 2000 units/day for 3 months or 50,000 units every month for 3 months

Serum 25(OH)D level 5-15 ng/mL: Children: 4000 units/day for 12 weeks or 50,000 units every other week for 12 weeks

Serum 25(OH)D level <5 ng/mL: Children: 8000 units/day for 4 weeks then 4000 units/day for 2 months for total therapy of 3 months or 50,000 units/week for 4 weeks followed by 50,000 units 2 times/month for a total therapy of 3 months

Maintenance dose [once repletion accomplished; serum 25(OH)D level >30 ng/mL]: 200-1000 units/day

Dosage adjustment: Monitor serum 25(OH)D, corrected total calcium and phosphorus levels 1 month following initiation of therapy, every 3 months during therapy and with any Vitamin D dose change.

Prevention and treatment of Vitamin D Deficiency in cystic fibrosis: Oral:

Recommended daily intake (Borowitz, 2002):

Infants <1 year: 400 units/day

Children >1 year: 400-800 units/day

Alternate dosing (Hall, 2010):

Infants <1 year: 8000 units/**week**

Children ≥1 year: 800 units/day

Note: If serum 25 hydroxyvitamin D [25(OH)D] level remains ≤30 ng/mL (75 nmol/L) and patient compliance established; then medium dose regimen may be used:

Medium Dose Regimen:

Patient <5 years: 12,000 units/week for 12 weeks

Patient ≥5 years: 50,000 units/week for 12 weeks

Note: If repeat 25 hydroxyvitamin D [25(OH)D] level remains ≤30 ng/mL (75 nmol/L) and patient compliance established; then high dose regimen may be used:

High Dose Regimen:

Patient <5 years: 12,000 units twice weekly for 12 weeks

Patient ≥5 years: 50,000 units twice weekly for 12 weeks

Adults:

Dietary Intake Reference for Vitamin D: Oral:

Adults 19-70 years: RDA: 600 units/day

Female: Pregnancy/lactating: RDA: 600 units/day (see Additional Information)

Osteoporosis prevention and treatment: 800-1000 units/day

Vitamin D deficiency treatment: 1000 units/day (Holick, 2007)

Administration May be administered without regard to meals; for oral liquid, use accompanying dropper for dosage measurements

Monitoring Parameters Children at increased risk of vitamin D deficiency (chronic fat malabsorption, chronic antiseizure medication use) require serum 25(OH)D, PTH, and bone-mineral status to evaluate. If vitamin D supplement is required, then 25(OH)D levels should be repeated at 3-month intervals until normal. PTH and bone mineral-status should be monitored every 6 months until normal.

Chronic kidney disease: Serum calcium and phosphorus levels (in CKD: After 1 month and then at least every 3 months); alkaline phosphatase, BUN; 25(OH)D (in CKD: After 3 months of treatment and as needed thereafter)

Reference Range Vitamin D status may be determined by serum 25(OH) D levels (Misra, 2008):

Severe deficiency: ≤5 ng/mL (12.5 nmol/L)

Deficiency: 15 ng/mL (37.5 nmol/L)

Insufficiency: 15-20 ng/mL (37.5-50 nmol/L)

Sufficiency: 20-100 ng/mL (50-250 nmol/L)*

Excess: >100 ng/mL (250 nmol/L)**

Intoxication: 150 ng/mL (375 nmol/L)

*Based on adult data a level of >32 ng/mL (80 nmol/L) is desirable

**Arbitrary designation

Target serum 25(OH) D: >30 ng/mL

Additional Information 1 mcg cholecalciferol provides 40 units of vitamin D activity

Biological potency may be greater with cholecalciferol (vitamin D_3) compared to ergocalciferol (vitamin D_2).

Maternal Supplementation of High Dose Vitamin D: Data has shown maternal doses of 2000 units/day will raise the antirachitic activity of breast milk and the serum 25(OH)D levels in exclusively breast-fed infants. Higher maternal doses of 4000-6400 units/day have been shown to produce significant satisfactory increases in these outcome measures without evidence of maternal vitamin D toxicity (Hollis 2004; Misra 2008; Taylor, 2008; Wagner, 2008). In geographical areas where rickets is frequently seen and baseline maternal and infant serum 25(OH)D levels are very low (eg, Middle East), concurrent maternal high dose supplementation (2000 units/day or 60,000 units/month) with infant supplementation (400 units/day) has been shown to produce a 64% reduction in prevalence of vitamin D deficiency in the study population (Saadi, 2009). Due to recent increase in number of reported cases of rickets, Canada has increased vitamin D recommendations for all full-term infants (400-800 units/day depending on month) and 2000 units/day maternal supplementation if lactating.

Chronic kidney disease (CKD) (KDIGO, 2013; KDOQI, 2002): Children ≥2 years, Adolescents, and Adults: GFR <60 mL/minute/1.73 m² or kidney damage for ≥3 months; stages of CKD are described below:

CKD Stage 1: Kidney damage with normal or increased GFR; GFR >90 mL/minute/1.73 m²

CKD Stage 2: Kidney damage with mild decrease in GFR; GFR 60-89 mL/minute/1.73 m²

CKD Stage 3: Moderate decrease in GFR; GFR 30-59 mL/minute/1.73 m²

CKD Stage 4: Severe decrease in GFR; GFR 15-29 mL/minute/1.73 m²

CKD Stage 5: Kidney failure; GFR <15 mL/minute/1.73 m² or dialysis

Dosage Forms Excipient information presented when available (limited, particularly for generics); consult specific product labeling.

Capsule, Oral:

D-3-5: 5000 units

Decara: 25,000 units [contains soybean oil]

Decara: 50,000 units [contains fd&c yellow #10 (quinoline yellow), fd&c yellow #6 (sunset yellow), soybean oil]

Dialyvite Vitamin D 5000: 5000 units

Pronutrients Vitamin D3: 1000 units [contains soybean oil]

Generic: 10,000 units

Capsule, Oral [preservative free]:

D-3-5: 5000 units [dye free]

D3-50: 50,000 units [dye free, sugar free, yeast free]

Generic: 2000 units, 5000 units

Liquid, Oral:

Aqueous Vitamin D: 400 units/mL (50 mL) [gluten free, lactose free, sugar free; contains methylparaben, polysorbate 80]

Bio-D-Mulsion: 400 units/0.03 mL (30 mL)

Bio-D-Mulsion Forte: 2000 units/0.03 mL (30 mL)

BProtected Pedia D-Vite: 400 units/mL (50 mL) [alcohol free, sugar free; contains polysorbate 80, propylene glycol, sodium benzoate; cherry flavor]

D-Vi-Sol: 400 units/mL (50 mL) [gluten free, lactose free, sugar free; contains polysorbate 80]

D-Vita: 400 units/mL (50 mL) [alcohol free, gluten free, lactose free, sugar free; contains polysorbate 80, propylene glycol, sodium benzoate; fruit flavor]

Generic: 400 units/mL (50 mL, 52.5 mL)

Liquid, Oral [preservative free]:

Generic: 5000 units/mL (52.5 mL)

Tablet, Oral:

Delta D3: 400 units [gelatin free, gluten free, lactose free, no artificial color(s), no artificial flavor(s), starch free, sugar free, yeast free]

Dialyvite Vitamin D3 Max: 50,000 units [scored]

Vitamin D3 Super Strength: 2000 units [gluten free]

Generic: 400 units, 1000 units, 3000 units, 5000 units

Tablet, Oral [preservative free]:

Generic: 400 units, 1000 units, 2000 units, 5000 units

Tablet Chewable, Oral:

Generic: 400 units

References

Borowitz D, Baker RD, and Stallings V, "Consensus Report on Nutrition for Pediatric Patients With Cystic Fibrosis," *J Pediatr Gastroenterol Nutr*, 2002, 35(3):246-59.

"Dietary Reference Intakes for Calcium, Phosphorus, Magnesium, Vitamin D, and Fluoride. Standing Committee on the Scientific Evaluation of Dietary Reference Intakes, Food and Nutrition Board, Institute of Medicine," National Academy of Sciences, Washington, DC: National Academy Press, 1997.

Gordon CM, Williams AL, Feldman HA, et al, "Treatment of Hypovitaminosis D in Infants and Toddlers," *J Clin Endocrinol Metab*, 2008, 93:2716-21.

Greer FR, "Vitamin Metabolism and Requirements in the Micropremie," *Clin Perinatol*, 2000, 27(1):95-118.

Hall WB, Sparks AA, and Aris RM, "Vitamin D Deficiency in Cystic Fibrosis," *Int J Endocrinol*, 2010, 218691.

Holick MF, "Vitamin D Deficiency," *N Engl J Med*, 2007, 357(3):266-81.

Hollis BW and Wagner CL, "Vitamin D Requirements During Lactation: High-Dose Maternal Supplementation as Therapy to Prevent Hypovitaminosis D for Both the Mother and the Nursing Infant," *Am J Clin Nutr*, 2004, 80(6 Suppl):1752S-8S.

KDOQI Work Group, "KDOQI Clinical Practice Guideline for Nutrition in Children with CKD: 2008 Update. Executive Summary," *Am J Kidney Dis*, 2009, 53(3 Suppl 2):S11-104.

Kidney Disease: Improving Global Outcomes (KDIGO) CKD Work Group. KDIGO 2012 clinical practice guideline for the evaluation and management of chronic kidney disease. *Kidney Inter.* 2013;3:1-150.

Misra M, Pacaud D, Petryk A, et al, "Vitamin D Deficiency in Children and Its Management: Review of Current Knowledge and Recommendations," *Pediatrics*, 2008, 122(2):398-417.

Saadi HF, Dawodu A, Afandi B, et al, "Effect of Combined Maternal and Infant Vitamin D Supplementation on Vitamin D Status of Exclusively Breastfed Infants," *Matern Child Nutr*, 2009, 5(1):25-32.

Taylor SN, Wagner CL, and Hollis BW, "Vitamin D Supplementation During Lactation to Support Infant and Mother," *J Am Coll Nutr*, 2008, 27(6):690-701.

Wagner CL, Greer FR, American Academy of Pediatrics Section on Breastfeeding, et al, "Prevention of Rickets and Vitamin D Deficiency in Infants, Children, and Adolescents," *Pediatrics*, 2008, 122 (5):1142-52.

Cholestyramine Resin (koe LES teer a meen REZ in)

Brand Names: U.S. Prevalite; Questran; Questran Light

Brand Names: Canada Novo-Cholamine; Novo-Cholamine Light; Olestyr; PMS-Cholestyramine; Questran; Questran Light Sugar Free; ZYM-Cholestyramine-Light; ZYM-Cholestyramine-Regular

Therapeutic Category Antilipemic Agent, Bile Acid Sequestrant

Generic Availability (U.S.) Yes

Use Adjunct in the management of primary hypercholesterolemia (FDA approved in adults); pruritus associated with elevated levels of bile acids (FDA approved in adults); has also been used to manage diarrhea associated with excess fecal bile acids; applied topically to treat diaper dermatitis and as a skin-protectant around enterostomy fistula sites.

Pregnancy Risk Factor C

Pregnancy Considerations Cholestyramine is not absorbed systemically, but may interfere with vitamin absorption; therefore, regular prenatal supplementation may not be adequate. There are no studies in pregnant women; use with caution.

Breast-Feeding Considerations Due to lack of systemic absorption cholestyramine is not expected to be excreted into breast milk; however, the tendency of cholestyramine to interfere with vitamin absorption may have an effect on the nursing infant.

Contraindications Hypersensitivity to cholestyramine or any component; complete biliary obstruction

Warnings Prevalite® and Questran® Light contain phenylalanine (~14 mg/5.5 g of cholestyramine); generic formulations may also contain phenylalanine; consult product specific labeling; avoid use or use with caution in patients with phenylketonuria.

Precautions Use with caution in patients with constipation or recent abdominal surgery; may produce or exacerbate constipation problems; initiate therapy at a reduced dose in patients with a history of constipation; ensure adequate fluid and possible fiber intake; hemorrhoids may be worsened.

Use with caution in patients susceptible to fat-soluble vitamin deficiencies; absorption of fat soluble vitamins A, D, E, and K and folic acid may be decreased; patients should take vitamins at least 1 hour before or ≥4 hours after cholestyramine; absorption of calcium, iron, zinc, and magnesium may also be decreased. Chronic use may be associated with bleeding problems due to hypoprothrombinemia, especially in high doses associated with vitamin K deficiency; may be prevented with use of oral vitamin K therapy. Some patients may also develop folate deficiency; supplementation with folic acid may be necessary with chronic use.

Use with caution in patients with renal impairment, volume depletion, or receiving concurrent spironolactone therapy; with prolonged use, may potentially cause hypochloremic acidosis due to the exchange of organic anions for chloride; risk may be higher in younger and smaller patients; growth failure and malnutrition may occur in these patients (ASPEN Core Curriculum, 2010).

May decrease absorption of other orally administered drugs; avoid taking cholestyramine simultaneously with many other medicines; ideally other medications should be taken at least 1 hour before or 4-6 hours after cholestyramine dose. Prolonged exposure to tooth enamel may result in discoloration or erosion; patients should be instructed to avoid sipping or slowly swallowing cholestyramine doses and to maintain good dental hygiene practices. May increase serum triglyceride concentrations; in a trial of children and adolescents (>10 years of age); the serum triglycerides increased 6% to 9% from baseline (not statistically significant) (McCrindle, 1997).

Adverse Reactions
Cardiovascular: Edema, syncope

Central nervous system: Anxiety, dizziness, drowsiness, eructation, fatigue, headache, vertigo

Dermatologic: Bruising, rash, skin irritation, urticaria

Endocrine & metabolic: Hyperchloremic acidosis (children), libido increased

Gastrointestinal: Abdominal pain, anorexia, biliary colic, black stools, constipation, dental bleeding, dental caries, dental erosion, diarrhea, diverticulitis, duodenal ulcer bleeding, dysphagia, eructation, flatulence, gallbladder calcification, GI hemorrhage, intestinal obstruction (rare), hemorrhoidal bleeding, nausea, pancreatitis, perianal irritation, rectal bleeding, rectal pain, steatorrhea, taste disturbance, tongue irritation, tooth discoloration, ulcer, vomiting, weight gain/loss

Hepatic: Hypothrombinemia, liver function abnormalities, prothrombin time increased

Hematologic: Anemia, bleeding

Neuromuscular & skeletal: Arthritis, backache, joint/muscle/nerve pain, osteoporosis, paresthesia

Ocular: Night blindness (rare), uveitis

Otic: Tinnitus

Renal: Diuresis, dysuria, hematuria

Respiratory: Asthma, dyspnea, wheezing

Miscellaneous: Hiccups, swollen glands

Drug Interactions
Metabolism/Transport Effects None known.

Avoid Concomitant Use
Avoid concomitant use of Cholestyramine Resin with any of the following: Deferasirox; Mycophenolate

Increased Effect/Toxicity
Cholestyramine Resin may increase the levels/effects of: Spironolactone

Decreased Effect
Cholestyramine Resin may decrease the levels/effects of: Acetaminophen; Amiodarone; AtorvaSTATin; Cardiac Glycosides; Chenodiol; Contraceptives (Estrogens); Contraceptives (Progestins); Corticosteroids (Oral); Deferasirox; Ezetimibe; Fibric Acid Derivatives; Fluvastatin; Leflunomide; Lomitapide; Loop Diuretics; Methotrexate; Methylfolate; Multivitamins/Fluoride (with ADE); Multivitamins/Minerals (with ADEK, Folate, Iron); Multivitamins/Minerals (with AE, No Iron); Mycophenolate; Niacin; Nonsteroidal Anti-Inflammatory Agents; PHENobarbital; Pravastatin; Propranolol; Raloxifene; Rosiglitazone; Teriflunomide; Tetracycline Derivatives; Thiazide Diuretics; Thyroid Products; Ursodiol; Vancomycin; Vitamin D Analogs; Vitamin K Antagonists

Food Interactions Cholestyramine (especially high doses or long-term therapy) may decrease the absorption of folic acid, calcium, fat-soluble vitamins (vitamins A, D, E, and K), and iron. Management: Supplementation of folic acid, calcium, fat-soluble vitamins (vitamins A, D, E, and K), and iron may be necessary.

Stability Store at 20°C to 25°C (68°F to 77°F); excursions permitted to 15°C to 30°C (59°F to 86°F).

Mechanism of Action Forms a nonabsorbable complex with bile acids in the intestine, releasing chloride ions in the process; inhibits enterohepatic reuptake of intestinal bile salts and thereby increases the fecal loss of bile salt-bound low density lipoprotein cholesterol

Pharmacodynamics Maximum effect on serum cholesterol levels: Within 4 weeks

Pharmacokinetics (Adult data unless noted)
Absorption: Not absorbed from the GI tract

Elimination: Forms an insoluble complex with bile acids which is excreted in feces

Dosing: Neonatal Diaper dermatitis: Limited data available: Topical: Apply to affected area with each diaper change; **Note:** Product not commercially available; may be prepared as an extemporaneously compounded ointment or paste in Aquaphor®; usual concentration: 5% to 10%; although higher concentrations (up to 20%) have been compounded; some centers have also used petrolatum as the base for compounding (White, 2003; Williams, 2011)

Dosing: Usual
Infants, Children, and Adolescents:

Diaper dermatitis: Limited data available: Infants and Children: Topical: Apply to affected area with each diaper change; **Note:** Product not commercially available; may be prepared as an extemporaneously compounded ointment or paste in Aquaphor® or polyethylene glycol; usual concentration 5% to 10%; although higher concentrations (up to 20%) have been compounded; some centers have also used petrolatum as the base for compounding (Preckshot, 2001; White, 2003; Williams, 2011)

Dyslipidemia: Limited data available: Oral: **Note:** Dosages are expressed in terms of anhydrous resin:

Age-directed (fixed-dosing): Children ≥6 years and Adolescents: Initial 2-4 g/day for 1 week, then increase as tolerated to 8 g/day; children <10 years of age may only tolerate doses of 4 g (McCrindle, 2007; Sprecher, 1996; Tonstad, 1996); lipid-lowering effects are better if dose is administered as a single daily dose with the evening meal (single daily morning doses are less effective); if patients cannot tolerate once daily dosing, the total daily dose may be divided into 2 doses and administered with the morning and evening meals; may also be administered in 3 divided doses daily (Daniels, 2002); doses >8 g/day may not provide additional significant cholesterol-lowering effects, but may increase adverse effects (Sprecher, 1996)

Weight-directed dosing: Children and Adolescents: 240 mg/kg/day in 3 divided doses; titrate to effect, maximum daily dose: 8 g/**day**

Pruritus secondary to cholestasis: Limited data available: Oral: **Note:** Dosages are expressed in terms of anhydrous resin:

Children ≤10 years: 240 mg/kg/day in 2 or 3 divided doses administered in the morning around breakfast and if necessary, the third dose at lunch; may titrate dose to effect. Some experts have suggested a maximum daily dose of 4 g/day; however, higher doses have been reported to treat pruritus in pediatric patients <10 years (in a case report (age: 9 years), the reported effective dose range was 3.3-6.6 g/day; in another case series (n=3; ages: 3-9 years), the reported range was 1.7-10 g/day; in some patients, higher doses were associated with increased steatorrhea and required dosage reduction (Cies, 2007; Sprecher, 1996)

Children >10 years and Adolescents: 240 mg/kg/day administered in the morning before breakfast; may titrate dose to effect. Some experts have suggested a maximum daily dose of 8 g/day; in adult patients, the AASLD guidelines recommend an initial dose of 4 g/day; may titrate up to 16 g/day; in some patients, higher doses have been associated with increased steatorrhea requiring dose reduction (Cies, 2007; Iman, 2012; Lindor, 2009; Sprecher, 1996).

Diarrhea secondary to intestinal failure, short-bowel syndrome: Limited data available: Children and Adolescents: Oral: 240 mg/kg/day in 3 divided doses; maximum daily dose: 8 g/day has been suggested (Ching, 2009); however, trials have not been completed in pediatric patients and others have recommended avoiding use at this time; further studies are needed (ASPEN Core Curriculum, 2010).

Adults: **Note:** Dosages are expressed in terms of anhydrous resin: **Dyslipidemia:** Oral: Initial: 4 g 1-2 times daily; increase gradually over ≥1-month intervals; maintenance: 8-16 g/day divided in 2 doses; maximum: 24 g/day

Dosing adjustment in renal impairment: There are no dosage adjustment provided in manufacturer's labeling; however, use with caution in renal impairment; may cause hyperchloremic acidosis.

Dosing adjustment in hepatic impairment: No dosage adjustment necessary; not absorbed from the gastrointestinal tract.

Administration Oral: Administer as prepared suspension; not to be taken in dry form orally; mix dry form with 2-6 ounces of water, noncarbonated liquid, or applesauce; suspension should not be sipped or held in mouth for prolonged periods. Administration at mealtime is recommended. Administer other drugs including vitamins or mineral supplements at least 1 hour before or at least 4-6 hours after cholestyramine.

Dyslipidemia: Administer as a single dose (preferably) with the evening meal; however, some patients may require divided doses; in pediatric patients, may use 2-3 divided doses and in adults up to 6 doses daily.

Pruritus; cholestasis: Administer before breakfast (gall bladder has highest concentration of bile acids available for binding); for patients with an intact gall bladder, it has been suggested to administer the first dose 30 minutes before breakfast, the second dose 30 minutes after breakfast, and the final dose with lunch (Cies, 2007)

Monitoring Parameters Serum cholesterol and triglycerides (4 weeks after initiation, then every 3-4 months the first year of therapy, every 6 months with second year, and whenever clinically indicated); with prolonged use: Prothrombin time, liver enzymes, CBC, electrolytes, number of stools/day, signs/symptoms of nutritional deficiency (fat soluble vitamins, folate, calcium, zinc, iron, or magnesium)

Test Interactions Increased prothrombin time

Dosage Forms Excipient information presented when available (limited, particularly for generics); consult specific product labeling. [DSC] = Discontinued product

Packet, Oral:

Prevalite: 4 g (1 ea, 42 ea, 60 ea) [contains aspartame; orange flavor]

Questran: 4 g (1 ea, 60 ea)

Questran Light: 4 g (1 ea [DSC], 60 ea [DSC]) [sugar free; contains aspartame; orange flavor]

Generic: 4 g (1 ea, 60 ea)

Powder, Oral:

Prevalite: 4 g/dose (231 g) [contains aspartame; orange flavor]

Questran: 4 g/dose (378 g)

Questran Light: 4 g/dose (210 g) [sugar free; contains aspartame]

Generic: 4 g/dose (210 g, 239.4 g, 378 g)

References

Btaiche IF and Khalidi N, "Parenteral Nutrition-Associated Liver Complications in Children," *Pharmacotherapy*, 2002, 22(2):188-211.

Carney LN, Nepa A, Cohen SS, et al, "Parenteral and Enteral Nutrition Support: Determining the Best Way to Feed," In: Corkins MR, Balint J, Bobo E, et al, eds, *The A.S.P.E.N Pediatric Nutrition Support Core Curriculum*, Silver Spring: MD: American Society of Parenteral and Enteral Nutrition, 2010, 433-47.

Ching YA, Gura K, and Modi B, "Pediatric Intestinal Failure: Nutrition, Pharmacologic, and Surgical Approaches," *Nutr Clin Pract*, 2007, 22 (6):653-63.

Cies JJ and Giamalis JN, "Treatment of Cholestatic Pruritus in Children," *Am J Health Syst Pharm*, 2007, 64(11):1157-62.

Daniels SR, personal communication, May 2002.

Imam MH, Gossard AA, and Sinakos E, "Pathogenesis and Management of Pruritus in Cholestatic Liver Disease," *J Gastroenterol Hepatol*, 2012, 27(7):1150-8.

Lindor KD, Gershwin ME, Poupon R, et al, "Primary Biliary Cirrhosis," *Hepatology*, 2009, 50(1):291-308.

McCrindle BW, O'Neill MB, Cullen-Dean G, et al, "Acceptability and Compliance With Two Forms of Cholestyramine in the Treatment of Hypercholesterolemia in Children: A Randomized, Crossover Trial," *J Pediatr*, 1997, 130(2):266-73.

McCrindle BW, Urbina EM, Dennison BA, et al, "Drug Therapy of High-Risk Lipid Abnormalities in Children and Adolescents: A Scientific Statement from the American Heart Association Atherosclerosis, Hypertension, and Obesity in Youth Committee, Council of Cardiovascular Disease in the Young, With the Council on Cardiovascular Nursing," *Circulation*, 2007, 115(14):1948-67.

Preckshot J, et al, "Cholestyramine 6.5% Ointment," *Int J Pharm Compound*, 2001, 5(1)42.

Sprecher DL and Daniels SR, "Rational Approach to Pharmacologic Reduction of Cholesterol Levels in Children," *J Pediatr*, 1996, 129 (1):4-7.

"Third Report of the National Cholesterol Education Program Expert Panel on Detection, Evaluation, and Treatment of High Blood Cholesterol in Adults (Adult Treatment Panel III)," May 2001. Available at http://www.nhlbi.nih.gov/guidelines/cholesterol.

Tonstad S, Knudtzon J, Sivertsen M, et al, "Efficacy and Safety of Cholestyramine Therapy in Peripubertal and Prepubertal Children With Familial Hypercholesterolemia," *J Pediatr*, 1996, 129(1):42-9.

White CM, Kalus JS, Caron MF, et al, "Cholestyramine Ointment Used on an Infant for Severe Buttocks Rash Resistant to Standard Therapeutic Modalities," *J Pharm Technol*, 2003, 19:11-3.

Williams KD and Williams L, "Diaper Rash Relief, Common Sense Remedies and Treatment," *Int J Pharm Compound*, 2011, 15 (6):464-9.

Choline Magnesium Trisalicylate

(KOE leen mag NEE zhum trye sa LIS i late)

Therapeutic Category Analgesic, Non-narcotic; Anti-inflammatory Agent; Antipyretic; Nonsteroidal Anti-inflammatory Drug (NSAID), Oral; Salicylate

Generic Availability (U.S.) Yes

Use Management of osteoarthritis, rheumatoid arthritis, and other arthritides; treatment of acute painful shoulder, mild to moderate pain, and fever

Pregnancy Risk Factor C/D (3rd trimester)

Pregnancy Considerations Animal reproduction studies have not been conducted. Due to the known effects of other salicylates (closure of ductus arteriosus), use during late pregnancy should be avoided.

Breast-Feeding Considerations Excreted in breast milk; peak levels occur 9-12 hours after dose. Use caution if used during breast-feeding.

Contraindications Hypersensitivity to salicylates, any component, or other nonacetylated salicylates; history of asthma, urticaria, or allergic-type reaction to aspirin, or other NSAIDs; patients with the "aspirin triad" [asthma, rhinitis (with or without nasal polyps), and aspirin intolerance] (fatal asthmatic and anaphylactoid reactions may occur in these patients)

Warnings Do not use salicylates in children and teenagers who have or who are recovering from chickenpox or flu symptoms (due to the association with Reye's syndrome); when using salicylates, changes in behavior (along with nausea and vomiting) may be an early sign of Reye's syndrome; instruct patients and caregivers to contact their healthcare provider if these symptoms occur.

Precautions Use with extreme caution in patients with impaired renal function, erosive gastritis or peptic ulcer

Adverse Reactions

Central nervous system: Dizziness, drowsiness, headache, lethargy, lightheadedness

Gastrointestinal: Constipation, diarrhea, dyspepsia, epigastric, heartburn, nausea, pain, vomiting

Otic: Hearing impairment, tinnitus

Rare but important or life-threatening: Anorexia, asthma, bruising, confusion, duodenal ulceration, dysgeusia, edema, epistaxis, erythema multiforme, esophagitis, hallucinations, hearing loss (irreversible), increased BUN, increased creatinine, increased hepatic enzymes, gastric ulceration, occult bleeding, pruritus, rash, weight gain

Drug Interactions

Metabolism/Transport Effects None known.

Avoid Concomitant Use

Avoid concomitant use of Choline Magnesium Trisalicylate with any of the following: Influenza Virus Vaccine (Live/Attenuated)

Increased Effect/Toxicity

Choline Magnesium Trisalicylate may increase the levels/effects of: Anticoagulants; Carbonic Anhydrase Inhibitors; Corticosteroids (Systemic); Hypoglycemic Agents; Methotrexate; PRALAtrexate; Salicylates; Thrombolytic Agents; Valproic Acid and Derivatives; Varicella Virus-Containing Vaccines; Vitamin K Antagonists

The levels/effects of Choline Magnesium Trisalicylate may be increased by: Agents with Antiplatelet Properties; Ammonium Chloride; Calcium Channel Blockers (Nondihydropyridine); Ginkgo Biloba; Herbs (Anticoagulant/Antiplatelet Properties); Influenza Virus Vaccine (Live/Attenuated); Loop Diuretics; Potassium Acid Phosphate; Treprostinil

Decreased Effect

Choline Magnesium Trisalicylate may decrease the levels/effects of: ACE Inhibitors; Hyaluronidase; Loop Diuretics; Probenecid

The levels/effects of Choline Magnesium Trisalicylate may be decreased by: Corticosteroids (Systemic)

Food Interactions Food may decrease the rate but not the extent of oral absorption. Curry powder, paprika, licorice, Benedictine liqueur, prunes, raisins, tea, and gherkins may cause salicylate accumulation. These foods contain 6 mg salicylate/100 g. Management: Administer with food or large volume of water or milk to minimize GI upset. Limit curry powder, paprika, licorice, Benedictine liqueur, prunes, raisins, tea, and gherkins.

Mechanism of Action Weakly inhibits cyclooxygenase enzymes, which results in decreased formation of prostaglandin precursors; antipyretic, analgesic, and anti-inflammatory properties.

Other proposed mechanisms not fully elucidated (and possibly contributing to the anti-inflammatory effect to varying degrees) include inhibiting chemotaxis, altering lymphocyte activity, inhibiting neutrophil aggregation/activation, and decreasing proinflammatory cytokine levels.

Pharmacokinetics (Adult data unless noted)

Absorption: From stomach and small intestine

Distribution: Readily distributes into most body fluids and tissues; crosses the placenta; appears in breast milk

Protein binding: 90% to 95%

Metabolism: Hepatic microsomal enzyme system

Half-life: Dose-dependent, ranging from 2-3 hours at low doses to 30 hours at high doses

Time to peak serum concentration: 20-35 minutes

Elimination: 10% excreted as unchanged drug

Dosing: Usual Oral (based on **total salicylate content**):

Children: 30-60 mg/kg/day given in 3-4 divided doses

Adults: 500 mg to 1.5 g 1-3 times/day

Administration Oral: Administer with food or milk to decrease GI upset; may be mixed with fruit juice just before drinking; do not administer with antacids

Monitoring Parameters Serum salicylate levels; serum magnesium with high doses or in patients with decreased renal function

Reference Range

Salicylate blood levels for anti-inflammatory effect: 150-300 mcg/mL

Analgesia and antipyretic effect: 30-50 mcg/mL

Test Interactions False-negative results for glucose oxidase urinary glucose tests (Clinistix®); false-positives using the cupric sulfate method (Clinitest®); also, interferes with Gerhardt test (urinary ketone analysis), VMA determination; 5-HIAA, xylose tolerance test, and T_3 and T_4; increased PBI

Additional Information Salicylate salts do not inhibit platelet aggregation and, therefore, should not be substituted for aspirin in the prophylaxis of thrombosis (ie, for aspirin's antiplatelet effects)

Dosage Forms Excipient information presented when available (limited, particularly for generics); consult specific product labeling.

Liquid, Oral:

Generic: 500 mg/5 mL (240 mL)

Tablet, Oral:

Generic: 1000 mg

References

Berde C, Ablin A, Glazer J, et al, "American Academy of Pediatrics Report of the Subcommittee on Disease-Related Pain in Childhood Cancer," *Pediatrics*, 1990, 86(5 Pt 2):818-25.

◆ **Chorionic Gonadotropin for Injection (Can)** *see* Chorionic Gonadotropin (Human) *on page 460*

Chorionic Gonadotropin (Human)

(kor ee ON ik goe NAD oh troe pin, HYU man)

Related Information

Safe Handling of Hazardous Drugs *on page 2419*

Brand Names: U.S. Novarel; Pregnyl

Brand Names: Canada Chorionic Gonadotropin for Injection; Pregnyl®

Therapeutic Category Gonadotropin; Ovulation Stimulator

Generic Availability (U.S.) Yes

Use Treatment of hypogonadotropic hypogonadism, prepubertal cryptorchidism; induce ovulation and pregnancy in anovulatory, infertile women

Pregnancy Risk Factor X

Pregnancy Considerations Teratogenic effects (forelimb, CNS) have been noted in animal studies at doses intended to induce superovulation (used in combination with gonadotropin). Testicular tumors in otherwise healthy men have been reported when treating secondary infertility.

Breast-Feeding Considerations It is not known if chorionic gonadotropin (human) is excreted in breast milk. The manufacturer recommends that caution be exercised when administering chorionic gonadotropin (human) to nursing women.

Contraindications Hypersensitivity to chorionic gonadotropin or any component; precocious puberty, prostatic carcinoma or other androgen-dependent neoplasms; pregnancy

Warnings Hazardous agent; use appropriate precautions for handling and disposal (NIOSH, 2012).

hCG is **not** effective in the treatment of obesity. hCG should only be used by clinicians who are experienced in the management of fertility disorders. May cause ovarian hyperstimulation syndrome (OHSS); if severe, treatment should be discontinued and patient should be hospitalized. OHSS results in a rapid (<24 hours to 7 days) accumulation of fluid in the peritoneal cavity, thorax, and possibly, the pericardium, which may become more severe if pregnancy occurs; monitor for ovarian enlargement. Use may lead to multiple births, arterial thromboembolism, enlargement or rupture of preexisting ovarian cysts with resultant hemoperitoneum.

Pregnyl® contains benzyl alcohol which may cause allergic reactions in susceptible individuals; large amounts of benzyl alcohol (≥99 mg/kg/day) have been associated with a potentially fatal toxicity ("gasping syndrome") in neonates; the "gasping syndrome" consists of metabolic acidosis, respiratory distress, gasping respirations, CNS dysfunction (including convulsions, intracranial hemorrhage), hypotension and cardiovascular collapse; avoid use of Pregnyl® in neonates. *In vitro* and animal studies have shown that benzoate, a metabolite of benzyl alcohol, displaces bilirubin from protein-binding sites.

Precautions Use with caution in patients with asthma, seizure disorders, migraine, cardiac or renal disease; may induce precocious puberty in children being treated for cryptorchidism; discontinue if signs of precocious puberty occur; safety and efficacy in children <4 years of age has not been established

Adverse Reactions
Cardiovascular: Edema
Central nervous system: Depression, fatigue, headache, irritability, restlessness
Endocrine & metabolic: Gynecomastia, precocious puberty
Local: Injection site reaction, pain at injection site
Miscellaneous: Hypersensitivity reaction (local or systemic)
Rare but important or life-threatening: Arterial thrombus, ovarian cyst rupture, ovarian hyperstimulation syndrome

Drug Interactions
Metabolism/Transport Effects None known.
Avoid Concomitant Use There are no known interactions where it is recommended to avoid concomitant use.
Increased Effect/Toxicity There are no known significant interactions involving an increase in effect.
Decreased Effect There are no known significant interactions involving a decrease in effect.

Stability Hazardous agent; use appropriate precautions for handling and disposal (NIOSH, 2012). Following reconstitution with provided diluent, stable for 30-90 days (depending upon preparation) when stored at 2°C to 15°C.

Mechanism of Action Luteinizing hormone obtained from the urine of pregnant women. Stimulates production of gonadal steroid hormones by causing production of androgen by the testes; as a substitute for luteinizing hormone (LH) to stimulate ovulation

Pharmacokinetics (Adult data unless noted)
Distribution: Distributes mainly into the testes in males and into the ovaries in females
Half-life, biphasic:
Initial: 11 hours
Terminal: 23 hours
Time to peak serum concentration: 6 hours
Elimination: Approximately 10% to 12% excreted unchanged in urine within 24 hours; detectable amounts may continue to be excreted in the urine for up to 3-4 days

Dosing: Usual
Children: I.M. (many regimens have been described):
Prepubertal cryptorchidism:
1000-2000 units/m^2/dose 3 times/week for 3 weeks or 4000 units 3 times/week for 3 weeks
or
5000 units every second day for 4 injections
or
500 units 3 times/week for 4-6 weeks
Hypogonadotropic hypogonadism:
500-1000 units 3 times/week for 3 weeks, followed by the same dose twice weekly for 3 weeks
or
1000-2000 units 3 times/week
or
4000 units 3 times/week for 6-9 months; reduce dosage to 2000 units 3 times/week for additional 3 months
Adults:
Induction of ovulation: Females: 5000-10,000 units the day following the last dose of menotropins
Spermatogenesis induction associated with hypogonadotropic hypogonadism: Male: Treatment regimens vary (range: 1000-2000 units 2-3 times a week). Administer hCG until serum testosterone levels are normal (may require 2-3 months of therapy), then may add follitropin alfa or menopausal gonadotropin if needed to induce spermatogenesis; continue hCG at the dose required to maintain testosterone levels.

Administration Hazardous agent; use appropriate precautions for handling and disposal (NIOSH, 2012).
Parenteral: Administer I.M. only.

Monitoring Parameters
Male: Serum testosterone levels, semen analysis
Female: Ultrasound and/or estradiol levels to assess follicle development; ultrasound to assess number and size of follicles; ovulation (basal body temperature, serum progestin level, menstruation, sonography)

Reference Range Depends on application and methodology; <3 milli international units/mL (SI: <3 units/L) usually normal (nonpregnant)

Test Interactions Cross-reacts with radioimmunoassay of gonadotropins, especially LH

Dosage Forms Excipient information presented when available (limited, particularly for generics); consult specific product labeling.
Solution Reconstituted, Intramuscular:
Novarel: 10,000 units (1 ea) [contains benzyl alcohol]
Pregnyl: 10,000 units (1 ea) [contains benzyl alcohol, sodium chloride]
Generic: 10,000 units (1 ea)

References
National Institute for Occupational Safety and Health (NIOSH), "NIOSH List of Antineoplastic and Other Hazardous Drugs in Healthcare Settings 2012." Available at http://www.cdc.gov/niosh/docs/2012-150/pdfs/2012-150.pdf. Accessed January 21, 2013.

◆ **Chromium** *see* Trace Elements *on page 2059*

Ciclesonide (Oral Inhalation) (sye KLES oh nide)

Brand Names: U.S. Alvesco
Brand Names: Canada Alvesco®
Therapeutic Category Adrenal Corticosteroid; Anti-inflammatory Agent; Antiasthmatic; Corticosteroid, Inhalant (Oral); Glucocorticoid
Generic Availability (U.S.) No
Use Maintenance treatment of asthma (prophylactic management) (FDA approved in ages ≥12 years and adults); **NOT** indicated for the relief of acute bronchospasm; has also been used as daily therapy to manage exercise-induced bronchoconstriction in patients who continue to have symptoms despite the use of short-acting beta$_2$-agonist before exercise (Parsons, 2013)

Pregnancy Risk Factor C

Pregnancy Considerations Adverse events were observed in some animal reproduction studies. Hypoadrenalism may occur in infants born to mothers receiving corticosteroids during pregnancy. Based on available data, an overall increased risk of congenital malformations or a decrease in fetal growth has not been associated with maternal use of inhaled corticosteroids during pregnancy (Bakhireva, 2005; NAEPP, 2005; Namazy, 2004). Uncontrolled asthma is associated with adverse events in pregnancy (increased risk of perinatal mortality, pre-eclampsia, preterm birth, low birth weight infants). Inhaled corticosteroids are recommended for the treatment of asthma during pregnancy (most information available using budesonide) (ACOG, 2008; NAEPP, 2005).

Breast-Feeding Considerations Systemic corticosteroids are excreted in human milk. It is not known if sufficient quantities of ciclesonide are absorbed following oral inhalation to produce detectable amounts in breast milk; however, oral absorption is limited (<1%). The manufacturer recommends that caution be exercised when administering ciclesonide to nursing women. The use of inhaled corticosteroids is not considered a contraindication to breast-feeding (NAEPP, 2005).

Contraindications Hypersensitivity to ciclesonide or any component; primary treatment of status asthmaticus or acute asthma episodes requiring intensive measures

Warnings Fatalities have occurred due to adrenal insufficiency in asthmatic patients during and after switching from systemic corticosteroids to aerosol steroids; several months may be required for full recovery of hypothalamic-pituitary-adrenal (HPA) function; patients receiving higher doses of systemic corticosteroids (eg, adults receiving ≥20 mg of prednisone per day) may be at greater risk; during this period of HPA suppression, aerosol steroids do not provide the systemic glucocorticoid or mineralocorticoid activity needed to treat patients requiring stress doses (ie, patients with major stress such as trauma, surgery, infections, or other conditions associated with severe electrolyte loss). When used at high doses, HPA suppression may occur; use with inhaled or systemic corticosteroids (even alternate-day dosing) may increase risk of HPA suppression. Acute adrenal insufficiency may occur with abrupt withdrawal after long-term use or with stress; withdrawal or discontinuation of corticosteroids should be done carefully; patients with HPA axis suppression may require doses of systemic glucocorticosteroids prior to, during, and after unusual stress (eg, surgery). Relative to other inhaled corticosteroids, ciclesonide may exhibit less effect on HPA function due to it being a prodrug which is activated in the lungs; in four pediatric patients, resolution of HPA suppression was reported after switching from fluticasone to ciclesonide therapy (Heller, 2010). Switching patients from systemic corticosteroids to aerosol steroids may unmask allergic conditions (eg, rhinitis, conjunctivitis, eczema, arthritis, and eosinophilic conditions) previously suppressed by the systemic steroid. Immunosuppression may occur; patients may be more susceptible to infections; avoid exposure to chickenpox and measles. Bronchospasm may occur after use of inhaled ciclesonide; if occurs, therapy should be discontinued, a fast-acting bronchodilator used to treat, and alternative treatment initiated.

C. albicans infections of the mouth and pharynx may occur with orally inhaled corticosteroid use, mostly mild to moderate in nature; interruption of therapy may be necessary at times while antifungal therapy is employed; advise patients to rinse mouth after use. The incidence of oral candidiasis and other localized oropharyngeal effects observed with ciclesonide use has been reported to be approximately one-half of that seen with other commonly inhaled corticosteroids such as budesonide and fluticasone. Small particle size, minimal activation, and deposition in the oropharynx may explain this decreased incidence. Hypersensitivity reactions with angioedema and swelling of the lips, tongue, and pharynx have been reported rarely.

Precautions Avoid using higher than recommended dosages; suppression of HPA function, suppression of linear growth (ie, reduction of growth velocity), reduced bone mineral density, or hypercorticism (Cushing's syndrome) may occur; titrate to lowest effective dose. Reduction in growth velocity [mean: 1 cm/year (range: 0.3-1.8 cm)] may occur when corticosteroids are administered to pediatric patients, even at recommended doses via inhaled route; reduction in growth velocity is related to dose and duration of exposure; monitor growth. Use ciclesonide with extreme caution in patients with respiratory tuberculosis, untreated systemic infections, or ocular herpes simplex. Rare cases of increased IOP, glaucoma, or cataracts have been reported with inhaled corticosteroids, including ciclesonide.

Adverse Reactions

Cardiovascular: Facial edema

Central nervous system: Dizziness, dysphonia, fatigue, headache

Dermatologic: Urticaria

Gastrointestinal: Gastroenteritis, oral candidiasis

Neuromuscular & Skeletal: Arthralgia, back pain, extremity pain, musculoskeletal chest pain

Ocular: Conjunctivitis

Otic: Ear pain

Respiratory: Hoarseness, nasal congestion, nasopharyngitis, paradoxical bronchospasm, pharyngolaryngeal pain, pneumonia, sinusitis, upper respiratory infection

Miscellaneous: Influenza

Rare but important or life-threatening: ALT increased, angioedema (with swelling of lip/pharynx/tongue), candidiasis (pharyngeal), cataract, chest discomfort, GGT increased, intraocular pressure increased, nausea, palpitation, rash, weight gain, xerostomia

Drug Interactions

Metabolism/Transport Effects Substrate of CYP3A4 (minor); **Note:** Assignment of Major/Minor substrate status based on clinically relevant drug interaction potential

Avoid Concomitant Use

Avoid concomitant use of Ciclesonide (Oral Inhalation) with any of the following: Aldesleukin

Increased Effect/Toxicity

Ciclesonide (Oral Inhalation) may increase the levels/effects of: Amphotericin B; Ceritinib; Deferasirox; Loop Diuretics; Thiazide Diuretics

The levels/effects of Ciclesonide (Oral Inhalation) may be increased by: Telaprevir

Decreased Effect

Ciclesonide (Oral Inhalation) may decrease the levels/effects of: Aldesleukin; Antidiabetic Agents; Corticorelin; Hyaluronidase; Telaprevir

Stability Store at 25°C (77°F), excursions to 15°C to 30°C (59°F to 86°F) permitted. Do not puncture. Do not use or store near open flame or heat; canister may burst if exposed to temperatures >49°C (120°F); do not throw canister into fire or incinerator.

Mechanism of Action Ciclesonide is a nonhalogenated, glucocorticoid prodrug that is hydrolyzed to the pharmacologically active metabolite des-ciclesonide following administration. Des-ciclesonide has a high affinity for the glucocorticoid receptor and exhibits anti-inflammatory activity. The mechanism of action for corticosteroids is believed to be a combination of three important properties − anti-inflammatory activity, immunosuppressive properties, and antiproliferative actions.

Pharmacodynamics Onset of action: >4 weeks for maximum benefit

Pharmacokinetics (Adult data unless noted)

Absorption: 52% (lung deposition)

Distribution: V_d: Ciclesonide: 2.9 L/kg; des-ciclesonide: 12.1 L/kg

Protein binding: ≥99%

Metabolism: Ciclesonide hydrolyzed to active metabolite, des-ciclesonide via esterases in nasal mucosa and lungs; further metabolism via hepatic CYP3A4 and 2D6

Half-life: Ciclesonide: 0.7 hours; des-ciclesonide: 6-7 hours

Time to peak serum concentration: ~1 hour (des-ciclesonide)

Elimination: Feces (66%)

Dosing: Usual

Children and Adolescents:

Asthma, maintenance therapy: Note: Doses should be titrated to the lowest effective dose once asthma is controlled: Oral inhalation:

Children 2-4 years: Limited data available; efficacy results variable: 40, 80, or 160 mcg once daily with spacer has been studied in 992 children 2-6 years of age clinically diagnosed with asthma; after 12 weeks of therapy, results showed exacerbation rates were lower in the pooled ciclesonide treatment groups versus placebo; and decreased utility of rescue medications compared to baseline for all groups, including placebo (however, a statistically significant difference was not shown between each ciclesonide group and placebo due to an unusually large and unexpected placebo response); in safety analysis, no untoward effects were observed (Brand, 2011)

Children 5-11 years: Limited data available: 40, 80, or 160 mcg once daily has been used in clinical trials; the majority of data showed statistically significant positive efficacy findings (Gelfand, 2006; Pedersen, 2010). Others have suggested the following (Global Strategy for Asthma Management and Prevention, 2011):

"Low" dose: 80-160 mcg/day

"Medium" dose: >160-320 mcg/day

"High" dose: >320 mcg/day; maximum daily dose: 640 mcg/**day**

Children ≥12 years and Adolescents:

Manufacturer's labeling:

Prior therapy with bronchodilators alone: Initial: 80 mcg twice daily, may increase dose after 4 weeks of therapy if response inadequate; maximum daily dose: 320 mcg/**day**

Prior therapy with inhaled corticosteroids: Initial: 80 mcg twice daily, may increase dose after 4 weeks of therapy if response inadequate; maximum daily dose: 640 mcg/**day**

Prior therapy with oral corticosteroids: Initial: 320 mcg twice daily, may increase dose after 4 weeks of therapy if response inadequate; maximum daily dose: 640 mcg/**day**

Alternate dosing (Global Strategy for Asthma Management and Prevention, 2011): **Note:** Other expert guideline recommendations suggest that doses >200 mcg/day may provide minimal additional benefit while increasing risks for adverse events; add-on therapy should be considered prior to dose increases >200 mcg/day (Lougheed, 2010).

"Low" dose: 80-160 mcg/day

"Medium" dose: >160-320 mcg/day

"High" dose: >320 mcg/day; maximum daily dose: 640 mcg/**day**

Adults:

Asthma, maintenance therapy: Note: Doses should be titrated to the lowest effective dose once asthma is controlled: Oral inhalation:

Manufacturer's labeling:

Prior therapy with bronchodilators alone: Initial: 80 mcg twice daily; maximum daily dose: 320 mcg/**day**

Prior therapy with inhaled corticosteroids: Initial: 80 mcg twice daily; maximum dose: 640 mcg/**day**

Prior therapy with oral corticosteroids: Initial: 320 mcg twice daily; maximum dose: 640 mcg/**day**

Alternate dosing (Global Strategy for Asthma Management and Prevention, 2011):

"Low" dose: 80-160 mcg/day

"Medium" dose: >160-320 mcg/day

"High" dose: >320 mcg/day

Administration Oral inhalation: Shaking inhaler before use is not necessary since drug is formulated as a solution aerosol. With initial use or if inhaler not in use for 7-10 days, prime the inhaler by releasing 3 puffs into the air. Do not spray into eyes or face while priming. Remove mouthpiece cover, place inhaler in mouth, close lips around mouthpiece, and inhale slowly and deeply. Press down on top of inhaler after slow inhalation has begun. Remove inhaler while holding breath for approximately 10 seconds. Breathe out slowly and replace mouthpiece on inhaler. Rinse mouth with water (and spit out) after use to reduce incidence of oral candidiasis. Do not wash any part of inhaler in water; clean mouthpiece using a dry cloth or tissue once weekly. Discard after the "discard by" date or after labeled number of doses has been used, even if container is not completely empty. Dose indicator will turn red when 20 puffs remain; if inhaler dropped, dose indicator may be inaccurate; manual tracking of inhaler actuations recommended.

Monitoring Parameters Check mucus membranes for signs of fungal infection; monitor growth in pediatric patients; monitor IOP with therapy >6 weeks. Monitor for symptoms of asthma, FEV_1, peak flow, and/or other pulmonary function tests

Additional Information When using ciclesonide oral inhalation to help reduce or discontinue oral corticosteroid therapy, begin corticosteroid taper after at least 1 week of ciclesonide inhalation therapy; reduce dose of oral corticosteroid gradually, with next decrease after 1-2 weeks depending on patient's response; do not decrease prednisone faster than 2.5 mg/day in adolescents and adults on a weekly basis; monitor patients for signs of asthma instability and adrenal insufficiency; decrease ciclesonide to lowest effective dose after prednisone reduction is complete.

Dosage Forms Considerations Alvesco 6.1 g canisters contain 60 inhalations.

Dosage Forms Excipient information presented when available (limited, particularly for generics); consult specific product labeling.

Aerosol Solution, Inhalation:

Alvesco: 80 mcg/actuation (6.1 g); 160 mcg/actuation (6.1 g)

References

ACOG Committee on Practice Bulletins-Obstetrics, "ACOG Practice Bulletin: Clinical Management Guidelines for Obstetrician-Gynecologists Number 90, February 2008: Asthma in Pregnancy," *Obstet Gynecol*, 2008, 111(2 Pt 1):457-64.

Bakhireva LN, Jones KL, Schatz M, et al, "Asthma Medication Use in Pregnancy and Fetal Growth," *J Allergy Clin Immunol*, 2005, 116 (3):503-9.

Brand PL, Luz García-García M, Morison A, et al. Ciclesonide in wheezy preschool children with a positive asthma predictive index or atopy. *Respir Med.* 2011;105:1588-1595.

Gelfand EW, Georgitis JW, Noonan M, et al, "Once-Daily Ciclesonide in Children: Efficacy and Safety in Asthma," *J Pediatr*, 2006, 148 (3):377-83.

Global Initiative for Asthma (GINA). *Global Strategy for Asthma Management and Prevention.* 2011. Available at http://www.ginasthma.org

Heller MK, Laks J, Kovesi TA, et al. Reversal of adrenal suppression with ciclesonide. *J Asthma.* 2010;47:337-339.

Lougheed MD, Lemière C, Dell SD, et al. Canadian Thoracic Society Asthma Management Continuum - 2010 consensus summary for children six years of age and over, and adults. *Can Respir J.* 2010;17(1):15-24.

Namazy J, Schatz M, Long L, et al, "Use of Inhaled Steroids by Pregnant Asthmatic Women Does Not Reduce Intrauterine Growth," *J Allergy Clin Immunol*, 2004, 113(3):427-32.

National Asthma Education and Prevention Program (NAEPP) Working Group Report on "Managing Asthma During Pregnancy: Recommendations for Pharmacologic Treatment," National Institutes of Health, National Heart, Lung, and Blood Institute, NIH Publication No. 05-5236, March 2005. Available at http://www.nhlbi.nih.gov/health/prof/lung/asthma/astpreg/astpreg_full.pdf

Parsons JP, Hallstrand TS, Mastronarde JG, et al. An official American Thoracic Society Clinical Practice Guideline: exercise-induced bronchoconstriction. *Am J Respir Crit Care Med*. 2013;187(9): 1016-1027.

Pedersen S, Engelstätter R, Weber HJ, et al, "Efficacy and Safety of Ciclesonide Once Daily and Fluticasone Propionate Twice Daily in Children With Asthma," *Pulm Pharmacol Ther*, 2009, 22(3):214-20.

Pedersen S, Potter P, Dachev S, et al, "Efficacy and Safety of Three Ciclesonide Doses vs Placebo in Children With Asthma: The RAINBOW Study," *Respir Med*, 2010, 104(11):1618-28.

Skoner DP, Maspero J, Banerji D, et al, "Assessment of the Long-Term Safety of Inhaled Ciclesonide on Growth in Children With Asthma," *Pediatrics*, 2008, 121(1):1-14.

von Berg A, Engelstätter R, Minic P, et al, "Comparison of the Efficacy and Safety of Ciclesonide 160 microg Once Daily vs Budesonide 400 microg Once Daily in Children With Asthma," *Pediatr Allergy Immunol*, 2007, 18(5):391-400.

Ciclesonide (Nasal) (sye KLES oh nide)

Brand Names: U.S. Omnaris; Zetonna
Brand Names: Canada Drymira; Omnaris; Omnaris HFA
Therapeutic Category Corticosteroid, Intranasal
Generic Availability (U.S.) No

Use
Omnaris: Management of seasonal allergic rhinitis (FDA approved in ages ≥6 years and adults); management of perennial allergic rhinitis (FDA approved in ages ≥12 years and adults)

Zetonna: Management of seasonal and perennial allergic rhinitis (FDA approved in ages ≥12 years and adults)

Intranasal corticosteroids have also been used as an adjunct to antibiotics in empiric treatment of acute bacterial rhinosinusitis primarily in patients with history of allergy rhinitis (Chow, 2012) and in pediatric patients with mild obstructive sleep apnea syndrome who cannot undergo adenotonsillectomy or who still have symptoms after surgery (Marcus, 2012)

Pregnancy Risk Factor C

Pregnancy Considerations Adverse events were observed in some animal reproduction studies. Hypoadrenalism may occur in newborns following maternal use of corticosteroids in pregnancy; monitor. Intranasal corticosteroids may be used in the treatment of rhinitis during pregnancy; the lowest effective dose should be used (NAEPP, 2005; Wallace, 2008).

Breast-Feeding Considerations Systemic corticosteroids are excreted in human milk. It is not known if sufficient quantities of ciclesonide are absorbed following nasal inhalation to produce detectable amounts in breast milk; however, oral absorption is limited (<1%). The use of inhaled corticosteroids is not considered a contraindication to breast-feeding (NAEPP, 2005). The manufacturer recommends caution be used if administered to a nursing woman.

Contraindications Hypersensitivity to ciclesonide or any component

Warnings HPA suppression or hypercorticism (Cushing's syndrome) may occur with use of higher than recommended doses or at typical doses in susceptible patients. Acute adrenal insufficiency may occur with abrupt withdrawal after long-term use, with stress, or when converting from systemic to topical corticosteroid therapy; withdrawal or discontinuation of corticosteroids should be done carefully; patients with HPA axis suppression may require doses of systemic glucocorticoids prior to, during, and after unusual stress (eg, surgery). Immunosuppression may occur; patients may be more susceptible to

infections; avoid exposure to chickenpox and measles. Epistaxis may occur.

Precautions Avoid using higher than recommended dosages; suppression of HPA function, suppression of linear growth (ie, reduction of growth velocity), reduced bone mineral density, or hypercorticism (Cushing's syndrome) may occur; titrate to lowest effective dose. Reduction in growth velocity may occur when corticosteroids are administered to pediatric patients, even at recommended doses via intranasal route (monitor growth). Use ciclesonide with extreme caution in patients with respiratory tuberculosis, untreated bacterial, fungal, systemic viral or parasitic infections, or ocular herpes simplex. Localized *Candida* infections of the nose and pharynx have been reported rarely; interruption of therapy may be necessary while antifungal therapy is employed. Corticosteroids impair wound healing; avoid use in patients with recent nasal ulcers, nasal surgery, or nasal trauma; allow healing to occur before use. Glaucoma, increased intraocular pressure, and cataracts have been reported following the intranasal application of corticosteroids; monitor patients who have change in vision and in patients with a history of increased ocular pressure, glaucoma, or cataracts. Use of nasal ciclesonide in place of systemic corticosteroids may unmask allergies (eg, eczema, rhinitis) that were previously controlled by the systemic corticosteroids. Rare cases of immediate hypersensitivity reactions or nasal septum perforation may occur with intranasal corticosteroids.

Adverse Reactions
Central nervous system: Dysphonia, fever (children), headache

Gastrointestinal: Nausea

Neuromuscular & skeletal: Back pain, muscle strain

Respiratory: Bronchitis, cough, epistaxis, hoarseness, nasal congestion, nasal discomfort, nasal septum disorder, nasopharyngitis, paradoxical bronchospasm, pharyngitis, pharyngolaryngeal pain, pneumonia, sinusitis, upper respiratory infection

Miscellaneous: Influenza

Rare but important or life-threatening: ALT increased, angioedema (with swelling of lip/pharynx/tongue), bruising, candidiasis (nasal/pharyngeal), cataract, chest discomfort, dizziness, dry throat, dysgeusia, dyspepsia, GGT increased, growth suppression, intraocular pressure increased, nasal ulcer, palpitation, rash, rhinorrhea, throat irritation, WBC increased, weight gain, wound healing impaired, xerostomia

Drug Interactions
Metabolism/Transport Effects Substrate of CYP3A4 (minor); **Note:** Assignment of Major/Minor substrate status based on clinically relevant drug interaction potential

Avoid Concomitant Use There are no known interactions where it is recommended to avoid concomitant use.

Increased Effect/Toxicity
Ciclesonide (Nasal) may increase the levels/effects of: Ceritinib

Decreased Effect There are no known significant interactions involving a decrease in effect.

Stability Store at 25°C (77°F), excursions to 15°C to 30°C (59°F to 86°F) permitted.
Omaris: Do not freeze; use within 4 months after opening aluminum pouch.
Zetonna: Protect from heat or open flame (>49°C [120°F]). Do not puncture.

Pharmacodynamics Onset of action: 24-48 hours; further improvement observed over 1-2 weeks in seasonal allergic rhinitis or 5 weeks in perennial allergic rhinitis

Pharmacokinetics (Adult data unless noted)
Absorption: Minimal systemic
Metabolism: Ciclesonide hydrolyzed to active metabolite, des-ciclesonide via esterases in nasal mucosa and lungs; further metabolism via hepatic CYP3A4 and 2D6

Bioavailability: Oral: <1%

Dosing: Usual Note: Product formulations are not inter-changeable: Omnaris®: One spray delivers 50 mcg; Zetonna: One spray delivers 37 mcg

Children and Adolescents:

Perennial allergic rhinitis: Intranasal:

Omnaris:

Children 2-11 years: Limited data available: 100 or 200 mcg once daily delivered as 50 mcg (1 spray) or 100 mg (2 sprays) **per nostril** (Berger, 2008; Kim, 2007)

Children ≥12 years and Adolescents: 200 mcg once daily delivered as 100 mcg (2 sprays) **per nostril**; maximum daily dose: 200 mcg/**day**

Zetonna: Children ≥12 years and Adolescents: 74 mcg once daily delivered as 37 mcg (1 spray) **per nostril**; maximum daily dose: 74 mcg/**day**

Seasonal allergic rhinitis: Intranasal:

Omnaris: Children ≥6 years and Adolescents: 200 mcg once daily delivered as 100 mcg (2 sprays) **per nostril**; maximum dose: 200 mcg/**day**

Zetonna: Children ≥12 years and Adolescents: 74 mcg once daily delivered as 37 mcg (1 spray) **per nostril**; maximum daily dose: 74 mcg/**day**

Adults: **Perennial allergic rhinitis, seasonal allergic rhinitis:** Intranasal:

Omnaris: 2 sprays (50 mcg/spray) **per nostril** once daily; maximum: 200 mcg/**day**

Zetonna: 74 mcg once daily delivered as 1 spray (37 mcg/spray) **per nostril** once daily; maximum: 74 mcg/**day**

Dosing adjustment in renal impairment: There are no dosage adjustments provided in the manufacturer's labeling; has not been studied.

Dosing adjustment in hepatic impairment: Children, Adolescents, and Adults: No dosage adjustment necessary.

Administration Intranasal: Blow nose to clear nostrils. Insert applicator into nostril, keeping bottle upright, and close off the other nostril. Breathe in through nose. While inhaling, press pump to release spray. Avoid spraying directly onto the nasal septum or into eyes. Discard after the "discard by" date or after labeled number of doses has been used, even if bottle is not completely empty.

Omnaris: Shake bottle gently before using. Prime pump prior to first use (press 8 times until fine mist appears) or if spray has not been used in 4 consecutive days (press 1 time or until a fine mist appears). Nasal applicator may be removed and rinsed with warm water to clean.

Zetonna: Use nasal canister with supplied nasal actuator only. Prime pump prior to first use (press 3 times until fine mist appears) or if spray has not been used in 10 consecutive days (press 3 times or until a fine mist appears). If canister and actuator become separated, spray 1 test spray in air before using. Clean outside of nose piece with a clean, dry tissue or cloth weekly; do not wash or put in water.

Monitoring Parameters Mucous membranes for signs of fungal infection, growth (pediatric patients), signs/symptoms of HPA axis suppression/adrenal insufficiency; ocular changes

Additional Information When used short term as adjunctive therapy in acute bacterial rhinosinusitis (ABRS), intranasal steroids show modest symptomatic improvement and few adverse effects; improvement is primarily due to increased sinus drainage. Use should be considered optional in ABRS; however, intranasal corticosteroids should be routinely prescribed to ABRS patients who have a history of or concurrent allergic rhinitis (Chow, 2012).

Dosage Forms Considerations

Omnaris 12.5 g bottles contain 120 actuations.

Zetonna 6.1 g canisters contain 60 actuations.

Dosage Forms Excipient information presented when available (limited, particularly for generics); consult specific product labeling.

Aerosol Solution, Nasal:

Zetonna: 37 mcg/actuation (6.1 g)

Suspension, Nasal:

Omnaris: 50 mcg/actuation (12.5 g) [contains edetate sodium (tetrasodium)]

References

Berger WE, Nayak A, Lanier BQ, et al, "Efficacy and Safety of Once-Daily Ciclesonide Nasal Spray in Children with Allergic Rhinitis," *Pediatr Asthma Allergy Immunol*, 2008, 21:73-82.

Chow AW, Benninger MS, Brook I, et al, "IDSA Clinical Practice Guideline for Acute Bacterial Rhinosinusitis in Children and Adults," *Clin Infect Dis*, 2012, 54(8):e72-e112.

Kim K, Weiswasser M, Nave R, et al, "Safety of Once-Daily Ciclesonide Nasal Spray in Children 2-5 Years of Age with Perennial Allergic Rhinitis," *Pediatr Asthma Allergy Immunol*, 2007, 20(4):229-42.

Marcus CL, Brooks LJ, Draper KA, et al, "Diagnosis and Management of Childhood Obstructive Sleep Apnea Syndrome," *Pediatrics*, 2012, 130(3):576-84.

NAEPP Working Group Report on "Managing Asthma During Pregnancy: Recommendations for Pharmacologic Treatment," National Institutes of Health, National Heart, Lung, and Blood Institute, NIH Publication No. 05-5236, March 2005. Available at http://www.nhlbi.nih.gov/health/prof/lung/asthma/astpreg/astpreg_full.pdf

Wallace DV, Dykewicz MS, Bernstein DI, et al, "The Diagnosis and Management of Rhinitis: An Updated Practice Parameter," *J Allergy Clin Immunol*, 2008, 122(2 Suppl):1-84.

◆ **Ciclodan** *see* Ciclopirox *on page 465*

◆ **Ciclodan Cream** *see* Ciclopirox *on page 465*

◆ **Ciclodan Solution** *see* Ciclopirox *on page 465*

Ciclopirox (sye kloe PEER oks)

Brand Names: U.S. Ciclodan; Ciclodan Cream; Ciclodan Solution; Ciclopirox Treatment; CNL8 Nail; Loprox; Pedipirox-4 Nail; Penlac

Brand Names: Canada Apo-Ciclopirox; Loprox; Penlac; PMS-Ciclopirox; Stieprox; Taro-Ciclopirox

Therapeutic Category Antifungal Agent, Topical

Generic Availability (U.S.) Yes

Use

Cream/lotion: Treatment of tinea pedis, tinea cruris, and tinea corporis caused by *Trichophyton mentagrophytes*, *T. rubrum*, *Epidermophyton floccosum*, or *Microsporum canis*; treatment of pityriasis versicolor caused by *Malassezia* species; treatment of cutaneous candidiasis caused by *Candida albicans*

Gel: Treatment of tinea corporis and interdigital tinea pedis; treatment of seborrheic dermatitis of the scalp

Shampoo: Treatment of seborrheic dermatitis of the scalp

Solution (lacquer): Treatment of mild to moderate onychomycosis of fingernails and toenails (not involving the lunula) and the immediately adjacent skin caused by *T. rubrum*

Pregnancy Risk Factor B

Pregnancy Considerations Teratogenic effects were not observed in animal studies, however, there are no adequate and well-controlled studies in pregnant women. Use during pregnancy only if clearly needed.

Breast-Feeding Considerations It is not known if ciclopirox is excreted in breast milk. The manufacturer recommends that caution be exercised when administering ciclopirox to nursing women.

Contraindications Hypersensitivity to ciclopirox or any component

Precautions Use with caution in immunocompromised patients and diabetics.

Adverse Reactions

Cardiovascular: Ventricular tachycardia (shampoo)

Central nervous system: Headache

Dermatologic: Acne, alopecia, contact dermatitis, dry skin, erythema, facial edema, hair discoloration (rare;

shampoo formulation in light-haired individuals), nail disorder (shape or color change with lacquer), pruritus, rash
Local: Burning sensation, irritation, pain, or redness
Ocular: Eye pain

Drug Interactions

Metabolism/Transport Effects None known.

Avoid Concomitant Use There are no known interactions where it is recommended to avoid concomitant use.

Increased Effect/Toxicity There are no known significant interactions involving an increase in effect.

Decreased Effect There are no known significant interactions involving a decrease in effect.

Stability Store at room temperature; protect from light. Store ciclopirox topical solution (nail lacquer) in a tight container, protected from heat; the solution's solvent is flammable.

Mechanism of Action Inhibiting transport of essential elements in the fungal cell disrupting the synthesis of DNA, RNA, and protein

Pharmacokinetics (Adult data unless noted)
Absorption: Topical: Rapid but minimal with intact skin
Distribution: Present in stratum corneum, dermis, sebaceous glands, nails
Protein binding: 94% to 98%
Metabolism: Conjugated with glucuronic acid
Half-life:
Ciclopirox olamine: 1.7 hours
Ciclopirox gel: 5.5 hours
Elimination: Urine

Dosing: Usual Topical:
Children >10 years, Adolescents, and Adults: Tinea pedis, tinea cruris, tinea corporis, tinea versicolor, and cutaneous candidiasis: Cream/suspension: Apply twice daily for 4 weeks (4-6 weeks for tinea cruris; 2 weeks for tinea versicolor if response is adequate). If no improvement after 4 weeks of treatment, re-evaluate diagnosis.
Children ≥12 years, Adolescents, and Adults: Solution (lacquer): Apply daily as part of a comprehensive management program for onychomycosis; remove with alcohol every 7 days; 48 weeks of continuous therapy may be needed to achieve clear nails
Children >16 years, Adolescents, and Adults:
Tinea pedis, tinea corporis: Gel: Apply twice daily. If no improvement after 4 weeks of treatment, re-evaluate diagnosis.
Seborrheic dermatitis of the scalp:
Gel: Apply twice daily. If no improvement after 4 weeks of treatment, re-evaluate diagnosis.
Shampoo: Apply ~5 mL to wet hair; may use up to 10 mL for longer hair; repeat twice weekly for 4 weeks; allow a minimum of 3 days between applications. If no improvement after 4 weeks of treatment, re-evaluate diagnosis.

Administration Topical:
Cream, gel, suspension: Gently massage into affected areas and surrounding skin.
Lotion: Shake lotion vigorously before application.
Shampoo: Apply to wet hair and scalp, lather, and leave in place ~3 minutes; rinse thoroughly.
Solution (lacquer): Apply evenly over the entire nail plate and 5 mm of surrounding skin using the applicator brush; allow to dry for 30 seconds; apply at bedtime (or allow 8 hours before washing). Solution can be reapplied daily over previous applications; remove with alcohol every 7 days. Avoid contact with eyes and mucous membranes; do not administer orally or intravaginally. Do not occlude affected area with dressings or wrappings.

Monitoring Parameters Resolution of skin or nail infection

Dosage Forms Excipient information presented when available (limited, particularly for generics); consult specific product labeling. [DSC] = Discontinued product

Cream, External, as olamine:
Ciclodan: 0.77% (90 g) [contains benzyl alcohol, cetyl alcohol]
Generic: 0.77% (15 g, 30 g, 90 g)
Gel, External:
Loprox: 0.77% (100 g [DSC]) [contains isopropyl alcohol]
Generic: 0.77% (30 g, 45 g, 100 g)
Kit, External:
Ciclodan Cream: 0.77% [contains benzyl alcohol, cetyl alcohol, edetate disodium, propylene glycol]
Ciclodan Solution: 8% [contains edetate disodium, isopropyl alcohol, menthol]
Ciclopirox Treatment: 8% [contains edetate disodium, isopropyl alcohol, menthol]
CNL8 Nail: 8% [contains isopropyl alcohol]
Pedipirox-4 Nail: 8% [contains isopropyl alcohol]
Generic: 8%
Shampoo, External:
Loprox: 1% (120 mL)
Generic: 1% (120 mL)
Solution, External:
Ciclodan: 8% (6.6 mL) [contains isopropyl alcohol]
Penlac: 8% (6.6 mL) [contains ethyl acetate, isopropyl alcohol]
Generic: 8% (6.6 mL)
Suspension, External, as olamine:
Generic: 0.77% (30 mL, 60 mL)

References
Barber K, Claveau J, and Thomas R, "Review of Treatment for Onychomycosis: Consideration for Special Populations," *J Cutan Med Surg*, 2006, 10(Suppl 2):S48-53.
Gallup E, Plott T, and Ciclopirox TS Investigators, "A Multicenter, Open-Label Study to Assess the Safety and Efficacy of Ciclopirox Topical Suspension 0.77% in the Treatment of Diaper Dermatitis Due to *Candida albicans*," *J Drugs Dermatol*, 2005, 4(1):29-34.

◆ **Ciclopirox Olamine** see Ciclopirox on page 465
◆ **Ciclopirox Treatment** see Ciclopirox on page 465
◆ **Ciclosporin** see CycloSPORINE (Ophthalmic) on page 569
◆ **Ciclosporin** see CycloSPORINE (Systemic) on page 564
◆ **Cidecin** see DAPTOmycin on page 589

Cidofovir (si DOF o veer)

Related Information
Safe Handling of Hazardous Drugs on page 2419
Brand Names: U.S. Vistide
Therapeutic Category Antiviral Agent, Parenteral
Generic Availability (U.S.) Yes
Use Treatment of cytomegalovirus (CMV) retinitis in patients with acquired immunodeficiency syndrome (AIDS) (FDA approved in adults). Has also been used for treatment of ganciclovir-resistant CMV, foscarnet-resistant CMV, and adenovirus infections in immunocompromised patients; has also been used intralesionally for the treatment of recurrent respiratory papillomatosis

Pregnancy Risk Factor C

Pregnancy Considerations [U.S. Boxed Warning]: Possibly carcinogenic and teratogenic based on animal data. May cause hypospermia. Cidofovir was shown to be teratogenic and embryotoxic in animal studies, some at doses which also produced maternal toxicity. Reduced testes weight and hypospermia were also noted in animal studies. There are no adequate and well-controlled studies in pregnant women; use during pregnancy only if the potential benefit to the mother outweighs the possible risk to the fetus. Women of childbearing potential should use effective contraception during therapy and for 1 month following treatment. Males should use a barrier contraceptive during therapy and for 3 months following treatment.

Breast-Feeding Considerations The CDC recommends **not** to breast-feed if diagnosed with HIV to avoid postnatal transmission of the virus.

Contraindications Hypersensitivity to cidofovir or any component; history of clinically severe hypersensitivity to probenecid or other sulfa-containing medications; initiation of therapy in patients with a serum creatinine >1.5 mg/dL, creatinine clearance ≤55 mL/minute, urine protein ≥100 mg/dL (≥2 plus proteinuria); patients who are receiving other nephrotoxic agents (discontinue at least 7 days prior to starting cidofovir); direct intraocular injection

Warnings Hazardous agent; use appropriate precautions for handling and disposal (NIOSH, 2012). Prepare admixture in a Class II laminar flow hood; administer and dispose according to guidelines issued for cytotoxic drugs. Possibly carcinogenic and teratogenic based on animal data and may cause hypospermia **[U.S. Boxed Warning]**; contraceptive precautions for female patients need to be used during and for 1 month following therapy; male patients should practice barrier contraceptive methods during and for 3 months following treatment. Administration in children warrants extreme caution due to risk of long-term carcinogenicity and reproductive toxicity. A case of invasive squamous cell cancer has been reported in a pediatric patient receiving intralesional cidofovir for severe, recurrent respiratory papillomatosis; causality not established (Lott, 2009).

May cause severe renal impairment **[U.S. Boxed Warning]**; acute renal failure resulting in dialysis and/or contributing to death has been reported to occur after as few as one or two cidofovir doses. Do not exceed recommended dose or frequency due to risk of nephrotoxicity. Dose-dependent nephrotoxicity requires dose adjustment or discontinuation if changes in renal function occur during therapy (eg, proteinuria, glycosuria, decreased serum phosphate, uric acid or bicarbonate, and elevated creatinine). Decreased serum bicarbonate associated with proximal tubule injury and renal wasting syndrome (including Fanconi's syndrome) has also been reported. Fatal cases of metabolic acidosis associated with liver dysfunction and pancreatitis have been reported; monitor for signs and symptoms of metabolic acidosis. Cidofovir administration must be accompanied by oral probenecid and intravenous saline. Probenecid may decrease the metabolic clearance of zidovudine; patients on concurrent zidovudine therapy should decrease dose by 50% or hold dose on days of cidofovir treatment.

May cause neutropenia **[U.S. Boxed Warning]**; not dose-related; occurs in up to 24% of AIDS patients; monitor blood counts during therapy. Ocular hypotony, iritis, and permanent impairment of vision have been reported in association with cidofovir treatment. Intraocular pressure may be decreased during therapy and has been associated with decreased visual acuity; monitor intraocular pressure.

Precautions Indicated only for CMV retinitis treatment in adult HIV patients **[U.S. Boxed Warning]**. For I.V. use only; do not administer via intraocular injection.

Adverse Reactions

Cardiovascular: Cardiomyopathy, cardiovascular disorder, CHF, edema, orthostatic hypotension, shock, syncope, tachycardia

Central nervous system: Agitation, amnesia, anxiety, chills, confusion, convulsion, dizziness, fever, hallucinations, headache, insomnia, malaise, pain, vertigo

Dermatologic: Alopecia, photosensitivity reaction, skin discoloration, urticaria

Endocrine & metabolic: Adrenal cortex insufficiency

Gastrointestinal: Abdominal pain, anorexia, aphthous stomatitis, colitis, constipation, diarrhea, dysphagia, fecal incontinence, gastritis, GI hemorrhage, gingivitis, melena, nausea, proctitis, splenomegaly, stomatitis, tongue discoloration, vomiting

Genitourinary: Urinary incontinence

Hematologic: Anemia, hypochromic anemia, leukocytosis, leukopenia, lymphadenopathy, lymphoma-like reaction, neutropenia, pancytopenia, thrombocytopenia, thrombocytopenic purpura

Local: Injection site reaction

Neuromuscular & skeletal: Tremor, weakness

Ocular: Amblyopia, blindness, cataract, conjunctivitis, corneal lesion, diplopia, intraocular pressure decreased, iritis, ocular hypotony, uveitis, vision abnormal

Otic: Hearing loss

Renal: Creatinine increased, Fanconi syndrome, proteinuria, renal toxicity

Respiratory: Cough, dyspnea, pneumonia

Rare but important or life-threatening: Hepatic failure, metabolic acidosis, pancreatitis

Miscellaneous: Allergic reaction, infection, oral moniliasis, sepsis, serum bicarbonate decreased

Drug Interactions

Metabolism/Transport Effects None known.

Avoid Concomitant Use There are no known interactions where it is recommended to avoid concomitant use.

Increased Effect/Toxicity

Cidofovir may increase the levels/effects of: Tenofovir

Decreased Effect There are no known significant interactions involving a decrease in effect.

Stability Store at 20°C to 25°C (68°F to 77°F); cidofovir admixture is stable for 24 hours under refrigeration.

Mechanism of Action Cidofovir is converted to cidofovir diphosphate which is the active intracellular metabolite; cidofovir diphosphate suppresses CMV replication by selective inhibition of viral DNA synthesis. Incorporation of cidofovir into growing viral DNA chain results in reductions in the rate of viral DNA synthesis.

Pharmacokinetics (Adult data unless noted) Note: Pharmacokinetic data is based on a combination of cidofovir administered with probenecid.

Distribution: V_d: 0.54 L/kg; does not cross significantly into the CSF

Protein binding: <6%

Metabolism: Minimal; Phosphorylated intracellularly to the active metabolite cidofovir diphosphate

Half-life: ~2.6 hours (cidofovir); 17 hours (cidofovir diphosphate)

Elimination: Renal tubular secretion and glomerular filtration

Renal clearance without probenecid: 150 ± 26.9 mL/minute/1.73 m²

Renal clearance with probenecid: 98.6 ± 27.9 mL/minute/1.73 m²

Dosing: Usual

Pediatric: **Note:** Administration of cidofovir should be accompanied by concomitant oral probenecid and intravenous normal saline hydration; various regimens have been reported (Anderson, 2008; Bhadri, 2009; Cesaro, 2005; Doan, 2007; Williams, 2009)

Hydration: I.V.: 20 mL/kg of 0.9% sodium chloride (maximum: 1000 mL) administered for 1 hour before cidofovir infusion and 20 mL/kg of 0.9% sodium chloride (maximum: 1000 mL) over 1 hour during cidofovir infusion, followed by 2 hours of maintenance fluids **or** increase the maintenance fluid infusion rate to 3 times the maintenance rate for 1 hour before cidofovir infusion and continuing until 1 hour after, then decrease to 2 times the maintenance fluid rate for the subsequent 2 hours

Probenecid: Oral: 25-40 mg/kg/dose (maximum dose: 2000 mg) administered 3 hours before cidofovir infusion and 10-20 mg/kg/dose (maximum dose: 1000 mg) at 2-3 hours and 8-9 hours after cidofovir infusion **or** 1-2 g/m^2/dose administered 3 hours prior to cidofovir, followed by 0.5-1.25 g/m^2/dose 1-2 hours and 8 hours after completion

Adenovirus infection, posthematopoietic stem cell transplant; treatment: I.V.: Limited data available; specific regimens may vary (Legrand, 2001; Ljungman, 2003; Yusuf, 2006): Infants, Children, and Adolescents:
Induction: 5 mg/kg/dose once weekly for 2 consecutive weeks (with hydration and probenecid)
Maintenance: 5 mg/kg/dose once every 2 weeks (with hydration and probenecid) until consecutive negative adenovirus samples. **Note:** Patients requiring longer treatment courses have been switched to 1 mg/kg/dose given 3 times/week (Bhadri, 2009)

Adenovirus infection, postlung transplant; treatment: Very limited data available: Infants ≥6 months and Children <3 years: I.V.: 1 mg/kg/dose every other day or 3 times weekly for 4 consecutive weeks (with hydration and probenecid); dosing from a case series (n=4, age range: 0.5-2.6 years) (Doan, 2007)

BK virus allograft nephropathy: Limited data available: Children and Adolescents: I.V.: Initial dose: 0.25 mg/kg/dose every 2-3 weeks; dose may be increased if BK virus PCR counts do not decrease 1 log fold to a maximum dose of 1 mg/kg/dose. Dosing based on reported experience from two case series of 11 renal transplant patients (ages 4-20 years). The reported hydration was D$_5$½NS or D$_5$¼NS for 2 hours before cidofovir and for 2 hours following the infusion; cidofovir was infused over 2 hours and no probenecid was used (Araya, 2008; Araya, 2010).

BK virus hemorrhagic cystitis after stem cell or bone marrow transplant: Limited data available; optimal dose not established: Children and Adolescents: I.V.: 5 mg/kg/dose once weekly for 2-4 weeks, followed by 5 mg/kg/dose every other week given with probenecid and adequate hydration until cystitis resolved is the most commonly reported dose (Cesaro, 2009; Gaziev, 2010; Megged, 2011). Others have described lower doses of 0.5-1 mg/kg/dose given once weekly with or without probenecid (Faraci, 2009; Cesaro, 2009; Cesaro, 2013).

Cytomegalovirus (CMV) infection: Limited data available. I.V.:
Allogeneic stem cell transplantation recipients: Treatment: Children and Adolescents: Dosing based on reported experience in 30 pediatric patients (2-14 years) as second-line therapy following allogeneic stem cell transplantation (Cesaro, 2005).
Induction: 5 mg/kg/dose once weekly for 2 consecutive weeks (with hydration, probenecid and antiemetic)
Maintenance: 3-5 mg/kg/dose once every 2 weeks for 2-4 doses (with hydration, probenecid and antiemetic)
HIV-exposed/-positive patients:
CMV retinitis:
Treatment: Adolescents [DHHS (adult), 2013]:
Induction: 5 mg/kg/dose once weekly for 2 consecutive weeks (with hydration and probenecid)
Maintenance: 5 mg/kg/dose every other week (with hydration and probenecid)
Secondary prophylaxis: 5 mg/kg/dose every other week (with hydration and probenecid) [DHHS (adult/pediatric), 2013]
Respiratory papillomatosis, recurrent: Intralesional: 7.5 mg/mL every 2 weeks until complete remission (Naiman, 2006)

Adults:
Cytomegalovirus (CMV) retinitis: Note: Administration of cidofovir should be accompanied by concomitant oral probenecid and intravenous normal saline hydration; administer 2000 mg probenecid orally 3 hours prior to each cidofovir dose and 1000 mg at 2 and 8 hours after completion of the cidofovir infusion (total probenecid dose: 4000 mg); infuse one liter NS over 1-2 hours prior to the cidofovir infusion; may administer second liter of NS over 1-3 hours with or immediately after the cidofovir infusion if tolerated
Induction: I.V.: 5 mg/kg/dose once weekly for 2 consecutive weeks
Maintenance: I.V.: 5 mg/kg/dose once every other week
Dosing adjustment in renal impairment: High flux hemodialysis removes ~75%
Infants ≥6 months, Children, and Adolescents If the S$_{cr}$ >1.5 mg/dL, CrCl <90 mL/minute/1.73 m^2, and >2+ proteinuria, the following dosing has been used for treatment of adenovirus post-transplant (Yusuf, 2006): I.V.:
Induction: 1 mg/kg/dose 3 times weekly on alternate days for 2 consecutive weeks
Maintenance: 1 mg/kg/dose every other week
Adults:
preexisting renal impairment: Initiation of cidofovir is contraindicated for Cr >1.5 mg/dL, CrCl ≤55 mL/minute or a urine protein ≥100 mg/dL (≥2+ proteinuria)
During therapy: If the serum creatinine increases by 0.3-0.4 mg/dL above baseline, reduce the cidofovir dose to 3 mg/kg; discontinue cidofovir therapy for increases ≥0.5 mg/dL above baseline or development of ≥3+ proteinuria.
Dosing adjustment in hepatic impairment: There are no dosage adjustments provided in the manufacturer's labeling.
Administration Hazardous agent; use appropriate precautions for handling and disposal (NIOSH, 2012). Do **not** administer by direct intraocular injection due to risk of iritis, ocular hypotony, and permanent visual impairment.
Parenteral: Administer by I.V. infusion over 1 hour. Dilute in 100 mL NS or D$_5$W or to a final concentration not to exceed 8 mg/mL.
Intralesional: In pediatric trials, has been administered as solution with final concentration of 5-10 mg/mL (Bielecki, 2009; Naiman, 2006).
Monitoring Parameters Monitor renal function (BUN, serum creatinine) within 48 hours prior to each dose, urinalysis (urine glucose and protein), CBC with differential (neutrophil count) prior to each dose, electrolytes (calcium, magnesium, phosphorus, uric acid), liver function tests (SGOT/SGPT), intraocular pressure and visual acuity
Dosage Forms Excipient information presented when available (limited, particularly for generics); consult specific product labeling.
Solution, Intravenous:
Vistide: 75 mg/mL (5 mL)
Solution, Intravenous [preservative free]:
Generic: 75 mg/mL (5 mL)

References

Anderson EJ, Guzman-Cottrill JA, Kletzel M, et al, "High-Risk Adenovirus-Infected Pediatric Allogeneic Hematopoietic Progenitor Cell Transplant Recipients and Preemptive Cidofovir Therapy," *Pediatr Transplant,* 2008, 12(2):219-27.

Araya CE, Garin EH, Neiberger RE, Dharnidharka VR. Leflunomide therapy for BK virus allograft nephropathy in pediatric and young adult kidney transplant recipients. *Pediatric Transplantation.* 2010;14:145-150.

Araya CE, Lew JF, Fennell RS, et al, "Intermediate Dose Cidofovir Does Not Cause Additive Nephrotoxicity in BK Virus Allograft Nephropathy," *Pediatr Transplant,* 2008, 12(7):790-5.

Bhadri VA, Lee-Horn L, Shaw PJ. Safety and tolerability of cidofovir in high-risk pediatric patients. *Transpl Infect Dis.* 2009;11(4):373-379.

Bielecki I, Mniszek J, Cofala M. Intralesional injection of cidofovir for recurrent respiratory papillomatosis in children. *International Journal of Pediatric Otorhinolaryngology.* 2009;73:681-684.

Cesaro S, Pillon M, Tridello G, et.al. Relationship between clinical and BK virological response in patients with late hemorrhagic cysteitis treated with cidofovir, a retrospective study from the European Group for Blood and Marrow Transplantation. *Bone Marrow Transplantation.* 2013;48:809-813.

Cesaro S, Zhou X, Manzardo C, et al, "Cidofovir for Cytomegalovirus Reactivation in Pediatric Patients After Hematopoietic Stem Cell Transplantation," *J Clin Virol*, 2005, 34(2):129-32.

DHHS. Guidelines for the prevention and treatment of opportunistic infections among HIV-exposed and HIV-infected children: recommendations from the National Institutes of Health, Centers for Disease Control and Prevention, the HIV Medicine Association of the Infectious Diseases Society of America, the Pediatric Infectious Diseases Society, and the American Academy of Pediatrics. November 6, 2013. Available at http://aidsinfo.nih.gov

DHHS Panel on Opportunistic Infections (OI) in HIV-Infected Adults and Adolescents. Guidelines for prevention and treatment of opportunistic infections in HIV-infected adults and adolescents: recommendations from the Centers for Disease Control and Prevention (CDC), the National Institutes of Health (NIH), and the HIV Medicine Association (HIVMA) of the Infectious Diseases Society of America (IDSA). May 7, 2013. Available at http://aidsinfo.nih.gov/contentfiles/lvguidelines/adult_oi.pdf

Doan ML, Mallory GB, Kaplan SL, et al, "Treatment of Adenovirus Pneumonia With Cidofovir in Pediatric Lung Transplant Recipients," *J Heart Lung Transplant*, 2007, 26(9):883-9.

Faraci M, Cuzzubbo D, Lanino E, et al, "Low Dosage Cidofovir Without Probenecid as Treatment for BK Virus Hamorrhagic Cystitis After Hemopoietic Stem Cell Transplant," *Pediatr Infect Dis J*, 2009, 28 (1):55-7.

Gaziev J, Paba P, Miano R, et.al. Late-onset hemorrhagic cystitis in children after hematopoietic stem cell transplantation for thalassemia and sickle cell anemia: a prospective evaluation of polyoma (BK) virus infection and treatment with cidofovir. *Biol Blood Marrow Transplant.* 2010;16:662-671.

Graupp M, Gugatschka M, Kiesler K, Reckenzaun E, Hammer G, Friedrich G. Experience of 11 years use of cidofovir in recurrent respiratory papillomatosis. *Eur Arch Otorhinolaryngol.* 2013;270:641-646.

Legrand F, Berrebi D, Houhou N, et al, "Early Diagnosis of Adenovirus Infection and Treatment With Cidofovir After Bone Marrow Transplantation in Children," *Bone Marrow Transplant*, 2001, 27(6):621-6.

Ljungman P, Ribaud P, Eyrich M, et al, "Cidofovir for Adenovirus Infections After Allogeneic Hematopoietic Stem Cell Transplantation: A Survey by the Infectious Diseases Working Party of the European Group for Blood and Marrow Transplantation," *Bone Marrow Transplant*, 2003, 31(6):481-6.

Lott DG, Krakovitz PR. Squamous cell carcinoma associated with intralesional injection of cidofovir for recurrent respiratory papillomatosis. *The Laryngoscope.* 2009;119:567-570.

Megged O, Stein J, Ben-Meir D, Shulman LM, Yaniv I, Shalit I, Levy I. BK-virus-associated hemorrhagic cystitis in children after hematopoietic stem cell transplantation. *J Pediatr Hematol Oncol.* 2011;33:190-193.

Naiman AN, Ayari S, Nicollas R, et al, "Intermediate-Term and Long-Term Results After Treatment by Cidofovir and Excision in Juvenile Laryngeal Papillomatosis," *Ann Otol Rhinol Laryngol*, 2006, 115 (9):667-72.

National Institute for Occupational Safety and Health (NIOSH), "NIOSH List of Antineoplastic and Other Hazardous Drugs in Healthcare Settings 2012." Available at http://www.cdc.gov/niosh/docs/2012-150/pdfs/2012-150.pdf. Accessed January 21, 2013.

Valera F, Maldonato L, Lima J, et.al. Efficacy of cidofovir in recurrent juvenile respiratory papillomatosis. *Braz J Otorhinolaryngol.* 2010;76 (6):713-717.

Wierzbicka M, Jackowska J, Bartochowska A, Józefiak A, Szyfter W, Kędzia W. Effectiveness of cidofovir intralesional treatment in recurrent respiratory papillomatosis. *Eur Arch Otorhinolaryngol.* 2011;268:1305-1311.

Williams KM, Agwu AL, Dabb AA, et al, "A Clinical Algorithm Identifies High Risk Pediatric Oncology and Bone Marrow Transplant Patients Likely to Benefit From Treatment of Adenoviral Infection," *J Pediatr Hematol Oncol*, 2009, 31(11):825-31.

Yusuf U, Hale GA, Carr J, et al, "Cidofovir for the Treatment of Adenoviral Infection in Pediatric Hematopoietic Stem Cell Transplant Patients," *Transplantation*, 2006, 81(10):1398-404.

◆ **Cilastatin and Imipenem** *see* Imipenem and Cilastatin *on page 1077*

◆ **Ciloxan** *see* Ciprofloxacin (Ophthalmic) *on page 475*

Cimetidine (sye MET i deen)

Medication Safety Issues
Sound-alike/look-alike issues:
Cimetidine may be confused with simethicone
Brand Names: U.S. Cimetidine Acid Reducer [OTC]; Tagamet HB [OTC]
Brand Names: Canada Apo-Cimetidine®; Dom-Cimetidine; Mylan-Cimetidine; Novo-Cimetidine; Nu-Cimet; PMS-Cimetidine
Therapeutic Category Gastrointestinal Agent, Gastric or Duodenal Ulcer Treatment; Histamine H_2 Antagonist
Generic Availability (U.S.) Yes
Use Short-term treatment of active duodenal ulcers and benign gastric ulcers; long-term prophylaxis of duodenal ulcer; gastric hypersecretory states; gastroesophageal reflux (GERD); over-the-counter (OTC) formulation for relief of acid indigestion, heartburn, or sour stomach
Pregnancy Risk Factor B
Pregnancy Considerations Teratogenic effects were not observed in animal reproduction studies; therefore, cimetidine is classified as pregnancy category B. Cimetidine crosses the placenta. An increased risk of congenital malformations or adverse events in the newborn has generally not been observed following maternal use of cimetidine during pregnancy. Histamine H_2 antagonists have been evaluated for the treatment of gastroesophageal reflux disease (GERD), as well as gastric and duodenal ulcers during pregnancy. Although if needed, cimetidine is not the agent of choice. Histamine H_2 antagonists may be used for aspiration prophylaxis prior to cesarean delivery.
Breast-Feeding Considerations Cimetidine is excreted into breast milk. The concentration of cimetidine in maternal serum in comparison to breast milk is highly variable. Breast-feeding is not recommended by the manufacturer. Consider the renal function of the breast-feeding infant.
Contraindications Hypersensitivity to cimetidine or any component
Warnings Use of gastric acid inhibitors including proton pump inhibitors and H_2 blockers has been associated with an increased risk for development of acute gastroenteritis and community-acquired pneumonia (Canani, 2006). A large epidemiological study has suggested an increased risk for developing pneumonia in patients receiving H_2 receptor antagonists; however, a causal relationship with cimetidine has not been demonstrated. A cohort analysis including over 11,000 neonates reported an association of H_2 blocker use and an increased incidence of NEC in VLBW neonates (Guillet, 2006). An ~sixfold increase in mortality, NEC, and infection (ie, sepsis, pneumonia, UTI) was reported in patients receiving an H_2 blocker (ranitidine) in a cohort analysis of 274 VLBW neonates (Terrin, 2011).
Precautions Modify dosage in patients with renal and/or hepatic impairment; multiple drug interactions exist requiring dose modifications of other medications or cimetidine.
Adverse Reactions
Cardiovascular: AV block, bradycardia, hypotension, tachycardia, vasculitis
Central nervous system: Agitation, confusion, dizziness, fever, headache, somnolence
Dermatologic: Alopecia, erythema multiforme, exfoliative dermatitis, Stevens-Johnson syndrome, toxic epidermal necrolysis, rash
Endocrine & metabolic: Edema of the breasts, gynecomastia, sexual ability decreased
Gastrointestinal: Diarrhea, nausea, pancreatitis, vomiting
Hematologic: Agranulocytosis, aplastic anemia, hemolytic anemia (immune-based), neutropenia, pancytopenia, thrombocytopenia

Hepatic: ALT increased, AST increased, hepatic fibrosis (case report)

Neuromuscular & skeletal: Arthralgia, myalgia, polymyositis

Renal: Creatinine increased, interstitial nephritis

Miscellaneous: Anaphylaxis, pneumonia (causal relationship not established)

Drug Interactions

Metabolism/Transport Effects Substrate of P-glycoprotein; **Inhibits** CYP1A2 (moderate), CYP2C19 (moderate), CYP2C9 (weak), CYP2D6 (moderate), CYP2E1 (weak), CYP3A4 (moderate)

Avoid Concomitant Use

Avoid concomitant use of Cimetidine with any of the following: Bosutinib; Dasatinib; Delavirdine; Dofetilide; EPIrubicin; Ibrutinib; Ivabradine; Lomitapide; PAZOPanib; Pimozide; Pirfenidone; PONATinib; Risedronate; Simeprevir; Thioridazine; Tolvaptan; Ulipristal

Increased Effect/Toxicity

Cimetidine may increase the levels/effects of: Agomelatine; Alfentanil; Amiodarone; Anticonvulsants (Hydantoin); ARIPiprazole; Avanafil; Benzodiazepines (metabolized by oxidation); Bosentan; Bosutinib; Bromazepam; Budesonide (Systemic, Oral Inhalation); Calcium Channel Blockers; Cannabis; Capecitabine; CarBAMazepine; Carmustine; Carvedilol; Cisapride; Citalopram; CloZAPine; Colchicine; CYP1A2 Substrates; CYP2C19 Substrates; CYP2D6 Substrates; CYP3A4 Substrates; Dalfampridine; Dexmethylphenidate; Dofetilide; DOXOrubicin (Conventional); Dronabinol; EPIrubicin; Eplerenone; Escitalopram; Everolimus; FentaNYL; Fesoterodine; Floxuridine; Fluorouracil (Systemic); Halofantrine; Ibrutinib; Imatinib; Ivabradine; Ivacaftor; Lomitapide; Lurasidone; Mebendazole; MetFORMIN; Methylphenidate; Metoprolol; Moclobemide; Nebivolol; Nicotine; OxyCODONE; Pentoxifylline; Pimecrolimus; Pimozide; Pirfenidone; Pramipexole; Praziquantel; Procainamide; Propafenone; QuiNIDine; QuiNINE; Ranolazine; Risedronate; Rivaroxaban; Roflumilast; Salmeterol; Saquinavir; Saxagliptin; Selective Serotonin Reuptake Inhibitors; Simeprevir; Sulfonylureas; Tegafur; Tetrahydrocannabinol; Theophylline Derivatives; Thioridazine; Tolvaptan; Tricyclic Antidepressants; Ulipristal; Varenicline; Vitamin K Antagonists; Zaleplon; ZOLMitriptan; Zuclopenthixol

The levels/effects of Cimetidine may be increased by: AtorvaSTATin; P-glycoprotein/ABCB1 Inhibitors

Decreased Effect

Cimetidine may decrease the levels/effects of: Atazanavir; Cefditoren; Cefpodoxime; Cefuroxime; Clopidogrel; Codeine; Dabrafenib; Dasatinib; Delavirdine; Erlotinib; Fosamprenavir; Gefitinib; Ifosfamide; Indinavir; Iron Salts; Itraconazole; Ketoconazole (Systemic); Mesalamine; Multivitamins/Minerals (with ADEK, Folate, Iron); Nelfinavir; Nilotinib; PAZOPanib; PONATinib; Posaconazole; Rilpivirine; Tamoxifen; TraMADol; Vismodegib

The levels/effects of Cimetidine may be decreased by: P-glycoprotein/ABCB1 Inducers

Food Interactions Prolonged treatment (≥2 years) may lead to malabsorption of dietary vitamin B_{12} and subsequent vitamin B_{12} deficiency (Lam, 2013).

Stability Protect from light; store at room temperature.

Mechanism of Action Competitive inhibition of histamine at H_2 receptors of the gastric parietal cells resulting in reduced gastric acid secretion, gastric volume and hydrogen ion concentration reduced

Pharmacokinetics (Adult data unless noted)

Distribution: Crosses the placenta; breast milk to plasma ratio: 4.6-11.76

Protein binding: 13% to 25%

Metabolism: Hepatic with a sulfoxide as the major metabolite

Bioavailability: 60% to 70%

Half-life:
Neonates: 3.6 hours
Children: 1.4 hours
Adults with normal renal function: 2 hours

Time to peak serum concentration: Oral: 45-90 minutes

Elimination: Primarily in urine (48% unchanged drug); some excretion in bile and feces

Dosing: Neonatal Oral: 5-10 mg/kg/day in divided doses every 8-12 hours

Dosing: Usual Oral:

Infants: 10-20 mg/kg/day divided every 6-12 hours

Children: 20-40 mg/kg/day in divided doses every 6 hours

Adults:

Short-term treatment of active ulcers: 300 mg 4 times/day or 800 mg at bedtime or 400 mg twice daily for up to 8 weeks

Duodenal ulcer prophylaxis: 400-800 mg at bedtime

Gastric hypersecretory conditions: 300-600 mg every 6 hours; dosage not to exceed 2.4 g/day

GERD: 800 mg twice daily or 400 mg 4 times/day for 12 weeks

Acid indigestion, heartburn, sour stomach relief (OTC use): 100 mg right before or up to 30 minutes before a meal; no more than 2 tablets per day

Dosing interval in renal impairment using 5-10 mg/kg/ dose in children or 300 mg in adults (titrate dose to gastric pH and CrCl):

CrCl >40 mL/minute: Administer every 6 hours

CrCl 20-40 mL/minute: Administer every 8 hours or reduce dose by 25%

CrCl <20 mL/minute: Administer every 12 hours or reduce dose by 50%

Hemodialysis: Administer after dialysis and every 12 hours during the interdialysis period

Dosing adjustment in hepatic impairment: Reduce dosage in severe liver disease

Administration Administer with food; do not administer with antacids

Monitoring Parameters CBC, gastric pH, occult blood with GI bleeding; monitor renal function to correct dose

Dosage Forms Excipient information presented when available (limited, particularly for generics); consult specific product labeling.

Solution, Oral, as hydrochloride [strength expressed as base]:
Generic: 300 mg/5 mL (237 mL, 240 mL)

Tablet, Oral:
Cimetidine Acid Reducer: 200 mg
Tagamet HB: 200 mg
Generic: 200 mg, 300 mg, 400 mg, 800 mg

Extemporaneous Preparations Note: Commercial oral solution is available (strength expressed as base: 60 mg/mL)

A 60 mg/mL oral suspension may be made with tablets. Place twenty-four 300 mg tablets in 5 mL of sterile water for ~3-5 minutes to dissolve film coating. Crush tablets in a mortar and reduce to a fine powder. Add 10 mL of glycerin and mix to a uniform paste; mix while adding Simple Syrup, NF in incremental proportions to **almost** 120 mL; transfer to a calibrated bottle, rinse mortar with vehicle, and add quantity of vehicle sufficient to make 120 mL. Label "shake well" and "refrigerate". Stable for 17 days.
Nahata MC, Pai VB, Hipple TF, *Pediatric Drug Formulations*, 5th ed, Cincinnati, OH: Harvey Whitney Books Co, 2004.

References

Canani RB, Cirillo P, Roggero P, et al, "Therapy With Gastric Acidity Inhibitors Increases the Risk of Acute Gastroenteritis and Community-Acquired Pneumonia in Children," *Pediatrics*, 2006, 117(5):e817-20.

Guillet R, Stoll BJ, Cotten CM, et al, "Association of H$_2$-Blocker Therapy and Higher Incidence of Necrotizing Enterocolitis in Very Low Birth Weight Infants," Pediatrics, 2006, 117(2):137-42.

Lambert J, Mobassaleh M, and Grand RJ, "Efficacy of Cimetidine for Gastric Acid Suppression in Pediatric Patients," J Pediatr, 1992, 120 (3):474-8.

Lloyd CW, Martin WJ, Taylor BD, et al, "Pharmacokinetics and Pharmacodynamics of Cimetidine and Metabolites in Critically Ill Children," J Pediatr, 1985, 107(2):295-300.

Lloyd CW, Martin WJ, and Taylor BD, "The Pharmacokinetics of Cimetidine and Metabolites in a Neonate," Drug Intell Clin Pharm, 1985, 19(3):203-5.

Somogyi A and Gugler R, "Clinical Pharmacokinetics of Cimetidine," Clin Pharmacokinet, 1983, 8(6):463-95.

Terrin G, Passariello A, De Curtis M, et al, "Ranitidine Is Associated With Infections, Necrotizing Enterocolitis, and Fatal Outcome in Newborns," Pediatrics, 2012, 129(1):40-5.

◆ **Cimetidine Acid Reducer [OTC]** see Cimetidine on page 469

◆ **Cinryze** see C1 Inhibitor (Human) on page 337

◆ **Cipralex (Can)** see Escitalopram on page 788

◆ **Cipralex MELTZ (Can)** see Escitalopram on page 788

◆ **Cipro** see Ciprofloxacin (Systemic) on page 471

◆ **Cipro XL (Can)** see Ciprofloxacin (Systemic) on page 471

◆ **Ciprodex** see Ciprofloxacin and Dexamethasone on page 477

Ciprofloxacin (Systemic) (sip roe FLOKS a sin)

Medication Safety Issues
Sound-alike/look-alike issues:
Ciprofloxacin may be confused with cephalexin
Cipro may be confused with Ceftin

Brand Names: U.S. Cipro; Cipro in D$_5$W; Cipro XR

Brand Names: Canada Apo-Ciproflox; Auro-Ciprofloxacin; Cipro; Cipro XL; Ciprofloxacin Injection; CO Ciprofloxacin; Dom-Ciprofloxacin; JAMP-Ciprofloxacin; Mar-Ciprofloxacin; Mint-Ciprofloxacin; Mylan-Ciprofloxacin; Novo-Ciprofloxacin; PHL-Ciprofloxacin; PMS-Ciprofloxacin; PMS-Ciprofloxacin XL; PRO-Ciprofloxacin; RAN-Ciprofloxacin; Riva-Ciprofloxacin; Sandoz-Ciprofloxacin; Septa-Ciprofloxacin; Taro-Ciprofloxacin

Therapeutic Category Antibiotic, Quinolone

Generic Availability (U.S.) Yes

Use Treatment of documented or suspected pseudomonal infection of the respiratory or urinary tract, skin and soft tissue, and bone and joint; treatment of complicated UTIs and pyelonephritis in children 1-17 years of age due to E. coli; documented multidrug-resistant, aerobic gram-negative bacilli, some gram-positive staphylococci, and Mycobacterium tuberculosis; documented infectious diarrhea due to Campylobacter jejuni, Shigella, or E. coli; typhoid fever caused by Salmonella typhi; osteomyelitis caused by susceptible organisms in which parenteral therapy is not feasible; uncomplicated cervical and urethral gonorrhea due to N. gonorrhoeae; chronic bacterial prostatitis caused by E. coli or Proteus mirabilis; pulmonary exacerbation of cystic fibrosis; empiric therapy for febrile neutropenia in combination with piperacillin; initial therapy or postexposure prophylaxis for inhalational anthrax; extended release tablet is used for the treatment of UTI and acute uncomplicated pyelonephritis caused by susceptible E. coli and Klebsiella pneumoniae

Medication Guide Available Yes

Pregnancy Risk Factor C

Pregnancy Considerations Adverse events have been observed in some animal reproduction studies. Ciprofloxacin crosses the placenta and produces measurable concentrations in the amniotic fluid and cord serum (Ludlam, 1997). An increased risk of teratogenic effects has not been observed in animals or humans following ciprofloxacin use during pregnancy; however, because of concerns of cartilage damage in immature animals, ciprofloxacin should only be used during pregnancy if a safer option is not available. Ciprofloxacin is recommended for prophylaxis and treatment of pregnant women exposed to anthrax (CDC, 2001a; CDC, 2001b). Serum concentrations of ciprofloxacin may be lower during pregnancy than in nonpregnant patients (Giamarellou, 1989).

Breast-Feeding Considerations Ciprofloxacin is excreted in breast milk. Due to the potential for serious adverse reactions in the nursing infant, the manufacturer recommends a decision be made whether to discontinue nursing or to discontinue the drug, taking into account the importance of treatment to the mother. However, due to the low concentrations in human milk, minimal toxicity would be expected in the nursing infant and infant serum levels were undetectable in one report (Gardner, 1992). Non-dose-related effects could include modification of bowel flora. There has been a single case report of perforated pseudomembranous colitis in a breast-feeding infant whose mother was taking ciprofloxacin (Harmon, 1992).

Contraindications Hypersensitivity to ciprofloxacin, any component, or other quinolones; concomitant administration with tizanidine; not recommended for use in pregnant women or during breast-feeding

Warnings Tendonitis and tendon rupture have been reported with fluoroquinolones in patients of all ages **[U.S. Boxed Warning]**; risk increased in patients taking concomitant corticosteroids, patients >60 years of age, and in solid organ transplant recipients. Rupture of the Achilles tendon sometimes requiring surgical repair has been reported most frequently; but other tendon sites (eg, rotator cuff, biceps) have also been reported; inflammation and rupture may occur bilaterally. Cases have been reported within the first 48 hours, during, and up to several months after discontinuation of therapy; strenuous physical activity may be an independent risk factor for tendonitis. Discontinue at first sign of tendon inflammation or pain. Use with caution in patients with a history of tendon disorder. Increased osteochondrosis in immature rats and dogs was observed with ciprofloxacin and fluoroquinolones have caused arthropathy with erosions of the cartilage in weight-bearing joints of immature animals. In an international safety data analysis of ciprofloxacin in approximately 700 pediatric patients (1-17 years), the follow-up arthropathy rate at 6 weeks and cumulative arthropathy rate at 1 year were higher in ciprofloxacin treatment group than comparative controls (6 weeks: 9.3% vs 6%; one-year: 13.7% to 9.5%). Safety of use in pediatric patients for >14 days of therapy has not reported; in available pediatric safety data, the typical duration of therapy was around 10 days (CAP, AOM) (Bradley, 2011).

CNS stimulation, increased intracranial pressure (including pseudotumor cerebri), and toxic psychosis may occur, resulting in tremors, restlessness, confusion, and very rarely hallucinations, depression, nightmares, suicidal ideation, or convulsive seizures. If these reactions occur, discontinue ciprofloxacin; use with caution in patients with known or suspected CNS disorders, seizure disorders, severe cerebral arteriosclerosis. Rare cases of polyneuropathy affecting small and/or large axons, resulting in paresthesias, hypoesthesias, dysesthesias, and weakness, have been reported in patients receiving ciprofloxacin. Discontinue ciprofloxacin if patient experiences pain, burning, tingling, numbness, or weakness or is found to have deficits in light touch, pain, temperature, position sense, vibrating sensation, or motor strength. Fluoroquinolones, including ciprofloxacin, may exacerbate muscle weakness associated with myasthenia gravis **[U.S. Boxed Warning]**; cases of severe exacerbations, including the need for ventilatory support and deaths, have been reported; avoid use in patients with myasthenia gravis.

Fluoroquinolones may prolong QT_c interval; avoid use in patients with a history of or at risk for QT_c prolongation, torsade de pointes, uncorrected hypokalemia, hypomagnesemia, cardiac disease (heart failure, myocardial infarction, bradycardia), or concurrent administration of other medications known to prolong the QT interval (including Class Ia and Class III antiarrhythmics, cisapride, erythromycin, antipsychotics, and tricyclic antidepressants).

Coadministration of ciprofloxacin with drugs metabolized by CYP1A2 (eg, theophylline, caffeine, tizanidine) may result in increased plasma concentrations of the coadministered drug with corresponding side effects. Serious and fatal reactions, including cardiac arrest, seizure, status epilepticus, and respiratory failure, have been reported in patients receiving ciprofloxacin and theophylline concurrently. Serum theophylline levels should be monitored and dosage adjustments made when concomitant use cannot be avoided. Hypotension and oversedation have been reported when ciprofloxacin and tizanidine were given concomitantly (concomitant administration of tizanidine and ciprofloxacin is contraindicated). Potentially significant interactions may exist, requiring dose or frequency adjustment, additional monitoring, and/or selection of alternative therapy. Consult drug interactions database for more detailed information.

Hepatocellular, cholestatic, or mixed liver injury has been reported, including hepatic necrosis, life-threatening hepatic events, and fatalities. Acute liver injury can be rapid onset (range: 1-39 days), often associated with hypersensitivity. Most fatalities occurred in patients >55 years of age. Discontinue immediately if signs/symptoms of hepatitis (abdominal tenderness, dark urine, jaundice, pruritus) occur. Additionally, temporary increases in transaminases or alkaline phosphatase, or cholestatic jaundice may occur (highest risk in patients with previous liver damage).

Severe hypersensitivity reactions, including anaphylaxis, have occurred with quinolone therapy. The spectrum of these reactions can vary widely; reactions may present as typical allergic symptoms (eg, itching, urticaria, rash, edema) after a single dose, or may manifest as severe idiosyncratic dermatologic (eg, Stevens-Johnson, toxic epidermal necrolysis), vascular (eg, vasculitis), pulmonary (eg, pneumonitis), renal (eg, nephritis), hepatic (eg, hepatitis, jaundice, hepatic failure or necrosis), and/or hematologic (eg, anemia, cytopenias) events, usually after multiple doses. Prompt discontinuation of drug should occur if skin rash or other symptoms arise.

Prolonged use may result in superinfection, including *C. difficile*-associated diarrhea and pseudomembranous colitis. Extended release tablets and immediate release formulations are **not** interchangeable.

Precautions Use with caution in renal impairment; modify dosage in patients with renal impairment. Avoid excessive sunlight and take precautions to limit exposure (eg, loose-fitting clothing, sunscreen); may rarely cause moderate-to-severe phototoxicity reactions. Discontinue use if phototoxicity occurs. Hemolytic reactions may (rarely) occur with fluoroquinolone use in patients with latent or actual G6PD deficiency. Fluoroquinolones have been associated with the development of serious, and sometimes fatal, hypoglycemia; these events have occurred most often in elderly patients with diabetes, but have also been reported in patients without a prior history of diabetes; prompt identification and treatment of hypoglycemia is essential; individual quinolones may differ in their potential to cause this effect [ie, most evident with gatifloxacin (no longer marketed as a systemic formulation)]. Hyperglycemia has also been associated with the use of fluoroquinolones; patients should be monitored closely for signs/symptoms of disordered glucose regulation. Patients consuming regular large quantities of caffeinated beverages may need to restrict caffeine intake if excessive cardiac or CNS stimulation occurs.

In pediatric patients, fluoroquinolones are not routinely first-line therapy, but after assessment of risks and benefits, can be considered a reasonable alternative for situations where no safe and effective substitute is available [eg, resistance (anthrax, common CF pathogens, multidrug resistant tuberculosis)] or in situations where the only alternative is parenteral therapy and ciprofloxacin offers an oral therapy option (Bradley, 2011).

Adverse Reactions

Central nervous system: Fever, headache (I.V. administration); neurologic events (includes dizziness, insomnia, nervousness, somnolence); restlessness (I.V. administration)

Dermatologic: Rash

Gastrointestinal: Abdominal pain, diarrhea, dyspepsia, nausea, vomiting

Hepatic: ALT increased, AST increased

Local: Injection site reactions (I.V. administration)

Respiratory: Rhinitis

Rare but important or life-threatening: Abnormal gait, acute generalized exanthemous pustulosis (AGEP), acute renal failure, agitation, agranulocytosis, albuminuria, alkaline phosphatase increase, allergic reactions, anaphylactic shock, anemia, angina pectoris, angioedema, anorexia, anxiety, arthralgia, ataxia, atrial flutter, bilirubin (serum) increase, bone marrow depression (life-threatening), bronchospasm, BUN increased, candidiasis, cardiopulmonary arrest, chills, cholestatic jaundice, chromatopsia, *Clostridium difficile*-associated diarrhea (CDAD), confusion, constipation, CPK increase, crystalluria (particularly in alkaline urine), cylindruria, delirium, depression (including self-injurious behavior), dizziness, drowsiness, dyspepsia (adults), dyspnea, edema, eosinophilia, erythema multiforme/nodosum, exfoliative dermatitis, fever (adults), fixed eruption, gastrointestinal bleeding, gout flare, hallucinations, headache (oral), hematocrit decreased, hematuria, hemoglobin decreased, hemolytic anemia, hepatic failure (some fatal), hepatic necrosis, hyper-/hypoglycemia, hyper-/hypotension, hyperesthesia, hyperpigmentation, hypertonia, insomnia, interstitial nephritis, intestinal perforation, intracranial pressure increased, irritability, joint pain, laryngeal edema, LDH increased, lightheadedness, lipase increased, lymphadenopathy, malaise, manic reaction, methemoglobinemia, MI, migraine, myalgia, myasthenia gravis exacerbation, myoclonus, nephritis, nightmares, nystagmus, palpitation, pancreatitis, pancytopenia (life-threatening or fatal), paranoia, peripheral neuropathy, petechiae, photosensitivity/toxicity, pneumonitis, polyneuropathy, prolongation of PT/INR (in patients treated with vitamin K antagonists), pseudotumor cerebri, psychosis (toxic), PT decrease, pulmonary edema, renal calculi, seizure (including grand mal), serum cholesterol increased, serum creatinine increased, serum sickness-like reactions, serum triglycerides increased, status epilepticus, Stevens-Johnson syndrome, suicidal thoughts/ideation/attempts and completions, syncope, tachycardia, taste loss, tendon rupture, tendonitis, thrombocytopenia, thrombocytosis, thrombophlebitis, tinnitus, torsade de pointes, toxic epidermal necrolysis, tremor, twitching, unresponsiveness, urethral bleeding, uric acid increased, vaginitis, vasculitis, ventricular arrhythmia, visual disturbance, weakness

Drug Interactions

Metabolism/Transport Effects Substrate of P-glycoprotein; **Inhibits** CYP1A2 (strong), CYP3A4 (weak)

Avoid Concomitant Use

Avoid concomitant use of Ciprofloxacin (Systemic) with any of the following: Agomelatine; BCG; CloZAPine;

Highest Risk QTc-Prolonging Agents; Ivabradine; Mifepristone; Pimozide; Pirfenidone; Pomalidomide; Strontium Ranelate; Tasimelteon; TiZANidine

Increased Effect/Toxicity

Ciprofloxacin (Systemic) may increase the levels/effects of: Agomelatine; ARIPiprazole; Bendamustine; CloZAPine; Corticosteroids (Systemic); CYP1A2 Substrates; Erlotinib; Highest Risk QTc-Prolonging Agents; Lomitapide; Methotrexate; Moderate Risk QTc-Prolonging Agents; Pentoxifylline; Pimozide; Pirfenidone; Pomalidomide; Porfimer; Roflumilast; ROPINIRole; Ropivacaine; Sulfonylureas; Tasimelteon; Theophylline Derivatives; TiZANidine; Varenicline; Vitamin K Antagonists

The levels/effects of Ciprofloxacin (Systemic) may be increased by: Fosphenytoin; Insulin; Ivabradine; Mifepristone; Nonsteroidal Anti-Inflammatory Agents; P-glycoprotein/ABCB1 Inhibitors; Probenecid; QTc-Prolonging Agents (Indeterminate Risk and Risk Modifying)

Decreased Effect

Ciprofloxacin (Systemic) may decrease the levels/effects of: BCG; Didanosine; Fosphenytoin; Mycophenolate; Phenytoin; Sodium Picosulfate; Sulfonylureas; Typhoid Vaccine

The levels/effects of Ciprofloxacin (Systemic) may be decreased by: Antacids; Calcium Salts; Didanosine; Iron Salts; Lanthanum; Magnesium Salts; Multivitamins/Minerals (with ADEK, Folate, Iron); Multivitamins/Minerals (with AE, No Iron); P-glycoprotein/ABCB1 Inducers; Quinapril; Sevelamer; Strontium Ranelate; Sucralfate; Zinc Salts

Food Interactions Food decreases rate, but not extent, of absorption. Ciprofloxacin serum levels may be decreased if taken with divalent or trivalent cations. Rarely, crystalluria may occur. Enteral feedings may decrease plasma concentrations of ciprofloxacin probably by >30% inhibition of absorption. Management: May administer with food to minimize GI upset. Avoid or take ciprofloxacin 2 hours before or 6 hours after antacids, dairy products, or calcium-fortified juices alone or in a meal containing >800 mg calcium, oral multivitamins, or mineral supplements containing divalent and/or trivalent cations. Ensure adequate hydration during therapy. Ciprofloxacin should not be administered with enteral feedings. The feeding would need to be discontinued for 1-2 hours prior to and after ciprofloxacin administration. Nasogastric administration produces a greater loss of ciprofloxacin bioavailability than does nasoduodenal administration.

Stability Premixed bags: Out of overwrap stability: 14 days at room temperature; reconstituted oral suspension: Stable for 14 days when stored at room temperature or refrigerated; store tablets, intact injection vial, and oral suspension prior to reconstitution at room temperature; protect from intense light; protect from freezing

Mechanism of Action Inhibits DNA-gyrase in susceptible organisms; inhibits relaxation of supercoiled DNA and promotes breakage of double-stranded DNA

Pharmacokinetics (Adult data unless noted)

Absorption: Oral: Well-absorbed; 500 mg orally every 12 hours produces an equivalent AUC to that produced by 400 mg I.V. over 60 minutes every 12 hours.

Distribution: Widely distributed into body tissues and fluids with high concentration in bile, saliva, urine, sputum, stool, lungs, liver, skin, muscle, prostate, genital tissue, and bone; low concentration in CSF; crosses the placenta

Protein binding: 16% to 43%

Metabolism: Partially in the liver to four active metabolites

Bioavailability: Oral: 50% to 85%; younger CF patients have a lower bioavailability of 68% vs CF patients >13 years of age with bioavailability of 95%

Half-life:

Children: 4 to 5 hours

Adults with normal renal function: 3 to 5 hours

Time to peak serum concentration: Oral: Immediate release tablet: Within 0.5-2 hours; Extended release tablet: 1 to 4 hours

Elimination: 30% to 50% excreted as unchanged drug in urine via glomerular filtration and active tubular secretion; 20% to 40% excreted in feces primarily from biliary excretion; <1% excreted in bile as unchanged drug

Clearance: After I.V.:

CF child: 0.84 L/hour/kg

Adult: 0.5 to 0.6 L/hour/kg

Dosing: Neonatal Note: In pediatric patients, ciprofloxacin is not routinely first-line therapy, but after assessment of risks and benefits, can be considered a reasonable alternative for some situations (Bradley, 2011).

Severe infection (eg, sepsis); usually multidrug resistant: Limited data available: I.V.: 10 mg/kg/dose every 12 hours (Kaguelidou, 2011). A study of 20 neonates (28-36 weeks) showed this dose produced serum concentrations sufficient to treat common gram-negative pathogens. A higher daily dose divided into shorter intervals may be required to achieve serum concentrations sufficient to treat *Staphylococcus aureus* or *Pseudomonas aeruginosa* (Aggarwal, 2004). Reported range: 10 to 60 mg/kg/day (Krcméry, 1999; Schaad, 1995; van den Oever, 1998).

Dosing: Usual Note: In pediatric patients, ciprofloxacin is not routinely first-line therapy, but after assessment of risks and benefits, can be considered a reasonable alternative for some situations [eg, anthrax, resistance (cystic fibrosis)] or in situations where the only alternative is parenteral therapy and ciprofloxacin offers an oral therapy option (Bradley, 2011). **Note:** Extended release tablets and immediate release formulations are not interchangeable. Unless otherwise specified, oral dosing reflects the use of **immediate release** formulation.

Infants, Children, and Adolescents:

General dosing, susceptible infection:

Oral: 20 to 30 mg/kg/day in 2 divided doses; maximum dose: 1.5 g/day

I.V.: 20 to 30 mg/kg/day divided every 12 hours; maximum dose: 800 mg/day

Inhalational anthrax (postexposure): Initial treatment:

I.V.: 20 mg/kg/day divided every 12 hours for 60 days; maximum dose: 800 mg/day (substitute oral antibiotics for I.V. antibiotics as soon as clinical condition improves)

Oral: 30 mg/kg/day divided every 12 hours for 60 days; maximum dose: 1000 mg/day

Complicated UTI or pyelonephritis:

I.V.: 18 to 30 mg/kg/day divided every 8 hours for 10 to 21 days; maximum dose: 1200 mg/day

Oral: 20 to 40 mg/kg/day divided every 12 hours for 10 to 21 days; maximum dose: 1500 mg/day

Cystic fibrosis:

Oral: 40 mg/kg/day divided every 12 hours; maximum dose: 2 g/day

I.V.: 30 mg/kg/day divided every 8 to 12 hours; maximum dose: 1.2 g/day

Adults:

Oral: 250 to 750 mg every 12 hours, depending on severity of infection and susceptibility

Acute sinusitis: Mild/moderate: 500 mg every 12 hours for 10 days

Uncomplicated UTI/acute cystitis:

Extended release tablet: 500 mg every 24 hours for 3 days

Immediate release formulation: Acute uncomplicated: 250 mg every 12 hours for 3 days; 250 mg every 12 hours for 7 to 14 days for mild to moderate UTI

Complicated UTI or acute uncomplicated pyelonephritis:
Extended release tablet: 1000 mg every 24 hours for 7 to 14 days
Immediate release formulation: 500 mg every 12 hours for 7 to 14 days
Bone and joint infections:
Mild/moderate: 500 mg every 12 hours for ≥4 to 6 weeks
Severe/complicated: 750 mg every 12 hours for ≥4 to 6 weeks
Chemoprophylaxis regimen for high-risk contacts of invasive meningococcal disease: 500 mg as a single dose
Chronic bacterial prostatitis: 500 mg every 12 hours for 28 days
Infectious diarrhea: 500 mg every 12 hours for 5 to 7 days
Skin and skin structure infections:
Mild/moderate: 500 mg every 12 hours for 7 to 14 days
Severe/complicated: 750 mg every 12 hours for 7 to 14 days
Uncomplicated gonorrhea: 500 mg as a single dose
Chancroid: 500 mg twice daily for 3 days
Lower respiratory tract infection:
Mild/moderate: 500 mg every 12 hours for 7 to 14 days
Severe/complicated: 750 mg every 12 hours for 7 to 14 days
Typhoid fever: 500 mg every 12 hours for 10 days
Inhalational anthrax (postexposure prophylaxis): 500 mg every 12 hours for 60 days
I.V.: 200-400 mg every 8-12 hours depending on severity of infection
Lower respiratory tract, skin and skin structure infection:
Mild/moderate: 400 mg every 12 hours for 7 to 14 days
Severe/complicated: 400 mg every 8 hours for 7 to 14 days
Treatment of anthrax infection: 400 mg every 12 hours for 60 days (substitute oral antibiotics for I.V. antibiotics as soon as clinical condition improves)
Empiric therapy in febrile neutropenic patients: 400 mg every 8 hours in combination with piperacillin for 7 to 14 days

Dosing adjustment in renal impairment:
Infants, Children, and Adolescents: Dosage adjustments are not provided in the manufacturer's labeling; however, the following guidelines have been used by some clinicians (Aronoff, 2007): I.V., Oral:
GFR ≥30 mL/minute/1.73 m²: No dosage adjustment necessary
GFR 10 to 29 mL/minute/1.73m²: 10 to 15 mg/kg/dose every 18 hours
GFR <10 mL/minute/1.73m²: 10 to 15 mg/kg/dose every 24 hours
Hemodialysis/peritoneal dialysis (PD) (after dialysis on dialysis days): 10 to 15 mg/kg/dose every 24 hours
CRRT: 10 to 15 mg/kg/dose every 12 hours
Adults:
Manufacturer's recommendations:
Oral, immediate release:
CrCl >50 mL/minute: No dosage adjustment necessary
CrCl 30 to 50 mL/minute: Oral: 250 to 500 mg every 12 hours
CrCl 5 to 29 mL/minute: 250 to 500 mg every 18 hours
Hemodialysis/peritoneal dialysis (PD) (administer after dialysis on dialysis days): 250 to 500 mg every 24 hours

Oral, extended release:
CrCl ≥30 mL/minute: No dosage adjustment necessary
CrCl <30 mL/minute: 500 mg every 24 hours
I.V.:
CrCl ≥30 mL/minute: No dosage adjustment necessary
CrCl 5 to 29 mL/minute: 200 to 400 mg every 18 to 24 hours
Alternate recommendations: Oral (immediate release), I.V.:
CrCl >50 mL/minute: No dosage adjustment necessary (Aronoff, 2007)
CrCl 10 to 50 mL/minute: Administer 50% to 75% of usual dose every 12 hours (Aronoff, 2007)
CrCl <10 mL/minute: Administer 50% of usual dose every 12 hours (Aronoff, 2007)
Intermittent hemodialysis (IHD) (administer after hemodialysis on dialysis days): Minimally dialyzable (<10%): Oral: 250 to 500 mg every 24 hours or I.V.: 200 to 400 mg every 24 hours (Heintz, 2009). **Note:** Dosing dependent on the assumption of 3 times/week, complete IHD sessions.
Continuous renal replacement therapy (CRRT) (Heintz, 2009; Trotman, 2005): Drug clearance is highly dependent on the method of renal replacement, filter type, and flow rate. Appropriate dosing requires close monitoring of pharmacologic response, signs of adverse reactions due to drug accumulation, as well as drug concentrations in relation to target trough (if appropriate). The following are general recommendations only (based on dialysate flow/ultrafiltration rates of 1-2 L/hour and minimal residual renal function) and should not supersede clinical judgment:
CVVH/CVVHD/CVVHDF: I.V.: 200 to 400 mg every 12 to 24 hours

Administration
Oral: May administer with food to minimize GI upset; divalent and trivalent cations [dairy foods (milk, yogurt) and mineral supplements (eg, iron, zinc, calcium) or calcium-fortified juices] decrease ciprofloxacin absorption; usual dietary calcium intake (including meals which include dairy products) has not been shown to interfere with ciprofloxacin absorption (per manufacturer). Administer immediate release ciprofloxacin and Cipro XR at least 2 hours before or 6 hours after any of these products.
Oral suspension: Should not be administered through feeding tubes (suspension is oil-based and adheres to the feeding tube). Patients should avoid chewing on the microcapsules.
Tablets:
Immediate release: Administering 2 hours after meals is preferable.
Extended release: Do not crush, split, or chew. May be administered with meals containing dairy products (calcium content <800 mg), but not with dairy products alone.
Nasogastric/orogastric tube: Crush immediate release tablet and mix with water. Flush feeding tube before and after administration. Hold tube feedings at least 1 hour before and 2 hours after administration.
Parenteral: Administer by slow I.V. infusion over 60 minutes to reduce the risk of venous irritation (burning, pain, erythema, and swelling); final concentration for administration should not exceed 2 mg/mL

Monitoring Parameters Monitor renal, hepatic, and hematopoietic function periodically; monitor number and type of stools/day for diarrhea. Patients receiving concurrent ciprofloxacin and theophylline should have serum levels of theophylline monitored; monitor INR in patients receiving warfarin; patients receiving concurrent ciprofloxacin and cyclosporine should have cyclosporine levels monitored.

Reference Range Therapeutic: 2.6 to 3 mcg/mL

Test Interactions Some quinolones may produce a false-positive urine screening result for opioids using commercially-available immunoassay kits. This has been demonstrated most consistently for levofloxacin and ofloxacin, but other quinolones have shown cross-reactivity in certain assay kits. Confirmation of positive opioid screens by more specific methods should be considered.

Additional Information Although fluoroquinolones are only FDA approved for use in children for complicated UTI, pyelonephritis, and postexposure treatment for inhalational anthrax, the AAP (Bradley, 2011) has identified other appropriate uses for fluoroquinolones once risks and benefits have been assessed to justify its use:

- UTI caused by *Pseudomonas aeruginosa* or other multidrug-resistant, gram-negative bacteria susceptible to fluoroquinolones
- Chronic suppurative otitis media or otitis externa caused by *P. aeruginosa*
- Chronic or acute osteomyelitis or osteochondritis caused by *P. aeruginosa*
- Mycobacterial infections caused by isolates sensitive to fluoroquinolones
- Gram-negative bacterial infections in immunocompromised hosts in which oral therapy is desired or resistance to alternative agents is present

Dosage Forms Excipient information presented when available (limited, particularly for generics); consult specific product labeling.

Solution, Intravenous:
Cipro in D₅W: 200 mg/100 mL (100 mL) [latex free]
Generic: 200 mg/100 mL (100 mL); 400 mg/200 mL (200 mL); 200 mg/20 mL (20 mL); 400 mg/40 mL (40 mL)
Solution, Intravenous [preservative free]:
Cipro in D₅W: 200 mg/100 mL (100 mL); 400 mg/200 mL (200 mL) [latex free]
Generic: 200 mg/100 mL (100 mL); 400 mg/200 mL (200 mL); 200 mg/20 mL (20 mL); 400 mg/40 mL (40 mL)
Suspension Reconstituted, Oral:
Cipro: 250 mg/5 mL (100 mL); 500 mg/5 mL (100 mL) [strawberry flavor]
Generic: 250 mg/5 mL (100 mL); 500 mg/5 mL (100 mL)
Tablet, Oral [strength expressed as base]:
Generic: 500 mg
Tablet, Oral, as hydrochloride [strength expressed as base]:
Cipro: 250 mg, 500 mg
Generic: 100 mg, 250 mg, 500 mg, 750 mg
Tablet Extended Release 24 Hour, Oral, as base and hydrochloride [strength expressed as base]:
Cipro XR: 500 mg, 1000 mg
Generic: 500 mg, 1000 mg

Extemporaneous Preparations A 50 mg/mL oral suspension may be made using 2 different vehicles (a 1:1 mixture of Ora-Sweet and Ora-Plus or a 1:1 mixture of Methylcellulose 1% and Simple Syrup, NF). Crush twenty 500 mg tablets and reduce to a fine powder. Add a small amount of vehicle and mix to a uniform paste; mix while adding the vehicle in geometric proportions to **almost** 200 mL; transfer to a calibrated bottle, rinse mortar with vehicle, and add quantity of vehicle sufficient to make 200 mL. Label "shake well" and "refrigerate". Stable 91 days refrigerated and 70 days at room temperature. **Note:** Microcapsules for oral suspension available (50 mg/mL; 100 mg/mL); not for use in feeding tubes.

Nahata MC, Pai VB, and Hipple TF, *Pediatric Drug Formulations*, 5th ed, Cincinnati, OH: Harvey Whitney Books Co, 2004.

References

Aggarwal P, Dutta S, Garg SK, et al, "Multiple Dose Pharmacokinetics of Ciprofloxacin in Preterm Babies," *Indian Pediatr*, 2004, 41 (10):1001-7.

Aronoff GR, Bennett WM, Berns JS, et al, *Drug Prescribing in Renal Failure: Dosing Guidelines for Adults and Children*, 5th ed, Philadelphia, PA: American College of Physicians, 2007, 66, 171.

Bradley JS, Byington CL, Shah SS, et al, "The Management of Community-Acquired Pneumonia in Infants and Children Older Than 3 Months of Age: Clinical Practice Guidelines by the Pediatric Infectious Diseases Society and the Infectious Diseases Society of America", *Clin Infect Dis*, 2011, 53(7):e25-76.

Bradley JS, Jackson MA, Committee on Infectious Diseases, American Academy of Pediatrics. The use of systemic and topical fluoroquinolones. *Pediatrics*. 2011;128:e1034-1045.

Campoli-Richards DM, Monk JP, Price A, et al, "Ciprofloxacin. A Review of Its Antibacterial Activity, Pharmacokinetic Properties and Therapeutic Use," *Drugs*, 1988, 35(4):373-447.

Centers for Disease Control and Prevention (CDC), "Guidelines for the Prevention and Treatment of Opportunistic Infections Among HIV-Exposed and HIV-Infected Children," *MMWR Recomm Rep*, 2009, 58(RR-11):1-166. Available at http://aidsinfo.nih.gov/contentfiles/Pediatric_OI.pdf

Centers for Disease Control and Prevention (CDC), "Updated Recommendations for Antimicrobial Prophylaxis Among Asymptomatic Pregnant Women After Exposure to *Bacillus anthracis*," *MMWR Morb Mortal Wkly Rep*, 2001a, 50(43):960.

Centers for Disease Control and Prevention (CDC), "Update: Investigation of Bioterrorism-Related Anthrax and Interim Guidelines for Exposure Management and Antimicrobial Therapy, October 2001," *MMWR*, October 26, 2001b, 50(42):909-19. Available at http://www.cdc.gov/mmwr/preview/mmwrhtml/mm5042a1.htm

Gardner DK, Gabbe SG, and Harter C, "Simultaneous Concentrations of Ciprofloxacin in Breast Milk and in Serum in Mother and Breast-Fed Infant," *Clin Pharm*, 1992, 11(4):352-4.

Giamarellou H, Kolokythas E, Petrikkos G, et al, "Pharmacokinetics of Three Newer Quinolones in Pregnant and Lactating Women," *Am J Med*, 1989, 87(Suppl 5A):49-51.

Harmon T, Burkhart G, and Applebaum H, "Perforated Pseudomembranous Colitis in the Breast-Fed Infant," *J Pediatr Surg*, 1992, 27 (6):744-6.

Inglesby TV, Henderson DA, Bartlett JG, et al, "Anthrax as a Biological Weapon: Medical and Public Health Management. Working Group on Civilian Biodefense," *JAMA*, 1999, 281(18):1735-45.

Kaguelidou F, Turner MA, Choonara I, et al, "Ciprofloxacin Use in Neonates: A Systematic Review of the Literature," *Pediatr Infect Dis J*, 2011, 30(2):e29-37.

Krcmëry V Jr, Filka J, Uher J, et al, "Ciprofloxacin in Treatment of Nosocomial Meningitis in Neonates and in Infants: Report of 12 Cases and Review," *Diagn Microbiol Infect Dis*, 1999, 35(1):75-80.

Ludlam H, Wreghitt TG, Thornton S, et al, "Q Fever in Pregnancy," *J Infect*, 34(1):75-8.

Rodriguez WJ and Wiedermann BL, "The Role of Newer Oral Cephalosporins, Fluoroquinolones, and Macrolides in the Treatment of Pediatric Infections," *Adv Pediatr Infect Dis*, 1994, 9:125-59.

Rubio TT, Miles MV, Lettieri JT, et al, "Pharmacokinetic Disposition of Sequential Intravenous/Oral Ciprofloxacin in Pediatric Cystic Fibrosis Patients With Acute Pulmonary Exacerbation," *Pediatr Infect Dis J*, 1997, 16(1):112-7.

Schaad UB, abdus Salam M, Aujard Y, et al, "Use of Fluoroquinolones in Pediatrics: Consensus Report of an International Society of Chemotherapy Commission," *Pediatr Infect Dis J*, 1995, 14(1):1-9.

van den Oever HL, Versteegh FG, Thewessen EA, et al, "Ciprofloxacin in Preterm Neonates: Case Report and Review of the Literature," *Eur J Pediatr*, 1998, 157(10):843-5.

Ciprofloxacin (Ophthalmic) (sip roe FLOKS a sin)

Medication Safety Issues
Sound-alike/look-alike issues:
Ciprofloxacin may be confused with cephalexin
Ciloxan may be confused with Cytoxan
Brand Names: U.S. Ciloxan
Brand Names: Canada Ciloxan
Therapeutic Category Antibiotic, Ophthalmic
Generic Availability (U.S.) May be product dependent
Use Treatment of bacterial conjunctivitis due to susceptible organisms (Ointment: FDA approved in ages ≥2 years and adults; Solution: FDA approved in ages ≥1 year and adults); treatment of corneal ulcers (Solution: FDA approved in ages ≥1 year and adults)
Pregnancy Risk Factor C
Pregnancy Considerations Adverse events have been observed in some animal reproduction studies. When administered orally or I.V., ciprofloxacin crosses the placenta. Refer to the Ciprofloxacin (Systemic) monograph for

details. The amount of ciprofloxacin available systemically following topical application of the ophthalmic drops is significantly less in comparison to oral or I.V. doses.

Breast-Feeding Considerations When administered orally or I.V., ciprofloxacin enters breast milk. Refer to the Ciprofloxacin (Systemic) monograph for details. The amount of ciprofloxacin available systemically following topical application of the ophthalmic drops is significantly less in comparison to oral or I.V. doses. The manufacturer recommends that caution be exercised when administering ciprofloxacin eye drops to nursing women.

Contraindications Hypersensitivity to ciprofloxacin, any component, or other quinolones

Warnings Severe hypersensitivity reactions, including anaphylaxis, have occurred with quinolone therapy (primarily with systemic use). Prompt discontinuation of drug should occur if skin rash or other symptoms arise. Prolonged use may result in fungal or bacterial superinfection. If superinfection is suspected, institute appropriate alternative therapy. Corneal healing may be delayed.

Precautions For ophthalmic use only. Not for subconjunctival injection or for introduction into the anterior chamber of the eye. To avoid contamination, do not touch tip of container to any surface. Some products contain benzalkonium chloride which may be absorbed by soft contact lenses; contact lenses should not be worn during treatment of ophthalmologic infections.

Adverse Reactions
Gastrointestinal: Unpleasant taste (immediately after instillation)
Ocular: Conjunctival hyperemia, crystal formation, burning, discomfort, foreign body sensation, itching, keratopathy (ointment), lid margin crusting, white crystalline precipitate (solution; in superficial portion of corneal defect; reversible after completion of therapy)
Rare but important or life-threatening: Corneal infiltrates, corneal staining, hypersensitivity reactions, keratitis, lid edema, nausea, photophobia, tearing, vision decreased

Drug Interactions
Metabolism/Transport Effects None known.
Avoid Concomitant Use There are no known interactions where it is recommended to avoid concomitant use.
Increased Effect/Toxicity There are no known significant interactions involving an increase in effect.
Decreased Effect There are no known significant interactions involving a decrease in effect.

Stability Store at 2°C to 25°C (36°F to 77°F); protect from light

Mechanism of Action Inhibits DNA-gyrase in susceptible organisms; inhibits relaxation of supercoiled DNA and promotes breakage of double-stranded DNA

Dosing: Usual
Children and Adolescents:
Bacterial conjunctivitis; treatment:
Ointment: Children ≥2 years and Adolescents: Apply 1/2" ointment ribbon into the conjunctival sac 3 times daily for 2 days, then twice daily for the next 5 days
Solution: Children ≥1 year and Adolescents: Instill 1-2 drops into the conjunctival sac of the affected eye(s) every 2 hours while awake for 2 days, then 1-2 drops every 4 hours while awake for the next 5 days
Corneal ulcers; treatment: Solution: Children ≥1 year and Adolescents: Instill 2 drops into the conjunctival sac every 15 minutes for the first 6 hours, then 2 drops every 30 minutes for the remainder of the first day; on the second day, 2 drops every hour; on the third day and for the duration of therapy, 2 drops every 4 hours thereafter. Treatment may continue after day 14 if re-epithelialization has not occurred.

Adults:
Bacterial conjunctivitis; treatment:
Ointment: Apply 1/2" ointment ribbon into the conjunctival sac 3 times daily for 2 days, then twice daily for the next 5 days
Solution: Instill 1-2 drops into the conjunctival sac of the affected eye(s) every 2 hours while awake for 2 days, then 1-2 drops every 4 hours while awake for the next 5 days
Corneal ulcers; treatment: Solution: Instill 2 drops into the conjunctival sac every 15 minutes for the first 6 hours, then 2 drops every 30 minutes for the remainder of the first day; on the second day, 2 drops every hour; on the third day and for the duration of therapy, 2 drops every 4 hours thereafter. Treatment may continue after day 14 if re-epithelialization has not occurred.

Administration Ophthalmic: For topical use only. Avoid contacting tip with skin or eye.
Ointment: Instill ointment in the lower conjunctival sac.
Solution: Apply finger pressure to lacrimal sac during and for 1-2 minutes after instillation to decrease risk of absorption and systemic effects.

Dosage Forms Excipient information presented when available (limited, particularly for generics); consult specific product labeling.
Ointment, Ophthalmic, as hydrochloride:
Ciloxan: 0.3% (3.5 g)
Solution, Ophthalmic, as hydrochloride:
Ciloxan: 0.3% (5 mL) [contains benzalkonium chloride, edetate disodium]
Generic: 0.3% (2.5 mL, 5 mL, 10 mL)

Ciprofloxacin (Otic) (sip roe FLOKS a sin)

Medication Safety Issues
Sound-alike/look-alike issues:
Cetraxal® may be confused with cefTRIAXone
Ciprofloxacin may be confused with cephalexin
Brand Names: U.S. Cetraxal
Therapeutic Category Antibiotic, Otic; Antibiotic, Quinolone
Generic Availability (U.S.) Yes
Use Treatment of acute otitis externa due to susceptible strains of *Pseudomonas aeruginosa* or *Staphylococcus aureus*
Pregnancy Risk Factor C
Pregnancy Considerations Adverse events have been observed in some animal studies; therefore, the manufacturer classifies ciprofloxacin otic as pregnancy category C. When administered orally or I.V., ciprofloxacin crosses the placenta. Refer to the Ciprofloxacin (Systemic) monograph for details. The amount of ciprofloxacin available systemically following topical application of the otic drops is expected to be significantly less in comparison to oral or I.V. doses.
Breast-Feeding Considerations When administered orally or I.V., ciprofloxacin enters breast milk. Refer to the Ciprofloxacin (Systemic) monograph for details. The amount of ciprofloxacin available systemically following topical application of the otic drops is expected to be significantly less in comparison to oral or I.V. doses; however, breast-feeding is not recommended by the manufacturer.
Contraindications Hypersensitivity to ciprofloxacin, any component, or other quinolones
Warnings There have been reports of tendon inflammation and/or rupture with systemic quinolone antibiotic use.
Precautions Hypersensitivity reaction may occur with quinolone therapy; prolonged use may result in superinfection
Adverse Reactions
Central nervous system: Headache
Local: Application site pain, fungal superinfection, pruritus

Drug Interactions

Metabolism/Transport Effects None known.

Avoid Concomitant Use There are no known interactions where it is recommended to avoid concomitant use.

Increased Effect/Toxicity There are no known significant interactions involving an increase in effect.

Decreased Effect There are no known significant interactions involving a decrease in effect.

Stability Protect from intense light; protect from freezing

Mechanism of Action Inhibits DNA-gyrase in susceptible organisms; inhibits relaxation of supercoiled DNA and promotes breakage of double-stranded DNA

Additional Information Although fluoroquinolones are only FDA approved for use in children for complicated UTI, pyelonephritis, and postexposure treatment for inhalational anthrax, the AAP has provided a list of other possible uses for fluoroquinolones once risks and benefits have been assessed to justify its use:

• Chronic suppurative otitis media or otitis externa caused by *P. aeruginosa*

Dosage Forms Excipient information presented when available (limited, particularly for generics); consult specific product labeling.

Solution, Otic, as hydrochloride [preservative free]:
Cetraxal: 0.2% (1 ea)
Generic: 0.2% (1 ea)

Ciprofloxacin and Dexamethasone
(sip roe FLOKS a sin & deks a METH a sone)

Brand Names: U.S. Ciprodex
Brand Names: Canada Ciprodex
Therapeutic Category Antibiotic/Corticosteroid, Otic
Generic Availability (U.S.) No
Use Treatment of acute otitis media in pediatric patients with tympanostomy tubes due to *S. aureus*, *S. pneumoniae*, *H. influenzae*, *M. catarrhalis*, or *P. aeruginosa*; acute otitis externa in children and adults due to *S. aureus* or *P. aeruginosa*

Pregnancy Risk Factor C

Pregnancy Considerations Animal reproduction studies have not been conducted with this combination. Refer to individual agents.

Breast-Feeding Considerations It is not known if serum levels of ciprofloxacin or dexamethasone are high enough following otic administration to produce detectable quantities in breast milk. Due to the potential for serious adverse reactions in the nursing infant, the manufacturer recommends a decision be made whether to discontinue nursing or to discontinue the drug, taking into account the importance of treatment to the mother. Refer to individual agents.

Contraindications Hypersensitivity to ciprofloxacin, other quinolones, dexamethasone, or any component; herpes simplex or other viral infections of the external ear canal

Warnings For otic use only; do not administer parenterally or ophthalmically

Adverse Reactions Also see individual agents.
Dermatologic: Pruritus of ear
Otic: Otalgia
Rare but important or life-threatening: Auditory impairment, oral candidiasis, superinfection

Drug Interactions

Metabolism/Transport Effects None known.

Avoid Concomitant Use There are no known interactions where it is recommended to avoid concomitant use.

Increased Effect/Toxicity There are no known significant interactions involving an increase in effect.

Decreased Effect There are no known significant interactions involving a decrease in effect.

Stability Store at room temperature; avoid freezing; protect from light

Mechanism of Action Ciprofloxacin is a fluoroquinolone antibiotic; dexamethasone is a corticosteroid used to decrease inflammation accompanying bacterial infections

Pharmacokinetics (Adult data unless noted) Time to peak serum concentration: 15 minutes to 2 hours post dose application

Dosing: Usual Otic: Children ≥6 months and Adults: Acute otitis media in patients with tympanostomy tubes or acute otitis externa: Instill 4 drops into affected ear(s) twice daily for 7 days

Administration To avoid dizziness which may result from the instillation of a cold solution, warm bottle in hand for 1-2 minutes. Shake suspension well before using; avoid contamination of the tip of the bottle to fingers, ear, or any surfaces. Patient should lie with affected ear upward and maintain position for 60 seconds after suspension is instilled.

Acute otitis media with tympanostomy tubes: Instill drops then gently press the tragus 5 times in a pumping motion to allow the drops to pass through the tube into the middle ear.

Acute otitis externa: Gently pull the outer ear lobe upward and backward to allow the drops to flow down into the ear canal.

Test Interactions See individual agents.

Dosage Forms Excipient information presented when available (limited, particularly for generics); consult specific product labeling.

Suspension, otic:
Ciprodex: Ciprofloxacin 0.3% and dexamethasone 0.1% (7.5 mL) [contains benzalkonium chloride]

References

Roland PS, Dohar JE, Lanier BJ, et al, "Topical Ciprofloxacin/Dexamethasone Otic Suspension is Superior to Ofloxacin Otic Solution in the Treatment of Granulation Tissue in Children With Acute Otitis Media With Otorrhea Through Tympanostomy Tubes," *Otolaryngol Head Neck Surg*, 2004, 130(6):736-41.

Ciprofloxacin and Hydrocortisone
(sip roe FLOKS a sin & hye droe KOR ti sone)

Related Information

Ciprofloxacin (Otic) *on page 476*
Hydrocortisone (Topical) *on page 1038*
Brand Names: U.S. Cipro® HC
Brand Names: Canada Cipro® HC
Therapeutic Category Antibiotic/Corticosteroid, Otic
Generic Availability (U.S.) No
Use Treatment of acute bacterial otitis externa due to susceptible strains of *S. aureus*, *P. aeruginosa*, or *Proteus mirabilis*

Pregnancy Risk Factor C

Pregnancy Considerations Animal reproduction studies have not been conducted with this combination. Refer to individual agents.

Breast-Feeding Considerations It is not known if serum levels of ciprofloxacin or hydrocortisone are high enough following otic administration to produce detectable quantities in breast milk. Refer to individual agents.

Contraindications Hypersensitivity to ciprofloxacin, hydrocortisone, any component, or other quinolones; patients with perforated tympanic membrane; patients with viral infections of the external ear canal

Adverse Reactions Central nervous system: Headache
Rare but important or life-threatening: Alopecia, fungal dermatitis, hypersensitivity reactions, migraine, paresthesia

Drug Interactions

Metabolism/Transport Effects None known.

Avoid Concomitant Use There are no known interactions where it is recommended to avoid concomitant use.

Increased Effect/Toxicity There are no known significant interactions involving an increase in effect.

Decreased Effect There are no known significant interactions involving a decrease in effect.

Dosing: Usual Children ≥1 year and Adults: Otic: Instill 3 drops into the affected ear(s) twice daily for 7 days

Administration Otic: Warm suspension by holding bottle in hand prior to instillation; shake well before use; patient should lie with affected ear upward and maintain position for 30-60 seconds after suspension is instilled into the ear canal

Test Interactions See individual agents.

Dosage Forms Excipient information presented when available (limited, particularly for generics); consult specific product labeling.

Suspension, otic:

Cipro® HC: Ciprofloxacin hydrochloride 0.2% and hydrocortisone 1% (10 mL) [contains benzyl alcohol]

◆ **Ciprofloxacin Hydrochloride** see Ciprofloxacin (Ophthalmic) on page 475

◆ **Ciprofloxacin Hydrochloride** see Ciprofloxacin (Otic) on page 476

◆ **Ciprofloxacin Hydrochloride** see Ciprofloxacin (Systemic) on page 471

◆ **Ciprofloxacin Hydrochloride and Dexamethasone** see Ciprofloxacin and Dexamethasone on page 477

◆ **Ciprofloxacin Hydrochloride and Hydrocortisone** see Ciprofloxacin and Hydrocortisone on page 477

◆ **Ciprofloxacin Injection (Can)** see Ciprofloxacin (Systemic) on page 471

◆ **Cipro® HC** see Ciprofloxacin and Hydrocortisone on page 477

◆ **Cipro in D₅W** see Ciprofloxacin (Systemic) on page 471

◆ **Cipro XR** see Ciprofloxacin (Systemic) on page 471

Cisapride (SIS a pride)

Medication Safety Issues
Sound-alike/look-alike issues:
Propulsid® may be confused with propranolol

Brand Names: U.S. Propulsid®

Therapeutic Category Gastrointestinal Agent, Prokinetic

Generic Availability (U.S.) No

Use Treatment of nocturnal symptoms of gastroesophageal reflux disease (GERD), also demonstrated effectiveness for gastroparesis, refractory constipation, and nonulcer dyspepsia in patients failing other therapies

Prescribing and Access Restrictions In U.S., available via limited-access protocol only. Call 877-795-4247 for more information.

Medication Guide Available Yes

Pregnancy Risk Factor C

Pregnancy Considerations Adverse events were observed in animal reproduction studies.

Breast-Feeding Considerations Cisapride is excreted into breast milk. The manufacturer recommends caution be used if administered to a nursing woman.

Contraindications Hypersensitivity to cisapride or any component; GI hemorrhage, mechanical obstruction, GI perforation, or other situations when GI motility stimulation is dangerous; patients with CHF, renal failure, multisystem organ failure, and COPD; patients at risk for developing or who have hypokalemia, hypocalcemia, or hypomagnesemia (eg, severe dehydration, vomiting, diarrhea, malnutrition, or receiving chronic diuretic therapy); patients with a known family history of congenital long-QT syndrome; prolonged QT intervals (QT_c >450), ventricular

arrhythmias, ischemic heart disease, sinus node dysfunction, clinically significant bradycardia, and second or third degree AV block; patients receiving medications known to prolong the QT interval such as quinidine, procainamide, sotalol, amitriptyline (and other tricyclic antidepressants), maprotiline, phenothiazines, sertindole, astemizole, bepridil, or sparfloxacin; serious cardiac arrhythmias including ventricular tachycardia, ventricular fibrillation, torsade de pointes, and QT prolongations have been reported in patients taking medications which inhibit cytochrome P450 3A4; some of these events have been fatal; do not coadminister with ketoconazole, itraconazole, fluconazole, miconazole, erythromycin, clarithromycin, nefazodone, delavirdine, indinavir, nelfinavir, ritonavir, saquinavir, or troleandomycin; do not coadminister with grapefruit juice

Warnings Serious cardiac arrhythmias including ventricular tachycardia, ventricular fibrillation, torsade de pointes, and QT prolongation have been reported in patients receiving cisapride **[U.S. Boxed Warning]**; more than 270 cases have been reported including 70 fatalities; 85% of these cases occurred in patients with known risk factors; for this reason, cisapride is available only for use in patients with severely debilitating conditions who meet specific criteria for a limited-access program directly through PRA International; for more information contact them at 877-795-4247

Precautions Use with caution in neonates, particularly if premature due to a potential increased risk of serious cardiac arrhythmias; decreased cisapride clearance found in neonates may result in increased serum levels; a 12-lead ECG (measuring QT intervals) should be done in all patients before beginning therapy

Adverse Reactions
Cardiovascular: Tachycardia

Central nervous system: Anxiety, extrapyramidal effects, fatigue, headache, insomnia, somnolence,

Dermatologic: Rash

Gastrointestinal: Abdominal cramping, constipation, diarrhea (dose dependent), nausea

Respiratory: Coughing, increased incidence of viral infection, rhinitis, sinusitis, upper respiratory tract infection

Rare but important or life-threatening: Apnea, bronchospasm, gynecomastia, hyperprolactinemia, methemoglobinemia, photosensitivity, psychiatric disturbances, seizure (have been reported only in patients with a history of seizure)

Drug Interactions
Metabolism/Transport Effects Substrate of CYP1A2 (minor), CYP2A6 (minor), CYP2B6 (minor), CYP2C19 (minor), CYP2C9 (minor), CYP3A4 (major); **Note:** Assignment of Major/Minor substrate status based on clinically relevant drug interaction potential; **Inhibits** CYP2D6 (weak), CYP3A4 (weak)

Avoid Concomitant Use
Avoid concomitant use of Cisapride with any of the following: Amitriptyline; Antifungal Agents (Azole Derivatives, Systemic); Aprepitant; Bepridil [Off Market]; Bicalutamide; Boceprevir; Cobicistat; Conivaptan; Fosaprepitant; Fusidic Acid (Systemic); Highest Risk QTc-Prolonging Agents; Ivabradine; Macrolide Antibiotics; Mifepristone; Moderate Risk QTc-Prolonging Agents; Nefazodone; Pimozide; Protease Inhibitors; Protriptyline; Simeprevir; Telaprevir

Increased Effect/Toxicity
Cisapride may increase the levels/effects of: Alcohol (Ethyl); Bepridil [Off Market]; Highest Risk QTc-Prolonging Agents; Lomitapide; NIFEdipine; Pimozide

The levels/effects of Cisapride may be increased by: Amitriptyline; Antifungal Agents (Azole Derivatives, Systemic); Aprepitant; Bicalutamide; Boceprevir; Cimetidine; Cobicistat; Conivaptan; CYP3A4 Inhibitors (Moderate); CYP3A4 Inhibitors (Strong); Fosaprepitant; Fusidic Acid (Systemic); Grapefruit Juice; Ivabradine; Ivacaftor; Luliconazole; Macrolide Antibiotics; Mifepristone; Moderate Risk QTc-Prolonging Agents; Nefazodone; Protease Inhibitors; Protriptyline; QTc-Prolonging Agents (Indeterminate Risk and Risk Modifying); Simeprevir; Stiripentol; Telaprevir

Decreased Effect There are no known significant interactions involving a decrease in effect.

Food Interactions Coadministration of grapefruit juice with cisapride increases the bioavailability of cisapride. Management: Avoid consumption of grapefruit/grapefruit juice during cisapride therapy.

Mechanism of Action Enhances the release of acetylcholine at the myenteric plexus. *In vitro* studies have shown cisapride to have serotonin-4 receptor agonistic properties which may increase gastrointestinal motility and cardiac rate; increases lower esophageal sphincter pressure and lower esophageal peristalsis; accelerates gastric emptying of both liquids and solids.

Pharmacodynamics Onset of action: 0.5-1 hour

Pharmacokinetics (Adult data unless noted)
Distribution: Breast milk to plasma ratio: 0.045
Protein binding: 98%
Metabolism: Extensive in liver via cytochrome P450 isoenzyme CYP 3A3/4 to norcisapride, which is eliminated in urine and feces
Bioavailability: 40% to 50%
Half-life: 7-10 hours
Elimination: <10% of dose excreted into feces and urine

Dosing: Neonatal Oral: 0.15-0.2 mg/kg/dose 3-4 times/day; maximum dose: 0.8 mg/kg/day

Dosing: Usual Oral:
Infants and Children: 0.15-0.3 mg/kg/dose 3-4 times/day; maximum dose: 10 mg/dose
Adults: Initial: 10 mg 4 times/day at least 15 minutes before meals and at bedtime; in some patients the dosage will need to be increased to 20 mg to obtain a satisfactory result

Dosage adjustment in liver dysfunction: Reduce daily dosage by 50%

Administration Oral: Administer 15 minutes before meals or feeding

Monitoring Parameters ECG (prior to beginning therapy), serum electrolytes in patients on diuretic therapy (prior to beginning therapy and periodically thereafter)

References

Cucchiara S, Staiano A, Boccieri A, et al, "Effects of Cisapride on Parameters of Oesophageal Motility and on the Prolonged Intra-oesophageal pH Test in Infants With Gastro-Oesophageal Reflux Disease," *Gut*, 1990, 31(1):21-5.

Hill SL, Evangelista KJ, Pizzi AM, et al, "Proarrhythmia Associated With Cisapride in Children," *Pediatrics*, 1998, 101(6):1053-6.

Hofmeyr GJ and Sonnendecker EW, "Secretion of the Gastrokinetic Agent Cisapride in Human Milk," *Eur J Clin Pharmacol*, 1986, 30 (6):735-6.

Khongphatthanayothin A, Lane J, Thomas D, et al, "Effects of Cisapride on QT Interval in Children," *J Pediatr*, 1998, 133(1):51-6.

Lander A, "The Risks and Benefits of Cisapride in Premature Neonates, Infants and Children," *Arch Dis Child*, 1998, 79:469-71.

Lewin MB, Bryant RM, Fenrich AL, et al, "Cisapride-Induced QT Interval," *J Pediatr*, 1996, 128(2):279-81.

Tolia V, "Long-Term Use of Cisapride in Premature Neonates of <34 Weeks Gestational Age," *J Pediatr Gastroenterol Nutr*, 1990, 11:420-2.

Van Eygen M and Van Ravensteyn H, "Effect of Cisapride on Excessive Regurgitation in Infants," *Clin Ther*, 1989, 11(5):669-77.

Cisapride (sis a tra KYOO ree um)

Medication Safety Issues
Sound-alike/look-alike issues:
Nimbex may be confused with NovoLOG
High alert medication:
The Institute for Safe Medication Practices (ISMP) includes this medication among its list of drugs which have a heightened risk of causing significant patient harm when used in error.
Other safety concerns:
United States Pharmacopeia (USP) 2006: The Interdisciplinary Safe Medication Use Expert Committee of the USP has recommended the following:
- Hospitals, clinics, and other practice sites should institute special safeguards in the storage, labeling, and use of these agents and should include these safeguards in staff orientation and competency training.
- Healthcare professionals should be on high alert (especially vigilant) whenever a neuromuscular-blocking agent (NMBA) is stocked, ordered, prepared, or administered.

Brand Names: U.S. Nimbex
Brand Names: Canada Nimbex
Therapeutic Category Neuromuscular Blocker Agent, Nondepolarizing; Skeletal Muscle Relaxant, Paralytic
Generic Availability (U.S.) Yes
Use Adjunct to general anesthesia, to facilitate endotracheal intubation, and provide skeletal muscle relaxation during surgery or mechanical ventilation (FDA approved in ages 1 month to 12 years and adults)
Pregnancy Risk Factor B
Pregnancy Considerations Adverse events have not been observed in animal reproduction studies.
Breast-Feeding Considerations It is not known if cisatracurium is excreted in breast milk. The manufacturer recommends that caution be exercised when administering cisatracurium to nursing women.
Contraindications Hypersensitivity to cisatracurium or any component
Warnings Ventilation must be supported during neuromuscular blockade; cisatracurium should only be administered by individuals who are experienced in the maintenance of an adequate airway and respiratory support. Due to its intermediate onset of action, cisatracurium is not recommended for rapid sequence intubation. Cisatracurium does not alter consciousness; use in conjunction with adequate sedation or anesthesia. Severe allergic reactions have been reported with neuromuscular blocking agents including cisatracurium; cross-sensitivity with other neuromuscular-blocking agents may occur; use extreme caution in patients with previous anaphylactic reactions.

Some multiple use vials (10 mL) may contain benzyl alcohol as a preservative; benzyl alcohol may cause allergic reactions in susceptible individuals; large amounts of benzyl alcohol (≥99 mg/kg/day) have been associated with a potentially fatal toxicity ("gasping syndrome") in neonates; the "gasping syndrome" consists of metabolic acidosis, respiratory distress, gasping respirations, CNS dysfunction (including convulsions, intracranial hemorrhage), hypotension, and cardiovascular collapse; avoid use of vials containing benzyl alcohol in neonates; *in vitro* and animal studies have shown that benzoate, a metabolite of benzyl alcohol, displaces bilirubin from protein-binding sites

Precautions Certain clinical conditions may result in potentiation or antagonism of neuromuscular blockade, see table. Increased sensitivity in patients with myasthenia gravis, Eaton-Lambert syndrome, resistance to neuromuscular blockade in burn patients (>30% of body) for period ▶

of 5-70 days postinjury; resistance to neuromuscular blockade in patients with muscle trauma, denervation, immobilization, infection. When used in conjunction with anesthetics, bradycardia may be more common with cisatracurium than with other neuromuscular-blocking agents; it has no clinically significant effects on heart rate to counteract the bradycardia produced by anesthetics.

Clinical Conditions Affecting Neuromuscular Blockade

Potentiation	Antagonism
Acidosis	Alkalosis
Acute intermittent porphyria	Demyelinating lesions
Electrolyte abnormalities	Diabetes mellitus
Hypermagnesemia	Hypercalcemia
Severe hypocalcemia	Peripheral neuropathies
Severe hypokalemia	
Severe hyponatremia	
Hepatic failure	
Neuromuscular diseases	
Renal failure	

Adverse Reactions Effects are minimal and transient: Acute quadriplegic myopathy syndrome (prolonged use), bradycardia, bronchospasm, flushing, hypotension, myositis ossificans (prolonged use), pruritus, rash

Drug Interactions

Metabolism/Transport Effects None known.

Avoid Concomitant Use

Avoid concomitant use of Cisatracurium with any of the following: QuiNINE

Increased Effect/Toxicity

Cisatracurium may increase the levels/effects of: Cardiac Glycosides; Corticosteroids (Systemic); OnabotulinumtoxinA; RimabotulinumtoxinB

The levels/effects of Cisatracurium may be increased by: AbobotulinumtoxinA; Aminoglycosides; Calcium Channel Blockers; Capreomycin; Clindamycin (Topical); Colistimethate; CycloSPORINE (Systemic); Fosphenytoin-Phenytoin; Inhalational Anesthetics; Ketorolac (Nasal); Ketorolac (Systemic); Lincosamide Antibiotics; Lithium; Loop Diuretics; Magnesium Salts; Polymyxin B; Procainamide; QuiNIDine; QuiNINE; Spironolactone; Tetracycline Derivatives; Vancomycin

Decreased Effect

The levels/effects of Cisatracurium may be decreased by: Acetylcholinesterase Inhibitors; Fosphenytoin-Phenytoin; Loop Diuretics

Stability Store intact vials at 2°C to 8°C (36°F to 46°F); protect from light; do not freeze. Use vials within 21 days upon removal from the refrigerator to room temperature (25°C to 77°F); unstable in alkaline solutions; **compatible** with D_5W, D_5NS, and NS; per the manufacturer, do not dilute in LR; dilutions of 0.1-0.2 mg/mL in NS or D_5W are stable for up to 24 hours at room temperature or under refrigeration and in D_5LR for up to 24 hours in the refrigerator. *Additional stability data:* Dilutions of 0.1, 2, and 5 mg/mL in D_5W or NS are stable in the refrigerator for up to 30 days; at room temperature (23°C), dilutions of 0.1 and 2 mg/mL began exhibiting substantial drug loss between 7-14 days; dilutions of 5 mg/mL in D_5W or NS are stable for up to 30 days at room temperature (23°C) (Xu, 1998); **incompatible** for Y-site administration with propofol or ketorolac; **compatible** for Y-site administration with sufentanil, alfentanil, fentanyl, midazolam, and droperidol.

Mechanism of Action Blocks neural transmission at the myoneural junction by binding with cholinergic receptor sites

Pharmacodynamics

Onset of action: I.V.: Within 2-3 minutes
Maximum effect: Within 3-5 minutes

Duration: Dose dependent, 35-45 minutes after a single 0.1 mg/kg dose; recovery begins in 20-35 minutes when anesthesia is balanced; recovery is attained in 90% of patients in 25-93 minutes

Pharmacokinetics (Adult data unless noted)

Distribution: V_d: Adults: 0.16 L/kg

Metabolism: Some metabolites are active; 80% of drug clearance is via a rapid nonenzymatic degradation (Hofmann elimination) in the bloodstream; additional metabolism occurs via ester hydrolysis

Half-life: 22-31 minutes

Elimination: <10% of dose excreted as unchanged drug in urine

Clearance:
Children: 5.9 mL/kg/minute
Adults: 5.1 mL/kg/minute

Dosing: Usual Paralysis/skeletal muscle relaxation: I.V.:

Infants and Children 1-23 months: 0.15 mg/kg over 5-10 seconds

Children ≥2 years and Adolescents: 0.1-0.15 mg/kg over 5-10 seconds (Martin, 1999; Playfor, 2007)

Adults: Initial: 0.15-0.2 mg/kg followed by maintenance dose of 0.03 mg/kg 40-65 minutes later or as needed to maintain neuromuscular blockade

Continuous I.V. infusion:

Infants, Children, and Adolescents: 1-4 mcg/kg/minute (0.06-0.24 mg/kg/hour); 3.9 ± 1.3 mcg/kg/minute (0.23 ± 0.08 mg/kg/hour) was the mean infusion rate needed to maintain neuromuscular blockade in 19 children (ages 3 months to 16 years) (Burnmester, 2005; Martin, 1999; Playfor, 2007)

Adults: 1-3 mcg/kg/minute (0.06-0.18 mg/kg/hour); **Note:** There may be wide interpatient variability in dosage (range: 0.5-10 mcg/kg/minute in adults) which may increase and decrease over time; optimize patient dosage by utilizing a peripheral nerve stimulator

Administration Parenteral: I.V. May be administered without further dilution by rapid I.V. injection over 5-10 seconds; for continuous I.V. infusions, dilute to a final concentration of 0.1-0.4 mg/mL in D_5W or NS; not for I.M. injection due to tissue irritation

Monitoring Parameters Muscle twitch response to peripheral nerve stimulation, heart rate, blood pressure, assisted ventilation status

Additional Information Neuromuscular blocking potency is 3 times that of atracurium; maximum block is up to 2 minutes longer than for equipotent doses of atracurium; laudanosine, a metabolite without neuromuscular blocking activity has been associated with hypotension and seizure activity in animal studies.

Dosage Forms Excipient information presented when available (limited, particularly for generics); consult specific product labeling.

Solution, Intravenous:
Nimbex: 10 mg/5 mL (5 mL)
Nimbex: 20 mg/10 mL (10 mL) [contains benzyl alcohol]
Nimbex: 10 mg/mL (20 mL)
Generic: 20 mg/10 mL (10 mL)
Solution, Intravenous [preservative free]:
Generic: 10 mg/5 mL (5 mL); 10 mg/mL (20 mL)

References

Burmester M and Mok Q, "Randomised Controlled Trial Comparing Cisatracurium and Vecuronium Infusions in a Paediatric Intensive Care Unit," *Intensive Care Med*, 2005, 31(5):686-92.

Martin LD, Bratton SL, and O'Rourke PP, "Clinical Uses and Controversies of Neuromuscular Blocking Agents in Infants and Children," *Crit Care Med*, 1999, 27(7):1358-68.

Playfor S, Jenkins I, Boyles C, et al, "Consensus Guidelines for Sustained Neuromuscular Blockade in Critically Ill Children," *Paediatr Anaesth*, 2007, 17(9):881-7.

Xu QA, Zhang YP, Trissel LA, et al, "Stability of Cisatracurium Besylate in Vials, Syringes, and Infusion Admixtures," *Am J Health Syst Pharm*, 1998, 55(10):1037-41.

◆ **Cisatracurium Besylate** see Cisatracurium on page 479

◆ **cis-DDP** see CISplatin on page 481

◆ **cis-Diamminedichloroplatinum** see CISplatin on page 481

CISplatin (SIS pla tin)

Medication Safety Issues
Sound-alike/look-alike issues:
CISplatin may be confused with CARBOplatin, oxaliplatin
High alert medication:
This medication is in a class the Institute for Safe Medication Practices (ISMP) includes among its list of drug classes which have a heightened risk of causing significant patient harm when used in error.
BEERS Criteria medication:
This drug may be potentially inappropriate for use in geriatric patients (Quality of evidence - moderate; Strength of recommendation - strong).
Administration issues:
Cisplatin doses >100 mg/m^2 once every 3 to 4 weeks are rarely used and should be verified with the prescriber.
Related Information
Emetogenic Potential of Antineoplastic Agents in Children on page 2327
Management of Drug Extravasations on page 2255
Safe Handling of Hazardous Drugs on page 2419
Brand Names: Canada AJ-Cisplatin; Cisplatin Injection; Cisplatin Injection BP
Therapeutic Category Antineoplastic Agent, Alkylating Agent; Antineoplastic Agent, Platinum Analog
Generic Availability (U.S.) Yes
Use Treatment of metastatic testicular cancer, advanced bladder cancer, and metastatic ovarian cancers (FDA approved in adults); has also been used in the treatment of central nervous system tumors, germ cell tumors, gestational trophoblastic disease (refractory), head and neck cancer, hepatobiliary cancer, hepatoblastoma, Hodgkin lymphoma, medulloblastoma, neuroblastoma, neuroendocrine tumors, non-Hodgkin lymphoma (NHL), osteosarcoma, soft tissue sarcomas, and unknown primary cancers
Pregnancy Risk Factor D
Pregnancy Considerations Adverse effects have been observed in animal reproduction studies. Women of childbearing potential should be advised to avoid pregnancy during treatment. May case fetal harm if administered during pregnancy.
Breast-Feeding Considerations Cisplatin is excreted in breast milk. Breast-feeding is not recommended by the manufacturer.
Contraindications Hypersensitivity to cisplatin, platinum-containing agents, or any component; preexisting renal impairment, hearing impairment, and myelosuppression
Warnings Hazardous agent; use appropriate precautions for handling and disposal (NIOSH, 2012). Anaphylactic reactions have been reported **[U.S. Boxed Warning]**; facial edema, bronchoconstriction, tachycardia, and hypotension may occur within minutes of administration. Epinephrine, corticosteroids, and antihistamines may be used to treat reactions. Doses >100 mg/m^2 once every 3-4 weeks are rarely used and should be verified with the prescriber **[U.S. Boxed Warning]**; use caution to prevent potential sound-alike/look-alike confusion between CISplatin and CARBOplatin, or prescribing practices that fail to differentiate daily dose versus total dose per cycle. Cumulative renal toxicity may be severe **[U.S. Boxed Warning]**; monitor serum creatinine, blood urea nitrogen, creatinine clearance, and serum electrolytes closely. According to the manufacturer's labeling, use is contraindicated in patients with preexisting renal impairment and renal function must return to normal prior to administering subsequent cycles;

some literature recommends reduced doses with renal impairment. Nephrotoxicity may be potentiated by aminoglycosides. Nausea and vomiting are dose-related toxicities **[U.S. Boxed Warning]**; may occur immediately and/or be delayed; occurs in >90% of pediatric patients (Dupuis, 2011); antiemetics are recommended. Diarrhea may also occur. Dose-related myelosuppression may occur **[U.S. Boxed Warning]**; manufacturer recommends that dose should not be repeated until platelets are ≥100,000/mm^3 and WBC ≥4,000/mm^3.

Ototoxicity, which may be especially pronounced in children, is manifested by tinnitus and/or loss of high frequency hearing, inability to hear normal conversational tone, and occasionally, deafness **[U.S. Boxed Warning]**; reported in 40% to 60% of pediatric patients with a single dose; may be unilateral or bilateral and may become more frequent and severe with repeated doses; may be immediate or delayed. Ototoxicity is cumulative and may be related to the peak plasma concentration. It is unclear whether ototoxity is reversible; risk is increased with prior or ongoing cranial irradiation, and may be more severe in patients less than 5 years old, those receiving concomitant ototoxic drugs (eg, aminoglycosides, vancomycin), and with renal impairment. Pediatric patients with certain genetic variations in the thiopurine S-methyltransferase (TPMT) gene may also be at increased risk of ototoxicity, even when conventional cisplatin doses are administered. Audiometric testing should be performed at baseline and prior to each dose. Pediatric patients should receive audiometric testing for several years after discontinuing therapy.

Severe (and possibly irreversible) neuropathies may occur with higher than recommended doses or more frequent administration; may require therapy discontinuation. Seizures, loss of motor function, loss of taste, leukoencephalopathy, and posterior reversible leukoencephalopathy syndrome (PRES [formerly RPLS]) have also been described. May cause ocular toxicity; optic neuritis, papilledema, cerebral blindness, blurred vision, and altered color perception have all been reported with use.

May cause electrolyte disturbances; serum electrolytes, particularly magnesium and potassium, should be monitored and replaced as needed during and after cisplatin therapy. May cause or exacerbate syndrome of inappropriate antidiuretic hormone secretion or hyponatremia; monitor sodium closely with initiation or dosage adjustments.

Hyperuricemia has been reported with cisplatin use, and is more pronounced with doses >50 mg/m^2; consider allopurinol therapy to reduce uric acid levels. Vascular toxicities have been reported when used in combination therapies; may include MI, cerebrovascular accident, thrombotic microangiopathy (hemolytic uremic syndrome), or cerebral arteritis. Secondary malignancies have been reported with cisplatin in combination with other chemotherapy agents. Local infusion site reactions may occur; cisplatin is a vesicant at higher concentrations, and an irritant at lower concentrations; ensure proper needle or catheter placement prior to and during infusion; avoid extravasation.
Precautions All patients should receive adequate hydration prior to (8-12 hours before dose) and for 24 hours after cisplatin administration; adequate urine output should also be maintained. Cisplatin should be administered under the supervision of an experienced cancer chemotherapy physician **[U.S. Boxed Warning]**.
Adverse Reactions
Central nervous system: Neurotoxicity, peripheral neuropathy
Gastrointestinal: Nausea and vomiting
Hematologic: Anemia, leukopenia, thrombocytopenia
Hepatic: Liver enzymes increased
Local: Tissue irritation

Renal: Nephrotoxicity (acute renal failure and chronic renal insufficiency)

Otic: Ototoxicity (as tinnitus, high frequency hearing loss; more common in children)

Rare but important or life-threatening: Alopecia (mild), anaphylactic reaction, arrhythmias, arterial vasospasm (acute), autonomic neuropathy, bradycardia, bronchoconstriction, cerebral arteritis, cerebrovascular accident, dehydration, extravasation injury, heart block, heart failure, hemolytic anemia (acute), hemolytic uremic syndrome, hypercholesterolemia, hyperuricemia, hypocalcemia, hypokalemia, hypomagnesemia, hyponatremia, hypophosphatemia, hypotension, leukoencephalopathy, Lhermitte's phenomenon, limb ischemia (acute), mesenteric ischemia (acute), mouth sores, myocardial infarction, myocardial ischemia, neutropenic typhlitis, optic neuritis, orthostatic hypotension, pancreatitis, papilledema, phlebitis, reversible posterior leukoencephalopathy syndrome (RPLS), seizures, serum amylase increased, SIADH, spinal cord injury, stroke, tachycardia, tetany, thrombophlebitis, thrombotic microangiopathy, thrombotic thrombocytopenic purpura, vision loss, visual color perception changes

Drug Interactions

Metabolism/Transport Effects None known.

Avoid Concomitant Use

Avoid concomitant use of CISplatin with any of the following: BCG; CloZAPine; Dipyrone; Natalizumab; Pimecrolimus; Tacrolimus (Topical); Tofacitinib; Vaccines (Live)

Increased Effect/Toxicity

CISplatin may increase the levels/effects of: Aminoglycosides; CloZAPine; Leflunomide; Natalizumab; Taxane Derivatives; Tofacitinib; Topotecan; Vaccines (Live); Vinorelbine

The levels/effects of CISplatin may be increased by: Denosumab; Dipyrone; Loop Diuretics; Pimecrolimus; Roflumilast; Tacrolimus (Topical); Trastuzumab

Decreased Effect

CISplatin may decrease the levels/effects of: BCG; Coccidioidin Skin Test; Fosphenytoin-Phenytoin; Sipuleucel-T; Vaccines (Inactivated); Vaccines (Live)

The levels/effects of CISplatin may be decreased by: Echinacea

Stability Store intact vials at 20°C to 25°C (68°F to 77°F); protect from light. Do not refrigerate solution as a precipitate may form. **Stability of diluted solutions is dependent on the chloride ion concentration** and should be mixed in solutions of NS (at least 0.3% NaCl). After initial entry into the vial, solution is stable for 28 days protected from light or for at least 7 days under fluorescent room light at room temperature.

Further dilutions in NS, $D_5/0.45\%$ NaCl or D_5/NS to a concentration of 0.05-2 mg/mL are stable for 72 hours at 4°C to 25°C. The infusion solution should have a final sodium chloride concentration $\geq 0.2\%$.

Mechanism of Action Inhibits DNA synthesis by the formation of DNA cross-links; denatures the double helix; covalently binds to DNA bases and disrupts DNA function; may also bind to proteins; the *cis*-isomer is 14 times more cytotoxic than the *trans*-isomer; both forms cross-link DNA but cis-platinum is less easily recognized by cell enzymes and, therefore, not repaired. Cisplatin can also bind two adjacent guanines on the same strand of DNA producing intrastrand cross-linking and breakage.

Pharmacokinetics (Adult data unless noted)

Distribution: I.V.: Rapid tissue distribution; high concentrations in kidneys, liver, uterus, and lungs

Protein binding: >90% (O'Dwyer, 2000)

Metabolism: Undergoes nonenzymatic metabolism; inactivated (in both cell and bloodstream) by sulfhydryl groups; covalently binds to glutathione and thiosulfate

Half-life, terminal:
Children:
Free drug: 1.3 hours
Total platinum: 44 hours
Adults: Initial: 14-49 minutes; Beta: 0.7-4.6 hours; Gamma: 24-127 hours (O'Dwyer, 2000)

Elimination: Urine and feces (minimal)

Dosing: Usual Note: Dosing and frequency may vary by protocol and/or treatment phase; refer to specific protocol.

Pediatric: **TO PREVENT POSSIBLE OVERDOSE, VERIFY ANY CISPLATIN DOSE EXCEEDING 100 mg/m^2 PER COURSE. Pretreatment hydration is recommended.**

Germ cell tumors: I.V.:
Infants: 0.7 mg/**kg**/dose every 3 weeks on days 1-5 in combination with bleomycin and etoposide (Cushing, 2004)

Children and Adolescents: 20 mg/m^2/dose every 3 weeks on days 1-5 in combination with bleomycin and etoposide (Cushing, 2004) **or** 100 mg/m^2 every 3 weeks on day 1 in combination with bleomycin and vinblastine or etoposide (Pinkerton, 1986)

Hepatoblastoma: I.V.:
Continuous I.V. infusion:
Infants and Children <10 kg: 2.7 mg/kg continuous infusion over 24 hours every 3 weeks on day 1 in combination with doxorubicin for 4-6 cycles (Pritchard, 2000)

Children ≥10 kg and Adolescents:
Monotherapy: **Note:** For use in standard-risk patients only: 80 mg/m^2 continuous infusion over 24 hours every 2 weeks on day 1

Combination therapy: 80 mg/m^2 continuous infusion over 24 hours every 3 weeks on day 1 in combination with doxorubicin (Perilongo, 2004; Perilongo, 2009; Pritchard, 2000).

Intermittent infusion (over 6 hours):
Infants and Children <10 kg: 3 mg/**kg**/dose given every 3 weeks on day 1 for 4-8 cycles in combination with vincristine and fluorouracil or continuous infusion doxorubicin (Douglass, 1993; Malogolowkin, 2008; Ortega, 2000)

Children and Adolescents: 90 mg/m^2/dose given every 3 weeks on day 1 for 4-8 cycles in combination with vincristine and fluorouracil or continuous infusion doxorubicin (Douglass, 1993; Malogolowkin, 2008; Ortega, 2000)

Medulloblastoma: Children ≥3 years and Adolescents: I.V.: 75 mg/m^2/dose every 6 weeks on either day 0 in combination with vincristine and cyclophosphamide or day 1 in combination with lomustine and vincristine of each chemotherapy cycle for 8 cycles (Packer, 2006; Packer, 2013)

Neuroblastoma, high-risk: Infants, Children, and Adolescents: I.V.: 50 mg/m^2/**day** on days 0-3 every 3 weeks in combination with etoposide (cycles 3 and 5) (Kreissman, 2013; Naranjo, 2011) or 50 mg/m^2/**day** on days 1-4 in combination with etoposide (cycles 3, 5, and 7) (Kushner, 1994)

Osteosarcoma: Children and Adolescents: I.V.: 60 mg/m^2/**day** for 2 days at weeks 2, 7, 25, and 28 (neoadjuvant) or weeks 5, 10, 25, and 28 (adjuvant) in combination with doxorubicin (Goorin, 2003) or 120 mg/m^2/**day** at weeks 0, 5, 12, and 17 in combination with doxorubicin (Meyers, 2005)

Adult: **TO PREVENT POSSIBLE OVERDOSE, VERIFY ANY CISPLATIN DOSE EXCEEDING 100 mg/m^2 PER COURSE. Pretreatment hydration is recommended.**
Note: Utilize patient's actual body weight (full weight) for calculation of body surface area- or weight-based dosing, particularly when the intent of therapy is curative; manage regimen-related toxicities in the same manner as for nonobese patients; if a dose reduction is utilized due to toxicity, consider resumption of full weight-based dosing with subsequent cycles, especially if cause of toxicity (eg, hepatic or renal impairment) is resolved (Griggs, 2012).

Bladder cancer, advanced: I.V.: 50-70 mg/m^2 every 3-4 weeks; heavily pretreated patients: 50 mg/m^2 every 4 weeks

Ovarian cancer, metastatic: I.V.:
Single agent: 100 mg/m^2 every 4 weeks
Combination therapy: 75-100 mg/m^2 every 4 weeks or 75 mg/m^2 every 3 weeks (Ozols, 2003)

Testicular cancer, metastatic: I.V.: 20 mg/m2/day for 5 days repeated every 3 weeks (Cushing, 2004; Saxman, 1998)

Dosing adjustment in renal impairment: Note: The manufacturer(s) recommend that repeat courses of cisplatin should not be given until serum creatinine is <1.5 mg/dL and/or BUN is <25 mg/dL and use is contraindicated in preexisting renal impairment. The following adjustments have been recommended:

Aronoff, 2007: All patients:
GFR >50 mL/minute/1.73 m^2: No dosage adjustment necessary
GFR 10-50 mL/minute/1.73 m^2: Administer 75% of dose
GFR <10 mL/minute/1.73 m^2: Administer 50% of dose
Hemodialysis: Partially cleared by hemodialysis: Administer 50% of dose posthemodialysis
Peritoneal dialysis: Administer 50% of dose
Continuous renal replacement therapy (CRRT): Administer 75% of dose

Kintzel, 1995: Adult:
CrCl 46-60 mL/minute: Administer 75% of dose
CrCl 31-45 mL/minute: Administer 50% of dose
CrCl ≤30 mL/minute: Consider use of alternative drug

Dosing adjustment in hepatic impairment: There are no dosage adjustments provided in the manufacturer's labeling; however, cisplatin undergoes nonenzymatic metabolism and predominantly renal elimination; therefore, dosage adjustment is likely not necessary.

Administration Hazardous agent; use appropriate precautions for handling and disposal (NIOSH, 2012).

Pretreatment hydration is recommended prior to cisplatin administration; adequate posthydration and urinary output (>100 mL/hour in adults) should be maintained for 24 hours after administration.

I.V.: Infuse over 6-8 hours; has also been infused over 30 minutes to 3 hours, at a rate of 1 mg/minute, or as a continuous infusion; infusion rate varies by protocol (refer to specific protocol for infusion details)

Needles or I.V. administration sets that contain aluminum should not be used in the preparation or administration; aluminum may react with cisplatin resulting in precipitate formation and loss of potency.

Vesicant (at higher concentrations); ensure proper needle or catheter placement prior to and during infusion; avoid extravasation. If extravasation occurs, stop infusion immediately and disconnect (leave cannula/needle in place); gently aspirate extravasated solution (do **NOT** flush the line); initiate sodium thiosulfate antidote; elevate extremity. Dimethyl sulfoxide (DMSO) may also be considered an option (See Management of Drug Extravasations for more details).

Vesicant/Extravasation Risk Vesicant (>0.4 mg/mL); Irritant (≤0.4 mg/mL)

Monitoring Parameters Renal function tests (serum creatinine, BUN, CrCl), electrolytes (particularly magnesium, calcium, potassium), audiography (baseline and prior to each subsequent dose and following treatment), neurologic exam (with high dose), liver function tests periodically, CBC with differential and platelet count (weekly), urine output, urinalysis

Dosage Forms Excipient information presented when available (limited, particularly for generics); consult specific product labeling.
Solution, Intravenous:
Generic: 50 mg/50 mL (50 mL); 100 mg/100 mL (100 mL)
Solution, Intravenous [preservative free]:
Generic: 50 mg/50 mL (50 mL); 100 mg/100 mL (100 mL); 200 mg/200 mL (200 mL)

References
Aronoff GR, Bennett WM, Berns JS, et al, *Drug Prescribing in Renal Failure: Dosing Guidelines for Adults and Children,* 5th ed. Philadelphia, PA: American College of Physicians; 2007.
Cisplatin [prescribing information]. New York, NY: Pfizer Labs; April 2012.
Cisplatin [prescribing information]. Rockford, IL: Mylan Institutional LLC; October 2013.
Cushing B, Giller R, Cullen JW, et al, "Randomized Comparison of Combination Chemotherapy With Etoposide, Bleomycin, and Either High-Dose or Standard-Dose Cisplatin in Children and Adolescents With High-Risk Malignant Germ Cell Tumors: A Pediatric Intergroup Study – Pediatric Oncology Group 9049 and Children's Cancer Group 8882," *J Clin Oncol,* 2004, 22(13):2691-700.
Dupuis LL, Boodhan S, Sung L, "Guideline for the Classification of the Acute Emetogenic Potential of Antineoplastic Medication in Pediatric Cancer Patients," *Pediatr Blood Cancer,* 2011, 57(2):191-8.
Goorin AM, Schwartzentruber DJ, Devidas M, et al, "Presurgical Chemotherapy Compared With Immediate Surgery and Adjuvant Chemotherapy for Nonmetastatic Osteosarcoma: Pediatric Oncology Group Study POG-8651," *J Clin Oncol,* 2003, 21(8):1574-80.
Kintzel PE and Dorr RT, "Anticancer Drug Renal Toxicity and Elimination: Dosing Guidelines for Altered Renal Function," *Cancer Treat Rev,* 1995, 21(1):33-64.
Kreismann SG, Seeger RC, Matthay KK, et al. Purged versus nonpurged peripheral blood stem-cell transplantation for high-risk neuroblastoma (COG A3973): a randomized phase 3 trial. *Lancet Oncol.* 2013;14:999-1008.
Kushner BH, LaQuaglia MP, Bonilla MA, et al, "Highly Effective Induction Therapy for Stage 4 Neuroblastoma in Children Over 1 Year of Age," *J Clin Oncol,* 1994, 12(12):2607-13.
Meyers PA, Schwartz CL, Krailo M, et al. Osteosarcoma: a randomized, prospective trial of the addition of ifosfamide and/or muramyl tripeptide to cisplatin, doxorubicin, and high-dose methotrexate. *J Clin Oncol.* 2005;23(9):2004-2011.
Naranjo A, Parisi MT, Shulkin BL, et al, "Comparison of ^{123}I-metaiodobenzylguanidine (MIBG) and ^{131}I-MIBG Semi-Quantitative Scores in Predicting Survival in Patients With Stage 4 Neuroblastoma: A Report from the Children's Oncology Group," *Pediatr Blood Cancer,* 2011, 56 (7):1041-5.
National Institute for Occupational Safety and Health (NIOSH), "NIOSH List of Antineoplastic and Other Hazardous Drugs in Healthcare Settings 2012." Available at http://www.cdc.gov/niosh/docs/2012-150/pdfs/2012-150.pdf. Accessed January 21, 2013.
O'Dwyer PJ, Stevenson JP and Johnson SW, "Clinical Pharmacokinetics and Administration of Established Platinum Drugs," *Drugs,* 2000, 59 (Suppl 4):19-27.
Ozols RF, Bundy BN, Greer BE, et al, "Phase III Trial of Carboplatin and Paclitaxel Compared With Cisplatin and Paclitaxel in Patients With Optimally Resected Stage III Ovarian Cancer: A Gynecologic Oncology Group Study," *J Clin Oncol,* 2003, 21(17):3194-200.
Packer RJ, Gajjar A, Vezina G, et al, "Phase III Study of Craniospinal Radiation Therapy Followed by Adjuvant Chemotherapy for Newly Diagnosed Average-Risk Medulloblastoma," *J Clin Oncol,* 2006, 24 (25):4202-8.
Packer RJ, Zhou T, Holmes E, Vezina G, Gajjar A. Survival and secondary tumors in children with medulloblastoma receiving radiotherapy and adjuvant chemotherapy: results of Chidlren's Oncology Group trial A9961. *Neuro-Oncology.* 2013;15(1):97-103.
Pegram MD, Pienkowski T, Northfelt DW, et al, "Results of Two Open-Label, Multicenter Phase II Studies of Docetaxel, Platinum Salts, and Trastuzumab in HER2-Positive Advanced Breast Cancer," *J Natl Cancer Inst,* 2004, 96(10):759-69.
Perilongo G, Maibach R, Shafford E, et al. Cisplatin versus cisplatin plus doxorubicin for standard-risk hepatoblastoma. *NEJM.* 2009;361:1662-1670.
Perilongo G, Shafford E, Maibach R, et al. Risk-adapted treatment for childhood hepatoblastoma: final report of the second study of the International Society of Paediatric Oncology – SIOPEL 2. *Eur J Cancer.* 2004;40(3):411-421.

Pinkerton CR, Pritchard J, and Spitz L, "High Complete Response Rate in Children With Advanced Germ Cell Tumors Using Cisplatin-Containing Combination Chemotherapy," *J Clin Oncol*, 1986, 4(2):194-9.

Pritchard J, Brown J, Shafford E, et al, "Cisplatin, Doxorubicin, and Delayed Surgery for Childhood Hepatoblastoma: A Successful Approach–Results of the First Prospective Study of the International Society of Pediatric Oncology," *J Clin Oncol*, 2000, 18(22):3819-28.

Reece PA, Stafford I, Abbott RL, et al, "Two-Versus 24-Hour Infusion of Cisplatin: Pharmacokinetic Considerations," *J Clin Oncol*, 1989, 7 (2):270-5.

Saxman SB, Finch D, Gonin R, et al, "Long-Term Follow-Up of a Phase III Study of Three Versus Four Cycles of Bleomycin, Etoposide, and Cisplatin in Favorable-Prognosis Germ-Cell Tumors: The Indian University Experience," *J Clin Oncol*, 1998, 16(2):702-6.

◆ **Cisplatin Injection (Can)** see CISplatin *on page 481*

◆ **Cisplatin Injection BP (Can)** see CISplatin *on page 481*

◆ *Cis*-**Retinoic Acid** see ISOtretinoin *on page 1161*

◆ **13-*cis*-Retinoic Acid** see ISOtretinoin *on page 1161*

◆ **13-*cis*-Vitamin A Acid** see ISOtretinoin *on page 1161*

Citalopram (sye TAL oh pram)

Medication Safety Issues
Sound-alike/look-alike issues:
CeleXA® may be confused with CeleBREX®, Cerebyx®, Ranexa™, ZyPREXA®

BEERS Criteria medication:
This drug may be potentially inappropriate for use in geriatric patients (Quality of evidence - moderate; Strength of recommendation - strong).

Related Information
Antidepressant Agents *on page 2219*

Brand Names: U.S. CeleXA

Brand Names: Canada
Apo-Citalopram®; Auro-Citalopram; Ava-Citalopram; Celexa®; Citalopram-Odan; CO Citalopram; CTP 30; Dom-Citalopram; JAMP-Citalopram; Manda-Citalopram; Mint-Citalopram; Mylan-Citalopram; PHL-Citalopram; PMS-Citalopram; Q-Citalopram; RAN™-Citalo; ratio-Citalopram; Riva-Citalopram; Sandoz-Citalopram; Septa-Citalopram; Teva-Citalopram

Therapeutic Category Antidepressant, Selective Serotonin Reuptake Inhibitor (SSRI)

Generic Availability (U.S.) Yes

Use Treatment of depression (FDA approved in adults); has also been used to treat obsessive-compulsive disorder (OCD)

Medication Guide Available Yes

Pregnancy Risk Factor C

Pregnancy Considerations
Adverse events have been observed in animal reproduction studies. Citalopram and its metabolites cross the human placenta. An increased risk of teratogenic effects, including cardiovascular defects, may be associated with maternal use of citalopram or other SSRIs; however, available information is conflicting. Nonteratogenic effects in the newborn following SSRI/SNRI exposure late in the third trimester include respiratory distress, cyanosis, apnea, seizures, temperature instability, feeding difficulty, vomiting, hypoglycemia, hypo- or hypertonia, hyper-reflexia, jitteriness, irritability, constant crying, and tremor. Symptoms may be due to the toxicity of the SSRIs/SNRIs or a discontinuation syndrome and may be consistent with serotonin syndrome associated with SSRI treatment. Persistent pulmonary hypertension of the newborn (PPHN) has also been reported with SSRI exposure. The long-term effects of *in utero* SSRI exposure on infant development and behavior are not known.

Due to pregnancy-induced physiologic changes, women who are pregnant may require adjusted doses of citalopram to achieve euthymia. The ACOG recommends that therapy with SSRIs or SNRIs during pregnancy be individualized; treatment of depression during pregnancy should incorporate the clinical expertise of the mental health clinician, obstetrician, primary healthcare provider, and pediatrician. According to the American Psychiatric Association (APA), the risks of medication treatment should be weighed against other treatment options and untreated depression. For women who discontinue antidepressant medications during pregnancy and who may be at high risk for postpartum depression, the medications can be restarted following delivery. Treatment algorithms have been developed by the ACOG and the APA for the management of depression in women prior to conception and during pregnancy.

Breast-Feeding Considerations
Citalopram and its metabolites are excreted in breast milk. According to the manufacturer, the decision to continue or discontinue breast-feeding during therapy should take into account the risk of exposure to the infant and the benefits of treatment to the mother. Excessive somnolence, decreased feeding, colic, irritability, restlessness, and weight loss have been reported in breast-fed infants. The long-term effects on development and behavior have not been studied; therefore, citalopram should be prescribed to a mother who is breast-feeding only when the benefits outweigh the potential risks. Maternal use of an SSRI during pregnancy may cause delayed milk secretion.

Contraindications
Hypersensitivity to citalopram or any component; use with MAO inhibitors within 14 days (potentially fatal reactions may occur); concurrent use of pimozide

Warnings
Clinical worsening of depression or suicidal ideation and behavior may occur in children and adults with major depressive disorder **[U.S. Boxed Warning]**. In clinical trials, antidepressants increased the risk of suicidal thinking and behavior (suicidality) in children, adolescents, and young adults (18-24 years of age) with major depressive disorder and other psychiatric disorders. This risk must be considered before prescribing antidepressants for any clinical use. Short-term studies did **not** show an increased risk of suicidality with antidepressant use in patients >24 years of age and showed a decreased risk in patients ≥65 years.

Patients of all ages who are treated with antidepressants for any indication require appropriate monitoring and close observation for clinical worsening of depression, suicidality, and unusual changes in behavior, especially during the first few months after antidepressant initiation or when the dose is adjusted. Family members and caregivers should be instructed to closely observe the patient (ie, daily) and communicate condition with healthcare provider. Patients should also be monitored for associated behaviors (eg, anxiety, agitation, panic attacks, insomnia, irritability, hostility, aggressiveness, impulsivity, akathisia, hypomania, mania) which may increase the risk for worsening depression or suicidality. Worsening depression or emergence of suicidality (or associated behaviors listed above) that is abrupt in onset, severe, or not part of the presenting symptoms, may require discontinuation or modification of drug therapy. Selective serotonin reuptake inhibitor (SSRI)-associated behavioral activation (ie, restlessness, hyperkinesis, hyperactivity, agitation) is two- to threefold more prevalent in children compared to adolescents; it is more prevalent in adolescents compared to adults. Somnolence (including sedation and drowsiness) is more common in adults compared to children and adolescents (Safer, 2006).

Avoid abrupt discontinuation; withdrawal syndrome with discontinuation symptoms (including agitation, dysphoria, anxiety, confusion, dizziness, hypomania, nightmares, irritability, sensory disturbances, headache, lethargy, emotional lability, insomnia, tinnitus, and seizures) may occur if therapy is abruptly discontinued or dose reduced; taper the dose to minimize risks of discontinuation symptoms. If intolerable symptoms occur following a decrease in dosage or upon discontinuation of therapy, consider resuming the previous dose with a more gradual taper. To reduce risk of intentional overdose, write prescriptions for the smallest quantity consistent with good patient care.

May worsen psychosis in some patients or precipitate a shift to mania or hypomania in patients with bipolar disorder. Monotherapy in patients with bipolar disorder should be avoided. Patients presenting with depressive symptoms should be screened for bipolar disorder. Citalopram is not FDA approved for the treatment of bipolar depression.

Citalopram use may result in a dose-dependent QT_c prolongation, which may be associated with torsade de pointes, ventricular tachycardia, or sudden death. Citalopram is not recommended in patients with congenital long QT syndrome, certain conditions (eg, bradycardia, heart failure, or recent acute MI), with concomitant medications which prolong the QT interval, or conditions that cause hypokalemia and/or hypomagnesemia; electrolyte and/or more frequent ECG monitoring is recommended if citalopram use is essential. Avoid doses >40 mg/day due to increased risk of QT_c prolongation; higher doses have also not been shown to be more effective in treating depression in clinical trials. Citalopram should be discontinued in patients with a persistent QT_c >500 msec. Patients experiencing symptoms of cardiac arrhythmias (dizziness, palpitations, or syncope) should be evaluated further including cardiac monitoring.

Potentially fatal serotonin syndrome (SS) or neuroleptic malignant syndrome (NMS)-like reactions have occurred with SSRIs and serotonin/norepinephrine reuptake inhibitors (SNRIs) when used alone and particularly when used in combination with serotonergic drugs (eg, triptans), drugs that impair the metabolism of serotonin (eg, MAO inhibitors, linezolid), or antidopaminergic agents (eg, antipsychotics). Identification and differentiation of SS (eg, tremor, myoclonus, agitation) and more severe NMS-like reactions (eg, hyperthermia, muscle rigidity, autonomic instability, mental status changes) can be complex; monitor patients closely for either syndrome. Discontinue treatment (and any concomitant serotonergic and/or antidopaminergic agents) immediately if signs or symptoms arise and initiate supportive symptomatic therapy. Tryptophan (which can be metabolized to serotonin) and the herbal medicine St John's wort (*Hypericum perforatum*) may increase serious side effects. Concomitant use of other SSRIs, SNRIs or tryptophan with citalopram is not recommended. Concurrent use or use within 2 weeks of discontinuing MAO inhibitors is contraindicated. In addition, allow at least 14 days after stopping citalopram before starting an MAO inhibitor.

Precautions Citalopram may impair platelet aggregation and cause abnormal bleeding (eg, ecchymosis, purpura, upper GI bleeding); risk may be increased in patients with impaired platelet aggregation and with concurrent use of aspirin, NSAIDs, warfarin, or other drugs that affect coagulation; bleeding related to SSRI or SNRI use has been reported to range from relatively minor bruising and epistaxis to life-threatening hemorrhage. Citalopram may impair cognitive or motor performance. Use with caution in patients with seizure disorders, concomitant illnesses that may effect hepatic metabolism or hemodynamic responses (eg, unstable cardiac disease, recent MI), and in suicidal patients; use with caution and decrease dose in patients with hepatic dysfunction; use with caution in patients with severe renal impairment.

Use with caution during third trimester of pregnancy [newborns may experience adverse effects or withdrawal symptoms (consider risk and benefits); exposure to SSRIs late in pregnancy may also be associated with an increased risk for persistent pulmonary hypertension of the newborn (Chambers, 2006)]; high doses of citalopram have been associated with teratogenicity in animals. Use with caution in patients receiving diuretics or those who are volume depleted (may cause hyponatremia or SIADH). SSRI-associated vomiting is two- to threefold more prevalent in children compared to adolescents and is more prevalent in adolescents compared to adults (Safer, 2006). No clinical studies have assessed the combined use of citalopram and electroconvulsive therapy; however, use with caution in patients receiving electroconvulsive therapy; may increase the risks associated with electroconvulsive therapy, consider discontinuing, when possible, prior to electroconvulsive therapy treatment.

Adverse Reactions

Cardiovascular: Bradycardia, hypotension, orthostatic hypotension, QT prolongation, tachycardia

Central nervous system: Agitation, amnesia, anorexia, anxiety, apathy, concentration impaired, confusion, depression, fatigue (dose related), fever, insomnia (dose related), migraine, somnolence (dose related), suicide attempt, yawning (dose related)

Dermatologic: Pruritus, rash

Endocrine & metabolic: Amenorrhea, dysmenorrhea, libido decreased

Gastrointestinal: Abdominal pain, anorexia, appetite increased, diarrhea, dyspepsia, flatulence, nausea, salivation increased, taste perversion, vomiting, weight gain/ loss, xerostomia

Genitourinary: Ejaculation disorder, impotence (dose related), polyuria

Neuromuscular & skeletal: Arthralgia, myalgia, paresthesia, tremor

Ocular: Abnormal accommodation

Respiratory: Cough, rhinitis, sinusitis, upper respiratory tract infection

Miscellaneous: Diaphoresis (dose related)

Rare but important or life-threatening: Allergic reaction, alopecia, anaphylaxis, anemia, angina pectoris, angioedema, arthritis, asthma, atrial fibrillation, bronchitis, bundle branch block, bursitis, cardiac arrest, cardiac failure, cataracts, catatonia, cerebrovascular accident, cholelithiasis, delirium, delusions, dependence, depersonalization, diplopia, diverticulitis, duodenal ulcer, eczema, epidermal necrolysis, erythema multiforme, extrapyramidal symptoms, extrasystoles, galactorrhea, gastric ulcer, gastrointestinal hemorrhage, glaucoma, granulocytopenia, gynecomastia, hallucinations, hemolytic anemia, hepatic necrosis, hepatitis, hyperpigmentation, hypertension, hypertrichosis, hypoglycemia, hypokalemia, hyponatremia, hypothyroidism, leukocytosis, leukopenia, lymphadenopathy, lymphocytosis, lymphopenia, muscle weakness, myocardial infarction, myocardial ischemia, neuroleptic malignant syndrome, obesity, osteoporosis, pancreatitis, phlebitis, photosensitivity, pneumonia, priapism, prolactinemia, prothrombin decreased, psoriasis, psychosis, ptosis, pulmonary embolism, renal calculi, renal failure, rhabdomyolysis, seizures, serotonin syndrome, SIADH, spontaneous abortion, syncope, thrombocytopenia, thrombosis, torsade de pointes, transient ischemic attack, urinary incontinence, urinary retention, vaginal bleeding, ventricular arrhythmia, withdrawal syndrome

Drug Interactions

Metabolism/Transport Effects Substrate of CYP2C19 (major), CYP2D6 (minor), CYP3A4 (major); **Note:** Assignment of Major/Minor substrate status based on clinically relevant drug interaction potential; **Inhibits** CYP1A2 (weak), CYP2B6 (weak), CYP2C19 (weak), CYP2D6 (weak)

Avoid Concomitant Use

Avoid concomitant use of Citalopram with any of the following: Conivaptan; Dosulepin; Fluconazole; Fusidic Acid (Systemic); Highest Risk QTc-Prolonging Agents; ▶

◄ Iobenguane I 123; Ivabradine; Linezolid; MAO Inhibitors; Methylene Blue; Mifepristone; Moderate Risk QTc-Prolonging Agents; Pimozide; Tryptophan; Urokinase

Increased Effect/Toxicity

Citalopram may increase the levels/effects of: Agents with Antiplatelet Properties; Anticoagulants; Antidepressants (Serotonin Reuptake Inhibitor/Antagonist); Antipsychotics; Apixaban; Aspirin; BusPIRone; CarBAMazepine; Collagenase (Systemic); Dabigatran Etexilate; Desmopressin; Dextromethorphan; Dosulepin; Highest Risk QTc-Prolonging Agents; Hypoglycemic Agents; Ibritumomab; Methylene Blue; Mexiletine; NSAID (COX-2 Inhibitor); NSAID (Nonselective); Pimozide; Rivaroxaban; Salicylates; Serotonin Modulators; Thiazide Diuretics; Thrombolytic Agents; Tositumomab and Iodine I 131 Tositumomab; TraMADol; Tricyclic Antidepressants; Urokinase; Vitamin K Antagonists

The levels/effects of Citalopram may be increased by: Alcohol (Ethyl); Analgesics (Opioid); Antiemetics (5HT3 Antagonists); Antipsychotics; BusPIRone; Cimetidine; CNS Depressants; Conivaptan; CYP2C19 Inhibitors (Moderate); CYP2C19 Inhibitors (Strong); CYP3A4 Inhibitors (Moderate); CYP3A4 Inhibitors (Strong); Fluconazole; Fusidic Acid (Systemic); Glucosamine; Herbs (Anticoagulant/Antiplatelet Properties); Ibrutinib; Ivabradine; Ivacaftor; Linezolid; Lithium; Luliconazole; MAO Inhibitors; Metoclopramide; Metyrosine; Mifepristone; Moderate Risk QTc-Prolonging Agents; Multivitamins/Fluoride (with ADE); Multivitamins/Minerals (with ADEK, Folate, Iron); Multivitamins/Minerals (with AE, No Iron); Nonsteroidal Anti-Inflammatory Agents; Omega-3 Fatty Acids; Pentosan Polysulfate Sodium; Pentoxifylline; Prostacyclin Analogues; QTc-Prolonging Agents (Indeterminate Risk and Risk Modifying); Simeprevir; Stiripentol; Tipranavir; TraMADol; Tricyclic Antidepressants; Tryptophan; Vitamin E

Decreased Effect

Citalopram may decrease the levels/effects of: Iobenguane I 123; Ioflupane I 123; Thyroid Products

The levels/effects of Citalopram may be decreased by: Bosentan; CarBAMazepine; CYP2C19 Inducers (Strong); CYP3A4 Inducers (Strong); Cyproheptadine; Dabrafenib; Deferasirox; Mitotane; Nonsteroidal Anti-Inflammatory Agents; NSAID (COX-2 Inhibitor); NSAID (Nonselective); Peginterferon Alfa-2b; Rifampin; Siltuximab; St Johns Wort; Tocilizumab

Stability Store at 25°C (77°F); excursions permitted to 15°C to 30°C (59°F to 86°F).

Mechanism of Action A racemic bicyclic phthalane derivative, citalopram selectively inhibits serotonin reuptake in the presynaptic neurons and has minimal effects on norepinephrine or dopamine. Uptake inhibition of serotonin is primarily due to the *S*-enantiomer of citalopram. Displays little to no affinity for serotonin, dopamine, adrenergic, histamine, GABA, or muscarinic receptor subtypes.

Pharmacodynamics

Onset of action: 1-2 weeks
Maximum effect: 8-12 weeks
Duration: 1-2 days

Pharmacokinetics (Adult data unless noted)

Distribution: V_d: Adults: 12 L/kg
Protein binding, plasma: ~80%
Metabolism: Extensively hepatic, primarily via CYP3A4 and CYP2C19; metabolized to N-demethylated, N-oxide, and deaminated metabolites
Bioavailability: 80%; tablets and oral solution are bioequivalent
Half-life elimination: Adults: Range: 24-48 hours; mean: 35 hours (doubled with hepatic impairment)
Time to peak serum concentration: 1 to 6 hours, average within 4 hours
Elimination: Urine (10% as unchanged drug)

Clearance: Hepatic impairment: Decreased by 37%; Mild to moderate renal impairment: Decreased by 17%; Severe renal impairment (CrCl <20 mL/minute): No information available

Dosing: Usual

Children and Adolescents: **Note:** Slower titration of dose every 2-4 weeks may minimize risk of SSRI associated behavioral activation, which has been shown to increase risk of suicidal behavior. Doses >40 mg are not recommended due to risk of QT$_c$ prolongation.

Depression: Note: Not FDA approved. Limited information is available; only one randomized, placebo controlled trial has shown citalopram to be effective for the treatment of depression in pediatric patients (Wagner, 2004); other controlled pediatric trials have **not** shown benefit (Sharp, 2006; von Knorring, 2006; Wagner, 2005). Some experts recommend the following doses (Dopheide, 2006):

Children ≤11 years: Initial: 10 mg/day given once daily; increase dose slowly by 5 mg/day as clinically needed; dosage range: 20-40 mg/day

Children and Adolescents ≥12 years: Initial: 20 mg/day given once daily; increase dose slowly by 10 mg/day every 2 weeks as clinically needed; dosage range: 20-40 mg/day

Obsessive-compulsive disorder: Note: Not FDA approved. Limited information is available; several open label trials have been published (Mukaddes, 2003; Thomsen, 1997; Thomsen, 2001). Some experts recommend the following doses:

Children ≤11 years: Initial: 5-10 mg/day given once daily; increase dose slowly by 5 mg/day every 2 weeks as clinically needed; dosage range: 10-40 mg/day.

Children and Adolescents ≥12 years: Initial: 10-20 mg/day given once daily; increase dose slowly by 10 mg/day every 2 weeks as clinically needed; dosage range: 10-40 mg/day.

Note: Higher mg/kg doses are needed in children compared to adolescents.

Adults: **Depression:**

Patients <60 years: Initial: 20 mg once daily; may increase dose in 20 mg increments at intervals of ≥1 week up to a maximum daily dose: 40 mg/day

Patients ≥60 years, poor metabolizers of CYP2C19 **or** concurrent use of moderate to strong CYP2C19 inhibitors (eg, cimetidine): 20 mg/day

Dosage adjustment in renal impairment: Adults:
Mild or moderate renal impairment: No dosage adjustment needed
Severe renal impairment (CrCl <20 mL/minute): Use with caution

Dosage adjustment in hepatic impairment: Adults: 20 mg once daily due to increased serum concentrations and the risk of QT prolongation

Administration May be administered without regard to meals

Monitoring Parameters ECG; electrolytes (potassium and magnesium concentrations); liver function tests and CBC with continued therapy; monitor patient periodically for symptom resolution; monitor for worsening depression, suicidality, and associated behaviors (especially at the beginning of therapy or when doses are increased or decreased). Monitor for anxiety, social functioning, mania, panic attacks; akathisia

Additional Information If used for an extended period of time, long-term usefulness of citalopram should be periodically re-evaluated for the individual patient. A recent report describes 5 children (age: 8-15 years) who developed epistaxis (n=4) or bruising (n=1) while receiving SSRI therapy (sertraline) (Lake, 2000).

Neonates born to women receiving SSRIs later during the third trimester may experience respiratory distress, apnea, cyanosis, temperature instability, vomiting, feeding difficulty, hypoglycemia, constant crying, irritability, hypotonia, hypertonia, hyper-reflexia, tremor, jitteriness, and seizures; these symptoms may be due to a direct toxic effect, withdrawal syndrome, or (in some cases) serotonin syndrome. Withdrawal symptoms occur in 30% of neonates exposed to SSRIs *in utero*; monitor newborns for at least 48 hours after birth; long-term effects of *in utero* exposure to SSRIs are unknown (Levinson-Castiel, 2006).

Dosage Forms Excipient information presented when available (limited, particularly for generics); consult specific product labeling.

Solution, Oral:
Generic: 10 mg/5 mL (240 mL)
Tablet, Oral:
CeleXA: 10 mg
CeleXA: 20 mg, 40 mg [scored]
Generic: 10 mg, 20 mg, 40 mg

References

Bernard L, Stern R, Lew D, et al, "Serotonin Syndrome After Concomitant Treatment With Linezolid and Citalopram," *Clin Infect Dis*, 2003, 36(9):1197.

Chambers CD, Hernandez-Diaz S, Van Marter LJ, et al, "Selective Serotonin-Reuptake Inhibitors and Risk of Persistent Pulmonary Hypertension of the Newborn," *N Engl J Med*, 2006, 354(6):579-87.

Dopheide JA, "Recognizing and Treating Depression in Children and Adolescents," *Am J Health Syst Pharm*, 2006, 63(3):233-43.

Lake MB, Birmaher B, Wassick S, et al, "Bleeding and Selective Serotonin Reuptake Inhibitors in Childhood and Adolescence," *J Child Adolesc Psychopharmacol*, 2000, 10(1):35-8.

Levinson-Castiel R, Merlob P, Linder N, et al, "Neonatal Abstinence Syndrome After *in utero* Exposure to Selective Serotonin Reuptake Inhibitors in Term Infants," *Arch Pediatr Adolesc Med*, 2006, 160 (2):173-6.

Mahlberg R, Kunz D, Sasse J, et al, "Serotonin Syndrome With Tramadol and Citalopram," *Am J Psychiatry*, 2004, 161(6):1129.

Mukaddes NM, Abali O, and Kaynak N, "Citalopram Treatment of Children and Adolescents With Obsessive-Compulsive Disorder: A Preliminary Report," *Psychiatry Clin Neurosci*, 2003, 57(4):405-8.

Pass SE and Simpson RW, "Discontinuation and Reinstitution of Medications During the Perioperative Period," *Am J Health Syst Pharm*, 2004, 61(9):899-912.

Reinblatt SP and Riddle MA, "Selective Serotonin Reuptake Inhibitors-Induced Apathy: A Pediatric Case Series," *J Child Adolesc Psychopharmacol*, 2006, 6(1/2):227-33.

Safer DJ and Zito JM, "Treatment Emergent Adverse Effects of Selective Serotonin Reuptake Inhibitors by Age Group: Children vs. Adolescents," *J Child Adolesc Psychopharmacol*, 2006, 16 (1/2):159-69.

Sharp SC and Hellings JA, "Efficacy and Safety of Selective Serotonin Reuptake Inhibitors in the Treatment of Depression in Children and Adolescents: Practitioner Review," *Clin Drug Investig*, 2006, 26 (5):247-55.

Tahir N, "Serotonin Syndrome as a Consequence of Drug-Resistant Infections: An Interaction Between Linezolid and Citalopram," *J Am Med Dir Assoc*, 2004, 5(2):111-3.

Thomsen PH, "Child and Adolescent Obsessive-Compulsive Disorder Treated With Citalopram: Findings From an Open Trial of 23 Cases," *J Child Adolesc Psychopharmacol*, 1997, 7(3):157-66.

Thomsen PH, Ebbesen C, and Persson C, "Long-Term Experience With Citalopram in the Treatment of Adolescent OCD," *J Am Acad Child Adolesc Psychiatry*, 2001, 40(8):895-902.

von Knorring AL, Olsson GI, Thomsen PH, et al, "A Randomized, Double-Blind, Placebo-Controlled Study of Citalopram in Adolescents With Major Depressive Disorder," *J Clin Psychopharmacol*, 2006, 26 (3):311-5.

Wagner KD, "Pharmacotherapy for Major Depression in Children and Adolescents," *Prog Neuropsychopharmacol Biol Psychiatry*, 2005, 29 (5):819-26.

Wagner KD, Robb AS, Findling RL, et al, "A Randomized, Placebo-Controlled Trial of Citalopram for the Treatment of Major Depression in Children and Adolescents," *Am J Psych*, 2004, 161(6):1079-83.

◆ **Citalopram Hydrobromide** see Citalopram on page 484

◆ **Citalopram-Odan (Can)** see Citalopram on page 484

◆ **Citrate of Magnesia** see Magnesium Citrate on page 1292

◆ **Citric Acid and Potassium Citrate** see Potassium Citrate and Citric Acid on page 1710

◆ **Citric Acid and Sodium Citrate** see Sodium Citrate and Citric Acid on page 1906

Citric Acid, Sodium Citrate, and Potassium Citrate
(SIT rik AS id, SOW dee um SIT rate, & poe TASS ee um SIT rate)

Medication Safety Issues
Sound-alike/look-alike issues:
Polycitra may be confused with Bicitra
Brand Names: U.S. Cytra-3; Tricitrates
Therapeutic Category Alkalinizing Agent, Oral
Generic Availability (U.S.) Yes
Use As long-term therapy to alkalinize the urine for control and/or dissolution of uric acid and cystine calculi of the urinary tract [FDA approved in pediatric patients (age not specified) and adults]; treatment of chronic metabolic acidosis secondary to renal tubule disorders [FDA approved in pediatric patients (age not specified) and adults]; treatment of gout as adjuvant therapy with uricosuric drugs [FDA approved in pediatric patients (age not specified) and adults]. Has also been used for treatment of chronic metabolic acidosis due chronic diarrhea and some inborn errors of metabolism.
Pregnancy Risk Factor Not established
Pregnancy Considerations Use caution with toxemia of pregnancy.
Contraindications Hypersensitivity to sodium or potassium citrate or any component; severe renal impairment with oliguria or azotemia, Addison's disease (untreated) or severe myocardial damage
Warnings Some oral solutions contain sodium benzoate; benzoic acid (benzoate) is a metabolite of benzyl alcohol; large amounts of benzyl alcohol (≥99 mg/kg/day) have been associated with a potentially fatal toxicity ("gasping syndrome") in neonates; the "gasping syndrome" consists of metabolic acidosis, respiratory distress, gasping respirations, CNS dysfunction (including convulsions, intracranial hemorrhage), hypotension and cardiovascular collapse; use oral solution containing sodium benzoate with caution in neonates; *in vitro* and animal studies have shown that benzoate displaces bilirubin from protein binding sites. Some oral solutions contain propylene glycol; in neonates large amounts of propylene glycol (eg, >3000 mg/day I.V.) have been associated with potentially fatal toxicities which can include metabolic acidosis, seizures, renal failure, and CNS depression; use oral solutions containing propylene glycol with caution in neonates.
Precautions Use caution in patients with cardiac disease, sodium- or fluid-retaining conditions (eg, cardiac failure, hypertension, peripheral/pulmonary edema, toxemia of pregnancy), patients receiving other potassium-sparing drugs or cardiac glycosides; patients on either a sodium- or potassium-restricted diet, use of single agent citrate formulation may be preferable; avoid use of aluminum-based antacids. Use with caution in patients with renal disease; may cause hyperkalemia or metabolic alkalosis. Undiluted solution can cause GI irritation; dilute with water prior to administration.

Adverse Reactions
Cardiovascular: Cardiac abnormalities
Endocrine & metabolic: Calcium levels, hyperkalemia, hypernatremia, metabolic alkalosis
Gastrointestinal: Diarrhea
Neuromuscular & skeletal: Tetany

Drug Interactions
Metabolism/Transport Effects None known.
Avoid Concomitant Use There are no known interactions where it is recommended to avoid concomitant use.
Increased Effect/Toxicity
Citric Acid, Sodium Citrate, and Potassium Citrate may increase the levels/effects of: ACE Inhibitors; Aluminum

Hydroxide; Angiotensin II Receptor Blockers; Potassium-Sparing Diuretics

The levels/effects of Citric Acid, Sodium Citrate, and Potassium Citrate may be increased by: Eplerenone; Heparin; Heparin (Low Molecular Weight)

Decreased Effect There are no known significant interactions involving a decrease in effect.

Stability Store at controlled room temperature of 20°C to 25°C (68°F to 77°F), protect from excessive heating or freezing.

Pharmacokinetics (Adult data unless noted)
Metabolism: ≥95% via hepatic oxidation to bicarbonate
Elimination: <5% unchanged in the urine

Dosing: Neonatal Oral: **Note:** 1 mL of oral solution contains 2 mEq of bicarbonate
Dosing per mEq of bicarbonate: 2-3 mEq bicarbonate/kg/**day** (1-1.5 mL/kg/day) in 3-4 divided doses

Dosing: Usual Oral: **Note:** 1 mL of oral solution contains 2 mEq of bicarbonate
Manufacturer's recommendation: Children: 5-15 mL (10-30 mEq bicarbonate) per dose after meals and at bedtime
Alternative recommendation: Dosing per mEq of bicarbonate:
Infants and Children: 2–3 mEq bicarbonate/kg/**day** (1-1.5 mL/kg/**day**) in 3-4 divided doses
Adults: 15-30 mL (30-60 mEq bicarbonate) per dose after meals and at bedtime
Note: When using to alkalinize the urine, 10-15 mL doses given 4 times daily typically maintain urinary pH 6.5-7.4; doses 15-20 mL4 times daily usually maintain urinary pH at 7.0-7.6

Administration Dose should be diluted in water; may follow dose with additional water if necessary. Administer after meals and at bedtime to prevent osmotic saline laxative effect; shake well before use.

Monitoring Parameters Periodic serum (sodium, potassium, calcium, bicarbonate); urine pH

Additional Information Prior to absorption, citrate ions effects are similar to chloride and therefore, does not affect gastrointestinal pH or disturb digestion.
Oral solution: 1 mL contains 1 mEq potassium, 1 mEq sodium, and 2 mEq of bicarbonate

Dosage Forms Excipient information presented when available (limited, particularly for generics); consult specific product labeling. [DSC] = Discontinued product
Solution, oral:
Cytra-3: Citric acid 334 mg, sodium citrate 500 mg, and potassium citrate 550 mg per 5 mL (480 mL [DSC]) [equivalent to potassium 1 mEq, sodium 1 mEq, and bicarbonate 2 mEq per 1 mL; alcohol free, sugar free; contains sodium benzoate and propylene glycol; raspberry flavor]
Tricitrates: Citric acid 334 mg, sodium citrate 500 mg, and potassium citrate 550 mg per 5 mL (480 mL) [equivalent to potassium 1 mEq, sodium 1 mEq, and bicarbonate 2 mEq per 1 mL; alcohol free, sugar free; contains sodiuim benzoate and propylene glycol; raspberry flavor]

References
American Academy of Pediatrics Committee on Drugs. "Inactive" ingredients in pharmaceutical products: update (subject review). *Pediatrics.* 1997;99(2):268-278.
Gal P and Reed M, "Medications," Kliegman: Nelson Textbook of Pediatrics, 18th ed, 2007.
Shehab N, Lewis CL, Streetman DD, Donn SM. Exposure to the pharmaceutical excipients benzyl alcohol and propylene glycol among critically ill neonates. *Pediatr Crit Care Med.* 2009;10 (2):256-259.

◆ **Citroma [OTC]** *see* Magnesium Citrate *on page 1292*

◆ **Citro-Mag (Can)** *see* Magnesium Citrate *on page 1292*

◆ **Citrovorum Factor** *see* Leucovorin Calcium *on page 1213*

◆ **CL-232315** *see* MitoXANtrone *on page 1427*

Cladribine (KLA dri been)

Medication Safety Issues
Sound-alike/look-alike issues:
Cladribine may be confused with clevidipine, clofarabine, cytarabine, fludarabine
Leustatin may be confused with lovastatin

High alert medication:
This medication is in a class the Institute for Safe Medication Practices (ISMP) includes among its list of drug classes which have a heightened risk of causing significant patient harm when used in error.

Related Information
Emetogenic Potential of Antineoplastic Agents in Children *on page 2327*
Management of Drug Extravasations *on page 2255*
Safe Handling of Hazardous Drugs *on page 2419*

Therapeutic Category Antineoplastic Agent, Antimetabolite (Purine Analog)

Generic Availability (U.S.) Yes

Use Treatment of active hairy cell leukemia (FDA approved in adults); has also been used for acute myeloid leukemia and refractory Langerhans cell histiocytosis (LCH)

Pregnancy Risk Factor D

Pregnancy Considerations Teratogenic effects and fetal mortality were observed in animal reproduction studies. May cause fetal harm if administered during pregnancy. Women of reproductive potential should use highly effective contraception during treatment.

Breast-Feeding Considerations Due to the potential for serious adverse reactions in the nursing infant, the decision to discontinue cladribine or to discontinue breast-feeding should take into account the importance of treatment to the mother.

Contraindications Hypersensitivity to cladribine or any component

Warnings Hazardous agent; use appropriate precautions for handling and disposal (NIOSH, 2012). Dose-dependent myelosuppression (neutropenia, anemia, and thrombocytopenia) is common and generally reversible **[U.S. Boxed Warning]**; use with caution in patients with preexisting hematologic or immunologic abnormalities; monitor blood counts, especially during the first 4-8 weeks after treatment. Cladribine therapy is associated with fever (>100°F), with or without neutropenia; more commonly observed in the first month. Infections (bacterial, viral, and fungal) were reported more commonly in the first month after treatment (generally mild or moderate in severity, although serious infections, including sepsis, have been reported); the incidence is reduced in the second month. Due to neutropenia and T-cell depletion, the risk versus benefit of treatment should be evaluated in patients with active infection. Administration of live vaccines is not recommended during treatment with cladribine; may increase the risk of infection due to immunosuppression.

Serious, dose-related neurologic toxicity, including irreversible paraparesis and quadriparesis, has been reported with continuous infusions of higher doses (4-9 times the FDA approved dose) **[U.S. Boxed Warning]**; may also occur at approved doses (rare); neurotoxicity may be delayed and may present as progressive, irreversible weakness; diagnostics with electromyography and nerve conduction studies were consistent with demyelinating disease.

Acute nephrotoxicity (eg, acidosis, anuria, increased serum creatinine), possibly requiring dialysis, has been reported with high doses (4-9 times the FDA approved dose) **[U.S. Boxed Warning]**; particularly when administered with other nephrotoxic agents or in patients with renal impairment. With high tumor burden, tumor lysis syndrome and subsequent hyperuricemia may occur (rare); consider allopurinol and hydrate accordingly.

Weekly (7-day) infusion preparation recommends further dilution of cladribine with bacteriostatic normal saline which contains benzyl alcohol and may cause allergic reactions in susceptible individuals; large amounts of benzyl alcohol (≥99 mg/kg/day) have been associated with a potentially fatal toxicity ("gasping syndrome") in neonates; use should be avoided in neonates.

Precautions Use with caution in patients with hepatic impairment; not adequately evaluated. Should be administered under the supervision of an experienced cancer chemotherapy physician **[U.S. Boxed Warning]**.

Adverse Reactions

Cardiovascular: Edema, tachycardia, thrombosis

Central nervous system: Anxiety, chills, dizziness, fatigue, fever, headache, insomnia, malaise, pain

Dermatologic: Bruising, erythema, hyperhidrosis, petechiae, pruritus, purpura, rash

Gastrointestinal: Abdominal pain, appetite decreased, constipation, diarrhea, flatulence, nausea, vomiting

Hematologic: Anemia, myelosuppression, neutropenia, neutropenic fever, thrombocytopenia

Local: Injection site reactions, phlebitis

Neuromuscular & skeletal: Arthralgia, muscle weakness, myalgia, weakness

Respiratory: Abnormal breath sounds, abnormal chest sounds, cough, dyspnea, epistaxis, rales

Miscellaneous: Diaphoresis, infection

Rare but important or life-threatening: Aplastic anemia, bacteremia, CD4 lymphocytopenia (nadir: 4-6 months), cellulitis, consciousness decreased, conjunctivitis, hemolytic anemia, hypereosinophilia, hypersensitivity, myelodysplastic syndrome, opportunistic infections (cytomegalovirus, fungal infections, herpes virus infections, listeriosis, *Pneumocystis jirovecii*), pancytopenia (prolonged), paraparesis, pneumonia, polyneuropathy (with high doses), progressive multifocal leukoencephalopathy (PML), pulmonary interstitial infiltrates, quadriparesis (reported at high doses), renal dysfunction (with high doses), renal failure, septic shock, Stevens-Johnson syndrome, stroke, toxic epidermal necrolysis, tuberculosis reactivation, tumor lysis syndrome

Drug Interactions

Metabolism/Transport Effects None known.

Avoid Concomitant Use

Avoid concomitant use of Cladribine with any of the following: BCG; CloZAPine; Dipyrone; Natalizumab; Pimecrolimus; Tacrolimus (Topical); Tofacitinib; Vaccines (Live)

Increased Effect/Toxicity

Cladribine may increase the levels/effects of: CloZAPine; Leflunomide; Natalizumab; Tofacitinib; Vaccines (Live)

The levels/effects of Cladribine may be increased by: Denosumab; Dipyrone; Pimecrolimus; Roflumilast; Tacrolimus (Topical); Trastuzumab

Decreased Effect

Cladribine may decrease the levels/effects of: BCG; Coccidioidin Skin Test; Sipuleucel-T; Vaccines (Inactivated); Vaccines (Live)

The levels/effects of Cladribine may be decreased by: Echinacea

Stability Hazardous agent; use appropriate precautions for handling and disposal (NIOSH, 2012). Store intact vials at 2°C to 8°C (36°F to 46°F); protect from light. A precipitate may develop at low temperatures and may be resolubilized at room temperature or by shaking the solution vigorously. Inadvertent freezing does not affect the solution; if freezing occurs prior to dilution, allow to thaw naturally prior to reconstitution; do not heat or microwave; do not refreeze.

24-hour continuous I.V. infusion: Dilutions for infusion should be used promptly; if not used promptly, the 24-hour infusion may be stored refrigerated for up to 8 hours prior to administration

7-day continuous I.V. infusion: Dilutions for infusion should be used promptly; if not used promptly, the 7-day infusion may be stored refrigerated for up to 8 hours prior to administration. Reconstituted solution is stable for 7 days (when diluted in bacteriostatic NS) in a CADD® medication cassette reservoir. For patients weighing >85 kg, the effectiveness of the preservative in the bacteriostatic diluent may be reduced (due to dilution).

Mechanism of Action A purine nucleoside analogue; prodrug which is activated via phosphorylation by deoxycytidine kinase to a 5'-triphosphate derivative (2-CaAMP). This active form incorporates into DNA to result in the breakage of DNA strand and shutdown of DNA synthesis and repair. This also results in a depletion of nicotinamide adenine dinucleotide and adenosine triphosphate (ATP). Cladribine is cell-cycle nonspecific.

Pharmacokinetics (Adult data unless noted)

Distribution: V_d:

Pediatric patients (8 months to 18 years): 12.7 ± 8.5 L/kg; penetrates CSF (CSF concentrations are ~18% of plasma concentration) (Kearns, 1994)

Adults: ~9 L/kg; penetrates CSF (CSF concentrations are ~25% of plasma concentration)

Protein binding: ~20%

Half-life:

Pediatric patients (8 months to 18 years): 19.7 ± 3.4 hours (Kearns, 1994)

Adults: After a 2-hour infusion (with normal renal function): 5.4 hours

Elimination: Urine (18%)

Dosing: Usual

Infants, Children, and Adolescents (details concerning dosing in combination regimens and protocols should be consulted):

Acute myeloid leukemia: Limited data available: I.V.: 8.9 mg/m²/day continuous infusion for 5 days for 1 or 2 courses (Krance, 2001) or 9 mg/m²/day over 30 minutes for 5 days for 1 course (in combination with cytarabine) (Crews, 2002; Rubnitz, 2009)

Langerhans cell histiocytosis, refractory: Limited data available: I.V.: 5 mg/m²/day over 2 hours for 5 days every 21 days for up to 6 cycles (Weitzman, 2009)

Adults: Details concerning dosing in combination regimens should also be consulted. **Hairy cell leukemia:** I.V.: 0.09 mg/kg/day continuous infusion for 7 days for 1 cycle

Dosing adjustment in renal impairment: There are no dosage adjustments provided in the manufacturer's labeling (due to inadequate data); use with caution. The following guidelines have been used by some clinicians (Aronoff, 2007):

Infants, Children, and Adolescents:

GFR >50 mL/minute/1.73 m²: No adjustment required

GFR 10-50 mL/minute/1.73 m²: Administer 50% of dose

GFR <10 mL/minute/1.73 m²: Administer 30% of dose

Hemodialysis: Administer 30% of dose

Continuous renal replacement therapy (CRRT): Administer 50% of dose

Adults:

CrCl 10-50 mL/minute: Administer 75% of dose

CrCl <10 mL/minute: Administer 50% of dose

Continuous ambulatory peritoneal dialysis (CAPD): Administer 50% of dose

Dosing adjustment in hepatic impairment: Adults: There are no dosage adjustments provided in the manufacturer's labeling (due to inadequate data); use with caution.

Administration Hazardous agent; use appropriate precautions for handling and disposal (NIOSH, 2012).

Parenteral: I.V.: Further dilute prior to use, may be administered over 24 hours as a continuous infusion, or as an intermittent infusion over 30 minutes or 2 hours; dependent upon indication and/or protocol.

24-hour continuous infusion: Further dilute dose in NS (Adults: 500 mL); the manufacturer recommends filtering with a 0.22 micron hydrophilic syringe filter prior to adding to infusion bag

7-day supply, continuous infusion: Further dilute dose in bacteriostatic NS (Adults: 100 mL); add to CADD® medication cassette reservoir; the manufacturer recommends filtering with 0.22 micron filter prior to adding to cassette/reservoir

Vesicant/Extravasation Risk May be an irritant.

Monitoring Parameters CBC with differential (particularly during the first 4-8 weeks post-treatment); baseline and periodic renal and hepatic function tests; body temperature (fever); bone marrow biopsy (after CBC has normalized; to confirm treatment response); signs and symptoms of neurotoxicity

Dosage Forms Excipient information presented when available (limited, particularly for generics); consult specific product labeling.

Solution, Intravenous [preservative free]:
  Generic: 1 mg/mL (10 mL)

References

Aronoff GR, Bennett WM, Berns JS, et al, *Drug Prescribing in Renal Failure: Dosing Guidelines for Adults and Children*, 5th ed. Philadelphia, PA: American College of Physicians; 2007, p 170.

Crews KR, Gandhi V, Srivastava DK, et al, "Interim Comparison of a Continuous Infusion versus a Short Daily Infusion of Cytarabine Given in Combination With Cladribine for Pediatric Acute Myeloid Leukemia," *J Clin Oncol*, 2002, 20(20):4217-24.

Kearns CM, Biakley RL, Santane VM, et al, "Pharmacokinetics of Cladribine (2-Chlorodeoxyadenosine) in Children with Acute Leukemia," *Cancer Research*, 1994, 54:1235-39.

Krance RA, Hurwitz CA, Head DR, et al, "Experience With 2-Chlorodeoxyadenosine in Previously Untreated Children With Newly Diagnosed Acute Myeloid Leukemia and Myelodysplastic Diseases," *J Clin Oncol*, 2001, 19(11):2804-11.

Larson RA, et al, "Dose Escalation Trial of Cladribine Using 5 Daily I.V. Infusions in Patients with Advanced Hematologic Malignancies," *J Clin Oncol*, 1996, 14(1):188-95.

Liliemark J, "The Clinical Pharmacokinetics of Cladribine," *Clin Pharmacokinet*, 1997, 32:120-131.

National Institute for Occupational Safety and Health (NIOSH), "NIOSH List of Antineoplastic and Other Hazardous Drugs in Healthcare Settings 2012." Available at http://www.cdc.gov/niosh/docs/2012-150/pdfs/2012-150.pdf. Accessed January 21, 2013.

Rodriguez-Galindo C, Kelly P, Jeng M, et al, "Treatment of Children With Langerhans Cell Histiocytosis With 2-Chlorodeoxyadenosine," *Am J Hematol*, 2002, 69(3):179-84.

Rubnitz JE, Crews KR, Pounds S, et al, "Combination of Cladribine and Cytarabine is Effective for Childhood Acute Myeloid Leukemia: Results of the St Jude AML97 Trial," *Leukemia*, 2009, 23(8):1410-6.

Stine KC, Saylors RL, Williams LL, et al, "2-Chlorodeoxyadenosine (2-CDA) for the Treatment of Refractory or Recurrent Langerhans Cell Histiocytosis (LCH) in Pediatric Patients," *Med Pediatr Oncol*, 1997, 29:288-92.

Weitzman S, Braier J, Donadieu J, et al, "2'-Chlorodeoxyadenosine (2-CdA) as Salvage Therapy for Langerhans Cell Histiocytosis (LCH). Results of the LCH-S-98 Protocol of the Histiocyte Society," *Pediatr Blood Cancer*, 2009, 53(7):1271-6.

◆ **Claforan** *see* Cefotaxime *on page 404*

◆ **Claforan in D₅W** *see* Cefotaxime *on page 404*

◆ **Claravis** *see* ISOtretinoin *on page 1161*

◆ **Clarinex** *see* Desloratadine *on page 611*

◆ **Clarinex Reditabs** *see* Desloratadine *on page 611*

Clarithromycin (kla RITH roe mye sin)

Medication Safety Issues

Sound-alike/look-alike issues:

Clarithromycin may be confused with Claritin, clindamycin, erythromycin

Related Information

H. pylori Treatment in Pediatric Patients *on page 2311*
Oral Medications That Should Not Be Crushed or Altered *on page 2438*
Prevention of Infective Endocarditis *on page 2336*

Brand Names: U.S. Biaxin; Biaxin XL; Biaxin XL Pac

Brand Names: Canada Accel-Clarithromycin; Apo-Clarithromycin; Ava-Clarithromycin; Biaxin; Biaxin BID; Biaxin XL; Dom-Clarithromycin; Mylan-Clarithromycin; PMS-Clarithromycin; RAN-Clarithromycin; ratio-Clarithromycin; Riva-Clarithromycin; Sandoz-Clarithromycin; Teva-Clarithromycin

Therapeutic Category Antibiotic, Macrolide

Generic Availability (U.S.) Yes

Use

Immediate release formulations: Treatment of upper and lower respiratory tract infections, community-acquired pneumonia, acute otitis media, and infections of the skin and skin structure due to susceptible organisms (FDA approved in ages ≥6 months and adults); prophylaxis and treatment of *Mycobacterium avium* complex (MAC) disease in patients with advanced HIV infection (FDA approved in ages ≥20 months and adults); treatment of *Helicobacter pylori* infection (FDA approved in adults); has also been used for infective endocarditis prophylaxis for dental procedures in penicillin-allergic patients; treatment of lyme disease, peritonitis prophylaxis, and post-exposure prophylaxis and treatment of pertussis

Extended release tablets: Treatment of acute maxillary sinusitis, acute bacterial exacerbation of chronic bronchitis, and community acquired pneumonia due to susceptible organisms (FDA approved in adults)

Pregnancy Risk Factor C

Pregnancy Considerations Adverse events have been documented in some animal reproduction studies. Clarithromycin crosses the placenta (Witt, 2003). The manufacturer recommends that clarithromycin not be used in a pregnant woman unless there are no alternative therapies. Clarithromycin is generally not recommended for the treatment or prophylaxis of *Mycobacterium avium* complex (MAC) or bacterial respiratory disease in HIV-infected pregnant patients (DHHS, 2013).

Breast-Feeding Considerations Clarithromycin and its active metabolite (14-hydroxy clarithromycin) are excreted into breast milk. The manufacturer recommends that caution be used if administered to nursing women. Decreased appetite, diarrhea, rash, and somnolence have been noted in nursing infants exposed to macrolide antibiotics (Goldstein, 2009).

Contraindications Hypersensitivity to clarithromycin, any component, erythromycin, or any macrolide antibiotic; concurrent use with ergot derivatives, pimozide, cisapride, astemizole, terfenadine, lovastatin, simvastatin, and colchicine (if patient has concomitant renal or hepatic impairment); history of cholestatic jaundice or hepatic dysfunction with prior clarithromycin use; history of QT prolongation or ventricular arrhythmia, including torsade de pointes

Warnings Severe acute hypersensitivity reactions have (rarely) been reported, including anaphylaxis, Stevens-Johnson syndrome, toxic epidermal necrolysis, drug rash with eosinophilia, and systemic symptoms (DRESS), and Henoch-Schönlein purpura (IgA vasculitis); discontinue therapy immediately and urgently initiate treatment.

Prolonged use may result in fungal or bacterial superinfection, including *C. difficile*-associated diarrhea (CDAD) and pseudomembranous colitis; CDAD has been observed >2 months postantibiotic treatment. Macrolides have been associated with QT prolongation and rare cardiac conduction alterations; use is contraindicated in patients with a history of QT_c prolongation and ventricular arrhythmias, including torsade de pointes; use with caution in patients at risk for prolonged cardiac repolarization; avoid use in patients with uncorrected hypokalemia or hypomagnesemia, clinically significant bradycardia, and patients receiving Class IA (eg, quinidine, procainamide) or Class III (eg, amiodarone, dofetilide, sotalol) antiarrhythmic agents. Use caution with any agents with substantial metabolism through the CYP3A4 pathway; high potential for drug interactions exists.

Tablets (immediate and extended release) contain propylene glycol; toxicities have been reported with use of products containing propylene glycol, including hyperosmolality, lactic acidosis, seizures, and respiratory depression; in neonates large amounts of propylene glycol delivered orally, intravenously (eg, >3000 mg/day), or topically have been associated with potentially fatal toxicities which can include metabolic acidosis, seizures, renal failure, and CNS depression; use tablets containing propylene glycol with caution (AAP, 1997; Shehab, 2009).

Precautions Use with caution in patients with hepatic or renal impairment; reduce dosage or prolong dosing interval in patients with severe renal impairment with or without coexisting hepatic impairment. Hepatic impairment including elevated liver enzymes and hepatocellular and/or cholestatic hepatitis with or without jaundice have been reported; usually reversible after discontinuation of clarithromycin. May lead to hepatic failure or death (rarely), especially in the presence of preexisting hepatic disease and/or concomitant use of hepatotoxic medications; discontinue immediately if symptoms of hepatitis occur. Use caution in patients with myasthenia gravis; may exacerbate symptoms and new onset of symptoms has occurred. Clarithromycin in combination with ranitidine bismuth citrate should not be used in patients with a history of acute porphyria nor in patients with significant renal impairment (CrCl <25 mL/minute).

When clarithromycin and colchicine are coadministered together, inhibition of CYP3A and p-glycoprotein may lead to increased exposure to colchicine (monitor for symptoms of colchicine toxicity); if coadministration is necessary, reduction of colchicine dose is recommended (concomitant use is contraindicated in patients with hepatic or renal impairment). Other potentially significant drug interactions may exist, requiring dose or frequency adjustment, additional monitoring, and/or selection of alternative therapy. Consult drug interactions database for more detailed information. In combination with high-dose rifabutin therapy, uveitis has been reported. Use with caution in patients with CAD; postmarketing safety trial suggests increased risk of cardiovascular mortality with short-term clarithromycin use (vs placebo) in patients with stable CAD; however, more smokers were randomized to the clarithromycin arm (Jespersen, 2006).

For used for *Helicobacter pylori* eradication, short-term combination therapy (≤7 days) in adults has been associated with a higher incidence of treatment failure; current guidelines recommend 10 to 14 days of therapy (triple or quadruple) for eradication of *H. pylori* in children and adults (ACG [Chey], 2007; NASPHGAN [Koletzko], 2011).

Children may experience some adverse effects not reported in adults, or more frequently than adults, including rash, and vomiting. The extended release formulation consists of drug within a nondeformable matrix; following drug release/absorption, the matrix/shell is expelled in the stool. The use of nondeformable products in patients with known stricture/narrowing of the GI tract has been associated with symptoms of obstruction.

Adverse Reactions

Central nervous system: Headache, insomnia

Dermatologic: Skin rash (children)

Gastrointestinal: Abdominal pain, diarrhea, dysgeusia (adults), dyspepsia (adults), nausea (adults), vomiting (children)

Hematologic & oncologic: Prolonged prothrombin time (adults)

Hepatic: Abnormal hepatic function tests

Hypersensitivity: Anaphylactoid reaction

Infection: Candidiasis (including oral)

Renal: Increased blood urea nitrogen

Rare but important or life-threatening: Abnormal albuminglobulin ratio, agranulocytosis, anaphylaxis, anorexia, anosmia, asthma, atrial fibrillation, behavioral changes, bullous dermatitis, cardiac arrest, cellulitis, chest pain, cholestasis, cholestatic hepatitis, *Clostridium difficile* associated diarrhea, *Clostridium difficile* (colitis), confusion, decreased white blood cell count, dental discoloration (reversible with dental cleaning), depersonalization, depression, DRESS syndrome, dyskinesia, eosinophilia, extrasystoles, gastroesophageal reflux disease, glossitis, hallucination, hearing loss (reversible), hemorrhage, hepatic failure, hepatic insufficiency, hepatitis, hypersensitivity, hypoglycemia, IgA vasculitis, increased gamma-glutamyl transferase, increased INR, increased lactate dehydrogenase, increased serum alkaline phosphatase, increased serum ALT, increased serum AST, increased serum bilirubin, increased serum creatinine, infection, interstitial nephritis, jaundice, leukopenia, loss of consciousness, maculopapular rash, manic behavior, neutropenia, nightmares, pancreatitis, prolonged QT interval on ECG, pseudomembranous colitis, psychosis, pulmonary embolism, renal failure, rhabdomyolysis, seizure, Stevens-Johnson syndrome, stomatitis, thrombocytopenia, tongue discoloration, torsades de pointes, toxic epidermal necrolysis, vaginal infection, ventricular arrhythmia, ventricular tachycardia

Drug Interactions

Metabolism/Transport Effects Substrate of CYP3A4 (major); **Note:** Assignment of Major/Minor substrate status based on clinically relevant drug interaction potential; **Inhibits** CYP1A2 (weak), CYP3A4 (strong), P-glycoprotein

Avoid Concomitant Use

Avoid concomitant use of Clarithromycin with any of the following: Ado-Trastuzumab Emtansine; Alfuzosin; Apixaban; Avanafil; Axitinib; BCG; Bosutinib; Cabozantinib; Ceritinib; Cisapride; Conivaptan; Crizotinib; Dihydroergotamine; Disopyramide; Dronedarone; Eplerenone; Ergotamine; Everolimus; Fusidic Acid (Systemic); Halofantrine; Highest Risk QTc-Prolonging Agents; Ibrutinib; Ivabradine; Lapatinib; Lomitapide; Lovastatin; Lurasidone; Macitentan; Mifepristone; Nilotinib; Nisoldipine; PAZOPanib; Pimozide; QuiNIDine; QuiNINE; Ranolazine; Red Yeast Rice; Regorafenib; Salmeterol; Silodosin; Simeprevir; Simvastatin; Tamsulosin; Terfenadine; Ticagrelor; Tolvaptan; Topotecan; Toremifene; Ulipristal; Vemurafenib; VinCRIStine (Liposomal); Vorapaxar

Increased Effect/Toxicity

Clarithromycin may increase the levels/effects of: Ado-Trastuzumab Emtansine; Afatinib; Alfentanil; Alfuzosin; Almotriptan; Alosetron; ALPRAZolam; Antifungal Agents (Azole Derivatives, Systemic); Antineoplastic Agents (Vinca Alkaloids); Apixaban; ARIPiprazole; AtorvaSTATin; Avanafil; Axitinib; Bedaquiline; Boceprevir; Bortezomib; Bosentan; Bosutinib; Brentuximab Vedotin; Brinzolamide; Budesonide (Nasal); Budesonide (Systemic, Oral Inhalation); BusPIRone; Cabozantinib; Calcium Channel Blockers; Cannabis; CarBAMazepine; Cardiac Glycosides; Ceritinib; Cilostazol; Cisapride; CloZAPine; Cobicistat; Colchicine; Conivaptan; Corticosteroids (Orally Inhaled); Corticosteroids (Systemic); Crizotinib; CYP3A4 Inducers (Strong); CYP3A4 Substrates; Dabigatran Etexilate; Dienogest; Dihydroergotamine; Disopyramide; DOXOrubicin (Conventional); ▶

Dronabinol; Dronedarone; Dutasteride; Eletriptan; Eplerenone; Ergot Derivatives; Ergotamine; Estazolam; Everolimus; FentaNYL; Fesoterodine; Fluticasone (Nasal); Fluticasone (Oral Inhalation); GlipiZIDE; GlyBURIDE; GuanFACINE; Halofantrine; Highest Risk QTc-Prolonging Agents; Ibrutinib; Imatinib; Ivabradine; Ivacaftor; Ixabepilone; Lacosamide; Lapatinib; Levomilnacipran; Lomitapide; Lovastatin; Lurasidone; Macitentan; Maraviroc; MethylPREDNISolone; Midazolam; Moderate Risk QTc-Prolonging Agents; Nilotinib; Nisoldipine; Ospemifene; OxyCODONE; Paricalcitol; PAZOPanib; P-glycoprotein/ABCB1 Substrates; Pimecrolimus; Pimozide; Pitavastatin; PONATinib; Pravastatin; Protease Inhibitors; Prucalopride; QuiNIDine; QuiNINE; Ranolazine; Red Yeast Rice; Regorafenib; Repaglinide; Rifaximin; Rilpivirine; Rivaroxaban; Ruxolitinib; Salmeterol; Saxagliptin; Selective Serotonin Reuptake Inhibitors; Sildenafil; Silodosin; Simeprevir; Simvastatin; Sirolimus; Tacrolimus (Topical); Tadalafil; Tamsulosin; Telaprevir; Temsirolimus; Terfenadine; Tetrahydrocannabinol; Theophylline Derivatives; Ticagrelor; Tofacitinib; Tolterodine; Tolvaptan; Topotecan; Toremifene; Triazolam; Ulipristal; Vardenafil; Vemurafenib; Vilazodone; VinCRIStine (Liposomal); Vitamin K Antagonists; Vorapaxar; Zidovudine; Zopiclone

The levels/effects of Clarithromycin may be increased by: Antifungal Agents (Azole Derivatives, Systemic); Boceprevir; Cobicistat; Conivaptan; CYP3A4 Inducers (Strong); CYP3A4 Inhibitors (Moderate); CYP3A4 Inhibitors (Strong); Fusidic Acid (Systemic); Ivabradine; Luliconazole; Mifepristone; Protease Inhibitors; QTc-Prolonging Agents (Indeterminate Risk and Risk Modifying); Stiripentol; Telaprevir

Decreased Effect

Clarithromycin may decrease the levels/effects of: BCG; Clopidogrel; Ifosfamide; Prasugrel; Sodium Picosulfate; Ticagrelor; Typhoid Vaccine; Zidovudine

The levels/effects of Clarithromycin may be decreased by: Bosentan; CYP3A4 Inducers (Strong); Dabrafenib; Deferasirox; Efavirenz; Etravirine; Mitotane; Protease Inhibitors; Siltuximab; St Johns Wort; Tocilizumab

Food Interactions Immediate release: Food delays rate, but not extent of absorption; Extended release: Food increases clarithromycin AUC by ~30% relative to fasting conditions. Management: Administer immediate release products without regard to meals. Administer extended release products with food.

Stability
Tablets:
Extended release: Store at 20°C to 25°C (68°F to 77°F); excursions are permitted between 15°C and 30°C (59°F and 86°F).
Immediate release:
250 mg: Store at 15°C to 30°C (59°F to 86°F); protect from light.
500 mg: Store at 20°C to 25°C (68°F to 77°F).
Granules for oral suspension: Store at 15°C to 30°C (59°F to 86°F) prior to and following reconstitution. Do not refrigerate. Use within 14 days of reconstitution.

Mechanism of Action Exerts its antibacterial action by binding to 50S ribosomal subunit resulting in inhibition of protein synthesis. The 14-OH metabolite of clarithromycin is twice as active as the parent compound against certain organisms.

Pharmacokinetics (Adult data unless noted)
Absorption:
Immediate release: Rapid; food delays rate, but not extent of absorption
Extended release: Fasting is associated with ~30% lower AUC relative to administration with food
Distribution: Widely distributed throughout the body with tissue concentrations higher than serum concentrations;

manufacturer reports no data in regards to CNS penetration
Protein binding: 42% to 70% (Peters, 1992)
Metabolism: Partially hepatic via CYP3A4; converted to 14-OH clarithromycin (active metabolite); undergoes extensive first-pass metabolism
Bioavailability: ~50%
Half-life: Dose-dependent, prolonged with renal dysfunction
Clarithromycin:
250 mg dose: 3 to 4 hours
500 mg dose: 5 to 7 hours
14-hydroxy metabolite:
250 mg dose: 5 to 6 hours
500 mg dose: 7 to 9 hours
Time to peak serum concentration: Immediate release formulations: 2 to 3 hours; Extended release: 5 to 8 hours
Elimination: After a 250 mg or 500 mg tablet dose, 20% or 30% is excreted unchanged in urine, respectively; 10% to 15% is excreted as active metabolite 14-OH clarithromycin; feces (29% to 40% mostly as metabolites) (Ferrero, 1990)

Dosing: Usual
Pediatric: **Note:** All pediatric dosing recommendations based on immediate release product formulations (tablet and oral suspension):
General dosing, susceptible infection: Infants, Children, and Adolescents: Oral: 15 mg/kg/day divided every 12 hours; maximum single dose: 500 mg; duration dependent on infection site and severity; usually 7 to 14 days (*Red Book* [AAP], 2012)
Acute otitis media (AOM): Infants ≥6 months and Children: Oral: 15 mg/kg/day divided every 12 hours for 10 days; maximum single dose: 500 mg; **Note:** Due to increased *S. pneumoniae* and *H. influenzae* resistance, clarithromycin is not routinely recommended as a treatment option (Lieberthal, 2013)
Bartonellosis, treatment and secondary prophylaxis in HIV-exposed/-positive patients (excluding CNS infections and endocarditis): Limited data available: Oral:
Infants and Children: 15 mg/kg/day divided every 12 hours for at least 3 months; maximum single dose: 500 mg (CDC, 2009)
Adolescents: 500 mg twice daily administered for at least 3 months (DHHS [adult], 2013)
Endocarditis, prophylaxis; dental procedures in patients allergic to penicillins: Limited data available: Children and Adolescents: Oral: 15 mg/kg; maximum single dose: 500 mg; administer 30 to 60 minutes before procedure. **Note:** As of April 2007, the American Heart Association guidelines now recommend prophylaxis only in patients undergoing invasive procedures and in whom underlying cardiac conditions may predispose to a higher risk of adverse outcomes should infection occur (Wilson, 2007).
Group A streptococcal infection; rheumatic fever, primary prevention and treatment of streptococcal tonsillopharyngitis: Infants, Children, and Adolescents: Oral: 15 mg/kg/day divided every 12 hours for 10 days; maximum single dose: 250 mg (Gerber, 2009; Shulman, 2012)
Helicobacter pylori **eradication:** Children and Adolescents: Oral: 20 mg/kg/day divided every 12 hours; maximum single dose: 500 mg; initial duration of treatment: 7 to 14 days; as part of triple or quadruple combination regimens with amoxicillin and proton pump inhibitor with or without metronidazole (Koletzko, 2011)
Lyme disease: Limited data available: Children and Adolescents: Oral: 7.5 mg/kg twice daily for 14 to 21 days; maximum single dose: 500 mg (Wormser, 2006)

Mycobacterium avium complex infection (MAC) (HIV-exposed/-positive):
Infants and Children (DHHS [pediatric], 2013)
Prophylaxis: Oral: 15 mg/kg/day divided every 12 hours; maximum single dose: 500 mg; to prevent first episode begin therapy at the following CD4+ T-lymphocyte counts (see below):
  Infants <12 months: <750 cells/mm^3
  Children 1 to 2 years: <500 cells/mm^3
  Children 2 to 5 years: <75 cells/mm^3
  Children ≥6 years: <50 cells/mm^3
Recurrence: Oral: 15 mg/kg/day divided every 12 hours; maximum single dose: 500 mg; use in combination with ethambutol with or without rifabutin
Treatment: Oral: 15 to 30 mg/kg/day divided every 12 hours; maximum single dose: 500 mg; use in combination with ethambutol and if severe infection, rifabutin; follow with chronic suppressive therapy
Adolescents (DHHS [adult], 2013):
Prophylaxis:
  Primary prophylaxis: Oral: 500 mg twice daily
  Secondary prophylaxis: Oral: 500 mg twice daily plus ethambutol; consider additional agents (eg, rifabutin, aminoglycoside, fluoroquinolone) for CD4 <50 cells/mm^3, high mycobacterial load, or ineffective antiretroviral therapy.
Treatment: Oral: 500 mg twice daily in combination with ethambutol: Consider additional agents (eg, rifabutin, aminoglycoside, fluoroquinolone) for CD4 <50 cells/mm^3, high mycobacterial load, or ineffective antiretroviral therapy.
Peritonitis, prophylaxis for patients receiving peritoneal dialysis who require dental procedures: Limited data available: Infants, Children, and Adolescents: Oral: 15 mg/kg 30 to 60 minutes before dental procedure; maximum single dose: 500 mg (Warady, 2012)
Pertussis: Infants, Children, and Adolescents: Oral: 15 mg/kg/day divided every 12 hours for 7 days; maximum single dose: 500 mg (CDC [Tiwari, 2005])
Pneumonia, community-acquired (CAP); presumed atypical pneumonia (*M. pneumoniae, C. pneumoniae, C. trachomatis*); mild infection or step-down therapy: Infants >3 months, Children, and Adolescents: Oral: 15 mg/kg/day every 12 hours for 10 days; shorter courses may be appropriate for mild disease; maximum single dose: 500 mg; **Note:** A beta-lactam antibiotic should be added if typical bacterial pneumonia cannot be ruled out (Bradley, 2011).
Adult:
General dosing, susceptible infection: Oral: 250 to 500 mg every 12 hours **or** 1000 mg (two 500 mg extended release tablets) once daily for 7 to 14 days
Acute exacerbation of chronic bronchitis: Oral:
M. catarrhalis and *S. pneumoniae:* 250 mg every 12 hours for 7 to 14 days **or** 1000 mg (two 500 mg extended release tablets) once daily for 7 days
H. influenzae: 500 mg every 12 hours for 7 to 14 days **or** 1000 mg (two 500 mg extended release tablets) once daily for 7 days
H. parainfluenzae: 500 mg every 12 hours for 7 days **or** 1000 mg (two 500 mg extended release tablets) once daily for 7 days
Acute maxillary sinusitis: Oral: 500 mg every 12 hours **or** 1000 mg (two 500 mg extended release tablets) once daily for 14 days
Mycobacterial infection (prevention and treatment): Oral: 500 mg twice daily (use with other antimycobacterial drugs (eg, ethambutol or rifampin). Continue therapy if clinical response is observed; may discontinue when patient is considered at low risk for disseminated infection.
Peptic ulcer disease: Eradication of *Helicobacter pylori:* Dual or triple combination regimens with bismuth subsalicylate, amoxicillin, an H$_2$-receptor antagonist, or proton pump inhibitor: Oral: 500 mg every 8 to 12 hours for 10-14 days
Pharyngitis, tonsillitis: Oral: 250 mg every 12 hours for 10 days
Pneumonia: Oral:
C. pneumoniae, M. pneumoniae, and *S. pneumoniae:* 250 mg every 12 hours for 7 to 14 days **or** 1000 mg (two 500 mg extended release tablets) once daily for 7 days
H. influenzae: 250 mg every 12 hours for 7 days **or** 1000 mg (two 500 mg extended release tablets) once daily for 7 days
H. parainfluenzae and *M. catarrhalis:* 1000 mg (two 500 mg extended release tablets) once daily for 7 days
Skin and skin structure infection, uncomplicated: Oral: 250 mg every 12 hours for 7 to 14 days
Dosing adjustment in renal impairment:
Infants, Children, and Adolescents: The following adjustments have been recommended (Aronoff, 2007). **Note:** Renally adjusted dose recommendations are based on a dose 15 mg/kg/day divided twice daily.
  GFR ≥30 mL/minute/1.73 m^2: No dosage adjustment necessary
  GFR 10 to 29 mL/minute/1.73 m^2: 8 mg/kg/day divided every 12 hours
  GFR <10 mL/minute/1.73 m^2: 4 mg/kg once daily
  Hemodialysis: Administer after HD session is completed: 4 mg/kg once daily
  Peritoneal dialysis: 4 mg/kg once daily
Adult:
  CrCl <30 mL/minute: Decrease clarithromycin dose by 50%
  Hemodialysis: Administer after HD session is completed (Aronoff, 2007)
  In combination with atazanavir or ritonavir:
    CrCl 30 to 60 mL/minute: Decrease clarithromycin dose by 50%
    CrCl <30 mL/minute: Decrease clarithromycin dose by 75%
Dosing adjustment in hepatic impairment: Adjustment not needed as long as renal function is normal
Administration
Immediate release tablets and oral suspension: May be administered with or without meals; give every 12 hours rather than twice daily to avoid peak and trough variation. Shake suspension well before each use.
Extended release tablets: Should be given with food. Do not crush or chew extended release tablet.
Monitoring Parameters CBC with differential, serum BUN and creatinine, liver function tests; serum concentration of drugs whose concentrations may be affected in patients receiving concomitant clarithromycin (ie, theophylline, carbamazepine, quinidine, digoxin, anticoagulants, triazolam); hearing (in patients receiving long-term treatment with clarithromycin); observe for changes in bowel frequency
Dosage Forms Excipient information presented when available (limited, particularly for generics); consult specific product labeling.
Suspension Reconstituted, Oral:
  Biaxin: 250 mg/5 mL (50 mL, 100 mL) [fruit punch flavor]
  Generic: 125 mg/5 mL (50 mL, 100 mL); 250 mg/5 mL (50 mL, 100 mL)
Tablet, Oral:
  Biaxin: 250 mg [contains brilliant blue fcf (fd&c blue #1), fd&c yellow #10 (quinoline yellow)]
  Biaxin: 500 mg [contains fd&c yellow #10 (quinoline yellow)]
  Generic: 250 mg, 500 mg

Tablet Extended Release 24 Hour, Oral:
Biaxin XL: 500 mg [contains fd&c yellow #10 (quinoline yellow)]
Biaxin XL Pac: 500 mg [contains fd&c yellow #10 (quinoline yellow)]
Generic: 500 mg

References

American Academy of Pediatrics (AAP). In: Pickering LK, Baker CJ, Kimberlin DW, Long SS, eds. *Red Book: 2012 Report of the Committee on Infectious Diseases.* 29th ed. Elk Grove Village, IL: American Academy of Pediatrics; 2012.

American Academy of Pediatrics Committee on Drugs. "Inactive" ingredients in pharmaceutical products: update (subject review). *Pediatrics.* 1997;99(2):268-278.

Aronoff GR, Bennett WM, Berns JS, et al, *Drug Prescribing in Renal Failure: Dosing Guidelines for Adults and Children,* 5th ed, Philadelphia, PA: American College of Physicians, 2007.

Biaxin Filmtab (clarithromycin tablets) [prescribing information]. Barceloneta, PR: AbbVie Inc; August 2013.

Bradley JS, Byington CL, Shah SS, et al, "The Management of Community-Acquired Pneumonia in Infants and Children Older Than 3 Months of Age: Clinical Practice Guidelines by the Pediatric Infectious Diseases Society and the Infectious Diseases Society of America", *Clin Infect Dis,* 2011, 53(7):e25-76.

Centers for Disease Control and Prevention (CDC). Guidelines for the prevention and treatment of opportunistic infections among HIV-exposed and HIV-infected children. *MMWR Recomm Rep.* 2009;58 (RR-11):1-166.

Chey WD, Wong BC, and Practice Parameters Committee of the American College of Gastroenterology, "American College of Gastroenterology Guideline on the Management of *Helicobacter pylori* Infection," *Am J Gastroenterol,* 2007, 102(8):1808-25.

DHHS. Guidelines for the prevention and treatment of opportunistic infections among HIV-exposed and HIV-infected children: recommendations from the National Institutes of Health, Centers for Disease Control and Prevention, the HIV Medicine Association of the Infectious Diseases Society of America, the Pediatric Infectious Diseases Society, and the American Academy of Pediatrics. November 6, 2013. Available at http://aidsinfo.nih.gov

DHHS Panel on Opportunistic Infections (OI) in HIV-Infected Adults and Adolescents, "Guidelines for Prevention and Treatment of Opportunistic Infections in HIV-Infected Adults and Adolescents: Recommendations From the Centers for Disease Control and Prevention (CDC), the National Institutes of Health (NIH), and the HIV Medicine Association (HIVMA) of the Infectious Diseases Society of America (IDSA)," May 7, 2013. Available at http://aidsinfo.nih.gov/contentfiles/lvguidelines/adult_oi.pdf

Ferrero JL, Bopp BA, Marsh KC, et al. Metabolism and disposition of clarithromycin in man. *Drug Metab Dispos.* 1990;18(4):441-446.

Gerber MA, Baltimore RS, Eaton CB, et al, "Prevention of Rheumatic Fever and Diagnosis and Treatment of Acute *Streptococcal pharyngitis*: A Scientific Statement From the American Heart Association Rheumatic Fever, Endocarditis, and Kawasaki Disease Committee of the Council on Cardiovascular Disease in the Young, the Interdisciplinary Council on Functional Genomics and Translational Biology, and the Interdisciplinary Council on Quality of Care and Outcomes Research: Endorsed by the American Academy of Pediatrics," *Circulation,* 2009, 119(11):1541-51.

Goldstein LH, Berlin M, Tsur L, et al, "The Safety of Macrolides During Lactation," *Breastfeed Med,* 2009, 4(4):197-200.

Guay DR and Craft JC, "Overview of the Pharmacology of Clarithromycin Suspension in Children and a Comparison With That in Adults," *Pediatr Infect Dis J,* 1993, 12(12 Suppl 3):S106-11.

Jespersen CM, Als-Nielsen B, Damgaard M, et al. Randomised placebo controlled multicentre trial to assess short term clarithromycin for patients with stable coronary heart disease: CLARICOR trial. *BMJ.* 2006; 332(7532):22-27.

Koletzko S, Jones NL, Goodman KJ, et al, "Evidence-Based Guidelines From ESPGHAN and NASPGHAN for *Helicobacter pylori* Infection in Children," *J Pediatr Gastroenterol Nutr,* 2011, 53(2):230-43.

Lieberthal AS, Carroll AE, Chonmaitree T, et al, "The Diagnosis and Management of Acute Otitis Media," *Pediatrics,* 2013, 131(3): e964-99.

Peters DH, Clissold SP. Clarithromycin: a review of its antimicrobial activity, pharmacokinetic properties, and therapeutic potential. *Drugs.* 1992; 44(1):117-164.

Shehab N, Lewis CL, Streetman DD, Donn SM. Exposure to the pharmaceutical excipients benzyl alcohol and propylene glycol among critically ill neonates. *Pediatr Crit Care Med.* 2009;10 (2):256-259.

Shulman ST, Bisno AL, Clegg HW, et al, "Clinical Practice Guideline for the Diagnosis and Management of Group A Streptococcal Pharyngitis: 2012 Update by the Infectious Diseases Society of America," *Clin Infect Dis,* 2012.

Tiwari T, Murphy TV, and Moran J, "Recommended Antimicrobial Agents for the Treatment and Postexposure Prophylaxis of Pertussis: 2005 CDC Guidelines," *MMWR Recomm Rep,* 2005, 54(RR-14):1-16.

Warady BA, Bakkaloglu S, Newland J, et al, "Consensus Guidelines for the Prevention and Treatment of Catheter-Related Infections and Peritonitis in Pediatric Patients Receiving Peritoneal Dialysis: 2012 Update," *Perit Dial Int,* 2012, 32(Suppl 2):S32-86.

Wilson W, Taubert KA, Gewitz M, et al, "Prevention of Infective Endocarditis. Guidelines From the American Heart Association," *Circulation,* 2007, 115:1-20.

Witt RA, Sommer EM, Cichna M, et al, "Placental Passage of Clarithromycin Surpasses Other Macrolide Antibiotics," *Am J Obstet Gynecol,* 2003, 188(3):816-9.

Wormser GP, Dattwyler RJ, Shapiro ED, et al, "The Clinical Assessment, Treatment, and Prevention of Lyme Disease, Human Granulocytic Anaplasmosis, and Babesiosis: Clinical Practice Guidelines by the Infectious Diseases Society of America," *Clin Infect Dis,* 2006, 43 (9):1089-134.

◆ **Claritin [OTC]** *see* Loratadine *on page 1278*

◆ **Claritin® (Can)** *see* Loratadine *on page 1278*

◆ **Claritin-D® 12 Hour Allergy & Congestion [OTC]** *see* Loratadine and Pseudoephedrine *on page 1279*

◆ **Claritin-D® 24 Hour Allergy & Congestion [OTC]** *see* Loratadine and Pseudoephedrine *on page 1279*

◆ **Claritin Allergic Decongestant (Can)** *see* Oxymetazoline (Nasal) *on page 1577*

◆ **Claritin® Extra (Can)** *see* Loratadine and Pseudoephedrine *on page 1279*

◆ **Claritin Eye [OTC]** *see* Ketotifen (Ophthalmic) *on page 1185*

◆ **Claritin® Kids (Can)** *see* Loratadine *on page 1278*

◆ **Claritin® Liberator (Can)** *see* Loratadine and Pseudoephedrine *on page 1279*

◆ **Claritin Reditabs [OTC]** *see* Loratadine *on page 1278*

◆ **Clarus™ (Can)** *see* ISOtretinoin *on page 1161*

◆ **Clavulanic Acid and Amoxicillin** *see* Amoxicillin and Clavulanate *on page 144*

◆ **Clavulanic Acid and Amoxycillin** *see* Amoxicillin and Clavulanate *on page 144*

◆ **Clavulin (Can)** *see* Amoxicillin and Clavulanate *on page 144*

◆ **Clear Away 1-Step Wart Remover [OTC]** *see* Salicylic Acid *on page 1860*

◆ **Clear Eyes Redness Relief [OTC]** *see* Naphazoline (Ophthalmic) *on page 1470*

◆ **Clearplex V [OTC]** *see* Benzoyl Peroxide *on page 275*

◆ **Clearplex X** *see* Benzoyl Peroxide *on page 275*

◆ **Clearskin [OTC]** *see* Benzoyl Peroxide *on page 275*

Clemastine (KLEM as teen)

Medication Safety Issues

BEERS Criteria medication:

This drug may be potentially inappropriate for use in geriatric patients (Quality of evidence - moderate; Strength of recommendation - strong).

Brand Names: U.S. Dayhist Allergy 12 Hour Relief [OTC]; Tavist Allergy [OTC]

Therapeutic Category Antihistamine

Generic Availability (U.S.) Yes

Use Perennial and seasonal allergic rhinitis and other allergic symptoms including urticaria (FDA approved in ages ≥6 years and adults)

Pregnancy Risk Factor B

Pregnancy Considerations Maternal clemastine use has generally not resulted in an increased risk of birth defects. Antihistamines are recommended for the treatment of rhinitis, urticaria, and pruritus with rash in pregnant women (although second generation antihistamines may be preferred). Antihistamines are not recommended for treatment of pruritus associated with intrahepatic cholestasis in pregnancy.

Breast-Feeding Considerations Small amounts of clemastine may be excreted in breast milk. Premature infants and newborns have a higher risk of intolerance to antihistamines. Adverse events were observed in single case report of a nursing infant. Use while breast-feeding is contraindicated by the manufacturer. Antihistamines may decrease maternal serum prolactin concentrations when administered prior to the establishment of nursing.

Contraindications Hypersensitivity to clemastine or any component; narrow-angle glaucoma; breast-feeding

Warnings May cause CNS depression, which may impair physical or mental abilities; effects may be potentiated when used with other sedative drugs or ethanol; patients must be cautioned about performing tasks which require mental alertness (eg, operating machinery or driving). Concomitant use with monoamine oxidase (MAO) inhibitors may prolong and intensify the anticholinergic effects of antihistamines; avoid concomitant therapy.

Precautions Use with caution in patients with stenosing peptic ulcer, GI or GU obstruction, asthma, prostatic hypertrophy, cardiovascular disease (including hypertension and ischemic heart disease), increased IOP, and thyroid dysfunction. May cause paradoxical excitation in young children.

Adverse Reactions

Cardiovascular: Hypotension, palpitation, tachycardia

Central nervous system: Confusion, dizziness increased, dyscoordination, fatigue, headache, insomnia, irritability, nervousness, restlessness, sedation, sleepiness, somnolence slight to moderate

Dermatologic: Photosensitivity, rash

Gastrointestinal: Constipation, diarrhea, epigastric distress, nausea, vomiting, xerostomia

Genitourinary: Difficult urination, urinary frequency, urinary retention

Hematologic: Agranulocytosis, hemolytic anemia, thrombocytopenia

Ocular: Blurred vision

Otic: Tinnitus

Respiratory: Thickening of bronchial secretions

Miscellaneous: Anaphylaxis

Drug Interactions

Metabolism/Transport Effects Inhibits CYP2D6 (weak), CYP3A4 (weak)

Avoid Concomitant Use

Avoid concomitant use of Clemastine with any of the following: Aclidinium; Azelastine (Nasal); Ipratropium (Oral Inhalation); Paraldehyde; Pimozide; Potassium Chloride; Thalidomide; Tiotropium; Umeclidinium

Increased Effect/Toxicity

Clemastine may increase the levels/effects of: AbobotulinumtoxinA; Alcohol (Ethyl); Analgesics (Opioid); Anticholinergic Agents; ARIPiprazole; Azelastine (Nasal); Buprenorphine; Cannabinoid-Containing Products; CNS Depressants; Dofetilide; Hydrocodone; Lomitapide; Methotrimeprazine; Metyrosine; Mirabegron; Mirtazapine; OnabotulinumtoxinA; Paraldehyde; Pimozide; Potassium Chloride; Pramipexole; RimabotulinumtoxinB; ROPINIRole; Rotigotine; Selective Serotonin Reuptake Inhibitors; Thalidomide; Thiazide Diuretics; Tiotropium; Topiramate; Zolpidem

The levels/effects of Clemastine may be increased by: Aclidinium; Brimonidine (Topical); Cannabis; Doxylamine; Dronabinol; Droperidol; HydrOXYzine; Ipratropium (Oral Inhalation); Kava Kava; Magnesium Sulfate; Methotrimeprazine; Nabilone; Perampanel; Pramlintide; Rufinamide; Sodium Oxybate; Tapentadol; Tetrahydrocannabinol; Umeclidinium

Decreased Effect

Clemastine may decrease the levels/effects of: Acetylcholinesterase Inhibitors (Central); Benzylpenicilloyl Polylysine; Betahistine; Hyaluronidase; Secretin

The levels/effects of Clemastine may be decreased by: Acetylcholinesterase Inhibitors (Central); Amphetamines

Mechanism of Action Competes with histamine for H_1-receptor sites on effector cells in the gastrointestinal tract, blood vessels, and respiratory tract

Pharmacodynamics

Onset of action: 2 hours after administration

Maximum effect: 5-7 hours

Duration: 10-12 hours

Pharmacokinetics (Adult data unless noted)

Absorption: Oral: Well absorbed

Distribution: Breast milk to plasma ratio: 0.25-0.5

Metabolism: In the liver

Time to peak serum concentration: 2-4 hours

Elimination: Majority of an oral dose eliminated in the urine

Dosing: Usual Oral:

Infants and Children <6 years: 0.05 mg/kg/day as **clemastine base** or 0.335-0.67 mg/day clemastine fumarate (0.25-0.5 mg base/day) divided into 2 or 3 doses; maximum daily dosage: 1.34 mg (1 mg base)

Children 6-12 years: 0.67-1.34 mg clemastine fumarate (0.5-1 mg base) twice daily; do not exceed 4.02 mg/day (3 mg/day base)

Children ≥12 years and Adults: 1.34 mg clemastine fumarate (1 mg base) twice daily to 2.68 mg (2 mg base) 3 times/day; do not exceed 8.04 mg/day (6 mg base)

Administration Oral: Administer with food

Monitoring Parameters Look for a reduction of rhinitis, urticaria, eczema, pruritus, or other allergic symptoms

Dosage Forms Excipient information presented when available (limited, particularly for generics); consult specific product labeling.

Syrup, Oral, as fumarate:
  Generic: 0.67 mg/5 mL (120 mL)

Tablet, Oral, as fumarate:
  Dayhist Allergy 12 Hour Relief: 1.34 mg [scored; sodium free]
  Tavist Allergy: 1.34 mg [scored; sodium free]
  Generic: 1.34 mg, 2.68 mg

◆ **Clemastine Fumarate** see Clemastine *on page 494*

◆ **Cleocin** see Clindamycin (Systemic) *on page 495*

◆ **Cleocin** see Clindamycin (Topical) *on page 500*

◆ **Cleocin in D₅W** see Clindamycin (Systemic) *on page 495*

◆ **Cleocin Phosphate** see Clindamycin (Systemic) *on page 495*

◆ **Cleocin-T** see Clindamycin (Topical) *on page 500*

◆ **Climara** see Estradiol (Systemic) *on page 796*

◆ **Clindacin ETZ** see Clindamycin (Topical) *on page 500*

◆ **Clindacin-P** see Clindamycin (Topical) *on page 500*

◆ **Clindacin Pac** see Clindamycin (Topical) *on page 500*

◆ **Clindagel** see Clindamycin (Topical) *on page 500*

◆ **ClindaMax** see Clindamycin (Topical) *on page 500*

Clindamycin (Systemic) (klin da MYE sin)

Medication Safety Issues

Sound-alike/look-alike issues:

Cleocin may be confused with bleomycin, Clinoril, Cubicin, Lincocin

Clindamycin may be confused with clarithromycin, Claritin, vancomycin

◀ **Related Information**
Prevention of Infective Endocarditis *on page 2336*
Brand Names: U.S. Cleocin; Cleocin in D$_5$W; Cleocin Phosphate
Brand Names: Canada Apo-Clindamycin; Ava-Clindamycin; Clindamycin Injection, USP; Clindamycine; Dalacin C; Mylan-Clindamycin; PMS-Clindamycin; Riva-Clindamycin; Teva-Clindamycin
Therapeutic Category Antibiotic, Anaerobic; Antibiotic, Miscellaneous
Generic Availability (U.S.) Yes
Use Treatment of infections involving the respiratory tract, skin and soft tissue, and female pelvis and genital tract; sepsis and intra-abdominal infections due to susceptible organisms (FDA approved in all ages); has also been used for endocarditis prophylaxis, preoperative prophylaxis, and treatment of babesiosis and malaria
Pregnancy Risk Factor B
Pregnancy Considerations Adverse events were not observed in animal reproduction studies. Clindamycin crosses the placenta and can be detected in the cord blood and fetal tissue (Philipson, 1973; Weinstein, 1976). Clindamycin pharmacokinetics are not affected by pregnancy (Philipson, 1976; Weinstein, 1976). Clindamycin therapy is recommended as an alternative treatment in certain pregnant patients for prophylaxis of group B streptococcal disease in newborns (ACOG 485, 2011); prophylaxis and treatment of *Toxoplasma gondii* encephalitis, or for the treatment of *Pneumocystis* pneumonia (PCP) (DHHS, 2013); bacterial vaginosis (CDC RR12, 2010); or malaria (CDC, 2013). Clindamycin is also one of the antibiotics recommended for prophylactic use prior to cesarean delivery and may be used in certain situations prior to vaginal delivery in women at high risk for endocarditis (ACOG 120, 2011).
Breast-Feeding Considerations Clindamycin can be detected in breast milk; reported concentrations range from 0.7 to 3.8 mcg/mL following maternal doses of 150 mg orally to 600 mg I.V. Due to the potential for serious adverse reactions in neonates, breast-feeding is not recommended by the manufacturer. Nondose-related effects could include modification of bowel flora. One case of bloody stools in an infant occurred after a mother received clindamycin while breast-feeding; however, a causal relationship was not confirmed (Mann, 1980).
Contraindications Hypersensitivity to clindamycin, lincomycin, or any component
Warnings Use can cause severe and possibly fatal colitis **[U.S. Boxed Warning]** characterized by severe persistent diarrhea, severe abdominal cramps, and possibly, the passage of blood and mucus; *C. difficile*-associated diarrhea (CDAD) has been observed >2 months postantibiotic treatment; use with caution in patients with a history of colitis; discontinue drug if significant diarrhea occurs. Antiperistaltic agents, such as opiates or diphenoxylate with atropine, may prolong and worsen the condition. Not appropriate for use in the treatment of meningitis due to inadequate penetration into the CSF.

Capsules may contain tartrazine which may cause allergic reactions in susceptible individuals. Injection contains benzyl alcohol which may cause allergic reactions in susceptible individuals; large amounts of benzyl alcohol (≥99 mg/kg/day) have been associated with a potentially fatal toxicity ("gasping syndrome") in neonates; the "gasping syndrome" consists of metabolic acidosis, respiratory distress, gasping respirations, CNS dysfunction (including convulsions, intracranial hemorrhage), hypotension, and cardiovascular collapse; use clindamycin injection products containing benzyl alcohol with caution in neonates; *in vitro* and animal studies have shown that benzoate, a metabolite of benzyl alcohol, displaces bilirubin from protein binding sites.

Precautions Use with caution in patients with severe renal and/or hepatic impairment; use with caution in atopic patients; use with caution in patients with previous pseudomembranous colitis, regional enteritis, or ulcerative colitis.
Adverse Reactions
Cardiovascular: Cardiac arrest (rare; I.V. administration), hypotension (rare; I.V. administration)
Dermatologic: Erythema multiforme (rare), exfoliative dermatitis (rare), pruritus, rash, Stevens-Johnson syndrome (rare), urticaria
Gastrointestinal: Abdominal pain, diarrhea, esophagitis, nausea, pseudomembranous colitis, vomiting
Genitourinary: Vaginitis
Hematologic: Agranulocytosis, eosinophilia (transient), neutropenia (transient), thrombocytopenia
Hepatic: Jaundice, liver function test abnormalities
Local: Induration/pain/sterile abscess (I.M.), thrombophlebitis (I.V.)
Neuromuscular & skeletal: Polyarthritis (rare)
Renal: Renal dysfunction (rare)
Miscellaneous: Anaphylactoid reactions (rare)
Drug Interactions
Metabolism/Transport Effects Substrate of CYP3A4 (minor); **Note:** Assignment of Major/Minor substrate status based on clinically relevant drug interaction potential
Avoid Concomitant Use
Avoid concomitant use of Clindamycin (Systemic) with any of the following: BCG; Erythromycin (Systemic)
Increased Effect/Toxicity
Clindamycin (Systemic) may increase the levels/effects of: Neuromuscular-Blocking Agents
Decreased Effect
Clindamycin (Systemic) may decrease the levels/effects of: BCG; Erythromycin (Systemic); Sodium Picosulfate; Typhoid Vaccine

The levels/effects of Clindamycin (Systemic) may be decreased by: Kaolin
Food Interactions Peak concentrations may be delayed with food. Management: May administer with food.
Stability
Oral capsule: Store at 20°C to 25°C (68°F to 77°F).
Oral solution: Store at 20°C to 25°C (68°F to 77°F). Do not refrigerate reconstituted oral solution (it will thicken). Following reconstitution, oral solution is stable for 2 weeks.
Parenteral: Store intact vials and premixed bags at 20°C to 25°C (68°F to 77°F). After initial use, discard any unused portion of vial after 24 hours. Infusion solution in NS or D$_5$W solution is stable for 16 days at room temperature, 32 days refrigerated, or 8 weeks frozen.
Peritoneal dialysis solutions: Stable in Dianeal PD1, PD2 3.86% at a concentration of 10 mg/L for 2 days at room temperature; stable in Dianeal PD2 at a concentration of 200 mg/L for 4 days refrigerated or at room temperature (Warady, 2012).
Mechanism of Action Reversibly binds to 50S ribosomal subunits preventing peptide bond formation thus inhibiting bacterial protein synthesis; bacteriostatic or bactericidal depending on drug concentration, infection site, and organism
Pharmacokinetics (Adult data unless noted)
Absorption: Oral: 90% of clindamycin hydrochloride is rapidly absorbed; clindamycin palmitate must be hydrolyzed in the GI tract before it is active
Distribution: No significant levels are seen in CSF, even with inflamed meninges; distributes into saliva, ascites fluid, pleural fluid, bone, and bile
Protein binding: 94%
Bioavailability: Oral: ~90%

Half-life:
  Neonates:
    Premature: 8.7 hours
    Full-term: 3.6 hours
  Infants 1 month to 1 year: 3 hours
  Children and Adults with normal renal function: 2-3 hours
Time to peak serum concentration:
  Oral: Within 60 minutes
  I.M.: Within 1-3 hours
Elimination: Most of the drug is eliminated by hepatic metabolism; 10% of an oral dose excreted in urine and 3.6% excreted in feces as active drug and metabolites

Dosing: Neonatal
  General dosing, susceptible infection (*Red Book* [AAP], 2012): I.M., I.V., Oral:
    Body weight <1 kg:
      PNA ≤14 days: 5 mg/kg/dose every 12 hours
      PNA 15-28 days: 5 mg/kg/dose every 8 hours
    Body weight 1-2 kg:
      PNA ≤7 days: 5 mg/kg/dose every 12 hours
      PNA 8-28 days: 5 mg/kg/dose every 8 hours
    Body weight >2 kg:
      PNA ≤7 days: 5 mg/kg/dose every 8 hours
      PNA 8-28 days: 5 mg/kg/dose every 6 hours
  Manufacturer's labeling: Term infant: I.M., I.V.: 15 to 20 mg/kg/day divided every 6 to 8 hours

Dosing: Usual
Infants, Children, and Adolescents:
  General dosing, susceptible infection:
    I.M., I.V.:
      Manufacturer's labeling: Infants, Children, and Adolescents 1 month to 16 years:
        Weight-directed dosing: 20 to 40 mg/kg/day divided every 6 to 8 hours
        BSA-directed dosing: 350 to 450 mg/m²/day divided every 6 to 8 hours
      Alternate dosing (*Red Book* [AAP], 2012): Infants, Children, and Adolescents:
        Mild to moderate infections: 20 mg/kg/day divided every 8 hours; maximum daily dose: 1800 mg/**day**
        Severe infections: 40 mg/kg/day divided every 6 to 8 hours; maximum daily dose: 2700 mg/**day**
    Oral:
      Manufacturer's labeling: Infants, Children, and Adolescents:
        Hydrochloride salt (capsule): 8 to 20 mg/kg/day divided every 6 to 8 hours
        Palmitate salt (solution): 8 to 25 mg/kg/day divided every 6 to 8 hours; minimum dose: 37.5 mg 3 times daily
      Alternate dosing (*Red Book* [AAP]; 2012): Infants, Children, and Adolescents:
        Mild to moderate infections: 10 to 25 mg/kg/day divided every 8 hours; maximum daily dose: 1800 mg/**day**
        Severe infections: 30 to 40 mg/kg/day divided every 6 to 8 hours; maximum daily dose: 1800 mg/**day**
  Acute otitis media: Oral: 30 to 40 mg/kg/day divided every 8 hours (Lieberthal, 2013)
  Babesiosis: Oral: 20 to 40 mg/kg/day divided every 8 hours for 7 to 10 days plus quinine; maximum single dose: 600 mg (*Red Book* [AAP], 2012)
  Bacterial endocarditis prophylaxis for dental and upper respiratory procedures in penicillin-allergic patients (*Red Book* [AAP], 2012; Wilson, 2007):
    I.M., I.V.: 20 mg/kg 30 minutes before procedure; maximum single dose: 600 mg
    Oral: 20 mg/kg 1 hour before procedure; maximum single dose: 600 mg
    Note: American Heart Association (AHA) guidelines now recommend prophylaxis only in patients undergoing invasive procedures and in whom underlying cardiac conditions may predispose to a higher risk of adverse outcomes should infection occur. As of April 2007, routine prophylaxis for GI/GU procedures is no longer recommended by the AHA.
  Intra-abdominal infection, complicated: I.V.: **Note:** Not recommended for community-acquired infections due to increasing *Bacteroides fragilis* resistance: 20 to 40 mg/kg/day divided every 6 to 8 hours in combination with gentamicin or tobramycin (Solomkin, 2010)
  Malaria, treatment:
    Uncomplicated: Oral: 20 mg/kg/day divided every 8 hours for 7 days plus quinine (CDC, 2011; *Red Book* [AAP], 2012)
    Severe: I.V.: Loading dose: 10 mg/kg once followed by 15 mg/kg/day divided every 8 hours plus I.V. quinidine gluconate; switch to oral therapy (clindamycin and quinine, see above) when able for total treatment duration of 7 days. **Note:** Quinine duration is region specific; consult CDC for current recommendations (CDC, 2011).
  Osteomyelitis, septic arthritis, due to MRSA: I.V., Oral: 40 mg/kg/day divided every 6 to 8 hours for at least 4 to 6 weeks (osteomyelitis) or 3 to 4 weeks (septic arthritis) (Liu, 2011)
  Peritonitis (CAPD):
    Prophylaxis (Warady, 2012):
      Invasive dental procedures: Oral: 20 mg/kg administered 30 to 60 minutes before procedure; maximum dose: 600 mg
      Gastrointestinal or genitourinary procedures: I.V.: 10 mg/kg administered 30 to 60 minutes before procedure; maximum dose: 600 mg
    Treatment:
      Exit-site and tunnel infection: Oral: 10 mg/kg/dose 3 times daily; maximum single dose: 600 mg (Warady, 2012)
      Intraperitoneal, continuous: Loading dose: 300 mg per liter of dialysate; maintenance dose: 150 mg per liter; **Note:** 125 mg/liter has also been recommended as a maintenance dose (Aronoff, 2007; Warady, 2012)
  Pharyngitis:
    AHA guidelines (Gerber, 2009): Children and Adolescents: Oral: 20 mg/kg/day in divided doses 3 times daily for 10 days; maximum single dose: 600 mg
    IDSA guidelines (Shulman, 2012): Children and Adolescents: Oral:
      Treatment and primary prevention of rheumatic fever: 21 mg/kg/day in divided doses 3 times daily for 10 days; maximum single dose: 300 mg
      Treatment of chronic carriers: 20 to 30 mg/kg/day in divided doses 3 times daily for 10 days; maximum single dose: 300 mg
  Pneumococcal disease, invasive: I.V.: 25 to 40 mg/kg/day divided every 6 to 8 hours (*Red Book* [AAP], 2012)
  ***Pneumocystis jirovecii* (formerly *carnii*) pneumonia (PCP):**
    Non HIV-exposed/-positive (*Red Book* [AAP], 2012):
      Mild to moderate disease: Oral: 10 mg/kg 3 to 4 times daily for 21 days; in combination with other agents; maximum single dose: 450 mg
      Moderate to severe disease: I.V.: 15 to 25 mg/kg 3 to 4 times daily for 21 days; give with pentamidine or primaquine; maximum single dose: 600 mg. May switch to oral dose after clinical improvement.
    HIV-exposed/-positive: Adolescents (DHHS [adult], 2013):
      Mild to moderate disease: Oral: 300 mg every 6 hours **or** 450 mg every 8 hours with primaquine for 21 days
      Moderate to severe disease:
        Oral: 300 mg every 6 hours **or** 450 mg every 8 hours with primaquine for 21 days
        I.V.: 600 mg every 6 hours **or** 900 mg every 8 hours with primaquine for 21 days

Pneumonia:

Community-acquired pneumonia (CAP) (IDSA/PIDS, Bradley, 2011): Infants ≥3 months, Children, and Adolescents: **Note:** In children ≥5 years, a macrolide antibiotic should be added if atypical pneumonia cannot be ruled out.

Moderate to severe infection: I.V.: 40 mg/kg/day divided every 6 to 8 hours

Mild infection, step-down therapy: Oral: 30 to 40 mg/kg/day divided every 6 to 8 hours

MRSA pneumonia: I.V.: 40 mg/kg/day divided every 6 to 8 hours for 7 to 21 days (Liu, 2011)

Rhinosinusitis, acute bacterial: Oral: 30 to 40 mg/kg/day divided every 8 hours with concomitant cefixime or cefpodoxime for 10 to 14 days. **Note:** Recommended in patients with nontype I penicillin allergy, after failure to initial therapy, or in patients at risk for antibiotic resistance (eg, daycare attendance, age <2 years, recent hospitalization, antibiotic use within the past month) (Chow, 2012).

Skin and soft tissue infection:

Impetigo: Oral: 10 to 20 mg/kg/day in divided doses 3 times daily; treatment duration: 7 days; maximum single dose: 400 mg (Stevens, 2005)

MRSA infection (Liu, 2011):

Cellulitis, nonpurulent or purulent: Oral: 40 mg/kg/day divided every 6 to 8 hours; maximum single dose: 450 mg; treatment duration based on clinical response, usually 7 to 14 days

Complicated SSTI infection: I.V., Oral: 40 mg/kg/day divided every 6 to 8 hours for 7 to 14 days; maximum single dose range: 450 to 600 mg

MSSA infection (Stevens, 2005): Duration of treatment dependent upon site and severity of infection; cellulitis and abscesses typically require 5 to 10 days of therapy

I.V.: 25 to 40 mg/kg/day in divided doses 3 times daily; maximum single dose: 600 mg

Oral: 10 to 20 mg/kg/day in divided doses 3 times daily; maximum single dose: 450 mg

Surgical prophylaxis: Children and Adolescents: I.V.: 10 mg/kg 30 to 60 minutes prior to the procedure; may repeat in 6 hours; maximum single dose: 900 mg (Bratzler, 2013)

Toxoplasmosis (HIV-exposed/positive or hematopoietic cell transplantation recipients):

Infants and Children (CDC, 2009; *Red Book* [AAP], 2012; Tomblyn, 2009):

Treatment, HIV-exposed/-positive: I.V., Oral: 5 to 7.5 mg/kg/dose 4 times daily with pyrimethamine and leucovorin; maximum single dose: 600 mg

Secondary prevention:

HIV-exposed/-positive: Oral: 7 to 10 mg/kg/dose every 8 hours and pyrimethamine plus leucovorin; maximum single dose: 600 mg (DHHS [pediatric], 2013)

Hematopoietic cell transplantation recipients: Oral: 5 to 7.5 mg/kg/dose every 6 hours and pyrimethamine plus leucovorin; maximum single dose: 450 mg

Adolescents (DHHS [adult], 2013; *Red Book* [AAP], 2012; Tomblyn, 2009):

Treatment: Oral, I.V.: 600 mg every 6 hours with pyrimethamine and leucovorin for at least 6 weeks; longer if clinical or radiologic disease is extensive or response is incomplete

Secondary prevention:

HIV-exposed/-positive: Oral: 600 mg every 8 hours with pyrimethamine and leucovorin

Hematopoietic cell transplantation recipients: Oral: 300 to 450 mg every 6 to 8 hours with pyrimethamine and leucovorin

Adults:

General dosing, susceptible infection:

Oral: 150 to 450 mg every 6 to 8 hours; maximum dose: 1800 mg daily

I.M., I.V.: 1200 to 2700 mg/day in 2 to 4 divided doses; maximum dose: 4800 mg daily

Amnionitis: I.V.: 450 to 900 mg every 8 hours

Bacterial vaginosis: Oral: 300 mg twice daily for 7 days (CDC, 2010)

Cellulitis due to MRSA: Oral: 300 to 450 mg 3 times daily for 5 to 10 days (Liu, 2011)

Complicated skin/soft tissue infection due to MRSA: I.V., Oral: 600 mg 3 times daily for 7 to 14 days (Liu, 2011)

Endocarditis prophylaxis (Wilson, 2007):

Oral: 600 mg 30 to 60 minutes before procedure with no follow-up dose needed

I.M., I.V.: 600 mg 30 to 60 minutes before procedure. Intramuscular injections should be avoided in patients who are receiving anticoagulant therapy. In these circumstances, orally administered regimens should be given whenever possible. Intravenously administered antibiotics should be used for patients who are unable to tolerate or absorb oral medications.

Note: American Heart Association (AHA) guidelines now recommend prophylaxis only in patients undergoing invasive procedures and in whom underlying cardiac conditions may predispose to a higher risk of adverse outcomes should infection occur. As of April 2007, routine prophylaxis for GI/GU procedures is no longer recommended by the AHA.

Gangrenous pyomyositis: I.V.: 900 mg every 8 hours with penicillin G

Group B Streptococcus (neonatal prophylaxis): I.V.: 900 mg every 8 hours until delivery (CDC, 2010a, *Red Book* [AAP], 2012)

Malaria, severe: I.V.: Load: 10 mg/kg followed by 15 mg/kg/day divided every 8 hours plus I.V. quinidine gluconate; switch to oral therapy (clindamycin plus quinine) when able for total clindamycin treatment duration of 7 days (**Note:** Quinine duration is region-specific, consult CDC for current recommendations) (CDC, 2011)

Malaria, uncomplicated treatment: Oral: 20 mg/kg/day divided every 8 hours for 7 days plus quinine (CDC, 2011)

Orofacial/peripharyngeal space infections:

Oral: 150 to 450 mg every 6 hours for at least 7 days; maximum daily dose: 1800 mg/**day**

I.V.: 600 to 900 mg every 8 hours

Osteomyelitis due to MRSA: I.V., Oral: 600 mg 3 times daily for a minimum of 8 weeks (some experts combine with rifampin) (Liu, 2011)

Pelvic inflammatory disease: I.V.: 900 mg every 8 hours with gentamicin (conventional or single daily dosing); 24 hours after clinical improvement may convert to oral clindamycin 450 mg 4 times daily or oral doxycycline to complete 14 days of total therapy. Avoid doxycycline if tubo-ovarian abscess is present (CDC, 2010).

Pharyngitis, group A streptococci (IDSA, Shulman, 2012): Oral:

Acute treatment in penicillin-allergic patients: 21 mg/kg/day divided every 8 hours for 10 days; maximum single dose: 300 mg

Chronic carrier treatment: 20 to 30 mg/kg/day divided every 8 hours for 10 days; maximum single dose: 300 mg

Pneumocystis jirovecii **pneumonia:**

I.V.: 600 mg every 6 hours **or** 900 mg every 8 hours with primaquine for 21 days (DHHS [adult], 2013)

Oral: 300 mg every 6 hours **or** 450 mg every 8 hours with primaquine for 21 days (DHHS [adult], 2013)

Pneumonia due to MRSA: I.V., Oral: 600 mg 3 times daily for 7 to 21 days (Liu, 2011)

Prophylaxis in total joint replacement patients undergoing dental procedures which produce bacteremia:

Oral: 600 mg 1 hour prior to procedure (ADA, 2003)

I.V.: 600 mg 1 hour prior to procedure (for patients unable to take oral medication) (ADA, 2003)

Prosthetic joint infection (Osmon, 2013):

Chronic antimicrobial suppression, staphylococci (oxacillin-susceptible): Oral: 300 mg every 6 hours

Propionibacterium acnes, treatment:

Oral: 300 to 450 mg every 6 hours for 4 to 6 weeks

I.V.: 600 to 900 mg every 8 hours for 4 to 6 weeks

Septic arthritis due to MRSA: I.V., Oral: 600 mg 3 times daily for 3 to 4 weeks (Liu, 2011)

Toxic shock syndrome: I.V.: 900 mg every 8 hours with penicillin G or ceftriaxone

Toxoplasmosis encephalitis, HIV-exposed/-positive (DHHS [adult], 2013):

Treatment: Oral, I.V.: 600 mg every 6 hours with pyrimethamine and leucovorin for at least 6 weeks; longer if clinical or radiologic disease is extensive or response is incomplete

Secondary prevention: Oral: 600 mg every 8 hours with pyrimethamine and leucovorin calcium

Dosing adjustment in renal impairment: No adjustment required. Not dialyzable (0% to 5%).

Dosing adjustment in hepatic impairment: No adjustment required. Use caution with severe hepatic impairment.

Administration

Oral: Capsule should be taken with a full glass of water to avoid esophageal irritation; shake oral solution well before use; may administer with or without meals

Parenteral:

I.M.: Deep I.M. injection; rotate sites. Do not exceed 600 mg in a single injection.

I.V.: Infuse over at least 10-60 minutes, at a rate not to exceed 30 mg/minute; hypotension and cardiopulmonary arrest have been reported following rapid I.V. administration; final concentration for administration should not exceed 18 mg/mL; pH: 6.0-6.3 (usual); 5.5-7.0 (range).

Monitoring Parameters Observe for changes in bowel frequency; during prolonged therapy, monitor CBC with differential, platelet count, and hepatic and renal function tests periodically.

Dosage Forms Excipient information presented when available (limited, particularly for generics); consult specific product labeling.

Capsule, Oral, as hydrochloride [strength expressed as base]:

Cleocin: 75 mg, 150 mg [contains brilliant blue fcf (fd&c blue #1), tartrazine (fd&c yellow #5)]

Cleocin: 300 mg [contains brilliant blue fcf (fd&c blue #1)]

Generic: 75 mg, 150 mg, 300 mg

Solution, Injection, as phosphate [strength expressed as base]:

Cleocin Phosphate: 300 mg/2 mL (2 mL) [contains benzyl alcohol]

Cleocin Phosphate: 300 mg/2 mL (2 mL); 600 mg/4 mL (4 mL) [contains benzyl alcohol, edetate disodium]

Cleocin Phosphate: 900 mg/6 mL (6 mL) [contains benzyl alcohol]

Cleocin Phosphate: 900 mg/6 mL (6 mL); 9 g/60 mL (60 mL) [contains benzyl alcohol, edetate disodium]

Generic: 300 mg/2 mL (2 mL); 600 mg/4 mL (4 mL); 900 mg/6 mL (6 mL); 9000 mg/60 mL (60 mL); 9 g/60 mL (60 mL)

Solution, Intravenous, as phosphate [strength expressed as base]:

Cleocin in D_5W: 300 mg/50 mL (50 mL); 600 mg/50 mL (50 mL); 900 mg/50 mL (50 mL) [contains edetate disodium]

Cleocin Phosphate: 600 mg/4 mL (4 mL) [contains benzyl alcohol, edetate disodium]

Cleocin Phosphate: 900 mg/6 mL (6 mL) [contains benzyl alcohol]

Generic: 300 mg/50 mL (50 mL); 600 mg/50 mL (50 mL); 900 mg/50 mL (50 mL); 300 mg/2 mL (2 mL); 600 mg/4 mL (4 mL); 900 mg/6 mL (6 mL)

Solution Reconstituted, Oral, as palmitate hydrochloride [strength expressed as base]:

Cleocin: 75 mg/5 mL (100 mL) [contains ethylparaben]

Generic: 75 mg/5 mL (100 mL)

References

American Academy of Pediatrics (AAP). In: Pickering LK, Baker CJ, Kimberlin DW, Long SS, eds. *Red Book: 2012 Report of the Committee on Infectious Diseases*. 29th ed. Elk Grove Village, IL: American Academy of Pediatrics; 2012.

American College of Obstetricians and Gynecologists. ACOG Practice Bulletin No. 120: use of prophylactic antibiotics in labor and delivery. *Obstet Gynecol.* 2011;117(6):1472-1483.

American College of Obstetricians and Gynecologists Committee on Obstetric Practice, "ACOG Committee Opinion No. 485: Prevention of Early-Onset Group B Streptococcal Disease in Newborns," *Obstet Gynecol*, 2011, 117(4):1019-27.

American Dental Association (ADA) and American Academy of Orthopedic Surgeons, "Antibiotic Prophylaxis for Dental Patients With Total Joint Replacements," *J Am Dent Assoc*, 2003, 134(7):895-9.

Aronoff GR, Bennett WM, Berns JS, et al, *Drug Prescribing in Renal Failure: Dosing Guidelines for Adults and Children*, 5th ed. Philadelphia, PA: American College of Physicians; 2007, p. 55, 149.

Bradley JS, Byington CL, Shah SS, et al, "The Management of Community-Acquired Pneumonia in Infants and Children Older Than 3 Months of Age: Clinical Practice Guidelines by the Pediatric Infectious Diseases Society and the Infectious Diseases Society of America", *Clin Infect Dis*, 2011, 53(7):e25-76.

Bratzler DW, Dellinger EP, Olsen KM, et al, "Clinical Practice Guidelines for Antimicrobial Prophylaxis in Surgery," *Am J Health Syst Pharm*, 2013, 70(3):195-283.

Centers for Disease Control and Prevention (CDC), "Diagnosis and Treatment of Malaria." Available at http://www.cdc.gov/malaria/diagnosis_treatment/index.html. Date accessed: October 21, 2011.

Centers for Disease Control and Prevention (CDC), "Prevention of Perinatal Group B Streptococcal Disease, Revised Guidelines From CDC, 2010," *MMWR Recomm Rep*, 2010a, 59(RR-10):1-32.

Centers for Disease Control and Prevention (CDC), "Sexually Transmitted Diseases Treatment Guidelines, 2010," *MMWR Recomm Rep*, 2010, 59(RR-12):1-110.

Chow AW, Benninger MS, Brook I, et al, "IDSA Clinical Practice Guideline for Acute Bacterial Rhinosinusitis in Children and Adults," *Clin Infect Dis*, 2012, 54(8):e72-112.

DHHS Panel on Opportunistic Infections (OI) in HIV-Infected Adults and Adolescents. Guidelines for prevention and treatment of opportunistic infections in HIV-infected adults and adolescents: recommendations from the Centers for Disease Control and Prevention (CDC), the National Institutes of Health (NIH), and the HIV Medicine Association (HIVMA) of the Infectious Diseases Society of America (IDSA)," May 7, 2013. Available at http://aidsinfo.nih.gov/contentfiles/lvguidelines/adult_oi.pdf

DHHS. Guidelines for the prevention and treatment of opportunistic infections among HIV-exposed and HIV-infected children: recommendations from the National Institutes of Health, Centers for Disease Control and Prevention, the HIV Medicine Association of the Infectious Diseases Society of America, the Pediatric Infectious Diseases Society, and the American Academy of Pediatrics. November 6, 2013. Available at http://aidsinfo.nih.gov

Gerber MA, Baltimore RS, Eaton CB, et al, "Prevention of Rheumatic Fever and Diagnosis and Treatment of Acute *Streptococcal pharyngitis*: A Scientific Statement From the American Heart Association Rheumatic Fever, Endocarditis, and Kawasaki Disease Committee of the Council on Cardiovascular Disease in the Young, the Interdisciplinary Council on Functional Genomics and Translational Biology, and the Interdisciplinary Council on Quality of Care and Outcomes Research: Endorsed by the American Academy of Pediatrics," *Circulation*, 2009, 119(11):1541-51.

Lieberthal AS, Carroll AE, Chonmaitree T, et al, "The Diagnosis and Management of Acute Otitis Media," *Pediatrics*, 2013, 131(3):e964-99.

Liu C, Bayer A, Cosgrove SE, et al, "Clinical Practice Guidelines by the Infectious Diseases Society of America for the Treatment of

Methicillin-Resistant *Staphylococcus aureus* Infections in Adults and Children: Executive Summary," *Clin Infect Dis*, 2011, 52(3):285-92.

Mann CF, "Clindamycin and Breast-Feeding," *Pediatrics*, 1980, 66 (6):1030-1.

Osmon DR, Berbari EF, Berendt AR, et al, "Diagnosis and Management of Prosthetic Joint Infection: Clinical Practice Guideline by the Infectious Diseases Society of America," *Clin Infect Dis*, 2013, 56(1):e1-25.

Philipson A, Sabath LD, and Charles D, "Transplacental Passage of Erythromycin and Clindamycin," *N Engl J Med*, 1973, 288 (23):1219-21.

Shulman ST, Bisno AL, Clegg HW, et al, "Clinical Practice Guideline for the Diagnosis and Management of Group A Streptococcal Pharyngitis: 2012 Update by the Infectious Diseases Society of America," *Clin Infect Dis*, 2012.

Solomkin JS, Mazuski JE, Bradley JS, et al, "Diagnosis and Management of Complicated Intra-abdominal Infection in Adults and Children: Guidelines by the Surgical Infection Society and the Infectious Diseases Society of America," *Clin Infect Dis*, 2010, 50(2):133-64.

Stevens DL, Bisno AL, Chambers HF, et al, "Practice Guidelines for the Diagnosis and Management of Skin and Soft-Tissue Infections," *Clin Infect Dis*, 2005, 41(10):1373-406.

Tomblyn M, Chiller T, Einsele H, et al, "Guidelines for Preventing Infectious Complications Among Hematopoietic Cell Transplantation Recipients: A Global Perspective," *Biol Blood Marrow Transplant*, 2009, 15(10):1143-238.

Trotman RL, Williamson JC, Shoemaker DM, et al, "Antibiotic Dosing in Critically Ill Adult Patients Receiving Continuous Renal Replacement Therapy," *Clin Infect Dis*, 2005, 41(8):1159-66.

Warady BA, Bakkaloglu S, Newland J, et al "Consensus Guidelines for the Prevention and Treatment of Catheter-Related Infections and Peritonitis in Pediatric Patients Receiving Peritoneal Dialysis: 2012 Update," *Perit Dial Int*, 2012, 32(Suppl 2):S32-86.

Weinstein AJ, Gibbs RS, and Gallagher M, "Placental Transfer of Clindamycin and Gentamicin in Term Pregnancy," *Am J Obstet Gynecol*, 1976, 124(7):688-91.

Wilson W, Taubert KA, Gewitz M, et al, "Prevention of Infective Endocarditis. Guidelines From the American Heart Association," *Circulation*, 2007, 115:1-20.

Wormser GP, Dattwyler RJ, Shapiro ED, et al, "The Clinical Assessment, Treatment, and Prevention of Lyme Disease, Human Granulocytic Anaplasmosis, and Babesiosis: Clinical Practice Guidelines by the Infectious Diseases Society of America," *Clin Infect Dis*, 2006, 43 (9):1089-134.

Clindamycin (Topical) (klin da MYE sin)

Medication Safety Issues
Sound-alike/look-alike issues:
Cleocin® may be confused with bleomycin, Clinoril®, Cubicin®, Lincocin®

Clindamycin may be confused with clarithromycin, Claritin®, vancomycin

Brand Names: U.S. Cleocin; Cleocin-T; Clindacin ETZ; Clindacin Pac; Clindacin-P; Clindagel; ClindaMax; Clindesse; Evoclin

Brand Names: Canada Clinda-T; Clindasol; Clindets; Dalacin T; Dalacin Vaginal; Taro-Clindamycin

Therapeutic Category Acne Products; Antibiotic, Anaerobic; Antibiotic, Miscellaneous

Generic Availability (U.S.) May be product dependent

Use
Topical: Treatment of acne vulgaris (FDA approved in ages ≥12 years and adults)

Vaginal:
Cleocin Vaginal Cream: Treatment of bacterial vaginosis (FDA approved in adults)

Cleocin Ovules, Clindesse cream: Treatment of bacterial vaginosis (FDA approved in nonpregnant, postmenarchal females)

Pregnancy Risk Factor B

Pregnancy Considerations Adverse effects were not observed in animal reproduction studies. Clindamycin has been shown to cross the placenta following oral and parenteral dosing. Refer to the Clindamycin (Systemic) monograph for details. The amount of clindamycin available systemically is less following topical and vaginal application than with I.V. or oral administration. Oral clindamycin is recommended in certain pregnant patients for the treatment of bacterial vaginosis; however, vaginal therapy is not recommended for use in the second half of pregnancy.

Various clindamycin vaginal products are available for the treatment of bacterial vaginosis. Recommendations for use in pregnant woman vary by product labeling. Current guidelines prefer the use of oral therapy for the treatment of bacterial vaginosis in pregnant women. The CDC notes that vaginal therapy with clindamycin may be associated with adverse outcomes if used in the latter half of pregnancy (CDC, 2010).

If treatment for acne is needed during pregnancy, topical clindamycin may be considered if an antibiotic is needed. To decrease systemic exposure, pregnant women should avoid application to inflamed skin for long periods of time, or to large body surface areas (Kong, 2013).

Breast-Feeding Considerations It is not known if clindamycin is excreted into breast milk following vaginal or topical administration. Due to the potential for serious adverse reactions in the nursing infant, most manufacturers recommend a decision be made whether to discontinue nursing or to discontinue the drug, taking into account the importance of treatment to the mother. If clindamycin is used topically to the chest for the treatment of acne in women who are nursing, care should be taken to avoid accidental ingestion by the infant. To decrease systemic exposure, breast-feeding women should avoid application to inflamed skin for long periods of time, or to large body surface areas (Kong, 2013).

Small amounts of clindamycin transfer to human milk following oral and I.V. dosing. Refer to the Clindamycin (Systemic) monograph for details. Systemic clindamycin concentrations are less following topical and vaginal application. This minimal absorption should minimize potential exposure to a nursing infant. Nondose-related effects could include modification of bowel flora.

Contraindications Hypersensitivity to clindamycin, lincomycin, or any component; history of regional enteritis, ulcerative colitis, or antibiotic-associated colitis

Warnings Prolonged use may result in fungal or bacterial superinfection, including *C. difficile*-associated diarrhea (CDAD); CDAD has been observed >2 months postantibiotic treatment. Discontinue drug if significant diarrhea, abdominal cramps, or passage of blood and mucus occurs. Clindamycin foam may cause skin irritation especially when used with abrasive, desquamating, or peeling agents; avoid contact with eyes, mouth, lips, mucous membranes, or broken skin.

Precautions Use topical clindamycin products with caution in atopic patients. Vaginal products may weaken condoms or contraceptive diaphragms; barrier contraceptives are not recommended concurrently or for 3-5 days (depending on the product) following treatment.

Adverse Reactions
Topical:
Central nervous system: Headache

Dermatologic: Dryness, burning, itching, scaliness, or peeling of skin (lotion, solution); erythema (foam, lotion, solution); oiliness (gel, lotion)

Rare but important or life-threatening: Abdominal pain, application site/skin pain, diarrhea (hemorrhagic or severe), dizziness, folliculitis, hypersensitivity reactions, nausea, pseudomembranous colitis, rash, seborrhea, urticaria, vomiting

Vaginal:
Central nervous system: Headache

Dermatologic: Pruritus

Gastrointestinal: Constipation

Genitourinary: Trichomonal vaginitis, urinary tract infection, vaginal moniliasis, vaginal pain, vulvovaginal disorder, vulvovaginal pruritus, vulvovaginitis

Neuromuscular & skeletal: Back pain

- Miscellaneous: Fungal infection
  Rare but important or life-threatening: Allergic reaction, atrophic vaginitis, bacterial infection, endometriosis, epistaxis, erythema, hematochezia, hypersensitivity, hyperthyroidism, local edema, metrorrhagia, pyelonephritis

Drug Interactions

Metabolism/Transport Effects None known.

Avoid Concomitant Use

Avoid concomitant use of Clindamycin (Topical) with any of the following: BCG; Erythromycin (Systemic); Erythromycin (Topical)

Increased Effect/Toxicity

Clindamycin (Topical) may increase the levels/effects of: Neuromuscular-Blocking Agents

Decreased Effect

Clindamycin (Topical) may decrease the levels/effects of: BCG; Sodium Picosulfate

The levels/effects of Clindamycin (Topical) may be decreased by: Erythromycin (Systemic); Erythromycin (Topical)

Stability

Topical:
  Foam (Evoclin): Store 20°C to 25°C (68°F to 77°F). Contents are flammable; do not puncture or incinerate container.
  Gel:
    Cleocin-T: Store at 20°C to 25°C (68°F to 77°F); protect from freezing.
    Clindagel: Store at 25°C (77°F); excursions permitted between 15°C to 30°C (59°F to 86°F). Do not store in direct sunlight.
  Lotion, solution, or pledgets: Store at 20°C to 25°C (68°F to 77°F); protect from freezing.
Vaginal:
  Cream:
    Cleocin: Store at 20°C to 25°C (68°F to 77°F); protect from freezing.
    Clindesse: Store at 20°C to 25°C (68°F to 77°F). Avoid heat >30°C (86°F).
  Ovule: Store at 25°C (77°F); excursions permitted between 15°C to 30°C (59°F to 86°F). Avoid heat >30°C (86°F) and high humidity.

Mechanism of Action Reversibly binds to 50S ribosomal subunits preventing peptide bond formation thus inhibiting bacterial protein synthesis; bacteriostatic or bactericidal depending on drug concentration, infection site, and organism

Pharmacokinetics (Adult data unless noted)

Absorption: Topical solution or foam, phosphate: Minimal; Vaginal cream, phosphate: ~5%; Vaginal suppository, phosphate: ~30%

Metabolism: Hepatic; forms metabolites (variable activity); Clindamycin phosphate is converted to clindamycin HCl (active)

Half-life elimination: Vaginal cream: 1.5-2.6 hours following repeated dosing; Vaginal suppository: 11 hours (range: 4-35 hours, limited by absorption rate)

Time to peak, serum: Vaginal cream: ~10-14 hours (range: 4-24 hours); Vaginal suppository: ~5 hours (range: 1-10 hours)

Excretion: Urine (<0.2% with topical foam and solution)

Dosing: Usual Children, Adolescents, and Adults:

Acne vulgaris: Children ≥12 years, Adolescents, and Adults: Topical:
  Gel (Clindagel), Foam (Evoclin): Apply to affected area once daily
  Gel (Cleocin T), pledget, lotion, solution: Apply a thin film twice daily

Bacterial vaginosis: Adolescents and Adults: Intravaginal:
  Cream:
    Adolescents: One full applicator inserted intravaginally at bedtime for 7 days (*Red Book*, 2012)
    Adults:
      Cleocin: One full applicator (100 mg clindamycin) inserted intravaginally once daily before bedtime for 3 or 7 consecutive days in nonpregnant patients and 7 consecutive days in pregnant patients
      Clindesse: One full applicator inserted intravaginally as a single dose at anytime during the day in nonpregnant patients
  Suppository: Insert one ovule (100 mg clindamycin) intravaginally once daily at bedtime for 3 days

Dosing adjustment in renal impairment: There are no dosage adjustments provided in the manufacturer's labeling; however, no dosage adjustments are required with systemic clindamycin use.

Dosing adjustment in hepatic impairment: There are no dosage adjustments provided in the manufacturer's labeling; however, no dosage adjustments are required with systemic clindamycin use; use caution with severe hepatic impairment.

Administration

Intravaginal: Do not use for topical therapy, instillation in the eye, or oral administration. Wash hands; insert applicator into vagina and expel suppository or cream. Remain lying down for 30 minutes following administration. Wash applicator with soap and water following suppository use; if administering the cream, use each disposable applicator only once.

Topical foam: Do not use intravaginally. Before applying foam, wash affected area with mild soap, then dry. Do not dispense foam directly onto hands or face. Remove cap, hold can at an upright angle, and dispense foam directly into the cap or onto a cool surface. If can is warm or foam is runny, run can under cold water. Use fingertips to pick up small amounts of foam and gently massage into affected area until foam disappears. Avoid fire, flame, or smoking during or immediately following application. Avoid contact with eyes, mouth, lips, mucous membranes, or broken skin.

Topical gel, pledget, solution: Do not use intravaginally, instill in the eye, or administer orally. Solution/pledget contains an alcohol base and if inadvertent contact with mucous membranes occurs, rinse with liberal amounts of water. Remove pledget from foil immediately before use; discard after single use. May use more than one pledget for each application to cover area.

Topical lotion: Shake well immediately before use; apply topically. Do not use intravaginally, instill in the eye, or administer orally.

Monitoring Parameters Observe for changes in bowel frequency.

Dosage Forms Excipient information presented when available (limited, particularly for generics); consult specific product labeling. [DSC] = Discontinued product

Cream, Vaginal, as phosphate [strength expressed as base]:
  Cleocin: 2% (40 g) [contains benzyl alcohol]
  Clindesse: 2% (5.8 g) [contains methylparaben, propylparaben]
  Generic: 2% (40 g)

Foam, External, as phosphate [strength expressed as base]:
  Evoclin: 1% (50 g, 100 g) [contains cetyl alcohol, propylene glycol]
  Generic: 1% (50 g, 100 g)

Gel, External, as phosphate [strength expressed as base]:
  Cleocin-T: 1% (30 g, 60 g) [contains methylparaben, propylene glycol]

◄

Clindagel: 1% (40 mL [DSC], 75 mL) [contains methylparaben, polyethylene glycol, propylene glycol]
ClindaMax: 1% (30 g, 60 g)
Generic: 1% (30 g, 60 g)
Kit, External, as phosphate [strength expressed as base]:
Clindacin ETZ: 1% [contains cetyl alcohol, isopropyl alcohol, propylene glycol]
Clindacin Pac: 1% [contains cetyl alcohol, isopropyl alcohol, propylene glycol]
Lotion, External, as phosphate [strength expressed as base]:
Cleocin-T: 1% (60 mL) [contains cetostearyl alcohol, methylparaben]
ClindaMax: 1% (60 mL)
Generic: 1% (60 mL)
Solution, External, as phosphate [strength expressed as base]:
Cleocin-T: 1% (30 mL, 60 mL) [contains isopropyl alcohol, propylene glycol]
Generic: 1% (30 mL, 60 mL)
Suppository, Vaginal, as phosphate [strength expressed as base]:
Cleocin: 100 mg (3 ea)
Swab, External, as phosphate [strength expressed as base]:
Cleocin-T: 1% (60 ea) [contains isopropyl alcohol, propylene glycol]
Clindacin ETZ: 1% (60 ea) [contains isopropyl alcohol, propylene glycol]
Clindacin-P: 1% (69 ea) [contains isopropyl alcohol, propylene glycol]
Generic: 1% (60 ea)

References

American Academy of Pediatrics (AAP). In: Pickering LK, Baker CJ, Kimberlin DW, Long SS, eds. Red Book: 2012 Report of the Committee on Infectious Diseases. 29th ed. Elk Grove Village, IL: American Academy of Pediatrics; 2012.
Centers for Disease Control and Prevention (CDC). 2010 STD Treatment Guidelines, 2010. MMWR Recomm Rep. 2010;59(RR-12):1-110. Available at http://www.cdc.gov/std/treatment/2010/
Kong YL, Tey HL. Treatment of acne vulgaris during pregnancy and lactation. Drugs. 2013;73(8):779-787.

Clindamycin and Benzoyl Peroxide
(klin da MYE sin & BEN zoe il peer OKS ide)

Brand Names: U.S. Acanya; BenzaClin; Duac
Brand Names: Canada BenzaClin; Clindoxyl
Therapeutic Category Acne Products; Topical Skin Product
Generic Availability (U.S.) Yes
Use Topical treatment of acne vulgaris (FDA approved in ages ≥12 years and adults)
Pregnancy Risk Factor C
Pregnancy Considerations Animal reproduction studies have not been conducted with this combination. Refer to individual monographs.
Breast-Feeding Considerations It is not known if clindamycin or benzoyl peroxide are excreted into breast milk following topical administration. Due to the potential for serious adverse reactions in the nursing infant, the manufacturers recommend a decision be made whether to discontinue nursing or to discontinue the drug, taking into account the importance of treatment to the mother. Also refer to individual monographs.
Contraindications Hypersensitivity to benzoyl peroxide, clindamycin, lincomycin, or any component; history of regional enteritis, ulcerative colitis, pseudomembranous colitis, or antibiotic-associated colitis
Warnings Use of topical clindamycin results in absorption from the skin surface; diarrhea, bloody diarrhea, and colitis (including pseudomembranous colitis) have been reported with the use of topical and systemic clindamycin; the colitis is usually characterized by severe persistent diarrhea and

severe abdominal cramps and may be associated with the passage of blood and mucus; discontinue drug if significant diarrhea occurs. Antiperistaltic agents such as opiates or diphenoxylate with atropine may prolong and worsen the condition. Use of antibiotic agents may be associated with the overgrowth of nonsusceptible organisms including fungi; if this occurs, discontinue use. May bleach hair or clothing. Concomitant use with topical or oral erythromycin-containing products is not recommended.
Precautions Avoid contact with eyes and mucous membranes. Concomitant topical acne therapy should be used with caution because a possible cumulative irritancy effect may occur, especially with the use of peeling, desquamating, or abrasive agents. Inform patients to use skin protection and minimize prolonged exposure to sun and avoid tanning beds.
Adverse Reactions Also see individual agents.
Dermatologic: Application site burning, application site erythema, application site itching, application site scaling, application site stinging, local desquamation, local dryness, sunburn (local)
Local: Application site reaction
Rare but important or life-threatening: Hypersensitivity reaction
Drug Interactions
Metabolism/Transport Effects None known.
Avoid Concomitant Use
Avoid concomitant use of Clindamycin and Benzoyl Peroxide with any of the following: BCG; Erythromycin (Systemic); Erythromycin (Topical)
Increased Effect/Toxicity
Clindamycin and Benzoyl Peroxide may increase the levels/effects of: Neuromuscular-Blocking Agents
Decreased Effect
Clindamycin and Benzoyl Peroxide may decrease the levels/effects of: BCG; Sodium Picosulfate

The levels/effects of Clindamycin and Benzoyl Peroxide may be decreased by: Erythromycin (Systemic); Erythromycin (Topical)
Stability
Acanya: Prior to dispensing, store in refrigerator between 2°C to 8°C (36°F to 46°F); do not freeze. Once dispensed, patient should store at room temperature of ≤25°C (≤77°F) for up to 10 weeks.
BenzaClin: Store at room temperature of 25°C (77°F); do not freeze. Once reconstituted and dispensed, patient should store at room temperature of ≤25°C (≤77°F) and use within 3 months.
Duac: Prior to dispensing, store in refrigerator, between 2°C to 8°C (36°F to 46°F); do not freeze. Once dispensed, patient should store at room temperature of ≤25°C (≤77°F) and use within 60 days.
Mechanism of Action Clindamycin and benzoyl peroxide have activity against *Propionibacterium acnes in vitro*. This organism has been associated with acne vulgaris. Benzoyl peroxide releases free-radical oxygen which oxidizes bacterial proteins in the sebaceous follicles decreasing the number of anaerobic bacteria and decreasing irritating-type free fatty acids. Clindamycin reversibly binds to 50S ribosomal subunits preventing peptide bond formation thus inhibiting bacterial protein synthesis; it is bacteriostatic or bactericidal depending on drug concentration, infection site, and organism.
Pharmacodynamics See individual agents.
Pharmacokinetics (Adult data unless noted) See individual agents.
Dosing: Usual Acne vulgaris: Topical: Children ≥12 years and Adults:
Acanya: Apply pea-sized amount of gel once daily; use >12 weeks has not been studied.
BenzaClin: Apply twice daily (morning and evening)
Duac: Apply once daily in the evening

Administration FOR EXTERNAL USE ONLY. Not for oral, ophthalmic, or intravaginal use.

Topical: Skin should be clean and dry before applying. Apply thin layer to affected areas avoiding contact with eyes, lips, inside of nose, mouth, and all mucous membranes.

BenzaClin: Add indicated amount of purified water to the mark on the vial; immediately shake to dissolve clindamycin. Add clindamycin solution to the gel and stir 1 1/2 minutes until homogenous.

Dosage Forms Excipient information presented when available (limited, particularly for generics); consult specific product labeling.

Gel, topical: Clindamycin 1% and benzoyl peroxide 5% (50 g); Clindamycin phosphate 1.2% and benzoyl peroxide 5% (45 g)

Acanya: Clindamycin phosphate 1.2% and benzoyl peroxide 2.5% (50 g)

BenzaClin: Clindamycin 1% and benzoyl peroxide 5% (25 g, 35 g, 50 g)

Duac: Clindamycin phosphate 1.2% and benzoyl peroxide 5% (45 g)

Clindamycin and Tretinoin
(klin da MYE sin & TRET i noyn)

Brand Names: U.S. Veltin™; Ziana®

Therapeutic Category Acne Products; Antibiotic, Miscellaneous; Retinoic Acid Derivative

Generic Availability (U.S.) No

Use Treatment of acne vulgaris (FDA approved in ages ≥12 years and adults)

Pregnancy Risk Factor C

Pregnancy Considerations Adverse events were observed in animal reproduction studies using this combination topically. Refer to individual monographs.

Breast-Feeding Considerations It is not known if clindamycin or tretinoin are excreted into breast milk following topical administration. Due to the potential for serious adverse reactions in the nursing infant, the manufacturer recommends a decision be made whether to discontinue nursing or to discontinue the drug, taking into account the importance of treatment to the mother. Refer to individual monographs.

Contraindications Hypersensitivity to clindamycin, tretinoin, or any component; regional enteritis, ulcerative colitis, or history of antibiotic-associated colitis

Warnings Clindamycin systemic absorption has been observed with topical use; prolonged use of clindamycin may result in fungal or bacterial superinfection, including *C. difficile*-associated diarrhea (CDAD) and pseudomembranous colitis; characterized by severe persistent diarrhea, severe abdominal cramps, and possibly, the passage of blood and mucus; CDAD has been observed >2 months postantibiotic treatment; discontinue drug if significant diarrhea occurs. Antiperistaltic agents, such as opiates or diphenoxylate with atropine, may prolong and worsen the condition.

Tretinoin use is associated with increased susceptibility/sensitivity to UV light; avoid sunlamps or excessive sunlight exposure. Daily sunscreen use and other protective measures are recommended. Tretinoin therapy can increase skin sensitivity to weather extremes of wind or cold. Also, concomitant topical medications (eg, medicated or abrasive soaps, cleansers, or cosmetics with a strong drying effect) should be used with caution due to increased skin irritation.

For external use only; avoid mucous membranes, eyes, mouth, and angles of nose.

Ziana™ topical gel contains polysorbate 80 (Tween 80) which may cause allergic reactions in susceptible individuals.

Precautions Use with caution or discontinue therapy in patients undergoing elective surgery. Use with caution in patients receiving erythromycin-containing products; may decrease effect of clindamycin.

Adverse Reactions

Dermatologic: Burning, dermatitis, dryness, erythema, exfoliation, irritation, pruritus, scaling, stinging, sunburn

Gastrointestinal: GI symptoms (unspecified)

Respiratory: Nasopharyngitis

Drug Interactions

Metabolism/Transport Effects None known.

Avoid Concomitant Use

Avoid concomitant use of Clindamycin and Tretinoin with any of the following: BCG; Erythromycin (Systemic); Erythromycin (Topical); Multivitamins/Fluoride (with ADE); Multivitamins/Minerals (with ADEK, Folate, Iron); Multivitamins/Minerals (with AE, No Iron)

Increased Effect/Toxicity

Clindamycin and Tretinoin may increase the levels/effects of: Neuromuscular-Blocking Agents; Porfimer

The levels/effects of Clindamycin and Tretinoin may be increased by: Multivitamins/Fluoride (with ADE); Multivitamins/Minerals (with ADEK, Folate, Iron); Multivitamins/Minerals (with AE, No Iron)

Decreased Effect

Clindamycin and Tretinoin may decrease the levels/effects of: BCG; Contraceptives (Progestins); Sodium Picosulfate

The levels/effects of Clindamycin and Tretinoin may be decreased by: Erythromycin (Systemic); Erythromycin (Topical)

Stability Store at 25°C (77°F); excursions permitted to 15°C to 30°C (59°F to 86°F); do not freeze. Protect from heat and light; when not in use, tube should be kept tightly closed.

Mechanism of Action Clindamycin reversibly binds to 50S ribosomal subunits preventing peptide chain elongation thus inhibiting bacterial protein synthesis. Clindamycin exhibits *in vitro* activity against *Propionibacterium acnes*, an organism associated with acne vulgaris. Topical tretinoin is believed to decrease follicular epithelial cells cohesiveness and increase follicular epithelial cell turnover resulting in decreased microcomedo formation and increased expulsion of comedones.

Pharmacokinetics (Adult data unless noted) Absorption: Tretinoin: Minimal systemic absorption; Clindamycin: Low and variable systemic absorption

Dosing: Usual Acne vulgaris: Children ≥12 years and Adults: Topical: Apply pea-size amount to entire face once daily at bedtime; **Note:** Higher dosages (larger amount or more frequent use) have not been shown to improve efficacy and are associated with increased adverse effects (eg, skin irritation)

Administration Prior to application, clean face with a mild soap and pat dry; place pea-size amount on one fingertip and then dot on chin, cheeks, nose, and forehead. Gently rub over entire face or entire affected area while avoiding eyes, lips, mouth, angles of nose, and mucous membranes. Wash hands after use.

Monitoring Parameters Observe for changes in bowel frequency.

Dosage Forms Excipient information presented when available (limited, particularly for generics); consult specific product labeling.

Gel, topical:

Veltin™: Clindamycin phosphate 1.2% and tretinoin 0.025% (30 g, 60 g)

Ziana®: Clindamycin phosphate 1.2% and tretinoin 0.025% (30 g, 60 g)

◆ **Clindamycine (Can)** *see* Clindamycin (Systemic) *on page 495*

◆ **Clindamycin Hydrochloride** *see* Clindamycin (Systemic) *on page 495*

◆ **Clindamycin Injection, USP (Can)** *see* Clindamycin (Systemic) *on page 495*

◆ **Clindamycin Palmitate** *see* Clindamycin (Systemic) *on page 495*

◆ **Clindamycin Phosphate** *see* Clindamycin (Topical) *on page 500*

◆ **Clindamycin Phosphate and Benzoyl Peroxide** *see* Clindamycin and Benzoyl Peroxide *on page 502*

◆ **Clindamycin Phosphate and Tretinoin** *see* Clindamycin and Tretinoin *on page 503*

◆ **Clindasol (Can)** *see* Clindamycin (Topical) *on page 500*

◆ **Clinda-T (Can)** *see* Clindamycin (Topical) *on page 500*

◆ **Clindesse** *see* Clindamycin (Topical) *on page 500*

◆ **Clindets (Can)** *see* Clindamycin (Topical) *on page 500*

◆ **Clindoxyl (Can)** *see* Clindamycin and Benzoyl Peroxide *on page 502*

◆ **Clinolipid** *see* Fat Emulsion (Plant Based) *on page 846*

◆ **Clinoril** *see* Sulindac *on page 1957*

◆ **Clinpro 5000** *see* Fluoride *on page 894*

CloBAZam (KLOE ba zam)

Medication Safety Issues
Sound-alike/look-alike issues:
CloBAZam may be confused with clonazePAM
Brand Names: U.S. Onfi
Brand Names: Canada Apo-Clobazam; Clobazam-10; Dom-Clobazam; Frisium; Novo-Clobazam; PMS-Clobazam
Therapeutic Category Anticonvulsant, Benzodiazepine
Generic Availability (U.S.) No
Use Adjunctive treatment of seizures associated with Lennox-Gastaut syndrome (FDA approved in ages ≥2 years and adults); has also been used as monotherapy and adjunctive treatment for other forms of epilepsy
Medication Guide Available Yes
Pregnancy Considerations Adverse events were observed in some animal reproduction studies. Clobazam crosses the placenta. An increased risk of fetal malformations may be associated with first trimester exposure. The Canadian labeling contraindicates use in the first trimester. The incidence of premature birth and low birth weights may be increased following maternal use of benzodiazepines; hypoglycemia and respiratory problems in the neonate may occur following exposure late in pregnancy. Neonatal withdrawal symptoms may occur within days to weeks after birth and "floppy infant syndrome" (which also includes withdrawal symptoms) has been reported with some benzodiazepines (Bergman, 1992; Iqbal, 2002; Wikner, 2007). A combination of factors influences the potential teratogenicity of anticonvulsant therapy. When treating women with epilepsy, monotherapy with the lowest effective dose and avoidance medications known to have a high incidence of teratogenic effects is recommended (Harden, 2009; Wlodarczyk, 2012).

Patients exposed to clobazam during pregnancy are encouraged to enroll themselves into the AED Pregnancy Registry by calling 1-888-233-2334. Additional information is available at www.aedpregnancyregistry.org.

Breast-Feeding Considerations Clobazam is excreted into breast milk. Use in nursing women is contraindicated in the Canadian labeling. Drowsiness, lethargy, or weight loss in nursing infants have been observed in case reports following maternal use of some benzodiazepines (Iqbal, 2002).

Contraindications Hypersensitivity to clobazam or any component

Warnings May cause CNS depression and dose-related somnolence and sedation (incidence: 32% with high doses); onset of somnolence and sedation occurs within first month of therapy and may lessen with continued treatment; patients must be cautioned about performing tasks which require mental alertness (eg, operating machinery or driving); use with caution in patients with severe respiratory insufficiency, sleep apnea, or who are receiving other CNS depressants, psychoactive agents, or ethanol as additive CNS depressant effects can occur; concomitant ethanol use can increase clobazam serum concentrations by 50%. May cause physical and psychological dependence with prolonged use; do not abruptly discontinue; rebound or withdrawal symptoms (including seizures) may occur following abrupt discontinuation or large decreases in dose; use caution when reducing dose or withdrawing therapy; decrease slowly (5-10 mg/day on a weekly basis) and monitor for withdrawal symptoms.

Antiepileptic drugs (AEDs) increase the risk of suicidal behavior and ideation in patients receiving these medications for any indication. Pooled analyses of placebo-controlled trials involving 11 different AEDs (regardless of indication) showed a twofold increased risk of suicidal thoughts or behavior (estimated incidence rate: 0.43% in AED treated patients compared to 0.24% of patients receiving placebo); increased risk was observed as early as 1 week after initiation of AED and continued through duration of trials (most trials ≤24 weeks); risk did not vary significantly by age (age range: 5-100 years). Consider risks and benefits of AEDs before prescribing. Monitor all patients receiving an AED for emergence of suicidal thoughts or behavior, thoughts of self-harm, any unusual changes in behavior or mood, or the emergence or worsening of depressive symptoms; notify healthcare provider immediately if symptoms or concerning behavior occur. **Note:** The FDA requires a Medication Guide for all antiepileptic drugs informing patients of this risk.

Does not have antidepressant, antipsychotic, or analgesic properties; benzodiazepines have been associated with anterograde amnesia. Paradoxical reactions, including hyperactive or aggressive behavior, have been reported with benzodiazepines, particularly in adolescent/pediatric or psychiatric patients. Hypotonia, hypothermia, withdrawal symptoms, and respiratory and feeding difficulties have been reported in the infant following maternal use of benzodiazepines near time of delivery.

Precautions Use with caution and adjust dose in patients with hepatic impairment; consider avoiding with severe hepatic impairment; no dosage recommendations exist. Use with caution and adjust dose in patients who are CYP2C19 poor metabolizers. Use with caution in patients at risk for falls, including elderly. May cause muscle weakness, use with caution in patients with preexisting muscle weakness, spinal or cerebellar ataxia, or myasthenia gravis. Use with caution in patients with impaired gag reflex; benzodiazepines may decrease the ability to manage secretions increasing risk for postictal aspiration pneumonia. Use with caution in patients with narrow-angle glaucoma. Tolerance and loss of seizure control have been reported with chronic administration. May decrease efficacy of hormonal contraceptives; female patients of childbearing potential should be counseled to use alternative nonhormonal contraception during therapy and for 28 days following clobazam discontinuation.

Decreased bone density and bone length and alterations in behavior have been reported in juvenile animal studies at levels of exposure greater than therapeutic doses; adverse bone effects were reversible upon discontinuation. Administration of high doses to rats for 2 years was associated with an increase in thyroid follicular cell adenomas; implications for human use are uncertain.

Adverse Reactions

Central nervous system: Aggressiveness, ataxia, fatigue, fever, insomnia, irritability, lethargy, psychomotor hyperactivity, sedation, somnolence

Gastrointestinal: Appetite increased, constipation, dysphagia, salivation increased, vomiting

Genitourinary: Urinary tract infection

Neuromuscular & skeletal: Dysarthria

Respiratory: Bronchitis, cough, pneumonia, upper respiratory tract infection

Postmarketing and/or case reports (Limited to important or life-threatening): Aspiration, behavior changes, blurred vision, confusion, delirium, delusions, depression, diplopia, eosinophilia, hallucinations, leukopenia, mood changes, respiratory depression, Stevens-Johnson syndrome, suicidal ideation, suicide attempts, thrombocytopenia, toxic epidermal necrolysis

Drug Interactions

Metabolism/Transport Effects Substrate of CYP2B6 (minor), CYP2C19 (major), CYP3A4 (minor), P-glycoprotein; **Note:** Assignment of Major/Minor substrate status based on clinically relevant drug interaction potential; **Inhibits** CYP2C9 (weak), CYP2D6 (moderate), UGT1A4, UGT1A6, UGT2B4; **Induces** CYP3A4 (weak/moderate)

Avoid Concomitant Use

Avoid concomitant use of CloBAZam with any of the following: Axitinib; Azelastine (Nasal); Methadone; OLANZapine; Paraldehyde; Simeprevir; Sodium Oxybate; Thalidomide; Thioridazine

Increased Effect/Toxicity

CloBAZam may increase the levels/effects of: Azelastine (Nasal); Buprenorphine; CloZAPine; CNS Depressants; CYP2D6 Substrates; Deferiprone; DOXOrubicin (Conventional); Fesoterodine; Hydrocodone; Methadone; Methotrimeprazine; Metoprolol; Metyrosine; Mirtazapine; Nebivolol; Paraldehyde; Pramipexole; ROPINIRole; Rotigotine; Selective Serotonin Reuptake Inhibitors; Sodium Oxybate; Stiripentol; Thalidomide; Thioridazine; Zolpidem

The levels/effects of CloBAZam may be increased by: Alcohol (Ethyl); Antifungal Agents (Azole Derivatives, Systemic); Aprepitant; Brimonidine (Topical); Calcium Channel Blockers (Nondihydropyridine); Cannabis; Cimetidine; CYP2C19 Inhibitors (Moderate); CYP2C19 Inhibitors (Strong); Doxylamine; Dronabinol; Droperidol; Fosaprepitant; Grapefruit Juice; HydrOXYzine; Isoniazid; Kava Kava; Luliconazole; Magnesium Sulfate; Methotrimeprazine; Nabilone; OLANZapine; Perampanel; Propafenone; Proton Pump Inhibitors; Rufinamide; Selective Serotonin Reuptake Inhibitors; Stiripentol; Tapentadol; Tetrahydrocannabinol

Decreased Effect

CloBAZam may decrease the levels/effects of: ARIPiprazole; Axitinib; Codeine; Contraceptives (Estrogens); Contraceptives (Progestins); Ibrutinib; Saxagliptin; Simeprevir; Tamoxifen; TraMADol

The levels/effects of CloBAZam may be decreased by: CarBAMazepine; CYP2C19 Inducers (Strong); Dabrafenib; Rifamycin Derivatives; Theophylline Derivatives; Yohimbine

Food Interactions

Ethanol: Concomitant administration may increase bioavailability of clobazam by 50%. Management: Monitor for increased effects with coadministration.

Food: Serum concentrations may be increased by grapefruit juice. Management: Keep grapefruit consumption consistent.

Stability Store at 20°C to 25°C (68°F to 77°F).

Mechanism of Action Clobazam is a 1,5 benzodiazepine which binds to stereospecific benzodiazepine receptors on the postsynaptic GABA neuron at several sites within the central nervous system, including the limbic system, reticular formation. Enhancement of the inhibitory effect of GABA on neuronal excitability results by increased neuronal membrane permeability to chloride ions. This shift in chloride ions results in hyperpolarization (a less excitable state) and stabilization.

Pharmacodynamics Maximum effect: 5-9 days

Pharmacokinetics (Adult data unless noted)

Absorption: Rapid and extensive; not affected by food or crushing tablet

Distribution: V_{dss}: 100 L; Protein binding: Clobazam: 80% to 90%; N-desmethylclobazam (NCLB): 70%

Metabolism: Hepatic via CYP3A4 and to a lesser extent via CYP2C19 and 2B6; N-demethylation to active metabolite (N-desmethyl) with ~20% activity of clobazam. CYP2C19 primarily mediates subsequent hydroxylation of the N-desmethyl metabolite; metabolic rate increased in children (53% to 69%) (Ng, 2007). Plasma concentrations of NCLB are 5 times higher in CYP2C19 poor metabolizers versus extensive metabolizers.

Bioavailability: 87% (Ng, 2007)

Half-life:

Children: Clobazam: 16 hours (Ng, 2007)

Adults: Clobazam: 36-42 hours

NCLB: 71-82 hours

Time to peak serum concentration: 0.5-4 hours

Elimination: Urine: 82% of dose; unchanged drug: 2%, NCLB and other metabolites: ~94%. Feces: 11% of dose; unchanged drug: 1%

Dosing: Usual Note: Dosage should be titrated according to patient tolerability and response.

Infants, Children, and Adolescents:

Lennox-Gastaut syndrome: Children ≥2 years and Adolescents: Oral:

≤30 kg: Initial: 5 mg once daily for ≥1 week, may then increase to 5 mg twice daily for ≥1 week, then increase to 10 mg twice daily thereafter (maximum daily dose: 20 mg/**day**)

>30 kg: Initial: 5 mg twice daily for ≥1 week, may then increase to 10 mg twice daily for ≥1 week, then increase to 20 mg twice daily thereafter (maximum daily dose: 40 mg/**day**)

Seizures, generalized or partial, monotherapy or adjunctive therapy: Oral: Limited data available [Frisium® prescribing information (U.K.; Canada), 2011; Canadian Study Group, 1998; Ng, 2007]:

Infants and Children <2 years: Initial: 0.5-1 mg/kg/**day** usually in divided doses twice daily; maximum initial daily dose: 5 mg/**day**; may increase dosage slowly (not more often than every 5-7 days); maximum daily dose: 10 mg/**day**

Children 2-16 years: Initial: 5 mg once daily; may increase dosage slowly (not more often than every 5 days), usual range: 10-20 mg/**day** or 0.3-1 mg/kg/**day** in divided doses twice daily; maximum daily dose: 40 mg/**day**

Adults:

Lennox-Gastaut, adjunctive: Oral:

≤30 kg: Initial: 5 mg once daily for ≥1 week, then increase to 5 mg twice daily for ≥1 week, then increase to 10 mg twice daily thereafter

>30 kg: Initial: 5 mg twice daily for ≥1 week, then increase to 10 mg twice daily for ≥1 week, then increase to 20 mg twice daily thereafter

Dosage adjustment in renal impairment: Children, Adolescents, and Adults:

CrCl ≥30 mL/minute: No dosage adjustment required
CrCl <30 mL/minute: Use with caution, has not been studied

Dosage adjustment in hepatic impairment: Children, Adolescents, and Adults:

Mild to moderate impairment (Child-Pugh Score 5-9):

≤30 kg: Initial: 5 mg once daily for ≥2 weeks, then increase to 5 mg twice daily for ≥1 week, may then increase to 10 mg twice daily based on patient tolerability and response

>30 kg: Initial: 5 mg once daily for ≥1 week, then increase to 5 mg twice daily for ≥1 week, then increase to 10 mg twice daily for ≥1 week, may then increase to 20 mg twice daily based on patient tolerability and response

Severe impairment: Use with extreme caution; has not been studied; undergoes extensive hepatic metabolism.

Dosage adjustment for CYP2C19 poor metabolizers: Children, Adolescents, and Adults:

≤30 kg: Initial: 5 mg once daily for ≥2 weeks, then increase to 5 mg twice daily for ≥1 week, may then increase to 10 mg twice daily based on patient tolerability and response

>30 kg: Initial: 5 mg once daily for ≥1 week, then increase to 5 mg twice daily for ≥1 week, may then increase to 10 mg twice daily for ≥1 week, may then increase to 20 mg twice daily based on patient tolerability and response

Administration May be administered with or without food. Tablets can be crushed and mixed in applesauce.

Monitoring Parameters Respiratory and mental status/suicidality (eg, suicidal thoughts, depression, behavioral changes); CBC, liver function, and renal function; some recommend periodic thyroid function tests

Controlled Substance C-IV

Dosage Forms Excipient information presented when available (limited, particularly for generics); consult specific product labeling. [DSC] = Discontinued product

Suspension, Oral:

Onfi: 2.5 mg/mL (120 mL) [contains methylparaben, polysorbate 80, propylene glycol, propylparaben; berry flavor]

Tablet, Oral:

Onfi: 5 mg [DSC]

Onfi: 10 mg, 20 mg [scored]

References

Bergman U, Rosa FW, Baum C, et al, "Effects of Exposure to Benzodiazepine During Fetal Life," *Lancet*, 1992, 340(8821):694-6.

Canadian Study Group for Childhood Epilepsy, "Clobazam Has Equivalent Efficacy to Carbamazepine and Phenytoin as Monotherapy for Childhood Epilepsy," *Epilepsia*, 1998, 39(9):952-9.

Harden CL, Meador KJ, Pennell PB, et al, "Practice Parameter Update: Management Issues for Women With Epilepsy-Focus on Pregnancy (an Evidence-Based Review): Teratogenesis and Perinatal Outcomes: Report of the Quality Standards Subcommittee and Therapeutics and Technology Assessment Subcommittee of the American Academy of Neurology and American Epilepsy Society," *Neurology*, 2009, 73(2):133-41.

Iqbal MM, Sobhan T, Ryals T, et al, "Effects of Commonly Used Benzodiazepines on the Fetus, the Neonate, and the Nursing Infant," *Psychiatr Serv*, 2002, 53(1):39-49.

Montenegro MA, Arif H, Nahm EA, et al, "Efficacy of Clobazam as Add-On Therapy for Refractory Epilepsy: Experience at a U.S. Epilepsy Center," *Clin Neuropharmacol*, 2008, 31(6):333-8.

Ng YT and Collins SD, "Clobazam," *Neurotherapeutics*, 2007, 4 (1):138-44.

Ng YT, Conry JA, Drummond R, et al, "Ranodmized, Phase III Study Results of Clobazam in Lennox-Gastaut Syndrome," *Neurology*, 2011, 77(15):1473-81.

Riss J, Cloyd J, Gates J, et al, "Benzodiazepines in Epilepsy: Pharmacology and Pharmacokinetics," *Acta Neurol Scand*, 2008, 118 (2):69-86.

Wikner BN, Stiller CO, Bergman U, et al, "Use of Benzodiazepines and Benzodiazepine Receptor Agonists During Pregnancy: Neonatal Outcome and Congenital Malformations," *Pharmacoepidemiol Drug Saf*, 2007, 16(11):1203-10.

Wlodarczyk BJ, Palacios AM, George TM, et al, "Antiepileptic Drugs and Pregnancy Outcomes," *Am J Med Genet A*, 2012, 158A (8):2071-90.

◆ **Clobazam-10 (Can)** see CloBAZam on page 504

Clobetasol (kloe BAY ta sol)

Medication Safety Issues

International issues:

Clobex [U.S., Canada, and multiple international markets] may be confused with Codex brand name for *Saccharomyces boulardii* [Italy]

Cloderm: Brand name for clobetasol [China, India, Malaysia, Singapore, Thailand], but also brand name for alclometasone [Indonesia]; clocortolone [U.S., Canada]; clotrimazole [Germany]

Related Information

Topical Corticosteroids on page 2224

Brand Names: U.S. Clobetasol Propionate E; Clobex; Clobex Spray; Clodan; Cormax Scalp Application; Olux; Olux-E; Temovate; Temovate E

Brand Names: Canada Clobex®; Dermovate®; Mylan-Clobetasol Cream; Mylan-Clobetasol Ointment; Mylan-Clobetasol Scalp Application; Novo-Clobetasol; PMS-Clobetasol; ratio-Clobetasol; Taro-Clobetasol

Therapeutic Category Adrenal Corticosteroid; Anti-inflammatory Agent; Corticosteroid, Topical; Glucocorticoid

Generic Availability (U.S.) May be product dependent

Use Short-term relief of inflammation and pruritus associated with corticosteroid-responsive dermatoses

Pregnancy Risk Factor C

Pregnancy Considerations Extensive use in pregnant women is not recommended. There are no adequate and well-controlled studies in pregnant women, however, teratogenic effects were observed in animal studies.

Breast-Feeding Considerations It is not known if topical application will result in detectable quantities in breast milk.

Contraindications Hypersensitivity to clobetasol propionate, other corticosteroids, or any component; the solution for scalp application is also contraindicated for use in patients with primary scalp infections

Warnings Hypothalamic-pituitary-adrenal (HPA) axis suppression may occur with topical clobetasol use, even at low doses; acute adrenal insufficiency may occur with abrupt withdrawal after long-term use or with stress; withdrawal or discontinuation should be done carefully; patients with HPA axis suppression may require increased doses of systemic glucocorticosteroids prior to, during, and after unusual stress (eg, surgery). Adverse systemic effects (including HPA axis suppression) may occur when topical steroids are used on large areas of the body, denuded areas, for prolonged periods of time, with an occlusive dressing, and/or in pediatric patients; infants and small children may be more susceptible to HPA axis suppression or other systemic toxicities due to a larger skin surface area to body mass ratio; use with caution in pediatric patients; due to the increased risk of HPA axis suppression and other systemic toxicities, the use of any clobetasol product for the treatment of steroid-responsive dermatoses is not recommended in children <12 years of age; use of clobetasol lotion or spray for moderate to severe plaque-type psoriasis in children <18 years is not recommended.

Do not use topical clobetasol for the treatment of rosacea or perioral dermatitis; do not apply to the face, groin, or axillae. Do not exceed maximum recommended dose or duration of therapy due to the potential development of HPA axis suppression.

Precautions Avoid using higher than recommended doses; suppression of HPA axis, suppression of linear growth (ie, reduction of growth velocity), reduced bone mineral, or hypercorticism (Cushing's syndrome) may occur. Discontinue treatment if local irritation develops. Use appropriate antibacterial or antifungal agents to treat concomitant skin infections; discontinue clobetasol treatment if infection does not resolve promptly.

Adverse Reactions May depend upon formulation used, length of application, surface area covered, and the use of occlusive dressings.

Central nervous system: Intracranial hypertension (systemic effect reported in children treated with topical corticosteroids), local pain, localized burning, numbness of fingers, stinging sensation

Dermatologic: Atrophic striae (children), eczema asteatotic, erythema, folliculitis, pruritus, skin atrophy, telangiectasia, xeroderma

Endocrine & metabolic: Adrenal suppression, Cushing's syndrome, glucosuria, growth suppression, HPA-axis suppression, hyperglycemia

Local: Local irritation, skin fissure

Respiratory: Nasopharyngitis, streptococcal pharyngitis, upper respiratory tract infection

Rare but important or life-threatening: Alopecia, exfoliation of skin, skin rash, urticaria

Drug Interactions

Metabolism/Transport Effects None known.

Avoid Concomitant Use

Avoid concomitant use of Clobetasol with any of the following: Aldesleukin

Increased Effect/Toxicity

Clobetasol may increase the levels/effects of: Ceritinib; Deferasirox

The levels/effects of Clobetasol may be increased by: Telaprevir

Decreased Effect

Clobetasol may decrease the levels/effects of: Aldesleukin; Corticorelin; Hyaluronidase; Telaprevir

Stability

Cream, emollient cream, ointment: Store at room temperature, between 15°C to 30°C (59°F to 86°F). Do not refrigerate.

Foam: Store at room temperature of 20°C to 25°C (68°F to 77°F); do not expose to heat or temperatures >49°C (120°F). Can is pressurized; do not puncture or incinerate. Contents are flammable; avoid flame, fire, or smoking during and immediately after application.

Gel: Store between 2°C to 30°C (36°F to 86°F)

Lotion: Store at room temperature of 20°C to 25°C (68°F to 77°F). Do not freeze.

Solution: Do not use near open flame.

Cormax® scalp application: Store at room temperature between 15°C to 30°C (59°F to 86°F); do not refrigerate.

Temovate® scalp application: Store between 4°C to 25°C (39°F to 77°F).

Spray: Store at controlled room temperature; do not refrigerate or freeze; do not store at >30°C; spray is flammable; avoid heat, do not use near open flame

Mechanism of Action Stimulates the synthesis of enzymes needed to decrease inflammation, suppress mitotic activity, and cause vasoconstriction

Pharmacokinetics (Adult data unless noted)

Absorption: Percutaneous absorption varies and depends on many factors including vehicle used, integrity of epidermis, dose, and use of occlusive dressing; absorption is increased by occlusive dressings or with decreased integrity of skin (eg, inflammation or skin disease); gel has greater absorption than cream

Metabolism: Hepatic

Elimination: Drug and metabolites are excreted in urine and bile

Dosing: Usual Topical: Use the smallest amount for the shortest period of time to avoid HPA suppression; discontinue therapy when control is achieved; reassess diagnosis if no improvement is seen within 2 weeks.

Children <12 years: Use not recommended (high risk of systemic adverse effects, eg, HPA axis suppression, Cushing's syndrome)

Children ≥12 years and Adults:

Steroid-responsive dermatoses:

Cream, emollient cream, gel, lotion, ointment: Apply sparingly twice daily for up to 2 weeks; maximum dose: 50 g/week or 50 mL/week

Foam, solution: Apply sparingly to affected area of scalp twice daily for up to 2 weeks; maximum dose: 50 g/week or 50 mL/week

Mild to moderate plaque-type psoriasis of nonscalp areas: Foam: Apply sparingly to affected area twice daily for up to 2 weeks; maximum dose: 50 g/week; do not apply to face or intertriginous areas

Moderate to severe plaque-type psoriasis: Emollient cream: Apply sparingly twice daily for up to 2 weeks; if response is not adequate, may be used for up to 2 more weeks if application is <10% of body surface area; use with caution; maximum dose: 50 g/week

Children ≥18 years and Adults: Moderate to severe plaque-type psoriasis:

Lotion: Apply sparingly twice daily for up to 2 weeks; if response is not adequate, may be used for up to 2 more weeks if application is <10% of body surface area; use with caution; maximum dose: 50 mL/week

Spray: Apply sparingly twice daily for up to 2 weeks; if response is not adequate, may be used for up to 2 more weeks, but use should be limited to skin lesions that have not sufficiently improved; maximum dose: 50 g (59 mL) per week

Administration

Topical: All products: Apply sparingly to clean dry skin of affected area, gently rub in until disappears; do not use on open skin; do not apply to face, underarms, or groin area; avoid contact with eyes and lips; do not occlude affected area; wash hands after applying

Foam: Turn can upside down and spray a small amount (maximum: 1 1/2 capful or about the size of a golf ball) of foam into the cap, other cool surface, or to affected area. If the can is warm or foam is runny, place can under cold, running water. If fingers are warm, rinse with cool water and dry prior to handling (foam will melt on contact with warm skin). Massage foam into affected area.

Monitoring Parameters Assess HPA axis suppression in patients using potent topical steroids applied to a large surface area or to areas under occlusion (eg, ACTH stimulation test, morning plasma cortisol test, urinary free cortisol test)

Additional Information Considered to be a super high potency topical corticosteroid; clobetasol is a prednisolone analog with a high level of glucocorticoid activity and slight degree of mineralocorticoid activity. Nine of 14 pediatric patients (12-17 years of age) with moderate to severe atopic dermatitis (involving ≥20% BSA), who were treated with clobetasol lotion 0.05% twice daily for 2 weeks, developed adrenal suppression (versus 2 of 10 patients treated with the cream). Due to this high incidence of adrenal suppression, the lotion is not approved for this indication in children <18 years of age.

Dosage Forms Excipient information presented when available (limited, particularly for generics); consult specific product labeling.

Cream, External, as propionate:

Clobetasol Propionate E: 0.05% (15 g, 30 g, 60 g) [contains cetostearyl alcohol, propylene glycol]

Clobetasol Propionate E: 0.05% (15 g, 30 g, 60 g) [contains propylene glycol]

Temovate: 0.05% (30 g, 60 g) [contains cetostearyl alcohol, chlorocresol (chloro-m-cresol), propylene glycol]

Temovate E: 0.05% (60 g)

Generic: 0.05% (15 g, 30 g, 45 g, 60 g)

Foam, External, as propionate:

Olux: 0.05% (50 g, 100 g) [contains cetyl alcohol, propylene glycol]

Olux-E: 0.05% (50 g, 100 g) [contains cetyl alcohol, propylene glycol]

Generic: 0.05% (50 g, 100 g)

Gel, External, as propionate:

Temovate: 0.05% (60 g) [contains propylene glycol]

Generic: 0.05% (15 g, 30 g, 60 g)

Kit, External, as propionate:

Clodan: 0.05% [contains alcohol, usp, cetyl alcohol, edetate disodium, propylene glycol]

Liquid, External, as propionate:

Clobex Spray: 0.05% (59 mL, 125 mL) [contains alcohol, usp]

Lotion, External, as propionate:

Clobex: 0.05% (59 mL, 118 mL)

Generic: 0.05% (59 mL, 118 mL)

Ointment, External, as propionate:

Temovate: 0.05% (15 g, 30 g) [contains propylene glycol]

Generic: 0.05% (15 g, 30 g, 45 g, 60 g)

Shampoo, External, as propionate:

Clobex: 0.05% (118 mL) [contains alcohol, usp]

Clodan: 0.05% (118 mL) [contains alcohol, usp]

Generic: 0.05% (118 mL)

Solution, External, as propionate:

Cormax Scalp Application: 0.05% (50 mL) [contains isopropyl alcohol]

Temovate: 0.05% (50 mL)

Generic: 0.05% (25 mL, 50 mL)

◆ **Clobetasol Propionate** see Clobetasol on page 506

◆ **Clobetasol Propionate E** see Clobetasol on page 506

◆ **Clobex** see Clobetasol on page 506

◆ **Clobex® (Can)** see Clobetasol on page 506

◆ **Clobex Spray** see Clobetasol on page 506

◆ **Clodan** see Clobetasol on page 506

Clofarabine (klo FARE a been)

Medication Safety Issues

Sound-alike/look-alike issues:

Clofarabine may be confused with cladribine, clevidipine, cytarabine, nelarabine

High alert medication:

This medication is in a class the Institute for Safe Medication Practices (ISMP) includes among its list of drug classes which have a heightened risk of causing significant patient harm when used in error.

Related Information

Emetogenic Potential of Antineoplastic Agents in Children on page 2327

Safe Handling of Hazardous Drugs on page 2419

Brand Names: U.S. Clolar

Brand Names: Canada Clolar®

Therapeutic Category Antineoplastic Agent, Antimetabolite; Antineoplastic Agent, Antimetabolite (Purine Antagonist)

Generic Availability (U.S.) No

Use Treatment of relapsed or refractory acute lymphoblastic leukemia (ALL) after at least two prior treatment regimens (FDA approved in ages 1-21 years); has also been used for the treatment of acute myelogenous leukemia (AML)

Pregnancy Risk Factor D

Pregnancy Considerations Teratogenic effects and resorptions were observed in animal reproduction studies. May cause fetal harm if administered to a pregnant woman. Women of childbearing potential should be advised to use effective contraception and avoid becoming pregnant during therapy.

Breast-Feeding Considerations Due to the potential for serious adverse reactions in the nursing infant, breast-feeding should be avoided during clofarabine treatment.

Contraindications Hypersensitivity to clofarabine or any component

Warnings Hazardous agent; use appropriate precautions for handling and disposal (NIOSH, 2012). Bone marrow suppression, which appears to be dose dependent and reversible, is common; may be severe and prolonged. Monitor blood counts and platelets daily during treatment, then 1-2 times weekly or as necessary. May be at increased risk for infection, including opportunistic infections or sepsis, due to prolonged neutropenia; monitor for signs and symptoms of infection and treat promptly if infection develops; may require clofarabine discontinuation.

Tumor lysis syndrome/hyperuricemia may occur as a result of leukemia treatment, including treatment with clofarabine, usually occurring in the first treatment cycle; may lead to life-threatening acute renal failure; adequate hydration and prophylactic antihyperuricemia throughout the 5 days of clofarabine treatment will reduce the risk/effects of tumor lysis syndrome; monitor closely. Cytokine release syndrome (eg, tachypnea, tachycardia, hypotension, pulmonary edema) may develop into capillary leak syndrome/systemic inflammatory response syndrome (SIRS) and organ dysfunction; discontinue with signs/symptoms of SIRS or capillary leak syndrome (rapid-onset respiratory distress, hypotension, pleural/pericardial effusion, and organ dysfunction) and consider supportive treatment with diuretics, corticosteroids, and/or albumin. Prophylactic corticosteroids may prevent or diminish the signs/symptoms of cytokine release. Monitor blood pressure during the 5 days of treatment; discontinue if hypotension develops. Monitor if on concomitant medications known to affect blood pressure.

Transaminases and bilirubin may be increased during treatment; in some cases, reported hepatotoxicity was severe and fatal; transaminase elevations generally occur within 10 days of administration and persist for ≤15 days; may require dosage modification or discontinuation of clofarabine. The risk for hepatotoxicity, including hepatic sinusoidal obstruction syndrome [SOS; formerly called veno-occlusive disease (VOD)], is increased in patients who have previously undergone a hematopoietic stem cell transplant; discontinue if SOS is suspected. Avoid the concomitant use of drugs that may cause hepatotoxicity; monitor liver function closely. Use with caution in patients with hepatic impairment; has not been studied.

Elevated creatinine, acute renal failure, and hematuria were observed in clinical studies; monitor renal function closely; may require dosage reduction or therapy discontinuation. Minimize the use of drugs known to cause renal toxicity during the 5-day treatment period.

Potentially significant interactions may exist, requiring dose or frequency adjustment, additional monitoring, and/or selection of alternative therapy. Consult drug interactions database for more detailed information.

Adverse Reactions

Cardiovascular: Edema, flushing, hyper-/hypotension, pericardial effusion, tachycardia

Central nervous system: Agitation, anxiety, chills, fatigue, fever, headache, irritability, lethargy, mental status change, pain, somnolence

Dermatologic: Cellulitis, erythema, palmar-plantar erythrodysesthesia syndrome, pruritic rash, pruritus, rash

Gastrointestinal: Abdominal pain, anorexia, cecitis, clostridium colitis, diarrhea, gingival bleeding, mouth hemorrhage, mucosal inflammation, nausea, oral candidiasis, oral mucosal petechiae, pancreatitis, proctalgia, stomatitis, vomiting

Hematologic: Anemia, febrile neutropenia, leukopenia, lymphopenia, neutropenia, thrombocytopenia

Hepatic: ALT increased, AST increased, bilirubin increased, jaundice

Neuromuscular & skeletal: Arthralgia, back pain, bone pain, limb pain, myalgia, weakness

Renal: Creatinine increased, hematuria

Respiratory: Dyspnea, epistaxis, pleural effusion, pneumonia, pulmonary edema, respiratory distress, respiratory tract infection, tachypnea

Miscellaneous: Bacteremia, candidiasis, capillary leak syndrome, catheter-related infection, herpes simplex, herpes zoster, hypersensitivity, infection (including bacterial, fungal, viral), sepsis, septic shock, staphylococcus bacteremia, tumor lysis syndrome

Rare but important or life-threatening: Bone marrow failure, dermatitis, gastrointestinal hemorrhage, hallucination, hepatic sinusoidal obstruction syndrome (SOS; venoocclusive disease), hepatomegaly, hypokalemia, hypophosphatemia, left ventricular systolic function decreased, right ventricular pressure increased, Stevens-Johnson syndrome, toxic epidermal necrolysis

Drug Interactions

Metabolism/Transport Effects None known.

Avoid Concomitant Use

Avoid concomitant use of Clofarabine with any of the following: BCG; CloZAPine; Dipyrone; Natalizumab; Pimecrolimus; Tacrolimus (Topical); Tofacitinib; Vaccines (Live)

Increased Effect/Toxicity

Clofarabine may increase the levels/effects of: CloZAPine; Leflunomide; Natalizumab; Tofacitinib; Vaccines (Live); Vitamin K Antagonists

The levels/effects of Clofarabine may be increased by: Denosumab; Dipyrone; Pimecrolimus; Roflumilast; Tacrolimus (Topical); Trastuzumab

Decreased Effect

Clofarabine may decrease the levels/effects of: BCG; Cardiac Glycosides; Coccidioidin Skin Test; Sipuleucel-T; Vaccines (Inactivated); Vaccines (Live); Vitamin K Antagonists

The levels/effects of Clofarabine may be decreased by: Echinacea

Stability Store intact vials at 25°C (77°F), excursions permitted to 15°C to 30°C (59°F to 86°F); diluted solution is stable for 24 hours at room temperature. To prevent drug incompatibilities, do not mix with other medications.

Mechanism of Action Clofarabine, a purine (deoxyadenosine) nucleoside analog, is metabolized to clofarabine 5'-triphosphate. Clofarabine 5'-triphosphate decreases cell replication and repair as well as causing cell death. To decrease cell replication and repair, clofarabine 5'-triphosphate competes with deoxyadenosine triphosphate for the enzymes ribonucleotide reductase and DNA polymerase. Cell replication is decreased when clofarabine 5'-triphosphate inhibits ribonucleotide reductase from reacting with deoxyadenosine triphosphate to produce deoxynucleotide triphosphate which is needed for DNA synthesis. Cell replication is also decreased when clofarabine 5'-triphosphate competes with DNA polymerase for incorporation into the DNA chain; when done during the repair process, cell repair is affected. To cause cell death, clofarabine 5'-triphosphate alters the mitochondrial membrane by releasing proteins, an inducing factor and cytochrome C.

Pharmacokinetics (Adult data unless noted)

Distribution: V_d : Decreased with increasing age, based on pharmacokinetic simulations: 5.8 L/kg (3 years old); 3.1 L/kg (30 years old); 2.7 L/kg (82 years old) (Bonate, 2011); Children and Adolescents 2-19 years: 172 L/m²

Protein binding: Children and Adolescents 2-19 years: 47%, primarily to albumin

Metabolism: Intracellularly by deoxycytidine kinase and mono- and di-phosphokinases to active metabolite clofarabine 5'-triphosphate; limited hepatic metabolism (0.2%)

Children and Adolescents 2-19 years: 5.2 hours

Adults: 7 hours; half-life may be increased in patients with renal impairment (Bonate, 2011)

Elimination: Children and Adolescents 2-19 years: 49% to 60% excreted in urine as unchanged drug

Dosing: Usual Dosing and frequency may vary by protocol and/or treatment phase; refer to specific protocol.

Note: Consider prophylactic corticosteroids (hydrocortisone 100 mg/m² on days 1-3) to prevent signs/symptoms of capillary leak syndrome or systemic inflammatory response syndrome (SIRS); provide I.V. hydration, antihyperuricemic agent, and alkalinize urine (to reduce the risk of tumor lysis syndrome/hyperuricemia); consider prophylactic antiemetics.

Pediatric:

Acute lymphocytic leukemia (ALL), relapsed or refractory:

Monotherapy: Children and Adolescents: I.V. infusion: 52 mg/m²/day once daily for days 1-5 of each cycle; repeat cycle every 2-6 weeks following recovery or return to baseline organ function; subsequent cycles should begin no sooner than 14 days from the start of the previous cycle and when ANC ≥750/mm³

Combination therapy: Limited data available: I.V. Infusion:

Infants: Dosing regimens variable with very limited data available:

Weight-directed dosing: 1.33 mg/kg/day for 5 days in combination with cyclophosphamide and etoposide (O'Connor, 2011)

BSA-directed dosing: 40 mg/m²/day for 5 days in combination with cyclophosphamide and etoposide (Inaba, 2012); and with topotecan, vinorelbine, thiotepa (TVTC regimen), and dexamethasone in a Phase I trial (Steinherz, 2010)

Children and Adolescents: Usual dose: 40 mg/m²/day for 5 days in combination with cyclophosphamide and etoposide has been most frequently studied (Hijiya, 2011; Hijiya, 2012; Inaba, 2012; Locatelli, 2009; O'Connor, 2011); and with topotecan, vinorelbine, thiotepa (TVTC regimen), and dexamethasone in a Phase I trial (Steinherz, 2010). In one trial, the protocol included 5 days of clofarabine therapy during induction and 4 days of therapy for consolidation; this study was also amended to exclude patients with prior hematopoietic stem cell transplantation due to a high incidence of venoocclusive disease (Hijiya, 2011).

Acute myeloid leukemia (AML), relapsed or refractory: Limited data available: Children and Adolescents: I.V. infusion:

Monotherapy: 52 mg/m²/day once daily for days 1-5 of each cycle; repeat cycle every 2-6 weeks for up to 12 cycles following recovery or return to baseline organ function; subsequent cycles should begin no sooner than 14 days from the start of the previous cycle and when ANC ≥750/mm³; the trial did not have minimum exclusion age (patient age ≤21 years at time of diagnosis); the youngest patient was 2 years of age (Jeha, 2009)

Combination therapy: 40 mg/m²/day once daily for days 1-5 of each cycle in combination with cyclophosphamide and etoposide (Inaba, 2012)

Adults ≤21 years: **Acute lymphocytic leukemia (ALL), relapsed or refractory:** I.V. infusion: 52 mg/m²/day once daily for days 1-5 of each cycle; repeat cycle every 2-6 weeks following recovery or return to baseline organ function; subsequent cycles should begin no sooner than 14 days from the start of the previous cycle and when ANC ≥750/mm³

Dosing adjustment for toxicity: Children, Adolescents, and Adults ≤21 years:

Hematologic toxicity: ANC <500/mm³ lasting ≥4 weeks: Reduce clofarabine dose by 25% for next cycle

Nonhematologic toxicity:

Clinically significant infection: Withhold treatment until infection is under control, then restart clofarabine at full dose

Grade 3 toxicity, excluding infection, nausea, and vomiting, and transient elevations in transaminases and bilirubin: Withhold treatment; may reinitiate clofarabine with a 25% dose reduction with resolution or return to baseline

Grade ≥3 increase in creatinine or bilirubin: Discontinue clofarabine; may reinitiate with 25% dosage reduction when creatinine or bilirubin return to baseline and patient is stable; administer allopurinol for hyperuricemia

Grade 4 toxicity (noninfectious): Discontinue clofarabine treatment

Capillary leak or systemic inflammatory response syndrome (SIRS) early signs/symptoms (eg, hypotension, tachycardia, tachypnea, pulmonary edema): Discontinue clofarabine; institute supportive measures. May consider reinitiating with a 25% dose-reduction after patient is stable and after organ function recovers to baseline.

Dosing adjustment for renal impairment: Children, Adolescents, and Adults ≤21 years:

CrCl >60 mL/minute: No dosage adjustment recommended

CrCl 30-60 mL/minute: Reduce dose by 50%

CrCl <30 mL/minute: There are no dosage adjustments provided in the manufacturer's labeling; use with caution (has not been studied).

Dosing adjustment for hepatic impairment: There are no dosage adjustments provided in the manufacturer's labeling.

Administration Hazardous agent; use appropriate precautions for handling and disposal (NIOSH, 2012).

Parenteral: I.V. infusion: Filter clofarabine through a 0.2 micron syringe filter prior to dilution, and further dilute dose with D₅W or NS to a final concentration of 0.15-0.4 mg/mL. Administer by I.V. infusion over 2 hours per the manufacturer's labeling and in most trials; a few trials have infused over 1 hour (Federl, 2005; Jeha, 2004; Kantarian, 2003. Do not administer with any other medications through the same intravenous line.

Monitoring Parameters CBC with differential and platelets (daily during treatment, then 1-2 times weekly or as necessary); liver and kidney function (during 5 days of clofarabine administration); blood pressure, cardiac function, and respiratory status during infusion; signs and symptoms of tumor lysis syndrome, infection, and cytokine release syndrome (tachypnea, tachycardia, hypotension, pulmonary edema); hydration status

Dosage Forms Excipient information presented when available (limited, particularly for generics); consult specific product labeling.

Solution, Intravenous [preservative free]:

Clolar: 1 mg/mL (20 mL)

References

Bonate PL, Cunningham CC, Gaynon P, et al, "Population Pharmacokinetics of Clofarabine and its Metabolite 6-Ketoclofarabine in Adult and Pediatric Patients With Cancer," *Cancer Chemother Pharmacol,* 2011, 67(4):875-90.

Federl S, Gandhi V, O'Brien S, et al. Results of a phase 1-2 study of clofarabine in combination with cytarabine (ara-C) in relapsed and refractory acute leukemias. *Blood.* 2005; 105:940-947.

Hijiya N, Barry E, Arceci R. Clofarabine in pediatric acute leukemia: current findings and issues. *Pediatr Blood Cancer.* 2012;59:417-422.

Hijiya N, Thomson B, Isakoff MS, et al. Phase 2 trial of clofarabine in combination with etoposide and cyclophosphamide in pediatric patients with refractory or relapsed acute lymphoblastic leukemia. *Blood.* 2001;118 6043-6049.

Inaba H, Bhojwani D, Pauley JL, et.al. Combination chemotherapy with clofarabine, cyclophosphamide, and etoposide in children with refractory or relapsed haematological malignancies. *Br J Haematol.* 2012;156(2):275-279.

Jeha S, Gandhi V, Chan KW, et al, "Clofarabine, a Novel Nucleoside Analog, Is Active in Pediatric Patients With Advanced Leukemia," *Blood,* 2004, 103(3):784-9.

Jeha S, Gaynon PS, Razzouk BI, et al, "Phase II Study of Clofarabine in Pediatric Patients With Refractory or Relapsed Acute Lymphoblastic Leukemia," *J Clin Oncol,* 2006, 24(12):1917-23.

Jeha S, Razzouk B, Rytting M, et.al. Phase II study of clofarabine in pediatric patients with refractory or relapsed acute myeloid leukemia. *J Clin Oncol.* 2009;27:4392-4397.

Kantarjian H, Gandhi V, Cortes J, et al, "Phase 2 Clinical and Pharmacologic Study of Clofarabine in Patients With Refractory or Relapsed Acute Leukemia," *Blood,* 2003, 102(7):2379-86.

Locatelli F, Testi AM, Bernardo ME, et al. Clofarabine, cyclophosphamide and etoposide as single-course re-induction therapy for children with refractory/multiple relapsed acute lymphoblastic leukaemia. *British Journal of Haematology.* 2009;147:371-378.

National Institute for Occupational Safety and Health (NIOSH), "NIOSH List of Antineoplastic and Other Hazardous Drugs in Healthcare Settings 2012." Available at http://www.cdc.gov/niosh/docs/2012-150/pdfs/2012-150.pdf. Accessed January 21, 2013.

O'Connor D, Sibson K, Caswell M, et al. Early UK experience in the use of clofarabine in the treatment of relapsed and refractory paediatric acute lymphoblastic leukaemia. *British Journal of Haematology.* 2011;154:482-485.

Steinherz PG, Shukla N, Kobos R, et al. Remission re-induction chemotherapy with clofarabine, topotecan, thiotepa and vinorelbine for patients with relapsed or refractory leukemia. *Pediatr Blood Cancer.* 2010;54:687-693.

◆ **Clofarex** *see* Clofarabine *on page 508*

◆ **Clolar** *see* Clofarabine *on page 508*

◆ **Clolar® (Can)** *see* Clofarabine *on page 508*

ClomiPRAMINE (kloe MI pra meen)

Medication Safety Issues

Sound-alike/look-alike issues:

ClomiPRAMINE may be confused with chlorproMAZINE, clevidipine, clomiPHENE, desipramine, Norpramin®

Anafranil® may be confused with alfentanil, enalapril, nafarelin

BEERS Criteria medication:

This drug may be potentially inappropriate for use in geriatric patients (Quality of evidence - high [moderate for SIADH]; Strength of recommendation - strong).

Related Information

Antidepressant Agents *on page 2219*

Brand Names: U.S. Anafranil

Brand Names: Canada Anafranil®; Apo-Clomipramine®; CO Clomipramine; Dom-Clomipramine; Novo-Clomipramine

Therapeutic Category Antidepressant, Tricyclic (Tertiary Amine)

Generic Availability (U.S.) Yes

Use Treatment of obsessive-compulsive disorder (OCD) (FDA approved in ages ≥10 years and adults)

Medication Guide Available Yes

Pregnancy Risk Factor C

Pregnancy Considerations Adverse events were observed in some animal reproduction studies. Clomipramine and its metabolite desmethylclomipramine cross the placenta and can be detected in cord blood and neonatal serum at birth (Loughhead, 2006; ter Horst, 2011). Data from five newborns found the half-life for clomipramine in the neonate to be 42 ± 16 hours following *in utero* exposure. Serum concentrations were not found to correlate to withdrawal symptoms (ter Horst, 2011). Withdrawal symptoms (including jitteriness, tremor, and seizures) have been observed in neonates whose mothers took clomipramine up to delivery.

The ACOG recommends that therapy for depression during pregnancy be individualized; treatment should incorporate the clinical expertise of the mental health clinician, obstetrician, primary healthcare provider, and pediatrician (ACOG, 2008). According to the American Psychiatric Association (APA), the risks of medication treatment should be weighed against other treatment options and untreated depression. For women who discontinue antidepressant medications during pregnancy and who may be at high risk for postpartum depression, the medications can be restarted following delivery (APA, 2010). Treatment algorithms have been developed by the ACOG and the APA for the management of depression in women prior to conception and during pregnancy (Yonkers, 2009).

Breast-Feeding Considerations Clomipramine is excreted in breast milk. Based on information from three mother-infant pairs, following maternal use of clomipramine 75-150 mg/day, the estimated exposure to the breast-feeding infant would be 0.4% to 4% of the weight-adjusted maternal dose. Adverse events have not been reported in nursing infants (information from seven cases). Infants should be monitored for signs of adverse events; routine monitoring of infant serum concentrations is not recommended (Fortinguerra, 2009). Due to the potential for serious adverse reactions in the nursing infant, the decision to continue or discontinue breast-feeding during therapy should take into account the risk of exposure to the infant and the benefits of treatment to the mother.

Contraindications Hypersensitivity to clomipramine, other tricyclic agents, or any component; use of MAO inhibitors within 14 days (potentially fatal reactions may occur); use in a patient during the acute recovery phase of MI

Warnings Clinical worsening of depression or suicidal ideation and behavior may occur in children and adults with major depressive disorder **[U.S. Boxed Warning]**. In clinical trials, antidepressants increased the risk of suicidal thinking and behavior (suicidality) in children, adolescents, and young adults (18-24 years of age) with major depressive disorder and other psychiatric disorders. This risk must be considered before prescribing antidepressants for any clinical use. Short-term studies did not show an increased risk of suicidality with antidepressant use in patients >24 years of age and showed a decreased risk in patients ≥65 years.

Patients of all ages who are treated with antidepressants for any indication require appropriate monitoring and close observation for clinical worsening of depression, suicidality, and unusual changes in behavior, especially during the first few months after antidepressant initiation or when the dose is adjusted. Family members and caregivers should be instructed to closely observe the patient (ie, daily) and communicate condition with healthcare provider. Patients should also be monitored for associated behaviors (eg, anxiety, agitation, panic attacks, insomnia, irritability, hostility, aggressiveness, impulsivity, akathisia, hypomania, mania) which may increase the risk for worsening depression or suicidality. Worsening depression or emergence of suicidality (or associated behaviors listed above) that is abrupt in onset, severe, or not part of the presenting symptoms, may require discontinuation or modification of drug therapy.

Do not discontinue abruptly in patients receiving high doses chronically (withdrawal symptoms may occur). To reduce risk of intentional overdose, write prescriptions for the smallest quantity consistent with good patient care. Screen individuals for bipolar disorder prior to treatment (using antidepressants alone may induce manic episodes in patients with this condition). May worsen psychosis in some patients. Clomipramine is not FDA approved for the treatment of bipolar depression.

Clomipramine may cause seizures (direct relationship to dose and/or duration of therapy); do not exceed maximum doses. Use with caution in patients with a previous seizure disorder or condition predisposing to seizures such as brain damage, alcoholism, or concurrent therapy with other drugs which lower the seizure threshold.

Precautions May cause sedation, resulting in impaired performance of tasks requiring alertness (eg, operating machinery or driving). Sedative effects may be additive with other CNS depressants and/or ethanol. The degree of sedation is very high relative to other antidepressants. Vomiting is two- to threefold more prevalent in children compared to adolescents and is more prevalent in adolescents compared to adults; to help minimize, divide the dose and give with food initially. Once titrated to maintenance therapy, can consolidate to once daily dosing at bedtime. Weight gain may occur. May increase the risks associated with electroconvulsive therapy; limit such treatment to patients in whom it is essential. Consider discontinuing, when possible, prior to elective surgery. Therapy should not be abruptly discontinued in patients receiving high doses for prolonged periods.

May cause tachycardia and orthostatic hypotension (risk is moderate to high relative to other antidepressants); use with caution in patients at risk of hypotension or in patients where transient tachycardia and hypotensive episodes would be poorly tolerated (cardiovascular disease or cerebrovascular disease). The degree of anticholinergic blockade produced by this agent is very high relative to other cyclic antidepressants; use with caution in patients with urinary retention, benign prostatic hyperplasia, narrow-angle glaucoma, increased IOP, xerostomia, visual problems, constipation, or history of bowel obstruction. Upon abrupt discontinuation, the effects of cholinergic rebound (eg, nausea, vomiting, diarrhea, salivation, lacrimation) may be more problematic in youth compared to adults. It is unknown what (if any) effects that long-term clomipramine treatment may have on growth and development in children.

Use with caution in patients with a history of cardiovascular disease (including previous MI, stroke, tachycardia, or conduction abnormalities). The risk of conduction abnormalities with this agent is high relative to other antidepressants. Use with caution in hyperthyroid patients or those receiving thyroid supplementation. Use with caution in patients with tumors of the adrenal medulla (hypertensive crisis may result). Use with caution in patients with hepatic or renal dysfunction.

Adverse Reactions
Cardiovascular: Chest pain (children), ECG abnormality, flushing, orthostatic hypotension, palpitation, syncope (children), tachycardia
Central nervous system: Abnormal dreaming (adults), abnormal thinking, aggressiveness (children), agitation (adults), anxiety (more common in adults), chills (adults), concentration impaired (adults), confusion, depersonalization, depression (adults), dizziness (more common in adults), emotional lability (adults), fatigue, fever (adults), headache (more common in adults), hypertonia, insomnia (more common in adults), irritability (children), memory impairment, migraine (adults), myasthenia, nervousness (more common in adults), pain, panic

reaction, psychosomatic disorder (adults), sleep disorder, somnolence, speech disorder (adults), twitching (adults), vertigo, yawning (adults)

Dermatologic: Body odor (children), dermatitis (adults), dry skin (adults), rash, pruritus (adults), purpura (adults), urticaria (adults)

Endocrine & metabolic: Amenorrhea (adults), breast enlargement (adults), breast pain (adults), hot flashes, lactation (nonpuerperal) (adults), libido changes (adults), menstrual disorder (adults)

Gastrointestinal: Abdominal pain, anorexia, appetite increased, constipation (more common in adults), diarrhea, dyspepsia, dysphagia (adults), esophagitis (adults), flatulence (adults), gastrointestinal disturbance (adults), halitosis (children), nausea (more common in adults), taste disturbance (adults), tooth disorder (adults), ulcerative stomatitis (children), vomiting, weight loss (children), weight gain (more common in adults), xerostomia (more common in adults)

Genitourinary: Cystitis (adults), ejaculation failure (more common in adults), impotence (adults), leukorrhea (adults), micturition disorder (more common in adults), micturition frequency (adults), urinary retention (more common in children), UTI (adults), vaginitis (adults)

Hepatic: Increased serum ALT (>3 x ULN), increased serum AST (>3 x ULN)

Hypersensitivity: Hypersensitivity reaction (children)

Neuromuscular & skeletal: Myalgia (adults), myoclonus (more common in adults), paresis (children), paresthesia (more common in adults), tremor (more common in adults), weakness (children)

Ophthalmic: Abnormal vision (more common in adults), anisocoria (children), blepharospasm (children), conjunctivitis (adults), lacrimation abnormal (adults), mydriasis (adults), ocular allergy (children)

Otic: Tinnitus

Respiratory: Bronchospasm (more common in children), dyspnea (children), epistaxis (adults), laryngitis (children), pharyngitis (adults), rhinitis (adults), sinusitis (adults)

Miscellaneous: Diaphoresis increased (more common in adults)

Rare but important or life-threatening: Accommodation abnormal, agranulocytosis, albuminuria, alopecia, anemia, aneurysm, anticholinergic syndrome, apathy, aphasia, apraxia, arrhythmia, ataxia, atrial flutter, blepharitis, blood in stool, bradycardia, breast fibroadenosis, bronchitis, bundle branch block, cardiac arrest, cardiac failure, catalepsy, cellulitis, cerebral hemorrhage, cervical dysplasia, cheilitis, chloasma, cholinergic syndrome, choreoathetosis, chromatopsia, chronic enteritis, colitis, coma, conjunctival hemorrhage, cyanosis, deafness, dehydration, delirium, delusion, diabetes mellitus, diplopia, duodenitis, dyskinesia, dysphonia, dystonia, eczema, edema, EEG abnormal, encephalopathy, endometrial hyperplasia, endometriosis, epididymitis, erythematous rash, exophthalmos, exostosis, extrapyramidal disorder, extrasystoles, gastric dilatation, gastric ulcer, gastroesophageal reflux disease, generalized spasm, glaucoma, glycosuria, goiter, gout, gynecomastia, hallucinations, heart block, hematuria, hemiparesis, hemoptysis, hepatitis, hostility, hyperacusis, hypercholesterolemia, hyper-/hypoesthesia, hyperglycemia, hyper-/hypokinesia, hyper-reflexia, hyperthermia, hyper-/hypothyroidism, hyperuricemia, hyper-/hypoventilation, hypnagogic hallucination, hypokalemia, ideation, intestinal obstruction, irritable bowel syndrome, keratitis, laryngismus, leukemoid reaction, leukopenia, liver injury (severe), lupus erythematosus rash, lymphadenopathy, lymphoma-like disorder, maculopapular rash, manic reaction, marrow depression, mutism, myocardial infarction, myocardial ischemia, myopathy, myositis, neuralgia, neuropathy, night blindness, oculogyric crisis, oculomotor nerve paralysis, oral/pharyngeal edema, ovarian cyst, pancytopenia, paralytic ileus, paranoia, parosmia, peptic ulcer, peripheral ischemia, phobic disorder, photophobia, photosensitivity reaction, pneumonia, polyarteritis nodosa, premature ejaculation, psoriasis, psychosis, pyelonephritis, pyuria, rectal hemorrhage, renal calculus, renal cyst, salivary gland enlargement, schizophrenic reaction, scleritis, seizure, sensory disturbance, serotonin syndrome, skin hypertrophy, skin ulceration, somnambulism, strabismus, stupor, suicidal ideation, suicide, suicide attempt, thrombocytopenia, thrombophlebitis, tongue ulceration, torticollis, urinary incontinence, uterine hemorrhage, uterine inflammation, vaginal hemorrhage, vasospasm, ventricular tachycardia, visual field defect, withdrawal syndrome

Drug Interactions

Metabolism/Transport Effects **Substrate** of CYP1A2 (major), CYP2C19 (major), CYP2D6 (major), CYP3A4 (minor); **Note:** Assignment of Major/Minor substrate status based on clinically relevant drug interaction potential; **Inhibits** CYP2D6 (moderate)

Avoid Concomitant Use

Avoid concomitant use of ClomiPRAMINE with any of the following: Aclidinium; Azelastine (Nasal); Iobenguane I 123; Ipratropium (Oral Inhalation); Linezolid; MAO Inhibitors; Methylene Blue; Moxonidine; Paraldehyde; Potassium Chloride; Thalidomide; Thioridazine; Tiotropium; Umeclidinium

Increased Effect/Toxicity

ClomiPRAMINE may increase the levels/effects of: AbobotulinumtoxinA; Alcohol (Ethyl); Alpha-/Beta-Agonists (Direct-Acting); Alpha1-Agonists; Amphetamines; Analgesics (Opioid); Anticholinergic Agents; Antipsychotics; ARIPiprazole; Aspirin; Azelastine (Nasal); Beta2-Agonists; Buprenorphine; Cannabinoid-Containing Products; Citalopram; CNS Depressants; CYP2D6 Substrates; Desmopressin; DOXOrubicin (Conventional); Escitalopram; Fesoterodine; Highest Risk QTc-Prolonging Agents; Hydrocodone; Methotrimeprazine; Methylene Blue; Metoprolol; Metyrosine; Milnacipran; Mirabegron; Moderate Risk QTc-Prolonging Agents; Nebivolol; NSAID (COX-2 Inhibitor); NSAID (Nonselective); OnabotulinumtoxinA; Paraldehyde; Potassium Chloride; Pramipexole; QuiNIDine; RimabotulinumtoxinB; ROPINIRole; Rotigotine; Serotonin Modulators; Sodium Phosphates; Sulfonylureas; Thalidomide; Thiazide Diuretics; Thioridazine; Tiotropium; Topiramate; TraMADol; Vitamin K Antagonists; Yohimbine; Zolpidem

The levels/effects of ClomiPRAMINE may be increased by: Abiraterone Acetate; Aclidinium; Altretamine; Antiemetics (5HT3 Antagonists); Antipsychotics; Brimonidine (Topical); BuPROPion; Cannabis; CarBAMazepine; Cimetidine; Cinacalcet; Citalopram; Cobicistat; CYP1A2 Inhibitors (Moderate); CYP1A2 Inhibitors (Strong); CYP2C19 Inhibitors (Moderate); CYP2C19 Inhibitors (Strong); CYP2D6 Inhibitors (Moderate); CYP2D6 Inhibitors (Strong); Darunavir; Deferasirox; Dexmethylphenidate; Doxylamine; Dronabinol; Droperidol; DULoxetine; Escitalopram; FLUoxetine; FluvoxaMINE; Grapefruit Juice; HydrOXYzine; Ipratropium (Oral Inhalation); Kava Kava; Linezolid; Lithium; Luliconazole; Magnesium Sulfate; MAO Inhibitors; Methotrimeprazine; Methylphenidate; Metoclopramide; Metyrosine; Mifepristone; Nabilone; PARoxetine; Perampanel; Pramlintide; Propafenone; Protease Inhibitors; QuiNIDine; Rufinamide; Sertraline; Sodium Oxybate; Tapentadol; Terbinafine (Systemic); Tetrahydrocannabinol; Thyroid Products; TraMADol; Umeclidinium; Valproic Acid and Derivatives; Vemurafenib

Decreased Effect

ClomiPRAMINE may decrease the levels/effects of: Acetylcholinesterase Inhibitors (Central); Alpha2-Agonists;

Alpha2-Agonists (Ophthalmic); Codeine; Iobenguane I 123; Moxonidine; Secretin; Tamoxifen

The levels/effects of ClomiPRAMINE may be decreased by: Acetylcholinesterase Inhibitors (Central); Barbiturates; Cannabis; CYP1A2 Inducers (Strong); CYP2C19 Inducers (Strong); Cyproterone; Dabrafenib; Peginterferon Alfa-2b; St Johns Wort

Food Interactions Serum concentrations/toxicity may be increased by grapefruit juice. Management: Avoid grapefruit juice.

Stability Store at controlled room temperature at 20°C to 25°C (68°F to 77°F). Dispense in tightly closed container; protect from moisture.

Mechanism of Action Clomipramine appears to affect serotonin uptake while its active metabolite, desmethylclomipramine, affects norepinephrine uptake

Pharmacodynamics
Onset of action: 1-2 weeks
Maximum effect: 8-12 weeks
Duration: 1-2 days

Pharmacokinetics (Adult data unless noted)
Absorption: Rapid
Distribution: Distributes into CSF, brain, and breast milk; active metabolite (desmethylclomipramine) also distributes into CSF with average CSF to plasma ratio: 2.6
Protein binding: 97%; primarily to albumin
Metabolism: Hepatic to desmethylclomipramine (DMI; active) and other metabolites; extensive first-pass effect; metabolites undergo glucuronide conjugation; metabolism of clomipramine and DMI may be capacity limited (ie, may display nonlinear pharmacokinetics); with multiple dosing, plasma concentrations of DMI are greater than clomipramine
Half-life: Adults (following a 150 mg dose): Clomipramine 19-37 hours (mean: 32 hours); DMI: 54-77 hours (mean: 69 hours)
Elimination: 50% to 60% of dose is excreted in the urine and 24% to 32% in feces; only 0.8% to 1.3% is excreted in urine as parent drug and active metabolite (combined amount)

Dosing: Usual Note: During initial dose titration, divide the dose and give with meals to minimize nausea and vomiting. During maintenance therapy, may administer total daily dose once daily at bedtime to minimize daytime sedation.
Children: **Note:** Controlled clinical trials have not shown tricyclic antidepressants to be superior to placebo for the treatment of depression in children and adolescents (Dopheide, 2006; Wagner, 2005).
<10 years: Safety and efficacy have not been established; specific recommendations cannot be made for use in this age group
≥10 years: OCD: Initial: 25 mg/day; gradually increase, as tolerated, to a maximum of 3 mg/kg/day or 100 mg/day (whichever is smaller) during the first 2 weeks; may then gradually increase, if needed, over the next several weeks to a maximum of 3 mg/kg/day or 200 mg/day (whichever is smaller)
Adults: OCD: Initial: 25 mg/day; gradually increase, as tolerated, to 100 mg/day during the first 2 weeks; may then gradually increase, if needed, over the next several weeks to a total of 250 mg/day maximum

Administration Oral: May administer with food to decrease GI upset.

Monitoring Parameters Monitor patient periodically for symptom resolution; monitor for worsening depression, suicidality, and associated behaviors (especially at the beginning of therapy or when doses are increased or decreased).

Monitor weight, pulse rate and blood pressure prior to and during therapy; ECG and cardiac status in patients with cardiac disease; periodic liver enzymes in patients with liver disease; CBC with differential in patients who develop fever and sore throat during treatment.

Test Interactions Increased glucose; may interfere with urine detection of methadone (false-positive)

Additional Information If used for an extended period of time, long-term usefulness of clomipramine should be periodically re-evaluated for the individual patient.

Dosage Forms Excipient information presented when available (limited, particularly for generics); consult specific product labeling.
Capsule, Oral, as hydrochloride:
Anafranil: 25 mg, 50 mg, 75 mg
Generic: 25 mg, 50 mg, 75 mg

References

ACOG Committee on Practice Bulletins-Obstetrics. ACOG practice bulletin: clinical management guidelines for obstetrician-gynecologists number 92, April 2008 (replaces practice bulletin number 87, November 2007). Use of psychiatric medications during pregnancy and lactation. *Obstet Gynecol.* 2008;111(4):1001-1020.

American Psychiatric Association (APA). Treatment recommendations for patients with major depressive disorder. 3rd ed, May 2010. Available at http://www.psychiatryonline.com/pracGuide/pracGuide-Topic_7.aspx

Braconnier A, LeCoent R, Cohen D, et al, "Paroxetine Versus Clomipramine in Adolescents With Severe Major Depression: A Double-Blind, Randomized, Multicenter Trial," *J Am Acad Child Adolesc Psychiatry,* 2003, 42(1):22-9.

Cano-Munoz JL, Montejo-Iglesias ML, Yanez-Saez RM, et al, "Possible Serotonin Syndrome Following the Combined Administration of Clomipramine and Alprazolam," *J Clin Psychiatry,* 1995, 56(3):122.

Dale O and Hole A, "Biphasic Time-Course of Serum Concentrations of Clomipramine and Desmethylclomipramine After a Near-Fatal Overdose," *Vet Hum Toxicol,* 1994, 36(4):309-10.

Dopheide JA, "Recognizing and Treating Depression in Children and Adolescents," *Am J Health Syst Pharm,* 2006, 63(3):233-43.

Fortinguerra F, Clavenna A, and Bonati M, "Psychotropic Drug Use During Breastfeeding: A Review of the Evidence," *Pediatrics,* 2009, 124(4):547-56.

Geller DA, "Obsessive Compulsive and Spectrum Disorders in Children and Adolescents," *Psychiatr Clin North Am,* 2006, 29(2):353-70.

Hernandez AF, Montero MN, Pla A, et al, "Fatal Moclobemide Overdose or Death Caused by Serotonin Syndrome?" *J Forensic Sci,* 1995, 40(1):128-30.

Kuisma MJ, "Fatal Serotonin Syndrome With Trismus," *Ann Emerg Med,* 1995, 26(1):108.

Larochelle P, Hamet P, and Enjalbert M, "Responses to Tyramine and Norepinephrine After Imipramine and Trazodone," *Clin Pharmacol Ther,* 1979, 26(1):24-30.

Larrey D, Rueff B, Pessayre D, et al, "Cross Hepatotoxicity Between Tricyclic Antidepressants," *Gut,* 1986, 27(6):726-7.

Lejoyeux M, et al, "Serotonin Syndrome: Incidence, Symptoms, and Treatment," *CNS Drugs,* 1994, 2:132-43.

Ljungren B and Bojs G, "A Case of Photosensitivity and Contact Allergy to Systemic Tricyclic Drugs, With Unusual Features," *Contact Dermatitis,* 1991, 24(4):259-65.

Loughhead AM, Stowe ZN, Newport DJ, et al. Placental passage of tricyclic antidepressants. *Biol Psychiatry.* 2006;59(3):287-290.

Pass SE and Simpson RW, "Discontinuation and Reinstitution of Medications During the Perioperative Period," *Am J Health Syst Pharm,* 2004, 61(9):899-912.

Roberge RJ, Martin TG, Hodgman M, et al, "Acute Chemical Pancreatitis Associated With a Tricyclic Antidepressant (Clomipramine) Overdose," *J Toxicol Clin Toxicol,* 1994, 32(4):425-9.

Safer DJ and Zito JM, "Treatment-Emergent Adverse Events From Selective Serotonin Reuptake Inhibitors by Age Group: Children vs Adolescents," *J Child and Adolesc Psychopharmacol,* 2006, 16(1/2):159-69.

Sternbach H, "Fluoxetine-Clomipramine Interaction," *J Clin Psychiatry,* 1995, 56(4):171-2.

Svedmyr N, "The Influence of a Tricyclic Antidepressive Agent (Protriptyline) on Some of the Circulatory Effects of Noradrenaline and Adrenalin® in Man," *Life Sci,* 1968, 7(1):77-84.

Swanson-Biearman B, Goetz CM, Dean BS, et al, "Anafranil® Overdose: A Fatal Outcome," *Vet Hum Toxicol,* 1989, 31:378.

ter Horst PG, van der Linde S, Smit JP, et al. Clomipramine concentration and withdrawal symptoms in 10 neonates. *Br J Clin Pharmacol.* 2012;73(2):295-302.

Tueth MJ, "The Serotonin Syndrome in the Emergency Department," *Ann Emerg Med,* 1993, 22(8):1369.

Wagner KD, "Pharmacotherapy for Major Depression in Children and Adolescents," *Prog Neuropsychopharmacol Biol Psychiatry,* 2005, 29(5):819-26.

Walsh KH and McDougle CJ, "Pharmacological Strategies for Trichotillomania," *Expert Opin Pharmacother,* 2005, 6(6):975-84.

- Yonkers KA, Wisner KL, Stewart DE, et al. The management of depression during pregnancy: a report from the American Psychiatric Association and the American College of Obstetricians and Gynecologists. *Obstet Gynecol.* 2009;114(3):703-713.

◆ **Clomipramine Hydrochloride** *see* ClomiPRAMINE *on page 510*

◆ **Clonapam (Can)** *see* ClonazePAM *on page 514*

ClonazePAM (kloe NA ze pam)

Medication Safety Issues
Sound-alike/look-alike issues:
ClonazePAM may be confused with cloBAZam, cloNIDine, clorazepate, cloZAPine, LORazepam

KlonoPIN® may be confused with cloNIDine, clorazepate, cloZAPine, LORazepam

BEERS Criteria medication:
This drug may be potentially inappropriate for use in geriatric patients (Quality of evidence - high; Strength of recommendation - strong).

Related Information
Safe Handling of Hazardous Drugs *on page 2419*

Brand Names: U.S. KlonoPIN

Brand Names: Canada Apo-Clonazepam; Clonapam; Clonazepam-R; CO Clonazepam; Dom-Clonazepam; Dom-Clonazepam-R; Mylan-Clonazepam; PHL-Clonazepam; PHL-Clonazepam-R; PMS-Clonazepam; PMS-Clonazepam-R; PRO-Clonazepam; ratio-Clonazepam; Riva-Clonazepam; Rivotril; Sandoz-Clonazepam; Teva-Clonazepam; ZYM-Clonazepam

Therapeutic Category Anticonvulsant, Benzodiazepine; Benzodiazepine

Generic Availability (U.S.) Yes

Use Alone or as an adjunct in the treatment of absence (petit mal), petit mal variant (Lennox-Gastaut), infantile spasms, akinetic, and myoclonic seizures; panic disorder with or without agoraphobia

Medication Guide Available Yes

Pregnancy Risk Factor D

Pregnancy Considerations Adverse events were observed in some animal reproduction studies. Clonazepam crosses the placenta. Teratogenic effects have been observed with some benzodiazepines; however, additional studies are needed. The incidence of premature birth and low birth weights may be increased following maternal use of benzodiazepines; hypoglycemia and respiratory problems in the neonate may occur following exposure late in pregnancy. Neonatal withdrawal symptoms may occur within days to weeks after birth and "floppy infant syndrome" (which also includes withdrawal symptoms) has been reported with some benzodiazepines, including clonazepam (Bergman, 1992; Iqbal, 2002; Wikner, 2007). A combination of factors influences the potential teratogenicity of anticonvulsant therapy. When treating women with epilepsy, monotherapy with the lowest effective dose and avoidance medications known to have a high incidence of teratogenic effects is recommended (Harden, 2009; Wlodarczyk, 2012).

Patients exposed to clonazepam during pregnancy are encouraged to enroll themselves into the AED Pregnancy Registry by calling 1-888-233-2334. Additional information is available at www.aedpregnancyregistry.org.

Breast-Feeding Considerations Clonazepam enters breast milk. Drowsiness, lethargy, or weight loss in nursing infants have been observed in case reports following maternal use of some benzodiazepines (Iqbal, 2002). The manufacturer states that women taking clonazepam should not breast-feed their infants.

Contraindications Hypersensitivity to clonazepam, any component, or other benzodiazepines; severe liver disease, acute narrow-angle glaucoma

Warnings Hazardous agent; use appropriate precautions for handling and disposal (NIOSH, 2012). Antiepileptic drugs (AEDs) increase the risk of suicidal behavior and ideation in patients receiving these medications for any indication. Pooled analyses of placebo-controlled trials involving 11 different AEDs (regardless of indication) showed a twofold increased risk of suicidal thoughts or behavior (estimated incidence rate: 0.43% in AED treated patients compared to 0.24% of patients receiving placebo); increased risk was observed as early as 1 week after initiation of AED and continued through duration of trials (most trials ≤24 weeks); risk did not vary significantly by age (age range: 5-100 years). Consider risks and benefits of AEDs before prescribing. Monitor all patients receiving an AED for emergence of suicidal thoughts or behavior, thoughts of self-harm, any unusual changes in behavior or mood, or the emergence or worsening of depressive symptoms; notify healthcare provider immediately if symptoms or concerning behavior occur. **Note:** The FDA is requiring that a Medication Guide be developed for all antiepileptic drugs informing patients of this risk.

Precautions Use with caution in patients with chronic respiratory disease, hepatic disease, or impaired renal function; abrupt discontinuance may precipitate withdrawal symptoms, status epilepticus or seizures (withdraw gradually when discontinuing therapy); worsening of seizures may occur when clonazepam is added to patients with multiple seizure types

Adverse Reactions Reactions reported in patients with seizure and/or panic disorder.

Cardiovascular: Edema (ankle or facial), palpitation

Central nervous system: Amnesia, ataxia, behavior problems, coma, confusion, coordination impaired, depression, dizziness, drowsiness, emotional lability, fatigue, fever, hallucinations, headache, hysteria, insomnia, intellectual ability reduced, memory disturbance, nervousness; paradoxical reactions (including aggressive behavior, agitation, anxiety, excitability, hostility, irritability, nervousness, nightmares, sleep disturbance, vivid dreams); psychosis, slurred speech, somnolence, vertigo

Dermatologic: Hair loss, hirsutism, skin rash

Endocrine & metabolic: Dysmenorrhea, libido increased/decreased

Gastrointestinal: Abdominal pain, anorexia, appetite increased/decreased, coated tongue, constipation, dehydration, diarrhea, encopresis, gastritis, gum soreness, nausea, weight changes (loss/gain), xerostomia

Genitourinary: Colpitis, dysuria, ejaculation delayed, enuresis, impotence, micturition frequency, nocturia, urinary retention, urinary tract infection

Hematologic: Anemia, eosinophilia, leukopenia, thrombocytopenia

Hepatic: Alkaline phosphatase increased (transient), hepatomegaly, transaminases increased (transient)

Neuromuscular & skeletal: Choreiform movements, coordination abnormal, dysarthria, hypotonia, muscle pain, muscle weakness, myalgia, tremor

Ocular: Blurred vision, eye movements abnormal, diplopia, nystagmus

Respiratory: Bronchitis, chest congestion, cough, hypersecretions, pharyngitis, respiratory depression, respiratory tract infection, rhinitis, rhinorrhea, shortness of breath, sinusitis

Miscellaneous: Allergic reaction, aphonia, dysdiadochokinesis, "glassy-eyed" appearance, hemiparesis, flu-like syndrome, lymphadenopathy

Rare but important or life-threatening: Apathy, burning skin, chest pain, depersonalization, dyspnea, excessive dreaming, hyperactivity, hypoesthesia, hypotension postural, infection, migraine, organic disinhibition, pain, paresthesia, paresis, periorbital edema, polyuria, suicidal attempt, suicide ideation, thick tongue, twitching, visual disturbance, xerophthalmia

Drug Interactions

Metabolism/Transport Effects Substrate of CYP3A4 (major); **Note:** Assignment of Major/Minor substrate status based on clinically relevant drug interaction potential

Avoid Concomitant Use

Avoid concomitant use of ClonazePAM with any of the following: Azelastine (Nasal); Conivaptan; Fusidic Acid (Systemic); Methadone; OLANZapine; Paraldehyde; Sodium Oxybate; Thalidomide

Increased Effect/Toxicity

ClonazePAM may increase the levels/effects of: Alcohol (Ethyl); Azelastine (Nasal); Buprenorphine; CloZAPine; CNS Depressants; Hydrocodone; Methadone; Methotrimeprazine; Metyrosine; Mirtazapine; Paraldehyde; Pramipexole; ROPINIRole; Rotigotine; Selective Serotonin Reuptake Inhibitors; Sodium Oxybate; Thalidomide; Zolpidem

The levels/effects of ClonazePAM may be increased by: Antifungal Agents (Azole Derivatives, Systemic); Aprepitant; Brimonidine (Topical); Calcium Channel Blockers (Nondihydropyridine); Cannabis; Ceritinib; Cimetidine; Cobicistat; Conivaptan; Contraceptives (Estrogens); Contraceptives (Progestins); Cosyntropin; CYP3A4 Inhibitors (Moderate); CYP3A4 Inhibitors (Strong); Dasatinib; Doxylamine; Dronabinol; Droperidol; Fosaprepitant; Fusidic Acid (Systemic); Grapefruit Juice; HydrOXYzine; Isoniazid; Ivacaftor; Kava Kava; Luliconazole; Magnesium Sulfate; Methotrimeprazine; Mifepristone; Nabilone; OLANZapine; Perampanel; Proton Pump Inhibitors; Rufinamide; Selective Serotonin Reuptake Inhibitors; Simeprevir; Stiripentol; Tapentadol; Tetrahydrocannabinol; Vigabatrin

Decreased Effect

The levels/effects of ClonazePAM may be decreased by: Bosentan; CarBAMazepine; CYP3A4 Inducers (Strong); Dabrafenib; Deferasirox; Mitotane; Rifamycin Derivatives; Siltuximab; St Johns Wort; Theophylline Derivatives; Tocilizumab; Yohimbine

Food Interactions Clonazepam serum concentration is unlikely to be increased by grapefruit juice because of clonazepam's high oral bioavailability.

Stability Hazardous agent; use appropriate precautions for handling and disposal (NIOSH, 2012). Store at 25°C (77°F); excursions permitted to 15°C to 30°C (59°F to 80°F).

Mechanism of Action The exact mechanism is unknown, but believed to be related to its ability to enhance the activity of GABA; suppresses the spike-and-wave discharge in absence seizures by depressing nerve transmission in the motor cortex

Pharmacodynamics

Onset of action: 20-60 minutes

Duration:
Infants and young children: Up to 6-8 hours
Adults: Up to 12 hours

Pharmacokinetics (Adult data unless noted)

Absorption: Oral: Well absorbed

Distribution: V_d: Adults: 1.5-4.4 L/kg

Protein binding: 85%

Metabolism: Extensively metabolized in the liver; undergoes nitroreduction to 7-aminoclonazepam, followed by acetylation to 7-acetamidoclonazepam; nitroreduction and acetylation are via cytochrome P450 enzyme system; metabolites undergo glucuronide and sulfate conjugation

Bioavailability: 90%

Half-life:
Children: 22-33 hours
Adults: Usual: 30-40 hours; range: 19-50 hours

Elimination: Metabolites excreted as glucuronide or sulfate conjugates; <2% excreted unchanged in urine

Dosing: Usual Oral:

Seizure disorders:
Infants and Children <10 years or 30 kg:
Initial daily dose: 0.01-0.03 mg/kg/day (maximum initial dose: 0.05 mg/kg/day) given in 2-3 divided doses; increase by no more than 0.5 mg every third day until seizures are controlled or adverse effects seen
Maintenance dose: 0.1-0.2 mg/kg/day divided 3 times/day; not to exceed 0.2 mg/kg/day

Children ≥10 years (>30 kg) and Adults:
Initial daily dose not to exceed 1.5 mg given in 3 divided doses; may increase by 0.5-1 mg every third day until seizures are controlled or adverse effects seen
Maintenance dose: 0.05-0.2 mg/kg/day; do not exceed 20 mg/day

Panic disorder: Adolescents ≥18 years and Adults: Initial: 0.25 mg twice daily; increase in increments of 0.125-0.25 mg twice daily every 3 days; target dose: 1 mg/day; maximum dose: 4 mg/day

Administration Hazardous agent; use appropriate precautions for handling and disposal (NIOSH, 2012).

Oral: May administer with food or water to decrease GI distress

Orally-disintegrating tablet: Open pouch and peel back foil on the blister; do not push tablet through foil. Use dry hands to remove tablet and place in mouth. May be swallowed with or without water. Use immediately after removing from package.

Monitoring Parameters Signs and symptoms of suicidality (eg, anxiety, depression, behavior changes). Long-term use: CBC with differential, platelets, liver enzymes

Reference Range Relationship between serum concentration and seizure control is not well established; measurement at random times postdose may contribute to this problem; predose concentrations are recommended

Proposed therapeutic levels: 20-80 ng/mL
Potentially toxic concentration: >80 ng/mL

Additional Information Ethosuximide or valproic acid may be preferred for treatment of absence (petit mal) seizures. Clonazepam-induced behavioral disturbances may be more frequent in mentally handicapped patients. When discontinuing therapy in children, the clonazepam dose may be safely reduced by ≤0.04 mg/kg/week and discontinued when the daily dose is ≤0.04 mg/kg/day. When discontinuing therapy in adults treated for panic disorder, the clonazepam dose may be decreased by 0.125 mg twice daily every 3 days, until the drug is completely withdrawn. Treatment of panic disorder for >9 weeks has not been studied; long-term usefulness of clonazepam for the treatment of panic disorder should be re-evaluated periodically.

Controlled Substance C-IV

Dosage Forms Excipient information presented when available (limited, particularly for generics); consult specific product labeling.

Tablet, Oral:
KlonoPIN: 0.5 mg [scored]
KlonoPIN: 1 mg, 2 mg
Generic: 0.5 mg, 1 mg, 2 mg

Tablet Dispersible, Oral:
Generic: 0.125 mg, 0.25 mg, 0.5 mg, 1 mg, 2 mg

Extemporaneous Preparations Hazardous agent: Use appropriate precautions for handling and disposal.

A 0.1 mg/mL oral suspension may be made with tablets and one of three different vehicles (cherry syrup; a 1:1 mixture of Ora-Sweet® and Ora-Plus®; or a 1:1 mixture of Ora-Sweet® SF and Ora-Plus®). Crush six 2 mg tablets in a mortar and reduce to a fine powder. Add 10 mL of the chosen vehicle and mix to a uniform paste; mix while adding the vehicle in incremental proportions to **almost** 120 mL; transfer to a calibrated bottle, rinse mortar with vehicle, and add quantity of vehicle sufficient to make 120 mL. Label "shake well" and "protect from light". Stable for 60 days when stored in amber prescription bottles in the dark at room temperature or refrigerated.

Allen LV Jr and Erickson MA 3rd, "Stability of Acetazolamide, Allopurinol, Azathioprine, Clonazepam, and Flucytosine in Extemporaneously Compounded Oral Liquids," *Am J Health Syst Pharm*, 1996, 53(16):1944-9.

References

Bergman U, Rosa FW, Baum C, et al, "Effects of Exposure to Benzodiazepine During Fetal Life," *Lancet*, 1992, 340(8821):694-6.

Harden CL, Meador KJ, Pennell PB, et al, "Practice Parameter Update: Management Issues for Women With Epilepsy-Focus on Pregnancy (an Evidence-Based Review): Teratogenesis and Perinatal Outcomes: Report of the Quality Standards Subcommittee and Therapeutics and Technology Assessment Subcommittee of the American Academy of Neurology and American Epilepsy Society," *Neurology*, 2009, 73(2):133-41.

Iqbal MM, Sobhan T, Ryals T, et al, "Effects of Commonly Used Benzodiazepines on the Fetus, the Neonate, and the Nursing Infant," *Psychiatr Serv*, 2002, 53(1):39-49.

National Institute for Occupational Safety and Health (NIOSH), "NIOSH List of Antineoplastic and Other Hazardous Drugs in Healthcare Settings 2012." Available at http://www.cdc.gov/niosh/docs/2012-150/pdfs/2012-150.pdf. Accessed January 21, 2013.

Sugai K, "Seizures With Clonazepam: Discontinuation and Suggestions for Safe Discontinuation Rates in Children," *Epilepsia*, 1993, 34 (6):1089-97.

Walson PD and Edge JH, "Clonazepam Disposition in Pediatric Patients," *Ther Drug Monit*, 1996, 18(1):1-5.

Wikner BN, Stiller CO, Bergman U, et al, "Use of Benzodiazepines and Benzodiazepine Receptor Agonists During Pregnancy: Neonatal Outcome and Congenital Malformations," *Pharmacoepidemiol Drug Saf*, 2007, 16(11):1203-10.

Wlodarczyk BJ, Palacios AM, George TM, et al, "Antiepileptic Drugs and Pregnancy Outcomes," *Am J Med Genet A*, 2012, 158A (8):2071-90.

◆ **Clonazepam-R (Can)** see ClonazePAM on page 514

CloNIDine (KLON i deen)

Medication Safety Issues

Sound-alike/look-alike issues:

CloNIDine may be confused with Clomid®, clomiPHENE, clonazePAM, cloZAPine, KlonoPIN®, quiNIDine

Catapres® may be confused with Cataflam®, Combipres

High alert medication:

The Institute for Safe Medication Practices (ISMP) includes this medication (epidural administration) among its list of drug classes which have a heightened risk of causing significant patient harm when used in error.

BEERS Criteria medication:

This drug may be potentially inappropriate for use in geriatric patients (Quality of evidence - low; Strength of recommendation - strong).

Administration issues:

Use caution when interpreting dosing information. Pediatric dose for epidural infusion expressed as mcg/kg/**hour**.

Other safety concerns:

Transdermal patch may contain conducting metal (eg, aluminum); remove patch prior to MRI. Errors have occurred when the inactive, optional adhesive cover has been applied instead of the active clonidine-containing patch.

Related Information

Oral Medications That Should Not Be Crushed or Altered *on page 2438*

Brand Names: U.S. Catapres; Catapres-TTS-1; Catapres-TTS-2; Catapres-TTS-3; Duraclon; Kapvay

Brand Names: Canada Apo-Clonidine®; Catapres®; Dixarit®; Dom-Clonidine; Novo-Clonidine

Therapeutic Category Adrenergic Agonist Agent; Alpha-Adrenergic Agonist; Analgesic, Non-narcotic (Epidural); Antihypertensive Agent

Generic Availability (U.S.) May be product dependent

Use

Oral:

Immediate release: Management of hypertension (monotherapy or as adjunctive therapy) (FDA approved in adults); has also been used for the treatment of attention-deficit/hyperactivity disorder, Tourette syndrome and tic disorders, neonatal abstinence syndrome (opioid withdrawal), and as an aid in the diagnosis of pheochromocytoma and growth hormone deficiency

Extended release: Kapvay™: Treatment of attention deficit hyperactivity disorder (ADHD) (monotherapy or as adjunctive therapy) (FDA approved in ages 6-17 years)

Parenteral: Epidural (Duraclon®): For continuous epidural administration as adjunctive therapy with opioids for treatment of severe cancer pain in patients tolerant to or unresponsive to opioids alone; epidural clonidine is generally more effective for neuropathic pain and less effective (or possibly ineffective) for somatic or visceral pain [FDA approved in pediatric patients (age not specified) and adults]

Transdermal patch: Management of hypertension (monotherapy or as adjunctive therapy) (FDA approved in adults)

Pregnancy Risk Factor C

Pregnancy Considerations Adverse events have been observed in some animal reproduction studies. Clonidine crosses the placenta; concentrations in the umbilical cord plasma are similar to those in the maternal serum and concentrations in the amniotic fluid may be 4 times those in the maternal serum. The pharmacokinetics of clonidine may be altered during pregnancy (Buchanan, 2009). Untreated chronic maternal hypertension is associated with adverse events in the fetus, infant, and mother. If treatment for hypertension during pregnancy is needed, other agents are preferred (ACOG, 2012; Chobanian, 2003). **[U.S. Boxed Warning]: Epidural clonidine is not recommended for obstetrical or postpartum pain** due to risk of hemodynamic instability.

Breast-Feeding Considerations Clonidine is excreted in breast milk. Concentrations have been noted as ~7% to 8% of those in the maternal plasma following oral dosing (Atkinson, 1988; Bunjes, 1993) and twice those in the maternal serum following epidural administration. The manufacturer recommends caution be used if administered to nursing women. Another source recommends avoiding use when nursing infants born <34 weeks gestation or when large maternal doses are needed (Atkinson, 1988). Breast-fed infants of mothers taking medications for hypertension should be monitored for adverse effects (Chobanian, 2003).

Contraindications Hypersensitivity to clonidine hydrochloride or any component; epidural injection is contraindicated in patients receiving anticoagulation therapy and in patients with a bleeding diathesis or an infection at the injection site. Administration of epidural clonidine above the C_4 dermatome is contraindicated.

Warnings Do not abruptly discontinue as rapid increase in blood pressure and symptoms of sympathetic overactivity (such as increased heart rate, tremors, agitation, anxiety, insomnia, sweating, palpitations) may occur. Since children commonly have gastrointestinal illnesses with vomiting, they are susceptible to hypertensive episodes due to abrupt inability to take oral medication. If need to discontinue clonidine, taper oral immediate release or epidural gradually over 2-4 days to avoid rebound hypertension. In patients receiving both a beta-blocker and clonidine, withdraw the beta-blocker several days before the gradual tapering of clonidine. In children and adolescents, extended release formulation (Kapvay™) should be tapered in decrements of ≤0.1 mg every 3-7 days. For surgical patients, discontinue oral immediate release formulations within 4 hours of surgery and restart as soon as possible afterwards; discontinue oral extended release formulations up to 28 hours prior to surgery, then restart the following day; monitor blood pressure closely during surgery; additional therapy to control blood pressure may be needed. Clonidine causes CNS depression, which may impair physical or mental abilities; patients must be cautioned about performing tasks which require mental alertness (eg, operating machinery, driving). Sedating effects may be potentiated when used with other CNS-depressant drugs or ethanol.

The American Heart Association recommends that all children diagnosed with ADHD who may be candidates for medication, such as clonidine, should have a thorough cardiovascular assessment prior to initiation of therapy. These recommendations are based upon reports of serious cardiovascular adverse events (including sudden death) in patients (both children and adults) taking usual doses of stimulant medications. Most of these patients were found to have underlying structural heart disease (eg, hypertrophic obstructive cardiomyopathy). This assessment should include a combination of thorough medical history, family history, and physical examination. An ECG is not mandatory but should be considered. **Note:** ECG abnormalities and 4 cases of sudden cardiac death have been reported in children receiving clonidine with methylphenidate; reduce dose of methylphenidate by 40% when used concurrently with clonidine; consider ECG monitoring. In patients with ADHD, clonidine may cause hypotension and bradycardia; use with caution in patients with history of hypotension, heart block, bradycardia, cardiovascular disease, syncope, conditions predisposing to syncope (including orthostatic hypotension, dehydration), or receiving concomitant antihypertensive therapy. Patients should be advised to avoid becoming dehydrated or overheated. Heart rate and blood pressure should be monitored at initiation of therapy, with any dose increase, and periodically during therapy.

Epidural clonidine is not recommended for perioperative, obstetrical, or postpartum pain [due to the risk of hemodynamic instability (hypotension, bradycardia)] **[U.S. Boxed Warning]**, in patients with severe cardiovascular disease, or those who are hemodynamically unstable. In all patients, use epidural clonidine with caution due to the potential for severe hypotension, especially in women and those of low body weight. Most hypotensive episodes occur within the first 4 days of initiation; however, episodes may occur throughout the duration of therapy. Epidural clonidine may cause bradycardia (symptomatic bradycardia may be treated with atropine); sedation, respiratory depression, and ventilatory abnormalities may occur with high epidural doses. Epidural formulation (500 mcg/mL) must be diluted prior to administration **[U.S. Boxed Warning]**; should be administered via continuous epidural infusion device; monitor closely for catheter-related infection, such as meningitis or epidural abscess.

Formulations of clonidine (immediate release vs extended release) are not interchangeable on a mg per mg basis due to different pharmacokinetic profiles.

Precautions Dosage modification is required in patients with renal impairment; use with caution in cerebrovascular disease, coronary insufficiency, recent MI, renal impairment, sinus node dysfunction, and conduction disturbances. Use with caution in patients concurrently receiving agents known to reduce SA node function and/or AV nodal conduction (eg, digoxin, diltiazem, metoprolol, verapamil); may increase risk of serious bradycardia. Monitor patients for signs of depression (especially those with a history of affective disorders). Transdermal patch may contain conducting metal (eg, aluminum) which may cause a burn to the skin during an MRI scan; remove patch prior to MRI; reapply patch after scan is completed. Due to the potential for altered electrical conductivity, remove transdermal patch before cardioversion or defibrillation. Localized contact sensitization to the transdermal system has been reported; in these patients, allergic reactions (eg, generalized rash, urticaria, angioedema) have also occurred following subsequent substitution of oral therapy. May cause significant xerostomia; may cause eye dryness in patients who wear contact lenses. In pediatric patients, epidural clonidine should be reserved for cancer patients with severe intractable pain, unresponsive to other analgesics, or epidural or spinal opioids.

Adverse Reactions

Oral, Transdermal:

Cardiovascular: Arrhythmia, atrioventricular block, bradycardia, chest pain, CHF, ECG abnormalities, flushing, orthostatic hypotension, pallor, palpitation, Raynaud's phenomenon, syncope, tachycardia

Central nervous system: Aggression, agitation, anxiety, behavioral changes, CVA, delirium, delusional perception, dizziness, drowsiness, fatigue, fever, hallucinations (visual and auditory), headache, insomnia, irritability, lethargy, malaise, mental depression, nervousness, nightmares, restlessness, sedation, vivid dreams

Dermatologic: Allergic contact sensitization (transdermal), alopecia, angioedema, blanching (transdermal), burning (transdermal), contact dermatitis (transdermal), edema, excoriation (transdermal), generalized macular rash, hives, hyperpigmentation (transdermal), localized hypopigmentation (transdermal), papules (transdermal), rash, throbbing (transdermal), transient localized skin reactions characterized by pruritus and erythema (transdermal), urticaria, vesiculation (transdermal)

Endocrine & metabolic: Creatine phosphokinase increased (transient; oral), gynecomastia, hyperglycemia (transient; oral), libido decreased, sexual dysfunction

Gastrointestinal: Abdominal pain (oral), anorexia, constipation, diarrhea, nausea, parotid gland pain (oral), parotitis (oral), pseudo-obstruction (oral), taste perversion, throat pain, vomiting, weight gain, xerostomia

Genitourinary: Dysuria, enuresis, erectile dysfunction, nocturia, urinary retention

Hematologic: Thrombocytopenia (oral)

Hepatic: Hepatitis, liver function test (mild transient abnormalities)

Neuromuscular & skeletal: Arthralgia, leg cramps, myalgia, numbness (localized, transdermal), pain in extremities, paresthesia, tremor, weakness

Ocular: Accommodation disorder, blurred vision, burning eyes, dry eyes, lacrimation decreased/increased

Otic: Ear pain, otitis media

Renal: Pollakiuria

Respiratory: Asthma, epistaxis, nasal congestion, nasal dryness, nasopharyngitis, respiratory tract infection, rhinorrhea

Miscellaneous: Flu-like syndrome, thirst, withdrawal syndrome

Epidural: Note: The following adverse events occurred more often than placebo in cancer patients with intractable pain being treated with concurrent epidural morphine.

Cardiovascular: Chest pain, hypotension, orthostatic hypotension

Central nervous system: Confusion, dizziness, hallucinations

Gastrointestinal: Nausea/vomiting, xerostomia

Otic: Tinnitus

Miscellaneous: Diaphoresis

Drug Interactions

Metabolism/Transport Effects None known.

Avoid Concomitant Use

Avoid concomitant use of CloNIDine with any of the following: Azelastine (Nasal); Ceritinib; Iobenguane I 123; Paraldehyde; Thalidomide

Increased Effect/Toxicity

CloNIDine may increase the levels/effects of: Alcohol (Ethyl); Amifostine; Antihypertensives; Azelastine (Nasal); Beta-Blockers; Bradycardia-Causing Agents; Buprenorphine; Calcium Channel Blockers (Nondihydropyridine); Cardiac Glycosides; Ceritinib; CNS Depressants; DULoxetine; Hydrocodone; Hypotensive Agents; Methotrimeprazine; Metyrosine; Obinutuzumab; Paraldehyde; Pramipexole; RiTUXimab; ROPINIRole; Rotigotine; Selective Serotonin Reuptake Inhibitors; Thalidomide; Zolpidem

The levels/effects of CloNIDine may be increased by: Alfuzosin; Barbiturates; Beta-Blockers; Brimonidine (Topical); Cannabis; Diazoxide; Doxylamine; Dronabinol; Droperidol; Herbs (Hypotensive Properties); HydrOXYzine; Kava Kava; Magnesium Sulfate; MAO Inhibitors; Methotrimeprazine; Methylphenidate; Nabilone; Pentoxifylline; Perampanel; Phosphodiesterase 5 Inhibitors; Prostacyclin Analogues; Rufinamide; Sodium Oxybate; Tapentadol; Tetrahydrocannabinol

Decreased Effect

CloNIDine may decrease the levels/effects of: Iobenguane I 123

The levels/effects of CloNIDine may be decreased by: Herbs (Hypertensive Properties); Mirtazapine; Serotonin/Norepinephrine Reuptake Inhibitors; Tricyclic Antidepressants; Yohimbine

Stability

Oral:

Immediate release tablets: Store at 25°C (77°F); excursions permitted to 15°C to 30°C (59°F to 86°F); dispense in tightly closed, light-resistant container.

Kapvey™ extended release tablets: Store at 20°C to 25°C (68°F to 77°F); dispense in tightly closed, light-resistant container.

Transdermal product: Store below 86°F (30°C)

Epidural formulation: Store at 25°C (77°F); excursions permitted to 15°C to 30°C (59°F to 86°F). **Preservative free:** Discard unused portion; do not admix with diluent (NS) containing preservative

Mechanism of Action Stimulates alpha$_2$-adrenoceptors in the brain stem, thus activating an inhibitory neuron, resulting in reduced sympathetic outflow from the CNS, producing a decrease in peripheral resistance, renal vascular resistance, heart rate, and blood pressure; epidural clonidine may produce pain relief at spinal presynaptic and postjunctional alpha$_2$-adrenoceptors by preventing pain signal transmission; pain relief occurs only for the body regions innervated by the spinal segments where analgesic concentrations of clonidine exist. For the treatment of ADHD, the mechanism of action is unknown; it has been proposed that postsynaptic alpha$_2$-agonist stimulation regulates subcortical activity in the prefrontal cortex, the area of the brain responsible for emotions, attentions, and behaviors and causes reduced hyperactivity, impulsiveness, and distractibility.

Pharmacodynamics

Antihypertensive effects:

Onset of action: Oral: Immediate release: 30-60 minutes; Transdermal: Initial application: 2-3 days

Maximum effect: Oral: Immediate release: Within 2-4 hours

Duration: Oral: Immediate release: 6-10 hours

Attention-deficit/hyperactivity disorder: Oral: Extended release: Onset of action: 1-2 weeks (AAP, 2011)

Pharmacokinetics (Adult data unless noted)

Absorption: Oral: Extended release tablets (Kapvay™) are not bioequivalent with immediate release formulations; peak plasma concentrations are 50% lower compared to immediate release formulations

Distribution: V$_d$: 2 L/kg; highly lipid soluble; distributes readily into extravascular sites; **Note:** Epidurally administered clonidine readily distributes into plasma via the epidural veins and attains clinically significant systemic concentrations.

Protein binding: 20% to 40%

Metabolism: Hepatic to inactive metabolites; undergoes enterohepatic recirculation

Bioavailability: Oral: Immediate release: 75% to 85%; extended release (Kapvay™): 89% (compared to immediate release formulation) (Cunningham, 1994)

Time to peak serum concentration: Oral: Immediate release: 3-5 hours; extended release: 7-8 hours

Half-life:

Oral: Serum half-life:

Neonates: 44-72 hours

Children: 8-12 hours

Adults:

Normal renal function: 12-16 hours

Renal impairment: ≤41 hours

Epidural administration: CSF half-life: 1.3 ± 0.5 hours

Elimination: Urine (40% to 60% as unchanged drug)

Dialysis: Not dialyzable (0% to 5%)

Dosing: Neonatal Neonatal abstinence syndrome (opioid withdrawal): Limited information; further studies needed. Oral: 0.5-1 **mcg**/kg/dose every 4-6 hours (Agthe, 2009; Hudak, 2012); for premature neonates, a dosing interval of every 6 hours was reported (median GA: 26 weeks and 2 days) and upon stabilization, clonidine doses were stopped or tapered by 0.25 **mcg**/kg every 6 hours if necessary (Leikin, 2009)

Dosing: Usual Note: Formulations of clonidine (immediate release vs extended release) are not interchangeable on a mg per mg basis due to different pharmacokinetic profiles.

Children and Adolescents:

Hypertension:

Oral: Immediate release:

Weight-directed dosing: Children and Adolescents 1-17 years: Initial: 5-10 **mcg**/kg/day in divided doses every 8-12 hours; increase gradually as needed; usual range: 5-25 **mcg**/kg/day in divided doses every 6 hours; maximum dose: 0.9 mg/day (Kavey, 2010; Rocchini, 1984)

Alternate dosing: Fixed dosing: Children and Adolescents ≥12 years: Initial: 0.1 mg twice daily; increase gradually, if needed, by 0.1 mg/day at weekly intervals; usual maintenance dose: 0.2-0.6 mg/day in divided doses; maximum recommended dose: 2.4 mg/day (rarely required) (NHBPEP, 2004)

Transdermal: Children and Adolescents: May be switched to the transdermal delivery system after oral therapy is titrated to an optimal and stable dose; a transdermal dose approximately equivalent to the total oral daily dose may be used (Hunt, 1990).

Hypertension, urgency and emergency: Oral: Immediate release: Children and Adolescents 1-17 years: 0.05-0.1 mg/dose; may repeat dose(s) up to a maximum total dose of 0.8 mg (NHBPEP, 2004)

ADHD: Children ≥6 years and Adolescents:
Oral:
Immediate release (Pliszka, 2007):
≤45 kg: Initial: 0.05 mg at bedtime; sequentially increase every 3-7 days in 0.05 mg/day increments given as 0.05 mg twice daily, then 3 times daily, then 4 times daily; maximum daily dose weight-dependent: Patient weight: 27-40.5 kg: 0.2 mg/day; patient weight: 40.5-45 kg: 0.3 mg/day
>45 kg: Initial: 0.1 mg at bedtime; sequentially increase every 3-7 days in 0.1 mg/day increments given as 0.1 mg twice daily, then 3 times daily, then 4 times daily; maximum daily dose: 0.4 mg/day
Extended release (Kapvay™): Initial: 0.1 mg at bedtime; increase in 0.1 mg/day increments every 7 days until desired response; doses should be administered twice daily (either split equally or with the higher split dosage given at bedtime); maximum: 0.4 mg/day. **Note:** Maintenance treatment for >5 weeks has not been evaluated. When discontinuing therapy, taper daily dose by ≤0.1 mg every 3-7 days.
Transdermal: Children may be switched to the transdermal delivery system after oral therapy is titrated to an optimal and stable dose; a transdermal dose approximately equivalent to the total oral daily dose may be used (Hunt, 1990).

Clonidine tolerance test (test of growth hormone release from the pituitary): Oral: 0.15 mg/m^2 or 5 **mcg**/kg as a single dose; maximum dose: 0.25 mg (250 mcg) (Lanes, 1982; Richmond, 2008)

Analgesia: Epidural: Continuous infusion: Initial: 0.5 **mcg**/kg/hour; adjust with caution, based on clinical effect; usual range: 0.5-2 **mcg**/kg/hour; do not exceed adult doses. Do not discontinue clonidine abruptly; if needed, gradually reduce dose over 2-4 days to avoid withdrawal symptoms. Manufacturer suggests use reserved for cancer patients with severe intractable pain, unresponsive to other opioid analgesics, or epidural or spinal opioids; has also been used for pediatric chronic pain syndromes.

Neuropathic pain:
Oral: Children and Adolescents: Some centers use the following doses (Galloway, 2000): Initial: 2 **mcg**/kg/dose every 4-6 hours; increase incrementally over several days; range: 2-4 **mcg**/kg/dose every 4-6 hours
Transdermal: Children and Adolescents: May be switched to the transdermal delivery system after oral therapy is titrated to an optimal and stable dose; a transdermal dose approximately equivalent to the total oral daily dose may be used (Galloway, 2000; Hunt, 1990).

Tic disorders and Tourette's syndrome: Oral: Initial: 0.025-0.05 mg/day; gradual titration to 3-4 times daily schedule using small increments (0.025 mg); target daily dose: 0.2-0.3 mg/day; doses up to 0.4 mg/day have been reported (Swain, 2007; The Tourette's Syndrome Study Group, 2002)
Adults:
Hypertension:
Oral:
Immediate release: Initial dose: 0.1 mg twice daily, usual maintenance dose: 0.2-1.2 mg/day in 2-4 divided doses; maximum recommended dose: 2.4 mg/day; usual dosage range (JNC 7): 0.1-0.8 mg/day in 2 divided doses
Conversion from transdermal to oral: After transdermal patch removal, therapeutic clonidine levels persist for ~8 hours and then slowly decrease over several days. Consider starting oral clonidine no sooner than 8 hours after patch removal.
Transdermal: Applied once weekly as transdermal delivery system; begin therapy with 0.1 mg/day patch applied once every 7 days; increase by 0.1 mg/day at

1-2 week intervals based on response; hypotensive action may not begin until 2-3 days after initial application; doses >0.6 mg/day do not improve efficacy; usual dosage range (JNC 7): 0.1-0.3 mg/day patch applied once weekly. **Note:** If transitioning from oral to transdermal therapy, overlap oral regimen for 1-2 days; transdermal route takes 2-3 days to achieve therapeutic effects.
Conversion from oral to transdermal:
Day 1: Place Catapres-TTS® 1; administer 100% of oral dose.
Day 2: Administer 50% of oral dose.
Day 3: Administer 25% of oral dose.
Day 4: Patch remains; no further oral supplement necessary

Analgesia: Epidural (continuous infusion): Reserved for cancer patients with severe intractable pain, unresponsive to other opioid analgesics: Initial: 30 **mcg**/hour; titrate as required for relief of pain or presence of side effects; minimal experience with doses >40 **mcg**/hour; should be considered an adjunct to intraspinal opioid therapy

Dosing adjustment in renal impairment:
Children and Adolescents: Oral [extended release (Kapvay)], epidural: The manufacturer recommends dosage adjustment according to degree of renal impairment; however, there are no specific dosage adjustment provided in the labeling (has not been studied). Bradycardia, sedation, and hypotension may be more likely to occur in patients with renal failure; drug is primarily eliminated unchanged in the urine; consider using doses at the lower end of the dosage range; monitor patients closely.
Adults: Oral (immediate release), transdermal, epidural: The manufacturer recommends dosage adjustment according to degree of renal impairment; however, no specific dosage adjustment provided. Bradycardia, sedation, and hypotension may be more likely to occur in patients with renal failure; half-life significantly prolonged in patients with severe renal failure; consider use of lower initial doses and monitor closely.
Hemodialysis: Not dialyzable (0% to 5%); supplemental dose is not necessary. Oral antihypertensive drugs given preferentially at night may reduce the nocturnal surge of blood pressure and minimize the intradialytic hypotension that may occur when taken the morning before a dialysis session (K/DOQI, 2005).

Dosing adjustment in hepatic impairment: There are no dosage adjustments provided in the manufacturer labeling.

Administration
Epidural: Not for I.V. use. Dilute the 500 mcg/mL product with preservative free NS to a final concentration of 100 mcg/mL prior to use; visually inspect for particulate matter and discoloration prior to administration (whenever permitted by container and solution). Do not discontinue clonidine abruptly; if needed, gradually reduce dose over 2-4 days to avoid withdrawal symptoms.
Oral: May be administered without regard to meals. Swallow extended release formulations whole; do not crush or chew. Kapvay™ should not be split. Do not discontinue clonidine abruptly; if needed, gradually reduce immediate release dose over 2-4 days to avoid rebound hypertension; extended release formulation (Kapvay™) should be tapered in decrements of ≤0.1 mg every 3-7 days.
Transdermal: Patches should be applied at bedtime to a clean, hairless area of the upper arm or chest; rotate patch sites weekly in adults; in children, the patch may need to be changed more frequently (eg, every 3-5 days); in adults, redness under patch may be reduced if a topical corticosteroid spray is applied to the area before placement of the patch (Tom,1994; **Note:** Transdermal patch is a membrane-controlled system; do **not** cut the

patch to deliver partial doses; rate of drug delivery, reservoir contents, and adhesion may be affected if cut; if partial dose is needed, surface area of patch can be blocked proportionally using adhesive bandage (Lee, 1997).

Monitoring Parameters Blood pressure, heart rate; consider ECG monitoring in patients with history of heart disease or concurrent use of medications affecting cardiac conduction. With epidural administration: Blood pressure, heart rate; pulse oximetry with large bolus doses; monitor infusion pump and catheter tubing for obstruction or dislodgment throughout the course of therapy to decrease risk of inadvertent abrupt discontinuation; monitor closely for catheter-related infection, such as meningitis or epidural abscess.

ADHD: Evaluate patients for cardiac disease prior to initiation of therapy for ADHD with thorough medical history, family history, and physical exam; consider ECG; perform ECG and echocardiogram if findings suggest cardiac disease; promptly conduct cardiac evaluation in patients who develop chest pain, unexplained syncope, or any other symptom of cardiac disease during treatment.

Clonidine tolerance test: In addition to growth hormone concentrations, monitor blood pressure and blood glucose (Huang, 2001)

Test Interactions Positive Coombs' test

Additional Information Clonidine-induced symptomatic bradycardia may be treated with atropine. Clonidine hydrochloride 0.1 mg is equal to 0.087 mg of the free base. Medications used to treat ADHD should be part of a total treatment program that may include other components, such as psychological, educational, and social measures. Long-term usefulness of clonidine for the treatment of ADHD should be periodically re-evaluated in patients receiving the drug for extended periods of time.

Dosage Forms Excipient information presented when available (limited, particularly for generics); consult specific product labeling. [DSC] = Discontinued product
Miscellaneous, Oral, as hydrochloride:
  Kapvay: 0.1 mg AM dose, 0.2 mg PM dose (60 ea [DSC])
Patch Weekly, Transdermal:
  Catapres-TTS-1: 0.1 mg/24 hr (4 ea)
  Catapres-TTS-2: 0.2 mg/24 hr (4 ea)
  Catapres-TTS-3: 0.3 mg/24 hr (4 ea)
  Generic: 0.1 mg/24 hr (1 ea, 4 ea); 0.2 mg/24 hr (1 ea, 4 ea); 0.3 mg/24 hr (1 ea, 4 ea)
Solution, Epidural, as hydrochloride:
  Duraclon: 100 mcg/mL (10 mL)
  Generic: 100 mcg/mL (10 mL); 500 mcg/mL (10 mL)
Solution, Epidural, as hydrochloride [preservative free]:
  Duraclon: 100 mcg/mL (10 mL)
  Duraclon: 500 mcg/mL (10 mL) [pyrogen free]
  Generic: 100 mcg/mL (10 mL); 500 mcg/mL (10 mL)
Tablet, Oral, as hydrochloride:
  Catapres: 0.1 mg [scored; contains brilliant blue fcf (fd&c blue #1), fd&c yellow #6 (sunset yellow)]
  Catapres: 0.2 mg, 0.3 mg [scored; contains fd&c yellow #6 (sunset yellow)]
  Generic: 0.1 mg, 0.2 mg, 0.3 mg
Tablet Extended Release 12 Hour, Oral, as hydrochloride:
  Kapvay: 0.1 mg
  Generic: 0.1 mg

Extemporaneous Preparations

0.01 mg/mL concentration
A **0.01** mg/mL oral suspension may be made from tablets. Crush twenty 0.1 mg tablets in a glass mortar and reduce to a fine powder. Slowly add Ora-Blend in ~15 mL increments while mixing to form a uniform paste until approximately half of the total volume (~100 mL) is added. Transfer the suspension to a graduated cylinder. Rinse the mortar and pestle with the remaining vehicle and add quantity to fill the volume within the graduated cylinder to

200 mL. Transfer this amount to a calibrated bottle. Label "shake well". When stored in clear plastic syringes, the suspension is stable for at least 91 days at room temperature (25°C) or refrigerated (4°C).
Ma C, Decarie D, Ensom MHH. Stability of clonidine oral suspension in oral plastic syringes. Am J Health-Syst Pharm. 2014;71:657-661.

0.1 mg/mL concentration
A **0.1** mg/mL oral suspension may be made from tablets. Crush thirty 0.2 mg tablets in a glass mortar and reduce to a fine powder. Slowly add 2 mL Purified Water USP and mix to a uniform paste. Slowly add Simple Syrup, NF in 15 mL increments; transfer to a calibrated bottle, rinse mortar with vehicle, and add quantity of vehicle sufficient to make 60 mL. Label "shake well" and "refrigerate". Stable for 28 days when stored in amber glass bottles and refrigerated.
Levinson ML and Johnson CE. Stability of an extemporaneously compounded clonidine hydrochloride oral liquid. Am J Hosp Pharm. 1992;49(1):122-125.

References

Agthe AG, Kim GR, Mathias KB, et al, "Clonidine as an Adjunct Therapy to Opioids for Neonatal Abstinence Syndrome: A Randomized, Controlled Trial," Pediatrics, 2009, 123(5):e849-56.

American Academy of Pediatrics, "ADHD: Clinical Practice Guideline for the Diagnosis, Evaluation, and Treatment of Attention-Deficit/ Hyperactivity Disorder in Children and Adolescents," Pediatrics, 2011; 128(5): 1-16.

American Academy of Pediatrics/American Heart Association Clarification of Statement on Cardiovascular Evaluation and Monitoring of Children and Adolescents With Heart Disease Receiving Medications for ADHD. Available at http://www.aap.org/pressroom/aap-ahastatement.htm

American College of Obstetricians and Gynecologists (ACOG), "ACOG Practice Bulletin No. 125: Chronic Hypertension in Pregnancy," Obstet Gynecol, 2012, 119(2 Pt 1):396-407.

Atkinson HC, Begg EJ, and Darlow BA, "Drugs in Human Milk. Clinical Pharmacokinetic Considerations," Clin Pharmacokinet, 1988, 14 (4):217-40.

Buchanan ML, Easterling TR, Carr DB, et al, "Clonidine Pharmacokinetics in Pregnancy," Drug Metab Dispos, 2009, 37(4):702-5.

Bunjes R, Schaefer C, and Holzinger D, "Clonidine and Breast-Feeding," Clin Pharm, 1993, 12(3):178-9.

Chafin CC, Hovinga CA, and Phelps SJ, "Clonidine in the Treatment of Attention Deficit Hyperactivity Disorder," Journal of Pediatric Pharmacy Practice, 1999, 4(6):308-15.

Chobanian AV, Bakris GL, Black HR, et al, "The Seventh Report of the Joint National Committee on Prevention, Detection, Evaluation, and Treatment of High Blood Pressure: The JNC 7 Report," JAMA, 2003, 289(19):2560-72.

Cunningham FE, Baughman VL, Peters J, et al, "Comparative Pharmacokinetics of Oral Versus Sublingual Clonidine," J Clin Anesth, 1994, 6(5):430-3.

Galloway KS and Yaster M, "Pain and Symptom Control in Terminally Ill Children," Pediatr Clin North Am, 2000, 47(3):711-46.

Hart-Santora D and Hart LL, "Clonidine in Attention Deficit Hyperactivity Disorder," Ann Pharmacother, 1992, 26(1):37-9.

Huang C, Banerjee K, Sochett E, et al, "Hypoglycemia Associated With Clonidine Testing for Growth Hormone Deficiency," J Pediatr, 2001, 139(2):323-4.

Hudak ML and Tan RC, "Neonatal Drug Withdrawal," Pediatrics, 2012, 129(2):e540-60.

Hunt RD, Capper L, and O'Connell P, "Clonidine in Child and Adolescent Psychiatry," J Child Adol Psychpharm, 1990, 1(1):87-102.

Hunt RD, Minderaa RB, and Cohen DJ, "The Therapeutic Effect of Clonidine in Attention Deficit Disorder With Hyperactivity: A Comparison With Placebo and Methylphenidate," Psychopharmacol Bull, 1986, 22(1):229-35.

Kavey RE, Daniels SR, and Flynn JT, "Management of High Blood Pressure in Children and Adolescents," Cardiol Clin, 2010, 28 (4):597-607.

K/DOQI Workgroup, "K/DOQI Clinical Practice Guidelines for Cardiovascular Disease in Dialysis Patients," Am J Kidney Dis, 2005, 45(4 Suppl 3):S46-57.

Lanes R and Hurtado E, "Oral Clonidine – An Effective Growth Hormone-Releasing Agent in Prepubertal Subjects," J Pediatr, 1982, 100(5):710-4.

Lee HA and Anderson PO, "Giving Partial Doses of Transdermal Patches," Am J Health Syst Pharm, 1997, 54(15):1759-60.

Leikin JB, Mackendrick WP, Maloney GE, et al, "Use of Clonidine in the Prevention and Management of Neonatal Abstinence Syndrome," Clin Toxicol (Phila), 2009, 47(6):551-5.

National Heart, Lung, and Blood Institute, "Expert Panel on Integrated Guidelines for Cardiovascular Health and Risk Reduction in Children and Adolescents," *Clinical Practice Guidelines*, 2011, National Institutes of Health. Available at http://www.nhlbi.nih.gov/guidelines/cvd_ped/peds_guidelines_full.pdf. Date accessed: June 11, 2012.

National High Blood Pressure Education Program (NHBPEP) Working Group on High Blood Pressure in Children and Adolescents, "The Fourth Report on the Diagnosis, Evaluation, and Treatment of High Blood Pressure in Children and Adolescents," *Pediatrics*, 2004, 114(2 Suppl 4th Report):555-76.

Pliszka S; AACAP Work Group on Quality Issues, "Practice Parameter for the Assessment and Treatment of Children and Adolescents With Attention-Deficit/Hyperactivity Disorder," *J Am Acad Child Adolesc Psychiatry*, 2007, 46(7):894-921.

Richmond EJ and Rogol AD, "Growth Hormone Deficiency in Children," *Pituitary*, 2008, 11(2):115-20.

Rocchini AP, "Childhood Hypertension: Etiology, Diagnosis, and Treatment," *Pediatr Clin North Am*, 1984, 31(6):1259-73.

Scahill L, "Alpha-2 Adrenergic Agonists in Attention Deficit Hyperactivity Disorder," *J Pediatr*, 2009, 154:S32-7.

Sinaiko AR, "Pharmacologic Management of Childhood Hypertension," *Pediatr Clin North Am*, 1993, 40(1):195-212.

Swain JE, Scahill L, Lombroso PJ, et al, "Tourette Syndrome and Tic Disorders: A Decade of Progress," *J Am Acad Child Adolesc Psychiatry*, 2007, 46(8):947-68.

Tom GR and Premer M, "Hydrocortisone Cream in Clonidine Patch Dermatitis," *Ann Pharmacother*, 1994, 28(7-8):889-90.

Tourette's Syndrome Study Group, "Treatment of ADHD in Children With Tics: A Randomized Controlled Trial," *Neurology*, 2002, 58 (4):527-36.

Vetter VL, Elia J, Erickson C, et al, "Cardiovascular Monitoring of Children and Adolescents With Heart Disease Receiving Stimulant Drugs: A Scientific Statement From the American Heart Association Council on Cardiovascular Disease in the Young Congenital Cardiac Defects Committee and the Council on Cardiovascular Nursing," *Circulation*, 2008, 117(18):2407-23.

◆ **Clonidine Hydrochloride** *see* CloNIDine *on page 516*

Clopidogrel (kloh PID oh grel)

Medication Safety Issues
Sound-alike/look-alike issues:
Plavix may be confused with Elavil, Paxil, Pradax (Canada), Pradaxa

Brand Names: U.S. Plavix

Brand Names: Canada Apo-Clopidogrel; CO Clopidogrel; Dom-Clopidogrel; JAMP-Clopidogrel; Mylan-Clopidogrel; Plavix; PMS-Clopidogrel; RAN-Clopidogrel; Sandoz-Clopidogrel; Teva-Clopidogrel

Therapeutic Category Antiplatelet Agent

Generic Availability (U.S.) Yes

Use Reduction of atherothrombotic events (MI, stroke, and vascular deaths) in patients with recent MI, stroke, or established peripheral arterial disease (FDA approved in adults); reduction of atherothrombotic events in patients with non-ST-segment elevation acute coronary syndrome (unstable angina and non-Q-wave MI) managed medically and through percutaneous coronary intervention (with or without stent) or CABG (FDA approved in adults); reduction of death rate and atherothrombotic events in patients with ST-segment elevation acute MI (STEMI) managed medically (FDA approved in adults).

Medication Guide Available Yes

Pregnancy Risk Factor B

Pregnancy Considerations Adverse events were not observed in animal reproduction studies. Information related to use during pregnancy is limited (Bauer, 2012; DeSantis, 2011; Myers, 2011).

Breast-Feeding Considerations It is not known if clopidogrel is excreted into breast milk. Due to the potential for serious adverse reactions in the nursing infant, the manufacturer recommends a decision be made whether to discontinue nursing or to discontinue the drug, taking into account the importance of treatment to the mother.

Contraindications Hypersensitivity to clopidogrel or any component; active pathological bleeding such as PUD or intracranial hemorrhage

Warnings Rare cases of thrombotic thrombocytopenic purpura (TTP) have been reported, sometimes with

exposure of <2 weeks; fatalities have occurred; urgent treatment including plasmapheresis (plasma exchange) is required

Clopidogrel is a prodrug requiring hepatic conversion to its active metabolite, in part via cytochrome P450 isoenzyme CYP2C19. Impaired clopidogrel conversion to its active metabolite (due to either genetic variations in CYP2C19 or concomitant medications that interfere with CYP2C19) will result in suboptimal antiplatelet activity and may lead to a higher rate of cardiovascular events following myocardial infarction or stent thrombosis following percutaneous coronary intervention (PCI) **[U.S. Boxed Warning]**. Although evidence is insufficient to recommended routine genetic testing, tests are available to determine CYP2C19 genotype and may be used to determine therapeutic strategy; alternative treatment or treatment strategies may be considered if patient is identified as a CYP2C19 poor metabolizer. Genetic testing may be considered prior to initiating clopidogrel in patients at moderate or high risk for poor outcomes (eg, PCI in patients with extensive and/or complex disease). The optimal dose for CYP2C19 poor metabolizers has yet to be determined. After initiation of clopidogrel, functional testing (eg, VerifyNow® P2Y12 assay) may also be done to determine clopidogrel responsiveness (Holmes, 2010). Patients of Chinese ancestry have a higher incidence of CYP2C19*2 and CYP2C19*3 alleles (which results in a higher incidence of CYP2C19 intermediate and poor metabolism and an increased risk of inadequate platelet inhibition with clopidogrel) compared to Caucasian or African-American patients.

Concurrent use with omeprazole, a proton pump inhibitor known to inhibit CYP2C19, significantly reduces concentrations of the active metabolite of clopidogrel and subsequently reduces clinical efficacy; this reduction in pharmacologic activity of clopidogrel occurs if omeprazole is given concomitantly with clopidogrel or 12 hours apart. No evidence exists that other drugs that decrease stomach acid, such as most Histamine-2 blockers (except cimetidine, which is a CYP2C19 inhibitor) or antacids, interfere with the antiplatelet activity of clopidogrel. If use of a proton pump inhibitor cannot be avoided, consider pantoprazole which has been shown to have less of an effect on the pharmacologic activity of clopidogrel. Avoid concurrent use of clopidogrel with CYP2C19 inhibitors, including omeprazole, esomeprazole, cimetidine, fluconazole, ketoconazole, voriconazole, etravirine, felbamate, fluoxetine, fluvoxamine, and ticlopidine.

Precautions Use with caution in patients with platelet disorders, bleeding disorders, or an increased risk for bleeding (eg, peptic ulcer disease, intraocular conditions, trauma, surgery, or patients receiving medications associated with ulcers or bleeding). Use with caution in patients receiving other platelet aggregation inhibitors; risk of bleeding may be increased. Use with caution in patients with impaired renal or hepatic function (experience is limited). Discontinue clopidogrel in patients 5 days prior to elective surgery **only** if antiplatelet effect is **not** required; patient-specific situations need to be discussed with cardiologist. Safety and efficacy have not been established in pediatric patients.

Adverse Reactions As with all drugs which may affect hemostasis, bleeding is associated with clopidogrel. Hemorrhage may occur at virtually any site. Risk is dependent on multiple variables, including the concurrent use of multiple agents which alter hemostasis and patient susceptibility.

Dermatologic: Pruritus, rash

Gastrointestinal: Bleeding, epistaxis, GI hemorrhage, purpura/bruising

Hematologic: Hematoma

Rare but important or life-threatening: Acute liver failure, agranulocytosis, anaphylactoid reaction, angioedema, aplastic anemia, arthritis, bronchospasm, bullous eruption, colitis (including ulcerative or lymphocytic), creatinine increased, diarrhea, DRESS syndrome, duodenal ulcer, eosinophilic pneumonia, erythema multiforme, gastric ulcer, glomerulopathy, hallucination, hemophilia A (acquired), hemorrhagic stroke (≤0.2%), hepatitis, hypersensitivity reaction, interstitial pneumonitis, intracranial hemorrhage (≤0.4%), lichen planus, musculoskeletal bleeding, myalgia, ocular bleeding (including conjunctival and retinal), pancreatitis, pancytopenia, pulmonary hemorrhage, respiratory tract hemorrhage, retroperitoneal hemorrhage, serum sickness, Stevens-Johnson syndrome, stomatitis, thrombotic thrombocytopenic purpura (TTP), toxic epidermal necrolysis, vasculitis, wound hemorrhage

Drug Interactions

Metabolism/Transport Effects Substrate of CYP2C19 (major), CYP3A4 (minor); **Note:** Assignment of Major/Minor substrate status based on clinically relevant drug interaction potential; **Inhibits** CYP2B6 (moderate), CYP2C9 (weak)

Avoid Concomitant Use

Avoid concomitant use of Clopidogrel with any of the following: Esomeprazole; Omeprazole; Urokinase

Increased Effect/Toxicity

Clopidogrel may increase the levels/effects of: Agents with Antiplatelet Properties; Anticoagulants; Apixaban; Collagenase (Systemic); CYP2B6 Substrates; Dabigatran Etexilate; Ibritumomab; Rivaroxaban; Salicylates; Thrombolytic Agents; Tositumomab and Iodine I 131 Tositumomab; Urokinase; Warfarin

The levels/effects of Clopidogrel may be increased by: Dasatinib; Glucosamine; Herbs (Anticoagulant/Antiplatelet Properties); Ibrutinib; Luliconazole; Multivitamins/Fluoride (with ADE); Multivitamins/Minerals (with ADEK, Folate, Iron); Multivitamins/Minerals (with AE, No Iron); Nonsteroidal Anti-Inflammatory Agents; Omega-3 Fatty Acids; Pentosan Polysulfate Sodium; Pentoxifylline; Prostacyclin Analogues; Rifamycin Derivatives; Tipranavir; Vitamin E

Decreased Effect

The levels/effects of Clopidogrel may be decreased by: Amiodarone; Calcium Channel Blockers; CYP2C19 Inhibitors (Moderate); CYP2C19 Inhibitors (Strong); Dexlansoprazole; Esomeprazole; Grapefruit Juice; Lansoprazole; Macrolide Antibiotics; Morphine (Liposomal); Morphine (Systemic); Nonsteroidal Anti-Inflammatory Agents; Omeprazole; Pantoprazole; RABEprazole

Food Interactions Consumption of three 200 mL glasses of grapefruit juice a day may substantially reduce clopidogrel antiplatelet effects. Management: Avoid or minimize the consumption of grapefruit or grapefruit juice (Holmberg, 2013).

Stability Store at controlled room temperature of 25°C (77°F); excursions permitted to 15°C to 30°C (59°F to 86°F).

Mechanism of Action Clopidogrel requires *in vivo* biotransformation to an active thiol metabolite. The active metabolite irreversibly blocks the $P2Y_{12}$ component of ADP receptors on the platelet surface, which prevents activation of the GPIIb/IIIa receptor complex, thereby reducing platelet aggregation. Platelets blocked by clopidogrel are affected for the remainder of their lifespan (~7-10 days).

Pharmacodynamics

Onset of action: Inhibition of platelet aggregation: Detected 2 hours after single oral dose

Maximum effect: Inhibition of platelet aggregation: 3-7 days; average inhibition level at steady-state in adults after receiving 75 mg/day: 40% to 60%.

Duration: Platelet aggregation and bleeding time gradually return to baseline after ~5 days after discontinuation.

Pharmacokinetics (Adult data unless noted)

Absorption: Rapid

Protein binding: Clopidogrel: 98%; main circulating metabolite (carboxylic acid derivative; inactive): 94%

Metabolism: Extensively hepatic via esterase-mediated hydrolysis to a carboxylic acid derivative (inactive) and via CYP450-mediated (CYP2C19 primarily) oxidation with a subsequent metabolism to a thiol metabolite (active).

Half-life: Parent drug: ~6 hours; thiol derivative (active metabolite): ~30 minutes; carboxylic acid derivative (inactive; main circulating metabolite): ~8 hours; **Note:** A clopidogrel radiolabeled study has shown that covalent binding to platelets accounts for 2% of radiolabel and has a half-life of 11 days

Time to peak serum concentration: ~0.75 hours

Elimination: Urine (50%) and feces (46%)

Dosing: Neonatal Note: Safety and efficacy have not been established in neonatal patients; optimal dose is not known; limited dosing information is available; further studies are needed: Oral: 0.2 mg/kg/dose once daily. A double-blind, placebo-controlled trial of 906 patients (n=461 neonates; n=445 infants ≤3 months) with cyanotic congenital heart disease surgically treated with a systemic-to-pulmonary artery shunt did not demonstrate a clinical benefit compared to placebo. Concomitant aspirin was used in 88% of patients (NCT00396877, 2011). In another trial, 0.2 mg/kg/dose once daily was found to achieve a mean inhibition of platelet aggregation similar to a standard adult dose; **Note:** This study (PICOLO Trial) included 73 evaluable patients [n=34 neonates (with exclusion of patients with weight <2 kg and GA <35 weeks); n=39 infants ≤24 months] with a systemic-to-pulmonary artery shunt, intracardiac or intravascular stent, Kawasaki disease, or arterial graft; 79% of patients received concomitant aspirin (Li, 2008).

Dosing: Usual Oral:

Infants, Children, and Adolescents: **Antiplatelet effect: Note:** Safety and efficacy have not been established in pediatric patients; optimal dose is not known; limited dosing information is available; further pediatric studies are needed:

Infants and Children ≤24 months: In the PICOLO trial, a dose of 0.2 mg/kg/dose once daily was found to achieve a mean inhibition of platelet aggregation similar to adults receiving the recommended dose; **Note:** This study included pediatric patients with a systemic-to-pulmonary artery shunt, intracardiac or intravascular stent, Kawasaki disease, or arterial graft; 79% of patients received concomitant aspirin (Li, 2008).

Children >2 years of age: Some centers use the following: Initial dose: 1 mg/kg once daily; titrate to response; in general, do not exceed adult dose (Finkelstein, 2005; Soman, 2006).

Adults:

Recent MI, recent stroke, or established peripheral arterial disease: 75 mg once daily

Acute coronary syndrome:

Unstable angina, non-ST-segment elevation myocardial infarction (UA/NSTEMI): Initial: 300 mg loading dose, followed by 75 mg once daily for at least 1 month and ideally up to 12 months (in combination with aspirin 75-162 mg once daily indefinitely) (Wright, 2011)

ST-segment elevation acute myocardial infarction (STEMI): 75 mg once daily (in combination with aspirin 162-325 mg initially, followed by 81-162 mg/day); **Note:** The CLARITY-TIMI 28 study used a 300 mg loading dose of clopidogrel (with thrombolysis) demonstrating an improvement in the patency rate of the infarct-related artery and reduction in ischemic complications. The duration of therapy was <28 days (usually until hospital discharge) unless nonprimary percutaneous coronary intervention (PCI) was performed (Sabatine, 2005).

The American College of Chest Physicians recommends (Goodman, 2008):

Patients ≤75 years: Initial: 300 mg loading dose, followed by 75 mg once daily for up to 28 days (in combination with aspirin)

Patients >75 years: 75 mg once daily for up to 28 days (with or without thrombolysis)

Percutaneous coronary intervention (PCI) for UA/ NSTEMI or STEMI: Loading dose: 300-600 mg (600 mg may be preferred for early invasive strategy with UA/NSTEMI) given as early as possible before or at the time of PCI followed by 75 mg once daily. **Note:** If an initial loading dose of 300 mg was given prior to PCI, a supplemental loading dose of 300 mg (total loading dose: 600 mg) may be administered (Kushner, 2009). For patients with UA/NSTEMI, it has been recommended that the loading dose be given at least 2 hours (or 24 hours in patients unable to take aspirin) prior to PCI (*Chest*, 2008).

Higher vs standard maintenance dosing: May consider a maintenance dose of 150 mg once daily for 6 days, then 75 mg once daily thereafter in patients not at high risk for bleeding (CURRENT-OASIS 7 Investigators, 2010; Wright, 2011); however, in another study, in patients with high on-treatment platelet reactivity, the use of 150 mg once daily for 6 months did not demonstrate a difference in 6-month incidence of death from cardiovascular causes, nonfatal MI, or stent thrombosis compared to standard dose therapy (Price, 2011).

Duration of clopidogrel (in combination with aspirin) after stent placement: **Premature interruption of therapy may result in stent thrombosis with subsequent fatal and nonfatal MI.** With STEMI, clopidogrel for at least 12 months regardless of stent type (ie, either bare metal or drug eluting stent) is recommended (Kushner, 2009). With UA/NSTEMI, at least 12 months of clopidogrel is recommended in patients receiving a drug eluting stent (DES) unless the risk of bleeding outweighs the benefits. For bare metal stent (BMS) placement, at least 1 month and ideally up to 12 months duration is recommended unless the risk of bleeding outweighs the benefits; then, a minimum of 2 weeks is recommended (Wright, 2011). In either setting, a duration >15 months may be considered in patients with DES placement (Kushner, 2009; Wright, 2011). For patients without ongoing ACS, clopidogrel should be continued for at least 1 month (for BMS) or at least 12 months (for DES) (Becker, 2008).

CYP2C19 poor metabolizers (ie, CYP2C19*2 or *3 carriers): Although routine genetic testing is not recommended in patients treated with clopidogrel undergoing PCI, testing may be considered to identify poor metabolizers who would be at risk for poor outcomes while receiving clopidogrel; if identified, these patients may be considered for an alternative P2Y12 inhibitor (Levine, 2011). An appropriate regimen for this patient population has not been established in clinical outcome trials. Although the manufacturer suggests a 600 mg loading dose, followed by 150 mg once daily, it does not appear that this dosing strategy improves outcomes for this patient population (Price, 2011).

Dosing adjustment in renal impairment: No dosage adjustment is required; use with caution; experience is limited; **Note:** Plasma concentrations of the main circulating metabolite were lower in adult patients with CrCl 5-15 mL/minute versus patients with CrCl 30-60 mL/minute or healthy adults. Inhibition of ADP-induced platelet aggregation was 25% lower compared to healthy adults; however, prolongation of bleeding time was similar.

Dosing adjustment in hepatic impairment: Use with caution; experience is limited; **Note:** Inhibition of ADP-induced platelet aggregation and mean bleeding time prolongation were similar in adult patients with severe hepatic impairment compared to healthy subjects after repeated doses of 75 mg once daily for 10 days.

Administration May be administered without regard to food.

Monitoring Parameters Signs of bleeding; hemoglobin and hematocrit periodically. Monitor mean inhibition of platelet aggregation: Goal of 30% to 50% inhibition (similar to adults receiving 75 mg/day). For unstable angina/non-ST-elevation MI in adults, platelet function testing has been used to determine platelet inhibitory response if results of testing may alter management (Wright, 2011).

Additional Information Overdose may lead to prolonged bleeding time with resultant bleeding complications; platelet transfusions may be an appropriate treatment when attempting to rapidly reverse the effects of clopidogrel

Dosage Forms Excipient information presented when available (limited, particularly for generics); consult specific product labeling.

Tablet, Oral:

Plavix: 75 mg, 300 mg

Generic: 75 mg, 300 mg

Extemporaneous Preparations A 5 mg/mL oral suspension may be made using tablets. Crush four 75 mg tablets and reduce to a fine powder. Add a small amount of a 1:1 mixture of Ora-Sweet® and Ora-Plus® and mix to a uniform paste; mix while adding the vehicle in geometric proportions to **almost** 60 mL; transfer to a calibrated bottle, rinse mortar with vehicle, and add quantity of vehicle sufficient to make 60 mL. Label "shake well". Stable 60 days at room temperature or under refrigeration.

Skillman KL, Caruthers RL, and Johnson CE, "Stability of an Extemporaneously Prepared Clopidogrel Oral Suspension," *Am J Health Syst Pharm*, 2010, 67(7):559-61.

References

Anderson JL, Adams CD, Antman EM, et al, "ACC/AHA 2007 Guidelines for the Management of Patients With Unstable Angina/Non-ST-Elevation Myocardial Infarction: A Report of the American College of Cardiology/American Heart Association Task Force on Practice Guidelines (Writing Committee to Revise the 2002 Guidelines for the Management of Patients With Unstable Angina/Non-ST-Elevation Myocardial Infarction) Developed in Collaboration With the American College of Emergency Physicians, the Society for Cardiovascular Angiography and Interventions, and the Society of Thoracic Surgeons Endorsed by the American Association of Cardiovascular and Pulmonary Rehabilitation and the Society for Academic Emergency Medicine," *J Am Coll Cardiol*, 2007, 50(7):1-157.

Angiolillo DJ, Fernandez-Ortiz A, Bernardo E, et al, "Contribution of Gene Sequence Variations of the Hepatic Cytochrome P450 3A4 Enzyme to Variability in Individual Responsiveness to Clopidogrel," *Arterioscler Thromb Vasc Biol*, 2006, 26(8):1895-900.

Antman EM, Anbe DT, Armstrong PW, et al, "ACC/AHA 2007 Guidelines for the Management of Patients With ST-Elevation Myocardial Infarction: A Report of the American College of Cardiology/American Heart Association Task Force on Practice Guidelines (Writing Committee to Revise the 1999 Guidelines for the Management of Patients With Acute Myocardial Infarction)," *J Am Coll Cardiol*, 2004, 44 (3):671-719.

Bauer ME, Bauer ST, Rabbani AB, et al, "Peripartum Management of Dual Antiplatelet Therapy and Neuraxial Labor Analgesia After Bare Metal Stent Insertion for Acute Myocardial Infarction," *Anesth Analg*, 2012, 115(3):613-5.

Becker RC, Meade TW, Berger PB, et al, "The Primary and Secondary Prevention of Coronary Artery Disease: American College of Chest Physicians Evidence-Based Clinical Practice Guidelines (8th Edition)," *Chest*, 2008, 133(6 Suppl):776-814.

Clarke TA and Waskell LA, "The Metabolism of Clopidogrel Is Catalyzed by Human Cytochrome P450 3A and Is Inhibited by Atorvastatin," *Drug Metab Dispos*, 2003, 31(1):53-9.

CURRENT-OASIS 7 Investigators, Mehta SR, Bassand JP, et al, "Dose Comparisons of Clopidogrel and Aspirin in Acute Coronary Syndromes," *N Engl J Med*, 2010, 363(10):930-42.

De Santis M, De Luca C, Mappa I, et al, "Clopidogrel Treatment During Pregnancy: A Case Report and a Review of Literature," *Intern Med*, 2011, 50(16):1769-73.

Douketis JD, Berger PB, Dunn AS, et al, "The Perioperative Management of Antithrombotic Therapy: American College of Chest

Physicians Evidence-Based Clinical Practice Guidelines (8th Edition)," *Chest*, 2008, 133(6 Suppl):299-339.

Finkelstein Y, Nurmohamed L, Avner M, et al, "Clopidogrel Use in Children," *J Pediatr*, 2005, 147(5):657.

Fraker TD, Fihn SD, Gibbons RJ, et al, "2007 Chronic Angina Focused Update of the ACC/AHA 2002 Guidelines for the Management of Patients With Chronic Stable Angina: A Report of the American College of Cardiology/American Heart Association Task Force on Practice Guidelines Writing Group to Develop the Focused Update of the 2002 Guidelines for the Management of Patients With Chronic Stable Angina," *Circulation*, 2007, 116(23):2762-72.

Goodman SG, Menon V, Cannon CP, et al, "Acute ST-Segment Elevation Myocardial Infarction: American College of Chest Physicians Evidence-Based Clinical Practice Guidelines (8th Edition)," *Chest*, 2008, 133(6 Suppl):707-75.

Grines CL, Bonow RO, Casey DE, et al, "AHA/ACC/SCAI/ACS/ADA Science Advisory, Prevention of Premature Discontinuation of Dual Antiplatelet Therapy in Patients With Coronary Artery Stents. A Science Advisory From the American Heart Association, American College of Cardiology, Society of Cardiovascular Angiography and Interventions, American College of Surgeons, and American Dental Association With Representation from the Amercian College of Physicians," *Circulation*, 2007, 115(6):813-8.

Kushner FG, Hand M, Smith SC, et al, "2009 Focused Updates: ACC/AHA Guidelines for the Management of Patients With ST-Elevation Myocardial Infarction (Updating the 2004 Guideline and 2007 Focused Update) and ACC/AHA/SCAI Guidelines on Percutaneous Coronary Intervention (Updating the 2005 Guideline and 2007 Focused Update): A Report of the American College of Cardiology Foundation/American Heart Association Task Force on Practice Guidelines," *J Am Coll Cardiol*, 2009, 54(23):2205-41.

Lau WC, Gurbel PA, Watkins PB, et al, "Contribution of Hepatic Cytochrome P450 3A4 Metabolic Activity to the Phenomenon of Clopidogrel Resistance," *Circulation*, 2004, 109(2):166-71.

Levine GN, Bates ER, Blankenship JC, et al, "2011 ACCF/AHA/SCAI Guideline for Percutaneous Coronary Intervention: A Report of the American College of Cardiology Foundation/American Heart Association Task Force on Practice Guidelines and the Society for Cardiovascular Angiography and Interventions," *Circulation*, 2011, 124(23):e574-651.

Li JS, Yow E, Berezny KY, et al, "Dosing of Clopidogrel for Platelet Inhibition in Infants and Young Children: Primary Results of the Platelet Inhibition in Children On cLOpidogrel (PICOLO) Trial," *Circulation*, 2008, 117(4):553-9.

Maltz LA, Gauvreau K, Connor JA, et al, "Clopidogrel in a Pediatric Population: Prescribing Practice and Outcomes From a Single Center," *Pediatr Cardiol*, 2009, 30(2):99-105.

Myers GR, Hoffman MK, and Marshall ES, "Clopidogrel Use Throughout Pregnancy in a Patient With a Drug-Eluting Coronary Stent," *Obstet Gynecol*, 2011, 118(2 Pt 2):432-3.

NCT00396877, "Efficacy and Safety of Clopidogrel in Neonates/Infants With Systemic to Pulmonary Artery Shunt Palliation (CLARINET)," Unpublished data. Available at http://clinicaltrials.gov/ct2/show/results/NCT00396877?term=clopidogrel&age=0&rank=3&sect=-X0125#all. Date accessed: April 14, 2011.

Price MJ, Berger PB, Teirstein PS, et al, "Standard- Vs High-Dose Clopidogrel Based on Platelet Function Testing After Percutaneous Coronary Intervention: The GRAVITAS Randomized Trial," *JAMA*, 2011, 305(11):1097-105.

Sabatine MS, Cannon CP, Gibson CM, et al, "Addition of Clopidogrel to Aspirin and Fibrinolytic Therapy for Myocardial Infarction With ST-Segment Elevation," *N Engl J Med*, 2005, 352(12):1179-89.

Savi P, Pereillo JM, Uzabiaga MF, et al, "Identification and Biological Activity of the Active Metabolite of Clopidogrel," *Thromb Haemost*, 2000, 84(5):891-6.

Scirica BM, Sabatine MS, Morrow DA, et al, "The Role of Clopidogrel in Early and Sustained Arterial Patency After Fibrinolysis for ST-Segment Elevation Myocardial Infarction: The ECG CLARITY-TIMI 28 Study," *J Am Coll Cardiol*, 2006, 48(1):37-42.

Society for Cardiovascular Angiography and Interventions, Society of Thoracic Surgeons, Writing Committee Members, et al, "ACCF/AHA Clopidogrel Clinical Alert: Approaches to the FDA "Boxed Warning": A Report of the American College of Cardiology Foundation Task Force on Clinical Expert Consensus Documents and the American Heart Association," *Circulation*, 2010, 122(5):537-57.

Soman T, Rafay MF, Hune S, et al, "The Risks and Safety of Clopidogrel in Pediatric Arterial Ischemic Stroke," *Stroke*, 2006, 37(4):1120-2.

Stanek EJ, Aubert RE, Flockhart DA, et al, "A National Study of the Effect of Individual Proton Pump Inhibitors on Cardiovascular Outcomes in Patients Treated With Clopidogrel Following Coronary Stenting: The Clopidogrel Medco Outcomes Study," Society for Cardiovascular Angiography and Interventions 2009 Scientific Sessions, Las Vegas, NV, May 6, 2009.

Wright RS, Anderson JL, Adams CD, et al, "2011 ACCF/AHA Focused Update of the Guidelines for the Management of Patients With Unstable Angina/Non-ST-Elevation Myocardial Infarction (Updating the 2007 Guideline) A Report of the American College of Cardiology Foundation/American Heart Association Task Force on Practice Guidelines," *J Am Coll Cardiol*, 2011, 57(18).

◆ **Clopidogrel Bisulfate** *see* Clopidogrel *on page 521*

Clorazepate (klor AZ e pate)

Medication Safety Issues
Sound-alike/look-alike issues:
Clorazepate may be confused with clofibrate, clonazepam, KlonoPIN®

BEERS Criteria medication:
This drug may be potentially inappropriate for use in geriatric patients (Quality of evidence - high; Strength of recommendation - strong).

Brand Names: U.S. Tranxene-T

Brand Names: Canada Apo-Clorazepate®; Novo-Clopate

Therapeutic Category Anticonvulsant, Benzodiazepine; Benzodiazepine; Sedative

Generic Availability (U.S.) Yes

Use Adjunct anticonvulsant in the management of partial seizures (FDA approved in ages ≥9 years and adults); treatment of anxiety disorders (FDA approved in adults); management of alcohol withdrawal (FDA approved in adults)

Medication Guide Available Yes

Pregnancy Considerations Nordiazepam, the active metabolite of clorazepate, crosses the placenta and is measurable in cord blood and amniotic fluid. Teratogenic effects have been observed with some benzodiazepines (including clorazepate); however, additional studies are needed. The incidence of premature birth and low birth weights may be increased following maternal use of benzodiazepines; hypoglycemia and respiratory problems in the neonate may occur following exposure late in pregnancy. Neonatal withdrawal symptoms may occur within days to weeks after birth and "floppy infant syndrome" (which also includes withdrawal symptoms) has been reported with some benzodiazepines (Bergman, 1992; Iqbal, 2002; Patel,1980; Rey, 1979; Wikner, 2007). A combination of factors influences the potential teratogenicity of anticonvulsant therapy. When treating women with epilepsy, monotherapy with the lowest effective dose and avoidance medications known to have a high incidence of teratogenic effects is recommended (Harden, 2009; Wlodarczyk, 2012).

Patients exposed to clorazepate during pregnancy are encouraged to enroll themselves into the AED Pregnancy Registry by calling 1-888-233-2334. Additional information is available at www.aedpregnancyregistry.org.

Breast-Feeding Considerations Nordiazepam, the active metabolite of clorazepate, is found in breast milk and is measurable in the serum of breast-feeding infants. Drowsiness, lethargy, or weight loss in nursing infants have been observed in case reports following maternal use of some benzodiazepines (Iqbal, 2002; Rey, 1979). The manufacturer states that women taking clorazepate should not breast-feed their infants.

Contraindications Hypersensitivity to clorazepate dipotassium or any component; cross-sensitivity with other benzodiazepines may exist; narrow-angle glaucoma; avoid using in patients with preexisting CNS depression or severe uncontrolled pain

Warnings Physical and psychological dependence may occur; abrupt discontinuation may cause withdrawal symptoms or seizures; use with caution in patients with a psychological predisposition for drug dependence. Clorazepate is not recommended for use in depressive neuroses or psychotic reactions.

Antiepileptic drugs (AEDs) increase the risk of suicidal behavior and ideation in patients receiving these medications for any indication. Pooled analyses of placebo-controlled trials involving 11 different AEDs (regardless of indication) showed a twofold increased risk of suicidal thoughts or behavior (estimated incidence rate: 0.43% in AED treated patients compared to 0.24% of patients receiving placebo); increased risk was observed as early as 1 week after initiation of AED and continued through duration of trials (most trials ≤24 weeks); risk did not vary significantly by age (age range: 5-100 years). Consider risks and benefits of AEDs before prescribing. Monitor all patients receiving an AED for emergence of suicidal thoughts or behavior, thoughts of self-harm, any unusual changes in behavior or mood, or the emergence or worsening of depressive symptoms; notify heathcare provider immediately if symptoms or concerning behavior occur. **Note:** The FDA is requiring that a Medication Guide be developed for all antiepileptic drugs informing patients of this risk.

Precautions Use with caution in patients with hepatic or renal disease. Clorazepate may cause CNS depression which may impair physical or mental abilities; patients must be cautioned about performing tasks which require mental alertness (eg, operating machinery or driving). Use with caution in patients receiving other CNS depressants or psychoactive medication (effects with other sedative drugs or ethanol may be potentiated) and in patients with depression.

Adverse Reactions
Cardiovascular: Hypotension

Central nervous system: Anxiety, ataxia, confusion, depression, dizziness, drowsiness, fatigue, headache, insomnia, irritability, lightheadedness, memory impairment, nervousness, slurred speech

Dermatologic: Rash

Endocrine & metabolic: Libido decreased

Gastrointestinal: Appetite increased/decreased, constipation, diarrhea, nausea, salivation decreased, vomiting, xerostomia

Hepatic: Jaundice, transaminase increased

Neuromuscular & skeletal: Dysarthria, tremor

Ocular: Blurred vision, diplopia

Drug Interactions
Metabolism/Transport Effects Substrate of CYP3A4 (major); **Note:** Assignment of Major/Minor substrate status based on clinically relevant drug interaction potential

Avoid Concomitant Use
Avoid concomitant use of Clorazepate with any of the following: Azelastine (Nasal); Conivaptan; Fusidic Acid (Systemic); Methadone; OLANZapine; Paraldehyde; Sodium Oxybate; Thalidomide

Increased Effect/Toxicity
Clorazepate may increase the levels/effects of: Alcohol (Ethyl); Azelastine (Nasal); Buprenorphine; CloZAPine; CNS Depressants; Hydrocodone; Methadone; Methotrimeprazine; Metyrosine; Mirtazapine; Paraldehyde; Pramipexole; ROPINIRole; Rotigotine; Selective Serotonin Reuptake Inhibitors; Sodium Oxybate; Thalidomide; Zolpidem

The levels/effects of Clorazepate may be increased by: Antifungal Agents (Azole Derivatives, Systemic); Aprepitant; Brimonidine (Topical); Calcium Channel Blockers (Nondihydropyridine); Cannabis; Ceritinib; Cimetidine; Conivaptan; Contraceptives (Estrogens); Contraceptives (Progestins); CYP3A4 Inhibitors (Moderate); CYP3A4 Inhibitors (Strong); Dasatinib; Doxylamine; Dronabinol; Droperidol; Fosamprenavir; Fosaprepitant; Fusidic Acid (Systemic); Grapefruit Juice; HydrOXYzine; Isoniazid; Ivacaftor; Kava Kava; Luliconazole; Magnesium Sulfate; MAO Inhibitors; Methotrimeprazine; Mifepristone; Nabilone; OLANZapine; Perampanel; Proton Pump Inhibitors; Ritonavir; Rufinamide; Saquinavir; Selective Serotonin

Reuptake Inhibitors; Simeprevir; Stiripentol; Tapentadol; Tetrahydrocannabinol

Decreased Effect
The levels/effects of Clorazepate may be decreased by: Bosentan; CarBAMazepine; CYP3A4 Inducers (Strong); Dabrafenib; Deferasirox; Mitotane; Rifamycin Derivatives; Siltuximab; St Johns Wort; Theophylline Derivatives; Tocilizumab; Yohimbine

Food Interactions Serum concentrations/toxicity may be increased by grapefruit juice. Management: Keep grapefruit consumption consistent.

Stability Unstable in water. Store at controlled room temperature at 20°C to 25°C (68°F to 77°F); protect from moisture; keep bottle tightly closed; dispense in tightly closed, light-resistant container

Mechanism of Action Binds to stereospecific benzodiazepine receptors on the postsynaptic GABA neuron at several sites within the central nervous system, including the limbic system, reticular formation. Enhancement of the inhibitory effect of GABA on neuronal excitability results by increased neuronal membrane permeability to chloride ions. This shift in chloride ions results in hyperpolarization (a less excitable state) and stabilization.

Pharmacokinetics (Adult data unless noted)
Distribution: Crosses the placenta

Protein binding: Nordiazepam: 97% to 98%

Metabolism: Rapidly decarboxylated to desmethyldiazepam (nordiazepam; primary metabolite; active) in acidic stomach prior to absorption; hepatically to oxazepam (active)

Half-life:
Nordiazepam: 40-50 hours
Oxazepam: 6-8 hours

Time to peak serum concentration: Oral: Within 1 hour

Elimination: Primarily in urine (62% to 67% of dose); feces (15% to 19%); found in urine as conjugated oxazepam (3-hydroxynordiazepam) (major urinary metabolite) and conjugated p-hydroxynordiazepam and nordiazepam (smaller amounts)

Dosing: Usual Oral:
Anticonvulsant:
Children: Initial dose: 0.3 mg/kg/day; maintenance dose: 0.5-3 mg/kg/day divided 2-4 times/day

or

Children 9-12 years: Initial: 3.75-7.5 mg/dose twice daily; increase dose by 3.75 mg at weekly intervals, not to exceed 60 mg/day in 2-3 divided doses

Children >12 years and Adults: Initial: Up to 7.5 mg/dose 2-3 times/day; increase dose by 7.5 mg at weekly intervals; usual dose: 0.5-1 mg/kg/day; not to exceed 90 mg/day

Anxiety: Adults: 7.5-15 mg 2-4 times/day; usual daily dose: 30 mg/day in divided doses; range: 15-60 mg/day; may be given as single dose of 15 mg at bedtime, with subsequent dosage adjustments based on patient response

Alcohol withdrawal: Adults: Initial: 30 mg, then 15 mg 2-4 times/day on first day; maximum daily dose: 90 mg; gradually decrease dose over subsequent days

Administration Oral: May administer with food or water to decrease GI upset

Monitoring Parameters Excessive CNS depression, respiratory rate, and cardiovascular status; with prolonged use: CBC, liver enzymes, renal function; signs and symptoms of suicidality (eg, anxiety, depression, behavior changes)

Reference Range Therapeutic: 0.12-1 mcg/mL (SI: 0.36-3.01 micromoles/L)

Test Interactions Decreased hematocrit; abnormal liver and renal function tests

Controlled Substance C-IV

Dosage Forms Excipient information presented when available (limited, particularly for generics); consult specific product labeling.

Tablet, Oral, as dipotassium:
Tranxene-T: 3.75 mg [scored; contains fd&c blue #2 (indigotine)]
Tranxene-T: 7.5 mg [scored; contains fd&c yellow #6 (sunset yellow)]
Tranxene-T: 15 mg [scored]
Generic: 3.75 mg, 7.5 mg, 15 mg

References
Bergman U, Rosa FW, Baum C, et al, "Effects of Exposure to Benzodiazepine During Fetal Life," *Lancet*, 1992, 340(8821):694-6.
Fenichel GM, *Clinical Pediatric Neurology: A Signs and Symptoms Approach*, 2nd ed, Philadelphia, PA: WB Saunders Co, 1993.
Fujii T, Okuno T, Go T, et al, "Clorazepate Therapy for Intractable Epilepsy," *Brain Dev*, 1987, 9(3):288-91.
Harden CL, Meador KJ, Pennell PB, et al, "Practice Parameter Update: Management Issues for Women With Epilepsy-Focus on Pregnancy (an Evidence-Based Review): Teratogenesis and Perinatal Outcomes: Report of the Quality Standards Subcommittee and Therapeutics and Technology Assessment Subcommittee of the American Academy of Neurology and American Epilepsy Society," *Neurology*, 2009, 73(2):133-41.
Iqbal MM, Sobhan T, Ryals T, et al, "Effects of Commonly Used Benzodiazepines on the Fetus, the Neonate, and the Nursing Infant," *Psychiatr Serv*, 2002, 53(1):39-49.
Mimaki T, Tagawa T, Ono J, et al, "Antiepileptic Effect and Serum Levels of Clorazepate on Children With Refractory Seizures," *Brain Dev*, 1984, 6(6):539-44.
Patel DA and Patel AR, "Clorazepate and Congenital Malformations," *JAMA*, 1980, 244(2):135-6.
Rey E, Giraux P, d'Athis P, et al, "Pharmacokinetics of the Placental Transfer and Distribution of Clorazepate and its Metabolite Nordiazepam in the Feto-Placental Unit and in the Neonate," *Eur J Clin Pharmacol*, 1979, 15(3):181-5.
Wikner BN, Stiller CO, Bergman U, et al, "Use of Benzodiazepines and Benzodiazepine Receptor Agonists During Pregnancy: Neonatal Outcome and Congenital Malformations," *Pharmacoepidemiol Drug Saf*, 2007, 16(11):1203-10.
Wlodarczyk BJ, Palacios AM, George TM, et al, "Antiepileptic Drugs and Pregnancy Outcomes," *Am J Med Genet A*, 2012, 158A (8):2071-90.

♦ **Clorazepate Dipotassium** see Clorazepate on page 524

♦ **Clotrimaderm (Can)** see Clotrimazole (Topical) on page 527

♦ **Clotrimazole 3 Day [OTC]** see Clotrimazole (Topical) on page 527

Clotrimazole (Oral) (kloe TRIM a zole)

Medication Safety Issues
Sound-alike/look-alike issues:
Clotrimazole may be confused with co-trimoxazole
Mycelex may be confused with Myoflex®

International issues:
Cloderm: Brand name for clotrimazole [Germany], but also brand name for alclomethasone [Indonesia]; clobetasol [China, India, Malaysia, Singapore, Thailand]; clocortolone [U.S., Canada]

Canesten [multiple international markets] may be confused with Canesten Bifonazol Comp brand name for bifonazole/urea [Austria]; Canesten Extra brand name for bifonazole [China, Germany]; Canesten Extra Nagelset brand name for bifonazole/urea [Denmark]; Canesten Fluconazole brand name for fluconazole [New Zealand]; Canesten Oasis brand name for sodium citrate [Great Britain]; Canesten Once Daily brand name for bifonazole [Australia]; Canesten Oral brand name for fluconazole [United Kingdom]; Cenestin brand name for estrogens (conjugated A/synthetic) [U.S., Canada]

Mycelex: Brand name for clotrimazole [U.S.] may be confused with Mucolex brand name for bromhexine [Malaysia]; carbocisteine [Thailand]

Therapeutic Category Antifungal Agent, Oral Nonabsorbed

Generic Availability (U.S.) Yes

Use Treatment of susceptible fungal infections, including oropharyngeal candidiasis; limited data suggests that the use of clotrimazole troches may be effective for prophylaxis against oropharyngeal candidiasis in neutropenic patients

Pregnancy Risk Factor C

Pregnancy Considerations In animal reproduction studies, adverse events were observed with oral administration of clotrimazole.

Contraindications Hypersensitivity to clotrimazole or any component

Warnings Clotrimazole troches should not be used for treatment of systemic fungal infection

Precautions Safety and effectiveness of clotrimazole lozenges (troches) in children <3 years of age have not been established

Adverse Reactions
Dermatologic: Pruritus
Gastrointestinal: Nausea, vomiting
Hepatic: Abnormal liver function tests

Drug Interactions
Metabolism/Transport Effects Inhibits CYP1A2 (weak), CYP2A6 (weak), CYP2B6 (weak), CYP2C19 (weak), CYP2C8 (weak), CYP2C9 (weak), CYP2D6 (weak), CYP2E1 (weak), CYP3A4 (moderate)

Avoid Concomitant Use
Avoid concomitant use of Clotrimazole (Oral) with any of the following: Bosutinib; Ibrutinib; Ivabradine; Lomitapide; Pimozide; Simeprevir; Tolvaptan; Ulipristal

Increased Effect/Toxicity
Clotrimazole (Oral) may increase the levels/effects of: ARIPiprazole; Avanafil; Bosentan; Bosutinib; Budesonide (Systemic, Oral Inhalation); Cannabis; Colchicine; CYP3A4 Substrates; Dofetilide; DOXOrubicin (Conventional); Dronabinol; Eplerenone; Everolimus; FentaNYL; Halofantrine; Ibrutinib; Imatinib; Ivabradine; Ivacaftor; Lomitapide; Lurasidone; OxyCODONE; Pimecrolimus; Pimozide; Propafenone; Ranolazine; Rivaroxaban; Salmeterol; Saxagliptin; Simeprevir; Tacrolimus (Systemic); Tetrahydrocannabinol; Tolvaptan; Ulipristal; Vilazodone; Zuclopenthixol

Decreased Effect
Clotrimazole (Oral) may decrease the levels/effects of: Ifosfamide

Mechanism of Action Binds to phospholipids in the fungal cell membrane altering cell wall permeability resulting in loss of essential intracellular elements

Pharmacokinetics (Adult data unless noted) Distribution: Following oral administration, clotrimazole is present in saliva for up to 3 hours following 30 minutes of dissolution time in the mouth

Dosing: Usual Children >3 years and Adults: Oral: 10 mg troche dissolved slowly 5 times/day

Administration Dissolve lozenge (troche) in mouth over 15-30 minutes

Monitoring Parameters Periodic liver function tests

Dosage Forms Excipient information presented when available (limited, particularly for generics); consult specific product labeling.

Lozenge, Mouth/Throat:
Generic: 10 mg (70 ea, 140 ea)
Troche, Mouth/Throat:
Generic: 10 mg

Clotrimazole (Topical) (kloe TRIM a zole)

Medication Safety Issues

Sound-alike/look-alike issues:

Clotrimazole may be confused with co-trimoxazole

Lotrimin® may be confused with Lotrisone®

International issues:

Cloderm: Brand name for clotrimazole [Germany], but also brand name for alclomethasone [Indonesia]; clobetasol [China, India, Malaysia, Singapore, Thailand]; clocortolone [U.S., Canada]

Canesten: Brand name for clotrimazole [multiple international markets] may be confused with Canesten Bifonazol Comp brand name for bifonazole/urea [Austria]; Canesten Extra brand name for bifonazole [China, Germany]; Canesten Extra Nagelset brand name for bifonazole/urea [Denmark]; Canesten Fluconazole brand name for fluconazole [New Zealand]; Canesten Oasis brand name for sodium citrate [Great Britain]; Canesten Once Daily brand name for bifonazole [Australia]; Canesten Oral brand name for fluconazole [United Kingdom]; Cenestin® brand name for estrogens (conjugated A/synthetic) [U.S., Canada]

Brand Names: U.S. Alevazol [OTC]; Clotrimazole 3 Day [OTC]; Clotrimazole Anti-Fungal [OTC]; Desenex [OTC]; Gyne-Lotrimin 3 [OTC]; Gyne-Lotrimin [OTC]; Lotrimin AF For Her [OTC]; Lotrimin AF [OTC]

Brand Names: Canada Canesten® Topical; Canesten® Vaginal; Clotrimaderm; Trivagizole-3®

Therapeutic Category Antifungal Agent, Topical; Antifungal Agent, Vaginal

Generic Availability (U.S.) Yes

Use Treatment of susceptible fungal infections, including dermatophytoses, superficial mycoses, cutaneous candidiasis, as well as vulvovaginal candidiasis

Pregnancy Considerations Following topical and vaginal administration, small amounts of imidazoles are absorbed systemically (Duhm, 1974). Vaginal products (7-day therapies) may be considered for the treatment of vulvovaginal candidiasis in pregnant women. This product may weaken latex condoms and diaphragms (CDC, 2010).

Contraindications Hypersensitivity to clotrimazole or any component

Adverse Reactions

Vaginal: Genitourinary: Vulvar/vaginal burning

Rare but important or life-threatening: Burning or itching of penis of sexual partner; polyuria; vulvar discharge, edema, itching, soreness

Drug Interactions

Metabolism/Transport Effects None known.

Avoid Concomitant Use There are no known interactions where it is recommended to avoid concomitant use.

Increased Effect/Toxicity

Clotrimazole (Topical) may increase the levels/effects of: Sirolimus; Tacrolimus (Systemic)

Decreased Effect There are no known significant interactions involving a decrease in effect.

Mechanism of Action Binds to phospholipids in the fungal cell membrane altering cell wall permeability resulting in loss of essential intracellular elements

Pharmacokinetics (Adult data unless noted) Absorption: Negligible through intact skin when administered topically; 3% to 10% of an intravaginal dose is absorbed

Dosing: Usual

Children >3 years and Adults: Topical: Apply twice daily

Children >12 years and Adults: Vaginal: 5 g (=1 applicatorful) of vaginal cream daily at bedtime for 3 days (2% vaginal cream) or 7 days (1% vaginal cream)

Administration

Topical: Apply sparingly and rub gently into the cleansed, affected area and surrounding skin; do not apply to the eye.

Vaginal: Wash hands before using. Insert full applicator into vagina gently and expel cream into vagina. Wash applicator with soap and water following use. Remain lying down for 30 minutes following administration.

Dosage Forms Excipient information presented when available (limited, particularly for generics); consult specific product labeling.

Cream, External:

Clotrimazole Anti-Fungal: 1% (15 g, 28.35 g) [contains benzyl alcohol]

Desenex: 1% (15 g, 30 g)

Lotrimin AF: 1% (12 g, 24 g)

Lotrimin AF For Her: 1% (24 g)

Generic: 1% (15 g, 30 g, 45 g)

Cream, Vaginal:

Clotrimazole 3 Day: 2% (22.2 g)

Gyne-Lotrimin: 1% (45 g) [contains benzyl alcohol]

Gyne-Lotrimin 3: 2% (21 g) [contains benzyl alcohol, cetyl alcohol]

Generic: 1% (45 g)

Ointment, External:

Alevazol: 1% (56.7 g)

Solution, External:

Generic: 1% (10 mL, 30 mL)

References

Centers for Disease Control and Prevention (CDC), "Sexually Transmitted Diseases Treatment Guidelines, 2010," *MMWR Recomm Rep*, 2010, 59(RR-12):1-110.

Duhm B, Medenwald H, Puetter J, et al, "The Pharmacokinetics of Clotrimazole 14C," *Postgrad Med J*, 1974, 50(Suppl 1):13-6.

◆ **Clotrimazole Anti-Fungal [OTC]** *see* Clotrimazole (Topical) *on page 527*

CloZAPine (KLOE za peen)

Medication Safety Issues

Sound-alike/look-alike issues:

CloZAPine may be confused with clonazePAM, cloNIDine, KlonoPIN

Clozaril may be confused with Clinoril, Colazal

BEERS Criteria medication:

This drug may be potentially inappropriate for use in geriatric patients (Quality of evidence - moderate; Strength of recommendation - strong).

Brand Names: U.S. Clozaril; FazaClo; Versacloz

Brand Names: Canada Apo-Clozapine; Clozaril; Gen-Clozapine

Therapeutic Category Antipsychotic Agent; Antipsychotic Agent, Atypical

Generic Availability (U.S.) May be product dependent

Use Treatment of refractory schizophrenia (FDA approved in adults); to reduce the risk of recurrent suicidal behavior in schizophrenia or schizoaffective disorder (FDA approved in adults)

Prescribing and Access Restrictions

U.S.: Versacloz has a REMS program; Clozaril is deemed to have a REMS program (approval pending from FDA). As a requirement of the REMS program, access to this medication is restricted. Patient-specific registration is required to dispense clozapine. Information specific to each monitoring program is available from the individual manufacturers. If a patient is switched from one brand/manufacturer of clozapine to another, the patient must be entered into a new registry (must be completed by the prescriber and delivered to the dispensing pharmacy). Healthcare providers, including pharmacists dispensing clozapine, should verify the patient's hematological status and qualification to receive clozapine with all existing registries. The manufacturers of clozapine request that health care providers submit all WBC/ANC values following discontinuation of therapy to the registry for all non-rechallengable patients until WBC is ≥3500/mm³ and ANC is ≥2000/mm³. Further information is available at 1-877-329-2256 or at the following websites:

Clozaril: http://www.clozarilregistry.com

Fazaclo: https://www.fazacloregistry.com

Versacloz: http://www.versaclozregistry.com

Canada: Currently, there are multiple manufacturers that distribute clozapine and each manufacturer has its own registry and distribution system. Patients must be registered in a database that includes their location, prescribing physician, testing laboratory, and dispensing pharmacist before using clozapine. Information specific to each monitoring program is available from the individual manufacturers.

Pregnancy Risk Factor B

Pregnancy Considerations Adverse events were not observed in animal reproduction studies. Clozapine crosses the placenta and can be detected in the fetal blood and amniotic fluid (Barnas, 1994). Antipsychotic use during the third trimester of pregnancy has a risk for abnormal muscle movements (extrapyramidal symptoms [EPS]) and/or withdrawal symptoms in newborns following delivery. Symptoms in the newborn may include agitation, feeding disorder, hypertonia, hypotonia, respiratory distress, somnolence, and tremor; these effects may be self-limiting or require hospitalization.

Clozapine may theoretically cause agranulocytosis in the fetus and should not routinely be used in pregnancy (NICE, 2007). The ACOG recommends that therapy during pregnancy be individualized; treatment with psychiatric medications during pregnancy should incorporate the clinical expertise of the mental health clinician, obstetrician, primary healthcare provider, and pediatrician. Safety data related to atypical antipsychotics during pregnancy is limited and routine use is not recommended. However, if a woman is inadvertently exposed to an atypical antipsychotic while pregnant, continuing therapy may be preferable to switching to a typical antipsychotic that the fetus has not yet been exposed to; consider risk:benefit (ACOG, 2008). An increased risk of exacerbation of psychosis should be considered when discontinuing or changing treatment during pregnancy and postpartum.

Healthcare providers are encouraged to enroll women 18-45 years of age exposed to clozapine during pregnancy in the Atypical Antipsychotics Pregnancy Registry (1-866-961-2388 or http://www.womensmentalhealth.org/pregnancyregistry).

Women with amenorrhea associated with use of other antipsychotic agents may return to normal menstruation when switching to clozapine therapy. Reliable contraceptive measures should be employed by women of childbearing potential switching to clozapine therapy.

Breast-Feeding Considerations Clozapine was found to accumulate in breast milk in concentrations higher than the maternal plasma (Barnas, 1994). Breast-feeding is not recommended by the manufacturer. Clozapine may theoretically cause agranulocytosis in the nursing infant and should not routinely be used in women who are breast-feeding (NICE, 2007).

Contraindications Hypersensitivity to clozapine or any component; history of agranulocytosis or granulocytopenia with clozapine; uncontrolled epilepsy; severe CNS depression or comatose state; paralytic ileus; myeloproliferative disorders; use with other agents which have a well-known risk of agranulocytosis or bone marrow suppression

Warnings Potentially life-threatening agranulocytosis may occur **[U.S. Boxed Warning]**. Due to the significant risk of agranulocytosis, it is strongly recommended that a patient must fail at least two trials of other primary medications for the treatment of schizophrenia (of adequate dose and duration) before initiating therapy with clozapine. Clozapine therapy should not be initiated in patients with WBC <3500/mm³ or ANC <2000/mm³, or history of myeloproliferative disorder, or clozapine induced agranulocytosis or granulocytopenia. WBC testing should occur periodically on an on-going basis (see prescribing information for monitoring details) to ensure that acceptable WBC/ANC counts are maintained. Initial episodes of moderate leukopenia or granulopoietic suppression confer up to a 12-fold increased risk for subsequent episodes of agranulocytosis. WBCs must be monitored weekly for at least 4 weeks after therapy discontinuation or until WBC is ≥3500/mm³ and ANC is ≥2000/mm³. Use with caution in patients receiving other marrow suppressive agents. Children and adolescents may be more sensitive to neutropenia compared to adults (Sporn, 2007); patients should be carefully monitored and counseled to report mouth sores, flu-like symptoms, or weakness. Eosinophilia has been reported to occur with clozapine; interrupt therapy for total eosinophil count >4000/mm³; may resume therapy when eosinophil count falls to <3000/mm³. The restricted distribution system ensures appropriate WBC and ANC monitoring.

Myocarditis, pericarditis, pericardial effusion, cardiomyopathy, CHF, ECG changes, arrhythmias, MI, and sudden death have also been reported with clozapine. Use clozapine with caution in patients with known cardiovascular or respiratory disease; carefully follow gradual dosage titration in these patients. Fatalities due to myocarditis have been reported; the highest incidence of fatal myocarditis occurs in the first month of therapy; however, later cases have also been reported **[U.S. Boxed Warning]**. Myocarditis or cardiomyopathy should be considered in patients who present with signs/symptoms of heart failure (dyspnea, fatigue, orthopnea, paroxysmal nocturnal dyspnea, peripheral edema), chest pain, palpitations, new ECG abnormalities (arrhythmias, ST-T wave abnormalities), or unexplained fever. Patients with tachycardia during the first month of therapy should be closely monitored for other signs of myocarditis. Discontinue clozapine if myocarditis is suspected; do not rechallenge in patients with clozapine-related myocarditis. The reported rate of myocarditis in clozapine-treated patients appears to be 17-322 times greater than in the general population.

May cause orthostatic hypotension (with or without syncope) and tachycardia **[U.S. Boxed Warning]**; collapse may rarely be profound and accompanied by respiratory and/or cardiac arrest; use with caution in patients at risk of this effect or in those who would not tolerate transient hypotensive episodes (eg, patients with cerebrovascular disease, cardiovascular disease, hypovolemia, or concurrent medication use which may predispose to hypotension/bradycardia). Collapse, respiratory arrest, and cardiac arrest during initiation of therapy have been reported in patients concurrently receiving benzodiazepines or other psychotropic drugs.

Clozapine is associated with QT prolongation and ventric-ular arrhythmias including torsades de pointes; cardiac arrest and sudden death may occur. Use with caution in patients with: History of long QT syndrome, conditions which may increase the risk of QT prolongation (eg, cardiovascular disease, recent MI, uncompensated heart failure, clinically significant arrhythmias, family history of long QT syndrome), concomitant use of medications known to prolong the QT interval [eg, certain antipsychotic medications (ziprasidone, iloperidone, chlorpromazine, thi-oridazine, mesoridazine, droperidol, pimozide), certain antibiotics (erythromycin, gatifloxacin, moxifloxacin, spar-floxacin), class Ia antiarrhythmics (quinidine, procaina-mide), class III antiarrhythmics (amiodarone, sotalol), or other medications known to prolong QT interval (pentam-idine, levomethadyl acetate, methadone, halofantrine, mefloquine, dolasetron, probucol or tacrolimus)]. Hypoka-lemia and/or hypomagnesemia may increase the risk of QT prolongation; correct electrolyte abnormalities prior to initiating therapy. Discontinue clozapine if QT_c interval >500 msec.

Seizures have been associated with clozapine use in a dose-dependent manner **[U.S. Boxed Warning]**; use with caution in patients at risk of seizures, including those with a history of seizures, head trauma, brain damage, alcohol-ism, or concurrent therapy with medications which may lower seizure threshold. Patients should be warned that a sudden loss of consciousness may occur with seizures.

Note: All of the above serious adverse effects have been reported in children and adolescents.

An increased risk of death has been reported with the use of antipsychotics in elderly patients with dementia-related psychosis **[U.S. Boxed Warning]**; most deaths seemed to be cardiovascular (eg, sudden death, heart failure) or infectious (eg, pneumonia) in nature. An increased inci-dence of cerebrovascular adverse events (eg, transient ischemic attack, stroke), including fatalities, has been reported with the use of atypical antipsychotics in elderly patients with dementia-related psychosis. Clozapine is not approved for the treatment of patients with dementia-related psychosis.

Precautions The possibility of a suicide attempt is inherent in psychotic illness or bipolar disorder; use with caution in high-risk patients during initiation of therapy. Prescriptions should be written for the smallest quantity consistent with good patient care.

May cause anticholinergic effects (constipation, xerosto-mia, blurred vision, urinary retention); use with caution in patients with decreased GI motility, paralytic ileus, urinary retention, benign prostatic hyperplasia, or visual problems. Use with caution in patients with narrow-angle glaucoma; condition may be exacerbated by cholinergic blockade; screening is recommended. Use with caution in patients with myasthenia gravis; condition may be exacerbated by cholinergic blockade. Impaired core body temperature regulation may occur; use with caution with strenuous exercise, heat exposure, dehydration, and concomitant medication possessing anticholinergic effects.

May cause extrapyramidal symptoms, including pseudo-parkinsonism, acute dystonic reactions, akathisia [may be as high as 15% in children and adolescents (Sporn, 2007)], and tardive dyskinesia (risk of these reactions is generally much lower relative to typical/conventional anti-psychotics, and is dose-dependent; risk of dystonia is increased with the use of high potency and higher doses of conventional antipsychotics and in males and younger patients).

Atypical antipsychotics have been associated with devel-opment of hyperglycemia; in some cases, this may be extreme and associated with ketoacidosis, hyperosmolar

coma, or death. Use with caution in patients with diabetes or other disorders of glucose regulation; monitor for wor-sening of glucose control. Patients with risk factors for diabetes should also be evaluated prior to therapy. Sig-nificant weight gain has been observed with clozapine; individual weight gain varies; monitor waist circumference and BMI. Use with caution in those at risk of aspiration pneumonia; dysphagia and esophageal dysmotility have been reported.

Clozapine has been associated with benign, self-limiting fever (<100.4°F, usually within first 3 weeks). However, clozapine may also be associated with severe febrile reactions, including neuroleptic malignant syndrome (NMS); monitor for mental status changes, fever, muscle rigidity, and/or autonomic instability. May be moderate to highly sedating; use with caution in disorders where CNS depression is a feature; patients must be cautioned about performing tasks which require mental alertness (eg, oper-ating machinery or driving). Use with caution in patients receiving general anesthesia (due to CNS effects). Rare cases of thromboembolism, including pulmonary embolism and stroke resulting in fatalities, have been associated with clozapine in patients with cardiovascular disease.

Clozapine is metabolized by CYP1A2, 2D6, and 3A4; use caution with medications which inhibit CYP activity.

Concurrent use with benzodiazepines may increase the risk of severe cardiopulmonary reactions. Cigarette smok-ing may enhance the metabolism of clozapine. Use with caution in patients with hepatic disease or impairment; hepatitis has been reported as a consequence of therapy. Use with caution in patients with renal impairment.

Clozapine should not be stopped abruptly; taper off over 1-2 weeks. If conditions warrant abrupt discontinuation (leukopenia, myocarditis, cardiomyopathy), monitor patient for psychosis and cholinergic rebound (headache, nausea, vomiting, diarrhea).

Orally disintegrating tablets contain aspartame which is metabolized to phenylalanine and must be avoided (or used with caution) in patients with phenylketonuria. **Note:** The allowable intake for aspartame in adults is 50 mg/kg/day.

Use caution when converting from brand to generic for-mulation; poor tolerability, including relapse, has been reported usually soon after product switch (1-3 months); monitor closely during this time (Bobo, 2010).

Adverse Reactions

Cardiovascular: Angina pectoris, ECG changes, hyper-/hypotension, syncope, tachycardia

Central nervous system: Agitation, akathisia, akinesia, anxiety, ataxia, confusion, depression, dizziness, drowsi-ness, fatigue, headache, insomnia, lethargy, myoclonic seizures, nightmares, pain, restlessness, seizure, slurred speech

Dermatologic: Skin rash

Gastrointestinal: Abdominal discomfort, anorexia, consti-pation, diarrhea, heartburn, nausea, sialorrhea, sore throat, vomiting, weight gain, xerostomia

Genitourinary: Urinary abnormalities (eg, abnormal ejacu-lation, retention, urgency, incontinence)

Hematologic: Agranulocytosis, eosinophilia, leukopenia

Hepatic: Abnormal liver function tests

Neuromuscular & skeletal: Hyper-/hypokinesia, muscle rigidity, muscle spasm, tremor, weakness

Ocular: Visual disturbances

Respiratory: Dyspnea, nasal congestion

Miscellaneous: Diaphoresis, numbness of tongue

Rare but important or life-threatening: Amentia, amnesia, anemia, arrhythmia (atrial or ventricular), aspiration, bra-dycardia, bronchitis, cardiomyopathy (usually dilated), cataplexy, CHF, cholestasis, CPK increased, cyanosis, delirium, delusions, dermatitis, diabetes mellitus, difficult urination, DVT, eczema, edema, EEG abnormal, erythema multiforme, ESR increased, fecal impaction, gastric ulcer, gastroenteritis, granulocytopenia, hallucinations, hematemesis, hepatitis, hypercholesterolemia (rare), hyperglycemia, hypersensitivity reaction, hypertriglyceridemia (rare), hyperuricemia, hyponatremia, hyperosmolar coma, hypothermia, impotence, interstitial nephritis (acute), intestinal obstruction, jaundice, ketoacidosis, loss of speech, metabolic syndrome (Lamberti, 2006), MI, mitral valve insufficiency, myasthenia syndrome, mydriasis, myocarditis, narrow-angle glaucoma, neuroleptic malignant syndrome, nocturnal enuresis, obsessive compulsive symptoms, orthostatic hypotension, pancreatitis (acute), paralytic ileus, paresthesia, pericardial effusion, pericarditis, periorbital edema, phlebitis, photosensitivity, pleural effusion, pneumonia, priapism, psychosis exacerbated, pulmonary embolism, rectal bleeding, respiratory arrest, rhabdomyolysis, salivary gland swelling, sepsis, status epilepticus, stroke, Stevens-Johnson syndrome, tardive dyskinesia, thrombocytopenia, thrombocytosis, thromboembolism, thrombophlebitis, torsade de pointes, vasculitis, weight loss

Drug Interactions

Metabolism/Transport Effects Substrate of CYP1A2 (major), CYP2A6 (minor), CYP2C19 (minor), CYP2C9 (minor), CYP2D6 (minor), CYP3A4 (minor); **Note:** Assignment of Major/Minor substrate status based on clinically relevant drug interaction potential; **Inhibits** CYP1A2 (weak), CYP2C19 (weak), CYP2C9 (weak), CYP2D6 (moderate), CYP2E1 (weak), CYP3A4 (weak)

Avoid Concomitant Use

Avoid concomitant use of CloZAPine with any of the following: Aclidinium; Amisulpride; Azelastine (Nasal); CarBAMazepine; Ciprofloxacin (Systemic); CYP3A4 Inducers (Strong); Highest Risk QTc-Prolonging Agents; Ipratropium (Oral Inhalation); Ivabradine; Metoclopramide; Mifepristone; Myelosuppressive Agents; Paraldehyde; Pimozide; Potassium Chloride; Sulpiride; Thalidomide; Thioridazine; Tiotropium; Umeclidinium

Increased Effect/Toxicity

CloZAPine may increase the levels/effects of: AbobotulinumtoxinA; Alcohol (Ethyl); Amisulpride; Analgesics (Opioid); Anticholinergic Agents; ARIPiprazole; Azelastine (Nasal); Buprenorphine; Cannabinoid-Containing Products; CNS Depressants; CYP2D6 Substrates; Fesoterodine; Highest Risk QTc-Prolonging Agents; Hydrocodone; Lomitapide; Methotrimeprazine; Methylphenidate; Metoprolol; Metyrosine; Mirabegron; Mirtazapine; Moderate Risk QTc-Prolonging Agents; Nebivolol; OnabotulinumtoxinA; Paraldehyde; Pimozide; Potassium Chloride; RimabotulinumtoxinB; Serotonin Modulators; Sulpiride; Thalidomide; Thiazide Diuretics; Thioridazine; Tiotropium; Topiramate; Zolpidem

The levels/effects of CloZAPine may be increased by: Abiraterone Acetate; Acetylcholinesterase Inhibitors (Central); Aclidinium; Benzodiazepines; Brimonidine (Topical); Cannabis; CarBAMazepine; Cimetidine; Ciprofloxacin (Systemic); CYP1A2 Inhibitors (Moderate); CYP1A2 Inhibitors (Strong); Deferasirox; Doxylamine; Dronabinol; Droperidol; HydrOXYzine; Ipratropium (Oral Inhalation); Ivabradine; Kava Kava; Lithium; Macrolide Antibiotics; Magnesium Sulfate; MAO Inhibitors; Methotrimeprazine; Methylphenidate; Metoclopramide; Metyrosine; Mifepristone; Myelosuppressive Agents; Nabilone; Nefazodone; Omeprazole; Perampanel; Pramlintide; QTc-Prolonging Agents (Indeterminate Risk and Risk Modifying); Rufinamide; Selective Serotonin Reuptake Inhibitors; Serotonin Modulators; Sodium Oxybate; Tapentadol; Tetrahydrocannabinol; Umeclidinium

Decreased Effect

CloZAPine may decrease the levels/effects of: Acetylcholinesterase Inhibitors (Central); Amphetamines; Anti-Parkinson's Agents (Dopamine Agonist); Codeine; Quinagolide; Secretin; Tamoxifen; TraMADol

The levels/effects of CloZAPine may be decreased by: Acetylcholinesterase Inhibitors (Central); Cannabis; CarBAMazepine; CYP3A4 Inducers (Strong); Cyproterone; Lithium; Omeprazole

Stability Clozaril®: Store at temperatures ≤30°C (86°F).

FazaClo®: Store at controlled room temperature at 25°C (77°F); excursions permitted to 15°C to 30°C (59°F to 86°F); protect from moisture; do not remove from package until ready to use

Dispensed in "clozapine patient system" packaging. **Note:** Drug is usually dispensed in a 1-week supply, unless patient is eligible for WBC and ANC testing at greater intervals (eg, every 2 or 4 weeks). Dispensing is contingent on WBC and ANC test results.

Mechanism of Action The therapeutic efficacy of clozapine (dibenzodiazepine antipsychotic) is proposed to be mediated through antagonism of the dopamine type 2 (D_2) and serotonin type 2A (5-HT_{2A}) receptors. In addition, it acts as an antagonist at alpha-adrenergic, histamine H_1, cholinergic, and other dopaminergic and serotonergic receptors.

Pharmacodynamics

Onset of action: Within 1 week for sedation, improvement in sleep; 6-12 weeks for antipsychotic effects

Adequate trial: 6-12 weeks at a therapeutic dose and blood level

Maximum effect: 6-12 months; improvement may continue 6-12 months after clozapine initiation (Meltzer, 2003)

Duration: Variable

Pharmacokinetics (Adult data unless noted)

Protein binding: 97% to serum proteins

Metabolism: Extensively hepatic; forms metabolites with limited (desmethyl metabolite) or no activity (hydroxylated and N-oxide derivative derivatives). **Note:** A pediatric pharmacokinetic study (n=6; age: 9-16 years) found higher concentrations of the desmethyl metabolite in comparison to clozapine (especially in females) when compared to data from adult studies; the authors suggest that both the parent drug and desmethyl metabolite contribute to the efficacy and adverse effect profile in children and adolescents (Frazier, 2003).

Bioavailability: 12% to 81% (not affected by food); orally disintegrating tablets are bioequivalent to the regular tablets

Half-life: Steady state: 12 hours (range: 4-66 hours)

Time to peak serum concentration: Tablets: 2.5 hours (range: 1-6 hours); orally disintegrating tablets: 2.3 hours (range: 1-6 hours)

Elimination: Urine (~50% of dose) and feces (30%); trace amounts of unchanged drug excreted in urine and feces

Dosing: Usual

Children and Adolescents: **Treatment of refractory childhood-onset schizophrenia or schizoaffective disorder:** Limited data available: Oral: Initial: 12.5 mg once or twice daily; increase daily dose as tolerated every 3-5 days (usually by 25 mg increments) to a target dose of 125-475 mg/day in divided doses (based on patient's age, size, and tolerability). Mean dose in most pediatric studies: 175-200 mg/day (Findling, 2007)

Adults:

Refractory schizophrenia or schizoaffective disorder: Oral: Initial: 12.5 mg once or twice daily; increase as tolerated, in increments of 25-50 mg/day to a target dose of 300-450 mg/day after 2-4 weeks; may increase further if needed, but no more than once or twice weekly, in increments ≤100 mg/day; some patients may require doses as high as 600-900 mg/day in divided doses. Do not exceed 900 mg/day. In some efficacy studies, total daily dosage was administered in three divided doses. **Note:** Due to significant adverse effects, patients who fail to adequately respond clinically, should not be normally continued on therapy for an extended period of time; responding patients should be maintained on the lowest effective dose; patients should be periodically assessed to determine if maintenance treatment is still required.

Reduction of the risk of suicidal behavior in schizophrenia or schizoaffective disorder: Oral: Initial: 12.5 mg once or twice daily; increased, as tolerated, in increments of 25-50 mg/day to a target dose of 300-450 mg/day after 2-4-weeks; may increase further if needed, but no more than once or twice weekly, in increments ≤100 mg/day; mean effective dose is ~300 mg/day (range: 12.5-900 mg). **Note:** A treatment course of at least 2 years is recommended to maintain the decreased risk for suicidal behavior; patients should be reassessed after 2 years for risk of suicidal behavior and periodically thereafter.

Termination of therapy: If dosing is interrupted for ≥48 hours, therapy must be reinitiated at 12.5-25 mg/day; if tolerated, the dose may be increased more rapidly than with initial titration, unless cardiopulmonary arrest occurred during initial titration.

In the event of planned termination of clozapine, gradual reduction in dose over a 1- to 2-week period is recommended. If conditions warrant abrupt discontinuation (eg, leukopenia, eosinophilia), monitor patient for psychosis and cholinergic rebound (headache, nausea, vomiting, diarrhea).

Dosing adjustment for toxicity: Adults: Oral:
Eosinophilia: Interrupt therapy for eosinophil count >4000/mm³; may resume therapy when eosinophil count <3000/mm³

Moderate leukopenia or granulocytopenia (WBC 2000-3000/mm³ and/or ANC 1000-1500/mm³): Discontinue therapy; may rechallenge patient when WBC is >3500/mm³ and ANC is >2000/mm³. **Note:** Patient is at greater risk for developing agranulocytosis.

Severe leukopenia or granulocytopenia (WBC <2000/mm³ and/or ANC <1000/mm³): Discontinue therapy and do not rechallenge patient.

Dosing adjustment in renal impairment: There are no dosage adjustments provided in manufacturer's labeling (has not been studied); use with caution.

Dosing adjustment in hepatic impairment: There are no dosage adjustments provided in manufacturer's labeling (has not been studied); use with caution.

Administration May be administered without regard to food.

Orally-disintegrating tablet: Should be removed from foil blister by peeling apart (do not push tablet through the foil). Remove immediately prior to use. Place tablet in mouth and allow to dissolve; swallow with saliva (no water is needed to take the dose). If dosing requires splitting tablet, throw unused portion away.

Monitoring Parameters Mental status, ECG, CBC (see below), liver function tests, vital signs, fasting lipid profile, and fasting blood glucose/Hgb A_{1c} (prior to treatment, at 3 months, then annually, or as symptoms warrant); height, weight, BMI, personal/family history of obesity, waist circumference (weight should be assessed prior to treatment, at 4 weeks, 8 weeks, 12 weeks, and then at quarterly intervals; consider titrating to a different antipsychotic agent for a weight gain ≥5% of the initial weight); blood pressure, pulse, abnormal involuntary movement scale (AIMS).

WBC and ANC should be obtained at baseline and at least weekly for the first 6 months of continuous treatment. If counts remain acceptable (WBC ≥3500/mm³, ANC ≥2000/mm³) during this time period, then they may be monitored every other week for the next 6 months. If WBC/ANC continue to remain within these acceptable limits after the second 6 months of therapy, monitoring can be decreased to every 4 weeks. If clozapine is discontinued, a weekly WBC should be conducted for an additional 4 weeks or until WBC is ≥3500/mm³ and ANC is ≥2000/mm³. If clozapine therapy is interrupted due to moderate leukopenia, weekly WBC/ANC monitoring is required for 12 months in patients restarted on clozapine treatment. If therapy is interrupted for reasons other than leukopenia/granulocytopenia, the 6-month time period for initiation of biweekly WBCs may need to be reset. This determination depends upon the treatment duration, the length of the break in therapy, and whether or not an abnormal blood event occurred. Consult manufacturer prescribing information for determination of appropriate WBC/ANC monitoring interval.

Interrupt therapy for eosinophil count >4000/mm³; may resume therapy when eosinophil count <3000/mm³.

Additional Information Clozapine produces little or no prolactin elevation; this is in contrast to other more typical antipsychotic drugs

Dosage Forms Excipient information presented when available (limited, particularly for generics); consult specific product labeling.

Suspension, Oral:
Versacloz: 50 mg/mL (100 mL) [contains methylparaben sodium, propylparaben sodium]
Tablet, Oral:
Clozaril: 25 mg, 100 mg [scored]
Generic: 25 mg, 50 mg, 100 mg, 200 mg
Tablet Dispersible, Oral:
FazaClo: 12.5 mg, 25 mg, 100 mg, 150 mg, 200 mg [contains aspartame]
Generic: 12.5 mg, 25 mg, 100 mg

References

ACOG Committee on Practice Bulletins-Obstetrics, "ACOG Practice Bulletin: Clinical Management Guidelines for Obstetrician-Gynecologists Number 92, April 2008 (Replaces Practice Bulletin Number 87, November 2007). Use of Psychiatric Medications During Pregnancy and Lactation," *Obstet Gynecol*, 2008, 111(4):1001-20.

Alfaro CL, Wudarsky M, Nicolson R, et al, "Correlation of Antipsychotic and Prolactin Concentrations in Children and Adolescents Acutely Treated With Haloperidol, Clozapine or Olanzapine," *J Child Adolesc Psychopharmacol*, 2002, 12(2):83-91.

American Diabetes Association; American Psychiatric Association; American Association of Clinical Endocrinologists; North American Association for the Study of Obesity, "Consensus Development Conference on Antipsychotic Drugs and Obesity and Diabetes," *Diabetes Care*, 2004, 27(2):596-601.

Baker RW and Chengappa KN, "Gastroesophageal Reflux as a Possible Result of Clozapine Treatment," *J Clin Psychiatry*, 1998, 59(5):257

Barnas C, Bergant A, Hummer M, et al, "Clozapine Concentrations in Maternal and Fetal Plasma, Amniotic Fluid, and Breast Milk," *Am J Psychiatry*, 1994, 151(6):945.

Bobo WV, Stovall JA, Knostman M, et al, "Converting From Brand-Name to Generic Clozapine: A Review of Effectiveness and Tolerability Trial," *Am J Health Syst Pharm*, 2010, 67(1):27-37.

Campellone JV, McCluskey LF, and Greenspan D, "Fatal Outcome From Neuroleptic Malignant Syndrome Associated With Clozapine," *Neuropsychiatry, Neuropsychology, and Behavioral Neurology*, 1995, 8:70-3.

Correll CU, Penzner JB, Parikh UH, et al, "Recognizing and Monitoring Adverse Events of Second-Generation Antipsychotics in Children and Adolescents," *Child Adolesc Psych Clin N Am*, 2006, 15(1):177-206.

Findling RL, Frazier JA, Gerbino-Rosen B, et al, "Is There a Role for Clozapine in the Treatment of Children and Adolescents?" *J Am Acad Child Adolesc Psych*, 2007, 46(3):423-8.

Frazier JA, Cohen LG, Jacobsen L, et al, "Clozapine Pharmacokinetics in Children and Adolescents With Childhood-Onset Schizophrenia," *J Clin Psychopharmacol*, 2003, 23(1):87-91.

Funderberg LG, Vertrees JE, True JE, et al, "Seizure Following Addition of Erythromycin to Clozapine Treatment," *Am J Psychiatry*, 1994, 151(12):1840-1.

Gerbino-Rosen G, Roofeh D, Tompkins DA, et al, "Hematological Adverse Events in Clozapine-Treated Children and Adolescents," *J Am Acad Child Adolesc Psychiatry*, 2005, 44(10):1024-31.

Gerson SL and Meltzer H, "Mechanisms of Clozapine-Induced Agranulocytosis," *Drug Saf*, 1992, 7(Suppl 1):17-25.

Hagg S, Spigset O, and Soderstrom TG, "Association of Venous Thromboembolism and Clozapine," *Lancet*, 2000, 355(9210):1155-6.

Kane J, Honigfeld G, Singer J, et al, "Clozapine for the Treatment-Resistant Schizophrenic. A Double-Blind Comparison With Chlorpromazine," *Arch Gen Psychiatry*, 1988, 45(9):789-96.

Kant R, Chalansani R, Chengappa KN, et al, "The Off-Label Use of Clozapine in Adolescents With Bipolar Disorder, Intermittent Explosive Disorder, or Posttraumatic Stress Disorder," *J Child Adolesc Psychopharmacol*, 2004, 14(1):57-63.

Kranzler HN, Kester HM, Gerbino-Rosen G, et al, "Treatment-Refractory Schizophrenia in Children and Adolescents: An Update on Clozapine and Other Pharmacologic Interventions," *Child Adolesc Psychiatr Clin N Am*, 2006, 15(1):135-59.

Kranzler H, Roofeh D, Gerbino-Rosen G, et al, "Clozapine: Its Impact on Aggressive Behavior Among Children and Adolescents With Schizophrenia," *J Am Acad Child Adolesc Psychiatry*, 2005, 44(1):55-63.

Kumra S, Frazier JA, Jacobsen LK, et al, "Childhood-Onset Schizophrenia. A Double-Blind Clozapine-Haloperidol Comparison," *Arch Gen Psychiatry*, 1996, 53(12):1090-7.

Lamberti JS, Olson D, Crilly JF, et al, "Prevalence of the Metabolic Syndrome Among Patients Receiving Clozapine," *Am J Psychiatry*, 2006, 163(7):1273-6.

Mady SP and Wax P, "Clozapine Intoxication in a Young Child," *Vet Hum Toxicol*, 1993, 35(4):338.

McCarthy RH and Terkelsen KG, "Esophageal Dysfunction in Two Patients After Clozapine Treatment," *J Clin Psychopharmacol*, 1994, 14(4):281-3.

Meltzer HY, Alphs L, Green AI, et al, "Clozapine Treatment for Suicidality in Schizophrenia: International Suicide Prevention Trial (InterSePT)," *Arch Gen Psychiatry*, 2003, 60(1):82-91.

National Institute for Health and Clinical Excellence (NICE), National Collaborating Centre for Mental Health, "Antenatal and Postnatal Mental Health," *National Clinical Practice Guideline Number 45*, 2007. Available at http://publications.nice.org.uk/antenatal-and-postnatal-mental-health-cg45

Pacia SV and Devinsky O, "Clozapine-Related Seizures: Experience With 5629 Patients," *Neurology*, 1994, 44(12):2247-9.

Radford JM, Brown TM, and Borison RL, "Unexpected Dystonia While Changing From Clozapine to Risperidone," *J Clin Psychopharmacol*, 1995, 15(3):225-6.

Shaw P, Sporn A, Gogtay N, et al, "Childhood-Onset Schizophrenia: A Double-Blind, Randomized, Clozapine-Olanzapine Comparison," *Arch Gen Psych*, 2006, 63(7):721-30.

Sporn AL, Vermani A, Greenstein DK, et al, "Clozapine Treatment of Childhood-Onset Schizophrenia: Evaluation of Effectiveness, Adverse Effects, and Long-Term Outcome," *J Am Acad Child Adolesc Psychiatry*, 2007, 46(10):1349-56.

Testani M, "Clozapine-Induced Orthostatic Hypotension Treated With Fludrocortisone," *J Clin Psychiatry*, 1994, 55(11):497-8.

Wheatley M, Plant J, Reader H, et al, "Clozapine Treatment of Adolescents With Posttraumatic Stress Disorder and Psychotic Symptoms," *J Clin Psychopharmacol*, 2004, 24(2):167-73.

Wilson WH and Claussen AM, "Seizures Associated With Clozapine Treatment in a State Hospital," *J Clin Psychiatry*, 1994, 55(5):184-8.

◆ **Clozaril** see CloZAPine *on page 527*

◆ **CMV Hyperimmune Globulin** see Cytomegalovirus Immune Globulin (Intravenous-Human) *on page 576*

◆ **CMV-IGIV** see Cytomegalovirus Immune Globulin (Intravenous-Human) *on page 576*

◆ **CNL8 Nail** see Ciclopirox *on page 465*

◆ **Coagulant Complex Inhibitor** see Anti-inhibitor Coagulant Complex (Human) *on page 180*

◆ **Coagulation Factor VIIa** see Factor VIIa (Recombinant) *on page 831*

Coal Tar (KOLE tar)

Medication Safety Issues
International issues:

Pentrax [U.S., Canada, Great Britain, Ireland] may be confused with Permax brand name for pergolide [multiple international markets]

Brand Names: U.S. Balnetar [OTC]; Beta Care Betatar Gel [OTC]; Cutar [OTC]; DHS Tar Gel [OTC]; DHS Tar [OTC]; Elta Lite Tar [OTC]; Elta Tar [OTC]; Ionil-T [OTC]; Neutrogena T/Gel Conditioner [OTC]; Neutrogena T/Gel Ex St [OTC]; PC-Tar [OTC]; Pentrax Gold [OTC]; Polytar [OTC]; Psoriasin [OTC]; Scytera [OTC]; Tera-Gel Tar [OTC]; Therapeutic [OTC]; Theraplex T [OTC]; X-Seb T Pearl [OTC]; X-Seb T Plus [OTC]

Brand Names: Canada Doak Oil Forte [OTC]; Doak Oil [OTC]; Emorex Gel [OTC]; Neuotrogena T/Gel Therapeutic Shampoo [OTC]; Odans Liquor Carbonis Detergens [OTC]; Pentrax Gold Shampoo [OTC]; Pentrax Tar Shampoo [OTC]; Psoriasin [OTC]; T/Gel Therapeutic Shampoo Extra Strength [OTC]; Targel® [OTC]; Tersa Tar Shp [OTC]

Therapeutic Category Antipsoriatic Agent, Topical; Antiseborrheic Agent, Topical

Generic Availability (U.S.) May be product dependent

Use Topically for controlling dandruff, seborrheic dermatitis, or psoriasis

Pregnancy Considerations Limited application of coal tar during pregnancy for the treatment of psoriasis appears to be safe in pregnant women (Gelmetti, 2009; Landau, 2011).

Breast-Feeding Considerations A case report describes the absorption of the components of a coal tar containing ointment by a nursing infant. The components were not detected in breast milk, but were assumed to be absorbed by the infant following skin-to-skin contact with the mother while nursing. If coal tar is used in a nursing mother, direct contact by the infant should be avoided (Scheepers, 2009).

Contraindications Hypersensitivity to coal tar or any ingredient in the formulation

Warnings Due to a potential carcinogenic risk, do not use around the rectum or in the genital area or groin

Precautions Do not apply to acutely inflamed skin; avoid exposure to sunlight for at least 24 hours

Adverse Reactions Dermatologic: Dermatitis, folliculitis, irritation, photosensitivity

Drug Interactions

Metabolism/Transport Effects None known.

Avoid Concomitant Use There are no known interactions where it is recommended to avoid concomitant use.

Increased Effect/Toxicity There are no known significant interactions involving an increase in effect.

Decreased Effect There are no known significant interactions involving a decrease in effect.

Dosing: Usual Children and Adults: Topical:

Bath: 60-90 mL of a 5% to 20% solution or 15-25 mL of 30% lotion is added to bath water; soak 5-20 minutes, then pat dry; use once daily to once every 3 days

Shampoo: Apply twice weekly for the first 2 weeks then once weekly or more often if needed

Skin: Apply to the affected area 1-4 times/day; decrease frequency to 2-3 times/week once condition has been controlled

Atopic dermatitis: 2% to 5% coal tar cream may be applied once daily or every other day to reduce inflammation

Scalp psoriasis: Tar oil bath or coal tar solution may be painted sparingly to the lesions 3-12 hours before each shampoo

Psoriasis of the body, arms, legs: Apply at bedtime; if thick scales are present, use product with salicylic acid and apply several times during the day

Administration Topical:

Bath: Add appropriate amount of coal tar to lukewarm bath water and mix thoroughly

Shampoo: Rub shampoo onto wet hair and scalp, rinse thoroughly; repeat; leave on 5 minutes; rinse thoroughly

Dosage Forms Excipient information presented when available (limited, particularly for generics); consult specific product labeling.

Bar, External:

Polytar: Coal tar 0.5% (1 ea)

Cream, External:
Elta Tar: 2% (107 g)
Emulsion, External:
Balnetar: 2.5% (221 mL)
Foam, External:
Scytera: 2% (100 g) [contains disodium edta]
Liquid, External:
Neutrogena T/Gel Conditioner: 0.5% (130 mL)
Lotion, External:
Elta Lite Tar: 10% (240 mL)
Oil, External:
Cutar: 7.5% (180 mL, 3840 mL)
Ointment, External:
Psoriasin: 2% (113 g) [contains alcohol, usp, polysorbate 80]
Shampoo, External:
Beta Care Betatar Gel: 2.5% (480 mL) [contains trolamine (triethanolamine)]
DHS Tar: 0.5% (120 mL, 240 mL)
DHS Tar Gel: 0.5% (240 mL)
Ionil-T: 1% (473 mL) [contains alcohol, usp, benzalkonium chloride, edetate sodium (tetrasodium), isopropyl alcohol]
Neutrogena T/Gel Ex St: 1% (177 mL) [contains methylparaben, propylparaben]
PC-Tar: 1% (180 mL)
Pentrax Gold: 4% (168 mL)
Polytar: Coal tar 0.5% (177 mL) [contains alcohol, usp, polysorbate 80, trolamine (triethanolamine)]
Tera-Gel Tar: 0.5% (114 mL, 235 mL) [contains edetate sodium (tetrasodium), methylparaben, polysorbate 80, propylparaben]
Therapeutic: 0.5% (251 mL)
Theraplex T: 1% (240 mL)
X-Seb T Pearl: 10% (236 mL) [contains brilliant blue fcf (fd&c blue #1), edetate disodium]
X-Seb T Plus: 10% (236 mL) [contains brilliant blue fcf (fd&c blue #1), edetate disodium]
Solution, External:
Generic: 20% (100 mL, 500 mL, 4000 mL)

References

Gelmetti C, "Therapeutic Moisturizers as Adjuvant Therapy for Psoriasis Patients," *Am J Clin Dermatol*, 2009, 10(Suppl 1):7-12.

Greaves MW, Weinstein GD, "Treatment of Psoriasis," *N Engl J Med*, 1995, 332(9):581-8.

Hanifin JM, "Atopic Dermatitis in Infants and Children," *Pediatr Clin North Am*, 1991, 38(4):763-89.

Landau JL, Moody MN, Kazakevich N, et al, "Psoriasis and the Pregnant Woman: What Are the Key Considerations?" *Skin Therapy Lett*, 2011, 16(9):1-3.

Scheepers PT, van Houtum JL, Anzion RB, et al, "Uptake of Pyrene in a Breast-Fed Child of a Mother Treated With Coal Tar," *Pediatr Dermatol*, 2009, 26(2):184-7.

◆ **CO Amlodipine (Can)** *see* AmLODIPine *on page 135*

◆ **Co-Amoxiclav** *see* Amoxicillin and Clavulanate *on page 144*

◆ **Coartem** *see* Artemether and Lumefantrine *on page 203*

◆ **CO Atenolol (Can)** *see* Atenolol *on page 222*

◆ **CO Atorvastatin (Can)** *see* AtorvaSTATin *on page 227*

◆ **CO Azithromycin (Can)** *see* Azithromycin (Systemic) *on page 247*

◆ **CO Bosentan (Can)** *see* Bosentan *on page 298*

Cocaine (koe KANE)

Therapeutic Category Analgesic, Topical; Local Anesthetic, Topical

Generic Availability (U.S.) Yes

Use Topical anesthesia for mucous membranes of the oral, laryngeal, and nasal cavities (FDA approved in children and adults); has also been used for its vasoconstrictive properties in nasal surgery

Pregnancy Risk Factor C

Pregnancy Considerations Animal reproduction studies have not been conducted with this product. Cocaine rapidly crosses the placenta in concentrations equal to those in the mother. Adverse events occur in the fetus (eg, congenital malformations, growth restriction), infant (neonatal abstinence syndrome), and mother (eg, preterm labor, placental abruption) following maternal abuse (Fajemirokun-Odudeyi, 2004).

Breast-Feeding Considerations Cocaine rapidly enters breast milk. Irritability, hypertension, tachypnea, tachycardia, and tremors have been reported in nursing infants (Chasnoff, 1987).

Contraindications Hypersensitivity to cocaine or any component; systemic use

Warnings For topical administration only; do not use intravenously; do not inject by any route. Not for intraocular use; causes sloughing of the corneal epithelium, causing clouding, pitting, and occasionally ulceration of the cornea. Use should be limited to appropriate healthcare settings. Resuscitative equipment and drugs should be immediately available when using local anesthetics. Debilitated, elderly patients, acutely ill patients, and children should be given reduced doses consistent with their age and physical status. Potential for drug dependency exists with systemic administration; consider assessment of risk for abuse prior to therapy; misuse may cause sudden death and serious cardiovascular adverse events; use with caution in patients with history of ethanol or drug abuse.

Precautions Use with caution in patients with cardiovascular disease and in infants; use with caution in patients with severely traumatized mucosa and sepsis in the region of intended application.

Adverse Reactions

Cardiovascular: Arrhythmias (ventricular), cardiac arrhythmia, cardiomyopathy, cerebral vasculitis, CHF, decreased heart rate (low doses), fibrillation (atrial), flutter (atrial), hypertension, myocarditis, pulmonary hypertension, QRS prolongation, Raynaud's phenomenon, sinus bradycardia, sinus tachycardia, tachycardia (moderate doses) tachycardia (supraventricular), thrombosis, vasoconstriction

Central nervous system: Agitation, cerebral vascular accident, clonic-tonic reactions, CNS stimulation, dystonic reactions, euphoria, excitation, fever, hallucinations, headache, hyperthermia, nervousness, paranoia, psychosis, restlessness, seizure, slurred speech, sympathetic storm, vasculitis

Dermatologic: Madarosis, pruritus, skin infarction

Gastrointestinal: Anorexia, colonic ischemia, loss of taste perception, nausea, spontaneous bowel perforation

Genitourinary: Priapism, uterine rupture

Hematologic: Thrombocytopenia

Neuromuscular & skeletal: Chorea (extrapyramidal), fasciculations, paresthesia, tremor

Ocular: Chemosis, iritis, Mydriasis (peak effect at 45 minutes; may last up to 12 hours), sloughing of the corneal epithelium, ulceration of the cornea

Renal: Myoglobinuria, necrotizing vasculitis

Respiratory: Bronchiolitis obliterans organizing pneumonia, hyposmia, nasal congestion, nasal mucosa damage (when snorting), rhinitis, tachypnea

Miscellaneous: Loss of smell, "washed-out" syndrome

Drug Interactions

Metabolism/Transport Effects Substrate of CYP3A4 (major); **Note:** Assignment of Major/Minor substrate status based on clinically relevant drug interaction potential; **Inhibits** CYP2D6 (strong), CYP3A4 (weak)

Avoid Concomitant Use

Avoid concomitant use of Cocaine with any of the following: Conivaptan; Fusidic Acid (Systemic); Iobenguane I 123; Pimozide; Tamoxifen; Thioridazine

Increased Effect/Toxicity

Cocaine may increase the levels/effects of: ARIPiprazole; AtoMOXetine; Cannabinoid-Containing Products; CYP2D6 Substrates; Dofetilide; DOXOrubicin (Conventional); Fesoterodine; Iloperidone; Lomitapide; Metoprolol; Nebivolol; Pimozide; Propafenone; Sympathomimetics; Tetrabenazine; Thioridazine; Vortioxetine

The levels/effects of Cocaine may be increased by: Ceritinib; Conivaptan; CYP3A4 Inhibitors (Moderate); CYP3A4 Inhibitors (Strong); Dasatinib; Fusidic Acid (Systemic); Ivacaftor; Linezolid; Luliconazole; Mifepristone; Simeprevir; Stiripentol

Decreased Effect

Cocaine may decrease the levels/effects of: Codeine; Iloperidone; Iobenguane I 123; Tamoxifen; TraMADol

Stability Store at 20°C to 25°C (68°F to 77°F); do not freeze.

Mechanism of Action Ester local anesthetic blocks both the initiation and conduction of nerve impulses by decreasing the neuronal membrane's permeability to sodium ions, which results in inhibition of depolarization with resultant blockade of conduction; interferes with the uptake of norepinephrine by adrenergic nerve terminals producing vasoconstriction

Pharmacodynamics Following topical administration to mucosa:

Onset of action: Within 1 minute

Maximum effect: Within 5 minutes

Duration: ≥30 minutes, depending upon route and dosage administered.

Pharmacokinetics (Adult data unless noted)

Absorption: Well absorbed through mucous membranes; ~35% absorbed when applied intranasally with cottonoid pledget (Liao, 1999); absorption is limited by drug-induced vasoconstriction and enhanced by inflammation

Distribution: V_d: ~2 L/kg

Metabolism: Hepatic; major metabolites are ecgonine methyl ester and benzoyl ecgonine

Half-life: 75 minutes

Elimination: Primarily in urine as metabolites and unchanged drug (<10%); cocaine metabolites may appear in the urine of neonates for up to 5 days after birth due to maternal cocaine use shortly before birth

Dosing: Usual Children, Adolescents, and Adults: Topical:

Topical anesthetic: Concentrations of 1% to 4% are used; use lowest effective dose; consider reduced dosages in children, elderly and debilitated patients; dose depends on patient tolerance, anesthetic technique, vascularity of tissue, and area to be anesthetized. Solutions >4% are not recommended due to increased risk and severity of systemic toxicities; maximum total dose: Children: 1-2 mg/kg/dose; Adolescents and Adults: 2-3 mg/kg **or** 200 mg, whichever is lower (Liao, 1999: McGee, 2010).

Administration Topical: Use only on mucous membranes of the oral, laryngeal, and nasal cavities; do not use on extensive areas of broken skin; do not apply commercially available products to the eye

Monitoring Parameters Heart rate, blood pressure, respiratory rate, temperature

Controlled Substance C-II

Dosage Forms Excipient information presented when available (limited, particularly for generics); consult specific product labeling.

Solution, External, as hydrochloride:

Generic: 4% (4 mL, 10 mL); 10% (4 mL)

References

Chasnoff IJ, Lewis DE, and Squires L, "Cocaine Intoxication in Breast-Fed Infants," *Pediatrics*, 1987, 80(6):836-8.

Fajemirokun-Odudeyi O and Lindow SW, "Obstetric Implications of Cocaine Use in Pregnancy: A Literature Review," *Eur J Obstet Gynecol Reprod Biol*, 2004, 112(1):2-8.

Greenglass EJ, "The Adverse Effects of Cocaine on the Developing Human," Yaffe SJ and Arana JV, eds, *Pediatric Pharmacology: Therapeutic Principles in Practice*, 2nd ed, Philadelphia, PA: WB Saunders Co, 1992, 598-604.

Liao BS, Hilsinger RL Jr, Rasgon BM, et al, "A Preliminary Study of Cocaine Absorption From the Nasal Mucosa," *Laryngoscope*, 1999, 109(1):98-102.

McGhee DL, "Local and Topical Anesthesia," Roberts JR and Hedges JR, eds, Clinical Procedures in Emergency Medicine, Philadelphia, PA: WB Saunders Co, 2010, 481-498.

Rezvani M and Hartfield D, "Cocaine Toxicity After Laryngoscopy in an Infant," *Can J Clin Pharmacol*, 2006, 13(2):e232-5.

◆ **Cocaine Hydrochloride** *see* Cocaine *on page* 533

◆ **CO Candesartan (Can)** *see* Candesartan *on page* 363

◆ **CO Ciprofloxacin (Can)** *see* Ciprofloxacin (Systemic) *on page* 471

◆ **CO Citalopram (Can)** *see* Citalopram *on page* 484

◆ **CO Clomipramine (Can)** *see* ClomiPRAMINE *on page* 510

◆ **CO Clonazepam (Can)** *see* ClonazePAM *on page* 514

◆ **CO Clopidogrel (Can)** *see* Clopidogrel *on page* 521

◆ **Codar GF** *see* Guaifenesin and Codeine *on page* 985

Codeine (KOE deen)

Medication Safety Issues

Sound-alike/look-alike issues:

Codeine may be confused with Cardene, Cordran, iodine, Lodine

High alert medication:

The Institute for Safe Medication Practices (ISMP) includes this medication among its list of drug classes which have a heightened risk of causing significant patient harm when used in error.

Related Information

Medications for Which a Single Dose May Be Fatal When Ingested by a Toddler *on page* 2408

Opioid Conversion Table *on page* 2242

Brand Names: Canada Codeine Contin; PMS-Codeine; ratio-Codeine

Therapeutic Category Analgesic, Narcotic; Antitussive; Cough Preparation

Generic Availability (U.S.) Yes

Use Treatment of mild to moderate pain where the use of an opioid is appropriate (FDA approved in adults)

Medication Guide Available Yes

Pregnancy Risk Factor C

Pregnancy Considerations Adverse events have been observed in animal reproduction studies. Opioid analgesics cross the placenta. In humans, birth defects (including some heart defects) have been associated with maternal use of codeine during the first trimester of pregnancy (Broussard, 2011). If chronic opioid exposure occurs in pregnancy, adverse events in the newborn (including withdrawal) may occur; monitoring of the neonate is recommended (Chou, 2009). The minimum effective dose should be used if opioids are needed (Chou, 2009). Neonatal abstinence syndrome following opioid exposure may present with autonomic (eg, fever, temperature instability), gastrointestinal (eg, diarrhea, vomiting, poor feeding/weight gain), or neurologic (eg, high pitched crying, increased muscle tone, irritability, seizure, tremor) symptoms (Dow, 2012; Hudak, 2012).

Breast-Feeding Considerations Codeine and its metabolite (morphine) are found in breast milk and can be detected in the serum of nursing infants. The relative dose to a nursing infant has been calculated to be ~1% of the weight-adjusted maternal dose (Spigset, 2000). Higher levels of morphine may be found in the breast milk of lactating mothers who are "ultrarapid metabolizers" of codeine; patients with two or more copies of the variant

CYP2D6*2 allele may have extensive conversion to morphine and thus increased opioid-mediated effects. In one case, excessively high serum concentrations of morphine were reported in a breast-fed infant following maternal use of acetaminophen with codeine. The mother was later found to be an "ultrarapid metabolizer" of codeine; symptoms in the infant included feeding difficulty and lethargy, followed by death. Caution should be used since most persons are not aware if they have the genotype resulting in "ultra-rapid metabolizer" status. When codeine is used in breast-feeding women, it is recommended to use the lowest dose for the shortest duration of time and observe the infant for increased sleepiness, difficulty in feeding or breathing, or limpness (FDA, 2007; Koren, 2006). The manufacturer recommends that caution be used if administered to a nursing woman. According to other guidelines, when treatment is needed for pain in nursing women, other agents should be used; if codeine cannot be avoided it should not be used for >4 days (Kahan, 2011; Wong, 2011).

Contraindications Hypersensitivity to codeine or any component; respiratory depression in the absence of resuscitative equipment; acute or severe bronchial asthma or hypercarbia; presence or suspicion of paralytic ileus; postoperative pain management in pediatric patients who have undergone tonsillectomy and/or adenoidectomy

Warnings Respiratory depression and death have occurred in children who received codeine following tonsillectomy and/or adenoidectomy and were found to have evidence of being ultrarapid metabolizers of codeine due to a CYP2D6 polymorphism **[U.S. Boxed Warning]**; patients with this phenotype may have extensive conversion of codeine to morphine with resultant increased serum morphine concentrations; this may result in increased opioid-mediated effects and possible life-threatening respiratory depression or signs of overdose (eg, extreme sleepiness, confusion, shallow breathing) at usual therapeutic doses of codeine; codeine is contraindicated in the postoperative pain management of children who have undergone tonsillectomy and/or adenoidectomy. Deaths have also occurred in nursing infants after being exposed to high concentrations of morphine because the mothers were ultrarapid metabolizers of codeine. Ultrarapid metabolizers of codeine [ie, patients with more than two copies of functional alleles (CYP2D6 genotype with gene duplications denoted as *1/*1xN or *1/*2xN)] are at increased risk of opioid toxicity; avoid the use of codeine in these patients; consider alternative analgesics such as morphine or a nonopioid agent (Crews, 2012). The observed occurrence of the CYP2D6 "ultrarapid" phenotype is: North Africans, Ethiopians, and Arabs: 16% to 28%; African-Americans: 3%; Caucasians: 1% to 10%; Hispanics: 0.5% to 1%; and Chinese and Japanese: 0.5% to 1%. Codeine should be prescribed in all patients in the lowest effective dose and for the shortest period of time; patients and caregivers should be informed about risks and signs of morphine overdose. Due to the incidence of serious side effects and fatalities associated with codeine use in children, Health Canada is no longer recommending codeine use in any child <12 years of age.

May cause CNS depression, which may impair physical or mental abilities; patients must be cautioned about performing tasks which require mental alertness (eg, operating machinery or driving). Effects may be potentiated when used with other sedative drugs including ethanol. Respiratory depression may occur even at therapeutic dosages; use with extreme caution in patients with respiratory diseases including asthma, emphysema, COPD, cor pulmonale, hypoxia, hypercapnia, preexisting respiratory depression, significantly decreased respiratory reserve, other obstructive pulmonary disease, kyphoscoliosis, or other skeletal disorder which may alter respiratory function.

Use with extreme caution in patients with head injury, intracranial lesions, or elevated intracranial pressure; exaggerated elevation of ICP may occur. May cause hypotension; use with caution in patients with circulatory shock, hypovolemia, impaired myocardial function, or those receiving drugs which may exaggerate hypotensive effects (including phenothiazines or general anesthetics). Codeine may obscure diagnosis or clinical course of patients with acute abdominal conditions.

Physical and psychological dependence may occur. Healthcare provider should be alert to problems of abuse, misuse, and diversion. Abrupt discontinuation after prolonged use may result in withdrawal symptoms or seizures. Concurrent use of agonist/antagonist analgesics may precipitate withdrawal symptoms and/or reduce analgesic efficacy in patients following prolonged therapy with mu opioid agonists. Infants born to women physically dependent on opioids will also be physically dependent and may experience respiratory difficulties or opioid withdrawal symptoms [neonatal abstinence syndrome (NAS)]. Onset, duration and severity of NAS depend upon the drug used (maternal), duration of use, maternal dose, and rate of drug elimination by the newborn. Symptoms of opioid withdrawal may include excessive crying, diarrhea, fever, hyper-reflexia, irritability, tremors, vomiting, or failure to gain weight. Opioid withdrawal syndrome in the neonate, unlike in adults, may be life-threatening and should be promptly treated. Some preparations contain sulfites which may cause allergic reactions in susceptible individuals.

Precautions Use with caution in patients with hypersensitivity reactions to other phenanthrene derivative opioid agonists (morphine, hydrocodone, hydromorphone, levorphanol, oxycodone, oxymorphone), adrenal insufficiency, biliary tract impairment, CNS depression/coma, morbid obesity, prostatic hyperplasia, urinary stricture, thyroid dysfunction, or severe liver or renal insufficiency.

Not recommended for use for cough control in patients with a productive cough; not recommended as an antitussive for children <2 years of age. Debilitated patients may be particularly susceptible to adverse effects of opioids.

Adverse Reactions

Cardiovascular: Bradycardia, cardiac arrest, circulatory depression, flushing, hyper-/hypotension, palpitation, shock, syncope, tachycardia

Central nervous system: Abnormal dreams, agitation, anxiety, apprehension, chills, coordination impaired, depression, disorientation, dizziness, drowsiness, dysphoria, euphoria, faintness, fatigue, hallucinations, headache, insomnia, intracranial pressure increased, lightheadedness, nervousness, sedation, shakiness, somnolence, vertigo

Dermatologic: Pruritus, rash, urticaria

Gastrointestinal: Abdominal cramps/pain, anorexia, biliary tract spasm, constipation, diarrhea, nausea, pancreatitis, taste disturbance, vomiting, xerostomia

Genitourinary: Urinary hesitancy/retention

Neuromuscular & skeletal: Paresthesia, rigidity, tremor, weakness

Ocular: Blurred vision, diplopia, miosis, nystagmus, visual disturbances

Respiratory: Bronchospasm, dyspnea, laryngospasm, respiratory arrest, respiratory depression

Miscellaneous: Allergic reaction, diaphoresis

Drug Interactions

Metabolism/Transport Effects Substrate of CYP2D6 (major); **Note:** Assignment of Major/Minor substrate status based on clinically relevant drug interaction potential

Avoid Concomitant Use

Avoid concomitant use of Codeine with any of the following: Azelastine (Nasal); Paraldehyde; Thalidomide

Increased Effect/Toxicity

Codeine may increase the levels/effects of: Alcohol (Ethyl); Alvimopan; Azelastine (Nasal); Buprenorphine; CNS Depressants; Desmopressin; Diuretics; Hydrocodone; Methotrimeprazine; Metyrosine; Mirtazapine; Paraldehyde; Pramipexole; ROPINIRole; Rotigotine; Selective Serotonin Reuptake Inhibitors; Thalidomide; Zolpidem

The levels/effects of Codeine may be increased by: Amphetamines; Anticholinergic Agents; Antipsychotic Agents (Phenothiazines); Brimonidine (Topical); Cannabis; Doxylamine; Dronabinol; Droperidol; HydrOXYzine; Kava Kava; Magnesium Sulfate; Methotrimeprazine; Nabilone; Perampanel; Rufinamide; Sodium Oxybate; Somatostatin Analogs; Succinylcholine; Tapentadol; Tetrahydrocannabinol

Decreased Effect

Codeine may decrease the levels/effects of: Pegvisomant

The levels/effects of Codeine may be decreased by: Ammonium Chloride; CYP2D6 Inhibitors (Moderate); CYP2D6 Inhibitors (Strong); Mixed Agonist / Antagonist Opioids; Naltrexone

Stability Oral solution, tablet: Store at controlled room temperature. Protect from light and moisture; dispense in tightly closed container.

Mechanism of Action Binds to opioid receptors in the CNS, causing inhibition of ascending pain pathways, altering the perception of and response to pain; causes cough suppression by direct central action in the medulla; produces generalized CNS depression

Pharmacodynamics

Onset of action: Oral: 30-60 minutes
Maximum effect: Oral: 60-90 minutes
Duration: 4-6 hours

Pharmacokinetics (Adult data unless noted)

Absorption: Oral: Adequate
Distribution: 3-6 L/kg
Protein binding: 7% to 25%
Metabolism: Hepatic via UGT2B7 and UGT2B4 to codeine-6-glucuronide, via CYP2D6 to morphine (active), and via CYP3A4 to norcodeine. Morphine is further metabolized via glucuronidation to morphine-3-glucuronide and morphine-6-glucuronide (active).
Bioavailability: 53%
Time to peak serum concentration: 1 hour
Half-life: 2.5-3.5 hours
Elimination: Urine (~90%, ~10% of the total dose as unchanged drug); feces

Dosing: Usual Doses should be titrated to appropriate analgesic effect; use the lowest effective dose for the shortest period of time:

Children and Adolescents: **Pain management; analgesia:** Limited data available: Oral: 0.5-1 mg/kg/dose every 4-6 hours as needed; maximum single dose: 60 mg (APS, 2008); **Note:** Do not use for postoperative tonsillectomy and/or adenoidectomy pain management.

Adults: **Pain management (analgesic):** Oral: Initial: 15-60 mg every 4 hours as needed; maximum total daily dose: 360 mg/**day**; patients with prior opioid exposure may require higher initial doses. **Note:** The American Pain Society recommends an initial dose of 30-60 mg for adults with moderate pain (American Pain Society, 2008).

Dosing adjustment in renal impairment:
Manufacturer's recommendations: Adults: There are no specific dosage adjustments provided in the manufacturer's labeling; however, clearance may be reduced; active metabolites may accumulate. Use with caution; initiate at lower doses or longer dosing intervals followed by careful titration.

Alternate recommendations: The following guidelines have been used by some clinicians (Aronoff, 2007):
Children and Adolescents:
GFR >50 mL/minute/1.73 m^2: No adjustment needed
GFR 10-50 mL/minute/1.73 m^2: Administer 75% of normal dose
GFR <10 mL/minute/1.73 m^2: Administer 50% of normal dose
Hemodialysis: Administer 50% of normal dose
Peritoneal dialysis (PD): Administer 50% of normal dose
CRRT: Administer 75% of normal dose
Adults:
CrCl >50 mL/minute: No adjustment needed
CrCl 10-50 mL/minute: Administer 75% of dose
CrCl <10 mL/minute: Administer 50% of dose

Dosing adjustment in hepatic impairment: Adults: There are no dosage adjustments provided in manufacturer's labeling (has not been studied); however, initial lower doses or longer dosing intervals followed by careful titration are recommended.

Administration Oral: Administer with food or water to decrease nausea and GI upset

Monitoring Parameters Respiratory rate, heart rate, blood pressure, pain relief, CNS status

Test Interactions Some quinolones may produce a false-positive urine screening result for opioids using commercially-available immunoassay kits. This has been demonstrated most consistently for levofloxacin and ofloxacin, but other quinolones have shown cross-reactivity in certain assay kits. Confirmation of positive opioid screens by more specific methods should be considered.

Controlled Substance C-II

Dosage Forms Excipient information presented when available (limited, particularly for generics); consult specific product labeling.

Solution, Oral, as sulfate:
Generic: 30 mg/5 mL (500 mL)
Tablet, Oral, as sulfate:
Generic: 15 mg, 30 mg, 60 mg

Extemporaneous Preparations A 3 mg/mL oral suspension may be made with codeine phosphate powder, USP. Add 600 mg of powder to a 400 mL beaker. Add 2.5 mL of Sterile Water for Irrigation, USP, and stir to dissolve the powder. Mix for 10 minutes while adding Ora-Sweet to make 200 mL; transfer to a calibrated bottle. Stable 98 days at room temperature.

Dentinger PJ and Swenson CF, "Stability of Codeine Phosphate in an Extemporaneously Compounded Syrup," *Am J Health Syst Pharm*, 2007, 64(24):2569-73.

References

Broussard CS, Rasmussen SA, Reefhuis J, et al, "Maternal Treatment With Opioid Analgesics and Risk for Birth Defects," *Am J Obstet Gynecol*, 2011, 204(4):314.e1-11.

Chou R, Fanciullo GJ, Fine PG, et al, "Clinical Guidelines For the Use of Chronic Opioid Therapy in Chronic Noncancer Pain," *J Pain*, 2009, 10 (2):113-30.

Crews KR, Gaedigk A, Dunnenberger HM, et al, "Clinical Pharmacogenetics Implementation Consortium (CPIC) Guidelines for Codeine Therapy in the Context of Cytochrome P450 2D6 (CYP2D6) Genotype," *Clin Pharmacol Ther*, 2012, 91(2):321-6.

Dow K, Ordean A, Murphy-Oikonen J, et al, "Neonatal Abstinence Syndrome Clinical Practice Guidelines For Ontario," *J Popul Ther Clin Pharmacol*, 2012, 19(3):e488-506.

Hudak ML, Tan RC, Committee On Drugs, et al, "Neonatal Drug Withdrawal," *Pediatrics*, 2012, 129(2):e540-60.

Kahan M, Wilson L, Mailis-Gagnon A, et al, "Canadian Guideline For Safe and Effective Use of Opioids For Chronic Noncancer Pain: Clinical Summary For Family Physicians. Part 2: Special Populations," *Can Fam Physician*, 2011, 57(11):1269-76, e419-28.

Khan K and Chang J, "Neonatal Abstinence Syndrome Due to Codeine," *Arch Dis Child Fetal Neonatal Ed*, 1997, 76(1):F59-60.

Koren G, Cairns J, Chitayat D, et al, "Pharmacogenetics of Morphine Poisoning in a Breastfed Neonate of a Codeine-Prescribed Mother," *Lancet*, 2006, 368(9536):704.

"Principles of Analgesic Use in the Treatment of Acute Pain and Cancer Pain," 6th ed, Glenview, IL: American Pain Society, 2008.

Reynolds EW, Riel-Romero RM, and Bada HS, "Neonatal Abstinence Syndrome and Cerebral Infarction Following Maternal Codeine Use During Pregnancy," *Clin Pediatr (Phila)*, 2007, 46(7):639-45.

Spigset O and Hägg S, "Analgesics and Breast-Feeding: Safety Considerations," *Paediatr Drugs*, 2000, 2(3):223-38.

U.S. Food and Drug Administration (FDA), Center for Drug Evaluation and Research, "FDA Public Health Advisory: Use of Codeine By Some Breastfeeding Mothers May Lead to Life-Threatening Side Effects in Nursing Babies," available at: http://www.fda.gov/cder/drug/advisory/codeine.htm.

Wong S, Ordean A, Kahan M, et al, "SOGC Clinical Practice Guidelines: Substance Use in Pregnancy: No. 256, April 2011," *Int J Gynaecol Obstet*, 2011, 114(2):190-202.

◆ **Codeine and Acetaminophen** see Acetaminophen and Codeine on page 53

◆ **Codeine and Guaifenesin** see Guaifenesin and Codeine on page 985

◆ **Codeine and Promethazine** see Promethazine and Codeine on page 1750

◆ **Codeine Contin (Can)** see Codeine on page 534

◆ **Codeine, Phenylephrine, and Promethazine** see Promethazine, Phenylephrine, and Codeine on page 1752

◆ **Codeine Phosphate** see Codeine on page 534

◆ **Codeine Sulfate** see Codeine on page 534

◆ **CO Diltiazem CD (Can)** see Diltiazem on page 667

◆ **CO Diltiazem T (Can)** see Diltiazem on page 667

◆ **Codulax [OTC] (Can)** see Bisacodyl on page 293

◆ **CO Enalapril (Can)** see Enalapril on page 744

◆ **Coenzyme R** see Biotin on page 292

◆ **Co-Etidronate (Can)** see Etidronate on page 810

◆ **CO Famciclovir (Can)** see Famciclovir on page 842

◆ **CO Fluconazole (Can)** see Fluconazole on page 877

◆ **CO Fluoxetine (Can)** see FLUoxetine on page 901

◆ **CO Fluvoxamine (Can)** see FluvoxaMINE on page 922

◆ **CO Gabapentin (Can)** see Gabapentin on page 950

◆ **Cogentin** see Benztropine on page 276

◆ **CO Irbesartan (Can)** see Irbesartan on page 1147

◆ **Colace [OTC]** see Docusate on page 701

◆ **Colazal** see Balsalazide on page 261

Colchicine (KOL chi seen)

Medication Safety Issues
Sound-alike/look-alike issues:
Colchicine may be confused with Cortrosyn
Related Information
Safe Handling of Hazardous Drugs on page 2419
Brand Names: U.S. Colcrys
Brand Names: Canada Jamp-Colchicine; PMS-Colchicine
Therapeutic Category Anti-inflammatory Agent; Antigout Agent
Generic Availability (U.S.) No
Use Treatment of familial Mediterranean fever (FMF) (FDA approved in ages ≥4 years and adults); prevention and treatment of acute gout flares (FDA approved in ages >16 years and adults); has also been used for prophylaxis of pseudogout, management of Behçet's disease
Medication Guide Available Yes
Pregnancy Risk Factor C
Pregnancy Considerations Adverse events were observed in animal reproduction studies. Colchicine crosses the human placenta. Use during pregnancy in the treatment of familial Mediterranean fever has not shown an increase in miscarriage, stillbirth, or teratogenic effects (limited data).
Breast-Feeding Considerations Colchicine enters breast milk; exclusively breast-fed infants are expected to receive <10% of the weight-adjusted maternal dose (limited data). The manufacturer recommends that caution be used if administered to a nursing woman.

Contraindications Hypersensitivity to colchicine or any component; fatal toxicity has been reported with concomitant use of colchicine with a P-glycoprotein (P-gp) inhibitor (eg, cyclosporine, ranolazine) or strong CYP3A4 inhibitor (eg, atazanavir, clarithromycin, indinavir, itraconazole, ketoconazole, nefazodone, nelfinavir, ritonavir, saquinavir, telithromycin) in presence of renal or hepatic impairment; concurrent use of colchicine and P-gp or strong CYP3A4 inhibitors is contraindicated in renal or hepatic impairment

Warnings Hazardous agent; use appropriate precautions for handling and disposal (NIOSH, 2012). Patients who become pregnant while receiving colchicine therapy may be at greater risk of producing trisomic offspring. Myelosuppression (eg, thrombocytopenia, leukopenia, granulocytopenia, pancytopenia) and aplastic anemia have been reported in patients receiving therapeutic doses. Myotoxicity (including rhabdomyolysis) has been reported in patients receiving therapeutic doses. Patients with renal dysfunction and elderly patients are at increased risk. Concomitant use of cyclosporine, diltiazem, verapamil, fibrates, and statins may increase the risk of myopathy.

Precautions Use with caution and consider dose modification if colchicine is given with a P-gp or strong CYP3A4 inhibitor in patients with normal renal and hepatic function.

Adverse Reactions
Central nervous system: Fatigue, headache
Endocrine & metabolic: Gout
Gastrointestinal: Abdominal cramps, abdominal pain, diarrhea, gastrointestinal disease, nausea, vomiting
Respiratory: Pharyngolaryngeal pain
Rare but important or life-threatening: Alopecia, aplastic anemia, azoospermia, bone marrow depression, generalized dermatosis, granulocytopenia, hepatotoxicity, hypersensitivity reaction, increased creatine phosphokinase, increased serum ALT, increased serum AST, lactose intolerance, leukopenia, maculopapular rash, myalgia, myasthenia, myopathy, myotonia, neuropathy, oligospermia, pancytopenia, peripheral neuritis, purpura, rhabdomyolysis, skin rash, thrombocytopenia

Drug Interactions
Metabolism/Transport Effects Substrate of CYP3A4 (major), P-glycoprotein; **Note:** Assignment of Major/Minor substrate status based on clinically relevant drug interaction potential; **Induces** CYP2C9 (weak/moderate), CYP2E1 (weak/moderate), CYP3A4 (weak/moderate)

Avoid Concomitant Use
Avoid concomitant use of Colchicine with any of the following: Axitinib; Conivaptan; Fusidic Acid (Systemic); Simeprevir

Increased Effect/Toxicity
Colchicine may increase the levels/effects of: HMG-CoA Reductase Inhibitors

The levels/effects of Colchicine may be increased by: Cobicistat; Conivaptan; CYP3A4 Inhibitors (Moderate); CYP3A4 Inhibitors (Strong); Dasatinib; Digoxin; Fibric Acid Derivatives; Fosamprenavir; Fusidic Acid (Systemic); Luliconazole; Mifepristone; P-glycoprotein/ABCB1 Inhibitors; Stiripentol; Telaprevir; Tipranavir

Decreased Effect
Colchicine may decrease the levels/effects of: ARIPiprazole; Axitinib; Cyanocobalamin; Ibrutinib; Multivitamins/Fluoride (with ADE); Multivitamins/Minerals (with ADEK, Folate, Iron); Multivitamins/Minerals (with AE, No Iron); Saxagliptin; Simeprevir

The levels/effects of Colchicine may be decreased by: P-glycoprotein/ABCB1 Inducers

Food Interactions Grapefruit juice may increase colchicine serum concentrations. Management: Administer orally ▶

with water and maintain adequate fluid intake. Dose adjustment may be required based on indication if ingesting grapefruit juice. Avoid grapefruit juice with hepatic or renal impairment.

Stability Hazardous agent; use appropriate precautions for handling and disposal (NIOSH, 2012). Store at controlled room temperature; protect from light.

Mechanism of Action Disrupts cytoskeletal functions by inhibiting β-tubulin polymerization into microtubules, preventing activation, degranulation, and migration of neutrophils associated with mediating some gout symptoms. In familial Mediterranean fever, may interfere with intracellular assembly of the inflammasome complex present in neutrophils and monocytes that mediate activation of interleukin-1β.

Pharmacodynamics Onset of action: Oral: Relief of pain and inflammation occurs after 18-24 hours

Pharmacokinetics (Adult data unless noted)
Bioavailability: <50%
Distribution: Concentrates in leukocytes, kidney, spleen, and liver; distributes into breast milk; crosses the placenta; does not distribute in heart, skeletal muscle, and brain; V_d: 5-8 L/kg
Protein binding: 39%
Metabolism: Hepatic via CYP3A4; three metabolites (2 primary, 1 minor); partially deacetylated and demethylated
Half-life, elimination: 27-31 hours
Time to peak serum concentration: Oral: 1-2 hours (range: 0.5-3 hours)
Excretion: Urine (40% to 65% as unchanged drug), enterohepatic recirculation and biliary excretion also possible
Dialysis: Not dialyzable (0% to 5%)

Dosing: Usual Oral:
Prophylaxis of familial Mediterranean fever (FMF):
Children:
4-6 years: 0.3-1.8 mg/day in 1-2 divided doses
6-12 years: 0.9-1.8 mg/day in 1-2 divided doses
Adolescents >12 years and Adults: 1.2-2.4 mg/day in 1-2 divided doses; titration: Increase or decrease dose in 0.3 mg/day increments based on efficacy or adverse effects; maximum dose: 2.4 mg/day
Gout: Children >16 years and Adults:
Flare treatment: Initial: 1.2 mg at the first sign of flare, followed in 1 hour with a single dose of 0.6 mg (maximum dosing: 1.8 mg over 1 hour); **Note:** Current FDA approved dose for gout flare is substantially lower than what has been used historically. Doses larger than the currently recommended dosage for gout flare have not been proven to be more effective. **Note:** Patients receiving prophylaxis treatment may receive treatment dosing; wait 12 hours before resuming prophylactic dose
Prophylaxis: 0.6 mg once or twice daily; maximum dose: 1.2 mg/day

Dosage adjustment for concomitant therapy with CYP3A4 or P-gp inhibitors: Dosage adjustment also required in patients receiving CYP3A4 or P-gp inhibitors up to 14 days prior to initiation of colchicine. **Note:** Treatment of gout flare with colchicine is not recommended in patients receiving prophylactic colchicine and CYP3A4 inhibitors. **Note:** Dosage adjustments may also apply to patients 12-18 years of age with FMF.
Coadministration of **strong** CYP3A4 inhibitor (eg, atazanavir, clarithromycin, indinavir, itraconazole, ketoconazole, nefazodone, nelfinavir, ritonavir, saquinavir, telithromycin):
FMF: Maximum dose: 0.6 mg/day **or** 0.3 mg twice daily
Gout prophylaxis:
If original dose is 0.6 mg twice daily, adjust dose to 0.3 mg once daily
If original dose is 0.6 mg once daily, adjust dose to 0.3 mg every other day

Gout flare treatment: Initial: 0.6 mg, followed in 1 hour by a single dose of 0.3 mg; wait at least 3 days to repeat
Coadministration of **moderate** CYP3A4 inhibitor (eg, amprenavir, aprepitant, diltiazem, erythromycin, fluconazole, fosamprenavir, grapefruit juice, verapamil):
FMF: Maximum dose: 1.2 mg/day **or** 0.6 mg twice daily
Gout prophylaxis:
If original dose is 0.6 mg twice daily, adjust dose to 0.3 mg twice daily **or** 0.6 mg once daily
If original dose is 0.6 mg once daily, adjust dose to 0.3 mg once daily
Gout flare treatment: 1.2 mg as a single dose; wait at least 3 days to repeat days
Coadministration of P-gp inhibitor (eg, cyclosporine, ranolazine):
FMF: Maximum dose: 0.6 mg/day **or** 0.3 mg twice daily
Gout prophylaxis:
If original dose is 0.6 mg twice daily, adjust dose to 0.3 mg once daily
If original dose is 0.6 mg once daily, adjust dose to 0.3 mg every other day
Gout flare treatment: Initial: 0.6 mg as a single dose; wait at least 3 days to repeat

Dosing adjustment in renal impairment: Concurrent use of colchicine and P-gp or strong CYP3A4 inhibitors is **contraindicated** in renal impairment. Use of colchicine to treat gout flares is not recommended in patients with renal impairment receiving prophylatic colchicine.
Children (Kallinich, 2007):
Moderate impairment (CrCl 10-50 mL/minute): Consider dose reduction
Severe impairment (CrCl <10 mL/minute): Reduce dose by 50% or consider discontinuation of therapy; maximum dose: 1 mg/day
Adults:
FMF:
CrCl 30-80 mL/minute: Monitor closely for adverse effects; dose adjustment may be necessary
CrCl <30 mL/minute: Initial dose: 0.3 mg/day; use caution if dose titrated; monitor for adverse effects
Dialysis: Initial dose: 0.3 mg/day; dosing can be increased with close monitoring; monitor for adverse effects. Not removed by dialysis.
Gout prophylaxis:
CrCl 30-80 mL/minute: Dosage adjustment not required; monitor closely for adverse effects
CrCl <30 mL/minute: Initial dose: 0.3 mg/day; use caution if dose titrated; monitor for adverse effects
Dialysis: 0.3 mg twice weekly; monitor closely for adverse effects
Gout flare treatment:
CrCl 30-80 mL/minute: Dosage adjustment not required; monitor closely for adverse effects
CrCl <30 mL/minute: Dosage adjustment may be considered; treatment course should not be repeated more frequently than every 14 days
Dialysis: 0.6 mg as a single dose; wait at least 14 days to repeat

Administration Hazardous agent; use appropriate precautions for handling and disposal (NIOSH, 2012).
Oral: Administer without regard to meals and maintain adequate fluid intake

Monitoring Parameters CBC with differential, urinalysis, and renal and hepatic function tests

Test Interactions May cause false-positive results in urine tests for erythrocytes or hemoglobin

Dosage Forms Excipient information presented when available (limited, particularly for generics); consult specific product labeling.
Tablet, Oral:
Colcrys: 0.6 mg [scored; contains fd&c blue #2 (indigotine), fd&c red #40]

References

Kallinich T, Haffner D, Niehues T, et al, "Colchicine Use in Children and Adolescents With Familial Mediterranean Fever: Literature Review and Consensus Statement," *Pediatrics*, 2007, 119(2):e474-83.

Levy M, Spino M, and Read SE, "Colchicine: A State-of-the-Art Review," *Pharmacotherapy*, 1991, 11(3):196-211.

Majeed HA, Carroll JE, Khuffash FA, et al, "Long-term Colchicine Prophylaxis in Children With Familial Mediterranean Fever (Recurrent Hereditary Polyserositis)," *J Pediatr*, 1990, 116(6):997-9.

National Institute for Occupational Safety and Health (NIOSH), "NIOSH List of Antineoplastic and Other Hazardous Drugs in Healthcare Settings 2012." Available at http://www.cdc.gov/niosh/docs/2012-150/pdfs/2012-150.pdf. Accessed January 21, 2013.

Terkeltaub RA, "Colchicine Update: 2008," *Semin Arthritis Rheum*, 2009, 38(6):411-9.

◆ **Colcrys** *see* Colchicine *on page 537*

Colesevelam (koh le SEV a lam)

Brand Names: U.S. Welchol
Brand Names: Canada Lodalis
Therapeutic Category Antilipemic Agent, Bile Acid Sequestrant
Generic Availability (U.S.) No
Use Management of heterozygous familial hypercholesterolemia if LDL-C remains ≥190 mg/dL, if ≥160 mg/dL with family history of premature cardiovascular disease, or presence of ≥2 cardiovascular risk factors in children and adolescent patients [FDA approved in ages 10-17 years (girls ≥1 year postmenarche)]; management of elevated LDL in primary hypercholesterolemia (Fredrickson type IIa) when used alone or in combination with an HMG-CoA reductase inhibitor (FDA approved in adults); improve glycemic control in type 2 diabetes mellitus (noninsulin dependent, NIDDM) in conjunction with diet, exercise, and insulin or oral antidiabetic agents (FDA approved in adults)

Pregnancy Risk Factor B
Pregnancy Considerations Adverse effects have not been observed in animal reproduction studies. Colesevelam is not absorbed systemically, but may interfere with vitamin absorption; therefore, regular supplementation may not be adequate.

Breast-Feeding Considerations Due to lack of systemic absorption, colesevelam is not expected to be excreted in breast milk; however, the tendency of colesevelam to interfere with the vitamin absorption may have an effect on the nursing infant.

Contraindications Hypersensitivity to bile acid sequestering resins or any component; history bowel obstruction; serum triglyceride concentration >500 mg/dL; history of hypertriglyceridemia-induced pancreatitis

Warnings Use in patients with gastroparesis, other severe GI motility disorders, or a history of major GI tract surgery is not recommended due to constipating effects of colesevelam. Patients with dysphagia or swallowing disorders should use the oral suspension form of colesevelam due to large tablet size and risk for esophageal obstruction. Avoid accidental inhalation or esophageal distress with colesevelam granules; always mix with other fluids prior to ingestion. May increase serum triglyceride concentrations (median increase 5% vs placebo in clinical trials); use caution if serum triglyceride levels are >300 mg/dL; discontinue if triglyceride concentrations exceed 500 mg/dL or hypertriglyceridemia-induced pancreatitis occurs. Granules for suspension contain phenylalanine (13.5 mg/1.875 g packet; 27 mg/3.75 g packet); avoid or use with caution in patients with phenylketonuria.

Precautions Use with caution in patients susceptible to fat-soluble vitamin deficiencies. Absorption of fat-soluble vitamins A, D, E, and K and folic acid may be decreased; patients should take vitamins ≥4 hours before colesevelam. Chronic use may be associated with bleeding problems due to hypoprothrombinemia, especially in high doses associated with vitamin K deficiency; may be prevented with use of oral vitamin K therapy. Some patients may also develop folate deficiency; supplementation with folic acid may be necessary. Secondary causes of hyperlipidemia should be ruled out prior to therapy; has not been studied in Fredrickson types I, III, IV, and V dyslipidemias.

May decrease absorption of many orally administered medications; avoid concomitant administration with other orally administered medications; separate administration of drug with known interaction by ≥4 hours. Colesevelam should not be used for glycemic control in type 1 diabetes mellitus or to treat diabetic ketoacidosis; also not indicated in type 2 diabetes mellitus as monotherapy or in combination with dipeptidyl peptidase 4 inhibitors or thiazolidinediones.

Adverse Reactions Unless otherwise noted, adverse effects are reported for adult patients.
Cardiovascular: Cardiovascular toxicity (including myocardial infarction, aortic stenosis, bradycardia), hypertension
Central nervous system: Fatigue (children), headache (children and adults)
Endocrine & metabolic: Hyperglycemia, hypertriglyceridemia, hypoglycemia
Gastrointestinal: Constipation, diarrhea, dyspepsia, gastroesophageal reflux disease, nausea (children and adults), periodontal abscess, vomiting (children)
Hematologic & oncologic: Change in serum protein (C-reactive protein increased)
Neuromuscular & skeletal: Back pain, increased creatine phosphokinase (children and adults), myalgia, weakness
Respiratory: Flu-like symptoms (children), nasopharyngitis (children), pharyngitis, rhinitis (children), upper respiratory tract infection (children and adults)
Rare but important or life-threatening: Dysphagia, esophageal obstruction, fecal impaction, hemorrhoids (exacerbation), increased serum transaminases, infection, intestinal obstruction, pancreatitis, unstable angina pectoris

Drug Interactions
Metabolism/Transport Effects None known.
Avoid Concomitant Use
Avoid concomitant use of Colesevelam with any of the following: Deferasirox; Mycophenolate
Increased Effect/Toxicity There are no known significant interactions involving an increase in effect.
Decreased Effect
Colesevelam may decrease the levels/effects of: Amiodarone; AtorvaSTATin; Chenodiol; Contraceptives (Estrogens); Contraceptives (Progestins); Corticosteroids (Oral); CycloSPORINE (Systemic); Deferasirox; Ethinyl Estradiol; Ezetimibe; Glimepiride; GlipiZIDE; GlyBURIDE; Leflunomide; Lomitapide; Loop Diuretics; Methotrexate; Multivitamins/Fluoride (with ADE); Multivitamins/Minerals (with ADEK, Folate, Iron); Multivitamins/Minerals (with AE, No Iron); Mycophenolate; Niacin; Nonsteroidal Anti-Inflammatory Agents; Norethindrone; Olmesartan; Phenytoin; Pravastatin; Propranolol; Raloxifene; Teriflunomide; Tetracycline Derivatives; Thiazide Diuretics; Thyroid Products; Ursodiol; Vancomycin; Vitamin D Analogs; Vitamin K Antagonists

Stability Store at 25°C (77°F); excursions permitted to 15°C to 30°C (59°F to 86°F). Protect from moisture.

Mechanism of Action Cholesterol is the major precursor of bile acid. Colesevelam binds with bile acids in the intestine to form an insoluble complex that is eliminated in feces. This increased excretion of bile acids results in an increased oxidation of cholesterol to bile acid and a lowering of the serum cholesterol.

Pharmacodynamics
Onset of action:
Lipid-lowering: Within 2 weeks (maximum effect)

Reduction HgA1C (Type II diabetes): 4-6 weeks initial onset, 12-18 weeks maximal effect

Pharmacokinetics (Adult data unless noted)

Absorption: Insignificant

Elimination: Urine (0.05%) after 1 month of chronic dosing

Dosing: Usual

Children and Adolescents: **Primary hyperlipidemia:** Children ≥10 years and Adolescents: Oral:

Once-daily dosing: 3.75 g (6 x 625 mg tablets or 1 packet)

Twice-daily dosing: 1.875 g (3 x 625 mg tablets)

Note: Due to large tablet size, oral suspension is recommended in pediatric patients. Do not administer granules in the dry form (to avoid GI distress).

Adults: **Dyslipidemia, type 2 diabetes (combination therapy with insulin or oral antidiabetic agents):** Oral:

Once-daily dosing: 3.75 g (oral suspension or 6 tablets)

Twice-daily dosing: 1.875 g (3 tablets)

Administration

Granules for oral suspension: Empty granules into glass; add 4-8 ounces of water, fruit juice or diet soft drink; mix well. Administer with meals. Do not take in dry form (to avoid GI distress).

Tablets: Due to tablet size, it is recommended that any patient who has trouble swallowing tablets should use the oral suspension form. Administer with meal(s) and a liquid.

Monitoring Parameters

Pediatric patients: Serum cholesterol and triglycerides (4 weeks after initiation, then every 3-4 months the first year of therapy, every 6 months with second year, and whenever clinically indicated); with prolonged use, prothrombin time, number of stools/day

Adults: Serum cholesterol, LDL, and triglyceride levels should be obtained before initiating treatment and periodically thereafter (in accordance with NCEP guidelines)

Test Interactions Increased prothrombin time

Dosage Forms Considerations

Welchol contains phenylalanine 27 mg per 3.75 gram packet

Dosage Forms Excipient information presented when available (limited, particularly for generics); consult specific product labeling:

Packet, Oral, as hydrochloride:

Welchol: 3.75 g (30 ea) [sugar free; contains aspartame]

Tablet, Oral, as hydrochloride:

Welchol: 625 mg

References

National Heart, Lung, and Blood Institute, "Expert Panel on Integrated Guidelines for Cardiovascular Health and Risk Reduction in Children and Adolescents," *Clinical Practice Guidelines*, 2011, National Institutes of Health. Available at http://www.nhlbi.nih.gov/guidelines/cvd_ped/peds_guidelines_full.pdf

Stein EA, Marais AD, Szamosi T, et al, "Colesevelam Hydrochloride: Efficacy and Safety in Pediatric Subjects With Heterozygous Familial Hypercholesterolemia," *J Pediatr*, 2010, 156(2):231-6.e1-3.

◆ **Colestid** see Colestipol *on page 540*

◆ **Colestid Flavored** see Colestipol *on page 540*

Colestipol (koe LES ti pole)

Medication Safety Issues

Sound-alike/look-alike issues:

Colestipol may be confused with calcitriol

Related Information

Oral Medications That Should Not Be Crushed or Altered *on page 2438*

Brand Names: U.S. Colestid; Colestid Flavored; Micronized Colestipol HCl

Brand Names: Canada Colestid

Therapeutic Category Antilipemic Agent, Bile Acid Sequestrant

Generic Availability (U.S.) Yes

Use Adjunct to dietary therapy to decrease elevated serum total and low density lipoprotein cholesterol (LDL-C) in primary hypercholesterolemia (FDA approved in adults)

Pregnancy Considerations Colestipol is not absorbed systemically (<0.17%), but may interfere with vitamin absorption; therefore, regular prenatal supplementation may not be adequate. There are no studies in pregnant women; use with caution.

Breast-Feeding Considerations Due to lack of systemic absorption (<0.17%), colestipol is not expected to be excreted into breast milk; however, the tendency of colestipol to interfere with vitamin absorption may have an effect on the nursing infant.

Contraindications Hypersensitivity to bile acid sequestering resins or any component

Warnings Colestid® Flavored formulations may contain phenylalanine (~18.2 mg/5 g of colestipol); avoid use or use with caution in patients with phenylketonuria. Avoid accidental inhalation or esophageal distress with colestipol powder and granules; always mix with other fluids prior to ingestion.

Precautions Use with caution in patients with constipation or recent abdominal surgery; may produce or exacerbate constipation problems; initiate therapy at a reduced dose in patients with a history of constipation; ensure adequate fluid and possible fiber intake; hemorrhoids may be worsened.

Use with caution in patients susceptible to fat soluble vitamin deficiencies. Absorption of fat soluble vitamins A, D, E, and K and folic acid may be decreased; patients should take vitamins ≥4 hours before cholestyramine. Chronic use may be associated with bleeding problems due to hypoprothrombinemia especially in high doses associated with vitamin K deficiency; may be prevented with use of oral vitamin K therapy. Some patients may also develop folate deficiency; supplementation with folic acid may be necessary.

Use caution in patients with renal impairment or volume depletion or receiving concurrent spironolactone therapy; with prolonged use, may potentially cause hypochoremic acidosis; risk may be higher in younger and smaller patients. May decrease absorption of other orally administered drugs; avoid taking colestipol simultaneously with many other medicines; ideally other medications should be taken 1 hour before or 4-6 hours after colestipol dose. May raise serum triglyceride concentrations; in a trial of combination therapy of colestipol and pravastatin in children and adolescents (>8 years of age); the serum triglycerides increased by 12% from baseline (McCrindle, 2002).

Adverse Reactions

Cardiovascular: Angina, chest pain, edema of hands or feet, tachycardia

Central nervous system: Dizziness, fatigue, headache (including migraine and sinus), lightheadedness, insomnia

Dermatologic: Dermatitis, rash, urticaria

Gastrointestinal: Abdominal pain and cramping, anorexia, bloating, constipation, cholecystitis, cholelithiasis, diarrhea, dysphagia, esophageal obstruction, flatulence, indigestion, heartburn, hemorrhoids (bleeding), nausea, peptic ulceration, vomiting

Hepatic: Alkaline phosphatase increased, ALT increased, AST increased

Neuromuscular & skeletal: Arthritis, backache, joint/muscle pain, weakness

Respiratory: Dyspnea

Drug Interactions

Metabolism/Transport Effects None known.

Avoid Concomitant Use

Avoid concomitant use of Colestipol with any of the following: Deferasirox; Mycophenolate

Increased Effect/Toxicity There are no known significant interactions involving an increase in effect.

Decreased Effect

Colestipol may decrease the levels/effects of: Amiodarone; AtorvaSTATin; Cardiac Glycosides; Chenodiol; Contraceptives (Estrogens); Contraceptives (Progestins); Corticosteroids (Oral); Deferasirox; Diltiazem; Ezetimibe; Fibric Acid Derivatives; Leflunomide; Lomitapide; Loop Diuretics; Methotrexate; Methylfolate; Multivitamins/Fluoride (with ADE); Multivitamins/Minerals (with ADEK, Folate, Iron); Multivitamins/Minerals (with AE, No Iron); Mycophenolate; Niacin; Nonsteroidal Anti-Inflammatory Agents; Pravastatin; Propranolol; Raloxifene; Teriflunomide; Tetracycline Derivatives; Thiazide Diuretics; Thyroid Products; Ursodiol; Vancomycin; Vitamin D Analogs; Vitamin K Antagonists

Stability Store at 20°C to 25°C (68°F to 77°F).

Mechanism of Action Binds with bile acids to form an insoluble complex that is eliminated in feces; it thereby increases the fecal loss of bile acid-bound low density lipoprotein cholesterol

Pharmacodynamics

Lowering of serum cholesterol: ~1 month
LDL-C reduction: ~19%

Pharmacokinetics (Adult data unless noted)

Absorption: None
Elimination: Feces

Dosing: Usual

Children and Adolescents: **Dyslipidemia:** Limited data available: Oral: Children >8 years and Adolescents: 2-12 g/day; the most recent study produced significant lowering of serum cholesterol utilizing either 10 g once daily or 5 g twice daily (McCrindle, 2002; Tonstad, 1996)

Adults: **Dyslipidemia:** Oral:
Granules: Initial: 5 g 1-2 times/day; maintenance: 5-30 g/day given once or in divided doses; increase by 5 g/day at 1- to 2-month intervals
Tablets: Initial: 2 g 1-2 times/day; maintenance: 2-16 g/day given once or in divided doses; increase by 2 g once or twice daily at 1- to 2-month intervals

Administration Oral: Other drugs should be administered at least 1 hour before or 4 hours after colestipol.

Granules: Do not administer in dry form (to avoid GI distress). Dry powder or granules should be added to at least 3 ounces (90 mL) of liquid and stirred until completely mixed. After administration, rinse glass with a small amount of liquid to ensure all medication is taken.

Tablets: Administer tablets one at a time, swallowed whole, with plenty of liquid. Do not cut, crush, or chew tablets.

Monitoring Parameters Serum cholesterol and triglycerides (4 weeks after initiation, then every 3-4 months the first year of therapy, every 6 months with second year, and whenever clinically indicated); with prolonged use, prothrombin time, electrolytes; number of stools/day

Test Interactions Increased prothrombin time

Dosage Forms Considerations

Colestid tablets contain micronized colestipol. Generic tablets are available in micronized and non-micronized formulations.

Dosage Forms Excipient information presented when available (limited, particularly for generics); consult specific product labeling.

Granules, Oral, as hydrochloride:
Colestid: 5 g (300 g, 500 g) [unflavored flavor]
Colestid Flavored: 5 g (450 g) [contains aspartame; orange flavor]
Generic: 5 g (500 g)
Packet, Oral, as hydrochloride:
Colestid: 5 g (30 ea, 90 ea) [unflavored flavor]
Colestid Flavored: 5 g (60 ea) [contains aspartame; orange flavor]
Generic: 5 g (30 ea, 90 ea)
Tablet, Oral, as hydrochloride:
Colestid: 1 g
Micronized Colestipol HCl: 1 g
Generic: 1 g

References

McCrindle BW, Helden E, Cullen-Dean G, et al, "A Randomized Crossover Trial of Combination Pharmacologic Therapy in Children With Familial Hyperlipidemia," *Pediatr Res*, 2002, 51(6):715-21.

McCrindle BW, Urbina EM, Dennison BA, et al, "Drug Therapy of High-Risk Lipid Abnormalities in Children and Adolescents: A Scientific Statement from the American Heart Association Atherosclerosis, Hypertension, and Obesity in Youth Committee, Council of Cardiovascular Disease in the Young, With the Council on Cardiovascular Nursing," *Circulation*, 2007, 115(14):1948-67.

National Heart, Lung, and Blood Institute, "Expert Panel on Integrated Guidelines for Cardiovascular Health and Risk Reduction in Children and Adolescents," Clinical Practice Guidelines, 2011, National Institutes of Health. Available at http://www.nhlbi.nih.gov/guidelines/cvd_ped/peds_guidelines_full.pdf

Tonstad S and Ose L, "Colestipol Tablets in Adolescents With Familial Hypercholesterolaemia," *Acta Paediatr*, 1996, 85(9):1080-2.

Tonstad S, Sivertsen M, Aksnes L, et al, "Low Dose Colestipol in Adolescents With Familial Hypercholesterolaemia," *Arch Dis Child*, 1996, 74(2):157-60.

◆ **Colestipol Hydrochloride** *see* Colestipol *on page 540*

◆ **CO Levetiracetam (Can)** *see* LevETIRAcetam *on page 1219*

◆ **CO Levofloxacin (Can)** *see* Levofloxacin (Systemic) *on page 1228*

◆ **CO Lisinopril (Can)** *see* Lisinopril *on page 1262*

Colistimethate (koe lis ti METH ate)

Medication Safety Issues

Other safety concerns:
Due to the potential for dosing errors, it is recommended that prescriptions for colistimethate be expressed as colistin base only.

Brand Names: U.S. Coly-Mycin M

Brand Names: Canada Coly-Mycin M

Therapeutic Category Antibiotic, Miscellaneous

Generic Availability (U.S.) Yes

Use Treatment of acute or chronic infections due to sensitive strains of certain gram-negative bacilli (particularly *Pseudomonas aeruginosa*) which are resistant to other antibacterials (FDA approved in all ages); has also been used as inhalation therapy to treat multidrug-resistant gram-negative pneumonia and in cystic fibrosis; intrathecal/intraventricular therapy to treat multidrug resistant gram-negative meningitis

Pregnancy Risk Factor C

Pregnancy Considerations Adverse events have been observed in animal reproduction studies. Colistimethate crosses the placenta in humans.

Breast-Feeding Considerations Colistin (the active form of colistimethate sodium) and colistin sulphate (another form of colistin) are excreted in human milk. The manufacturer recommends caution if giving colistimethate sodium to a breast-feeding woman. Nondose-related effects could include modification of bowel flora.

Contraindications Hypersensitivity to colistimethate or any component

Warnings Colistimethate, an inactive prodrug, is converted to the bioactive colistin by spontaneous hydrolysis once colistimethate is mixed into aqueous solution. Potential for dosing errors exist due to lack of standardization when referring to product and dose; colistimethate (inactive prodrug) and colistin base strengths are not interchangeable; prior to dispensing verify which terms (colistimethate or colistin base) the prescribed dose is expressed.

Manufacturer recommends a maximum **colistin base** dose of 5 mg/kg/**day** in patients with normal renal function.

Use only to prevent or treat infections strongly suspected or proven to be caused by susceptible bacteria to minimize development of bacterial drug-resistance; reserve use for life-threatening infections caused by organisms resistant to the preferred drugs. Colistimethate can cause serious nephrotoxicity and/or neurotoxicity. Neurotoxic reactions may be manifested by circumoral paresthesia, numbness, tingling of the extremities, pruritus, vertigo, dizziness, and slurring of speech; patients must be cautioned about performing tasks which require mental alertness (eg, operating machinery or driving); dosage reduction may alleviate symptoms. Nephrotoxicity is dose-dependent and reversible upon discontinuation and has been observed to occur within the first 4 days of therapy in patients with cystic fibrosis (Bosso, 1991). Avoid concurrent or sequential use of other nephrotoxic and neurotoxic drugs, particularly bacitracin, kanamycin, streptomycin, paromomycin, polymyxin B, tobramycin, neomycin, gentamicin, and amikacin. Neuromuscular blockade resulting in respiratory arrest has been reported in patients with neuromuscular disease (ie, myasthenia gravis) and patients receiving neuromuscular blocking agents; impaired renal function increases the possibility of apnea and neuromuscular blockade. Prolonged use may result in fungal or bacterial superinfection, including *C. difficile*-associated diarrhea (CDAD) and pseudomembranous colitis; CDAD has been observed >2 months postantibiotic treatment; use with caution in patients with a history of colitis.

The Cystic Fibrosis Foundation recommends that patients not use colistimethate for inhalation premixed by pharmacies; patients should prepare their colistimethate nebulizer inhalation solutions immediately prior to use. Colistin is comprised of two components: Colistin A (polymyxin E1) and colistin B (polymyxin E2). Polymyxin E1 has been shown to cause localized airway inflammation in animal studies and may result in lung toxicity in humans. Clinicians who continue to prescribe colistimethate for inhalation should be aware of this potentially life-threatening effect and should administer solutions for inhalation promptly following preparation of solution.

Precautions Use with caution in patients with impaired renal function; dosage adjustments are recommended.

Adverse Reactions

Central nervous system: Dizziness, fever, headache, slurred speech, vertigo

Dermatologic: Pruritus, rash, urticaria

Gastrointestinal: GI upset

Neuromuscular & skeletal: Paresthesia (extremities, oral); weakness (lower limb)

Renal: BUN increased, creatinine increased, nephrotoxicity, proteinuria, urine output decreased

Respiratory: Apnea, respiratory distress

Rare but important or life-threatening: Lung toxicity (bronchoconstriction, bronchospasm, chest tightness, respiratory distress, acute respiratory failure following inhalation)

Drug Interactions

Metabolism/Transport Effects None known.

Avoid Concomitant Use

Avoid concomitant use of Colistimethate with any of the following: BCG

Increased Effect/Toxicity

Colistimethate may increase the levels/effects of: Neuromuscular-Blocking Agents

The levels/effects of Colistimethate may be increased by: Aminoglycosides; Amphotericin B; Capreomycin; Polymyxin B; Vancomycin

Decreased Effect

Colistimethate may decrease the levels/effects of: BCG; Sodium Picosulfate; Typhoid Vaccine

Stability Store intact vials (prior to reconstitution) at 20°C to 25°C (68°F to 77°F); excursions permitted to 15°C to 30°C (59°F to 86°F). Reconstituted vials may be refrigerated at 2°C to 8°C (36°F to 46°F) or stored at 20°C to 25°C (68°F to 77°F) for up to 7 days. Solutions for infusion should be freshly prepared; do not use beyond 24 hours. For inhalation, use reconstituted solution immediately after preparation.

Mechanism of Action Colistimethate (or the sodium salt [colistimethate sodium]) is the inactive prodrug which is hydrolyzed to colistin, which acts as a cationic detergent and damages the bacterial cytoplasmic membrane causing leaking of intracellular substances and cell death

Pharmacokinetics (Adult data unless noted)

Absorption: Not absorbed from the GI tract, mucous membranes, or intact skin (**Note:** GI absorption has been observed in infants.)

Distribution: Widely distributed to body tissues, such as liver, kidney, heart, and lungs; does not penetrate into CSF, synovial, pleural, or pericardial fluids

V_d: Adolescents and Adults with cystic fibrosis: 0.09 ± 0.03 L/kg (Reed, 2001)

Protein binding: 50%

Half-life:

Infants (including premature infants), Children, Adolescents, and Adults: 2-3 hours

Adolescents and Adults with cystic fibrosis: 3.5 ± 1 hour (Reed, 2001)

Time to peak serum concentration: I.M.: ~2 hours

Elimination: Primarily by the kidney through glomerular filtration and urinary excretion as unchanged drug

Dosing: Neonatal Note: Dosage expressed in terms of colistin **base**.

General dosing, susceptible infection: I.M., I.V.: 2.5-5 mg/kg/**day** divided every 6-12 hours

Pulmonary infection: Limited data available: Inhalation: 4 mg/kg/dose every 12 hours has been used to treat ventilator-associated pneumonia in neonates [n=8, gestational age: 28-41 weeks; median treatment duration: 9 days (range: 4-14 days)] (Nakwan, 2011)

Dosing: Usual Note: Doses should be based on ideal body weight in obese patients; **Dosage expressed in terms of colistin base:**

Infants, Children, and Adolescents:

General dosing, susceptible infection: Infants, Children, and Adolescents: I.M., I.V.: 2.5-5 mg/kg/**day** divided every 6-12 hours

Cystic fibrosis, pulmonary infection: Limited data available: Children ≥5 years and Adolescents: I.V.: Usual reported range: 3-5 mg/kg/**day** divided every 8 hours; maximum dose: 100 mg/dose (Bosso, 1991; Reed, 2001; Young, 2013); doses >5 mg/kg/day (up to 8 mg/kg/day) may be required in some situations; however, higher doses are associated with more severe toxicity (Bosso, 1991; Reed, 2001).

Pulmonary infection: Limited data available: Infants, Children, and Adolescents: Inhalation: Usual dose: 75-150 mg in 3 mL of NS (4 mL total volume) via nebulizer twice daily is most frequently reported in clinical practice; reported range: 30-150 mg/dose (Le, 2010; Tramper, 2010)

Adults: Susceptible infections: I.M., I.V.: 2.5-5 mg/kg/**day** in 2-4 divided doses

Dosing interval in renal impairment: Adults: I.M., I.V.:

CrCl >80 mL/minute: No dosage adjustment necessary

CrCl 50-79 mL/minute: 2.5-3.8 mg/kg/day in 2 divided doses

CrCl 30-49 mL/minute: 2.5 mg/kg/day in 1-2 divided doses

CrCl 10-29 mL/minute: 1.5 mg/kg every 36 hours

Intermittent hemodialysis (IHD) (administer after hemodialysis on dialysis days): 1.5 mg/kg every 24-48 hours (Heintz, 2009). **Note:** Dosing dependent on the assumption of 3 times/week, complete IHD sessions.

Continuous renal replacement therapy (CRRT) (Heintz, 2009; Trotman, 2005): Drug clearance is highly dependent on the method of renal replacement, filter type, and flow rate. Appropriate dosing requires close monitoring of pharmacologic response, signs of adverse reactions due to drug accumulation, as well as drug concentrations in relation to target trough (if appropriate). The following are general recommendations only (based on dialysate flow/ultrafiltration rates of 1-2 L/hour and minimal residual renal function) and should not supersede clinical judgment:

CVVH/CVVHD/CVVHDF: 2.5 mg/kg every 24-48 hours (frequency dependent upon site or severity of infection or susceptibility of pathogen)

Note: A single case report has demonstrated that the use of 2.5 mg/kg every 48 hours with a dialysate flow rate of 1 L/hour may be inadequate and that dosing every 24 hours was well-tolerated. Based on pharmacokinetic analysis, the authors recommend dosing as frequent as every 12 hours in patients receiving CVVHDF (Li, 2005).

Dosing adjustment in hepatic impairment: There are no dosage adjustments provided in manufacturer's labeling.

Dosing adjustment for toxicity:

CNS toxicity: Dose reduction may reduce neurologic symptoms.

Nephrotoxicity: Withhold treatment if signs of renal impairment occur during treatment.

Administration

Parenteral: Reconstitute vial containing 150 mg of colistin base activity with 2 mL SWI resulting in a concentration of 75 mg colistin base activity/mL; swirl gently to avoid frothing.

I.M.: No further dilution required; administer deep into a large muscle mass (eg, gluteal muscle or lateral part of the thigh).

Intermittent I.V. injection: No further dilution required; administer over 3-5 minutes.

Intermittent infusion: Further dilute in an appropriate volume; administer over 30 minutes.

Continuous I.V. infusion: Initially, one-half of the total daily dose is administered by direct I.V. injection over 3-5 minutes followed 1-2 hours later by the remaining one-half of the total daily dose diluted in a compatible I.V. solution infused over 22-23 hours. The final concentration for continuous infusion administration should be based on the patient's fluid needs; infusion should be completed within 24 hours of preparation.

Inhalation: Reconstitute vial containing 150 mg of colistin base activity with 2 mL SWI resulting in a concentration of 75 mg colistin base activity/mL. Further dilute dose to a total volume of 4 mL in NS and administer solution via nebulizer promptly following preparation of solution.

Monitoring Parameters CBC with differential, renal function tests, urine output; number and type of stools/day for diarrhea; for inhalation therapy: Pre- and post-treatment spirometry; signs of bronchospasm

Additional Information Colistimethate dosing differs between the U.S. and European countries. In the U.S. doses should be expressed as **colistin base**. In European countries, the dose is often expressed as colistimethate sodium and is expressed in terms of units rather than mg:

1 mg colistin base = 2.67 mg colistimethate sodium

1 mg colistimethate sodium = 12,500 units of colistimethate sodium

Dosage Forms Excipient information presented when available (limited, particularly for generics); consult specific product labeling.

Solution Reconstituted, Injection [strength expressed as base]:

Coly-Mycin M: 150 mg (1 ea)

Generic: 150 mg (1 ea)

References

Beringer P, "The Clinical Use of Colistin in Patients With Cystic Fibrosis," *Curr Opin Pulm Med*, 2001, 7(6):434-40.

Bosso JA, Liptak CA, Seilheimer DK, et al, "Toxicity of Colistin in Cystic Fibrosis Patients," *DICP*, 1991, 25(11):1168-70.

Cunningham S, Prasad A, Collyer L, et al, "Bronchoconstriction Following Nebulised Colistin in Cystic Fibrosis," *Arch Dis Child*, 2001, 84 (5):432-3.

Falagas ME and Kasiakou SK, "Use of International Units When Dosing Colistin Will Help Decrease Confusion Related to Various Formulations of the Drug Around the World," *Antimicrob Agents Chemother*, 2006, 50(6):2274-5.

Falagas ME, Sideri G, Korbila IP, et al, "Inhaled Colistin for the Treatment of Tracheobronchitis and Pneumonia in Critically Ill Children Without Cystic Fibrosis," *Pediatr Pulmonol*, 2010, 45(11):1135-40.

Heintz BH, Matzke GR, and Dager WE, "Antimicrobial Dosing Concepts and Recommendations for Critically Ill Adult Patients Receiving Continuous Renal Replacement Therapy or Intermittent Hemodialysis," *Pharmacotherapy*, 2009, 29(5):562-77.

Iosifidis E, Antachopoulos C, Ioannidou M, et al, "Colistin Administration to Pediatric and Neonatal Patients," *Eur J Pediatr*, 2010, 169 (7):867-74.

Jajoo M, Kumar V, Jain M, et al, "Intravenous Colistin Administration in Neonates," *Pediatr Infect Dis J*, 2011, 30(3):218-21.

Katragkou A and Roilides E, "Successful Treatment of Multidrug-Resistant *Acinetobacter baumannii* Central Nervous System Infections With Colistin," *J Clin Microbiol*, 2005, 43(9):4916-7.

Le J, Ashley ED, Neuhauser MM, et al, "Consensus Summary of Aerosolized Antimicrobial Agents: Application of Guideline Criteria. Insights From the Society of Infectious Diseases Pharmacists," *Pharmacotherapy*, 2010, 30(6):562-84.

Li J, Rayner CR, Nation RL, et al, "Pharmacokinetics of Colistin Methanesulfonate and Colistin in a Critically Ill Patient Receiving Continuous Venovenous Hemodiafiltration," *Antimicrob Agents Chemother*, 2005, 49(11):4814-5.

Lim LM, Ly N, Anderson D, et al, "Resurgence of Colistin: A Review of Resistance, Toxicity, Pharmacodynamics, and Dosing," *Pharmacotherapy*, 2010, 30(12):1279-91.

Nakwan N, Wannaro J, Thongmak T, et al, "Safety in Treatment of Ventilator-Associated Pneumonia Due to Extensive Drug-Resistant *Acinetobacter baumannii* With Aerosolized Colistin in Neonates: A Preliminary Report," *Pediatr Pulmonol*, 2011, 46(1):60-6.

Reed MD, Stern RC, O'Riordan MA, et al, "The Pharmacokinetics of Colistin in Patients With Cystic Fibrosis," *J Clin Pharmacol*, 2001, 41 (6):645-54.

Sabuda DM, Laupland K, Pitout J, et al, "Utilization of Colistin for Treatment of Multidrug-Resistant *Pseudomonas aeruginosa*," *Can J Infect Dis Med Microbiol*, 2008, 19(6):413-8.

Tramper-Stranders GA, Wolfs TF, van Haren Noman S, et al, "Controlled Trial of Cycled Antibiotic Prophylaxis to Prevent Initial *Pseudomonas aeruginosa* Infection in Children With Cystic Fibrosis," *Thorax*, 2010, 65(10):915-20.

Trotman RL, Williamson JC, Shoemaker DM, et al, "Antibiotic Dosing in Critically Ill Adult Patients Receiving Continuous Renal Replacement Therapy," *Clin Infect Dis*, 2005, 41:1159-66.

Young DC, Zobell JT, Waters CD, et al, "Optimization of Anti-pseudomonal Antibiotics for Cystic Fibrosis Pulmonary Exacerbations: IV. Colistimethate Sodium," *Pediatr Pulmonol*, 2013, 48(1):1-7.

◆ **Colistimethate Sodium** see Colistimethate *on page 541*

◆ **Colistin Methanesulfonate** see Colistimethate *on page 541*

◆ **Colistin Sulfomethate** see Colistimethate *on page 541*

◆ **Colocort** see Hydrocortisone (Topical) *on page 1038*

◆ **CO Losartan (Can)** see Losartan *on page 1283*

◆ **CO Lovastatin (Can)** see Lovastatin *on page 1286*

◆ **Coly-Mycin M** see Colistimethate *on page 541*

◆ **Colyte** see Polyethylene Glycol-Electrolyte Solution *on page 1697*

◆ **Combantrin (Can)** see Pyrantel Pamoate *on page 1774*

◆ **Combivir®** see Lamivudine and Zidovudine *on page 1198*

◆ **CO Meloxicam (Can)** see Meloxicam *on page 1325*

◆ **CO Metformin (Can)** see MetFORMIN *on page 1353*

◆ **Compazine** see Prochlorperazine *on page 1745*

- **Complete Allergy Medication [OTC]** *see* Diphenhydr-AMINE (Systemic) *on page 673*
- **Complete Allergy Relief [OTC]** *see* DiphenhydrAMINE (Systemic) *on page 673*
- **Compound E** *see* Cortisone *on page 548*
- **Compound F** *see* Hydrocortisone (Systemic) *on page 1034*
- **Compound F** *see* Hydrocortisone (Topical) *on page 1038*
- **Compound S** *see* Zidovudine *on page 2168*
- **Compound S, Abacavir, and Lamivudine** *see* Abacavir, Lamivudine, and Zidovudine *on page 41*
- **Compro** *see* Prochlorperazine *on page 1745*
- **Comvax®** *see* Haemophilus b Conjugate and Hepatitis B Vaccine *on page 993*
- **CO Mycophenolate (Can)** *see* Mycophenolate *on page 1453*
- **Concerta** *see* Methylphenidate *on page 1379*
- **Congest (Can)** *see* Estrogens (Conjugated/Equine, Systemic) *on page 799*
- **Conjugated Estrogen** *see* Estrogens (Conjugated/Equine, Systemic) *on page 799*
- **Conjugated Estrogen** *see* Estrogens (Conjugated/Equine, Topical) *on page 801*
- **Constulose** *see* Lactulose *on page 1193*
- **Contac® Cold 12 Hour Relief Non Drowsy (Can)** *see* Pseudoephedrine *on page 1770*
- **ControlRx** *see* Fluoride *on page 894*
- **ControlRx Multi** *see* Fluoride *on page 894*
- **Conventional Amphotericin B** *see* Amphotericin B (Conventional) *on page 147*
- **Conventional Cytarabine** *see* Cytarabine (Conventional) *on page 573*
- **Conventional Daunomycin** *see* DAUNOrubicin (Conventional) *on page 599*
- **Conventional Doxorubicin** *see* DOXOrubicin (Conventional) *on page 718*
- **Conventional Paclitaxel** *see* PACLitaxel *on page 1579*
- **Conventional Vincristine** *see* VinCRIStine *on page 2138*
- **ConZip** *see* TraMADol *on page 2060*
- **CO Olanzapine (Can)** *see* OLANZapine *on page 1525*
- **CO Olanzapine ODT (Can)** *see* OLANZapine *on page 1525*
- **CO Ondansetron (Can)** *see* Ondansetron *on page 1544*
- **CO Oxycodone CR (Can)** *see* OxyCODONE *on page 1569*
- **CO Pantoprazole (Can)** *see* Pantoprazole *on page 1595*
- **CO Paroxetine (Can)** *see* PARoxetine *on page 1609*
- **Copegus** *see* Ribavirin *on page 1818*

Copper (KOP er)

Medication Safety Issues
Sound-alike/look-alike issues:
Cupric sulfate may be confused with calcium gluconate
Brand Names: U.S. Coppermin [OTC]; Cu-5 [OTC]
Therapeutic Category Trace Element, Parenteral
Generic Availability (U.S.) May be product dependent
Use Supplement to total parenteral nutrition (TPN) to maintain copper serum concentrations and to prevent depletion of endogenous stores and subsequent deficiency [FDA approved in pediatric patients (age not specified) and adults]
Pregnancy Risk Factor C

Pregnancy Considerations Animal reproduction studies have not been conducted. It is not known whether administration to a pregnant woman can cause fetal harm or can affect reproductive capacity.
Breast-Feeding Considerations It is unknown whether this drug is excreted in human milk. Because many drugs are excreted in human milk, caution should be exercised.
Contraindications Hypersensitivity to copper or any component; direct intravenous or intramuscular injection of 0.4 mg/mL copper solution (cupric chloride, USP)
Warnings Copper may accumulate in patients with liver and/or biliary tract dysfunction; consider dosage reduction or avoidance of copper in patients with biliary obstruction; avoid copper use in patients with Wilson's disease. Direct I.V. or I.M. injection of 0.4 mg/mL solution may cause tissue necrosis due to acidic nature (pH: 1.5-2.5).
Precautions Patients with high output intestinal fistulae may require a larger dose than the recommended daily allowance (ASPEN, 2002). Copper ion may degrade ascorbic acid in TPN solutions; to avoid loss, add multivitamin additives to TPN solutions immediately prior to infusion or add to separate TPN solution container.

May contain aluminum; toxic aluminum concentrations may be seen with high doses, prolonged use, or renal dysfunction. Premature neonates are at higher risk due to immature renal function and aluminum intake from other parenteral sources. Parenteral aluminum exposure of >4-5 mcg/kg/day is associated with CNS and bone toxicity and tissue loading may occur at lower doses.
Adverse Reactions Note: Generally well tolerated; excessive copper levels may result in the following adverse effects:
Hepatic: Hepatic dysfunction (including hepatic necrosis)
Drug Interactions
Metabolism/Transport Effects None known.
Avoid Concomitant Use There are no known interactions where it is recommended to avoid concomitant use.
Increased Effect/Toxicity There are no known significant interactions involving an increase in effect.
Decreased Effect
Copper may decrease the levels/effects of: Ascorbic Acid
Stability Store at controlled room temperature of 20°C to 25°C (68°F to 77°F).
Mechanism of Action Copper is an essential nutrient which serves as a cofactor for serum ceruloplasmin, an oxidase necessary for proper formation of the iron carrier protein, transferrin. It also helps maintain normal rates of red and white blood cell formation and helps prevent development of deficiency symptoms: Leukopenia, neutropenia, anemia, depressed ceruloplasmin levels, impaired transferring formation, secondary iron deficiency and osteoporosis.
Pharmacokinetics (Adult data unless noted) Elimination: Bile (primarily, 80%); intestinal wall (16%); urine (4%)
Dosing: Neonatal
Adequate intake (AI): 200 mcg/day
I.V.: **Note:** Incorporated into parenteral nutrition solution.
Parenteral nutrition supplementation:
ASPEN Guidelines (Mirtallo, 2004): Preterm and term: 20 mcg/kg/day
Manufacturer recommendation: 20 mcg/kg/day; **Note:** Premature neonates weighing <1.5 kg may have higher daily requirements due to low body reserves and accelerated growth rate.
Dosing: Usual
Infants, Children, and Adolescents:
Adequate intake (AI):
1-6 months: 200 mcg/day
6-12 months: 220 mcg/day
Recommended daily allowances (RDA):
1-3 years: 340 mcg/day
4-8 years: 440 mcg/day

9-13 years: 700 mcg/day
14-18 years: 890 mcg/day
≥19 years: 900 mcg/day
I.V.: **Note:** Incorporated into parenteral nutrition solution.
Parenteral nutrition supplementation:
ASPEN Guidelines (Mirtallo, 2004):
Infants <10 kg: 20 mcg/kg/day
Infants ≥10 kg and Children ≤40 kg or <12 years: 5-20 mcg/kg/day (maximum dose: 500 mcg/day)
Children ≥12 years or >40 kg and Adolescents: 200-500 mcg/day
Manufacturer recommendation: 20 mcg/kg/day
Adults: **Parenteral nutrition supplementation:** ASPEN Guidelines (Mirtallo, 2004): 0.3-0.5 **mg**/day; manufacturer recommendation: 0.5-1.5 **mg**/day; high output intestinal fistula: Some clinicians may use twice the recommended daily allowance (ASPEN, 2002)
Dosing adjustment in renal impairment: Use caution; contains aluminum
Dosing adjustment in hepatic impairment: Use caution; dosage reduction may be required
Administration Not for direct I.V. or I.M. injection; must be diluted in a volume ≥100 mL; direct administration of 0.4 mg/mL solution causes tissue irritation; pH: 1.5-2.5
Dosage Forms Excipient information presented when available (limited, particularly for generics); consult specific product labeling.
Capsule, Oral [preservative free]:
Cu-5: 5 mg [dye free]
Solution, Intravenous:
Generic: 0.4 mg/mL (10 mL)
Tablet, Oral:
Coppermin: 5 mg [corn free, rye free, wheat free]

References

ASPEN Board of Directors and the Clinical Guidelines Task Force, "Guidelines for the Use of Parenteral and Enteral Nutrition in Adult and Pediatric Patients," *JPEN J Parenter Enteral Nutr*, 2002, 26(1 Suppl):1-138.

Department of Health and Human Services, Food and Drug Administration, "Aluminum in Large and Small Volume Parenterals Used in Total Parenteral Nutrition," *Fed Regist*, 2000, 65(17):4103-11.

Institute of Medicine of the National Academies, "Dietary Reference Intakes (DRIs): Recommended Dietary Allowances and Adequate Intakes, Vitamins." Available at http://iom.edu/Activities/Nutrition/SummaryDRIs/~/media/Files/Activity%20Files/Nutrition/DRIs/RDA%20and%20AIs_Vitamin%20and%20Elements.pdf. Accessed August 24, 2011.

Mirtallo J, Canada T, Johnson D, et al, "Safe Practices for Parenteral Nutrition," *JPEN J Parenter Enteral Nutr*, 2004, 28(6):S39-70.

◆ **Copper** see Trace Elements on page 2059
◆ **Coppermin [OTC]** see Copper on page 544
◆ **CO Pravastatin (Can)** see Pravastatin on page 1720
◆ **CO Quetiapine (Can)** see QUEtiapine on page 1783
◆ **CO Ranitidine (Can)** see Ranitidine on page 1805
◆ **Cordarone** see Amiodarone on page 127
◆ **Coreg** see Carvedilol on page 385
◆ **Coreg CR** see Carvedilol on page 385
◆ **Corgard** see Nadolol on page 1460
◆ **Coricidin HBP Chest Congestion and Cough [OTC]** see Guaifenesin and Dextromethorphan on page 987
◆ **CO Risperidone (Can)** see RisperiDONE on page 1831
◆ **CO Rizatriptan (Can)** see Rizatriptan on page 1845
◆ **CO Rizatriptan ODT (Can)** see Rizatriptan on page 1845
◆ **Corlopam** see Fenoldopam on page 852
◆ **Cormax Scalp Application** see Clobetasol on page 506
◆ **Corn Remover One Step [OTC]** see Salicylic Acid on page 1860
◆ **Corn Remover Ultra Thin [OTC]** see Salicylic Acid on page 1860
◆ **CO Rosuvastatin (Can)** see Rosuvastatin on page 1853

◆ **Correct [OTC]** see Bisacodyl on page 293
◆ **Correctol Stool Softener [OTC] (Can)** see Docusate on page 701
◆ **CortAlo** see Hydrocortisone (Topical) on page 1038
◆ **Cortamed® (Can)** see Hydrocortisone (Topical) on page 1038
◆ **Cortef** see Hydrocortisone (Systemic) on page 1034
◆ **Cortef® (Can)** see Hydrocortisone (Systemic) on page 1034
◆ **Cortenema** see Hydrocortisone (Topical) on page 1038
◆ **Cortenema® (Can)** see Hydrocortisone (Topical) on page 1038
◆ **Corticool [OTC]** see Hydrocortisone (Topical) on page 1038

Corticotropin (kor ti koe TROE pin)

Medication Safety Issues
Sound-alike/look-alike issues:
Corticotropin may be confused with corticorelin, cosyntropin
Brand Names: U.S. Acthar HP
Therapeutic Category Adrenal Corticosteroid; Infantile Spasms, Treatment
Generic Availability (U.S.) No
Use Treatment of infantile spasms as monotherapy (FDA approved in ages <2 years); treatment of acute exacerbations of multiple sclerosis (FDA approved in adults); adjunctive therapy for exacerbations/acute episodes of rheumatic disorders (eg, psoriatic arthritis, rheumatoid arthritis, juvenile idiopathic arthritis, ankylosing spondylitis) (FDA approved in ages >2 years and adults); exacerbations or maintenance therapy for collagen diseases (eg, systemic lupus erythematosus, systemic dermatomyositis) (FDA approved in ages >2 years and adults); treatment of dermatologic (severe erythema multiforme, Stevens-Johnson syndrome) and allergic (serum sickness) states (FDA approved in ages >2 years and adults); treatment of severe acute/chronic allergic and inflammatory ophthalmic disease (eg, keratitis, iritis, iridocyclitis, diffuse posterior uveitis and choroiditis, optic neuritis, chorioretinitis, anterior segment inflammation) and symptomatic sarcoidosis (FDA approved in ages >2 years and adults); to induce diuresis or remission of proteinuria in patients with nephrotic syndrome without idiopathic uremia or due to lupus erythematosus (FDA approved in ages >2 years and adults)
Prescribing and Access Restrictions H.P. Acthar® Gel is only available through specialty pharmacy distribution and not through traditional distribution sources (eg, wholesalers, retail pharmacies). Hospitals wishing to acquire H.P. Acthar® Gel should contact CuraScript Specialty Distribution (1-877-599-7748).

After treatment is initiated, discharge or outpatient prescriptions should be submitted to the Acthar Support and Access Program (A.S.A.P.) in order to ensure an uninterrupted supply of the medication. The Acthar Referral/Prescription form is available online at http://www.acthar.com/files/Acthar-Prescription-Referral-Form.pdf.

Additional information is available for the A.S.A.P. at http://www.acthar.com/healthcare-professionals/physician-patient-referrals or by calling 1-888-435-2284.
Medication Guide Available Yes
Pregnancy Considerations Embryocidal effects may be observed following corticotropin use during pregnancy. Endogenous corticotropin concentrations are increased near delivery (Smith, 2007).

Some studies have shown an association between first trimester systemic corticosteroid use and oral clefts (Park-Wyllie, 2000; Pradat, 2003). Systemic corticosteroids may also influence fetal growth (decreased birth weight); however, information is conflicting (Lunghi, 2010). When systemic corticosteroids are needed in pregnancy, it is generally recommended to use the lowest effective dose for the shortest duration of time, avoiding high doses during the first trimester (Leachman, 2006; Lunghi, 2010; Makol, 2011; Østensen, 2009).

Breast-Feeding Considerations Corticosteroids are excreted in human milk; information specific to corticotropin has not been located. Due to the potential for serious adverse reactions in the nursing infant, the manufacturer recommends a decision be made whether to discontinue nursing or to discontinue the drug, taking into account the importance of treatment to the mother.

Contraindications Hypersensitivity to corticotropin, porcine proteins, or any component; scleroderma, osteoporosis, systemic fungal infections, ocular herpes simplex, peptic ulcer, uncontrolled hypertension, CHF; recent surgery; primary adrenocortical insufficiency; adrenocortical hyperfunction; infants with suspected congenital infections; concomitant administration of live or live attenuated vaccines; intravenous administration

Warnings Hypothalamic-pituitary-adrenal (HPA) suppression may occur, particularly in younger children or in patients receiving high doses for prolonged periods; in infants being treated for infantile spasms, symptoms of HPA suppression may be nonspecific and include anorexia, fatigue, lethargy, weakness, excessive weight loss, hypotension, and abdominal pain. Acute adrenal insufficiency (adrenal crisis) may occur with abrupt withdrawal after long-term therapy or with stress; withdrawal and discontinuation of corticotropin should be tapered slowly and carefully; patients with HPA axis suppression may require doses of systemic glucocorticosteroids prior to, during, and after unusual stress (eg, surgery). Additionally, when used for infantile spasm, therapy should not be discontinued abruptly; withdraw gradually to lessen chance for increased seizure frequency.

Immunosuppression may occur; patients may be more susceptible to infections; prolonged use of corticotropin and corticosteroids may also increase the incidence of secondary infection, mask acute infection (including fungal infections), prolong or exacerbate viral or fungal infections, activate latent opportunistic infections, or limit response to vaccines; live or attenuated live vaccines should not be used during corticotropin therapy; exposure to chickenpox should be avoided. Close observation is required in patients with latent tuberculosis and/or TB reactivity; restrict use in active TB (only in conjunction with antituberculosis treatment).

May cause osteoporosis (at any age) or inhibition of bone growth in pediatric patients. Use with caution in patients with osteoporosis; underlying clinical condition may also impact bone health and osteoporotic effect of corticosteroids and corticotropin (Leonard, 2006).

Corticosteroid use may cause psychiatric disturbances, including depression, euphoria, insomnia, mood swings, personality changes, and irritability (especially in infants). Antibodies may develop following prolonged use and increase the risk of hypersensitivity reactions.

Precautions Avoid using higher than recommended doses; suppression of HPA function, suppression of linear growth (ie, reduction of growth velocity), reduced bone mineral density, hypercorticism (Cushing's syndrome), hyperglycemia, or glucosuria may occur; titrate to lowest effective dose. Reduction in growth velocity may occur when corticosteroids or corticotropin are administered to pediatric patients by any route (monitor growth). Use with extreme caution in patients with respiratory tuberculosis or untreated systemic infections. Use with caution in patients with controlled hypertension or renal impairment; long-term use has been associated with fluid retention, increased excretion of potassium and calcium, and hypertension. Use with caution in patients with GI diseases (diverticulitis, peptic ulcer, ulcerative colitis) due to risk of GI bleeding and perforation. Use with caution in patients with myasthenia gravis; exacerbation of symptoms has occurred, especially during initial treatment with corticosteroids. Use with caution in patients with hepatic impairment, including cirrhosis; enhanced pharmacologic effect due to decreased metabolism and long-term use has been associated with fluid retention.

Use with caution in patients with diabetes; corticosteroids may alter glucose regulation, leading to hyperglycemia. Use with caution in patients with cataracts and/or glaucoma; increased intraocular pressure, open-angle glaucoma, and cataracts have occurred with prolonged use; consider routine eye exams in chronic users. Use with caution in patients with a history of seizure disorder; seizures have been reported with adrenal crisis. Use with caution in patients with thyroid dysfunction; changes in thyroid status may necessitate dosage adjustments; metabolic clearance of corticosteroids increases in hyperthyroid patients and decreases in hypothyroid patients. Use with caution in patients with thromboembolic tendencies or thrombophlebitis.

Adverse Reactions

Adverse events associated with cortisol elevation; frequency not defined:

Cardiovascular: Blood pressure increased

Central nervous system: Behavioral changes, mood changes

Endocrine & metabolic: Fluid retention, glucose intolerance

Gastrointestinal: Appetite increased, weight gain

Adverse events associated with infantile spasm treatment:

Cardiovascular: Cardiac hypertrophy, hypertension

Central nervous system: Irritability, pyrexia, seizure

Endocrine & metabolic: Cushingoid syndrome

Gastrointestinal: Appetite decreased, diarrhea, vomiting, weight gain

Respiratory: Nasal congestion

Miscellaneous: Infection

Postmarketing and/or case reports (other adverse events associated with corticosteroids may also occur): Abdominal distension, allergic reactions, carbohydrate intolerance (infants), congestive heart failure, diaphoresis (adults), facial erythema, headache (adults), hirsutism, hypokalemic alkalosis (infants), intracranial hemorrhage (adults), muscle weakness, necrotizing angiitis (adults), pancreatitis (adults), reversible brain shrinkage (secondary to hypertension; infants), skin thinning (adults), subdural hematoma, ulcerative esophagitis, vertebral compression fractures (infants), vertigo (adults)

Drug Interactions

Metabolism/Transport Effects None known.

Avoid Concomitant Use

Avoid concomitant use of Corticotropin with any of the following: Aldesleukin; BCG; Indium 111 Capromab Pendetide; Mifepristone; Natalizumab; Pimecrolimus; Tacrolimus (Topical); Tofacitinib

Increased Effect/Toxicity

Corticotropin may increase the levels/effects of: Acetylcholinesterase Inhibitors; Amphotericin B; Androgens; Ceritinib; Deferasirox; Leflunomide; Loop Diuretics; Natalizumab; NSAID (COX-2 Inhibitor); NSAID (Nonselective); Thiazide Diuretics; Tofacitinib; Vaccines (Live); Warfarin

The levels/effects of Corticotropin may be increased by:
Antifungal Agents (Azole Derivatives, Systemic); Aprepitant; Calcium Channel Blockers (Nondihydropyridine); Denosumab; Estrogen Derivatives; Fluconazole; Fosaprepitant; Indacaterol; Macrolide Antibiotics; Mifepristone; Neuromuscular-Blocking Agents (Nondepolarizing); Pimecrolimus; Quinolone Antibiotics; Roflumilast; Salicylates; Tacrolimus (Topical); Telaprevir; Trastuzumab

Decreased Effect

Corticotropin may decrease the levels/effects of: Aldesleukin; Antidiabetic Agents; BCG; Calcitriol; Coccidioidin Skin Test; Corticorelin; Hyaluronidase; Indium 111 Capromab Pendetide; Isoniazid; Salicylates; Sipuleucel-T; Telaprevir; Urea Cycle Disorder Agents; Vaccines (Inactivated)

The levels/effects of Corticotropin may be decreased by: Aminoglutethimide; Barbiturates; Echinacea; Mifepristone; Mitotane; Primidone; Rifamycin Derivatives

Stability Store in the refrigerator at 2°C to 8°C (36°F to 46°F).

Mechanism of Action Stimulates the adrenal cortex to secrete adrenal steroids (including hydrocortisone, cortisone), androgenic substances, and a small amount of aldosterone

Pharmacodynamics

Maximum effect: Cortisol serum concentration: I.M., SubQ: 3-12 hours

Duration: Repository: 10-25 hours, up to 3 days

Pharmacokinetics (Adult data unless noted)

Absorption: I.M.: Over 8-16 hours

Half-life: ACTH: 15 minutes

Elimination: In urine

Dosing: Usual Note: Sudden withdrawal may lead to adrenal insufficiency or recurrent symptoms; tapering the dose prior to discontinuation of therapy may be necessary following prolonged administration.

Infants, Children, and Adolescents:

Infants and Children <2 years: **Infantile spasms:** Various regimens have been used; optimal dose and duration of treatment are not established (Go, 2012; Mackey, 2004; Pellock, 2010). Some neurologists recommend low-dose ACTH (5-40 units/day) for short periods (1-6 weeks), while others recommend larger doses of ACTH (40-160 units/day) for long periods of treatment (3-12 months); current guidelines recommend consideration to a low-dose ACTH regimen (as an alternative to high-dose); however, literature suggests that the two dosing regimens are probably equally effective for short-term treatment (Go, 2012); a recent U.S. consensus report recommends short duration (~2 weeks), followed by a taper (Pellock, 2010).

Manufacturer labeling: I.M.: 75 units/m^2/dose twice daily for 2 weeks, followed by a 2-week taper: 30 units/m^2/dose once daily in the morning for 3 days, followed by 15 units/m^2/dose once daily in the morning for 3 days, followed by 10 units/m^2/dose once daily in the morning for 3 days and 10 units/m^2/dose every other morning for 6 days

Alternative dosing: I.M.: A prospective, single-blind study (Hrachovy, 1994) found no major difference in effectiveness between high-dose long-duration versus low-dose short-duration ACTH therapy. Hypertension, however, occurred more frequently in the high-dose group. Further studies comparing long-term outcomes are needed. Low-dose regimen used in this study: Initial: 20 units/day for 2 weeks, if patient responds, taper and discontinue over a 1-week period; if patient does not respond, increase dose to 30 units/day for 4 weeks then taper and discontinue over a 1-week period.

Children >2 years and Adolescents: **Anti-inflammatory/immunosuppression:**

Manufacturer labeling: I.M., SubQ: 40-80 units/dose every 24-72 hours

Alternative dosing: I.M.: 0.8 units/kg/**day or** 25 units/m^2/**day** divided every 12-24 hours

Adults:

Acute exacerbation of multiple sclerosis: I.M., SubQ: 80-120 units/**day** for 2-3 weeks

All other indications: I.M., SubQ: 40-80 units/dose every 24-72 hours

Administration Parenteral: Warm gel before administration; do not over-pressurize vial when withdrawing product. May be administered I.M. or SubQ; I.M. route is recommended for the treatment of infantile spasms; do not administer I.V.

Monitoring Parameters Blood pressure, serum glucose, potassium, and calcium and clinical presence of adverse effects. Monitor intraocular pressure (if therapy >6 weeks) for signs of secondary ocular infections; linear growth of pediatric patients (with chronic use), assess HPA suppression; for infantile spasms, monitor seizure frequency, type, and duration

Test Interactions May suppress the wheal and flare reactions to skin test antigens

Additional Information Cosyntropin is preferred over corticotropin for diagnostic test of adrenocortical insufficiency (cosyntropin is less allergenic and test is shorter in duration).

Dosage Forms Excipient information presented when available (limited, particularly for generics); consult specific product labeling.

Gel, Injection:

Acthar HP: 80 units/mL (5 mL) [contains phenol]

References

Go CY, Mackay MT, Weiss SK, et al, "Evidence-Based Guideline Update: Medical Treatment of Infantile Spasms: Report of the Guideline Development Subcommittee of the American Academy of Neurology and the Practice Committee of the Child Neurology Society," *Neurology*, 2012, 78(24):1974-80.

Haines ST and Casto DT, "Treatment of Infantile Spasms," *Ann Pharmacother*, 1994, 28(6):779-91.

Hrachovy RA and Frost JD Jr, "Infantile Spasms," *Pediatr Clin North Am*, 1989, 36(2):311-29.

Hrachovy RA, Frost JD Jr, and Glaze DG, "High-Dose, Long-Duration Versus Low-Dose, Short-Duration Corticotropin Therapy for Infantile Spasms," *J Pediatr*, 1994, 124(5 Pt 1):803-6.

Hrachovy RA, Frost JD Jr, Kellaway P, et al, "Double-Blind Study of ACTH vs Prednisone Therapy in Infantile Spasms," *J Pediatr*, 1983, 103(4):641-5.

Leachman SA and Reed BR, "The Use of Dermatologic Drugs in Pregnancy and Lactation," *Dermatol Clin*, 2006, 24(2):167-97, vi.

Lunghi L, Pavan B, Biondi C, et al, "Use of Glucocorticoids in Pregnancy," *Curr Pharm Des*, 2010, 16(32):3616-37.

Mackay MT, Weiss SK, Adams-Webber T, et al, "Practice Parameter: Medical Treatment of Infantile Spasms: Report of the American Academy of Neurology and the Child Neurology Society," *Neurology*, 2004, 62(10):1668-81.

Makol A, Wright K, and Amin S, "Rheumatoid Arthritis and Pregnancy: Safety Considerations in Pharmacological Management," *Drugs*, 2011, 71(15):1973-87.

Østensen M and Forger F, "Management of RA Medications in Pregnant Patients," *Nat Rev Rheumatol*, 2009, 5(7):382-90.

Park-Wyllie L, Mazzotta P, Pastuszak A, et al, "Birth defects After Maternal Exposure to Corticosteroids: Prospective Cohort Study and Meta-Analysis of Epidemiological Studies," *Teratology*, 2000, 62(6):385-92.

Pellock JM, Hrachovy R, Shinnar S, et al, "Infantile Spasms: A U.S. Consensus Report," *Epilepsia*, 2010, 51(10):2175-89.

Pradat P, Robert-Gnansia E, Di Tanna GL, et al, "First Trimester Exposure to Corticosteroids and Oral Clefts," *Birth Defects Res A Clin Mol Teratol*, 2003, 67(12):968-70.

Smith R, "Parturition," *N Engl J Med*, 2007, 356(3):271-83.

◆ **Corticotropin, Repository** *see* Corticotropin *on page 545*

◆ **Cortifoam** *see* Hydrocortisone (Topical) *on page 1038*

◆ **Cortifoam™ (Can)** *see* Hydrocortisone (Topical) *on page 1038*

◆ **Cortimyxin (Can)** *see* Neomycin, Polymyxin B, and Hydrocortisone *on page 1485*

◆ **Cortisol** *see* Hydrocortisone (Systemic) *on page 1034*

◆ **Cortisol** *see* Hydrocortisone (Topical) *on page 1038*

Cortisone (KOR ti sone)

Medication Safety Issues
Sound-alike/look-alike issues:
Cortisone may be confused with Cardizem, Cortizone
Related Information
Corticosteroids Systemic Equivalencies *on page 2222*
Therapeutic Category Adrenal Corticosteroid; Anti-inflammatory Agent; Corticosteroid, Systemic; Glucocorticoid
Generic Availability (U.S.) Yes
Use Management of adrenocortical insufficiency
Pregnancy Considerations Adequate reproduction studies have not been conducted. Cortisone crosses the placenta (Migeon, 1957). Some studies have shown an association between first trimester systemic corticosteroid use and oral clefts (Park-Wyllie, 2000; Pradat, 2003). Systemic corticosteroids may also influence fetal growth (decreased birth weight); however, information is conflicting (Lunghi, 2010). Hypoadrenalism may occur in newborns following maternal use of corticosteroids in pregnancy; monitor. When systemic corticosteroids are needed in pregnancy, it is generally recommended to use the lowest effective dose for the shortest duration of time, avoiding high doses during the first trimester (Leachman, 2006; Lunghi, 2010; Makol, 2011; Østensen, 2009).

Women exposed to cortisone during pregnancy for the treatment of an autoimmune disease may contact the OTIS Autoimmune Diseases Study at 877-311-8972.

Breast-Feeding Considerations Corticosteroids are excreted in human milk. The manufacturer notes that when used systemically, maternal use of corticosteroids have the potential to cause adverse events in a nursing infant (eg, growth suppression, interfere with endogenous corticosteroid production). Breast-feeding is not recommended by the manufacturer in women taking pharmacologic doses. If there is concern about exposure to the infant, some guidelines recommend waiting 4 hours after the maternal dose of an oral systemic corticosteroid before breast-feeding in order to decrease potential exposure to the nursing infant (based on a study using prednisolone) (Bae, 2011; Leachman, 2006; Makol, 2011; Ost, 1985).

Contraindications Hypersensitivity to cortisone, any component, or corticosteroids; serious infections, except septic shock or tuberculous meningitis; systemic fungal or viral infections

Warnings Hypothalamic-pituitary-adrenal (HPA) suppression may occur, particularly in younger children or in patients receiving high doses for prolonged periods; acute adrenal insufficiency (adrenal crisis) may occur with abrupt withdrawal after long-term therapy or with stress; withdrawal and discontinuation of corticosteroids should be tapered slowly and carefully; patients with HPA axis suppression may require doses of systemic glucocorticosteroids prior to, during, and after unusual stress (eg, surgery).

Immunosuppression may occur; patients may be more susceptible to infections; prolonged use of corticosteroids may also increase the incidence of secondary infection, mask acute infection (including fungal infections), prolong or exacerbate viral or fungal infections, activate latent opportunistic infections, or limit response to vaccines. Exposure to chickenpox should be avoided; corticosteroids should not be used to treat ocular herpes simplex; use caution in patients with a history of ocular herpes simplex. Corticosteroids should not be used for cerebral malaria or viral hepatitis. Close observation is required in patients with latent tuberculosis and/or TB reactivity; restrict use in active TB (only in conjunction with antituberculosis treatment).

May cause osteoporosis (at any age) or inhibition of bone growth in pediatric patients. Use with caution in patients with osteoporosis. In a population-based study of children, risk of fracture was shown to be increased with >4 courses of corticosteroids; underlying clinical condition may also impact bone health and osteoporotic effect of corticosteroids (Leonard, 2006).

Corticosteroid use may cause psychiatric disturbances, including depression, euphoria, insomnia, mood swings, and personality changes. Pre-exisiting psychiatric conditions may be exacerbated by corticosteroid use. Acute myopathy may occur with high doses, usually in patients with neuromuscular transmission disorders; myopathy may involve ocular and/or respiratory muscles; monitor creatine kinase; recovery may be delayed. Increased IOP may occur, especially with prolonged use; in children, increased IOP has been shown to be dose-dependent and produce a greater IOP in children <6 years than older children (Lam, 2005). Rare cases of anaphylactoid reactions have been reported with corticosteroids.

Precautions Avoid using higher than recommended doses; suppression of HPA function, suppression of linear growth (ie, reduction of growth velocity), reduced bone mineral density, hypercorticism (Cushing's syndrome), hyperglycemia, or glucosuria may occur; titrate to lowest effective dose. Reduction in growth velocity may occur when corticosteroids are administered to pediatric patients by any route (monitor growth). Use with extreme caution in patients with respiratory tuberculosis or untreated systemic infections. Use with caution in patients with hypertension, heart failure, or renal impairment; long-term use has been associated with fluid retention and hypertension. Use with caution in patients with GI diseases (diverticulitis, peptic ulcer, ulcerative colitis) due to risk of GI bleeding and perforation. High-dose corticosteroids should not be used for management of head injury; increased mortality was observed in patients receiving high-dose I.V. methylprednisolone. Use with caution in patients with myasthenia gravis; exacerbation of symptoms has occurred, especially during initial treatment with corticosteroids. Use with caution in patients with hepatic impairment, including cirrhosis; enhanced pharmacologic effect due to decreased metabolism and long-term use has been associated with fluid retention. Use with caution following acute MI; corticosteroids have been associated with myocardial rupture.

Use with caution in patients with diabetes; corticosteroids may alter glucose regulation, leading to hyperglycemia. Use with caution in patients with cataracts and/or glaucoma; increased intraocular pressure, open-angle glaucoma, and cataracts have occurred with prolonged use; consider routine eye exams in chronic users. Use with caution in patients with a history of seizure disorder; seizures have been reported with adrenal crisis. Use with caution in patients with thyroid dysfunction; changes in thyroid status may necessitate dosage adjustments; metabolic clearance of corticosteroids increases in hyperthyroid patients and decreases in hypothyroid patients. Prolonged treatment with corticosteroids has been associated with the development of Kaposi's sarcoma (case reports); if noted, discontinuation of therapy should be considered. Use with caution in patients with thromboembolic tendencies or thrombophlebitis.
Adverse Reactions
Central nervous system: Insomnia, nervousness

Dermatologic: Hirsutism
Endocrine & metabolic: Diabetes mellitus
Gastrointestinal: Increased appetite, indigestion
Neuromuscular & skeletal: Arthralgia
Ocular: Cataracts, glaucoma
Respiratory: Epistaxis
Rare but important or life-threatening: Alkalosis, Cushing's syndrome, delirium, edema, euphoria, fractures, hallucinations, hypersensitivity reactions, hypertension, hypokalemia, muscle wasting, myalgia, osteoporosis, pancreatitis, peptic ulcer, pituitary-adrenal axis suppression, pseudotumor cerebri, psychoses, seizure, skin atrophy, ulcerative esophagitis

Drug Interactions
Metabolism/Transport Effects None known.
Avoid Concomitant Use
Avoid concomitant use of Cortisone with any of the following: Aldesleukin; BCG; Indium 111 Capromab Pendetide; Mifepristone; Natalizumab; Pimecrolimus; Tacrolimus (Topical); Tofacitinib

Increased Effect/Toxicity
Cortisone may increase the levels/effects of: Acetylcholinesterase Inhibitors; Amphotericin B; Androgens; Ceritinib; Deferasirox; Leflunomide; Loop Diuretics; Natalizumab; NSAID (COX-2 Inhibitor); NSAID (Nonselective); Thiazide Diuretics; Tofacitinib; Vaccines (Live); Warfarin

The levels/effects of Cortisone may be increased by: Antifungal Agents (Azole Derivatives, Systemic); Aprepitant; Calcium Channel Blockers (Nondihydropyridine); Denosumab; Estrogen Derivatives; Fluconazole; Fosaprepitant; Indacaterol; Macrolide Antibiotics; Mifepristone; Neuromuscular-Blocking Agents (Nondepolarizing); Pimecrolimus; Quinolone Antibiotics; Roflumilast; Salicylates; Tacrolimus (Topical); Telaprevir; Trastuzumab

Decreased Effect
Cortisone may decrease the levels/effects of: Aldesleukin; Antidiabetic Agents; BCG; Calcitriol; Coccidioidin Skin Test; Corticorelin; Hyaluronidase; Indium 111 Capromab Pendetide; Isoniazid; Salicylates; Sipuleucel-T; Telaprevir; Urea Cycle Disorder Agents; Vaccines (Inactivated)

The levels/effects of Cortisone may be decreased by: Aminoglutethimide; Antacids; Barbiturates; Bile Acid Sequestrants; Echinacea; Mifepristone; Mitotane; Primidone; Rifamycin Derivatives; Somatropin; Tesamorelin

Mechanism of Action Decreases inflammation by suppression of migration of polymorphonuclear leukocytes and reversal of increased capillary permeability

Pharmacodynamics
Maximum effect: Oral: Within 2 hours
Duration: 30-36 hours

Pharmacokinetics (Adult data unless noted)
Distribution: Crosses the placenta; appears in breast milk; distributes to muscles, liver, skin, intestines, and kidneys
Metabolism: In the liver to inactive metabolites
Half-life: 30 minutes
Elimination: In bile and urine

Dosing: Usual Depends upon the condition being treated and the response of the patient. Supplemental doses may be warranted during times of stress in the course of withdrawing therapy. Oral:
Children:
  Anti-inflammatory or immunosuppressive: 2.5-10 mg/kg/day or 20-300 mg/m²/day in divided doses every 6-8 hours
  Physiologic replacement: 0.5-0.75 mg/kg/day or 20-25 mg/m²/day in divided doses every 8 hours
Adults: 20-300 mg/day divided every 12-24 hours

Administration Oral: Administer with meals, food, or milk to decrease GI effects

Monitoring Parameters Long-term use: Electrolytes, glucose, blood pressure, height, weight

Test Interactions May suppress the wheal and flare reactions to skin test antigens

Additional Information Insoluble in water

Dosage Forms Excipient information presented when available (limited, particularly for generics); consult specific product labeling.
Tablet, Oral, as acetate:
  Generic: 25 mg

References

Bae YS, Van Voorhees AS, Hsu S, et al, "Review of Treatment Options For Psoriasis in Pregnant or Lactating Women: From the Medical Board of the National Psoriasis Foundation," J Am Acad Dermatol, 2012, 67(3):459-77.

Lam DS, Fan DS, Ng JS, et al, "Ocular Hypertensive and Anti-Inflammatory Responses to Different Dosages of Topical Dexamethasone in Children: A Randomized Trial," Clin Experiment Ophthalmol, 2005, 33 (3):252-8.

Leachman SA and Reed BR, "The Use of Dermatologic Drugs in Pregnancy and Lactation," Dermatol Clin, 2006, 24(2):167-97, vi.

Leonard MB, "Glucocorticoid-Induced Osteoporosis in Children: Impact of the Underlying Disease," Pediatrics, 2007, 119 Suppl 2:S166-74.

Lunghi L, Pavan B, Biondi C, et al, "Use of Glucocorticoids in Pregnancy," Curr Pharm Des, 2010, 16(32):3616-37.

Makol A, Wright K, and Amin S, "Rheumatoid Arthritis and Pregnancy: Safety Considerations in Pharmacological Management," Drugs, 2011, 71(15):1973-87.

Migeon CJ, Bertrand J, and Wall PE, "Physiological Disposition of 4-C14-Cortisol During Late Pregnancy," J Clin Invest, 1957, 36 (9):1350-62.

Østensen M and Forger F, "Management of RA Medications in Pregnant Patients," Nat Rev Rheumatol, 2009, 5(7):382-90.

Ost L, Wettrell G, Bjorkhem I, et al, "Prednisolone Excretion in Human Milk," J Pediatr, 1985, 106(6):1008-11.

Park-Wyllie L, Mazzotta P, Pastuszak A, et al, "Birth defects After Maternal Exposure to Corticosteroids: Prospective Cohort Study and Meta-Analysis of Epidemiological Studies," Teratology, 2000, 62 (6):385-92.

Pradat P, Robert-Gnansia E, Di Tanna GL, et al, "First Trimester Exposure to Corticosteroids and Oral Clefts," Birth Defects Res A Clin Mol Teratol, 2003, 67(12):968-70.

◆ **Cortisone Acetate** see Cortisone on page 548

◆ **Cortisporin** see Neomycin, Polymyxin B, and Hydrocortisone on page 1485

◆ **Cortisporin® Ointment** see Bacitracin, Neomycin, Polymyxin B, and Hydrocortisone on page 258

◆ **Cortisporin Otic (Can)** see Neomycin, Polymyxin B, and Hydrocortisone on page 1485

◆ **Cortisporin® Topical Ointment (Can)** see Bacitracin, Neomycin, Polymyxin B, and Hydrocortisone on page 258

◆ **Cortomycin** see Neomycin, Polymyxin B, and Hydrocortisone on page 1485

◆ **Cortrosyn** see Cosyntropin on page 549

◆ **CO Sertraline (Can)** see Sertraline on page 1879

◆ **CO Sildenafil (Can)** see Sildenafil on page 1884

◆ **CO Simvastatin (Can)** see Simvastatin on page 1892

◆ **Cosmegen** see DACTINomycin on page 580

◆ **CO Sotalol (Can)** see Sotalol on page 1925

◆ **CO Sumatriptan (Can)** see SUMAtriptan on page 1958

Cosyntropin (koe sin TROE pin)

Medication Safety Issues
Sound-alike/look-alike issues:
Cortrosyn® may be confused with colchicine, corticorelin, corticotropin, Cotazym®
Cosyntropin may be confused with corticorelin, corticotropin

Brand Names: U.S. Cortrosyn

Brand Names: Canada Cortrosyn; Synacthen Depot

Therapeutic Category Adrenal Corticosteroid; Diagnostic Agent, Adrenocortical Insufficiency

Generic Availability (U.S.) Yes

Use Diagnostic test to differentiate primary adrenal from secondary (pituitary) adrenocortical insufficiency [FDA approved in pediatric patients (age not specified) and adults]; has also been used in the diagnosis of congenital adrenal hyperplasia

Pregnancy Risk Factor C

Pregnancy Considerations Animal reproduction studies have not been conducted with cosyntropin; adverse events have been observed with corticosteroids in animal reproduction studies. Some studies have shown an association between first trimester systemic corticosteroid use and oral clefts (Park-Wyllie, 2000; Pradat, 2003). Systemic corticosteroids may also influence fetal growth (decreased birth weight); however, information is conflicting (Lunghi, 2010). When systemic corticosteroids are needed in pregnancy, it is generally recommended to use the lowest effective dose for the shortest duration of time, avoiding high doses during the first trimester (Leachman, 2006; Lunghi, 2010; Makol, 2011; Østensen, 2009).

Breast-Feeding Considerations It is not known if cosyntropin is excreted into breast milk. The manufacturer recommends that caution be exercised when administering cosyntropin to nursing women.

Contraindications Hypersensitivity to cosyntropin or any component

Precautions Use with caution in patients with preexisting allergic disease or a history of allergic reactions to corticotropin

Adverse Reactions Note: Adverse events associated with other corticosteroids may be observed when Synacthen Depot [Canadian product] is used for therapeutic purposes. Refer to corticosteroid monographs for comprehensive lists.

Cardiovascular: Bradycardia, hypertension, peripheral edema, tachycardia

Dermatologic: Rash

Local: Whealing with redness at the injection site

Miscellaneous: Anaphylaxis, hypersensitivity reaction

Rare but important or life-threatening: Synacthen Depot [Canadian product]: Adrenal hemorrhage

Drug Interactions

Metabolism/Transport Effects None known.

Avoid Concomitant Use

Avoid concomitant use of Cosyntropin with any of the following: Valproic Acid and Derivatives

Increased Effect/Toxicity

Cosyntropin may increase the levels/effects of: ClonazePAM; Diazepam; Nitrazepam; PHENobarbital; Phenytoin; Primidone; Valproic Acid and Derivatives

Decreased Effect There are no known significant interactions involving a decrease in effect.

Stability

Powder for injection: Store at controlled room temperature of 15°C to 30°C (59°F to 86°F).

I.V. infusion: Stable for 12 hours at room temperature.

Solution for injection: Store refrigerated between 2°C to 8°C (36°F to 46°F); protect from light and freezing.

I.V. infusion: Stable for 12 hours at room temperature.

Suspension for injection: Synacthen® Depot (Canadian availability): Store refrigerated between 2°C to 8°C (36°F to 46°F); protect from light.

Mechanism of Action Stimulates the adrenal cortex to secrete adrenal steroids (including hydrocortisone, cortisone), androgenic substances, and a small amount of aldosterone

Pharmacodynamics

Onset of action: I.M., I.V.: Within 5 minutes increases in plasma cortisol concentrations are observed in healthy individuals

Maximum effect: I.M., I.V.: 45-60 minutes peak plasma cortisol concentration

Dosing: Neonatal Adrenocortical insufficiency, diagnostic test: Note: Cosyntropin injection solution formulation is not recommended for I.M. administration; use powder for injection formulation.

Preterm neonates: Limited data available; reported range: I.M., I.V.: 0.1-3.5 **mcg**/kg/dose. In 276 ELBW neonates, a dose of 1 **mcg**/kg was found to be superior to 0.1 **mcg**/kg in assessing adrenal function; in addition, the 0.1 **mcg**/kg/dose given I.M. produced a significantly lower response than when given I.V. (mean GA: 25.5 weeks; mean birth weight: 743 g) (Watterberg, 2005). Physiologic doses of 0.1 **mcg**/kg were used to test adrenal function in VLBW neonates [mean birth weight 900 g; mean GA: 27 weeks (range: 23-32 weeks)]; only 36% of neonates responded; increasing the dose to 0.2 **mcg**/kg resulted in 67% of the neonates responding, but sensitivity of the test was decreased (Korte, 1996). Doses of 3.5 **mcg**/kg were administered to test adrenal function in 44 preterm neonates (mean birth weight: 823 g; mean GA: 26.2 weeks; mean postmenstrual age: 30.1 weeks) during inhaled beclomethasone therapy (Cole, 1999).

Full-term neonates: I.M., I.V.: 15 **mcg**/kg/dose

Dosing: Usual

Infants, Children, and Adolescents:

Adrenocortical insufficiency, diagnostic test: Note: Cosyntropin injection solution formulation is not recommended for I.M. administration; use powder for injection formulation.

Infants and Children ≤2 years: I.M., I.V.:

Manufacturer's labeling: 0.125 mg

Alternate dosing: 15 **mcg**/kg

Children >2 years and Adolescents:

Manufacturer's labeling:

I.M., I.V.: 0.25 mg; **Note:** Doses in the range of 0.25-0.75 mg have been used in clinical studies; however, maximal response is seen with 0.25 mg dose

I.V. infusion: 0.25 mg administered over 6 hours (rate: 0.04 mg/hour); may be useful when greater cortisol stimulation required

Alternate dosing (low-dose): Children ≥5 years and Adolescents: I.V.: 1 **mcg** (Cemeroglu, 2011; Kazlauskaite, 2008)

Congenital adrenal hyperplasia, evaluation: Infants and Children: I.M., I.V.: 0.125-0.25 mg (Speiser, 2010)

Adults: **Adrenocortical insufficiency, diagnostic test: Note:** Cosyntropin injection solution formulation is not recommended for I.M. administration; use powder for injection formulation.

Conventional dose: I.M., I.V.: 0.25 mg; **Note:** Doses in the range of 0.25-0.75 mg have been used in clinical studies; however, maximal response is seen with 0.25 mg dose

I.V. infusion: 0.25 mg administered over 6 hours (rate: 0.04 mg/hour); may be useful when greater cortisol stimulation required

Low-dose protocol: I.M., I.V.: 1 **mcg** (Abdu, 1999); **Note:** The use of the low-dose protocol has been advocated by some clinicians, particularly in mild or secondary adrenal insufficiency. The low-dose protocol is not recommended in critically ill patients (Marik, 2008).

Administration Parenteral: For powder for injection, reconstitute vial with 1 mL NS (concentration: 0.25 mg/mL); visually inspect solution for discoloration and particulate matter prior to injection. Contains no preservatives; discard unused portion of vial after use.

I.M.:

Powder for injection: Administer as 0.25 mg/mL concentration

Injection solution: Not recommended for I.M. administration per manufacturer

I.V.:

I.V. push: For standard doses, administer dose in 2-5 mL of NS over 2 minutes. For low doses, cosyntropin 1 **mcg**/mL (final volume: 1 mL) and 0.5 **mcg**/mL (final volume: 2 mL) have been reported (Abdu, 1999; Cemeroglu, 2011).

I.V. infusion: Dilute dose in D_5W or NS; infuse over 4-8 (~0.04 mg/hour over 6 hours)

Reference Range Plasma cortisol concentrations should be measured immediately before and exactly 30 minutes after the dose; dose should be given in the early morning; normal morning baseline cortisol >5 mcg/dL (SI: >138 nmol/L); normal response 30 minutes after cosyntropin injection: an increase in serum cortisol concentration of ≥7 mcg/dL (SI: ≥193 nmol/L) or peak response >18 mcg/dL (SI: >497 nmol/L). If increase in plasma cortisol levels at 30 minutes is equivocal, consider repeat cortisol sampling at 60 and/or 90 minutes.

Test Interactions Concurrent or recent use of spironolactone, hydrocortisone, cortisone, etomidate, estrogens

Additional Information Each 0.25 mg of cosyntropin is equivalent to 25 units of corticotropin.

Dosage Forms Excipient information presented when available (limited, particularly for generics); consult specific product labeling.

Solution, Intravenous:
Generic: 0.25 mg/mL (1 mL)
Solution Reconstituted, Injection:
Cortrosyn: 0.25 mg (1 ea)
Generic: 0.25 mg (1 ea)
Solution Reconstituted, Injection [preservative free]:
Generic: 0.25 mg (1 ea)

References

Abdu TA, Elhadd TA, Neary R, et al, "Comparison of the Low Dose Short Synacthen Test (1 Microg), the Conventional Dose Short Synacthen Test (250 Microg), and the Insulin Tolerance Test for Assessment of the Hypothalamo-Pituitary-Adrenal Axis in Patients With Pituitary Disease," *J Clin Endocrinol Metab*, 1999, 84(3):838-43.

Cemeroglu AP, Kleis L, Postellon DC, et al, "Comparison of Low-Dose and High-Dose Cosyntropin Stimulation Testing in Children," *Pediatr Int*, 2011, 53(2):175-80.

Cole CH, Shah B, Abbasi S, et al, "Adrenal Function in Premature Infants During Inhaled Beclomethasone Therapy," *J Pediatr*, 1999, 135(1):65-70.

Kazlauskaite R, Evans AT, Villabona CV, et al, "Corticotropin Tests for Hypothalamic-Pituitary-Adrenal Insufficiency: A Metaanalysis," *J Clin Endocrinol Metab*, 2008, 93(11):4245-53.

Korte C, Styne D, Merritt TA, et al, "Adrenocortical Function in the Very Low Birth Weight Infant: Improved Testing Sensitivity and Association With Neonatal Outcome," *J Pediatr*, 1996, 128(2):257-63.

Leachman SA and Reed BR, "The Use of Dermatologic Drugs in Pregnancy and Lactation," *Dermatol Clin*, 2006, 24(2):167-97, vi.

Lunghi L, Pavan B, Biondi C, et al, "Use of Glucocorticoids in Pregnancy," *Curr Pharm Des*, 2010, 16(32):3616-37.

Makol A, Wright K, and Amin S, "Rheumatoid Arthritis and Pregnancy: Safety Considerations in Pharmacological Management," *Drugs*, 2011, 71(15):1973-87.

Marik PE, Pastores SM, Annane D, et al, "Recommendations for the Diagnosis and Management of Corticosteroid Insufficiency in Critically Ill Adult Patients: Consensus Statements From an International Task Force by the American College of Critical Care Medicine," *Crit Care Med*, 2008, 36(6):1937-49.

Østensen M and Forger F, "Management of RA Medications in Pregnant Patients," *Nat Rev Rheumatol*, 2009, 5(7):382-90.

Park-Wyllie L, Mazzotta P, Pastuszak A, et al, "Birth defects After Maternal Exposure to Corticosteroids: Prospective Cohort Study and Meta-Analysis of Epidemiological Studies," *Teratology*, 2000, 62 (6):385-92.

Pradat P, Robert-Gnansia E, Di Tanna GL, et al, "First Trimester Exposure to Corticosteroids and Oral Clefts," *Birth Defects Res A Clin Mol Teratol*, 2003, 67(12):968-70.

Speiser PW, Azziz R, Baskin LS, et al, "Congenital Adrenal Hyperplasia Due to Steroid 21-Hydroxylase Deficiency: An Endocrine Society Clinical Practice Guideline," *J Clin Endocrinol Metab*, 2010, 95 (9):4133-60.

Thaler LM and Blevins LS Jr, "The Low Dose (1-Microg) Adrenocorticotropin Stimulation Test in the Evaluation of Patients With Suspected Central Adrenal Insufficiency," *J Clin Endocrinol Metab*, 1998, 83 (8):2726-9.

Watterberg KL, Shaffer ML, Garland JS, et al, "Effect of Dose on Response to Adrenocorticotropin in Extremely Low Birth Weight Infants," *J Clin Endocrinol Metab*, 2005, 90(12):6380-5.

◆ **Cotazym (Can)** *see* Pancrelipase *on page 1591*

◆ **Co-Temozolomide (Can)** *see* Temozolomide *on page 1972*

◆ **CO Terbinafine (Can)** *see* Terbinafine (Systemic) *on page 1982*

◆ **CO Topiramate (Can)** *see* Topiramate *on page 2046*

◆ **Co-Trimoxazole** *see* Sulfamethoxazole and Trimethoprim *on page 1948*

◆ **Cough DM [OTC]** *see* Dextromethorphan *on page 636*

◆ **Cough Syrup [OTC]** *see* GuaiFENesin *on page 984*

◆ **Coumadin** *see* Warfarin *on page 2156*

◆ **Coumadin® (Can)** *see* Warfarin *on page 2156*

◆ **CO Valacyclovir (Can)** *see* ValACYclovir *on page 2097*

◆ **CO Valsartan (Can)** *see* Valsartan *on page 2108*

◆ **CO Venlafaxine XR (Can)** *see* Venlafaxine *on page 2125*

◆ **Covera (Can)** *see* Verapamil *on page 2129*

◆ **Covera-HS (Can)** *see* Verapamil *on page 2129*

◆ **Co-Vidarabine** *see* Pentostatin *on page 1644*

◆ **Coviracil** *see* Emtricitabine *on page 738*

◆ **Cozaar** *see* Losartan *on page 1283*

◆ **CPDG2** *see* Glucarpidase *on page 972*

◆ **CPG2** *see* Glucarpidase *on page 972*

◆ **CPM** *see* Cyclophosphamide *on page 561*

◆ **CPT-11** *see* Irinotecan *on page 1149*

◆ **CPZ** *see* ChlorproMAZINE *on page 450*

◆ **13-CRA** *see* ISOtretinoin *on page 1161*

◆ **Creomulsion Adult [OTC]** *see* Dextromethorphan *on page 636*

◆ **Creomulsion for Children [OTC]** *see* Dextromethorphan *on page 636*

◆ **Creon** *see* Pancrelipase *on page 1591*

◆ **Crestor** *see* Rosuvastatin *on page 1853*

◆ **Critic-Aid Clear AF [OTC]** *see* Miconazole (Topical) *on page 1410*

◆ **Critic-Aid Skin Care® [OTC]** *see* Zinc Oxide *on page 2176*

◆ **Crixivan** *see* Indinavir *on page 1093*

◆ **Crixivan® (Can)** *see* Indinavir *on page 1093*

◆ **CroFab** *see* Crotalidae Polyvalent Immune Fab (Ovine) *on page 553*

◆ **Crolom** *see* Cromolyn (Ophthalmic) *on page 553*

◆ **Cromoglicate** *see* Cromolyn (Nasal) *on page 553*

◆ **Cromoglicate** *see* Cromolyn (Ophthalmic) *on page 553*

◆ **Cromoglicate** *see* Cromolyn (Systemic, Oral Inhalation) *on page 551*

◆ **Cromoglycic Acid** *see* Cromolyn (Nasal) *on page 553*

◆ **Cromoglycic Acid** *see* Cromolyn (Ophthalmic) *on page 553*

◆ **Cromoglycic Acid** *see* Cromolyn (Systemic, Oral Inhalation) *on page 551*

Cromolyn (Systemic, Oral Inhalation)
(KROE moe lin)

Brand Names: U.S. Gastrocrom
Brand Names: Canada Nalcrom; Nu-Cromolyn; PMS-Sodium Cromoglycate
Therapeutic Category Antiasthmatic; Inhalation, Miscellaneous

Generic Availability (U.S.) Yes

Use

Nebulization: Prophylactic agent used for long-term (chronic) control of persistent asthma; **NOT** indicated for the relief of acute bronchospasm; also used for the prevention of allergen- or exercise-induced bronchospasm (**Note:** Cromolyn is not as effective as inhaled short-acting beta$_2$-agonists for exercise-induced bronchospasm; NAEPP, 2007)

Systemic: Mastocytosis, food allergy, and treatment of inflammatory bowel disease

Pregnancy Risk Factor B

Pregnancy Considerations Adverse events were not observed in animal reproduction studies. No data available on whether cromolyn crosses the placenta or clinical effects on the fetus. Available evidence suggests safe use during pregnancy.

Breast-Feeding Considerations No data available on whether cromolyn enters into breast milk or clinical effects on the infant. Use of cromolyn is not considered a contraindication to breast-feeding.

Contraindications Hypersensitivity to cromolyn or any component; primary treatment of status asthmaticus

Warnings Cromolyn is a prophylactic drug with no benefit for acute situations; rare but severe anaphylactic reactions can occur; discontinue if eosinophilic pneumonia occurs.

Precautions Use with caution and decrease dose in patients with renal and hepatic impairment; use with caution when tapering the dose or withdrawing the drug since symptoms may reoccur.

Oral cromolyn increased mortality in neonatal rats when administered at ~9 times the maximum recommended daily dose for infants, but not at ~3 times the maximum recommended daily dose; use of oral cromolyn in infants and children <2 years is not recommended and should be reserved for patients with severe mastocytosis in whom potential benefits clearly outweigh the risks.

Adverse Reactions

Cardiovascular: Angioedema, chest pain, edema, flushing, palpitation, premature ventricular contractions, tachycardia

Central nervous system: Anxiety, behavior changes, convulsions, depression, dizziness, fatigue, hallucinations, headache, irritability, insomnia, lethargy, migraine, nervousness, hypoesthesia, postprandial lightheadedness, psychosis

Dermatologic: Erythema, photosensitivity, pruritus, purpura, rash, urticaria

Gastrointestinal: Abdominal pain, constipation, diarrhea, dyspepsia, dysphagia, esophagospasm, flatulence, glossitis, nausea, stomatitis, vomiting

Genitourinary: Dysuria, urinary frequency

Hematologic: Neutropenia, pancytopenia, polycythemia

Hepatic: Liver function test abnormal

Local: Burning

Neuromuscular & skeletal: Arthralgia, leg weakness, leg stiffness, myalgia, paresthesia

Otic: Tinnitus

Respiratory: Dyspnea, pharyngitis

Miscellaneous: Lupus erythematosus

Drug Interactions

Metabolism/Transport Effects None known.

Avoid Concomitant Use There are no known interactions where it is recommended to avoid concomitant use.

Increased Effect/Toxicity There are no known significant interactions involving an increase in effect.

Decreased Effect There are no known significant interactions involving a decrease in effect.

Stability Protect from direct light and heat; nebulization solution is compatible with beta-agonists, anticholinergic solutions, acetylcysteine, and NS; incompatible with alkaline solutions and calcium and magnesium salts; store oral concentrate ampuls in foil pouch until ready for use

Mechanism of Action Prevents the mast cell release of histamine, leukotrienes, and slow-reacting substance of anaphylaxis by inhibiting degranulation after contact with antigens

Pharmacodynamics Not effective for immediate relief of symptoms in acute asthmatic attacks; must be used at regular intervals for 2-4 weeks to be effective; **Note:** Therapeutic response may occur within 2 weeks; however, a trial of 4-6 weeks may be needed to determine maximum benefits.

Pharmacokinetics (Adult data unless noted)

Absorption:

Oral: 0.5% to 2%

Inhalation: ~8% reaches lungs upon inhalation; well absorbed

Half-life: 80-90 minutes

Time to peak serum concentration: Within 15 minutes after inhalation

Elimination: Equally excreted unchanged in urine and feces (via bile); small amounts after inhalation are exhaled

Dosing: Usual

Inhalation, nebulization solution:

Chronic control of asthma: Children ≥2 years and Adults: Initial: 20 mg 4 times/day; usual dose: 20 mg 3-4 times/day; **Note:** Once control is achieved, taper frequency to the lowest effective dose (ie, 4 times/day to 3 times/day to twice daily)

Prevention of allergen- or exercise-induced bronchospasm: Children ≥2 years and Adults: Single dose of 20 mg; **Note:** Administer 10-15 minutes prior to exercise or allergen exposure but no longer than 1 hour before

NIH Asthma Guidelines (NAEPP, 2007): Children ≥2 years and Adults: 20 mg 4 times/day

Oral:

Systemic mastocytosis:

Neonates and Preterm Infants: Not recommended

Infants and Children <2 years: Not recommended; reserve use for patients with severe disease in whom potential benefits outweigh risks; 20 mg/kg/day in 4 divided doses; may increase in patients 6 months to 2 years of age if benefits not seen after 2-3 weeks; do not exceed 30 mg/kg/day

Children 2-12 years: 100 mg 4 times/day; not to exceed 40 mg/kg/day

Children >12 years and Adults: 200 mg 4 times/day

Food allergy and inflammatory bowel disease:

Infants and Children <2 years: Not recommended

Children 2-12 years: Initial dose: 100 mg 4 times/day; may double the dose if effect is not satisfactory within 2-3 weeks; not to exceed 40 mg/kg/day

Children >12 years and Adults: Initial dose: 200 mg 4 times/day; may double the dose if effect is not satisfactory within 2-3 weeks; up to 400 mg 4 times/day

Once desired effect is achieved, dose may be tapered to lowest effective dose

Administration Oral concentrate: Open ampul and squeeze contents into glass of water; stir well; administer at least 30 minutes before meals and at bedtime; do not mix with juice, milk, or food

Monitoring Parameters Asthma: Periodic pulmonary function tests; signs and symptoms of disease state when tapering dose

Additional Information The 2007 Expert Panel Report of the National Asthma Education and Prevention Program (NAEPP, 2007) does not recommend cromolyn for initial treatment of persistent asthma in children; inhaled corticosteroids are the preferred agents; cromolyn is considered an alternative medication for the treatment of mild persistent asthma in children. Reserve systemic use in children

<2 years of age for severe disease; avoid systemic use in premature infants.

Dosage Forms Excipient information presented when available (limited, particularly for generics); consult specific product labeling.

Concentrate, Oral, as sodium:
  Gastrocrom: 100 mg/5 mL (5 mL)
Concentrate, Oral, as sodium [preservative free]:
  Generic: 100 mg/5 mL (5 mL)
Nebulization Solution, Inhalation, as sodium:
  Generic: 20 mg/2 mL (2 mL)

References

National Asthma Education and Prevention Program (NAEPP), "Expert Panel Report 3 (EPR-3): Guidelines for the Diagnosis and Management of Asthma," *Clinical Practice Guidelines*, National Institutes of Health, National Heart, Lung, and Blood Institute, NIH Publication No. 08-4051, prepublication 2007; available at http://www.nhlbi.nih.gov/guidelines/asthma/asthgdln.htm.

Cromolyn (Nasal) (KROE moe lin)

Medication Safety Issues
  Sound-alike/look-alike issues:
    NasalCrom® may be confused with Nasacort®, Nasalide®
Brand Names: U.S. NasalCrom [OTC]
Brand Names: Canada Apo-Cromolyn Nasal Spray [OTC]; Rhinaris-CS Anti-Allergic Nasal Mist
Therapeutic Category Inhalation, Miscellaneous
Generic Availability (U.S.) Yes
Use Management of seasonal or perennial allergic rhinitis
Pregnancy Considerations Animal reproduction studies have not been conducted; however, studies in pregnant women have not shown signs of adverse effects or increased teratogenicity with use during pregnancy (Gilbert, 2005; Mazzotta, 1999).
Breast-Feeding Considerations Use of cromolyn is not considered a contraindication to breast-feeding (NAEPP, 2005).
Contraindications Hypersensitivity to cromolyn or any component
Adverse Reactions
Central nervous system: Headache
Gastrointestinal: Unpleasant taste
Respiratory: Coughing; hoarseness; increase in burning, irritation, sneezing, or stinging inside of nose; postnasal drip
Rare but important or life-threatening: Epistaxis
Drug Interactions
  Metabolism/Transport Effects None known.
  Avoid Concomitant Use There are no known interactions where it is recommended to avoid concomitant use.
  Increased Effect/Toxicity There are no known significant interactions involving an increase in effect.
  Decreased Effect There are no known significant interactions involving a decrease in effect.
Stability Protect from light.
Dosing: Usual Intranasal: Children ≥2 years and Adults: 1 spray in each nostril 3-4 times/day; maximum dose: 1 spray in each nostril 6 times/day
Administration Clear nasal passages by blowing nose prior to use.
Dosage Forms Excipient information presented when available (limited, particularly for generics); consult specific product labeling.
Aerosol Solution, Nasal, as sodium:
  NasalCrom: 5.2 mg/actuation (13 mL, 26 mL) [contains benzalkonium chloride, edetate disodium]
  Generic: 5.2 mg/actuation (26 mL)
References

Gilbert C, Mazzotta P, Loebstein R, et al, "Fetal Safety of Drugs Used in the Treatment of Allergic Rhinitis: A Critical Review," *Drug Saf*, 2005, 28(8):707-19.

Mazzotta P, Loebstein R, and Koren G, "Treating Allergic Rhinitis in Pregnancy. Safety Considerations," *Drug Saf*, 1999, 20(4):361-75.
NAEPP Working Group Report on "Managing Asthma During Pregnancy: Recommendations for Pharmacologic Treatment," National Institutes of Health, National Heart, Lung, and Blood Institute, NIH Publication No. 05-5236, March 2005. Available at http://www.nhlbi.nih.gov/health/prof/lung/asthma/astpreg/astpreg_full.pdf

Cromolyn (Ophthalmic) (KROE moe lin)

Brand Names: Canada Opticrom®
Generic Availability (U.S.) Yes
Use Vernal conjunctivitis, vernal keratoconjunctivitis, and vernal keratitis
Pregnancy Risk Factor B
Pregnancy Considerations Adverse events were not observed in animal reproduction studies.
Breast-Feeding Considerations Use of cromolyn is not considered a contraindication to breast-feeding.
Contraindications Hypersensitivity to cromolyn or any component
Precautions Patients should not wear contact lenses during treatment with ophthalmic solution.
Adverse Reactions
Ocular: Conjunctival injection, dryness around the eye, edema, eye irritation, immediate hypersensitivity reactions, itchy eyes, puffy eyes, rash, styes, watery eyes
Respiratory: Dyspnea
Drug Interactions
  Metabolism/Transport Effects None known.
  Avoid Concomitant Use There are no known interactions where it is recommended to avoid concomitant use.
  Increased Effect/Toxicity There are no known significant interactions involving an increase in effect.
  Decreased Effect There are no known significant interactions involving a decrease in effect.
Stability Protect from light.
Pharmacokinetics (Adult data unless noted)
Half-life: 80-90 minutes
Elimination: Equally excreted unchanged in urine and feces (via bile)
Dosing: Usual Ophthalmic: Children >4 years and Adults: Instill 1-2 drops 4-6 times/day
Dosage Forms Excipient information presented when available (limited, particularly for generics); consult specific product labeling.
Solution, Ophthalmic, as sodium:
  Generic: 4% (10 mL)

◆ **Cromolyn Sodium** see Cromolyn (Nasal) *on page 553*
◆ **Cromolyn Sodium** see Cromolyn (Ophthalmic) *on page 553*
◆ **Cromolyn Sodium** see Cromolyn (Systemic, Oral Inhalation) *on page 551*

Crotalidae Polyvalent Immune Fab (Ovine) (kroe TAL ih die pol i VAY lent i MYUN fab (oh vine))

Brand Names: U.S. CroFab
Therapeutic Category Antivenin
Generic Availability (U.S.) No
Use Management of patients with North American crotalid envenomations [eg, rattlesnakes (*Crotalus, Sistrurus*), copperheads, and cottonmouth/water moccasins (*Agkistrodon*)] [FDA approved in pediatric patients (age not specified) and adults]
Pregnancy Risk Factor C
Pregnancy Considerations Animal reproduction studies have not been conducted. Products contain thimerosal which may be associated with mercury-related toxicities, including neurological and renal toxicities in the fetus and very young children. In general, medications used as ▶

antidotes should take into consideration the health and prognosis of the mother; antidotes should be administered to pregnant women if there is a clear indication for use and should not be withheld because of fears of teratogenicity (Bailey, 2003).

Breast-Feeding Considerations It is not known if this product is excreted into breast milk. The manufacturer recommends caution be used if administered to a nursing woman.

Contraindications Hypersensitivity to *Crotalidae* Polyvalent Immune Fab (Ovine) or any component, including papaya or papain, unless the benefits outweigh the risks and appropriate management for anaphylaxis is readily available

Warnings Coagulopathy, characterized by decreased fibrinogen, decreased platelets, and elevated prothrombin time, may recur following treatment with CroFab® possibly due to leaching of retained venom at the envenomation site; reported incidence ~50% in clinical trials; repeat dosing may be necessary. Recurrent coagulopathy may persist for 1-2 weeks or longer and may require repeat dosing (Miller, 2010; Ruha, 2011); typically reported in patients who experienced coagulopathy during the initial treatment, but may occur in any patient; consider additional monitoring for at least 1 week following initial treatment and evaluate for other preexisting conditions associated with bleeding disorders.

Anaphylaxis and anaphylactoid reactions are possible due to sheep proteins in the antivenin. Immediate treatment (including epinephrine 1:1000) for anaphylactoid and/or hypersensitivity reactions should be available prior to administration. Incidence of acute hypersensitivity reactions may be lower than previously thought (Buchanan, 2009; Cannon, 2008; Lavonas, 2011). This product lacks the immunogenic Fc fragments and proteins found in the older equine-derived product. Sensitization to proteins may occur; use caution when administering repeat courses for subsequent envenomations.

Contains thimerosal (0.03 mg of mercury per vial; maximum dose of 18 vials would deliver ≤0.6 mg mercury); accumulation of thimerosal has been associated with neurological and renal toxicity; developing fetuses and young children are most susceptible; the presence of thimerosal should not deter use as the risks of untreated crotalid envenomations far outweigh the risk of thimerosal exposure.

Precautions Use caution in patients with allergies to papaya, other papaya extracts, papain, chymopapain, or the pineapple-enzyme bromelain since papain is used in the manufacturing process; may also have cross allergenicity with dust mite and latex allergens.

Adverse Reactions
Cardiovascular: Hypotension
Central nervous system: Chills, fever
Dermatologic: Pruritus, rash, urticaria
Gastrointestinal: Anorexia, nausea
Respiratory: Asthma, cough, dyspnea, wheezing
Miscellaneous: Anaphylaxis, anaphylactoid reaction, hypersensitivity reactions, serum sickness
Rare but important or life-threatening: Angioedema, chest discomfort, dizziness, erythema, headache, hyperhidrosis, lip swelling, musculoskeletal chest pain, tachycardia, tachypnea, tongue swelling, tracheal edema

Drug Interactions
Avoid Concomitant Use There are no known interactions for which it is recommended to avoid concomitant use.

Increased Effect/Toxicity There are no known significant interactions involving an increase in effect.

Decreased Effect There are no known significant interactions involving a decrease in effect.

Stability Store between 2°C to 8°C (36°F to 46°F); do not freeze; use within 4 hours of reconstitution.

Mechanism of Action A venom-specific fragment of IgG, which binds and neutralizes venom toxin, helping to remove the toxin from the target tissue and eliminate it from the body.

Pharmacodynamics Onset of action: Stability of patient or reduction in symptoms may be seen within 1 hour of administration

Pharmacokinetics (Adult data unless noted)
Distribution: V_d: Unbound Fab: 110 mL/kg (Seifert, 2001)
Half-life: 12-23 hours (based on limited data)
Elimination: Speculated to occur via reticuloendothelial system (Dart, 1997)
Clearance: Unbound Fab: 5.9 mL/h/kg (Seifert, 2001)

Dosing: Usual I.V.: Children, Adolescents, and Adults: **Note:** Antivenom dosage is based on venom load and severity of symptoms and not on patient size; therefore, a reduced, weight-based antivenom dose in pediatric patients is **not** recommended (Behm, 2003; Lavonas, 2011a; Offerman, 2002). Clinicians are encouraged to contact their local poison control center or clinical toxicologist for consultation when treating any envenomed patient.

Crotalid envenomation:
Initial dose: 4-6 vials as soon as possible and ideally within 6 hours of snakebite; monitor for 1 hour following infusion to determine if control of envenomation is achieved (arrest of local manifestations and normalization of coagulation studies and other systemic signs). If control is not achieved, repeat with additional dose of 4-6 vials until initial control is achieved. Some experts recommend doubling the initial dose in patients presenting with life-threatening symptoms such as respiratory distress, cardiovascular collapse, significant hemorrhage, or severe neurologic toxicity (Goto, 2009; Lavonas, 2011a).
Maintenance dose (begin once control of envenomation achieved): 2 vials every 6 hours for up to 18 hours. Optimal dosing beyond 18 hours has not been established; however, treatment may be continued if deemed necessary based on patient condition.

Administration Reconstitute each vial with 18 mL NS and mix by continuous manual inversion until no solid material is visible. Do not shake. A faster dissolution has been shown using 25 mL SWI for reconstitution and hand rolling/inverting which may allow for more rapid administration (Quan, 2010). After reconstitution, further dilute **total** dose (4-6 vials) in 250 mL NS; lower infusion volumes may be considered for patients <10 kg or fluid sensitive patients, such as those with congestive heart failure, chronic lung disease, or renal insufficiency (Goto, 2009; Johnson, 2008; Offerman, 2002; Pizon, 2007). Administer I.V. at an initial rate of 25-50 mL/hour for the first 10 minutes; if tolerated and no allergic reaction observed, then increase rate so that total dose infuses over 60 minutes, usually to 250 mL/hour. Continue to monitor closely. Epinephrine and diphenhydramine should be available during the infusion. Decreasing the rate of infusion may help control some adverse effects, such as fever, nausea, low back pain, and wheezing.

Monitoring Parameters Vital signs; CBC, platelet count, prothrombin time, aPTT, fibrinogen levels, fibrin split products, clot retraction, bleeding and coagulation times, BUN, electrolytes, bilirubin; size of bite area (repeat every 15-30 minutes); intake and output; signs and symptoms of anaphylaxis/allergy. CBC, platelet counts, and clotting studies should be evaluated at 6-hour intervals until patient is stable.

Additional Information Envenomation Category:
Minimal: Swelling, pain, and bruising are limited to immediate bite site; no systemic signs and symptoms; normal coagulation parameters; no clinical evidence of bleeding

Moderate: Swelling, pain, and bruising are limited to less than a full extremity (or <50 cm if bite was on head or trunk); systemic signs and symptoms are not life-threatening (nausea, vomiting, oral paresthesia, unusual taste, mild hypotension, mild tachycardia, tachypnea); coagulation parameters may be abnormal; no bleeding other than minor hematuria, gum bleeding, or nosebleeds, if not severe

Severe: Swelling, pain, and bruising involve more than the entire extremity or threaten the airway; systemic signs and symptoms are markedly abnormal (severe alteration of mental status, severe hypotension, severe tachycardia, tachypnea, respiratory insufficiency); coagulation parameters are abnormal; serious bleeding or severe threat of bleeding

Dosage Forms Excipient information presented when available (limited, particularly for generics); consult specific product labeling.

Solution Reconstituted, Intravenous:
CroFab: (1 ea) [contains thimerosal]

References

Bailey B, "Are There Teratogenic Risks Associated With Antidotes Used in the Acute Management of Poisoned Pregnant Women?" *Birth Defects Res A Clin Mol Teratol*, 2003, 67(2):133-40.

Behm MO and Kearns GL, "Crotaline Fab Antivenom for Treatment of Children With Rattlesnake Envenomation," *Pediatrics*, 2003, 112(6 Pt 1):1458-9.

Buchanan JA, Varney SM, Mlynarchek SL, et al, "Immediate Adverse Events (AEs) After Administration of Crotalidae Polyvalent Immune Fab (Fav AV)," *Clin Toxicol*, 2009, 47(7):703.

Cannon R, Ruha AM, and Kashani J, "Acute Hypersensitivity Reactions Associated With Administration of Crotalidae Polyvalent Immune Fab Antivenom," *Ann Emerg Med*, 2008, 51(4):407-11.

Dart RC, Seifert SA, Carroll L, et al, "Affinity-Purified, Mixed Monospecific Crotalid Antivenom Ovine Fab for the Treatment of Crotalid Venom Poisoning," *Ann Emerg Med*, 1997, 30(1):33-9.

Goto CS and Feng SY, "Crotalidae Polyvalent Immune Fab for the Treatment of Pediatric Crotaline Envenomation," *Pediatr Emer Care* 2009, 25(4):273-82.

Johnson PN, McGoodwin L, and Banner W Jr, "Utilisation of Crotalidae Polyvalent Immune Fab (Ovine) for Viperidae Envenomations in Children," *Emerg Med J*, 2008, 25(12):793-8.

Lavonas EJ, Kokko J, Schaeffer TH, et al, "Short-Term Outcomes After Fab Antivenom Therapy for Severe Crotaline Snakebite," *Ann Emerg Med*, 2011, 579(2):128-37.

Lavonas EJ, Ruha AM, Banner W, et al, "Unified Treatment Algorithm for the Management of Crotaline Snakebite in the United States: Results of an Evidence-Informed Consensus Workshop," *BMC Emerg Med*, 2011a, 11:2.

Miller AD, Young MC, DeMott MC, et al, "Recurrent Coagulopathy and Thrombocytopenia in Children Treated With Crotalidae Polyvalent Immune Fab: A Case Series," *Pediatr Emerg Care*, 2010, 26 (8):576-82.

Offerman SR, Bush SP, Moynihan JA, et al, "Crotaline Fab Antivenom for the Treatment of Children With Rattlesnake Envenomation," *Pediatrics*, 2002, 110(5):968-71.

Pizon AF, Riley BD, LoVecchio F, et al, "Safety and Efficacy of Crotalidae Polyvalent Immune Fab in Pediatric Crotaline Envenomations," *Acad Emerg Med*, 2007, 14(4):373-6.

Quan AN, Quan D, and Curry SC, "Improving Crotalidae Polyvalent Immune Fab Reconstitution Times," *Am J Emerg Med*, 2010, 28 (5):593-5.

Ruha AM, Curry SC, Albrecht C, et al, "Late Hematologic Toxicity Following Treatment of Rattlesnake Envenomation With Crotalidae Polyvalent Immune Fab Antivenom," *Toxicon*, 2011, 57(1):53-9.

Seifert SA and Boyer LV, "Recurrence Phenomena After Immunoglobulin Therapy for Snake Envenomations: Part 1. Pharmacokinetics and Pharmacodynamics of Immunoglobulin Antivenoms and Related Antibodies," *Ann Emerg Med*, 2001, 37(2):189-95.

◆ **Crotaline Antivenin, Polyvalent, FAB (Ovine)** *see Crotalidae* Polyvalent Immune Fab (Ovine) *on page 553*

◆ **Crotaline Antivenom, Polyvalent, FAB (Ovine)** *see Crotalidae* Polyvalent Immune Fab (Ovine) *on page 553*

Crotamiton (kroe TAM i tonn)

Medication Safety Issues
Sound-alike/look-alike issues:
Eurax® may be confused with Efudex®, Eulexin, Evoxac®, Serax, Urex
International issues:
Eurax [U.S., Canada, and multiple international markets] may be confused with Urex brand name for furosemide [Australia, China,Turkey] and methenamine [U.S., Canada]

Brand Names: U.S. Eurax
Brand Names: Canada Eurax Cream
Therapeutic Category Scabicidal Agent
Generic Availability (U.S.) No
Use Treatment of scabies (*Sarcoptes scabiei*) in infants and children; symptomatic treatment of pruritic skin
Pregnancy Risk Factor C
Pregnancy Considerations Animal reproduction studies have not been conducted; use during pregnancy only if clearly needed.
Breast-Feeding Considerations It is not known if crotamiton is excreted in breast milk.
Contraindications Hypersensitivity to crotamiton or any component; patients who manifest a primary irritation response to topical medications
Precautions Avoid contact with face, eyes, mucous membranes, and urethral meatus; do not apply to acutely inflamed or raw skin
Adverse Reactions
Dermatologic: Contact dermatitis, pruritus, rash
Local: Local irritation
Miscellaneous: Allergic sensitivity reactions, warm sensation
Drug Interactions
Metabolism/Transport Effects None known.
Avoid Concomitant Use There are no known interactions where it is recommended to avoid concomitant use.
Increased Effect/Toxicity There are no known significant interactions involving an increase in effect.
Decreased Effect There are no known significant interactions involving a decrease in effect.
Stability Store at room temperature.
Mechanism of Action Crotamiton has scabicidal activity against *Sarcoptes scabiei*; mechanism of action unknown
Pharmacokinetics (Adult data unless noted) Absorption: Amount of systemic absorption following topical use has not been determined
Dosing: Usual Topical: Infants, Children, and Adults:
Scabicide: Apply over entire body below the head; apply once daily for 2 days followed by a cleansing bath 48 hours after the last application; treatment may be repeated after 7-10 days if mites reappear
Pruritus: Massage into affected areas until medication is completely absorbed; may repeat as necessary
Administration Topical: Wash thoroughly and scrub away loose scales, then towel dry; apply a thin layer and gently massage drug onto skin of the entire body from the neck to the toes (with special attention to skin folds, creases, and interdigital spaces); also apply cream or lotion under fingernails after trimming nails short; since scabies can affect the head, scalp, and neck in infants and young children, apply to scalp, neck, and body of this age group; do not apply to the face, eyes, mouth, mucous membranes, or urethral meatus; shake lotion well before use
Additional Information Treatment may be repeated after 7-10 days if live mites are still present
Dosage Forms Excipient information presented when available (limited, particularly for generics); consult specific product labeling.

Cream, External:
Eurax: 10% (60 g)
Lotion, External:
Eurax: 10% (60 g, 454 g)

References
Eichenfield LF, Honig PJ, "Blistering Disorders in Childhood," *Pediatr Clin North Am*, 1991, 38(4):959-76.
Hogan DJ, Schachner L, Tanglertsampan C, "Diagnosis and Treatment of Childhood Scabies and Pediculosis," *Pediatr Clin North Am*, 1991, 38(4):941-57.

◆ **Crude Coal Tar** see Coal Tar on page 532
◆ **Cruex Prescription Strength [OTC]** see Miconazole (Topical) on page 1410
◆ **Crystalline Penicillin** see Penicillin G (Parenteral/Aqueous) on page 1631
◆ **Crystal Violet** see Gentian Violet on page 968
◆ **Crystapen® (Can)** see Penicillin G (Parenteral/Aqueous) on page 1631
◆ **CsA** see CycloSPORINE (Ophthalmic) on page 569
◆ **CsA** see CycloSPORINE (Systemic) on page 564
◆ **C-Time [OTC]** see Ascorbic Acid on page 206
◆ **CTLA-4Ig** see Abatacept on page 44
◆ **CTM** see Chlorpheniramine on page 448
◆ **CTP 30 (Can)** see Citalopram on page 484
◆ **CTX** see Cyclophosphamide on page 561
◆ **Cu-5 [OTC]** see Copper on page 544
◆ **Cubicin** see DAPTOmycin on page 589
◆ **Culturelle® [OTC]** see Lactobacillus on page 1191
◆ **Cupric Chloride** see Copper on page 544
◆ **Cupric Chloride Dihydrate** see Copper on page 544
◆ **Cuprimine** see PenicillAMINE on page 1627
◆ **Cuprimine® (Can)** see PenicillAMINE on page 1627
◆ **Curosurf** see Poractant Alfa on page 1702
◆ **Curosurf® (Can)** see Poractant Alfa on page 1702
◆ **Cutar [OTC]** see Coal Tar on page 532
◆ **Cutivate** see Fluticasone (Topical) on page 915
◆ **Cutivate™ (Can)** see Fluticasone (Topical) on page 915
◆ **Cuvposa** see Glycopyrrolate on page 977
◆ **CyA** see CycloSPORINE (Ophthalmic) on page 569
◆ **CyA** see CycloSPORINE (Systemic) on page 564

Cyanocobalamin (sye an oh koe BAL a min)

Brand Names: U.S. Nascobal; Physicians EZ Use B-12
Therapeutic Category Nutritional Supplement; Vitamin, Water Soluble
Generic Availability (U.S.) Yes
Use Treatment of pernicious anemia; vitamin B_{12} deficiency due to dietary deficiencies or malabsorption diseases; inadequate secretion of intrinsic factor, inadequate utilization of B_{12} (eg, during neoplastic treatment); increased B_{12} requirements due to pregnancy, thyrotoxicosis, hemorrhage, malignancy, liver or kidney disease; nutritional supplement
Pregnancy Considerations Animal reproduction studies have not been conducted. Water soluble vitamins cross the placenta. Absorption of vitamin B_{12} may increase during pregnancy. Vitamin B_{12} requirements may be increased in pregnant women compared to nonpregnant women. Serum concentrations of vitamin B_{12} are higher in the neonate at birth than the mother (IOM, 1998).
Breast-Feeding Considerations Vitamin B_{12} is found in breast milk. Milk concentrations are similar to maternal serum concentrations and concentrations may be decreased in women who are vegetarians. Vitamin B_{12}

requirements may be increased in nursing women compared to non-nursing women (IOM, 1998).
Contraindications Hypersensitivity to cyanocobalamin, any component, or cobalt; patients with hereditary optic nerve atrophy (Leber's disease)
Warnings Only I.M./SubQ routes are used to treat pernicious anemia; oral and intranasal administration are not indicated until hematologic remission and there are no signs of nervous system involvement. Avoid the I.V. route as it has been associated with anaphylaxis. Vitamin B_{12} deficiency for >3 months results in irreversible degenerative CNS lesions; neurologic manifestations will not be prevented with folic acid unless vitamin B_{12} is also given; spinal cord degeneration might also occur when folic acid is used as a substitute for vitamin B_{12} in anemia prevention. Vegetarian diets may result in vitamin B_{12} deficiency.

Injection may contain benzyl alcohol which may cause allergic reactions in susceptible individuals; large amounts of benzyl alcohol (≥99 mg/kg/day) have been associated with a potentially fatal toxicity ("gasping syndrome") in neonates; the "gasping syndrome" consists of metabolic acidosis, respiratory distress, gasping respirations, CNS dysfunction (including convulsions, intracranial hemorrhage), hypotension and cardiovascular collapse; avoid use of benzyl alcohol containing injections in neonates; *in vitro* and animal studies have shown that benzoate, a metabolite of benzyl alcohol, displaces bilirubin from protein-binding sites.

Intranasal therapy is only for use in patients who are in remission following injectable treatment. Efficacy of intranasal treatment in patients with nasal pathology or with other concomitant intranasal therapy has not been determined. Patients with early Leber's disease (hereditary optic nerve atrophy) who were treated with vitamin B_{12} suffered severe and swift optic atrophy. These patients should not receive cyanocobalamin therapy.
Precautions Serum potassium concentrations and platelet counts should be monitored early as severe hypokalemia (sometimes fatal) and thrombocytosis have occurred after the conversion of megaloblastic anemia to normal erythropoiesis; an intradermal test dose of parenteral cyanocobalamin is recommended before initiating the nasal spray in patients suspected to be sensitive to cyanocobalamin. Vitamin B_{12} deficiency masks signs of polycythemia vera; use caution in other conditions where folic acid or vitamin B_{12} administration alone might mask true diagnosis despite hematologic response. The parenteral product may contain aluminum; toxic aluminum concentrations may be seen with high doses, prolonged use, or renal dysfunction. Premature neonates are at higher risk due to immature renal function and aluminum intake from other parenteral sources. Parenteral aluminum exposure of >4-5 mcg/kg/day is associated with CNS and bone toxicity and tissue loading may occur at lower doses.
Adverse Reactions
Cardiovascular: CHF, peripheral vascular disorder, peripheral vascular thrombosis
Central nervous system: Anxiety, dizziness, headache, hypoesthesia, incoordination, pain, nervousness
Dermatologic: Itching, urticaria, exanthema (transient)
Gastrointestinal: Diarrhea, dyspepsia, glossitis, nausea, sore throat, vomiting
Hematologic: Polycythemia vera
Neuromuscular & skeletal: Abnormal gait, arthritis, back pain, myalgia, paresthesia, weakness
Respiratory: Dyspnea, pulmonary edema, rhinitis
Miscellaneous: Anaphylaxis (parenteral) and infection
Drug Interactions
Metabolism/Transport Effects None known.
Avoid Concomitant Use There are no known interactions where it is recommended to avoid concomitant use.

Increased Effect/Toxicity There are no known significant interactions involving an increase in effect.

Decreased Effect

The levels/effects of Cyanocobalamin may be decreased by: Chloramphenicol; Colchicine

Food Interactions Heavy ethanol consumption >2 weeks may impair vitamin B_{12} absorption.

Stability Store at room temperature; protect from light

Mechanism of Action Coenzyme for various metabolic functions, including fat and carbohydrate metabolism and protein synthesis, used in cell replication and hematopoiesis

Pharmacodynamics Onset of action:

Megaloblastic anemia: I.M.:

Conversion of megaloblastic to normoblastic erythroid hyperplasia within bone marrow: 8 hours

Increased reticulocytes: 2-5 days

Complicated vitamin B_{12} deficiency: I.M., SubQ: Resolution of:

Psychiatric sequelae: 24 hours

Thrombocytopenia: 10 days

Granulocytopenia: 2 weeks

Pharmacokinetics (Adult data unless noted)

Absorption: Oral: Drug is absorbed from the terminal ileum in the presence of calcium; for absorption to occur, gastric "intrinsic factor" must be present to transfer the compound across the intestinal mucosa

Distribution: Principally stored in the liver, also stored in the kidneys and adrenals

Protein binding: Bound to transcobalamin II

Metabolism: Converted in the tissues to active coenzymes methylcobalamin and deoxyadenosylcobalamin

Bioavailability:

Oral: Pernicious anemia: 1.2%

Intranasal gel: 8.9% (relative to I.M. formulation)

Intranasal spray: Nascobal®: 6.1% (relative to I.M. formulation)

Time to peak serum concentration:

I.M., SubQ: 30 minutes to 2 hours

Intranasal: 1.6 hours

Elimination: 50% to 98% unchanged in the urine

Dosing: Neonatal

Adequate intake (AI): Oral, sublingual: 0.4 mcg/day (~0.05 mcg/kg/day); **Note:** Neonates born to vegan mothers should be supplemented with the AI for vitamin B_{12} from birth; they may have low vitamin B_{12} stores at birth and, if breast-feeding, may only receive a small amount of the vitamin from the mother's milk (Mangels, 2001).

Anemia of prematurity: I.M.: Limited data available; 100 mcg once monthly for 4 months with concomitant folic acid administration produced higher hemoglobin in 34 preterm neonates (GA <36 weeks; birth weight <1800 g) when compared to placebo or folate monotherapy; all patients received vitamin E and iron supplementation (Worthington-White, 1994).

Pernicious anemia; treatment of deficiency: Limited data available: I.M., SubQ: Initial: 1000 mcg/day for 2-7 days based upon clinical response; maintenance: 100 mcg/month; **Note:** For severe anemia, a lower initial dose of 0.2 mcg/kg/dose for 2 days followed by the above regimen has been recommended due to potential hypokalemia observed during initial treatment of adults with severe anemia; additional potassium supplementation may also be required (Rasmussen, 2001).

Dosing: Usual

Infants, Children, and Adolescents:

Adequate intake (AI): Oral, sublingual: **Note:** Neonates born to vegan mothers should be supplemented with the AI for vitamin B_{12} from birth; they may have low vitamin B_{12} stores at birth and, if breast-feeding, may

only receive a small amount of the vitamin from the mother's milk (Mangels, 2001).

Infants 1-6 months: 0.4 mcg/day (0.05 mcg/kg/day)

Infants 7-12 months: 0.5 mcg/day (0.05 mcg/kg/day)

Recommended daily allowance (RDA): Oral, Sublingual:

Children and Adolescents:

1-3 years: 0.9 mcg/day

4-8 years: 1.2 mcg/day

9-13 years: 1.8 mcg/day

Adolescents ≥14 years: 2.4 mcg/day

Pernicious anemia: Limited data available: I.M., SubQ: Initial: 1000 mcg/day for 2-7 days based upon clinical response; maintenance: 100 mcg/month; for severe anemia, a lower initial dose of 0.2 mcg/kg/dose for 2 days followed by the above regimen has been recommended; initial low dosage recommended due to potential hypokalemia observed during initial treatment of adults with severe anemia (Rasmussen, 2001). Concurrent folic acid supplementation may also be needed.

Vitamin B_{12} deficiency: Dosing regimens variable: I.M., SubQ: 1000 mcg/day for 2-7 days based upon clinical response followed by 100 mcg/week for a month; for severe deficiency, a lower initial dose of 0.2 mcg/kg/dose for 2 days followed by the above regimen has been recommended due to potential hypokalemia observed during initial treatment of adults with severe anemia; additional potassium supplementation may also be required (Rasmussen, 2001); for malabsorptive causes of B_{12} deficiency, monthly maintenance doses of 100 mcg have been recommended or as an alternative 100 mcg/day for 10-15 days (total dose of 1-1.5 mg), then once or twice weekly for several months; may taper to 60 mcg every month

Adults:

Recommended intake: 2.4 mcg/day

Pregnancy: 2.6 mcg/day

Lactation: 2.8 mcg/day

Pernicious anemia:

Manufacturer's labeling: I.M., deep SubQ: 100 mcg/day for 6-7 days; if improvement, give same dose on alternate days for 7 doses; then every 3-4 days for 2-3 weeks; once hematologic values have returned to normal, maintenance dosage: 100 mcg/month

Alternate dosing: I.M., deep SubQ: Initial: 1000 mcg/day for 5 days followed by 500-1000 mcg/month

Hematologic remission (without evidence of nervous system involvement):

I.M., SubQ: 100-1000 mcg/month

Intranasal (Nascobal®): 500 mcg (1 spray) in one nostril once weekly

Oral: 1000-2000 mcg/day

Vitamin B_{12} deficiency:

I.M., deep SubQ: Initial: 30 mcg/day for 5-10 days; maintenance: 100-200 mcg monthly

Intranasal (Nascobal®): 500 mcg (1 spray) in one nostril once weekly

Oral: 250 mcg/day

Administration

Intranasal: Nascobal® nasal spray: Prior to initial dose, activate (prime) spray nozzle by pumping unit quickly and firmly until first appearance of spray, then prime twice more. The unit must be reprimed once immediately before each use. Administer at least one hour before or after ingestion of hot foods or liquids; hot foods can cause nasal secretions and a resulting loss of medication

Oral: Not generally recommended for treatment of severe vitamin B_{12} deficiency due to poor oral absorption (lack of intrinsic factor); oral administration may be used in less severe deficiencies and maintenance therapy; may be administered without regard to food

Parenteral: I.M. or deep SubQ: Avoid I.V. administration due to a more rapid system elimination with resulting decreased utilization

Sublingual: Place under the tongue and allow to dissolve; do not swallow whole, chew, or crush

Monitoring Parameters Serum potassium (particularly during initial treatment of deficiency), erythrocyte and reticulocyte count, hemoglobin, hematocrit, platelets, serum cyanocobalamin and folate concentrations; methylmalonate (MMA) and total homocysteine (elevated in Vitamin B_{12} deficiency)

Reference Range Serum vitamin B_{12} levels: Normal: >300 pg/mL; vitamin B_{12} deficiency: <200 pg/mL (200-300 pg/mL borderline result, possible deficiency); megaloblastic anemia: <100 pg/mL

Test Interactions Methotrexate, pyrimethamine, and most antibiotics invalidate folic acid and vitamin B_{12} diagnostic blood assays

Product Availability Nascobal Nasal Spray single-use device: FDA approved June 2014; availability anticipated in September 2014. The device requires no priming or assembly and will replace the currently available multi-use product.

Dosage Forms Excipient information presented when available (limited, particularly for generics); consult specific product labeling.

Kit, Injection:
Physicians EZ Use B-12: 1000 mcg/mL [contains benzyl alcohol]

Liquid, Sublingual:
Generic: 3000 mcg/mL (52 mL)

Lozenge, Oral:
Generic: 50 mcg (100 ea); 100 mcg (100 ea); 250 mcg (100 ea, 250 ea); 500 mcg (100 ea, 250 ea)

Solution, Injection:
Generic: 1000 mcg/mL (1 mL, 10 mL, 30 mL)

Solution, Nasal:
Nascobal: 500 mcg/0.1 mL (1.3 mL) [contains benzalkonium chloride]

Tablet, Oral:
Generic: 100 mcg, 250 mcg, 500 mcg, 1000 mcg

Tablet, Oral [preservative free]:
Generic: 100 mcg, 500 mcg, 1000 mcg

Tablet Extended Release, Oral:
Generic: 1000 mcg

Tablet Sublingual, Sublingual:
Generic: 2500 mcg

Tablet Sublingual, Sublingual [preservative free]:
Generic: 2500 mcg

References

Department Health and Human Services, Food Drug Administration, "Aluminum in Large and Small Volume Parenterals Used in Total Parenteral Nutrition," *Federal Register,* 2000, 65(17):4103-11.

"Dietary Reference Intakes for Thiamin, Riboflavin, Niacin, Vitamin B_6, Folate, Vitamin B_{12}, Pantothenic Acid, Biotin, and Choline," (Chapter 9) available at http://books.nap.edu/openbook/0309065542/html/306.html. Last accessed February 22, 2005.

Lane LA and Rojas-Fernandez C, "Treatment of Vitamin B(12)-Deficiency Anemia: Oral Versus Parenteral Therapy," *Ann Pharmacother,* 2002, 36(7):1268-72.

Mangels AR and Messina V, "Considerations in Planning Vegan Diets: Infants," *J Am Diet Assoc,* 2001, 101(6):670-7.

Rasmussen SA, Fernhoff PM, and Scanlon KS, "Vitamin B_{12} Deficiency in Children and Adolescents," *J Pediatr,* 2001, 138(1):10-7.

Worthington-White DA, Behnke M, and Gross S, "Premature Infants Require Additional Folate and Vitamin B_{12} to Reduce the Severity of the Anemia of Prematurity," *Am J Clin Nutr,* 1994, 60(6):930-5.

◆ **Cyanokit** *see* Hydroxocobalamin *on page 1045*

Cyclobenzaprine (sye kloe BEN za preen)

Medication Safety Issues

Sound-alike/look-alike issues:
Cyclobenzaprine may be confused with cycloSERINE, cyproheptadine
Flexeril may be confused with Floxin

BEERS Criteria medication:
This drug may be potentially inappropriate for use in geriatric patients (Quality of evidence - moderate; Strength of recommendation - strong).

International issues:
Flexin: Brand name for cyclobenzaprine [Chile], but also the brand name for diclofenac [Argentina] and orphenadrine [Israel]

Flexin [Chile] may be confused with Floxin brand name for flunarizine [Thailand], norfloxacin [South Africa], ofloxacin [U.S., Canada], and perfloxacin [Philippines]; Fluoxine brand name for fluoxetine [Thailand]; Flexinol brand name for methocarbamol and paracetamol [India]

Related Information
Oral Medications That Should Not Be Crushed or Altered *on page 2438*

Brand Names: U.S. Active-Cyclobenzaprine; Amrix; EnovaRX-Cyclobenzaprine HCl; Fexmid

Brand Names: Canada Apo-Cyclobenzaprine; Auro-Cyclobenzaprine; Ava-Cyclobenzaprine; Dom-Cyclobenzaprine; JAMP-Cyclobenzaprine; Mylan-Cyclobenzaprine; Novo-Cycloprine; PHL-Cyclobenzaprine; PMS-Cyclobenzaprine; Q-Cyclobenzaprine; ratio-Cyclobenzaprine; Riva-Cycloprine; ZYM-Cyclobenzaprine

Therapeutic Category Skeletal Muscle Relaxant, Nonparalytic

Generic Availability (U.S.) May be product dependent

Use Treatment of muscle spasm associated with acute painful musculoskeletal conditions (immediate release tablets: FDA approved in ages ≥15 years and adults; extended release capsules: FDA approved in adults); has also been used for treatment of muscle spasm associated with acute temporomandibular joint pain (TMJ)

Pregnancy Risk Factor B

Pregnancy Considerations Adverse events have not been observed in animal reproduction studies. The manufacturer recommends avoiding use during pregnancy unless clearly needed.

Breast-Feeding Considerations It is not known if cyclobenzaprine is excreted in breast milk. The manufacturer recommends that caution be exercised when administering cyclobenzaprine to nursing women.

Contraindications Hypersensitivity to cyclobenzaprine or any component; hyperthyroidism; acute recovery phase of MI; CHF; arrhythmias; heart block or conduction disturbances; do not use concomitantly or within 14 days of MAO inhibitors

Warnings Not effective in the treatment of spasticity due to cerebral or spinal cord disease or in children with cerebral palsy; shares the toxic potentials of the tricyclic antidepressants, including prolongation of conduction time, arrhythmias, and tachycardia; the usual precautions of tricyclic antidepressant therapy should be observed; hyperpyretic crisis seizures and death have occurred when used in combination with MAO inhibitors

Precautions Use with caution in patients with urinary retention, angle-closure glaucoma, increased intraocular pressure, and patients receiving anticholinergic medications. Use with caution in patients with mild hepatic impairment; consider dosage reduction; avoid use in patients with moderate to severe hepatic dysfunction; extended release capsules not recommended in patients with hepatic impairment of any severity (mild, moderate, or severe). May cause CNS depression which may impair physical or mental abilities; patients must be cautioned about performing tasks which require mental alertness (eg, operating machinery or driving)

Adverse Reactions

Central nervous system: Confusion, decreased mental acuity, dizziness, drowsiness, fatigue, headache, irritability, nervousness

Gastrointestinal: Abdominal pain, acid regurgitation, constipation, diarrhea, dyspepsia, nausea, unpleasant taste, xerostomia

Neuromuscular & skeletal: Weakness

Ophthalmic: Blurred vision

Respiratory: Pharyngitis, upper respiratory tract infection

Rare but important or life-threatening: Anaphylaxis, angioedema, cardiac arrhythmia, convulsions, hepatitis (rare), hypertonia, hypotension, paresthesia, psychosis, seizure, serotonin syndrome, skin rash, syncope, tachycardia

Drug Interactions

Metabolism/Transport Effects Substrate of CYP1A2 (major), CYP2D6 (minor), CYP3A4 (minor); **Note:** Assignment of Major/Minor substrate status based on clinically relevant drug interaction potential

Avoid Concomitant Use

Avoid concomitant use of Cyclobenzaprine with any of the following: Aclidinium; Azelastine (Nasal); Ipratropium (Oral Inhalation); MAO Inhibitors; Paraldehyde; Potassium Chloride; Thalidomide; Tiotropium; Umeclidinium

Increased Effect/Toxicity

Cyclobenzaprine may increase the levels/effects of: AbobotulinumtoxinA; Alcohol (Ethyl); Analgesics (Opioid); Anticholinergic Agents; Antipsychotics; Azelastine (Nasal); Buprenorphine; Cannabinoid-Containing Products; CNS Depressants; Hydrocodone; MAO Inhibitors; Methotrimeprazine; Metoclopramide; Metyrosine; Mirabegron; OnabotulinumtoxinA; Paraldehyde; Potassium Chloride; Pramipexole; RimabotulinumtoxinB; ROPINIRole; Rotigotine; Serotonin Modulators; Thalidomide; Thiazide Diuretics; Tiotropium; Topiramate; TraMADol; Zolpidem

The levels/effects of Cyclobenzaprine may be increased by: Abiraterone Acetate; Aclidinium; Antiemetics (5HT3 Antagonists); Antipsychotics; Brimonidine (Topical); Cannabis; CYP1A2 Inhibitors (Moderate); CYP1A2 Inhibitors (Strong); Deferasirox; Doxylamine; Dronabinol; Droperidol; HydrOXYzine; Ipratropium (Oral Inhalation); Kava Kava; Magnesium Sulfate; Methotrimeprazine; Nabilone; Perampanel; Pramlintide; Rufinamide; Sodium Oxybate; Tapentadol; Tetrahydrocannabinol; Umeclidinium; Vemurafenib

Decreased Effect

Cyclobenzaprine may decrease the levels/effects of: Acetylcholinesterase Inhibitors (Central); Secretin

The levels/effects of Cyclobenzaprine may be decreased by: Acetylcholinesterase Inhibitors (Central); Peginterferon Alfa-2b

Food Interactions Food increases bioavailability (peak plasma concentrations increased by 35% and area under the curve by 20%) of the extended release capsule. Management: Monitor for increased effects if taken with food.

Stability Oral: Store at 20°C to 25°C (68°F to 77°F)

Amrix®, Flexeril®: Store at 25°C (77°F); excursions permitted to 15°C to 30°C (59°F to 86°F)

Mechanism of Action Centrally-acting skeletal muscle relaxant pharmacologically related to tricyclic antidepressants; reduces tonic somatic motor activity influencing both alpha and gamma motor neurons

Pharmacodynamics

Onset of action: Immediate release tablet: Within 1 hour

Duration: Immediate release tablet: 12-24 hours

Pharmacokinetics (Adult data unless noted)

Metabolism: Hepatic via CYP3A4, 1A2, and 2D6; may undergo enterohepatic recirculation

Bioavailability: 33% to 55%

Half-life: Normal hepatic function: Range: 8-37 hours; immediate release tablet: 18 hours; extended release capsule: 32 hours; impaired hepatic function: 46.2 hours (range: 22.4-188 hours) (Winchell, 2002)

Time to peak serum concentration: Immediate release tablet: ~4 hours (Winchell, 2002); extended release capsule: 7-8 hours

Elimination: Primarily renal as inactive metabolites and in the feces (via bile) as unchanged drug

Clearance: 0.7 L/minute

Dosing: Usual Oral: **Note:** Do not use longer than 2-3 weeks

Muscle spasm, treatment:

Adolescents ≥15 years: Immediate release tablet: 5 mg 3 times daily; may increase to 7.5-10 mg 3 times daily

Adults:

Immediate release tablet: 5 mg 3 times daily; may increase to 7.5-10 mg 3 times daily

Extended release capsule: 15 mg once daily; may increase to 30 mg once daily

Dosage adjustment in hepatic impairment:

Immediate release tablet:

Mild: 5 mg 3 times daily

Moderate to severe: Use not recommended

Extended release capsule: Mild to severe impairment: Use not recommended

Administration Oral:

Immediate release tablet: May be administered without regard to meals

Extended release capsule: Administer at the same time daily; do not crush or chew

Monitoring Parameters Relief of muscle spasms and pain; improvement in physical activities

Test Interactions May cause false-positive serum TCA screen (Wong, 1995)

Dosage Forms Considerations

EnovaRX-Cyclobenzaprine and Active-Cyclobenzaprine are compounding kits. Refer to manufacturer's package insert for compounding instructions.

Dosage Forms Excipient information presented when available (limited, particularly for generics); consult specific product labeling.

Capsule Extended Release 24 Hour, Oral, as hydrochloride:

Amrix: 15 mg

Amrix: 30 mg [contains brilliant blue fcf (fd&c blue #1), fd&c blue #2 (indigotine), fd&c red #40, fd&c yellow #6 (sunset yellow)]

Cream, Transdermal, as hydrochloride:

Active-Cyclobenzaprine: 5% (120 g) [contains chlorocresol (chloro-m-cresol)]

EnovaRX-Cyclobenzaprine HCl: 20 mg/g (120 g) [contains cetearyl alcohol]

Tablet, Oral, as hydrochloride:

Fexmid: 7.5 mg

Generic: 5 mg, 7.5 mg, 10 mg

References

Winchell GA, King JD, Chavez-Eng CM, et al, "Cyclobenzaprine Pharmacokinetics, Including the Effects of Age, Gender, and Hepatic Insufficiency," *J Clin Pharmacol*, 2002, 42(1):61-9.

◆ **Cyclobenzaprine Hydrochloride** *see* Cyclobenzaprine *on page 558*

◆ **Cyclogyl** *see* Cyclopentolate *on page 560*

◆ **Cyclogyl® (Can)** *see* Cyclopentolate *on page 560*

◆ **Cyclomen® (Can)** *see* Danazol *on page 582*

◆ **Cyclomydril®** *see* Cyclopentolate and Phenylephrine *on page 560*

Cyclopentolate (sye kloe PEN toe late)

Brand Names: U.S. Cyclogyl
Brand Names: Canada AK Pentolate Oph Soln; Cyclogyl®; Diopentolate®; Minims Cyclopentolate; PMS-Cyclopentolate
Therapeutic Category Anticholinergic Agent, Ophthalmic; Ophthalmic Agent, Mydriatic
Generic Availability (U.S.) Yes
Use Diagnostic procedures requiring mydriasis and cycloplegia
Pregnancy Risk Factor C
Pregnancy Considerations Animal reproduction studies have not been conducted.
Breast-Feeding Considerations It is not known if cyclopentolate is excreted in breast milk. The manufacturer recommends that caution be exercised when administering cyclopentolate to nursing women.
Contraindications Hypersensitivity to cyclopentolate or any component; narrow-angle glaucoma
Warnings Use of cyclopentolate has been associated with psychotic reactions and behavioral disturbances in pediatric patients, especially with the 2% solution; increased susceptibility to these effects has been reported in young infants, young children, and in children with spastic paralysis or brain damage; effects usually occur ~30-45 minutes after instillation. Observe neonates and infants closely for at least 30 minutes following instillation. Feeding intolerance may occur in infants; withhold feeding for 4 hours after examination. May cause transient elevation of intraocular pressure
Precautions Use with caution in patients with Down syndrome (predisposition to angle-closure glaucoma); cyclopentolate may cause transient increases in intraocular pressure. Contains benzalkonium chloride which may be adsorbed by contact lenses; remove contacts prior to administration and wait 15 minutes before reinserting.
Adverse Reactions
Cardiovascular: Tachycardia
Central nervous system: Ataxia, hallucinations, hyperactivity, incoherent speech, psychosis, restlessness, seizure
Dermatologic: Burning sensation
Ocular: Intraocular pressure increased, loss of visual accommodation
Miscellaneous: Allergic reaction
Drug Interactions
Metabolism/Transport Effects None known.
Avoid Concomitant Use
Avoid concomitant use of Cyclopentolate with any of the following: Aclidinium; Ipratropium (Oral Inhalation); Potassium Chloride; Tiotropium; Umeclidinium
Increased Effect/Toxicity
Cyclopentolate may increase the levels/effects of: AbobotulinumtoxinA; Analgesics (Opioid); Anticholinergic Agents; Cannabinoid-Containing Products; Mirabegron; OnabotulinumtoxinA; Potassium Chloride; RimabotulinumtoxinB; Thiazide Diuretics; Tiotropium; Topiramate

The levels/effects of Cyclopentolate may be increased by: Aclidinium; Ipratropium (Oral Inhalation); Pramlintide; Umeclidinium
Decreased Effect
Cyclopentolate may decrease the levels/effects of: Acetylcholinesterase Inhibitors (Central); Secretin

The levels/effects of Cyclopentolate may be decreased by: Acetylcholinesterase Inhibitors (Central)
Mechanism of Action Prevents the muscle of the ciliary body and the sphincter muscle of the iris from responding to cholinergic stimulation, causing mydriasis and cycloplegia

Pharmacodynamics
Maximum effect:
Cycloplegia: 15-60 minutes
Mydriasis: Within 15-60 minutes, with recovery taking up to 24 hours
Dosing: Neonatal Ophthalmic: See Cyclopentolate and Phenylephrine monograph (preferred agent for use in neonates and infants due to lower cyclopentolate concentration and reduced risk for systemic reactions)
Dosing: Usual Ophthalmic:
Infants: See Cyclopentolate and Phenylephrine monograph (preferred agent for use in neonates and infants due to lower cyclopentolate concentration and reduced risk for systemic reactions)
Children: 1 drop of 0.5% or 1% in eye followed by 1 drop of 0.5% or 1% in 5 minutes, if necessary, approximately 40-50 minutes before procedure
Adults: 1 drop of 1% followed by another drop in 5 minutes; approximately 40-50 minutes prior to the procedure, may use 2% solution in heavily pigmented iris
Administration Ophthalmic: Instill drops into conjunctival sac of affected eye(s); avoid contact of bottle tip with skin or eye; to avoid excessive systemic absorption, finger pressure should be applied on the lacrimal sac during and for 1-2 minutes following application
Additional Information Pilocarpine ophthalmic drops applied after the examination may reduce recovery time to 3-6 hours
Dosage Forms Excipient information presented when available (limited, particularly for generics); consult specific product labeling.
Solution, Ophthalmic, as hydrochloride:
Cyclogyl: 0.5% (15 mL); 1% (2 mL, 5 mL, 15 mL); 2% (2 mL, 5 mL, 15 mL)
Generic: 1% (2 mL, 15 mL); 2% (2 mL, 5 mL, 15 mL)

Cyclopentolate and Phenylephrine
(sye kloe PEN toe late & fen il EF rin)

Brand Names: U.S. Cyclomydril®
Therapeutic Category Adrenergic Agonist Agent, Ophthalmic; Anticholinergic Agent, Ophthalmic; Ophthalmic Agent, Mydriatic
Generic Availability (U.S.) No
Use Diagnostic procedures requiring mydriasis and cycloplegia; preferred agent for use in neonates and infants
Pregnancy Risk Factor C
Pregnancy Considerations Animal reproduction studies have not been conducted with this combination.
Contraindications Hypersensitivity to cyclopentolate, phenylephrine, or any component; narrow-angle glaucoma or untreated anatomically narrow angles
Warnings Use of cyclopentolate has been associated with psychotic reactions and behavioral disturbances in pediatric patients; increased susceptibility to these effects has been reported in young infants, young children, and in children with spastic paralysis or brain damage, particularly with concentrations >1%; observe neonates and infants closely for at least 30 minutes after administration; may cause transient elevation of intraocular pressure. The preservative, benzalkonium chloride, may be absorbed by soft contact lenses. Wait at least 10 minutes after instillation before reinserting lenses.
Precautions Use with caution in patient's with Down's syndrome, cardiovascular disease, hypertension, and hyperthyroidism; feeding intolerance may follow ophthalmic use of this product in neonates and infants; withhold feedings for 4 hours after examination
Adverse Reactions See individual agents.
Drug Interactions
Metabolism/Transport Effects None known.

Avoid Concomitant Use

Avoid concomitant use of Cyclopentolate and Phenyl-ephrine with any of the following: Ergot Derivatives; Iobenguane I 123; MAO Inhibitors

Increased Effect/Toxicity

Cyclopentolate and Phenylephrine may increase the levels/effects of: Sympathomimetics

The levels/effects of Cyclopentolate and Phenylephrine may be increased by: AtoMOXetine; Cannabinoid-Containing Products; Ergot Derivatives; Linezolid; MAO Inhibitors; Tricyclic Antidepressants

Decreased Effect

Cyclopentolate and Phenylephrine may decrease the levels/effects of: Iobenguane I 123

The levels/effects of Cyclopentolate and Phenylephrine may be decreased by: Alpha1-Blockers

Stability Store at room temperature

Pharmacodynamics Onset of action and duration of effect are partially dependent upon eye pigment; dark eyes have a prolonged onset of action and shorter duration than blue eyes

Onset of action: 15-60 minutes

Duration: 4-12 hours

Dosing: Neonatal Ophthalmic: Instill 1 drop into the eye every 5-10 minutes, for up to 3 doses, ~45 minutes before the examination

Dosing: Usual Ophthalmic: Infants, Children, and Adults: Instill 1 drop into the eye every 5-10 minutes, for up to 3 doses, ~40-50 minutes before the examination

Administration Ophthalmic: Instill drops into conjunctival sac of affected eye(s); avoid contact of bottle tip with skin or eye; to avoid excessive systemic absorption, finger pressure should be applied on the lacrimal sac during and for 1-2 minutes following application; preservative absorbed by soft contact lenses; wait at least 10 minutes before reinserting

Additional Information Cyclomydril® is the preferred agent for use in neonates and infants because lower concentrations of both cyclopentolate and phenylephrine provide optimal dilation while minimizing the systemic side effects noted with a higher concentration of each agent used alone

Dosage Forms Excipient information presented when available (limited, particularly for generics); consult specific product labeling.

Solution, ophthalmic:

Cyclomydril®: Cyclopentolate hydrochloride 0.2% and phenylephrine hydrochloride 1% (2 mL, 5 mL) [contains benzalkonium chloride]

References

Chew C, Rahman RA, Shafie SM, et al, "Comparison of Mydriatic Regimens Used in Screening for Retinopathy of Prematurity in Preterm Infants With Dark Irides," *J Pediatr Ophthalmol Strabismus,* 2005, 42(3):166-73.

♦ **Cyclopentolate Hydrochloride** *see* Cyclopentolate *on page 560*

Cyclophosphamide (sye kloe FOS fa mide)

Medication Safety Issues

Sound-alike/look-alike issues:

Cyclophosphamide may be confused with cycloSPOR-INE, ifosfamide

Cytoxan may be confused with cefOXitin, Ciloxan, cytarabine, CytoGam, Cytosar, Cytosar-U, Cytotec

High alert medication:

This medication is in a class the Institute for Safe Medication Practices (ISMP) includes among its list of drug classes which have a heightened risk of causing significant patient harm when used in error.

Related Information

Emetogenic Potential of Antineoplastic Agents in Children *on page 2327*

Management of Drug Extravasations *on page 2255*

Oral Medications That Should Not Be Crushed or Altered *on page 2438*

Safe Handling of Hazardous Drugs *on page 2419*

Brand Names: Canada Procytox

Therapeutic Category Antineoplastic Agent, Alkylating Agent; Antineoplastic Agent, Alkylating Agent (Nitrogen Mustard); Antirheumatic Miscellaneous; Immunosuppressant Agent

Generic Availability (U.S.) Yes

Use

Oncology: Treatment of Hodgkin's lymphoma, non-Hodgkin's lymphoma (including Burkitt's lymphoma), chronic lymphocytic leukemia (CLL), chronic myelocytic leukemia (CML), acute myelocytic leukemia (AML), acute lymphocytic leukemia (ALL), mycosis fungoides, multiple myeloma, neuroblastoma, retinoblastoma, breast cancer, ovarian adenocarcinoma [FDA approved in pediatrics (age not specified) and adults]; has also been used for Ewing's sarcoma, rhabdomyosarcoma, Wilms tumor, ovarian germ cell tumors, small cell lung cancer, testicular cancer, pheochromocytoma, bone marrow transplantation conditioning regimen

Nononcology: Treatment of nephrotic syndrome in children [FDA approved in pediatrics (age not specified) and adults]; has also been used for severe rheumatoid disorders, Wegener's granulomatosis, myasthenia gravis, multiple sclerosis, systemic lupus erythematosus, lupus nephritis, autoimmune hemolytic anemia, idiopathic thrombocytic purpura (ITP), and antibody-induced pure red cell aplasia

Pregnancy Risk Factor D

Pregnancy Considerations Cyclophosphamide crosses the placenta and can be detected in amniotic fluid (D'Incalci, 1982). Based on the mechanism of action, cyclophosphamide may cause fetal harm if administered during pregnancy. Adverse events (including ectrodactylia) were observed in human studies following exposure to cyclophosphamide. Women of childbearing potential should avoid pregnancy while receiving cyclophosphamide and for up to 1 year after completion of treatment. Males with female partners who are or may become pregnant should use a condom during and for at least 4 months after cyclophosphamide treatment. Cyclophosphamide may cause sterility in males and females (may be irreversible) and amenorrhea in females. When treatment is needed for lupus nephritis, cyclophosphamide should be avoided in women who are pregnant or those who wish to preserve their fertility (Hahn, 2012). Chemotherapy, if indicated, may be administered to pregnant women with breast cancer as part of a combination chemotherapy regimen (common regimens administered during pregnancy include doxorubicin (or epirubicin), cyclophosphamide, and fluorouracil); chemotherapy should not be administered during the first trimester, after 35 weeks gestation, or within 3 weeks of planned delivery (Amant, 2010; Loibl, 2006).

Breast-Feeding Considerations Cyclophosphamide is excreted into breast milk. Leukopenia and thrombocytopenia were noted in an infant exposed to cyclophosphamide while nursing. The mother was treated with one course of cyclophosphamide 6 weeks prior to delivery then cyclophosphamide I.V. 6 mg/kg (300 mg) once daily for 3 days beginning 20 days postpartum. Complete blood counts were obtained in the breast-feeding infant on each day of therapy; WBC and platelets decreased by day 3 (Durodola, 1979). Due to the potential for serious adverse effects in the nursing infant, a decision should be made to discontinue cyclophosphamide or to discontinue breast-feeding, ▶

taking into account the importance of treatment to the mother.

Contraindications Hypersensitivity to cyclophosphamide or any component

Warnings Hazardous agent; use appropriate precautions for handling and disposal (NIOSH, 2012). Cardiotoxicity has been reported, usually with high doses associated with transplant conditioning regimens, although may rarely occur with lower doses. Cardiac abnormalities do not appear to persist. Cardiotoxicities reported include arrhythmia, congestive heart failure, heart block, hemorrhagic myocarditis, hemopericardium (secondary to hemorrhagic myocarditis and myocardial necrosis), pericarditis, and tachyarrhythmias. Cardiotoxicity is related to endothelial capillary damage; symptoms may be managed with diuretics, ACE inhibitors, beta-blockers, or inotropics (Floyd, 2005). Use with caution in patients with preexisting cardiovascular disease. For patients with multiple cardiac risk factors, consider monitoring during treatment (Floyd, 2005). Cyclophosphamide is associated with the development of hemorrhagic cystitis; may rarely be severe and even fatal. Discontinue cyclophosphamide with severe hemorrhagic cystitis. Bladder injury is due to excretion of cyclophosphamide metabolites in the urine and appears to be dose- and treatment duration-dependent. Bladder fibrosis may also occur, either with or without cystitis. Increased hydration and frequent voiding is recommended to help prevent cystitis; some protocols utilize mesna to protect against hemorrhagic cystitis. Monitor urinalysis for hematuria. Severe or prolonged hemorrhagic cystitis may require medical or surgical treatment. Hematuria generally resolves within a few days after treatment is withheld, although it may persist. Secondary malignancies (bladder cancer and myeloproliferative and lymphoproliferative malignancies) have been reported with both single-agent and combination chemotherapy regimens; onset may be delayed (up to several years after treatment). Bladder malignancy usually occurs in patients previously experiencing hemorrhagic cystitis.

May impair fertility; interferes with oogenesis and spermatogenesis. Effect on fertility is generally dependent on dose and duration of treatment and may be irreversible. The age at treatment initiation and cumulative dose were determined to be risk factors for ovarian failure in cyclophosphamide use for the treatment of systemic lupus erythematosus (SLE) (Mok, 1998).

Nausea and vomiting commonly occur; premedication with antiemetics is recommended. Stomatitis/mucositis may also occur. Anaphylactic reactions have been reported. Cross-sensitivity with other alkylating agents may occur.

Dose-related neutropenia is common; thrombocytopenia and anemia may also occur; immunosuppression and serious infections may occur; infections may require dose reduction or interruption or discontinuation of treatment.

Pulmonary toxicities, including pneumonitis and acute respiratory distress syndrome, have been reported. Consider pulmonary function testing to assess the severity of pneumonitis (Morgan, 2011). Cyclophosphamide-induced pneumonitis is rare and may present as early (within 1-6 months) or late onset (several months to years); early onset has been reversible with discontinuation; late onset is associated with pleural thickening and may persist chronically (Malik, 1996).

Precautions Use with caution in hepatic or renal impairment; dosage adjustment may be necessary.

Adverse Reactions

Dermatologic: Alopecia (reversible; onset: 3-6 weeks after start of treatment)

Endocrine & metabolic: Amenorrhea, azoospermia, gonadal suppression, oligospermia, oogenesis impaired, sterility

Gastrointestinal: Abdominal pain, anorexia, diarrhea, mucositis, nausea/vomiting (dose-related), stomatitis

Genitourinary: Hemorrhagic cystitis

Hematologic: Anemia, leukopenia (dose-related; recovery: 7-10 days after cessation), myelosuppression, neutropenia, neutropenic fever, thrombocytopenia

Miscellaneous: Infection

Rare but important or life-threatening: Acute respiratory distress syndrome, anaphylactic reactions, anaphylaxis, arrhythmias (with high-dose [HSCT] therapy), bladder/urinary fibrosis, blurred vision, cardiac tamponade (with high-dose [HSCT] therapy), cardiotoxicity, confusion, dyspnea, ejection fraction decreased, erythema multiforme, gastrointestinal hemorrhage, hearing disorders, heart block, heart failure (with high-dose [HSCT] therapy), hematuria, hemopericardium, hemorrhagic colitis, hemorrhagic myocarditis (with high-dose [HSCT] therapy), hemorrhagic ureteritis, hepatic sinusoidal obstruction syndrome (SOS; formerly called veno-occlusive liver disease), hepatitis, hepatotoxicity, hypersensitivity reactions, hyperuricemia, hypokalemia, hyponatremia, interstitial pneumonitis, interstitial pulmonary fibrosis (with high doses), jaundice, latent infection reactivation, mesenteric ischemia (acute), methemoglobinemia (with high-dose [HSCT] therapy), multiorgan failure, myocardial necrosis (with high-dose [HSCT] therapy), neurotoxicity, neutrophilic eccrine hidradenitis, ovarian fibrosis, pancreatitis, pericarditis, pigmentation changes (skin/fingernails), pneumonia, pulmonary hypertension, pulmonary infiltrates, pulmonary veno-occlusive disease, pyelonephritis, radiation recall, renal tubular necrosis, reversible posterior leukoencephalopathy syndrome (RPLS), rhabdomyolysis, secondary malignancy, septic shock, sepsis, SIADH, Stevens-Johnson syndrome, testicular atrophy, thrombocytopenia (immune mediated), thrombotic disorders (arterial and venous), toxic epidermal necrolysis, toxic megacolon, tumor lysis syndrome, wound healing impaired

Drug Interactions

Metabolism/Transport Effects Substrate of CYP2A6 (minor), CYP2B6 (major), CYP2C19 (minor), CYP2C9 (minor), CYP3A4 (minor); **Note:** Assignment of Major/Minor substrate status based on clinically relevant drug interaction potential; **Inhibits** CYP3A4 (weak); **Induces** CYP2B6 (weak/moderate), CYP2C9 (weak/moderate)

Avoid Concomitant Use

Avoid concomitant use of Cyclophosphamide with any of the following: BCG; Belimumab; CloZAPine; Dipyrone; Etanercept; Natalizumab; Pimecrolimus; Pimozide; Tacrolimus (Topical); Tofacitinib; Vaccines (Live)

Increased Effect/Toxicity

Cyclophosphamide may increase the levels/effects of: Amiodarone; Antineoplastic Agents (Anthracycline, Systemic); ARIPiprazole; CloZAPine; CycloSPORINE (Systemic); Dofetilide; Leflunomide; Lomitapide; Natalizumab; Pimozide; Sargramostim; Succinylcholine; Tofacitinib; Vaccines (Live); Vitamin K Antagonists

The levels/effects of Cyclophosphamide may be increased by: Allopurinol; AzaTHIOprine; Belimumab; CYP2B6 Inhibitors (Moderate); CYP2B6 Inhibitors (Strong); Denosumab; Dipyrone; Etanercept; Filgrastim; Pentostatin; Pimecrolimus; Protease Inhibitors; Quazepam; Roflumilast; Tacrolimus (Topical); Thiazide Diuretics; Trastuzumab

Decreased Effect

Cyclophosphamide may decrease the levels/effects of: BCG; Cardiac Glycosides; Coccidioidin Skin Test; CycloSPORINE (Systemic); Sipuleucel-T; Vaccines (Inactivated); Vaccines (Live); Vitamin K Antagonists

The levels/effects of Cyclophosphamide may be decreased by: CYP2B6 Inducers (Strong); Dabrafenib; Echinacea

Stability Hazardous agent; use appropriate precautions for handling and disposal (NIOSH, 2012). Reconstituted I.V. solution is stable for 24 hours at room temperature or 6 days if refrigerated.

Mechanism of Action Cyclophosphamide is an alkylating agent that prevents cell division by cross-linking DNA strands and decreasing DNA synthesis. It is a cell cycle phase nonspecific agent. Cyclophosphamide also possesses potent immunosuppressive activity. Cyclophosphamide is a prodrug that must be metabolized to active metabolites in the liver.

Pharmacokinetics (Adult data unless noted)
Absorption: 75% to 95% with low doses
Distribution: Crosses the placenta; appears in breast milk; distributes throughout the body including the brain and CSF, but not in concentrations high enough to treat meningeal leukemia
Protein binding: 20%; metabolite: 60%
Metabolism: Inactive prodrug must undergo hydroxylation to form active alkylating mustards; further oxidation leads to formation of inactive metabolites
Half-life: Range 3-12 hours
  Children: 4 hours
  Adults: 6-8 hours
Time to peak serum concentration: Oral: Within 1 hour
Elimination: In urine as unchanged drug (<20%) and as metabolites (85% to 90%)
Dialysis: Moderately dialyzable (20% to 50%)

Dosing: Usual Refer to individual protocols
Children and Adults with no hematologic problems:
  Induction:
    Oral, I.V.: Children: 2-8 mg/kg or 60-250 mg/m^2/day
    I.V.: 40-50 mg/kg (1.5-1.8 g/m^2) in divided doses over 2-5 days
  Maintenance:
    Oral: Children: 2-5 mg/kg or 50-150 mg/m^2 twice weekly
    Oral: Adults: 1-5 mg/kg/day
    I.V.: 10-15 mg/kg (350-550 mg/m^2) every 7-10 days or 3-5 mg/kg (110-185 mg/m^2) twice weekly
Children:
  SLE: I.V.: 500-750 mg/m^2 every month; maximum dose: 1 g/m^2
  JRA/vasculitis: I.V.: 10 mg/kg every 2 weeks
  BMT conditioning regimen: I.V.: 50 mg/kg/day once daily for 3-4 days
  Nephrotic syndrome: Oral: 2-3 mg/kg/day every day for up to 12 weeks when corticosteroids are unsuccessful

Dosing adjustment in renal impairment:
CrCl >10 mL/minute: Administer 100% of normal dose
CrCl ≤10 mL/minute: Administer 75% of normal dose

Administration Hazardous agent; use appropriate precautions for handling and disposal (NIOSH, 2012).
Oral: Administer with food only if GI distress occurs
Parenteral: May administer IVP, I.V. intermittent, or continuous infusion at a final maximum concentration for administration of 20-25 mg/mL; usually administered as a single bolus dose or in fractionated doses over 2-3 days. Most protocols use a 30-60 minute infusion time; doses >1800 mg/m^2 need to be infused over a longer period (ie, 4- or 6-hour infusions)

Vesicant/Extravasation Risk May be an irritant

Monitoring Parameters CBC with differential and platelet count, ESR, BUN, urinalysis, serum electrolytes, serum creatinine, urine specific gravity, urine output

Additional Information Aggressive hydration using fluid containing at least 0.45% sodium chloride at 125 mL/m^2/hour, frequent emptying of the bladder, and concurrent administration of mesna are used to reduce the potential of hemorrhagic cystitis (use mesna with cyclophosphamide doses >1 g/m^2/day; doses ≤1 g/m^2/day may not require use of mesna)

Myelosuppressive effects:
  WBC: Moderate
  Platelets: Moderate
  Onset (days): 7
  Nadir (days): 8-14
  Recovery (days): 21

Product Availability Cyclophosphamide capsules: FDA approved September 2013; anticipated availability is currently unknown. Refer to the prescribing information for additional information.

Dosage Forms Excipient information presented when available (limited, particularly for generics); consult specific product labeling.
Capsule, Oral:
  Generic: 25 mg, 50 mg
Solution Reconstituted, Injection:
  Generic: 500 mg (1 ea); 1 g (1 ea); 2 g (1 ea)
Tablet, Oral:
  Generic: 25 mg, 50 mg

Extemporaneous Preparations Hazardous agent: Use appropriate precautions for handling and disposal.

Liquid solutions for oral administration may be prepared by dissolving cyclophosphamide injection in Aromatic Elixir, N.F. Store refrigerated (in glass container) for up to 14 days.
Cyclophosphamide Prescribing Information, Baxter Healthcare Corporation, Deerfield, Il, May, 2013.

A 10 mg/mL oral suspension may be prepared by reconstituting one 2 g vial for injection with 100 mL of NaCl 0.9%, providing an initial concentration of 20 mg/mL. Mix this solution in a 1:1 ratio with either Simple Syrup, NF or Ora-Plus® to obtain a final concentration of 10 mg/mL. Label "shake well" and "refrigerate". Stable for 56 days refrigerated.
Kennedy R, Groepper D, Tagen M, et al, "Stability of Cyclophosphamide in Extemporaneous Oral Suspensions," Ann Pharmacother, 2010, 44(2):295-301.

References
Amant F, Deckers S, Van Calsteren K, et al. Breast cancer in pregnancy: recommendations of an international consensus meeting. Eur J Cancer. 2010;46(18):3158-3168.
Bostrom BC, Weisdorf DJ, Kim TH, et al, "Bone Marrow Transplantation for Advanced Acute Leukemia: A Pilot Study of High-Energy Total Body Irradiation, Cyclophosphamide and Continuous Infusion Etoposide," Bone Marrow Transplant, 1990, 5(2):83-9.
D'Incalci M, Sessa C, Colombo N, et al. Transplacental passage of cyclophosphamide. Cancer Treat Rep. 1982;66(8):1681-1682.
Durodola JI. Administration of cyclophosphamide during late pregnancy and early lactation: a case report. J Natl Med Assoc. 1979;71(2):165-166.
Floyd JD, Nguyen DT, Lobins RL, et al, "Cardiotoxicity of Cancer Therapy," J Clin Oncol, 2005, 23(30):7685-96.
Loibl S, von Minckwitz G, Gwyn K, et al. Breast carcinoma during pregnancy. International recommendations from an expert meeting. Cancer. 2006;106(2):237-246.
Malik SW, Myers JL, DeRemee RA, et al, "Lung Toxicity Associated With Cyclophosphamide Use. Two Distinct Patterns," Am J Respir Crit Care Med, 1996, 154(6 Pt 1):1851-6.
McCune WJ, Golbus J, Zeldes W, et al, "Clinical and Immunologic Effects of Monthly Administration of Intravenous Cyclophosphamide in Severe Systemic Lupus Erythematosus," N Engl J Med, 1988, 318(22):1423-31.
Mok CC, Lau CS, and Wong RW, "Risk Factors for Ovarian Failure in Patients With Systemic Lupus Erythematosus Receiving Cyclophosphamide Therapy," Arthritis Rheum, 1998, 41(5):831-7.
National Institute for Occupational Safety and Health (NIOSH), "NIOSH List of Antineoplastic and Other Hazardous Drugs in Healthcare Settings 2012." Available at http://www.cdc.gov/niosh/docs/2012-150/pdfs/2012-150.pdf. Accessed January 21, 2013.

CycloSERINE (sye kloe SER een)

Medication Safety Issues
Sound-alike/look-alike issues:
  CycloSERINE may be confused with cyclobenzaprine, cycloSPORINE

Brand Names: U.S. Seromycin [DSC]

Therapeutic Category Antibiotic, Miscellaneous; Antitubercular Agent

Generic Availability (U.S.) Yes

Use Adjunctive treatment in pulmonary or extrapulmonary tuberculosis; treatment of acute urinary tract infections caused by *E. coli* or *Enterobacter* species when less toxic conventional therapy has failed or is contraindicated

Pregnancy Risk Factor C

Pregnancy Considerations Teratogenic effects have not been observed in animal reproduction studies. Cycloserine crosses the placenta and can be detected in the fetal blood and amniotic fluid. The American Thoracic Society recommends use in pregnant women only if there are no alternatives (CDC, 2003).

Breast-Feeding Considerations Cycloserine levels in breast milk are similar to those found in the maternal serum.

Contraindications Hypersensitivity to cycloserine or any component; epilepsy, depression, severe anxiety or psychosis, severe renal insufficiency, chronic alcoholism

Precautions Dosage must be adjusted in patients with renal impairment

Adverse Reactions Frequency not defined.
Cardiovascular: Cardiac arrhythmia, heart failure
Central nervous system: Coma, confusion, dizziness, drowsiness, headache, paresis, psychosis, restlessness, seizures, vertigo
Dermatologic: Rash
Endocrine & metabolic: Vitamin B_{12} deficiency
Hematologic: Folate deficiency
Hepatic: Liver enzymes increased
Neuromuscular & skeletal: Dysarthria, hyperreflexia, paresthesia, tremor
Miscellaneous: Allergic manifestations

Drug Interactions
Metabolism/Transport Effects None known.
Avoid Concomitant Use
Avoid concomitant use of CycloSERINE with any of the following: Alcohol (Ethyl); BCG
Increased Effect/Toxicity
The levels/effects of CycloSERINE may be increased by: Alcohol (Ethyl); Ethionamide; Isoniazid
Decreased Effect
CycloSERINE may decrease the levels/effects of: BCG; Sodium Picosulfate; Typhoid Vaccine

Food Interactions May increase vitamin B_{12} and folic acid dietary requirements. Management: Vitamin B_{12} and folic acid supplementation may be needed.

Mechanism of Action Inhibits bacterial cell wall synthesis by competing with amino acid (D-alanine) for incorporation into the bacterial cell wall; bacteriostatic or bactericidal

Pharmacokinetics (Adult data unless noted)
Absorption: ~70% to 90% from the GI tract
Distribution: Crosses the placenta; appears in breast milk, bile, sputum, synovial fluid and CSF
Protein binding: Not plasma protein bound
Half-life: Patients with normal renal function: 10 hours
Time to peak serum concentration: Within 3-4 hours
Elimination: 60% to 70% of an oral dose excreted unchanged in urine by glomerular filtration within 72 hours, small amounts excreted in feces, remainder is metabolized

Dosing: Usual Oral:
Tuberculosis:
Children: 10-20 mg/kg/day divided every 12 hours up to 1000 mg/day
Adults: Initial: 250 mg every 12 hours for 14 days, then give 500 mg to 1 g/day in 2 divided doses
Urinary tract infection: Adults: 250 mg every 12 hours for 14 days
Dosing adjustment in renal impairment:
CrCl 10-50 mL/minute: Administer every 24 hours

CrCl <10 mL/minute: Administer every 36-48 hours

Administration Oral: May administer without regard to meals

Monitoring Parameters Periodic renal, hepatic, hematological tests, and plasma cycloserine concentrations

Reference Range Adjust dosage to maintain blood cycloserine concentrations <30 mcg/mL

Dosage Forms Excipient information presented when available (limited, particularly for generics); consult specific product labeling. [DSC] = Discontinued product
Capsule, Oral:
Seromycin: 250 mg [DSC] [contains brilliant blue fcf (fd&c blue #1), fd&c yellow #10 (quinoline yellow), fd&c yellow #6 (sunset yellow)]
Generic: 250 mg

References
Centers for Disease Control and Prevention (CDC), "Guidelines for the Prevention and Treatment of Opportunistic Infections Among HIV-Exposed and HIV-Infected Children," *MMWR Recomm Rep*, 2009, 58(RR-11):1-166. Available at http://aidsinfo.nih.gov/contentfiles/Pediatric_OI.pdf
Centers for Disease Control and Prevention (CDC), "Treatment of Tuberculosis. American Thoracic Society, CDC, and Infectious Diseases Society of America," *MMWR Recomm Rep*, 2003, 52 (RR11):3-5. Available at http://www.cdc.gov/mmwr/preview/mmwrhtml/rr5211a1.htm

◆ **Cycloset®** *see* Bromocriptine *on page 304*

◆ **Cycloset** *see* Bromocriptine *on page 304*

◆ **Cyclosporin A** *see* CycloSPORINE (Ophthalmic) *on page 569*

◆ **Cyclosporin A** *see* CycloSPORINE (Systemic) *on page 564*

CycloSPORINE (Systemic) (SYE kloe spor een)

Medication Safety Issues
Sound-alike/look-alike issues:
CycloSPORINE may be confused with cyclophosphamide, Cyklokapron, cycloSERINE
CycloSPORINE modified (Neoral, Gengraf) may be confused with cycloSPORINE non-modified (SandIMMUNE)
Gengraf may be confused with Prograf
Neoral may be confused with Neurontin, Nizoral
SandIMMUNE may be confused with SandoSTATIN

Related Information
Oral Medications That Should Not Be Crushed or Altered *on page 2438*
Safe Handling of Hazardous Drugs *on page 2419*

Brand Names: U.S. Gengraf; Neoral; SandIMMUNE

Brand Names: Canada Apo-Cyclosporine; Neoral; Sandimmune I.V.; Sandoz-Cyclosporine

Therapeutic Category Immunosuppressant Agent

Generic Availability (U.S.) Yes

Use Immunosuppressant used with corticosteroids to prevent organ rejection in patients with kidney, liver, lung, heart, and bone marrow transplants; treatment of nephrotic syndrome in patients with documented focal glomerulosclerosis when corticosteroids and cyclophosphamide are unsuccessful; severe psoriasis; severe rheumatoid arthritis not responsive to methotrexate alone; severe autoimmune disease that is resistant to corticosteroids and other therapy; prevention and treatment of graft-versus-host disease in bone marrow transplant patients

Pregnancy Risk Factor C

Pregnancy Considerations Adverse events were not observed following the use of oral cyclosporine in animal reproduction studies (using doses that were not maternally toxic). In humans, cyclosporine crosses the placenta; maternal concentrations do not correlate with those found in the umbilical cord. Cyclosporine may be detected in the serum of newborns for several days after birth (Claris,

1993). Based on clinical use, premature births and low birth weight were consistently observed in pregnant transplant patients (additional pregnancy complications also present). Formulations may contain alcohol; the alcohol content should be taken into consideration in pregnant women.

The pharmacokinetics of cyclosporine may be influenced by pregnancy (Grimer, 2007). Cyclosporine may be used in pregnant renal, liver, or heart transplant patients (Cowan, 2012; EBPG Expert Group on Renal Transplantation, 2002; McGuire, 2009; Parhar 2012). If therapy is needed for psoriasis, other agents are preferred; however, cyclosporine may be used as an alternative agent along with close clinical monitoring; use should be avoided during the first trimester if possible (Bae, 2012). If treatment is needed for lupus nephritis, other agents are recommended to be used in pregnant women (Hahn, 2012).

Following transplant, normal menstruation and fertility may be restored within months; however, appropriate contraception is recommended to prevent pregnancy until 1-2 years following the transplant to improve pregnancy outcomes (Cowan, 2012; EBPG Expert Group on Renal Transplantation, 2002; McGuire, 2009; Parhar 2012).

A pregnancy registry has been established for pregnant women taking immunosuppressants following any solid organ transplant (National Transplantation Pregnancy Registry, Temple University, 877-955-6877).

A pregnancy registry has also been established for pregnant women taking Neoral for psoriasis or rheumatoid arthritis (Neoral Pregnancy Registry for Psoriasis and Rheumatoid Arthritis, Thomas Jefferson University, 888-522-5581).

Breast-Feeding Considerations Cyclosporine is excreted in breast milk. Concentrations of cyclosporine in milk vary widely and breast-feeding during therapy is generally not recommended (Bae, 2012; Cowan, 2012). Due to the potential for serious adverse in the nursing infant, the decision to discontinue cyclosporine or to discontinue breast-feeding should take into account the importance of treatment to the mother. Formulations may contain alcohol which may be present in breast milk and could be absorbed orally by the nursing infant.

Contraindications Hypersensitivity to cyclosporine or any component (ie, polyoxyl 35 castor oil is an ingredient of the parenteral formulation and polyoxyl 40 hydrogenated castor oil is an ingredient of the cyclosporine capsules and solution for microemulsion). AAP considers cyclosporine to be contraindicated during breast-feeding. Concurrent therapy with PUVA or UVB, methotrexate, coal tar, or radiation therapy for use in patients with psoriasis; presence of uncontrolled hypertension, abnormal renal function, or malignancies in treatment of psoriasis or rheumatoid arthritis.

Warnings Hazardous agent; use appropriate precautions for handling and disposal (NIOSH, 2012). Immunosuppression with cyclosporine may result in an increased susceptibility to infection **[U.S. Boxed Warning]**; fatal infections have been reported. May increase the risk of malignancy (lymphomas, lymphoproliferative disorders, and squamous cell carcinoma) **[U.S. Boxed Warning]**; closely monitor and be prepared to treat anaphylaxis in patients receiving I.V. cyclosporine. Renal impairment, including structural kidney damage, has occurred (when used at high doses) **[U.S. Boxed Warning]**; serious nephrotoxicity, hepatotoxicity, hypertension, and/or seizures may occur in children receiving cyclosporine; **monitor renal function and adjust dosage to avoid toxicity or possible organ rejection via cyclosporine blood or plasma concentration monitoring.** Use caution when using with other nephrotoxic drugs. Immunosuppressed patients are at increased risk for opportunistic infections

(eg, activation of latent viral infection, including BK virus-associated nephropathy, which may impair renal function and cause graft loss). Consider decreasing immunosuppressive burden if renal function deteriorates and BK nephropathy is suspected.

Transplant patients: Cyclosporine may cause significant hyperkalemia and hyperuricemia. May cause seizures, particularly if used with high-dose corticosteroids. Predisposing factors associated with neurological disorders include hypertension, hypomagnesemia, hypocholesterolemia, high-dose corticosteroids, high cyclosporine serum concentration, and graft-versus-host disease. Risk of skin cancer may be increased in psoriasis patients with a history of PUVA and possibly methotrexate or other immunosuppressants, UVB, coal tar, or radiation **[U.S. Boxed Warning]**.

Precautions Close monitoring and dosage adjustment is required in patients with renal and hepatic impairment. Cyclosporine (modified) has increased bioavailability as compared to cyclosporine (non-modified) and cannot be used interchangeably without close monitoring **[U.S. Boxed Warning]**; use caution when changing dosage forms since products cannot be used interchangeably. Should only be prescribed by physicians experienced in the management of systemic immunosuppressants **[U.S. Boxed Warning]**.

Adverse Reactions Adverse reactions reported with systemic use, including rheumatoid arthritis, psoriasis, and transplantation (kidney, liver, and heart).

Any indication:
Cardiovascular: Edema, hypertension
Central nervous system: Headache, paresthesia
Dermatologic: Hypertrichosis
Endocrine & metabolic: Female genital tract disease, hirsutism, increased serum triglycerides
Gastrointestinal: Abdominal distress, diarrhea, dyspepsia, gingival hyperplasia, nausea
Infection: Increased susceptibility to infection
Neuromuscular & skeletal: Leg cramps, tremor
Renal: Increased serum creatinine, renal insufficiency
Respiratory: Upper respiratory tract infection

Kidney, liver, and heart transplant only:
Cardiovascular: Chest pain, flushing, glomerular capillary thrombosis, myocardial infarction
Central nervous system: Anxiety, confusion, convulsions, lethargy, tingling sensation
Dermatologic: Acne vulgaris, nail disease (brittle fingernails), hair breakage, night sweats, pruritus, skin infection
Endocrine & metabolic: Gynecomastia, hyperglycemia, hypomagnesemia, weight loss
Gastrointestinal: Anorexia, aphthous stomatitis, constipation, dysphagia, gastritis, hiccups, pancreatitis, vomiting
Genitourinary: Hematuria, urinary tract infection (kidney transplant)
Hematologic & oncologic: Anemia, leukopenia, lymphoma, thrombocytopenia, upper gastrointestinal hemorrhage
Hepatic: Hepatotoxicity
Infection: Abscess, cytomegalovirus disease, fungal infection (systemic), localized fungal infection, septicemia, viral infection (kidney transplant)
Neuromuscular & skeletal: Arthralgia, myalgia, weakness
Ophthalmic: Conjunctivitis, visual disturbance
Otic: Hearing loss, tinnitus
Respiratory: Pneumonia, sinusitis
Miscellaneous: Fever

Rheumatoid arthritis only:
Cardiovascular: Abnormal heart sounds, cardiac arrhythmia, cardiac failure, chest pain, myocardial infarction, peripheral ischemia

Central nervous system: Anxiety, depression, dizziness, drowsiness, emotional lability, hypoesthesia, insomnia, lack of concentration, malaise, migraine, neuropathy, nervousness, pain, paranoia, vertigo

Dermatologic: Cellulitis, dermatological reaction, dermatitis, diaphoresis, dyschromia, eczema, enanthema, folliculitis, nail disease, pruritus, urticaria, xeroderma

Endocrine & metabolic: Decreased libido, diabetes mellitus, goiter, hot flash, hyperkalemia, hyperuricemia, hypoglycemia, increased libido, menstrual disease, weight gain, weight loss

Gastrointestinal: Constipation, dysgeusia, dysphagia, enlargement of salivary glands, eructation, esophagitis, flatulence, gastric ulcer, gastritis, gastroenteritis, gingival hemorrhage, gingivitis, glossitis, peptic ulcer, tongue disease, vomiting, xerostomia

Genitourinary: Breast fibroadenosis, hematuria, leukorrhea, mastalgia, nocturia, urine abnormality, urinary incontinence, urinary urgency, uterine hemorrhage

Hematologic & oncologic: Anemia, carcinoma, leukopenia, lymphadenopathy, purpura

Hepatic: Hyperbilirubinemia

Infection: Abscess (including renal), bacterial infection, candidiasis, fungal infection, herpes simplex infection, herpes zoster, viral infection

Neuromuscular & skeletal: Arthralgia, bone fracture, dislocation, myalgia, stiffness, synovial cyst, tendon disease, weakness

Ophthalmic: Cataract, conjunctivitis, eye pain, visual disturbance

Otic: Tinnitus, deafness, vestibular disturbance

Renal: Abscess (renal), increased blood urea nitrogen, polyuria, pyelonephritis

Respiratory: Abnormal breath sounds, bronchospasm, cough, dyspnea, epistaxis, sinusitis, tonsillitis

Psoriasis only:

Cardiovascular: Chest pain, flushing

Central nervous system: Dizziness, insomnia, nervousness, pain, psychiatric disturbance, vertigo

Dermatologic: Acne vulgaris, folliculitis, hyperkeratosis, pruritus, skin rash, xeroderma

Endocrine & metabolic: Hot flash

Gastrointestinal: Abdominal distention, constipation, gingival hemorrhage, increased appetite

Genitourinary: Urinary frequency

Hematologic & oncologic: Abnormal erythrocytes, altered platelet function, blood coagulation disorder, carcinoma, hemorrhagic diathesis

Hepatic: Hyperbilirubinemia

Neuromuscular & skeletal: Arthralgia

Ophthalmic: Visual disturbance

Respiratory: Bronchospasm, cough, dyspnea, flu-like symptoms, respiratory tract infection, rhinitis

Miscellaneous: Fever

Rare but important or life-threatening; any indication:
Anaphylaxis/anaphylactoid reaction (possibly associated with Cremophor EL vehicle in injection formulation), brain disease, central nervous system toxicity, cholestasis, cholesterol increased, exacerbation of psoriasis (transformation to erythrodermic or pustular psoriasis), gout, haemolytic uremic syndrome, hepatic insufficiency, hepatitis, hyperbilirubinemia, hyperkalemia, hyperlipidemia, hypertrichosis, hyperuricemia, hypomagnesemia, impaired consciousness, increased susceptibility to infection (including JC virus and BK virus), jaundice, malignant lymphoma, migraine, myalgia, myopathy, myositis, papilledema, progressive multifocal leukoencephalopathy, pseudotumor cerebri, pulmonary edema (noncardiogenic), renal disease (polyoma virus-associated), reversible posterior leukoencephalopathy syndrome, rhabdomyolysis, thrombotic microangiopathy

Drug Interactions

Metabolism/Transport Effects Substrate of CYP3A4 (major), P-glycoprotein; **Note:** Assignment of Major/Minor substrate status based on clinically relevant drug interaction potential; **Inhibits** CYP2C9 (weak), CYP3A4 (moderate), P-glycoprotein

Avoid Concomitant Use

Avoid concomitant use of CycloSPORINE (Systemic) with any of the following: Aliskiren; AtorvaSTATin; BCG; Bosentan; Bosutinib; Conivaptan; Crizotinib; Dronedarone; Enzalutamide; Eplerenone; Fusidic Acid (Systemic); Ibrutinib; Ivabradine; Lomitapide; Lovastatin; Mifepristone; Natalizumab; PAZOPanib; Pimecrolimus; Pimozide; Pitavastatin; Potassium-Sparing Diuretics; Silodosin; Simvastatin; Sitaxentan; Tacrolimus (Systemic); Tacrolimus (Topical); Tofacitinib; Tolvaptan; Topotecan; Ulipristal; Vaccines (Live); VinCRIStine (Liposomal)

Increased Effect/Toxicity

CycloSPORINE (Systemic) may increase the levels/ effects of: Afatinib; Aliskiren; Ambrisentan; ARIPiprazole; AtorvaSTATin; Avanafil; Boceprevir; Bosentan; Bosutinib; Brentuximab Vedotin; Budesonide (Systemic, Oral Inhalation); Calcium Channel Blockers (Dihydropyridine); Calcium Channel Blockers (Nondihydropyridine); Cannabis; Cardiac Glycosides; Caspofungin; Colchicine; CYP3A4 Substrates; Dabigatran Etexilate; Dexamethasone (Systemic); Dofetilide; DOXOrubicin (Conventional); Dronabinol; Dronedarone; Etoposide; Etoposide Phosphate; Everolimus; Ezetimibe; FentaNYL; Fibric Acid Derivatives; Fluvastatin; Halofantrine; Ibrutinib; Imipenem; Ivabradine; Ivacaftor; Leflunomide; Lomitapide; Loop Diuretics; Lovastatin; Lurasidone; Methotrexate; MethylPREDNISolone; Minoxidil (Systemic); Minoxidil (Topical); MitoXANtrone; Natalizumab; Neuromuscular-Blocking Agents; Nonsteroidal Anti-Inflammatory Agents; OxyCODONE; PAZOPanib; P-glycoprotein/ABCB1 Substrates; Pimozide; Pitavastatin; Pravastatin; PrednisoLONE (Systemic); PredniSONE; Propafenone; Protease Inhibitors; Prucalopride; Ranolazine; Repaglinide; Rifaximin; Rivaroxaban; Rosuvastatin; Salmeterol; Saxagliptin; Silodosin; Simvastatin; Sirolimus; Sitaxentan; Tacrolimus (Systemic); Tacrolimus (Topical); Tetrahydrocannabinol; Ticagrelor; Tofacitinib; Tolvaptan; Topotecan; Ulipristal; Vaccines (Live); Vilazodone; VinCRIStine (Liposomal); Zuclopenthixol

The levels/effects of CycloSPORINE (Systemic) may be increased by: ACE Inhibitors; AcetaZOLAMIDE; Aminoglycosides; Amiodarone; Amphotericin B; Androgens; Angiotensin II Receptor Blockers; Antifungal Agents (Azole Derivatives, Systemic); Boceprevir; Bromocriptine; Calcium Channel Blockers (Nondihydropyridine); Carvedilol; Ceritinib; Chloramphenicol; Conivaptan; Crizotinib; Cyclophosphamide; CYP3A4 Inhibitors (Moderate); CYP3A4 Inhibitors (Strong); Dasatinib; Denosumab; Dexamethasone (Systemic); Eplerenone; Ezetimibe; Fluconazole; Fusidic Acid (Systemic); GlyBURIDE; Grapefruit Juice; Imatinib; Imipenem; Luliconazole; Macrolide Antibiotics; Melphalan; Methotrexate; MethylPREDNISolone; Metoclopramide; Metreleptin; MetroNIDAZOLE (Systemic); Mifepristone; Nonsteroidal Anti-Inflammatory Agents; Norfloxacin; Omeprazole; P-glycoprotein/ABCB1 Inhibitors; Pimecrolimus; Potassium-Sparing Diuretics; Pravastatin; PrednisoLONE (Systemic); PredniSONE; Protease Inhibitors; Pyrazinamide; Quinupristin; Roflumilast; Sirolimus; Stiripentol; Sulfonamide Derivatives; Tacrolimus (Systemic); Tacrolimus (Topical); Telaprevir; Temsirolimus; Ticagrelor; Trastuzumab

Decreased Effect

CycloSPORINE (Systemic) may decrease the levels/ effects of: BCG; Coccidioidin Skin Test; GlyBURIDE;

Ifosfamide; Mycophenolate; Sipuleucel-T; Vaccines (Inactivated); Vaccines (Live)

The levels/effects of CycloSPORINE (Systemic) may be decreased by: Adalimumab; Armodafinil; Ascorbic Acid; Barbiturates; Bosentan; CarBAMazepine; Colesevelam; Cyclophosphamide; CYP3A4 Inducers (Strong); Dabrafenib; Deferasirox; Dexamethasone (Systemic); Echinacea; Efavirenz; Enzalutamide; Fibric Acid Derivatives; Fosphenytoin; Griseofulvin; Imipenem; MethylPREDNISolone; Metreleptin; Mitotane; Modafinil; Multivitamins/Fluoride (with ADE); Multivitamins/Minerals (with ADEK, Folate, Iron); Multivitamins/Minerals (with AE, No Iron); Nafcillin; Orlistat; P-glycoprotein/ABCB1 Inducers; Phenytoin; PrednisoLONE (Systemic); PredniSONE; Rifamycin Derivatives; Siltuximab; Somatostatin Analogs; St Johns Wort; Sulfinpyrazone [Off Market]; Sulfonamide Derivatives; Tocilizumab; Vitamin E

Food Interactions Grapefruit juice increases cyclosporine serum concentrations. Management: Avoid grapefruit juice.

Stability Hazardous agent; use appropriate precautions for handling and disposal (NIOSH, 2012). Do not store oral solution or oral solution for emulsion in the refrigerator; store oral solutions in original container only and use contents within 2 months after opening; store ampuls and ophthalmic emulsion-containing vials at room temperature; protect from light; I.V. cyclosporine prepared in NS is stable 6 hours in a polyvinyl chloride container or 12 hours in a glass container; I.V. cyclosporine diluted in D_5W to a final concentration of 2 mg/mL is stable for 24 hours in glass or polyvinyl chloride containers; I.V. cyclosporine may bind to the plastic tubing in I.V. administration sets and to polyvinyl chloride bags. Polyoxyethylated castor oil (Cremophor El®) surfactant in cyclosporine injection may leach phthalate from polyvinyl chloride containers, such as bags and tubing.

Mechanism of Action Inhibition of production and release of interleukin II and inhibits interleukin II-induced activation of resting T-lymphocytes.

Pharmacokinetics (Adult data unless noted)
Absorption: Oral:
Cyclosporine (nonmodified) solution or soft gelatin capsule: Erratically and incompletely absorbed; dependent on the presence of food, bile acids, and GI motility; larger oral doses of cyclosporine are needed in pediatric patients vs adults due to a shorter bowel length resulting in limited intestinal absorption
Cyclosporine (modified) solution in a microemulsion or soft gelatin capsule in a microemulsion: Erratically and incompletely absorbed; increased absorption, up to 30% when compared to cyclosporine (nonmodified); absorption is less dependent on food intake, bile, or GI motility when compared to cyclosporine (nonmodified)
Distribution: Widely distributed in tissues and body fluids including the liver, pancreas, and lungs
V_{dss}: 4-6 L/kg in renal, liver, and marrow transplant recipients (slightly lower values in cardiac transplant patients; children <10 years of age have higher values)
Protein binding: 90% to 98% of dose binds to blood lipoproteins
Metabolism: Undergoes extensive first-pass metabolism following oral administration; extensively metabolized by the cytochrome P450 system in the liver; forms at least 25 metabolites
Bioavailability:
Cyclosporine (nonmodified): Dependent on patient population and transplant type (<10% in adult liver transplant patients and as high as 89% in renal patients). The bioavailability of Sandimmune® capsules and oral solution are equivalent; bioavailability of oral solution is ~30% of the I.V. solution.

Children: 28% (range: 17% to 42%); with gut dysfunction commonly seen in BMT recipients, oral bioavailability is further reduced
Cyclosporine (modified): Bioavailability of Neoral® capsules and oral solution are equivalent:
Children: 43% (range: 30% to 68%)
Adults: 23% greater than with Sandimmune® in renal transplant patients, 50% greater in liver transplant patients
Half-life: May be prolonged in patients with hepatic impairment and lower in pediatric patients due to a higher metabolic rate
Cyclosporine (nonmodified): Biphasic
Alpha phase: 1.4 hours
Terminal phase: 6-24 hours
Cyclosporine (modified): Biphasic; Terminal: 8.4 hours (range: 5-18 hours)
Time to peak serum concentration:
Cyclosporine (nonmodified): 2-6 hours; some patients have a second peak at 5-6 hours
Cyclosporine (modified): 1.5-2 hours (in renal transplant patients)
Elimination: Primarily biliary with 6% of the dose excreted in urine as unchanged drug (0.1%) and metabolites; clearance is more rapid in pediatric patients than in adults
Dosing: Usual Children and Adults (oral dosage is ~3 times the I.V. dosage):
Transplantations:
I.V.: Cyclosporine (non-modified):
Initial: 5-6 mg/kg/dose (1/3 the oral dose) administered 4-12 hours prior to organ transplantation
Maintenance: 2-10 mg/kg/day in divided doses every 8-24 hours; patients should be switched to oral cyclosporine as soon as possible; cyclosporine doses should be adjusted to maintain whole blood HPLC trough concentrations in the reference range
Oral: Cyclosporine (non-modified):
Initial: 14-18 mg/kg/dose administered 4-12 hours prior to organ transplantation; lower initial doses of 10-14 mg/kg/day have been used for renal transplants
Maintenance, postoperative: 5-15 mg/kg/day divided every 12-24 hours; maintenance dose is usually tapered to 3-10 mg/kg/day
When using non-modified formulation, cyclosporine levels may increase in liver transplant patients when the T-tube is closed; may need to decrease dose
Oral: Cyclosporine (modified): Based on the organ transplant population:
Initial: Same as the initial dose for solution or soft gelatin capsule
or
Renal: 9 mg/kg/day (range: 6-12 mg/kg/day) divided every 12 hours
Liver: 8 mg/kg/day (range: 4-12 mg/kg/day) divided every 12 hours
Heart: 7 mg/kg/day (range: 4-10 mg/kg/day) divided every 12 hours
Note: A 1:1 ratio conversion from Sandimmune® to Neoral® has been recommended initially; however, lower doses of Neoral® may be required after conversion to prevent overdose. Total daily doses should be adjusted based on the cyclosporine trough blood concentration and clinical assessment of organ rejection. Cyclosporine blood trough levels should be determined prior to conversion. After conversion to Neoral®, cyclosporine trough levels should be monitored every 4-7 days. **Neoral® and Sandimmune® are not bioequivalent and cannot be used interchangeably.**
Focal segmental glomerulosclerosis: Oral: Initial: 3 mg/kg/day divided every 12 hours
Rheumatoid arthritis: Oral: Cyclosporine (modified): Initial: 2.5 mg/kg/day divided every 12 hours; may increase dose by 0.5-0.75 mg/kg/day if insufficient response is

567

seen after 8 weeks of treatment; maximum dose: 4 mg/kg/day

Psoriasis: Oral: Cyclosporine (modified): Initial: 2.5 mg/kg/day divided every 12 hours; may increase dose by 0.5 mg/kg/day if insufficient response is seen after 4 weeks of treatment; maximum dose: 4 mg/kg/day

Autoimmune diseases: Oral: 1-3 mg/kg/day

Administration Hazardous agent; use appropriate precautions for handling and disposal (NIOSH, 2012).

Oral: Administer consistently at the same time twice daily; use oral syringe, glass dropper, or glass container (not plastic or styrofoam cup); to improve palatability, oral solution may be mixed with milk, chocolate milk, orange juice, or apple juice that is at room temperature; dilution of Neoral® with milk can be unpalatable; stir well and drink at once; do not allow to stand before drinking; rinse with more diluent to ensure that the total dose is taken; after use, dry outside of glass dropper; do not rinse with water or other cleaning agents

Parenteral: May administer by I.V. intermittent infusion or continuous infusion; for intermittent infusion, administer over 2-6 hours at a final concentration not to exceed 2.5 mg/mL. Anaphylaxis has been reported with I.V. use. Patients should be continuously monitored for at least the first 30 minutes of the infusion and should be monitored frequently thereafter

Monitoring Parameters Blood/serum drug concentration (trough), blood drug concentration (C_2), renal and hepatic function tests, serum electrolytes, lipid profile, blood pressure, heart rate

Reference Range Reference ranges are method- and specimen-dependent; use the same analytical method consistently; trough levels should be obtained immediately prior to next dose

Therapeutic: Not well-defined; dependent on organ transplanted, time after transplant, organ function, and cyclosporine toxicity. Empiric therapeutic concentration ranges for trough cyclosporine concentrations:

Kidney: 100-200 ng/mL (serum, RIA)

BMT: 100-250 ng/mL (serum, RIA)

Heart: 100-200 ng/mL (serum, RIA)

Liver: 100-400 ng/mL (blood, HPLC)

Method-dependent (optimum cyclosporine trough concentrations):

Serum, RIA: 150-300 ng/mL; 50-150 ng/mL (late post-transplant period)

Whole blood, RIA: 250-800 ng/mL; 150-450 ng/mL (late post-transplant period)

Whole blood, HPLC: 100-500 ng/mL

C_2 (cyclosporine concentration 2 hours after dose):

Blood, Fluorescence Polarization Immunoassay (FPIA): 1000-1500 ng/mL (in first 6 months after transplantation)

Blood, FPIA: 800-900 ng/mL (in second 6 months after transplantation)

Test Interactions Specific whole blood assay for cyclosporine may be falsely elevated if sample is drawn from the same central venous line through which dose was administered (even if flush has been administered and/or dose was given hours before); cyclosporine metabolites cross-react with radioimmunoassay and fluorescence polarization immunoassay

Additional Information Diltiazem has been used to prevent cyclosporine nephrotoxicity, to reduce the frequency of delayed graft function when administered before and after surgery, and to treat the mild hypertension that occurs in most patients after transplantation; diltiazem increases cyclosporine blood concentration by delaying its clearance, resulting in decreased dosage requirements for cyclosporine.

Dosage Forms Considerations

Cyclosporine (modified): Gengraf and Neoral

Cyclosporine (non-modified): SandIMMUNE

Dosage Forms Excipient information presented when available (limited, particularly for generics); consult specific product labeling.

Capsule, Oral:

Gengraf: 25 mg, 100 mg [contains cremophor el, fd&c blue #2 (indigotine)]

Neoral: 25 mg, 100 mg [contains alcohol, usp]

SandIMMUNE: 25 mg [contains alcohol, usp]

SandIMMUNE: 100 mg

Generic: 25 mg, 50 mg, 100 mg

Solution, Intravenous:

SandIMMUNE: 50 mg/mL (5 mL) [contains alcohol, usp, cremophor el]

Generic: 50 mg/mL (5 mL)

Solution, Oral:

Gengraf: 100 mg/mL (50 mL) [contains propylene glycol]

Neoral: 100 mg/mL (50 mL) [contains alcohol, usp]

SandIMMUNE: 100 mg/mL (50 mL) [contains alcohol, usp]

Generic: 100 mg/mL (50 mL)

References

Bae YS, Van Voorhees AS, Hsu S, et al. National Psoriasis Foundation. Review of treatment options for psoriasis in pregnant or lactating women: from the Medical Board of the National Psoriasis Foundation. *J Am Acad Dermatol.* 2012;67(3):459-477.

Burckart GJ, Canafax DM, and Yee GC, "Cyclosporine Monitoring," *Drug Intell Clin Pharm*, 1986, 20(9):649-52.

Claris O, Picaud JC, Brazier JL, et al, "Pharmacokinetics of Cyclosporin A in 16 Newborn Infants of Renal or Cardiac Transplant Mothers," *Dev Pharmacol Ther*, 1993, 20(3-4):180-5.

Cowan SW, Davison JM, Doria C, et al. Pregnancy after cardiac transplantation. *Cardiol Clin.* 2012;30(3):441-452.

EBPG Expert Group on Renal Transplantation. European best practice guidelines for renal transplantation. Section IV: Long-term management of the transplant recipient. IV.10. Pregnancy in renal transplant recipients. *Nephrol Dial Transplant.* 2002;(17 Suppl 4):50-55.

Grimer M; Caring for Australians with Renal Impairment (CARI). The CARI guidelines. Calcineurin inhibitors in renal transplantation: pregnancy, lactation and calcineurin inhibitors. *Nephrology (Carlton).* 2007;(12 Suppl 1):S98-S105.

Hahn BH, McMahon MA, Wilkinson A, et al, "American College of Rheumatology Guidelines for Screening, Treatment, and Management of Lupus Nephritis," *Arthritis Care Res (Hoboken)*, 2012, 64 (6):797-808.

Hardinger KL, Koch MJ, and Brennan DC, "Current and Future Immunosuppressive Strategies in Renal Transplantation," *Pharmacotherapy*, 2004, 24(9):1159-76.

Holt DW, Mueller EA, Kovarik JM, et al, "Sandimmune® Neoral® Pharmacokinetics: Impact of the New Oral Formulation," *Transplant Proc*, 1995, 27(1):1434-7.

Lin CY and Lee SF, "Comparison of Pharmacokinetics Between CsA Capsules and Sandimmune® Neoral® in Pediatric Patients," *Transplant Proc*, 1994, 26(5):2973-4.

McGuire BM, Rosenthal P, Brown CC, et al; American Society of Transplantation. Long-term management of the liver transplant patient: recommendations for the primary care doctor. *Am J Transplant.* 2009;9(9):1988-2003.

National Institute for Occupational Safety and Health (NIOSH), "NIOSH List of Antineoplastic and Other Hazardous Drugs in Healthcare Settings 2012." Available at http://www.cdc.gov/niosh/docs/2012-150/pdfs/2012-150.pdf. Accessed January 21, 2013.

Niese D, "A Double-Blind Randomized Study of Sandimmune® Neoral® vs Sandimmune® in New Renal Transplant Recipients: Results After 12 Months," *Transplant Proc*, 1995, 27(2):1849-56.

Parhar KS, Gibson PS, Coffin CS. Pregnancy following liver transplantation: review of outcomes and recommendations for management. *Can J Gastroenterol.* 2012;26(9):621-626.

Taesch S, Niese D, and Mueller EA, "Sandimmune® Neoral®, A New Oral Formulation of Cyclosporine With Improved Pharmacokinetic Characteristics: Safety and Tolerability in Renal Transplant Patients," *Transplant Proc*, 1994, 26(6):3147-9.

Wandstrat TL, Schroeder TJ, and Myre SA, "Cyclosporine Pharmacokinetics in Pediatric Transplant Recipients," *Ther Drug Monit*, 1989, 11 (5):493-6.

Yee GC, "Recent Advances in Cyclosporine Pharmacokinetics," *Pharmacotherapy*, 1991, 11(5):130S-134S.

CycloSPORINE (Ophthalmic)

(SYE kloe spor een)

Medication Safety Issues

Sound-alike/look-alike issues:

CycloSPORINE may be confused with cyclophospha-mide, Cyklokapron®, cycloSERINE

Related Information

Safe Handling of Hazardous Drugs *on page 2419*

Brand Names: U.S. Restasis

Brand Names: Canada Restasis®

Therapeutic Category Immunosuppressant Agent

Generic Availability (U.S.) No

Use Increase tear production in patients with moderate to severe keratoconjunctivitis sicca-associated ocular inflammation

Pregnancy Risk Factor C

Pregnancy Considerations Adverse events were not observed following the use of oral cyclosporine in animal reproduction studies when using doses that were approximately 300,000 times greater than a human ophthalmic dose (assuming complete absorption).

Breast-Feeding Considerations Cyclosporine is found in breast milk following oral administration. Serum concentrations are below the limit of detection (<0.1 ng/mL) following ophthalmic use.

Contraindications Hypersensitivity to cyclosporine or any component; active ocular infections

Warnings Hazardous agent; use appropriate precautions for handling and disposal (NIOSH, 2012).

Adverse Reactions Ocular: Blurred vision, burning, conjunctival hyperemia, discharge, epiphora, eye pain, foreign body sensation, pruritus, stinging, visual disturbance

Drug Interactions

Metabolism/Transport Effects None known.

Avoid Concomitant Use There are no known interactions where it is recommended to avoid concomitant use.

Increased Effect/Toxicity There are no known significant interactions involving an increase in effect.

Decreased Effect There are no known significant interactions involving a decrease in effect.

Stability Hazardous agent; use appropriate precautions for handling and disposal (NIOSH, 2012). Store at room temperature; protect from light.

Dosing: Usual Children ≥16 years and Adults: Ophthalmic: Instill one drop in affected eye(s) every 12 hours

Administration Hazardous agent; use appropriate precautions for handling and disposal (NIOSH, 2012). Invert vial prior to use to obtain a uniform emulsion. Avoid contact of vial tip with skin or eye; remove contact lenses prior to administration; lenses may be inserted 15 minutes after instillation. May be used with artificial tears; separate administration by at least 15 minutes.

Dosage Forms Excipient information presented when available (limited, particularly for generics); consult specific product labeling.

Emulsion, Ophthalmic [preservative free]:

Restasis: 0.05% (1 ea) [contains polysorbate 80]

References

National Institute for Occupational Safety and Health (NIOSH), "NIOSH List of Antineoplastic and Other Hazardous Drugs in Healthcare Settings 2012." Available at http://www.cdc.gov/niosh/docs/2012-150/pdfs/2012-150.pdf. Accessed January 21, 2013.

◆ **Cyklokapron** *see* Tranexamic Acid *on page 2063*

Cyproheptadine (si proe HEP ta deen)

Medication Safety Issues

Sound-alike/look-alike issues:

Cyproheptadine may be confused with cyclobenzaprine

Periactin may be confused with Percodan®, Persantine®

BEERS Criteria medication:

This drug may be potentially inappropriate for use in geriatric patients (Quality of evidence - moderate; Strength of recommendation - strong).

International issues:

Periactin brand name for cyproheptadine [U.S., multiple international markets] may be confused with Perative brand name for an enteral nutrition preparation [multiple international markets] and brand name for ketoconazole [Argentina]

Related Information

Serotonin Syndrome *on page 2405*

Brand Names: Canada Euro-Cyproheptadine; PMS-Cyproheptadine

Therapeutic Category Antihistamine

Generic Availability (U.S.) Yes

Use Perennial and seasonal allergic rhinitis and other allergic symptoms including cold urticaria (FDA approved in ages ≥2 years and adults); has also been used to promote weight gain by appetite stimulation in various disease states (eg, cystic fibrosis, cancer-related cachexia); migraine prophylaxis; prevention of episodes of cyclic vomiting; management of dyspeptic symptoms; treatment of spasticity associated with spinal cord damage; and management of serotonin syndrome (eg, following acute SSRI ingestions)

Pregnancy Risk Factor B

Pregnancy Considerations Adverse events have been observed in some animal reproduction studies. Maternal antihistamine use has generally not resulted in an increased risk of birth defects; however, information specific to cyproheptadine is limited. Antihistamines are recommended for the treatment of rhinitis, urticaria, and pruritus with rash in pregnant women (although second generation antihistamines may be preferred). Antihistamines are not recommended for treatment of pruritus associated with intrahepatic cholestasis in pregnancy.

Breast-Feeding Considerations It is not known if cyproheptadine is excreted into breast milk. Premature infants and newborns have a higher risk of intolerance to antihistamines. Use while breast-feeding is contraindicated by the manufacturer. Antihistamines may decrease maternal serum prolactin concentrations when administered prior to the establishment of nursing.

Contraindications Hypersensitivity to cyproheptadine or any component; newborns or premature infants; nursing mothers; elderly or debilitated patients; narrow-angle glaucoma; bladder neck obstruction; stenosing peptic ulcer; pyloroduodenal obstruction; symptomatic prostatic hypertrophy; concurrent MAO inhibitor therapy

Warnings May cause CNS depression, which may impair physical or mental abilities; patients must be cautioned about performing tasks which require mental alertness (eg, operating machinery or driving). Effects may be potentiated when used with other sedating drugs or ethanol. Excessive dosages of antihistamine in infants and young children may cause hallucinations, CNS depression, seizures, and death; use is contraindicated in newborns and premature infants; safety and efficacy has not been established in pediatric patients <2 years; use with caution and use the lowest effective dose in children ≥2 years of age and avoid concomitant use with other medications having respiratory depressant effects. In elderly patients, use of this potent anticholinergic agent is contraindicated due to increased risk of confusion, dry mouth, constipation, and other anticholinergic effects; clearance decreases in patients of advanced age (Beers Criteria).

Precautions Antihistamines may cause paradoxical excitation in young children. Use with caution in renal impairment; clearance is decreased. Use with caution in patients with cardiovascular disease, including hypertension and ischemic heart disease. Use with caution in patients with increased intraocular pressure. Use with caution in patients with asthma or other chronic breathing disorders. Use with caution in patients with thyroid dysfunction.

Adverse Reactions

Cardiovascular: Extrasystoles, hypotension, palpitation, tachycardia

Central nervous system: Confusion, coordination disturbed, dizziness, excitation, euphoria, faintness, hallucinations, headache, hysteria, insomnia, irritability, nervousness, neuritis, restlessness, sedation, seizure, sleepiness, tremor, vertigo

Dermatologic: Angioedema, photosensitivity, rash, urticaria

Gastrointestinal: Abdominal pain, anorexia, appetite increased, constipation, diarrhea, nausea, vomiting, xerostomia

Genitourinary: Difficult urination, urinary frequency, urinary retention

Hematologic: Agranulocytosis, hemolytic anemia, leukopenia, thrombocytopenia

Hepatic: Cholestasis, hepatic failure, hepatitis, jaundice

Neuromuscular & skeletal: Paresthesia

Ocular: Blurred vision, diplopia

Otic: Labyrinthitis (acute), tinnitus

Respiratory: Bronchial secretions (thickening), nasal congestion, pharyngitis

Miscellaneous: Allergic reactions, anaphylactic shock, chills, diaphoresis, fatigue

Drug Interactions

Metabolism/Transport Effects None known.

Avoid Concomitant Use

Avoid concomitant use of Cyproheptadine with any of the following: Aclidinium; Azelastine (Nasal); Ipratropium (Oral Inhalation); MAO Inhibitors; Paraldehyde; Potassium Chloride; Thalidomide; Tiotropium; Umeclidinium

Increased Effect/Toxicity

Cyproheptadine may increase the levels/effects of: AbobotulinumtoxinA; Alcohol (Ethyl); Analgesics (Opioid); Anticholinergic Agents; Azelastine (Nasal); Buprenorphine; Cannabinoid-Containing Products; CNS Depressants; Hydrocodone; Methotrimeprazine; Metyrosine; Mirabegron; Mirtazapine; OnabotulinumtoxinA; Paraldehyde; Potassium Chloride; Pramipexole; RimabotulinumtoxinB; ROPINIRole; Rotigotine; Thalidomide; Thiazide Diuretics; Tiotropium; Topiramate; Zolpidem

The levels/effects of Cyproheptadine may be increased by: Aclidinium; Brimonidine (Topical); Cannabis; Doxylamine; Dronabinol; Droperidol; HydrOXYzine; Ipratropium (Oral Inhalation); Kava Kava; Magnesium Sulfate; MAO Inhibitors; Methotrimeprazine; Nabilone; Perampanel; Pramlintide; Rufinamide; Sodium Oxybate; Tapentadol; Tetrahydrocannabinol; Umeclidinium

Decreased Effect

Cyproheptadine may decrease the levels/effects of: Acetylcholinesterase Inhibitors (Central); Benzylpenicilloyl Polylysine; Betahistine; Hyaluronidase; MAO Inhibitors; Secretin; Selective Serotonin Reuptake Inhibitors

The levels/effects of Cyproheptadine may be decreased by: Acetylcholinesterase Inhibitors (Central); Amphetamines

Stability

Oral solution: Store at 15°C to 30°C (59°F to 86°F); protect from light.

Oral syrup: Store at 20°C to 25°C (68°F to 77°F); excursions permitted to 15°C to 30°C (59°F to 86°F); protect from light.

Oral tablets: Store at 20°C to 25°C (68°F to 77°F).

Mechanism of Action A potent antihistamine and serotonin antagonist, competes with histamine for H_1-receptor sites on effector cells in the gastrointestinal tract, blood vessels, and respiratory tract

Pharmacokinetics (Adult data unless noted)

Absorption: Well absorbed

Metabolism: Primarily by hepatic glucuronidation via UGT1A (Walker, 1996)

Half-life: 1-4 hours; metabolites: ~16 hours (Paton, 1985)

Time to peak serum concentration: 6-9 hours (Paton, 1985)

Elimination: Urine (~40% primarily as metabolites); feces (2% to 20%, <6% as unchanged drug)

Dosing: Usual

Infants, Children, and Adolescents

Allergic conditions: Oral: Children ≥2 years and Adolescents: 0.25 mg/kg/day or 8 mg/m^2/day in 2-3 divided doses

Alternate (fixed dosing):

2-6 years: 2 mg every 8-12 hours; maximum daily dose: 12 mg/**day**

7-14 years: 4 mg every 8-12 hours; maximum daily dose: 16 mg/**day**

≥15 years: Initial: 4 mg every 8 hours; titrate to effect; usual range: 12-16 mg/day although some patients may require up to 32 mg; maximum daily dose: 0.5 mg/kg/**day**

Appetite stimulation: Limited data available; dosing regimens variable; further studies are needed: Oral:

Weight-directed dosing: Children ≥2 years and Adolescents: 0.25 mg/kg/day divided twice daily; age-dependent maximum daily dose: ≤6 years: 12 mg/day; 7-14 years: 16 mg/**day**; ≥15 years: 32 mg/**day**. Dosing based on an open-label trial of 66 pediatric cancer patients (median age: 11.7 years; range: 3-19 years) which reported 76% response rate (either weight gained or stabilized); mean weight gain: 2.6 kg (range: -0.1 to 10 kg); in a subset analysis, patients >9 years showed a greater response than younger patients as did patients with hematologic malignancies (Couluris, 2008).

Fixed dosing: Children ≥5 years and Adolescents: Initial: 2 mg every 6 hours (4 times daily) for 1 week; if tolerated, increase dose to 4 mg every 6 hours; dosing based on a short-term (12-week) double-blind, placebo-controlled trial (n=8 treatment group) and a long-term (1-year) open-label trial (n=12) in cystic fibrosis patients; results showed significant increases in weight gain (3.4 kg vs 1.1 kg in placebo); long-term results showed a generally sustained effect (eg, no further weight loss or some additional weight gain) over study duration (Homnick, 2004; Homnick, 2005).

Cyclic vomiting syndrome; prevention: Limited data available: Oral: Children 2-5 years: 0.25-0.5 mg/kg/day in divided doses 2-3 times daily; maximum daily dose: 12 mg/**day**; some clinicians have used once daily dose at bedtime to prevent day time sedation (Andersen, 1997; Li, 2008)

Dyspeptic syndrome; refractory: Limited data available: Oral: Infants ≥9 months and Children <12 years: Reported range: 0.04-0.6 mg/kg/day in divided doses 2-3 times daily; median effective dose: 0.22 mg/kg/day; dosing based on a retrospective, open-label trial of 80 pediatric patients (median age: 9.8 years; range: 9 months to 20 years) with dyspeptic symptoms (eg, nausea, early satiety, abdominal pain, retching after fundoplication and vomiting) which failed to respond to conventional therapy (eg, diet changes, H_2-blockers, proton pump inhibitors); observed response rate was 55%; a higher response rate (86%) was seen with retching post-Nissen fundoplication (Rodriguez, 2013).

Migraine; prophylaxis: Limited data available: Oral: Children ≥3 years and Adolescents: 0.2-0.4 mg/kg/day divided twice daily; reported daily dose range: 2-8 mg/day; maximum daily dose: 0.5 mg/kg/**day**; experience suggests younger patients more tolerant of common cyproheptadine side effects (ie, sedation and increased appetite) (Lewis, 2004; Lewis, 2004a)

Spasticity associated with spinal cord damage: Limited data available; efficacy results variable: Oral: Children ≥12 years and Adolescents: 4 mg at bedtime; increase by a 4 mg dose every 3-4 days; mean daily dose: 16 mg/day in divided doses; maximum daily dose: 36 mg/**day** (Gracie, 1997). In the most rigorous evaluation, a double-blind, placebo-controlled, cross-over trial of 16 hemiplegic pediatric patients (age range: 4-18 years), cyproheptadine (relatively low dose: 1-2 mg/day) had no statistical evidence of an effect on gait nor improvement in spasticity parameters (Khodadadeh, 1998); further studies are needed

Adults: **Allergic conditions:** Oral: 4-20 mg/day divided every 8 hours (not to exceed 0.5 mg/kg/day); some patients may require up to 32 mg/day for adequate control of symptoms

Dosing adjustment in renal impairment: There are no dosage adjustments provided in manufacturer's labeling; however, elimination is diminished in renal insufficiency.

Dosing adjustment in hepatic impairment: There are no dosage adjustments provided in manufacturer's labeling

Administration Oral: Usually administered in 2-4 divided doses (eg, every 6-12 hours); for some uses (eg, cyclic vomiting syndrome), once daily administration at bedtime has been used for some indications to improve tolerability of sedative effects.

Test Interactions Diagnostic antigen skin test results may be suppressed; false positive serum TCA screen

Dosage Forms Excipient information presented when available (limited, particularly for generics); consult specific product labeling.

Syrup, Oral, as hydrochloride:
Generic: 2 mg/5 mL (10 mL, 473 mL)
Tablet, Oral, as hydrochloride:
Generic: 4 mg

References

Andersen JM, Sugerman KS, Lockhart JR, et al, "Effective Prophylactic Therapy for Cyclic Vomiting Syndrome in Children Using Amitriptyline or Cyproheptadine," *Pediatrics*, 1997, 100(6):977-81.

Couluris M, Mayer JL, Freyer DR, et al, "The Effect of Cyproheptadine Hydrochloride (Periactin) and Megestrol Acetate (Megace) on Weight in Children With Cancer/Treatment-Related Cachexia," *J Pediatr Hematol Oncol*, 2008, 30(11):791-7.

Gracies JM, Nance P, Elovic E, et al, "Traditional Pharmacological Treatments for Spasticity. Part II: General and Regional Treatments," *Muscle Nerve Suppl*, 1997, 6:S92-120.

Homnick DN, Homnick BD, Reeves AJ, et al, "Cyproheptadine Is an Effective Appetite Stimulant in Cystic Fibrosis," *Pediatr Pulmonol*, 2004, 38(2):129-34.

Homnick DN, Marks JH, Hare KL, et al, "Long-Term Trial of Cyproheptadine as an Appetite Stimulant in Cystic Fibrosis," *Pediatr Pulmonol*, 2005, 40(3):251-6.

Khodadadeh S, Holstein H, Purushothaman S, et al, "A Study of the Effect of Cyproheptadine on Gait in Hemiplegic Children," *Gait Posture*, 1998, 8(3):205-213.

Lewis D, Ashwal S, Hershey A, et al, "Practice Parameter: Pharmacological Treatment of Migraine Headache in Children and Adolescents: Report of the American Academy of Neurology Quality Standards Subcommittee and the Practice Committee of the Child Neurology Society," *Neurology*, 2004, 63(12):2215-24.

Lewis DW, Diamond S, Scott D, et al, "Prophylactic Treatment of Pediatric Migraine," *Headache*, 2004, 44(3):230-7.

Li BU, Lefevre F, Chelimsky GG, et al, "North American Society for Pediatric Gastroenterology, Hepatology, and Nutrition Consensus Statement on the Diagnosis and Management of Cyclic Vomiting Syndrome," *J Pediatr Gastroenterol Nutr*, 2008, 47(3):379-93.

Paton DM and Webster DR, "Clinical Pharmacokinetics of H1-Receptor Antagonists (The Antihistamines)," *Clin Pharmacokinet*, 1985, 10(6):477-97.

Rodriguez L, Diaz J, and Nurko S, "Safety and Efficacy of Cyproheptadine for Treating Dyspeptic Symptoms in Children," *J Pediatr*, 2013, Feb 16.

Wainberg M, Barbeau H, and Gauthier S, "The Effects of Cyproheptadine on Locomotion and on Spasticity in Patients With Spinal Cord Injuries," *J Neurol Neurosurg Psychiatry*, 1990, 53(9):754-63.

Walker RB and Kanfer I, "Pharmacokinetics of Cyclizine Following Intravenous Administration to Human Volunteers," *Eur J Pharm Sci*, 1996, 4(5):301-6.

Wians FH, Norton JT, and Wirebaugh, "False-Positive Serum Tricyclic Antidepressant Screen With Cyproheptadine," *Clin Chem*, 1993, 39(6):1355-6.

◆ **Cyproheptadine Hydrochloride** *see* Cyproheptadine *on page* 569

◆ **Cystadane** *see* Betaine *on page* 281

◆ **Cystadane® (Can)** *see* Betaine *on page* 281

◆ **Cystagon** *see* Cysteamine (Systemic) *on page* 571

Cysteamine (Systemic) (sis TEE a meen)

Brand Names: U.S. Cystagon; Procysbi

Therapeutic Category Anticystine Agent; Urinary Tract Product

Generic Availability (U.S.) No

Use Management of nephropathic cystinosis

Pregnancy Risk Factor C

Pregnancy Considerations Use only when the potential benefits outweigh the potential hazards to the fetus; in animal studies, cysteamine is teratogenic and fetotoxic. There are no adequate and well-controlled studies in pregnant women.

Breast-Feeding Considerations It is unknown whether cysteamine is excreted in breast milk. Discontinue nursing or discontinue drug during lactation.

Contraindications Hypersensitivity to cysteamine, penicillamine, or any component

Warnings Leukocyte cystine levels should be monitored during oral cysteamine therapy (at least every 3 months); cysteamine should be given in the lowest dose possible to achieve adequate leukocyte cystine depletion; toxicity may be reduced by initiating therapy with a slowly increasing dose schedule; if skin rash develops, discontinue treatment until rash clears; may then resume treatment at a lower dose with a slow titration to the therapeutic dose; if severe rash develops (eg, erythema multiforme bullosa or toxic epidermal necrolysis), immediately discontinue and do not resume therapy. High doses of cysteamine salts have been associated with purplish hemorrhagic lesions over the elbow area on both arms and have been described as molluscoid pseudotumors. Skin striae, bone lesions (described as osteopenia, compression fractures, scoliosis, and genu valgum) along with leg pain and joint hyperextension may also be present. Reduce dosage if this reaction occurs. Routine monitoring of skin and bones is recommended.

CNS symptoms such as seizures, lethargy, somnolence, depression, and encephalopathy have been associated with cysteamine therapy; patients who develop these symptoms should be carefully evaluated and the dosage adjusted as necessary; use with caution in patients with neurological disorder. Benign intracranial hypertension (or pseudotumor cerebri) and/or papilledema with cysteamine therapy has resolved with diuretic therapy.

Precautions Use with caution in patients with a history of gastric or duodenal ulcer; gastrointestinal ulcers and bleeding have been reported; promptly evaluate if signs and symptoms occur; adjust dose downward if severe GI symptoms develop (most common during initiation of therapy). Use with caution in patients with a history of blood dyscrasias.

Adverse Reactions

Cardiovascular: Hypertension

Central nervous system: Abnormal thinking, ataxia, confusion, depression, dizziness, emotional lability, encephalopathy, fever, hallucinations, headache, impaired cognition, jitteriness, lethargy, nervousness, nightmares, seizure, somnolence

Dermatologic: Rash, urticaria

Endocrine & metabolic: Dehydration

Gastrointestinal: Abdominal pain, constipation, duodenal ulceration, duodenitis, dyspepsia, gastroenteritis, gastrointestinal bleeding, gastrointestinal ulcers, halitosis, nausea

Hematologic: Anemia, leukopenia

Hepatic: Abnormal LFTs

Neuromuscular & skeletal: Hyperkinesia, tremor

Otic: Hearing decreased

Rare but important or life-threatening: Compression fracture, genu valgum, hyperthermia, interstitial nephritis, intracranial hypertension (benign), joint hyperextension, leg pain, molluscoid pseudotumor, osteopenia, papilledema, pseudotumor cerebri, renal failure, scoliosis, skin fragility, skin lesion, skin striae

Drug Interactions

Metabolism/Transport Effects None known.

Avoid Concomitant Use There are no known interactions where it is recommended to avoid concomitant use.

Increased Effect/Toxicity There are no known significant interactions involving an increase in effect.

Decreased Effect There are no known significant interactions involving a decrease in effect.

Food Interactions Concurrent ingestion of food and the delayed release formulation of cysteamine can reduce the systemic exposure of cysteamine. Management: Administer ≥30 minutes before and ≥2 hours after meals; if necessary, patients may eat only a small amount (~4 ounces or $1/2$ cup) of food between 1 hour before and 1 hour after administration.

Stability Store at room temperature; protect from light

Mechanism of Action Reacts with cystine within the lysosome to convert it to cysteine and to a cysteine-cysteamine mixed disulfide, both of which can then exit the lysosome in patients with cystinosis, an inherited defect of lysosomal transport

Pharmacodynamics

Peak effect: 1.8 hours

Duration: 6 hours

Pharmacokinetics (Adult data unless noted)

Absorption: Rapid

Distribution: V_d: Children: 156 L

Protein binding: Mean: 52%

Half-life: 1 hour

Time to peak serum concentration: 1.4 hours

Elimination: Clearance: Children: 1.2 L/minute

Dosing: Usual Dose-related side effects resulting in withdrawal from research studies occurred more frequently in those patients receiving 1.95 g/m²/day as compared to 1.3 g/m²/day; start at the lowest dose and titrate gradually to prevent intolerance.

Oral: Initiate therapy with 1/4 to 1/6 of maintenance dose and titrate slowly over 4-6 weeks:

Children <12 years: Initial: 1.3 g/m²/day in 4 divided doses; may increase gradually to a maximum of 1.95 g/m²/day

Children ≥12 years (>110 lbs) and Adults (>110 lbs): 2 g/day in 4 divided doses; dosage may be increased gradually to 1.95 g/m²/day

Approximate Cysteamine Initial Dose

(to achieve ~1.3 g/m²/day)

Weight (lbs)	Dose (mg every 6 h)
≤10	100
11-20	150
21-30	200
31-40	250
41-50	300
51-70	350
71-90	400
91-110	450
>110	500

Administration Oral: Contents of capsule may be sprinkled over food; if a dose is missed, take it as soon as possible then return to normal dosing schedule; if identified within 2 hours of next scheduled dose, skip dose; do **not** double the next dose

Monitoring Parameters Blood counts and liver enzymes during therapy; blood pressure; monitor leukocyte cystine measurements to determine adequate dosage and compliance (measure 5-6 hours after administration); monitor skin and bone

Reference Range Leukocyte cystine level goal (measured 5-6 hours after cysteamine dose): <1 nmol of half-cystine/mg protein (some measurable benefits have been seen with levels <2); routine measurements are recommended every 3 months

Dosage Forms Excipient information presented when available (limited, particularly for generics); consult specific product labeling.

Capsule, Oral:

Cystagon: 50 mg, 150 mg

Capsule Delayed Release, Oral:

Procysbi: 25 mg, 75 mg

◆ **Cysteamine Bitartrate** see Cysteamine (Systemic) *on page 571*

◆ **Cystech [OTC]** see Cysteine *on page 572*

Cysteine (SIS te een)

Brand Names: U.S. Cystech [OTC]

Therapeutic Category Nutritional Supplement

Generic Availability (U.S.) May be product dependent

Use Supplement to crystalline amino acid solutions, in particular the specialized pediatric formulas (eg, Aminosyn® PF, TrophAmine®) to meet the intravenous amino acid nutritional requirements of infants receiving parenteral nutrition (PN)

Pregnancy Considerations Cysteine is generally considered to be a nonessential amino acid in adults because it can be synthesized from methionine (an essential amino acid). The RDA for methionine + cysteine is increased in pregnant women (IOM, 2005).

Breast-Feeding Considerations Cysteine is found in breast milk. The RDA for methionine + cysteine is increased in breast-feeding women (IOM, 2005).

Contraindications Hypersensitivity to cysteine or any component; patients with hepatic coma or metabolic disorders involving impaired nitrogen utilization

Warnings Metabolic acidosis has occurred in infants related to the "hydrochloride" component of cysteine; each 1 mmol cysteine (175 mg) delivers 1 mEq chloride and 1 mEq hydrogen ion; to balance the extra hydrochloride ions and prevent acidosis, addition to the PN solution of a 1 mEq acetate electrolyte salt for each mmol (175 mg) of cysteine may be needed; each 40 mg cysteine (equal to every 1 g amino acid when used in the recommended ratio) adds 0.228 mEq chloride and hydrogen

Precautions Use with caution in patients with renal dysfunction and hepatic insufficiency

Adverse Reactions
Cardiovascular: Flushing
Central nervous system: Fever
Endocrine & metabolic: Metabolic acidosis
Gastrointestinal: Nausea
Local: Erythema, phlebitis, thrombosis, warm sensation
Renal: Azotemia, BUN increased

Stability Avoid excessive heat, do not freeze; when combined with parenteral amino acid solutions, cysteine is relatively unstable; it is intended to be added immediately prior to administration to the patient; infusion of the admixture should begin within 1 hour of mixing or refrigerated until use; stable 24 hours in PN solution; opened vials must be used within 4 hours of entry

Mechanism of Action Cysteine is a sulfur-containing amino acid synthesized from methionine via the transulfuration pathway. It is a precursor of the tripeptide glutathione and also of taurine. Newborn infants have a relative deficiency of the enzyme necessary to affect this conversion. Cysteine may be considered an essential amino acid in infants.

Dosing: Neonatal I.V.: Added as a fixed ratio to crystalline amino acid solution: 40 mg cysteine per g of amino acids; dosage will vary with the daily amino acid dosage (eg, 0.5-2.5 g/kg/day amino acids would result in 20-100 mg/kg/day cysteine); individual doses of cysteine of 0.8-1 mmol/kg/day have also been added directly to the daily PN solution; the duration of treatment relates to the need for PN

Dosing: Usual I.V.: Infants: Added as a fixed ratio to crystalline amino acid solution: 40 mg cysteine per g of amino acids; dosage will vary with the daily amino acid dosage (eg, 0.5-2.5 g/kg/day amino acids would result in 20-100 mg/kg/day cysteine); individual doses of cysteine of 0.8-1 mmol/kg/day have also been added directly to the daily PN solution; the duration of treatment relates to the need for PN; patients on chronic PN therapy have received cysteine until 6 months of age and in some cases until 2 years of age

Administration Parenteral: Use only after dilution into PN solution; dilute with amino acid solution in a ratio of 40 mg cysteine to 1 g amino acid: eg, 500 mg cysteine is added to 12.5 g (250 mL) of 5% amino acid solution

Monitoring Parameters BUN, ammonia, electrolytes, pH, acid-base balance, serum creatinine, liver function tests, growth curve

Additional Information Addition of cysteine to PN solutions enhances the solubility of calcium and phosphate by lowering the overall pH of the solution

Dosage Forms Excipient information presented when available (limited, particularly for generics); consult specific product labeling.
Capsule, Oral, as hydrochloride [preservative free]:
Cystech: 500 mg [dye free]
Solution, Intravenous, as hydrochloride:
Generic: 50 mg/mL (10 mL, 50 mL)

References
IOM (Institute of Medicine), *Dietary Reference Intakes for Energy, Carbohydrate, Fiber, Fat, Fatty Acids, Cholesterol, Protein, and Amino Acids (Macronutrients)*, Washington, DC: The National Academies Press, 2005.

◆ **Cysteine Hydrochloride** see Cysteine on page 572
◆ **CYT** see Cyclophosphamide on page 561
◆ **Cytarabine** see Cytarabine (Conventional) on page 573

Cytarabine (Conventional)
(sye TARE a been con VEN sha nal)

Medication Safety Issues
Sound-alike/look-alike issues:
Cytarabine may be confused with clofarabine, Cytosar, Cytoxan, vidarabine
Cytarabine (conventional) may be confused with cytarabine liposomal
Cytosar-U may be confused with cytarabine, Cytovene, Cytoxan, Neosar

High alert medication:
This medication is in a class the Institute for Safe Medication Practices (ISMP) includes among its list of drugs classes which have a heightened risk of causing significant patient harm when used in error.

Administration issues:
Intrathecal medication safety: The American Society of Clinical Oncology (ASCO)/Oncology Nursing Society (ONS) chemotherapy administration safety standards (Jacobson, 2009) encourage the following safety measures for intrathecal chemotherapy:
• Intrathecal medication should not be prepared during the preparation of any other agents
• After preparation, store in an isolated location or container clearly marked with a label identifying as "intrathecal" use only
• Delivery to the patient should only be with other medications also intended for administration into the central nervous system

Related Information
Emetogenic Potential of Antineoplastic Agents in Children on page 2327
Safe Handling of Hazardous Drugs on page 2419

Brand Names: Canada Cytarabine Injection; Cytosar

Therapeutic Category Antineoplastic Agent, Antimetabolite

Generic Availability (U.S.) Yes

Use Remission induction in acute myeloid leukemia (AML), treatment of acute lymphocytic leukemia (ALL) and chronic myelocytic leukemia (CML; blast phase) (FDA approved in children and adults); prophylaxis and treatment of meningeal leukemia (FDA approved in children and adults); has also been used in postinduction, postremission consolidation, and salvage treatment of AML, treatment of primary central nervous system lymphoma, treatment of relapsed or refractory Hodgkin's lymphoma, treatment of non-Hodgkin's lymphomas (NHL)

Pregnancy Risk Factor D

Pregnancy Considerations Adverse effects were demonstrated in animal reproduction studies. Limb and ear defects have been noted in case reports of cytarabine exposure during the first trimester of pregnancy. The following have also been noted in the neonate: Pancytopenia, WBC depression, electrolyte abnormalities, prematurity, low birth weight, decreased hematocrit or platelets. Risk to the fetus is decreased if treatment can be avoided during the first trimester; however, women of childbearing potential should be advised of the potential risks.

Breast-Feeding Considerations It is not known if cytarabine is excreted in breast milk. Due to the potential for serious adverse reactions in the nursing infant, the decision to discontinue cytarabine or to discontinue breast-feeding should take into account the importance of treatment to the mother.

Contraindications Hypersensitivity to cytarabine or any component

◄ **Warnings** Hazardous agent; use appropriate precautions for handling and disposal (NIOSH, 2012). Causes significant bone marrow depression (leukopenia, thrombocytopenia, and anemia) **[U.S. Boxed Warning]**; use with caution in patients with prior bone marrow suppression; monitor for signs of febrile neutropenia. Must monitor for drug toxicity; high dose regimens have been associated with GI, CNS, pulmonary, ocular (prophylaxis with ophthalmic corticosteroids is recommended) toxicities, and cardiomyopathy. Neurotoxicity associated with high-dose treatment may present as acute cerebellar toxicity or may be severe with seizure and/or coma; may be delayed, occurring up to 3-8 days after treatment has begun; possibly irreversible. Risk factors for neurotoxicity include cumulative cytarabine dose, prior CNS disease, and renal impairment (incidence may be up to 55% in patients with renal impairment). Cytarabine syndrome which is characterized by fever, myalgia, bone pain, chest pain, maculopapular rash, conjunctivitis, and malaise may occur 6-12 hours following administration; may be managed with corticosteroids. May cause nausea, vomiting, diarrhea, abdominal pain, oral ulceration, and hepatic dysfunction; irreversible cerebellar toxicity may occur. There have been reports of acute pancreatitis in patients receiving continuous infusion and in patients previously treated with L-asparaginase.

When used for intrathecal administration, should not be prepared during the preparation of any other agents; after preparation, store intrathecal medications in an isolated location or container clearly marked with a label identifying as "intrathecal" use only; delivery of intrathecal medications to the patient should only be with other medications intended for administration into the central nervous system (Jacobson, 2009). Some parenteral products contain benzyl alcohol; do not use products containing benzyl alcohol or products reconstituted with bacteriostatic diluent intrathecally or for high-dose cytarabine regimens. Benzyl alcohol may cause allergic reactions in susceptible individuals; large amounts of benzyl alcohol (≥99 mg/kg/day) have been associated with a potentially fatal toxicity ("gasping syndrome") in neonates.

Precautions Marked bone marrow suppression necessitates dosage reduction or a reduction in the number of days of administration; use with caution in patients with severe hepatic dysfunction; dosage reduction may be necessary. Use high-dose cytarabine with caution in patients with impaired renal function; patients are at higher risk (up to 55%) for cerebellar toxicity and other CNS toxicities; dosage adjustment may be required. With high-dose therapy, tumor lysis syndrome and subsequent hyperuricemia may occur; consider allopurinol and hydrate accordingly. Should be administered under the supervision of an experienced cancer chemotherapy physician. Adequate facilities must be available **[U.S. Boxed Warning]**.

Adverse Reactions

Cardiovascular: Chest pain, pericarditis
Central nervous system: Dizziness, fever, headache, neural toxicity, neuritis
Dermatologic: Alopecia, pruritus, rash, skin freckling, skin ulceration, urticaria
Gastrointestinal: Abdominal pain, anal inflammation, anal ulceration, anorexia, bowel necrosis, diarrhea, esophageal ulceration, esophagitis, mucositis, nausea, pancreatitis, sore throat, vomiting
Genitourinary: Urinary retention
Hematologic: Myelosuppression, neutropenia (onset: 1 to 7 days; nadir [biphasic]: 7 to 9 days and at 15 to 24 days; recovery [biphasic]: 9 to 12 and at 24 to 34 days), thrombocytopenia (onset: 5 days; nadir: 12 to 15 days; recovery 15 to 25 days), anemia, bleeding, leukopenia, megaloblastosis, reticulocytes decreased

Hepatic: Hepatic dysfunction, jaundice, transaminases increased (acute)
Local: Injection site cellulitis, thrombophlebitis
Ocular: Conjunctivitis
Renal: Renal dysfunction
Respiratory: Dyspnea
Miscellaneous: Allergic edema, anaphylaxis, sepsis
Rare but important or life-threatening: Acute respiratory distress syndrome, amylase increased, angina, aseptic meningitis, cardiopulmonary arrest (acute), cerebral dysfunction, cytarabine syndrome (bone pain, chest pain, conjunctivitis, fever, maculopapular rash, malaise, myalgia); exanthematous pustulosis, hepatic sinusoidal obstruction syndrome (SOS; veno-occlussive disease), hyperuricemia, injection site inflammation (SubQ injection), injection site pain (SubQ injection), interstitial pneumonitis, lipase increased, paralysis (intrathecal and I.V. combination therapy), reversible posterior leukoencephalopathy syndrome (RPLS), rhabdomyolysis, toxic megacolon

Adverse events associated with high-dose cytarabine (CNS, gastrointestinal, ocular, and pulmonary toxicities are more common with high-dose regimens):
Cardiovascular: Cardiomegaly, cardiomyopathy (in combination with cyclophosphamide)
Central nervous system: Cerebellar toxicity, coma, neurotoxicity, personality change, somnolence
Dermatologic: Alopecia (complete), desquamation, rash (severe)
Gastrointestinal: Gastrointestinal ulcer, pancreatitis, peritonitis, pneumatosis cystoides intestinalis
Hepatic: Hyperbilirubinemia, liver abscess, liver damage, necrotizing colitis
Neuromuscular & skeletal: Peripheral neuropathy (motor and sensory)
Ocular: Corneal toxicity, hemorrhagic conjunctivitis
Respiratory: Pulmonary edema, syndrome of sudden respiratory distress
Miscellaneous: Sepsis

Adverse events associated with intrathecal cytarabine administration:
Central nervous system: Accessory nerve paralysis, fever, necrotizing leukoencephalopathy (with concurrent cranial irradiation, intrathecal methotrexate, and intrathecal hydrocortisone), neurotoxicity, paraplegia
Gastrointestinal: Dysphagia, nausea, vomiting
Ocular: Blindness (with concurrent systemic chemotherapy and cranial irradiation), diplopia
Respiratory: Cough, hoarseness
Miscellaneous: Aphonia

Drug Interactions

Metabolism/Transport Effects None known.

Avoid Concomitant Use
Avoid concomitant use of Cytarabine (Conventional) with any of the following: BCG; CloZAPine; Dipyrone; Natalizumab; Pimecrolimus; Tacrolimus (Topical); Tofacitinib; Vaccines (Live)

Increased Effect/Toxicity
Cytarabine (Conventional) may increase the levels/effects of: CloZAPine; Leflunomide; Natalizumab; Tofacitinib; Vaccines (Live)

The levels/effects of Cytarabine (Conventional) may be increased by: Denosumab; Dipyrone; Pimecrolimus; Roflumilast; Tacrolimus (Topical); Trastuzumab

Decreased Effect
Cytarabine (Conventional) may decrease the levels/effects of: BCG; Cardiac Glycosides; Coccidioidin Skin Test; Flucytosine; Sipuleucel-T; Vaccines (Inactivated); Vaccines (Live)

The levels/effects of Cytarabine (Conventional) may be decreased by: Echinacea

Stability Hazardous agent; use appropriate precautions for handling and disposal (NIOSH, 2012). Use appropriate precautions for handling and disposal. Store intact vials of powder for injection at room temperature of 20°C to 25°C (68°F to 77°F); store intact vials of solution at room temperature of 15°C to 30°C (59°F to 86°F).

I.V.: Powder for reconstitution: Reconstitute with bacteriostatic water for injection [for standard dose (100-200 mg/m^2)]; do not use a diluent containing benzyl alcohol to prepare high-dose I.V. therapies. After reconstitution, store at room temperature and use within 48 hours.

For I.V. infusion: Further dilutions in NS or D$_5$W are stable for 7 days at room temperature.

Intrathecal: Powder for reconstitution: Reconstitute with preservative-free NS; administer as soon as possible after preparation. Do **not** use a diluent containing benzyl alcohol to prepare.

Intrathecal triple therapy (ITT): Cytarabine 30-50 mg with hydrocortisone sodium succinate 15-25 mg and methotrexate 12 mg; compatible together for up to 24 hours in a syringe; however, should be administered as soon as possible after preparation because intrathecal preparations are preservative free

Mechanism of Action Inhibits DNA synthesis. Cytosine gains entry into cells by a carrier process, and then must be converted to its active compound, aracytidine triphosphate. Cytosine is a pyrimidine analog and is incorporated into DNA; however, the primary action is inhibition of DNA polymerase resulting in decreased DNA synthesis and repair. The degree of cytotoxicity correlates linearly with incorporation into DNA; therefore, incorporation into the DNA is responsible for drug activity and toxicity. Cytarabine is specific for the S phase of the cell cycle (blocks progression from the G$_1$ to the S phase).

Pharmacokinetics (Adult data unless noted)

Distribution:: V$_d$: Total body water; widely and rapidly since it enters the cells readily; crosses blood-brain barrier achieving CSF concentrations 40% to 50% of plasma concentration

Protein binding: 13%

Metabolism: Primarily hepatic; metabolized by deoxycytidine kinase and other nucleotide kinases to aracytidine triphosphate (active); about 86% to 96% of dose is metabolized to inactive uracil arabinoside (ARA-U); intrathecal administration results in little conversion to ARA-U due to the low amount of deaminase in the CSF

Half-life, terminal: 1-3 hours; intrathecal: 2-6 hours

Time to peak serum concentration: SubQ: 20-60 minutes

Elimination: Urine (~80%; 90% as metabolite ARA-U) within 24 hours

Dosing: Usual

I.V.: Children and Adults (refer to individual protocols):

AML remission induction: Manufacturer's recommendation: Standard dose: 100 mg/m^2/day continuous infusion for 7 days **or** 100 mg/m^2/dose continuous infusion (over 12 hours) every 12 hours for 7 days

Remission maintenance:

I.V.: 70-200 mg/m^2/day for 2-5 days at monthly intervals

SubQ: 1-1.5 mg/kg single dose for maintenance at 1- to 4-week intervals

High-dose therapy for refractory or secondary leukemias or refractory non-Hodgkin's lymphoma: I.V. infusion: 1-3 g/m^2/dose every 12 hours for up to 12 doses

Intrathecal: Infants, Children, and Adults (refer to individual protocols):

Meningeal leukemia: Manufacturer's recommendation: Usual dose: 30 mg/m^2 intrathecally every 4 days; range: 5-75 mg/m^2 once daily for 4 days or once every 4 days until CNS findings normalize, followed by one additional treatment. **Note:** Optimal intrathecal chemotherapy dosing should be based on age (see following information) rather than on body surface area (BSA); CSF volume correlates with age and not to BSA (Bleyer, 1983; Kerr, 2001). Age based dosing: Age in years:

CNS prophylaxis: I.T.:

<1 years: 20 mg per dose

1 to <2 years: 30 mg per dose

2 to <3 years: 50 mg per dose

≥3 years: 70 mg per dose

CNS prophylaxis (ALL): Other age-specific regimens reported from literature:

Gaynon, 1993: Administer on day 0 of induction therapy:

<2 years: 30 mg per dose

2-3 years: 50 mg per dose

≥3 years: 70 mg per dose

Matloub, 2006: Administer on day 0 of induction therapy, then as part of ITT on days 7, 14, and 21 during consolidation therapy; as part of ITT on days 0, 28, and 35 for 2 cycles of delayed intensification therapy, and then maintenance treatment as part of ITT on day 0 every 12 weeks for 38 months (boys) or 26 months (girls) from initial induction treatment:

<2 years: 16 mg per dose

2 to <3 years: 20 mg per dose

3-8 years: 24 mg per dose

>8 years: 30 mg per dose

Pieters, 2007: Administer on day 15 of induction therapy, days 1 and 15 of reinduction phase; and day 1 of cycle 2 of maintenance 1A phase:

<1 year: 15 mg per dose

≥1 years: 20 mg per dose

Lin, 2007: Administer as part of intrathecal triple therapy (ITT) on days 1 and 15 of induction therapy; days 1, 15, 50, and 64 (standard risk patients) or days 1, 15, 29, and 43 (high-risk patients) during consolidation therapy; day 1 of reinduction therapy, and during maintenance therapy (very high risk patients receive on days 1, 22, 45, and 59 of induction, days 8, 22, 36, and 50 of consolidation therapy, days 8 and 38 of reinduction therapy, and during maintenance):

<1 year: 18 mg per dose

1 to <2 years: 24 mg per dose

2 to <3 years: 30 mg per dose

>3 years: 36 mg per dose

Treatment, CNS leukemia (ALL): Administer as part of ITT weekly until CSF remission, then every 4 weeks throughout continuation treatment (Lin, 2007):

<1 year: 18 mg per dose

1 to <2 years: 24 mg per dose

2 to <3 years: 30 mg per dose

≥3 years: 36 mg per dose

Dosing adjustment in renal impairment: I.V.: The following guidelines have been used by some clinicians:

Aronoff, 2007 (cytarabine 100-200 mg/m^2): Children and Adults: No adjustment necessary

Smith, 1997 (high-dose cytarabine ≥2 g/m^2/dose): For serum creatinine 1.5-1.9 mg/dL or increase (from baseline) of 0.5-1.2 mg/dL: Reduce dose to 1 g/m^2/dose

Dosing adjustment for hepatic impairment: I.V.: Dose may need to be adjusted in patients with liver failure since cytarabine is partially detoxified in the liver. The following guideline has been used by some clinicians:

Floyd, 2006: Transaminases (any elevation): Administer 50% of dose; may increase subsequent doses in the absence of toxicity

Koren, 1992 (dose not specified): Bilirubin >2 mg/dL: Administer 50% of dose; may increase subsequent doses in the absence of toxicity

Administration Hazardous agent; use appropriate precautions for handling and disposal (NIOSH, 2012).

Parenteral: May administer SubQ, IVP, I.V. infusion, or I.T.; pH: 5-7.4

I.V. infusion: After reconstitution, further dilute in 250-1000 mL NS or D$_5$W. Infuse as a continuous infusion (standard dose) or infuse over 1-3 hours (infusion rate based on protocol). GI adverse effects may be more pronounced with divided I.V. bolus doses than with continuous infusion.

High-dose regimens or for use in neonates: Diluents containing benzyl alcohol should not be used to reconstitute the drug for high-dose regimens; high-dose regimens (dose >1 g/m^2) are usually administered by I.V. infusion over ~2-3 hours

IVP: May administer over 15 minutes

I.T. administration: Reconstitute with preservative-free NS; may be further diluted to preferred final volume with Elliott's B solution, or preservative-free NS or LR solution, do **not** use diluents containing benzyl alcohol; the final volume generally based on institution or practitioner preferences; volume range is 3-10 mL and may be up to 12 mL and should correspond to an equivalent volume of CSF removed; filter through a 0.22 micron filter; antiemetic therapy should be administered prior to intrathecal doses of cytarabine. Administer as soon as possible after preparation. Intrathecal medications should not be prepared during the preparation of any other agents. After preparation, store intrathecal medications in an isolated location or container clearly marked with a label identifying as "intrathecal" use only.

SubQ administration: Rotate injection sites to thigh, abdomen, and flank regions; avoid repeated administration to a single site

Monitoring Parameters Liver function tests, CBC with differential and platelet count, serum creatinine, BUN, serum uric acid; signs of neurotoxicity

Additional Information Consider corticosteroid eye drops for prophylaxis of conjunctivitis prior to, during, and for 2-7 days after high-dose cytarabine; pyridoxine has been administered on days of high-dose cytarabine therapy for prophylaxis of CNS toxicity.

Dosage Forms Excipient information presented when available (limited, particularly for generics); consult specific product labeling.

Solution, Injection:
Generic: 20 mg/mL (25 mL); 100 mg/mL (20 mL)
Solution, Injection [preservative free]:
Generic: 20 mg/mL (5 mL, 50 mL); 100 mg/mL (20 mL)
Solution Reconstituted, Injection:
Generic: 100 mg (1 ea); 500 mg (1 ea); 1 g (1 ea)

References

Aronoff GR, Bennett WM, Berns JS, et al, *Drug Prescribing in Renal Failure: Dosing Guidelines for Adults and Children*, 5th ed. Philadelphia, PA: American College of Physicians; 2007, p 98, 170.

Baker WJ, Royer GL, and Weiss RB, "Cytarabine and Neurologic Toxicity," *J Clinical Oncology*, 1991, 9(4):679-93.

Bleyer WA, Coccia PF, Sather HN, et al, "Reduction in Central Nervous System Leukemia With a Pharmacokinetically Derived Intrathecal Methotrexate Dosage Regimen," *J Clin Oncol*, 1983, 1(5):317-25.

Capizzi RL, White JC, Powell BL, et al, "Effect of Dose on the Pharmacokinetic and Pharmacodynamic Effects of Cytarabine," *Semin Hematol*, 1991, 28(3 Suppl 4):54-69.

de Lemos ML, Monfared S, Denyssevych T, et al, "Evaluation of Osmolality and pH of Various Concentrations of Methotrexate,

Cytarabine, and Thiotepa Prepared in Normal Saline, Sterile Water for Injection, and Lactated Ringers's Solution for Intrathecal Administration," *J Oncol Pharm Pract*, 2009, 15(1):45-52.

Floyd J, Mirza I, Sachs B, et al, "Hepatotoxicity of Chemotherapy," *Semin Oncol*, 2006, 33(1):50-67.

Gaynon PS, Steinherz PG, Bleyer WA, et al, "Improved Therapy for Children With Acute Lymphoblastic Leukemia and Unfavorable Presenting Features: A Follow-Up Report of the Childrens Cancer Group Study CCG-106," *J Clin Oncol*, 1993, 11(11):2234-42.

Grossman L, Baker MA, Sutton DM, et al, "Central Nervous System Toxicity of High-Dose Cytosine Arabinoside," *Med Pediatr Oncol*, 1983, 11(4):246-50.

Jacobson JO, Polovich M, McNiff KK, et al, "American Society of Clinical Oncology/Oncology Nursing Society Chemotherapy Administration Safety Standards," *J Clin Oncol*, 2009, 27(32):5469-75.

Kerr JZ, Berg S, and Blaney SM, "Intrathecal Chemotherapy," *Crit Rev Oncol Hematol*, 2001, 37(3):227-36.

Koren G, Beatty K, Seto A, et al, "The Effects of Impaired Liver Function on the Elimination of Antineoplastic Agents," *Ann Pharmacother*, 1992, 26(3):363-71.

Lin WY, Liu HC, Yeh TC, et al, "Triple Intrathecal Therapy Without Cranial Irradiation for Central Nervous System Preventive Therapy in Childhood Acute Lymphoblastic Leukemia," *Pediatr Blood Cancer*, 2008, 50(3):523-7.

Matloub Y, Lindemulder S, Gaynon PS, et al, "Intrathecal Triple Therapy Decreases Central Nervous System Relapse but Fails to Improve Event-Free Survival When Compared With Intrathecal Methotrexate: Results of the Children's Cancer Group (CCG) 1952 Study for Standard-Risk Acute Lymphoblastic Leukemia, Reported by the Children's Oncology Group," *Blood*, 2006, 108(4):1165-73.

National Institute for Occupational Safety and Health (NIOSH), "NIOSH List of Antineoplastic and Other Hazardous Drugs in Healthcare Settings 2012." Available at http://www.cdc.gov/niosh/docs/2012-150/pdfs/2012-150.pdf. Accessed January 21, 2013.

Pease CL, Horton TM, McClain KL, et al, "Aseptic Meningitis in a Child After Systemic Treatment With High Dose Cytarabine," *Pediatr Infect Dis J*, 2001, 20(1):87-9.

Pieters R, Schrappe M, De Lorenzo P, et al, "A Treatment Protocol for Infants Younger Than 1 Year With Acute Lymphoblastic Leukaemia (Interfant-99): An Observational Study and a Multicentre Randomised Trial," *Lancet*, 2007, 370(9583):240-50.

Smith G, Damon LE, Rugo HS, et al. "High-Dose Cytarabine Dose Modification Reduces the Incidence of Neurotoxicity in Patients With Renal Insufficiency," *J Clin Oncol*, 1997, 15(2): 833-9.

♦ **Cytarabine Hydrochloride** *see* Cytarabine (Conventional) *on page 573*

♦ **Cytarabine Injection (Can)** *see* Cytarabine (Conventional) *on page 573*

♦ **CytoGam®** *see* Cytomegalovirus Immune Globulin (Intravenous-Human) *on page 576*

Cytomegalovirus Immune Globulin (Intravenous-Human)

(sye toe meg a low VYE rus i MYUN GLOB yoo lin in tra VEE nus HYU man)

Medication Safety Issues
Sound-alike/look-alike issues:
CytoGam® may be confused with Cytoxan, Gamimune® N

Related Information
Immunization Administration Recommendations *on page 2368*

Immunization Guidelines *on page 2373*

Brand Names: U.S. CytoGam®

Brand Names: Canada CytoGam®

Therapeutic Category Immune Globulin

Generic Availability (U.S.) No

Use Prophylaxis of cytomegalovirus (CMV) disease associated with kidney, lung, liver, pancreas, or heart transplantation [FDA approved in pediatric patients (age not specified) and adults]; concomitant use with ganciclovir should be considered in organ transplants other than kidney from CMV seropositive donors to CMV seronegative recipients; has also been used for CMV treatment in hematopoietic stem cell transplantation

Pregnancy Risk Factor C

Pregnancy Considerations Animal reproduction studies have not been conducted.

Contraindications Hypersensitivity to cytomegalovirus immune globulin (CMV-IGIV), other immune globulin preparations, or any component; selective IgA deficiency

Warnings Hypersensitivity and anaphylactic reactions can occur; monitor vital signs during infusion; discontinue immediately for hypotension or anaphylaxis; immediate treatment (including epinephrine 1:1000) should be available. Systemic allergic reactions are rare; may be treated with epinephrine and diphenhydramine

Acute renal dysfunction with increased serum creatinine, oliguria, osmotic nephrosis, and/or acute renal failure can rarely occur with administration of immune globulin products; usually within 7 days of use and more likely with products stabilized with sucrose; CytoGam® contains sucrose as a stabilizing agent. Patients at risk for renal failure include the elderly, patients with preexisting renal disease, diabetes mellitus, volume depletion, sepsis, paraproteinemia, and nephrotoxic medications. In patients at risk for renal dysfunction, the rate of infusion and concentration of solution should be minimized. Discontinue if renal function deteriorates. Correct any volume depletion prior to therapy.

Aseptic meningitis syndrome (AMS) has been reported with intravenous immune globulin administration (rare); may occur with high doses (≥2 g/kg); patients with history of migraines may be at a higher risk. Symptoms include severe headache, nuchal rigidity, drowsiness, fever, photophobia, painful eye movements, and nausea and vomiting. Syndrome usually appears within several hours to 2 days following treatment; usually resolves within several days after discontinuation.

Pulmonary events including transfusion-related acute lung injury (TRALI) have been reported; noncardiogenic pulmonary edema has been reported with intravenous immune globulin use. TRALI is characterized by severe respiratory distress, pulmonary edema, hypoxemia, and fever in the presence of normal left ventricular function and usually occurs within 1-6 hours after infusion; monitor closely; may be managed with oxygen and respiratory support.

Thrombotic events have been reported with administration of intravenous immune globulin; patients at risk include those with advanced age or a history of atherosclerosis, cardiovascular and/or thrombotic risk factors, or known/suspected hyperviscosity; use with caution in these patients; consider a baseline assessment of blood viscosity in patients at risk for hyperviscosity. Rapid infusion may be a possible risk factor for vascular occlusive events. Intravenous immune globulin has been associated with antiglobulin hemolysis; monitor for signs of hemolytic anemia.

Precautions Product of human plasma; may potentially contain infectious agents which could transmit disease. Screening of donors, as well as testing and/or inactivation or removal of certain viruses, reduces the risk. Infections thought to be transmitted by this product should be reported to the manufacturer. Product is stabilized with albumin. Response to live vaccines may be reduced following immune globulin treatment; refer to package insert or current practice guidelines for recommendations on separation intervals.

Adverse Reactions

Cardiovascular: Flushing

Central nervous system: Chills, fever

Gastrointestinal: Nausea, vomiting

Neuromuscular & skeletal: Arthralgia, back pain, muscle cramps

Respiratory: Wheezing

Rare but important or life-threatening: Abdominal pain, acute renal failure, acute respiratory distress syndrome (ARDS), acute tubular necrosis, allergic reactions (systemic), anaphylactic shock, angioneurotic edema, anuria, apnea, aseptic meningitis syndrome (AMS), blood pressure decreased, bronchospasm, bullous dermatitis, BUN increased, cardiac arrest, coma, Coomb's test positive, cyanosis, dyspnea, epidermolysis, erythema multiforme, hemolysis, hypotension, hypoxemia, leukopenia, liver dysfunction, loss of consciousness, oliguria, osmotic nephrosis, pancytopenia, proximal tubular nephropathy, pulmonary edema, renal dysfunction, rigors, seizure, serum creatinine increased, Stevens-Johnson syndrome, thromboembolism, transfusion-related acute lung injury (TRALI), tremor, vascular collapse

Drug Interactions

Metabolism/Transport Effects None known.

Avoid Concomitant Use There are no known interactions where it is recommended to avoid concomitant use.

Increased Effect/Toxicity There are no known significant interactions involving an increase in effect.

Decreased Effect

Cytomegalovirus Immune Globulin (Intravenous-Human) may decrease the levels/effects of: Vaccines (Live)

Stability Store at 2°C to 8°C (36°F to 46°F); do not freeze. Infusion should begin within 6 hours after entering the vial.

Mechanism of Action CMV-IGIV is a preparation of immunoglobulin G (and trace amounts of IgA and IgM) derived from pooled healthy blood donors and contains a high titer of CMV antibodies; administration provides a passive source of antibodies against cytomegalovirus to attenuate or reduce the incidence of serious CMV disease

Pharmacokinetics (Adult data unless noted) Half-life: 8-24 days

Dosing: Usual

Infants, Children, and Adolescents: **Note:** Refer to individual protocols.

Prophylaxis of CMV disease in kidney transplant: Initial: I.V.: 150 mg/kg within 72 hours of transplant; 100 mg/kg at weeks 2, 4, 6, and 8 after transplant and 50 mg/kg at weeks 12 and 16 after transplant

Prophylaxis of CMV disease in liver, lung, pancreas, or heart transplant (CMV (+) donor and CMV (-) recipient): I.V.: 150 mg/kg within 72 hours of transplant, 150 mg/kg at weeks 2, 4, 6, and 8 after transplant; 100 mg/kg at weeks 12 and 16 after transplant

Treatment, CMV disease: Limited data available:

Ganciclovir-resistant infection and disease: I.V.: 100 mg/kg/dose weekly in combination with other antivirals (eg, ganciclovir, foscarnet, cidofovir); duration of therapy dependent upon CMV antigenemia assay (pp65) or PCR (Bueno, 2002)

Pneumonitis, severe: Children and Adolescents: I.V.: 400 mg/kg on days 1, 2, and 7 followed by 200 mg/kg on days 14; if still symptomatic, may administer an additional 200 mg/kg on day 21; use in combination with ganciclovir (Reed, 1988)

Adults:

Prophylaxis of CMV disease in kidney transplant: I.V.: Initial dose (within 72 hours of transplant): 150 mg/kg/dose

2-, 4-, 6-, and 8 weeks after transplant: 100 mg/kg/dose 12 and 16 weeks after transplant: 50 mg/kg/dose

Prophylaxis of CMV disease in liver, lung, pancreas, or heart transplant: I.V.:

Initial dose (within 72 hours of transplant): 150 mg/kg/dose

2-, 4-, 6-, and 8 weeks after transplant: 150 mg/kg/dose 12 and 16 weeks after transplant: 100 mg/kg/dose

Dosage adjustment in renal impairment: No dosage adjustment provided in manufacturer's labeling; use with caution. Infuse at minimum rate.

Administration Parenteral: I.V. infusion: Does not require further dilution; administer as a 50 mg/mL solution through a dedicated I.V. line containing an in-line 15 micron filter (a 0.2 micron filter is also acceptable) using an infusion pump. Do not mix with other infusions; do not use if turbid. Begin infusion within 6 hours of entering vial, complete infusion within 12 hours of vial entry. Infusion with other products is not recommended; however, if unavoidable, may be piggybacked into an I.V. line of NS, D_5W, $D_{10}W$, or dextrose 20% in water. Do not dilute more than 1:2.

Initial infusion: Begin at 15 mg/kg/hour; if there are no infusion-related reactions after 30 minutes, increase to 30 mg/kg/hour; if no infusion-related reactions after 30 minutes, increase to 60 mg/kg/hour for the remainder of the infusion; infusion rate should not exceed 75 mL/hour. Monitor closely after each rate change. If patient develops nausea, back pain, or flushing during infusion, slow the rate or temporarily stop the infusion. Discontinue if blood pressure drops or in case of anaphylactic reaction.

Subsequent infusions: Initiate at 15 mg/kg/hour for the first 15 minutes, if no infusion-related reactions, increase to 30 mg/kg/hour for the next 15 minutes; if rate is tolerated, increase to 60 mg/kg/hour and maintain this rate until completion of dose; maximum infusion rate: 60 mg/kg/hour or not to exceed 75 mL/hour.

Monitoring Parameters Renal function (BUN, serum creatinine prior to initial infusion and periodically thereafter); urine output; vital signs, including blood pressure (throughout infusion); signs/symptoms of infusion-related adverse reactions, anaphylaxis; signs and symptoms of hemolytic anemia; blood viscosity (baseline; in patients at risk for hyperviscosity); presence of antineutrophil antibodies (if TRALI is suspected); volume status; weight gain; clinical response

Additional Information
IgA content: Trace
Plasma Source: 2000-5000 donors (5% with top CMV titers)
IgG subclass (%):
IgG$_1$: 65
IgG$_2$: 28
IgG$_3$: 5.2
IgG$_4$: 1.7
Monomers + dimer (%): ≥95 monomers + dimers
Gamma globulin (%): 99
Albumin: 10 mg/mL
Sodium content: 20-30 mEq/L
Sugar content: 5% sucrose
Osmolality: >200 mOsm/L

Dosage Forms Excipient information presented when available (limited, particularly for generics); consult specific product labeling.
Injection, solution [preservative free]:
CytoGam®: 50 mg (± 10 mg)/mL (50 mL) [contains sodium 20-30 mEq/L, human albumin, and sucrose 50 mg/mL]

References
Bowden RA, Fisher LD, Rogers K, et al, "Cytomegalovirus (CMV)-Specific Intravenous Immunoglobulin for the Prevention of Primary CMV Infection and Disease After Marrow Transplant," J Infect Dis, 1991, 164(3):483-7.

Bueno J, Ramil C, and Green M, "Current Management Strategies for the Prevention and Treatment of Cytomegalovirus Infection in Pediatric Transplant Recipients," Paediatr Drugs, 2002, 4(5):279-90.

Reed EC, Bowden RA, Dandliker PS, et al, "Treatment of Cytomegalovirus Pneumonia With Ganciclovir and Intravenous Cytomegalovirus Immunoglobulin in Patients With Bone Marrow Transplants," Ann Intern Med, 1988, 109(10):783-8.

Snydman DR, Werner BG, Dougherty NN, et al, "Cytomegalovirus Immune Globulin Prophylaxis in Liver Transplantation. A Randomized, Double-Blind, Placebo-Controlled Trial," Ann Intern Med, 1993, 119(10):984-91.

Valantine HA, Luikart H, Doyle R, et al, "Impact of Cytomegalovirus Hyperimmune Globulin on Outcome After Cardiothoracic Transplantation: A Comparative Study of Combined Prophylaxis With CMV Hyperimmune Globulin Plus Ganciclovir Versus Ganciclovir Alone," Transplantation, 2001, 72(10):1647-52.

◆ **Cytomel** see Liothyronine on page 1256

◆ **Cytomel® (Can)** see Liothyronine on page 1256

◆ **Cytosar (Can)** see Cytarabine (Conventional) on page 573

◆ **Cytosar-U** see Cytarabine (Conventional) on page 573

◆ **Cytosine Arabinosine Hydrochloride** see Cytarabine (Conventional) on page 573

◆ **Cytotec** see Misoprostol on page 1423

◆ **Cytovene** see Ganciclovir (Systemic) on page 955

◆ **Cytovene® (Can)** see Ganciclovir (Systemic) on page 955

◆ **Cytoxan** see Cyclophosphamide on page 561

◆ **Cytra-2** see Sodium Citrate and Citric Acid on page 1906

◆ **Cytra-3** see Citric Acid, Sodium Citrate, and Potassium Citrate on page 487

◆ **Cytra-K** see Potassium Citrate and Citric Acid on page 1710

◆ **D2** see Ergocalciferol on page 774

◆ **D2E7** see Adalimumab on page 70

◆ **D3** see Cholecalciferol on page 455

◆ **D-3-5 [OTC]** see Cholecalciferol on page 455

◆ **D3-50 [OTC]** see Cholecalciferol on page 455

◆ **D-3-Mercaptovaline** see PenicillAMINE on page 1627

◆ **d4T** see Stavudine on page 1932

◆ **D_5W** see Dextrose on page 637

◆ **$D_{10}W$** see Dextrose on page 637

◆ **$D_{25}W$** see Dextrose on page 637

◆ **$D_{30}W$** see Dextrose on page 637

◆ **$D_{40}W$** see Dextrose on page 637

◆ **$D_{50}W$** see Dextrose on page 637

◆ **$D_{60}W$** see Dextrose on page 637

◆ **$D_{70}W$** see Dextrose on page 637

Dacarbazine (da KAR ba zeen)

Medication Safety Issues
Sound-alike/look-alike issues:
Dacarbazine may be confused with procarbazine
High alert medication:
This medication is in a class the Institute for Safe Medication Practices (ISMP) includes among its list of drugs which have a heightened risk of causing significant patient harm when used in error.

Related Information
Emetogenic Potential of Antineoplastic Agents in Children on page 2327
Safe Handling of Hazardous Drugs on page 2419

Brand Names: Canada Dacarbazine for Injection

Therapeutic Category Antineoplastic Agent, Miscellaneous

Generic Availability (U.S.) Yes

Use Treatment of malignant melanoma, Hodgkin's disease (FDA approved in adults); has also been used in the treatment of soft tissue sarcomas (fibrosarcomas, rhabdomyosarcoma), islet cell carcinoma, pheochromocytoma, and medullary carcinoma of the thyroid

Pregnancy Risk Factor C

Pregnancy Considerations [U.S. Boxed Warning]: This agent is carcinogenic and/or teratogenic when used in animals; adverse effects have been observed in animal studies. There are no adequate and well-controlled trials in pregnant women; use in pregnancy only if the potential benefit outweighs the potential risk to the fetus.

Breast-Feeding Considerations Due to the potential for serious adverse reactions in the nursing infant, breast-feeding is not recommended.

Contraindications Hypersensitivity to dacarbazine or any component

Warnings Hazardous agent; use appropriate precautions for handling and disposal (NIOSH, 2012). Hematopoietic depression is common **[U.S. Boxed Warning]**. Leukopenia and thrombocytopenia may be life-threatening; temporary cessation of drug may be required with bone marrow suppression. Hepatotoxicity with hepatocellular necrosis and hepatic vein thrombosis has been reported **[U.S. Boxed Warning]**; hepatotoxicity usually occurs with combination chemotherapy, but may occur with dacarbazine alone; may be carcinogenic and/or teratogenic **[U.S. Boxed Warning]**; dacarbazine has been reported to cause sterility and is mutagenic and teratogenic in rats.

Precautions Use with caution in patients with bone marrow suppression, renal and/or hepatic impairment; dosage reduction may be necessary in patients with renal or hepatic insufficiency; avoid extravasation of the drug; extravasation may result in tissue damage and severe pain. Administer under the supervision of a physician experienced in cancer chemotherapy. Physician should weigh risk to benefit ratio **[U.S. Boxed Warning]**.

Adverse Reactions

Dermatologic: Alopecia

Gastrointestinal: Anorexia, nausea and vomiting

Hematologic: Myelosuppression (onset: 5-7 days; nadir: 7-10 days; recovery: 21-28 days), leukopenia, thrombocytopenia

Local: Pain on infusion

Infrequent, postmarketing, and/or case reports: Anaphylactic reactions, anemia, diarrhea, eosinophilia, erythema, facial flushing, facial paresthesia, flu-like syndrome (fever, myalgia, malaise), hepatic necrosis, hepatic vein occlusion, liver enzymes increased (transient), paresthesia, photosensitivity, rash, renal functions test abnormalities, taste alteration, urticaria

Drug Interactions

Metabolism/Transport Effects Substrate of CYP1A2 (major), CYP2E1 (major); **Note:** Assignment of Major/Minor substrate status based on clinically relevant drug interaction potential

Avoid Concomitant Use

Avoid concomitant use of Dacarbazine with any of the following: BCG; CloZAPine; Dipyrone; Natalizumab; Pimecrolimus; Tacrolimus (Topical); Tofacitinib; Vaccines (Live)

Increased Effect/Toxicity

Dacarbazine may increase the levels/effects of: CloZAPine; Leflunomide; Natalizumab; Tofacitinib; Vaccines (Live)

The levels/effects of Dacarbazine may be increased by: Abiraterone Acetate; CYP1A2 Inhibitors (Moderate); CYP1A2 Inhibitors (Strong); CYP2E1 Inhibitors (Moderate); CYP2E1 Inhibitors (Strong); Deferasirox; Denosumab; Dipyrone; MAO Inhibitors; Pimecrolimus; Roflumilast; Tacrolimus (Topical); Trastuzumab; Vemurafenib

Decreased Effect

Dacarbazine may decrease the levels/effects of: BCG; Coccidioidin Skin Test; Sipuleucel-T; Vaccines (Inactivated); Vaccines (Live)

The levels/effects of Dacarbazine may be decreased by: Cannabis; CYP1A2 Inducers (Strong); Cyproterone; Echinacea; SORAfenib

Stability Hazardous agent; use appropriate precautions for handling and disposal (NIOSH, 2012). Store intact vials at 2°C to 8°C (36°F to 46°F); protect from light; reconstituted dacarbazine solution 10 mg/mL is stable for 72 hours when refrigerated or 8 hours at room temperature; dacarbazine solution further diluted in D_5W or NS is stable for 24 hours when refrigerated or 8 hours at room temperature; drug decomposition has occurred if the solution turns pink; dacarbazine is incompatible with hydrocortisone sodium succinate.

Mechanism of Action Alkylating agent which is converted to the active alkylating metabolite MTIC [(methyl-triazene-1-yl)-imidazole-4-carboxamide] via the cytochrome P450 system. The cytotoxic effects of MTIC are manifested through alkylation (methylation) of DNA at the O^6, N^7 guanine positions which lead to DNA double strand breaks and apoptosis. Non-cell cycle specific.

Pharmacokinetics (Adult data unless noted)

Distribution: Distributes to the liver; very little distribution into CSF with CSF concentrations ~14% of plasma concentrations

V_{dss}: Adults: 17 L/m^2

Protein binding: Minimal, 5%

Metabolism: N-demethylated in the liver by microsomal enzymes; metabolites may also have an antineoplastic effect

Half-life, biphasic: Initial: 20-40 minutes; terminal: 5 hours (in patients with normal renal/hepatic function)

Elimination: ~30% to 50% of dose excreted in urine by tubular secretion, 15% to 25% is excreted in urine as unchanged drug

Dosing: Usual I.V. (refer to individual protocols):

Children:

Pediatric solid tumors: 200-470 mg/m^2/day over 5 days every 21-28 days

Hodgkin's disease: 375 mg/m^2 on days 1 and 15 of treatment course, repeat every 28 days

Adults:

Malignant melanoma: 2-4.5 mg/kg/day for 10 days, repeat in 4 weeks or may use 250 mg/m^2/day for 5 days, repeat in 3 weeks

Hodgkin's disease: 150 mg/m^2/day for 5 days, repeat every 4 weeks **or** 375 mg/m^2 on day 1, repeat in 15 days of each 28-day cycle in combination with other agents

Administration Hazardous agent; use appropriate precautions for handling and disposal (NIOSH, 2012).

Parenteral: Reconstitute 100 mg vial with 9.9 mL SWI or 200 mg vial with 19.7 mL SWI, resulting in a concentration of 10 mg/mL; may further dilute in D_5W or NS and administer by slow IVP over 2-3 minutes or by I.V. infusion over 15-120 minutes at a concentration not to exceed 10 mg/mL

Vesicant/Extravasation Risk May be an irritant

Monitoring Parameters CBC with differential, erythrocytes and platelet count; liver function tests

Dosage Forms Excipient information presented when available (limited, particularly for generics); consult specific product labeling.

Solution Reconstituted, Intravenous:

Generic: 100 mg (1 ea); 200 mg (1 ea)

Solution Reconstituted, Intravenous [preservative free]:

Generic: 200 mg (1 ea)

References

Berg SL, Grisell DL, DeLaney TF, et al, "Principles of Treatment of Pediatric Solid Tumors," *Pediatr Clin North Am*, 1991, 38(2):249-67.

Finklestein JZ, Albo V, Ertel I, et al, "5-(3,3-Dimethyl-l-triazeno) imidazole-4-carboxamide (NSC-45388) in the Treatment of Solid Tumors in Children," *Cancer Chemother Rep*, 1975, 59(2 Pt 1):351-7.

Marchesi F, Turriziani M, Tortorelli G, et al, "Triazene Compounds: Mechanism of Action and Related DNA Repair Systems," *Pharmacol Res*, 2007, 56(4):275-87.

Mutz ID and Urban CE, "Dimethyl-triazeno-imidazole-carboxamide (DTIC) in Combination Chemotherapy for Childhood Neuroblastoma," *Wien Klin Wochenschr*, 1978, 90(24):867-70.

National Institute for Occupational Safety and Health (NIOSH), "NIOSH List of Antineoplastic and Other Hazardous Drugs in Healthcare Settings 2012." Available at http://www.cdc.gov/niosh/docs/2012-150/pdfs/2012-150.pdf. Accessed January 21, 2013.

◆ **Dacarbazine for Injection (Can)** *see* Dacarbazine *on page 578*

◆ **DACT** *see* DACTINomycin *on page 580*

DACTINomycin (dak ti noe MYE sin)

Medication Safety Issues
Sound-alike/look-alike issues:
DACTINomycin may be confused with Dacogen, DAP-TOmycin, DAUNOrubicin

Actinomycin may be confused with achromycin

High alert medication:
This medication is in a class the Institute for Safe Medication Practices (ISMP) includes among its list of drug classes which have a heightened risk of causing significant patient harm when used in error.

Related Information
Management of Drug Extravasations *on page 2255*
Safe Handling of Hazardous Drugs *on page 2419*

Brand Names: U.S. Cosmegen

Brand Names: Canada Cosmegen

Therapeutic Category Antineoplastic Agent, Antibiotic

Generic Availability (U.S.) No

Use Management (either alone or in combination with other treatment modalities) of Wilms' tumor, childhood rhabdomyosarcoma, Ewing's sarcoma, gestational trophoblastic neoplasms, and metastatic nonseminomatous testicular tumors (FDA approved in ages >6 months and adults); used in regional perfusion (palliative or adjunctive) of locally recurrent or locoregional solid tumors (sarcomas, carcinomas, and adenocarcinomas) (FDA approved in adults). Has also been used for treatment of soft tissue sarcoma (other than rhabdomyosarcoma).

Pregnancy Risk Factor D

Pregnancy Considerations Adverse effects have been observed in animal reproduction studies. Women of child-bearing potential are advised not to become pregnant. Use only when potential benefit justifies potential risk to the fetus. **[U.S. Boxed Warning]: Avoid exposure during pregnancy.**

Breast-Feeding Considerations It is not known if dactinomycin is excreted in human breast milk. According to the manufacturer labeling, due to the potential for serious adverse reactions in the nursing infant, the decision to discontinue dactinomycin or to discontinue breast-feeding during therapy should take into account the benefits of treatment to the mother.

Contraindications Hypersensitivity to dactinomycin or any component; patients with chickenpox or herpes zoster

Warnings Hazardous agent; use appropriate precautions for handling and disposal (NIOSH, 2012).

Dactinomycin is extremely toxic; avoid inhalation of vapors/powder or contact with skin, mucous membrane, or eyes **[U.S. Boxed Warning]**; if accidental exposure occurs, immediately irrigate area with water, normal saline, or balanced salt ophthalmic irrigating solution for at least 15 minutes; prompt ophthalmic or medical consultation is also recommended. Contaminated clothing should be destroyed and shoes thoroughly cleaned prior to reuse. Dactinomycin is extremely irritating to tissues **[U.S. Boxed Warning]**. If extravasation occurs during I.V. use, severe damage to soft tissue will occur leading to pain, swelling, ulceration, and necrosis. Extravasation leading to contracture of the arms has also been reported. Recommended for I.V. administration only. The manufacturer recommends intermittent ice (15 minutes 4 times daily) for suspected extravasation. Toxic effects may be delayed in onset (2-4 days following a course of treatment) and may require 1-2 weeks to reach maximum severity. Discontinue treatment with severe myelosuppression, diarrhea, or stomatitis.

Avoid exposure during pregnancy **[U.S. Boxed Warning]**; dactinomycin may cause fetal harm when administered to pregnant women. Women of childbearing potential must be warned to avoid becoming pregnant. Avoid use in infants <6 months of age; toxic effects may occur more frequently.

Reports of secondary malignancies (including leukemia) following treatment with radiation and dactinomycin have occurred; long-term observation of cancer survivors is recommended. May cause potentially fatal hepatic sinusoidal obstruction syndrome [SOS; formerly called veno-occlusive disease (VOD)]; reported incidence of veno-occlusive disease across different clinical studies is 2% to 13.5% with increased risk in children <4 years of age; use with caution in hepatobiliary dysfunction. Monitor for signs or symptoms of hepatic VOD, including bilirubin >1.4 mg/dL, unexplained weight gain, ascites, hepatomegaly, or unexplained right upper quadrant pain (Arndt, 2004).

Precautions Use with caution in patients receiving radiation therapy; may potentiate the effects of radiation therapy; patients receiving radiation therapy are at increased risk for gastrointestinal and myelosuppressive effects. Reduce dosages in patients who are receiving dactinomycin and radiation therapy simultaneously. Erythema from prior radiation therapy may be reactivated by dactinomycin. Avoid dactinomycin use within 2 months of radiation treatment for right-sided Wilms' tumor; may increase the risk of hepatotoxicity. Regional perfusion therapy may result in local limb edema, soft tissue damage, and possible venous thrombosis; dactinomycin leakage into systemic circulation may result in hematologic toxicity, infection, impaired wound healing, and mucositis. Avoid administering live virus vaccinations during therapy with dactinomycin. Administer under the supervision of a physician experienced in cancer chemotherapy **[U.S. Boxed Warning]**.

Adverse Reactions
Central nervous system: Fatigue, fever, lethargy, malaise
Dermatologic: Acne, alopecia (reversible), cheilitis, erythema multiforme, increased pigmentation, sloughing, or erythema of previously irradiated skin; skin eruptions, Stevens-Johnson syndrome, toxic epidermal necrolysis
Endocrine & metabolic: Growth retardation, hyperuricemia, hypocalcemia
Gastrointestinal: Abdominal pain, anorexia, diarrhea, dysphagia, esophagitis, GI ulceration, mucositis, nausea, pharyngitis, proctitis, stomatitis, vomiting
Hematologic: Agranulocytosis, anemia, aplastic anemia, febrile neutropenia, leukopenia, myelosuppression (onset: 7 days, nadir: 14-21 days, recovery: 21-28 days), neutropenia, pancytopenia, reticulocytopenia, thrombocytopenia, thrombocytopenia (immune mediated)
Hepatic: Ascites, bilirubin increased, hepatic failure, hepatitis, hepatomegaly, hepatopathy thrombocytopenia syndrome, hepatotoxicity, liver function test abnormality, hepatic sinusoidal obstruction syndrome (SOS; veno-occlusive liver disease)
Local: Erythema, edema, epidermolysis, pain, tissue necrosis, and ulceration (following extravasation)
Neuromuscular & skeletal: Myalgia
Renal: Renal function abnormality
Respiratory: Pneumonitis
Miscellaneous: Anaphylactoid reaction, infection, sepsis (including neutropenic sepsis)

Drug Interactions
Metabolism/Transport Effects None known.

Avoid Concomitant Use
Avoid concomitant use of DACTINomycin with any of the following: BCG; CloZAPine; Dipyrone; Natalizumab; Pimecrolimus; Tacrolimus (Topical); Tofacitinib; Vaccines (Live)

Increased Effect/Toxicity

DACTINomycin may increase the levels/effects of: Clo-ZAPine; Leflunomide; Natalizumab; Tofacitinib; Vaccines (Live)

The levels/effects of DACTINomycin may be increased by: Denosumab; Dipyrone; Pimecrolimus; Roflumilast; Tacrolimus (Topical); Trastuzumab

Decreased Effect

DACTINomycin may decrease the levels/effects of: BCG; Coccidioidin Skin Test; Sipuleucel-T; Vaccines (Inactivated); Vaccines (Live)

The levels/effects of DACTINomycin may be decreased by: Echinacea

Stability Hazardous agent; use appropriate precautions for handling and disposal (NIOSH, 2012). Store at 20°C to 25°C (68°F to 77°F); protect from light and humidity. According to the manufacturer's labeling, recommended final concentrations (≥10 mcg/mL) are stable for 10 hours at room temperature but should be administered within 4 hours due to the lack of preservative.

Mechanism of Action Binds to the guanine portion of DNA intercalating between guanine and cytosine base pairs inhibiting DNA and RNA synthesis and protein synthesis

Pharmacokinetics (Adult data unless noted)

Distribution: Children: Extensive extravascular distribution (59-714 L) (Veal, 2005); does not penetrate blood-brain barrier

Metabolism: Minimal

Half-life, terminal:

Children: 14-43 hours (Veal, 2005)

Adults: 36 hours

Elimination: ~30% in urine and feces within 1 week

Dosing: Usual Details concerning dosing in combination regimens should be consulted. **Note: Medication orders for dactinomycin are commonly written in MICROgrams (eg, 150 mcg) although many regimens list the dose in MILLIgrams (eg, mg/kg or mg/m^2).** The dose intensity per 2-week cycle for adults and children should not exceed 15 mcg/kg/day for 5 days or 400-600 mcg/m^2/day for 5 days. Some practitioners recommend calculation of the dosage for obese or edematous adult patients on the basis of body surface area in an effort to relate dosage to lean body mass.

Infants ≥6 months, Children, and Adolescents:

Ewing's sarcoma: I.V.: 15 mcg/kg/day for 5 days (in various combination regimens and schedules)

Osteosarcoma: I.V.: Limited data available: 600 mcg/m^2/day days 1, 2, and 3 of weeks 15, 31, 34, 39, and 42 (as part of a combination chemotherapy regimen) (Goorin, 2003)

Rhabdomyosarcoma: I.V.:

Manufacturer's labeling: 15 mcg/kg/day for 5 days (in various combination regimens and schedules)

Alternate dosing: Limited data available: VAC regimen: Infants ≥6 months: 25 mcg/kg every 3 weeks, weeks 0 to 45 (in combination with vincristine and cyclophosphamide, and mesna); dose omission required following radiation therapy (Raney, 2011)

Children and Adolescents: 45 mcg/kg (maximum dose: 2500 mcg) every 3 weeks, weeks 0 to 45 (in combination with vincristine and cyclophosphamide, and mesna); dose omission required following radiation therapy (Raney, 2011)

Wilms' tumor: I.V.:

Manufacturer's labeling: 15 mcg/kg/day for 5 days (in various combination regimens and schedules)

Alternate dosing: Limited data available:

DD-4A regimen: Children and Adolescents: 45 mcg/kg on day 1 every 6 weeks for 54 weeks (in combination with doxorubicin and vincristine) (Green, 1998)

EE-4A regimen: Children and Adolescents: 45 mcg/kg on day 1 every 3 weeks for 18 weeks (in combination with vincristine) (Green, 1998)

VAD regimen:

Infants ≥6 months: 750 mcg/m^2 every 6 weeks for 1 year (stage III disease) (in combination with vincristine and doxorubicin) (Pritchard, 1995)

Children and Adolescents: 1500 mcg/m^2 every 6 weeks for 1 year (stage III disease) (in combination with vincristine and doxorubicin) (Pritchard, 1995)

Adults:

Testicular cancer: I.V.: 1000 mcg/m^2 on day 1 (as part of a combination chemotherapy regimen)

Gestational trophoblastic neoplasm: I.V.: 12 mcg/kg/day for 5 days (monotherapy) **or** 500 mcg/dose days 1 and 2 (as part of a combination chemotherapy regimen)

Wilms' tumor, Ewing's sarcoma, rhabdomyosarcoma: I.V.: 15 mcg/kg/day for 5 days (in various combination regimens and schedules)

Regional perfusion (dosages and techniques may vary by institution; obese patients and patients with prior chemotherapy or radiation therapy may require lower doses): Lower extremity or pelvis: 50 mcg/kg; upper extremity: 35 mcg/kg

Dosing adjustment in renal impairment: There are no dosage adjustments provided in the manufacturer's labeling; however, based on the amount of urinary excretion, dosage adjustments may not be necessary.

Dosing adjustment in hepatic impairment: There are no dosage adjustments provided in the manufacturer's labeling; however, the following adjustments have been recommended: Children, Adolescents and Adults: Any transaminase increase: Reduce dose by 50%; may increase by monitoring toxicities (Floyd, 2006).

Administration Hazardous agent; use appropriate precautions for handling and disposal (NIOSH, 2012).

Reconstitute initially with 1.1 mL of preservative-free SWFI to yield a concentration of 500 mcg/mL (diluent containing preservatives will cause precipitation). May administer undiluted into the side-port of a free flowing I.V. infusion by slow IVP over a few minutes; or may further dilute in D$_5$W or NS in glass or polyvinyl chloride (PVC) containers to a recommended concentration of ≥10 mcg/mL; final concentrations <10 mcg/mL are not recommended; administer as I.V. infusion over 10-15 minutes; consider a D$_5$W or NS flush before and after a dactinomycin dose to ensure venous patency. Cellulose ester membrane filters may partially remove dactinomycin from solution and should not be used during preparation or administration. Avoid extravasation; do not give I.M. or SubQ.

Vesicant/Extravasation Risk Vesicant

Monitoring Parameters CBC with differential and platelet count, liver function tests and renal function tests; monitor for signs/symptoms of hepatic SOS, including unexplained weight gain, ascites, hepatomegaly, or unexplained right upper quadrant pain (Arndt, 2004); monitor serum beta-hCG (management of gestational trophoblastic neoplasms)

Test Interactions May interfere with bioassays of antibacterial drug levels

Dosage Forms Excipient information presented when available (limited, particularly for generics); consult specific product labeling.

Solution Reconstituted, Intravenous:

Cosmegen: 0.5 mg (1 ea)

References

Arndt C, Hawkins D, Anderson JR, et al, "Age Is a Risk Factor for Chemotherapy-Induced Hepatopathy With Vincristine, Dactinomycin, and Cyclophosphamide," *J Clin Oncol*, 2004, 22(10):1894-90.

Bagshawe KD, "High-Risk Metastatic Trophoblastic Disease," *Obstet Gynecol Clin North Am*, 1988, 15(3):531-43.

Berg SL, Grisell DL, DeLaney TF, et al, "Principles of Treatment of Pediatric Solid Tumors," *Pediatr Clin North Am*, 1991, 38(2):249-67.

Berkowitz RS and Goldstein DP, "Gestational Trophoblastic Disease," *Cancer*, 1995, 76(10 Suppl):2079-85.

Carli M, Pastore G, Perilongo G, et al, "Tumor Response and Toxicity After Single High-Dose Versus Standard Five-Day Divided Dose Dactinomycin in Childhood Rhabdomyosarcoma," *J Clin Oncol*, 1988, 6(4):654-8.

Floyd J, Mirza I, Sachs B, et al, "Hepatotoxicity of Chemotherapy," *Semin Oncol*, 2006, 33(1):50-67.

Gershenson DM, Copeland LJ, Kavanagh JJ, et al, "Treatment of Malignant Nondysgerminomatous Germ Cell Tumors of the Ovary With Vincristine, Dactinomycin, and Cyclophosphamide," *Cancer*, 1985, 56(12):2756-6.

Goorin AM, Schwartzentruber DJ, Devidas M, et al, "Presurgical Chemotherapy Compared With Immediate Surgery and Adjuvant Chemotherapy for Nonmetastatic Osteosarcoma: Pediatric Oncology Group Study POG-8651," *J Clin Oncol*, 2003, 21(8):1574-80.

Green DM, Breslow NE, Beckwith JB, et al, "Effect of Duration of Treatment on Treatment Outcome and Cost of Treatment for Wilms' Tumor: A Report From the National Wilms' Tumor Study Group," *J Clin Oncol*, 1998, 16(12):3744-51.

National Institute for Occupational Safety and Health (NIOSH), "NIOSH List of Antineoplastic and Other Hazardous Drugs in Healthcare Settings 2012." Available at http://www.cdc.gov/niosh/docs/2012-150/pdfs/2012-150.pdf. Accessed January 21, 2013.

Pritchard J, Imeson J, Barnes J, et al, "Results of the United Kingdom Children's Cancer Study Group First Wilms' Tumor Study," *J Clin Oncol*, 1995, 13(1):124-33.

Raney RB, Walterhouse DO, Meza JL, et al, "Results of the Intergroup Rhabdomyosarcoma Study Group D9602 Protocol, Using Vincristine and Dactinomycin With or Without Cyclophosphamide and Radiation Therapy, for Newly Diagnosed Patients With Low-Risk Embryonal Rhabdomyosarcoma: A Report From the Soft Tissue Sarcoma Committee of the Children's Oncology Group," *J Clin Oncol*, 2011, 29 (10):1312-8.

Veal GJ, Cole M, Errington J, et al, "Pharmacokinetics of Dactinomycin in a Pediatric Patient Population: A United Kingdom Children's Cancer Study Group Study," *Clin Cancer Res*, 2005, 11(16):5893-9.

◆ **Dalacin C (Can)** *see* Clindamycin (Systemic) *on page 495*

◆ **Dalacin T (Can)** *see* Clindamycin (Topical) *on page 500*

◆ **Dalacin Vaginal (Can)** *see* Clindamycin (Topical) *on page 500*

◆ **Dalfopristin and Quinupristin** *see* Quinupristin and Dalfopristin *on page 1796*

◆ **Dalmane® (Can)** *see* Flurazepam *on page 907*

◆ **d-Alpha Tocopherol** *see* Vitamin E *on page 2148*

Danazol (DA na zole)

Medication Safety Issues
Sound-alike/look-alike issues:
Danazol may be confused with Dantrium®
Brand Names: Canada Cyclomen®
Therapeutic Category Androgen
Generic Availability (U.S.) Yes
Use Treatment of endometriosis amenable to hormonal management; fibrocystic breast disease; hereditary angioedema
Pregnancy Risk Factor X
Pregnancy Considerations [U.S. Boxed Warning]: Pregnancy should be ruled out prior to treatment using a sensitive test (beta subunit test, if available). Nonhormonal contraception should be used during therapy. May cause androgenic effects to the female fetus; clitoral hypertrophy, labial fusion, urogenital sinus defect, vaginal atresia, and ambiguous genitalia have been reported. Therapy should be discontinued for 2 months prior to attempting pregnancy (Caballero, 2012).
Breast-Feeding Considerations
Use of danazol in nursing women is contraindicated.
Contraindications Hypersensitivity to danazol or any component; pregnancy; undiagnosed abnormal genital bleeding; breast-feeding; porphyria; markedly impaired renal, hepatic, or cardiac function

Warnings Use of danazol in pregnancy is contraindicated **[U.S. Boxed Warning]**; exposure to danazol *in utero* may result in androgenic effects on the female fetus; clitoral hypertrophy, labial fusion, urogenital sinus defect, vaginal atresia, and ambiguous genitalia have been reported; a sensitive test capable of determining early pregnancy is recommended immediately prior to initiation of therapy; nonhormonal method of contraception should be used during treatment if indicated. Thromboembolism, thrombotic, and thrombophlebitic events have been reported (including life-threatening or fatal stroke) **[U.S. Boxed Warning]**. Long-term use has been associated with peliosis hepatis and hepatic adenoma **[U.S. Boxed Warning]**; these conditions may be complicated by acute, potentially life-threatening intra-abdominal hemorrhage; monitor liver function. Danazol has been associated with benign intracranial hypertension (pseudotumor cerebri) **[U.S. Boxed Warning]**; monitor for early signs and symptoms including papilledema, headache, nausea, vomiting, and visual disturbances. May increase risk of atherosclerosis and CAD due to decreased HDL and possible increase LDL. May cause nonreversible androgenic effects; patients should be watched closely for signs of androgenic effects.

Precautions Use with caution in patients with seizure disorders, migraine headaches, or conditions influenced by edema

Adverse Reactions
Cardiovascular: Benign intracranial hypertension (rare), edema, flushing, hypertension, MI, palpitation, tachycardia

Central nervous system: Anxiety (rare), chills (rare), convulsions (rare), depression, dizziness, emotional lability, fainting, fatigue, fever (rare), Guillain-Barré syndrome (rare), headache, nervousness, sleep disorders

Dermatologic: Acne, alopecia, erythema multiforme (rare), mild hirsutism, maculopapular rash, papular rash, petechial rash, pruritus, purpuric rash, seborrhea, Stevens-Johnson syndrome (rare), photosensitivity (rare), urticaria, vesicular rash

Endocrine & metabolic: Amenorrhea (which may continue post therapy), breast size reduction, clitoris hypertrophy (rare), glucose intolerance/glucagon changes, HDL decreased, LDL increased, libido changes, nipple discharge (rare), menstrual disturbances (spotting, altered timing of cycle), semen abnormalities (changes in volume, viscosity, sperm count/motility), sex hormone-binding globulin changes, spermatogenesis reduction, thyroid binding globulin changes

Gastrointestinal: Appetite changes (rare), bleeding gums (rare), constipation, gastroenteritis, nausea, pancreatitis (rare), splenic peliosis (rare), vomiting, weight gain

Genitourinary: Vaginal dryness, vaginal irritation, pelvic pain (rare)

Hematologic: Eosinophilia, erythrocytosis (reversible), leukocytosis, leukopenia, platelet count increased, polycythemia, RBC increased, thrombocytopenia

Hepatic: Cholestatic jaundice, hepatic adenoma, jaundice, liver enzymes increased, malignant tumors (after prolonged use), peliosis hepatis

Neuromuscular & skeletal: Back pain, carpal tunnel syndrome (rare), CPK changes, extremity pain, joint lockup, joint pain, joint swelling, muscle cramps, neck pain, paresthesia, spasms, tremor, weakness

Ocular: Cataracts (rare), visual disturbances

Renal: Hematuria

Respiratory: Interstitial pneumonitis, nasal congestion (rare)

Miscellaneous: Diaphoresis, voice change (hoarseness, sore throat, instability, deepening of pitch)

Drug Interactions

Metabolism/Transport Effects Inhibits CYP3A4 (weak)

Avoid Concomitant Use

Avoid concomitant use of Danazol with any of the following: Pimozide

Increased Effect/Toxicity

Danazol may increase the levels/effects of: ARIPiprazole; CarBAMazepine; CycloSPORINE (Systemic); Dofetilide; HMG-CoA Reductase Inhibitors; Lomitapide; Pimozide; Tacrolimus (Systemic); Tacrolimus (Topical); Vitamin D Analogs; Vitamin K Antagonists

The levels/effects of Danazol may be increased by: Corticosteroids (Systemic)

Decreased Effect

Danazol may decrease the levels/effects of: Antidiabetic Agents

Food Interactions Food delays time to peak levels. A high-fat meal increases plasma concentration and extent of availability.

Stability Store at room temperature.

Mechanism of Action Suppresses pituitary output of follicle-stimulating hormone and luteinizing hormone that causes regression and atrophy of normal and ectopic endometrial tissue; decreases rate of growth of abnormal breast tissue; reduces attacks associated with hereditary angioedema by increasing levels of C4 component of complement

Pharmacodynamics

Endometriosis:
Onset of action: 3 weeks

Fibrocystic breast disease:
Onset of action: 1 month
Maximum effect: 4-6 months
Duration: Symptoms recur in 50% of patients within one year after discontinuation of treatment

Pharmacokinetics (Adult data unless noted)

Absorption: Well absorbed

Metabolism: Extensive hepatic metabolism to inactive metabolites

Half-life: Adults: 4.5 hours

Time to peak serum concentration: 2 hours

Dosing: Usual Adolescents and Adults: Oral: **Note:** Begin treatment during menstruation or obtain appropriate tests to ensure patient is not pregnant:

Endometriosis:
Mild case: 100-200 mg twice daily for 3-6 months; may be continued up to 9 months if necessary
Moderate to severe case: 400 mg twice daily for 3-6 months; may be continued up to 9 months if necessary
Note: A gradual downward titration to a dose sufficient to maintain amenorrhea may be considered depending upon the patient's response

Fibrocystic breast disease: 50-200 mg twice daily

Hereditary angioedema: Initial: 200 mg 2-3 times/day depending upon the patient's response; after a favorable response is obtained, decrease the dosage by 50% or less at intervals of 1-3 months or longer. If an attack occurs, the daily dosage may be increased by up to 200 mg.

Administration Oral: Avoid administration with fatty meals.

Monitoring Parameters Liver function tests, symptomatology and site of disease; serum glucose (if diabetic); HDL and LDL cholesterol; signs and symptoms of pseudotumor cerebri; androgenic effects

Test Interactions Estradiol (Kishino, 2010); testosterone, androstenedione, dehydroepiandrosterone

Additional Information Danazol has seen limited use for treatment of ITP in children refractory to steroids. Ten children, 2.5-17 years of age were treated with 20-30 mg/kg/day in divided doses (maximum: 800 mg/day). Treatment was tapered off after patients responded to therapy (Weinblatt, 1988). Danazol has also been evaluated in hemophilia A in a randomized, double-blind placebo-controlled crossover trial in 19 children. Children <15 years received 150 mg/day and >15 years received 300 mg/day for 3 months. Factor VIII:C levels were increased (Mehta, 1992).

Dosage Forms Excipient information presented when available (limited, particularly for generics); consult specific product labeling.

Capsule, Oral:
Generic: 50 mg, 100 mg, 200 mg

References

Caballero T, Farkas H, Bouillet L, et al, "International Consensus and Practical Guidelines on the Gynecologic and Obstetric Management of Female Patients With Hereditary Angioedema Caused by C1 Inhibitor Deficiency," *J Allergy Clin Immunol*, 2012, 129(2):308-20.

Mehta J, Singhal S, Kamath MV, et al, "A Randomized Placebo-Controlled Double-Blind Study of Danazol in Hemophilia A," *Acta Haematol*, 1992, 88(1):14-6.

Weinblatt ME, Kochen J, and Ortega J, "Danazol for Children With Immune Thrombocytopenic Purpura," *Am J Dis Child*, 1988, 142 (12):1317-9.

◆ **Dandrex [OTC]** *see* Selenium Sulfide *on page* 1877

◆ **Danocrine** *see* Danazol *on page* 582

◆ **Dantrium** *see* Dantrolene *on page* 583

◆ **Dantrium® (Can)** *see* Dantrolene *on page* 583

Dantrolene (DAN troe leen)

Medication Safety Issues

Sound-alike/look-alike issues:
Dantrium® may be confused with danazol, Daraprim®
Revonto® may be confused with Revatio®

Related Information

Management of Drug Extravasations *on page* 2255
Serotonin Syndrome *on page* 2405

Brand Names: U.S. Dantrium; Revonto

Brand Names: Canada Dantrium®

Therapeutic Category Antidote, Malignant Hyperthermia; Hyperthermia, Treatment; Skeletal Muscle Relaxant, Nonparalytic

Generic Availability (U.S.) May be product dependent

Use

Parenteral: Management of the fulminant hypermetabolism of skeletal muscle characteristic of malignant hyperthermia (FDA approved in all ages); preoperative/postoperative prevention and attenuation of malignant hyperthermia in susceptible individuals (FDA approved in all ages)

Oral: Treatment of spasticity associated with upper motor neuron disorders such as spinal cord injury, stroke, cerebral palsy, or multiple sclerosis (FDA approved in ages ≥5 years and adults); preoperative/postoperative prevention and attenuation of malignant hyperthermia in susceptible individuals (FDA approved in ages ≥5 years and adults)

Note: Dantrolene prophylaxis is not routinely recommended for most malignant hyperthermia susceptible patients, provided there is immediate availability of parenteral dantrolene and adequate perioperative patient management [eg, avoiding known trigger agents (eg, anesthetics) in susceptible patients]

Pregnancy Risk Factor C

Pregnancy Considerations Adverse events were observed in animal reproduction studies. Dantrolene crosses the human placenta. Cord blood concentrations are similar to those in the maternal plasma at term and dantrolene can be detected in the newborn serum at delivery. Adverse events were not observed in the newborn following maternal doses of 100 mg/day administered orally prior to delivery (Shime, 1988). Uterine atony has been reported following dantrolene injection after delivery; however, this may be due in part to the mannitol contained in the I.V. preparation (Shin, 1995; Weingarten, 1987). Prophylactic use of dantrolene is not routinely recommended in pregnant women susceptible to MH prior to obstetric surgery, if use is needed, close monitoring of the mother and newborn is recommended (Krause, 2004; Norman, 1995).

Breast-Feeding Considerations Low amounts of dantrolene are excreted into breast milk. Due to the potential for serious adverse reactions in the nursing infant, the manufacturer recommends that a decision be made whether to discontinue nursing or to discontinue the drug, taking into account the importance of treatment to the mother. In a case report, the half-life of dantrolene in breast milk was calculated to be 9 hours; the highest milk concentration was 1.2 mcg/mL following a maternal I.V. dose; however, the maternal serum concentrations were not reported (Fricker, 1998).

Contraindications Hypersensitivity to dantrolene or any component. Additional contraindications: Oral: Active hepatic disease (eg, hepatitis and cirrhosis); spasticity that is utilized to maintain posture or balance or to maintain increased function

Warnings With oral therapy, the potential for hepatotoxicity including symptomatic hepatitis (fatal and nonfatal) exists **[U.S. Boxed Warning]**; avoid use in clinical conditions for which dantrolene is not recommended. Hepatic injury is associated with higher doses (ie, ≥800 mg/day) of chronic therapy and sporadic short courses; incidence is lower at doses <400 mg/day but may still occur. Overt hepatitis has been most frequently observed between the third and twelfth month of therapy; risk of hepatic injury appears to be greater in females, in patients >35 years of age (especially elderly patients) and in those with concomitant medication therapy that is also potentially hepatotoxic. Monitor LFTs at baseline and regularly throughout therapy, use lowest effective dose. Discontinue if no benefit is observed after a total of 45 days of therapy, abnormal LFTs or signs and symptoms of jaundice occur.

Injection is an alkaline solution and extremely irritating to peripheral veins; may cause severe tissue necrosis if extravasation occurs; administer in a fast moving I.V. solution into a large vein or into a central line.

Precautions Oral: Use with caution in patients with severely impaired cardiac or pulmonary function or history of liver disease. Lightheadedness and vertigo may occur with therapy; patients must be cautioned about performing tasks which require mental alertness (eg, operating machinery or driving). May cause photosensitivity; discontinue if skin erythema occurs; use skin protection and avoid prolonged exposure to sunlight; do not use tanning equipment.

Parenteral: Use of calcium channel blockers with I.V. dantrolene may increase risk for hyperkalemia and subsequent cardiac arrest. The combination of I.V. dantrolene and calcium channel blockers is not recommended. Contains 3 g mannitol/vial for isotonicity; therefore, the patient will receive 0.375 g/kg of mannitol with the initial I.V. dantrolene dose of 2.5 mg/kg; use caution if additional mannitol therapy. Dantrolene I.V. is not the only therapeutic approach for management of malignant hyperthermia; supportive measures including discontinuing trigger agents (eg, anesthetic agents); administering oxygen; utilizing cooling methods; and monitoring blood gases, urinary output, urine color, and electrolytes must also be utilized and individualized.

Adverse Reactions

Cardiovascular: Blood pressure (altered), heart failure, tachycardia

Central nervous system: Chills, confusion, dizziness, drowsiness, fatigue, fever, headache, insomnia, lightheadedness, malaise, mental depression, nervousness, seizure, speech disturbance

Dermatologic: Eczematoid eruption, hair growth (abnormal), pruritus, rash, urticaria

Gastrointestinal: Abdominal cramps, anorexia, constipation, diarrhea, dysphagia, gastric irritation, gastrointestinal hemorrhage, nausea, taste change, vomiting

Genitourinary: Crystalluria, difficult erection, difficult urination, nocturia, polyuria, urinary incontinence, urinary retention

Hematologic: Anemia, aplastic anemia, leukopenia, thrombocytopenia

Hepatic: Hepatitis

Local: Injection site reaction (pain, erythema, swelling), thrombophlebitis, tissue necrosis

Neuromuscular & skeletal: Back pain, muscle weakness, myalgia

Ocular: Blurred vision, diplopia, tearing (excessive)

Renal: Hematuria

Respiratory: Feeling of suffocation, pleural effusion (associated with pericarditis), pulmonary edema, respiratory depression

Miscellaneous: Anaphylaxis, diaphoresis, lymphocytic lymphoma, sialorrhea

Drug Interactions

Metabolism/Transport Effects Substrate of CYP3A4 (major); **Note:** Assignment of Major/Minor substrate status based on clinically relevant drug interaction potential

Avoid Concomitant Use

Avoid concomitant use of Dantrolene with any of the following: Azelastine (Nasal); Calcium Channel Blockers (Nondihydropyridine); Conivaptan; Fusidic Acid (Systemic); Paraldehyde; Thalidomide

Increased Effect/Toxicity

Dantrolene may increase the levels/effects of: Alcohol (Ethyl); Azelastine (Nasal); Buprenorphine; Calcium Channel Blockers (Nondihydropyridine); CNS Depressants; Hydrocodone; Methotrimeprazine; Metyrosine; Mirtazapine; Paraldehyde; Pramipexole; ROPINIRole; Rotigotine; Selective Serotonin Reuptake Inhibitors; Thalidomide; Vecuronium; Zolpidem

The levels/effects of Dantrolene may be increased by: Brimonidine (Topical); Cannabis; Ceritinib; Conivaptan; CYP3A4 Inhibitors (Moderate); CYP3A4 Inhibitors (Strong); Dasatinib; Doxylamine; Dronabinol; Droperidol; Fusidic Acid (Systemic); HydrOXYzine; Ivacaftor; Kava Kava; Luliconazole; Magnesium Sulfate; Methotrimeprazine; Mifepristone; Nabilone; Perampanel; Rufinamide; Simeprevir; Sodium Oxybate; Stiripentol; Tapentadol; Tetrahydrocannabinol

Decreased Effect

The levels/effects of Dantrolene may be decreased by: Bosentan; CYP3A4 Inducers (Strong); Dabrafenib; Deferasirox; Mitotane; Siltuximab; St Johns Wort; Tocilizumab

Stability

Oral: Store at 20°C to 25°C (68°F to 77°F).

Parenteral: Protect from light; use reconstituted injection within 6 hours; incompatible with dextrose and sodium chloride solutions and bacteriostatic water for injection; precipitates when placed in glass containers for infusion

Dantrium®: Store intact vials and reconstituted solutions at 15°C to 30°C (59°F to 86°F).

Revonto®: Store intact vials and reconstituted solutions at 20°C to 25°C (68°F to 77°F).

Mechanism of Action Acts directly on skeletal muscle by interfering with release of calcium ion from the sarcoplasmic reticulum; prevents or reduces the increase in myoplasmic calcium ion concentration that activates the acute catabolic processes associated with malignant hyperthermia

Pharmacokinetics (Adult data unless noted)

Absorption: Oral: 70% (Allen, 1988)

Metabolism: Extensive; metabolized to active metabolite: 5-hydroxydantrolene

Half-life:

Neonates (at birth): ~20 hours (Shime, 1988)

Children 2-7 years: 10 hours (range: 8.1-14.8 hours) (Lerman, 1989)

Adults: 4-8 hours

Elimination: 25% excreted in urine as metabolites and unchanged drug; 45% to 50% excreted in feces via bile

Dosing: Usual

Infants, Children, and Adolescents:

Spasticity: Oral: Note: Titrate to desired effect; if no further benefit is observed at a higher dosage, decrease dose to previous lower dose.

Manufacturer's labeling: Children and Adolescents ≥5 years:

Patient weight <50 kg: Initial: 0.5 mg/kg/dose once daily for 7 days, increase to 0.5 mg/kg/dose 3 times per day for 7 days, increase to 1 mg/kg/dose 3 times/day for 7 days, and then increase to 2 mg/kg/dose 3 times/day; some patients may require 2 mg/kg/dose 4 times/day; maximum daily dose: 400 mg/day

Patient weight ≥50 kg: Initial: 25 mg once daily for 7 days, then increase to 25 mg 3 times/daily for 7 days, then increase to 50 mg 3 times/daily for 7 days, and then increase to 100 mg 3 times/daily; some patients may require 100 mg 4 times/daily; maximum daily dose: 400 mg/day

Alternate dosing: Children and Adolescents: Initial: 0.5 mg/kg/dose twice daily (maximum dose: 25 mg); titrate frequency at 4-7 days to 3-4 times daily; then increase dose by 0.5 mg/kg increments at weekly intervals to effect; maximum daily dose: 12 mg/kg/day, or 400 mg/day, whichever is lower (Krause, 2004)

Malignant hyperthermia:

Preoperative prophylaxis: Note: Routine use not recommended provided that there is immediate availability of parenteral dantrolene and adequate perioperative patient management (eg, avoiding known trigger agents in susceptible patients):

Oral: 4-8 mg/kg/day in 3-4 divided doses for 1-2 days prior to surgery with the last dose administered approximately 3-4 hours before scheduled surgery

I.V.: 2.5 mg/kg/dose administered approximately 1.25 hours prior to surgery (infuse over 1 hour)

Crisis: I.V.: 2.5 mg/kg (MHAUS recommendation, available at www.mhaus.org); continuously repeat dose until symptoms subside or a cumulative dose of 10 mg/kg is reached (rarely, some patients may require up to 30 mg/kg for initial treatment). Note: Manufacturer's labeling suggests an initial dose of 1 mg/kg.

24-hour MH Hotline (for emergencies only):

United States: 1-800-644-9737

Outside the U.S.: 00-1-209-417-3722

Postcrisis follow-up:

MHAUS protocol suggestion: 1 mg/kg every 4-6 hours (route not specified) or a continuous I.V. infusion of 0.25 mg/kg/hour for at least 24 hours; further doses may be indicated

Manufacturer's recommendation: Oral: 4-8 mg/kg/day in 4 divided doses for 1-3 days; I.V. dantrolene may be used to prevent or attenuate recurrence of MH signs when oral therapy is not practical; individualize dosage beginning with 1 mg/kg or more as the clinical situation dictates

Adults:

Spasticity: Oral: Initial: 25 mg once daily for 7 days, increase to 25 mg 3 times/day for 7 days, increase to 50 mg 3 times/day for 7 days, and then increase to 100 mg 3 times/day; some patients may require 100 mg 4 times/day; maximum daily dose: 400 mg/day. Note: Titrate to desired effect; if no further benefit is observed at a higher dosage, decrease dose to previous lower dose.

Malignant hyperthermia:

Preoperative prophylaxis: Note: Dantrolene prophylaxis is not recommended for most MH-susceptible patients, provided nontriggering anesthetics are used and an adequate supply of dantrolene is available.

Oral: 4-8 mg/kg/day in 3-4 divided doses for 1-2 days prior to surgery with the last dose administered approximately 3-4 hours before scheduled surgery

I.V.: 2.5 mg/kg/dose administered approximately 1.25 hours prior to surgery (infuse over 1 hour) with additional doses as needed

Crisis: I.V.: 2.5 mg/kg (MHAUS recommendation, available at www.mhaus.org); continuously repeat dose until symptoms subside or a cumulative dose of 10 mg/kg is reached (rarely, some patients may require up to 30 mg/kg for initial treatment). Note: Manufacturer's labeling suggests an initial dose of 1 mg/kg.

24-hour MH Hotline (for emergencies only):

United States: 1-800-644-9737

Outside the U.S.: 00-1-209-417-3722

Postcrisis follow-up:

MHAUS protocol suggestion: 1 mg/kg every 4-6 hours (route not specified) or a continuous I.V. infusion of 0.25 mg/kg/hour for at least 24 hours; further doses may be indicated

Manufacturer's recommendation: Oral: 4-8 mg/kg/day in 4 divided doses for 1-3 days; I.V. dantrolene may be used to prevent or attenuate recurrence of MH signs when oral therapy is not practical; individualize dosage beginning with 1 mg/kg or more as the clinical situation dictates

Dosing adjustment in renal impairment: There are no dosage adjustments provided in the manufacturer's labeling.

Dosing adjustments in hepatic impairment: There are no dosage adjustments provided in the manufacturer's labeling; use of oral dantrolene in patients with active liver disease (hepatitis or cirrhosis) is contraindicated.

Administration

Oral: Contents of capsule may be mixed with juice or liquid

Parenteral: Reconstitute by adding 60 mL SWI to 20 mg vial, resultant concentration 0.333 mg/mL; shake vial for ~20 seconds or until solution is clear; no further dilution required; administer crisis doses by rapid I.V. injection; preferably in large-bore I.V. or central line; for intermittent infusion (prophylaxis doses) or continuous I.V. infusion, may transfer dose to sterile plastic bag and administer over 1 hour

Vesicant/Extravasation Risk Vesicant; because of the high pH (~9.5), may cause tissue necrosis if extravasated.

Monitoring Parameters

Spasticity: Motor performance should be monitored for therapeutic outcomes; nausea, vomiting, and liver function tests (baseline and at appropriate intervals thereafter) should be monitored for potential hepatotoxicity

Malignant hyperthermia: Cardiac and blood pressure monitoring; during and postacute phase: Per MHAUS protocol, patient should be observed in an ICU for at least 24 hours since recrudescence may occur; monitor for arrhythmias; monitor vital signs (including core temperature), electrolytes, ABG, CK, end tidal CO_2 ($EtCO_2$)/ capnography, urine output, urine myoglobin

◄ **Additional Information** MHAUS (www.mhaus.org) provides educational and technical information to patients and healthcare providers; contact at 607-674-7920 or email from the "contact" page of the website. Triggers for the development of malignant hyperthermia in susceptible individuals include: All volatile inhalation anesthetics (desflurane, sevoflurane, isoflurane, halothane, enflurane, ether, methoxyflurane, and cyclopropane) and succinylcholine.

Dantrolene has been used successfully to treat neuroleptic malignant syndrome associated with antipsychotic agents such as prochlorperazine, promethazine, clozapine, and risperidone and also non-neuroleptic agents such as metoclopramide, amoxapine, and lithium. The recommended dose for this indication has not been established. Published case reports have used doses ranging from 1-10 mg/kg/day in divided doses both I.V. and orally.

Although dantrolene is FDA approved in all ages for malignant hyperthermia, it does not usually occur in patients <12 months of age and has not been reported at <4 months of age (Chamley, 2000; Larach, 2010, Silva, 1999).

Dosage Forms Excipient information presented when available (limited, particularly for generics); consult specific product labeling.

Capsule, Oral, as sodium:

Dantrium: 25 mg, 50 mg, 100 mg [contains fd&c yellow #6 (sunset yellow)]

Generic: 25 mg, 50 mg, 100 mg

Solution Reconstituted, Intravenous, as sodium:

Dantrium: 20 mg (1 ea)

Revonto: 20 mg (1 ea)

Extemporaneous Preparations A 5 mg/mL oral suspension may be made with dantrolene capsules, a citric acid solution, and either simple syrup or syrup BP (containing 0.15% w/v methylhydroxybenzoate). Add the contents of five 100 mg dantrolene capsules to a citric acid solution (150 mg citric acid powder in 10 mL water); mix while adding the chosen vehicle in incremental proportions to **almost** 100 mL. Transfer to a calibrated bottle and add quantity of vehicle sufficient to make 100 mL. Label "shake well" and "refrigerate". Simple syrup suspension is stable for 2 days refrigerated; syrup BP suspension is stable for 30 days refrigerated.

Nahata MC, Pai VB, and Hipple TF, *Pediatric Drug Formulations*, 5th ed, Cincinnati, OH: Harvey Whitney Books Co, 2004.

References

Allen GC, Cattran CB, Peterson RG, et al, "Plasma Levels of Dantrolene Following Oral Administration in Malignant Hyperthermia-Susceptible Patients," *Anesthesiology*, 1988, 69(6):900-4.

Chamley D, Pollock NA, Stowell KM, et al, "Malignant Hyperthermia in Infancy and Identification of Novel RYR1 Mutation," *Br J Anaesth*, 2000, 84(4):500-4.

Delgado MR, Hirtz D, Aisen M, et al, "Practice Parameter: Pharmacologic Treatment of Spasticity in Children and Adolescents With Cerebral Palsy (an Evidence-Based Review): Report of the Quality Standards Subcommittee of the American Academy of Neurology and the Practice Committee of the Child Neurology Society," *Neurology*, 2010, 74(4):336-43.

Fricker RM, Hoerauf KH, Drewe J, et al, "Secretion of Dantrolene Into Breast Milk After Acute Therapy of a Suspected Malignant Hyperthermia Crisis During Cesarean Section," *Anesthesiology*, 1998, 89(4):1023-5.

Glahn KP, Ellis FR, Halsall PJ, et al, "Recognizing and Managing a Malignant Hyperthermia Crisis: Guidelines From the European Malignant Hyperthermia Group," *Br J Anaesth*, 2010, 105(4):417-20.

Krause T, Gerbershagen MU, Fiege M, et al, "Dantrolene - A Review of Its Pharmacology, Therapeutic Use and New Developments," *Anaesthesia*, 2004, 59(4):364-73.

Larach MG, Gronert GA, Allen GC, et al, "Clinical Presentation, Treatment, and Complications of Malignant Hyperthermia in North America From 1987 to 2006," *Anesth Analg*, 2010, 110(2):498-507.

Lerman J, McLeod ME, and Strong HA, "Pharmacokinetics of Intravenous Dantrolene in Children," *Anesthesiology*, 1989, 70(4):625-9.

Malignant Hyperthermia Association of the United States (MHAUS), "Guidelines and 24-Hour Hotline." Available at http://www.mhaus.org/healthcare-professionals/#.T6rV3VI2cTY

Norman PF and Eichhorn JH, "Management of Anesthetic Complications and Emergencies in the Obstetric Patient," *Obstet Gynecol Clin North Am*, 1995, 22(1):1-12.

Podranski T, Bouillon T, Schumacher PM, et al, "Compartmental Pharmacokinetics of Dantrolene in Adults: Do Malignant Hyperthermia Association Dosing Guidelines Work?" *Anesth Analg*, 2005, 101(6):1695-9.

Shime J, Gare D, Andrews J, et al, "Dantrolene in Pregnancy: Lack of Adverse Effects on the Fetus and Newborn Infant," *Am J Obstet Gynecol*, 1988, 159(4):831-4.

Shin YK, Kim YD, Collea JV, et al, "Effect of Dantrolene Sodium on Contractility of Isolated Human Uterine Muscle," *Int J Obstet Anesth*, 1995, 4(4):197-200.

Silva RR, Munoz DM, Alpert M, et al, "Neuroleptic Malignant Syndrome in Children and Adolescents," *J Am Acad Child Adolesc Psychiatry*, 1999, 38(2):187-94.

Weingarten AE, Korsh JI, Neuman GG, et al, "Postpartum Uterine Atony After Intravenous Dantrolene," *Anesth Analg*, 1987, 66(3):269-70.

♦ **Dantrolene Sodium** see Dantrolene *on page 583*

♦ **Dapcin** see DAPTOmycin *on page 589*

Dapsone (Systemic) (DAP sone)

Medication Safety Issues

Sound-alike/look-alike issues:

Dapsone may be confused with Diprosone

Therapeutic Category Antibiotic, Sulfone; Leprostatic Agent

Generic Availability (U.S.) Yes

Use Treatment of leprosy due to susceptible strains [FDA approved in pediatric patients (age not specified) and adults]; treatment of dermatitis herpetiformis [FDA approved in pediatric patients (age not specified) and adults]; has also been used for prophylaxis and treatment of *Pneumocystis jirovecii* pneumonia (PCP); prophylaxis against toxoplasmic encephalitis; treatment of linear IgA bullous dermatosis (LABD) and refractory idiopathic thrombocytopenia purpura (ITP)

Pregnancy Risk Factor C

Pregnancy Considerations Because of adverse events observed in some animal studies, dapsone is classified as pregnancy category C. Per the manufacturer, dapsone has not shown an increased risk of congenital anomalies when given during all trimesters of pregnancy. Several reports have described adverse effects in the newborn after *in utero* exposure to dapsone, including neonatal hemolytic disease, methemoglobinemia, and hyperbilirubinemia. Dapsone is an alternative for prophylaxis and treatment of *Pneumocystis jirovecii* pneumonia (PCP) in pregnant, HIV-infected patients. Dapsone is also recommended for pregnant women requiring maintenance therapy of either leprosy or dermatitis herpetiformis

Breast-Feeding Considerations Dapsone is excreted in breast milk and can be detected in the serum of nursing infants. Hemolytic anemia has been reported in a breast-fed infant. Breast-feeding is not recommended by the manufacturer due to the potential for carcinogenicity observed in animal studies and the potential for hemolysis in the neonate, especially if there is a family history of G6PD deficiency.

Contraindications Hypersensitivity to dapsone, its derivatives, or any component

Warnings May cause aplastic anemia, agranulocytosis, or other severe and potentially fatal blood dyscrasias; monitor carefully; incidence may be increased if coadministered with a folic acid antagonist; if used concomitantly, increase monitoring. Use with caution in patients with severe anemia; severe anemia should be treated prior to initiation of dapsone therapy. Toxic hepatitis and cholestatic jaundice have been reported early in therapy; monitor liver function tests. Motor loss and muscle weakness have been reported with use.

May rarely cause serious dermatologic reactions, including toxic epidermal necrolysis; if new or toxic dermatologic reactions occur, promptly discontinue and institute appropriate therapy. Use with caution in patients with hypersensitivity to other sulfonamides. Leprosy reactional states do not require discontinuation. Potentially significant interactions may exist, requiring dose or frequency adjustment, additional monitoring, and/or selection of alternative therapy. Consult drug interactions database for more detailed information. Prolonged use may result in fungal or bacterial superinfection, including *C. difficile*-associated diarrhea (CDAD); CDAD has been observed >2 months postantibiotic treatment.

Precautions Use with caution in patients with G-6-PD deficiency, methemoglobin reductase deficiency or hemoglobin M; hemolysis and Heinz body formation may be exaggerated (dose-related); obtain G-6-PD levels prior to initiating dapsone therapy. Use with caution in severe cardiopulmonary disease; hemolysis and methemoglobin effects may be poorly tolerated. Use with caution in patients with altered acetylation rates; patients with high acetylation rates, or who are receiving treatment affecting acetylation may require an adjustment in dosage.

Adverse Reactions

Cardiovascular: Tachycardia

Central nervous system: Fever, headache, insomnia, psychosis (oral/topical), vertigo

Dermatologic: Bullous and exfoliative dermatitis, erythema nodosum, exfoliative dermatitis, morbilliform and scarlatiniform reactions, phototoxicity, Stevens-Johnson syndrome, toxic epidural necrolysis, urticaria

Endocrine & metabolic: Hypoalbuminemia (without proteinuria), male infertility

Gastrointestinal: Abdominal pain, nausea, pancreatitis, vomiting

Hematologic: Agranulocytosis, anemia, leukopenia, pure red cell aplasia (case report); hemolysis (dose related; seen in patients with and without G6PD deficiency), hemoglobin decrease (1-2 g/dL), reticulocyte increase, methemoglobinemia, red cell life span shortened

Hepatic: Cholestatic jaundice, hepatitis

Neuromuscular & skeletal: Drug-induced lupus erythematosus, lower motor neuron toxicity (prolonged therapy), peripheral neuropathy (rare, nonleprosy patients)

Ocular: Blurred vision

Otic: Tinnitus

Renal: Albuminuria, nephrotic syndrome, renal papillary necrosis

Respiratory: Interstitial pneumonitis, pulmonary eosinophilia

Miscellaneous: Infectious mononucleosis-like syndrome (rash, fever, lymphadenopathy, hepatic dysfunction)

Drug Interactions

Metabolism/Transport Effects Substrate of CYP2C19 (minor), CYP2C8 (minor), CYP2C9 (major), CYP2E1 (minor), CYP3A4 (major); **Note:** Assignment of Major/Minor substrate status based on clinically relevant drug interaction potential

Avoid Concomitant Use

Avoid concomitant use of Dapsone (Systemic) with any of the following: BCG; Conivaptan; Fusidic Acid (Systemic)

Increased Effect/Toxicity

Dapsone (Systemic) may increase the levels/effects of: Antimalarial Agents; Prilocaine; Sodium Nitrite; Trimethoprim

The levels/effects of Dapsone (Systemic) may be increased by: Antimalarial Agents; Ceritinib; Conivaptan; CYP2C9 Inhibitors (Moderate); CYP2C9 Inhibitors (Strong); CYP3A4 Inhibitors (Moderate); CYP3A4 Inhibitors (Strong); Dasatinib; Fusidic Acid (Systemic); Ivacaftor; Luliconazole; Mifepristone; Nitric Oxide; Probenecid; Simeprevir; Stiripentol; Trimethoprim

Decreased Effect

Dapsone (Systemic) may decrease the levels/effects of: BCG; Sodium Picosulfate; Typhoid Vaccine

The levels/effects of Dapsone (Systemic) may be decreased by: Bosentan; CYP2C9 Inducers (Strong); CYP3A4 Inducers (Strong); Dabrafenib; Deferasirox; Mitotane; Peginterferon Alfa-2b; Rifamycin Derivatives; Siltuximab; St Johns Wort; Tocilizumab

Stability Store at 20°C to 25°C (68°F to 77°F); protect from light.

Mechanism of Action Competitive antagonist of para-aminobenzoic acid (PABA) and prevents normal bacterial utilization of PABA for the synthesis of folic acid

Pharmacokinetics (Adult data unless noted)

Absorption: Rapid and almost complete

Distribution: Distributes into skin, muscle, kidneys, liver, sweat, sputum, saliva, tears, and bile

V_d: 1.5 L/kg

Protein binding: Dapsone: 70% to 90%; Metabolite: ~99%

Metabolism: Hepatic (acetylated and hydroxylated)

Half-life:

Children: 15.1 hours (Mirochnick, 1993)

Adults: 28 hours (range: 10-50 hours)

Time to peak serum concentration: Within 4-8 hours

Elimination: ~85% excreted in urine as metabolites

Dosing: Neonatal Linear IgA bullous dermatosis

(LABD): Very limited data available: Term infants: Oral: 0.5 or 1 mg/kg/day; dosing based on experience from two case reports (PNA: 9 days and 20 days) which showed a positive response to dapsone therapy; however, adverse effects hindered treatment course. In the case report involving the youngest patient (PNA: 9 days), the initial dose was 1 mg/kg/day with concurrent prednisolone; the dose was increased to 2 mg/kg/day at which point the neonate developed methemoglobinemia by day 14 of treatment and dapsone was temporarily discontinued; a second course was initiated at 9 months of age for another disease flare at 0.5 mg/kg/day (Gluth, 2004). In the other case report (PNA: 20 days), initial therapy was 0.5 mg/kg/day; the dose was later increased to 1 mg/kg/day; while LABD improved on dapsone therapy, the patient developed pneumonia (highly resistant) which required discontinuation of dapsone (Kishida, 2004).

Dosing: Usual

Pediatric:

Dermatitis herpetiformis: Infants, Children, and Adolescents: Oral: 0.5 to 2 mg/kg/day in 1 to 2 divided doses; maximum initial daily dose in adults: 50 mg/**day**; once lesions controlled, the dose may be decreased as tolerated for chronic therapy; usual range: 0.125 to 0.5 mg/kg/day (Ermacora, 1986; Kliegman, 2011)

Idiopathic thrombocytopenic purpura (ITP), refractory: Limited data available: Children ≥3 years and Adolescents: Oral: 1 to 2 mg/kg/day for at least 2 months. Dosing based on two retrospective reviews. The first was a retrospective cohort analysis of adult and pediatric (age range: 3-61 years, including 35 patients <16 years) with chronic ITP (>6 months with diagnosis) who failed steroid therapy and observed an overall similar response rate for children (65.7%) and adults (Damodar, 2005). Adverse effects occurred in three patients (one with acute hemolysis and two with an erythematous rash). The second was a small retrospective report of seven pediatric patients with acute or chronic refractory, symptomatic ITP (age range: 6-15 years) which also showed a similar response rate (60%); however, a higher incidence [two of seven patients (29%)] of methemoglobinemia was observed (Meeker, 2003).

◄ **Leprosy:** Infants, Children, and Adolescents: Oral:
Multibacillary leprosy (6 patches or more):
Weight-based: 1 mg/kg/dose once daily; continue for 24 months in combination with other leprosy agents; maximum single dose: 100 mg (*Red Book* [AAP], 2012)
Fixed-dose (WHO, 2010):
Children <10 years: 25 mg once daily; continue treatment for 12 months
Children 10-12 years: 50 mg once daily; continue treatment for 12 months
Paucibacillary leprosy (1-5 patches):
Weight-based: 1 to 2 mg/kg/dose once daily; continue for 12 months in combination with other leprosy agents; maximum single dose: 100 mg (*Red Book* [AAP], 2012)
Fixed-dose (WHO, 2010):
Children <10 years: 25 mg once daily; continue treatment for 6 months
Children 10-12 years: 50 mg once daily; continue treatment for 6 months
Linear IgA bullous dermatosis (LABD): Limited data available: Infants, Children, and Adolescents: Oral: 0.5 to 2 mg/kg/day in 1 to 2 divided doses with or without prednisone; maximum initial daily dose in adults for other indications: 50 to 100 mg/day; may increase if needed at weekly intervals; maximum reported daily dose: 4 mg/kg/**day** (Kenani, 2009; Kliegman, 2011; Thappa, 2003)
***Pneumocystis jirovecii* pneumonia (PCP):** Oral:
Prophylaxis (primary or secondary):
Infants and Children (independent of HIV status including HSCT recipient): 2 mg/kg/dose once daily (maximum single dose: 100 mg) **or** 4 mg/kg/dose once **weekly**; maximum single weekly dose: 200 mg) (CDC/IDSA [Tomblyn], 2009; DHHS [pediatric], 2013; *Red Book* [AAP], 2012)
Adolescents (HIV-exposed/-positive or HSCT recipient): 100 mg/day in 1 or 2 divided doses as monotherapy **or** 50 mg once daily in combination with weekly pyrimethamine and leucovorin **or** 200 mg once **weekly** in combination with weekly pyrimethamine and leucovorin; monotherapy should not be used in patients who are seropositive for *Toxoplasma gondii* (CDC/IDSA [Tomblyn], 2009; DHHS [adult], 2013)
Treatment, mild to moderate disease: Infants, Children, and Adolescents (independent of HIV status): 2 mg/kg/dose once daily in combination with trimethoprim for 21 days; maximum single dose: 100 mg (DHHS [adult], 2013; *Red Book* [AAP], 2012)
***Toxoplasma gondii*, primary prophylaxis:** Oral:
Infants and Children (independent of HIV status): 2 mg/kg/dose **or** 15 mg/m²/dose once daily in combination with pyrimethamine and leucovorin; maximum single dose: 25 mg; a weekly regimen typically used for PCP prophylaxis but which also covers toxoplasma is 4 mg/kg/dose once **weekly** in combination with weekly pyrimethamine and leucovorin; maximum single weekly dose: 200 mg (DHHS [pediatric], 2013; *Red Book* [AAP], 2012)
Adolescents (HIV-exposed/-positive): 50 mg once daily in combination with weekly pyrimethamine and leucovorin or 200 mg once **weekly** in combination with weekly pyrimethamine and leucovorin (DHHS [adult], 2013)
Adult:
Dermatitis herpetiformis: Oral: Initial: 50 mg once daily; increase to 300 mg daily or higher to achieve full control; reduce dosage to minimal level as soon as possible
Leprosy: Oral: 100 mg once daily in combination with other antileprosy drugs; duration of therapy is variable

Dosing adjustment in renal impairment: There are no dosage adjustments provided in the manufacturer's labeling; however, some clinicians have used the following: Infants, Children, and Adolescents: No adjustment necessary (Aronoff, 2007).
Dosing adjustment in hepatic impairment: There are no dosage adjustments provided in the manufacturer's labeling.
Administration Oral: May administer with meals if GI upset occurs.
Monitoring Parameters CBC with differential (weekly for the first month, monthly for 6 months, then semiannually), reticulocyte count, and liver function tests; check G-6-PD levels prior to initiation of dapsone; monitor for signs of jaundice, hemolysis, or methemoglobinemia.
Additional Information The National Hansen's Disease (Leprosy) Programs (NHDP) may be contacted for further information regarding disease consultation and acquisition of necessary medication (http://www.hrsa.gov/hansensdisease/index.htm)
Dosage Forms Excipient information presented when available (limited, particularly for generics); consult specific product labeling.
Tablet, Oral:
Generic: 25 mg, 100 mg
Extemporaneous Preparations A 2 mg/mL oral suspension may be made with tablets and a 1:1 mixture of Ora-Sweet® and Ora-Plus®. Crush eight 25 mg tablets in a mortar and reduce to a fine powder. Add small portions of vehicle and mix to a uniform paste; mix while adding the vehicle in incremental proportions to almost 100 mL; transfer to a calibrated bottle, rinse mortar with vehicle, and add quantity of vehicle sufficient to make 100 mL. Label "shake well". Stable for 90 days at room temperature or refrigerated.

Jacobus Pharmaceutical Company makes a 2 mg/mL proprietary liquid formulation available under an IND for the prophylaxis of *Pneumocystis jirovecii* pneumonia.
Nahata MC, Morosco RS, and Trowbridge JM, "Stability of Dapsone in Two Oral Liquid Dosage Forms," *Ann Pharmacother*, 2000, 34 (7-8):848-50.

References

American Academy of Pediatrics (AAP). In: Pickering LK, Baker CJ, Kimberlin DW, Long SS, eds. *Red Book: 2012 Report of the Committee on Infectious Diseases*. 29th ed. Elk Grove Village, IL: American Academy of Pediatrics; 2012.
Aronoff GR, Bennett WM, Berns JS, et al, *Drug Prescribing in Renal Failure: Dosing Guidelines for Adults and Children*, 5th ed. Philadelphia, PA: American College of Physicians; 2007.
Barnett ED, Pelton SI, Mirochnick M, et al, "Dapsone for Prevention of Pneumocystis Pneumonia in Children With Acquired Immunodeficiency Syndrome" *Pediatr Infect Dis J*, 1994, 13(1):72-4.
Damodar S, Viswabandya A, George B, Mathews V, Chandy M, Srivastava A. Dapsone for chronic idiopathic thrombocytopenic purpura in children and adults – a report on 90 patients. *Eur J Haematol*. 2005;75:328-331.
DHHS. Guidelines for the Prevention and Treatment of Opportunistic Infections Among HIV-Exposed and HIV-Infected Children: Recommendations From the National Institutes of Health, Centers for Disease Control and Prevention, the HIV Medicine Association of the Infectious Diseases Society of America, the Pediatric Infectious Diseases Society, and the American Academy of Pediatrics. http://aidsinfo.nih.gov. Published November 2013.
DHHS Panel on Opportunistic Infections (OI) in HIV-Infected Adults and Adolescents, "Guidelines for Prevention and Treatment of Opportunistic Infections in HIV-Infected Adults and Adolescents: Recommendations from the Centers for Disease Control and Prevention (CDC), the National Institutes of Health (NIH), and the HIV Medicine Association (HIVMA) of the Infectious Diseases Society of America (IDSA)," May 7, 2013. Available at http://aidsinfo.nih.gov/contentfiles/lvguidelines/adult_oi.pdf
Ermacora E, Prampolini L, Tribbia G, et.al. Long-term follow-up of dermatitis herpetiformis in children. *J Am Acad Dermatol*. 1986;15:24-30.
Gluth MB, Witman PM, Thompson DM. Upper aerodigestive tract complications in a neonate with linear IgA bullous dermatosis. *Int J Pediatr Otorhinolaryngol*. 2004;68(7):965-970.

Human Resources and Services Administration, U.S. Department of Health and Human Services. National Hansens Disease (Leprosy) Program. Available at http://www.hrsa.gov/hansensdisease/

Kenani N, Mebazaa A, Denguezli M, et al. Childhood linear IgA bullous dermatosis in Tunisia. *Pediatric Dermatology* . 2009;26(1):28-33.

Kishida Y, Kameyama J, Nei M, Hashimoto T, Baba K. Linear IgA bullous dermatosis of neonatal onset: case report and review of the literature. *Acta Paediatr.* 2004;93:850-854.

Kliegman RM, Stanton BF, St. Gemell JW, et al, eds. *Nelson Textbook of Pediatrics.* 19th ed. Philadelphia, PA: Saunders Elsevier;2011.

Meeker ND, Goldsby R, Terrill KR, Delaney KS, Slayton WB. Dapsone therapy for children with immune thrombocytopenic purpura. *J Pediatr Hematol Oncol.* 2003;25(2):173-175.

Mirochnick M, Michaels M, Clarke D, et al, "Pharmacokinetics of Dapsone in Children," *J Pediatr,* 1993, 122(5 Pt 1):806-9.

Stavola JJ and Noel GJ, "Efficacy and Safety of Dapsone Prophylaxis Against *Pneumocystis carinii* Pneumonia in Human Immunodeficiency Virus-Infected Children," *Pediatr Infect Dis J,* 1993, 12 (8):644-7.

Thappa DM, Jeevankumar B. Chronic bullous dermatosis of childhood. *Postgrad Med J.* 2003;79(934):437.

Tomblyn M, Chiller T, Einsele H, et al. Guidelines for preventing infectious complications among hematopoietic cell transplantation recipients: a global perspective. *Biol Blood Marrow Transplant.* 2009;15:1143-1238.

World Health Organization. WHO model formulary for children. 2010.

Dapsone (Topical) (DAP sone)

Medication Safety Issues
Sound-alike/look-alike issues:
Dapsone may be confused with Diprosone®
Brand Names: U.S. Aczone
Brand Names: Canada Aczone™
Generic Availability (U.S.) No
Use Topical treatment of acne vulgaris (FDA approved in ages 12-17 years and adults)
Pregnancy Risk Factor C
Pregnancy Considerations Because of adverse events observed in some animal studies, dapsone is classified as pregnancy category C. Dapsone has not shown an increased risk of congenital anomalies when given orally during pregnancy; however, adverse effects in the newborn have been reported following *in utero* exposure. Refer to the Dapsone (Systemic) monograph for details. The amount of dapsone available systemically is less following topical application than with oral administration. During pregnancy, treatment for acne is often discontinued. If treatment is deemed necessary due to the risk of significant scarring or severe disease, dapsone is generally not the topical antibiotic of choice.
Breast-Feeding Considerations Dapsone is excreted in breast milk following oral administration. Refer to the Dapsone (Systemic) monograph for details. The amount of dapsone available systemically is less following topical application than with oral administration; however, because of the potential for adverse events in a nursing infant, the manufacturer states that the decision to continue dapsone or discontinue breast-feeding during therapy should take into account the risk of exposure to the infant and the benefits of treatment to the mother.
Contraindications Hypersensitivity to dapsone or any component
Precautions Changes suggestive of mild hemolysis have been observed in some patients with glucose-6-phosphate dehydrogenase (G-6-PD) deficiency and using dapsone gel; discontinue use with signs/symptoms of hemolytic anemia. Do not use concomitantly with oral dapsone, trimethoprim/sulfamethoxazole, or antimalarial medications; may increase the risk of hemolysis in patients with G-6-PD deficiency. Localized discoloration (yellow or orange) of the skin or facial hair may occur if benzoyl peroxide is used subsequent to dapsone gel; typically resolves in ~1-8 weeks. Vehicle used for product formulation may cause skin dryness, erythema, oiliness, and peeling; patients should be counseled about these effects.

Adverse Reactions
Cardiovascular: Facial edema
Central nervous system: Depression, psychosis, suicide attempt, tonic-clonic movement
Gastrointestinal: Abdominal pain, pancreatitis, vomiting
Local: Application site reactions including burning, dryness, erythema, oiliness/peeling, and pruritus were reported at an incidence similar to or less than placebo
Respiratory: Pharyngitis, sinusitis
Drug Interactions
Metabolism/Transport Effects Substrate of CYP2C19 (minor), CYP2C8 (minor), CYP2C9 (minor), CYP2E1 (minor), CYP3A4 (minor); **Note:** Assignment of Major/Minor substrate status based on clinically relevant drug interaction potential
Avoid Concomitant Use
Avoid concomitant use of Dapsone (Topical) with any of the following: BCG
Increased Effect/Toxicity
The levels/effects of Dapsone (Topical) may be increased by: Antimalarial Agents; Trimethoprim
Decreased Effect
Dapsone (Topical) may decrease the levels/effects of: BCG; Sodium Picosulfate
Stability Store at 20°C to 25°C (68°F to 77°F); excursions permitted to 15°C to 30°C (59°F to 86°F). Protect from freezing.
Dosing: Usual Acne vulgaris: Children ≥12 years, Adolescents, and Adults: Topical: Apply a pea-sized amount of gel to the acne-affected areas twice daily; re-evaluate patient if no improvement after 12 weeks of therapy
Dosage adjustment in renal impairment: No dosage adjustment provided in manufacturer's labeling; has not been studied.
Dosage adjustment in hepatic impairment: No dosage adjustment provided in manufacturer's labeling; has not been studied.
Administration Topical: Wash skin and pat dry then rub in thin layer of gel gently and completely. Wash hands after application.
Dosage Forms Excipient information presented when available (limited, particularly for generics); consult specific product labeling.
Gel, External:
Aczone: 5% (30 g, 60 g, 90 g) [contains methylparaben]

◆ **Daptacel** see Diphtheria and Tetanus Toxoids, and Acellular Pertussis Vaccine on page 686

DAPTOmycin (DAP toe mye sin)

Medication Safety Issues
Sound-alike/look-alike issues:
Cubicin may be confused with Cleocin
DAPTOmycin may be confused with DACTINomycin
Brand Names: U.S. Cubicin
Brand Names: Canada Cubicin
Therapeutic Category Antibiotic, Cyclic Lipopeptide
Generic Availability (U.S.) No
Use Treatment of complicated skin and skin structure infections caused by susceptible aerobic gram-positive organisms including *S. aureus* [methicillin-susceptible *Staph. aureus* (MSSA) and methicillin-resistant *Staph. aureus* (MRSA)], *S. pyogenes, S. agalactiae, S. dysgalactiae,* and *E. faecalis* (FDA approved in ages ≥18 years). Treatment of *S. aureus* bacteremia, including right-sided infective endocarditis caused by MSSA or MRSA (FDA approved in ages ≥18 years). Daptomycin is active against bacteria resistant to methicillin, vancomycin, and linezolid.
Pregnancy Risk Factor B
Pregnancy Considerations Adverse events were not observed in animal reproduction studies. Successful use

of daptomycin during the second and third trimesters of pregnancy has been described; however, only limited information is available from case reports.

Breast-Feeding Considerations Low concentrations of daptomycin have been detected in breast milk; however, daptomycin is poorly absorbed orally. The manufacturer recommends caution if daptomycin is used during breast-feeding. Per the Canadian product labeling, daptomycin should be discontinued while breast-feeding. Nondose-related effects could include modification of bowel flora.

Contraindications Hypersensitivity to daptomycin or any component

Warnings Hypersensitivity reactions and anaphylaxis have been reported with use; discontinue use immediately with signs/symptoms of hypersensitivity and initiate appropriate treatment. May be associated with an increased incidence of myopathy; discontinue daptomycin in patients with unexplained signs and symptoms of myopathy in conjunction with CPK elevation >5 times ULN or >1000 units/L or in asymptomatic patients who have CPK elevations ≥10 x ULN. Myopathy may occur more frequently when daptomycin dose and/or frequency exceeds the recommended dose. Symptoms suggestive of peripheral neuropathy have been observed with treatment; monitor for new-onset or worsening neuropathy. Use with caution in patients receiving other drugs associated with myopathy and rhabdomyolysis (eg, HMG-CoA reductase inhibitors); monitor CPK levels; consider temporarily suspending the use of HMG-CoA reductase inhibitors in patients receiving daptomycin. Prolonged use may result in fungal or bacterial superinfection, including *C. difficile*-associated diarrhea and pseudomembranous colitis.

Eosinophilic pneumonia, a rare condition of eosinophil accumulation in the lungs with typical pneumonia presentation that if left unrecognized or treated may lead to respiratory failure, has been reported with use; generally develops 2-4 weeks after therapy initiation. Monitor for signs and symptoms of eosinophilic pneumonia, including new onset or worsening fever, dyspnea, difficulty breathing, new infiltrates on chest imaging studies, and/or >25% eosinophils present in bronchoalveolar lavage; discontinue use immediately with signs/symptoms of eosinophilic pneumonia and initiate appropriate treatment (ie, corticosteroids); may reoccur with re-exposure.

Daptomycin is not indicated for treatment of pneumonia due to its inactivation by pulmonary surfactant and its poor lung penetration.

Precautions Use with caution in patients with renal impairment; dosage adjustment required in severe renal impairment (CrCl <30 mL/minute). Limited data (eg, subgroup analysis) from complicated skin and soft tissue infections and endocarditis trials suggest possibly reduced clinical efficacy (relative to comparators) in patients with baseline moderate renal impairment (<50 mL/minute).

Adverse Reactions

Cardiovascular: Chest pain, hypertension, hypotension, peripheral edema

Central nervous system: Anxiety, dizziness, headache, insomnia

Dermatologic: Diaphoresis, erythema, pruritus, skin rash

Endocrine & metabolic: Hyperkalemia, hyperphosphatemia, hypokalemia

Gastrointestinal: Abdominal pain, constipation, diarrhea, dyspepsia, gastrointestinal hemorrhage, loose stools, nausea, vomiting

Genitourinary: Urinary tract infection

Hematologic & oncologic: Anemia, eosinophilia, increased INR

Hepatic: Increased serum alkaline phosphatase, increased serum transaminases

Infection: Bacteremia, fungal infection, gram-negative organism infection, sepsis

Local: Injection site reaction

Neuromuscular & skeletal: Arthralgia, back pain, increased creatine phosphokinase, limb pain, osteomyelitis, weakness

Renal: Renal failure

Respiratory: Cough, dyspnea, pneumonia, pharyngolaryngeal pain, pleural effusion

Miscellaneous: Fever

Rare but important or life-threatening: Anaphylaxis, atrial fibrillation, atrial flutter, candidiasis, cardiac arrest, *Clostridium difficile* associated diarrhea, coma (post anaesthesia/surgery), eczema, eosinophilic pneumonitis, hallucination, hypomagnesemia, hypersensitivity, jaundice, increased lactate dehydrogenase, lymphadenopathy, mental status changes, neutropenia (Knoll, 2013), oral candidiasis, peripheral neuropathy, proteinuria, prolonged prothrombin time, renal insufficiency, rhabdomyolysis, increased serum bicarbonate, Stevens-Johnson syndrome, stomatitis, supraventricular cardiac arrhythmia, thrombocytopenia, thrombocythemia

Drug Interactions

Metabolism/Transport Effects None known.

Avoid Concomitant Use There are no known interactions where it is recommended to avoid concomitant use.

Increased Effect/Toxicity

The levels/effects of DAPTOmycin may be increased by: HMG-CoA Reductase Inhibitors

Decreased Effect There are no known significant interactions involving a decrease in effect.

Stability Store intact vials at 2°C to 8°C (36°F to 46°F); may also be stored at room temperature for up to 12 months [data on file (Cubist Pharmaceuticals, 2011)]. However, the manufacturer recommends storage under refrigeration. Room temperature stability information should only be utilized in situations where the drug has been inadvertently exposed to prolonged room temperature. Reconstituted solution (either in vial or in infusion bag) is stable for a cumulative time of 12 hours at room temperature and 48 hours if refrigerated [2°C to 8°C (36°F to 46°F)]. Daptomycin is incompatible with dextrose-containing solutions.

Mechanism of Action Daptomycin binds to components of the cell membrane of susceptible organisms and causes rapid depolarization, inhibiting intracellular synthesis of DNA, RNA, and protein. Daptomycin is bactericidal in a concentration-dependent manner.

Pharmacokinetics (Adult data unless noted)

Distribution: V_d:

Neonates and Infants <3 months: Median: 0.21 L/kg (range: 0.11-0.34 L/kg) (Cohen-Wolkowiez, 2012)

Children 2-6 years: 0.14 L/kg (Abdel-Rahman, 2008; Abdel-Rahman, 2011)

Children 7-17 years: 0.11 ± 0.02 L/kg (Abdel-Rahman, 2008)

Adults: 0.1 L/kg; Critically ill: V_{ss}: 0.23 ± 0.14 L/kg (Vilay, 2010)

Protein binding: 90% to 93%; patients with renal impairment (CrCl <30 mL/minute): 84% to 88%

Metabolism: Minor amounts of oxidative metabolites have been detected; does not induce or inhibit cytochrome P450 enzymes

Half-life:

Neonates and Infants <3 months: Median: 6.2 hours (range: 3.7-9 hours) (Cohen-Wolkowiez, 2012)

Children 2-6 years: Mean range: 5.3-5.7 hours (Abdel-Rahman, 2008; Abdel-Rahman, 2011)

Children 7-11 years: 5.6 ± 2.2 hours (Abdel-Rahman, 2008)

Children 12-17 years: 6.7 ± 2.2 hours (Abdel-Rahman, 2008)

Adults: 8-9 hours; prolonged with renal impairment up to 28 hours

Elimination: 78% of the dose excreted in urine primarily as unchanged drug; feces (6%)

Clearance:

Neonates and Infants <3 months: Median: 21 mL/hour/kg (range: 16-34 mL/hour/kg) (Cohen-Wolkowiez, 2012)

Children 2-6 years: 19-20 mL/hour/kg (Abdel-Rahman, 2008; Abdel-Rahman, 2011)

Children 7-11 years: 17 mL/hour/kg (Abdel-Rahman, 2008)

Children 12-17 years: 11 mL/hour/kg (Abdel-Rahman, 2008)

Adults: 8.3-9 mL/hour/kg

Dialysis: 15% removed by 4-hour hemodialysis session; high permeability intermittent hemodialysis removes ~50% during a 4-hour session (Salama, 2010)

Dosing: Neonatal

Gram-positive infection, severe: Very limited data available: PMA ≥32 weeks: I.V.: 6 mg/kg/dose every 12 hours for 10-14 days was used in two neonates [patient age: PMA 32 weeks (PNA: 8 weeks) and PMA: 35 weeks (PNA: 3 weeks)] with normal renal function (Cohen-Wolkowiez, 2008). A pharmacokinetic study of 20 neonates and infants [GA: Median: 32 weeks (range: 23-40 weeks); PNA: Median: 3 days (range: 1-85 days)] evaluated a single 6 mg/kg dose and reported median AUC exposure ~60% of that achieved in adults with standard adult dosing and a faster clearance than adults and adolescents (Cohen-Wolkowiez, 2012). Further studies are needed.

Dosage adjustment in renal impairment: Data limited to a single case report: A full-term neonate (PNA: 41 days) with decreased renal function (S_{cr}: 0.9 mg/dL), an initial dose of 4 mg/kg/dose every 48 hours was used and increased to 6 mg/kg/dose every 36 hours upon a decrease in serum creatinine (S_{cr}: 0.6 mg/dL) and daptomycin serum concentration evaluation which showed a subtherapeutic peak value (Beneri, 2008). Further studies are needed.

Dosing: Usual

Children and Adolescents:

General dosing, susceptible organisms (severe infection): Limited data available:

Children 2-6 years: I.V.: 8-10 mg/kg/dose once daily (*Red Book*, 2012); in a pharmacokinetic study of 12 children (age: 2-6 years) dosages presented showed similar serum concentrations to standard adult doses (4-6 mg/kg) (Abdel-Rahman, 2011; *Red Book*, 2012)

Children ≥6 years to <12 years: I.V.: 7 mg/kg/dose once daily (*Red Book*, 2012)

Children ≥12 years and Adolescents: I.V.: 4-6 mg/kg/dose once daily (*Red Book*, 2012)

MRSA Infection: Limited data available (Lui, 2011):

Bacteremia: Children and Adolescents: I.V.: 6-10 mg/kg/dose once daily

Endocarditis, infective (prosthetic valve): Children and Adolescents: I.V.: 6-10 mg/kg/dose once daily

Osteomyeolitis, or septic arthritis: Children and Adolescents: I.V.: 6-10 mg/kg/dose once daily

Note: IDSA guidelines state ongoing pediatric daptomycin clinical trials focus on an inverse relationship between age and required per kg dose; the following daily doses are under investigation in children and adolescents (Clinicaltrials.gov NCT 00711802)

Children 2-6 years: I.V.: 9 mg/kg/dose once daily

Children 7-11 years: I.V.: 7 mg/kg/dose once daily

Children and Adolescents 12-17 years: I.V.: 5 mg/kg/dose once daily

Adults:

Skin and/or skin structure infections (complicated): I.V.: 4 mg/kg/dose once daily for 7-14 days

Bacteremia, right-sided native valve endocarditis caused by MSSA or MRSA: I.V.: 6 mg/kg/dose once daily for 2-6 weeks [some experts recommend 8-10 mg/kg once daily for complicated bacteremia or infective endocarditis (Liu, 2011)]

Dosage adjustment in renal impairment:

Children ≥2 years and Adolescents: The following dosage adjustments have been recommended (Aronoff, 2007): I.V.:

GFR >30 mL/minute/1.73 m^2: Administer full dose

GFR 10-29 mL/minute/1.73 m^2: Administer 67% of a full dose every 24 hours

GFR <10 mL/minute/1.73 m^2: Administer 67% of a full dose every 48 hours

Hemodialysis: Administer 67% of a full dose every 48 hours after dialysis

Peritoneal dialysis: Administer 67% of a full dose every 48 hours

Adults: I.V.:

CrCl <30 mL/minute:

Skin and soft tissue infections: 4 mg/kg/dose every 48 hours

Staphylococcal bacteremia: 6 mg/kg/dose every 48 hours

Intermittent hemodialysis or peritoneal dialysis (PD): Dose as in CrCl <30 mL/minute (administer after hemodialysis on dialysis days) **or** (unlabeled dosing) may administer 6 mg/kg/dose after hemodialysis 3 times weekly (Salama, 2010)

Note: High permeability intermittent hemodialysis removes ~50% during a 4-hour session (Salama, 2010)

Continuous renal replacement therapy (CRRT) (Heintz, 2009; Trotman, 2005): Drug clearance is highly dependent on the method of renal replacement, filter type, and flow rate. Appropriate dosing requires close monitoring of pharmacologic response, signs of adverse reactions due to drug accumulation, as well as drug concentrations in relation to target trough (if appropriate). The following are general recommendations only (based on dialysate flow/ultrafiltration rates of 1-2 L/hour and minimal residual renal function) and should not supersede clinical judgment:

Continuous veno-venous hemodialysis (CVVHD): 8 mg/kg/dose every 48 hours (Vilay, 2010)

Note: For other forms of CRRT (eg, CVVH or CVVHDF), dosing as with CrCl <30 mL/minute may result in low C_{max}. May consider 4-6 mg/kg/dose every 24 hours (or 8 mg/kg every 48 hours) depending on site or severity of infection or if not responding to standard dosing; therapeutic drug monitoring and/or more frequent serum CPK levels may be necessary (Heintz, 2009).

Slow extended daily dialysis (or extended dialysis): 6 mg/kg/dose every 24 hours (Kielstein, 2010). **Note:** Dialysis should be initiated within 8 hours of administering daptomycin dose to avoid dose accumulation.

Dosage adjustment in hepatic impairment: No adjustment required for mild-to-moderate impairment (Child-Pugh Class A or B); not evaluated in severe hepatic impairment (Child-Pugh Class C)

Administration I.V.: Reconstitute vial with 10 mL NS by gently rotating vial to wet powder; allow vial to stand for 10 minutes, then gently swirl to obtain completely reconstituted solution. Do not shake or agitate vial vigorously.

Neonates: Dilution information has not been reported; infuse over 60 minutes (Cohen-Wolkowiez, 2012)

Children 2-6 years: Further dilute in 25 mL of NS and infuse over 60 minutes (Abdel-Rahman, 2011)

Children and Adolescents 7-17 years: Further dilute in 50 mL of NS and infuse over 30 minutes (Abdel-Rahman, 2008)

Adults: May administer I.V. push over 2 minutes at a final concentration of 50 mg/mL or infuse IVPB over 30 minutes at a final concentration not to exceed 20 mg/mL

Do not use in conjunction with ReadyMED® elastomeric infusion pumps (Cardinal Health, Inc) due to an impurity (2-mercaptobenzothiazole) which leaches from the pump system into the daptomycin solution.

Monitoring Parameters Signs and symptoms of myopathy (muscle pain or weakness, particularly of the distal extremities), weekly CPK levels during therapy (more frequent monitoring if history of current or prior statin therapy and/or renal impairment), signs of peripheral neuropathy; observe for changes in bowel frequency; monitor renal function periodically

Reference Range Adults:
Trough concentrations at steady-state:
4 mg/kg once daily: 5.9 ± 1.6 mcg/mL
6 mg/kg once daily: 6.7 ± 1.6 mcg/mL
Note: Trough concentrations are not predictive of efficacy/toxicity. Daptomycin exhibits concentration-dependent bactericidal activity, so C_{max}:MIC ratios may be a more useful parameter.

Test Interactions Daptomycin may cause false prolongation of the PT and increase of INR with certain recombinant thromboplastin reagents. This appears to be a dose-dependent phenomenon. If PT/INR is elevated, repeat PT/INR immediately prior to next daptomycin dose (eg, trough). If PT/INR remains elevated, repeat PT/INR using alternate reagents (if available) and evaluate for other causes of elevated PT/INR.

Dosage Forms Excipient information presented when available (limited, particularly for generics); consult specific product labeling.
Solution Reconstituted, Intravenous [preservative free]:
Cubicin: 500 mg (1 ea)

References

Abdel-Rahman SM, Benziger DP, Jacobs RF, et al, "Single-Dose Pharmacokinetics of Daptomycin in Children With Suspected or Proved Gram-Positive Infections," *Pediatr Infect Dis J*, 2008, 27 (4):330-4.
Abdel-Rahman SM, Chandorkar G, Akins RL, et al, "Single-Dose Pharmacokinetics and Tolerability of Daptomycin 8 to 10 mg/kg in Children Aged 2 to 6 Years With Suspected or Proved Gram-Positive Infections," *Pediatr Infect Dis J*, 2011, 30(8):712-4.
American Academy of Pediatrics (AAP). In: Pickering LK, Baker CJ, Kimberlin DW, Long SS, eds. *Red Book: 2012 Report of the Committee on Infectious Diseases.* 29th ed. Elk Grove Village, IL: American Academy of Pediatrics; 2012.
Ardura MI, Mejías A, Katz KS, et al, "Daptomycin Therapy for Invasive Gram-Positive Bacterial Infections in Children," *Pediatr Infect Dis J*, 2007, 26(12):1128-32.
Aronoff GR, Bennett WM, Berns JS, et al, *Drug Prescribing in Renal Failure: Dosing Guidelines for Adults and Children*, 5th ed. Philadelphia, PA: American College of Physicians, 2007.
Beneri CA, Nicolau DP, Seiden HS, et al, "Successful Treatment of a Neonate With Persistent Vancomycin-Resistant Enterococcal Bacteremia With a Daptomycin-Containing Regimen," *Infect Drug Resist*, 2008, 1:9-11.
Cohen-Wolkowiez M, Smith PB, Benjamin DK Jr, et al, "Daptomycin Use in Infants: Report of Two Cases With Peak and Trough Drug Concentrations," *J Perinatol*, 2008, 28(3):233-4.
Cohen-Wolkowiez M, Watt KM, Hornik CP, et al, "Pharmacokinetics and Tolerability of Single-Dose Daptomycin in Young Infants," *Pediatr Infect Dis J*, 2012.
Heintz BH, Matzke GR, Dager WE, "Antimicrobial Dosing Concepts and Recommendations for Critically Ill Adult Patients Receiving Continuous Renal Replacement Therapy or Intermittent Hemodialysis," *Pharmacotherapy*, 2009, 29(5):562-77.
Kielstein JT, Eugbers C, Bode-Boeger SM, et al, "Dosing of Daptomycin in Intensive Care Unit Patients With Acute Kidney Injury Undergoing Extended Dialysis – A Pharmacokinetic Study," *Nephrol Dial Transplant*, 2010, 25(5):1537-41.
Knoll BM, Spieler PJ, Kubiak DW, et al, "Neutropenia Associated With Prolonged Daptomycin Use," *Clin Infect Dis*, 2013, 56(9):1353-4.
Liu C, Bayer A, Cosgrove SE, et al, "Clinical Practice Guidelines by the Infectious Diseases Society of America for the Treatment of Methicillin-Resistant *Staphylococcus aureus* Infections in Adults and Children: Executive Summary," *Clin Infect Dis*, 2011, 52(3):285-92.
NCT00711802, "Safety and Efficacy Study of Daptomycin in Pediatric Subjects (2-17 Years) With Skin and Skin Structure Infections," Unpublished data. Available at http://clinicaltrials.gov/ct2/show/NCT00711802?term=NCT+00711802&rank=1
Salama NN, Segal JH, Churchwell MD, et al, "Single-Dose Daptomycin Pharmacokinetics in Chronic Haemodialysis Patients," *Nephrol Dial Transplant*, 2010, 25(4):1279-84.
Trotman RL, Williamson JC, Shoemaker DM, et al, "Antibiotic Dosing in Critically Ill Adult Patients Receiving Continuous Renal Replacement Therapy," *Clin Infect Dis*, 2005, 41(8):1159-66.
Vilay MA, Grio M, DePestel DD, et al, "Daptomycin Pharmacokinetics in Critically Ill Patients Receiving Continuous Venovenous Hemodialysis," *Crit Care Med*, 2011, 39(1):19-25.

◆ **Daraprim** *see* Pyrimethamine *on page 1780*

◆ **Daraprim® (Can)** *see* Pyrimethamine *on page 1780*

Darbepoetin Alfa (dar be POE e tin AL fa)

Medication Safety Issues
Sound-alike/look-alike issues:
Aranesp may be confused with Aralast, Aricept
Darbepoetin alfa may be confused with dalteparin, epoetin alfa, epoetin beta

Brand Names: U.S. Aranesp (Albumin Free)

Brand Names: Canada Aranesp

Therapeutic Category Colony-Stimulating Factor; Erythropoiesis Stimulating Protein; Hematopoietic Agent

Generic Availability (U.S.) No

Use Treatment of anemia due to chronic kidney disease (FDA approved in ages ≥1 year and adults) or anemia associated with concurrent myelosuppressive chemotherapy for nonmyeloid malignancies receiving chemotherapy (palliative intent) for a planned minimum of 2 additional months of chemotherapy (FDA approved in adults)

Prescribing and Access Restrictions As a requirement of the REMS program, access to this medication is restricted. Healthcare providers and hospitals must be enrolled in the ESA APPRISE (Assisting Providers and Cancer Patients with Risk Information for the Safe use of ESAs) Oncology Program (866-284-8089; http://www.esa-apprise.com) to prescribe or dispense ESAs (ie, darbepoetin alfa, epoetin alfa) to patients with cancer.

Medication Guide Available Yes

Pregnancy Risk Factor C

Pregnancy Considerations Adverse events were observed in animal reproduction studies. Women who become pregnant during treatment with darbepoetin are encouraged to enroll in Amgen's Pregnancy Surveillance Program (800-772-6436).

Breast-Feeding Considerations It is not known if darbepoetin alfa is excreted in breast milk. The manufacturer recommends that caution be exercised when administering darbepoetin alfa to nursing women.

Contraindications Hypersensitivity to darbepoetin alfa or any component; uncontrolled hypertension; pure red cell aplasia (due to darbepoetin or other erythropoietin protein drugs)

Warnings Patients with chronic kidney disease (CKD) are at greater risk for death, serious cardiovascular events, and stroke with a rapid rise in hemoglobin (>1 g/dL over 2 weeks) or when using erthyropoiesis-stimulating agents (ESAs) to target higher hemoglobin concentrations (≥11 g/dL); use the lowest dose sufficient to reduce the need for RBC transfusions **[U.S. Boxed Warning]**. Hemoglobin rising >1 g/dL in a 2-week period may contribute to the risk. An optimal target hemoglobin concentration, dose, or dosing strategy to reduce these risks has not been identified in clinical trials. CKD patients who exhibit an inadequate hemoglobin response to ESA therapy may be at a higher risk for cardiovascular events and mortality compared to other patients. In clinical trials, ~40% of CKD patients required initiation or intensification of antihypertensive therapy; blood pressure should be controlled adequately before initiation of darbepoetin alfa therapy; close blood pressure monitoring is recommended. ESA therapy may reduce dialysis efficacy (due to increase in red blood cells and decrease in plasma volume); adjustments in dialysis parameters may be needed. Patients treated with ESAs may require increased heparinization during dialysis to prevent clotting of the extracorporeal circuit.

ESAs shortened survival and/or time-to-tumor progression in studies of advanced breast, head and neck, lymphoid, and nonsmall cell lung cancer in patients receiving ESAs dosed to a target hemoglobin of ≥12 g/dL **[U.S. Boxed Warning]**. This risk has not been excluded when a lower target hemoglobin is used. Because of the risks of decreased survival and increased risk of tumor growth or progression, all healthcare providers and hospitals are required to enroll and comply with the ESA APPRISE (Assisting Providers and Cancer Patients with Risk Information for the Safe use of ESAs) Oncology Program prior to prescribing or dispensing ESAs to cancer patients, ESA APPRISE Oncology Program **[U.S. Boxed Warning]**. Prescribers and patients will have to provide written documentation of discussed risks with each darbepoetin course. For patients with cancer, use only for the treatment of anemia due to concomitant myelosuppressive chemotherapy, use the lowest dose needed to avoid transfusions, and discontinue following completion of chemotherapy course; ESAs are **not** indicated for patients receiving myelosuppressive chemotherapy when the anticipated outcome is curative **[U.S. Boxed Warning]**. Darbepoetin alfa is not approved for use in patients with myeloid malignancies or in patients with cancer-related anemia who are not receiving concurrent chemotherapy.

The risk of thrombotic events (eg, pulmonary emboli, thrombophlebitis, thrombosis) is increased with ESA therapy. Increased mortality (due to thrombotic events) was observed in patients undergoing coronary artery bypass surgery who received ESAs; these deaths were associated with thrombotic events. An increased risk of DVT has been observed in patients treated with ESAs undergoing surgical orthopedic procedures. Darbepoetin alfa is not approved for reduction in allogeneic RBC transfusions in patients scheduled for surgical procedures.

Cases of pure red cell aplasia (PRCA) and severe anemia with or without other cytopenias associated with neutralizing antibodies to erythropoietin have been reported in CKD patients and patients receiving subcutaneous ESAs. Cases have also been reported in patients with hepatitis C who were receiving ESAs, interferon, and ribavirin. Patients who develop a sudden loss of responsiveness to darbepoetin therapy along with a severe anemia and low reticulocyte count should be evaluated for the presence of these antibodies. Withhold darbepoetin until the etiology is confirmed; evaluate for PRCA with associated neutralizing antibodies to epoetin; discontinue epoetin (permanently) if these antibodies are detected. Safety and efficacy in patients with underlying hematologic diseases (eg, porphyria, thalassemia, hemolytic anemia, and sickle cell disease) have not been established.

Injection contains polysorbate 80 (Tween 80®) which may cause allergic reactions in susceptible individuals. In premature neonates, thrombocytopenia, ascites, pulmonary deterioration, and renal and hepatic failure have been reported after receiving parenteral products containing polysorbate 80 (Alade, 1986; MMWR, 1984). Infusion of polysorbate 80-containing solutions through polyvinyl chloride tubing may cause DEHP to leach into the solution; in immature animals, exposure to DEHP may adversely affect the development of the male reproductive tract.

Precautions Use with caution in patients with a history of seizures or hypertension; an excessive rate of rise of hematocrit may possibly be associated with the exacerbation of hypertension or seizures. Decrease the darbepoetin alfa dosage if the hemoglobin increase exceeds 1 g/dL in any 2-week period. Blood pressure should be controlled prior to the start of therapy and monitored closely throughout treatment. Hypertensive encephalopathy has been reported with patients receiving erythropoietic therapy. Seizures have occurred during ESA therapy; monitor closely for premonitory neurologic symptoms during the first several months of therapy. Potentially serious allergic reactions have been reported (rarely). Discontinue immediately (and permanently) in patients who experience serious allergic/anaphylactic reactions.

Darbepoetin alfa is not intended for patients who require acute corrections of anemia and is not a substitute for emergency blood transfusion. Allow sufficient time (an interval of 4-6 weeks) to determine the patient's response to a particular dosage; patients with CKD not yet requiring dialysis may require lower maintenance doses. Assessment of iron stores and therapeutic iron supplementation is essential for optimal therapy. Iron supplementation is necessary to provide for increased requirements during expansion of the red cell mass secondary to marrow stimulation unless iron stores are already in excess. Optimal iron stores are demonstrated by a transferrin saturation of 20% or more and a serum ferritin of 100-150 mcg/L. Some products contain albumin, which confers a theoretical risk of transmission of viral disease or Creutzfeldt-Jakob disease. Factors which may impair erythropoiesis include inflammatory conditions, infections, and bleeding; poor response to therapy should prompt evaluation of potential factors impairing erythropoiesis, as well as possible malignant processes and hematologic disease (thalassemia, refractory anemia, myeloblastic disorder), occult blood loss, hemolysis, osteitis fibrosa cystic, and/or bone marrow fibrosis.

Adverse Reactions

Cardiovascular: Angina, edema, fluid overload, hyper-/hypotension, MI, peripheral edema, thromboembolic events

Central nervous system: Cerebrovascular disorder

Dermatologic: Rash/erythema

Gastrointestinal: Abdominal pain

Local: AV graft thrombosis, vascular access complications

Respiratory: Cough, dyspnea, pulmonary embolism

Rare but important or life-threatening: Allergic reaction, anaphylactic reactions, anemia associated with neutralizing antibodies (severe; with or without other cytopenias), angioedema, bronchospasm, hypertensive encephalopathy, pure red cell aplasia (PRCA), seizure, stroke, tumor progression/recurrence (cancer patients), urticaria

Drug Interactions

Metabolism/Transport Effects None known.

Avoid Concomitant Use There are no known interactions where it is recommended to avoid concomitant use.

Increased Effect/Toxicity

The levels/effects of Darbepoetin Alfa may be increased by: Nandrolone

Decreased Effect There are no known significant interactions involving a decrease in effect.

Stability Store at 2°C to 8°C (36°F to 46°F); protect from light; store in original container until use; contains no preservatives; discard after entry

Mechanism of Action Induces erythropoiesis by stimulating the division and differentiation of committed erythroid progenitor cells; induces the release of reticulocytes from the bone marrow into the bloodstream, where they mature to erythrocytes. There is a dose response relationship with this effect. This results in an increase in reticulocyte counts followed by a rise in hematocrit and hemoglobin levels. When administered SubQ or I.V., darbepoetin's half-life is ~3 times that of epoetin alfa concentrations.

Pharmacodynamics
Onset of action: Several days
Maximum effect: 4-6 weeks

Pharmacokinetics (Adult data unless noted)
Absorption: SubQ: Slow and rate-limiting
Distribution: V_d:
 Children: 51.6 mL/kg (range: 21-73 mL/kg)
 Adults: 52.4 ± 6.6 mL/kg
Bioavailability: SubQ: CKD:
 Children: 54% (range:32% to 70%)
 Adults: ~37% (range: 30% to 50%)
Half-life:
 Children:
  I.V.: Terminal: 22.1 hours (range: 12-30 hours)
  SubQ: Terminal: 42.8 hours (range: 16-86 hours); Children with cancer: 49.4 hours
 Adults: CKD:
  I.V.: Terminal: 21 hours
  SubQ: Terminal: 49 ± 12.7 hours
Time to peak serum concentration: SubQ:
 CKD patients: 34 hours (range: 24-72 hours)
 Cancer patients:
  Children: 71.4 hours (median time)
  Adults: 90 hours (range: 71-123 hours)
Elimination:
 Clearance: I.V.:
  Children: 2.29 mL/hour/kg (range: 1.6-3.5 mL/hour/kg)
  Adults: 1.6 ± 1.0 mL/hour/kg

Dosing: Usual
Children and Adolescents: **Anemia associated with chronic kidney disease (CKD):** Individualize dosing and use the lowest dose necessary to reduce the need for RBC transfusions.
Initial dosing:
 Manufacturer labeling:
  CKD patients **ON** dialysis (initiate treatment when hemoglobin is <10 g/dL; reduce or interrupt treatment if hemoglobin approaches or exceeds 11 g/dL): Children ≥1 year and Adolescents: Conversion from epoetin alfa: I.V. (preferred), SubQ: Initial: Epoetin alfa doses of 1500 to ≥90,000 units per week may be converted to doses ranging from 6.25-200 mcg/dose darbepoetin alfa per week (see pediatric column in conversion table).
 Alternate dosing: CKD patients darbepoetin alfa-naive (either on dialysis or not on dialysis): Children ≥11 years and Adolescents: I.V., SubQ: Initial dose: ~0.45 mcg/kg/dose once weekly; titrate to hemoglobin response (André, 2007)
 Dosage adjustment in CKD (either on dialysis or not on dialysis): Children ≥1 year and Adolescents: Do not increase dose more frequently than every 4 weeks (dose decreases may occur more frequently).
  If hemoglobin increases >1 g/dL in any 2-week period: Decrease dose by ≥25%
  If hemoglobin does not increase by >1 g/dL after 4 weeks: Increase dose by 25%

Inadequate or lack of response: If adequate response is not achieved over 12 weeks, further increases are unlikely to be of benefit and may increase the risk for adverse events; use the minimum effective dose that will maintain a hemoglobin level sufficient to avoid red blood cell transfusions **and** evaluate patient for other causes of anemia; discontinue treatment if responsiveness does not improve

Adults:
Anemia associated with chronic kidney disease (CKD): Individualize dosing and use the lowest dose necessary to reduce the need for RBC transfusions.
 CKD patients **ON** dialysis (I.V. route is preferred for hemodialysis patients; initiate treatment when hemoglobin is <10 g/dL; reduce dose or interrupt treatment if hemoglobin approaches or exceeds 11 g/dL): I.V. (preferred), SubQ: Initial: 0.45 mcg/kg/dose once weekly or 0.75 mcg/kg/dose once every 2 weeks or epoetin alfa doses of <1500 to ≥90,000 units per week may be converted to doses ranging from 6.25-200 mcg darbepoetin per week (see adult column in conversion table)
 CKD patients **NOT** on dialysis (consider initiating treatment when hemoglobin is <10 g/dL; use only if rate of hemoglobin decline would likely result in RBC transfusion and desire is to reduce risk of alloimmunization or other RBC transfusion-related risks; reduce or interrupt dose if hemoglobin exceeds 10 g/dL): I.V., SubQ: Initial: 0.45 mcg/kg/dose once every 4 weeks
 Dosage adjustment in CKD (either on dialysis or not on dialysis): Do not increase dose more frequently than every 4 weeks (dose decreases may occur more frequently).
  If hemoglobin increases >1 g/dL in any 2-week period: Decrease dose by ≥25%
  If hemoglobin does not increase by >1 g/dL after 4 weeks: Increase dose by 25%
  Inadequate or lack of response: If adequate response is not achieved over 12 weeks, further increases are unlikely to be of benefit and may increase the risk for adverse events; use the minimum effective dose that will maintain a hemoglobin level sufficient to avoid red blood cell transfusions and evaluate patient for other causes of anemia; discontinue treatment if responsiveness does not improve

Anemia due to chemotherapy in cancer patients: Initiate treatment only if hemoglobin <10 g/dL and anticipated duration of myelosuppressive chemotherapy is ≥2 months. Titrate dosage to use the minimum effective dose that will maintain a hemoglobin concentration sufficient to avoid red blood cell transfusions. Discontinue darbepoetin following completion of chemotherapy. SubQ: Initial: 2.25 mcg/kg/dose once weekly **or** 500 mcg once every 3 weeks until completion of chemotherapy
 Dosage adjustments:
  Increase dose: If hemoglobin does not increase by 1 g/dL **and** remains below 10 g/dL after initial 6 weeks (for patients receiving weekly therapy only), increase dose to 4.5 mcg/kg/dose once weekly (no dosage adjustment if using every-3-week dosing).
  Reduce dose by 40% if hemoglobin increases >1 g/dL in any 2-week period **or** hemoglobin reaches a level sufficient to avoid red blood cell transfusion.
  Withhold dose if hemoglobin exceeds a level needed to avoid red blood cell transfusion. Resume treatment with a 40% dose reduction when hemoglobin approaches a level where transfusions may be required.
  Discontinue: On completion of chemotherapy or if after 8 weeks of therapy there is no hemoglobin response or RBC transfusions still required

Conversion from epoetin alfa to darbepoetin alfa: See table.

Conversion From Epoetin Alfa to Darbepoetin Alfa (I.V. or SubQ)

(maintain the same route of administration for the conversion)

Previous Weekly Epoetin Alfa Dose (units/wk)	Weekly Darbepoetin Alfa Dosage	
	Pediatric (mcg/wk)	Adults (mcg/wk)
<1500	Not established	6.25
1500-2499	6.25	6.25
2500-4999	10	12.5
5000-10,999	20	25
11,000-17,999	40	40
18,000-33,999	60	60
34,000-89,999	100	100
≥90,000	200	200

Note: Due to the longer serum half-life of darbepoetin alfa, when converting from epoetin alfa, administer darbepoetin alfa once weekly if the patient was receiving epoetin alfa 2-3 times weekly and administer darbepoetin alfa once every two weeks if the patient was receiving epoetin alfa once weekly.

Administration May be administered I.V. or SubQ. Do not shake as this may denature the glycoprotein rendering the drug biologically inactive; only use SureClick™ autoinjectors if administering the full dose. Autoinjectors are for subcutaneous administration only. I.V.: Infuse over 1-3 minutes; I.V. route preferred for hemodialysis patients.

Monitoring Parameters Hemoglobin (at least once per week until maintenance dose established and after dosage changes; monitor less frequently once hemoglobin is stabilized); CKD patients should be also be monitored at least monthly following hemoglobin stability); iron stores (transferrin saturation and ferritin) prior to and during therapy; serum chemistry (CKD patients)

Cancer patients: Examinations recommended by the ASCO/ASH guidelines (Rizzo, 2010) prior to treatment include peripheral blood smear (in some situations a bone marrow exam may be necessary), assessment for iron, folate, or vitamin B_{12} deficiency, reticulocyte count, renal function status, and occult blood loss; during ESA treatment, assess baseline and periodic iron, total iron-binding capacity, and transferrin saturation or ferritin concentrations.

Additional Information Optimal response is achieved when iron stores are maintained with supplemental iron if necessary; evaluate iron stores prior to and during therapy. Use of ESAs in anemic patients with HIV who have been treated with zidovudine has not been demonstrated in controlled clinical trials to improve the symptoms of anemia, quality of life, fatigue, or well-being.

1 mcg darbepoetin alfa is equivalent to 200 units epoetin alfa.

Dosage Forms Excipient information presented when available (limited, particularly for generics); consult specific product labeling.

Solution, Injection [preservative free]:
Aranesp (Albumin Free): 25 mcg/mL (1 mL); 40 mcg/mL (1 mL); 25 mcg/0.42 mL (0.42 mL); 60 mcg/mL (1 mL); 40 mcg/0.4 mL (0.4 mL); 100 mcg/mL (1 mL); 60 mcg/0.3 mL (0.3 mL); 100 mcg/0.5 mL (0.5 mL); 150 mcg/0.75 mL (0.75 mL); 200 mcg/mL (1 mL); 300 mcg/mL (1 mL); 200 mcg/0.4 mL (0.4 mL); 300 mcg/0.6 mL (0.6 mL) [albumin free; contains polysorbate 80]

Aranesp (Albumin Free): 150 mcg/0.3 mL (0.3 mL); 500 mcg/mL (1 mL) [contains polysorbate 80]

References
Alade SL, Brown RE, and Paquet A Jr, "Polysorbate 80 and E-Ferol Toxicity," *Pediatrics*, 1986, 77(4):593-7.
André JL, Deschênes G, Boudailliez B, et al, "Darbepoetin, Effective Treatment of Anaemia in Paediatric Patients With Chronic Renal Failure," *Pediatr Nephrol*, 2007, 22(5):708-14.
Blumer J, Berg S, Adamson PC, et al, "Pharmacokinetic Evaluation of Darbepoetin Alfa for the Treatment of Pediatric Patients With Chemotherapy-Induced Anemia," *Pediatr Blood Cancer*, 2007, 49(5):687-93.
Joy MS, "Darbepoetin Alfa: A Novel Erythropoiesis-Stimulating Protein," *Ann Pharmacother*, 2002, 36(7):1183-92.
KDOQI, "KDOQI Clinical Practice Guideline and Clinical Practice Recommendations for Anemia in Chronic Kidney Disease: 2007 Update of Hemoglobin Target," *Am J Kidney Dis*, 2007, 50(3):471-530.
Lerner J, Kale AS, Warady BA, et al, "Pharmacokinetics of Darbepoetin Alfa in Pediatric Patients With Chronic Kidney Disease," *Pediatr Nephrol*, 2002, 17(11):933-7.
Rizzo JD, Brouwers M, Hurley P, et al, "American Society of Clinical Oncology/American Society of Hematology Clinical Practice Guideline Update on the Use of Epoetin and Darbepoetin in Adult Patients With Cancer," *J Clin Oncol*, 2010, 28(33):4996-5010.
Rizzo JD, Somerfield MR, Hagerty KL, et al, "Use of Epoetin and Darbepoetin in Patients With Cancer: 2007 American Society of Hematology/American Society of Clinical Oncology Clinical Practice Guideline Update," *Blood*, 2008, 111(1):25-41.

Darunavir (dar OO na veer)

Related Information
Adult and Adolescent HIV *on page 2348*
Pediatric HIV *on page 2338*
Perinatal HIV *on page 2356*
Brand Names: U.S. Prezista
Brand Names: Canada Prezista®
Therapeutic Category Antiretroviral Agent; HIV Agents (Anti-HIV Agents); Protease Inhibitor
Generic Availability (U.S.) No
Use Treatment of HIV-1 infection in combination with ritonavir and other antiretroviral agents (FDA approved in ages ≥3 years and adults). **Note:** HIV regimens consisting of **three** antiretroviral agents are strongly recommended.
Pregnancy Risk Factor C
Pregnancy Considerations Teratogenic effects have not been observed in animal reproduction studies. Darunavir has a low level of transfer across the human placenta. Serum concentrations are decreased during pregnancy; therefore, once-daily dosing is not recommended; twice-daily dosing should be used. The DHHS Perinatal HIV Guidelines consider darunavir to be an alternative protease inhibitor (PI) for use in antiretroviral-naïve pregnant patients when combined with low-dose ritonavir boosting. A small increased risk of preterm birth has been associated with maternal use of protease inhibitor-based combination antiretroviral (ARV) therapy during pregnancy; however, the benefits of use generally outweigh this risk and PIs should not be withheld if otherwise recommended. Hyperglycemia, new onset of diabetes mellitus, or diabetic ketoacidosis have been reported with PIs; it is not clear if pregnancy increases this risk.

Regardless of CD4 count or HIV RNA copy number, all HIV-infected pregnant women should receive a combination ARV drug regimen combination of antepartum, intrapartum, and infant ARV prophylaxis. ARV therapy should be started as soon as possible in women with symptomatic infection. Although earlier initiation may be more effective in reducing the perinatal transmission of HIV, initiation may be delayed until after 12 weeks gestation in women who do not require immediate treatment after careful consideration of maternal conditions (eg, nausea and vomiting) and the potential risks of first trimester fetal exposure for specific agents. A scheduled cesarean delivery at 38 weeks gestation is recommended for all women with HIV RNA >1000 copies/mL or unknown concentrations near delivery in order to decrease transmission. If ARV therapy must be interrupted for <24 hours during the peripartum period, stop then restart all medications simultaneously in order to decrease the chance of developing resistance. Long-term follow-up is recommended for all infants exposed to ARV medications. In couples who want to conceive, the HIV-infected partner should attain maximum viral suppression prior to conception.

Healthcare providers are encouraged to enroll pregnant women exposed to antiretroviral medications in the Antiretroviral Pregnancy Registry (1-800-258-4263 or www.-APRegistry.com). Healthcare providers caring for HIV-infected women and their infants may contact the National Perinatal HIV Hotline (888-448-8765) for clinical consultation (DHHS [perinatal], 2014).

Breast-Feeding Considerations It is not known if darunavir is excreted into breast milk. Maternal or infant antiretroviral therapy does not completely eliminate the risk of postnatal HIV transmission. In addition, multiclass-resistant virus has been detected in breast-feeding infants despite maternal therapy. Therefore, in the United States, where formula is accessible, affordable, safe, and sustainable, and the risk of infant mortality due to diarrhea and respiratory infections is low, complete avoidance of breast-feeding by HIV-infected women is recommended to decrease potential transmission of HIV (DHHS [perinatal], 2014).

Contraindications Hypersensitivity to darunavir or any component; coadministration of darunavir plus ritonavir with alfuzosin, cisapride, ergot alkaloids (eg, dihydroergotamine, ergonovine, ergotamine, methylergonovine), lovastatin, midazolam (oral), pimozide, rifampin, sildenafil [for pulmonary artery hypertension (eg, Revatio)], simvastatin, St John's wort, triazolam

Warnings Do not use without ritonavir; use without ritonavir will result in low plasma levels, altering both therapeutic effect and drug interactions. Drug-induced hepatitis (including acute and cytolytic) has been reported during use of darunavir plus ritonavir. Liver injury has also been reported (including some fatalities); risk may be higher in patients receiving multiple medications, with advanced HIV disease, hepatitis B or C coinfection, and/or immune reconstitution syndrome. Monitor patients closely; consider interrupting or discontinuing therapy if signs/symptoms of liver impairment occur. May exacerbate preexisting hepatic dysfunction; use with caution in patients with underlying hepatic disease, such as hepatitis B or C or cirrhosis. Use is not recommended in severe hepatic impairment.

Skin rash may occur with darunavir plus ritonavir use; usually mild to moderate; reported incidence: 10.3% (all grades); onset generally in the first 4 weeks of therapy; treatment may be continued if rash is mild to moderate (rash may resolve). Stevens-Johnson syndrome, toxic epidermal necrolysis, acute generalized exanthematous pustulosis, and drug rash with eosinophilia and systemic symptoms (DRESS) have been reported rarely; discontinue treatment if severe rash or moderate symptoms accompanied by other systemic symptoms occur. Use with caution in patients with sulfonamide allergy; darunavir contains sulfonamide moiety; cross-sensitivity may occur.

Darunavir plus ritonavir is an inhibitor of cytochrome P450 isoenzyme CYP3A and CYP2D6. Administration with drugs that are primarily metabolized by CYP3A or CYP2D6 may result in increased serum concentrations of the other drug and lead to an increase or prolongation of adverse effects. Due to potential serious and/or life-threatening drug interactions, some drugs are contraindicated or not recommended for concurrent use; other drug interactions require dosage or regimen adjustment or monitoring of serum concentrations of drugs coadministered with darunavir.

Do not use darunavir in children <3 years of age or weighing <10 kg; seizures and death associated with immaturity of the blood-brain barrier and immature hepatic metabolic pathways were observed in juvenile rats (DHHS [pediatric], 2014). Although once daily dosing in treatment-naïve pediatric patients or treatment-experienced pediatric patients with no darunavir resistance-associated viral mutations was FDA approved in February 2013, once daily dosing is **not** recommended in the current DHHS guidelines for any patient <12 years, patients 12 to 18 years who are treatment-experienced with prior treatment failure, or patients ≥18 years with darunavir resistance-associated viral mutations (DHHS [pediatric], 2014). Darunavir resistance-associated viral mutations include: V11I, V32I, L33F, I47V, I50V, I54L, I54M, T74P, L76V, I84V, and L89V.

Precautions Use with caution in patients with diabetes mellitus; hyperglycemia, changes in glucose tolerance, exacerbation of diabetes, DKA, and new-onset diabetes mellitus have been reported in patients receiving protease inhibitors. Use with caution in patients with hemophilia A or B; increased bleeding during protease inhibitor therapy has been reported.

Fat redistribution and accumulation [ie, central obesity, peripheral wasting, facial wasting, breast enlargement, dorsocervical fat enlargement (buffalo hump), and cushingoid appearance] have been observed in patients receiving antiretroviral agents (causal relationship not established). Increases in total cholesterol and triglycerides have been reported; screening should be done prior to therapy and periodically throughout treatment.

Immune reconstitution syndrome (an acute inflammatory response to residual or indolent opportunistic infections) may occur in HIV patients during initial treatment with combination antiretroviral agents; this syndrome may require further patient assessment and therapy. Autoimmune disorders (eg, Graves' disease, Guillain-Barré syndrome, and polymyositis) have been reported in patients experiencing immune reconstitution; time to onset is variable and may occur many months after antiretroviral treatment is initiated.

Some adverse effects have been reported more frequently in pediatric patients (6 to 18 years) than adults including: Vomiting (13% to 33% vs 2% to 5%); headache (9% vs 3% to 7%); pruritus (8% vs <2%); decreased appetite (8% vs 2%).

Adverse Reactions As a class, protease inhibitors potentially cause dyslipidemias which includes elevated cholesterol and triglycerides and a redistribution of body fat centrally to cause increased abdominal girth, buffalo hump, facial atrophy, and breast enlargement. These agents also cause hyperglycemia. See also Ritonavir monograph.

Central nervous system: Fatigue (more common in children), headache (more common in children)

Dermatologic: Pruritus (more common in children), skin rash (more common in children)

Endocrine & metabolic: Diabetes mellitus, hypercholesterolemia (more common in adults), hyperglycemia, increased amylase (more common in adults), increased LDL cholesterol (more common in adults), increased serum triglycerides

Gastrointestinal: Abdominal distention, abdominal pain (more common in children), anorexia (more common in children), decreased appetite (more common in children), diarrhea (more common in children), dyspepsia, increased serum lipase (more common in adults), nausea (more common in children), vomiting (more common in children)

Hepatic: Increased serum ALT (more common in adults), increased serum AST (more common in adults)

Neuromuscular & skeletal: Weakness

Rare but important or life-threatening: Acute renal failure, alopecia, arthritis, bradycardia, cerebrovascular accident, depression, dermatitis (including dermatitis medicamentosa), DRESS syndrome, facial paralysis, folliculitis, gynecomastia, hematuria, hepatic failure, hepatic neoplasm (malignant), hepatitis (acute and cytolytic), hepatotoxicity, hyperlipidemia, hypersensitivity, hyperthermia, immune reconstitution syndrome, impaired consciousness, infection (including clostridium infection, parasitic infection [cryptosporidiosis], cytomegalovirus disease [encephalitis], hepatitis B, esophageal candidiasis), malignant lymphoma, myocardial infarction, nephrolithiasis, neutropenia, obesity, oropharyngeal ulcer, osteoporosis, pancreatitis, pancytopenia, peripheral neuropathy, pneumothorax, progressive multifocal leukoencephalopathy, pulmonary edema, rectal hemorrhage, redistribution of body fat (eg, buffalo hump, increased abdominal girth, breast engorgement, facial atrophy), respiratory failure, rhabdomyolysis (coadministration with HMG-CoA reductase inhibitors), seizure, sepsis, skin rash (toxic), tachycardia, uveitis

Drug Interactions

Metabolism/Transport Effects Substrate of CYP3A4 (major); **Note:** Assignment of Major/Minor substrate status based on clinically relevant drug interaction potential; **Inhibits** CYP2D6 (weak), CYP3A4 (strong), P-glycoprotein

Avoid Concomitant Use

Avoid concomitant use of Darunavir with any of the following: Ado-Trastuzumab Emtansine; Alfuzosin; Amiodarone; Apixaban; Avanafil; Axitinib; Bosutinib; Cabozantinib; Ceritinib; Cisapride; Conivaptan; Crizotinib; Dronedarone; Eplerenone; Ergot Derivatives; Everolimus; Fosphenytoin; Fusidic Acid (Systemic); Halofantrine; Ibrutinib; Ivabradine; Lapatinib; Lomitapide; Lopinavir; Lovastatin; Lurasidone; Macitentan; Midazolam; Nilotinib; Nisoldipine; PAZOPanib; PHENobarbital; Phenytoin; Pimozide; QuiNIDine; Ranolazine; Red Yeast Rice; Regorafenib; Rifampin; Rivaroxaban; Salmeterol; Saquinavir; Silodosin; Simeprevir; Simvastatin; St Johns Wort; Tamsulosin; Telaprevir; Ticagrelor; Tipranavir; Tolvaptan; Topotecan; Toremifene; Triazolam; Ulipristal; Vemurafenib; VinCRIStine (Liposomal); Vorapaxar; Voriconazole

Increased Effect/Toxicity

Darunavir may increase the levels/effects of: Ado-Trastuzumab Emtansine; Afatinib; Alfuzosin; Almotriptan; Alosetron; ALPRAZolam; Amiodarone; Apixaban; ARIPiprazole; AtorvaSTATin; Avanafil; Axitinib; Bedaquiline; Bortezomib; Bosentan; Bosutinib; Brentuximab Vedotin; Brinzolamide; Budesonide (Nasal); Budesonide (Systemic, Oral Inhalation); Cabozantinib; Calcium Channel Blockers (Dihydropyridine); Calcium Channel Blockers (Nondihydropyridine); Cannabis; CarBAMazepine; Ceritinib; Cisapride; Clarithromycin; Colchicine; Conivaptan; Corticosteroids (Orally Inhaled); Crizotinib; Cyclophosphamide; CycloSPORINE (Systemic); CYP2D6 Substrates; CYP3A4 Substrates; Dabigatran Etexilate; Digoxin; Dofetilide; DOXOrubicin (Conventional); Dronabinol; Dronedarone; Dutasteride; Efavirenz; Enfuvirtide; Eplerenone; Ergot Derivatives; Everolimus; FentaNYL; Fesoterodine; Fluticasone (Nasal); Fluticasone (Oral Inhalation); GuanFACINE; Halofantrine; Ibrutinib; Iloperidone; Imatinib; Itraconazole; Ivabradine; Ivacaftor; Ixabepilone; Ketoconazole (Systemic); Lacosamide; Lapatinib; Levomilnacipran; Lomitapide; Lovastatin; Lumefantrine; Lurasidone; Macitentan; Maraviroc; Meperidine; MethylPREDNISolone; Midazolam; Mifepristone; Nefazodone; Nilotinib; Nisoldipine; Ospemifene; OxyCODONE; Paricalcitol; PAZOPanib; P-glycoprotein/ABCB1 Substrates; Pimecrolimus; Pimozide; PONATinib; Pravastatin; Propafenone; Protease Inhibitors; Prucalopride; QUEtiapine; QuiNIDine; Ranolazine; Red Yeast Rice; Regorafenib; Repaglinide; Rifabutin; Rifaximin; Rilpivirine; Riociguat; Rivaroxaban; RomiDEPsin; Rosuvastatin; Ruxolitinib; Salmeterol; Saxagliptin; Sildenafil; Silodosin; Simeprevir; Simvastatin; SORAfenib; Tacrolimus (Systemic); Tacrolimus (Topical); Tadalafil; Tamsulosin; Temsirolimus; Tenofovir; Tetrahydrocannabinol; Ticagrelor; Tofacitinib; Tolterodine; Tolvaptan; Topotecan; Toremifene; TraZODone; Triazolam; Tricyclic Antidepressants; Ulipristal; Vardenafil; Vemurafenib; Vilazodone; VinCRIStine (Liposomal); Vorapaxar; Zuclopenthixol

The levels/effects of Darunavir may be increased by: Clarithromycin; Conivaptan; CycloSPORINE (Systemic); CYP3A4 Inhibitors (Moderate); CYP3A4 Inhibitors (Strong); Delavirdine; Enfuvirtide; Etravirine; Fusidic Acid (Systemic); Itraconazole; Ketoconazole (Systemic); Luliconazole; Mifepristone; Rifabutin; Simeprevir; Stiripentol; Tenofovir

Decreased Effect

Darunavir may decrease the levels/effects of: Abacavir; Boceprevir; Clarithromycin; Contraceptives (Estrogens); Contraceptives (Progestins); Delavirdine; Didanosine; Etravirine; Ifosfamide; Meperidine; Methadone; Norethindrone; PARoxetine; Prasugrel; Sertraline; Telaprevir; Ticagrelor; Valproic Acid and Derivatives; Voriconazole; Warfarin; Zidovudine

The levels/effects of Darunavir may be decreased by: Boceprevir; Bosentan; CYP3A4 Inducers (Strong); Dabrafenib; Deferasirox; Efavirenz; Fosphenytoin; Garlic; Lopinavir; Mitotane; PHENobarbital; Phenytoin; Rifampin; Saquinavir; Siltuximab; St Johns Wort; Telaprevir; Tipranavir; Tocilizumab

Food Interactions Absorption and bioavailability are increased when administered with food. Management: Take with meals.

Stability

Oral suspension: Store at 25°C (77°F); excursions permitted to 15°C to 30°C (59°F to 86°F); do not refrigerate or freeze; avoid exposure to excessive heat; store in original container.

Oral tablets: Store at 25°C (77°F); excursions permitted to 15°C to 30°C (59°F to 86°F).

Mechanism of Action Binds to the site of HIV-1 protease activity and inhibits cleavage of viral Gag-Pol polyprotein precursors into individual functional proteins required for infectious HIV. This results in the formation of immature, noninfectious viral particles.

Pharmacokinetics (Adult data unless noted) Note: All pharmacokinetic parameters derived in the presence of ritonavir coadministration; pharmacokinetic data in pediatric patients (6 to 18 years) reported to be similar to adult data.

Protein binding: ~95%; primarily to alpha$_1$ acid glycoprotein

Metabolism: Hepatic, primarily via CYP3A4 to minimally active metabolites

Bioavailability: Absolute oral: 82% (with ritonavir); bioavailability is increased 30% to 40% with food

Half-life elimination: ~15 hours

Time to peak, serum concentration: 2.5 to 4 hours

Elimination: Feces (~80%, 41% as unchanged drug); urine (~14%, 8% as unchanged drug)

Dosing: Usual

Pediatric: **HIV infection, treatment: Note:** Genotypic testing for viral resistance is recommended in therapy experienced patients; coadministration with ritonavir is required; use in combination with other antiretroviral agents.

Note: Darunavir resistance-associated viral mutations include: V11I, V32I, L33F, I47V, I50V, I54L, I54M, T74P, L76V, I84V, and L89V.

Infants and Children <3 years of age or weighing <10 kg: Do not use; seizures and death associated with immaturity of the blood-brain barrier and immature hepatic metabolic pathways were observed in juvenile rats (DHHS [pediatric], 2014)

Treatment-naïve patients or treatment-experienced patients, without darunavir resistance-associated mutation: Children ≥3 years weighing ≥10 kg and Adolescents:

AIDS*info* recommendations (DHHS [pediatric], 2014):

Oral:

Weight-directed dosing: Body weight 10 to 15 kg: Darunavir 20 mg/kg (maximum dose: 600 mg) twice daily **plus** ritonavir 3 mg/kg (maximum dose: 100 mg) twice daily

Fixed-dosing:

Twice-daily regimen: Children and Adolescents 3 to <18 years weighing ≥10 kg:

10 kg to <11 kg: Darunavir 200 mg **plus** ritonavir 32 mg twice daily

11 kg to <12 kg: Darunavir 220 mg **plus** ritonavir 32 mg twice daily

12 kg to <13 kg: Darunavir 240 mg **plus** ritonavir 40 mg twice daily

13 kg to <14 kg: Darunavir 260 mg **plus** ritonavir 40 mg twice daily

14 kg to <15 kg: Darunavir 280 mg **plus** ritonavir 48 mg twice daily

15 kg to <30 kg: Darunavir 375 mg **plus** ritonavir 48 twice daily

30 kg to <40 kg: Darunavir 450 mg **plus** ritonavir 100 mg twice daily

≥40 kg: Darunavir 600 mg **plus** ritonavir 100 mg twice daily

Once-daily regimen: Children and Adolescents ≥12 years

30 kg to <40 kg: Darunavir 675 mg **plus** ritonavir 100 mg once daily

≥40 kg: Darunavir 800 mg **plus** ritonavir 100 mg once daily

Manufacturer's labeling: Oral: **Note:** Although FDA approved, the Pediatric AIDS*info* guidelines do not recommend once-daily dosing in children <12 years. Alternate weight-directed and fixed-dosing regimens with twice daily dosing are recommended for children >3 year to <12 years of age (see above AIDS*info* recommendations); once-daily dosing is only recommended in patients ≥12 years of age or ≥30 k g without resistant-associated mutations. If once-daily dosing is used in children <12 years of age, therapeutic drug monitoring with measurement of plasma concentrations and inhibitory quotient should be performed (DHHS [pediatric], 2014).

Weight-directed dosing: Body weight 10 to <15 kg: Darunavir 35 mg/kg (maximum dose 800mg) twice daily **plus** ritonavir 7 mg/kg (maximum dose: 100 mg) once daily

Fixed-dosing:

10 kg to <11 kg: Darunavir 350 mg **plus** ritonavir 64 mg once daily

11 kg to <12 kg: Darunavir 385 mg **plus** ritonavir 64 mg once daily

12 kg to <13 kg: Darunavir 420 mg **plus** ritonavir 80 mg once daily

13 kg to <14 kg: Darunavir 455 mg **plus** ritonavir 80 mg once daily

14 kg to <15 kg: Darunavir 490 mg **plus** ritonavir 96 mg once daily

15 kg to <30 kg: Darunavir 600 mg **plus** ritonavir 100 mg once daily

30 kg to <40 kg: Darunavir 675 mg **plus** ritonavir 100 mg once daily

≥40 kg: Darunavir 800 mg **plus** ritonavir 100 mg once daily

Treatment-experienced patients, with at least one darunavir resistance-associated mutation: Children ≥3 years of age weighing ≥10 kg and Adolescents:

Weight-directed dosing: Body weight 10 kg to <15 kg: Darunavir 20 mg/kg (maximum dose: 600 mg) twice daily **plus** ritonavir 3 mg/kg (maximum dose: 100 mg) twice daily

Fixed-dosing:

10 kg to <11 kg: Darunavir 200 mg **plus** ritonavir 32 mg twice daily

11 kg to <12 kg: Darunavir 220 mg **plus** ritonavir 32 mg twice daily

12 kg to <13 kg: Darunavir 240 mg **plus** ritonavir 40 mg twice daily

13 kg to <14 kg: Darunavir 260 mg **plus** ritonavir 40 mg twice daily

14 kg to <15 kg: Darunavir 280 mg **plus** ritonavir 48 mg twice daily

15 kg to <30 kg: Darunavir 375 mg **plus** ritonavir 48 twice daily; **Note:** If weight ≥20 kg, the ritonavir 100 mg tablet may be substituted for liquid formulation to enhance palatability (DHHS [pediatric], 2014).

30 kg to <40 kg: Darunavir 450 mg **plus** ritonavir 60 mg twice daily; **Note:** The ritonavir 100 mg tablet may be substituted for the liquid formulation to enhance palatability (DHHS [pediatric], 2014).

≥40 kg: Darunavir 600 mg **plus** ritonavir 100 mg twice daily

Adult: **HIV infection, treatment:** Oral: **Note:** Genotypic testing for viral resistance is recommended in therapy experienced patients; coadministration with ritonavir is required; use in combination with other antiretroviral agents.

Therapy-naïve: Darunavir 800 mg **plus** ritonavir 100 mg once daily

Therapy-experienced:

With no darunavir resistance-associated substitutions: Darunavir 800 mg **plus** ritonavir 100 mg once daily

With ≥1 darunavir resistance-associated substitution or no genotypic testing: Darunavir 600 mg **plus** ritonavir 100 mg twice daily

Dosing adjustment in renal impairment:

Children ≥3 years of age and Adolescents (DHHS [pediatric], 2014):

CrCl ≥30 mL/minute: No dosage adjustment required

CrCl <30 mL/minute: There are no dosage adjustments provided in manufacturer's labeling (has not been studied).

Adults: No dosage adjustment required (DHHS [adult], 2014).

Dialysis: Darunavir is highly bound to plasma proteins; therefore, removal by hemodialysis or peritoneal dialysis is expected to be minimal.

Dosing adjustment in hepatic impairment:

Mild to moderate impairment (Child-Pugh class A or B): No dosage adjustment necessary

Severe impairment (Child-Pugh class C): Use not recommended

Administration Coadministration with ritonavir and food is required (bioavailability is increased). Shake suspension well prior to each dose; use manufacturer-provided oral dosing syringe to measure dose. In patients taking darunavir once daily, if a dose of darunavir or ritonavir is missed by >12 hours, the next dose should be taken at the regularly scheduled time. If a dose of darunavir or ritonavir is missed by <12 hours, the dose should be taken immediately and then the next dose should be taken at the regularly scheduled time. In patients taking darunavir twice daily, if a dose of darunavir or ritonavir is missed by >6 hours, the next dose should be taken at the regularly scheduled time. If a dose of darunavir or ritonavir is missed by <6 hours, the dose should be taken immediately and then the next dose should be taken at the regularly scheduled time.

Monitoring Parameters Note: Monitor CD4 percentage (if <5 years of age) or CD4 count (if ≥5 years of age) at least every 3 to 4 months (DHHS [pediatric], 2014).

Prior to initiation of therapy: Genotypic resistance testing, CD4 and viral load (every 3 to 4 months), CBC with differential, LFTs, BUN, creatinine, electrolytes, glucose, rinalysis (every 6 to 12 months), and assessment for readiness for adherence with medication regimen. At initiation and with any change in treatment regimen: CBC with differential, electrolytes, calcium, phosphate, glucose, LFTs, bilirubin, urinalysis (at initiation), BUN, creatinine, albumin, total protein, lipid panel (at initiation), CD4, and viral load. After 1 to 2 weeks of therapy: Signs of medication toxicity and adherence. After 2 to 4 weeks of therapy: CBC with differential, viral load, signs of medication toxicity, and adherence; then every 3 to 4 months: CBC with differential, electrolytes, glucose, LFTs, bilirubin, BUN, creatinine, CD4, viral load, signs of medication toxicity, and adherence. Every 6 to 12 months: Lipid panel and urinalysis. CD4 monitoring frequency may be decreased to every 6 to 12 months in children who are adherent to therapy if the value is well above the threshold for opportunistic infections, viral suppression is sustained, and the clinical status is stable for more than 2 to 3 years (DHHS [pediatric], 2014). Monitor for growth and development, signs of HIV-specific physical conditions, HIV disease progression, opportunistic infections, hepatitis, and skin rash.

Reference Range Trough concentration (Limited data available; data is from adult clinical trials that utilized 600 mg twice daily dosing; range utilized in trials): Median: 3300 mg/mL (range: 1255 to 7368 ng/mL) (DHHS [adult, pediatric], 2014)

Dosage Forms Excipient information presented when available (limited, particularly for generics); consult specific product labeling. [DSC] = Discontinued product

Suspension, Oral:

Prezista: 100 mg/mL (200 mL) [contains methylparaben sodium; strawberry cream flavor]

Tablet, Oral:

Prezista: 75 mg, 150 mg

Prezista: 400 mg [DSC], 600 mg [contains fd&c yellow #6 (sunset yellow)]

Prezista: 800 mg

References

DHHS Panel on Antiretroviral Guidelines for Adults and Adolescents. Guidelines for the use of antiretroviral agents in HIV-1-infected adults and adolescents, Department of Health and Human Services. May 1, 2014. Available at http://www.aidsinfo.nih.gov/ContentFiles/AdultandAdolescentGL.pdf

DHHS Panel on Antiretroviral Therapy and Medical Management of HIV-Infected Children. Guidelines for the use of antiretroviral agents in pediatric HIV infection. February 12, 2014. Available at http://aidsinfo.nih.gov

DHHS Panel on Treatment of HIV-Infected Pregnant Women and Prevention of Perinatal Transmission. Recommendations for the use of antiretroviral drugs in pregnant HIV-1-infected women for maternal health and interventions to reduce perinatal HIV-1 transmission in the United States. March 28, 2014. Available at http://aidsinfo.nih.gov

Prezista (darunavir) [prescribing information]. Titusville NJ: Janssen Pharmaceuticals, Inc; April 2014.

◆ **Darunavir Ethanolate** *see* Darunavir *on page 595*

◆ **Daunomycin** *see* DAUNORubicin (Conventional) *on page 599*

DAUNOrubicin (Conventional)
(daw noe ROO bi sin con VEN sha nal)

Medication Safety Issues
Sound-alike/look-alike issues:

DAUNOrubicin may be confused with DACTINomycin, DOXOrubicin, DOXOrubicin liposomal, epirubicin, IDArubicin, valrubicin

Conventional formulation (Cerubidine, DAUNOrubicin hydrochloride) may be confused with the liposomal formulation (DaunoXome®)

High alert medication:

The Institute for Safe Medication Practices (ISMP) includes this medication among its list of drug classes which have a heightened risk of causing significant patient harm when used in error.

Related Information

Emetogenic Potential of Antineoplastic Agents in Children *on page 2327*

Management of Drug Extravasations *on page 2255*

Safe Handling of Hazardous Drugs *on page 2419*

Brand Names: Canada Cerubidine; Daunorubicin Hydrochloride for Injection

Therapeutic Category Antineoplastic Agent, Anthracycline; Antineoplastic Agent, Antibiotic; Antineoplastic Agent, Topoisomerase II Inhibitor

Generic Availability (U.S.) Yes

Use In combination with other agents in the treatment of leukemias (ALL, AML)

Pregnancy Risk Factor D

Pregnancy Considerations Adverse events have been observed in animal reproduction studies. Daunorubicin crosses the placenta. Women of reproductive potential should avoid pregnancy.

Breast-Feeding Considerations It is not known if daunorubicin is excreted into breast milk. Due to the potential for serious adverse reactions in the nursing infant, the manufacturer recommends a decision be made whether to discontinue nursing or to discontinue the drug, taking into account the importance of treatment to the mother.

Contraindications Hypersensitivity to daunorubicin or any component; CHF, left ventricular ejection fraction <30% to 40%, or arrhythmias; preexisting bone marrow suppression

Warnings Hazardous agent; use appropriate precautions for handling and disposal (NIOSH, 2012); I.V. use only; severe local tissue necrosis will result if extravasation occurs **[U.S. Boxed Warning]**. May cause severe myelosuppression, dose-limiting, primarily leukopenia and neutropenia **[U.S. Boxed Warning]**; irreversible myocardial toxicity may occur as total dosage approaches 550 mg/m^2 in adults, 400 mg/m^2 in patients receiving chest radiation, 300 mg/m^2 in children ≥2 years of age, or 10 mg/kg in children <2 years **[U.S. Boxed Warning]**; this may occur during therapy or several months after therapy; total cumulative dose should take into account previous or concomitant treatment with cardiotoxic agents or irradiation of chest; infants and children may be more susceptible to anthracycline-induced cardiotoxicity than adults; monitor left ventricular (LV) function (baseline and periodic) with ECHO or MUGA scan; monitor ECG. Secondary leukemias may occur when used with combination chemotherapy or radiation therapy.

Precautions Reduce dosage in patients with hepatic, or renal impairment **[U.S. Boxed Warning]**, or in patients with biliary impairment. Should be administered under the supervision of an experienced cancer chemotherapy physician **[U.S. Boxed Warning]**.

Adverse Reactions

Cardiovascular: Transient ECG abnormalities (supraventricular tachycardia, S-T wave changes, atrial or ventricular extrasystoles); generally asymptomatic and self-limiting. CHF, dose related, may be delayed for 7-8 years after treatment

Dermatologic: Alopecia (reversible); discoloration of saliva, sweat, or tears, radiation recall, skin "flare" at injection site

Endocrine & metabolic: Hyperuricemia

Gastrointestinal: Abdominal pain, diarrhea, GI ulceration, diarrhea, mild nausea or vomiting, stomatitis

Genitourinary: Discoloration of urine (red)

Hematologic: Myelosuppression (onset: 7 days; nadir: 10-14 days; recovery: 21-28 days), primarily leukopenia; thrombocytopenia and anemia

Rare but important or life-threatening: Anaphylactoid reaction, arrhythmia, bilirubin increased, cardiomyopathy, hepatitis, infertility; local (cellulitis, pain, thrombophlebitis at injection site); MI, myocarditis, neutropenic typhlitis, pericarditis, secondary leukemia, skin rash, sterility, systemic hypersensitivity (including urticaria, pruritus, angioedema, dysphagia, dyspnea); transaminases increased

Drug Interactions

Metabolism/Transport Effects Substrate of P-glycoprotein

Avoid Concomitant Use

Avoid concomitant use of DAUNOrubicin (Conventional) with any of the following: BCG; CloZAPine; Dipyrone; Natalizumab; Pimecrolimus; Tacrolimus (Topical); Tofacitinib; Vaccines (Live)

Increased Effect/Toxicity

DAUNOrubicin (Conventional) may increase the levels/ effects of: CloZAPine; Leflunomide; Natalizumab; Tofacitinib; Vaccines (Live)

The levels/effects of DAUNOrubicin (Conventional) may be increased by: Bevacizumab; Cyclophosphamide; Denosumab; Dipyrone; P-glycoprotein/ABCB1 Inhibitors; Pimecrolimus; Roflumilast; Tacrolimus (Topical); Taxane Derivatives; Trastuzumab

Decreased Effect

DAUNOrubicin (Conventional) may decrease the levels/ effects of: BCG; Cardiac Glycosides; Coccidioidin Skin Test; Sipuleucel-T; Vaccines (Inactivated); Vaccines (Live)

The levels/effects of DAUNOrubicin (Conventional) may be decreased by: Cardiac Glycosides; Echinacea; P-glycoprotein/ABCB1 Inducers

Stability Hazardous agent; use appropriate precautions for handling and disposal (NIOSH, 2012). Protect from light; reconstituted solution is stable for 48 hours when refrigerated and 24 hours at room temperature; a color change from red to blue/purple indicates decomposition of the drug; unstable in solutions with a pH >8; incompatible with heparin, sodium bicarbonate, fluorouracil, and dexamethasone.

Mechanism of Action Inhibition of DNA and RNA synthesis by intercalation between DNA base pairs and by steric obstruction. Daunomycin intercalates at points of local uncoiling of the double helix. Although the exact mechanism is unclear, it appears that direct binding to DNA (intercalation) and inhibition of DNA repair (topoisomerase II inhibition) result in blockade of DNA and RNA synthesis and fragmentation of DNA.

Pharmacokinetics (Adult data unless noted)

Distribution: Widely distributed in tissues such as spleen, heart, kidneys, liver, and lungs; does not cross the blood-brain barrier; crosses the placenta

Metabolism: To daunorubicinol (active)

Half-life, terminal: 14-18.5 hours

Daunorubicinol, active metabolite: 26.7 hours

Elimination: 40% of dose excreted in bile; ~14% to 23% excreted in urine as metabolite and unchanged drug

Dosing: Usual I.V. (refer to individual protocols):

Children <2 years or <0.5 m^2: Dosage should be calculated on the basis of body weight rather than body surface area: 1 mg/kg or per protocol with frequency dependent on regimen employed

Children:

ALL combination therapy: Remission induction: 25-45 mg/m^2 on days 1 and 8 of cycle, or 30-45 mg/m^2/day for 3 days every 3-4 weeks, or 25 mg/m^2 every week for 4 weeks

AML combination therapy: Induction: I.V. continuous infusion: 30-60 mg/m^2/day on days 1-3 of cycle, or 20 mg/m^2/day for 4 days every 14 days

Adults: 30-60 mg/m^2/day for 3-5 days, repeat dose in 3-4 weeks; total cumulative dose should not exceed 400-600 mg/m^2

AML: Single agent induction: 60 mg/m^2/day for 3 days; repeat every 3-4 weeks

AML: Combination therapy induction: 45 mg/m^2/day for 3 days of the first course of induction therapy; subsequent courses: Every day for 2 days

ALL: Combination therapy: Remission induction: 45 mg/m^2 on days 1, 2, and 3 of induction course

Dosing adjustment in hepatic or renal impairment: Reduce dose by 25% in patients with serum bilirubin of 1.2-3 mg/dL; reduce dose by 50% in patients with serum bilirubin and/or creatinine >3 mg/dL

Administration Hazardous agent; use appropriate precautions for handling and disposal (NIOSH, 2012).

Parenteral: Drug is very irritating, do not inject I.M. or SubQ; administer IVP diluting the reconstituted dose in 10-15 mL NS and administering over 2-3 minutes into the tubing of a rapidly infusing I.V. solution of D$_5$W or NS; daunorubicin has also been diluted in 100 mL of D$_5$W or NS and infused over 30-45 minutes or as a continuous 24-hour infusion

Vesicant/Extravasation Risk Vesicant

Monitoring Parameters CBC with differential and platelet count, serum bilirubin, serum uric acid, liver function test, ECG, ventricular ejection fraction, renal function test; patency of I.V. line

Additional Information Myelosuppressive effects:

WBC: Severe

Platelets: Severe

Onset (days): 7

Nadir (days): 10-14

Recovery (days): 21-28

Dosage Forms Excipient information presented when available (limited, particularly for generics); consult specific product labeling.

Injectable, Intravenous:

Generic: 5 mg/mL (4 mL)

Injectable, Intravenous [preservative free]:

Generic: 5 mg/mL (4 mL, 10 mL)

References

Crom WR, Glynn-Barnhart AM, Rodman JH, et al, "Pharmacokinetics of Anticancer Drugs in Children," *Clin Pharmacokinet*, 1987, 12 (3):168-213.

National Institute for Occupational Safety and Health (NIOSH), "NIOSH List of Antineoplastic and Other Hazardous Drugs in Healthcare Settings 2012." Available at http://www.cdc.gov/niosh/docs/2012-150/pdfs/2012-150.pdf. Accessed January 21, 2013.

◆ **DAUNOrubicin Hydrochloride** *see* DAUNOrubicin (Conventional) *on page 599*

◆ **Daunorubicin Hydrochloride for Injection (Can)** *see* DAUNOrubicin (Conventional) *on page 599*

◆ **Dayhist Allergy 12 Hour Relief [OTC]** *see* Clemastine *on page 494*

◆ **Daypro** *see* Oxaprozin *on page 1562*

◆ **Daytrana** *see* Methylphenidate *on page 1379*

◆ **dCF** *see* Pentostatin *on page 1644*

◆ **DDAVP** *see* Desmopressin *on page 612*

◆ **DDAVP® (Can)** *see* Desmopressin *on page 612*

◆ **DDAVP® Melt (Can)** *see* Desmopressin *on page 612*

◆ **DDAVP Rhinal Tube** *see* Desmopressin *on page 612*

◆ **ddI** *see* Didanosine *on page 654*

◆ **1-Deamino-8-D-Arginine Vasopressin** *see* Desmopressin *on page 612*

◆ **Debrox [OTC]** *see* Carbamide Peroxide *on page 377*

◆ **Decadron** *see* Dexamethasone (Systemic) *on page 615*

◆ **Decara** *see* Cholecalciferol *on page 455*

◆ **Declomycin** *see* Demeclocycline *on page 607*

◆ **Decongestant 12Hour Max St [OTC]** *see* Pseudoephedrine *on page 1770*

◆ **Deep Sea Nasal Spray [OTC]** *see* Sodium Chloride *on page 1902*

Deferasirox (de FER a sir ox)

Medication Safety Issues
Sound-alike/look-alike issues:
Deferasirox may be confused with deferiprone, deferoxamine

Brand Names: U.S. Exjade

Brand Names: Canada Exjade

Therapeutic Category Chelating Agent, Oral

Generic Availability (U.S.) No

Use Treatment of chronic iron overload due to blood transfusions (FDA approved in ages ≥2 years and adults); treatment of chronic iron overload due to nontransfusion-dependent thalassemia syndromes with a liver iron concentration (LIC) of at least 5 mg iron per gram of liver dry weight (mg Fe/g dw) and serum ferritin >300 mcg/L (FDA approved in ages ≥10 years and adults)

Prescribing and Access Restrictions Deferasirox (Exjade) is only available through a restricted distribution program called EPASS Complete Care. Prescribers must enroll patients in this program in order to obtain the medication. For patient enrollment, contact 1-888-90-EPASS (1-888-903-7277).

Pregnancy Risk Factor C

Pregnancy Considerations Teratogenic effects were observed in animal reproduction studies. Use during pregnancy only if the potential benefit justifies the potential risk to the fetus.

Breast-Feeding Considerations It is not known if deferasirox is excreted in breast milk. The decision to discontinue deferasirox or to discontinue breast-feeding during therapy should take into account the benefits of treatment to the mother.

Contraindications Hypersensitivity to deferasirox or any component; platelet counts <50,000/mm³; poor performance status; high-risk myelodysplastic syndromes; advanced malignancies; creatinine clearance <40 mL/minute or serum creatinine >2 times the age-appropriate ULN

Warnings Acute renal failure (including fatalities and cases requiring dialysis) may occur **[U.S. Boxed Warning]**; observed more frequently in patients with comorbid conditions and advanced hematologic malignancies. In clinical trials, dose-dependent increases in serum creatinine were observed; reported incidence was 36% to 38% which was higher than the incidence in the comparative deferoxamine treatment group (14% to 22%). Obtain serum creatinine and calculate creatinine clearance in duplicate at baseline prior to initiation, and monitor at least monthly thereafter; consider more frequent monitoring if serum concentrations

are increasing. Use with caution in patients with renal impairment; in patients with underlying renal dysfunction or at risk for acute renal failure; dosage modification or treatment discontinuation may be required; reductions in initial dose are recommended for patients with CrCl 40-60 mL/minute; use is contraindicated in patients with a creatinine clearance <40 mL/minute or serum creatinine >2 times age-appropriate ULN. May cause proteinuria; monitor monthly although the clinical significance of proteinuria is unknown. Renal tubular damage, including Fanconi's syndrome, has also been reported, primarily in pediatric/adolescent patients with β-thalassemia and serum ferritin levels <1500 mcg/L.

Hepatic injury and failure (including fatalities) may occur **[U.S. Boxed Warning]**; monitor transaminases and bilirubin at baseline, every 2 weeks for 1 month, then at least monthly thereafter. Hepatitis and elevated transaminases have also been reported. Hepatotoxicity is more common in patients >55 years and in patients with significant comorbidities (eg, cirrhosis, multiorgan failure). Reduce dose or temporarily interrupt treatment for severe or persistent increases in transaminases/bilirubin. Avoid use in patients with severe (Child-Pugh class C) hepatic impairment; a dose reduction is required in patients with moderate (Child-Pugh class B) hepatic impairment. Monitor patients with mild (Child-Pugh class A) or moderate (Child-Pugh class B) impairment closely for efficacy and for adverse reactions requiring dosage reduction.

Gastrointestinal hemorrhage, including fatalities, may occur **[U.S. Boxed Warning]**; observed more frequently in elderly patients with advanced hematologic malignancies and/or low platelets; discontinue treatment for suspected GI hemorrhage or ulceration. Other GI effects including irritation and ulceration have been reported. Use caution with concurrent medications that may increase risk of adverse GI effects (eg, NSAIDs, corticosteroids, anticoagulants, oral bisphosphonates). Monitor patients closely for signs/symptoms of GI ulceration/bleeding.

Auditory disturbances of decreased hearing and high frequency hearing loss have been reported (rare) with use; perform auditory testing prior to initiation and regularly (every 12 months) during use; if abnormalities develop, monitor more closely and consider dose reduction or treatment interruption. Ocular disturbances including lens opacities, cataracts, intraocular pressure elevation, and retinal disorders have been reported (rare) with use; perform ophthalmic testing prior to initiation and regularly (every 12 months) during use; if abnormalities develop, monitor more closely and consider dose reduction or treatment interruption.

May cause bone marrow suppression including agranulocytosis, neutropenia, worsening anemia, and thrombocytopenia have been reported (some fatal); risk may be increased in patients with preexisting hematologic disorders; monitor blood counts regularly. Interrupt treatment in patients who develop cytopenias; may reinitiate once cause of cytopenia has been determined; use contraindicated if platelet count <50,000/mm³.

Hypersensitivity reactions including severe reactions (eg, anaphylaxis and angioedema) have been reported; usual onset is within the first month of treatment; discontinue if severe. May cause skin rash (dose-related); mild to moderate rashes may resolve without treatment interruption; for severe rash, interrupt treatment and consider restarting at a lower dose with dose escalation in combination with a short period of oral steroid administration. Severe skin reactions, including Stevens-Johnson syndrome (SJS) and erythema multiforme, have also been reported; discontinue and evaluate if suspected.

Potent UDP-glucuronosyltransferase (UGT) inducers (eg, rifampin) or bile acid sequestrants (eg, cholestyramine) may decrease the efficacy of deferasirox; avoid concomitant use. If coadministration necessary, dosage modifications may be needed; monitor serum ferritin and clinical response. Other potentially significant interactions may exist, requiring dose or frequency adjustment, additional monitoring, and/or selection of alternative therapy; consult drug interactions database for more detailed information.

Precautions May cause overchelation. For patients with transfusion-associated chronic iron overload, treatment should be initiated for transfusion volume ≥100 mL/kg of packed RBCs (eg, ≥20 units for a 40 kg individual) and serum ferritin consistently >1000 mcg/L. For patients with nontransfusion-dependent chronic iron overload, treatment should be initiated for a liver iron concentration of at least 5 mg iron per gram of liver (dry weight) (mg Fe/g dry weight) and serum ferritin >300 mcg/L. Prior to use, consider risk versus anticipated benefit with respect to individual patient's life expectancy, prognosis, and comorbidities. An improvement in survival or disease-related symptoms due to the therapy has not been established in clinical trials. Overchelation of iron may increase development of toxicity; temporary interruption of treatment should be considered if serum ferritin <500 mcg/L. Do not combine with other iron chelation therapies; safety of combinations has not been established. Controlled studies in myelodysplastic syndromes (MDS) and chronic iron overload due to blood transfusions have not been conducted.

Adverse Reactions

Central nervous system: Fatigue, fever, headache

Dermatologic: Rash, urticaria

Gastrointestinal: Abdominal pain, diarrhea, nausea, vomiting

Hepatic: ALT increased, transaminitis

Neuromuscular & skeletal: Arthralgia, back pain

Otic: Ear infection

Renal: Proteinuria, serum creatinine increased (dose related)

Respiratory: Acute, bronchitis, cough, nasopharyngitis, pharyngitis, pharyngolaryngeal pain, respiratory tract infection, rhinitis

Miscellaneous: Influenza

Rare but important or life-threatening: Acute renal failure, agranulocytosis, anaphylaxis, anemia (worsening), angioedema, ascites, cataract, cholecystitis, cholelithiasis, cytopenias, drug fever, duodenal ulcer, edema, erythema multiforme, Fanconi's syndrome, gastric ulcer, gastritis, gastrointestinal bleeding, gastrointestinal hemorrhage, glomerulonephritis, glucosuria, hearing loss (including high frequency), hematuria, Henoch-Schönlein purpura (IgA vasculitis), hepatic dysfunction, hepatic encephalopathy, hepatic failure, hepatic transaminases increased, hepatitis, hyperactivity, hypersensitivity reaction, hypocalcemia, intraocular pressure increased, jaundice, lens opacities, leukocytoclastic vasculitis, maculopathy, neutropenia, optic neuritis, pigment disorder, purpura, renal tubular necrosis, renal tubulopathy, retinal disorder, sleep disorder, Stevens-Johnson syndrome, thrombocytopenia, tubulointerstitial nephritis, visual disturbance

Drug Interactions

Metabolism/Transport Effects Substrate of UGT1A1; **Inhibits** CYP1A2 (moderate), CYP2C8 (moderate); **Induces** CYP3A4 (weak/moderate)

Avoid Concomitant Use

Avoid concomitant use of Deferasirox with any of the following: Aluminum Hydroxide; Axitinib; Bile Acid Sequestrants; Pirfenidone; Simeprevir; Theophylline

Increased Effect/Toxicity

Deferasirox may increase the levels/effects of: Agomelatine; CYP1A2 Substrates; CYP2C8 Substrates; Pirfenidone; Repaglinide; Theophylline

The levels/effects of Deferasirox may be increased by: Anticoagulants; Bisphosphonate Derivatives; Corticosteroids; Corticosteroids (Systemic); Nonsteroidal Anti-Inflammatory Agents

Decreased Effect

Deferasirox may decrease the levels/effects of: ARIPiprazole; Axitinib; CYP3A4 Substrates; Ibrutinib; Saxagliptin; Simeprevir

The levels/effects of Deferasirox may be decreased by: Aluminum Hydroxide; Bile Acid Sequestrants; Fosphenytoin; PHENobarbital; Phenytoin; Rifampin; Ritonavir

Food Interactions Bioavailability is increased variably when taken with food. Management: Take on an empty stomach at the same time each day at least 30 minutes before food. Maintain adequate hydration, unless instructed to restrict fluid intake.

Stability Store at 25°C (77°F); excursions permitted to 15°C to 30°C (59°F to 86°F). Protect from moisture.

Mechanism of Action Selectively binds iron, forming a complex which is excreted primarily through the feces.

Pharmacokinetics (Adult data unless noted) Note: Systemic exposure has been shown to be less in pediatric patients (2-16 years) compared to adults; in children 2-6 years, exposure was reduced by ~50% compared to adults; however, results of safety and efficacy trials using the same dose were similar in pediatric and adult patients. Patients with myelodysplastic syndromes (MDS) and CrCl of 40-60 mL/minute had 50% higher mean deferasirox trough concentrations compared to patients with MDS and CrCl >60 mL/minute.

Distribution: 14.4 ± 2.7 L

Protein binding: 99% to serum albumin

Metabolism: Hepatic via glucuronidation by UGT1A1 and UGT1A3; minor oxidation by CYP450; undergoes enterohepatic recirculation

Bioavailability: 70%

Half-life: 8-16 hours

Time to peak serum concentration: Median range: 1.5-4 hours

Elimination: Feces (84%), urine (8%)

Clearance: Females have moderately lower clearance than males (17.5% lower)

Dosing: Usual Note: Calculate dose to the nearest whole tablet size.

Pediatric:

Blood transfusion; chronic iron overload: Children ≥2 years and Adolescents: Oral: **Note:** Treatment should only be initiated with evidence of chronic iron overload [ie, transfusion of 100 mL/kg of packed RBCs (eg, ≥20 units for a 40 kg individual) and serum ferritin consistently >1000 mcg/L].

Initial: 20 mg/kg once daily

Maintenance: Adjust dose every 3 to 6 months based on serum ferritin levels; increase dose by 5 or 10 mg/kg/day increments; usual range: 20 to 30 mg/kg/day; for serum ferritin levels persistently >2500 mcg/L without evidence of a decreasing trend, may consider a dose of 40 mg/kg/day; doses >40 mg/kg/day are not recommended. If serum ferritin is <500 mcg/L, interrupt therapy.

Nontransfusion-dependent chronic iron overload; thalassemia syndromes: Children ≥10 years and Adolescents: Oral: **Note:** Treatment should only be initiated with evidence of chronic iron overload (hepatic iron concentration ≥5 mg Fe/g dry weight and serum ferritin >300 mcg/L).

Initial: 10 mg/kg once daily; after 4 weeks; if baseline hepatic iron concentration was >15 mg Fe/g dry weight, may increase to 20 mg/kg once daily

Maintenance: Dependent upon serum ferritin measurements (monthly) and hepatic iron concentrations (every 6 months).

If serum ferritin is <300 mcg/L: Interrupt therapy and obtain hepatic iron concentration

If hepatic iron concentration:
  <3 mg Fe/g dry weight: Interrupt therapy; resume treatment when hepatic iron concentration is >5 mg Fe/g dry weight
  >7 mg Fe/g dry weight: Consider dose increase to 20 mg/kg/day; repeat measurement and if remains >7 mg Fe/g dry weight, continue current dose; if repeat measurement is 3 to 7 mg Fe/g dry weight, then decrease dose to 10 mg/kg/day

Adult:
Chronic iron overload due to blood transfusion: Oral:
Initial: 20 mg/kg once daily; **Note:** Treatment should only be initiated with evidence of chronic iron overload (ie, transfusion of ≥100 mL/kg of packed red blood cells [eg, ≥20 units for a 40 kg individual] and serum ferritin consistently >1000 mcg/L).
Initial: 20 mg/kg once daily
Maintenance: Adjust dose every 3 to 6 months based on serum ferritin trends; adjust by 5 or 10 mg/kg/day; titrate to individual response and treatment goals. Usual range: 20 to 30 mg/kg/day; doses up to 40 mg/kg/day may be considered for serum ferritin levels persistently >2500 mcg/L (doses above 40 mg/kg/day are not recommended). **Note:** Consider interrupting therapy for serum ferritin <500 mcg/L (risk of toxicity may be increased).

Chronic iron overload in nontransfusion-dependent thalassemia syndromes: Oral: **Note:** Treatment should only be initiated with evidence of chronic iron overload (hepatic iron concentration ≥5 mg Fe/g dry weight and serum ferritin >300 mcg/L).
Initial: 10 mg/kg once daily. Consider increasing to 20 mg/kg once daily after 4 weeks if baseline hepatic iron concentration is >15 mg Fe/g dry weight.
Maintenance: Monitor serum ferritin monthly; if serum ferritin is <300 mcg/L, interrupt therapy and obtain hepatic iron concentration. Monitor hepatic iron concentration every 6 months; interrupt therapy when hepatic iron concentration <3 mg Fe/g dry weight. After 6 months of therapy, consider dose adjustment to 20 mg/kg/day if hepatic iron concentration >7 mg Fe/g dry weight. Reduce dose to ≤10 mg/kg when hepatic iron concentration is 3 to 7 mg Fe/g dry weight. Doses above 20 mg/kg/day are not recommended. After interruption, resume treatment when hepatic iron concentration >5 mg Fe/g dry weight.

Dosing adjustment with concomitant bile acid sequestrants (eg, cholestyramine, colesevelam, colestipol) or potent UGT inducers (eg, rifampin, phenytoin, phenobarbital, ritonavir): Children ≥2 years, Adolescents, and Adults: Avoid concomitant use; if coadministration necessary, consider increasing the initial deferasirox dose by 50%; monitor serum ferritin and clinical response.

Dosing adjustment in renal impairment:
Baseline: Children ≥2 years, Adolescents, and Adults:
CrCl >60 mL/minute: No dosage adjustment necessary
CrCl 40-60 mL/minute: Reduce initial dose by 50%
CrCl <40 mL/minute or serum creatinine >2 x age-appropriate ULN: Use is contraindicated
During therapy: Adjustment dependent upon indication for use.
Transfusional iron overload:
Children ≥2 years and Adolescents <16 years: For increase in serum creatinine ≥33% above the

average baseline level and above the age-appropriate ULN: Reduce daily dose by 10 mg/kg/day
Adolescents ≥16 years and Adults: If increase in serum creatinine ≥33% above the average baseline: Repeat serum creatinine measurement in 1 week; if still elevated by ≥33%: Reduce daily dose by 10 mg/kg/day
All patients: If serum creatinine >2 times age-appropriate ULN or CrCl <40 mL/minute: Discontinue therapy
Nontransfusion-dependent thalassemia syndromes:
Children ≥10 years and Adolescents <16 years: For increase in serum creatinine ≥33% above the average baseline level and above the age-appropriate ULN: Reduce daily dose by 5 mg/kg/day
Adolescents ≥16 years and Adults: If increase in serum creatinine ≥33% above the average baseline; repeat serum creatinine measurement in 1 week; if still elevated by ≥33%: If current dose is: 5 mg/kg/day: Interrupt therapy; or if current dose is 10-20 mg/kg/day: Reduce dose by 50%
All patients: If serum creatinine >2 times age-appropriate ULN or CrCl <40 mL/minute: Discontinue therapy

Dosing adjustment in hepatic impairment: Children ≥2 years, Adolescents, and Adults:
Baseline:
Mild impairment (Child-Pugh class A): No adjustment necessary; monitor closely for efficacy and for adverse reactions requiring dosage reduction
Moderate impairment (Child-Pugh class B): Reduce dose by 50%; monitor closely for efficacy and for adverse reactions requiring dosage reduction
Severe impairment (Child-Pugh class C): Avoid use
During therapy: Severe or persistent increases in transaminases/bilirubin: Reduce dose or temporarily interrupt treatment

Dosing adjustment for toxicity:
Bone marrow suppression: Interrupt treatment; may reinitiate once cause of cytopenia has been determined; contraindicated if platelet count <50,000/mm^3
Dermatologic toxicity:
  Rash (severe): Interrupt treatment; may reintroduce at a lower dose (with future dose escalation) and short-term oral corticosteroids
  Severe skin reaction (Stevens-Johnson syndrome, erythema multiforme): Discontinue and evaluate.
Gastrointestinal: Discontinue treatment for suspected GI ulceration or hemorrhage.
Hearing loss or visual disturbance: Consider dose reduction or treatment interruption

Administration Oral: **Do not chew or swallow whole tablets;** administer as an oral suspension. Completely disperse tablets in water, orange juice, or apple juice; use 3.5 ounces for total doses <1 g and 7 ounces for doses ≥1 g; stir to form suspension and drink entire contents. Rinse remaining residue with more fluid; drink. Avoid dispersion of tablets in milk (due to slowed dissolution) or carbonated drinks (due to foaming) (Séchaud, 2008). Administer at same time each day on an empty stomach, at least 30 minutes before food. Do not administer simultaneously with aluminum-containing antacids or cholestyramine.

Monitoring Parameters Serum ferritin (baseline, then monthly), iron levels (baseline), CBC with differential, serum creatinine, and/or creatinine clearance [two baseline assessments, then at least monthly; for patients who are at increased risk of complications (eg, preexisting renal conditions, elderly, comorbid conditions, or receiving other potentially nephrotoxic medications): Two baseline assessments, weekly for the first month then at least monthly thereafter]; urine protein (monthly), serum transaminases (ALT/AST) and bilirubin at baseline, every 2 weeks for 1 month, then monthly; baseline and annual auditory and ophthalmic function (including slit lamp examinations and dilated fundoscopy); performance status (in patients with hematologic malignancies); signs and symptoms of GI ulcers or hemorrhage; cumulative number of RBC units received

Dosage Forms Excipient information presented when available (limited, particularly for generics); consult specific product labeling.

Tablet Soluble, Oral:

Exjade: 125 mg, 250 mg, 500 mg

References

Bacon BR, Adams PC, Kowdley KV, et al, "Diagnosis and Management of Hemochromatosis: 2011 Practice Guideline by the American Association for the Study of Liver Diseases," *Hepatology*, 2011, 54 (1):328-43.

Cappellini MD, Bejaoui M, Agaoglu L, et al, "Iron Chelation With Deferasirox in Adult and Pediatric Patients With Thalassemia Major: Efficacy and Safety During 5 Years' Follow-Up," *Blood*, 2011, 118 (4):884-93.

Galanello R, Piga A, Alberti D, et al, "Safety, Tolerability, and Pharmacokinetics of ICL670, a New Orally Active Iron-Chelating Agent in Patients With Transfusion-Dependent Iron Overload Due to Beta-Thalassemia," *J Clin Pharmacol*, 2003, 43(6):565-72.

Nisbet-Brown E, Olivieri NF, Giardina PJ, et al, "Effectiveness and Safety of ICL670 in Iron-Loaded Patients With Thalassaemia: A Randomised, Double-Blind, Placebo-Controlled, Dose-Escalation Trial," *Lancet*, 2003, 361(9369):1597-602.

Raphael JL, Bernhardt MB, Mahoney DH, et al, "Oral Iron Chelation and the Treatment of Iron Overload in a Pediatric Hematology Center," *Pediatr Blood Cancer*, 2009, 52(5):616-20.

Rund D and Rachmilewitz E, "Beta-Thalassemia," *N Engl J Med*, 2005, 353(11):1135-46.

Séchaud R, Dutreix C, Balez S, et al. Relative bioavailability of deferasirox tablets administered without dispersion and dispersed in various drinks. *Int J Clin Pharmacol Ther*. 2008;46(2):102-108.

Yusuf B, McPhedran P, and Brewster UC, "Hypocalcemia in a Dialysis Patient Treated With Deferasirox for Iron Overload," *Am J Kidney Dis*, 2008, 52(3):587-90.

Deferoxamine (de fer OKS a meen)

Medication Safety Issues

Sound-alike/look-alike issues:

Deferoxamine may be confused with cefuroxime, deferasirox, deferiprone

Desferal® may be confused with desflurane, Desyrel®, Dexferrum®

International issues:

Desferal [U.S., Canada, and multiple international markets] may be confused with Deseril brand name for methysergide [Australia, Belgium, Great Britain, Netherlands]; Disophrol brand name for dexbrompheniramine and pseudoephedrine [Czech Republic, Poland, Turkey]

Brand Names: U.S. Desferal

Brand Names: Canada Desferal®; PMS-Deferoxamine

Therapeutic Category Antidote, Aluminum Toxicity; Antidote, Iron Toxicity; Chelating Agent, Parenteral

Generic Availability (U.S.) Yes

Use Adjunct treatment of acute iron intoxication and treatment of chronic iron overload secondary to multiple transfusions (FDA approved in ages ≥3 years and adults); has also been used in the diagnosis and treatment of aluminum accumulation in chronic renal failure

Pregnancy Risk Factor C

Pregnancy Considerations Skeletal anomalies and delayed ossification were observed in some but not all animal reproduction studies. Toxic amounts of iron or deferoxamine have not been noted to cross the placenta. In case of acute iron toxicity, treatment during pregnancy should not be withheld.

Breast-Feeding Considerations It is not known if deferoxamine is excreted in human milk; the manufacturer recommends that caution be used if administered to a breast-feeding woman.

Contraindications Hypersensitivity to deferoxamine or any component; patients with severe renal disease, anuria

Warnings Ocular disturbances (blurred vision, cataracts, corneal opacities, decreased visual acuity, impaired peripheral and color vision, impaired night vision, optic neuritis, retinal pigmentary abnormalities, scotoma, visual loss/deficit) have been reported following prolonged administration, at high doses, or in patients with low ferritin levels; generally reversible with early detection and immediate discontinuation; periodic eye exams are recommended with long-term therapy.

Auditory disturbances (tinnitus and high-frequency hearing loss) have been reported with prolonged administration, at high doses, or in patients with low ferritin levels; effects are generally reversible with early detection and immediate discontinuation; periodic auditory exams are recommended.

Deferoxamine has been associated with ARDS following treatment of acute iron intoxication or thalassemia with high doses of deferoxamine. Flushing of the skin, urticaria, hypotension, and shock have been reported after rapid I.V. administration; may administer I.M., by slow subcutaneous infusion or slow I.V. infusion only. Increases in serum creatinine, acute renal failure, and renal tubular disorders have been reported; when iron is chelated with deferoxamine, the chelate is excreted renally. Rare and serious cases of mucormycosis (including fatalities) have been reported in chronic renal failure patients receiving deferoxamine. Ferrioxamine (chelated form of iron with deferoxamine) enhances the growth and pathogenicity of certain species of *Mucor*.

Growth retardation in pediatric patients especially in patients ≤3 years has been associated with high doses (>60 mg/kg) and concurrent low ferritin levels; a reduction in deferoxamine dosage may partially improve growth velocity; monitor growth in children receiving chronic therapy closely.

Treatment with deferoxamine in patients with aluminum toxicity may cause hypocalcemia and aggravate hyperparathyroidism; deferoxamine may cause neurological symptoms (including seizure) in patients with aluminum-related encephalopathy receiving dialysis; deferoxamine may precipitate the onset of dialysis dementia. Avoid deferoxamine use in patients with serum aluminum levels >200 mcg/L.

Patients with severe chronic iron overload treated with deferoxamine and high dose vitamin C have been reported to develop impaired cardiac function which is reversed after discontinuation of vitamin C; vitamin C increases the availability of iron for chelation with deferoxamine. To decrease the risk of impaired cardiac function, the manufacturer recommends: Avoiding vitamin C in patients with preexisting cardiac failure; start vitamin C supplementation only after the first month of deferoxamine therapy; use vitamin C only if the patient is regularly receiving deferoxamine; monitor cardiac function; do not exceed vitamin C doses of: children <10 years: 50 mg/day, older children and adolescents: 100 mg/day, and adults: 200 mg/day.

Precautions Patients with iron overload are at increased susceptibility to *Yersinia enterocolitica* and *Yersinia pseudotuberculosis* infections; treatment with deferoxamine may enhance this risk; if infection develops, discontinue therapy until resolved.

Deferoxamine is **not** indicated for the treatment of primary hemochromatosis (treatment of choice is phlebotomy). Patients should be informed that urine may have a reddish color.

Local injection site reactions may be minimized by daily rotation of subcutaneous injection sites and by applying topical corticosteroids; painful lumps formed under the skin may indicate that the rate of SubQ administration exceeds the rate of absorption from the injection site or the needle is inserted too close to the dermis.

Adverse Reactions

Cardiovascular: Flushing, hypotension, shock, tachycardia

Central nervous system: Dizziness, encephalopathy (aluminum toxicity/dialysis-related), fever, headache, seizure

Dermatologic: Angioedema, rash, urticaria

Endocrine & metabolic: Growth retardation (children), hyperparathyroidism (aggravated), hypocalcemia

Gastrointestinal: Abdominal discomfort, abdominal pain, diarrhea, nausea, vomiting

Genitourinary: Dysuria, urine discoloration (reddish color)

Hematologic: Leukopenia, thrombocytopenia

Hepatic: Hepatic dysfunction, transaminases increased

Local: Injection site: Burning, crust, edema, erythema, eschar, induration, infiltration, irritation, pain, pruritus, swelling, vesicles, wheal formation

Neuromuscular & skeletal: Arthralgia, metaphyseal dysplasia (children <3 years; dose related), muscle spasms, myalgia, neuropathy (peripheral, sensory, motor, or mixed), paresthesia

Ocular: Blurred vision, cataract, corneal opacities, dyschromatopsia, loss of vision, night blindness, optic neuritis, peripheral vision impaired, retinal pigment abnormalities, scotoma, visual acuity decreased, visual field defects

Otic: Hearing loss, tinnitus

Renal: Acute renal failure, renal tubular disorders, serum creatinine increased

Respiratory: Acute respiratory distress syndrome (dyspnea, cyanosis, and/or interstitial infiltrates), asthma

Miscellaneous: Anaphylaxis (with or without shock), hypersensitivity reaction, infections (*Yersinia*, mucormycosis)

Drug Interactions

Metabolism/Transport Effects None known.

Avoid Concomitant Use There are no known interactions where it is recommended to avoid concomitant use.

Increased Effect/Toxicity

Deferoxamine may increase the levels/effects of: Prochlorperazine

The levels/effects of Deferoxamine may be increased by: Ascorbic Acid; Multivitamins/Fluoride (with ADE); Multivitamins/Minerals (with ADEK, Folate, Iron); Multivitamins/Minerals (with AE, No Iron)

Decreased Effect There are no known significant interactions involving a decrease in effect.

Stability Store intact vials at ≤25°C (77°F). Following reconstitution, solutions may be stored for 24 hours at room temperature, although the manufacturer recommends use begin within 3 hours of reconstitution. Do not refrigerate solutions as it may cause precipitation. When stored at 30°C in polypropylene infusion pump syringes, deferoxamine 250 mg/mL in sterile water for injection retained 95% of initial concentration for 14 days (Stiles, 1996).

Mechanism of Action Complexes with trivalent ions (ferric ions) to form ferrioxamine, which is removed by the kidneys; slows accumulation of hepatic iron and retards or eliminates progression of hepatic fibrosis. Also known to inhibit DNA synthesis *in vitro*.

Pharmacokinetics (Adult data unless noted)

Absorption: I.M., SubQ: Well absorbed

Distribution: Distributed throughout body fluids

Metabolism: Plasma enzymes; binds with iron to form ferrioxamine (iron complex)

Half-life: 14 hours; plasma: 20-30 minutes (Brittenham, 2011)

Elimination: Primarily urine (as unchanged drug and ferrioxamine); feces (via bile)

Dialysis: Dialyzable

Dosing: Neonatal

Acute iron intoxication: Very limited data available: I.V. infusion: 5 mg/kg/hour; dosing based on a case report of an oral ferrous sulfate overdose in a former premature neonate (GA: 27 weeks and age at time of treatment PCA: 34 weeks); further studies needed (Valentine, 2009).

Dosing: Usual

Children and Adolescents:

Acute iron intoxication: Limited data available: **Note:** The I.V. route is used when severe toxicity is evidenced by cardiovascular collapse or systemic symptoms (coma, shock, metabolic acidosis, or gastrointestinal bleeding) or potentially severe intoxications (peak serum iron level >500 mcg/dL) (Perrone, 2011). When severe symptoms are not present, the I.M. route may be used.

Continuous I.V. infusion: Initial: 15 mg/kg/hour and reduce rate as clinically indicated; maximum daily dose: 80 mg/kg/**day** and not to exceed 6 g/**day** [Desferal® prescribing information (Canada; UK), 2011]

I.V.: Initial: 20 mg/kg (maximum dose: 1000 mg) administered no faster than 15 mg/kg/hour followed by 10 mg/kg (maximum dose: 500 mg) over 4-hour intervals for 2 doses; subsequent doses of 10 mg/kg (maximum dose: 500 mg) over 4-12 hours may be repeated depending upon the clinical response; maximum dose: 6 g/**day**; this dosing may also be used I.M. if symptoms not severe.

I.M.: 90 mg/kg/dose for one dose, then 45 mg/kg/dose every 4-12 hours as needed; maximum single dose: Children: 1000 mg; Adults: 2000 mg; maximum daily dose: 6 g/day [Desferal® prescribing information (Canada; UK), 2011]; others have used 50 mg/kg/dose every 6 hours with maximum daily dose: 6 g/**day** (Chang, 2011); may also use intermittent I.V. dosing (see above)

Chronic iron overload:

General dosing: Manufacturer's labeling: Children ≥3 years and Adolescents:

I.V.:

Children and Growing Adolescents: 20-40 mg/kg/day over 8-12 hours, 5-7 days per week, usual maximum daily dose: 40 mg/kg/**day**

Adolescents once growth has ceased: 40-50 mg/kg/day over 8-12 hours, 5-7 days per week, usual maximum daily dose: 60 mg/kg/**day**

SubQ infusion via a portable, controlled infusion device: 20-40 mg/kg/day over 8-12 hours 3-7 days per week; maximum daily dose: 2000 mg/**day**. Doses >60 mg/kg/day have not been shown to provide additional benefit (Vlachos, 2008).

Sickle cell disease, chronic iron overload: Children and Adolescents: SubQ infusion: 25 mg/kg/day over 8 hours; dose and duration may be increased as needed (NHLBI, 2005)

Thalassemia, chronic iron overload: **Note:** A lower dose may be required if the ferritin levels are low. In general, the therapeutic index should be kept <0.025 at all times. Therapeutic index = mean daily deferoxamine dose (mg/kg)/ferritin (mcg/L) (Cappellini, 2008):

Children and Growing Adolescents: SubQ infusion: 20-40 mg/kg/day over 8-12 hours, 6-7 nights per week, maximum daily dose: 40 mg/kg/**day**

Adolescents once growth has ceased:

SubQ infusion (preferred): 40-60 mg/kg/day over 8-12 hours, 6-7 nights per week, maximum daily dose: 2000 mg/**day**

SubQ bolus: 45 mg/kg/dose, 5 times per week.

Aluminum-induced bone disease in chronic renal failure: Note: Intended for predialysis serum aluminum concentration of 60-200 mcg/L; do not start chelation therapy if serum aluminum concentration >200 mcg/L; intensive dialysis (6 days per week with a high flux dialysis membrane) should be used until serum aluminum concentration decreases below 200 mcg/L (National Kidney Foundation, 2003):

Test (diagnostic) dose: I.V.: 5 mg/kg as a single dose infused over the last hour of dialysis; measure serum aluminum concentration 2 days later; depending upon the change in serum aluminum concentration, treatment with deferoxamine may be indicated (see Treatment below)

Treatment: I.V.: Monitor serum aluminum levels closely. See National Kidney Foundation guidelines for additional details on treatment algorithms.

Aluminum rise ≥300 mcg/L or adverse effects with test dose: 5 mg/kg once a week 5 hours before dialysis for 4 months

Aluminum rise <300 mcg/L: 5 mg/kg once a week during the last hour of dialysis for 2 months

Adults:

Acute iron intoxication: Note: The I.V. route is used when severe toxicity is evidenced by cardiovascular collapse or systemic symptoms (coma, shock, metabolic acidosis, or gastrointestinal bleeding) or potentially severe intoxications (peak serum iron level >500 mcg/dL) (Perrone, 2011). When severe symptoms are not present, the I.M. route may be used.

I.M., I.V.: 1000 mg stat, then 500 mg every 4 hours for 2 doses, additional doses of 500 mg every 4-12 hours may be needed depending upon the clinical response; maximum daily dose: 6 **g/day**

Chronic iron overload:

I.M.: 500-1000 mg/dose; maximum daily dose: 1000 mg/**day**

I.V.: 40-50 mg/kg/day over 8-12 hours for 5-7 days per week; maximum daily dose: 6 **g/day**

SubQ via portable, controlled infusion device: 1000-2000 mg/day or 20-40 mg/kg/day over 8-24 hours

Dosage adjustment in renal impairment:

Manufacturer's labeling: Severe renal disease or anuria: Use is contraindicated.

Alternate recommendations: The following adjustments have been recommended (Aronoff, 2007): Adults:

CrCl >50 mL/minute: No adjustment required

CrCl 10-50 mL/minute or CRRT: Administer 25% to 50% of normal dose

CrCl <10 mL/minute, hemodialysis, or peritoneal dialysis: Avoid use

Dosage adjustment in hepatic impairment: There are no dosage adjustments provided in the manufacturer's labeling (not studied).

Administration

Intramuscular: Reconstitute 500 mg vial with 2 mL SWI or 2000 mg vial with 8 mL SWI; resulting concentration: 213 mg/mL; no further dilution required.

Intravenous: May reconstitute 500 mg vial with 5 mL SWI or 2000 mg vial with 20 mL SWI, resulting concentration: 95 mg/mL; further dilute in D$_5$W, NS, 0.45% NS, or LR; may administer as intermittent I.V. infusion or as continuous I.V. infusion; maximum rate: 15 mg/kg/hour; may consider reducing infusion rate to <125 mg/hour after the first 1000 mg have been infused.

Subcutaneous: Reconstitute 500 mg vial with 5 mL SWI or 2000 mg vial with 20 mL SWI; resulting concentration: 95 mg/mL; no further dilution required; local reactions at the site of subcutaneous infusion may be minimized by diluting the deferoxamine in 5-10 mL SWI and adding 1 mg hydrocortisone to each mL of deferoxamine solution (Kirking, 1991)

Monitoring Parameters Serum ferritin, iron, total iron binding capacity; CBC with differential, renal function tests, liver function tests, growth velocity (including weight and height) every 3 months, ophthalmologic exam, and audiometry (with chronic use); blood pressure (with I.V. infusions)

Dialysis patients: Serum aluminum (yearly; every 3 months in patients on aluminum-containing medications)

Aluminum-induced bone disease: Serum aluminum 2 days following test dose; test is considered positive if serum aluminum increases ≥50 mcg/L

Reference Range

Iron, serum: Normal: 50-160 mcg/dL; peak levels >500 mcg/dL associated with toxicity. Consider treatment in symptomatic patients with levels ≥350 mcg/dL; toxicity cannot be excluded with serum iron levels <350 mcg/dL.

Aluminum, serum: <20 mcg/L (National Kidney Foundation, 2003)

Test Interactions TIBC may be falsely elevated with high serum iron concentrations or deferoxamine therapy. Imaging results may be distorted due to rapid urinary excretion of deferoxamine-bound gallium-67; discontinue deferoxamine 48 hours prior to scintigraphy.

Dosage Forms Excipient information presented when available (limited, particularly for generics); consult specific product labeling.

Solution Reconstituted, Injection, as mesylate:

Desferal: 500 mg (1 ea); 2 g (1 ea)

Generic: 500 mg (1 ea); 2 g (1 ea)

References

Aronoff GR, Bennett WM, Berns JS, et al, *Drug Prescribing in Renal Failure: Dosing Guidelines for Adults and Children*, 5th ed, Philadelphia, PA: American College of Physicians, 2007, 116.

Brittenham GM, "Iron-Chelating Therapy for Transfusional Iron Overload," *N Engl J Med*, 2011, 364(2):146-56.

Cappellini MD, Cohen A, Eleftheriou A, et al, "Guidelines for the Clinical Management of Thalassemia," 2nd ed, Nicosia, Cyprus: Thalassaemia International Federation, November 2008. Available at http://www.thalassaemia.org.cy/pdf/Guidelines_2nd_revised_edition_EN.-pdf

Chang TPY and Rangan C, "Iron Poisoning-A Literature-Based Review of Epidemiology, Diagnosis, and Management," *Pediatr Emerg Care*, 2011, 27(10):978-85.

Division of Blood Diseases and Resources, NHLBI, "The Management of Sickle Cell Disease," Bethesda, MD: National Heart, Lung, and Blood Insitute, 2002. Available at http://www.nhlbi.nih.gov/health/prof/blood/sickle/sc_mngt.pdf

Kirking MH, "Treatment of Chronic Iron Overload," *Clin Pharm*, 1991, 10 (10):775-83.

Manoguerra AS, Erdman AR, Booze LL, et al, "Iron Ingestion: An Evidence-Based Consensus Guideline for Out-of-Hospital Management," *Clin Toxicol (Phila)*, 2005, 43(6):553-70.

National Kidney Foundation, "K/DOQI Clinical Practice Guidelines for Bone Metabolism and Disease in Chronic Kidney Failure," *Am J Kidney Dis*, 2003, 42(4 Suppl 3):1-201.

Perrone J, "Iron," *Goldfrank's Toxicologic Emergencies*, 9th ed, Nelson LS, Hoffman RS, Lewin NA, et al, eds, New York, NY: McGraw-Hill Companies, Inc, 2011.

Stiles ML, Allen LV, and Prince SJ, "Stability of Deferoxamine Mesylate, Floxuridine, Fluorouracil, Hydromorphone Hydrochloride, Lorazepam, and Midazolam Hydrochloride in Polypropylene Infusion-Pump Syringes," *Am J Health Syst Pharm*, 1996, 53(13):1583-8.

Valentine K, Mastropietro C, and Sarnaik AP, "Infantile Iron Poisoning: Challenges in Diagnosis and Management," *Pediatr Crit Care Med*, 2009, 10(3):e31-3.

Vlachos A, Ball S, Dahl N, et al, "Diagnosing and Treating Diamond Blackfan Anaemia: Results of an International Clinical Consensus Conference," *Br J Haematol*, 2008, 142(6):859-76.

◆ **Deferoxamine Mesylate** see Deferoxamine on page 604

◆ **Dehydral® (Can)** see Methenamine on page 1361

◆ **Dehydrobenzperidol** see Droperidol on page 725

◆ **Delatestryl (Can)** see Testosterone on page 1986

◆ **Delestrogen** see Estradiol (Systemic) on page 796

◆ **Delsym [OTC]** see Dextromethorphan on page 636

◆ **Delta-9-tetrahydro-cannabinol** see Dronabinol on page 725

◆ **Delta-9 THC** *see* Dronabinol *on page 725*
◆ **Deltacortisone** *see* PredniSONE *on page 1732*
◆ **Delta D3 [OTC]** *see* Cholecalciferol *on page 455*
◆ **Deltadehydrocortisone** *see* PredniSONE *on page 1732*
◆ **Delzicol** *see* Mesalamine *on page 1347*
◆ **Demadex** *see* Torsemide *on page 2057*

Demeclocycline (dem e kloe SYE kleen)

Therapeutic Category Antibiotic, Tetracycline Derivative
Generic Availability (U.S.) Yes
Use Treatment of susceptible bacterial infections (acne, gonorrhea, pertussis, chronic bronchitis, and urinary tract infections) caused by both gram-negative and gram-positive organisms; treatment of chronic syndrome of inappropriate antidiuretic hormone (SIADH) secretion
Pregnancy Risk Factor D
Pregnancy Considerations Tetracyclines, including demeclocycline, cross the placenta and accumulate in developing teeth and long tubular bones. Tetracyclines may discolor fetal teeth following maternal use during pregnancy; the specific teeth involved and the portion of the tooth affected depends on the timing and duration of exposure relative to tooth calcification. As a class, tetracyclines are generally considered second-line antibiotics in pregnant women and their use should be avoided (Gibbons, 1960; Mylonas, 2011).
Breast-Feeding Considerations Tetracyclines are excreted into breast milk. According to the manufacturer, the decision to continue or discontinue breast-feeding during therapy should take into account the risk of exposure to the infant and the benefits of treatment to the mother.

Tetracyclines, including demeclocycline, bind to calcium (Mitrano, 2009). The calcium in maternal milk will significantly decrease the amount of demeclocycline absorbed by the breast-feeding infant. Nondose-related effects could include modification of bowel flora.
Contraindications Hypersensitivity to demeclocycline, tetracyclines, or any component
Warnings Photosensitivity reactions, characterized as severe burns of exposed surfaces, occur frequently with this drug; avoid prolonged exposure to sunlight; do not use tanning equipment. Do not administer to children <8 years of age; use of tetracyclines during tooth development (last half of pregnancy, infancy, and children <8 years of age) may cause permanent discoloration of the teeth and enamel hypoplasia. Do not administer to pregnant women; use of tetracyclines in pregnant women may result in retardation of bone growth and skeletal development of the fetus. Prolonged use may result in fungal or bacterial superinfection, including *C. difficile*-associated diarrhea (CDAD) and pseudomembranous colitis; CDAD has been observed >2 months postantibiotic treatment. Avoid use when possible in patients with hepatic disease. Demeclocycline may cause a reversible, dose-related diabetes insipidus syndrome. Use of outdated tetracyclines has caused a Fanconi-like syndrome.
Precautions Use with caution in patients with impaired renal or hepatic function; modify dose in patients with renal impairment

Adverse Reactions
Cardiovascular: Pericarditis
Central nervous system: Bulging fontanels (infants), dizziness, headache, pseudotumor cerebri (adults)
Dermatologic: Angioedema, anogenital inflammatory lesions (with monilial overgrowth), erythema multiforme, erythematous rash, exfoliative dermatitis (rare), maculopapular rash, photosensitivity, pigmentation of skin, Stevens-Johnson syndrome (rare), urticaria

Endocrine & metabolic: Microscopic discoloration of thyroid gland (brown/black), nephrogenic diabetes insipidus, thyroid dysfunction (rare)
Gastrointestinal: Anorexia, diarrhea, dysphagia, enterocolitis, esophageal ulcerations, glossitis, nausea, pancreatitis, vomiting
Genitourinary: Balanitis
Hematologic: Eosinophilia, neutropenia, hemolytic anemia, thrombocytopenia
Hepatic: Hepatitis (rare), hepatotoxicity (rare), liver enzymes increased, liver failure (rare)
Neuromuscular & skeletal: Myasthenic syndrome, polyarthralgia, tooth discoloration (children <8 years, rarely in adults)
Ocular: Visual disturbances
Otic: Tinnitus
Renal: Acute renal failure, BUN increased
Respiratory: Pulmonary infiltrates
Miscellaneous: Anaphylaxis, anaphylactoid purpura, fixed drug eruptions (rare), lupus-like syndrome, superinfection, systemic lupus erythematosus exacerbation
Drug Interactions
Metabolism/Transport Effects None known.
Avoid Concomitant Use
Avoid concomitant use of Demeclocycline with any of the following: BCG; Retinoic Acid Derivatives; Strontium Ranelate
Increased Effect/Toxicity
Demeclocycline may increase the levels/effects of: Mipomersen; Neuromuscular-Blocking Agents; Porfimer; Retinoic Acid Derivatives; Vitamin K Antagonists
Decreased Effect
Demeclocycline may decrease the levels/effects of: BCG; Desmopressin; Penicillins; Sodium Picosulfate; Typhoid Vaccine

The levels/effects of Demeclocycline may be decreased by: Antacids; Bile Acid Sequestrants; Bismuth; Bismuth Subsalicylate; Calcium Salts; Iron Salts; Lanthanum; Magnesium Salts; Multivitamins/Minerals (with ADEK, Folate, Iron); Multivitamins/Minerals (with AE, No Iron); Quinapril; Strontium Ranelate; Sucralfate; Sucroferric Oxyhydroxide; Zinc Salts
Food Interactions Demeclocycline serum levels may be decreased if taken with food, milk, or dairy products. Management: Administer 1 hour before or 2 hours after food, milk, or dairy products.
Mechanism of Action Inhibits protein synthesis by binding with the 30S and possibly the 50S ribosomal subunit(s) of susceptible bacteria; may also cause alterations in the cytoplasmic membrane; inhibits the action of ADH in patients with chronic SIADH
Pharmacodynamics Onset of action for diuresis in SIADH: Within 5 days
Pharmacokinetics (Adult data unless noted)
Absorption: ~60% to 80% of dose absorbed from the GI tract; food and dairy products reduce absorption by 50% or more
Distribution: Distributes into pleural fluid, bronchial secretions, sputum, prostatic and seminal fluids, and to body tissues; crosses into breast milk
Protein binding: 36% to 91%
Metabolism: Small amounts metabolized in the liver to inactive metabolites; enterohepatically recycled
Half-life: Adults: 10-17 hours (prolonged with reduced renal function)
Time to peak serum concentration: Oral: Within 3-4 hours
Elimination: Excreted as unchanged drug (42% to 50%) in urine and 31% in feces
Dosing: Usual Oral:
Children >8 years: 8-12 mg/kg/day divided every 6-12 hours
Adults: 150 mg 4 times/day or 300 mg twice daily

▶

Uncomplicated gonorrhea: 600 mg stat, 300 mg every 12 hours for 4 days (3 g total)

SIADH: Initial: 600-1200 mg/day or 13-15 mg/kg/day divided every 6-8 hours; then decrease to 600-900 mg/day

Dosing adjustment in renal impairment: Dose and/or frequency should be modified in response to the degree of renal impairment

Dosing adjustment in hepatic impairment: Not recommended for use

Administration Oral: Administer 1 hour before or 2 hours after food or milk with plenty of fluids; do not administer with food, milk, dairy products, antacids, zinc, or iron supplements

Monitoring Parameters CBC, renal and hepatic function tests, I & O, urine output, serum sodium; observe for changes in bowel frequency

Dosage Forms Excipient information presented when available (limited, particularly for generics); consult specific product labeling.

Tablet, Oral, as hydrochloride:
Generic: 150 mg, 300 mg

References
Abdi EA and Bishop S, "The Syndrome of Inappropriate Antidiuretic Hormone Secretion With Carcinoma of the Tongue," *Med Pediatr Oncol*, 1988, 16(3):210-5.

De Troyer AD, "Demeclocycline. Treatment for Syndrome of Inappropriate Antidiuretic Hormone Secretion," *JAMA*, 1977, 237(25):2723-6.

Gibbons RJ and Reichelderfer TE, "Transplacental Transmission of Demethylchlortetracycline and Toxicity Studies in Premature and Full Term, Newly Born Infants," *Antibiotic Med Clin Ther*, 1960, 7:618-22.

Mitrano JA, Spooner LM, and Belliveau P, "Excretion of Antimicrobials Used to Treat Methicillin-Resistant *Staphylococcus aureus* Infections During Lactation: Safety in Breastfeeding Infants," *Pharmacotherapy*, 2009, 29(9):1103-9.

◆ **Demeclocycline Hydrochloride** *see* Demeclocycline *on page 607*

◆ **Demerol** *see* Meperidine *on page 1337*

◆ **4-Demethoxydaunorubicin** *see* IDArubicin *on page 1067*

◆ **Demethylchlortetracycline** *see* Demeclocycline *on page 607*

◆ **Denavir** *see* Penciclovir *on page 1627*

◆ **Denta 5000 Plus** *see* Fluoride *on page 894*

◆ **DentaGel** *see* Fluoride *on page 894*

◆ **Dentapaine [OTC]** *see* Benzocaine *on page 273*

◆ **Dent-O-Kain/20 [OTC]** *see* Benzocaine *on page 273*

◆ **Deodorized Tincture of Opium (error-prone synonym)** *see* Opium Tincture *on page 1548*

◆ **2′-Deoxycoformycin** *see* Pentostatin *on page 1644*

◆ **Deoxycoformycin** *see* Pentostatin *on page 1644*

◆ **Depacon** *see* Valproic Acid and Derivatives *on page 2102*

◆ **Depakene** *see* Valproic Acid and Derivatives *on page 2102*

◆ **Depakote** *see* Valproic Acid and Derivatives *on page 2102*

◆ **Depakote ER** *see* Valproic Acid and Derivatives *on page 2102*

◆ **Depakote Sprinkles** *see* Valproic Acid and Derivatives *on page 2102*

◆ **Depen Titratabs** *see* PenicillAMINE *on page 1627*

◆ **DepoDur** *see* Morphine (Liposomal) *on page 1449*

◆ **Depo-Estradiol** *see* Estradiol (Systemic) *on page 796*

◆ **Depo-Medrol** *see* MethylPREDNISolone *on page 1386*

◆ **Depo-Prevera® (Can)** *see* MedroxyPROGESTERone *on page 1318*

◆ **Depo-Provera** *see* MedroxyPROGESTERone *on page 1318*

◆ **Depo-Provera® (Can)** *see* MedroxyPROGESTERone *on page 1318*

◆ **Depo-SubQ Provera 104** *see* MedroxyPROGESTERone *on page 1318*

◆ **Depotest 100 (Can)** *see* Testosterone *on page 1986*

◆ **Depo-Testosterone** *see* Testosterone *on page 1986*

◆ **DermaFungal [OTC]** *see* Miconazole (Topical) *on page 1410*

◆ **DermaMed [OTC]** *see* Aluminum Hydroxide *on page 110*

◆ **Derma-Smoothe/FS® (Can)** *see* Fluocinolone (Topical) *on page 892*

◆ **Derma-Smoothe/FS Body** *see* Fluocinolone (Topical) *on page 892*

◆ **Derma-Smoothe/FS Scalp** *see* Fluocinolone (Topical) *on page 892*

◆ **Dermasorb HC** *see* Hydrocortisone (Topical) *on page 1038*

◆ **Dermasorb TA** *see* Triamcinolone (Topical) *on page 2078*

◆ **Dermatop** *see* Prednicarbate *on page 1725*

◆ **Dermatop® (Can)** *see* Prednicarbate *on page 1725*

◆ **Dermazole (Can)** *see* Miconazole (Topical) *on page 1410*

◆ **DermOtic** *see* Fluocinolone (Otic) *on page 892*

◆ **Dermovate® (Can)** *see* Clobetasol *on page 506*

◆ **Desenex [OTC]** *see* Clotrimazole (Topical) *on page 527*

◆ **Desenex [OTC]** *see* Miconazole (Topical) *on page 1410*

◆ **Desenex Jock Itch [OTC]** *see* Miconazole (Topical) *on page 1410*

◆ **Desenex Spray [OTC]** *see* Miconazole (Topical) *on page 1410*

◆ **Desferal** *see* Deferoxamine *on page 604*

◆ **Desferal® (Can)** *see* Deferoxamine *on page 604*

◆ **Desferrioxamine** *see* Deferoxamine *on page 604*

◆ **Desiccated Thyroid** *see* Thyroid, Desiccated *on page 2018*

Desipramine (des IP ra meen)

Medication Safety Issues
Sound-alike/look-alike issues:
Desipramine may be confused with clomiPRAMINE, dalfampridine, diphenhydrAMINE, disopyramide, imipramine, nortriptyline
Norpramin® may be confused with clomiPRAMINE, imipramine, Normodyne®, Norpace®, nortriptyline, Tenormin®

BEERS Criteria medication:
This drug may be potentially inappropriate for use in geriatric patients (SIADH: Quality of evidence - moderate; Strength of recommendation - strong).

International issues:
Norpramin: Brand name for desipramine [U.S., Canada], but also the brand name for enalapril/hydrochlorothiazide [Portugal]; omeprazole [Spain]

Related Information
Antidepressant Agents *on page 2219*
Medications for Which a Single Dose May Be Fatal When Ingested by a Toddler *on page 2408*

Brand Names: U.S. Norpramin

Brand Names: Canada Dom-Desipramine; Novo-Desipramine; Nu-Desipramine; PMS-Desipramine

Therapeutic Category Antidepressant, Tricyclic (Secondary Amine)

Generic Availability (U.S.) Yes

Use Treatment of depression (FDA approved in adults); has also been used as an analgesic in chronic pain; treatment of peripheral neuropathies

Medication Guide Available Yes

Pregnancy Considerations Animal reproduction studies are inconclusive. Tricyclic antidepressants may be associated with irritability, jitteriness, and convulsions (rare) in the neonate (Yonkers, 2009).

The ACOG recommends that therapy for depression during pregnancy be individualized; treatment should incorporate the clinical expertise of the mental health clinician, obstetrician, primary healthcare provider, and pediatrician (ACOG, 2008). According to the American Psychiatric Association (APA), the risks of medication treatment should be weighed against other treatment options and untreated depression. For women who discontinue antidepressant medications during pregnancy and who may be at high risk for postpartum depression, the medications can be restarted following delivery (APA, 2010). Treatment algorithms have been developed by the ACOG and the APA for the management of depression in women prior to conception and during pregnancy (Yonkers, 2009).

Breast-Feeding Considerations Desipramine is excreted into breast milk. Based on information from one mother-infant pair, following maternal use of desipramine 300 mg/day, the estimated exposure to the breast-feeding infant would be 2% of the weight-adjusted maternal dose. Adverse events were not reported. Infants should be monitored for signs of adverse events; routine monitoring of infant serum concentrations is not recommended (Fortinguerra, 2009).

Contraindications Hypersensitivity to desipramine (cross-sensitivity with other tricyclic antidepressants may occur) or any component; use of MAO inhibitors within 14 days (potentially fatal reactions may occur); use in patients during the acute recovery phase following MI; narrow-angle glaucoma

Warnings Clinical worsening of depression or suicidal ideation and behavior may occur in children and adults with major depressive disorder **[U.S. Boxed Warning]**. In clinical trials, antidepressants increased the risk of suicidal thinking and behavior (suicidality) in children, adolescents, and young adults (18-24 years of age) with major depressive disorder and other psychiatric disorders. This risk must be considered before prescribing antidepressants for any clinical use. Short-term studies did **not** show an increased risk of suicidality with antidepressant use in patients >24 years of age and showed a decreased risk in patients ≥65 years.

Patients of all ages who are treated with antidepressants for any indication require appropriate monitoring and close observation for clinical worsening of depression, suicidality, and unusual changes in behavior, especially during the first few months after antidepressant initiation or when the dose is adjusted. Family members and caregivers should be instructed to closely observe the patient (ie, daily) and communicate condition with healthcare provider. Patients should also be monitored for associated behaviors (eg, anxiety, agitation, panic attacks, insomnia, irritability, hostility, aggressiveness, impulsivity, akathisia, hypomania, mania) which may increase the risk for worsening depression or suicidality. Worsening depression or emergence of suicidality (or associated behaviors listed above) that is abrupt in onset, severe, or not part of the presenting symptoms, may require discontinuation or modification of drug therapy.

Do not discontinue abruptly in patients receiving high doses chronically (withdrawal symptoms may occur). To reduce risk of intentional overdose, write prescriptions for the smallest quantity consistent with good patient care. Screen individuals for bipolar disorder prior to treatment (using antidepressants alone may induce manic episodes in patients with this condition). Hypertensive episodes have been reported during surgery in patients receiving desipramine (discontinue desipramine use as soon as possible prior to elective surgery).

The American Heart Association recommends that all children diagnosed with ADHD who may be candidates for medication, such as desipramine, should have a thorough cardiovascular assessment prior to initiation of therapy. These recommendations are based upon reports of serious cardiovascular adverse events (including sudden death) in patients (both children and adults) taking usual doses of stimulant medications. Most of these patients were found to have underlying structural heart disease (eg, hypertrophic obstructive cardiomyopathy). Asymptomatic ECG changes and minor increases in diastolic blood pressure and heart rate have been noted in children receiving >3.5 mg/kg/day; four cases of sudden death have been reported in children 5-14 years of age; an association between desipramine and sudden death was not shown to be significant in one retrospective study. Pretreatment cardiovascular assessment should include a combination of thorough medical history, family history, and physical examination. An ECG is not mandatory but should be considered.

Precautions Use with extreme caution in the following patients: Patients with cardiovascular disease (due to the possibility of conduction defects, arrhythmias, tachycardias, strokes, and acute MI); patients who have a family history of sudden death, dysrhythmias, or conduction abnormalities; patients with thyroid disease or taking thyroid medications (due to the possibility of cardiovascular toxicity and arrhythmias); patients with a history of seizure disorders (desipramine may lower the seizure threshold; in some patients, seizures may precede cardiac dysrhythmias and death); patients with a history of urinary retention or glaucoma (due to the anticholinergic effects of the medication). Desipramine causes less sedation and fewer anticholinergic adverse effects than amitriptyline or imipramine; it should be noted that overdose of desipramine has resulted in a higher death rate compared to other tricyclic antidepressants.

Adverse Reactions

Cardiovascular: Arrhythmias, edema, flushing, heart block, hyper-/hypotension, MI, palpitation, stroke, tachycardia

Central nervous system: Agitation, anxiety, ataxia, confusion, delusions, disorientation, dizziness, drowsiness, EEG alterations, exacerbation of psychosis, extrapyramidal symptoms, fatigue, fever, hallucinations, headache, hypomania, incoordination, insomnia, neuroleptic malignant syndrome, nightmares, restlessness, seizure, suicidal thinking and behavior

Dermatologic: Alopecia, itching, petechiae, photosensitivity, skin rash, urticaria

Endocrine & metabolic: Breast enlargement, galactorrhea, gynecomastia, hyper-/hypoglycemia, impotence, libido changes, SIADH

Gastrointestinal: Abdominal cramps, anorexia, black tongue, constipation, diarrhea, epigastric distress, nausea, parotid edema, paralytic ileus, stomatitis, sublingual adenitis, unpleasant taste, vomiting, weight gain/loss, xerostomia

Genitourinary: Micturition delayed, nocturia, painful ejaculation, polyuria, testicular edema, urinary retention

Hematologic: Agranulocytosis, eosinophilia, purpura, thrombocytopenia

Hepatic: Alkaline phosphatase increased, cholestatic jaundice, hepatitis, liver enzymes increased

Neuromuscular & skeletal: Falling, numbness, paresthesia of extremities, peripheral neuropathy, tingling, tremor, weakness

Ocular: Blurred vision, disturbances of accommodation, intraocular pressure increased, mydriasis

Otic: Tinnitus

Miscellaneous: Allergic reaction, diaphoresis (excessive), withdrawal symptoms

Drug Interactions

Metabolism/Transport Effects Substrate of CYP1A2 (minor), CYP2D6 (major); **Note:** Assignment of Major/Minor substrate status based on clinically relevant drug interaction potential; **Inhibits** CYP2A6 (moderate), CYP2B6 (moderate), CYP2D6 (moderate), CYP2E1 (weak), CYP3A4 (moderate)

Avoid Concomitant Use

Avoid concomitant use of Desipramine with any of the following: Aclidinium; Azelastine (Nasal); Bosutinib; Ibrutinib; Iobenguane I 123; Ipratropium (Oral Inhalation); Ivabradine; Linezolid; Lomitapide; MAO Inhibitors; Methylene Blue; Moxonidine; Paraldehyde; Pimozide; Potassium Chloride; Simeprevir; Tegafur; Thalidomide; Thioridazine; Tiotropium; Tolvaptan; Ulipristal; Umeclidinium

Increased Effect/Toxicity

Desipramine may increase the levels/effects of: Abobotulinumtoxina; Alcohol (Ethyl); Alpha-/Beta-Agonists (Direct-Acting); Alpha1-Agonists; Amphetamines; Analgesics (Opioid); Anticholinergic Agents; Antipsychotics; ARIPiprazole; Avanafil; Azelastine (Nasal); Beta2-Agonists; Bosentan; Bosutinib; Budesonide (Systemic, Oral Inhalation); Buprenorphine; Cannabinoid-Containing Products; Cannabis; Citalopram; CNS Depressants; Colchicine; CYP2B6 Substrates; CYP2D6 Substrates; CYP3A4 Substrates; Desmopressin; DOXOrubicin (Conventional); Dronabinol; Eplerenone; Escitalopram; Everolimus; FentaNYL; Fesoterodine; Halofantrine; Highest Risk QTc-Prolonging Agents; Hydrocodone; Ibrutinib; Imatinib; Ivabradine; Ivacaftor; Lomitapide; Lurasidone; Methotrimeprazine; Methylene Blue; Metoprolol; Metyrosine; Moderate Risk QTc-Prolonging Agents; Nebivolol; OnabotulinumtoxinA; OxyCODONE; Paraldehyde; Pimecrolimus; Pimozide; Potassium Chloride; Pramipexole; Propafenone; QuiNIDine; Ranolazine; Rimabotulinumtoxin B; Rivaroxaban; ROPINIRole; Rotigotine; Salmeterol; Saxagliptin; Serotonin Modulators; Simeprevir; Sodium Phosphates; Sulfonylureas; Tetrahydrocannabinol; Thalidomide; Thiazide Diuretics; Thioridazine; Tiotropium; Tolvaptan; Topiramate; TraMADol; Ulipristal; Vitamin K Antagonists; Yohimbine; Zolpidem

The levels/effects of Desipramine may be increased by: Abiraterone Acetate; Aclidinium; Altretamine; Antiemetics (5HT3 Antagonists); Antipsychotics; Boceprevir; Brimonidine (Topical); BuPROPion; Cannabis; Cimetidine; Cinacalcet; Citalopram; Cobicistat; CYP2D6 Inhibitors (Moderate); CYP2D6 Inhibitors (Strong); Darunavir; Dexmethylphenidate; Doxylamine; Dronabinol; Droperidol; DULoxetine; Escitalopram; FLUoxetine; FluvoxaMINE; HydrOXYzine; Ipratropium (Oral Inhalation); Kava Kava; Linezolid; Lithium; Magnesium Sulfate; MAO Inhibitors; Methotrimeprazine; Methylphenidate; Metoclopramide; Metyrosine; Mifepristone; Mirabegron; Nabilone; PARoxetine; Perampanel; Pramlintide; Propafenone; Protease Inhibitors; QuiNIDine; Rufinamide; Sertraline; Sodium Oxybate; Tapentadol; Terbinafine (Systemic); Tetrahydrocannabinol; Thyroid Products; TraMADol; Umeclidinium; Valproic Acid and Derivatives

Decreased Effect

Desipramine may decrease the levels/effects of: Acetylcholinesterase Inhibitors (Central); Alpha2-Agonists; Alpha2-Agonists (Ophthalmic); Codeine; Ifosfamide; Iobenguane I 123; Moxonidine; Secretin; Tamoxifen; Tegafur

The levels/effects of Desipramine may be decreased by: Acetylcholinesterase Inhibitors (Central); Barbiturates; CarBAMazepine; Peginterferon Alfa-2b; St Johns Wort

Mechanism of Action Traditionally believed to increase the synaptic concentration of norepinephrine (and to a lesser extent, serotonin) in the central nervous system by inhibition of its reuptake by the presynaptic neuronal membrane. However, additional receptor effects have been found including desensitization of adenyl cyclase, down regulation of beta-adrenergic receptors, and down regulation of serotonin receptors.

Pharmacodynamics Antidepressant effects:

Onset of action: Occasionally seen in 2-5 days

Maximum effect: After more than 2 weeks

Pharmacokinetics (Adult data unless noted)

Absorption: Rapidly and well absorbed from the GI tract

Distribution: V_d: 21 L/kg; distributes into breast milk (concentrations approximately equal to maternal plasma)

Protein binding: 90%

Metabolism: In the liver

Half-life: 12-57 hours

Elimination: 70% in urine

Dosing: Usual Oral: Depression: **Note:** Not FDA approved for use in pediatric patients; controlled clinical trials have not shown tricyclic antidepressants to be superior to placebo for the treatment of depression in children and adolescents (Dopheide, 2006; Wagner, 2005).

Children 6-12 years: 1-3 mg/kg/day in divided doses; monitor carefully with doses >3 mg/kg/day; maximum dose: 5 mg/kg/day

Adolescents: Initial: 25-50 mg/day; gradually increase to 100 mg/day in single or divided doses; maximum dose: 150 mg/day

Adults: Initial: 75 mg/day in divided doses; increase gradually to 150-200 mg/day in divided or single dose; maximum dose: 300 mg/day

Administration Oral: Administer with food to decrease GI upset

Monitoring Parameters Blood pressure, heart rate, ECG, mental status, weight. Monitor patient periodically for symptom resolution; monitor for worsening of depression, suicidality, and associated behaviors (especially at the beginning of therapy or when doses are increased or decreased)

ADHD: Evaluate patients for cardiac disease prior to initiation of therapy for ADHD with thorough medical history, family history, and physical exam; consider ECG; perform ECG and echocardiogram if findings suggest cardiac disease; promptly conduct cardiac evaluation in patients who develop chest pain, unexplained syncope, or any other symptom of cardiac disease during treatment.

Long-term use: Also monitor CBC with differential, liver enzymes, serum concentrations

Reference Range Plasma concentrations do not always correlate with clinical effectiveness.

Timing of serum samples: Draw trough just before next dose

Therapeutic: 50-300 ng/mL (SI: 188-1125 nmol/L)

Possible toxicity: >300 ng/mL (SI: >1070 nmol/L)

Toxic: >1000 ng/mL (SI: >3750 nmol/L)

Test Interactions Increased glucose; decreased glucose has also been reported. May interfere with urine detection of amphetamines/methamphetamines (false-positive).

Dosage Forms Excipient information presented when available (limited, particularly for generics); consult specific product labeling.

Tablet, Oral, as hydrochloride:

Norpramin: 10 mg, 25 mg, 50 mg, 75 mg, 100 mg, 150 mg

Generic: 10 mg, 25 mg, 50 mg, 75 mg, 100 mg, 150 mg

References

American Academy of Pediatrics/American Heart Association Clarification of Statement on Cardiovascular Evaluation and Monitoring of Children and Adolescents With Heart Disease Receiving Medications for ADHD; available at: http://americanheart.mediaroon.com/index.php?s=43&item=422.

ACOG Committee on Practice Bulletins-Obstetrics. ACOG practice bulletin: clinical management guidelines for obstetrician-gynecologists number 92, April 2008 (replaces practice bulletin number 87, November 2007). Use of psychiatric medications during pregnancy and lactation. *Obstet Gynecol.* 2008;111(4):1001-1020.

American Psychiatric Association (APA). Treatment recommendations for patients with major depressive disorder. 3rd ed, May 2010. Available at http://www.psychiatryonline.com/pracGuide/pracGuideTopic_7.aspx

Biederman J, Thisted RA, Greenhill LL, et al, "Estimation of the Association Between Desipramine and the Risk for Sudden Death in 5-14 Year-Old Children," *J Clin Psychiatry*, 1995, 56(3):87-93.

Dopheide JA, "Recognizing and Treating Depression in Children and Adolescents," *Am J Health Syst Pharm*, 2006, 63(3):233-43.

Fortinguerra F, Clavenna A, and Bonati M, "Psychotropic Drug Use During Breastfeeding: A Review of the Evidence," *Pediatrics*, 2009, 124(4):547-56.

Levy HB, Harper CR, and Weinberg WA, "A Practical Approach to Children Failing in School," *Pediatr Clin North Am*, 1992, 39 (4):895-928.

Vetter VL, Elia J, Erickson C, et al, "Cardiovascular Monitoring of Children and Adolescents With Heart Disease Receiving Stimulant Drugs: A Scientific Statement From the American Heart Association Council on Cardiovascular Disease in the Young Congenital Cardiac Defects Committee and the Council on Cardiovascular Nursing," *Circulation*, 2008, 117(18):2407-23.

Wagner KD, "Pharmacotherapy for Major Depression in Children and Adolescents," *Prog Neuropsychopharmacol Biol Psychiatry*, 2005, 29 (5):819-26.

Yonkers KA, Wisner KL, Stewart DE, et al. The management of depression during pregnancy: a report from the American Psychiatric Association and the American College of Obstetricians and Gynecologists. *Obstet Gynecol.* 2009;114(3):703-713.

◆ **Desipramine Hydrochloride** *see* Desipramine *on page 608*

◆ **Desitin® [OTC]** *see* Zinc Oxide *on page 2176*

◆ **Desitin® Creamy [OTC]** *see* Zinc Oxide *on page 2176*

Desloratadine (des lor AT a deen)

Medication Safety Issues
Sound-alike/look-alike issues:
Clarinex® may be confused with Celebrex®

Brand Names: U.S. Clarinex; Clarinex Reditabs

Brand Names: Canada Aerius®; Aerius® Kids; Desloratadine Allergy Control

Therapeutic Category Antihistamine

Generic Availability (U.S.) May be product dependent

Use Symptomatic relief of nasal and non-nasal symptoms of allergic rhinitis; chronic idiopathic urticaria

Pregnancy Risk Factor C

Pregnancy Considerations Adverse events have been observed in animal reproduction studies; therefore, the manufacturer classifies desloratadine as pregnancy category C. The use of antihistamines for the treatment of rhinitis during pregnancy is generally considered to be safe at recommended doses. Information related to the use of desloratadine during pregnancy is limited; therefore, other agents may be preferred. Desloratadine is the primary metabolite of loratadine; refer to the Loratadine monograph for additional information.

Breast-Feeding Considerations Desloratadine is excreted into breast milk. According to the manufacturer, the decision to continue or discontinue breast-feeding during therapy should take into account the risk of exposure to the infant and the benefits of treatment to the mother.

Contraindications Hypersensitivity to desloratadine, loratadine, or any component

Warnings Use with caution and adjust dosage in patients with liver or renal impairment. Syrup contains sodium

benzoate; benzoic acid (benzoate) is a metabolite of benzyl alcohol; large amounts of benzyl alcohol (≥99 mg/kg/day) have been associated with a potentially fatal toxicity ("gasping syndrome") in neonates; the "gasping syndrome" consists of metabolic acidosis, respiratory distress, gasping respirations, CNS dysfunction (including convulsions, intracranial hemorrhage), hypotension and cardiovascular collapse; avoid use in neonates; *in vitro* and animal studies have shown that benzoate displaces bilirubin from protein binding sites

Precautions A subset of the general population (7% in clinical trials) are slow metabolizers of desloratadine; the frequency of slow metabolism appears to be higher in African Americans; patients who are slow metabolizers may be more susceptible to dose-related side effects; use with caution in "slow metabolizers." Use cautiously in patients who are also taking ketoconazole, itraconazole, fluconazole, erythromycin, clarithromycin, or other drugs which may impair desloratadine's hepatic metabolism; although increased plasma levels of desloratadine have been observed, no adverse effects with concomitant administration have been reported, including QT interval prolongation which has occurred when similar antihistamines, terfenadine and astemizole, were combined with these agents. While less sedating than other antihistamines, desloratadine may cause drowsiness and impair ability to perform hazardous activities requiring mental alertness. Use cautiously in breast-feeding women as desloratadine passes into breast milk. RediTabs® contain aspartame which is metabolized to phenylalanine and must be used with caution in patients with phenylketonuria.

Adverse Reactions Note: Reported in children, unless otherwise noted.

Central nervous system: Dizziness (adults), drowsiness (more common in children), emotional lability, fatigue (adults), headache (adults), irritability, insomnia

Gastrointestinal: Anorexia, appetite increased, diarrhea, dyspepsia (adults), nausea (children and adults), vomiting, xerostomia (adults)

Dermatologic: Erythema, maculopapular rash

Genitourinary: Dysmenorrhea (adults), urinary tract infection

Infection: Parasitic infection, varicella

Neuromuscular & skeletal: Myalgia (adults)

Otic: Otitis media

Respiratory: Bronchitis, cough, epistaxis, pharyngitis (children and adults), rhinorrhea, upper respiratory tract infection

Miscellaneous: Fever

Rare but important or life-threatening: Hepatitis (rare), hypersensitivity reactions (including anaphylaxis, dyspnea, edema, pruritus, rash, urticaria), psychomotor agitation, seizure, tachycardia

Drug Interactions

Metabolism/Transport Effects Substrate of P-glycoprotein

Avoid Concomitant Use
Avoid concomitant use of Desloratadine with any of the following: Aclidinium; Azelastine (Nasal); Ipratropium (Oral Inhalation); Paraldehyde; Potassium Chloride; Thalidomide; Tiotropium; Umeclidinium

Increased Effect/Toxicity
Desloratadine may increase the levels/effects of: AbobotulinumtoxinA; Alcohol (Ethyl); Analgesics (Opioid); Anticholinergic Agents; Azelastine (Nasal); Buprenorphine; Cannabinoid-Containing Products; CNS Depressants; Hydrocodone; Methotrimeprazine; Metyrosine; Mirabegron; Mirtazapine; OnabotulinumtoxinA; Paraldehyde; Potassium Chloride; Pramipexole; RimabotulinumtoxinB; ROPINIRole; Rotigotine; Selective Serotonin Reuptake Inhibitors; Thalidomide; Thiazide Diuretics; Tiotropium; Topiramate; Zolpidem

The levels/effects of Desloratadine may be increased by: Aclidinium; Brimonidine (Topical); Cannabis; Doxylamine; Dronabinol; Droperidol; HydrOXYzine; Ipratropium (Oral Inhalation); Kava Kava; Magnesium Sulfate; Methotrimeprazine; Nabilone; Perampanel; P-glycoprotein/ABCB1 Inhibitors; Pramlintide; Rufinamide; Sodium Oxybate; Tapentadol; Tetrahydrocannabinol; Umeclidinium

Decreased Effect
Desloratadine may decrease the levels/effects of: Acetylcholinesterase Inhibitors (Central); Benzylpenicilloyl Polylysine; Betahistine; Hyaluronidase; Secretin

The levels/effects of Desloratadine may be decreased by: Acetylcholinesterase Inhibitors (Central); Amphetamines; P-glycoprotein/ABCB1 Inducers

Food Interactions Food does not affect bioavailability.

Stability Store at room temperature; avoid excessive heat and moisture; RediTabs® must be used immediately after removal from blister pack

Mechanism of Action Desloratadine, a major active metabolite of loratadine, is a long-acting tricyclic antihistamine with selective peripheral histamine H_1 receptor antagonistic activity.

Pharmacodynamics
Onset of action: 1 hour
Duration: 24 hours

Pharmacokinetics (Adult data unless noted)
Distribution: Distributes into breast milk

Protein binding: 82% to 87% (desloratadine), 85% to 89% (metabolite)

Metabolism: Metabolized to an active metabolite (3-hydroxydesloratadine); subset of population are slow metabolizers of desloratadine (7% of patients in clinical trials were slow-metabolizers)

Half-life: 27 hours (both desloratadine and active metabolite)

Time to peak serum concentration: 3 hours

Elimination: 87% eliminated via urine and feces as metabolic products

Dosing: Usual Oral:
Children 6-11 months: 1 mg once daily
Children 1-5 years: 1.25 mg once daily
Children 6-11 years: 2.5 mg once daily
Children ≥12 years and Adults: 5 mg once daily

Dosage adjustment in renal/hepatic impairment: Administer dosage every other day

Administration Oral: May administer without regard to food. Place RediTabs® directly on the tongue; tablet will disintegrate immediately; may be taken with or without water

Monitoring Parameters Improvement in signs and symptoms of allergic rhinitis

Reference Range Therapeutic serum levels (not used clinically): Desloratadine: 2.5-4 ng/mL

Test Interactions May suppress the wheal and flare reactions to skin test antigens

Dosage Forms Excipient information presented when available (limited, particularly for generics); consult specific product labeling.
Syrup, Oral:
Clarinex: 0.5 mg/mL (473 mL) [contains edetate disodium, fd&c yellow #6 (sunset yellow), propylene glycol, sodium benzoate; bubble-gum flavor]
Tablet, Oral:
Clarinex: 5 mg [contains fd&c blue #2 aluminum lake]
Generic: 5 mg

Tablet Dispersible, Oral:
Clarinex Reditabs: 2.5 mg, 5 mg [contains aspartame; tutti-frutti flavor]
Generic: 2.5 mg, 5 mg

References
Murdoch D, Goa KL, and Keam SJ, "Desloratadine: An Update of Its Efficacy in the Management of Allergic Disorders," *Drugs*, 2003, 63 (19):2051-77.

♦ **Desloratadine Allergy Control (Can)** see Desloratadine on page 611

♦ **Desmethylimipramine Hydrochloride** see Desipramine on page 608

Desmopressin (des moe PRES in)

Brand Names: U.S. DDAVP; DDAVP Rhinal Tube; Stimate

Brand Names: Canada Apo-Desmopressin®; DDAVP®; DDAVP® Melt; Minirin®; Novo-Desmopressin; Octostim®; PMS-Desmopressin

Therapeutic Category Antihemophilic Agent; Hemostatic Agent; Hormone, Posterior Pituitary; Vasopressin Analog, Synthetic

Generic Availability (U.S.) Yes

Use Treatment of diabetes insipidus (tablets: FDA approved in ages ≥4 years and adults; injection: FDA approved in ages >12 years and adults); control of bleeding in hemophilia A (with factor VIII levels >5%), mild to moderate type I von Willebrand disease (injection: FDA approved in ages >3 months and adults; nasal spray: FDA approved in ages >12 months and adults), and thrombocytopenia; primary nocturnal enuresis (tablets only: FDA approved in ages ≥6 years)

Pregnancy Risk Factor B

Pregnancy Considerations Adverse events were not observed in animal reproduction studies. Anecdotal reports suggest congenital anomalies and low birth weight. However, causal relationship has not been established. Desmopressin has been used safely throughout pregnancy for the treatment of diabetes insipidus (Brewster, 2005; Schrier, 2010). The use of desmopressin is limited for the treatment of von Willebrand disease in pregnant women (NHLBI, 2007).

Breast-Feeding Considerations It is not known if desmopressin is excreted in breast milk. The manufacturer recommends that caution be exercised when administering desmopressin to nursing women.

Contraindications Hypersensitivity to desmopressin or any component; avoid using in patients with severe type I, type IIB, or platelet-type (pseudo) von Willebrand disease, hemophilia A with factor VIII levels ≤5% or hemophilia B; moderate-to-severe renal impairment (CrCl <50 mL/minute); patients with hyponatremia or history of hyponatremia

Warnings Desmopressin in combination with excessive fluid consumption can result in hyponatremia, an imbalance between intracellular and extracellular sodium. This imbalance can lead to seizures, brain swelling, coma, and death. The FDA has reviewed 61 postmarketing cases of hyponatremia-related seizures associated with the use of desmopressin acetate. Intranasal desmopressin was used in the majority of cases. Many of the patients were children being treated for primary nocturnal enuresis (PNE). An association with at least one concomitant drug or disease that also may cause hyponatremia and/or seizures was noted. As a result, **intranasal** desmopressin is no longer indicated for the treatment of PNE. In addition, **intranasal** desmopressin should not be used in patients with hyponatremia or a history of hyponatremia. Desmopressin acetate **tablets** may be used for the treatment of PNE; however, treatment should be interrupted if the patient experiences an acute illness (eg, fever, recurrent vomiting, diarrhea), vigorous exercise, or any condition associated with an increase in water consumption. Patients and caregivers should also be instructed to restrict fluid intake 1 hour prior to dose until the next morning, or for at least 8 hours after administration.

Avoid intranasal use in patients with nasal mucosa changes (scarring, edema, discharge, obstruction, or severe atopic rhinitis)

Precautions Use with caution in patients with predisposition to thrombus formation, conditions associated with fluid and electrolyte imbalance (eg, cystic fibrosis, CHF, renal disorders), in patients with habitual or psychogenic polydipsia or using medications known to either increase thirst or cause syndrome of inappropriate antidiuretic hormone secretion (SIADH) (eg, carbamazepine, SSRIs), and in patients with coronary artery disease and/or hypertensive cardiovascular disease; fluid intake may need to be reduced to decrease potential for development of water intoxication

Adverse Reactions

Cardiovascular: Blood pressure increased/decreased (I.V.), facial flushing

Central nervous system: Chills (intranasal), dizziness (intranasal), headache

Dermatologic: Rash

Endocrine & metabolic: Hyponatremia, water intoxication

Gastrointestinal: Abdominal cramps, abdominal pain (intranasal), gastrointestinal disorder (intranasal), nausea (intranasal), sore throat

Hepatic: Transient increases in liver transaminases (associated primarily with tablets)

Local: Injection: Burning pain, erythema, and swelling at the injection site

Neuromuscular & Skeletal: Weakness (intranasal)

Ocular: Conjunctivitis (intranasal), eye edema (intranasal), lacrimation disorder (intranasal)

Respiratory: Cough, epistaxis (intranasal), nasal congestion, nostril pain (intranasal), rhinitis (intranasal), upper respiratory infection

Rare but important or life-threatening: Acute cerebrovascular thrombosis (I.V.), acute MI (I.V.), agitation, allergic reactions (rare), anaphylaxis (rare), balanitis, chest pain, coma, diarrhea, dyspepsia, edema, insomnia, itching eyes, light-sensitive eyes, pain, palpitation, seizure, somnolence, tachycardia, thinking abnormal, vomiting, vulval pain, warmth

Drug Interactions

Metabolism/Transport Effects None known.

Avoid Concomitant Use There are no known interactions where it is recommended to avoid concomitant use.

Increased Effect/Toxicity

Desmopressin may increase the levels/effects of: Lithium

The levels/effects of Desmopressin may be increased by: Analgesics (Opioid); CarBAMazepine; ChlorproMAZINE; LamoTRIgine; Nonsteroidal Anti-Inflammatory Agents; Selective Serotonin Reuptake Inhibitors; Tricyclic Antidepressants

Decreased Effect

The levels/effects of Desmopressin may be decreased by: Demeclocycline; Lithium

Stability

DDAVP:

Nasal spray: Store at 20°C to 25°C (68°F to 77°F). Keep nasal spray in upright position.

Rhinal Tube solution: Store refrigerated at 2°C to 8°C (36°F to 46°F). May store at controlled room temperature of 20°C to 25°C (68°F to 77°F) for up to 3 weeks.

Solution for injection: Store at 2°C to 8°C (36°F to 46°F).

Tablet: Store at controlled room temperature of 20°C to 25°C (68°F to 77°F).

Stimate nasal spray: Store at room temperature not to exceed 25°C (77°F). Discard 6 months after opening bottle.

Mechanism of Action In a dose dependent manner, desmopressin increases cyclic adenosine monophosphate (cAMP) in renal tubular cells which increases water permeability resulting in decreased urine volume and increased urine osmolality; increases plasma levels of von Willebrand factor, factor VIII, and t-PA contributing to a shortened activated partial thromboplastin time (aPTT) and bleeding time.

Pharmacodynamics

Oral administration:
Onset of ADH action: 1 hour
Maximum effect: 2 to 7 hours
Duration: 6 to 8 hours; **Note:** 0.4 mcg doses have had antidiuretic effects for up to 12 hours

Intranasal administration:
Onset of ADH action: Within 1 hour
Maximum effect: Within 1.5 hours
Duration: 5 to 21 hours

I.V. infusion:
Onset of increased factor VIII activity: Within 15 to 30 minutes
Maximum effect: 90 minutes to 3 hours

Pharmacokinetics (Adult data unless noted) Note: Due to large differences in bioavailability between product formulations and patient variability in response, dosage conversions between product formulations should be done conservatively titrating to clinical improvement.

Absorption:
Oral tablets: 0.08% to 0.16%; **Note:** Bioavailability of tablet is ~5% of nasal spray.
Nasal solution: 10% to 20%
Nasal spray (1.5 mg/mL concentration): 3.3% to 4.1%

Metabolism: Unknown

Half-life:
Oral: 1.5 to 2.5 hours
I.V.:
Initial: 7.8 minutes
Terminal: 75.5 minutes (range: 0.4 to 4 hours); severe renal impairment: 9 hours
Intranasal: 3.3 to 3.5 hours

Time to peak serum concentration:
Oral: 0.9 hours
Intranasal: 1.5 hours

Excretion: Primarily in urine

Dosing: Usual

Diabetes insipidus:

Oral:
Children ≤12 years: Initial: 0.05 mg twice daily; titrate to desired response (range: 0.1 to 0.8 mg daily)
Children >12 years and Adults: 0.05 mg twice daily; titrate to desired response (range: 0.1 to 1.2 mg divided 2 to 3 times/day)

Intranasal: **Note:** Use nasal solution in patients whose dosage needs are <10 mcg or are not met with 10 mcg per spray increments in spray formulation.
Children 3 months to ≤12 years: Initial: 5 mcg/day (0.05 mL/day nasal solution) divided 1 to 2 times/day; range: 5 to 30 mcg/day (0.05 to 0.3 mL/day nasal solution); adjust morning and evening doses separately for an adequate diurnal rhythm of water turnover
Children >12 years and Adults: Initial: 5 to 40 mcg (0.05-0.4 mL nasal solution) divided 1 to 3 times/day; most patients require 0.2 mL daily in 2 divided doses; adjust morning and evening doses separately for an adequate diurnal rhythm of water turnover

I.V., SubQ: Children <12 years: No definitive dosing available. Adult dosing should not be used in this age group; adverse events such as hyponatremia-induced seizures may occur. Dose should be reduced. Some have suggested an initial dosage range of 0.1 to 1 mcg in 1 or 2 divided doses (Cheetham, 2002). Initiate at low dose and increase as necessary. Closely monitor serum sodium levels and urine output; fluid restriction is recommended.

I.V., SubQ: Children ≥12 years and Adults: 2 to 4 mcg/day in 2 divided doses or $^1/_{10}$ of the maintenance intranasal dose; adjust morning and evening doses separately for an adequate diurnal rhythm of water turnover

Hemophilia:

I.V.: Children ≥3 months and Adults: 0.3 mcg/kg beginning 30 minutes before procedure; may repeat dose if needed. **Note:** Adverse events such as hyponatremia-induced seizures have been reported especially in young children using this dosing regimen (Das, 2005; Molnár, 2005; Smith, 1989; Thumfart, 2005; Weinstein, 1989). Fluid restriction and careful monitoring of serum sodium levels and urine output are necessary.

Intranasal: Children >12 years and Adults: Using high concentration Stimate nasal spray:

≤50 kg: 150 mcg (1 spray)

>50 kg: 300 mcg (1 spray each nostril)

Repeat use is determined by the patient's clinical condition and laboratory work; if using preoperatively, administer 2 hours before surgery

Nocturnal enuresis (short-term treatment, 4 to 8 weeks); intranasal formulations are not recommended for nocturnal enuresis treatment:

Oral: Children ≥6 years: Initial dose: 0.2 mg once before bedtime; titrate as needed to a maximum of 0.6 mg; fluid intake should be limited to a minimum from 1 hour before desmopressin administration until the next morning, or at least 8 hours after administration

Administration

Intranasal: Using rhinal tube delivery system, draw solution into flexible, calibrated rhinal tube; insert one end into nostril; blow on the other end to deposit the solution deep into the nasal cavity. The Stimate® spray pump must be primed prior to first use; to prime pump, press down 4 times. Avoid spray use in children <6 years of age due to difficulty in titrating dosage; discard any solution remaining after 25 or 50 doses (2.5 or 5 mL vials, respectively) because the amount delivered may be substantially less than prescribed

Parenteral: I.V.: Dilute to a maximum concentration of 0.5 mcg/mL in NS (recommended: Children <10 kg: 10 mL diluent; Children >10 kg and Adults: 50 mL diluent); infuse over 15 to 30 minutes; if desmopressin I.V. is given preoperatively, administer 30 minutes prior to surgery

Monitoring Parameters Note: For all indications, fluid intake, urine volume, and signs and symptoms of hyponatremia should be closely monitored especially in high risk patient subgroups (eg, young children, elderly, patients with heart failure).

I.V. infusion: Blood pressure and pulse should be monitored

Diabetes insipidus: Urine specific gravity, plasma and urine osmolality, serum electrolytes

Hemophilia: Factor VIII antigen levels, APTT, Factor VIII activity level

Additional Information 1 mcg of desmopressin acetate injection is approximately equal to 4 units of antidiuretic activity; desmopressin acetate injection has an antidiuretic effect about ten times that of an equivalent dose administered intranasally

Dosage Forms Considerations

DDAVP and Minirin 5 mL bottles contain 50 sprays. Stimate 2.5 mL bottles contain 25 sprays.

Dosage Forms Excipient information presented when available (limited, particularly for generics); consult specific product labeling.

Solution, Injection, as acetate:

DDAVP: 4 mcg/mL (1 mL, 10 mL)

Generic: 4 mcg/mL (1 mL, 10 mL)

Solution, Nasal, as acetate:

DDAVP: 0.01% (5 mL)

DDAVP Rhinal Tube: 0.01% (2.5 mL)

Stimate: 1.5 mg/mL (2.5 mL) [contains benzalkonium chloride]

Generic: 0.01% (2.5 mL, 5 mL)

Tablet, Oral, as acetate:

DDAVP: 0.1 mg, 0.2 mg [scored]

Generic: 0.1 mg, 0.2 mg

References

Brewster UC and Hayslett JP, "Diabetes Insipidus in the Third Trimester of Pregnancy," *Obstet Gynecol*, 2005, 105(5 Pt 2):1173-6.

Cheetham T and Baylis PH, "Diabetes Insipidus in Children: Pathophysiology, Diagnosis and Management," *Paediatr Drugs*, 2002, 4 (12):785-96.

Das P, Carcao M, and Hitzler J, "DDAVP-Induced Hyponatremia in Young Children," *J Pediatr Hematol Oncol*, 2005, 27(6):330-2.

Eller N, Kollenz CJ, and Hitzenberger G, "A Comparative Study of Pharmacodynamics and Bioavailability of 2 Different Desmopressin Nasal Sprays," *Int J Clin Pharmacol Ther*, 1998, 36(3):139-45.

Eller N, Kollenz CJ, Bauer P, et al, "The Duration of Antidiuretic Response of Two Desmopressin Nasal Sprays," *Int J Clin Pharmacol Ther*, 1998, 36(9):494-500.

Molnár Z, Farkas V, Nemes L, et al, "Hyponatraemic Seizures Resulting From Inadequate Post-Operative Fluid Intake Following a Single Dose of Desmopressin," *Nephrol Dial Transplant*, 2005, 20 (10):2265-7.

National Heart, Lung, and Blood Institute, "The Diagnosis, Evaluation, and Management of von Willebrand Disease," NIH Publication No. 08-5832. Bethesda, MD: U.S. Department of Health and Human Services, Public Health Service, National Institutes of Health, National Heart, Lung, and Blood, 2007.

Robson WL, Leung AK, and Norgaard JP, "The Comparative Safety of Oral Versus Intranasal Desmopressin for the Treatment of Children With Nocturnal Enuresis," *J Urol*, 2007, 178(1):24-30.

Schrier RW, "Systemic Arterial Vasodilation, Vasopressin, and Vasopressinase in Pregnancy," *J Am Soc Nephrol*, 2010, 21(4):570-2.

Smith TJ, Gill JC, Ambruso DR, et al, "Hyponatremia and Seizures in Young Children Given DDAVP," *Am J Hematol*, 1989, 31(3):199-202.

Stenberg A and Läckgren G, "Desmopressin Tablets in the Treatment of Severe Nocturnal Enuresis in Adolescents," *Pediatrics*, 1994, 94(6 Pt 1):841-46.

Thumfart J, Roehr CC, Kapelari K, et al, "Desmopressin Associated Symptomatic Hyponatremic Hypervolemia in Children. Are There Predictive Factors?" *J Urol*, 2005, 174(1):294-8.

Weinstein RE, Bona RD, Altman AJ, et al, "Severe Hyponatremia After Repeated Intravenous Administration of Desmopressin," *Am J Hematol*, 1989, 32(4):258-61.

◆ **Desmopressin Acetate** *see* Desmopressin *on page 612*

◆ **Desoxyephedrine Hydrochloride** *see* Methamphetamine *on page 1359*

◆ **Desoxyn** *see* Methamphetamine *on page 1359*

◆ **Desoxyphenobarbital** *see* Primidone *on page 1737*

◆ **Desquam-X® (Can)** *see* Benzoyl Peroxide *on page 275*

◆ **Desquam-X Wash [OTC]** *see* Benzoyl Peroxide *on page 275*

◆ **Desyrel** *see* TraZODone *on page 2065*

◆ **Detemir Insulin** *see* Insulin Detemir *on page 1119*

◆ **Detrol** *see* Tolterodine *on page 2045*

◆ **Detrol® (Can)** *see* Tolterodine *on page 2045*

◆ **Detrol LA** *see* Tolterodine *on page 2045*

◆ **Detrol® LA (Can)** *see* Tolterodine *on page 2045*

Dexamethasone (Systemic)
(deks a METH a sone)

Medication Safety Issues
Sound-alike/look-alike issues:
Dexamethasone may be confused with desoximetasone, dextroamphetamine

Decadron may be confused with Percodan

Related Information
Corticosteroids Systemic Equivalencies *on page 2222*

Brand Names: U.S. Baycadron; Dexamethasone Intensol; DexPak 10 Day; DexPak 13 Day; DexPak 6 Day

Brand Names: Canada Apo-Dexamethasone; Dexasone; Dom-Dexamethasone; PHL-Dexamethasone; PMS-Dexamethasone; PRO-Dexamethasone; ratio-Dexamethasone

Therapeutic Category Adrenal Corticosteroid; Anti-inflammatory Agent; Antiemetic; Corticosteroid, Systemic; Glucocorticoid

Generic Availability (U.S.) May be product dependent

Use Oral, parenteral: Primarily as an anti-inflammatory or immunosuppressant agent in the treatment of a variety of diseases, including those of allergic, hematologic, dermatologic, neoplastic, rheumatic, autoimmune, nervous system, renal, and respiratory origin [FDA approved in pediatric patients (age not specified) and adults]; primary or secondary adrenocorticoid deficiency (not first line) [FDA approved in pediatric patients (age not specified) and adults]; management of cerebral edema, shock, and as a diagnostic agent [FDA approved in pediatric patients (age not specified) and adults]. Has also been used as adjunctive antiemetic agent in the treatment of chemotherapy-induced emesis, treatment of croup (laryngotracheobronchitis), treatment of airway edema prior to extubation, treatment of acute mountain sickness (AMS) and high altitude cerebral edema (HACE), and in neonates with bronchopulmonary dysplasia to facilitate ventilator weaning

Pregnancy Risk Factor C

Pregnancy Considerations Adverse events have been observed with corticosteroids in animal reproduction studies. Betamethasone crosses the placenta (Brownfoot, 2013); and is partially metabolized by placental enzymes to an inactive metabolite (Murphy, 2007). Some studies have shown an association between first trimester systemic corticosteroid use and oral clefts (Park-Wyllie, 2000; Pradat, 2003). Systemic corticosteroids may have an effect on fetal growth (decreased birth weight); however, information is conflicting (Lunghi, 2010). Hypoadrenalism may occur in newborns following maternal use of corticosteroids during pregnancy; monitor.

Because antenatal corticosteroid administration may reduce the incidence of intraventricular hemorrhage, necrotizing enterocolitis, neonatal mortality, and respiratory distress syndrome, the injection is often used in patients with preterm premature rupture of membranes (membrane rupture between 24 0/7 weeks and 34 0/7 weeks of gestation) who are at risk of preterm delivery (ACOG, 2013). When systemic corticosteroids are needed in pregnancy, it is generally recommended to use the lowest effective dose for the shortest duration of time, avoiding high doses during the first trimester (Leachman, 2006; Lunghi, 2010; Makol, 2011; Østensen, 2009).

Women exposed to dexamethasone during pregnancy for the treatment of an autoimmune disease may contact the OTIS Autoimmune Diseases Study at 877-311-8972.

Breast-Feeding Considerations Corticosteroids are excreted in human milk; information specific to dexamethasone has not been located. The manufacturer notes that when used systemically, maternal use of corticosteroids have the potential to cause adverse events in a nursing infant (eg, growth suppression, interfere with endogenous corticosteroid production). Due to the potential for serious adverse reactions in the nursing infant, the manufacturer recommends a decision be made whether to discontinue nursing or to discontinue the drug, taking into account the importance of treatment to the mother. If there is concern about exposure to the infant, some guidelines recommend waiting 4 hours after the maternal dose of an oral systemic corticosteroid before breast feeding in order to decrease potential exposure to the nursing infant (based on a study using prednisolone) (Bae, 2011; Leachman, 2006; Makol, 2011; Ost, 1985).

Contraindications Hypersensitivity to dexamethasone or any component, active untreated infections, systemic fungal infections, cerebral malaria

Warnings Hypothalamic-pituitary-adrenal (HPA) suppression may occur, particularly in younger children or in patients receiving high doses for prolonged periods; acute adrenal insufficiency (adrenal crisis) may occur with abrupt withdrawal after long-term therapy or with stress; withdrawal and discontinuation of corticosteroids should be tapered slowly and carefully; patients with HPA axis suppression may require doses of systemic glucocorticosteroids prior to, during, and after unusual stress (eg, surgery).

Immunosuppression may occur; patients may be more susceptible to infections; prolonged use of corticosteroids may also increase the incidence of secondary infection, mask acute infection (including fungal infections), prolong or exacerbate viral or fungal infections, activate latent opportunistic infections, or limit response to vaccines. Exposure to chickenpox should be avoided; corticosteroids should not be used to treat ocular herpes simplex; use caution in patients with a history of ocular herpes simplex. Corticosteroids should not be used for cerebral malaria or viral hepatitis. Close observation is required in patients with latent tuberculosis and/or TB reactivity; restrict use in active TB (only in conjunction with antituberculosis treatment).

May cause osteoporosis (at any age) or inhibition of bone growth in pediatric patients. Use with caution in patients with osteoporosis. In a population-based study of children, risk of fracture was shown to be increased with >4 courses of corticosteroids; underlying clinical condition may also impact bone health and osteoporotic effect of corticosteroids (Leonard, 2006).

Corticosteroid use may cause psychiatric disturbances, including depression, euphoria, insomnia, mood swings, and personality changes. preexisting psychiatric conditions may be exacerbated by corticosteroid use. In premature neonates, the use of high-dose dexamethasone (approximately >0.5 mg/kg/day) for the prevention or treatment of BPD has been associated with adverse neurodevelopmental outcomes, including higher rates of cerebral palsy without additional clinical benefit over lower doses; current data does not support use of high doses, further studies are needed (Watterberg, 2010).

Acute myopathy may occur with high doses, usually in patients with neuromuscular transmission disorders; myopathy may involve ocular and/or respiratory muscles; monitor creatine kinase; recovery may be delayed. Increased IOP may occur especially with prolonged use; in children, increased IOP has been shown to be dose-dependent and produce a greater IOP in children <6 years than older children (Lam, 2005).

Rare cases of anaphylactoid reactions have been reported with corticosteroids.

Injection may contain sulfites and 0.5 mg tablet may contain tartrazine, either may cause allergic reactions in susceptible individuals. Concentrated oral solution ▶

(Intensol™) and elixir may contain ethanol (30% and 5.1%, respectively).

Concentrated oral solution (Intensol) and elixir contain propylene glycol; toxicities have been reported with use of products containing propylene glycol, including hyperosmolality, lactic acidosis, seizures, and respiratory depression; in neonates large amounts of propylene glycol delivered orally, intravenously (eg, >3000 mg/day), or topically have been associated with potentially fatal toxicities which can include metabolic acidosis, seizures, renal failure, and CNS depression; use products containing propylene glycol with caution (AAP, 1997; Shehab, 2009).

Elixir may contain benzoic acid; benzoic acid (benzoate) is a metabolite of benzyl alcohol; large amounts of benzyl alcohol (≥99 mg/kg/day) have been associated with a potentially fatal toxicity ("gasping syndrome") in neonates; the "gasping syndrome" consists of metabolic acidosis, respiratory distress, gasping respirations, CNS dysfunction (including convulsions, intracranial hemorrhage), hypotension and cardiovascular collapse; use dexamethasone products containing benzoic acid with caution in neonates; *in vitro* and animal studies have shown that benzoate displaces bilirubin from protein binding sites.

Precautions Avoid using higher than recommended doses; suppression of HPA function, suppression of linear growth (ie, reduction of growth velocity), reduced bone mineral density, hypercorticism (Cushing's syndrome), hyperglycemia, or glucosuria may occur; titrate to lowest effective dose. Reduction in growth velocity may occur when corticosteroids are administered to pediatric patients by any route (monitor growth). Use with extreme caution in patients with respiratory tuberculosis or untreated systemic infections. Use with caution in patients with hypertension, heart failure, or renal impairment; long-term use has been associated with fluid retention and hypertension. Use with caution in patients with GI diseases (diverticulitis, peptic ulcer, ulcerative colitis) due to risk of GI bleeding and perforation. High-dose corticosteroids should not be used for management of head injury; increased mortality was observed in patients receiving high-dose I.V. methylprednisolone. Use with caution in patients with myasthenia gravis; exacerbation of symptoms has occurred especially during initial treatment with corticosteroids. Use with caution in patients with hepatic impairment, including cirrhosis; enhanced pharmacologic effect due to decreased metabolism and long-term use has been associated with fluid retention. Use with caution following acute MI; corticosteroids have been associated with myocardial rupture; hypertrophic cardiomyopathy has been reported in premature neonates.

Use with caution in patients with diabetes; corticosteroids may alter glucose regulation leading to hyperglycemia. Use with caution in patients with cataracts and/or glaucoma; increased intraocular pressure, open-angle glaucoma, and cataracts have occurred with prolonged use, consider routine eye exams in chronic users. Use with caution in patients with a history of seizure disorder; seizures have been reported with adrenal crisis. Use with caution in patients with thyroid dysfunction; changes in thyroid status may necessitate dosage adjustments; metabolic clearance of corticosteroids increases in hyperthyroid patients and decreases in hypothyroid ones. Dexamethasone does not provide adequate mineralocorticoid activity in adrenal insufficiency (may be employed as a single dose while cortisol assays are performed). Prolonged treatment with corticosteroids has been associated with the development of Kaposi's sarcoma (case reports); if noted, discontinuation of therapy should be considered. Use with caution in patients with thromboembolic tendencies or thrombophlebitis.

Adverse Reactions

Cardiovascular: Arrhythmia, bradycardia, cardiac arrest, cardiomyopathy, CHF, circulatory collapse, edema, hypertension, myocardial rupture (post-MI), syncope, thromboembolism, vasculitis

Central nervous system: Depression, emotional instability, euphoria, headache, intracranial pressure increased, insomnia, malaise, mood swings, neuritis, personality changes, pseudotumor cerebri (usually following discontinuation), psychic disorders, seizure, vertigo

Dermatologic: Acne, allergic dermatitis, alopecia, angioedema, bruising, dry skin, erythema, fragile skin, hirsutism, hyper-/hypopigmentation, hypertrichosis, perianal pruritus (following I.V. injection), petechiae, rash, skin atrophy, skin test reaction impaired, striae, urticaria, wound healing impaired

Endocrine & metabolic: Adrenal suppression, carbohydrate tolerance decreased, Cushing's syndrome, diabetes mellitus, glucose intolerance decreased, growth suppression (children), hyperglycemia, hypokalemic alkalosis, menstrual irregularities, negative nitrogen balance, pituitary-adrenal axis suppression, protein catabolism, sodium retention

Gastrointestinal: Abdominal distention, appetite increased, gastrointestinal hemorrhage, gastrointestinal perforation, nausea, pancreatitis, peptic ulcer, ulcerative esophagitis, weight gain

Genitourinary: Altered (increased or decreased) spermatogenesis

Hepatic: Hepatomegaly, transaminases increased

Local: Postinjection flare (intra-articular use), thrombophlebitis

Neuromuscular & skeletal: Arthropathy, aseptic necrosis (femoral and humoral heads), fractures, muscle mass loss, myopathy (particularly in conjunction with neuromuscular disease or neuromuscular-blocking agents), neuropathy, osteoporosis, parasthesia, tendon rupture, vertebral compression fractures, weakness

Ocular: Cataracts, exophthalmos, glaucoma, intraocular pressure increased

Renal: Glucosuria

Respiratory: Pulmonary edema

Miscellaneous: Abnormal fat deposition, anaphylactoid reaction, anaphylaxis, avascular necrosis, diaphoresis, hiccups, hypersensitivity, impaired wound healing, infections, Kaposi's sarcoma, moon face, secondary malignancy

Drug Interactions

Metabolism/Transport Effects Substrate of CYP3A4 (major), P-glycoprotein; **Note:** Assignment of Major/Minor substrate status based on clinically relevant drug interaction potential; **Inhibits** P-glycoprotein; **Induces** CYP2A6 (weak/moderate), CYP2B6 (weak/moderate), CYP2C9 (weak/moderate), CYP3A4 (strong), P-glycoprotein

Avoid Concomitant Use

Avoid concomitant use of Dexamethasone (Systemic) with any of the following: Abiraterone Acetate; Aldesleukin; Apixaban; Apremilast; Artemether; Axitinib; BCG; Bedaquiline; Boceprevir; Bosutinib; Cabozantinib; Ceritinib; CloZAPine; Conivaptan; Crizotinib; Dabigatran Etexilate; Dienogest; Dronedarone; Enzalutamide; Everolimus; Fusidic Acid (Systemic); Ibrutinib; Indium 111 Capromab Pendetide; Itraconazole; Ivacaftor; Lapatinib; Lumefantrine; Lurasidone; Macitentan; Mifepristone; Natalizumab; NIFEdipine; Nilotinib; Nisoldipine; PAZOPanib; Perampanel; Pimecrolimus; PONATinib; Praziquantel; Ranolazine; Regorafenib; Rilpivirine; Rivaroxaban; Roflumilast; RomiDEPsin; Simeprevir; Sofosbuvir; SORAfenib; Tacrolimus (Topical); Tasimelteon; Telaprevir; Ticagrelor; Tofacitinib; Tolvaptan; Toremifene; Ulipristal; Vandetanib; Vemurafenib; VinCRIStine (Liposomal); Vorapaxar

Increased Effect/Toxicity

Dexamethasone (Systemic) may increase the levels/ effects of: Acetylcholinesterase Inhibitors; Amphotericin B; Androgens; Clarithromycin; CycloSPORINE (Systemic); Deferasirox; Ifosfamide; Leflunomide; Lenalidomide; Loop Diuretics; Natalizumab; NSAID (COX-2 Inhibitor); NSAID (Nonselective); Thalidomide; Thiazide Diuretics; Tofacitinib; Vaccines (Live); Warfarin

The levels/effects of Dexamethasone (Systemic) may be increased by: Aprepitant; Asparaginase (E. coli); Asparaginase (Erwinia); Clarithromycin; Conivaptan; CycloSPORINE (Systemic); CYP3A4 Inhibitors (Moderate); CYP3A4 Inhibitors (Strong); Denosumab; Estrogen Derivatives; Fluconazole; Fosaprepitant; Fusidic Acid (Systemic); Indacaterol; Luliconazole; Macrolide Antibiotics; Mifepristone; Neuromuscular-Blocking Agents (Nondepolarizing); P-glycoprotein/ABCB1 Inhibitors; Pimecrolimus; Quinolone Antibiotics; Salicylates; Stiripentol; Tacrolimus (Topical); Trastuzumab

Decreased Effect

Dexamethasone (Systemic) may decrease the levels/ effects of: Abiraterone Acetate; Afatinib; Aldesleukin; Antidiabetic Agents; Apixaban; Apremilast; ARIPiprazole; Artemether; Axitinib; BCG; Bedaquiline; Boceprevir; Bosutinib; Brentuximab Vedotin; Cabozantinib; Cannabidiol; Cannabis; Caspofungin; Ceritinib; Clarithromycin; CloZAPine; Cobicistat; Coccidioidin Skin Test; Corticorelin; Crizotinib; CycloSPORINE (Systemic); CYP3A4 Substrates; Dabigatran Etexilate; Dasatinib; Dienogest; DOXOrubicin (Conventional); Dronabinol; Dronedarone; Elvitegravir; Enzalutamide; Everolimus; Exemestane; FentaNYL; Gefitinib; GuanFACINE; Hyaluronidase; Ibrutinib; Imatinib; Indium 111 Capromab Pendetide; Isoniazid; Itraconazole; Ivacaftor; Ixabepilone; Lapatinib; Linagliptin; Lumefantrine; Lurasidone; Macitentan; Maraviroc; Mifepristone; NIFEdipine; Nilotinib; Nisoldipine; PAZOPanib; Perampanel; P-glycoprotein/ABCB1 Substrates; PONATinib; Praziquantel; QUEtiapine; Ranolazine; Regorafenib; Rilpivirine; Rivaroxaban; Roflumilast; RomiDEPsin; Salicylates; Saxagliptin; Simeprevir; Sipuleucel-T; Sofosbuvir; SORAfenib; SUNItinib; Tadalafil; Tasimelteon; Telaprevir; Tetrahydrocannabinol; Ticagrelor; Tofacitinib; Tolvaptan; Toremifene; Triazolam; Ulipristal; Urea Cycle Disorder Agents; Vaccines (Inactivated); Vandetanib; Vemurafenib; Vilazodone; VinCRIStine (Liposomal); Vorapaxar; Vortioxetine; Zuclopenthixol

The levels/effects of Dexamethasone (Systemic) may be decreased by: Aminoglutethimide; Antacids; Barbiturates; Bile Acid Sequestrants; Bosentan; CYP3A4 Inducers (Strong); Dabrafenib; Deferasirox; Echinacea; Mifepristone; Mitotane; P-glycoprotein/ABCB1 Inducers; Siltuximab; St Johns Wort; Tocilizumab

Stability

Elixir: Store at 15°C to 30°C (59°F to 86°F); avoid freezing; dispense in tightly closed container

Injection: Store at 20°C to 25°C (68°F to 77°F), excursions permitted to 15°C to 30°C (59°F to 86°F); protect from light and freezing; dilution with D_5W or NS is stable for at least 24 hours at room temperature or 2 days under refrigeration temperature (4°C).

Oral concentrated solution (Intensol™): Store at 20°C to 25°C (68°F to 77°F); do not freeze; do not use if precipitate is present; dispense only in original bottle and only with manufacturer-supplied calibrated dropper; discard open bottle after 90 days.

Oral solution: Store at 20°C to 25°C (68°F to 77°F); dispense in tightly closed, light-resistant container.

Tablets: Store at 20°C to 25°C (68°F to 77°F); protect from moisture; dispense in tightly closed, light-resistant container.

Mechanism of Action Decreases inflammation by suppression of neutrophil migration, decreased production of inflammatory mediators, and reversal of increased capillary permeability; suppresses normal immune response. Dexamethasone's mechanism of antiemetic activity is unknown.

Pharmacodynamics Duration: Metabolic effects can last for 72 hours

Pharmacokinetics (Adult data unless noted)

Metabolism: In the liver

Half-life: Terminal:

Extremely low birth-weight infants with BPD: 9.3 hours

Children 3 months to 16 years: 4.3 hours

Healthy adults: 3 hours

Time to peak serum concentration:

Oral: Within 1-2 hours

I.M.: Within 8 hours

Elimination: In urine and bile

Dosing: Neonatal

Airway edema or extubation: I.V.: 0.25 mg/kg/dose given ~4 hours prior to scheduled extubation then every 8 hours for a total of 3 doses (Couser, 1992); others have used 0.5 mg/kg/dose every 8 hours for 3 doses with last dose administered 1 hour prior to scheduled extubation (Davis, 2001); range: 0.25-0.5 mg/kg/dose for 1-3 doses; maximum dose: 1.5 mg/kg/day; limited data available, reported dosing regimens variable. **Note:** A longer duration of therapy may be needed with more severe cases. A recent meta-analysis concluded that future neonatal clinical trials should study a multiple dose strategy with initiation of dexamethasone at least 12 hours before extubation (Khemani, 2009).

Bronchopulmonary dysplasia, facilitation of ventilator wean: PNA ≥7 days: Oral, I.V.: Initial: 0.15 mg/kg/day given in divided doses every 12 hours for 3 days, then tapered every 3 days over 7 days; total dexamethasone dose: 0.89 mg/kg given over 10 days (Doyle, 2006); others have used 0.2 mg/kg/day given once daily and tapered every 3 days over 7 days (total dexamethasone dose: 1 mg/kg) (Durand, 2002) or tapered over 14 days (total dexamethasone dose: 1.9 mg/kg) (Walther, 2003). **Note:** High doses (~0.5 mg/kg/day) do not confer additional benefit over lower doses, are associated with higher incidence of adverse effects (including adverse neurodevelopmental outcomes), and are not recommended for use (Watterberg, 2010). However, a meta-analysis reported total cumulative doses >4 mg/kg reduced the relative risk for the combined outcome, mortality, or bronchopulmonary dysplasia; further studies are needed (Onland, 2009).

Dosing: Usual

Infants and Children:

Acute mountain sickness (AMS) (moderate)/high altitude cerebral edema (HACE); treatment: Oral, I.M., I.V.: 0.15 mg/kg/dose every 6 hours; consider using for high altitude pulmonary edema because of associated HACE with this condition (Luks, 2010; Pollard, 2001)

Airway edema or extubation: Oral, I.M., I.V.: 0.5 mg/kg/ dose given at 6-12 hours prior to extubation then every 6 hours for 6 doses (total dexamethasone dose: 3 mg/kg); maximum dose: 10 mg (Anene, 1996; Khemani, 2009; Tellez, 1991)

Antiemetic (chemotherapy-induced): Refer to individual protocols and emetogenic potential: I.V.: Severely emetogenic chemotherapy: Usual: 10 mg/m²/dose once daily on days of chemotherapy; some patients may require every 12 hour dosing; usual range: 8-14 mg/m²/dose (Holdsworth, 2006; Jordan, 2010; Phillips, 2010); others have used: Initial: 10 mg/m²/dose (maximum dose: 20 mg) then 5 mg/m²/dose every 6 hours

Anti-inflammatory: Oral, I.M., I.V.: 0.08-0.3 mg/kg/day or 2.5-10 mg/m²/day in divided doses every 6-12 hours

Asthma exacerbation: Oral, I.M., I.V.: 0.6 mg/kg once (maximum dose: 16 mg) (Hegenbarth, 2008)

Bacterial meningitis (*H. influenzae* type b): Infants and Children >6 weeks: I.V.: 0.15 mg/kg/dose every 6 hours for the first 2-4 days of antibiotic treatment; start dexamethasone 10-20 minutes before or with the first dose of antibiotic; if antibiotics have already been administered, dexamethasone use has not been shown to improve patient outcome and is not recommended (Tunkel, 2004). **Note:** For pneumococcal meningitis, data has not shown clear benefit from dexamethasone administration; risk and benefits should be considered prior to use (*Red Book*, 2009).

Cerebral edema: Oral, I.M., I.V.: Loading dose: 1-2 mg/kg/dose as a single dose; maintenance: 1-1.5 mg/kg/day (maximum dose: 16 mg/day) in divided doses every 4-6 hours

Croup (laryngotracheobronchitis): Oral, I.M., I.V.: 0.6 mg/kg once; usual maximum dose: 16 mg (doses as high as 20 mg have been used) (Bjornson, 2004; Hegenbarth, 2008; Rittichier, 2000); **Note:** A single oral dose of 0.15 mg/kg has been shown effective in children with mild to moderate croup (Russell, 2004; Sparrow, 2006)

Physiologic replacement: Oral, I.M., I.V.: 0.03-0.15 mg/kg/day or 0.6-0.75 mg/m²/day in divided doses every 6-12 hours

Adults:

Acute mountain sickness (AMS)/high altitude cerebral edema (HACE):

Prevention: Oral: 2 mg every 6 hours or 4 mg every 12 hours starting on the day of ascent; may be discontinued after staying at the same elevation for 2-3 days or if descent is initiated; do not exceed a 10-day duration (Luks, 2010). **Note:** In situations of rapid ascent to altitudes >3500 meters (such as rescue or military operations), 4 mg every 6 hours may be considered (Luks, 2010).

Treatment: Oral, I.M., I.V.:

AMS: 4 mg every 6 hours (Luks, 2010)

HACE: Initial: 8 mg as a single dose; Maintenance: 4 mg every 6 hours until symptoms resolve (Luks, 2010)

Anti-inflammatory:

Oral, I.M., I.V.: 0.75-9 mg/day in divided doses every 6-12 hours

Intra-articular, intralesional, or soft tissue: 0.4-6 mg/day

Extubation or airway edema: Oral, I.M., I.V.: 0.5-2 mg/kg/day in divided doses every 6 hours beginning 24 hours prior to extubation and continuing for 4-6 doses afterwards

Antiemetic:

Prophylaxis: Oral, I.V.: 10-20 mg 15-30 minutes before treatment on each treatment day; continuous infusion regimen: Oral or I.V.: 10 mg every 12 hours on each treatment day

Mildly emetogenic therapy: Oral, I.M., I.V.: 4 mg every 4-6 hours

Delayed nausea/vomiting: Oral: 4-10 mg 1-2 times/day for 2-4 days **or**

8 mg every 12 hours for 2 days; then

4 mg every 12 hours for 2 days **or**

20 mg 1 hour before chemotherapy; then

10 mg 12 hours after chemotherapy; then

8 mg every 12 hours for 4 doses; then

4 mg every 12 hours for 4 doses

Multiple myeloma: Oral, I.V.: 40 mg/day, days 1-4, 9-12, and 17-20, repeated every 4 weeks (alone or as part of a regimen)

Cerebral edema: I.V.: 10 mg stat, then 4 mg I.M./I.V. (should be given as sodium phosphate) every 6 hours until response is maximized, then switch to oral regimen, then taper off if appropriate; dosage may be reduced after 2-4 days and gradually discontinued over 5-7 days

Cushing's syndrome, diagnostic: Oral: 1 mg at 11 PM, draw blood at 8 AM; greater accuracy for Cushing's syndrome may be achieved by the following:

Dexamethasone: 0.5 mg by mouth every 6 hours for 48 hours (with 24-hour urine collection for 17-hydroxycorticosteroid excretion)

Differentiation of Cushing's syndrome due to ACTH excess from Cushing's due to other causes: Oral: Dexamethasone 2 mg every 6 hours for 48 hours (with 24-hour urine collection for 17-hydroxycorticosteroid excretion)

Multiple sclerosis (acute exacerbation): Oral: 30 mg/day for 1 week, followed by 4-12 mg/day for 1 month

Shock, treatment:

Addisonian crisis/shock (eg, adrenal insufficiency/responsive to steroid therapy): I.V.: 4-10 mg as a single dose, which may be repeated if necessary

Unresponsive shock (eg, unresponsive to steroid therapy): I.V.: 1-6 mg/kg as a single I.V. dose or up to 40 mg initially followed by repeat doses every 2-6 hours while shock persists

Physiological replacement: Oral, I.M., I.V. (should be given as sodium phosphate): 0.03-0.15 mg/kg/day **or** 0.6-0.75 mg/m²/day in divided doses every 6-12 hours

Administration

Oral: May administer with food or milk to decrease GI adverse effects; in some pediatric croup trials, dose was prepared using a parenteral dexamethasone formulation and mixing it with an oral flavored syrup (Bjornson, 2004)

Parenteral: Use preservative-free dosage forms in neonates.

I.M.: May administer 4 mg/mL or 10 mg/mL undiluted

I.V.: May administer as undiluted solution (4 mg/mL or 10 mg/mL) slow I.V. push, usually over 1-4 minutes; rapid administration is associated with perineal discomfort (burning, tingling) (Allan, 1986; Neff, 2002); may consider further dilution of high doses in D₅W or NS and administration by I.V. intermittent infusion over 15-30 minutes (Allan, 1986; Bernini, 1998)

Monitoring Parameters Hemoglobin, occult blood loss, blood pressure, serum potassium and glucose; IOP with systemic use >6 weeks; weight and height in children

Reference Range Dexamethasone suppression test: 8 AM cortisol <6 mcg/100 mL in adults given dexamethasone 1 mg at 11 PM the previous night

Test Interactions May suppress the wheal and flare reactions to skin test antigens

Additional Information Systemic: Due to the long duration of effect (36-54 hours), alternate day dosing does not allow time for adrenal recovery between doses.

Dosage Forms Excipient information presented when available (limited, particularly for generics); consult specific product labeling.

Concentrate, Oral:

Dexamethasone Intensol: 1 mg/mL (30 mL) [contains alcohol, usp; unflavored flavor]

Elixir, Oral:

Baycadron: 0.5 mg/5 mL (237 mL) [contains alcohol, usp, benzoic acid, fd&c red #40, propylene glycol; raspberry flavor]

Generic: 0.5 mg/5 mL (237 mL)

Solution, Oral:

Generic: 0.5 mg/5 mL (240 mL, 500 mL)

Solution, Injection, as sodium phosphate:

Generic: 4 mg/mL (1 mL, 5 mL, 30 mL); 20 mg/5 mL (5 mL); 120 mg/30 mL (30 mL); 10 mg/mL (1 mL, 10 mL); 100 mg/10 mL (10 mL)

Solution, Injection, as sodium phosphate [preservative free]:

Generic: 10 mg/mL (1 mL)

Tablet, Oral:

DexPak 10 Day: 1.5 mg [scored; contains fd&c red #40 aluminum lake]

DexPak 13 Day: 1.5 mg [scored; contains fd&c red #40 aluminum lake]

DexPak 6 Day: 1.5 mg [scored; contains fd&c red #40 aluminum lake]

Generic: 0.5 mg, 0.75 mg, 1 mg, 1.5 mg, 2 mg, 4 mg, 6 mg

References

ACOG Committee on Obstetric Practice, "ACOG Committee Opinion No. 475: Antenatal Corticosteroid Therapy for Fetal Maturation," *Obstet Gynecol*, 2011, 117(2 Pt 1):422-4.

Allan SG, Leonard RCF. Dexamethasone antiemesis and side-effects. *Lancet*. 1986;8488:1035.

American Academy of Pediatrics Committee on Drugs. "Inactive" ingredients in pharmaceutical products: update (subject review). *Pediatrics*. 1997;99(2):268-278.

American Academy of Pediatrics Committee on Infectious Diseases, "Dexamethasone Therapy for Bacterial Meningitis in Infants and Children," *Pediatrics*, 1990, 86(1):130-3.

Anene O, Meert KL, Uy H, et al, "Dexamethasone for the Prevention of Postextubation Airway Obstruction: A Prospective, Randomized, Double-Blind, Placebo-Controlled Trial," *Crit Care Med*, 1996, 24 (10):1666-9.

Bae YS, Van Voorhees AS, Hsu S, et al, "Review of Treatment Options For Psoriasis in Pregnant or Lactating Women: From the Medical Board of the National Psoriasis Foundation," *J Am Acad Dermatol*, 2012, 67(3):459-77.

Bernini JC, Rogers ZR, Sandler ES, et al. Beneficial effect of intravenous dexamethasone in children with mild to moderately severe acute chest syndrome complicating sickle cell disease. *Blood*. 1998;92:3082-3089.

Bjornson CL, Klassen TP, Williamson J, et al, "A Randomized Trial of a Single Dose of Oral Dexamethasone for Mild Croup," *N Engl J Med*, 2004, 351(13):1306-13.

Couser RJ, Ferrara TB, Falde B, et al, "Effectiveness of Dexamethasone in Preventing Extubation Failure in Preterm Infants at Increased Risk for Airway Edema," *J Pediatr*, 1992, 121(4):591-6.

Davis PG and Henderson-Smart DJ, "Intravenous Dexamethasone for Extubation of Newborn Infants," *Cochrane Database Syst Rev*, 2001, (4):CD000308.

Doyle LW, Davis PG, Morley CJ, et al, "Low-Dose Dexamethasone Facilitates Extubation Among Chronically Ventilator-Dependent Infants: A Multicenter, International, Randomized, Controlled Trial," *Pediatrics*, 2006, 117(1):75-83.

Durand M, Mendoza ME, Tantivit P, et al, "A Randomized Trial of Moderately Early Low-Dose Dexamethasone Therapy in Very Low Birth Weight Infants: Dynamic Pulmonary Mechanics, Oxygenation, and Ventilation," *Pediatrics*, 2002, 109(2):262-8.

Durand M, Sardesai S, and McEvoy C, "Effects of Early Dexamethasone Therapy on Pulmonary Mechanics and Chronic Lung Disease in Very Low Birth Weight Infants: A Randomized, Controlled Trial," *Pediatrics*, 1995, 95(4):584-90.

Hegenbarth MA and American Academy of Pediatrics Committee on Drugs, "Preparing for Pediatric Emergencies: Drugs to Consider," *Pediatrics*, 2008, 121(2):433-43.

Holdsworth MT, Raisch DW, and Frost J, "Acute and Delayed Nausea and Emesis Control in Pediatric Oncology Patients," *Cancer*, 2006, 106(4):931-40.

Jordan K, Roila F, Molassiotis A, et al, "Antiemetics in Children Receiving Chemotherapy. MASCC/ESMO Guideline Update 2009," *Support Care Cancer*, 2010.

Khemani RG, Randolph A, and Markovitz B, "Corticosteroids for the Prevention and Treatment of Post-Extubation Stridor in Neonates, Children and Adults," *Cochrane Database Syst Rev*, 2009, (3): CD001000.

Kris MG, Hesketh PJ, Somerfield MR, et al, "American Society of Clinical Oncology Guideline for Antiemetics in Oncology: Update 2006," *J Clin Oncol*, 2006, 2024(18):2932-47.

Leachman SA and Reed BR, "The Use of Dermatologic Drugs in Pregnancy and Lactation," *Dermatol Clin*, 2006, 24(2):167-97, vi.

Leonard MB, "Glucocorticoid-Induced Osteoporosis in Children: Impact of the Underlying Disease," *Pediatrics*, 2007, 119 Suppl 2:S166-74.

Lunghi L, Pavan B, Biondi C, et al, "Use of Glucocorticoids in Pregnancy," *Curr Pharm Des*, 2010, 16(32):3616-37.

Luks AM, McIntosh SE, Grissom CK, et al, "Wilderness Medical Society Consensus Guidelines for the Prevention and Treatment of Acute Altitude Illness," *Wilderness Environ Med*, 2010, 21(2):146-55.

Makol A, Wright K, and Amin S, "Rheumatoid Arthritis and Pregnancy: Safety Considerations in Pharmacological Management," *Drugs*, 2011, 71(15):1973-87.

Mongelluzzo J, Mohamad Z, Ten Have TR, et al, "Corticosteroids and Mortality in Children With Bacterial Meningitis," *JAMA*, 2008, 299 (17):2048-55.

Murphy VE, Fittock RJ, Zarzycki PK, et al, "Metabolism of Synthetic Steroids by the Human Placenta," *Placenta*, 2007, 28(1):39-46.

Neff SPW, Stapelberg F, Warmington A. Excruciating perineal pain after intravenous dexamethasone. *Anaesth Intensive Care*. 2002;30:370-371.

Onland W, Offringa M, De Jaegere AP, et al, "Finding the Optimal Postnatal Dexamethasone Regimen for Preterm Infants at Risk of Bronchopulmonary Dysplasia: A Systematic Review of Placebo-Controlled Trials," *Pediatrics*, 2009, 123(1):367-77.

Østensen M and Forger F, "Management of RA Medications in Pregnant Patients," *Nat Rev Rheumatol*, 2009, 5(7):382-90.

Ost L, Wettrell G, Bjorkhem I, et al, "Prednisolone Excretion in Human Milk," *J Pediatr*, 1985, 106(6):1008-11.

Park-Wyllie L, Mazzotta P, Pastuszak A, et al, "Birth defects After Maternal Exposure to Corticosteroids: Prospective Cohort Study and Meta-Analysis of Epidemiological Studies," *Teratology*, 2000, 62 (6):385-92.

Phillips RS, Gopaul S, Gibson F, et al, "Antiemetic Medication for Prevention and Treatment of Chemotherapy Induced Nausea and Vomiting in Childhood," *Cochrane Database Syst Rev*, 2010, (9): CD007786.

Pollard AJ, Niermeyer S, Barry P, et al, "Children at High Altitude: An International Consensus Statement by an Ad Hoc Committee of the International Society for Mountain Medicine, March 12, 2001," *High Alt Med Biol*, 2001, 2(3):389-403.

Pradat P, Robert-Gnansia E, Di Tanna GL, et al, "First Trimester Exposure to Corticosteroids and Oral Clefts," *Birth Defects Res A Clin Mol Teratol*, 2003, 67(12):968-70.

Red Book: 2009 Report of the Committee on Infectious Diseases, 28th ed, Pickering LK, ed, Elk Grove Village, IL: American Academy of Pediatrics, 2009.

Rittichier KK and Ledwith CA, "Outpatient Treatment of Moderate Croup With Dexamethasone: Intramuscular Versus Oral Dosing," *Pediatrics*, 2000, 106(6):1344-8.

Russell K, Wiebe N, Saenz A, et al, "Glucocorticoids for Croup," *Cochrane Database Syst Rev*, 2004, (1):CD001955.

Shehab N, Lewis CL, Streetman DD, Donn SM. Exposure to the pharmaceutical excipients benzyl alcohol and propylene glycol among critically ill neonates. *Pediatr Crit Care Med*. 2009;10 (2):256-259.

Sparrow A and Geelhoed G, "Prednisolone Versus Dexamethasone in Croup: A Randomised Equivalence Trial," *Arch Dis Child*, 2006, 91 (7):580-3.

Tellez DW, Galvis AG, Storgion SA, et al, "Dexamethasone in the Prevention of Postextubation Stridor in Children," *J Pediatr*, 1991, 118(2):289-94.

Tunkel AR, Hartman BJ, Kaplan SL, et al, "Practice Guidelines for the Management of Bacterial Meningitis," *Clin Infect Dis*, 2004, 39 (9):1267-84.

van de Beek D, Farrar JJ, de Gans J, et al, "Adjunctive Dexamethasone in Bacterial Meningitis: A Meta-analysis of Individual Patient Data," *Lancet Neurol*, 2010, 9(3):254-63.

Walther FJ, Findlay RD, and Durand M, "Adrenal Suppression and Extubation Rate After Moderately Early Low-Dose Dexamethasone Therapy in Very Preterm Infants," *Early Hum Dev*, 2003, 74(1):37-45.

Watterberg KL and American Academy of Pediatrics. Committee on Fetus and Newborn, "Policy Statement–Postnatal Corticosteroids to Prevent or Treat Bronchopulmonary Dysplasia," *Pediatrics*, 2010, 126 (4):800-8.

Dexamethasone (Ophthalmic)

(deks a METH a sone)

Medication Safety Issues

Sound-alike/look-alike issues:

Dexamethasone may be confused with desoximetasone, dextroamphetamine

Maxidex® may be confused with Maxzide®

Brand Names: U.S. Maxidex; Ozurdex

Brand Names: Canada Diodex®; Maxidex®; Ozurdex®

Therapeutic Category Anti-inflammatory Agent, Ophthalmic; Corticosteroid, Ophthalmic

Generic Availability (U.S.) May be product dependent

Use

Ophthalmic: Management of steroid responsive inflammatory conditions such as allergic conjunctivitis, acne rosacea, superficial punctuate keratitis, herpes zoster keratitis, iritis, cyclitis, or select infective conjunctivitis when benefit of reduced edema and inflammation exceeds steroid use risks (FDA approved in adults); symptomatic treatment of corneal injury from chemical, radiation, or thermal burns, or from penetration of foreign bodies (FDA approved in adults)

Ophthalmic intravitreal implant (Ozurdex®): Treatment of macular edema following branch retinal vein occlusion (BRVO) or central retinal vein occlusion (CRVO) (FDA approved in adults); noninfective uveitis of the posterior segment of the eye (FDA approved in adults)

Otic (using ophthalmic solution): Management of steroid responsive inflammatory conditions such as allergic otitis externa and select infective purulent and nonpurulent otitis externa when benefit of reduced edema and inflammation exceeds steroid use risks (FDA approved in adults)

Pregnancy Risk Factor C

Pregnancy Considerations Adverse events were observed in animal reproduction studies following use of ophthalmic dexamethasone.

Breast-Feeding Considerations Although it is not known if detectable concentrations are found in breast milk following application of ophthalmic dexamethasone, the manufacturer recommends caution be used if administered to a nursing woman.

Contraindications Hypersensitivity to dexamethasone or any component; active untreated periocular infections

Suspension/solution: Viral disease of the cornea and conjunctiva (including epithelial herpes simplex keratitis, vaccinia, varicella); mycobacterial or fungal infection of the eye; otic use (solution): Perforation of the eardrum membrane

Intravitreal implant: Advanced glaucoma; active or suspected ocular or periocular infections; anterior chamber intraocular lens (ACIOL) and aphakic eyes with rupture of posterior lens capsule

Warnings Immunosuppression may occur; patients may be more susceptible to infections; prolonged use of corticosteroids may also increase the incidence of secondary infection, mask acute infection (including fungal infections), prolong or exacerbate viral or fungal infections, activate latent opportunistic infections, or limit response to vaccines. Exposure to chickenpox should be avoided; corticosteroids should not be used to treat ocular herpes simplex; use caution in patients with a history of ocular herpes simplex. Close observation is required in patients with latent tuberculosis and/or TB reactivity; restrict use in active TB (only in conjunction with antituberculosis treatment). Increased IOP may occur especially with prolonged use; in children, increased IOP has been shown to be dose-dependent and produce a greater IOP in children <6 years than older children (Lam, 2005).

Ophthalmic solution (drops) may contain sulfites, which may cause allergic reactions in susceptible individuals.

Precautions Use with caution in patients with cataracts and/or glaucoma; increased intraocular pressure, open-angle glaucoma, and cataracts have occurred with prolonged use, consider routine eye exams in chronic users. Avoid prolonged use of ophthalmic corticosteroids, which may result in ocular hypertension and/or glaucoma, with damage to the optic nerve, defects in visual acuity and fields of vision, and posterior subcapsular cataract formation. Monitor intraocular pressure if ophthalmic solution/suspension used for 10 days or longer.

Following intravitreal injection of the ocular implant formulation, endophthalmitis, ocular inflammation, increased intraocular pressure, and retinal detachments may occur. Intraocular pressure elevations usually peak 60 days following intravitreal injection and return to baseline by day 180; prolonged monitoring of intraocular pressure may be required. A risk of implant migration into the anterior chamber may be present if the posterior capsule of the lens is absent or torn. Temporary blurring may occur following intravitreal injections; patients should not drive or perform other high-risk activities until this resolves.

Prolonged use of ophthalmic corticosteroids may increase the risk of secondary ocular infections, including persistent fungal infections or bacterial keratitis. Avoid wearing contact lenses during therapy; ophthalmic solution and suspension may contain benzalkonium chloride which may be absorbed by contact lenses.

Adverse Reactions

Intravitreal implant (Ozurdex®):

Central nervous system: Headache

Ocular: Cataract, conjunctival hemorrhage, conjunctival hyperemia, pain, hypertension, intraocular pressure increased, vitreous detachment

Rare but important or life-threatening: Corneal edema, device dislocation, endophthalmitis, hypotony, implant misplacement, retinal detachment

Ophthalmic solution/suspension: Ocular: Burning, cataract formation, filtering blebs, glaucoma (with optic nerve damage), perforation of globe, secondary ocular infections, stinging, visual acuity defects, visual field defects

Drug Interactions

Metabolism/Transport Effects None known.

Avoid Concomitant Use There are no known interactions where it is recommended to avoid concomitant use.

Increased Effect/Toxicity

Dexamethasone (Ophthalmic) may increase the levels/ effects of: Ceritinib

Decreased Effect There are no known significant interactions involving a decrease in effect.

Stability

Ophthalmic ointment/suspension: Store at 8°C to 27°C (46°F to 80°F).

Ophthalmic solution, ocular implant: Store at 15°C to 30°C (59°F to 86°F).

Mechanism of Action Decreases inflammation by suppression of neutrophil migration, decreased production of inflammatory mediators, and reversal of increased capillary permeability; suppresses normal immune response.

Dosing: Usual

Infants, Children, and Adolescents: **Anti-inflammatory:**

Solution: Limited data available: Ophthalmic: Instill 1-2 drops into conjunctival sac every hour during the day and every other hour during the night; gradually reduce dose to every 3-4 hours, then to 3-4 times/day (Cassidy, 2001)

Suspension: Limited data available: Ophthalmic: Instill 1-2 drops into conjunctival sac up to 4-6 times per day; may use hourly in severe disease in older children; taper prior to discontinuation; others have used 2-4 times/day dosing in children following strabismus surgery; in one study twice daily eye drops controlled inflammation equally well as 4 times daily dosing, but with less increase in IOP (Lam, 2005; Ng, 2000)

Adults:

Ocular inflammation:

Solution: Ophthalmic: Instill 1-2 drops into conjunctival sac every hour during the day and every other hour during the night; gradually reduce dose to every 4 hours, then to 3-4 times/day

Suspension: Ophthalmic: Instill 1-2 drops into conjunctival sac up to 4-6 times per day; may use hourly in severe disease; taper prior to discontinuation

Macular edema (following BRVO or CRVO): Ophthalmic intravitreal implant (Ozurdex®): Intravitreal: 0.7 mg implant injected in affected eye

Noninfective uveitis: Ophthalmic intravitreal implant (Ozurdex®): Intravitreal: 0.7 mg implant injected in affected eye

Otic inflammation: Ophthalmic solution: Initial: Instill 3-4 drops into the aural canal 2-3 times a day; reduce dose gradually once a favorable response is obtained. Alternately, may pack the aural canal with a gauze wick saturated with the solution; remove from the ear after 12-24 hours. Repeat as necessary.

Administration

Ophthalmic: Avoid contact of container tip with skin or eye; remove soft contact lenses prior to using solutions containing benzalkonium chloride. Shake suspension well prior to use.

Intravitreal injection (Ozurdex®): Administer under controlled aseptic conditions (eg, sterile gloves, sterile drape, sterile eyelid speculum). Adequate anesthesia and a broad-spectrum bactericidal agent should be administered prior to injection. In sterile field, open foil pouch, remove applicator, and pull the safety tab straight off of the applicator (do not twist or flex the tab). See package insert for further administration details. If administration is required in the second eye, a new applicator should be used and the sterile field, syringe, gloves, drapes, and eyelid speculum should be changed.

Solution and suspension: Apply finger pressure to lacrimal sac during and for 1-2 minutes after instillation to decrease risk of absorption and systemic effects.

Otic: May use ophthalmic solution otically. Prior to use, clean the aural canal thoroughly and sponge dry.

Monitoring Parameters

Ophthalmic, topical: Intraocular pressure (Lam, 2005)

Ophthalmic intravitreal implant: Following intravitreal injection, monitor for increased IOP and endophthalmitis; check for perfusion of optic nerve head immediately after injection, tonometry within 30 minutes, biomicroscopy between 2-7 days after injection

Dosage Forms Excipient information presented when available (limited, particularly for generics); consult specific product labeling.

Implant, Intraocular [preservative free]:
Ozurdex: 0.7 mg (1 ea)
Solution, Ophthalmic, as phosphate:
Generic: 0.1% (5 mL)
Suspension, Ophthalmic:
Maxidex: 0.1% (5 mL)

References

American Academy of Pediatrics Committee on Drugs, "'Inactive' Ingredients in Pharmaceutical Products: Update (Subject Review)," *Pediatrics*, 1997, 99(2):268-78.

Cassidy L, Rahi J, Nischal K, et al, "Outcome of Lens Aspiration and Intraocular Lens Implantation in Children Aged 5 Years and Under," *Br J Ophthalmol*, 2001, 85(5):540-2.

Lam DS, Fan DS, Ng JS, et al, "Ocular Hypertensive and Anti-Inflammatory Responses to Different Dosages of Topical Dexamethasone in Children: A Randomized Trial," *Clin Experiment Ophthalmol*, 2005, 33 (3):252-8.

Ng JS, Fan DS, Young AL, et al, "Ocular Hypertensive Response to Topical Dexamethasone in Children: A Dose-Dependent Phenomenon," *Ophthalmology*, 2000, 107(11):2097-100.

◆ **Dexamethasone and Ciprofloxacin** *see* Ciprofloxacin and Dexamethasone *on page 477*

◆ **Dexamethasone Intensol** *see* Dexamethasone (Systemic) *on page 615*

◆ **Dexamethasone, Neomycin, and Polymyxin B** *see* Neomycin, Polymyxin B, and Dexamethasone *on page 1484*

◆ **Dexamethasone Sodium Phosphate** *see* Dexamethasone (Ophthalmic) *on page 619*

◆ **Dexamethasone Sodium Phosphate** *see* Dexamethasone (Systemic) *on page 615*

◆ **Dexasone (Can)** *see* Dexamethasone (Systemic) *on page 615*

◆ **Dexedrine** *see* Dextroamphetamine *on page 629*

◆ **Dexedrine® (Can)** *see* Dextroamphetamine *on page 629*

◆ **Dexferrum** *see* Iron Dextran Complex *on page 1153*

◆ **Dexiron (Can)** *see* Iron Dextran Complex *on page 1153*

Dexmedetomidine (deks MED e toe mi deen)

Medication Safety Issues

Sound-alike/look-alike issues:
Precedex may be confused with Peridex

High alert medication:
The Institute for Safe Medication Practices (ISMP) includes this medication among its list of drug classes which have a heightened risk of causing significant patient harm when used in error.

Administration issues:
Errors have occurred due to misinterpretation of dosing information; use caution. Maintenance dose expressed as mcg/kg/**hour**.

Brand Names: U.S. Precedex

Brand Names: Canada Precedex

Therapeutic Category Adrenergic Agonist Agent; Alpha-Adrenergic Agonist; Sedative

Generic Availability (U.S.) No

Use Sedation of initially intubated and mechanically ventilated patients during treatment in an intensive care setting; sedation prior to and/or during surgical or other procedures of nonintubated patients; duration of infusion should not exceed 24 hours. Other uses include premedication prior to anesthesia induction with thiopental; relief of pain and reduction of opioid dose following laparoscopic tubal ligation; as an adjunct anesthetic in ophthalmic surgery; treatment of shivering; premedication to attenuate the cardiostimulatory and postanesthetic delirium of ketamine. FDA approved in ages ≥18 years.

Pregnancy Risk Factor C

Pregnancy Considerations Adverse effects were observed in some animal reproduction studies. Dexmedetomidine is expected to cross the placenta. Information related to use during pregnancy is limited (El-Tahan, 2012).

Breast-Feeding Considerations It is not known if dexmedetomidine is excreted in breast milk. The manufacturer recommends that caution be exercised when administering dexmedetomidine to nursing women.

Contraindications Hypersensitivity to dexmedetomidine or any component; use outside of an intensive care setting

Warnings Should be administered only by persons skilled in management of patients in intensive care setting or operating room. Patients should be continuously monitored. Episodes of bradycardia and sinus arrest have been associated with dexmedetomidine when administered rapidly I.V. (eg, bolus administration) or to patients with high vagal tone. Hypotension and bradycardia have been associated with dexmedetomidine infusion; treatment may include the use of atropine or glycopyrrolate, stopping or decreasing the infusion, increasing the rate of I.V. fluid administration, use of pressor agents, and elevation of the lower extremities. Transient hypertension has been primarily observed during the loading dose in association with the initial peripheral vasoconstrictive effects of dexmedetomidine. Treatment is usually unnecessary; however, reduction of infusion rate may be required.

Usage for >24 hours is not recommended; abrupt discontinuation, if used for prolonged periods may result in withdrawal symptoms similar to those reported for another alpha$_2$ adrenergic agent, clonidine.

Precautions Use with caution in patients with advanced heart block, severe ventricular dysfunction, hypovolemia, diabetes mellitus, and chronic hypertension. Use with caution in patients receiving vasodilators or drugs which decrease heart rate. Patients may be arousable and alert when stimulated. This alone should not be considered as lack of efficacy in the absence of other clinical signs/ symptoms.

Adverse Reactions

Cardiovascular: Atrial fibrillation, bradycardia, edema, hypertension, hypertension (diastolic), hypotension, hypovolemia, peripheral edema, systolic hypertension, tachycardia

Central nervous system: Agitation, anxiety

Endocrine & metabolic: Hyperglycemia, hypocalcemia, hypokalemia, hypoglycemia, hypomagnesemia, increased thirst

Gastrointestinal: Constipation, nausea, xerostomia

Genitourinary: Oliguria

Hematologic & oncologic: Anemia

Renal: Acute renal failure, decreased urine output

Respiratory: Pleural effusion, respiratory depression, wheezing

Miscellaneous: Fever, withdrawal syndrome (ICU sedation)

Rare but important or life-threatening: Acidosis, apnea, atrioventricular block, bronchospasm, cardiac arrest, cardiac arrhythmia, confusion, delirium, diaphoresis, drug tolerance (use >24 hours), extrasystoles, hallucination, heart block, hemorrhage, hepatic insufficiency, hyperbilirubinemia, hypercapnia, hyperkalemia, hyperpyrexia, hypoventilation, hypoxia, illusion, increased blood urea nitrogen, increased gamma-glutamyl transferase, increased serum alkaline phosphatase, increased serum ALT, increased serum AST, inversion T wave on ECG, myocardial infarction, neuralgia, neuritis, oliguria, photopsia, pulmonary congestion, respiratory acidosis, rigors, seizure, sinoatrial arrest, speech disturbance, supraventricular tachycardia, tachyphylaxis (use >24 hours), ventricular arrhythmia, ventricular tachycardia, visual disturbance

Drug Interactions

Metabolism/Transport Effects Substrate of CYP2A6 (major); **Note:** Assignment of Major/Minor substrate status based on clinically relevant drug interaction potential; **Inhibits** CYP1A2 (weak), CYP2C9 (weak), CYP3A4 (weak)

Avoid Concomitant Use

Avoid concomitant use of Dexmedetomidine with any of the following: Ceritinib; Iobenguane I 123; Pimozide

Increased Effect/Toxicity

Dexmedetomidine may increase the levels/effects of: ARIPiprazole; Beta-Blockers; Bradycardia-Causing Agents; Ceritinib; Dofetilide; DULoxetine; Hypotensive Agents; Lomitapide; Pimozide

The levels/effects of Dexmedetomidine may be increased by: Barbiturates; Beta-Blockers; CYP2A6 Inhibitors (Moderate); CYP2A6 Inhibitors (Strong); MAO Inhibitors

Decreased Effect

Dexmedetomidine may decrease the levels/effects of: Iobenguane I 123

The levels/effects of Dexmedetomidine may be decreased by: Mirtazapine; Serotonin/Norepinephrine Reuptake Inhibitors; Tricyclic Antidepressants

Stability Store at room temperature; compatible when administered with LR, D_5W, NS, 20% mannitol, thiopental, etomidate, vecuronium, pancuronium, succinylcholine, atracurium, mivacurium, glycopyrrolate, phenylephrine, atropine, midazolam, morphine, and fentanyl (see manufacturer's information for more extensive compatibility listings). Incompatible when administered with amphotericin B and diazepam.

May adsorb to certain types of natural rubber; use components made with synthetic or coated natural rubber gaskets whenever possible.

Mechanism of Action Selective alpha$_2$-adrenoceptor agonist with anesthetic and sedative properties thought to be due to activation of G-proteins by alpha$_{2a}$-adrenoceptors in the brainstem resulting in inhibition of norepinephrine release; peripheral alpha$_{2b}$-adrenoceptors are activated at high doses or with rapid I.V. administration resulting in vasoconstriction.

Pharmacokinetics (Adult data unless noted)

Distribution: V_{dss}: Approximately 118 L

Bioavailability: I.M.: 73%

Protein binding: 94%

Metabolism: Hepatic via N-glucuronidation, N-methylation, and CYP2A6

Half-life: Distribution: 6 minutes; Terminal: 2 hours

Elimination: Urine (95%); feces (4%)

Clearance: Adults: 39 L/hour; hepatic impairment (Child-Pugh Class A, B, or C): mean clearance values were 74%, 64%, and 53% respectively, of those observed in healthy adults; clearance at birth is approximately 30% of adults, reaching adult values between 6-12 months of age

Dosing: Usual Note: Errors have occurred due to misinterpretation of dosing information. Maintenance dose expressed as mcg/kg/**hour**. **Note:** Individualize and titrate to desired clinical effect: I.V.:

Children (limited data): Loading dose: 0.5-1 mcg/kg; followed by a maintenance infusion of 0.2-0.7 mcg/kg/**hour**; children <1 year may require higher infusion rates; average infusion range: 0.4 mcg/kg/**hour** vs 0.29 mcg/kg/**hour** in children >1 year; doses as high as 0.75 mcg/kg/**hour** were used (Chrysostomou, 2006). Other studies have used maintenance doses as high as 1 mcg/kg/**hour** (Munro, 2007; Nichols, 2005).

Adults:

ICU sedation: Initial: Loading dose: 1 mcg/kg, followed by a maintenance infusion of 0.2-0.7 mcg/kg/**hour**; adjust rate to desired level of sedation

Procedural sedation: Initial: Loading infusion of 1 mcg/kg [or 0.5 mcg/kg for less invasive procedures (eg, ophthalmic)] over 10 minutes, followed by a maintenance infusion of 0.6 mcg/kg/**hour**, titrate to desired effect; usual range: 0.2-1 mcg/kg/**hour**

Fiberoptic intubation (awake): Initial: Loading infusion of 1 mcg/kg over 10 minutes, followed by a maintenance infusion of 0.7 mcg/kg/**hour** until endotracheal tube is secured

Note: The manufacturer does not recommend that the duration of infusion exceed 24 hours; however, there have been a few studies in adults demonstrating that dexmedetomidine was well tolerated in treatment periods >24 hours; titrate infusion rate so patient awakens slowly; abrupt discontinuation, particularly after prolonged infusions may result in withdrawal symptoms.

Dosage adjustment in hepatic impairment: Dosage reduction may need to be considered. No specific guidelines available.

Usual Infusion Concentrations: Pediatric I.V. infusion: 4 mcg/mL

Administration I.V.: Administer using a controlled infusion device. Dilute 200 mcg (2 mL) in 48 mL NS to achieve a final concentration of 4 mcg/mL. Infuse loading dose over 10 minutes; rapid infusions are associated with severe side effects. Dexmedetomidine may adhere to natural rubber; use administration components made with synthetic or coated natural rubber gaskets.

Monitoring Parameters Level of sedation, heart rate, respiration, ECG, blood pressure, pain control

Additional Information As an adjunct to anesthesia, dexmedetomidine has been administered I.M. 0.5-1.5 mcg/kg/dose, 60 minutes prior to anesthesia.

Dosage Forms Excipient information presented when available (limited, particularly for generics); consult specific product labeling.

Solution, Intravenous [preservative free]:
Precedex: 200 mcg/2 mL (2 mL) [additive free]
Precedex: 200 mcg/50 mL (50 mL); 400 mcg/100 mL (100 mL) [latex free]

References

Berkenbosch JW, Wankum PC, and Tobias JD, "Prospective Evaluation of Dexmedetomidine for Noninvasive Procedural Sedation in Children," *Pediatr Crit Care Med*, 2005, 6(4):435-9.

Buck ML, "Dexmedetomidine for Sedation in the Pediatric Intensive Care Setting," *Pedatr Pharm*, 2006, 12(1).

Chrysostomou C, Di Filippo S, Manrique AM, et al, "Use of Dexmedetomidine in Children After Cardiac and Thoracic Surgery," *Pediatr Crit Care Med*, 2006, 7(2):126-31.

El-Tahan MR, Mowafi HA, Al Sheikh IH, et al, "Efficacy of Dexmedetomidine in Suppressing Cardiovascular and Hormonal Responses to General Anaesthesia for Caesarean Delivery: A Dose-Response Study," *Int J Obstet Anesth*, 2012, 21(3):222-9.

Munro HM, Tirotta CF, Felix DE, et al, "Initial Experience With Dexmedetomidine for Diagnostic and Interventional Cardiac Catheterization in Children," *Paediatr Anaesth*, 2007, 17(2):109-12.

Nichols DP, Berkenbosch JW, and Tobias JD, "Rescue Sedation With Dexmedetomidine for Diagnostic Imaging: A Preliminary Report," *Paediatr Anaesth*, 2005, 15(3):199-203.

Phan H and Nahata MC, "Clinical Uses of Dexmedetomidine in Pediatric Patients," *Paediatr Drugs*, 2008, 10(1):49-69.

Walker J, Maccalum M, Fischer C, et al, "Sedation Using Dexmedetomidine in Pediatric Burn Patients," *J Burn Care Res*, 2006, 27 (2):206-10.

◆ **Dexmedetomidine Hydrochloride** *see* Dexmedetomidine *on page 621*

Dexmethylphenidate (dex meth il FEN i date)

Medication Safety Issues

Sound-alike/look-alike issues:
Dexmethylphenidate may be confused with methadone
Focalin® may be confused with Folotyn®

Related Information
Oral Medications That Should Not Be Crushed or Altered *on page 2438*

Brand Names: U.S. Focalin; Focalin XR

Therapeutic Category Central Nervous System Stimulant

Generic Availability (U.S.) Yes

Use Treatment of attention-deficit/hyperactivity disorder (ADHD) (FDA approved in ages ≥6 years and adults)

Medication Guide Available Yes

Pregnancy Risk Factor C

Pregnancy Considerations Teratogenic effects were noted in animal studies. There are no adequate and well-controlled studies in pregnant women. Use only if the potential benefit to the mother outweighs the possible risks to the fetus.

Breast-Feeding Considerations It is not known if dexmethylphenidate is excreted into breast milk. Dexmethylphenidate is the more active *d-threo*-enantiomer of racemic methylphenidate, and methylphenidate is excreted into breast milk. Refer to Methylphenidate monograph for additional information.

Contraindications Hypersensitivity to dexmethylphenidate, methylphenidate, or any component; glaucoma; motor tics; Tourette's syndrome (diagnosis or family history); patients with marked agitation, tension, and anxiety; concurrent use or use within 14 days of MAO inhibitors (hypertensive crisis may occur)

Warnings Serious cardiovascular events including sudden death may occur in patients with preexisting structural cardiac abnormalities or other serious heart problems. Sudden death has been reported in children and adolescents; sudden death, stroke, and MI have been reported in adults. Avoid the use of CNS stimulants in patients with known serious structural cardiac abnormalities, cardiomyopathy, serious heart rhythm abnormalities, coronary artery disease, or other serious cardiac problems that could place patients at an increased risk to the sympathomimetic effects of a stimulant drug. Patients should be carefully evaluated for cardiac disease prior to initiation of therapy. The American Heart Association recommends that all children diagnosed with ADHD who may be candidates for medication, such as dexmethylphenidate, should have a thorough cardiovascular assessment prior to initiation of therapy. This assessment should include a combination of medical history, family history, and physical examination focusing on cardiovascular disease risk factors. An ECG is not mandatory but should be considered. **Note:** ECG abnormalities and four cases of sudden cardiac death have been reported in children receiving clonidine with methylphenidate; this problem may potentially occur with dexmethylphenidate; consider ECG monitoring and reduction of dexmethylphenidate dose when used concurrently with clonidine.

If a child displays symptoms of cardiovascular disease, including chest pain, dyspnea, or fainting, parents should seek immediate medical care for the child. In a recent retrospective study on the possible association between stimulant medication use and sudden death in children, 564 previously healthy children who died suddenly in motor vehicle accidents were compared to a group of 564 previously healthy children who died suddenly. Two of the 564 (0.4%) children in motor vehicle accidents were taking stimulant medications compared to 10 of 564 (1.8%) children who died suddenly. While the authors of this study conclude there may be an association between stimulant use and sudden death in children, there were a number of limitations to the study and the FDA cannot conclude this information impacts the overall risk:benefit profile of these medications (Gould, 2009). In a large retrospective cohort study involving 1,200,438 children and young adults (aged 2-24 years), none of the currently available stimulant medications or atomoxetine were shown to increase the risk of serious cardiovascular events (ie, acute MI, sudden cardiac death, or stroke) in current (adjusted hazard ratio: 0.75; 95% CI: 0.31-1.85) or former (adjusted hazard ratio: 1.03; 95% CI: 0.57-1.89) users compared to nonusers. It should be noted that due to the upper limit of the 95% CI, the study could not rule out a doubling of the risk, albeit low (Cooper, 2011).

Stimulant medications may increase blood pressure (average increase 2-4 mm Hg) and heart rate (average increase 3-6 bpm); some patients may experience greater increases; use stimulant medications with caution in patients with hypertension and other cardiovascular conditions that may be exacerbated by increases in blood pressure or heart rate.

Psychiatric adverse events may occur. Stimulants may exacerbate symptoms of behavior disturbance and thought disorder in patients with preexisting psychosis. New-onset psychosis or mania may occur with stimulant use in patients without a prior history of psychotic illness or mania, even at standard doses. Stimulants may induce mixed/manic episodes in patients with bipolar disorder; patients should be screened for bipolar disorder prior to treatment; consider discontinuation if such symptoms (eg, delusional thinking, hallucinations, or mania) occur. May be associated with aggressive behavior or hostility (causal relationship not established); monitor for development or worsening of these behaviors.

Long-term effects in pediatric patients have not been determined. Use of stimulants in children has been associated with growth suppression; monitor growth; treatment interruption may be needed. Appetite suppression may occur; monitor weight during therapy, particularly in children. Stimulants may lower seizure threshold leading to new onset or breakthrough seizure activity; use with caution in patients with a history of seizure disorder. Visual disturbances, such as difficulty in accommodation and blurred vision, have been reported.

CNS stimulants possess a high potential for abuse **[U.S. Boxed Warning]**; misuse may cause sudden death and serious cardiovascular adverse events; prolonged administration may lead to drug dependence; abrupt discontinuation following high doses or for prolonged periods may result in symptoms of withdrawal; avoid abrupt discontinuation in patients who have received dexmethylphenidate for prolonged periods; use with caution in patients with history of ethanol or drug abuse. Do not use for severe depression or normal fatigue states.

Prolonged and painful erections (priapism), sometimes requiring surgical intervention, have been reported with methylphenidate use in pediatric and adult patients. Priapism has been reported to develop after some time on the drug, often subsequent to an increase in dose and also during a period of drug withdrawal (drug holidays or discontinuation). Patients who develop abnormally sustained or frequent and painful erections should seek immediate medical attention.

Hypersensitivity reactions (angioedema and anaphylactic reactions) have been reported with methylphenidate; similar reactions could occur with dexmethylphenidate use.

Precautions Use with caution in patients with heart failure, recent MI, hyperthyroidism, acute stress reactions, emotional instability. Hematological monitoring is advised with long-term use.

Adverse Reactions

Central nervous system: Anxiety, depression (children), dizziness (adults), fever (children), headache, insomnia (children), irritability (children), mood swings (children), restlessness (adults)

Dermatologic: Pruritus (children)

Gastrointestinal: Abdominal pain (children), anorexia (children), appetite decreased (children), dyspepsia, nausea (children), pharyngolaryngeal pain (adults), vomiting (children), xerostomia (adults)

Respiratory: Nasal congestion (children)

Rare but important or life-threatening: Accommodation difficulties, anaphylaxis, hypersensitivity reactions

Also refer to Methylphenidate for adverse effects seen with other methylphenidate products.

Drug Interactions

Metabolism/Transport Effects None known.

Avoid Concomitant Use

Avoid concomitant use of Dexmethylphenidate with any of the following: Iobenguane I 123; MAO Inhibitors

Increased Effect/Toxicity

Dexmethylphenidate may increase the levels/effects of: Fosphenytoin; PHENobarbital; Phenytoin; Primidone; Sympathomimetics; Tricyclic Antidepressants; Vitamin K Antagonists

The levels/effects of Dexmethylphenidate may be increased by: Antacids; AtoMOXetine; Cannabinoid-Containing Products; H2-Antagonists; MAO Inhibitors; Proton Pump Inhibitors

Decreased Effect

Dexmethylphenidate may decrease the levels/effects of: Iobenguane I 123; Ioflupane I 123

Food Interactions High-fat meal may increase time to peak concentration. Management: Administer without regard to meals.

Stability

Immediate release tablets: Store at 25°C (77°F); excursions permitted to 15°C to 30°C (59°F to 86°F). Protect from light and moisture.

Extended release capsule: Store at 25°C (77°F); excursions permitted to 15°C to 30°C (59°F to 86°F). Dispense in tight container.

Mechanism of Action Dexmethylphenidate is the more active, *d-threo*-enantiomer, of racemic methylphenidate. It is a CNS stimulant; blocks the reuptake of norepinephrine and dopamine, and increases their release into the extraneuronal space.

Pharmacodynamics

Onset of action: Rapid, within 1-2 hours of an effective dose

Maximum effect: Variable

Duration: Immediate release: 3-5 hours; extended release: 9-12 hours (Dopheide, 2009)

Pharmacokinetics (Adult data unless noted)

Absorption: Immediate release: Rapid; Extended release: Bimodal (with 2 peak concentrations ~4 hours apart)

Distribution: V_d: 2.65 ± 1.11 L/kg

Protein binding: Unknown; racemic methylphenidate: 12% to 15%

Metabolism: Via de-esterification to inactive metabolite, *d*-α-phenyl-piperidine acetic acid (*d*-ritalinic acid)

Bioavailability: 22% to 25%

Half-life:

Children: 2-3 hours

Adults: 2-4.5 hours; **Note:** A few subjects displayed a half-life between 5-7 hours

Time to peak serum concentration:

Immediate release: Fasting: 1-1.5 hours; after a high-fat meal: 2.9 hours

Extended release: First peak: 1.5 hours (range: 1-4 hours); second peak: 6.5 hours (range: 4.5-7 hours)

Elimination: Urine (90%, primarily as inactive metabolite)

Dosing: Usual Note: Reduce dose or discontinue in patients with paradoxical aggravation of symptoms or other adverse events. Discontinue if no improvement is seen after appropriate dosage adjustment over a 1-month period of time.

Children and Adolescents:

Attention-deficit/hyperactivity disorder: Children ≥6 years and Adolescents: Oral:

Patients not currently taking methylphenidate:

Immediate release: Initial: 2.5 mg twice daily; doses should be taken at least 4 hours apart; dosage may be adjusted in increments of 2.5-5 mg at weekly intervals; maximum daily dose: 20 mg/**day** (manufacturer labeling); some experts recommend maximum daily dose: 50 mg/**day** (Dopheide, 2009; Pliszka, 2007)

Extended release: Initial: 5 mg once daily; dosage may be adjusted in increments of 5 mg/day at weekly intervals; maximum daily dose: 30 mg/**day** (manufacturer labeling); some experts recommend maximum daily dose: 50 mg/**day** (Dopheide, 2009; Pliszka, 2007)

Conversion to dexmethylphenidate from methylphenidate:

Immediate release: Initial: Half the total daily dose of racemic methylphenidate; maximum daily dexmethylphenidate dose: 20 mg/**day** (manufacturer labeling); some experts recommend maximum daily dose: 50 mg/**day** (Dopheide, 2009; Pliszka, 2007)

Extended release: Initial: Half the total daily dose of racemic methylphenidate; maximum daily dexmethylphenidate dose: 30 mg/**day** (manufacturer labeling); some experts recommend maximum daily dose: 50 mg/**day** (Dopheide, 2009; Pliszka, 2007)

Conversion from dexmethylphenidate immediate release to dexmethylphenidate extended release: When changing from Focalin® tablets to Focalin® XR capsules, switch to the same daily dose using Focalin® XR; maximum daily dose: 30 mg/**day** (manufacturer labeling); some experts recommend maximum daily dose: 50 mg/**day** (Dopheide, 2009; Pliszka, 2007)

Adults: **Attention-deficit/hyperactivity disorder:** Oral:

Patients not currently taking methylphenidate:

Immediate release: Initial: 2.5 mg twice daily; dosage may be adjusted in increments of 2.5-5 mg at weekly intervals; maximum daily dose: 20 mg/**day**; doses should be taken at least 4 hours apart

Extended release: Initial: 10 mg once daily; dosage may be adjusted in increments of 10 mg/**day** at weekly intervals; maximum daily dose: 40 mg/**day**

Conversion to dexmethylphenidate from methylphenidate:

Immediate release: Initial: Half the total daily dose of racemic methylphenidate; maximum daily dexmethylphenidate dose: 20 mg/**day**

Extended release: Initial: Half the total daily dose of racemic methylphenidate; maximum daily dexmethylphenidate dose: 40 mg/**day**

Conversion from dexmethylphenidate immediate release to dexmethylphenidate extended release: When changing from Focalin® tablets to Focalin® XR capsules, switch to the same daily dose using Focalin® XR; maximum daily dose: 40 mg/**day**

Dosage adjustment in renal impairment: No dosage adjustments provided in the manufacturer's labeling; however, since very little unchanged drug is eliminated in the urine, dosage adjustment in renal impairment is not expected to be required.

Dosage adjustment in hepatic impairment: No dosage adjustments provided in the manufacturer's labeling (not studied); use with caution.

Administration

Immediate release: Twice daily dosing should be administered at least 4 hours apart; may be taken with or without food.

Extended release: Administer once daily in the morning. Do not crush, chew, or divide capsule; swallow whole. Capsule may be opened and contents sprinkled over a spoonful of applesauce; consume immediately and entirely; do not store for future use.

Monitoring Parameters Evaluate patients for cardiac disease prior to initiation of therapy with thorough medical history, family history, and physical exam; consider ECG; perform ECG and echocardiogram if findings suggest cardiac disease; promptly conduct cardiac evaluation in patients who develop chest pain, unexplained syncope, or any other symptom of cardiac disease during treatment. Monitor CNS activity; CBC with differential, platelet count; blood pressure and heart rate (baseline following dose increases and periodically during treatment), sleep, appetite, abnormal movements, height, weight, BMI, growth in children. Patients should be re-evaluated at appropriate intervals to assess continued need of the medication. Observe for signs/symptoms of aggression or hostility, or depression. Monitor for visual disturbances.

Additional Information Treatment with dexmethylphenidate should include "drug holidays" or periodic discontinuation in order to assess the patient's requirements, decrease tolerance, and limit suppression of linear growth and weight. Medications used to treat ADHD should be part of a total treatment program that may include other components such as psychological, educational, and social measures. Long-term use of the immediate release tablets (ie, >6 weeks) and extended release capsules (>7 weeks) has not been studied; long-term usefulness should be periodically re-evaluated for the individual patient.

Focalin® XR capsules use a bimodal release where 1/2 the dose is provided in immediate release beads and 1/2 the dose is in delayed release beads. A single, once-daily dose of a capsule provides the same amount of dexmethylphenidate as two tablets given 4 hours apart. The modified release properties of Focalin® XR capsules are pH dependent; thus, concomitant administration of antacids or acid suppressants might alter the release of dexmethylphenidate.

Controlled Substance C-II

Dosage Forms Excipient information presented when available (limited, particularly for generics); consult specific product labeling.

Capsule Extended Release 24 Hour, Oral, as hydrochloride:

Focalin XR: 5 mg [contains fd&c blue #2 (indigotine)]

Focalin XR: 10 mg

Focalin XR: 15 mg [contains fd&c blue #2 (indigotine)]

Focalin XR: 20 mg

Focalin XR: 25 mg [contains fd&c blue #2 (indigotine)]

Focalin XR: 30 mg

Focalin XR: 35 mg, 40 mg [contains fd&c blue #2 (indigotine)]

Generic: 15 mg, 30 mg, 40 mg

Tablet, Oral, as hydrochloride:

Focalin: 2.5 mg, 5 mg, 10 mg

Generic: 2.5 mg, 5 mg, 10 mg

References

American Academy of Pediatrics, "ADHD: Clinical Practice Guideline for the Diagnosis, Evaluation, and Treatment of Attention-Deficit/Hyperactivity Disorder in Children and Adolescents," *Pediatrics*, 2011, 128(5):1007-22.

American Academy of Pediatrics/American Heart Association Clarification of Statement on Cardiovascular Evaluation and Monitoring of Children and Adolescents With Heart Disease Receiving Medications for ADHD; available at: http://americanheart.mediaroon.com/index.php?s=43&item=422.

Cooper WO, Habel LA, Sox CM, et al, "ADHD Drugs and Serious Cardiovascular Events in Children and Young Adults," *N Engl J Med*, 2011, 365(20):1896-904.

Dopheide JA and Pliszka SR, "Attention-Deficit-Hyperactivity Disorder: An Update," *Pharmacotherapy*, 2009, 29(6):656-79.

Gelperin K, "Cardiovascular Risk With Drug Treatments of ADHD," available at: http://www.fda.gov/ohrms/dockets/ac/06/slides/2006-4210s-index.htm. Accessed May 25, 2006.

Gelperin K, "Psychiatric Adverse Events With Drug Treatments of ADHD," available at: http://www.fda.gov/ohrms/dockets/ac/06/slides/2006-4210s-index.htm. Accessed May 25, 2006.

Gould MS, Walsh BT, Munfakh JL, et al, "Sudden Death and Use of Stimulant Medications in Youths," *Am J Psychiatry*, 2009, 166(9):992-1001.

Greenhill LL, Muniz R, Ball RR, et al, "Efficacy and Safety of Dexmethylphenidate Extended-Release Capsules in Children With Attention-Deficit/Hyperactivity Disorder," *J Am Acad Child Adolesc Psychiatry*, 2006, 45(7):817-23.

"National Institute of Mental Health Multimodal Treatment Study of ADHD Follow-Up: Changes in Effectiveness and Growth After the End of Treatment," *Pediatrics*, 2004, 113(4):762-9.

Nissen SE, "ADHD Drugs and Cardiovascular Risk," *New Eng J Med*, 2006, 354(14):1445-8.

Pliszka S and AACAP Work Group on Quality Issues, "Practice Parameter for the Assessment and Treatment of Children and Adolescents With Attention-Deficit/Hyperactivity Disorder," *J Am Acad Child Adolesc Psychiatry*, 2007, 46(7):894-921.

Poulton A, "Growth on Stimulant Medication; Clarifying the Confusion: A Review," *Arch Dis Child*, 2005, 90(8):801-6.

Prince JB, "Pharmacotherapy of Attention-Deficit Hyperactivity Disorder in Children and Adolescents: Update on New Stimulant Preparations, Atomoxetine, and Novel Treatments," *Child Adolesc Psych Clin N Am*, 2006, 15(1):13-50.

Robinson DM and Keating GM, "Dexmethylphenidate Extended Release: In Attention-Deficit Hyperactivity Disorder," *Drugs*, 2006, 66(5):661-8.

Silva RR, Muniz R, Pestreich L, et al, "Dexmethylphenidate Extended-Release Capsules in Children With Attention-Deficit/Hyperactivity Disorder," *J Am Acad Child Adolesc Psychiatry*, 2008, 47(2):199-208.

Silva RR, Muniz R, Pestreich L, et al, "Efficacy and Duration of Effect of Extended-Release Dexmethylphenidate Versus Placebo in Schoolchildren With Attention-Deficit/Hyperactivity Disorder," *J Child Adolesc Psychopharmacol*, 2006, 16(3):239-51.

Vetter VL, Elia J, Erickson C, et al, "Cardiovascular Monitoring of Children and Adolescents With Heart Disease Receiving Stimulant Drugs: A Scientific Statement From the American Heart Association Council on Cardiovascular Disease in the Young Congenital Cardiac Defects Committee and the Council on Cardiovascular Nursing," *Circulation*, 2008, 117(18):2407-23.

Wilens TE, "Mechanism of Action of Agents Used in Attention-deficit Hyperactivity Disorder," *J Clin Psychiatry*, 2006, 67(suppl 8):32-8.

◆ **Dexmethylphenidate Hydrochloride** *see* Dexmethyl-phenidate *on page 623*

◆ **DexPak 6 Day** *see* Dexamethasone (Systemic) *on page 615*

◆ **DexPak 10 Day** *see* Dexamethasone (Systemic) *on page 615*

◆ **DexPak 13 Day** *see* Dexamethasone (Systemic) *on page 615*

Dexrazoxane (deks ray ZOKS ane)

Medication Safety Issues
Sound-alike/look-alike issues:
Zinecard may be confused with Gemzar
Related Information
Emetogenic Potential of Antineoplastic Agents in Children *on page 2327*
Management of Drug Extravasations *on page 2255*
Safe Handling of Hazardous Drugs *on page 2419*
Brand Names: U.S. Totect; Zinecard
Brand Names: Canada Zinecard
Therapeutic Category Antidote; Cardioprotective Agent; Chelating Agent; Chemoprotectant Agent
Generic Availability (U.S.) Yes
Use
Zinecard®: Reduction of anthracycline-induced (ie, doxor-ubicin-induced) cardiotoxicity in women with metastatic breast cancer (FDA approved in adults). Not recom-mended for use with initial anthracycline therapy; most dexrazoxane studies have been done in women with metastatic breast cancer who had received a cumulative doxorubicin dose of 300 mg/m^2. Has also been used for prevention of doxorubicin cardiomyopathy associated with treatment of acute lymphoblastic leukemia (ALL).
Totect®: Treatment of anthracycline extravasation (FDA approved in adults)
Pregnancy Risk Factor D
Pregnancy Considerations Adverse events were observed in animal reproduction studies using doses less than the equivalent human dose (based on BSA).
Breast-Feeding Considerations Due to the potential for serious adverse reactions in the nursing infant, discontinue nursing during dexrazoxane therapy.
Contraindications Hypersensitivity to dexrazoxane or any component; Zinecard® should only be used with chemo-therapy regimens containing an anthracycline
Warnings Hazardous agent; use appropriate precautions for handling and disposal (NIOSH, 2012). Based on limited experience, the possibility of dexrazoxane interference with antineoplastic efficacy may exist; use Zinecard® only in those patients who have received a cumulative doxor-ubicin dose of 300 mg/m^2 and are continuing with doxor-ubicin therapy. Does not eliminate the potential for anthracycline-induced cardiac toxicity; carefully monitor cardiac function. May cause mild myelosuppression activ-ity (leukopenia, neutropenia, and thrombocytopenia); may be additive with concurrently administered chemothera-peutic agents. Secondary malignant neoplasms (SMN) have been reported with dexrazoxane and razoxane use [racemic mixture of which dexrazoxane is the S(+) enan-tiomer]; a multicenter review of pediatric trials reported the incidence of SMN to be very rare; a single case was reported out of 533 pediatric patients evaluated throughout 5-year follow-up (Vrooman, 2011).
Precautions Do not give doxorubicin prior to dexrazox-ane administration. Doxorubicin should be given within 30 minutes after the beginning of a dexrazoxane infusion when used for the prevention of cardiomyopathy. For I.V. administration; **not** for local infiltration into extravasation

site. Do not use dimethylsulfoxide (DMSO) in patients receiving dexrazoxane for anthracycline-induced extrava-sation; may diminish dexrazoxane efficacy.

Use with caution in patients for hepatic impairment; adjust dosage; a proportional dose reduction in dexrazoxane is recommended to maintain the dosage ratio of 10:1. Use with caution in patients with renal impairment; dosage adjustment required for CrCl <40 mL/minute.
Adverse Reactions Note: Most adverse reactions are thought to be attributed to chemotherapy, except for increased myelosuppression, pain at injection site, and phlebitis.

Prevention of doxorubicin cardiomyopathy (reactions listed are those which were greater in the dexrazoxane arm in a comparison of chemotherapy plus dexrazoxane vs chemotherapy alone):
Central nervous system: Fatigue/malaise, fever
Dermatologic: Alopecia, streaking/erythema
Gastrointestinal: Serum amylase increased
Hematologic: Granulocytopenia, leukopenia, myelosup-pression, thrombocytopenia
Local: Extravasation, injection site pain, phlebitis
Neuromuscular & skeletal: Neurotoxicity
Miscellaneous: Infection, sepsis

Anthracycline extravasation:
Cardiovascular: Peripheral edema
Central nervous system: Depression, dizziness, fatigue, fever, headache, insomnia
Dermatologic: Alopecia
Endocrine & metabolic: Hypercalcemia, hyponatremia
Gastrointestinal: Abdominal pain, anorexia, constipation, diarrhea, nausea, vomiting
Hematologic: Anemia, leukopenia, neutropenia, neutro-penic fever, thrombocytopenia
Hepatic: Alkaline phosphatase increased, ALT increased, AST increased, bilirubin increased, LDH increased
Local: Injection site pain/discomfort, phlebitis
Renal: Creatinine increased
Respiratory: Cough, dyspnea, pneumonia
Miscellaneous: Infection
Drug Interactions
Metabolism/Transport Effects None known.
Avoid Concomitant Use
Avoid concomitant use of Dexrazoxane with any of the following: CloZAPine; Dimethyl Sulfoxide; Dipyrone
Increased Effect/Toxicity
Dexrazoxane may increase the levels/effects of: CloZA-Pine

The levels/effects of Dexrazoxane may be increased by: Dipyrone
Decreased Effect
Dexrazoxane may decrease the levels/effects of: DOX-Orubicin (Conventional)

The levels/effects of Dexrazoxane may be decreased by: Dimethyl Sulfoxide
Stability Note: Preparation and storage are product spe-cific; refer to individual product labeling for further details. Hazardous agent; use appropriate precautions for han-dling and disposal (NIOSH, 2012). Discard unused solu-tions.
Totect®: Store intact vials at room temperature of 25°C (77°F); excursions permitted to 15°C to 30°C (59°F to 86°F); protect from light. When reconstituted with the supplied diluent to a final concentration of 10 mg/mL, the reconstituted solution is stable for 2 hours. Solutions for infusion are stable for 4 hours when stored <25°C (<77°F).
Zinecard®: Store intact vials at room temperature of 25°C (77°F); excursions permitted to 15°C to 30°C (59°F to 86°F). When reconstituted with SWI, the reconstituted

solution is stable for 30 minutes at room temperature or 3 hours under refrigeration. Solutions for infusion are stable for 1 hour when stored at room temperature or 4 hours under refrigeration at 2°C to 8°C (36°F to 46°F).

Dexrazoxane generic formulation (Bedford Laboratories; Mylan, Inc): Store intact vials at room temperature of 20°C to 25°C (68°F to 77°F). Reconstituted solutions and solutions diluted for infusion are stable for 6 hours when stored at room temperature or under refrigeration 2°C to 8°C (36°F to 46°F).

Additional stability information: When studied as a 24-hour continuous infusion for the prevention of cardiomyopathy, solutions prepared with sodium lactate diluent and diluted to a final concentration of 0.1 or 0.5 mg/mL in D_5W were found to retain ≥90% of their initial concentration when stored at room temperature (ambient light conditions) for ≤24 hours (Tetef, 2001).

Mechanism of Action Derivative of ethylenediaminetetraacetic acid (EDTA); potent intracellular chelating agent. The mechanism of cardioprotectant activity is not fully understood. Appears to be converted intracellularly to a ring-opened chelating agent that interferes with iron-mediated oxygen free radical generation thought to be responsible, in part, for anthracycline-induced cardiomyopathy. In the management of anthracycline-induced extravasation, dexrazoxane may act by reversibly inhibiting topoisomerase II, protecting tissue from anthracycline cytotoxicity, thereby decreasing tissue damage.

Pharmacokinetics (Adult data unless noted)
Distribution: Distributes to heart, liver, and kidneys
V_d:
  Children: 0.96 L/kg
  Adults: 22-25 L/m^2
Protein binding: Insignificant
Metabolism: Hydrolyzed by dihydropyrimidine aminohydrolase and dihydrocrotase
Half-life: Biphasic: Adults:
  Distribution half-life: 8-21 minutes
  Elimination half-life: 2-3 hours
Elimination: 40% to 60% of dose excreted renally within 24 hours

Dosing: Usual
Infants, Children, and Adolescents: **Prevention of anthracycline cardiomyopathy associated with acute lymphoblastic leukemia (ALL):** I.V.: A 10:1 dose ratio of dexrazoxane:doxorubicin (example: 300 mg/m² dexrazoxane: 30 mg/m² doxorubicin) (Lipshultz, 2010; Moghrabi, 2007; Silverman, 2010). **Note:** Cardiac monitoring should continue during dexrazoxane therapy; anthracycline/dexrazoxane should be discontinued in patients who develop a decline in LVEF or clinical CHF.

Adults:
Prevention of doxorubicin cardiomyopathy: I.V.: A 10:1 ratio of dexrazoxane:doxorubicin (dexrazoxane 500 mg/m²:doxorubicin 50 mg/m²). **Note:** Cardiac monitoring should continue during dexrazoxane therapy; doxorubicin/dexrazoxane should be discontinued in patients who develop a decline in LVEF or clinical CHF.

Treatment of extravasation: I.V.: 1000 mg/m² on days 1 and 2 (maximum dose: 2000 mg), followed by 500 mg/m² on day 3 (maximum dose: 1000 mg); begin treatment as soon as possible, within 6 hours of extravasation

Dosage adjustment in renal impairment: Adults: **Note:** Renal function may be estimated using the Cockcroft-Gault formula.

Moderate-to-severe (CrCl<40 mL/minute):
  Prevention of cardiomyopathy: Reduce dose by 50%, using a 5:1 dexrazoxane:doxorubicin ratio (Example: 250 mg/m² dexrazoxane: 50 mg/m² doxorubicin)
  Anthracycline-induced extravasation: Reduce dose by 50%

Dosage adjustment in hepatic impairment:
Prevention of cardiomyopathy: Since doxorubicin dosage is reduced in hyperbilirubinemia, a proportional reduction in dexrazoxane dosage is recommended (maintain a 10:1 ratio of dexrazoxane:doxorubicin)
Anthracycline-induced extravasation: Use has not been evaluated in patients with hepatic dysfunction

Administration I.V.:
Prevention of doxorubicin cardiomyopathy: Administer doxorubicin within 30 minutes after beginning the infusion with dexrazoxane.
  Zinecard®: Reconstitute vial with SWI to a concentration of dexrazoxane 10 mg/mL. Prior to infusion, further dilute reconstituted dexrazoxane solution in lactated Ringer's injection to a final concentration of 1.3-3 mg/mL. Administer by rapid drip infusion; do **not** administer by I.V. push.
  Dexrazoxane generic formulation (Bedford Laboratories, Mylan, Inc): Reconstitute with the supplied diluent (0.167 Molar sodium lactate injection) to a final concentration of 10 mg/mL. Prior to infusion, further dilute reconstituted dexrazoxane solution with D_5W or NS to a final concentration of 1.3-5 mg/mL. Administer by slow I.V push or rapid drip infusion
Treatment of anthracycline extravasation: Reconstitute 500 mg vial with 50 mL of the supplied diluent (0.167 Molar sodium lactate injection) to a final concentration of 10 mg/mL. Prior to infusion, further dilute reconstituted dexrazoxane solution in NS 1000 mL. Administer I.V. over 1-2 hours; begin infusion as soon as possible, within 6 hours of extravasation. Infusion solution should be at room temperature prior to administration. Infuse in a large vein in an area remote from the extravasation. If extravasation is also being managed with cooling, withhold cooling beginning 15 minutes before dexrazoxane infusion; continue withholding cooling until 15 minutes after infusion is completed. Day 2 and 3 doses should be administered at approximately the same time (± 3 hours) as the dose on day 1. For I.V. administration; not for local infiltration into extravasation.

Hazardous agent; use appropriate precautions for handling and disposal (NIOSH, 2012).

Monitoring Parameters CBC with differential (frequent); liver function; serum creatinine; cardiac function (for adults: repeat monitoring at 400 mg/m², 500 mg/m², and with every 50 mg/m² of doxorubicin thereafter); monitor site of extravasation

Dosage Forms Excipient information presented when available (limited, particularly for generics); consult specific product labeling.
Solution Reconstituted, Intravenous:
  Totect: 500 mg (1 ea) [pyrogen free]
  Zinecard: 250 mg (1 ea); 500 mg (1 ea) [pyrogen free]
  Generic: 250 mg (1 ea); 500 mg (1 ea)

References
Brier ME, Gaylor SK, McGovren JP, et al, "Pharmacokinetics of Dexrazoxane in Subjects With Impaired Kidney Function," *J Clin Pharmacol*, 2011, 51(5):731-8.

Hensley ML, Hagerty KL, Kewalramani T, et al, "American Society of Clinical Oncology 2008 Clinical Practice Guideline Update: Use of Chemotherapy and Radiation Therapy Protectants," *J Clin Oncol*, 2009, 27(1):127-45.

Holcenberg JS, Tutsch KD, Earhart RH, et al, "Phase I Study of ICRF-187 in Pediatric Cancer Patients and Comparison of Its Pharmacokinetics in Children and Adults," *Cancer Treat Rep*, 1986, 70(6):703-9.

Lipshultz SE, Rifai N, Dalton VM, et al, "The Effect of Dexrazoxane on Myocardial Injury in Doxorubicin-Treated Children With Acute Lymphoblastic Leukemia," *N Engl J Med*, 2004, 351(2):145-53.

Lipshultz SE, Scully RE, Lipsitz SR, et al, "Assessment of Dexrazoxane as a Cardioprotectant in Doxorubicin-Treated Children With High-Risk Acute Lymphoblastic Leukemia: Long-Term Follow-Up of a Prospective, Randomised, Multicentre Trial," *Lancet Oncol*, 2010, 11 (10):950-61.

Moghrabi A, Levy DE, Asselin B, et al, "Results of the Dana-Farber Cancer Institute ALL Consortium Protocol 95-01 for Children With Acute Lymphoblastic Leukemia," *Blood*, 2007, 109(3):896-904.

National Institute for Occupational Safety and Health (NIOSH), "NIOSH List of Antineoplastic and Other Hazardous Drugs in Healthcare Settings 2012." Available at http://www.cdc.gov/niosh/docs/2012-150/pdfs/2012-150.pdf. Accessed January 21, 2013.

Sehested M, Holm B, and Jensen PB, "Dexrazoxane for Protection Against Cardiotoxic Effects of Anthracyclines," *J Clin Oncol*, 1996, 14:2884.

Silverman LB, Stevenson KE, O'Brien JE, et al, "Long-Term Results of Dana-Farber Cancer Institute ALL Consortium Protocols for Children With Newly Diagnosed Acute Lymphoblastic Leukemia (1985-2000)," *Leukemia*, 2010, 24(2):320-34.

Swain SM, Whaley FS, Gerber MC, et al, "Cardioprotection With Dexrazoxane in Doxorubicin-Containing Therapy in Advanced Breast Cancer," *J Clin Oncol*, 1997, 15:1318-32.

Swain SM, Whaley FS, Gerber MC, et al, "Delayed Administration of Dexrazoxane Provides Cardioprotection for Patients With Advanced Breast Cancer Treated With Doxorubicin-Containing Therapy," *J Clin Oncol*, 1997, 15:1333-40.

Tetef ML, Synold TW, Chow W, et al, "Phase I Trial of 96-Hour Continuous Infusion of Dexrazoxane in Patients With Advanced Malignancies," *Clin Cancer Res*, 2001, 7(6):1569-76.

Vrooman LM, Neuberg DS, Stevenson KE, et al, "The Low Incidence of Secondary Acute Myelogenous Leukaemia in Children and Adolescents Treated With Dexrazoxane for Acute Lymphoblastic Leukaemia: A Report From the Dana-Farber Cancer Institute ALL Consortium," *Eur J Cancer*, 2011, 47(9):1373-9.

Wexler LH, Andrich MP, Venzon D, et al, "Randomized Trial of the Cardioprotective Agent ICRF-187 in Pediatric Sarcoma Patients Treated With Doxorubicin," *J Clin Oncol*, 1996, 14:362-72.

Dextran (DEKS tran)

Medication Safety Issues
Sound-alike/look-alike issues:
Dextran may be confused with Dexedrine
Brand Names: U.S. LMD in D_5W; LMD in NaCl
Therapeutic Category Plasma Volume Expander
Generic Availability (U.S.) No
Use Adjunctive treatment of shock or impending shock due to trauma (eg, burns, hemorrhage, surgery, surgical complications), a priming fluid in pump oxygenators during extracorporeal circulation, and for venous thrombosis and pulmonary embolism prophylaxis in patients undergoing surgery associated with a high incidence of thromboembolic complications (eg, hip surgery) (All indications: FDA approved in infants, children, adolescents, and adults), **Note:** This is not a substitute for blood or plasma; does not have oxygen-carrying capacity.
Pregnancy Risk Factor C
Pregnancy Considerations Animal reproduction studies have not been conducted.
Breast-Feeding Considerations It is not known if dextran is excreted in breast milk. The manufacturer recommends that caution be exercised when administering dextran to nursing women.
Contraindications Hypersensitivity to dextran or any component; marked cardiac decompensation, renal disease with severe oliguria or anuria, marked hemostatic defects of all types (eg, severe thrombocytopenia; hypofibrinogenemia) including those caused by medications (eg, heparin, warfarin)
Warnings Severe and fatal anaphylactoid reactions have been reported; discontinue use immediately with signs of hypersensitivity and administer appropriate therapy. Patients receiving dextran for the first time should be closely monitored during the first few minutes of the infusion. Large volumes of dextran (doses >1000 mL in adults) may cause reduction in hemoglobin concentration and excessive dilution of plasma proteins due to hemodilution; transient prolongation of bleeding time or an increase in bleeding tendency may occur with large volumes; use caution to prevent a decrease in hematocrit <30%. Administration of dextran may cause fluid overload; use with caution in patients at risk from overexpansion of

blood volume (eg, very young, elderly patients, or those with heart failure). Dose-related wound hematoma and seroma and pulmonary edema have been observed; recommended doses should not be exceeded.
Precautions Use with caution in patients with renal impairment; fluid status including urine output should be monitored closely; consider impact of sodium load and possible retention from use of dextran products in normal saline; in patients with reduced urine output, urine viscosity and specific gravity may be increased; monitor urine osmolality as part of hydration status assessment. Excessive dosing may precipitate renal failure in patients with advanced renal disease; use in severe oliguria or anuria is contraindicated; tubular vacuolization (osmotic nephrosis) has been reported in patients with renal failure while on dextran; causality not fully established. Use with caution in heart failure patients; monitor closely for fluid overload; contraindicated in patients with marked cardiac decompensation. Use with caution in patients with active hemorrhage; may increase the risk of bleeding. Use with caution in patients with thrombocytopenia; may interfere with platelet function.

Adverse Reactions
Cardiovascular: Cardiac arrest, hypotension, tightness of chest
Dermatologic: Urticaria
Gastrointestinal: Nausea, vomiting
Hematologic (all dose related): Bleeding time (prolonged), wound bleeding, wound hematoma
Hepatic: Liver function tests (abnormal)
Renal: Acute renal failure
Respiratory: Pulmonary edema (dose related), wheezing
Miscellaneous: Anaphylactoid reaction

Drug Interactions
Metabolism/Transport Effects None known.
Avoid Concomitant Use
Avoid concomitant use of Dextran with any of the following: Abciximab
Increased Effect/Toxicity
Dextran may increase the levels/effects of: Abciximab
Decreased Effect There are no known significant interactions involving a decrease in effect.
Stability Store at 20°C to 25°C (68°F to 77°F); do not freeze; do not use if crystallization has occurred; discard partially used containers
Mechanism of Action Produces plasma volume expansion by virtue of its highly colloidal starch structure.
Pharmacodynamics
Duration: Plasma expanding effect lasts 3-4 hours
Pharmacokinetics (Adult data unless noted)
Metabolism: Molecules with molecular weight ≥50,000 are metabolized to glucose
Elimination: Dextran 40: ~75% excreted in urine (unchanged) within 24 hours
Dosing: Usual
Infants, Children, Adolescents: **Note:** Dose and infusion rate are dependent upon the patient's fluid status and must be individualized:
Volume expansion/shock: I.V.:
Infants: Infuse 5 mL/kg as rapidly as necessary; maximum daily dose: 20 mL/kg/**day** for first 24 hours, 10 mL/kg/**day** thereafter; therapy should not be continued beyond 5 days
Children and Adolescents <50 kg: Infuse 10 mL/kg as rapidly as necessary; maximum daily dose: 20 mL/kg/**day** for first 24 hours, 10 mL/kg/**day** thereafter; therapy should not be continued beyond 5 days
Adolescents ≥50 kg: Infuse 500-1000 mL (~10 mL/kg) as rapidly as necessary; maximum daily dose: 20 mL/kg/**day** for first 24 hours; 10 mL/kg/**day** thereafter; therapy should not be continued beyond 5 days

Pump prime: I.V.: **Note:** Dose will vary with the volume of the pump oxygenator; doses usually added to the perfusion circuit.

Infants: 5 mL/kg; usual maximum total dose: 20 mL/kg/**day**

Children: 10 mL/kg; usual maximum total dose: 20 mL/kg/**day**

Adolescents: 10-20 mL/kg; usual maximum total dose: 20 mL/kg/**day**

Postoperative prophylaxis of venous thrombosis/pulmonary embolism: I.V.: **Note:** Current ACCP guidelines for the prevention of venous thromboembolism in surgical patients do not recommend the use of dextran; consider the use of other anticoagulants (Falck-Ytter, 2012; Gould, 2012):

Infants: Begin during surgical procedure and give 5 mL/kg; continue daily for 2-3 days; an additional 5 mL/kg should be administered every 2-3 days during the period of risk (up to 2 weeks postoperatively)

Children and Adolescents (<50 kg): Begin during surgical procedure and give 10 mL/kg; continue daily for 2-3 days; an additional 10 mL/kg should be administered every 2-3 days during the period of risk (up to 2 weeks postoperatively)

Adolescents (≥50 kg): I.V.: Begin during surgical procedure and give 500-1000 mL (~10 mL/kg); an additional 500 mL should be administered every 2-3 days during the period of risk (up to 2 weeks postoperatively)

Adults:

Volume expansion/shock: I.V.: Infuse 500-1000 mL (~10 mL/kg) as rapidly as possible; maximum: 20 mL/kg/day for first 24 hours; 10 mL/kg/day thereafter; therapy should not be continued beyond 5 days

Pump prime: I.V.: Varies with the volume of the pump oxygenator; generally, the solution is added in a dose of 10-20 mL/kg; usual maximum total dose: 20 mL/kg

Postoperative prophylaxis of venous thrombosis/pulmonary embolism: I.V.: **Note:** Current ACCP guidelines for the prevention of venous thromboembolism in surgical patients do not recommend the use of dextran; consider the use of other anticoagulants (Falck-Ytter, 2012; Gould, 2012): Per the manufacturer, begin during surgical procedure and give 500-1000 mL (~10 mL/kg); continue treatment with 500 mL once daily for 2-3 additional days. Additional 500 mL should be administered every 2-3 days during the period of risk (up to 2 weeks postoperatively)

Administration Parenteral: Do not use if crystalline precipitate forms. For I.V. infusion only (use an infusion pump or pressure infusion). For volume expansion/shock, may infuse initial volume as rapidly as possible. **Monitor closely for anaphylactic reaction; have epinephrine and resuscitative equipment available.**

Monitoring Parameters Vital signs, signs of allergic/anaphylactoid reaction especially for 30 minutes after starting infusions; coagulation parameters, hemoglobin, hematocrit, acid-base balance, electrolytes, serum protein, signs of circulatory overload (ie, heart rate, blood pressure, central venous pressure, hematocrit), renal function, urine output; urine specific gravity; platelets

Test Interactions Falsely elevated serum glucose when determined by methods that use high concentrations of acid (eg, sulfuric acid, acetic acid); may interfere with bilirubin assays that use alcohol and total protein assays using biuret reagents; dextran 70 may produce erythrocyte aggregation and interfere with blood typing and cross matching of blood

Additional Information Dextran in sodium chloride 0.9% contains sodium chloride 154 mEq/L

Dosage Forms Excipient information presented when available (limited, particularly for generics); consult specific product labeling.

Solution, Intravenous:
LMD in D₅W: 10% Dextran 40 (500 mL) [latex free]
LMD in NaCl: 10% Dextran 40 (500 mL) [latex free]

References

Falck-Ytter Y, Francis CW, Johanson NA, et al. Prevention of VTE in orthopedic surgery patients: Antithrombotic Therapy and Prevention of Thrombosis, 9th ed: American College of Chest Physicians Evidence-Based Clinical Practice Guidelines. *Chest.* 2012;141(Suppl 2) e278S-325S.

Gould MK, Garcia DA, Wren SM, et al. Prevention of VTE in non-orthopedic surgical patients: antithrombotic therapy and prevention of thrombosis, 9th ed: American College of Chest Physicians Evidence-Based Clinical Practice Guidelines. *Chest.* 2012;141(2 Suppl): e227-277.

◆ **Dextran 40** *see* Dextran *on page 628*
◆ **Dextran, Low Molecular Weight** *see* Dextran *on page 628*

Dextroamphetamine (deks troe am FET a meen)

Medication Safety Issues
Sound-alike/look-alike issues:
Dexedrine® may be confused with dextran, Excedrin®
Dextroamphetamine may be confused with dexamethasone

Related Information
Oral Medications That Should Not Be Crushed or Altered *on page 2438*

Brand Names: U.S. Dexedrine; ProCentra; Zenzedi

Brand Names: Canada Dexedrine®

Therapeutic Category Amphetamine; Anorexiant; Central Nervous System Stimulant

Generic Availability (U.S.) Yes

Use
Immediate release tablets, oral solution (ProCentra®): Treatment of attention-deficit/hyperactivity disorder (ADHD) (FDA approved in ages 3-16 years); treatment of narcolepsy (FDA approved in ages ≥6 years and adults); has also been used for treatment of obesity secondary to hypothalamic-pituitary dysfunction

Extended/sustained release capsules (Dexedrine® Spansule®): Treatment of attention-deficit/hyperactivity disorder (ADHD) (FDA approved in ages 6-16 years); treatment of narcolepsy (FDA approved in ages ≥6 years and adults)

Medication Guide Available Yes

Pregnancy Risk Factor C

Pregnancy Considerations Adverse effects have been observed in animal reproduction studies. The majority of human data is based on illicit amphetamine/methamphetamine exposure and not from therapeutic maternal use (Golub, 2005). Use of amphetamines during pregnancy may result in an increased risk of premature birth and low birth weight; newborns may experience symptoms of withdrawal. Behavioral problems may also occur later in childhood (LaGasse, 2012).

Breast-Feeding Considerations The majority of human data is based on illicit amphetamine/methamphetamine exposure and not from therapeutic maternal use (Golub, 2005). Amphetamines are excreted into breast milk and use may decrease milk production. Increased irritability, agitation, and crying have been reported in nursing infants (ACOG, 2011). The manufacturer recommends that mothers taking dextroamphetamine refrain from nursing.

Contraindications Hypersensitivity or idiosyncrasy to dextroamphetamine, other sympathomimetic amines, or any component; advanced arteriosclerosis, symptomatic cardiovascular disease, moderate to severe hypertension, hyperthyroidism, glaucoma, agitated states, history of drug abuse; concurrent use or use within 14 days of MAO inhibitors (hypertensive crisis may occur)

Warnings Serious cardiovascular events including sudden death may occur in patients with preexisting structural cardiac abnormalities or other serious heart problems. Sudden death has been reported in children and adolescents; sudden death, stroke, and MI have been reported in adults. Avoid the use of amphetamines in patients with known serious structural cardiac abnormalities, cardiomyopathy, serious heart rhythm abnormalities, coronary artery disease, or other serious cardiac problems that could place patients at an increased risk to the sympathomimetic effects of amphetamines. Patients should be carefully evaluated for cardiac disease prior to initiation of therapy. The American Heart Association recommends that all children diagnosed with ADHD who may be candidates for medication, such as dextroamphetamine, should have a thorough cardiovascular assessment prior to initiation of therapy. This assessment should include a combination of medical history, family history, and physical examination focusing on cardiovascular disease risk factors. An ECG is not mandatory but should be considered. If a child displays symptoms of cardiovascular disease, including chest pain, dyspnea, or fainting, parents should seek immediate medical care for the child. In a recent retrospective study on the possible association between stimulant medication use and sudden death in children, 564 previously healthy children who died suddenly in motor vehicle accidents were compared to a group of 564 previously healthy children who died suddenly. Two of the 564 (0.4%) children in motor vehicle accidents were taking stimulant medications compared to 10 of 564 (1.8%) children who died suddenly. While the authors of this study conclude there may be an association between stimulant use and sudden death in children, there were a number of limitations to the study and the FDA cannot conclude this information impacts the overall risk:benefit profile of these medications (Gould, 2009). In a large retrospective cohort study involving 1,200,438 children and young adults (aged 2-24 years), none of the currently available stimulant medications or atomoxetine were shown to increase the risk of serious cardiovascular events (ie, acute MI, sudden cardiac death, or stroke) in current (adjusted hazard ratio: 0.75; 95% CI: 0.31-1.85) or former (adjusted hazard ratio: 1.03; 95% CI: 0.57-1.89) users compared to nonusers. It should be noted that due to the upper limit of the 95% CI, the study could not rule out a doubling of the risk, albeit low (Cooper, 2011).

Stimulant medications may increase blood pressure (average increase: 2-4 mm Hg) and heart rate (average increase: 3-6 bpm); some patients may experience greater increases; use stimulant medications with caution in patients with hypertension and other cardiovascular conditions that may be exacerbated by increases in blood pressure or heart rate; use is contraindicated in patients with moderate to severe hypertension.

Psychiatric adverse events may occur. Stimulants may exacerbate symptoms of behavior disturbance and thought disorder in patients with preexisting psychosis. New-onset psychosis or mania may occur with stimulant use in patients without a prior history of psychotic illness or mania, even at standard doses. Stimulants may induce mixed/manic episode in patients with bipolar disorder; patients should be screened for bipolar disorder prior to treatment; consider discontinuation if such symptoms (eg, delusional thinking, hallucinations, or mania) occur. May be associated with aggressive behavior or hostility (causal relationship not established); monitor for development or worsening of these behaviors.

Long-term effects in pediatric patients have not been determined. Use of stimulants in children has been associated with growth suppression; monitor growth; treatment interruption may be needed. Appetite suppression may

occur; monitor weight during therapy, particularly in children. Stimulants may lower seizure threshold leading to new onset or breakthrough seizure activity; use with caution in patients with a history of seizure disorder. Visual disturbances (difficulty in accommodation and blurred vision) have been reported.

Amphetamines possess a high potential for abuse **[U.S. Boxed Warning]**; misuse may cause sudden death and serious cardiovascular adverse events **[U.S. Boxed Warning]**; use in weight reduction programs only when alternative therapy has been ineffective; prolonged administration may lead to drug dependence; abrupt discontinuation following high doses or for prolonged periods may result in symptoms of withdrawal; avoid abrupt discontinuation in patients who have received amphetamines for prolonged periods. Amphetamines may impair the ability to engage in potentially hazardous activities. May exacerbate motor and phonic tics and Tourette's syndrome.

Some tablets may contain tartrazine which may cause allergic reactions in susceptible individuals. Oral solution contains benzoic acid; benzoic acid (benzoate) is a metabolite of benzyl alcohol; large amounts of benzyl alcohol (≥99 mg/kg/day) have been associated with a potentially fatal toxicity ("gasping syndrome") in neonates; avoid use of dextroamphetamine products containing benzoic acid in neonates; *in vitro* and animal studies have shown that benzoate displaces bilirubin from protein binding sites.

Precautions Use with caution in patients receiving other sympathomimetic agents. Prescriptions should be written for the smallest quantity consistent with good patient care to minimize possibility of overdose.

Adverse Reactions Frequency not defined.

Cardiovascular: Cardiomyopathy, hypertension, palpitations, tachycardia

Central nervous system: Aggressive behavior, dizziness, dysphoria, euphoria, exacerbation of tics, Gilles de la Tourette's syndrome, headache, insomnia, mania, overstimulation, psychosis, restlessness

Dermatologic: Urticaria

Endocrine & metabolic: Change in libido, weight loss

Gastrointestinal: Anorexia, constipation, diarrhea, unpleasant taste, xerostomia

Genitourinary: Frequent erections, impotence, prolonged erection

Neuromuscular & skeletal: Dyskinesia, tremor

Ophthalmic: Accommodation disturbances, blurred vision

Drug Interactions

Metabolism/Transport Effects Substrate of CYP2D6 (minor); **Note:** Assignment of Major/Minor substrate status based on clinically relevant drug interaction potential

Avoid Concomitant Use

Avoid concomitant use of Dextroamphetamine with any of the following: Iobenguane I 123; MAO Inhibitors

Increased Effect/Toxicity

Dextroamphetamine may increase the levels/effects of: Analgesics (Opioid); Sympathomimetics

The levels/effects of Dextroamphetamine may be increased by: Alkalinizing Agents; Antacids; AtoMOXetine; Cannabinoid-Containing Products; Carbonic Anhydrase Inhibitors; Linezolid; MAO Inhibitors; Proton Pump Inhibitors; Tricyclic Antidepressants

Decreased Effect

Dextroamphetamine may decrease the levels/effects of: Antihistamines; Ethosuximide; Iobenguane I 123; Ioflupane I 123; PHENobarbital; Phenytoin

The levels/effects of Dextroamphetamine may be decreased by: Ammonium Chloride; Antipsychotics; Ascorbic Acid; Gastrointestinal Acidifying Agents; Lithium; Methenamine; Multivitamins/Fluoride (with ADE);

Multivitamins/Minerals (with ADEK, Folate, Iron); Multivitamins/Minerals (with AE, No Iron); Peginterferon Alfa-2b; Urinary Acidifying Agents

Food Interactions Amphetamine serum levels may be reduced if taken with acidic food, juices, or vitamin C. Management: Monitor response when taken concurrently.

Stability Store at 20°C to 25°C (68°F to 77°F); protect from light; dispense in tightly closed container.

Mechanism of Action Amphetamines are noncatecholamine, sympathomimetic amines that promote release of catecholamines (primarily dopamine and norepinephrine) from their storage sites in the presynaptic nerve terminals. A less significant mechanism may include their ability to block the reuptake of catecholamines by competitive inhibition.

Pharmacodynamics
Onset of action: Oral: 60-90 minutes
Duration of action: Immediate release: 4-6 hours; extended release: 8 hours (Dopheide, 2009)

Pharmacokinetics (Adult data unless noted)
Distribution: V_d: 3.5-4.6 L/kg; distributes into CNS; mean CSF concentrations are 80% of plasma
Metabolism: Hepatic via CYP monooxygenase and glucuronidation
Half-life: 12 hours
Time to peak serum concentration: Oral: Immediate release: 3 hours; sustained release: 8 hours
Elimination: In urine as unchanged drug and inactive metabolites; urinary excretion is pH dependent and is increased with acid urine (low pH)

Dosing: Usual Note: Use lowest effective individualized dose.
Children and Adolescents:
Attention-deficit/hyperactivity disorder:
Immediate release tablets; oral solution:
Children 3-5 years: Oral: Initial: 2.5 mg once daily in the morning; increase daily dose by 2.5 mg increments at weekly intervals until optimal response is obtained; maximum daily dose: 40 mg/day in 2-3 divided doses; use intervals of 4-6 hours between doses. **Note:** Although FDA approved, current guidelines do not recommend use in children ≤5 years due to insufficient evidence (AAP, 2011).
Children ≥6 years and Adolescents: Oral: Initial: 5 mg once or twice daily with first dose in the morning; increase daily dose by 5 mg increments at weekly intervals until optimal response is obtained, usual range 5-20 mg/day; maximum daily dose: 40 mg/day in 2-3 divided doses; use intervals of 4-6 hours between doses
Extended/sustained release capsules: Children ≥6 years and Adolescents: Oral: Initial: 5 mg once or twice daily with first dose in the morning; increase daily dose by 5 mg increments at weekly intervals until optimal response is obtained, usual range: 5-20 mg/day; maximum daily dose: 40 mg/day in 1-2 divided doses; use intervals of 6-8 hours between doses; in patients >50 kg, a maximum daily dose of 60 mg/day in divided doses has been used (Dopheide, 2009; Pliszka, 2007)
Narcolepsy:
Immediate release tablets, oral solution:
Children 6-12 years: Oral: Initial: 5 mg daily, may increase at 5 mg increments at weekly intervals until optimal response is obtained; maximum daily dose: 60 mg/day in 1-3 divided doses: use intervals of 4-6 hours between doses
Adolescents: Oral: Initial: 10 mg daily, may increase at 10 mg increments at weekly intervals until optimal response is obtained; maximum daily dose: 60 mg/day in 1-3 divided doses; use intervals of 4-6 hours between doses

Extended/sustained release capsules:
Children 6-12 years: Oral: Initial: 5 mg daily, may increase at 5 mg increments at weekly intervals until optimal response is obtained; maximum daily dose: 60 mg/day in 1-2 divided doses; use intervals of 6-8 hours between doses
Adolescents: Oral: Initial: 10 mg daily, may increase at 10 mg increments at weekly intervals until optimal response is obtained; maximum daily dose: 60 mg/day in 1-2 divided doses; use intervals of 6-8 hours between doses
Obesity secondary to hypothalamic-pituitary dysfunction: Limited data available: Children ≥6 years and Adolescents: Immediate release tablet; oral solution: Oral: Initial: 5 mg once daily in the morning; may increase daily dose at 2.5 mg increments at weekly intervals until optimal response is obtained; additional daily doses may be given before lunch and dinner if necessary; dosing based on a small, open-label trial of five children (age: 6-9 years) postsurgical resection for management of craniopharyngioma (Mason, 2002); maximum daily dose: 20 mg/day in 3 divided doses; further studies are needed.
Adults: **Narcolepsy:** Extended/sustained release capsules; immediate release tablets; oral solution: Oral: Initial: 10 mg daily, may increase at 10 mg increments in weekly intervals until optimal response is obtained; maximum daily dose: 60 mg/day

Administration Oral: Administer initial dose upon awakening; do not administer doses late in the evening due to potential for insomnia. Do not crush or chew extended/sustained release preparations.

Monitoring Parameters Evaluate patients for cardiac disease prior to initiation of therapy with thorough medical history, family history, and physical exam; consider ECG; perform ECG and echocardiogram if findings suggest cardiac disease; promptly conduct cardiac evaluation in patients who develop chest pain, unexplained syncope, or any other symptom of cardiac disease during treatment. Monitor CNS activity, blood pressure, heart rate, sleep, appetite, abnormal movements, height, weight, BMI, growth in children. Patients should be re-evaluated at appropriate intervals to assess continued need of the medication. Observe for signs/symptoms of aggression or hostility, or depression. Monitor for visual disturbances.

Test Interactions Amphetamines may elevate plasma corticosteroid levels; may interfere with urinary steroid determinations.

Additional Information Treatment for ADHD should include "drug holiday" or periodic discontinuation in order to assess the patient's requirements, decrease tolerance, and limit suppression of linear growth and weight. Medications used to treat ADHD should be part of a total treatment program that may include other components such as psychological, educational, and social measures. Sustained release capsule (Dexedrine® Spansule®) is formulated to release an initial dose promptly with the remaining medication gradually released over a prolonged time.

Controlled Substance C-II

Dosage Forms Excipient information presented when available (limited, particularly for generics); consult specific product labeling.
Capsule Extended Release 24 Hour, Oral, as sulfate:
Dexedrine: 5 mg, 10 mg, 15 mg [contains brilliant blue fcf (fd&c blue #1), fd&c blue #1 aluminum lake, fd&c red #40, fd&c yellow #10 (quinoline yellow), fd&c yellow #6 (sunset yellow)]
Generic: 5 mg, 10 mg, 15 mg
Solution, Oral, as sulfate:
ProCentra: 5 mg/5 mL (473 mL) [contains benzoic acid, saccharin sodium; bubble-gum flavor]
Generic: 5 mg/5 mL (473 mL)

Tablet, Oral, as sulfate:
Zenzedi: 2.5 mg
Zenzedi: 5 mg [scored; contains fd&c yellow #6 (sunset yellow)]
Zenzedi: 7.5 mg [contains brilliant blue fcf (fd&c blue #1), fd&c yellow #10 (quinoline yellow)]
Zenzedi: 10 mg [scored; contains fd&c blue #2 (indigotine), fd&c red #40, fd&c yellow #6 (sunset yellow)]
Zenzedi: 15 mg [contains brilliant blue fcf (fd&c blue #1), fd&c blue #2 (indigotine), fd&c red #40]
Zenzedi: 20 mg [contains brilliant blue fcf (fd&c blue #1)]
Zenzedi: 30 mg [contains fd&c yellow #10 (quinoline yellow)]
Generic: 5 mg, 10 mg

References

American Academy of Pediatrics, "ADHD: Clinical Practice Guideline for the Diagnosis, Evaluation, and Treatment of Attention-Deficit/Hyperactivity Disorder in Children and Adolescents," *Pediatrics*, 2011, 128(5):1007-22.

American Academy of Pediatrics/American Heart Association Clarification of Statement on Cardiovascular Evaluation and Monitoring of Children and Adolescents With Heart Disease Receiving Medications for ADHD; available at: http://americanheart.mediaroon.com/index.-php?s=43&item=422.

American College of Obstetricians and Gynecologists (ACOG) Committee Opinion: No. 479, "Methamphetamine Abuse in Women of Reproductive Age," *Obstet Gynecol*, 2011, 117(3):751-5.

August GP, Caprio S, Fennoy I, et al, "Prevention and Treatment of Pediatric Obesity: An Endocrine Society Clinical Practice Guideline Based on Expert Opinion," *J Clin Endocrinol Metab*, 2008, 93 (12):4576-99.

Cooper WO, Habel LA, Sox CM, et al, "ADHD Drugs and Serious Cardiovascular Events in Children and Young Adults," *N Engl J Med*, 2011, 365(20):1896-904.

Dopheide JA and Pliszka SR, "Attention-Deficit-Hyperactivity Disorder: An Update," *Pharmacotherapy*, 2009, 29(6):656-79.

Golub M, Costa L, Crofton K, et al, "NTP-CERHR Expert Panel Report on the Reproductive and Developmental Toxicity of Amphetamine and Methamphetamine," *Birth Defects Res B Dev Reprod Toxicol*, 2005, 74(6):471-584.

Gould MS, Walsh BT, Munfakh JL, et al, "Sudden Death and Use of Stimulant Medications in Youths," *Am J Psychiatry*, 2009, 166 (9):992-1001.

Habel LA, Cooper WO, Sox CM, et al, "ADHD Medications and Risk of Serious Cardiovascular Events in Young and Middle-Aged Adults," *JAMA*, 2011, 306(24):2673-83.

LaGasse LL, Derauf C, Smith LM, et al, "Prenatal Methamphetamine Exposure and Childhood Behavior Problems at 3 and 5 Years of Age," *Pediatrics*, 2012, 129(4):681-8.

Mason PW, Krawiecki N, and Meacham LR, "The Use of Dextroamphetamine to Treat Obesity and Hyperphagia in Children Treated for Craniopharyngioma," *Arch Pediatr Adolesc Med*, 2002, 156 (9):887-92.

Pliszka S and AACAP Work Group on Quality Issues, "Practice Parameter for the Assessment and Treatment of Children and Adolescents With Attention-Deficit/Hyperactivity Disorder," *J Am Acad Child Adolesc Psychiatry*, 2007, 46(7):894-921.

Vetter VL, Elia J, Erickson C, et al, "Cardiovascular Monitoring of Children and Adolescents With Heart Disease Receiving Stimulant Drugs: A Scientific Statement From the American Heart Association Council on Cardiovascular Disease in the Young Congenital Cardiac Defects Committee and the Council on Cardiovascular Nursing," *Circulation*, 2008, 117(18):2407-23.

Dextroamphetamine and Amphetamine
(deks troe am FET a meen & am FET a meen)

Medication Safety Issues
Sound-alike/look-alike issues:
Adderall may be confused with Inderal

Related Information
Dextroamphetamine *on page 629*
Oral Medications That Should Not Be Crushed or Altered *on page 2438*

Brand Names: U.S. Adderall; Adderall XR
Brand Names: Canada Adderall XR
Therapeutic Category Amphetamine; Anorexiant; Central Nervous System Stimulant
Generic Availability (U.S.) Yes

Use
Immediate release tablets (Adderall®): Treatment of attention-deficit/hyperactivity disorder (ADHD) (FDA approved in ages ≥3 years and adults); treatment of narcolepsy (FDA approved in ages ≥6 years and adults)
Extended release capsules (Adderall XR®): Treatment of attention-deficit/hyperactivity disorder (ADHD) (FDA approved in ages ≥6 years and adults)

Medication Guide Available Yes
Pregnancy Risk Factor C
Pregnancy Considerations Adverse effects have been observed in animal reproduction studies. The majority of human data is based on illicit amphetamine/methamphetamine exposure and not from therapeutic maternal use (Golub, 2005). Use of amphetamines during pregnancy may lead to an increased risk of premature birth and low birth weight; newborns may experience symptoms of withdrawal. Behavioral problems may also occur later in childhood (LaGasse, 2012).

Breast-Feeding Considerations The majority of human data is based on illicit amphetamine/methamphetamine exposure and not from therapeutic maternal use (Golub, 2005). Amphetamines are excreted into breast milk and use may decrease milk production. Increased irritability, agitation, and crying have been reported in nursing infants (ACOG, 2011). A case report describes maternal use of amphetamine 20 mg/day throughout pregnancy and while breast-feeding. Milk concentrations were higher in breast milk than the maternal serum. The milk/plasma ratio ranged from 2.8-7.5 when measured on days 10 and 42 following delivery (Steiner, 1984). The manufacturer recommends that mothers taking dextroamphetamine/amphetamine refrain from nursing.

Contraindications Hypersensitivity or idiosyncrasy to dextroamphetamine, amphetamine, sympathomimetic amines, or any component; advanced arteriosclerosis, moderate to severe hypertension, symptomatic cardiovascular disease, hyperthyroidism, glaucoma, agitated states, history of drug abuse; concurrent use or use within 14 days of MAO inhibitors (hypertensive crisis may occur)

Warnings Serious cardiovascular events including sudden death may occur in patients with preexisting structural cardiac abnormalities or other serious heart problems. Sudden death has been reported in children and adolescents; sudden death, stroke, and MI have been reported in adults. Avoid the use of amphetamines in patients with known serious structural cardiac abnormalities, cardiomyopathy, serious heart rhythm abnormalities, coronary artery disease, or other serious cardiac problems that could place patients at an increased risk to the sympathomimetic effects of amphetamines. Patients should be carefully evaluated for cardiac disease prior to initiation of therapy. The American Heart Association recommends that all children diagnosed with ADHD who may be candidates for medication, such as dextroamphetamine and amphetamine, should have a thorough cardiovascular assessment prior to initiation of therapy. This assessment should include a combination of medical history, family history, and physical examination focusing on cardiovascular disease risk factors. An ECG is not mandatory but should be considered. If a child displays symptoms of cardiovascular disease, including chest pain, dyspnea, or fainting, parents should seek immediate medical care for the child. In a recent retrospective study on the possible association between stimulant medication use and sudden death in children, 564 previously healthy children who died suddenly in motor vehicle accidents were compared to a group of 564 previously healthy children who died suddenly. Two of the 564 (0.4%) children in motor vehicle accidents were taking stimulant medications compared to 10 of 564 (1.8%) children who died suddenly. While the authors of this study conclude there may be an association between stimulant use and sudden death in children, there were a number of limitations to the study and the FDA cannot conclude this information impacts the overall risk: benefit profile of these medications (Gould, 2009). In a large retrospective cohort study involving 1,200,438 children and young adults (aged 2-24 years), none of the currently available stimulant medications or atomoxetine were shown to increase the risk of serious cardiovascular events (ie, acute MI, sudden cardiac death, or stroke) in current (adjusted hazard ratio: 0.75; 95% CI: 0.31-1.85) or former (adjusted hazard ratio: 1.03; 95% CI: 0.57-1.89) users compared to nonusers. It should be noted that due to the upper limit of the 95% CI, the study could not rule out a doubling of the risk, albeit low (Cooper, 2011).

Stimulant medications may increase blood pressure (average increase 2-4 mm Hg) and heart rate (average increase 3-6 bpm); some patients may experience greater increases; use stimulant medications with caution in patients with hypertension and other cardiovascular conditions that may be exacerbated by increases in blood pressure or heart rate. Use is contraindicated in patients with moderate to severe hypertension.

Psychiatric adverse events may occur. Stimulants may exacerbate symptoms of behavior disturbance and thought disorder in patients with preexisting psychosis. New-onset psychosis or mania may occur with stimulant use in patients without a prior history of psychotic illness or mania, even at standard doses. Stimulants may induce mixed/manic episode in patients with bipolar disorder; patients should be screened for bipolar disorder prior to treatment; consider discontinuation if such symptoms (eg, delusional thinking, hallucinations, or mania) occur. May be associated with aggressive behavior or hostility (causal relationship not established); monitor for development or worsening of these behaviors.

Long-term effects in pediatric patients have not been determined. Use of stimulants in children has been associated with growth suppression; monitor growth; treatment interruption may be needed. Appetite suppression may occur; monitor weight during therapy, particularly in children. Stimulants may lower seizure threshold leading to new onset or breakthrough seizure activity; use with caution in patients with a history of seizure disorder.

Amphetamines possess a high potential for abuse **[U.S. Boxed Warning]**; misuse may cause sudden death and serious cardiovascular adverse events **[U.S. Boxed Warning]**; prolonged administration may lead to drug dependence; abrupt discontinuation following high doses or for prolonged periods may result in symptoms of withdrawal; avoid abrupt discontinuation in patients who have received amphetamines for prolonged periods. Amphetamines may impair the ability to engage in potentially hazardous activities. May exacerbate motor and phonic tics and Tourette's syndrome. Visual disturbances (difficulty in accommodation and blurred vision) have been reported.

Precautions Use with caution in patients receiving other sympathomimetic agents. Prescribe or dispense least amount feasible to minimize chance of overdose.

Adverse Reactions

As reported with Adderall XR:

Cardiovascular: Palpitation, tachycardia (adults)

Central nervous system: Agitation (adults), anxiety (adults), dizziness, drowsiness, emotional lability, headache (adults), insomnia, nervousness, speech disturbance

Dermatologic: Diaphoresis, skin photosensitivity

Endocrine & metabolic: Decreased libido, dysmenorrhea

Gastrointestinal: Abdominal pain, anorexia, constipation, decreased appetite, diarrhea, dyspepsia, nausea, teeth clenching, vomiting, weight loss, xerostomia

Genitourinary: Impotence, urinary tract infection

Infection: Increased susceptibility to infection, tooth infection

Neuromuscular & skeletal: Twitching

Respiratory: Dyspnea

Miscellaneous: Fever

Rare but important or life-threatening: Alopecia, anaphylaxis, angioedema, anorexia, cardiomyopathy, cerebrovascular accident, depression, dyskinesia, dysphoria, euphoria, frequent erections, Gilles de la Tourette's syndrome, hypertension, motor tics (exacerbation), mydriasis, myocardial infarction, prolonged erections, psychosis, Raynaud's phenomenon, seizure, Steven-Johnson syndrome, toxic epidermal necrolysis, vocal tics (exacerbation)

Drug Interactions

Metabolism/Transport Effects Refer to individual components.

Avoid Concomitant Use

Avoid concomitant use of Dextroamphetamine and Amphetamine with any of the following: Iobenguane I 123; MAO Inhibitors

Increased Effect/Toxicity

Dextroamphetamine and Amphetamine may increase the levels/effects of: Analgesics (Opioid); Sympathomimetics

The levels/effects of Dextroamphetamine and Amphetamine may be increased by: Alkalinizing Agents; Antacids; AtoMOXetine; Cannabinoid-Containing Products; Carbonic Anhydrase Inhibitors; Linezolid; MAO Inhibitors; Proton Pump Inhibitors; Tricyclic Antidepressants

Decreased Effect

Dextroamphetamine and Amphetamine may decrease the levels/effects of: Antihistamines; Ethosuximide; Iobenguane I 123; Ioflupane I 123; PHENobarbital; Phenytoin

The levels/effects of Dextroamphetamine and Amphetamine may be decreased by: Ammonium Chloride; Antipsychotics; Ascorbic Acid; Gastrointestinal Acidifying Agents; Lithium; Methenamine; Multivitamins/Fluoride (with ADE); Multivitamins/Minerals (with ADEK, Folate, Iron); Multivitamins/Minerals (with AE, No Iron); Peginterferon Alfa-2b; Urinary Acidifying Agents

Food Interactions Amphetamine serum levels may be reduced if taken with acidic food, juices, or vitamin C. Management: Monitor response when taken concurrently.

Stability

Immediate release tablets (Adderall®): Store at 20°C to 25°C (68°F to 77°F); dispense in tight, light-resistant container

Extended release capsules (Adderall XR®): Store at 25°C (77°F); excursions permitted to 15°C to 30°C (59°F to 86°F); dispense in tight, light-resistant container

Mechanism of Action Amphetamines are noncatecholamine, sympathomimetic amines that promote release of catecholamines (primarily dopamine and norepinephrine) from their storage sites in the presynaptic nerve terminals. A less significant mechanism may include their ability to block the reuptake of catecholamines by competitive inhibition.

Pharmacodynamics Oral:

Onset of action: Tablet: 30-60 minutes

Duration: Tablet: 4-6 hours

Pharmacokinetics (Adult data unless noted)

Absorption: Oral: Well-absorbed

Distribution: V_d: 3.5-4.6 L/kg; distributes into CNS, mean CSF concentrations are 80% of plasma

Metabolism: Hepatic via cytochrome P450 mono-oxygenase and glucuronidation; two active metabolites (norephedrine and 4-hydroxyamphetamine) are formed via oxidation

Half-life:
d-amphetamine:
Children 6-12 years: 9 hours
Adolescents 13-17 years: 11 hours
Adults: 10 hours
l-amphetamine:
Children 6-12 years: 11 hours
Adolescents 13-17 years: 13-14 hours
Adults: 13 hours
Time to peak serum concentration:
Tablet (immediate release): 3 hours
Capsule (extended release): 7 hours
Elimination: 70% of a single dose is eliminated within 24 hours; excreted as unchanged amphetamine (30%), benzoic acid, hydroxyamphetamine, hippuric acid, norephedrine and p-hydroxynorephedrine; **Note:** Urinary recovery of amphetamine is highly dependent on urine flow rates and urinary pH; urinary recovery of amphetamine may range from 1% in alkaline urine to 75% in acidic urine
Clearance: Children have a higher clearance (on a mg/kg basis) than adolescents and adults

Dosing: Usual Note: Use lowest effective individualized dose; administer first dose as soon as awake

Children and Adolescents:
Attention-deficit/hyperactivity disorder:
Immediate release tablets:
Children 3-5 years: Oral: Initial 2.5 mg daily given every morning; increase daily dose by 2.5 mg at weekly intervals until optimal response is obtained; maximum daily dose: 40 mg/**day** given in 1-2 divided doses per day; use intervals of 4-6 hours between doses. **Note:** Select patients may require daily dose to be given in 3 divided doses per day. Although FDA approved, current guidelines do not recommend dextroamphetamine/amphetamine use in children ≤5 years due to insufficient evidence (AAP, 2011).
Children ≥6 years and Adolescents: Oral: Initial: 5 mg once or twice daily; increase daily dose by 5 mg at weekly intervals until optimal response is obtained; usual maximum dose: 40 mg/**day** given in 1-2 divided doses per day; use intervals of 4-6 hours between doses; in patients >50 kg a maximum daily dose of 60 mg/**day** in divided doses has been used (Dopheide, 2009; Pliszka, 2007). **Note:** Select patients may require daily dose to be given in 3 divided doses per day.
Extended release capsules: **Note:** Patients taking divided doses of immediate release tablets may be switched to extended release capsule using the same total daily dose (taken once daily); titrate dose at weekly intervals to achieve optimal response.
Children 6-12 years: Oral: Initial: 5-10 mg daily given every morning; increase daily dose by 5 mg or 10 mg at weekly intervals until optimal response is obtained; usual maximum daily dose: 30 mg/**day**; in patients >50 kg a maximum daily dose of 60 mg/**day** has been used (Dopheide, 2009; Pliszka, 2007)
Adolescents 13-17 years: Oral: Initial: 10 mg daily given every morning; may increase to 20 mg daily after 1 week if symptoms are not controlled; usual maximum daily dose: 20 mg/**day**; in patients >50 kg a maximum daily dose of 60 mg/**day** has been used (Dopheide, 2009; Pliszka, 2007)

Narcolepsy:
Children 6-12 years: Immediate release tablets: Oral: Initial: 5 mg daily; increase daily dose by 5 mg at weekly intervals until optimal response is obtained; maximum daily dose: 60 mg/**day** given in 1-3 divided doses per day; use intervals of 4-6 hours between doses

Adolescents: Immediate release tablets: Oral: Initial: 10 mg daily; increase daily dose by 10 mg at weekly intervals until optimal response is obtained; maximum daily dose: 60 mg/**day** given in 1-3 divided doses per day; use intervals of 4-6 hours between doses

Adults:
Attention-deficit/hyperactivity disorder:
Immediate release tablets: Oral: Initial: 5 mg once or twice daily; increase daily dose in 5 mg increments at weekly intervals until optimal response is obtained; usual maximum dose: 40 mg/**day** given in 1-3 divided doses per day; use intervals of 4-6 hours between doses
Extended release capsules: Oral: Initial: 20 mg once daily in the morning; higher doses (up to 60 mg once daily) have been evaluated; however, there is not adequate evidence that higher doses provide additional benefit. **Note:** Patients taking divided doses of immediate release tablets may be switched to extended release capsule using the same total daily dose (taken once daily); titrate dose at weekly intervals to achieve optimal response.
Narcolepsy: Immediate release tablets: Oral: Initial: 10 mg daily; increase daily dose by 10 mg at weekly intervals until optimal response is obtained; maximum daily dose: 60 mg/**day** given in 1-3 divided doses per day; use intervals of 4-6 hours between doses
Dosage adjustment in renal impairment: No dosage adjustments provided in the manufacturer's labeling; use with caution; elimination may be decreased with renal impairment.
Dosage adjustment in hepatic impairment: No dosage adjustments provided in the manufacturer's labeling; use with caution; elimination may be decreased with hepatic impairment.

Administration
Immediate release tablet: To avoid insomnia, last daily dose should be administered no less than 6 hours before retiring
Extended release capsule: Avoid afternoon doses to prevent insomnia. Swallow capsule whole; do not chew or divide. May be administered with or without food. May open capsule and sprinkle contents on applesauce; consume applesauce/medication mixture immediately; do not store; do not chew sprinkled beads from capsule
Monitoring Parameters Evaluate patients for cardiac disease prior to initiation of therapy with thorough medical history, family history, and physical exam; consider ECG; perform ECG and echocardiogram if findings suggest cardiac disease; promptly conduct cardiac evaluation in patients who develop chest pain, unexplained syncope, or any other symptom of cardiac disease during treatment. Monitor CNS activity, blood pressure, heart rate, sleep, appetite, abnormal movements, height, weight, BMI, growth in children. Patients should be re-evaluated at appropriate intervals to assess continued need of the medication. Observe for signs/symptoms of aggression or hostility, or depression. Monitor for visual disturbances.
Test Interactions May interfere with urinary steroid testing
Additional Information Treatment of ADHD should include "drug holidays" or periodic discontinuation of medication in order to assess the patient's requirements, decrease tolerance, and limit suppression of linear growth and weight. Medications used to treat ADHD should be part of a total treatment program that may include other components such as psychological, educational, and social measures. The combination of equal parts of d, l-amphetamine aspartate, d, l-amphetamine sulfate, dextroamphetamine saccharate and dextroamphetamine sulfate results in a 3:1 ratio of the dextro- and levo-isomers of amphetamine.

The duration of action of Adderall® is longer than methylphenidate; behavioral effects of a single morning dose of Adderall® may last throughout the school day; a single morning dose of Adderall® has been shown in several studies to be as effective as twice daily dosing of methylphenidate for the treatment of ADHD (Manos, 1999; Pelham, 1999; Pliszka, 2000).

Controlled Substance C-II

Dosage Forms Excipient information presented when available (limited, particularly for generics); consult specific product labeling.

Capsule, extended release, oral:

5 mg [dextroamphetamine sulfate 1.25 mg, dextroamphetamine saccharate 1.25 mg, amphetamine aspartate monohydrate 1.25 mg, amphetamine sulfate 1.25 mg (equivalent to amphetamine base 3.1 mg)]

10 mg [dextroamphetamine sulfate 2.5 mg, dextroamphetamine saccharate 2.5 mg, amphetamine aspartate monohydrate 2.5 mg, amphetamine sulfate 2.5 mg (equivalent to amphetamine base 6.3 mg)]

15 mg [dextroamphetamine sulfate 3.75 mg, dextroamphetamine saccharate 3.75 mg, amphetamine aspartate monohydrate 3.75 mg, amphetamine sulfate 3.75 mg (equivalent to amphetamine base 9.4 mg)]

20 mg [dextroamphetamine sulfate 5 mg, dextroamphetamine saccharate 5 mg, amphetamine aspartate monohydrate 5 mg, amphetamine sulfate 5 mg (equivalent to amphetamine base 12.5 mg)]

25 mg [dextroamphetamine sulfate 6.25 mg, dextroamphetamine saccharate 6.25 mg, amphetamine aspartate monohydrate 6.25 mg, amphetamine sulfate 6.25 mg (equivalent to amphetamine base 15.6 mg)]

30 mg [dextroamphetamine sulfate 7.5 mg, dextroamphetamine saccharate 7.5 mg, amphetamine aspartate monohydrate 7.5 mg, amphetamine sulfate 7.5 mg (equivalent to amphetamine base 18.8 mg)]

Adderall XR

5 mg [dextroamphetamine sulfate 1.25 mg, dextroamphetamine saccharate 1.25 mg, amphetamine aspartate monohydrate 1.25 mg, amphetamine sulfate 1.25 mg (equivalent to amphetamine base 3.1 mg)]

10 mg [dextroamphetamine sulfate 2.5 mg, dextroamphetamine saccharate 2.5 mg, amphetamine aspartate monohydrate 2.5 mg, amphetamine sulfate 2.5 mg (equivalent to amphetamine base 6.3 mg)]

15 mg [dextroamphetamine sulfate 3.75 mg, dextroamphetamine saccharate 3.75 mg, amphetamine aspartate monohydrate 3.75 mg, amphetamine sulfate 3.75 mg (equivalent to amphetamine base 9.4 mg)]

20 mg [dextroamphetamine sulfate 5 mg, dextroamphetamine saccharate 5 mg, amphetamine aspartate monohydrate 5 mg, amphetamine sulfate 5 mg (equivalent to amphetamine base 12.5 mg)]

25 mg [dextroamphetamine sulfate 6.25 mg, dextroamphetamine saccharate 6.25 mg, amphetamine aspartate monohydrate 6.25 mg, amphetamine sulfate 6.25 mg (equivalent to amphetamine base 15.6 mg)]

30 mg [dextroamphetamine sulfate 7.5 mg, dextroamphetamine saccharate 7.5 mg, amphetamine aspartate monohydrate 7.5 mg, amphetamine sulfate 7.5 mg (equivalent to amphetamine base 18.8 mg)]

Tablet, oral:

5 mg [dextroamphetamine sulfate 1.25 mg, dextroamphetamine saccharate 1.25 mg, amphetamine aspartate monohydrate 1.25 mg, amphetamine sulfate 1.25 mg (equivalent to amphetamine base 3.13 mg)]

7.5 mg [dextroamphetamine 1.875 mg, dextroamphetamine saccharate 1.875 mg, amphetamine aspartate monohydrate 1.875 mg, amphetamine sulfate 1.875 mg (equivalent to amphetamine base 4.7 mg)]

10 mg [dextroamphetamine sulfate 2.5 mg, dextroamphetamine saccharate 2.5 mg, amphetamine aspartate

monohydrate 2.5 mg, amphetamine sulfate 2.5 mg (equivalent to amphetamine base 6.3 mg)]

12.5 mg [dextroamphetamine sulfate 3.125 mg, dextroamphetamine saccharate 3.125 mg, amphetamine aspartate monohydrate 3.125 mg, amphetamine sulfate 3.125 mg (equivalent to amphetamine base 7.8 mg)]

15 mg [dextroamphetamine sulfate 3.75 mg, dextroamphetamine saccharate 3.75 mg, amphetamine aspartate monohydrate 3.75 mg, amphetamine sulfate 3.75 mg (equivalent to amphetamine base 9.4 mg)]

20 mg [dextroamphetamine sulfate 5 mg, dextroamphetamine saccharate 5 mg, amphetamine aspartate monohydrate 5 mg, amphetamine sulfate 5 mg (equivalent to amphetamine base 12.6 mg)]

30 mg [dextroamphetamine sulfate 7.5 mg, dextroamphetamine saccharate 7.5 mg, amphetamine aspartate monohydrate 7.5 mg, amphetamine sulfate 7.5 mg (equivalent to amphetamine base 18.8 mg)]

Adderall:

5 mg [dextroamphetamine sulfate 1.25 mg, dextroamphetamine saccharate 1.25 mg, amphetamine aspartate monohydrate 1.25 mg, amphetamine sulfate 1.25 mg (equivalent to amphetamine base 3.13 mg)]

7.5 mg [dextroamphetamine sulfate 1.875 mg, dextroamphetamine saccharate 1.875 mg, amphetamine aspartate monohydrate 1.875 mg, amphetamine sulfate 1.875 mg (equivalent to amphetamine base 4.7 mg)]

10 mg [dextroamphetamine sulfate 2.5 mg, dextroamphetamine saccharate 2.5 mg, amphetamine aspartate monohydrate 2.5 mg, amphetamine sulfate 2.5 mg (equivalent to amphetamine base 6.3 mg)]

12.5 mg [dextroamphetamine sulfate 3.125 mg, dextroamphetamine saccharate 3.125 mg, amphetamine aspartate monohydrate 3.125 mg, amphetamine sulfate 3.125 mg (equivalent to amphetamine base 7.8 mg)]

15 mg [dextroamphetamine sulfate 3.75 mg, dextroamphetamine saccharate 3.75 mg, amphetamine aspartate monohydrate 3.75 mg, amphetamine sulfate 3.75 mg (equivalent to amphetamine base 9.4 mg)]

20 mg [dextroamphetamine sulfate 5 mg, dextroamphetamine saccharate 5 mg, amphetamine aspartate monohydrate 5 mg, amphetamine sulfate 5 mg (equivalent to amphetamine base 12.6 mg)]

30 mg [dextroamphetamine sulfate 7.5 mg, dextroamphetamine saccharate 7.5 mg, amphetamine aspartate monohydrate 7.5 mg, amphetamine sulfate 7.5 mg (equivalent to amphetamine base 18.8 mg)]

Extemporaneous Preparations A 1 mg/mL oral suspension may be made with tablets. Crush ten 10 mg tablets in a mortar and reduce to a fine powder. Add small portions of Ora-Sweet and mix to a uniform paste; mix while adding the vehicle in equal proportions to **almost** 100 mL; transfer to a calibrated bottle, rinse mortar with vehicle, and add sufficient quantity of vehicle to make 100 mL. Label "shake well". Stable 30 days at room temperature.

Justice J, Kupiec TC, Matthews P, et al, "Stability of Adderall in Extemporaneously Compounded Oral Liquids," *Am J Health Syst Pharm*, 2001, 58(15):1418-21.

References

American Academy of Pediatrics/American Heart Association Clarification of Statement on Cardiovascular Evaluation and Monitoring of Children and Adolescents With Heart Disease Receiving Medications for ADHD; available at: http://americanheart.mediaroon.com/index.-php?s=43&item=422.

American College of Obstetricians and Gynecologists Committee on Health Care for Underserved Women, "Committee Opinion No. 479: Methamphetamine Abuse in Women of Reproductive Age," *Obstet Gynecol*, 2011, 117(3):751-5.

Cooper WO, Habel LA, Sox CM, et al, "ADHD Drugs and Serious Cardiovascular Events in Children and Young Adults," *N Engl J Med*, 2011, 365(20):1896-904.

Dopheide JA and Pliszka SR, "Attention-Deficit-Hyperactivity Disorder: An Update," *Pharmacotherapy*, 2009, 29(6):656-79.

Golub M, Costa L, Crofton K, et al, "NTP-CERHR Expert Panel Report on the Reproductive and Developmental Toxicity of Amphetamine and Methamphetamine," *Birth Defects Res B Dev Reprod Toxicol*, 2005, 74(6):471-584.

Gould MS, Walsh BT, Munfakh JL, et al, "Sudden Death and Use of Stimulant Medications in Youths," *Am J Psychiatry*, 2009, 166 (9):992-1001.

LaGasse LL, Derauf C, Smith LM, et al, "Prenatal Methamphetamine Exposure and Childhood Behavior Problems at 3 and 5 Years of Age," *Pediatrics*, 2012, 129(4):681-8.

Manos MJ, Short EJ, and Findling RL, "Differential Effectiveness of Methylphenidate and Adderall® in School-Age Youths With Attention-Deficit/Hyperactivity Disorder," *J Am Acad Child Adolesc Psychiatry*, 1999, 38(7):813-9.

Pelham WE, Gnagy EM, Chronis AM, et al, "A Comparison of Morning-Only and Morning/Late Afternoon Adderall to Morning-Only, Twice-Daily, and Three Times-Daily Methylphenidate in Children With Attention-Deficit/Hyperactivity Disorder," *Pediatrics*, 1999, 104(6):1300-11.

Pliszka S and AACAP Work Group on Quality Issues, "Practice Parameter for the Assessment and Treatment of Children and Adolescents With Attention-Deficit/Hyperactivity Disorder," *J Am Acad Child Adolesc Psychiatry*, 2007, 46(7):894-921.

Pliszka SR, Browne RG, Olvera RL, et al, "A Double-Blind, Placebo-Controlled Study of Adderall® and Methylphenidate in the Treatment of Attention-Deficit/Hyperactivity Disorder," *J Am Acad Child Adolesc Psychiatry*, 2000, 39(5):619-26.

Steiner E, Villén T, Hallberg M, et al, "Amphetamine Secretion in Breast Milk," *Eur J Clin Pharmacol*, 1984, 27(1):123-4.

Swanson JM, Wigal S, Greenhill LL, et al, "Analog Classroom Assessment of Adderall® in Children With ADHD," *J Am Acad Child Adolesc Psychiatry*, 1998, 37(5):519-26.

Vetter VL, Elia J, Erickson C, et al, "Cardiovascular Monitoring of Children and Adolescents With Heart Disease Receiving Stimulant Drugs: A Scientific Statement From the American Heart Association Council on Cardiovascular Disease in the Young Congenital Cardiac Defects Committee and the Council on Cardiovascular Nursing," *Circulation*, 2008, 117(18):2407-23.

◆ **Dextroamphetamine Sulfate** *see* Dextroamphetamine *on page 629*

Dextromethorphan (deks troe meth OR fan)

Medication Safety Issues
Sound-alike/look-alike issues:
Benylin may be confused with Benadryl, Ventolin
Delsym may be confused with Delfen, Desyrel

Brand Names: U.S. Cough DM [OTC]; Creomulsion Adult [OTC]; Creomulsion for Children [OTC]; Delsym [OTC]; ElixSure Cough [OTC]; Hold [OTC]; Little Colds Cough Formula [OTC]; Nycoff [OTC]; PediaCare Childrens Long-Act [OTC]; Robafen Cough [OTC]; Robitussin Childrens Cough LA [OTC]; Robitussin CoughGels [OTC]; Robitussin Lingering CoughGels [OTC]; Robitussin Lingering LA Cough [OTC]; Robitussin Maximum Strength [OTC]; Scot-Tussin Diabetes CF [OTC]; Silphen DM Cough [OTC]; Simply Cough [OTC]; Triaminic Long Acting Cough [OTC]; Trocal Cough Suppressant [OTC]; Vicks Nature Fusion Cough [OTC]

Therapeutic Category Antitussive; Cough Preparation

Generic Availability (U.S.) May be product dependent

Use Symptomatic relief of coughs caused by minor viral upper respiratory tract infections or inhaled irritants

Pregnancy Considerations Maternal use of standard OTC doses of dextromethorphan when used as an antitussive during the first trimester of pregnancy has not been found to increase the risk of teratogenic effects. Dextromethorphan is metabolized in the liver via CYP2D6 and CYP3A enzymes. The activity of both enzymes is increased in the mother during pregnancy. In the fetus, CYP2D6 activity is low in the fetal liver and CYP3A4 activity is present by ~17 weeks gestation.

Contraindications Hypersensitivity to dextromethorphan or any component; concurrent administration with or within 14 days of discontinuing an MAO inhibitor

Warnings Do not use for persistent or chronic cough, or for cough accompanied by excessive secretions; Creo-Terpin® contains tartrazine which may cause allergic

reactions in susceptible individuals; some products may contain sodium benzoate which may cause allergic reactions in susceptible individuals; sodium benzoate has been associated with a potentially fatal toxicity ("gasping syndrome") in neonates; *in vitro* and animal studies have shown that benzoate, a metabolite of benzyl alcohol, displaces bilirubin from protein binding sites; avoid use of products containing sodium benzoate in neonates. Serotonin syndrome may occur when administered with concomitant proserotonergic drugs (ie, SSRIs/SNRIs or triptans); especially with higher dextromethorphan doses.

Precautions Anecdotal reports of abuse of dextromethorphan-containing cough/cold products have increased, especially among teenagers. Healthcare providers should be alert to problems of abuse or misuse as abuse can cause death, brain damage, seizure, loss of consciousness, and irregular heartbeat.

Adverse Reactions Central nervous system: Confusion, excitement, irritability, nervousness, serotonin syndrome

Drug Interactions
Metabolism/Transport Effects Substrate of CYP2B6 (minor), CYP2C19 (minor), CYP2C9 (minor), CYP2D6 (major), CYP2E1 (minor), CYP3A4 (minor); **Note:** Assignment of Major/Minor substrate status based on clinically relevant drug interaction potential; **Inhibits** CYP2D6 (weak)

Avoid Concomitant Use
Avoid concomitant use of Dextromethorphan with any of the following: MAO Inhibitors

Increased Effect/Toxicity
Dextromethorphan may increase the levels/effects of: Antipsychotics; ARIPiprazole; Metoclopramide; Serotonin Modulators

The levels/effects of Dextromethorphan may be increased by: Abiraterone Acetate; Antiemetics (5HT3 Antagonists); Antipsychotics; CYP2D6 Inhibitors (Moderate); CYP2D6 Inhibitors (Strong); Darunavir; MAO Inhibitors; QuiNIDine; Selective Serotonin Reuptake Inhibitors

Decreased Effect
The levels/effects of Dextromethorphan may be decreased by: Peginterferon Alfa-2b

Mechanism of Action Decreases the sensitivity of cough receptors and interrupts cough impulse transmission by depressing the medullary cough center through sigma receptor stimulation; structurally related to codeine

Pharmacodynamics
Onset of antitussive action: Within 15-30 minutes
Duration: Up to 6 hours

Pharmacokinetics (Adult data unless noted)
Metabolism: In the liver
Half-Life: 1.4-3.9 hours
Time to peak serum concentration: 2-2.5 hours
Elimination: Principally in urine

Dosing: Usual Dosage in children <4 years of age is not well established; Oral:
Children:
1-3 months: 0.5-1 mg every 6-8 hours
3-6 months: 1-2 mg every 6-8 hours
7 months to 1 year: 2-4 mg every 6-8 hours
≥2-6 years: 2.5-7.5 mg every 4-8 hours; extended release formulation: 15 mg twice daily (maximum: 30 mg/24 hours)
7-12 years: 5-10 mg every 4 hours or 15 mg every 6-8 hours; extended release formulation: 30 mg twice daily (maximum: 60 mg/24 hours)
Children >12 years and Adults: 10-30 mg every 4-8 hours or extended release formulation: 60 mg twice daily (maximum: 120 mg/24 hours)

Administration Oral: May administer without regard to meals

Monitoring Parameters Cough, mental status

Test Interactions False-positive phencyclidine, opioids and heroin urine drug screen

Additional Information Dextromethorphan 15-30 mg equals 8-15 mg codeine as an antitussive

Dosage Forms Excipient information presented when available (limited, particularly for generics); consult specific product labeling.

Capsule, Oral, as hydrobromide:
  Robafen Cough: 15 mg [contains brilliant blue fcf (fd&c blue #1), fd&c red #40]
  Robitussin CoughGels: 15 mg [contains brilliant blue fcf (fd&c blue #1)]
  Robitussin Lingering CoughGels: 15 mg [contains brilliant blue fcf (fd&c blue #1), fd&c red #40, polyethylene glycol, propylene glycol]

Gel, Oral, as hydrobromide:
  ElixSure Cough: 7.5 mg/5 mL (120 mL) [alcohol free; contains carbomer 934p, propylene glycol, propylparaben; cherry bubblegum flavor]

Liquid, Oral, as hydrobromide:
  Little Colds Cough Formula: 7.5 mg/mL (30 mL) [alcohol free, dye free, saccharin free; contains sodium benzoate; grape flavor]
  PediaCare Childrens Long-Act: 7.5 mg/5 mL (118 mL) [contains brilliant blue fcf (fd&c blue #1), saccharin sodium, sodium benzoate]
  Robitussin Lingering LA Cough: 15 mg/5 mL (118 mL) [contains alcohol, usp, fd&c red #40, menthol, saccharin sodium, sodium benzoate]
  Scot-Tussin Diabetes CF: 10 mg/5 mL (118.3 mL, 480 mL, 3780 mL) [alcohol free, dye free, fructose free, sodium free, sorbitol free, sugar free]
  Triaminic Long Acting Cough: 7.5 mg/5 mL (118 mL) [alcohol free, dye free, pseudoephedrine free; contains benzoic acid, propylene glycol]
  Vicks Nature Fusion Cough: 15 mg/15 mL (236 mL) [alcohol free, dye free, gluten free; contains polyethylene glycol, propylene glycol; honey flavor]

Liquid Extended Release, Oral:
  Cough DM: 30 mg/5 mL (89 mL) [alcohol free; contains fd&c yellow #10 aluminum lake, methylparaben, polysorbate 80, propylparaben, sodium metabisulfite; orange flavor]
  Delsym: 30 mg/5 mL (89 mL, 148 mL) [alcohol free; contains brilliant blue fcf (fd&c blue #1), disodium edta, methylparaben, polyethylene glycol, polysorbate 80, propylene glycol, propylparaben; grape flavor]
  Delsym: 30 mg/5 mL (89 mL, 148 mL) [alcohol free; contains edetate disodium, fd&c yellow #6 (sunset yellow), methylparaben, polyethylene glycol, polysorbate 80, propylene glycol, propylparaben; orange flavor]
  Generic: 30 mg/5 mL (89 mL)

Lozenge, Mouth/Throat, as hydrobromide:
  Hold: 5 mg (10 ea)
  Hold: 5 mg (10 ea) [cherry flavor]
  Nycoff: 15 mg (500 ea)
  Trocal Cough Suppressant: 7.5 mg (1 ea) [cherry flavor]

Strip, Oral, as hydrobromide:
  Triaminic Long Acting Cough: 7.5 mg (14 ea, 16 ea) [contains alcohol, usp, fd&c red #40; cherry flavor]
  Triaminic Long Acting Cough: 7.5 mg (14 ea) [contains alcohol, usp, fd&c red #40, isopropyl alcohol]

Syrup, Oral, as hydrobromide:
  Creomulsion Adult: 20 mg/15 mL (118 mL)
  Creomulsion for Children: 5 mg/5 mL (118 mL) [cherry flavor]
  Robitussin Childrens Cough LA: 7.5 mg/5 mL (118 mL) [contains fd&c red #40, propylene glycol, saccharin sodium, sodium benzoate]
  Robitussin Maximum Strength: 15 mg/5 mL (118 mL) [contains alcohol, usp, fd&c red #40, menthol, saccharin sodium, sodium benzoate; pleasant-tasting flavor]

Silphen DM Cough: 10 mg/5 mL (118 mL) [contains alcohol, usp; strawberry flavor]
Simply Cough: 5 mg/5 mL (120 mL) [alcohol free; cherry-berry flavor]
Triaminic Long Acting Cough: 7.5 mg/5 mL (118 mL) [alcohol free, dye free; contains benzoic acid, edetate disodium, propylene glycol]

♦ **Dextromethorphan and Guaifenesin** *see* Guaifenesin and Dextromethorphan *on page 987*

Dextrose (DEKS trose)

Medication Safety Issues
Sound-alike/look-alike issues:
  Glutose™ may be confused with Glutofac®
High alert medication:
  The Institute for Safe Medication Practices (ISMP) includes this medication (hypertonic solutions ≥20%) among its list of drugs which have a heightened risk of causing significant patient harm when used in error.
Other safety concerns:
  Inappropriate use of low sodium or sodium-free intravenous fluids (eg D_5W, hypotonic saline) in pediatric patients can lead to significant morbidity and mortality due to hyponatremia (ISMP, 2009).

Related Information
  Management of Drug Extravasations *on page 2255*
  Pediatric Parenteral Nutrition *on page 2312*

Brand Names: U.S. Dextrose Thermoject System; Glucose Nursette [OTC]; Glutol [OTC]; Glutose 15 [OTC]; Glutose 45 [OTC]; Insta-Glucose [OTC]

Therapeutic Category Antidote, Insulin; Antidote, Oral Hypoglycemic; Fluid Replacement, Enteral; Fluid Replacement, Parenteral; Hyperglycemic Agent; Hyperkalemia, Adjunctive Treatment Agent; Intravenous Nutritional Therapy

Generic Availability (U.S.) May be product dependent

Use
I.V.:
  5% and 10% solutions: Peripheral infusion to provide calories and fluid replacement
  10% solution: Treatment of hypoglycemia in neonates
  25% (hypertonic) solution: Treatment of acute symptomatic episodes of hypoglycemia to restore depressed blood glucose levels; adjunctive treatment of hyperkalemia when combined with insulin (FDA approved in neonates and older infants)
  50% (hypertonic) solution: Treatment of insulin-induced hypoglycemia (hyperinsulinemia or insulin shock) and adjunctive treatment of hyperkalemia in adolescents and adults
  ≥10% solutions: Infusion after admixture with amino acids for nutritional support
  Oral: Treatment of hypoglycemia

Pregnancy Risk Factor C (injection, infusion)

Pregnancy Considerations In patients who require parenteral nutrition for treatment of hyperemesis gravidarum, dextrose is part of the parenteral nutrition regimen (ASPEN, 2002).

Contraindications Hypersensitivity to corn or corn products; diabetic coma with hyperglycemia; hypertonic solutions in patients with intracranial or intraspinal hemorrhage; patients with delirium tremens and dehydration; patients with anuria, hepatic coma, or glucose-galactose malabsorption syndrome

Warnings Hypertonic solutions (>10%) may cause thrombosis if infused via peripheral veins; administer hypertonic solutions via a central venous catheter; rapid administration of hypertonic solutions may produce significant hyperglycemia, glycosuria, and shifts in electrolytes; this may result in dehydration, hyperosmolar syndrome, coma, and death especially in patients with chronic uremia or carbohydrate intolerance; excessive or rapid dextrose administration in very low birth weight infants has been associated with increased serum osmolality and possible intracerebral hemorrhage; hyperglycemia and glycosuria may be functions of the rate of administration of dextrose; to minimize these effects, reduce the rate of infusion; addition of insulin may be necessary; administration of potassium free I.V. dextrose solutions may result in significant hypokalemia, particularly if highly concentrated dextrose solutions are used; add potassium to dextrose solutions for patients with adequate renal function; administration of low sodium or sodium free I.V. dextrose solutions may result in significant hyponatremia or water intoxication in pediatric patients; monitor serum sodium concentration; abrupt withdrawal of dextrose solution may be associated with rebound hypoglycemia; an unexpected rise in blood glucose level in an otherwise stable patient may be an early symptom of infection; glucose is not absorbed from the buccal cavity; it must be swallowed to be effective; do not use oral forms in unconscious patients

Parenteral dextrose solutions contain aluminum which may accumulate to toxic levels with prolonged administration particularly in patients with impaired renal function. Patients with impaired renal function including premature neonates who receive aluminum at >4-5 mcg/kg/day accumulate aluminum at levels associated with CNS and bone toxicity.

Precautions Use with caution in premature infants, especially very low birth weight infants, as rapid changes is osmolality may produce profound effects on the brain, including intraventricular hemorrhage; small incremental changes in infusion rates are necessary in these patients; use with caution also in patients with diabetes mellitus.

Adverse Reactions Note: Most adverse effects are associated with excessive dosage or rate of infusion.

Cardiovascular: Edema, dehydration, hyper-/hypovolemia, phlebitis, venous thrombosis

Central nervous system: Fever, hyperosmolar syndrome, mental confusion, unconsciousness

Endocrine & metabolic: Acidosis, hyperglycemia, hypokalemia, hypophosphatemia, hypomagnesemia

Genitourinary: Ketonuria, glycosuria, polyuria

Gastrointestinal: Diarrhea (oral), nausea, polydipsia

Local: Pain, tissue necrosis, vein irritation

Respiratory: Pulmonary edema, tachypnea

Drug Interactions

Metabolism/Transport Effects None known.

Avoid Concomitant Use There are no known interactions where it is recommended to avoid concomitant use.

Increased Effect/Toxicity There are no known significant interactions involving an increase in effect.

Decreased Effect There are no known significant interactions involving a decrease in effect.

Stability Stable at room temperature; protect from freezing and extreme heat; store oral dextrose in airtight containers

Mechanism of Action Dextrose, a monosaccharide, is a source of calories and fluid for patients unable to obtain an adequate oral intake; may decrease body protein and nitrogen losses; promotes glycogen deposition in the liver. When used in the treatment of hyperkalemia (combined with insulin), dextrose stimulates the uptake of potassium by cells, especially in muscle tissue, lowering serum potassium.

Pharmacodynamics

Onset of action: Treatment of hypoglycemia: Oral: 10 minutes

Maximum effect: Treatment of hyperkalemia: I.V.: 30 minutes

Pharmacokinetics (Adult data unless noted)

Absorption: Rapidly from the small intestine by an active mechanism

Metabolism: Metabolized to carbon dioxide and water

Time to peak serum concentration: Oral: 40 minutes

Dosing: Neonatal

Hypoglycemia: Note: Doses may be repeated in severe cases:

Age-directed dosing:

GA <34 weeks: I.V.: 0.1-0.2 g/kg/dose (1-2 mL/kg/dose of $D_{10}W$); followed by continuous I.V. infusion at a rate of 4-6 **mg**/kg/minute

GA ≥34 weeks: I.V.: 0.2 g/kg/dose (2 mL/kg/dose of $D_{10}W$) and/or a continuous I.V. infusion at a rate of 5-8 **mg**/kg/minute to maintain serum glucose concentration to maintain plasma glucose ≥40-50 mg/dL (Adamkin, 2011)

PALS Guidelines (PALS, 2010): I.V., I.O.: Newborns: 0.5-1 g/kg/dose (5-10 mL/kg/dose of $D_{10}W$)

Parenteral nutrition: I.V.: Dextrose component (ASPEN Guidelines, 2002; ASPEN Pediatric Nutrition Support Core Curriculum, 2010):

Preterm neonates: Initial:5-7 **mg**/kg/minute; daily increase: 1-2.5 **mg**/kg/minute or 1% to 2.5% increments; maximum: 18 **mg**/kg/minute

Term neonates: Initial: 6-9 **mg**/kg/minute; daily increase: 1-2 **mg**/kg/minute or 2.5% to 5% increments; maximum: 18 **mg**/kg/minute

Dosing: Usual

Hypoglycemia: Note: Doses may be repeated in severe cases:

Infants and Children:

PALS Guidelines (PALS, 2010): I.V., I.O.: Infants and Children: 0.5-1 g/kg/dose (2–4 mL/kg/dose of 25% solution)

Infants 1-6 months: I.V.: 0.25-0.5 g/kg/dose (1-2 mL/kg/dose of 25% solution; 2.5-5 mL/kg of 10% solution; 0.5-1 mL/kg of 50% solution); maximum: 25 g/dose

Infants >6 months and Children: I.V.: 0.5-1 g/kg/dose (2-4 mL/kg/dose of 25% solution; 5-10 mL/kg of 10% solution; 1-2 mL/kg of 50% solution); maximum: 25 g/dose

Children >2 years: Oral: 10-20 g as single dose; repeat in 10 minutes if necessary

Adolescents and Adults:

PALS Guidelines (PALS, 2010): I.V., I.O.: 0.5-1 g/kg/dose (1-2 mL/kg of 50% solution)

Alternate dosing: I.V.: 10-25 g (40-100 mL of 25% solution or 20-50 mL of 50% solution)

Oral: 10-20 g as single dose; repeat in 10 minutes if necessary

Hyperkalemia, treatment: I.V. (in combination with insulin):

Infants and Children: 0.5-1 g/kg (using 25% or 50% solution) combined with regular insulin 1 unit for every 4-5 g dextrose given; infuse over 2 hours (infusions as short as 30 minutes have been recommended); repeat as needed

Adolescents and Adults: 25-50 g dextrose (250-500 mL $D_{10}W$) combined with 10 units regular insulin administered over 30-60 minutes; repeat as needed or as an alternative 25 g dextrose (50 mL $D_{50}W$) combined with 5-10 units regular insulin infused over 5 minutes; repeat as needed

Note: More rapid infusions (<30 minutes) may be associated with hyperglycemia and hyperosmolality and will exacerbate hyperkalemia; avoid use in patients who are already hyperglycemic

Parenteral nutrition: I.V.: Dextrose component (ASPEN Guidelines, 2002; ASPEN Pediatric Nutrition Support Core Curriculum, 2010):

Infants <1 year: Initial: 6-9 **mg**/kg/minute; daily increase: 1-2.5 **mg**/kg/minute or 1% to 2.5% increments; maximum: 18 **mg**/kg/minute

Children 1-10 years: Initial: 10%; daily increase 1-2 **mg**/kg/minute or 5% increments; maximum: 8-10 **mg**/kg/minute

Children >10 years and Adolescents: Initial: 3.5 **mg**/kg/minute or 10%; daily increase: 1-2 **mg**/kg/minute or 5% increments; maximum: 5-6 **mg**/kg/minute

Administration

Oral: Must be swallowed to be absorbed

Parenteral: For I.V. administration only, not SubQ or I.M. Further dilute concentrated dextrose solutions for peripheral venous administration to a maximum concentration of 12.5%; in emergency situations, 25% dextrose has been used peripherally; for direct I.V. infusion, administer over 1 minute at a rate not to exceed 200 mg/kg; continuous infusion rates vary with tolerance and range from 4.5-15 **mg**/kg/minute; hyperinsulinemic neonates may require up to 15-25 **mg**/kg/minute infusion rates

Vesicant/Extravasation Risk Vesicant (at concentrations >10%)

Monitoring Parameters Serum and urine glucose concentrations; serum electrolytes, I & O, caloric intake

Additional Information

1 g dextrose I.V. = 3.4 kcal

1 g glucose monohydrate = 1 g anhydrous dextrose

Osmolarity: Dextrose 10%: 505 mOsm/L; Dextrose 25%: 1330 mOsm/L; Normal body fluid: 310 mOsm/L

Dosage Forms Excipient information presented when available (limited, particularly for generics); consult specific product labeling. [DSC] = Discontinued product

Crystals, Oral:
Generic: (120 g [DSC])

Gel, Oral:
Glutose 15: 40% (37.5 g)
Glutose 15: 40% (37.5 g) [lemon flavor]
Glutose 45: 40% (112.5 g) [lemon flavor]
Insta-Glucose: 40% (31 g) [cherry flavor]

Liquid, Oral:
Glutol: 55% (180 mL) [lemon flavor]

Solution, Injection:
Dextrose Thermoject System: 5% (10 mL)

Solution, Intravenous:
Generic: 250 mg/mL (10 mL); 5% (25 mL, 50 mL, 100 mL, 150 mL, 250 mL, 500 mL, 1000 mL); 10% (250 mL, 500 mL, 1000 mL); 20% (500 mL); 30% (500 mL); 40% (500 mL); 50% (50 mL, 500 mL, 1000 mL, 2000 mL); 70% (500 mL, 1000 mL, 2000 mL)

Solution, Oral:
Glucose Nursette: 5% (59 mL)

Tablet Chewable, Oral:
Generic: 4 g

References

Adamkin DH and Committee on Fetus and Newborn, "Postnatal Glucose Homeostasis in Late-Preterm and Term Infants," *Pediatrics*, 2011, 127(3):575-9.

ASPEN Board of Directors and the Clinical Guidelines Task Force, "Guidelines for the Use of Parenteral and Enteral Nutrition in Adult and Pediatric Patients," *JPEN J Parenter Enteral Nutr*, 2002, 26(1 Suppl):1-138.

Carney LN, Nepa A, Cohen SS, et al, "Parenteral and Enteral Nutrition Support: Determining the Best Way to Feed," In: Corkins MR, Balint J, Bobo E, et al, eds, The A.S.P.E.N Pediatric Nutrition Support Core Curriculum, Silver Spring: MD: American Society of Parenteral and Enteral Nutrition, 2010, 433-47.

Department Health and Human Services, Food Drug Administration, "Aluminum in Large and Small Volume Parenterals Used in Total Parenteral Nutrition," *Federal Register*, 2000, 65(17):4103-11.

Institute for Safe Medication Practice, "Plain D₅W or Hypotonic Saline Solutions Post-Op Could Result in Acute Hyponatremia and Death in Healthy Children," ISMP Medication Safety Alert, August 13, 2009.

Available at http://www.ismp.org/Newsletters/acutecare/articles/20090813.asp

Kleinman ME, Chameides L, Schexnayder SM, et al, "Part 14: Pediatric Advanced Life Support: 2010 American Heart Association Guidelines for Cardiopulmonary Resuscitation and Emergency Cardiovascular Care," *Circulation*, 2010, 122(18 Suppl 3):876-908.

Mirtallo J, Canada T, Johnson D, et al, "Safe Practices for Parenteral Nutrition," *JPEN J Parenter Enteral Nutr*, 2004, 28(6):S39-70.

◆ **Dextrose Monohydrate** *see* Dextrose *on page* 637

◆ **Dextrose Thermoject System** *see* Dextrose *on page* 637

◆ **Dex-Tuss** *see* Guaifenesin and Codeine *on page* 985

◆ **dFdC** *see* Gemcitabine *on page* 959

◆ **dFdCyd** *see* Gemcitabine *on page* 959

◆ **DFM** *see* Deferoxamine *on page* 604

◆ **DHAD** *see* MitoXANtrone *on page* 1427

◆ **DHAQ** *see* MitoXANtrone *on page* 1427

◆ **DHE** *see* Dihydroergotamine *on page* 665

◆ **D.H.E. 45** *see* Dihydroergotamine *on page* 665

◆ **DHPG Sodium** *see* Ganciclovir (Systemic) *on page* 955

◆ **DHS Sal [OTC]** *see* Salicylic Acid *on page* 1860

◆ **DHS Tar [OTC]** *see* Coal Tar *on page* 532

◆ **DHS Tar Gel [OTC]** *see* Coal Tar *on page* 532

◆ **Diabeta** *see* GlyBURIDE *on page* 974

◆ **DiaBeta (Can)** *see* GlyBURIDE *on page* 974

◆ **DiabetAid® Pain and Tingling Relief [OTC]** *see* Capsaicin *on page* 367

◆ **Diabetic Siltussin DAS-Na [OTC]** *see* GuaiFENesin *on page* 984

◆ **Diabetic Siltussin-DM DAS-Na [OTC]** *see* Guaifenesin and Dextromethorphan *on page* 987

◆ **Diabetic Siltussin-DM DAS-Na Maximum Strength [OTC]** *see* Guaifenesin and Dextromethorphan *on page* 987

◆ **Diabetic Tussin [OTC]** *see* GuaiFENesin *on page* 984

◆ **Diabetic Tussin DM [OTC]** *see* Guaifenesin and Dextromethorphan *on page* 987

◆ **Diabetic Tussin DM Maximum Strength [OTC]** *see* Guaifenesin and Dextromethorphan *on page* 987

◆ **Diabetic Tussin Mucus Relief [OTC]** *see* GuaiFENesin *on page* 984

◆ **Dialyvite Vitamin D 5000 [OTC]** *see* Cholecalciferol *on page* 455

◆ **Dialyvite Vitamin D3 Max [OTC]** *see* Cholecalciferol *on page* 455

◆ **Diaminocyclohexane Oxalatoplatinum** *see* Oxaliplatin *on page* 1557

◆ **Diaminodiphenylsulfone** *see* Dapsone (Systemic) *on page* 586

◆ **Diaminodiphenylsulfone** *see* Dapsone (Topical) *on page* 589

◆ **Diamode [OTC]** *see* Loperamide *on page* 1270

◆ **Diamox® (Can)** *see* AcetaZOLAMIDE *on page* 56

◆ **Diamox Sequels** *see* AcetaZOLAMIDE *on page* 56

◆ **Diarr-Eze (Can)** *see* Loperamide *on page* 1270

◆ **Diastat® (Can)** *see* Diazepam *on page* 640

◆ **Diastat AcuDial** *see* Diazepam *on page* 640

◆ **Diastat Pediatric** *see* Diazepam *on page* 640

◆ **Diazemuls® (Can)** *see* Diazepam *on page* 640

Diazepam (dye AZ e pam)

Medication Safety Issues
Sound-alike/look-alike issues:
Diazepam may be confused with diazoxide, diltiazem, Ditropan, LORazepam

Valium® may be confused with Valcyte®

BEERS Criteria medication:
This drug may be potentially inappropriate for use in geriatric patients (Quality of evidence - high; Strength of recommendation - strong).

Related Information
Management of Drug Extravasations *on page 2255*
Patient Information for Disposal of Unused Medications *on page 2412*
Preprocedure Sedatives in Children *on page 2402*
Serotonin Syndrome *on page 2405*

Brand Names: U.S. Diastat AcuDial; Diastat Pediatric; Diazepam Intensol; Valium

Brand Names: Canada Apo-Diazepam®; Bio-Diazepam; Diastat®; Diazemuls®; Diazepam Auto Injector; Diazepam Injection USP; Novo-Dipam; PMS-Diazepam; Valium®

Therapeutic Category Antianxiety Agent; Anticonvulsant, Benzodiazepine; Benzodiazepine; Hypnotic; Sedative

Generic Availability (U.S.) May be product dependent

Use
Oral: Management of general anxiety disorders, ethanol withdrawal symptoms, relief of skeletal muscle spasms, muscle spasticity, and tetany; adjunct in the treatment of convulsive disorders (FDA approved in ages ≥6 months and adults)

Parenteral: Management of general anxiety disorders, ethanol withdrawal symptoms, relief of skeletal muscle spasms, muscle spasticity, and tetany; to provide preoperative or preprocedural sedation and amnesia; adjunct treatment of status epilepticus and severe recurrent convulsive disorders (FDA approved in ages >30 days and adults)

Rectal gel: Management of intermittent bouts of increased seizure activity in refractory epilepsy patients on stable AED therapy (FDA approved in ages ≥2 years and adults)

Pregnancy Risk Factor D
Pregnancy Considerations Teratogenic effects have been reported in animal reproduction studies. In humans, diazepam and its metabolites (N-desmethyldiazepam, temazepam, and oxazepam) cross the placenta. Teratogenic effects have been observed with diazepam; however, additional studies are needed. The incidence of premature birth and low birth weights may be increased following maternal use of benzodiazepines; hypoglycemia and respiratory problems in the neonate may occur following exposure late in pregnancy. Neonatal withdrawal symptoms may occur within days to weeks after birth and "floppy infant syndrome" (which also includes withdrawal symptoms) has been reported with some benzodiazepines (including diazepam) (Bergman, 1992; Iqbal, 2002; Wikner, 2007). A combination of factors influences the potential teratogenicity of anticonvulsant therapy. When treating women with epilepsy, monotherapy with the lowest effective dose and avoidance of medications known to have a high incidence of teratogenic effects is recommended (Harden, 2009; Wlodarczyk, 2012).

Breast-Feeding Considerations Diazepam and N-desmethyldiazepam can be found in breast milk; the oxazepam metabolite has also been detected in the urine of a nursing infant. Drowsiness, lethargy, or weight loss in nursing infants have been observed in case reports following maternal use of some benzodiazepines, including diazepam (Iqbal, 2002). Because diazepam and its metabolites may be present in breast milk for prolonged periods following administration, one manufacturer recommends discontinuing breast-feeding for an appropriate period of time.

Contraindications Hypersensitivity to diazepam or any component; possible cross-sensitivity with other benzodiazepines; do not use in a comatose patient, in those with preexisting CNS depression, respiratory depression, acute narrow-angle glaucoma, severe uncontrolled pain, myasthenia gravis, severe respiratory insufficiency, severe hepatic insufficiency, or sleep apnea syndrome; oral dosage forms are listed by manufacturer as being contraindicated in patients <6 months of age (due to lack of adequate clinical experience).

Warnings Abrupt discontinuation may cause withdrawal symptoms or seizures. Rapid I.V. push may cause sudden respiratory depression, apnea, hypotension, or cardiac arrest. Appropriate resuscitative equipment and qualified personnel should be available during parenteral administration with appropriate monitoring. Do not administer injection to patients in coma, shock, or acute ethanol intoxication with depression of vital signs. Tonic status epilepticus may occur in patients with petit mal status or petit mal variant status who are treated with diazepam. Administration of rectal gel should only be performed by individuals trained to recognize characteristic seizure activity for which the product is indicated and who are capable of monitoring patient's response to determine need for additional medical intervention.

Psychiatric and paradoxical reactions, including hyperactive or aggressive behavior, hallucinations, and psychoses, have been reported with benzodiazepines, particularly in adolescent/pediatric or elderly patients; discontinue diazepam if such reactions occur. Diazepam is not recommended for the treatment of psychotic patients, in place of appropriate therapy. Teratogenic effects have been reported in animal studies. In humans, diazepam crosses the placenta. An increased risk of congenital malformations and other developmental abnormalities have been associated with diazepam; epilepsy itself may also increase the risk. Hypotonia, hypothermia, withdrawal symptoms, and respiratory and feeding difficulties have been reported in the infant following maternal use of benzodiazepines near time of delivery.

Injection and rectal gel contain benzoic acid, benzyl alcohol, and sodium benzoate; benzyl alcohol may cause allergic reactions in susceptible individuals; benzoic acid (benzoate) is a metabolite of benzyl alcohol; large amounts of benzyl alcohol (≥99 mg/kg/day) have been associated with a potentially fatal toxicity ("gasping syndrome") in neonates; the "gasping syndrome" consists of metabolic acidosis, respiratory distress, gasping respirations, CNS dysfunction (including convulsions, intracranial hemorrhage), hypotension and cardiovascular collapse; use diazepam products containing benzoic acid, benzyl alcohol, or sodium benzoate with caution in neonates; *in vitro* and animal studies have shown that benzoate displaces bilirubin from protein binding sites. Parenteral formulation contains propylene glycol; toxicities have been reported with use of products containing propylene glycol, including hyperosmolality, lactic acidosis, seizures, and respiratory depression; in neonates large amounts of propylene glycol delivered orally, intravenously (eg, >3000 mg/day), or topically have been associated with potentially fatal toxicities which can include metabolic acidosis, seizures, renal failure, and CNS depression; use products containing propylene glycol with caution (AAP, 1997; Shehab, 2009). Oral liquid products contain polyethylene glycol, which may have adverse effects.

Precautions Use with caution in patients receiving other CNS depressants or psychoactive medication (effects with other sedative drugs or ethanol may be potentiated) and in patients with depression. Use with caution in patients with hypoalbuminemia, renal or hepatic dysfunction, and in neonates and young infants; neonates have decreased metabolism of diazepam and desmethyldiazepam (active metabolite), both can accumulate with repeated use and cause increased toxicity. Modify dosage in patients with hepatic impairment or chronic respiratory insufficiency, and in debilitated patients. Use with extreme caution in patients with a history of drug or alcohol abuse. Vesicant; ensure proper needle or catheter placement prior to and during I.V. administration; avoid extravasation.

Adverse Reactions Reactions may vary by route of administration.

Cardiovascular: Hypotension, vasodilatation

Central nervous system: Amnesia, ataxia, confusion, depression, drowsiness, fatigue, headache, slurred speech, paradoxical reactions (eg, aggressiveness, agitation, anxiety, delusions, hallucinations, inappropriate behavior, increased muscle spasms, insomnia, irritability, psychoses, rage, restlessness, sleep disturbances, stimulation), vertigo

Dermatologic: Rash

Endocrine & metabolic: Libido changes

Gastrointestinal: Constipation, diarrhea, nausea, salivation changes (dry mouth or hypersalivation)

Genitourinary: Incontinence, urinary retention

Hepatic: Jaundice

Local: Phlebitis, pain with injection

Neuromuscular & skeletal: Dysarthria, tremor, weakness

Ocular: Blurred vision, diplopia

Respiratory: Apnea, asthma, respiratory rate decreased

Drug Interactions

Metabolism/Transport Effects Substrate of CYP1A2 (minor), CYP2B6 (minor), CYP2C19 (major), CYP2C9 (minor), CYP3A4 (major); **Note:** Assignment of Major/Minor substrate status based on clinically relevant drug interaction potential; **Inhibits** CYP2C19 (weak), CYP3A4 (weak)

Avoid Concomitant Use

Avoid concomitant use of Diazepam with any of the following: Azelastine (Nasal); Conivaptan; Fusidic Acid (Systemic); Methadone; OLANZapine; Paraldehyde; Pimozide; Sodium Oxybate; Thalidomide

Increased Effect/Toxicity

Diazepam may increase the levels/effects of: Alcohol (Ethyl); Alfentanil; ARIPiprazole; Azelastine (Nasal); Buprenorphine; CloZAPine; CNS Depressants; Dofetilide; Hydrocodone; Lomitapide; Methadone; Methotrimeprazine; Metyrosine; Mirtazapine; Paraldehyde; Pimozide; Pramipexole; ROPINIRole; Rotigotine; Selective Serotonin Reuptake Inhibitors; Sodium Oxybate; Thalidomide; Zolpidem

The levels/effects of Diazepam may be increased by: Antifungal Agents (Azole Derivatives, Systemic); Aprepitant; Brimonidine (Topical); Calcium Channel Blockers (Nondihydropyridine); Cannabis; Ceritinib; Cimetidine; Conivaptan; Contraceptives (Estrogens); Contraceptives (Progestins); Cosyntropin; CYP2C19 Inhibitors (Moderate); CYP2C19 Inhibitors (Strong); CYP3A4 Inhibitors (Moderate); CYP3A4 Inhibitors (Strong); Dasatinib; Disulfiram; Doxylamine; Dronabinol; Droperidol; Etravirine; Fosamprenavir; Fosaprepitant; Fusidic Acid (Systemic); Grapefruit Juice; HydrOXYzine; Isoniazid; Ivacaftor; Kava Kava; Luliconazole; Magnesium Sulfate; Methotrimeprazine; Mifepristone; Nabilone; OLANZapine; Perampanel; Proton Pump Inhibitors; Ritonavir; Rufinamide; Saquinavir; Selective Serotonin Reuptake Inhibitors; Simeprevir; Stiripentol; Tapentadol; Tetrahydrocannabinol

Decreased Effect

The levels/effects of Diazepam may be decreased by: Bosentan; CarBAMazepine; CYP2C19 Inducers (Strong); CYP3A4 Inducers (Strong); Dabrafenib;

Deferasirox; Etravirine; Mitotane; Rifamycin Derivatives; Siltuximab; St Johns Wort; Theophylline Derivatives; Tocilizumab; Yohimbine

Food Interactions Diazepam serum concentrations may be decreased if taken with food. Grapefruit juice may increase diazepam serum concentrations. Management: Avoid concurrent use of grapefruit juice. Maintain adequate hydration, unless instructed to restrict fluid intake.

Stability

Injection: Store at 20°C to 25°C (68°F to 77°F); excursions permitted to 15°C to 30°C (59°F to 86°F); protect from light; potency is retained for up to 3 months when kept at room temperature; most stable at pH 4-8; hydrolysis occurs at pH <3; do not mix injection with other medications

Oral solution: Store at 25°C (77°F); excursions permitted to 15°C to 30°C (59°F to 86°F); dispense in light-resistant, tightly closed container

Oral concentrated solution: Store at 25°C (77°F); excursions permitted to 15°C to 30°C (59°F to 86°F); protect from light; discard opened bottle after 90 days

Tablet: Store at 15°C to 30°C (59°F to 86°F); dispense in tightly closed, light-resistant container

Rectal gel: Store at 25°C (77°F); excursion permitted to 15°C to 30°C (59°F to 86°F)

Mechanism of Action Binds to stereospecific benzodiazepine receptors on the postsynaptic GABA neuron at several sites within the central nervous system, including the limbic system, reticular formation. Enhancement of the inhibitory effect of GABA on neuronal excitability results by increased neuronal membrane permeability to chloride ions. This shift in chloride ions results in hyperpolarization (a less excitable state) and stabilization.

Pharmacodynamics Status epilepticus:

Onset of action:

I.V.: 1-3 minutes

Rectal: 2-10 minutes

Duration: 15-30 minutes

Pharmacokinetics (Adult data unless noted)

Absorption:

Oral: 85% to 100%

I.M.: Poor

Rectal (gel): Well absorbed

Distribution: Widely distributed; crosses blood-brain barrier and placenta; distributes into breast milk; V_d: Adults: 0.8-1 L/kg

Protein binding:

Neonates: 84% to 86%

Adults: 98%

Metabolism: In the liver to desmethyldiazepam (active metabolite) and N-methyloxazepam (active metabolite); these are metabolized to oxazepam (active) which undergoes glucuronide conjugation before being excreted

Bioavailability: Rectal (gel): 90%

Half-life:

Diazepam:

Neonates: 50-95 hours

Infants 1 month to 2 years: 40-50 hours

Children 2-12 years: 15-21 hours

Children 12-16 years: 18-20 hours

Adults: 20-50 hours

Increased half-life in those with severe hepatic disorders

Desmethyldiazepam (active metabolite): Adults: 50-100 hours; may be further prolonged in neonates

Time to peak serum concentration:

Oral: Mean: 1-1.5 hours; range: 0.25-2.5 hours

Rectal (gel): 1.5 hours

Elimination: In urine, primarily as conjugated oxazepam (75%), desmethyldiazepam, and N-methyloxazepam

Dialysis: Not dialyzable (0% to 5%)

Dosing: Neonatal Status epilepticus: I.V: (Not recommended as first-line agent; use only after multiple agents have failed; injection contains benzoic acid, sodium benzoate, and benzyl alcohol): 0.1 to 0.3 mg/kg/dose given over 3 to 5 minutes, every 15 to 30 minutes, to a maximum total dose of 2 mg

Rectal gel formulation: Not recommended; product contains benzoic acid, sodium benzoate, benzyl alcohol, ethanol 10%, and propylene glycol; prolonged CNS depression has been reported in neonates receiving diazepam

Dosing: Usual
Anxiety:
Children:
Oral: 0.12 to 0.8 mg/kg/day in divided doses every 6 to 8 hours
I.M., I.V.: 0.04 to 0.3 mg/kg/dose every 2 to 4 hours to a maximum of 0.6 mg/kg within an 8-hour period if needed
Adults:
Oral: 2 to 10 mg 2 to 4 times/day
I.M., I.V.: 2 to 10 mg, may repeat in 3 to 4 hours if needed
Convulsive disorders:
Adjunct: Adults: Oral: 2 to 10 mg 2 to 4 times/day
Acute treatment:
Rectal gel formulation:
Infants 1 to <6 months: Not recommended; product contains benzoic acid, sodium benzoate, benzyl alcohol, ethanol 10%, and propylene glycol
Infants and Children 6 months to 2 years: Dose not established
Children 2 to 5 years: 0.5 mg/kg
Children 6 to 11 years: 0.3 mg/kg
Children ≥12 years and Adults: 0.2 mg/kg
Note: Round dose to the nearest 2.5 mg increment, not exceeding a 20 mg/dose; dose may be repeated in 4 to 12 hours if needed; do not use more than 5 times per month or more than once every 5 days
Rectal: Undiluted 5 mg/mL parenteral formulation (filter if using ampul): 0.5 mg/kg/dose then 0.25 mg/kg/dose in 10 minutes if needed
Febrile seizure prophylaxis: Children: Oral: 1 mg/kg/day divided every 8 hours; initiate therapy at first sign of fever and continue for 24 hours after fever resolves (Rosman, 1993; Steering Committee, 2008)
Status epilepticus:
Infants >30 days and Children: I.V: 0.1 to 0.3 mg/kg/dose given over 3 to 5 minutes, every 5 to 10 minutes (maximum: 10 mg/dose) (Hegenbarth, 2008)
Manufacturer's recommendations:
Infants >30 days and Children <5 years: I.V: 0.2 to 0.5 mg slow I.V. every 2 to 5 minutes up to a maximum total dose of 5 mg; repeat in 2-4 hours if needed
Children ≥5 years: I.V: 1 mg slow I.V. every 2 to 5 minutes up to a maximum of 10 mg; repeat in 2 to 4 hours if needed
Adult: I.V: Initial: 5 to 10 mg; may repeat every 10 to 15 minutes up to a maximum dose of 30 mg; may repeat in 2 to 4 hours if needed, but residual active metabolites may still be present
Ethanol withdrawal (acute): Adults: Oral: 10 mg 3 to 4 times during first 24 hours, then decrease to 5 mg 3 to 4 times/day as needed
Muscle spasms:
Cerebral palsy-associated spasticity: Note: Limited information exists; further studies are needed. Dose should be individualized and titrated to effect and tolerability.
Oral:
Children <12 years and <15 kg (Delgado, 2010; Mathew, 2005):
<8.5 kg: 0.5 to 1 mg at bedtime

8.5 to 15 kg: 1 to 2 mg at bedtime
Children 5 to 16 years and ≥15 kg: Initial: 1.25 mg 3 times daily; may titrate to 5 mg 4 times daily (Engle, 1966)
General muscle spasms: Adults: I.V., I.M.: Initial: 5 to 10 mg; then 5 to 10 mg in 3 to 4 hours, if necessary. Larger doses may be required if associated with tetanus.
Tetanus-associated:
Infants >30 days: I.V., I.M.: 1 to 2 mg/dose every 3 to 4 hours as needed
Children ≥5 years: I.V., I.M.: 5 to 10 mg/dose every 3 to 4 hours as needed
Preoperative medication: Adults: I.M.: 10 mg before surgery
Sedation or muscle relaxation: Children:
Oral: 0.12 to 0.8 mg/kg/day in divided doses every 6 to 8 hours
I.M., I.V.: 0.04 to 0.3 mg/kg/dose every 2 to 4 hours to a maximum of 0.6 mg/kg within an 8-hour period if needed
Moderate sedation for procedures:
Children:
Oral: 0.2 to 0.3 mg/kg (maximum dose: 10 mg) 45 to 60 minutes prior to procedure
I.V.: Initial: 0.05 to 0.1 mg/kg over 3 to 5 minutes, titrate slowly to effect (maximum total dose: 0.25 mg/kg) (Krauss, 2006)
Adolescents:
Oral: 10 mg
I.V.: 5 mg; may repeat with 2.5 mg if needed
Skeletal muscle relaxant (adjunct therapy): Adults:
Oral: 2 to 10 mg 3 to 4 times/day
Administration
Oral: Administer with food or water. Oral concentrate solution (5 mg/mL): Measure dose only with calibrated dropper provided; dose should be diluted or mixed with water, juice, soda, applesauce, or pudding before use
Parenteral: I.V.: Rapid injection may cause respiratory depression or hypotension; infants and children: Do not exceed 1-2 mg/minute I.V. push; adults: Maximum infusion rate: 5 mg/minute; maximum concentration for administration: 5 mg/mL.
Vesicant; ensure proper needle or catheter placement prior to and during infusion; avoid extravasation. If extravasation occurs, stop I.V. administration immediately and disconnect (leave cannula/needle in place); gently aspirate extravasated solution (do NOT flush the line); remove needle/cannula; elevate extremity. Apply dry cold compresses (Hurst, 2004).
Rectal: Diastat AcuDial: Prior to administration, confirm that the syringe is properly set to the correct dose and that the green "ready" band is visible.
Diastat AcuDial and Diastat: Place patient on side (facing person responsible for monitoring), with top leg bent forward. Insert rectal tip (lubricated) gently into rectum until rim fits snug against rectal opening; push plunger gently over 3 seconds. After additional 3 seconds, remove syringe; hold buttocks together while slowly counting to 3 to prevent leakage; keep patient on side, facing towards you and continue to observe patient; discard any unused medication, syringe, and all used materials safely away from children; do not reuse; see Administration and Disposal Instructions that come with product.
Vesicant/Extravasation Risk Vesicant
Monitoring Parameters Heart rate, respiratory rate, blood pressure, mental status; with long-term therapy: Liver enzymes, CBC
Reference Range Effective therapeutic range not well established
Proposed therapeutic:
Diazepam: 0.2-1.5 mcg/mL (SI: 0.7-5.3 micromoles/L)

N-desmethyldiazepam (nordiazepam): 0.1-0.5 mcg/mL (SI: 0.35-1.8 micromoles/L)

Test Interactions False-negative urinary glucose determinations when using Clinistix® or Diastix®

Additional Information Diazepam does not have any analgesic effects. Diarrhea in a 9 month old infant receiving high-dose oral diazepam was attributed to the diazepam oral solution that contained polyethylene glycol and propylene glycol (both are osmotically active); diarrhea resolved when crushed tablets were substituted for the oral solution (Marshall, 1995).

Diastat® AcuDial™: Prescribed dose must be "dialed in" and locked before dispensing; consult package insert for directions on setting prescribed dose; confirm green "ready" band is visible prior to dispensing product.

Controlled Substance C-IV

Dosage Forms Excipient information presented when available (limited, particularly for generics); consult specific product labeling.

Concentrate, Oral:

Diazepam Intensol: 5 mg/mL (30 mL) [contains alcohol, usp; unflavored flavor]

Device, Intramuscular:

Generic: 10 mg/2 mL (2 mL)

Gel, Rectal:

Diastat AcuDial: 10 mg (1 ea); 20 mg (1 ea) [contains alcohol, usp, benzoic acid, sodium benzoate]

Diastat Pediatric: 2.5 mg (1 ea) [contains alcohol, usp]

Generic: 2.5 mg (1 ea); 10 mg (1 ea); 20 mg (1 ea)

Solution, Injection:

Generic: 5 mg/mL (2 mL, 10 mL)

Solution, Oral:

Generic: 1 mg/mL (5 mL, 500 mL)

Tablet, Oral:

Valium: 2 mg, 5 mg, 10 mg [scored]

Generic: 2 mg, 5 mg, 10 mg

References

American Academy of Pediatrics Committee on Drugs. "Inactive" ingredients in pharmaceutical products: update (subject review). *Pediatrics.* 1997;99(2):268-278.

American Academy of Pediatrics; American Academy of Pediatric Dentistry, Coté CJ, et al, "Guidelines for Monitoring and Management of Pediatric Patients During and After Sedation for Diagnostic and Therapeutic Procedures: An Update," *Pediatrics*, 2006, 118 (6):2587-602.

Bergman U, Rosa FW, Baum C, et al, "Effects of Exposure to Benzodiazepine During Fetal Life," *Lancet*, 1992, 340(8821):694-6.

Delgado MR, Hirtz D, Aisen M, et al, "Practice Parameter: Pharmacologic Treatment of Spasticity in Children and Adolescents With Cerebral Palsy (An Evidence-Based Review): Report of the Quality Standards Subcommittee of the American Academy of Neurology and the Practice Committee of the Child Neurology Society," *Neurology*, 2010, 74(4):336-43.

Dreifuss FE, Rosman NP, Cloyd JC, et al, "A Comparison of Rectal Diazepam Gel and Placebo for Acute Repetitive Seizures," *N Engl J Med*, 1998, 338(26):1869-75.

Engle HA, "The Effect of Diazepam (Valium) in Children With Cerebral Palsy: A Double-Blind Study," *Dev Med Child Neurol*, 1966, 8 (6):661-7.

Harden CL, Meador KJ, Pennell PB, et al, "Practice Parameter Update: Management Issues for Women With Epilepsy-Focus on Pregnancy (an Evidence-Based Review): Teratogenesis and Perinatal Outcomes: Report of the Quality Standards Subcommittee and Therapeutics and Technology Assessment Subcommittee of the American Academy of Neurology and American Epilepsy Society," *Neurology*, 2009, 73(2):133-41.

Hegenbarth MA and American Academy of Pediatrics Committee on Drugs, "Preparing for Pediatric Emergencies: Drugs to Consider," *Pediatrics*, 2008, 121(2):433-43.

Hurst S, McMillan M. Innovative solutions in critical care units: extravasation guidelines. *Dimens Crit Care Nurs.* 2004;23(3):125-128.

Iqbal MM, Sobhan T, Ryals T, et al, "Effects of Commonly Used Benzodiazepines on the Fetus, the Neonate, and the Nursing Infant," *Psychiatr Serv*, 2002, 53(1):39-49.

Krauss B and Green SM, "Procedural Sedation and Analgesia in Children," *Lancet*, 2006, 367(9512):766-80.

Marshall JD, Farrar HC, and Kearns GL, "Diarrhea Associated With Enteral Benzodiazepine Solutions," *J Pediatr*, 1995, 126(4):657-9.

Mathew A, Mathew MC, Thomas M, et al, "The Efficacy of Diazepam in Enhancing Motor Function in Children With Spastic Cerebral Palsy," *J Trop Pediatr*, 2005, 51(2):109-13.

Rosman NP, Colton T, Labazzo J, et al, "A Controlled Trial of Diazepam Administered During Febrile Illnesses to Prevent Recurrence of Febrile Seizures," *N Engl J Med*, 1993, 329(2):79-84.

Shehab N, Lewis CL, Streetman DD, Donn SM. Exposure to the pharmaceutical excipients benzyl alcohol and propylene glycol among critically ill neonates. *Pediatr Crit Care Med.* 2009;10 (2):256-259.

Steering Committee on Quality Improvement and Management, Subcommittee on Febrile Seizures American Academy of Pediatrics, "Febrile Seizures: Clinical Practice Guideline for the Long-Term Management of the Child With Simple Febrile Seizures," *Pediatrics*, 2008, 121(6):1281-6.

Wikner BN, Stiller CO, Bergman U, et al, "Use of Benzodiazepines and Benzodiazepine Receptor Agonists During Pregnancy: Neonatal Outcome and Congenital Malformations," *Pharmacoepidemiol Drug Saf*, 2007, 16(11):1203-10.

Wlodarczyk BJ, Palacios AM, George TM, et al, "Antiepileptic Drugs and Pregnancy Outcomes," *Am J Med Genet A*, 2012, 158A (8):2071-90.

Zeltzer LK, Altman A, Cohen D, et al, "Report of the Subcommittee on the Management of Pain Associated With Procedures in Children With Cancer," *Pediatrics*, 1990, 86(5 Pt 2):826-31.

◆ **Diazepam Auto Injector (Can)** see Diazepam on page 640

◆ **Diazepam Injection USP (Can)** see Diazepam on page 640

◆ **Diazepam Intensol** see Diazepam on page 640

Diazepam Intensol see Diazepam on page 640

Diazoxide (dye az OKS ide)

Medication Safety Issues

Sound-alike/look-alike issues:

Diazoxide may be confused with diazepam, Dyazide®

Brand Names: U.S. Proglycem

Brand Names: Canada Proglycem®

Therapeutic Category Antihypoglycemic Agent; Vasodilator

Generic Availability (U.S.) No

Use

Management of hypoglycemia related to hyperinsulinism secondary to the following conditions: Islet cell adenoma, adenomatosis, or hyperplasia; extrapancreatic malignancy; nesidioblastosis (persistent hyperinsulinemic hypoglycemia of infancy); leucine sensitivity (All indications: FDA approved in neonates, infants, and children)

Management of hypoglycemia related to hyperinsulinism secondary to the following conditions: Inoperable islet cell adenoma or carcinoma; extrapancreatic malignancy (FDA approved in adults)

Pregnancy Risk Factor C

Pregnancy Considerations Adverse events have been observed in animal studies. Diazoxide crosses the human placenta. Altered carbohydrate metabolism, hyperbilirubinemia, or thrombocytopenia have been reported in the fetus or neonate. Alopecia and hypertrichosis lanuginosa have also been reported in infants following maternal use of diazoxide during the last 19-60 days of pregnancy.

Breast-Feeding Considerations It is not known if diazoxide is excreted in breast milk. Due to the potential for serious adverse reactions in the nursing infant, a decision should be made whether to discontinue nursing or to discontinue the drug, taking into account the importance of treatment to the mother.

Contraindications Hypersensitivity to diazoxide, any component, or other thiazides; functional hypoglycemia

Warnings Diazoxide use may lead to increased fluid retention and precipitate CHF in patients with compromised cardiac reserve; used with caution in patients with heart failure; diuretics may be used to treat fluid retention. Ketoacidosis or nonketotic hyperosmolar coma may occur during treatment, usually in patients with concomitant illness; prompt recognition and treatment are essential (especially due to the long half-life of the drug). Transient cataracts have been reported in an infant in association with hyperosmolar coma; cataracts subsided following correction of hyperosmolarity. Abnormal facial features have been reported in four children who received diazoxide for >4 years for the treatment of hypoglycemia hyperinsulinism.

Suspension contains ethanol (~7.25%) and sodium benzoate. Benzoic acid (benzoate) is a metabolite of benzyl alcohol; large amounts of benzyl alcohol (≥99 mg/kg/day) have been associated with a potentially fatal toxicity ("gasping syndrome") in neonates; the "gasping syndrome" consists of metabolic acidosis, respiratory distress, gasping respirations, CNS dysfunction (including convulsions, intracranial hemorrhage), hypotension, and cardiovascular collapse; use solution containing sodium benzoate with caution in neonates; in vitro and animal studies have shown that benzoate displaces bilirubin from protein binding sites.

Suspension contains propylene glycol; toxicities have been reported with use of products containing propylene glycol, including hyperosmolality, lactic acidosis, seizures, and respiratory depression; in neonates large amounts of propylene glycol delivered orally, intravenously (eg, >3000 mg/day), or topically have been associated with potentially fatal toxicities which can include metabolic acidosis, seizures, renal failure, and CNS depression; use suspension products containing propylene glycol with caution (AAP, 1997; Shehab, 2009).

Precautions Use with caution and consider dosage reduction in patients with renal impairment. Use with caution in patients with diabetes mellitus, hepatic impairment, hyperuricemia, or history of gout. May displace bilirubin from albumin; use caution in newborns with hyperbilirubinemia.

Initiate treatment with diazoxide under close clinical supervision; carefully monitor blood glucose and clinical response until patient's condition becomes stable (usually several days); discontinue diazoxide if drug is not effective after 2-3 weeks of therapy. Regular monitoring of urine for glucose and ketones (especially under conditions of stress) are required with prolonged therapy; abnormal results should be reported to physician promptly. Periodic monitoring of blood glucose is required for dosage adjustment.

Use with caution when administered concomitantly with antihypertensives; diazoxide may enhance the antihypertensive effects.

Adverse Reactions

Cardiovascular: Cardiac failure (due to sodium and water retention), chest pain (rare), hyperosmolar coma (nonketotic), hypertension (transient), hypotension, palpitations, tachycardia

Central nervous system: Anxiety, dizziness, extrapyramidal reaction, headache, insomnia, malaise, paresthesia, peripheral neuritis (poly)

Dermatologic: Cutaneous candidiasis, loss of scalp hair, pruritus, purpura, skin rash

Endocrine & metabolic: Albuminuria, diabetic ketoacidosis, fluid retention, galactorrhea, glycosuria, gout, hirsutism, hyperglycemia, sodium retention

Gastrointestinal: Abdominal pain, acute pancreatitis, ageusia (transient), anorexia, diarrhea, intestinal obstruction, nausea, pancreatic necrosis, vomiting

Genitourinary: Azotemia, decreased urine output, hematuria, lump in breast (enlargement), nephrotic syndrome (reversible), uricosuria

Hematologic & oncologic: Decreased hematocrit, decreased hemoglobin, decreased serum immunoglobulins (IgG), eosinophilia, hemorrhage (excessive), lymphadenopathy, neutropenia (transient), thrombocytopenia

Hepatic: Increased serum alkaline phosphatase, increased serum AST

Infection: Herpes virus infection

Neuromuscular & skeletal: Accelerated bone maturation, craniofacial abnormality (children with chronic use), weakness

Ophthalmic: Blurred vision, cataract (transient), diplopia, lacrimation, scotoma (ring), subconjunctival hemorrhage

Renal: Decreased creatinine clearance

Miscellaneous: Fever

Drug Interactions

Metabolism/Transport Effects None known.

Avoid Concomitant Use There are no known interactions where it is recommended to avoid concomitant use.

Increased Effect/Toxicity

Diazoxide may increase the levels/effects of: Antihypertensives

The levels/effects of Diazoxide may be increased by: MAO Inhibitors; Thiazide Diuretics; Thiopental

Decreased Effect

Diazoxide may decrease the levels/effects of: Fosphenytoin; Phenytoin

Stability Suspension: Store at 25°C (77°F); excursions permitted to 15°C to 30°C (59°F to 86°F). Protect from light. Store in carton until ready to use.

Mechanism of Action Opens ATP-dependent potassium channels on pancreatic beta cells in the presence of ATP and Mg^{2+}, resulting in hyperpolarization of the cell and inhibition of insulin release. Diazoxide binds to a different site on the potassium channel than the sulfonylureas (Doyle, 2003).

Pharmacodynamics

Hyperglycemic effects (oral):

Onset of action: Within 1 hour

Duration (normal renal function): 8 hours

Pharmacokinetics (Adult data unless noted)

Protein binding: >90%

Half-life:

Children: 9-24 hours

Adults: 24-36 hours

Elimination: 50% excreted unchanged in urine

Dosing: Neonatal Hyperinsulinemic hypoglycemia: Oral: Initial: 10 mg/kg/day in divided doses every 8 hours; usual range: 5-15 mg/kg/day in divided doses every 8 hours (Hussain, 2004; Kapoor, 2009); **Note:** Often given in conjunction with chlorothiazide

Dosing: Usual Note: Dose should be individualized based on the severity of the hypoglycemic condition, blood glucose concentration, and clinical response of patient. Use the least amount of drug that achieves the desired clinical and laboratory results.

Infants, Children, and Adolescents: **Hyperinsulinemic hypoglycemia:**

Infants: Oral: Initial: 10 mg/kg/day in divided doses every 8 hours; usual range: 8-15 mg/kg/day in divided doses every 8-12 hours; range of 5-20 mg/kg/day in divided doses every 8 hours has been used (Kapoor, 2009)

Children and Adolescents: Oral: Initial: 3 mg/kg/day in divided doses every 8 hours; usual range: 3-8 mg/kg/day in divided doses every 8-12 hours. **Note:** In certain instances, patients with refractory hypoglycemia may require higher doses.

Adults: **Hyperinsulinemic hypoglycemia:** Oral: Initial: 3 mg/kg/day in divided doses every 8 hours; usual range: 3-8 mg/kg/day in divided doses every 8-12 hours. **Note:** In certain instances, patients with refractory hypoglycemia may require higher doses.

Dosing adjustment in renal impairment: Half-life may be prolonged with renal impairment; a reduced dose should be considered.

Dosing adjustment in hepatic impairment: There are no dosage adjustments provided in the manufacturer's labeling.

Administration Shake suspension well before use; suspension comes with calibrated dropper (to deliver dose of 10-50 mg, in 10 mg increments).

Monitoring Parameters Blood glucose, serum uric acid, electrolytes, BUN; renal function; AST, CBC with differential, platelets; urine glucose and ketones; blood pressure, heart rate

Test Interactions Serum renin concentrations may be increased. Serum cortisol concentrations may be decreased.

Additional Information The injectable form of diazoxide, which was used for the emergency treatment of hypertension, is no longer available.

Dosage Forms Excipient information presented when available (limited, particularly for generics); consult specific product labeling.

Suspension, Oral:
Proglycem: 50 mg/mL (30 mL) [chocolate mint flavor]

References
American Academy of Pediatrics Committee on Drugs. "Inactive" ingredients in pharmaceutical products: update (subject review). *Pediatrics.* 1997;99(2):268-278.

Hussain K and Aynsley-Green A, "Hyperinsulinaemic Hypoglycaemia in Preterm Neonates," *Arch Dis Child Fetal Neonatal Ed,* 2004, 89(1): F65-7.

Kapoor RR, Flanagan SE, James C, et al, "Hyperinsulinaemic Hypoglycaemia," *Arch Dis Child,* 2009, 94(6):450-7.

Shehab N, Lewis CL, Streetman DD, Donn SM. Exposure to the pharmaceutical excipients benzyl alcohol and propylene glycol among critically ill neonates. *Pediatr Crit Care Med.* 2009;10 (2):256-259.

◆ **Dibenzyline** *see* Phenoxybenzamine *on page 1655*

Dibucaine (DYE byoo kane)

Brand Names: U.S. Nupercainal [OTC]

Therapeutic Category Analgesic, Topical; Local Anesthetic, Topical

Generic Availability (U.S.) Yes

Use Fast, temporary relief of pain and itching due to hemorrhoids, minor burns, other minor skin conditions

Pregnancy Considerations Dibucaine is not absorbed systemically following topical administration on intact skin. Systemic absorption would be required in order for dibucaine to cross the placenta and reach the fetus.

Breast-Feeding Considerations No data reported; however, topical administration is probably compatible.

Contraindications Hypersensitivity to dibucaine, other amide-type anesthetics, or any component

Warnings Some products may contain sulfites which may cause allergic reactions in susceptible individuals

Adverse Reactions
Dermatologic: Angioedema, contact dermatitis
Local: Burning

Drug Interactions

Metabolism/Transport Effects None known.

Avoid Concomitant Use There are no known interactions where it is recommended to avoid concomitant use.

Increased Effect/Toxicity There are no known significant interactions involving an increase in effect.

Decreased Effect There are no known significant interactions involving a decrease in effect.

Mechanism of Action Local anesthetics bind selectively to the intracellular surface of sodium channels to block influx of sodium into the axon. As a result, depolarization necessary for action potential propagation and subsequent nerve function is prevented. The block at the sodium channel is reversible. When drug diffuses away from the axon, sodium channel function is restored and nerve propagation returns.

Pharmacodynamics
Onset of action: Within 15 minutes
Duration: 2-4 hours

Pharmacokinetics (Adult data unless noted) Absorption: Poor through intact skin, but well absorbed through mucous membranes and excoriated skin

Dosing: Usual Children and Adults:
Rectal: Hemorrhoids: Administer each morning, evening, and after each bowel movement
Topical: Apply gently to the affected areas; no more than 30 g for adults or 7.5 g for children should be used in any 24-hour period

Administration
Rectal: Insert ointment into rectum using a rectal applicator
Topical: Apply gently to affected areas; do not use near the eyes or over denuded surfaces or blistered areas

Dosage Forms Excipient information presented when available (limited, particularly for generics); consult specific product labeling.

Ointment, External:
Nupercainal: 1% (56.7 g)
Generic: 1% (28 g, 28.35 g)
Ointment, Rectal:
Nupercainal: 1% (28.4 g, 56.7 g, 60 g)

◆ **DIC** *see* Dacarbazine *on page 578*

Diclofenac (Systemic) (dye KLOE fen ak)

Medication Safety Issues
Sound-alike/look-alike issues:
Diclofenac may be confused with Diflucan
Cataflam may be confused with Catapres
Voltaren may be confused with traMADol, Ultram, Verelan

BEERS Criteria medication:
This drug may be potentially inappropriate for use in geriatric patients (Quality of evidence - moderate; Strength of recommendation - strong).

International issues:
Diclofenac may be confused with Duphalac brand name for lactulose [multiple international markets]
Flexin: Brand name for diclofenac [Argentina], but also the brand name for cyclobenzaprine [Chile] and orphenadrine [Israel]
Flexin [Argentina] may be confused with Floxin brand name for flunarizine [Thailand], norfloxacin [South Africa], and ofloxacin [U.S.]

Related Information
Oral Medications That Should Not Be Crushed or Altered *on page 2438*

Brand Names: U.S. Cambia; Cataflam; Voltaren-XR; Zipsor; Zorvolex

Brand Names: Canada Apo-Diclo; Apo-Diclo Rapide; Apo-Diclo SR; Ava-Diclofenac; Ava-Diclofenac SR; Cambia; Diclofenac EC; Diclofenac ECT; Diclofenac K; Diclofenac SR; Diclofenac-SR; Dom-Diclofenac; Dom-Diclofenac SR; PMS-Diclofenac; PMS-Diclofenac K; PMS-Diclofenac-SR; PRO-Diclo-Rapide; Sandoz-Diclofenac; Sandoz-Diclofenac Rapide; Sandoz-Diclofenac SR; Teva-Diclofenac; Teva-Diclofenac EC; Teva-Diclofenac K; Teva-Diclofenac SR; Voltaren; Voltaren Rapide; Voltaren SR

Therapeutic Category Analgesic, Non-narcotic; Anti-inflammatory Agent; Nonsteroidal Anti-inflammatory Drug (NSAID), Oral

Generic Availability (U.S.) May be product dependent

Use Oral:
Capsule: Relief of mild to moderate acute pain (FDA approved in ages ≥18 years and adults)
Immediate release tablet: Relief of mild to moderate pain; primary dysmenorrhea; acute and chronic treatment of

rheumatoid arthritis and osteoarthritis (all indications: FDA approved in adults); has also been used for juvenile idiopathic arthritis

Delayed release tablet: Acute and chronic treatment of rheumatoid arthritis, osteoarthritis, and ankylosing spondylitis (FDA approved in adults)

Extended release tablet: Chronic treatment of osteoarthritis and rheumatoid arthritis (FDA approved in adults)

Oral solution: Treatment of acute migraine with or without aura (FDA approved in ages ≥18 years and adults)

Medication Guide Available Yes

Pregnancy Risk Factor C (oral)/D (≥30 weeks gestation [oral])

Pregnancy Considerations Adverse events were not observed in the initial animal reproduction studies; therefore, manufacturers classify most dosage forms of diclofenac as pregnancy category C (oral: Category D ≥30 weeks gestation). Diclofenac crosses the placenta and can be detected in fetal tissue and amniotic fluid. NSAID exposure during the first trimester is not strongly associated with congenital malformations; however, cardiovascular anomalies and cleft palate have been observed following NSAID exposure in some studies. The use of a NSAID close to conception may be associated with an increased risk of miscarriage. Nonteratogenic effects have been observed following NSAID administration during the third trimester including: Myocardial degenerative changes, prenatal constriction of the ductus arteriosus, fetal tricuspid regurgitation, failure of the ductus arteriosus to close postnatally; renal dysfunction or failure, oligohydramnios; gastrointestinal bleeding or perforation, increased risk of necrotizing enterocolitis; intracranial bleeding (including intraventricular hemorrhage), platelet dysfunction with resultant bleeding; pulmonary hypertension. Because they may cause premature closure of the ductus arteriosus, use of NSAIDs in pregnancy (particularly late pregnancy) should be avoided. Product labeling for Cambia, Zipsor, and Zorvolex specifically notes that use at ≥30 weeks' gestation should be avoided. Use in the third trimester is contraindicated in the Canadian labeling. The chronic use of NSAIDs in women of reproductive age may be associated with infertility that is reversible upon discontinuation of the medication. A registry is available for pregnant women exposed to autoimmune medications including diclofenac. For additional information contact the Organization of Teratology Information Specialists, OTIS Autoimmune Diseases Study, at 877-311-8972

Breast-Feeding Considerations Low concentrations of diclofenac can be found in breast milk. Breast-feeding is not recommended by most manufacturers. Use while breast-feeding is contraindicated in Canadian labeling.

Contraindications Hypersensitivity to diclofenac or any component; history of asthma, urticaria, or allergic-type reaction to aspirin or other NSAIDs; patients with the "aspirin triad" [asthma, rhinitis (with or without nasal polyps), and aspirin intolerance] (fatal asthmatic and anaphylactoid reactions may occur in these patients); perioperative pain in the setting of coronary artery bypass graft (CABG)

Warnings NSAIDs are associated with an increased risk of adverse cardiovascular thrombotic events, including potentially fatal MI and stroke **[U.S. Boxed Warning]**; risk may be increased with duration of use or preexisting cardiovascular risk factors or disease; carefully evaluate cardiovascular risk profile prior to prescribing; use the lowest effective dose for the shortest duration of time, taking into consideration individual patient treatment goals; alternate therapies should be considered for patients at high risk. Use is contraindicated for treatment of perioperative pain in the setting of CABG surgery **[U.S. Boxed Warning]**; an increased incidence of MI and stroke was found in patients receiving COX-2 selective NSAIDs for the treatment of pain within the first 10-14 days after CABG surgery. NSAIDs may cause fluid retention, edema, and new onset or worsening of preexisting hypertension; use with caution in patients with hypertension, CHF, or fluid retention. Concurrent administration of ibuprofen, and potentially other nonselective NSAIDs; may interfere with aspirin's cardioprotective effect.

NSAIDs may increase the risk of gastrointestinal inflammation, ulceration, bleeding, and perforation **[U.S. Boxed Warning]**. These events, which can be potentially fatal, may occur at any time during therapy, and without warning. Avoid the use of NSAIDs in patients with active GI bleeding or ulcer disease. Use NSAIDs with extreme caution in patients with a history of GI bleeding or ulcers (these patients have a 10-fold increased risk for developing a GI bleed). Use NSAIDs with caution in patients with other risk factors which may increase GI bleeding (eg, concurrent therapy with aspirin, anticoagulants, and/or corticosteroids, longer duration of NSAID use, smoking, use of alcohol, and poor general health). Use the lowest effective dose for the shortest duration of time, taking into consideration individual patient treatment goals; alternate therapies should be considered for patients at high risk.

NSAIDs may compromise existing renal function. Renal toxicity may occur in patients with impaired renal function, dehydration, heart failure, liver dysfunction, and those taking diuretics and ACE inhibitors; use with caution in these patients; monitor renal function closely. NSAIDs are not recommended for use in patients with advanced renal disease. Long-term use of NSAIDs may cause renal papillary necrosis and other renal injury.

Fatal asthmatic and anaphylactoid reactions may occur in patients with the "aspirin triad" who receive NSAIDs. NSAIDs may cause serious dermatologic adverse reactions, including exfoliative dermatitis, Stevens-Johnson syndrome, and toxic epidermal necrolysis. Avoid use of NSAIDs in late pregnancy as they may cause premature closure of the ductus arteriosus. Avoid the use of diclofenac in patients with hepatic porphyria (eg, variegate porphyria, acute intermittent porphyria, porphyria cutanea tarda); acute attacks of porphyria may occur.

Cases of drug-induced hepatotoxicity, including hepatic failure, resulting in death or requiring transplantation, have been reported. A potential for liver function test elevation exists with use of any diclofenac-containing product. Transaminase elevations generally occur within the first 2 months of therapy but may occur at any time; initiate monitoring after 4-8 weeks of therapy. Discontinue therapy immediately if abnormal liver tests persist or worsen, if clinical signs and/or symptoms consistent with liver disease develop, or if systemic manifestations occur (eg, eosinophilia, rash, abdominal pain, diarrhea, dark urine).

Oral solution is only indicated for acute treatment of migraine; not indicated for migraine prophylaxis or cluster headache. The oral solution is not bioequivalent to other forms of diclofenac (even if same dose); do not interchange products.

Precautions Use with caution and decrease the dose in patients with decreased hepatic function; closely monitor patients with abnormal LFTs; severe hepatic reactions (eg, fulminant hepatitis, liver failure) have occurred. Use with caution in patients with asthma; asthmatic patients may have aspirin-sensitive asthma which may be associated with severe and potentially fatal bronchospasm when aspirin or NSAIDs are administered. Anemia (due to occult or gross blood loss from the GI tract, fluid retention, or other effect on erythropoiesis) may occur; monitor hemoglobin and hematocrit in patients receiving long-term therapy. Use with caution and monitor carefully in patients with coagulation disorders or those receiving anticoagulants; NSAIDs inhibit platelet aggregation and may prolong bleeding time. Oral solution contains phenylalanine (25 mg/packet); use with caution in patients with phenylketonuria.

Adverse Reactions
Oral:
Cardiovascular: Edema

Central nervous system: Dizziness, headache

Dermatologic: Pruritus, rash

Endocrine & metabolic: Fluid retention

Gastrointestinal: Abdominal distension, abdominal pain, constipation, diarrhea, dyspepsia, flatulence, GI perforation, heartburn, nausea, peptic ulcer/GI bleed, vomiting

Hematologic: Anemia, bleeding time increased

Hepatic: Liver enzyme abnormalities

Otic: Tinnitus

Renal: Renal function abnormal

Rare but important or life-threatening: Agranulocytosis, alopecia, anaphylactoid reactions, anaphylaxis, angioedema, aplastic anemia, anxiety, appetite changes, arrhythmia, aseptic meningitis, asthma, azotemia, blurred vision, chest pain, CHF, colitis, coma, confusion, conjunctivitis, cystitis, depression, diplopia, disorientation, dreams abnormal, drowsiness, dyspnea, dysuria, ecchymosis, eosinophilia, eructation, erythema multiforme, esophageal lesions, esophagitis, exfoliative dermatitis, fever, fulminant hepatitis, gastritis, glossitis, hallucination, hearing impairment, hearing loss, hematemesis, hematuria, hemoglobin decreased, hemolytic anemia, hepatic failure, hepatic necrosis, hepatitis, hepatotoxicity, hyper-/hypotension, hyper-/hypoglycemia, infection, insomnia, interstitial nephritis, intestinal perforation, jaundice, laryngeal edema, leukopenia, lymphadenopathy, malaise, melena, memory disturbance, meningitis, MI, nephrotic syndrome, nervousness, oliguria, palpitation, pancreatitis, pancytopenia, paresthesia, pharynx edema, photosensitivity, pneumonia, polyuria, proteinuria, psychotic reactions, purpura, rectal bleeding, renal failure, renal papillary necrosis, respiratory depression, seizure, sepsis, somnolence, Stevens-Johnson syndrome, stomatitis, stroke, swelling of lips and tongue, syncope, tachycardia, taste disorder, thrombocytopenia, toxic epidermal necrolysis, tremor, urticaria, vasculitis, vertigo, weight change, weakness, xerostomia

Rectal suppository [Canadian product]:
Also refer to adverse reactions associated with oral formulations.

Rare but important or life-threatening: Local: Bleeding, hemorrhoid exacerbation, proctitis, rectal irritation

Drug Interactions
Metabolism/Transport Effects Substrate of CYP1A2 (minor), CYP2B6 (minor), CYP2C19 (minor), CYP2C8 (minor), CYP2C9 (minor), CYP2D6 (minor), CYP3A4 (minor); **Note:** Assignment of Major/Minor substrate status based on clinically relevant drug interaction potential; **Inhibits** CYP1A2 (weak), CYP2C9 (weak), CYP2E1 (weak), CYP3A4 (weak), UGT1A6

Avoid Concomitant Use
Avoid concomitant use of Diclofenac (Systemic) with any of the following: Floctafenine; Ketorolac (Nasal); Ketorolac (Systemic); NSAID (COX-2 Inhibitor); Omacetaxine; Pimozide; Urokinase

Increased Effect/Toxicity
Diclofenac (Systemic) may increase the levels/effects of: 5-ASA Derivatives; Agents with Antiplatelet Properties; Aliskiren; Aminoglycosides; Anticoagulants; Apixaban; ARIPiprazole; Bisphosphonate Derivatives; Collagenase (Systemic); CycloSPORINE (Systemic); Dabigatran Etexilate; Deferasirox; Deferiprone; Desmopressin; Digoxin; Dofetilide; Eplerenone; Haloperidol; Ibritumomab; Lithium; Lomitapide; Methotrexate; Nonsteroidal Anti-Inflammatory Agents; NSAID (COX-2 Inhibitor);

Omacetaxine; PEMEtrexed; Pimozide; Porfimer; Potassium-Sparing Diuretics; PRALAtrexate; Quinolone Antibiotics; Rivaroxaban; Salicylates; Tenofovir; Thrombolytic Agents; Tositumomab and Iodine I 131 Tositumomab; Urokinase; Vancomycin; Vitamin K Antagonists

The levels/effects of Diclofenac (Systemic) may be increased by: ACE Inhibitors; Angiotensin II Receptor Blockers; Antidepressants (Tricyclic, Tertiary Amine); Corticosteroids (Systemic); CycloSPORINE (Systemic); CYP2C9 Inhibitors (Strong); Dasatinib; Floctafenine; Glucosamine; Herbs (Anticoagulant/Antiplatelet Properties); Ibrutinib; Ketorolac (Nasal); Ketorolac (Systemic); Multivitamins/Fluoride (with ADE); Multivitamins/Minerals (with ADEK, Folate, Iron); Multivitamins/Minerals (with AE, No Iron); Nonsteroidal Anti-Inflammatory Agents; Omega-3 Fatty Acids; Pentosan Polysulfate Sodium; Pentoxifylline; Probenecid; Prostacyclin Analogues; Selective Serotonin Reuptake Inhibitors; Serotonin/Norepinephrine Reuptake Inhibitors; Sodium Phosphates; Tipranavir; Treprostinil; Vitamin E; Voriconazole

Decreased Effect
Diclofenac (Systemic) may decrease the levels/effects of: ACE Inhibitors; Agents with Antiplatelet Properties; Aliskiren; Angiotensin II Receptor Blockers; Beta-Blockers; Eplerenone; HydrALAZINE; Loop Diuretics; Potassium-Sparing Diuretics; Prostaglandins (Ophthalmic); Salicylates; Selective Serotonin Reuptake Inhibitors; Thiazide Diuretics

The levels/effects of Diclofenac (Systemic) may be decreased by: Bile Acid Sequestrants; CYP2C9 Inducers (Strong); Nonsteroidal Anti-Inflammatory Agents; Peginterferon Alfa-2b; Salicylates

Stability
Capsule, oral solution: Store at 25°C (77°F); excursions permitted from 15°C to 30°C (59°F to 86°F)

Tablets: Store at ≤30°C (86°F); protect from moisture; dispense in tight container

Mechanism of Action Reversibly inhibits cyclooxygenase-1 and 2 (COX-1 and 2) enzymes, which results in decreased formation of prostaglandin precursors; has antipyretic, analgesic, and anti-inflammatory properties

Other proposed mechanisms not fully elucidated (and possibly contributing to the anti-inflammatory effect to varying degrees), include inhibiting chemotaxis, altering lymphocyte activity, inhibiting neutrophil aggregation/activation, and decreasing proinflammatory cytokine levels.

Pharmacokinetics (Adult data unless noted)
Distribution: V_d: 1.4 L/kg

Protein binding: >99%

Metabolism: Hepatic; undergoes first-pass metabolism; in the liver, undergoes hydroxylation then glucuronide and sulfate conjugation

Bioavailability: 50%

Half-life: 2.3 hours

Time to peak serum concentration:

Cambia™: 0.25 hours

Cataflam®: 1 hour

Voltaren®: 2.22 hours

Voltaren®-XR: 5.25 hours

Elimination: About 65% of the dose is eliminated in the urine and ~35% in the bile (primarily as conjugated forms); little or no unchanged drug is excreted in urine or bile

Dosing: Usual Note: Different oral formulations are not bioequivalent; do not interchange products.

Children and Adolescents <18 years: **Juvenile idiopathic arthritis:** Limited data available: Oral: Immediate release tablet: 2-3 mg/kg/day divided 2-4 times/day; maximum daily dose: 200 mg/**day** (Haapasaari, 1983; Hashkes, 2005)

Adolescents ≥18 years and Adults:

Analgesia: Oral:

Immediate release capsule: 25 mg 4 times/day

Immediate release tablet: Adults: Initial: 50 mg 3 times/day [maximum dose: 150 mg/day]; may administer 100 mg loading dose, followed by 50 mg every 8 hours; initial maximum daily dose (day 1): 200 mg/day; maximum dose day 2 and thereafter: 150 mg/day]

Ankylosing spondylitis: Adults: Oral: Delayed release tablet: 100-125 mg/day in 4-5 divided doses

Migraine: Oral: Oral solution: 50 mg (one packet) as a single dose at the time of migraine onset; safety and efficacy of a second dose have not been established

Osteoarthritis: Adults: Oral:

Immediate release tablet: 150-200 mg/day in 3-4 divided doses

Delayed release tablet: 150-200 mg/day in 2-4 divided doses

Extended release tablet: 100 mg/day; may increase dose to 200 mg/day in 2 divided doses

Primary dysmenorrhea: Adults: Oral: Immediate release tablet: Initial: 50 mg 3 times/day (maximum dose: 150 mg/day); may administer 100 mg loading dose, followed by 50 mg every 8 hours

Rheumatoid arthritis: Adults: Oral:

Immediate release tablet: 150-200 mg/day in 3-4 divided doses

Delayed release tablet: 150-200 mg/day in 2-4 divided doses

Extended release tablet: 100 mg/day; may increase dose to 200 mg/day in 2 divided doses

Dosing adjustment in renal impairment: Not recommended in patients with advanced renal disease or significant renal impairment.

Dosing adjustment in hepatic impairment: May require dosage adjustment; use oral solution only if benefits outweigh risks.

Administration Administer with milk or food to decrease GI upset; take with full glass of water to enhance absorption.

Delayed or extended release dosage form: Do not chew or crush delayed release or extended release tablets, swallow whole.

Oral solution: Empty contents of packet into 1-2 ounces (30-60 mL) of water (do not use other liquids); mix well and administer right away. Food may reduce effectiveness.

Monitoring Parameters CBC, liver enzymes (periodically during chronic therapy starting 4-8 weeks after initiation); monitor urine output, BUN, serum creatinine in patients receiving diuretics

Additional Information Diclofenac potassium = Cataflam®; potassium content: 5.8 mg (0.15 mEq) per 50 mg tablet

Dosage Forms Excipient information presented when available (limited, particularly for generics); consult specific product labeling.

Capsule, Oral, as base:

Zorvolex: 18 mg, 35 mg [contains brilliant blue fcf (fd&c blue #1), fd&c blue #2 (indigotine)]

Capsule, Oral, as potassium:

Zipsor: 25 mg [contains gelatin (bovine)]

Packet, Oral, as potassium:

Cambia: 50 mg (1 ea, 9 ea) [contains aspartame, saccharin sodium; flavored flavor]

Tablet, Oral, as potassium:

Cataflam: 50 mg

Generic: 50 mg

Tablet Delayed Release, Oral, as sodium:

Generic: 25 mg, 50 mg, 75 mg

Tablet Extended Release 24 Hour, Oral, as sodium:

Voltaren-XR: 100 mg

Generic: 100 mg

References

Brogden RN, Heel RC, Pakes GE, et al, "Diclofenac Sodium: A Review of Its Pharmacological Properties and Therapeutic Use in Rheumatic Diseases and Pain of Varying Origin," Drugs, 1980, 20(1):24-48.

Haapasaari J, Wuolijoki E, and Ylijoki H, "Treatment of Juvenile Rheumatoid Arthritis With Diclofenac Sodium," Scand J Rheumatol, 1983, 12(4):325-30.

Hashkes PJ and Laxer RM, "Medical Treatment of Juvenile Idiopathic Arthritis," JAMA, 2005, 294(13):1671-84.

Diclofenac (Ophthalmic) (dye KLOE fen ak)

Medication Safety Issues

Sound-alike/look-alike issues:

Diclofenac may be confused with Diflucan

International Issues:

Diclofenac may be confused with Duphalac brand name for lactulose [multiple international markets]

Flexin: Brand name for diclofenac [Argentina], but also the brand name for cyclobenzaprine [Chile] and orphenadrine [Israel]

Flexin [Argentina] may be confused with Floxin brand name for flunarizine [Thailand], norfloxacin [South Africa], ofloxacin [U.S., Canada], and pefloxacin [Philippines]

Brand Names: Canada Voltaren Ophtha

Therapeutic Category Analgesic, Non-narcotic; Anti-inflammatory Agent; Nonsteroidal Anti-inflammatory Drug (NSAID), Ophthalmic

Generic Availability (U.S.) Yes

Use Treatment of postoperative inflammation after cataract extraction; temporary relief of pain and photophobia in patients undergoing corneal refractive surgery (FDA approved in adults)

Pregnancy Risk Factor C

Pregnancy Considerations Adverse events have not been observed in animal studies; therefore, the manufacturer classifies diclofenac ophthalmic as pregnancy category C. When administered orally, diclofenac crosses the placenta. Refer to the Diclofenac (Systemic) monograph for details. The amount of diclofenac available systemically following topical application of the ophthalmic drops is significantly less in comparison to oral doses; however, because it may cause prenatal constriction of the ductus arteriosus, the manufacturer recommends that the use of diclofenac ophthalmic drops late in pregnancy be avoided.

Breast-Feeding Considerations When administered orally, low concentrations of diclofenac can be found in breast milk. Refer to the Diclofenac (Systemic) monograph for details. The amount of diclofenac available systemically following topical application of the ophthalmic drops is significantly less in comparison to oral doses.

Contraindications Hypersensitivity to diclofenac or any component

Warnings Refractive stability is not established in patients undergoing corneal refractive procedures; monitor patients for 1 year following application of ophthalmic drops. May cause increased bleeding time following surgery; increased bleeding of ocular tissues (including hyphemas) has been reported with other ophthalmic NSAID use.

Precautions Use with caution in patients with previous sensitivity to acetylsalicylic acid and phenylacetic acid derivatives, including patients who experience bronchospasm, asthma, rhinitis, or urticaria following NSAID or aspirin therapy. Use with caution in patients with complicated ocular surgeries, corneal denervation, epithelial defects, diabetes, rheumatoid arthritis, ocular surface diseases (eg, dry eye syndrome), or ocular surgeries repeated within short periods of time; corneal thinning, erosion, or ulceration leading to possible loss of vision have been reported; discontinue if corneal epithelial breakdown occurs. Use of ophthalmic NSAIDs may be associated with keratitis; continued use may be associated with sight-threatening complications, including corneal perforation. Use of topical ophthalmic NSAIDs for more than 24 hours prior to surgery and more than 14 days after ocular surgery has been associated with an increased risk of more frequent and severe corneal adverse events. Ophthalmic drops may slow or delay healing time following surgery. Patients using ophthalmic drops should not wear soft contact lenses. To minimize the risk of infection following surgery of both eyes, two separate bottles of eye drops (one for each eye) should be used for postsurgical patients; instruct patients not to use the same bottle for both eyes.

Adverse Reactions

Cardiovascular: Facial edema

Central nervous system: Chills, dizziness, fever, headache, insomnia, pain

Gastrointestinal: Abdominal pain, nausea, vomiting

Neuromuscular & skeletal: Pain, weakness

Ocular: Abnormal vision, blurred vision, conjunctivitis, corneal deposits, corneal edema, corneal lesions, corneal opacity, discharge, eyelid swelling, injection, intraocular pressure increased, iritis, irritation, itching, keratitis, lacrimation, lacrimation disorder, ocular allergy, transient burning/stinging

Respiratory: Rhinitis

Miscellaneous: Viral infection

Rare but important or life-threatening: Corneal erosion, corneal infiltrates, corneal perforation, corneal thinning, corneal ulceration, epithelial breakdown

Drug Interactions

Metabolism/Transport Effects None known.

Avoid Concomitant Use There are no known interactions where it is recommended to avoid concomitant use.

Increased Effect/Toxicity There are no known significant interactions involving an increase in effect.

Decreased Effect There are no known significant interactions involving a decrease in effect.

Stability Store at 15°C to 25°C (59°F to 77°F).

Mechanism of Action Reversibly inhibits cyclooxygenase-1 and 2 (COX-1 and 2) enzymes, which results in decreased formation of prostaglandin precursors; has antipyretic, analgesic, and anti-inflammatory properties.

Other proposed mechanisms not fully elucidated (and possibly contributing to the anti-inflammatory effect to varying degrees), include inhibiting chemotaxis, altering lymphocyte activity, inhibiting neutrophil aggregation/activation, and decreasing proinflammatory cytokine levels.

Dosing: Usual Adults:

Cataract surgery: Instill 1 drop into affected eye 4 times/day beginning 24 hours after cataract surgery and continuing for 2 weeks

Corneal refractive surgery: Instill 1-2 drops into operative eye within the hour prior to surgery, within 15 minutes after surgery, and continuing 4 times/day for up to 3 days

Administration For ophthalmic use only; avoid contact of bottle tip with skin or eye; apply finger pressure to lacrimal sac during and for 1-2 minutes after instillation to decrease risk of absorption and systemic effects. Wait at least 5 minutes before administering other types of eye drops.

Dosage Forms Excipient information presented when available (limited, particularly for generics); consult specific product labeling.

Solution, Ophthalmic, as sodium:

Generic: 0.1% (2.5 mL, 5 mL)

Diclofenac (Topical) (dye KLOE fen ak)

Medication Safety Issues

Sound-alike/look-alike issues:

Diclofenac may be confused with Diflucan

Voltaren may be confused with traMADol, Ultram, Verelan

Other safety concerns:

Transdermal patch (Flector) contains conducting metal (eg, aluminum); remove patch prior to MRI.

International issues:

Diclofenac may be confused with Duphalac brand name for lactulose [multiple international markets]

Flexin: Brand name for diclofenac [Argentina], but also the brand name for cyclobenzaprine [Chile] and orphenadrine [Israel]

Flexin [Argentina] may be confused with Floxin brand name for flunarizine [Thailand], norfloxacin [South Africa], ofloxacin [U.S., Canada], and perfloxacin [Philippines]

Brand Names: U.S. Flector; Pennsaid; Solaraze; Voltaren

Brand Names: Canada Pennsaid; Voltaren Emulgel

Therapeutic Category Analgesic, Non-narcotic; Anti-inflammatory Agent

Generic Availability (U.S.) May be product dependent

Use

Topical gel 1%: Relief of osteoarthritis pain in joints amenable to topical therapy (eg, ankle, elbow, foot, hand, knee, wrist) in adults (FDA approved in adults)

Topical gel 3%: Treatment of actinic keratosis in adults (in conjunction with sun avoidance) (FDA approved in adults)

Topical patch: Acute pain due to minor strains, sprains, and contusions (FDA approved in adults)

Topical solution: Relief of osteoarthritis pain of the knee (FDA approved in adults)

Medication Guide Available Yes

Pregnancy Risk Factor B (topical gel 3%) / C (topical gel 1%, topical solution, topical patch) / D (topical solution ≥30 weeks gestation)

Pregnancy Considerations Adverse events have been observed in some animal reproduction studies. When administered orally, diclofenac crosses the placenta. The amount of diclofenac available systemically following topical application is less in comparison to oral doses. Because it may cause prenatal constriction of the ductus arteriosus, the use of diclofenac topical late in pregnancy should be avoided. Reversible constriction of the ductus arteriosus *in utero* has been observed following topical application of diclofenac. Additional adverse fetal and maternal effects have been observed following oral use of diclofenac. Refer to the Diclofenac (Systemic) monograph for details. A registry is available for pregnant women exposed to autoimmune medications including diclofenac. For additional information contact the Organization of Teratology Information Specialists, OTIS Autoimmune Diseases Study, at 877-311-8972.

Breast-Feeding Considerations It is not known if topical diclofenac is excreted in breast milk; however, when administered orally, low concentrations of diclofenac can be found in breast milk. Refer to the Diclofenac (Systemic) monograph for details. Due to the potential for serious adverse reactions in the nursing infant, the manufacturer recommends a decision be made whether to discontinue nursing or to discontinue the drug, taking into account the importance of treatment to the mother.

Contraindications Hypersensitivity to diclofenac, any component, aspirin, or NSAIDs; patients with the "aspirin triad" [asthma, rhinitis (with or without nasal polyps) and aspirin intolerance] (fatal asthmatic and anaphylactoid reactions may occur in these patients); perioperative pain in the setting of coronary artery bypass graft (CABG). Do not apply to nonintact or damaged skin (eg, exudative dermatitis, eczema, infected lesions, burns, or wounds)

Warnings NSAIDs are associated with an increased risk of adverse cardiovascular thrombotic events, including potentially fatal MI and stroke **[U.S. Boxed Warning]**; risk may be increased with duration of use or preexisting cardiovascular risk factors or disease; carefully evaluate cardiovascular risk profile prior to prescribing; use the lowest effective dose for the shortest duration of time, taking into consideration individual patient treatment goals; alternate therapies should be considered for patients at high risk. Use is contraindicated for treatment of perioperative pain in the setting of CABG surgery **[U.S. Boxed Warning]**; an increased incidence of MI and stroke was found in patients receiving COX-2 selective NSAIDs for the treatment of pain within the first 10-14 days after CABG surgery. NSAIDs may cause fluid retention, edema, and new onset or worsening of preexisting hypertension; use with caution in patients with hypertension, CHF, or fluid retention. Concurrent administration of ibuprofen, and potentially other nonselective NSAIDs, may interfere with aspirin's cardioprotective effect.

Transdermal patch (used and unused) contains a large amount of medication which can cause serious adverse effects in children or pets if patch is chewed or ingested; fold used patches so the adhesive side sticks to itself; store and dispose used patches properly and out of the reach of children and pets. Transdermal patch contains conducting metal (aluminum) which may cause a burn to the skin during an MRI scan; remove patch prior to MRI; reapply patch after scan is completed. Due to the potential for altered electrical conductivity, remove transdermal patch before cardioversion or defibrillation. Apply transdermal patch only to intact skin. Do not apply topical patch to the eyes, mucous membranes, open wounds, infected areas, or to exudative dermatitis. Patch should not be worn during bathing or showering.

Topical gel 3% contains benzyl alcohol which may cause allergic reactions in susceptible individuals; large amounts of benzyl alcohol (≥99 mg/kg/day) have been associated with a potentially fatal toxicity ("gasping syndrome") in neonates; avoid use of diclofenac products containing benzyl alcohol in neonates; *in vitro* and animal studies have shown that benzoate, a metabolite of benzyl alcohol, displaces bilirubin from protein binding sites. Topical get 1% and transdermal patch contain propylene glycol; toxicities have been reported with use of products containing propylene glycol, including hyperosmolality, lactic acidosis, seizures, and respiratory depression; in neonates large amounts of propylene glycol delivered orally, intravenously (eg, >3000 mg/day), or topically have been associated with potentially fatal toxicities which can include metabolic acidosis, seizures, renal failure, and CNS depression; use products containing propylene glycol with caution (AAP, 1997; Shehab, 2009).

Precautions Do not apply topical gel or solution to open skin wounds, infected areas, mucous membranes, or exfoliative dermatitis; do not allow gel or topical solution to come in contact with eyes; do not use topical gel or solution in neonates, infants, or children. Avoid use of occlusive dressings. Avoid sunlight exposure to treated areas. Combination use with oral NSAIDs is not recommended due to increased risk of adverse reactions.

Adverse Reactions
Topical gel:
Cardiovascular: Chest pain, hypertension

Central nervous system: Headache, hyperesthesia, migraine, pain, paresthesia

Dermatologic: Acne vulgaris (application site), alopecia (application site), application site pain, application site paresthesia, application site rash, contact dermatitis, dermal ulcer, desquamation (application site), pruritus, skin photosensitivity (application site), skin rash, vesiculobullous dermatitis (application site), xeroderma

Endocrine & metabolic: Application site edema, hypercholesterolemia, hyperglycemia

Gastrointestinal: Abdominal pain, diarrhea, dyspepsia

Genitourinary: Hematuria

Hepatic: Increased liver enzymes, increased serum ALT, increased serum AST, increased serum transaminases

Neuromuscular and skeletal: Arthralgia, arthropathy, back pain, hypokinesia, increased creatine phosphokinase, myalgia, neck pain, weakness

Ophthalmic: Conjunctivitis, eye pain

Respiratory: Asthma, dyspnea, flu-like symptoms, pneumonia, sinusitis

Miscellaneous: Accidental injury

Rare but important or life-threatening: Application site irritation, application site papules, application site reaction (skin carcinoma, hypertonia, skin hypertrophy lacrimation disorder, maculopapular rash, purpuric rash, vasodilation), application site vesicles, edema, hepatic failure, hepatitis (fulfillment; with and without jaundice), seborrhea, skin hypertrophy, urticaria

Topical solution:
Cardiovascular: Edema

Dermatologic: Application site erythema, application site induration, application site pain, application site rash, contact dermatitis, desquamation (application site), pruritus, skin rash, xeroderma

Gastrointestinal: Abdominal pain, constipation, diarrhea, dyspepsia, flatulence, halitosis, nausea

Genitourinary: Urinary tract infection

Hematologic & oncologic: Bruise

Infection: Infection

Respiratory: Sinus congestion, sinusitis

Rare but important or life-threatening: Accidental injury, aphthous stomatitis, asthma, body odor, burning sensation of skin, cardiovascular disease, cataract, chest pain, depression, eczema, eye disease, gastroenteritis, hypersensitivity reaction, hypertension, increased serum creatinine, laryngismus, oral mucosa ulcer, palpitations, rectal hemorrhage, skin discoloration, visual disturbance

Transdermal patch:
Central nervous system: Dizziness, hypoesthesia

Dermatologic: Dermatitis, hyperhidrosis, hypersensitivity reaction (dermal), local dryness, localized erythema, localized vesiculation, skin discoloration

Gastrointestinal: Constipation, diarrhea, dysgeusia, gastritis, nausea, upper abdominal pain, vomiting, xerostomia

Local: Application site atrophy, local irritation, localized edema, local pruritus

Neuromuscular & skeletal: Hyperkinesia

Rare but important or life-threatening: Cerebrovascular accident, edema, myocardial infarction, Stevens-Johnson syndrome

Drug Interactions
Metabolism/Transport Effects Substrate of CYP1A2 (minor), CYP2B6 (minor), CYP2C19 (minor), CYP2C8 (minor), CYP2C9 (minor), CYP2D6 (minor), CYP3A4 (minor); **Note:** Assignment of Major/Minor substrate status based on clinically relevant drug interaction potential; **Inhibits** CYP1A2 (weak), CYP2C9 (weak), CYP2E1 (weak), CYP3A4 (weak)

Avoid Concomitant Use
Avoid concomitant use of Diclofenac (Topical) with any of the following: Floctafenine; Ketorolac (Nasal); Ketorolac (Systemic); NSAID (COX-2 Inhibitor); Omacetaxine; Pimozide; Urokinase

Increased Effect/Toxicity

Diclofenac (Topical) may increase the levels/effects of: 5-ASA Derivatives; Agents with Antiplatelet Properties; Aliskiren; Aminoglycosides; Anticoagulants; Apixaban; ARIPiprazole; Bisphosphonate Derivatives; Collagenase (Systemic); CycloSPORINE (Systemic); Dabigatran Etexilate; Deferasirox; Desmopressin; Digoxin; Dofetilide; Eplerenone; Haloperidol; Ibritumomab; Lithium; Lomitapide; Methotrexate; Nonsteroidal Anti-Inflammatory Agents; NSAID (COX-2 Inhibitor); Omacetaxine; PEMEtrexed; Pimozide; Porfimer; Potassium-Sparing Diuretics; PRALAtrexate; Quinolone Antibiotics; Rivaroxaban; Salicylates; Tenofovir; Thrombolytic Agents; Tositumomab and Iodine I 131 Tositumomab; Urokinase; Vancomycin; Vitamin K Antagonists

The levels/effects of Diclofenac (Topical) may be increased by: ACE Inhibitors; Angiotensin II Receptor Blockers; Antidepressants (Tricyclic, Tertiary Amine); Corticosteroids (Systemic); CycloSPORINE (Systemic); Dasatinib; Floctafenine; Glucosamine; Herbs (Anticoagulant/Antiplatelet Properties); Ibrutinib; Ketorolac (Nasal); Ketorolac (Systemic); Multivitamins/Fluoride (with ADE); Multivitamins/Minerals (with ADEK, Folate, Iron); Multivitamins/Minerals (with ADEK, No Iron); Nonsteroidal Anti-Inflammatory Agents; Omega-3 Fatty Acids; Pentosan Polysulfate Sodium; Pentoxifylline; Probenecid; Prostacyclin Analogues; Selective Serotonin Reuptake Inhibitors; Serotonin/Norepinephrine Reuptake Inhibitors; Sodium Phosphates; Tipranavir; Treprostinil; Vitamin E; Voriconazole

Decreased Effect

Diclofenac (Topical) may decrease the levels/effects of: ACE Inhibitors; Agents with Antiplatelet Properties; Aliskiren; Angiotensin II Receptor Blockers; Beta-Blockers; Eplerenone; HydrALAZINE; Loop Diuretics; Potassium-Sparing Diuretics; Prostaglandins (Ophthalmic); Salicylates; Selective Serotonin Reuptake Inhibitors; Thiazide Diuretics

The levels/effects of Diclofenac (Topical) may be decreased by: Bile Acid Sequestrants; Nonsteroidal Anti-Inflammatory Agents; Peginterferon Alfa-2b; Salicylates

Stability

Topical gel: Store at controlled room temperature of 20°C to 25°C (68°F to 77°F); do not freeze.

Topical solution: Store at controlled room temperature of 25°C (77°F); excursions permitted to 15°C to 30°C (59°F to 86°F).

Transdermal patch: Store at controlled room temperature 25°C (77°F); excursions permitted to 15°C to 30°C (59°F to 86°F). Keep envelope sealed when not being used.

Mechanism of Action

Reversibly inhibits cyclooxygenase-1 and 2 (COX-1 and 2) enzymes, which results in decreased formation of prostaglandin precursors; has antipyretic, analgesic, and anti-inflammatory properties

Other proposed mechanisms not fully elucidated (and possibly contributing to the anti-inflammatory effect to varying degrees), include inhibiting chemotaxis, altering lymphocyte activity, inhibiting neutrophil aggregation/activation, and decreasing proinflammatory cytokine levels.

Pharmacokinetics (Adult data unless noted)

Absorption: Topical gel: 6% to 10%; Topical solution: ~2% to 3%

Half-life elimination: Patch: ~12 hours

Time to peak serum concentration: Flector®: 10-20 hours; Pennsaid®: 5-17 hours; Solaraze® Gel: ~5 hours; Voltaren® Gel: 10-14 hours

Dosing: Usual Adults:

Actinic keratosis: (Solaraze® Gel): Apply 3% gel to lesions twice daily; recommended duration of therapy: 60-90 days

Acute pain (strains, sprains, contusions): Patch: Apply 1 patch twice daily to most painful area of skin

Osteoarthritis:

Topical gel: (Voltaren® Gel): **Note:** Maximum total body dose of 1% gel should not exceed 32 g per day

Lower extremities: Apply 4 g of 1% gel to affected area 4 times daily (maximum: 16 g per joint per day)

Upper extremities: Apply 2 g of 1% gel to affected area 4 times daily (maximum: 8 g per joint per day)

Topical solution: Knee: Apply 40 drops to each affected knee(s) 4 times daily

Administration

Topical gel: Do not cover with occlusive dressings or apply sunscreens, cosmetics, lotions, moisturizers, insect repellents, or other topical medications to affected area. Do not wash area for 1 hour following application. Wash hands immediately after application (unless hands are treated joint). Avoid sunlight to exposure areas.

1% formulation: Use dosing card supplied with product to measure correct amount of medication. Apply gel to affected joint and rub into skin gently, making sure to apply to entire joint.

3% formulation: Apply a small amount of gel to affected area; smooth gently over lesion; usually 0.5 g of gel is used per 5 x 5 cm lesion site.

Topical solution: Apply to clean, dry, intact skin; do not apply to eyes, mucous membranes, or open wounds. Wash hands before and after use. Apply 10 drops at a time either directly onto knee or into hand then onto knee (helps avoid spillage). Repeat procedure until total dose has been applied. Spread evenly around knee (front, back, sides). Allow knee to dry before applying clothing. Do not shower or bathe for at least 30 minutes after applying. Do not apply heat or occlusive dressing to treated knee; protect treated knee from sunlight. Cosmetics, insect repellant, lotion, moisturizer, sunscreens, or other topical medication may be applied to treated knee once solution has dried.

Transdermal patch: Apply to intact, nondamaged skin. Remove transparent liner prior to applying to skin. Wash hands after applying, handling, or removal of patch. Avoid contact with eyes. May tape down edges of patch, if peeling occurs. Should not be worn while bathing or showering. Fold used patches so the adhesive side sticks to itself; dispose of used patches out of reach of children and pets.

Additional Information The safety of concurrent use of cosmetics, sunscreens, or other topical agents with diclofenac gel is not known.

Dosage Forms Excipient information presented when available (limited, particularly for generics); consult specific product labeling.

Gel, Transdermal, as sodium:

Solaraze: 3% (100 g) [contains benzyl alcohol, polyethylene glycol, sodium hyaluronate]

Voltaren: 1% (100 g) [contains isopropyl alcohol, propylene glycol]

Generic: 3% (100 g)

Patch, Transdermal, as epolamine:

Flector: 1.3% (5 ea, 30 ea) [contains edetate disodium, methylparaben, polysorbate 80, propylparaben]

Solution, Transdermal, as sodium:

Pennsaid: 1.5% (150 mL); 2% (112 g) [contains propylene glycol]

Generic: 1.5% (150 mL)

References

American Academy of Pediatrics Committee on Drugs. "Inactive" ingredients in pharmaceutical products: update (subject review). *Pediatrics.* 1997;99(2):268-278.

Shehab N, Lewis CL, Streetman DD, Donn SM. Exposure to the pharmaceutical excipients benzyl alcohol and propylene glycol among critically ill neonates. *Pediatr Crit Care Med.* 2009;10 (2):256-259.

◆ **Diclofenac Diethylamine [CAN]** *see* Diclofenac (Topical) *on page 649*

◆ **Diclofenac EC (Can)** *see* Diclofenac (Systemic) *on page 645*

◆ **Diclofenac ECT (Can)** *see* Diclofenac (Systemic) *on page 645*

◆ **Diclofenac Epolamine** *see* Diclofenac (Topical) *on page 649*

◆ **Diclofenac K (Can)** *see* Diclofenac (Systemic) *on page 645*

◆ **Diclofenac Potassium** *see* Diclofenac (Systemic) *on page 645*

◆ **Diclofenac Sodium** *see* Diclofenac (Ophthalmic) *on page 648*

◆ **Diclofenac Sodium** *see* Diclofenac (Systemic) *on page 645*

◆ **Diclofenac Sodium** *see* Diclofenac (Topical) *on page 649*

◆ **Diclofenac SR (Can)** *see* Diclofenac (Systemic) *on page 645*

Dicloxacillin (dye kloks a SIL in)

Therapeutic Category Antibiotic, Penicillin (Antistaphylococcal)

Generic Availability (U.S.) Yes

Use Treatment of skin and soft tissue infections, pneumonia and follow-up therapy of osteomyelitis caused by susceptible penicillinase-producing staphylococci

Pregnancy Risk Factor B

Pregnancy Considerations Adverse events have not been observed in animal studies; therefore, dicloxacillin is classified as pregnancy category B. Dicloxacillin crosses the placenta. Teratogenic effects have not been reported with dicloxacillin, but adequate and well-controlled studies of dicloxacillin have not been completed in pregnant women. Other penicillins are considered safe for use in pregnancy.

Breast-Feeding Considerations It is not known if dicloxacillin crosses into human milk. The manufacturer recommends that caution be exercised when administering dicloxacillin to nursing women. Other penicillins distribute into human milk and are considered safe for use during breast-feeding. Nondose-related effects could include modification of bowel flora.

Contraindications Hypersensitivity to dicloxacillin, penicillin, or any component

Warnings Elimination is prolonged in neonates

Adverse Reactions

Gastrointestinal: Abdominal pain, diarrhea, nausea

Rare but important or life-threatening: Agranulocytosis, eosinophilia, hemolytic anemia, hepatotoxicity, hypersensitivity, interstitial nephritis, leukopenia, neutropenia, prolonged PT, pseudomembranous colitis, rash (maculopapular to exfoliative), seizure with extremely high doses and/or renal failure, serum sickness-like reactions, thrombocytopenia, vaginitis, vomiting

Drug Interactions

Metabolism/Transport Effects Induces CYP3A4 (weak/moderate)

Avoid Concomitant Use

Avoid concomitant use of Dicloxacillin with any of the following: Axitinib; BCG; Probenecid; Simeprevir

Increased Effect/Toxicity

Dicloxacillin may increase the levels/effects of: Methotrexate

The levels/effects of Dicloxacillin may be increased by: Probenecid

Decreased Effect

Dicloxacillin may decrease the levels/effects of: ARIPiprazole; Axitinib; BCG; Ibrutinib; Mycophenolate; Saxagliptin; Simeprevir; Sodium Picosulfate; Typhoid Vaccine; Vitamin K Antagonists

The levels/effects of Dicloxacillin may be decreased by: Tetracycline Derivatives

Food Interactions Food decreases drug absorption rate and serum concentration. Management: Administer around-the-clock on an empty stomach with a large glass of water 1 hour before or 2 hours after meals.

Mechanism of Action Inhibits bacterial cell wall synthesis by binding to one or more of the penicillin-binding proteins (PBPs) which in turn inhibits the final transpeptidation step of peptidoglycan synthesis in bacterial cell walls, thus inhibiting cell wall biosynthesis. Bacteria eventually lyse due to ongoing activity of cell wall autolytic enzymes (autolysins and murein hydrolases) while cell wall assembly is arrested.

Pharmacokinetics (Adult data unless noted)

Absorption: 35% to 76% absorbed from the GI tract

Distribution: Into bone, bile, pleural fluid, synovial fluid, and amniotic fluid; appears in breast milk

Protein binding: 96% to 98%

Half-life: Adults: 0.6-0.8 hours; slightly prolonged in patients with renal impairment

Time to peak serum concentration: Within 0.5-2 hours

Elimination: Partially eliminated by the liver and excreted in bile; 31% to 65% eliminated in urine as unchanged drug and active metabolite

Neonates: Prolonged

CF patients: More rapid elimination than healthy patients

Dialysis: Not dialyzable (0% to 5%)

Dosing: Usual Oral:

Children <40 kg: 25-50 mg/kg/day divided every 6 hours; doses of 50-100 mg/kg/day in divided doses every 6 hours have been used for follow-up therapy of osteomyelitis; maximum dose: 2 g/day

Children >40 kg and Adults: 125-500 mg every 6 hours; maximum dose: 2 g/day

Administration Oral: Administer with water 1 hour before or 2 hours after meals on an empty stomach

Monitoring Parameters Periodic monitoring of CBC, platelet count, BUN, serum creatinine, urinalysis, and liver enzymes during prolonged therapy

Test Interactions False-positive urine and serum proteins; false-positive in uric acid, urinary steroids; may interfere with urinary glucose tests using cupric sulfate (Benedict's solution, Clinitest®); may inactivate aminoglycosides *in vitro*

Additional Information Sodium content of 250 mg capsule: 0.6 mEq

Dosage Forms Excipient information presented when available (limited, particularly for generics); consult specific product labeling.

Capsule, Oral:

Generic: 250 mg, 500 mg

◆ **Dicloxacillin Sodium** *see* Dicloxacillin *on page 652*

Dicyclomine (dye SYE kloe meen)

Medication Safety Issues

Sound-alike/look-alike issues:

Dicyclomine may be confused with diphenhydrAMINE, doxycycline, dyclonine

Bentyl may be confused with Aventyl, Benadryl, Bontril, Cantil, Proventil, TRENtal

BEERS Criteria medication:

This drug may be potentially inappropriate for use in geriatric patients (Quality of evidence - moderate; Strength of recommendation - strong).

Brand Names: U.S. Bentyl

Brand Names: Canada Bentylol; Dicyclomine Hydrochloride Injection; Formulex; Jamp-Dicyclomine; Protylol; Riva-Dicyclomine

Therapeutic Category Anticholinergic Agent; Antispasmodic Agent, Gastrointestinal

Generic Availability (U.S.) Yes

Use Treatment of functional bowel/irritable bowel syndrome

Pregnancy Risk Factor B

Pregnancy Considerations Adverse events have not been observed in animal reproduction studies. In epidemiologic studies, birth defects were not observed in pregnant women taking doses up to 40 mg daily throughout the first trimester; information has not been located when used in pregnant women at recommended doses (80-160 mg daily). Use for the treatment of irritable bowel syndrome (IBS) is not recommended during pregnancy (Mahadevan, 2006).

Breast-Feeding Considerations Dicyclomine is excreted in breast milk. Due to the potential for serious adverse reactions in the nursing infant, use in nursing women and infants <6 months of age is contraindicated. In addition, anticholinergics may suppress lactation.

Contraindications Hypersensitivity to dicyclomine or any component; narrow-angle glaucoma, tachycardia, GI obstruction, obstruction of the urinary tract, severe ulcerative colitis, myasthenia gravis; should not be used in infants <6 months of age (due to reports of respiratory distress, seizures, syncope, asphyxia, pulse rate fluctuations, muscular hypotonia, and coma), nursing mothers

Warnings Heat prostration may occur in the presence of increased environmental temperature; use caution in hot weather and/or exercise. Psychosis has been reported in patients with an extreme sensitivity to anticholinergic effects. Injectable formulation is for I.M. administration only; inadvertent I.V. administration may cause thrombosis/thrombophlebitis and injection site reactions (eg, pain, edema, skin color change, reflex sympathetic dystrophy).

Precautions Use with caution in children with Down's syndrome, spastic paralysis, or brain damage; increased sensitivity to toxic effects compared to adults has been reported. Use with caution in patients with hepatic or renal disease, mild-moderate ulcerative colitis, hyperthyroidism, coronary heart disease, CHF, cardiac tachyarrhythmias, hypertension, hiatal hernia, autonomic neuropathy

Adverse Reactions

Central nervous system: Dizziness, nervousness, somnolence

Gastrointestinal: Nausea, xerostomia

Neuromuscular & skeletal: Weakness

Ocular: Blurred vision

Postmarketing and/or case reports with dicyclomine: Abdominal distension, abdominal pain, anaphylactic shock, angioedema, confusional state, constipation, cycloplegia, delirium, dermatitis (allergic), hypersensitivity, dyspepsia, dyspnea, erythema, facial edema, fatigue, hallucinations, headache, insomnia, lactation suppressed, malaise, mydriasis, nasal congestion, palpitation, rash, syncope, tachyarrhythmias, vomiting

Postmarketing and/or case reports with similar anticholinergic drugs: Anorexia, apnea, diaphoresis decreased, diplopia, focal coagulation necrosis (I.M. injection), dyskinesia, hypertension, impotence, itching, lightheadedness (transient), numbness, ocular tension increased, sneezing, speech disorder, throat congestion, tingling, urinary hesitancy, urinary retention (in patients with prostatic hypertrophy), urticaria

Drug Interactions

Metabolism/Transport Effects None known.

Avoid Concomitant Use

Avoid concomitant use of Dicyclomine with any of the following: Aclidinium; Ipratropium (Oral Inhalation); Potassium Chloride; Tiotropium; Umeclidinium

Increased Effect/Toxicity

Dicyclomine may increase the levels/effects of: AbobotulinumtoxinA; Analgesics (Opioid); Anticholinergic Agents; Cannabinoid-Containing Products; Mirabegron; OnabotulinumtoxinA; Potassium Chloride; RimabotulinumtoxinB; Thiazide Diuretics; Tiotropium; Topiramate

The levels/effects of Dicyclomine may be increased by: Aclidinium; Ipratropium (Oral Inhalation); Pramlintide; Umeclidinium

Decreased Effect

Dicyclomine may decrease the levels/effects of: Acetylcholinesterase Inhibitors (Central); Secretin

The levels/effects of Dicyclomine may be decreased by: Acetylcholinesterase Inhibitors (Central)

Stability Protect from light

Mechanism of Action Blocks the action of acetylcholine at parasympathetic sites in smooth muscle, secretory glands and the CNS

Pharmacodynamics

Onset of action: 1-2 hours

Duration: Up to 4 hours

Pharmacokinetics (Adult data unless noted)

Absorption: Oral: Well absorbed

Distribution: V_d: 3.65 L/kg

Bioavailability: 67%

Half-life:

Initial phase: 1.8 hours

Terminal phase: 9-10 hours

Time to peak serum concentration: Oral: 1-1.5 hours

Elimination: 80% in urine; 10% in feces

Dosing: Usual

Infants >6 months: Oral: 5 mg/dose 3-4 times/day

Children: Oral: 10 mg/dose 3-4 times/day

Adults:

Oral: Initial: 20 mg 4 times/day, then increase up to 40 mg 4 times/day

I.M.: 20 mg/dose 4 times/day; oral therapy should replace I.M. therapy as soon as possible

Administration

Oral: Administer 30 minutes before eating

Parenteral: I.M. only; not for I.V. use

Dosage Forms Excipient information presented when available (limited, particularly for generics); consult specific product labeling.

Capsule, Oral, as hydrochloride:

Bentyl: 10 mg [contains brilliant blue fcf (fd&c blue #1), fd&c red #40]

Generic: 10 mg

Solution, Intramuscular, as hydrochloride:

Bentyl: 10 mg/mL (2 mL) [pyrogen free]

Solution, Oral, as hydrochloride:

Generic: 10 mg/5 mL (473 mL)

Tablet, Oral, as hydrochloride:

Bentyl: 20 mg

Generic: 20 mg

References

Mahadevan U and Kane S, "American Gastroenterological Association Institute Medical Position Statement on the Use of Gastrointestinal Medications in Pregnancy," *Gastroenterology*, 2006, 131(1):278-82.

◆ **Dicyclomine Hydrochloride** see Dicyclomine on page 652

◆ **Dicyclomine Hydrochloride Injection (Can)** see Dicyclomine on page 652

◆ **Dicycloverine Hydrochloride** see Dicyclomine on page 652

Didanosine (dye DAN oh seen)

Medication Safety Issues

Sound-alike/look-alike issues:
Videx® may be confused with Lidex®

Related Information
Adult and Adolescent HIV *on page 2348*
Oral Medications That Should Not Be Crushed or Altered *on page 2438*
Pediatric HIV *on page 2338*
Perinatal HIV *on page 2356*

Brand Names: U.S. Videx; Videx EC
Brand Names: Canada Videx®; Videx® EC
Therapeutic Category Antiretroviral Agent; HIV Agents (Anti-HIV Agents); Nucleoside Reverse Transcriptase Inhibitor (NRTI)
Generic Availability (U.S.) May be product dependent
Use Treatment of HIV infection in combination with other antiretroviral agents (Oral solution: FDA approved in ages ≥2 weeks and adults; Delayed release capsule: FDA approved in ages ≥6 years weighing ≥20 kg and adults); **Note:** HIV regimens consisting of **three** antiretroviral agents are strongly recommended
Medication Guide Available Yes
Pregnancy Risk Factor B
Pregnancy Considerations Adverse events have not been observed in animal reproduction studies. Didanosine has a low to moderate level of transfer across the human placenta. Based on data from the Antiretroviral Pregnancy Registry, an increased rate of birth defects has been observed following maternal use of didanosine during the first trimester and later during pregnancy; no pattern of defects has been observed and clinical relevance is uncertain. Pharmacokinetics are not significantly altered during pregnancy; dose adjustments are not needed. Cases of lactic acidosis/hepatic steatosis syndrome related to mitochondrial toxicity have been reported in pregnant women with prolonged use of nucleoside analogues. It is not known if pregnancy itself potentiates this known side effect; however, women may be at increased risk of lactic acidosis and liver damage. In addition, these adverse events are similar to other rare but life-threatening syndromes which occur during pregnancy (eg, HELLP syndrome). Hepatic enzymes and electrolytes should be monitored in women receiving nucleoside analogues and clinicians should watch for early signs of the syndrome. In addition, mitochondrial dysfunction may develop in infants following in utero exposure. Due to the reports of lactic acidosis, maternal, and neonatal mortality, didanosine and stavudine should not be used in combination during pregnancy. The DHHS Perinatal HIV Guidelines recommend didanosine to be used only in special circumstances during pregnancy; not recommended for initial therapy in antiretroviral-naïve pregnant women due to toxicity (DHHS [perinatal], 2014).

Regardless of CD4 count or HIV RNA copy number, all HIV-infected pregnant women should receive a combination antiretroviral (ARV) drug regimen. A combination of antepartum, intrapartum, and infant ARV prophylaxis is recommended. ARV therapy should be started as soon as possible in women with symptomatic infection.Although earlier initiation may be more effective in reducing the perinatal transmission of HIV, initiation may be delayed until after 12 weeks gestation in women who do not require immediate treatment after careful consideration of maternal conditions (eg, nausea and vomiting) and the potential risks of first trimester fetal exposure for specific agents. A scheduled cesarean delivery at 38 weeks gestation is recommended for all women with HIV RNA >1000 copies/mL or unknown concentrations near delivery in order to decrease transmission. If ARV therapy must be interrupted for <24 hours during the peripartum period, stop then restart all medications simultaneously in order to decrease the chance of developing resistance. Long-term follow-up is recommended for all infants exposed to ARV medications. In couples who want to conceive, the HIV-infected partner should attain maximum viral suppression prior to conception.

Healthcare providers are encouraged to enroll pregnant women exposed to antiretroviral medications in the Antiretroviral Pregnancy Registry (1-800-258-4263 or www.APRegistry.com). Healthcare providers caring for HIV-infected women and their infants may contact the National Perinatal HIV Hotline (888-448-8765) for clinical consultation (DHHS [perinatal], 2014).

Breast-Feeding Considerations Maternal or infant antiretroviral therapy does not completely eliminate the risk of postnatal HIV transmission. In addition, multiclass-resistant virus has been detected in breast-feeding infants despite maternal therapy. Therefore, in the United States, where formula is accessible, affordable, safe, and sustainable, and the risk of infant mortality due to diarrhea and respiratory infections is low, complete avoidance of breast-feeding by HIV-infected women is recommended to decrease potential transmission of HIV (DHHS [perinatal], 2014).

Contraindications Hypersensitivity to didanosine or any component; concurrent therapy with allopurinol or ribavirin

Warnings Fatal and nonfatal pancreatitis have been reported during therapy **[U.S. Boxed Warning]**; more common in adults than children [1% to 7% vs 3% (normal doses)]; other risk factors for developing pancreatitis include a previous history of the condition, higher doses (eg, >10 mg/kg/day), renal impairment without dose adjustment, concurrent CMV or MAC infection, advanced HIV infection, and concomitant use of stavudine with or without hydroxyurea; use didanosine with extreme caution and only if clearly indicated in patients with risk factors for pancreatitis; discontinue didanosine if clinical signs of pancreatitis occur; only after pancreatitis has been ruled out should dosing be resumed. Dose-related (treatment-limiting) peripheral neuropathy occurs most often after 2 to 6 months of continuous didanosine administration; may occur more frequently in patients with a history of neuropathy, advanced HIV disease, or concurrent treatment with neurotoxic drugs, including stavudine or hydroxyurea; consider discontinuation of didanosine in patients who develop peripheral neuropathy. Retinal depigmentation in children receiving doses >300 mg/m^2/day may occur; retinal changes and optic neuritis have been reported in pediatric and adult patients; perform periodic retinal examinations.

Cases of lactic acidosis, severe hepatomegaly with steatosis, and death have been reported in patients receiving nucleoside analogs **[U.S. Boxed Warning]**; most of these cases have been in women; prolonged nucleoside use, obesity, and prior liver disease may be risk factors; use with extreme caution in patients with other risk factors for liver disease; discontinue therapy in patients who develop laboratory or clinical evidence of lactic acidosis or pronounced hepatotoxicity. Fatal lactic acidosis has occurred in pregnant women who received didanosine plus stavudine with other antiretroviral agents; use didanosine plus stavudine with caution during pregnancy and only if benefit outweighs risks.

Didanosine-associated noncirrhotic portal hypertension may occur; cases leading to liver transplantation or death have been reported. Onset of signs and symptoms of portal hypertension occurred within months to years of initiating didanosine. Patients may present with increased liver enzymes, hematemesis, esophageal varices, splenomegaly, and ascites. Monitor patients for early signs of portal hypertension (eg, splenomegaly, thrombocytopenia);

consider appropriate laboratory testing; discontinue didanosine in patients with evidence of noncirrhotic portal hypertension.

Precautions Use with caution in patients with renal or hepatic impairment. Adjust dosage in patients with renal impairment. Monitor patients with hepatic impairment closely; these patients may be at risk for didanosine-associated liver function abnormalities, including severe and potentially fatal hepatic adverse events. Avoid using the combination of didanosine, stavudine, and hydroxyurea; fatal hepatic events were reported most often in HIV patients receiving this combination. Due to an increased risk of serious toxicities, the combined use of stavudine and didanosine is **not** recommended for use in adults and adolescents (DHHS [adult], 2014) and is not recommended as part of an initial antiretroviral regimen in pediatric patients; however, it may be considered for use in pediatric regimens if the potential benefit clearly outweighs the risks (DHHS [pediatric], 2014).

Fat redistribution and accumulation [ie, central obesity, peripheral wasting, facial wasting, breast enlargement, dorsocervical fat enlargement (buffalo hump), and cushingoid appearance] have been observed in patients receiving antiretroviral agents (causal relationship not established).

Immune reconstitution syndrome (an acute inflammatory response to residual or indolent opportunistic infections) may occur in HIV patients during initial treatment with combination antiretroviral agents, including didanosine; this syndrome may require further patient assessment and therapy. Autoimmune disorders (eg, Grave's disease, Guillain-Barré syndrome, and polymyositis) have been reported in patients experiencing immune reconstitution; time to onset is variable and may occur many months after antiretroviral treatment is initiated.

Adverse Reactions As reported in monotherapy studies; risk of toxicity may increase when combined with other agent.

Dermatologic: Pruritus, rash

Endocrine & metabolic: Uric acid increased

Gastrointestinal: Abdominal pain, amylase increased, diarrhea, pancreatitis (patients >65 years of age had a higher frequency of pancreatitis than younger patients)

Hepatic: Alkaline phosphatase increased, ALT increased, AST increased

Neuromuscular & skeletal: Peripheral neuropathy

Rare but important or life-threatening: Acute renal impairment, alopecia, anaphylactoid reaction, anemia, anorexia, arthralgia, chills/fever, diabetes mellitus, dry eyes, dyspepsia, flatulence, granulocytopenia, hepatic steatosis, hepatitis, hyper-/hypoglycemia, hyperlactatemia (symptomatic), hypersensitivity, immune reconstitution syndrome, lactic acidosis/hepatomegaly, leukopenia, lipodystrophy, liver failure, myalgia, myopathy, optic neuritis, pain, parotid gland enlargement, portal hypertension (noncirrhotic), retinal depigmentation, rhabdomyolysis, sialoadenitis, Stevens-Johnson syndrome, thrombocytopenia, weakness, xerostomia

Drug Interactions

Metabolism/Transport Effects None known.

Avoid Concomitant Use

Avoid concomitant use of Didanosine with any of the following: Alcohol (Ethyl); Allopurinol; Febuxostat; Hydroxyurea; Ribavirin; Tenofovir

Increased Effect/Toxicity

Didanosine may increase the levels/effects of: Hydroxyurea

The levels/effects of Didanosine may be increased by: Alcohol (Ethyl); Allopurinol; Febuxostat; Ganciclovir-Valganciclovir; Hydroxyurea; Ribavirin; Stavudine; Tenofovir

Decreased Effect

Didanosine may decrease the levels/effects of: Antifungal Agents (Azole Derivatives, Systemic); Atazanavir; Indinavir; Quinolone Antibiotics; Rilpivirine

The levels/effects of Didanosine may be decreased by: Atazanavir; Darunavir; Lopinavir; Methadone; Quinolone Antibiotics; Rilpivirine; Tenofovir; Tipranavir

Food Interactions Food decreases AUC and C_{max}; serum levels may be decreased by 55%. Management: Administer on an empty stomach at least 30 minutes before or 2 hours after eating depending on dosage form.

Stability Undergoes rapid degradation when exposed to an acidic environment; 10% of the drug decomposes to hypoxanthine in <2 minutes at pH <3 at 37°C.

Delayed release capsules: Store in tightly closed bottles at 25°C (77°F); excursions permitted to 15°C to 30°C (59°F to 86°F).

Powder for oral solution: Unreconstituted powder should be stored at 15°C to 30°C (59°F to 86°F). Powder for oral solution is unbuffered and must be reconstituted with water and mixed with an equal volume of double-strength antacid at time of preparation. Reconstituted solution (10 mg/mL) is stable for 30 days if refrigerated; discard unused portion after 30 days. When unbuffered powder for oral solution is reconstituted and admixed with a double-strength antacid to make a 20 mg/mL solution for adult once-daily dosing, the admixture is stable for 24 hours at room temperature and for 30 days if refrigerated

Mechanism of Action Didanosine, a purine nucleoside (adenosine) analog and the deamination product of dideoxyadenosine (ddA), inhibits HIV replication *in vitro* in both T cells and monocytes. Didanosine is converted within the cell to the mono-, di-, and triphosphates of ddA. These ddA triphosphates act as substrate and inhibitor of HIV reverse transcriptase substrate and inhibitor of HIV reverse transcriptase thereby blocking viral DNA synthesis and suppressing HIV replication.

Pharmacokinetics (Adult data unless noted)

Absorption: Subject to degradation by acidic pH of stomach; some formulations are buffered to resist acidic pH. Delayed release capsules contain enteric-coated beadlets which dissolve in the small intestine.

Distribution: Extensive intracellular distribution

CSF/plasma ratio:

Infants 8 months to Adolescents 19 years: 46% (range: 12% to 85%)

Adults: 21%

V_d (apparent):

Age-based:

Infants 8 months to Adolescents 19 years: 28 ± 15 L/m²

Adults: 43.7 ± 8.9 L/m²

Weight-based:

Children 20 kg to <25 kg: 98 ± 30 L

Children 25 kg to <60 kg: 155 ± 55 L

Children ≥60 kg: 363 ± 138 L

Adults ≥60 kg: 308 ± 164 L

Protein binding: <5%

Metabolism: Converted intracellularly to active triphosphate form; presumed to be metabolized via the same metabolic pathway as endogenous purines

Bioavailability: Variable and affected by the presence of food in the GI tract, gastric pH, and the dosage form administered

Infants 8 months to Adolescents 19 years: 25% ± 20%

Adults: 42% ± 12%

Half-life:

Plasma:

Newborns (1 day old): 2 ± 0.7 hours

Infants 2 weeks to 4 months: 1.2 ± 0.3 hours

Infants 8 months to Adolescents 19 years: 0.8 ± 0.3 hours

Adults with normal renal function: 1.5 ± 0.4 hours

Intracellular: Adults: 25 to 40 hours

Elimination:

Children 20 kg to <25 kg: 0.75 ± 0.13 hours

Children 25 kg to <60 kg: 0.92 ± 0.09 hours

Children ≥60 kg: 1.26 ± 0.19 hours

Adults ≥60 kg: 1.19 ± 21 hours

Time to peak serum concentration: Delayed release capsules: 2 hours; Oral solution: 0.25 to 1.5 hours

Elimination: Unchanged drug excreted in urine

Infants 8 months to Adolescents 19 years: 18% ± 10%

Adults: 18% ± 8%

Dosing: Neonatal

HIV infection, treatment: Use in combination with other antiretroviral agents:

PNA <14 days: Dose not established; pharmacokinetic parameters are too variable to determine appropriate dosage

PNA ≥14 days: Oral solution:

AIDS*info* recommendation (DHHS [pediatric], 2014): 50 mg/m²/dose every 12 hours.

Manufacturer's labeling: 100 mg/m²/dose every 12 hours. **Note:** Not recommended based on pharmacokinetic data; expert panel members suggest toxicity may occur using this dose in this age group (DHHS [pediatric]; 2014).

Dosing adjustment in renal impairment: Insufficient data exists to recommend a specific dosage adjustment; however, a decrease in the dose should be considered in pediatric patients with renal impairment.

Dosing: Usual

Pediatric: **HIV infection, treatment:** Oral: Use in combination with other antiretroviral agents:

Infants 1 to 8 months: Oral solution:

AIDS*info* recommendation (DHHS [pediatric], 2014):

Infants 1 to <3 months: 50 mg/m²/dose every 12 hours

Infants ≥3 to 8 months: Oral solution: 100 mg/m²/dose every 12 hours

Manufacturer's labeling: 100 mg/m²/dose every 12 hours. **Note:** Based on pharmacokinetic data, expert panel members suggest toxicity may occur using manufacturer dosing in infants <3 months (DHHS [pediatric], 2014).

Infants >8 months and Children:

Oral solution:

Manufacturer's labeling: 120 mg/m²/dose every 12 hours; do not exceed adult dose; once-daily dosing of the oral solution is not FDA approved in children; limited data is available

AIDS*info* recommendation (DHHS [pediatric], 2014): 120 mg/m²/dose every 12 hours; maximum dose: 200 mg/dose

Alternate once-daily dosing for treatment-naive children ≥3 years: 240 mg/m²/dose once daily; maximum dose: 400 mg/dose; may also use the delayed release capsule if calculated dose is appropriate and child is able to swallow a capsule whole

Delayed release capsule: Children ≥6 years and ≥20 kg who are able to swallow a capsule whole:

20 kg to <25 kg: 200 mg once daily

25 kg to <60 kg: 250 mg once daily

≥60 kg: 400 mg once daily

Adolescents:

Oral solution: **Note:** Although once-daily dosing is available, it should only be considered for adolescent/adult patients whose management requires once-daily administration (eg, to enhance compliance); the preferred dosing frequency of didanosine oral solution is twice daily because there is more evidence to support the effectiveness of this dosing frequency:

<60 kg: 125 mg every 12 hours **or** 250 mg once daily

≥60 kg: 200 mg every 12 hours or 400 mg once daily using a special Videx solution in double strength antacid which provides 400 mg/20 mL for once-daily dosing

Delayed release capsule:

20 kg to <25 kg: 200 mg once daily

25 kg to <60 kg: 250 mg once daily

≥60 kg: 400 mg once daily

Adult: **HIV infection, treatment:** Oral:

Dosing based on patient weight:

Pediatric powder for oral solution (Videx):

<60 kg: 125 mg twice daily (preferred) or 250 mg once daily

≥60 kg: 200 mg twice daily (preferred) or 400 mg once daily

Delayed release capsule (Videx EC):

25 kg to <60 kg: 250 mg once daily

≥60 kg: 400 mg once daily

When taken with tenofovir: **Note:** Combined use of tenofovir with didanosine is no longer recommended (DHHS [adult], 2014).

<60 kg and CrCl ≥60 mL/minute: 200 mg once daily

≥60 kg and CrCl ≥60 mL/minute: 250 mg once daily

CrCl <60 mL/minute: Dose has not been established

Dosing adjustment in renal impairment:

Infants and Children: Insufficient data exists to recommend a specific dosage adjustment; however, a decrease in the dose should be considered in pediatric patients with renal impairment. The following guidelines have been used by some clinicians (Aronoff, 2007):

GFR >50 mL/minute/1.73 m²: No adjustment required

GFR 30 to 50 mL/minute/1.73 m²: 75 mg/m²/dose every 12 hours

GFR 10 to 29 mL/minute/1.73 m²: 90 mg/m²/dose every 24 hours

GFR <10 mL/minute/1.73 m²: 75 mg/m²/dose every 24 hours

Hemodialysis: 75 mg/m²/dose every 24 hours after dialysis

Peritoneal dialysis: 75 mg/m²/dose every 24 hours

Continuous renal replacement therapy (CRRT): 75 mg/m²/dose every 12 hours

Adolescents and Adults: Dosing based on patient weight, creatinine clearance, and dosage form:

Dosing for patients <60 kg:

CrCl ≥60 mL/minute: No dosage adjustment required

CrCl 30 to 59 mL/minute:

Oral solution: 75 mg twice daily or 150 mg once daily

Delayed release capsule: 125 mg once daily

CrCl 10 to 29 mL/minute:

Oral solution: 100 mg once daily

Delayed release capsule: 125 mg once daily

CrCl <10 mL/minute:

Oral solution: 75 mg once daily

Delayed release capsule: Use alternate formulation

Dosing for patients ≥60 kg:

CrCl ≥60 mL/minute: No dosage adjustment required

CrCl 30 to 59 mL/minute:

Oral solution: 100 mg twice daily or 200 mg once daily

Delayed release capsule: 200 mg once daily

CrCl 10 to 29 mL/minute:
Oral solution: 150 mg once daily
Delayed release capsule: 125 mg once daily
CrCl <10 mL/minute:
Oral solution: 100 mg once daily
Delayed release capsule: 125 mg once daily

Dosing adjustment in patients requiring continuous ambulatory peritoneal dialysis (CAPD) or hemodialysis: Use dosing recommendations for patients with CrCl <10 mL/minute; supplemental doses following hemodialysis are not needed

Dosing adjustment in hepatic impairment: No adjustment recommended; Adults: In a single-dose study, mean AUC and peak serum concentrations of didanosine were 13% and 19% higher, respectively, in adults with moderate to severe hepatic impairment (Child-Pugh Class B or C). However, a similar range and distribution of AUC and peak concentrations were observed. It is important to monitor patients with hepatic impairment closely for didanosine toxicity. Patients with hepatic impairment may be at increased risk for didanosine toxicities.

Administration Oral: Administer oral solution and delayed release capsule on an empty stomach 30 minutes before or at least 2 hours after a meal. Some experts have recommended giving without regard to meals in order to improve compliance (DHHS [pediatric], 2014). Swallow capsule whole; do not break open or chew. If administered with tenofovir, the delayed release capsule may be administered with a light meal or in the fasted state. Administer didanosine at least 1 hour apart from indinavir. Administer didanosine at least 2 hours apart from ritonavir or atazanavir. Didanosine should be given at least 1 hour before or 2 hours after lopinavir/ritonavir. Nelfinavir should be administered 2 hours before or 1 hour after didanosine. Administer buffered formulations of didanosine at least 1 hour apart from fosamprenavir.

Unbuffered pediatric powder should be reconstituted with water and admixed in equal parts with a double-strength antacid to provide a final concentration of 10 mg/mL; unbuffered pediatric powder has also been reconstituted and admixed with a double-strength antacid to provide a final concentration of 20 mg/mL to be used for once-daily dosing in adults; shake oral solution well before use.

Monitoring Parameters Note: Monitor CD4 percentage (if <5 years of age) or CD4 count (if ≥5 years of age) at least every 3-4 months (DHHS [pediatric], 2014).

Prior to initiation of therapy: Genotypic resistance testing, CD4 and viral load (every 3 to 4 months), CBC with differential, LFTs, BUN, creatinine, electrolytes, glucose, urinalysis (every 6 to 12 months), and assessment of readiness for adherence with medication regimen. At initiation and with any change in treatment regimen: CBC with differential, electrolytes, calcium, phosphate, glucose, LFTs, bilirubin, urinalysis (at initiation), BUN, creatinine, albumin, total protein, lipid panel (at initiation), CD4, and viral load. After 1 to 2 weeks of therapy: Signs of medication toxicity and adherence. After 2 to 4 weeks of therapy: CBC with differential, viral load, signs of medication toxicity, and adherence; then every 3 to 4 months: CBC with differential, electrolytes, glucose, LFTs, bilirubin, BUN, creatinine, CD4, viral load, signs of medication toxicity, and adherence. Lipid panel and urinalysis every 6 to 12 months. CD4 monitoring frequency may be decreased to every 6 to 12 months in children who are adherent to therapy if the value is well above the threshold for opportunistic infections, viral suppression is sustained, and the clinical status is stable for more than 2 to 3 years (DHHS [pediatric], 2014). Monitor for growth and development, signs of HIV-specific physical conditions, HIV disease progression, opportunistic infections, peripheral neuropathy, pancreatitis, or lactic acidosis

To monitor for portal hypertension: CBC with platelet count, splenomegaly on physical exam, liver enzymes, serum bilirubin, albumin, INR, ultrasound

Additional Information Once daily, didanosine delayed-release capsules have been approved for use in children 6 to 18 years of age who are ≥20 kg. This approval was based on pharmacokinetic studies; however, limited published literature exists. In a single-dose pharmacokinetic study in children 4 to 11.5 years of age (n=10; median age: 7.6 years), a dose of 240 mg/m^2 was shown to have a similar plasma AUC as compared to the buffered formulation. However, two patients were excluded from data analysis, one due to extremely low didanosine serum concentrations throughout the dosing interval (King, 2002). Doses of 240 mg/m^2 once daily, with a maximum of 400 mg once daily, are being studied in pediatric clinical trials. **Note:** In PACTG 1021, treatment-naive children (3 to 21 years of age) received 240 mg/m^2/dose once daily (maximum: 400 mg/dose) with good viral suppression (DHHS [pediatric], 2014). Children with a surface area ≥0.45 m^2 who could swallow capsules received the delayed-release capsule; the oral suspension was used for smaller children (McKinney, 2007).

The relative bioavailability of didanosine suspension administered once daily versus twice daily was studied in 24 children, 4.8 ± 2.9 years of age. Didanosine was administered in doses of 90 mg/m^2/dose every 12 hours and 180 mg/m^2/dose once daily. The relative bioavailability of once-daily dosing compared to twice daily dosing was 0.95 ± 0.49 (range: 0.22 to 1.97). The authors suggest these results support the potential clinical use of once-daily dosing in pediatric patients. However, due to the large inter- and intrasubject variability, these 2 regimens would **not** be considered to be bioequivalent based on FDA criteria (Abreu, 2000). Further studies are needed.

A high rate of early virologic failure in therapy-naive adult HIV patients has been observed with the once-daily three-drug combination therapy of didanosine enteric-coated beadlets (Videx EC), lamivudine, and tenofovir and the once-daily three-drug combination therapy of abacavir, lamivudine, and tenofovir. These combinations should not be used or offered at any time. Any patient currently receiving either of these regimens should be closely monitored for virologic failure and considered for treatment modification. Early virologic failure was also observed in therapy-naive adult HIV patients treated with tenofovir, didanosine enteric-coated beadlets (Videx EC), and either efavirenz or nevirapine; rapid emergence of resistant mutations has also been reported with this combination; the combination of tenofovir, didanosine, and any non-nucleoside reverse transcriptase inhibitor is **not** recommended as initial antiretroviral therapy. **Note:** Didanosine plus tenofovir is **not** recommended as a component of an initial antiretroviral therapy regimen in pediatric patients and is no longer recommended as part of any antiretroviral regimen in adults and adolescents (DHHS [pediatric, adult], 2014).

One major study found an increased risk of MI in patients receiving didanosine; however, other cohort studies did not find an increased cardiovascular risk (DHHS [adult], 2014).

Dosage Forms Excipient information presented when available (limited, particularly for generics); consult specific product labeling.

Capsule Delayed Release, Oral:
Videx EC: 125 mg, 200 mg, 250 mg, 400 mg
Generic: 125 mg, 200 mg, 250 mg, 400 mg
Solution Reconstituted, Oral:
Videx: 2 g (100 mL); 4 g (200 mL)

References

Abreu T, Plaisance K, Rexroad V, et al, "Bioavailability of Once- and Twice-Daily Regimens of Didanosine in Human Immunodeficiency Virus-Infected Children," *Antimicrob Agents Chemother*, 2000, 44 (5):1375-6.

Aronoff GR, Bennett WM, Berns JS, et al, *Drug Prescribing in Renal Failure: Dosing Guidelines for Adults and Children*, 5th ed. Philadelphia, PA: American College of Physicians, 2007.

Balis FM, Pizzo PA, Butler KM, et al, "Clinical Pharmacology of 2', 3'-Dideoxyinosine in Human Immunodeficiency Virus-Infected Children," *J Infect Dis*, 1992, 165(1):99-104.

Butler KM, Husson RN, Balis FM, et al, "Dideoxyinosine in Children With Symptomatic Human Immunodeficiency Virus Infection," *N Engl J Med*, 1991, 324(3):137-44.

DHHS Panel on Antiretroviral Guidelines for Adults and Adolescents, "Guidelines for the Use of Antiretroviral Agents in HIV-Infected Adults and Adolescents," May 1, 2014. Available at http://www.aidsinfo.nih.gov

DHHS Panel on Antiretroviral Therapy and Medical Management of HIV-Infected Children, "Guidelines for the Use of Antiretroviral Agents in Pediatric HIV Infection," February 12, 2014. Available at http://aidsinfo.nih.gov

DHHS Panel on Treatment of HIV-Infected Pregnant Women and Prevention of Perinatal Transmission, "Recommendations for the Use of Antiretroviral Drugs in Pregnant HIV-1-Infected Women for Maternal Health and Interventions to Reduce Perinatal HIV-1 Transmission in the United States," March 28, 2014. Available at http://aidsinfo.nih.gov

King JR, Nachman S, Yogev R, et al, "Single-Dose Pharmacokinetics of Enteric-Coated Didanosine in HIV-Infected Children," *Antivir Ther*, 2002, 7(4):267-70.

Kovari H, Ledergerber B, Peter U, et al, "Association of Noncirrhotic Portal Hypertension in HIV-Infected Persons and Antiretroviral Therapy With Didanosine: A Nested Case-Control Study," *Clin Infect Dis*, 2009, 49(4):626-35.

McKinney RE Jr, Rodman J, Hu C, et al, "Long-Term Safety and Efficacy of a Once-Daily Regimen of Emtricitabine, Didanosine, and Efavirenz in HIV-Infected, Therapy-Naive Children and Adolescents: Pediatric AIDS Clinical Trials Group Protocol P1021," *Pediatrics*, 2007, 120(2):e416-23.

◆ **Dideoxyinosine** see Didanosine on page 654

◆ **Dietary Fiber Laxative [OTC]** see Psyllium on page 1773

◆ **Differin** see Adapalene on page 73

◆ **Differin® (Can)** see Adapalene on page 73

◆ **Differin® XP (Can)** see Adapalene on page 73

◆ **Diflucan** see Fluconazole on page 877

◆ **Difluorodeoxycytidine Hydrochlorothiazide** see Gemcitabine on page 959

◆ **Digestive Enzyme** see Pancrelipase on page 1591

◆ **Digibind** see Digoxin Immune Fab on page 663

◆ **DigiFab** see Digoxin Immune Fab on page 663

◆ **DigiFab® (Can)** see Digoxin Immune Fab on page 663

◆ **Digitalis** see Digoxin on page 658

◆ **Digox** see Digoxin on page 658

Digoxin (di JOKS in)

Medication Safety Issues

Sound-alike/look-alike issues:

Digoxin may be confused with Desoxyn, doxepin

Lanoxin may be confused with Lasix, levothyroxine, Levoxyl, Levsinex, Lomotil, Mefoxin, naloxone, Xanax

High alert medication:

The Institute for Safe Medication Practices (ISMP) includes this medication among its list of drugs which have a heightened risk of causing significant patient harm when used in error.

BEERS Criteria medication:

This drug may be potentially inappropriate for use in geriatric patients (Quality of evidence - moderate; Strength of recommendation - strong).

International issues:

Lanoxin [U.S., Canada, and multiple international markets] may be confused with Limoxin brand name for ambroxol [Indonesia] and amoxicillin [Mexico]

Related Information

Management of Drug Extravasations on page 2255

Brand Names: U.S. Digox; Lanoxin; Lanoxin Pediatric

Brand Names: Canada Apo-Digoxin; Digoxin Injection CSD; Lanoxin; Pediatric Digoxin CSD; PMS-Digoxin; Toloxin

Therapeutic Category Antiarrhythmic Agent, Miscellaneous; Cardiac Glycoside

Generic Availability (U.S.) Yes

Use Treatment of mild to moderate heart failure (HF) (Injection, oral solution: FDA approved in all ages; Tablets: FDA approved in ages ≥5 years and adults); chronic atrial fibrillation (rate-control) (all dosage forms: FDA approved in adults). Has also been used for fetal tachycardia with or without hydrops; to slow ventricular rate in supraventricular tachyarrhythmias such as supraventricular tachycardias (SVT), excluding atrioventricular reciprocating tachycardia (AVRT)

Pregnancy Risk Factor C

Pregnancy Considerations Animal reproduction studies have not been conducted. Digoxin crosses the placenta and serum concentrations are similar in the mother and fetus at delivery. Digoxin is recommended as first-line in the treatment of fetal tachycardia determined to be SVT. In pregnant women with atrial fibrillation or SVT, use of digoxin is recommended (Anderson, 2013; Blomström-Lundqvist, 2003).

Breast-Feeding Considerations Digoxin is excreted into breast milk and similar concentrations are found within mother's serum and milk. The manufacturer recommends that caution be used when administered to nursing women.

Contraindications Hypersensitivity to digoxin (rare), other forms of digitalis, or any component; ventricular fibrillation

Warnings Use with extreme caution in patients with hypoxia, hypothyroidism, acute myocarditis, electrolyte disorders, acute MI. Correct electrolyte disturbances, especially hypokalemia or hypomagnesemia, prior to use and throughout therapy. Hypercalcemia may increase the risk of digoxin toxicity; maintain normocalcemia. Monitor for proarrhythmic effects (especially with toxicity); monitor and adjust dose to prevent QT_c prolongation.

Injectable product contains propylene glycol; toxicities have been reported with use of products containing propylene glycol, including hyperosmolality, lactic acidosis, seizures, and respiratory depression; in neonates large amounts of propylene glycol delivered orally, intravenously (eg, >3000 mg/day), or topically have been associated with potentially fatal toxicities which can include metabolic acidosis, seizures, renal failure, and CNS depression; use injectable products containing propylene glycol with caution (AAP, 1997; Shehab, 2009).

Precautions Use with caution and reduce dosage in patients with renal impairment. Use with caution in patients with sinus nodal disease (may worsen condition). Withdrawal of digoxin in patients with heart failure may lead to recurrence of heart failure symptoms (monitor carefully). Atrial arrhythmias associated with hypermetabolic states are difficult to treat (use with caution). Use with caution in patients with an acute MI (within 6 months); may increase myocardial oxygen demand. During the immediate post-MI period, digoxin administered I.V. may be used in the acute treatment of refractory atrial fibrillation/flutter (especially when HF or LV dysfunction coexists) or refractory reentrant PSVT (Antman, 2004).

During an episode of atrial fibrillation or flutter in patients with an accessory bypass tract [eg, Wolff-Parkinson-White (WPW) syndrome], digoxin use has been associated with a greater slowing of conduction in the atrioventricular node than in accessory pathways leading to ventricular fibrillation; avoid use in such patients. Avoid use in patients with second- or third-degree heart block (except in patients with a functioning artificial pacemaker); incomplete AV block (eg, Stokes-Adams attacks) may progress to complete block with digoxin administration.

HF patients with preserved left ventricular function, including patients with restrictive cardiomyopathy, constrictive pericarditis, and amyloid heart disease, may be susceptible to digoxin toxicity; avoid use unless used to control ventricular response with atrial fibrillation. Digoxin should not be used in patients with low ejection fraction, sinus rhythm, and no HF symptoms since the risk of harm may be greater than clinical benefit (Hunt, 2009). Outflow obstruction may worsen due to the positive inotropic effects of digoxin; avoid use unless used to control ventricular response with atrial fibrillation.

Children are more likely to experience cardiac arrhythmia as a sign of excessive dosing. The most common are conduction disturbances or tachyarrhythmia (atrial tachycardia with or without block) and junctional tachycardia. Ventricular tachyarrhythmias are less common. In infants, sinus bradycardia may be a sign of digoxin toxicity. Any arrhythmia seen in a child on digoxin should be considered as digoxin toxicity. The gastrointestinal and central nervous system symptoms are not frequently seen in children.

Use with caution in patients with hypothyroidism; higher digoxin concentrations may result. Use with caution in patients with hyperthyroidism; lower digoxin concentrations may result due to decreased absorption. **Note:** New-onset atrial fibrillation or exacerbation of ventricular arrhythmias should prompt evaluation of thyroid status. Avoid rapid I.V. administration of calcium in digitalized patients; may produce serious arrhythmias. Use with caution in patients taking strong inducers or inhibitors of P-glycoprotein (eg, cyclosporine). Upon initiation of amiodarone, propafenone, quinidine, or verapamil, the need for digoxin should be evaluated and the digoxin dose should be reduced (eg, by 50%) to avoid toxicity.

Adverse Reactions

Cardiovascular: Accelerated junctional rhythm, asystole, atrial tachycardia with or without block, AV dissociation, first-, second- (Wenckebach), or third-degree heart block, facial edema, PR prolongation, PVCs (especially bigeminy or trigeminy), ST segment depression, ventricular tachycardia or ventricular fibrillation

Central nervous system: Apathy, anxiety, confusion, delirium, depression, dizziness, fever, hallucinations, headache, mental disturbances

Dermatologic: Rash (erythematous, maculopapular [most common], papular, scarlatiniform, vesicular or bullous), pruritus, urticaria, angioneurotic edema

Gastrointestinal: Abdominal pain, anorexia, diarrhea, nausea, vomiting

Neuromuscular & skeletal: Weakness

Ocular: Visual disturbances (blurred or yellow vision)

Respiratory: Laryngeal edema

Rare but important or life-threatening: Asymmetric chorea, gynecomastia, thrombocytopenia, palpitation, intestinal ischemia, hemorrhagic necrosis of the intestines, vaginal cornification, eosinophilia, sexual dysfunction, diaphoresis

Drug Interactions

Metabolism/Transport Effects Substrate of CYP3A4 (minor), P-glycoprotein; **Note:** Assignment of Major/Minor substrate status based on clinically relevant drug interaction potential

Avoid Concomitant Use

Avoid concomitant use of Digoxin with any of the following: Ceritinib

Increased Effect/Toxicity

Digoxin may increase the levels/effects of: Adenosine; Bradycardia-Causing Agents; Carvedilol; Ceritinib; Colchicine; Dronedarone; Midodrine

The levels/effects of Digoxin may be increased by: Aminoquinolines (Antimalarial); Amiodarone; Antithyroid Agents; AtorvaSTATin; Beta-Blockers; Boceprevir; Brimonidine (Topical); Calcium Channel Blockers (Nondihydropyridine); Calcium Polystyrene Sulfonate; Carvedilol; CloNIDine; Conivaptan; CycloSPORINE (Systemic); Dronedarone; Epoprostenol; Etravirine; Ezogabine; Flecainide; Glycopyrrolate; Itraconazole; Lenalidomide; Licorice; Loop Diuretics; Macrolide Antibiotics; Mifepristone; Milnacipran; Mirabegron; Multivitamins/Fluoride (with ADE); Multivitamins/Minerals (with ADEK, Folate, Iron); Multivitamins/Minerals (with AE, No Iron); Nefazodone; Neuromuscular-Blocking Agents; NIFEdipine; Nonsteroidal Anti-Inflammatory Agents; Paricalcitol; P-glycoprotein/ABCB1 Inhibitors; Posaconazole; Potassium-Sparing Diuretics; Propafenone; Protease Inhibitors; QuiNIDine; QuiNINE; Ranolazine; Regorafenib; Reserpine; Simeprevir; SitaGLIPtin; Sodium Polystyrene Sulfonate; Spironolactone; Telaprevir; Telmisartan; Ticagrelor; Tolvaptan; Trimethoprim; Vandetanib; Vitamin D Analogs

Decreased Effect

Digoxin may decrease the levels/effects of: Antineoplastic Agents (Anthracycline, Systemic)

The levels/effects of Digoxin may be decreased by: 5-ASA Derivatives; Acarbose; Aminoglycosides; Antineoplastic Agents; Antineoplastic Agents (Anthracycline, Systemic); Bile Acid Sequestrants; Kaolin; PenicillAMINE; P-glycoprotein/ABCB1 Inducers; Polyethylene Glycol 3350; Polyethylene Glycol 4000; Potassium-Sparing Diuretics; St Johns Wort; Sucralfate

Food Interactions Digoxin peak serum concentrations may be decreased if taken with food. Meals containing increased fiber (bran) or foods high in pectin may decrease oral absorption of digoxin.

Stability Store at 25°C (77°F); excursions permitted to 15°C to 30°C (59°F to 86°F); protect from light; may precipitate if diluted less than fourfold.

◄ ## Mechanism of Action

Heart failure: Inhibition of the sodium/potassium ATPase pump in myocardial cells results in a transient increase of intracellular sodium, which in turn promotes calcium influx via the sodium-calcium exchange pump leading to increased contractility.

Supraventricular arrhythmias: Direct suppression of the AV node conduction to increase effective refractory period and decrease conduction velocity - positive inotropic effect, enhanced vagal tone, and decreased ventricular rate to fast atrial arrhythmias. Atrial fibrillation may decrease sensitivity and increase tolerance to higher serum digoxin concentrations.

Pharmacodynamics

Onset of action: Heart rate control:
Oral: 1-2 hours
I.V.: 5-60 minutes; dependent upon rate of infusion
Maximum effect: Heart rate control:
I.V.: 1-6 hours; Note: In adult patients with atrial fibrillation, median time to ventricular rate control in one study was 6 hours (range: 3-15 hours) (Siu, 2009)
Duration: Adults: 3-4 days

Pharmacokinetics (Adult data unless noted)

Absorption: By passive nonsaturable diffusion in the upper small intestine; food may delay but does not affect extent of absorption

Distribution: Distribution phase: 6-8 hours

V_d: Extensive to peripheral tissues; concentrates in heart, liver, kidney, skeletal muscle, and intestines. Heart/serum concentration is 70:1. Pharmacologic effects are delayed and do not correlate well with serum concentrations during distribution phase

Neonates, full-term: 7.5-10 L/kg
Children: 16 L/kg
Adults: 7 L/kg
Disease-related changes:
Hyperthyroidism: Increased V_d
Hyperkalemia, hyponatremia: Decreased digoxin distribution to heart and muscle
Hypokalemia: Increased digoxin distribution to heart and muscles
Chronic renal failure: Decreased V_d: 4-6 L/kg
Decreased sodium/potassium ATPase activity: Decreased tissue binding

Protein binding: ~25%; in uremic patients, digoxin is displaced from plasma protein binding sites

Metabolism: Via sequential sugar hydrolysis in the stomach or by reduction of lactone ring by intestinal bacteria (in ~10% of population, gut bacteria may metabolize up to 40% of digoxin dose); once absorbed, only ~16% is metabolized to 3-beta-digoxigenin, 3-keto-digoxigenin, and glucuronide and sulfate conjugates; metabolites may contribute to therapeutic and toxic effects of digoxin; metabolism is reduced with decompensated heart failure

Bioavailability:
Oral solution: 70% to 85%
Tablets: 60% to 80%
Half-life, elimination:
Premature: 61-170 hours
Neonates, full-term: 35-45 hours
Infants: 18-25 hours
Children: 35 hours
Adults: 36-48 hours
Anuric adults: 3.5-5 days
Metabolites: Digoxigenin: 4 hours; Monodigitoxoside: 3-12 hours

Time to peak serum concentration: Oral tablets: 1-3 hours; oral solution: 30-90 minutes

Elimination: Urine (50% to 70% as unchanged drug)

Dialysis: Nondialyzable (0% to 5%)

Dosing: Neonatal Heart failure, atrial dysrhythmias:

Injection, Oral solution: Dosage must be individualized due to substantial individual variation. For management of heart failure, a lower serum digoxin concentration may be adequate compared to treatment of cardiac arrhythmias; consider doses at the lower end of the recommended range for treatment of heart failure; a digitalizing dose (loading dose) may not be necessary when treating heart failure (Ross, 2001). For management of atrial dysrhythmias, dose should be titrated to the lowest effective dose.

The dosage tables below list dosage recommendations for normal renal function and are based upon average patient response. Total digitalizing dose should be decreased by 50% in patients with end-stage renal disease. Note: Total digitalizing dose should be divided (see below). If changing from oral solution to I.V. therapy, dosage should be reduced by 20% to 25%.

Initial Dosage Recommendations for Digoxin[A] (Digitalizing)

Age	Total Digitalizing Dose Administer in three divided doses[B] (mcg/kg)	
	Oral	I.V.[C]
Preterm neonates	20-30	15-25
Full-term neonates	25-35	20-30

[A]Based on lean body weight and normal renal function for age

[B]Do not give full total digitalizing dose (TDD) at once. Give one-half of the TDD for the initial dose, then give one-quarter of the TDD for each of two subsequent doses at 6- to 8-hour intervals; prior to additional doses, clinical response should be fully evaluated (eg, ECG).

[C]May also be administered I.M.; however, not usually recommended.

Maintenance Dosage Recommendations for Digoxin[A]

Age	Total Daily Maintenance Dose Administer in equal divided doses every 12 hours (mcg/kg/day)	
	Oral	I.V.[B,C]
Preterm neonates	5-7.5	4-6
Full-term neonates	8-10	5-8

[A]Based on lean body weight and normal renal function for age. Decrease maintenance dose in patients with decreased renal function.

[B]Daily maintenance I.V. dose is typically 20% to 30% of total I.V. digitalizing dose.

[C]May also be administered I.M.; however, not usually recommended.

Dosing: Usual

Infants, Children, and Adolescents: Dosage must be individualized due to substantial individual variation; for management of heart failure, a lower serum digoxin concentration may be adequate compared to treatment of cardiac arrhythmias; consider doses at the lower end of the recommended range for treatment of heart failure; a digitalizing dose (loading dose) may not be necessary when treating heart failure (Ross, 2001). For management of atrial dysrhythmias, dose should be titrated to the lowest effective dose.

The dosage tables below list dosage recommendations for normal renal function and are based on average patient response. Total digitalizing dose should be decreased by 50% in patients with end-stage renal disease. **Note:** Total digitalizing dose should be divided. If changing from oral solution or tablets to I.V. therapy, dosage should be reduced by 20% to 25%.

Initial Dosage Recommendations for Digoxin[A] (Digitalizing)

Age	Total Digitalizing Dose Administer in three divided doses[B] (mcg/kg)		
	Oral Solution	Tablets	I.V.[C]
1-24 months	35-60	–	30-50
2-5 years	30-45	–	25-35
5-10 years	20-35	20-45	15-30
>10 years	10-15	10-15	8-12

[A]Based on lean body weight and normal renal function for age

[B]**Do not give full total digitalizing dose (TDD) at once.** Give one-half of the TDD for the initial dose, then give one-quarter of the TDD for each of two subsequent doses at 6- to 8-hour intervals; prior to additional doses, clinical response should be fully evaluated (eg, ECG).

[C]May also be administered by I.M; however, not recommended.

Maintenance Dosage Recommendations for Digoxin[A]

Age	Daily Maintenance Dose If ≤10 years, administer in equal divided doses twice daily If >10 years, administer once daily (mcg/kg/day)		
	Oral Solution	Tablets	I.V.[B,C]
1-24 months	10-15	–	7.5-12
2-5 years	8-10	–	6-9
5-10 years	5-10	6-11	4-8
>10 years	2.5-5	2.5-5	2-3

[A]Based on lean body weight and normal renal function for age. Decrease maintenance dose in patients with decreased renal function.

[B]May also be administered by I.M; however, not recommended.

[C]Daily maintenance I.V. dose is typically 20% to 30% of total digitalizing I.V. dose in pediatric patients ≤24 months and 25% to 35% in older pediatric patients.

Adults:

Atrial fibrillation (rate control) in patients with heart failure: Loading dose: I.V.: 0.25 mg every 2 hours, up to 1.5 mg within 24 hours; for nonacute situations, may administer 0.5 mg orally once daily for 2 days, followed by oral maintenance dose. Maintenance dose: I.V., Oral: 0.125-0.375 mg once daily (Fuster, 2006)

Heart failure: Note: Loading dose not recommended; Daily maintenance dose: Oral: 0.125-0.25 mg once daily; higher daily doses (up to 0.5 mg/day) are rarely necessary. If patient is >70 years old, has impaired renal function, or has a low lean body mass, low doses (eg, 0.125 mg daily or every other day) should be used (Hunt, 2009).

Supraventricular tachyarrhythmias (rate control):
Initial: Total digitalizing dose:
Oral: 0.75-1.5 mg
I.V., I.M: 0.5-1 mg (**Note:** I.M. not preferred due to severe injection site pain.)
Give ½ of the total digitalizing dose (TDD) as the initial dose, then give ¼ of the TDD in each of two subsequent doses at 6- to 8-hour intervals. Obtain ECG 6 hours after each dose to assess potential toxicity.
Daily maintenance dose:
Oral: 0.125-0.5 mg once daily

I.V., I.M: 0.1-0.4 mg once daily (**Note:** I.M. not preferred due to severe injection site pain.)

Dosing adjustment in renal impairment:
Infants, Children, and Adolescents:
Loading dose: Reduce by 50% in end-stage renal disease
Maintenance dose:
Manufacturer's labeling: Dosage reductions and close monitoring recommended; see product labeling for CrCl-specific dosage recommendation
Alternate dosing: The following adjustments have been recommended (Aronoff, 2007):
GFR: 30-50 mL/minute/1.73 m²: Administer 75% of normal dose at normal intervals
GFR: 10-29 mL/minute/1.73 m²: Administer 50% of normal dose at normal intervals or administer normal dose every 36 hours
GFR: <10 mL/minute/1.73 m²: Administer 25% of normal dose at normal intervals or administer normal dose every 48 hours
Intermittent hemodialysis: Administer 25% of normal dose at normal intervals or administer normal dose every 48 hours
Peritoneal dialysis (PD): Administer 25% of normal dose at normal intervals or administer normal dose every 48 hours
Continuous renal replacement therapy (CRRT): Administer 75% of normal dose at normal intervals; titrate to desired effect; monitor serum concentrations
Adults:
Loading dose:
ESRD: If loading dose necessary, reduce by 50%
Acute renal failure: Based on expert opinion, if patient in acute renal failure requires ventricular rate control (eg, in atrial fibrillation), consider alternative therapy. If loading digoxin becomes necessary, patient volume of distribution may be increased and reduction in loading dose may not be necessary; however, maintenance dosing will require adjustment as long as renal failure persists.
Maintenance dose:
CrCl 10-50 mL/minute: Administer 25% to 75% of normal daily dose (divided and given at normal intervals) or administer normal dose every 36 hours
CrCl <10 mL/minute: Administer 10% to 25% of normal daily dose (divided and given at normal intervals) or give normal dose every 48 hours

Administration
Oral: Administer consistently with relationship to meals; avoid concurrent administration (ie, administer digoxin 1 hour before or 2 hours after) with meals high in fiber or pectin and with drugs that decrease oral absorption of digoxin
Oral solution: Only the calibrated manufacturer-provided dropper or a calibrated oral syringe should be used to measure the dose. For doses <0.2 mL the manufacturer-provided dropper is not accurate and should not be used; use a calibrated oral syringe.
Parenteral: I.V.: May be administered undiluted or diluted at least fourfold in D₅W, D₁₀W, NS, or SWI (less than a fourfold dilution could lead to precipitation) and slowly administered I.V. over ≥5 minutes (usually 5-10 minutes); avoid rapid I.V. infusion since this may result in systemic and coronary arteriolar vasoconstriction; I.M. route not usually recommended due to local irritation, pain, and tissue damage.

Vesicant/Extravasation Risk Vesicant
Monitoring Parameters Heart rate and rhythm, periodic ECG; follow serum potassium, magnesium, and calcium closely (especially in patients receiving diuretics or amphotericin); decreased serum potassium and magnesium, or

increased serum magnesium and calcium may increase digoxin toxicity; assess renal function (serum BUN, S_{cr}) in order to adjust dose; obtain serum drug concentrations at least 8-12 hours after a dose, preferably prior to next scheduled dose.

Therapeutic drug monitoring: Digoxin serum concentrations are monitored because digoxin possesses a narrow therapeutic serum concentration range; the therapeutic endpoint is difficult to quantify and digoxin toxicity may be life-threatening. Digoxin serum concentrations should be drawn **at least 6-8 hours after the previous dose, regardless of route of administration (optimally 12-24 hours after a dose)**. Note: Serum digoxin concentrations may decrease in response to exercise due to increased skeletal muscle uptake; a period of rest (eg, ~2 hours) after exercise may be necessary prior to drawing serum digoxin concentrations.

Initiation of therapy:

If a loading dose is given: Digoxin serum concentration may be drawn within 12-24 hours after the initial loading dose administration. Concentrations drawn this early may confirm the relationship of digoxin plasma concentrations and response but are of little value in determining maintenance doses.

If a loading dose is not given: Digoxin serum concentration should be obtained after 3-5 days of therapy.

Maintenance therapy:

Trough concentrations should be followed just prior to the next dose or at a minimum of 6-8 hours after last dose.

Digoxin serum concentrations should be obtained within 5-7 days (approximate time to steady-state) after any dosage changes. Continue to obtain digoxin serum concentrations 7-14 days after any change in maintenance dose. Note: Time to steady state will be longer in patients with decreased renal function (eg, premature neonates or patients with renal impairment). In patients with end-stage renal disease, it may take 15-20 days to reach steady-state.

Patients who are receiving electrolyte-altering medications such as diuretics, serum potassium, magnesium, and calcium should be monitored closely.

Digoxin serum concentrations should be obtained whenever any of the following conditions occur:
Questionable patient compliance or to evaluate clinical deterioration following an initial good response
Changing renal function
Suspected digoxin toxicity
Initiation or discontinuation of therapy with drugs (eg, amiodarone, quinidine, verapamil) which potentially interact with digoxin.
Any disease changes (eg, thyroid disease)

Reference Range Digoxin therapeutic serum trough concentrations:
Heart failure: 0.5-0.8 ng/mL
Adults: <0.5 ng/mL (SI: <0.6 nmol/L); probably indicates underdigitalization unless there are special circumstances
Toxic: >2 ng/mL; (SI: >2.6 nmol/L). Note: Serum concentration must be used in conjunction with clinical symptoms and ECG to confirm diagnosis of digoxin intoxication.
Digoxin-like immunoreactive substance (DLIS) may cross-react with digoxin immunoassay and falsely increase serum concentrations. DLIS has been found in patients with renal and liver disease, heart failure, neonates, and pregnant women (3rd trimester).

Test Interactions Spironolactone may interfere with digoxin radioimmunoassay.

Dosage Forms Excipient information presented when available (limited, particularly for generics); consult specific product labeling.
Solution, Injection:
Lanoxin: 0.25 mg/mL (2 mL) [contains alcohol, usp, propylene glycol]
Lanoxin Pediatric: 0.1 mg/mL (1 mL) [contains alcohol, usp, propylene glycol]
Generic: 0.25 mg/mL (1 mL, 2 mL)
Solution, Oral:
Generic: 0.05 mg/mL (60 mL)
Tablet, Oral:
Digox: 125 mcg [scored; contains fd&c yellow #10 aluminum lake]
Digox: 250 mcg [scored]
Lanoxin: 62.5 mcg [contains fd&c yellow #6 (sunset yellow)]
Lanoxin: 125 mcg [scored; contains fd&c yellow #10 (quinoline yellow), fd&c yellow #6 (sunset yellow)]
Lanoxin: 187.5 mcg
Lanoxin: 250 mcg [scored]
Generic: 125 mcg, 250 mcg

References
American Academy of Pediatrics Committee on Drugs. "Inactive" ingredients in pharmaceutical products: update (subject review). *Pediatrics*. 1997;99(2):268-278.
Antman EM, Anbe DT, Armstrong PW, et al, "ACC/AHA Guidelines for the Management of Patients With ST-Elevation Myocardial Infarction: A Report of the American College of Cardiology/American Heart Association Task Force on Practice Guidelines (Committee to Revise the 1999 Guidelines for the Management of Patients with Acute Myocardial Infarction)," *Circulation*, 2004, 110(9):e82-292.
Bakir M and Bilgic A, "Single Daily Dose of Digoxin for Maintenance Therapy of Infants and Children With Cardiac Disease: Is It Reliable?" *Pediatr Cardiol*, 1994, 15(5):229-32.
Bendayan R and McKenzie MW, "Digoxin Pharmacokinetics and Dosage Requirements in Pediatric Patients," *Clin Pharm*, 1983, 2 (3):224-35.
Blomström-Lundqvist C, Scheinman MM, Aliot EM, et al, "ACC/AHA/ESC Guidelines for the Management of Patients With Supraventricular Arrhythmias–Executive Summary. A Report of the American College of Cardiology/American Heart Association Task Force on Practice Guidelines and the European Society of Cardiology Committee for Practice Guidelines (Writing Committee to Develop Guidelines for the Management of Patients With Supraventricular Arrhythmias)," *Circulation*, 2003, 108(15):1871-909.
European Heart Rhythm Association; Heart Rhythm Society, Fuster V, et al, "ACC/AHA/ESC 2006 Guidelines for the Management of Patients With Atrial Fibrillation – Executive Summary: A Report of the American College of Cardiology/American Heart Association Task Force on Practice Guidelines and the European Society of Cardiology Committee for Practice Guidelines (Writing Committee to Revise the 2001 Guidelines for the Management of Patients With Atrial Fibrillation)," *J Am Coll Cardiol*, 2006, 48(4):854-906.
Fuster V, Ryden LE, Cannom DS, et al, "ACC/AHA/ESC 2006 Guidelines for the Management of Patients With Atrial Fibrillation-Executive Summary. A Report of the American College of Cardiology/American Heart Association Task Force on Practice Guidelines and the European Society of Cardiology Committee for Practice Guidelines (Writing Committee to Revise the 2001 Guidelines for the Management of Patients With Atrial Fibrillation). Developed in Collaboration With the European Heart Rhythm Association and the Heart Rhythm Society," *J Am Coll Cardiol*, 2006, 48(4):854-906.
Hunt SA, Abraham WT, Chin MH, et al, "2009 Focused Update Incorporated Into the ACC/AHA 2005 Guidelines for the Diagnosis and Management of Heart Failure in Adults: A Report of the American College of Cardiology Foundation/American Heart Association Task Force on Practice Guidelines Developed in Collaboration With the International Society for Heart and Lung Transplantation," *J Am Coll Cardiol*, 2009, 53(15):e1-e90.
Johne A, Brockmoller J, Bauer S, et al, "Pharmacokinetic Interaction of Digoxin With an Herbal Extract From St John's Wort (*Hypericum perforatum*)," *Clin Pharmacol Ther*, 1999, 66(4):338-45.
Latifi S, Lidsky K, and Blumer JL, "Pharmacology of Inotropic Agents in Infants and Children," *Prog Pediatr Cardiol*, 2000, 12(1):57-79.

Packer M, Gheorghiade M, Young JB, et al, "Withdrawal of Digoxin From Patients With Chronic Heart Failure Treated With Angiotensin-Converting-Enzyme Inhibitors. RADIANCE Study," *N Engl J Med*, 1993, 329(1):1-7.

Park MK, "Use of Digoxin in Infants and Children With Specific Emphasis on Dosage," *J Pediatr*, 1986, 108(6):871-7.

Ross RD, "Medical Management of Chronic Heart Failure in Children," *Am J Cardiovasc Drugs*, 2001, 1(1):37-44.

Shehab N, Lewis CL, Streetman DD, Donn SM. Exposure to the pharmaceutical excipients benzyl alcohol and propylene glycol among critically ill neonates. *Pediatr Crit Care Med*. 2009;10 (2):256-259.

Siu CW, Lau CP, Lee WL, et al, "Intravenous Diltiazem Is Superior to Intravenous Amiodarone or Digoxin for Achieving Ventricular Rate Control in Patients With Acute Uncomplicated Atrial Fibrillation," *Crit Care Med*, 2009, 37(7):2174-9.

Digoxin Immune Fab (di JOKS in i MYUN fab)

Brand Names: U.S. DigiFab
Brand Names: Canada DigiFab®
Therapeutic Category Antidote, Digoxin
Generic Availability (U.S.) No

Use Treatment of potentially life-threatening digoxin or digitoxin intoxication in carefully selected patients; acute digoxin ingestion (ie, >10 mg in adults; >0.1 mg/kg or >4 mg in children; ingestions resulting in serum concentrations >10 ng/mL), chronic ingestions leading to steady-state digoxin concentrations >6 ng/mL in adults or >4 ng/ mL in children; patients experiencing manifestations of digoxin toxicity due to overdose (eg, life-threatening ventricular arrhythmias, progressive bradycardia, second- or third-degree heart block not responsive to atropine, serum potassium >5.5 mEq/L in adults or >6 mEq/L in children) [FDA approved in pediatric patients (age not specified) and adults]

Pregnancy Risk Factor C

Pregnancy Considerations Animal reproduction studies have not been conducted. Safety and efficacy in pregnant women have not been established. Use during pregnancy only if clearly needed. In general, medications used as antidotes should take into consideration the health and prognosis of the mother; antidotes should be administered to pregnant women if there is a clear indication for use and should not be withheld because of fears of teratogenicity (Bailey, 2003).

Breast-Feeding Considerations It is not known if digoxin immune fab is excreted into breast milk. The manufacturer recommends caution be used if administered to a nursing woman. Also consider the presence of digoxin in breast milk.

Contraindications Hypersensitivity to digoxin immune Fab or any component

Warnings Patients experiencing acute digitalis toxicity may present with significant hyperkalemia due to shifting of potassium into the extracellular space. Upon treatment with digoxin immune Fab, potassium shifts back into the intracellular space; therefore, hypokalemia may rapidly develop. Monitor potassium closely, especially during the first few hours after administration; treat hypokalemia cautiously when clinically indicated. Total serum digoxin concentrations will rise precipitously following administration of digoxin immune Fab due to the presence of the Fab-digoxin complex; because digoxin bound to Fab fragments is not physiologically active this rise has no clinical meaning. Therefore, avoid monitoring total serum digoxin concentrations until the Fab fragments have been eliminated completely. The Fab-digoxin complex will be eliminated more slowly in patients with renal failure (experience limited). Toxicity may recur due to dissociation of the Fab-digoxin complex; prolonged monitoring for recurrence of symptoms and evaluation of free (unbound) digoxin concentrations (if test available) may be warranted in this patient population. In patients chronically maintained on digoxin for heart failure, administration of digoxin immune

Fab may result in exacerbation of heart failure symptoms due to a reduction in digoxin serum concentration. If redigitalization is required, consider postponing until Fab fragments have been eliminated completely; elimination may take several days or longer, especially in patients with renal impairment.

Precautions Use with caution in renal or cardiac failure. Digoxin immune Fab is derived from ovine (sheep) Fab immunoglobulin fragments; hypersensitivity reactions (eg, anaphylactic or anaphylactoid reactions, delayed allergic reactions) are possible. Patients with allergies to sheep proteins and patients with prior exposure to ovine antibodies or ovine Fab may be at a higher risk for hypersensitivity reactions. In patients who develop an anaphylactic reaction, discontinue the infusion and administer emergency care. Immediate treatment (eg, epinephrine 1:1000, corticosteroids, diphenhydramine) should be available; the benefit of epinephrine in this situation must be weighed against the potential risk in digoxin toxicity. Digoxin immune Fab is processed with papain and may cause hypersensitivity reactions in patients allergic to papaya, other papaya extracts, papain, chymopapain, or the pineapple-enzyme bromelain. There may also be cross allergenicity with dust mite and latex allergens.

Adverse Reactions
Cardiovascular: Heart failure exacerbation (due to withdrawal of digoxin), orthostatic hypotension, rapid ventricular response (patients with atrial fibrillation; due to withdrawal of digoxin)
Endocrine & metabolic: Hypokalemia
Local: Phlebitis
Miscellaneous: Allergic reactions, serum sickness

Drug Interactions
Metabolism/Transport Effects None known.
Avoid Concomitant Use There are no known interactions where it is recommended to avoid concomitant use.
Increased Effect/Toxicity There are no known significant interactions involving an increase in effect.
Decreased Effect There are no known significant interactions involving a decrease in effect.

Stability Store vials at 2°C to 8°C (36°F to 46°F); do not freeze. The following stability information has also been reported: May be stored at room temperature for up to 30 days (Cohen, 2007). Reconstituted solutions are stable for 4 hours when stored at 2°C to 8°C (36°F to 46°F).

Mechanism of Action Digoxin immune antigen-binding fragments (Fab) are specific antibodies for the treatment of digitalis intoxication in carefully selected patients; binds with molecules of digoxin or DIGIToxin and is then excreted by the kidneys and removed from the body

Pharmacodynamics Onset of action: Improvement in signs and symptoms occurs within 2-30 minutes following I.V. infusion

Pharmacokinetics (Adult data unless noted)
Distribution: V_d: 0.3 L/kg
Half-life: 15 hours; renal impairment prolongs half-life
Elimination: Renal with concentrations declining to undetectable amounts within 5-7 days

Dosing: Neonatal Acute ingestion of known amount: I.V.:
Based on amount (in mg) of digoxin ingested:
Step 1: Calculate total body load (mg)
Total body load (mg) = 0.8 x [amount (mg) digoxin tablets or elixir ingested]
Step 2: Calculate number of vials needed
Digoxin Immune Fab Dose (vials) = Total body load (mg) / (0.5)

◄ **Based on steady-state serum digoxin concentration:**
Consider dilution of the reconstituted vial with NS and administer the dose via a tuberculin syringe.

Digoxin Immune Fab Dose (mg) = [(serum digoxin concentration [ng/mL] x weight [kg]) / 100] x 40 mg/vial

Dose Estimates of Digoxin Immune Fab (in mg) From Serum Digoxin Concentration

Patient Weight (kg)	Serum Digoxin Concentration (ng/mL)						
	1	2	4	8	12	16	20
1	0.4 mg^A	1 mg^A	1.5mg^A	3 mg	5 mg	6.5 mg	8 mg
3	1 mg^A	2.5 mg^A	5 mg	10 mg	14 mg	19 mg	24 mg
5	2 mg^A	4 mg	8 mg	16 mg	24 mg	32 mg	40 mg

^ADilution of reconstituted vial to 1 mg/mL may be desirable.

Dosing: Usual Infants, Children, Adolescents, and Adults:
Note: Estimation of the dose is based on the body burden of digitalis. This may be calculated if the amount ingested is known or the postdistribution serum drug concentration is known (round the dose up to the nearest whole vial). If the amount ingested is unknown, general dosing guidelines should be used.
Acute ingestion of unknown amount: I.V.: 20 vials is adequate to treat most life-threatening ingestions. In small children, it is important to monitor for fluid overload. May give as a single dose or give 10 vials, observe the response, and give a second dose of 10 vials if indicated.
Acute ingestion of known amount: I.V.:
Based on amount of digoxin ingested:
Step 1: Calculate total body load (mg)
Total body load (mg) = 0.8 x [amount (mg) digoxin tablets or elixir ingested]
Step 2: Calculate number of vials needed
Digoxin Immune Fab Dose (vials) = Total body load (mg) / (0.5)
Based on steady-state serum digoxin concentration: I.V.:
Digoxin Immune Fab Dose (mg) = [(serum digoxin concentration [ng/mL] x weight [kg]) / 100] x 40 mg/vial
Digoxin Immune Fab Dose (vials) = (serum digoxin concentration [ng/mL] x weight [kg]) / 100
Note: Infants and Children ≤20 kg may require smaller doses; calculate the dose in milligrams (mg), consider dilution of the reconstituted vial with NS, and administer the dose via a tuberculin syringe.
Alternatively, the following table gives an estimation of the amount of Digoxin Immune Fab needed based on the steady-state serum digoxin concentration.

Infants and Children Dose Estimates of Digoxin Immune Fab (in mg) From Serum Digoxin Concentration

Patient Weight (kg)	Serum Digoxin Concentration (ng/mL)						
	1	2	4	8	12	16	20
3	1 mg^A	2.5 mg^A	5 mg	10 mg	14 mg	19 mg	24 mg
5	2 mg^A	4 mg	8 mg	16 mg	24 mg	32 mg	40 mg
10	4 mg	8 mg	16 mg	32 mg	48 mg	64 mg	80 mg
20	8 mg	16 mg	32 mg	64 mg	96 mg	128 mg	160 mg

^ADilution of reconstituted vial to 1 mg/mL may be desirable.

Adult Dose Estimate of Digoxin Immune Fab (in # of Vials) From Serum Digoxin Concentration

Patient Weight (kg)	Serum Digoxin Concentration (ng/mL)						
	1	2	4	8	12	16	20
40	0.5 vial	1 vial	2 vials	3 vials	5 vials	7 vials	8 vials
60	0.5 vial	1 vial	3 vials	5 vials	7 vials	10 vials	12 vials
70	1 vial	2 vials	3 vials	6 vials	9 vials	11 vials	14 vials
80	1 vial	2 vials	3 vials	7 vials	10 vials	13 vials	16 vials
100	1 vial	2 vials	4 vials	8 vials	12 vials	16 vials	20 vials

Chronic toxicity (serum digoxin concentration unavailable): I.V.:
Infants and Children ≤20 kg: 1 vial is adequate to reverse most cases of toxicity
Children >20 kg, Adolescents, and Adults: 6 vials is adequate to reverse most cases of toxicity
Dosing adjustment in renal impairment: No dosage adjustment necessary; however, use with caution since digoxin-digoxin immune Fab complex is renally eliminated. Patients should undergo prolonged monitoring for recurrence of toxicity.
Administration Parenteral: I.V.: Reconstitute with 4 mL SWI, resulting in an 10 mg/mL concentration for I.V. infusion. I.V. infusion over at least 30 minutes is preferred. May also be given by bolus injection if cardiac arrest is imminent (infusion-related reaction may occur). Small doses (eg, those required in infants or small children) may be administered using a tuberculin syringe as undiluted digoxin immune Fab or diluted with NS to a concentration of 1 mg/mL digoxin immune Fab. Discontinue the infusion and reinitiate at a slower rate if an infusion-related reaction occurs.
Monitoring Parameters Prior to the first dose of digoxin immune Fab evaluate serum potassium, serum digoxin concentration, and serum creatinine; closely monitor serum potassium (eg, hourly for 4-6 hours; at least daily thereafter), temperature, blood pressure, and electrocardiogram after administration. Total serum digoxin concentrations will rise precipitously following administration of digoxin immune Fab due to the presence of the Fab-digoxin complex; because digoxin bound to Fab fragments is not physiologically active this rise has no clinical meaning. Therefore, avoid monitoring total serum digoxin concentrations until the Fab fragments have been eliminated completely; this may be several days to weeks in patients with renal impairment (Ujhelyi, 1995).

Patients with renal failure may experience a recurrence of toxicity; prolonged monitoring for recurrence of symptoms and evaluation of free (unbound) digoxin concentrations (if test available) may be warranted in this patient population.
Test Interactions Digoxin immune fab will interfere with digitalis immunoassay measurements, thereby resulting in clinically misleading total serum digoxin concentrations until all Fab fragments are eliminated from the body (may take several days to >1 week after administration).
Additional Information Each 40 mg vial (DigiFab™) will bind approximately 0.5 mg digoxin or digitoxin; for individuals at increased risk of sensitivity an intradermal or scratch technique skin test using a 1:100 dilution of reconstituted digoxin immune Fab diluted in NS has been used. Skin test volume is 0.1 mL of 1:100 dilution; evaluate after 20 minutes.

Dosage Forms Excipient information presented when available (limited, particularly for generics); consult specific product labeling.

Solution Reconstituted, Intravenous [preservative free]:
DigiFab: 40 mg (1 ea)

References

Bailey B, "Are There Teratogenic Risks Associated With Antidotes Used in the Acute Management of Poisoned Pregnant Women?" *Birth Defects Res A Clin Mol Teratol*, 2003, 67(2):133-40.

Cohen V, Jellinek SP, Teperikidis L, et al, "Room-Temperature Storage of Medications Labeled for Refrigeration," *Am J Health Syst Pharm*, 2007, 64(16):1711-5.

Hickey AR, Wenger TL, Carpenter VP, et al, "Digoxin Immune Fab Therapy in the Management of Digitalis Intoxication: Safety and Efficacy Results of an Observational Surveillance Study," *J Am Coll Cardiol*, 1991, 17(3):590-8.

Schneider PJ, McCollam PL, and Osborn JJ, "Possible Dissociation of the Digibind-Digoxin Complex in Renal Failure," *DICP*, 1991, 25 (11):1269.

Ujhelyi MR and Robert S, "Pharmacokinetic Aspects of Digoxin-Specific Fab Therapy in the Management of Digitalis Toxicity," *Clin Pharmacokinet*, 1995, 28(6):483-93.

◆ **Digoxin Injection CSD (Can)** *see* Digoxin *on page 658*

Dihydroergotamine (dye hye droe er GOT a meen)

Related Information

Safe Handling of Hazardous Drugs *on page 2419*
Brand Names: U.S. D.H.E. 45; Migranal
Brand Names: Canada Migranal®
Therapeutic Category Alpha-Adrenergic Blocking Agent, Intranasal; Alpha-Adrenergic Blocking Agent, Parenteral; Antimigraine Agent; Ergot Alkaloid and Derivative
Generic Availability (U.S.) Yes
Use

Intranasal: Treatment of migraine headache with or without aura (FDA approved in adults)
Parenteral: Treatment of headache with or without aura and cluster headaches (FDA approved in adults)
Pregnancy Risk Factor X
Pregnancy Considerations Dihydroergotamine is oxytocic and should not be used during pregnancy.
Breast-Feeding Considerations Ergot derivatives inhibit prolactin and it is known that ergotamine is excreted in breast milk (vomiting, diarrhea, weak pulse, and unstable blood pressure have been reported in nursing infants). It is not known if dihydroergotamine would also cause these effects, however, it is likely that it is excreted in human breast milk. Do not use in nursing women.
Contraindications Hypersensitivity to dihydroergotamine, other ergot alkaloids, or any component; pregnancy; breast-feeding; uncontrolled hypertension, ischemic heart disease, angina pectoris, history of MI, silent ischemia, or coronary artery vasospasm including Prinzmetal's angina; hemiplegic or basilar migraine; peripheral vascular disease, sepsis, severe hepatic or renal dysfunction, and following vascular surgery; concurrent therapy with potent CYP3A4 inhibitors (eg, protease inhibitors, azole antifungals, and certain macrolide antibiotics); do not use within 24 hours of sumatriptan, zolmitriptan, other serotonin agonists, ergot-like agents or methysergide; concurrent use of peripheral and central vasoconstrictors
Warnings Hazardous agent; use appropriate precautions for handling and disposal (NIOSH, 2012).

Concomitant use with potent inhibitors of CYP3A4 (including protease inhibitors, azole antifungals, and some macrolide antibiotics) has been associated with acute ergot toxicity (ergotism) characterized by serious and/or life-threatening cerebral and peripheral ischemia **[U.S. Boxed Warning]**; some cases have resulted in amputation; less potent CYP3A4 inhibitors (eg, metronidazole, fluoxetine, nefazodone, and zileuton) may carry the same risk.

Vasospasm or vasoconstriction can occur, possibly resulting in decreased cerebral blood flow, ECG changes, and hypertension; sustained vasoconstriction may also lead to ischemic colitis, intermittent claudication, aggravation of angina, or precipitation of MI. Do not use in any patient at risk or predisposed to vascular effects of ergot alkaloids. Ergot alkaloid use may result in ergotism (intense vasoconstriction) resulting in peripheral vascular ischemia and possible gangrene. Ergotism is usually associated with overdosage or prolonged chronic use; do not exceed dosing guidelines and avoid prolonged administration. Patients with risk factors for CAD should have a baseline cardiovascular evaluation prior to first dose; if evaluation is satisfactory, the healthcare provider should administer the first dose and cardiovascular status should be periodically evaluated.

Injection: Rare reports of adverse cardiac events (acute MI, life-threatening arrhythmias, death) have been reported; cerebral hemorrhage, subarachnoid hemorrhage, and stroke have also occurred. Injection is not intended for prolonged use; pleural and retroperitoneal fibrosis have been reported with daily use. Cardiac valvular fibrosis has been associated with ergot alkaloid use.

Nasal spray (Migranal®): Local irritation to nose and throat (usually transient and mild-moderate in severity) can occur; long-term consequences on nasal or respiratory mucosa have not been extensively evaluated
Precautions May cause nausea; in pediatric patients, antiemetic prophylaxis (prochlorperazine or metoclopramide) 30 minutes prior to initial dihydroergotamine dose has been used (O'Brien, 2011).
Adverse Reactions
Nasal spray:
Central nervous system: Dizziness, somnolence
Endocrine & metabolic: Hot flashes
Gastrointestinal: Diarrhea, nausea, taste disturbance, vomiting
Local: Application site reaction
Neuromuscular & skeletal: Stiffness, weakness
Respiratory: Pharyngitis, rhinitis
Rare but important or life-threatening: Injection and nasal spray: Cerebral hemorrhage, coronary artery vasospasm, dyspnea, hypertension, MI, paresthesia, peripheral cyanosis, peripheral ischemia, stroke, subarachnoid hemorrhage, ventricular fibrillation, ventricular tachycardia. Pleural and retroperitoneal fibrosis have been reported following prolonged use of the injection; cardiac valvular fibrosis has been associated with ergot alkaloids.
Drug Interactions
Metabolism/Transport Effects Substrate of CYP3A4 (major); **Note:** Assignment of Major/Minor substrate status based on clinically relevant drug interaction potential; **Inhibits** CYP3A4 (weak)
Avoid Concomitant Use

Avoid concomitant use of Dihydroergotamine with any of the following: Alpha-/Beta-Agonists; Alpha1-Agonists; Boceprevir; Clarithromycin; Cobicistat; Conivaptan; Crizotinib; Enzalutamide; Fusidic Acid (Systemic); Itraconazole; Ketoconazole (Systemic); Lorcaserin; Mifepristone; Nitroglycerin; Pimozide; Posaconazole; Protease Inhibitors; Serotonin 5-HT1D Receptor Agonists; Telaprevir; Voriconazole

Increased Effect/Toxicity

Dihydroergotamine may increase the levels/effects of: Alpha-/Beta-Agonists; Alpha1-Agonists; Antipsychotics; ARIPiprazole; Dofetilide; Lomitapide; Metoclopramide; Pimozide; Serotonin 5-HT1D Receptor Agonists; Serotonin Modulators

The levels/effects of Dihydroergotamine may be increased by: Antiemetics (5HT3 Antagonists); Antipsychotics; Beta-Blockers; Boceprevir; Ceritinib;

Clarithromycin; Cobicistat; Conivaptan; Crizotinib; CYP3A4 Inhibitors (Moderate); CYP3A4 Inhibitors (Strong); Dasatinib; Fusidic Acid (Systemic); Itraconazole; Ivacaftor; Ketoconazole (Systemic); Lorcaserin; Luliconazole; Macrolide Antibiotics; Mifepristone; Nitroglycerin; Posaconazole; Protease Inhibitors; Serotonin 5-HT1D Receptor Agonists; Simeprevir; Stiripentol; Telaprevir; Voriconazole

Decreased Effect

Dihydroergotamine may decrease the levels/effects of: Nitroglycerin

The levels/effects of Dihydroergotamine may be decreased by: Enzalutamide

Stability Hazardous agent; use appropriate precautions for handling and disposal (NIOSH, 2012).

Injection: Store at 20°C to 25°C (68°F to 77°F); do not refrigerate or freeze; protect the vials from light and heat.

Nasal spray: Store below 25°C (77°F); do not refrigerate or freeze; once the nasal spray applicator has been prepared, use within 8 hours; discard any unused nasal solution.

Mechanism of Action Ergot alkaloid alpha-adrenergic blocker directly stimulates vascular smooth muscle to vasoconstrict peripheral and cerebral vessels; also has effects on serotonin receptors

Pharmacodynamics

Onset of action:
I.M.: 15-30 minutes
Intranasal: 30 minutes
I.V.: Immediate
Duration: I.M.: 3-4 hours

Pharmacokinetics (Adult data unless noted)

Distribution: V_d: ~800 L
Bioavailability: Intranasal: 32%
Protein binding: 93%
Metabolism: Extensively in the liver; one active metabolite
Half-life: Biphasic: terminal half-life: ~9-10 hours
Time to peak serum concentration: I.M.: Within 15-30 minutes; intranasal: 0.5-1 hour; I.V.: 15 minutes; SubQ: 15-45 minutes
Elimination: Predominately into bile and feces and 10% excreted in urine, mostly as metabolites
Clearance: 1.5 L/minute

Dosing: Usual

Children and Adolescents: **Intractable migraine >72 hours (status migrainosus):** Limited data available; optimal dose not established:
I.V.: Premedicate with antiemetic (metoclopramide or prochlorperazine have been used)
Low dose regimen:
Children 6 to <10 years: 0.1 mg/dose every 6 hours; improvement usually seen after 5 doses; if improvement noted, continue therapy until headache-free up to a maximum of 16 doses; if no improvement after 5 doses, discontinue therapy (O'Brien, 2011)
Children ≥10 to 12 years: 0.15 mg/dose every 6 hours; improvement usually seen after 5 doses; if improvement noted, continue therapy until headache-free up to a maximum of 16 doses; if no improvement after 5 doses, discontinue therapy. One study reported increasing the dose by 0.05 mg increments as tolerated (ie, no abdominal discomfort). Postmenarche female patients should complete pregnancy screening prior to first dose (Linder, 1994; O'Brien, 2011).
Adolescents ≤16 years: 0.2 mg/dose every 6 hours; improvement usually seen after 5 doses; if improvement noted, continue therapy until headache-free up to a maximum of 16 doses; if no improvement after 5 doses, discontinue therapy. Postmenarche female patients should complete pregnancy screening prior to first dose (O'Brien, 2011).

High dose regimen:
Children 6-9 years or Children ≥10 years and <25 kg: 0.5 mg/dose every 8 hours; improvement usually seen after 5 doses; if improvement noted, continue therapy until headache-free up to a maximum of 20 doses; if no improvement after 5 doses, discontinue therapy; an additional dose after headache subsides has also been suggested (Kabbouche, 2009; O'Brien, 2011). **Note:** An initial test dose (half of the appropriate dose for age and weight) has been used; if test dose tolerated, remainder of dose administered 30 minutes later (Kabbouche, 2009).
Children ≥10 years and >25 kg and Adolescents: 1 mg/dose every 8 hours; improvement usually seen after 5 doses; if improvement noted, continue therapy until headache-free up to a maximum of 20 doses; if no improvement after 5 doses, discontinue therapy (Kabbouche, 2009; O'Brien, 2011). **Note:** An initial test dose (half of the appropriate dose for age and weight) has been used; if test dose tolerated, remainder of dose administered 30 minutes later (Kabbouche, 2009).
Intranasal: Adolescents: 1 spray (0.5 mg) into each nostril (total dose: 1 mg); repeat if needed within 15 minutes up to a total of 4 sprays (2 mg); maximum daily dose: 6 sprays (3 mg)/24-hour period; **Note:** Do not exceed 8 sprays (4 mg)/week.

Adults: **Migraine, cluster headache:**
I.M., SubQ: 1 mg at first sign of headache; repeat hourly to a maximum dose of 3 mg/day; maximum dose: 6 mg/week
I.V.: 1 mg at first sign of headache; repeat hourly up to a maximum of 2 mg/day; maximum dose: 6 mg/week
Intranasal: 1 spray (0.5 mg) of nasal spray should be administered into each nostril; if needed, repeat after 15 minutes, up to a total of 4 sprays (2 mg). **Note:** Do not exceed 6 sprays (3 mg) in a 24-hour period and no more than 8 sprays (4 mg) in a week.

Dosing adjustment in renal impairment: Contraindicated in severe renal impairment

Dosing adjustment in hepatic impairment: Dosage reductions are probably necessary but specific guidelines are not available; contraindicated in severe hepatic dysfunction

Administration

Intranasal: Prior to administration, the nasal spray applicator must be primed (pumped 4 times); spray once into each nostril; avoid deep inhalation through the nose while spraying or immediately after spraying; do not tilt head back. For further information, consult manufacturer labeling.

I.M., SubQ: Administer without dilution
I.V.: Administer without dilution slowly over 2-3 minutes

Hazardous agent; use appropriate precautions for handling and disposal (NIOSH, 2012).

Dosage Forms Considerations

Migranal nasal solution contains caffeine 10 mg/mL

Dosage Forms Excipient information presented when available (limited, particularly for generics); consult specific product labeling.

Solution, Injection, as mesylate:
D.H.E. 45: 1 mg/mL (1 mL)
Generic: 1 mg/mL (1 mL)
Solution, Nasal, as mesylate:
Migranal: 4 mg/mL (1 mL)
Generic: 4 mg/mL (1 mL)

References

National Institute for Occupational Safety and Health (NIOSH), "NIOSH List of Antineoplastic and Other Hazardous Drugs in Healthcare Settings 2012." Available at http://www.cdc.gov/niosh/docs/2012-150/pdfs/2012-150.pdf. Accessed January 21, 2013.

◆ **Dihydroergotamine Mesylate** see Dihydroergotamine on page 665

◆ **Dihydrohydroxycodeinone** see OxyCODONE on page 1569

◆ **Dihydromorphinone** see HYDROmorphone on page 1041

◆ **Dihydroxyanthracenedione** see MitoXANtrone on page 1427

◆ **Dihydroxyanthracenedione Dihydrochloride** see MitoXANtrone on page 1427

◆ **1,25 Dihydroxycholecalciferol** see Calcitriol on page 342

◆ **Dihydroxydeoxynorvinkaleukoblastine** see Vinorelbine on page 2143

◆ **Diiodohydroxyquin** see Iodoquinol on page 1144

◆ **Dilacor XR [DSC]** see Diltiazem on page 667

◆ **Dilantin** see Phenytoin on page 1663

◆ **Dilantin Infatabs** see Phenytoin on page 1663

◆ **Dilaudid** see HYDROmorphone on page 1041

◆ **Dilaudid-HP** see HYDROmorphone on page 1041

◆ **Dilt-CD [DSC]** see Diltiazem on page 667

Diltiazem (dil TYE a zem)

Medication Safety Issues
Sound-alike/look-alike issues:
Cardizem may be confused with Cardene, Cardene SR, Cardizem CD, Cardizem SR, cortisone

Cartia XT may be confused with Procardia XL

Diltiazem may be confused with Calan, diazepam, Dilantin

Tiazac may be confused with Tigan, Tiazac XC [CAN], Ziac

High alert medication:
The Institute for Safe Medication Practices (ISMP) includes this medication (I.V. formulation) among its list of drug classes which have a heightened risk of causing significant patient harm when used in error.

Administration issues:
Significant differences exist between oral and I.V. dosing. Use caution when converting from one route of administration to another.

International issues:
Cardizem [U.S., Canada, and multiple international markets] may be confused with Cardem brand name for celiprolol [Spain]

Cartia XT [U.S.] may be confused with Cartia brand name for aspirin [multiple international markets]

Dilacor XR [U.S.] may be confused with Dilacor brand name for verapamil [Brazil]

Dipen [Greece] may be confused with Depen brand name for penicillamine [U.S.]; Depin brand name for nifedipine [India]; Depon brand name for acetaminophen [Greece]

Tiazac: Brand name for diltiazem [U.S, Canada], but also the brand name for pioglitazone [Chile]

Related Information
Medications for Which a Single Dose May Be Fatal When Ingested by a Toddler on page 2408

Oral Medications That Should Not Be Crushed or Altered on page 2438

Brand Names: U.S. Cardizem; Cardizem CD; Cardizem LA; Cartia XT; Dilacor XR [DSC]; Dilt-CD [DSC]; Dilt-XR; Diltiazem HCl CD; Diltzac [DSC]; Matzim LA; Taztia XT; Tiazac

Brand Names: Canada Apo-Diltiaz; Apo-Diltiaz CD; Apo-Diltiaz Injectable; Apo-Diltiaz SR; Apo-Diltiaz TZ; Ava-Diltiazem; Cardizem CD; CO Diltiazem CD; CO Diltiazem T; Diltiazem HCl ER; Diltiazem Hydrochloride Injection; Diltiazem TZ; Diltiazem-CD; Nu-Diltiaz; Nu-Diltiaz-CD; PMS-Diltiazem CD; ratio-Diltiazem CD; Sandoz-Diltiazem CD; Sandoz-Diltiazem T; Teva-Diltiazem; Teva-Diltiazem CD; Teva-Diltiazem HCL ER Capsules; Tiazac; Tiazac XC

Therapeutic Category Antianginal Agent; Antihypertensive Agent; Calcium Channel Blocker; Calcium Channel Blocker, Nondihydropyridine

Generic Availability (U.S.) Yes

Use
Oral: Treatment of chronic stable angina or angina from coronary artery spasm; hypertension (**Note:** Only extended release products are FDA approved for the treatment of hypertension) (FDA approved in adults)

Injection: Management of atrial fibrillation or atrial flutter; paroxysmal supraventricular tachycardias (PSVT) (FDA approved in adults); has also been used for stable narrow-complex tachycardia uncontrolled or unconverted by adenosine or vagal maneuvers or if SVT is recurrent

Pregnancy Risk Factor C

Pregnancy Considerations Adverse events have been observed in animal reproduction studies. Untreated chronic maternal hypertension is associated with adverse events in the fetus, infant, and mother. If treatment for hypertension during pregnancy is needed, other agents are preferred (ACOG, 2013). The Canadian labeling contraindicates use in pregnant women or women of childbearing potential. Diltiazem may be used to control atrial fibrillation in pregnant women (Fuster, 2006). Women with hypertrophic cardiomyopathy who are controlled with diltiazem prior to pregnancy may continue therapy, but increased fetal monitoring is recommended (Gersh, 2011).

Breast-Feeding Considerations Diltiazem is excreted into breastmilk in concentrations similar to those in the maternal plasma (Okada, 1985). Breast-feeding is not recommended by the manufacturer.

Contraindications Hypersensitivity to diltiazem or any component; severe hypotension; second or third degree heart block (except in patients with a functioning artificial pacemaker); sick-sinus syndrome (except in patients with a functioning artificial pacemaker); acute MI with pulmonary congestion; cardiogenic shock; I.V. administration concomitantly or within a few hours of the administration of I.V. beta-blockers; atrial fibrillation or flutter associated with accessory bypass tract (eg, Wolff-Parkinson-White syndrome or short PR syndrome); ventricular tachycardia (with wide-complex tachycardia, must determine whether origin is supraventricular or ventricular)

Warnings May cause bradycardia, second or third degree heart block, hypotension, or rarely, acute hepatic injury (with significant elevations in hepatic transaminases); may worsen CHF. The risk of first-, second-, or third-degree heart block or sinus bradycardia is increased when used with agents that slow cardiac conduction. Concomitant use of diltiazem and a beta-blocker may result in conduction disturbances, hypotension, and worsened LV function. Use with other agents known to either reduce SA node function and/or AV nodal conduction (eg, digoxin) or reduce sympathetic outflow (eg, clonidine) may increase the risk of serious bradycardia.

Precautions Use with caution in patients with CHF or impaired renal or hepatic function. Dermatologic reactions may occur; these may be transient or disappear with continued therapy; however, erythema multiforme or exfoliative dermatitis have been reported; discontinue diltiazem if skin rash persists or is severe. Use Dilacor® XR with caution in patients with preexisting severe GI narrowing; this product uses a slowly disintegrating matrix; **Note:** No reports of obstructive symptoms in patients with strictures have been reported, but caution is advised.

Adverse Reactions

Cardiovascular: AV block, bradycardia, edema, extrasystoles, flushing, hypotension, pain, palpitation, vasodilation

Central nervous system: Dizziness, headache, nervousness

Dermatologic: Rash

Endocrine & metabolic: Gout

Gastrointestinal: Constipation, diarrhea, dyspepsia, vomiting

Local: Injection site reactions: Burning, itching

Neuromuscular & skeletal: Myalgia, weakness

Respiratory: Bronchitis, dyspnea, pharyngitis, rhinitis sinus congestion

Rare but important or life-threatening: Alkaline phosphatase increased, allergic reaction, ALT increased, AST increased, amblyopia, amnesia, arrhythmia, AV block (second or third degree), bundle branch block, CHF, depression, dysgeusia, extrapyramidal symptoms, gingival hyperplasia, hemolytic anemia, petechiae, photosensitivity, Stevens-Johnson syndrome, syncope, tachycardia, thrombocytopenia, tremor, toxic epidermal necrolysis

Drug Interactions

Metabolism/Transport Effects Substrate of CYP2C9 (minor), CYP2D6 (minor), CYP3A4 (major), P-glycoprotein; **Note:** Assignment of Major/Minor substrate status based on clinically relevant drug interaction potential; **Inhibits** CYP2C9 (weak), CYP2D6 (weak), CYP3A4 (moderate)

Avoid Concomitant Use

Avoid concomitant use of Diltiazem with any of the following: Bosutinib; Ceritinib; Conivaptan; Dantrolene; Fusidic Acid (Systemic); Ibrutinib; Ivabradine; Lomitapide; Pimozide; Simeprevir; Tolvaptan; Ulipristal

Increased Effect/Toxicity

Diltiazem may increase the levels/effects of: Alfentanil; Amifostine; Amiodarone; Antihypertensives; Aprepitant; ARIPiprazole; AtorvaSTATin; Atosiban; Avanafil; Benzodiazepines (metabolized by oxidation); Beta-Blockers; Bosentan; Bosutinib; Bradycardia-Causing Agents; Budesonide (Systemic, Oral Inhalation); BusPIRone; Calcium Channel Blockers (Dihydropyridine); Cannabis; CarBAMazepine; Cardiac Glycosides; Ceritinib; Colchicine; Corticosteroids (Systemic); CycloSPORINE (Systemic); CYP3A4 Substrates; Dofetilide; DOXOrubicin (Conventional); Dronabinol; Dronedarone; DULoxetine; Eletriptan; Eplerenone; Everolimus; FentaNYL; Fingolimod; Fosaprepitant; Fosphenytoin; Halofantrine; Hypotensive Agents; Ibrutinib; Imatinib; Ivabradine; Ivacaftor; Lithium; Lomitapide; Lovastatin; Lurasidone; Magnesium Salts; Midodrine; Neuromuscular-Blocking Agents (Nondepolarizing); Nitroprusside; Obinutuzumab; OxyCODONE; Phenytoin; Pimecrolimus; Pimozide; Propafenone; QuiNIDine; Ranolazine; Red Yeast Rice; RiTUXimab; Rivaroxaban; Salicylates; Salmeterol; Saxagliptin; Simeprevir; Simvastatin; Tacrolimus (Systemic); Tacrolimus (Topical); Tetrahydrocannabinol; Tolvaptan; Ulipristal; Vilazodone; Zuclopenthixol

The levels/effects of Diltiazem may be increased by: Alfuzosin; Alpha1-Blockers; Anilidopiperidine Opioids; Antifungal Agents (Azole Derivatives, Systemic); Aprepitant; AtorvaSTATin; Barbiturates; Brimonidine (Topical); Calcium Channel Blockers (Dihydropyridine); Cimetidine; CloNIDine; Conivaptan; CycloSPORINE (Systemic); CYP3A4 Inhibitors (Moderate); CYP3A4 Inhibitors (Strong); Dantrolene; Dasatinib; Diazoxide; Dronedarone; Fluconazole; Fosaprepitant; Fusidic Acid (Systemic); Grapefruit Juice; Herbs (Hypotensive Properties); Ivabradine; Lovastatin; Luliconazole; Macrolide Antibiotics; Magnesium Salts; MAO Inhibitors; Mifepristone; Pentoxifylline; P-glycoprotein/ABCB1 Inhibitors; Phosphodiesterase 5 Inhibitors; Prostacyclin Analogues; Protease Inhibitors; Regorafenib; Simvastatin; Stiripentol

Decreased Effect

Diltiazem may decrease the levels/effects of: Clopidogrel; Ifosfamide

The levels/effects of Diltiazem may be decreased by: Barbiturates; Bosentan; Calcium Salts; CarBAMazepine; Colestipol; CYP3A4 Inducers (Strong); Dabrafenib; Deferasirox; Efavirenz; Herbs (Hypertensive Properties); Methylphenidate; Mitotane; Nafcillin; Peginterferon Alfa-2b; P-glycoprotein/ABCB1 Inducers; Rifamycin Derivatives; Siltuximab; St Johns Wort; Tocilizumab; Yohimbine

Food Interactions Diltiazem serum levels may be elevated if taken with food. Serum concentrations were not altered by grapefruit juice in small clinical trials.

Stability

Oral: Dispense oral formulations in a tight, light-resistant container; avoid excess humidity.

Capsule: Extended release:

Cardizem® CD, Tiazac®: Store at 25°C (77°F); excursions permitted to 15°C to 30°C (59°F to 86°F).

Cartia XT®, Dilacor XR® Dilt-CD, Diltia XT®, Taztia XT®: Store at 20°C to 25°C (68°F to 77°F).

Dilt-XR: Store at 20°C to 25°C (68°F to 77°F); excursions permitted to 15°C to 30°C (59°F to 86°F).

Tablet: Immediate release:

Cardizem: Store at 25°C (77°F); excursions permitted to 15°C to 30°C (59°F to 86°F).

Diltiazem: Store at 20°C to 25°C (68°F to 77°F).

Tablet: Extended release:

Cardizem LA: Store at 25°C (77°F); excursions permitted to 15°C to 30°C (59°F to 86°F).

Matzim® LA: Store at 20°C to 25°C (68°F to 77°F); avoid temperatures above 30°C (86°F).

Injection: Store vials under refrigeration at 2°C to 8°C (36°F to 46°F); do not freeze. Contains no preservatives, discard unused portion. May store unopened at room temperature for up to 1 month; destroy after 1 month at room temperature. Compatible in D_5W, NS, and $D_5^{1}/_2$NS at a maximum concentration of 1 mg/mL for 24 hours when stored at room temperature or under refrigeration. Do not mix with other drugs in the same container; do not coinfuse with other drugs in the same I.V. line; **not** physically compatible with acetazolamide, acyclovir, aminophylline, ampicillin, ampicillin and sulbactam, cefamandole, cefoperazone, diazepam, furosemide, hydrocortisone, insulin, methylprednisolone, mezlocillin, nafcillin, phenytoin, rifampin, and sodium bicarbonate.

Mechanism of Action Nondihydropyridine calcium channel blocker which inhibits calcium ion from entering the "slow channels" or select voltage-sensitive areas of vascular smooth muscle and myocardium during depolarization, producing a relaxation of coronary vascular smooth muscle and coronary vasodilation; increases myocardial oxygen delivery in patients with vasospastic angina

Pharmacodynamics

Onset of action:

Oral: Tablet: Immediate release: 30-60 minutes

Parenteral (I.V. bolus): Within 3 minutes

Maximum effect:

Antiarrhythmic (I.V. bolus): 2-7 minutes

Antihypertensive (Oral; multiple dosing): Within 2 weeks

Pharmacokinetics (Adult data unless noted)

Absorption: 80%

Distribution: V_d: 1.7 L/kg; appears in breast milk

Protein binding: 70% to 80%

Metabolism: Extensive first-pass effect; metabolized in the liver; desacetyldiltiazem is an active metabolite (25% to 50% as potent as diltiazem based on coronary vasodilation effects); desacetyldiltiazem may accumulate with plasma concentrations 10% to 20% of diltiazem levels

Bioavailability: Oral: ~40%

Half-life: 3-4.5 hours, up to 8 hours with chronic high dosing

Time to peak serum concentration:
Tablet: Immediate release: 2-4 hours
Cardizem® CD: 10-14 hours
Cardizem® LA, Matzim® LA: 11-18 hours
Cardizem® SR: 6-11 hours
Dilacor® XR: 4-6 hours

Elimination: In urine and bile mostly as metabolites; 2% to 4% excreted as unchanged drug in urine

Dialysis: Not dialyzable

Dosing: Usual

Hypertension: Oral:
Children: Minimal information available; some centers use the following: Initial: 1.5-2 mg/kg/day in 3-4 divided doses (extended release formulations may be dosed once or twice daily); maximum dose: 3.5 mg/kg/day; some centers use a maximum dose of 6 mg/kg/day up to 360 mg/day (Flynn, 2000); **Note:** Doses up to 8 mg/kg/day given in 4 divided doses have been used for investigational therapy of Duchenne muscular dystrophy.

Adolescents ≥18 years and Adults:
Capsule, extended release (once-daily dosing): **Note:** Usual dosage range (JNC 7): 180-420 mg once daily
Cardizem® CD, Cartia XT®, Dilt-CD: Initial: 180-240 mg once daily; may increase dose after 14 days; usual: 240-360 mg once daily; maximum: 480 mg once daily
Dilacor® XR, Diltia XT®, Dilt-XR: Initial: 180-240 mg once daily; may increase after 14 days; usual: 180-480 mg once daily; maximum: 540 mg once daily
Taztia XT® Tiazac®: Initial: 120-240 mg once daily; may increase dose after 14 days; maximum: 540 mg once daily

Capsule, extended release (twice-daily dosing): Initial: 60-120 mg twice daily; may increase dose after 14 days; usual: 240-360 mg/day
Note: Diltiazem is available as a generic intended for either once- or twice-daily dosing, depending on the formulation; verify appropriate extended release capsule formulation is administered.

Tablet, extended release: Cardizem® LA, Matzim® LA: Initial: 180-240 mg once daily; may increase dose after 14 days; limited clinical experience with doses >360 mg/day; maximum dose: 540 mg once daily; usual dosage range (JNC 7): 120-540 mg once daily
Tablet, immediate release: 30-120 mg 3-4 times/day; dosage should be increased gradually, at 1- to 2-day intervals until optimum response is obtained; usual maintenance dose: 180-360 mg/day

Angina: Adults: Oral:
Capsule, extended release:
Dilacor XR®, Dilt-XR, Diltia XT®: Initial: 120 mg once daily; titrate over 7-14 days; usual dose range: 120-320 mg/day; maximum: 480 mg/day
Cardizem® CD, Cartia XT®, Dilt-CD: Initial: 120-180 mg once daily; titrate over 7-14 days; usual dose range: 120-320 mg/day; maximum: 480 mg/day
Tiazac®, Taztia XT®: Initial: 120-180 mg once daily; titrate over 7-14 days; usual dose range: 120-320 mg/day; maximum: 540 mg/day
Tablet, extended release (Cardizem® LA, Matzim® LA): 180 mg once daily; may increase at 7- to 14-day intervals; usual dose range: 120-320 mg/day; maximum: 360 mg/day
Tablet, immediate release (Cardizem®): Usual starting dose: 30 mg 4 times/day; titrate dose gradually at 1- to 2-day intervals; usual dose range: 120-320 mg/day

Atrial fibrillation, atrial flutter, PSVT: Adults: I.V.:
Initial bolus dose: 0.25 mg/kg actual body weight over 2 minutes (average adult dose: 20 mg); ACLS guideline recommends 15-20 mg
Repeat bolus dose (may be administered after 15 minutes if the response is inadequate): 0.35 mg/kg actual body weight over 2 minutes (average adult dose: 25 mg); ACLS guideline recommends 20-25 mg
Continuous infusion (infusions >24 hours or infusion rates >15 mg/hour are not recommended): Initial infusion rate of 10 mg/hour; rate may be increased in 5 mg/hour increments up to 15 mg/hour as needed; some patients may respond to an initial rate of 5 mg/hour.
If diltiazem injection is administered by continuous infusion for >24 hours, the possibility of decreased diltiazem clearance, prolonged elimination half-life, and increased diltiazem and/or diltiazem metabolite plasma concentrations should be considered.

Conversion from I.V. diltiazem to oral diltiazem: Start first oral dose approximately 3 hours after bolus dose

Oral dose (mg/day) is approximately equal to [(rate in mg/hour x 3) + 3] x 10; Note: Dose per day may need to be divided depending on formulation used
3 mg/hour = 120 mg/day
5 mg/hour = 180 mg/day
7 mg/hour = 240 mg/day
11 mg/hour = 360 mg/day (maximum recommended dose)

Usual Infusion Concentrations: Pediatric I.V. infusion: 1 mg/mL

Administration

Oral:
Tablet, immediate release (Cardizem®): Administer before meals and at bedtime
Extended release preparations (CD, LA, XR, XT, Tiazac): Swallow whole; do not chew, break, or crush. Do not open Dilacor XR® capsules.
Dilacor XR®, Dilt-XR, Diltia XT®: Take in the morning on an empty stomach
Cardizem® CD, Cardizem® LA, Cartia XT®, Dilt-CD, Matzim® LA: May be administered with or without food, but should be administered consistently with relation to meals; administer with a full glass of water
Taztia XT® and Tiazac® capsules (extended release) may be opened and sprinkled on applesauce; swallow applesauce immediately, do not chew; follow with some cool water (adults: 1 glass) to ensure complete swallowing; do not use hot applesauce; do not divide capsule contents (ie, do not administer partial doses); do not store mixture of applesauce and capsule contents, use immediately
Parenteral:
I.V. bolus: Adults: Infuse over 2 minutes
I.V. continuous infusion: May dilute with NS, D_5W, or $D_5\frac{1}{2}NS$; maximum final concentration: 1 mg/mL

Monitoring Parameters Blood pressure, heart rate, renal function, liver enzymes; ECG with I.V. therapy

Additional Information Cartia XT® and Dilt CD are the generic versions of Cardizem® CD; Diltia XT® and Dilt-XR are the generic versions of Dilacor XR®; Taztia XT® is the generic version of Tiazac®; Matzim® LA is the generic version of Cardizem® LA.

Dosage Forms Excipient information presented when available (limited, particularly for generics); consult specific product labeling. [DSC] = Discontinued product
Capsule Extended Release 12 Hour, Oral, as hydrochloride:
Generic: 60 mg, 90 mg, 120 mg
Capsule Extended Release 24 Hour, Oral, as hydrochloride:
Cardizem CD: 120 mg, 180 mg, 240 mg, 300 mg, 360 mg [contains brilliant blue fcf (fd&c blue #1)]
Cartia XT: 120 mg, 180 mg, 240 mg, 300 mg

Dilacor XR: 240 mg [DSC]
Dilt-CD: 120 mg [DSC]
Dilt-CD: 180 mg [DSC], 240 mg [DSC] [contains brilliant blue fcf (fd&c blue #1)]
Dilt-CD: 300 mg [DSC]
Dilt-XR: 120 mg, 180 mg, 240 mg [contains brilliant blue fcf (fd&c blue #1), fd&c red #40, fd&c yellow #10 (quinoline yellow)]
Diltiazem HCl CD: 360 mg [contains brilliant blue fcf (fd&c blue #1)]
Diltzac: 120 mg [DSC] [contains brilliant blue fcf (fd&c blue #1)]
Diltzac: 180 mg [DSC]
Diltzac: 240 mg [DSC], 300 mg [DSC] [contains brilliant blue fcf (fd&c blue #1)]
Diltzac: 360 mg [DSC]
Taztia XT: 120 mg, 180 mg, 240 mg, 300 mg, 360 mg
Tiazac: 120 mg, 180 mg, 240 mg, 300 mg, 360 mg, 420 mg
Generic: 120 mg, 180 mg, 240 mg, 300 mg, 360 mg, 420 mg
Solution, Intravenous, as hydrochloride:
Generic: 25 mg/5 mL (5 mL); 50 mg/10 mL (10 mL); 125 mg/25 mL (25 mL)
Solution, Intravenous, as hydrochloride [preservative free]:
Generic: 50 mg/10 mL (10 mL); 125 mg/25 mL (25 mL)
Solution Reconstituted, Intravenous, as hydrochloride:
Generic: 100 mg (1 ea)
Tablet, Oral, as hydrochloride:
Cardizem: 30 mg
Cardizem: 30 mg [contains fd&c blue #1 aluminum lake, fd&c yellow #10 aluminum lake]
Cardizem: 60 mg [scored]
Cardizem: 60 mg [scored; contains fd&c blue #1 aluminum lake, fd&c yellow #10 aluminum lake, fd&c yellow #6 aluminum lake, methylparaben]
Cardizem: 90 mg [DSC] [scored]
Cardizem: 120 mg [scored; contains fd&c yellow #10 aluminum lake, fd&c yellow #6 aluminum lake, methylparaben]
Generic: 30 mg, 60 mg, 90 mg, 120 mg
Tablet Extended Release 24 Hour, Oral, as hydrochloride:
Cardizem LA: 120 mg, 180 mg, 240 mg, 300 mg, 360 mg, 420 mg
Matzim LA: 180 mg, 240 mg, 300 mg, 360 mg, 420 mg
Generic: 180 mg, 240 mg, 300 mg, 360 mg, 420 mg

Extemporaneous Preparations A 12 mg/mL oral suspension may be made from tablets (regular, not extended release) and one of three different vehicles (cherry syrup, a 1:1 mixture of Ora-Sweet® and Ora-Plus®, or a 1:1 mixture of Ora-Sweet® SF and Ora-Plus®). Crush sixteen 90 mg tablets in a mortar and reduce to a fine powder. Add 10 mL of the chosen vehicle and mix to a uniform paste; mix while adding the vehicle in incremental proportions to **almost** 120 mL; transfer to a calibrated bottle, rinse mortar with vehicle, and add quantity of vehicle sufficient to make 120 mL. Label "shake well" and "protect from light". Stable for 60 days when stored in amber plastic prescription bottles in the dark at room temperature or refrigerated.

Allen LV and Erickson MA, "Stability of Baclofen, Captopril, Diltiazem Hydrochloride, Dipyridamole, and Flecainide Acetate in Extemporaneously Compounded Oral Liquids," *Am J Health Syst Pharm*, 1996, 53(18):2179-84.

References

American College of Obstetricians and Gynecologists (ACOG), "ACOG Practice Bulletin No. 125: Chronic Hypertension in Pregnancy," *Obstet Gynecol*, 2012, 119(2 Pt 1):396-407.

Bertorini TE, Palmieri GMA, Griffin JW, et al, "Effect of Chronic Treatment With the Calcium Antagonist Diltiazem in Duchenne Muscular Dystrophy," *Neurology*, 1988, 38(4):609-13.

Chobanian AV, Bakris GL, Black HR, et al, "The Seventh Report of the Joint National Committee on Prevention, Detection, Evaluation, and Treatment of High Blood Pressure: The JNC 7 report," *JAMA*, 2003, 289(19):2560-72.

Field JM, Hazinski MF, Sayre MR, et al, "Part 1: Executive Summary: 2010 American Heart Association Guidelines for Cardiopulmonary Resuscitation and Emergency Cardiovascular Care," *Circulation*, 2010, 122(18 Suppl 3):640-56.

Flynn JT and Pasko DA, "Calcium Channel Blockers: Pharmacology and Place in Therapy of Pediatric Hypertension," *Pediatr Nephrol*, 2000, 15(3-4):302-16.

Fuster V, Ryden LE, Cannom DS, et al, "ACC/AHA/ESC 2006 Guidelines for the Management of Patients With Atrial Fibrillation-Executive Summary. A Report of the American College of Cardiology/American Heart Association Task Force on Practice Guidelines and the European Society of Cardiology Committee for Practice Guidelines (Writing Committee to Revise the 2001 Guidelines for the Management of Patients With Atrial Fibrillation). Developed in Collaboration With the European Heart Rhythm Association and the Heart Rhythm Society," *J Am Coll Cardiol*, 2006, 48(4):854-906.

Gersh BJ, Maron BJ, Bonow RO, et al, "2011 ACCF/AHA Guideline for the Diagnosis and Treatment of Hypertrophic Cardiomyopathy: A Report of the American College of Cardiology Foundation/American Heart Association Task Force on Practice Guidelines," *Circulation*, 2011, 124(24):e783-831.

Neumar RW, Otto CW, Link MS, et al, "Part 8: Adult Advanced Cardiovascular Life Support: 2010 American Heart Association Guidelines for Cardiopulmonary Resuscitation and Emergency Cardiovascular Care," *Circulation*, 2010, 122(18 Suppl 3):729-67.

Okada M, Inoue H, Nakamura Y, et al, "Excretion of Diltiazem in Human Milk," *N Engl J Med*, 1985, 312(15):992-3.

Pass RH, Liberman L, Al-Fayaddh M, et al, "Continuous Intravenous Diltiazem Infusion for Short-Term Ventricular Rate Control in Children," *Am J Cardiol*, 2000, 86(5):559-62, A9.

◆ **Diltiazem-CD (Can)** see Diltiazem on page 667

◆ **Diltiazem HCl CD** see Diltiazem on page 667

◆ **Diltiazem HCl ER (Can)** see Diltiazem on page 667

◆ **Diltiazem Hydrochloride** see Diltiazem on page 667

◆ **Diltiazem Hydrochloride Injection (Can)** see Diltiazem on page 667

◆ **Diltiazem TZ (Can)** see Diltiazem on page 667

◆ **Dilt-XR** see Diltiazem on page 667

◆ **Diltzac [DSC]** see Diltiazem on page 667

DimenhyDRINATE (dye men HYE dri nate)

Medication Safety Issues
Sound-alike/look-alike issues:
DimenhyDRINATE may be confused with diphenhydrAMINE

BEERS Criteria medication:
This drug may be potentially inappropriate for use in geriatric patients (Quality of evidence - varies based on comorbidity; Strength of recommendation - varies based on comorbidity)

Brand Names: U.S. Dramamine [OTC]; Driminate [OTC]; Motion Sickness [OTC]

Brand Names: Canada Apo-Dimenhydrinate® [OTC]; Children's Motion Sickness Liquid [OTC]; Dimenhydrinate Injection [OTC]; Dinate® [OTC]; Gravol IM; Gravol® [OTC]; Jamp-Dimenhydrinate [OTC]; Nauseatol [OTC]; Novo-Dimenate [OTC]; PMS-Dimenhydrinate [OTC]; Sandoz-Dimenhydrinate [OTC]; Travel Tabs [OTC]

Therapeutic Category Antiemetic; Antihistamine

Generic Availability (U.S.) May be product dependent

Use Treatment and prevention of nausea, vertigo, and vomiting associated with motion sickness (oral tablets: FDA approved in children ≥2 years and adults; I.V. product: FDA approved in infants, children, and adults)

Pregnancy Risk Factor B

Pregnancy Considerations Adverse events have not been observed in animal reproduction studies. The risk of fetal abnormalities was not increased following maternal use of dimenhydrinate during any trimester of pregnancy. Dimenhydrinate is recommended for the treatment of nausea and vomiting of pregnancy. Dimenhydrinate may have an oxytocic effect if used during labor.

Breast-Feeding Considerations Small amounts of dimenhydrinate are excreted into breast milk. Irritability in a breast-feeding infant was noted in one study. According to the manufacturer, the decision to continue or discontinue breast-feeding during therapy should take into account the risk of exposure to the infant and the benefits of treatment to the mother. Antihistamines may decrease maternal serum prolactin concentrations when administered prior to the establishment of nursing.

Contraindications Hypersensitivity to dimenhydrinate or any component, neonates (injection contains benzyl alcohol)

Warnings Chewable tablets contain tartrazine which may cause allergic reactions in susceptible individuals

Precautions Use with caution in patients with a history of seizure disorder; may produce excitation in the young child; use with caution in any condition which may be aggravated by anticholinergic symptoms such as prostatic hypertrophy, asthma, bladder neck obstruction, narrow-angle glaucoma, etc; chewable tablets contain aspartame which is metabolized to phenylalanine and must be used with caution in patients with phenylketonuria; use caution if used in conjunction with antibiotics that have the potential to cause ototoxicity (dimenhydrinate may mask symptoms of ototoxicity); do not inject intra-arterially; vials contain benzyl alcohol as a preservative; benzyl alcohol may cause allergic reactions in susceptible individuals; large amounts of benzyl alcohol (≥99 mg/kg/day) have been associated with a potentially fatal toxicity ("gasping syndrome") in neonates; the "gasping syndrome" consists of metabolic acidosis, respiratory distress, gasping respirations, CNS dysfunction (including convulsions, intracranial hemorrhage), hypotension, and cardiovascular collapse; avoid use of vials containing benzyl alcohol in neonates

Adverse Reactions
Cardiovascular: Tachycardia
Central nervous system: Dizziness, drowsiness, excitation, headache, insomnia, lassitude, nervousness, restlessness
Dermatologic: Rash
Gastrointestinal: Anorexia, epigastric distress, nausea, xerostomia
Genitourinary: Dysuria
Ocular: Blurred vision
Respiratory: Thickening of bronchial secretions

Drug Interactions
Metabolism/Transport Effects None known.
Avoid Concomitant Use
Avoid concomitant use of DimenhyDRINATE with any of the following: Aclidinium; Azelastine (Nasal); Ipratropium (Oral Inhalation); Paraldehyde; Potassium Chloride; Thalidomide; Tiotropium; Umeclidinium
Increased Effect/Toxicity
DimenhyDRINATE may increase the levels/effects of: AbobotulinumtoxinA; Alcohol (Ethyl); Analgesics (Opioid); Anticholinergic Agents; Azelastine (Nasal); Buprenorphine; Cannabinoid-Containing Products; CNS Depressants; Hydrocodone; Methotrimeprazine; Metyrosine; Mirabegron; Mirtazapine; OnabotulinumtoxinA; Paraldehyde; Potassium Chloride; Pramipexole; RimabotulinumtoxinB; ROPINIRole; Rotigotine; Selective Serotonin Reuptake Inhibitors; Thalidomide; Thiazide Diuretics; Tiotropium; Topiramate; Zolpidem

The levels/effects of DimenhyDRINATE may be increased by: Aclidinium; Brimonidine (Topical); Cannabis; Doxylamine; Dronabinol; Droperidol; HydrOXYzine; Ipratropium (Oral Inhalation); Kava Kava; Magnesium Sulfate; Methotrimeprazine; Nabilone; Perampanel; Pramlintide; Rufinamide; Sodium Oxybate; Tapentadol; Tetrahydrocannabinol; Umeclidinium

Decreased Effect
DimenhyDRINATE may decrease the levels/effects of: Acetylcholinesterase Inhibitors (Central); Benzylpenicilloyl Polylysine; Betahistine; Hyaluronidase; Secretin

The levels/effects of DimenhyDRINATE may be decreased by: Acetylcholinesterase Inhibitors (Central); Amphetamines

Mechanism of Action Competes with histamine for H_1-receptor sites on effector cells in the gastrointestinal tract, blood vessels, and respiratory tract; blocks chemoreceptor trigger zone, diminishes vestibular stimulation, and depresses labyrinthine function through its central anticholinergic activity

Pharmacodynamics
Onset of action: Oral: Within 15-30 minutes
Duration: ~3-6 hours

Pharmacokinetics (Adult data unless noted)
Absorption: Well absorbed from the GI tract
Metabolism: Extensive in the liver

Dosing: Usual
Children 2-5 years:
Oral:
12.5-25 mg every 6-8 hours; maximum dose: 75 mg/day
or
5 mg/kg/day or 150 mg/m²/day in 4 divided doses, not to exceed 75 mg/day
I.M.:
1.25 mg/kg
or
37.5 mg/m² 4 times/day; maximum: 75 mg/day
Children: 6-12 years:
Oral:
25-50 mg every 6-8 hours; maximum dose: 150 mg/day
or
5 mg/kg/day or 150 mg/m²/day in 4 divided doses, not to exceed 150 mg/day
I.M.:
1.25 mg /kg
or
37.5 mg/m² 4 times/day; maximum: 150 mg/day
Children ≥12 years and Adults:
Oral: 50-100 mg every 4-6 hours, not to exceed 400 mg/day
I.M., I.V.: 50-100 mg every 4 hours

Administration
Oral: Administer with food or water
Parenteral: Using the I.V. route in children is not recommended by the manufacturer; administer I.M. Do not inject intra-arterially. Must dilute each 50 mg in 10 mL of NS for I.V. administration.

Dosage Forms Excipient information presented when available (limited, particularly for generics); consult specific product labeling.
Solution, Injection:
Generic: 50 mg/mL (1 mL)
Tablet, Oral:
Dramamine: 50 mg
Dramamine: 50 mg [scored]
Driminate: 50 mg [scored]
Motion Sickness: 50 mg [scored]
Generic: 50 mg
Tablet Chewable, Oral:
Dramamine: 50 mg [contains aspartame, fd&c yellow #6 aluminum lake]
Dramamine: 50 mg [scored; contains aspartame, fd&c yellow #6 aluminum lake]

◆ **Dimenhydrinate Injection (Can)** *see* DimenhyDRINATE *on page 670*

Dimercaprol (dye mer KAP role)

Brand Names: U.S. Bal in Oil

Therapeutic Category Antidote, Arsenic Toxicity; Antidote, Gold Toxicity; Antidote, Lead Toxicity; Antidote, Mercury Toxicity; Chelating Agent, Parenteral

Generic Availability (U.S.) Yes

Use Antidote to gold, arsenic (except arsine), or acute mercury poisoning (except nonalkyl mercury); adjunct to edetate CALCIUM disodium in acute lead poisoning [FDA approved in pediatric patients (age not specified) and adults]

Pregnancy Risk Factor C

Pregnancy Considerations Animal reproduction studies have not been conducted. There are no adequate and well-controlled studies in pregnant women.

Lead poisoning: Lead is known to cross the placenta in amounts related to maternal plasma levels. Prenatal lead exposure may be associated with adverse events such as spontaneous abortion, preterm delivery, decreased birth weight, and impaired neurodevelopment. Some adverse outcomes may occur with maternal blood lead levels <10 mcg/dL. In addition, pregnant women exposed to lead may have an increased risk of gestational hypertension. Consider chelation therapy in pregnant women with confirmed blood lead levels ≥45 mcg/dL (pregnant women with blood lead levels ≥70 mcg/dL should be considered for chelation regardless of trimester); consultation with experts in lead poisoning and high-risk pregnancy is recommended. Encephalopathic pregnant women should be chelated regardless of trimester (CDC, 2010).

Breast-Feeding Considerations It is not known if dimercaprol is excreted in breast milk; however, it is not absorbed orally, which would limit the exposure to a nursing infant. When used for the treatment of lead poisoning, the amount of lead in breast milk may range from 0.6% to 3% of the maternal serum concentration. Women with confirmed blood lead levels ≥40 mcg/dL should not initiated breast-feeding; pumping and discarding breast milk is recommended until blood lead levels are <40 mcg/dL, at which point breast-feeding may resume (CDC, 2010). Calcium supplementation may reduce the amount of lead in breast milk.

Contraindications Hypersensitivity to dimercaprol; hepatic insufficiency (unless due to arsenic poisoning)

Warnings Product contains peanut oil; use with caution in patients with peanut allergy; medication for the treatment of hypersensitivity reactions should be available for immediate use. In children, fevers may occur; incidence is ~30%; may persist for the duration of therapy. Potentially a nephrotoxic drug; use with caution in patients with oliguria. Keep urine alkaline to protect the kidneys (prevents dimercaprol-metal complex breakdown). Discontinue or use with extreme caution if renal insufficiency develops during treatment. Hemodialysis may be used to remove dimercaprol-metal chelate in patients with renal dysfunction. May cause dose-dependent increases in blood pressure with tachycardia.

Precautions Use with caution in patients with glucose 6-phosphate dehydrogenase deficiency; may increase the risk of hemolytic anemia. When treating for lead poisoning, investigate, identify, and remove sources of lead exposure prior to treatment; do not permit patients to re-enter the contaminated environment until lead abatement has been completed. For heavy metal poisoning, primary care providers should consult experts in the chemotherapy of heavy metal toxicity before using chelation drug therapy. Not indicated for the treatment of iron, cadmium, or selenium poisoning; use in these patients may result in toxic dimercaprol-metal complexes.

Adverse Reactions

Cardiovascular: Chest pain, hypertension (dose related), tachycardia (dose related)

Central nervous system: Anxiety, fever, headache, nervousness

Dermatologic: Abscess

Gastrointestinal: Abdominal pain, burning sensation (lips, mouth, throat), nausea, salivation, throat irritation/pain, vomiting

Genitourinary: Burning sensation (penis)

Hematologic: Leukopenia (polymorphonuclear)

Local: Injection site pain

Neuromuscular & skeletal: Paresthesias (hand), weakness

Ocular: Blepharospasm, conjunctivitis, lacrimation

Renal: Acute renal insufficiency

Respiratory: Rhinorrhea, throat constriction

Miscellaneous: Diaphoresis

Drug Interactions

Metabolism/Transport Effects None known.

Avoid Concomitant Use

Avoid concomitant use of Dimercaprol with any of the following: Iron Salts; Multivitamins/Minerals (with ADEK, Folate, Iron)

Increased Effect/Toxicity

Dimercaprol may increase the levels/effects of: Iron Salts; Multivitamins/Minerals (with ADEK, Folate, Iron)

Decreased Effect There are no known significant interactions involving a decrease in effect.

Stability Store at 20°C to 25°C (68°F to 77°F); incompatible in same syringe with edetate CALCIUM sodium.

Mechanism of Action Sulfhydryl group combines with ions of various heavy metals to form relatively stable, nontoxic, soluble chelates which are excreted in urine

Pharmacokinetics (Adult data unless noted)

Absorption: I.M.: Rapid; Oral: Not absorbed

Distribution: To all tissues including the brain

Metabolism: Hepatic; rapid to inactive metabolites

Time to peak serum concentration: 30-60 minutes

Elimination: Urine and feces via bile

Dosing: Usual Infants, Children, Adolescents, and Adults:

Note: Premedication with a histamine H_1 antagonist (eg, diphenhydramine) is recommended.

Arsenic or gold poisoning (acute, mild): I.M.: 2.5 mg/kg/dose every 6 hours for 2 days, then every 12 hours on the third day, and once daily thereafter for 10 days

Arsenic or gold poisoning (acute, severe): I.M.: 3 mg/kg/dose every 4 hours for 2 days then every 6 hours on the third day, then every 12 hours thereafter for 10 days

Mercury poisoning (acute): I.M.: 5 mg/kg initially followed by 2.5 mg/kg/dose 1-2 times/day for 10 days

Lead poisoning: I.M.: **Note:** For the treatment of high blood lead levels in children, the CDC recommends chelation treatment when blood lead levels are >45 mcg/dL (CDC, 2002); however, dimercaprol is only recommended for use (in combination with edetate CALCIUM disodium) in children whose blood lead levels are >70 mcg/dL or in children with lead encephalopathy (AAP, 2005; Chandran, 2010). In adults, available guidelines recommend chelation therapy with blood lead levels >50 mcg/dL and significant symptoms; chelation therapy may also be indicated with blood lead levels ≥100 mcg/dL and/or symptoms (Kosnett, 2007).

Blood lead levels ≥70 mcg/dL, symptomatic lead poisoning, or lead encephalopathy (in conjunction with edetate CALCIUM disodium): 4 mg/kg/dose every 4 hours for 2-7 days; duration of therapy of at least 3 days is recommended by some experts (Chandran, 2010). **Note:** Begin treatment with edetate CALCIUM disodium with the second dimercaprol dose.

Dosing adjustment in renal impairment: There are no adjustments provided in manufacturer's labeling. Use with extreme caution or discontinue if acute renal insufficiency develops during therapy.

Dosing adjustment in hepatic impairment: Use is contraindicated in hepatic insufficiency (except in cases of postarsenical jaundice).

Administration Parenteral: Administer undiluted, **deep** I.M.; rotate injection sites. Keep urine alkaline to protect renal function. When used in the treatment of lead poisoning, administer in a separate site from edetate CALCIUM disodium

Monitoring Parameters Renal function, urine pH, infusion-related reactions

For lead poisoning: Blood lead levels (baseline and 7-21 days after completing chelation therapy); hemoglobin or hematocrit, iron status, free erythrocyte protoporphyrin, or zinc protoporphyrin; neurodevelopmental changes

For arsenic poisoning: Urine arsenic concentration

Test Interactions Iodine I^{131} thyroidal uptake values may be decreased

Dosage Forms Excipient information presented when available (limited, particularly for generics); consult specific product labeling.

Solution, Intramuscular:

Bal in Oil: 100 mg/mL (3 mL) [contains benzyl benzoate, peanut oil]

References

American Academy of Pediatrics Committee on Environmental Health, "Lead Exposure in Children: Prevention, Detection, and Management," *Pediatrics*, 2005, 116(4):1036-46.

Cantilena LR Jr and Klaassen CD, "The Effect of Chelating Agents on the Excretion of Endogenous Metals," *Toxicol Appl Pharmacol*, 1982, 63(3):344-50.

Centers for Disease Control and Prevention (CDC), "Guidelines For the Identification and Management of Lead Exposure in Pregnant and Lactating Women," Atlanta: CDC, 2010.

Centers for Disease Control and Prevention (CDC), "Interpreting and Managing Blood Lead Levels <10 microg/dL in Children and Reducing Childhood Exposures to Lead," *MMWR Recomm Rep*, 2007, 56 (RR-8):1-16.

Centers for Disease Control and Prevention (CDC), " Managing Elevated Blood Lead Levels Among Young Children: Recommendations From the Advisory Committee on Childhood Lead Poisoning Prevention," Atlanta: CDC, 2002.

Chandran L and Cataldo R, "Lead Poisoning: Basics and New Developments," *Pediatr Rev*, 2010, 31(10):399-405.

Gardella C, "Lead Exposure in Pregnancy: A Review of the Literature and Argument For Routine Prenatal Screening," *Obstet Gynecol Surv*, 2001, 56(4):231-8.

Kosnett MJ, "Chelation For Heavy Metals (Arsenic, Lead, and Mercury): Protective or Perilous?" *Clin Pharmacol Ther*, 2010, 88(3):412-5.

Kosnett MJ, "Unanswered Questions in Metal Chelation," *J Toxicol Clin Toxicol*, 1992, 30(4):529-47.

Kosnett MJ, Wedeen RP, Rothenberg SJ, et al, "Recommendations For Medical Management of Adult Lead Exposure," *Environ Health Perspect*, 2007, 115(3):463-71.

Shannon M, "Severe Lead Poisoning in Pregnancy," *Ambul Pediatr*, 2003, 3(1):37-9.

◆ **2,3-Dimercapto-1-Propanol** see Dimercaprol on page 672

◆ **2,3-Dimercaptopropan-1-Ol** see Dimercaprol on page 672

◆ **2,3-Dimercaptopropanol** see Dimercaprol on page 672

◆ **Dimethyl Triazeno Imidazole Carboxamide** see Dacarbazine on page 578

◆ **Dinate® [OTC] (Can)** see DimenhyDRINATE on page 670

◆ **Diocaine® (Can)** see Proparacaine on page 1755

◆ **Diocarpine (Can)** see Pilocarpine (Ophthalmic) on page 1675

◆ **Diochloram® (Can)** see Chloramphenicol on page 439

◆ **Diocto [OTC]** see Docusate on page 701

◆ **Dioctyl Calcium Sulfosuccinate** see Docusate on page 701

◆ **Dioctyl Sodium Sulfosuccinate** see Docusate on page 701

◆ **Diodex® (Can)** see Dexamethasone (Ophthalmic) on page 619

◆ **Diodoquin® (Can)** see Iodoquinol on page 1144

◆ **Diogent® (Can)** see Gentamicin (Ophthalmic) on page 966

◆ **Diomycin® (Can)** see Erythromycin (Ophthalmic) on page 784

◆ **Dionephrine® (Can)** see Phenylephrine (Ophthalmic) on page 1661

◆ **Diopentolate® (Can)** see Cyclopentolate on page 560

◆ **Dioptic's Atropine Solution (Can)** see Atropine on page 234

◆ **Dioptrol® (Can)** see Neomycin, Polymyxin B, and Dexamethasone on page 1484

◆ **Diosulf™ (Can)** see Sulfacetamide (Ophthalmic) on page 1943

◆ **Diotame [OTC]** see Bismuth on page 294

◆ **Diotrope® (Can)** see Tropicamide on page 2092

◆ **Diovan** see Valsartan on page 2108

◆ **Diovol® (Can)** see Aluminum Hydroxide and Magnesium Hydroxide on page 111

◆ **Diovol® Ex (Can)** see Aluminum Hydroxide and Magnesium Hydroxide on page 111

◆ **Dipentum** see Olsalazine on page 1532

◆ **Dipentum® (Can)** see Olsalazine on page 1532

◆ **Diphen [OTC]** see DiphenhydrAMINE (Systemic) on page 673

◆ **Diphenhist [OTC]** see DiphenhydrAMINE (Systemic) on page 673

DiphenhydrAMINE (Systemic)
(dye fen HYE dra meen)

Medication Safety Issues

Sound-alike/look-alike issues:

DiphenhydrAMINE may be confused with desipramine, dicyclomine, dimenhyDRINATE

Benadryl® may be confused with benazepril, Bentyl®, Benylin®, Caladryl®

BEERS Criteria medication:

This drug may be potentially inappropriate for use in geriatric patients (Quality of evidence - moderate; Strength of recommendation - strong).

International issues:

Benadryl brand name for diphenhydramine [U.S., Canada], but also the brand name for cetirizine [Great Britain, Phillipines] and acrivastine and pseudoephedrine [Great Britain]

Sominex brand name for diphenhydramine [U.S., Canada], but also the brand name for promethazine [Great Britain]; valerian [Chile]

Brand Names: U.S. Aler-Dryl [OTC]; Allergy Relief Childrens [OTC]; Allergy Relief [OTC]; Altaryl [OTC]; Anti-Hist Allergy [OTC]; Banophen [OTC]; Benadryl Allergy Childrens [OTC]; Benadryl Allergy [OTC]; Benadryl Dye-Free Allergy [OTC]; Benadryl [OTC]; Complete Allergy Medication [OTC]; Complete Allergy Relief [OTC]; Diphen [OTC]; Diphenhist [OTC]; Genahist [OTC]; Geri-Dryl [OTC]; Nighttime Sleep Aid [OTC]; Nytol Maximum Strength [OTC]; Nytol [OTC]; PediaCare Childrens Allergy [OTC]; Pharbedryl [OTC]; Q-Dryl [OTC]; Quenalin [OTC]; Scot-Tussin Allergy Relief [OTC]; Siladryl Allergy [OTC]; Silphen Cough [OTC]; Simply Allergy [OTC]; Simply Sleep [OTC]; Sleep Tabs [OTC]; Sominex Maximum Strength [OTC]; Sominex [OTC]; Tetra-Formula Nighttime Sleep [OTC]; Total Allergy

Medicine [OTC]; Total Allergy [OTC]; Triaminic Cough/Runny Nose [OTC]; ZzzQuil [OTC]

Brand Names: Canada Allerdryl®; Allernix; Benadryl®; Nytol®; Nytol® Extra Strength; PMS-Diphenhydramine; Simply Sleep®; Sominex®

Therapeutic Category Antidote, Drug-induced Dystonic Reactions; Antidote, Hypersensitivity Reactions; Antihistamine; Sedative

Generic Availability (U.S.) May be product dependent

Use

Prescription products:

Oral (Liquid: 12.5 mg per 5 mL): Treatment of allergic reactions caused by histamine release, adjunct to epinephrine in anaphylaxis after acute symptoms have been controlled, relief of other uncomplicated acute allergic conditions including urticaria and angioedema, treatment and prophylaxis of motion sickness, management of Parkinsonian syndrome including drug-induced extrapyramidal symptoms (dystonic reactions) alone or in combination with centrally acting anticholinergic agents, treatment of allergic conjunctivitis, and dermatographism (FDA approved in ages ≥28 days and adults); treatment of occasional insomnia (FDA approved in ages ≥12 years and adults)

Parenteral: Treatment of allergic reactions caused by histamine release; adjunct to epinephrine in anaphylaxis after acute symptoms have been controlled; relief of other uncomplicated acute allergic conditions including urticaria and angioedema; treatment of motion sickness; management of Parkinsonian syndrome including drug-induced extrapyramidal symptoms (dystonic reactions) alone or in combination with centrally acting anticholinergic agents (All indications: FDA approved in ages ≥28 days and adults)

OTC products: Relief of symptoms of hay fever or other respiratory allergies [OTC products: Capsules, tablets, liquid (12.5 mg per 5 mL): FDA approved in ages ≥6 years and adults]; relief of symptoms of common cold (OTC products: Capsules and tablets: FDA approved in ages ≥6 years and adults); treatment of occasional insomnia [OTC products: Capsules, liquid (50 mg per 30 mL): FDA approved in ages ≥12 years and adults].

Note: Approved uses for generic products may vary; consult labeling for specific information.

Pregnancy Risk Factor B

Pregnancy Considerations Adverse events have not been observed in animal reproduction studies. Diphenhydramine crosses the placenta. Maternal diphenhydramine use has generally not resulted in an increased risk of birth defects; however, adverse events (withdrawal symptoms, respiratory depression) have been reported in newborns exposed to diphenhydramine *in utero*. Antihistamines are recommended for the treatment of rhinitis, urticaria, and pruritus with rash in pregnant women (although second generation antihistamines may be preferred). Antihistamines are not recommended for treatment of pruritus associated with intrahepatic cholestasis in pregnancy.

Breast-Feeding Considerations Diphenhydramine is excreted into breast milk; drowsiness has been reported in a breast-feeding infant. Premature infants and newborns have a higher risk of intolerance to antihistamines. Breast-feeding is contraindicated by the manufacturer. Antihistamines may decrease maternal serum prolactin concentrations when administered prior to the establishment of nursing.

Contraindications Hypersensitivity to diphenhydramine, other structurally similar antihistamines, or any component; neonates or premature infants; breast-feeding (infants may be more sensitive to the effects of antihistamines)

Additional contraindications: Parenteral: Use as a local anesthetic

OTC labeling: When used for self-medication (OTC), do not use with any other diphenhydramine-containing products including topical products; oral solution (12.5 mg per 5 mL) to make children sleepy

Warnings Safety and efficacy for the use of cough and cold products in children <2 years of age is limited. Serious adverse effects, including death, have been reported. The FDA notes that there are no approved OTC uses for these products in children <2 years of age. Healthcare providers are reminded to ask caregivers about the use of OTC cough and cold products in order to avoid exposure to multiple medications containing the same ingredient.

Diphenhydramine may cause drowsiness; alcohol, sedatives, and tranquilizers may increase this effect; patients must be cautioned about performing tasks which require mental alertness (eg, operating machinery or driving). Antihistamines may cause paradoxical excitation in young children. Toxicity (overdosage) in pediatric patients can result in hallucinations, convulsions, or death. Neonates and infants are highly sensitive to depressive effects of diphenhydramine; use is contraindicated in neonates (premature and term); use with extreme caution in infants and young children.

Subcutaneous or intradermal use has been associated with tissue necrosis; should be administered I.V. or I.M. only.

Some products may contain propylene glycol; toxicities have been reported with use of products containing propylene glycol, including hyperosmolality, lactic acidosis, seizures, and respiratory depression; in neonates, large amounts of propylene glycol delivered orally, intravenously (eg, >3000 mg/day), or topically have been associated with potentially fatal toxicities which can include metabolic acidosis, seizures, renal failure, and CNS depression; use liquids containing propylene glycol with caution (AAP, 1997; Shehab, 2009). Some products contain polysorbate 80 (Tween 80) which may cause allergic reactions in susceptible individuals. Some oral liquids contain alcohol (14% for some products) and some contain sodium benzoate; benzoic acid (benzoate) is a metabolite of benzyl alcohol; large amounts of benzyl alcohol (≥99 mg/kg/day) have been associated with a potentially fatal toxicity ("gasping syndrome") in neonates. Some products contain soy protein; avoid use in patients with soy allergy. Some products may contain aspartame; use with caution in phenylketonuric patients. Consult detailed product-specific labeling for additional information.

Oral solutions are available in two concentrations [ie, 12.5 mg/5 mL and 50 mg/30 mL (eg, ZzzQuil)]; precautions should be taken to verify and avoid confusion between the different concentrations; dose should be clearly presented as "mg"; the 50 mg/30 mL oral solution is indicated for the occasional treatment of insomnia.

Precautions Use with caution in patients with narrow angle glaucoma, increased intraocular pressure, asthma or a history of asthma, stenosing peptic ulcer, symptomatic prostatic hyperplasia, bladder neck obstruction, pyloroduodenal obstruction, cardiovascular disease including hypertension and ischemic heart disease, or thyroid dysfunction due to potential for anticholinergic effects.

Adverse Reactions

Cardiovascular: Chest tightness, extrasystoles, hypotension, palpitation, tachycardia

Central nervous system: Chills, confusion, convulsion, disturbed coordination, dizziness, euphoria, excitation, fatigue, headache, insomnia, irritability, nervousness, paradoxical excitement, restlessness, sedation, sleepiness, vertigo

Endocrine & metabolic: Menstrual irregularities (early menses)

Gastrointestinal: Anorexia, constipation, diarrhea, dry mucous membranes, epigastric distress, nausea, throat tightness, vomiting, xerostomia

Genitourinary: Difficult urination, urinary frequency, urinary retention

Hematologic: Agranulocytosis, hemolytic anemia, thrombocytopenia

Neuromuscular & skeletal: Neuritis, paresthesia, tremor

Ocular: Blurred vision, diplopia

Otic: Labyrinthitis (acute), tinnitus

Respiratory: Nasal stuffiness, thickening of bronchial secretions, wheezing

Miscellaneous: Anaphylactic shock, diaphoresis

Drug Interactions

Metabolism/Transport Effects Inhibits CYP2D6 (moderate)

Avoid Concomitant Use

Avoid concomitant use of DiphenhydrAMINE (Systemic) with any of the following: Aclidinium; Azelastine (Nasal); Ipratropium (Oral Inhalation); Paraldehyde; Potassium Chloride; Thalidomide; Thioridazine; Tiotropium; Umeclidinium

Increased Effect/Toxicity

DiphenhydrAMINE (Systemic) may increase the levels/effects of: AbobotulinumtoxinA; Alcohol (Ethyl); Analgesics (Opioid); Anticholinergic Agents; ARIPiprazole; Azelastine (Nasal); Buprenorphine; Cannabinoid-Containing Products; CNS Depressants; CYP2D6 Substrates; DOXOrubicin (Conventional); Fesoterodine; Highest Risk QTc-Prolonging Agents; Hydrocodone; Methotrimeprazine; Metoprolol; Metyrosine; Mirabegron; Mirtazapine; Moderate Risk QTc-Prolonging Agents; Nebivolol; OnabotulinumtoxinA; Paraldehyde; Potassium Chloride; Pramipexole; RimabotulinumtoxinB; ROPINIRole; Rotigotine; Selective Serotonin Reuptake Inhibitors; Thalidomide; Thiazide Diuretics; Thioridazine; Tiotropium; Topiramate; Zolpidem

The levels/effects of DiphenhydrAMINE (Systemic) may be increased by: Aclidinium; Brimonidine (Topical); Cannabis; Doxylamine; Dronabinol; Droperidol; HydrOXYzine; Ipratropium (Oral Inhalation); Kava Kava; Magnesium Sulfate; Methotrimeprazine; Mifepristone; Nabilone; Perampanel; Pramlintide; Propafenone; Rufinamide; Sodium Oxybate; Tapentadol; Tetrahydrocannabinol; Umeclidinium

Decreased Effect

DiphenhydrAMINE (Systemic) may decrease the levels/effects of: Acetylcholinesterase Inhibitors (Central); Benzylpenicilloyl Polylysine; Betahistine; Codeine; Hyaluronidase; Secretin; Tamoxifen; TraMADol

The levels/effects of DiphenhydrAMINE (Systemic) may be decreased by: Acetylcholinesterase Inhibitors (Central); Amphetamines

Stability

Injection: Store at 15°C to 30°C (59°F to 86°F); protect from freezing. Protect from light.

Oral: Store at room temperature; protect from light. Protect capsules and tablets from moisture. Consult product-specific labeling for details.

Mechanism of Action Competes with histamine for H_1-receptor sites on effector cells in the gastrointestinal tract, blood vessels, and respiratory tract; anticholinergic and sedative effects are also seen

Pharmacodynamics

Maximum sedative effect: 1-3 hours after administration

Duration: 4-7 hours

Pharmacokinetics (Adult data unless noted)

Absorption: Oral: Well-absorbed but 40% to 60% of an oral dose reaches the systemic circulation due to first-pass metabolism

Distribution: V_d: 3-22 L/kg

Protein-binding: 78%

Metabolism: Extensive hepatic n-demethylation via CYP2D6; minor demethylation via CYP1A2, 2C9, and 2C19; significant first-pass effect

Bioavailability: ~40% to 70%

Half-life: 2-8 hours

Time to peak serum concentration: 2-4 hours

Elimination: Urine (as unchanged drug)

Dosing: Usual Note: Oral solutions are available in two concentrations [ie, 12.5 mg/5 mL and 50 mg/30 mL (eg, ZzzQuil)]; precautions should be taken to verify and avoid confusion between the different concentrations; dose should be clearly presented as "mg;" the 50 mg/30 mL oral solution is indicated for the occasional treatment of insomnia.

Pediatric:

Allergies; hay fever: Infants, Children, and Adolescents: Oral:

Weight-directed dosing: 5 mg/kg/day divided into 3-4 doses; maximum daily dose: 300 mg/day; age-related maximum daily doses may also be considered: <6 years: 37.5 mg/day; 6-11 years: 150 mg/day; ≥12 years: 300 mg/day

Fixed dosing:

Children 2 to <6 years: Limited data available: 6.25 mg every 4-6 hours; maximum daily dose: 37.5 mg/day (Kliegman, 2011)

Children 6 to <12 years: 12.5-25 mg every 4-6 hours; maximum daily dose: 150 mg/day

Children ≥12 years and Adolescents: 25-50 mg every 4-6 hours; maximum daily dose: 300 mg/day

Allergic reaction (severe)/anaphylaxis (adjunct to epinephrine): Infants, Children, and Adolescents:

Manufacturer's labeling: I.V., I.M., Oral: 1.25 mg/kg/dose given every 6 hours; maximum daily dose: 300 mg/day

Alternate dosing: I.V., I.M., Oral: 1-2 mg/kg/dose; maximum single dose: 50 mg/**dose** (Hegenbarth, 2008; Kliegman, 2011; Liberman, 2008; Lieberman, 2010; Simons, 2011)

Rhinitis, sneezing due to common cold: Oral:

Children 6 to <12 years: 25 mg every 4-6 hours; maximum daily dose: 150 mg/day

Children ≥12 years and Adolescents: 25-50 mg every 4-6 hours; maximum daily dose: 300 mg/day

Dystonic reactions: Infants, Children, and Adolescents: I.V., I. M.: 1-2 mg/kg/dose; maximum single dose: 50 mg (Hegenbarth, 2008; Kliegman, 2011); may repeat in 20-30 minutes if necessary

Motion sickness: Infants, Children, and Adolescents: Prophylaxis: Oral:

Manufacturer's labeling: First dose should be administered 30 minutes before travel.

Weight-directed dosing: 5 mg/kg/day divided into 3-4 doses; maximum daily dose: 300 mg/day

Fixed dosing: 12.5-25 mg 3-4 times daily

Alternate dosing: Children 2-12 years: Limited data available: 0.5-1 mg/kg/dose every 6 hours; maximum single dose: 25 mg. First dose should be administered 1 hour before travel (CDC, 2014).

Treatment:

I.V., I.M.: 1.25 mg/kg/dose every 6 hours; maximum daily dose: 300 mg/day

Oral:

Weight-directed dosing: 5 mg/kg/day divided into 3-4 doses; maximum daily dose: 300 mg/day

Fixed dosing: 12.5-25 mg 3-4 times daily

Insomnia; occasional: Oral:

Children 2-12 years, weighing 10-50 kg: Limited data available: 1 mg/kg administered 30 minutes before bedtime; maximum single dose: 50 mg (Russo, 1976)

Children ≥12 years and Adolescents: 50 mg administered 30 minutes before bedtime

◄

Pruritis (opioid-induced): Limited data available: Infants, Children, and Adolescents: I.M., I.V., Oral: 0.5-1 mg/kg/dose every 6 hours; maximum daily dose: 100/day (Kliegman, 2011)

Urticaria: Infants, Children, and Adolescents: Oral: Weight-directed dosing: 5 mg/kg/day divided into 3-4 doses; maximum daily dose: 300 mg/day
Fixed dosing: 12.5-25 mg 3-4 times daily

Adult:

Allergic reactions:
Oral: 25-50 mg every 6-8 hours
I.M., I.V.: 10-50 mg per dose; single doses up to 100 mg may be used if needed; not to exceed 400 mg/day

Antitussive: Oral: 25 mg every 4 hours; maximum: 150 mg/24 hours

Motion sickness:
Oral: 25-50 mg every 6-8 hours
I.M., I.V.: 10-50 mg per dose; single doses up to 100 mg may be used if needed; not to exceed 400 mg/day

Insomnia; occasional: Oral: 50 mg at bedtime

Dystonic reactions: I.M., I.V.: 50 mg in a single dose; may repeat in 20-30 minutes if necessary

Administration

Oral: May administer without regards to meals; when used to prevent motion sickness, first dose should be given 30-60 minutes prior to exposure

Parenteral:
I.V.: Dilute with compatible I.V. fluid to a maximum concentration of 25 mg/mL and infuse over 10-15 minutes (maximum rate of infusion: 25 mg/minute)
I.M.: 50 mg/mL concentration by deep I.M. injection

Test Interactions May interfere with urine detection of methadone and phencyclidine (false-positives); may cause false-positive serum TCA screen; may suppress the wheal and flare reactions to skin test antigens

Dosage Forms Excipient information presented when available (limited, particularly for generics); consult specific product labeling.

Capsule, Oral, as hydrochloride:
Allergy Relief: 25 mg [contains brilliant blue fcf (fd&c blue #1), butylparaben, edetate calcium disodium, fd&c blue #2 (indigotine), fd&c red #40, fd&c yellow #10 (quinoline yellow), methylparaben, polysorbate 80, propylparaben]
Banophen: 25 mg [contains brilliant blue fcf (fd&c blue #1), fd&c red #40, fd&c yellow #6 (sunset yellow), methylparaben, propylparaben]
Banophen: 50 mg [contains brilliant blue fcf (fd&c blue #1), fd&c red #40]
Benadryl: 25 mg
Benadryl Allergy: 25 mg [dye free]
Benadryl Dye-Free Allergy: 25 mg [dye free]
Diphenhist: 25 mg [contains brilliant blue fcf (fd&c blue #1), butylparaben, fd&c red #40, methylparaben, propylparaben]
Genahist: 25 mg
Geri-Dryl: 25 mg
Pharbedryl: 25 mg, 50 mg [contains brilliant blue fcf (fd&c blue #1), fd&c red #40]
Q-Dryl: 25 mg [contains brilliant blue fcf (fd&c blue #1), butylparaben, fd&c red #40, methylparaben, propylparaben]
ZzzQuil: 25 mg [contains brilliant blue fcf (fd&c blue #1), fd&c red #40]
Generic: 25 mg, 50 mg

Elixir, Oral, as hydrochloride:
Altaryl: 12.5 mg/5 mL (120 mL, 480 mL, 3840 mL) [contains alcohol, usp]
Generic: 12.5 mg/5 mL (5 mL, 10 mL)

Liquid, Oral, as hydrochloride:
Allergy Relief Childrens: 12.5 mg/5 mL (118 mL, 480 mL) [alcohol free; contains fd&c red #40, sodium benzoate]

Banophen: 12.5 mg/5 mL (118 mL) [alcohol free; cherry flavor]
Banophen: 12.5 mg/5 mL (473 mL) [alcohol free, sugar free; cherry flavor]
Benadryl Allergy Childrens: 12.5 mg/5 mL (118 mL, 236 mL) [alcohol free; contains fd&c red #40, sodium benzoate]
Benadryl Allergy Childrens: 12.5 mg/5 mL (5 mL, 236 mL) [alcohol free; contains fd&c red #40, sodium benzoate; cherry flavor]
Benadryl Allergy Childrens: 12.5 mg/5 mL (118 mL) [alcohol free, dye free, sugar free; contains saccharin sodium, sodium benzoate]
Diphenhist: 12.5 mg/5 mL (118 mL, 473 mL) [alcohol free; contains fd&c red #40, saccharin sodium, sodium benzoate; fruit flavor]
PediaCare Childrens Allergy: 12.5 mg/5 mL (118 mL) [alcohol free; contains fd&c red #40, sodium benzoate]
Q-Dryl: 12.5 mg/5 mL (118 mL, 237 mL, 473 mL) [alcohol free; contains fd&c red #40, saccharin sodium, sodium benzoate; cherry flavor]
Scot-Tussin Allergy Relief: 12.5 mg/5 mL (118.3 mL, 240 mL, 480 mL, 3780 mL) [alcohol free, dye free, saccharin free, sodium free, sorbitol free, sugar free]
Siladryl Allergy: 12.5 mg/5 mL (118 mL, 237 mL, 473 mL) [alcohol free, sugar free; contains fd&c red #40, methylparaben, propylene glycol, propylparaben, saccharin sodium; cherry flavor]
Total Allergy Medicine: 12.5 mg/5 mL (118 mL) [alcohol free]
ZzzQuil: 50 mg/30 mL (177 mL, 354 mL) [contains alcohol, usp, brilliant blue fcf (fd&c blue #1), fd&c red #40, propylene glycol, saccharin sodium, sodium benzoate; berry flavor]

Solution, Injection, as hydrochloride:
Generic: 50 mg/mL (1 mL, 10 mL)

Solution, Injection, as hydrochloride [preservative free]:
Generic: 50 mg/mL (1 mL)

Strip, Oral, as hydrochloride:
Triaminic Cough/Runny Nose: 12.5 mg (14 ea) [contains alcohol, usp, brilliant blue fcf (fd&c blue #1), fd&c red #40]
Triaminic Cough/Runny Nose: 12.5 mg (16 ea) [contains alcohol, usp, brilliant blue fcf (fd&c blue #1), fd&c red #40; grape flavor]

Syrup, Oral, as hydrochloride:
Altaryl: 12.5 mg/5 mL (120 mL, 480 mL, 3785 mL) [alcohol free; cherry flavor]
Quenalin: 12.5 mg/5 mL (120 mL) [fruit flavor]
Silphen Cough: 12.5 mg/5 mL (118 mL, 237 mL, 473 mL) [contains alcohol, usp, fd&c red #40, menthol, methylparaben, propylene glycol, propylparaben; strawberry flavor]

Tablet, Oral, as hydrochloride:
Aler-Dryl: 50 mg
Allergy Relief: 25 mg [contains polysorbate 80]
Anti-Hist Allergy: 25 mg
Banophen: 25 mg
Benadryl: 25 mg
Benadryl Allergy: 25 mg
Benadryl Allergy: 25 mg [contains edetate calcium disodium, fd&c red #40, methylparaben, polysorbate 80, propylparaben]
Complete Allergy Medication: 25 mg
Complete Allergy Relief: 25 mg
Diphen: 25 mg
Diphenhist: 25 mg
Geri-Dryl: 25 mg
Nighttime Sleep Aid: 25 mg [contains fd&c blue #1 aluminum lake, fd&c blue #2 aluminum lake, polysorbate 80]
Nighttime Sleep Aid: 50 mg [contains fd&c blue #1 aluminum lake]

Nytol: 25 mg

Nytol Maximum Strength: 50 mg

Simply Allergy: 25 mg

Simply Sleep: 25 mg [contains brilliant blue fcf (fd&c blue #1)]

Sleep Tabs: 25 mg [scored; contains fd&c blue #1 aluminum lake]

Sominex: 25 mg [contains fd&c blue #1 aluminum lake]

Sominex Maximum Strength: 50 mg [contains fd&c blue #1 aluminum lake, polysorbate 80]

Tetra-Formula Nighttime Sleep: 50 mg [contains fd&c blue #1 aluminum lake]

Total Allergy: 25 mg

Generic: 25 mg

Tablet Chewable, Oral, as hydrochloride:

Benadryl Allergy Childrens: 12.5 mg [contains aspartame, fd&c blue #1 aluminum lake; cherry flavor]

Benadryl Allergy Childrens: 12.5 mg [contains aspartame, fd&c blue #1 aluminum lake; grape flavor]

References

Centers for Disease Control and Prevention (CDC). *CDC Health Information for International Travel 2014.* New York: Oxford University Press; 2014; Chapter 2. http://wwwnc.cdc.gov/travel/page/yellow-book-home-2014

Hegenbarth MA, American Academy of Pediatrics Committee on Drugs. Preparing for pediatric emergencies: drugs to consider. *Pediatrics.* 2008; 121(2):433-443.

Kliegman RM, Stanton BF, St. Gemell JW, et al, eds. *Nelson Textbook of Pediatrics.* 19th ed. Philadelphia, PA: Saunders Elsevier;2011.

Liberman DB, Teach SJ. Management of anaphylaxis in children. *Pediatr Emerg Care.* 2008;24:861-869.

Lieberman P, Nicklas RA, Oppenheimer J, et al. The diagnosis and management of anaphylaxis practice parameter: 2010 update. *J Allergy Clin Immunol.* 2010;126(3):477-480.

Russo RM, Guraraj VJ, Allen JE. The effectiveness of diphenhydramine HCl in pediatric sleep disorders. *J Clin Pharmacol.* 1976;16: 284-288.

Simons FE, Ardusso LR, Bilo MB, et al. World allergy organization guidelines for the assessment and management of anaphylaxis. *World Allergy Organ J.* 2011;4:13-37.

DiphenhydrAMINE (Topical)
(dye fen HYE dra meen)

Medication Safety Issues

Sound-alike/look-alike issues:

DiphenhydrAMINE may be confused with desipramine, dicyclomine, dimenhyDRINATE

Benadryl® may be confused with benazepril, Bentyl®, Benylin®, Caladryl®

Administration issues:

Institute for Safe Medication Practices (ISMP) has reported cases of patients mistakenly *swallowing* Benadryl® Itch Stopping [OTC] gel intended for topical application. Unclear labeling and similar packaging of the topical gel in containers resembling an oral liquid are factors believed to be contributing to the administration errors. The topical gel contains camphor which can be toxic if swallowed. ISMP has requested the manufacturer to make the necessary changes to prevent further confusion.

Brand Names: U.S. Anti-Itch Maximum Strength [OTC]; Anti-Itch [OTC]; Banophen [OTC]; Benadryl Itch Relief [OTC]; Benadryl Itch Stopping [OTC]; Benadryl Maximum Strength [OTC]; Itch Relief [OTC]

Brand Names: Canada Benadryl® Cream; Benadryl® Itch Relief Stick; Benadryl® Spray

Therapeutic Category Antihistamine

Generic Availability (U.S.) May be product dependent

Use Relief of pain and itching associated with insect bites, minor cuts and burns, or rashes

Pregnancy Considerations When administered orally, diphenhydramine crosses the placenta. Diphenhydramine can also be measurable in the serum following topical administration to large areas of the body. Refer to the Diphenhydramine (Systemic) monograph.

Breast-Feeding Considerations When administered orally, diphenhydramine can be detected in breast milk. Diphenhydramine can also be measurable in the serum following topical administration to large areas of the body. Refer to the Diphenhydramine (Systemic) monograph.

Contraindications Hypersensitivity to diphenhydramine or any component; breast-feeding (infants may be more sensitive to the effects of antihistamines)

Warnings Should not be used to treat chickenpox, poison ivy, or sunburn; on large areas of the body; or on blistered or oozing skin, due to potential for causing toxic psychosis, particularly in children.

Adverse Reactions Dermatologic: Photosensitivity, rash, urticaria

Drug Interactions

Metabolism/Transport Effects None known.

Avoid Concomitant Use

Avoid concomitant use of DiphenhydrAMINE (Topical) with any of the following: Aclidinium; Azelastine (Nasal); Ipratropium (Oral Inhalation); Paraldehyde; Potassium Chloride; Thalidomide; Tiotropium; Umeclidinium

Increased Effect/Toxicity

DiphenhydrAMINE (Topical) may increase the levels/effects of: AbobotulinumtoxinA; Alcohol (Ethyl); Analgesics (Opioid); Anticholinergic Agents; Azelastine (Nasal); Buprenorphine; Cannabinoid-Containing Products; CNS Depressants; Hydrocodone; Methotrimeprazine; Metyrosine; Mirabegron; Mirtazapine; OnabotulinumtoxinA; Paraldehyde; Potassium Chloride; Pramipexole; RimabotulinumtoxinB; ROPINIRole; Rotigotine; Selective Serotonin Reuptake Inhibitors; Thalidomide; Thiazide Diuretics; Tiotropium; Topiramate; Zolpidem

The levels/effects of DiphenhydrAMINE (Topical) may be increased by: Aclidinium; Brimonidine (Topical); Cannabis; Doxylamine; Dronabinol; Droperidol; HydrOXYzine; Ipratropium (Oral Inhalation); Kava Kava; Magnesium Sulfate; Methotrimeprazine; Nabilone; Perampanel; Pramlintide; Rufinamide; Sodium Oxybate; Tapentadol; Tetrahydrocannabinol; Umeclidinium

Decreased Effect

DiphenhydrAMINE (Topical) may decrease the levels/effects of: Acetylcholinesterase Inhibitors (Central); Benzylpenicilloyl Polylysine; Betahistine; Hyaluronidase; Secretin

The levels/effects of DiphenhydrAMINE (Topical) may be decreased by: Acetylcholinesterase Inhibitors (Central); Amphetamines

Dosing: Usual Topical cream, gel, spray, or stick:

Children ≥2 to 12 years: Apply 1% concentration not more than 3-4 times/day

Children ≥12 years and Adults: Apply 1% or 2% concentration not more than 3-4 times/day

Administration Shake well (gel); apply thin coat to affected area

Test Interactions May suppress the wheal and flare reactions to skin test antigens

Dosage Forms Excipient information presented when available (limited, particularly for generics); consult specific product labeling.

Cream, External, as hydrochloride:

Anti-Itch: 2% (28.4 g) [contains cetyl alcohol, methylparaben, propylene glycol, propylparaben]

Anti-Itch: 2% (28.4 g) [contains methylparaben, propylparaben]

Anti-Itch Maximum Strength: 2% (30 g)

Banophen: 2% (28 g) [contains cetyl alcohol, methylparaben, propylene glycol, propylparaben]

Benadryl Itch Stopping: 1% (28.3 g) [contains cetyl alcohol]

Itch Relief: 2% (15 g, 30 g, 56.8 g)

Gel, External, as hydrochloride:
Benadryl Itch Stopping: 2% (118 mL) [contains alcohol, usp, methylparaben, propylparaben]
Solution, External, as hydrochloride:
Benadryl Maximum Strength: 2% (60 mL) [contains alcohol, usp]
Stick, External, as hydrochloride:
Benadryl Itch Relief: 2% (14 mL) [contains alcohol, usp]

◆ **Diphenhydramine Citrate** see DiphenhydrAMINE (Systemic) on page 673

◆ **Diphenhydramine Hydrochloride** see DiphenhydrAMINE (Systemic) on page 673

◆ **Diphenhydramine Hydrochloride** see DiphenhydrAMINE (Topical) on page 677

◆ **Diphenhydramine Tannate** see DiphenhydrAMINE (Systemic) on page 673

Diphenoxylate and Atropine
(dye fen OKS i late & A troe peen)

Medication Safety Issues
Sound-alike/look-alike issues:
Lomotil® may be confused with LaMICtal®, LamISIL®, lamoTRIgine, Lanoxin®, Lasix®, loperamide
International issues:
Lomotil [U.S., Canada, and multiple international markets] may be confused with Ludiomil brand name for maprotiline [multiple international markets]
Lomotil: Brand name for diphenoxylate [U.S., Canada, and multiple international markets], but also the brand name for loperamide [Mexico, Philippines]
Brand Names: U.S. Lomotil®
Brand Names: Canada Lomotil®
Therapeutic Category Antidiarrheal
Generic Availability (U.S.) Yes
Use Treatment of diarrhea
Pregnancy Risk Factor C
Pregnancy Considerations Teratogenic effects were not noted in animal studies; decreased maternal weight, fertility and litter sizes were observed. There are no adequate and well-controlled studies in pregnant women.
Breast-Feeding Considerations Atropine is excreted in breast milk (refer to Atropine monograph); the manufacturer states that diphenoxylic acid may be excreted in breast milk.
Contraindications Hypersensitivity to diphenoxylate, atropine, or any component; severe liver disease, obstructive jaundice, dehydration, narrow-angle glaucoma, diarrhea associated with pseudomembranous enterocolitis or enterotoxin-producing bacteria. Do not use in children <2 years of age.
Warnings Use in conjunction with fluid and electrolyte therapy in children and in adults when appropriate. In case of severe dehydration or electrolyte imbalance, withhold diphenoxylate/atropine treatment until corrective therapy has been initiated. Inhibiting peristalsis may lead to fluid retention in the intestine aggravating dehydration and electrolyte imbalance. Reduction of intestinal motility may be deleterious in diarrhea resulting from Shigella, Salmonella, toxigenic strains of E. coli and from pseudomembranous enterocolitis associated with broad spectrum antibiotics; use is not recommended.

Use with caution in children. Younger children (especially those with Down syndrome) may develop signs of atropinism (dry skin and mucous membranes, thirst, hyperthermia, tachycardia, urinary retention, flushing) even at the recommended dosages. Overdose in children may result in severe respiratory depression (young children may be at greater risk), coma, and possibly permanent brain damage.

If acute diarrhea does not clinically improve within 48 hours, this medication is unlikely to be effective and should be discontinued; if chronic diarrhea is not improved symptomatically within 10 days at maximum dosage, control is unlikely with further use. Prolonged use may result in tolerance to antidiarrheal effects and physical or psychological dependence; abrupt discontinuation may cause withdrawal symptoms.
Precautions Use with extreme caution in patients with dehydration, cirrhosis, hepatorenal disease, renal dysfunction, and acute ulcerative colitis
Adverse Reactions
Cardiovascular: Tachycardia
Central nervous system: Confusion, depression, dizziness, drowsiness, euphoria, flushing, headache, hyperthermia, lethargy, malaise, restlessness, sedation
Dermatologic: Angioneurotic edema, dry skin, pruritus, urticaria
Gastrointestinal: Abdominal discomfort, anorexia, gum swelling, nausea, pancreatitis, paralytic ileus, toxic megacolon, vomiting, xerostomia
Genitourinary: Urinary retention
Neuromuscular & skeletal: Numbness
Miscellaneous: Anaphylaxis
Drug Interactions
Metabolism/Transport Effects None known.
Avoid Concomitant Use
Avoid concomitant use of Diphenoxylate and Atropine with any of the following: Aclidinium; Azelastine (Nasal); Ipratropium (Oral Inhalation); Paraldehyde; Potassium Chloride; Thalidomide; Tiotropium; Umeclidinium
Increased Effect/Toxicity
Diphenoxylate and Atropine may increase the levels/effects of: AbobotulinumtoxinA; Alcohol (Ethyl); Analgesics (Opioid); Anticholinergic Agents; Azelastine (Nasal); Buprenorphine; Cannabinoid-Containing Products; CNS Depressants; Hydrocodone; Methotrimeprazine; Metyrosine; Mirabegron; Mirtazapine; OnabotulinumtoxinA; Paraldehyde; Potassium Chloride; Pramipexole; RimabotulinumtoxinB; ROPINIRole; Rotigotine; Selective Serotonin Reuptake Inhibitors; Thalidomide; Thiazide Diuretics; Tiotropium; Topiramate; Zolpidem

The levels/effects of Diphenoxylate and Atropine may be increased by: Aclidinium; Brimonidine (Topical); Cannabis; Doxylamine; Dronabinol; Droperidol; HydrOXYzine; Ipratropium (Oral Inhalation); Kava Kava; Magnesium Sulfate; Methotrimeprazine; Nabilone; Perampanel; Pramlintide; Rufinamide; Sodium Oxybate; Tapentadol; Tetrahydrocannabinol; Umeclidinium
Decreased Effect
Diphenoxylate and Atropine may decrease the levels/effects of: Acetylcholinesterase Inhibitors (Central); Secretin

The levels/effects of Diphenoxylate and Atropine may be decreased by: Acetylcholinesterase Inhibitors (Central)
Stability Protect from light; dispense liquid only in original container
Mechanism of Action Diphenoxylate inhibits excessive GI motility and GI propulsion; commercial preparations contain a subtherapeutic amount of atropine to discourage abuse
Pharmacodynamics Antidiarrheal effects:
Onset of action: Within 45-60 minutes
Maximum effect: Within 2 hours
Duration: 3-4 hours
Tolerance to antidiarrheal effects may occur with prolonged use
Pharmacokinetics (Adult data unless noted)
Atropine: See Atropine
Diphenoxylate:
Absorption: Oral: Well absorbed

Distribution: Major metabolite (diphenoxylic acid) may be excreted in breast milk

Metabolism: Extensive in the liver via ester hydrolysis to diphenoxylic acid (active)

Half-life:

Diphenoxylate: 2.5 hours

Diphenoxylic acid: 12-24 hours

Time to peak serum concentration: ~2 hours

Elimination: Primarily (49%) in feces (via bile); ~14% is excreted in urine; <1% excreted unchanged in urine

Dosing: Usual Oral (as diphenoxylate):

Children 2-12 years: **Liquid: Note:** Only the liquid product is recommended for children under 13 years of age; do not exceed recommended doses; reduce dose as soon as symptoms are initially controlled; maintenance doses may be as low as 25% of initial dose; if no improvement within 48 hours of therapy, diphenoxylate is not likely to be effective

Initial: 0.3-0.4 mg/kg/day in 4 divided doses (maximum: 10 mg/day) **or**

Manufacturer's recommendations: Initial:

<2 years: Not recommended

2 years (11-14 kg): 1.5-3 mL 4 times/day

3 years (12-16 kg): 2-3 mL 4 times/day

4 years (14-20 kg): 2-4 mL 4 times/day

5 years (16-23 kg): 2.5-4.5 mL 4 times/day

6-8 years (17-32 kg): 2.5-5 mL 4 times/day

9-12 years (23-55 kg): 3.5-5 mL 4 times/day

Alternative pediatric dosing: Initial:

<2 years: Not recommended

2-5 years: 2 mg 3 times/day

5-8 years: 2 mg 4 times/day

8-12 years: 2 mg 5 times/day

Adults: Initial: 5 mg (2 tablets or 10 mL) 4 times/day until control achieved (maximum: 20 mg/day); then reduced dose as needed; maintenance: 5-15 mg/day in 2-3 divided doses; some patients may be controlled on doses as low as 5 mg/day

Note: Do not exceed recommended doses; reduce dose once symptoms are initially controlled; acute diarrhea usually improves within 48 hours; if chronic diarrhea dose not improve within 10 days at maximum daily doses of 20 mg, diphenoxylate is not likely to be effective.

Administration Oral: May be administered with food to decrease GI upset; use plastic dropper provided when measuring liquid; **Note:** Dropper has a 2 mL (1 mg) capacity and is calibrated in increments of 1/2 mL (0.25 mg)

Monitoring Parameters Bowel frequency, signs and symptoms of atropinism, fluid and electrolytes

Additional Information Naloxone reverses toxicity due to diphenoxylate; Lomotil® solution also contains sorbitol

Controlled Substance C-V

Dosage Forms Excipient information presented when available (limited, particularly for generics); consult specific product labeling. [DSC] = Discontinued product

Solution, oral: Diphenoxylate hydrochloride 2.5 mg and atropine sulfate 0.025 mg per 5 mL (5 mL, 10 mL, 60 mL)

Lomotil®: Diphenoxylate hydrochloride 2.5 mg and atropine sulfate 0.025 mg per 5 mL (60 mL) [contains alcohol 15%; cherry flavor] [DSC]

Tablet, oral: Diphenoxylate hydrochloride 2.5 mg and atropine sulfate 0.025 mg

Lomotil®: Diphenoxylate hydrochloride 2.5 mg and atropine sulfate 0.025 mg

◆ **Diphenylhydantoin** see Phenytoin on page 1663

Diphtheria and Tetanus Toxoids
(dif THEER ee a & TET a nus TOKS oyds)

Medication Safety Issues

Sound-alike/look-alike issues:

Diphtheria and Tetanus Toxoids (Td) may be confused with tuberculin purified protein derivative (PPD)

Pediatric diphtheria and tetanus (DT) may be confused with adult tetanus and diphtheria (Td)

Related Information

Immunization Administration Recommendations on page 2368

Immunization Guidelines on page 2373

Brand Names: U.S. Tenivac

Brand Names: Canada Td Adsorbed

Therapeutic Category Vaccine

Generic Availability (U.S.) Yes

Use

Diphtheria and tetanus toxoids adsorbed for pediatric use (DT): Active immunity against diphtheria and tetanus and tetanus prophylaxis in wound management when pertussis vaccine is contraindicated (FDA approved in ages ≥6 weeks to <7 years)

Tetanus and diphtheria toxoids adsorbed for adult use (Td) (Tenivac): Active immunity against diphtheria and tetanus; tetanus prophylaxis in wound management (FDA approved in ages ≥7 years and adults)

The Advisory Committee on Immunization Practices (ACIP) recommends routine vaccination for the following:

• Children ≥7 years, Adolescents, and Adults should receive a booster dose of Td every 10 years; may substitute a single Td booster dose with Tdap (CDC, 60 [1], 2011)

• Children 7-10 years, Adolescents, Adults, and the Elderly (≥65 years) who are wounded in bombings or similar mass casualty events who have penetrating injuries or nonintact skin exposure and who cannot confirm receipt of a tetanus booster within the previous 5 years, may also receive a single dose of Td; children ≥11 years, adolescents and adults may also receive Td if Tdap is unavailable (CDC [Chapman, 2008])

Pregnancy Risk Factor C

Pregnancy Considerations Reproduction studies have not been conducted. DT is not recommended for use in persons ≥7 years of age. Inactivated bacterial vaccines have not been shown to cause increased risks to the fetus (CDC, 60[2], 2011). The Advisory Committee on Immunization Practices (ACIP) recommends booster injections for previously vaccinated pregnant women who have not had Td vaccination within the past 10 years. Pregnant women who are not immunized or are only partially immunized should complete the primary series. Vaccination may be deferred until the postpartum period in women who are likely to have sufficient diphtheria and tetanus protection until delivery; Tdap may be substituted for Td after delivery to add extra protection against pertussis. Td should be administered during pregnancy to women who do not have sufficient tetanus immunity to protect against maternal and neonatal tetanus, and if booster protection for diphtheria is required (eg, travel to where diphtheria is endemic). Tetanus immune globulin and a tetanus toxoid containing vaccine are recommended by the ACIP as part of the standard wound management to prevent tetanus in pregnant women; the use of Td during pregnancy is recommended for wound management if ≥5 years have passed since the last Td vaccination (CDC, 2008).

Breast-Feeding Considerations It is not known if this vaccine is excreted into breast milk. The manufacturer recommends that caution be used if administered to breast-feeding women. Inactivated vaccines do not affect the safety of breast-feeding for the mother or the infant. Breast-feeding infants should be vaccinated according to the recommended schedules (CDC, 60[2], 2011).

Contraindications Hypersensitivity to diphtheria, tetanus toxoid, or any component

Warnings Diphtheria and tetanus toxoid is available in two formulations which contain different amounts of the diphtheria toxoid; DT or "pediatric" formulation has twice the diphtheria toxoid as Td or "adult" toxoid; use of DT in children >7 years and adults is associated with more severe adverse reactions to the diphtheria toxoid than in infants and younger children. Immediate treatment (including epinephrine 1:1000) for anaphylactic and/or hypersensitivity reactions should be available during vaccine use. Patients with a history of severe local reaction (Arthus-type) following a previous tetanus toxoid dose should not be given further routine or emergency doses of Td more frequently than every 10 years, even if using for wound management with wounds that are not clean or minor; these patients generally have high serum antitoxin levels. Guillain-Barré syndrome, occurring within 6 weeks of tetanus toxoid vaccination, has been reported. Apnea has occurred following intramuscular vaccine administration in premature infants; consider clinical status implications. Syncope has been reported with use of injectable vaccines and may be accompanied by transient visual disturbances, weakness, or tonic-clonic movements. Procedures should be in place to avoid injuries from falling and to restore cerebral perfusion if syncope occurs (CDC, 57[17], 2008).

Precautions The decision to administer or delay vaccination because of current or recent febrile illness depends on the severity of symptoms and the etiology of the disease. Immunization should be delayed during the course of an acute severe febrile illness; may administer to patients with mild acute illness (with or without fever). Use with caution in severely immunocompromised patients (eg, patients receiving chemo/radiation therapy or other immunosuppressive therapy, including high-dose corticosteroids); may have a reduced response to vaccination; inactivated vaccines should be administered ≥2 weeks prior to planned immunosuppression when feasible (IDSA [Rubin, 2013]). In general, household and close contacts of persons with altered immunocompetence may receive all age-appropriate vaccines. Vaccination may not result in effective immunity in all patients. Response depends upon multiple factors (eg, type of vaccine, age of patient) and may be improved by administering the vaccine at the recommended dose, route, and interval (CDC/ACIP [Kroger, 2011]).

Use with caution in patients with coagulation disorders, including thrombocytopenia, due to an increased risk for bleeding following I.M. injection; if the patient receives antihemophilia or other similar therapy, I.M. injection can be scheduled shortly after such therapy is administered. Antipyretics have not been shown to prevent febrile seizures; antipyretics may be used to treat fever or discomfort following vaccination (CDC/ACIP [Kroger, 2011]). One study reported that routine prophylactic administration of acetaminophen to prevent fever prior to vaccination decreased the immune response of some vaccines; the clinical significance of this reduction in immune response has not been established (Prymula, 2009).

Use of this vaccine for specific medical and/or other indications (eg, immunocompromising conditions, hepatic or kidney disease, diabetes) is also addressed in the ACIP Recommended Immunization Schedule (CDC/ACIP [Akinsanya-Beysolow, 2014]; CDC/ACIP [Bridges, 2014]).

Specific recommendations for use of this vaccine in immunocompromised patients with asplenia, cancer, HIV infection, cerebrospinal fluid leaks, cochlear implants, hematopoietic stem cell transplant (prior to or after), sickle cell disease, solid organ transplant (prior to or after), or those receiving immunosuppressive therapy for chronic conditions as well as contacts of immunocompromised patients are available from the IDSA (Rubin, 2014).

Some products may contain natural latex/natural rubber; use with caution in patients who may be susceptible to hypersensitivity reactions. Some products may contain thimerosal.

Adverse Reactions All serious adverse reactions must be reported to the U.S. Department of Health and Human Services (DHHS) Vaccine Adverse Event Reporting System (VAERS) 1-800-822-7967 or online at https://vaers.hhs.gov/esub/index. In Canada, adverse reactions may be reported to local provincial/territorial health agencies or to the Vaccine Safety Section at Public Health Agency of Canada (1-866-844-0018).

Central nervous system: Chills, fever, headache, tiredness

Endocrine & metabolic: Lymph node swelling

Gastrointestinal: Diarrhea, nausea, vomiting

Local: Injection site: Erythema, pain, swelling

Neuromuscular & skeletal: Body ache/muscle weakness, sore/swollen joints

Dermatologic: Rash

Rare but important or life-threatening: Allergic reactions (angioedema, rash, urticaria), anaphylactic reactions, arthralgia, chills, dizziness, fatigue, injection site reactions (cellulitis, induration, nodules, warmth), lymphadenopathy, musculoskeletal stiffness, myalgia, pain, pain in extremities, paresthesia, peripheral edema, seizure, syncope, weakness

Drug Interactions

Metabolism/Transport Effects None known.

Avoid Concomitant Use There are no known interactions where it is recommended to avoid concomitant use.

Increased Effect/Toxicity There are no known significant interactions involving an increase in effect.

Decreased Effect

The levels/effects of Diphtheria and Tetanus Toxoids may be decreased by: Belimumab; Fingolimod; Immunosuppressants; Meningococcal Polysaccharide (Groups A / C / Y and W-135) Tetanus Toxoid Conjugate Vaccine

Stability Store at 2°C to 8°C (35°F to 46°F). Do not freeze; discard if product has been frozen.

Dosing: Usual

Primary Immunization:

Infants and Children 6 weeks to <7 years (prior to 7th birthday) with contraindication to immunization containing pertussis: **Note:** Preterm infants should be vaccinated according to their chronological age from birth; Pediatric formulation (DT): I.M.: 0.5 mL per dose for a total of 5 doses administered as follows:

Three doses, usually given at 2-, 4-, and 6 months of age; may be given as early as 6 weeks of age and repeated every 4 to 8 weeks

Fourth dose: Given at ~15 to 18 months of age, but at least 6 months after third dose. The fourth dose may be given as early as 12 months of age, but at least 6 months must have elapsed between the third dose and the fourth dose.

Fifth dose: Given at 4 to 6 years of age, prior to starting school or kindergarten; if the fourth dose is given at ≥4 years of age, the fifth dose may be omitted

Catch-up immunization:

CDC (ACIP) Recommendations (Akinsanya-Beysolow, 2014): **Note:** Do not restart the series. If doses have been given, begin the below schedule at the applicable dose number.

Infants and Children who start primary immunization series ≥4 months of age through 6 years (prior to seventh birthday): Pediatric formulation (DT): I.M.: 0.5 mL per dose for a total of 4 to 5 doses administered as follows: 3 doses at least 4 weeks apart followed 6 months later with dose 4; a fifth dose may be given 6 months later (the fifth dose is not necessary if the child received the fourth dose after 4 years of age)

Children 7 to 10 years not fully, or never vaccinated against diphtheria, or tetanus, or pertussis, or whose vaccination status is not known: I.M.: 0.5 mL per dose for a total of 3 to 4 doses given as follows:

First dose given on the elected date: Use Td only if contraindication to vaccine containing pertussis, Tdap (Adacel, Boostrix) is preferred for this dose

Second dose (tetanus and diphtheria, Td) given at least 4 weeks after the first dose

Third dose (tetanus and diphtheria, Td) given at least 4 weeks after the second dose (if first DTaP/DT at <12 months of age) **or** given at least 6 months after the second dose (if first dose DTaP/DT at ≥12 months)

Fourth dose (tetanus and diphtheria, Td) given at least 6 months after the third dose; fourth dose is not needed if the first DTaP/DT dose was given at ≥12 months of age.

Manufacturer's labeling: Tenivac: Children ≥7 years, Adolescents, and Adults: I.M.: Patients previously not immunized should receive 2 primary doses of 0.5 mL each, given at an interval of 8 weeks; plus a third (reinforcing) dose of 0.5 mL given 6 to 8 months later

Booster immunization: For routine booster in patients who have completed primary immunization series. The ACIP prefers Tdap for use in in some situations if no contraindications exist; refer to Diphtheria and Tetanus Toxoids, and Acellular Pertussis Vaccine monograph for additional information.

Children 11 to 12 years: I.M.: 0.5 mL as a single dose when at least 5 years have elapsed since last dose of toxoid-containing vaccine. Subsequent routine doses are not recommended more often than every 10 years.

Adolescents and Adults: I.M. 0.5 mL as a single dose every 10 years

Tetanus prophylaxis in wound management: Infants, Children, Adolescents, and Adults: Tetanus prophylaxis in patients with wounds should consider if the wound is clean or contaminated, the immunization status of the patient, proper use of tetanus toxoid and/or tetanus immune globulin (TIG), wound cleaning, and (if required) surgical debridement and the proper use of antibiotics. Patients with an uncertain or incomplete tetanus immunization status should have additional follow-up to ensure a series is completed. Patients with a history of Arthus reaction following a previous dose of a tetanus toxoid-containing vaccine should not receive a tetanus toxoid-containing vaccine until >10 years after the most recent dose even if they have a wound that is neither clean nor minor. See table.

Tetanus Prophylaxis Wound Management

History of Tetanus Immunization (Doses)	Clean, Minor Wounds		All Other Wounds[1]	
	Tetanus toxoid[2]	TIG	Tetanus toxoid[2]	TIG
Uncertain or <3 doses	Yes	No	Yes	Yes
3 or more doses	No[3]	No	No[4]	No

[1]Such as, but not limited to, wounds contaminated with dirt, feces, soil, and saliva; puncture wounds; wounds from crushing, tears, burns, and frostbite.

[2]Tetanus toxoid in this chart refers to a tetanus toxoid containing vaccine. For children <7 years old DTaP (DT, if pertussis vaccine contraindicated) is preferred to tetanus toxoid alone. For children ≥7 years of age and Adults, Td preferred to tetanus toxoid alone; Tdap may be preferred if the patient has not previously been vaccinated with Tdap.

[3]Yes, if ≥10 years since last dose.

[4]Yes, if ≥5 years since last dose.

Abbreviations: **DT** = Diphtheria and Tetanus Toxoids (formulation for age ≤6 years); **DTaP** = Diphtheria and Tetanus Toxoids, and Acellular Pertussis (formulation for age ≤6 years; Daptacel®, Infanrix®); **Td** = Diphtheria and Tetanus Toxoids (formulation for age ≥7 years; Tenivac™); **TT** = Tetanus toxoid (adsorbed [formulation for age ≥7 years]); **Tdap** = Diphtheria and Tetanus Toxoids, and Acellular Pertussis (Adacel® or Boostrix® [formulations for age ≥7 years]); **TIG** = Tetanus Immune Globulin

Adapted from the Yellow Book 2010, Chapter 2, *Routine Vaccine-Preventable Diseases, Tetanus*; Available at www.cdc.gov/yellowbook; and *MMWR*, 2006, 55:RR-17.

Dosing adjustment in renal impairment: There are no dosage adjustments provided in the manufacturer's labeling.

Dosing adjustment in hepatic impairment: There are no dosage adjustments provided in the manufacturer's labeling.

Administration I.M. Prior to use, shake suspension well; **not for I.V. or SubQ administration**. Adolescents and adults should be vaccinated while seated or lying down:

DT (pediatric use): Administer in either the anterolateral aspect of the thigh or the deltoid muscle; do not inject in the gluteal area

Td: Administer in the deltoid muscle; do not inject in the gluteal area.

U.S. law requires that the date of administration, the vaccine manufacturer, lot number of vaccine, and the administering person's name, title, and address be entered into the patient's permanent medical record.

Monitoring Parameters Observe for syncope for 15 minutes following administration. If seizure-like activity associated with syncope occurs, maintain patient in supine or Trendelenburg position to re-establish adequate cerebral perfusion.

Additional Information In order to maximize vaccination rates, the ACIP recommends simultaneous administration (ie, >1 vaccine on the same day at different anatomic sites) of all age-appropriate vaccines (live or inactivated) for which a person is eligible at a single visit, unless contraindications exist. If available, the use of combination vaccine is generally preferred over separate injections, taking into consideration provider assessment, patient preference, and potential adverse events. If separate vaccines are being used, evaluate product information regarding same syringe compatibility of vaccines. Separate needles and syringes should be used for each injection. The ACIP prefers each dose of specific vaccine in a series come from the same manufacturer if possible (CDC/ACIP, [Kroger, 2011]).

For additional information, please refer to the following website: http://www.cdc.gov/vaccines/vpd-vac/.

Dosage Forms Excipient information presented when available (limited, particularly for generics); consult specific product labeling. [DSC] = Discontinued product

◀ Injection, suspension [Td, adult; preservative free]: Diphtheria 2 Lf units and tetanus 2 Lf units per 0.5 mL (0.5 mL)
Tenivac: Diphtheria 2 Lf units and tetanus 5 Lf units per 0.5 mL (0.5 mL) [contains aluminum, may contain natural rubber/natural latex in prefilled syringe]
Injection, suspension [DT, pediatric; preservative free]: Diphtheria 6.7 Lf units and tetanus 5 Lf units per 0.5 mL (0.5 mL) [DSC]; Diphtheria 25 Lf units and tetanus 5 Lf units per 0.5 mL (0.5 mL) [contains aluminum]

References

AAP Steering Committee on Quality Improvement and Management, Subcommittee on Febrile Seizures American Academy of Pediatrics, "Febrile Seizures: Clinical Practice Guideline for the Long-Term Management of the Child With Simple Febrile Seizures," *Pediatrics*, 2008, 121(6):1281-6.

Akinsanya-Beysolow I, Advisory Committee on Immunization Practices (ACIP), ACIP Child/Adolescent Immunization Work Group, et al. Advisory committee on immunization practices recommended immunization schedules for persons 0 through 18 years - United States, 2014. *MMWR Morb Mortal Wkly Rep.* 2014; 63(5):108-109. Full schedule available at http://www.cdc.gov/vaccines/schedules/downloads/child/0-18yrs-child-combined-schedule.pdf

Bridges CB, Coyne-Beasley T, et.al. Advisory committee on immunization practices recommended immunization schedule for adults aged 19 years or older - United States, 2014. *MMWR Morb Mortal Wkly Rep.* 2014;63(5):108-109. Full schedule available at http://www.cdc.gov/vaccines/schedules/downloads/adult/adult-combined-schedule.pdf

Broder KR, Cortese MM, Iskander JK, et al. Preventing tetanus, diphtheria, and pertussis among adolescents: use of tetanus toxoid, reduced diphtheria toxoid and acellular pertussis vaccines: recommendations of the Advisory Committee on Immunization Practices (ACIP). *MMWR Recomm Rep.* 2006;55(RR-3):1-34.

Centers for Disease Control and Prevention (CDC), "Syncope After Vaccination-United States, January 2005-July 2007," *MMWR Morb Mortal Wkly Rep*, 2008, 2;57(17):457-60.

Centers for Disease Control and Prevention (CDC). Updated recommendations for use of tetanus toxoid, reduced diphtheria toxoid and acellular pertussis (Tdap) vaccine from the Advisory Committee on Immunization Practices, 2010. *MMWR Morb Mortal Wkly Rep.* 2011;60(1):13-15.

Chapman LE, Sullivent EE, Grohskopf LA, et al. Recommendations for postexposure interventions to prevent infection with hepatitis B virus, hepatitis C virus, or human immunodeficiency virus, and tetanus in persons wounded during bombings and other mass-casualty events-United States, 2008: recommendations of the Centers For Disease Control and Prevention (CDC). *MMWR Recomm Rep.* 2008;57(RR-6):1-21.

Kretsomger K, Broder K, Cortese MM, et al. Preventing tetanus, diphtheria, and pertussis among adults: use of tetanus toxoid, reduced diphtheria toxoid and acellular pertussis vaccine, recommendations of the Advisory Committee on Immunization Practices (ACIP) and recommendation of ACIP, supported by the Healthcare Infection Control Practices Advisory Committee (HICPAC), for use of Tdap among health-care personnel. *MMWR Recomm Rep.* 2006;55(RR-17):1-37.

Kroger AT, Atkinson WL, Marcuse EK, Pickering LK. General recommendations on immunization - recommendations of the Advisory Committee on Immunization Practices (ACIP). *MMWR Recomm Rep.* 2011;60(RR-2):1-64.

Prymula R, Siegrist CA, Chlibek R, et al, "Effect of Prophylactic Paracetamol Administration at Time of Vaccination on Febrile Reactions and Antibody Responses in Children: Two Open-Label, Randomised Controlled Trials," *Lancet*, 2009, 374(9698):1339-50.

Rubin LG, Levin MJ, Ljungman P, et al. 2013 IDSA clinical practice guideline for vaccination of the immunocompromised host. *Clin Infect Dis.* 2014;58(3):e44-e100.

Diphtheria and Tetanus Toxoids, Acellular Pertussis, and Poliovirus Vaccine

(dif THEER ee a & TET a nus TOKS oyds, ay CEL yoo lar per TUS sis & POE lee oh VYE rus vak SEEN)

Medication Safety Issues

Sound-alike/look-alike issues:

Adacel® (trade name for Diphtheria and Tetanus Toxoids, and Acellular Pertussis Vaccine) should not be confused with Adacel®-Polio (trade name for Diphtheria and Tetanus Toxoids, Acellular Pertussis, and Poliovirus Vaccine in Canada)

Related Information

Immunization Administration Recommendations *on page 2368*
Immunization Guidelines *on page 2373*
Brand Names: U.S. Kinrix®
Brand Names: Canada Adacel®-Polio
Therapeutic Category Vaccine
Generic Availability (U.S.) No
Use Active immunization in children 4 to 6 years of age against diphtheria, tetanus, pertussis, and poliomyelitis; used as the 5th dose in the DTaP series and the 4th dose in the IPV series (FDA approved in ages 4 to 6 years)

The Advisory Committee on Immunization Practices (ACIP) recommends this as routine vaccination for use as the fifth dose in the DTaP series and the fourth dose in the IPV series in children who received DTaP (Infanrix) and/or DTaP-Hepatitis B-IPV (Pediarix) as the first 3 doses and DTaP (Infanrix) as the fourth dose. Whenever feasible, the same manufacturer should be used to provide the pertussis component; however, vaccination should not be deferred if a specific brand is not known or is not available.

Pregnancy Risk Factor C
Pregnancy Considerations Reproduction studies have not been conducted; Kinrix® is not indicated for women of childbearing age. Adacel®-Polio is not recommended for use in pregnant women unless a definite risk of pertussis exists.

Breast-Feeding Considerations Kinrix® is not indicated for use in patients ≥7 years of age. Use of Adacel®-Polio in lactating women has not been studied.

Contraindications Hypersensitivity to any component including neomycin and polymyxin B; encephalopathy occurring within 7 days of administration of a previous dose of a pertussis-containing vaccine that is not attributable to another cause; progressive neurological disorder, including infantile spasms, uncontrolled epilepsy, or progressive encephalopathy (pertussis vaccine should be withheld until the clinical condition is stabilized)

Warnings Immediate treatment (including epinephrine 1:1000) for anaphylactic and/or hypersensitivity reactions should be available during vaccine use. Subsequent vaccination with a pertussis-containing vaccine should be carefully considered if the following reactions occur with a temporal relationship to a previous dose of DTaP: Temperature ≥40.5°C (105°F) within 48 hours, not attributable to another identifiable cause; collapse or shock-like state (hypotonic-hyporesponsive episode) within 48 hours; persistent crying lasting ≥3 hours within 48 hours; or convulsions with or without fever, occurring within 3 days. Guillain Barré syndrome occurring within 6 weeks of vaccines containing tetanus toxoid has been reported. Patients with a history of severe local reaction (Arthustype) following a previous tetanus toxoid dose should not be given further routine or emergency doses of Td more frequently than every 10 years, even if using for wound management with wounds that are not clean or minor; these patients generally have high serum antitoxin levels. Syncope has been reported with use of injectable vaccines and may be accompanied by transient visual disturbances, weakness, or tonic-clonic movements. Procedures should be in place to avoid injuries from falling and to restore cerebral perfusion if syncope occurs (CDC, 57[17], 2008). Product may contain aluminum, neomycin, polymyxin B, and polysorbate 80 (Tween 80) which may cause allergic reactions in susceptible individuals.

Precautions The decision to administer or delay vaccination because of current or recent febrile illness depends on the severity of symptoms and the etiology of the disease. Immunization should be delayed during the course of an acute severe febrile illness; may administer to patients with mild acute illness (with or without fever). Use with caution in severely immunocompromised patients (eg, patients receiving chemo-/radiation therapy or other immunosuppressive therapy including high-dose corticosteroids); may have a reduced response to vaccination; inactivated vaccines should be administered ≥2 weeks prior to planned immunosuppression when feasible (IDSA [Rubin, 2013]). In general, household and close contacts of persons with altered immunocompetence may receive all age-appropriate vaccines. Vaccination may not result in effective immunity in all patients. Response depends upon multiple factors (eg, type of vaccine, age of patient) and may be improved by administering the vaccine at the recommended dose, route, and interval (CDC/ACIP [Kroger, 2011]).

A family history of seizures is not a contraindication to use of DTaP; however, use in patients with a history of seizure disorder, progressive neurologic disease, or conditions predisposing to seizures should be deferred until health status can be assessed and condition stabilized. Antipyretics may be considered at the time of and for 24 hours following vaccination to patients at high risk for seizures to reduce the possibility of postvaccination fever. Antipyretics have not been shown to prevent febrile seizures. Antipyretics may be used to treat fever or discomfort following vaccination (CDC/ACIP [Kroger, 2011]). One study reported that routine prophylactic administration of acetaminophen to prevent fever due to vaccines has been shown to decrease the immune response of some vaccines; the clinical significance of this reduction in immune response has not been established (Prymula, 2009). Use with caution in patients with coagulation disorders, including thrombocytopenia, due to an increased risk for bleeding following I.M. administration; if the patient receives antihemophilia or other similar therapy, I.M. injection can be scheduled shortly after such therapy is administered.

If Kinrix is inadvertently administered to children ≥7 years of age earlier than the fifth dose in the series, it may be counted as a valid dose, provided the minimum interval requirements were met. Patients with latex allergy should not handle the needle cover or plunger of the prefilled syringes since they contain latex.

Adverse Reactions All serious adverse reactions must be reported to the U.S. Department of Health and Human Services (DHHS) Vaccine Adverse Event Reporting System (VAERS) 1-800-822-7967 or online at https://vaers.hhs.gov/esub/index. In Canada, adverse reactions may be reported to local provincial/territorial health agencies or to the Vaccine Safety Section at Public Health Agency of Canada (1-866-844-0018).

Adverse events reported within 4 days of vaccination:

Central nervous system: Drowsiness, fever

Gastrointestinal: Loss of appetite

Local: Injection site: Arm circumference increase, pain, redness, swelling

Rare but important or life-threatening: Cellulitis, cerebrovascular accident, constipation, dehydration, gastroenteritis, hypernatremia, injection site vesicles, pruritus

Additional postmarketing events associated with Infanrix®: Allergic reactions, anaphylactoid reactions, anaphylaxis, angioedema, apnea, hypotonic-hyporesponsive episode, lymphadenopathy, seizures, thrombocytopenia, urticaria

Drug Interactions

Metabolism/Transport Effects None known.

Avoid Concomitant Use There are no known interactions where it is recommended to avoid concomitant use.

Increased Effect/Toxicity There are no known significant interactions involving an increase in effect.

Decreased Effect

The levels/effects of Diphtheria and Tetanus Toxoids, Acellular Pertussis, and Poliovirus Vaccine may be decreased by: Belimumab; Fingolimod; Immunosuppressants; Meningococcal Polysaccharide (Groups A / C / Y and W-135) Tetanus Toxoid Conjugate Vaccine

Stability Store at 2°C to 8°C (36°F to 46°F); do not freeze. Discard if frozen.

Mechanism of Action Promotes active immunity to diphtheria, tetanus, pertussis, and poliovirus (types 1, 2 and 3) by inducing production of specific antibodies and antitoxins.

Pharmacodynamics Onset of action: Immune response observed to all components ~1 month following vaccination

Dosing: Usual Pediatric: **Immunization:** Children 4 to 6 years: I.M.: 0.5 mL as a single dose; **Note:** For use as the fifth dose in the DTaP series and the fourth dose in the IPV series

Dosing adjustment in renal impairment: There are no dosage adjustments provided in the manufacturer's labeling.

Dosing adjustment in hepatic impairment: There are no dosage adjustments provided in the manufacturer's labeling.

Administration Shake well; do not use unless a homogeneous, turbid, white suspension forms; administer I.M. the deltoid muscle of the upper arm; **not for I.V. or SubQ administration**. U.S. law requires that the date of administration, name of the vaccine manufacturer, lot number of vaccine, and the administering person's name, title, and address be entered into the patient's permanent medical record.

Monitoring Parameters Observe for syncope for 15 minutes following administration. If seizure-like activity associated with syncope occurs, maintain patient in supine or Trendelenburg position to reestablish adequate cerebral perfusion.

Additional Information Contains the following three pertussis antigens: Inactivated pertussis toxin (PT), filamentous hemagglutinin (FHA), and pertactin. Contains the same diphtheria, tetanus toxoids, and pertussis antigens found in Infanrix and Pediarix. Contains the same poliovirus antigens found in Infanrix.

In order to maximize vaccination rates, the ACIP recommends simultaneous administration of all age-appropriate vaccines (live or inactivated) for which a person is eligible at a single visit, unless contraindications exist. The use of combination vaccines is generally preferred over separate injections, taking into consideration provider assessment, patient preference, and potential adverse events.

For additional information, please refer to the following website: http://www.cdc.gov/vaccines/vpd-vac/.

Dosage Forms Excipient information presented when available (limited, particularly for generics); consult specific product labeling.

Injection, suspension [preservative free]:

Kinrix®: Diphtheria toxoid 25 Lf, tetanus toxoid 10 Lf, acellular pertussis antigens [inactivated pertussis toxin 25 mcg, filamentous hemagglutinin 25 mcg, pertactin 8 mcg], type 1 poliovirus 40 D-antigen units, type 2 poliovirus 8 D-antigen units, and type 3 poliovirus 32 D-antigen units per 0.5 mL (0.5 mL) [contains aluminum, neomycin sulfate, polymyxin B, polysorbate 80; may contain natural rubber/natural latex in prefilled syringe]

References

Akinsanya-Beysolow I; Advisory Committee on Immunization Practices (ACIP); ACIP Child/Adolescent Immunization Work Group; Centers for Disease Control and Prevention (CDC). Advisory Committee on Immunization Practices recommended immunization schedules for persons aged 0 through 18 years – United States, 2014. *MMWR Morb Mortal Wkly Rep.* 2014;63(5):108-109. Available at http://www.cdc.gov/vaccines/schedules/downloads/child/0-18yrs-child-combined-schedule.pdf

Centers for Disease Control and Prevention (CDC). Licensure of a diphtheria and tetanus toxoids and acellular pertussis adsorbed and inactivated poliovirus vaccine and guidance for use as a booster dose. *MMWR Morb Mortal Wkly Rep.* 2008;57(39):1078-1079.

Kroger AT, Atkinson WL, Marcuse EK, Pickering LK. General recommendations on immunization - recommendations of the Advisory

Committee on Immunization Practices (ACIP). *MMWR Recomm Rep.* 2011;60(RR-2):1-64.

Prymula R, Siegrist CA, Chlibek R, et al. Effect of prophylactic paracetamol administration at time of vaccination on febrile reactions and antibody responses in children: two open-label, randomised controlled trials. *Lancet.* 2009;374(9698):1339-1350.

Rubin LG, Levin MJ, Ljungman P, et al. 2013 IDSA clinical practice guideline for vaccination of the immunocompromised host. *Clin Infect Dis.* 2014;58(3):e44-e100.

Diphtheria and Tetanus Toxoids, Acellular Pertussis, Poliovirus and *Haemophilus* b Conjugate Vaccine

(dif THEER ee a & TET a nus TOKS oyds ay CEL yoo lar per TUS sis POE lee oh VYE rus & hem OF fi lus bee KON joo gate vak SEEN)

Medication Safety Issues
Administration issues:
Pentacel® is supplied in two vials, one containing DTaP-IPV liquid and one containing Hib powder, which must be mixed together in order to administer the recommended vaccine components.

Related Information
Immunization Administration Recommendations *on page 2368*

Immunization Guidelines *on page 2373*

Brand Names: U.S. Pentacel®

Brand Names: Canada Pediacel®; Pentacel®

Therapeutic Category Vaccine

Generic Availability (U.S.) No

Use Active immunization against diphtheria, tetanus, pertussis, poliomyelitis, and invasive disease caused by *H. influenzae* type b in infants (at least 6 weeks of age) and children (prior to fifth birthday) (FDA approved in ages 6 weeks through 4 years)

Advisory Committee on Immunization Practices (ACIP) states that Pentacel (DTaP-IPV/Hib) may be used to provide the recommended DTaP, IPV, and Hib immunization in children <5 years of age. Whenever feasible, the same manufacturer should be used to provide the pertussis component; however, vaccination should not be deferred if a specific brand is not known or is not available. The Hib component in Pentacel contains a tetanus toxoid conjugate. A Hib vaccine containing the PRP-OMP conjugate (PedvaxHIB) may provide a more rapid seroconversion following the first dose and may be preferable to use in certain populations (eg, American Indian or Alaska Native children).

Pregnancy Risk Factor C

Pregnancy Considerations Animal reproduction studies have not been conducted for this combination product. This product is not indicated for use in women of child-bearing age.

Contraindications Hypersensitivity to any component including neomycin, polymyxin B; encephalopathy occurring within 7 days of administration of a previous dose of a pertussis-containing vaccine that is not attributable to another cause; progressive neurological disorder, including infantile spasms, uncontrolled epilepsy, or progressive encephalopathy (pertussis vaccine may be withheld until the clinical condition has stabilized)

Warnings Immediate treatment (including epinephrine 1:1000) for anaphylactic and/or hypersensitivity reactions should be available during vaccine use. Subsequent vaccination with a pertussis-containing vaccine should be carefully considered if the following reactions occur with a temporal relationship to a previous dose of DTaP: Temperature ≥40.5°C (105°F) within 48 hours, not attributable to another identifiable cause; collapse or shock-like state (hypotonic-hyporesponsive episode) within 48 hours; persistent crying lasting ≥3 hours within 48 hours; or convulsions with or without fever occurring within 3 days.

Guillain-Barré syndrome occurring within 6 weeks of vaccines containing tetanus toxoid has been reported. Patients with a history of severe local reaction (Arthus-type) following a previous tetanus toxoid dose should not be given further routine or emergency doses of Td more frequently than every 10 years, even if using for wound management with wounds that are not clean or minor; these patients generally have high serum antitoxin levels. Syncope has been reported with use of injectable vaccines and may be accompanied by transient visual disturbances, weakness, or tonic-clonic movements. Procedures should be in place to avoid injuries from falling and to restore cerebral perfusion if syncope occurs. Apnea has occurred following intramuscular vaccine administration in premature infants; consider clinical status implications (CDC, 57 [17], 2008). Injection contains polysorbate 80 (Tween 80) which may cause allergic reactions in susceptible individuals. In premature neonates, thrombocytopenia, ascites, pulmonary deterioration, and renal and hepatic failure have been reported after receiving parenteral products containing polysorbate 80 (Alade, 1986; CDC, 1984).

Precautions The decision to administer or delay vaccination because of current or recent febrile illness depends on the severity of symptoms and the etiology of the disease. Immunization should be delayed during the course of an acute severe febrile illness; may administer to patients with mild acute illness (with or without fever). Use with caution in severely immunocompromised patients (eg, patients receiving chemo/radiation therapy or other immunosuppressive therapy, including high-dose corticosteroids); may have a reduced response to vaccination; inactivated vaccines should be administered ≥2 weeks prior to planned immunosuppression when feasible (IDSA [Rubin, 2013]). In general, household and close contacts of persons with altered immunocompetence may receive all age-appropriate vaccines. Vaccination may not result in effective immunity in all patients. Response depends upon multiple factors (eg, type of vaccine, age of patient) and may be improved by administering the vaccine at the recommended dose, route, and interval (CDC/ACIP [Kroger, 2011]).

Use with caution in patients with coagulation disorders, including thrombocytopenia, due to an increased risk for bleeding following I.M. administration; if the patient receives antihemophilia or other similar therapy, I.M. injection can be scheduled shortly after such therapy is administered. A family history of seizures is not a contraindication to use of DTaP; however, use in patients with or history of seizure disorder, progressive neurologic disease, or conditions predisposing to seizures should be deferred until health status can be assessed and condition stabilized. Antipyretics have not been shown to prevent febrile seizures. Antipyretics may be used to treat fever or discomfort following vaccination (CDC/ACIP [Kroger, 2011]). One study reported that routine prophylactic administration of acetaminophen to prevent fever due to vaccines has been shown to decrease the immune response of some vaccines; the clinical significance of this reduction in immune response has not been established (Prymula, 2009).

Adverse Reactions All serious adverse reactions must be reported to the U.S. Department of Health and Human Services (DHHS) Vaccine Adverse Event Reporting System (VAERS) 1-800-822-7967 or online at https://vaers.hhs.gov/esub/index. In Canada, adverse reactions may be reported to local provincial/territorial health agencies or to the Vaccine Safety Section at Public Health Agency of Canada (1-866-844-0018).

Central nervous system: Crying (inconsolable), fever ≥38°C, fussiness/irritability, lethargy/decreased activity

Local: Injection site reactions: Arm circumference increase >5 mm, redness >5 mm, swelling >5 mm, tenderness

Rare but important or life-threatening: Anaphylaxis/anaphylactic reaction, apnea, appetite decreased, asthma, bronchiolitis, consciousness decreased, cough, cyanosis, dehydration, diarrhea, encephalopathy, erythema, gastroenteritis, hypersensitivity reactions, hypotonia, hypotonic-hyporesponsive episodes, injection site reactions (abscess, extensive swelling of injected limb, inflammation, mass), pallor, pneumonia, screaming, seizure, skin discoloration, somnolence, vomiting

Drug Interactions
Metabolism/Transport Effects None known.

Avoid Concomitant Use There are no known interactions where it is recommended to avoid concomitant use.

Increased Effect/Toxicity There are no known significant interactions involving an increase in effect.

Decreased Effect
The levels/effects of Diphtheria and Tetanus Toxoids, Acellular Pertussis, Poliovirus and Haemophilus b Conjugate Vaccine may be decreased by: Belimumab; Fingolimod; Immunosuppressants; Meningococcal Polysaccharide (Groups A / C / Y and W-135) Tetanus Toxoid Conjugate Vaccine

Stability Store at 2°C to 8°C (35°F to 46°F); do not freeze. Discard if frozen. Use immediately after reconstitution.

Dosing: Usual
Pediatric: Primary immunization:

Infants and Children 6 weeks to ≤4 years: I.M.: 0.5 mL per dose for a total of 4 doses administered as follows: 2, 4, 6, and 15 to 18 months of age. The first dose may be administered as early as 6 weeks of age. Following completion of the 4-dose series, children should receive a dose of DTaP vaccine at 4 to 6 years of age (Daptacel recommended due to same pertussis antigen used in both products).

Note: Per the ACIP, polio vaccine should not be administered more frequently than 4 weeks apart. Use of the minimum age and minimum intervals during the first 6 months of life should only be done when the vaccine recipient is at risk for imminent exposure to circulating poliovirus (shorter intervals and earlier start dates may lead to lower seroconversion). Pentacel is not indicated for the polio booster dose given at 4 to 6 years of age; Kinrix or IPV should be used.

Children previously vaccinated with ≥1 dose of Daptacel or IPV vaccines: Pentacel may be used to complete the first 4 doses of the DTaP or IPV series in children scheduled to receive the other components in the vaccine.

Children previously vaccinated with ≥1 dose of *Haemophilus b* Conjugate vaccine: Pentacel may be used to complete the series in children scheduled to receive the other components in the vaccine; however, if different brands of *Haemophilus b* Conjugate vaccine are administered to complete the series, 3 primary immunizing doses are needed, followed by a booster dose.

Note: Completion of 3 doses of Pentacel provides primary immunization against diphtheria, tetanus, *H. influenzae* type B, and poliomyelitis. Completion of the 4-dose series with Pentacel provides primary immunization against pertussis. It also provides a booster vaccination against diphtheria, tetanus, *H. influenzae* type B, and poliomyelitis.

Administration Pentacel® is supplied in two vials, one containing DTaP-IPV liquid and one containing Hib powder. First, gently shake vial containing DTaP-IPV component; withdraw liquid contents, and inject into vial containing Hib powder; gently swirl until uniform, cloudy suspension results.

Administer I.M. in the anterolateral aspect of thigh in children <1 year of age or deltoid muscle of upper arm in older children. Do not administer to gluteal area or areas near a major nerve trunk; **not for I.V. or SubQ administration**. Do not administer additional vaccines or immunoglobulins at the same site or using the same syringe.

U.S. law requires that the date of administration, name of the vaccine manufacturer, lot number of vaccine, and the administering person's name, title, and address be entered into the patient's permanent medical record.

Monitoring Parameters Observe for syncope for 15 minutes following administration. If seizure-like activity associated with syncope occurs, maintain patient in supine or Trendelenburg position to reestablish adequate cerebral perfusion.

Additional Information Contains the following three pertussis antigens: Inactivated pertussis toxin (PT), filamentous hemagglutinin (FHA), and pertactin. Contains the same diphtheria, tetanus toxoids, and pertussis antigens found in Daptacel; the same poliovirus antigens found in IPOL; the same Hib-PRP found in ActHIB.

In order to maximize vaccination rates, the ACIP recommends simultaneous administration (ie, >1 vaccine on the same day at different anatomic sites) of all age-appropriate vaccines (live or inactivated) for which a person is eligible at a single visit, unless contraindications exist. If available, the use of combination vaccine is generally preferred over separate injections, taking into consideration provider assessment, patient preference, and potential adverse events. If separate vaccines are being used, evaluate product information regarding same-syringe compatibility of vaccines. Separate needles and syringes should be used for each injection. The ACIP prefers each dose of specific vaccine in a series come from the same manufacturer if possible (CDC/ACIP [Kroger, 2011]).

For additional information, please refer to the following website: http://www.cdc.gov/vaccines/vpd-vac/.

Dosage Forms Excipient information presented when available (limited, particularly for generics); consult specific product labeling.

Injection, suspension:

Pentacel®: Diphtheria toxoid 15 Lf, tetanus toxoid 5 Lf, acellular pertussis antigens [pertussis toxin detoxified 20 mcg, filamentous hemagglutinin 20 mcg, pertactin 3 mcg, fimbriae (types 2 and 3) 5 mcg], type 1 poliovirus 40 D-antigen units; type 2 poliovirus 8 D-antigen units; type 3 poliovirus 32 D-antigen units, and *Haemophilus* b capsular polysaccharide 10 mcg [bound to tetanus toxoid 24 mcg] per 0.5 mL (0.5 mL) [contains albumin, aluminum, neomycin, polymyxin B sulfate, and polysorbate 80; supplied in two vials, one containing DTaP-IPV liquid and one containing Hib powder]

References
AAP Steering Committee on Quality Improvement and Management, Subcommittee on Febrile Seizures American Academy of Pediatrics, "Febrile Seizures: Clinical Practice Guideline for the Long-Term Management of the Child With Simple Febrile Seizures," *Pediatrics*, 2008, 121(6):1281-6.

Akinsanya-Beysolow I, Advisory Committee on Immunization Practices (ACIP), ACIP Child/Adolescent Immunization Work Group, et al. Advisory committee on immunization practices recommended immunization schedules for persons aged 0 through 18 years - United States, 2014. *MMWR Morb Mortal Wkly Rep*. 2014; 63(5):108-109. Full schedule available at http://www.cdc.gov/vaccines/schedules/downloads/child/0-18yrs-child-combined-schedule.pdf

Alade SL, Brown RE, and Paquet A Jr, "Polysorbate 80 and E-Ferol Toxicity," *Pediatrics*, 1986, 77(4):593-7.

Centers for Disease Control and Prevention (CDC), "Licensure of a Diphtheria and Tetanus Toxoids and Acellular Pertussis Adsorbed, Inactivated Poliovirus, and *Haemophilus* B Conjugate Vaccine and Guidance for Use in Infants and Children," *MMWR Morb Mortal Wkly Rep*, 2008, 57(39):1079-80.

Centers for Disease Control and Prevention (CDC), "Unusual Syndrome With Fatalities Among Premature Infants: Association With a New Intravenous Vitamin E Product," *MMWR Morb Mortal Wkly Rep*, 1984, 33(14):198-9.

Centers for Disease Control and Prevention (CDC), "Syncope After Vaccination-United States, January 2005-July 2007," *MMWR Morb Mortal Wkly Rep*, 2008, 2;57(17):457-60.

Centers for Disease Control and Prevention (CDC), "Updated Recommendations of the Advisory Committee on Immunization Practices (ACIP) Regarding Routine Poliovirus Vaccination," *MMWR Morb Mortal Wkly Rep*, 2009, 58(30):829-30.

Kroger AT, Atkinson WL, Marcuse EK, Pickering LK. General recommendations on immunization - recommendations of the Advisory Committee on Immunization Practices (ACIP). *MMWR Recomm Rep*. 2011;60(RR-2):1-64.

Prymula R, Siegrist CA, Chlibek R, et al, "Effect of Prophylactic Paracetamol Administration at Time of Vaccination on Febrile Reactions and Antibody Responses in Children: Two Open-Label, Randomised Controlled Trials," *Lancet*, 2009, 374(9698):1339-50.

Rubin LG, Levin MJ, Ljungman P, et al. 2013 IDSA clinical practice guideline for vaccination of the immunocompromised host. *Clin Infect Dis.* 2014;58(3):e44-e100.

◆ **Diphtheria and Tetanus Toxoids and Acellular Pertussis Adsorbed, and Inactivated Poliovirus Vaccine Combined** *see* Diphtheria and Tetanus Toxoids, Acellular Pertussis, and Poliovirus Vaccine *on page 682*

◆ **Diphtheria and Tetanus Toxoids and Acellular Pertussis Adsorbed, Hepatitis B (Recombinant) and Inactivated Poliovirus Vaccine Combined** *see* Diphtheria, Tetanus Toxoids, Acellular Pertussis, Hepatitis B (Recombinant), and Poliovirus (Inactivated) Vaccine *on page 690*

Diphtheria and Tetanus Toxoids, and Acellular Pertussis Vaccine

(dif THEER ee a & TET a nus TOKS oyds & ay CEL yoo lar per TUS sis vak SEEN)

Medication Safety Issues

Sound-alike/look-alike issues:

Adacel (Tdap) may be confused with Daptacel (DTaP)

Tdap (Adacel, Boostrix) may be confused with DTaP (Daptacel, Infanrix, Tripedia)

Administration issues:

Carefully review product labeling to prevent inadvertent administration of Tdap when DTaP is indicated. Tdap contains lower amounts of diphtheria toxoid and some pertussis antigens than DTaP.

Tdap is not indicated for use in children <10 years of age

DTaP is not indicated for use in persons ≥7 years of age

Guidelines are available in case of inadvertent administration of these products; refer to ACIP recommendations, February 2006 available at http://www.cdc.gov/mmwr/preview/mmwrhtml/rr55e223a1.htm

Other safety concerns:

DTaP: Diphtheria and tetanus toxoids and acellular pertussis vaccine

DTP: Diphtheria and tetanus toxoids and pertussis vaccine (unspecified pertussis antigens)

DTwP: Diphtheria and tetanus toxoids and whole-cell pertussis vaccine (no longer available on U.S. market)

Tdap: Tetanus toxoid, reduced diphtheria toxoid, and acellular pertussis vaccine

Related Information

Immunization Administration Recommendations *on page 2368*

Immunization Guidelines *on page 2373*

Brand Names: U.S. Adacel; Boostrix; Daptacel; Infanrix

Brand Names: Canada Adacel; Boostrix

Therapeutic Category Vaccine

Generic Availability (U.S.) No

Use

DTaP (Daptacel, Infanrix): Active immunization for prevention of diphtheria, tetanus, and pertussis (FDA approved in ages 6 weeks through 6 years); has also been used for wound management for the prevention of tetanus

Tdap:

Adacel: Active booster immunization for prevention of diphtheria, tetanus, and pertussis (FDA approved in ages 10 to 64 years)

Boostrix: Active booster immunization for prevention of diphtheria, tetanus, and pertussis (FDA approved in ages ≥10 years); has also been used for wound management for the prevention of tetanus

The Advisory Committee on Immunization Practices (ACIP) recommends routine vaccination for the following:

Infants and Children 6 weeks to <7 years (DTaP):

• For primary immunization against diphtheria, tetanus, and pertussis (CDC/ACIP [Rennels, 2000])

• Pediatric patients wounded in bombings or similar mass casualty events, have penetrating injuries or nonintact skin exposure, and have an uncertain vaccination history should receive a tetanus booster with DTaP if no contraindications exist (CDC [Chapman, 2008])

Children 7 to 10 years (Tdap):

• Children not fully vaccinated against pertussis should receive a single dose of Tdap if no contraindications exist (CDC, 60[1], 2011)

• Children never vaccinated against diphtheria, tetanus, or pertussis, or whose vaccination status is not known should receive a series of three vaccinations containing tetanus and diphtheria toxoids and the first dose should be with Tdap (CDC, 60[1], 2011)

Children ≥11 years and Adolescents (Tdap):

• A single dose of Tdap as a booster dose in adolescents who have completed the recommended childhood DTaP vaccination series (preferred age of administration is 11 to 12 years) (CDC, 60[1], 2011)

Children ≥11 years, Adolescents, and Adults (Tdap):

• Persons wounded in bombings or similar mass casualty events and who cannot confirm receipt of a tetanus booster within the previous 5 years and who have penetrating injuries or nonintact skin exposure should receive a single dose of Tdap (CDC [Chapman, 2008])

Adolescent and Adult females: Pregnant females should receive a single dose with each pregnancy, preferably between 27 to 36 weeks gestation (CDC, 62[7], 2013)

Adults ≥19 years (including adults ≥65 years) (Tdap): A single dose of Tdap should be given to all patients who have not previously received Tdap or for whom their vaccine status is unknown. Following administration of Tdap, Td vaccine should be used for routine boosters (CDC/ACIP [Bridges, 2014]). The following patients, who have not yet received Tdap or for whom vaccine status is not known, should receive a single dose of Tdap as soon as feasible:

• Close contacts of children <12 months of age: Tdap should ideally be administered at least 2 weeks prior to beginning close contact (CDC/ACIP, 60[41], 2011; CDC [Kretsinger, 2006])

• Healthcare providers with direct patient contact (CDC [Kretsinger, 2006])

Note: Tdap is currently recommended for a single dose only (all age groups) (CDC, 60[1], 2011; CDC/ACIP, 61 [25], 2012) except pregnant females (CDC, 62 [7], 2013)

Pregnancy Risk Factor B/C (manufacturer specific)

Pregnancy Considerations Animal reproduction studies have not been conducted with all products; when conducted, adverse effects to the fetus were not observed in developmental toxicity studies. Inactivated bacterial vaccines have not been shown to cause increased risks to the fetus (CDC, 60[2], 2011). Daptacel and Infanrix are not recommended for use in a pregnant woman or any patient ≥7 years of age. Using data collected from 2005-2010 VAERS, there were not any patterns of adverse maternal, fetal, or neonatal outcomes identified following maternal use of the Tdap vaccine (Zheteyeva, 2012). All pregnant females should receive a single dose of Tdap during each pregnancy, regardless of previous vaccination status, preferably between 27-36 weeks gestation. Alternately, administration of Tdap can be given immediately postpartum to all women who have not previously been vaccinated with Tdap in order to protect the mother and infant from pertussis (CDC, 62[7], 2013). In case of an ongoing local pertussis epidemic, pregnant women should be vaccinated with Tdap for their own protection as is recommended for nonpregnant women, regardless of fetal gestational age. In addition, if a tetanus toxoid–containing vaccine is needed as standard care for wound management, Tdap may be given regardless of fetal gestational age if otherwise indicated. However, if Tdap is used prior to 27-36 weeks gestation in these instances, women should not receive more than 1 dose during the same pregnancy (ACOG, 2013).

Pregnancy registries have been established for women who may become exposed to Boostrix® (888-452-9622) or Adacel® (800-822-2463) while pregnant.

Breast-Feeding Considerations It is not known if this vaccine is excreted into breast milk. The manufacturer recommends that caution be used if administered to a nursing woman. Breast-feeding is not a contraindication to vaccine administration. Women who have not previously had a dose of Tdap should receive a dose postpartum to help prevent pertussis in infants <12 months of age (CDC, 62[7], 2013). Inactivated vaccines do not affect the safety of breast-feeding for the mother or the infant. Breast-feeding infants should be vaccinated according to the recommended schedules (CDC, 60[2], 2011).

Contraindications Severe allergic reaction to diphtheria toxoid, tetanus toxoid, pertussis-containing vaccine, or any component; encephalopathy occurring within 7 days of administration of a previous dose of a pertussis-containing vaccine that is not attributable to another cause; progressive neurological disorder, including infantile spasms, uncontrolled epilepsy, or progressive encephalopathy; (pertussis vaccine should be withheld until the clinical condition has stabilized)

Warnings Immediate treatment (including epinephrine 1:1000) for anaphylactic and/or acute hypersensitivity reactions should be available during vaccine use. Subsequent vaccination with a pertussis containing vaccine should be carefully considered if any of the following reactions occur with a temporal relationship to a previous dose of any pertussis-containing vaccine: Temperature ≥40.5°C (105°F) within 48 hours, not attributable to another identifiable cause; collapse or shock-like state (hypotonic-hyporesponsive episode) within 48 hours, persistent crying lasting ≥3 hours within 48 hours, or convulsions with or without fever occurring within 3 days. Guillain-Barré syndrome occurring within 6 weeks of vaccines containing tetanus toxoid has been reported. Patients with a history of severe local reaction (Arthustype) following a previous tetanus toxoid dose should not be given further routine or emergency doses of Td more frequently than every 10 years, even if using for wound management with wounds that are not clean or minor; these patients generally have high serum antitoxin levels. Boostrix and Adacel contain reduced antigens and are not indicated for use in the primary vaccine series (ages 6 weeks to 6 years). Apnea has occurred following intramuscular vaccine administration in premature infants; consider clinical status implications.

Syncope has been reported with use of injectable vaccines and may be accompanied by transient visual disturbances, weakness, or tonic-clonic movements. Procedures should be in place to avoid injuries from falling and to restore cerebral perfusion if syncope occurs (CDC, 57[17], 2008).

Injection may contain polysorbate 80 (Tween 80) which may cause allergic reactions in susceptible individuals. In premature neonates, thrombocytopenia, ascites, pulmonary deterioration, and renal and hepatic failure have been reported after receiving parenteral products containing polysorbate 80 (Alade, 1986; CDC, 1984).

Precautions The decision to administer or delay vaccination because of current or recent febrile illness depends on the severity of symptoms and the etiology of the disease. Immunization should be delayed during the course of an acute severe febrile illness; may administer to patients with mild acute illness (with or without fever). Use with caution in severely immunocompromised patients (eg, patients receiving chemo/radiation therapy or other immunosuppressive therapy, including high-dose corticosteroids); may have a reduced response to vaccination; inactivated vaccines should be administered ≥2 weeks prior to planned immunosuppression when feasible (IDSA [Rubin, 2013]). In general, household and close contacts of persons with altered immunocompetence may receive all age-appropriate vaccines. Vaccination may not result in effective immunity in all patients. Response depends upon multiple factors (eg, type of vaccine, age of patient) and may be improved by administering the vaccine at the recommended dose, route, and interval (CDC/ACIP [Kroger, 2011]).

A family history of seizures is not a contraindication to use of DTaP; however, use in patients with a history of seizure disorder, progressive neurologic disease, or conditions predisposing to seizures should be deferred until health status can be assessed and condition stabilized. Antipyretics have not been shown to prevent febrile seizures; antipyretics may be used to treat fever or discomfort following vaccination (CDC/ACIP [Kroger, 2011]). One study reported that routine prophylactic administration of acetaminophen to prevent fever prior to vaccination decreased the immune response of some vaccines; the clinical significance of this reduction in immune response has not been established (Prymula, 2009). Use with caution in patients with coagulation disorders, including thrombocytopenia, due to an increased risk for bleeding following I.M. injection; if the patient receives antihemophilia or other similar therapy, I.M. injection can be scheduled shortly after such therapy is administered.

Use of this vaccine for specific medical and/or other indications (eg, immunocompromising conditions, hepatic or kidney disease, diabetes) is also addressed in the ACIP Recommended Immunization Schedule (CDC/ACIP [Akinsanya-Beysolow, 2014]; CDC/ACIP [Bridges, 2014]). Specific recommendations for use of this vaccine in immunocompromised patients with asplenia, cancer, HIV infection, cerebrospinal fluid leaks, cochlear implants, hematopoietic stem cell transplant (prior to or after), sickle cell disease, solid organ transplant (prior to or after), or those receiving immunosuppressive therapy for chronic conditions, as well as contacts of immunocompromised patients, are available from the IDSA (Rubin, 2014). Some products may contain natural latex/natural rubber; use with caution in patients who may be susceptible to hypersensitivity reactions.

Adverse Reactions All serious adverse reactions must be reported to the U.S. Department of Health and Human Services (DHHS) Vaccine Adverse Event Reporting System (VAERS) 1-800-822-7967 or online at https://vaers.hhs.gov/esub/index. In Canada, adverse reactions may be reported to local provincial/territorial health agencies or to the Vaccine Safety Section at Public Health Agency of Canada (1-866-844-0018).

Daptacel®, Infanrix® (incidence of erythema, swelling, and fever increases with successive doses):
Central nervous system: Drowsiness, fever, fussiness, irritability, lethargy
Gastrointestinal: Appetite decreased, vomiting
Local: Pain, redness, swelling, tenderness

Miscellaneous: Prolonged or persistent crying, refusal to play

Rare but important or life-threatening: Allergic reaction, anaphylactic reactions, angioedema, apnea, bronchitis, cellulitis, cough, cyanosis, diarrhea, ear pain, encephalopathy, erythema, fatigue, headache, hypersensitivity, hypotonia, hypotonic-hyporesponsive episode, immune thrombocytopenia (ITP), infantile spasm, injection site reaction (abscess, cellulitis, induration, mass, nodule, rash), intussusception, limb swelling, lymphadenopathy, nausea, pruritus, rash, respiratory tract infection, seizure, screaming, somnolence, sudden infant death syndrome, thrombocytopenia, urticaria

Adacel®; Boostrix®:

Central nervous system: Chills, fatigue/tiredness, headache

Dermatologic: Rash

Gastrointestinal: Gastrointestinal symptoms, includes abdominal pain, diarrhea, nausea and/or vomiting

Local: Arm circumference increased, injection site pain, redness, swelling

Neuromuscular & skeletal: Body aches/muscle weakness, soreness/swollen joints

Miscellaneous: Lymph node swelling

Rare but important or life-threatening: Anaphylactic reaction, arthralgia, back pain, diabetes mellitus, encephalitis, exanthema, facial palsy, GBS, Henoch-Schönlein purpura (IgA vasculitis), hypersensitivity reactions, hypoesthesia, injection site reaction (bruising, induration, inflammation, mass, nodule, pruritus, sterile abscess, warmth), limb swelling (extensive), lymphadenitis, lymphadenopathy, myalgia, myocarditis, myositis, nerve compression, paresthesia, pruritus, seizure, syncope, urticaria

Drug Interactions

Metabolism/Transport Effects None known.

Avoid Concomitant Use There are no known interactions where it is recommended to avoid concomitant use.

Increased Effect/Toxicity There are no known significant interactions involving an increase in effect.

Decreased Effect

The levels/effects of Diphtheria and Tetanus Toxoids, and Acellular Pertussis Vaccine may be decreased by: Belimumab; Fingolimod; Immunosuppressants; Meningococcal Polysaccharide (Groups A / C / Y and W-135) Tetanus Toxoid Conjugate Vaccine

Stability Store at 2°C to 8°C (35°F to 46°F); do not freeze; discard if frozen. The following stability information has also been reported for Infanrix: May be stored at room temperature for up to 72 hours (Cohen, 2007). Tripedia may be used to reconstitute ActHIB for children ≥15 months of age

Mechanism of Action Promotes active immunity to diphtheria, tetanus, and pertussis by inducing production of specific antibodies.

Dosing: Usual

Primary immunization: Infants and Children 6 weeks to <7 years: **Note:** Whenever possible, the same product should be used for all doses. Preterm infants should be vaccinated according to their chronological age from birth. DTaP (Daptacel, Infanrix): I.M.: 0.5 mL per dose for a total of 5 doses administered as follows:

Three doses, usually given at 2-, 4-, and 6 months of age; may be given as early as 6 weeks of age and repeated every 4 to 8 weeks

Fourth dose: Given at ~15 to 20 months of age but at least 6 months after third dose. The fourth dose may be given as early as 12 months of age but at least 6 months must have elapsed between the third dose and the fourth dose.

Fifth dose: Given at 4 to 6 years of age, prior to starting school or kindergarten; if the fourth dose is given at ≥4 years of age, the fifth dose may be omitted

Catch-up immunization: CDC (ACIP) Recommendations (Akinsany-Beysolow, 2014): **Note:** Do not restart the series. If doses have been given, begin the below schedule at the applicable dose number.

Infants and children who start primary immunization series ≥4 months of age through 6 years (prior to 7th birthday): DTaP (Daptacel, Infanrix): I.M.: 0.5 mL per dose for a total of 4 to 5 doses administered as follows: 3 doses at least 4 weeks apart, followed 6 months later with dose 4; a 5th dose may be given 6 months later (the 5th dose is not necessary if the child received the 4th dose after 4 years of age)

Children 7 to 8 years of age not fully vaccinated against pertussis, or never vaccinated against diphtheria, tetanus, or pertussis, or whose vaccination status is not known: I.M.: 0.5 mL per dose; first dose: Tdap (Adacel, Boostrix) given on the elected date, followed by a series of 2 vaccinations containing tetanus and diphtheria toxoids (Td product, see monograph for specific details) (CDC, 60[1], 2011). Tdap can be administered regardless of the interval between the last tetanus or diphtheria toxoid-containing vaccine.

Booster immunization (Adacel, Boostrix): Children ≥10 years, Adolescents, and Adults: **Note:** Tdap can be administered regardless of the interval between the last tetanus or diphtheria toxoid-containing vaccine. Tdap is currently recommended for a single dose only (CDC, 60 [1], 2011; CDC/ACIP, 61[25], 2012), except pregnant females (CDC, 62[7], 2013). **Note:** If Tdap was received as part of a catch-up series, Tdap should not be administered as the booster dose; use Td instead.

CDC (ACIP) recommendations:

Children and Adolescents 10 to 18 years: Tdap (Adacel, Boostrix): I.M.: 0.5 mL per dose as a single dose. Tdap should be given as a single booster dose at age 11 or 12 years in children who have completed a childhood vaccination series, followed by booster doses of Td every 10 years. Children who have not received Tdap at age 11 or 12 should receive a single dose of Tdap in place of a single Td booster dose (CDC/ACIP [Broder, 2006]; CDC, 60[1], 2011]).

Adults ≥19 years: Tdap (Adacel, Boostrix): I.M.: 0.5 mL per dose. A single dose of Tdap should be given to replace a single dose of the 10 year Td booster in patients who have not previously received Tdap or for whom vaccine status is not known. A single dose of Tdap is recommended for healthcare personnel who have not previously received Tdap and who have direct patient contact (CDC/ACIP [Kretsinger, 2006]). Tdap should be administered regardless of interval since last tetanus- or diphtheria-containing vaccine (CDC/ACIP, 61[25], 2012).

Manufacturer's labeling: Tdap (Adacel, Boostrix): Children ≥10 years, Adolescents, and Adults: I.M.: 0.5 mL as a single dose, administered 5 years after last dose of tetanus toxoid, diphtheria toxoid, and/or pertussis-containing vaccine

Tetanus prophylaxis in wound management: Children ≥7 years, Adolescents, and Adults: Tdap (Adacel, Boostrix): I.M.: 0.5 mL as a single dose may be used as an alternative to Td vaccine when a tetanus toxoid-containing vaccine is needed for wound management, and in whom the pertussis component is also indicated. Tetanus prophylaxis in patients with wounds should consider if the wound is clean or contaminated, the immunization status of the patient, proper use of tetanus toxoid and/or tetanus immune globulin (TIG), wound cleaning, and (if required) surgical debridement and the proper use of antibiotics. Patients with an uncertain or incomplete tetanus immunization status should have additional follow-up to ensure a series is completed. Patients with a history of Arthus reaction following a previous dose of a tetanus toxoid-containing vaccine should not receive a tetanus toxoid-containing vaccine until >10 years after the most recent dose even if they have a wound that is neither clean nor minor. See table.

Tetanus Prophylaxis Wound Management

History of Tetanus Immunization (Doses)	Clean, Minor Wounds		All Other Wounds[1]	
	Tetanus toxoid[2]	TIG	Tetanus toxoid[2]	TIG
Uncertain or <3 doses	Yes	No	Yes	Yes
3 or more doses	No[3]	No	No[4]	No

[1]Such as, but not limited to, wounds contaminated with dirt, feces, soil, and saliva; puncture wounds; wounds from crushing, tears, burns, and frostbite.

[2]Tetanus toxoid in this chart refers to a tetanus toxoid containing vaccine. For children <7 years old DTaP (DT, if pertussis vaccine contraindicated) is preferred to tetanus toxoid alone. For children ≥7 years of age and Adults, Td preferred to tetanus toxoid alone; Tdap may be preferred if the patient has not previously been vaccinated with Tdap.

[3]Yes, if ≥10 years since last dose.

[4]Yes, if ≥5 years since last dose.

Abbreviations: **DT** = Diphtheria and Tetanus Toxoids (formulation for age ≤6 years); **DTaP** = Diphtheria and Tetanus Toxoids, and Acellular Pertussis (formulation for age ≤6 years; Daptacel, Infanrix); **Td** = Diphtheria and Tetanus Toxoids (formulation for age ≥7 years; Tenivac™); **TT** = Tetanus toxoid (adsorbed [formulation for age ≥7 years]); **Tdap** = Diphtheria and Tetanus Toxoids, and Acellular Pertussis (Adacel or Boostrix [formulations for age ≥7 years]); **TIG** = Tetanus Immune Globulin

Adapted from the Yellow Book 2010, Chapter 2, *Routine Vaccine-Preventable Diseases, Tetanus*; Available at www.cdc.gov/yellowbook; and *MMWR*, 2006, 55:RR-17.

Dosing adjustment in renal impairment: There are no dosage adjustments provided in the manufacturer's labeling.

Dosing adjustment in hepatic impairment: There are no dosage adjustments provided in the manufacturer's labeling.

Administration Shake vial well before withdrawing the dose; administer I.M. into midlateral aspect of the thigh in infants and small children; administer in the deltoid area to older children and adults; **not for I.V., intradermal, or SubQ administration.** Adolescents and adults should be vaccinated while seated or lying down. U.S. law requires that the date of administration, the vaccine manufacturer, lot number of vaccine, and the administering person's name, title, and address be entered into the patient's permanent medical record.

Monitoring Parameters Observe for syncope for 15 minutes following administration. If seizure-like activity associated with syncope occurs, maintain patient in supine or Trendelenburg position to reestablish adequate cerebral perfusion.

Additional Information Adacel is formulated with the same antigens found in Daptacel but with reduced quantities of tetanus and pertussis; Boostrix is formulated with the same antigens found in Infanrix but in reduced quantities. Use of Adacel or Boostrix in the primary immunization series or to complete the primary series has not been evaluated.

The ACIP considers Adacel and Boostrix to be interchangeable when administered to adolescents for childhood vaccination according to the Child and Adolescent Immunization Schedule.

In order to maximize vaccination rates, the ACIP recommends simultaneous administration (ie, >1 vaccine on the same day at different anatomic sites) of all age-appropriate vaccines (live or inactivated) for which a person is eligible at a single visit, unless contraindications exist. If available, the use of combination vaccines is generally preferred over separate injections, taking into consideration provider assessment, patient preference, and potential adverse events. If separate vaccines being used, evaluate product information regarding same syringe compatibility of vaccines. Separate needles and syringes should be used for each injection. The ACIP prefers each dose of specific vaccine in a series come from the same manufacturer if possible (CDC/ACIP [Kroger, 2011]).

For additional information, please refer to the following website: http://www.cdc.gov/vaccines/vpd-vac/.

Dosage Forms Excipient information presented when available (limited, particularly for generics); consult specific product labeling.

Injection, suspension [Tdap, booster formulation]:

Adacel®: Diphtheria 2 Lf units, tetanus 5 Lf units, and acellular pertussis antigens [detoxified pertussis toxin 2.5 mcg, filamentous hemagglutinin 5 mcg, pertactin 3 mcg, fimbriae (types 2 and 3) 5 mcg] per 0.5 mL (0.5 mL) [contains aluminum; may contain natural rubber/natural latex in prefilled syringe]

Boostrix®: Diphtheria 2.5 Lf units, tetanus 5 Lf units, and acellular pertussis antigens [inactivated pertussis toxin 8 mcg, filamentous hemagglutinin 8 mcg, pertactin 2.5 mcg] per 0.5 mL (0.5 mL) [contains aluminum and polysorbate 80; may contain natural rubber/natural latex in prefilled syringe]

Injection, suspension [DTaP, active immunization formulation]:

Daptacel®: Diphtheria 15 Lf units, tetanus 5 Lf units, and acellular pertussis antigens [detoxified pertussis toxin 10 mcg, filamentous hemagglutinin 5 mcg, pertactin 3 mcg, fimbriae (types 2 and 3) 5 mcg] per 0.5 mL (0.5 mL) [preservative free; contains aluminum]

Infanrix®: Diphtheria 25 Lf units, tetanus 10 Lf units, and acellular pertussis antigens [inactivated pertussis toxin 25 mcg, filamentous hemagglutinin 25 mcg, pertactin 8 mcg] per 0.5 mL (0.5 mL) [preservative free; contains aluminum and polysorbate 80]

Infanrix®: Diphtheria 25 Lf units, tetanus 10 Lf units, and acellular pertussis antigens [inactivated pertussis toxin 25 mcg, filamentous hemagglutinin 25 mcg, pertactin 8 mcg] per 0.5 mL (0.5 mL) [preservative free; contains aluminum and polysorbate 80; prefilled syringes contain natural rubber/natural latex] [DSC]

References

AAP Steering Committee on Quality Improvement and Management, Subcommittee on Febrile Seizures American Academy of Pediatrics. Febrile seizures: clinical practice guideline for the long-term management of the child with simple febrile seizures. *Pediatrics.* 2008;121 (6):1281-1286.

Adacel (tetanus toxoid, reduced diphtheria toxoid and acellular pertussis vaccine adsorbed) [prescribing information]. Swiftwater, PA: Sanofi Pasteur Inc; March 2014.

Akinsanya-Beysolow I; Advisory Committee on Immunization Practices (ACIP); ACIP Child/Adolescent Immunization Work Group; Centers for Disease Control and Prevention (CDC). Advisory Committee on Immunization Practices recommended immunization schedules for persons aged 0 through 18 years – United States, 2014. *MMWR Morb Mortal Wkly Rep.* 2014;63(5):108-109. Available at http://www.cdc.gov/vaccines/schedules/downloads/child/0-18yrs-child-combined-schedule.pdf

Alade SL, Brown RE, Paquet A Jr. Polysorbate 80 and e-ferol toxicity. *Pediatrics.* 1986;77(4):593-597.

Bridges CB, Coyne-Beasley T; Advisory Committee on Immunization Practices (ACIP); ACIP Adult Immunization Work Group; Centers for Disease Control and Prevention (CDC). Advisory Committee on Immunization Practices recommended immunization schedule for adults aged 19 years or older – United States, 2014. *MMWR Morb Mortal Wkly Rep.* 2014;63(5):110-112. Available at http://www.cdc.gov/vaccines/schedules/downloads/adult/adult-combined-schedule.pdf

Broder KR, Cortese MM, Iskander JK, et al. Preventing tetanus, diphtheria, and pertussis among adolescents: use of tetanus toxoid, reduced diphtheria toxoid and acellular pertussis vaccines recommendations of the Advisory Committee on Immunization Practices (ACIP). *MMWR Recomm Rep.* 2006;55(RR-3):1-34.

Centers for Disease Control and Prevention (CDC). Syncope after vaccination – United States, January 2005-July 2007. *MMWR Morb Mortal Wkly Rep.* 2008;57(17):457-460.

Centers for Disease Control and Prevention (CDC). Updated recommendations for use of tetanus toxoid, reduced diphtheria toxoid and acellular pertussis (Tdap) vaccine from the Advisory Committee on Immunization Practices, 2010. *MMWR Morb Mortal Wkly Rep.* 2011;60(1):13-15.

Centers for Disease Control and Prevention (CDC). Updated recommendations for use of tetanus toxoid, reduced diphtheria toxoid, and acellular pertussis vaccine (Tdap) in pregnant women – Advisory Committee on Immunization Practices (ACIP), 2012. *MMWR Morb Mortal Wkly Rep.* 2013;62(7):131-135.

Centers for Disease Control and Prevention (CDC). Updated recommendations for use of tetanus toxoid, reduced diphtheria toxoid, and acellular pertussis (Tdap) vaccine in adults aged 65 years and older – Advisory Committee on Immunization Practices (ACIP). *MMWR Morb Mortal Wkly Rep.* 2012;61(25):468-470.

Centers for Disease Control and Prevention (CDC). Updated recommendations for use of tetanus toxoid, reduced diphtheria toxoid, and acellular pertussis vaccine (Tdap) in pregnant women and persons who have or anticipate having close contact with an infant aged <12 months – Advisory Committee on Immunization Practices (ACIP), 2011. *MMWR Morb Mortal Wkly Rep.* 2011;60(41):1424-1426.

Centers for Disease Control and Prevention (CDC). Unusual syndrome with fatalities among premature infants: association with a new intravenous vitamin E product. *MMWR Morb Mortal Wkly Rep.* 1984;33 (14):198-199.

Centers for Disease Control and Prevention (CDC). Vaccines for children program, vaccines to prevent diphtheria, tetanus and pertussis. Resolution no. 6/11-2. Available at http://www.cdc.gov/vaccines/programs/vfc/downloads/resolutions/0611dtap.pdf

Chapman LE, Sullivent EE, Grohskopf LA, et al. Recommendations for postexposure interventions to prevent infection with hepatitis B virus, hepatitis C virus, or human immunodeficiency virus, and tetanus in persons wounded during bombings and other mass-casualty events – United States, 2008: recommendations of the Centers for Disease Control and Prevention (CDC). *MMWR Recomm Rep.* 2008;57(RR-6):1-21.

Cohen V, Jellinek SP, Teperikidis L, Berkovits E, Goldman WM. Room-temperature storage of medications labeled for refrigeration. *Am J Health-Syst Pharm.* 2007;64(16):1711-1715.

Daptacel (diphtheria and tetanus toxoids and acellular pertussis vaccine adsorbed) [prescribing information]. Swiftwater, PA: Sanofi Pasteur Inc; October 2013.

Kretsinger K, Broder KR, Cortese MM, et al. Preventing tetanus, diphtheria, and pertussis among adults: use of tetanus toxoid, reduced diphtheria toxoid and acellular pertussis vaccine. *MMWR Recomm Rep.* 2006;55(RR-17):1-37.

Kroger AT, Atkinson WL, Marcuse EK, Pickering LK. General recommendations on immunization - recommendations of the Advisory Committee on Immunization Practices (ACIP). *MMWR Recomm Rep.* 2011;60(RR-2):1-64.

Prymula R, Siegrist CA, Chlibek R, et al. Effect of prophylactic paracetamol administration at time of vaccination on febrile reactions and antibody responses in children: two open-label, randomised controlled trials. *Lancet.* 2009;374(9698):1339-1350.

Rubin LG, Levin MJ, Ljungman P, et al. 2013 IDSA clinical practice guideline for vaccination of the immunocompromised host. *Clin Infect Dis.* 2014;58(3):e44-e100.

Use of diphtheria toxoid-tetanus toxoid-acellular pertussis vaccine as a five-dose series. Supplemental recommendations of the Advisory Committee on Immunization Practices (ACIP). *MMWR Recomm Rep.* 2000;49(RR-13):1-8.

Zheteyeva YA, Moro PL, Tepper NK, et al, "Adverse Event Reports After Tetanus Toxoid, Reduced Diphtheria Toxoid, and Acellular Pertussis Vaccines in Pregnant Women," *Am J Obstet Gynecol*, 2012, 207 (1):59.e1-7.

◆ **Diphtheria, Tetanus Toxoids, Acellular Pertussis (DTaP)** *see* Diphtheria and Tetanus Toxoids, Acellular Pertussis, and Poliovirus Vaccine *on page 682*

◆ **Diphtheria, Tetanus Toxoids, Acellular Pertussis (DTaP)** *see* Diphtheria and Tetanus Toxoids, Acellular Pertussis, Poliovirus and *Haemophilus* b Conjugate Vaccine *on page 684*

Diphtheria, Tetanus Toxoids, Acellular Pertussis, Hepatitis B (Recombinant), and Poliovirus (Inactivated) Vaccine

(dif THEER ee a, TET a nus TOKS oyds, ay CEL yoo lar per TUS sis, hep a TYE tis bee ree KOM be nant, & POE lee oh VYE rus in ak ti VAY ted vak SEEN)

Related Information

Immunization Administration Recommendations *on page 2368*

Immunization Guidelines *on page 2373*

Brand Names: U.S. Pediarix®

Brand Names: Canada Pediarix®

Therapeutic Category Vaccine

Generic Availability (U.S.) No

Use Combination vaccine for the active immunization against diphtheria, tetanus, pertussis, hepatitis B virus (all known subtypes), and poliomyelitis (caused by poliovirus types 1, 2, and 3) (FDA approved in ages 6 weeks through 6 years)

The Advisory Committee on Immunization Practices (ACIP) recommends Pediarix for the following (CDC, 52 [10], 2003):

• Primary vaccination for DTaP, Hep B, and IPV in children at 2, 4, and 6 months of age.

• To complete the primary vaccination series in children who have received DTaP (Infanrix) or a birth-dose of hepatitis B and who are scheduled to receive the other components of the vaccine. Whenever feasible, the same manufacturer should be used to provide the pertussis component; however, vaccination should not be deferred if a specific brand is not known or is not available. HepB and IPV from different manufacturers are interchangeable.

Pregnancy Risk Factor C

Pregnancy Considerations Reproduction studies have not been conducted; not indicated for women of child-bearing age.

Breast-Feeding Considerations Not indicated for women of childbearing age.

Contraindications Hypersensitivity to any component including yeast, neomycin, and polymyxin B; encephalopathy occurring within 7 days of administration of a previous dose of a pertussis-containing vaccine that is not attributable to another cause; progressive neurological disorder, including infantile spasms, uncontrolled epilepsy, or progressive encephalopathy (pertussis vaccine should be withheld until the clinical condition has stabilized).

Warnings Immediate treatment (including epinephrine 1:1000) for anaphylactic and/or hypersensitivity reactions should be available during vaccine use. Subsequent vaccination with a pertussis-containing vaccine should be carefully considered if the following reactions occur with a temporal relationship to a previous dose of any pertussis-containing vaccine: Temperature ≥40.5°C (105°F) within 48 hours not attributable to another identifiable cause, collapse or shock-like state (hypotonic-hyporesponsive episode) within 48 hours, persistent crying lasting ≥3 hours within 48 hours, or convulsions with or without fever occurring within 3 days. Guillain-Barré syndrome occurring within 6 weeks of vaccines containing tetanus toxoid has been reported. A family history of seizures is not a contraindication to use of DTaP; however, use in patients with or history of seizure disorder, progressive neurologic disease, or conditions predisposing to seizures should be deferred until health status can be assessed and condition stabilized. Due to a higher rate of fever with this combination formulation than with individual vaccines, antipyretic prophylaxis at the time of and following vaccination may be considered for patients at high risk for seizures (per the manufacturer). However, antipyretics have not been shown to prevent febrile seizures; antipyretics may be used to treat fever or discomfort following vaccination (CDC/ACIP [Kroger, 2011]). One study reported that routine prophylactic administration of acetaminophen to prevent fever prior to vaccination decreased the immune response of some vaccines; the clinical significance of this reduction in immune response has not been established (Prymula, 2009). Apnea has occurred following intramuscular vaccine administration in premature infants; consider clinical status implications. Syncope has been reported with use of injectable vaccines and may be accompanied by transient visual disturbances, weakness, or tonic-clonic movements. Procedures should be in place to avoid injuries from falling and to restore cerebral perfusion if syncope occurs (CDC, 57[17], 2008). Injection contains polysorbate 80 (Tween 80) which may cause allergic reactions in susceptible individuals. In premature neonates, thrombocytopenia, ascites, pulmonary deterioration, and renal and hepatic failure have been reported after receiving parenteral products containing polysorbate 80 (Alade, 1986; CDC, 1984).

Precautions The decision to administer or delay vaccination because of current or recent febrile illness depends on the severity of symptoms and the etiology of the disease. Immunization should be delayed during the course of an acute severe febrile illness; may administer to patients with mild acute illness (with or without fever). Use with caution in severely immunocompromised patients (eg, patients receiving chemo/radiation therapy or other immunosuppressive therapy, including high-dose corticosteroids); may have a reduced response to vaccination; inactivated vaccines should be administered ≥2 weeks prior to planned immunosuppression when feasible (IDSA [Rubin, 2014]). In general, household and close contacts of persons with altered immunocompetence may receive all age-appropriate vaccines. Vaccination may not result in effective immunity in all patients. Response depends upon multiple factors (eg, type of vaccine, age of patient) and may be improved by administering the vaccine at the recommended dose, route, and interval (CDC/ACIP [Kroger, 2011]).

Use with caution in patients with coagulation disorders, including thrombocytopenia, due to an increased risk for bleeding following I.M. administration; if the patient receives antihemophilia or other similar therapy, I.M. injection can be scheduled shortly after such therapy is administered.

Infants born of HBsAg-positive mothers should receive monovalent hepatitis B vaccine for birth-dose and hepatitis B immune globulin; infants born of HBsAg-unknown mothers should receive monovalent hepatitis B vaccine for birth-dose; data on use of combination product in these patients to complete the hepatitis B vaccination series is limited but is considered acceptable by the ACIP.

Adverse Reactions All serious adverse reactions must be reported to the U.S. Department of Health and Human Services (DHHS) Vaccine Adverse Event Reporting System (VAERS) 1-800-822-7967 or online at https://vaers.hhs.gov/esub/index. In Canada, adverse reactions may be reported to local provincial/territorial health agencies or to the Vaccine Safety Section at Public Health Agency of Canada (1-866-844-0018).

Adverse events reported within 4 days of vaccination at 2-, 4-, and 6 months of age in patients given Pediarix® concomitantly with Hib conjugate vaccine and PCV7 vaccine.

Central nervous system: Drowsiness, fever, irritability/fussiness

Gastrointestinal: Loss of appetite

Local: Injection site: Pain, redness, swelling

Additional and postmarketing events: Anaphylactic/anaphylactoid reaction, angioedema, anorexia, apnea, arthus-type hypersensitivity reactions, brachial neuritis, bulging fontanelle, consciousness depressed, cough, cranial mononeuropathy, crying, cyanosis, demyelinating disease, diarrhea, dyspnea, encephalitis, erythema, fatigue, febrile convulsion, Guillain-Barré syndrome, hypersensitivity reaction, hypotonia, hypotonic-hyporesponsive episode, injection site reactions (cellulitis, induration, itching, nodule, warmth, vesicles), insomnia, lethargy, limb pain, limb swelling, liver function test abnormalities, nervousness, pallor, peripheral mononeuropathy, petechiae, rash, restlessness, screaming, seizure, SIDS, somnolence, upper respiratory tract infection, urticaria, vomiting

Drug Interactions

Metabolism/Transport Effects None known.

Avoid Concomitant Use There are no known interactions where it is recommended to avoid concomitant use.

Increased Effect/Toxicity There are no known significant interactions involving an increase in effect.

Decreased Effect

The levels/effects of Diphtheria, Tetanus Toxoids, Acellular Pertussis, Hepatitis B (Recombinant), and Poliovirus (Inactivated) Vaccine may be decreased by: Belimumab; Fingolimod; Immunosuppressants; Meningococcal Polysaccharide (Groups A / C / Y and W-135) Tetanus Toxoid Conjugate Vaccine

Stability Store at 2°C to 8°C (36°F to 46°F); do not freeze. Discard if frozen. The following stability information has also been reported for Pediarix: May be stored at room temperature for up to 24 hours (Cohen, 2007).

Mechanism of Action Promotes active immunity to diphtheria, tetanus, pertussis, hepatitis B and poliovirus (types 1, 2 and 3) by inducing production of specific antibodies and antitoxins.

Dosing: Usual

Pediatric: **Primary immunization:** Infants ≥6 weeks and Children <7 years: I.M.: 0.5 mL per dose for a total of three doses administered as follows: 2, 4, and 6 months. Vaccination usually begins at 2 months, but may be started as early as 6 weeks of age. Preterm infants should be vaccinated according to their chronological age from birth.

Note: Infants ≥6 weeks and children previously vaccinated with one or more components of this combination vaccine and who are also scheduled to receive all vaccine components may use Pediarix to complete the series.

Dosing adjustment in renal impairment: There are no dosage adjustments provided in the manufacturer's labeling.

Dosing adjustment in hepatic impairment: There are no dosage adjustments provided in the manufacturer's labeling

Administration Shake well; administer I.M. in either the anterolateral aspect of the thigh or in the deltoid muscle of the upper arm; **not for I.V. or SubQ administration.**

U.S. law requires that the date of administration, name of the vaccine manufacturer, lot number of vaccine, and the administering person's name, title, and address be entered into the patient's permanent medical record.

Monitoring Parameters Observe for syncope for 15 minutes following administration. If seizure-like activity associated with syncope occurs, maintain patient in supine or Trendelenburg position to reestablish adequate cerebral perfusion.

Additional Information Contains the following three pertussis antigens: Inactivated pertussis toxin (PT), filamentous hemagglutinin (FHA), and pertactin. Contains the same diphtheria and tetanus toxoids and pertussis antigens found in Infanrix. Contains the same hepatitis B ▶

surface antigen (HB$_s$Ag) found in Engerix-B (recombinant vaccine). Thimerosal is used during manufacturing, but removed to less than detectable levels in the final suspension.

In order to maximize vaccination rates, the ACIP recommends simultaneous administration (ie, >1 vaccine on the same day at different anatomic sites) of all age-appropriate vaccines (live or inactivated) for which a person is eligible at a single visit, unless contraindications exist. If available, the use of combination vaccine is generally preferred over separate injections, taking into consideration provider assessment, patient preference, and potential adverse events. If separate vaccines being used, evaluate product information regarding same syringe compatibility of vaccines. Separate needles and syringes should be used for each injection. The ACIP prefers each dose of specific vaccine in a series come from the same manufacturer if possible (CDC/ACIP [Kroger, 2011]).

For additional information, please refer to the following website: http://www.cdc.gov/vaccines/vpd-vac/.

Dosage Forms Excipient information presented when available (limited, particularly for generics); consult specific product labeling.

Injection, suspension [preservative free]:

Pediarix®: Diphtheria toxoid 25 Lf, tetanus toxoid 10 Lf, acellular pertussis antigens [inactivated pertussis toxin 25 mcg, filamentous hemagglutin 25 mcg, pertactin 8 mcg, HBsAg 10 mcg, type 1 poliovirus 40 D antigen units, type 2 poliovirus 8 D antigen units and type 3 poliovirus 32 D antigen units] per 0.5 mL (0.5 mL) [contains aluminum, neomycin sulfate (trace amounts), polymyxin B (trace amounts), polysorbate 80, and yeast protein ≤5%; may contain natural rubber/natural latex in prefilled syringe]

References

AAP Steering Committee on Quality Improvement and Management, Subcommittee on Febrile Seizures American Academy of Pediatrics, "Febrile Seizures: Clinical Practice Guideline for the Long-Term Management of the Child With Simple Febrile Seizures," *Pediatrics,* 2008, 121(6):1281-6.

Akinsanya-Beysolow I, Advisory Committee on Immunization Practices (ACIP), ACIP Child/Adolescent Immunization Work Group, et al. Advisory committee on immunization practices recommended immunization schedules for persons 0 through 18 years - United States, 2014. *MMWR Morb Mortal Wkly Rep.* 2014; 63(5):108-109. Full schedule available at http://www.cdc.gov/vaccines/schedules/downloads/child/0-18yrs-child-combined-schedule.pdf

Alade SL, Brown RE, and Paquet A Jr, "Polysorbate 80 and E-Ferol Toxicity," *Pediatrics,* 1986, 77(4):593-7.

Centers for Disease Control and Prevention (CDC). FDA licensure of diphtheria and tetanus toxoids and acellular pertussis adsorbed, hepatitis B (recombinant), and poliovirus vaccine combined, (Pediarix) for use in infants. *MMWR Morb Mortal Wkly Rep.* 2003;52 (10):203-204.

Centers for Disease Control (CDC), "Unusual Syndrome With Fatalities Among Premature Infants: Association With a New Intravenous Vitamin E Product," *MMWR Morb Mortal Wkly Rep,* 1984, 33 (14):198-9.

Centers for Disease Control and Prevention (CDC), "Syncope After Vaccination – United States, January 2005-July 2007," *MMWR Morb Mortal Wkly Rep,* 2008, 57(17):457-60.

Cohen V, Jellinek SP, Teperikidis L, Berkovits E, Goldman WM. Room-temperature storage of medications labeled for refrigeration. *Am J Health-Syst Pharm.* 2007;64(16):1711-1715.

Kroger AT, Atkinson WL, Marcuse EK, Pickering LK. General recommendations on immunization - recommendations of the Advisory Committee on Immunization Practices (ACIP). *MMWR Recomm Rep.* 2011;60(RR-2):1-64.

Prymula R, Siegrist CA, Chlibek R, et al, "Effect of Prophylactic Paracetamol Administration at Time of Vaccination on Febrile Reactions and Antibody Responses in Children: Two Open-Label, Randomised Controlled Trials," *Lancet,* 2009, 374(9698):1339-50.

Rubin LG, Levin MJ, Ljungman P, et al. 2013 IDSA clinical practice guideline for vaccination of the immunocompromised host. *Clin Infect Dis.* 2014;58(3):e44-e100.

◆ **Diphtheria, Tetanus Toxoids, Acellular Pertussis, Hepatitis B (Recombinant), and Poliovirus (Inactivated)**

Vaccine *see* Diphtheria, Tetanus Toxoids, Acellular Pertussis, Hepatitis B (Recombinant), and Poliovirus (Inactivated) Vaccine *on page 690*

◆ **Diphtheria, Tetanus Toxoids, Acellular Pertussis, Hepatitis B (Recombinant), and Poliovirus Vaccine** *see* Diphtheria, Tetanus Toxoids, Acellular Pertussis, Hepatitis B (Recombinant), and Poliovirus (Inactivated) Vaccine *on page 690*

◆ **Diphtheria Toxoid** *see* Diphtheria and Tetanus Toxoids, Acellular Pertussis, Poliovirus and *Haemophilus* b Conjugate Vaccine *on page 684*

◆ **Dipivalyl Epinephrine** *see* Dipivefrin *on page 692*

Dipivefrin (dye PI ve frin)

Brand Names: Canada Ophtho-Dipivefrin™; PMS-Dipivefrin; Propine®

Therapeutic Category Adrenergic Agonist Agent, Ophthalmic; Ophthalmic Agent, Vasoconstrictor

Generic Availability (U.S.) No

Use Reduces elevated IOP in chronic open-angle glaucoma; treatment of ocular hypertension

Pregnancy Risk Factor B

Pregnancy Considerations Adverse events have not been observed in animal reproduction studies when administered orally. Systemic adverse events (eg, arrhythmias, hypertension) have been reported following ophthalmic application; use is not recommended in pregnancy (Razeghinejad, 2011).

Breast-Feeding Considerations Systemic adverse events (eg, arrhythmias, hypertension) have been reported following ophthalmic application; use is not recommended in breast-feeding women (Razeghinejad, 2011).

Contraindications Hypersensitivity to dipivefrin, any component, or epinephrine; contraindicated in patients with angle-closure glaucoma

Warnings Commercial preparation contains sodium metabisulfate which may cause allergic reactions in susceptible individuals

Precautions Use with caution in patients with vascular hypertension or cardiac disorders and in aphakic patients (dipivefrin may cause cystoid macular edema in aphakic patients)

Adverse Reactions

Central nervous system: Headache

Local: Burning, stinging

Ocular: Blepharoconjunctivitis, blurred vision, bulbar conjunctival follicles, cystoid macular edema, ocular congestion, ocular pain, mydriasis, photophobia

Rare but important or life-threatening: Arrhythmias, hypertension

Drug Interactions

Metabolism/Transport Effects None known.

Avoid Concomitant Use

Avoid concomitant use of Dipivefrin with any of the following: Ergot Derivatives; Iobenguane I 123

Increased Effect/Toxicity

Dipivefrin may increase the levels/effects of: Sympathomimetics

The levels/effects of Dipivefrin may be increased by: AtoMOXetine; Cannabinoid-Containing Products; Ergot Derivatives; Linezolid; Serotonin/Norepinephrine Reuptake Inhibitors

Decreased Effect

Dipivefrin may decrease the levels/effects of: Iobenguane I 123

The levels/effects of Dipivefrin may be decreased by: Alpha1-Blockers; Spironolactone

Stability Protect from light and avoid exposure to air; discolored or darkened solutions indicate loss of potency

Mechanism of Action Dipivefrin is a prodrug of epinephrine which is the active agent that stimulates alpha- and/or beta-adrenergic receptors increasing aqueous humor outflow

Pharmacodynamics
Onset of action:
Ocular pressure effects: Within 30 minutes
Mydriasis: Within 30 minutes
Maximum effect: Ocular pressure effects: Within 1 hour
Duration:
Ocular pressure effects: 12 hours or longer
Mydriasis: Several hours

Pharmacokinetics (Adult data unless noted) Absorption: Rapid into the aqueous humor; converted to epinephrine

Dosing: Usual Children and Adults: Ophthalmic: Initial: Instill 1 drop every 12 hours

Administration Ophthalmic: Instill drop into eye; apply finger pressure to lacrimal sac during and for 1-2 minutes after instillation to decrease risk of absorption and systemic effects; avoid contacting bottle tip with skin or eye

Monitoring Parameters IOP

Dosage Forms Excipient information presented when available (limited, particularly for generics); consult specific product labeling. [DSC] = Discontinued product
Solution, ophthalmic, as hydrochloride [drops]:
Propine®: 0.1% (10 mL [DSC]) [contains benzalkonium chloride]

References
Razeghinejad MR, Tania Tai TY, Fudemberg SJ, et al, "Pregnancy and Glaucoma," *Surv Ophthalmol*, 2011, 56(4):324-35.

◆ **Dipivefrin Hydrochloride** *see* Dipivefrin *on page 692*

◆ **Diprivan** *see* Propofol *on page 1755*

◆ **Diprolene** *see* Betamethasone (Topical) *on page 285*

◆ **Diprolene AF** *see* Betamethasone (Topical) *on page 285*

◆ **Dipropylacetic Acid** *see* Valproic Acid and Derivatives *on page 2102*

◆ **Diprosone (Can)** *see* Betamethasone (Topical) *on page 285*

Dipyridamole (dye peer ID a mole)

Medication Safety Issues
Sound-alike/look-alike issues:
Dipyridamole may be confused with disopyramide
Persantine® may be confused with Periactin
BEERS Criteria medication:
This drug may be potentially inappropriate for use in geriatric patients (Quality of evidence - moderate; Strength of recommendation - strong).
International issues:
Persantine [U.S., Canada, Belgium, Denmark, France] may be confused with Permitil brand name for sildenafil [Argentina]

Brand Names: U.S. Persantine

Brand Names: Canada Apo-Dipyridamole FC®; Dipyridamole For Injection; Persantine®

Therapeutic Category Antiplatelet Agent; Vasodilator, Coronary

Generic Availability (U.S.) Yes

Use Maintain patency after surgical grafting procedures including coronary artery bypass; with warfarin to decrease thrombosis in patients after artificial heart valve replacement; for chronic management of angina pectoris; with aspirin to prevent coronary artery thrombosis; in combination with aspirin or warfarin to prevent other thromboembolic disorders; dipyridamole may also be given 2 days prior to heart surgery to prevent platelet activation by extracorporeal bypass pump; diagnostic agent I.V. (dipyridamole stress test) for coronary artery disease

Pregnancy Risk Factor B

Pregnancy Considerations Teratogenic effects were not observed in animal studies.

Breast-Feeding Considerations Excretion in breast milk is reported to be minimal.

Contraindications Hypersensitivity to dipyridamole or any component

Precautions Use with caution in patients with hypotension (may further decrease blood pressure due to peripheral vasodilation); use with caution in patients with CAD (may aggravate chest pain)

Adverse Reactions
Oral:
Cardiovascular: Angina pectoris, flushing
Central nervous system: Headache, dizziness
Dermatologic: Pruritus, rash
Gastrointestinal: Abdominal distress, diarrhea, vomiting
Hepatic: Liver dysfunction
Postmarketing and/or case reports: Alopecia, arthritis, cholelithiasis, dyspepsia, fatigue, hepatitis, hypersensitivity reaction, hypotension, larynx edema, malaise, myalgia, nausea, palpitation, paresthesia, tachycardia, thrombocytopenia
I.V.:
Cardiovascular: Blood pressure lability, ECG abnormalities (ST-T changes, extrasystoles), pain, exacerbation of angina pectoris, hyper-/hypotension, tachycardia
Central nervous system: Dizziness, fatigue, flushing, headache
Gastrointestinal: Nausea
Neuromuscular & skeletal: Paresthesia
Respiratory: Dyspnea
Rare but important or life-threatening: Abdominal pain, abnormal coordination, allergic reaction (pruritus, rash, urticaria), appetite increased, arrhythmia (ventricular tachycardia, bradycardia, AV block, SVT, atrial fibrillation, asystole), arthralgia, asthenia, back pain, breast pain, bronchospasm, cardiomyopathy, cough, depersonalization, diaphoresis, dry mouth, dysgeusia, dyspepsia, dysphagia, earache, ECG abnormalities (unspecified), edema, eructation, flatulence, hypertonia, hyperventilation, injection site reaction, intermittent claudication leg cramping, malaise, MI, myalgia, orthostatic hypotension, palpitation, perineal pain, pharyngitis, pleural pain, renal pain, rhinitis, rigor, syncope, tenesmus, thirst, tinnitus, tremor, vertigo, vision abnormalities, vomiting

Drug Interactions
Metabolism/Transport Effects Inhibits BCRP, P-glycoprotein
Avoid Concomitant Use
Avoid concomitant use of Dipyridamole with any of the following: Bosutinib; PAZOPanib; Riociguat; Silodosin; Topotecan; Urokinase; VinCRIStine (Liposomal)
Increased Effect/Toxicity
Dipyridamole may increase the levels/effects of: Adenosine; Afatinib; Agents with Antiplatelet Properties; Anticoagulants; Apixaban; Beta-Blockers; Bosutinib; Brentuximab Vedotin; Colchicine; Collagenase (Systemic); Dabigatran Etexilate; DOXOrubicin (Conventional); DULoxetine; Everolimus; Hypotensive Agents; Ibritumomab; PAZOPanib; P-glycoprotein/ABCB1 Substrates; Prucalopride; Regadenoson; Rifaximin; Riociguat; Rivaroxaban; Salicylates; Silodosin; Thrombolytic Agents; Topotecan; Tositumomab and Iodine I 131 Tositumomab; Urokinase; VinCRIStine (Liposomal)

The levels/effects of Dipyridamole may be increased by: Barbiturates; Dasatinib; Glucosamine; Herbs (Anticoagulant/Antiplatelet Properties); Ibrutinib; Multivitamins/Fluoride (with ADE); Multivitamins/Minerals (with ADEK, Folate, Iron); Multivitamins/Minerals (with AE, No Iron); Nonsteroidal Anti-Inflammatory Agents; Omega-3 Fatty

Acids; Pentosan Polysulfate Sodium; Pentoxifylline; Prostacyclin Analogues; Tipranavir; Vitamin E

Decreased Effect

Dipyridamole may decrease the levels/effects of: Acetyl-cholinesterase Inhibitors

The levels/effects of Dipyridamole may be decreased by: Nonsteroidal Anti-Inflammatory Agents

Stability Do not freeze; protect I.V. preparation from light

Mechanism of Action Inhibits the activity of adenosine deaminase and phosphodiesterase, which causes an accumulation of adenosine, adenine nucleotides, and cyclic AMP; these mediators then inhibit platelet aggregation and may cause vasodilation; may also stimulate release of prostacyclin or PGD_2; causes coronary vasodilation

Pharmacokinetics (Adult data unless noted) Oral:

Absorption: Slow and variable

Distribution: Distributes to breast milk

V_d: Adults: 2-3 L/kg

Protein binding: 91% to 99%

Metabolism: In the liver to glucuronide conjugate

Bioavailability: 27% to 66%

Half-life, terminal: 10-12 hours

Time to peak serum concentration: Oral: 75 minutes

Elimination: In feces via bile as glucuronide conjugates and unchanged drug

Dosing: Usual

Children:

Oral: 3-6 mg/kg/day in 3 divided doses

Doses of 4-10 mg/kg/day have been used investigationally to treat proteinuria in pediatric renal disease

Mechanical prosthetic heart valves: 2-5 mg/kg/day [used in combination with an oral anticoagulant in children who have systemic embolism despite adequate oral anticoagulant therapy (INR 2.5-3.5), and used in combination with low-dose oral anticoagulation (INR 2-3) plus aspirin in children in whom full-dose oral anticoagulation is contraindicated] (Monagle, 2001). **Note:** The *Chest* guidelines (Monagle, 2004) do not mention the use of dipyridamole for prophylaxis for mechanical prosthetic heart valves in children; an oral anticoagulant plus aspirin is recommended for the patient groups mentioned above.

Adults:

Prophylaxis of thromboembolism after cardiac valve replacement (adjunctive use): Oral: 75-100 mg 4 times/day

Dipyridamole stress test (for evaluation of myocardial perfusion): I.V.: 0.142 mg/kg/minute for a total of 4 minutes (0.57 mg/kg total); maximum dose: 60 mg; inject thallium 201 within 5 minutes after end of injection of dipyridamole

Administration

Oral: Administer with water on an empty stomach 1 hour before or 2 hours after meals; may take with milk or food to decrease GI upset

Parenteral: I.V.: Dilute in at least a 1:2 ratio with NS, ½NS, or D_5W; infusion of undiluted dipyridamole may cause local irritation; see Dosing: Usual for infusion rates

Monitoring Parameters Blood pressure, heart rate

Test Interactions Concurrent caffeine or theophylline use may demonstrate a false-negative result with dipyridamole-thallium myocardial imaging.

Dosage Forms Excipient information presented when available (limited, particularly for generics); consult specific product labeling.

Solution, Intravenous:

Generic: 5 mg/mL (2 mL, 10 mL)

Tablet, Oral:

Persantine: 25 mg, 50 mg, 75 mg [contains fd&c yellow #10 aluminum lake, methylparaben, propylparaben, sodium benzoate]

Generic: 25 mg, 50 mg, 75 mg

Extemporaneous Preparations A 10 mg/mL oral suspension may be made with tablets and one of three different vehicles (cherry syrup, a 1:1 mixture of Ora-Sweet® and Ora-Plus®, or a 1:1 mixture of Ora-Sweet® SF and Ora-Plus®). Crush twenty-four 50 mg tablets in a mortar and reduce to a fine powder. Add 20 mL of the chosen vehicle and mix to a uniform paste; mix while adding the vehicle in incremental proportions to **almost** 120 mL; transfer to a calibrated bottle, rinse mortar with vehicle, and add quantity of vehicle sufficient to make 120 mL. Label "shake well" and "protect from light". Stable for 60 days when stored in amber plastic prescription bottles in the dark at room temperature or refrigerated.

Allen LV and Erickson III MA, "Stability of Baclofen, Captopril, Diltiazem, Hydrochloride, Dipyridamole, and Flecainide Acetate in Extemporaneously Compounded Oral Liquids," *Am J Health Syst Pharm*, 1996, 53:2179-84.

References

Monagle P, Chan A, Massicotte P, et al, "Antithrombotic Therapy in Children: The Seventh ACCP Conference on Antithrombotic and Thrombolytic Therapy," *Chest*, 2004, 126(3 Suppl):645S-687S.

Monagle P, Michelson AD, Bovill E, et al, "Antithrombotic Therapy in Children," *Chest*, 2001, 119(1 Suppl):344S-370S.

Rao PS, Solymar L, Mardini MK, et al, "Anticoagulant Therapy in Children With Prosthetic Valves," *Ann Thorac Surg*, 1989, 47 (4):589-92.

Stanek EJ, Melko GP, and Charland SL, "Xanthine Interference With Dipyridamole-Thallium-201 Myocardial Imaging," *Ann Pharmacother*, 1995, 29(4):425-7.

Ueda N, Kawaguchi S, Niinomi Y, et al, "Effect of Dipyridamole Treatment on Proteinuria in Pediatric Renal Disease," *Nephron*, 1986, 44 (3):174-9.

♦ **Dipyridamole For Injection (Can)** *see* Dipyridamole *on page 693*

♦ **Disodium Cromoglycate** *see* Cromolyn (Nasal) *on page 553*

♦ **Disodium Cromoglycate** *see* Cromolyn (Ophthalmic) *on page 553*

♦ **Disodium Cromoglycate** *see* Cromolyn (Systemic, Oral Inhalation) *on page 551*

♦ **Disodium Thiosulfate Pentahydrate** *see* Sodium Thiosulfate *on page 1919*

♦ **d-Isoephedrine Hydrochloride** *see* Pseudoephedrine *on page 1770*

Disopyramide (dye soe PEER a mide)

Medication Safety Issues

Sound-alike/look-alike issues:

Disopyramide may be confused with desipramine, dipyridamole

Norpace® may be confused with Norpramin®

BEERS Criteria medication:

This drug may be potentially inappropriate for use in geriatric patients (Quality of evidence - low; Strength of recommendation - strong).

Related Information

Medications for Which a Single Dose May Be Fatal When Ingested by a Toddler *on page 2408*

Oral Medications That Should Not Be Crushed or Altered *on page 2438*

Brand Names: U.S. Norpace; Norpace CR

Brand Names: Canada Norpace®; Rythmodan®; Rythmodan®-LA

Therapeutic Category Antiarrhythmic Agent, Class I-A

Generic Availability (U.S.) May be product dependent

Use Treatment of life-threatening ventricular arrhythmias; suppression and prevention of unifocal and multifocal ventricular premature complexes, coupled ventricular premature complexes, and/or paroxysmal ventricular tachycardia; also effective in the conversion and prevention of recurrence of atrial fibrillation, atrial flutter, and paroxysmal atrial tachycardia

Pregnancy Risk Factor C

Pregnancy Considerations Adverse events have been observed in animal reproduction studies. Disopyramide levels have been reported in human fetal blood. Disopyramide may stimulate contractions in pregnant women. In a case report, disopyramide use in the third trimester resulted in painful uterine contractions after the first dose and hemorrhage after the second dose (Abbi, 1999).

Breast-Feeding Considerations Disopyramide is excreted in breast milk. Due to the potential for serious adverse reactions in nursing infants, the manufacturer recommends a decision be made whether to discontinue nursing or to discontinue the drug, taking into account the importance of the treatment to the mother.

Contraindications Hypersensitivity to disopyramide or any component; preexisting second or third degree A-V block (except in patients with a functioning artificial pacemaker); congenital QT prolongation; cardiogenic shock

Warnings Antiarrhythmic agents should be reserved for patients with life-threatening ventricular arrhythmias **[U.S. Boxed Warning]**. In the Cardiac Arrhythmia Suppression Trial (CAST), recent (>6 days but <2 years ago) myocardial infarction patients with asymptomatic, nonlife-threatening ventricular arrhythmias did not benefit and may have been harmed by attempts to suppress the arrhythmia with flecainide or encainide. An increased mortality or nonfatal cardiac arrest rate (7.7%) was seen in the active treatment group compared with patients in the placebo group (3%). The applicability of the CAST results to other populations is unknown.

May cause or worsen CHF; may cause severe hypotension; not recommended for use in patients with uncompensated or marginally compensated CHF or hypotension unless caused by an arrhythmia. May cause significant widening (>25%) of QRS complex; discontinue disopyramide if this occurs. Lengthening of QT interval and worsening of arrhythmia (including ventricular tachycardia or ventricular fibrillation) may occur; patients with quinidine-associated QT prolongation may be at higher risk; torsade de pointes may occur. Monitor patients carefully and consider discontinuation of disopyramide if QT prolongation is >25% and ectopy continues. May cause heart block; reduce dosage if first-degree heart block develops; discontinue drug if second or third degree AV block or unifascicular, bifascicular, or trifascicular block develops (unless pacemaker is present).

Disopyramide may cause hypoglycemia. Significant anticholinergic activity occurs; avoid use in patients with glaucoma, myasthenia gravis, or urinary retention unless appropriate overriding measures are taken.

Serious and potentially fatal drug interactions may occur. Avoid concurrent use with other drugs known to prolong QT$_c$ interval or decrease myocardial contractility. Life-threatening interactions have been reported with concomitant use of disopyramide with clarithromycin and erythromycin. Disopyramide is not recommended for use 48 hours before or 24 hours after verapamil.

Precautions Use with caution in patients with sick sinus syndrome, Wolf Parkinson White syndrome (WPW) or bundle-branch block. May increase ventricular rate in patients with atrial fibrillation or flutter who have not received digoxin. Use with caution and do not give loading dose in patients with myocarditis or other cardiomyopathy; may cause significant hypotension. Use with caution and decrease dose in patients with renal or hepatic impairment; extended release form is not recommended for patients

with severe renal impairment (CrCl <40 mL/minute). Correct electrolyte disturbances, especially hypokalemia or hypomagnesemia, prior to use and throughout therapy.

Adverse Reactions The most common adverse effects are related to cholinergic blockade. The most serious adverse effects of disopyramide are CHF and hypotension.

Cardiovascular: Cardiac conduction disturbance, chest pain CHF, edema, hypotension, syncope

Central nervous system: Dizziness, fatigue, headache, malaise, nervousness

Dermatologic: Generalized dermatoses, pruritus, rash

Endocrine & metabolic: Cholesterol increased, hypokalemia, triglycerides increased

Gastrointestinal: Abdominal bloating, abdominal distension, anorexia, constipation, diarrhea, dry throat, flatulence, nausea, vomiting, weight gain, xerostomia

Genitourinary: Impotence, urinary frequency, urinary hesitancy, urinary retention, urinary urgency

Neuromuscular & skeletal: Muscular pain, muscle weakness

Ocular: Blurred vision, dry eyes

Respiratory: Dyspnea

Rare but important or life-threatening: Agranulocytosis, AV block, BUN increased, cholestatic jaundice, creatinine increased, depression, dysuria, gynecomastia, hepatotoxicity, hypoglycemia, insomnia, new or worsened arrhythmia (proarrhythmic effect), paresthesia, psychotic reaction, respiratory distress, thrombocytopenia, transaminases increased. Rare cases of lupus have been reported (generally in patients previously receiving procainamide), peripheral neuropathy, psychosis, toxic cutaneous blisters.

Drug Interactions

Metabolism/Transport Effects Substrate of CYP3A4 (major); **Note:** Assignment of Major/Minor substrate status based on clinically relevant drug interaction potential

Avoid Concomitant Use

Avoid concomitant use of Disopyramide with any of the following: Aclidinium; Amiodarone; Conivaptan; Fingolimod; Fusidic Acid (Systemic); Highest Risk QTc-Prolonging Agents; Ipratropium (Oral Inhalation); Itraconazole; Ivabradine; Ketoconazole (Systemic); Macrolide Antibiotics; Mifepristone; Moderate Risk QTc-Prolonging Agents; Potassium Chloride; Propafenone; Tiotropium; Umeclidinium; Verapamil

Increased Effect/Toxicity

Disopyramide may increase the levels/effects of: AbobotulinumtoxinA; Analgesics (Opioid); Anticholinergic Agents; Beta-Blockers; Cannabinoid-Containing Products; Fosphenytoin; Highest Risk QTc-Prolonging Agents; Lidocaine (Systemic); Lidocaine (Topical); OnabotulinumtoxinA; Potassium Chloride; RimabotulinumtoxinB; Thiazide Diuretics; Tiotropium; Topiramate

The levels/effects of Disopyramide may be increased by: Aclidinium; Amiodarone; Conivaptan; CYP3A4 Inhibitors (Moderate); CYP3A4 Inhibitors (Strong); Fingolimod; Fusidic Acid (Systemic); Ipratropium (Oral Inhalation); Itraconazole; Ivabradine; Ivacaftor; Ketoconazole (Systemic); Luliconazole; Lurasidone; Macrolide Antibiotics; Mifepristone; Moderate Risk QTc-Prolonging Agents; Pramlintide; Propafenone; QTc-Prolonging Agents (Indeterminate Risk and Risk Modifying); Simeprevir; Stiripentol; Umeclidinium; Verapamil

Decreased Effect

Disopyramide may decrease the levels/effects of: Acetylcholinesterase Inhibitors (Central); Secretin

The levels/effects of Disopyramide may be decreased by: Acetylcholinesterase Inhibitors (Central); Bosentan; CYP3A4 Inducers (Strong); Dabrafenib; Deferasirox; Etravirine; Fosphenytoin; Mitotane; PHENobarbital; Phenytoin; Rifampin; Siltuximab; St Johns Wort; Tocilizumab

◀ **Mechanism of Action** Class Ia antiarrhythmic: Decreases myocardial excitability and conduction velocity; reduces disparity in refractory between normal and infarcted myocardium; possesses anticholinergic, peripheral vasoconstrictive, and negative inotropic effects

Pharmacodynamics
Capsules, regular:
Onset of action: 30-210 minutes
Duration: 1.5-8.5 hours

Pharmacokinetics (Adult data unless noted)
Protein binding: Concentration dependent, stereoselective, and ranges from 20% to 60%
Distribution: V_d: Children: 1 L/kg
Metabolism: In the liver; major metabolite has anticholinergic and antiarrhythmic effects
Bioavailability: 60% to 83%
Half-life:
Children: 3.15 hours
Adults: 4-10 hours (mean: 6.7 hours), increased half-life with hepatic or renal disease
Elimination: 40% to 60% excreted unchanged in urine and 10% to 15% in feces
Clearance is greater and half-life shorter in children vs adults; clearance (children): 3.76 mL/minute/kg

Dosing: Usual Oral:
Children (start with lower dose listed):
<1 year: 10-30 mg/kg/day in 4 divided doses
1-4 years: 10-20 mg/kg/day in 4 divided doses
4-12 years: 10-15 mg/kg/day in 4 divided doses
12-18 years: 6-15 mg/kg/day in 4 divided doses
Adults: **Note:** Some patients may require initial loading dose; see product information for details
<50 kg: 100 mg every 6 hours **or** 200 mg every 12 hours (controlled release)
>50 kg: 150 mg every 6 hours **or** 300 mg every 12 hours (controlled release); if no response, may increase to 200 mg every 6 hours; maximum dose required for patients with severe refractory ventricular tachycardia is 400 mg every 6 hours. **Note:** Use lower doses (100 mg of nonsustained release every 6-8 hours) in adults with cardiomyopathy or cardiac decompensation.

Adult dosing adjustment in renal impairment: 100 mg (nonsustained release) given at the following intervals: See table.

Creatinine Clearance (mL/min)	Dosage Interval
30-40	Every 8 h
15-30	Every 12 h
<15	Every 24 h

Administration Oral: Administer on an empty stomach; do not crush, break, or chew controlled release capsules, swallow whole

Monitoring Parameters Blood pressure, ECG, drug level; serum potassium, glucose, cholesterol, triglycerides, and liver enzymes; especially important to monitor ECG in patients with hepatic or renal disease, heart disease, or others with increased risk of adverse effects

Reference Range Therapeutic:
Atrial arrhythmias: 2.8-3.2 mcg/mL (SI: 8.3-9.4 micromoles/L)
Ventricular arrhythmias: 3.3-7.5 mcg/mL (SI: 9.7-22 micromoles/L)
Toxic: >7 mcg/mL (SI: >20.7 micromoles/L)

Dosage Forms Excipient information presented when available (limited, particularly for generics); consult specific product labeling.
Capsule, Oral:
Norpace: 100 mg, 150 mg
Generic: 100 mg, 150 mg

Capsule Extended Release 12 Hour, Oral:
Norpace CR: 100 mg, 150 mg

Extemporaneous Preparations A 1 mg/mL oral suspension may be made with a tablet and Simple Syrup, NF. Crush one 100 mg tablet in a mortar and reduce to a fine powder. Add small portions of the vehicle and mix to a uniform paste; mix while adding the vehicle in incremental proportions to **almost** 100 mL; transfer to a calibrated bottle, rinse mortar with vehicle, and add quantity of vehicle sufficient to make 100 mL. Label "shake well" and "refrigerate". Stable for 28 days.

A 10 mg/mL oral suspension may be made with tablets and Simple Syrup, NF. Crush ten 100 mg tablets in a mortar and reduce to a fine powder. Add small portions of the vehicle and mix to a uniform paste; mix while adding the vehicle in incremental proportions to **almost** 100 mL; transfer to a calibrated bottle, rinse mortar with vehicle, and add quantity of vehicle sufficient to make 100 mL. Label "shake well" and "refrigerate". Stable for 28 days.
Nahata MC, Pai VB, and Hipple TF, *Pediatric Drug Formulations*, 5th ed, Cincinnati, OH: Harvey Whitney Books Co, 2004.

References
Chiba K, Koike K, Nakamoto M, et al, "Steady-State Pharmacokinetics and Bioavailability of Total and Unbound Disopyramide in Children With Cardiac Arrhythmias," *Ther Drug Monit*, 1992, 14(2):112-8.
Echizen H, Takahashi H, Nakamura H, et al, "Stereoselective Disposition and Metabolism of Disopyramide in Pediatric Patients," *J Pharmacol Exp Ther*, 1991, 259(3):953-60.

◆ **Disopyramide Phosphate** *see* Disopyramide *on page 694*

◆ **Dithioglycerol** *see* Dimercaprol *on page 672*

◆ **Ditropan** *see* Oxybutynin *on page 1568*

◆ **Ditropan XL** *see* Oxybutynin *on page 1568*

◆ **Diuril** *see* Chlorothiazide *on page 446*

◆ **Divalproex Sodium** *see* Valproic Acid and Derivatives *on page 2102*

◆ **Divigel** *see* Estradiol (Systemic) *on page 796*

◆ **Dixarit® (Can)** *see* CloNIDine *on page 516*

◆ **5071-1DL(6)** *see* Megestrol *on page 1324*

◆ ***dl*-Alpha Tocopherol** *see* Vitamin E *on page 2148*

◆ **D-Mannitol** *see* Mannitol *on page 1301*

◆ **4-DMDR** *see* IDArubicin *on page 1067*

◆ **DMSA** *see* Succimer *on page 1937*

◆ **Doak Oil [OTC] (Can)** *see* Coal Tar *on page 532*

◆ **Doak Oil Forte [OTC] (Can)** *see* Coal Tar *on page 532*

DOBUTamine (doe BYOO ta meen)

Medication Safety Issues
Sound-alike/look-alike issues:
DOBUTamine may be confused with DOPamine
High alert medication:
The Institute for Safe Medication Practices (ISMP) includes this medication among its list of drugs which have a heightened risk of causing significant patient harm when used in error.

Related Information
Emergency Drip Calculations *on page 2191*
Management of Drug Extravasations *on page 2255*

Brand Names: Canada Dobutamine Injection, USP; Dobutrex®

Therapeutic Category Adrenergic Agonist Agent; Sympathomimetic

Generic Availability (U.S.) Yes

Use Short-term management of patients with cardiac decompensation

Pregnancy Risk Factor B

Pregnancy Considerations Adverse events have not been observed in animal reproduction studies.

Breast-Feeding Considerations It is not known if dobutamine is excreted in breast milk. The manufacturer recommends that caution be exercised when administering dobutamine to nursing women.

Contraindications Hypersensitivity to dobutamine or any component; patients with idiopathic hypertrophic subaortic stenosis (IHSS)

Warnings Potent drug; must be diluted prior to use; patient's hemodynamic status should be monitored; contains sulfites which may cause allergic reactions in susceptible individuals

Precautions Hypovolemia should be corrected prior to use; infiltration causes local inflammatory changes, extravasation may cause dermal necrosis

Adverse Reactions

Cardiovascular: Anginal pain, hypotension, increased blood pressure, increased heart rate, increased ventricular ectopic activity, nonspecific chest pain, palpitation, premature ventricular beats (dose related)

Central nervous system: Fever, headache, paresthesia

Endocrine & metabolic: Slight decrease in serum potassium

Gastrointestinal: Nausea

Hematologic: Thrombocytopenia (isolated cases)

Local: Cutaneous necrosis (isolated cases), local inflammatory changes and pain from infiltration, phlebitis

Neuromuscular & skeletal: Mild leg cramps

Respiratory: Dyspnea

Drug Interactions

Metabolism/Transport Effects Substrate of COMT

Avoid Concomitant Use

Avoid concomitant use of DOBUTamine with any of the following: Iobenguane I 123

Increased Effect/Toxicity

DOBUTamine may increase the levels/effects of: Sympathomimetics

The levels/effects of DOBUTamine may be increased by: AtoMOXetine; Cannabinoid-Containing Products; COMT Inhibitors; Linezolid

Decreased Effect

DOBUTamine may decrease the levels/effects of: Iobenguane I 123

The levels/effects of DOBUTamine may be decreased by: Calcium Salts

Stability Stable in various parenteral solutions for 24 hours; incompatible with alkaline solutions, do not give through same I.V. line as heparin, sodium bicarbonate, ethacrynic acid, cefazolin, or penicillin; compatible when coadministered with dopamine, nitroprusside, potassium chloride, protamine sulfate, tobramycin, epinephrine, atracurium, vecuronium, isoproterenol, and lidocaine; pink discoloration of dobutamine hydrochloride indicates slight oxidation, but no significant loss of potency if administered within the recommended time period

Mechanism of Action Stimulates beta$_1$-adrenergic receptors, causing increased contractility and heart rate, with little effect on beta$_2$- or alpha-receptors

Pharmacodynamics

Onset of action: I.V.: 1-10 minutes

Maximum effect: Within 10-20 minutes

Pharmacokinetics (Adult data unless noted)

Metabolism: In tissues and the liver to inactive metabolites

Half-life: 2 minutes

Dosing: Neonatal Continuous I.V. infusion: 2-20 mcg/kg/minute; titrate to desired response

Dosing: Usual Continuous I.V. infusion: Infants, Children, and Adults: 2.5-15 mcg/kg/minute, titrate to desired response; maximum dose: 40 mcg/kg/minute

Usual Infusion Concentrations: Neonatal Note: Premixed solutions available.

I.V. infusion: 1000 mcg/mL, 2000 mcg/mL, or 4000 mcg/mL

Usual Infusion Concentrations: Pediatric Note: Premixed solutions available.

I.V. infusion: 1000 mcg/mL, 2000 mcg/mL, or 4000 mcg/mL

Administration Parenteral: Dilute in dextrose or NS; maximum recommended concentration: 5000 mcg/mL (5 mg/mL); rate of infusion (mL/hour) = dose (mcg/kg/minute) x weight (kg) x 60 minutes/hour divided by the concentration (mcg/mL); administer into large vein; use infusion device to control rate of flow

Monitoring Parameters ECG, heart rate, CVP, MAP, urine output; if pulmonary artery catheter is in place, monitor CI, PCWP, RAP, and SVR. Dobutamine lowers central venous pressure and wedge pressure but has little effect on pulmonary vascular resistance.

Dosage Forms Excipient information presented when available (limited, particularly for generics); consult specific product labeling.

Solution, Intravenous, as hydrochloride:

Generic: 1 mg/mL (250 mL); 2 mg/mL (250 mL); 4 mg/mL (250 mL); 250 mg/20 mL (20 mL); 500 mg/40 mL (40 mL)

References

Hegenbarth MA and American Academy of Pediatrics Committee on Drugs, "Preparing for Pediatric Emergencies: Drugs to Consider," *Pediatrics*, 2008, 121(2):433-43.

Institute for Safe Medication Practices (ISMP), "Standard Concentrations of Neonatal Drug Infusions," *ISMP*, 2011.

Kleinman ME, Chameides L, Schexnayder SM, et al, "Part 14: Pediatric Advanced Life Support: 2010 American Heart Association Guidelines for Cardiopulmonary Resuscitation and Emergency Cardiovascular Care," *Circulation*, 2010, 122(18 Suppl 3):876-908.

Phillips MS, "Standardizing I.V. Infusion Concentrations: National Survey Results," *Am J Health Syst Pharm*, 2011, 68(22):2176-82.

Subhedar NV, "Treatment of Hypotension in Newborns," *Semin Neonatol*, 2003, 8(6):413-23.

◆ **Dobutamine Hydrochloride** *see* DOBUTamine *on page 696*

◆ **Dobutamine Injection, USP (Can)** *see* DOBUTamine *on page 696*

◆ **Dobutrex® (Can)** *see* DOBUTamine *on page 696*

◆ **Docefrez** *see* DOCEtaxel *on page 697*

DOCEtaxel (doe se TAKS el)

Medication Safety Issues

Sound-alike/look-alike issues:

DOCEtaxel may be confused with cabazitaxel, PACLitaxel

Taxotere may be confused with Taxol

High alert medication:

This medication is in a class the Institute for Safe Medication Practices (ISMP) includes among its list of drug classes which have a heightened risk of causing significant patient harm when used in error.

Administration issues:

Multiple concentrations: Docetaxel is available as a one-vial formulation at concentrations of 10 mg/mL (generic formulation) and 20 mg/mL (concentrate; Taxotere), and as a lyophilized powder (Docefrez) which is reconstituted (with provided diluent) to 20 mg/0.8 mL (20 mg vial) or 24 mg/mL (80 mg vial). Docetaxel was previously available as a two-vial formulation (a concentrated docetaxel solution vial and a diluent vial) resulting in a reconstituted concentration of 10 mg/mL. The two-vial formulation has been discontinued by the Taxotere manufacturer (available generically). Admixture errors have occurred due to the availability of various docetaxel concentrations.

Related Information

Emetogenic Potential of Antineoplastic Agents in Children *on page 2327*

Management of Drug Extravasations *on page 2255*

Safe Handling of Hazardous Drugs *on page 2419*

Brand Names: U.S. Docefrez; Taxotere

Brand Names: Canada Docetaxel for Injection; Taxotere

Therapeutic Category Antineoplastic Agent, Antimicrotubular; Antineoplastic Agent, Taxane Derivative

Generic Availability (U.S.) May be product dependent

Use Treatment of breast cancer (locally advanced/metastatic or adjuvant treatment of operable node-positive); locally advanced or metastatic nonsmall cell lung cancer (NSCLC); and hormone refractory, metastatic prostate cancer (Docefrez, Taxotere: FDA approved in adults); advanced gastric adenocarcinoma; locally advanced squamous cell head and neck cancer (Taxotere: FDA approved in adults); has also been used in the treatment of soft tissue sarcoma, Ewing's sarcoma, osteosarcoma, and unknown primary adenocarcinoma

Pregnancy Risk Factor D

Pregnancy Considerations Adverse events have been observed in animal reproduction studies. An *ex vivo* human placenta perfusion model illustrated that docetaxel crossed the placenta at term. Placental transfer was low and affected by the presence of albumin; higher albumin concentrations resulted in lower docetaxel placental transfer (Berveiller, 2012). Women of childbearing potential should avoid becoming pregnant. A pregnancy registry is available for all cancers diagnosed during pregnancy at Cooper Health (877-635-4499).

Breast-Feeding Considerations It is not known if docetaxel is excreted into breast milk. Due to the potential for serious adverse reactions in nursing the infant, the decision to discontinue docetaxel or to discontinue breast-feeding should take into account the importance of treatment to the mother.

Contraindications Severe hypersensitivity to docetaxel or any component; prior severe hypersensitivity to other medications containing polysorbate 80; neutrophil count <1500/mm^3

Warnings Hazardous agent; use appropriate precautions for handling and disposal (NIOSH, 2012).

Avoid use in patients with bilirubin exceeding upper limit of normal (ULN) or AST and/or ALT >1.5 times ULN in conjunction with alkaline phosphatase >2.5 times ULN **[U.S. Boxed Warning]**; patients with isolated transaminase elevations >1.5 times ULN also had a higher rate of neutropenic fever, although no increased incidence of toxic death. Patients with abnormal liver function are also at increased risk of other treatment-related adverse events, including grade 4 neutropenia, infections, and severe thrombocytopenia, stomatitis, skin toxicity, or toxic death. Obtain liver function tests prior to each treatment cycle.

Severe fluid retention characterized by pleural effusion (requiring immediate drainage), ascites, peripheral edema (poorly tolerated), dyspnea at rest, cardiac tamponade, generalized edema, and weight gain has been reported **[U.S. Boxed Warning]**. In adults, the incidence (13% to 60%) and severity of the syndrome is dose-dependent and increases sharply at cumulative doses ≥400 mg/m^2. Patients should be premedicated with a corticosteroid (starting 1 day prior to administration) to prevent or reduce the severity of fluid retention. Closely monitor patients with existing effusions.

Severe hypersensitivity reactions characterized by generalized rash/erythema, hypotension, bronchospasms, or anaphylaxis may occur (may be fatal; has occurred in patients receiving corticosteroid premedication); do not administer to patients with a history of severe hypersensitivity to docetaxel or polysorbate 80 **[U.S. Boxed Warning]**; reported incidence is 1% to 21%; observe for hypersensitivity, especially with the first two infusions; discontinue for severe reactions; do not rechallenge if severe; minor reactions including flushing or localized skin reactions may also occur. Patients should be premedicated with a corticosteroid (starting 1 day prior to administration) to prevent or reduce severity of hypersensitivity reactions; however, severe reactions may still occur (incidence: 15%). Patients should be observed closely for hypersensitivity reactions, especially during the first and second infusions. Infusion of polysorbate 80-containing solutions through polyvinyl chloride tubing may cause DEHP to leach into the solution; in immature animals, exposure to DEHP may adversely affect the development of the male reproductive tract.

The dose-limiting toxicity is neutropenia and frequent WBCs should be monitored. Patients with increased liver function tests experienced more episodes of neutropenia with a greater number of severe infections. Patients with an absolute neutrophil count <1500/mm^3 should not receive docetaxel **[U.S. Boxed Warning]**. Platelets should recover to >100,000/mm^3 prior to treatment. When administered as sequential infusions, taxane derivatives (docetaxel, paclitaxel) should be administered before platinum derivatives (carboplatin, cisplatin) to limit myelosuppression and to enhance efficacy.

Patients with abnormal liver function, those receiving higher doses, and patients with nonsmall cell lung cancer and a history of prior treatment with platinum derivatives who receive single-agent docetaxel at a dose >100 mg/m^2 are at higher risk for treatment-related mortality **[U.S. Boxed Warning]**.

Cutaneous reactions including erythema (with edema) and desquamation have been reported; may require dose reduction. Dosage adjustment is recommended with severe neurosensory symptoms (paresthesia, dysesthesia, pain); persistent symptoms may require discontinuation; reversal of symptoms may be delayed after discontinuation.

Docetaxel is an irritant with vesicant-like properties; ensure proper needle or catheter placement prior to and during infusion; avoid extravasation.

Precautions Treatment-related acute myeloid leukemia or myelodysplasia occurred in patients receiving docetaxel in combination with anthracyclines and/or cyclophosphamide. Ocular adverse effects may occur; in a study of adult patients receiving docetaxel for the adjuvant treatment of breast cancer, a majority of patients experienced lacrimation (tearing), which occurred in patients with and without lacrimal duct obstruction at baseline. Onset was generally after cycle 1, but subsided in most patients within 4 months after therapy completion (Chan, 2013).

Fatigue and weakness have been reported (incidence: 53% to 66%); may be severe in some cases (incidence: 13% to 18%); symptoms may last a few days up to several weeks; in patients with progressive disease, weakness may be associated with a decrease in performance status. Should be administered under the supervision of an experienced cancer chemotherapy physician. Avoid concomitant use with strong CYP3A4 inhibitors; although data are limited, a 50% dose reduction is suggested if concomitant therapy with a CYP3A4 inhibitor is required. Potentially significant interactions may exist, requiring dose or frequency adjustment, additional monitoring, and/or selection of alternative therapy. Consult drug interactions database for more detailed information.

Adverse Reactions Frequency of adverse effects may vary depending on diagnosis, dose, liver function, prior treatment, and premedication. The incidence of adverse events was usually higher in patients with elevated liver function tests.

Cardiovascular: Decreased left ventricular ejection fraction, hypotension

Central nervous system: Central nervous system toxicity (including neuropathy), peripheral motor neuropathy (mainly distal extremity weakness)

Dermatologic: Alopecia, dermatological reaction, nail disease

Endocrine & metabolic: Fluid retention (dose dependent)

Gastrointestinal: Diarrhea, dysgeusia, nausea, stomatitis, vomiting

Hematologic & oncologic: Anemia (dose dependent), febrile neutropenia (dose dependent), leukopenia, neutropenia (nadir [median]: 7 days, duration [severe neutropenia]: 7 days; dose dependent), thrombocytopenia (dose dependent)

Hepatic: Increased serum alkaline phosphatase, increased serum bilirubin, increased serum transaminases

Hypersensitivity: Hypersensitivity

Infection: Infection (dose dependent)

Local: Infusion site reactions (including hyperpigmentation, inflammation, redness, dryness, phlebitis, extravasation, swelling of the vein)

Neuromuscular & skeletal: Arthralgia, myalgia, neuromuscular reaction, weakness

Ophthalmic: Epiphora (associated with canalicular stenosis)

Respiratory: Pulmonary reaction

Miscellaneous: Hypersensitivity (including with premedication), infection (dose dependent)

Rare but important or life-threatening: Acute myelocytic leukemia, acute respiratory distress, anaphylactic shock, anorexia, ascites, atrial fibrillation, atrial flutter, atrioventricular block, bradycardia, bronchospasm, cardiac arrhythmia, cardiac failure, cardiac tamponade, chest pain, chest tightness, colitis, confusion, conjunctivitis, constipation, cystoid macular edema, deep vein thrombosis, dehydration, disease of the lacrimal apparatus (duct obstruction), disseminated intravascular coagulation, drug fever, duodenal ulcer, dyspnea, ECG abnormality, erythema multiforme, esophagitis, gastrointestinal hemorrhage, gastrointestinal obstruction, gastrointestinal perforation, hearing loss, hemorrhagic diathesis, hepatitis, hypertension, hyponatremia, intestinal obstruction, interstitial pulmonary disease, ischemic colitis, ischemic heart disease, loss of consciousness (transient), lymphedema (peripheral), multiorgan failure, myelodysplastic syndrome, myocardial infarction, neutropenic enterocolitis, ototoxicity, palmar-plantar erythrodysesthesia, pericardial effusion, pleural effusion, pneumonia, pneumonitis, pruritus, pulmonary edema, pulmonary embolism, pulmonary fibrosis, radiation pneumonitis, radiation recall phenomenon, renal failure, renal insufficiency, respiratory failure, skin changes (scleroderma-like), seizure, sepsis, sinus tachycardia, Stevens-Johnson syndrome, subacute cutaneous lupus erythematosus, syncope, toxic epidermal necrolysis, tachycardia, thrombophlebitis, unstable angina pectoris, visual disturbance (transient)

Drug Interactions

Metabolism/Transport Effects Substrate of CYP3A4 (major), P-glycoprotein; **Note:** Assignment of Major/Minor substrate status based on clinically relevant drug interaction potential; **Inhibits** CYP3A4 (weak)

Avoid Concomitant Use

Avoid concomitant use of DOCEtaxel with any of the following: BCG; CloZAPine; Conivaptan; Dipyrone; Fusidic Acid (Systemic); Natalizumab; Pimecrolimus; Pimozide; Tacrolimus (Topical); Tofacitinib; Vaccines (Live)

Increased Effect/Toxicity

DOCEtaxel may increase the levels/effects of: Antineoplastic Agents (Anthracycline, Systemic); ARIPiprazole;

CloZAPine; Dofetilide; Leflunomide; Lomitapide; Natalizumab; Pimozide; Tofacitinib; Vaccines (Live)

The levels/effects of DOCEtaxel may be increased by: Antifungal Agents (Azole Derivatives, Systemic); Ceritinib; Conivaptan; CYP3A4 Inhibitors (Moderate); CYP3A4 Inhibitors (Strong); Dasatinib; Denosumab; Dipyrone; Dronedarone; Fusidic Acid (Systemic); Ivacaftor; Luliconazole; Mifepristone; P-glycoprotein/ABCB1 Inhibitors; Pimecrolimus; Platinum Derivatives; Roflumilast; Simeprevir; SORAfenib; Stiripentol; Tacrolimus (Topical); Trastuzumab

Decreased Effect

DOCEtaxel may decrease the levels/effects of: BCG; Coccidioidin Skin Test; Sipuleucel-T; Vaccines (Inactivated); Vaccines (Live)

The levels/effects of DOCEtaxel may be decreased by: Bosentan; CYP3A4 Inducers (Strong); Dabrafenib; Deferasirox; Echinacea; Mitotane; P-glycoprotein/ABCB1 Inducers; Siltuximab; St Johns Wort; Tocilizumab

Stability Hazardous agent; use appropriate precautions for handling and disposal (NIOSH, 2012).

Docetaxel 10 mg/mL: Store intact vials between 2°C to 25°C (36°F to 77°F) (actual recommendations may vary by generic manufacturer; consult manufacturer's labeling). Protect from bright light. Freezing does not adversely affect the product. Multiuse vials (80 mg/8 mL and 160 mg/16 mL) are stable for up to 28 days after first entry when stored between 2°C to 8°C (36°F to 46°F) and protected from light.

Docetaxel concentrate; Taxotere 20 mg/mL: Store intact vials between 2°C to 25°C (36°F to 77°F). Protect from bright light. Freezing does not adversely affect the product.

Docetaxel lyophilized powder (Docefrez): Store intact vials between 2°C to 8°C (36°F to 46°F). Protect from light. Allow vials (and provided diluent) to stand at room temperature for 5 minutes prior to reconstitution. After reconstitution, may be stored refrigerated or at room temperature for up to 8 hours.

Solutions diluted for infusion should be used within 4 hours of preparation, including infusion time.

Mechanism of Action Docetaxel promotes the assembly of microtubules from tubulin dimers, and inhibits the depolymerization of tubulin which stabilizes microtubules in the cell. This results in inhibition of DNA, RNA, and protein synthesis. Most activity occurs during the M phase of the cell cycle.

Pharmacokinetics (Adult data unless noted) Exhibits linear pharmacokinetics at the recommended dosage range

Distribution: Extensive extravascular distribution and/or tissue binding; V_d: 80-90 L/m^2, V_{dss}: 113 L (mean steady state)

Protein binding: ~94% to 97%, primarily to alpha$_1$-acid glycoprotein, albumin, and lipoproteins

Metabolism: Hepatic; oxidation via CYP3A4 to metabolites

Half-life: Terminal: 11 hours

Elimination: Feces (75%, <8% as unchanged drug); urine (6%)

Dosing: Usual Refer to individual protocols: **Note:** Premedicate with corticosteroids, beginning the day before docetaxel administration (administer corticosteroids for 1-3 days), to reduce the severity of hypersensitivity reactions and pulmonary/peripheral edema

Children and Adolescents: **Ewing's Sarcoma; osteosarcoma (recurrent or progressive):** Limited data available: I.V.: 75-125 mg/m^2 every 21 days; administer on day 8 of treatment cycle if given in combination with other chemotherapy (Mora, 2009; Navid, 2008; Zwerdling, 2006)

Adults:
Breast cancer: I.V.:
Locally-advanced or metastatic: 60-100 mg/m^2 every 3 weeks as a single agent
Operable, node-positive (adjuvant treatment): 75 mg/m^2 every 3 weeks for 6 courses (in combination with doxorubicin and cyclophosphamide)
Nonsmall cell lung cancer: I.V.: 75 mg/m^2 every 3 weeks (as monotherapy or in combination with cisplatin)
Prostate cancer (hormone-refractory, metastatic): I.V.: 75 mg/m^2 every 3 weeks (in combination with prednisone)
Gastric adenocarcinoma: I.V.: 75 mg/m^2 every 3 weeks (in combination with cisplatin and fluorouracil)
Head and neck cancer: I.V.: 75 mg/m^2 every 3 weeks (in combination with cisplatin and fluorouracil) for 3 or 4 cycles, followed by radiation therapy

Dosing adjustment for toxicity: Adults: **Note:** Toxicity includes febrile neutropenia, neutrophils ≤500/mm^3 for >1 week, severe or cumulative cutaneous reactions; in nonsmall cell lung cancer, this may also include platelets <25,000/mm^3 and other grade 3/4 nonhematologic toxicities.

Breast cancer (single agent): Patients dosed initially at 100 mg/m^2; reduce dose to 75 mg/m^2; **Note:** If the patient continues to experience these adverse reactions, the dosage should be reduced to 55 mg/m^2 or therapy should be discontinued; discontinue for peripheral neuropathy ≥grade 3. Patients initiated at 60 mg/m^2 who do not develop toxicity may tolerate higher doses.
Breast cancer, adjuvant treatment (combination chemotherapy): TAC regimen should be administered when neutrophils are ≥1500/mm^3. Patients with persistent febrile neutropenia (while on G-CSF), patients experiencing severe/cumulative cutaneous reactions, moderate neurosensory effects (signs/symptoms), or grade 3 or 4 stomatitis should receive a reduced dose (60 mg/m^2) of docetaxel. Discontinue therapy with persistent toxicities after dosage reduction.
Nonsmall cell lung cancer:
Monotherapy: Patients dosed initially at 75 mg/m^2 should have dose held until toxicity is resolved, then resume at 55 mg/m^2; discontinue for peripheral neuropathy ≥grade 3.
Combination therapy (with cisplatin): Patients dosed initially at 75 mg/m^2 should have the docetaxel dosage reduced to 65 mg/m^2 in subsequent cycles; if further adjustment is required, dosage may be reduced to 50 mg/m^2
Prostate cancer: Reduce dose to 60 mg/m^2; discontinue therapy if toxicities persist at lower dose.
Gastric cancer, head and neck cancer: Note: Cisplatin may require dose reductions/therapy delays for peripheral neuropathy, ototoxicity, and/or nephrotoxicity. Patients experiencing febrile neutropenia, documented infection with neutropenia or neutropenia >7 days should receive G-CSF in all subsequent cycles. For neutropenic complications despite G-CSF use, further reduce dose to 60 mg/m^2. Dosing with neutropenic complications in subsequent cycles should be further reduced to 45 mg/m^2. Patients who experience grade 4 thrombocytopenia should receive a dose reduction from 75 mg/m^2 to 60 mg/m^2. Discontinue therapy for persistent toxicities.
Gastrointestinal toxicity for docetaxel in combination with cisplatin and fluorouracil for treatment of gastric cancer or head and neck cancer:
Diarrhea, grade 3:
First episode: Reduce fluorouracil dose by 20%
Second episode: Reduce docetaxel dose by 20%

Diarrhea, grade 4:
First episode: Reduce fluorouracil and docetaxel doses by 20%
Second episode: Discontinue treatment
Stomatitis, grade 3:
First episode: Reduce fluorouracil dose by 20%
Second episode: Discontinue fluorouracil for all subsequent cycles
Third episode: Reduce docetaxel dose by 20%
Stomatitis, grade 4:
First episode: Discontinue fluorouracil for all subsequent cycles
Second episode: Reduce docetaxel dose by 20%

Dosing adjustment in renal impairment: Adults: Renal excretion is minimal; therefore, the need for dosage adjustments for renal dysfunction is unlikely (Janus, 2010; Li, 2007). Not removed by hemodialysis; may be administered before or after hemodialysis (Janus, 2010).
Dosing adjustment in hepatic impairment: Adults:
Manufacturer's labeling:
Total bilirubin greater than the ULN, or AST/ALT >1.5 times ULN concomitant with alkaline phosphatase >2.5 times ULN: Use is not recommended.
Hepatic impairment dosing adjustment specific for gastric or head and neck cancer:
AST/ALT >2.5 to ≤5 times ULN and alkaline phosphatase ≤2.5 times ULN: Administer 80% of dose
AST/ALT >1.5 to ≤5 times ULN and alkaline phosphatase >2.5 to ≤5 times ULN: Administer 80% of dose
AST/ALT >5 times ULN and /or alkaline phosphatase >5 times ULN: Discontinue docetaxel
The following guidelines have been used by some clinicians (Floyd, 2006):
AST/ALT 1.6-6 times ULN: Administer 75% of dose
AST/ALT >6 times ULN: Use clinical judgment
Administration Hazardous agent; use appropriate precautions for handling and disposal (NIOSH, 2012). **Note: Multiple concentrations:** Docetaxel is available as a one-vial formulation at concentrations of 10 mg/mL (generic formulation) and 20 mg/mL (concentrate; Taxotere), and as a lyophilized powder (Docefrez), which is reconstituted (with provided diluent) to 20 mg/0.8 mL (20 mg vial) or 24 mg/mL (80 mg vial). Admixture errors have occurred due to the availability of various concentrations. Docetaxel was previously available as a two-vial formulation which included two vials (a concentrated docetaxel vial and a diluent vial), resulting in a reconstituted concentration of 10 mg/mL; the two-vial formulation has been discontinued by the manufacturer.
Preparation:
One-vial formulations: Product can be directly added to solution for infusion; further dilute for infusion in 250-500 mL of NS or D$_5$W in a non-DEHP container (eg, glass, polypropylene, polyolefin) to a final concentration of 0.3-0.74 mg/mL. Gently rotate to mix thoroughly; avoid shaking or vigorous agitation. **Note:** For docetaxel injection concentrate 20 mg/mL (Taxotere), use **only** a 21-gauge needle to withdraw docetaxel from the vial (larger bore needles, such as 18-gauge or 19-gauge needles may cause stopper coring and rubber precipitates).
Lyophilized powder: Allow vials (and provided diluent) to stand at room temperature for 5 minutes prior to reconstitution. Reconstitute with the provided diluent (contains ethanol in polysorbate 80); add 1 mL of diluent to each 20 mg vial (resulting concentration is 20 mg/0.8 mL) and 4 mL of diluent to each 80 mg vial (resulting concentration is 24 mg/mL). Shake well to dissolve completely. If air bubbles are present, allow to stand for a few minutes while air bubbles dissipate. Further dilute in 250 mL of NS or D$_5$W in a non-DEHP container (eg, glass, polypropylene, polyolefin) to a final

concentration of 0.3-0.74 mg/mL (for doses >200 mg, use a larger volume of NS or D_5W, not to exceed a final concentration of 0.74 mg/mL). Mix thoroughly by manual agitation.

Administration: Administer as an I.V. infusion over 1 hour through nonsorbing polyethylene lined (non-DEHP) tubing; in-line filter is not necessary. Infusion should be completed within 4 hours of preparation. **Note:** Premedication with corticosteroids for 3 days, beginning the day before docetaxel administration, is recommended to prevent hypersensitivity reactions and pulmonary/peripheral edema. Irritant with vesicant-like properties; avoid extravasation. Assure proper needle or catheter position prior to administration.

Extravasation management: If extravasation occurs, stop infusion immediately and disconnect (leave cannula/needle in place); gently aspirate extravasated solution (do **NOT** flush the line); remove needle/cannula; elevate extremity. Information conflicts regarding the use of warm or cold compresses (Pérez Fidalgo, 2012; Polovich, 2009).

Vesicant/Extravasation Risk Irritant with vesicant-like properties

Monitoring Parameters CBC with differential, liver function tests, bilirubin, alkaline phosphatase, renal function; monitor for hypersensitivity reactions, neurosensory symptoms, gastrointestinal toxicity (eg, diarrhea, stomatitis), cutaneous reactions, fluid retention, epiphora, and canalicular stenosis

Additional Information Premedication with oral corticosteroids is recommended to decrease the incidence and severity of fluid retention and severity of hypersensitivity reactions. The manufacturer recommends dexamethasone 16 mg (8 mg twice daily) orally for 3 days. In one pediatric clinical trial, dexamethasone 3 mg/m^2 orally or I.V. every 6 hours for 2 doses, starting 12 hours before docetaxel administration has been described (Zwerdling, 2006).

Dosage Forms Excipient information presented when available (limited, particularly for generics); consult specific product labeling.

Concentrate, Intravenous:
Taxotere: 20 mg/mL (1 mL); 80 mg/4 mL (4 mL) [contains alcohol, usp, polysorbate 80]
Generic: 20 mg/mL (1 mL); 80 mg/4 mL (4 mL); 160 mg/8 mL (8 mL); 20 mg/0.5 mL (0.5 mL); 80 mg/2 mL (2 mL)

Concentrate, Intravenous [preservative free]:
Generic: 20 mg/mL (1 mL); 80 mg/4 mL (4 mL); 140 mg/7 mL (7 mL)

Solution, Intravenous:
Generic: 20 mg/2 mL (2 mL); 80 mg/8 mL (8 mL); 160 mg/16 mL (16 mL)

Solution Reconstituted, Intravenous:
Docefrez: 20 mg (1 ea); 80 mg (1 ea) [contains alcohol, usp, polysorbate 80]

References
Berveiller P, Vinot C, Mir O, et al, "Comparative Transplacental Transfer of Taxanes Using the Human Perfused Cotyledon Placental Model," *Am J Obstet Gynecol,* 2012, 207(6):514.e1-514.e7.
Chan A, Su C, de Boer RH, et al. Prevalence of excessive tearing in women with early breast cancer receiving adjuvant docetaxel-based chemotherapy. *J Clin Oncol.* 2013;31(17):2123-2127.
Clarke SJ and Rivory LP, "Clinical Pharmacokinetics of Docetaxel," *Clin Pharmacokinet,* 1999, 36(2):99-114.
Floyd J, Mirza I, Sachs B, et al, "Hepatotoxicity of Chemotherapy," *Semin Oncol,* 2006, 33(1):50-67.
Janus N, Thariat J, Boulanger H, et al, "Proposal for Dosage Adjustment and Timing of Chemotherapy in Hemodialyzed Patients," *Ann Oncol,* 2010, 21(7):1395-403.
Li YF, Fu S, Hu W, et al, "Systemic Anticancer Therapy in Gynecological Cancer Patients With Renal Dysfunction," *Int J Gynecol Cancer,* 2007, 17(4):739-63.
Mora J, Cruz CO, Parareda A, et al, "Treatment of Relapsed/Refractory Pediatric Sarcomas With Gemcitabine and Docetaxel," *J Pediatr Hematol Oncol,* 2009, 31(10):723-9.
National Institute for Occupational Safety and Health (NIOSH), "NIOSH List of Antineoplastic and Other Hazardous Drugs in Healthcare Settings 2012." Available at http://www.cdc.gov/niosh/docs/2012-150/pdfs/2012-150.pdf. Accessed January 21, 2013.
Navid F, Willert JR, McCarville MB, et al, "Combination of Gemcitabine and Docetaxel in the Treatment of Children and Young Adults With Refractory Bone Sarcoma," *Cancer,* 2008, 113(2):419-25.
Pérez Fidalgo JA, García Fabregat L, Cervantes A, et al. Management of chemotherapy extravasation: ESMO-EONS clinical practice guidelines. *Ann Oncol.* 2012;23(Suppl 7):167-173.
Polovich M, Whitford JN, Olsen M. *Chemotherapy and Biotherapy Guidelines and Recommendations for Practice.* 3rd ed. Pittsburgh, PA: Oncology Nursing Society; 2009.
Thiesen J and Kramer I, "Physico-Chemical Stability of Docetaxel Premix Solution and Docetaxel Infusion Solutions in PVC Bags and Polyolefine Containers," *Pharm World Sci,* 1999, 21(3):137-41.
Zwerdling T, Krailo M, Monteleone P, et al, "Phase II Investigation of Docetaxel in Pediatric Patients With Recurrent Solid Tumors: A Report From the Children's Oncology Group," *Cancer,* 2006, 106 (8):1821-8.

◆ **Docetaxel for Injection (Can)** *see* DOCEtaxel *on page 697*

◆ **DocQLace [OTC]** *see* Docusate *on page 701*

◆ **Doc-Q-Lax [OTC]** *see* Docusate and Senna *on page 702*

◆ **Docu [OTC]** *see* Docusate *on page 701*

◆ **Docuprene [OTC]** *see* Docusate *on page 701*

Docusate (DOK yoo sate)

Medication Safety Issues
Sound-alike/look-alike issues:
Colace® may be confused with Calan®, Cozaar®
Dulcolax® (docusate) may be confused with Dulcolax® (bisacodyl)
International issues:
Docusate may be confused with Doxinate brand name for doxylamine and pyridoxine [India]

Related Information
Oral Medications That Should Not Be Crushed or Altered *on page 2438*

Brand Names: U.S. Colace [OTC]; D.O.S. [OTC]; Diocto [OTC]; DocQLace [OTC]; Docu Soft [OTC]; Docu [OTC]; Docuprene [OTC]; Docusil [OTC]; DocuSol Kids [OTC]; DocuSol Mini [OTC]; DOK [OTC]; Dulcolax Stool Softener [OTC]; Enemeez Mini [OTC]; Healthy Mama Move It Along [OTC]; Kao-Tin [OTC]; KS Stool Softener [OTC]; Laxa Basic [OTC]; Pedia-Lax [OTC]; Promolaxin [OTC]; Silace [OTC]; Sof-Lax [OTC]; Stool Softener Laxative DC [OTC]; Stool Softener [OTC]; Sur-Q-Lax [OTC]; Vacuant Mini-Enema [OTC] [DSC]

Brand Names: Canada Apo-Docusate Calcium [OTC]; Apo-Docusate Sodium [OTC]; Calax [OTC]; Colace [OTC]; Correctol Stool Softener [OTC]; Docusate Sodium Odan [OTC]; Dom-Docusate Sodium [OTC]; Dosolax [OTC]; Euro-Docusate C [OTC]; Jamp-Docusate [OTC]; Novo-Docusate Calcium [OTC]; Novo-Docusate Sodium [OTC]; PHL-Docusate Sodium [OTC]; PMS-Docusate Calcium [OTC]; PMS-Docusate Sodium [OTC]; ratio-Docusate Sodium [OTC]; Selax [OTC]; Silace [OTC]; Sirop Docusate De Sodium [OTC]; Soflax C [OTC]; Soflax Pediatric Drops [OTC]; Soflax [OTC]; Taro-Docusate [OTC]; Teva-Docusate Sodium [OTC]

Therapeutic Category Laxative, Surfactant; Stool Softener

Generic Availability (U.S.) May be product dependent

Use Stool softener in patients who should avoid straining during defecation; constipation associated with hard, dry stools; ceruminolytic

Pregnancy Considerations The short-term use of docusate for the treatment of constipation is generally considered safe during pregnancy (Mahadevan, 2006). Hypomagnesemia was reported in a newborn following chronic maternal overuse throughout pregnancy (Schindler, 1984).

Breast-Feeding Considerations Maternal use of docusate is considered to be compatible with breast-feeding (Mahadevan, 2006).

Contraindications Hypersensitivity to docusate or any component; concomitant use of mineral oil; intestinal obstruction, acute abdominal pain, nausea, vomiting

Adverse Reactions

Gastrointestinal: Abdominal cramping, diarrhea, Intestinal obstruction

Miscellaneous: Throat irritation

Drug Interactions

Metabolism/Transport Effects None known.

Avoid Concomitant Use There are no known interactions where it is recommended to avoid concomitant use.

Increased Effect/Toxicity There are no known significant interactions involving an increase in effect.

Decreased Effect There are no known significant interactions involving a decrease in effect.

Mechanism of Action Reduces surface tension of the oil-water interface of the stool resulting in enhanced incorporation of water and fat allowing for stool softening

Pharmacodynamics Onset of action: 12-72 hours

Dosing: Usual

Infants and Children: Oral: 5 mg/kg/day in 1-4 divided doses **or** dose by age:

<3 years: 10-40 mg/day in 1-4 divided doses

3-6 years: 20-60 mg/day in 1-4 divided doses

6-12 years: 40-150 mg/day in 1-4 divided doses

Adolescents and Adults: Oral: 50-400 mg/day in 1-4 divided doses

Older Children and Adults: Rectal: Add 50-100 mg of docusate liquid (not syrup) to enema fluid (NS or water)

Administration

Oral: Administer docusate liquid (not syrup) with milk, fruit juice, or infant formula to mask the bitter taste; ensure adequate fluid intake

Rectal: Administer as a retention or flushing enema

Test Interactions Decreased potassium (S), decreased chloride (S)

Additional Information Docusate sodium 5-10 mg/mL **liquid** instilled in the ear as a ceruminolytic produces substantial ear wax disintegration within 15 minutes and complete disintegration after 24 hours

Dosage Forms Excipient information presented when available (limited, particularly for generics); consult specific product labeling. [DSC] = Discontinued product

Capsule, Oral, as calcium:

Kao-Tin: 240 mg [sodium free; contains fd&c red #40]

Stool Softener Laxative DC: 240 mg [contains fd&c red #40]

Sur-Q-Lax: 240 mg

Generic: 240 mg

Capsule, Oral, as sodium:

Colace: 50 mg, 100 mg

D.O.S.: 250 mg

DocQLace: 100 mg [contains fd&c red #40, fd&c yellow #6 (sunset yellow)]

Docu Soft: 100 mg

Docusil: 100 mg

DOK: 100 mg, 250 mg

Dulcolax Stool Softener: 100 mg [contains fd&c red #40, fd&c yellow #6 (sunset yellow)]

KS Stool Softener: 100 mg [stimulant free; contains brilliant blue fcf (fd&c blue #1), fd&c red #40, methylparaben, propylparaben, tartrazine (fd&c yellow #5)]

Laxa Basic: 100 mg

Sof-Lax: 100 mg

Stool Softener: 100 mg

Stool Softener: 100 mg, 250 mg [contains fd&c red #40, fd&c yellow #6 (sunset yellow)]

Stool Softener: 100 mg [stimulant free; contains brilliant blue fcf (fd&c blue #1), fd&c red #40, fd&c yellow #6 (sunset yellow)]

Generic: 100 mg, 250 mg

Enema, Rectal, as sodium:

DocuSol Kids: 100 mg/5 mL (5 ea) [contains polyethylene glycol]

DocuSol Mini: 283 mg (5 ea)

Enemeez Mini: 283 mg (5 mL)

Vacuant Mini-Enema: 283 mg (5 mL [DSC])

Liquid, Oral, as sodium:

Diocto: 50 mg/5 mL (473 mL) [contains fd&c red #40, methylparaben, polyethylene glycol, propylene glycol, propylparaben; vanilla flavor]

Diocto: 50 mg/5 mL (473 mL) [contains parabens, polyethylene glycol]

Docu: 50 mg/5 mL (10 mL, 473 mL) [contains methylparaben, polyethylene glycol, propylene glycol, propylparaben, sodium benzoate; vanilla flavor]

Pedia-Lax: 50 mg/15 mL (118 mL) [contains edetate disodium, methylparaben, polyethylene glycol, propylene glycol, propylparaben; fruit punch flavor]

Silace: 150 mg/15 mL (473 mL) [lemon-vanilla flavor]

Generic: 50 mg/5 mL (10 mL)

Syrup, Oral, as sodium:

Diocto: 60 mg/15 mL (473 mL) [contains fd&c red #40, menthol, methylparaben, polyethylene glycol, propylparaben, sodium benzoate; peppermint flavor]

Diocto: 60 mg/15 mL (473 mL [DSC]) [contains fd&c red #40, methylparaben, propylene glycol, propylparaben, sodium benzoate; peppermint flavor]

Diocto: 60 mg/15 mL (473 mL) [contains fd&c red #40, propylene glycol, saccharin sodium, sodium benzoate]

Silace: 60 mg/15 mL (473 mL) [contains alcohol, usp; peppermint flavor]

Tablet, Oral, as sodium:

Docuprene: 100 mg [contains sodium benzoate]

DOK: 100 mg [scored]

Healthy Mama Move It Along: 100 mg [scored; stimulant free; contains sodium benzoate]

Promolaxin: 100 mg [scored; contains sodium benzoate]

Stool Softener: 100 mg [contains sodium benzoate]

Generic: 100 mg

References

Chen DA and Caparosa RJ, "A Nonprescription Cerumenolytic," *Am J Otol*, 1991, 12(6):475-6.

Mahadevan U and Kane S, "American Gastroenterological Association Institute Medical Position Statement on the Use of Gastrointestinal Medications in Pregnancy," *Gastroenterology*, 2006, 131(1):278-82.

Schindler AM, "Isolated Neonatal Hypomagnesaemia Associated With Maternal Overuse of Stool Softener," *Lancet*, 1984, 2(8406):822.

Docusate and Senna (DOK yoo sate & SEN na)

Medication Safety Issues

Sound-alike/look-alike issues:

Senokot® may be confused with Depakote®

Brand Names: U.S. Doc-Q-Lax [OTC]; Dok™ Plus [OTC]; Geri-Stool [OTC]; Peri-Colace® [OTC]; Senexon®-S [OTC]; Senna Plus [OTC]; SennaLax-S [OTC]; Senokot-S® [OTC]; SenoSol™-SS [OTC]

Therapeutic Category Laxative, Stimulant; Laxative, Surfactant; Stool Softener

Generic Availability (U.S.) Yes

Use Treatment of constipation generally associated with dry, hard stools and decreased intestinal motility; prevention of opiate-induced constipation

Pregnancy Considerations See individual agents.

Breast-Feeding Considerations See individual agents.

Contraindications Hypersensitivity to docusate, senna, or any component; concomitant use of mineral oil; undiagnosed abdominal pain; appendicitis, intestinal obstruction or perforation; acute abdominal pain; nausea, vomiting

Warnings Do not use when abdominal pain, rectal bleeding, nausea, or vomiting are present

Precautions Avoid prolonged use (>1 week); chronic use may lead to dependency, fluid and electrolyte imbalance, vitamin and mineral deficiencies

Adverse Reactions

Gastrointestinal: Abdominal cramps, diarrhea, nausea, vomiting

Genitourinary: Urine discoloration (red/brown)

Mechanism of Action Docusate is a stool softener; sennosides are laxatives

Pharmacodynamics Onset of action: Within 6-12 hours

Pharmacokinetics (Adult data unless noted) Senna:

Metabolism: Senna is metabolized in the liver

Elimination: In the feces (via bile) and in urine

Dosing: Usual Oral:

Children 2 to <6 years: 1/2 tablet once daily at bedtime; maximum: 1 tablet twice daily

Children 6 to <12 years: 1 tablet once daily at bedtime; maximum: 2 tablets twice daily

Children ≥12 years, Adolescents, and Adults: 2 tablets once daily at bedtime; maximum: 4 tablets twice daily

Administration Administer with water, preferably in the evening

Monitoring Parameters I & O, frequency of bowel movements, serum electrolytes if severe diarrhea develops

Dosage Forms Excipient information presented when available (limited, particularly for generics); consult specific product labeling.

Tablet, oral: Docusate sodium 50 mg and sennosides 8.6 mg

Doc-Q-Lax: Docusate sodium 50 mg and sennosides 8.6 mg

Dok™ Plus: Docusate sodium 50 mg and sennosides 8.6 mg [contains sodium benzoate]

Geri-Stool: Docusate sodium 50 mg and sennosides 8.6 mg

Peri-Colace®: Docusate sodium 50 mg and sennosides 8.6 mg

Senexon®-S: Docusate sodium 50 mg and sennosides 8.6 mg [contains calcium 20 mg/tablet, sodium 6 mg/tablet]

SennaLax-S: Docusate sodium 50 mg and sennosides 8.6 mg [contains sodium benzoate]

Senna Plus: Docusate sodium 50 mg and sennosides 8.6 mg

Senokot-S®: Docusate sodium 50 mg and sennosides 8.6 mg [sugar free; contains sodium 4 mg/tablet]

SenoSol™-SS: Docusate sodium 50 mg and sennosides 8.6 mg [contains sodium 3 mg/tablet]

References

Baker SS, Liptak GS, Colletti RB, et al, "Constipation in Infants and Children: Evaluation and Treatment. A Medical Position Statement of the North American Society for Pediatric Gastroenterology and Nutrition," *J Pediatr Gastroenterol Nutr*, 1999, 29(5):612-26.

Herndon CM, Jackson KC II, and Hallin PA, "Management of Opioid-Induced Gastrointestinal Effects in Patients Receiving Palliative Care," *Pharmacotherapy*, 2002, 22(2):240-50.

◆ **Docusate Calcium** see Docusate on page 701

◆ **Docusate Potassium** see Docusate on page 701

◆ **Docusate Sodium** see Docusate on page 701

◆ **Docusate Sodium Odan [OTC] (Can)** see Docusate on page 701

◆ **Docusil [OTC]** see Docusate on page 701

◆ **Docu Soft [OTC]** see Docusate on page 701

◆ **DocuSol Kids [OTC]** see Docusate on page 701

◆ **DocuSol Mini [OTC]** see Docusate on page 701

◆ **Dofus [OTC]** see Lactobacillus on page 1191

◆ **DOK [OTC]** see Docusate on page 701

◆ **Dok™ Plus [OTC]** see Docusate and Senna on page 702

Dolasetron (dol A se tron)

Medication Safety Issues

Sound-alike/look-alike issues:

Anzemet may be confused with Aldomet, Antivert, Avandamet

Dolasetron may be confused with granisetron, ondansetron, palonosetron

Brand Names: U.S. Anzemet

Brand Names: Canada Anzemet

Therapeutic Category Antiemetic; Selective 5-HT$_3$ Receptor Antagonist

Generic Availability (U.S.) No

Use

Parenteral solution: Prevention and treatment of postoperative nausea and vomiting (FDA approved in ages ≥2 years and adults)

Tablets: Prevention of nausea and vomiting associated with emetogenic cancer chemotherapy (initial and repeat courses) (FDA approved in ages ≥2 years and adults)

Pregnancy Risk Factor B

Pregnancy Considerations Adverse events have not been observed in animal reproduction studies.

Breast-Feeding Considerations It is not known if dolasetron is excreted in breast milk. The manufacturer recommends that caution be exercised when administering dolasetron to nursing women.

Contraindications Hypersensitivity to dolasetron or any component

Dosage form specific: Parenteral (intravenous administration): Use for prevention of chemotherapy-associated nausea and vomiting

Warnings Dolasetron is associated with a number of dose-dependent increases in ECG intervals (eg, PR, QT/QT$_c$, JT prolongation, and QRS widening) usually occurring 1-2 hours after I.V. administration and usually lasting 6-8 hours; however, may last ≥24 hours. May rarely lead to cardiovascular consequences, such as heart block or cardiac arrhythmias. Clinically relevant QT interval prolongation may occur, resulting in torsade de pointes, when used in conjunction with other agents that prolong the QT interval (eg, Class I and III antiarrhythmics). Avoid use in patients at greater risk for QT prolongation, including patients with congenital long QT syndrome, concurrent medication known to prolong QT interval (eg, Class I and III antiarrhythmics), electrolyte abnormalities (ie, hypokalemia, hypomagnesemia) or medications known to reduce potassium or magnesium concentrations (eg, diuretics), and cumulative high-dose anthracycline therapy. Correct potassium or magnesium abnormalities prior to initiating therapy; ECG monitoring is recommended in patient with renal impairment and geriatric patients. Parenteral formulation of 5-HT$_3$ antagonists has a greater association with ECG interval changes, compared to oral formulation. Reduction in heart rate may also occur with the 5-HT$_3$ antagonists. Use with caution in children and adolescents who have or may develop QT$_c$ prolongation due to rare reports of supraventricular and ventricular arrhythmias, MI, and cardiac arrest in pediatric and adolescent patients. Canadian healthcare officials have deemed dolasetron contraindicated for the treatment of children and adolescents <18 years of age.

Precautions Use with caution in patients allergic to other 5-HT$_3$ receptor antagonists; cross reactivity has been reported with other 5-HT$_3$ receptor antagonists. For chemotherapy associated nausea and vomiting, dolasetron should be used on a scheduled basis, not on an "as needed" (PRN) basis, since data support the use of this drug only in the prevention of nausea and vomiting (due to antineoplastic therapy) and not in the rescue of nausea and vomiting; not intended for treatment of nausea and vomiting or for chronic continuous therapy. For postoperative nausea and vomiting, if the prophylaxis dolasetron dose has failed, a repeat dose should not be administered as rescue or treatment.

Potentially significant interactions may exist, requiring dose or frequency adjustment, additional monitoring, and/or selection of alternative therapy. Consult drug interactions database for more detailed information.

Adverse Reactions Adverse events may vary according to indication

Cardiovascular: Bradycardia, hypertension, tachycardia

Central nervous system: Chills/shivering, dizziness, fatigue, fever, headache, pain

Gastrointestinal: Abdominal pain, diarrhea, dyspepsia

Hepatic: Abnormal hepatic function

Renal: Oliguria, urinary retention

Rare but important or life-threatening: Abnormal vision, abnormal dreams, acute renal failure, alkaline phosphatase increased, ALT increased, anaphylactic reaction, anemia, anxiety, AST increased, ataxia, bronchospasm, cardiac arrest, chest pain, confusion, constipation, diaphoresis, dyspnea, dysuria, edema, epistaxis, facial edema, flushing, GGT increased, hematuria, hyperbilirubinemia, hypotension, ischemia (peripheral), local injection site reaction (pain/burning), MI, myocardial ischemia, orthostatic hypotension, palpitation, pancreatitis, paresthesia, peripheral edema, photophobia, polyuria, prothrombin time increased, PTT increased, purpura/hematoma, rash, syncope, taste alteration, thrombocytopenia, thrombophlebitis/phlebitis, tinnitus, tremor, twitching, urticaria, vertigo

Note: Cardiac conduction abnormalities (including arrhythmia [sinus, supraventricular and ventricular], atrial flutter/fibrillation, AV block, bundle branch block, extrasystoles, poor R wave progression, prolonged PR, QRS, JT, and QT_c intervals, ST, T and U wave changes, torsade de pointes, ventricular tachycardia, wide complex tachycardia and ventricular fibrillation) have also been reported.

Drug Interactions

Metabolism/Transport Effects Substrate of CYP2C9 (minor), CYP3A4 (minor); **Note:** Assignment of Major/Minor substrate status based on clinically relevant drug interaction potential; **Inhibits** CYP2D6 (weak)

Avoid Concomitant Use

Avoid concomitant use of Dolasetron with any of the following: Apomorphine; Highest Risk QTc-Prolonging Agents; Ivabradine; Mifepristone

Increased Effect/Toxicity

Dolasetron may increase the levels/effects of: Apomorphine; ARIPiprazole; Highest Risk QTc-Prolonging Agents; Moderate Risk QTc-Prolonging Agents; Serotonin Modulators

The levels/effects of Dolasetron may be increased by: Ivabradine; Mifepristone; QTc-Prolonging Agents (Indeterminate Risk and Risk Modifying)

Decreased Effect

Dolasetron may decrease the levels/effects of: Tapentadol; TraMADol

Food Interactions Food does not affect the bioavailability of oral doses.

Stability

Injection: Store intact vials at 20°C to 25°C (68°F to 77°F); excursions are permitted to 15°C to 30°C (59°F to 86°F). Protect from light. Solutions diluted for infusion in compatible solution (NS, D_5W, $D_5\frac{1}{2}NS$, D_5LR, LR, and 10% mannitol solution) are stable under normal lighting conditions at room temperature for 24 hours or under refrigeration for 48 hours.

Tablets: Store at 20°C to 25°C (68°F to 77°F). Protect from light.

Mechanism of Action Selective serotonin receptor ($5\text{-}HT_3$) antagonist, blocking serotonin both peripherally (primary site of action) and centrally at the chemoreceptor trigger zone

Pharmacokinetics (Adult data unless noted) Due to the rapid metabolism of dolasetron to hydrodolasetron (primary active metabolite), the majority of the following pharmacokinetic parameters relate to hydrodolasetron:

Absorption: Oral: Rapid and complete

Distribution:

Children: 5.9-7.4 L/kg

Adults: 4.15-5.5 L/kg

Metabolism: Hepatic; rapidly converted by carbonyl reductase to active major metabolite, hydrodolasetron; hydrodolasetron is metabolized by the cytochrome P450 CYP2D6 and CYP3A enzyme systems and flavin mono-oxygenase

Bioavailability: Oral: Children: 59% (formulation not specified), adults: 70% to 80% (not affected by food)

Protein binding: 69% to 77% (active metabolite)

Half-life, elimination:

Dolasetron: <10 minutes

Hydrodolasetron:

Oral: Children: 5.7 hours, adults: 8.1 hours (range: 5-10 hours)

I.V.: Children: 4.8 hours, adults: 7.3 hours (range: 4-8 hours)

Time to peak serum concentration:

Oral: 1-1.5 hours

I.V.: 0.6 hours

Elimination: Dolasetron: <1% excreted unchanged in urine; hydrodolasetron: 53% to 61% of total dose excreted unchanged in urine within 36 hours

Dosing: Usual

Children ≥2 years and Adolescents:

Chemotherapy-induced nausea and vomiting (CINV); prevention: Note: Due to increased risk of QT_c prolongation, the use of I.V. dolasetron for CINV is contraindicated:

Children and Adolescents 2-16 years: Oral: 1.8 mg/kg as a single dose (maximum dose: 100 mg) within 1 hour before chemotherapy

Adolescents >16 years: Oral: 100 mg as a single dose within 1 hour before chemotherapy

Postoperative nausea and vomiting: Note: If the prophylaxis dolasetron dose has failed, a repeat dose should not be administered as rescue or treatment.

Prevention:

Oral (using parenteral formulation administered orally): Children and Adolescents 2-16 years: 1.2 mg/kg administered within 2 hours before surgery; maximum dose: 100 mg

I.V.:

Children and Adolescents 2-16 years: 0.35 mg/kg ~15 minutes before cessation of anesthesia; maximum dose: 12.5 mg

Adolescents >16 years: 12.5 mg ~15 minutes before cessation of anesthesia (do not exceed the recommended dose)

Treatment: I.V.:

Children and Adolescents 2-16 years: 0.35 mg/kg as soon as nausea or vomiting present; maximum dose: 12.5 mg

Adolescents >16 years: 12.5 mg as soon as nausea or vomiting present (do not exceed the recommended dose)

Adults:

Prevention of chemotherapy-associated nausea and vomiting (including initial and repeat courses): Oral: 100 mg within 1 hour before chemotherapy

Postoperative nausea and vomiting:
Prevention: I.V.: 12.5 mg ~15 minutes before cessation of anesthesia (do not exceed the recommended dose)
Treatment: I.V.: 12.5 mg as soon as nausea or vomiting present (do not exceed the recommended dose)

Dosing adjustment in renal impairment: No dosage adjustment necessary; however, ECG monitoring is recommended in patients with renal impairment.

Dosing adjustment in hepatic impairment: No dosage adjustment necessary.

Administration

Oral: May be administered with or without food; parenteral solution may be administered orally, diluted in apple or apple-grape juice; dilution is stable for 2 hours at room temperature

Parenteral: I.V.: May infuse undiluted over 30 seconds or dilute in 50 mL compatible I.V. fluid and infuse over ≤15 minutes; do not mix with other medications; flush line before and after dolasetron administration

Monitoring Parameters ECG (in patients with cardiovascular disease, elderly, renally impaired, those at risk of developing hypokalemia and/or hypomagnesemia); serum potassium and magnesium

Dosage Forms Excipient information presented when available (limited, particularly for generics); consult specific product labeling.

Solution, Intravenous, as mesylate:
Anzemet: 20 mg/mL (0.625 mL, 5 mL, 25 mL)
Tablet, Oral, as mesylate:
Anzemet: 50 mg, 100 mg

Extemporaneous Preparations Dolasetron injection may be diluted in apple or apple-grape juice and taken orally; this dilution is stable for 2 hours at room temperature (Anzemet prescribing information, 2013).

A 10 mg/mL oral suspension may be prepared with tablets and either a 1:1 mixture of Ora-Plus and Ora-Sweet SF or a 1:1 mixture of strawberry syrup and Ora-Plus. Crush twelve 50 mg tablets in a mortar and reduce to a fine powder. Slowly add chosen vehicle to **almost** 60 mL; transfer to a calibrated bottle, rinse mortar with vehicle, and add quantity of vehicle sufficient to make 60 mL. Label "shake well" and "refrigerate". Stable for 90 days refrigerated.

Anzemet® prescribing information, sanofi-aventis U.S. LLC, Bridgewater, NJ, 2013.

Johnson CE, Wagner DS, and Bussard WE, "Stability of Dolasetron in Two Oral Liquid Vehicles," *Am J Health Syst Pharm*, 2003, 60 (21):2242-4.

References

American Society of Clinical Oncology, Kris MG, Hesketh PJ, et al, "American Society of Clinical Oncology Guideline for Antiemetics in Oncology: Update 2006," *J Clin Oncol*, 2006, 24(18):2932-47.

"ASHP Therapeutic Guidelines on the Pharmacologic Management of Nausea and Vomiting in Adult and Pediatric Patients Receiving Chemotherapy or Radiation Therapy or Undergoing Surgery," *Am J Health Syst Pharm*, 1999, 56(8):729-64.

National Comprehensive Cancer Network® (NCCN), "Clinical Practice Guidelines in Oncology™: Antiemesis," Version 4.2009. Available at: http://www.nccn.org/professionals/physician_gls/PDF/antiemesis.pdf.

Olutoye O, Jantzen EC, Alexis R, et al, "A Comparison of the Costs and Efficacy of Ondansetron and Dolasetron in the Prophylaxis of Postoperative Vomiting in Pediatric Patients Undergoing Ambulatory Surgery," *Anesth Analg*, 2003, 97(2):390-6.

◆ **Dolasetron Mesylate** *see* Dolasetron *on page 703*

◆ **Dolophine** *see* Methadone *on page 1355*

◆ **Doloral (Can)** *see* Morphine (Systemic) *on page 1440*

Dolutegravir (doe loo TEG ra vir)

Related Information
Adult and Adolescent HIV *on page 2348*
Pediatric HIV *on page 2338*
Perinatal HIV *on page 2356*

Brand Names: U.S. Tivicay
Brand Names: Canada Tivicay
Therapeutic Category Antiretroviral, Integrase Inhibitor (Anti-HIV); Antiviral Agent; HIV Agents (Anti-HIV Agents); Integrase Inhibitor
Generic Availability (U.S.) No

Use
Treatment of HIV-1 infection in combination with other antiretroviral agents (FDA approved in ages ≥12 years weighing ≥40 kg and adults). **Note:** HIV regimens consisting of **three** antiretroviral agents are strongly recommended.

Medication Guide Available Yes
Pregnancy Risk Factor B
Pregnancy Considerations Adverse events were not observed in animal reproduction studies. It is not known if dolutegravir crosses the placenta. The DHHS Perinatal HIV Guidelines note there are insufficient data to recommend use in pregnancy.

Regardless of CD4 count or HIV RNA copy number, all HIV-infected pregnant women should receive a combination antiretroviral (ARV) drug regimen. A combination of antepartum, intrapartum, and infant ARV prophylaxis is recommended. ARV therapy should be started as soon as possible in women with symptomatic infection. Although earlier initiation may be more effective in reducing the perinatal transmission of HIV, initiation may be delayed until after 12 weeks gestation in women who do not require immediate treatment after careful consideration of maternal conditions (eg, nausea and vomiting) and the potential risks of first trimester fetal exposure for specific agents. A scheduled cesarean delivery at 38 weeks gestation is recommended for all women with HIV RNA >1000 copies/mL or unknown concentrations near delivery in order to decrease transmission. If ARV therapy must be interrupted for <24 hours during the peripartum period, stop then restart all medications simultaneously in order to decrease the chance of developing resistance. Long-term follow-up is recommended for all infants exposed to ARV medications. In couples who want to conceive, the HIV-infected partner should attain maximum viral suppression prior to conception.

Health care providers are encouraged to enroll pregnant women exposed to antiretroviral medications in the Antiretroviral Pregnancy Registry (1-800-258-4263 or www.APRegistry.com). Health care providers caring for HIV-infected women and their infants may contact the National Perinatal HIV Hotline (888-448-8765) for clinical consultation (DHHS [perinatal], 2014).

Breast-Feeding Considerations It is not known if dolutegravir is excreted into breast milk. Maternal or infant antiretroviral therapy does not completely eliminate the risk of postnatal HIV transmission. In addition, multiclass-resistant virus has been detected in breast-feeding infants despite maternal therapy. Therefore, in the United States, where formula is accessible, affordable, safe, and sustainable, and the risk of infant mortality due to diarrhea and respiratory infections is low, complete avoidance of breast-feeding by HIV-infected women is recommended to decrease potential transmission of HIV (DHHS [perinatal], 2014).The manufacturer notes that women should be instructed not to breast-feed their infants while on dolutegravir therapy.

▶

◄ **Contraindications** Hypersensitivity to dolutegravir or any component; concurrent use with dofetilide

Warnings Hypersensitivity reactions including rash, constitutional findings, and organ dysfunction (including liver injury) have been reported. Discontinue immediately if signs of hypersensitivity (including severe rash, rash with fever, malaise, fatigue, muscle/joint aches, blistering or peeling of skin, oral blisters/lesions, conjunctivitis, facial edema, hepatitis, eosinophilia, angioedema, difficulty breathing) occur. Monitor clinical status and liver function tests, and initiate supportive therapy as appropriate. If hypersensitivity occurs, do not reinitiate therapy with dolutegravir.

Precautions Patients with underlying hepatic disease (such as hepatitis B or C coinfection) may be at increased risk of development or worsening of transaminase elevations; use with caution. Elevation in transaminases may be concurrent with development of immune reconstitution syndrome or hepatitis B reactivation (especially if antihepatitis therapy has been discontinued). Monitor transaminases at baseline and during therapy. Immune reconstitution syndrome (an acute inflammatory response to residual or indolent opportunistic infections) may occur in HIV patients during initial treatment with combination antiretroviral agents; this syndrome may require further patient assessment and therapy. Autoimmune disorders (eg, Graves' disease, Guillain-Barré syndrome, and polymyositis) have been reported in patients experiencing immune reconstitution; time to onset is variable and may occur many months after antiretroviral treatment is initiated.

Fat redistribution and accumulation (ie, central obesity, peripheral wasting, facial wasting, breast enlargement, dorsocervical fat enlargement [buffalo hump], and cushingoid appearance) have been observed in patients receiving antiretroviral agents (causal relationship not established).

Potentially significant interactions may exist, requiring dose or frequency adjustment, additional monitoring, and/or selection of alternative therapy. Consult drug interactions database for more detailed information.

Adverse Reactions Adverse reactions reported with combination therapy.
Central nervous system: Fatigue, headache, insomnia
Dermatologic: Pruritus
Endocrine & metabolic: Hyperbilirubinemia, hyperglycemia
Gastrointestinal: Abdominal distress, abdominal pain, diarrhea, elevated serum lipase, flatulence, nausea, upper abdominal pain, vomiting
Hematologic & oncologic: Leukopenia, neutropenia
Hepatic: Hepatitis, increased serum ALT, increased serum AST
Hypersensitivity: Hypersensitivity reaction
Neuromuscular & skeletal: Increased creatine phosphokinase, myositis
Renal: Renal insufficiency
Rare but important or life-threatening: Immune reconstitution syndrome

Drug Interactions
Metabolism/Transport Effects Substrate of BCRP, CYP3A4 (minor), P-glycoprotein, UGT1A1, UGT1A3, UGT1A9; **Note:** Assignment of Major/Minor substrate status based on clinically relevant drug interaction potential

Avoid Concomitant Use
Avoid concomitant use of Dolutegravir with any of the following: CarBAMazepine; Dofetilide; Fosphenytoin-Phenytoin; Nevirapine; OXcarbazepine; PHENobarbital; Primidone; St Johns Wort

Increased Effect/Toxicity
Dolutegravir may increase the levels/effects of: Dofetilide; MetFORMIN
Decreased Effect
The levels/effects of Dolutegravir may be decreased by: Aluminum Hydroxide; Calcium Salts; CarBAMazepine; Efavirenz; Etravirine; Fosamprenavir; Fosphenytoin-Phenytoin; Iron Salts; Magnesium Salts; Multivitamins/Minerals (with ADEK, Folate, Iron); Multivitamins/Minerals (with AE, No Iron); Nevirapine; OXcarbazepine; PHENobarbital; Primidone; Rifampin; Selenium; St Johns Wort; Sucralfate; Tipranavir; Zinc Salts

Stability Store at 25°C (77°F); excursions permitted to 15°C to 30°C (59°F to 86°F).
Mechanism of Action Binds to the integrase active site and inhibits the strand transfer step of HIV-1 DNA integration necessary for the HIV replication cycle.
Pharmacokinetics (Adult data unless noted) Note: The pharmacokinetics of dolutegravir in HIV-1-infected pediatric patients aged 12 to <18 years were similar to those observed in HIV-1-infected adults.
Absorption: Food increased the extent of absorption and slowed the rate of absorption of dolutegravir. Low-, moderate-, and high-fat meals increased dolutegravir AUC by 33%, 41%, and 66%, respectively; increased C_{max} by 46%, 52%, and 67%, respectively; and prolonged T_{max} to 3, 4, and 5 hours from 2 hours under fasted conditions, respectively.
Distribution: $V_d/F = ~17.4$ L
Protein binding: ≥98.9%
Metabolism: Primarily metabolized via UGT1A1 with some contribution from CYP3A
Bioavailability: Has not been established
Half-life elimination: ~14 hours
Time to peak serum concentration: 2 to 3 hours
Elimination: Feces (53% as unchanged drug); urine (~31% as metabolites, <1% as unchanged drug)
Dosing: Usual
Pediatric: **HIV infection, treatment:** Children ≥12 years and Adolescents weighing ≥40 kg: Oral: **Note:** Use in combination with other antiretroviral agents.
Treatment-naive or treatment-experienced integrase strand transfer inhibitor (INSTI)-naive: 50 mg once daily
Treatment-naive or treatment-experienced INSTI-naive when coadministered with efavirenz, fosamprenavir/ritonavir, tipranavir/ritonavir or rifampin: 50 mg twice daily
Adult: **HIV treatment:** Oral: **Note:** Use in combination with other antiretroviral agents.
Treatment-naive or treatment-experienced integrase strand transfer inhibitor (INSTI)-naive: 50 mg once daily
Treatment-naive or treatment-experienced INSTI-naive when coadministered with efavirenz, fosamprenavir/ritonavir, tipranavir/ritonavir, or rifampin: 50 mg twice daily
INSTI-experienced with certain INSTI-associated resistance substitutions or clinically suspected INSTI resistance (**Note:** Consult prescribing information for details): 50 mg twice daily
Dosing adjustment in renal impairment:
Treatment-naive or treatment-experienced INSTI-naive: Children ≥12 years, Adolescents, and Adults: Mild, moderate, or severe impairment: No dosage adjustment required.
INSTI-experienced with certain INSTI-associated resistance substitutions or clinically suspected INSTI resistance: Adults:
CrCl ≥30 mL/minute: No dosage adjustment necessary.
CrCl <30 mL/minute: Use with caution since the reduction in dolutegravir concentrations may result in loss of therapeutic effect and development of resistance to dolutegravir or other coadministered antiretroviral agents.

ESRD including hemodialysis: Has not been studied.

Dosing adjustment in hepatic impairment: Children ≥12 years, Adolescents, and Adults:

Mild to moderate impairment (Child-Pugh class A or B): No dosage adjustment necessary.

Severe impairment (Child-Pugh class C): Not recommended (has not been studied).

Administration Oral: May be administered without regard to meals. Take 2 hours before or 6 hours after cation-containing antacids or laxatives, sucralfate, oral supplements containing iron or calcium, or buffered medications. Alternatively, dolutegravir and supplements containing calcium or iron can be taken together with food.

Monitoring Parameters Note: Monitor CD4 percentage (if <5 years of age) or CD4 count (if ≥5 years of age) at least every 3 to 4 months (DHHS [pediatric], 2014).

Prior to initiation of therapy: Genotypic resistance testing, CD4 and viral load (every 3 to 4 months), CBC with differential, LFTs, BUN, creatinine, electrolytes, glucose, urinalysis (every 6 to 12 months), and assessment of readiness for adherence with mediation regimen. At initiation and with any change in treatment regimen: CBC with differential, electrolytes, calcium, phosphate, glucose, LFTs, bilirubin, urinalysis (at initiation), BUN, creatinine, albumin, total protein, lipid panel (at initiation), CD4, and viral load. After 1 to 2 weeks of therapy: Signs of medication toxicity and adherence. After 2 to 4 weeks of therapy: CBC with differential, viral load, signs of medication toxicity, and adherence; then every 3 to 4 months: CBC with differential, electrolytes, glucose, LFTs, bilirubin, BUN, creatinine, CD4, viral load, signs of medication toxicity, and adherence. Every 6 to 12 months: Lipid panel and urinalysis. CD4 monitoring frequency may be decreased to every 6 to 12 months in children who are adherent to therapy if the value is well above the threshold for opportunistic infections, viral suppression is sustained, and the clinical status is stable for more than 2 to 3 years (DHHS [pediatric], 2014). Monitor for growth and development, signs of HIV-specific physical conditions, HIV disease progression, opportunistic infections and hypersensitivity.

Additional Information In clinical trials, poor virologic response was observed in patients with an INSTI-resistance Q148 substitution (Q148H/R) plus ≥2 additional INSTI-resistance substitutions including L741/M, E138A/D/K/T, G140A/S, Y143H/R, E157Q, G163E/K/Q/R/S, or G193E/R treated with dolutegravir 50 mg twice daily.

Dosage Forms Excipient information presented when available (limited, particularly for generics); consult specific product labeling.

Tablet, Oral:

Tivicay: 50 mg

References

DHHS Panel on Antiretroviral Guidelines for Adults and Adolescents. Guidelines for the Use of Antiretroviral Agents in HIV-1-Infected Adults and Adolescents, Department of Health and Human Services. Updated May 1, 2014. Available at http://www.aidsinfo.nih.gov/ContentFiles/AdultandAdolescentGL.pdf.

DHHS Panel on Antiretroviral Guidelines for Adults and Adolescents, "Recommendation on Integrase Inhibitor (INSTI) Use in Antiretroviral Treatment-Naive HIV-Infected Individuals from the HHS Panel on Antiretroviral Guidelines for Adults and Adolescents", October 2013. Available at http://aidsinfo.nih.gov

DHHS Panel on Antiretroviral Therapy and Medical Management of HIV-Infected Children. Guidelines for the use of antiretroviral agents in pediatric HIV infection. February 12, 2014. Available at http://aidsinfo.nih.gov

DHHS Panel on Treatment of HIV-Infected Pregnant Women and Prevention of Perinatal Transmission. Recommendations for Use of Antiretroviral Drugs in Pregnant HIV-1-Infected Women for Maternal Health and Interventions to Reduce Perinatal HIV Transmission in the United States. July 31, 2012. Available at http://aidsinfo.nih.gov/contentfiles/lvguidelines/perinatalgl.pdf

Tivicay (dolutegravir) [prescribing information]. Research Triangle Park, NC: GlaxoSmithKline; May 2014.

◆ **Dolutegravir Sodium** see Dolutegravir on page 705
◆ **Dom-Amantadine (Can)** see Amantadine on page 112
◆ **Dom-Amiodarone (Can)** see Amiodarone on page 127
◆ **Dom-Amlodipine (Can)** see AmLODIPine on page 135
◆ **Dom-Anagrelide (Can)** see Anagrelide on page 166
◆ **Dom-Atenolol (Can)** see Atenolol on page 222
◆ **DOM-Atomoxetine (Can)** see AtoMOXetine on page 224
◆ **Dom-Atorvastatin (Can)** see AtorvaSTATin on page 227
◆ **Dom-Azithromycin (Can)** see Azithromycin (Systemic) on page 247
◆ **Dom-Baclofen (Can)** see Baclofen on page 259
◆ **Dom-Bromocriptine (Can)** see Bromocriptine on page 304
◆ **Dom-Buspirone (Can)** see BusPIRone on page 332
◆ **DOM-Candesartan (Can)** see Candesartan on page 363
◆ **Dom-Captopril (Can)** see Captopril on page 368
◆ **Dom-Carbamazepine (Can)** see CarBAMazepine on page 372
◆ **Dom-Carvedilol (Can)** see Carvedilol on page 385
◆ **Dom-Cephalexin (Can)** see Cephalexin on page 429
◆ **Dom-Cimetidine (Can)** see Cimetidine on page 469
◆ **Dom-Ciprofloxacin (Can)** see Ciprofloxacin (Systemic) on page 471
◆ **Dom-Citalopram (Can)** see Citalopram on page 484
◆ **Dom-Clarithromycin (Can)** see Clarithromycin on page 490
◆ **Dom-Clobazam (Can)** see CloBAZam on page 504
◆ **Dom-Clomipramine (Can)** see ClomiPRAMINE on page 510
◆ **Dom-Clonazepam (Can)** see ClonazePAM on page 514
◆ **Dom-Clonazepam-R (Can)** see ClonazePAM on page 514
◆ **Dom-Clonidine (Can)** see CloNIDine on page 516
◆ **Dom-Clopidogrel (Can)** see Clopidogrel on page 521
◆ **Dom-Cyclobenzaprine (Can)** see Cyclobenzaprine on page 558
◆ **Dom-Desipramine (Can)** see Desipramine on page 608
◆ **Dom-Dexamethasone (Can)** see Dexamethasone (Systemic) on page 615
◆ **Dom-Diclofenac (Can)** see Diclofenac (Systemic) on page 645
◆ **Dom-Diclofenac SR (Can)** see Diclofenac (Systemic) on page 645
◆ **Dom-Divalproex (Can)** see Valproic Acid and Derivatives on page 2102
◆ **Dom-Docusate Sodium [OTC] (Can)** see Docusate on page 701
◆ **Dom-Doxazosin (Can)** see Doxazosin on page 712
◆ **Dom-Doxycycline (Can)** see Doxycycline on page 721
◆ **Domeboro [OTC]** see Aluminum Acetate on page 110
◆ **Dom-Fluconazole (Can)** see Fluconazole on page 877
◆ **Dom-Fluoxetine (Can)** see FLUoxetine on page 901
◆ **Dom-Fluvoxamine (Can)** see FluvoxaMINE on page 922
◆ **Dom-Furosemide (Can)** see Furosemide on page 948
◆ **Dom-Gabapentin (Can)** see Gabapentin on page 950
◆ **Dom-Glyburide (Can)** see GlyBURIDE on page 974
◆ **Dom-Irbesartan (Can)** see Irbesartan on page 1147
◆ **Dom-Levetiracetam (Can)** see LevETIRAcetam on page 1219

- ◆ **Dom-Lisinopril (Can)** see Lisinopril on page 1262
- ◆ **Dom-Loperamide (Can)** see Loperamide on page 1270
- ◆ **Dom-Lorazepam (Can)** see LORazepam on page 1280
- ◆ **Dom-Lovastatin (Can)** see Lovastatin on page 1286
- ◆ **Dom-Medroxyprogesterone (Can)** see MedroxyPRO-GESTERone on page 1318
- ◆ **Dom-Meloxicam (Can)** see Meloxicam on page 1325
- ◆ **Dom-Metformin (Can)** see MetFORMIN on page 1353
- ◆ **Dom-Methimazole (Can)** see Methimazole on page 1362
- ◆ **Dom-Metoprolol-L (Can)** see Metoprolol on page 1396
- ◆ **Dom-Metoprolol-B (Can)** see Metoprolol on page 1396
- ◆ **Dom-Minocycline (Can)** see Minocycline on page 1420
- ◆ **Dom-Montelukast (Can)** see Montelukast on page 1438
- ◆ **Dom-Montelukast FC (Can)** see Montelukast on page 1438
- ◆ **Dom-Nortriptyline (Can)** see Nortriptyline on page 1512
- ◆ **Dom-Omeprazole DR (Can)** see Omeprazole on page 1535
- ◆ **Dom-Ondansetron (Can)** see Ondansetron on page 1544
- ◆ **Dom-Oxybutynin (Can)** see Oxybutynin on page 1568
- ◆ **Dom-Pantoprazole (Can)** see Pantoprazole on page 1595
- ◆ **Dom-Paroxetine (Can)** see PARoxetine on page 1609
- ◆ **Dom-Piroxicam (Can)** see Piroxicam on page 1683
- ◆ **Dom-Pravastatin (Can)** see Pravastatin on page 1720
- ◆ **Dom-Propranolol (Can)** see Propranolol on page 1759
- ◆ **Dom-Quetiapine (Can)** see QUEtiapine on page 1783
- ◆ **Dom-Ranitidine (Can)** see Ranitidine on page 1805
- ◆ **Dom-Risperidone (Can)** see RisperiDONE on page 1831
- ◆ **Dom-Rosuvastatin (Can)** see Rosuvastatin on page 1853
- ◆ **Dom-Salbutamol (Can)** see Albuterol on page 84
- ◆ **Dom-Sertraline (Can)** see Sertraline on page 1879
- ◆ **Dom-Simvastatin (Can)** see Simvastatin on page 1892
- ◆ **Dom-Sotalol (Can)** see Sotalol on page 1925
- ◆ **Dom-Sucralfate (Can)** see Sucralfate on page 1940
- ◆ **Dom-Sumatriptan (Can)** see SUMAtriptan on page 1958
- ◆ **Dom-Terazosin (Can)** see Terazosin on page 1981
- ◆ **Dom-Terbinafine (Can)** see Terbinafine (Systemic) on page 1982
- ◆ **Dom-Timolol (Can)** see Timolol (Ophthalmic) on page 2028
- ◆ **Dom-Topiramate (Can)** see Topiramate on page 2046
- ◆ **Dom-Trazodone (Can)** see TraZODone on page 2065
- ◆ **Dom-Ursodiol C (Can)** see Ursodiol on page 2095
- ◆ **DOM-Valacyclovir (Can)** see ValACYclovir on page 2097
- ◆ **Dom-Valproic Acid (Can)** see Valproic Acid and Derivatives on page 2102
- ◆ **Dom-Valproic Acid E.C. (Can)** see Valproic Acid and Derivatives on page 2102
- ◆ **Dom-Venlafaxine XR (Can)** see Venlafaxine on page 2125
- ◆ **Dom-Verapamil SR (Can)** see Verapamil on page 2129
- ◆ **Donnatal®** see Hyoscyamine, Atropine, Scopolamine, and Phenobarbital on page 1058
- ◆ **Donnatal Extentabs®** see Hyoscyamine, Atropine, Scopolamine, and Phenobarbital on page 1058

DOPamine (DOE pa meen)

Medication Safety Issues
Sound-alike/look-alike issues:
DOPamine may be confused with DOBUTamine, Dopram
High alert medication:
The Institute for Safe Medication Practices (ISMP) includes this medication among its list of drugs which have a heightened risk of causing significant patient harm when used in error.

Related Information
Adult ACLS Algorithms on page 2198
Emergency Drip Calculations on page 2191
Management of Drug Extravasations on page 2255

Therapeutic Category Adrenergic Agonist Agent; Sympathomimetic

Generic Availability (U.S.) Yes

Use Increase cardiac output, blood pressure, and urine flow as an adjunct in the treatment of shock or hypotension which persists after adequate fluid volume replacement; in low dosage to increase renal perfusion

Pregnancy Risk Factor C

Pregnancy Considerations Adverse events have been observed in some animal reproduction studies. It is not known if dopamine crosses the placenta.

Breast-Feeding Considerations It is not known if dopamine is excreted in breast milk. The manufacturer recommends that caution be exercised when administering dopamine to nursing women.

Contraindications Hypersensitivity to dopamine or any component; pheochromocytoma, or ventricular fibrillation

Warnings Potent drug; must be diluted prior to use; patient's hemodynamic status should be monitored; injection solution contains sulfites which may cause allergic reactions in susceptible individuals

Precautions Blood volume depletion should be corrected, if possible, before starting dopamine therapy. Dopamine must not be used as sole therapy in hypovolemic patients. Extravasation may cause tissue necrosis (treat extravasation with phentolamine) **[U.S. Boxed Warning]**; due to potential gangrene of extremities, use with caution in patients with occlusive vascular disease.

Adverse Reactions
Cardiovascular: Aberrant conduction, anginal pain, atrial fibrillation, bradycardia, ectopic beats, gangrene (high dose), hyper-/hypotension, palpitation, tachycardia, vasoconstriction, ventricular arrhythmia, widened QRS complex
Central nervous system: Anxiety, headache
Endocrine & metabolic: Piloerection, serum glucose increased (usually not above normal limits)
Gastrointestinal: Nausea, vomiting
Local: Extravasation of dopamine can cause tissue necrosis and sloughing of surrounding tissues
Ocular: Dilated pupils, intraocular pressure increased
Renal: Azotemia, polyuria
Respiratory: Dyspnea

Drug Interactions
Metabolism/Transport Effects Substrate of COMT
Avoid Concomitant Use
Avoid concomitant use of DOPamine with any of the following: Ergot Derivatives; Inhalational Anesthetics; Iobenguane I 123; Lurasidone
Increased Effect/Toxicity
DOPamine may increase the levels/effects of: Lurasidone; Sympathomimetics

The levels/effects of DOPamine may be increased by: AtoMOXetine; Beta-Blockers; Cannabinoid-Containing Products; COMT Inhibitors; Ergot Derivatives; Hyaluronidase; Inhalational Anesthetics; Linezolid; Serotonin/Norepinephrine Reuptake Inhibitors; Tricyclic Antidepressants

Decreased Effect

DOPamine may decrease the levels/effects of: Benzyl-penicilloyl Polylysine; Iobenguane I 123

The levels/effects of DOPamine may be decreased by: Alpha1-Blockers; Spironolactone

Stability Protect from light; solutions that are darker than slightly yellow should not be used; incompatible with alkaline solutions or iron salts; compatible when coadministered with dobutamine, epinephrine, isoproterenol, lidocaine, atracurium, vecuronium

Mechanism of Action Stimulates both adrenergic and dopaminergic receptors, lower doses are mainly dopaminergic stimulating and produce renal and mesenteric vasodilation, higher doses also are both dopaminergic and beta$_1$-adrenergic stimulating and produce cardiac stimulation and renal vasodilation; large doses stimulate alpha-adrenergic receptors

Pharmacodynamics

Onset of action: Adults: 5 minutes

Duration: Due to its short duration of action (<10 minutes) a continuous infusion must be used

Pharmacokinetics (Adult data unless noted)

Metabolism: In plasma, kidneys, and liver; 75% to inactive metabolites by monoamine oxidase and catechol-o-methyltransferase and 25% to norepinephrine (active)

Half-life: 2 minutes

Clearance: Neonatal clearance varies and appears to be age related. Clearance is more prolonged with combined hepatic and renal dysfunction. Dopamine has exhibited nonlinear kinetics in children; dose changes in children may not achieve steady-state for approximately 1 hour rather than 20 minutes seen in adults.

Dosing: Neonatal Continuous I.V. infusion: 1-20 mcg/kg/minute; titrate to desired response

The hemodynamic effects of dopamine are dose-dependent:

Low dosage: 1-5 mcg/kg/minute, increased renal blood flow and urine output

Intermediate dosage: 5-15 mcg/kg/minute, increased renal blood flow, heart rate, cardiac contractility, cardiac output, and blood pressure

High dosage: >15 mcg/kg/minute, alpha-adrenergic effects begin to predominate, vasoconstriction, increased blood pressure

Dosing: Usual Continuous I.V. infusion:

The hemodynamic effects of dopamine are dose-dependent:

Low dosage: 1-5 mcg/kg/minute, increased renal blood flow and urine output

Intermediate dosage: 5-15 mcg/kg/minute, increased renal blood flow, heart rate, cardiac contractility, cardiac output, and blood pressure

High dosage: >15 mcg/kg/minute, alpha-adrenergic effects begin to predominate, vasoconstriction, increased blood pressure

Infants and Children: 1-20 mcg/kg/minute, maximum dose: 50 mcg/kg/minute continuous infusion, titrate to desired response

Adults: 1 mcg/kg/minute up to 50 mcg/kg/minute, titrate to desired response

If dosages >20-30 mcg/kg/minute are needed, a more direct-acting pressor may be beneficial (ie, epinephrine, norepinephrine)

Usual Infusion Concentrations: Neonatal Note: Premixed solutions available.

I.V. infusion: 1600 **mcg**/mL or 3200 **mcg**/mL

Usual Infusion Concentrations: Pediatric Note: Premixed solutions available.

I.V. infusion: 1600 **mcg**/mL or 3200 **mcg**/mL

Administration Parenteral: Must be diluted prior to administration; maximum concentration: 3200 mcg/mL (3.2 mg/mL); (concentrations as high as 6000 mcg/mL have been infused into large veins, safely and with efficacy, in cases of extreme fluid restriction); rate of infusion (mL/hour) = dose (mcg/kg/minute) x weight (kg) x 60 minutes/hour divided by concentration (mcg/mL); administer into large vein to prevent the possibility of extravasation; use infusion device to control rate of flow; administration into an umbilical arterial catheter is **not** recommended

Vesicant/Extravasation Risk Vesicant

Monitoring Parameters ECG, heart rate, CVP, MAP, urine output; if pulmonary artery catheter is in place, monitor Cl, PWCP, SVR, RAP, and PVR

Dosage Forms Excipient information presented when available (limited, particularly for generics); consult specific product labeling.

Solution, Intravenous, as hydrochloride:

Generic: 0.8 mg/mL (250 mL, 500 mL); 1.6 mg/mL (250 mL, 500 mL); 3.2 mg/mL (250 mL); 40 mg/mL (5 mL, 10 mL); 80 mg/mL (5 mL); 160 mg/mL (5 mL)

References

Banner W, Jr, Vernon DD, Dean JM, et al, "Nonlinear Dopamine Pharmacokinetics in Pediatric Patients," *J Pharmacol Exp Ther,* 1989, 249(1):131-3.

Hegenbarth MA and American Academy of Pediatrics Committee on Drugs, "Preparing for Pediatric Emergencies: Drugs to Consider," *Pediatrics,* 2008, 121(2):433-43.

Institute for Safe Medication Practices (ISMP), "Standard Concentrations of Neonatal Drug Infusions," *ISMP,* 2011.

Kleinman ME, Chameides L, Schexnayder SM, et al, "Part 14: Pediatric Advanced Life Support: 2010 American Heart Association Guidelines for Cardiopulmonary Resuscitation and Emergency Cardiovascular Care," *Circulation,* 2010, 122(18 Suppl 3):876-908.

Phillips MS, "Standardizing I.V. Infusion Concentrations: National Survey Results," *Am J Health Syst Pharm,* 2011, 68(22):2176-82.

Subhedar NV, "Treatment of Hypotension in Newborns," *Semin Neonatol,* 2003, 8(6):413-23.

◆ **Dopamine Hydrochloride** see DOPamine on page 708

◆ **Dopram** see Doxapram on page 711

Dornase Alfa (DOOR nase AL fa)

Brand Names: U.S. Pulmozyme

Brand Names: Canada Pulmozyme®

Therapeutic Category Enzyme, Inhalant; Mucolytic Agent

Generic Availability (U.S.) No

Use Management of cystic fibrosis patients to reduce the frequency of respiratory infections that require parenteral antibiotics in patients with FVC ≥40% of predicted; in conjunction with standard therapies to improve pulmonary function (FDA approved in ages ≥5 years and adults)

Pregnancy Risk Factor B

Pregnancy Considerations Teratogenic effects were not observed in animal reproduction studies.

Breast-Feeding Considerations Measurable amounts would not be expected in breast milk following inhalation; however, it is not known if dornase alfa is excreted in human milk.

Contraindications Hypersensitivity to dornase alfa, Chinese hamster ovary cell products (eg, epoetin alfa), or any component

Precautions Use with caution in infants and children <5 years of age; safety studies included infants down to 3 months; limit use to those infants and children <5 years to those with potential for benefit in pulmonary function or in risk of respiratory tract infection; some adverse effects were reported more frequently in infants and children <5 years of age than older children (5-10 years of age) including: Cough (45% vs 30%) and rhinitis (35% vs 27%). In patients with pulmonary function <40% of normal, dornase alfa does not significantly reduce the risk of respiratory infections that require parenteral antibiotics; fever reported in 32% of these patients.

Adverse Reactions Adverse events were similar in children using the PARI BABY™ nebulizer (facemask as opposed to mouthpiece) with the addition of cough.

Cardiovascular: Chest pain

Central nervous system: Fever

Dermatologic: Rash

Gastrointestinal: Dyspepsia

Ocular: Conjunctivitis

Respiratory: Dyspnea, FVC decrease ≥10% of predicted, laryngitis, pharyngitis, rhinitis

Miscellaneous: Dornase alfa serum antibodies, voice alteration

Rare but important or life-threatening: Headache, urticaria

Drug Interactions

Metabolism/Transport Effects None known.

Avoid Concomitant Use There are no known interactions where it is recommended to avoid concomitant use.

Increased Effect/Toxicity There are no known significant interactions involving an increase in effect.

Decreased Effect There are no known significant interactions involving a decrease in effect.

Stability Must be stored in the refrigerator at 2°C to 8°C (36°F to 46°F) and protected from strong light; unopened vials left at room temperature for a total time of 24 hours should be discarded; discard solution if cloudy or discolored

Mechanism of Action The hallmark of cystic fibrosis lung disease is the presence of abundant, purulent airway secretions composed primarily of highly polymerized DNA. The principal source of this DNA is the nuclei of degenerating neutrophils, which is present in large concentrations in infected lung secretions. The presence of this DNA produces a viscous mucous that may contribute to the decreased mucociliary transport and persistent infections that are commonly seen in this population. Dornase alfa is a deoxyribonuclease (DNA) enzyme produced by recombinant gene technology. Dornase selectively cleaves DNA, thus reducing mucous viscosity and as a result, airflow in the lung is improved and the risk of bacterial infection may be decreased.

Pharmacodynamics Onset of improved pulmonary function tests (PFTs): 3-8 days; PFTs will return to baseline 2-3 weeks after discontinuation of therapy

Pharmacokinetics (Adult data unless noted) Following nebulization, enzyme levels are measurable in the sputum within 15 minutes and decline rapidly thereafter

Dosing: Usual

Infants and Children ≤5 years: Not approved for use, however studies using this therapy in small numbers of children as young as 3 months of age have reported efficacy and similar side effects.

Children >5 years and Adults: Inhalation: 2.5 mg/day through selected nebulizers in conjunction with a Pulmo-Aide®, Pari-Proneb®, Mobilaire™, Porta-Neb®, or Pari Baby™ compressor system

Note: While some patients, especially older than 21 years of age or with forced vital capacity (FVC) >85%, may benefit from twice daily administration, another study (Fuchs, 1994) reported no difference between once or twice daily therapy; in a randomized crossover trial involving 48 children, alternate day treatment was as effective as daily treatment over a 12-week period (Suri, 2001).

Administration Nebulization: Should not be diluted or mixed with any other drugs in the nebulizer, this may inactivate the drug

Dosage Forms Excipient information presented when available (limited, particularly for generics); consult specific product labeling.

Solution, Inhalation:

Pulmozyme: 1 mg/mL (2.5 mL)

References

Fuchs HJ, Borowitz DS, Christiansen DH, et al, "Effect of Aerosolized Recombinant Human DNase on Exacerbations of Respiratory Symptoms and on Pulmonary Function in Patients With Cystic Fibrosis," *N Engl J Med*, 1994, 331(10):637-42.

Mueller GA, Rubins G, Wessel D, et al, "Effects of Dornase Alfa on Pulmonary Function Tests in Infants with Cystic Fibrosis," *Am J Respir Crit Care Med*, 1996, 153:A70.

Rock M, Kirchner K, McCubbin M, et al, "Aerosol Delivery and Safety of rhDNASE in Young Children With Cystic Fibrosis: A Bronchoscopic Study," *Pediatr Pulmonol*, 1996, 13(Suppl):A268.

Suri R, Metcalfe C, Lees B, et al, "Comparison of Hypertonic Saline and Alternate-Day or Daily Recombinant Human Deoxyribonuclease in Children With Cystic Fibrosis: A Randomised Trial," *Lancet*, 2001, 358 (9290):1316-21.

Suri R, "The Use of Human Deoxyribonuclease (rhDNase) in the Management of Cystic Fibrosis," *BioDrugs*, 2005, 19(3):135-44.

Wagener JS, Rock MJ, McCubbin MM, et al, "Aerosol Delivery and Safety of Recombinant Human Deoxyribonuclease in Young Children With Cystic Fibrosis: A Bronchoscopic Study. Pulmozyme Pediatric Broncoscopy Study Group," *J Pediatr*, 1998, 133(4):486-91.

◆ **Doryx** see Doxycycline on page 721

Dorzolamide (dor ZOLE a mide)

Brand Names: U.S. Trusopt

Brand Names: Canada Sandoz-Dorzolamide; Trusopt®

Therapeutic Category Carbonic Anhydrase Inhibitor, Ophthalmic

Generic Availability (U.S.) Yes

Use Treatment of elevated intraocular pressure in patients with ocular hypertension or open-angle glaucoma [FDA approved in pediatric patients (age not specified) and adults]

Pregnancy Risk Factor C

Pregnancy Considerations Adverse events have been observed in animal reproduction studies following systemic administration. IOP is usually lower during pregnancy. If topical medications for the treatment of glaucoma in pregnant women cannot be discontinued because small increases in IOP cannot be tolerated, the minimum effective dose should be used in combination with punctual occlusion to decrease exposure to the fetus (Johnson, 2001).

Breast-Feeding Considerations It is not known if dorzolamide is excreted in breast milk. Due to the potential for serious adverse reactions in the nursing infant, a decision should be made whether to discontinue nursing or to discontinue the drug, taking into account the importance of treatment to the mother.

Contraindications Hypersensitivity to dorzolamide, sulfonamides, or any component

Warnings Dorzolamide, a sulfonamide, is absorbed systemically and may produce the same adverse effects seen with other sulfonamides; avoid use in patients with severe renal dysfunction (CrCl <30 mL/minute); contains the preservative benzalkonium chloride which may be absorbed by soft contact lenses; contact lenses should be removed prior to administration of the solution and may be reinserted 15 minutes following administration; concomitant use with other carbonic anhydrase inhibitors is not recommended

Precautions Use with caution in patients with hepatic impairment

Adverse Reactions

Gastrointestinal: Bitter taste following administration

Ocular: Blurred vision; burning, stinging, or discomfort immediately following administration; conjunctivitis; dryness; lid reactions; photophobia; signs and symptoms of ocular allergic reaction; superficial punctate keratitis; redness; tearing

Rare but important or life-threatening: Allergic reaction (systemic), angioedema, bronchospasm, choriodal detachment (following filtration procedures), dyspnea, epistaxis, myopia (transient), ocular pain, paresthesia, pharyngitis, Stevens-Johnson syndrome, throat irritation, toxic epidermal necrolysis

Drug Interactions
Metabolism/Transport Effects Substrate of CYP2C9 (minor), CYP3A4 (minor); **Note:** Assignment of Major/Minor substrate status based on clinically relevant drug interaction potential

Avoid Concomitant Use
Avoid concomitant use of Dorzolamide with any of the following: Carbonic Anhydrase Inhibitors

Increased Effect/Toxicity
Dorzolamide may increase the levels/effects of: Alpha-/Beta-Agonists (Indirect-Acting); Carbonic Anhydrase Inhibitors

Decreased Effect There are no known significant interactions involving a decrease in effect.

Stability Store at room temperature.

Mechanism of Action Reversible inhibition of the enzyme carbonic anhydrase resulting in reduction of hydrogen ion secretion at renal tubule and an increased renal excretion of sodium, potassium, bicarbonate, and water to decrease production of aqueous humor; also inhibits carbonic anhydrase in central nervous system to retard abnormal and excessive discharge from CNS neurons

Pharmacodynamics
Maximum effect: 2 hours
Duration: 8-12 hours
Average lowering of intraoptic pressure: 3-5 mm Hg or at least 15% decrease from unmedicated baseline value

Pharmacokinetics (Adult data unless noted)
Absorption: Reaches systemic circulation
Distribution: Accumulates in RBCs during chronic administration
Protein binding: 33%
Metabolism: In liver to active but less potent metabolite, N-desethyl dorzolamide
Half-life: Terminal RBC half-life: 147 days
Elimination: Primarily unchanged in the urine

Dosing: Usual Glaucoma: Children and Adults: 1 drop into the affected eye(s) 3 times/day

Administration Ophthalmic: Apply gentle pressure to lacrimal sac during and immediately following instillation (1 minute) or instruct patient to gently close eyelid after administration to decrease systemic absorption of ophthalmic drops; avoid contact of bottle tip with skin or eye; remove contact lenses prior to administration; lenses may be inserted 15 minutes after instillation; if more than one topical ophthalmic drug is being used, separate administration by at least 10 minutes

Monitoring Parameters Intraoptic pressure

Dosage Forms Excipient information presented when available (limited, particularly for generics); consult specific product labeling.
Solution, Ophthalmic:
Trusopt: 2% (10 mL)
Generic: 2% (10 mL)

References
Johnson SM, Martinez M, and Freedman S, "Management of Glaucoma in Pregnancy and Lactation," *Surv Ophthalmol*, 2001, 45(5):449-54.
Portellos M, Buckley EG, and Freedman SF, "Topical Versus Oral Carbonic Anhydrase Inhibitor Therapy for Pediatric Glaucoma," *J AAPOS*, 1998, 2(1):43-7.

♦ **Dorzolamide Hydrochloride** *see* Dorzolamide *on page 710*

♦ **D.O.S. [OTC]** *see* Docusate *on page 701*

♦ **Dosolax [OTC] (Can)** *see* Docusate *on page 701*

♦ **DOSS** *see* Docusate *on page 701*

♦ **Double Tussin DM [OTC]** *see* Guaifenesin and Dextromethorphan *on page 987*

Doxapram (DOKS a pram)

Medication Safety Issues
Sound-alike/look-alike issues:
Doxapram may be confused with doxazosin, doxepin, DOXOrubicin
Dopram® may be confused with DOPamine
International issues:
Doxapram may be confused with Doxinate brand name for doxylamine and pyridoxine [Italy]

Brand Names: U.S. Dopram

Therapeutic Category Central Nervous System Stimulant; Respiratory Stimulant

Generic Availability (U.S.) Yes

Use Respiratory and CNS stimulant for treatment of respiratory depression secondary to anesthesia, drug-induced CNS depression, and acute hypercapnia secondary to COPD (FDA approved in ages ≥12 years and adults); has also been used for idiopathic apnea of prematurity refractory to xanthines

Pregnancy Risk Factor B

Pregnancy Considerations Adverse events have not been observed in animal reproduction studies.

Breast-Feeding Considerations It is not known if doxapram is excreted in breast milk. The manufacturer recommends that caution be exercised when administering doxapram to nursing women.

Contraindications Hypersensitivity to doxapram or any component; epilepsy, cerebral edema, head injury, suspected or proven pulmonary embolism, pheochromocytoma, cardiovascular or coronary artery disease, severe hypertension, hyperthyroidism, cardiac arrhythmias; concomitant use with mechanical ventilation in COPD patients; patients with mechanical disorders of ventilation such as bronchial obstruction, muscle paresis (including NM blockade), flail chest, pneumothorax, pulmonary fibrosis, asthma, or other conditions resulting in restriction of chest wall muscles of respiration or alveolar expansion

Warnings Avoid use in conjunction with mechanical ventilation.

Doxapram contains benzyl alcohol which may cause allergic reactions in susceptible individuals; large amounts of benzyl alcohol (≥99 mg/kg/day) have been associated with a potentially fatal toxicity ("gasping syndrome") in neonates; the "gasping syndrome" consists of metabolic acidosis, respiratory distress, gasping respirations, CNS dysfunction (including convulsions, intracranial hemorrhage), hypotension and cardiovascular collapse. Recommended doses of doxapram for treatment of neonatal apnea will deliver 5.4-27 mg/kg/day of benzyl alcohol; the use of doxapram should be reserved for neonates who are unresponsive to the treatment of apnea with therapeutic serum concentrations of theophylline or caffeine. *In vitro* and animal studies have shown that benzoate, a metabolite of benzyl alcohol, displaces bilirubin from protein-binding sites.

Doxapram is not an antagonist to muscle relaxant drugs nor a specific opioid antagonist; doxapram alone may not stimulate adequate spontaneous breathing or provide sufficient arousal in patients who are severely depressed; use as an adjunct to establish supportive measures; since respiratory depression may recur after stimulation with doxapram, monitor closely until the patient has been fully alert for 30-60 minutes; to reduce the potential for arrhythmias, including VT and VF, in patients who have received general anesthesia with a volatile agent known to sensitize the myocardium to catecholamines, administration of ▶

doxapram should be delayed until the complete excretion of anesthetic has occurred.

Precautions Use with caution in premature neonates and infants; hypertension (dose-related), irritability, seizures, excessive crying, sleep disturbances, abdominal distention, vomiting, NEC, increased gastric residuals, bloody stools, hyperglycemia, and glycosuria have been reported. Oxygen, resuscitative equipment, and anticonvulsants should be readily available to manage excessive CNS stimulation. Frequent arterial blood gas measurements are recommended to identify and prevent the development of CO_2 retention and acidosis in COPD patients with acute hypercapnia; infusion of doxapram in premature neonates has been associated with a statistically significant but moderate lengthening of QT_c interval; cardiac monitoring during treatment is suggested (Maillard, 2001); use caution in patients with impaired hepatic or renal function or receiving MAOIs or sympathomimetic drugs

Adverse Reactions

Cardiovascular: Arrhythmia, blood pressure increased, chest pain, chest tightness, flushing, heart rate changes, T waves lowered, ventricular tachycardia, ventricular fibrillation

Central nervous system: Apprehension, Babinski turns positive, disorientation, dizziness, hallucinations, headache, hyperactivity, pyrexia, seizure

Dermatologic: Burning sensation, pruritus

Gastrointestinal: Defecation urge, diarrhea, nausea, vomiting

Genitourinary: Spontaneous voiding, urinary retention

Hematologic: Hematocrit decreased, hemoglobin decreased, hemolysis, red blood cell count decreased

Local: Phlebitis

Neuromuscular & skeletal: Clonus, deep tendon reflexes increase, fasciculations, involuntary muscle movement, muscle spasm, paresthesia

Ocular: Pupillary dilatation

Renal: Albuminuria, BUN increased

Respiratory: Bronchospasm, cough, dyspnea, hiccups, hyperventilation, laryngospasm, rebound hypoventilation, tachypnea

Miscellaneous: Diaphoresis

Rare but important or life-threatening: Emergence agitation, second-degree AV block (premature neonates), QT-interval prolonged (premature neonates)

Drug Interactions

Metabolism/Transport Effects None known.

Avoid Concomitant Use

Avoid concomitant use of Doxapram with any of the following: Iobenguane I 123

Increased Effect/Toxicity

Doxapram may increase the levels/effects of: Sympathomimetics

The levels/effects of Doxapram may be increased by: AtoMOXetine; Cannabinoid-Containing Products; Linezolid; MAO Inhibitors

Decreased Effect

Doxapram may decrease the levels/effects of: Iobenguane I 123

Stability Stable at room temperature; incompatible with aminophylline, sodium bicarbonate, thiopental sodium, and other alkaline solutions

Mechanism of Action Stimulates respiration through action on peripheral carotid chemoreceptors; respiratory center in medulla is also directly stimulated as dosage is increased

Pharmacodynamics Following a single I.V. injection:

Onset of respiratory stimulation: Within 20-40 seconds

Maximum effect: Within 1-2 minutes

Duration: 5-12 minutes

Pharmacokinetics (Adult data unless noted)

Metabolism: Extensive in the liver to active metabolite (keto-doxapram)

Distribution: V_d: Neonates: 4-7.3 L/kg

Half-life:

Neonates, premature: 6.6-12 hours

Adults: Mean: 3.4 hours (range: 2.4-4.1 hours)

Clearance: Neonates, premature: 0.44-0.7 L/hour/kg

Dosing: Neonatal I.V.: Apnea of prematurity: Initial loading dose: 2.5-3 mg/kg followed by a continuous I.V. infusion of 1 mg/kg/hour; titrate to the lowest rate at which apnea is controlled (maximum dose: 2.5 mg/kg/hour); **Note:** Typically considered third-line agent.

Dosing: Usual I.V.:

Respiratory depression following anesthesia: Adults: Titrate to sustain the desired level of respiratory stimulation with a minimum of side effects:

Initial: 0.5-1 mg/kg; may repeat at 5-minute intervals; maximum total dose: 2 mg/kg

Continuous I.V. infusion: Initial: 5 mg/minute until adequate response or adverse effects seen; decrease to 1-3 mg/minute; usual total infusion dose: 0.5-4 mg/kg or 300 mg

Drug-induced CNS depression: Adults: Mild to moderate depression: Initial: 1-2 mg/kg; may repeat in 5 minutes; may repeat at 1-2 hour intervals (until sustained consciousness); maximum dose: 3 g/day; if depression recurs, may repeat in 24 hours. As an alternative, after the initial doses, a continuous infusion of 1-3 mg/minute may be used. Discontinue if patient begins to waken; do not infuse for more than 2 hours.

Hypercapnia associated with COPD: Adults: Continuous infusion of 1-2 mg/minute for 2 hours; may increase to 3 mg/minute if needed. Do not infuse for more than 2 hours. Monitor arterial blood gases closely (in a minimum of 30-minute intervals)

Administration Parenteral: I.V. use only: Dilute loading dose to a maximum concentration of 2 mg/mL and infuse over 15-30 minutes; for infusion, dilute in NS or dextrose (D_5W or $D_{10}W$) to 1 mg/mL (maximum concentration: 2 mg/mL); irritating to tissues; avoid extravasation

Monitoring Parameters Pulse oximetry, blood pressure, heart rate, arterial blood gases, deep tendon reflexes; for apnea: number, duration, and severity of apneic episodes

Reference Range Initial studies suggest a therapeutic serum level of at least 1.5 mg/L; toxicity becomes frequent at serum levels >5 mg/L

Dosage Forms Excipient information presented when available (limited, particularly for generics); consult specific product labeling.

Solution, Intravenous, as hydrochloride:

Dopram: 20 mg/mL (20 mL) [contains benzyl alcohol]

Generic: 20 mg/mL (20 mL)

References

Barrington KJ, Finer NN, Torok-Both G, et al, "Dose-Response Relationship of Doxapram in the Therapy for Refractory Idiopathic Apnea of Prematurity," *Pediatrics*, 1987, 80(1):22-7.

Bhatt-Mehta V and Schumacher RE, "Treatment of Apnea of Prematurity," *Paediatr Drugs*, 2003, 5(3):195-210.

Maillard C, Boutroy MJ, Fresson J, et al, "QT Interval Lengthening in Premature Infants Treated With Doxapram," *Clin Pharmacol Ther*, 2001, 70(6):540-5.

♦ **Doxapram Hydrochloride** see Doxapram on page 711

Doxazosin (doks AY zoe sin)

Medication Safety Issues

Sound-alike/look-alike issues:

Doxazosin may be confused with doxapram, doxepin, DOXOrubicin

Cardura may be confused with Cardene, Cordarone, Cordran, Coumadin, K-Dur, Ridaura

BEERS Criteria medication:
This drug may be potentially inappropriate for use in geriatric patients (Quality of evidence - moderate; Strength of recommendation - strong).

Related Information
Oral Medications That Should Not Be Crushed or Altered on page 2438

Brand Names: U.S. Cardura; Cardura XL

Brand Names: Canada Apo-Doxazosin; Cardura-1; Cardura-2; Cardura-4; Dom-Doxazosin; Mylan-Doxazosin; PMS-Doxazosin; Teva-Doxazosin

Therapeutic Category Alpha-Adrenergic Blocking Agent, Oral; Antihypertensive Agent; Vasodilator

Generic Availability (U.S.) May be product dependent

Use
Immediate release tablets: Treatment of hypertension alone or in combination with diuretics, beta-blockers, calcium channel blockers, or ACE inhibitors (FDA approved in adults); treatment of urinary outflow obstruction and/or obstructive and irritative symptoms associated with benign prostatic hyperplasia (BPH) (FDA approved in adults); has also been used for treatment of dysfunctional voiding and primary bladder neck dysfunction

Extended release tablets: Treatment of signs and symptoms of benign prostatic hyperplasia (BPH) (FDA approved in adults)

Pregnancy Risk Factor C

Pregnancy Considerations Adverse events were observed in some animal reproduction studies. Untreated chronic maternal hypertension is associated with adverse events in the fetus, infant, and mother. If treatment for hypertension during pregnancy is needed, other agents are generally preferred (ACOG, 2013).

Breast-Feeding Considerations Doxazosin is excreted into breast milk. Information is available from a single case report following a maternal dose of doxazosin 4 mg every 24 hours for 2 doses. Milk samples were obtained at various intervals over 24 hours, beginning ~17 hours after the first dose. Maternal serum samples were obtained at nearly the same times, beginning ~1 hour later. The highest serum and milk concentrations of doxazosin were observed ~1 hour after the dose. Using the highest milk concentration (4.15 mcg/L), the estimated dose to the nursing infant was calculated to be <1% of the weight-adjusted maternal dose (Jensen, 2013). The manufacturer recommends that caution be used if administered to nursing women.

Contraindications Hypersensitivity to doxazosin, quinazolines (prazosin, terazosin), or any component

Warnings Marked orthostatic hypotension, syncope, and loss of consciousness may occur with first dose or within first few days of therapy; syncope usually occurs 30-90 minutes after initial dose; occasionally preceded with severe tachycardia (120-160 bpm in adults); anticipate a similar effect if therapy is interrupted for a few days, if dosage is rapidly increased, if large initial dose (≥2 mg in adults), or if another antihypertensive drug (eg, beta-blockers, diuretics, and particularly vasodilators) or a PDE-5 inhibitor (eg, sildenafil, tadalafil, vardenafil) is introduced. Patients should be cautioned about performing hazardous tasks when starting new therapy or adjusting dosage upward. May cause priapism (rarely).

Precautions Use with caution in patients with mild to moderate hepatic impairment or receiving medications known to affect hepatic function; use is not recommended if severe hepatic impairment. Use with caution with concomitant use of strong CYP3A4 inhibitor, such as atanazavir, clarithromycin, indinavir, itraconazole, ketoconazole, nefazodone, nelfinavir, ritonavir, saquinavir, telithromycin,

or voriconazole; *in vitro* data suggests doxazosin is a CYP3A4 substrate. Use with caution in patients with cataracts or undergoing corrective cataract surgery; intraoperative floppy iris syndrome (IFIS) has been observed in cataract surgery patients receiving or previously treated with alpha$_1$-blockers; there appears to be no benefit in discontinuing alpha$_1$-blockers prior to surgery. Use with caution in patients with coronary insufficiency; discontinue drug if angina occurs or worsens.

The extended release tablet consists of drug within a nondeformable matrix; following drug release/absorption, the matrix/shell is expelled in the stool. The use of nondeformable products in patients with known stricture/narrowing of the GI tract has been associated with symptoms of obstruction. Use with caution in patients with increased GI retention (eg, chronic constipation) as doxazosin exposure may be increased.

Adverse Reactions
Cardiovascular: Arrhythmia, edema, facial edema, flushing, hypotension, orthostatic hypotension

Central nervous system: Anxiety, ataxia, dizziness, fatigue, headache, hypertonia, insomnia, malaise, movement disorder, pain, somnolence, vertigo

Endocrine & metabolic: Sexual dysfunction

Gastrointestinal: Abdominal pain, dyspepsia, nausea, xerostomia

Genitourinary: Impotence, incontinence, polyuria, urinary tract infection

Neuromuscular & skeletal: Arthritis, muscle cramps, muscle weakness, myalgia

Ocular: Abnormal vision

Otic: Tinnitus

Respiratory: Dyspnea, epistaxis, respiratory disorder, rhinitis

Rare but important or life-threatening: Abnormal lacrimation, abnormal thinking, agitation, allergic reaction, alopecia, amnesia, angina, anorexia, appetite increased, arthralgia, back pain, blurred vision, bradycardia, breast pain, bronchospasm, cerebrovascular accident, chest pain, cholestasis, confusion, cough, depersonalization, diaphoresis increased, diarrhea, dry skin, dysuria, earache, eczema, emotional lability, fecal incontinence, fever, gastroenteritis, gout, gynecomastia, hematuria, hepatitis, hot flashes, hypoesthesia, hypokalemia, impaired concentration, impotence, infection, influenza-like syndrome, intraoperative floppy iris syndrome (cataract surgery), jaundice, leukopenia, liver function tests increased, libido decreased, lymphadenopathy, micturition abnormality, migraine, MI, neutropenia, nocturia, pallor, palpitation, paranoia, paresis, parosmia, peripheral ischemia, pharyngitis, photophobia, priapism, pruritus, purpura, renal calculus, rigors, sinusitis, skin rash, syncope, taste perversion, thirst, thrombocytopenia, tremor, twitching, urticaria, vomiting, weight gain/loss

Drug Interactions
Metabolism/Transport Effects Substrate of CYP2C19 (minor), CYP2D6 (minor), CYP3A4 (major); **Note:** Assignment of Major/Minor substrate status based on clinically relevant drug interaction potential

Avoid Concomitant Use
Avoid concomitant use of Doxazosin with any of the following: Alpha1-Blockers; Boceprevir; Conivaptan; Fusidic Acid (Systemic)

Increased Effect/Toxicity
Doxazosin may increase the levels/effects of: Alpha1-Blockers; Amifostine; Antihypertensives; Calcium Channel Blockers; DULoxetine; Hypotensive Agents; Obinutuzumab; RiTUXimab

The levels/effects of Doxazosin may be increased by: Barbiturates; Beta-Blockers; Boceprevir; Brimonidine (Topical); Ceritinib; Conivaptan; CYP3A4 Inhibitors (Moderate); CYP3A4 Inhibitors (Strong); Dasatinib; Diazoxide;

Fusidic Acid (Systemic); Herbs (Hypotensive Properties); Ivacaftor; Luliconazole; MAO Inhibitors; Mifepristone; Pentoxifylline; Phosphodiesterase 5 Inhibitors; Prostacyclin Analogues; Simeprevir; Stiripentol

Decreased Effect

Doxazosin may decrease the levels/effects of: Alpha-/Beta-Agonists; Alpha1-Agonists

The levels/effects of Doxazosin may be decreased by: Bosentan; CYP3A4 Inducers (Strong); Dabrafenib; Deferasirox; Herbs (Hypertensive Properties); Methylphenidate; Mitotane; Peginterferon Alfa-2b; Siltuximab; St Johns Wort; Tocilizumab; Yohimbine

Stability Store at 25°C (77°F); excursions permitted to 15°C to 30°C (59°F to 86°F).

Mechanism of Action

Hypertension: Competitively inhibits postsynaptic alpha$_1$-adrenergic receptors which results in vasodilation of veins and arterioles and a decrease in total peripheral resistance and blood pressure; ~50% as potent on a weight by weight basis as prazosin.

BPH: Competitively inhibits postsynaptic alpha$_1$-adrenergic receptors in prostatic stromal and bladder neck tissues. This reduces the sympathetic tone-induced urethral stricture causing BPH symptoms.

Pharmacodynamics

Onset of action: Urinary outflow effects (immediate release): 1-2 weeks

Maximum effect: Antihypertensive effect (immediate release): 2-6 hours

Duration: Antihypertensive effect (immediate release): >24 hours

Pharmacokinetics (Adult data unless noted)

Protein binding: ~98%

Metabolism: Extensively hepatic to active metabolites; primarily via CYP3A4; secondary pathways involve CYP2D6 and 2C19; may undergo enterohepatic recycling

Bioavailability: Immediate release: ~65%; Extended release relative to immediate release: 54% to 59%

Half-life: Immediate release: ~22 hours; Extended release: 15-19 hours; prolonged in patients with hepatic impairment

Time to peak serum concentration: Immediate release: 2-3 hours; Extended release: 8-9 hours

Elimination: Feces (63%, primarily as metabolites); urine (9%, primarily as metabolites; trace amounts as unchanged drug)

Dosing: Usual Note: If drug is discontinued for greater than several days, consider beginning with initial dose and retitrate as needed.

Children and Adolescents:

Dysfunctional voiding: Limited data available, efficacy results variable: Children ≥3 years and Adolescents: Oral: Immediate release: Initial: 0.5 mg once daily at bedtime; some trials maintained a fixed dose; others titrated at weekly or biweekly intervals to effect as tolerated (maximum daily dose: 2 mg/**day**) (Austin, 1999; Cain, 2003; El-Hefnawy, 2012; Yucel, 2005). In some trials, a larger initial dose (1 mg/**day**) was used in patients weighing >40-50 kg (Austin, 1999; Yucel, 2005).

Hypertension: Limited data available: Children and Adolescents: Oral: Immediate release: Initial: 1 mg/**day**; maximum daily dose: 4 mg/**day** (NHBPEP, 2004; NHLBI, 2011)

Adults:

Benign prostatic hypertrophy (BPH): Oral:

Immediate release: 1 mg once daily in morning or evening; may be increased to 2 mg once daily. Thereafter titrate upwards, if needed, over several weeks, balancing therapeutic benefit with doxazosin-induced postural hypotension. Usual range: 4-8 mg/day; maximum dose: 8 mg/day

Reinitiation of therapy: If therapy is discontinued for several days, restart at 1 mg dose and titrate as before

Extended release: 4 mg once daily with breakfast; titrate based on response and tolerability every 3-4 weeks to maximum recommended dose of 8 mg/day

Reinitiation of therapy: If therapy is discontinued for several days, restart at 4 mg dose and titrate as before

Note: Conversion to extended release from immediate release: Omit final evening dose of immediate release prior to starting morning dosing with extended release product; initiate extended release product using 4 mg once daily

Hypertension: Oral: Immediate release: 1 mg once daily in morning or evening; may be increased to 2 mg once daily. Thereafter titrate upwards, if needed, over several weeks, balancing therapeutic benefit with doxazosin-induced postural hypotension. Maximum dose: 16 mg/day

Reinitiation of therapy: If therapy is discontinued for several days, restart at 1 mg dose and titrate as before

Dosing adjustment in hepatic impairment: Adults: Use with caution in mild-to-moderate hepatic dysfunction. Do not use with severe impairment.

Dosing adjustment in renal impairment: There are no dosage adjustments provided in manufacturer's labeling; however, limited data suggest renal impairment does not significantly alter pharmacokinetic parameters.

Administration Oral:

Immediate release: Administer without regard to meals at the same time each day

Extended release (Cardura® XL): Tablets should be swallowed whole; do not crush, chew, or divide. Administer with morning meal.

Monitoring Parameters Standing and sitting/supine blood pressure, especially 2-6 hours after the initial dose, then prior to doses (to ensure adequate control throughout the dosing interval); urinary symptoms if used for dysfunctional voiding or BPH treatment.

Dosage Forms Excipient information presented when available (limited, particularly for generics); consult specific product labeling.

Tablet, Oral:

Cardura: 1 mg, 2 mg, 4 mg, 8 mg [scored]

Generic: 1 mg, 2 mg, 4 mg, 8 mg

Tablet Extended Release 24 Hour, Oral:

Cardura XL: 4 mg, 8 mg

References

Austin PF, Homsy YL, Masel JL, et al, "Alpha-Adrenergic Blockade in Children With Neuropathic and Nonneuropathic Voiding Dysfunction," *J Urol*, 1999, 162(3 Pt 2):1064-7.

Cain MP, Wu SD, Austin PF, et al, "Alpha Blocker Therapy for Children With Nonneurogenic Voiding and Urinary Retention," *J Urol*, 2003, 170 (4 Pt 2):1514-5.

Chase J, Austin P, Hoebeke P, et al, "The Management of Dysfunctional Voiding in Children: A Report From the Standardisation Committee of the International Children's Continence Society," *J Urol*, 2010, 183 (4):1296-302.

Chobanian AV, Bakris GL, Black HR, et al, "The Seventh Report of the Joint National Committee on Prevention, Detection, Evaluation, and Treatment of High Blood Pressure: The JNC 7 Report," *JAMA*, 2003, 289(19):2560-71.

El-Hefnawy AS, Helmy T, El-Assmy MM, et al, "Doxazosin Versus Tizanidine for Treatment of Dysfunctional Voiding in Children: A Prospective Randomized Open-Labeled Trial," *Urology*, 2012, 79 (2):428-33.

Jensen BP, Dalrymple JM, and Begg EJ, "Transfer of Doxazosin Into Breast Milk," *J Hum Lact*, 2013, 29(2):150-3.

National Heart, Lung, and Blood Institute, "Expert Panel on Integrated Guidelines for Cardiovascular Health and Risk Reduction in Children and Adolescents," Clinical Practice Guidelines, 2011, National Institutes of Health. Available at http://www.nhlbi.nih.gov/guidelines/cvd_ped/peds_guidelines_full.pdf

National High Blood Pressure Education Program Working Group on High Blood Pressure in Children and Adolescents, "The Fourth Report on the Diagnosis, Evaluation, and Treatment of High Blood Pressure in Children and Adolescents," *Pediatrics*, 2004, 114(2 Suppl 4th Report):555-76.

Yucel S, Akkaya E, Guntekin E, et al, "Can Alpha-Blocker Therapy be an Alternative to Biofeedback for Dysfunctional Voiding and Urinary Retention? A prospective Study," *J Urol*, 2005, 174(4 Pt 2):1612-5.

◆ **Doxazosin Mesylate** *see* Doxazosin *on page 712*

Doxepin (Systemic) (DOKS e pin)

Medication Safety Issues
Sound-alike/look-alike issues:
Doxepin may be confused with digoxin, doxapram, doxazosin, Doxidan, doxycycline

SINEquan may be confused with saquinavir, SEROquel, Singulair, Zonegran

BEERS Criteria medication:
This drug may be potentially inappropriate for use in geriatric patients (Quality of evidence - high [moderate for SIADH]; Strength of recommendation - strong).

International issues:
Doxal [Finland] may be confused with Doxil brand name for doxorubicin (liposomal) [U.S., Israel]

Doxal brand name for doxepin [Finland] but also brand name for pyridoxine/thiamine [Brazil]

Related Information
Antidepressant Agents *on page 2219*

Brand Names: U.S. Silenor

Brand Names: Canada Apo-Doxepin; Novo-Doxepin; Silenor; Sinequan; Zonalon

Therapeutic Category Antianxiety Agent; Antidepressant, Tricyclic (Tertiary Amine)

Generic Availability (U.S.) May be product dependent

Use Treatment of various forms of depression and anxiety disorders associated with psychoneurosis, alcoholism, organic disease, and manic-depressive disorders (FDA approved in ages ≥12 years and adults); treatment of insomnia with difficulty of sleep maintenance (Silanor®: FDA approved in adults)

Medication Guide Available Yes

Pregnancy Risk Factor C

Pregnancy Considerations Adverse events were observed in animal reproduction studies. Tricyclic antidepressants may be associated with irritability, jitteriness, and convulsions (rare) in the neonate (Yonkers, 2009).

The ACOG recommends that therapy for depression during pregnancy be individualized; treatment should incorporate the clinical expertise of the mental health clinician, obstetrician, primary healthcare provider, and pediatrician (ACOG, 2008). According to the American Psychiatric Association (APA), the risks of medication treatment should be weighed against other treatment options and untreated depression. For women who discontinue antidepressant medications during pregnancy and who may be at high risk for postpartum depression, the medications can be restarted following delivery (APA, 2010). Treatment algorithms have been developed by the ACOG and the APA for the management of depression in women prior to conception and during pregnancy (Yonkers, 2009).

Breast-Feeding Considerations Doxepin and N-desmethyldoxepin are excreted into breast milk (Frey, 1999; Kemp, 1985). Drowsiness, vomiting, poor feeding, and muscle hypotonia were noted in a nursing infant following maternal use of doxepin. Symptoms began to resolve 24 hours after feedings with breast milk were discontinued (Frey, 1999). In addition, product labeling notes that drowsiness and apnea have been reported in a nursing infant following maternal use of doxepin for depression. The manufacturer recommends that caution be used if administered to a nursing woman.

Contraindications Hypersensitivity to doxepin, any component, or drugs from similar chemical class; narrow-angle glaucoma; urinary retention; use of MAO inhibitors within 14 days

Warnings Clinical worsening of depression or suicidal ideation and behavior may occur in children and adults with major depressive disorder (MDD) **[U.S. Boxed Warning]**. In clinical trials, antidepressants increased the risk of suicidal thinking and behavior (suicidality) in children, adolescents, and young adults (18-24 years of age) with major depressive disorder (MDD) and other psychiatric disorders. This risk must be considered before prescribing antidepressants for any clinical use. Short-term studies did **not** show an increased risk of suicidality with antidepressant use in patients >24 years of age and showed a decreased risk in patients ≥65 years of age.

Patients of all ages who are treated with antidepressants for any indication require appropriate monitoring and close observation for clinical worsening of depression, suicidality, and unusual changes in behavior, especially during the first few months after antidepressant initiation or when the dose is adjusted. Family members and caregivers should be instructed to closely observe the patient (ie, daily) and communicate condition with healthcare provider. Patients should also be monitored for associated behaviors (eg, anxiety, agitation, panic attacks, insomnia, irritability, hostility, aggressiveness, impulsivity, akathisia, hypomania, mania) which may increase the risk for worsening depression or suicidality. Worsening depression or emergence of suicidality (or associated behaviors listed above) that are abrupt in onset, severe, or not part of the presenting symptoms, may require discontinuation or modification of drug therapy. Risk of suicidal behavior may be increased regardless of doxepin dose; antidepressant doses of doxepin are 10- to 100-fold higher than doses for insomnia.

Avoid abrupt discontinuation; discontinuation symptoms (including headache, nausea, and malaise) may occur if therapy is abruptly discontinued or dose is reduced; taper the dose to minimize risks of discontinuation symptoms. To reduce risk of intentional overdose, write prescriptions for the smallest quantity consistent with good patient care. Screen individuals for bipolar disorder prior to treatment (using antidepressants alone may induce manic episodes in patients with this condition). May worsen psychosis or precipitate mania or hypomania in patients with bipolar disease; monotherapy in patients with bipolar disorder should be avoided. Patients presenting with depressive symptoms should be screened for bipolar disorder. Doxepin is not FDA approved for the treatment of bipolar depression. May increase the risks associated with electroconvulsive therapy. Discontinue therapy, when possible, prior to elective surgery (do not discontinue abruptly).

Doxepin causes a high degree of sedation (relative to other antidepressants); may result in impaired performance of tasks requiring alertness. Patients who take doxepin for insomnia should confine their activities to those necessary to prepare for bed after taking the dose; a residual pharmacologic effect may also occur the next day. Hazardous, sleep-related activities, such as sleep-driving (driving while not fully awake), cooking or eating food, and making phone calls while asleep have also been noted; an increased risk of these type of events has been reported with the use of hypnotic agents taken in greater than recommended dosages, as well as with concomitant ethanol or CNS depressant use; amnesia may also occur; discontinue treatment in patients who report any sleep-related episodes. Use with caution in patients receiving other CNS depressants; effects with other sedative drugs or ethanol may be potentiated. Failure of sleep disturbance to resolve after 7-10 days, exacerbation of insomnia, or emergence of new cognitive or behavioral abnormalities may indicate psychiatric or medical illness.

Precautions Use with caution in patients with hepatic impairment; higher doxepin concentrations may occur. May cause orthostatic hypotension (risk is moderate relative to other antidepressants); use with caution in patients at risk of this effect or in those who would not tolerate transient hypotensive episodes (cerebrovascular disease, cardiovascular disease, hypovolemia, or concurrent medication use which may predispose to hypotension/bradycardia). Use with caution in patients with a history of cardiovascular disease (including previous MI, stroke, tachycardia, or conduction abnormalities); the risk of conduction abnormalities with this agent is moderate relative to other antidepressants. Use with caution in patients with respiratory compromise or sleep apnea; use is generally not recommended in patients with severe sleep apnea. Use with caution in patients at risk of seizures, including those with a history of seizures, head trauma, brain damage, alcoholism, or concurrent therapy with medications which may lower seizure threshold. Use with caution in patients with hyperthyroidism or those receiving thyroid supplementation. Use with caution in patients with renal impairment. May cause anticholinergic effects (constipation, xerostomia, blurred vision, urinary retention); use with caution in patients with decreased gastrointestinal motility, paralytic ileus, urinary retention, BPH, xerostomia, or visual problems. The degree of anticholinergic blockade produced by this agent is high relative to other antidepressants.

Adverse Reactions May be dependent on diagnosis.

Cardiovascular: Edema, flushing, hypertension (chronic insomnia patients), hypotension, tachycardia

Central nervous system: Ataxia, chills, confusion, disorientation, dizziness (chronic insomnia patients), drowsiness, extrapyramidal reaction, fatigue, hallucination, headache, numbness, paresthesia, sedation (chronic insomnia patients), seizure, tardive dyskinesia

Dermatologic: Alopecia, diaphoresis (excessive), pruritus, skin photosensitivity, skin rash

Endocrine & metabolic: Altered serum glucose, change in libido, galactorrhea, gynecomastia, SIADH, weight gain

Gastrointestinal: Anorexia, aphthous stomatitis, constipation, diarrhea, dysgeusia, dyspepsia, gastroenteritis (chronic insomnia patients), nausea (chronic insomnia patients), vomiting, xerostomia

Genitourinary: Breast hypertrophy, testicular swelling, urinary retention

Hematologic & oncologic: Agranulocytosis, eosinophilia, leukopenia, purpura, thrombocytopenia, purpura

Hepatic: Jaundice

Neuromuscular & skeletal: Tremor, weakness

Ophthalmic: Blurred vision

Otic: Tinnitus

Respiratory: Exacerbation of asthma, upper respiratory tract infection (chronic insomnia patients)

Rare but important or life-threatening: Adenocarcinoma (lung, stage I), adjustment disorder, anemia, atrioventricular block, bone fracture, breast cyst, cerebrovascular accident, chest pain, decreased neutrophils, decreased performance on neuropsychometrics, decreased range of motion (joints), depression, ECG abnormality (ST-T segment, QRS complex, QRS axis), eye infection, fungal infection, gastroesophageal reflux disease, hematochezia, hematoma, hemoglobinuria, hyperbilirubinemia, hyperkalemia, hypermagnesemia, hypersensitivity, hypoacusis, hypokalemia, increased serum ALT, increased serum transaminases, malignant melanoma, migraine, peripheral edema, pneumonia, sleep paralysis, somnambulism (complex sleep-related behavior [sleep-driving, cooking or eating food, making phone calls]), staphylococcal cellulitis, syncope, tenosynovitis, tooth infection, urinary incontinence, urinary tract infection, viral infection

Drug Interactions

Metabolism/Transport Effects Substrate of CYP1A2 (minor), CYP2C19 (minor), CYP2D6 (major), CYP3A4 (minor). **Note:** Assignment of Major/Minor substrate status based on clinically relevant drug interaction potential

Avoid Concomitant Use

Avoid concomitant use of Doxepin (Systemic) with any of the following: Aclidinium; Azelastine (Nasal); Iobenguane I 123; Ipratropium (Oral Inhalation); Linezolid; MAO Inhibitors; Methylene Blue; Moxonidine; Paraldehyde; Potassium Chloride; Thalidomide; Tiotropium; Umeclidinium

Increased Effect/Toxicity

Doxepin (Systemic) may increase the levels/effects of: AbobotulinumtoxinA; Alcohol (Ethyl); Alpha-/Beta-Agonists (Direct-Acting); Alpha1-Agonists; Amphetamines; Analgesics (Opioid); Anticholinergic Agents; Antipsychotics; Aspirin; Azelastine (Nasal); Beta2-Agonists; Buprenorphine; Cannabinoid-Containing Products; Citalopram; CNS Depressants; Desmopressin; Escitalopram; Highest Risk QTc-Prolonging Agents; Hydrocodone; Methotrimeprazine; Methylene Blue; Metyrosine; Mirabegron; Moderate Risk QTc-Prolonging Agents; NSAID (COX-2 Inhibitor); NSAID (Nonselective); OnabotulinumtoxinA; Paraldehyde; Potassium Chloride; Pramipexole; QuiNIDine; RimabotulinumtoxinB; ROPINIRole; Rotigotine; Serotonin Modulators; Sodium Phosphates; Sulfonylureas; Thalidomide; Thiazide Diuretics; Tiotropium; Topiramate; TraMADol; Vitamin K Antagonists; Yohimbine; Zolpidem

The levels/effects of Doxepin (Systemic) may be increased by: Abiraterone Acetate; Aclidinium; Altretamine; Antiemetics (5HT3 Antagonists); Antipsychotics; Brimonidine (Topical); BuPROPion; Cannabis; Cimetidine; Cinacalcet; Citalopram; Cobicistat; CYP2D6 Inhibitors (Moderate); CYP2D6 Inhibitors (Strong); Darunavir; Dexmethylphenidate; Doxylamine; Dronabinol; Droperidol; DULoxetine; Escitalopram; FLUoxetine; FluvoxaMINE; HydrOXYzine; Ipratropium (Oral Inhalation); Kava Kava; Linezolid; Lithium; Magnesium Sulfate; MAO Inhibitors; Methotrimeprazine; Methylphenidate; Metoclopramide; Metyrosine; Mifepristone; Nabilone; PARoxetine; Perampanel; Pramlintide; Protease Inhibitors; QuiNIDine; Rufinamide; Sertraline; Sodium Oxybate; Tapentadol; Terbinafine (Systemic); Tetrahydrocannabinol; Thyroid Products; TraMADol; Umeclidinium; Valproic Acid and Derivatives

Decreased Effect

Doxepin (Systemic) may decrease the levels/effects of: Acetylcholinesterase Inhibitors (Central); Alpha2-Agonists; Alpha2-Agonists (Ophthalmic); Iobenguane I 123; Moxonidine; Secretin

The levels/effects of Doxepin (Systemic) may be decreased by: Acetylcholinesterase Inhibitors (Central); Barbiturates; CarBAMazepine; Peginterferon Alfa-2b; St Johns Wort

Food Interactions Administration with a high-fat meal increases the bioavailability of Silenor and delays the peak plasma concentration by ~3 hours. Management: Silenor should not be taken during or within 3 hours of a meal.

Stability Store at 20°C to 25°C (68°F to 77°F); protect from light.

Mechanism of Action Increases the synaptic concentration of serotonin and norepinephrine in the central nervous system by inhibition of their reuptake by the presynaptic neuronal membrane (Pinder, 1977); antagonizes the histamine (H_1) receptor for sleep maintenance

Pharmacodynamics

Onset: Sedation: ~30 minutes

Maximum effects: Antidepressant: Usually >2 weeks; anxiolytic: May occur sooner

Pharmacokinetics (Adult data unless noted)

Distribution: Widely throughout body tissues; V_d: ~12,000 L

Protein binding: 80% to 85%

Metabolism: Hepatic primarily via CYP2C19 and 2D6 to metabolites, including N-desmethyldoxepin (active); N-desmethyldoxepin undergoes glucuronide conjugation

Half-life: Doxepin: ~15 hours; N-desmethyldoxepin: 31 hours

Time to peak serum concentration: Fasting: Silenor®: 3.5 hours

Elimination: Urine (mainly excreted as glucuronide conjugates; <3% as unchanged drug or N-desmethyl-doxepin)

Dosing: Usual

Children and Adolescents: **Depression and/or anxiety:** Oral:

Children 7-11 years: Limited data available; efficacy results variable; controlled clinical trials have not shown tricyclic antidepressants to be superior to placebo for the treatment of depression in children and have not recommended them for use (Dopheide, 2006; USPTF, 2009; Wagner, 2005); some centers have used the following doses: 1-3 mg/kg/day in single or divided doses

Children ≥12 years and Adolescents: **Note:** Controlled clinical trials have not shown tricyclic antidepressants to be superior to placebo for the treatment of depression in adolescents and have not recommended them for use (Dopheide, 2006; USPTF, 2009; Wagner, 2005); Initial: 25-75 mg/day at bedtime or in 2-3 divided doses; begin at the low end of range and gradually titrate; select patients may respond to 25-50 mg/day; maximum single dose: 150 mg; maximum daily dose: 300 mg/**day**

Adults:

Depression and/or anxiety: Oral: Initial: 25-150 mg/day at bedtime or in 2-3 divided doses; may gradually increase up to 300 mg/day; single dose should not exceed 150 mg; select patients may respond to 25-50 mg/day

Insomnia (Silenor®): Oral: 3-6 mg once daily 30 minutes prior to bedtime; maximum dose: 6 mg/day

Administration

Depression/anxiety: Administer with food to decrease GI upset; oral concentrate should be diluted in water, milk, or juice (orange, grapefruit, tomato, prune, or pineapple; but not grape juice) prior to administration (use 120 mL for adults); do not mix with carbonated beverages.

Insomnia (Silenor®): Administer within 30 minutes prior to bedtime; do not take within 3 hours of a meal; **Note:** Not taking Silenor® within 3 hours of a meal will give a faster onset and help minimize the risk for next day effects.

Monitoring Parameters Blood pressure, heart rate, mental status, weight, liver enzymes, and CBC with differential. Monitor patient periodically for symptom resolution; monitor for worsening depression, suicidality, and associated behaviors (especially at the beginning of therapy or when doses are increased or decreased).

Reference Range Utility of serum concentration monitoring is controversial

Doxepin plus desmethyldoxepin:

Proposed therapeutic concentration: 110-250 ng/mL (394-895 nmol/L)

Toxic concentration: >500 ng/mL (>1790 nmol/L) (toxicities may be seen at lower concentrations in some patients)

Additional Information For treatment of insomnia, use beyond 3 months has not been evaluated.

Dosage Forms Excipient information presented when available (limited, particularly for generics); consult specific product labeling.

Capsule, Oral:

Generic: 10 mg, 25 mg, 50 mg, 75 mg, 100 mg, 150 mg

Concentrate, Oral:

Generic: 10 mg/mL (118 mL, 120 mL)

Tablet, Oral:

Silenor: 3 mg [contains brilliant blue fcf (fd&c blue #1)]

Silenor: 6 mg [contains brilliant blue fcf (fd&c blue #1), fd&c yellow #10 (quinoline yellow)]

References

AACAP Work Group on Quality Issues, "Practice Parameter for the Assessment and Treatment of Children and Adolescents With Depressive Disorders," *J Am Acad Child Adolesc Psychiatry*, 2007, 46(11):1503-26.

ACOG Committee on Practice Bulletins-Obstetrics. ACOG practice bulletin: clinical management guidelines for obstetrician-gynecologists number 92, April 2008 (replaces practice bulletin number 87, November 2007). Use of psychiatric medications during pregnancy and lactation. *Obstet Gynecol*. 2008;111(4):1001-1020.

American Psychiatric Association (APA). Treatment recommendations for patients with major depressive disorder. 3rd ed, May 2010. Available at http://www.psychiatryonline.com/pracGuide/pracGuide-Topic_7.aspx

Dopheide JA, "Recognizing and Treating Depression in Children and Adolescents," *Am J Health Syst Pharm*, 2006, 63(3):233-43.

Frey OR, Scheidt P, von Brenndorff Al. Adverse effects in a newborn infant breast-fed by a mother treated with doxepin. *Ann Pharmacother*. 1999;33(6):690-693.

Kemp J, Ilett KF, Booth J, et al. Excretion of doxepin and N-desmethyldoxepin in human milk. *Br J Clin Pharmacol*. 1985;20(5):497-499.

Levy HB, Harper CR, and Weinberg WA, "A Practical Approach to Children Failing in School," *Pediatr Clin North Am*, 1992, 39 (4):895-928.

US Preventive Services Task Force (USPTF), "Screening and Treatment for Major Depressive Disorder in Children and Adolescents: US Preventive Services Task Force Recommendation Statement," *Pediatrics*, 2009, 123(4):1223-8.

Wagner KD, "Pharmacotherapy for Major Depression in Children and Adolescents," *Prog Neuropsychopharmacol Biol Psychiatry*, 2005, 29 (5):819-26.

Yonkers KA, Wisner KL, Stewart DE, et al. The management of depression during pregnancy: a report from the American Psychiatric Association and the American College of Obstetricians and Gynecologists. *Obstet Gynecol*. 2009;114(3):703-713.

Doxepin (Topical) (DOKS e pin)

Medication Safety Issues

Sound-alike/look-alike issues:

Doxepin may be confused with digoxin, doxapram, doxazosin, Doxidan®, doxycycline

Zonalon® may be confused with Zone-A®

International issues:

Doxal [Finland] may be confused with Doxil brand name for doxorubicin (liposomal) [U.S., Israel]

Doxal brand name for doxepin [Finland] but also brand name for pyridoxine/thiamine [Brazil]

Brand Names: U.S. Prudoxin; Zonalon

Brand Names: Canada Zonalon®

Generic Availability (U.S.) No

Use Adults: Short-term (<8 days) therapy of moderate pruritus due to atopic dermatitis or lichen simplex chronicus

Pregnancy Risk Factor B

Pregnancy Considerations Adverse effects were not observed in animal reproduction studies. Following topical application, plasma levels may be similar to those achieved with oral administration. Also refer to the Doxepin (Systemic) monograph.

Breast-Feeding Considerations Doxepin is excreted into breast milk following oral administration. Following topical application, plasma levels may be similar to those achieved with oral administration. Due to the potential for serious adverse reactions in the nursing infant, the manufacturer recommends a decision be made whether to discontinue nursing or to discontinue the drug, taking into account the importance of treatment to the mother. Also refer to the Doxepin (Systemic) monograph.

◄ **Contraindications** Hypersensitivity to doxepin or any component; cross-sensitivity with other tricyclic antidepressants may occur; narrow-angle glaucoma; patients with urinary retention

Warnings Doxepin causes a high degree of sedation (relative to other antidepressants); may cause orthostatic hypotension and anticholinergic side effects; may worsen psychosis or precipitate mania or hypomania in patients with bipolar disease; may increase the risks associated with electroconvulsive therapy. Cream contains benzyl alcohol which may cause allergic reactions in susceptible individuals; large amounts of benzyl alcohol (≥99 mg/kg/day) have been associated with a potentially fatal toxicity ("gasping syndrome") in neonates; avoid use of doxepin products containing benzyl alcohol in neonates; *in vitro* and animal studies have shown that benzoate, a metabolite of benzyl alcohol, displaces bilirubin from protein binding sites.

Precautions Use with caution in patients with cardiovascular disease, conduction disturbances, seizure disorders, urinary retention, hyperthyroidism, or those receiving thyroid replacement; avoid use during lactation; use with caution during pregnancy.

Drowsiness may occur with topical use; incidence with cream is 22%, especially if applied to >10% of BSA; occlusive dressings may increase absorption of doxepin; if drowsiness or sedation occurs, dosage adjustment may be needed (eg, reduction in area treated, number of applications per day, amount of cream used); discontinue therapy is excessive drowsiness occurs. Allergic contact dermatitis may occur with topical use; risk may be increased with use >8 days. **Note:** Cream is not recommended for use in pediatric patients; overdoses from topical administration in children have been reported.

Adverse Reactions
Cardiovascular: Edema:
Central nervous system: Dizziness, drowsiness, emotional changes
Dermatologic: Stinging/burning
Gastrointestinal: Taste alteration, xerostomia
Rare but important or life-threatening: Anxiety, contact dermatitis, tongue numbness

Drug Interactions
Metabolism/Transport Effects Substrate of CYP1A2 (minor), CYP2C19 (minor), CYP2D6 (major), CYP3A4 (minor); **Note:** Assignment of Major/Minor substrate status based on clinically relevant drug interaction potential

Avoid Concomitant Use
Avoid concomitant use of Doxepin (Topical) with any of the following: Aclidinium; Azelastine (Nasal); Iobenguane I 123; Ipratropium (Oral Inhalation); Linezolid; MAO Inhibitors; Methylene Blue; Moxonidine; Paraldehyde; Potassium Chloride; Thalidomide; Tiotropium; Umeclidinium

Increased Effect/Toxicity
Doxepin (Topical) may increase the levels/effects of: AbobotulinumtoxinA; Alcohol (Ethyl); Alpha-/Beta-Agonists (Direct-Acting); Alpha1-Agonists; Amphetamines; Analgesics (Opioid); Anticholinergic Agents; Antipsychotics; Aspirin; Azelastine (Nasal); Beta2-Agonists; Buprenorphine; Cannabinoid-Containing Products; Citalopram; CNS Depressants; Desmopressin; Escitalopram; Highest Risk QTc-Prolonging Agents; Hydrocodone; Methotrimeprazine; Methylene Blue; Metyrosine; Mirabegron; Moderate Risk QTc-Prolonging Agents; NSAID (COX-2 Inhibitor); NSAID (Nonselective); OnabotulinumtoxinA; Paraldehyde; Potassium Chloride; Pramipexole; QuiNIDine; RimabotulinumtoxinB; ROPINIRole; Rotigotine; Serotonin Modulators; Sodium Phosphates; Sulfonylureas; Thalidomide; Thiazide Diuretics; Tiotropium; Topiramate; TraMADol; Vitamin K Antagonists; Yohimbine; Zolpidem

The levels/effects of Doxepin (Topical) may be increased by: Abiraterone Acetate; Aclidinium; Altretamine; Antiemetics (5HT3 Antagonists); Antipsychotics; Brimonidine (Topical); BuPROPion; Cannabis; Cimetidine; Cinacalcet; Citalopram; Cobicistat; CYP2D6 Inhibitors (Moderate); CYP2D6 Inhibitors (Strong); Darunavir; Dexmethylphenidate; Doxylamine; Dronabinol; Droperidol; DULoxetine; Escitalopram; FLUoxetine; FluvoxaMINE; HydrOXYzine; Ipratropium (Oral Inhalation); Kava Kava; Linezolid; Lithium; Magnesium Sulfate; MAO Inhibitors; Methotrimeprazine; Methylphenidate; Metoclopramide; Metyrosine; Mifepristone; Nabilone; PARoxetine; Perampanel; Pramlintide; Protease Inhibitors; QuiNIDine; Rufinamide; Sertraline; Sodium Oxybate; Tapentadol; Terbinafine (Systemic); Tetrahydrocannabinol; Thyroid Products; TraMADol; Umeclidinium; Valproic Acid and Derivatives

Decreased Effect
Doxepin (Topical) may decrease the levels/effects of: Acetylcholinesterase Inhibitors (Central); Alpha2-Agonists; Alpha2-Agonists (Ophthalmic); Iobenguane I 123; Moxonidine; Secretin

The levels/effects of Doxepin (Topical) may be decreased by: Acetylcholinesterase Inhibitors (Central); Barbiturates; CarBAMazepine; Peginterferon Alfa-2b; St Johns Wort

Dosing: Usual Topical: Adults: Apply to affected area 4 times/day

Administration Apply thin film of cream to affected area with at least 3-4 hours between applications; do not use occlusive dressings; do not use for >8 days; avoid contact with eyes.

Additional Information Safety and effectiveness of topical cream when used for >8 days has not been established; use >8 days may result in an increase in serum concentrations and systemic effects.

Dosage Forms Excipient information presented when available (limited, particularly for generics); consult specific product labeling.
Cream, External, as hydrochloride:
Prudoxin: 5% (45 g)
Zonalon: 5% (30 g, 45 g)

◆ **Doxepin Hydrochloride** *see* Doxepin (Systemic) *on page 715*

◆ **Doxepin Hydrochloride** *see* Doxepin (Topical) *on page 717*

DOXOrubicin (Conventional)
(doks oh ROO bi sin con VEN sha nal)

Medication Safety Issues
Sound-alike/look-alike issues:
DOXOrubicin may be confused with DACTINomycin, DAUNOrubicin, DAUNOrubicin liposomal, doxapram, doxazosin, DOXOrubicin liposomal, epirubicin, IDArubicin, valrubicin
Adriamycin PFS may be confused with achromycin, Aredia, Idamycin
Conventional formulation (Adriamycin PFS, Adriamycin RDF) may be confused with the liposomal formulation (Doxil)

High alert medication:
This medication is in a class the Institute for Safe Medication Practices (ISMP) includes among its list of drug classes which have a heightened risk of causing significant patient harm when used in error.

Administration issues:
Use caution when selecting product for preparation and dispensing; indications, dosages and adverse event profiles differ between conventional DOXOrubicin hydrochloride solution and DOXOrubicin liposomal.

Both formulations are the same concentration. As a result, serious errors have occurred.

Other safety concerns:

ADR is an error-prone abbreviation

International issues:

Doxil may be confused with Doxal which is a brand name for doxepin in Finland, a brand name for doxycycline in Austria, and a brand name for pyridoxine/thiamine combination in Brazil

Rubex, a discontinued brand name for DOXOrubicin in the U.S, is a brand name for ascorbic acid in Ireland

Related Information

Emetogenic Potential of Antineoplastic Agents in Children on page 2327

Management of Drug Extravasations on page 2255

Safe Handling of Hazardous Drugs on page 2419
Injection

Brand Names: U.S. Adriamycin

Brand Names: Canada Adriamycin PFS; Doxorubicin Hydrochloride For Injection, USP; Doxorubicin Hydrochloride Injection

Therapeutic Category Antineoplastic Agent, Anthracycline; Antineoplastic Agent, Antibiotic; Antineoplastic Agent, Topoisomerase II Inhibitor

Generic Availability (U.S.) Yes

Use Treatment of acute lymphocytic leukemia (ALL), acute myeloid leukemia (AML), Hodgkin's disease, malignant lymphoma, soft tissue and bone sarcomas, thyroid cancer, small cell lung cancer, breast cancer, gastric cancer, ovarian cancer, bladder cancer, neuroblastoma, and Wilms' tumor [FDA approved in pediatrics (age not specified) and adults]; has also been used for the treatment of multiple myeloma, endometrial carcinoma, uterine sarcoma, head and neck cancer, liver cancer, and kidney cancer

Pregnancy Risk Factor D

Pregnancy Considerations Adverse events have been observed in animal reproduction studies. Based on the mechanism of action, doxorubicin may cause fetal harm if administered during pregnancy (according to the manufacturer's labeling). Advise patients (females of reproductive potential and males with female partners of reproductive potential) to use effective nonhormonal contraception during and for 6 months following therapy. The National Comprehensive Cancer Network (NCCN) breast cancer guidelines (v3.2013) state that chemotherapy, if indicated, may be administered to pregnant women with breast cancer as part of a combination chemotherapy regimen (common regimens administered during pregnancy include doxorubicin, cyclophosphamide, and fluorouracil); chemotherapy should not be administered during the first trimester, after 35 weeks gestation, or within 3 weeks of planned delivery.

Breast-Feeding Considerations Doxorubicin and its metabolites are excreted in breast milk. Due to the potential for serious adverse reactions in the nursing infant, the manufacturer recommends a decision be made whether to discontinue nursing or to discontinue the drug, taking into account the importance of treatment to the mother. Per the NCCN guidelines (v3.2013), breast-feeding after breast-conserving treatment for breast cancer is not contraindicated; however, the quantity and quality of breast milk may not be sufficient or may be lacking some nutrients needed.

Contraindications Hypersensitivity to doxorubicin or any component; severe CHF, cardiomyopathy, preexisting myelosuppression; patients who have received a total dose of 550 mg/m^2 of doxorubicin or 400 mg/m^2 in patients with previous or concomitant treatment with daunorubicin, idarubicin, mitoxantrone, cyclophosphamide, or irradiation of the cardiac region; patients who have received previous treatment with complete cumulative doses of daunorubicin, idarubicin, or other anthracycline derivatives; pregnancy

Warnings Hazardous agent; use appropriate precautions for handling and disposal (NIOSH, 2012). **I.V. use only,** severe local tissue necrosis will result if extravasation occurs **[U.S. Boxed Warning].** May cause severe myelosuppression; dose-limiting, primarily leukopenia and neutropenia **[U.S. Boxed Warning]**; irreversible myocardial toxicity, including potentially fatal CHF, may occur during therapy or months to years after therapy termination **[U.S. Boxed Warning].** The probability of developing myocardial toxicity is estimated to be 1% to 2% at a total cumulative dose of 300 mg/m^2 of doxorubicin, 3% to 5% at a total cumulative dose of 400 mg/m^2, 5% to 8% at a total cumulative dose of 450 mg/m^2, and 6% to 20% at 500 mg/m^2. Myocardial toxicity may occur at lower cumulative doses in patients with prior mediastinal irradiation, concurrent cyclophosphamide therapy, or preexisting heart disease. Pediatric patients are at increased risk for developing delayed cardiac toxicity and CHF during early adulthood due to an increasing census of long-term survivors; periodic long-term monitoring of cardiac function is recommended. Doxorubicin may contribute to prepubertal growth failure in pediatric patients. Secondary acute myelogenous leukemia and myelodysplastic syndrome have been reported following treatment **[U.S. Boxed Warning].**

Precautions Use with caution and modify dosage in patients with impaired hepatic function **[U.S. Boxed Warning].** Should be administered under the supervision of an experienced cancer chemotherapy physician **[U.S. Boxed Warning].**

Adverse Reactions

Cardiovascular:

Acute cardiotoxicity: Atrioventricular block, bradycardia, bundle branch block, ECG abnormalities, extrasystoles (atrial or ventricular), sinus tachycardia, ST-T wave changes, supraventricular tachycardia, tachyarrhythmia, ventricular tachycardia

Delayed cardiotoxicity: LVEF decreased, CHF (manifestations include ascites, cardiomegaly, dyspnea, edema, gallop rhythm, hepatomegaly, oliguria, pleural effusion, pulmonary edema, tachycardia); myocarditis, pericarditis

Central nervous system: Malaise

Dermatologic: Alopecia, itching, photosensitivity, radiation recall, rash; discoloration of saliva, sweat, or tears

Endocrine & metabolic: Amenorrhea, dehydration, infertility (may be temporary), hyperuricemia

Gastrointestinal: Abdominal pain, anorexia, colon necrosis, diarrhea, GI ulceration, mucositis, nausea, vomiting

Genitourinary: Discoloration of urine

Hematologic: Leukopenia/neutropenia (nadir: 10-14 days; recovery: by day 21); thrombocytopenia and anemia

Local: Skin "flare" at injection site, urticaria

Neuromuscular & skeletal: Weakness

Rare but important or life-threatening: Anaphylaxis, azoospermia, bilirubin increased, coma (when in combination with cisplatin or vincristine), conjunctivitis, fever, gonadal impairment (children), growth failure (prepubertal), hepatitis, hyperpigmentation (nail, skin & oral mucosa), infection, keratitis, lacrimation, myelodysplastic syndrome, neutropenic fever, neutropenic typhlitis, oligospermia, peripheral neurotoxicity (with intra-arterial doxorubicin), phlebosclerosis, radiation recall pneumonitis (children), secondary acute myelogenous leukemia (when in combination with cisplatin or vincristine), seizure (when in combination with cisplatin or vincristine), sepsis, shock, Stevens-Johnson syndrome, systemic hypersensitivity (including urticaria, pruritus, angioedema, dysphagia, and dyspnea), toxic epidermal necrolysis, transaminases increased, urticaria

Drug Interactions

Metabolism/Transport Effects Substrate of CYP2D6 (major), CYP3A4 (major), P-glycoprotein; **Note:** Assignment of Major/Minor substrate status based on clinically relevant drug interaction potential; **Inhibits** CYP2B6

(moderate), CYP2D6 (weak), CYP3A4 (weak); **Induces** P-glycoprotein

Avoid Concomitant Use

Avoid concomitant use of DOXOrubicin (Conventional) with any of the following: BCG; CloZAPine; Conivaptan; Dabigatran Etexilate; Dipyrone; Fusidic Acid (Systemic); Natalizumab; Pimecrolimus; Pimozide; Sofosbuvir; Tacrolimus (Topical); Tofacitinib; Vaccines (Live); Vin-CRIStine (Liposomal)

Increased Effect/Toxicity

DOXOrubicin (Conventional) may increase the levels/effects of: ARIPiprazole; CloZAPine; CYP2B6 Substrates; Dofetilide; Leflunomide; Lomitapide; Mercaptopurine; Natalizumab; Pimozide; Tofacitinib; Vaccines (Live); Vitamin K Antagonists; Zidovudine

The levels/effects of DOXOrubicin (Conventional) may be increased by: Abiraterone Acetate; Bevacizumab; Conivaptan; Cyclophosphamide; CycloSPORINE (Systemic); CYP2D6 Inhibitors (Moderate); CYP2D6 Inhibitors (Strong); CYP3A4 Inhibitors (Moderate); CYP3A4 Inhibitors (Strong); Dasatinib; Denosumab; Dipyrone; Fusidic Acid (Systemic); Luliconazole; Mifepristone; P-glycoprotein/ABCB1 Inhibitors; Pimecrolimus; Roflumilast; SORAfenib; Stiripentol; Tacrolimus (Topical); Taxane Derivatives; Trastuzumab

Decreased Effect

DOXOrubicin (Conventional) may decrease the levels/effects of: Afatinib; BCG; Brentuximab Vedotin; Cardiac Glycosides; Coccidioidin Skin Test; Dabigatran Etexilate; Linagliptin; P-glycoprotein/ABCB1 Substrates; Sipuleucel-T; Sofosbuvir; Stavudine; Vaccines (Inactivated); Vaccines (Live); VinCRIStine (Liposomal); Vitamin K Antagonists; Zidovudine

The levels/effects of DOXOrubicin (Conventional) may be decreased by: Bosentan; Cardiac Glycosides; CYP3A4 Inducers (Strong); Dabrafenib; Deferasirox; Dexrazoxane; Echinacea; Mitotane; Peginterferon Alfa-2b; P-glycoprotein/ABCB1 Inducers; Siltuximab; St Johns Wort; Tocilizumab

Stability Hazardous agent; use appropriate precautions for handling and disposal (NIOSH, 2012). Protect from light; store vials containing powder at room temperature, refrigerate vials containing liquid; reconstituted vials stable for 7 days at room temperature and 15 days if refrigerated and protected from light. Discard unused portion of preservative free injection vial. Incompatible with hydrocortisone, fluorouracil, furosemide, sodium bicarbonate, aminophylline, heparin, cephalothin, dexamethasone; unstable in solutions with a pH <3 or >7. Color change from red to purple indicates decomposition of drug.

Mechanism of Action Inhibition of DNA and RNA synthesis by intercalation between DNA base pairs by inhibition of topoisomerase II and by steric obstruction. Doxorubicin intercalates at points of local uncoiling of the double helix. Although the exact mechanism is unclear, it appears that direct binding to DNA (intercalation) and inhibition of DNA repair (topoisomerase II inhibition) result in blockade of DNA and RNA synthesis and fragmentation of DNA. Doxorubicin is also a powerful iron chelator; the iron-doxorubicin complex can bind DNA and cell membranes and produce free radicals that immediately cleave the DNA and cell membranes.

Pharmacokinetics (Adult data unless noted)

Distribution: Into breast milk; does not penetrate into CSF; distributes into cells rapidly with high concentrations in lung, kidney, muscle, spleen, and liver

Protein binding: 75%

Metabolism: In both the liver and in plasma to both active and inactive metabolites

Half-life, triphasic:

Primary: 30 minutes

Secondary: 3-3.5 hours for its metabolites

Terminal: 17-30 hours for doxorubicin and its metabolites

Elimination: Undergoes triphasic elimination; 40% to 60% eventually excreted in bile and feces; <5% excreted in urine, primarily as unchanged drug and metabolites

Clearance:

Infants <2 years: 813 mL/minute/m^2

Children >2 years: 1540 mL/minute/m^2

Dosing: Usual Patient's ideal weight should be used to calculate body surface area. Lower dose regimens should be given to patients with decreased bone marrow reserve, prior radiation therapy, or marrow infiltration with malignant cells.

I.V. (refer to individual protocols):

Children: 35-75 mg/m^2 as a single dose, repeat every 21 days; or 20-30 mg/m^2 once weekly; or 60-90 mg/m^2 given as a continuous infusion over 96 hours every 3-4 weeks

Adults: 60-75 mg/m^2 as a single dose, repeat every 21 days; or 20-30 mg/m^2/day for 2-3 days, repeat in 4 weeks or 20 mg/m^2 once weekly

Dosing adjustment in hepatic impairment:

Bilirubin 1.2-3 mg/dL: Reduce dose by 50%

Bilirubin >3 mg/dL: Reduce dose by 75%

Administration Hazardous agent; use appropriate precautions for handling and disposal (NIOSH, 2012).

Parenteral: I.V. use only; reconstitute IVP doses with D$_5$W or NS to ensure isotonicity of the final solution; administer slow IVP at a rate no faster than over 3-5 minutes or by I.V. infusion over 1-4 hours at a concentration not to exceed 2 mg/mL, or by I.V. continuous infusion

Vesicant/Extravasation Risk Vesicant

Monitoring Parameters CBC with differential, erythrocyte and platelet count; serum uric acid, echocardiogram, radionuclide left ventricular ejection fraction, liver enzymes, and bilirubin; observe I.V. injection site for infiltration and vein irritation

Additional Information Myelosuppressive effects:

WBC: Moderate

Platelets: Moderate

Onset (days): 7

Nadir (days): 10-14

Recovery (days): 21-28

Dosage Forms Excipient information presented when available (limited, particularly for generics); consult specific product labeling. [DSC] = Discontinued product

Solution, Intravenous, as hydrochloride:

Adriamycin: 2 mg/mL (5 mL, 10 mL, 25 mL, 100 mL)

Generic: 2 mg/mL (5 mL, 10 mL, 25 mL, 100 mL)

Solution, Intravenous, as hydrochloride [preservative free]:

Generic: 2 mg/mL (5 mL, 10 mL, 25 mL, 75 mL, 100 mL)

Solution Reconstituted, Intravenous, as hydrochloride:

Adriamycin: 10 mg (1 ea); 20 mg (1 ea); 50 mg (1 ea)

Generic: 50 mg (1 ea)

Solution Reconstituted, Intravenous, as hydrochloride [preservative free]:

Generic: 10 mg (1 ea); 50 mg (1 ea [DSC])

References

Berg SL, Grisell DL, DeLaney TF, et al, "Principles of Treatment of Pediatric Solid Tumors," *Pediatr Clin North Am*, 1991, 38(2):249-67.

Ishii E, Hara T, Ohkubo K, et al, "Treatment of Childhood Acute Lymphoblastic Leukemia With Intermediate Dose Cytosine Arabinoside and Adriamycin," *Med Pediatr Oncol*, 1986, 14(2):73-7.

Legha SS, Benjamin RS, Mackay B, et al, "Reduction of Doxorubicin Cardiotoxicity by Prolonged Continuous Intravenous Infusion," *Ann Intern Med*, 1982, 96(2):133-9.

National Institute for Occupational Safety and Health (NIOSH), "NIOSH List of Antineoplastic and Other Hazardous Drugs in Healthcare Settings 2012." Available at http://www.cdc.gov/niosh/docs/2012-150/pdfs/2012-150.pdf. Accessed January 21, 2013.

◆ **Doxorubicin HCl** *see* DOXOrubicin (Conventional) *on page 718*

◆ **Doxorubicin Hydrochloride** *see* DOXOrubicin (Conventional) *on page 718*

♦ **Doxorubicin Hydrochloride For Injection, USP (Can)**
see DOXOrubicin (Conventional) *on page 718*

♦ **Doxorubicin Hydrochloride Injection (Can)** *see* DOX-Orubicin (Conventional) *on page 718*

♦ **Doxy 100** *see* Doxycycline *on page 721*

♦ **Doxycin (Can)** *see* Doxycycline *on page 721*

Doxycycline (doks i SYE kleen)

Medication Safety Issues
Sound-alike/look-alike issues:
Doxycycline may be confused with dicyclomine, doxepin, doxylamine
Doxy100 may be confused with Doxil
Monodox may be confused with Maalox
Oracea may be confused with Orencia
Vibramycin may be confused with vancomycin, Vibativ
International issues:
Oracea (U.S brand name) is marketed in Canada under the brand name Apprilon

Related Information
Oral Medications That Should Not Be Crushed or Altered *on page 2438*

Brand Names: U.S. Adoxa; Adoxa Pak 1/100; Adoxa Pak 1/150; Adoxa Pak 2/100; Alodox Convenience; Avidoxy; Doryx; Doxy 100; Monodox; Morgidox; NicAzelDoxy 30; NicAzelDoxy 60; Ocudox; Oracea; Vibramycin

Brand Names: Canada Apo-Doxy; Apo-Doxy Tabs; Apprilon; Dom-Doxycycline; Doxycin; Doxytab; Periostat; PHL-Doxycycline; PMS-Doxycycline; Teva-Doxycycline; Vibra-Tabs; Vibramycin

Therapeutic Category Antibiotic, Tetracycline Derivative

Generic Availability (U.S.) May be product dependent

Use Treatment of infections caused by susceptible *Rickettsia*, *Chlamydia*, and *Mycoplasma*; alternative to mefloquine for malaria prophylaxis; treatment for syphilis, uncomplicated *Neisseria gonorrhoeae*, *Listeria*, *Actinomyces israelii*, *Fusobacterium fusiforme*, and *Clostridium* infections in penicillin-allergic patients; used for community-acquired pneumonia and other common infections due to susceptible organisms; anthrax due to *Bacillus anthracis*, including inhalational anthrax (postexposure); treatment of infections caused by uncommon susceptible gram-negative and gram-positive organisms, including *Borrelia recurrentis*, *Ureaplasma urealyticum*, *Haemophilus ducreyi*, *Yersinia pestis*, *Francisella tularensis*, *Vibrio cholerae*, *Campylobacter fetus*, *Brucella* spp, *Bartonella bacilliformis*, and *Calymmatobacterium granulomatis*, Q fever, Lyme disease; treatment of inflammatory lesions associated with rosacea; adjunct to amebicides for intestinal amebiasis; adjunct for treatment of severe acne (FDA approved in ages ≥8 years and adults); treatment of inflammatory lesions (papules and pustules) associated with rosacea (Oracea®; FDA approved in adults). Has also been used for community-acquired MRSA cellulitis, in ehrlichiosis and management of malignant pleural effusions with intrapleural administration.

Pregnancy Risk Factor D

Pregnancy Considerations Tetracyclines cross the placenta and accumulate in developing teeth and long tubular bones. Therapeutic doses of doxycycline during pregnancy are unlikely to produce substantial teratogenic risk, but data are insufficient to say that there is no risk. In general, reports of exposure have been limited to short durations of therapy in the first trimester. Tetracyclines may discolor fetal teeth following maternal use during pregnancy; the specific teeth involved and the portion of the tooth affected depends on the timing and duration of exposure relative to tooth calcification. As a class, tetracyclines are generally considered second-line antibiotics in pregnant women and their use should be avoided.

Tetracycline medications should be used during pregnancy only when other medications are contraindicated or ineffective (Mylonas, 2011).

Breast-Feeding Considerations Doxycycline is excreted in breast milk (Chung, 2002). According to the manufacturer, the decision to continue or discontinue breast-feeding during therapy should take into account the risk of exposure to the infant and the benefits of treatment to the mother. Although nursing is not specifically contraindicated, the effects of long-term exposure via breast milk are not known. Oral absorption of doxycycline is not markedly influenced by simultaneous ingestion of milk; therefore, oral absorption of doxycycline by the breast-feeding infant would not be expected to be diminished by the calcium in the maternal milk. Nondose-related effects could include modification of bowel flora.

Contraindications Hypersensitivity to doxycycline, tetracycline, or any component

Warnings Syrup contains sodium metabisulfite which may cause allergic reactions in susceptible individuals. Oracea® should not be used for the treatment or prophylaxis of bacterial infections since the lower dose of drug per capsule may be subtherapeutic and promote resistance.

Photosensitivity reaction may occur with this drug; avoid prolonged exposure to sunlight or tanning equipment. Do not administer to children <8 years of age (except in treatment of anthrax exposure, tickborne rickettsial diseases, or ehrlichiosis); administration of tetracycline 25 mg/kg/day was associated with decreased fibular growth rate in premature infants (reversible with discontinuation of drug); retardation of skeletal development has been observed in fetal animal studies. Use of tetracyclines during tooth development may cause permanent discoloration of the teeth and enamel hypoplasia; staining of teeth is dose-related so that duration of therapy should be minimized; doxycycline may be less likely to stain developing teeth than tetracycline since it binds less strongly to calcium; pseudomembranous colitis has been reported with doxycycline; prolonged use may result in superinfection. Autoimmune syndromes have been reported. Tetracyclines may induce hyperpigmentation in many organs, including nails, bone, skin (diffuse pigmentation as well as over sites of scars and injury), eyes, thyroid, visceral tissue, oral cavity (teeth, mucosa, alveolar bone), sclerae, and heart valves independently of time or amount of drug administration. Prolonged use may result in fungal or bacterial superinfection, including *C. difficile*-associated diarrhea (CDAD) and pseudomembranous colitis; CDAD has been observed >2 months postantibiotic treatment.

Precautions Use with caution in patients with renal impairment; increased BUN secondary to antianabolic effects may occur. Hepatotoxicity rarely occurs; if symptomatic, assess liver function tests and discontinue drug. Pseudotumor cerebri has been (rarely) reported with tetracycline use; usually resolves with discontinuation; bulging fontanels have been reported in infants.

Adverse Reactions
Central nervous system: Bulging fontanel (infants), headache, intracranial hypertension (adults), pericarditis
Dermatologic: Discoloration of thyroid gland (brown/black, no dysfunction reported), erythema multiforme, erythematous rash, exfoliative dermatitis, maculopapular rash, skin hyperpigmentation, skin photosensitivity, Stevens-Johnson syndrome, toxic epidermal necrolysis, urticaria
Endocrine & metabolic: Hypoglycemia
Gastrointestinal: Anorexia, *Clostridium difficile* associated diarrhea, dental discoloration (children), diarrhea, dysphagia, enterocolitis, esophageal ulcer, esophagitis, glossitis, nausea, upper abdominal pain, vomiting
Genitourinary: Vaginitis (bacterial, 3%), vulvovaginal disease (mycotic infection, 2%), inflammatory anogenital lesion

Hematologic & oncologic: Anaphylactoid purpura, eosinophilia, hemolytic anemia, neutropenia, thrombocytopenia

Hepatic: Hepatotoxicity (rare)

Hypersensitivity: Anaphylaxis, angioedema, serum sickness

Neuromuscular & skeletal: Exacerbation of systemic lupus erythematosus

Renal: Increased blood urea nitrogen (dose related)

Note: Additional adverse reactions not listed above that have been reported with Oracea or Periostat (Canadian availability; not available in the U.S.):

Periostat: Arthralgia (6%), dyspepsia (6%), dysmenorrhea (4%), pain (4%), bronchitis (3%)

Oracea: Nasopharyngitis (5%), hypertension (3%), sinusitis (3%), anxiety (2%), fungal infection (2%), increased blood pressure (2%), increased lactate dehydrogenase (2%), increased serum AST (2%), influenza (2%), pain (2%), abdominal pain (1% to 2%), back pain (1%), hyperglycemia (1%), sinus headache (1%), xerostomia (1%)

Drug Interactions

Metabolism/Transport Effects Inhibits CYP3A4 (weak)

Avoid Concomitant Use

Avoid concomitant use of Doxycycline with any of the following: BCG; Pimozide; Retinoic Acid Derivatives; Strontium Ranelate

Increased Effect/Toxicity

Doxycycline may increase the levels/effects of: ARIPiprazole; Dofetilide; Lomitapide; Mipomersen; Neuromuscular-Blocking Agents; Pimozide; Porfimer; Retinoic Acid Derivatives; Vitamin K Antagonists

Decreased Effect

Doxycycline may decrease the levels/effects of: BCG; Penicillins; Sodium Picosulfate; Typhoid Vaccine

The levels/effects of Doxycycline may be decreased by: Antacids; Barbiturates; Bile Acid Sequestrants; Bismuth; Bismuth Subsalicylate; Calcium Salts; CarBAMazepine; Fosphenytoin; Iron Salts; Lanthanum; Magnesium Salts; Multivitamins/Minerals (with ADEK, Folate, Iron); Multivitamins/Minerals (with AE, No Iron); Phenytoin; Quinapril; Rifampin; Strontium Ranelate; Sucralfate; Sucroferric Oxyhydroxide

Food Interactions

Ethanol: Chronic ethanol ingestion may reduce the serum concentration of doxycycline.

Food: Doxycycline serum levels may be slightly decreased if taken with food or milk. Administration with iron or calcium may decrease doxycycline absorption. May decrease absorption of calcium, iron, magnesium, zinc, and amino acids. Management: Doryx® tablets can be administered without regard to meals.

Stability Store below 30°C (86°F); protect from light. Reconstituted oral doxycycline suspension is stable for 2 weeks at room temperature; I.V. doxycycline solutions must be protected from direct sunlight

Mechanism of Action Inhibits protein synthesis by binding with the 30S and possibly the 50S ribosomal subunit(s) of susceptible bacteria; may also cause alterations in the cytoplasmic membrane

Periostat® capsules (Canadian availability; not available in the U.S.): Proposed mechanism: Has been shown to inhibit collagenase activity *in vitro*. Also has been noted to reduce elevated collagenase activity in the gingival crevicular fluid of patients with periodontal disease. Systemic levels do not reach inhibitory concentrations against bacteria.

Pharmacokinetics (Adult data unless noted)

Absorption: Almost completely from the GI tract; absorption can be reduced by food or milk by 20%

Distribution: Widely distributed into body tissues and fluids including synovial and pleural fluid, bile, bronchial secretions; poor penetration into the CSF; appears in breast milk

Protein binding: 80% to 85%

Metabolism: Not metabolized in the liver; partially inactivated in the GI tract by chelate formation

Bioavailability: Reduced at high pH; may be clinically significant in patients with gastrectomy, gastric bypass surgery, or who are otherwise deemed achlorhydric

Half-life: 12-15 hours (usually increases to 22-24 hours with multiple dosing); Oracea®: 21hours

Time to peak serum concentration: Oral: Within 1.5-4 hours

Elimination: In the urine (23%) and feces (30%)

Dialysis: Not dialyzable (0% to 5%)

Dosing: Usual

Children <8 years:

Anthrax: Note: In the presence of systemic involvement, extensive edema, and/or lesions on head/neck, doxycycline should initially be administered I.V. Initial treatment should include two or more agents per CDC recommendations. Agents suggested for use in conjunction with doxycycline include rifampin, vancomycin, penicillin, ampicillin, chloramphenicol, imipenem, clindamycin, or clarithromycin. For bioterrorism postexposure, continue combined therapy for 60 days; if natural exposure, 7-10 days of therapy.

Treatment: I.V.: 2.2 mg/kg/dose every 12 hours (maximum dose: 100 mg/dose); may switch to oral therapy (same dosing) when clinically appropriate (CDC, 2001)

Prophylaxis; postexposure (inhalation or cutaneous): Oral: 2.2 mg/kg/dose every 12 hours for 60 days (maximum dose: 100 mg/dose) (CDC, 2001; *Red Book*, 2009)

Ehrlichiosis: Oral, I.V.: 2 mg/kg/dose every 12 hours (maximum dose: 100 mg/dose) for 3 days after defervescence and at least 7 days total (*Red Book*, 2009)

Tickborne rickettsial disease: Oral, I.V.: 2.2 mg/kg/dose every 12 hours (maximum dose: 100 mg/dose) for 5-7 days. Severe or complicated disease may require longer treatment; human granulocytotropic anaplasmosis (HGA) should be treated for 10-14 days (CDC, 2006)

Children ≥8 years:

General dosing: Oral, I.V.: 2-4 mg/kg/**day** divided every 12-24 hours, maximum daily dose: 200 mg/**day**

Anthrax (if strain is proven susceptible): Note: In the presence of systemic involvement, extensive edema, and/or lesions on head/neck, doxycycline should initially be administered I.V. Initial treatment should include two or more agents per CDC recommendations. Agents suggested for use in conjunction with doxycycline include rifampin, vancomycin, penicillin, ampicillin, chloramphenicol, imipenem, clindamycin, or clarithromycin. For bioterrorism postexposure, continue combined therapy for 60 days; if natural exposure, administer 7-10 days of therapy.

Treatment: I.V.: 2.2 mg/kg/dose every 12 hours (maximum dose: 100 mg/dose); may switch to oral therapy (same dosing) when clinically appropriate

Prophylaxis; postexposure (inhalation or cutaneous): Oral: 2.2 mg/kg/dose every 12 hours for 60 days (maximum dose: 100 mg/dose)

Brucellosis: Oral: 1-2 mg/kg/dose twice daily for 6 weeks (maximum dose: 100 mg/dose); use in combination with rifampin

Chlamydial infections, uncomplicated: Oral: 100 mg/dose twice daily for 7 days

Lyme disease, Q fever, or Tularemia: Oral: 100 mg/dose twice daily for 14-21 days

Malaria:
Treatment: Oral, I.V.: 2.2 mg/kg/dose twice daily for 7 days (maximum dose: 100 mg/dose) (CDC, 2011); for uncomplicated cases, combination therapy with quinine sulfate is recommended; in severe cases, combination therapy with quinidine gluconate should be used; **Note:** Duration of either quinine sulfate or quinidine gluconate is region-specific; consult CDC for current recommendations.
Prophylaxis: Oral: 2.2 mg/kg/dose once daily (maximum dose: 100 mg/day) starting 1-2 days before travel to the area with endemic infection, continuing daily during travel and for 4 weeks after leaving endemic area; maximum duration of prophylaxis: 4 months

MRSA, community-acquired cellulitis (purulent); skin/soft tissue infections: Oral:
≤45 kg: 2 mg/kg/dose every 12 hours for 5-10 days
>45 kg: 100 mg twice daily for 5-10 days (Liu, 2011)
Tickborne rickettsial disease or Ehrlichiosis: >45 kg: Oral, I.V.: 100 mg every 12 hours. Severe or complicated disease may require longer treatment; HGA should be treated for 10-14 days

Adolescents and Adults:
General dosing: Oral, I.V.: 100-200 mg/day in 1-2 divided doses
Anthrax (if strain is proven susceptible): Refer to Children's dosing for **"Note"** on route, combined therapy, and duration
Treatment: I.V.: 100 mg every 12 hours for 60 days (substitute oral antibiotics for I.V. antibiotics as soon as clinical condition improves)
Prophylaxis; postexposure (inhalation or cutaneous): Oral: 100 mg every 12 hours for 60 days
Chlamydial infections, uncomplicated: Oral: 100 mg/dose twice daily for 7 days
Lyme disease, Q fever, or Tularemia: Oral: 100 mg/dose twice daily for 14-21 days
Malaria:
Treatment: Oral, I.V.: 100 mg twice daily for 7 days (CDC, 2011); for uncomplicated cases, combination therapy with quinine sulfate is recommended; in severe cases, combination therapy with quinidine gluconate should be used; **Note:** Duration of either quinine sulfate or quinidine gluconate is region-specific; consult CDC for current recommendations.
Prophylaxis: Oral: 100 mg/dose once daily starting 1-2 days before travel to the area with endemic infection, continuing daily during travel, and for 4 weeks after leaving endemic area; maximum duration of prophylaxis: 4 months
MRSA, community-acquired cellulitis (purulent): Oral: 100 mg twice daily for 5-10 days (Liu, 2011)
Nongonococcal urethritis caused by *C. trachomatis* or *U. urealyticum*: Oral: 100 mg/dose twice daily for 7 days
Pelvic inflammatory disease:
Treatment, inpatient: Oral, I.V.: 100 mg every 12 hours for 14 days administered with cefoxitin or cefotetan; may transition to oral doxycycline (add clindamycin or metronidazole if tubo-ovarian abscess present) to complete the 14 days of therapy (CDC, 2010)
Treatment, outpatient: Oral: 100 mg every 12 hours for 14 days (with or without metronidazole); preceded by a single I.M. dose of cefoxitin (plus oral probenecid) or ceftriaxone (CDC, 2010)
Periodontitis: Oral (Periostat®): 20 mg twice daily as an adjunct following scaling and root planing; may be administered for up to 9 months
Rosacea: Oral (Oracea®): 40 mg once daily in the morning. **Note:** Oracea® capsules are not bioequivalent to other doxycycline products.

Sclerosing agent for pleural effusion: 500 mg in 25-30 mL of NS instilled into the pleural space to control pleural effusions associated with metastatic tumors; or for recurrent malignant pleural effusions: 500 mg in 250 mL NS
Tickborne rickettsial disease or ehrlichiosis: Oral, I.V.: 100 mg every 12 hours. Severe or complicated disease may require longer treatment; HGA should be treated for 10-14 days
Dosing adjustment in renal impairment: No adjustment necessary

Administration
Oral: Administer capsules or tablets with adequate amounts of fluid; avoid antacids, infant formula, milk, dairy products, and iron for 1 hour before or 2 hours after administration of doxycycline (unless extemporaneously prepared in the instance of public health emergency when milk or pudding is appropriate); may be administered with food to decrease GI upset; shake suspension well before use
Doryx®: May break up the tablet and sprinkle the delayed release pellets on a spoonful of applesauce. Do **not** crush or damage the delayed release pellets; loss or damage of pellets prevents using the dose. Swallow the Doryx®/applesauce mixture immediately without chewing. Discard mixture if it cannot be used immediately.
Parenteral: For I.V. use only; administer by slow I.V. intermittent infusion over a minimum of 1-2 hours at a concentration not to exceed 1 mg/mL (may be infused over 1-4 hours); concentrations <0.1 mg/mL are not recommended
Sclerosing agent:
To control pleural effusions associated with metastatic tumors: Instill into the pleural space through a thoracostomy tube following drainage of the accumulated pleural fluid; clamp the tube then remove the fluid
For recurrent malignant pleural effusions: Administer via chest tube lavage, clamp tube for 24 hours then drain

Monitoring Parameters Periodic monitoring of renal, hematologic, and hepatic function tests; observe for changes in bowel frequency

Test Interactions Injectable tetracycline formulations (if they contain large amounts of ascorbic acid) may result in a false-negative urine glucose using glucose oxidase tests (eg, Clinistix®, Diastix, Tes-Tape®); false elevations of urinary catecholamines with fluorescence

Additional Information Injection contains ascorbic acid. According to the CDC, staining of the teeth is negligible with short courses of doxycycline and is of minimal consequence in children >6 or 7 years of age because visible tooth formation is complete by this age. Benefits outweigh the risks for rickettsial infections, ehrlichiosis, anthrax, and cholera (CDC, 2006; *Red Book*, 2009). Oracea® capsules are not bioequivalent to other doxycycline products.

Dosage Forms Considerations
Alodox Convenience kits contain doxycycline tablets 20 mg, plus eyelid cleanser
Morgidox kits contain doxycycline capsules 100 mg, plus AcuWash moisturizing Daily Cleanser
NizAzel Doxy kits contain doxycycline tablets 100 mg, plus NicAzel FORTE dietary supplement tablets
Ocudox kits contain doxycycline capsules 50 mg, plus eyelid cleanser and Tears Again Advanced eyelid spray

Dosage Forms Excipient information presented when available (limited, particularly for generics); consult specific product labeling.
Capsule, Oral, as hyclate [strength expressed as base]:
Morgidox: 100 mg [contains brilliant blue fcf (fd&c blue #1)]
Vibramycin: 100 mg [contains brilliant blue fcf (fd&c blue #1)]
Generic: 50 mg, 100 mg

Capsule, Oral, as monohydrate [strength expressed as base]:

Adoxa: 150 mg [contains fd&c red #40, fd&c yellow #6 (sunset yellow)]

Monodox: 75 mg, 100 mg

Generic: 50 mg, 75 mg, 100 mg, 150 mg

Capsule Delayed Release, Oral, as monohydrate [strength expressed as base]:

Oracea: 40 mg

Kit, Combination, as hyclate [strength expressed as base]:

Alodox Convenience: 20 mg

Morgidox: 1 x 100 mg, 2 x 100 mg [contains brilliant blue fcf (fd&c blue #1), cetyl alcohol, edetate disodium]

Ocudox: 50 mg [contains brilliant blue fcf (fd&c blue #1)]

Kit, Oral, as monohydrate [strength expressed as base]:

NicAzelDoxy 30: 100 mg [contains brilliant blue fcf (fd&c blue #1), fd&c yellow #10 aluminum lake, fd&c yellow #6 (sunset yellow), fd&c yellow #6 aluminum lake, tartrazine (fd&c yellow #5)]

NicAzelDoxy 60: 100 mg [contains brilliant blue fcf (fd&c blue #1), fd&c yellow #10 aluminum lake, fd&c yellow #6 (sunset yellow), fd&c yellow #6 aluminum lake, tartrazine (fd&c yellow #5)]

Solution Reconstituted, Intravenous, as hyclate [strength expressed as base, preservative free]:

Doxy 100: 100 mg (1 ea)

Generic: 100 mg (1 ea)

Suspension Reconstituted, Oral, as monohydrate [strength expressed as base]:

Vibramycin: 25 mg/5 mL (60 mL) [contains brilliant blue fcf (fd&c blue #1), methylparaben, propylparaben; raspberry flavor]

Generic: 25 mg/5 mL (60 mL)

Syrup, Oral, as calcium [strength expressed as base]:

Vibramycin: 50 mg/5 mL (473 mL) [contains butylparaben, propylene glycol, propylparaben, sodium metabisulfite; raspberry-apple flavor]

Tablet, Oral, as hyclate [strength expressed as base]:

Generic: 20 mg, 100 mg

Tablet, Oral, as monohydrate [strength expressed as base]:

Adoxa: 50 mg

Adoxa: 75 mg [contains fd&c yellow #10 aluminum lake, fd&c yellow #6 (sunset yellow)]

Adoxa: 100 mg

Adoxa Pak 1/100: 100 mg [contains fd&c yellow #10 aluminum lake, fd&c yellow #6 (sunset yellow)]

Adoxa Pak 2/100: 100 mg [contains fd&c yellow #10 aluminum lake, fd&c yellow #6 (sunset yellow)]

Adoxa Pak 1/150: 150 mg [scored; contains fd&c yellow #6 (sunset yellow)]

Avidoxy: 100 mg [contains fd&c yellow #10 aluminum lake, fd&c yellow #6 aluminum lake]

Generic: 50 mg, 75 mg, 100 mg, 150 mg

Tablet Delayed Release, Oral, as hyclate [strength expressed as base]:

Doryx: 150 mg, 200 mg [scored]

Generic: 75 mg, 100 mg, 150 mg

Extemporaneous Preparations If a public health emergency is declared and liquid doxycycline is unavailable for the treatment of anthrax, emergency doses may be prepared for children or adults who cannot swallow tablets.

Add 20 mL of water to one 100 mg tablet. Allow tablet to soak in the water for 5 minutes to soften. Crush into a fine powder and stir until well mixed. Appropriate dose should be taken from this mixture. To increase palatability, mix with food or drink. If mixing with drink, add 15 mL of milk, chocolate milk, chocolate pudding, or apple juice to the appropriate dose of mixture. If using apple juice, also add 4 teaspoons of sugar. Doxycycline and water mixture may be stored at room temperature for up to 24 hours.

U.S. Food and Drug Administration, Center for Drug Evaluation and Research, "Public Health Emergency Home Preparation Instructions for Doxycycline." Available at http://www.fda.gov/Drugs/Emergency-Preparedness/BioterrorismandDrugPreparedness/ucm130996.htm

References

Bradley JS, Byington CL, Shah SS, et al, "The Management of Community-Acquired Pneumonia in Infants and Children Older Than 3 Months of Age: Clinical Practice Guidelines by the Pediatric Infectious Diseases Society and the Infectious Diseases Society of America", *Clin Infect Dis*, 2011, 53(7):e25-76.

Centers for Disease Control and Prevention (CDC), "Guidelines for the Prevention and Treatment of Opportunistic Infections Among HIV-Exposed and HIV-Infected Children," *MMWR Recomm Rep*, 2009, 58(RR-11):1-166. Available at http://aidsinfo.nih.gov/contentfiles/Pediatric_OI.pdf

Centers for Disease Control and Prevention (CDC), "Guidelines for Treatment of Malaria in the United States," Treatment Table Update, September 23, 2011. Available at http://www.cdc.gov/malaria/pdf/treatmenttable.pdf

Centers for Disease Control and Prevention, "Update: Investigation of Anthrax Associated with Intentional Exposure and Interim Public Health Guidelines, October 2001," *MMWR Morb Mortal Wkly Rep*, 2001, 50(41):889-93.

Chapman AS, Bakken JS, Folk SM, et al, "Diagnosis and Management of Tickborne Rickettsial Diseases: Rocky Mountain Spotted Fever, Ehrlichioses, and Anaplasmosis–United States: A Practical Guide for Physicians and Other Health-Care and Public Health Professionals," *MMWR Recomm Rep*, 2006, 55(RR-4):1-27.

Inglesby TV, Henderson DA, Bartlett JG, et al, "Anthrax as a Biological Weapon: Medical and Public Health Management. Working Group on Civilian Biodefense," *JAMA*, 1999, 281(18):1735-45.

Liu C, Bayer A, Cosgrove SE, et al, "Clinical Practice Guidelines by the Infectious Diseases Society of America for the Treatment of Methicillin-Resistant *Staphylococcus Aureus* Infections in Adults and Children: Executive Summary," *Clin Infect Dis*, 2011, 52(3):285-92.

Mylonas I, "Antibiotic Chemotherapy During Pregnancy and Lactation Period: Aspects for Consideration," *Arch Gynecol Obstet*, 2011, 283 (1):7-18.

Red Book: 2009 Report of the Committee on Infectious Diseases, "*Ehrlichia* and *Anaplasma* Infections (Human Ehrlichiosis and Anaplasmosis)," 28th ed, Pickering LK, ed, Elk Grove Village, IL: American Academy of Pediatrics, 2009, 284-7.

Red Book: 2009 Report of the Committee on Infectious Diseases, "Tetracyclines," 28th ed, Pickering LK, ed, Elk Grove Village, IL: American Academy of Pediatrics, 2009, 739.

Stern EJ, Uhde KB, Shadomy SV, et al, "Conference Report on Public Health and Clinical Guidelines for Anthrax," *Emerg Infect Dis*, 2008, 14(4). Available at http://wwwnc.cdc.gov/eid/article/14/4/07-0969.htm

Workowski KA, Berman S, and Centers for Disease Control and Prevention (CDC), "Sexually Transmitted Diseases Treatment Guidelines, 2010," *MMWR Recomm Rep*, 2010, 59(RR-12):1-110.

◆ **Doxycycline Calcium** *see* Doxycycline *on page 721*

◆ **Doxycycline Hyclate** *see* Doxycycline *on page 721*

◆ **Doxycycline Monohydrate** *see* Doxycycline *on page 721*

◆ **Doxytab (Can)** *see* Doxycycline *on page 721*

◆ **DPA** *see* Valproic Acid and Derivatives *on page 2102*

◆ **DPE** *see* Dipivefrin *on page 692*

◆ **D-Penicillamine** *see* PenicillAMINE *on page 1627*

◆ **DPH** *see* Phenytoin *on page 1663*

◆ **Dramamine [OTC]** *see* DimenhyDRINATE *on page 670*

◆ **Dramamine Less Drowsy [OTC]** *see* Meclizine *on page 1317*

◆ **Dr Gs Clear Nail [OTC]** *see* Tolnaftate *on page 2044*

◆ **Driminate [OTC]** *see* DimenhyDRINATE *on page 670*

◆ **Drisdol** *see* Ergocalciferol *on page 774*

◆ **Drisdol® (Can)** *see* Ergocalciferol *on page 774*

◆ **Dristan Long Lasting Nasal (Can)** *see* Oxymetazoline (Nasal) *on page 1577*

◆ **Dristan Spray [OTC]** *see* Oxymetazoline (Nasal) *on page 1577*

◆ **Drixoral Nasal (Can)** *see* Oxymetazoline (Nasal) *on page 1577*

◆ **Drixoral® ND (Can)** *see* Pseudoephedrine *on page 1770*

Dronabinol (droe NAB i nol)

Medication Safety Issues
Sound-alike/look-alike issues:
Dronabinol may be confused with droperidol
Brand Names: U.S. Marinol
Brand Names: Canada Marinol®
Therapeutic Category Antiemetic
Generic Availability (U.S.) Yes
Use Treatment of nausea and vomiting secondary to cancer chemotherapy in patients who have not responded to conventional antiemetics; treatment of anorexia associated with weight loss in AIDS patients
Pregnancy Risk Factor C
Pregnancy Considerations Adverse events have been observed in animal reproduction studies.
Breast-Feeding Considerations Dronabinol is excreted in breast milk. Breast-feeding is not recommended by the manufacturer.
Contraindications Hypersensitivity to dronabinol, sesame oil, or any component, marijuana, or cannabinoids; should not be used in patients with a history of schizophrenia
Warnings Dronabinol has a high potential for abuse; limit antiemetic therapy availability to current cycle of chemotherapy
Precautions Use with caution in patients with heart disease, history of substance abuse, hepatic disease, or seizure disorders (may lower seizure threshold); reduce dosage in patients with severe hepatic impairment; tolerance to CNS side effects usually occurs in 1-3 days of continued use; tachyphylaxis and tolerance does not appear to develop when used as an appetite stimulant as efficacy has been documented in clinical trials for up to 5 months of treatment. Use with caution in patients with mania or depression as dronabinol may exacerbate these conditions

Adverse Reactions
Cardiovascular: Palpitations, tachycardia, vasodilation/facial flushing
Central nervous system: Abnormal thinking, amnesia, anxiety, ataxia, depersonalization, dizziness, euphoria, hallucination, paranoia, somnolence
Gastrointestinal: Abdominal pain, nausea, vomiting
Neuromuscular & skeletal: Weakness
Rare but important or life-threatening: Conjunctivitis, depression, diarrhea, fatigue, fecal incontinence, flushing, hypotension, myalgia, nightmares, seizure, speech difficulties, tinnitus, vision difficulties

Drug Interactions
Metabolism/Transport Effects Substrate of CYP2C9 (minor), CYP3A4 (minor); **Note:** Assignment of Major/Minor substrate status based on clinically relevant drug interaction potential
Avoid Concomitant Use There are no known interactions where it is recommended to avoid concomitant use.
Increased Effect/Toxicity
Dronabinol may increase the levels/effects of: Alcohol (Ethyl); CNS Depressants; Sympathomimetics

The levels/effects of Dronabinol may be increased by: Anticholinergic Agents; Cocaine; CYP2C9 Inhibitors (Moderate); CYP2C9 Inhibitors (Strong); CYP3A4 Inhibitors (Moderate); CYP3A4 Inhibitors (Strong); MAO Inhibitors; Ritonavir
Decreased Effect
The levels/effects of Dronabinol may be decreased by: CYP3A4 Inducers (Strong)
Food Interactions Administration with high-lipid meals may increase absorption.
Stability Store in a cool environment (46°F to 59°F); may be refrigerated; do not freeze

Mechanism of Action Unknown, may inhibit endorphins in the brain's emetic center, suppress prostaglandin synthesis, and/or inhibit medullary activity through an unspecified cortical action. Some pharmacologic effects appear to involve sympathomometic activity; tachyphylaxis to some effect (eg, tachycardia) may occur, but appetite-stimulating effects do not appear to wane over time. Antiemetic activity may be due to effect on cannabinoid receptors (CB1) within the central nervous system.

Pharmacodynamics
Onset of action: 30 minutes to 1 hour
Maximum effect: 2-4 hours
Duration:
Psychoactive effects: 4-6 hours
Appetite stimulation: 24 hours

Pharmacokinetics (Adult data unless noted)
Absorption: Oral: 90% to 95%; first-pass metabolism results in low systemic bioavailability
Distribution: V_d: ~10L/kg
Protein binding: ~97%
Metabolism: Extensive first-pass; metabolized in the liver to several metabolites some of which are active
Bioavailability: 10% to 20%
Half-life:
Biphasic: Alpha: 4 hours
Terminal: 25-36 hours
Dronabinol metabolites: 44-59 hours
Time to peak serum concentration: Within 0.5-4 hours
Elimination: Biliary excretion is the major route of elimination; 50% excreted in feces within 72 hours; 10% to 15% excreted in urine within 72 hours
Clearance: Adults: Mean 0.2 L/kg/hour (highly variable)

Dosing: Usual Oral:
Antiemetic: Children and Adults: 5 mg/m² 1-3 hours before chemotherapy, then give 5 mg/m²/dose every 2-4 hours after chemotherapy for a total of 4-6 doses/day; dose may be increased in 2.5 mg/m² increments to a maximum of 15 mg/m² per dose if needed
Alternative dosing: Adults: 5 mg 3-4 times/day; dosage may be escalated during a chemotherapy cycle or at subsequent cycles depending upon response
Appetite stimulant: Adults: 2.5 mg twice daily before lunch and dinner; if intolerant, a dosage of 2.5 mg once daily at night may be tried; maximum dosage (escalating): 10 mg twice daily
Administration May be administered without regard to meals; take before meals if used to stimulate appetite
Monitoring Parameters Heart rate, blood pressure
Test Interactions Decreased FSH, LH, growth hormone, and testosterone
Controlled Substance C-III
Dosage Forms Excipient information presented when available (limited, particularly for generics); consult specific product labeling.
Capsule, Oral:
Marinol: 2.5 mg, 5 mg, 10 mg [contains sesame oil]
Generic: 2.5 mg, 5 mg, 10 mg
References
Lane M, Smith FE, Sullivan RA, et al, "Dronabinol and Prochlorperazine Alone and in Combination as Antiemetic Agents for Cancer Chemotherapy," *Am J Clin Oncol*, 1990, 13(6):480-4.

Droperidol (droe PER i dole)

Medication Safety Issues
Sound-alike/look-alike issues:
Droperidol may be confused with dronabinol
Brand Names: Canada Droperidol Injection, USP
Therapeutic Category Antiemetic
Generic Availability (U.S.) Yes
Use Reduce the incidence of nausea and vomiting associated with surgical and diagnostic procedures in patients

for whom other treatments are ineffective or inappropriate (FDA approved in ages ≥2 years and adults)

Pregnancy Risk Factor C

Pregnancy Considerations Adverse events were observed in some animal reproduction studies. Although use in pregnancy has been reported, due to cases of QT prolongation and torsade de pointes (some fatal), use of other agents in pregnant women is preferred (ACOG, 2004).

Breast-Feeding Considerations It is not known if droperidol is excreted in breast milk. The manufacturer recommends that caution be exercised when administering droperidol to nursing women.

Contraindications Hypersensitivity to droperidol or any component; known or suspected QT prolongation (ie, in adults, prolonged QT_c is defined as >440 msec in males or >450 msec in females); congenital long QT syndrome

Warnings Cases of QT prolongation and torsade de pointes in patients treated with droperidol in doses within or even below the approved dosage range have been reported **[U.S. Boxed Warning]**. Some cases occurred in patients with no underlying risk factors for QT prolongation; fatalities have occurred. Droperidol should be reserved for patients who fail other treatments. Prior to its use, all patients should undergo a 12-lead ECG. If the QT interval is prolonged, droperidol should not be used. Droperidol should be used with extreme caution in patients with risk factors for prolonged QT syndrome, including: CHF; bradycardia; cardiac hypertrophy; any clinically significant cardiac disease; hypokalemia; hypomagnesemia; concomitant use of Class I or Class III antiarrhythmics, MAO inhibitors, or medications known to prolong the QT interval; age >65 years; concomitant use of medication known to induce hypokalemia or hypomagnesemia [eg, diuretics, laxatives, corticosteroids (supraphysiologic doses)]; alcohol abuse; and use of medications such as benzodiazepines, volatile anesthetics, and I.V. opiates.

The dosage of droperidol should be individualized; dosages should be started low and titrated upward. Not recommended for routine use in children for ambulatory operative procedures unless patient is being admitted to the hospital and other antiemetic therapies have failed (Gan, 2007). Continuous ECG monitoring should be done prior to treatment and for 2-3 hours after treatment to monitor for arrhythmias. I.V. fluids and other therapy to treat hypotension should be readily available; monitor patients carefully. Use reduced initial doses of opioids, if needed. May be sedating; use with caution in disorders where CNS depression is a feature; patients must be cautioned about performing tasks which require mental alertness (eg, operating machinery or driving). Neuromalignant syndrome may rarely occur; monitor for mental status changes, fever, muscle rigidity, and/or autonomic instability.

Precautions Use with caution in patients with impaired hepatic or renal function. Severe hypertension and tachycardia may occur in patients with pheochromocytoma. Use with caution in patients with decreased gastrointestinal motility, urinary retention, BPH, xerostomia, or visual problems; may cause anticholinergic effects (constipation, xerostomia, blurred vision, urinary retention); relative to other neuroleptics, droperidol has a low potency of cholinergic blockade

Adverse Reactions

Cardiovascular: Cardiac arrest, hypertension, hypotension (especially orthostatic), QT_c prolongation (dose dependent), tachycardia, torsade de pointes, ventricular tachycardia

Central nervous system: Anxiety, chills, depression (postoperative, transient), dizziness, drowsiness (postoperative) increased, dysphoria, extrapyramidal symptoms (akathisia, dystonia, oculogyric crisis), hallucinations

(postoperative), hyperactivity, neuroleptic malignant syndrome (NMS) (rare), restlessness

Respiratory: Bronchospasm, laryngospasm

Miscellaneous: Anaphylaxis, shivering

Drug Interactions

Metabolism/Transport Effects None known.

Avoid Concomitant Use

Avoid concomitant use of Droperidol with any of the following: Aclidinium; Amisulpride; Azelastine (Nasal); Highest Risk QTc-Prolonging Agents; Ipratropium (Oral Inhalation); Ivabradine; Metoclopramide; Mifepristone; Paraldehyde; Potassium Chloride; Sulpiride; Thalidomide; Tiotropium; Umeclidinium

Increased Effect/Toxicity

Droperidol may increase the levels/effects of: AbobotulinumtoxinA; Alcohol (Ethyl); Amisulpride; Anticholinergic Agents; Azelastine (Nasal); Buprenorphine; Cannabinoid-Containing Products; CNS Depressants; Highest Risk QTc-Prolonging Agents; Hydrocodone; Methotrimeprazine; Methylphenidate; Metoclopramide; Mirabegron; Moderate Risk QTc-Prolonging Agents; OnabotulinumtoxinA; Paraldehyde; Potassium Chloride; RimabotulinumtoxinB; Selective Serotonin Reuptake Inhibitors; Serotonin Modulators; Sulpiride; Thalidomide; Thiazide Diuretics; Tiotropium; Zolpidem

The levels/effects of Droperidol may be increased by: Acetylcholinesterase Inhibitors (Central); Aclidinium; Brimonidine (Topical); Cannabis; Dronabinol; Ipratropium (Oral Inhalation); Ivabradine; Kava Kava; Lithium; Magnesium Sulfate; MAO Inhibitors; Methotrimeprazine; Methylphenidate; Metyrosine; Mifepristone; Nabilone; Perampanel; Pramlintide; QTc-Prolonging Agents (Indeterminate Risk and Risk Modifying); Rufinamide; Serotonin Modulators; Sodium Oxybate; Tapentadol; Tetrahydrocannabinol; Umeclidinium

Decreased Effect

Droperidol may decrease the levels/effects of: Acetylcholinesterase Inhibitors (Central); Amphetamines; Anti-Parkinson's Agents (Dopamine Agonist); Quinagolide; Secretin

The levels/effects of Droperidol may be decreased by: Acetylcholinesterase Inhibitors (Central); Anti-Parkinson's Agents (Dopamine Agonist); Lithium

Stability Store at 20°C to 25°C (68°F to 77°F); excursions permitted to 15°C to 30°C (59°F to 86°F). Protect from light; store in carton until time of use. Solutions diluted in NS or D_5W (20 mg/L) are stable at room temperature for up to 7 days in polyvinyl chloride bags or glass bottles. Solutions diluted in LR are stable at room temperature for 24 hours in polyvinyl chloride bags and up to 7 days in glass bottles.

Mechanism of Action Droperidol is a butyrophenone antipsychotic; antiemetic effect is a result of blockade of dopamine stimulation of the chemoreceptor trigger zone. Other effects include alpha-adrenergic blockade, peripheral vascular dilation, and reduction of the pressor effect of epinephrine resulting in hypotension and decreased peripheral vascular resistance; may also reduce pulmonary artery pressure

Pharmacodynamics

Onset of action: 3-10 minutes

Maximum effect: Within 30 minutes

Duration: 2-4 hours (up to 12 hours)

Pharmacokinetics (Adult data unless noted)

V_d: Children: ~0.6 L/kg; Adults: ~1.5 L/kg (McKeage, 2006)

Absorption: I.M.: Rapid (Cressman, 1973)

Protein binding: 85% to 90% (McKeage, 2006)

Metabolism: Hepatic, to p-fluorophenylacetic acid, benzimidazolone, p-hydroxypiperidine

Half-life: Children: 1.7 hours; adults: 1.7-2.2 hours (McKeage, 2006)

Elimination: In urine (75%; <1% as unchanged drug) and feces (22%) (Cressman, 1973; McKeage, 2006)

Dosing: Usual Dosage must be individualized, based on age, body weight, underlying medical conditions, physical status, concomitant medications, type of anesthesia, and surgical procedure

Children 2-12 years:

Postoperative nausea and vomiting (PONV):

Prevention, if high risk for PONV: I.M., I.V.: 0.01-0.015 mg/kg/dose given near the end of surgery (Gan, 2007); maximum dose: 1.25 mg; administer additional doses after at least 6 hours with caution and only if potential benefit outweighs risks; **Note:** Previous reports suggested a higher dose of 0.075 mg/kg as effective; however, due to side-effects associated with the higher doses, doses >0.05 mg/kg are considered excessive and no longer recommended (Gan, 2007; Henzi, 2000).

Treatment (not first line): I.V.:

Manufacturer's labeling: **Maximum** initial dose: 0.1 mg/kg/dose; administer additional doses with extreme caution and only if potential benefit outweighs risks

Alternate dosing: Doses as low as 0.01-0.015 mg/kg/dose (up to 0.03 mg/kg) may be effective for breakthrough nausea and vomiting; maximum initial dose: 0.1 mg/kg; administer additional doses after at least 6 hours with caution and only if potential benefit outweighs risks

Adults:

Prevention of PONV: I.M., I.V.:

Manufacturer labeling: Maximum initial dose: 2.5 mg; additional doses of 1.25 mg may be administered with caution to achieve desired effect

Consensus guideline recommendations: 0.625-1.25 mg I.V. administered at the end of surgery (Gan, 2007)

Dosage adjustment in renal impairment: Specific dosing recommendations are not provided; use with caution.

Dosage adjustment in hepatic impairment: Specific dosing recommendations are not provided; use with caution.

Administration Parenteral: Administer by slow I.V. injection over 2-5 minutes; maximum concentration: 2.5 mg/mL (I.M. or I.V.); pH: 3-3.8.

Monitoring Parameters Prior to use: 12-lead ECG to identify patients with QT prolongation (use is contraindicated); continuous ECG during and for 2-3 hours after dosage administration is recommended. Blood pressure, heart rate, respiratory rate; serum potassium and magnesium; observe for dystonias, extrapyramidal side effects; temperature

Dosage Forms Excipient information presented when available (limited, particularly for generics); consult specific product labeling.

Solution, Injection:

Generic: 2.5 mg/mL (2 mL)

References

American College of Obstetrics and Gynecology (ACOG), "ACOG (American College of Obstetrics and Gynecology) Practice Bulletin: Nausea and Vomiting of Pregnancy," *Obstet Gynecol*, 2004, 103 (4):803-14.

Cressman WA, Plostnieks J, and Johnson PC, "Absorption, Metabolism and Excretion of Droperidol by Human Subjects Following Intramuscular and Intravenous Administration," *Anesthesiology*, 1973, 38 (4):363-9.

Gan TJ, Meyer TA, Apfel CC, et al, "Society for Ambulatory Anesthesia Guidelines for the Management of Postoperative Nausea and Vomiting," *Anesth Analg*, 2007, 105(6):1615-28.

Henzi I, Sonderegger J, and Tramer MR, "Efficacy, Dose-Response, and Adverse Effects of Droperidol for Prevention of Postoperative Nausea and Vomiting," *Can J Anaesth*, 2000, 47(6):537-51.

McKeage K, Simpson D, and Wagstaff AJ, "Intravenous Droperidol: A Review of Its Use in the Management of Postoperative Nausea and Vomiting," *Drugs*, 2006, 66(16):2123-47.

Yaster M, Sola JE, Pegoli W Jr, et al, "The Night After Surgery: Postoperative Management of the Pediatric Outpatient - Surgical and Anesthetic Aspects," *Pediatr Clin North Am*, 1994, 41(1):199-220.

◆ **Droperidol Injection, USP (Can)** *see* Droperidol *on page 725*

◆ **Droxia** *see* Hydroxyurea *on page 1051*

◆ **DRV** *see* Darunavir *on page 595*

◆ **Drymira (Can)** *see* Ciclesonide (Nasal) *on page 464*

◆ **DSCG** *see* Cromolyn (Nasal) *on page 553*

◆ **DSCG** *see* Cromolyn (Ophthalmic) *on page 553*

◆ **DSCG** *see* Cromolyn (Systemic, Oral Inhalation) *on page 551*

◆ **DSS** *see* Docusate *on page 701*

◆ **DT** *see* Diphtheria and Tetanus Toxoids *on page 679*

◆ **DTaP** *see* Diphtheria and Tetanus Toxoids, and Acellular Pertussis Vaccine *on page 686*

◆ **DTaP-HepB-IPV** *see* Diphtheria, Tetanus Toxoids, Acellular Pertussis, Hepatitis B (Recombinant), and Poliovirus (Inactivated) Vaccine *on page 690*

◆ **DTaP-IPV** *see* Diphtheria and Tetanus Toxoids, Acellular Pertussis, and Poliovirus Vaccine *on page 682*

◆ **DTaP-IPV/Hib** *see* Diphtheria and Tetanus Toxoids, Acellular Pertussis, Poliovirus and *Haemophilus* b Conjugate Vaccine *on page 684*

◆ **DTIC** *see* Dacarbazine *on page 578*

◆ **DTIC-Dome** *see* Dacarbazine *on page 578*

◆ **DTO (error-prone abbreviation)** *see* Opium Tincture *on page 1548*

◆ **Duac** *see* Clindamycin and Benzoyl Peroxide *on page 502*

◆ **Ducodyl [OTC]** *see* Bisacodyl *on page 293*

◆ **Dulcolax [OTC]** *see* Bisacodyl *on page 293*

◆ **Dulcolax For Women [OTC] (Can)** *see* Bisacodyl *on page 293*

◆ **Dulcolax Milk of Magnesia [OTC]** *see* Magnesium Hydroxide *on page 1294*

◆ **Dulcolax Stool Softener [OTC]** *see* Docusate *on page 701*

◆ **Dulera®** *see* Mometasone and Formoterol *on page 1436*

◆ **Duofilm® (Can)** *see* Salicylic Acid *on page 1860*

◆ **Duoforte® 27 (Can)** *see* Salicylic Acid *on page 1860*

◆ **DuP 753** *see* Losartan *on page 1283*

◆ **Duraclon** *see* CloNIDine *on page 516*

◆ **Duragesic** *see* FentaNYL *on page 853*

◆ **Duragesic MAT (Can)** *see* FentaNYL *on page 853*

◆ **Duralith® (Can)** *see* Lithium *on page 1266*

◆ **Duramorph** *see* Morphine (Systemic) *on page 1440*

◆ **Durela (Can)** *see* TraMADol *on page 2060*

◆ **Duricef** *see* Cefadroxil *on page 392*

◆ **Duvoid® (Can)** *see* Bethanechol *on page 288*

◆ **D-Vi-Sol [OTC]** *see* Cholecalciferol *on page 455*

◆ **D-Vi-Sol® (Can)** *see* Cholecalciferol *on page 455*

◆ **D-Vita [OTC]** *see* Cholecalciferol *on page 455*

Dyclonine (DYE kloe neen)

Medication Safety Issues

Sound-alike/look-alike issues:

Dyclonine may be confused with dicyclomine

Brand Names: U.S. Sucrets® Children's [OTC]; Sucrets® Maximum Strength [OTC]; Sucrets® Regular Strength [OTC]

Therapeutic Category Local Anesthetic, Oral
Generic Availability (U.S.) No
Use Used topically for temporary relief of pain associated with oral mucosa
Contraindications Hypersensitivity to chlorobutanol (preservative used in dyclonine), dyclonine, or any component
Warnings When used for self-medication (OTC), patients should contact healthcare provider if symptoms worsen or last for >7 days. When treating a severe sore throat, patients should contact healthcare provider if symptoms lasts >2 days, occur with fever, headache, rash, nausea, or vomiting. Not for OTC use in children <2 years of age.
Adverse Reactions
Local: Irritation, numbness, pain, stinging
Miscellaneous: Allergic reactions, cold/heat sensation
Drug Interactions
Metabolism/Transport Effects None known.
Avoid Concomitant Use There are no known interactions where it is recommended to avoid concomitant use.
Increased Effect/Toxicity There are no known significant interactions involving an increase in effect.
Decreased Effect There are no known significant interactions involving a decrease in effect.
Stability Store in tight, light-resistant container; avoid freezing
Dosing: Usual
Children >3 years: Topical: Slowly dissolve 1 lozenge (1.2 mg) in mouth every 2 hours, if necessary
Children >12 years and Adults: Topical: Slowly dissolve 1 lozenge (3 mg) in mouth every 2 hours, if necessary
Administration Topical: Apply to mucous membranes of the mouth or throat area: food should not be ingested for 60 minutes following application in the mouth or throat area
Dosage Forms Excipient information presented when available (limited, particularly for generics); consult specific product labeling. [DSC] = Discontinued product
Lozenge, oral, as hydrochloride:
Sucrets® Children's: 1.2 mg (18s) [cherry flavor]
Sucrets® Maximum Strength: 3 mg (18s) [black-cherry flavor]
Sucrets® Maximum Strength: 3 mg (18s) [wintergreen flavor]
Sucrets® Regular Strength: 2 mg (18s)
Sucrets® Regular Strength: 2 mg (18s [DSC]) [wild cherry flavor]
References
Carnel SB, Blakeslee DB, Oswald SG, et al, "Treatment of Radiation- and Chemotherapy-Induced Stomatitis," *Otolaryngol Head Neck Surg*, 1990, 102(4):326-30.

◆ **Dyclonine Hydrochloride** *see* Dyclonine *on page* 727

◆ **Dyrenium** *see* Triamterene *on page* 2079

◆ **Dyspel [OTC]** *see* Ibuprofen *on page* 1059

◆ **E-400 [OTC]** *see* Vitamin E *on page* 2148

◆ **E-400-Clear [OTC]** *see* Vitamin E *on page* 2148

◆ **E-400-Mixed [OTC]** *see* Vitamin E *on page* 2148

◆ **E 2080** *see* Rufinamide *on page* 1858

◆ **EACA** *see* Aminocaproic Acid *on page* 122

◆ **Ear Drops Earwax Aid [OTC]** *see* Carbamide Peroxide *on page* 377

◆ **Ear Wax Remover [OTC]** *see* Carbamide Peroxide *on page* 377

◆ **Earwax Treatment Drops [OTC]** *see* Carbamide Peroxide *on page* 377

◆ **EC-Naprosyn** *see* Naproxen *on page* 1470

◆ **E. coli Asparaginase** *see* Asparaginase (E. coli) *on page* 208

Econazole (e KONE a zole)

Brand Names: U.S. Ecoza
Therapeutic Category Antifungal Agent, Topical
Generic Availability (U.S.) May be product dependent
Use Topical treatment of tinea pedis, tinea cruris, tinea corporis, tinea versicolor, and cutaneous candidiasis
Pregnancy Risk Factor C
Pregnancy Considerations Adverse events were observed in some animal reproduction studies. The manufacturer recommends avoiding use during pregnancy, especially during the first trimester.
Breast-Feeding Considerations It is not known if econazole is excreted in breast milk. The manufacturer recommends that caution be exercised when administering econazole to nursing women.
Contraindications Hypersensitivity to econazole or any component
Warnings Not for ophthalmic or intravaginal use
Precautions Discontinue the drug if sensitivity or chemical irritation occurs; cross-sensitization may occur with other imidazole derivatives (ie, clotrimazole, miconazole)
Adverse Reactions
Dermatologic: Burning sensation of skin, erythema, pruritus, stinging of the skin
Rare but important or life-threatening: Application site reaction, pruritic rash
Drug Interactions
Metabolism/Transport Effects Inhibits CYP2E1 (weak)
Avoid Concomitant Use There are no known interactions where it is recommended to avoid concomitant use.
Increased Effect/Toxicity
Econazole may increase the levels/effects of: Vitamin K Antagonists
Decreased Effect There are no known significant interactions involving a decrease in effect.
Mechanism of Action Alters fungal cell wall membrane permeability; may interfere with RNA and protein synthesis, and lipid metabolism
Pharmacokinetics (Adult data unless noted)
Absorption: Following topical administration, <10% is percutaneously absorbed
Metabolism: In the liver to >20 metabolites
Elimination: <1% of an applied dose recovered in urine or feces
Dosing: Usual Children and Adults: Topical:
Tinea cruris, corporis, pedis, and tinea versicolor: Apply once daily
Cutaneous candidiasis: Apply twice daily
Administration Topical: Apply a sufficient amount of cream to cover affected areas; do not apply to the eye or intravaginally
Additional Information Candidal infections and tinea cruris, versicolor, and corporis should be treated for 2 weeks and tinea pedis for 1 month; occasionally, longer treatment periods may be required
Product Availability Ecoza topical foam: FDA approved October 2013; anticipated availability currently unknown
Dosage Forms Excipient information presented when available (limited, particularly for generics); consult specific product labeling.
Cream, External, as nitrate:
Generic: 1% (15 g, 30 g, 85 g)
Foam, External, as nitrate:
Ecoza: 1% (70 g) [contains propylene glycol, trolamine (triethanolamine)]

◆ **Econazole Nitrate** *see* Econazole *on page* 728

◆ **Econopred** *see* PrednisoLONE (Ophthalmic) *on page* 1730

- ◆ **Ecotrin [OTC]** *see* Aspirin *on page 212*
- ◆ **Ecotrin Arthritis Strength [OTC]** *see* Aspirin *on page 212*
- ◆ **Ecotrin Low Strength [OTC]** *see* Aspirin *on page 212*
- ◆ **Ecoza** *see* Econazole *on page 728*
- ◆ **Ed ChlorPed** *see* Chlorpheniramine *on page 448*
- ◆ **Ed Chlorped Jr [OTC]** *see* Chlorpheniramine *on page 448*
- ◆ **Ed-Chlor-Tan** *see* Chlorpheniramine *on page 448*
- ◆ **Edecrin** *see* Ethacrynic Acid *on page 806*

Edetate CALCIUM Disodium
(ED e tate KAL see um dye SOW dee um)

Medication Safety Issues
Sound-alike look-alike issues:
To avoid potentially serious errors, the abbreviation "EDTA" should **never** be used.

Edetate CALCIUM disodium (CaEDTA) may be confused with edetate disodium (Na₂EDTA) (not commercially available in the U.S. or Canada). CDC recommends that edetate disodium should **never** be used for chelation therapy in children. Fatal hypocalcemia may result if edetate disodium is used for chelation therapy instead of edetate calcium disodium. ISMP recommends confirming the diagnosis to help distinguish between the two drugs prior to dispensing and/or administering either drug.

Edetate CALCIUM disodium may be confused with etomidate

Therapeutic Category Antidote, Lead Toxicity; Chelating Agent, Parenteral

Generic Availability (U.S.) Yes

Use Treatment of acute and chronic lead poisoning; also used as an aid in the diagnosis of lead poisoning

Pregnancy Risk Factor B

Pregnancy Considerations Adverse events were observed in some animal reproduction studies; there are no well controlled studies of edetate CALCIUM disodium in pregnant women. Lead is known to cross the placenta in amounts related to maternal plasma levels. Prenatal lead exposure may be associated with adverse events such as spontaneous abortion, preterm delivery, decreased birth weight, and impaired neurodevelopment. Some adverse outcomes may occur with maternal blood lead levels <10 mcg/dL. In addition, pregnant women exposed to lead may have an increased risk of gestational hypertension. Consider chelation therapy in pregnant women with confirmed blood lead levels ≥45 mcg/dL (pregnant women with blood lead levels ≥70 mcg/dL should be considered for chelation regardless of trimester); consultation with experts in lead poisoning and high-risk pregnancy is recommended. Encephalopathic pregnant women should be chelated regardless of trimester (CDC, 2010).

Breast-Feeding Considerations If present in breast milk, oral absorption of edetate CALCIUM disodium is poor (<5%) which would limit exposure to a nursing infant. However, edetate CALCIUM disodium is not used orally because it may increase lead absorption from the GI tract. The amount of lead in breast milk may range from 0.6% to 3% of the maternal serum concentration. Women with confirmed blood lead levels ≥40 mcg/dL should not initiate breast-feeding; pumping and discarding breast milk is recommended until blood lead levels are <40 mcg/dL, at which point breast-feeding may resume (CDC, 2010). Calcium supplementation may reduce the amount of lead in breast milk.

Contraindications Hypersensitivity to edetate calcium disodium or any component; active renal disease, anuria, hepatitis

Warnings Patients with lead encephalopathy and cerebral edema may experience a lethal increase in intracranial pressure following I.V. infusion of edetate CALCIUM EDTA **[U.S. Boxed Warning]**; avoid rapid I.V. infusion, particularly in the management of lead encephalopathy; I.M. administration is the preferred route in these patients, if the I.V. route is necessary, infuse slowly (over at least 3 hours) **[U.S. Boxed Warning]**; do not exceed recommended daily dose **[U.S. Boxed Warning]**; if anuria, increasing proteinuria, or hematuria occurs during therapy, discontinue calcium EDTA.

Precautions Renal tubular necrosis and fatal nephrosis may occur, especially with high doses; establish urine flow prior to administration

Adverse Reactions
Cardiovascular: Arrhythmia, ECG changes, hypotension

Central nervous system: Chills, fatigue, fever, headache, malaise

Dermatologic: Cheilosis, dermatitis, rash

Endocrine & metabolic: Hypercalcemia, hypokalemia

Gastrointestinal: Anorexia, GI upset, nausea, thirst (excessive), vomiting

Hematologic: Anemia, bone marrow suppression (transient)

Hepatic: Alkaline phosphatase decreased, liver function test increased (mild)

Local: Pain at injection site (I.M. injection), thrombophlebitis (I.V. infusion when concentration >5 mg/mL)

Neuromuscular & skeletal: Arthralgia, myalgia, numbness, paresthesia, tremor

Ocular: Lacrimation

Renal: Glucosuria, microscopic hematuria, nephrosis, nephrotoxicity, proteinuria, renal tubular necrosis, urinary frequency/urgency

Respiratory: Nasal congestion, sneezing

Miscellaneous: Iron, magnesium, and/or zinc deficiency (with chronic therapy)

Drug Interactions
Metabolism/Transport Effects None known.

Avoid Concomitant Use
Avoid concomitant use of Edetate CALCIUM Disodium with any of the following: CloZAPine; Dipyrone

Increased Effect/Toxicity
Edetate CALCIUM Disodium may increase the levels/effects of: CloZAPine; Insulin

The levels/effects of Edetate CALCIUM Disodium may be increased by: Dipyrone

Decreased Effect There are no known significant interactions involving a decrease in effect.

Stability Dilute with NS or D₅W; physically incompatible with D₁₀W, LR; do not mix in the same syringe with dimercaprol

Mechanism of Action Calcium is displaced by divalent and trivalent heavy metals, forming a nonionizing soluble complex that is excreted in urine

Pharmacodynamics
Onset of chelation with I.V. administration: 1 hour
Maximum excretion of chelated lead with I.V. administration: 24-48 hours

Pharmacokinetics (Adult data unless noted)
Absorption: I.M., SubQ: Well absorbed

Distribution: Into extracellular fluid; minimal CSF penetration

Half-life, plasma:
I.M.: 1.5 hours
I.V.: 20 minutes

Elimination: Rapid in urine as metal chelates or unchanged drug ▶

729

Dosing: Usual Several regimens have been recommended:

Diagnosis of lead poisoning: Mobilization test (not recommended by AAP guidelines): I.M., I.V.:

Children: 500 mg/m^2/dose, (maximum dose: 1 g) as a single dose or divided into 2 doses

Adults: 500 mg/m^2/dose

Note: Urine is collected for 24 hours after first EDTA dose and analyzed for lead content; if the ratio of mcg of lead in urine to mg calcium EDTA given is >1, then test is considered positive; for convenience, an 8-hour urine collection may be done after a single 50 mg/kg I.M. (maximum dose: 1 g) or 500 mg/m^2 I.V. dose; a positive test occurs if the ratio of lead excretion to mg calcium EDTA >0.5-0.6.

Treatment of lead poisoning: Children and Adults (each regimen is specific for route):

Symptoms of lead encephalopathy and/or blood lead level >70 mcg/dL: Treat 5 days; give in conjunction with dimercaprol; wait a minimum of 2 days with no treatment before considering a repeat course:

I.M.: 250 mg/m^2/dose every 4 hours

I.V.: 50 mg/kg/day as 24-hour continuous I.V. infusion or 1-1.5 g/m^2 I.V. as either an 8- to 24-hour infusion or divided into 2 doses every 12 hours

Symptomatic lead poisoning without encephalopathy or asymptomatic with blood lead level >70 mcg/dL: Treat 3-5 days; treatment with dimercaprol is recommended until the blood lead level concentration <50 mcg/dL:

I.M.: 167 mg/m^2 every 4 hours

I.V.: 1 g/m^2 as an 8- to 24-hour infusion or divided every 12 hours

Asymptomatic children with blood lead level 45-69 mcg/dL: I.V.: 25 mg/kg/day for 5 days as an 8- to 24-hour infusion or divided into 2 doses every 12 hours

Depending upon the blood lead level, additional courses may be necessary; repeat at least 2-4 days and preferably 2-4 weeks apart

Adults with lead nephropathy: An alternative dosing regimen reflecting the reduction in renal clearance is based upon the serum creatinine (adapted from Morgan, 1975; see table):

Alternative Dosing I.V. Regimen for Adults With Lead Nephropathy

Serum Creatinine (mg/dL)	Ca EDTA Dosage
>2-3	Reduce recommended dosage by 50%
>3-4	Reduce recommended dosage by 50% and administer every other day
>4	Reduce recommended dosage by 50% and administer once weekly

Adapted from Morgan, 1975.

Repeat these regimens monthly until lead excretion is reduced toward normal.

Administration Parenteral:

Intermittent I.V. infusion: Administer the dose I.V. over at least 1 hour in asymptomatic patients, 2 hours in symptomatic patients

Single daily I.V. continuous infusion: Dilute to 2-4 mg/mL in D$_5$W or NS and infuse over at least 8 hours, usually over 12-24 hours

I.M. injection: To minimize pain at the injection site, 1.67 mL of 2% procaine may be added to 5 mL calcium EDTA, resulting in 150 mg/mL concentration with 0.5% procaine (stable 3 months; Nahata, 1997)

Monitoring Parameters BUN, serum creatinine, urinalysis, fluid balance, ECG, blood and urine lead concentrations

Test Interactions If edetate CALCIUM disodium is given as a continuous I.V. infusion, stop the infusion for at least 1 hour before blood is drawn for lead concentration to avoid a falsely elevated value

Dosage Forms Excipient information presented when available (limited, particularly for generics); consult specific product labeling. [DSC] = Discontinued product

Solution, Injection:

Generic: 500 mg/2.5 mL (2.5 mL [DSC]); 1 g/5 mL (5 mL)

References

American Academy of Pediatrics Committee on Drugs, "Treatment Guidelines for Lead Exposure in Children," *Pediatrics*, 1995, 96(1 Pt 1):155-60.

Centers for Disease Control and Prevetion (CDC), *Guidelines for the Identification and Management of Lead Exposure in Pregnant and Lactating Women*, Atlanta: CDC; 2010.

Gracia RC and Snodgrass WR, "Lead Toxicity and Chelation Therapy," *Am J Health Syst Pharm*, 2007, 64(1):45-53.

Morgan JM, "Chelation Therapy in Lead Nephropathy," *South Med J*, 1975, 68(8):1001-6.

Nahata MC and Hipple TF, *Pediatric Drug Formulations*, 3rd ed, Cincinnati, OH: Harvey Whitney Books Co, 1997.

◆ **Edetate Disodium CALCIUM** *see* Edetate CALCIUM Disodium *on page 729*

◆ **Edex** *see* Alprostadil *on page 103*

◆ **Edluar** *see* Zolpidem *on page 2182*

Edrophonium (ed roe FOE nee um)

Brand Names: U.S. Enlon

Brand Names: Canada Enlon®; Tensilon®

Therapeutic Category Antidote, Neuromuscular Blocking Agent; Cholinergic Agent; Diagnostic Agent, Myasthenia Gravis

Generic Availability (U.S.) No

Use Diagnosis of myasthenia gravis; differentiation of cholinergic crises from myasthenia crises; reversal of nondepolarizing neuromuscular blockers; treatment of paroxysmal atrial tachycardia

Pregnancy Considerations Animal reproduction studies have not been conducted.

Breast-Feeding Considerations It is not known if edrophonium is excreted in breast milk. According to the manufacturer, if administration is required, avoid breast-feeding the infant immediately after use due to the potential for adverse events in the nursing infant.

Contraindications Hypersensitivity to edrophonium or any component; GI or GU mechanical obstruction

Warnings Overdosage can cause cholinergic crisis which may be fatal; I.V. atropine should be readily available for treatment of cholinergic reactions; injection contains sulfites which may cause allergic reactions in susceptible individuals

Precautions Use with caution in asthmatic patients, patients with cardiac dysrhythmias, and those receiving a cardiac glycoside

Adverse Reactions

Cardiovascular: Arrhythmias (especially bradycardia), AV block, carbon monoxide decreased, cardiac arrest, ECG changes (nonspecific), flushing, hypotension, nodal rhythm, syncope, tachycardia

Central nervous system: Convulsions, dizziness, drowsiness, dysarthria, dysphonia, headache, loss of consciousness

Dermatologic: Skin rash, thrombophlebitis (I.V.), urticaria

Gastrointestinal: Diarrhea, dysphagia, flatulence, hyperperistalsis, nausea, salivation, stomach cramps, vomiting

Genitourinary: Urinary urgency

Neuromuscular & skeletal: Arthralgias, fasciculations, muscle cramps, spasms, weakness

Ocular: Lacrimation, small pupils

Respiratory: Bronchiolar constriction, bronchospasm, dyspnea, bronchial secretions increased, laryngospasm, respiratory arrest, respiratory depression, respiratory muscle paralysis

Miscellaneous: Allergic reactions, anaphylaxis, diaphoresis increased

Drug Interactions

Metabolism/Transport Effects None known.

Avoid Concomitant Use There are no known interactions where it is recommended to avoid concomitant use.

Increased Effect/Toxicity

Edrophonium may increase the levels/effects of: Beta-Blockers; Cholinergic Agonists; Succinylcholine

The levels/effects of Edrophonium may be increased by: Corticosteroids (Systemic)

Decreased Effect

Edrophonium may decrease the levels/effects of: Neuromuscular-Blocking Agents (Nondepolarizing)

The levels/effects of Edrophonium may be decreased by: Dipyridamole

Mechanism of Action Inhibits destruction of acetylcholine by acetylcholinesterase. This facilitates transmission of impulses across myoneural junction and results in increased cholinergic responses such as miosis, increased tonus of intestinal and skeletal muscles, bronchial and ureteral constriction, bradycardia, and increased salivary and sweat gland secretions.

Pharmacodynamics

Onset of action:
 I.M.: 2-10 minutes
 I.V.: 30-60 seconds
Duration:
 I.M.: 5-30 minutes
 I.V.: 5-10 minutes

Pharmacokinetics (Adult data unless noted)

Distribution: V_d:
 Infants: 1.18 ± 0.2 L/kg
 Children: 1.22 ± 0.74 L/kg
 Adults: 0.9 ± 0.13 L/kg
Half-life:
 Infants: 73 ± 30 minutes
 Children: 99 ± 31 minutes
 Adults: 126 ± 59 minutes
Elimination: Clearance:
 Infants: 17.8 mL/kg/minute
 Children: 14.2 mL/kg/minute
 Adults: 8.3 ± 2.9 mL/kg/minute

Dosing: Usual Usually administered I.V., however, if not possible, I.M. or SubQ may be used

Infants: Diagnosis of myasthenia gravis: Initial:
 I.M., SubQ: 0.5-1 mg
 I.V.: Initial: 0.1 mg, followed by 0.4 mg (if no response); total dose = 0.5 mg
Children:
 Diagnosis of myasthenia gravis: Initial:
  I.M., SubQ: ≤34 kg: 2 mg; >34 kg: 5 mg
  I.V.: 0.04 mg/kg given over 1 minute followed by 0.16 mg/kg given within 45 seconds (if no response) (maximum dose: 10 mg total)
  or
  Alternative (manufacturer's recommendations):
   ≤34 kg: 1 mg; if no response after 45 seconds, it may be repeated in 1 mg increments every 30-45 seconds to a total of 5 mg
   >34 kg: 2 mg; if no response after 45 seconds, it may be repeated in 1 mg increments every 30-45 seconds to a total of 10 mg
 Titration of oral anticholinesterase therapy: I.V.: 0.04 mg/kg once given 1 hour after oral intake of the drug being used in treatment; if strength improves, an increase in neostigmine or pyridostigmine dose is indicated

Adults:
 Diagnosis of myasthenia gravis: Initial:
  I.M., SubQ: Initial: 10 mg; if no cholinergic reaction occurs, administer 2 mg 30 minutes later to rule out false-negative reaction
  I.V.: 2 mg test dose administered over 15-30 seconds; 8 mg given 45 seconds later (if no response is seen); test dose may be repeated after 30 minutes.
 Titration of oral anticholinesterase therapy: I.V.: 1-2 mg given 1 hour after oral dose of anticholinesterase; if strength improves, an increase in neostigmine or pyridostigmine dose is indicated
 Differentiation of cholinergic from myasthenic crisis: I.V.: 1 mg, may repeat after 1 minute (**Note:** Intubation and controlled ventilation may be required if patient has cholinergic crises.)
 Reversal of nondepolarizing neuromuscular blocking agents (neostigmine with atropine usually preferred): I.V.: 10 mg over 30-45 seconds, may repeat every 5-10 minutes up to 40 mg total dose
 Termination of paroxysmal atrial tachycardia: I.V.: 5-10 mg

Dosing adjustment in renal impairment: Dose may need to be reduced in patients with chronic renal failure

Administration Parenteral: Edrophonium is administered by direct I.V. or I.M. injection

Monitoring Parameters Pre- and postinjection strength (cranial musculature is most useful); heart rate, respiratory rate, blood pressure, changes in fasciculations

Test Interactions Increased aminotransferase [ALT/AST] (S), amylase (S)

Dosage Forms Excipient information presented when available (limited, particularly for generics); consult specific product labeling.
 Solution, Injection, as chloride:
  Enlon: 10 mg/mL (15 mL) [contains phenol]

◆ **Edrophonium Chloride** *see* Edrophonium *on page 730*

◆ **Ed-Spaz** *see* Hyoscyamine *on page 1056*

◆ **EDTA (CALCIUM Disodium) (error-prone abbreviation)** *see* Edetate CALCIUM Disodium *on page 729*

◆ **EES (Can)** *see* Erythromycin (Systemic) *on page 780*

◆ **E.E.S. 400** *see* Erythromycin (Systemic) *on page 780*

◆ **E.E.S. Granules** *see* Erythromycin (Systemic) *on page 780*

Efavirenz (e FAV e renz)

Related Information

Adult and Adolescent HIV *on page 2348*
Oral Medications That Should Not Be Crushed or Altered *on page 2438*
Pediatric HIV *on page 2338*
Perinatal HIV *on page 2356*

Brand Names: U.S. Sustiva

Brand Names: Canada Mylan-Efavirenz; Sustiva; Teva-Efavirenz

Therapeutic Category Antiretroviral Agent; HIV Agents (Anti-HIV Agents); Non-nucleoside Reverse Transcriptase Inhibitor (NNRTI)

Generic Availability (U.S.) No

Use Treatment of HIV-1 infection in combination with other antiretroviral agents (FDA approved in ages ≥3 months weighing at least 3.5 kg and adults). **Note:** HIV regimens consisting of **three** antiretroviral agents are strongly recommended.

Prescribing and Access Restrictions Efavirenz oral solution is available only through an expanded access (compassionate use) program. Enrollment information may be obtained by calling 877-372-7097.

Pregnancy Risk Factor D

▶

Pregnancy Considerations Teratogenic effects have been observed in primates receiving efavirenz. Efavirenz crosses the placenta. Based on data from the Antiretroviral Pregnancy Registry, an increased risk of overall birth defects has not been observed following first trimester exposure to efavirenz; however, neural tube and other CNS defects have been reported. Due to the low number of first trimester exposures and the low incidence of neural tube defects in the general population, available data are insufficient to evaluate risk. Other antiretroviral agents should strongly be considered for use in women of childbearing potential who are planning to become pregnant or who are sexually active and not using effective contraception. Nonpregnant women of reproductive age should undergo pregnancy testing prior to initiation of efavirenz. Barrier contraception should be used in combination with other (hormonal) methods of contraception during therapy and for 12 weeks after efavirenz is discontinued. Neural tube defects would occur following exposure during the first 5 to 6 weeks of gestation (most pregnancies are not detected before 4 to 6 weeks gestation). For women who present in the first trimester already on an efavirenz-containing regimen and who have adequate viral suppression, efavirenz may be continued; changing regimens may lead to loss of viral control and increase the risk of perinatal transmission. Pharmacokinetic data from available studies do not suggest dose alterations are needed during pregnancy. Hypersensitivity reactions (including hepatic toxicity and rash) are more common in women on NNRTI therapy; it is not known if pregnancy increases this risk

Regardless of CD4 count or HIV RNA copy number, all HIV-infected pregnant women should receive a combination antepartum antiretroviral (ARV) drug regimen; this includes women who require therapy for their own health, as well as women who do not yet require therapy for their own health. ARV therapy should be started as soon as possible if required for the woman's health. Although earlier initiation may be more effective in reducing the perinatal transmission of HIV, also consider maternal conditions (eg, nausea and vomiting) and the potential risks of first trimester fetal exposure for specific agents. Plasma HIV RNA levels should be assessed at ~34 to 36 weeks gestation in order to help determine mode of delivery. If ARV therapy must be interrupted for <24 hours during the peripartum period, stop then restart all medications simultaneously in order to decrease the chance of developing resistance. Long-term follow-up is recommended for all infants exposed to ARV medications.

Healthcare providers are encouraged to enroll pregnant women exposed to antiretroviral medications in the Antiretroviral Pregnancy Registry (1-800-258-4263 or www.-APRegistry.com). Healthcare providers caring for HIV-infected women and their infants may contact the National Perinatal HIV Hotline (888-448-8765) for clinical consultation (DHHS [perinatal], 2012).

Breast-Feeding Considerations Efavirenz is excreted into breast milk. Although breast-feeding is not recommended, plasma concentrations of efavirenz in nursing infants have been reported as ~13% of maternal plasma concentrations.

Maternal or infant antiretroviral therapy does not completely eliminate the risk of postnatal HIV transmission. In addition, multiclass-resistant virus has been detected in breast-feeding infants despite maternal therapy. Therefore, in the United States, where formula is accessible, affordable, safe, and sustainable, and the risk of infant mortality due to diarrhea and respiratory infections is low, complete avoidance of breast-feeding by HIV-infected women is recommended to decrease potential transmission of HIV (DHHS [perinatal], 2014).

Contraindications Hypersensitivity (eg, Stevens-Johnson syndrome, erythema multiforme, or toxic skin eruptions) to efavirenz or any component; concurrent therapy with bepridil, cisapride, midazolam, pimozide, triazolam, ergot derivatives, or St John's wort

Warnings Efavirenz is a mixed inducer/inhibitor of CYP450 enzymes and numerous drug interactions occur. Due to potential serious and/or life-threatening drug interactions, certain drugs are contraindicated. Other drug interactions require dosage adjustment; standard doses of efavirenz and voriconazole must **not** be coadministered; however, **adjusted** doses may be administered concurrently.

Resistance emerges rapidly if administered as monotherapy; always use efavirenz in combination with at least two other antiretroviral agents; do not add efavirenz as a single agent to antiretroviral regimens that are failing; initiate in combination with at least one other antiretroviral agent to which the patient is naïve. Do not administer efavirenz with other efavirenz-containing products (eg, Atripla), unless needed for dosage adjustment with concomitant rifampin treatment.

Efavirenz may cause CNS effects (eg, abnormal dreams, insomnia, impaired concentration, hallucinations, dizziness, or drowsiness). The overall reported incidence of CNS adverse effects was 53% vs 25% in controls; nervous system symptoms in children were reported to be 18%. Fever has been reported with use (children: 21%). CNS symptoms usually begin within 1 to 2 days after starting efavirenz, and generally resolve within 2 to 4 weeks of continued therapy. Patients must be cautioned about performing tasks which require mental alertness (eg, operating machinery or driving). Tolerability of CNS effects may be improved by dosing at bedtime. CNS effects may be potentiated when used with other sedative drugs or ethanol.

Teratogenic effects have been observed in primates receiving efavirenz; human birth defects following efavirenz exposure in the first trimester have been reported, including cases of neural tube defects (including meningomyelocele and Dandy-Walker malformation) and one case of anophthalmia. Women of childbearing potential should be tested for pregnancy before starting efavirenz; women receiving efavirenz should avoid pregnancy while receiving this drug and for 12 weeks after discontinuation of this drug (due to long half-life of efavirenz); barrier contraception in combination with other (hormonal) methods of contraception should be used. Avoid use of efavirenz during the first trimester of pregnancy and in women with significant childbearing potential; women who use this drug during the first trimester or who become pregnant while taking this drug should be apprised of the potential harm to the fetus.

Efavirenz is hepatically metabolized, primarily via highly polymorphic CYP2B6 enzymes; individuals with the CYP2B6 516 T/T genotype have been shown to have reduced metabolism, resulting in greater exposure compared to the G/G or G/T genotypes (extensive metabolizers); this has particularly been demonstrated in infants and children <3 years of age. The T/T genotype has an allele frequency of 20% in African-Americans. Although FDA approved in pediatric patients ≥3 months of age and weighing ≥3.5 kg, current guidelines recommend that efavirenz not be used in infants and children <3 years of age in general; pharmacokinetic data suggest that FDA approved dosing may result in subtherapeutic levels in extensive metabolizers and supratherapeutic in slow metabolizers. In infants and children 3 months to <3 years of age and weighing ≥3 kg, evaluate CYP2B6 genotype prior to efavirenz therapy; in those with T/T genotype (slow metabolizer), dosage reduction and therapeutic drug level monitoring recommended (DHHS [pediatric], 2014).

Precautions Use with caution in patients with a history of mental illness; serious psychiatric side effects have been associated with use including aggressive behavior, severe depression, suicidal ideation, suicide, paranoia, and mania. Use with caution in patients with a history of substance abuse due to a predisposition to psychological reactions. Patients should be instructed to contact healthcare provider if serious psychiatric effects occur. Use with caution in patients with a history of seizures; convulsions may occur; efavirenz may decrease the serum concentrations of antiepileptic agents that are metabolized by the liver; monitor anticonvulsant serum concentrations periodically.

Efavirenz may cause a rash, which usually presents as pruritic maculopapular skin eruptions; incidence is more common and more severe in children than in adults [incidence: Adults 26%, children 32%; median onset: Adults: 11 days, children: 28 days (range: 3 to 1642 days)]. In adults, most rashes appear within 14 days after starting therapy and the mean duration was 16 days; rash may be treated with antihistamines and corticosteroids and usually resolves within 1 month while continuing therapy. Discontinue efavirenz if severe rash (involving blistering, desquamation, mucosal involvement, ulceration, or fever) occurs. **Consider prophylaxis with antihistamines in children due to frequency and severity of rash reported in children.**

Use with caution in patients with known or suspected hepatitis B or C, those receiving other hepatotoxic medications, and those with mild hepatic impairment; weigh risk versus benefit in patients with persistent elevations of serum transaminases (ie, >5 times normal); not recommended in moderate to severe hepatic impairment. Cross resistance with other non-nucleoside reverse transcriptase inhibitors may occur. Elevations of serum cholesterol and triglyceride concentrations may occur; monitor during therapy. Fat redistribution and accumulation [ie, central obesity, peripheral wasting, facial wasting, breast enlargement, dorsocervical fat enlargement (buffalo hump), and cushingoid appearance] have been observed in patients receiving antiretroviral agents (causal relationship not established). May cause diarrhea or loose stools; reported incidence in children is 39%. Cough may occur; reported incidence in children is 16%.

Immune reconstitution syndrome (an acute inflammatory response to residual or indolent opportunistic infections) may occur in HIV patients during initial treatment with combination antiretroviral agents; this syndrome may require further patient assessment and therapy. Autoimmune disorders (eg, Grave's disease, Guillain-Barré syndrome, and polymyositis) have been reported in patients experiencing immune reconstitution; time to onset is variable and may occur many months after antiretroviral treatment is initiated.

Adverse Reactions

Central nervous system: Abnormal dreams, anxiety, depression, dizziness, fatigue, fever, hallucinations, headache, impaired concentration, insomnia, nervousness, pain, severe depression, somnolence

Dermatologic: Pruritus, rash

Endocrine & metabolic: HDL increased, hyperglycemia, total cholesterol increased, triglycerides increased

Gastrointestinal: Abdominal pain, amylase increased, anorexia, diarrhea, dyspepsia, nausea, vomiting

Hematologic: Neutropenia

Hepatic: ALT increased, AST increased

Respiratory: Cough

Rare but important or life-threatening: Allergic reaction, ataxia, body fat accumulation/redistribution, cerebellar coordination disturbances, delusions, dermatitis (photoallergic), erythema multiforme, gynecomastia, hepatic

failure, hepatitis, immune reconstitution syndrome, malabsorption, mania, neuropathy, neurosis, palpitations, pancreatitis, paranoia, psychosis, seizures, Stevens-Johnson syndrome, suicide attempts, suicidal ideation, visual abnormalities

Drug Interactions

Metabolism/Transport Effects Substrate of CYP2B6 (major), CYP3A4 (major); **Note:** Assignment of Major/Minor substrate status based on clinically relevant drug interaction potential; **Inhibits** CYP2C19 (moderate), CYP2C9 (moderate); **Induces** CYP2B6 (weak/moderate), CYP3A4 (weak/moderate)

Avoid Concomitant Use

Avoid concomitant use of Efavirenz with any of the following: Atovaquone; Axitinib; Azelastine (Nasal); Boceprevir; CarBAMazepine; Etravirine; Itraconazole; Ketoconazole (Systemic); Nevirapine; Paraldehyde; Posaconazole; Reverse Transcriptase Inhibitors (Non-Nucleoside); Rilpivirine; Simeprevir; St Johns Wort; Thalidomide

Increased Effect/Toxicity

Efavirenz may increase the levels/effects of: Alcohol (Ethyl); Azelastine (Nasal); Bosentan; Cannabis; Carvedilol; Citalopram; CNS Depressants; CYP2C19 Substrates; CYP2C9 Substrates; Dronabinol; Etravirine; Fosphenytoin; Hydrocodone; Methotrimeprazine; Metyrosine; Mirtazapine; Nevirapine; Paraldehyde; Phenytoin; Pramipexole; Rilpivirine; Ritonavir; ROPINIRole; Rotigotine; Selective Serotonin Reuptake Inhibitors; Tetrahydrocannabinol; Thalidomide; Vitamin K Antagonists; Zolpidem

The levels/effects of Efavirenz may be increased by: Boceprevir; Brimonidine (Topical); Cannabis; CYP2B6 Inhibitors (Moderate); CYP2B6 Inhibitors (Strong); Darunavir; Doxylamine; Dronabinol; Droperidol; HydrOXYzine; Kava Kava; Magnesium Sulfate; Methotrimeprazine; Mifepristone; Nabilone; Nevirapine; Perampanel; Quazepam; Reverse Transcriptase Inhibitors (Non-Nucleoside); Ritonavir; Rufinamide; Saquinavir; Sodium Oxybate; Tapentadol; Tetrahydrocannabinol; Voriconazole

Decreased Effect

Efavirenz may decrease the levels/effects of: Alcohol (Ethyl); ARIPiprazole; Artemether; Atazanavir; AtorvaSTATin; Atovaquone; Axitinib; Boceprevir; Buprenorphine; BuPROPion; Calcium Channel Blockers; Canagliflozin; CarBAMazepine; Caspofungin; Clarithromycin; Clopidogrel; Contraceptives (Progestins); CycloSPORINE (Systemic); Darunavir; Diltiazem; Dolutegravir; Etonogestrel; Etravirine; Everolimus; Fosamprenavir; Ibrutinib; Indinavir; Itraconazole; Ketoconazole (Systemic); Lopinavir; Lovastatin; Maraviroc; Methadone; Norgestimate; Posaconazole; Pravastatin; Proguanil; Raltegravir; Rifabutin; Rilpivirine; Saquinavir; Saxagliptin; Sertraline; Simeprevir; Simvastatin; Sirolimus; Tacrolimus (Systemic); Telaprevir; Vitamin K Antagonists; Voriconazole

The levels/effects of Efavirenz may be decreased by: Bosentan; CarBAMazepine; CYP2B6 Inducers (Strong); CYP3A4 Inducers (Strong); Dabrafenib; Deferasirox; Fosphenytoin; Mitotane; Nevirapine; Phenytoin; Reverse Transcriptase Inhibitors (Non-Nucleoside); Rifabutin; Rifampin; Siltuximab; St Johns Wort; Telaprevir; Tocilizumab

Food Interactions High-fat meals increase the absorption of efavirenz. CNS effects are possible. Management: Avoid high-fat meals. Administer at or before bedtime on an empty stomach unless using capsule sprinkle method in patients unable to swallow capsules or tablets. If capsule sprinkle method is used, patient should not consume additional food for 2 hours after administration.

Stability Store at 25°C (77°F); excursions permitted to 15°C to 30°C (59°F to 86°F)

Mechanism of Action As a non-nucleoside reverse transcriptase inhibitor, efavirenz has activity against HIV-1 by binding to reverse transcriptase. It consequently blocks the RNA-dependent and DNA-dependent DNA polymerase activities including HIV-1 replication. It does not require intracellular phosphorylation for antiviral activity.

Pharmacokinetics (Adult data unless noted)
Absorption: Increased by fatty meals
Distribution: CSF concentrations are 0.69% of plasma (range: 0.26% to 1.2%); however, CSF:plasma concentration ratio is 3 times higher than free fraction in plasma
Protein binding: 99.5% to 99.8%, primarily to albumin
Metabolism: Hepatic via CYP3A4 and CYP2B6 to hydroxylated metabolites which then undergo glucuronidation; induces P450 enzymes and its own metabolism
Bioavailability: 42%
Half-life:
Single dose: 52 to 76 hours
Multiple doses: 40 to 55 hours
Time to peak serum concentration: 3 to 5 hours
Elimination: <1% excreted unchanged in the urine; 14% to 34% excreted as metabolites in the urine and 16% to 61% in feces (primarily as unchanged drug)

Dosing: Neonatal Not recommended for use; limited pharmacokinetic data demonstrate that target trough concentrations are difficult to achieve (DHHS [pediatric], 2014); additional studies are needed to determine the appropriate dosage.

Dosing: Usual
Pediatric: **HIV infection, treatment:** Use in combination with other antiretroviral agents; dosage adjustments for concomitant drug administration may be required; see below Dosage adjustment for concomitant drugs:
Infants <3 months or <3 kg: Not recommended for use
Infants ≥3 months weighing ≥3 kg and Children <3 years:
Oral:
AIDSinfo recommendation: Very limited data available:
Note: In general, current guidelines do not recommend efavirenz use in patients <3 years of age unless use is unavoidable due to the clinical situation; CYP2B6 genotype testing should be performed prior to therapy initiation. The following doses are under investigation and have been suggested by the expert panel based on pharmacokinetic data (DHHS [pediatric], 2014)
Extensive metabolizers (CYP2B6 516 G/G or G/T genotypes):
3 kg to <5 kg: 200 mg once daily
5 kg to <7 kg: 300 mg once daily
7 kg to <14 kg: 400 mg once daily
14 kg to <17 kg: 500 mg once daily
≥17 kg: 600 mg once daily
Slow metabolizer (CYP 2B6 516 T/T genotype):
3.3 kg to <7 kg: 50 mg once daily
7 kg to <14 kg: 100 mg once daily
≥14 kg: 150 mg once daily
Manufacturer's labeling: **Note:** Although FDA approved in pediatric patients ≥3 months of age and weighing ≥3.5 kg, pharmacokinetic data suggest that the FDA approved dosing may result in subtherapeutic levels in extensive metabolizers and supratherapeutic in slow metabolizers and use should be avoided.
3.5 kg to <5 kg: 100 mg once daily
5 kg to <7.5 kg: 150 mg once daily
7.5 kg to <15 kg: 200 mg once daily
15 kg to <20 kg: 250 mg once daily
Children ≥3 years and Adolescents:
Weight-directed dosing: Oral:
10 kg to <15 kg: 200 mg once daily
15 kg to <20 kg: 250 mg once daily
20 kg to <25 kg: 300 mg once daily
25 kg to <32.5 kg: 350 mg once daily
32.5 kg to <40 kg: 400 mg once daily

≥40 kg: 600 mg once daily
BSA-directed dosing: Oral: 367 mg/m^2/dose once daily, maximum dose: 600 mg; recommended by some experts due to concern of underdosing at the upper end of each weight range (DHHS [pediatric], 2014)
Adult: **HIV infection, treatment: Note:** Use in combination with other antiretroviral agents: Oral: 600 mg once daily (DHHS [adult], 2014)

Dosage adjustment for concomitant rifampin:
Pediatric patients weighing ≤50 kg and Adults ≤50 kg: There are no dosage adjustments provided in manufacturer's labeling; however, efavirenz dosage increase may be considered.
Pediatric patients weighing >50 kg and Adults >50 kg: Oral: Increase efavirenz dose to 800 mg once daily

Dosage adjustment for concomitant voriconazole:
Infants ≥3 months, Children, and Adolescents: There are no dosage adjustments provided in manufacturer's labeling; however, efavirenz dose reduction and voriconazole dosage increase may be considered.
Adults: Oral: Reduce efavirenz dose to 300 mg once daily (use capsule formulation) and increase voriconazole dose to 400 mg every 12 hours

Dosing adjustment in renal impairment: Infants >3 months, Children, Adolescents, and Adults: There are no dosage adjustments provided in manufacturer's labeling; however, drug undergoes minimal renal excretion.

Dosing adjustment in hepatic impairment: Infants >3 months, Children, Adolescents, and Adults:
Mild impairment (Child-Pugh class A): No dosage adjustment recommended; use with caution
Moderate to severe impairment (Child-Pugh class B or C): Use not recommended; not studied

Administration Administer dose at bedtime to decrease CNS adverse effects; administer with water on an empty stomach (administration with food may increase efavirenz concentrations and adverse effects). Capsules and tablets should be swallowed intact. For patients who cannot swallow capsules or tablets, the capsules may be opened and added to 1 to 2 teaspoons of age-appropriate soft food (eg, applesauce, grape jelly, or yogurt) or 10 mL of room temperature infant formula. **Note:** Efavirenz tastes peppery (grape jelly may be used to improve taste). After administration, an additional small amount (2 teaspoons) of food or formula must be added to the empty mixing container, stirred to disperse any remaining efavirenz residue, and administered to the patient. Administer the efavirenz food or formula mixture within 30 minutes of mixing; do not save for future use. No additional food should be consumed for 2 hours after administration. Refer to the detailed "Instructions of Use" (found in the product labeling) for preparing a dose of efavirenz using the capsule sprinkle method.

Monitoring Parameters Note: Monitor CD4 percentage (if <5 years of age) or CD4 count (if ≥5 years of age) at least every 3 to 4 months (DHHS [pediatric], 2014).

Prior to initiation of therapy: Genotypic resistance testing, CD4 and viral load (every 3 to 4 months), CBC with differential, LFTs, BUN, creatinine, electrolytes, glucose, urinalysis (every 6 to 12 months), and assessment of readiness for adherence with medication regimen. At initiation and with any change in treatment regimen: CBC with differential, electrolytes, calcium, phosphate, glucose, LFTs, bilirubin, urinalysis (at initiation), BUN, creatinine, albumin, total protein, lipid panel (at initiation), CD4, and viral load. After 1 to 2 weeks of therapy: Signs of medication toxicity and adherence. After 2 to 4 weeks of therapy: CBC with differential, viral load, and signs of medication toxicity, and adherence; then every 3 to 4 months: CBC with differential, electrolytes, glucose, LFTs, bilirubin, BUN, creatinine, CD4, viral load, signs of medication toxicity, and adherence. Every 6 to 12 months: Lipid panel and urinalysis. CD4 monitoring frequency may be decreased to every 6 to 12 months in children who are adherent to therapy if the value is well above the threshold for opportunistic infections, viral suppression is sustained, and the clinical status is stable for more than 2 to 3 years (DHHS [pediatric], 2014). Monitor for growth and development, signs of HIV-specific physical conditions, HIV disease progression, opportunistic infections, signs and symptoms of rash, serum amylase, and CNS and psychiatric effects.

Additional monitoring for patients 3 months to <3 years of age weighing ≥3kg: CYP 2B6 genotype prior to therapy; efavirenz serum trough concentrations 2 weeks after initiation and at 3 years of age (DHHS [pediatric], 2014)

Reference Range Trough concentration: >1000 ng/mL (DHHS [adult, pediatric], 2014)

Test Interactions False-positive tests for cannabinoids have been reported when the CEDIA DAU Multilevel THC assay is used. False-positive results with other assays for cannabinoids have not been observed. False-positive tests for benzodiazepines have been reported and are likely due to the 8-hydroxy-efavirenz major metabolite.

Additional Information An oral liquid formulation of efavirenz (strawberry/mint-flavored solution) is available on an investigational basis from Bristol-Myers Squibb Company as part of an expanded access program for HIV-infected children and adolescents 3 to 16 years of age; for further details call 877-372-7097. **Note:** The bioavailability of the investigational liquid was found to be 20% lower than that of the capsules in adult volunteers; a recent pediatric study used initial doses of the liquid formulation that were 20% higher than pediatric capsule doses; these higher doses resulted in AUC values that were similar to AUCs achieved with the capsules (Starr, 2002).

Early virologic failure and rapid emergence of resistant mutations have been observed in therapy-naïve adult HIV patients treated with tenofovir, didanosine enteric-coated beadlets (Videx® EC), and either efavirenz or nevirapine; the combination of tenofovir, didanosine, and any non-nucleoside reverse transcriptase inhibitor is **not** recommended as initial antiretroviral therapy.

Dosage Forms Excipient information presented when available (limited, particularly for generics); consult specific product labeling.

Capsule, Oral:
  Sustiva: 50 mg, 200 mg
Tablet, Oral:
  Sustiva: 600 mg

References
Adkins JC, Noble S. Efavirenz. *Drugs.* 1998;56(6):1055-1064.
Aronoff GR, Bennett WM, Berns JS, et al. *Drug Prescribing in Renal Failure: Dosing Guidelines for Adults and Children.* 5th ed. Philadelphia, PA: American College of Physicians; 2007;77.
DHHS Panel on Antiretroviral Guidelines for Adults and Adolescents, "Guidelines for the Use of Antiretroviral Agents in HIV-Infected Adults and Adolescents," May 1, 2014. Available at http://www.aidsinfo.nih.gov
DHHS Panel on Antiretroviral Therapy and Medical Management of HIV-Infected Children, "Guidelines for the Use of Antiretroviral Agents in Pediatric HIV Infection," February 12, 2014. Available at http://aidsinfo.nih.gov
DHHS Panel on Treatment of HIV-Infected Pregnant Women and Prevention of Perinatal Transmission, "Recommendations for the Use of Antiretroviral Drugs in Pregnant HIV-1-Infected Women for Maternal Health and Interventions to Reduce Perinatal HIV-1 Transmission in the United States," March 28, 2014. Available at http://aidsinfo.nih.gov
Maddocks S, Dwyer D. The role of non-nucleoside reverse transcriptase inhibitors in children with HIV-1 infection. *Paediatr Drugs.* 2001;3(9):681-702.
Naidoo P, Chetty VV, Chetty M. Impact of CYP polymorphisms, ethnicity and sex differences in metabolism on dosing strategies: the case of efavirenz. *Eur J Clin Pharmacol.* 2014;70(4):379-389.
Piscitelli SC, Burstein AH, Chaitt D, Alfaro RM, Falloon J. Indinavir concentrations and St John's wort. *Lancet.* 2000;355(9203):547-548.
Starr SE, Fletcher CV, Spector SA, et al. Combination therapy with efavirenz, nelfinavir, and nucleoside reverse-transcriptase inhibitors in children infected with human immunodeficiency virus type 1. Pediatric AIDS Clinical Trials Group 382 Team. *N Engl J Med.* 1999;341(25):1874-1881.
Starr SE, Fletcher CV, Spector SA, et al. Efavirenz liquid formulation in human immunodeficiency virus-infected children. *Pediatr Infect Dis J.* 2002;21(7):659-663.

Efavirenz, Emtricitabine, and Tenofovir
(e FAV e renz, em trye SYE ta been, & ten OF oh vir)

Related Information
Adult and Adolescent HIV *on page 2348*
Pediatric HIV *on page 2338*
Perinatal HIV *on page 2356*
Brand Names: U.S. Atripla
Brand Names: Canada Atripla
Therapeutic Category Antiretroviral Agent; HIV Agents (Anti-HIV Agents); Non-nucleoside Reverse Transcriptase Inhibitor (NNRTI); Nucleoside Reverse Transcriptase Inhibitor (NRTI); Nucleotide Reverse Transcriptase Inhibitor (NRTI)
Generic Availability (U.S.) No
Use Treatment of HIV infection either alone or in combination with other antiretroviral agents (FDA approved in ages ≥12 years weighing at least 40 kg and adults)
Pregnancy Risk Factor D
Pregnancy Considerations Adverse events have been observed in some animal reproduction studies. The manufacturer of this combination recommends pregnancy testing prior to therapy and effective contraception in women of reproductive potential during treatment and for 12 weeks after therapy is discontinued. See individual agents.
Breast-Feeding Considerations Efavirenz, emtricitabine, and tenofovir are excreted into breast milk. See individual agents.
Contraindications Hypersensitivity to efavirenz (including a history of clinically significant hypersensitivity, such as Stevens-Johnson syndrome, erythema multiforme, or toxic skin eruptions), emtricitabine, tenofovir, or any component; concurrent therapy with bepridil, cisapride, midazolam, pimozide, triazolam, ergot derivatives, voriconazole, or St John's wort
Warnings Cases of lactic acidosis, severe hepatomegaly with steatosis, and death have been reported in patients receiving nucleoside analogues (including tenofovir) **[U.S. Boxed Warning]**; most of these cases have been in women; prolonged nucleoside use, obesity, and prior liver disease may be risk factors; use with extreme caution in patients with other risk factors for liver disease; discontinue therapy in patients who develop laboratory or clinical evidence of lactic acidosis or pronounced hepatotoxicity. Testing for hepatitis B is recommended prior to the initiation of efavirenz, emtricitabine, and tenofovir therapy; HIV-infected patients who are coinfected with hepatitis B may experience severe acute exacerbations of hepatitis (ie, clinical symptoms or laboratory evidence of hepatitis) when emtricitabine or tenofovir is discontinued **[U.S. Boxed Warning]**; liver decompensation and hepatic failure have been associated with exacerbation of hepatitis B in patients treated with emtricitabine or tenofovir following discontinuation; monitor patients closely (with both clinical and laboratory follow-up) for at least several months after discontinuation of efavirenz, emtricitabine, and tenofovir; initiate antihepatitis B therapy if needed.

Efavirenz is a mixed inducer/inhibitor of CYP450 enzymes and numerous drug interactions occur. Due to potential serious and/or life-threatening drug interactions, certain drugs are contraindicated (significant drug interactions may also occur with tenofovir). Emtricitabine and tenofovir are primarily eliminated by the kidney; while efavirenz is not; do not use this fixed dose combination of efavirenz, emtricitabine, and tenofovir in patients with moderate or severe renal impairment (CrCl <50 mL/minute); monitor renal function closely; renal dysfunction, including acute renal failure and Fanconi syndrome (renal tubular injury with severe hypophosphatemia) has been reported with tenofovir use; this may occur especially in patients with renal disease, underlying systemic disease, or those taking nephrotoxic medications; adults with a low body weight and those taking medications that increase tenofovir serum concentration may also be at increased risk for tenofovir-associated nephrotoxicity; avoid tenofovir in patients with concomitant or recent use of nephrotoxic agents; cases of nephrotoxicity have been reported in adolescents receiving tenofovir-containing regimens; evaluate and monitor renal function in all patients receiving tenofovir (regardless of age).

Efavirenz may cause CNS effects (eg, abnormal dreams, insomnia, impaired concentration, hallucinations, dizziness, or drowsiness). The overall reported incidence of CNS adverse effects was 53% vs 25% in controls; nervous system symptoms in children were reported to be 18%. Fever has been reported with use (children: 21%). CNS symptoms usually begin within 1 to 2 days after starting efavirenz, and generally resolve within 2 to 4 weeks of continued therapy. Patients must be cautioned about performing tasks which require mental alertness (eg, operating machinery or driving). Tolerability of CNS effects may be improved by dosing at bedtime. CNS effects may be potentiated when used with other sedative drugs or ethanol.

Efavirenz may cause a rash, which usually presents as pruritic maculopapular skin eruptions; incidence is more common and more severe in children than in adults [incidence: Adults 26%, children 46%; median onset: Adults: 11 days, children: 9 days (range: 6 to 205 days)]. Most rashes in children appeared within 14 days after starting therapy [median duration: Adults: 16 days, children: 6 days (range: 2 to 37 days)]. Median duration of rash in children who continued therapy was 9 days; rash may be treated with antihistamines and corticosteroids and usually resolves within 1 month while continuing therapy. Discontinue if severe rash (involving blistering, desquamation, mucosal involvement, ulceration, or fever) occurs. **Consider prophylaxis with antihistamines in children due to frequency and severity of rash reported in children.**

Teratogenic effects have been observed in primates receiving efavirenz; human birth defects following efavirenz exposure in the first trimester have been reported, including cases of neural tube defects (including meningomyelocele and Dandy-Walker malformation); women of childbearing potential should be tested for pregnancy before starting efavirenz; women receiving efavirenz should avoid pregnancy while receiving this drug and for 12 weeks after discontinuation of this drug (due to long half-life of efavirenz); barrier contraception in combination with other (hormonal) methods of contraception should be used; avoid use of efavirenz during the first trimester of pregnancy and in women with significant childbearing potential; women who use this drug during the first trimester or who become pregnant while taking this drug should be apprised of the potential harm to the fetus.

Atripla contains efavirenz, emtricitabine, and tenofovir as a fixed-dose combination; do not administer Atripla with other efavirenz-, emtricitabine-, or tenofovir-containing medications (eg, Complera, Emtriva, Stribild, Sustiva, Truvada, or Viread) or with medications that contain lamivudine (eg, Epivir, Epivir-HBV, Combivir, Epzicom, or Trizivir). Do not coadminister with adefovir; may diminish efficacy of tenofovir. Coadministration with efavirenz may be required for dose adjustment with concomitant rifampin therapy.

Precautions Use efavirenz, emtricitabine, and tenofovir with caution in patients with mild hepatic impairment; product is not recommended for patients with moderate or severe hepatic impairment, marked transaminase elevations, known or suspected hepatitis B or C, and in those receiving other hepatotoxic medications; monitor liver enzymes before and during treatment in these patients; weigh risk versus benefit in patients with persistent elevations of serum transaminases (ie, >5 times normal). Hepatic failure (including fatalities and cases requiring liver transplantation) has been reported in patients with no preexisting liver disease or other known risk factors; consider liver enzyme monitoring in patients without preexisting liver disease or other known risk factors. Elevations of serum cholesterol and triglycerides may occur; monitor during therapy.

Use efavirenz with caution in patients with a history of mental illness or substance abuse (predisposition to psychological reactions); serious psychiatric side effects have been associated with use including aggressive behavior, severe depression, suicidal ideation, suicide, paranoia, and mania; patients should be instructed to contact healthcare provider if serious psychiatric effects occur. Use with caution in patients with a history of seizures; convulsions may occur. Efavirenz may decrease the serum concentrations of antiepileptic agents that are metabolized by the liver; monitor anticonvulsant concentrations periodically. Cross-resistance with other non-nucleoside reverse transcriptase inhibitors may occur.

Emtricitabine-associated hyperpigmentation may occur at a higher frequency in pediatric patients compared to adults. Tenofovir-associated osteomalacia and reduced bone mineral density (BMD) may occur; long-term effects in humans are not known. Postmarketing cases of osteomalacia which may increase risk of bone fractures have also been reported in association with proximal renal tubulopathy. Recent studies suggest that tenofovir-related bone loss may be greater in children who are less mature (eg, Tanner stage 1 to 2) than in those who are more physically mature (Tanner ≥3). A significant decrease in lumbar spine BMD (>6%) was reported in five of 15 pediatric patients who received a tenofovir-containing regimen for 48 weeks. No orthopedic fractures occurred, but two patients required discontinuation of tenofovir. All five patients with a decrease in BMD were virologic responders and prepubertal (Tanner Stage 1). This study found a moderately strong correlation between decreases in bone mineral density z scores at week 48 and age at baseline. No correlation between decreases in bone mineral density z scores and tenofovir dose or pharmacokinetics was observed; BMD loss may limit the usefulness of tenofovir in prepubertal children [DHHS (pediatric), 2012; Giacomet, 2005; Hazra, 2005; Purdy, 2008]. Monitor BMD for potential bone toxicities during therapy; supplementation with calcium and vitamin D may be beneficial but has not been studied.

Fat redistribution and accumulation [ie, central obesity, peripheral wasting, facial wasting, breast enlargement, dorsocervical fat enlargement (buffalo hump), and cushingoid appearance] have been observed in patients receiving antiretroviral agents (causal relationship not established).

Immune reconstitution syndrome (an acute inflammatory response to residual or indolent opportunistic infections) may occur in HIV patients during initial treatment with combination antiretroviral agents; this syndrome may require further patient assessment and therapy. Autoimmune disorders (eg, Graves' disease, Guillain-Barré syndrome, and polymyositis) have been reported in patients experiencing immune reconstitution; time to onset is variable and may occur many months after antiretroviral treatment is initiated.

Adverse Reactions The complete adverse reaction profile of combination therapy has not been established. **See individual agents.** The following adverse effects were noted in clinical trials with combination therapy:

Central nervous system: Abnormal dreams, anxiety, depression, dizziness, fatigue, headache, insomnia, somnolence

Dermatologic: Rash

Endocrine & metabolic: Bone mineral density decreased, hypercholesterolemia, hyperglycemia, triglycerides increased

Gastrointestinal: Diarrhea, nausea, serum amylase increased, vomiting

Hematologic: Neutropenia

Hepatic: Alkaline phosphatase increased, ALT increased, AST increased

Neuromuscular & skeletal: Creatine increased

Renal: Hematuria

Respiratory: Nasopharyngitis, sinusitis, upper respiratory infection

Rare but important or life-threatening: Glycosuria

Drug Interactions

Metabolism/Transport Effects Refer to individual components.

Avoid Concomitant Use

Avoid concomitant use of Efavirenz, Emtricitabine, and Tenofovir with any of the following: Adefovir; Atovaquone; Axitinib; Azelastine (Nasal); Boceprevir; CarBAMazepine; Dabigatran Etexilate; Didanosine; Etravirine; Itraconazole; Ketoconazole (Systemic); LamiVUDine; Nevirapine; Paraldehyde; Posaconazole; Reverse Transcriptase Inhibitors (Non-Nucleoside); Rilpivirine; Simeprevir; St Johns Wort; Thalidomide; VinCRIStine (Liposomal)

Increased Effect/Toxicity

Efavirenz, Emtricitabine, and Tenofovir may increase the levels/effects of: Adefovir; Alcohol (Ethyl); Aminoglycosides; Azelastine (Nasal); Bosentan; Cannabis; Carvedilol; Citalopram; CNS Depressants; CYP2C19 Substrates; CYP2C9 Substrates; Darunavir; Didanosine; Dronabinol; Etravirine; Fosphenytoin; Hydrocodone; Methotrimeprazine; Metyrosine; Mirtazapine; Nevirapine; Paraldehyde; Phenytoin; Pramipexole; Rilpivirine; Ritonavir; ROPINIRole; Rotigotine; Selective Serotonin Reuptake Inhibitors; Tetrahydrocannabinol; Thalidomide; Vitamin K Antagonists; Zolpidem

The levels/effects of Efavirenz, Emtricitabine, and Tenofovir may be increased by: Acyclovir-Valacyclovir; Adefovir; Aminoglycosides; Atazanavir; Boceprevir; Brimonidine (Topical); Cannabis; Cidofovir; CYP2B6 Inhibitors (Moderate); CYP2B6 Inhibitors (Strong); Darunavir; Diclofenac (Systemic); Doxylamine; Dronabinol; Droperidol; Ganciclovir-Valganciclovir; HydrOXYzine; Kava Kava; LamiVUDine; Magnesium Sulfate; Methotrimeprazine; Mifepristone; Nabilone; Nevirapine; Nonsteroidal Anti-Inflammatory Agents; Perampanel; Quazepam; Reverse Transcriptase Inhibitors (Non-Nucleoside); Ribavirin; Ritonavir; Rufinamide; Saquinavir; Sodium Oxybate; Tapentadol; Tetrahydrocannabinol; Voriconazole

Decreased Effect

Efavirenz, Emtricitabine, and Tenofovir may decrease the levels/effects of: Afatinib; Alcohol (Ethyl); ARIPiprazole; Artemether; Atazanavir; AtorvaSTATin; Atovaquone; Axitinib; Boceprevir; Brentuximab Vedotin; Buprenorphine; BuPROPion; Calcium Channel Blockers; Canagliflozin; CarBAMazepine; Caspofungin; Clarithromycin; Clopidogrel; Contraceptives (Progestins); CycloSPORINE (Systemic); Dabigatran Etexilate; Darunavir; Didanosine; Diltiazem; Dolutegravir; DOXOrubicin (Conventional);

Etonogestrel; Etravirine; Everolimus; Fosamprenavir; Ibrutinib; Indinavir; Itraconazole; Ketoconazole (Systemic); Linagliptin; Lopinavir; Lovastatin; Maraviroc; Methadone; Norgestimate; P-glycoprotein/ABCB1 Substrates; Posaconazole; Pravastatin; Proguanil; Raltegravir; Rifabutin; Rilpivirine; Saquinavir; Saxagliptin; Sertraline; Simeprevir; Simvastatin; Sirolimus; Tacrolimus (Systemic); Telaprevir; Tipranavir; VinCRIStine (Liposomal); Vitamin K Antagonists; Voriconazole

The levels/effects of Efavirenz, Emtricitabine, and Tenofovir may be decreased by: Adefovir; Bosentan; CarBAMazepine; CYP2B6 Inducers (Strong); CYP3A4 Inducers (Strong); Dabrafenib; Deferasirox; Fosphenytoin; Mitotane; Nevirapine; Phenytoin; Reverse Transcriptase Inhibitors (Non-Nucleoside); Rifabutin; Rifampin; Siltuximab; St Johns Wort; Telaprevir; Tipranavir; Tocilizumab

Food Interactions See individual agents.

Stability Store tablets at 25°C (77°F); excursions permitted to 15°C to 30°C (59°F to 86°F). Keep container tightly closed; do not use if seal on bottle is broken or missing. Dispense only in original container.

Mechanism of Action See individual agents.

Pharmacokinetics (Adult data unless noted) One Atripla® tablet is bioequivalent to one efavirenz 600 mg tablet plus one emtricitabine 200 mg capsule plus one tenofovir 300 mg tablet (single dose study); see individual agents

Dosing: Usual

Pediatric: **HIV infection, treatment:** May be used alone or in combination with other antiretroviral agents:

Children <12 years or <40 kg: Product is a fixed-dose combination; safety and efficacy have not been established; use in patients <40 kg would result in an excessive efavirenz dose

Children ≥12 years and Adolescents; weighing ≥40 kg: Oral: 1 tablet once daily

Adult: **HIV infection, treatment:** Oral: 1 tablet once daily

Dosing adjustment in renal impairment: Children ≥12 years, Adolescents, and Adults: CrCl <50 mL/minute: Use not recommended.

Dosing adjustment in hepatic impairment: Children ≥12 years, Adolescents, and Adults:

Mild hepatic impairment (Child-Pugh class A): Use with caution; limited clinical experience

Moderate to severe hepatic impairment (Child-Pugh class B, C): Not recommended

Administration Administer dose at bedtime to decrease CNS adverse effects. Administer with water on an empty stomach; administration with food may increase efavirenz concentrations and adverse effects.

Monitoring Parameters Note: Monitor CD4 percentage (if <5 years of age) or CD4 count (if ≥5 years of age) at least every 3 to 4 months (DHHS [pediatric], 2014).

Patients should be screened for hepatitis B infection before starting therapy. Prior to initiation of therapy: Genotypic resistance testing, CD4 and viral load (every 3 to 4 months), CBC with differential, LFTs, BUN, creatinine, creatinine clearance, electrolytes, glucose, urinalysis (every 6 to 12 months), and assessment of readiness for adherence with medication regimen. At initiation and with any change in treatment regimen: CBC with differential, electrolytes, calcium, phosphorus, glucose, LFTs, bilirubin, urinalysis (at initiation), BUN, creatinine, albumin, total protein, lipid panel (at initiation), CD4, and viral load. After 1 to 2 weeks of therapy: Signs of medication toxicity and adherence. After 2 to 4 weeks of therapy: CBC with differential, viral load, and signs of medication toxicity, and adherence; then every 3 to 4 months: CBC with differential, electrolytes, glucose, LFTs, bilirubin, BUN, creatinine, CD4, viral load, signs of medication toxicity, and adherence. Every 6 to 12 months: Lipid panel and urinalysis. CD4 monitoring frequency may be decreased to every 6 to 12 months in children who are adherent to therapy if the value is well above the threshold for opportunistic infections, viral suppression is sustained, and the clinical status is stable for more than 2 to 3 years (DHHS [pediatric], 2014). Monitor for growth and development, signs of HIV-specific physical conditions, HIV disease progression, opportunistic infections, rash, CNS and psychiatric effects, bone abnormalities, hyperpigmentation, or lactic acidosis. Consider bone mineral density assessment for all patients with a history of pathologic bone fractures or other risk factors for osteoporosis or bone loss. Some experts recommend obtaining a DXA scan prior to therapy and 6 months into therapy, especially for patients in pre- and early puberty (Tanner stages 1 and 2) (DHHS [pediatric], 2014).

Reference Range Efavirenz: Trough concentration: >1000 ng/mL (DHHS [adult, pediatric], 2014)

Test Interactions False-positive test for cannabinoids have been reported when the CEDIA DAU Multilevel THC assay is used in patients receiving efavirenz. False-positive results with other assays for cannabinoids have not been observed.

Dosage Forms Excipient information presented when available (limited, particularly for generics); consult specific product labeling.

Tablet, oral:
Atripla®: Efavirenz 600 mg, emtricitabine 200 mg, and tenofovir disoproxil fumarate 300 mg

References

DHHS Panel on Antiretroviral Guidelines for Adults and Adolescents. Guidelines for the use of antiretroviral agents in HIV-1-infected adults and adolescents, Department of Health and Human Services. May 1, 2014. Available at http://www.aidsinfo.nih.gov/ContentFiles/AdultandAdolescentGL.pdf

DHHS Panel on Antiretroviral Therapy and Medical Management of HIV-Infected Children. Guidelines for the use of antiretroviral agents in pediatric HIV infection. February 12, 2014. Available at http://aidsinfo.nih.gov

DHHS Panel on Treatment of HIV-Infected Pregnant Women and Prevention of Perinatal Transmission. Recommendations for the use of antiretroviral drugs in pregnant HIV-1-infected women for maternal health and interventions to reduce perinatal HIV-1 transmission in the United States. March 28, 2014. Available at http://aidsinfo.nih.gov

Giacomet V, Mora S, Martelli L, Merlo M, Sciannamblo M, Viganò A. A 12-month treatment with tenofovir does not impair bone mineral accrual in HIV-infected children. *J Acquir Immune Defic Syndr.* 2005;40(4):448-450.

Hazra R, Gafni RI, Maldarelli F, et al. Tenofovir disoproxil fumarate and an optimized background regimen of antiretroviral agents as salvage therapy for pediatric HIV infection. *Pediatrics.* 2005;116(6):e846-e854.

Purdy JB, Gafni RI, Reynolds JC, Zeichner S, Hazra R. Decreased bone mineral density with off-label use of tenofovir in children and adolescents infected with human immunodeficiency virus. *J Pediatr.* 2008;152(4):582-584.

◆ **Effer-K** see Potassium Bicarbonate on page 1707

◆ **Effexor XR** see Venlafaxine on page 2125

◆ **Eformoterol and Budesonide** see Budesonide and Formoterol on page 314

◆ **Efudex** see Fluorouracil (Topical) on page 900

◆ **Efudex® (Can)** see Fluorouracil (Topical) on page 900

◆ **EHDP** see Etidronate on page 810

◆ **Elavil** see Amitriptyline on page 133

◆ **Electrolyte Lavage Solution** see Polyethylene Glycol-Electrolyte Solution on page 1697

◆ **Elestat** see Epinastine on page 761

◆ **Elestrin** see Estradiol (Systemic) on page 796

◆ **Elidel** see Pimecrolimus on page 1675

◆ **Eligard** see Leuprolide on page 1215

◆ **Elimite** see Permethrin on page 1647

◆ **Eliphos** see Calcium Acetate on page 344

◆ **Elitek** see Rasburicase on page 1808

◆ **Elixophyllin** see Theophylline on page 2005

◆ **ElixSure Congestion [OTC]** see Pseudoephedrine on page 1770

◆ **ElixSure Cough [OTC]** see Dextromethorphan on page 636

◆ **Elocom (Can)** see Mometasone (Topical) on page 1435

◆ **Elocon** see Mometasone (Topical) on page 1435

◆ **Eloctate** see Antihemophilic Factor (Recombinant) on page 172

◆ **Eloxatin** see Oxaliplatin on page 1557

◆ **Elspar [DSC]** see Asparaginase (E. coli) on page 208

◆ **Elta Lite Tar [OTC]** see Coal Tar on page 532

◆ **Elta Tar [OTC]** see Coal Tar on page 532

◆ **Eltor® (Can)** see Pseudoephedrine on page 1770

◆ **Eltroxin (Can)** see Levothyroxine on page 1234

◆ **E-Max-1000 [OTC]** see Vitamin E on page 2148

◆ **Emend** see Aprepitant on page 190

◆ **Emend** see Fosaprepitant on page 934

◆ **Emend® (Can)** see Aprepitant on page 190

◆ **Emend® IV (Can)** see Fosaprepitant on page 934

◆ **EMLA®** see Lidocaine and Prilocaine on page 1246

◆ **Emo-Cort® (Can)** see Hydrocortisone (Topical) on page 1038

◆ **Emorex Gel [OTC] (Can)** see Coal Tar on page 532

◆ **Emtec** see Acetaminophen and Codeine on page 53

Emtricitabine (em trye SYE ta been)

Related Information
Adult and Adolescent HIV on page 2348
Pediatric HIV on page 2338
Perinatal HIV on page 2356

Brand Names: U.S. Emtriva

Brand Names: Canada Emtriva®

Therapeutic Category Antiretroviral Agent; HIV Agents (Anti-HIV Agents); Nucleoside Reverse Transcriptase Inhibitor (NRTI)

Generic Availability (U.S.) No

Use Treatment of HIV infection in combination with other antiretroviral agents (FDA approved in all ages). **Note:** HIV regimens consisting of **three** antiretroviral agents are strongly recommended.

Pregnancy Risk Factor B

Pregnancy Considerations Adverse events were not observed in animal studies. Emtricitabine has a high level of transfer across the human placenta; no increased risk of overall birth defects has been observed according to data collected by the antiretroviral pregnancy registry. Cases of lactic acidosis/hepatic steatosis syndrome related to mitochondrial toxicity have been reported in pregnant women with prolonged use of nucleoside analogues. It is not known if pregnancy itself potentiates this known side effect; however, women may be at increased risk of lactic acidosis and liver damage. In addition, these adverse events are similar to other rare but life-threatening syndromes which occur during pregnancy (eg, HELLP syndrome). Hepatic enzymes and electrolytes should be monitored in women receiving nucleoside analogues and clinicians should watch for early signs of the syndrome. In addition, mitochondrial dysfunction may develop in infants following in utero exposure. A pharmacokinetic study shows a slight decrease in emtricitabine serum levels during the third trimester and immediately postpartum; however, there is no clear need to adjust the dose. The

DHHS Perinatal HIV Guidelines consider emtricitabine with tenofovir to be a preferred NRTI backbone in antiretroviral-naïve pregnant women. The DHHS Perinatal HIV Guidelines consider emtricitabine plus tenofovir a recommended dual NRTI/NtRTI backbone for HIV/HBV coinfected pregnant women.

Regardless of CD4 count or HIV RNA copy number, all HIV-infected pregnant women should receive a combination antiretroviral (ARV) drug regimen. A combination of antepartum, intrapartum, and infant ARV prophylaxis is recommended. ARV therapy should be started as soon as possible in women with symptomatic infection. Although earlier initiation may be more effective in reducing the perinatal transmission of HIV, initiation may be delayed until after 12 weeks gestation in women who do not require immediate treatment after careful consideration of maternal conditions (eg, nausea and vomiting) and the potential risks of first trimester fetal exposure for specific agents. A scheduled cesarean delivery at 38 weeks gestation is recommended for all women with HIV RNA >1000 copies/mL or unknown concentrations near delivery in order to decrease transmission. If ARV therapy must be interrupted for <24 hours during the peripartum period, stop then restart all medications simultaneously in order to decrease the chance of developing resistance. Long-term follow-up is recommended for all infants exposed to ARV medications. In couples who want to conceive, the HIV-infected partner should attain maximum viral suppression prior to conception.

Healthcare providers are encouraged to enroll pregnant women exposed to antiretroviral medications in the Antiretroviral Pregnancy Registry (1-800-258-4263 or www.APRegistry.com). Healthcare providers caring for HIV-infected women and their infants may contact the National Perinatal HIV Hotline (888-448-8765) for clinical consultation (DHHS [perinatal], 2014).

Breast-Feeding Considerations Emtricitabine is excreted into breast milk. Maternal or infant antiretroviral therapy does not completely eliminate the risk of postnatal HIV transmission. In addition, multiclass-resistant virus has been detected in breast-feeding infants despite maternal therapy. Therefore, in the United States, where formula is accessible, affordable, safe, and sustainable, and the risk of infant mortality due to diarrhea and respiratory infections is low, complete avoidance of breast-feeding by HIV-infected women is recommended to decrease potential transmission of HIV (DHHS [perinatal], 2014).

Contraindications Hypersensitivity to emtricitabine or any component

Warnings Cases of lactic acidosis, severe hepatomegaly with steatosis, and death have been reported in patients receiving nucleoside analogues **[U.S. Boxed Warning]**; most of these cases have been in women; prolonged nucleoside use, obesity, and prior liver disease may be risk factors; use with extreme caution in patients with other risk factors for liver disease; discontinue therapy in patients who develop laboratory or clinical evidence of lactic acidosis or pronounced hepatotoxicity. Safety and efficacy during coinfection of HIV and HBV have not been established; acute, severe exacerbations of HBV have been reported following discontinuation of antiretroviral therapy **[U.S. Boxed Warning]**; monitor hepatic function closely for several months after discontinuation; initiate antihepatitis B therapy if needed. Not indicated for treatment of chronic hepatitis B. All patients with HIV should be tested for HBV prior to initiation of treatment. Use with caution in patients with known or suspected hepatitis B or C infection; monitoring of liver function is recommended.

The oral solution formulation contains propylene glycol; toxicities have been reported with use of products containing propylene glycol, including hyperosmolality, lactic acidosis, seizures, and respiratory depression; in neonates, large amounts of propylene glycol delivered orally, intravenously (eg, >3000 mg/day), or topically have been associated with potentially fatal toxicities which can include metabolic acidosis, seizures, renal failure, and CNS depression; use the oral solution containing propylene glycol with caution (AAP, 1997; Shehab, 2009).

Precautions Use with caution and reduce dosage in patients with impaired renal function. Fat redistribution and accumulation [ie, central obesity, peripheral wasting, facial wasting, breast enlargement, dorsocervical fat enlargement (buffalo hump), and cushingoid appearance] have been observed in patients receiving antiretroviral agents (causal relationship not established).

Immune reconstitution syndrome (an acute inflammatory response to residual or indolent opportunistic infections) may occur in HIV patients during initial treatment with combination antiretroviral agents; this syndrome may require further patient assessment and therapy. Autoimmune disorders (eg, Grave's disease, Guillain-Barré syndrome, and polymyositis) have been reported in patients experiencing immune reconstitution; time to onset is variable and may occur many months after antiretroviral treatment is initiated.

Hyperpigmentation may occur at a higher frequency in pediatric patients compared to adults [children: 32%; adults: 2% to 6% (may be higher in African-Americans)]; occurs primarily on palms and/or soles but may include tongue, arms, lips, and nails; generally mild, asymptomatic, nonprogressive, and without associated local reactions, such as pruritus or rash. Do not administer Emtriva with other emtricitabine-containing medications (eg, Atripla, Complera, Stribild or Truvada) or with medications that contain lamivudine (eg, Epivir, Epivir-HBV, Combivir, Epzicom, or Trizivir).

Adverse Reactions

Central nervous system: Abnormal dreams, depression, dizziness, headache, insomnia, neuropathy/neuritis

Dermatologic: Hyperpigmentation (primarily of palms and/or soles but may include tongue, arms, lip and nails; generally mild and nonprogressive without associated local reactions such as pruritus or rash), rash (includes pruritus, maculopapular rash, vesiculobullous rash, pustular rash, and allergic reaction)

Endocrine & metabolic: Disordered glucose homeostasis, serum amylase increased, serum triglycerides increased

Gastrointestinal: Abdominal pain, diarrhea, dyspepsia, nausea, serum amylase increased, vomiting

Genitourinary: Hematuria

Hematologic: Anemia, neutropenia

Hepatic: Alkaline phosphatase increased, bilirubin increased, transaminases increased

Neuromuscular & skeletal: Arthralgia, CPK increased, creatinine kinase increased, myalgia, paresthesia, weakness

Respiratory: Cough, respiratory tract infection (upper), pharyngitis, rhinitis, sinusitis

Rare but important or life-threatening: Immune reconstitution syndrome

Drug Interactions

Metabolism/Transport Effects None known.

Avoid Concomitant Use

Avoid concomitant use of Emtricitabine with any of the following: LamiVUDine

Increased Effect/Toxicity

The levels/effects of Emtricitabine may be increased by: Ganciclovir-Valganciclovir; LamiVUDine; Ribavirin

Decreased Effect There are no known significant interactions involving a decrease in effect.

Food Interactions Food decreases peak plasma concentrations, but does not alter the extent of absorption or ▶

overall systemic exposure. Management: Administer without regard to meals.

Stability

Capsules: Store at 25°C (77°F); excursions permitted to 15°C to 30°C (59°F to 86°F).

Oral solution: Store at 2°C to 8°C (36°F to 46°F). Use within 3 months if stored at 25°C (77°F) with excursions permitted to 15°C to 30°C (59°F to 86°F).

Mechanism of Action Nucleoside reverse transcriptase inhibitor; emtricitabine is a cytosine analogue which is phosphorylated intracellularly to emtricitabine 5'-triphosphate which interferes with HIV viral RNA dependent DNA polymerase resulting in inhibition of viral replication.

Pharmacokinetics (Adult data unless noted)

Absorption: Rapid, extensive

Protein binding: <4%

Metabolism: Converted intracellularly to the active triphosphate form; undergoes minimal biotransformation via oxidation and glucuronide conjugation

Bioavailability:

Capsules: 93%

Oral solution: 75%

Note: Relative bioavailability of solution to capsule: 80%

Half-life: Normal renal function:

Infants, Children, and Adolescents: Elimination half-life (emtricitabine):

Single dose: 11 hours

Multiple dose: 7.9 to 9.5 hours

Infants 0 to 3 months (n=20; median age: 26 days): 12.1 ± 3.1 hours

Infants 3 to 24 months (n=14): 8.9 ± 3.2 hours

Children 25 months to 6 years (n=19): 11.3 ± 6.4 hours

Children 7 to 12 years (n=17): 8.2 ± 3.2 hours

Adolescents 13 to 17 years (n=27): 8.9 ± 3.3 hours

Adults:

Elimination half-life (emtricitabine): 10 hours

Intracellular half-life (emtricitabine 5'-triphosphate): 39 hours

Time to peak serum concentration: 1 to 2 hours

Elimination: Urine (86% of dose, primarily as unchanged drug; 13% as metabolites; 9% of dose as oxidative metabolite; 4% as glucuronide metabolite); feces (14% of dose)

Clearance: Renal clearance is greater than creatinine clearance; thus, emtricitabine may be eliminated by both glomerular filtration and active tubular secretion

Dosing: Neonatal HIV infection, treatment: Note: Use in combination with other antiretroviral agents. Oral solution: 3 mg/kg/dose once daily

Dosing adjustment in renal impairment: Monitor clinical response and renal function closely. There are no dosage adjustments provided in the manufacturer's labeling (not studied); however, consider a reduction in the dose and/or an increase in the dosing interval similar to dosage adjustments for adults.

Dosing: Usual

Pediatric: **HIV infection, treatment: Note:** Use in combination with other antiretroviral agents. Oral:

Infants 1 to <3 months: Oral solution: 3 mg/kg/dose once daily

Infants ≥3 months, Children, and Adolescents:

Oral solution: 6 mg/kg/dose once daily; maximum daily dose: 240 mg/**day**

Capsules: Patient weight >33 kg and able to swallow capsule whole: 200 mg once daily

Adolescents ≥18 years:

Capsules: 200 mg once daily

Oral solution: 240 mg once daily

Adult: **HIV infection, treatment: Note:** Use in combination with other antiretroviral agents. Oral:

Capsules: 200 mg once daily

Oral solution: 240 mg once daily

Dosing adjustment in renal impairment: Monitor clinical response and renal function closely. Dialysis: 30% of the dose is removed by hemodialysis (over 3 hours)

Infants, Children, and Adolescents <18 years: There are no dosage adjustments provided in the manufacturer's labeling; however, may consider a reduction in the dose and/or an increase in the dosing interval similar to dosage adjustments for adults.

Adolescents ≥18 years and Adults:

CrCl ≥50 mL/minute: No dosage adjustment necessary

CrCl 30 to 49 mL/minute: Capsule: 200 mg every 48 hours; oral solution: 120 mg every 24 hours

CrCl 15 to 29 mL/minute: Capsule: 200 mg every 72 hours; oral solution: 80 mg every 24 hours

CrCl <15 mL/minute (including hemodialysis patients): **Note:** If dose is given on day of dialysis, administer dose after dialysis: Capsule: 200 mg every 96 hours; oral solution: 60 mg every 24 hours

Dosing adjustment in hepatic impairment: There are no dosage adjustments provided in the manufacturer's labeling; however, emtricitabine is not metabolized by liver enzymes so the impact of liver impairment should be minimal; monitor patients closely.

Administration May be administered without regard to food

Monitoring Parameters Note: Monitor CD4 percentage (if <5 years of age) or CD4 count (if ≥5 years of age) at least every 3 to 4 months (DHHS [pediatric], 2014)

Patients should be screened for hepatitis B infection before starting therapy. Prior to initiation of therapy: Genotypic resistance testing, CD4 and viral load (every 3 to 4 months), CBC with differential, LFTs, BUN, creatinine, electrolytes, glucose, urinalysis (every 6 to 12 months), and assessment of readiness for adherence with medication regimen. At initiation and with any change in treatment regimen: CBC with differential, electrolytes, calcium, phosphorus, glucose, LFTs, bilirubin, urinalysis (at initiation), BUN, creatinine, albumin, total protein, lipid panel (at initiation), CD4, and viral load. After 1 to 2 weeks of therapy: Signs of medication toxicity and adherence. After 2 to 4 weeks of therapy: CBC with differential, viral load, signs of medication toxicity, and adherence; then every 3 to 4 months: CBC with differential, electrolytes, glucose, LFTs, bilirubin, BUN, creatinine, CD4, viral load, signs of medication toxicity, and adherence. Every 6 to 12 months: Lipid panel and urinalysis. CD4 monitoring frequency may be decreased to every 6 to 12 months in children who are adherent to therapy if the value is well above the threshold for opportunistic infections, viral suppression is sustained, and the clinical status is stable for more than 2 to 3 years (DHHS [pediatric], 2014). Monitor for growth and development, signs of HIV-specific physical conditions, HIV disease progression, opportunistic infections, skin rash, or hyperpigmentation.

Additional Information Emtricitabine is the (-) enantiomer of 2', 3'-dideoxy-5-fluoro-3'-thiacytidine (FTC), a fluorinated derivative of lamivudine.

Mutation in the HIV reverse transcriptase gene at codon 184, M184V/I (ie, substitution of methionine by valine or isoleucine) is associated with resistance to emtricitabine. Emtricitabine-resistant isolates (M184V/I) are cross-resistant to lamivudine and zalcitabine. HIV-1 isolates containing the K65R mutation show reduced susceptibility to emtricitabine.

Dosage Forms Excipient information presented when available (limited, particularly for generics); consult specific product labeling.

Capsule, Oral:

Emtriva: 200 mg [contains fd&c blue #2 (indigotine)]

Solution, Oral:
Emtriva: 10 mg/mL (170 mL) [contains edetate disodium, fd&c yellow #6 (sunset yellow), methylparaben, propylene glycol, propylparaben; cotton candy flavor]

References

American Academy of Pediatrics Committee on Drugs. "Inactive" ingredients in pharmaceutical products: update (subject review). *Pediatrics.* 1997;99(2):268-278.

Bang LM, Scott LJ. Emtricitabine: an antiretroviral agent for HIV infection. *Drugs.* 2003;63(22):2413-2424.

DHHS Panel on Antiretroviral Guidelines for Adults and Adolescents. Guidelines for the use of antiretroviral agents in HIV-1-infected adults and adolescents, Department of Health and Human Services. May 1, 2014. Available at http://www.aidsinfo.nih.gov/ContentFiles/AdultandAdolescentGL.pdf

DHHS Panel on Antiretroviral Therapy and Medical Management of HIV-Infected Children. Guidelines for the use of antiretroviral agents in pediatric HIV infection. February 12, 2014. Available at http://aidsinfo.nih.gov

DHHS Panel on Treatment of HIV-Infected Pregnant Women and Prevention of Perinatal Transmission. Recommendations for the use of antiretroviral drugs in pregnant HIV-1-infected women for maternal health and interventions to reduce perinatal HIV-1 transmission in the United States. March 28, 2014. Available at http://aidsinfo.nih.gov

Frampton JE, Perry CM. Emtricitabine: a review of its use in the management of HIV infection. *Drugs.* 2005;65(10):1427-1448.

Morris JL, Kraus DM. New antiretroviral therapies for pediatric HIV infection. *J Pediatr Pharmacol Ther.* 2005;10:215-247.

Shehab N, Lewis CL, Streetman DD, Donn SM. Exposure to the pharmaceutical excipients benzyl alcohol and propylene glycol among critically ill neonates. *Pediatr Crit Care Med.* 2009;10 (2):256-259.

Wang LH, Wiznia AA, Rathore MH, et al. Pharmacokinetics and safety of single oral doses of emtricitabine in human immunodeficiency virus-infected children. *Antimicrob Agents Chemother.* 2004;48 (1):183-191.

Emtricitabine and Tenofovir
(em trye SYE ta been & ten OF oh vir)

Related Information

Adult and Adolescent HIV *on page 2348*
Pediatric HIV *on page 2338*
Perinatal HIV *on page 2356*

Brand Names: U.S. Truvada

Brand Names: Canada Truvada

Therapeutic Category Antiretroviral Agent; HIV Agents (Anti-HIV Agents); Nucleoside Reverse Transcriptase Inhibitor (NRTI); Nucleotide Reverse Transcriptase Inhibitor (NRTI)

Generic Availability (U.S.) No

Use Treatment of HIV infection in combination with other antiretroviral agents (FDA approved in ages ≥12 years weighing at least 35 kg and adults); **Note:** HIV regimens consisting of **three** antiretroviral agents are strongly recommended; pre-exposure prophylaxis (PrEP) in combination with safer sex practices for prevention of HIV infection in adults at high risk (FDA approved in adults)

Medication Guide Available Yes

Pregnancy Risk Factor B

Pregnancy Considerations Animal reproduction studies have not been conducted with this combination. Although approved for use in combination with safer sex practices for the prevention of HIV-1 infection in adults who are at high risk for acquiring HIV (pre-exposure prophylaxis [PrEP]), data on use in heterosexual HIV serodiscordant couples wishing to conceive is under study. Women of reproductive age should have a pregnancy test prior to starting PrEP and at regular intervals during therapy. In addition to pregnancy testing, uninfected women considering PrEP therapy should also undergo screening for HIV and other sexually transmitted diseases. Serodiscordant couples wishing to conceive should seek expert consultation to determine the safest approach for their specific situation. If HIV infection is documented during PrEP therapy, the antiretroviral agents should be discontinued in order to minimize drug resistance. If pregnancy is

detected during therapy, the potential risks and benefits of continuing PrEP during pregnancy should be discussed (DHHS [perinatal], 2014). Refer to individual monographs for additional information.

The DHHS Perinatal HIV Guidelines consider emtricitabine in combination with tenofovir to be a preferred NRTI backbone for use in antiretroviral-naive pregnant women (DHHS [perinatal], 2014).

Healthcare providers are encouraged to enroll pregnant women exposed to antiretroviral medications in the Antiretroviral Pregnancy Registry (1-800-258-4263 or www.APRegistry.com). Healthcare providers caring for HIV-infected women and their infants may contact the National Perinatal HIV Hotline (888-448-8765) for clinical consultation (DHHS [perinatal], 2014).

Breast-Feeding Considerations Emtricitabine and tenofovir are excreted into breast milk. Refer to individual monographs. Use in combination with safer sex practices for pre-exposure prophylaxis (PrEP) in lactating women who are HIV-uninfected is limited (DHHS [perinatal], 2014).

Contraindications Hypersensitivity to emtricitabine, tenofovir, or any component
Additional contraindications:
Pre-exposure prophylaxis: Use in a patient with unknown or positive HIV-1 status
HIV treatment: Monotherapy

Warnings Cases of lactic acidosis, severe hepatomegaly with steatosis, and death have been reported in patients receiving nucleoside analogues, including emtricitabine and tenofovir **[U.S. Boxed Warning]**; most of these cases have been in women; prolonged nucleoside use, obesity, and prior liver disease may be risk factors; use with extreme caution in patients with other risk factors for liver disease; discontinue therapy in patients who develop laboratory or clinical evidence of lactic acidosis or pronounced hepatotoxicity.

Safety and efficacy during coinfection of HIV and HBV have not been established; acute, severe exacerbations of HBV have been reported following discontinuation of emtricitabine and tenofovir **[U.S. Boxed Warning]**; monitor hepatic function closely for several months after discontinuing; initiate antihepatitis B therapy if needed. Not indicated for treatment of chronic hepatitis B. All patients with HIV should be tested for HBV prior to initiation of treatment. Use with caution in patients with known or suspected hepatitis B or C infection; monitoring of liver function is recommended.

Both emtricitabine and tenofovir are primarily eliminated by the kidney; when used for treatment of HIV, dosage adjustment is required in patients with CrCl <50 mL/minute; do not use in patients with severe renal impairment (CrCl <30 mL/minute or patients requiring hemodialysis); for pre-exposure prophylaxis, use should be avoided in patients with CrCl <60 mL/minute. Renal toxicity including acute renal failure and/or Fanconi syndrome (renal tubular injury with severe hypophosphatemia) have been reported with tenofovir use; risk may be increased in patients with preexisting renal disease, underlying systemic disease, or those taking nephrotoxic medications; adults with a low body weight and those taking medications that increase tenofovir serum concentration may also be at increased risk for nephrotoxicity; cases of nephrotoxicity have been reported in adolescents receiving tenofovir-containing regimens. Avoid use with concurrent or recent nephrotoxic therapy. Evaluate and monitor renal function, including calculation of creatinine clearance, at baseline and during therapy in all patients (regardless of age); monitor serum phosphorus. Use with caution in patients with low body weight or concurrent medications which increase tenofovir levels.

◄ Truvada contains emtricitabine and tenofovir as a fixed-dose combination; do not administer Truvada with other emtricitabine- or tenofovir-containing medications (eg, Atripla, Complera, Emtriva, Stribild, or Viread) or with medications that contain lamivudine (eg, Epivir, Epivir-HBV, Combivir, Epzicom, or Trizivir). Do not coadminister with adefovir; may diminish efficacy of tenofovir.

Precautions Use with caution in patients with hepatic impairment. Significant drug interactions may occur. Fat redistribution and accumulation [ie, central obesity, peripheral wasting, facial wasting, breast enlargement, dorsocervical fat enlargement (buffalo hump), and cushingoid appearance] have been observed in patients receiving antiretroviral agents (causal relationship not established).

Immune reconstitution syndrome (an acute inflammatory response to residual or indolent opportunistic infections) may occur in HIV patients during initial treatment with combination antiretroviral agents; this syndrome may require further patient assessment and therapy. Autoimmune disorders (eg, Graves' disease, Guillain-Barré syndrome, and polymyositis) have been reported in patients experiencing immune reconstitution; time to onset is variable and may occur many months after antiretroviral treatment is initiated.

Emtricitabine-associated hyperpigmentation may occur at a higher frequency in pediatric patients compared to adults [children: 32%; adults: 2% to 6% (may be higher in African-Americans)]; occurs primarily on palms and/or soles but may include tongue, arms, lips, and nails; generally mild, asymptomatic, nonprogressive, and without associated local reactions, such as pruritus or rash. Safety and efficacy have not been established in patients <12 years of age.

Tenofovir-associated osteomalacia and reduced bone mineral density (BMD) may occur; long-term effects in humans are not known. Postmarketing cases of osteomalacia which may increase risk of bone fractures have also been reported in association with proximal renal tubulopathy. Recent studies suggest that tenofovir-related bone loss may be greater in children who are less mature (eg, Tanner stage 1-2) than in those who are more physically mature (Tanner ≥3). A significant decrease in lumbar spine BMD (>6%) was reported in five of 15 pediatric patients who received a tenofovir-containing regimen for 48 weeks. No orthopedic fractures occurred, but two patients required discontinuation of tenofovir. All five patients with a decrease in BMD were virologic responders and prepubertal (Tanner Stage 1). This study found a moderately strong correlation between decreases in bone mineral density z scores at week 48 and age at baseline. No correlation between decreases in bone mineral density z scores and tenofovir dose or pharmacokinetics was observed; BMD loss may limit the usefulness of tenofovir in prepubertal children [DHHS (pediatric), 2014; Giacomet, 2005; Hazra, 2005; Purdy, 2008]. Monitor BMD for potential bone toxicities during therapy; supplementation with calcium and vitamin D may be beneficial but has not been studied.

When used for pre-exposure prophylaxis (PrEP), confirm HIV-1 negative status immediately before and at least every 3 months during therapy **[U.S. Boxed Warning]**; increased risk of drug resistant HIV-1 variants with PrEP use if patient has undetected acute HIV-1 infection. Some HIV-1 tests (eg, rapid tests/HIV antibody test) do not detect acute HIV-1 infection; screen PrEP candidates for acute viral infections and potential exposure events ≤1 month of starting PrEP; if infections or events exist, wait 1 month to start PrEP and reconfirm HIV-1 negative status. Do not start PrEP if signs or symptoms of acute HIV-1 infection are present unless HIV-1 negative status is confirmed by a test approved by the Food and Drug Administration (FDA)

as an aid to detect HIV-1 infection (including acute or primary infection). PrEP should be accompanied by a comprehensive HIV-1 prevention program (eg, risk reduction counseling, access to condoms), with particular emphasis on medication adherence; regular monitoring [eg, HIV status of patient and partner(s), risk behavior, adherence, adverse effects, sexually transmitted infections that facilitate HIV-1 transmission] is highly recommended.

The use of antiretroviral regimens that only contain triple nucleoside reverse transcriptase inhibitors (NRTIs) are generally less effective than regimens containing two NRTIs and either a non-nucleoside reverse transcriptase inhibitor or protease inhibitor; use triple NRTI-containing regimens with great caution; early virological failure and high rates of resistance may occur; closely monitor for virologic failure and consider treatment modification.

Adverse Reactions The adverse reaction profile of combination therapy has not been established. See individual agents.

Drug Interactions

Metabolism/Transport Effects Refer to individual components.

Avoid Concomitant Use

Avoid concomitant use of Emtricitabine and Tenofovir with any of the following: Adefovir; Dabigatran Etexilate; Didanosine; LamiVUDine; VinCRIStine (Liposomal)

Increased Effect/Toxicity

Emtricitabine and Tenofovir may increase the levels/effects of: Adefovir; Aminoglycosides; Darunavir; Didanosine

The levels/effects of Emtricitabine and Tenofovir may be increased by: Acyclovir-Valacyclovir; Adefovir; Aminoglycosides; Atazanavir; Cidofovir; Darunavir; Diclofenac (Systemic); Ganciclovir-Valganciclovir; LamiVUDine; Lopinavir; Nonsteroidal Anti-Inflammatory Agents; Ribavirin; Simeprevir; Telaprevir

Decreased Effect

Emtricitabine and Tenofovir may decrease the levels/effects of: Afatinib; Atazanavir; Brentuximab Vedotin; Dabigatran Etexilate; Didanosine; DOXOrubicin (Conventional); Linagliptin; P-glycoprotein/ABCB1 Substrates; Simeprevir; Tipranavir; VinCRIStine (Liposomal)

The levels/effects of Emtricitabine and Tenofovir may be decreased by: Adefovir; Tipranavir

Food Interactions See individual agents.

Stability Store tablets at 25°C (77°F); excursions permitted to 15°C to 30°C (59°F to 86°F). Keep container tightly closed; do not use if seal on bottle is broken or missing. Dispense only in original container.

Mechanism of Action Nucleoside and nucleotide reverse transcriptase inhibitor combination; emtricitabine is a cytosine analogue while tenofovir disoproxil fumarate (TDF) is an analog of adenosine 5'-monophosphate. Each drug interferes with HIV viral RNA dependent DNA polymerase resulting in inhibition of viral replication.

Pharmacokinetics (Adult data unless noted) One Truvada tablet is bioequivalent to one emtricitabine 200 mg capsule and one tenofovir 300 mg tablet (single dose study); see individual agents

Dosing: Usual

Pediatric: **HIV infection, treatment:** Use in combination with other antiretroviral agents.

Children and Adolescents <12 years or <35 kg: Not intended for use; product is a fixed-dose combination; safety and efficacy have not been established in these patients

Children and Adolescents ≥12 years and ≥35 kg: Oral: One tablet once daily

Adult:

HIV infection, treatment: Oral: One tablet once daily

Pre-exposure prophylaxis (PrEP) for prevention of HIV infection in uninfected high-risk individuals:
Oral: One tablet once daily

Dosing adjustment in renal impairment: Note: Closely monitor clinical response and renal function in these patients; clinical effectiveness and safety of these guidelines have not been evaluated.

HIV infection, treatment:

Children ≥12 years and Adolescents: CrCl <30 mL/minute or patients requiring hemodialysis: Use not recommended (DHHS [pediatric], 2014).

Adults: Manufacturer's labeling:

CrCl ≥50 mL/minute: No adjustment necessary.

CrCl 30-49 mL/minute: Administer every 48 hours.

CrCl <30 mL/minute or patients requiring hemodialysis: Use not recommended.

Pre-exposure prophylaxis (PrEP): Adults:

CrCl >60 mL/minute: No adjustment necessary.

CrCl <60 mL/minute: Use not recommended.

Dosing adjustment in hepatic impairment: There are no dosage adjustments provided in the manufacturer's labeling; however, no dosing adjustments are necessary for tenofovir in hepatic impairment. No specific data is available on emtricitabine in hepatic impairment, but given its limited hepatic metabolism, the impact of liver impairment should be minimal; need for dose adjustment is unlikely.

Administration May be administered without regard to food

Monitoring Parameters

HIV treatment: Note: Monitor CD4 percentage (if <5 years of age) or CD4 count (if ≥5 years of age) at least every 3 to 4 months (DHHS [pediatric], 2014).

Patients should be screened for hepatitis B infection before starting therapy. Prior to initiation of therapy: HIV genotypic resistance testing, CD4 and viral load (every 3 to 4 months), CBC with differential, LFTs, BUN, creatinine, urine dipstick for protein and glucose, electrolytes, glucose, urinalysis (every 6 to 12 months), and assessment of readiness for adherence with medication regimen. At initiation and with any change in treatment regimen: CBC with differential, electrolytes, calcium, phosphate, glucose, LFTs, bilirubin, urinalysis (at initiation), BUN, creatinine, albumin, total protein, lipid panel (at initiation), CD4, and viral load. After 1 to 2 weeks of therapy: Signs of medication toxicity and adherence. After 2 to 4 weeks of therapy: CBC with differential, viral load, signs of medication toxicity, and adherence; then every 3 to 4 months: CBC with differential, electrolytes, glucose, LFTs, bilirubin, BUN, creatinine, CD4, viral load, signs of medication toxicity, and adherence. Every 6 to 12 months: Lipid panel and urinalysis. CD4 monitoring frequency may be decreased to every 6 to 12 months in children who are adherent to therapy if the value is well above the threshold for opportunistic infections, viral suppression is sustained, and the clinical status is stable for more than 2 to 3 years (DHHS [pediatric], 2014). Monitor for growth and development, signs of HIV-specific physical conditions, HIV disease progression, opportunistic infections, lactic acidosis, hyperpigmentation, or bone abnormalities. Consider bone mineral density assessment for all patients with a history of pathologic bone fractures or other risk factors for osteoporosis or bone loss. Some experts recommend obtaining a DXA scan prior to therapy and 6 months into therapy, especially for patients in pre- and early puberty (Tanner stages 1 and 2) (DHHS [pediatric], 2014). In patients coinfected with HBV, monitor hepatic function closely (clinically and with laboratory tests) for at least several months after discontinuing emtricitabine and tenofovir therapy.

HIV-1 pre-exposure prophylaxis (PrEP): Pregnancy test for women receiving PrEP (every visit); documented negative HIV test (immediately prior to use, every 2 to 3 months, and following discontinuation of PrEP), assess risk behaviors and symptoms of sexually transmitted infections (STIs) or acute HIV-1 infection and provide condoms (immediately prior to use, then every 2 to 3 months during therapy); BUN and serum creatinine (prior to initiation, 3 months after initiation, then every 6 months); testing for HBV (prior to initiation) and STIs (prior to initiation, then at least every 6 months, even if asymptomatic) (CDC, 2011; CDC, 2012).

Additional Information Emtricitabine is the (-) enantiomer of 2', 3'-dideoxy-5-fluoro-3'-thiacytidine (FTC), a fluorinated derivative of lamivudine.

Mutation in the HIV reverse transcriptase gene at codon 184, M184V/I (ie, substitution of methionine by valine or isoleucine) is associated with resistance to emtricitabine. Emtricitabine-resistant isolates (M184V/I) are cross-resistant to lamivudine and zalcitabine. HIV-1 isolates containing the K65R mutation show reduced susceptibility to emtricitabine.

Dosage Forms Excipient information presented when available (limited, particularly for generics); consult specific product labeling.

Tablet:

Truvada: Emtricitabine 200 mg and tenofovir disoproxil fumarate 300 mg

References

Centers for Disease Control and Prevention (CDC). Interim guidance for clinicians considering the use of preexposure prophylaxis for the prevention of HIV infection in heterosexually active adults. *MMWR Morb Mortal Wkly Rep*. 2012;61(31):586-589.

Centers for Disease Control and Prevention (CDC). Interim guidance: preexposure prophylaxis for the prevention of HIV infection in men who have sex with men. *MMWR Morb Mortal Wkly Rep*. 2011;60 (3):65-68.

DHHS Panel on Antiretroviral Guidelines for Adults and Adolescents. Guidelines for the use of antiretroviral agents in HIV-1-infected adults and adolescents, Department of Health and Human Services. May 1, 2014. Available at http://www.aidsinfo.nih.gov/ContentFiles/AdultandAdolescentGL.pdf

DHHS Panel on Antiretroviral Therapy and Medical Management of HIV-Infected Children. Guidelines for the use of antiretroviral agents in pediatric HIV infection. February 12, 2014. Available at http://aidsinfo.nih.gov

DHHS Panel on Treatment of HIV-Infected Pregnant Women and Prevention of Perinatal Transmission. Recommendations for the use of antiretroviral drugs in pregnant HIV-1-infected women for maternal health and interventions to reduce perinatal HIV-1 transmission in the United States. March 28, 2014. Available at http://aidsinfo.nih.gov

Giacomet V, Mora S, Martelli L, Merlo M, Sciannamblo M, Viganò A. A 12-month treatment with tenofovir does not impair bone mineral accrual in HIV-infected children. *J Acquir Immune Defic Syndr*. 2005;40(4):448-450.

Hazra R, Gafni RI, Maldarelli F, et al. Tenofovir disoproxil fumarate and an optimized background regimen of antiretroviral agents as salvage therapy for pediatric HIV infection. *Pediatrics*. 2005;116(6):e846-e854.

Purdy JB, Gafni RI, Reynolds JC, Zeichner S, Hazra R. Decreased bone mineral density with off-label use of tenofovir in children and adolescents infected with human immunodeficiency virus. *J Pediatr*. 2008;152(4):582-584.

◆ **Emtricitabine, Efavirenz, and Tenofovir** see Efavirenz, Emtricitabine, and Tenofovir *on page 735*

◆ **Emtriva** see Emtricitabine *on page 738*

◆ **Emtriva® (Can)** see Emtricitabine *on page 738*

Enalapril (e NAL a pril)

Medication Safety Issues

Sound-alike/look-alike issues:

Enalapril may be confused with Anafranil, Elavil, Eldepryl, ramipril

Administration issues:

Significant differences exist between oral and I.V. dosing. Use caution when converting from one route of administration to another.

International issues:

Acepril [Hungary, Switzerland] may be confused with Accupril which is a brand name for quinapril [U.S., Canada, multiple international markets]

Acepril: Brand name for enalapril [Hungary, Switzerland], but also brand name for captopril [Great Britain]; lisinopril [Malaysia]

Brand Names: U.S. Epaned; Vasotec

Brand Names: Canada Apo-Enalapril; Ava-Enalapril; CO Enalapril; Mylan-Enalapril; PMS-Enalapril; PRO-Enalapril; RAN-Enalapril; ratio-Enalapril; Riva-Enalapril; Sandoz-Enalapril; Sig-Enalapril; Taro-Enalapril; Teva-Enalapril; Vasotec

Therapeutic Category Angiotensin-Converting Enzyme (ACE) Inhibitor

Generic Availability (U.S.) May be product dependent

Use Management of mild to severe hypertension (FDA approved in ages 1 month to 16 years and adults), CHF (FDA approved in adults), and asymptomatic left ventricular dysfunction (FDA approved in adults); has also been used to treat proteinuria in steroid-resistant nephrotic syndrome patients

Pregnancy Risk Factor D

Pregnancy Considerations [U.S. Boxed Warning]: Drugs that act on the renin-angiotensin system can cause injury and death to the developing fetus. Discontinue as soon as possible once pregnancy is detected. Enalaprilat, the active metabolite of enalapril, crosses the placenta; teratogenic effects may occur following maternal use during pregnancy. Drugs that act on the renin-angiotensin system are associated with oligohydramnios. Oligohydramnios, due to decreased fetal renal function, may lead to fetal lung hypoplasia and skeletal malformations. The use of these drugs in pregnancy is also associated with anuria, hypotension, renal failure, skull hypoplasia, and death in the fetus/neonate. Chronic maternal hypertension itself is also associated with adverse events in the fetus/infant. ACE inhibitors are not recommended during pregnancy to treat maternal hypertension or heart failure. Use of an ACE inhibitor should also be avoided in any woman of reproductive age. Women who are planning a pregnancy should be considered for other medication options if an ACE inhibitor is currently prescribed or the ACE inhibitor should be discontinued as soon as possible once pregnancy is detected. The exposed fetus should be monitored for fetal growth, amniotic fluid volume, and organ formation. Infants exposed to an ACE inhibitor *in utero* should be monitored for hyperkalemia, hypotension, and oliguria (exchange transfusions or dialysis may be needed). These adverse events are generally associated with maternal use in the second and third trimesters.

Untreated chronic maternal hypertension is also associated with adverse events in the fetus, infant, and mother. The use of ACE inhibitors is not recommended to treat chronic uncomplicated hypertension in pregnant women and should generally be avoided in women of reproductive potential (ACOG, 2013).

Breast-Feeding Considerations Enalapril and enalaprilat are excreted in breast milk. Breast-feeding is not recommended by the manufacturer.

Contraindications Hypersensitivity to enalapril, enalaprilat, any component, or other ACE inhibitors; patients with idiopathic or hereditary angioedema or a history of angioedema with ACE inhibitors; in patients with diabetes, concurrent use with aliskiren

Warnings Angioedema can occur at any time during treatment (especially following first dose). The relative risk of angioedema with ACE inhibitors is higher within the first 30 days of use (compared to >1 year of use), for Black Americans (compared to Whites), for lisinopril or enalapril (compared to captopril), and for patients previously hospitalized within 30 days (Brown, 1996). Angioedema may occur in the head, neck, extremities, or intestines; patients with angioedema of the intestines may present with abdominal pain (with or without nausea or vomiting); angioedema of the larynx, glottis, or tongue may cause airway obstruction, especially in patients with a history of airway surgery. Prolonged monitoring may be required, even in patients with swelling of only the tongue (ie, without respiratory distress) because treatment with corticosteroids and antihistamines may not be sufficient; very rare fatalities have occurred with angioedema of the larynx or tongue; appropriate treatment (eg, establishing patent airway and/or SubQ epinephrine) should be readily available for patients with angioedema of larynx, glottis, or tongue, in whom airway obstruction is likely to occur.

Anaphylactic/anaphylactoid reactions can occur with ACE inhibitors. Life-threatening anaphylactoid reactions may be seen during hemodialysis (eg, CVVHD) with high-flux dialysis membranes (eg, AN69), and rarely, during low density lipoprotein apheresis with dextran sulfate cellulose. Rare cases of anaphylactoid reactions have been reported in patients undergoing sensitization treatment with hymenoptera (bee, wasp) venom while receiving ACE inhibitors.

Enalapril has been associated with rare but potentially fatal cases of agranulocytosis, neutropenia, or leukopenia with myeloid hypoplasia; higher risk for development of neutropenia is associated with renal impairment; risk is further increased in patients with both renal impairment and collagen vascular disease (eg, systemic lupus erythematosus); onset of neutropenia is usually within 3 months of captopril treatment; closely monitor CBC with differential for the first 3 months of therapy and periodically thereafter in these patients; neutrophil count generally returns to baseline within 2 weeks of discontinuation.

ACE inhibitor use has been associated with deterioration of renal function and/or increases in serum creatinine, particularly in patients with low renal blood flow (eg, renal artery stenosis, heart failure) whose glomerular filtration rate (GFR) is dependent on efferent arteriolar vasoconstriction by angiotensin II; deterioration may result in oliguria, acute renal failure, and progressive azotemia. Small increases in serum creatinine may occur following initiation; consider discontinuation only in patients with progressive and/or significant deterioration in renal function.

A rare toxicity associated with ACE inhibitors includes cholestatic jaundice, which may progress to fulminant hepatic necrosis; discontinue if marked elevation of hepatic transaminases or jaundice occurs and initiate appropriate medical treatment.

Drugs that act on the renin-angiotensin system can cause injury and death to the developing fetus. Discontinue as soon as possible once pregnancy is detected **[U.S. Boxed Warning]**. Concomitant use of an ARB or renin inhibitor (eg, aliskiren) is associated with an increased risk of hypotension, hyperkalemia, and renal dysfunction. Concomitant use with aliskiren should be avoided in patients with GFR <60 mL/minute and is contraindicated in patients with diabetes mellitus (regardless of GFR).

Precautions Use with caution in patients with renal impairment; dosage reduction may be necessary; avoid rapid dosage escalation which may lead to further renal impairment. Use with caution in patients with unstented unilateral/bilateral renal artery stenosis. When unstented bilateral renal artery stenosis is present, use is generally avoided due to the elevated risk of deterioration in renal function unless possible benefits outweigh risks.

Use with caution when initiating therapy and in volume-depleted patients; may cause symptomatic hypotension with or without syncope, usually with the first several doses; correct volume depletion prior to initiation; initiate lower doses in patients with sodium or volume depletion; close monitoring of patient is required especially with initial dosing and dosing increases; blood pressure must be lowered at a rate appropriate for the patient's clinical condition. Although dose reduction may be necessary, hypotension alone is not a reason for discontinuation of future ACE inhibitor use especially in patients with heart failure where a reduction in systolic blood pressure is a desirable observation. Use caution in patients with ischemic heart disease or cerebrovascular disease during therapy initiation; observe closely due to the potential consequences posed by falling blood pressure (eg, MI, stroke); fluid replacement, may be required to restore blood pressure; therapy may then be resumed; discontinue therapy in patients whose hypotension recurs. Use with caution in patients with severe aortic stenosis; may reduce coronary perfusion resulting in ischemia. Use with caution in patients with hypertrophic cardiomyopathy (HCM) and outflow tract obstruction since reduction in afterload may worsen symptoms associated with this condition.

May cause hyperkalemia; risk factors include renal dysfunction, diabetes mellitus, concomitant use of potassium-sparing diuretics, potassium supplements, and/or potassium-containing salts; use with caution, if at all, with these agents, and monitor potassium closely.

Use with caution before, during, or immediately after major surgery; cardiopulmonary bypass, intraoperative blood loss or vasodilating anesthesia increases endogenous renin release; use of ACE inhibitors perioperatively will blunt angiotensin II formation and may result in hypotension.

An ACE inhibitor cough is a dry, hacking, nonproductive one that usually occurs within the first few months of treatment and should generally resolve within 1-4 weeks after discontinuation of the ACE inhibitor. In pediatric patients, an isolated dry hacking cough lasting >3 weeks was reported in seven of 42 pediatric patients (17%) receiving ACE inhibitors (von Vigier, 2000); a review of pediatric randomized-controlled ACE inhibitor trials reported a lower incidence of 3.2% (Baker-Smith, 2010). Other causes of cough should be considered (eg, pulmonary congestion in patients with heart failure) and excluded prior to discontinuation.

Adverse Reactions

Cardiovascular: Chest pain, hypotension, orthostatic effect, orthostatic hypotension, syncope

Central nervous system: Dizziness, fatigue, headache

Dermatologic: Skin rash

Gastrointestinal: Abdominal pain, anorexia, constipation, diarrhea, dysgeusia, nausea, vomiting

Neuromuscular & skeletal: Weakness

Renal: Increased serum creatinine, renal insufficiency (in patients with bilateral renal artery stenosis or hypovolemia)

Respiratory: Bronchitis, cough, dyspnea

Rare but important or life-threatening: Acute generalized exanthematous pustulosis, agranulocytosis, alopecia, anaphylactoid reaction, angina pectoris, angioedema, anosmia, arthritis, asthma, ataxia, atrial fibrillation, atrial tachycardia, bone marrow depression, bradycardia, cardiac arrest, cardiac arrhythmia, cerebrovascular accident, cholestatic jaundice, confusion, conjunctivitis, depression, eosinophilia, eosinophilic pneumonitis, erythema multiforme, exfoliative dermatitis, giant-cell arteritis, gynecomastia, hallucination, hemolysis (with G6PD), herpes zoster, IgA vasculitis, increased erythrocyte sedimentation rate, intestinal obstruction, insomnia, interstitial nephritis, leukocytosis, lichenoid eruption, melena, myocardial infarction, myositis, neutropenia, ototoxicity, pancreatitis, pemphigus, pemphigus foliaceus, peripheral neuropathy, positive ANA titer, psychosis, pulmonary edema, pulmonary embolism, pulmonary infarct, pulmonary infiltrates, Raynaud's phenomenon, serositis, Sjogren's syndrome, skin photosensitivity, Stevens-Johnson syndrome, stomatitis, systemic lupus erythematosus, thrombocytopenia, toxic epidermal necrolysis, upper respiratory tract infection, vasculitis, visual hallucination (Doane, 2013)

Drug Interactions

Metabolism/Transport Effects None known.

Avoid Concomitant Use There are no known interactions where it is recommended to avoid concomitant use.

Increased Effect/Toxicity

Enalapril may increase the levels/effects of: Allopurinol; Amifostine; Antihypertensives; AzaTHIOprine; CycloSPORINE (Systemic); DULoxetine; Ferric Gluconate; Gold Sodium Thiomalate; Grass Pollen Allergen Extract (5 Grass Extract); Hypotensive Agents; Iron Dextran Complex; Lithium; Nonsteroidal Anti-Inflammatory Agents; Obinutuzumab; RiTUXimab; Sodium Phosphates

The levels/effects of Enalapril may be increased by: Alfuzosin; Aliskiren; Angiotensin II Receptor Blockers; Barbiturates; Brimonidine (Topical); Canagliflozin; Diazoxide; DPP-IV Inhibitors; Eplerenone; Everolimus; Heparin; Heparin (Low Molecular Weight); Herbs (Hypotensive Properties); Loop Diuretics; MAO Inhibitors; Pentoxifylline; Phosphodiesterase 5 Inhibitors; Potassium Salts; Potassium-Sparing Diuretics; Prostacyclin Analogues; Sirolimus; Temsirolimus; Thiazide Diuretics; TiZANidine; Tolvaptan; Trimethoprim

Decreased Effect

The levels/effects of Enalapril may be decreased by: Antacids; Aprotinin; Herbs (Hypertensive Properties); Icatibant; Lanthanum; Methylphenidate; Nonsteroidal Anti-Inflammatory Agents; Salicylates; Yohimbine

Stability Store at 20°C to 25°C (68°F to 77°F); excursions permitted to 15°C to 30°C (59°F to 86°F); protect from light and moisture.

Mechanism of Action Competitive inhibitor of angiotensin-converting enzyme (ACE); prevents conversion of angiotensin I to angiotensin II, a potent vasoconstrictor; results in lower levels of angiotensin II which causes an increase in plasma renin activity and a reduction in aldosterone secretion

Pharmacodynamics Antihypertensive effect:

Onset of action: Within 1 hour

Maximum effect: Within 4-8 hours

Duration: 12-24 hours

Pharmacokinetics (Adult data unless noted)

Absorption: 55% to 75%

Protein binding: 50% to 60%

Metabolism: Enalapril is a prodrug (inactive) and undergoes biotransformation to enalaprilat (active) in the liver

Half-life:

Enalapril:

CHF: Neonates (n=3, PNA: 10-19 days): 10.3 hours (range: 4.2-13.4 hours) (Nakamura, 1994)

CHF: Infants and Children ≤6.5 years of age (n=11): 2.7 hours (range: 1.3-6.3 hours) (Nakamura, 1994)

Healthy Adults: 2 hours

CHF: Adults: 3.4-5.8 hours
Enalaprilat (active metabolite):
CHF: Neonates (n=3, PNA: 10-19 days): 11.9 hours (range: 5.9-15.6 hours) (Nakamura, 1994)
CHF: Infants and Children ≤6.5 years of age (n=11): 11.1 hours (range: 5.1-20.8 hours) (Nakamura, 1994)
Infants 6 weeks to 8 months: 6-10 hours
Adults: 35-38 hours
Time to peak serum concentration:
Enalapril: Within 0.5-1.5 hours
Enalaprilat (active): Within 3-4.5 hours
Elimination: Principally in urine (60% to 80%) with some fecal excretion

Dosing: Neonatal Use lower listed initial dose in patients with hyponatremia, hypovolemia, severe CHF, decreased renal function, or in those receiving diuretics.
Hypertension: Oral: Initial: 0.04-0.1 mg/kg/day every 24 hours; initiate at the lower end of the range and titrate to effect as required every few days; hypotension and oliguria have been associated with initial doses of 0.1 mg/kg (Dutta, 2003; Schilder, 1995); maximum reported dose: 0.27 mg/kg/day (Leversha, 1994)
Dosing adjustment in renal impairment: Use in neonates with GFR <30 mL/minute/1.73 m^2 is not recommended; no dosing data available

Dosing: Usual Use lower listed initial dose in patients with hyponatremia, hypovolemia, severe CHF, decreased renal function, or in those receiving diuretics.
Infants, Children, and Adolescents:
Heart Failure: Limited data available: Oral: Initial: 0.1 mg/kg/day in 1-2 divided doses; increase as required over 2 weeks to maximum of 0.5 mg/kg/day; mean dose required for CHF improvement in 39 children (mean age: 4 years) was 0.36 mg/kg/day; select individuals have been treated with doses up to 0.94 mg/kg/day (Leversha, 1994; Momma, 2006)
Hypertension: Oral: Initial: 0.08 mg/kg once daily (maximum dose: 5 mg); adjust dose according to blood pressure readings; doses >0.58 mg/kg (or >40 mg) have not been studied
Proteinuria, nephrotic syndrome: Limited data available; further studies are needed: Oral:
Fixed dosing: Children ≥7 years and Adolescents: 2.5-5 mg/day was reported in a retrospective study in normotensive pediatric patients as either monotherapy (n=17; mean age: 13.7 years; range: 8-17 years) or with prednisone (n=11; mean age: 12.6 years; range: 7-16 years); significant decrease in proteinuria (with or without nephrotic syndrome) occurred; no significant change in blood pressure was observed (Sasinka, 1999); a case series of three adolescents with sickle anemia nephropathy reported an initial dose of 5 mg/day; one patient required an increase to 7.5 mg/day (Fitzhugh, 2005)
Weight-based directed dosing: Children and Adolescents: Initial: 0.2 mg/kg/day; titrate to response at 4- to 12-week intervals; range: 0.2-0.6 mg/kg/day; maximum daily dose: 20 mg/**day**; a crossover dose comparison trial showed effects on proteinuria were dose-dependent (Bagga, 2004; Chandar, 2007; Delucchi, 2000; Lama, 2000; White, 2003); if combined with other angiotensin blockade (ARB), lower doses have been reported (0.1-0.16 mg/kg/day) (Chandar, 2007)
Adults:
Asymptomatic left ventricular dysfunction: Oral: Initial: 2.5 mg twice daily; increase as tolerated; usual dose: 20 mg/day in 2 divided doses
Heart failure: Oral: Initial: 2.5 mg once or twice daily (usual range: 5-40 mg/day in 2 divided doses); titrate slowly at 1- to 2-week intervals. Target dose: 10-20 mg twice daily (ACC/AHA 2009 Heart Failure Guidelines)
Hypertension: Oral: 2.5-5 mg/day then increase as required, usually at 1- to 2-week intervals; usual dose range (JNC 7): 2.5-40 mg/day in 1-2 divided doses.
Note: Initiate with 2.5 mg if patient is taking a diuretic which cannot be discontinued. May add a diuretic if blood pressure cannot be controlled with enalapril alone.

Dosing adjustment in renal impairment:
Infants, Children, and Adolescents:
Manufacturer's labeling: Use in infants, children, and adolescents ≤16 years of age with GFR <30 mL/minute/1.73 m^2 is not recommended; no dosing data available in this population
Alternate recommendations (Aronoff, 2007):
GFR >50 mL/minute/1.73m^2: No dosage adjustment necessary
GFR 10-50 mL/minute/1.73m^2: Administer 75% of usual dose
GFR <10 mL/minute/1.73m^2: Administer 50% of usual dose
Adults:
Manufacturer's labeling:
CrCl >30 mL/minute: No dosage adjustment necessary
CrCl ≤30 mL/minute: Administer 2.5 mg/day; titrate upward until blood pressure is controlled
Alternate recommendations (Aronoff, 2007):
GFR >50 mL/minute: No dosage adjustment necessary
GFR 10-50 mL/minute: Administer 50% to 100% of usual dose
GFR <10 mL/minute: Administer 25% of usual dose
Peritoneal dialysis: Supplemental dose is not necessary, although some removal of drug occurs

Administration May administer without regard to food
Monitoring Parameters Blood pressure, renal function, WBC, serum potassium, serum glucose; monitor for angioedema and anaphylactoid reactions
Test Interactions Positive Coombs' [direct]; may cause false-positive results in urine acetone determinations using sodium nitroprusside reagent
Additional Information Severe hypotension was reported in a **preterm** neonate (birth weight: 835 g, gestational age: 26 weeks, postnatal age: 9 days) who was treated with enalapril 0.1 mg/kg orally; hypotension responded to I.V. plasma and dopamine; the authors suggest starting enalapril in preterm infants at 0.01 mg/kg and increasing upwards in a stepwise fashion with very close monitoring of blood pressure and urine output. However, in this case report, oral enalapril at doses of 0.01 mg/kg to 0.04 mg/kg did not adequately control blood pressure. Further studies are needed (Schilder, 1995).
Dosage Forms Excipient information presented when available (limited, particularly for generics); consult specific product labeling.
Solution Reconstituted, Oral, as maleate:
Epaned: 1 mg/mL (150 mL) [contains methylparaben, propylparaben, saccharin sodium; berry-citrus flavor]
Tablet, Oral, as maleate:
Vasotec: 2.5 mg, 5 mg, 10 mg, 20 mg [scored]
Generic: 2.5 mg, 5 mg, 10 mg, 20 mg
Extemporaneous Preparations Note: Commercial oral solution kit is available (1 mg/mL).

A 1 mg/mL oral suspension may be made with tablets, Bicitra [discontinued] or equivalent, and Ora-Sweet SF. Place ten 20 mg tablets in a 200 mL polyethylene terephthalate bottle; add 50 mL of Bicitra [discontinued] or equivalent and shake well for at least 2 minutes. Let stand for 1 hour then shake for 1 additional minute; add 150 mL of Ora-Sweet SF and shake well. Label "shake well" and "refrigerate". Stable for 30 days when stored in a polyethylene terephthalate bottle and refrigerated (Vasotec prescribing information, 2011).

A 1 mg/mL oral suspension may be made with tablets and one of three different vehicles (cherry syrup, a 1:1 mixture of Ora-Sweet and Ora-Plus, or a 1:1 mixture of Ora-Sweet SF and Ora-Plus). Crush six 20 mg tablets in a mortar and reduce to a fine powder. Add 15 mL of the chosen vehicle and mix to a uniform paste; mix while adding the vehicle in incremental proportions to **almost** 120 mL; transfer to a calibrated bottle, rinse mortar with vehicle, and add quantity of vehicle sufficient to make 120 mL. Label "shake well" and "protect from light". Stable for 60 days when stored in amber plastic prescription bottles in the dark at room temperature or refrigerated (Allen, 1998).

A 1 mg/mL oral suspension may be made with tablets and one of three different vehicles (deionized water, citrate buffer solution at pH 5.0, or a 1:1 mixture of Ora-Sweet and Ora-Plus). Crush twenty 10 mg tablets in a mortar and reduce to a fine powder. Add small portions of the chosen vehicle and mix to a uniform paste; mix while adding vehicle in incremental proportions to **almost** 200 mL; transfer to a graduated cylinder, rinse mortar with vehicle, and add quantity of vehicle sufficient to make 200 mL. Label "shake well" and "protect from light". Preparations made in citrate buffer solution at pH 5.0 and the 1:1 mixture of Ora-Sweet and Ora-Plus are stable for 91 days when stored in plastic prescription bottles in the dark at room temperature or refrigerated. Preparation made in deionized water is stable for 91 days refrigerated or 56 days at room temperature when stored in plastic prescription bottles in the dark. **Note:** To prepare the isotonic citrate buffer solution (pH 5.0), see reference (Nahata, 1998).

A more dilute, 0.1 mg/mL oral suspension may be made with tablets and an isotonic buffer solution at pH 5.0. Grind one 20 mg tablet in a glass mortar and reduce to a fine powder; mix with isotonic citrate buffer (pH 5.0) and filter; add quantity of buffer solution sufficient to make 200 mL. Label "shake well", "protect from light", and "refrigerate". Stable for 90 days (Boulton, 1994).

Allen LV Jr and Erickson MA 3rd, "Stability of Alprazolam, Chloroquine Phosphate, Cisapride, Enalapril Maleate, and Hydralazine Hydrochloride in Extemporaneously Compounded Oral Liquids," *Am J Health Syst Pharm*, 1998, 55(18):1915-20.

Boulton DW, Woods DJ, Fawcett JP, et al, "The Stability of an Enalapril Maleate Oral Solution Prepared From Tablets," *Aust J Hosp Pharm*, 1994, 24(2):151-6.

Nahata MC, Morosco RS, and Hipple TF, "Stability of Enalapril Maleate in Three Extemporaneously Prepared Oral Liquids," *Am J Health Syst Pharm*, 1998, 55(11):1155-7.

Vasotec® prescribing information, Valeant Pharmaceuticals North America LLC, Bridgewater, NJ; 2011.

References

Aronoff GR, Bennett WM, Berns JS, et al, *Drug Prescribing in Renal Failure: Dosing Guidelines for Adults and Children*, 5th ed, Philadelphia, PA: American College of Physicians; 2007.

Bagga A, Mudigoudar BD, Hari P, et al, "Enalapril Dosage in Steroid-Resistant Nephrotic Syndrome," *Pediatr Nephrol*, 2004, 19(1):45-50.

Baker-Smith CM, Benjamin DK Jr, Califf RM, et al, "Cough in Pediatric Patients Receiving Angiotensin-Converting Enzyme Inhibitor Therapy or Angiotensin Receptor Blocker Therapy in Randomized Controlled Trials," *Clin Pharmacol Ther*, 2010, 87(6):668-71.

Brown NJ, Ray WA, Snowden M, et al, "Black Americans Have an Increased Rate of Angiotensin Converting Enzyme Inhibitor-Associated Angioedema," *Clin Pharmacol Ther*, 1996, 60(1):8-13.

Bult Y and van den Anker J, "Hypertension in a Preterm Infant Treated With Enalapril," *J Pediatr Pharm Pract*, 1997, 2(4):229-31.

Chandar J, Abitbol C, Montané B, et al, "Angiotensin Blockade as Sole Treatment for Proteinuric Kidney Disease in Children," *Nephrol Dial Transplant*, 2007, 22(5):1332-7.

Chobanian AV, Bakris GL, Black HR, et al, "The Seventh Report of the Joint National Committee on Prevention, Detection, Evaluation, and Treatment of High Blood Pressure: The JNC 7 Report," *JAMA*, 2003, 289(19):2560-71.

Delucchi A, Cano F, Rodriguez E, et al, "Enalapril and Prednisone in Children With Nephrotic-Range Proteinuria," *Pediatr Nephrol*, 2000, 14(12):1088-91.

Dutta S and Narang A, "Enalapril-Induced Acute Renal Failure in a Newborn Infant," *Pediatr Nephrol*, 2003, 18(6):570-2.

Fitzhugh CD, Wigfall DR, and Ware RE, "Enalapril and Hydroxyurea Therapy for Children With Sickle Nephropathy," *Pediatr Blood Cancer*, 2005, 45(7):982-5.

Frenneaux M, Stewart RA, Newman CM, et al, "Enalapril for Severe Heart Failure in Infancy," *Arch Dis Child*, 1989, 64(2):219-23.

Hogg RJ, Portman RJ, Milliner D, et al, "Evaluation and Management of Proteinuria and Nephrotic Syndrome in Children: Recommendations From a Pediatric Nephrology Panel Established at the National Kidney Foundation Conference on Proteinuria, Albuminuria, Risk, Assessment, Detection, and Elimination (PARADE)," *Pediatrics*, 2000, 105(6):1242-9.

Hunt SA, Abraham WT, Chin MH, et al, "2009 Focused Update Incorporated Into the ACC/AHA 2005 Guidelines for the Diagnosis and Management of Heart Failure in Adults: A Report of the American College of Cardiology Foundation/American Heart Association Task Force on Practice Guidelines Developed in Collaboration With the International Society for Heart and Lung Transplantation," *J Am Coll Cardiol*, 2009, 53(15):1-90.

Lama G, Luongo I, Piscitelli A, et al, "Enalapril: Antiproteinuric Effect in Children With Nephrotic Syndrome," *Clin Nephrol*, 2000, 53(6):432-6.

Leversha AM, Wilson NJ, Clarkson PM, et al, "Efficacy and Dosage of Enalapril in Congenital and Acquired Heart Disease," *Arch Dis Child*, 1994, 70(1):35-9.

Lloyd TR, Mahoney LT, Knoedel D, et al, "Orally Administered Enalapril for Infants With Congestive Heart Failure: A Dose-Finding Study," *J Pediatr*, 1989, 114(4):650-4.

Momma K, "ACE Inhibitors in Pediatric Patients With Heart Failure," *Paediatr Drugs*, 2006, 8(1):55-69.

Nakamura H, Ishii M, Sugimura T, et al, "The Kinetic Profiles of Enalapril and Enalaprilat and Their Possible Developmental Changes in Pediatric Patients With Congestive Heart Failure," *Clin Pharmacol Ther*, 1994, 56(2):160-8.

National High Blood Pressure Education Program Working Group on High Blood Pressure in Children and Adolescents, "The Fourth Report on the Diagnosis, Evaluation, and Treatment of High Blood Pressure in Children and Adolescents," *Pediatrics*, 2004, 114(2 Suppl):555-76.

Sasinka MA, Podracka L, Boor A, et al, "Enalapril Treatment of Proteinuria in Normotensive Children," *Bratisl Lek Listy*, 1999, 100 (9):476-80.

Schilder JL and Van den Anker JN, "Use of Enalapril in Neonatal Hypertension," *Acta Paediatr*, 1995, 84(12):1426-8.

von Vigier RO, Mozzettini S, Truttmann AC, et al, "Cough is Common in Children Prescribed Converting Enzyme Inhibitors," *Nephron*, 2000, 84(1):98.

Wells TG, Bunchman TE, and Kearns GL, "Treatment of Neonatal Hypertension With Enalaprilat," *J Pediatr*, 1990, 117(4):664-7.

White CT, Macpherson CF, Hurley RM, et al, "Antiproteinuric Effects of Enalapril and Losartan: A Pilot Study," *Pediatr Nephrol*, 2003, 18 (10):1038-43.

Enalaprilat (en AL a pril at)

Medication Safety Issues
Administration issues:
Significant differences exist between oral and I.V. dosing. Use caution when converting from one route of administration to another.

Brand Names: Canada Vasotec I.V

Therapeutic Category Angiotensin-Converting Enzyme (ACE) Inhibitor

Generic Availability (U.S.) Yes

Use Treatment of hypertension when oral therapy is not practical (FDA approved in adults); has also been used for heart failure

Pregnancy Risk Factor C (1st trimester); D (2nd and 3rd trimesters)

Pregnancy Considerations [U.S. Boxed Warning]: Drugs that act on the renin-angiotensin system can cause injury and death to the developing fetus. Discontinue as soon as possible once pregnancy is detected. Enalaprilat, the active metabolite of enalapril, crosses the placenta; teratogenic effects may occur following maternal use during pregnancy. Drugs that act on the renin-angiotensin system are associated with oligohydramnios. Oligohydramnios, due to decreased fetal renal function, may lead to fetal lung hypoplasia and skeletal malformations. The use of these drugs in pregnancy is also associated with anuria, hypotension, renal failure, skull hypoplasia, and death in the fetus/neonate. Chronic maternal hypertension itself is also associated with adverse events in the fetus/infant. ACE inhibitors are not recommended during pregnancy to treat maternal hypertension or heart failure. Use of an ACE inhibitor should also be avoided in any woman of reproductive age. Women who are planning a pregnancy should be considered for other medication options if an ACE inhibitor is currently prescribed or the ACE inhibitor should be discontinued as soon as possible once pregnancy is detected. The exposed fetus should be monitored for fetal growth, amniotic fluid volume, and organ formation. Infants exposed to an ACE inhibitor *in utero* should be monitored for hyperkalemia, hypotension, and oliguria (exchange transfusions or dialysis may be needed). These adverse events are generally associated with maternal use in the second and third trimesters.

Untreated chronic maternal hypertension is also associated with adverse events in the fetus, infant, and mother. The use of ACE inhibitors is not recommended to treat chronic uncomplicated hypertension in pregnant women and should generally be avoided in women of reproductive potential (ACOG, 2013).

Breast-Feeding Considerations Enalapril and enalaprilat are excreted in breast milk. Breast-feeding is not recommended by the manufacturer.

Contraindications Hypersensitivity to enalapril, enalaprilat, any component, or other ACE inhibitors; patients with idiopathic or hereditary angioedema or a history of angioedema with ACE inhibitors

Warnings Angioedema can occur at any time during treatment (especially following first dose). The relative risk of angioedema with ACE inhibitors is higher within the first 30 days of use (compared to >1 year of use), for Black Americans (compared to Whites), for lisinopril or enalapril (compared to captopril), and for patients previously hospitalized within 30 days (Brown, 1996). Angioedema may occur in the head, neck, extremities, or intestines; patients with angioedema of the intestines may present with abdominal pain (with or without nausea or vomiting); angioedema of the larynx, glottis, or tongue may cause airway obstruction, especially in patients with a history of airway surgery. Prolonged monitoring may be required, even in patients with swelling of only the tongue (ie, without respiratory distress) because treatment with corticosteroids and antihistamines may not be sufficient; very rare fatalities have occurred with angioedema of the larynx or tongue; appropriate treatment (eg, establishing patent airway and/or SubQ epinephrine) should be readily available for patients with angioedema of larynx, glottis, or tongue, in whom airway obstruction is likely to occur.

Anaphylactic/anaphylactoid reactions can occur with ACE inhibitors. Life-threatening anaphylactoid reactions may be seen during hemodialysis (eg, CVVHD) with high-flux dialysis membranes (eg, AN69), and rarely, during low density lipoprotein apheresis with dextran sulfate cellulose. Rare cases of anaphylactoid reactions have been reported in patients undergoing sensitization treatment with hymenoptera (bee, wasp) venom while receiving ACE inhibitors.

Enalapril has been associated with rare but potentially fatal cases of agranulocytosis, neutropenia, or leukopenia with myeloid hypoplasia; higher risk for development of neutropenia is associated with renal impairment; risk is further increased in patients with both renal impairment and collagen vascular disease (eg, systemic lupus erythematosus). Onset of neutropenia is usually within 3 months of enalapril initiation; closely monitor CBC with differential for the first 3 months of therapy and periodically thereafter in these patients; neutrophil count generally returns to baseline within 2 weeks of discontinuation.

ACE inhibitor use has been associated with deterioration of renal function and/or increases in serum creatinine, particularly in patients with low renal blood flow (eg, renal artery stenosis, heart failure) whose glomerular filtration rate (GFR) is dependent on efferent arteriolar vasoconstriction by angiotensin II; deterioration may result in oliguria, acute renal failure, and progressive azotemia. Small increases in serum creatinine may occur following initiation; consider discontinuation only in patients with progressive and/or significant deterioration in renal function.

A rare toxicity associated with ACE inhibitors includes cholestatic jaundice, which may progress to fulminant hepatic necrosis; discontinue if marked elevation of hepatic transaminases or jaundice occurs and initiate appropriate medical treatment.

Drugs that act on the renin-angiotensin system can cause injury and death to the developing fetus. Discontinue as soon as possible once pregnancy is detected **[U.S. Boxed Warning]**. Concomitant use of an ARB or renin inhibitor (eg, aliskiren) is associated with an increased risk of hypotension, hyperkalemia, and renal dysfunction. Concomitant use with aliskiren should be avoided in patients with GFR <60 mL/minute and is contraindicated in patients with diabetes mellitus (regardless of GFR).

Injectable product contains benzyl alcohol (9 mg/mL) which may cause allergic reactions in susceptible individuals; large amounts of benzyl alcohol (≥99 mg/kg/day) have been associated with a potentially fatal toxicity ("gasping syndrome") in neonates; the "gasping syndrome" consists of metabolic acidosis, respiratory distress, gasping respirations, CNS dysfunction (including convulsions, intracranial hemorrhage), hypotension, and cardiovascular collapse; use enalaprilat products containing benzyl alcohol with caution in neonates; *in vitro* and animal studies have shown that benzoate, a metabolite of benzyl alcohol, displaces bilirubin from protein binding sites.

Precautions Use with caution in patients with renal impairment; dosage reduction may be necessary; avoid rapid dosage escalation which may lead to further renal impairment. Use with caution in patients with unstented unilateral/bilateral renal artery stenosis. When unstented bilateral renal artery stenosis is present, use is generally avoided due to the elevated risk of deterioration in renal function unless possible benefits outweigh risks.

Use with caution when initiating therapy and in volume-depleted patients; may cause symptomatic hypotension with or without syncope, usually with the first several doses; correct volume depletion prior to initiation; initiate lower doses in patients with sodium or volume depletion; close monitoring of patient is required especially with initial dosing and dosing increases; blood pressure must be lowered at a rate appropriate for the patient's clinical condition. Although dose reduction may be necessary, hypotension alone is not a reason for discontinuation of future ACE inhibitor use especially in patients with heart failure where a reduction in systolic blood pressure is a desirable observation. Use caution in patients with ischemic heart disease or cerebrovascular disease during therapy initiation; observe closely due to the potential consequences posed by falling blood pressure (eg, MI, stroke); fluid replacement may be required to restore blood pressure; therapy may then be resumed; discontinue therapy in patients whose hypotension recurs. Use with caution in patients with severe aortic stenosis; may reduce coronary perfusion resulting in ischemia. Use with caution in patients with hypertrophic cardiomyopathy (HCM) and outflow tract obstruction since reduction in afterload may worsen symptoms associated with this condition.

May cause hyperkalemia; risk factors include renal dysfunction, diabetes mellitus, concomitant use of potassium-sparing diuretics, potassium supplements, and/or potassium-containing salts; use with caution, if at all, with these agents, and monitor potassium closely.

Use with caution before, during, or immediately after major surgery; cardiopulmonary bypass, intraoperative blood loss, or vasodilating anesthesia increases endogenous renin release; use of ACE inhibitors perioperatively will blunt angiotensin II formation and may result in hypotension.

An ACE inhibitor cough is a dry, hacking, nonproductive one that usually occurs within the first few months of treatment and should generally resolve within 1-4 weeks after discontinuation of the ACE inhibitor. In pediatric patients, an isolated dry hacking cough lasting >3 weeks was reported in seven of 42 pediatric patients (17%) receiving ACE inhibitors (von Vigier, 2000); a review of pediatric randomized-controlled ACE inhibitor trials reported a lower incidence of 3.2% (Baker-Smith, 2010). Other causes of cough should be considered (eg, pulmonary congestion in patients with heart failure) and excluded prior to discontinuation.

Adverse Reactions Note: Since enalapril is converted to enalaprilat, adverse reactions associated with enalapril may also occur with enalaprilat (also refer to Enalapril monograph).

Cardiovascular: Hypotension

Central nervous system: Headache

Gastrointestinal: Nausea

Rare but important or life-threatening: Angioedema, constipation, cough, dizziness, fatigue, fever, MI, rash

Drug Interactions

Metabolism/Transport Effects None known.

Avoid Concomitant Use There are no known interactions where it is recommended to avoid concomitant use.

Increased Effect/Toxicity

Enalaprilat may increase the levels/effects of: Allopurinol; Amifostine; Antihypertensives; AzaTHIOprine; CycloSPORINE (Systemic); DULoxetine; Ferric Gluconate; Gold Sodium Thiomalate; Grass Pollen Allergen Extract (5 Grass Extract); Hypotensive Agents; Iron Dextran Complex; Lithium; Nonsteroidal Anti-Inflammatory Agents; Obinutuzumab; RiTUXimab; Sodium Phosphates

The levels/effects of Enalaprilat may be increased by: Alfuzosin; Aliskiren; Angiotensin II Receptor Blockers; Barbiturates; Brimonidine (Topical); Canagliflozin; Diazoxide; DPP-IV Inhibitors; Eplerenone; Everolimus; Heparin; Heparin (Low Molecular Weight); Herbs (Hypotensive Properties); Loop Diuretics; MAO Inhibitors; Pentoxifylline; Phosphodiesterase 5 Inhibitors; Potassium Salts; Potassium-Sparing Diuretics; Prostacyclin Analogues; Sirolimus; Temsirolimus; Thiazide Diuretics; TiZANidine; Tolvaptan; Trimethoprim

Decreased Effect

The levels/effects of Enalaprilat may be decreased by: Aprotinin; Herbs (Hypertensive Properties); Icatibant; Methylphenidate; Nonsteroidal Anti-Inflammatory Agents; Salicylates; Yohimbine

Stability Store intact vials below 30°C (86°F); solutions for I.V. infusion mixed in NS, D_5W, D_5NS, or D_5LR are stable for 24 hours at room temperature

Mechanism of Action Competitive inhibitor of angiotensin-converting enzyme (ACE); prevents conversion of angiotensin I to angiotensin II, a potent vasoconstrictor; results in lower levels of angiotensin II which causes an increase in plasma renin activity and a reduction in aldosterone secretion

Pharmacodynamics Antihypertensive effect:

Onset of action: Within 15 minutes

Maximum effect: Within 1-4 hours

Duration: Dose dependent, usually 4-6 hours

Pharmacokinetics (Adult data unless noted)

Protein binding: 50% to 60%

Half-life:

CHF: Neonates (n=3; PNA: 10-19 days): 11.9 hours (range: 5.9-15.6 hours) (Nakamura, 1994)

CHF: Infants and Children ≤6.5 years of age (n=11): 11.1 hours (range: 5.1-20.8 hours) (Nakamura, 1994)

Infants 6 weeks to 8 months: 6-10 hours

Adults: 35-38 hours

Elimination: Principally in urine (60% to 80%) with some fecal excretion

Dosing: Neonatal Use lower listed initial dose in patients with hyponatremia, hypovolemia, severe CHF, decreased renal function, or in those receiving diuretics

Hypertension: I.V.: 5-10 **mcg**/kg/dose every 8-24 hours as determined by clinical response (eg, blood pressure readings); monitor patients carefully; some patients may require higher doses

Dosing adjustment in renal impairment: Note: Use in neonates with GFR <30 mL/minute/1.73 m^2 is not recommended; no dosing data available

Dosing: Usual Use lower listed initial dose in patients with hyponatremia, hypovolemia, severe CHF, decreased renal function, or in those receiving diuretics

Infants and Children: **Hypertension:** I.V.: 5-10 **mcg**/kg/dose every 8-24 hours; maximum dose:1.25 mg/dose; frequency determined by clinical response (eg, blood pressure readings); monitor patients carefully; some patients may require higher doses (NHBPEP, 2005)

Adolescents and Adults: **Hypertension:** I.V.: 0.625-1.25 mg/dose every 6 hours; doses as high as 5 mg/dose every 6 hours have been tolerated for up to 36 hours; little experience with doses >20 mg/day

Dosing adjustment in renal impairment:

Infants, Children, and Adolescents:

Aronoff, 2007:

GFR >50 mL/minute/1.73 m^2: No dosage adjustment necessary

GFR 10-50 mL/minute/1.73 m^2: Administer 75% of usual dose

GFR <10 mL/minute/1.73 m^2: Administer 50% of usual dose

Alternate recommendations: Others suggest avoiding use in infants, children, and adolescents ≤16 years of age with GFR <30 mL/minute/1.73 m^2.

Adults:

Manufacturer's labeling:

CrCl >30 mL/minute: No dosage adjustment necessary

CrCl ≤30 mL/minute: Initiate with 0.625 mg; if after 1 hour clinical response is unsatisfactory, may repeat. May then administer 1.25 mg every 6 hours

Alternate recommendations (Aronoff, 2007):

GFR >50 mL/minute: No dosage adjustment necessary

GFR 10-50 mL/minute: Administer 50% to 100% of usual dose

GFR <10 mL/minute: Administer 25% to 50% of usual dose

Peritoneal dialysis: Supplemental dose is not necessary, although some removal of drug occurs.

Administration Administer as I.V. infusion (undiluted or further diluted) over 5 minutes; to deliver small I.V. doses, a dilution with NS to a final concentration of 25 mcg/mL can be used

Monitoring Parameters Blood pressure, renal function, WBC, serum potassium, serum glucose; monitor for angioedema and anaphylactoid reactions

Dosage Forms Excipient information presented when available (limited, particularly for generics); consult specific product labeling.

Injectable, Intravenous:

Generic: 1.25 mg/mL (1 mL, 2 mL)

References

Baker-Smith CM, Benjamin DK Jr, Califf RM, et al, "Cough in Pediatric Patients Receiving Angiotensin-Converting Enzyme Inhibitor Therapy or Angiotensin Receptor Blocker Therapy in Randomized Controlled Trials," *Clin Pharmacol Ther*, 2010, 87(6):668-71.

Brown NJ, Ray WA, Snowden M, et al, "Black Americans Have an Increased Rate of Angiotensin Converting Enzyme Inhibitor-Associated Angioedema," *Clin Pharmacol Ther*, 1996, 60(1):8-13.

Chobanian AV, Bakris GL, Black HR, et al, "The Seventh Report of the Joint National Committee on Prevention, Detection, Evaluation, and Treatment of High Blood Pressure: The JNC 7 Report," *JAMA*, 2003, 289(19):2560-71.

Marcadis ML, Kraus DM, Hatzopoulos FK, et al, "Use of Enalaprilat for Neonatal Hypertension," *J Pediatr*, 1991, 119(3):505-6.

Nakamura H, Ishii M, Sugimura T, et al, "The Kinetic Profiles of Enalapril and Enalaprilat and Their Possible Developmental Changes in Pediatric Patients With Congestive Heart Failure," *Clin Pharmacol Ther*, 1994, 56(2):160-8.

National High Blood Pressure Education Program Working Group on High Blood Pressure in Children and Adolescents, "The Fourth Report on the Diagnosis, Evaluation, and Treatment of High Blood Pressure in Children and Adolescents," *Pediatrics*, 2004, 114(2 Suppl):555-76.

von Vigier RO, Mozzettini S, Truttmann AC, et al, "Cough is Common in Children Prescribed Converting Enzyme Inhibitors," *Nephron*, 2000, 84(1):98.

Wells TG, Bunchman TE, and Kearns GL, "Treatment of Neonatal Hypertension With Enalaprilat," *J Pediatr*, 1990, 117(4):664-7.

◆ **Enalapril Maleate** *see* Enalapril *on page 744*

◆ **Enbrel** *see* Etanercept *on page 803*

◆ **Enbrel SureClick** *see* Etanercept *on page 803*

◆ **Endocet** *see* Oxycodone and Acetaminophen *on page 1573*

◆ **Endodan®** *see* Oxycodone and Aspirin *on page 1575*

◆ **Enemeez Mini [OTC]** *see* Docusate *on page 701*

◆ **Enerjets [OTC]** *see* Caffeine *on page 338*

Enfuvirtide (en FYOO vir tide)

Related Information

Adult and Adolescent HIV *on page 2348*
Pediatric HIV *on page 2338*
Perinatal HIV *on page 2356*
Brand Names: U.S. Fuzeon
Brand Names: Canada Fuzeon®
Therapeutic Category Antiretroviral Agent; Fusion Inhibitor; HIV Agents (Anti-HIV Agents)
Generic Availability (U.S.) No
Use Treatment of HIV-1 infection in combination with other antiretroviral agents in treatment-experienced patients who are failing current antiretroviral therapy (FDA approved in ages ≥6 years and adults). **Note:** HIV regimens consisting of **three** antiretroviral agents are strongly recommended. However, in published studies, enfuvirtide was added onto a new optimized background regimen of 3 to 5 antiretroviral agents, in patients failing their current antiretroviral regimen. Selection of the new optimized regimen was based on medication history, genotyping, and phenotyping. Due to the lack of studies, enfuvirtide cannot be recommended as initial therapy in patients who are antiretroviral naïve.

Pregnancy Risk Factor B

Pregnancy Considerations Teratogenic effects were not observed in animal studies. Enfuvirtide has minimal to low transfer across the human placenta. The DHHS Perinatal HIV Guidelines note that data are insufficient to recommend use during pregnancy.

Regardless of CD4 count or HIV RNA copy number, all HIV-infected pregnant women should receive a combination antiretroviral (ARV) drug regimen. A combination of antepartum, intrapartum, and infant ARV prophylaxis is recommended. ARV therapy should be started as soon as possible in women with symptomatic infection. Although earlier initiation may be more effective in reducing the perinatal transmission of HIV, initiation may be delayed until after 12 weeks gestation in women who do not require immediate treatment after careful consideration of maternal conditions (eg, nausea and vomiting) and the potential risks of first trimester fetal exposure for specific agents. A scheduled cesarean delivery at 38 weeks gestation is recommended for all women with HIV RNA >1000 copies/mL or unknown concentrations near delivery in order to decrease transmission. If ARV therapy must be interrupted for <24 hours during the peripartum period, stop then restart all medications simultaneously in order to decrease the chance of developing resistance. Long-term follow-up is recommended for all infants exposed to ARV medications. In couples who want to conceive, the HIV-infected partner should attain maximum viral suppression prior to conception.

Healthcare providers are encouraged to enroll pregnant women exposed to antiretroviral medications in the Antiretroviral Pregnancy Registry (1-800-258-4263 or www.APRegistry.com). Healthcare providers caring for HIV-infected women and their infants may contact the National Perinatal HIV Hotline (888-448-8765) for clinical consultation (DHHS [perinatal], 2014).

Breast-Feeding Considerations It is not known if enfuvirtide is excreted into breast milk. Maternal or infant antiretroviral therapy does not completely eliminate the risk of postnatal HIV transmission. In addition, multiclass-resistant virus has been detected in breast-feeding infants despite maternal therapy. Therefore, in the United States, where formula is accessible, affordable, safe, and sustainable, and the risk of infant mortality due to diarrhea and respiratory infections is low, complete avoidance of breast-feeding by HIV-infected women is recommended to decrease potential transmission of HIV (DHHS [perinatal], 2014).

Contraindications Hypersensitivity to enfuvirtide or any component

Warnings Local injection site reactions occur in the majority of patients (98% incidence); most patients have first injection site reaction during initial week of therapy; reactions are usually mild to moderate in severity, but may be more severe; symptoms may include discomfort, ecchymosis, erythema, induration, pain, pruritus, and nodule or cyst formation; infection, including cellulitis or abscess, occurs more frequently in adolescent patients than adults (11% vs 1.7%); some patients require analgesics (11%) or limitation of usual activities; reactions often occur at >1 injection site; 26% of patients have 6 to 14 injection site reactions and 1.3% have >14 injection site reactions at any given time; average duration of single injection site reaction is 3 to 7 days in 41% of patients and >7 days in 24%; 7% of patients discontinue therapy either due to injection site reactions (4%) or problems with administering injections (3%). Instruct patient or caregiver on proper injection method; monitor patients for local infection or cellulitis. Administration using a needle-free device (Biojector 2000) has been associated with nerve pain (including neuralgia and/or paresthesia lasting up to 6 months) when administered at sites where large nerves are close to the skin, bruising, and hematomas; administer medication only in recommended sites. A higher risk of postinjection bleeding may occur in patients receiving anticoagulants and in those with hemophilia or other coagulation disorders.

Bacterial pneumonia was observed at a higher rate in patients receiving enfuvirtide during clinical trials (6.7 events per 100 patient years vs 0.6 events per 100 patient years in control group; about 50% of patients with pneumonia required hospitalization); certain patients may be at greater risk (eg, those with a history of lung disease, low CD4 cell count, high initial viral load, I.V. drug use, or smoking); monitor patients closely for signs and symptoms of pneumonia. Systemic hypersensitivity reactions may occur; symptoms may include rash, fever, nausea, vomiting, chills, rigor, hypotension, and elevated transaminases; discontinue enfuvirtide and do not restart in patients with systemic hypersensitivity reactions.

Precautions Use of enfuvirtide may theoretically result in the production of anti-enfuvirtide antibodies, which may cross react with HIV-1 gp41; this could potentially result in a false positive ELISA test in noninfected HIV individuals; the western blot test would be expected to be negative; use of enfuvirtide in non-HIV infected individuals has not been studied.

Immune reconstitution syndrome (an acute inflammatory response to residual or indolent opportunistic infections) may occur in HIV patients during initial treatment with combination antiretroviral agents, including enfuvirtide; this syndrome may require further patient assessment and therapy. Autoimmune disorders (eg, Graves' disease, Guillain-Barré syndrome, and polymyositis) have been reported in patients experiencing immune reconstitution; time to onset is variable and may occur many months after antiretroviral treatment is initiated.

Adverse Reactions

Central nervous system: Fatigue, insomnia

Dermatologic: Folliculitis

Gastrointestinal: Abdominal pain, anorexia, appetite decreased, diarrhea, nausea, pancreatitis, weight loss, xerostomia

Hematologic: Eosinophilia

Hepatic: Transaminases increased

Local: Injection site infection, injection site reactions (may include rash, erythema, induration, pruritus, ecchymosis, nodule or cyst formation)

Neuromuscular & skeletal: CPK increased, limb pain, myalgia

Ocular: Conjunctivitis

Respiratory: Bacterial pneumonia, cough, sinusitis

Miscellaneous: Flu-like syndrome, herpes simplex, infection, lymphadenopathy

Rare but important or life-threatening: Abacavir hypersensitivity worsening, amylase increased, angina, anxiety, constipation, depression, GGT increased, glomerulonephritis, Guillain-Barré syndrome, hepatic steatosis, hyperglycemia; hypersensitivity reactions (symptoms may include rash, fever, nausea, vomiting, hypotension, and transaminase increases); insomnia, lipase increased, lymphadenopathy, neutropenia, peripheral neuropathy, pneumopathy, renal failure, renal insufficiency, respiratory distress, sepsis, sixth nerve palsy, suicide attempt, taste disturbances, thrombocytopenia, toxic hepatitis, triglycerides increased, tubular necrosis, weakness

Drug Interactions

Metabolism/Transport Effects None known.

Avoid Concomitant Use There are no known interactions where it is recommended to avoid concomitant use.

Increased Effect/Toxicity

Enfuvirtide may increase the levels/effects of: Protease Inhibitors

The levels/effects of Enfuvirtide may be increased by: Protease Inhibitors

Decreased Effect There are no known significant interactions involving a decrease in effect.

Stability Store intact vials at 25°C (77°F); excursions permitted to 15°C to 30°C (59°F to 86°F). Store reconstituted solution in the original vial at 2°C to 8°C (36°F to 46°F); use within 24 hours.

Mechanism of Action Binds to the first heptad-repeat (HR1) in the gp41 subunit of the viral envelope glycoprotein. Inhibits the fusion of HIV-1 virus with CD4 cells by blocking the conformational change in gp41 required for membrane fusion and entry into CD4 cells

Pharmacokinetics (Adult data unless noted)

Absorption: SubQ: Absorption is comparable when injected into abdomen, arm, or thigh

Distribution: V_d (mean ± SD): 5.5 ± 1.1 L

CSF concentrations (2 to 18 hours after administration; n=4): Nondetectable (<0.025 mcg/mL)

Protein Binding: 92%; primarily to albumin, but also to alpha-1 acid glycoprotein (to a lesser extent)

Metabolism: Expected to undergo catabolism via peptidases and proteinases in the liver and kidneys to amino acids; amino acids would then be recycled in the body pool. A deaminated metabolite (with 20% activity compared to parent drug) was formed via hydrolysis during *in vitro* human microsomal and hepatocyte studies.

Bioavailability:

Oral: Not bioavailable by this route

SubQ: Absolute: 84.3% ± 15.5%; **Note:** Bioequivalence was found to be similar in a study comparing standard administration using a needle versus a needle-free device.

Half-life: 3.8 ± 0.6 hours

Time to peak serum concentration: SubQ:

Single dose: Median: 8 hours (range: 3 to 12 hours)

Multiple dosing: Median: 4 hours (range: 4 to 8 hours)

Clearance:

Plasma clearance is decreased in adults with lower body weight and in females after adjusting for body weight (clearance in adults females is 20% lower compared to adults males). However, no adjustment in dose is recommended for gender or weight.

Compared to patients with normal renal function, enfuvirtide clearance is decreased by 38% in patients with severe renal impairment (CrCl 11 to 35 mL/minute) and by 14% to 28% in patients with end-stage renal disease who are maintained on dialysis. However, no adjustment in dose is recommended for patients with renal impairment.

Apparent clearance: Multiple dosing:

Children: 40 ± 17 mL/hour/kg

Adults: 30.6 ± 10.6 mL/hour/kg

Dosing: Usual

Pediatric: **HIV infection, treatment:** Treatment-experienced patients only. Use not recommended in antiretroviral therapy naïve patients (DHHS [pediatric, adult], 2014): **Note:** Use in combination with other antiretroviral agents:

Age-directed dosing:

Children and Adolescents 6 to 16 years: SubQ: 2 mg/kg twice daily; maximum dose: 90 mg/dose

Adolescents >16 years: SubQ: 90 mg twice daily (DHHS [pediatric], 2014)

Weight-directed, fixed dosing: Children ≥6 years and Adolescents: SubQ:

11 to 15.5 kg: 27 mg twice daily

15.6 to 20 kg: 36 mg twice daily

20.1 to 24.5 kg: 45 mg twice daily

24.6 to 29 kg: 54 mg twice daily

29.1 to 33.5 kg: 63 mg twice daily

33.6 to 38 kg: 72 mg twice daily

38.1 to 42.5 kg: 81 mg twice daily

≥42.6 kg: 90 mg twice daily

Adult: **HIV infection, treatment:** Treatment-experienced patients only. Use not recommended in antiretroviral therapy naïve patients (DHHS [adult], 2014): **Note:** Use in combination with other antiretroviral agents: SubQ: 90 mg twice daily

Dosing adjustment in renal impairment: Adults:

CrCl >35 mL/minute: Clearance of enfuvirtide is not affected; no dosage adjustment required.

CrCl ≤35 mL/minute: Limited data showed decreased clearance; however, no dosage adjustment recommended.

End-stage renal disease (on dialysis): Limited data showed decreased clearance; however, no dosage adjustment recommended. **Note:** Hemodialysis does not significantly affect clearance of enfuvirtide.

Dosing adjustment in hepatic impairment: No dosage adjustment required.

Administration Reconstitute vial with 1.1 mL SWI to result in delivery of 90 per 1 mL; to avoid foaming, do not shake; gently tap vial for 10 seconds and roll gently between hands to ensure contact of drug with liquid; allow vial to stand until lyophilized powder goes completely into solution; this may require up to 45 minutes; to reduce reconstitution time, may gently roll vial between hands until drug is completely dissolved; visually inspect vial to ensure complete dissolution of drug; solution should be clear, colorless, and without particulate matter or bubbles; if the solution is foamy or jelled, allow more time for it to dissolve; do not use vials that contain particulate matter.

Vial does not contain preservatives; reconstituted solutions should be injected immediately or refrigerated and used within 24 hours; bring refrigerated reconstituted vials to room temperature before injection and visually inspect vial again as outlined above.

Inject SubQ into upper arm, abdomen, or anterior thigh. Do not inject I.M. (severity of reactions is increased). Do not inject into skin abnormalities including directly over a blood vessel, into moles, bruises, scar tissue, near the navel, surgical scars, burn sites, or tattoos. Do not inject in or near sites where large nerves are close to the skin including near the elbow, knee, groin, and inferior or medial sections of the buttocks. Rotate injection site (ie, give injections at a site different from the preceding injection site); do not inject into any site where an injection site reaction is present. After injection, apply heat or ice to injection site or gently massage area to better disperse the dose, to minimize local injection reactions (DHHS [pediatric], 2014); discard unused portion of the vial (vial is for single use only).

Monitoring Parameters Note: Monitor CD4 percentage (if <5 years of age) or CD4 count (if ≥5 years of age) at least every 3 to 4 months (DHHS [pediatric], 2014).

Prior to initiation of therapy: Genotypic resistance testing, CD4 and viral load (every 3 to 4 months), CBC with differential, LFTs, BUN, creatinine, electrolytes, glucose, and urinalysis (every 6 to 12 months), and assessment of readiness for adherence with medication regimen. At initiation and with any change in treatment regimen: CBC with differential, electrolytes, calcium, phosphate, glucose, LFTs, bilirubin, urinalysis (at initiation), BUN, creatinine, albumin, total protein, lipid panel (at initiation), CD4, and viral load. After 1 to 2 weeks of therapy: Signs of medication toxicity and adherence. After 2 to 4 weeks of therapy: CBC with differential, viral load, signs of medication toxicity, and adherence; then every 3 to 4 months: CBC with differential, electrolytes, glucose, LFTs, bilirubin, BUN, creatinine, CD4, viral load, signs of medication toxicity, and adherence. Every 6 to 12 months: Lipid panel and urinalysis. CD4 monitoring frequency may be decreased to every 6 to 12 months in children who are adherent to therapy if the value is well above the threshold for opportunistic infections, viral suppression is sustained, and the clinical status is stable for more than 2 to 3 years (DHHS [pediatric], 2014). Monitor for growth and development, signs of HIV-specific physical conditions, HIV disease progression, opportunistic infections, local injection site reactions, local infection, cellulitis, and signs and symptoms of pneumonia, especially in patients at risk.

Additional Information Reconstituted injection has a pH ~9.0.

Dosage Forms Excipient information presented when available (limited, particularly for generics); consult specific product labeling.
Solution Reconstituted, Subcutaneous:
Fuzeon: 90 mg (1 ea)

References

Church JA, Cunningham C, Hughes M, et al. Safety and antiretroviral activity of chronic subcutaneous administration of T-20 in human immunodeficiency virus 1-infected children. *Pediatr Infect Dis J.* 2002;21(7):653-659.

DHHS Panel on Antiretroviral Guidelines for Adults and Adolescents. Guidelines for the use of antiretroviral agents in HIV-1-infected adults and adolescents, Department of Health and Human Services. May 1, 2014. Available at http://www.aidsinfo.nih.gov/ContentFiles/AdultandAdolescentGL.pdf

DHHS Panel on Antiretroviral Therapy and Medical Management of HIV-Infected Children. Guidelines for the use of antiretroviral agents in pediatric HIV infection. February 12, 2014. Available at http://aidsinfo.nih.gov

DHHS Panel on Treatment of HIV-Infected Pregnant Women and Prevention of Perinatal Transmission. Recommendations for the use of antiretroviral drugs in pregnant HIV-1-infected women for maternal health and interventions to reduce perinatal HIV-1 transmission in the United States. March 28, 2014. Available at http://aidsinfo.nih.gov

Hardy H, Skolnik PR. Enfuvirtide, a new fusion inhibitor for therapy of human immunodeficiency virus infection. *Pharmacotherapy.* 2004;24(2):198-211.

Morris JL, Kraus DM. New antiretroviral therapies for pediatric HIV infection. *J Pediatr Pharmacol Ther.* 2005;10:215-247.

Soy D, Aweeka FT, Church JA, et al. Population pharmacokinetics of enfuvirtide in pediatric patients with human immunodeficiency virus: searching for exposure-response relationships. *Clin Pharmacol Ther.* 2003;74(6):569-580.

◆ **Engerix-B** *see* Hepatitis B Vaccine (Recombinant) *on page 1009*

◆ **Enhanced-Potency Inactivated Poliovirus Vaccine** *see* Poliovirus Vaccine (Inactivated) *on page 1694*

◆ **Enlon** *see* Edrophonium *on page 730*

◆ **Enlon® (Can)** *see* Edrophonium *on page 730*

◆ **EnovaRX-Baclofen** *see* Baclofen *on page 259*

◆ **EnovaRX-Cyclobenzaprine HCl** *see* Cyclobenzaprine *on page 558*

◆ **EnovaRX-Ibuprofen** *see* Ibuprofen *on page 1059*

◆ **EnovaRX-Lidocaine HCl** *see* Lidocaine (Topical) *on page 1242*

◆ **EnovaRX-Naproxen** *see* Naproxen *on page 1470*

◆ **EnovaRX-Tramadol** *see* TraMADol *on page 2060*

Enoxaparin (ee noks a PA rin)

Medication Safety Issues
Sound-alike/look-alike issues:
Lovenox may be confused with Lasix, Levaquin, Lotronex, Protonix

High alert medication:
The Institute for Safe Medication Practices (ISMP) includes this medication among its list of drugs which have a heightened risk of causing significant patient harm when used in error.

National Patient Safety Goals:
The Joint Commission (TJC) requires healthcare organizations that provide anticoagulant therapy to have a process in place to reduce the risk of anticoagulant-associated patient harm. Patients receiving anticoagulants should receive individualized care through a defined process that includes standardized ordering, dispensing, administration, monitoring and education. This does not apply to routine short-term use of anticoagulants for prevention of venous thromboembolism when the expectation is that the patient's laboratory values will remain within or close to normal values (NPSG.03.05.01).

Brand Names: U.S. Lovenox

Brand Names: Canada Enoxaparin Injection; Lovenox; Lovenox HP

Therapeutic Category Anticoagulant; Low Molecular Weight Heparin (LMWH)

Generic Availability (U.S.) Yes

Use Prophylaxis and treatment of thromboembolic disorders, specifically prevention of DVT following hip or knee replacement surgery, abdominal surgery in patients at thromboembolic risk (ie, >40 years of age, obese, general anesthesia >30 minutes, malignancy, history of DVT, or pulmonary embolism), and in medical patients at thromboembolic risk due to severely restricted mobility during acute illness (FDA approved in adults). Administered with warfarin: For inpatient treatment of acute DVT (with or without pulmonary embolism) and outpatient treatment of acute DVT (without pulmonary embolism) (FDA approved in adults). Administered with aspirin: For prevention of ischemic complications of non-Q-wave MI and unstable angina and for the treatment of acute ST-segment elevation myocardial infarction (STEMI) (FDA approved in adults)

Pregnancy Risk Factor B

Pregnancy Considerations Adverse events were not observed in animal reproduction studies. Low molecular weight heparin (LMWH) does not cross the placenta; increased risks of fetal bleeding or teratogenic effects have not been reported.

LMWH is recommended over unfractionated heparin for the treatment of acute venous thromboembolism (VTE) in pregnant women. LMWH is also recommended over unfractionated heparin for VTE prophylaxis in pregnant women with certain risk factors (eg, homozygous factor V Leiden, antiphospholipid antibody syndrome with ≥3 previous pregnancy losses). Prophylaxis is not routinely recommended for women undergoing assisted reproduction therapy; however, LMWH therapy is recommended for women who develop severe ovarian hyperstimulation syndrome. LMWH should be discontinued at least 24 hours prior to induction of labor or a planned cesarean delivery. For women undergoing cesarean section and who have additional risk factors for developing VTE, the prophylactic use of LMWH may be considered.

LMWH may also be used in women with mechanical heart valves (consult current ACCP guidelines for details). Women who require long-term anticoagulation with warfarin and who are considering pregnancy, LMWH substitution should be done prior to conception when possible. When choosing therapy, fetal outcomes (ie, pregnancy loss, malformations), maternal outcomes (ie, VTE, hemorrhage), burden of therapy, and maternal preference should be considered (Guyatt, 2012). Monitoring antifactor Xa levels is recommended.

Multiple-dose vials contain benzyl alcohol (avoid in pregnant women due to association with gasping syndrome in premature infants); use of preservative-free formulations is recommended.

Breast-Feeding Considerations Small amounts of LMWH have been detected in breast milk; however, because it has a low oral bioavailability, it is unlikely to cause adverse events in a nursing infant. Enoxaparin product labeling does not recommend use in nursing women; however, antithrombotic guidelines state that use of LMWH may be continued in breast-feeding women (Guyatt, 2012).

Contraindications Hypersensitivity to enoxaparin, heparin, any component, or pork products (enoxaparin is derived from porcine intestinal mucosa); active major bleeding; acute heparin-induced or low molecular weight heparin-induced thrombocytopenia

Warnings Bleeding or thrombocytopenia may occur; major hemorrhages (eg, intracranial and retroperitoneal bleeding) may be fatal; thrombocytopenia with thrombosis may occur and may be complicated by limb ischemia, organ infarction, or death; discontinue therapy and consider alternative treatment if platelets are <100,000/mm^3 and/or thrombosis develops. Use with extreme caution in patients with an increased risk of hemorrhage (eg, active GI ulceration or bleeding, angiodysplastic GI disease, bacterial endocarditis, bleeding disorders, hemorrhagic stroke); recent brain, spinal, or ophthalmic surgery; concomitant platelet inhibitor therapy; or a history of heparin-induced thrombocytopenia. Do not use unit-for-unit in place of heparin or other low molecular weight heparins (units are not equivalent). Enoxaparin is **not** recommended for prophylaxis of thromboembolic disorders in patients with prosthetic heart valves, especially pregnant women (prosthetic heart valve thrombosis may occur; several cases occurred in pregnant women and resulted in maternal and fetal deaths; pregnant women with prosthetic heart valves may be at a higher risk for thromboembolism; use with extreme caution and monitor peak and trough anti-Factor Xa levels frequently in these patients; adjust dosage accordingly)

Epidural or spinal hematoma resulting in long-term or permanent paralysis may occur in patients receiving low molecular weight heparins or heparinoids during epidural/spinal anesthesia or spinal puncture **[U.S. Boxed Warning]**; these patients must be monitored frequently for neurological impairment and treated immediately if compromised. The risk of epidural/spinal hematoma is increased with the following: The use of indwelling epidural catheters for analgesia; concomitant use of platelet inhibitors, NSAIDs, or other anticoagulants; history of spinal deformity or spinal surgery; and repeated or traumatic epidural/spinal puncture. Potential benefits must be weighed against the risks. Enoxaparin should be withheld (at least 2 doses) and antifactor Xa activity should be determined (if possible), prior to lumbar or epidural procedures.

To minimize the risk of bleeding following percutaneous coronary revascularization procedures (eg, vascular instrumentation during treatment of unstable angina, non-Q-wave MI and acute STEMI), strictly adhere to the recommended dosing intervals. Hemostasis must be achieved at the puncture site after percutaneous coronary interventions (PCI). See product labeling for further information. Cases of hyperkalemia have been reported, usually in patients with risk factors for the development of hyperkalemia (eg, renal dysfunction, concomitant use of potassium-sparing diuretics or potassium supplements, hematoma in body tissues); monitor serum potassium.

Enoxaparin multidose vial contains benzyl alcohol which may cause allergic reactions in susceptible individuals; large amounts of benzyl alcohol (≥99 mg/kg/day) have been associated with a potentially fatal toxicity ("gasping syndrome") in neonates; the "gasping syndrome" consists of metabolic acidosis, respiratory distress, gasping respirations, CNS dysfunction (including convulsions, intracranial hemorrhage), hypotension and cardiovascular collapse; avoid use of enoxaparin products containing benzyl alcohol in neonates; use the preservative free injection; in vitro and animal studies have shown that benzoate, a metabolite of benzyl alcohol, displaces bilirubin from protein binding sites. Use multidose vial with caution in pregnant women and only if clearly needed (benzyl alcohol may cross the placenta).

▶

Precautions Use with caution in patients with uncontrolled arterial hypertension, bleeding diathesis, pregnancy, history of recent GI ulceration, diabetic retinopathy, and hemorrhage. Use with caution in patients with renal impairment; decrease dose in patients with severe renal dysfunction (CrCl <30 mL/minute). Use with caution and monitor carefully in low-weight patients (ie, women <45 kg and men <57 kg) receiving nonweight-adjusted doses (an increase in enoxaparin AUC has been reported). Institute appropriate therapy if thromboembolism occurs despite enoxaparin prophylaxis

Adverse Reactions As with all anticoagulants, bleeding is the major adverse effect of enoxaparin. Hemorrhage may occur at virtually any site. Risk is dependent on multiple variables. At the recommended doses, single injections of enoxaparin do not significantly influence platelet aggregation or affect global clotting time (ie, PT or aPTT).

Central nervous system: Confusion, pain

Gastrointestinal: Diarrhea, nausea

Hematologic & oncologic: Anemia, bruise, major hemorrhage (includes cases of intracranial, retroperitoneal, or intraocular hemorrhage; incidence varies with indication/population), thrombocytopenia

Hepatic: Increased serum ALT, increased serum AST

Local: Bruising at injection site, erythema at injection site, hematoma at injection site, irritation at injection site, pain at injection site

Renal: Hematuria

Miscellaneous: Fever

Rare but important or life-threatening: Alopecia, anaphylaxis, anaphylactoid reaction, eczematous rash (plaques), eosinophilia, epidural hematoma (spinal; after neuroaxial anesthesia or spinal puncture; risk may be increased with indwelling epidural catheter or concomitant use of other drugs affecting hemostasis), headache, hepatic injury (hepatocellular and cholestatic), hyperkalemia, hyperlipidemia (very rare), hypersensitivity angiitis, hypersensitivity reaction, hypertriglyceridemia, intracranial hemorrhage (up to 0.8%), osteoporosis (following long-term therapy), pruritic erythematous rash (patches), pruritus, purpura, retroperitoneal hemorrhage, severe anemia (hemorrhagic), shock, skin necrosis, thrombocythemia, thrombocytopenia, thrombosis (prosthetic value [in pregnant females] or associated with enoxaparin-induced thrombocytopenia; can cause limb ischemia or organ infarction), urticaria, vesicobullous rash

Drug Interactions

Metabolism/Transport Effects None known.

Avoid Concomitant Use

Avoid concomitant use of Enoxaparin with any of the following: Apixaban; Dabigatran Etexilate; Omacetaxine; Rivaroxaban; Urokinase; Vorapaxar

Increased Effect/Toxicity

Enoxaparin may increase the levels/effects of: ACE Inhibitors; Aliskiren; Angiotensin II Receptor Blockers; Anticoagulants; Canagliflozin; Collagenase (Systemic); Deferasirox; Eplerenone; Ibritumomab; Omacetaxine; Palifermin; Potassium Salts; Potassium-Sparing Diuretics; Rivaroxaban; Tositumomab and Iodine I 131 Tositumomab

The levels/effects of Enoxaparin may be increased by: 5-ASA Derivatives; Agents with Antiplatelet Properties; Apixaban; Dabigatran Etexilate; Dasatinib; Herbs (Anticoagulant/Antiplatelet Properties); Ibrutinib; Nonsteroidal Anti-Inflammatory Agents; Omega-3 Fatty Acids; Pentosan Polysulfate Sodium; Pentoxifylline; Prostacyclin Analogues; Salicylates; Sugammadex; Thrombolytic Agents; Tibolone; Tipranavir; Urokinase; Vitamin E; Vorapaxar

Decreased Effect

The levels/effects of Enoxaparin may be decreased by: Estrogen Derivatives; Progestins

Stability Store at 25°C (77°F); excursions permitted to 15°C to 30°C (59°F to 86°F). Prefilled syringes do not contain preservatives, discard unused portions; multidose vials should be discarded within 28 days after first use. For SubQ use, do not mix with other injections or infusions. For I.V. use (treatment of acute STEMI only), multidose vials may be mixed with NS or D₅W; do not mix with other drugs.

Mechanism of Action Standard heparin consists of components with molecular weights ranging from 4000-30,000 daltons with a mean of 16,000 daltons. Heparin acts as an anticoagulant by enhancing the inhibition rate of clotting proteases by antithrombin III impairing normal hemostasis and inhibition of factor Xa. Low molecular weight heparins have a small effect on the activated partial thromboplastin time and strongly inhibit factor Xa. Enoxaparin is derived from porcine heparin that undergoes benzylation followed by alkaline depolymerization. The average molecular weight of enoxaparin is 4500 daltons which is distributed as (≤20%) 2000 daltons (≥68%) 2000-8000 daltons, and (≤15%) >8000 daltons. Enoxaparin has a higher ratio of antifactor Xa to antifactor IIa activity than unfractionated heparin.

Pharmacodynamics Antifactor Xa and antithrombin (antifactor IIa) activities:

Maximum effect: SubQ: 3-5 hours

Duration: ~12 hours following a 40 mg daily dose given SubQ

Pharmacokinetics (Adult data unless noted) Based on antifactor Xa activity

Distribution: Does not cross the placental barrier

Mean V_d: Adults: 4.3 L

Protein binding: Does not bind to most heparin binding proteins

Metabolism: Primarily in the liver via desulfation and depolymerization to lower molecular weight molecules with very low biological activity

Bioavailability: Adults: SubQ: ~100%

Half-life: SubQ: Adults: Single dose: 4.5 hours; repeat dosing: 7 hours

Elimination: 40% of I.V. dose is excreted in urine as active and inactive fragments; 10% of dose is excreted by kidneys as active enoxaparin fragments; 8% to 20% of antifactor Xa activity is recovered within 24 hours in the urine

Clearance: Decreased by 30% in patients with CrCl <30 mL/minute

Dosing: Neonatal SubQ:

Initial therapy:

Chest, 2008 recommendations (Monagle, 2008):

Prophylaxis: 0.75 mg/kg/dose every 12 hours

Treatment: 1.5 mg/kg/dose every 12 hours

Alternate dosing: Treatment: **Note:** Several recent studies suggest that doses higher than those recommended in the *Chest* guidelines are required in neonates (Malowany, 2007; Malowany, 2008; Sanchez de Toledo, 2010). Some centers are using the following; however, further studies are needed to validate these proposed higher initial doses.

Premature neonates: 2 mg/kg/dose every 12 hours

Full-term neonates: 1.7 mg/kg/dose every 12 hours

Maintenance therapy: *Chest,* 2008 recommendations (Monagle, 2008): See **Dosage Titration** table on next page; **Note:** In a prospective study of 177 courses of enoxaparin in pediatric patients (146 treatment courses; 31 prophylactic courses) considerable variation in maintenance dosage requirements was observed (Dix, 2000).

Enoxaparin Dosage Titration

Antifactor Xa	Dose Titration	Time to Repeat Antifactor Xa Level
<0.35 units/mL	Increase dose by 25%	4 h after next dose
0.35-0.49 units/mL	Increase dose by 10%	4 h after next dose
0.5-1 unit/mL	Keep same dosage	Next day, then 1 wk later, then monthly (4 h after dose)
1.1-1.5 units/mL	Decrease dose by 20%	Before next dose
1.6-2 units/mL	Hold dose for 3 h and decrease dose by 30%	Before next dose, then 4 h after next dose
>2 units/mL	Hold all doses until antifactor Xa is 0.5 units/mL, then decrease dose by 40%	Before next dose and every 12 h until antifactor Xa <0.5 units/mL

Modified from Monagle P, Michelson AD, Bovill E, et al, "Antithrombotic Therapy in Children," *Chest*, 2001, 119:344S-70S.

Dosing: Usual

Infants and Children: SubQ:

Initial therapy:

Chest, 2008 recommendations (Monagle, 2008):

Infants 1 to <2 months:

Prophylaxis: 0.75 mg/kg/dose every 12 hours

Treatment: 1.5 mg/kg/dose every 12 hours

Infants ≥2 months and Children ≤18 years:

Prophylaxis: 0.5 mg/kg/dose every 12 hours

Treatment: 1 mg/kg/dose every 12 hours

Alternate dosing: Treatment: **Note:** Several recent studies suggest that doses higher than those recommended in the *Chest* guidelines are required in pediatric patients (especially in young infants) (Bauman, 2009; Malowany, 2007; Malowany, 2008). Some centers are using the following; however, further studies are needed to validate these proposed higher initial doses.

1 to <3 months: 1.8 mg/kg/dose every 12 hours

3-12 months: 1.5 mg/kg/dose every 12 hours

1-5 years: 1.2 mg/kg/dose every 12 hours

6-18 years: 1.1 mg/kg/dose every 12 hours

Maintenance therapy: *Chest*, 2008 recommendations (Monagle, 2008): See **Dosage Titration** table: **Note:** In a prospective study of 177 courses of enoxaparin in pediatric patients (146 treatment courses; 31 prophylactic courses) considerable variation in maintenance dosage requirements was observed (Dix, 2000).

Enoxaparin Dosage Titration

Antifactor Xa	Dose Titration	Time to Repeat Antifactor Xa Level
<0.35 units/mL	Increase dose by 25%	4 h after next dose
0.35-0.49 units/mL	Increase dose by 10%	4 h after next dose
0.5-1 unit/mL	Keep same dosage	Next day, then 1 wk later, then monthly (4 h after dose)
1.1-1.5 units/mL	Decrease dose by 20%	Before next dose
1.6-2 units/mL	Hold dose for 3 h and decrease dose by 30%	Before next dose, then 4 h after next dose
>2 units/mL	Hold all doses until antifactor Xa is 0.5 units/mL, then decrease dose by 40%	Before next dose and every 12 h until antifactor Xa <0.5 units/mL

Modified from Monagle P, Michelson AD, Bovill E, et al, "Antithrombotic Therapy in Children," *Chest*, 2001, 119:344S-70S.

Adults: **Note:** Consider lower doses for patients <45 kg

Prevention of DVT: SubQ:

Knee replacement surgery: 30 mg every 12 hours; give first dose 12-24 hours after surgery (provided hemostasis has been established); average duration 7-10 days, up to 14 days

Hip replacement surgery: Initial phase: 30 mg every 12 hours with first dose 12-24 hours after surgery (provided hemostasis has been established) or consider 40 mg once daily with first dose given 12 ± 3 hours prior to surgery; average duration of initial phase: 7-10 days, up to 14 days; after initial phase, give 40 mg once daily for 3 weeks

Abdominal surgery in patients at risk: 40 mg once daily; give first dose 2 hours prior to surgery; average duration: 7-10 days, up to 12 days

Medical patients at risk due to severely restricted mobility during acute illness: 40 mg once daily; average duration: 6-11 days, up to 14 days

Treatment of acute DVT and pulmonary embolism: SubQ: **Note:** Initiate warfarin therapy on the same day of starting enoxaparin; continue enoxaparin for a minimum of 5 days (average 7 days) until INR is therapeutic (between 2 and 3) for 24 hours (Kearon, 2008).

Inpatient treatment of acute DVT with or without pulmonary embolism: 1 mg/kg every 12 hours or 1.5 mg/kg once daily

Outpatient treatment of acute DVT without pulmonary embolism: 1 mg/kg every 12 hours

Prevention of ischemic complications of non-Q-wave MI or unstable angina: SubQ: 1 mg/kg every 12 hours in conjunction with oral aspirin (100-325 mg once daily); continue treatment for a minimum of 2 days until patient is clinically stabilized (usually 2-8 days; up to 12.5 days)

Treatment of acute ST-segment elevation myocardial infarction (STEMI): Note: Optimal duration is not defined; in the major clinical trial, therapy was continued for 8 days or until hospital discharge; optimal duration may be >8 days. All patients should receive aspirin (75-325 mg once daily) as soon as they are identified as having STEMI. In patients with STEMI receiving thrombolytics, initiate enoxaparin dosing between 15 minutes before and 30 minutes after fibrinolytic therapy. In patients undergoing percutaneous coronary intervention (PCI), if balloon inflation occurs ≤8 hours after the last SubQ enoxaparin dose, no additional dosing is needed. If balloon inflation occurs 8-12 hours after last SubQ enoxaparin dose, a single I.V. dose of 0.3 mg/kg should be administered (Hirsh, 2008; King, 2007).

Adults <75 years of age: Initial: 30 mg single I.V. bolus **plus** 1 mg/kg (maximum: 100 mg/dose for the first 2 doses only) SubQ every 12 hours. The first SubQ dose should be administered with the I.V. bolus. Maintenance: After first 2 doses, administer 1 mg/kg SubQ every 12 hours.

Adults ≥75 years of age: Dosage adjustment required; see package insert

Dosage adjustment in renal impairment:

CrCl ≥30 mL/minute: No specific adjustment recommended; monitor patients closely for bleeding

CrCl <30 mL/minute: **Note:** Monitor antifactor Xa activity closely. Adults:

DVT prophylaxis in abdominal surgery, hip replacement, knee replacement, or in medical patients during acute illness: SubQ: 30 mg once daily

DVT treatment in conjunction with warfarin (in inpatients with or without pulmonary embolism and in outpatients without pulmonary embolism): SubQ: 1 mg/kg once daily

Prevention of ischemic complications of non-Q-wave MI or unstable angina (with aspirin): SubQ: 1 mg/kg once daily

Treatment of STEMI:

Adults <75 years: Initial: 30 mg single I.V. bolus **plus** 1 mg/kg SubQ (administered at the same time as the I.V. bolus); maintenance: SubQ: 1 mg/kg once daily

Adults ≥75 years: See package insert

Dosage adjustment in hepatic impairment: Dosage adjustment not established; use with caution in patients with hepatic impairment

Administration Parenteral: Do not administer I.M. For SubQ use, administer by deep SubQ injection; do not rub injection site after SubQ administration as bruising may occur. When administering 30 mg or 40 mg SubQ from a commercially prefilled syringe, do not expel the air bubble from the syringe prior to injection (in order to avoid loss of drug). I.V. administration is indicated as part of treatment of STEMI only; flush I.V. access with NS or D_5W before and after enoxaparin I.V. bolus administration (to clear drug from port)

Monitoring Parameters CBC with platelets, stool occult blood tests, serum creatinine and potassium; antifactor Xa activity in select patients (eg, neonates, infants, children, obese patients, and patients with significant renal impairment, active bleeding, or abnormal coagulation parameters); **Note**: Routine monitoring of PT and APTT is not warranted since PT and APTT are relatively insensitive measures of low molecular weight heparin activity; consider monitoring bone density in infants and children with long-term use

Reference Range Antifactor Xa: **Note:** The following are suggested peak values of antifactor Xa. Once daily dosing in pediatric patients is not feasible due to faster enoxaparin clearance and lower drug exposure in pediatric patients compared to adults (O'Brien, 2007).

Therapeutic:

Neonates and Children: 0.5-1.0 units/mL, measured 4-6 hours after SubQ administration **or** 0.5-0.8 units/mL, measured 2-6 hours after SubQ administration (Monagle, 2012)

Adults:

Once-daily dosing: >1 anti-Xa units/mL (Garcia, 2012); the manufacturer recommends a range of 1-2 anti-Xa units/mL

Twice-daily dosing: 0.6-1 anti-Xa units/mL (Garcia, 2012)

Prophylactic:

Children: Prevention of central venous access device related DVT: 0.1-0.3 units/mL (Monagle, 2012)

Adults: 0.2-0.4 units/mL (Nutescu, 2009)

Additional Information Each 10 mg of enoxaparin sodium equals ~1000 units of antifactor Xa activity.

Enoxaparin contains fragments of unfractionated heparin produced by alkaline degradation (depolymerization) of heparin benzyl ester; enoxaparin has mean molecular weights of 3500-5600 daltons, which are much lower than mean molecular weights of unfractionated heparin (12,000-15,000 daltons). Low molecular weight heparins (LMWH) have several advantages over unfractionated heparin: Better SubQ bioavailability, more convenient administration (SubQ versus I.V.), longer half-life (longer dosing interval), more predictable pharmacokinetics and pharmacodynamic (anticoagulant) effect, less intensive laboratory monitoring, reduced risk of heparin-induced thrombocytopenia, potential for outpatient use, and probable reduced risk of osteoporosis (further studies are needed).

Accidental overdosage of enoxaparin may be treated with protamine sulfate; 1 mg protamine sulfate neutralizes 1 mg enoxaparin; first dose of protamine sulfate should equal the dose of enoxaparin injected, if enoxaparin was given in the previous 8 hours; use 0.5 mg protamine sulfate per 1 mg enoxaparin if enoxaparin was given >8 hours prior to protamine or if a second dose of protamine is needed; a second dose of protamine sulfate (0.5 mg per 1 mg enoxaparin) may be given if APTT remains prolonged 2-4 hours after first dose; protamine may not be required ≥12 hours after enoxaparin administration; avoid overdosage with protamine

Some centers dispense pediatric doses in an insulin syringe for greater delivery accuracy and to avoid errors associated with dilutions. Each 1 unit on a 30, 50, or 100 unit graduated insulin syringe is 0.01 mL; using a **100 mg/mL** enoxaparin injection, each "1 unit" on the insulin syringe would provide 1 mg of enoxaparin (Bauman, 2009a).

Dosage Forms Excipient information presented when available (limited, particularly for generics); consult specific product labeling.

Solution, Injection, as sodium:

Lovenox: 300 mg/3 mL (3 mL) [contains benzyl alcohol]

Generic: 300 mg/3 mL (3 mL)

Solution, Subcutaneous, as sodium:

Lovenox: 30 mg/0.3 mL (0.3 mL); 40 mg/0.4 mL (0.4 mL); 60 mg/0.6 mL (0.6 mL); 80 mg/0.8 mL (0.8 mL); 100 mg/mL (1 mL); 120 mg/0.8 mL (0.8 mL); 150 mg/mL (1 mL)

Generic: 30 mg/0.3 mL (0.3 mL); 40 mg/0.4 mL (0.4 mL); 60 mg/0.6 mL (0.6 mL); 80 mg/0.8 mL (0.8 mL); 100 mg/mL (1 mL); 120 mg/0.8 mL (0.8 mL); 150 mg/mL (1 mL)

Solution, Subcutaneous, as sodium [preservative free]:

Lovenox: 30 mg/0.3 mL (0.3 mL); 40 mg/0.4 mL (0.4 mL); 60 mg/0.6 mL (0.6 mL); 80 mg/0.8 mL (0.8 mL); 100 mg/mL (1 mL); 120 mg/0.8 mL (0.8 mL); 150 mg/mL (1 mL)

Generic: 30 mg/0.3 mL (0.3 mL); 40 mg/0.4 mL (0.4 mL); 60 mg/0.6 mL (0.6 mL); 80 mg/0.8 mL (0.8 mL); 100 mg/mL (1 mL); 120 mg/0.8 mL (0.8 mL); 150 mg/mL (1 mL)

References

Bauman ME, Belletrutti MJ, Bajzar L, et al, "Evaluation of Enoxaparin Dosing Requirements in Infants and Children. Better Dosing to Achieve Therapeutic Levels," *Thromb Haemost*, 2009, 101(1):86-92.

Bauman ME, Black KL, Bauman ML, "Novel Uses of Insulin Syringes to Reduce Dosing Errors: A Retrospective Chart Review of Enoxaparin Whole Milligram Dosing," *Thromb Res*, 2009a, 123(6):845-7.

Bontadelli J, Moeller A, Schmugge M, et al, "Enoxaparin Therapy for Arterial Thrombosis in Infants With Congenital Heart Disease," *Intensive Care Med*, 2007, 33(11):1978-84.

deVeber G, Chan A, Monagle P, et al, "Anticoagulation Therapy in Pediatric Patients With Sinovenous Thrombosis: A Cohort Study," *Arch Neurol*, 1998, 55(12):1533-7.

Dix D, Andrew M, Marzinotto V, et al, "The Use of Low Molecular Weight Heparin in Pediatric Patients: A Prospective Cohort Study," *J Pediatr*, 2000, 136(4):439-45.

Dunaway KK, Gal P, and Ransom JL, "Use of Enoxaparin in a Preterm Infant," *Ann Pharmacother*, 2000, 34(12):1410-3.

Guyatt GH, Akl EA, Crowther M, et al, "Executive Summary: Antithrombotic Therapy and Prevention of Thrombosis, 9th ed: American College of Chest Physicians Evidence-Based Clinical Practice Guidelines," *Chest*, 2012, 141(2 Suppl):7-47.

Hirsh J, Guyatt G, Albers GW, et al, "Executive Summary: American College of Chest Physicians Evidence-Based Clinical Practice Guidelines (8th Edition)," *Chest*, 2008, 133(6 Suppl):71-109.

Hirsh J, Warkentin TE, Shaughnessy SG, et al, "Heparin and Low-Molecular-Weight Heparin: Mechanisms of Action, Pharmacokinetics, Dosing, Monitoring, Efficacy, and Safety," *Chest*, 2001, 119:64S-94S.

Kearon C, Kahn SR, Agnelli G, et al, "Antithrombotic Therapy for Venous Thromboembolic Disease: American College of Chest Physicians Evidence-Based Clinical Practice Guidelines (8th Edition)," *Chest*, 2008, 33(6 Suppl):454-545.

King SB 3rd, Smith SC Jr, Hirshfeld JW JR, et al, "2007 Focused Update of the ACC/AHA/SCAI 2005 Guideline Update for Percutaneous Coronary Intervention. A Report of the American College of Cardiology/American Heart Association Task Force on Practice Guidelines: 2007 Writing Group to Review New Evidence and Update the ACC/AHA/SCAI 2005 Guideline Update for Percutaneous Coronary Intervention, Writing on Behalf of the 2005 Writing Committee," *Circulation*, 2008, 117(2):261-95.

Malowany JI, Knoppert DC, Chan AK, et al, "Enoxaparin Use in the Neonatal Intensive Care Unit: Experience Over 8 Years," *Pharmacotherapy*, 2007, 27(9):1263-71.

Malowany JI, Monagle P, Knoppert DC, et al, "Enoxaparin for Neonatal Thrombosis: A Call for a Higher Dose for Neonates," *Thromb Res*, 2008, 122(6):826-30.

Martineau P and Tawil N, "Low-Molecular-Weight Heparins in the Treatment of Deep-Vein Thrombosis," *Ann Pharmacother*, 1998, 32 (5):588-98, 601.

Massicotte P, Adams M, Marzinotto V, et al, "Low-Molecular-Weight Heparin in Pediatric Patients With Thrombotic Disease: A Dose Finding Study," *J Pediatr*, 1996, 128(3):313-8.

Michaels LA, Gurian M, Hegyi T, et al, "Low Molecular Weight Heparin in the Treatment of Venous and Arterial Thromboses in the Premature Infant," *Pediatrics*, 2004, 114(3):703-7.

Monagle P, Chalmers E, Chan A, et al, "Antithrombotic Therapy in Neonates and Children: American College of Chest Physicians Evidence-Based Clinical Practice Guidelines (8th Edition)," *Chest*, 2008, 133(6 Suppl):887S-968S.

Monagle P, Michelson AD, Bovill E, et al, "Antithrombotic Therapy in Children," *Chest*, 2001, 119:344S-70S.

Nutescu EA, Spinler SA, Wittkowsky A, et al, "Low-Molecular-Weight Heparins in Renal Impairment and Obesity: Available Evidence and Clinical Practice Recommendations Across Medical and Surgical Settings," *Ann Pharmacother*, 2009, 43(6):1064-83.

O'Brien SH, Lee H, and Ritchey AK, "Once-Daily Enoxaparin in Pediatric Thromboembolism: A Dose Finding and Pharmacodynamics/Pharmacokinetics Study," *J Thromb Haemost*, 2007, 5(9):1985-7.

Sanchez de Toledo J, Gunawardena S, Munoz R, et al, "Do Neonates, Infants and Young Children Need a Higher Dose of Enoxaparin in the Cardiac Intensive Care Unit?" *Cardiol Young*, 2010, 20(2):138-43.

♦ **Enoxaparin Injection (Can)** *see* Enoxaparin *on page 752*

♦ **Enoxaparin Sodium** *see* Enoxaparin *on page 752*

Entecavir (en TE ka veer)

Related Information
Safe Handling of Hazardous Drugs *on page 2419*
Brand Names: U.S. Baraclude
Brand Names: Canada Baraclude
Therapeutic Category Antiviral Agent
Generic Availability (U.S.) No
Use Treatment of chronic hepatitis B infection with evidence of active viral replication and either evidence of persistent transaminase elevations or histologically active disease (FDA approved in ages ≥16 years and adults)
Pregnancy Risk Factor C
Pregnancy Considerations Teratogenic effects have been observed in animal studies. Information related to use in pregnancy is limited; use only if other options are inappropriate (DHHS [OI], 2013). Pregnant women taking entecavir should enroll in the pregnancy registry by calling 1-800-258-4263.
Breast-Feeding Considerations It is not known if entecavir is excreted in breast milk. Due to the potential for serious adverse reactions in the nursing infant, the manufacturer recommends a decision be made whether to discontinue nursing or to discontinue the drug, taking into account the importance of treatment to the mother.
Contraindications Hypersensitivity to entecavir or any component
Warnings Hazardous agent; use appropriate precautions for handling and disposal (NIOSH, 2012). Severe, acute exacerbation of hepatitis B may occur upon discontinuation of entecavir **[U.S. Boxed Warning]**. Monitor liver function several months after stopping treatment; reinitiation of antihepatitis B therapy may be required. May cause the development of HIV resistance in chronic hepatitis B patients with unrecognized or untreated HIV infection **[U.S. Boxed Warning]**. Determine HIV status prior to initiating treatment with entecavir. Not recommended for use in HIV/HBV coinfected patients unless also receiving highly active antiretroviral therapy (HAART). According to manufacturer labeling, entecavir does not exhibit any clinically relevant activity against human immunodeficiency virus (HIV type 1); however, a small number of case reports have indicated declines in virus levels during entecavir therapy. Reports of

HIV resistance to a common HIV drug has been reported in an HIV/HBV-infected patient receiving entecavir as monotherapy for HBV. Cross-resistance may develop in patients failing previous therapy with lamivudine. Lactic acidosis and severe hepatomegaly with steatosis have been reported with nucleoside analogues, including fatal cases **[U.S. Boxed Warning]**; use with caution in patients with risk factors for liver disease (risk may be increased with female gender, obesity, pregnancy, or prolonged exposure) and suspend treatment in any patient who develops clinical or laboratory findings suggestive of lactic acidosis or hepatotoxicity (transaminase elevation may/may not accompany hepatomegaly and steatosis).

The 0.5 mg tab contains polysorbate 80 (Tween 80) which may cause allergic reactions in susceptible individuals.

Precautions Use with caution in patients with renal impairment or patients receiving concomitant therapy which may reduce renal function; dose adjustment recommended for CrCl <50 mL/minute. Safety and efficacy have not been established in liver transplant patients; limited data available; monitor renal function before and during treatment in liver transplant patients receiving concurrent therapy of cyclosporine or tacrolimus; entecavir dosage may need to be adjusted.

Adverse Reactions Adverse reactions are generally similar in adult and pediatric patients.

Cardiovascular: Peripheral edema (with decompensated liver disease)

Central nervous system: Dizziness, fatigue, headache

Dermatologic: Skin rash

Endocrine & metabolic: Decreased serum bicarbonate (with decompensated liver disease), glycosuria, hyperglycemia

Gastrointestinal: Abdominal pain, diarrhea, dyspepsia, increased serum amylase, increased serum lipase, nausea, unpleasant taste, vomiting

Genitourinary: Hematuria

Hepatic: Ascites (with decompensated liver disease), increased serum ALT, increased serum bilirubin, hepatic encephalopathy

Hematologic & oncologic: Hepatic carcinoma (with decompensated liver disease)

Renal: Increased serum creatinine

Respiratory: Upper respiratory tract infection (with decompensated liver disease)

Miscellaneous: Fever (with decompensated liver disease)

Rare but important or life-threatening: Alopecia, anaphylactoid reaction, hepatomegaly, insomnia, lactic acidosis, macular edema (Muqit, 2011), renal failure, thrombocytopenia

Drug Interactions
Metabolism/Transport Effects None known.
Avoid Concomitant Use There are no known interactions where it is recommended to avoid concomitant use.
Increased Effect/Toxicity
The levels/effects of Entecavir may be increased by: Ganciclovir-Valganciclovir; Ribavirin
Decreased Effect There are no known significant interactions involving a decrease in effect.
Food Interactions Food delays absorption and reduces AUC by 18% to 20%. Management: Administer on an empty stomach 2 hours before or after a meal.
Stability
Oral solution: Store at 25°C (77°F); excursions permitted to 15°C to 30°C (59°F to 86°F). Store in original carton; protect from light. After opening, solution may be used up to expiration date on the container.
Tablets: Store at 25°C (77°F); excursions permitted to 15°C to 30°C (59°F to 86°F). Store in original container; protect from light
Mechanism of Action Entecavir is intracellularly phosphorylated to guanosine triphosphate which competes with ▶

natural substrates to effectively inhibit hepatitis B viral polymerase; enzyme inhibition blocks reverse transcriptase activity thereby reducing viral DNA synthesis.

Pharmacokinetics (Adult data unless noted)

Distribution: Extensive to tissues (V_d in excess of total body water)

Protein binding: ~13%

Metabolism: Minor hepatic glucuronide/sulfate conjugation

Bioavailability: Tablet and oral solution are bioequivalent.

Half-life elimination: Terminal: 5-6 days; accumulation: 24 hours

Time to peak serum concentration: 0.5-1.5 hours

Elimination: Urine (60% to 73% as unchanged drug); undergoes glomerular filtration and tubal secretion

Dosing: Usual Note: Oral tablets and solution may be used interchangeably on a mg:mg basis.

Children and Adolescents:

Hepatitis B infection (HBV), chronic: Oral: **Note:** Optimal duration of treatment not established for nucleoside analogs, a minimum of 12 months and typically longer required; consolidation therapy of at least 6 months after seroconversion and complete viral suppression has been suggested (Jonas, 2010).

Children and Adolescents <16 years: Limited data available:

Nucleoside treatment naïve with compensated liver disease: Children ≥2 years and Adolescents <16 years: No data available; currently under investigation in two separate trials assessing pharmacokinetics and efficacy; see Additional Information.

Lamivudine refractory or resistant or previous antihepatitis therapy: Children ≥4 years and Adolescents <16 years: Limited data available: 0.03 mg/kg once daily (maximum dose: 1 mg) **or** 0.5 mg or 1 mg once daily; dosing based on experience in 38 patients (age range: 4-17 years); in the largest trial (n=30) after 24 weeks of therapy, patients showed statistically significant decrease in HBV-DNA levels and 12 patients had undetectable levels; in the smaller trial (n=8), undetectable HBV-DNA levels were reported in 37.5% of patients (Chu, 2012; Pawlowska, 2012); further studies are needed.

Adolescents ≥16 years:

Nucleoside treatment naïve with compensated liver disease: 0.5 mg once daily

Lamivudine-refractory or known lamivudine or telbivudine-resistant mutations: 1 mg once daily

HIV/Hepatitis B virus coinfection: Limited data available: **Note:** Only recommended in patients who cannot take tenofovir; must be used in addition to a fully suppressive antiretroviral therapy regimen (DHHS [adult/pediatric], 2013): Oral:

Nucleoside treatment naive: Adolescents: 0.5 mg once daily (DHHS [adult], 2013)

Lamivudine-refractory or -resistant with decompensated liver disease:

Children 12 years of age: 0.5 mg once daily (DHHS [pediatric], 2013)

Adolescents: 1 mg once daily (DHHS [adult], 2013)

HBV reinfection prophylaxis, postliver transplant (with or without HBIG): Limited data available: Adolescents ≥16 years: Oral: 1 mg once daily has been reported in an open-label trial of 65 patients (age range: 16 years and older); however, a lower dose of 0.5 mg once daily has also been used in adult patients (age range: 23-65 years); further studies are needed (Fung, 2011; Perrillo, 2012).

Adults: **Hepatitis B virus (HBV) infection, treatment:** Oral:

Nucleoside treatment naive: 0.5 mg once daily

Lamivudine-refractory or -resistant viremia (or known lamivudine- or telbivudine-resistant mutations): 1 mg once daily

Decompensated liver disease: 1 mg once daily

Treatment duration (AASLD Practice Guidelines, 2009):

Hepatitis Be antigen (HBeAg) positive chronic hepatitis: Treat ≥1 year until HBeAg seroconversion and undetectable serum HBV DNA; continue therapy for ≥6 months after HBeAg seroconversion

HBeAg negative chronic hepatitis: Treat >1 year until hepatitis B surface antigen (HBsAg) clearance

Decompensated liver disease: Lifelong treatment is recommended.

Note: Patients not achieving a primary response (<2 log decrease in serum HBV DNA) after at least 6 months of therapy should either receive additional treatment or be switched to an alternative therapy.

Dosing adjustment in renal impairment: Adolescents ≥16 years and Adults: Daily dosage regimen preferred:

CrCl ≥50 mL/minute: No adjustment necessary

CrCl 30-49 mL/minute: Administer 50% of usual dose once daily or administer the normal dose every 48 hours

CrCl 10-29 mL/minute: Administer 30% of usual dose once daily or administer the normal dose every 72 hours

CrCl <10 mL/minute: Administer 10% of usual dose once daily or administer the normal dose every 7 days; administer after hemodialysis

Hemodialysis and peritoneal dialysis (CAPD): Minimally removed by hemodialysis (13% over 4 hours) and CAPD (0.3% over 7 days): Administer 10% of usual dose once daily or administer the normal dose every 7 days; administer after hemodialysis

Dosing adjustment in hepatic impairment: No adjustment necessary.

Administration Hazardous agent; use appropriate precautions for handling and disposal (NIOSH, 2012). Administer on an empty stomach (2 hours before or after a meal).

Oral solution: Do not dilute or mix oral solution with water or other beverages; use calibrated oral dosing syringe.

Monitoring Parameters HIV status (prior to initiation of therapy); liver function tests, renal function; in HBV/HIV-coinfected patients, monitor HIV viral load and CD4 count; HBeAg, HBV DNA; in patients with lamivudine-refractory or -resistant viremia (or known lamivudine- or telbivudine-resistance mutations) entecavir resistance can develop rapidly. Monitor HBV DNA every 3 months (DHHS [adults], 2013).

Additional Information The use of entecavir for the treatment of chronic hepatitis B in pediatric patients 2-15 years who are nucleoside treatment naïve with compensated liver disease is currently under investigation in two separate trials which are assessing pharmacokinetics and efficacy. In both trials, the investigational protocol (0.015 mg/kg once daily; maximum dose: 0.5 mg) being evaluated is similar to adult regimen where dose is 50% less in nucleoside naïve patients relative to those patients with lamivudine resistance; results are pending (NCT00423891; NCT01079806).

Dosage Forms Excipient information presented when available (limited, particularly for generics); consult specific product labeling.

Solution, Oral:

Baraclude: 0.05 mg/mL (210 mL) [contains methylparaben, propylparaben; orange flavor]

Tablet, Oral:

Baraclude: 0.5 mg, 1 mg

References

Chu M, Cho SM, Choe B, et al. Virologic responses to add-on adefovir dipivoxil treatment versus entecavir monotherapy in children with lamivudine-resistant chronic hepatitis B. *J Pediatr Gastroenterol Nutr.* 2012;55:648-652.

DHHS. Guidelines for the prevention and treatment of opportunistic infections among HIV-exposed and HIV-infected children: recommendations from the National Institutes of Health, Centers for Disease Control and Prevention, the HIV Medicine Association of the

Infectious Diseases Society of America, the Pediatric Infectious Diseases Society, and the American Academy of Pediatrics. Available at http://aidsinfo.nih.gov

DHHS Panel on Antiretroviral Guidelines for Adults and Adolescents. Guidelines for the use of antiretroviral agents in HIV-1-infected adults and adolescents, Department of Health and Human Services. February 12, 2013;1-267. Available at http://www.aidsinfo.nih.gov

DHHS Panel on Opportunistic Infections (OI) in HIV-Infected Adults and Adolescents. Guidelines for prevention and treatment of opportunistic infections in HIV-infected adults and adolescents: recommendations from the Centers for Disease Control and Prevention (CDC), the National Institutes of Health (NIH), and the HIV Medicine Association (HIVMA) of the Infectious Diseases Society of America (IDSA)," May 7, 2013. Available at http://aidsinfo.nih.gov/contentfiles/lvguidelines/adult_oi.pdf

Fung J, Cheung C, Chan SC, et al. Entecavir monotherapy is effective in suppressing hepatitis B virus after liver transplantation. Gastroenterology. 2011;141(4):1212-1219.

Jonas MM, Block JM, Haber BA, et al. Treatment of children with chronic hepatitis B virus infection in the United States: patient selection and therapeutic options. Hepatology. 2010;52(6):2192-2205.

Lok AS, McMahon BJ. Chronic hepatitis B: update 2009. Hepatology. 2009;50(3):661-662.

Muqit MK, Stanga PE, Vilar FJ, et al. Presumed entecavir-induced ocular toxicity. Eye (Lond). 2011;25(12):1665-1668.

National Institute for Occupational Safety and Health (NIOSH). NIOSH list of antineoplastic and other hazardous drugs in healthcare settings 2012. Available at http://www.cdc.gov/niosh/docs/2012-150/pdfs/2012-150.pdf

NCT00423891. A study of entecavir in pediatric patients with chronic hepatitis B virus (HBV)-infection. Unpublished data. Available at http://clinicaltrials.gov/ct2/show/NCT00423891?term=00423891&rank=1

NCT01079806. A phase III study of the safety and efficacy of entecavir in pediatric patients with chronic HBV-infection. Unpublished data. Available at http://clinicaltrials.gov/ct2/show/NCT01079806?term=01079806&rank=1

Pawlowska M, Halota W, Smukalska E, et al. HBV DNA suppression during entecavir treatment in previously treated children with chronic hepatitis B. Eur J Clin Microbiol Infect Dis. 2012;31:571-574.

Perrillo R, Buti M, Durand F, et al. Entecavir and hepatitis B immune globulin in patients undergoing liver transplantation for chronic hepatitis B. Liver Transplant. 2013;19:887-895.

♦ **Entocort (Can)** see Budesonide (Systemic, Oral Inhalation) on page 308

♦ **Entocort EC** see Budesonide (Systemic, Oral Inhalation) on page 308

♦ **Entrophen (Can)** see Aspirin on page 212

♦ **Entsol [OTC]** see Sodium Chloride on page 1902

♦ **Entsol Nasal [OTC]** see Sodium Chloride on page 1902

♦ **Entsol Nasal Wash [OTC]** see Sodium Chloride on page 1902

♦ **Enulose** see Lactulose on page 1193

♦ **Epaned** see Enalapril on page 744

♦ **EPEG** see Etoposide on page 815

EPHEDrine (Systemic) (e FED rin)

Medication Safety Issues
Sound-alike/look-alike issues:
EPHEDrine may be confused with Epifrin®, EPINEPHrine

Therapeutic Category Adrenergic Agonist Agent; Sympathomimetic

Generic Availability (U.S.) Yes

Use
Oral: Temporary relief of bronchial asthma symptoms (shortness of breath, tightness of chest, and wheezing) (OTC labeling: FDA approved in ages ≥12 years and adults); **Note:** Not recommended for routine management and treatment of asthma (NAEPP, 2007); has also been used for nasal decongestion and congenital myasthenic syndromes

Parenteral: Treatment of anesthesia-induced hypotension; treatment of hypotension following induced sympathectomy or following overdosage of antihypertensive drugs

[FDA approved in pediatric patients (age not specified) and adults]; has also been used for idiopathic orthostatic hypotension and bronchodilation; **Note:** Not recommended for routine management and treatment of asthma (NAEPP, 2007) nor septic shock (Brierley, 2009).

Pregnancy Risk Factor C

Pregnancy Considerations Animal reproduction studies have not been conducted. Ephedrine crosses the placenta (Hughes, 1985). Ephedrine injection is used at delivery for the prevention and/or treatment of maternal hypotension associated with spinal anesthesia in women undergoing cesarean section (ASA, 2007).

Contraindications Hypersensitivity to ephedrine, any component, or sympathomimetic amines; angle-closure glaucoma

Warnings Use of ephedrine as a pressor is not a substitute for replacement of blood, plasma, fluids, and electrolytes; blood volume should be corrected as fully as possible before ephedrine therapy; must not be used as sole therapy in hypovolemic patients; hypoxia, hypercapnia, and acidosis may reduce the effectiveness and increase the incidence of side effects of ephedrine. May cause hypertension which may result in intracranial hemorrhage; use should generally be avoided or used with extreme caution in situations where vasopressor therapy is contraindicated [eg, thyrotoxicosis, diabetes, hypertension (including pregnancy-related), and other cardiovascular disorders]. May induce angina symptoms and potentially fatal arrhythmias in patients with cardiac disease (eg, coronary insufficiency, ischemia heart disease) or are receiving drugs that may sensitize myocardium to adrenergic stimulation; avoid use in these patients; concomitant use with anesthetics, such as cyclopropane or halothane should be avoided; agents may sensitize heart to arrhythmic effects of other sympathomimetics. Initial parenteral administration may cause temporary decrease in urine formation due to renal vasoconstriction.

Ephedrine should only be used in patients who have been diagnosed with asthma by a physician. Generally, ephedrine should not be used as a bronchodilator since other beta₂-agonists are less toxic; do not use in patients that have been hospitalized due to asthma or use other prescription medications to control asthma symptoms; if asthma symptoms do not improve within 1 hour after dose, patients should be instructed to call prescriber.

Long-term use has been associated with anxiety and symptoms of paranoid schizophrenia; the FDA has issued warnings concerning ephedrine-containing nonprescription products with claims of producing effects, such as euphoria, increased sexual sensation, increased energy, and weight loss; healthcare professionals are urged to be aware of these products and counsel patients, when appropriate, about the potential adverse effects of ephedrine, such as headache, dizziness, heart irregularities, seizures, and possibly death.

Precautions Use with caution in patients with hyperthyroidism, prostatic hypertrophy, and/or urinary stricture. Use with extreme caution in patients taking MAO inhibitors; prolonged hypertension may result from concurrent use. Safety and efficacy for the use of cough and cold products in children <2 years of age is limited. Serious adverse effects including death have been reported. The FDA notes that there are no approved OTC uses for these products in children <2 years of age. Healthcare providers are reminded to ask caregivers about the use of OTC cough and cold products in order to avoid exposure to multiple medications containing the same ingredient.

Adverse Reactions
Cardiovascular: Arrhythmias, chest pain, elevation or depression of blood pressure, hypertension, palpitation, tachycardia, unusual pallor

Central nervous system: Agitation, anxiety, apprehension, CNS stimulating effects, dizziness, excitation, fear, headache hyperactivity, insomnia, irritability, nervousness, restlessness, tension

Gastrointestinal: Anorexia, GI upset, nausea, vomiting, xerostomia

Genitourinary: Painful urination

Neuromuscular & skeletal: Trembling, tremor (more common in the elderly), weakness

Respiratory: Dyspnea

Miscellaneous: Diaphoresis increased

Drug Interactions

Metabolism/Transport Effects None known.

Avoid Concomitant Use

Avoid concomitant use of EPHEDrine (Systemic) with any of the following: Ergot Derivatives; Inhalational Anesthetics; Iobenguane I 123; MAO Inhibitors

Increased Effect/Toxicity

EPHEDrine (Systemic) may increase the levels/effects of: Droxidopa; Inhalational Anesthetics; Sympathomimetics

The levels/effects of EPHEDrine (Systemic) may be increased by: Alkalinizing Agents; AtoMOXetine; Cannabinoid-Containing Products; Carbonic Anhydrase Inhibitors; Ergot Derivatives; Hyaluronidase; Linezolid; MAO Inhibitors; Serotonin/Norepinephrine Reuptake Inhibitors

Decreased Effect

EPHEDrine (Systemic) may decrease the levels/effects of: Benzylpenicilloyl Polylysine; FentaNYL; Iobenguane I 123

The levels/effects of EPHEDrine (Systemic) may be decreased by: Alpha1-Blockers; Spironolactone; Urinary Acidifying Agents

Stability

Oral: Store at 20°C to 25°C (68°F to 77°F); protect from light and moisture

Parenteral: Store at 15°C to 30°C (59°F to 86°F); protect from light

Mechanism of Action Releases tissue stores of norepinephrine and thereby produces an alpha- and beta-adrenergic stimulation; longer-acting and less potent than epinephrine

Pharmacodynamics Pressor/cardiac effects: Duration:

Oral: 4 hours

SubQ: 1 hour

Pharmacokinetics (Adult data unless noted)

Absorption: Oral: Complete

Metabolism: Minimally hepatic by oxidative deamination, demethylation, aromatic hydroxylation, and conjugation

Bioavailability: Oral: 85%

Half-life: 3-6 hours

Elimination: Dependent upon urinary pH with greatest excretion in acid pH; urine pH 5: 74% to 99% excreted unchanged; urine pH 8: 22% to 25% excreted unchanged

Dosing: Neonatal Myasthenic syndromes, congenital: Limited data available: Oral: Initial: 1 mg/kg/**day** in 3 divided doses, may increase to 3 mg/kg/**day** in 3 divided doses (Kliegman, 2011)

Dosing: Usual

Pediatric:

Asthma, bronchodilation: Children ≥12 years and Adolescents: Oral: 12.5-25 mg every 4 hours; if symptoms do not improve after 1 hour from initial dose, physician should be contacted and continuation of therapy evaluated; maximum daily dose: 150 mg/**day**; **Note:** Not recommended for routine management and treatment of asthma and **NOT** indicated for the relief of acute bronchospasm (NAEPP, 2007)

Hypotension, anesthesia-induced: Use the smallest effective dose for the shortest time; **Note:** Not recommended for use in management of septic shock (Brierley, 2009):

Infants, Children, and Adolescents ≤15 years: Limited data available: Slow I.V. push: 0.1-0.3 mg/kg/dose every 4-6 hours; maximum dose: 25 mg (Taguchi, 1996)

Adolescents >15 years: I.V.: 5-25 mg/dose slow I.V. push repeated after 5-10 minutes as needed, then every 3-4 hours; maximum dose: 150 mg/24 hours

Myasthenic syndromes, congenital: Infants, Children, and Adolescents: Limited data available: Oral: Initial: 1 mg/kg/**day** in 3 divided doses, may increase to 3 mg/kg/**day** in 3 divided doses (Engel, 2007; Kliegman, 2011)

Adult:

Hypotension, anesthesia-induced: I.V.: 5-25 mg/dose slow I.V. push repeated after 5-10 minutes as needed, then every 3-4 hours (maximum: 150 mg/24 hours)

Idiopathic orthostatic hypotension: Oral: 25-50 mg 3 times/**day**; maximum daily dose: 150 mg/**day**; **Note:** Not considered first-line for this indication.

Administration

Oral: May be administered without regard to food

Parenteral: I.V.: Administer by slow I.V. push; in a pediatric hypotension trial, ephedrine doses of 0.1 mg/kg and 0.2 mg/kg were diluted to 1 mg/mL and 2 mg/mL, respectively, prior to administration (Taguchi, 1996)

Monitoring Parameters Blood pressure, pulse, respiratory symptoms

Test Interactions Can cause a false-positive amphetamine EMIT assay

Additional Information Because ephedrine and pseudoephedrine have been used to synthesize methamphetamine, the DEA has placed them in the category of "Schedule Listed Products"; restrictions are in place to reduce the potential for misuse (diversion) and abuse (eg, storage requirements, additional documentation of sale); the DEA limit for a single transaction to a single individual for drug products containing ephedrine or pseudoephedrine is 3.6 g/24 hours, 9 g/30 days, or if mail-order transaction 7.5 g/30 days.

Dosage Forms Excipient information presented when available (limited, particularly for generics); consult specific product labeling.

Capsule, Oral, as sulfate:

Generic: 25 mg

Solution, Injection, as sulfate:

Generic: 50 mg/mL (1 mL)

Solution, Injection, as sulfate [preservative free]:

Generic: 50 mg/mL (1 mL)

References

American Society of Anesthesiologists Task Force on Obstetric Anesthesia, "Practice Guidelines for Obstetric Anesthesia: An Updated Report by the American Society of Anesthesiologists Task Force on Obstetric Anesthesia," *Anesthesiology*, 2007, 106(4):843-63.

Brierley J, Carcillo JA, Choong K, et al, "Clinical Practice Parameters for Hemodynamic Support of Pediatric and Neonatal Septic Shock: 2007 Update From the American College of Critical Care Medicine," *Crit Care Med*, 2009, 37(2):666-88.

Engel AG, "The Therapy of Congenital Myasthenic Syndromes," *Neurotherapeutics*, 2007, 4(2):252-7.

Ephedrine sulfate [prescribing information]. Eatontown, NJ: West-ward Pharmaceutical Corp; October 2009

Ephedrine sulfate [prescribing information]. Princeton, NJ: Sandoz, Inc.

Hughes SC, Ward MG, Levinson G, et al, "Placental Transfer of Ephedrine Does Not Affect Neonatal Outcome," *Anesthesiology*, 1985, 63(2):217-9.

Kliegman RM, Stanton BF, St. Gemell JW, et al, eds. *Nelson Textbook of Pediatrics*. 19th ed. Philadelphia, PA: Saunders Elsevier;2011.

National Asthma Education and Prevention Program (NAEPP), "Expert Panel Report 3 (EPR-3): Guidelines for the Diagnosis and Management of Asthma," *Clinical Practice Guidelines*, National Institutes of Health, National Heart, Lung, and Blood Institute, NIH Publication No. 08-4051, 2007. Available at http://www.nhlbi.nih.gov/guidelines/asthma/asthgdln.htm

Taguchi N, Nishikawa T, Inomata S, et al, "Hemodynamic Effects of Intravenous Ephedrine in Infants and Children Anesthetized With Halothane and Nitrous Oxide," *Anesth Analg*, 1996, 82(3):568-73.

◆ **Ephedrine Sulfate** *see* EPHEDrine (Systemic) *on page 759*

◆ **E-Pherol [OTC]** *see* Vitamin E *on page 2148*

◆ **Epi-Clenz™ [OTC]** *see* Alcohol (Ethyl) *on page 88*

◆ **Epiduo®** *see* Adapalene and Benzoyl Peroxide *on page 74*

◆ **Epi E-Z Pen (Can)** *see* EPINEPHrine (Systemic, Oral Inhalation) *on page 761*

Epinastine (ep i NAS teen)

Brand Names: U.S. Elestat
Therapeutic Category Antiallergic, Ophthalmic
Generic Availability (U.S.) Yes
Use Prevention of itching associated with allergic conjunctivitis (FDA approved in ages ≥2 years and adults)
Pregnancy Risk Factor C
Pregnancy Considerations Teratogenic effects were not observed in animal studies. There are no adequate and well-controlled studies in pregnant women.
Breast-Feeding Considerations It is not known if epinastine is excreted in breast milk. The manufacturer recommends that caution be exercised when administering epinastine to nursing women.
Contraindications Hypersensitivity to epinastine or any component
Warnings Inadvertent contamination of multiple-dose ophthalmic solutions has caused bacterial keratitis. Not for the treatment of contact lens irritation. Solution contains the preservative benzalkonium chloride, which may be absorbed by soft contact lenses; wait at least 10 minutes after instillation before inserting soft contact lenses. Do not wear contact lenses if eyes are red.
Adverse Reactions
Central nervous system: Headache
Ocular: Burning sensation, folliculosis, hyperemia, pruritus
Respiratory: Cough, pharyngitis, rhinitis, sinusitis
Miscellaneous: Infection (defined as cold symptoms and upper respiratory infection)
Rare but important or life-threatening: Lacrimation increased
Drug Interactions
Metabolism/Transport Effects None known.
Avoid Concomitant Use There are no known interactions where it is recommended to avoid concomitant use.
Increased Effect/Toxicity There are no known significant interactions involving an increase in effect.
Decreased Effect There are no known significant interactions involving a decrease in effect.
Stability Store at 15°C to 25°C (59°F to 77°F). Keep tightly closed.
Mechanism of Action Selective H_1-receptor antagonist; inhibits release of histamine from the mast cell; also has affinity for the H_2, alpha$_1$, alpha$_2$, and the 5-HT$_2$ receptors
Pharmacodynamics
Onset of action: 3-5 minutes
Duration: 8 hours
Pharmacokinetics (Adult data unless noted)
Absorption: Low systemic absorption following topical application
Distribution: Does not cross blood-brain barrier
Protein binding: 64%

Metabolism: <10% metabolized
Half-life: 12 hours
Elimination: I.V.: Urine (55%); feces (30%)
Dosing: Usual Children ≥2 years, Adolescents, and Adults: **Allergic Conjunctivitis:** Ophthalmic: Instill 1 drop into each eye twice daily; continue throughout period of exposure, even in the absence of symptoms
Dosing adjustment in renal impairment: There are no dosage adjustments provided in the manufacturer's labeling; however, dosage adjustment unlikely necessary due to low systemic absorption.
Dosing adjustment in hepatic impairment: There are no dosage adjustments provided in the manufacturer's labeling; however, dosage adjustment unlikely necessary due to low systemic absorption.
Administration For ophthalmic use only; avoid touching tip of applicator to eye or other surfaces. Contact lenses should be removed prior to application; may be reinserted after 10 minutes. Do not wear contact lenses if eyes are red.
Dosage Forms Excipient information presented when available (limited, particularly for generics); consult specific product labeling.
Solution, Ophthalmic, as hydrochloride:
Elestat: 0.05% (5 mL) [contains benzalkonium chloride]
Generic: 0.05% (5 mL)

◆ **Epinastine Hydrochloride** *see* Epinastine *on page 761*

EPINEPHrine (Systemic, Oral Inhalation)
(ep i NEF rin)

Medication Safety Issues
Sound-alike/look-alike issues:
EPINEPHrine may be confused with ePHEDrine
Epifrin may be confused with ephedrine, EpiPen
High alert medication:
The Institute for Safe Medication Practices (ISMP) includes this medication among its list of drugs which have a heightened risk of causing significant patient harm when used in error.
Administration issues:
Medication errors have occurred due to confusion with epinephrine products expressed as ratio strengths (eg, 1:1000 vs 1:10,000).
Epinephrine 1:1000 = 1 mg/mL and is most commonly used I.M.
Epinephrine 1:10,000 = 0.1 mg/mL and is used I.V.
Medication errors have occurred when topical epinephrine 1 mg/mL (1:1000) has been inadvertently injected. Vials of injectable and topical epinephrine look very similar. Epinephrine should always be appropriately labeled with the intended administration.
International issues:
EpiPen [U.S., Canada, and multiple international markets] may be confused with Epigen brand name for glycyrrhizinic acid [Argentina, Mexico, Russia] and Epopen brand name for epoetin alfa [Spain]
Related Information
Adult ACLS Algorithms *on page 2198*
Emergency Drip Calculations *on page 2191*
Management of Drug Extravasations *on page 2255*
Newborn Resuscitation Algorithm *on page 2193*
Pediatric ALS (PALS) Algorithms *on page 2195*
Safe Handling of Hazardous Drugs *on page 2419*
Serotonin Syndrome *on page 2405*
Brand Names: U.S. Adrenaclick; Adrenalin; Asthmanefrin Refill [OTC]; Asthmanefrin Starter Kit [OTC]; Auvi-Q; EpiPen 2-Pak; EpiPen Jr 2-Pak; Micronefrin [OTC]; S2 [OTC]
Brand Names: Canada Adrenalin; Epi E-Z Pen; EpiPen; EpiPen Jr; Twinject

◀ **Therapeutic Category** Adrenergic Agonist Agent; Anti-asthmatic; Antidote, Hypersensitivity Reactions; Broncho-dilator; Sympathomimetic

Generic Availability (U.S.) May be product dependent

Use

Parenteral:

Injection: Treatment of bronchospasms, bronchial asthma, anaphylactic reactions, cardiac arrest, and attacks of transitory atrioventricular (AV) heart block with syncopal seizures (Stokes-Adams Syndrome); added to local anesthetics to decrease systemic absorption of intraspinal and local anesthetics and increase duration of action; induction and maintenance of mydriasis during intraocular surgery [FDA approved in pediatric patients (age not specified) and adults]

Autoinjectors (eg, Auvi-Q™, EpiPen®): Emergency treatment (immediate administration) of severe allergic reactions including anaphylaxis in patient at increased risk or previous history of anaphylactic reactions (FDA approved in patients weighing ≥15 kg)

Oral inhalation (nebulization): Racemic epinephrine: Treatment of bronchial asthma (OTC labeling: FDA approved in ages ≥4 years and adults); has also been used to treat upper airway obstruction and croup

Pregnancy Risk Factor C

Pregnancy Considerations Teratogenic effects have been observed in animal reproduction studies. Epinephrine crosses the placenta and may cause fetal anoxia. Use during pregnancy when the potential benefit to the mother outweighs the possible risk to the fetus.

Breast-Feeding Considerations It is not known if epinephrine is excreted in breast milk. The manufacturer recommends that caution be exercised when administering epinephrine to nursing women.

Contraindications Note: There are no absolute contraindications to the use of injectable epinephrine (including Auvi-Q™, EpiPen®, EpiPen® Jr, and Twinject®) in a life-threatening situation. Hypersensitivity to epinephrine or any component; general anesthesia with halogenated hydrocarbons (eg, halothane) or cyclopropane; narrow angle glaucoma; nonanaphylactic shock; organic brain damage; cardiac dilatation and coronary insufficiency; labor, in combination with local anesthesia of certain areas such as fingers, toes, and ears

Oral inhalation: Concurrent use or within 2 weeks of MAO inhibitors

Warnings Due to direct catecholamine effect, administration of epinephrine may cause high arterial blood pressure (may cause angina pectoris, aortic rupture, or cerebral hemorrhage); induce potentially serious cardiac arrhythmias; and produce constriction of renal blood vessels and decrease urine formation initially (with parenteral administration). Rapid I.V. administration may cause death from cerebrovascular hemorrhage or cardiac arrhythmias; however, rapid I.V. administration during pulseless arrest is necessary. Use of undiluted epinephrine intraocularly may cause corneal epithelial damage; must dilute 1:**1000** (1 mg/mL) solution to a concentration of 1:**100,000** to 1:**1,000,000** (10 mcg/mL to 1 **mcg**/mL) prior to intraocular use. Self-medication of the oral inhalation (OTC use) should be avoided if any of the following are present: Heart disease, high blood pressure, thyroid disease, diabetes, seizures, narrow angle glaucoma, psychiatric/emotional condition, or difficulty urinating due to an enlarged prostate.

Autoinjectors should be injected only into the anterolateral aspect of the thigh; injection into the buttocks may not provide effective treatment; accidental injection into digits, hands, or feet may result in local reactions including injection site pallor, coldness, and hypoesthesia or injury resulting in bruising, bleeding, discoloration, erythema, or skeletal injury. Patient should seek immediate medical attention if occurs.

Some products contain sulfites as preservatives which may cause allergic reactions in susceptible individuals; the presence of sulfites should not deter administration during a serious allergic or other emergency situation even if the patient is sulfite-sensitive.

For self-medication (OTC use), oral inhalation should only be used in patients with diagnosis of asthma who are not currently on asthma therapy nor have ever required hospitalization for asthma symptoms; patients should contact healthcare provider prior to therapy initiation; if symptoms are not relieved in 20 minutes or worsen, discontinue and seek immediate medical assistance. OTC use of oral inhalation should not be used more frequently or at higher doses than recommended unless directed by a healthcare provider.

Precautions Use with caution in patients with diabetes mellitus; may increase blood glucose levels. Use with caution in cardiovascular disease (coronary artery disease, hypertension), thyroid disease, and cerebrovascular disease due to direct catecholamine effect of epinephrine. Use with caution in Parkinson's disease; may cause temporary increase in symptoms. Use with extreme caution in patients taking MAO inhibitors and tricyclic antidepressants; effects of epinephrine may be potentiated.

Adverse Reactions

Cardiovascular: Angina, cardiac arrhythmia, chest pain, flushing, hypertension, pallor, palpitation, sudden death, tachycardia (parenteral), vasoconstriction, ventricular ectopy, ventricular fibrillation

Central nervous system: Anxiety (transient), apprehensiveness, cerebral hemorrhage, dizziness, headache, insomnia, lightheadedness, nervousness, restlessness

Gastrointestinal: Dry throat, loss of appetite, nausea, vomiting, xerostomia

Genitourinary: Acute urinary retention in patients with bladder outflow obstruction

Neuromuscular & skeletal: Tremor, weakness

Ocular: Allergic lid reaction, burning, corneal endothelial damage (intraocular use), eye pain, ocular irritation, precipitation of or exacerbation of narrow-angle glaucoma, transient stinging

Respiratory: Dyspnea, pulmonary edema

Miscellaneous: Diaphoresis

Drug Interactions

Metabolism/Transport Effects Substrate of COMT

Avoid Concomitant Use

Avoid concomitant use of EPINEPHrine (Systemic, Oral Inhalation) with any of the following: Ergot Derivatives; Iobenguane I 123; Lurasidone

Increased Effect/Toxicity

EPINEPHrine (Systemic, Oral Inhalation) may increase the levels/effects of: Lurasidone; Sympathomimetics

The levels/effects of EPINEPHrine (Systemic, Oral Inhalation) may be increased by: AtoMOXetine; Beta-Blockers; Cannabinoid-Containing Products; COMT Inhibitors; Ergot Derivatives; Hyaluronidase; Inhalational Anesthetics; Linezolid; MAO Inhibitors; Serotonin/Norepinephrine Reuptake Inhibitors; Tricyclic Antidepressants

Decreased Effect

EPINEPHrine (Systemic, Oral Inhalation) may decrease the levels/effects of: Benzylpenicilloyl Polylysine; Iobenguane I 123

The levels/effects of EPINEPHrine (Systemic, Oral Inhalation) may be decreased by: Alpha1-Blockers; Promethazine; Spironolactone

Stability Epinephrine is sensitive to light and air. Protection from light is recommended. Oxidation turns drug pink, then a brown color. **Solutions should not be used if they are discolored or contain a precipitate.**

Parenteral: Store between 20°C to 25°C (68°F to 77°F); excursions permitted to 15°C to 30°C (59°F to 86°F); do not freeze. Protect from light; stability of injection in parenteral admixture at room temperature (25°C) or refrigeration (4°C) is 24 hours.

Parenteral (autoinjectors): Auvi-Q™, EpiPen® and Epi-Pen® Jr, Twinject®: Store at 20°C to 25°C (68°F to 77°F); excursions permitted to 15°C to 30°C (59°F to 86°F); do not freeze or refrigerate. Protect from light by storing in carrier tube provided.

Oral inhalation (solution):

Asthmanefrin™: Store between 20°C to 25°C (68°F to 77°F); protect from light and excessive heat.

S2®: Store between 2°C to 25°C (36°F to 68°F); protect from light and excessive heat.

Mechanism of Action Stimulates alpha-, beta$_1$-, and beta$_2$-adrenergic receptors resulting in relaxation of smooth muscle of the bronchial tree, cardiac stimulation (increasing myocardial oxygen consumption), and dilation of skeletal muscle vasculature; small doses can cause vasodilation via beta$_2$-vascular receptors; large doses may produce constriction of skeletal and vascular smooth muscle

Pharmacodynamics

Local vasoconstriction:
Onset of action: 5 minutes
Duration: <1 hour

Onset of bronchodilation:
Inhalation: Within 1 minute
SubQ.: Within 5-10 minutes

Pharmacokinetics (Adult data unless noted)

Absorption: Orally ingested doses are rapidly metabolized in GI tract and liver; pharmacologically active concentrations are not achieved

Distribution: Does not cross blood-brain barrier

Metabolism: Taken up into the adrenergic neuron and metabolized by monoamine oxidase and catechol-o-methyltransferase; circulating drug hepatically metabolized

Excretion: Urine (as inactive metabolites, metanephrine, and sulfate and hydroxy derivatives of mandelic acid; small amounts as unchanged drug)

Dosing: Neonatal Cardiopulmonary resuscitation (Kattwinkel, 2010):

I.V.: 0.01-0.03 mg/kg (0.1-0.3 mL/kg of **1:10,000** solution) every 3-5 minutes as needed

Endotracheal: **Note:** I.V. route preferred: E.T.: 0.05-0.1 mg/kg (0.5-1 mL/kg of **1:10,000** solution) every 3-5 minutes until I.V. access established or return of spontaneous circulation

Dosing: Usual

Infants, Children, and Adolescents:

Asthma, bronchodilation:

Nebulization: Racemic epinephrine (2.25% solution): Children ≥4 years and Adolescents: Manufacturer labeling: 0.5 mL diluted with 3-5 mL of NS; administer with jet nebulizer every ~15 minutes every 3-4 hours as needed. **Note:** Not recommended for routine management and treatment of asthma (NAEPP, 2007).

Asystole or pulseless arrest (AHA, 2010):

I.V., I.O.: 0.01 mg/kg (0.1 mL/kg of **1:10,000** solution) (maximum single dose: 1 mg); every 3-5 minutes until return of spontaneous circulation

Endotracheal: 0.1 mg/kg (0.1 mL/kg of **1:1000** solution) (maximum single dose: 2.5 mg) every 3-5 minutes until return of spontaneous circulation or I.V./I.O. access established. **Note:** Recent clinical studies suggest that lower epinephrine concentrations delivered by endotracheal administration may produce transient β-adrenergic effects which may be detrimental (eg, hypotension, lower coronary artery perfusion

pressure). I.V. or I.O. are the preferred methods of administration.

Bradycardia (AHA, 2010):

I.V., I.O.: 0.01 mg/kg (0.1 mL/kg of **1:10,000** solution) (maximum dose: 1 mg or 10 mL); may repeat every 3-5 minutes as needed

Endotracheal: 0.1 mg/kg (0.1 mL/kg of **1:1000** solution) (maximum single dose: 2.5 mg); doses as high as 0.2 mg/kg may be effective; may repeat every 3-5 minutes as needed until I.V./I.O. access established

Continuous infusion: I.V., I.O.: 0.1-1 **mcg**/kg/**minute**; titrate dosage to desired effect

Croup (laryngotracheobronchitis), airway edema:

Nebulization: Infants, Children, and Adolescents: **Note:** Typically relief of symptoms occurs within 10-30 minutes and lasts 2-3 hours; patients should be observed for rapid symptom recurrence and possible repeat treatment.

Racemic epinephrine (2.25% solution): 0.05-0.1 mL/kg (maximum dose: 0.5 mL) diluted in 2 mL NS, may repeat dose every 20 minutes; others have reported use of 0.5 mL as a fixed dose for all patients; use lower end of dosing range for younger infants (Hegenbarth, 2008; Rosekrans, 1998; Rotta, 2003; Wright, 2002)

L-epinephrine: 0.5 mL/kg of **1:1000** solution (maximum dose: 5 mL) diluted in NS, may repeat dose every 20 minutes; **Note:** Racemic epinephrine 10 mg = 5 mg L-epinephrine (Hegenbarth, 2008)

Hypersensitivity/Allergic reactions: Note: SubQ administration results in slower absorption and is less reliable. I.M. administration in the anterolateral aspect of the middle third of the thigh is preferred in the setting of anaphylaxis (ACLS guidelines, 2010; Kemp, 2008). For self-administration following severe allergic reactions (eg, insect stings, food), the World Health Organization (WHO) and Anaphylaxis Canada recommend the availability of one dose for every 10-20 minutes of travel time to a medical emergency facility.

I.M., SubQ: 0.01 mg/kg (0.01 mL/kg/dose of **1:1000** solution) not to exceed 0.3-0.5 mg every 5-15 minutes (Hegenbarth, 2008; Kemp, 2008)

I.M.: Autoinjector dose:

AAP/World Allergy Organization recommendations (Kemp, 2008; Sicherer, 2007):

10-25 kg: 0.15 mg
>25 kg: 0.3 mg

Manufacturer labeling (Auvi-Q™, EpiPen® Jr, Epi-Pen®, Twinject®):

15-29 kg: 0.15 mg; if anaphylactic symptoms persist, dose may be repeated in 5-15 minutes

≥30 kg: 0.3 mg; if anaphylactic symptoms persist, dose may be repeated in 5-15 minutes

I.V.: 0.01 mg/kg (0.1 mL/kg of **1:10,000** solution) not to exceed 0.5 mg every 20 minutes; may use continuous infusion (0.1 mcg/kg/minute) to prevent frequent doses in more severe reactions

Hypotension/shock, fluid-resistant: Continuous I.V. infusion: 0.1-1 **mcg**/kg/**minute**; doses up to 5 mcg/kg/minute may rarely be necessary, may be combined with inotropic support (Hegenbarth, 2008)

SubQ: 0.01 mg/kg (0.01 mL/kg of **1:1000** solution) (maximum single dose: 0.5 mg) every 20 minutes for 3 doses (Hegenbarth, 2008)

Inotropic support: Continuous I.V. infusion: 0.1-1 **mcg**/kg/**minute**; titrate dosage to desired effect

Postresuscitation infusion to maintain cardiac output or stabilize: Continuous I.V./I.O. infusion rate: 0.1-1 mcg/kg/minute; doses <0.3 mcg/kg/minute generally produce β-adrenergic effects and higher doses (>0.3 mcg/kg/minute) generally produce alpha-adrenergic vasoconstriction; titrate dosage to desired effect

Adults:

Asystole/pulseless arrest, pulseless VT/VF (ACLS, 2010):

I.V., I.O.: 1 mg every 3-5 minutes until return of spontaneous circulation; if this approach fails, higher doses of epinephrine (up to 0.2 mg/kg) have been used for treatment of specific problems (eg, beta-blocker or calcium channel blocker overdose)

Endotracheal: 2-2.5 mg every 3-5 minutes until I.V./I.O. access established or return of spontaneous circulation; dilute in 5-10 mL NS or sterile water. **Note:** Absorption may be greater with sterile water (Naganobu, 2000).

Bradycardia (symptomatic; unresponsive to atropine or pacing): I.V. infusion: 2-10 mcg/minute **or** 0.1-0.5 mcg/kg/minute (7-35 mcg/minute in a 70 kg patient); titrate to desired effect (ACLS, 2010)

Bronchodilator:

Nebulization: S2® (racemic epinephrine, OTC labeling): 0.5 mL: Repeat no more frequently than every 3-4 hours as needed.

SubQ: 0.3-0.5 mg (**1:1000** solution) every 20 minutes for 3 doses

Hypersensitivity reactions: Note: SubQ administration results in slower absorption and is less reliable. I.M. administration in the anterolateral aspect of the middle third of the thigh is preferred in the setting of anaphylaxis (ACLS guidelines, 2010; Kemp, 2008).

I.M., SubQ: 0.2-0.5 mg (**1:1000** solution) every 5-15 minutes in the absence of clinical improvement (ACLS, 2010; Kemp, 2008; Lieberman, 2010). If clinician deems appropriate, the 5-minute interval between injections may be shortened to allow for more frequent administration (Lieberman, 2010).

I.V.: 0.1 mg (**1:10,000** solution) over 5 minutes; may infuse at 1-4 mcg/minute to prevent the need to repeat injections frequently **or** may initiate with an infusion at 5-15 mcg/minute (with crystalloid administration) (ACLS, 2010; Brown, 2004). In general, I.V. administration should only be done in patients who are profoundly hypotensive or are in cardiopulmonary arrest refractory to volume resuscitation and several epinephrine injections (Lieberman, 2010).

Self-administration following severe allergic reactions (eg, insect stings, food): **Note:** The World Health Organization (WHO) and Anaphylaxis Canada recommend the availability of one dose for every 10-20 minutes of travel time to a medical emergency facility. More than 2 doses should only be administered under direct medical supervision.

Auvi-Q™: I.M., SubQ: 0.3 mg; if anaphylactic symptoms persist, dose may be repeated

Twinject®: I.M., SubQ: 0.3 mg; if anaphylactic symptoms persist, dose may be repeated in 5-15 minutes using the same device after partial disassembly

EpiPen®: I.M., SubQ: 0.3 mg; if anaphylactic symptoms persist, dose may be repeated in 5-15 minutes using an additional EpiPen®

Hypotension/shock, severe and fluid resistant: I.V. infusion: Initial: 0.1-0.5 mcg/kg/minute (7-35 mcg/minute in a 70 kg patient); titrate to desired response (ACLS, 2010)

Induction and maintenance of mydriasis during intraocular surgery: Intraocular: Must dilute 1:**1000** (1 mg/mL) solution to a concentration of 1:**100,000** to 1:**1,000,000** (10 **mcg**/mL to 1 **mcg**/mL) prior to intraocular use: May use as an irrigation solution as needed during the procedure or may administer intracamerally (ie, directly into the anterior chamber of the eye) with a bolus dose of 0.1 mL of a 1:**100,000** to 1:**400,000** (10 **mcg**/mL to 2.5 **mcg**/mL) dilution.

Dosing adjustment in renal impairment: There are no dosage adjustment provided in manufacturer's labeling.

Dosing adjustment in hepatic impairment: There are no dosage adjustment provided in manufacturer's labeling.

Usual Infusion Concentrations: Neonatal I.V. infusion: 10 **mcg**/mL, 16 **mcg**/mL, 32 **mcg**/mL, or 64 **mcg**/mL

Usual Infusion Concentrations: Pediatric I.V. infusion: 16 **mcg**/mL, 32 **mcg**/mL, or 64 **mcg**/mL

Administration

Endotracheal:

Neonates: Use 0.1 mg/mL (**1:10,000**) solution

Infants, Children, and Adolescents: Use 1 mg/mL solution (**1:1000**); administer and flush with a minimum of 5 mL NS, followed by 5 manual ventilations

Nebulization: Dilute in 2-3 mL NS; if using jet nebulizer: Administer over ~15 minutes; must be diluted. If using handheld rubber bulb nebulizer; dilution is not required.

Parenteral:

Direct I.V. or I.O. administration: Dilute to a maximum concentration of 100 mcg/mL; if using **1:10,000** concentration, no dilution is necessary; pH: 2.5-5.0

Continuous I.V. infusion: Rate of infusion (mL/hour) = dose (mcg/kg/minute) x weight (kg) x 60 minutes/hour divided by the concentration (mcg/mL); maximum concentration: 64 mcg/mL

I.M. (Auvi-Q™, EpiPen®, EpiPen® Jr, Twinject®): Intramuscularly into anterolateral aspect of the middle third of the thigh; Auvi-Q™ and EpiPen® products are single-use products and a new device should be used for each dose; Twinject® device contains two doses; second dose is available after partial disassembly; **Note:** In overweight or obese children, because skin surface to muscle depth is greater in the upper half of the thigh, administration into the lower half of the thigh may be preferred. In very obese children, injection into the calf will provide an even greater chance of intramuscular administration (Arkwright, 2013).

SubQ: Use only **1:1000** solution

Vesicant/Extravasation Risk Vesicant

Monitoring Parameters ECG, heart rate, blood pressure, site of infusion for excessive blanching/extravasation, rebound respiratory symptoms, cardiac monitor and blood pressure monitor required during continuous infusion

Dosage Forms Excipient information presented when available (limited, particularly for generics); consult specific product labeling. [DSC] = Discontinued product

Device, Injection:

Auvi-Q: 0.15 mg/0.15 mL (2 ea); 0.3 mg/0.3 mL (2 ea) [contains sodium bisulfite]

EpiPen 2-Pak: 0.3 mg/0.3 mL (2 ea) [latex free; contains sodium metabisulfite]

EpiPen Jr 2-Pak: 0.15 mg/0.3 mL (2 ea) [contains sodium metabisulfite]

Nebulization Solution, Inhalation:

Asthmanefrin Refill: 2.25% (1 ea) [contains edetate disodium]

Asthmanefrin Starter Kit: 2.25% (1 ea) [contains edetate disodium]

Micronefrin: 2.25% (15 mL, 30 mL)

Nebulization Solution, Inhalation [preservative free]:

S2: 2.25% (1 ea) [sulfite free; contains edetate disodium]

Solution, Injection:

Adrenalin: 1 mg/mL (1 mL) [contains sodium metabisulfite]

Adrenalin: 30 mg/30 mL (30 mL) [contains chlorobutanol (chlorobutol), sodium metabisulfite]

Generic: 0.1 mg/mL (10 mL); 1 mg/mL (1 mL)

Solution, Injection, as hydrochloride:

Adrenalin: 1 mg/mL (30 mL [DSC]) [contains chlorobutanol (chlorobutol), sodium bisulfite]

Adrenalin: 1 mg/mL (1 mL [DSC]) [contains sodium bisulfite]

Generic: 1 mg/mL (1 mL, 30 mL)

Solution Auto-injector, Injection:
Adrenaclick: 0.15 mg/0.15 mL (2 ea); 0.3 mg/0.3 mL (2 ea) [latex free; contains chlorobutanol (chlorobutol), sodium bisulfite]
Generic: 0.15 mg/0.15 mL (2 ea); 0.3 mg/0.3 mL (1 ea, 2 ea)
Solution Prefilled Syringe, Injection:
Generic: 0.1 mg/mL (10 mL)

References

Arkwright P, Wright N, and Bewick D, "Anatomical and Anthropometric Determinants of Intramuscular Versus Subcutaneous Administration in Children With Epinephrine Auto-injectors," *J Allergy Clin Immunol*, 2013, 131(2):199.

Brown SG, Blackman KE, Stenlake V, et al, "Insect Sting Anaphylaxis: Prospective Evaluation of Treatment With Intravenous Adrenaline and Volume Resuscitation," *Emerg Med J*, 2004, 21(2):149-54.

Field JM, Hazinski MF, Sayre MR, et al, "Part 1: Executive Summary: 2010 American Heart Association Guidelines for Cardiopulmonary Resuscitation and Emergency Cardiovascular Care," *Circulation*, 2010, 122 (Suppl 3):640-56.

Hegenbarth MA and the American Academy of Pediatrics Committee on Drugs, "Preparing for Pediatric Emergencies: Drugs to Consider," *Pediatrics*, 2008, 121(2):433-43.

Institute for Safe Medication Practices (ISMP), "Standard Concentrations of Neonatal Drug Infusions," *ISMP*, 2011.

Kattwinkel J, Perlman JM, Aziz K, et al, "Neonatal Resuscitation: 2010 American Heart Association Guidelines for Cardiopulmonary Resuscitation and Emergency Cardiovascular Care," *Pediatrics*, 2010, 126 (5):e1400-13.

Kemp SF, Lockey RF, Simons FE, et al, "Epinephrine: The Drug of Choice for Anaphylaxis. A Statement of the World Allergy Organization," *Allergy*, 2008, 63(8):1061-70.

Kleinman ME, Chameides L, Schexnayder SM, et al, "Part 14: Pediatric Advanced Life Support: 2010 American Heart Association Guidelines for Cardiopulmonary Resuscitation and Emergency Cardiovascular Care," *Circulation*, 2010, 122(18 Suppl 3):876-908.

Lieberman P, Nicklas RA, Oppenheimer J, et al, "The Diagnosis and Management of Anaphylaxis Practice Parameter: 2010 Update," *J Allergy Clin Immunol*, 2010, 126(3):477-80.

Naganobu K, Hasebe Y, Uchiyama Y, et al, "A Comparison of Distilled Water and Normal Saline as Diluents for Endobronchial Administration of Epinephrine in the Dog," *Anesth Analg*, 2000, 91(2):317-21.

Neumar RW, Otto CW, Link MS, et al, "Part 8: Adult Advanced Cardiovascular Life Support: 2010 American Heart Association Guidelines for Cardiopulmonary Resuscitation and Emergency Cardiovascular Care," *Circulation*, 2010, 122(18 Suppl 3):729-67.

Peberdy MA, Callaway CW, Neumar RW, et al, "Part 9: Post Cardiac Arrest Care: 2010 American Heart Association Guidelines for Cardiopulmonary Resuscitation and Emergency Cardiovascular Care," *Circulation*, 2010, 122(18 Suppl 3):768-86.

Phillips MS, "Standardizing I.V. Infusion Concentrations: National Survey Results," *Am J Health Syst Pharm*, 2011, 68(22):2176-82.

Rosekrans JA, "Viral Croup: Current Diagnosis and Treatment," *Mayo Clin Proc*, 1998, 73(11):1102-6.

Rotta AT and Wiryawan B, "Respiratory Emergencies in Children," *Respir Care*, 2003, 48(3):248-58.

Sicherer S, Simons F, et al, "Self-Injectable Epinephrine for First-Aid Management of Anaphylaxis," *Pediatrics*, 2007,119(3):638-46.

Vanden Hoek TL, Morrison LJ, Shuster M, et al, "Part 12: Cardiac Arrest in Special Situations: 2010 American Heart Association Guidelines for Cardiopulmonary Resuscitation and Emergency Cardiovascular Care," *Circulation*, 2010, 122(18 Suppl 3):829-61.

Waisman Y, Klein BL, Boenning DA, et al, "Prospective Randomized Double-Blind Study Comparing L-Epinephrine and Racemic Epinephrine Aerosols in the Treatment of Laryngotracheitis (Croup)," *Pediatrics*, 1992, 89(2):302-6.

Wright RB, Pomerantz WJ, and Luria JW, "New Approaches to Respiratory Infections in Children. Bronchiolitis and Croup," *Emerg Med Clin North Am*, 2002, 20(1):93-114.

EPINEPHrine (Nasal) (ep i NEF rin)

Medication Safety Issues
Sound-alike/look-alike issues:
EPINEPHrine may be confused with ePHEDrine

Related Information
Safe Handling of Hazardous Drugs *on page 2419*

Brand Names: U.S. Adrenalin
Brand Names: Canada Adrenalin®
Therapeutic Category Decongestant, Nasal
Generic Availability (U.S.) No
Use Nasal decongestant, decrease superficial hemorrhage

Pregnancy Considerations Refer to the EPINEPHrine (Systemic) monograph.
Breast-Feeding Considerations Refer to the EPINEPHrine (Systemic) monograph.
Contraindications Hypersensitivity to epinephrine or any component; concurrent use or within 2 weeks of MAO inhibitors
Warnings Some products contain sulfites as preservatives which may cause allergic reactions in susceptible individuals; the presence of sulfites in some products (eg, EpiPen® and Twinject®) should not deter administration during a serious allergic or other emergency situation even if the patient is sulfite-sensitive. Due to direct catecholamine effect, administration of epinephrine may cause high arterial blood pressure (may cause angina pectoris, aortic rupture, or cerebral hemorrhage); induce potentially serious cardiac arrhythmias; and produce constriction of renal blood vessels and decrease urine formation initially (with parenteral administration)
Precautions Use with caution in patients with diabetes mellitus or cardiovascular disease (coronary artery disease, hypertension, diabetes mellitus, Parkinson's disease, thyroid disease, or cerebrovascular disease. Use with extreme caution in patients taking MAO inhibitors and tricyclic antidepressants; effects of epinephrine may be potentiated. Rebound nasal congestion may occur after frequent nasal use.

Adverse Reactions
Cardiovascular: Angina, cardiac arrhythmia, chest pain, flushing, hypertension, pallor, palpitation, sudden death, tachycardia (parenteral), vasoconstriction, ventricular ectopy
Central nervous system: Anxiety (transient), apprehensiveness, cerebral hemorrhage, dizziness, headache, insomnia, lightheadedness, nervousness, restlessness
Gastrointestinal: Dry throat, loss of appetite, nausea, vomiting, xerostomia
Genitourinary: Acute urinary retention in patients with bladder outflow obstruction
Neuromuscular & skeletal: Tremor, weakness
Ocular: Allergic lid reaction, burning, eye pain, ocular irritation, precipitation of or exacerbation of narrow-angle glaucoma, transient stinging
Respiratory: Dyspnea, pulmonary edema
Miscellaneous: Diaphoresis

Drug Interactions
Metabolism/Transport Effects Substrate of COMT
Avoid Concomitant Use
Avoid concomitant use of EPINEPHrine (Nasal) with any of the following: Ergot Derivatives; Iobenguane I 123
Increased Effect/Toxicity
EPINEPHrine (Nasal) may increase the levels/effects of: Sympathomimetics

The levels/effects of EPINEPHrine (Nasal) may be increased by: AtoMOXetine; Beta-Blockers; Cannabinoid-Containing Products; COMT Inhibitors; Ergot Derivatives; Inhalational Anesthetics; Linezolid; MAO Inhibitors; Serotonin/Norepinephrine Reuptake Inhibitors; Tricyclic Antidepressants
Decreased Effect
EPINEPHrine (Nasal) may decrease the levels/effects of: Iobenguane I 123

The levels/effects of EPINEPHrine (Nasal) may be decreased by: Alpha1-Blockers; Promethazine; Spironolactone
Mechanism of Action Stimulates alpha-, beta$_1$-, and beta$_2$-adrenergic receptors resulting in local vasoconstriction and relief of nasal congestion
Pharmacodynamics Local vasoconstriction (topical):
Onset of action: 5 minutes
Duration: <1 hour

Pharmacokinetics (Adult data unless noted)

Distribution: Crosses placenta but not blood-brain barrier

Metabolism: Extensive in the liver and other tissues by the enzymes catechol-o-methyltransferase and monoamine oxidase

Dosing: Usual Children ≥6 years and Adults: Apply drops locally as needed; do not exceed 1 mL every 15 minutes

Administration Apply as drops or with sterile swab.

Monitoring Parameters Heart rate, blood pressure

Dosage Forms Excipient information presented when available (limited, particularly for generics); consult specific product labeling.

Solution, Nasal, as hydrochloride:

Adrenalin: 0.1% (30 mL)

◆ **Epinephrine and Lidocaine** see Lidocaine and Epinephrine on page 1245

◆ **Epinephrine Bitartrate** see EPINEPHrine (Systemic, Oral Inhalation) on page 761

◆ **Epinephrine Hydrochloride** see EPINEPHrine (Nasal) on page 765

◆ **Epinephrine Hydrochloride** see EPINEPHrine (Systemic, Oral Inhalation) on page 761

◆ **EpiPen (Can)** see EPINEPHrine (Systemic, Oral Inhalation) on page 761

◆ **EpiPen 2-Pak** see EPINEPHrine (Systemic, Oral Inhalation) on page 761

◆ **EpiPen Jr (Can)** see EPINEPHrine (Systemic, Oral Inhalation) on page 761

◆ **EpiPen Jr 2-Pak** see EPINEPHrine (Systemic, Oral Inhalation) on page 761

◆ **Epipodophyllotoxin** see Etoposide on page 815

◆ **Epitol** see CarBAMazepine on page 372

◆ **Epival (Can)** see Valproic Acid and Derivatives on page 2102

◆ **Epivir** see LamiVUDine on page 1194

◆ **Epivir HBV** see LamiVUDine on page 1194

◆ **EPO** see Epoetin Alfa on page 766

Epoetin Alfa (e POE e tin AL fa)

Medication Safety Issues

Sound-alike/look-alike issues:

Epoetin alfa may be confused with darbepoetin alfa, epoetin beta

Epogen may be confused with Neupogen

International issues:

Epopen [Spain] may be confused with EpiPen brand name for epinephrine [U.S., Canada, and multiple international markets]

Brand Names: U.S. Epogen; Procrit

Brand Names: Canada Eprex

Therapeutic Category Colony-Stimulating Factor; Growth Factor; Hematopoietic Agent; Recombinant Human Erythropoietin

Generic Availability (U.S.) No

Use Treatment of anemia associated with chronic kidney disease (CKD) in patients on dialysis (FDA approved in ages 1 month to 16 years and adults); treatment of anemia associated with CKD without dialysis (FDA approved in adults); anemia in cancer patients with nonmyeloid malignancies receiving concurrent myelosuppressive chemotherapy (palliative intent) when chemotherapy is a planned for a minimum of 2 months (FDA approved in ages ≥5 years and adults); anemia related to HIV therapy with zidovudine (FDA approved in ages ≥8 months and adults); reduction of allogeneic RBC transfusion for elective, noncardiac, nonvascular surgery when perioperative hemoglobin is >10 to ≤13 g/dL and with high risk for blood loss (FDA approved in adults); has also been used for anemia of prematurity; treatment of symptomatic anemia in myelodysplastic syndrome

Prescribing and Access Restrictions As a requirement of the REMS program, access to this medication is restricted. Healthcare providers and hospitals must be enrolled in the ESA APPRISE (Assisting Providers and Cancer Patients with Risk Information for the Safe use of ESAs) Oncology Program (866-284-8089; http://www.esa-apprise.com) to prescribe or dispense ESAs (ie, epoetin alfa, darbepoetin alfa) to patients with cancer.

Medication Guide Available Yes

Pregnancy Risk Factor C

Pregnancy Considerations Adverse events were observed in animal reproduction studies. In vitro studies suggest that recombinant erythropoietin does not cross the human placenta (Reisenberger, 1997). Polyhydramnios and intrauterine growth retardation have been reported with use in women with chronic kidney disease (adverse effects also associated with maternal disease). Hypospadias and pectus excavatum have been reported with first trimester exposure (case report).

Recombinant erythropoietin alfa has been evaluated as adjunctive treatment for severe pregnancy associated iron deficiency anemia (Breymann, 2001; Krafft, 2009) and has been used in pregnant women with iron-deficiency anemia associated with chronic kidney disease (CKD) (Furaz-Czerpak 2012; Josephson, 2007).

Amenorrheic premenopausal women should be cautioned that menstruation may resume following treatment with recombinant erythropoietin (Furaz-Czerpak, 2012). Multidose formulations containing benzyl alcohol are contraindicated for use in pregnant women; if treatment during pregnancy is needed, single dose preparations should be used.

Women who become pregnant during treatment with epoetin are encouraged to enroll in Amgen's Pregnancy Surveillance Program (1-800-772-6436).

Breast-Feeding Considerations Endogenous erythropoietin is found in breast milk (Semba, 2002). It is not known if recombinant erythropoietin alfa is excreted into breast milk. The manufacturer recommends caution be used if the single dose vial preparation is administered to nursing women; use of the multiple dose vials containing benzyl alcohol is contraindicated in breast-feeding women. When administered enterally to neonates (mixed with human milk or infant formula), recombinant erythropoietin did not significantly increase serum EPO concentrations. If passage via breast milk does occur, risk to a nursing infant appears low (Juul, 2003).

Contraindications Hypersensitivity to epoetin alfa or any component, uncontrolled hypertension, pure red cell aplasia (due to epoetin alfa or other erythropoietin protein drugs); multidose vials contain benzyl alcohol and are contraindicated in neonates, infants, pregnant women, and nursing women

Warnings Clinical trials have not shown that epoetin alfa improves quality of life, fatigue, or well-being. Patients with chronic kidney disease are at greater risk for death, serious cardiovascular events, and stroke when using erythropoiesis-stimulating agents (ESAs) to target hemoglobin concentrations >11 g/dL; use the lowest dose sufficient to reduce the need for RBC transfusions **[U.S. Boxed Warning]**. Hemoglobin rising >1 g/dL in a 2-week period may contribute to the risk. An optimal target hemoglobin level, dose, or dosing strategy to reduce these risks has not been identified in clinical trials. Chronic kidney disease patients who exhibit an inadequate hemoglobin response to ESA therapy may be at a higher risk for cardiovascular events and mortality compared to other patients. Blood pressure should be controlled adequately before initiation of epoetin alfa therapy particularly in CKD patients; ~25% of CKD patients on dialysis may require increased antihypertensive medications while receiving epoetin alfa; hypertensive encephalopathy and seizures have been observed in CKD patients treated with epoetin alfa; close blood pressure monitoring is recommended. ESA therapy may reduce dialysis efficacy (due to increase in red blood cells and decrease in plasma volume); adjustments in dialysis parameters may be needed. Patients treated with epoetin alfa may require increased heparinization during dialysis to prevent clotting of the extracorporeal circuit.

ESAs shortened survival and/or time-to-tumor progression in studies of advanced breast, cervical, head and neck, lymphoid, and nonsmall cell lung cancer in patients receiving ESAs when dosed to target a hemoglobin of ≥12 g/dL **[U.S. Boxed Warning]**. This risk has not been excluded when a lower target hemoglobin is used. Because of the risks of decreased survival and increased risk of tumor growth or progression, all healthcare providers and hospitals are required to enroll and comply with the ESA APPRISE (Assisting Providers and Cancer Patients with Risk Information for the Safe use of ESAs) Oncology Program prior to prescribing or dispensing ESAs to cancer patients **[U.S. Boxed Warning]**. Prescribers and patients will have to provide written documentation of discussed risks with each epoetin alfa course. For patients with cancer, use only for the treatment of anemia due to concomitant myelosuppressive chemotherapy, use the lowest dose needed to avoid RBC transfusions, and discontinue following completion of chemotherapy course; ESAs are not indicated for patients receiving myelosuppressive therapy when the anticipated outcome is curative **[U.S. Boxed Warning]**. Epoetin alfa is not approved for use in patients with myeloid malignancies or in patients with cancer-related anemia who are not receiving concurrent myelosuppressive chemotherapy.

DVT prophylaxis is recommended in perisurgery patients due to the risk of DVT **[U.S. Boxed Warning]**. Increased mortality (due to thrombotic events) has been reported in coronary artery bypass surgery patients using epoetin alfa; an increased risk of DVT in patients undergoing orthopedic procedures has been reported; epoetin alfa is **not** approved for reduction of red blood cell transfusion in patients undergoing cardiac or vascular surgery; for surgical patients willing to donate autologous blood; for cancer patients receiving hormonal therapy, therapeutic biologic products, or radiation therapy unless also receiving concurrent myelosuppressive chemotherapy.

Seizures have occurred during therapy in patients with CKD; monitor closely for premonitory neurologic symptoms during the first several months of therapy in these patients. Pure red cell aplasia (PRCA) and severe anemia have been reported, predominantly in patients with CKD and patients receiving subcutaneous ESAs; cases have also been reported in patients with hepatitis C who were receiving ESAs, interferon, and ribavirin. Should a sudden loss of responsiveness to epoetin alfa combined with a severe anemia and low reticulocyte count occur, temporarily discontinue epoetin alfa and evaluate for PRCA with associated neutralizing antibodies to epoetin alfa. Discontinue epoetin alfa permanently if these antibodies are detected. Prior to and during epoetin alfa therapy, assess the patient's iron stores utilizing serum ferritin, TIBC; supplemental iron therapy is recommended to support erythropoiesis and avoid depletion of iron stores.

Potentially serious allergic reactions have been reported (rarely); discontinue immediately (and permanently) in patients who experience serious allergic/anaphylactic reactions. The multidose formulation contains benzyl alcohol which may cause allergic reactions in susceptible individuals; large amounts of benzyl alcohol (≥99 mg/kg/day)

have been associated with a potentially fatal toxicity ("gasping syndrome") in neonates; the "gasping syndrome" consists of metabolic acidosis, respiratory distress, gasping respirations, CNS dysfunction (including convulsions, intracranial hemorrhage), hypotension and cardiovascular collapse; avoid use of multidose formulation in neonates; *in vitro* and animal studies have shown that benzoate, a metabolite of benzyl alcohol, displaces bilirubin from protein-binding sites. Pooled use of unused portions of preservative-free epoetin alfa has resulted in microbial contamination, bacteremia, and pyrogenic reactions. Preservative-free formulations are intended for single use only.

Precautions Use with caution in patients with porphyria as exacerbations of porphyria have been reported in patients with CKD. Use with caution in patients with a history of seizures or hypertension; an excessive rate of rise of hematocrit may possibly be associated with the exacerbation of hypertension or seizures. Decrease the epoetin alfa dosage if the hemoglobin increase exceeds 1g/dL in any 2-week period. Blood pressure should be controlled prior to the start of therapy and monitored closely throughout treatment. Hypertensive encephalopathy has been reported with patients receiving erythropoietic therapy. Seizures have occurred during ESA therapy; monitor closely for premonitory neurologic symptoms during the first several months of therapy.

Epoetin alfa is not intended for patients who require acute corrections of anemia and is not a substitute for emergency blood transfusion. Epoetin alfa contains albumin, which confers a theoretical risk of transmission of viral disease or Creutzfeldt-Jakob disease. Factors which may impair erythropoiesis include inflammatory conditions, infections, and bleeding; poor response to therapy should prompt evaluation of potential factors impairing erythropoiesis, as well as possible malignant processes and hematologic disease (thalassemia, refractory anemia, myelodysplastic disorder), occult blood loss, hemolysis, osteitis fibrosa cystic, and/or bone marrow fibrosis. Additional factors that may limit response to epoetin alfa include iron deficiency; aluminum overload; hyperparathyroidism; folic acid or vitamin B_{12} deficiency; or patient nonadherence.

Assessment of iron stores and therapeutic iron supplementation is essential to optimal epoetin alfa therapy. Iron supplementation is necessary to provide for increased requirements during expansion of the red cell mass secondary to marrow stimulation by epoetin alfa, unless iron stores are already in excess. Supplemental iron is recommended if serum ferritin <100 mcg/mL or serum transferrin saturation <20%.

Adverse Reactions

Cardiovascular: Deep vein thrombosis, edema, hypertension, thrombosis

Central nervous system: Chills, depression, dizziness, fever, headache, insomnia

Dermatologic: Pruritus, rash,urticaria

Endocrine & metabolic: Hyperglycemia, hypokalemia

Gastrointestinal: Dysphagia, nausea, stomatitis, vomiting, weight loss

Hematologic: Leukopenia

Local: Clotted vascular access, injection site reaction

Neuromuscular & skeletal: Arthralgia, bone pain, muscle spasm, myalgia

Respiratory: Cough, pulmonary embolism, respiratory congestion, upper respiratory infection

Rare but important or life-threatening: Allergic reaction, anaphylactic reaction, angioedema, bronchospasm, erythema, hypersensitivity reactions, hypertensive encephalopathy, microvascular thrombosis, MI, neutralizing antibodies, porphyria, pure red cell aplasia (PRCA), renal vein thrombosis, retinal artery thrombosis, seizure, ▸

stroke, tachycardia, temporal vein thrombosis, thrombophlebitis, TIA, tumor progression

Drug Interactions

Metabolism/Transport Effects None known.

Avoid Concomitant Use There are no known interactions where it is recommended to avoid concomitant use.

Increased Effect/Toxicity

The levels/effects of Epoetin Alfa may be increased by:
Nandrolone

Decreased Effect There are no known significant interactions involving a decrease in effect.

Stability Vials should be stored at 2°C to 8°C (36°F to 46°F); **do not freeze or shake.** Protect from light.

Single-dose vials contain no preservatives; discard after entry. Multiple-dose vials contain benzyl alcohol preservative and may be used up to 21 days after initial entry when stored between 2°C to 8°C (36°F to 46°F). Prefilled syringes containing the preservative formulation are stable for 6 weeks refrigerated [2°C to 8°C (36°F to 46°F)] (Naughton, 2003). Epoetin alfa is stable for 24 hours when diluted in dextrose I.V. fluid which contains at least 0.05% human albumin or parenteral nutrition solutions containing at least 0.5% amino acids.

Mechanism of Action Induces erythropoiesis by stimulating the division and differentiation of committed erythroid progenitor cells; induces the release of reticulocytes from the bone marrow into the bloodstream, where they mature to erythrocytes. There is a dose response relationship with this effect. This results in an increase in reticulocyte counts followed by a rise in hematocrit and hemoglobin levels.

Pharmacodynamics

Onset of action: Several days

Maximum effect: 2-6 weeks

Pharmacokinetics (Adult data unless noted)

Absorption: SubQ: 31.9%

Distribution: Adults: V_d: 9 L; rapid in the plasma compartment; majority of drug is taken up by the liver, kidneys, and bone marrow

Bioavailability: SubQ: ~21% to 31%

Half-life:

Neonates: SubQ: 17.6 hours on day 3 of therapy, 11.2 hours on day 10 of therapy

Children and Adults: I.V.: 4-13 hours in patients with chronic kidney disease (CKD); half-life is 20% shorter in patients with normal renal function; Cancer: Adults: SubQ: 16-67 hours

Time to peak serum concentration: SubQ: 5-24 hours

Elimination: Some metabolic degradation does occur with small amounts recovered in the urine

Clearance: Neonates: SubQ or continuous I.V. infusion: 26-35 mL/hour/kg on day 3 of therapy and 65-87 mL/hour/kg on day 10 of therapy

Note: While a much higher peak plasma concentration is achieved after I.V. bolus administration, it declines at a more rapid rate (over 2-3 days) than after subcutaneous administration (plasma concentrations greater than endogenous are maintained for at least 4 days). Subcutaneous administration is associated with a 30% to 50% lower EPO dose requirement.

Dosing: Neonatal

Anemia of prematurity: I.V., SubQ: Dosing range: 500-1250 units/kg/**week** divided into 2-5 doses for 10 doses; commonly used dose: 250 units/kg/dose 3 times weekly for 10 doses; supplement with oral iron therapy 3-8 mg/kg/day

Neuroprotective/hypoxic ischemia encephalopathy (HIE): Limited data available, dosing regimens variable; further studies needed:

Low dose: Initial dose: SubQ: 300 or 500 units/kg/dose; maintenance dose: I.V.: 300 or 500 units/kg/dose every other day for 2 weeks beginning within first 48 hours of life was used in 73 neonates diagnosed with moderate

HIE; improved neurologic outcomes were reported at 18 months of age (Zhu, 2009)

High dose: I.V., SubQ: 1000 or 2500 units/kg/dose once daily for 3-5 days beginning within first 24 hours of life; dosing based on a Phase I/II safety and pharmacokinetic, case-control study of 30 ELBW neonates (mean GA: 26.1 weeks, birth weight: 745 g) which showed dosing ≥1000 units/kg I.V. provided proposed target serum concentration for neuroprotective effects (>6000 mIU/mL) and reported a diminished severity of ICH in treatment groups (Juul, 2008). In a prospective, case-controlled pilot efficacy trial, 15 term neonates diagnosed with HIE received SubQ administration of 2500 units/kg/dose for 5 days beginning within first 24 hours of life; short-term findings (PNA: 2 weeks) included decreased nitric oxide serum concentrations and fewer seizures; long-term finding (PNA: 6 months) included fewer neurologic abnormalities (Elmahdy, 2010)

Dosing: Usual Dosing schedules need to be individualized and careful monitoring of patients receiving the drug is recommended. Use has not been demonstrated in controlled clinical trials to improve symptoms of anemia, quality of life, fatigue, or patient well-being.

Infants, Children, and Adolescents:

Anemia in chronic kidney disease (ON dialysis):

Note: I.V. route is preferred for hemodialysis patients; initiate treatment when hemoglobin is <10 g/dL; reduce dose or interrupt treatment if hemoglobin approaches or exceeds 11 g/dL:

Initial dose: Infants, Children, and Adolescents ≤16 years: I.V., SubQ: 50 units/kg/dose 3 times weekly

Dosage adjustments:

If hemoglobin does not increase by >1 g/dL after 4 weeks: Increase dose by 25%; do not increase the dose more frequently than once every 4 weeks

If hemoglobin increases >1 g/dL in any 2-week period: Reduce dose by ≥25%; dose reductions can occur more frequently than once every 4 weeks; avoid frequent dosage adjustments

Inadequate or lack of response over a 12-week escalation period: Further increases are unlikely to improve response and may increase risks; use the minimum effective dose that will maintain an Hgb level sufficient to avoid RBC transfusions and evaluate patient for other causes of anemia. Discontinue therapy if responsiveness does not improve.

Anemia due to myelosuppressive chemotherapy (palliative) in cancer patients: Note: Initiate treatment only if hemoglobin <10 g/dL and anticipated duration of myelosuppressive chemotherapy is ≥2 months. Titrate dosage to use the minimum effective dose that will maintain a hemoglobin level sufficient to avoid red blood cell transfusions. Children ≥5 years and Adolescents: I.V.:

Initial dose: 600 units/kg/dose once weekly until completion of chemotherapy

Dosage adjustments:

If hemoglobin does not increase by >1 g/dL **and** remains <10 g/dL after initial 4 weeks: Increase to 900 units/kg/dose (maximum dose: 60,000 units); discontinue after 8 weeks of treatment if RBC transfusions are still required or there is no hemoglobin response

If hemoglobin exceeds a level needed to avoid red blood cell transfusion: Withhold dose; resume treatment with a 25% dose reduction when hemoglobin approaches a level where transfusions may be required

If hemoglobin increases >1 g/dL in any 2-week period **or** hemoglobin reaches a level sufficient to avoid red blood cell transfusion: Reduce dose by 25%

Anemia due to zidovudine in HIV-infected patients: Titrate dosage to use the minimum effective dose that will maintain a hemoglobin level sufficient to avoid red blood cell transfusions. Infants ≥8 months, Children, and Adolescents ≤17 years: I.V., SubQ: Limited data available; doses ranging from 50-400 units/kg/dose 2-3 times weekly have been reported; withhold dose if hemoglobin exceeds 12 g/dL, may resume treatment with a 25% dose reduction once hemoglobin <11 g/dL

Adults:

Anemia associated with chronic kidney disease: Individualize dosing and use the lowest dose necessary to reduce the need for RBC transfusions.

Chronic kidney disease patients **ON dialysis** (I.V. route is preferred for hemodialysis patients; initiate treatment when hemoglobin is <10 g/dL; reduce dose or interrupt treatment if hemoglobin approaches or exceeds 11 g/dL): I.V., SubQ: Initial dose: 50-100 units/kg/dose 3 times weekly

Chronic kidney disease patients **NOT on dialysis** (consider initiating treatment when hemoglobin is <10 g/dL; use only if rate of hemoglobin decline would likely result in RBC transfusion and desire is to reduce risk of alloimmunization or other RBC transfusion-related risks; reduce dose or interrupt treatment if hemoglobin exceeds 10 g/dL): I.V., SubQ: Initial dose: 50-100 units/kg/dose 3 times weekly

Dosage adjustments for chronic kidney disease patients (either on dialysis or not on dialysis):

If hemoglobin does not increase by >1 g/dL after 4 weeks: Increase dose by 25%; do not increase the dose more frequently than once every 4 weeks

If hemoglobin increases >1 g/dL in any 2-week period: Reduce dose by ≥25%; dose reductions can occur more frequently than once every 4 weeks; avoid frequent dosage adjustments

Inadequate or lack of response over a 12-week escalation period: Further increases are unlikely to improve response and may increase risks; use the minimum effective dose that will maintain an Hgb level sufficient to avoid RBC transfusions and evaluate patient for other causes of anemia. Discontinue therapy if responsiveness does not improve.

Anemia due to chemotherapy in cancer patients: Initiate treatment only if hemoglobin <10 g/dL and anticipated duration of myelosuppressive chemotherapy is ≥2 months. Titrate dosage to use the minimum effective dose that will maintain a hemoglobin level sufficient to avoid red blood cell transfusions. Discontinue erythropoietin following completion of chemotherapy. SubQ: Initial dose: 150 units/kg/dose 3 times weekly or 40,000 units once weekly until completion of chemotherapy.

Dosage adjustments:

If hemoglobin does not increase by >1 g/dL **and** remains below 10 g/dL after initial 4 weeks: Increase to 300 units/kg 3 times/week or 60,000 units weekly; discontinue after 8 weeks of treatment if RBC transfusions are still required or there is no hemoglobin response

If hemoglobin exceeds a level needed to avoid red blood cell transfusion: Withhold dose; resume treatment with a 25% dose reduction when hemoglobin approaches a level where transfusions may be required

If hemoglobin increases >1 g/dL in any 2-week period **or** hemoglobin reaches a level sufficient to avoid red blood cell transfusion: Reduce dose by 25%

Anemia due to zidovudine in HIV-infected patients: Titrate dosage to use the minimum effective dose that will maintain a hemoglobin level sufficient to avoid red blood cell transfusions. Hemoglobin levels should not exceed 12 g/dL.

Serum erythropoietin levels ≤500 mUnits/mL and zidovudine doses ≤4200 mg/week): I.V., SubQ: Initial: 100 units/kg/dose 3 times weekly; if hemoglobin does not increase after 8 weeks, increase dose by ~50-100 units/kg/dose at 4-8 week intervals until hemoglobin reaches a level sufficient to avoid RBC transfusion; maximum dose: 300 units/kg. Withhold dose if hemoglobin exceeds 12 g/dL, may resume treatment with a 25% dose reduction once hemoglobin <11 g/dL. Discontinue if hemoglobin increase is not achieved with 300 units/kg/dose for 8 weeks.

Surgery patients (perioperative hemoglobin should be >10 g/dL and ≤13 g/dL; DVT prophylactic anticoagulation is recommended): SubQ: Initial dose:

300 units/kg/day beginning 10 days before surgery, on the day of surgery, and for 4 days after surgery **or**

600 units/kg once weekly for 4 doses, given 21, 14, and 7 days before surgery, and on the day of surgery

Administration Parenteral: Do not shake as this may denature the glycoprotein rendering the drug biologically inactive

SubQ is the preferred route of administration; 1:1 dilution with bacteriostatic NS (containing benzyl alcohol) acts as a local anesthetic to reduce pain at the injection site. Multiple-dose vials already contain benzyl alcohol.

I.V.: Manufacturer recommends administering without dilution; some institutions may wish to dilute with an equal volume of NS; infuse over 1-3 minutes; it may be administered into the venous line at the end of the dialysis procedure; may be infused in dextrose solution when diluted with albumin

Monitoring Parameters Careful monitoring of blood pressure is indicated; problems with hypertension have been noted especially in kidney disease patients treated with epoetin alfa. Other patients are less likely to develop this complication. Monitor for premonitory neurologic symptoms during the first several months of therapy.

Monitor transferrin saturation and serum ferritin (prior to and during treatment); hemoglobin (weekly after initiation and following dose adjustments until stable and sufficient to minimize need for RBC transfusion); blood pressure

Reference Range Zidovudine-treated HIV patients: Available evidence indicates patients with endogenous serum erythropoietin concentrations >500 mIU/mL are unlikely to respond

Dosage Forms Excipient information presented when available (limited, particularly for generics); consult specific product labeling.

Solution, Injection:

Epogen: 10,000 units/mL (2 mL); 20,000 units/mL (1 mL) [contains benzyl alcohol]

Procrit: 10,000 units/mL (2 mL); 20,000 units/mL (1 mL) [contains benzyl alcohol]

Solution, Injection [preservative free]:

Epogen: 2000 units/mL (1 mL); 3000 units/mL (1 mL); 4000 units/mL (1 mL); 10,000 units/mL (1 mL)

Procrit: 2000 units/mL (1 mL); 3000 units/mL (1 mL); 4000 units/mL (1 mL); 10,000 units/mL (1 mL); 40,000 units/mL (1 mL)

References

Blanche S, Caniglia M, Fischer A, et al, "Zidovudine Therapy in Children With Acquired Immunodeficiency Syndrome," *Am J Med*, 1988, 85 (2A):203-7.

Breymann C, Visca E, Huch R, et al, "Efficacy and Safety of Intravenously Administered Iron Sucrose With and Without Adjuvant Recombinant Human Erythropoietin for the Treatment of Resistant Iron-Deficiency Anemia During Pregnancy," *Am J Obstet Gynecol*, 2001, 184(4):662-7.

Brown MS, Eichorst D, Lala-Black B, et al, "Higher Cumulative Doses of Erythropoietin and Developmental Outcomes in Preterm Infants," *Pediatrics*, 2009, 124(4):681-7.

Elmahdy H, El-Mashad AR, El-Bahrawy H, et al, "Human Recombinant Erythropoietin in Asphyxia Neonatorum: Pilot Trial," *Pediatrics*, 2010, 125(5):1135-42.

Furaz-Czerpak KR, Fernández-Juárez G, Moreno-de la Higuera MÁ, et al, "Pregnancy in Women on Chronic Dialysis: A Review," *Nefrologia*, 2012, 32(3):287-94.

Halperin DS, Wacker P, Lacourt G, et al, "Effects of Recombinant Human Erythropoietin in Infants With the Anemia of Prematurity: A Pilot Study," *J Pediatr*, 1990, 116(5):779-86.

Josephson MA and McKay DB, "Considerations in the Medical Management of Pregnancy in Transplant Recipients, *Adv Chronic Kidney Dis*, 2007, 14(2):156-67.

Juul SE, McPherson RJ, Bauer LA, et al, "A Phase I/II Trial of High-Dose Erythropoietin in Extremely Low Birth Weight Infants: Pharmacokinetics and Safety," *Pediatrics*, 2008, 122(2):383-91.

KDOQI, "KDOQI Clinical Practice Guideline and Clinical Practice Recommendations for Anemia in Chronic Kidney Disease: 2007 Update of Hemoglobin Target," *Am J Kidney Dis*, 2007, 50(3):471-530.

Krafft A, Bencaiova G, and Breymann C, "Selective Use of Recombinant Human Erythropoietin in Pregnant Patients With Severe Anemia or Nonresponsive to Iron Sucrose Alone," *Fetal Diagn Ther*, 2009, 25 (2):239-45.

Naughton CA, Duppong LM, Forbes KD, et al, "Stability of Multidose, Preserved Formulation Epoetin Alfa in Syringes for Three and Six Weeks," *Am J Health Syst Pharm*, 2003, 60(5):464-8.

Neubauer AP, Voss W, Wachtendorf M, et al, "Erythropoietin Improves Neurodevelopmental Outcome of Extremely Preterm Infants," *Ann Neurol*, 2010, 67(5):657-66.

Ohls RK and Christensen, RD, "Stability of Human Recombinant Epoetin Alfa in Commonly Used Neonatal Intravenous Solutions," *Ann Pharmacother*, 1996, 30(5):466-468.

Ohls RK, Veerman MW, and Christensen RD, "Pharmacokinetics and Effectiveness of Recombinant Erythropoietin Administered to Preterm Infants by Continuous Infusion in Total Parenteral Nutrition Solution," *J Pediatr*, 1996, 128(4):518-23.

Reisenberger K, Egarter C, Kapiotis S, et al, "Transfer of Erythropoietin Across the Placenta Perfused *in vitro*," *Obstet Gynecol*, 1997, 89(5 Pt 1):738-42.

Rhondeau SM, Christensen RD, Ross MP, et al, "Responsiveness to Recombinant Human Erythropoietin of Marrow Erythroid Progenitors From Infants With the Anemia of Prematurity," *J Pediatr*, 1988, 112 (6):935-40.

Rizzo JD, Brouwers M, Hurley P, et al, "American Society of Clinical Oncology/American Society of Hematology Clinical Practice Guideline Update on the Use of Epoetin and Darbepoetin in Adult Patients With Cancer," *J Clin Oncol*, 2010, 28(33):4996-5010.

Semba RD and Juul SE, "Erythropoietin in Human Milk: Physiology and Role in Infant Health," *J Hum Lact*, 2002, 18(3):252-61.

Shannon KM, Keith JF 3rd, Mentzer WC, et al, "Recombinant Human Erythropoietin Stimulates Erythropoiesis and Reduces Erythrocyte Transfusions in Very Low Birth Weight Preterm Infants," *Pediatrics*, 1995, 95(1):1-8.

Sinai-Trieman L, Salusky IB, and Fine RN, "Use of Subcutaneous Recombinant Human Erythropoietin in Children Undergoing Continuous Cycling Peritoneal Dialysis," *J Pediatr*, 1989, 114(4 Pt 1):550-4.

Zhu C, Kang W, Xu F, et al, "Erythropoietin Improved Neurologic Outcomes in Newborns With Hypoxic-Ischemic Encephalopathy," *Pediatrics*, 2009, 124(2):e218-26.

◆ **Epogen** *see* Epoetin Alfa *on page 766*

Epoprostenol (e poe PROST en ole)

Medication Safety Issues
High alert medication:
The Institute for Safe Medication Practices (ISMP) includes this medication among its list of drugs which have a heightened risk of causing significant patient harm when used in error.

Brand Names: U.S. Flolan; Veletri

Brand Names: Canada Caripul; Flolan

Therapeutic Category Prostaglandin

Generic Availability (U.S.) Yes

Use Treatment of pulmonary arterial hypertension (PAH) (WHO Group I) to improve exercise capacity. **Note:** Efficacy has been established in patients with NYHA Class III or IV symptoms with idiopathic or heritable PAH or PAH associated with connective tissue diseases (FDA approved in adults)

Has also been used diagnostically as a short-term I.V. infusion in patients with pulmonary hypertension in the cardiac catheterization laboratory to screen for responsiveness to other oral vasodilating agents (eg, calcium channel blockers). **Note:** Responsiveness to short-term (acute) I.V. infusions of epoprostenol predicts responsiveness to long-term treatment with oral calcium channel blockers; however, it does not predict responsiveness to long-term I.V. epoprostenol therapy. Patients who do not respond acutely to epoprostenol may respond to the drug when used chronically.

Other potential uses include treatment of secondary pulmonary hypertension associated with ARDS, SLE, congenital heart disease, congenital diaphragmatic hernia, neonatal pulmonary hypertension, cardiopulmonary bypass surgery, hemodialysis, peripheral vascular disorders, portal hypertension, and neonatal purpura fulminans.

Prescribing and Access Restrictions Orders for epoprostenol are distributed by two sources in the United States. Information on orders or reimbursement assistance may be obtained from either Accredo Health, Inc (1-866-344-4874) or CVS Caremark (1-877-242-2738).

Pregnancy Risk Factor B

Pregnancy Considerations Adverse events were not observed in animal reproduction studies. Women with PAH are encouraged to avoid pregnancy (McLaughlin, 2009).

Breast-Feeding Considerations It is not known if epoprostenol is excreted in breast milk. The manufacturer recommends that caution be exercised when administering epoprostenol to nursing women.

Contraindications Hypersensitivity to epoprostenol, any component, or structurally-related compounds; chronic use in patients with CHF due to severe left ventricular systolic dysfunction. **Note:** Do not use epoprostenol chronically in patients who develop pulmonary edema during dose initiation.

Warnings Epoprostenol **must** only be reconstituted with a product-specific diluent (Flolan®: manufacturer-supplied diluent; Veletri®: SWI or NS); do **not** reconstitute or mix with other I.V. fluids or I.V. medications prior to or during administration. Abrupt withdrawal, interruptions in drug delivery, or sudden reductions in epoprostenol dosage may result in symptoms associated with rebound pulmonary hypertension (eg, asthenia, dizziness, dyspnea) and can be potentially fatal; avoid abrupt withdrawal, interruptions in drug delivery, and sudden large reductions in dosage. Immediate access to back up infusion pump and I.V. infusion sets is essential to prevent treatment interruptions. Pulmonary edema, which may be associated with pulmonary veno-occlusive disease may develop in patients with pulmonary hypertension during epoprostenol dose initiation (do not use epoprostenol chronically in these patients).

Symptoms of overdose include headache, hypotension, tachycardia, nausea, vomiting, diarrhea, and flushing. Reduce the infusion rate to decrease symptoms. If symptoms do not subside or worsen, consider drug discontinuation. Fatalities due to hypoxemia, hypotension, and respiratory arrest have been reported following overdose with epoprostenol.

Precautions Use with caution and appropriately monitor patients; epoprostenol is a potent pulmonary and systemic vasodilator; it should be used only by clinicians who are experienced in the diagnosis and treatment of pulmonary hypertension; dose initiation must occur in a setting with adequately trained personnel and proper equipment for physiologic monitoring and emergency care. Asymptomatic increases in pulmonary artery pressure, associated with increases in cardiac output, may rarely occur during dose initiation; consider dosage reduction in these patients. During chronic use, unless contraindicated, anticoagulants should be coadministered in adult patients to reduce the risk of thromboembolism [**Note:** The use of anticoagulants in **adult** patients with primary pulmonary hypertension has been shown to improve survival. Although such efficacy has **not** been demonstrated in pediatric patients, some studies have reported the routine use of warfarin in pediatric patients receiving long-term (chronic) infusions of epoprostenol for pulmonary hypertension (Barst, 1999; Rosenzweig, 1999), while other studies have routinely discontinued anticoagulants prior to the initiation of epoprostenol therapy (Higenbottam, 1993). Epoprostenol is a potent inhibitor of platelet aggregation; monitor patients for bleeding, especially those with other risk factors or medications which may increase the risk for hemorrhage. Further studies are needed to assess the risks and benefits of routine anticoagulation in pediatric patients treated with epoprostenol.]

Adverse Reactions

Note: Adverse events reported during dose initiation and escalation include flushing, headache, nausea/vomiting, hypotension, anxiety/nervousness/agitation, chest pain; dizziness, abdominal pain, bradycardia, musculoskeletal pain, dyspnea, back pain, diaphoresis, dyspepsia, hypoesthesia/paresthesia, and tachycardia are also reported. Although some adverse reactions may be related to the underlying disease state, abdominal pain, anxiety/nervousness/agitation, arthralgia, bleeding, bradycardia, diarrhea, diaphoresis, flu-like syndrome, flushing, headache, hypotension, jaw pain, nausea, pain, pulmonary edema, rash, tachycardia, thrombocytopenia, and vomiting are clearly contributed to epoprostenol. The following adverse events have been reported during chronic administration for idiopathic or heritable PAH:

Cardiovascular: Flushing, hypotension, tachycardia
Central nervous system: Anxiety, chills, dizziness, fever, flu-like syndrome, nervousness, sepsis, tremor
Dermatologic: Eczema, rash, skin ulcer, urticaria
Gastrointestinal: Anorexia, diarrhea, nausea, vomiting
Local: Injection site reactions: Infection, pain

Neuromuscular & skeletal: Arthralgia, arthritis, hyper-/hypoesthesia, jaw pain, musculoskeletal pain, myalgia, neck pain, pain, paresthesia
Rare but important or life-threatening: Anemia, fatigue, hepatic failure, hypersplenism, hyperthyroidism, pallor, pancytopenia, pulmonary embolism, splenomegaly, thrombocytopenia

Drug Interactions

Metabolism/Transport Effects None known.

Avoid Concomitant Use There are no known interactions where it is recommended to avoid concomitant use.

Increased Effect/Toxicity
Epoprostenol may increase the levels/effects of: Agents with Antiplatelet Properties; Anticoagulants; Antihypertensives; Digoxin

Decreased Effect There are no known significant interactions involving a decrease in effect.

Stability

Flolan®: Store unopened vials of drug and sterile diluent at room temperature of 15°C to 25°C (59°F to 77°F); protect drug vials from light; do not freeze diluent. Following reconstitution, solution must be stored under refrigeration at 2°C to 8°C (36°F to 46°F) if not used immediately; reconstituted solution is stable for up to 48 hours when refrigerated; protect from light; do not freeze (discard if solution has been frozen). Total storage and infusion time must not exceed 48 hours for reconstituted solutions. Reconstituted solution (pH 10.2-10.8) is increasingly unstable at a lower pH and drug is rapidly hydrolyzed at the pH of I.V. fluids.

Following dilution, each reservoir of solution may be refrigerated for ≤40 hours and infused at room temperature not to exceed 25°C (77°F) for ≤8 hours; alternatively, each reservoir may be refrigerated for ≤24 hours and infused with the use of a cold pouch for ≤24 hours. Cold pouch should be changed every 12 hours and must be capable of maintaining the reconstituted solution at a temperature between 2°C to 8°C (36°F to 46°F) for 12 hours. Protect diluted solution from light.

Veletri®: Store unopened vials at 20°C to 25°C (68°F to 77°F); do not freeze (discard if solution has been frozen). Protect from light. Following reconstitution, solution may be stored under refrigeration at 2°C to 8°C (36°F to 46°F) up to 5 days or at room temperature of 25°C (77°F) up to 48 hours if not used immediately; do not freeze (discard if solution has been frozen). Protect from light. Discard if refrigerated for >5 days or if at room temperature for >48 hours. Discard unused portion of vial (vial is for single use only).

Following dilution, solutions which have been **immediately** added to a drug delivery reservoir may be administered immediately or stored at 2°C to 8°C (36°F to 46°F) for 1-7 days (dependent on concentration and time to initiation of infusion).

Mechanism of Action Epoprostenol is also known as prostacyclin and PGI_2. It is a strong vasodilator of all vascular beds. In addition, it is a potent endogenous inhibitor of platelet aggregation. The reduction in platelet aggregation results from epoprostenol's activation of intracellular adenylate cyclase and the resultant increase in cyclic adenosine monophosphate concentrations within the platelets. Additionally, it is capable of decreasing thrombogenesis and platelet clumping in the lungs by inhibiting platelet aggregation.

◄ **Pharmacokinetics (Adult data unless noted)**

Metabolism: Rapidly hydrolyzed at a neutral pH in blood; also metabolized by enzymatic degradation; two primary metabolites with pharmacologic activity less than epoprostenol are formed: 6-keto-PGF$_{1alpha}$ (via spontaneous degradation) and 6,15-diketo-13,14-dihydro-PGF$_{1alpha}$ (via enzymatic degradation); 14 minor metabolites have also been isolated in the urine

Half-life: ≤6 minutes

Elimination: Urine (84% of dose); feces (4%)

Dosing: Neonatal Note: Doses are expressed in units of **nanograms** (ng)/kg/minute.

Pulmonary hypertension: Very limited data available; efficacy results variable; optimal dose not established; further studies are needed. **Note:** Avoid abrupt withdrawal or sudden large dose reductions when discontinuing therapy to prevent rebound pulmonary hypertension.

Continuous I.V. infusion:

Low-dose regimen: Initial: 2 ng/kg/minute slowly titrated to 20 ng/kg/minute over ~3 hours was described in a single case report; epoprostenol was used in a full-term neonate (PNA: 72 hours) for PPHN refractory to inhaled nitric oxide and showed initial improvement in oxygenation index (Golzand, 2005)

High-dose regimen: Initial: 20 ng/kg/minute, slowly titrated (according to oxygenation) at 30-minute intervals over 4-12 hours to a mean dose of 60 ng/kg/minute (range: 30-120 ng/kg/minute) and continued for a mean of 5.3 days (range: 3-10.5 days) was used in an open-label trial of eight neonates (GA: 34-42 weeks; PNA: 3-32 hours) with PPHN (excluding CHD and congenital diaphragmatic hernia) (Eronen, 1997)

Dosing: Usual Note: Doses are expressed in units of **nanograms** (ng)/kg/minute.

Pulmonary hypertension: Infants, Children, Adolescents, and Adults: Continuous I.V. infusion:

Initial: 1-2 ng/kg/minute, increase dose in increments of 1-2 ng/kg/minute every 15 minutes or longer until dose-limiting side effects are noted or tolerance limit to epoprostenol is observed

Dose adjustment:

Increase dose: 1-2 ng/kg/minute increments at intervals of at least 15 minutes if symptoms of pulmonary hypertension persist or recur following improvement. In clinical trials, dosing increases occurred at intervals of 24-48 hours or longer.

Decrease dose: 2 ng/kg/minute decrements at intervals of at least 15 minutes in case of dose-limiting pharmacologic (adverse) events. Avoid abrupt withdrawal or sudden large dose reductions.

Chronic dosing: The need for increased doses should be expected with chronic use; incremental increases occur more frequently during the first few months after the drug is initiated. The optimal dose in children is not well defined. The mean chronic dose at 1 year of therapy is 20-40 ng/kg/minute in adults, but is 50-80 ng/kg/minute in children (particularly younger children); significant variability in optimal dose occurs in pediatric patients (Barst, 1999; Rosenweig, 1999; Widlitz, 2003).

Administration Continuous I.V. infusion: Administer through a central venous catheter; peripheral infusion may be used temporarily until central line is established. Epoprostenol should be infused in a dedicated lumen exclusive of any other drugs; consider a multilumen catheter if other I.V. medications are routinely administered. Avoid abrupt withdrawal, interruptions in delivery, or sudden large reductions in dosing. Patients should have access to a backup infusion pump and infusion sets. The final concentration of epoprostenol solution is determined by the minimum and maximum flow rates of the infusion pump and desired duration of infusion from the specific reservoir volume. Do not reconstitute or mix with other I.V. fluids or I.V. medications prior to or during administration as epoprostenol is very unstable in neutral or acidic pH solutions. Patients may be discharged using an ambulatory infusion pump. Appropriate ambulatory infusion pump should be small and lightweight; be able to adjust infusion rates in 2 ng/kg/minute increments; have occlusion, end of infusion, and low battery alarms; have ±6% accuracy of the programmed rate; and be positive continuous or pulsatile pressure-driven with intervals ≤3 minutes between pulses. The reservoir should be made of polypropylene, polyvinyl chloride, or glass.

Flolan®: Reconstitute with the manufacturer-supplied sterile diluent only (see "Preparation of Epoprostenol Infusion" table). The final volume (usually 100 mL) is a 24-hour supply and may be divided into 3 equal parts (ie, three 8-hour infusion aliquots); one portion to be administered at present and the two other portions should be stored in the refrigerator until time of administration. During use, a single reservoir of solution may be used at room temperature for a total duration of 8 hours, or used with a cold pouch for administration up to 24 hours (change cold pack every 12 hours).

Veletri®: Reconstitute with SWI or NS (see "Preparation of Epoprostenol Infusion" table on next page).

Immediate dilution: Diluted solutions which have been **immediately** added to a drug delivery reservoir may be administered immediately or stored at 2°C to 8°C (36°F to 46°F) for 1-7 days dependent on concentration and time to initiation of therapy (see below).

Immediate use following reconstitution: If administered immediately, the following maximum infusion duration at room temperature according to solution concentration is recommended:

• ≥3,000 to <6,000 ng/mL: 12 hours
• ≥6,000 to <30,000 ng/mL: 24 hours
• ≥30,000 ng/mL: 72 hours

Stored in a drug delivery reservoir following reconstitution and dilution:

If stored at 2°C to 8°C (36°F to 46°F) for 1 day, the following maximum infusion duration at room temperature according to the solution concentration is recommended:

• <6,000 ng/mL: Do not use
• ≥6,000 to <12,000 ng/mL: 12 hours
• ≥12,000 to <30,000 ng/mL: 24 hours
• ≥30,000 ng/mL: 48 hours

If stored at 2°C to 8°C (36°F to 46°F) for >1 to 7 days, the following maximum infusion duration at room temperature according to the solution concentration is recommended:

• <9,000 ng/mL: Do not use
• ≥9,000 to <30,000 ng/mL: 12 hours
• ≥30,000 ng/mL: 24 hours

Delayed dilution: Stored [≤5 days under refrigeration at 2°C to 8°C (36°F to 46°F) **or** ≤48 hours at room temperature of 25°C (77°F)] **in the original vial following reconstitution:** If using **previously reconstituted and stored** Veletri® vials, each vial must be further diluted prior to adding to the drug delivery reservoir.

Each reservoir diluted to a concentration ≥15,000 ng/mL can be administered at room temperature for up to 24 hours; if lower concentrations are used, pump reservoirs should be changed every 12 hours.

Preparation of Epoprostenol (Flolan® or Veletri®) Infusion

To make solution with concentration:	Flolan® Instructions	Veletri® Instructions
	Note: Flolan® may only be prepared with sterile diluent provided.	Note: Veletri® may only be prepared with SWI or NS.
3000 ng/mL	Reconstitute one 0.5 mg vial with 5 mL supplied diluent to prepare a 100,000 ng/mL solution. Withdraw 3 mL (300,000 ng) and add to 97 mL of supplied diluent to make a total of 100 mL.	Reconstitute one 1.5 mg vial with 5 mL of SWI or NS to prepare a 300,000 ng/mL solution. Withdraw 1 mL (300,000 ng) and further dilute in 99 mL of the same diluent use to reconstitute to make a total of 100 mL.
5000 ng/mL	Reconstitute one 0.5 mg vial with 5 mL supplied diluent to prepare a 100,000 ng/mL solution. Withdraw 5 mL (500,000 ng) and add to 95 mL of supplied diluent to make a total of 100 mL.	
6000 ng/mL		Reconstitute one 1.5 mg vial with 5 mL of SWI or NS to prepare a 300,000 ng/mL solution. Withdraw 2 mL (600,000 ng/mL) and further dilute in 98 mL of the same diluent used to reconstitute to make a total of 100 mL.
9000 ng/mL		Reconstitute one 1.5 mg vial with 5 mL of SWI or NS to prepare a 300,000 ng/mL solution. Withdraw 3 mL (900,000 ng) and further dilute in 97 mL of the same diluent used to reconstitute to make a total of 100 mL.
10,000 ng/mL	Reconstitute two 0.5 mg vials each with 5 mL supplied diluent to prepare a 100,000 ng/mL solution per vial. Withdraw 10 mL (1,000,000 ng) and add to 90 mL of supplied diluent to make a total of 100 mL.	
12,000 ng/mL		Reconstitute one 1.5 mg vial with 5 mL of SWI or NS to prepare a 300,000 ng/mL solution. Withdraw 4 mL (1,200,000 ng) and further dilute in 96 mL of the same diluent used to reconstitute to make a total of 100 mL.
15,000 ng/mL	Reconstitute one 1.5 mg vial with 5 mL supplied diluent to prepare a 300,000 ng/mL solution. Withdraw 5 mL (1,500,000 ng) and add to 95 mL of supplied diluent to make a total of 100 mL.	Reconstitute one 1.5 mg vial with 5 mL of SWI or NS to prepare a 300,000 ng/mL solution. Withdraw 5 mL (1,500,000 ng) and further dilute in 95 mL of the same diluent used to reconstitute to make a total of 100 mL.

(continued)

To make solution with concentration:	Flolan® Instructions	Veletri® Instructions
20,000 ng/mL	Reconstitute two 0.5 mg vials each with 5 mL supplied diluent to prepare a 100,000 ng/mL solution per vial. Withdraw 10 mL (1,000,000 ng) and add to 40 mL of supplied diluent to make a total of 50 mL (DeWet, 2004).	
30,000 ng/mL		Reconstitute two 1.5 mg vials each with 5 mL of SWI or NS to prepare a 300,000 ng/mL solution. Withdraw 10 mL (3,000,000 ng) and further dilute in 90 mL of the same diluent used to reconstitute to make a total of 100 mL.

Monitoring Parameters Hemodynamic effects (pulmonary vascular resistance, pulmonary arterial pressure, systemic blood pressure, heart rate). Monitor blood pressure (standing and supine) and heart rate closely for several hours following dosage adjustments. Monitor for improvements in exercise capacity, exertional dyspnea, fatigue, syncope, chest pain, and quality of life. Monitor the infusion pump device and catheters to avoid drug delivery system related failures. Monitor weight; serum potassium.

Additional Information The primary role of epoprostenol is in the treatment of primary pulmonary hypertension in patients unresponsive to other therapy. Response to initial therapy is evaluated in a controlled setting before chronic therapy is administered. The role of epoprostenol in the treatment of heart failure confers a negative impact on cardiovascular morbidity and mortality. Clinical trials in adults showed improvement of heart failure symptoms and exercise tolerance, but an increase in mortality.

Dosage Forms Excipient information presented when available (limited, particularly for generics); consult specific product labeling.

Solution Reconstituted, Intravenous:

Flolan: 0.5 mg (1 ea); 1.5 mg (1 ea)

Veletri: 0.5 mg (1 ea); 1.5 mg (1 ea)

Generic: 0.5 mg (1 ea); 1.5 mg (1 ea)

References

Barst RJ, "Pharmacologically Induced Pulmonary Vasodilatation in Children and Young Adults With Primary Pulmonary Hypertension," *Chest*, 1986, 89(4):497-503.

Barst RJ, Maislin G, and Fishman AP, "Vasodilator Therapy for Primary Pulmonary Hypertension in Children," *Circulation*, 1999, 99 (9):1197-208.

Barst RJ, Rubin LJ, Long WA, et al, "A Comparison of Continuous Intravenous Epoprostenol (Prostacyclin) With Conventional Therapy for Primary Pulmonary Hypertension. The Primary Pulmonary Hypertension Study Group," *N Engl J Med*, 1996, 334(5):296-302.

De Wet CJ, Affleck DG, Jacobsohn E, et al, "Inhaled Prostacyclin Is Safe, Effective, and Affordable in Patients With Pulmonary Hypertension, Right Heart Dysfunction, and Refractory Hypoxemia After Cardiothoracic Surgery," *J Thorac Cardiovasc Surg*, 2004, 127 (4):1058-67.

Eronen M, Pohjavuori M, Andersson S, et al, "Prostacyclin Treatment for Persistent Pulmonary Hypertension of the Newborn," *Pediatr Cardiol*, 1997, 18(1):3-7.

Golzand E, Bar-Oz B, and Arad I, "Intravenous Prostacyclin in the Treatment of Persistent Pulmonary Hypertension of the Newborn Refractory to Inhaled Nitric Oxide," *Isr Med Assoc J*, 2005, 7(6):408-9.

Higenbottam TW, Spiegelhalter D, Scott JP, et al, "Prostacyclin (Epoprostenol) and Heart-Lung Transplantation as Treatments for Severe Pulmonary Hypertension," *Br Heart J*, 1994, 70:366-70.

Kermode J, Butt W, and Shann F, "Comparison Between Prostaglandin E1 and Epoprostenol (Prostacyclin) in Infants After Heart Surgery," *Br Heart J*, 1991, 66(2):175-8.

McLaughlin VV, Archer SL, Badesch DB, et al, "ACCF/AHA 2009 Expert Consensus Document on Pulmonary Hypertension. A Report of the American College of Cardiology Foundation Task Force on Expert Consensus Documents and the American Heart Association," *Circulation*, 2009, 119(16):2250-94.

Rosenzweig EB, Kerstein D, and Barst RJ, "Long-Term Prostacyclin for Pulmonary Hypertension With Associated Congenital Heart Defects," *Circulation*, 1999, 99(14):1858-65.

Widlitz A and Barst RJ, "Pulmonary Arterial Hypertension in Children," *Eur Respir J*, 2003, 21(1):155-76.

- **Epoprostenol Sodium** *see* Epoprostenol *on page 770*
- **Eprex (Can)** *see* Epoetin Alfa *on page 766*
- **Epsilon Aminocaproic Acid** *see* Aminocaproic Acid *on page 122*
- **Epsom Salt [OTC]** *see* Magnesium Sulfate *on page 1297*
- **Epsom Salts** *see* Magnesium Sulfate *on page 1297*
- **EPT** *see* Teniposide *on page 1976*
- **Eptacog Alfa (Activated)** *see* Factor VIIa (Recombinant) *on page 831*
- **Epzicom®** *see* Abacavir and Lamivudine *on page 39*
- **Equalizer Gas Relief [OTC]** *see* Simethicone *on page 1891*
- **Equetro** *see* CarBAMazepine *on page 372*

Ergocalciferol (er goe kal SIF e role)

Medication Safety Issues
Sound-alike/look-alike issues:
Calciferol™ may be confused with calcitriol
Drisdol® may be confused with Drysol™
Ergocalciferol may be confused with alfacalcidol, cholecalciferol

Administration issues:
Liquid vitamin D preparations have the potential for dosing errors when administered to infants. Droppers should be clearly marked to easily provide 400 international units. For products intended for infants, the FDA recommends that accompanying droppers deliver no more than 400 international units per dose.

Related Information
Oral Medications That Should Not Be Crushed or Altered *on page 2438*

Brand Names: U.S. Calcidol [OTC]; Calciferol [OTC]; Drisdol; Drisdol [OTC]

Brand Names: Canada Drisdol®; Ostoforte®

Therapeutic Category Nutritional Supplement; Vitamin D Analog; Vitamin, Fat Soluble

Generic Availability (U.S.) Yes

Use Prevention and treatment of vitamin D deficiency and/or rickets or osteomalacia (FDA approved in all ages); treatment of familial hypophosphatemia; treatment of hypoparathyroidism; prevention and treatment of vitamin D deficiency and insufficiency in patients with chronic kidney disease (CKD); dietary supplement

Pregnancy Risk Factor C (manufacturer); A/C (dose exceeding RDA recommendation; per expert analysis)

Pregnancy Considerations Abnormalities have been observed in animal studies with maternal doses causing hypervitaminosis D. Doses larger than the RDA should be avoided during pregnancy.

Breast-Feeding Considerations Small quantities of vitamin D are found in breast milk following normal maternal exposure via sunlight and diet. The amount in breast milk does not correlate with serum levels in the infant. Therefore, vitamin D supplementation is recommended in all infants who are partially or exclusively breast fed. Hypercalcemia has been noted in a breast-feeding infant following maternal use of large doses of ergocalciferol; high doses should be avoided in lactating women.

Contraindications Hypersensitivity to ergocalciferol or any component; hypercalcemia; malabsorption syndrome; evidence of vitamin D toxicity

Warnings Some products contain tartrazine which may cause allergic reactions in susceptible individuals. Oral solution contains propylene glycol; toxicities have been reported with use of products containing propylene glycol, including hyperosmolality, lactic acidosis, seizures, and respiratory depression; in neonates large amounts of propylene glycol delivered orally, intravenously (eg, >3000 mg/day), or topically have been associated with potentially fatal toxicities which can include metabolic acidosis, seizures, renal failure, and CNS depression; use oral solution containing propylene glycol with caution (AAP, 1997; Shehab, 2009).

Precautions Use with caution in patients with coronary artery disease, renal stones, and impaired renal function; adequate calcium intake is necessary for clinical response to ergocalciferol therapy; maintain adequate fluid intake; avoid hypercalcemia

Adverse Reactions Endocrine & metabolic: Hypervitaminosis D (signs and symptoms include hypercalcemia, resulting in headache, nausea, vomiting, lethargy, confusion, sluggishness, abdominal pain, bone pain, polyuria, polydipsia, weakness, cardiac arrhythmias [eg, QT shortening, sinus tachycardia], soft tissue calcification, calciuria, and nephrocalcinosis)

Drug Interactions
Metabolism/Transport Effects None known.

Avoid Concomitant Use
Avoid concomitant use of Ergocalciferol with any of the following: Aluminum Hydroxide; Multivitamins/Fluoride (with ADE); Multivitamins/Minerals (with ADEK, Folate, Iron); Sucralfate; Sucroferric Oxyhydroxide; Vitamin D Analogs

Increased Effect/Toxicity
Ergocalciferol may increase the levels/effects of: Aluminum Hydroxide; Cardiac Glycosides; Sucralfate; Vitamin D Analogs

The levels/effects of Ergocalciferol may be increased by: Calcium Salts; Danazol; Multivitamins/Fluoride (with ADE); Multivitamins/Minerals (with ADEK, Folate, Iron); Thiazide Diuretics

Decreased Effect
The levels/effects of Ergocalciferol may be decreased by: Bile Acid Sequestrants; Mineral Oil; Orlistat; Sucroferric Oxyhydroxide

Stability Store at room temperature; protect from light

Mechanism of Action Stimulates calcium and phosphate absorption from the small intestine, promotes secretion of calcium from bone to blood; promotes renal tubule phosphate resorption

Pharmacodynamics Maximum effect occurs in ~1 month following daily doses

Pharmacokinetics (Adult data unless noted)
Absorption: Readily absorbed from GI tract; absorption requires intestinal presence of bile
Metabolism: Inactive until hydroxylated in the liver and the kidney to calcifediol and then to calcitriol (most active form)

Dosing: Neonatal
Note: 1 mcg = 40 USP units
Adequate Intake (AI): Oral: 10 mcg/day (400 units)
Prevention of Vitamin D deficiency (Greer, 2000; Wagner, 2008): Oral:
Premature neonates: 10-20 mcg/day (400-800 units), up to 750 mcg/day (30,000 units)
Breast-fed neonates (fully or partially): 10 mcg/day (400 units/day) beginning in the first few days of life. Continue supplementation until infant is weaned to ≥1000 mL/day or 1 qt/day of vitamin D-fortified formula (after 12 months of age)

Formula-fed neonates ingesting <1000 mL of vitamin D-fortified formula: 10 mcg/day (400 units/day)

Vitamin D-dependent rickets: In addition to calcium supplementation: Oral: 25 mcg/day (1000 units) for 2-3 months; once radiologic evidence of healing is observed, dose should be decreased to 10 mcg/day (400 units/day)

Dosing: Usual Note: 1 mcg = 40 USP units

Infants, Children, and Adolescents:

Adequate Intake (AI): Oral: Infants: 10 mcg/day (400 units)

Recommended Daily Allowance (RDA): Oral: Children and Adolescents: 15 mcg/day (600 units)

Prevention of Vitamin D Deficiency (Greer, 2000; Wagner, 2008): Oral:

Breast-fed infants (fully or partially): 10 mcg/day (400 units/day) beginning in the first few days of life. Continue supplementation until infant is weaned to ≥1000 mL/day or 1 qt/day of vitamin D-fortified formula or whole milk (after 12 months of age)

Formula-fed infants ingesting <1000 mL of vitamin D-fortified formula or milk: 10 mcg/day (400 units/day)

Children ingesting <1000 mL of vitamin D-fortified milk: 10 mcg/day (400 units/day)

Children with increased risk of vitamin D deficiency (chronic fat malabsorption, maintained on chronic antiseizure medications): Higher doses may be required. Use laboratory testing [25(OH)D, PTH, bone mineral status] to evaluate.

Adolescents without adequate intake: 10 mcg/day (400 units/day)

Vitamin D insufficiency or deficiency associated with CKD (stages 2-5, 5D); serum 25 hydroxyvitamin D (25[OH]D) level <30 ng/mL: (K/DOQI Guidelines, 2009): Oral:

Serum 25(OH)D level 16-30 ng/mL: Children: 2000 units/day for 3 months or 50,000 units every month for 3 months

Serum 25(OH)D level 5-15 ng/mL: Children: 4000 units/day for 12 weeks or 50,000 units every other week for 12 weeks

Serum 25(OH)D level <5 ng/mL: Children: 8000 units/day for 4 weeks then 4000 units/day for 2 months for total therapy of 3 months or 50,000 units/week for 4 weeks followed by 50,000 units 2 times/month for a total therapy of 3 months

Maintenance dose [once repletion accomplished; serum 25(OH)D level >30 ng/mL]: 200-1000 units/day

Dosage adjustment: Monitor 25(OH)D, corrected total calcium and phosphorus levels 1 month following initiation of therapy, every 3 months during therapy and with any Vitamin D dose change.

Hypoparathyroidism: Oral: Children: 1.25-5 mg/day (50,000-200,000 units) with calcium supplements

Vitamin D-dependent rickets: Oral: **Note:** In addition to calcium supplementation:

Infants 1-12 months: 25-125 mcg/day (1000-5000 units) for 2-3 months; once radiologic evidence of healing is observed, dose should be decreased to 10 mcg/day (400 units/day)

Children >12 months: 125-250 mcg/day (5000-10,000 units) for 2-3 months; once radiologic evidence of healing is observed, dose should be decreased to 10 mcg/day (400 units/day)

Prevention and treatment vitamin D Deficiency in cystic fibrosis: Oral: Recommended daily intake (Borowitz 2002):

Infants <1 year: 400 units/day

Children >1 year: 400-800 units/day

Nutritional rickets and osteomalacia: Oral:

Children with normal absorption: 25-125 mcg/day (1000-5000 units) for 6-12 weeks

Children with malabsorption: 250-625 mcg/day (10,000-25,000 units)

Familial hypophosphatemia: Oral: Children: Initial: 1000-2000 mcg/day (40,000-80,000 units) with phosphate supplements; daily dosage is increased at 3- to 4-month intervals in 250-500 mcg (10,000-20,000 units) increments

Adults:

Dietary Reference Intake for Vitamin D: Oral:

Adults 19-70 years: RDA: 600 units/day

Female: Pregnancy/lactating: RDA: 600 units/day

Vitamin D deficiency treatment: Oral: 50,000 units once per week for 8 weeks, followed by 50,000 units every 2-4 weeks thereafter for maintenance of adequate levels (Holick, 2007) **or** 50,000 units twice per week for 5 weeks (Stechschulte, 2009)

Vitamin D deficiency/insufficiency in patients with CKD stages 3-4 (K/DOQI guidelines): Oral: Dose is based on 25-hydroxyvitamin D serum level [25(OH)D]: Treatment duration should be a total of 6 months:

Serum 25(OH)D 16-30 ng/mL: 50,000 units/month

Serum 25(OH)D 5-15 ng/mL: 50,000 units/week for 4 weeks, then 50,000 units/month

Serum 25(OH)D <5 ng/mL: 50,000 units/week for 12 weeks, then 50,000 units/month

Hypoparathyroidism: Oral: 625 mcg to 5 mg/day (25,000-200,000 units) and calcium supplements

Nutritional rickets and osteomalacia: Oral:

Adults with normal absorption: 25-125 mcg/day (1000-5000 units)

Adults with malabsorption: 250-7500 mcg (10,000-300,000 units)

Vitamin D-dependent rickets: Oral: 250 mcg to 1.5 mg/day (10,000-60,000 units)

Vitamin D-resistant rickets: Oral: 12,000-500,000 units/day

Familial hypophosphatemia: Oral: 10,000-60,000 units plus phosphate supplements

Administration Oral: May be administered without regard to meals; for oral liquid, use accompanying dropper for dosage measurements

Monitoring Parameters Children at increased risk of vitamin D deficiency (chronic fat malabsorption, chronic antiseizure medication use) require serum 25(OH)D, PTH, and bone-mineral status to evaluate. If vitamin D supplement is required, then 25(OH)D levels should be repeated at 3-month intervals until normal. PTH and bone mineral-status should be monitored every 6 months until normal.

Chronic kidney disease: Serum calcium and phosphorus levels (in CKD: After 1 month and then at least every 3 months); alkaline phosphatase, BUN; bone x-ray (hypophosphatemia or hypoparathyroidism); 25(OH)D (in CKD: After 3 months of treatment and as needed thereafter)

Reference Range Vitamin D status may be determined by serum 25(OH) D levels (Misra, 2008):

Severe deficiency: ≤5 ng/mL (12.5 nmol/L)

Deficiency: 15 ng/mL (37.5 nmol/L)

Insufficiency: 15-20 ng/mL (37.5-50 nmol/L)

Sufficiency: 20-100 ng/mL (50-250 nmol/L)*

Excess: >100 ng/mL (250 nmol/L)**

Intoxication: 150 ng/mL (375 nmol/L)

*Based on adult data a level of >32 ng/mL (80 nmol/L) is desirable

**Arbitrary designation

Target serum 25(OH) D: >30 ng/mL

Additional Information 1.25 mg ergocalciferol provides 50,000 units of vitamin D activity; 1 drop of 8000 units/mL = 200 units (40 drops = 1 mL)

Chronic kidney disease (CKD) (KDIGO, 2013; KDOQI, 2002): Children ≥2 years, Adolescents, and Adults: GFR <60 mL/minute/1.73 m^2 or kidney damage for ≥3 months; stages of CKD are described below:

CKD Stage 1: Kidney damage with normal or increased GFR; GFR >90 mL/minute/1.73 m^2

CKD Stage 2: Kidney damage with mild decrease in GFR; GFR 60-89 mL/minute/1.73 m^2

CKD Stage 3: Moderate decrease in GFR; GFR 30-59 mL/minute/1.73 m^2

CKD Stage 4: Severe decrease in GFR; GFR 15-29 mL/minute/1.73 m^2

CKD Stage 5: Kidney failure; GFR <15 mL/minute/1.73 m^2 or dialysis

Dosage Forms Excipient information presented when available (limited, particularly for generics); consult specific product labeling.

Capsule, Oral:

Drisdol: 50,000 units [contains brilliant blue fcf (fd&c blue #1), soybean oil, tartrazine (fd&c yellow #5)]

Generic: 50,000 units

Solution, Oral:

Calcidol: 8000 units/mL (60 mL) [contains propylene glycol]

Calciferol: 8000 units/mL (60 mL)

Drisdol: 8000 units/mL (60 mL)

Generic: 8000 units/mL (60 mL)

Tablet, Oral:

Generic: 400 units, 2000 units

References

American Academy of Pediatrics Committee on Drugs. "Inactive" ingredients in pharmaceutical products: update (subject review). *Pediatrics.* 1997;99(2):268-278.

Borowitz D, Baker RD, and Stallings V, "Consensus Report on Nutrition for Pediatric Patients With Cystic Fibrosis," *J Pediatr Gastroenterol Nutr,* 2002, 35(3):246-59.

"Dietary Reference Intakes for Calcium, Phosphorus, Magnesium, Vitamin D, and Fluoride. Standing Committee on the Scientific Evaluation of Dietary Reference Intakes, Food and Nutrition Board, Institute of Medicine," National Academy of Sciences, Washington, DC: National Academy Press, 1997.

Holick MF, "Vitamin D Deficiency," *N Engl J Med,* 2007, 357(3):266-81.

"K/DOQI Clinical Practice Guidelines for Chronic Kidney Disease: Evaluation, Classification, and Stratification, Part 4. Definition and Classification of Stages of Chronic Kidney Disease," *Am J Kidney Dis,* 2002, 39(2 Suppl 1):46-75.

KDOQI Work Group, "KDOQI Clinical Practice Guideline for Nutrition in Children with CKD: 2008 Update. Executive Summary," *Am J Kidney Dis,* 2009, 53(3 Suppl 2):S11-104.

Kidney Disease: Improving Global Outcomes (KDIGO) CKD Work Group. KDIGO 2012 clinical practice guideline for the evaluation and management of chronic kidney disease. *Kidney Inter.* 2013;3:1-150.

Misra M, Pacaud D, Petryk A, et al, "Vitamin D Deficiency in Children and Its Management: Review of Current Knowledge and Recommendations," *Pediatrics,* 2008, 122(2):398-417.

Sanchez CP, "Secondary Hyperparathyroidism in Children With Chronic Renal Failure: Pathogenesis and Treatment," *Paediatr Drugs,* 2003, 5 (11): 763-76.

Shehab N, Lewis CL, Streetman DD, Donn SM. Exposure to the pharmaceutical excipients benzyl alcohol and propylene glycol among critically ill neonates. *Pediatr Crit Care Med.* 2009;10 (2):256-259.

Stechschulte SA, Kirsner RS, and Federman DG, "Vitamin D: Bone and Beyond, Rationale and Recommendations for Supplementation," *Am J Med,* 2009, 122(9):793-802.

Wagner CL, Greer FR; American Academy of Pediatrics Section on Breastfeeding, et al, "Prevention of Rickets and Vitamin D Deficiency in Infants, Children, and Adolescents," *Pediatrics,* 2008, 122 (5):1142-52.

Ziolkowska H, "Minimizing Bone Abnormalities in Children With Renal Failure," *Paediatr Drugs,* 2006, 8(4):205-22.

◆ **Ergomar** *see* Ergotamine *on page 776*

Ergotamine (er GOT a meen)

Related Information

Oral Medications That Should Not Be Crushed or Altered *on page 2438*

Safe Handling of Hazardous Drugs *on page 2419*

Brand Names: U.S. Ergomar

Therapeutic Category Alpha-Adrenergic Blocking Agent, Oral; Antimigraine Agent; Ergot Alkaloid

Generic Availability (U.S.) No

Use Prevent or abort vascular headaches, such as migraine and migraine variants also known as "histaminic cephalalgia"

Pregnancy Risk Factor X

Pregnancy Considerations May cause prolonged constriction of the uterine vessels and/or increased myometrial tone leading to reduced placental blood flow. This has contributed to fetal growth retardation in animals.

Breast-Feeding Considerations Ergotamine is excreted in breast milk and may cause vomiting, diarrhea, weak pulse, and unstable blood pressure in the nursing infant. Consider discontinuing the drug or discontinuing nursing.

Contraindications Hypersensitivity to ergotamine or any component; pregnancy; peripheral vascular disease, hepatic or renal disease, hypertension, peptic ulcer disease, sepsis, coronary heart disease; concurrent therapy with potent CYP3A4 inhibitors (eg, protease inhibitors and macrolide antibiotics).

Warnings Hazardous agent; use appropriate precautions for handling and disposal (NIOSH, 2012). Long-term use is associated with fibrotic changes to heart, pulmonary valves, and rare cases of retroperitoneal fibrosis; chronic usage may also be harmful due to a reduction in cerebral blood flow, ECG changes, and hypertension; sustained vasoconstriction may precipitate angina or MI, aggravate intermittent claudication, or lead to ischemic colitis. Concomitant use with potent inhibitors of CYP3A4 (including protease inhibitors and macrolide antibiotics) has been associated with acute ergot toxicity characterized by serious and/or life-threatening cerebral and peripheral ischemia **[U.S. Boxed Warning]**; some cases have resulted in amputation; less potent CYP3A4 inhibitors (eg, metronidazole, nefazodone, fluoxetine, zileuton, and azole antifungals) may carry the same risk. Patients who take ergotamine for extended periods of time may become dependent on it and discontinuation may result in withdrawal symptoms (eg, rebound headache). Safety and efficacy have not been established in children.

Adverse Reactions

Cardiovascular: Absence of pulse, bradycardia, cardiac valvular fibrosis, cyanosis, ECG changes, edema, gangrene, hypertension, ischemia, precordial distress and pain, tachycardia, vasospasm

Central nervous system: Vertigo

Dermatologic: Itching

Gastrointestinal: Nausea, vomiting

Genitourinary: Retroperitoneal fibrosis

Neuromuscular & skeletal: Muscle pain, numbness, paresthesia, weakness

Respiratory: Pleuropulmonary fibrosis

Miscellaneous: Cold extremities

Drug Interactions

Metabolism/Transport Effects Substrate of CYP3A4 (major); **Note:** Assignment of Major/Minor substrate status based on clinically relevant drug interaction potential; **Inhibits** CYP3A4 (weak)

Avoid Concomitant Use

Avoid concomitant use of Ergotamine with any of the following: Alpha-/Beta-Agonists; Alpha1-Agonists; Boceprevir; Clarithromycin; Cobicistat; Conivaptan; Crizotinib; Enzalutamide; Fusidic Acid (Systemic); Itraconazole; Ketoconazole (Systemic); Lorcaserin; Mifepristone; Nitroglycerin; Pimozide; Posaconazole; Protease Inhibitors; Serotonin 5-HT1D Receptor Agonists; Telaprevir; Voriconazole

Increased Effect/Toxicity

Ergotamine may increase the levels/effects of: Alpha-/Beta-Agonists; Alpha1-Agonists; Antipsychotics; ARIPiprazole; Dofetilide; Lomitapide; Metoclopramide; Pimozide; Serotonin 5-HT1D Receptor Agonists; Serotonin Modulators

The levels/effects of Ergotamine may be increased by: Antiemetics (5HT3 Antagonists); Antipsychotics; Beta-Blockers; Boceprevir; Ceritinib; Clarithromycin; Cobicistat; Conivaptan; Crizotinib; CYP3A4 Inhibitors (Moderate); CYP3A4 Inhibitors (Strong); Dasatinib; Fusidic Acid (Systemic); Itraconazole; Ivacaftor; Ketoconazole (Systemic); Lorcaserin; Luliconazole; Macrolide Antibiotics; Mifepristone; Nitroglycerin; Posaconazole; Protease Inhibitors; Serotonin 5-HT1D Receptor Agonists; Simeprevir; Stiripentol; Telaprevir; Voriconazole

Decreased Effect

Ergotamine may decrease the levels/effects of: Nitroglycerin

The levels/effects of Ergotamine may be decreased by: Enzalutamide

Food Interactions Grapefruit juice may cause increased blood levels of ergotamine, leading to increased toxicity. Management: Avoid grapefruit juice.

Stability Hazardous agent; use appropriate precautions for handling and disposal (NIOSH, 2012).

Mechanism of Action Has partial agonist and/or antagonist activity against tryptaminergic, dopaminergic and alpha-adrenergic receptors depending upon their site; is a highly active uterine stimulant; it causes constriction of peripheral and cranial blood vessels and produces depression of central vasomotor centers

Pharmacokinetics (Adult data unless noted)

Absorption: Oral, rectal: Erratic

Distribution: V_d: Adults: 1.85 L/kg

Metabolism: Extensive in the liver

Bioavailability: Poor overall (<5%)

Half-life: Adults: 2-2.5 hours

Time to peak serum concentration: Oral: Within 0.5-3 hours

Elimination: In bile as metabolites (90%)

Dosing: Usual Adolescents and Adults: **Note:** Not for chronic daily administration: Sublingual: 1 tablet under tongue at first sign, then 1 tablet every 30 minutes; maximum: 3 tablets/24 hours, 5 tablets/week

Administration Hazardous agent; use appropriate precautions for handling and disposal (NIOSH, 2012).

Sublingual: Place tablet under the tongue; do not crush; may administer without regard to meals.

Dosage Forms Excipient information presented when available (limited, particularly for generics); consult specific product labeling.

Tablet Sublingual, Sublingual, as tartrate:

Ergomar: 2 mg [contains fd&c blue #1 aluminum lake, fd&c yellow #10 aluminum lake, saccharin sodium]

References

National Institute for Occupational Safety and Health (NIOSH), "NIOSH List of Antineoplastic and Other Hazardous Drugs in Healthcare Settings 2012." Available at http://www.cdc.gov/niosh/docs/2012-150/pdfs/2012-150.pdf. Accessed January 21, 2013.

Ergotamine and Caffeine

(er GOT a meen & KAF een)

Medication Safety Issues

Sound-alike/look-alike issues:

Cafergot may be confused with Carafate

Brand Names: U.S. Cafergot; Migergot

Brand Names: Canada Cafergor

Therapeutic Category Alpha-Adrenergic Blocking Agent, Oral; Antimigraine Agent; Ergot Alkaloid

Generic Availability (U.S.) Yes: Tablet

Use Prevent or abort vascular headaches, such as migraine and migraine variants also known as "histaminic cephalalgia"

Pregnancy Risk Factor X

Pregnancy Considerations May cause prolonged constriction of the uterine vessels and/or increased myometrial tone leading to reduced placental blood flow. This has contributed to fetal growth retardation in animals.

Breast-Feeding Considerations Ergotamine is excreted in breast milk and may cause vomiting, diarrhea, weak pulse, and unstable blood pressure in the nursing infant. Consider discontinuing the drug or discontinuing nursing.

Contraindications Hypersensitivity to ergotamine, caffeine, or any component; pregnancy; peripheral vascular disease, hepatic or renal disease, hypertension, peptic ulcer disease, sepsis, coronary heart disease; concurrent therapy with potent CYP3A4 inhibitors (eg, protease inhibitors and macrolide antibiotics)

Warnings Long-term use is associated with fibrotic changes to heart, pulmonary valves, and rare cases of retroperitoneal fibrosis; chronic usage may also be harmful due to a reduction in cerebral blood flow, ECG changes, and hypertension; sustained vasoconstriction may precipitate angina or MI, aggravate intermittent claudication, or lead to ischemic colitis. Concomitant use with potent inhibitors of CYP3A4 (including protease inhibitors and macrolide antibiotics) has been associated with acute ergot toxicity characterized by serious and/or life-threatening cerebral and peripheral ischemia **[U.S. Boxed Warning]**; some cases have resulted in amputation; less potent CYP3A4 inhibitors (eg, metronidazole, fluoxetine, nefazodone, zileuton, and azole antifungals) may carry the same risk. Patients who take ergotamine for extended periods of time may become dependent on it and discontinuation may result in withdrawal symptoms (eg, rebound headache). Safety and efficacy have not been established in children.

Adverse Reactions

Cardiovascular: Absence of pulse, bradycardia, cardiac valvular fibrosis, cyanosis, ECG changes, edema, gangrene, hypertension, ischemia, precordial distress and pain, tachycardia, vasospasm

Central nervous system: Vertigo

Dermatologic: Itching

Gastrointestinal: Anal or rectal ulcer (with overuse of suppository), nausea, vomiting

Genitourinary: Retroperitoneal fibrosis

Neuromuscular & skeletal: Muscle pain, numbness, paresthesia, weakness

Respiratory: Pleuropulmonary fibrosis

Miscellaneous: Cold extremities

Drug Interactions

Metabolism/Transport Effects Refer to individual components.

Avoid Concomitant Use

Avoid concomitant use of Ergotamine and Caffeine with any of the following: Alpha-/Beta-Agonists; Alpha1-Agonists; Boceprevir; Clarithromycin; Cobicistat; Conivaptan; Crizotinib; Enzalutamide; Fusidic Acid (Systemic); Iobenguane I 123; Itraconazole; Ketoconazole (Systemic); Lorcaserin; Mifepristone; Nitroglycerin; Pimozide; Posaconazole; Protease Inhibitors; Serotonin 5-HT1D Receptor Agonists; Stiripentol; Telaprevir; Voriconazole

Increased Effect/Toxicity

Ergotamine and Caffeine may increase the levels/effects of: Alpha-/Beta-Agonists; Alpha1-Agonists; Antipsychotics; ARIPiprazole; Dofetilide; Formoterol; Indacaterol; Lomitapide; Metoclopramide; Pimozide; Serotonin 5-HT1D Receptor Agonists; Serotonin Modulators; Sympathomimetics

The levels/effects of Ergotamine and Caffeine may be increased by: Antiemetics (5HT3 Antagonists); Antipsychotics; AtoMOXetine; Beta-Blockers; Boceprevir; Cannabinoid-Containing Products; Ceritinib; Clarithromycin; Cobicistat; Conivaptan; Crizotinib; CYP1A2 Inhibitors (Moderate); CYP1A2 Inhibitors (Strong); CYP3A4 Inhibitors (Moderate); CYP3A4 Inhibitors (Strong); Dasatinib; Deferasirox; Fusidic Acid

(Systemic); Itraconazole; Ivacaftor; Ketoconazole (Systemic); Linezolid; Lorcaserin; Luliconazole; Macrolide Antibiotics; Mifepristone; Nitroglycerin; Norfloxacin; Posaconazole; Protease Inhibitors; Serotonin 5-HT1D Receptor Agonists; Simeprevir; Stiripentol; Telaprevir; Vemurafenib; Voriconazole

Decreased Effect

Ergotamine and Caffeine may decrease the levels/effects of: Adenosine; Iobenguane I 123; Nitroglycerin; Regadenoson

The levels/effects of Ergotamine and Caffeine may be decreased by: Enzalutamide; Peginterferon Alfa-2b; Teriflunomide

Food Interactions See individual agents.

Mechanism of Action Has partial agonist and/or antagonist activity against tryptaminergic, dopaminergic and alpha-adrenergic receptors depending upon their site; is a highly active uterine stimulant; it causes constriction of peripheral and cranial blood vessels and produces depression of central vasomotor centers

Pharmacokinetics (Adult data unless noted)

Absorption: Oral, rectal: Erratic; absorption is enhanced by caffeine coadministration

Metabolism: Extensive in the liver

Bioavailability: Poor overall (<5%)

Half-life: 2-2.5 hours

Time to peak serum concentration: Oral: Within 0.5-3 hours

Elimination: In bile as metabolites (90%)

Dosing: Usual Adolescents and Adults: **Note:** Not for chronic daily administration:

Oral: 2 mg at onset of attack; then 1-2 mg every 30 minutes as needed; maximum dose: 6 mg per attack; do not exceed 10 mg/week

Rectal, suppositories: 1 suppository at first sign of an attack; follow with second dose after 1 hour, if needed; maximum dose: 2 per attack; do not exceed 5/week

Administration Oral: Tablets may be taken without regard to meals.

Dosage Forms Excipient information presented when available (limited, particularly for generics); consult specific product labeling.

Suppository, rectal:

Migergot: Ergotamine tartrate 2 mg and caffeine 100 mg (12s)

Tablet, oral: Ergotamine tartrate 1 mg and caffeine 100 mg

Cafergot: Ergotamine tartrate 1 mg and caffeine 100 mg

◆ **Ergotamine Tartrate** *see* Ergotamine *on page 776*

◆ **Ergotamine Tartrate and Caffeine** *see* Ergotamine and Caffeine *on page 777*

◆ **E-R-O Ear Drops [OTC]** *see* Carbamide Peroxide *on page 377*

◆ **E-R-O Ear Wax Removal System [OTC]** *see* Carbamide Peroxide *on page 377*

◆ **Errin** *see* Norethindrone *on page 1511*

Ertapenem (er ta PEN em)

Medication Safety Issues

Sound-alike/look-alike issues:

Ertapenem may be confused with doripenem, imipenem, meropenem

INVanz may be confused with AVINza, I.V. vancomycin

Brand Names: U.S. INVanz

Brand Names: Canada Invanz

Therapeutic Category Antibiotic, Carbapenem

Generic Availability (U.S.) No

Use Treatment of moderate to severe, complicated intra-abdominal infections, acute pelvic infections, complicated skin and skin structure infections (including diabetic foot infections without osteomyelitis), community-acquired pneumonia, and complicated urinary tract infections (including pyelonephritis) caused by susceptible organisms (FDA approved in ages ≥3 months and adults); prophylaxis of surgical site infection following colorectal surgery (FDA approved in adults)

Pregnancy Risk Factor B

Pregnancy Considerations Teratogenic effects were not observed in animal reproduction studies. Ertapenem is approved for the treatment of postpartum endomyometritis, septic abortion, and postsurgical infections. Information related to use during pregnancy has not been located.

Breast-Feeding Considerations Ertapenem is excreted in breast milk. The low concentrations in milk and low oral bioavailability suggest minimal exposure risk to the infant. The manufacturer recommends that caution be exercised when administering ertapenem to nursing women. Non-dose-related effects could include modification of bowel flora.

Contraindications Hypersensitivity to ertapenem, carbapenems, or any component; patients who have had an anaphylactoid reaction to beta-lactams; hypersensitivity to local anesthetics of the amide type for patients receiving I.M. injections

Warnings Serious and occasionally fatal hypersensitivity reactions have been reported in patients receiving beta-lactam therapy; careful inquiry should be made concerning previous hypersensitivity reactions to penicillins, cephalosporins, or other beta-lactams before initiating ertapenem; administration to patients with a history of anaphylactoid reaction to beta-lactams is contraindicated. I.M. administration preparations are mixed with lidocaine; use is contraindicated in patients with hypersensitivity to amide local anesthetics.

Carbapenems have been associated with CNS adverse effects, including confusional states and seizures (myoclonic); use caution in patients with CNS disorders (eg, brain lesions and history of seizures) and adjust dose in renal impairment to avoid drug accumulation, which may increase seizure risk; seizures have been reported with ertapenem therapy. Valproic acid (VPA) serum concentrations may be significantly decreased by concurrent carbapenem use leading to breakthrough seizures; VPA dosage adjustment may not adequately compensate for this interaction; concurrent use with valproic acid/divalproex sodium not recommended.

Pseudomembranous colitis has been reported in patients receiving ertapenem; prolonged use may result in superinfection, including *C. difficile*-associated diarrhea (CDAD); CDAD has been observed >2 months postantibiotic treatment.

Precautions Use with caution in patients with severe renal impairment (CrCl ≤30 mL/minute/1.73 m^2); dosage adjustment required.

Adverse Reactions

Cardiovascular: Chest pain, edema, hypertension, hypotension, phlebitis, tachycardia, thrombophlebitis

Central nervous system: Altered mental status (ie, agitation, confusion, disorientation, mental acuity decreased, somnolence, stupor); anxiety, dizziness, fatigue, headache, hypothermia (infants, children, and adolescents), insomnia

Dermatologic: Diaper rash (infants and children), erythema, genital rash (infants, children, and adolescents), pruritus, skin lesion (infants, children, and adolescents), skin rash

Endocrine & metabolic: Decreased serum albumin, hyperglycemia, hyperkalemia, hypokalemia

Gastrointestinal: Abdominal pain, acid regurgitation, constipation, decreased appetite (infants, children, and adolescents), diarrhea, dyspepsia, nausea, oral candidiasis, vomiting

Genitourinary: Erythrocyturia, vaginitis

Hematologic & oncologic: Decreased hematocrit, decreased hemoglobin, decreased neutrophils, eosinophilia, leukocyturia, leukopenia, prolonged prothrombin time, thrombocythemia, thrombocytopenia

Hepatic: Increased liver enzymes, increased serum alkaline, increased serum bilirubin (total)

Infection: Herpes simplex infection (infants, children, and adolescents)

Local: Extravasation, infused vein complication

Neuromuscular & skeletal: Arthralgia (infants, children, and adolescents), leg pain, weakness

Otic: Otitis media (infants, children, and adolescents)

Renal: Increased serum creatinine

Respiratory: Cough, dyspnea, nasopharyngitis (infants, children, and adolescents), pharyngitis, rales, respiratory distress, rhinitis (infants, children, and adolescents), rhinorrhea (infants, children, and adolescents), rhonchi, upper respiratory tract infection (infants, children, and adolescents), wheezing (infants, children, and adolescents)

Miscellaneous: Fever

Rare but important or life-threatening: Anaphylactoid reaction, anaphylaxis, asthma, asystole, atrial fibrillation, bradycardia, bronchoconstriction, cardiac arrest, cardiac arrhythmia, cardiac failure, cholelithiasis, *Clostridium difficile*-associated diarrhea, delirium, DRESS syndrome, gastrointestinal hemorrhage, gout, heart murmur, hemoptysis, hypoxemia, impaired consciousness, intestinal obstruction, jaundice, oliguria/anuria, pancreatitis, pleural effusion, renal insufficiency, seizure, septicemia, septic shock, subdural hematoma, ventricular tachycardia

Drug Interactions

Metabolism/Transport Effects None known.

Avoid Concomitant Use

Avoid concomitant use of Ertapenem with any of the following: BCG

Increased Effect/Toxicity

Ertapenem may increase the levels/effects of: Tacrolimus (Systemic)

The levels/effects of Ertapenem may be increased by: Probenecid

Decreased Effect

Ertapenem may decrease the levels/effects of: BCG; Sodium Picosulfate; Typhoid Vaccine; Valproic Acid and Derivatives

Stability Store intact vial at ≤25°C (77°F).

Reconstituted I.V. ertapenem solution further diluted in NS or following activation of ertapenem in ADD-Vantage® vials with ADD-Vantage® diluent: Stable for 6 hours at room temperature or 24 hours if refrigerated and used within 4 hours after removal from refrigeration; do not freeze.

Reconstituted I.M. ertapenem solution should be used within 1 hour after preparation.

Mechanism of Action Inhibits bacterial cell wall synthesis by binding to one or more of the penicillin-binding proteins; which in turn inhibits the final transpeptidation step of peptidoglycan synthesis in bacterial cell walls, thus inhibiting cell wall biosynthesis. Bacteria eventually lyse due to ongoing activity of cell wall autolytic enzymes (autolysins and murein hydrolases) while cell wall assembly is arrested.

Pharmacokinetics (Adult data unless noted)

Absorption: I.M.: Almost complete

Distribution: V_d:

Infants ≥3 months and Children: ~0.2 L/kg

Adolescents: 0.16 L/kg

Adults: 0.12 L/kg

Protein binding: 85% to 95% (concentration-dependent, primarily to albumin)

Metabolism: Non-CYP-mediated hydrolysis to inactive metabolite

Bioavailability: I.M.: 90%

Half-life:

Infants ≥3 months and Children: 2.5 hours

Adolescents and Adults: 4 hours

Time to peak serum concentration: I.M.: 2.3 hours

Elimination: Urine [80% (38% as unchanged drug)] and feces (10%)

Dosing: Usual Note: I.V. therapy may be administered for up to 14 days; I.M. for up to 7 days.

Infants, Children, and Adolescents:

General dosing, susceptible infection: I.M., I.V.:

Infants and Children (*Red Book* [AAP], 2012): Severe infections: 15 mg/kg/dose twice daily; maximum single dose: 500 mg

Adolescents: 1000 mg once daily

Intra-abdominal infection, complicated: I.M., I.V.: **Note:** IDSA guidelines recommend a treatment duration of 4-7 days (provided source controlled) for community-acquired, mild to moderate infections (Solomkin, 2010)

Infants <3 months: 15 mg/kg/dose twice daily (*Red Book* [AAP], 2012)

Infants ≥3 months and Children: 15 mg/kg/dose twice daily for 5-14 days; maximum single dose: 500 mg

Adolescents: 1000 mg once daily for 5-14 days

Pelvic infections, acute: I.M., I.V.:

Infants <3 months: 15 mg/kg/dose twice daily (*Red Book* [AAP], 2012)

Infants ≥3 months and Children: 15 mg/kg/dose twice daily for 3-10 days; maximum single dose: 500 mg

Adolescents: 1000 mg once daily for 3-10 days

Pneumonia, community acquired: I.M., I.V.: **Note:** Duration includes possible switch to appropriate oral step-down therapy after at least 3 days of parenteral treatment, once clinical improvement demonstrated.

Infants <3 months: 15 mg/kg/dose twice daily (*Red Book* [AAP], 2012)

Infants ≥3 months and Children: 15 mg/kg/dose twice daily for 10-14 days; maximum single dose: 500 mg

Adolescents: 1000 mg once daily for 10-14 days

Skin and skin structure infections, complicated: I.M., I.V.:

Infants <3 months: 15 mg/kg/dose twice daily (*Red Book* [AAP], 2012)

Infants ≥3 months and Children: 15 mg/kg/dose twice daily for 7-14 days; maximum single dose: 500 mg

Adolescents: 1000 mg once daily for 7-14 days

Surgical prophylaxis: I.V.: Children and Adolescents: 15 mg/kg 60 minutes before procedure; maximum dose: 1000 mg (Bratzler, 2013)

Urinary tract infections (including pyelonephritis): I.M., I.V.: **Note:** Duration includes possible switch to appropriate oral therapy after at least 3 days of parenteral treatment, once clinical improvement demonstrated.

Infants <3 months: 15 mg/kg/dose twice daily (*Red Book* [AAP], 2012)

Infants ≥3 months and Children: 15 mg/kg/dose twice daily for 10-14 days; maximum single dose: 500 mg

Adolescents: 1000 mg once daily for 10-14 days

Adults:

General dosing, susceptible infection: I.M., I.V.: 1000 mg once daily

Prophylaxis of surgical site infection following colorectal surgery: I.V.: Single 1000 mg dose administered 1 hour prior to surgical procedure

Dosing adjustment in renal impairment: Adults:

CrCl >30 mL/minute/1.73 m²: No dosage adjustment required.

CrCl ≤30 mL/minute/1.73 m²: 500 mg once daily

Continuous Ambulatory Peritoneal Dialysis (CAPD): 500 mg daily (Cardone, 2011)
Hemodialysis: ~30% removed by hemodialysis (Curran, 2003). If daily dose is given within 6 hours prior to hemodialysis, a supplementary dose of 150 mg should be given following hemodialysis.

Dosing adjustment in hepatic impairment: There are no dosage adjustments provided in the manufacturer's labeling.

Administration Parenteral:

I.M. injection: Reconstitute 1 g vial with 3.2 mL of 1% lidocaine immediately prior to administration with a resultant concentration of 312.5 mg/mL. Shake vial well. Administer deep into a large muscle mass such as the gluteus maximus or lateral part of the thigh. Avoid injection into a blood vessel.

I.V. intermittent infusion: Reconstitute 1 g vial with 10 mL SWI, NS, or bacteriostatic water for injection with a resultant concentration of 100 mg/mL. Further dilute dose with NS to a final maximum concentration of 20 mg/mL and administer over 30 minutes. Do not coinfuse with other medications. **Do not infuse with dextrose-containing solutions.**

Monitoring Parameters Periodic renal, hepatic, and hematologic function tests; neurological assessment

Additional Information Sodium content: 1000 mg ertapenem contains 6 mEq

Dosage Forms Excipient information presented when available (limited, particularly for generics); consult specific product labeling.

Solution Reconstituted, Injection:
INVanz: 1 g (1 ea)

Solution Reconstituted, Intravenous:
INVanz: 1 g (1 ea)

References

American Academy of Pediatrics (AAP). In: Pickering LK, Baker CJ, Kimberlin DW, Long SS, eds. *Red Book: 2012 Report of the Committee on Infectious Diseases.* 29th ed. Elk Grove Village, IL: American Academy of Pediatrics; 2012.

Arguedas A, Cespedes J, Botet FA, et al, "Safety and Tolerability of Ertapenem Versus Ceftriaxone in a Double-Blind Study Performed in Children With Complicated Urinary Tract Infection, Community-Acquired Pneumonia or Skin and Soft-Tissue Infection," *Int J Antimicrob Agents,* 2009, 33(2):163-7.

Bratzler DW, Dellinger EP, Olsen KM, et al. Clinical practice guidelines for antimicrobial prophylaxis in surgery. *Am J Health Syst Pharm.* 2013;70(3):195-283.

Cardone KE, Grabe DW, Kulawy RW, et al. Ertapenem pharmacokinetics and pharmacodynamics during continuous ambulatory peritoneal dialysis. *Antimicrob Agents Chemother.* 2012;56(2):725-730.

Curran M, Simpson D, and Perry C, "Ertapenem: A Review of Its Use in the Management of Bacterial Infections," *Drugs,* 2003, 63 (17):1855-78.

Keating GM and Perry CM, "Ertapenem: A Review of Its Use in the Treatment of Bacterial Infections," Drugs, 2005, 65(15):2151-78.

Nix DE, Majumdar AK, and DiNubile MJ, "Pharmacokinetics and Pharmacodynamics of Ertapenem: An Overview for Clinicians," *J Antimicrob Chemother,* 2004, 53(Suppl 2):ii23-8.

Solomkin JS, Mazuski JE, Bradley JS, et al. Diagnosis and management of complicated intra-abdominal infection in adults and children: guidelines by the Surgical Infection Society and the Infectious Diseases Society of America. *Clin Infect Dis.* 2010;50(2):133-164.

◆ **Ertapenem Sodium** *see Ertapenem on page 778*

◆ **Erwinase (Can)** *see Asparaginase (Erwinia) on page 211*

◆ **Erwinaze** *see Asparaginase (Erwinia) on page 211*

◆ *Erwinia chrysanthemi see Asparaginase (Erwinia) on page 211*

◆ **Ery** *see Erythromycin (Topical) on page 785*

◆ **Erybid (Can)** *see Erythromycin (Systemic) on page 780*

◆ **Eryc (Can)** *see Erythromycin (Systemic) on page 780*

◆ **Erygel** *see Erythromycin (Topical) on page 785*

◆ **EryPed 200** *see Erythromycin (Systemic) on page 780*

◆ **EryPed 400** *see Erythromycin (Systemic) on page 780*

◆ **Erysol (Can)** *see Erythromycin (Topical) on page 785*

◆ **Ery-Tab** *see Erythromycin (Systemic) on page 780*

◆ **Erythrocin Lactobionate** *see Erythromycin (Systemic) on page 780*

◆ **Erythrocin Stearate** *see Erythromycin (Systemic) on page 780*

Erythromycin (Systemic) (er ith roe MYE sin)

Medication Safety Issues

Sound-alike/look-alike issues:

Erythromycin may be confused with azithromycin, clarithromycin

Eryc may be confused with Emcyt, Ery-Tab

Related Information

Oral Medications That Should Not Be Crushed or Altered *on page 2438*

Brand Names: U.S. E.E.S. 400; E.E.S. Granules; Ery-Tab; EryPed 200; EryPed 400; Erythrocin Lactobionate; Erythrocin Stearate; PCE

Brand Names: Canada Apo-Erythro Base; Apo-Erythro E-C; Apo-Erythro-ES; Apo-Erythro-S; EES; Erybid; Eryc; Novo-Rythro Estolate; Novo-Rythro Ethylsuccinate; Nu-Erythromycin-S; PCE

Therapeutic Category Antibiotic, Macrolide

Generic Availability (U.S.) May be product dependent

Use Treatment of mild to moderately severe infections of the upper and lower respiratory tract and skin infections due to susceptible *streptococcus* and *staphylococcus* sp. and *Haemophilus influenzae;* other susceptible bacterial infections, including *Mycoplasma pneumoniae, Legionella pneumonia,* nongonococcal urethritis, Lyme disease, diphtheria, pertussis, chancroid, *Chlamydia, Ureaplasma,* and *Campylobacter* gastroenteritis, syphilis, prophylaxis of recurrent rheumatic fever in penicillin- or sulfa-allergic patients (all indications: FDA approved in all ages); has also been used in conjunction with neomycin for decontaminating the bowel for surgery; prophylaxis of pneumococcal infections in children with sickle cell disease (SCD), and functional or anatomic asplenia who are penicillin allergic

Pregnancy Risk Factor B

Pregnancy Considerations Adverse events were not observed in animal reproduction studies. Erythromycin crosses the placenta and low concentrations are found in the fetal serum. Cardiovascular anomalies following exposure in early pregnancy have been reported in some observational studies. Serum concentrations of erythromycin may be variable in pregnant women (Kiefer, 1955; Philipson, 1976).

In patients with acute infections during pregnancy, erythromycin may be given if an antibiotic is required and appropriate based on bacterial sensitivity (ACOG No. 120, 2011). Erythromycin is the antibiotic of choice for preterm premature rupture of membranes (with membrane rupture between 24 0/7 to 33 6/7 weeks gestation) (ACOG 2013), the treatment of granuloma inguinale, and lymphogranuloma venereum in pregnancy (CDC [RR-12], 2010), and the treatment of or long-term suppression of *Bartonella* infection in HIV-infected pregnant patients [DHHS, 2013]. Erythromycin may be appropriate as an alternative agent for the treatment of chlamydial infections in pregnant women (consult current guidelines) (CDC [RR-12], 2010).

Breast-Feeding Considerations Erythromycin is excreted in breast milk; therefore, the manufacturer recommends that caution be exercised when administering erythromycin to breast-feeding women. Decreased appetite, diarrhea, rash, and somnolence have been reported in nursing infants exposed to macrolide antibiotics (Goldstein, 2009).

One case report and a cohort study raise the possibility for a connection with pyloric stenosis in neonates exposed to erythromycin via breast milk and an alternative antibiotic may be preferred for breast-feeding mothers of infants in this age group (Sorensen, 2003; Stang, 1986).

Contraindications Hypersensitivity to erythromycin, other macrolides, or any component; concomitant administration with pimozide, astemizole, terfenadine, cisapride, ergotamine, or dihydroergotamine

Contraindications from other product labeling: Concomitant administration with lovastatin or simvastatin

Warnings Hepatic impairment with or without jaundice has occurred primarily in older children and adults; reported incidence in children is ~0.1% and in adults is 0.25%; it may be accompanied by malaise, nausea, vomiting, abdominal colic, and fever; discontinue use if these occur. Infantile hypertrophic pyloric stenosis with symptoms of nonbilious vomiting or irritability with feeding has been reported in 5% of infants who received erythromycin for pertussis prophylaxis. Prolonged use may result in fungal or bacterial superinfection, including *C. difficile*-associated diarrhea (CDAD) and pseudomembranous colitis; CDAD has been observed >2 months postantibiotic treatment.

Risk of serious cardiac arrhythmias exist in patients receiving erythromycin and pimozide, astemizole, terfenadine, or cisapride; do not use concurrently with erythromycin. Erythromycin has been associated with rare QT_c prolongation and ventricular arrhythmias, including torsade de pointes; avoid use in patients with prolonged QT interval, uncorrected hypokalemia or hypomagnesemia, clinically significant bradycardia, or concurrent use of Class IA (eg, quinidine, procainamide) or Class III (eg, amiodarone, dofetilide, sotalol) antiarrhythmic agents. Use caution with other medication relying on CYP3A4 metabolism (eg, fluconazole, ketoconazole, itraconazole, diltiazem, verapamil); high potential for drug interactions exists. Avoid concurrent use with strong CYP3A inhibitors due to increased risk of sudden cardiac death (Ray, 2004). Rhabdomyolysis has been reported in seriously ill patients receiving erythromycin and lovastatin or simvastatin concomitantly; concurrent use is contraindicated (per manufacturer labeling of lovastatin and simvastatin.

Erythromycin lactobionate injection may contain benzyl alcohol which may cause allergic reactions in susceptible individuals; large amounts of benzyl alcohol (≥99 mg/kg/day) have been associated with a potentially fatal toxicity ("gasping syndrome") in neonates; the "gasping syndrome" consists of metabolic acidosis, respiratory distress, gasping respirations, CNS dysfunction (including convulsions, intracranial hemorrhage), hypotension and cardiovascular collapse; use erythromycin lactobionate injection products containing benzyl alcohol with caution in neonates; *in vitro* and animal studies have shown that benzoate, a metabolite of benzyl alcohol, displaces bilirubin from protein binding sites.

Precautions Use with caution in patients with hepatic impairment. Use with caution in patients with myasthenia gravis; erythromycin has been associated with aggravation of weakness.

Adverse Reactions

Cardiovascular: QT_c prolongation, torsade de pointes, ventricular arrhythmia, ventricular tachycardia

Central nervous system: Seizure

Dermatologic: Erythema multiforme, pruritus, rash, Stevens-Johnson syndrome, toxic epidermal necrolysis

Gastrointestinal: Abdominal pain, anorexia, diarrhea, infantile hypertrophic pyloric stenosis, nausea, oral candidiasis, pancreatitis, pseudomembranous colitis, vomiting

Hepatic: Cholestatic jaundice (most common with estolate), hepatitis, liver function tests abnormal

Local: Phlebitis at the injection site, thrombophlebitis

Neuromuscular & skeletal: Weakness

Otic: Hearing loss

Miscellaneous: Allergic reactions, anaphylaxis, hypersensitivity reactions, interstitial nephritis, urticaria

Drug Interactions

Metabolism/Transport Effects Substrate of CYP2B6 (minor), CYP3A4 (major), P-glycoprotein; **Note:** Assignment of Major/Minor substrate status based on clinically relevant drug interaction potential; **Inhibits** CYP3A4 (moderate), P-glycoprotein

Avoid Concomitant Use

Avoid concomitant use of Erythromycin (Systemic) with any of the following: BCG; Bosutinib; Cisapride; Clindamycin (Topical); Conivaptan; Disopyramide; Fluconazole; Fusidic Acid (Systemic); Highest Risk QTc-Prolonging Agents; Ibrutinib; Ivabradine; Lincosamide Antibiotics; Lomitapide; Lovastatin; Mifepristone; PAZOPanib; Pimozide; QuiNIDine; QuiNINE; Silodosin; Simeprevir; Simvastatin; Terfenadine; Tolvaptan; Topotecan; Ulipristal; VinCRIStine (Liposomal)

Increased Effect/Toxicity

Erythromycin (Systemic) may increase the levels/effects of: Afatinib; Alfentanil; ALPRAZolam; Antifungal Agents (Azole Derivatives, Systemic); Antineoplastic Agents (Vinca Alkaloids); ARIPiprazole; AtorvaSTATin; Avanafil; Bosentan; Bosutinib; Brentuximab Vedotin; Budesonide (Systemic, Oral Inhalation); BusPIRone; Calcium Channel Blockers; Cannabis; CarBAMazepine; Cardiac Glycosides; Cilostazol; Cisapride; CloZAPine; Colchicine; Corticosteroids (Systemic); CycloSPORINE (Systemic); CYP3A4 Substrates; Dabigatran Etexilate; Disopyramide; DOXOrubicin (Conventional); Dronabinol; Eletriptan; Eplerenone; Ergot Derivatives; Estazolam; Everolimus; FentaNYL; Fexofenadine; Highest Risk QTc-Prolonging Agents; Ibrutinib; Imatinib; Ivabradine; Ivacaftor; Lomitapide; Lovastatin; Lurasidone; Midazolam; Moderate Risk QTc-Prolonging Agents; OxyCODONE; PAZOPanib; P-glycoprotein/ABCB1 Substrates; Pimecrolimus; Pimozide; Pitavastatin; Pravastatin; QuiNIDine; QuiNINE; Ranolazine; Repaglinide; Rifamycin Derivatives; Rifaximin; Rilpivirine; Rivaroxaban; Salmeterol; Saxagliptin; Selective Serotonin Reuptake Inhibitors; Sildenafil; Silodosin; Simeprevir; Simvastatin; Sirolimus; Tacrolimus (Systemic); Tacrolimus (Topical); Telaprevir; Temsirolimus; Terfenadine; Tetrahydrocannabinol; Theophylline Derivatives; Tolvaptan; Topotecan; Triazolam; Ulipristal; Vardenafil; Vilazodone; VinCRIStine (Liposomal); Vitamin K Antagonists; Zopiclone

The levels/effects of Erythromycin (Systemic) may be increased by: Antifungal Agents (Azole Derivatives, Systemic); Conivaptan; CYP3A4 Inhibitors (Moderate); CYP3A4 Inhibitors (Strong); Dasatinib; Fluconazole; Fusidic Acid (Systemic); Ivabradine; Luliconazole; Mifepristone; P-glycoprotein/ABCB1 Inhibitors; QTc-Prolonging Agents (Indeterminate Risk and Risk Modifying); Stiripentol; Telaprevir

Decreased Effect

Erythromycin (Systemic) may decrease the levels/effects of: BCG; Clindamycin (Topical); Clopidogrel; Ifosfamide; Sodium Picosulfate; Typhoid Vaccine; Zafirlukast

The levels/effects of Erythromycin (Systemic) may be decreased by: Bosentan; CYP3A4 Inducers (Strong); Dabrafenib; Deferasirox; Etravirine; Lincosamide Antibiotics; Mitotane; P-glycoprotein/ABCB1 Inducers; Siltuximab; St Johns Wort; Tocilizumab

Food Interactions

Ethanol: Ethanol may decrease absorption of erythromycin or enhance effects of ethanol. Management: Avoid ethanol.

Food: Erythromycin serum levels may be altered if taken with food (formulation-dependent). GI upset, including diarrhea, is common. Management: May be taken with food to decrease GI upset, otherwise take around-the-clock with a full glass of water. Do not give with milk or acidic beverages (eg, soda, juice).

Stability

Injection: Store vial at 20°C to 25°C (68°F to 77°F); after reconstitution with SWI, solution is stable for 2 weeks under refrigeration or 24 hours at room temperature. Stability of lactobionate is pH-dependent; stable at pH 6-8; longest stability in NS. Stability of parenteral admixture at room temperature and at refrigeration temperature is 24 hours.

Tablets, capsules, powder for reconstitution, or granules for suspension: Store at <30°C (<86°F); after mixing the powder for suspension, store at ≤25°C (77°F) and use within 35 days; after mixing the granules for suspension, refrigerate and use within 10 days.

Mechanism of Action Inhibits RNA-dependent protein synthesis at the chain elongation step; binds to the 50S ribosomal subunit resulting in blockage of transpeptidation

Pharmacokinetics (Adult data unless noted)

Absorption: Variable, but better with salt forms than with base; 18% to 45% absorbed orally; ethylsuccinate may be better absorbed with food

Distribution: Poor penetration into the CSF
V_d: 0.64 L/kg

Protein binding: 73% to 81%

Metabolism: In the liver by demethylation via CYP3A4

Half-life:
Neonates (≤15 days of age): 2.1 hours
Adults: 1.5-2 hours
ESRD: 5-6 hours

Time to peak serum concentration: Oral:
Base: 4 hours
Stearate: 3 hours
Ethylsuccinate: 0.5-2.5 hours

Elimination: 2% to 5% unchanged drug excreted in urine, major excretion in feces (via bile)

Dialysis: Not removed by peritoneal dialysis or hemodialysis

Dosing: Neonatal

General dosing: Oral (ethylsuccinate); I.V. (lactobionate): (*Red Book*, 2012):
Body weight <1 kg:
PNA ≤14 days: 10 mg/kg/dose every 12 hours
PNA 15-28 days: 10 mg/kg/dose every 8 hours
Body weight 1-2 kg:
PNA ≤7 days: 10 mg/kg/dose every 12 hours
PNA 8-28 days: 10 mg/kg/dose every 8 hours
Bodyweight >2 kg:
PNA ≤7 days: 10 mg/kg/dose every 12 hours
PNA 8-28 days: 10 mg/kg/dose every 8 hours

Chlamydial conjunctivitis or chlamydial pneumonia: Oral: Ethylsuccinate or base: Full-term neonates: 50 mg/kg/**day** divided every 6 hours for 14 days; a repeat course may be necessary (*Red Book*, 2012)

Pertussis; treatment or postexposure prophylaxis: Oral: Ethylsuccinate: 10 mg/kg/dose 4 times daily for 14 days; **Note:** Due to association of erythromycin and infantile hypertrophic pyloric stenosis in neonates, azithromycin is considered first-line agent in infants <1 month of age (*Red Book*, 2012)

Prokinetic (GI motility) agent: Limited data available; efficacy results variable; optimal dose not established; further studies are needed: PNA ≥14 days:
Low-dose regimen: Oral: 1.5-2.5 mg/kg/dose every 6 hours; therapy started after initiation of enteral feeds; has been studied in GA <32 weeks (Chicella, 2005; Oei, 2001)
Intermediate-dose regimen: Oral: 5 mg/kg/dose every 6 hours; therapy started after initiation of enteral feeds;

dosing based on a randomized, controlled trial of 45 VLBW neonates (n=19 treatment group; mean GA: 28.4 weeks); treatment was initiated at a mean PNA: 21.9 + 7.7 days and continued for 14 days (Ng, 2012)
High-dose regimens (antimicrobial doses): Oral: 10-12.5 mg/kg/dose every 6-8 hours orally have been used after initiation of enteral feeds; efficacy has not been demonstrated in the majority of trials. Exposure to these doses in neonates with PNA ≤14 days has been associated with a 10-fold increase in the risk of hypertrophic pyloric stenosis (Chicella, 2005)

Dosing: Usual

Infants, Children, and Adolescents:
General dosing, susceptible infection:
Manufacturer's labeling:
Oral: Base, ethylsuccinate, stearate: 30-50 mg/kg/**day** divided every 6-8 hours usually; for severe infection may double dose; maximum daily dose: Mild to moderate infection: 2000 mg/**day**; severe infection: 4000 mg/**day**
I.V.: Lactobionate: 15-20 mg/kg/**day** divided every 6 hours; maximum daily dose: 4000 mg/**day**
Alternate dosing (*Red Book*, 2012):
Mild to moderate infection: Oral: 50 mg/kg/**day** divided every 6-8 hours; maximum daily dose: 2000 mg/**day**
Severe infection: I.V.: Lactobionate: 5 mg/kg/dose every 6 hours, maximum daily dose: 4000 mg/**day**

Acne, moderate to severe; treatment: Children and Adolescents: Oral: 250-500 mg 1-2 times daily in conjunction with topical therapy (eg, benzoyl peroxide); maximum daily dose: 50 mg/kg/**day**; duration of 4-8 weeks of therapy usually necessary to evaluate initial clinical response with a longer duration for a maximum effect (3-6 months); resistance problematic with therapy, use typically reserved for patients <8 years who cannot receive tetracycline derivatives (Eichenfield, 2013)

Anthrax, cutaneous, community-acquired (Stevens, 2005): Oral: 10 mg/kg/dose every 6 hours; treatment duration of 5-9 days usually adequate in most cases
I.V.: 20-40 mg/kg/**day** divided every 6 hours; maximum daily dose: 4000 mg; treatment duration of 5-9 days usually adequate in most cases

Bartonella sp infections [bacillary angiomatosis (BA), peliosis hepatis (PH)]:
Non-HIV-exposed/-positive; treatment: Oral: Ethylsuccinate: 10 mg/kg/ dose 4 times daily; maximum daily dose: 2000 mg/day; treatment duration: BA: 3 months; PH: 4 months (Rolain, 2004)
HIV-exposed/-positive:
Prophylaxis: Infants and Children (CDC, 2009): Oral: 30-50 mg/kg/day divided into 2-4 doses daily; maximum daily dose: 2000 mg/**day**
Treatment: Duration of therapy: ≥3 months (of sufficient duration to prevent relapse)
Infants and Children (CDC, 2009):
Oral: 30-50 mg/kg/day divided into 2-4 doses daily; maximum daily dose: 2000 mg/**day**
I.V.: 15-50 mg/kg/day divided into 4 doses daily; maximum daily dose: 2000 mg/**day**
Adolescents: I.V., Oral: 500 mg every 6 hours with or without rifampin (DHHS [adult], 2013)

Chlamydia trachomatis infection (CDC, 2010; *Red Book*, 2012):
Conjunctivitis or pneumonia: Oral (base or ethylsuccinate): 50 mg/kg/**day** divided every 6 hours for 14 days; maximum daily dose: 2000 mg/**day**; a repeat course may be necessary; for severe trachoma, longer durations may be necessary (40 days)
Anogenital tract infection:
Children and Adolescents <45 kg: Oral (base or ethylsuccinate): 50 mg/kg/**day** divided every 6 hours for 14 days; maximum daily dose: 2000 mg/**day**

Adolescents ≥45 kg: Oral:
Base: 500 mg 4 times daily for 7 days
Ethylsuccinate: 800 mg 4 times daily for 7 days
Lymphogranuloma venereum (LGV): Adolescents ≥45 kg: Oral (base): 500 mg 4 times daily for 21 days
Impetigo: Oral: 10 mg/kg/dose 4 times daily (Stevens, 2005)
Lyme Disease: Oral: 50 mg/kg/day divided every 6 hours for 14-21 days; maximum dose: 500 mg (Wormser, 2006)
Peritonitis, exit-site and tunnel infection: Oral (base): 30-50 mg/kg/day divided 3-4 times daily; maximum single dose: 500 mg (Warady, 2012)
Pertussis (CDC, 2005; *Red Book*, 2012):
Infants 1-5 months: Oral: 10 mg/kg/dose 4 times daily for 14 days
Infants ≥6 months and Children: Oral: 10 mg/kg/dose 4 times daily for 7-14 days; maximum daily dose: 2000 mg/**day**
Adolescents: Oral: 500 mg 4 times daily for 7-14 days
Pneumonia, community-acquired (CAP) (Bradley, 2011): Infants >3 months, Children, and Adolescents:
Note: A beta-lactam antibiotic should be added if typical bacterial pneumonia cannot be ruled out.
Presumed atypical (*M. pneumoniae, C. pneumoniae, C. trachomatis*); mild infection or step-down therapy: Oral: 10 mg/kg/dose every 6 hours; maximum daily dose: 2000 mg/**day**
Moderate to severe atypical infection: I.V.: Lactobionate: 5 mg/kg/dose every 6 hours; maximum daily dose: 4000 mg/**day**
Preoperative bowel preparation: Children and Adolescents: Oral: Base: 20 mg/kg; maximum dose: 1000 mg administered at 1, 2, and 11 PM on the day before surgery combined with mechanical cleansing of the large intestine and oral neomycin (Bratzler, 2013)
Prokinetic (GI motility) agent: Limited data available:
Diagnosis; gastric emptying study (provocative testing): I.V.: 2.8 mg/kg infused over 20 minutes was reported from one center's experience; maximum dose: 250 mg (Waseem, 2012)
Treatment: Oral: 3 mg/kg/dose 4 times daily; may increase as needed to effect; maximum dose: 10 mg/kg or 250 mg (Rodriguez, 2012)
Pneumococcal, prophylaxis in penicillin-allergic patients with sickle cell disease (SCD) and functional or anatomic asplenia (Knight-Madden, 2001): Oral:
Infants and Children: 4 months to <3 years: 125 mg twice daily; salt not specified
Children 3-4 years: 250 mg twice daily; salt not specified
Adults:
General dosing: Note: Due to differences in absorption, 400 mg erythromycin ethylsuccinate produces the same serum levels as 250 mg erythromycin base or stearate.
I.V.: Lactobionate: 15-20 mg/kg/day divided every 6 hours or given as a continuous infusion over 24 hours, not to exceed 4 g/day
Oral:
Base, delayed release: 333 mg every 8 hours
Stearate or base: 250-500 mg every 6-12 hours
Ethylsuccinate: 400-800 mg every 6-12 hours
Chancroid: Oral: Base: 500 mg 3 times/day for 7 days
Chlamydia trachomatis: Oral:
Base: 500 mg 4 times/day for 7 days **or**
Ethylsuccinate: 800 mg 4 times/day for 7 days
Pertussis: Oral: 500 mg every 6 hours for 14 days
Preoperative bowel preparation: Oral: 1 g erythromycin base at 1, 2, and 11 PM on the day before surgery combined with mechanical cleansing of the large intestine and oral neomycin

Dosing adjustment in renal impairment: Infants, Children, and Adolescents: The following adjustments have been recommended (Aronoff, 2007). **Note:** Renally adjusted dose recommendations are based on oral doses of 30-50 mg/kg/**day** divided every 6-8 hours.
GFR ≥10 mL/minute/1.73 m^2: No adjustment required
GFR <10 mL/minute/1.73 m^2: Intermittent hemodialysis, peritoneal dialysis: Not removed by peritoneal dialysis or hemodialysis: 10-17 mg/kg/dose every 8 hours
Dosing adjustment in hepatic impairment: There are no dosage adjustments provided in the manufacturer's labeling.

Administration

Oral: Avoid milk and acidic beverages 1 hour before or after a dose; administer after food to decrease GI discomfort; ethylsuccinate chewable tablets should not be swallowed whole; do not chew or break delayed release capsule or enteric coated tablets, swallow whole
Parenteral: Administer by I.V. intermittent or continuous infusion diluted in either dextrose or saline solutions to a concentration of 1-2.5 mg/mL; maximum concentration: 5 mg/mL; I.V. intermittent infusions may be administered over 20-60 minutes; to decrease vein irritation, administer as a continuous infusion at a concentration ≤1 mg/mL; prolonging the infusion duration over 60 minutes or longer has been recommended to decrease the cardiotoxic effects of erythromycin; pH (lactobionate): 6.5-7.5 (reconstituted with SW or D$_5$W to a 50 mg/mL concentration)

Monitoring Parameters Assess results of culture and sensitivity tests and patient's previous allergy history prior to therapy; liver function tests, observe for changes in bowel frequency; with I.V. use: Blood pressure, heart rate

Test Interactions False-positive urinary catecholamines, 17-hydroxycorticosteroids and 17-ketosteroids

Additional Information Treatment of erythromycin-associated cardiac toxicity with prolongation of the QT interval and ventricular tachydysrhythmias includes discontinuing erythromycin and administering magnesium.

Dosage Forms Excipient information presented when available (limited, particularly for generics); consult specific product labeling.
Capsule Delayed Release Particles, Oral, as base:
Generic: 250 mg
Solution Reconstituted, Intravenous, as lactobionate:
Erythrocin Lactobionate: 500 mg (1 ea); 1000 mg (1 ea)
Suspension Reconstituted, Oral, as ethylsuccinate:
E.E.S. Granules: 200 mg/5 mL (100 mL, 200 mL) [cherry flavor]
EryPed 200: 200 mg/5 mL (100 mL) [fruit flavor]
EryPed 400: 400 mg/5 mL (100 mL) [banana flavor]
Tablet, Oral, as base:
Generic: 250 mg, 500 mg
Tablet, Oral, as ethylsuccinate:
E.E.S. 400: 400 mg [contains fd&c red #40, fd&c yellow #10 (quinoline yellow)]
Generic: 400 mg
Tablet, Oral, as stearate:
Erythrocin Stearate: 250 mg
Tablet Delayed Release, Oral, as base:
Ery-Tab: 250 mg, 333 mg, 500 mg
PCE: 333 mg
PCE: 500 mg [dye free, no artificial color(s)]

References

American Academy of Pediatrics (AAP). In: Pickering LK, Baker CJ, Kimberlin DW, Long SS, eds. *Red Book: 2012 Report of the Committee on Infectious Diseases*. 29th ed. Elk Grove Village, IL: American Academy of Pediatrics; 2012.
American College of Obstetricians and Gynecologists (ACOG). Practice bulletin no. 139: premature rupture of membranes. *Obstet Gynecol*. 2013;122(4):918-930.
Bradley JS, Byington CL, Shah SS, et al, "The Management of Community-Acquired Pneumonia in Infants and Children Older Than 3 Months of Age: Clinical Practice Guidelines by the Pediatric

Infectious Diseases Society and the Infectious Diseases Society of America", *Clin Infect Dis*, 2011, 53(7):e25-76.

Bratzler DW, Dellinger EP, Olsen KM, et al, "Clinical Practice Guidelines For Antimicrobial Prophylaxis in Surgery," *Am J Health Syst Pharm*, 2013, 70(3):195-283.

Camilleri M, Parkman HP, Shafi MA, et al, "Clinical Guideline: Management of Gastroparesis," *Am J Gastroenterol*, 2013, 108(1):18-37.

Centers for Disease Control and Prevention (CDC). Guidelines for the prevention and treatment of opportunistic infections among HIV-exposed and HIV-infected children. *MMWR Recomm Rep*. 2009;58 (RR-11):1-166. Available at http://aidsinfo.nih.gov/contentfiles/Pediatric_OI.pdf

Centers for Disease Control and Prevention (CDC), "Sexually Transmitted Diseases Treatment Guidelines, 2010," *MMWR Recomm Rep*, 2010, 59(RR-12):1-110.

Chicella MF, Batres LA, Heesters MS, et al, "Prokinetic Drug Therapy in Children: A Review of Current Options," *Ann Pharmacother*, 2005, 39 (4):706-11.

Costalos C, Gounaris A, Varhalama E, et al, "Erythromycin as a Prokinetic Agent in Preterm Infants," *J Pediatr Gastroenterol Nutr*, 2002, 34(1):23-5.

Curry JI, Lander TD, and Stringer MD, "Review Article: Erythromycin as a Prokinetic Agent in Infants and Children," *Aliment Pharmacol Ther*, 2001, 15(5):595-603.

DHHS Panel on Opportunistic Infections (OI) in HIV-Infected Adults and Adolescents. Guidelines for prevention and treatment of opportunistic infections in HIV-infected adults and adolescents: recommendations from the Centers for Disease Control and Prevention (CDC), the National Institutes of Health (NIH), and the HIV Medicine Association (HIVMA) of the Infectious Diseases Society of America (IDSA). May 7, 2013. Available at http://aidsinfo.nih.gov/contentfiles/lvguidelines/adult_oi.pdf

Di Lorenzo C, Lachman R, and Hyman PE, "Intravenous Erythromycin for Postpyloric Intubation," *J Pediatr Gastroenterol Nutr*, 1990, 11 (1):45-7.

Eichenfield LF, Krakowski AC, Piggott C, et al, "Evidence-Based Recommendations For the Diagnosis and Treatment of Pediatric Acne," *Pediatrics*, 2013, 131 Suppl 3:S163-86.

Goldstein LH, Berlin M, Tsur L, et al, "The Safety of Macrolides During Lactation," *Breastfeed Med*, 2009, 4(4):197-200.

Jadcherla SR and Berseth CL, "Effect of Erythromycin on Gastroduodenal Contractile Activity in Developing Neonates," *J Pediatr Gastroenterol Nutr*, 2002, 34(1):16-22.

Kiefer L, Rubin A, McCoy JB, et al, "The Placental Transfer of Erythromycin," *Am J Obstet Gynecol*, 1955, 69(1):174-7.

Knight-Madden J and Serjeant GR, "Invasive Pneumococcal Disease in Homozygous Sickle Cell Disease: Jamaican Experience 1973-1997," *J Pediatr*, 2001, 138(1):65-70.

Ng YY, Su PH, Chen JY, et al, "Efficacy of Intermediate-Dose Oral Erythromycin on Very Low Birth Weight Infants With Feeding Intolerance," *Pediatr Neonatol*, 2012, 53(1):34-40.

Oei J and Lui K, "A Placebo-Controlled Trial of Low-Dose Erythromycin to Promote Feed Tolerance in Preterm Infants," *Acta Paediatr*, 2001, 90(8):904-8.

Patole S, Rao S, and Doherty D, "Erythromycin as a Prokinetic Agent in Preterm Neonates: A Systematic Review," *Arch Dis Child Fetal Neonatal Ed*, 2005, 90(4):F301-6.

Philipson A, Sabath LD, and Charles D, "Erythromycin and Clindamycin Absorption and Elimination in Pregnant Women," *Clin Pharmacol Ther*, 1976, 19(1):68-77.

Ray WA, Murray KT, Meredith S, et al, "Oral Erythromycin and the Risk of Sudden Death From Cardiac Causes," *N Engl J Med*, 2004, 351 (11):1089-96.

Red Book: 2009 Report of the Committee on Infectious Diseases, 28th ed, Pickering LK, ed, Elk Grove Village, IL: American Academy of Pediatrics, 2009.

Reid D, DiLorenzo C, Travis L, et al, "Diabetic Gastroparesis Due to Postprandial Antral Hypomotility in Childhood," *Pediatrics*, 1992, 90(1 Pt 1):43-6.

Rodriguez L, Irani K, Jiang H, et al, "Clinical presentation, Response to Therapy, and outcome of Gastroparesis in Children," *J Pediatr Gastroenterol Nutr*, 2012, 55(2):185-90.

Rolain JM, Brouqui P, Koehler JE, et al, "Recommendations for Treatment of Human Infections Caused by Bartonella Species," *Antimicrob Agents Chemother*, 2004, 48(6):1921-33.

Sorensen HT, Skriver MV, Pedersen L, et al, "Risk of Infantile Hypertrophic Pyloric Stenosis After Maternal Postnatal Use of Macrolides," *Scand J Infect Dis*, 2003, 35(2):104-6.

Stang H, "Pyloric Stenosis Associated With Erythromycin Ingested Through Breastmilk," *Minn Med*, 1986, 69(11):669-70, 682.

Stevens DL, Bisno AL, Chambers HF, et al, "Practice Guidelines for the Diagnosis and Management of Skin and Soft-Tissue Infections," *Clin Infect Dis*, 2005, 41(10):1373-406.

Tiwari T, Murphy TV, and Moran J, "Recommended Antimicrobial Agents for the Treatment and Postexposure Prophylaxis of Pertussis: 2005 CDC Guidelines," *MMWR*, 2005, 54(RR-14):1-16.

Vanderhoof JA, Young R, Kaufman SS, et al, "Treatment of cyclic vomiting in childhood with erythromycin," *J Pediatr Gastroenterol Nutr*, 1995, 21(Suppl 1):S60-2.

Waites KB, Sims PJ, Crouse DT, et al, "Serum Concentrations of Erythromycin After Intravenous Infusion in Preterm Neonates Treated for *Ureaplasma urealyticum* Infection," *Pediatr Infect Dis J*, 1994, 13 (4):287-93.

Warady BA, Bakkaloglu S, Newland J, et al, "Consensus Guidelines for the Prevention and Treatment of Catheter-Related Infections and Peritonitis in Pediatric Patients Receiving Peritoneal Dialysis: 2012 Update," *Perit Dial Int*, 2012, 32(Suppl 2):S32-86.

Waseem S, Islam S, Kahn G, et al, "Spectrum of Gastroparesis in Children," *J Pediatr Gastroenterol Nutr*, 2012, 55(2):166-72.

Wormser GP, Dattwyler RJ, Shapiro ED, et al, "The Clinical Assessment, Treatment, and Prevention of Lyme Disease, Human Granulocytic Anaplasmosis, and Babesiosis: Clinical Practice Guidelines by the Infectious Diseases Society of America," *Clin Infect Dis*, 2006, 43 (9):1089-134.

Erythromycin (Ophthalmic) (er ith roe MYE sin)

Medication Safety Issues
Sound-alike/look-alike issues:
Erythromycin may be confused with azithromycin

Brand Names: U.S. Ilotycin; Romycin

Brand Names: Canada Diomycin®; PMS-Erythromycin

Therapeutic Category Antibiotic, Macrolide; Antibiotic, Ophthalmic

Generic Availability (U.S.) Yes

Use Treatment of superficial eye infections involving the conjunctiva or cornea; prevention of ophthalmia neonatorum due to *Neisseria gonorrhoeae* or *Chlamydia trachomatis* [FDA approved in pediatric patients (all ages) and adults]; has also been used for the treatment of chlamydial ophthalmic infections

Pregnancy Risk Factor B

Pregnancy Considerations Adverse events were not observed in animal reproduction studies. Erythromycin has been shown to cross the placenta following oral dosing. Refer to the Erythromycin (Systemic) monograph for details. The amount of erythromycin available systemically following ophthalmic application is not known. Systemic absorption would be required in order for erythromycin to cross the placenta and reach the fetus.

Breast-Feeding Considerations It is not known of erythromycin is excreted into breast milk following ophthalmic application. The manufacturer recommends that caution be exercised when administering erythromycin ophthalmic ointment to nursing women. Erythromycin has been shown to enter breast milk following oral dosing. Refer to the Erythromycin (Systemic) monograph for details. Systemic absorption would be required in order for erythromycin to enter breast milk and reach the nursing infant.

Contraindications Hypersensitivity to erythromycin or any component

Adverse Reactions Ocular: Hypersensitivity, minor ocular irritation, redness

Drug Interactions
Metabolism/Transport Effects None known.
Avoid Concomitant Use There are no known interactions where it is recommended to avoid concomitant use.
Increased Effect/Toxicity
Erythromycin (Ophthalmic) may increase the levels/effects of: Vitamin K Antagonists
Decreased Effect There are no known significant interactions involving a decrease in effect.

Stability Store at 20°C to 25°C (68°F to 77°F); protect from freezing and excessive heat.

Mechanism of Action Inhibits RNA-dependent protein synthesis at the chain elongation step; binds to the 50S ribosomal subunit resulting in blockage of transpeptidation

Dosing: Neonatal Ophthalmic: Prophylaxis of neonatal gonococcal or chlamydial ophthalmia: Ointment: Instill 1 cm ribbon into each conjunctival sac once

Dosing: Usual Ophthalmic: Conjunctivitis: Infants, Children, and Adults: Ointment: Instill 1 cm ribbon one or more times daily up to 6 times daily depending on the severity of the infection

Administration Ophthalmic ointment for prevention of neonatal ophthalmia: Wipe each eyelid gently with sterile cotton; instill 1 cm ribbon of ointment in each lower conjunctival sac; massage eyelids gently to spread the ointment; after 1 minute, excess ointment can be wiped away with sterile cotton. Avoid contact of applicator tip with skin or eye.

Dosage Forms Excipient information presented when available (limited, particularly for generics); consult specific product labeling.

Ointment, Ophthalmic:

Ilotycin: 5 mg/g (1 g)

Romycin: 5 mg/g (3.5 g)

Generic: 5 mg/g (1 g, 3.5 g)

Erythromycin (Topical) (er ith roe MYE sin)

Medication Safety Issues

Sound-alike/look-alike issues:

Erythromycin may be confused with azithromycin, clarithromycin

Brand Names: U.S. Akne-Mycin; Ery; Erygel

Brand Names: Canada Erysol

Therapeutic Category Antibiotic, Macrolide; Antibiotic, Topical

Generic Availability (U.S.) May be product dependent

Use Treatment of acne vulgaris

Pregnancy Risk Factor B

Pregnancy Considerations Adverse events were not observed in animal reproduction studies. Erythromycin has been shown to cross the placenta following oral dosing. Refer to the Erythromycin (Systemic) monograph for details. The amount of erythromycin available systemically following topical application is considered to be very low (Akhavan, 2003). Systemic absorption would be required in order for erythromycin to cross the placenta and reach the fetus. Topical erythromycin may be used for the treatment of acne in pregnancy (Dréno, 2013; Eichenfield, 2013; Gollnick, 2003).

Breast-Feeding Considerations It is not known if erythromycin is excreted into breast milk following topical application. The manufacturer recommends that caution be exercised when administering to nursing women. Erythromycin has been shown to enter breast milk following oral dosing. Refer to the Erythromycin (Systemic) monograph for details. The amount of erythromycin available systemically following topical application is considered to be very low (Akhavan, 2003). Systemic absorption would be required in order for erythromycin to enter breast milk and reach the nursing infant.

Contraindications Hypersensitivity to erythromycin or any component

Adverse Reactions

Dermatologic: Erythema, dryness, oiliness, peeling, pruritus, tenderness, urticaria

Ocular: Eye irritation

As reported with Erysol [Canadian product]:

Dermatologic: Coriaceousness, desquamation, fissure (around mouth), oiliness, scaling

Local: Application site: Irritation (burning, dryness, erythema, stinging, tenderness)

Rare but important or life-threatening: Abdominal discomfort/pain, allergic reaction, diarrhea, facial edema, pruritus, rash, skin exfoliation, urticaria

Drug Interactions

Metabolism/Transport Effects None known.

Avoid Concomitant Use

Avoid concomitant use of Erythromycin (Topical) with any of the following: BCG; Clindamycin (Topical)

Increased Effect/Toxicity There are no known significant interactions involving an increase in effect.

Decreased Effect

Erythromycin (Topical) may decrease the levels/effects of: BCG; Clindamycin (Topical); Sodium Picosulfate

Mechanism of Action Antibacterial activity is due to inhibition of RNA-dependent protein synthesis at the chain elongation step; binds to the 50S ribosomal subunit resulting in blockage of transpeptidation. Alcohol component induces skin drying and peeling.

Dosing: Usual Children and Adults: Apply 2% solution over the affected area twice daily after the skin has been thoroughly washed and patted dry

Administration Apply thin film to the cleansed, affected area.

Dosage Forms Excipient information presented when available (limited, particularly for generics); consult specific product labeling.

Gel, External:

Erygel: 2% (30 g, 60 g)

Generic: 2% (30 g, 60 g)

Ointment, External:

Akne-Mycin: 2% (25 g) [contains cetostearyl alcohol]

Pad, External:

Ery: 2% (60 ea) [contains propylene glycol]

Generic: 2% (60 ea)

Solution, External:

Generic: 2% (60 mL)

References

Akhavan A and Bershad S, "Topical Acne Drugs: Review of Clinical Properties, Systemic Exposure, and Safety," *Am J Clin Dermatol*, 2003, 4(7):473-92.

Dréno B, Layton A, Zouboulis CC, et al. Adult female acne: a new paradigm. *J Eur Acad Dermatol Venereol*. 2013;27(9):1063-1070.

Eichenfield LF, Krakowski AC, Piggott C, et al. Evidence-based recommendations for the diagnosis and treatment of pediatric acne. *Pediatrics*. 2013;131 (Suppl 3):S163-186.

Gollnick H, Cunliffe W, Berson D, et al, "Management of Acne: A Report From a Global Alliance to Improve Outcomes in Acne," *J Am Acad Dermatol*, 2003, 49(1 Suppl):S1-37.

Erythromycin and Sulfisoxazole

(er ith roe MYE sin & sul fi SOKS a zole)

Medication Safety Issues

Sound-alike/look-alike issues:

Pediazole® may be confused with Pediapred®

Brand Names: U.S. E.S.P.®

Brand Names: Canada Pediazole®

Therapeutic Category Antibiotic, Macrolide; Antibiotic, Sulfonamide Derivative

Generic Availability (U.S.) Yes

Use Treatment of otitis media caused by susceptible strains of *Haemophilus influenzae* (FDA approved in ages 2 months to 12 years)

Pregnancy Risk Factor C

Pregnancy Considerations Animal reproduction studies have not been conducted with this combination. Erythromycin and sulfisoxazole cross the placenta. Most reports do not identify an increase in risk for congenital abnormalities due to prenatal exposure to erythromycin. Cardiovascular anomalies following exposure in early pregnancy have been reported in some observational studies; see Erythromycin (Systemic) monograph for additional information. Based on available information, an increased risk for congenital malformations has not been observed after use of sulfisoxazole during pregnancy (Aselton, 1985; Heinonen, 1977; Hibbard, 1967; Jick 1981); however, studies with sulfonamides as a class have shown mixed results (ACOG No. 494, 2011).

Individually, erythromycin and sulfonamides may be used to treat infections in pregnant women when clinically appropriate for confirmed infections caused by susceptible organisms. Use of sulfonamides during the first trimester should be limited to situations where no alternative therapies are available (ACOG No. 120, 2011; ACOG No. 494, 2011). Erythromycin/sulfisoxazole is contraindicated in late pregnancy because sulfonamides may cause kernicterus in the newborn. Neonatal healthcare providers should be informed if maternal sulfonamide therapy is used near the time of delivery (DHHS, 2013).

Breast-Feeding Considerations Erythromycin and sulfisoxazole are both excreted into breast milk. Per the manufacturer, this combination is contraindicated in mothers nursing infants <2 months of age because sulfonamides distribute into breast milk and may cause kernicterus in the newborn. Sulfonamides should not be used while nursing an infant with G6PD deficiency or hyperbilirubinemia (Della-Giustina, 2003). See Erythromycin (Systemic) monograph for information specific to the use of erythromycin in nursing women. Nondose-related effects could include modification of bowel flora.

Contraindications Hypersensitivity to erythromycin, any component, or sulfonamides; hepatic dysfunction; infants <2 months of age and mothers nursing infants who are <2 months of age (sulfas compete with bilirubin for binding sites which may result in kernicterus in newborns); pregnant women at term

Additional contraindications of erythromycin (systemic): Concomitant use with pimozide, cisapride, ergotamine or dihydroergotamine, terfenadine, astemizole, lovastatin, or simvastatin

Warnings Macrolides have been associated with rare QT_c prolongation and ventricular arrhythmias, including torsade de pointes; use with caution in patients at risk of prolonged cardiac repolarization. Rhabdomyolysis has been reported in seriously ill patients receiving erythromycin and lovastatin or simvastatin concomitantly; concurrent use is contraindicated (per manufacturer labeling of lovastatin and simvastatin).

Fatalities associated with hepatic necrosis have occurred with sulfonamides; discontinue use at first sign of rash or signs of serious adverse reactions. Use with caution in patients with preexisting liver disease; hepatic impairment, including hepatocellular and/or cholestatic hepatitis, with or without jaundice, has been observed with erythromycin. Discontinue if symptoms of malaise, nausea, vomiting, abdominal colic, and fever. Fatalities associated with severe reactions including agranulocytosis, aplastic anemia, and other blood dyscrasias have occurred with sulfonamides; discontinue use at first sign of rash or signs of serious adverse reactions. Fatalities associated with severe reactions including Stevens-Johnson syndrome and toxic epidermal necrolysis have occurred with sulfonamides; discontinue use at first sign of rash. Chemical similarities are present among sulfonamides, sulfonylureas, carbonic anhydrase inhibitors, thiazides, and loop diuretics (except ethacrynic acid); potential for cross-reaction exists in patients with allergy to any of these compounds; avoid use when previous reaction has been severe. In an established infection, sulfonamides do not eradicate streptococcus nor prevent sequelae, such as rheumatic fever, and should not be used for the treatment of group A beta-hemolytic streptococcal infection.

Prolonged use may result in fungal or bacterial superinfection, including *C. difficile*-associated diarrhea (CDAD) and pseudomembranous colitis; CDAD has been observed >2 months postantibiotic treatment.

Contains polysorbate 80 (Tween 80®) which may cause allergic reaction in susceptible individuals.

Precautions Use with caution in patients with renal impairment; clearance of sulfisoxazole may be prolonged. Use with caution in patients with G6PD deficiency; hemolysis may occur. Use with caution in myasthenia gravis; erythromycin has been associated with aggravation of weakness associated with myasthenia gravis. Use with caution in patients with allergies or asthma.

Adverse Reactions Adverse events specific to this combination have not been identified.

Cardiovascular: Allergic myocarditis, arteritis, cyanosis, edema (including periorbital), flushing, intracranial hypertension, palpitations, periarteritis nodosa, syncope, tachycardia, torsade de pointes, vasculitis, ventricular arrhythmia

Central nervous system: Anxiety, ataxia, depression, disorientation, dizziness, drowsiness, fatigue, fever, hallucinations, headache, insomnia, psychosis, seizure, vertigo

Dermatologic: Angioedema, erythema multiforme, exfoliative dermatitis, photosensitivity, pruritus, purpura, rash, Stevens-Johnson syndrome, toxic epidermal necrolysis, urticaria

Endocrine & metabolic: Goiter (rare), hypoglycemia (rare)

Gastrointestinal: Abdominal pain, anorexia, diarrhea, flatulence, gastrointestinal hemorrhage, glossitis, hypertrophic pyloric stenosis, melena, nausea, oral candidiasis, pancreatitis, pseudomembranous colitis, salivary gland swelling, stomatitis, vomiting

Genitourinary: Urinary retention

Hematologic: Agranulocytosis, anemia, aplastic anemia, clotting disorders (including hypoprothrombinemia, hypofibrinogenemia, sulfhemoglobinemia, methemoglobinemia), eosinophilia, hemolytic anemia, leukopenia, thrombocytopenia

Hepatic: Hepatotoxicity (including hepatitis, hepatic necrosis, and cholestatic jaundice), liver enzymes increased

Neuromuscular & skeletal: Paresthesia, peripheral neuritis, rigors, weakness

Otic: Hearing loss (reversible), tinnitus

Renal: Acute renal failure, blood urea nitrogen increased, crystalluria, diuresis (rare), hematuria, nephritis, serum creatinine increased, toxic nephrosis (with oliguria and anuria)

Respiratory: Cough, dyspnea, pneumonitis, pulmonary infiltrates

Miscellaneous: Anaphylaxis, hypersensitivity reactions, serum sickness, systemic lupus erythematosus (SLE)

Drug Interactions

Metabolism/Transport Effects Refer to individual components.

Avoid Concomitant Use

Avoid concomitant use of Erythromycin and Sulfisoxazole with any of the following: BCG; Bosutinib; Cisapride; Clindamycin (Topical); Conivaptan; Disopyramide; Fluconazole; Fusidic Acid (Systemic); Highest Risk QTc-Prolonging Agents; Ibrutinib; Ivabradine; Lincosamide Antibiotics; Lomitapide; Lovastatin; Methenamine; Mifepristone; PAZOPanib; Pimozide; Potassium P-Aminobenzoate; Procaine; QuiNIDine; QuiNINE; Silodosin; Simeprevir; Simvastatin; Terfenadine; Tolvaptan; Topotecan; Ulipristal; VinCRIStine (Liposomal)

Increased Effect/Toxicity

Erythromycin and Sulfisoxazole may increase the levels/effects of: Afatinib; Alfentanil; ALPRAZolam; Antifungal Agents (Azole Derivatives, Systemic); Antineoplastic Agents (Vinca Alkaloids); ARIPiprazole; AtorvaSTATin; Avanafil; Bosentan; Bosutinib; Brentuximab Vedotin; Budesonide (Systemic, Oral Inhalation); BusPIRone; Calcium Channel Blockers; Cannabis; CarBAMazepine; Cardiac Glycosides; Carvedilol; Cilostazol; Cisapride; CloZAPine; Colchicine; Corticosteroids (Systemic); CycloSPORINE (Systemic); CYP2C9 Substrates; CYP3A4 Substrates; Dabigatran Etexilate; Diclofenac

(Systemic); Disopyramide; DOXOrubicin (Conventional); Dronabinol; Eletriptan; Eplerenone; Ergot Derivatives; Estazolam; Everolimus; FentaNYL; Fexofenadine; Highest Risk QTc-Prolonging Agents; Ibrutinib; Imatinib; Ivabradine; Ivacaftor; Lacosamide; Lomitapide; Lovastatin; Lurasidone; Methotrexate; Midazolam; Moderate Risk QTc-Prolonging Agents; Ospemifene; OxyCODONE; PAZOPanib; P-glycoprotein/ABCB1 Substrates; Pimecrolimus; Pimozide; Pitavastatin; Porfimer; Pravastatin; QuiNIDine; QuiNINE; Ranolazine; Repaglinide; Rifamycin Derivatives; Rifaximin; Rilpivirine; Rivaroxaban; Salmeterol; Saxagliptin; Selective Serotonin Reuptake Inhibitors; Sildenafil; Silodosin; Simeprevir; Simvastatin; Sirolimus; Sulfonylureas; Tacrolimus (Systemic); Tacrolimus (Topical); Telaprevir; Temsirolimus; Terfenadine; Tetrahydrocannabinol; Theophylline Derivatives; Thiopental; Tolvaptan; Topotecan; Triazolam; Ulipristal; Vardenafil; Vilazodone; VinCRIStine (Liposomal); Vitamin K Antagonists; Zopiclone

The levels/effects of Erythromycin and Sulfisoxazole may be increased by: Antifungal Agents (Azole Derivatives, Systemic); Cannabis; Conivaptan; CYP2C9 Inhibitors (Moderate); CYP2C9 Inhibitors (Strong); CYP3A4 Inhibitors (Moderate); CYP3A4 Inhibitors (Strong); Dasatinib; Fluconazole; Fusidic Acid (Systemic); Ivabradine; Luliconazole; Methenamine; Mifepristone; P-glycoprotein/ABCB1 Inhibitors; QTc-Prolonging Agents (Indeterminate Risk and Risk Modifying); Stiripentol; Telaprevir

Decreased Effect

Erythromycin and Sulfisoxazole may decrease the levels/effects of: BCG; Clindamycin (Topical); Clopidogrel; CycloSPORINE (Systemic); Ifosfamide; Sodium Picosulfate; Typhoid Vaccine

The levels/effects of Erythromycin and Sulfisoxazole may be decreased by: Bosentan; CYP2C9 Inducers (Strong); CYP3A4 Inducers (Strong); Dabrafenib; Deferasirox; Etravirine; Lincosamide Antibiotics; Mitotane; Peginterferon Alfa-2b; P-glycoprotein/ABCB1 Inducers; Potassium P-Aminobenzoate; Procaine; Siltuximab; St Johns Wort; Tocilizumab

Stability Prior to reconstitution, store at room temperature; after reconstitution, store in refrigerator for up to 14 days.

Mechanism of Action Erythromycin inhibits bacterial protein synthesis; sulfisoxazole competitively inhibits bacterial synthesis of folic acid from para-aminobenzoic acid

Pharmacokinetics (Adult data unless noted)

Erythromycin ethylsuccinate:
Absorption: Well absorbed from the GI tract; improved in presence of food
Distribution: Widely distributed into most body tissues and fluids; poor penetration into CSF
Protein binding: 75% to 90%
Metabolism: In the liver by demethylation via CYP3A4
Half-life: 1-1.5 hours
Elimination: Unchanged drug is excreted and concentrated in bile; <5% of dose eliminated in urine
Dialysis: Not removed by peritoneal dialysis or hemodialysis

Sulfisoxazole acetyl:
Absorption: Rapid and complete; the small intestine is the major site of absorption
Distribution: Into extracellular space; CSF concentration ranges from 8% to 57% of blood concentration in patients with normal meninges
Protein binding: 85%; primarily to albumin
Metabolism: Undergoes N-acetylation and N-glucuronide conjugation in the liver
Half-life: 4.6-7.8 hours, prolonged in renal impairment
Time to peak serum concentration: 2.5 hours (range: 1-4 hours)
Elimination: Urine (97%; 52% as unchanged drug)
Dialysis: >50% removed by hemodialysis

Dosing: Usual Infants ≥2 months and Children: **Otitis media:** 40-50 mg/kg/day of erythromycin in divided doses every 6-8 hours; maximum daily dose: 2000 mg/**day** of erythromycin; if dosing based on sulfisoxazole component: 150 mg/kg/day of sulfisoxazole in divided doses every 6-8 hours; maximum daily dose: 6 g/**day** sulfisoxazole

Dosing adjustment in renal impairment: There are no dosage adjustments provided in manufacturer's labeling.

Dosing adjustment in hepatic impairment: There are no dosage adjustments provided in manufacturer's labeling; use with caution.

Administration Oral suspension: Administer without regard to food; shake suspension well before use

Monitoring Parameters CBC with differential and platelet count, urinalysis; periodic liver function and renal function tests; urinalysis, observe patient for diarrhea

Test Interactions False-positive urinary protein; false-positive urinary catecholamines, 17-hydroxycorticosteroids and 17-ketosteroids

Dosage Forms Excipient information presented when available (limited, particularly for generics); consult specific product labeling.

Powder for oral suspension: Erythromycin ethylsuccinate 200 mg and sulfisoxazole acetyl 600 mg per 5 mL (100 mL, 150 mL, 200 mL)
E.S.P.®: Erythromycin ethylsuccinate 200 mg and sulfisoxazole acetyl 600 mg per 5 mL (100 mL, 150 mL, 200 mL) [cheri beri flavor]

References

American College of Obstetricians and Gynecologists (ACOG), "ACOG Practice Bulletin No. 120: Use of Prophylactic Antibiotics in Labor and Delivery," *Obstet Gynecol,* 2011, 117(6):1472-83.

American College of Obstetricians and Gynecologists (ACOG) Committee on Obstetric Practice, "ACOG Committee Opinion No. 494: Sulfonamides, Nitrofurantoin, and Risk of Birth Defects," *Obstet Gynecol,* 2011, 117(6):1484-5.

Aselton P, Jick H, Milunsky A, et al, "First-Trimester Drug Use and Congenital Disorders," *Obstet Gynecol,* 1985, 65(4):451-5.

Della-Giustina K and Chow G, "Medications in Pregnancy and Lactation," *Emerg Med Clin North Am,* 2003, 21(3):585-613.

DHHS Panel on Opportunistic Infections (OI) in HIV-Infected Adults and Adolescents, "Guidelines for Prevention and Treatment of Opportunistic Infections in HIV-Infected Adults and Adolescents; Recommendations From the Centers for Disease Control and Prevention (CDC), the National Institutes of Health (NIH) and the HIV Medicine Association (HIVMA) of the Infectious Diseases Society of America (IDSA)," May 7, 2013. Available at http://aidsinfo.nih.gov/contentfiles/lvguidelines/adult_oi.pdf

Heinonen OP, Sloane D, and Shapiro S, *Birth Defects and Drugs in Pregnancy,* Littleton, MA: Publishing Sciences Group, Inc, 1977.

Hibbard L, Thrupp L, Summeril S, et al, "Treatment of Pyelonephritis in Pregnancy," *Am J Obstet Gynecol,* 1967, 98(5):609-15.

Jick H, Holmes LB, Hunter JR, et al, "First-Trimester Drug Use and Congenital Disorders," *JAMA,* 1981, 246(4):343-6.

♦ **Erythromycin Base** *see* Erythromycin (Ophthalmic) *on page 784*

♦ **Erythromycin Base** *see* Erythromycin (Systemic) *on page 780*

♦ **Erythromycin Ethylsuccinate** *see* Erythromycin (Systemic) *on page 780*

♦ **Erythromycin Lactobionate** *see* Erythromycin (Systemic) *on page 780*

♦ **Erythromycin Stearate** *see* Erythromycin (Systemic) *on page 780*

♦ **Erythropoiesis-Stimulating Agent (ESA)** *see* Darbepoetin Alfa *on page 592*

♦ **Erythropoiesis-Stimulating Agent (ESA)** *see* Epoetin Alfa *on page 766*

♦ **Erythropoiesis-Stimulating Protein** *see* Darbepoetin Alfa *on page 592*

♦ **Erythropoietin** *see* Epoetin Alfa *on page 766*

Escitalopram (es sye TAL oh pram)

Medication Safety Issues
Sound-alike/look-alike issues:
Lexapro may be confused with Loxitane
BEERS Criteria medication:
This drug may be potentially inappropriate for use in geriatric patients (Quality of evidence - moderate; Strength of recommendation - strong).
International issues:
Zavesca: Brand name for escitalopram [in multiple international markets; ISMP April 21, 2010], but also brand name for miglustat [Canada, U.S., and multiple international markets]

Related Information
Antidepressant Agents on page 2219

Brand Names: U.S. Lexapro

Brand Names: Canada Cipralex; Cipralex MELTZ

Therapeutic Category Antidepressant, Selective Serotonin Reuptake Inhibitor (SSRI)

Generic Availability (U.S.) Yes

Use Treatment of major depressive disorder (FDA approved in ages 12-17 years and adults); treatment of generalized anxiety disorders (GAD) (FDA approved in adults); has also been studied in children and adolescents with social anxiety disorders and pervasive developmental disorders (PDD) including autism

Medication Guide Available Yes

Pregnancy Risk Factor C

Pregnancy Considerations Adverse events have been observed in animal reproduction studies. Escitalopram crosses the placenta and is distributed into the amniotic fluid. An increased risk of teratogenic effects, including cardiovascular defects, may be associated with maternal use of escitalopram or other SSRIs; however, available information is conflicting. Nonteratogenic effects in the newborn following SSRI/SNRI exposure late in the third trimester include respiratory distress, cyanosis, apnea, seizures, temperature instability, feeding difficulty, vomiting, hypoglycemia, hypo- or hypertonia, hyper-reflexia, jitteriness, irritability, constant crying, and tremor. Symptoms may be due to the toxicity of the SSRIs/SNRIs or a discontinuation syndrome and may be consistent with serotonin syndrome associated with SSRI treatment. Persistent pulmonary hypertension of the newborn (PPHN) has also been reported with SSRI exposure. The long-term effects of in utero SSRI exposure on infant development and behavior are not known. Escitalopram is the S-enantiomer of the racemic derivative citalopram; also refer to the Citalopram monograph.

Due to pregnancy-induced physiologic changes, some pharmacokinetic parameters of escitalopram may be altered. The ACOG recommends that therapy with SSRIs or SNRIs during pregnancy be individualized; treatment of depression during pregnancy should incorporate the clinical expertise of the mental health clinician, obstetrician, primary healthcare provider, and pediatrician. According to the American Psychiatric Association (APA), the risks of medication treatment should be weighed against other treatment options and untreated depression. For women who discontinue antidepressant medications during pregnancy and who may be at high risk for postpartum depression, the medications can be restarted following delivery. Treatment algorithms have been developed by the ACOG and the APA for the management of depression in women prior to conception and during pregnancy.

Breast-Feeding Considerations Escitalopram and its metabolite are excreted into breast milk. Limited data is available concerning the effects escitalopram may have in the nursing infant and the long-term effects on development and behavior have not been studied. Adverse effects have been reported in nursing infants exposed to some SSRIs. According to the manufacturer, the decision to continue or discontinue breast-feeding during therapy should take into account the risk of exposure to the infant and the benefits of treatment to the mother. Maternal use of an SSRI during pregnancy may cause delayed milk secretion. Escitalopram is the S-enantiomer of the racemic derivative citalopram; also refer to the Citalopram monograph.

Contraindications Hypersensitivity to escitalopram, citalopram, or any component; use with MAO inhibitors within 14 days (potentially fatal reactions may occur); concurrent use of pimozide

Warnings Clinical worsening of depression or suicidal ideation and behavior may occur in children and adults with major depressive disorder **[U.S. Boxed Warning]**. In clinical trials, antidepressants increased the risk of suicidal thinking and behavior (suicidality) in children, adolescents, and young adults (18-24 years of age) with major depressive disorder and other psychiatric disorders. This risk must be considered before prescribing antidepressants for any clinical use. Short-term studies did **not** show an increased risk of suicidality with antidepressant use in patients >24 years of age and showed a decreased risk in patients ≥65 years.

Patients of all ages who are treated with antidepressants for any indication require appropriate monitoring and close observation for clinical worsening of depression, suicidality, and unusual changes in behavior, especially during the first few months after antidepressant initiation or when the dose is adjusted. Family members and caregivers should be instructed to closely observe the patient (ie, daily) and communicate condition with healthcare provider. Patients should also be monitored for associated behaviors (eg, anxiety, agitation, panic attacks, insomnia, irritability, hostility, aggressiveness, impulsivity, akathisia, hypomania, mania) which may increase the risk for worsening depression or suicidality. Worsening depression or emergence of suicidality (or associated behaviors listed above) that is abrupt in onset, severe, or not part of the presenting symptoms may require discontinuation or modification of drug therapy. SSRI-associated behavioral activation (ie, restlessness, hyperkinesis, hyperactivity, agitation) is two- to threefold more prevalent in children compared to adolescents; it is more prevalent in adolescents compared to adults. Somnolence (including sedation and drowsiness) is more common in adults compared to children and adolescents (Safer, 2006).

Avoid abrupt discontinuation; withdrawal syndrome with discontinuation symptoms (including agitation, dysphoria, anxiety, confusion, dizziness, hypomania, nightmares, irritability, sensory disturbances, headache, lethargy, emotional lability, insomnia, tinnitus, and seizures) may occur if therapy is abruptly discontinued or dose is reduced; taper the dose to minimize risks of discontinuation symptoms. If intolerable symptoms occur following a decrease in dosage or upon discontinuation of therapy, consider resuming the previous dose with a more gradual taper. To reduce risk of intentional overdose, write prescriptions for the smallest quantity consistent with good patient care.

May worsen psychosis in some patients or precipitate a shift to mania or hypomania in patients with bipolar disorder. Monotherapy in patients with bipolar disorder should be avoided. Patients presenting with depressive symptoms should be screened for bipolar disorder. Use with caution in patients with a history of mania. Escitalopram is not FDA approved for the treatment of bipolar depression.

Potentially fatal serotonin syndrome (SS) or neuroleptic malignant syndrome (NMS)-like reactions have occurred with selective serotonin reuptake inhibitors (SSRIs) and serotonin/norepinephrine reuptake inhibitors (SNRIs)

when used alone and particularly when used in combination with serotonergic drugs (eg, triptans), drugs that impair the metabolism of serotonin (eg, MAO inhibitors, linezolid), or antidopaminergic agents (eg, antipsychotics). Identification and differentiation of SS (eg, tremor, myoclonus, agitation) and more severe NMS-like reactions (eg, hyperthermia, muscle rigidity, autonomic instability, mental status changes) can be complex; monitor patients closely for either syndrome. Discontinue treatment (and any concomitant serotonergic and/or antidopaminergic agents) immediately if signs or symptoms arise and initiate supportive symptomatic therapy. Tryptophan (which can be metabolized to serotonin) and the herbal medicine St John's wort (*Hypericum perforatum*) may increase serious side effects (concomitant use of these agents with escitalopram is not recommended).

Precautions Escitalopram may impair platelet aggregation and cause abnormal bleeding (eg, ecchymosis, purpura, upper GI bleeding); risk may be increased in patients with impaired platelet aggregation and with concurrent use of aspirin, NSAIDs, warfarin, or other drugs that affect coagulation; bleeding related to SSRI or SNRI use has been reported to range from relatively minor bruising and epistaxis to life-threatening hemorrhage. Escitalopram may impair cognitive or motor performance. SSRI-associated vomiting is two- to threefold more prevalent in children compared to adolescents and more prevalent in adolescents compared to adults (Safer, 2006). Use with caution in patients with seizure disorders, concomitant illnesses that may affect hepatic metabolism or hemodynamic responses (eg, unstable cardiac disease, recent MI), and suicidal ideation; use with caution and decrease dose in patients with hepatic dysfunction; use with caution in patients with severe renal impairment.

Use with caution during third trimester of pregnancy [newborns may experience adverse effects or withdrawal symptoms (consider risk:benefits); exposure to SSRIs late in pregnancy may also be associated with an increased risk for persistent pulmonary hypertension of the newborn (Chambers, 2006)]; high doses of escitalopram have been associated with teratogenicity in animals. Use with caution in patients receiving diuretics or those who are volume-depleted (may cause hyponatremia or SIADH). No clinical studies have assessed the combined use of escitalopram and electroconvulsive therapy; however, use with caution in patients receiving electroconvulsive therapy; may increase the risks associated with electroconvulsive therapy; consider discontinuing, when possible, prior to electroconvulsive therapy treatment. Oral solution contains propylene glycol and sorbitol.

Adverse Reactions

Central nervous system: Abnormal dreams, dizziness, fatigue, headache, insomnia, lethargy, somnolence, yawning

Endocrine & metabolic: Anorgasmia, libido decreased, menstrual disorder

Gastrointestinal: Abdominal pain, appetite decreased, constipation, diarrhea, flatulence, indigestion, nausea, toothache, vomiting, xerostomia

Genitourinary: Ejaculation disorder, impotence, urinary tract infection

Neuromuscular & skeletal: Back pain, neck/shoulder pain, paresthesia

Respiratory: Nasal congestion, rhinitis, sinusitis

Miscellaneous: Diaphoresis, flu-like syndrome

Rare but important or life-threatening: Abdominal cramps, acute renal failure, aggression, agitation, agranulocytosis, akathisia, allergic reaction, allergy, alopecia, amnesia, anaphylaxis, anemia, angioedema, anxiety, apathy, aplastic anemia, appetite increased, arthralgia, ataxia, atrial fibrillation, bilirubin increased, blurred vision, bradycardia, bronchitis, cardiac failure, cerebrovascular accident, chest pain, choreoathetosis, concentration impaired delirium, delusion, depersonalization, depression aggravated, dermatitis, diabetes mellitus, diplopia, DVT, dyskinesia, dysphagia, dyspnea, dystonia, dysuria, ecchymosis, edema, epistaxis, erythema multiforme, extrapyramidal symptoms, fever, flushing, gait abnormal, gastroenteritis, GERD, GI hemorrhage, glaucoma, hallucination, heartburn, hemolytic anemia, hepatic necrosis, hepatitis, hot flashes, hypercholesterolemia, hyper-/hypoglycemia, hypertensive crisis, hypertension, hypoesthesia, hypokalemia, hyponatremia, hypotension, INR increased, irritability, jaw stiffness, leukopenia, lightheadedness, limb pain, liver enzymes increased, liver failure, menorrhagia, menstrual cramps, migraine, muscle weakness, myalgia, mydriasis, myocardial infarction, myoclonus, nasal congestion, neuroleptic malignant syndrome, nightmares, nystagmus, orthostasis, palpitation, pancreatitis, panic reaction, paranoia, Parkinsonism, phlebitis, photosensitivity, priapism, prolactinemia, prothrombin decreased, psychosis, pulmonary embolism, QT prolonged, rash, rectal hemorrhage, rhabdomyolysis, seizures, serotonin syndrome, SIADH, sinus congestion, sinus headache, spontaneous abortion, Stevens-Johnson syndrome, suicidal tendency, suicide attempt, syncope, tachycardia, tardive dyskinesia, thrombocytopenia, thrombocytopenic purpura (idiopathic), thrombosis, tinnitus, torsade de pointes, toxic epidermal necrolysis, tremor, urinary frequency, urinary retention, urticaria, ventricular arrhythmia, ventricular tachycardia, vertigo, visual disturbance, withdrawal syndrome

Drug Interactions

Metabolism/Transport Effects Substrate of CYP2C19 (major), CYP3A4 (major); **Note:** Assignment of Major/Minor substrate status based on clinically relevant drug interaction potential; **Inhibits** CYP2D6 (weak)

Avoid Concomitant Use

Avoid concomitant use of Escitalopram with any of the following: Conivaptan; Dosulepin; Fusidic Acid (Systemic); Highest Risk QTc-Prolonging Agents; Iobenguane I 123; Ivabradine; Linezolid; MAO Inhibitors; Methylene Blue; Mifepristone; Moderate Risk QTc-Prolonging Agents; Pimozide; Tryptophan; Urokinase

Increased Effect/Toxicity

Escitalopram may increase the levels/effects of: Agents with Antiplatelet Properties; Anticoagulants; Antidepressants (Serotonin Reuptake Inhibitor/Antagonist); Antipsychotics; Apixaban; Aspirin; BusPIRone; CarBAMazepine; Collagenase (Systemic); Dabigatran Etexilate; Desmopressin; Dextromethorphan; Dosulepin; Highest Risk QTc-Prolonging Agents; Hypoglycemic Agents; Ibritumomab; Methylene Blue; Mexiletine; NSAID (COX-2 Inhibitor); NSAID (Nonselective); Pimozide; Rivaroxaban; Salicylates; Serotonin Modulators; Thiazide Diuretics; Thrombolytic Agents; Tositumomab and Iodine I 131 Tositumomab; TraMADol; Tricyclic Antidepressants; Urokinase; Vitamin K Antagonists

The levels/effects of Escitalopram may be increased by: Alcohol (Ethyl); Analgesics (Opioid); Antiemetics (5HT3 Antagonists); Antipsychotics; BusPIRone; Cimetidine; CNS Depressants; Conivaptan; CYP2C19 Inhibitors (Moderate); CYP2C19 Inhibitors (Strong); CYP3A4 Inhibitors (Moderate); CYP3A4 Inhibitors (Strong); Fusidic Acid (Systemic); Glucosamine; Herbs (Anticoagulant/Antiplatelet Properties); Ibrutinib; Ivabradine; Ivacaftor; Linezolid; Lithium; Luliconazole; MAO Inhibitors; Metoclopramide; Metyrosine; Mifepristone; Moderate Risk QTc-Prolonging Agents; Multivitamins/Fluoride (with ADE); Multivitamins/Minerals (with ADEK, Folate, Iron); Multivitamins/Minerals (with AE, No Iron); Nonsteroidal Anti-Inflammatory Agents; Omega-3 Fatty Acids; Omeprazole; Pentosan Polysulfate Sodium; Pentoxifylline; Prostacyclin Analogues; QTc-Prolonging Agents ▶

(Indeterminate Risk and Risk Modifying); Stiripentol; Tipranavir; TraMADol; Tricyclic Antidepressants; Tryptophan; Vitamin E

Decreased Effect

Escitalopram may decrease the levels/effects of: lobenguane I 123; Ioflupane I 123; Simeprevir; Thyroid Products

The levels/effects of Escitalopram may be decreased by: Boceprevir; Bosentan; CarBAMazepine; CYP2C19 Inducers (Strong); CYP3A4 Inducers (Strong); Cyproheptadine; Dabrafenib; Deferasirox; Mitotane; Nonsteroidal Anti-Inflammatory Agents; NSAID (COX-2 Inhibitor); NSAID (Nonselective); Siltuximab; St Johns Wort; Telaprevir; Tocilizumab

Stability Store at 25°C (77°F); excursions permitted to 15°C to 30°C (59°F to 86°F)

Mechanism of Action Escitalopram is the S-enantiomer of the racemic derivative citalopram, which selectively inhibits the reuptake of serotonin with little to no effect on norepinephrine or dopamine reuptake. It has no or very low affinity for 5-HT_{1-7}, alpha- and beta-adrenergic, D_{1-5}, H_{1-3}, M_{1-5}, and benzodiazepine receptors. Escitalopram does not bind to or has low affinity for Na^+, K^+, Cl^-, and Ca^{++} ion channels.

Pharmacodynamics

Onset of action: 1-2 weeks

Maximum effect: 8-12 weeks

Pharmacokinetics (Adult data unless noted)

Distribution: V_d: Adults: 12 L/kg

Protein binding, plasma: ~56%

Metabolism: Extensively hepatic via CYP2C19 and 3A4 to S-demethylcitalopram (S-DCT; $1/7$ the activity of escitalopram); S-DCT is metabolized to S-didemethylcitalopram (S-DDCT; active; $1/27$ the activity of escitalopram) via CYP2D6

Bioavailability: 80%; tablets and oral solution are bioequivalent

Half-life elimination: Mean:

Adults: 27-32 hours

Adolescents: 19 hours

Time to peak serum concentration: Adults: 5 hours; Adolescents: 2.9 hours

Elimination: Urine (8% as unchanged drug)

Clearance (citalopram):

Hepatic impairment: Decreased by 37%

Mild-to-moderate renal impairment: Decreased by 17%

Severe renal impairment (CrCl <20 mL/minute): No information available

Dosing: Usual Oral:

Children and Adolescents:

Depression:

Children <12 years: Limited data available; only one randomized, placebo-controlled trial has been published; efficacy was not demonstrated for children <12 years of age (Wagner, 2006)

Adolescents ≥12 years: Initial: 10 mg once daily; may be increased to 20 mg/day after at least 3 weeks

Autism and PDD: Limited data available; based on one published prospective, 10-week, open-labeled, forced dose-titration trial of 28 children and adolescents 6-17 years of age (mean age: 10.4 years) (Owley, 2005). Mean severity outcome scores showed significant improvement; mean final dose: 11.1 ± 6.5 mg/day (range: 0-20 mg/day); no significant correlation between final tolerated dose and weight was shown; 10 of 28 treated subjects could not tolerate a 10 mg/day dose; further studies are needed

Children and Adolescents 6-17 years: Initial: 2.5 mg once daily; may increase if needed to 5 mg/day after 1 week; may then increase at weekly intervals by 5 mg/day if needed and as tolerated; maximum dose: 20 mg/day

Social anxiety disorder: Limited data available; based on one prospective, 12-week, open-labeled trial of 20 children and adolescents 10-17 years of age (mean age: 15 years) (Isolan, 2007). At the end of the 12 weeks, 65% of patients met overall response criteria and all symptomatic and quality of life outcome measures showed significant improvements; mean final dose: 13 ± 4.1 mg/day; further studies are needed

Children and Adolescents 10-17 years: Initial: 5 mg once daily for 7 days, then 10 mg/day for 7 days; may then increase at weekly intervals by 5 mg/day if needed, based on clinical response and tolerability; maximum dose: 20 mg/day

Adults: **Depression, generalized anxiety disorder:** Initial: 10 mg once daily; dose may be increased to 20 mg/day after at least 1 week

Dosage adjustment in renal impairment:

Mild-to-moderate impairment: No dosage adjustment needed

Severe impairment: CrCl <20 mL/minute: Use with caution

Dosage adjustment in hepatic impairment: Adolescents >12 years and Adults: 10 mg/day

Administration Administer once daily (morning or evening); may be administered with or without food.

Monitoring Parameters Monitor patient periodically for symptom resolution; monitor for worsening depression, suicidality, and associated behaviors (especially at the beginning of therapy or when doses are increased or decreased). Monitor for anxiety, social functioning, mania, panic attacks; akathisia. Monitor for signs and symptoms of serotonin syndrome or neuroleptic malignant syndrome-like reactions.

Additional Information If used for an extended period of time, long-term usefulness of escitalopram should be periodically re-evaluated for the individual patient. A recent report describes 5 children (age: 8-15 years) who developed epistaxis (n=4) or bruising (n=1) while receiving SSRI therapy (sertraline) (Lake, 2000).

Neonates born to women receiving SSRIs later during the third trimester may experience respiratory distress, apnea, cyanosis, temperature instability, vomiting, feeding difficulty, hypoglycemia, constant crying, irritability, hypotonia, hypertonia, hyper-reflexia, tremor, jitteriness, and seizures; these symptoms may be due to a direct toxic effect, withdrawal syndrome, or (in some cases) serotonin syndrome. Withdrawal symptoms occur in 30% of neonates exposed to SSRIs *in utero*; monitor newborns for at least 48 hours after birth; long-term effects of *in utero* exposure to SSRIs are unknown (Levinson-Castiel, 2006).

Dosage Forms Excipient information presented when available (limited, particularly for generics); consult specific product labeling.

Solution, Oral:

Lexapro: 5 mg/5 mL (240 mL) [contains methylparaben; propylene glycol, propylparaben; peppermint flavor]

Generic: 5 mg/5 mL (240 mL)

Tablet, Oral:

Lexapro: 5 mg

Lexapro: 10 mg, 20 mg [scored]

Generic: 5 mg, 10 mg, 20 mg

References

Boyer EW and Shannon M, "The Serotonin Syndrome," *New Engl J Med*, 2005, 352:1112-20.

Chambers CD, Hernandez-Diaz S, Van Marter LJ, et al, "Selective Serotonin-Reuptake Inhibitors and Risk of Persistent Pulmonary Hypertension of the Newborn," *N Engl J Med*, 2006, 354(6):579-87.

Isolan L, Pheula G, Salum GA Jr, et al, "An Open-Label Trial of Escitalopram in Children and Adolescents With Social Anxiety Disorder," *J Child Adolesc Psychopharmacol*, 2007, 17(6):751-60.

Lake MB, Birmaher B, Wassick S, et al, "Bleeding and Selective Serotonin Reuptake Inhibitors in Childhood and Adolescence," *J Child Adolesc Psychopharmacol*, 2000, 10(1):35-8.

Levinson-Castiel R, Merlob P, Linder N, et al, "Neonatal Abstinence Syndrome After *in utero* Exposure to Selective Serotonin Reuptake Inhibitors in Term Infants," *Arch Pediatr Adolesc Med*, 2006, 160 (2):173-6.

Murdoch D and Keam SJ, "Escitalopram: A Review of Its Use in the Management of Major Depressive Disorder," *Drugs*, 2005, 65 (16):2379-404.

Owley T, Walton L, Salt J, et al, "An Open-Label Trial of Escitalopram in Pervasive Developmental Disorders," *J Am Acad Child Adolesc Psychiatry*, 2005, 44(4):343-8.

Rao N, "The Clinical Pharmacokinetics of Escitalopram," *Clin Pharmacokinet*, 2007, 46(4):281-90.

Safer DJ and Zito JM, "Treatment Emergent Adverse Effects of Selective Serotonin Reuptake Inhibitors by Age Group: Children vs. Adolescents," *J Child Adolesc Psychopharmacol*, 2006, 16 (1-2):159-69.

Wagner KD, Jonas J, Findling RL, et al, "A Double-Blind, Randomized, Placebo-Controlled Trial of Escitalopram in the Treatment of Pediatric Depression," *J Am Acad Child Adolesc Psychiatry*, 2006, 45(3):280-8.

◆ **Escitalopram Oxalate** *see* Escitalopram *on page 788*

◆ **Eserine Salicylate** *see* Physostigmine *on page 1670*

◆ **Eskalith** *see* Lithium *on page 1266*

Esmolol (ES moe lol)

Medication Safety Issues
Sound-alike/look-alike issues:
Esmolol may be confused with Osmitrol®
Brevibloc® may be confused with Brevital®, Bumex®, Buprenex®

High alert medication:
The Institute for Safe Medication Practices (ISMP) includes this medication among its list of drugs which have a heightened risk of causing significant patient harm when used in error.

Related Information
Management of Drug Extravasations *on page 2255*
Serotonin Syndrome *on page 2405*

Brand Names: U.S. Brevibloc; Brevibloc in NaCl

Brand Names: Canada Brevibloc®; Brevibloc® Premixed

Therapeutic Category Antiarrhythmic Agent, Class II; Antihypertensive Agent; Beta-Adrenergic Blocker

Generic Availability (U.S.) Yes

Use Treatment of supraventricular tachycardia (primarily to control ventricular rate in patients with atrial fibrillation or flutter) (FDA approved in adults); noncompensatory sinus tachycardia (FDA approved in adults); perioperative tachycardia and hypertension (FDA approved in adults)

Pregnancy Risk Factor C

Pregnancy Considerations Adverse events were observed in some animal reproduction studies. Esmolol has been shown to decrease fetal heart rate. Adverse fetal/neonatal events have also been observed with the chronic use of beta-blockers during pregnancy. Esmolol is a short-acting beta-blocker and not indicated for the chronic treatment of hypertension. Esmolol may be considered for the acute management of atrial fibrillation in pregnant women (Fuster, 2006). Esmolol has been evaluated for use during intubation as an agent to offset the exaggerated pressor response observed in pregnant women with hypertension undergoing surgery (Bansal, 2002).

Breast-Feeding Considerations It is not known if esmolol is excreted into breast milk. Due to the potential for serious adverse reactions in the nursing infant, the manufacturer recommends a decision be made whether to discontinue nursing or to discontinue the drug, taking into account the importance of treatment to the mother. The short half-life and the fact that it is not intended for chronic use should limit any potential exposure to the nursing infant.

Contraindications Hypersensitivity to esmolol, any component, or other beta-blockers; sinus bradycardia or heart block, uncompensated CHF, cardiogenic shock

Warnings Caution should be exercised when discontinuing esmolol infusions to avoid withdrawal effects. Hypotension can commonly occur; especially with doses >200 mcg/kg/minute; monitor patients closely.

Precautions Use with extreme caution in patients with hyper-reactive airway disease; in general, patients with bronchospastic disease should not receive beta-blockers; however, esmolol, with B_1 selectivity, has been used cautiously with close monitoring; use lowest dose possible and discontinue infusion if bronchospasm occurs; incidence less than compared to propranolol but more likely with higher doses. Use with caution in diabetes mellitus or hypoglycemia; may potentiate hypoglycemia and/or mask signs and symptoms. Use with caution in patients with renal impairment; active metabolite retained. Avoid extravasation, can lead to skin necrosis and sloughing. Use caution with history of severe anaphylaxis to allergens; patients taking beta-blockers may become more sensitive to repeated challenges. Treatment of anaphylaxis (eg, epinephrine) in patients taking beta-blockers may be ineffective or promote undesirable effects.

Adverse Reactions
Cardiovascular: Asymptomatic hypotension, blood pressure decreased, peripheral ischemia, symptomatic hypotension

Central nervous system: Agitation, confusion, dizziness, headache, somnolence

Gastrointestinal: Nausea, vomiting

Local: Infusion site reaction (including irritation, inflammation, and severe reactions associated with extravasation [eg, thrombophlebitis, necrosis, and blistering])

Rare but important or life-threatening: Abdominal discomfort, abnormal thinking, angioedema, anorexia, anxiety, bradycardia, bronchospasm, cardiac arrest, constipation, coronary arteriospasm, decompensated heart failure, depression, dyspepsia, flushing, heart block, hyperkalemia, lightheadedness, pallor, paresthesia, psoriasis, renal tubular acidosis, seizure, severe bradycardia/asystole (rare), syncope, urinary retention, urticaria, xerostomia

Drug Interactions

Metabolism/Transport Effects None known.

Avoid Concomitant Use
Avoid concomitant use of Esmolol with any of the following: Ceritinib; Floctafenine; Methacholine

Increased Effect/Toxicity
Esmolol may increase the levels/effects of: Alpha-/Beta-Agonists (Direct-Acting); Alpha1-Blockers; Alpha2-Agonists; Amifostine; Antihypertensives; Antipsychotic Agents (Phenothiazines); Bradycardia-Causing Agents; Bupivacaine; Cardiac Glycosides; Ceritinib; Cholinergic Agonists; DULoxetine; Ergot Derivatives; Fingolimod; Grass Pollen Allergen Extract (5 Grass Extract); Hypotensive Agents; Insulin; Lidocaine (Systemic); Lidocaine (Topical); Mepivacaine; Methacholine; Midodrine; Obinutuzumab; RiTUXimab; Sulfonylureas

The levels/effects of Esmolol may be increased by: Acetylcholinesterase Inhibitors; Alpha2-Agonists; Aminoquinolines (Antimalarial); Amiodarone; Anilidopiperidine Opioids; Antipsychotic Agents (Phenothiazines); Barbiturates; Brimonidine (Topical); Calcium Channel Blockers (Dihydropyridine); Calcium Channel Blockers (Nondihydropyridine); Diazoxide; Dipyridamole; Disopyramide; Dronedarone; Floctafenine; Herbs (Hypotensive Properties); MAO Inhibitors; Pentoxifylline; Phosphodiesterase 5 Inhibitors; Propafenone; Prostacyclin Analogues; Regorafenib; Reserpine

Decreased Effect
Esmolol may decrease the levels/effects of: Beta2-Agonists; Theophylline Derivatives

The levels/effects of Esmolol may be decreased by: Barbiturates; Herbs (Hypertensive Properties); Methylphenidate; Nonsteroidal Anti-Inflammatory Agents; Rifamycin Derivatives; Yohimbine

Stability Store at controlled room temperature at 25°C (77°F); excursions permitted to 15°C to 30°C (59°F to 86°F); protect from freezing and excessive heat. Stable for at least 24 hours (under refrigeration or at controlled room temperature) at a final concentration of 10 mg/mL in the following solutions: D_5W, D_5LR, $D_5^{1/2}NS$, D_5NS, LR, NS, $^{1/2}NS$, D_5W with KCl 40 mEq/L; **not** compatible with sodium bicarbonate 5%

Mechanism of Action Class II antiarrhythmic: Competitively blocks response to beta$_1$-adrenergic stimulation with little or no effect of beta$_2$-receptors except at high doses, no intrinsic sympathomimetic activity, no membrane stabilizing activity

Pharmacodynamics

Onset of action: I.V.: Beta blockade occurs within 2-10 minutes (onset of effects is quickest when loading doses are administered)

Duration: Short (10-30 minutes)

Pharmacokinetics (Adult data unless noted)

Protein binding: 55%

Distribution: V_d:

Children: 2 L/kg

Adults: 3.5 L/kg (range: 2-5 L/kg)

Metabolism: In blood by esterases

Half-life, elimination:

Children:

18 months to 14 years (n=12): 2.88 ± 2.67 minutes

2.5-16 years (n=20): 4.5 ± 2.1 minutes

Adults: 9 minutes

Elimination: ~69% of dose excreted in urine as metabolites and 2% as unchanged drug

Dosing: Neonatal Note: Must be adjusted to individual response and tolerance.

Postoperative hypertension: Limited data available; further studies are needed. An open-label trial used the following dosing guidelines to treat postoperative hypertension following cardiac surgery; dose was titrated until blood pressure was ≤90th percentile for age; final dose required was significantly higher in patients with aortic coarctation repair than in patients with repair of other congenital heart defects (Wiest, 1998):

Term neonates: PNA 0-7 days: Initial: 50 mcg/kg/minute; titrate dose by 25-50 mcg/kg/minute every 20 minutes

Term neonates: PNA 8-28 days: Initial: 75 mcg/kg/minute; titrate dose by 50 mcg/kg/minute every 20 minutes

Note: Maximum dose: 1000 mcg/kg/minute; higher doses have not been evaluated

Dosing: Usual Note: Must be adjusted to individual response and tolerance.

Infants and Children: I.V.: Limited data available:

Supraventricular tachycardia (SVT): Some centers have utilized initial doses of 100-500 mcg/kg given over 1 minute followed by a continuous infusion for control of SVT. One electrophysiologic study assessing esmolol-induced beta-blockade (n=20, 2-16 years of age) used an initial dose of 600 mcg/kg over 2 minutes followed by an infusion of 200 mcg/kg/minute; the infusion was titrated upward by 50-100 mcg/kg/minute every 5-10 minutes until a reduction >10% in heart rate or mean blood pressure occurred. Mean dose required: 550 mcg/kg/minute with a range of 300-1000 mcg/kg/minute (Trippel, 1991).

Postoperative hypertension: Loading doses of 500 mcg/kg/minute over 1 minute followed by a continuous infusion with doses of 50-250 mcg/kg/minute (mean: 173) have been used in addition to nitroprusside in a small number of patients (7 patients, 7-19 years of age,

median age: 13 years) after coarctation of aorta repair (Vincent, 1990).

An open-label trial of 20 infants and children (1 month to 12 years of age; median age: 25.6 months) used the following dosing guidelines to treat postoperative hypertension following cardiac surgery: Age >1 month to 1 year: Initial: 100 mcg/kg/minute; titrate dose by 50 mcg/kg/minute every 10 minutes; age >1 year to 12 years: Initial: 150 mcg/kg/minute; titrate dose by 50-100 mcg/kg/minute every 10 minutes; dose was titrated until blood pressure was ≤90th percentile for age or until maximum dose of 1000 mcg/kg/minute was reached; mean required dose: 700 mcg/kg/minute (range: 300-1000 mcg/kg/minute); final dose required was significantly higher in patients with aortic coarctation repair (mean ± SD: 830 ± 153 mcg/kg/minute) than in patients with repair of other congenital heart defects (mean ± SD: 570 ± 230 mcg/kg/minute) (Wiest, 1998)

Adults: I.V.:

Intraoperative tachycardia and/or hypertension (immediate control): Loading dose: 80 mg (~1 mg/kg) over 30 seconds; follow with a 150 mcg/kg/minute infusion, if necessary; adjust infusion rate as needed to maintain desired heart rate and/or blood pressure; maximum dose: 300 mcg/kg/minute.

Supraventricular tachycardia or gradual control of postoperative tachycardia and hypertension: Loading dose: 500 mcg/kg over 1 minute; follow with a 50 mcg/kg/minute infusion for 4 minutes; if response is inadequate, rebolus with another 500 mcg/kg loading dose over 1 minute, and increase the maintenance infusion to 100 mcg/kg/minute. Repeat this process until a therapeutic effect has been achieved or to a maximum recommended maintenance dose of 200 mcg/kg/minute. Usual dosage range: 50-200 mcg/kg/minute with average dose = 100 mcg/kg/minute.

Usual Infusion Concentrations: Pediatric Note: Premixed solutions available.

I.V. infusion: 10,000 **mcg**/mL or 20,000 **mcg**/mL

Administration Parenteral: I.V.: Commercially available concentrations (10 mg/mL and 20 mg/mL) are iso-osmotic and can be used for direct I.V. use; infuse I.V. loading dose over 1-2 minutes. **Note:** Parenteral drug products are for single patient use only; products do **not** contain preservatives. Do not introduce additives into the premixed bags. Medication port of premixed bag should be used to withdraw only the initial bolus; do not use medication port to withdraw additional bolus doses (sterility cannot be assured).

Vesicant/Extravasation Risk Vesicant

Monitoring Parameters Blood pressure, ECG, heart rate, respiratory rate, I.V. site

Dosage Forms Excipient information presented when available (limited, particularly for generics); consult specific product labeling.

Solution, Intravenous, as hydrochloride:

Brevibloc: 10 mg/mL (10 mL)

Brevibloc in NaCl: 2000 mg (100 mL); 2500 mg (250 mL)

Generic: 10 mg/mL (10 mL)

Solution, Intravenous, as hydrochloride [preservative free]:

Generic: 10 mg/mL (10 mL); 100 mg/10 mL (10 mL)

References

Bansal S and Pawar M, "Haemodynamic Responses to Laryngoscopy and Intubation in Patients With Pregnancy-Induced Hypertension: Effect of Intravenous Esmolol With or Without Lidocaine," *Int J Obstet Anesth*, 2002, 11(1):4-8.

Cuneo BF, Zales VR, Blahunka PC, et al, "Pharmacodynamics and Pharmacokinetics of Esmolol, A Short-Acting Beta-Blocking Agent in Children," *Pediatr Cardiol*, 1994, 15(6):296-301.

Fuster V, Rydén LE, Cannom DS, et al, "ACC/AHA/ESC 2006 Guidelines for the Management of Patients With Atrial Fibrillation-Executive Summary: A Report of the American College of Cardiology/American Heart Association Task Force on Practice Guidelines and the European Society of Cardiology Committee for Practice Guidelines

(Writing Committee to Revise the 2001 Guidelines for the Management of Patients With Atrial Fibrillation)," *J Am Coll Cardiol*, 2006, 48 (4):854-906.

Phillips MS, "Standardizing I.V. Infusion Concentrations: National Survey Results," *Am J Health Syst Pharm*, 2011, 68(22):2176-82.

Trippel DL, Wiest DB, and Gillette PC, "Cardiovascular and Antiarrhythmic Effects of Esmolol in Children," *J Pediatr*, 1991, 119 (1):142-7.

Vincent RN, Click LA, Williams HM, et al, "Esmolol As an Adjunct in the Treatment of Systemic Hypertension After Operative Repair of Coarctation of the Aorta," *Am J Cardiol*, 1990, 65(13):941-3.

Wiest DB, Garner SS, Uber WE, et al, "Esmolol for the Management of Pediatric Hypertension After Cardiac Operations," *J Thorac Cardiovasc Surg*, 1998, 115(4):890-7.

Wiest DB, Trippel DL, Gillette PC, et al, "Pharmacokinetics of Esmolol in Children," *Clin Pharmacol Ther*, 1991, 49(6):618-23.

◆ **Esmolol Hydrochloride** see Esmolol *on page 791*

Esomeprazole (es oh ME pray zol)

Medication Safety Issues
Sound-alike/look-alike issues:
Esomeprazole may be confused with ARIPiprazole, omeprazole

NexIUM may be confused with NexAVAR

Related Information
Oral Medications That Should Not Be Crushed or Altered *on page 2438*

Brand Names: U.S. NexIUM; NexIUM I.V.

Brand Names: Canada Apo-Esomeprazole; Mylan-Esomeprazole; Nexium

Therapeutic Category Gastric Acid Secretion Inhibitor; Gastrointestinal Agent, Gastric or Duodenal Ulcer Treatment; Proton Pump Inhibitor

Generic Availability (U.S.) May be product dependent

Use
Oral: Short-term treatment (up to 6 weeks) of erosive esophagitis associated with gastroesophageal reflux disease (GERD) (FDA approved in ages 1 month to <1 year); short-term treatment (4-8 weeks) and maintenance of healing of severe erosive esophagitis (FDA approved in ages ≥1 year and adults); short-term treatment (4-8 weeks) of symptomatic gastroesophageal reflux disease (GERD) (FDA approved in children ≥1 year and adults); adjunctive treatment of duodenal ulcers associated with *Helicobacter pylori*; prevention of gastric ulcers associated with continuous NSAID therapy in patients at high risk; long-term treatment of pathological hypersecretory conditions including Zollinger-Ellison syndrome (FDA approved in adults)

I.V.: Short-term alternative treatment (≤10 days) of GERD with erosive esophagitis when oral therapy is not possible or appropriate (FDA approved in ages ≥1 month and adults)

Medication Guide Available Yes

Pregnancy Risk Factor C

Pregnancy Considerations Adverse events were observed in some animal reproduction studies. An increased risk of hypospadias was reported following maternal use of proton pump inhibitors (PPIs) during pregnancy (Anderka, 2012), but this was based on a small number of exposures and the same association was not found in another study (Erichsen, 2012). An increased risk of major birth defects following maternal use of PPIs during pregnancy was not observed in an additional study (Pasternak, 2010). Esomeprazole is the s-isomer of omeprazole; refer to the Omeprazole monograph for additional information. When treating GERD in pregnancy, PPIs may be used when clinically indicated (Katz, 2013).

Breast-Feeding Considerations Esomeprazole and strontium (limited data) are excreted in breast milk. The manufacturer of esomeprazole recommends that caution be exercised when administering to nursing women. The manufacturer of esomeprazole strontium recommends a

decision be made whether to discontinue nursing or to discontinue the drug, taking into account the importance of treatment to the mother. Esomeprazole is the s-isomer of omeprazole and omeprazole is excreted in breast milk; refer to Omeprazole monograph for additional information.

Contraindications Hypersensitivity to esomeprazole, substituted benzimidazole proton pump inhibitors (eg, omeprazole, lansoprazole, pantoprazole), or any component

Warnings Esomeprazole is an enantiomer of omeprazole and may share the same potential long-term side effects as omeprazole. Benign and malignant neoplasia has been observed in long-term rodent studies using omeprazole; while not reported in humans, the relevance of these findings in regards to tumorigenicity in humans is not known. Symptomatic response to therapy does not preclude the presence of GI malignancy. Atrophic gastritis has been reported occasionally in gastric corpus biopsies from patients treated long-term with omeprazole.

An increased incidence of osteoporosis-related bone fractures of the hip, spine, or wrist may occur with proton pump inhibitor (PPI) therapy; patients on high-dose (multiple daily doses) or long-term therapy (≥1 year) should be monitored. Use the lowest effective dose for the shortest duration of time, use vitamin D and calcium supplementation, and follow appropriate guidelines to reduce risk of fractures in patients at risk. Hypomagnesemia has been reported rarely, usually with prolonged PPI use of >3 months (most cases >1 year of therapy), and may be symptomatic or asymptomatic; severe cases may cause tetany, seizures, and cardiac arrhythmias. Consider obtaining serum magnesium concentrations prior to beginning long-term therapy, especially if taking concomitant digoxin, diuretics, or other drugs known to cause hypomagnesemia; and periodically thereafter. Hypomagnesemia may be corrected by magnesium supplementation, although discontinuation of esomeprazole may be necessary; magnesium concentrations typically return to normal within 1 week of stopping.

Use of gastric acid inhibitors including proton pump inhibitors and H_2 blockers has been associated with an increased risk for development of acute gastroenteritis and community-acquired pneumonia (Canani, 2006). Use of PPIs may also increase the risk of *Clostridium difficile*-associated diarrhea (CDAD), especially in hospitalized patients; consider CDAD diagnosis in patients with persistent diarrhea that does not improve. Use the lowest dose and shortest duration of PPI therapy appropriate for the condition being treated.

Proton pump inhibitors (PPIs) may diminish the therapeutic effect of clopidogrel, thought to be due to reduced formation of the active metabolite of clopidogrel. The manufacturer of clopidogrel recommends either avoidance of both omeprazole (even when scheduled 12 hours apart) and esomeprazole or use of a PPI with comparatively less effect on the active metabolite of clopidogrel (eg, pantoprazole). In contrast to these warnings, others have recommended the continued use of PPIs, regardless of the degree of inhibition, in patients with a history of GI bleeding or multiple risk factors for GI bleeding who are also receiving clopidogrel since no evidence has established clinically meaningful differences in outcome; however, a clinically significant interaction cannot be excluded in those who are poor metabolizers of clopidogrel (Abraham, 2010; Levine, 2011). Concomitant use of PPIs with high-dose methotrexate may lead to increased and prolonged serum concentrations of methotrexate and/or its metabolite, possibly causing methotrexate toxicities; temporary discontinuation of PPIs may be considered.

Serum chromogranin A (CgA) levels increase secondary to drug-induced decreases in gastric acid; may cause false-positive results in diagnostic investigations for neuroendocrine tumors. Stop esomeprazole treatment temporarily before CgA test; if CgA level high, repeat to confirm. Use same commercial laboratory for testing to prevent variable results.

Precautions Bioavailability may be increased in patients with hepatic dysfunction or patients of Asian descent; consider dosage reductions, especially for maintenance healing of erosive esophagitis

Adverse Reactions

Central nervous system: Dizziness, drowsiness, headache

Dermatologic: Pruritus

Gastrointestinal: Abdominal pain, constipation, diarrhea, flatulence, nausea, xerostomia

Local: Injection site reaction (I.V.)

Rare but important or life-threatening: Aggression, agranulocytosis, alopecia, anaphylaxis, anemia, angioedema, anorexia, benign polyps/nodules, blurred vision, bone fracture, cervical lymphadenopathy, chest pain, *Clostridium difficile*-associated diarrhea (CDAD), conjunctivitis, cyanocobalamin deficiency, cystitis, depression, dermatitis, dysgeusia, dysmenorrhea, epistaxis, erythema multiforme, exacerbation of arthritis, exacerbation of asthma, fibromyalgia syndrome, fungal infection, gastric carcinoid tumor, gastroenteritis, GI dysplasia, GI moniliasis, goiter, gynecomastia, hallucinations, hematuria, hepatic encephalopathy, hepatic failure, hepatitis, hernia, hyperhidrosis, hyperparathyroidism, hypersensitivity reactions, hypertension, hypertonia, hyperuricemia, hypoesthesia, hypokalemia, hypomagnesemia (with or without hypocalcemia and/or hypokalemia), hyponatremia, impotence, increased gastrin, increased serum alkaline phosphatase, increased serum ALT, increased serum AST, increased serum creatinine, increased thyroid-stimulating hormone, insomnia, interstitial nephritis, jaundice, laryngeal edema, leukocytosis, leukopenia, microscopic colitis, migraine, moniliasis, myasthenia, otitis media, pancreatitis, pancytopenia, parosmia, pathological fracture due to osteoporosis, phlebitis, photosensitivity, pneumonia, polymyalgia rheumatica, proteinuria, pruritus ani, rigors, skin rash (erythematous and maculopapular), Stevens-Johnson syndrome, stomatitis, tachycardia, thrombocytopenia, thrombophlebitis, toxic epidermal necrolysis, vaginitis, visual field defect, weight changes

Drug Interactions

Metabolism/Transport Effects Substrate of CYP2C19 (major), CYP3A4 (minor); **Note:** Assignment of Major/Minor substrate status based on clinically relevant drug interaction potential; **Inhibits** CYP2C19 (moderate)

Avoid Concomitant Use

Avoid concomitant use of Esomeprazole with any of the following: Clopidogrel; Dasatinib; Delavirdine; Erlotinib; Nelfinavir; PAZOPanib; PONATinib; Rifampin; Rilpivirine; Risedronate; St Johns Wort

Increased Effect/Toxicity

Esomeprazole may increase the levels/effects of: Amphetamine; Benzodiazepines (metabolized by oxidation); Cilostazol; Citalopram; CYP2C19 Substrates; Dexmethylphenidate; Dextroamphetamine; Methotrexate; Methylphenidate; Raltegravir; Risedronate; Saquinavir; Tacrolimus (Systemic); Vitamin K Antagonists; Voriconazole

The levels/effects of Esomeprazole may be increased by: Fluconazole; Ketoconazole (Systemic); Voriconazole

Decreased Effect

Esomeprazole may decrease the levels/effects of: Atazanavir; Bisphosphonate Derivatives; Bosutinib; Cefditoren; Clopidogrel; Dabigatran Etexilate; Dabrafenib; Dasatinib; Delavirdine; Erlotinib; Gefitinib; Indinavir; Iron Salts; Itraconazole; Ketoconazole (Systemic); Mesalamine; Multivitamins/Minerals (with ADEK, Folate, Iron); Mycophenolate; Nelfinavir; Nilotinib; PAZOPanib;

PONATinib; Posaconazole; Rilpivirine; Riociguat; Risedronate; Vismodegib

The levels/effects of Esomeprazole may be decreased by: CYP2C19 Inducers (Strong); Dabrafenib; Rifampin; St Johns Wort; Tipranavir

Food Interactions Prolonged treatment (≥2 years) may lead to malabsorption of dietary vitamin B_{12} and subsequent vitamin B_{12} deficiency (Lam, 2013).

Stability Esomeprazole stability is a function of pH; it is rapidly degraded in acidic media, but has acceptable stability under alkaline conditions. Each capsule of esomeprazole contains enteric-coated granules to prevent esomeprazole degradation by gastric acidity.

Capsule, granules: Store at 25°C (77°F); excursions permitted to 15°C to 30°C (59°F to 86°F). Keep container tightly closed.

Powder for injection: Store at 25°C (77°F); excursions permitted to 15°C to 30°C (59°F to 86°F). Protect from light. Per the manufacturer, following reconstitution, solution for injection prepared in NS, and solution for infusion prepared in NS or LR should be used within 12 hours. Following reconstitution, solution for infusion prepared in D_5W should be used within 6 hours. Refrigeration is not required following reconstitution. Additional stability testing has shown that following reconstitution, solutions for infusion prepared in D_5W, NS, or LR in polyvinyl chloride bags are chemically and physically stable for 48 hours at room temperature (25°C) and for at least 120 hours under refrigeration (4°C) (Kupiec, 2008).

Mechanism of Action Proton pump inhibitor suppresses gastric acid secretion by inhibition of the H^+/K^+-ATPase in the gastric parietal cell. Esomeprazole is the S-isomer of omeprazole.

Pharmacokinetics (Adult data unless noted)

Distribution: V_d: 16 L

Protein binding: 97%

Metabolism: Hepatic via CYP2C19 primarily and to a lesser extent via 3A3/4 isoenzymes to hydroxy, desmethyl, and sulfone metabolites (all inactive)

Bioavailability: 64% after a single dose; 90% with repeated administration

Half-life:

Infants: 0.93 hours

Children 1-5 years: 0.42-0.74 hours (Zhao, 2006)

Children 6-11 years: 0.73-0.88 hours (Zhao, 2006)

Adolescents 12-17 years: 0.82-1.22 hours (Li, 2006)

Adults: 1-1.5 hours

Time to peak serum concentration: Oral:

Infants: Median: 3 hours

Children 1-5 years: 1.33-1.44 hours (Zhao, 2006)

Children 6-11 years: 1.75-1.79 hours (Zhao, 2006)

Adolescents 12-17 years: 1.96-2.04 hours (Li, 2006)

Adults: 1.6 hours

Elimination: Urine (80%, primarily as inactive metabolites; <1% excreted as active drug); feces (20%)

Clearance (with repeated dosing):

Children 1-5 years: 6-19.44 L/hour (Zhao, 2006)

Children 6-11 years: 7.84-9.22 L/hour (Zhao, 2006)

Adolescents 12-17 years: 8.36-15.88 L/hour (Li, 2006)

Dosing: Neonatal GERD: Oral: 0.5 mg/kg/dose given once daily for 7 days; has been shown to reduce esophageal acid exposure and gastric acidity, but did not decrease bolus reflux in 26 preterm and term infants with symptoms of GERD (GA: 23-41 weeks) (Omari, 2009)

Dosing: Usual

Infants, Children, and Adolescents:

Erosive esophagitis associated with GERD:

Oral:

Infants: **Note:** Safety and efficacy of doses >1.33 mg/kg/**day** and/or therapy beyond 6 weeks have not been studied.

3-5 kg: 2.5 mg once daily
>5-7.5 kg: 5 mg once daily
>7.5 kg: 10 mg once daily
Children 1-11 years: **Note:** Safety and efficacy of doses >1 mg/kg/**day** and/or therapy beyond 8 weeks have not been established.
<20 kg: 10 mg once daily
>20 kg: 10 or 20 mg once daily
Children ≥12 years and Adolescents: 20-40 mg once daily for 4 to 8 weeks
I.V.: **Note:** Indicated only in cases where oral therapy is inappropriate or not possible; safety and efficacy >10 days has not been established.
Infants: 0.5 mg/kg/dose once daily
Children 1-17 years:
<55 kg: 10 mg once daily
≥55 kg: 20 mg once daily
GERD, symptomatic: Oral:
Manufacturer's labeling:
Children 1-11 years: 10 mg once daily for up to 8 weeks. **Note:** Safety and efficacy of doses >1 mg/kg/**day** and/or therapy beyond 8 weeks have not been established.
Children ≥12 years and Adolescents: 20 mg once daily for 4-8 weeks
Alternate dosing (AAP recommendation): Infants, Children, and Adolescents: 0.7-3.3 mg/kg/**day** (Lightdale, 2013)
Adults:
Erosive esophagitis (healing): Oral: Initial: 20-40 mg once daily for 4-8 weeks; if incomplete healing, continue for an additional 4-8 weeks; maintenance: 20 mg once daily (controlled studies did not extend beyond 6 months)
GERD, short-term treatment: I.V.: 20 mg or 40 mg once daily. **Note:** Indicated only in cases where oral therapy is inappropriate or not possible; safety and efficacy ≥10 days has not been established.
GERD, symptomatic: Oral: 20 mg once daily for 4 weeks; may consider an additional 4 weeks of treatment if symptoms do not resolve
***Helicobacter pylori* eradication:** Oral: 40 mg once daily (in combination with antibiotic therapy) for 10 days
Pathological hypersecretory conditions including Zollinger-Ellison syndrome: Oral: 40 mg twice daily; adjust regimen to individual patient needs; doses up to 240 mg daily have been administered
Prevention of NSAID-induced gastric ulcers: Oral: 20-40 mg once daily for up to 6 months. **Note:** 40 mg daily did not show additional benefit over 20 mg daily in clinical trials.
Dosing adjustment in renal impairment: Infants, Children, Adolescents, and Adults: Oral, I.V.: No dosage adjustments are recommended.
Dosing adjustment in hepatic impairment: Adults: Oral, I.V.:
Mild to moderate liver impairment (Child-Pugh Class A or B): No dosage adjustments are recommended.
Severe liver impairment (Child-Pugh Class C): Use with caution; do not exceed 20 mg daily.
Usual Infusion Concentrations: Pediatric I.V. infusion: 0.4 mg/mL **or** 0.8 mg/mL
Administration
Oral: Administer at least 1 hour before food or meals
Capsule: Swallow whole, do not chew or crush. For patients with difficulty swallowing the capsule, capsule may be opened and the enteric coated pellets may be mixed with 1 tablespoon of applesauce (applesauce should not be hot) and swallowed immediately; do not chew or crush granules; do not store mixture for future use.
Nasogastric tube administration: Open capsule and place intact granules into a 60 mL catheter-tipped

syringe; mix with 50 mL of water. Replace plunger and shake vigorously for 15 seconds. Ensure that no granules remain in syringe tip. Do not administer if pellets dissolve or disintegrate. Use immediately after preparation. After administration, flush nasogastric tube with additional water.
Granules: Mix contents of the 2.5 mg or 5 mg packet with 5 mL of water or the 10 mg, 20 mg, or 40 mg packet with 15 mL water and stir; leave for 2-3 minutes to thicken; stir and drink within 30 minutes. If any medicine remains after drinking, add more water, stir and drink immediately.
Nasogastric or gastric tube administration: If using a 2.5 mg or 5 mg packet, first add 5 mL of water to a catheter-tipped syringe, then add granules from packet. If using a 10 mg, 20 mg, or 40 mg packet, first add 15 mL of water to a catheter-tipped syringe, then add granules from packet. Shake the syringe, leave 2-3 minutes to thicken. Shake the syringe and administer through nasogastric or gastric tube (French size 6 or greater) within 30 minutes. Refill the syringe with an equal amount (5 mL or 15 mL) of water, shake and flush tube.
I.V.: Flush line prior to and after administration with NS, LR, or D_5W.
Infants, Children, and Adolescents: Reconstitute vial (20 mg or 40 mg) with 5 mL of NS; further dilute to a final volume of 50 mL to achieve a final concentration of 0.4 mg/mL or 0.8 mg/mL, respectively; administer desired dose by intermittent infusion over 10-30 minutes. The manufacturer recommends that children receive intravenous esomeprazole by intermittent infusion only.
Adults: Reconstitute vial (20 mg or 40 mg) with 5 mL D_5W, NS, or LR. May administer dosage without further dilution over at least 3 minutes. May also be diluted in 50 mL D_5W, NS, or LR (0.4-0.8 mg/mL) and infused over 10-30 minutes.
Test Interactions Esomeprazole may falsely elevate serum chromogranin A (CgA) levels. The increased CgA level may cause false-positive results in the diagnosis of a neuroendocrine tumor. Temporarily stop esomeprazole ≥14 days prior to assessing CgA level; repeat level if initially elevated; use the same laboratory for all testing of CgA levels.
Dosage Forms Considerations
Esomeprazole strontium 24.65 mg is equivalent to 20 mg of esomeprazole base; esomeprazole strontium 49.3 mg is equivalent to 40 mg of esomeprazole base.
Dosage Forms Excipient information presented when available (limited, particularly for generics); consult specific product labeling. [DSC] = Discontinued product
Capsule Delayed Release, Oral, as magnesium [strength expressed as base]:
NexIUM: 20 mg, 40 mg [contains brilliant blue fcf (fd&c blue #1), fd&c red #40, fd&c yellow #10 (quinoline yellow)]
Capsule Delayed Release, Oral, as strontium:
Generic: 24.65 mg [DSC], 49.3 mg
Packet, Oral, as magnesium [strength expressed as base]:
NexIUM: 2.5 mg (30 ea); 5 mg (30 ea); 10 mg (30 ea); 20 mg (30 ea); 40 mg (30 ea)
Solution Reconstituted, Intravenous, as sodium [strength expressed as base]:
NexIUM I.V.: 20 mg (1 ea [DSC]); 40 mg (1 ea)
Generic: 20 mg (1 ea); 40 mg (1 ea)
References
Abraham NS, Hlatky MA, Antman EM, et al, "ACCF/ACG/AHA 2010 Expert Consensus Document on the Concomitant Use of Proton Pump Inhibitors and Thienopyridines: A Focused Update of the ACCF/ACG/AHA 2008 Expert Consensus Document on Reducing the Gastrointestinal Risks of Antiplatelet Therapy and NSAID Use: A Report of the American College of Cardiology Foundation Task

Force on Expert Consensus Documents," *Circulation*, 2010, 122 (24):2619-33.

Anderka M, Mitchell AA, Louik C, et al, "Medications Used to Treat Nausea and Vomiting of Pregnancy and the Risk of Selected Birth Defects," *Birth Defects Res A Clin Mol Teratol*, 2012, 94(1):22-30.

Canani RB, Cirillo P, Roggero P, et al, "Therapy With Gastric Acidity Inhibitors Increases the Risk of Acute Gastroenteritis and Community-Acquired Pneumonia in Children," *Pediatrics*, 2006, 117(5):e817-20.

Dohil R, Fidler M, Barshop B, et al, "Esomeprazole Therapy for Gastric Acid Hypersecretion in Children With Cystinosis," *Pediatr Nephrol*, 2005, 20(12):1786-93.

Erichsen R, Mikkelsen E, Pedersen L, et al, "Maternal Use of Proton Pump Inhibitors During Early Pregnancy and the Prevalence of Hypospadias in Male Offspring," *Am J Ther*, 2012.

Gibbons TE and Gold BD, "The Use of Proton Pump Inhibitors in Children: A Comprehensive Review," *Paediatr Drugs*, 2003, 5 (1):25-40.

Katz PO, Gerson LB, and Vela MF, "Guidelines for the Diagnosis and Management of Gastroesophageal Reflux Disease," *Am J Gastroenterol*, 2013, 108(3):308-28.

Kupiec TC, Aloumanis V, Ben M, et al, "Physical and Chemical Stability of Esomeprazole Sodium Solutions," *Ann Pharmacother*, 2008, 42 (9):1247-51.

Levine GN, Bates ER, Blankenship JC, et al, "2011 ACCF/AHA/SCAI Guideline for Percutaneous Coronary Intervention: A Report of the American College of Cardiology Foundation/American Heart Association Task Force on Practice Guidelines and the Society for Cardiovascular Angiography and Interventions," *Circulation*, 2011, 124(23): e574-651.

Lightdale JR, Gremse DA, and the Section on Gastroenterology, Hepatology, and Nutrition, "Gastroesophageal Reflux: Management Guidance for the Pediatrician," *Pediatrics*, 2013, 131(5):e1684-95.

Li J, Zhao J, Hamer-Maansson JE, et al, "Pharmacokinetic Properties of Esomeprazole in Adolescent Patients Aged 12 to 17 Years With Symptoms of Gastroesophageal Reflux Disease: A Randomized, Open-Label Study," *Clin Ther*, 2006, 28(3):419-27.

Omari T, Davidson G, Bondarov P, et al, "Pharmacokinetics and Acid-Suppressive Effects of Esomeprazole in Infants 1-24 Months Old With Symptoms of Gastroesophageal Reflux Disease," *J Pediatr Gastroenterol Nutr*, 2007, 45(5):530-7.

Omari T, Lundborg P, Sandström M, et al, "Pharmacodynamics and Systemic Exposure of Esomeprazole in Preterm Infants and Term Neonates With Gastroesophageal Reflux Disease," *J Pediatr*, 2009, 155(2):222-8.

Pasternak B and Hviid A, "Use of Proton-Pump Inhibitors in Early Pregnancy and the Risk of Birth Defects," *N Engl J Med*, 2010, 363 (22):2114-23.

White CM, Kalus JS, Quercia R, et al, "Delivery of Esomeprazole Magnesium Enteric-Coated Pellets Through Small Caliber and Standard Nasogastric Tubes and Gastrostomy Tubes *In Vitro*," *Am J Health Syst Pharm*, 2002, 59(21):2085-8.

Zhao J, Li J, Hamer-Maansson JE, et al, "Pharmacokinetic Properties of Esomeprazole in Children Aged 1 to 11 Years With Symptoms of Gastroesophageal Reflux Disease: A Randomized, Open-Label Study," *Clin Ther*, 2006, 28(11):1868-76.

♦ **Esomeprazole Magnesium** see Esomeprazole on page 793

♦ **Esomeprazole Sodium** see Esomeprazole on page 793

♦ **Esomeprazole Strontium** see Esomeprazole on page 793

♦ **E.S.P.®** see Erythromycin and Sulfisoxazole on page 785

♦ **Ester-C [OTC]** see Ascorbic Acid on page 206

♦ **Estrace** see Estradiol (Systemic) on page 796

♦ **Estradiol** see Estradiol (Systemic) on page 796

Estradiol (Systemic) (es tra DYE ole)

Medication Safety Issues

Sound-alike/look-alike issues:

Alora may be confused with Aldara

Elestrin may be confused with alosetron

BEERS Criteria medication:

This drug may be potentially inappropriate for use in geriatric patients (Quality of evidence - high [oral and transdermal patch]; Strength of recommendation - strong [oral and transdermal patch]).

Other safety issues:

Transdermal patch may contain conducting metal (eg, aluminum); remove patch prior to MRI.

International issues:

Vivelle: Brand name for estradiol [U.S. and multiple international markets, but also the brand name for ethinyl estradiol and norgestimate [Austria]

Related Information

Contraceptive Comparison Table on page 2266

Safe Handling of Hazardous Drugs on page 2419

Brand Names: U.S. Alora; Climara; Delestrogen; Depo-Estradiol; Divigel; Elestrin; Estrace; Estrasorb [DSC]; Estrogel; Evamist; Femring; Menostar; Minivelle; Vivelle-Dot

Brand Names: Canada Climara; Depo-Estradiol; Divigel; Estradot; EstroGel; Menostar; Oesclim; Sandoz-Estradiol Derm 100; Sandoz-Estradiol Derm 50; Sandoz-Estradiol Derm 75

Therapeutic Category Estrogen Derivative

Generic Availability (U.S.) May be product dependent

Use Treatment of hypoestrogenism (due to hypogonadism, castration, or primary ovarian failure), moderate to severe vasomotor symptoms of menopause, and moderate to severe symptoms of vulvar and vaginal atrophy due to menopause; palliative treatment of breast cancer in select patients; palliative treatment of androgen-dependent prostate cancer; prevention of osteoporosis in postmenopausal women; FDA approved in adults

Pregnancy Risk Factor X

Pregnancy Considerations In general, the use of estrogen and progestin as in combination hormonal contraceptives has not been associated with teratogenic effects when inadvertently taken early in pregnancy. These products are contraindicated for use during pregnancy.

Breast-Feeding Considerations Estrogens are excreted in breast milk and have been shown to decrease the quantity and quality of human milk. The manufacturer recommends that caution be used if administered to breast-feeding women. Monitor the growth of the infant closely.

Contraindications Hypersensitivity to estradiol or any component; history of or current DVT or PE; recent (eg, within past year) or current arterial thromboembolic disease (eg, MI, stroke); undiagnosed vaginal bleeding; pregnancy; known, suspected, or history of breast cancer (except in select patients being treated for metastatic disease); estrogen-dependent neoplasia; liver disease or dysfunction

Warnings Hazardous agent; use appropriate precautions for handling and disposal (NIOSH, 2012).

Estrogens have been reported to increase the risk of endometrial carcinoma **[U.S. Boxed Warning]**; adequate diagnostic measures, including endometrial sampling, if indicated, should be performed to rule out malignancy in all cases of undiagnosed abnormal vaginal bleeding; the addition of a progestin has been shown to decrease the risk of estrogen-induced endometrial hyperplasia, a condition thought to be a precursor to endometrial cancer. Do not use estrogens (with or without progestins) for the prevention of cardiovascular disease **[U.S. Boxed Warning]**; a significantly increased risk of MI, stroke, PE, DVT, and invasive breast cancer was reported in postmenopausal women receiving conjugated equine estrogens combined with medroxyprogesterone acetate (Rossouw, 2002); use of conjugated estrogens alone significantly increased the risk of stroke in postmenopausal women, but did not affect the risk of coronary heart disease (Women's Health Initiative Steering Committee, 2004); due to these risks, use estrogens (with or without progestins) at the lowest effective doses and for the shortest duration possible that is consistent with an individual's treatment goals and risks **[U.S. Boxed Warning]**; periodic risk:benefit assessments should be conducted; discontinue estrogens immediately if MI, stroke, PE, or DVT occur; in order to minimize the risk of thromboembolism in patients receiving estrogens, other risk factors for venous thromboembolism (eg, obesity, SLE, personal or family history of venous thromboembolism) and arterial vascular disease (eg, diabetes mellitus, hypertension, tobacco use, obesity, hypercholesterolemia) should be appropriately managed.

Since estrogens may increase the risk of venous thromboembolism, discontinue therapy, if possible, at least 4-6 weeks before surgery that is associated with an increased risk of thromboembolism, or during times of prolonged immobilization. Estrogens may increase the risk of breast cancer, gallbladder disease, hypercalcemia, and retinal vascular thrombosis (discontinue estrogen therapy in patients with sudden partial or complete loss of vision, sudden onset of diplopia, proptosis, or migraine, or if eye exam reveals retinal vascular lesions or papilledema). The combined use of conjugated equine estrogens and medroxyprogesterone acetate was reported to significantly increase the risk of probable dementia in postmenopausal women **[U.S. Boxed Warning]**; it is currently not known if these findings apply to younger women or to patients receiving estrogen alone.

Transdermal patch may contain conducting metal (eg, aluminum) which may cause a burn to the skin during an MRI scan; remove and dispose of patch prior to MRI. Apply new patch after scan is completed. Due to the potential for altered electrical conductivity, remove transdermal patch before cardioversion or defibrillation. Injection may contain benzyl alcohol and oral tablet may contain tartrazine, both of which may cause allergic reactions in susceptible individuals; large amounts of benzyl alcohol (≥99 mg/kg/day) have been associated with a potentially fatal toxicity ("gasping syndrome") in neonates; avoid use of estradiol products containing benzyl alcohol in neonates; *in vitro* and animal studies have shown that benzoate, a metabolite of benzyl alcohol, displaces bilirubin from protein binding sites.

Estradiol may be absorbed by others upon physical contact with topical emulsion application site. Topical gel is alcohol based and is flammable; patients should avoid fire, flame, or smoking until the gel has dried (gel dries in 2-5 minutes after application); photosensitivity after gel application and effects of concurrent application of sunscreen with gel have not been evaluated; estradiol was **not** absorbed by others after physical contact with topical gel application site 1 hour after application.

Precautions Use with caution in patients with asthma, epilepsy, migraines, diabetes, hypothyroidism, hypocalcemia, hypercalcemia, endometriosis, porphyria, SLE, hepatic hemangioma, history of cholestatic jaundice due to past estrogen use or pregnancy, or cardiac, liver, or renal dysfunction. Estrogens may cause premature closure of the epiphyses in young individuals (with large and repeated doses over an extended period of time); may cause premature breast development in prepubertal girls or gynecomastia in boys; may include vaginal bleeding or vaginal cornification in girls; may increase risk of ovarian cancer; may increase blood pressure; may cause fluid retention; may greatly increase triglycerides and lead to pancreatitis and other problems in patients with familial defects of lipoprotein metabolism.

Adverse Reactions Some adverse reactions observed with estrogen and/or progestin combination therapy.

Cardiovascular: Chest pain, DVT, edema, hypertension, MI, stroke, syncope, TIA, vasodilation, venous thromboembolism

Central nervous system: Anxiety, dementia, dizziness, epilepsy exacerbation, headache, insomnia, irritability, mental depression, migraine, mood disturbances, nervousness

Dermatologic: Angioedema, chloasma, dermatitis, erythema multiforme, erythema nodosum, hemorrhagic eruption, hirsutism, loss of scalp hair, melasma, rash, pruritus, urticaria

Endocrine & metabolic: Breast cancer, breast enlargement, breast pain, breast tenderness, carbohydrate intolerance, fibrocystic breast changes, fluid retention, galactorrhea, hot flashes, hypocalcemia, libido changes, nipple discharge, nipple pain

Gastrointestinal: Abdominal cramps, abdominal pain, bloating, cholecystitis, cholelithiasis, constipation, diarrhea, dyspepsia, flatulence, gallbladder disease, gastritis, nausea, pancreatitis, vomiting, weight gain/loss

Genitourinary: Alterations in frequency and flow of bleeding patterns, breakthrough bleeding, cervical ectropion changes, cervical secretion changes, cystitis, dysmenorrhea, endometrial cancer, endometrial hyperplasia, genital eruption, menorrhagia, metrorrhagia, ovarian cancer, ovarian cyst, Pap smear suspicious, spotting, uterine leiomyomata size increased, leukorrhea, uterine cancer, uterine enlargement, uterine pain, urinary incontinence, urogenital pruritus, vaginal candidiasis, vaginal discharge, vaginal moniliasis, vaginitis

Hematologic: Aggravation of porphyria

Hepatic: Cholestatic jaundice, hepatic hemangioma enlargement

Local: Thrombophlebitis

Gel, spray: Application site reaction

Transdermal patches: Erythema, irritation

Neuromuscular & skeletal: Arthralgia, back pain, chorea, leg cramps, myalgia, muscle cramps, skeletal pain, weakness

Ocular: Blindness, contact lens intolerance, corneal curvature steepening, retinal vascular thrombosis

Respiratory: Asthma exacerbation, pulmonary thromboembolism

Miscellaneous: Anaphylactoid/anaphylactic reactions, hypersensitivity reactions

Rare but important or life-threatening: Vaginal ring: Bowel obstruction, ring adherence to vaginal wall, toxic shock syndrome

Drug Interactions

Metabolism/Transport Effects Substrate of CYP1A2 (major), CYP2A6 (minor), CYP2B6 (minor), CYP2C19 (minor), CYP2C9 (minor), CYP2D6 (minor), CYP2E1 (minor), CYP3A4 (major), P-glycoprotein; **Note:** Assignment of Major/Minor substrate status based on clinically relevant drug interaction potential; **Inhibits** CYP1A2 (weak), CYP2C8 (weak); **Induces** CYP3A4 (weak/moderate)

Avoid Concomitant Use

Avoid concomitant use of Estradiol (Systemic) with any of the following: Anastrozole; Axitinib; Dehydroepiandrosterone; Exemestane; Indium 111 Capromab Pendetide; Ospemifene; Simeprevir

Increased Effect/Toxicity

Estradiol (Systemic) may increase the levels/effects of: Corticosteroids (Systemic); Ospemifene; ROPINIRole; Theophylline Derivatives; Tipranavir

The levels/effects of Estradiol (Systemic) may be increased by: Ascorbic Acid; Dehydroepiandrosterone; Herbs (Estrogenic Properties); NSAID (COX-2 Inhibitor); P-glycoprotein/ABCB1 Inhibitors

Decreased Effect

Estradiol (Systemic) may decrease the levels/effects of: Anastrozole; Anticoagulants; ARIPiprazole; Axitinib; Chenodiol; Exemestane; Hyaluronidase; Ibrutinib; Indium 111

Capromab Pendetide; Ospemifene; Saxagliptin; Simeprevir; Somatropin; Thyroid Products; Ursodiol

The levels/effects of Estradiol (Systemic) may be decreased by: Bosentan; Cannabis; CYP1A2 Inducers (Strong); CYP3A4 Inducers (Strong); Cyproterone; Dabrafenib; Deferasirox; Mitotane; Peginterferon Alfa-2b; P-glycoprotein/ABCB1 Inducers; Siltuximab; St Johns Wort; Tipranavir; Tocilizumab

Food Interactions Folic acid absorption may be decreased. Routine use of ethanol increases estrogen level and risk of breast cancer; may also increase the risk of osteoporosis. Management: Avoid ethanol.

Stability Hazardous agent; use appropriate precautions for handling and disposal (NIOSH, 2012).

Mechanism of Action Estrogens are responsible for the development and maintenance of the female reproductive system and secondary sexual characteristics. Estradiol is the principle intracellular human estrogen and is more potent than estrone and estriol at the receptor level; it is the primary estrogen secreted prior to menopause. Following menopause, estrone and estrone sulfate are more highly produced. Estrogens modulate the pituitary secretion of gonadotropins, luteinizing hormone, and follicle-stimulating hormone through a negative feedback system; estrogen replacement reduces elevated levels of these hormones in postmenopausal women.

Pharmacokinetics (Adult data unless noted)

Absorption: Oral: Well-absorbed

Distribution: Widely distributes throughout the body; sex hormone target organs contain higher concentrations; distributes into breast milk

Protein binding: Primarily bound to sex hormone-binding globulin and albumin

Metabolism: Hepatic, via cytochrome P450 isoenzyme CYP3A4; estradiol is converted to estrone and estriol; estrone is also converted to estriol and is converted to estradiol (**Note:** A dynamic equilibrium of metabolic interconversions between estrogens exists in the circulation); estrogens also undergo hepatic sulfate and glucuronide conjugation and enterohepatic recirculation

Elimination: Excreted in the urine as estradiol, estrone, and estriol and glucuronide and sulfate conjugates

Dosing: Usual Adolescents and Adults: **Note:** Use lowest effective dose for shortest duration possible that is consistent with an individual's treatment goals and risks; all dosage needs to be adjusted based upon the patient's response

Female hypogonadism:
I.M.:
Cypionate: 1.5-2 mg given once each month
Valerate: 10-20 mg given once each month
Oral: 0.5-2 mg/day in a cyclic regimen (3 weeks on drug, 1 week off)
Transdermal:
Once-weekly patch (Climara®): Initial: 0.025 mg/day patch applied once weekly (titrate dosage to response)
Twice-weekly patch: Alora®, Estraderm®: Initial: 0.05 mg patch; Vivelle Dot®: Initial: 0.0375 mg patch; titrate dosage to response; apply patch twice weekly in a cyclic regimen (3 weeks on drug, 1 week off) in patients with intact uterus and continuously in patients without a uterus
Vaginal ring: Moderate to severe vasomotor symptoms associated with menopause; vulvar/vaginal atrophy:
Femring™: 0.05 mg intravaginally; following insertion, ring should remain in place for 3 months; dose may be increased to 0.1 mg if needed
Topical emulsion: Moderate to severe vasomotor symptoms associated with menopause: 3.48 g (contents of 2 pouches) applied once daily in the morning

Topical gel: Moderate to severe vasomotor symptoms associated with menopause or vulvar and vaginal atrophy
Divigel®: 0.25-1 g/day
Elestrin®: 0.87 g applied once daily at the same time each day; adjust dose based on patient response. Dosing range: 0.87-1.7 g/day
EstroGel®: 1.25 g applied once daily at the same time each day
Topical spray: Evamist™: Initial: One spray (1.53 mg) per day. Adjust dose based on patient response. Dosing range: 1-3 sprays per day

Administration

Oral: Administer with food or after a meal to reduce GI upset
Parenteral: Injection for I.M. use only
Transdermal: Apply to clean, dry area; do not apply to breasts; do not apply to waistline (may loosen patch); rotate application sites

Hazardous agent; use appropriate precautions for handling and disposal (NIOSH, 2012).

Monitoring Parameters Blood pressure, weight, serum calcium, glucose, liver enzymes; bone maturation and epiphyseal effects in young patients in whom bone growth is not complete; breast exam, mammogram, Papanicolaou smear, signs for endometrial cancer in female patients with a uterus; bone density measurement if used for prevention of osteoporosis

Test Interactions Reduced response to metyrapone test.

Additional Information See package insert for doses related to postmenopausal symptoms, prevention of osteoporosis in postmenopausal women, and palliative treatment of breast cancer or androgen-dependent prostate cancer in adults.

Dosage Forms Excipient information presented when available (limited, particularly for generics); consult specific product labeling. [DSC] = Discontinued product

Emulsion, Transdermal, as hemihydrate:
Estrasorb: 4.35 mg/1.74 g (1.74 g [DSC]) [contains polysorbate 80, soybean oil]
Gel, Transdermal:
Divigel: 0.25 mg/0.25 g (1 ea); 0.5 mg/0.5 g (1 ea); 1 mg/g (1 g) [contains alcohol, usp, trolamine (triethanolamine)]
Elestrin: 0.06% (26 g) [contains alcohol, usp, edetate disodium, propylene glycol, trolamine (triethanolamine)]
Estrogel: 0.06% (50 g) [contains alcohol, usp, trolamine (triethanolamine)]
Oil, Intramuscular, as cypionate:
Depo-Estradiol: 5 mg/mL (5 mL)
Oil, Intramuscular, as valerate:
Delestrogen: 10 mg/mL (5 mL) [contains chlorobutanol (chlorobutol), sesame oil]
Delestrogen: 20 mg/mL (5 mL); 40 mg/mL (5 mL) [contains benzyl alcohol]
Generic: 10 mg/mL (5 mL); 20 mg/mL (5 mL); 40 mg/mL (5 mL)
Patch Biweekly, Transdermal:
Alora: 0.025 mg/24 hr (1 ea, 8 ea); 0.05 mg/24 hr (1 ea, 8 ea); 0.075 mg/24 hr (1 ea, 8 ea); 0.1 mg/24 hr (1 ea, 8 ea)
Minivelle: 0.0375 mg/24 hr (8 ea); 0.05 mg/24 hr (8 ea); 0.075 mg/24 hr (8 ea); 0.1 mg/24 hr (8 ea)
Vivelle-Dot: 0.025 mg/24 hr (8 ea); 0.0375 mg/24 hr (1 ea, 8 ea); 0.05 mg/24 hr (1 ea, 8 ea); 0.075 mg/24 hr (1 ea, 8 ea); 0.1 mg/24 hr (1 ea, 8 ea)
Patch Weekly, Transdermal:
Climara: 0.025 mg/24 hr (4 ea); 0.0375 mg/24 hr (4 ea); 0.05 mg/24 hr (1 ea, 4 ea); 0.06 mg/24 hr (4 ea); 0.075 mg/24 hr (4 ea); 0.1 mg/24 hr (1 ea, 4 ea)
Menostar: 14 mcg/24 hr (4 ea)

Generic: 0.025 mg/24 hr (4 ea); 0.0375 mg/24 hr (4 ea); 0.05 mg/24 hr (4 ea); 0.06 mg/24 hr (4 ea); 0.075 mg/24 hr (4 ea); 0.1 mg/24 hr (4 ea)

Ring, Vaginal, as acetate:
Femring: 0.05 mg/24 hr (1 ea); 0.1 mg/24 hr (1 ea)

Solution, Transdermal:
Evamist: 1.53 mg/spray (8.1 mL) [contains alcohol, usp, octyl salicylate]

Tablet, Oral:
Estrace: 0.5 mg, 1 mg, 2 mg [scored]
Generic: 0.5 mg, 1 mg, 2 mg

References

National Institute for Occupational Safety and Health (NIOSH), "NIOSH List of Antineoplastic and Other Hazardous Drugs in Healthcare Settings 2012." Available at http://www.cdc.gov/niosh/docs/2012-150/pdfs/2012-150.pdf. Accessed January 21, 2013.

Rossouw JE, Anderson GL, Prentice RL, et al, "Risks and Benefits of Estrogen Plus Progestin in Healthy Postmenopausal Women: Principal Results From the Women's Health Initiative Randomized Controlled Trial," *JAMA*, 2002, 288(3):321-33.

Women's Health Initiative Steering Committee, "Effects of Conjugated Equine Estrogen in Postmenopausal Women With Hysterectomy: The Women's Health Initiative Randomized Controlled Trial," *JAMA*, 2004, 291(14):1701-12.

◆ **Estradiol Acetate** *see* Estradiol (Systemic) *on page 796*

◆ **Estradiol Transdermal** *see* Estradiol (Systemic) *on page 796*

◆ **Estradiol Valerate** *see* Estradiol (Systemic) *on page 796*

◆ **Estradot (Can)** *see* Estradiol (Systemic) *on page 796*

◆ **Estrasorb [DSC]** *see* Estradiol (Systemic) *on page 796*

◆ **Estrogel** *see* Estradiol (Systemic) *on page 796*

◆ **EstroGel (Can)** *see* Estradiol (Systemic) *on page 796*

◆ **Estrogenic Substances, Conjugated** *see* Estrogens (Conjugated/Equine, Systemic) *on page 799*

◆ **Estrogenic Substances, Conjugated** *see* Estrogens (Conjugated/Equine, Topical) *on page 801*

Estrogens (Conjugated/Equine, Systemic) (ES troe jenz KON joo gate ed, EE kwine)

Medication Safety Issues
Sound-alike/look-alike issues:
Premarin® may be confused with Primaxin®, Provera®, Remeron®

BEERS Criteria medication:
This drug may be potentially inappropriate for use in geriatric patients (Quality of evidence - high [oral]; Strength of recommendation - strong [oral]).

Related Information
Contraceptive Comparison Table *on page 2266*
Safe Handling of Hazardous Drugs *on page 2419*

Brand Names: U.S. Premarin

Brand Names: Canada C.E.S.®; Congest; PMS-Conjugated Estrogens C.S.D.; Premarin®

Therapeutic Category Estrogen Derivative

Generic Availability (U.S.) No

Use Treatment of dysfunctional uterine bleeding, hypoestrogenism (due to hypogonadism, castration, or primary ovarian failure), moderate to severe vasomotor symptoms of menopause; moderate to severe symptoms of vulvar and vaginal atrophy due to menopause; palliative treatment of breast cancer in select patients; palliative treatment of androgen-dependent prostate cancer; prevention of osteoporosis in postmenopausal women; **Note:** Intravenous product is indicated for short-term use only

Pregnancy Considerations Estrogens are not indicated for use during pregnancy or immediately postpartum. In general, the use of estrogen and progestin as in combination hormonal contraceptives have not been associated with teratogenic effects when inadvertently taken early in pregnancy. These products are contraindicated for use during pregnancy.

Breast-Feeding Considerations Estrogen has been shown to decrease the quantity and quality of human milk. Use only if clearly needed. Monitor the growth of the infant closely.

Contraindications Hypersensitivity to estrogens or any component; history of or current DVT or PE; recent (eg, within past year) or current arterial thromboembolic disease (eg, MI, stroke); undiagnosed vaginal bleeding; pregnancy; known, suspected, or history of breast cancer (except in select patients being treated for metastatic disease); estrogen-dependent neoplasia; liver disease or dysfunction

Warnings Hazardous agent; use appropriate precautions for handling and disposal (NIOSH, 2012).

Estrogens have been reported to increase the risk of endometrial carcinoma **[U.S. Boxed Warning]**; adequate diagnostic measures, including endometrial sampling, if indicated, should be performed to rule out malignancy in all cases of undiagnosed abnormal vaginal bleeding; the addition of a progestin has been shown to decrease the risk of estrogen-induced endometrial hyperplasia, a condition thought to be a precursor to endometrial cancer. Do not use estrogens (with or without progestins) for the prevention of cardiovascular disease **[U.S. Boxed Warning]**; a significantly increased risk of MI, stroke, PE, DVT, and invasive breast cancer was reported in postmenopausal women receiving conjugated equine estrogens combined with medroxyprogesterone acetate (Rossouw, 2002); use of conjugated estrogens alone significantly increased the risk of stroke in postmenopausal women, but did not affect the risk of coronary heart disease (Women's Health Initiative Steering Committee, 2004); due to these risks, use estrogens (with or without progestins) at the lowest effective doses and for the shortest duration possible that is consistent with an individual's treatment goals and risks; periodic risk:benefit assessments should be conducted; discontinue estrogens immediately if MI, stroke, PE, or DVT occur; in order to minimize the risk of thromboembolism in patients receiving estrogens, other risk factors for venous thromboembolism (eg, obesity, SLE, personal or family history of venous thromboembolism) and arterial vascular disease (eg, diabetes mellitus, hypertension, tobacco use, obesity, and hypercholesterolemia) should be appropriately managed.

Since estrogens may increase the risk of venous thromboembolism, discontinue therapy, if possible, at least 4-6 weeks before surgery that is associated with an increased risk of thromboembolism, or during times of prolonged immobilization. Estrogens may increase the risk of breast cancer, gallbladder disease, hypercalcemia, and retinal vascular thrombosis (discontinue estrogen therapy in patients with sudden partial or complete loss of vision, sudden onset of diplopia, proptosis, or migraine, or if eye exam reveals retinal vascular lesions or papilledema). The combined use of conjugated equine estrogens and medroxyprogesterone acetate was reported to significantly increase the risk of probable dementia in postmenopausal women; it is currently not known if these findings apply to younger women or to patients receiving estrogen alone.

Precautions Use with caution in patients with asthma, epilepsy, migraines, diabetes, hypothyroidism, hypocalcemia, hypercalcemia, endometriosis, porphyria, SLE, hepatic hemangioma, history of cholestatic jaundice due to past estrogen use or pregnancy, cardiac, liver, or renal dysfunction. Estrogens may cause premature closure of the epiphyses in young individuals (with large and repeated doses over an extended period of time); may cause premature breast development in prepubertal girls or gynecomastia in boys; may induce vaginal bleeding or vaginal cornification in girls; may increase risk of ovarian cancer. May increase blood pressure; may cause fluid retention; may greatly increase triglycerides and lead to pancreatitis and other problems in patients with familial defects of lipoprotein metabolism.

Adverse Reactions

Central nervous system: Depression, dizziness, headache, nervousness, pain

Dermatologic: Pruritus

Endocrine & metabolic: Breast pain

Gastrointestinal: Abdominal pain, diarrhea, flatulence

Genitourinary: Leukorrhea, vaginal hemorrhage, vaginal moniliasis, vaginitis

Neuromuscular & skeletal: Arthralgia, back pain, leg cramps, weakness

Respiratory: Cough increased, pharyngitis, sinusitis

Additional adverse reactions reported with injection; frequency not defined: Local: injection site: Edema, pain, phlebitis

Rare but important or life-threatening: Alopecia, anaphylaxis, angioedema, asthma exacerbation, benign meningioma (possible growth), bloating, breast cancer, breast discharge/enlargement/tenderness, cervical secretion changes, chloasma, cholestatic jaundice, contact lens intolerance, dementia, deep vein thrombosis (DVT), dysmenorrhea, edema, endometrial cancer, endometrial hyperplasia, epilepsy exacerbation, erythema multiforme, erythema nodosum, fibrocystic breast changes, galactorrhea, gallbladder disease, glucose intolerance, gynecomastia (males), hepatic hemangiomas (enlargement), hirsutism, hypersensitivity reactions, hypertension, irritability, ischemic colitis, libido changes, melasma, MI, migraine, mood disturbances, nausea, ovarian cancer, pancreatitis, pulmonary emboli (PE), pelvic pain, porphyria exacerbation, rash, retinal vascular thrombosis, stroke, superficial venous thrombosis, thrombophlebitis, triglyceride increase, urticaria, uterine bleeding (abnormal), uterine leiomyomata (increase in size), vaginal candidiasis, vomiting, weight changes

Drug Interactions

Metabolism/Transport Effects Substrate of CYP1A2 (major), CYP2A6 (minor), CYP2B6 (minor), CYP2C19 (minor), CYP2C9 (minor), CYP2D6 (minor), CYP2E1 (minor), CYP3A4 (major); **Note:** Assignment of Major/Minor substrate status based on clinically relevant drug interaction potential; **Inhibits** CYP1A2 (weak); **Induces** CYP3A4 (weak/moderate)

Avoid Concomitant Use

Avoid concomitant use of Estrogens (Conjugated/Equine, Systemic) with any of the following: Anastrozole; Axitinib; Dehydroepiandrosterone; Exemestane; Indium 111 Capromab Pendetide; Ospemifene; Simeprevir

Increased Effect/Toxicity

Estrogens (Conjugated/Equine, Systemic) may increase the levels/effects of: Corticosteroids (Systemic); Ospemifene; ROPINIRole; Theophylline Derivatives; Tipranavir

The levels/effects of Estrogens (Conjugated/Equine, Systemic) may be increased by: Ascorbic Acid; Dehydroepiandrosterone; Herbs (Estrogenic Properties); NSAID (COX-2 Inhibitor)

Decreased Effect

Estrogens (Conjugated/Equine, Systemic) may decrease the levels/effects of: Anastrozole; Anticoagulants; ARIPiprazole; Axitinib; Chenodiol; Exemestane; Hyaluronidase; Ibrutinib; Indium 111 Capromab Pendetide; Ospemifene; Saxagliptin; Simeprevir; Somatropin; Thyroid Products; Ursodiol

The levels/effects of Estrogens (Conjugated/Equine, Systemic) may be decreased by: Bosentan; Cannabis; CYP1A2 Inducers (Strong); CYP3A4 Inducers (Strong); Cyproterone; Dabrafenib; Deferasirox; Mitotane; Peginterferon Alfa-2b; Siltuximab; St Johns Wort; Tipranavir; Tocilizumab

Food Interactions Folic acid absorption may be decreased. Routine use of ethanol increases estrogen level and risk of breast cancer; may also increase the risk of osteoporosis. Management: Avoid ethanol.

Stability Hazardous agent; use appropriate precautions for handling and disposal (NIOSH, 2012).

Injection: Store unreconstituted vials in the refrigerator at 2°C to 8°C (36°F to 46°F); if reconstituted solution is not used within a few hours, store under refrigeration; reconstituted solution is stable for 60 days when stored under refrigeration; compatible with NS, dextrose, and invert sugar solutions; not compatible with ascorbic acid, protein hydrolysate, or acidic pH

Mechanism of Action Conjugated estrogens contain a mixture of estrone sulfate, equilin sulfate, 17 alpha-dihydroequilin, 17 alpha-estradiol and 17 beta-dihydroequilin. Estrogens are responsible for the development and maintenance of the female reproductive system and secondary sexual characteristics. Estradiol is the principle intracellular human estrogen and is more potent than estrone and estriol at the receptor level; it is the primary estrogen secreted prior to menopause. Following menopause, estrone and estrone sulfate are more highly produced. Estrogens modulate the pituitary secretion of gonadotropins, luteinizing hormone, and follicle-stimulating hormone through a negative feedback system; estrogen replacement reduces elevated levels of these hormones in postmenopausal women.

Pharmacokinetics (Adult data unless noted)

Absorption: Oral, transmucosal, transdermal: Well absorbed

Distribution: Widely distributes throughout the body; sex hormone target organs contain higher concentrations; distributes into breast milk

Protein binding: Primarily bound to sex hormone-binding globulin and albumin

Metabolism: Hepatic, via cytochrome P450 isoenzyme CYP3A4; estradiol is converted to estrone and estriol; estrone is also converted to estriol and is converted to estradiol (**Note:** A dynamic equilibrium of metabolic interconversions between estrogens exists in the circulation); estrogens also undergo hepatic sulfate and glucuronide conjugation and enterohepatic recirculation

Elimination: Excreted in the urine as estradiol, estrone, estriol (major urinary metabolite), and glucuronide and sulfate conjugates

Dosing: Usual

Adolescents and Adults: **Note:** Use lowest effective dose for the shortest duration possible that is consistent with an individual's treatment goals and risks:

Female castration or primary ovarian failure: Oral: Cyclic regimen: 1.25 mg/day for 3 weeks, then no drug for the 4th week per cycle; repeat; titrate dose to response; use lowest effective dose

Female hypogonadism: Oral:

Manufacturer's recommendation: Cyclic regimen: 0.3-0.625 mg/day for 3 weeks, then no drug for the 4th week per cycle; titrate dose to response; use lowest effective dose

Alternative dosing: 2.5-7.5 mg/day in divided doses for 20 days, off 10 days and repeat until menses occur

Dysfunctional uterine bleeding:

Stable hematocrit: Oral: 1.25 mg twice daily for 21 days; if bleeding persists after 48 hours, increase to 2.5 mg twice daily; if bleeding persists after 48 more hours, increase to 2.5 mg 4 times/day; some recommend starting at 2.5 mg 4 times/day (**Note:** Medroxyprogesterone acetate 10 mg/day is also given on days 17-21; Neistein, 1991)

Alternatively: Oral: 2.5-5 mg/day for 7-10 days; then decrease to 1.25 mg/day for 2 weeks

Unstable hematocrit: Oral, I.V.: 5 mg 2-4 times/day; if bleeding is profuse, 20-40 mg every 4 hours up to 24 hours may be used; **Note:** A progestational-weighted contraception pill should also be given (eg, Ovral® 2 tablets stat and 1 tablet 4 times/day or medroxyprogesterone acetate 5-10 mg 4 times/day; Neistein, 1991)

Alternatively: I.M., I.V.: 25 mg every 6-12 hours until bleeding stops

Administration

Oral: Administer with food or after eating to reduce GI upset; administration of dose at bedtime may decrease adverse effects

Parenteral: Add 5 mL SWI slowly against the side of the vial and shake gently; use immediately after reconstitution. I.V.: Administer slow I.V. to avoid vascular flushing; I.M.: may be administered I.M. for dysfunctional uterine bleeding, but I.V. use is preferred (more rapid response)

Hazardous agent; use appropriate precautions for handling and disposal (NIOSH, 2012).

Monitoring Parameters Blood pressure, weight, serum calcium, glucose, liver enzymes; dysfunctional uterine bleeding: Hematocrit, hemoglobin, PT; bone maturation and epiphyseal effects in young patients in whom bone growth is not complete; breast exam, mammogram, Papanicolaou smear, signs for endometrial cancer in female patients with a uterus; bone density measurement if used for prevention of osteoporosis

Test Interactions Reduced response to metyrapone test.

Additional Information See package insert for doses related to postmenopausal symptoms, prevention of osteoporosis in postmenopausal women, and palliative treatment of breast cancer or androgen-dependent prostate cancer in adults.

Dosage Forms Excipient information presented when available (limited, particularly for generics); consult specific product labeling.

Solution Reconstituted, Injection:
Premarin: 25 mg (1 ea) [contains benzyl alcohol]

Tablet, Oral:
Premarin: 0.3 mg [contains fd&c blue #2 (indigotine), fd&c yellow #10 (quinoline yellow)]

Premarin: 0.45 mg [contains fd&c blue #2 (indigotine)]

Premarin: 0.625 mg [contains fd&c blue #2 (indigotine), fd&c red #40]

Premarin: 0.9 mg

Premarin: 1.25 mg [contains fd&c yellow #10 (quinoline yellow), fd&c yellow #6 (sunset yellow)]

References

Minjarez DA and Bradshaw KD, "Abnormal Uterine Bleeding in Adolescents," *Obstet Gynecol Clin North Am*, 2000, 27(1):63-78.

Mitan LA and Slap GB, "Adolescent Menstrual Disorders. Update," *Med Clin North Am*, 2000, 84(4):851-68.

National Institute for Occupational Safety and Health (NIOSH), "NIOSH List of Antineoplastic and Other Hazardous Drugs in Healthcare Settings 2012." Available at http://www.cdc.gov/niosh/docs/2012-150/pdfs/2012-150.pdf. Accessed January 21, 2013.

Neistein LS, *Adolescent Health Care - A Practical Guide*, 2nd ed, Baltimore: Urban & Schwarzenberg, 1991, 661-6.

Rossouw JE, Anderson GL, Prentice RL, et al, "Risks and Benefits of Estrogen Plus Progestin in Healthy Postmenopausal Women: Principal Results From the Women's Health Initiative Randomized Controlled Trial," *JAMA*, 2002, 288(3):321-33.

Women's Health Initiative Steering Committee, "Effects of Conjugated Equine Estrogen in Postmenopausal Women With Hysterectomy: The Women's Health Initiative Randomized Controlled Trial," *JAMA*, 2004, 291(14):1701-12.

Estrogens (Conjugated/Equine, Topical)
(ES troe jenz KON joo gate ed, EE kwine)

Medication Safety Issues
Sound-alike/look-alike issues:
Premarin® may be confused with Primaxin®, Provera®, Remeron®

BEERS Criteria medication:
This drug may be potentially inappropriate for use in geriatric patients (Quality of evidence - moderate [topical]; Strength of recommendation - weak [topical]).

Related Information
Contraceptive Comparison Table *on page 2266*
Safe Handling of Hazardous Drugs *on page 2419*

Brand Names: U.S. Premarin
Brand Names: Canada Premarin®
Therapeutic Category Estrogen Derivative; Estrogen Derivative, Vaginal
Generic Availability (U.S.) No

Use Treatment of vulvar and vaginal atrophy; moderate to severe dyspareunia (pain during intercourse) due to vaginal/vulvar atrophy of menopause

Pregnancy Considerations Estrogens are not indicated for use during pregnancy or immediately postpartum. In general, the use of estrogen and progestin as in combination hormonal contraceptives have not been associated with teratogenic effects when inadvertently taken early in pregnancy. These products are contraindicated for use during pregnancy. Use of the vaginal cream may weaken latex found in condoms, diaphragms, or cervical caps.

Breast-Feeding Considerations Estrogen has been shown to decrease the quantity and quality of human milk. Use only if clearly needed. Monitor the growth of the infant closely.

Contraindications Hypersensitivity to estrogens or any component; history of or current DVT or PE; recent (eg, within past year) or current arterial thromboembolic disease (eg, MI, stroke); undiagnosed vaginal bleeding; pregnancy; known, suspected, or history of breast cancer (except in select patients being treated for metastatic disease); estrogen-dependent neoplasia; liver disease or dysfunction

Warnings Hazardous agent; use appropriate precautions for handling and disposal (NIOSH, 2012).

Estrogens have been reported to increase the risk of endometrial carcinoma **[U.S. Boxed Warning]**; adequate diagnostic measures, including endometrial sampling, if indicated, should be performed to rule out malignancy in all cases of undiagnosed abnormal vaginal bleeding; the addition of a progestin has been shown to decrease the risk of estrogen-induced endometrial hyperplasia, a condition thought to be a precursor to endometrial cancer. Do not use estrogens (with or without progestins) for the prevention of cardiovascular disease **[U.S. Boxed Warning]**; a significantly increased risk of MI, stroke, PE, DVT, and invasive breast cancer was reported in postmenopausal women receiving conjugated equine estrogens combined with medroxyprogesterone acetate (Rossouw, 2002); use of conjugated estrogens alone significantly increased the risk of stroke in postmenopausal women, but did not affect the risk of coronary heart disease (Women's Health Initiative Steering Committee, 2004); due to these risks, use estrogens (with or without progestins) at the lowest effective doses and for the shortest duration possible that is consistent with an individual's treatment goals and risks; periodic risk:benefit assessments should be conducted; discontinue estrogens immediately if MI, stroke, PE, or DVT occur; in order to minimize the risk of thromboembolism in patients receiving estrogens, other risk factors for venous thromboembolism (eg, obesity, SLE, personal or family history of venous thromboembolism) and arterial vascular disease (eg, diabetes mellitus, hypertension, tobacco use, obesity, and hypercholesterolemia) should be appropriately managed.

Since estrogens may increase the risk of venous thromboembolism, discontinue therapy, if possible, at least 4-6 weeks before surgery that is associated with an increased risk of thromboembolism, or during times of prolonged immobilization. Estrogens may increase the risk of breast cancer, gallbladder disease, hypercalcemia, and retinal vascular thrombosis (discontinue estrogen therapy in patients with sudden partial or complete loss of vision, sudden onset of diplopia, proptosis, or migraine, or if eye exam reveals retinal vascular lesions or papilledema). The combined use of conjugated equine estrogens and medroxyprogesterone acetate was reported to significantly increase the risk of probable dementia in postmenopausal women; it is currently not known if these findings apply to younger women or to patients receiving estrogen alone.

Systemic absorption may occur with intravaginal or topical use.

Precautions Use with caution in patients with asthma, epilepsy, migraines, diabetes, hypothyroidism, hypocalcemia, hypercalcemia, endometriosis, porphyria, SLE, hepatic hemangioma, history of cholestatic jaundice due to past estrogen use or pregnancy, cardiac, liver, or renal dysfunction. Estrogens may cause premature closure of the epiphyses in young individuals; may cause premature breast development in prepubertal girls or gynecomastia in boys; may induce vaginal bleeding or vaginal cornification in girls; may increase risk of ovarian cancer. May increase blood pressure; may cause fluid retention; may greatly increase triglycerides and lead to pancreatitis and other problems in patients with familial defects of lipoprotein metabolism. Estrogen vaginal creams may contribute to the failure of barrier contraceptives by weakening condoms, diaphragms, or cervical caps made of latex or rubber.

Adverse Reactions Due to systemic absorption, other adverse effects associated with systemic therapy may also occur. Reported with daily use:
Cardiovascular: Vasodilatation
Central nervous system: Pain
Endocrine & metabolic: Breast pain
Gastrointestinal: Abdominal pain
Genitourinary: Vaginitis
Neuromuscular & skeletal: Back pain, weakness
Rare but important or life-threatening: Anaphylactic reactions, breast cancer, deep vein thrombosis (DVT), dementia, depression, endometrial cancer, gallbladder disease, gynecomastia (males), hypertension, leukorrhea, MI, pulmonary emboli (PE), retinal vascular thrombosis, stroke, uterine leiomyomata (increase in size)

Drug Interactions

Metabolism/Transport Effects Substrate of CYP1A2 (major), CYP2A6 (minor), CYP2B6 (minor), CYP2C19 (minor), CYP2C9 (minor), CYP2D6 (minor), CYP2E1 (minor), CYP3A4 (major); **Note:** Assignment of Major/Minor substrate status based on clinically relevant drug interaction potential; **Inhibits** CYP1A2 (weak); **Induces** CYP3A4 (weak/moderate)

Avoid Concomitant Use

Avoid concomitant use of Estrogens (Conjugated/Equine, Topical) with any of the following: Anastrozole; Axitinib; Dehydroepiandrosterone; Exemestane; Indium 111 Capromab Pendetide; Ospemifene; Simeprevir

Increased Effect/Toxicity

Estrogens (Conjugated/Equine, Topical) may increase the levels/effects of: Corticosteroids (Systemic); Ospemifene; ROPINIRole; Theophylline Derivatives; Tipranavir

The levels/effects of Estrogens (Conjugated/Equine, Topical) may be increased by: Ascorbic Acid;

Dehydroepiandrosterone; Herbs (Estrogenic Properties); NSAID (COX-2 Inhibitor)

Decreased Effect

Estrogens (Conjugated/Equine, Topical) may decrease the levels/effects of: Anastrozole; Anticoagulants; ARIPiprazole; Axitinib; Chenodiol; Exemestane; Hyaluronidase; Ibrutinib; Indium 111 Capromab Pendetide; Ospemifene; Saxagliptin; Simeprevir; Somatropin; Thyroid Products; Ursodiol

The levels/effects of Estrogens (Conjugated/Equine, Topical) may be decreased by: Bosentan; Cannabis; CYP1A2 Inducers (Strong); CYP3A4 Inducers (Strong); Cyproterone; Dabrafenib; Deferasirox; Mitotane; Peginterferon Alfa-2b; Siltuximab; St Johns Wort; Tipranavir; Tocilizumab

Stability Hazardous agent; use appropriate precautions for handling and disposal (NIOSH, 2012).

Mechanism of Action Conjugated estrogens contain a mixture of estrone sulfate, equilin sulfate, 17 alpha-dihydroequilin, 17 alpha-estradiol and 17 beta-dihydroequilin. Estrogens are responsible for the development and maintenance of the female reproductive system and secondary sexual characteristics. Estradiol is the principle intracellular human estrogen and is more potent than estrone and estriol at the receptor level; it is the primary estrogen secreted prior to menopause. Following menopause, estrone and estrone sulfate are more highly produced. Estrogens modulate the pituitary secretion of gonadotropins, luteinizing hormone, and follicle-stimulating hormone through a negative feedback system; estrogen replacement reduces elevated levels of these hormones in postmenopausal women.

Pharmacokinetics (Adult data unless noted) Absorption: Transmucosal, transdermal: Well absorbed

Dosing: Usual Adults: Female:
Moderate to severe dyspareunia: Intravaginal: 0.5 g twice weekly (eg, Monday and Thursday) or once daily cyclically*
Vulvar and vaginal atrophy: Intravaginal: 0.5-2 g/day given cyclically*
*Cyclic administration: Either 3 weeks on, 1 week off or 25 days on, 5 days off

Administration Intravaginal: Use marked stopping points on applicator to measure prescribed dose; to administer, lay down on back and draw knees up; gently insert applicator into vagina and press plunger downward to deliver medication; wash plunger and barrel with mild soap and water after use; do not boil or use hot water.

Hazardous agent; use appropriate precautions for handling and disposal (NIOSH, 2012).

Monitoring Parameters Blood pressure, weight, serum calcium, glucose, liver enzymes; dysfunctional uterine bleeding; hematocrit, hemoglobin, PT; bone maturation and epiphyseal effects in young patients in whom bone growth is not complete; breast exam, mammogram, Papanicolaou smear, signs for endometrial cancer in female patients with a uterus

Test Interactions Reduced response to metyrapone test.

Dosage Forms Excipient information presented when available (limited, particularly for generics); consult specific product labeling.
Cream, Vaginal:
Premarin: 0.625 mg/g (30 g) [contains benzyl alcohol, cetyl alcohol, propylene glycol monostearate]

References
National Institute for Occupational Safety and Health (NIOSH), "NIOSH List of Antineoplastic and Other Hazardous Drugs in Healthcare Settings 2012." Available at http://www.cdc.gov/niosh/docs/2012-150/pdfs/2012-150.pdf. Accessed January 21, 2013.

Etanercept (et a NER sept)

Medication Safety Issues
Sound-alike/look-alike issues:
Enbrel may be confused with Levbid
Brand Names: U.S. Enbrel; Enbrel SureClick
Brand Names: Canada Enbrel
Therapeutic Category Antirheumatic, Disease Modifying; Tumor Necrosis Factor (TNF) Blocking Agent
Generic Availability (U.S.) No
Use Treatment of moderately- to severely-active polyarticular juvenile idiopathic arthritis (FDA approved in ages ≥2 years);treatment of signs and symptoms of moderately- to severely-active rheumatoid arthritis, psoriatic arthritis, and active ankylosing spondylitis (FDA approved in ages ≥18 years and adults); treatment of chronic (moderate to severe) plaque psoriasis in patients who are candidates for systemic therapy or phototherapy (FDA approved in ages ≥18 years and adults); has also been used as adjunctive therapy Kawasaki disease and for treatment of familial Mediterranean fever (colchicine refractory or colchicine intolerant), scleroderma, and chronic nonbacterial osteomyelitis
Medication Guide Available Yes
Pregnancy Risk Factor B
Pregnancy Considerations Adverse events were not observed in animal reproduction studies. Etanercept crosses the placenta. Following in utero exposure, concentrations in the newborn at delivery are 3-32% of the maternal serum concentration.

A pregnancy registry has been established to monitor outcomes of women exposed to etanercept during pregnancy (800-772-6436).

Breast-Feeding Considerations Etanercept is excreted into breast milk in low concentrations and is minimally absorbed by a nursing infant (limited data). The manufacturer recommends that caution be used if administered to a nursing woman, taking into account the importance of the drug to the mother and potential effects to the nursing infant. A lactation surveillance program has been established to monitor outcomes of breastfed infants exposed to etanercept (800-772-6436).

Contraindications Hypersensitivity to etanercept or any component; sepsis

Warnings Patients receiving etanercept are at increased risk for serious infections which may result in hospitalization and/or fatality **[U.S. Boxed Warning]**; risk factors for infection include age >65 years, comorbidities, and concomitant immunosuppressive therapy (eg, methotrexate or corticosteroids) and may present as disseminated (rather than local) disease. Active tuberculosis (or reactivation of latent tuberculosis); invasive fungal (including aspergillosis, blastomycosis, candidiasis, coccidioidomycosis, histoplasmosis, and pneumocystosis); and bacterial, viral, or other opportunistic infections (including legionellosis and listeriosis) have been reported in patients receiving TNF-blocking agents, including etanercept. Monitor closely for signs/symptoms of infection. Discontinue for serious infection or sepsis. Consider risks versus benefits prior to use in patients with a history of chronic or recurrent infection. Consider empiric antifungal therapy in patients who are at risk for invasive fungal infection and develop severe systemic illness. Caution should be exercised when considering use in the elderly or in patients with conditions that predispose them to infections (eg, diabetes) or residence/travel from areas of endemic mycoses (blastomycosis, coccidioidomycosis, histoplasmosis) or with latent or localized infections. Do not initiate etanercept therapy with clinically important active infection. Patients who develop a new infection while undergoing treatment should be monitored closely. Discontinue etanercept in a child who develops varicella infection or who has a significant exposure to varicella virus and consider prophylactic treatment with varicella-zoster immune globulin. Due to higher incidence of serious infections, etanercept should not be used in combination with anakinra or abatacept.

Tuberculosis (disseminated or extrapulmonary) has been reported in patients receiving etanercept **[U.S. Boxed Warning]**; both reactivation of latent infection and new infections have been reported. Patients should be evaluated for tuberculosis risk factors and for latent tuberculosis with a tuberculin skin test prior to starting and periodically during therapy. Treatment of latent tuberculosis should be initiated before etanercept is used; consider antituberculosis treatment if adequate course of treatment cannot be confirmed in patients with a history of latent or active tuberculosis or with risk factors despite negative skin test. Some patients who tested negative prior to therapy have developed active infection; monitor for signs and symptoms of tuberculosis in all patients.

Rare reactivation of hepatitis B (HBV) has occurred in chronic carriers of the virus, usually in patients receiving concomitant immunosuppressants; evaluate for HBV prior to initiation in all patients. Monitor during and for several months following discontinuation of treatment in HBV carriers; interrupt therapy if reactivation occurs and treat appropriately with antiviral therapy; if resumption of therapy is deemed necessary, exercise caution and monitor patient closely.

Hypersensitivity reactions may occur; if an anaphylactic reaction or other serious allergic reaction occurs, administration should be discontinued immediately and appropriate therapy initiated.

Rare (<0.1%) cases of CNS demyelinating disorders, such as multiple sclerosis, transverse myelitis, optic neuritis, Guillain-Barré syndrome, other peripheral demyelinating neuropathies, and seizure disorders have been reported in patients undergoing etanercept therapy; cases may present with mental status changes and some may be associated with permanent disability. Use with caution in patients with preexisting or recent onset CNS demyelinating disorders.

In children and adolescents, lymphomas and other malignancies, some fatal, have been reported with use of TNF blockers **[U.S. Boxed Warning]**. Use may affect defenses against malignancies; impact on the development and course of malignancies is not fully defined. In an analysis of children and adolescents who had received TNF blockers (etanercept and infliximab), the FDA identified 48 cases of malignancy. Of the 48 cases, ~50% were lymphomas (eg, Hodgkin's and non-Hodgkin's lymphoma) and other malignancies, such as leukemia, melanoma, and solid organ tumors, were also reported; malignancies rarely seen in children (eg, leiomyosarcoma, hepatic malignancies, and renal cell carcinoma) were also observed. Overall, in pediatric patients, the median onset of malignancy was after 30 months of therapy (range: 1-84 months); most of these cases (88%) were receiving other immunosuppressive medications (eg, azathioprine and methotrexate). As compared to the general population, an increased risk of lymphoma has been noted in clinical trials; however, rheumatoid arthritis has been previously associated with an increased rate of lymphoma. The role of TNF blockers in the development of malignancies in children cannot be excluded. The FDA also reviewed 147 postmarketing reports of leukemia (including acute myeloid leukemia, chronic lymphocytic leukemia, and chronic myeloid leukemia) in patients (children and adults) using TNF blockers. Average onset time to development of leukemia was within the first 1-2 years of TNF blocker initiation. Although most patients were receiving other

803

immunosuppressive agents, the role of TNF blockers in the development of leukemia could not be excluded. The FDA concluded that there is a possible association with the development of leukemia and the use of TNF blockers. Patients should be monitored closely for signs and symptoms suggestive of malignancy, evidence of which should result in prompt discontinuation of the medication and appropriate diagnostic evaluation.

Effect on fertility is unknown. Use is not recommended in patients with Wegener's granulomatosis receiving immunosuppressive therapy due to higher incidence of non-cutaneous solid malignancies. Positive antinuclear antibody titers have been detected in patients (with negative baselines). Rare cases of autoimmune disorders, including lupus-like syndrome or autoimmune hepatitis, have been reported; in JIA patients, rare inflammatory bowel disease has also been reported (vanDijken, 2011); monitor and discontinue therapy if symptoms develop.

Diluent for etanercept injection contains benzyl alcohol which may cause allergic reactions in susceptible individuals; large amounts of benzyl alcohol (≥99 mg/kg/day) have been associated with a potentially fatal toxicity ("gasping syndrome") in neonates; patients with latex allergy should not handle the needle cap on the prefilled syringe and on the SureClick autoinjector since it contains latex.

Precautions Use with caution in patients with moderate to severe alcoholic hepatitis; compared to placebo, the mortality rate in patients treated with etanercept was similar at one month but significantly higher after 6 months. Use with caution in patients with heart failure or decreased left ventricular function; worsening and new-onset heart failure has been reported. Use with caution in patients with a history of significant hematologic abnormalities; has been associated with pancytopenia and aplastic anemia (rare cases in postmarketing experience). Patients must be advised to seek medical attention if they develop signs and symptoms suggestive of blood dyscrasias; discontinue if significant hematologic abnormalities are confirmed. Patients should be brought up to date with all immunizations before initiating therapy. Live vaccines should not be given concurrently; there is no data available concerning secondary transmission of live vaccines in patients receiving therapy.

Adverse Reactions
Central nervous system: Dizziness, headache
Dermatologic: Pruritus, skin rash
Gastrointestinal: Abdominal pain (more common in children), diarrhea, nausea (children), vomiting
Infection: Infection
Local: Injection site reaction (bleeding, bruising, erythema, itching, pain, or swelling)
Neuromuscular & skeletal: Weakness
Respiratory: Cough, pharyngitis, respiratory distress, respiratory tract infection, rhinitis, sinusitis, upper respiratory tract infection
Miscellaneous: Antibody development (positive antidouble-stranded DNA antibodies), fever, positive ANA titer
Rare but important or life-threatening: Abscess, adenopathy, anemia, angioedema, anorexia, aplastic anemia, appendicitis, aseptic meningitis, aspergillosis, autoimmune hepatitis, blood coagulation disorder, bursitis, cardiac failure, cerebral ischemia, cerebrovascular accident, cholecystitis, cutaneous lupus erythematous, deep vein thrombosis, demyelinating disease of the central nervous system (suggestive of multiple sclerosis, transverse myelitis, or optic neuritis), depression, dermal ulcer, erythema multiforme, gastritis, gastroenteritis, gastrointestinal hemorrhage, glomerulopathy (membranous), herpes zoster, hydrocephalus (with normal pressure), hypersensitivity, hypersensitivity reaction, hypertension, hypotension, inflammatory bowel disease, interstitial pulmonary

disease, intestinal perforation, ischemic heart disease, leukemia, leukopenia, lupus-like syndrome, lymphadenopathy, malignant lymphoma, malignant melanoma, malignant neoplasm, Merkel cell carcinoma, myocardial infarction, multiple sclerosis, nephrolithiasis, neutropenia, optic neuritis, oral mucosa ulcer, pancreatitis, pancytopenia, pneumonia due to *Pneumocystis carinii*, polymyositis, psoriasis (including new onset, palmoplantar, pustular, or exacerbation), pulmonary disease, pulmonary embolism, reactivation of HBV, sarcoidosis, scleritis, seizure, skin carcinoma, Stevens-Johnson syndrome, subcutaneous nodule, thrombocytopenia, thrombophlebitis, toxic epidermal necrolysis, tuberculosis, tuberculous arthritis, urinary tract infection, uveitis, varicella zoster infection, vasculitis (cutaneous and systemic), weight gain

Drug Interactions
Metabolism/Transport Effects None known.
Avoid Concomitant Use
Avoid concomitant use of Etanercept with any of the following: Abatacept; Anakinra; BCG; Belimumab; Canakinumab; Certolizumab Pegol; Cyclophosphamide; InFLIXimab; Natalizumab; Pimecrolimus; Rilonacept; Tacrolimus (Topical); Tocilizumab; Tofacitinib; Vaccines (Live); Vedolizumab
Increased Effect/Toxicity
Etanercept may increase the levels/effects of: Abatacept; Anakinra; Belimumab; Canakinumab; Certolizumab Pegol; Cyclophosphamide; InFLIXimab; Leflunomide; Natalizumab; Rilonacept; Tofacitinib; Vaccines (Live); Vedolizumab

The levels/effects of Etanercept may be increased by: Denosumab; Pimecrolimus; Roflumilast; Tacrolimus (Topical); Tocilizumab; Trastuzumab
Decreased Effect
Etanercept may decrease the levels/effects of: BCG; Coccidioidin Skin Test; Sipuleucel-T; Vaccines (Inactivated); Vaccines (Live)

The levels/effects of Etanercept may be decreased by: Echinacea
Stability
Prefilled syringes, autoinjectors: Store at 2°C to 8°C (36°F to 46°F); do not freeze; protect from light; do not shake. The following stability information has also been reported: May be stored at room temperature for up to 4 days (Cohen, 2007).
Powder for reconstitution: Store at 2°C to 8°C (36°F to 46°F); do not freeze. Reconstituted solution prepared with bacteriostatic water for injection is stable for 14 days if refrigerated.
Mechanism of Action Etanercept is a recombinant DNA-derived protein composed of tumor necrosis factor receptor (TNFR) linked to the Fc portion of human IgG1. Etanercept binds tumor necrosis factor (TNF) and blocks its interaction with cell surface receptors. TNF plays an important role in the inflammatory processes and the resulting joint pathology of rheumatoid arthritis (RA), polyarticular-course juvenile idiopathic arthritis (JIA), ankylosing spondylitis (AS), and plaque psoriasis.
Pharmacodynamics
Onset of action: RA: 1-2 weeks
Maximum effect: RA: Full effect is usually seen within 3 months
Pharmacokinetics (Adult data unless noted)
Absorption: Absorbed slowly after SubQ injection
Distribution: V_d: 1.78-3.39 L/m^2
Bioavailability: SubQ: 60%
Half-life:
Children: 70-94.8 hours
Adults: 102 ± 30 hours
Time to peak serum concentration: SubQ: 69 ± 34 hours

Elimination: Clearance:
Children and Adolescents 4-17 years: 46 mL/hour/m^2
Adults: 160 ± 80 mL/hour

Dosing: Usual

Children and Adolescents:

Juvenile idiopathic arthritis: Children ≥2 years and Adolescents: SubQ:
Once-weekly dosing: 0.8 mg/kg/dose once weekly; maximum dose: 50 mg
Twice-weekly dosing: 0.4 mg/kg/dose twice weekly, given 72-96 hours apart; maximum dose: 25 mg (Lovell, 2000)

Kawasaki disease; acute, adjunct therapy: Limited data available: Infants ≥6 months and Children <6 years: SubQ: 0.8 mg/kg/dose for 3 doses; administer first dose within 24 hours after completion of I.V. immunoglobulin (day 0), the second dose at day 7, and third dose at day 14; maximum dose: 50 mg. Dosing based on an open-labeled pilot trial of 15 pediatric patients (mean age: 2.6 years); all patients also received standard aspirin therapy; no patients required retreatment or rescue therapy for signs/symptoms of Kawasaki disease (Choueiter, 2010). A large double-blind, placebo-controlled trial is ongoing [EATAK trial (NCT00841789)] utilizing the same dosage regimen; results pending (Portman, 2011).

Mediterranean fever; familial (FMF) (intolerance or resistance to colchicine): Very limited data available; efficacy results variable: Children ≥11 years and Adolescents: SubQ: 0.8 mg/kg once weekly; maximum dose: 50 mg; dosing based on a case series (n=3); results showed fewer attacks with treatment, median duration of therapy was 3 months and all patients continued colchicine therapy if able; over time, therapy was eventually changed to anakinra due to clinician determined unsatisfactory response (Akgul, 2012; Özen, 2011; Sakallioglu, 2006; Soriano, 2013); a case series in adult patients (n=5, age range: 20-40 years) reported no further attacks (80%) or decrease frequency (20%) with etanercept (25 mg twice weekly) therapy (Bilgen, 2011); further studies needed.

Plaque psoriasis: Limited data available: Children and Adolescents 4-17 years: SubQ: 0.8 mg/kg/dose once weekly; maximum dose: 50 mg; results of a long-term study (96 weeks) showed efficacy maintained and therapy generally well-tolerated (Paller, 2008; Paller, 2010; Siegfried, 2010)

Adolescents ≥18 years and Adults:

Plaque psoriasis: SubQ: Initial: 50 mg twice weekly (administered 72-96 hours apart) for 3 months; **Note:** Initial doses of 25 mg or 50 mg per week were also shown to be efficacious; maintenance dose: 50 mg once weekly

Rheumatoid arthritis, psoriatic arthritis, ankylosing spondylitis: SubQ:
Once-weekly dosing: 50 mg once weekly
Twice-weekly dosing: 25 mg given twice weekly (individual doses should be separated by 72-96 hours); maximum amount administered at a single injection site: 25 mg

Dosing adjustment in renal impairment: There are no dosage adjustment provided in manufacturer's labeling (has not been studied).

Dosing adjustment in hepatic impairment: There are no dosage adjustment provided in manufacturer's labeling (has not been studied).

Administration

Administer subcutaneously into thigh, abdomen, or upper arm. Rotate injection sites. New injections should be given at least one inch from an old site and never into areas where the skin is tender, bruised, red, or hard. **Note:** If the prescriber determines that it is appropriate, patients may self-inject after proper training in injection technique.

Multiple-use vial: To avoid foaming, add 1 mL of bacteriostatic water for injection slowly to 25 mg vial, gently swirl; do not shake or agitate vigorously; dissolution generally complete in <10 minutes; resulting solution is 25 mg/mL. Do not administer >25 mg at a single injection site if the multiple-use vial is used to prepare the dose.

Single-use prefilled syringe or autoinjector: Allow injection to reach room temperature (approximately 15-30 minutes); do not remove needle cover or needle shield during this period; solution may have small white particles of protein, which is normal for a proteinaceous solution; should not be used if cloudy, discolored or if foreign matter is present.

Monitoring Parameters Monitor improvement of symptoms and physical function assessments (eg, joint swelling, pain, and tenderness; ESR or C-reactive protein level). Latent TB screening prior to initiating and during therapy; signs/symptoms of infection (prior to, during, and following therapy); CBC with differential; signs/symptoms/worsening of heart failure; HBV screening prior to initiating (all patients), HBV carriers (during and for several months following therapy); signs and symptoms of hypersensitivity reaction; symptoms of lupus-like syndrome; signs/symptoms of malignancy (eg, splenomegaly, hepatomegaly, abdominal pain, persistent fever, night sweats, weight loss).

Dosage Forms Excipient information presented when available (limited, particularly for generics); consult specific product labeling.

Kit, Subcutaneous [preservative free]:
Enbrel: 25 mg [contains benzyl alcohol, tromethamine]
Solution, Subcutaneous [preservative free]:
Enbrel: 25 mg/0.5 mL (0.51 mL); 50 mg/mL (0.98 mL)
Enbrel SureClick: 50 mg/mL (0.98 mL)

References

Akgul O, Kilic E, Kilic G, et al, "Efficacy and Safety of Biologic Treatments in Familial Mediterranean Fever," *Am J Med Sci*, 2012, Dec 28.

Bilgen SA, Kilic L, Akdogan A, et al, "Effects of Anti-tumor Necrosis Factor Agents for Familial Mediterranean Fever Patients With Chronic Arthritis and/or Sacroiliitis Who Were Resistant to Colchicine Treatment," *J Clin Rheumatol*, 2011, 17(7):358-62.

Borzutzky A, Stern S, Reiff A, et al, "Pediatric Chronic Nonbacterial Osteomyelitis," *Pediatrics*, 2012, 130(5):e1190-7.

Choueiter NF, Olson AK, Shen DD, et al, "Prospective Open-Label Trial of Etanercept as Adjunctive Therapy for Kawasaki Disease," *J Pediatr*, 2010, 157(6):960-6.

Cohen V, Jellinek SP, Teperikidis L, et al, "Room-Temperature Storage of Medications Labeled for Refrigeration," *Am J Health-Syst Pharm*, 2007, 64(16):1711-15.

Lovell DJ, Reiff A, Jones OY, et al, "Long-Term Safety and Efficacy of Etanercept in Children With Polyarticular-Course Juvenile Rheumatoid Arthritis," *Arthritis Rheum*, 2006, 54(6):1987-94.

Moreland LW, Baumgartner SW, Schiff MH, et al, "Treatment of Rheumatoid Arthritis With a Recombinant Human Tumor Necrosis Factor Receptor (p75)-Fc Fusion Protein," *N Engl J Med*, 1997, 337 (3):141-7.

Özen S, Bilginer Y, Aktay Ayaz N, et al, "Anti-interleukin 1 Treatment for Patients With Familial Mediterranean Fever Resistant to Colchicine," *J Rheumatol*, 2011, 38(3):516-8.

Paller AS, Siegfried EC, Eichenfield LF, et al, "Long-Term Etanercept in Pediatric Patients With Plaque Psoriasis," *J Am Acad Dermatol*, 2010, 63(5):762-8.

Paller AS, Siegfried EC, Langley RG, et al, "Etanercept Treatment for Children and Adolescents With Plaque Psoriasis," *N Engl J Med*, 2008, 358(3):241-51.

Portman MA, Olson A, Soriano B, et al, "Etanercept as Adjunctive Treatment for Acute Kawasaki Disease: Study Design and Rationale," *Am Heart J*, 2011, 161(3):494-9.

Sakallioglu O, Duzova A, and Ozen S, "Enercept in the Treatment of Arthritis in a Patient With Familial Mediterranean Fever," *Clin Exp Rheumatol*, 2006, 24(4):435-7.

Siegfried EC, Eichenfield LF, Paller AS, et al, "Intermittent Etanercept Therapy in Pediatric Patients With Psoriasis," *J Am Acad Dermatol*, 2010, 63(5):769-74.

Soriano A, Verecchia E, Afeltra A, et al, "IL-1β Biological Treatment of Familial Mediterranean Fever," *Clin Rev Allergy Immunol*, 2013, Jan 16.

van Dijken TD, Vastert SJ, Gerloni VM, et al, "Development of Inflammatory Bowel Disease in Patients With Juvenile Idiopathic Arthritis Treated With Etanercept," *J Rheumatol*, 2011, 38(7):1441-6.

◆ **Ethacrynate Sodium** *see* Ethacrynic Acid *on page 806*

Ethacrynic Acid (eth a KRIN ik AS id)

Medication Safety Issues
Sound-alike/look-alike issues:
Edecrin may be confused with Eulexin, Ecotrin
Brand Names: U.S. Edecrin; Sodium Edecrin
Brand Names: Canada Edecrin; Sodium Edecrin
Therapeutic Category Antihypertensive Agent; Diuretic, Loop
Generic Availability (U.S.) No
Use Management of edema secondary to CHF, hepatic or renal disease; hypertension
Pregnancy Risk Factor B
Pregnancy Considerations Adverse events were not observed in animal reproduction studies.
Breast-Feeding Considerations It is not known if ethacrynic acid is excreted in breast milk. Due to the potential for serious adverse reactions in the nursing infant, a decision should be made whether to discontinue nursing or to discontinue the drug, taking into account the importance of treatment to the mother.
Contraindications Hypersensitivity to ethacrynic acid or any component; hypotension, hyponatremic dehydration, metabolic alkalosis with hypokalemia, or anuria
Warnings Loop diuretics are potent diuretics; excess amounts can lead to profound diuresis with fluid and electrolyte loss; close medical supervision and dose evaluation is required; may increase risk of gastric hemorrhage associated with corticosteroid treatment
Precautions Avoid use in patients with severe renal dysfunction (CrCl <10 mL/minute)
Adverse Reactions
Central nervous system: Apprehension, chills, confusion, encephalopathy (patients with preexisting liver disease), fatigue, fever, headache, vertigo
Dermatologic: Henoch-Schönlein purpura (IgA vasculitis) (in patient with rheumatic heart disease), skin rash
Endocrine & metabolic: Gout; hyperglycemia; hypoglycemia (occurred in two uremic patients who received doses above those recommended); hyponatremia; reversible hyperuricemia; variations in phosphorus, CO_2 content, bicarbonate, and calcium
Gastrointestinal: Abdominal discomfort or pain, acute pancreatitis (rare), anorexia, diarrhea, dysphagia, gastrointestinal bleeding, malaise, nausea, vomiting
Genitourinary: Hematuria
Hepatic: Abnormal liver function tests, jaundice
Hematology: Agranulocytosis, severe neutropenia, thrombocytopenia
Local: Local irritation and pain, thrombophlebitis (with intravenous use)
Ocular: Blurred vision
Otic: Temporary or permanent deafness, tinnitus
Renal: Increased serum creatinine
Drug Interactions
Metabolism/Transport Effects None known.
Avoid Concomitant Use
Avoid concomitant use of Ethacrynic Acid with any of the following: Furosemide
Increased Effect/Toxicity
Ethacrynic Acid may increase the levels/effects of: ACE Inhibitors; Allopurinol; Amifostine; Aminoglycosides; Antihypertensives; Cardiac Glycosides; CISplatin; Dofetilide; DULoxetine; Hypotensive Agents; Ivabradine; Lithium; Methotrexate; Neuromuscular-Blocking Agents; Obinutuzumab; RisperiDONE; RiTUXimab; Salicylates; Sodium Phosphates; Topiramate; Vitamin K Antagonists

The levels/effects of Ethacrynic Acid may be increased by: Alfuzosin; Analgesics (Opioid); Barbiturates; Beta2-Agonists; Brimonidine (Topical); Canagliflozin; Corticosteroids (Orally Inhaled); Corticosteroids (Systemic); CycloSPORINE (Systemic); Diazoxide; Furosemide; Herbs (Hypotensive Properties); Licorice; MAO Inhibitors; Methotrexate; Pentoxifylline; Phosphodiesterase 5 Inhibitors; Probenecid; Prostacyclin Analogues
Decreased Effect
Ethacrynic Acid may decrease the levels/effects of: Hypoglycemic Agents; Lithium; Neuromuscular-Blocking Agents

The levels/effects of Ethacrynic Acid may be decreased by: Bile Acid Sequestrants; Fosphenytoin; Herbs (Hypertensive Properties); Methotrexate; Methylphenidate; Nonsteroidal Anti-Inflammatory Agents; Phenytoin; Probenecid; Salicylates; Yohimbine
Stability When reconstituted with 50 mL D_5W or NS, resultant solution (1 mg/mL) is stable for 24 hours at room temperature
Mechanism of Action Inhibits reabsorption of sodium and chloride in the ascending loop of Henle and distal renal tubule, interfering with the chloride-binding cotransport system, thus causing increased excretion of water, sodium, chloride, magnesium, and calcium
Pharmacodynamics
Onset of action:
Oral: Within 30 minutes
I.V.: 5 minutes
Peak effect:
Oral: 2 hours
I.V.: 15-30 minutes
Duration:
Oral: 6-8 hours
I.V.: 2 hours
Pharmacokinetics (Adult data unless noted)
Absorption: Oral: Rapid
Protein binding: >90%
Metabolism: In the liver to active cysteine conjugate (35% to 40%)
Elimination: In bile, 30% to 60% excreted unchanged in urine
Dosing: Usual
Children:
Oral: 1 mg/kg/dose once daily, increase at intervals of 2-3 days to a maximum of 3 mg/kg/day
I.V.: 1 mg/kg/dose; repeat doses are not routinely recommended, however if indicated, repeat doses every 8-12 hours
Adults:
Oral: 25-400 mg/day in 1-2 divided doses
I.V.: 0.5-1 mg/kg/dose (maximum dose: 100 mg/dose); repeat doses not routinely recommended, however if indicated, repeat every 8-12 hours
Administration
Oral: Administer with food or milk
Parenteral: Dilute injection with 50 mL D_5W or NS (1 mg/mL concentration resulting); maximum concentration 2 mg/mL; may be injected without further dilution over a period of several minutes or infused over 20-30 minutes; tissue irritant; not to be administered I.M. or SubQ
Monitoring Parameters Serum electrolytes, blood pressure, renal function, hearing
Additional Information Injection contains thimerosal
Dosage Forms Excipient information presented when available (limited, particularly for generics); consult specific product labeling.
Solution Reconstituted, Intravenous, as ethacrynate sodium:
Sodium Edecrin: 50 mg (1 ea)

Tablet, Oral:
Edecrin: 25 mg [scored]

Extemporaneous Preparations A 1 mg/mL oral suspension may be made with ethacrynic acid powder. Dissolve 120 mg ethacrynic acid powder in a small amount of 10% alcohol. Add a small amount of 50% sorbitol solution and stir. Adjust pH to 7 with 0.1N sodium hydroxide solution. Add sufficient quantity of 50% sorbitol solution to make a final volume of 120 mL. Add methylparaben 6 mg and propylparaben 2.4 mg as preservatives. Stable for 220 days at room temperature.

Das Gupta V, Gibbs CW Jr, and Ghanekar AG, "Stability of Pediatric Liquid Dosage Forms of Ethacrynic Acid, Indomethacin, Methyldopate Hydrochloride, Prednisone and Spironolactone," *Am J Hosp Pharm,* 1978, 35(11):1382-5.

Handbook on Extemporaneous Formulations, Bethesda, MD: American Society of Hospital Pharmacists, 1987.

Ethambutol (e THAM byoo tole)

Medication Safety Issues

Sound-alike/look-alike issues:
Myambutol® may be confused with Nembutal®

Brand Names: U.S. Myambutol

Brand Names: Canada Etibi®

Therapeutic Category Antitubercular Agent

Generic Availability (U.S.) Yes

Use Treatment of pulmonary tuberculosis (FDA approved in ages ≥13 years and adults) and other mycobacterial diseases in conjunction with other antimycobacterial agents

Pregnancy Risk Factor C

Pregnancy Considerations Teratogenic effects have been seen in animals. There are no adequate and well-controlled studies in pregnant women; there have been reports of ophthalmic abnormalities in infants born to women receiving ethambutol as a component of antituberculous therapy. Use only during pregnancy if benefits outweigh risks.

Breast-Feeding Considerations The manufacturer suggests use during breast-feeding only if benefits to the mother outweigh the possible risk to the infant. Some references suggest that exposure to the infant is low and does not produce toxicity, and breast-feeding should not be discouraged. Other references recommend if breast-feeding, monitor the infant for rash, malaise, nausea, or vomiting.

Contraindications Hypersensitivity to ethambutol or any component; optic neuritis, unless clinical judgment determines that it may be used; use in patients unable to discern and report visual changes (eg, very young, unconscious patients)

Warnings Optic neuropathy including optic neuritis or retrobulbar neuritis characterized by decreased visual acuity, scotoma, color blindness, and/or visual defect has been reported with ethambutol therapy and may be related to dose and treatment duration; irreversible blindness has also been reported. Loss of visual acuity is generally reversible when ethambutol is discontinued promptly, but reversal may require up to a year. Some patients have received ethambutol again after such recovery without recurrence of visual acuity loss. Use only in children whose visual acuity can accurately be determined and monitored; fatal hepatotoxicity has been reported; not recommended for use in children <13 years of age unless benefit outweighs risk of therapy

Precautions Use with caution in patients with ocular defects or impaired renal function; modify dose in patients with renal impairment

Adverse Reactions

Cardiovascular: Myocarditis, pericarditis

Central nervous system: Confusion, disorientation, dizziness, fever, hallucinations, headache, malaise

Dermatologic: Dermatitis, erythema multiforme, exfoliative dermatitis, pruritus, rash

Endocrine & metabolic: Acute gout or hyperuricemia

Gastrointestinal: Abdominal pain, anorexia, GI upset, nausea, vomiting

Hematologic: Eosinophilia, leukopenia, lymphadenopathy, neutropenia, thrombocytopenia

Hepatic: Hepatitis, hepatotoxicity (possibly related to concurrent therapy), LFTs abnormal

Neuromuscular & skeletal: Arthralgia, peripheral neuritis

Ocular: Optic neuritis; symptoms may include decreased acuity, scotoma, color blindness, or visual defects (usually reversible with discontinuation, irreversible blindness has been described)

Renal: Nephritis

Respiratory: Infiltrates (with or without eosinophilia), pneumonitis

Miscellaneous: Anaphylaxis, anaphylactoid reaction; hypersensitivity syndrome (cutaneous reactions, eosinophilia, and organ-specific inflammation)

Drug Interactions

Metabolism/Transport Effects None known.

Avoid Concomitant Use There are no known interactions where it is recommended to avoid concomitant use.

Increased Effect/Toxicity There are no known significant interactions involving an increase in effect.

Decreased Effect
The levels/effects of Ethambutol may be decreased by: Aluminum Hydroxide

Stability Store tablets at controlled room temperature 20°C to 25°C (68°F to 77°F)

Mechanism of Action Inhibits arabinosyl transferase resulting in impaired mycobacterial cell wall synthesis

Pharmacokinetics (Adult data unless noted)

Absorption: Oral: ~80%

Distribution: Well distributed throughout the body with high concentrations in kidneys, lungs, saliva, and red blood cells; concentrations in CSF are low; crosses the placenta; excreted into breast milk

Protein binding: 20% to 30%

Metabolism: 20% by the liver to inactive metabolite

Half-life: 2.5-3.6 hours (up to 7 hours or longer with renal impairment)

Time to peak serum concentration: Within 2-4 hours

Elimination: ~50% in urine and 20% excreted in feces as unchanged drug

Dialysis: Slightly dialyzable (5% to 20%)

Dosing: Usual Oral:

Infants and Children:

Tuberculosis, active: **Note:** Used as part of a multidrug regimen; treatment regimens consist of an initial 2-month phase, followed by a continuation phase of 4 or 7 additional months; frequency of dosing may differ depending on phase of therapy

HIV negative: 15-20 mg/kg/day once daily (maximum: 1 g/day) **or** 50 mg/kg/dose twice weekly (maximum: 2.5 g/dose) (*MMWR,* 2003)

HIV-exposed/-infected: 15-25 mg/kg/day once daily (maximum: 2.5 g/day) (CDC, 2009)

MAC, secondary prophylaxis or treatment in HIV-exposed/-infected: 15-25 mg/kg/day once daily (maximum: 2.5 g/day) with clarithromycin (or azithromycin) with or without rifabutin (CDC, 2009)

Nontuberculous mycobacterial infection: 15-25 mg/kg/day once daily (maximum: 2.5 g/day)

Adolescents and Adults:

Disseminated *Mycobacterium avium* (MAC) treatment in patients with advanced HIV infection: 15 mg/kg ethambutol in combination with clarithromycin or azithromycin with/without rifabutin (Griffith, 2007)

Nontuberculous mycobacterium (*M. kansasii*): Adults: 15 mg/kg/day ethambutol for duration to include 12 months of culture-negative sputum; typically used in combination with rifampin and isoniazid; **Note:** Previous recommendations stated to use 25 mg/kg/day for the initial 2 months of therapy; however, IDSA guidelines state this may be unnecessary given the success of rifampin-based regimens with ethambutol 15 mg/kg/day or omitted altogether (Griffith, 2007)

Tuberculosis, active: **Note:** Used as part of a multidrug regimen; treatment regimens consist of an initial 2-month phase, followed by a continuation phase of 4 or 7 additional months; frequency of dosing may differ depending on phase of therapy.

Initial: 15 mg/kg once daily; Retreatment (previous antituberculosis therapy): 25 mg/kg once daily

Suggested doses by lean body weight (*MMWR*, 2003):
Daily therapy: 15-25 mg/kg
  40-55 kg: 800 mg
  56-75 kg: 1200 mg
  76-90 kg: 1600 mg (maximum dose regardless of weight)
Twice weekly directly observed therapy (DOT): 50 mg/kg
  40-55 kg: 2000 mg
  56-75 kg: 2800 mg
  76-90 kg: 4000 mg (maximum dose regardless of weight)
Three times/week DOT: 25-30 mg/kg (maximum: 2.5 g)
  40-55 kg: 1200 mg
  56-75 kg: 2000 mg
  76-90 kg: 2400 mg (maximum dose regardless of weight)

Dosing interval in renal impairment: Aronoff, 2007:
CrCl 10-50 mL/minute: Administer every 24-36 hours
CrCl <10 mL/minute: Administer every 48 hours
Hemodialysis: Slightly dialyzable (5% to 20%); Administer dose postdialysis
Peritoneal dialysis: Dose for CrCl <10 mL/minute: Administer every 48 hours
Continuous arteriovenous or venovenous hemofiltration: Dose for CrCl 10-50 mL/minute: Administer every 24-36 hours
MMWR, 2003: Adults: CrCl <30 mL/minute and hemodialysis: 15-25 mg/kg/dose 3 times weekly

Administration Oral: Administer with or without food; if GI upset occurs, administer with food. Tablet may be pulverized and mixed with apple juice or apple sauce. Do not mix with other juices or syrups since they do not mask ethambutol's bitter taste or are not stable. Administer ethambutol at least 4 hours before aluminum hydroxide.

Monitoring Parameters Monthly examination of visual acuity and color discrimination in patients receiving >15 mg/kg/day; periodic renal, hepatic, and hematologic function tests

Dosage Forms Excipient information presented when available (limited, particularly for generics); consult specific product labeling.
Tablet, Oral, as hydrochloride:
  Myambutol: 100 mg
  Myambutol: 400 mg [scored]
  Generic: 100 mg, 400 mg

References

American Academy of Pediatrics, Committee on Infectious Diseases, "Chemotherapy for Tuberculosis in Infants and Children," *Pediatrics*, 1992, 89(1):161-5.

American Thoracic Society, CDC, and Infectious Diseases Society of America, "Treatment of Tuberculosis," *MMWR Recomm Rep*, 2003, 52(RR-11):1-77.

Aronoff GR, Bennett WM, Berns JS, et al, *Drug Prescribing in Renal Failure: Dosing Guidelines for Adults and Children*, 5th ed. Philadelphia, PA: American College of Physicians, 2007.

Centers for Disease Control and Prevention (CDC), "Guidelines for the Prevention and Treatment of Opportunistic Infections Among HIV-Exposed and HIV-Infected Children," *MMWR Recomm Rep*, 2009, 58(RR-11):1-166. Available at http://aidsinfo.nih.gov/contentfiles/Pediatric_OI.pdf

Graham SM, Bell DJ, Nyirongo S, et al, "Low Levels of Pyrazinamide and Ethambutol in Children With Tuberculosis and Impact of Age, Nutritional Status, and Human Immunodeficiency Virus Infection," *Antimicrob Agents Chemother*, 2006, 50(2):407-13.

Griffith DE, Aksamit T, Brown-Elliott BA, et al, "An Official ATS/IDSA Statement: Diagnosis, Treatment, and Prevention of Nontuberculous Mycobacterial Diseases," *Am J Respir Crit Care Med*, 2007, 175 (4):367-416.

Hill S, Regondi I, Grzemska M, et al, "Children and Tuberculosis Medicines: Bridging the Research Gap," *Bull World Health Organ*, 2008, 86(9):658.

Starke JR and Correa AG, "Management of Mycobacterial Infection and Disease in Children," *Pediatr Infect Dis J*, 1995, 14:455-70.

◆ **Ethambutol Hydrochloride** *see* Ethambutol *on page 807*

◆ **Ethanoic Acid** *see* Acetic Acid *on page 58*

◆ **Ethanol** *see* Alcohol (Ethyl) *on page 88*

◆ **Etherified Starch** *see* Tetrastarch *on page 1998*

◆ **Ethiofos** *see* Amifostine *on page 116*

Ethionamide (e thye on AM ide)

Brand Names: U.S. Trecator
Brand Names: Canada Trecator®
Therapeutic Category Antitubercular Agent
Generic Availability (U.S.) No
Use In conjunction with other antituberculosis agents in the treatment of tuberculosis and other mycobacterial diseases
Pregnancy Risk Factor C
Pregnancy Considerations Ethionamide crosses the placenta; teratogenic effects were observed in animal studies. Use during pregnancy is not recommended.
Breast-Feeding Considerations If ethionamide is used while breast-feeding, monitor the infant for adverse effects.
Contraindications Hypersensitivity to ethionamide or any component; severe hepatic impairment
Warnings May cause hepatotoxicity; monitor liver function tests monthly. Drug-resistant tuberculosis develops rapidly if ethionamide is used alone; must administer with at least one other antituberculosis agent.
Precautions Use with caution in patients with diabetes mellitus; may cause hypoglycemia. Use not recommended in patients with porphyria; porphyria-inducing in animal and *in vitro* studies (WHO, 2008). Use with caution in patients with thyroid dysfunction; hypothyroidism (reversible) has been reported. Use with caution in patients receiving isoniazid; temporarily increases isoniazid levels. Some cross-resistance has been reported if inhA mutation is present (WHO, 2008). Use with caution in patients receiving cycloserine; seizures have been reported. Periodic eye exams are recommended.
Adverse Reactions
Cardiovascular: Orthostatic hypotension
Central nervous system: Depression, dizziness, drowsiness, headache, psychiatric disturbances, restlessness, seizure
Dermatologic: Acne, alopecia, photosensitivity, purpura, rash
Endocrine & metabolic: Gynecomastia, hypoglycemia, hypothyroidism or goiter, menstrual irregularities, pellagra-like syndrome
Gastrointestinal: Abdominal pain, anorexia, diarrhea, excessive salivation, metallic taste, nausea, stomatitis, vomiting, weight loss
Genitourinary: Impotence
Hematologic: Leukopenia, thrombocytopenia
Hepatic: Bilirubin increased, hepatitis, jaundice, liver function tests increased
Neuromuscular & skeletal: Arthralgia, peripheral neuritis
Ocular: Blurred vision, diplopia, optic neuritis
Respiratory: Olfactory disturbances

Miscellaneous: Hypersensitivity reaction

Drug Interactions

Metabolism/Transport Effects None known.

Avoid Concomitant Use There are no known interactions where it is recommended to avoid concomitant use.

Increased Effect/Toxicity
Ethionamide may increase the levels/effects of: Cyclo-SERINE; Isoniazid

The levels/effects of Ethionamide may be increased by: Alcohol (Ethyl)

Decreased Effect There are no known significant interactions involving a decrease in effect.

Mechanism of Action Inhibits peptide synthesis; bacteriostatic

Pharmacokinetics (Adult data unless noted)
Absorption: ~80% is rapidly absorbed from the GI tract
Distribution: Crosses the placenta; widely distributed into body tissues and fluids including liver, kidneys, and CSF
Protein binding: 10%
Metabolism: In the liver to active and inactive metabolites
Bioavailability: 80%
Half-life: 2-3 hours
Time to peak serum concentration: Oral: Within 3 hours
Elimination: As metabolites (active and inactive) and parent drug in the urine

Dosing: Usual Oral:
Children: 15-20 mg/kg/day in 2-3 divided doses, not to exceed 1 g/day
Adults: 500-1000 mg/day in 1-3 divided doses

Administration Oral: Administer with meals to decrease GI distress

Monitoring Parameters Initial and periodic serum AST and ALT, blood glucose, thyroid function tests, periodic ophthalmologic exams

Dosage Forms Excipient information presented when available (limited, particularly for generics); consult specific product labeling.
Tablet, Oral:
Trecator: 250 mg [contains fd&c yellow #6 (sunset yellow)]

References
Centers for Disease Control and Prevention (CDC), "Guidelines for the Prevention and Treatment of Opportunistic Infections Among HIV-Exposed and HIV-Infected Children," *MMWR Recomm Rep*, 2009, 58(RR-11):1-166. Available at http://aidsinfo.nih.gov/contentfiles/Pediatric_OI.pdf

Donald PR and Seifart HI,"Cerebrospinal Fluid Concentrations of Ethionamide in Children With Tuberculous Meningitis," *J Pediatr*, 1989, 115(3):483-6.

Starke JR and Correa AG, "Management of Mycobacterial Infection and Disease in Children," *Pediatr Infect Dis J*, 1995, 14(6):455-69.

World Health Organization, "Guidelines for the Programmatic Management of Drug-Resistant Tuberculosis, Emergency Update 2008," 2008, World Health Organization, Geneva. Available at http://whqlibdoc.who.int/publications/2008/9789241547581_eng.pdf

---

Ethosuximide (eth oh SUKS i mide)

Medication Safety Issues
Sound-alike/look-alike issues:
Ethosuximide may be confused with methsuximide
Zarontin® may be confused with Neurontin®, Xalatan®, Zantac®, Zaroxolyn®

Brand Names: U.S. Zarontin

Brand Names: Canada Zarontin®

Therapeutic Category Anticonvulsant, Succinimide

Generic Availability (U.S.) Yes

Use Management of absence (petit mal) epilepsy (FDA approved in ages ≥3 years and adults); also used for management of myoclonic seizures and akinetic epilepsy

Medication Guide Available Yes

Pregnancy Considerations Ethosuximide crosses the placenta. Cases of birth defects have been reported in infants. Epilepsy itself, the number of medications, genetic factors, or a combination of these probably influence the teratogenicity of anticonvulsant therapy.

Patients exposed to ethosuximide during pregnancy are encouraged to enroll themselves into the NAAED Pregnancy Registry by calling 1-888-233-2334. Additional information is available at www.aedpregnancyregistry.org.

Breast-Feeding Considerations Ethosuximide is excreted into breast milk. The manufacturer recommends caution be used if administered to a nursing woman.

Contraindications Hypersensitivity to succinimides or any component

Warnings Blood dyscrasias (sometimes fatal) have been reported (monitor hematologic function periodically or if signs/symptoms of infection develop); SLE has been reported.

Antiepileptic drugs (AEDs) increase the risk of suicidal behavior and ideation in patients receiving these medications for any indication. Pooled analyses of placebo-controlled trials involving 11 different AEDs (regardless of indication) showed a two-fold increased risk of suicidal thoughts or behavior (estimated incidence rate: 0.43% in AED-treated patients compared to 0.24% in patients receiving placebo); increased risk was observed as early as one week after initiation of AED and continued through duration of trials (most trials ≤24 weeks); risk did not vary significantly by age (age range: 5–100 years). Consider risks and benefits of AEDs before prescribing. Monitor all patients receiving an AED for emergence of suicidal thoughts or behavior, thoughts of self-harm, any unusual changes in behavior or mood, or the emergence or worsening of depressive symptoms; notify healthcare provider immediately if symptoms or concerning behavior occur. **Note:** The FDA is requiring that a Medication Guide be developed for all antiepileptic drugs, informing patients of this risk. Severe dermatologic reactions, including Stevens-Johnson syndrome, have been reported with an onset usually within 28 days, but may be observed later. Ethosuximide should be discontinued if there are any signs of rash. If SJS is suspected do not resume ethosuximide and consider alternative therapy.

Oral solution may contain sodium benzoate; benzoic acid (benzoate) is a metabolite of benzyl alcohol; large amounts of benzyl alcohol (≥99 mg/kg/day) have been associated with a potentially fatal toxicity ("gasping syndrome") in neonates; the "gasping syndrome" consists of metabolic acidosis, respiratory distress, gasping respirations, CNS dysfunction (including convulsions, intracranial hemorrhage), hypotension and cardiovascular collapse; use ethosuximide products containing sodium benzoate with caution in neonates; *in vitro* and animal studies have shown that benzoate displaces bilirubin from protein binding sites

Precautions Use with caution in patients with hepatic or renal disease. Avoid abrupt withdrawal (may precipitate absence status). When used alone, ethosuximide may increase tonic-clonic seizures in patients with mixed seizure disorders; ethosuximide must be used in combination with other anticonvulsants in patients with both absence and tonic-clonic seizures. May cause CNS depression, which may impair physical or mental abilities; patients must be cautioned about performing tasks which require mental alertness.

Adverse Reactions
Central nervous system: Aggressiveness, ataxia, concentration impaired, dizziness, drowsiness, euphoria, fatigue, headache, hyperactivity, irritability, lethargy, mental depression (with cases of overt suicidal intentions), night terrors, paranoid psychosis, sleep disturbance
Dermatologic: Hirsutism, pruritus, rash, Stevens-Johnson syndrome, urticaria

Endocrine & metabolic: Libido increased

Gastrointestinal: Abdominal pain, anorexia, cramps, diarrhea, epigastric pain, gastric upset, gum hypertrophy, nausea, tongue swelling, vomiting, weight loss

Genitourinary: Hematuria (microscopic), vaginal bleeding

Hematologic: Agranulocytosis, eosinophilia, leukopenia, pancytopenia

Ocular: Myopia

Miscellaneous: Allergic reaction, drug rash with eosinophilia and systemic symptoms (DRESS), hiccups, systemic lupus erythematosus

Drug Interactions

Metabolism/Transport Effects Substrate of CYP3A4 (major); **Note:** Assignment of Major/Minor substrate status based on clinically relevant drug interaction potential

Avoid Concomitant Use

Avoid concomitant use of Ethosuximide with any of the following: Azelastine (Nasal); Conivaptan; Fusidic Acid (Systemic); Paraldehyde; Thalidomide

Increased Effect/Toxicity

Ethosuximide may increase the levels/effects of: Alcohol (Ethyl); Azelastine (Nasal); Buprenorphine; CNS Depressants; Fosphenytoin; Hydrocodone; Methotrimeprazine; Metyrosine; Mirtazapine; Paraldehyde; Phenytoin; Pramipexole; ROPINIRole; Rotigotine; Selective Serotonin Reuptake Inhibitors; Thalidomide; Zolpidem

The levels/effects of Ethosuximide may be increased by: Brimonidine (Topical); Cannabis; Ceritinib; Cobicistat; Conivaptan; CYP3A4 Inhibitors (Moderate); CYP3A4 Inhibitors (Strong); Dasatinib; Doxylamine; Dronabinol; Droperidol; Fusidic Acid (Systemic); HydrOXYzine; Ivacaftor; Kava Kava; Luliconazole; Magnesium Sulfate; Methotrimeprazine; Mifepristone; Nabilone; Perampanel; Rufinamide; Simeprevir; Sodium Oxybate; Stiripentol; Tapentadol; Tetrahydrocannabinol; Valproic Acid and Derivatives

Decreased Effect

Ethosuximide may decrease the levels/effects of: Valproic Acid and Derivatives

The levels/effects of Ethosuximide may be decreased by: Amphetamines; Bosentan; CYP3A4 Inducers (Strong); Dabrafenib; Deferasirox; Fosphenytoin; Ketorolac (Nasal); Ketorolac (Systemic); Mefloquine; Mitotane; Orlistat; Phenytoin; Siltuximab; St Johns Wort; Tocilizumab

Stability

Capsules: Store at controlled room temperature

Solution: Store below 30°C (86°F) in tightly-closed container. Protect from light; do not freeze.

Mechanism of Action Increases the seizure threshold and suppresses paroxysmal spike-and-wave pattern in absence seizures; depresses nerve transmission in the motor cortex

Pharmacokinetics (Adult data unless noted)

Distribution: V_d: Adults: 0.62-0.72 L/kg; crosses the placenta; excreted in human breast milk

Protein binding: <10%

Metabolism: ~80% metabolized in the liver to three inactive metabolites

Half-life:

Children: 30 hours

Adults: 50-60 hours

Time to peak serum concentration:

Capsule: Within 2-4 hours

Solution: <2-4 hours

Elimination: Slow in urine as metabolites (50%) and as unchanged drug (10% to 20%); small amounts excreted in feces

Dialysis: Removed by hemodialysis and peritoneal dialysis

Dosing: Usual

Children and Adolescents: **Management of absence (petit mal) seizures:** Oral:

Children <6 years (Limited data available in children <3 years): Initial: 15 mg/kg/day in 2 divided doses; maximum single dose: 250 mg; may increase every 4-7 days; usual maintenance dose: 15-40 mg/kg/day in 2 divided doses; maximum daily dose: 1500 mg/**day**

Children ≥6 years and Adolescents: Initial: 250 mg twice daily; may increase every 4-7 days in 250 mg/**day** increments; maximum daily dose: 1500 mg/**day** in 2 divided doses; usual maintenance dose: 20-40 mg/kg/day in 2 divided doses

Adults: **Management of absence (petit mal) seizures:** Oral: Initial: 500 mg/day; increase by 250 mg as needed every 4-7 days up to 1500 mg/day in divided doses

Dosing adjustment in renal impairment: There are no dosage adjustment provided in manufacturer's labeling; use with caution.

Dosing adjustment in hepatic impairment: There are no dosage adjustment provided in manufacturer's labeling; use with caution.

Administration Oral: Administer with food or milk to decrease GI upset

Monitoring Parameters Seizure frequency, trough serum concentrations; CBC with differential, platelets, liver enzymes, urinalysis, renal function; signs and symptoms of suicidality (eg, anxiety, depression, behavior changes)

Reference Range

Therapeutic: 40-100 mcg/mL (SI: 280-710 micromoles/L)

Toxic: >150 mcg/mL (SI: >1062 micromoles/L)

Additional Information Considered to be a drug of choice for simple absence seizures

Dosage Forms Excipient information presented when available (limited, particularly for generics); consult specific product labeling.

Capsule, Oral:

Zarontin: 250 mg [contains fd&c yellow #10 (quinoline yellow)]

Generic: 250 mg

Solution, Oral:

Zarontin: 250 mg/5 mL (474 mL) [raspberry flavor]

Generic: 250 mg/5 mL (473 mL, 474 mL)

References

Marquardt ED, Ishisaka DY, Batra KK, et al, "Removal of Ethosuximide and Phenobarbital by Peritoneal Dialysis in a Child," *Clin Pharm*, 1992, 11(12):1030-1.

◆ **Ethoxynaphthamido Penicillin Sodium** *see* Nafcillin *on page 1462*

◆ **Ethyl Alcohol** *see* Alcohol (Ethyl) *on page 88*

◆ **Ethyl Aminobenzoate** *see* Benzocaine *on page 273*

◆ **Ethyol** *see* Amifostine *on page 116*

◆ **Ethyol® (Can)** *see* Amifostine *on page 116*

◆ **Etibi® (Can)** *see* Ethambutol *on page 807*

Etidronate (e ti DROE nate)

Medication Safety Issues

Sound-alike/look-alike issues:

Etidronate may be confused with etomidate

Brand Names: Canada Co-Etidronate; Mylan-Etidronate

Therapeutic Category Antidote, Hypercalcemia; Bisphosphonate Derivative

Generic Availability (U.S.) Yes

Use Symptomatic treatment of Paget's disease of bone and prevention and treatment of heterotopic ossification following spinal cord injury or total hip replacement (FDA approved in adults)

Pregnancy Risk Factor C

Pregnancy Considerations Adverse events were observed in some animal reproduction studies. It is not known if bisphosphonates cross the placenta, but fetal exposure is expected (Djokanovic, 2008; Stathopoulos, 2011). Bisphosphonates are incorporated into the bone matrix and gradually released over time. The amount available in the systemic circulation varies by dose and duration of therapy. Theoretically, there may be a risk of fetal harm when pregnancy follows the completion of therapy; however, available data have not shown that exposure to bisphosphonates during pregnancy significantly increases the risk of adverse fetal events (Djokanovic, 2008; Levy, 2009; Stathopoulos, 2011). Until additional data is available, most sources recommend discontinuing bisphosphonate therapy in women of reproductive potential as early as possible prior to a planned pregnancy; use in premenopausal women should be reserved for special circumstances when rapid bone loss is occurring (Bhalla, 2010; Pereira, 2012; Stathopoulos, 2011). Because hypocalcemia has been described following *in utero* bisphosphonate exposure, exposed infants should be monitored for hypocalcemia after birth (Djokanovic, 2008; Stathopoulos, 2011).

Breast-Feeding Considerations It is not known if etidronate is excreted into breast milk. The manufacturer recommends caution be exercised when administering etidronate to nursing women.

Contraindications Hypersensitivity to etidronate, biphosphonates, or any component; clinically overt osteomalacia; patients with abnormalities of the esophagus which delay esophageal emptying, such as stricture or achalasia

Warnings Response to therapy in Paget's disease may be slow in onset and continue for months after therapy is discontinued; do not increase dosage rapidly; treatment >6 months or at doses >20 mg/kg/day have been associated with osteomalacia and increased risk of fracture; long bones with predominantly lytic lesions may be prone to fracture, particularly in patients unresponsive to treatment; hyperphosphatemia may occur at doses of 10-20 mg/kg/day due to drug-related increases in the tubular reabsorption of phosphate; serum phosphate levels usually return to normal 2-4 weeks after discontinuation of therapy; monitor serum phosphate closely

Precautions Use with caution in patients with restricted calcium and vitamin D intake; use with caution in patients with enterocolitis due to etidronate's potential to cause diarrhea particularly when using high dosages. Use with caution in patients with renal impairment; may require dose reduction. May cause irritation to upper gastrointestinal mucosa. Esophagitis, dysphagia, esophageal ulcers, esophageal erosions, and esophageal stricture (rare) have been reported with oral bisphosphonates; risk increases in patients unable to comply with dosing instructions. Use with caution in patients with dysphagia, esophageal disease, gastritis, duodenitis, or ulcers; may worsen underlying condition. Discontinue use if new or worsening symptoms develop.

Osteonecrosis of the jaw (ONJ) has been reported in patients receiving bisphosphonates, including etidronate. Risk factors include invasive dental procedures (eg, tooth extraction, dental implants, bone surgery), a diagnosis of cancer with concomitant chemotherapy or corticosteroids, poor oral hygiene, ill-fitting dentures, and comorbid disorders (anemia, coagulopathy, infection, preexisting dental disease). Most reported cases occurred after I.V. bisphosphonate therapy; however, cases have been reported following oral therapy. A dental exam and preventive dentistry should be performed prior to placing patients with risk factors on chronic bisphosphonate therapy. The manufacturer's labeling states that discontinuing bisphosphonates in patients requiring invasive dental procedures may reduce the risk of ONJ; however, other experts suggest that there is no evidence that discontinuing therapy reduces the risk of developing ONJ (Assael, 2009). The benefit:risk must be assessed by the treating physician and/or dentist/surgeon prior to any invasive dental procedure. Patients developing ONJ while on bisphosphonates should receive care by an oral surgeon.

Adverse Reactions
Gastrointestinal: Diarrhea, nausea
Neuromuscular & skeletal: Bone pain
Postmarketing and/or case reports: Agranulocytosis, alopecia, amnesia, angioedema, arthralgia, arthritis, asthma exacerbation, bone fracture, confusion, depression, esophageal cancer, esophagitis, follicular eruption, gastritis, glossitis, hallucination, headache, hypersensitivity reactions, leg cramps, leukopenia, macular rash, maculopapular rash, musculoskeletal pain (sometimes severe and/or incapacitating), osteomalacia, pancytopenia, paresthesia, peptic ulcer disease exacerbation, pruritus, Stevens-Johnson syndrome, urticaria

Drug Interactions
Metabolism/Transport Effects None known.
Avoid Concomitant Use There are no known interactions where it is recommended to avoid concomitant use.
Increased Effect/Toxicity
Etidronate may increase the levels/effects of: Deferasirox; Phosphate Supplements

The levels/effects of Etidronate may be increased by: Aminoglycosides; Nonsteroidal Anti-Inflammatory Agents; Systemic Angiogenesis Inhibitors
Decreased Effect
The levels/effects of Etidronate may be decreased by: Antacids; Calcium Salts; Iron Salts; Magnesium Salts; Multivitamins/Minerals (with ADEK, Folate, Iron); Multivitamins/Minerals (with AE, No Iron); Proton Pump Inhibitors; Sucroferric Oxyhydroxide

Food Interactions Food and/or supplements decrease the absorption and bioavailability of the drug. Management: Administer tablet on an empty stomach with a full glass of plain water or fruit juice (6-8 oz) 2 hours before food. Avoid administering foods/supplements with calcium, iron, or magnesium within 2 hours of drug. Do not take with mineral water or other beverages.

Stability Store at controlled room temperature of 25°C (77°F).

Mechanism of Action Decreases bone resorption by inhibiting osteocystic osteolysis; decreases mineral release and matrix or collagen breakdown in bone

Pharmacodynamics
Onset of therapeutic effects: Within 1-3 months of therapy
Duration: Persists for 12 months without continuous therapy

Pharmacokinetics (Adult data unless noted)
Absorption: ~3%
Half-life: 1-6 hours
Elimination: Primarily as unchanged drug in urine (50%) with unabsorbed drug eliminated in feces

Dosing: Usual Oral:
Heterotopic ossification: Children and Adults:
Spinal cord injury: 20 mg/kg once daily (or in divided doses if GI discomfort occurs) for 2 weeks, then 10 mg/kg/day for 10 weeks
Total hip replacement: 20 mg/kg/day 1 month before and 3 months after surgery
Note: This dosage when used in children for >1 year has been associated with a rachitic syndrome.
Paget's disease: Adults: Initial: 5-10 mg/kg/day (not to exceed 6 months) or 11-20 mg/kg/day (not to exceed 3 months). Doses >20 mg/kg/day are **not** recommended. Higher doses should be used only when lower doses are ineffective or there is a need to suppress rapid bone turnover (eg, potential for irreversible neurologic damage)

◄ or reduce elevated cardiac output. Daily dose may be divided if adverse GI effects occur; courses of therapy should be separated by drug-free periods of at least 3 months.

Dosing adjustment in renal impairment: Adult:
S_{cr} 2.5-4.9 mg/dL: Use with caution
S_{cr} ≥5 mg/dL: **Not recommended**

Administration Oral: Administer on an empty stomach with a full glass of plain water (6-8 oz), 2 hours before meals. Patients should be instructed to stay upright (not to lie down) after taking the medication.

Monitoring Parameters Serum calcium, phosphate, creatinine, BUN, alkaline phosphatase, 25(OH)D, pain

Test Interactions Bisphosphonates may interfere with diagnostic imaging agents such as technetium-99m-diphosphonate in bone scans.

Dosage Forms Excipient information presented when available (limited, particularly for generics); consult specific product labeling.
Tablet, Oral, as disodium:
Generic: 200 mg, 400 mg

References

Assael LA, "Oral Bisphosphonates as a Cause of Bisphosphonate-Related Osteonecrosis of the Jaws: Clinical Findings, Assessment of Risks, and Preventive Strategies," *J Oral Maxillofac Surg*, 2009, 67 (5 Suppl):35-43.

Bhalla AK, "Management of Osteoporosis in a Pre-menopausal Woman," *Best Pract Res Clin Rheumatol*, 2010, 24(3):313-27.

Djokanovic N, Klieger-Grossmann C, and Koren G, "Does Treatment With Bisphosphonates Endanger the Human Pregnancy?" *J Obstet Gynaecol Can*, 2008, 30(12):1146-8.

Levy S, Fayez I, Taguchi N, et al, "Pregnancy Outcome Following in utero Exposure to Bisphosphonates," *Bone*, 2009, 44(3):428-30.

Mital MA, Garber JE, and Stinson JT, "Ectopic Bone Formation in Children and Adolescents With Head Injuries: Its Management," *J Pediatr Orthop*, 1987, 7(1):83-90.

Pereira RM, Carvalho JF, Paula AP, et al, "Guidelines for the Prevention and Treatment of Glucocorticoid-Induced Osteoporosis," *Rev Bras Reumatol*, 2012, 52(4):580-93.

Silverman SL, Hurvitz EA, Nelson VS, et al, "Rachitic Syndrome After Disodium Etidronate Therapy in an Adolescent," *Arch Phys Med Rehabil*, 1994, 75(1):118-20.

Stathopoulos IP, Liakou CG, Katsalira A, et al, "The Use of Bisphosphonates in Women Prior to or During Pregnancy and Lactation," *Hormones (Athens)*, 2011, 10(4):280-91.

Wysowski DK, "Reports of Esophageal Cancer With Oral Bisphosphonate Use," *N Engl J Med*, 2009, 360(1):89-90.

◆ **Etidronate Disodium** see Etidronate on page 810

Etodolac (ee toe DOE lak)

Medication Safety Issues
Sound-alike/look-alike issues:
Lodine may be confused with codeine, iodine, Lopid®
BEERS Criteria medication:
This drug may be potentially inappropriate for use in geriatric patients (Quality of evidence - moderate; Strength of recommendation - strong).

Brand Names: Canada Apo-Etodolac; Utradol

Therapeutic Category Analgesic, Non-narcotic; Anti-inflammatory Agent; Nonsteroidal Anti-inflammatory Drug (NSAID), Oral

Generic Availability (U.S.) Yes

Use Oral:
Immediate release: Acute and long-term management of osteoarthritis and rheumatoid arthritis; management of acute pain (All indications: FDA approved in ages ≥18 years and adults)
Extended release: Relief of the signs and symptoms of JIA (FDA approved in ages 6-16 years weighing at least 20 kg); relief of signs and symptoms of osteoarthritis and rheumatoid arthritis (FDA approved in adults)

Medication Guide Available Yes

Pregnancy Risk Factor C

Pregnancy Considerations Adverse events were not observed in the initial animal reproduction study; therefore, the manufacturer classifies etodolac as pregnancy category C. NSAID exposure during the first trimester is not strongly associated with congenital malformations; however, cardiovascular anomalies and cleft palate have been observed following NSAID exposure in some studies. The use of an NSAID close to conception may be associated with an increased risk of miscarriage. Nonteratogenic effects have been observed following NSAID administration during the third trimester including: Myocardial degenerative changes, prenatal constriction of the ductus arteriosus, fetal tricuspid regurgitation, failure of the ductus arteriosus to close postnatally; renal dysfunction or failure, oligohydramnios; gastrointestinal bleeding or perforation, increased risk of necrotizing enterocolitis; intracranial bleeding (including intraventricular hemorrhage), platelet dysfunction with resultant bleeding; pulmonary hypertension. Because they may cause premature closure of the ductus arteriosus, use of NSAIDs late in pregnancy should be avoided (use after 31 or 32 weeks gestation is not recommended by some clinicians). The chronic use of NSAIDs in women of reproductive age may be associated with infertility that is reversible upon discontinuation of the medication.

Breast-Feeding Considerations It is not known if etodolac is excreted into breast milk. Use of etodolac while breast-feeding is not recommended by the manufacturer.

Contraindications Hypersensitivity to etodolac or any component; history of asthma, urticaria, or allergic-type reaction to aspirin or other NSAIDs; patients with the "aspirin triad" [asthma, rhinitis (with or without nasal polyps), and aspirin intolerance] (fatal asthmatic and anaphylactoid reactions may occur in these patients); perioperative pain in the setting of coronary artery bypass graft (CABG)

Warnings NSAIDs are associated with an increased risk of adverse cardiovascular thrombotic events, including potentially fatal MI and stroke **[U.S. Boxed Warning]**. Risk may be increased with duration of use or preexisting cardiovascular risk factors or disease. Carefully evaluate individual cardiovascular risk profiles prior to prescribing. To reduce the risk of cardiovascular events, use the lowest effective dose for the shortest duration of time, taking into consideration individual patient treatment goals; alternate therapies should be considered for patients at high risk. Use is contraindicated for treatment of perioperative pain in the setting of CABG surgery **[U.S. Boxed Warning]**; an increased incidence of MI and stroke was found in patients receiving COX-2 selective NSAIDs for the treatment of pain within the first 10-14 days after CABG surgery. NSAIDs may cause fluid retention, edema, and new-onset or worsening of preexisting hypertension; use with caution in patients with hypertension, CHF, or fluid retention. Concurrent administration of ibuprofen, and potentially other nonselective NSAIDs, may interfere with aspirin's cardioprotective effect.

NSAIDs may increase the risk of gastrointestinal inflammation, ulceration, bleeding, and perforation **[U.S. Boxed Warning]**. These events, which can be potentially fatal, may occur at any time during therapy and without warning. Avoid the use of NSAIDs in patients with active GI bleeding or ulcer disease. Use NSAIDs with extreme caution in patients with a history of GI bleeding or ulcers (these patients have a 10-fold increased risk for developing a GI bleed). Use NSAIDs with caution in patients with other risk factors which may increase GI bleeding (eg, concurrent therapy with aspirin, anticoagulants, and/or corticosteroids, longer duration of NSAID use, smoking, use of alcohol, and poor general health). Use the lowest effective dose for the shortest duration of time, taking into consideration individual patient treatment goals; alternate therapies should be considered for patients at high risk.

NSAIDs may compromise existing renal function; dose-dependent decreases in prostaglandin synthesis may result from NSAID use, reducing renal blood flow which may cause renal decompensation. Patients with impaired renal function, dehydration, heart failure, liver dysfunction, and in those taking diuretics and ACE inhibitors are at greatest risk of renal toxicity; use with caution in these patients; monitor renal function closely. Rehydrate patient before starting therapy. NSAIDs are not recommended for use in patients with advanced renal disease. Long-term use of NSAIDs may cause renal papillary necrosis and other renal injury.

Anaphylactoid reactions may occur, even in patients without prior exposure; patients with "aspirin triad" [bronchial asthma, aspirin intolerance, and rhinitis (with or without nasal polyps)] are at increased risk; use is contraindicated in these patients. Do not use in patients who experience bronchospasm, asthma, rhinitis, or urticaria with NSAID or aspirin therapy. NSAIDs may cause serious and potentially fatal dermatologic adverse reactions including exfoliative dermatitis, Stevens-Johnson syndrome, and toxic epidermal necrolysis; discontinue use at first sign of skin rash or hypersensitivity. Avoid use of NSAIDs in late pregnancy (beginning at 30 weeks gestation) as they may cause premature closure of the ductus arteriosus. NSAIDs may mask fever and inflammation and thus decrease the ability of these signs to help diagnose infectious conditions.

Use of extended release product consisting of a non-deformable matrix should be avoided in patients with stricture/narrowing of the GI tract; symptoms of obstruction have been associated with nondeformable products.

Precautions Use with caution in patients with decreased hepatic function; etodolac is significantly metabolized in the liver; closely monitor patients with abnormal LFTs; severe hepatic reactions [eg, fulminant hepatitis, jaundice, liver failure (some cases fatal)] have occurred with NSAID use, rarely; discontinue if signs or symptoms of liver disease develop, or if systemic manifestations (eg, eosinophilia, rash, abdominal pain, diarrhea, dark urine) occur. Use with caution in patients with asthma; asthmatic patients may have aspirin-sensitive asthma which may be associated with severe and potentially fatal bronchospasm when aspirin or NSAIDs are administered. Anemia (due to occult or gross blood loss from the GI tract, fluid retention, or other effect on erythropoiesis) may occur; monitor hemoglobin and hematocrit in patients receiving long-term therapy. Use with caution and monitor carefully in patients with coagulation disorders or those receiving anticoagulants; NSAIDs inhibit platelet aggregation and may prolong bleeding time.

Adverse Reactions

Central nervous system: Chills/fever, depression, dizziness, nervousness

Dermatologic: Pruritus, rash

Gastrointestinal: Abdominal cramps, constipation, diarrhea, dyspepsia, flatulence, gastritis, melena, nausea, vomiting

Genitourinary: Dysuria

Neuromuscular & skeletal: Weakness

Ocular: Blurred vision

Otic: Tinnitus

Renal: Polyuria

Rare but important or life-threatening: Agranulocytosis, allergic reaction, allergic/necrotizing vasculitis, alopecia, anaphylactic/anaphylactoid reactions, anemia, angioedema, anorexia, arrhythmia, aseptic meningitis, asthma, bleeding time increased, CHF, confusion, conjunctivitis, CVA, cystitis, duodenitis, dyspnea, ecchymosis, edema, erythema multiforme, esophagitis (+/- stricture or cardiospasm), exfoliative dermatitis, GI ulceration, hallucination, headache, hearing decreased, hematemesis, hematuria, hepatic failure, hepatitis, hyperglycemia (in controlled patients with diabetes), hyperpigmentation, hypertension, infection, insomnia, interstitial nephritis, irregular uterine bleeding, jaundice, LFTs increased, leukopenia, MI, palpitation, pancreatitis, pancytopenia, paresthesia, peptic ulcer (+/- bleeding/perforation), peripheral neuropathy, photophobia, photosensitivity, pulmonary infiltration (eosinophilia), rectal bleeding, renal calculus, renal failure, renal insufficiency, shock, Stevens-Johnson syndrome, syncope, thrombocytopenia, toxic epidermal necrolysis, ulcerative stomatitis, urticaria, vesiculobullous rash, renal papillary necrosis, visual disturbances

Drug Interactions

Metabolism/Transport Effects None known.

Avoid Concomitant Use

Avoid concomitant use of Etodolac with any of the following: Floctafenine; Ketorolac (Nasal); Ketorolac (Systemic); NSAID (COX-2 Inhibitor); Omacetaxine; Urokinase

Increased Effect/Toxicity Etodolac may increase effect/toxicity of aspirin (GI irritation), lithium, methotrexate, digoxin, cyclosporine (nephrotoxicity), and warfarin (bleeding).

Decreased Effect Decreased effect with aspirin. May reduce effect of some diuretics and antihypertensive effect of B-blockers.

Food Interactions Etodolac peak serum levels may be decreased if taken with food. Management: Administer with food to decrease GI upset.

Stability

Immediate release: Store at 20°C to 25°C (68°F to 77°F); protect from moisture and light.

Extended release: Store at 20°C to 25°C (68°F to 77°F); protect from excessive heat, humidity, and light.

Mechanism of Action Reversibly inhibits cyclooxygenase-1 and 2 (COX-1 and 2) enzymes, which results in decreased formation of prostaglandin precursors; has antipyretic, analgesic, and anti-inflammatory properties

Other proposed mechanisms not fully elucidated (and possibly contributing to the anti-inflammatory effect to varying degrees), include inhibiting chemotaxis, altering lymphocyte activity, inhibiting neutrophil aggregation/activation, and decreasing proinflammatory cytokine levels.

Pharmacodynamics

Acute pain: Immediate release:

Onset of action: 30 minutes

Maximum effect: 1-2 hours

Duration of action: Mean range: 4-6 hours

Arthritis (chronic management): Onset of action: Typically within 2 weeks

Pharmacokinetics (Adult data unless noted)

Absorption: Immediate release: Rapid

Distribution:

Immediate release: Pediatric patients (6-16 years; n=11): Terminal V_d: 0.49 L/kg (Boni, 1999); Adults: Apparent V_d: 0.49 L/kg

Extended release: Apparent V_d: 0.57 L/kg

Protein binding: ≥99%, primarily albumin

Metabolism: Hepatic to several hydroxylated metabolites and etodolac glucuronide; hydroxylated metabolites undergo further glucuronidation

Bioavailability: ≥80%

Half-life elimination: Terminal:

Immediate release: Pediatric patients (6-16 years, n=11): 6.5 hours (Boni, 1999); Adults: 6.4 hours

Extended release: Pediatric patients (6-16 years, n=72): 12 hours; Adults: 8.4 hours

Time to peak serum concentration:
Immediate release: Pediatric patients (6-16 years, n=11): 1.4 hours (Boni, 1999); Adults: 1-2 hours
Extended release: 6-7 hours
Elimination: Urine 73% (1% unchanged); feces 16%; clearance similar in pediatric patients and adults (~0.05 L/hour/kg) (Boni, 1999)

Dosing: Usual Note: Dosage should be titrated to the lowest effective dose for the shortest duration possible. For chronic conditions, therapeutic response may take 1-2 weeks of treatment.

Children and Adolescents:
Analgesia, acute pain: Limited data available in ages <18 years: Oral: Immediate release capsules or tablets: Manufacturer's labeling: Adolescents ≥18 years: 200-400 mg every 6-8 hours, as needed; maximum daily dose: 1000 mg/**day**
Alternate dosing (American Pain Society, 2008): Children and Adolescents:
Patient weight <50 kg: 7.5-10 mg/kg/dose every 12 hours; maximum daily dose: 1000 mg/**day**
Patient weight ≥50 kg: 300-400 mg every 8-12 hours; maximum daily dose: 1000 mg/**day**

Juvenile idiopathic arthritis: Children and Adolescents:
Oral: Extended release tablets:
20-30 kg: 400 mg once daily
31-45 kg: 600 mg once daily
46-60 kg: 800 mg once daily
>60 kg: 1000 mg once daily

Rheumatoid arthritis, osteoarthritis: Oral: Adolescents ≥18 years:
Immediate release capsules and tablets: 300-500 mg twice daily or 300 mg 3 times daily; maximum daily dose: 1000 mg/**day**
Extended release tablets: 400-1000 mg once daily

Adults:
Acute pain: Oral: Immediate release capsules or tablets: 200-400 mg every 6-8 hours, as needed; maximum daily dose: 1000 mg/**day**
Rheumatoid arthritis, osteoarthritis: Oral:
Immediate release capsules or tablets: 400 mg 2 times/day **or** 300 mg 2-3 times/day **or** 500 mg 2 times/day; doses >1000 mg/day have not been evaluated
Extended release tablets: 400-1000 mg once daily

Dosing adjustment in renal impairment:
Immediate release: Adolescents ≥18 years and Adults:
Mild to moderate: No adjustment required.
Severe: No dosing adjustment necessary.
Hemodialysis: Not removed; dosing adjustment not necessary.
Extended release: There are no dosing adjustments provided in the manufacturer's labeling; has not been studied.

Dosing adjustment in hepatic impairment: No adjustment required.

Administration May be administered with food to decrease GI upset.

Monitoring Parameters Periodic CBC, liver enzymes, serum BUN and creatinine, signs and symptoms of GI bleeding

Test Interactions False-positive for urinary bilirubin and ketone

Dosage Forms Excipient information presented when available (limited, particularly for generics); consult specific product labeling.
Capsule, Oral:
Generic: 200 mg, 300 mg
Tablet, Oral:
Generic: 400 mg, 500 mg
Tablet Extended Release 24 Hour, Oral:
Generic: 400 mg, 500 mg, 600 mg

References
Boni JP, Korth-Bradley JM, Martin P, et al. Pharmacokinetics of etodolac in patients with stable juvenile rheumatoid arthritis. *Clin Therap.* 1999;21(10): 1715-1724.
Ji P, Chowdhury BA, Yim S, et al. Dosing regimen determination for juvenile idiopathic arthritis: a review of studies during drug development. *J Pharm Sci.* 2012;101(8):2621-2634.
Principles of Analgesic Use in the Treatment of Acute Pain and Cancer Pain, 6th ed, Glenview, IL: American Pain Society, 2008.

◆ **Etodolic Acid** *see* Etodolac *on page 812*
◆ **EtOH** *see* Alcohol (Ethyl) *on page 88*

Etomidate (e TOM i date)

Medication Safety Issues
Sound-alike/look-alike issues:
Etomidate may be confused with etidronate
High alert medication:
The Institute for Safe Medication Practices (ISMP) includes this medication among its list of drugs which have a heightened risk of causing significant patient harm when used in error.

Brand Names: U.S. Amidate
Therapeutic Category General Anesthetic
Generic Availability (U.S.) Yes
Use Induction and maintenance of general anesthesia particularly in patients with diminished cardiovascular function; sedation for short procedures
Pregnancy Risk Factor C
Pregnancy Considerations Adverse events have been observed in animal reproduction studies.
Breast-Feeding Considerations It is not known if etomidate is excreted in breast milk. The manufacturer recommends that caution be exercised when administering etomidate to nursing women.
Contraindications Hypersensitivity to etomidate or any component of the formulation
Warnings Etomidate inhibits 11-B-hydroxylase, an enzyme necessary for the production of cortisol, aldosterone, and corticosterone. A single induction dose blocks the normal stress-induced increase in adrenal cortisol production for 4-8 hours and up to 24 hours in elderly and debilitated patients. This suppression does not appear to be dose related and is unresponsive to ACTH stimulation. Since prolonged infusion of etomidate for sedation particularly in critically ill patients may prevent the response to stress, use of prolonged continuous infusions is not recommended. Consider exogenous corticosteroid replacement in patients undergoing severe stress. Etomidate does not possess analgesic activity; use in combination with opioid analgesics to blunt the hemodynamic response to endotracheal intubation or for painful procedures.
Precautions Use with caution in patients with renal failure and hepatic cirrhosis as the duration of effect may be prolonged; use with caution in patients with seizure disorder due to its ability to increase EEG activation with epileptiform spikes; high doses of etomidate have been associated with EEG slowing and isoelectricity; involuntary muscles movements or myoclonus occur in up to 30% of patients; this may be minimized by pretreatment with benzodiazepines or fentanyl
Adverse Reactions
Gastrointestinal: Hiccups, nausea, vomiting on emergence from anesthesia
Local: Pain at injection site
Neuromuscular & skeletal: Myoclonus, transient skeletal movements, uncontrolled eye movements
Rare but important or life-threatening: Apnea, arrhythmia, bradycardia, decreased cortisol synthesis, hyper-/hypotension, hyper-/hypoventilation, laryngospasm, tachycardia

Drug Interactions

Metabolism/Transport Effects None known.

Avoid Concomitant Use There are no known interactions where it is recommended to avoid concomitant use.

Increased Effect/Toxicity There are no known significant interactions involving an increase in effect.

Decreased Effect There are no known significant interactions involving a decrease in effect.

Stability Store at room temperature. Compatible when administered by Y-site injection with: Alfentanil, atracurium, atropine, doxacurium, ephedrine, fentanyl, lidocaine, lorazepam, midazolam, mivacurium, morphine, pancuronium, phenylephrine, succinylcholine, sufentanil. Incompatible with ascorbic acid, vecuronium

Mechanism of Action Ultrashort-acting nonbarbiturate hypnotic (benzylimidazole) used for the induction of anesthesia; chemically, it is a carboxylated imidazole which produces a rapid induction of anesthesia with minimal cardiovascular effects; produces EEG burst suppression at high doses

Pharmacodynamics

Onset of action: 30-60 seconds

Maximum effect: 1 minute

Duration: Dose dependent: 2-3 minutes (0.15 mg/kg dose); 4-10 minutes (0.3 mg/kg dose); rapid recovery is due to rapid redistribution

Pharmacokinetics (Adult data unless noted)

Distribution: V_d: 3.6-4.5 L/kg

Protein binding: 76%; decreased protein binding resulting in an increased percentage of "free" etomidate in patients with renal failure or hepatic cirrhosis

Metabolism: Hepatic and plasma esterases

Half-life, elimination: Terminal: 2.6-3.5 hours

Time to peak serum concentration: 7 minutes

Excretion: 75% excreted in urine over 24 hours; 2% excreted unchanged

Dosing: Usual I.V.:

Induction & maintenance of anesthesia: Children >10 years and Adults: Initial: 0.2-0.6 mg/kg over 30-60 seconds; maintenance: 10-20 mcg/kg/minute; smaller doses may be used to supplement subpotent anesthetic agents

Procedural sedation: Limited data in children; initial doses 0.1-0.3 mg/kg have been used; repeat doses may be needed depending upon the duration of the procedure and the response of the patient

Administration I.V.: Administer I.V. push over 30-60 seconds; very irritating; avoid administration into small vessels on the dorsum of the head or hand; preadministration of lidocaine may be beneficial

Monitoring Parameters Cardiac monitoring, blood pressure, respiratory rate, sedation score (procedural sedation)

Dosage Forms Excipient information presented when available (limited, particularly for generics); consult specific product labeling.

Solution, Intravenous:

Amidate: 2 mg/mL (10 mL, 20 mL) [contains propylene glycol]

Generic: 2 mg/mL (10 mL, 20 mL)

Solution, Intravenous [preservative free]:

Generic: 2 mg/mL (10 mL, 20 mL)

References

Falk J and Zed PJ, "Etomidate for Procedural Sedation in the Emergency Department," *Ann Pharmacother*, 2004, 38(7-8):1272-7.

Kienstra AJ, Ward MA, Sasan F, et al, "Etomidate Versus Pentobarbital for Sedation of Children for Head and Neck CT Imaging," *Pediatr Emerg Care*, 2004, 20(8):499-506.

Tobias JD, "Etomidate: Applications in Pediatric Critical Care and Pediatric Aanesthesiology," *Pediatr Crit Care Med*, 2000, 1(2):100-6.

Etoposide (e toe POE side)

Medication Safety Issues

Sound-alike/look-alike issues:

Etoposide may be confused with teniposide

Etoposide may be confused with etoposide phosphate (a prodrug of etoposide which is rapidly converted in the plasma to etoposide)

VePesid may be confused with Versed

High alert medication:

This medication is in a class the Institute for Safe Medication Practices (ISMP) includes among its list of drug classes which have a heightened risk of causing significant patient harm when used in error.

Related Information

Emetogenic Potential of Antineoplastic Agents in Children *on page 2327*

Management of Drug Extravasations *on page 2255*

Oral Medications That Should Not Be Crushed or Altered *on page 2438*

Safe Handling of Hazardous Drugs *on page 2419*

Brand Names: U.S. Toposar

Brand Names: Canada Etoposide Injection USP; Vepesid™

Therapeutic Category Antineoplastic Agent, Mitotic Inhibitor; Antineoplastic Agent, Topoisomerase Inhibitor

Generic Availability (U.S.) Yes

Use Treatment of refractory testicular tumors (Parenteral: FDA approved in adults) and small cell lung cancer (Oral and parenteral: FDA approved in adults); has also been used for malignant lymphoma, Hodgkin's disease, leukemias (ALL, ANLL, AML), neuroblastoma; treatment of Ewing's sarcoma, rhabdomyosarcoma, osteosarcoma, Wilms' tumor, CNS tumors; conditioning regimen with hematopoietic stem cell transplantation

Pregnancy Risk Factor D

Pregnancy Considerations Animal reproduction studies have demonstrated teratogenicity and fetal loss. There are no adequate and well-controlled studies in pregnant women. Women of childbearing potential should be advised to avoid pregnancy.

Breast-Feeding Considerations Due to the potential for serious adverse reactions in the nursing infant, the decision to discontinue etoposide or to discontinue breast-feeding during treatment should take into account the benefits of treatment to the mother.

Contraindications Hypersensitivity to etoposide or any component

Warnings Hazardous agent; use appropriate precautions for handling and disposal (NIOSH, 2012). Etoposide is mutagenic, potentially carcinogenic, teratogenic, and embryotoxic. Secondary acute leukemias have been reported with etoposide, either as monotherapy or in combination with other chemotherapy agents. Severe dose-limiting and dose-related myelosuppression with resulting infection or bleeding may occur **[U.S. Boxed Warning]**; treatment should be withheld for platelets <50,000/mm^3 or absolute neutrophil count (ANC) <500/mm^3 until counts recover. Hypotension may occur due to rapid infusion of etoposide; infuse slowly over at least 30-60 minutes. If hypotension occurs, interrupt infusion and administer I.V. hydration and supportive care; decrease infusion rate upon reinitiation.

Etoposide injection contains benzyl alcohol which may cause allergic reactions in susceptible individuals; large amounts of benzyl alcohol (≥99 mg/kg/day) have been associated with a potentially fatal toxicity ("gasping syndrome") in neonates; the "gasping syndrome" consists of metabolic acidosis, respiratory distress, gasping respirations, CNS dysfunction (including convulsions, intracranial hemorrhage), hypotension and cardiovascular collapse;

use etoposide injection containing benzyl alcohol with caution in neonates; *in vitro* and animal studies have shown that benzoate, a metabolite of benzyl alcohol, displaces bilirubin from protein binding sites. Benzyl alcohol may also play a role in the development of hypersensitivity reactions occurring with intravenous administration. Injectable formulation also contains alcohol (~33% v/v); may contribute to adverse reactions, especially with higher etoposide doses. Etoposide injection also contains polysorbate 80 (Tween 80) which may cause allergic reactions in susceptible individuals. In premature neonates, thrombocytopenia, ascites, pulmonary deterioration, and renal and hepatic failure have been reported after receiving parenteral products containing polysorbate 80 (Alade, 1986; CDC, 1984). Infusion of polysorbate 80-containing solutions through PVC tubing may cause DEHP to leach into the solution; in immature animals, exposure to DEHP may adversely affect the development of the male reproductive tract. Polysorbate 80 may also play a role in the development of hypersensitivity reactions occurring with intravenous administration.

Anaphylactic reactions including chills, fever, tachycardia, bronchospasm, dyspnea and hypotension have been reported with etoposide. In addition, facial/tongue swelling, coughing, chest tightness, cyanosis, laryngospasm, diaphoresis, hypertension, and flushing have also been reported less commonly. Incidence is primarily associated with intravenous administration (up to 2%) compared to oral administration (<1%); concentration and rate of infusion may contribute to anaphylactic reactions. Higher rates of anaphylactoid reactions have been reported in children who received I.V. infusions of etoposide at higher than recommended concentrations. If a reaction occurs, discontinue infusion and provide appropriate supportive care. High drug concentration and rate of infusion, as well as presence of polysorbate 80 and benzyl alcohol in the etoposide intravenous formulation, have been suggested as contributing factors to the development of hypersensitivity reactions. Unlike etoposide injection, the water soluble prodrug formulation (etoposide phosphate) does not contain either benzyl alcohol or polysorbate 80; case reports describe etoposide phosphate success in patients with previous hypersensitivity reactions to etoposide (Collier, 2008; Siderov, 2002).

Precautions Use with caution and consider dosage reduction in patients with hepatic impairment, bone marrow suppression, and renal impairment. Use with caution in patients with low serum albumin; may increase risk for toxicities. Should be administered under the supervision of an experienced cancer chemotherapy physician **[U.S. Boxed Warning]**.

Adverse Reactions Note: The following may occur with higher doses used in stem cell transplantation: Alopecia, ethanol intoxication, hepatitis, hypotension (infusion-related), metabolic acidosis, mucositis, nausea and vomiting (severe), secondary malignancy, skin lesions (resembling Stevens-Johnson syndrome).

Cardiovascular: Hypotension (due to rapid infusion)
Dermatologic: Alopecia
Gastrointestinal: Abdominal pain, anorexia, diarrhea, nausea/vomiting, stomatitis
Hematologic: Anemia, leukopenia (nadir: 7-14 days; recovery: by day 20), thrombocytopenia (nadir 9-16 days; recovery: by day 20)
Hepatic: Hepatic toxicity
Neuromuscular & skeletal: Peripheral neuropathy
Miscellaneous: Anaphylactic-like reaction (including chills, fever, tachycardia, bronchospasm, dyspnea)
Rare but important or life-threatening: Amenorrhea, blindness (transient/cortical), cyanosis, extravasation (induration/necrosis), facial swelling, hypersensitivity, hypersensitivity-associated apnea, interstitial

pneumonitis, laryngospasm, maculopapular rash, metabolic acidosis, MI, mucositis, myocardial ischemia, optic neuritis, perivasculitis, pruritus, pulmonary fibrosis, radiation-recall dermatitis, rash, reversible posterior leukoencephalopathy syndrome (RPLS), seizure, Stevens-Johnson syndrome, tongue swelling, toxic epidermal necrolysis, toxic megacolon, vasospasm

Drug Interactions

Metabolism/Transport Effects Substrate of CYP1A2 (minor), CYP2E1 (minor), CYP3A4 (major), P-glycoprotein; **Note:** Assignment of Major/Minor substrate status based on clinically relevant drug interaction potential; **Inhibits** CYP2C9 (weak), CYP3A4 (weak)

Avoid Concomitant Use
Avoid concomitant use of Etoposide with any of the following: BCG; CloZAPine; Conivaptan; Dipyrone; Fusidic Acid (Systemic); Natalizumab; Pimecrolimus; Pimozide; Tacrolimus (Topical); Tofacitinib; Vaccines (Live)

Increased Effect/Toxicity
Etoposide may increase the levels/effects of: ARIPiprazole; CloZAPine; Dofetilide; Leflunomide; Lomitapide; Natalizumab; Pimozide; Tofacitinib; Vaccines (Live); Vitamin K Antagonists

The levels/effects of Etoposide may be increased by: Atovaquone; Ceritinib; Conivaptan; CycloSPORINE (Systemic); CYP3A4 Inhibitors (Moderate); CYP3A4 Inhibitors (Strong); Dasatinib; Denosumab; Dipyrone; Fusidic Acid (Systemic); Ivacaftor; Luliconazole; Mifepristone; P-glycoprotein/ABCB1 Inhibitors; Pimecrolimus; Roflumilast; Simeprevir; Stiripentol; Tacrolimus (Topical); Trastuzumab

Decreased Effect
Etoposide may decrease the levels/effects of: BCG; Coccidioidin Skin Test; Sipuleucel-T; Vaccines (Inactivated); Vaccines (Live)

The levels/effects of Etoposide may be decreased by: Barbiturates; Bosentan; CYP3A4 Inducers (Strong); Dabrafenib; Deferasirox; Fosphenytoin; Mitotane; P-glycoprotein/ABCB1 Inducers; Phenytoin; Siltuximab; St Johns Wort; Tocilizumab

Stability
Capsules: Store oral capsules at 2°C to 8°C (36°F to 46°F); do not freeze.
Injection: Store unopened vials at 20°C to 25°C (68°F to 77°F); do not freeze. Undiluted etoposide injection may cause cracks and leaking when stored in acrylic or ABS (acrylonitrile, butadiene, and styrene) plastic containers. Stability of diluted injection is concentration dependent; more concentrated solutions have shorter stability (0.2 mg/mL: 96 hours; 0.4 mg/mL: 24 hours); incidence of precipitation increases with final concentrations >0.4 mg/mL; at a concentration of 1 mg/mL in D_5W or NS, crystallization has occurred within 30 minutes.

Mechanism of Action Etoposide has been shown to delay transit of cells through the S phase and arrest cells in late S or early G_2 phase. The drug may inhibit mitochondrial transport at the NADH dehydrogenase level or inhibit uptake of nucleosides into HeLa cells. It is a topoisomerase II inhibitor and appears to cause DNA strand breaks. Etoposide does not inhibit microtubular assembly.

Pharmacokinetics (Adult data unless noted)
Absorption: Oral: Large variability
Distribution: CSF concentration is <5% of plasma concentration
Children: V_{dss}: 10 L/m^2
Adults: V_{dss}: 7-17 L/m^2
Protein binding: 94% to 97%
Metabolism: In the liver (with a biphasic decay)
Bioavailability: Averages 50% (range: 25% to 75%)

Half-life, terminal:

Children: 6-8 hours

Adults: 4-15 hours with normal renal and hepatic function

Elimination: Both unchanged drug and metabolites are excreted in urine and a small amount (2% to 16%) in feces; up to 55% of an I.V. dose is excreted unchanged in urine in children

Dosing: Usual

Pediatric: **Note:** Dose, frequency, number of doses, and start date may vary by protocol and treatment phase; refer to individual protocols; limited data available:

Acute lymphocytic leukemia (ALL), relapsed: Children and Adolescents: I.V.: *Consolidation:* 100 mg/m^2/dose once daily on days 15-19 (in combination with other chemotherapeutic agents) (Parker, 2010)

Acute myeloid leukemia (AML):

Induction:

Age-directed dosing (Gibson, 2011):

Infants <1 year: 75 mg/m^2/dose once daily on days 1-5 (in combination with cytarabine and daunorubicin or mitoxantrone)

Children ≥1 year and Adolescents: I.V.: 100 mg/m^2/dose once daily on days 1-5 (in combination with cytarabine and daunorubicin or mitoxantrone)

BSA-directed dosing (Cooper, 2012): Infants, Children, and Adolescents: I.V.:

BSA <0.6 m^2: 3.3 mg/**kg**/dose once daily on days 1-5 (in combination with other chemotherapeutic agents)

BSA ≥0.6 m^2: 100 mg/m^2/dose once daily on days 1-5 (in combination with other chemotherapeutic agents)

Intensification: BSA-directed dosing (Cooper, 2012): Infants, Children, and Adolescents: I.V.:

BSA <0.6 m^2: 5 mg/**kg**/dose once daily on days 1-5 (in combination with cytarabine)

BSA ≥0.6 m^2: 150 mg/m^2/dose once daily on days 1-5 (in combination with cytarabine)

Consolidation: Infants, Children, and Adolescents: I.V.: 100 mg/m^2/dose once daily for 4-5 days, administered over 1 hour (in combination with cytarabine and daunorubicin or amsacrine) (Gibson, 2012; Perel, 2002); 75 mg/m^2/dose once daily on days 1-5 (in combination with cytarabine and amsacrine) was administered to infants <1 year in one study (Gibson, 2012)

CNS tumor:

Infants and Children <3 years: I.V.: 6.5 mg/**kg**/dose administered on days 3 and 4 (in combination with cisplatin as Cycle B regimen) for 28 day cycle alternating with Cycle A regimen (cyclophosphamide and vincristine); therapy initiated 2-4 weeks after tumor resection (Duffner, 1993)

Children ≥3 years and Adolescents: I.V.: 100 mg/m^2/dose once daily on days 1, 2, and 3 (in combination with vincristine and carboplatin or cyclophosphamide) every 3 weeks for 4 cycles prior to radiation (Taylor, 2003)

Children ≥6 years and Adolescents: I.V.: 150 mg/m^2/dose once daily on days 3 and 4 (in combination with cisplatin) every 3 weeks for 4 cycles prior to radiation (Kovnar, 1990)

Hematopoietic stem cell transplantation (HSCT), conditioning regimen: Children ≥1 year and Adolescents: I.V.: 30 **or** 60 mg/kg/dose administered over 4-8 hours as a single dose 3 or 4 days prior to transplantation (Biagi, 2000; Duerst, 2000; Horning, 1994; Snyder, 1993; Zander, 1997)

Hodgkin's lymphoma, advanced stage (BEACOPP regimen): *Induction:* Children ≥4 years and Adolescents: I.V.: 200 mg/m^2/dose once daily on days 0-2 (3 doses) every 3 weeks for 4 cycles (in combination with bleomycin, doxorubicin, cyclophosphamide, vincristine,

procarbazine, and prednisone); 4 additional cycles may be given to slow early responders (Kelly, 2002; Kelly, 2011)

Neuroblastoma, high-risk: Children ≥1 year and Adolescents:

Induction: I.V.: 100-200 mg/m^2/dose infused over 1-2 hours once daily for 3-5 consecutive days (in combination with other chemotherapy agents) (Kaneko, 2002; Kushner, 2004; Simon, 2007; Simon, 2007a); other reported regimens include 100 mg/m^2/dose on day 2 and 5 (in combination with cisplatin, doxorubicin, and cyclophosphamide) every 28 days for 5 cycles (Matthay, 1999)

Myeloablative therapy with stem cell rescue:

I.V.: 100-200 mg/m^2/day for 4-5 days beginning 8-9 days prior to transplantation was used in 301 patients (Kaneko, 2002)

Continuous I.V. infusion: 640 mg/m^2 infused over 96 hours beginning 8 days prior to transplant (Matthany, 1999; Park, 2009)

Sarcoma: Children ≥1 year and Adolescents: I.V.: 100 mg/m^2/dose once daily for 5 doses on days 0-4 every 3 weeks [in combination with ifosfamide and carboplatin (ICE regimen)] (Van Winkle, 2005); other reported regimens include: 150 mg/m^2/dose once daily for 3 doses on days 1-3 in combination with vincristine, doxorubicin, cyclophosphamide, and ifosfamide (VACIE regimen) (Navid, 2006)

Wilms tumor (ICE Regimen): Children and Adolescents: I.V.: 100 mg/m^2/dose once daily for 3-5 doses (in combination with ifosfamide and carboplatin); repeat cycle every 21 days (Abu-Ghosh, 2002; Daw, 2009)

Adult: **Note:** Utilize patient's actual body weight (full weight) for calculation of body surface area- or weight-based dosing, particularly when the intent of therapy is curative (excludes HSCT dosing); manage regimen-related toxicities in the same manner as for nonobese patients; if a dose reduction is utilized due to toxicity, consider resumption of full weight-based dosing with subsequent cycles, especially if cause of toxicity (eg, hepatic or renal impairment) is resolved (Griggs, 2012).

Small cell lung cancer (in combination with other chemotherapy agents):

I.V.: 35 mg/m^2/day for 4 days, up to 50 mg/m^2/day for 5 days every 3-4 weeks

Oral: Due to poor bioavailability, oral doses should be twice the I.V. dose (and rounded to the nearest 50 mg)

Testicular cancer (in combination with other chemotherapy agents): I.V.: 50-100 mg/m^2/day on days 1-5 or 100 mg/m^2/day on days 1, 3, and 5 repeated every 3-4 weeks

Dosing adjustment in renal impairment:

Infants, Children, and Adolescents: Dosage adjustments are not provided in the manufacturer's labeling; however, the following adjustments have been recommended (Aronoff, 2007):

GFR >50 mL/minute/1.73 m^2: No dosage adjustment necessary

GFR 10-50 mL/minute/1.73m^2: Administer 75% of dose

GFR <10 mL/minute/1.73m^2: Administer 50% of dose

Hemodialysis/peritoneal dialysis (PD) (after dialysis on dialysis days): Administer 50% of dose

Continuous renal replacement therapy (CRRT): Administer 75% of dose and reduce for hyperbilirubinemia

Adults:

Manufacturer's labeling:

CrCl >50 mL/minute: No adjustment required.

CrCl 15-50 mL/minute: Administer 75% of dose

CrCl <15 mL minute: Data not available; consider further dose reductions

The following guidelines have been used by some clinicians:

Aronoff, 2007:

CrCl >50 mL/minute: No adjustment required.

CrCl 10-50 mL/minute: Administer 75% of normal dose

CrCl <10 mL/minute: Administer 50% of normal dose

Hemodialysis: Administer 50% of dose; supplemental posthemodialysis dose is not necessary

Peritoneal dialysis: Administer 50% of dose; supplemental dose is not necessary

Continuous renal replacement therapy (CRRT): Administer 75% of dose

Janus, 2010: Hemodialysis: Reduce dose by 50%; not removed by hemodialysis so may be administered before or after dialysis

Kintzel, 1995:

CrCl 46-60 mL/minute: Administer 85% of dose

CrCl 31-45 mL/minute: Administer 80% of dose

CrCl ≤30 mL/minute: Administer 75% of dose

Dosing adjustment in hepatic impairment:

Infants, Children, and Adolescents: The following adjustments have been recommended (Floyd, 2006): Bilirubin 1.5-3 mg/dL or AST >3 times ULN: Administer 50% of dose

Adults: There are no dosage adjustments provided in manufacturer's labeling; however, the following adjustments have been recommended.

Donelli, 1998: Liver dysfunction may reduce the metabolism and increase the toxicity of etoposide. Normal doses of I.V. etoposide should be given to patients with liver dysfunction (dose reductions may result in subtherapeutic concentrations); however, use caution with concomitant liver dysfunction (severe) and renal dysfunction as the decreased metabolic clearance cannot be compensated by increased renal clearance.

Floyd, 2006: Bilirubin 1.5-3 mg/dL or AST >3 times ULN: Administer 50% of dose

King, 2001; Koren, 1992: Bilirubin 1.5-3 mg/dL or AST >180 units/L: Administer 50% of dose

Dosage adjustment for toxicity: Adults:

Infusion (hypersensitivity) reactions: Interrupt infusion

ANC <500/mm^3 or platelets <50,000/mm^3: Withhold treatment until recovery

Severe adverse reactions (nonhematologic): Reduce dose or discontinue treatment

Administration Hazardous agent; use appropriate precautions for handling and disposal (NIOSH, 2012).

Oral: In adults, doses ≤200 mg/day should be given as a single daily dose; doses >400 mg should be given in 2-4 divided doses. If necessary, the injection may be used for oral administration either as an extemporaneous preparation or by mixing dose with orange juice, apple juice, or lemonade at a final concentration not to exceed 0.4 mg/mL.

Parenteral: I.V.: Further dilute in NS or D$_5$W to a typical final concentration of 0.2-0.4 mg/mL to minimize hypotension risk; however, more concentrated I.V. solutions (0.6-1 mg/mL) may be used. For high-dose etoposide infusions, undiluted etoposide (20 mg/mL) has been infused as a single dose from a glass syringe via syringe pump through a central venous catheter over 1-4 hours. Higher than recommended concentrations of etoposide infusions may crack hard plastic in chemo venting pins and infusion lines; inspect infusion solution for particulate matter and plastic devices for cracks and leaks; pH:3-4

For I.V. infusion only; do not administer by rapid I.V. injection or by intrathecal, intraperitoneal, or intrapleural routes due to possible severe toxicity. Administer by continuous I.V. infusion or I.V. intermittent infusion via an in-line 0.22 micron filter over at least 60 minutes at a rate not to exceed 100 mg/m^2/hour (or 3.3 mg/**kg**/hour).

Vesicant/Extravasation Risk May be an irritant

Monitoring Parameters CBC with differential and platelet count, hemoglobin, vital signs (blood pressure), albumin, bilirubin, liver and renal function tests

Dosage Forms Excipient information presented when available (limited, particularly for generics); consult specific product labeling.

Capsule, Oral:

Generic: 50 mg

Solution, Intravenous:

Toposar: 100 mg/5 mL (5 mL); 500 mg/25 mL (25 mL); 1 g/50 mL (50 mL) [contains alcohol, usp, polyethylene glycol 300, polysorbate 80]

Generic: 100 mg/5 mL (5 mL); 500 mg/25 mL (25 mL); 1 g/50 mL (50 mL)

Extemporaneous Preparations Hazardous agent: Use appropriate precautions for handling and disposal.

Etoposide 10 mg/mL oral solution: Dilute etoposide for injection 1:1 with normal saline to a concentration of 10 mg/mL. This solution is stable in plastic oral syringes for 22 days at room temperature. Prior to oral administration, further mix with fruit juice (orange, apple, or lemon; **NOT** grapefruit juice) to a concentration of <0.4 mg/mL; once mixed with fruit juice, use within 3 hours.

McLeod HL and Relling MV, "Stability of Etoposide Solution for Oral Use," *Am J Hosp Pharm*, 1992, 49(11):2784-5.

References

Abu-Ghosh AM, Krailo MD, Goldman SC, et al, "Ifosfamide, Carboplatin and Etoposide in Children With Poor-Risk Relapsed Wilms' Tumor: A Children's Cancer Group Report," *Ann Oncol*, 2002, 13(3):460-9.

Alade SL, Brown RE, and Paquet A Jr, "Polysorbate 80 and E-Ferol Toxicity," *Pediatrics*, 1986, 77(4):593-7.

Aronoff GR, Bennett WM, Berns JS, et al, *Drug Prescribing in Renal Failure: Dosing Guidelines for Adults and Children*, 5th ed, Philadelphia, PA: American College of Physicians; 2007.

Berg SL, Grisell DL, DeLaney TF, et al, "Principles of Treatment of Pediatric Solid Tumors," *Pediatr Clin North Am*, 1991, 38(2):249-67.

Biagi E, Rovelli A, Balduzzi A, et al, "TBI, Etoposide and Cyclophosphamide as a Promising Conditioning Regimen for BMT in Childhood ALL in Second Remission," *Bone Marrow Transplant*, 2000, 26 (11):1260-2.

Boos J, Krümpelmann S, Schulze-Westhoff P, et al, "Steady-State Levels and Bone Marrow Toxicity of Etoposide in Children and Infants: Does Etoposide Require Age-Dependent Dose Calculation?" *J Clin Oncol*, 1995, 13(12):2954-60.

Centers for Disease Control (CDC), "Unusual Syndrome With Fatalities Among Premature Infants: Association With a New Intravenous Vitamin E Product," *MMWR Morb Mortal Wkly Rep*, 1984, 33 (14):198-9.

Clark PI and Slevin ML, "The Clinical Pharmacology of Etoposide and Teniposide," *Clin Pharmacokinet*, 1987, 12(4):223-52.

Collier K, Schink C, Young AM, et al, "Successful Treatment With Etoposide Phosphate in Patients With Previous Etoposide Hypersensitivity," *J Oncol Pharm Pract*, 2008, 14(1):51-5.

Cooper TM, Franklin J, Gerbing RB, et al, "AAML03P1, A Pilot Study of the Safety of Gemtuzumab Ozogamicin in Combination With Chemotherapy for Newly Diagnosed Childhood Acute Myeloid Leukemia: A Report From the Children's Oncology Group," *Cancer*, 2012, 118 (3):761-9.

Daw NC, Gregornik D, Rodman J, et al, "Renal Function After Ifosfamide, Carboplatin and Etoposide (ICE) Chemotherapy, Nephrectomy and Radiotherapy in Children With Wilms Tumour," *Eur J Cancer*, 2009, 45(1):99-106.

Donelli MG, Zucchetti M, Munzone E, D'Incalci M, Crosignani A. Pharmacokinetics of anticancer agents in patients with impaired liver function. *Eur J Cancer*. 1998;34(1):33-46.

Duerst RE, Horan JT, Liesveld JL, et al, "Allogeneic Bone Marrow Transplantation for Children With Acute Leukemia: Cytoreduction With Fractionated Total Body Irradiation, High-Dose Etoposide and Cyclophosphamide," *Bone Marrow Transplant*, 2000, 25(5):489-94.

Duffner PK, Horowitz ME, Krischer JP, et al, "Postoperative Chemotherapy and Delayed Radiation in Children Less Than Three Years of Age With Malignant Brain Tumors," *N Engl J Med*, 1993, 328 (24):1725-31.

Floyd J, Mirza I, Sachs B, et al, "Hepatotoxicity of Chemotherapy," *Semin Oncol*, 2006, 33(1):50-67.

Gibson BE, Webb DK, Howman AJ, et al, "Results of a Randomized Trial in Children With Acute Myeloid Leukaemia: Medical Research Council AML12 Trial," *Br J Haematol*, 2011, 155(3):366-76.

Griggs JJ, Mangu PB, Anderson H, et al. Appropriate chemotherapy dosing for obese adult patients with cancer: American Society of

Clinical Oncology Clinical Practice Guideline. *J Clin Oncol*. 2012,30 (13):1553-1561.

Horning SJ, Negrin RS, Chao JC, et al, "Fractionated Total-Body Irradiation, Etoposide, and Cyclophosphamide Plus Autografting in Hodgkin's Disease and Non-Hodgkin's Lymphoma," *J Clin Oncol*, 1994, 12(12):2552-8.

Janus N, Thariat J, Boulanger H, Deray G, Launay-Vacher V. Proposal for dosage adjustment and timing of chemotherapy in hemodialyzed patients. *Ann Onco*. 2010;21(7):1395-1403.

Kaneko M, Tsuchida Y, Mugishima H, et al, "Intensified Chemotherapy Increases the Survival Rates in Patients With Stage 4 Neuroblastoma With MYCN Amplification," *J Pediatr Hematol Oncol*, 2002, 24 (8):613-21.

Kelly KM, Hutchinson RJ, Sposto R, et al, "Feasibility of Upfront Dose-Intensive Chemotherapy in Children With Advanced-Stage Hodgkin's Lymphoma: Preliminary Results From the Children's Cancer Group Study CCG-59704," *Ann Oncol*, 2002,13 Suppl 1:107-11.

Kelly KM, Sposto R, Hutchinson R, et al, "BEACOPP Chemotherapy is a Highly Effective Regimen in Children and Adolescents With High-Risk Hodgkin Lymphoma: A Report From the Children's Oncology Group," *Blood*, 2011, 117(9):2596-603.

King PD, Perry MC. Hepatotoxicity of chemotherapy. *Oncologist*. 2001;6(2):162-176.

Kintzel PE and Dorr RT, "Anticancer Drug Renal Toxicity and Elimination: Dosing Guidelines for Altered Renal Function," *Cancer Treat Rev*, 1995, 21(1):33-64.

Koren G, Beatty K, Seto A, Einarson TR, Lishner M. The effects of impaired liver function on the elimination of antineoplastic agents. *Ann Pharmacother*. 1992;26(3):363-371.

Kovnar EH, Kellie SJ, Horowitz ME, et al, "Preirradiation Cisplatin and Etoposide in the Treatment of High-Risk Medulloblastoma and Other Malignant Embryonal Tumors of the Central Nervous System: A Phase II Study," *J Clin Oncol*, 1990, 8(2):330-6.

Kushner BH, Kramer K, LaQuaglia MP, et al, "Reduction From Seven to Five Cycles of Intensive Induction Chemotherapy in Children With High-Risk Neuroblastoma," *J Clin Oncol*, 2004, 22(24):4888-92.

Lazarus HM, Creger RJ, and Diaz D, "Simple Method for the Administration of High-Dose Etoposide During Autologous Bone Marrow Transplantation," *Cancer Treat Rep*, 1986, 70(6):819-20.

Matthay KK, Villablanca JG, Seeger RC, et al, "Treatment of High-Risk Neuroblastoma With Intensive Chemotherapy, Radiotherapy, Autologous Bone Marrow Transplantation, and 13-Cis-Retinoic Acid. Children's Cancer Group," *N Engl J Med*, 1999, 341(16):1165-73.

National Institute for Occupational Safety and Health (NIOSH), "NIOSH List of Antineoplastic and Other Hazardous Drugs in Healthcare Settings 2012." Available at http://www.cdc.gov/niosh/docs/2012-150/pdfs/2012-150.pdf. Accessed January 21, 2013.

Navid F, Santana VM, Billups CA, et al, "Concomitant Administration of Vincristine, Doxorubicin, Cyclophosphamide, Ifosfamide, and Etoposide for High-Risk Sarcomas: The St. Jude Children's Research Hospital Experience," *Cancer*, 2006, 106(8):1846-56.

Nishikawa A, Nakamura Y, Nobori U, et al, "Acute Monocytic Leukemia in Children. Response to VP-16-213 as a Single Agent," *Cancer*, 1987, 60(9):2146-9.

O'Dwyer PJ, Leyland-Jones B, Alonso MT, et al, "Etoposide (VP-16-213): Current Status of an Active Anticancer Drug," *N Engl J Med*, 1985, 312(11):692-700.

Park JR, Villablanca JG, London WB, et al, "Outcome of High-Risk Stage 3 Neuroblastoma With Myeloablative Therapy and 13-Cis-Retinoic Acid: A Report From the Children's Oncology Group," *Pediatr Blood Cancer*, 2009, 52(1):44-50.

Parker C, Waters R, Leighton C, "Effect of Mitoxantrone on Outcome of Children With First Relapse of Acute Lymphoblastic Leukaemia (ALL R3): An Open-Label Randomised Trial," *Lancet*, 2010, 376 (9757):2009-17.

Perel Y, Auvrignon A, Leblanc T, et al, "Impact of Addition of Maintenance Therapy to Intensive Induction and Consolidation Chemotherapy for Childhood Acute Myeloblastic Leukemia: Results of a Prospective Randomized Trial, LAME 89/91. Leucámie Aiqüe Myéloïde Enfant," *J Clin Oncol*, 2002, 20(12):2774-82.

Siderov J, Prasad P, De Boer R, et al, "Safe Administration of Etoposide Phosphate After Hypersensitivity Reaction to Intravenous Etoposide," *Br J Cancer*, 2002, 86(1):12-3.

Simon T, Längler A, Berthold F, et al, "Topotecan and Etoposide in the Treatment of Relapsed High-Risk Neuroblastoma: Results of a Phase 2 Trial," *J Pediatr Hematol Oncol*, 2007, 29(2):101-6.

Simon T, Längler A, Harnischmacher U, et al, "Topotecan, Cyclophosphamide, and Etoposide (TCE) in the Treatment of High-Risk Neuroblastoma. Results of a Phase-II Trial," *J Cancer Res Clin Oncol*, 2007a, 133(9):653-61.

Snyder DS, Chao NJ, Amylon MD, et al, "Fractionated Total Body Irradiation and High-Dose Etoposide as a Preparatory Regimen for Bone Marrow Transplantation for 99 Patients With Acute Leukemia in First Complete Remission," *Blood*, 1993, 82(9):2920-8.

Superfin D, Iannucci AA, and Davies AM, "Commentary: Oncologic Drugs in Patients With Organ Dysfunction: A Summary," *Oncologist*, 2007, 12(9):1070-83.

Taylor RE, Bailey CC, Robinson K, et al, "Results of a Randomized Study of Preradiation Chemotherapy Versus Radiotherapy Alone for Nonmetastatic Medulloblastoma: The International Society of Paediatric Oncology/United Kingdom Children's Cancer Study Group PNET-3 Study," *J Clin Oncol*, 2003, 21(8):1581-91.

Van Winkle P, Angiolillo A, Krailo M, et al, "Ifosfamide, Carboplatin, and Etoposide (ICE) Reinduction Chemotherapy in a Large Cohort of Children and Adolescents With Recurrent/Refractory Sarcoma: The Children's Cancer Group (CCG) Experience," *Pediatr Blood Cancer*, 2005, 44(4):338-47.

Zander AR, Berger C, Kröger N, et al, "High Dose Chemotherapy With Busulfan, Cyclophosphamide, and Etoposide as Conditioning Regimen for Allogeneic Bone Marrow Transplantation for Patients With Acute Myeloid Leukemia in First Complete Remission," *Clin Cancer Res*, 1997, 3(12 Pt 2):2671-5.

◆ **Etoposide Injection USP (Can)** *see* Etoposide *on page 815*

◆ **ETR** *see* Etravirine *on page 819*

Etravirine (et ra VIR een)

Medication Safety Issues
International issues:
Etravirine [U.S. and multiple international markets] may be confused with ethaverine [multiple international markets]

Related Information
Adult and Adolescent HIV *on page 2348*
Oral Medications That Should Not Be Crushed or Altered *on page 2438*
Pediatric HIV *on page 2338*
Perinatal HIV *on page 2356*

Brand Names: U.S. Intelence
Brand Names: Canada Intelence®
Therapeutic Category Antiretroviral Agent; HIV Agents (Anti-HIV Agents); Non-nucleoside Reverse Transcriptase Inhibitor (NNRTI)
Generic Availability (U.S.) No
Use Treatment of HIV-1 infection in combination with other antiretroviral agents (FDA approved in ages ≥6 years weighing at least 16 kg and adults); **Note:** HIV regimens consisting of **three** antiretroviral agents are strongly recommended.
Pregnancy Risk Factor B
Pregnancy Considerations Adverse events have not been noted in animal reproduction studies. Etravirine crosses the placenta. Based on limited data, dose adjustments are not needed in pregnant women. However, because available data in pregnant women are insufficient, the DHHS Perinatal HIV Guidelines do not recommend use in antiretroviral-naive women unless other alternatives are not available. Hypersensitivity reactions (including hepatic toxicity and rash) are more common in women on NNRTI therapy; it is not known if pregnancy increases this risk.

Regardless of CD4 count or HIV RNA copy number, all HIV-infected pregnant women should receive a combination antiretroviral (ARV) drug regimen. A combination of antepartum, intrapartum, and infant ARV prophylaxis is recommended. ARV therapy should be started as soon as possible in women with symptomatic infection. Although earlier initiation may be more effective in reducing the perinatal transmission of HIV, initiation may be delayed until after 12 weeks gestation in women who do not require immediate treatment after careful consideration of maternal conditions (eg, nausea and vomiting) and the potential risks of first trimester fetal exposure for specific agents. A scheduled cesarean delivery at 38 weeks gestation is recommended for all women with HIV RNA >1000 copies/mL or unknown concentrations near delivery in order to decrease transmission. If ARV therapy must be interrupted for <24 hours during the peripartum period, stop then restart all medications simultaneously in order to decrease the chance of developing resistance. Long-term follow-up is recommended for all infants exposed to ARV medications. In couples who want to conceive, the HIV-infected partner should attain maximum viral suppression prior to conception.

Health care providers are encouraged to enroll pregnant women exposed to antiretroviral medications in the Antiretroviral Pregnancy Registry (1-800-258-4263 or www.-APRegistry.com). Health care providers caring for HIV-infected women and their infants may contact the National Perinatal HIV Hotline (888-448-8765) for clinical consultation (DHHS [perinatal], 2014).

Breast-Feeding Considerations It is not known if etravirine is excreted into breast milk. Maternal or infant antiretroviral therapy does not completely eliminate the risk of postnatal HIV transmission. In addition, multiclass-resistant virus has been detected in breast-feeding infants despite maternal therapy. Therefore, in the United States, where formula is accessible, affordable, safe, and sustainable, and the risk of infant mortality due to diarrhea and respiratory infections is low, complete avoidance of breast-feeding by HIV-infected women is recommended to decrease potential transmission of HIV (DHHS [perinatal], 2014).

Contraindications Hypersensitivity to etravirine or any component

Warnings Severe, life-threatening, and fatal cases of skin reactions (including Stevens-Johnson syndrome, toxic epidermal necrolysis, and erythema multiforme). Hypersensitivity reactions (including drug rash with eosinophilia and systemic symptoms [DRESS]) have also been reported and were characterized by rash, constitutional symptoms, and occasional organ dysfunction including hepatic failure; discontinue immediately with signs or symptoms of severe skin reaction or hypersensitivity including rash, fever, blistering, oral lesions, conjunctivitis, facial edema, muscle or joint aches, general malaise, fatigue, hepatitis, eosinophilia, or angioedema and monitor clinical status including liver function; initiate appropriate therapy. Rash, including serious (Grade 3 or 4) events and discontinuations, were more frequently observed in female subjects compared to male subjects.

Rash is more common and severe in pediatric patients (6 years to <18 years) than in adults; usually described as pruritic, maculopapular skin eruptions (incidence: Pediatric patients: 15%, adults 10%). In pediatric patients, rashes usually appeared within 14 days of starting therapy and generally resolved within a week. Discontinue etravirine if severe rash (involving blistering, desquamation, mucosal involvement, ulceration, or fever) occurs.

Etravirine is a mixed inducer/inhibitor of CYP450 enzymes and numerous drug interactions occur. Due to potential serious and/or life-threatening drug interactions, certain drugs must be avoided; other drug interactions may require dosage adjustment.

Resistance emerges rapidly if administered as monotherapy; always use etravirine in combination with at least two other antiretroviral agents; do not add etravirine as a single agent to antiretroviral regimens that are failing; initiate in combination with at least one other antiretroviral agent to which the patient is naive.

Precautions Use with caution in patients with severe hepatic dysfunction (Child-Pugh class C); use has not been evaluated. Cross-resistance with other non-nucleoside reverse transcriptase inhibitors may occur. Fat redistribution and accumulation [ie, central obesity, peripheral wasting, facial wasting, breast enlargement, dorsocervical fat enlargement (buffalo hump), and cushingoid appearance] have been observed in patients receiving antiretroviral agents (causal relationship not established).

Immune reconstitution syndrome (an acute inflammatory response to residual or indolent opportunistic infections) may occur in HIV patients during initial treatment with combination antiretroviral agents; this syndrome may require further patient assessment and therapy. Autoimmune disorders (eg, Grave's disease, Guillain-Barré syndrome, and polymyositis) have been reported in patients experiencing immune reconstitution; time to onset is variable and may occur many months after antiretroviral treatment is initiated.

Adverse Reactions
Dermatologic: Rash

Endocrine & metabolic: Cholesterol (total) increased, hyperglycemia, LDL increased, triglycerides increased

Gastrointestinal: Amylase increased, diarrhea (children and adolescents), nausea

Hepatic: ALT increased, AST increased

Neuromuscular & skeletal: Peripheral neuropathy

Renal: Creatinine increased

Rare but important or life-threatening: Amnesia, anemia (including hemolytic), angina, angioedema, anorexia, atrial fibrillation, diabetes mellitus, drug rash with eosinophilia and systemic symptoms (DRESS), erythema multiforme, GERD, gynecomastia, hemorrhagic stroke, hematemesis, hepatic failure, hepatic steatosis, hepatitis, hepatomegaly, hypersensitivity reaction, hypersomnia, hypoesthesia, immune reconstitution syndrome, insomnia, lipohypertrophy/dystrophy, MI, pancreatitis, paresthesia, renal failure, rhabdomyolysis, seizure, Stevens-Johnson syndrome, syncope, toxic epidermal necrolysis

Drug Interactions
Metabolism/Transport Effects Substrate of CYP2C19 (major), CYP2C9 (major), CYP3A4 (major); **Note:** Assignment of Major/Minor substrate status based on clinically relevant drug interaction potential; **Inhibits** CYP2C19 (moderate), CYP2C9 (moderate); **Induces** CYP3A4 (weak/moderate)

Avoid Concomitant Use
Avoid concomitant use of Etravirine with any of the following: Atazanavir; Axitinib; CarBAMazepine; Efavirenz; Fosamprenavir; Fosphenytoin; PHENobarbital; Phenytoin; Primidone; Reverse Transcriptase Inhibitors (Non-Nucleoside); Rifamycin Derivatives; Rilpivirine; Ritonavir; Simeprevir; St Johns Wort; Tipranavir

Increased Effect/Toxicity
Etravirine may increase the levels/effects of: Antifungal Agents (Azole Derivatives, Systemic); Artemether; Bosentan; Cannabis; Carvedilol; Citalopram; CYP2C19 Substrates; CYP2C9 Substrates; Diazepam; Digoxin; Dronabinol; Efavirenz; Fosamprenavir; Protease Inhibitors; Rilpivirine; Tetrahydrocannabinol

The levels/effects of Etravirine may be increased by: Antifungal Agents (Azole Derivatives, Systemic); Artemether; Atazanavir; Reverse Transcriptase Inhibitors (Non-Nucleoside)

Decreased Effect
Etravirine may decrease the levels/effects of: Amiodarone; Antifungal Agents (Azole Derivatives, Systemic); ARIPiprazole; Artemether; Atazanavir; Axitinib; Bepridil [Off Market]; Buprenorphine; CarBAMazepine; Clopidogrel; Diazepam; Disopyramide; Dolutegravir; Efavirenz; Flecainide; HMG-CoA Reductase Inhibitors; Ibrutinib; Lidocaine (Systemic); Macrolide Antibiotics; Maraviroc; Methadone; Mexiletine; Phosphodiesterase 5 Inhibitors; Propafenone; QuiNIDine; Rilpivirine; Saxagliptin; Simeprevir; Telaprevir

The levels/effects of Etravirine may be decreased by: Bosentan; CarBAMazepine; CYP2C19 Inducers (Strong); CYP2C9 Inducers (Strong); CYP3A4 Inducers (Strong); Dabrafenib; Deferasirox; Fosphenytoin; Mitotane; Peginterferon Alfa-2b; PHENobarbital; Phenytoin; Primidone; Protease Inhibitors; Reverse Transcriptase

Inhibitors (Non-Nucleoside); Rifabutin; Rifamycin Derivatives; Ritonavir; Siltuximab; St Johns Wort; Tipranavir; Tocilizumab

Food Interactions Food increases absorption of etravirine by ~50%. Management: Take after meals and maintain adequate hydration, unless instructed to restrict fluid intake.

Stability Store at 25°C (77°F); excursions permitted to 15°C to 30°C (59°F to 86°F). Store in the original bottle; keep tightly closed. Protect from moisture and do not remove the desiccant pouches.

Mechanism of Action As a non-nucleoside reverse transcriptase inhibitor, etravirine has activity against HIV-1 by binding to reverse transcriptase. It consequently blocks the RNA-dependent and DNA-dependent DNA polymerase activities, including HIV-1 replication. It does not require intracellular phosphorylation for antiviral activity.

Pharmacokinetics (Adult data unless noted) Note: Pharmacokinetic data suggests that with comparable dosing, exposure in pediatric patients ≥6 years is similar to adult patients.

Absorption: Decreased under fasting conditions

Protein binding: ~99.9%; primarily to albumin and alpha$_1$-acid glycoprotein

Metabolism: Hepatic, primarily by CYP3A4, 2C9, and 2C19; major metabolites exhibit ~10% of parent drug activity against wild-type HIV

Half-life elimination: 41 hours ± 20 hours

Time to peak serum concentration: 2.5-4 hours

Elimination: Feces (up to 86% as unchanged drug)

Hemodialysis: Due to extensive protein binding, significant removal by hemodialysis or peritoneal dialysis is unlikely

Dosing: Usual

Pediatric: **HIV infection, treatment:** Use in combination with other antiretroviral agents.

Children <6 years or pediatric patients <16 kg: Not recommended for use; no dosing recommendations available.

Children ≥6 years and Adolescents, antiretroviral-experienced: Oral:

16 kg to <20 kg: 100 mg twice daily

20 kg to <25 kg: 125 mg twice daily

25 kg to <30 kg: 150 mg twice daily

≥30 kg: 200 mg twice daily

Adult: **HIV infection, treatment:** Use in combination with other antiretroviral agents.

Oral: Antiretroviral-experienced: 200 mg twice daily

Dosing adjustment in renal impairment: Children, Adolescents, and Adults: No dosage adjustments required (DHHS [adult, pediatric], 2014).

Dosing adjustment in hepatic impairment:

Mild to moderate impairment (Child-Pugh class A or B): Children, Adolescents, and Adults: No dosage adjustments required (DHHS [adult, pediatric], 2014).

Severe impairment (Child-Pugh class C): Adolescents and Adults: There are no dosage adjustments provided in manufacturer's labeling (has not been studied).

Administration Oral: Administer after meals. Swallow tablet whole with water; do not chew. If unable to swallow tablets, may disperse tablets in 5 mL water (enough to cover tablets), stir well (until milky appearance), add additional water (or may add milk or orange juice), and drink immediately. Rinse glass several times (with water, milk, or orange juice) and swallow entire contents to ensure administration of full dose. Do not use grapefruit juice, carbonated beverages, or warm (>40°C) drinks (including warm water).

Monitoring Parameters Note: Monitor CD4 percentage (if <5 years of age) or CD4 count (if ≥5 years of age) at least every 3 to 4 months (DHHS [pediatric], 2014).

Prior to initiation of therapy: Genotypic resistance testing, CD4 and viral load (every 3 to 4 months), CBC with

differential, LFTs, BUN, creatinine, electrolytes, glucose, urinalysis (every 6 to 12 months), and assessment of readiness for adherence with medication regimen. At initiation and with any change in treatment regimen: CBC with differential, electrolytes, calcium, phosphate, glucose, LFTs, bilirubin, urinalysis (at initiation), BUN, creatinine, albumin, total protein, lipid panel, CD4, and viral load. After 1 to 2 weeks of therapy: Signs of medication toxicity and adherence. After 2 to 4 weeks of therapy: CBC with differential, viral load, signs of medication toxicity, and adherence; then every 3 to 4 months: CBC with differential, electrolytes, glucose, LFTs, bilirubin, BUN, creatinine, CD4, viral load, signs of medication toxicity, and adherence. Every 6 to 12 months: Lipid panel and urinalysis. CD4 monitoring frequency may be decreased to every 6 to 12 months in children who are adherent to therapy if the value is well above the threshold for opportunistic infections, viral suppression is sustained, and the clinical status is stable for more than 2 to 3 years (DHHS [pediatric], 2014). Monitor for growth and development, signs of HIV-specific physical conditions, HIV disease progression, opportunistic infections, skin rash, or hypersensitivity.

Reference Range Trough concentration (Limited data available; range utilized in trials): Adolescents and Adults: Median: 275 ng/mL (range: 81 to 2980 ng/mL) (DHHS [adult], 2014)

Dosage Forms Excipient information presented when available (limited, particularly for generics); consult specific product labeling.

Tablet, Oral:

Intelence: 25 mg [scored]

Intelence: 100 mg, 200 mg

References

DHHS Panel on Antiretroviral Guidelines for Adults and Adolescents. Guidelines for the use of antiretroviral agents in HIV-1-infected adults and adolescents, Department of Health and Human Services. May 1, 2014. Available at http://www.aidsinfo.nih.gov/ContentFiles/AdultandAdolescentGL.pdf

DHHS Panel on Antiretroviral Therapy and Medical Management of HIV-Infected Children. Guidelines for the use of antiretroviral agents in pediatric HIV infection. February 12, 2014. Available at http://aidsinfo.nih.gov

DHHS Panel on Treatment of HIV-Infected Pregnant Women and Prevention of Perinatal Transmission. Recommendations for the use of antiretroviral drugs in pregnant HIV-1-infected women for maternal health and interventions to reduce perinatal HIV-1 transmission in the United States. March 28, 2014. Available at http://aidsinfo.nih.gov

◆ **Euglucon (Can)** see GlyBURIDE on page 974

◆ **Eurax** see Crotamiton on page 555

◆ **Eurax Cream (Can)** see Crotamiton on page 555

◆ **Euro-Cyproheptadine (Can)** see Cyproheptadine on page 569

◆ **Euro-Docusate C [OTC] (Can)** see Docusate on page 701

◆ **Euro-Lithium (Can)** see Lithium on page 1266

◆ **Eutectic Mixture of Lidocaine and Tetracaine** see Lidocaine and Tetracaine on page 1248

◆ **Evac [OTC]** see Psyllium on page 1773

◆ **Evamist** see Estradiol (Systemic) on page 796

Everolimus (e ver OH li mus)

Medication Safety Issues

Sound-alike/look-alike issues:

Everolimus may be confused with sirolimus, tacrolimus, temsirolimus

Afinitor may be confused with afatinib

High alert medication:

This medication is in a class the Institute for Safe Medication Practices (ISMP) includes among its list of

drug classes which have a heightened risk of causing significant patient harm when used in error.

Administration issues:
Tablets (Afinitor, Zortress) and tablets for oral suspension (Afinitor Disperz) are not interchangeable; do not combine formulations to achieve total desired dose.

Related Information
Emetogenic Potential of Antineoplastic Agents in Children *on page 2327*
Oral Medications That Should Not Be Crushed or Altered *on page 2438*
Safe Handling of Hazardous Drugs *on page 2419*

Brand Names: U.S. Afinitor; Afinitor Disperz; Zortress
Brand Names: Canada Afinitor
Therapeutic Category Antineoplastic Agent, mTOR Kinase Inhibitor; Immunosuppressant Agent
Generic Availability (U.S.) No

Use
Afinitor®: Treatment of subependymal giant cell astrocytoma (SEGA) associated with tuberous sclerosis which requires intervention, but cannot be curatively resected (FDA approved in ages ≥1 year and adults); treatment of advanced hormone receptor-positive, HER2-negative breast cancer in postmenopausal women (in combination with exemestane and after letrozole or anastrozole failure (FDA approved in adults); treatment of advanced renal cell cancer (RCC), after sunitinib or sorafenib failure (FDA approved in adults); treatment of renal angiomyolipoma with tuberous sclerosis complex (TSC) not requiring immediate surgery (FDA approved in adults); treatment of advanced, metastatic, or unresectable pancreatic neuroendocrine tumors (PNET) (FDA approved in adults)
Afinitor® Disperz: Treatment of SEGA associated with TSC which requires intervention, but cannot be curatively resected (FDA approved in ages ≥1 year and adults)
Zortress®: Prophylaxis of organ rejection in patients at low-moderate immunologic risk receiving renal transplants (FDA approved in adults)

Medication Guide Available Yes
Pregnancy Risk Factor D (Afinitor) / C (Zortress)
Pregnancy Considerations Adverse events were observed in animal reproduction studies with exposures lower than expected with human doses. Based on the mechanism of action, may cause fetal harm if administered during pregnancy. Women of reproductive potential should be advised to avoid pregnancy and use highly effective birth control during treatment and for up to 8 weeks after everolimus discontinuation.

The National Transplantation Pregnancy Registry (NTPR) (Temple University) is a registry for pregnant women taking immunosuppressants following any solid organ transplant. The NTPR encourages reporting of all immunosuppressant exposures during pregnancy in transplant recipients at 877-955-6877.

Breast-Feeding Considerations It is not known if everolimus is excreted in breast milk. Due to the potential for serious adverse reactions in the nursing infant, breast-feeding should be avoided.

Contraindications Hypersensitivity to everolimus or any component; hypersensitivity to sirolimus or other rapamycin derivatives

Warnings Hazardous agent; use appropriate precautions for handling and disposal (NIOSH, 2012). Everolimus has immunosuppressant properties which may result in infection **[U.S. Boxed Warning]**; the risk of developing bacterial (including mycobacterial), viral, fungal, and protozoal infections and for local, opportunistic (including polyomavirus infection), systemic infections, and/or sepsis is increased. Polyomavirus infection in transplant patients may be serious and/or fatal. Polyoma virus-associated nephropathy (due to BK virus), which may result in serious cases of

deteriorating renal function and renal graft loss, has been observed with use in renal transplantation. JC virus-associated progressive multiple leukoencephalopathy (PML) may also be associated with everolimus use in transplantation. Reduced immunosuppression should be considered with evidence of polyoma virus infection or PML. Reactivation of hepatitis B has been observed in patients with RCC. Resolve preexisting invasive fungal infections prior to treatment initiation. Monitor for signs and symptoms of infection during treatment. Discontinue if invasive systemic fungal infection is diagnosed (and manage with appropriate antifungal therapy). Everolimus use may delay wound healing and increase the occurrence of wound-related complications (eg, wound dehiscence, infection, incisional hernia, lymphocele, seroma); may require surgical intervention. Decreases in hemoglobin, neutrophils, platelets, and lymphocytes have been reported with use.

Noninfectious pneumonitis (sometimes fatal) has been observed with mTOR inhibitors, including everolimus; symptoms include dyspnea, cough, hypoxia, and/or pleural effusion; promptly evaluate worsening respiratory symptoms. Moderate symptoms may require treatment interruption followed by dose reduction or corticosteroid therapy; severe symptoms may require discontinuation.

Immunosuppressant use may result in the development of malignancy, including lymphoma and skin cancer **[U.S. Boxed Warning]**; the risk is associated with treatment intensity and the duration of therapy. To minimize the risk for skin cancer, exposure to sunlight and ultraviolet light should be limited, protective clothing worn, and sunscreen used.

Due to the increased risk for nephrotoxicity in renal transplantation, avoid standard doses of cyclosporine in combination with everolimus; reduced cyclosporine doses are recommended when everolimus is used in combination with cyclosporine **[U.S. Boxed Warning]**. Therapeutic monitoring of cyclosporine and everolimus concentrations is recommended. Monitor for proteinuria; the risk of proteinuria is increased when everolimus is used in combination with cyclosporine and with higher serum everolimus concentrations. Everolimus and cyclosporine combination therapy may increase the risk for thrombotic microangiopathy/thrombotic thrombocytopenic purpura/hemolytic uremic syndrome (TMA/TTP/HUS) syndrome; monitor blood counts. An increased risk of renal arterial and venous thrombosis has been reported with use in renal transplantation, generally within the first 30 days after transplant; may result in graft loss **[U.S. Boxed Warning]**.

Elevations in serum creatinine and acute renal failure (some cases fatal) have been also observed with everolimus use for renal cell cancer; monitor renal function. An increased incidence of rash, infection, and dose interruptions have been reported in patients with renal insufficiency (CrCl ≤60 mL/minute) who received mTOR inhibitors for the treatment of renal cell cancer (Gupta, 2011); pharmacokinetic studies have not been conducted; dosage adjustments are not required based on renal impairment. The safety and efficacy of everolimus in patients with high-immunologic risk in renal transplantation or in solid organ transplant other than renal have not been established.

Avoid concomitant use with strong CYP3A4 inducers (eg, dexamethasone, phenytoin, carbamazepine, rifampin, rifabutin, rifapentine, phenobarbital) and strong CYP3A4 inhibitors (eg, ketoconazole, itraconazole, voriconazole, clarithromycin, telithromycin, atazanavir, saquinavir, ritonavir, indinavir, delavirdine, fosamprenavir, nelfinavir, nefazodone, grapefruit juice). Everolimus dosage modification and therapeutic drug monitoring may be needed if concomitant use with strong CYP3A4 inducers cannot be avoided. Use with caution with concomitant moderate CYP3A4 inhibitors and/or P-gp inhibitors; decreased everolimus doses are recommended. In renal transplant patients, avoid the use of certain HMG-CoA reductase inhibitors (eg, simvastatin and lovastatin); may increase the risk for rhabdomyolysis due to the potential interaction with cyclosporine (which is given in combination with everolimus for renal transplantation).

Use is associated with mouth ulcers, mucositis, and stomatitis; avoid the use of alcohol-, peroxide, iodine, or thyme-based mouthwashes. Due to the high potential for drug interactions, avoid the use of systemic antifungals unless fungal infection has been diagnosed.

Everolimus is associated with the development of angioedema; concomitant use with other agents known to cause angioedema (eg, ACE inhibitors) may increase the risk. Generalized edema, including peripheral edema and lymphedema, and local fluid accumulation (eg, pericardial effusion, pleural effusion, ascites) may also occur.

Increased mortality (usually associated with infections) within the first 3 months after transplant was noted in a study of patients with *de novo* heart transplant receiving immunosuppressive regimens containing everolimus (with or without induction therapy); use in heart transplantation is not recommended [U.S. Boxed Warning].

Tablets (Afinitor®, Zortress®) and tablets for oral suspension (Afinitor® Disperz) are not interchangeable; do not combine formulations to achieve desired dose.

Precautions Use with caution in patients with hepatic impairment; everolimus exposure is increased in patients with moderate hepatic impairment; consider dosage reductions; use is not recommended in patients with severe impairment (has not been studied). For patients with breast cancer, PNET, RCC, or renal angiomyolipoma with mild and moderate hepatic impairment, reduced doses are recommended; in patients with severe hepatic impairment, use is recommended (at reduced doses) if the potential benefit outweighs risks. For patients with SEGA, reduced doses may be needed (based on therapeutic drug monitoring) for mild and moderate hepatic impairment, and are recommended in severe hepatic impairment; monitor trough levels. Reduced doses are also recommended in renal transplant patients with moderate hepatic impairment; pharmacokinetic information does not exist for renal transplant patients with severe impairment, although an AUC increase greater than observed in moderate impairment is likely.

Use with caution in patients with hyperlipidemia; may increase serum lipids (cholesterol and triglycerides); higher everolimus serum concentrations are associated with an increased risk for hyperlipidemia; use has not been studied in patients with baseline cholesterol >350 mg/dL; antihyperlipidemic therapy may not normalize levels.

Increases in serum glucose are common; may alter insulin and/or oral hypoglycemic therapy requirements in patients with diabetes; the risk for new onset diabetes is increased with everolimus use after transplantation. Patients should not be immunized with live virus vaccines during or shortly after treatment and should avoid close contact with individuals recently vaccinated with live virus vaccines; consider the timing of routine immunizations prior to the start of therapy in pediatric patients treated for SEGA.

Azoospermia and oligospermia have been observed in males. Avoid use in patients with hereditary galactose intolerance, Lapp lactase deficiency, or glucose-galactose malabsorption; may result in diarrhea and malabsorption. In renal transplantation, everolimus should only be used by physicians experienced in immunosuppressive therapy and management of transplant patients [U.S. Boxed Warning]; adequate laboratory and supportive medical resources must be readily available.

Adverse Reactions

Cardiovascular: Angina pectoris, atrial fibrillation, cardiac failure, chest discomfort, chest pain, deep vein thrombosis, edema (generalized), hypertension (including hypertensive crisis), hypotension, palpitations, peripheral edema, pulmonary embolism, renal artery thrombosis, syncope, tachycardia, venous thromboembolism

Central nervous system: Agitation, behavioral changes (anxiety/aggression/behavioral disturbance; SEGA), chills, depression, dizziness, drowsiness, fatigue, hallucination, headache, hemiparesis, hypoesthesia, insomnia, lethargy, malaise, migraine, neuralgia, paresthesia, seizure

Dermatologic: Acneiform eruption, acne vulgaris, alopecia, cellulitis (SEGA), contact dermatitis, eczema, erythema, excoriation, hyperhidrosis, hypertrichosis, nail disease (including onychoclasis), night sweats, palmar-plantar erythrodysesthesia (hand-foot syndrome), papule, pityriasis rosea, pruritus, skin lesion, skin rash, xeroderma

Endocrine & metabolic: Amenorrhea, cushingoid appearance, cyanocobalamin deficiency, decreased serum albumin, decreased serum bicarbonate, dehydration, diabetes mellitus (new onset; more common in liver transplant), exacerbation of diabetes mellitus, gout, hirsutism, hypercalcemia, hypercholesterolemia, hyperglycemia, hyperkalemia (renal transplant), hyperlipidemia (renal, liver transplant), hypermenorrhea, hyperparathyroidism, hyperphosphatemia, hypertriglyceridemia, hyperuricemia, hypocalcemia, hypoglycemia, hypokalemia, hypomagnesemia (renal transplant), hyponatremia, hypophosphatemia, increased follicle-stimulating hormone, increased luteinizing hormone, iron deficiency, irregular menses, lipid metabolism disorder (renal transplant), menstrual disease, ovarian cyst

Gastrointestinal: Abdominal distention, abdominal pain, ageusia, anorexia, constipation, decreased appetite, diarrhea, dysgeusia, dyspepsia, dysphagia, epigastric distress, flatulence, gastritis, gastroenteritis, gastroesophageal reflux disease, gingival hyperplasia, hematemesis, hemorrhoids, intestinal obstruction, mucositis, nausea, oral herpes, peritonitis, stomatitis (more common in oncology uses), vomiting, weight loss, xerostomia

Genitourinary: Bladder spasm, dysmenorrhea, dysuria (renal transplant), erectile dysfunction, hematuria (renal transplant), irregular menses, pollakiuria, proteinuria, pyuria, scrotal edema, urinary retention, urinary tract infection, urinary urgency, vaginal hemorrhage

Hematologic & oncologic: Anemia, hemorrhage, leukocytosis, leukopenia (more common in oncology uses), lymphadenopathy, lymphocytopenia, neoplasm (liver transplant), neutropenia, pancytopenia (renal, liver transplant), prolonged partial thromboplastin time (SEGA), thrombocytopenia (more common in oncology uses)

Hepatic: Abnormal hepatic function tests (liver transplant), ascites (liver transplant), increased serum alkaline phosphatase (more common in oncology uses), increased serum ALT, increased serum AST, increased serum bilirubin, increased serum transaminases

Hypersensitivity: Hypersensitivity (including anaphylaxis, dyspnea, flushing, chest pain, angioedema)

Infection: BK virus, candidiasis, herpes virus infection, infection, sepsis

Neuromuscular & skeletal: Arthralgia, back pain, jaw pain, joint swelling, limb pain, muscle spasm, musculoskeletal pain, myalgia, osteonecrosis, osteopenia, osteoporosis, spondylitis, tremor, weakness

Ophthalmic: Blurred vision, cataract, conjunctivitis, eyelid edema, ocular hyperemia

Otic: Otitis

Renal: Hydronephrosis, increased blood urea nitrogen, increased serum creatinine, interstitial nephritis, polyuria, renal failure, renal insufficiency

Respiratory: Atelectasis, bronchitis, cough, dyspnea, epistaxis, lower respiratory tract infection, nasal congestion, nasopharyngitis, oropharyngeal pain, pharyngolaryngeal pain, pharyngitis, pleural effusion, pneumonia, pneumonitis (including alveolitis, interstitial lung disease, lung infiltrate, pulmonary alveolar hemorrhage, pulmonary toxicity), pulmonary edema, rhinitis, rhinorrhea, sinus congestion, sinusitis, upper respiratory tract infection, wheezing

Miscellaneous: Fever, postoperative wound complication (including incisional hernia), wound healing impairment (more common in renal and liver transplant)

Rare but important or life-threatening: Aspergillosis, azoospermia, cardiac arrest, decreased plasma testosterone, fluid retention, hepatic artery thrombosis, influenza, intrahepatic cholestasis, malignant lymphoma, oligospermia, pancreatitis, progressive multifocal leukoencephalopathy, reactivation of HBV, respiratory distress, skin neoplasm, synovitis (severe), thrombosis of vascular graft, thrombotic microangiopathy/thrombotic thrombocytopenic purpura/hemolytic uremic syndrome

Drug Interactions

Metabolism/Transport Effects Substrate of CYP3A4 (major), P-glycoprotein; **Note:** Assignment of Major/Minor substrate status based on clinically relevant drug interaction potential

Avoid Concomitant Use

Avoid concomitant use of Everolimus with any of the following: BCG; CloZAPine; Conivaptan; CYP3A4 Inducers (Strong); CYP3A4 Inhibitors (Strong); Dipyrone; Fusidic Acid (Systemic); Grapefruit Juice; Natalizumab; Pimecrolimus; St Johns Wort; Tacrolimus (Topical); Tofacitinib; Vaccines (Live); Voriconazole

Increased Effect/Toxicity

Everolimus may increase the levels/effects of: ACE Inhibitors; CloZAPine; Leflunomide; Natalizumab; Tofacitinib; Vaccines (Live)

The levels/effects of Everolimus may be increased by: Conivaptan; CycloSPORINE (Systemic); CYP3A4 Inhibitors (Moderate); CYP3A4 Inhibitors (Strong); Dasatinib; Denosumab; Dipyrone; Fusidic Acid (Systemic); Grapefruit Juice; Luliconazole; Mifepristone; P-glycoprotein/ABCB1 Inhibitors; Pimecrolimus; Roflumilast; Tacrolimus (Topical); Trastuzumab; Voriconazole

Decreased Effect

Everolimus may decrease the levels/effects of: BCG; Coccidioidin Skin Test; Sipuleucel-T; Vaccines (Inactivated); Vaccines (Live)

The levels/effects of Everolimus may be decreased by: Bosentan; CYP3A4 Inducers (Strong); Dabrafenib; Deferasirox; Echinacea; Efavirenz; P-glycoprotein/ABCB1 Inducers; Siltuximab; St Johns Wort; Tocilizumab

Food Interactions Grapefruit juice may increase levels of everolimus. Absorption with food may be variable. Management: Avoid grapefruit juice. Take with or without food, but be consistent with regard to food.

Stability Hazardous agent; use appropriate precautions for handling and disposal (NIOSH, 2012). Tablets and tablets for suspension: Store at 25°C (77°F); excursions permitted to 15°C to 30°C (59°F to 86°F). Protect from light; protect from moisture.

Mechanism of Action Everolimus is a macrolide immunosuppressant and a mammalian target of rapamycin (mTOR) inhibitor which has antiproliferative and antiangiogenic properties, and also reduces lipoma volume in patients with angiomyolipoma. Reduces protein synthesis and cell proliferation by binding to the FK binding protein-12 (FKBP-12), an intracellular protein, to form a complex that inhibits activation of mTOR (mammalian target of rapamycin) serine-threonine kinase activity. Also reduces angiogenesis by inhibiting vascular endothelial growth factor (VEGF) and hypoxia-inducible factor (HIF-1) expression. Angiomyolipomas may occur due to unregulated mTOR activity in TSC-associated renal angiomyolipoma (Budde, 2012); everolimus reduces lipoma volume (Bissler, 2012).

Pharmacokinetics (Adult data unless noted)

Absorption: Rapid but moderate

Distribution: V_d apparent: 128-589 L; volume of distribution in pediatric patients (3-16 years) lower than adults (Van-Damme-Lombaerts, 2002)

Protein binding: ~74%

Metabolism: Extensively metabolized via CYP3A4; forms 6 weak metabolites

Bioavailability: ~30%

Half-life elimination: ~30 hours; in pediatric patients (3-16 years), half-life similar to adult data (Van-Damme-Lombaerts, 2002)

Time to peak serum concentration: 1-2 hours

Elimination: Feces (80%, based on solid organ transplant studies); urine (~5%, based on solid organ transplant studies); clearance in pediatric patients lower than adults possibly due to distributive differences (Van-Damme-Lombaerts, 2002)

Dosing: Usual

Children ≥1 year and Adolescents: **Note:** Tablets (Afinitor®, Zortress®) and tablets for oral suspension (Afinitor® Disperz) are not interchangeable. Afinitor® Disperz is only indicated for the treatment of subependymal giant cell astrocytoma (SEGA), in conjunction with therapeutic monitoring. Do not combine formulations to achieve desired dose.

Subependymal giant cell astrocytoma (SEGA): Afinitor®; Afinitor® Disperz: Oral: Initial: 4.5 mg/m² once daily; round to nearest tablet (tablet or tablet for oral suspension) size; assess trough concentrations 2 weeks after initiation or dosage modification; adjust maintenance dose if needed at 2-week intervals to achieve and maintain serum trough concentrations between 5 and 15 ng/mL; monitor trough concentrations routinely; once stable dose is attained and BSA is stable throughout treatment, monitor trough concentrations every 6-12 months; monitor every 3-6 months if BSA is changing. Continue until disease progression or unacceptable toxicity. Serum trough concentrations should also be assessed if dosage form switched (tablets or tablets for oral suspension), hepatic function changes or therapy with a CYP3A4 or P-gp inducer or inhibitor is modified (initiated, dose change, or discontinued).

If trough <5 ng/mL: Increase dose by 2.5 mg/day (tablets) or 2 mg/day (tablets for oral suspension).

If trough >15 ng/mL: Reduce dose by 2.5 mg/day (tablets) or 2 mg/day (tablets for oral suspension).

If dose reduction necessary in patients receiving the lowest strength available, administer every other day.

Transplantation; renal, rejection prophylaxis: Zortress®: Limited data available: Initial: 0.8 mg/m²/dose twice daily (maximum single dose: 1.5 mg) to maintain serum concentration: 3-6 ng/mL; reported start time of therapy variable: Within 48 hours post-transplantation was used in a multicenter, international trial of 19 pediatric patients; another trial began at 2 weeks after transplantation (single center, n=20 pediatric patients); a trial evaluating use for 3 years in pediatric patients (<16 years), the mean reported dose was 1.53 mg/m²/day and no untoward adverse effects were noted (Ettenger, 2008; Hoyer, 2003; Pape, 2007; Pape, 2010; Pape, 2011; Van-Damme-Lombaerts, 2002; Vester, 2002). Further studies are needed.

Adults: **Note:** Tablets (Afinitor®, Zortress®) and tablets for oral suspension (Afinitor® Disperz) are not interchangeable; Afinitor® Disperz is only indicated for the treatment of subependymal giant cell astrocytoma (SEGA), in conjunction with therapeutic monitoring. Do not combine formulations to achieve desired dose.

Breast cancer, advanced, hormone receptor-positive, HER2-negative: Afinitor®: Oral: 10 mg once daily (in combination with exemestane); continue treatment until no longer clinically beneficial or until unacceptable toxicity

Pancreatic neuroendocrine tumors, advanced (PNET): Afinitor®: 10 mg once daily; continue treatment until no longer clinically benefiting or until unacceptable toxicity

Renal cell cancer (RCC), advanced: Afinitor®: 10 mg once daily; continue treatment until no longer clinically benefiting or until unacceptable toxicity

Renal angiomyolipoma: Afinitor®: Oral: 10 mg once daily; continue treatment until no longer clinically beneficial or until unacceptable toxicity

Subependymal giant cell astrocytoma (SEGA): Afinitor®: Body surface area-based dosing: Oral: Initial dose: 4.5 mg/m^2 once daily; round to nearest tablet (tablet or tablet for oral suspension) size. Assess trough concentrations 2 weeks after initiation or dosage modification; adjust maintenance dose if needed at 2-week intervals to achieve and maintain serum trough concentrations between 5 and 15 ng/mL; monitor trough concentrations routinely; once stable dose is attained and BSA is stable throughout treatment, monitor trough concentrations every 6-12 months; monitor every 3-6 months if BSA is changing. Continue until disease progression or unacceptable toxicity.

If trough <5 ng/mL: Increase dose by 2.5 mg/day (tablets) or 2 mg/day (tablets for oral suspension).

If trough >15 ng/mL: Reduce dose by 2.5 mg/day (tablets) or 2 mg/day (tablets for oral suspension).

If dose reduction necessary in patients receiving the lowest strength available, administer every other day.

Transplantation; renal, rejection prophylaxis: Zortress®: Initial: 0.75 mg twice daily; adjust maintenance dose if needed at a 4- to 5-day interval (from prior dose adjustment) based on serum concentrations, tolerability, and response; goal serum concentration is between 3 and 8 ng/mL (based on an LCMSMS assay method). **Note:** For use in renal transplantation, administer in combination with basiliximab induction and concurrently with cyclosporine (dose adjustment required) and corticosteroids.

Dosage adjustment for concomitant CYP3A4 inhibitors/inducers and/or P-gp inhibitors:

Breast cancer, PNET, RCC, renal angiomyolipoma: Adults:

CYP3A4 inducers: Strong inducers: Avoid concomitant administration with strong CYP3A4 inducers; if concomitant use cannot be avoided, consider adjusting everolimus dose upward in 5 mg increments up to 20 mg daily, with careful monitoring. If the strong CYP3A4 enzyme inducer is discontinued, reduce the everolimus to the dose used prior to initiation of the CYP3A4 inducer.

CYP3A4 or P-gp inhibitors:

Strong inhibitors: Avoid concomitant administration with strong CYP3A4 inhibitors.

Moderate inhibitors: Reduce dose to 2.5 mg once daily; may consider increasing from 2.5 mg to 5 mg once daily based on patient tolerance. When the moderate inhibitor is discontinued, allow ~2-3 days to elapse prior to adjusting the everolimus upward to the dose used prior to initiation of the moderate inhibitor.

SEGA: Children, Adolescents, and Adults:

CYP3A4 inducers: Strong inducers: Avoid concomitant administration with strong CYP3A4 inducers; if concomitant cannot be avoided, an initial starting everolimus dose of 9 mg/m^2 once daily is recommended, or double the everolimus dose; individualize subsequent doses based on therapeutic drug monitoring. If the strong CYP3A4 enzyme inducer is discontinued, reduce the everolimus to the dose used prior to initiation of the CYP3A4 inducer; reassess trough concentration after 2 weeks.

CYP3A4 or P-gp inhibitors:

Strong inhibitors: Avoid concomitant administration with strong CYP3A4 inhibitors.

Moderate inhibitors: Initial everolimus dose: 2.5 mg/m^2 once daily or reduce dose by 50% (if dose reduction is required for patients receiving the lowest strength available, consider alternate day dosing); assess trough concentrations after 2 weeks; individualize dosing based on therapeutic drug monitoring. When the moderate inhibitor is discontinued, adjust the everolimus upward to the dose used prior to initiation of the moderate inhibitor; reassess trough concentrations after 2 weeks.

Transplantation; renal: Children, Adolescents, and Adults: Dosage adjustments may be necessary based on everolimus serum concentrations.

Dosage adjustment in renal impairment: No adjustment necessary

Dosage adjustment in hepatic impairment:

Mild hepatic impairment (Child-Pugh class A):

Breast cancer, PNET, RCC, renal angiomyolipoma: Adults: Reduce dose to 7.5 mg once daily; if not tolerated, may further reduce to 5 mg once daily.

SEGA: Children, Adolescents, and Adults: Adjustment to initial dose may not be necessary; subsequent dosing is based on therapeutic drug monitoring (monitor 2 weeks after initiation, dosage modifications, or after any change in hepatic status; target trough concentration: 5-15 ng/mL).

Transplantation, renal: No adjustment necessary.

Moderate hepatic impairment (Child-Pugh class B):

Breast cancer, PNET, RCC, renal angiomyolipoma: Adults: Reduce dose to 5 mg once daily if not tolerated, may further reduce to 2.5 mg once daily.

SEGA: Children, Adolescents, and Adults: Adjustment to initial dose may not be necessary; subsequent dosing is based on therapeutic drug monitoring (monitor 2 weeks after initiation, dosage modifications, or after any change in hepatic status; target trough concentration: 5-15 ng/mL).

Transplantation, renal: Adults: Reduce initial dose by 50%; individualize subsequent dosing based on therapeutic drug monitoring.

Severe hepatic impairment (Child-Pugh class C):

Breast cancer, PNET, RCC, renal angiomyolipoma: Adults: If potential benefit outweighs risks, a maximum dose of 2.5 mg once daily may be used.

SEGA: Children, Adolescents, and Adults: Reduce initial dose to 2.5 mg/m^2 once daily (or current dose by ~50%); subsequent dosing is based on therapeutic drug monitoring.

Transplantation, renal: No dosage adjustment provided in the manufacturer's labeling (pharmacokinetics have not been studied in severe hepatic impairment).

Dosage adjustment for toxicity: Children, Adolescents and Adults:

Breast cancer (adjustments apply to everolimus), PNET, RCC, renal angiomyolipoma, SEGA: Reduce everolimus dose by ~50% if dosage adjustment is necessary.

Noninfectious pneumonitis:

Grade 1 (asymptomatic radiological changes suggestive of pneumonitis): No dosage adjustment necessary; monitor appropriately.

Grade 2 [symptomatic but not interfering with activities of daily living (ADL)]: Consider interrupting treatment, rule out infection, and consider corticosteroids until symptoms improve to ≤grade 1; reinitiate at a lower dose. Discontinue if recovery does not occur within 4 weeks.

Grade 3 (symptomatic, interferes with ADL; oxygen indicated): Interrupt treatment until symptoms improve to ≤grade 1; rule out infection and consider corticosteroid treatment; may reinitiate at a lower dose. If grade 3 toxicity recurs, consider discontinuing.

Grade 4 (life-threatening; ventilatory support indicated): Discontinue treatment; rule out infection; consider corticosteroid treatment.

Stomatitis (avoid the use of products containing alcohol, hydrogen peroxide, iodine, or thyme derivatives):

Grade 1 (minimal symptoms, normal diet): No dosage adjustment necessary; manage with mouth wash (nonalcoholic or salt water) several times a day.

Grade 2 (symptomatic but can eat and swallow modified diet): Interrupt treatment until symptoms improve to ≤grade 1; reinitiate at same dose; if stomatitis recurs at grade 2, interrupt treatment until symptoms improve to ≤grade 1 and then reinitiate at a lower dose. Also manage with topical (oral) analgesics (eg, benzocaine, butyl aminobenzoate, tetracaine, menthol, or phenol) ± topical (oral) corticosteroids (eg, triamcinolone).

Grade 3 (symptomatic and unable to orally aliment or hydrate adequately): Interrupt treatment until symptoms improve to ≤grade 1; then reinitiate at a lower dose. Also manage with topical (oral) analgesics (eg, benzocaine, butyl aminobenzoate, tetracaine, menthol, or phenol) ± topical (oral) corticosteroids (eg, triamcinolone).

Grade 4 (life-threatening symptoms): Discontinue treatment; initiate appropriate medical intervention.

Metabolic toxicity (eg, hyperglycemia, dyslipidemia):

Grade 1: No dosage adjustment necessary; initiate appropriate medical intervention and monitor.

Grade 2: No dosage adjustment necessary; manage with appropriate medical intervention and monitor.

Grade 3: Temporarily interrupt treatment; reinitiate at a lower dose; manage with appropriate medical intervention and monitor.

Grade 4: Discontinue treatment; manage with appropriate medical intervention.

Nonhematologic toxicities (excluding pneumonitis, stomatitis, and metabolic toxicity):

Grade 1: If toxicity is tolerable, no dosage adjustment necessary; initiate appropriate medical intervention and monitor.

Grade 2: If toxicity is tolerable, no dosage adjustment necessary; initiate appropriate medical intervention and monitor. If toxicity becomes intolerable, temporarily interrupt treatment until improvement to ≤grade 1 and reinitiate at the same dose; if toxicity recurs at grade 2, temporarily interrupt treatment until improvement to ≤grade 1 and then reinitiate at a lower dose.

Grade 3: Temporarily interrupt treatment until improvement to ≤grade 1; initiate appropriate medical

intervention and monitor. May reinitiate at a lower dose; if toxicity recurs at grade 3, consider discontinuing.

Grade 4 (life-threatening symptoms): Discontinue treatment; initiate appropriate medical intervention.

SEGA: *Other severe/intolerable adverse reactions:* Temporarily reduce dose (by ~50% from prior dose) and/or temporarily interrupt treatment; if dose reduction is required for patients receiving the lowest available strength, consider alternate day dosing.

Transplantation, renal: *Evidence of polyoma virus infection or PML:* Consider reduced immunosuppression (taking into account the allograft risks associated with decreased immunosuppression).

Administration Hazardous agent; use appropriate precautions for handling and disposal (NIOSH, 2012).

Oral: May be taken with or without food; to reduce variability, take consistently with regard to food; if using for SEGA, breast cancer, PNET, renal angiolipoma, or RCC, administer at the same time each day; if using for renal transplantation, administer consistently ~12 hours apart and at the same time as cyclosporine.

Tablets: Swallow tablet whole with a glass of water; do not chew or crush; do not use tablets that are crushed or broken; avoid contact with or exposure to crushed or broken tablets.

Tablets for oral suspension: Administer as a suspension only. Administer immediately after preparation; discard if not administered within 60 minutes after preparation. Prepare suspension in water only. Do not break or crush tablets.

Preparation in an oral syringe: Place dose into 10 mL oral syringe (maximum 10 mg/syringe; use an additional syringe for doses >10 mg). Draw ~5 mL of water and ~4 mL of air into oral syringe; allow to sit (tip up) in a container until tablets are in suspension (3 minutes). Gently invert syringe 5 times immediately prior to administration; administer contents (dose), and then add ~5 mL water and ~4 mL of air to same syringe, swirl to suspend remaining particles, and administer entire contents.

Preparation in a small glass: Place dose into a small glass (≤100 mL) containing ~25 mL water (maximum 10 mg/glass; use an additional glass for doses >10 mg); allow to sit until tablets are in suspension (3 minutes). Stir gently with spoon immediately prior to administration; administer contents, then add ~25 mL water to same glass, swirl with same spoon to suspend remaining particles and administer entire contents.

Monitoring Parameters CBC with differential (baseline and periodic), liver function, serum creatinine, urinary protein, and BUN (baseline and periodic); fasting serum glucose and lipid profile (baseline and periodic); monitor for signs and symptoms of infection, noninfectious pneumonitis, or malignancy

SEGA: Monitor everolimus serum trough concentrations approximately 2 weeks after treatment initiation, 2 weeks after dose modifications, and after initiation or dose modification of concomitant CYP3A4 and/or P-gp inducers or inhibitors.

Transplantation; renal: Monitor serum trough concentrations (based on an LCMSMS assay method), especially in patients with hepatic impairment, with concomitant CYP3A4 inhibitors and inducers, and when cyclosporine formulations or doses are changed; dosage adjustments should be made on trough concentrations obtained 4-5 days after previous dosage adjustment; monitor cyclosporine concentrations and proteinuria.

Reference Range Recommended range for everolimus serum concentrations:

SEGA: 5-15 ng/mL (high concentrations may be associated with larger reductions in SEGA volumes; responses have been observed at concentrations as low as 5 ng/mL)

Transplantation; renal: 3-8 ng/mL (based on LCMSMS assay method); in pediatric studies, reported target range: 3-6 ng/mL

Dosage Forms Excipient information presented when available (limited, particularly for generics); consult specific product labeling.

Tablet, Oral:

Afinitor: 2.5 mg, 5 mg, 7.5 mg, 10 mg

Zortress: 0.25 mg, 0.5 mg, 0.75 mg

Tablet Soluble, Oral:

Afinitor Disperz: 2 mg, 3 mg, 5 mg

Extemporaneous Preparations Hazardous agent: Use appropriate precautions for handling and disposal.

Tablets: An oral liquid may be prepared using tablets. Disperse tablet in ~30 mL (1 oz) of water; gently stir. Administer and rinse container with additional 30 mL (1 oz) water and administer to ensure entire dose is administered. Administer immediately after preparation.

Afinitor (everolimus) [prescribing information]. East Hanover, NJ: Novartis Pharmaceuticals Corporation; July 2012.

Tablets for oral suspension: Administer as a suspension only. Administer immediately after preparation; discard if not administered within 60 minutes after preparation. Prepare suspension in water only. Do not break or crush tablets.

Preparation in an oral syringe: Place dose into 10 mL oral syringe (maximum 10 mg/syringe; use an additional syringe for doses >10 mg). Draw ~5 mL of water and ~4 mL of air into oral syringe; allow to sit (tip up) in a container until tablets are in suspension (3 minutes). Gently invert syringe 5 times immediately prior to administration; administer contents, then add ~5 mL water and ~4 mL of air to same syringe, swirl to suspend remaining particles and administer entire contents.

Preparation in a small glass: Place dose into a small glass (≤100 mL) containing ~25 mL water (maximum 10 mg/glass; use an additional glass for doses >10 mg); allow to sit until tablets are in suspension (3 minutes). Stir gently with spoon immediately prior to administration; administer contents, then add ~25 mL water to same glass, swirl with same spoon to suspend remaining particles and administer entire contents. Administer immediately after preparation; discard if not administered within 60 minutes after preparation.

Afinitor and Afinitor Disperz (everolimus) [prescribing information]. East Hanover, NJ: Novartis Pharmaceuticals Corporation; August 2012.

References

Bissler JJ, Kingswood JC, Zonnenberg BA, et al, "Everolimus Therapy for Angiomyolipoma in Patients With Tuberous Sclerosis Complex or Sporadic Lymphangioleiomyomatosis: Results From EXIST-2," J Clin Oncology, 2012, 30(Supp 5):356.

Budde K and Gaedeke J, "Tuberous Sclerosis Complex-Associated Angiomyolipomas: Focus on mTOR Inhibition," Am J Kidney Dis, 2012, 59(2):276-83.

Ettenger R, Hoyer PF, Grimm P, et al, "Multicenter Trial of Everolimus in Pediatric Renal Transplant Recipients: Results at Three Year," Pediatr Transplant, 2008, (4):456-63.

Hoyer PF, Ettenger R, Kovarik JM, et al, "Everolimus in Pediatric de nova Renal Transplant Patients," Transplantation, 2003, 75 (12):2082-5.

Kirchner GI, Meier-Wiedenbach I, and Manns MP, "Clinical Pharmacokinetics of Everolimus," Clin Pharmacokinet, 2004, 43(2):83-95.

Kovarik JM, Sabia HD, Figueiredo J, et al, "Influence of Hepatic Impairment on Everolimus Pharmacokinetics: Implications for Dose Adjustment," Clin Pharmacol Ther, 2001, 70(5):425-30.

Krueger DA, Care MM, Holland K, et al, "Everolimus for Subependymal Giant-Cell Astrocytomas in Tuberous Sclerosis," N Engl J Med, 2010, 363(19):1801-11.

Lorber MI, Ponticelli C, Whelchel J, et al, "Therapeutic Drug Monitoring for Everolimus in Kidney Transplantation Using 12-Month Exposure, Efficacy, and Safety Data," Clin Transplant, 2005, 19(2):145-52.

National Institute for Occupational Safety and Health (NIOSH), "NIOSH List of Antineoplastic and Other Hazardous Drugs in Healthcare Settings 2012." Available at http://www.cdc.gov/niosh/docs/ 2012-150/pdfs/2012-150.pdf. Accessed January 21, 2013.

O'Donnell A, Faivre S, Burris HA 3rd, et al, "Phase I Pharmacokinetic and Pharmacodynamic Study of the Oral Mammalian Target of Rapamycin Inhibitor Everolimus in Patients With Advanced Solid Tumors," J Clin Oncol, 2008, 26(10):1588-95.

Pape L, Ahlenstiel T, Ehrich JH, et al, "Reversal of Loss of Glomerular Filtration Rate in Children With Transplant Nephropathy After Switch to Everolimus and Low-Dose Cyclosporine A," Pediatr Transplant, 2007, 11(3):291-5.

Pape L, Lehner F, Blume C, et al, "Pediatric Kidney Transplantation Followed by de novo Therapy With Everolimus, Low-Dose Cyclosporine A, and Steroid Elimination: 3-Year Data," Transplantation, 2011, 92(6):658-62.

Pape L, Offner G, Kreuzer M, et al, "De novo Therapy With Everolimus, Low-Dose Ciclosporine A, Basiliximab and Steroid Elimination in Pediatric Kidney Transplantation," Am J Transplant, 2010, 10 (10):2349-54.

Tabernero J, Rojo F, Calvo E, et al, "Dose- and Schedule-Dependent Inhibition of the Mammalian Target of Rapamycin Pathway With Everolimus: A Phase I Tumor Pharmacodynamic Study in Patients With Advanced Solid Tumors," J Clin Oncol. 2008 Apr 1;26 (10):1603-10.

Van Damme-Lombaerts R, Webb NA, Hoyer PF, et al, "Single-Dose Pharmacokinetics and Tolerability of Everolimus in Stable Pediatric Renal Transplant Patients," Pediatr Transplant, 2002, 6(2):147-52.

Vester U, Kranz B, Wehr S, et al, "Everolimus (Certican) in Combination With Neoral in Pediatric Renal Transplant Recipients: Interim Analysis After 3 Months," Transplant Proc, 2002, 34(6):2209-10.

◆ **Everone 200 (Can)** see Testosterone on page 1986

◆ **Evithrom®** see Thrombin (Topical) on page 2017

◆ **Evoclin** see Clindamycin (Topical) on page 500

◆ **Evzio** see Naloxone on page 1466

◆ **Exalgo** see HYDROmorphone on page 1041

◆ **Excedrin Tension Headache [OTC]** see Acetaminophen on page 47

◆ **Exjade** see Deferasirox on page 601

◆ **Ex-Lax [OTC]** see Senna on page 1877

◆ **Ex-Lax Maximum Strength [OTC]** see Senna on page 1877

◆ **Ex-Lax Ultra [OTC]** see Bisacodyl on page 293

◆ **Extended Release Epidural Morphine** see Morphine (Liposomal) on page 1449

◆ **Extina** see Ketoconazole (Topical) on page 1179

◆ **Extra Strength Allergy Relief [OTC] (Can)** see Cetirizine on page 431

◆ **Exuviance Blemish Treatment [OTC]** see Salicylic Acid on page 1860

◆ **Eye-Sed [OTC]** see Zinc Sulfate on page 2176

◆ **EZ Char [OTC]** see Charcoal, Activated on page 432

Ezetimibe (ez ET i mibe)

Medication Safety Issues

Sound-alike/look-alike issues:

Ezetimibe may be confused with ezogabine

Zetia may be confused with Zebeta, Zestril

Brand Names: U.S. Zetia

Brand Names: Canada Ezetrol

Therapeutic Category Antilipemic Agent; Cholesterol Absorption Inhibitor

Generic Availability (U.S.) No

Use Adjunct to dietary therapy in combination with simvastatin in patients with heterozygous familial hypercholesterolemia (FDA approved in boys and postmenarchal girls 10-17 years of age); adjunct to dietary therapy (monotherapy or in combination with HMG-CoA reductase inhibitor in patients with primary hypercholesterolemia (heterozygous familial and nonfamilial) (FDA approved in adults); in combination with atorvastatin or simvastatin in the treatment of homozygous familial hypercholesterolemia (FDA approved in adults); in combination with fenofibrate in the treatment of mixed hyperlipidemia (FDA approved in adults); adjunct to dietary therapy for the reduction of elevated sitosterol and campesterol levels in patients with homozygous familial sitosterolemia (FDA approved in adults)

Pregnancy Risk Factor C

Pregnancy Considerations Use is contraindicated in women who are or who may become pregnant.

Breast-Feeding Considerations It is not known if ezetimibe is excreted in breast milk. According to the manufacturer, the decision to continue or discontinue breastfeeding during therapy should take into account the risk of exposure to the infant and the benefits of treatment to the mother. Use is contraindicated in nursing women who require combination therapy with an HMG-CoA reductase inhibitor.

Contraindications Hypersensitivity to ezetimibe or any component; active liver disease; unexplained persistent elevations of serum transaminases; women who are pregnant or who may become pregnant; nursing mothers

Warnings The incidence of rhabdomyolysis or myopathy in clinical trials with ezetimibe was no different than that of placebo; however, rhabdomyolysis and myopathy are known adverse effects of HMG-CoA reductase inhibitors which are often used in combination with ezetimibe; follow rhabdomyolysis and myopathy monitoring recommendations for HMG-CoA reductase inhibitors when used in combination; also when ezetimibe is used in combination with HMG-CoA reductase inhibitors, the incidence of elevated serum transaminases was higher than when the HMG-CoA reductase inhibitors were used alone; monitor serum transaminases when used in combination with HMG-CoA reductase inhibitors. When studied in combination with fenofibrate, an increase in cholecystectomy rate (0.6% vs 1.7%) when compared with monotherapy was observed; monitor for signs and symptoms of cholelithiasis when used with fenofibrate.

Precautions Use with caution in renal or mild hepatic impairment; use is not recommended in patients with moderate to severe hepatic impairment. If using concurrent simvastatin in patients with moderate to severe renal impairment (GFR <60 mL/minute/1.73 m^2), the manufacturer of ezetimibe recommends that simvastatin doses exceeding 20 mg be used with caution and monitor closely for adverse events (eg, myopathy). Secondary causes of hyperlipidemia should be ruled out prior to therapy; has not been studied in Fredrickson types I, III, IV, and V dyslipidemias.

Adverse Reactions

Central nervous system: Fatigue

Gastrointestinal: Diarrhea

Hepatic: Transaminases increased (with HMG-CoA reductase inhibitors) (≥3 x ULN)

Neuromuscular & skeletal: Arthralgia, pain in extremity

Respiratory: Sinusitis, upper respiratory tract infection

Miscellaneous: Influenza

Rare but important or life-threatening: Abdominal pain, anaphylaxis, angioedema, autoimmune hepatitis (Stolk, 2006), cholecystitis, cholelithiasis, cholestatic hepatitis (Stolk, 2006), CPK increased, depression, dizziness, erythema multiforme, headache, hepatitis, hypersensitivity reactions, myalgia, myopathy, nausea, pancreatitis, paresthesia, rash, rhabdomyolysis, thrombocytopenia, urticaria

Drug Interactions

Metabolism/Transport Effects Substrate of SLCO1B1

Avoid Concomitant Use There are no known interactions where it is recommended to avoid concomitant use.

Increased Effect/Toxicity

Ezetimibe may increase the levels/effects of: CycloSPORINE (Systemic)

The levels/effects of Ezetimibe may be increased by: CycloSPORINE (Systemic); Eltrombopag; Fibric Acid Derivatives

Decreased Effect

The levels/effects of Ezetimibe may be decreased by: Bile Acid Sequestrants

Stability Store at 25°C (77°F), excursions permitted to 15°C to 30°C (59°F to 86°F); protect from moisture.

Mechanism of Action Inhibits absorption of cholesterol at the brush border of the small intestine via the sterol transporter, Niemann-Pick C1-Like1 (NPC1L1). This leads to a decreased delivery of cholesterol to the liver, reduction of hepatic cholesterol stores and an increased clearance of cholesterol from the blood; decreases total C, LDL-cholesterol (LDL-C), ApoB, and triglycerides (TG) while increasing HDL-cholesterol (HDL-C).

Pharmacodynamics

Onset of action: Within 1 week

Maximum effect: 2-4 weeks

Pharmacokinetics (Adult data unless noted) Note: Pharmacokinetic data in children and adolescents ≥10 years of age are reported to be similar to that in adult patients.

Protein binding: >90%

Metabolism: Extensive glucuronide conjugation in the small intestine and liver to a pharmacologically active metabolite; may undergo enterohepatic recycling

Bioavailability: Variable

Hepatic impairment: Moderate hepatic impairment (Child-Pugh score 7-9): AUC increased 3-4 times; severe hepatic impairment (Child-Pugh 10-15): AUC increased 5-6 times

Renal impairment: Severe renal dysfunction (CrCl <30 mL/minute/1.73 m^2): AUC increased 1.5 times

Half-life: 22 hours (ezetimibe and metabolite)

Time to peak serum concentration: 4-12 hours (ezetimibe); 1-2 hours (active metabolite)

Elimination: Feces (78%, 69% as ezetimibe): urine (11%, 9% as metabolite)

Dosing: Usual

Children and Adolescents: **Hyperlipidemia:**

Children 5-9 years: Limited data available: Oral: 10 mg once daily; dosing based on two studies of monotherapy; a prospective trial (n=17 including six patients ≤9 years) and a retrospective review (n=36, age range: 8-17 years) showed significant decreases in total cholesterol and LDL-C; patients were followed up to a mean of 13.6 months, no untoward effects were noted; further studies are needed (Clauss, 2009; Yeste, 2009)

Children ≥10 years and Adolescents: Oral: 10 mg once daily in combination with simvastatin. Has also been shown in small pediatric trials to decrease TC and LDL-C when used as monotherapy as adjunct to dietary changes (Clauss, 2009; Yeste, 2009)

Adults: **Hyperlipidemias, sitosterolemia:** Oral: 10 mg once daily

Dosing adjustment in renal impairment: No dosage adjustments are recommended.

Dosing adjustment in hepatic impairment:

Mild hepatic impairment (Child-Pugh score 5-6): No dosage adjustments are recommended.

Moderate to severe impairment (Child-Pugh score 7-15): Use is not recommended.

Administration Oral: May be taken without regard to meals or time of day; may be administered with an HMG-CoA reductase inhibitor (eg, atorvastatin, simvastatin) or fenofibrate. Administer ≥2 hours before or ≥4 hours after bile acid sequestrants.

Monitoring Parameters Serum cholesterol (total and fractionated) prior to therapy and when clinically indicated and/or periodically thereafter. When used in combination with fenofibrate, monitor LFTs and signs and symptoms of cholelithiasis.

Note: When used in combination with an HMG-CoA reductase inhibitor (ie, simvastatin), also monitor: Baseline: ALT, AST, and creatine phosphokinase levels (CPK); if no myopathy symptoms or laboratory abnormalities, then monitor ALT and AST every 3-4 months during the first year and then every 6 months thereafter (NHLBI, 2011)

Dosage Forms Excipient information presented when available (limited, particularly for generics); consult specific product labeling.

Tablet, Oral:

Zetia: 10 mg

References

Clauss S, Wall K, Kavey RW, et al. Ezetimibe treatment of pediatric patients with hypercholesterolemia. *J Pediatr.* 2009;154:869-872.

Daniels SR, Greer FR, and Committee on Nutrition, "Lipid Screening and Cardiovascular Health in Childhood," *Pediatrics*, 2008, 122 (1):198-208.

Gagne C, Gaudet D, Bruckert E, et al, "Efficacy and Safety of Ezetimibe Coadministered With Atorvastatin or Simvastatin in Patients With Homozygous Familial Hypercholesterolemia," *Circulation*, 2002, 105 (21):2469-75.

McCrindle BW, Urbina EM, Dennison BA, et al, "Drug Therapy of High-Risk Lipid Abnormalities in Children and Adolescents: A Scientific Statement from the American Heart Association Atherosclerosis, Hypertension, and Obesity in Youth Committee, Council of Cardiovascular Disease in the Young, With the Council on Cardiovascular Nursing," *Circulation*, 2007, 115(14):1948-67.

National Heart, Lung, and Blood Institute. Expert panel on Integrated Guidelines for Cardiovascular Health and Risk Reduction in Children and Adolescents. Clinical Practice Guidelines, 2011, National Institutes of Health. Available at http://www.nhlbi.nih.gov/guidelines/cvd_ped/peds_guidelines_full.pdf

Stolk MF, Becx MC, Kuypers KC, et al, "Severe Hepatic Side Effects of Ezetimibe," *Clin Gastroenterol Hepatol*, 2006, 4(7):908-11.

"Third Report of the National Cholesterol Education Program Expert Panel on Detection, Evaluation, and Treatment of High Blood Cholesterol in Adults (Adult Treatment Panel III)," May 2001, www.nhlbi.nih.gov/guidelines/cholesterol.

Yeste D, Chacon P, Clemente M, et al. Ezetimibe as monotherapy in the treatment of hypercholesterolemia in children and adolescents. *J Pediatr Endocrinol Metabl.* 2009;22(6):487-492.

Ezetimibe and Simvastatin
(ez ET i mibe & SIM va stat in)

Medication Safety Issues

Sound-alike/look-alike issues:

Vytorin may be confused with Vyvanse

Brand Names: U.S. Vytorin

Therapeutic Category Antilipemic Agent; Cholesterol Absorption Inhibitor; HMG-CoA Reductase Inhibitor

Generic Availability (U.S.) No

Use Adjunct to dietary therapy to decrease elevated serum total (total-C), low density lipoprotein cholesterol (LDL-C), and apolipoprotein B (apo-B) in patients with heterozygous familial hypercholesterolemia (FDA approved in boys and postmenarchal girls 10-17 years of age); adjunct to dietary therapy to decrease elevated serum total and low density lipoprotein cholesterol (LDL-C), apolipoprotein B (apo-B), non-high-density lipoprotein cholesterol (non-HDL-C) and triglyceride levels, and to increase high density lipoprotein cholesterol (HDL-C) in patients with primary hypercholesterolemia (heterozygous, familial, and nonfamilial) and mixed dyslipidemia (Fredrickson types IIa and IIb) (FDA approved in adults); treatment of homozygous familial hypercholesterolemia (FDA approved in adults).

Pregnancy Risk Factor X

Pregnancy Considerations Use is contraindicated in pregnant women or women who may become pregnant. See individual agents.

Breast-Feeding Considerations It is not known if ezetimibe or simvastatin are excreted into breast milk. Use is contraindicated in nursing women. See individual agents.

Contraindications Hypersensitivity to simvastatin, ezetimibe, or any component; active liver disease; unexplained persistent elevations of serum transaminases; pregnancy; breast-feeding; concomitant use of strong CYP3A4 inhibitors (eg, boceprevir, clarithromycin, erythromycin, HIV protease inhibitors, itraconazole, ketoconazole, nefazodone, posaconazole, telaprevir, telithromycin), cyclosporine, danazol, and gemfibrozil

Warnings Patients receiving HMG-CoA reductase inhibitors have developed rhabdomyolysis with or without acute renal failure and/or myopathy; patients should be monitored closely; risk is dose-related and greater in patients receiving simvastatin 80 mg than those receiving other HMG-CoA reductase inhibitors at similar efficacy dose. **High-dose (80 mg) is limited to patients who have been taking this dose for >12 consecutive months without evidence of myopathy and are not currently taking or beginning to take a simvastatin dose-limiting or contraindicated interacting medication.** Risk is also increased with concurrent use of other lipid-lowering medications (eg, fibric acid derivatives or niacin at doses >1 g/day) or during concurrent use with potent CYP3A4 inhibitor (some are contraindicated) or large quantities of grapefruit juice (>1 quart/day). With concurrent use of verapamil, diltiazem, dronedarone, amiodarone, amlodipine, and ranolazine; dosage reductions of simvastatin recommended. Concomitant use of high-dose simvastatin (80 mg) with niacin ≥1 g/day may increase risk of myopathy in Chinese patients. Ensure patient is on the lowest effective atorvastatin dose in all circumstances. Discontinue in any patient in which CPK levels are markedly elevated (>10 times ULN) or if myopathy is suspected/diagnosed; monitoring of CPK may be warranted, but may not prevent severe myopathy. The manufacturer recommends temporary discontinuation for elective major surgery, acute medical or surgical conditions, or in any patient experiencing an acute or serious condition predisposing to renal failure (eg, sepsis, hypotension, trauma, uncontrolled seizures). However, based upon current evidence, HMG-CoA reductase inhibitor therapy should be continued in the perioperative period unless risk outweighs cardioprotective benefit. Use caution in patients with renal impairment, inadequately treated hypothyroidism, and those taking other drugs associated with myopathy (eg, colchicine); these patients are predisposed to myopathy. Patients should be instructed to report unexplained muscle pain, tenderness, weakness, or brown urine.

An autoimmune-mediated myopathy (IMNM), has been reported (rarely) with HMG-CoA reductase inhibitor therapy; presents as proximal muscle weakness with elevated CPK levels, which persists despite discontinuation of HMG-CoA reductase inhibitor therapy; additionally, muscle biopsy may show necrotizing myopathy with limited inflammation; immunosuppressive therapy (eg, corticosteroids, azathioprine) may be used for treatment.

Postmarketing reports of fatal and nonfatal hepatic failure with simvastatin therapy are rare; if serious hepatotoxicity with clinical symptoms and/or hyperbilirubinemia or jaundice occurs during treatment, interrupt therapy. If an alternate etiology is not identified, do not restart simvastatin. Liver enzyme tests should be obtained at baseline and as clinically indicated; routine periodic monitoring of liver enzymes is not necessary. Use simvastatin with caution in patients with history of heavy alcohol use or a previous history of liver disease. Use ezetimibe with caution in patients with mild hepatic impairment; not recommended for use with moderate or severe hepatic impairment.

Precautions Increases in Hb A_{1c} and fasting blood glucose have been reported with HMG-CoA reductase inhibitors; however, the benefits of statin therapy far outweigh the risk of dysglycemia. Secondary causes of hyperlipidemia should be ruled out prior to therapy; has not been studied in Fredrickson types I, III, IV, and V dyslipidemia.

Although rare, reversible cognitive impairment (including confusion, forgetfulness, amnesia, and memory loss) can occur with HMG-CoA reductase inhibitors. These cognitive symptoms have been reported at variable times during therapy (1 day to years after initiation) and are reversible with discontinuation; resolution usually occurs within ~3 weeks. Cases have not been associated with fixed or progressive dementia; nor have they been associated with age, specific HMG CoA reductase inhibitor, dose, or concomitant medication use.

Use with caution in patients with renal impairment; avoid use in patients with severe renal impairment (creatinine clearance not defined) unless patient has already tolerated simvastatin at a dose ≥5 mg; **use doses of simvastatin >20 mg/day with caution and monitor closely for adverse events (eg, myopathy) in patients with moderate to severe renal impairment (ie, CrCl <60 mL/minute/1.73 m^2).** Initial dosage adjustment is not necessary in mild to moderate impairment. Renal impairment may also increase risk for myopathy.

Adverse Reactions Also see individual agents.
Central nervous system: Headache
Gastrointestinal: Diarrhea
Hepatic: ALT increased
Neuromuscular & skeletal: Myalgia, myopathy, pain in extremity
Respiratory: Upper respiratory infection
Miscellaneous: Influenza

Drug Interactions
Metabolism/Transport Effects Refer to individual components.
Avoid Concomitant Use
Avoid concomitant use of Ezetimibe and Simvastatin with any of the following: Boceprevir; Clarithromycin; Conivaptan; CycloSPORINE (Systemic); CYP3A4 Inhibitors (Strong); Erythromycin (Systemic); Fusidic Acid (Systemic); Gemfibrozil; Mifepristone; Protease Inhibitors; Red Yeast Rice; Telaprevir; Telithromycin
Increased Effect/Toxicity
Ezetimibe and Simvastatin may increase the levels/effects of: ARIPiprazole; DAPTOmycin; Diltiazem; PAZOPanib; Trabectedin; Vitamin K Antagonists

The levels/effects of Ezetimibe and Simvastatin may be increased by: Amiodarone; AmLODIPine; Azithromycin (Systemic); Bezafibrate; Boceprevir; Ceritinib; Clarithromycin; Colchicine; Conivaptan; CycloSPORINE (Systemic); CYP3A4 Inhibitors (Moderate); CYP3A4 Inhibitors (Strong); Cyproterone; Danazol; Dasatinib; Diltiazem; Dronedarone; Eltrombopag; Erythromycin (Systemic); Fenofibrate and Derivatives; Fibric Acid Derivatives; Fluconazole; Fusidic Acid (Systemic); Gemfibrozil; Grapefruit Juice; Green Tea; Imatinib; Ivacaftor; Lomitapide; Luliconazole; Mifepristone; Niacin; Niacinamide; Protease Inhibitors; QuiNINE; Raltegravir; Ranolazine; Red Yeast Rice; Sildenafil; Simeprevir; Telaprevir; Telithromycin; Ticagrelor; Verapamil
Decreased Effect
Ezetimibe and Simvastatin may decrease the levels/effects of: Lanthanum

The levels/effects of Ezetimibe and Simvastatin may be decreased by: Antacids; Bile Acid Sequestrants; Bosentan; CYP3A4 Inducers (Strong); Dabrafenib; Deferasirox; Efavirenz; Eslicarbazepine; Etravirine; Fosphenytoin; Mitotane; Phenytoin; Rifamycin Derivatives; Siltuximab; St Johns Wort; Tocilizumab
Food Interactions See individual agents.
Stability Store at 20°C to 25°C (68°F to 77°F); keep container tightly closed.
Mechanism of Action
Ezetimibe: Inhibits absorption of cholesterol at the brush border of the small intestine, leading to a decreased delivery of cholesterol to the liver. Ezetimibe inhibits the

enzyme Niemann-Pick C1-Like1 (NPC1L1), a sterol transporter.
Simvastatin: A methylated derivative of lovastatin that acts by competitively inhibiting 3-hydroxy-3-methylglutaryl-coenzyme A (HMG-CoA) reductase, the enzyme that catalyzes the rate-limiting step in cholesterol biosynthesis.

Pharmacodynamics
Onset of action: >3 days
Maximum effect: After 2-4 weeks
Pharmacokinetics (Adult data unless noted) See individual agents.
Bioavailability: Vytorin® is equivalent to coadministered ezetimibe and simvastatin.

Dosing: Usual
Children and Adolescents: **Note:** A lower, conservative dosing regimen may be necessary in patient populations predisposed to myopathy, including patients of Chinese descent or those concurrently receiving other lipid-lowering agents (eg, niacin, fibric acid derivatives), amiodarone, amlodipine, diltiazem, dronedarone, ranolazine, verapamil (see the following conservative, maximum adult doses)
Heterozygous familial hypercholesterolemia: Children ≥10 years and Adolescents: Oral: Initial: Ezetimibe 10 mg and simvastatin 10-20 mg once daily in the evening; maximum dose: Ezetimibe 10 mg and simvastatin 40 mg
Adults: **Note: Dosing limitation: Simvastatin 80 mg is limited to patients that have been taking this dose for >12 consecutive months without evidence of myopathy and are not currently taking or beginning to take a simvastatin dose-limiting or contraindicated interacting medication.** If patient is unable to achieve low-density lipoprotein-cholesterol (LDL-C) goal using the 40 mg dose of simvastatin, increasing to 80 mg dose is not recommended. Instead, switch patient to an alternative LDL-C-lowering treatment providing greater LDL-C reduction. After initiation or titration, monitor lipid response after ≥2 weeks and adjust dose as necessary.
Homozygous familial hypercholesterolemia: Oral: Ezetimibe 10 mg and simvastatin 40 mg once daily in the evening
Hyperlipidemias: Oral: Initial: Ezetimibe 10 mg and simvastatin 10-20 mg once daily in the evening. Dosing range: Ezetimibe 10 mg and simvastatin 10-40 mg once daily
Patients who require less aggressive reduction in LDL-C: Initial: Ezetimibe 10 mg and simvastatin 10 mg once daily in the evening
Patients who require >55% reduction in LDL-C: Initial: Ezetimibe 10 mg and simvastatin 40 mg once daily in the evening
Dosing adjustment with concomitant medications: Oral: Adults: **Note:** Patients currently tolerating and requiring a dose of simvastatin 80 mg who require initiation of an interacting drug with a dose cap for simvastatin should be switched to an alternative statin with less potential for drug-drug interaction.
Amiodarone, amlodipine, or ranolazine: Simvastatin dose should **not** exceed 20 mg once daily
Diltiazem, dronedarone, or verapamil: Simvastatin dose should **not** exceed 10 mg once daily
Dosing adjustment in Chinese patients on niacin doses ≥1 g/day: Adults: Oral: Use caution with simvastatin doses exceeding 20 mg/day; because of an increased risk of myopathy, do not administer simvastatin 80 mg.
Dosing adjustment in renal impairment: Adults:
GFR ≥60 mL/minute/1.73 m^2: No adjustment required.
GFR <60 mL/minute/1.73 m^2: Maximum dose: 10 mg ezetimibe/20 mg simvastatin daily; use with caution and monitor closely if higher doses are needed.

Dosing adjustment for hepatic impairment:
Mild impairment: No adjustment required.
Moderate to severe impairment: Use not recommended.
Administration Oral: May be taken without regard to meals. Administration with the evening meal or at bedtime has been associated with somewhat greater LDL-C reduction. Ezetimibe/simvastatin should be taken ≥2 hours before or ≥4 hours after administration of a bile acid sequestrant.

Monitoring Parameters
Pediatric patients: Baseline: ALT, AST, and creatine phosphokinase levels (CPK); fasting lipid panel (FLP) and repeat ALT and AST should be checked after 4 weeks of therapy; if no myopathy symptoms or laboratory abnormalities, then monitor FLP, ALT, and AST every 3-4 months during the first year and then every 6 months thereafter (NHLBI, 2011).

Adults: Baseline CPK (recheck CPK in any patient with symptoms suggestive of myopathy; discontinue therapy if markedly elevated); baseline liver function tests (LFTs) and repeat when clinically indicated thereafter. Patients with elevated transaminase levels should have a second (confirmatory) test and frequent monitoring until values normalize; discontinue if increase in ALT/AST is persistently >3 times ULN (NCEP, 2002).

Lipid panel (total cholesterol, HDL, LDL, triglycerides):
ATP III recommendations (NCEP, 2002): Baseline; 6-8 weeks after initiation of drug therapy; if dose increased, then at 6-8 weeks until final dose determined. Once treatment goal achieved, follow up intervals may be reduced to every 4-6 months. Lipid panel should be assessed at least annually, and preferably at each clinic visit.

Manufacturer recommendation: Upon initiation or titration, lipid panel should be analyzed after ≥2 weeks.

Dosage Forms Excipient information presented when available (limited, particularly for generics); consult specific product labeling.
Tablet:
Vytorin 10/10: Ezetimibe 10 mg and simvastatin 10 mg
Vytorin 10/20: Ezetimibe 10 mg and simvastatin 20 mg
Vytorin 10/40: Ezetimibe 10 mg and simvastatin 40 mg
Vytorin 10/80: Ezetimibe 10 mg and simvastatin 80 mg

References

Daniels SR, Greer FR, and Committee on Nutrition, "Lipid Screening and Cardiovascular Health in Childhood," *Pediatrics*, 2008, 122 (1):198-208.

Dejongh S, Stalenhoef AF, Tuohy MB, et al, "Efficacy, Safety, and Tolerability of Simvastatin in Children With Familial Hypercholesterolemia: Rational, Design and Baseline Characterisitics," *Clin Drug Invest*, 2002, 22(8):533-40.

Ducobu J, Brasseur D, Chaudron JM, et al, "Simvastatin Use in Children," *Lancet*, 1992, 339(8807):1488.

Gagne C, Gaudet D, Bruckert E, et al, "Efficacy and Safety of Ezetimibe Coadministered With Atorvastatin or Simvastatin in Patients With Homozygous Familial Hypercholesterolemia," *Circulation*, 2002, 105 (21):2469-75.

McCrindle BW, Urbina EM, Dennison BA, et al, "Drug Therapy of High-Risk Lipid Abnormalities in Children and Adolescents: A Scientific Statement from the American Heart Association Atherosclerosis, Hypertension, and Obesity in Youth Committee, Council of Cardiovascular Disease in the Young, With the Council on Cardiovascular Nursing," *Circulation*, 2007, 115(14):1948-67.

National Heart, Lung, and Blood Institute, "Expert Panel on Integrated Guidelines for Cardiovascular Health and Risk Reduction in Children and Adolescents," Clinical Practice Guidelines, 2011, National Institutes of Health. Available at http://www.nhlbi.nih.gov/guidelines/cvd_ped/peds_guidelines_full.pdf

"Third Report of the National Cholesterol Education Program (NCEP) Expert Panel on Detection, Evaluation, and Treatment of High Blood Cholesterol in Adults (Adult Treatment Panel III) Final Report," *Circulation*, 2002, 106(25):3143-421.

◆ **Ezetrol (Can)** *see* Ezetimibe *on page 827*

◆ **EZFE 200 [OTC]** *see* Polysaccharide-Iron Complex *on page 1701*

◆ **F₃T** *see* Trifluridine *on page 2084*

◆ **FA-8 [OTC]** *see* Folic Acid *on page 925*

◆ **FabAV, FAB (Ovine)** *see* Crotalidae Polyvalent Immune Fab (Ovine) *on page 553*

◆ **Fabior** *see* Tazarotene *on page 1971*

◆ **Fabrazyme** *see* Agalsidase Beta *on page 79*

◆ **Fabrazyme® (Can)** *see* Agalsidase Beta *on page 79*

Factor VIIa (Recombinant)
(FAK ter SEV en aye ree KOM be nant)

Brand Names: U.S. NovoSeven RT
Brand Names: Canada Niastase®; Niastase® RT
Therapeutic Category Antihemophilic Agent
Generic Availability (U.S.) No
Use Treatment of bleeding episodes and prevention of bleeding in surgical interventions in patients with either hemophilia A or B when inhibitors to factor VIII or factor IX are present, acquired hemophilia, or congenital factor VII deficiency [FDA approved in pediatrics (age not specified) and adults]
Pregnancy Risk Factor C
Pregnancy Considerations Adverse events were observed in animal reproduction studies.
Breast-Feeding Considerations It is not known if factor VIIa (recombinant) is excreted in breast milk. Due to the potential for serious adverse reactions in the nursing infant, a decision should be made whether to discontinue nursing or to discontinue the drug, taking into account the importance of treatment to the mother.
Contraindications Hypersensitivity to factor VII or any component
Warnings Serious and sometimes fatal thrombotic events have been associated with the use of factor VIIa outside labeled indications **[U.S. Boxed Warning]**. Arterial and venous thrombotic and thromboembolic events, some fatal, following administration of factor VIIa have been reported during postmarketing surveillance. Thrombotic events have also been reported when used within labeled indications; thrombotic events may be increased in patients with disseminated intravascular coagulation (DIC), advanced atherosclerotic disease, sepsis, crush injury, or concomitant treatment with prothrombin complex concentrates. All patients receiving factor VIIa should be monitored for signs and symptoms of activation of the coagulation system or thrombosis. Efficacy with prolonged infusions and data evaluating long-term adverse effects are limited. Contains polysorbate 80 (Tween 80®) which may cause allergic reactions in susceptible individuals. In premature neonates, thrombocytopenia, ascites, pulmonary deterioration, and renal and hepatic failure have been reported after receiving parenteral products containing polysorbate 80 (Alade, 1986; *MMWR*, 1984). Infusion of polysorbate 80-containing solutions through polyvinyl chloride tubing may cause DEHP to leach into the solution; in immature animals, exposure to DEHP may adversely affect the development of the male reproductive tract.
Precautions Use with caution in patients with hypersensitivity to mouse, hamster, bovine proteins. Monitor PT and factor VII coagulant activity in factor VII deficient patients; if no response, may consider testing for antibody formation.
Adverse Reactions
Cardiovascular: Bradycardia, edema, hyper-/hypotension
Central nervous system: Fever, headache, pain
Dermatologic: Pruritus, purpura, rash
Gastrointestinal: Vomiting
Hematologic: Disseminated intravascular coagulation, fibrinolysis increased, plasma fibrinogen decreased, prothrombin decreased
Local: Injection site reaction
Neuromuscular & skeletal: Arthrosis
Renal: Abnormal renal function

Respiratory: Pneumonia

Miscellaneous: Allergic reactions

Rare but important or life-threatening: Anaphylactic shock, angina, angioedema, antibody formation, arterial thrombosis, arterial thrombosis (limb), arthralgia, bowel infarction, cerebral artery occlusion, cerebral infarction and/or ischemia, consumptive coagulopathy, CVA, D-dimer elevation, deep vein thrombosis, fibrin degradation products increased, flushing, hepatic artery thrombosis, hypersensitivity, hypersensitivity reaction, injection site pain, intestinal infarction, I.V. site thrombosis, localized phlebitis, MI, myocardial ischemia, nausea, peripheral ischemia, portal vein thrombosis, pulmonary embolism, renal artery thrombosis, retinal artery embolism, retinal artery thrombosis, shock, thrombophlebitis, thrombosis, urticaria

Drug Interactions

Metabolism/Transport Effects None known.

Avoid Concomitant Use There are no known interactions where it is recommended to avoid concomitant use.

Increased Effect/Toxicity
The levels/effects of Factor VIIa (Recombinant) may be increased by: Factor XIII A-Subunit (Recombinant)

Decreased Effect There are no known significant interactions involving a decrease in effect.

Stability NovoSeven® RT: Prior to reconstitution, store under refrigeration or between 2°C to 25°C (36°F to 77°F). Do not freeze. Protect from light. Reconstituted solutions may be stored at room temperature or under refrigeration but must be infused within 3 hours of reconstitution. Do not freeze reconstituted solutions. Do not store reconstituted solutions in syringes.

Mechanism of Action Recombinant factor VIIa, a vitamin K-dependent glycoprotein, promotes hemostasis by activating the extrinsic pathway of the coagulation cascade. It replaces deficient activated coagulation factor VII, which complexes with tissue factor and may activate coagulation factor X to Xa and factor IX to IXa. When complexed with other factors, coagulation factor Xa converts prothrombin to thrombin, a key step in the formation of a fibrin-platelet hemostatic plug.

Pharmacodynamics

Onset of action: 10-20 minutes

Maximum effect: 6 hours

Pharmacokinetics (Adult data unless noted)

Distribution: V_d: Children: 130 mL/kg; Adults: 103-105 mL/kg (range: 78-139 mL/kg)

Half-life: Elimination: Children: 1.32 hours; Adults: 2.3 hours (range: 1.7-2.7 hours)

Time to peak serum concentration: 15 minutes

Elimination: Clearance: Children: 67 mL/kg/hour; Adults: 30-36 mL/kg/hour (range: 27-49 mL/kg/hour)

Dosing: Usual I.V.: Children and Adults:

Hemophilia A or B with inhibitors:

Bleeding episodes: 90 mcg/kg every 2 hours until hemostasis is achieved or until the treatment is judged ineffective. The dose and interval may be adjusted based upon the severity of bleeding and the degree of hemostasis achieved. Doses between 35-120 mcg/kg have been used successfully in clinical trials. The dose, interval, and duration of therapy may be adjusted based on severity of bleeding and the degree of hemostasis achieved. For patients treated for joint or muscle bleeds, a decision on the outcome of treatment was reached within 8 doses in the majority of patients, although more doses were required for severe bleeds; adverse effects were reported most commonly in patients treated with 12 or more doses. For patients experiencing severe bleeds to maintain the hemostatic plug, dosing should be continued at 3- to 6-hour intervals; the duration of posthemostatic dosing should be minimized.

Surgical interventions: 90 mcg/kg immediately before surgery; repeat at 2-hour intervals for the duration of surgery. Continue every 2 hours for 48 hours, then every 2-6 hours until healed for minor surgery; continue every 2 hours for 5 days, then every 4 hours until healed for major surgery

Congenital factor VII deficiency: Bleeding episodes and surgical interventions: 15-30 mcg/kg every 4-6 hours until hemostasis is achieved. Doses as low as 10 mcg/kg have been effective; individualized dosing is recommended.

Acquired hemophilia: 70-90 mcg/kg every 2-3 hours until hemostasis is achieved

Administration Parenteral: I.V.: NovoSeven® RT: Prior to reconstitution, bring to room temperature. Add recommended diluent along wall of vial; do not inject directly onto powder. Gently swirl until dissolved. Reconstitute each vial to a final concentration of 1 mg/mL using the provided histidine diluent as follows:

1 mg vial: 1.1 mL histidine diluent

2 mg vial: 2.1 mL histidine diluent

5 mg vial: 5.2 mL histidine diluent

8 mg vial: 8.1 mL histidine diluent

Administer as a slow bolus over 2-5 minutes.

Monitoring Parameters Monitor for evidence of hemostasis; although the prothrombin time/INR, aPTT, and factor VII clotting activity have no correlation with achieving clinical hemostasis, these parameters may be useful as adjunct tests to evaluate efficacy and guide dose or interval adjustments

Additional Information Each mg factor VIIa contains 0.4 mEq sodium and 0.01 mEq calcium; "off-label" uses in limited patient populations have been reported (primarily adult patients) including reversal of anticoagulant over dose and reduction in bleeding associated with thrombocytopenia, trauma, hepatic dysfunction, and cardiac bypass surgery; further randomized, blinded clinical trials are needed to determine efficacy, dosage, and safety for these indications (Ghorashian, 2004; Tobias, 2004)

Dosage Forms Excipient information presented when available (limited, particularly for generics); consult specific product labeling.

Solution Reconstituted, Intravenous [preservative free]:

NovoSeven RT: 1 mg (1 ea); 2 mg (1 ea); 5 mg (1 ea); 8 mg (1 ea) [contains polysorbate 80]

References

Alade SL, Brown RE, and Paquet A Jr, "Polysorbate 80 and E-Ferol Toxicity," *Pediatrics*, 1986, 77(4):593-7.

Centers for Disease Control (CDC), "Unusual Syndrome With Fatalities Among Premature Infants: Association With a New Intravenous Vitamin E Product," *MMWR Morb Mortal Wkly Rep*, 1984, 33 (14):198-9.

Ghorashian S and Hunt BJ, "'Off-License' Use of Recombinant Activated Factor VII," *Blood Rev*, 2004, 18(4):245-59.

Goodnough LT, Lublin DM, Zhang L, et al, "Transfusion Medicine Service Policies for Recombinant Factor VIIa Administration," *Transfusion*, 2004, 44(9):1325-31.

Tobias JD, Simsic JM, Weinstein S, et al, "Recombinant Factor VIIa to Control Excessive Bleeding Following Surgery for Congenital Heart Disease in Pediatric Patients," *J Intensive Care Med*, 2004, 19 (5):270-3.

♦ **Factor VIII Concentrate** *see* Antihemophilic Factor/von Willebrand Factor Complex (Human) *on page 177*

♦ **Factor VIII (Human)** *see* Antihemophilic Factor (Human) *on page 170*

♦ **Factor VIII (Human)** *see* Antihemophilic Factor/von Willebrand Factor Complex (Human) *on page 177*

♦ **Factor VIII Inhibitor Bypassing Activity** *see* Anti-inhibitor Coagulant Complex (Human) *on page 180*

♦ **Factor VIII (Recombinant)** *see* Antihemophilic Factor (Recombinant) *on page 172*

Factor IX Complex (Human) [(Factors II, IX, X)] (FAK ter nyne KOM pleks HYU man FAKter too nyne ten)

Medication Safety Issues
Sound-alike/look-alike issues:
Factor IX Complex may be confused with Factor IX
Safety concern:
Factor IX Complex may be confused with Factor IX
The term "Prothrombin Complex Concentrate" or "PCC" has been used to describe both Factor IX Complex (Human) [Factors II, IX, X] and Prothrombin Complex Concentrate (Human) [(Factors II, VII, IX, X), Protein C, Protein S]. **Factor IX Complex (Human) [Factors II, IX, X] (Bebulin, Profilnine) contains low or nontherapeutic levels of factor VII component** and should not be confused with Prothrombin Complex Concentrate (Human) [(Factors II, VII, IX, X), Protein C, Protein S] (Kcentra, Octaplex) which contains therapeutic levels of factor VII.

Brand Names: U.S. Bebulin VH; Profilnine SD

Therapeutic Category Antihemophilic Agent; Blood Product Derivative

Generic Availability (U.S.) No

Use Prevention and control of bleeding in patients with factor IX deficiency (hemophilia B or Christmas disease) (Profilnine® SD: FDA approved in ages >16 years and adults; Bebulin® VH: FDA approved in adults)

Pregnancy Risk Factor C

Pregnancy Considerations Animal reproduction studies have not been conducted. Factor IX concentrations do not change significantly in pregnant women with coagulation disorders and women with factor IX deficiency may be at increased risk of postpartum hemorrhage. Pregnant women should have clotting factors monitored, particularly at 28 and 34 weeks gestation and prior to invasive procedures. Prophylaxis may be needed if factor IX concentrations are <50 units/mL at term and treatment should continue for 3-5 days postpartum depending on route of delivery. Because parvovirus infection may cause hydrops fetalis or fetal death, a recombinant product is preferred if prophylaxis or treatment is needed. The neonate may also be at an increased risk of bleeding following delivery and should be tested for the coagulation disorder (Chi, 2012; Kadir, 2009; Lee, 2006).

Contraindications Hypersensitivity to factor IX complex or any component

Warnings Human factor IX complex is prepared from human plasma and even with heat treated or other viral attenuated processes, the risk of viral transmission (ie, viral hepatitis, HIV, parvovirus B19, and theoretically, Creutzfeldt-Jacob disease agent) is not totally eradicated. Hepatitis B vaccination and hepatitis A vaccination are recommended for patients with hemophilia (at birth or at diagnosis). Serious and potentially fatal thrombosis or DIC may occur in patients with hepatic impairment and in patients undergoing surgery (risk is greater following surgery); use with caution in these patients; consider risk versus benefit before prescribing.

Hypersensitivity and anaphylactic reactions have been reported with use. Delayed reactions (up to 20 days after infusion) in previously untreated patients may also occur. Due to potential allergic reactions, the initial ~10-20 administrations should be performed under appropriate medical supervision. Patients experiencing allergic reactions should be evaluated for factor IX inhibitors. The development of factor IX inhibitors (or antibodies) usually occurs within the first 10-20 exposure days to factor IX therapy; the presence of inhibitors increases the risk of severe hypersensitivity reactions. Patients with severe gene defects (eg, gene deletion or inversion) are more likely to develop inhibitors. When clinical response is suboptimal or patient is to undergo surgical procedure, screening for inhibitors should be completed (WFH, 2013).

Precautions Observe closely for signs or symptoms of intravascular coagulation or thrombosis. Use with caution when administering to patients with liver disease, postoperatively, or patients at risk of thromboembolic phenomena, disseminated intravascular coagulation, or patients with signs of fibrinolysis due to the potential risk of thromboembolic complications. Products do not contain therapeutic levels of factor VII and should not be used for the treatment of factor VII deficiency. Some products (eg, Bebulin® VH) contain natural rubber latex (in certain components of the product packaging) which may cause allergic reactions in susceptible individuals; avoid use in patients with allergy to latex. Some products contain heparin; use with caution in patients with a history of heparin-induced thrombocytopenia.

Adverse Reactions
Cardiovascular: Flushing, thrombosis (sometimes fatal)
Central nervous system: Chills, fever, headache, lethargy, somnolence
Dermatologic: Rash, urticaria
Gastrointestinal: Nausea, vomiting
Hematologic: DIC
Neuromuscular & skeletal: Paresthesia
Respiratory: Dyspnea
Miscellaneous: Anaphylactic shock, clotting factor antibodies (development of), heparin-induced thrombocytopenia (with products containing heparin)

Drug Interactions
Metabolism/Transport Effects None known.
Avoid Concomitant Use
Avoid concomitant use of Factor IX Complex (Human) [(Factors II, IX, X)] with any of the following: Aminocaproic Acid
Increased Effect/Toxicity
The levels/effects of Factor IX Complex (Human) [(Factors II, IX, X)] may be increased by: Aminocaproic Acid
Decreased Effect There are no known significant interactions involving a decrease in effect.

Stability Store unopened vials at 2°C to 8°C (35°F to 46°F); do not freeze. Profilnine® SD: May store unopened vials at room temperature (<30°C) for up to 3 months. Administer within 3 hours after reconstitution; **do not refrigerate after reconstitution;** discard unused portion.

Mechanism of Action Replaces deficient clotting factor including factor X; hemophilia B, or Christmas disease, is an X-linked recessively inherited disorder of blood coagulation characterized by insufficient or abnormal synthesis of the clotting protein factor IX. Factor IX is a vitamin K-dependent coagulation factor which is synthesized in the liver. Factor IX is activated by factor XIa in the intrinsic coagulation pathway. Activated factor IX (IXa), in combination with factor VII:C, activates factor X to Xa, resulting ultimately in the conversion of prothrombin to thrombin and the formation of a fibrin clot. The infusion of exogenous factor IX to replace the deficiency present in hemophilia B temporarily restores hemostasis.

Pharmacokinetics (Adult data unless noted) Half-life: Cleared rapidly from the serum in two phases:
First phase: 4-6 hours
Terminal: 22.5 hours

Dosing: Usual
Hemophilia B: Children, Adolescents, and Adults: I.V.: Dosage is expressed in units of factor IX activity and must be individualized based on severity of factor IX deficiency, extent and location of bleeding, and clinical status of patient (WHF, 2013). When multiple doses are required, administer at 24-hour intervals unless otherwise specified.

Formula for units required to raise blood level%:
Bebulin® VH: In general, 1 unit/kg of factor IX will increase the plasma factor IX level by 0.8%

Number of Factor IX units required = body weight (kg) x desired factor IX increase (as% of normal) x 1.2 units/kg

For example, to increase factor IX level to 25% of normal in a 70 kg patient: Number of factor IX units needed = 70 kg x 25 x 1.2 unit/kg = 2100 units

Profilnine® SD: In general, 1 unit/kg of factor IX will increase the plasma factor IX level by 1%:

Number of factor IX units required = bodyweight (kg) x desired factor IX increase (as% of normal) x 1 unit/kg

For example, to increase factor IX level to 25% of normal in a 70 kg patient: Number of factor IX units needed = 70 kg x 25 x 1 unit/kg = 1750 units

As a general rule, the level of factor IX required for treatment of different conditions is listed below:

Hemorrhage:

Minor bleeding (early hemarthrosis, minor epistaxis, gingival bleeding, mild hematuria):

Bebulin® VH: Raise factor IX level to 20% of normal [typical initial dose: 25-35 units/kg]; generally a single dose is sufficient

Profilnine® SD: Mild to moderate bleeding: Raise factor IX level to 20% to 30% of normal; generally a single dose is sufficient

Moderate bleeding (severe joint bleeding, early hematoma, major open bleeding, minor trauma, minor hemoptysis, hematemesis, melena, major hematuria):

Bebulin® VH: Raise factor IX level to 40% of normal [typical initial dose: 40-55 units/kg]; average duration of treatment is 2 days or until adequate wound healing

Profilnine® SD: Mild to moderate bleeding: Raise factor IX level to 20% to 30% of normal

Major bleeding (severe hematoma, major trauma, severe hemoptysis, hematemesis, melena):

Bebulin® VH: Raise factor IX level to ≥60% of normal [typical initial dose: 60-70 units/kg]; average duration of treatment is 2-3 days or until adequate wound healing. Do not raise >60% in patients who may be predisposed to thrombosis.

Profilnine® SD: Raise factor IX level to 30% to 50% of normal; daily infusions are usually required

Surgical procedures:

Dental surgery:

Bebulin® VH: Raise factor IX level to 40% to 60% of normal on day of surgery [typical dose: 50-60 units/kg]. One infusion, administered 1 hour prior to surgery, is generally sufficient for the extraction of one tooth; for the extraction of multiple teeth, replacement therapy may be required for up to 1 week (see dosing guidelines for Minor Surgery).

Profilnine® SD: Raise factor IX level to 50% of normal immediately prior to procedure; administer additional doses if bleeding recurs

Minor surgery:

Bebulin® VH: Raise factor IX level to 40% to 60% of normal on day of surgery [typical initial dose: 50-60 units/kg]. Decrease factor IX level from 40% of normal to 20% of normal during initial postoperative period (1-2 weeks or until adequate wound healing) [typical dose: 55 units/kg decreasing to 25 units/kg]. The preoperative dose should be given 1 hour prior to surgery. The average dosing interval may be every 12 hours initially, then every 24 hours later in the postoperative period.

Profilnine® SD: Raise factor IX level to 30% to 50% of normal for at least 1 week following surgery

Major surgery:

Bebulin® VH: Raise factor IX level to ≥60% of normal on day of surgery [typical initial dose: 70-95 units/kg]; do not raise >60% in patients who may be predisposed to thrombosis. Decrease factor IX level from

60% of normal to 20% of normal during initial postoperative period (1-2 weeks) [typical dose: 70 units/kg decreasing to 35 units/kg]; further decrease to maintain a factor IX level of 20% of normal during late postoperative period (≥3 weeks) and continuing until adequate wound healing is achieved [typical dose: 35 units/kg decreasing to 25 units/kg]. The preoperative dose should be given 1 hour prior to surgery. The average dosing interval may be every 12 hours initially, then every 24 hours later in the postoperative period.

Profilnine® SD: Raise factor IX level to 30% to 50% of normal for at least 1 week following surgery

Prophylaxis, hemorrhage (long-term management):

Bebulin® VH: 20-30 units/kg/dose once or twice a week may reduce frequency of spontaneous hemorrhage; dosing regimen should be individualized.

Administration Parenteral: I.V. administration only; infuse slowly; rate of administration should be individualized for patient's comfort; rapid I.V. administration may cause vasomotor reactions; maximum rates of administration: Bebulin® VH: 2 mL/minute; Profilnine® SD: 10 mL/minute; visually inspect for particulate matter and discoloration prior to administration whenever permitted by solution or container. **Note:** Slowing the rate of infusion, changing the lot of medication, or administering antihistamines may relieve some adverse reactions

Monitoring Parameters Levels of factors II, IX, and X; signs/symptoms of hypersensitivity reactions and bleeding; hemoglobin, hematocrit; screen for factor IX inhibitors by measuring inhibitor titers (children: Every 3-12 months or 10-20 exposure days)

Reference Range Patients with severe hemophilia will have factor IX levels <1%, often undetectable. Moderate forms of the disease have levels of 1% to 5% while some mild cases may have 5% to 49% of normal factor IX. Plasma concentration is about 4 mg/L.

Dosage Forms Excipient information presented when available (limited, particularly for generics); consult specific product labeling. [DSC] = Discontinued product

Injection, powder for reconstitution:

Bebulin® VH: Exact potency labeled on each vial [vapor heated; contains heparin and natural rubber/natural latex in packaging]

Profilnine® SD: ~500 units, ~1000 units, ~1500 units [exact potency labeled on each vial; solvent/detergent treated]

References

Chi C and Kadir RA, "Inherited Bleeding Disorders in Pregnancy," *Best Pract Res Clin Obstet Gynaecol*, 2012, 26(1):103-17.

Kadir R, Chi C, and Bolton-Maggs P, "Pregnancy and Rare Bleeding Disorders," *Haemophilia*, 2009, 15(5):990-1005.

Lee CA, Chi C, Pavord SR, et al, "The Obstetric and Gynaecological Management of Women With Inherited Bleeding Disorders-Review With Guidelines Produced by a Taskforce of UK Haemophilia Centre Doctors' Organization," *Haemophilia*, 2006, 12(4):301-36.

Lee JW, "Von Willebrand Disease, Hemophilia A and B, and Other Factor Deficiencies," *Int Anesthesiol Clin*, 2004, 42(3):59-76.

Lusher JM, "Thrombogenicity Associated With Factor IX Complex Concentrates," *Semin Hematol*, 1991, 28(3 Suppl 6):3-5.

National Hemophilia Foundation, "Guidelines for Emergency Department Management of Individuals With Hemophilia," 2006. Available at http://www.hemophilia.org/NHFWeb/Resource/StaticPages/menu0/menu5/menu57/175.pdf

National Hemophilia Foundation, "MASAC Recommendations Concerning Products Licensed for the Treatment of Hemophilia and Other Bleeding Disorders," 2010. Available at http://www.hemophilia.org/NHFWeb/Resource/StaticPages/menu0/menu5/menu57/masac190.pdf

National Hemophilia Foundation, "MASAC Recommendations Concerning Prophylaxis (Regular Administration of Clotting Factor Concentrate to Prevent Bleeding)," 2007. Available at http://www.hemophilia.org/NHFWeb/Resource/StaticPages/menu0/menu5/menu57/masac179.pdf

Shord SS and Lindley CM, "Coagulation Products and Their Uses," *Am J Health Syst Pharm*, 2000, 57(15):1403-20.

Srivastava A, Brewer AK, Mauser-Bunschoten EP, et al, "Guidelines for the Management of Hemophilia," *Haemophilia*, 2013, 19(1):e1-47.

◆ **Factor Eight Inhibitor Bypassing Activity** *see* Antiinhibitor Coagulant Complex (Human) *on page 180*

◆ **Factor IX Concentrate** *see* Factor IX (Human) *on page 835*

◆ **Factor IX Concentrate** *see* Factor IX (Recombinant) *on page 838*

Factor IX (Human) (FAK ter nyne HYU man)

Medication Safety Issues
Sound-alike/look-alike issues:
Factor IX may be confused with Factor IX Complex
Brand Names: U.S. AlphaNine SD; Mononine
Brand Names: Canada Immunine® VH
Therapeutic Category Antihemophilic Agent; Blood Product Derivative
Generic Availability (U.S.) No
Use
AlphaNine SD: Prevention and control of bleeding in factor IX deficiency (hemophilia B or Christmas disease) (FDA approved in ages ≥16 years and adults)

Mononine: Prevention and control of bleeding in factor IX deficiency (hemophilia B or Christmas disease) (FDA approved in all ages)

NOTE: Contains **nondetectable levels of factors II, VII, and X**; therefore, **NOT INDICATED** for replacement therapy of any other clotting factor besides factor IX or for reversal of anticoagulation due to either vitamin K antagonists or other anticoagulants (eg, dabigatran), for hemophilia A patients with factor VIII inhibitors, or for patients in a hemorrhagic state caused by reduced production of liver-dependent coagulation factors (eg, hepatitis, cirrhosis).

Pregnancy Risk Factor C
Pregnancy Considerations Animal reproduction studies have not been conducted. Factor IX concentrations do not change significantly in pregnant women with coagulation disorders and women with factor IX deficiency may be at increased risk of postpartum hemorrhage. Pregnant women should have clotting factors monitored, particularly at 28 and 34 weeks gestation and prior to invasive procedures. Prophylaxis may be needed if factor IX concentrations are <50 units/mL at term and treatment should continue for 3-5 days postpartum depending on route of delivery. Because parvovirus infection may cause hydrops fetalis or fetal death, a recombinant product is preferred if prophylaxis or treatment is needed. The neonate may also be at an increased risk of bleeding following delivery and should be tested for the coagulation disorder (Chi, 2012; Kadir, 2009; Lee, 2006).

Contraindications Hypersensitivity to mouse protein (Mononine) or any component

Warnings Product of human plasma. Despite purification methods (AlphaNine SD: Solvent detergent treated/virus filtered; Mononine: Virus filtered), products may potentially contain infectious agents (eg, viruses) which could transmit disease. Screening of donors, as well as testing and/or inactivation or removal of certain viruses, reduces the risk. Infections thought to be transmitted by this product should be reported to the manufacturer. Hepatitis B vaccination and hepatitis A vaccination are recommended for patients with hemophilia (at birth or at diagnosis).

Hypersensitivity and anaphylactic reactions have been reported. Delayed reactions (up to 20 days after infusion) in previously untreated patients may also occur. Due to potential allergic reactions, the initial ~10-20 administrations should be performed under appropriate medical

supervision. Hypersensitivity reactions may be associated with factor IX inhibitor development; patients experiencing allergic reactions should be evaluated for factor IX antibodies (or inhibitors). The development of factor IX inhibitors usually occurs within the first 10-20 exposure days to factor IX therapy; the presence of inhibitors increases the risk of severe hypersensitivity reactions. When clinical response is suboptimal or patient is to undergo surgical procedure, screen for inhibitors. Patients with severe hemophilia are more likely to develop inhibitors [WFH guidelines (Srivastava, 2013)].

Response to factor IX administration may vary. If bleeding is not controlled with the recommended dose, determine plasma level of factor IX and follow with a sufficient dose to achieve satisfactory clinical response. If plasma levels of factor IX fail to increase as expected or bleeding continues, suspect the presence of an inhibitor; test as appropriate. In the presence of an inhibitor, higher factor IX doses may be required to control bleeding.

Plasma-derived products contain **nondetectable levels of factors II, VII, and X** (<0.0025 units per factor IX unit using standard coagulation assays; therefore, factor IX products are **NOT INDICATED** for replacement therapy of any other clotting factor besides factor IX or for reversal of anticoagulation due to either vitamin K antagonists or other anticoagulants (eg, dabigatran), for hemophilia A patients with factor VIII inhibitors, or for patients in a hemorrhagic state caused by reduced production of liver-dependent coagulation factors (eg, hepatitis, cirrhosis).

Observe closely for signs or symptoms of intravascular coagulation or thrombosis; risk is generally associated with the use of factor IX complex concentrates (containing therapeutic amounts of additional factors); however, potential risk exists with use of factor IX products (containing only factor IX). Use with caution when administering to patients with liver disease, postoperatively, neonates, or patients at risk of thromboembolic phenomena, disseminated intravascular coagulation, or patients with signs of fibrinolysis due to the potential risk of thromboembolic complications. The safety and efficacy of continuous infusion administration has not been established; thrombotic events have been reported in patients receiving continuous infusion of recombinant Factor IX through a central venous catheter, including life-threatening superior vena cava syndrome in neonates.

Safety and efficacy have not been established in immune tolerance induction with factor IX products. Nephrotic syndrome has occurred following immune tolerance induction in patients with factor IX inhibitors and a history of allergic reactions to therapy.

Products contain polysorbate 80 (Tween 80) which may cause allergic reactions in susceptible individuals. In premature neonates, thrombocytopenia, ascites, pulmonary deterioration, and renal and hepatic failure have been reported after receiving parenteral products containing polysorbate 80 (Alade, 1986; CDC, 1984). Infusion of polysorbate 80-containing solutions through PVC tubing may cause DEHP to leach into the solution; in immature animals, exposure to DEHP may adversely affect the development of the male reproductive tract.

Adverse Reactions
Cardiovascular: Chest tightness, flushing, hypotension, thrombosis

Central nervous system: Burning sensation (in jaw/skull), chills, dizziness, drowsiness, headache, lethargy, paresthesia, rigors

Dermatologic: Skin photosensitivity, skin rash, urticaria

Gastrointestinal: Diarrhea, dysgeusia, nausea, vomiting

Hematologic & Oncologic: Disseminated intravascular coagulation, factor IX inhibitor development

▶

Hepatic: Increased serum alkaline phosphatase, increased serum ALT, increased serum AST

Hypersensitivity: Anaphylaxis, angioedema, hypersensitivity reaction

Local: Injection site reaction: Cellulitis at injection site, discomfort at injection site, injection site phlebitis, pain at injection site

Miscellaneous: Fever (including transient fever following rapid administration)

Neuromuscular & skeletal: Neck tightness

Ophthalmic: Visual disturbance

Respiratory: Allergic rhinitis, asthma, cough, cyanosis, dyspnea, hypoxia, laryngeal edema, pulmonary disease

Rare, but important or life-threatening: Decreased therapeutic response, HAV (hepatitis A virus) seroconversion, nephrotic syndrome (associated with immune tolerance induction), parvovirus B19 seroconversion, renal infarction, superior vena cava syndrome (neonates)

Drug Interactions

Metabolism/Transport Effects None known.

Avoid Concomitant Use

Avoid concomitant use of Factor IX (Human) with any of the following: Aminocaproic Acid

Increased Effect/Toxicity

The levels/effects of Factor IX (Human) may be increased by: Aminocaproic Acid

Decreased Effect There are no known significant interactions involving a decrease in effect.

Stability When stored at refrigerator temperature, 2°C to 8°C (36°F to 46°F), factor IX is stable for the period indicated by the expiration date on its label. Avoid freezing which may damage container for the diluent.

AlphaNine SD: May also be stored at room temperature not to exceed 30°C (86°F) for up to 1 month. Reconstitute with provided diluent; reconstituted solution should be used within 3 hours of preparation.

Mononine: May also be stored at room temperature not to exceed 25°C (77°F) for up to 1 month. Reconstitute with provided diluent; reconstituted solution should be stored at room temperature and used within 3 hours of preparation.

Mechanism of Action Replaces deficient clotting factor IX. Hemophilia B, or Christmas disease, is an X-linked inherited disorder of blood coagulation characterized by insufficient or abnormal synthesis of the clotting protein factor IX. Factor IX is a vitamin K-dependent coagulation factor which is synthesized in the liver. Factor IX is activated by factor XIa in the intrinsic coagulation pathway. Activated factor IX (IXa), in combination with factor VII:C activates factor X to Xa, resulting ultimately in the conversion of prothrombin to thrombin and the formation of a fibrin clot. The infusion of exogenous factor IX to replace the deficiency present in hemophilia B temporarily restores hemostasis.

Pharmacokinetics (Adult data unless noted) Half-life: Factor IX component: ~21-25 hours

Dosing: Neonatal NOTE: Contains **nondetectable levels of factors II, VII, and X**; therefore, **NOT INDICATED** for replacement therapy of any other clotting factor besides factor IX or for reversal of anticoagulation due to either vitamin K antagonists or other anticoagulants (eg, dabigatran), for hemophilia A patients with factor VIII inhibitors, or for patients in a hemorrhagic state caused by reduced production of liver-dependent coagulation factors (eg, hepatitis, cirrhosis).

Control or prevention of bleeding in patients with factor IX deficiency (hemophilia B or Christmas disease): I.V.: Dosage is expressed in units of factor IX activity and must be individualized based on formulation, severity of factor IX deficiency, extent and location of bleed, and clinical situation of patient.

Formula for units required to raise blood level:

Mononine:

Number of Factor IX Units Required = body weight (in kg) x desired Factor IX level increase (% or units/dL) x 1 unit/kg

For example, for a 100% level in a 3 kg patient who has an actual level of 20%: Number of Factor IX Units needed = 3 kg x 80% x 1 unit/kg = 240 units

Dosing: Usual NOTE: Contains **nondetectable levels of factors II, VII, and X**; therefore, **NOT INDICATED** for replacement therapy of any other clotting factor besides factor IX or for reversal of anticoagulation due to either vitamin K antagonists or other anticoagulants (eg, dabigatran), for hemophilia A patients with factor VIII inhibitors, or for patients in a hemorrhagic state caused by reduced production of liver-dependent coagulation factors (eg, hepatitis, cirrhosis).

Pediatric:

Control or prevention of bleeding in patients with factor IX deficiency (hemophilia B or Christmas disease): Infants, Children, and Adolescents: I.V.: Dosage is expressed in units of factor IX activity and must be individualized based on formulation, severity of factor IX deficiency, extent and location of bleed, and clinical situation of patient.

Formula for units required to raise blood level:

Number of Factor IX Units Required = body weight (in kg) x desired Factor IX level increase (% or units/dL) x 1 unit/kg

For example, for a 100% level in a 25 kg patient who has an actual level of 20%: Number of Factor IX Units needed = 25 kg x 80% x 1 unit/kg = 2000 units

Manufacturer's labeling: AlphaNine SD, Mononine: Infants, Children, and Adolescents: Intermittent I.V.:

Desired Factor IX Level, Dosing Interval and Duration based on Hemorrhage Type:

Minor hemorrhage (eg, bruising, cuts/scrapes, uncomplicated joint hemorrhage):

Desired factor IX levels (% or units/dL): 15-30

Frequency of dosing: Every 12-24 hours

Duration of treatment: 1-2 days

Moderate hemorrhage (eg, epistaxis, oropharyngeal bleeds, dental extractions, hematuria):

Desired factor IX levels (% or units/dL): 25-50

Frequency of dosing: Every 12-24 hours

Duration of treatment: 2-7 days

Major hemorrhage [eg, joint and muscle (especially large muscles) hemorrhage, intracranial or intraperitoneal hemorrhage], major trauma, or surgical prophylaxis:

Desired factor IX levels (% or units/dL): 50-100 (depending on the clinical situation, desired Factor IX level may be reduced following active treatment period for hemorrhage or >48 hours postop)

Frequency of dosing: Every 12-24 hours (AlphaNine SD) or 18-30 hours (Mononine), interval dependent upon product used, half-life, and measured factor IX levels (after 3-5 days, maintain at least 20% activity)

Duration of treatment: 7-10 days, depending upon nature of insult

Alternate dosing: **Note:** The following recommendations reflect general dosing requirements; may vary from those found within prescribing information or practitioner preference:

Prophylaxis, primary: Infants, Children, and Adolescents: I.V.: 15-30 units/kg twice weekly [WFH guidelines (Srivastava, 2013) (Utrecht protocol)] **or** 25-40 units/kg twice weekly [WFH guidelines (Srivastava, 2013) (Malmö protocol)] **or** 40-100 units/kg 2-3 times weekly (National Hemophilia Foundation, MASAC recommendation, 2007); however, the optimum regimen has yet to be defined.

Hemorrhage, treatment (when no significant resource constraints exist) [WFH guidelines (Srivastava, 2013)]: **Note:** Factor IX level may either be expressed as units/dL or as%. Dosing frequency most commonly corresponds to the half-life of factor IX but should be determined based on an assessment of factor IX levels before the next dose. Infants, Children, and Adolescents:

Intermittent I.V.: Desired Factor IX Level to Maintain and Duration Based on Site of Hemorrhage/Clinical Situation:

Joint: 40-60 units/dL for 1-2 days, may be longer if response is inadequate

Superficial muscle (no neurovascular compromise): 40-60 units/dL for 2-3 days, sometimes longer if response is inadequate

Iliopsoas and deep muscle with neurovascular injury, or substantial blood loss: Initial: 60-80 units/dL for 1-2 days; Maintenance: 30-60 units/dL for 3-5 days, sometimes longer as secondary prophylaxis during physiotherapy

CNS/head: Initial: 60-80 units/dL for 1-7 days; Maintenance: 30 units/dL for 8-21 days

Throat and neck: Initial: 60-80 units/dL for 1-7 days; Maintenance: 30 units/dL for 8-14 days

Gastrointestinal: Initial: 60-80 units/dL for 7-14 days; Maintenance: 30 units/dL (duration not specified)

Renal: 40 units/dL for 3-5 days

Deep laceration: 40 units/dL for 5-7 days

Surgery (major):

Preop: 60-80 units/dL

Postop: 40-60 units/dL for 1-3 days, then 30-50 units/dL for 4-6 days, then 20-40 units/dL for 7-14 days

Surgery (minor):

Preop: 50-80 units/dL

Postop: 30-80 units/dL for 1-5 days depending on procedure type

Continuous I.V. infusion: Very limited data available; only data with Mononine product available: **Note:** Used for patients who require prolonged periods of treatment (eg, intracranial hemorrhage or surgery) to avoid peaks and troughs associated with intermittent infusions [Batorova, 2002; Hoots, 2003; Morfini, 2008; Poon, 2012; WFH guidelines (Srivastava, 2013)]:

Following initial bolus to achieve the desired factor IX level: Initial dosing: 4-6 units/kg/hour; adjust dose based on frequent factor IX assays and calculation of factor IX clearance at steady-state using the following equations:

Factor IX clearance (mL/kg/hour) = (current infusion rate in units/kg/hour)/(plasma Factor IX level in units/**mL**)

New infusion rate (units/kg/hour) = (factor IX clearance in mL/kg/hour) x (desired plasma level in units/**mL**)

The median reported dose in post-operative patients (7-85 years) was 3.84 units/kg/hour (range: 1.74-7.3 units/kg/hour) (Hoots, 2003)

Adult: Control or prevention of bleeding in patients with factor IX deficiency (hemophilia B or Christmas disease): I.V.: AlphaNine SD, Mononine: Dosage is expressed in units of factor IX activity; dosing must be individualized based on severity of factor IX deficiency, extent and location of bleeding, and clinical status of patient. Refer to product information for specific manufacturer recommended dosing. Alternatively, the WFH has recommended general dosing for factor IX products.

Formula for units required to raise blood level: **Note:** If patient has severe hemophilia (ie, baseline factor IX level is or presumed to be <1%), then may just use "desired factor IX level" instead of "desired factor IX level increase".

Number of factor IX units required = patient weight (in kg) x desired factor IX level increase (as% or units/dL) x 1 unit/kg

For example, to attain an 80% level in a 70 kg patient who has a baseline level of 20%: Number of factor IX units needed = 70 kg x 60% x 1 unit/kg = 4200 units

WFH guidelines (Srivastava, 2013): **Note:** The following recommendations may vary from those found within prescribing information or practitioner preference.

Prophylaxis: I.V.: 15-30 units/kg twice weekly [WFH guidelines (Srivastava, 2013) (Utrecht protocol)] **or** 25-40 units/kg twice weekly [WFH guidelines (Srivastava, 2013) (Malmo protocol)] **or** 40-100 units/kg administered 2-3 times weekly (National Hemophilia Foundation, MASAC recommendation, 2007); optimum regimen has yet to be defined.

Treatment:

Intermittent I.V.: 2013 World Federation of Hemophilia Treatment Recommendations (When No Significant Resource Constraint Exists): **Note:** Factor IX level may either be expressed as units/dL or as%. Dosing frequency most commonly corresponds to the half-life of factor IX but should be determined based on an assessment of factor IX levels before the next dose.

Desired Factor IX Level to Maintain and Duration Based on Site of Hemorrhage/Clinical Situation:

Joint: 40-60 units/dL for 1-2 days, may be longer if response is inadequate

Superficial muscle (no neurovascular compromise): 40-60 units/dL for 2-3 days, sometimes longer if response is inadequate

Iliopsoas and deep muscle with neurovascular injury, or substantial blood loss: Initial: 60-80 units/dL for 1-2 days; Maintenance: 30-60 units/dL for 3-5 days, sometimes longer as secondary prophylaxis during physiotherapy

CNS/head: Initial: 60-80 units/dL for 1-7 days; Maintenance: 30 units/dL for 8-21 days

Throat and neck: Initial: 60-80 units/dL for 1-7 days; Maintenance: 30 units/dL for 8-14 days

Gastrointestinal: Initial: 60-80 units/dL for 7-14 days; Maintenance: 30 units/dL (duration not specified)

Renal: 40 units/dL for 3-5 days

Deep laceration: 40 units/dL for 5-7 days

Surgery (major):

Preop: 60-80 units/dL

Postop: 40-60 units/dL for 1-3 days, then 30-50 units/dL for 4-6 days, then 20-40 units/dL for 7-14 days

Surgery (minor):

Preop: 50-80 units/dL

Postop: 30-80 units/dL for 1-5 days depending on procedure type

Continuous I.V. infusion: **Note:** For patients who require prolonged periods of treatment (eg, intracranial hemorrhage or surgery) to avoid peaks and troughs associated with intermittent infusion [Batorova, 2002; Poon, 2012; Rickard, 1995; WFH guidelines (Srivastava, 2013)]: Following initial bolus to achieve the desired factor IX level: Initiate 4-6 units/kg/hour; adjust dose based on frequent factor assays and calculation of factor IX clearance at steady-state using the following equations:

Factor IX clearance (mL/kg/hour) = (current infusion rate in units/kg/hour) divided by (plasma level in units/**mL**)

New infusion rate (units/kg/hour) = (factor IX clearance in mL/kg/hour) x (desired plasma level in units/mL)

Administration Solution should be infused at room temperature.

I.V. bolus: Should be infused **slowly over several minutes**: Rate of administration should be determined by the response and comfort of the patient.

AlphaNine SD: Administer I.V. at a rate not exceeding 10 mL/minute

Mononine: Administer I.V. at a rate of ~2 mL/minute. Administration rates of up to 225 **units**/minute have been regularly tolerated without incident (when reconstituted as directed to ~100 units/mL).

WFH recommendations: Infuse at a rate determined by age: Young children: 100 **units**/minute; Adults: 3 mL/minute. With patients who have had allergic reactions during factor IX infusion, administration of hydrocortisone prior to infusion may be necessary [WFH guidelines (Srivastava, 2013)].

Continuous I.V. infusion: In an open-label, multicenter trial (age range: 7-85 years), Mononine was reconstituted to 100 units/mL and then infused undiluted or was further diluted in NS to either 5 units/mL or 10 units/mL. The preparation of solution for infusion is dependent upon prescriber discretion and should be replaced every 12 hours (Hoots, 2003).

Monitoring Parameters Factor IX levels [measure 15 minutes after infusion to verify calculated doses [WFH guidelines (Srivastava, 2013)], aPTT, BP, HR, signs of hypersensitivity reactions; screen for factor IX inhibitors if the patient experiences hypersensitivity reaction or when patient is to undergo surgery, if suboptimal response to treatment occurs, if patient is being intensively treated for >5 days within 4 weeks of the last infusion, or at the following intervals [WFH guidelines (Srivastava, 2013)]:

Children: Screen for inhibitors every 5 exposure days until 20 exposure days, every 10 exposure days between 21-50 exposure days, and at a minimum of twice a year until 150 exposure days is reached.

Adults (with >150 exposure days apart from a 6-12 monthly review): Screen for inhibitors when suboptimal response occurs.

Reference Range Average normal factor IX levels are 50% to 150%; patients with severe hemophilia B will have levels <1%, often undetectable. Moderate forms of the disease have levels of 1% to 5% while some mild cases may have 5% to 49% of normal factor IX.

Additional Information In absence of inhibitors, 1 unit/kg factor IX human administered will increase plasma factor IX level by 1 unit/dL [WFH guidelines (Srivastava, 2013)].

Dosage Forms Excipient information presented when available (limited, particularly for generics); consult specific product labeling.

Solution Reconstituted, Intravenous [preservative free]:

AlphaNine SD: 500 units (1 ea); 1000 units (1 ea); 1500 units (1 ea) [contains polysorbate 80]

Mononine: 250 units (1 ea); 500 units (1 ea) [contains polysorbate 80]

References

Alade SL, Brown RE, Paquet A Jr. Polysorbate 80 and e-ferol toxicity. *Pediatrics.* 1986;77(4):593-597.

Batorova A, Martinowitz U. Continuous infusion of coagulation factors. *Haemophilia.* 2002;8(3):170-177.

Centers for Disease Control and Prevention (CDC). Unusual syndrome with fatalities among premature infants: association with a new intravenous vitamin E product. *MMWR Morb Mortal Wkly Rep.*1984;33 (14):198-199.

Chi C, Kadir RA. Inherited bleeding disorders in pregnancy. *Best Pract Res Clin Obstet Gynaecol.* 2012;26(1):103-117.

Hoots WK, Leissinger C, Stabler S, et al. Continuous intravenous infusion of a plasma-derived factor IX concentrate (Mononine) in haemophilia B. *Haemophilia.* 2003;9(2):164-172.

Kadir R, Chi C, Bolton-Maggs P. Pregnancy and rare bleeding disorders. *Haemophilia.* 2009;15(5):990-1005.

Lee CA, Chi C, Pavord SR, et al. The obstetric and gynaecological management of women with inherited bleeding disorders-review with guidelines produced by a Taskforce of UK Haemophilia Centre Doctors' Organization. *Haemophilia.* 2006;12(4):301-336.

Morfini M. Secondary prophylaxis with factor IX concentrates: continuous infusion. *Blood Transfus.* 2008;6(Suppl 2):21–25.

Poon MC, Card R. Hemophilia management in transfusion medicine. *Transfus Apher Sci.* 2012;46(3):299-307.

Rickard KA. Guidelines for therapy and optimal dosages of coagulation factors for treatment of bleeding and surgery in haemophilia. *Haemophilia.* 1995;1(Suppl 1):8-13.

Srivastava A, Brewer AK, Mauser-Bunschoten EP, et al. Guidelines for the management of hemophilia. *Haemophilia.* 2013;19(1):e1-47.

Factor IX (Recombinant)

(FAK ter nyne ree KOM be nant)

Medication Safety Issues

Sound-alike/look-alike issues:

Factor IX may be confused with Factor IX Complex

Brand Names: U.S. BeneFIX; Rixubis

Brand Names: Canada BeneFix

Therapeutic Category Antihemophilic Agent

Generic Availability (U.S.) Yes

Use

BeneFIX: Prevention and control of bleeding in patients with hemophilia B (congenital factor IX deficiency or Christmas disease); perioperative management in patients with hemophilia B [All indications: FDA approved in pediatric patients (age not specified) and adults]

Rixubis: Prevention and control of bleeding episodes in patients with hemophilia B (congenital factor IX deficiency or Christmas disease); perioperative management in patients with hemophilia B; routine prophylaxis to prevent or reduce the frequency of bleeding episodes in patients with hemophilia B (All indications: FDA approved in adults)

NOTE: Contains **only factor IX**. Therefore, **NOT INDICATED** for replacement therapy of any other clotting factor besides factor IX or for reversal of anticoagulation due to either vitamin K antagonists or other anticoagulants (eg, dabigatran), for hemophilia A patients with factor VIII inhibitors, or for patients in a hemorrhagic state caused by reduced production of liver-dependent coagulation factors (eg, hepatitis, cirrhosis).

Pregnancy Risk Factor C

Pregnancy Considerations Animal reproduction studies have not been conducted. Factor IX concentrations do not change significantly in pregnant women with coagulation disorders and women with factor IX deficiency may be at increased risk of postpartum hemorrhage. Pregnant women should have clotting factors monitored, particularly at 28 and 34 weeks gestation and prior to invasive procedures. Prophylaxis may be needed if factor IX concentrations are <50 units/mL at term and treatment should continue for 3 to 5 days postpartum depending on route of delivery. Because parvovirus infection may cause hydrops fetalis or fetal death, a recombinant product is preferred if prophylaxis or treatment is needed. The neonate may also be at an increased risk of bleeding following delivery and should be tested for the coagulation disorder (Chi, 2012; Kadir, 2009; Lee, 2006).

Breast-Feeding Considerations It is not known if factor IX (recombinant) is excreted in breast milk. The manufacturer recommends that caution be exercised when administering factor IX (recombinant) to nursing women.

Contraindications Life-threatening, immediate hypersensitivity reactions (including anaphylaxis) to factor IX, hamster protein, or any component; additional product specific contraindications: Rixubis: Disseminated intravascular coagulation, signs of fibrinolysis

Warnings Hypersensitivity and anaphylactic reactions have been reported. Risk is highest during the early phases of initial exposure in previously untreated patients, especially those with high-risk gene mutations. Delayed reactions (up to 20 days after infusion) in previously untreated patients may also occur. Due to potential allergic reactions, the initial 10-20 administrations should be performed under appropriate medical supervision. Hypersensitivity reactions may be associated with factor IX inhibitor development; patients experiencing allergic reactions should be evaluated for factor IX antibodies (or inhibitors). The development of factor IX inhibitors usually occurs within the first 10-20 exposure days to factor IX therapy; the presence of inhibitors increases the risk of severe hypersensitivity reactions. When clinical response is suboptimal or patient is to undergo surgical procedure, screen for inhibitors. Patients with severe hemophilia are more likely to develop inhibitors [WFH guidelines (Srivastava, 2013)].

Response to factor IX administration may vary. If bleeding is not controlled with the recommended dose, determine plasma level of factor IX and follow with a sufficient dose to achieve satisfactory clinical response. If plasma levels of factor IX fail to increase as expected or bleeding continues, suspect the presence of an inhibitor; test as appropriate. In the presence of an inhibitor, higher factor IX doses may be required to control bleeding.

Recombinant products contain **only factor IX**. Therefore, factor IX products are **NOT INDICATED** for replacement therapy of any other clotting factor besides factor IX or for reversal of anticoagulation due to either vitamin K antagonists or other anticoagulants (eg, dabigatran), for hemophilia A patients with factor VIII inhibitors, or for patients in a hemorrhagic state caused by reduced production of liver-dependent coagulation factors (eg, hepatitis, cirrhosis).

Observe closely for signs or symptoms of intravascular coagulation or thrombosis; risk is generally associated with the use of factor IX complex concentrates (containing therapeutic amounts of additional factors); however, potential risk exists with use of factor IX products (containing only factor IX). Use with caution when administering to patients with liver disease, postoperatively, neonates, patients at risk of thromboembolic phenomena or disseminated intravascular coagulation, or patients with signs of fibrinolysis due to the potential risk of thromboembolic complications. Rixubis is contraindicated in patients with disseminated intravascular coagulation and signs of fibrinolysis. The safety and efficacy of continuous infusion administration has not been established; thrombotic events have been reported in patients receiving continuous infusion through a central venous catheter, including life-threatening superior vena cava syndrome in neonates. Safety and efficacy have not been established in immune tolerance induction with factor IX products. Nephrotic syndrome has occurred following immune tolerance induction in patients with factor IX inhibitors and a history of allergic reactions to therapy.

Products contain polysorbate 80 (Tween 80) which may cause allergic reactions in susceptible individuals. In premature neonates, thrombocytopenia, ascites, pulmonary deterioration, and renal and hepatic failure have been reported after receiving parenteral products containing polysorbate 80 (Alade, 1986; CDC, 1984). Infusion of polysorbate 80 containing solutions through PVC tubing may cause DEHP to leach into the solution; in immature animals, exposure to DEHP may adversely affect the development of the male reproductive tract.

Adverse Reactions

Cardiovascular: Chest tightness, flushing

Central nervous system: Chills, dizziness, drowsiness, headache, oral paresthesia

Dermatologic: Skin rash, urticaria

Gastrointestinal: Dysgeusia, nausea, vomiting

Immunologic: Antibody development (furin), factor IX inhibitor development

Local: Injection site reaction (including cellulitis, pain, phlebitis)

Neuromuscular & skeletal: Limb pain, tremor

Ophthalmic: Blurred vision

Renal: Renal infarction

Respiratory: Cough, dyspnea, hypoxia

Miscellaneous: Fever (including transient fever following rapid administration)

Rare but important or life-threatening: Anaphylaxis, angioedema, arterial thrombosis, deep vein thrombosis, hypersensitivity reaction, hypotension, nephrotic syndrome (associated with immune tolerance induction), obstructive uropathy, palpitations, peripheral thrombophlebitis, pulmonary embolism, superior vena cava syndrome (neonates), thrombosis

Drug Interactions

Metabolism/Transport Effects None known.

Avoid Concomitant Use

Avoid concomitant use of Factor IX (Recombinant) with any of the following: Aminocaproic Acid

Increased Effect/Toxicity

The levels/effects of Factor IX (Recombinant) may be increased by: Aminocaproic Acid

Decreased Effect There are no known significant interactions involving a decrease in effect.

Stability

BeneFIX:

Product labeled for room temperature storage: May either store at 2°C to 30°C (36°F to 86°F) or refrigerated at 2°C to 8°C (36°F to 46°F). Avoid freezing, which may damage the diluent syringe. Reconstitute with provided diluent; reconstituted solution should be stored at room temperature and used within 3 hours of preparation.

Product labeled for refrigerated storage: Store at 2°C to 8°C (36°F to 46°F). May be stored at room temperature [not to exceed 30°C (86°F)] for up to 6 months; do not use after this 6-month period has elapsed even if the expiration date on the carton has not been exceeded. If date of removal from refrigeration is not recorded on the carton, the assigned expiration date (printed on the end flap of the carton) **must be reduced by 12 months**. Avoid freezing, which may damage the diluent syringe. Reconstitute with provided diluent; reconstituted solution should be stored at room temperature and used within 3 hours of preparation.

Rixubis: Store at 2°C to 8°C (36°F to 46°F) for up to 18 months; do not freeze. After removal from refrigeration, may store at room temperature not to exceed 30°C (86°F) for up to 6 months within the 18-month time period; do not return to refrigerator. Following reconstitution, use within 3 hours and do not refrigerate.

Mechanism of Action

Replaces deficient clotting factor IX. Hemophilia B, or Christmas disease, is an X-linked inherited disorder of blood coagulation characterized by insufficient or abnormal synthesis of the clotting protein factor IX. Factor IX is a vitamin K-dependent coagulation factor which is synthesized in the liver. Factor IX is activated by factor XIa in the intrinsic coagulation pathway. Activated factor IX (IXa) in combination with factor VII:C activates factor X to Xa, resulting ultimately in the conversion of prothrombin to thrombin and the formation of a fibrin clot. The infusion of exogenous factor IX to replace the deficiency present in hemophilia B temporarily restores hemostasis.

Pharmacokinetics (Adult data unless noted)

Half-life elimination:

BeneFIX:

Children ≥2 years and Adolescents ≤15 years: 14-28 hours

Adolescents ≥16 years and Adults: 11-36 hours

Rixubis: Adolescents ≥15 years and Adults: 16-52 hours

Dosing: Neonatal NOTE: Contains **only factor IX**. Therefore, **NOT INDICATED** for replacement therapy of any other clotting factor besides factor IX or for reversal of anticoagulation due to either vitamin K antagonists or other anticoagulants (eg, dabigatran), for hemophilia A patients with factor VIII inhibitors, or for patients in a hemorrhagic state caused by reduced production of liver-dependent coagulation factors (eg, hepatitis, cirrhosis).

Control or prevention of bleeding in patients with factor IX deficiency (hemophilia B or Christmas disease): I.V.: Dosage is expressed in units of factor IX activity and must be individualized based on formulation, severity of factor IX deficiency, extent and location of bleed, and clinical situation of patient.

Formula for units required to raise blood level:
BeneFIX:
Number of Factor IX Units Required = body weight (in kg) x desired factor IX level increase (% or units/dL) x 1.4 units/kg per units/dL
For example, for a 100% level in a 3 kg patient who has an actual level of 20%: Number of Factor IX Units needed = 3 kg x 80% x 1.4 units/kg per units/dL = 336 units

Dosing: Usual NOTE: Contains **only factor IX**; therefore, **NOT INDICATED** for replacement therapy of any other clotting factor besides factor IX or for reversal of anticoagulation due to either vitamin K antagonists or other anticoagulants (eg, dabigatran), for hemophilia A patients with factor VIII inhibitors, or for patients in a hemorrhagic state caused by reduced production of liver-dependent coagulation factors (eg, hepatitis, cirrhosis).

Pediatric: **Control or prevention of bleeding in patients with factor IX deficiency (hemophilia B or Christmas disease):** I.V.: Dosage is expressed in units of factor IX activity and must be individualized based on formulation, severity of factor IX deficiency, extent and location of bleeding, and clinical status of patient.

Formula for units required to raise blood level:
Infants, Children, and Adolescents <15 years: BeneFIX: Number of factor IX units required = patient weight (in kg) x desired factor IX level increase (as% or units/dL) x 1.4 units/kg per units/dL
For example, for a 100% level in a 25 kg patient who has an actual level of 20%: Number of factor IX Units needed = 25 kg x 80% x 1.4 units/kg per units/dL = 2800 units
Adolescents ≥15 years: BeneFIX: Number of factor IX units required = patient weight (in kg) x desired factor IX level increase (as% or units/dL) x 1.3 units/kg per units/dL
For example, for a 100% level in a 70 kg patient who has an actual level of 20%: Number of factor IX Units needed = 70 kg x 80% x 1.3 units/kg per units/dL = 7280 units

Manufacturer's labeling: BeneFIX: Infants, Children, and Adolescents: Intermittent I.V.:
Desired factor IX level, dosing interval and duration based on hemorrhage type:
Minor hemorrhage (uncomplicated joint hemorrhage, superficial muscle, or soft tissue):
Desired factor IX levels (% or units/dL): 20-30
Frequency of dosing: Every 12-24 hours
Duration of treatment: 1-2 days
Moderate hemorrhage (intramuscular or soft tissue with dissection, mucous membrane, dental extractions, or hematuria):
Desired factor IX levels (% or units/dL): 25-50
Frequency of dosing: Every 12-24 hours
Duration of treatment: Until bleeding stops and healing begins, ~2-7 days
Major hemorrhage (pharynx, retorpharnynx, retroperitoneum, CNS, surgery):
Desired factor IX levels (% or units/dL): 50-100

Frequency of dosing: Every 12-24 hours
Duration of treatment: 7-10 days
Alternative dosing: **Note:** The following recommendations reflect general dosing requirements; may vary from those found within prescribing information or practitioner preference:
Prophylaxis, primary: Infants, Children, and Adolescents: I.V.: 15-30 units/kg twice weekly [WFH guidelines (Srivastava, 2013) (Utrecht protocol)] **or** 25-40 units/kg twice weekly [WFH guidelines (Srivastava, 2013) (Malmö protocol)] **or** 40-100 units/kg administered 2-3 times weekly (National Hemophilia Foundation, MASAC recommendation, 2007); optimum regimen has yet to be defined.
Hemorrhage, treatment: **Note:** Factor IX level may either be expressed as units/dL or as %. Dosing frequency most commonly corresponds to the half-life of factor IX but should be determined based on an assessment of factor IX levels before the next dose.
Infants, Children, and Adolescents: I.V:
Desired Factor IX Level to Maintain and Duration Based on Site of Hemorrhage/Clinical Situation (when no significant resource constraints exist) [WFH guidelines (Srivastava, 2013)]:
Joint: 40-60 units/dL for 1-2 days, may be longer if response is inadequate
Superficial muscle (no neurovascular compromise): 40-60 units/dL for 2-3 days, sometimes longer if response is inadequate
Iliopsoas and deep muscle with neurovascular injury, or substantial blood loss: Initial: 60-80 units/dL for 1-2 days; Maintenance: 30-60 units/dL for 3-5 days, sometimes longer as secondary prophylaxis during physiotherapy
CNS/head: Initial: 60-80 units/dL for 1-7 days; Maintenance: 30 units/dL for 8-21 days
Throat and neck: Initial: 60-80 units/dL for 1-7 days; Maintenance: 30 units/dL for 8-14 days
Gastrointestinal: Initial: 60-80 units/dL for 7-14 days; Maintenance: 30 units/dL (duration not specified)
Renal: 40 units/dL for 3-5 days
Deep laceration: 40 units/dL for 5-7 days
Surgery (major):
Preop: 60-80 units/dL
Postop: 40-60 units/dL for 1-3 days; then 30-50 units/dL for 4-6 days; then 20-40 units/dL for 7-14 days
Surgery (minor):
Preop: 50-80 units/dL
Postop: 30-80 units/dL for 1-5 days depending on procedure type
Adult:
Control or prevention of bleeding in patients with factor IX deficiency (hemophilia B or Christmas disease): I.V.: Dosage is expressed in units of factor IX activity; dosing must be individualized based on severity of factor IX deficiency, extent and location of bleeding, and clinical status of patient. Refer to product information for specific manufacturer recommended dosing. Alternatively, the World Federation of Hemophilia (WFH) has recommended general dosing for factor IX products.
Formula for units required to raise blood level: **Note:** If patient has severe hemophilia (ie, baseline factor IX level is or presumed to be <1%), then may just use "desired factor IX level" instead of "desired factor IX level increase".
Number of factor IX units required = patient weight (in kg) x desired factor IX level increase (as% or units/dL) x 1.3 units/kg per units/dL
World Federation of Hemophilia (WFH) Guidelines (Srivastava, 2013): **Note:** The following recommendations

may vary from those found within prescribing information or practitioner preference.

Prophylaxis, primary: I.V.: 15-30 units/kg twice weekly [WFH guidelines (Srivastava, 2013) (Utrecht protocol)] **or** 25-40 units/kg twice weekly [WFH guidelines (Srivastava, 2013) (Malmö protocol)] **or** 40-100 units/kg 2 or 3 times weekly (National Hemophilia Foundation, MASAC recommendation, 2007); however, the optimum regimen has yet to be defined.

Treatment: Intermittent I.V.: 2013 World Federation of Hemophilia Treatment Recommendations (When No Significant Resource Constraint Exists): **Note:** Factor IX level may either be expressed as units/dL or as %. Dosing frequency most commonly corresponds to the half-life of factor IX but should be determined based on an assessment of factor IX levels before the next dose.

Desired Factor IX Level to Maintain and Duration Based on Site of Hemorrhage/Clinical Situation:

Joint: 40-60 units/dL for 1-2 days, may be longer if response is inadequate

Superficial muscle (no neurovascular compromise): 40-60 units/dL for 2-3 days, sometimes longer if response is inadequate

Iliopsoas and deep muscle with neurovascular injury, or substantial blood loss: Initial: 60-80 units/dL for 1-2 days; Maintenance: 30-60 units/dL for 3-5 days, sometimes longer as secondary prophylaxis during physiotherapy

CNS/head: Initial: 60-80 units/dL for 1-7 days; Maintenance: 30 units/dL for 8-21 days

Throat and neck: Initial: 60-80 units/dL for 1-7 days; Maintenance: 30 units/dL for 8-14 days

Gastrointestinal: Initial: 60-80 units/dL for 7-14 days; Maintenance: 30 units/dL (duration not specified)

Renal: 40 units/dL for 3-5 days

Deep laceration: 40 units/dL for 5-7 days

Surgery (major):
Preop: 60-80 units/dL
Postop: 40-60 units/dL for 1-3 days; then 30-50 units/dL for 4-6 days; then 20-40 units/dL for 7-14 days

Surgery (minor):
Preop: 50-80 units/dL
Postop: 30-80 units/dL for 1-5 days depending on procedure type

Continuous I.V. infusion: **Note:** For patients who require prolonged periods of treatment (eg, intracranial hemorrhage or surgery) to avoid peaks and troughs associated with intermittent infusions [Batorova, 2002; Poon, 2012; Rickard, 1995; WFH guidelines (Srivastava, 2013)]: Following initial bolus to achieve the desired factor IX level: Initiate 4-6 units/kg/hour; adjust dose based on frequent factor assays and calculation of factor IX clearance at steady-state using the following equations:

Factor IX clearance (mL/kg/hour) = (current infusion rate in units/kg/hour)/(plasma level in units/**mL**)

Factor IX clearance (mL/kg/hour) = (current infusion rate in units/kg/hour)/(plasma level in units/mL)

New infusion rate (units/kg/hour) = (factor IX clearance in mL/kg/hour) x (desired plasma level in units/mL)

New infusion rate (units/kg/hour) = (factor IX clearance in mL/kg/hour) x (desired plasma level in units/**mL**)

Routine prophylaxis to prevent bleeding episodes in patients with factor IX deficiency (hemophilia B or Christmas disease): Rixubis: I.V.: 40-60 units/kg twice weekly; may titrate dose depending upon age, bleeding pattern, and physical activity

Administration Solution should be infused at room temperature. Safety and efficacy of continuous infusion administration have not been determined.

I.V. bolus:

BeneFIX: Should be infused **slowly over several minutes**. Rate of administration should be determined by the response and comfort of the patient.

Rixubis: Bolus infusion; maximum rate of administration is 10 mL/minute

WFH recommendations: Infuse at a rate determined by age: Young children: 100 **units**/minute; Adults: 3 mL/minute; may also administer as a continuous infusion in select patients. With patients who have had allergic reactions during factor IX infusion, administration of hydrocortisone prior to infusion may be necessary [WFH guidelines (Srivastava, 2013)].

Continuous I.V. infusion: Limited data available: One study reconstituted with SWFI to a final concentration of 100 units/mL for continuous administration; some patients also had heparin added to the infusion at a final concentration of 4 units/mL; solutions with or without heparin retained 90% clotting activity for 14 days when stored at 4°C; when stored at room temperature nonheparin-containing solutions retained over 90% activity until day 7 and heparin-containing solutions were the least stable and fell below 90% activity after 4 days (Chowdary, 2001).

Monitoring Parameters

Factor IX levels [measure 15 minutes after infusion to verify calculated doses [WFH guidelines (Srivastava, 2013)], aPTT, BP, HR, signs of hypersensitivity reactions; screen for factor IX inhibitors if the patient experiences hypersensitivity reaction or when patient is to undergo surgery, if suboptimal response to treatment occurs, if patient is being intensively treated for >5 days within 4 weeks of the last infusion, or at the following intervals [WFH guidelines (Srivastava, 2013)]:

Children: Screen for inhibitors every 5 exposure days until 20 exposure days, every 10 exposure days between 21-50 exposure days, and at a minimum of twice a year until 150 exposure days is reached.

Adults (with >150 exposure days apart from a 6-12 monthly review): Screen for inhibitors when suboptimal response occurs.

Reference Range Average normal factor IX levels are 50% to 150%; patients with severe hemophilia will have levels <1%, often undetectable. Moderate forms of the disease have levels of 1% to 5% while some mild cases may have 5% to 49% of normal factor IX.

Additional Information In absence of inhibitors, 1 unit/kg of factor IX *recombinant* will increase plasma factor IX level by 0.7 unit/dL in children <15 years and 0.8 units/dL in adults (WFH guidelines [Srivastava, 2013]).

Product Availability Alprolix: FDA approved March 2014; availability anticipated in May 2014.

Dosage Forms Excipient information presented when available (limited, particularly for generics); consult specific product labeling.

Solution Reconstituted, Intravenous [preservative free]:
BeneFIX: 250 units (1 ea); 500 units (1 ea); 1000 units (1 ea); 2000 units (1 ea) [contains polysorbate 80]

Rixubis: 250 units (1 ea); 500 units (1 ea); 1000 units (1 ea); 2000 units (1 ea); 3000 units (1 ea) [contains polysorbate 80]

References

Alade SL, Brown RE, Paquet A Jr. Polysorbate 80 and e-ferol toxicity. *Pediatrics*. 1986;77(4):593-597.

Batorova A, Martinowitz U. Continuous infusion of coagulation factors. *Haemophilia.* 2002;8(3):170-177.

Centers for Disease Control (CDC). Unusual syndrome with fatalities among premature infants: association with a new intravenous vitamin E product. *MMWR Morb Mortal Wkly Rep.*1984;33(14):198-199.

Chi C, Kadir RA. Inherited bleeding disorders in pregnancy. *Best Pract Res Clin Obstet Gynaecol.* 2012;26(1):103-117.

Chowdary P, Dasani H, Jones JA, et al. Recombinant factor IX (BeneFix) by adjusted continuous infusion: a study of stability, sterility and clinical experience. *Haemophilia.* 2001;7(2):140-145.

Kadir R, Chi C, Bolton-Maggs P. Pregnancy and rare bleeding disorders. *Haemophilia.* 2009;15(5):990-1005.

Lee CA, Chi C, Pavord SR, et al. The obstetric and gynaecological management of women with inherited bleeding disorders-review with guidelines produced by a Taskforce of UK Haemophilia Centre Doctors' Organization. *Haemophilia.* 2006;12(4):301-336.

Poon MC, Card R. Hemophilia management in transfusion medicine. *Transfus Apher Sci.* 2012;46(3):299-307.

Rickard KA. Guidelines for therapy and optimal dosages of coagulation factors for treatment of bleeding and surgery in haemophilia. *Haemophilia.* 1995;1(Suppl 1):8-13.

Srivastava A, Brewer AK, Mauser-Bunschoten EP, et al. Guidelines for the management of hemophilia. *Haemophilia.* 2013;19(1):e1-47.

◆ **3 Factor PCC** *see* Factor IX Complex (Human) [(Factors II, IX, X)] *on page 833*

Famciclovir (fam SYE kloe veer)

Medication Safety Issues
Sound-alike/look-alike issues:
Famvir® may be confused with Femara®
Brand Names: U.S. Famvir
Brand Names: Canada Apo-Famciclovir®; Ava-Famciclovir; CO Famciclovir; Famvir®; PMS-Famciclovir; Sandoz-Famciclovir
Therapeutic Category Antiviral Agent, Oral
Generic Availability (U.S.) Yes
Use Treatment of acute herpes zoster (shingles); treatment or suppression of recurrent episodes of genital herpes in immunocompetent patients; treatment of recurrent episodes of herpes labialis (cold sores) in immunocompetent patients; treatment of recurrent episodes of mucocutaneous herpes simplex infections in HIV patients (FDA approved in ages ≥18 years)
Pregnancy Risk Factor B
Pregnancy Considerations Teratogenic effects were not observed in animal reproduction studies. Data in pregnant women is limited. A registry has been established for women exposed to famciclovir during pregnancy (888-669-6682).
Breast-Feeding Considerations There is no specific data describing the excretion of famciclovir in breast milk. Breast-feeding is not recommended by the manufacturer unless the potential benefits outweigh any possible risk. If herpes lesions are on breast, breast-feeding should be avoided in order to avoid transmission to infant.
Contraindications Hypersensitivity to famciclovir, penciclovir, or any component
Precautions Use with caution and decrease dose in patients with renal dysfunction; acute renal failure has been reported in patients with renal dysfunction who received inappropriately high doses of famciclovir for their level of renal function. Dosage adjustment may be needed in patients with poorly compensated hepatic impairment. Tablets contain lactose; do not use in patients with galactose intolerance, severe lactase deficiency, or glucose-galactose malabsorption syndromes. Efficacy has not been established in adults for treatment of initial episodes of genital herpes infection, ophthalmic zoster, disseminated zoster, or in immunocompromised patients with herpes zoster.
Adverse Reactions
Central nervous system: Fatigue, headache, migraine
Dermatologic: Pruritus, rash
Endocrine & metabolic: Dysmenorrhea

Gastrointestinal: Abdominal pain, diarrhea, flatulence, nausea, vomiting
Hematologic: Neutropenia
Hepatic: Bilirubin increased, transaminases increased
Neuromuscular & skeletal: Paresthesia
Rare but important or life-threatening: Anemia, angioedema (eyelid, face, periorbital, pharyngeal edema), cholestatic jaundice, confusion, delirium, disorientation, dizziness, erythema multiforme, hallucinations, leukocytoclastic vasculitis, palpitations, somnolence, Stevens-Johnson syndrome, thrombocytopenia, toxic epidermal necrolysis, urticaria
Drug Interactions
Metabolism/Transport Effects None known.
Avoid Concomitant Use
Avoid concomitant use of Famciclovir with any of the following: Zoster Vaccine
Increased Effect/Toxicity There are no known significant interactions involving an increase in effect.
Decreased Effect
Famciclovir may decrease the levels/effects of: Zoster Vaccine
Food Interactions Rate of absorption and/or conversion to penciclovir and peak concentration are reduced with food, but bioavailability is not affected. Management: Administer without regard to meals.
Mechanism of Action Famciclovir undergoes rapid biotransformation to the active compound, penciclovir (prodrug), which is phosphorylated by viral thymidine kinase in HSV-1, HSV-2, and VZV-infected cells to a monophosphate form; this is then converted to penciclovir triphosphate and competes with deoxyguanosine triphosphate to inhibit HSV-2 polymerase, therefore, herpes viral DNA synthesis/replication is selectively inhibited.
Pharmacokinetics (Adult data unless noted) Penciclovir:
Absorption: Rapid
Distribution: V_{dss}: Healthy adults: 1.08 ± 0.17 L/kg
Protein binding: <20%
Metabolism: Famciclovir is a prodrug which is metabolized via deacetylation and oxidation in the intestinal wall and liver to penciclovir (active) during extensive first-pass metabolism
Bioavailability: $77\% \pm 8\%$
Half-life:
Serum: Mean: 2-3 hours; increased with renal dysfunction
Mean half-life, terminal:
CrCl >80 mL/minute: 2.15 hours
CrCl 60-80 mL/minute: 2.47 hours
CrCl 30-59 mL/minute: 3.87 hours
CrCl <29 mL/minute: 9.85 hours
Intracellular penciclovir triphosphate: HSV 1: 10 hours; HSV 2: 20 hours; VZV: 7 hours
Time to peak serum concentration: ~1 hour
Elimination: Primarily excreted via the kidneys; after oral administration, 73% is excreted in the urine (predominantly as penciclovir) and 27% in feces; penciclovir undergoes tubular secretion; requires dosage adjustment with renal impairment
Dialysis: Hemodialysis: May enhance elimination of penciclovir
Dosing: Usual Oral:
Children and Adolescents: Insufficient clinical data exists to identify an appropriate pediatric dose (AAP, 2006):
Adults:
Herpes zoster: 500 mg every 8 hours for 7 days; initiate as soon as diagnosed; initiation of therapy within 48 hours of rash onset may be more beneficial; no efficacy data available for treatment initiated >72 hours after onset of rash

Genital herpes: Treatment of initial clinical episode: 250 mg 3 times/day for 7-10 days; **Note:** Treatment may be continued if healing is not complete after 10 days of therapy (CDC, 2006)

Recurrent genital herpes in immunocompetent patients: Treatment: 1000 mg twice daily for 1 day or 125 mg twice daily for 5 days (CDC, 2006); initiate at first sign or symptom; efficacy is not established if treatment is started >6 hours after onset of lesions or symptoms

Suppression: 250 mg twice daily for up to 1 year

Recurrent herpes labialis (cold sores): 1500 mg as a single dose; initiate at first sign or symptom such as tingling, burning, or itching; efficacy established for initiation of treatment within 1 hour of symptom onset

Recurrent orolabial or genital herpes in HIV patients: Treatment: 500 mg twice daily for 7 days

Recurrent genital herpes in HIV patients: Suppression: 500 mg twice daily (CDC, 2006)

Dosing interval in renal impairment: Adults:

Herpes zoster:

CrCl ≥60 mL/minute: Administer 500 mg every 8 hours

CrCl 40-59 mL/minute: Administer 500 mg every 12 hours

CrCl 20-39 mL/minute: Administer 500 mg every 24 hours

CrCl <20 mL/minute: Administer 250 mg every 24 hours

Patients on hemodialysis: Administer 250 mg after each dialysis session

Recurrent genital herpes: Treatment (single day regimen):

CrCl ≥60 mL/minute: Administer 1000 mg every 12 hours for 1 day

CrCl 40-59 mL/minute: Administer 500 mg every 12 hours for 1 day

CrCl 20-39 mL/minute: Administer 500 mg as a single dose

CrCl <20 mL/minute: Administer 250 mg as a single dose

Patients on hemodialysis: Administer 250 mg as a single dose after dialysis session

Recurrent genital herpes: Suppression:

CrCl ≥40 mL/minute: Administer 250 mg every 12 hours

CrCl 20-39 mL/minute: Administer 125 mg every 12 hours

CrCl <20 mL/minute: Administer 125 mg every 24 hours

Patients on hemodialysis: Administer 125 mg after each dialysis session

Recurrent herpes labialis: Treatment (single dose regimen):

CrCl ≥60 mL/minute: Administer 1500 mg as a single dose

CrCl 40-59 mL/minute: Administer 750 mg as a single dose

CrCl 20-39 mL/minute: Administer 500 mg as a single dose

CrCl <20 mL/minute: Administer 250 mg as a single dose

Patients on hemodialysis: Administer 250 mg as a single dose after dialysis session

Recurrent orolabial or genital herpes in HIV infected patients:

CrCl ≥40 mL/minute: Administer 500 mg every 12 hours

CrCl 20-39 mL/minute: Administer 500 mg every 24 hours

CrCl <20 mL/minute: Administer 250 mg every 24 hours

Patients on hemodialysis: Administer 250 mg after each dialysis session

Administration Oral: May be administered without regard to meals; may be administered with food to decrease GI upset

Monitoring Parameters Resolution of rash, renal function, WBC, liver enzymes

Dosage Forms Excipient information presented when available (limited, particularly for generics); consult specific product labeling.

Tablet, Oral:

Famvir: 125 mg, 250 mg, 500 mg

Generic: 125 mg, 250 mg, 500 mg

References

Boike SC, Pue MA, and Freed MI, "Pharmacokinetics of Famciclovir in Subjects With Varying Degrees of Renal Impairment," *Clin Pharmacol Ther*, 1994, 55(4):418-26.

Centers for Disease Control and Prevention (CDC), "Sexually Transmitted Diseases Treatment Guidelines, 2006," *MMWR Recomm Rep*, 2006, 55(RR-11):1-94.

Red Book: 2006 Report of the Committee on Infectious Diseases, 27th ed, Pickering LK, ed, Elk Grove Village IL: American Academy of Pediatrics, 2006, 787.

Spruance SL, Bodsworth N, Resnick H, et al, "Single-Dose, Patient-Initiated Famciclovir: A Randomized, Double-Blind, Placebo-Controlled Trial for Episodic Treatment of Herpes Labialis," *J Am Acad Dermatol*, 2006, 55(1):47-53.

Famotidine (fa MOE ti deen)

Medication Safety Issues

Sound-alike/look-alike issues:

Famotidine may be confused with FLUoxetine, furosemide

Brand Names: U.S. Acid Reducer Maximum Strength [OTC]; Acid Reducer [OTC]; Heartburn Relief Max St [OTC]; Heartburn Relief [OTC]; Pepcid

Brand Names: Canada Acid Control; Apo-Famotidine®; Apo-Famotidine® Injectable; Famotidine Omega; Mylan-Famotidine; Novo-Famotidine; Nu-Famotidine; Pepcid®; Pepcid® AC; Pepcid® I.V.; Ulcidine

Therapeutic Category Gastrointestinal Agent, Gastric or Duodenal Ulcer Treatment; Histamine H_2 Antagonist

Generic Availability (U.S.) Yes

Use Short-term therapy and treatment of duodenal ulcer, active benign gastric ulcer, gastroesophageal reflux disease (GERD) (FDA approved in ages 1-16 and adults); pathological hypersecretory conditions (eg, Zollinger-Ellison syndrome, multiple endocrine adenomas) (FDA approved in adults); OTC formulation for use in the relief of heartburn, acid indigestion, and sour stomach (FDA approved in children >12 years and adults); has also been used for stress ulcer prophylaxis and gastric acid suppression in critically ill patients, and symptomatic relief in gastritis.

Pregnancy Risk Factor B

Pregnancy Considerations Adverse events have not been observed in animal reproduction studies; therefore, famotidine is classified as pregnancy category B. Famotidine crosses the placenta. An increased risk of congenital malformations or adverse events in the newborn has generally not been observed following maternal use of famotidine during pregnancy. Histamine H_2 antagonists have been evaluated for the treatment of gastroesophageal reflux disease (GERD), as well as gastric and duodenal ulcers, during pregnancy. Although if needed, famotidine is not the agent of choice. Histamine H_2 antagonists may be used for aspiration prophylaxis prior to cesarean delivery.

Breast-Feeding Considerations Famotidine is excreted into breast milk with peak concentrations occurring ~6 hours after the maternal dose. According to the manufacturer, the decision to continue or discontinue breast-feeding during therapy should take into account the risk of exposure to the infant and the benefits of treatment to the mother.

◀ **Contraindications** Hypersensitivity to famotidine, any component, or other H_2 antagonists

Warnings QT prolongation has been reported in patients with renal dysfunction. Use of gastric acid inhibitors, including proton pump inhibitors and H_2 blockers, has been associated with an increased risk for development of acute gastroenteritis and community-acquired pneumonia (Canani, 2006). A large epidemiological study has suggested an increased risk for developing pneumonia in patients receiving H_2 receptor antagonists; however, a causal relationship has not been demonstrated. A cohort analysis including over 11,000 neonates reported an association of H_2 blocker use and an increased incidence of NEC in VLBW neonates (Guillet, 2006). An approximate sixfold increase in mortality, NEC, and infection (ie, sepsis, pneumonia, UTI) was reported in patients receiving an H_2 blocker (ranitidine) in a cohort analysis of 274 VLBW neonates (Terrin, 2011).

Multidose injection contains benzyl alcohol which may cause allergic reactions in susceptible individuals; large amounts of benzyl alcohol (≥99 mg/kg/day) have been associated with a potentially fatal toxicity ("gasping syndrome") in neonates; the "gasping syndrome" consists of metabolic acidosis, respiratory distress, gasping respirations, CNS dysfunction (including convulsions, intracranial hemorrhage), hypotension and cardiovascular collapse; avoid use of the multidose injection in neonates. The oral suspension contains sodium benzoate; *in vitro* and animal studies have shown that benzoate, a metabolite of benzyl alcohol, displaces bilirubin from protein binding sites; avoid use in neonates.

Precautions Use with caution in renal impairment; seizures have been reported; dosage modification necessary. Relief of symptoms does not preclude the presence of a gastric malignancy. Reversible confusional states, usually clearing within 3-4 days after discontinuation, have been linked to use; increased age (>50 years) and renal or hepatic impairment are thought to be associated.

When used for self-medication, patients should be instructed not to use if they have difficulty swallowing, are vomiting blood, or have bloody or black stools and not to extend use >14 days without consulting their physician.

Adverse Reactions
Central nervous system: Dizziness, headache
Gastrointestinal: Constipation, diarrhea, necrotizing enterocolitis (VLBW neonates; Guillet, 2006)
Rare but important or life-threatening: Abdominal discomfort, acne, agitation, agranulocytosis, allergic reaction, alopecia, anaphylaxis, angioedema, anorexia, anxiety, arrhythmia, arthralgia, AV block, bronchospasm, cholestatic jaundice, confusion, conjunctival injection, depression, dry skin, facial edema, fatigue, fever, flushing, hallucinations, hepatitis, injection site reactions, insomnia, interstitial pneumonia, leukopenia, libido decreased, liver function tests increased, muscle cramps, nausea, palpitation, pancytopenia, paresthesia, pruritus, QT-interval prolongation, rash, rhabdomyolysis, seizure, somnolence, Stevens-Johnson syndrome, taste disorder, tinnitus, thrombocytopenia, torsade de pointes, toxic epidermal necrolysis, urticaria, vomiting, weakness, xerostomia

Drug Interactions
Metabolism/Transport Effects None known.
Avoid Concomitant Use
Avoid concomitant use of Famotidine with any of the following: Dasatinib; Delavirdine; PAZOPanib; PONATinib; Risedronate
Increased Effect/Toxicity
Famotidine may increase the levels/effects of: Dexmethylphenidate; Highest Risk QTc-Prolonging Agents;

Methylphenidate; Moderate Risk QTc-Prolonging Agents; Risedronate; Saquinavir; Varenicline

The levels/effects of Famotidine may be increased by: Mifepristone
Decreased Effect
Famotidine may decrease the levels/effects of: Atazanavir; Bosutinib; Cefditoren; Cefpodoxime; Cefuroxime; Dabrafenib; Dasatinib; Delavirdine; Erlotinib; Fosamprenavir; Gefitinib; Indinavir; Iron Salts; Itraconazole; Ketoconazole (Systemic); Mesalamine; Multivitamins/Minerals (with ADEK, Folate, Iron); Nelfinavir; Nilotinib; PAZOPanib; PONATinib; Posaconazole; Rilpivirine; Vismodegib

Food Interactions Prolonged treatment (≥2 years) may lead to malabsorption of dietary vitamin B_{12} and subsequent vitamin B_{12} deficiency (Lam, 2013).

Stability
Oral:
Powder for oral suspension: Prior to mixing, dry powder should be stored at controlled room temperature of 25°C (77°F). Reconstituted oral suspension is stable for 30 days at room temperature; do not freeze
Tablet: Store controlled room temperature. Protect from moisture
Parenteral:
Solution for injection: Prior to use, store at 2°C to 8°C (36°F to 46°F). If solution freezes, allow to solubilize at controlled room temperature. May be stored at room temperature for up to 3 months [data on file (Bedford Laboratories, 2011)].
I.V. push: Following preparation, solutions for I.V. push should be used immediately or may be stored in refrigerator and used within 48 hours.
Infusion: Following preparation, the manufacturer states may be stored for up to 48 hours under refrigeration; however, solutions for infusion have been found to be physically and chemically stable for 7 days at room temperature; injection is compatible with D_5W, NS, $D_{10}W$, LR injection, 5% bicarbonate injection, and standard parenteral nutrition solutions with electrolytes, multivitamins, and trace minerals
Solution for injection, premixed bags: Store at controlled room temperature of 25°C (77°F); avoid excessive heat; stable at room temperature for 15 months

Mechanism of Action Competitive inhibition of histamine at H_2 receptors of the gastric parietal cells, which inhibits gastric acid secretion

Pharmacodynamics Antisecretory effect:
Onset: I.V.; Oral: Within 1 hour
Maximum effect:
I.V.: 30 minutes
Oral: 1-4 hours
Duration: 10-12 hours

Pharmacokinetics (Adult data unless noted)
Absorption: Oral: Incompletely
Distribution: V_d:
Infants:
0-3 months: 1.4-1.8 ± 0.3-0.4 L/kg
>3 to 12 months: 2.3 ± 0.7 L/kg
Children: 2 ± 1.5 L/kg
Adolescents: 1.5 ± 0.4 L/kg
Adults: 0.94-1.33 L/kg
Protein binding: 15% to 20%
Metabolism: 30% to 35%; minimal first-pass metabolism; forms one metabolite (S-oxide)
Bioavailability: Oral: 40% to 45%
Half-life:
Infants:
0-3 months: 8.1-10.5 ± 3.5-5.4 hours
>3 to 12 months: 4.5 ± 1.1 hours
Children: 3.3 ± 2.5 hours
Adolescents: 2.3 ± 0.4 hours

Adults: 2.5-3.5 hours; increases with renal impairment; if CrCl <10 mL/minute, half-life ≥20 hours

Anuria: 24 hours

Time to peak serum concentration: Oral: 1-3 hours; orally disintegrating tablet: 2.5 hours

Elimination: 65% to 70% unchanged drug in urine

Clearance:

Infants:

0-3 months: 0.13-0.21 ± 0.06 L/hour/kg

>3-12 months: 0.49 ± 0.17 L/hour/kg

Children 1-11 years: 0.54 ± 0.34 L/hour/kg

Adolescents: 0.48 ± 0.14 L/hour/kg

Adults: 0.39 ± 0.14 L/hour/kg

Dosing: Neonatal

Gastric acid suppression, GERD: Oral: 0.5 mg/kg/dose once daily

Stress ulcer prophylaxis, gastric acid suppression: I.V.: 0.5 mg/kg/dose once daily (Crill, 1999; James, 1998; Wenning, 2005)

Dosing: Usual

Infants, Children and Adolescent ≤16 years:

GERD, esophagitis: Oral:

Infants 1-3 months: 0.5 mg/kg/dose once daily for up to 8 weeks

Infants ≥3 months to 1 year: 0.5 mg/kg/dose twice daily for up to 8 weeks

Children and Adolescents 1-16 years: 0.5 mg/kg/dose twice daily (maximum dose: 40 mg/dose); doses up to 1 mg/kg/dose twice daily have been reported

Patients unable to take oral medication: I.V.:

Infants: 0.25-0.5 mg/kg/dose once daily (Crill, 1999; James, 1998; Wenning, 2005)

Children and Adolescents 1-16 years: Initial: 0.25 mg/kg/dose every 12 hours (maximum dose: 20 mg/dose); doses up to 0.5 mg/kg/dose every 12 hours have been reported

Peptic ulcer disease: Oral: Children and Adolescents 1-16 years: 0.5 mg/kg/**day** once daily at bedtime or divided twice daily (maximum daily dose: 40 mg/day); doses up to 1 mg/kg/**day** have been used

Stress ulcer prophylaxis, gastric acid suppression: I.V.: 0.5-1 mg/kg/dose every 12 hours (maximum dose: 20 mg/dose) (Crill, 1999)

Hypersecretory conditions: Oral: Adolescents: Initial: 20 mg every 6 hours, may increase up to 160 mg every 6 hours

Heartburn, acid indigestion, or sour stomach (OTC use): Oral: Adolescents: 10-20 mg 15-60 minutes before eating; not more than 2 tablets/day

Adults:

Duodenal ulcer: Oral: Acute therapy: 40 mg/day at bedtime (or 20 mg twice daily) for 4-8 weeks; maintenance therapy: 20 mg/day at bedtime

Gastric ulcer: Oral: Acute therapy: 40 mg/day at bedtime

Hypersecretory conditions: Oral: Initial: 20 mg every 6 hours, may increase in increments up to 160 mg every 6 hours

GERD: Oral: 20 mg twice daily for 6 weeks

Esophagitis and accompanying symptoms due to GERD: Oral: 20 mg or 40 mg twice daily for up to 12 weeks

Patients unable to take oral medication: I.V.: 20 mg every 12 hours

Heartburn, indigestion, sour stomach: OTC labeling: Oral: 10-20 mg every 12 hours; dose may be taken 15-60 minutes before eating foods known to cause heartburn

Dosing adjustment in renal impairment: CrCl <50 mL/minute: Manufacturer recommendation: Administer 50% of dose or increase the dosing interval to every 36-48 hours (to limit potential CNS adverse effects)

Administration

Oral: May administer with food and antacids; shake suspension vigorously for 10-15 seconds prior to each use

Parenteral:

I.V. push: May be administered at a maximum concentration of 4 mg/mL at a rate of ≤10 mg/minute over at least 2 minutes

I.V. infusion: Dilute to 0.2 mg/mL in an appropriate diluent, infuse over 15-30 minutes

Dosage Forms Excipient information presented when available (limited, particularly for generics); consult specific product labeling. [DSC] = Discontinued product

Solution, Intravenous:

Generic: 20 mg (50 mL); 20 mg/2 mL (2 mL); 40 mg/4 mL (4 mL); 200 mg/20 mL (20 mL); 500 mg/50 mL (50 mL)

Solution, Intravenous [preservative free]:

Generic: 20 mg/2 mL (2 mL)

Suspension Reconstituted, Oral:

Pepcid: 40 mg/5 mL (50 mL) [contains methylparaben sodium, propylparaben sodium, sodium benzoate; cherry banana mint flavor]

Generic: 40 mg/5 mL (50 mL)

Tablet, Oral:

Acid Reducer: 10 mg

Acid Reducer Maximum Strength: 20 mg

Heartburn Relief: 10 mg

Heartburn Relief Max St: 20 mg

Pepcid: 20 mg [scored]

Pepcid: 40 mg

Pepcid: 40 mg [DSC] [scored]

Generic: 10 mg, 20 mg, 40 mg

Extemporaneous Preparations An 8 mg/mL oral suspension may be made with tablets. Crush seventy 40 mg tablets in a mortar and reduce to a fine powder. Add small portions of sterile water and mix to a uniform paste. Mix while adding a 1:1 mixture of Ora-Plus® and Ora-Sweet® in incremental proportions to almost 350 mL; transfer to a calibrated bottle, rinse mortar with vehicle, and add quantity of vehicle sufficient to make 350 mL. Label "shake well". Stable for 95 days at room temperature.

Dentinger PJ, Swenson CF, and Anaizi NH, "Stability of Famotidine in an Extemporaneously Compounded Oral Liquid," *Am J Health Syst Pharm*, 2000, 57(14):1340-2.

References

Canani RB, Cirillo P, Roggero P, et al, "Therapy With Gastric Acidity Inhibitors Increases the Risk of Acute Gastroenteritis and Community-Acquired Pneumonia in Children," *Pediatrics*, 2006, 117(5):e817-20.

Crill CM and Hak EB, "Upper Gastrointestinal Tract Bleeding in Critically Ill Pediatric Patients," *Pharmacotherapy*, 1999, 19(2):162-80.

Guillet R, Stoll BJ, Cotten CM, et al, "Association of H₂-Blocker Therapy and Higher Incidence of Necrotizing Enterocolitis in Very Low Birth Weight Infants," *Pediatrics*, 2006, 117(2):137-42.

James LP and Kearns GL, "Pharmacokinetics and Pharmacodynamics of Famotidine in Paediatric Patients," *Clin Pharmacokinet*, 1996, 31 (2):103-10.

James LP, Marotti T, Stowe CD, et al, "Pharmacokinetics and Pharmacodynamics of Famotidine in Infants," *J Clin Pharmacol*, 1998, 38 (12):1089-95.

Rudolph CD, Mazur LJ, Liptak GS, et al, "Guidelines for Evaluation and Treatment of Gastroesophageal Reflux in Infants and Children: Recommendations of the North American Society for Pediatric Gastroenterology and Nutrition," *J Pediatr Gastroenterol Nutr*, 2001, 32 (Suppl 2):1-31.

Terrin G, Passariello A, De Curtis M, et al, "Ranitidine Is Associated With Infections, Necrotizing Enterocolitis, and Fatal Outcome in Newborns," *Pediatrics*, 2012, 129(1):40-5.

Treem WR, Davis PM, and Hyams JS, "Suppression of Gastric Acid Secretion by Intravenous Administration of Famotidine in Children," *J Pediatr*, 1991, 118(5):812-6.

Wenning LA, Murphy MG, James LP, et al, "Pharmacokinetics of Famotidine in Infants," *Clin Pharmacokinet*, 2005, 44(4):395-406.

◆ **Famotidine Omega (Can)** see Famotidine on page 843

◆ **Famvir** see Famciclovir on page 842

◆ **Famvir® (Can)** see Famciclovir on page 842

◆ **Fansidar® [DSC]** see Sulfadoxine and Pyrimethamine on page 1947

♦ **2F-ara-AMP** *see* Fludarabine *on page 885*

♦ **Faslodex** *see* Fulvestrant *on page 946*

♦ **Faslodex® (Can)** *see* Fulvestrant *on page 946*

♦ **Fasturtec® (Can)** *see* Rasburicase *on page 1808*

Fat Emulsion (Plant Based)
(fat e MUL shun plant baste)

Medication Safety Issues
Sound-alike/look-alike issues:
Intralipid may be confused with ViperSlide (lubricant used during atherectomy procedures)

Related Information
Pediatric Parenteral Nutrition *on page 2312*

Brand Names: U.S. Intralipid; Liposyn III

Brand Names: Canada Intralipid

Therapeutic Category Caloric Agent; Intravenous Nutritional Therapy

Generic Availability (U.S.) No

Use Source of calories and essential fatty acids for patients requiring parenteral nutrition of extended duration (FDA approved in all ages); prevention and treatment of essential fatty acid deficiency (EFAD) (FDA approved in all ages); has also been used for treatment of local anesthetic-induced cardiac arrest unresponsive to conventional resuscitation

Pregnancy Risk Factor C

Pregnancy Considerations Animal reproductive studies have not been conducted. Indications for fat emulsion therapy in pregnant women are the same as in nonpregnant women. The ASPEN guidelines for parenteral and enteral nutrition state that intravenous fat emulsion may be used safely in pregnant women to provide calories and prevent essential fatty acid deficiency (ASPEN Guidelines, 2002).

Breast-Feeding Considerations The fatty acids found in fat emulsion (eg, linoleic acid, linolenic acid) are endogenous to human milk and concentrations are influenced by maternal diet (IOM, 2005). The manufacturers recommend that caution be exercised when administering fat emulsion therapy to nursing women.

Contraindications Hypersensitivity to fat emulsion or any component; disturbances of normal fat metabolism (eg, pathologic hyperlipidemia, lipoid nephrosis, pancreatitis with hyperlipemia)

Warnings Deaths in preterm neonates after infusion of I.V. fat emulsion have been reported **[U.S. Boxed Warning]**. Autopsy findings included intravascular fat accumulation in the lungs. I.V. fat emulsion should be used carefully in preterm neonates adhering to maximum daily dosages and infusing as slowly as possible. Preterm infants have a decreased ability to eliminate infused fat and must be monitored closely using triglyceride or plasma free fatty acid concentrations. Avoid use of 10% fat emulsion in preterm infants as a greater accumulation of plasma lipids occurs with the greater phospholipid load of the 10% fat emulsion. Frequent platelet counts (some advise daily) should also be obtained in neonatal patients receiving fat emulsion. Monitor liver function tests when using as long-term therapy.

Fat emulsion in a 3-in-1 mixture may obscure the presence of a precipitate; follow compounding guidelines, especially regarding calcium and phosphate compatibility. Thirty percent fat emulsions are not intended for direct I.V. infusion and dilution with another I.V. fluid (eg, NS or SWI) does not produce a dilution equivalent to 10% or 20% I.V. fat emulsion; such dilutions should not be administered by direct I.V. infusion.

Precautions Use with caution in patients with severe liver damage, pulmonary disease, anemia, or blood coagulation disorders or when there is risk for fat embolism; use with caution in cholestatic patients or in those at risk for parenteral nutrition-associated cholestasis. When cholestatsis occurs, fat emulsion may be temporarily decreased or stopped. Use with caution in patients with severe egg or soybean allergies.

Fat emulsions contain aluminum; toxic aluminum concentrations may be seen with high doses, prolonged use, or renal dysfunction. Premature neonates are at higher risk due to immature renal function and aluminum intake from other parenteral sources. Parenteral aluminum exposure of >4-5 mcg/kg/day is associated with CNS and bone toxicity and tissue loading may occur at lower doses.

Adverse Reactions
Endocrine & metabolic: Hyperglycemia, hyperlipidemia

Gastrointestinal: Gallbladder disorder, nausea and vomiting

Genitourinary: Urinary tract infection

Hematologic & oncologic: Hypoproteinemia

Hepatic: Abnormal hepatic function tests, hepatic abnormality

Infection: Septicemia

Miscellaneous: Fever

Rare but important or life-threatening: Cholestasis, cyanosis, decreased INR, hepatic effects (brown pigment deposition in the reticuloendothelial system ["intravenous fat pigment"]), hepatomegaly, hypercoagulability state, hypersensitivity reaction, infusion site irritation, jaundice, leukopenia, liver steatosis, overloading syndrome (focal seizures, fever, leukocytosis, hepatomegaly, splenomegaly, shock), pancreatitis, thrombocytopenia, thrombophlebitis

Stability
Intralipid®: Store below 25°C (77°F).

Liposyn® III: Store at 20°C to 25°C (68°F to 77°F).

Do not freeze; do not store in partly used containers; fat emulsion can support the growth of various organisms. Do not use if emulsion appears to be layering out; exposure to light, particularly phototherapy light, used in treatment or prevention of hyperbilirubinemia has been associated with increased lipid oxidation; the clinical significance remains to be established; do not mix other drugs with fat emulsion; only heparin at a concentration of 1-2 units/mL may be added to fat emulsion

Mechanism of Action Fat emulsion is metabolized and utilized as an energy source; provides the essential fatty acids, linoleic acid, and alpha linolenic acid necessary for normal structure and function of cell membranes; in local anesthetic toxicity, lipid emulsion probably extracts lipophilic local anesthesia from cardiac muscle

In local anesthetic toxicity, exogenous lipids provide an alternative source of binding of lipid-soluble local anesthetics (Rowlingson, 2008), commonly known as the "lipid sink" effect. This is more relevant to bupivacaine, levobupivacaine, and ropivacaine than mepivacaine and prilocaine. High lipid partition constant and large volumes of distribution are good predictors of success when using lipid therapy (French, 2011). Lipid administration may also affect the heart in a metabolically advantageous way by improving fatty acid transport (Weinberg, 2006).

Dosing: Neonatal
Parenteral nutrition: Note: Fat emulsion should not exceed 60% of the total daily calories. At the onset of therapy, the patient should be observed for any immediate allergic reactions such as dyspnea, cyanosis, and fever.

Premature neonates: I.V.: Initial dose: 1-2 g/kg/day, increase by 0.5-1 g/kg/day to a maximum of 3-3.5 g/kg/day depending upon the needs/nutritional goals; daily dose infused over 24 hours; total infusion time may be incrementally increased (ie, cycled) to a maximum daily infusion over 12 hours (ASPEN Guidelines,

2002; ASPEN Pediatric Nutrition Support Core Curriculum, 2010); do not exceed 1 g/kg in 4 hours

Term neonates: I.V.: Initial dose: 1-2 g/kg/day, increase by 0.5-1 g/kg/day to a maximum of 3 g/kg/day depending upon the needs/nutritional goals; daily dose infused over 24 hours; total infusion time may be incrementally increased (ie, cycled) to a maximum daily infusion over 12 hours (ASPEN Guidelines, 2002; ASPEN Pediatric Nutrition Support Core Curriculum, 2010)

Localized anesthetic toxicity: Full-term neonate: Very limited data available: 20% fat emulsion: I.V.: 1 **mL**/kg was reported in a single case report in a 2-day-old neonate undergoing caudal epidural block for a urologic procedure (Lin, 2010)

Dosing: Usual

Parenteral nutrition: Note: Fat emulsion should not exceed 60% of the total daily calories. At the onset of therapy, the patient should be observed for any immediate allergic reactions such as dyspnea, cyanosis, and fever.

Infants: I.V.: Initial dose: 1-2 g/kg/day, increase by 0.5-1 g/kg/day to a maximum of 3 g/kg/day depending upon the needs/nutritional goals; daily dose infused over 24 hours; total infusion time may be incrementally increased (ie, cycled) to a maximum daily infusion over 12 hours (ASPEN Guidelines, 2002; ASPEN Pediatric Nutrition Support Core Curriculum, 2010)

Children 1-10 years: I.V.: Initial dose: 1-2 g/kg/day, increase by 0.5-1 g/kg/day to a maximum of 2-3 g/kg/day depending upon the needs/nutritional goals; daily dose infused over 24 hours; total infusion time may be incrementally increased (ie, cycled) to a maximum daily infusion over 12 hours (ASPEN Guidelines, 2002; ASPEN Pediatric Nutrition Support Core Curriculum, 2010)

Children ≥11 years, Adolescents, and Adults: I.V.: Initial dose: 1 g/kg/day; not to exceed 500 mL 20% fat emulsion on the first day of therapy, increase by 1 g/kg/day to a maximum of 2.5 g/kg/day; daily dose infused over 24 hours; total infusion time may be incrementally increased (ie, cycled) to a maximum daily infusion over 12 hours (ASPEN Guidelines, 2002; ASPEN Pediatric Nutrition Support Core Curriculum, 2010)

Essential fatty acid deficiency (EFAD), prevention: Children, Adolescents, and Adults: I.V.: Administer 8% to 10% of total caloric intake as fat emulsion; infuse 2-3 times weekly; may need to increase dose during stress

Local anesthetic toxicity:

Infants, Children, and Adolescents: Limited data available: 20% fat emulsion: I.V.: 0.8-3 **mL**/kg bolus has been used successfully in several pediatric case reports (1 month-13 years) (Fuzaylov, 2010; Ludot, 2008; Shah, 2009; Wong, 2010); a single case report in a 6-year-old described use of a continuous I.V. infusion at 0.25 **mL**/kg/minute to a total dose of 8 **mL**/kg following the bolus dose (Wong, 2010)

Adults: 20% fat emulsion: I.V.: Infuse 1.5 mL/kg over 1 minute, followed immediately by an infusion of 0.25 mL/kg/minute; continue chest compressions (lipid must circulate). Repeat the bolus 1-2 times as needed for persistent asystole, pulseless electrical activity, or re-emergence of hemodynamic instability. Continue I.V. infusion for at least 10 minutes after hemodynamic stability is restored; discontinue within 1 hour, if possible. Increase the infusion rate to 0.5 mL/kg/minute if hemodynamic instability persists or recurs (ACMT, 2010; Neal, 2012).

Administration Parenteral:

Parenteral nutrition:

10% and 20% emulsions: May be simultaneously infused with amino acid and dextrose mixtures by means of Y-connector located near infusion site into either central or peripheral line or administered in total nutrient mixtures (3-in-1) with amino acids, dextrose, and other nutrients. At the bedside, fat emulsion solution should be elevated higher than other parenteral fluids to prevent it running up into other I.V. lines due to its low specific gravity. For Intralipid®: Do not use <1.2 micron filter; for Liposyn® III: Do not use a filter.

30% emulsion: **Intended only for use as component of 3-in-1 or total nutrient admixture;** not intended for direct infusion; must be further diluted to a final concentration not to exceed 20%

Neonates, Infants, and Children: **Note:** Premature and/or septic infants may require reduced infusion rates; do not exceed 1 g/kg in 4 hours in this population.

10% emulsions: Avoid use of 10% fat emulsion in preterm infants as a greater accumulation of plasma lipids occurs with the greater phospholipid load of the 10% fat emulsion

Intralipid®: Initiate at ≤0.1 **mL**/minute for 10-15 minutes; if no untoward effects occur, the infusion rate may be increased to 1 **mL**/kg/**hour.**

Liposyn® III: Initiate at 0.1 **mL**/minute for 15 minutes, may increase to ≤100 **mL/hour** if tolerated

20% emulsions:

Intralipid®: Initiate at ≤0.05 **mL**/minute for 10-15 minutes; if no untoward effects occur, the infusion rate may be increased to 0.5 **mL/kg/hour**

Liposyn® III: Initiate at 0.1 **mL**/minute for 15 minutes, may increase to ≤50 **mL/hour** if tolerated

Adults:

10% emulsions (Intralipid®; Liposyn® III): Initiate at 1 **mL**/minute for 15-30 minutes; if no untoward effects occur, the infusion rate may be increased to 2 **mL**/minute.

20% emulsions (Intralipid®; Liposyn® III): Initiate at 0.5 **mL**/minute for 15-30 minutes; if no untoward effects occur, the infusion rate may be increased to 1 **mL**/minute.

Local anesthetic toxicity: 20% emulsion: Administer initial bolus undiluted over 1 minute; may be administered either peripherally or centrally; bolus may be followed by a continuous infusion depending on clinical scenario. Chest compressions should continue during administration if patient is in cardiac arrest. Continue the infusion for at least 10 minutes after hemodynamic stability is restored. The infusion rate may be increased if hemodynamic instability recurs (ACMT, 2010; Neal, 2012).

Monitoring Parameters Serum triglycerides, free fatty acids, platelets (neonates), liver enzymes

Additional Information Fat emulsion has been used successfully as a treatment in a pediatric patient experiencing local anesthetic cardiovascular toxicity (Ludot, 2008) and also in animal studies and several human case reports in which cardiovascular toxicity was unresponsive to conventional resuscitation and antidotal measures. May consider use of 20% fat emulsion when local anesthetic toxicity is likely and conventional methods are unsuccessful. Continue CPR throughout treatment with lipid emulsion. Additional information is available at http://www.lipidrescue.org.

Caloric content: 10% emulsion = 1.1 Kcal/mL; 20% emulsion = 2 Kcal/mL; 30% emulsion = 3 Kcal/mL

Phosphorus: ~1.5 mMol/100 mL of emulsion

10% and 20% emulsions are isotonic and may be administered peripherally

Product Availability Clinolipid: FDA approved October 2013; anticipated availability is currently unknown. Refer to the prescribing information for additional information.

Dosage Forms Considerations

Product oil source for Intralipid and Liposyn III: soybean

Dosage Forms Excipient information presented when available (limited, particularly for generics); consult specific product labeling.

Emulsion, Intravenous:
Intralipid: 20% (100 mL, 250 mL, 500 mL, 1000 mL); 30% (500 mL) [contains egg yolk phospholipids]
Liposyn III: 10% (200 mL, 250 mL, 500 mL); 20% (200 mL, 250 mL, 500 mL); 30% (500 mL) [contains egg phosphatides]

References

American College of Medical Toxicology (ACMT), "Interim Guidance for the Use of Lipid Resuscitation Therapy," 2010. Available at http://www.acmt.net/cgi/page.cgi?aid=3384&_id=52&zine=show

ASPEN Board of Directors and the Clinical Guidelines Task Force, "Guidelines for the Use of Parenteral and Enteral Nutrition in Adult and Pediatric Patients," JPEN J Parenter Enteral Nutr, 2002, 26(1 Suppl):1SA-138SA.

Carney LN, Nepa A, Cohen SS, et al, "Parenteral and Enteral Nutrition Support: Determining the Best Way to Feed," In: Corkins MR, Balint J, Bobo E, et al, eds, The A.S.P.E.N Pediatric Nutrition Support Core Curriculum, Silver Spring: MD: American Society of Parenteral and Enteral Nutrition, 2010, 440-1.

Colomb V, Jobert-Giraud A, Lacaille F, et al, "Role of Lipid Emulsions in Cholestasis Associated With Long-Term Parenteral Nutrition in Children," JPEN J Parenter Enteral Nutr, 2000, 24(6):345-50.

Corcoran W, Butterworth J, Weller RS, et al, "Local Anesthetic-Induced Cardiac Toxicity: A Survey of Contemporary Practice Strategies Among Academic Anesthesiology Departments," Anesth Analg, 2006, 103(5):1322-6.

Department of Health & Human Services, Food and Drug Administration, "Aluminum in Large and Small Volume Parenterals Used in Total Parenteral Nutrition," Federal Register, 2000, 65(17):4103-11.

Foxall G, McCahon R, Lamb J, et al, "Levobupivacaine-Induced Seizures and Cardiovascular Collapse Treated With Intralipid," Anaesthesia, 2007, 62(5):516-8.

French D, Smollin C, Ruan W, et al, "Partition Constant and Volume of Distribution as Predictors of Clinical Efficacy of Lipid Rescue for Toxicological Emergencies," Clin Toxicol, 2011, 49(9):801-9.

Fuzaylov G, Ying B, Tang Y, et al, "Successful Resuscitation After Inadvertent Intravenous Injection of Bupivacaine in an Adolescent," Paediatr Anaesth, 2010, 20(10):958-9.

Haumont D, Richelle M, Deckelbaum RJ, et al, "Effect of Liposomal Content of Lipid Emulsions of Plasma Lipid Concentrations in Low Birth Weight Infants Receiving Parenteral Nutrition," J Pediatr, 1992, 121(5 Pt 1):759-63.

IOM (Institute of Medicine), Dietary Reference Intakes for Energy, Carbohydrate, Fiber, Fat, Fatty Acids, Cholesterol, Protein, and Amino Acids (Macronutrients), Washington, DC: The National Academies Press, 2005.

Lin EP and Aronson LA, "Successful Resuscitation of Bupivacaine-Induced Cardiotoxicity in a Neonate," Paediatr Anaesth, 2010, 20 (10):955-7.

Litz RJ, Popp M, Stehr SN, et al, "Successful Resuscitation of a Patient With Ropivacaine-Induced Asystole After Axillary Plexus Block Using Lipid Infusion," Anaesthesia, 2006, 61(8):800-1.

Ludot H, Tharin JY, Belouadah M, et al, "Successful Resuscitation After Ropivacaine and Lidocaine-Induced Ventricular Arrhythmia Following Posterior Lumbar Plexus Block in a Child," Anesth Analg, 2008, 106 (5):1572-4.

Mirtallo J, Canada T, Johnson D, et al, "Safe Practices for Parenteral Nutrition. Task Force for the Revision of Safe Practices for Parenteral Nutrition," JPEN J Parenter Enteral Nutr, 2004, 28(6):S39-70.

Neal JM, Mulroy MF, and Weinberg GL, "American Society of Regional Anesthesia and Pain Medicine Checklist for Managing Local Anesthetic Systemic Toxicity: 2012 Version," Reg Anesth Pain Med, 2012, 37(1):16-8.

Neuzil J, Darlow BA, Inder TE, et al, "Oxidation of Parenteral Lipid Emulsion by Ambient and Phototherapy Light: Potential Toxicity of Routine Parenteral Feeding," J Pediatr, 1995, 126(5 Pt 1):785-90.

Rowlingson JC, "Lipid Rescue: A Step Forward in Patient Safety? Likely So!" Anesth Analg, 2008, 106(5):1333-6.

Shah S, Gopalakrishnan S, Apuya J, et al, "Use of Intralipid in an Infant With Impending Cardiovascular Collapse Due to Local Anesthetic Toxicity," J Anesth, 2009, 23(3):439-41.

Shin JI, Namgung R, Park MS, et al, "Could Lipid Infusion Be a Risk for Parenteral Nutrition-Associated Cholestasis in Low Birth Weight Neonates?" Eur J Pediatr, 2008, 167(2):197-202.

Weinberg GL, Ripper R, Murphy P, et al, "Lipid Infusion Accelerates Removal of Bupivacaine and Recovery From Bupivacaine Toxicity in the Isolated Rat Heart," Reg Anesth Pain Med, 2006, 31(4):296-303.

Wong GK, Joo DT, and McDonnell C, "Lipid Resuscitation in a Carnitine Deficient Child Following Intravascular Migration of an Epidural Catheter," Anaesthesia, 2010, 65(2):192-5.

♦ **FazaClo** see CloZAPine on page 527

♦ **5-FC** see Flucytosine on page 882

♦ **Feiba NF** see Anti-inhibitor Coagulant Complex (Human) on page 180

♦ **FEIBA NF (Can)** see Anti-inhibitor Coagulant Complex (Human) on page 180

♦ **FEIBA VH** see Anti-inhibitor Coagulant Complex (Human) on page 180

Felbamate (FEL ba mate)

Brand Names: U.S. Felbatol
Therapeutic Category Anticonvulsant, Miscellaneous
Generic Availability (U.S.) Yes
Use Not a first-line agent; reserved for patients who do not adequately respond to alternative agents and whose epilepsy is so severe that the benefit outweighs the risk of liver failure or aplastic anemia; used as monotherapy and adjunctive therapy in patients with partial seizures with and without secondary generalization (FDA approved in ages ≥14 years and adults); adjunctive therapy in children who have partial and generalized seizures associated with Lennox-Gastaut syndrome (FDA approved in ages 2-14 years)
Prescribing and Access Restrictions A patient "informed consent" form should be completed and signed by the patient and physician. Copies are available from MEDA Pharmaceuticals by calling 800-526-3840.
Medication Guide Available Yes
Pregnancy Risk Factor C
Pregnancy Considerations Adverse events were not observed in animal reproduction studies. Postmarketing case reports in humans include fetal death, genital malformation, anencephaly, encephalocele, and placental disorder.

Patients exposed to felbamate during pregnancy are encouraged to enroll themselves into the North American Antiepileptic Drug (AED) Pregnancy Registry by calling 1-888-233-2334. Additional information is available at www.aedpregnancyregistry.org.
Breast-Feeding Considerations Felbamate has been detected in human milk.
Contraindications Hypersensitivity to felbamate, any component, or other carbamates (eg, meprobamate); history of or current blood dyscrasia or hepatic dysfunction
Warnings Felbamate is associated with a significant increased risk of aplastic anemia **[U.S. Boxed Warning]**. Risk may be more than 100-fold greater than in untreated population. Current estimates of aplastic anemia-related fatality are 20% to 30%, but higher rates (up to 70%) have been reported in the past. It is not known if dose, duration, or use of concomitant medications affects risk. Aplastic anemia can develop at any point during therapy. Routine blood monitoring is recommended to potentially allow for detection of hematologic changes, although aplastic anemia can occur without warning.

Use is associated with acute hepatic failure **[U.S. Boxed Warning]**. The overall postmarketing reported rate of hepatic failure leading to transplant or death is 6 cases per 75,000 patient years of use; this rate is underestimated due to under reporting (eg, the true rate could be as high as 1 case per 1250 patient years of use if the reporting rate is only 10%). Approximately 67% of the reported cases of hepatic failure led to liver transplantation or death, usually within 5 weeks of the onset of signs and symptoms of hepatic failure; the earliest onset of severe liver dysfunction was 3 weeks after starting felbamate; in some cases, dark urine and nonspecific prodromal symptoms (eg, malaise, anorexia, GI symptoms) preceded the onset of jaundice. It is not known if dose, duration, or use of concomitant medications affects risk of hepatic failure.

Felbamate should not be used in any patient with a history of hepatic dysfunction.

All patients receiving felbamate must be monitored closely; in addition, a CBC with differential and platelet count should be taken before, during, and for a significant time after discontinuing felbamate therapy; liver enzyme tests and bilirubin should be obtained before initiation and periodically during therapy. Felbamate should be immediately withdrawn if abnormal liver function tests or bone marrow suppression occur. Do not restart felbamate in patients who experience hematologic or hepatic adverse reactions.

Felbamate should only be used in patients who have severe, refractory seizures that are unresponsive to other medications. The FDA and the manufacturer strongly recommend that physicians discuss the risks of felbamate with each patient and a written informed consent be obtained from the patient prior to starting therapy or before continuing therapy. A patient information consent form is included as part of the package insert and is available from the local Wallace representative or by calling 800-526-3840.

Antiepileptic drugs (AEDs) increase the risk of suicidal behavior and ideation in patients receiving these medications for any indication. Pooled analyses of placebo-controlled trials involving 11 different AEDs (regardless of indication) showed a twofold increased risk of suicidal thoughts or behavior (estimated incidence rate: 0.43% in AED treated patients compared to 0.24% of patients receiving placebo); increased risk was observed as early as 1 week after initiation of AED and continued through duration of trials (most trials ≤24 weeks); risk did not vary significantly by age (age range: 5-100 years). Consider risks and benefits of AEDs before prescribing. Monitor all patients receiving an AED for emergence of suicidal thoughts or behavior, thoughts of self-harm, any unusual changes in behavior or mood, or the emergence or worsening of depressive symptoms; notify healthcare provider immediately if symptoms or concerning behavior occur. **Note:** The FDA is requiring that a Medication Guide be developed for all antiepileptic drugs informing patients of this risk.

Precautions Use with caution in patients concurrently receiving other antiepileptic drugs due to the potential for drug interactions; felbamate may increase the serum concentrations of phenytoin, valproic acid, phenobarbital, and carbamazepine epoxide (active metabolite of carbamazepine); a 20% to 33% reduction in the dose of these concomitant medications is recommended when felbamate is added to the regimen; further dosage reductions may be needed when felbamate doses are titrated upward; monitor serum levels of concomitant antiepileptic drug therapy.

Use with caution and reduce dose in patients with renal dysfunction. Anticonvulsants should not be discontinued abruptly because of the possibility of increasing seizure frequency; felbamate should be withdrawn gradually to minimize the potential of increased seizure frequency, unless safety concerns require a more rapid withdrawal.

Adverse Reactions
Cardiovascular: Chest pain, facial edema, palpitation, tachycardia
Central nervous system: Abnormal thinking, agitation, aggressive reaction, ataxia, depression, dizziness, emotional lability, euphoria, fatigue, fever, hallucinations, headache, insomnia, malaise, migraine, nervousness, psychological disturbances, somnolence, stupor, suicide attempt
Dermatologic: Acne, bullous eruption, pruritus, purpura, skin rash, urticaria

Endocrine and metabolic: Hypokalemia, hyponatremia, hypophosphatemia, intramenstrual bleeding
Gastrointestinal: Abdominal pain, anorexia, appetite increased, constipation, diarrhea, dyspepsia, esophagitis, hiccup, nausea, taste perversion, vomiting, weight gain/loss, xerostomia
Genitourinary: Urinary tract infection
Hematologic: Granulocytopenia, leukocytosis, leukopenia, lymphadenopathy, thrombocytopenia
Hepatic: Alkaline phosphatase increased, liver function tests increased
Neuromuscular & skeletal: Abnormal gait, dystonia, myalgia, pain, paresthesia, tremor, weakness
Ocular: Abnormal vision, diplopia, miosis
Otic: Otitis media
Respiratory: Cough, pharyngitis, rhinitis, sinusitis, upper respiratory infection
Miscellaneous: Flu-like syndrome, LDH increased
Rare but important or life-threatening: Acute renal failure, agranulocytosis, allergic reaction, alopecia, anaphylactoid reaction, anemia, aplastic anemia, atrial arrhythmia, atrial fibrillation, bradycardia, cardiac arrest, cardiac failure, cerebrovascular disorder, cerebral edema, choreoathetosis, coagulation disorder, coma, concentration impaired, confusion, CPK increased, delusion, diaphoresis, DIC, dysphagia, dyspnea, dysarthria, dyskinesia, dysuria, embolism, encephalopathy, enteritis, eosinophilia, epistaxis, extrapyramidal disorder, flushing, gastric ulcer, gastritis, gastroesophageal reflux, GI hemorrhage, gingival bleeding, glossitis, hematemesis, hematuria, hemolytic anemia, Henoch-Schönlein vasculitis, hepatic failure, hepatitis, hepatorenal syndrome, hyperammonemia, hyper-/hypoglycemia, hyper-/hypotension, hypernatremia, hypocalcemia, hypomagnesemia, hypoxia, ileus, ischemic necrosis, jaundice, manic reaction, mononeuritis, nephrosis, nystagmus, pancreatitis, pancytopenia, paralysis, paranoid reaction, peripheral ischemia, photosensitivity, platelet disorder, pleural effusion, pneumonitis, psychosis, pulmonary hemorrhage, rectal hemorrhage, renal function abnormal, respiratory depression, rhabdomyolysis, SIADH, status epilepticus, Stevens-Johnson syndrome, sudden death, suicidal behavior/ideation, SVT, thrombophlebitis, torsade de pointes, toxic epidermal necrolysis, ulcerative stomatitis, urinary retention, urticaria

Drug Interactions
Metabolism/Transport Effects Substrate of CYP2E1 (minor), CYP3A4 (major); **Note:** Assignment of Major/Minor substrate status based on clinically relevant drug interaction potential; **Inhibits** CYP2C19 (weak); **Induces** CYP3A4 (weak/moderate)

Avoid Concomitant Use
Avoid concomitant use of Felbamate with any of the following: Axitinib; Azelastine (Nasal); Conivaptan; Fusidic Acid (Systemic); Paraldehyde; Simeprevir; Thalidomide

Increased Effect/Toxicity
Felbamate may increase the levels/effects of: Alcohol (Ethyl); Azelastine (Nasal); Barbiturates; Buprenorphine; CNS Depressants; Fosphenytoin; Highest Risk QTc-Prolonging Agents; Hydrocodone; Methotrimeprazine; Metyrosine; Mirtazapine; Moderate Risk QTc-Prolonging Agents; Paraldehyde; PHENobarbital; Phenytoin; Pramipexole; Primidone; ROPINIRole; Rotigotine; Selective Serotonin Reuptake Inhibitors; Thalidomide; Valproic Acid and Derivatives; Zolpidem

The levels/effects of Felbamate may be increased by: Brimonidine (Topical); Cannabis; Ceritinib; Conivaptan; CYP3A4 Inhibitors (Moderate); CYP3A4 Inhibitors (Strong); Dasatinib; Doxylamine; Dronabinol; Droperidol; Fusidic Acid (Systemic); HydrOXYzine; Ivacaftor; Kava Kava; Luliconazole; Magnesium Sulfate;

Methotrimeprazine; Mifepristone; Nabilone; Perampanel; Rufinamide; Sodium Oxybate; Stiripentol; Tapentadol; Tetrahydrocannabinol

Decreased Effect

Felbamate may decrease the levels/effects of: ARIPiprazole; Axitinib; CarBAMazepine; Contraceptives (Estrogens); Contraceptives (Progestins); Ibrutinib; Saxagliptin; Simeprevir

The levels/effects of Felbamate may be decreased by: Barbiturates; Bosentan; CarBAMazepine; CYP3A4 Inducers (Strong); Dabrafenib; Deferasirox; Fosphenytoin; Ketorolac (Nasal); Ketorolac (Systemic); Mefloquine; Mitotane; Orlistat; PHENobarbital; Phenytoin; Primidone; Siltuximab; St Johns Wort; Tocilizumab

Food Interactions Tablet: Food does not affect absorption. Management: Administer without regard to meals.

Stability Store in tightly closed container at room temperature of 20°C to 25°C (68°F to 77°F).

Mechanism of Action Mechanism of action is unknown but has properties in common with other marketed anticonvulsants; has weak inhibitory effects on GABA-receptor binding, benzodiazepine receptor binding, and is devoid of activity at the MK-801 receptor binding site of the NMDA receptor-ionophore complex.

Pharmacokinetics (Adult data unless noted)

Absorption: Oral: Rapid and almost complete

Distribution: V_d: Adults: Mean: 0.75 L/kg; range: 0.7-1.1 L/kg

Protein binding: 20% to 25%, primarily to albumin

Metabolism: In the liver via hydroxylation and conjugation

Bioavailability: >90%

Half-life: Adults: Mean: 20-30 hours; shorter (ie, 14 hours) with concomitant enzyme-inducing drugs; half-life is prolonged (by 9-15 hours) in patients with renal dysfunction

Time to peak serum concentration: 1-4 hours

Elimination: 40% to 50% excreted as unchanged drug and 40% as inactive metabolites in urine

Clearance, apparent: Clearance is decreased (by 40% to 50%) in patients with renal impairment

Children 2-9 years: 61.3 ± 8.2 mL/kg/hour

Children 10-12 years: 34.3 ± 4.3 mL/kg/hour

Dosing: Usual See Precautions regarding concomitant antiepileptic drugs

Children 2-14 years with Lennox-Gastaut: Adjunctive therapy: Initial: 15 mg/kg/day in 3-4 divided doses; increase dose by 15 mg/kg/day increments at weekly intervals; maximum dose: 45 mg/kg/day or 3600 mg/day (whichever is less). Decrease dose of concomitant anticonvulsants (ie, carbamazepine, phenytoin, phenobarbital, valproic acid) by 20% at initiation of felbamate; further dosage reductions of concurrent anticonvulsants may be needed.

Children ≥14 years and Adults:

Adjunctive therapy: Initial: 1200 mg/day in 3-4 divided doses; increase daily dose by 1200 mg increments every week to a maximum dose of 3600 mg/day. Decrease dose of concomitant anticonvulsants (ie, carbamazepine, phenytoin, phenobarbital, valproic acid) by 20% at initiation of felbamate; further dosage reductions of concurrent anticonvulsants may be needed.

Conversion to monotherapy: Initial: 1200 mg/day in 3 or 4 divided doses; at week 2, increase daily dose by 1200 mg increments every week up to a maximum dose of 3600 mg/day. Decrease dose of other anticonvulsants by 1/3 their original dose at initiation of felbamate, and when felbamate dose is increased at week 2; continue to reduce other anticonvulsants as clinically needed.

Monotherapy: Initial: 1200 mg/day in 3 or 4 divided doses; titrate dosage upward according to clinical response and monitor patients closely; increase daily dose in 600 mg increments every 2 weeks to 2400 mg/day; maximum dose: 3600 mg/day

Dosage adjustment in renal impairment: Use with caution; reduce initial and maintenance doses by 50%

Administration Oral: May be administered without regard to meals; shake suspension well before use

Monitoring Parameters Serum concentrations of concomitant anticonvulsant therapy; CBC with differential and platelet count before, during, and for a significant time after discontinuing felbamate therapy; liver enzyme tests and bilirubin before initiation and periodically during therapy; signs and symptoms of suicidality (eg, anxiety, depression, behavior changes)

Reference Range Not necessary to routinely monitor serum drug levels; dose should be titrated to clinical response; therapeutic range not fully determined; proposed 30-100 mcg/mL

Additional Information Monotherapy has not been associated with gingival hyperplasia, impaired concentration, weight gain, or abnormal thinking; felbamate has also been used in a small number of patients with infantile spasms (Pellock, 1999); an open-label study in children with refractory partial seizures (n=30; mean age: 9 years; range: 2-17 years) found that children >10 years of age had a more favorable response; this was thought to be related to the higher felbamate serum concentrations (and lower apparent clearance) in children >10 years of age compared to those <10 years; the faster apparent clearance in children <10 years of age should be considered when using this agent (Carmant, 1994)

Dosage Forms Excipient information presented when available (limited, particularly for generics); consult specific product labeling.

Suspension, Oral:

Felbatol: 600 mg/5 mL (237 mL, 946 mL)

Generic: 600 mg/5 mL (237 mL, 240 mL, 473 mL, 946 mL)

Tablet, Oral:

Felbatol: 400 mg, 600 mg [scored]

Generic: 400 mg, 600 mg

References

Carmant L, Holmes GL, Sawyer S, et al, "Efficacy of Felbamate in Therapy for Partial Epilepsy in Children," *J Pediatr*, 1994, 125 (3):481-6.

Dodson WE, "Felbamate in the Treatment of Lennox-Gastaut Syndrome: Results of a 12-Month Open-Label Study Following a Randomized Clinical Trial," *Epilepsia*, 1993, 34(Suppl 7):518-24.

French J, Smith M, Faught E, et al, "Practice Advisory: The Use of Felbamate in the Treatment of Patients With Intractable Epilepsy: Report of the Quality Standards Subcommittee of the American Academy of Neurology and the American Epilepsy Society," *Neurology*, 1999, 52(8):1540-5.

Kaufman DW, Kelly JP, Anderson T, et al, "Evaluation of Case Reports of Aplastic Anemia Among Patients Treated With Felbamate," *Epilepsia*, 1997, 38(12):1265-9.

Leppik IE, "Felbamate," *Epilepsia*, 1995, 36(Suppl 2):S66-72.

Pellock JM, "Felbamate in Epilepsy Therapy: Evaluating the Risks," *Drug Saf*, 1999, 21(3):225-39.

Pellock JM, "Managing Pediatric Epilepsy Syndromes With New Antiepileptic Drugs," *Pediatrics*, 1999, 104(5 Pt 1):1106-16.

Perucca E, "Clinically Relevant Drug Interactions With Antiepileptic Drugs," *Br J Clin Pharmacol*, 2006, 61(3):246-55.

The Felbamate Study Group in Lennox-Gastaut Syndrome, "Efficacy of Felbamate in Childhood Epileptic Encephalopathy (Lennox-Gastaut Syndrome)," *N Engl J Med*, 1993, 328(1):29-33.

◆ **Felbatol** *see* Felbamate *on page 848*

◆ **Feldene** *see* Piroxicam *on page 1683*

Felodipine (fe LOE di peen)

Medication Safety Issues

Sound-alike/look-alike issues:

Plendil may be confused with Isordil®, pindolol, Pletal, PriLOSEC, Prinivil

Related Information
Oral Medications That Should Not Be Crushed or Altered *on page 2438*

Brand Names: Canada Plendil; Renedil; Sandoz-Felodipine

Therapeutic Category Antihypertensive Agent; Calcium Channel Blocker; Calcium Channel Blocker, Dihydropyridine

Generic Availability (U.S.) Yes

Use Treatment of hypertension alone or in combination with other antihypertensives (FDA approved in adults)

Pregnancy Risk Factor C

Pregnancy Considerations Adverse events were observed in animal reproduction studies. Untreated chronic maternal hypertension is associated with adverse events in the fetus, infant, and mother. If treatment for hypertension during pregnancy is needed, other agents are preferred (ACOG, 2013).

Breast-Feeding Considerations It is not known if felodipine is excreted in breast milk. Due to the potential for serious adverse reactions in the nursing infant, the manufacturer recommends a decision be made whether to discontinue nursing or to discontinue the drug, taking into account the importance of treatment to the mother.

Contraindications Hypersensitivity to felodipine or any component

Warnings Symptomatic hypotension may occur with use; syncope may rarely occur; blood pressure must be lowered at a rate appropriate for the patient's clinical condition. Increased angina and/or MI has occurred with initiation or dosage titration of dihydropyridine calcium channel blockers; reflex tachycardia may occur resulting in angina and/or MI in patients with obstructive coronary disease especially in the absence of concurrent beta-blockade. May cause peripheral edema; usually occurs within 2-3 weeks of starting therapy.

Precautions
Use with caution in patients with hepatic impairment; clearance is reduced by ~60% and requires lower initial dose. Use with extreme caution in patients with severe aortic stenosis; may reduce coronary perfusion resulting in ischemia. Use with caution in patients with heart failure; safety and efficacy have not been established. Use with caution in patients with hypertrophic cardiomyopathy (HCM) and outflow tract obstruction since reduction in afterload may worsen symptoms associated with this condition. Use with caution in patients taking CYP3A4 inhibitors; may result in increased felodipine concentrations; monitor for adverse effects/toxicity and consider dose adjustments. May cause mild gingival hyperplasia; incidence and severity may be decreased with good oral hygiene.

Adverse Reactions
Cardiovascular: Flushing, peripheral edema, tachycardia
Central nervous system: Headache
Rare but important or life-threatening: Angina, angioedema, anxiety, arrhythmia, CHF, CVA, decreased libido, depression, dizziness, gingival hyperplasia, dyspnea, dysuria, gynecomastia, hypotension, impotence, insomnia, irritability, leukocytoclastic vasculitis, MI, nervousness, paresthesia, somnolence, syncope, urticaria, vomiting

Drug Interactions
Metabolism/Transport Effects Substrate of CYP3A4 (major); **Note:** Assignment of Major/Minor substrate status based on clinically relevant drug interaction potential; **Inhibits** CYP2C8 (moderate), CYP2C9 (weak), CYP2D6 (weak), CYP3A4 (weak)

Avoid Concomitant Use
Avoid concomitant use of Felodipine with any of the following: Conivaptan; Fusidic Acid (Systemic); Itraconazole; Ketoconazole (Systemic); Pimozide

Increased Effect/Toxicity
Felodipine may increase the levels/effects of: Amifostine; Antihypertensives; ARIPiprazole; Atosiban; Beta-Blockers; Calcium Channel Blockers (Nondihydropyridine); CYP2C8 Substrates; Dofetilide; DULoxetine; Fosphenytoin; Hypotensive Agents; Lomitapide; Magnesium Salts; Neuromuscular-Blocking Agents (Nondepolarizing); Nitroprusside; Obinutuzumab; Phenytoin; Pimozide; RiTUXimab; Tacrolimus (Systemic)

The levels/effects of Felodipine may be increased by: Alfuzosin; Alpha1-Blockers; Antifungal Agents (Azole Derivatives, Systemic); Barbiturates; Brimonidine (Topical); Calcium Channel Blockers (Nondihydropyridine); Ceritinib; Cimetidine; Conivaptan; CycloSPORINE (Systemic); CYP3A4 Inhibitors (Moderate); CYP3A4 Inhibitors (Strong); Dasatinib; Diazoxide; Fluconazole; Fusidic Acid (Systemic); Grapefruit Juice; Herbs (Hypotensive Properties); Itraconazole; Ivacaftor; Ketoconazole (Systemic); Luliconazole; Macrolide Antibiotics; Magnesium Salts; MAO Inhibitors; Mifepristone; Pentoxifylline; Phosphodiesterase 5 Inhibitors; Prostacyclin Analogues; Protease Inhibitors; Simeprevir; Stiripentol

Decreased Effect
Felodipine may decrease the levels/effects of: Clopidogrel

The levels/effects of Felodipine may be decreased by: Barbiturates; Bosentan; Calcium Salts; CarBAMazepine; CYP3A4 Inducers (Strong); Dabrafenib; Deferasirox; Efavirenz; Herbs (Hypertensive Properties); Melatonin; Methylphenidate; Mitotane; Nafcillin; Rifamycin Derivatives; Siltuximab; St Johns Wort; Tocilizumab; Yohimbine

Food Interactions
Ethanol: Ethanol increases felodipine absorption. Management: Monitor for a greater hypotensive effect if ethanol is consumed.

Food: Compared to a fasted state, felodipine peak plasma concentrations are increased up to twofold when taken after a meal high in fat or carbohydrates. Grapefruit juice similarly increases felodipine C_{max} by twofold. Increased therapeutic and vasodilator side effects, including severe hypotension and myocardial ischemia, may occur. Management: May be taken with a small meal that is low in fat and carbohydrates; avoid grapefruit juice during therapy.

Stability Store at 20°C to 25°C (68°F to 77°F); excursions permitted to 15°C to 30°C (59°F to 86°F); protect from light.

Mechanism of Action Inhibits calcium ions from entering the "slow channels" or select voltage-sensitive areas of vascular smooth muscle and myocardium during depolarization, producing a relaxation of coronary vascular smooth muscle and coronary vasodilation; increases myocardial oxygen delivery in patients with vasospastic angina

Pharmacodynamics
Onset of action: Antihypertensive: 2-5 hours
Duration: Antihypertensive: 24 hours

Pharmacokinetics (Adult data unless noted)
Absorption: ~100%
Distribution: V_d: 10 L/kg
Protein binding: >99%
Metabolism: Hepatic; CYP3A4 substrate (major); extensive first-pass effect
Bioavailability: 20%; extensive first-pass metabolism
Half-life: 11-16 hours
Time to peak serum concentration: 2.5-5 hours
Elimination: Urine (70% as metabolites); feces 10%

Dosing: Usual
Children ≥6 years and Adolescents: **Hypertension:** Oral: Initial: 2.5 mg once daily; may increase as needed at 2-week intervals to a maximum daily dose: 10 mg/**day** (NHLBI, 2011)

Adults: **Hypertension:** Oral: 2.5-10 mg once daily; increase by 5 mg at 2-week intervals, as needed, to a maximum of 20 mg/day; usual dose range (JNC 7): 2.5-20 mg once daily

Dosing adjustment for renal impairment: Adults: Usually not required

Dosing adjustment for hepatic impairment: Adults: Initial dose: 2.5 mg/day; **Note:** Clearance is reduced to ~60% of normal in patients with hepatic disease; monitor closely

Administration Oral: Must be swallowed whole; do not crush or chew; should be taken either without food or with a light meal.

Monitoring Parameters Blood pressure, peripheral edema, liver enzymes

Dosage Forms Excipient information presented when available (limited, particularly for generics); consult specific product labeling.

Tablet Extended Release 24 Hour, Oral:
Generic: 2.5 mg, 5 mg, 10 mg

References

American College of Obstetricians and Gynecologists (ACOG), "ACOG Practice Bulletin No. 125: Chronic Hypertension in Pregnancy," *Obstet Gynecol*, 2012, 119(2 Pt 1):396-407.

Chobanian AV, Bakris GL, Black HR, et al, "The Seventh Report of the Joint National Committee on Prevention, Detection, Evaluation, and Treatment of High Blood Pressure: The JNC 7 Report," *JAMA*, 2003, 289(19):2560-71.

National Heart, Lung, and Blood Institute, "Expert Panel on Integrated Guidelines for Cardiovascular Health and Risk Reduction in Children and Adolescents," Clinical Practice Guidelines, 2011, National Institutes of Health. Available at http://www.nhlbi.nih.gov/guidelines/cvd_ped/peds_guidelines_full.pdf.

National High Blood Pressure Education Program Working Group on High Blood Pressure in Children and Adolescents, "The Fourth Report on the Diagnosis, Evaluation, and Treatment of High Blood Pressure in Children and Adolescents," *Pediatrics*, 2004, 114(2 Suppl):555-76.

◆ **Femara** *see* Letrozole *on page 1211*

◆ **Femring** *see* Estradiol (Systemic) *on page 796*

◆ **Fenesin DM IR [OTC]** *see* Guaifenesin and Dextromethorphan *on page 987*

◆ **Fenesin IR [OTC]** *see* GuaiFENesin *on page 984*

Fenoldopam (fe NOL doe pam)

Brand Names: U.S. Corlopam
Therapeutic Category Dopamine Agonist
Generic Availability (U.S.) Yes
Use Short-term reduction in blood pressure (up to 4 hours) [FDA approved in ages <1 month (full term or ≥2 kg) to 12 years and adults]; treatment of severe hypertension (up to 48 hours), including in patients with renal compromise (FDA approved in adults); has also been used for augmentation of urine output and prevention of acute renal injury in critically ill patients (for 24 hours)
Pregnancy Risk Factor B
Pregnancy Considerations Fetal harm was not observed in animal studies; however, safety and efficacy have not been established for use during pregnancy. Use during pregnancy only if clearly needed.
Breast-Feeding Considerations It is not known if fenoldopam is excreted in breast milk. The manufacturer recommends that caution be exercised when administering fenoldopam to nursing women.
Contraindications Hypersensitivity of fenoldopam or any component
Warnings May cause hypokalemia; monitor serum potassium at 6 hour intervals during therapy. Contains sulfites which may cause allergic reaction in susceptible individuals, including anaphylactic symptoms or asthmatic episodes. Fenoldopam contains propylene glycol; toxicities have been reported with use of products containing propylene glycol, including hyperosmolality, lactic acidosis,

seizures, and respiratory depression; in neonates large amounts of propylene glycol delivered orally, intravenously (eg, >3000 mg/day), or topically have been associated with potentially fatal toxicities which can include metabolic acidosis, seizures, renal failure, and CNS depression; use products containing propylene glycol with caution (AAP, 1997; Shehab, 2009).
Precautions Use with caution in patients with glaucoma or intraocular hypertension; dose-dependent increases in intraocular pressure has been reported. A dose-related tachycardia can occur, especially at infusion rates >0.1 mcg/kg/minute; in pediatric patients at doses >0.8 mcg/kg/minute, tachycardia has been shown to persist for at least 4 hours. Close monitoring of blood pressure is necessary; hypotension can occur. For continuous infusion only; no bolus doses. Use caution in patients with increased intracranial pressure; use has not been studied in this population.
Adverse Reactions
Cardiovascular: Angina, bradycardia, chest pain, cutaneous flushing, extrasystoles, heart failure, hypotension, MI, orthostatic hypotension, palpitation, ST-T abnormalities, T-wave inversion, tachycardia
Central nervous system: Anxiety, dizziness, fever, headache, insomnia
Endocrine & metabolic: Hyperglycemia, hypokalemia, LDH increased
Gastrointestinal: Abdominal pain/fullness, constipation, diarrhea, nausea, vomiting
Genitourinary: Urinary tract infection
Hematologic: Bleeding, leukocytosis
Hepatic: Transaminases increased
Local: Injection site reactions
Neuromuscular & skeletal: Back pain, limb cramps
Ocular: Intraocular pressure increased
Renal: BUN increased, creatinine increased, oliguria
Respiratory: Dyspnea, nasal congestion
Miscellaneous: Diaphoresis
Drug Interactions
Metabolism/Transport Effects None known.
Avoid Concomitant Use There are no known interactions where it is recommended to avoid concomitant use.
Increased Effect/Toxicity There are no known significant interactions involving an increase in effect.
Decreased Effect There are no known significant interactions involving a decrease in effect.
Stability Store at 2°C to 30°C (35°F to 86°F). Must be diluted prior to infusion. Following dilution, store at room temperature and use solution within 24 hours.
Mechanism of Action A selective postsynaptic dopamine agonist (D_1-receptors) which exerts hypotensive effects by decreasing peripheral vasculature resistance with increased renal blood flow, diuresis, and natriuresis; 6 times as potent as dopamine in producing renal vasodilatation; has minimal adrenergic effects
Pharmacodynamics
Onset of action: Children: 5 minutes; Adults: 10 minutes; **Note:** Majority of effect of a given infusion rate is attained within 15 minutes.
Duration of effect (after stopping infusion): 30-60 minutes
Pharmacokinetics (Adult data unless noted)
Distribution: V_d: 0.6 L/kg
Metabolism: Hepatic via methylation, glucuronidation, and sulfation; the 8-sulfate metabolite may have some activity; extensive first-pass effect
Half-life, elimination: Children: 3-5 minutes; Adults: ~5 minutes
Elimination: Urine (90%); feces (10%)
Clearance: Children: 3 L/hour/kg

Dosing: Usual I.V.:

Children: Initial: 0.2 mcg/kg/minute; may be increased every 20-30 minutes to 0.3-0.5 mcg/kg/minute; maximum dose: 0.8 mcg/kg/minute (higher doses have been shown to worsen tachycardia without any additional blood pressure benefits)

Adults: Initial: 0.1-0.3 mcg/kg/minute (lower initial doses may be associated with less reflex tachycardia); may be increased in increments of 0.05-0.1 mcg/kg/minute every 15 minutes until target blood pressure is reached; the maximal infusion rate reported in clinical studies was 1.6 mcg/kg/minute

Dosage adjustment for renal impairment: No guidelines are available.

Usual Infusion Concentrations: Pediatric I.V. infusion: 60 mcg/mL

Administration For continuous I.V. infusion using an infusion pump; dilute ampule contents in NS or D$_5$W to a maximum final concentration of 60 mcg/mL for children and 40 mcg/mL for adults.

Monitoring Parameters Blood pressure, heart rate, ECG, renal/hepatic function tests

Additional Information Fenoldopam infusion can be abruptly discontinued or gradually tapered prior to discontinuation.

Dosage Forms Excipient information presented when available (limited, particularly for generics); consult specific product labeling.

Solution, Intravenous:
Corlopam: 10 mg/mL (1 mL); 20 mg/2 mL (2 mL) [contains propylene glycol, sodium metabisulfite]
Generic: 10 mg/mL (1 mL); 20 mg/2 mL (2 mL)

References

American Academy of Pediatrics Committee on Drugs. "Inactive" ingredients in pharmaceutical products: update (subject review). *Pediatrics.* 1997;99(2):268-278.

Hammer GB, Verghese ST, Drover DR, et al, "Pharmacokinetics and Pharmacodynamics of Fenoldopam Mesylate for Blood Pressure Control in Pediatric Patients," *BMC Anesthesiol,* 2008, 8:6.

Moffett BS, Mott AR, Nelson DP, et al, "Renal Effects of Fenoldopam in Critically Ill Pediatric Patients: A Retrospective Review," *Pediatr Crit Care Med,* 2008, 9(4):403-6.

Shehab N, Lewis CL, Streetman DD, Donn SM. Exposure to the pharmaceutical excipients benzyl alcohol and propylene glycol among critically ill neonates. *Pediatr Crit Care Med.* 2009;10 (2):256-259.

◆ **Fenoldopam Mesylate** *see* Fenoldopam *on page 852*

FentaNYL (FEN ta nil)

Medication Safety Issues

Sound-alike/look-alike issues:
FentaNYL may be confused with alfentanil, SUFentanil

High alert medication:
The Institute for Safe Medication Practices (ISMP) includes this medication among its list of drug classes which have a heightened risk of causing significant patient harm when used in error.

Administration issues:
Fentanyl transdermal system patches: Leakage of fentanyl gel from the patch has been reported; patch may be less effective; do not use. Thoroughly wash any skin surfaces coming into direct contact with gel with water (do not use soap). May contain conducting metal (eg, aluminum); remove patch prior to MRI.

Other safety concerns:
Fentanyl transdermal system patches:
Dosing of transdermal fentanyl patches may be confusing. Transdermal fentanyl patches should always be prescribed in mcg/hour, not size. Patch dosage form of Duragesic-12 actually delivers 12.5 mcg/hour of fentanyl. Use caution, as orders may be written as "Duragesic 12.5" which can be erroneously interpreted as a 125 mcg dose.

Patches should be stored and disposed of with care to avoid accidental exposure to children. The FDA has issued numerous safety advisories to warn users of the possible consequences (including hospitalization and death) of inappropriate storage or disposal of patches.

Abstral, Actiq, Fentora, Onsolis, and Subsys are not interchangeable; do not substitute doses on a mcg-per-mcg basis.

Related Information

Opioid Conversion Table *on page 2242*

Oral Medications That Should Not Be Crushed or Altered *on page 2438*

Patient Information for Disposal of Unused Medications *on page 2412*

Preprocedure Sedatives in Children *on page 2402*

Brand Names: U.S. Abstral; Actiq; Duragesic; Fentora; Lazanda; Onsolis; Subsys

Brand Names: Canada Abstral; Actiq; Apo-Fentanyl Matrix; Duragesic; Duragesic MAT; Fentanyl Citrate Injection, USP; Novo-Fentanyl; Onsolis; PMS-Fentanyl MTX; RAN-Fentanyl Matrix Patch; RAN-Fentanyl Transdermal System; ratio-Fentanyl; Sandoz Fentanyl Patch; Teva-Fentanyl

Therapeutic Category Analgesic, Narcotic; General Anesthetic

Generic Availability (U.S.) Yes: Injection, lozenge, patch

Use

Parenteral: Relief of pain; preoperative medication; adjunct to general or regional anesthesia (FDA approved in ages ≥2 years and adults); has also been used for sedation and intranasally for analgesia

Transdermal patch (Duragesic®): Treatment of persistent, moderate-to-severe chronic pain in opioid-tolerant patients who are currently receiving opioids (FDA approved in ages ≥2 years and adults); see **Note**

Transmucosal products:

Buccal film (Onsolis®): Breakthrough cancer pain in opioid-tolerant patients who are currently receiving around-the-clock opioids for persistent cancer pain (FDA approved in ≥18 years and adults); see **Note**

Buccal tablet (Fentora®): Breakthrough cancer pain in opioid-tolerant patients who are currently receiving around-the-clock opioids for persistent cancer pain (FDA approved in ≥18 years and adults); see **Note**

Nasal spray (Lazanda®): Breakthrough cancer pain in opioid-tolerant patients who are currently receiving around-the-clock opioids for persistent cancer pain (FDA approved in ≥18 years and adults); see **Note**

Oral lozenge (Actiq®): Breakthrough cancer pain in opioid-tolerant patients who are currently receiving around-the-clock opioids for persistent cancer pain (FDA approved in ages ≥16 years and adults); see **Note**

Sublingual spray (Subsys®): Breakthrough cancer pain in opioid-tolerant patients who are currently receiving around-the-clock opioids for persistent cancer pain (FDA approved in ≥18 years and adults); see **Note**

Sublingual tablet (Abstral®): Breakthrough cancer pain in opioid-tolerant patients who are currently receiving around-the-clock opioids for persistent cancer pain (FDA approved in ≥18 years and adults); see **Note**

Note: Patients are considered opioid-tolerant if they are receiving around-the-clock opioids at a dose of at least 60 mg/day of morphine, 25 mcg/hour of transdermal fentanyl, 30 mg/day of oral oxycodone, 8 mg/day of oral hydromorphone, or an equivalent dose of another opioid for 1 week or longer.

Prescribing and Access Restrictions As a requirement of the REMS program, access is restricted.

Transmucosal immediate-release fentanyl products (eg, sublingual tablets and spray, oral lozenges, buccal tablets and soluble film, nasal spray) are only available through the Transmucosal Immediate-Release Fentanyl (TIRF) REMS ACCESS program. Enrollment in the program is required for outpatients, prescribers for outpatient use, pharmacies (inpatient and outpatient), and distributors. Enrollment is not required for inpatient administration (eg, hospitals, hospices, long-term care facilities), inpatients, and prescribers who prescribe to inpatients. Further information is available at 1-866-822-1483 or at www.TIRFREMSaccess.com

Note: Effective December, 2011, individual REMs programs for TIRF products were combined into a single access program (TIRF REMS Access). Prescribers and pharmacies that were enrolled in at least one individual REMS program for these products will automatically be transitioned to the single access program.

Medication Guide Available Yes

Pregnancy Risk Factor C

Pregnancy Considerations Adverse events were observed in some animal reproduction studies. Fentanyl crosses the placenta.

Fentanyl injection may be used for the management of pain during labor (ACOG, 2002). When used for pain relief during labor, opioids may temporarily affect the heart rate of the fetus (ACOG, 2002). Transient muscular rigidity has been observed in the neonate with fentanyl; symptoms of respiratory or neurological depression were not different than those observed in infants of untreated mothers.

If chronic opioid exposure occurs in pregnancy, adverse events in the newborn (including withdrawal) may occur; monitoring of the neonate is recommended. The minimum effective dose should be used if opioids are needed (Chou, 2009). Symptoms characteristic of neonatal abstinence syndrome have been observed following chronic fentanyl use in pregnant women. Neonatal abstinence syndrome following opioid exposure may present with autonomic (eg, fever, temperature instability), gastrointestinal (eg, diarrhea, vomiting, poor feeding/weight gain), or neurologic (eg, high pitched crying, increased muscle tone, irritability, seizure, tremor) symptoms (Dow, 2012; Hudak, 2012).

Transdermal patch, transmucosal lozenge, nasal spray (Lazanda), sublingual tablet, sublingual spray (Subsys), buccal tablet (Fentora), and buccal film (Onsolis) are not recommended for analgesia during labor and delivery.

Breast-Feeding Considerations Fentanyl is excreted in low concentrations into breast milk and breast-feeding is not recommended by the manufacturers.

Parenteral opioids used during labor have the potential to interfere with a newborn's natural reflex to nurse within the first few hours after birth. When needed, a short-acting opioid, such as fentanyl, is preferred for women who will be nursing (Montgomery, 2012)

Breast-feeding is considered acceptable following single doses to the mother; however, limited information is available when used long-term (Spigset, 2000). Nursing infants exposed to large doses of opioids should be monitored for apnea and sedation (Montgomery, 2012).

Note: Transdermal patch, transmucosal lozenge, sublingual tablet, sublingual spray (Subsys), buccal tablet (Fentora), and buccal film (Onsolis) are not recommended in nursing women due to potential for sedation and/or respiratory depression.

Contraindications Hypersensitivity or intolerance to fentanyl, other opioid agonists, or any component
Additional product-specific contraindications:
Transdermal patches (eg, Duragesic): Severe respiratory disease or depression including acute asthma (unless patient is mechanically ventilated); paralytic ileus; patients requiring short-term therapy; management of

pain following outpatient or day surgery, intermittent pain, or mild pain
Transdermal patches (eg, Duragesic) and transmucosal products [buccal film (eg, Onsolis), buccal tablets (Fentora), lozenges (eg, Actiq), nasal spray (Lazanda), sublingual spray (Subsys), sublingual tablet (Abstral)]: Additional contraindications: Patients who are not opioid-tolerant (see **Note** in Use field) and in the management of acute or postoperative pain (including headache, migraine, or dental pain). Abstral and Onsolis are also contraindicated for acute pain management in the emergency room.

Warnings High potential for abuse; physical and psychological dependence may occur with prolonged use [**U.S. Boxed Warning**]; abrupt discontinuation may result in withdrawal or seizures; potent opioids have a high risk of fatal overdose due to respiratory depression. Symptoms of opioid withdrawal may occur in patients after conversion of one dosage form to another or after dosage adjustment. With prolonged use, taper dose to prevent withdrawal symptoms. Neonates who receive a total fentanyl dose >1.6 mg/kg or continuous infusion duration >5 days are more likely to develop opioid withdrawal symptoms; for infants and children 1 week to 22 months of age, those who receive a total dose of 1.5 mg/kg or duration >5 days have a 50% chance of developing opioid withdrawal and those receiving a total dose >2.5 mg/kg or duration of infusion >9 days have a 100% chance of developing withdrawal. Use with CYP3A4 inhibitors may result in increased effects and potentially fatal respiratory depression [**U.S. Boxed Warning**]. Use with alcohol and other CNS depressants may increase risk of respiratory depression, hypotension, sedation or coma; dosage reduction may be needed.

Dosage form specific warnings:

Parenteral: Rapid I.V. infusion may result in skeletal muscle and chest wall rigidity, impaired ventilation, respiratory distress, apnea, bronchoconstriction, laryngospasm; inject slowly over 3-5 minutes; nondepolarizing skeletal muscle relaxant may be required

Transdermal patch: May cause potentially life-threatening hypoventilation, respiratory depression, and/or death [**U.S. Boxed Warning**]; should only be prescribed for opioid-tolerant patients. Transdermal patch is contraindicated in the management of short-term analgesia, in the management of postoperative pain, and in patients who are opioid-nontolerant; should only be prescribed by healthcare professionals who are knowledgeable in the use of potent opioids in the management of chronic pain [**U.S. Boxed Warning**]. Monitor closely for respiratory depression during use, particularly during first two applications after initiation of therapy or after dose increases [**U.S. Boxed Warning**]. Use in pediatric patients **only** if they are opioid-tolerant, receiving at least 60 mg oral morphine equivalents per day, and ≥2 years of age. Patients should be monitored carefully, especially 24-72 hours after initial patch application (when peak fentanyl serum levels occur) and following increases in dosage. Monitor patients who experience adverse reactions for at least 24 hours after removal of the patch (apparent transdermal half-life is 17 hours).

Accidental exposure may lead to severe respiratory depression, including death, in children and adults; proper procedures for handling and disposal of patches should be followed [**U.S. Boxed Warning**]. Keep used and unused patches out of the reach of children. Avoid unclothed/unwashed application site exposure, inadvertent person-to-person patch transfer (eg, while hugging), incidental exposure (eg, sharing same bed, sitting on patch), intentional exposure (eg, chewing, swallowing), or accidental exposure by caregivers when applying/removing patch.

Avoid exposure of application site and surrounding area to direct external heat sources. Patients who experience fever or increase in core body temperature should be monitored closely **[U.S. Boxed Warning]**; serum fentanyl concentrations may increase by approximately one-third for patients with a body temperature of 40°C (104°F) secondary to a temperature-dependent increase in fentanyl release from the patch and increased skin permeability. Transdermal patch should be applied only to intact skin. Use of a patch that has been cut, damaged, or altered in any way may result in potentially fatal overdosage. Transdermal patch may contain conducting metal (eg, aluminum) which may cause a burn to the skin during an MRI scan; remove patch prior to MRI; reapply patch after scan is completed. Due to the potential for altered electrical conductivity, remove transdermal patch before cardioversion or defibrillation.

Transmucosal products:

Buccal film (Onsolis®): May cause potentially life-threatening hypoventilation, respiratory depression, and/or death **[U.S. Boxed Warning]**; should only be prescribed for opioid-tolerant patients; risk of respiratory depression increased in elderly patients, debilitated patients, and patients with conditions associated with hypoxia or hypercapnia; usually occurs after administration of initial dose in nontolerant patients or when given with other drugs that depress respiratory function. Use is contraindicated in the management of acute or postoperative pain and in opioid-nontolerant patients **[U.S. Boxed Warning]**. Should be used only for the care of opioid-tolerant cancer patients with breakthrough pain and is intended for use by specialists who are knowledgeable in treating cancer pain **[U.S. Boxed Warning]**. Due to the risk for misuse, abuse, and overdose, Onsolis® is available only through a restricted distribution program, called the FOCUS Program **[U.S. Boxed Warning]**. Substantial differences exist in the pharmacokinetic profile of fentanyl products; do not convert patients on a mcg-per-mcg basis from one fentanyl product to another fentanyl product; the substitution of one fentanyl product for another fentanyl product may result in a fatal overdose **[U.S. Boxed Warning]**; appropriate dosage adjustments must be made; use caution and monitor closely when changing patients from one product to another. Patients using Onsolis® who experience breakthrough pain must wait at least 2 hours before taking another dose **[U.S. Boxed Warning]**. Preparation contains an amount of medication that can be fatal to children; keep all used and unused products out of the reach of children at all times and discard products properly **[U.S. Boxed Warning]**; patients and caregivers should be counseled on the dangers to children including the risk of exposure to partially consumed products.

Buccal tablet (Fentora®): May cause potentially life-threatening hypoventilation, respiratory depression, and/or death **[U.S. Boxed Warning]**; should only be prescribed for opioid-tolerant patients; risk of respiratory depression increased in elderly patients, debilitated patients, and patients with conditions associated with hypoxia or hypercapnia; usually occurs after administration of initial dose in nontolerant patients or when given with other drugs that depress respiratory function. Use is contraindicated in the management of acute or postoperative pain (including headache/migraine) and in opioid-nontolerant patients **[U.S. Boxed Warning]**. Should be used only for the care of opioid-tolerant cancer patients with breakthrough pain and is intended for use by specialists who are knowledgeable in treating

cancer pain **[U.S. Boxed Warning]**. Due to the risk for misuse, abuse, and overdose, Fentora® is available only through a restricted distribution program, called the FENTORA REMS program **[U.S. Boxed Warning]**. Substantial differences exist in the pharmacokinetic profile of fentanyl products; do not convert patients on a mcg-per-mcg basis from one fentanyl product to another fentanyl product; the substitution of one fentanyl product for another fentanyl product may result in a fatal overdose **[U.S. Boxed Warning]**; appropriate dosage adjustments must be made; use caution and monitor closely when changing patients from one product to another. Patients using Fentora® who experience breakthrough pain may only take **one** additional dose (if pain not relieved after 30 minutes) using the same strength tablet and must wait 4 hours before taking another dose **[U.S. Boxed Warning]**. Preparation contains an amount of medication that can be fatal to children; keep all used and unused products out of the reach of children at all times and discard products properly **[U.S. Boxed Warning]**; patients and caregivers should be counseled on the dangers to children including the risk of exposure to partially consumed products.

Nasal spray (Lazanda®): May cause potentially life-threatening hypoventilation, respiratory depression, and/or death **[U.S. Boxed Warning]**; should be used only for opioid-tolerant patients; risk of respiratory depression increased in elderly patients, debilitated patients, and patients with conditions associated with hypoxia or hypercapnia; usually occurs after administration of initial dose in nontolerant patients or when given with other drugs that depress respiratory function. Use is contraindicated in opioid nontolerant patients or in the management of acute or postoperative pain, including headache/migraine, dental pain, or use in the emergency room **[U.S. Boxed Warning]**. Should be used only for the care of opioid-tolerant cancer patients with breakthrough pain and is intended for use by specialists who are knowledgeable in treating cancer pain **[U.S. Boxed Warning]**. Due to the risk for misuse, abuse, and overdose, Lazanda® is available only through a restricted distribution program, called the Lazanda® REMS program **[U.S. Boxed Warning]**. Substantial differences exist in the pharmacokinetic profile of fentanyl products; do not convert patients on a mcg-per-mcg basis from one fentanyl product to another fentanyl product; the substitution of one fentanyl product for another fentanyl product may result in a fatal overdose **[U.S. Boxed Warning]**; appropriate dosage adjustments must be made; use caution and monitor closely when changing patients from one product to another. Patients using Lazanda® must begin therapy with a 100 mcg dose and titrate, if needed; during therapy, patients must wait at least 2 hours before taking another dose of nasal spray. Preparation contains an amount of medication that can be fatal to children; keep all used and unused products out of the reach of children at all times and discard products properly **[U.S. Boxed Warning]**; patients and caregivers should be counseled on the dangers to children including the risk of exposure to partially consumed products

Oral lozenge (Actiq®): May cause potentially life-threatening hypoventilation, respiratory depression, and/or death **[U.S. Boxed Warning]**; should be used only for opioid-tolerant patients; risk of respiratory depression increased in elderly patients, debilitated patients, and patients with conditions associated with hypoxia or hypercapnia; usually occurs after administration of initial dose in nontolerant patients or when given with other drugs that depress respiratory function.

Use is contraindicated in opioid-nontolerant patients or in the management of acute or postoperative pain, including headache/migraine, dental pain, or use in the emergency room **[U.S. Boxed Warning]**. Should be used only for the care of opioid-tolerant cancer patients with breakthrough pain and is intended for use by specialists who are knowledgeable in treating cancer pain **[U.S. Boxed Warning]**. Due to the risk for misuse, abuse, and overdose, Actiq® is available only through a restricted distribution program, called the ACTIQ® REMS program **[U.S. Boxed Warning]**. Substantial differences exist in the pharmacokinetic profile of fentanyl products; do not convert patients on a mcg-per-mcg basis from one fentanyl product to another fentanyl product; the substitution of one fentanyl product for another fentanyl product may result in a fatal overdose **[U.S. Boxed Warning]**; appropriate dosage adjustments must be made; use caution and monitor closely when changing patients from one product to another. Patients using Actiq® must begin therapy with an initial dose of 200 mcg and titrate, if needed; during therapy, patients must wait at least 4 hours before taking another dose of the same strength. Preparation contains an amount of medication that can be fatal to children; keep all used and unused products out of the reach of children at all times and discard products properly **[U.S. Boxed Warning]**; patients and caregivers should be counseled on the dangers to children including the risk of exposure to partially consumed products. Safety and efficacy have not been established for patients <16 years of age; 15 opioid-tolerant pediatric patients (age: 5-15 years) with breakthrough pain were treated with Actiq® in a clinical study; 12 of the 15 patients received doses of 200 mcg to 600 mcg; no conclusions about safety and efficacy could be drawn due to the small sample size.

Sublingual spray (Subsys®): May cause potentially life-threatening hypoventilation, respiratory depression, and/or death **[U.S. Boxed Warning]**; should be used only for opioid-tolerant patients; risk of respiratory depression increased in elderly patients, debilitated patients, and patients with conditions associated with hypoxia or hypercapnia; usually occurs after administration of initial dose in nontolerant patients or when given with other drugs that depress respiratory function. Use is contraindicated in opioid-nontolerant patients or in the management of acute or postoperative pain, including headache/migraine **[U.S. Boxed Warning]**. Should be used only for the care of opioid-tolerant cancer patients with breakthrough pain and is intended for use by specialists who are knowledgeable in treating cancer pain **[U.S. Boxed Warning]**. Due to the risk for misuse, abuse, and overdose, Subsys® is available only through a restricted distribution program, called the TIRF REMS ACCESS program **[U.S. Boxed Warning]**. Substantial differences exist in the pharmacokinetic profile of fentanyl products; do not convert patients on a mcg-per-mcg basis from one fentanyl product to another fentanyl product; the substitution of one fentanyl product for another fentanyl product may result in a fatal overdose **[U.S. Boxed Warning]**; appropriate dosage adjustments must be made; use caution and monitor closely when changing patients from one product to another. Patients using Subsys® must begin therapy with an initial dose of 100 mcg and titrate, if needed; during therapy, patients must wait at least 4 hours before taking another dose of the same strength. Preparation contains an amount of medication that can be fatal to children; keep all used and unused products out of the reach of children at all times and discard products properly **[U.S. Boxed Warning]**; patients and caregivers should be counseled on the dangers to

children including the risk of exposure to partially consumed products. Cancer patients with oral mucositis experienced increased fentanyl exposure following sublingual spray administration; avoid use in patients with grade 2 or higher mucositis; use with caution in patients with grade 1 mucositis, and closely monitor for respiratory and CNS depression.

Sublingual tablet (Abstral®): May cause potentially life-threatening hypoventilation, respiratory depression, and/or death **[U.S. Boxed Warning]**; should be used only for opioid-tolerant patients; risk of respiratory depression increased in elderly patients, debilitated patients, and patients with conditions associated with hypoxia or hypercapnia; usually occurs after administration of initial dose in nontolerant patients or when given with other drugs that depress respiratory function. Use is contraindicated in opioid-nontolerant patients or in the management of acute or postoperative pain **[U.S. Boxed Warning]**. Should be used only for the care of opioid-tolerant cancer patients with breakthrough pain and is intended for use by specialists who are knowledgeable in treating cancer pain **[U.S. Boxed Warning]**. Due to the risk for misuse, abuse, and overdose, Subsys® is available only through a restricted distribution program, called the ABSTRAL REMS program **[U.S. Boxed Warning]**. Substantial differences exist in the pharmacokinetic profile of fentanyl products; do not convert patients on a mcg-per-mcg basis from one fentanyl product to another fentanyl product; the substitution of one fentanyl product for another fentanyl product may result in a fatal overdose **[U.S. Boxed Warning]**; appropriate dosage adjustments must be made; use caution and monitor closely when changing patients from one product to another. Patients using Subsys® must begin therapy with an initial dose of 100 mcg and titrate, if needed; during therapy, patients must wait at least 2 hours before taking another dose of the same strength. Preparation contains an amount of medication that can be fatal to children; keep all used and unused products out of the reach of children at all times and discard products properly **[U.S. Boxed Warning]**; patients and caregivers should be counseled on the dangers to children including the risk of exposure to partially consumed products.

Precautions Use with extreme caution in patients with bradycardia; hepatic, biliary tract, renal, or respiratory disease; acute pancreatitis; cor pulmonale; significant COPD; other chronic respiratory conditions; or those with increased ICP, head injuries, or impaired consciousness. Patients must be monitored until fully recovered; decrease dose in patients with hepatic and/or renal disease; not recommended if patient received MAO inhibitors within 14 days. Use transdermal patch with caution in cachectic or debilitated patients; these patients may have altered pharmacokinetics due to muscle wasting, poor fat stores, or altered clearance. Frequent use of Actiq® or generic lozenge may increase risk of dental caries; Actiq® and generic lozenge contain 2 g of sugar/unit, as hydrated dextrates; patients should maintain good oral hygiene; inform diabetic patients of sugar content. Use buccal tablets with caution in patients with mucositis (no dose adjustment is needed in patients with Grade I mucositis; safety and efficacy in patients with more severe mucositis have not been studied).

Fentanyl is not recommended for analgesia during labor and delivery; transient muscular rigidity has been observed in neonates born to women who were treated with I.V. fentanyl

Adverse Reactions
Cardiovascular: Bradycardia, cardiac arrhythmia, cardiorespiratory arrest, chest pain, DVT, edema, flushing, hyper-/hypotension, orthostatic hypotension, pallor,

palpitation, peripheral edema, sinus tachycardia, syncope, tachycardia, vasodilation

Central nervous system: Abnormal dreams, abnormal thinking, agitation, amnesia, anxiety, attention disturbance, chills, CNS depression, confusion, depression, disorientation, dizziness, drowsiness, dysphoria, euphoria, fatigue, fever, hallucinations, headache, hypoesthesia, insomnia, irritability, lethargy, malaise, mental status change, migraine, nervousness, paranoid reaction, restlessness, sedation, somnolence, stupor, vertigo

Dermatologic: Alopecia, bruising, cellulitis, decubitus ulcer, erythema, hyperhidrosis, papules, pruritus, rash

Endocrine & metabolic: Breast pain, dehydration, hot flashes, hyper-/hypocalcemia, hyper-/hypoglycemia, hypoalbuminemia, hypokalemia, hypomagnesemia, hyponatremia

Gastrointestinal: Abdominal distension, abdominal pain, abnormal taste, anorexia, appetite decreased, biliary tract spasm, constipation, diarrhea, dyspepsia, dysphagia (buccal tablet/film/sublingual spray), flatulence, gastritis, gastroenteritis, gastroesophageal reflux, GI hemorrhage, gingival pain (buccal tablet), gingivitis (lozenge), glossitis (lozenge), hematemesis, ileus, intestinal obstruction (buccal film), nausea, periodontal abscess (lozenge/buccal tablet), proctalgia, stomatitis (lozenge/buccal tablet/sublingual tablet/sublingual spray), tongue disorder (sublingual tablet), ulceration (gingival, lip, mouth; transmucosal use/nasal spray), vomiting, weight loss, xerostomia

Genitourinary: Dysuria, erectile dysfunction, urinary incontinence, urinary retention, urinary tract infection, vaginitis, vaginal hemorrhage

Hematologic: Anemia, leukopenia, neutropenia, thrombocytopenia

Hepatic: Alkaline phosphatase increased, ascites, AST increased, jaundice

Local: Application-site erythema/irritation/pain

Neuromuscular & skeletal: Abnormal coordination, abnormal gait, arthralgia, back pain, Chest wall rigidity (high dose I.V.), limb pain, muscle rigidity, myalgia, neuropathy, paresthesia, rigors, tremor, weakness

Ocular: Blurred vision, diplopia, dry eye, miosis, swelling, ptosis, strabismus

Renal: Renal failure

Respiratory: Apnea, asthma, bronchitis, cough, dyspnea (exertional), epistaxis, hemoptysis, hypoventilation, hypoxia, laryngitis, nasal congestion (nasal spray), nasal discomfort (nasal spray), nasopharyngitis, pharyngolaryngeal pain, pharyngitis, pneumonia, postnasal drip (nasal spray), pulmonary embolism (nasal spray), respiratory depression, rhinitis, rhinorrhea (nasal spray), sinusitis, upper respiratory infection, wheezing

Miscellaneous: Diaphoresis, flu-like syndrome, hiccups, hypersensitivity, lymphadenopathy, night sweats, parosmia, speech disorder, withdrawal syndrome

Rare but important or life-threatening: Amblyopia, allergic reaction, anaphylaxis, angina, aphasia, bladder pain, bronchospasm, CNS excitation or delirium, depersonalization, dysesthesia, emotional lability, esophageal stenosis, exfoliative dermatitis, fecal impaction, gum line erosion (lozenge), gum hemorrhage (lozenge), hematuria, hostility, hyper-/hypotonia, laryngospasm, myasthenia, nocturia, oliguria, pancytopenia, paradoxical dizziness, physical and psychological dependence with prolonged use, pleural effusion, polyuria, pustules, speech disorder, stertorous breathing, seizure, tooth loss (lozenge), urinary tract spasm, urticaria, vertigo

Drug Interactions

Metabolism/Transport Effects Substrate of CYP3A4 (major); **Note:** Assignment of Major/Minor substrate status based on clinically relevant drug interaction potential; **Inhibits** CYP3A4 (weak)

Avoid Concomitant Use
Avoid concomitant use of FentaNYL with any of the following: Azelastine (Nasal); Conivaptan; Crizotinib; Enzalutamide; Fusidic Acid (Systemic); MAO Inhibitors; Mifepristone; Paraldehyde; Pimozide; Thalidomide

Increased Effect/Toxicity
FentaNYL may increase the levels/effects of: Alcohol (Ethyl); Alvimopan; ARIPiprazole; Azelastine (Nasal); Beta-Blockers; Buprenorphine; Calcium Channel Blockers (Nondihydropyridine); CNS Depressants; Desmopressin; Diuretics; Dofetilide; Hydrocodone; Lomitapide; MAO Inhibitors; Methotrimeprazine; Metyrosine; Mirtazapine; Paraldehyde; Pimozide; Pramipexole; ROPINIRole; Rotigotine; Selective Serotonin Reuptake Inhibitors; Thalidomide; Zolpidem

The levels/effects of FentaNYL may be increased by: Amphetamines; Anticholinergic Agents; Antipsychotic Agents (Phenothiazines); Brimonidine (Topical); Cannabis; Conivaptan; Crizotinib; CYP3A4 Inhibitors (Moderate); CYP3A4 Inhibitors (Strong); Dasatinib; Doxylamine; Dronabinol; Droperidol; Fusidic Acid (Systemic); HydrOXYzine; Ivacaftor; Kava Kava; Luliconazole; Magnesium Sulfate; Methotrimeprazine; Mifepristone; Nabilone; Perampanel; Rufinamide; Simeprevir; Sodium Oxybate; Stiripentol; Succinylcholine; Tapentadol; Tetrahydrocannabinol

Decreased Effect
FentaNYL may decrease the levels/effects of: Ioflupane I 123; Pegvisomant

The levels/effects of FentaNYL may be decreased by: Alpha-/Beta-Agonists (Indirect-Acting); Alpha1-Agonists; Ammonium Chloride; CYP3A4 Inducers (Strong); Enzalutamide; Mixed Agonist / Antagonist Opioids; Naltrexone; St Johns Wort

Food Interactions Fentanyl concentrations may be increased by grapefruit juice. Management: Avoid concurrent intake of large quantities (>1 quart/day) of grapefruit juice.

Stability

Injection formulation: Store at 20°C to 25°C (66°F to 77°F); protect from light.

Nasal spray: Do not store above 25°C (77°F); do not freeze. Protect from light. Bottle should be stored in the provided child-resistant container when not in use and kept out of reach of children at all times.

Transdermal patch: Do not store above 25°C (77°F). Store in protective pouch until ready to use. Keep out of reach of children.

Transmucosal buccal film, buccal tablets, oral lozenge, sublingual spray, sublingual tablet: Store at 20°C to 25°C (68°F to 77°F); protect from freezing and moisture. Store in original child-resistant blister packaging until ready to use; do not use if blister package has been opened. Keep out of reach of children.

Mechanism of Action Binds with stereospecific receptors at many sites within the CNS, increases pain threshold, alters pain reception, inhibits ascending pain pathways

Pharmacodynamics Respiratory depressant effect may last longer than analgesic effect

Onset of action: Analgesia:
I.M.: 7-8 minutes
Intranasal: Children 3-12 years: 5-10 minutes (Borland, 2002)
I.V.: Almost immediate
Transdermal patch (initial placement): 6 hours
Transmucosal: 5-15 minutes

Maximum effect:
Transdermal patch (initial placement): 24 hours
Transmucosal: 15-30 minutes

Duration:
I.M.: 1-2 hours
I.V.: 0.5-1 hour

Transdermal patch (removal of patch/no placement): 17 hours

Transmucosal: Related to blood level; respiratory depressant effect may last longer than analgesic effect

Pharmacokinetics (Adult data unless noted) Note:
Fentanyl serum concentrations are ~twofold higher in children 1.5-5 years old who are not opioid-tolerant and are receiving the transdermal patch. Pharmacokinetic parameters in older pediatric patients are similar to adults.

Absorption:
Transdermal: Drug is released at a nearly constant rate from the transdermal matrix system into the skin, where it accumulates; this results in a depot of fentanyl in the outer layer of the skin. Fentanyl is absorbed into the systemic circulation from the depot. This results in a gradual increase in serum concentrations over the first 12-24 hours, followed by a fairly constant concentration for the remainder of the dosing interval. Absorption is decreased in cachectic patients (compared to normal size patients). Pharmacokinetics of transdermal patch with or without Bioclusive™ overlay (polyurethane film dressing) were bioequivalent. Exposure to external heat increases drug absorption from patch.

Transmucosal:
Buccal film and buccal tablet: Rapid; ~50% from the buccal mucosa; 50% swallowed with saliva and slowly absorbed from GI tract

Transmucosal lozenge: Rapid; ~25% absorbed from buccal mucosa; 75% swallowed with saliva and slowly absorbed from GI tract

Distribution: Highly lipophilic, redistributes into muscle and fat; crosses placenta; Note: I.V. fentanyl exhibits a 3-compartment distribution model. Changes in blood pH may alter ionization of fentanyl and affect its distribution between plasma and CNS

V_{dss}: Children: 0.05-14 years of age (after long-term continuous infusion): ~15 L/kg (range: 5-30 L/kg)

V_{dss}: Adults: 4-6 L/kg

Protein binding: 80% to 85%, primarily to alpha-1-acid glycoprotein; also binds to albumin and erythrocytes; Note: Free fraction increases with acidosis

Metabolism: >90% metabolized in the liver via cytochrome P450 isoenzyme CYP3A4 by N-dealkylation (to norfentanyl) and hydroxylation to other inactive metabolites

Bioavailability: Note: Comparative studies have found the buccal film to have a 40% greater systemic exposure (ie, AUC) than the transmucosal lozenge, and the buccal tablet to have a 30% to 50% greater exposure than the transmucosal lozenge

Buccal film: 71% (mucositis did not have a clinically significant effect on peak concentration and AUC; however, bioavailability is expected to decrease if film is inappropriately chewed and swallowed)

Buccal tablet: 65%

Oral lozenge: 47%

Sublingual spray: 76%

Sublingual tablet: 54%

Half-life:
I.V.:
Pediatric patients 5 months to 4.5 years: 2.4 hours

Pediatric patients 6 months to 14 years (after long-term continuous infusion): ~21 hours (range: 11-36 hours)

Adults: 2-4 hours; Note: Using a 3-compartment model, fentanyl displayed an initial distribution half-life of 6 minutes; second distribution half-life of 1 hour and terminal half-life of 16 hours

Transdermal patch: 17 hours (range: 13-22 hours, apparent half-life is influenced by extended absorption)

Transmucosal products: 3-14 hours (dose-dependent)

Buccal film: ~14 hours

Buccal tablet: 100-200 mcg: 3-4 hours; 400-800 mcg: 11-12 hours

Nasal spray: 15-25 hours (based on a multiple-dose pharmacokinetic study when doses are administered in the same nostril and separated by a 1-, 2-, or 4-hour time lapse)

Time to peak serum concentration:
Transdermal patch: 24-72 hours, after several sequential 72-hour applications, steady state serum concentrations are reached

Transmucosal products:
Buccal film: Median: 1 hour (range: 0.75-4 hours)

Buccal tablet: Median: 47 minutes (range: 20-240 minutes)

Nasal spray: Median: 15-21 minutes

Oral lozenge: Median: 20-40 minutes (range: 20-480 minutes), measured after the start of dose administration

Sublingual spray: Median: 90 minutes (range: 10-120 minutes)

Sublingual tablet: Median: 30-60 minutes (range: 15-240 minutes)

Elimination: Urine 75% (primarily as metabolites, <7% to 10% as unchanged drug); feces ~9%

Clearance: Newborn infants: Clearance may be significantly correlated to gestational age and birth weight (Saarenmaa, 2000)

Dosing: Neonatal Note: Doses should be titrated to appropriate effects; wide range of doses exist, dependent upon desired degree of analgesia/anesthesia, clinical environment, patient's status, and presence of opioid tolerance. Lower initial doses are recommended for nonventilated patients (WHO, 2012).

Analgesia: Limited data available:
International Evidence-Based Group for Neonatal Pain recommendations (Anand, 2001): Opioid-naive:
Intermittent doses: Slow I.V. push: 0.5-3 mcg/kg/dose

Continuous I.V. infusion: 0.5-2 mcg/kg/**hour**

WHO Guidelines for Pediatric Pain (WHO, 2012): Opioid-naive:
Intermittent doses: Slow I.V. push: Initial: 1-2 mcg/kg/dose; may repeat every 2-4 hours, titrate dose to effectiveness

Continuous I.V. infusion: Initial I.V. bolus: Slow I.V. push: 1-2 mcg/kg, then 0.5-1 mcg/kg/**hour**; titrate upward; usual range: 1-3 mcg/kg/**hour**

Alternate dosing: Intermittent doses: Some centers have used the following: Slow I.V. push: 1-4 mcg/kg/dose; may repeat every 2-4 hours (Nelson, 1996)

Continuous analgesia/sedation; mechanically ventilated patient: Limited data available: Initial I.V. bolus: 1-2 mcg/kg, then 0.5-1 mcg/kg/**hour**; titrate carefully to effect. Dosing based on a trial of 20 neonates ventilated for respiratory distress syndrome; mean required dose was age-dependent: GA <34 weeks (n=12): 0.64 mcg/kg/**hour** and for GA ≥34 weeks (n=8): 0.75 mcg/kg/**hour** (Roth, 1991).

Continuous analgesia/sedation during ECMO: Limited data available: Initial I.V. bolus: 5-10 mcg/kg slow I.V. push over 10 minutes, then 1-5 mcg/kg/**hour**; titrate carefully to effect; tolerance may develop; higher doses (up to 20 mcg/kg/**hour**) may be needed by day 6 of ECMO (Arnold, 1991; Leuschen, 1993).

Endotracheal intubation: Limited data available: I.V.: 1-4 mcg/kg slow I.V. push (Cloherty, 2012; Kumar, 2010)

Dosing: Usual Note: Doses should be titrated to appropriate effects; wide range of doses exist, dependent upon desired degree of analgesia/anesthesia, clinical environment, patient's status, and presence of opioid tolerance.

Infants and Children:
Acute pain: I.V.: Opioid-naive:
Infants: Limited data available: Initial: 1-2 mcg/kg/dose; may repeat at 2-4 hour intervals; in opioid-tolerant or younger infants, titration to higher doses may be

required (up to 4 mcg/kg/dose) (Hegenbarth, 2008; Nelson, 1996; WHO, 2012)

Children: Limited data available in children <2 years: Initial: 1-2 mcg/kg/dose; may repeat at 30- to 60-minute intervals; in opioid-tolerant children, titration to higher doses may be required (Hegenbarth, 2008; Nelson, 1996; WHO, 2012)

Analgesia for minor procedures/sedation: Limited data available in children <2 years:

I.M., I.V.: 1-2 mcg/kg/dose; administer 3 minutes before the procedure; maximum dose: 50 mcg; may repeat ¹/₂ original dose every 3-5 minutes if necessary; titrate to effect (Cramton, 2012; Krauss, 2006; Zeltzer, 1990)

Intranasal (using parenteral preparation): Limited data available: Infants and Children ≥10 kg: 1.5 mcg/kg once (maximum: 100 mcg/dose); reported range: 1-2 mcg/kg; some studies that used an initial dose of 1.5 mcg/kg allowed for additional incremental doses of 0.3-0.5 mcg/kg to be administered every 5 minutes, not to exceed a total dose of 3 mcg/kg depending on pain type and severity (Borland, 2002; Borland, 2005; Borland, 2007; Chung, 2010; Cole, 2009; Crellin, 2010; Herd, 2009; Manjushree, 2002; Saunders, 2010)

Anesthesia, adjunct: I.M., I.V.: Children 2-12 years: 2-3 mcg/kg/ dose

Continuous analgesia/sedation: Limited data available in children <2 years: Initial I.V. bolus: 1-2 mcg/kg then 1 mcg/kg/**hour**; titrate to effect; usual: 1-3 mcg/kg/**hour**; some require 5 mcg/kg/**hour** (WHO, 2012)

Chronic pain, moderate to severe: Transdermal patch: Children ≥2 years who are opioid-tolerant receiving at least 60 mg oral morphine equivalents per day: Initial: 25 mcg/**hour** system or higher, based on conversion to fentanyl equivalents and administration of equianalgesic dosage (see package insert for further information); use short-acting analgesics for first 24 hours with supplemental PRN doses thereafter (for breakthrough pain); dose may be increased after 3 days, based on the daily dose of supplementary PRN opioids required; use the ratio of 45 mg of oral morphine equivalents per day to a 12.5 mcg/**hour** increase in transdermal patch dosage; change patch every 72 hours; **Note:** Dosing intervals less than every 72 hours are **not** recommended for children and adolescents. Initiation of the transdermal patch in children taking <60 mg of oral morphine equivalents per day has not been studied in controlled clinical trials; in open-label trials, children 2-18 years of age who were receiving at least 45 mg of oral morphine equivalents per day were started with an initial transdermal dose of 25 mcg/**hour** (or higher, depending upon equianalgesic dose of opioid received).

Endotracheal intubation, emergent: Limited data available: I.V.: 1-5 mcg/kg/dose (Hegenbarth, 2008)

Patient-controlled analgesia (PCA): Limited data available: I.V.: Children ≥5 years; opioid-naïve: **Note:** PCA has been used in children as young as 5 years of age; however, clinicians need to assess children 5-8 years of age to determine if they are able to use the PCA device correctly. All patients should receive an initial loading dose of an analgesic (to attain adequate control of pain) before starting PCA for maintenance. Adjust doses, lockouts, and limits based on required loading dose, age, state of health, and presence of opioid tolerance. Use lower end of dosing range for opioid-naïve. Assess patient and pain control at regular intervals and adjust settings if needed (American Pain Society, 2008):

Patient weight ≤50 kg:
Usual concentration: Determined by weight; some centers use the following:
Children <12 kg: 10 mcg/mL
Children 12-30 kg: 25 mcg/mL
Children >30 kg: 50 mcg/mL

Demand dose: Usual initial: 0.5-1 mcg/kg/dose; usual range: 0.5-1 mcg/kg/dose
Lockout: Usual initial: 5 doses/hour
Lockout interval: Range: 6-8 minutes
Usual basal rate: 0-0.5 mcg/kg/**hour**
Patient weight >50 kg:
Usual concentration: 50 mcg/mL
Demand dose: Usual initial: 20 mcg; usual range: 10-50 mcg
Lockout interval: Usual initial: 6 minutes; usual range: 5-8 minutes
Usual basal rate: ≤50 mcg/**hour**

Adolescents and Adults:

Analgesia for minor procedures/sedation: I.V.: 0.5-1 mcg/kg/dose; may repeat after 30-60 minutes; or 25-50 mcg, repeat full dose in 5 minutes if needed, may repeat 4-5 times with 25 mcg at 5-minute intervals if needed.
Note: Higher doses are used for major procedures.

Continuous analgesia/sedation:
<50 kg: Initial I.V. bolus: 1-2 mcg/kg; continuous infusion rate: 1-2 mcg/kg/**hour**
>50 kg: Initial I.V. bolus: 1-2 mcg/kg **or** 25-100 mcg/dose; continuous infusion rate: 1-2 mcg/kg/**hour or** 25-200 mcg/**hour**

Patient-controlled analgesia (PCA): I.V.: **Note:** All patients should receive an initial loading dose of an analgesic (to attain adequate control of pain) before starting PCA for maintenance. Adjust doses, lockouts, and limits based on required loading dose, age, state of health, and presence of opioid tolerance. Use lower end of dosing range for opioid-naïve. Assess patient and pain control at regular intervals and adjust settings if needed (American Pain Society, 2008):

Adolescents ≤50 kg; opioid-naïve:
Usual concentration: 50 mcg/mL
Demand dose: Usual initial: 0.5-1 mcg/kg/dose; usual range: 0.5-1 mcg/kg/dose
Lockout: Usual initial: 5 doses/hour
Lockout interval: Range: 6-8 minutes
Usual basal rate: 0-0.5 mcg/kg/**hour**
Adolescents >50 kg and Adults; opioid-naïve:
Usual concentration: 50 mcg/mL
Demand dose: Usual initial: 20 mcg; usual range: 10-50 mcg
Lockout interval: Usual initial: 6 minutes; usual range: 5-8 minutes
Usual basal rate: ≤50 mcg/**hour**

Preoperative sedation, adjunct to regional anesthesia, postoperative pain: I.M., I.V.: 25-100 mcg/dose

Adjunct to general anesthesia: Slow I.V.:
Low dose: 0.5-2 mcg/kg/dose depending on the indication
Moderate dose: Initial: 2-20 mcg/kg/dose; Maintenance (bolus or infusion): 1-2 mcg/kg/**hour**. Discontinuing fentanyl infusion 30-60 minutes prior to the end of surgery will usually allow adequate ventilation upon emergence from anesthesia. For "fast-tracking" and early extubation following major surgery, total fentanyl doses are limited to 10-15 mcg/kg.
High dose: 20-50 mcg/kg/dose; **Note:** High dose fentanyl as an adjunct to general anesthesia is rarely used, but is still described in the manufacturer's label.

General anesthesia without additional anesthetic agents: I.V.: 50-100 mcg/kg/dose with O₂ and skeletal muscle relaxant

Moderate to severe chronic pain: Transdermal patch: Opioid-tolerant patients receiving at least 60 mg oral morphine equivalents per day: Initial: 25 mcg/**hour** system or higher, based on conversion to fentanyl equivalents and administration of equianalgesic dosage (see manufacturer labeling for further information); use short-acting analgesics for first 24 hours with supplemental PRN doses thereafter (for breakthrough pain);

dose may be increased after 3 days based on the daily dose of supplementary PRN opioids required; use the ratio of 45 mg of oral morphine equivalents per day to a 12.5 mcg/**hour** increase in transdermal patch dosage; transdermal patch is usually administered every 72 hours but select **adult** patients may require every 48-hour administration; dosage increase administered every 72 hours should be tried before 48-hour schedule is used

Breakthrough cancer pain: Adolescents ≥16 years and Adults: Transmucosal lozenge (Actiq®): Opioid-tolerant patients: Titrate dose to provide adequate analgesia: Initial: 200 mcg; may repeat dose only once, 15 minutes after completion of first dose if needed. Do not exceed a maximum of 2 doses per each breakthrough cancer pain episode; patient must wait at least 4 hours before treating another episode. Titrate dose up to next higher strength if treatment of several consecutive breakthrough episodes requires >1 Actiq® per episode; evaluate each new dose over several breakthrough cancer pain episodes (generally 1-2 days) to determine proper dose of analgesia with acceptable side effects. Once dose has been determined, consumption should be limited to ≤4 units/day. Re-evaluate maintenance (around-the-clock) opioid dose if patient requires >4 units/day. If signs of excessive opioid effects occur before a dose is complete, the unit should be removed from the mouth immediately, and subsequent doses decreased.

Adolescents 18 years of age and Adults:
Severe pain:
I.M, I.V.: 50-100 mcg/dose every 1-2 hours as needed; patients with prior opioid exposure may tolerate higher initial doses

Intrathecal (American Pain Society, 2008): **Note: Must use preservative-free.** Doses must be adjusted for age, injection site, and patient's medical condition and degree of opioid tolerance.
Single dose: 5-25 mcg/dose; may provide adequate relief for up to 6 hours
Continuous infusion: Not recommended in acute pain management due to risk of excessive accumulation. For chronic cancer pain, infusion of very small doses may be practical (American Pain Society, 2008).

Epidural (American Pain Society, 2008): **Note: Must use preservative-free.** Doses must be adjusted for age, injection site, and patient's medical condition and degree of opioid tolerance.
Single dose: 25-100 mcg/dose; may provide adequate relief for up to 8 hours
Continuous infusion: 25-100 mcg/**hour**

Breakthrough cancer pain: Opioid-tolerant patients: For patients who are tolerant to and currently receiving opioid therapy for persistent cancer pain; dosing should be individually titrated to provide adequate analgesia with minimal side effects. Dose titration should be done if patient requires more than 1 dose/breakthrough pain episode for several consecutive episodes. Patients experiencing >4 breakthrough pain episodes/day should have the dose of their long-term opioid re-evaluated.

Buccal film (Onsolis®): Initial dose: 200 mcg for all patients; **Note:** Patients previously using another transmucosal product should be initiated at doses of 200 mcg; do **not** switch patients using any other fentanyl product on a mcg-per-mcg basis.
Dose titration: If titration of dose is required, increase dose in 200 mcg increments once per episode using multiples of the 200 mcg film; do not redose within a single episode of breakthrough pain and separate single doses by ≥2 hours. During titration, do not exceed 4 simultaneous applications of the 200 mcg films (800 mcg). If >800 mcg required, treat next

episode with one 1200 mcg film (maximum dose: 1200 mcg). Once maintenance dose is determined, all other unused films should be disposed of and that strength (using a single film) should be used. During any pain episode, if adequate relief is not achieved after 30 minutes following buccal film application, a rescue medication (as determined by healthcare provider) may be used.
Maintenance: Determined dose applied as a single film once per episode and separated by ≥2 hours (dose range: 200-1200 mcg); limit to 4 applications/day. Consider increasing the around-the-clock opioid therapy in patients experiencing >4 breakthrough pain episodes/day.

Buccal tablets (Fentora®): Initial dose: 100 mcg; a second 100 mcg dose, if needed, may be administered 30 minutes after the start of the first dose; **Note:** For patients previously using the transmucosal lozenge (Actiq®), the initial dose should be selected using the conversions listed below (maximum: 2 doses per breakthrough pain episode every 4 hours).
Dose titration: If required, should be done using multiples of the 100 mcg tablets. Patient can take two 100 mcg tablets (one on each side of mouth). If that dose is not successful, can use four 100 mcg tablets (two on each side of mouth). If titration requires >400 mcg/dose, then use 200 mcg tablets. **Note:** Buccal tablet may be administered sublingually once an effective maintenance dose has been established.
Conversion from transmucosal lozenge to buccal tablet (Fentora®): Initial dose:
Lozenge dose 200-400 mcg, then use buccal tablet 100 mcg
Lozenge dose 600-800 mcg, then use buccal tablet 200 mcg
Lozenge dose 1200-1600 mcg, then use buccal tablet 400 mcg
Note: Four 100 mcg buccal tablets deliver approximately 12% and 13% higher values of C_{max} and AUC, respectively, compared to one 400 mcg buccal tablet. To prevent confusion, patient should only have one strength of tablets available at a time. Using more than four buccal tablets at a time has not been studied.

Nasal spray (Lazanda®):
Initial dose: 100 mcg (one 100 mcg spray in one nostril) for all patients. **Note:** Patients previously using another fentanyl product should be initiated at a dose of 100 mcg; do not convert patients from other fentanyl products to Lazanda® on a mcg-per-mcg basis.
Dose titration: If pain is relieved within 30 minutes, that same dose should be used to treat subsequent episodes. If pain is unrelieved, may increase to a higher dose using the recommended titration steps. **Must wait at least 2 hours before treating another episode with nasal spray.** Dose titration steps: If no relief with 100 mcg dose, increase to 200 mcg dose per episode (one 100 mcg spray in each nostril); if no relief with 200 mcg dose, increase to 400 mcg per episode (one 400 mcg spray in one nostril); if no relief with 400 mcg dose, increase to 800 mcg dose per episode (one 400 mcg spray in each nostril). **Note:** Single doses >800 mcg have not been evaluated. There are no data supporting the use of a combination of dose strengths.
Maintenance dose: Once maintenance dose for breakthrough pain episode has been determined, use that dose for subsequent episodes. For pain that is not relieved after 30 minutes of Lazanda® administration or if a separate breakthrough pain episode occurs within the 2 hour window before the next Lazanda® dose is permitted, a rescue medication

may be used. Limit Lazanda® use to ≤4 episodes of breakthrough pain per day. If response to maintenance dose changes (increase in adverse reactions or alterations in pain relief), dose readjustment may be necessary. If patient is experiencing >4 breakthrough pain episodes/day, consider increasing the around-the-clock, long-acting opioid therapy; if long-acting opioid therapy dose is altered, re-evaluate and retitrate Lazanda® dose as needed.

Sublingual spray (Subsys®):

Initial dose: 100 mcg for all patients. If pain is unrelieved, one additional 100 mcg dose may be given 30 minutes after administration of the first dose. A maximum of two doses can be given per breakthrough pain episode; must wait at least 4 hours before treating another episode. **Note:** Patients must remain on around-the-clock opioids during use. Patients previously using other fentanyl products should be initiated at a dose of 100 mcg; do not convert patients from any other fentanyl product (transmucosal, transdermal, or parenteral) to Subsys® on a mcg-per-mcg basis.

Dose titration: If pain is relieved within 30 minutes, that same dose should be used to treat subsequent episodes and no titration is necessary. If pain is unrelieved, may increase to a higher dose using the recommended titration steps. Goal is to determine the dose that provides adequate analgesia (with tolerable side effects) using a single dose per breakthrough pain episode. For each breakthrough pain episode, if pain unrelieved after 30 minutes only one additional dose using the same strength may be given (maximum: Two doses per breakthrough pain episode). **Must wait at least 4 hours before treating another episode with Subsys®.**

Dose titration steps: If no relief with 100 mcg dose, increase to 200 mcg dose per episode (one 200 mcg unit); if no relief with 200 mcg dose, increase to 400 mcg per episode (one 400 mcg unit); if no relief with 400 mcg dose, increase to 600 mcg dose per episode (one 600 mcg unit); if no relief with 600 mcg dose, increase to 800 mcg dose per episode (one 800 mcg unit); if no relief with 800 mcg dose, increase to 1200 mcg dose per episode (two 600 mcg units); if no relief with 1200 mcg dose, increase to 1600 mcg per episode (two 800 mcg units).

Maintenance dose: Once maintenance dose for breakthrough pain episode has been determined, use that dose for subsequent episodes. If occasional episodes of unrelieved breakthrough pain occur following 30 minutes of Subsys® administration, one additional dose using the same strength may be administered (maximum: Two doses per breakthrough pain episode); patient must wait 4 hours before treating another breakthrough pain episode with Subsys®. Once maintenance dose is determined, limit Susbsys® use to ≤4 episodes of breakthrough pain per day. If response to maintenance dose changes (increase in adverse reactions or alterations in pain relief), dose readjustment may be necessary. If patient is experiencing >4 breakthrough pain episodes/day, consider increasing the around-the-clock, long-acting opioid therapy.

Sublingual tablet (Abstral®):

Initial dose: 100 mcg for all patients; if pain is unrelieved, a second dose may be given 30 minutes after administration of the first dose. A maximum of two doses can be given per breakthrough pain episode; must wait at least 2 hours before treating another episode. **Note:** Patients previously using another fentanyl product should be initiated at a dose of 100 mcg; do not convert patients from other fentanyl products to Abstral® on a mcg-per-mcg basis.

Dose titration: If titration required, increase in 100 mcg increments (up to 400 mcg) over consecutive breakthrough episodes. If titration requires >400 mcg/dose, increase in increments of 200 mcg, starting with 600 mcg dose. During titration, patients may use multiples of 100 mcg and/or 200 mcg tablets for any single dose; do not exceed 4 tablets at one time; safety and efficacy of doses >800 mcg have not been evaluated.

Maintenance dose: Once maintenance dose for breakthrough pain episode has been determined, use only one tablet in the appropriate strength per episode; if pain is unrelieved with maintenance dose. A second dose may be given after 30 minutes; maximum of two doses/episode of breakthrough pain; separate treatment of subsequent episodes by ≥2 hours; limit treatment to ≤4 breakthrough episodes/day. Consider increasing the around-the-clock, long-acting opioid therapy in patients experiencing >4 breakthrough pain episodes/day; if long-acting opioid therapy dose altered, re-evaluate and retitrate Abstral® dose as needed.

Dosing adjustment in renal impairment:

Infants, Children, and Adolescents: There are no dosage adjustments provided in the manufacturer's labeling; however, the following guidelines have been used by some clinicians (Aronoff, 2007): The following assumes dosages of 0.5-2 mcg/kg/dose or 1-5 mcg/kg/**hour** in normal renal function: I.V.:

GFR >50 mL/minute/1.73 m^2: No adjustment required

GFR 10-50 mL/minute/1.73m^2: Administer 75% of usual dose

GFR <10 mL/minute/1.73m^2: Administer 50% of usual dose

Intermittent hemodialysis: Administer 50% of usual dose

Peritoneal dialysis (PD): Administer 50% of usual dose

Continuous renal replacement therapy (CRRT): Administer 75% of usual dose

Adolescents ≥16 years and Adults: Transdermal (patch): Degree of impairment (ie, CrCl) not defined in manufacturer's labeling.

Mild to moderate impairment: Initial: Reduce dose by 50%; monitor patient closely

Severe impairment: Use not recommended

Adolescents ≥18 years and Adults: Transmucosal (buccal film/tablet, sublingual spray/tablet, lozenge) and nasal spray: Although fentanyl pharmacokinetics may be altered in renal disease, fentanyl can be used successfully in the management of breakthrough cancer pain. Use with caution; reduce initial dose and titrate to reach clinical effect with careful monitoring of patients, especially those with severe renal disease.

Dosing adjustment in hepatic impairment:

Transdermal (patch): Adolescents ≥16 years and Adults: Mild to moderate impairment: Initial: Reduce dose by 50%

Severe impairment: Use not recommended

Transmucosal (buccal film/tablet, sublingual spray/tablet, lozenge) and nasal spray: Adolescents ≥18 years and Adults: Although fentanyl pharmacokinetics may be altered in hepatic disease, fentanyl can be used successfully in the management of breakthrough cancer pain. Use with caution; reduce initial dose and titrate to reach clinical effect with careful monitoring of patients, especially those with severe hepatic disease.

Usual Infusion Concentrations: Neonatal I.V. infusion: 10 **mcg/mL**

Usual Infusion Concentrations: Pediatric I.V. infusion: 10 **mcg/mL**

Administration

Parenteral: I.V.: Administer by slow I.V. push over 3-5 minutes or by continuous infusion. Larger bolus doses ▶

(>5 mcg/kg) should be given by slow I.V. push over 5-10 minutes.

Transdermal patch: Apply to nonhairy, clean, dry, non-irritated, intact skin of the flat area of front or back of upper torso, flank area, or upper arm; apply to upper back in young children or in people with cognitive impairment to decrease the potential of the patient removing the patch. Monitor the adhesion of the system closely in children. Clip hair prior to application, do **not** shave area; prior to application, skin may be cleaned with clear water (do not use soaps, lotions, alcohol, oils, or other substances which may irritate the skin); allow skin to dry thoroughly prior to application. Apply patch immediately after removing from package; firmly press in place and hold for at least 30 seconds; change patch every 72 hours; remove old patch before applying new patch; do not apply new patch to same place as old patch; wash hands after applying patch. If there is difficulty with patch adhesion, the edges of the system may be taped in place with first-aid tape; if difficulty with adhesion persists, an adhesive film dressing (eg, Bioclusive™, Tegaderm™) may be applied over the system. If patch falls off before 72 hours, a new patch may be applied to a different skin site.

Note: Transdermal patch is a membrane-controlled system; do **not** cut the patch to deliver partial doses; do **not** use patches that are cut, damaged, or leaking; do **not** use if seal of package is broken; rate of drug delivery may be significantly increased if patch is cut, damaged, or leaking and result in absorption of a potentially fatal dose; reservoir contents and adhesion may be affected if cut; if partial dose is needed, surface area of patch can be blocked proportionally using adhesive bandage (Lee, 1997). Do **not** use soap, alcohol, or other solvents to remove transdermal gel if it accidentally touches skin as they may increase transdermal absorption; use copious amounts of water. Avoid exposing application site to external heat sources (eg, electric blanket, heating pad, heat lamp, tanning lamp, sauna, heated water bed, hot tub, hot baths, sunbathing). Dispose of properly.

Transmucosal products:

Buccal film (Onsolis®): Foil overwrap should be removed just prior to administration. Prior to placing film, wet inside of cheek using tongue or by rinsing with water. Place film inside mouth with the pink side of the unit against the inside of the moistened cheek. With finger, press the film against cheek and hold for 5 seconds. The film should stick to the inside of cheek after 5 seconds. The film should be left in place until it dissolves (usually within 15-30 minutes after application). Liquids may be consumed after 5 minutes of application. Food can be eaten after film dissolves. If using more than one film simultaneously (during titration period), apply films on either side of mouth (do not apply on top of each other). Do not chew or swallow film. Do not cut or tear the film.

Buccal tablet (Fentora®): Do not use if blister package has been opened or tampered with. Blister package should be opened just prior to administration. Peel back the blister backing to expose the tablet; do not push tablet through the blister (damage to the tablet may occur). Administer tablet immediately after removal from blister. Place entire tablet in the buccal cavity (above a rear molar, between the upper cheek and gum) or under the tongue; should dissolve in about 14-25 minutes. If remnants remain after 30 minutes they may be swallowed with a glass of water. Use alternate side of mouth for subsequent doses. Do not break, split, suck, chew, or swallow tablet (this will result in decreased effect). If excessive opioid effects appear before tablet is completely dissolved (eg, dizziness, sedation, nausea), instruct patient to rinse mouth with water and spit remaining pieces of tablet into sink or toilet immediately; rinse the sink or flush toilet to dispose of tablet particles.

Intranasal:

Solution (injectable product): Pediatric patients ≥10 kg: If congested, suction nostrils prior to administration. Using a 50 mcg/mL solution, administer half of the dose to each nostril using an atomizer such as the MAD® Nasal Drug delivery device or drip into the nostril slowly with a syringe; higher concentrations (150 mcg/mL and 300 mcg/mL) have been studied to prevent excess volume administration and decrease leakage, but comparative trials have not been performed.

Nasal spray (Lazanda®): Prior to initial use, prime device by spraying 4 sprays into the provided pouch (the counting window will show a green bar when the bottle is ready for use). Insert nozzle a short distance into the nose (~1/2 inch or 1 cm) and point towards the bridge of the nose (while closing off the other nostril using one finger). Press on finger grips until a "click" sound is heard and the number in the counting window advances by one. The "click" sound and dose counter are the only reliable methods for ensuring a dose has been administered (spray is not always felt on the nasal mucosa). Patient should remain seated for at least 1 minute following administration. Do not blow nose for ≥30 minutes after administration. Wash hands before and after use. There are 8 full therapeutic sprays in each bottle; do not continue to use bottle after "8" sprays have been used. Dispose of bottle and contents if ≥5 days have passed since last use or if it has been ≥4 days since bottle was primed. Spray the remaining contents into the provided pouch, seal in the child-resistant container, and dispose of in the trash.

Oral lozenge (Actiq®): Oral: Do not use if blister package has been opened. Blister package should be opened with scissors just prior to administration; once removed, patient should place the lozenge in mouth and suck it; do not bite or chew lozenge. Place lozenge in mouth between cheek and lower gum; occasionally move lozenge from one side of the mouth to the other; consume lozenge over 15 minutes; remove lozenge from mouth if signs of excessive opioid effects appear before lozenge is totally consumed. Remove handle after lozenge is consumed or patient achieves adequate response.

Sublingual spray (Subsys®): Open sealed blister unit with scissors immediately prior to administration. Contents of unit should be sprayed into mouth under the tongue. Dispose of unit immediately after use, using disposal bottle provided.

Sublingual tablet (Abstral®): Remove from the blister unit immediately prior to administration. Place tablet directly under the tongue on the floor of the mouth and allow to completely dissolve; do not chew, suck, or swallow. Do not eat or drink anything until tablet is completely dissolved. In patients with a dry mouth, water may be used to moisten the buccal mucosa just before administration.

Monitoring Parameters Respiratory rate, blood pressure, heart rate, oxygen saturation, bowel sounds, abdominal distention; signs of misuse, abuse, or addiction

Transdermal patch: Monitor patient for at least 24 hours after application of first dose

Additional Information Fentanyl is 50-100 times as potent as morphine; morphine 10 mg I.M. = fentanyl 0.1-0.2 mg I.M. Fentanyl has less hypotensive effects than morphine or meperidine due to minimal or no histamine release. I.V. product has a pH of 4.0-7.5.

Controlled Substance C-II

Dosage Forms Excipient information presented when available (limited, particularly for generics); consult specific product labeling.

Film, for buccal application, as citrate [strength expressed as base]:
Onsolis: 200 mcg (30s); 400 mcg (30s); 600 mcg (30s); 800 mcg (30s); 1200 mcg (30s)

Injection, solution, as citrate [strength expressed as base, preservative free]: 0.05 mg/mL (2 mL, 5 mL, 10 mL, 20 mL, 50 mL)

Liquid, sublingual, as base [spray]:
Subsys: 100 mcg (30s); 200 mcg (30s); 400 mcg (30s); 600 mcg (30s); 800 mcg (30s) [contains dehydrated ethanol 63.6%, propylene glycol]

Lozenge, oral, as citrate [strength expressed as base, transmucosal]: 200 mcg (30s); 400 mcg (30s); 600 mcg (30s); 800 mcg (30s); 1200 mcg (30s); 1600 mcg (30s)
Actiq: 200 mcg (30s); 400 mcg (30s); 600 mcg (30s); 800 mcg (30s); 1200 mcg (30s); 1600 mcg (30s) [contains sugar 2 g/lozenge; berry flavor]

Patch, transdermal, as base: 12 [delivers 12.5 mcg/hr] (5s); 25 [delivers 25 mcg/hr] (5s); 50 [delivers 50 mcg/hr] (5s); 75 [delivers 75 mcg/hr] (5s); 100 [delivers 100 mcg/hr] (5s)
Duragesic: 12 [delivers 12.5 mcg/hr] (5s) [contains ethanol 0.1 mL/10 cm^2; 5 cm^2]
Duragesic: 25 [delivers 25 mcg/hr] (5s) [contains ethanol 0.1 mL/10 cm^2; 10 cm^2]
Duragesic: 50 [delivers 50 mcg/hr] (5s) [contains ethanol 0.1 mL/10 cm^2; 20 cm^2]
Duragesic: 75 [delivers 75 mcg/hr] (5s) [contains ethanol 0.1 mL/10 cm^2; 30 cm^2]
Duragesic: 100 [delivers 100 mcg/hr] (5s) [contains ethanol 0.1 mL/10 $cm^{2;}$ 40 cm^2]

Powder, for prescription compounding, as citrate: USP: 100% (1 g)

Solution, intranasal, as citrate [strength expressed as base, spray]:
Lazanda: 100 mcg/spray (5 mL); 400 mcg/spray (5 mL) [delivers 8 metered sprays]

Tablet, for buccal application, as citrate [strength expressed as base]:
Fentora: 100 mcg (28s); 200 mcg (28s); 400 mcg (28s); 600 mcg (28s); 800 mcg (28s)

Tablet, sublingual, as citrate [strength expressed as base]:
Abstral: 100 mcg (12s, 32s); 200 mcg (12s, 32s); 300 mcg (12s, 32s); 400 mcg (12s, 32s); 600 mcg (32s); 800 mcg (32s)

References

ACOG Committee on Practice Bulletins-Obstetrics, "ACOG Practice Bulletin. Clinical Management Guidelines for Obstetrician-Gynecologists Number 36, July 2002. Obstetric Analgesia and Anesthesia," *Obstet Gynecol*, 2002, 100(1):177-91.

Anand KJ and International Evidence-Based Group for Neonatal Pain, "Consensus Statement for the Prevention and Management of Pain in the Newborn," *Arch Pediatr Adolesc Med*, 2001, 155(2):173-80.

Arnold JH, Truog RD, Scavone JM, et al. Changes in the pharmacodynamics response to fentanyl in neonates during continuous infusion. *Journal of Pediatrics*. 1991;119:639-643.

Billmire DA, Neale HW, and Gregory RO, "Use of I.V. Fentanyl in the Outpatient Treatment of Pediatric Facial Trauma," *J Trauma*, 1985, 25 (11):1079-80.

Borland M, Jacobs I, King B, et al, "A Randomized Controlled Trial Comparing Intranasal Fentanyl to Intravenous Morphine for Managing Acute Pain in Children in the Emergency Department," *Ann Emerg Med*, 2007, 49(3):335-40.

Borland ML, Bergesio R, Pascoe EM, et al, "Intranasal Fentanyl Is an Equivalent Analgesic to Oral Morphine in Paediatric Burns Patients for Dressing Changes: A Randomised Double Blind Crossover Study," *Burns*, 2005, 31(7):831-7.

Borland ML, Jacobs I, and Geelhoed G, "Intranasal Fentanyl Reduces Acute Pain in Children in the Emergency Department: A Safety and Efficacy Study," *Emerg Med (Fremantle)*, 2002, 14(3):275-80.

Chou R, Fanciullo GJ, Fine PG, et al, "Clinical Guidelines for the Use of Chronic Opioid Therapy in Chronic Noncancer Pain," *J Pain*, 2009, 10 (2):113-30.

Chung S, Lim R, and Goldman RD, "Intranasal Fentanyl Versus Placebo for Pain in Children During Catheterization for Voiding Cystourethrography," *Pediatr Radiol*, 2010, 40(7):1236-40.

Cloherty JP, Eichenwald EC, Stark AR, eds. *Manual of Neonatal Care*. 7th ed. Philadelphia, PA: Lippincott Williams & Wilkins; 2012.

Cole J, Shepherd M, and Young P, "Intranasal Fentanyl in 1-3-Year-Olds: A Prospective Study of the Effectiveness of Intranasal Fentanyl as Acute Analgesia," *Emerg Med Australas*, 2009, 21(5):395-400.

Cramton RE, Gruchala NE. Managing procedural pain in pediatric patients. *Curr Opin Pediatr*. 2012;24(4):530-538.

Crellin D, Ling RX, and Babl F, "Does the Standard Intravenous Solution of Fentanyl (50 microg/mL) Administered Intranasally Have Analgesic Efficacy?" *Emerg Med Australas*, 2010, 22(1):62-7.

Dow K, Ordean A, Murphy-Oikonen J, et al, "Neonatal Abstinence Syndrome Clinical Practice Guidelines For Ontario," *J Popul Ther Clin Pharmacol*, 2012, 19(3):e488-506.

Finn M and Harris D, "Intranasal Fentanyl for Analgesia in the Paediatric Emergency Department," *Emerg Med J*, 2010, 27(4):300-1.

Gomar C and Fernandez C, "Epidural Analgesia-Anaesthesia in Obstetrics," *Eur J Anaesthesiol*, 2000, 17(9):542-58.

Hegenbarth MA. Preparing for pediatric emergencies: drugs to consider. *Pediatrics*. 2008;121:433-443.

Herd D and Borland M, "Intranasal Fentanyl Paediatric Clinical Practice Guidelines," *Emerg Med Australas*, 2009, 21(4):335.

Hudak M, Tan RC, Committee On Drugs, et al, "Neonatal Drug Withdrawal," *Pediatrics*, 2012, 129(2):e540-60.

Institute for Safe Medication Practices (ISMP), "Standard Concentrations of Neonatal Drug Infusions," *ISMP*, 2011.

Katz R, Kelly HW, and Hsi A, "Prospective Study on the Occurrence of Withdrawal in Critically Ill Children Who Receive Fentanyl by Continuous Infusion," *Crit Care Med*, 1994, 22(5):763-7.

Krauss B, Green SM. Procedural sedation and analgesia in children. *Lancet*. 2006;367(9512):766-780.

Kumar P, Denson SE, Mancuso TJ. Clinical report – premedication for nonemergency endotracheal intubation in the neonate. *Pediatrics*. 2010;125:608-615.

Lee HA and Anderson PO, "Giving Partial Doses of Transdermal Patches," *Am J Health Syst Pharm*, 1997, 54(15):1759-60.

Leuschen MP, Willett LD, Hoie EB, et al, "Plasma Fentanyl Levels in Infants Undergoing Extracorporeal Membrane Oxygenation," *J Thorac Cardiovasc Surg*, 1993, 105(5):885-91.

Lim S, Paech MJ, Sunderland VB, et al, "Pharmacokinetics of Nasal Fentanyl," *J Pharm Pract Res*, 2003, 33:59-63.

Manjushree R, Lahiri A, Ghosh BR, et al, "Intranasal Fentanyl Provides Adequate Postoperative Analgesia in Pediatric Patients," *Can J Anaesth*, 2002, 49(2):190-3.

Nelson WE, Behrman RE, Kliegman RM, et al, eds. *Nelson Textbook of Pediatrics*. 15th ed. Philadelphia, PA: WB Saunders Company; 1996.

Phillips MS, "Standardizing I.V. Infusion Concentrations: National Survey Results," *Am J Health Syst Pharm*, 2011, 68(22):2176-82.

"Principles of Analgesic Use in the Treatment of Acute Pain and Cancer Pain," 6th ed, Glenview, IL: American Pain Society, 2008.

Roth B, Schlunder C, Houben F, et al, "Analgesia and Sedation in Neonatal Intensive Care Using Fentanyl by Continuous Infusion," *Dev Pharmacol Ther*, 1991, 17(3-4):121-7.

Saarenmaa E, Neuvonen PJ, and Fellman V, "Gestational Age and Birth Weight Effects on Plasma Clearance of Fentanyl in Newborn Infants," *J Pediatr*, 2000, 136(6):767-70.

Saunders M, Adelgais K, and Nelson D, "Use of Intranasal Fentanyl for the Relief of Pediatric Orthopedic Trauma Pain," *Acad Emerg Med*, 2010, 17(11):1155-61.

Schechter NL, Weisman SJ, Rosenblum M, et al, "The Use of Oral Transmucosal Fentanyl Citrate for Painful Procedures in Children," *Pediatrics*, 1995, 95(3):335-9.

Spigset O and Hagg S, "Analgesics and Breast-feeding: Safety Considerations," *Paediatr Drugs*, 2000, 2(3):223-38.

Toussaint S, Maidl J, Schwagmeier R, et al, "Patient-Controlled Intranasal Analgesia: Effective Alternative to Intravenous PCA for Postoperative Pain Relief," *Can J Anaesth*, 2000, 47(4):299-302.

World Health Organization (WHO). *WHO guidelines on the pharmacological treatment of persisting pain in children with medical illnesses*. 2012.

Zeltzer LK, Altman A, Cohen D, et al, "Report of the Subcommittee on the Management of Pain Associated With Procedures in Children With Cancer," *Pediatrics*, 1990, 86(5 Pt 2):826-31.

◆ **Fentanyl Citrate** see FentaNYL *on page 853*

◆ **Fentanyl Citrate Injection, USP (Can)** see FentaNYL *on page 853*

◆ **Fentanyl Hydrochloride** see FentaNYL *on page 853*

◆ **Fentanyl Patch** see FentaNYL *on page 853*

◆ **Fentora** see FentaNYL *on page 853*

◆ **Ferate [OTC]** see Ferrous Gluconate *on page 866*

◆ **Fergon [OTC]** *see* Ferrous Gluconate *on page 866*

◆ **Fer-In-Sol [OTC]** *see* Ferrous Sulfate *on page 868*

◆ **Fer-In-Sol® (Can)** *see* Ferrous Sulfate *on page 868*

◆ **Fer-Iron [OTC]** *see* Ferrous Sulfate *on page 868*

◆ **Fermalac (Can)** *see* Lactobacillus *on page 1191*

◆ **Ferodan™ (Can)** *see* Ferrous Sulfate *on page 868*

◆ **FeroSul [OTC]** *see* Ferrous Sulfate *on page 868*

◆ **Ferretts [OTC]** *see* Ferrous Fumarate *on page 865*

◆ **Ferrex 150 [OTC]** *see* Polysaccharide-Iron Complex *on page 1701*

◆ **Ferrex 150 Plus [OTC]** *see* Polysaccharide-Iron Complex *on page 1701*

Ferric Gluconate (FER ik GLOO koe nate)

Medication Safety Issues
Sound-alike/look-alike issues:
   Ferric gluconate may be confused with ferric carboxymaltose, ferumoxytol
Brand Names: U.S. Ferrlecit
Brand Names: Canada Ferrlecit
Therapeutic Category Iron Salt, Parenteral; Mineral, Parenteral
Generic Availability (U.S.) Yes
Use Treatment of microcytic, hypochromic anemia resulting from iron deficiency in combination with erythropoietin in hemodialysis patients when iron administration is not feasible or ineffective
Pregnancy Risk Factor B
Pregnancy Considerations Adverse events were not observed in animal reproduction studies. It is recommended that pregnant women meet the dietary requirements of iron with diet and/or supplements in order to prevent adverse events associated with iron deficiency anemia in pregnancy. Treatment of iron deficiency anemia in pregnant women is the same as in nonpregnant women and in most cases, oral iron preparations may be used. Except in severe cases of maternal anemia, the fetus achieves normal iron stores regardless of maternal concentrations.
Breast-Feeding Considerations Iron is normally found in breast milk. Breast milk or iron fortified formulas generally provide enough iron to meet the recommended dietary requirements of infants. The amount of iron in breast milk is generally not influenced by maternal iron status.
Contraindications Hypersensitivity to the iron formulation or any component; anemias that are not associated with iron deficiency; hemochromatosis; hemolytic anemia; iron overload
Warnings Deaths associated with parenteral iron administration following anaphylactic-type reactions have been reported; treatment agents for anaphylactic reactions (eg, epinephrine, steroids, diphenhydramine) should be immediately available; a test dose is recommended prior to initial therapy; rapid I.V. administration is associated with flushing, fatigue, weakness, hypotension, and chest, back, groin, or flank pain; use parenteral iron only in patients where the iron deficient state is not amenable to oral iron therapy; ferric gluconate is not approved for I.M. administration.

Ferric gluconate contains benzyl alcohol which may cause allergic reactions in susceptible individuals; large amounts of benzyl alcohol (≥99 mg/kg/day) have been associated with a potentially fatal toxicity ("gasping syndrome") in neonates; the "gasping syndrome" consists of metabolic acidosis, respiratory distress, gasping respirations, CNS dysfunction (including convulsions, intracranial hemorrhage), hypotension and cardiovascular collapse; *in vitro*

and animal studies have shown that benzoate, a metabolite of benzyl alcohol, displaces bilirubin from protein-binding sites; avoid use of ferric gluconate formulation in neonates.
Precautions Use with caution in patients with histories of significant allergies, asthma, hepatic impairment, rheumatoid arthritis
Adverse Reactions
   Cardiovascular: Angina pectoris, bradycardia, chest pain, edema, hyper-/hypotension, hypervolemia, MI, peripheral edema, syncope, tachycardia, vasodilation
   Central nervous system: Agitation, chills, consciousness decreased, dizziness, fatigue, fever, headache, lightheadedness, malaise, rigors, somnolence
   Dermatologic: Pruritus, rash
   Endocrine & metabolic: Hyper-/hypokalemia, hypoglycemia
   Gastrointestinal: Abdominal pain, anorexia, diarrhea, dyspepsia, eructation, flatulence, GI disorder, melena, nausea, rectal disorder, vomiting
   Genitourinary: Menorrhagia, UTI
   Hematologic: Anemia, erythrocytes abnormal (changes in morphology/color/number), leukocytosis, lymphadenopathy
   Local: Injection site reaction
   Neuromuscular & skeletal: Arm pain, arthralgia, back pain, cramps, leg cramps, leg edema, paresthesia, weakness
   Ocular: Arcus senilis, conjunctivitis, diplopia, puffy eyelids, redness of eyes, rolling of eyes, watery eyes
   Otic: Deafness
   Respiratory: Cough, dyspnea, pharyngitis, pneumonia, pulmonary edema, rhinitis, upper respiratory infections
   Miscellaneous: Abscess, carcinoma, diaphoresis, flu-like symptoms, infection, sepsis
   Rare but important or life-threatening: Allergic reaction, anaphylactic reactions, convulsion, facial flushing, hemorrhage, hypertonia, hypoesthesia, loss of consciousness, shock, skin discoloration
Drug Interactions
   Metabolism/Transport Effects None known.
   Avoid Concomitant Use
      Avoid concomitant use of Ferric Gluconate with any of the following: Dimercaprol
   Increased Effect/Toxicity
      The levels/effects of Ferric Gluconate may be increased by: ACE Inhibitors; Dimercaprol
   Decreased Effect
      Ferric Gluconate may decrease the levels/effects of: Cefdinir; Eltrombopag; Levothyroxine; Phosphate Supplements; Trientine

      The levels/effects of Ferric Gluconate may be decreased by: Pancrelipase; Trientine
Stability Store at room temperature; do not freeze; use immediately after dilution in NS. Product literature states parenteral iron formulations should not be mixed with other medications or in parenteral nutrition solutions.
Mechanism of Action Supplies a source to elemental iron necessary to the function of hemoglobin, myoglobin and specific enzyme systems; allows transport of oxygen via hemoglobin
Pharmacodynamics
   Onset of action: Hematologic response to either oral or parenteral iron salts is essentially the same; red blood cell form and color changes within 3-10 days
   Maximum effect: Peak reticulocytosis occurs in 5-10 days, and hemoglobin values increase within 2-4 weeks
Pharmacokinetics (Adult data unless noted) Following I.V. doses, the uptake of iron by the reticuloendothelial system appears to be constant at about 40-60 mg/hour
   Half-life: 1.31 hours
   Elimination: By the reticuloendothelial system and excreted in urine and feces (via bile)

Dialysis: Not dialyzable

Dosing: Usual Multiple forms for parenteral iron exist; close attention must be paid to the specific product when ordering and administering; incorrect selection or substitution of one form for another without proper dosage adjustment may result in serious over- or under-dosing; test doses are recommended before starting therapy. **Note:** Per National Kidney Foundation DOQI Guidelines, initiation of iron therapy, determination of dose, and duration of therapy should be guided by results of iron status tests combined with the Hb level and the dose of the erythropoietin stimulating agent. There is insufficient evidence to recommend I.V. iron if ferritin level >500 ng/mL.

Dosage expressed in mg **elemental** iron: I.V.:

Children ≥6 years: 1.5 mg/kg (0.12 mL/kg Ferrlecit®) repeated at each of 8 sequential dialysis sessions not to exceed 125 mg (10 mL) per dose

Adults: 125 mg (10 mL) during hemodialysis; most patients will require a cumulative dose of 1 g over ~8 sequential dialysis treatments to achieve a favorable response

Note: A test dose (25 mg in adult patients) previously recommended in product literature is no longer listed. No pediatric test dose has been recommended by the manufacturer.

Administration Parenteral: Avoid dilution in dextrose due to an increased incidence of local pain and phlebitis

I.V. infusion: If a test dose is used, dilute in 50 mL NS and infuse over 1 hour; dilute repletion dose in 25-100 mL NS and infuse over at least 1 hour; do not exceed 12.5 mg/minute; not for I.M. administration

Slow I.V. injection: 1 mL (12.5 mg iron) of undiluted solution per minute (5 minutes/vial)

Monitoring Parameters Vital signs and other symptoms of anaphylactoid reactions (during I.V. infusion); reticulocyte count, serum ferritin, hemoglobin, serum iron concentrations, and transferrin saturation (TSAT). Ferritin and TSAT may be inaccurate if measured within 14 days of receiving a large single dose (1000 mg in adults).

Reference Range

Serum iron:

Newborns: 110-270 mcg/dL

Infants: 30-70 mcg/dL

Children: 55-120 mcg/dL

Adults: Male: 75-175 mcg/dL; female: 65-165 mcg/dL

Total iron binding capacity:

Newborns: 59-175 mcg/dL

Infants: 100-400 mcg/dL

Children and Adults: 230-430 mcg/dL

Transferrin: 204-360 mg/dL

Percent transferrin saturation (TSAT): 20% to 50%

Iron levels >300 mcg/dL may be considered toxic; should be treated as an overdosage

Ferritin: 13-300 ng/mL

Chronic kidney disease (CKD): Targets for iron therapy (KDOQI Guidelines, 2007) to maintain Hgb 11-12 g/dL:

Children: Nondialysis CKD, hemodialysis, or peritoneal dialysis: Ferritin: >100 ng/mL and TSAT >20%

Adults: Nondialysis (CKD) or peritoneal dialysis: Ferritin: >100 ng/mL and TSAT >20%

Hemodialysis: Ferritin >200 ng/mL and TSAT >20% or CHr (content of hemoglobin in reticulocytes) >29 pg/cell

Test Interactions Serum or transferrin bound iron levels may be falsely elevated if assessed within 24 hours of ferric gluconate administration. Serum ferritin levels may be falsely elevated for 5 days after ferric gluconate administration.

Additional Information Iron storage may lag behind the appearance of normal red blood cell morphology; use periodic hematologic determination to assess therapy

Dosage Forms Considerations Strength of ferric gluconate injection is expressed as elemental iron.

Dosage Forms Excipient information presented when available (limited, particularly for generics); consult specific product labeling.

Solution, Intravenous:

Ferrlecit: 12.5 mg/mL (5 mL) [contains benzyl alcohol, sucrose]

Generic: 12.5 mg/mL (5 mL)

References

"KDOQI Clinical Practice Guideline and Clinical Practice Recommendations for Anemia in Chronic Kidney Disease: 2007 Update of Hemoglobin Target," *Am J Kidney Dis*, 2007, 50(3):471-530.

Seligman PA, Dahl NV, Strobos J, et al, "Single-Dose Pharmacokinetics of Sodium Ferric Gluconate Complex in Iron-Deficient Subjects," *Pharmacotherapy*, 2004, 24(5):574-83.

Warady BA, Zobrist RH, Wu J, et al, "Sodium Ferric Gluconate Complex Therapy in Anemic Children on Hemodialysis," *Pediatr Nephrol*, 2005, 20(9):1320-7.

◆ **Ferrimin 150 [OTC]** *see* Ferrous Fumarate *on page 865*

◆ **Ferrlecit** *see* Ferric Gluconate *on page 864*

◆ **Ferro-Bob [OTC]** *see* Ferrous Sulfate *on page 868*

◆ **Ferrocite [OTC]** *see* Ferrous Fumarate *on page 865*

Ferrous Fumarate (FER us FYOO ma rate)

Related Information

Oral Medications That Should Not Be Crushed or Altered *on page 2438*

Brand Names: U.S. Ferretts [OTC]; Ferrimin 150 [OTC]; Ferrocite [OTC]; Hemocyte [OTC]

Brand Names: Canada Palafer®

Therapeutic Category Iron Salt; Mineral, Oral

Generic Availability (U.S.) Yes

Use Prevention and treatment of iron deficiency anemias (OTC: FDA approved in adults; see product specific labeling for pediatric approval ages); has also been used as supplemental therapy for patients receiving epoetin alfa

Pregnancy Considerations It is recommended that pregnant women meet the dietary requirements of iron with diet and/or supplements in order to prevent adverse events associated with iron deficiency anemia in pregnancy. Treatment of iron deficiency anemia in pregnant women is the same as in nonpregnant women and in most cases, oral iron preparations may be used. Except in severe cases of maternal anemia, the fetus achieves normal iron stores regardless of maternal concentrations.

Breast-Feeding Considerations Iron is normally found in breast milk. Breast milk or iron-fortified formulas generally provide enough iron to meet the recommended dietary requirements of infants. The amount of iron in breast milk is generally not influenced by maternal iron status.

Contraindications Hypersensitivity to iron salts or any component; hemochromatosis, hemolytic anemia

Warnings Accidental iron overdose is a leading cause of fatal poisoning in children under 6 years of age **[U.S. Boxed Warning]**; in case of accidental overdose, contact poison control center immediately; ingestions of ≥40 mg/kg elemental iron or who have persistent symptoms should seek immediate care. Consider all iron sources when evaluating the dose of iron, including combination products, infant formulas, and liquid nutritional supplements; store out of children's reach and in child-resistant containers. Some products may contain tartrazine which may cause allergic reactions in susceptible individuals.

Precautions Routine use for longer than 6 months is not recommended; some patients may require prolonged therapy (eg, continuous bleeding or menorrhagia). Avoid use in patients with peptic ulcer, enteritis, or ulcerative colitis. Avoid in patients receiving frequent blood transfusions; patients already prone to chronic iron overload.

◄ **Adverse Reactions**
Gastrointestinal: Constipation, dark stools, diarrhea, heart-
burn, nausea, staining of teeth, stomach cramping, vomit-
ing
Genitourinary: Discoloration of urine
Rare but important or life-threatening: Contact irritation

Drug Interactions
Metabolism/Transport Effects None known.
Avoid Concomitant Use
Avoid concomitant use of Ferrous Fumarate with any of
the following: Dimercaprol
Increased Effect/Toxicity
The levels/effects of Ferrous Fumarate may be increased
by: Dimercaprol
Decreased Effect
Ferrous Fumarate may decrease the levels/effects of:
Bisphosphonate Derivatives; Cefdinir; Deferiprone; Dolu-
tegravir; Eltrombopag; Levodopa; Levothyroxine; Methyl-
dopa; PenicillAMINE; Phosphate Supplements;
Quinolone Antibiotics; Tetracycline Derivatives; Trientine

The levels/effects of Ferrous Fumarate may be
decreased by: Antacids; H2-Antagonists; Pancrelipase;
Proton Pump Inhibitors; Trientine
Food Interactions Cereals, dietary fiber, tea, coffee, eggs,
and milk may decrease absorption.
Stability Store at 15°C to 30°C (59°F to 86°F) in child-
resistant container and out of reach of children.
Mechanism of Action Replaces iron found in hemoglobin, myoglobin, and enzymes; allows the transportation of
oxygen via hemoglobin
Pharmacodynamics
Onset of action: Hematologic response: Red blood cells
form within 3-10 days; similar onset as parenteral iron
salts
Maximum effect: Peak reticulocytosis occurs in 5-10 days,
and hemoglobin values increase within 2-4 weeks
Pharmacokinetics (Adult data unless noted)
Absorption: Oral: Iron is absorbed in the duodenum and
upper jejunum; in persons with normal iron stores 10% of
an oral dose is absorbed, this is increased to 20% to 30%
in persons with inadequate iron stores; food and achlo-
rhydria will decrease absorption
Protein binding: To transferrin
Elimination: Excreted in the urine, sweat, sloughing of
intestinal mucosa, and by menses
Dosing: Usual Note: Doses expressed as **elemental** iron.
Children and Adolescents:
Recommended daily allowance (RDA): Oral:
Children 4-8 years: 10 mg /day
Children and Adolescents 9-13 years: 8 mg /day
Adolescents 14-18 years:
Male: 11 mg /day
Female: 15 mg /day
Iron deficiency, prevention: Oral:
Children ≥5 years in areas where anemia prevalence is
>40%: 30 mg/day with folic acid (WHO, 2001)
Adolescents in areas where anemia prevalence is
>40%: 60 mg/day with folic acid (WHO, 2001)
Iron deficiency, treatment of iron deficiency: Oral:
Severe iron deficiency anemia: 4-6 mg/kg/day in 3
divided doses (Carney, 2010)
Mild to moderate iron deficiency anemia: 3 mg/kg/day in
1-2 divided doses (CDC, 1998; IOM, 1993)
Adults:
Recommended daily allowance (RDA): Oral
19-50 years:
Males: 8 mg/day
Females 18 mg/day
>50 years: 8 mg/day
Iron deficiency, prevention: Oral: 60-100 mg iron/day

Iron deficiency, treatment: Oral: Usual range:
150-200 mg elemental iron/day in divided doses;
60-100 mg iron twice daily, up to 60 mg iron 4 times/day
Note: To avoid GI upset, start with a single daily dose
and increase by 1 tablet/day each week or as tolerated
until desired daily dose is achieved.
Administration Oral: Do not chew or crush sustained
release preparations; administer with water or juice
between meals for maximum absorption; may administer
with food if GI upset occurs; do not administer with milk or
milk products
Monitoring Parameters Serum iron, total iron binding
capacity, reticulocyte count, hemoglobin, ferritin
Reference Range
Serum iron: 22-184 mcg/dL
Total iron binding capacity:
Infants: 100-400 mcg/dL
Children and Adults: 250-400 mcg/dL
Additional Information When treating iron deficiency
anemias, treat for 3-4 months after hemoglobin/hematocrit
return to normal in order to replenish total body stores

Elemental Iron Content of Iron Salts

Iron Salt	Elemental Iron Content (% of salt form)	Approximate Equivalent Doses (mg of iron salt)
Ferrous fumarate	33	197
Ferrous gluconate	11.6	560
Ferrous sulfate	20	324
Ferrous sulfate, exsiccated	30	217

Dosage Forms Excipient information presented when
available (limited, particularly for generics); consult specific
product labeling.
Tablet, Oral:
Ferretts: 325 mg [scored]
Ferrimin 150: 150 mg
Ferrocite: 324 mg [contains fd&c blue #1 aluminum lake,
fd&c yellow #5 aluminum lake]
Hemocyte: 324 mg
Generic: 29 mg, 90 mg, 324 mg
References

Carney LN, Nepa A, Cohen SS, et al, "Parenteral and Enteral Nutrition
Support: Determining the Best Way to Feed," In: Corkins MR, Balint J,
Bobo E, et al, eds, The A.S.P.E.N Pediatric Nutrition Support Core
Curriculum, Silver Spring: MD: American Society of Parenteral and
Enteral Nutrition, 2010, 440-1.
Centers for Disease Control and Prevention (CDC), "Recommendations
to Prevent and Control Iron Deficiency in the United States," MMWR
REcomm Rep, 1998, 47(RR-3):1-36.
Institute of Medicine, National Research Council, "Iron Deficiency
Anemia: Recommended Guidelines for the Prevention, Detection,
and Management Among U.S. Children and Women of Childbearing
Age," Washington, D.C.: The National Academies Press, 1993.
World Health Organization (WHO), "Iron Deficiency Anaemia: Assess-
ment, Prevention, and Control. A Guide for Programme Managers,"
2001.

Ferrous Gluconate (FER us GLOO koe nate)

Related Information
Oral Medications That Should Not Be Crushed or Altered
on page 2438
Brand Names: U.S. Ferate [OTC]; Fergon [OTC]
Brand Names: Canada Apo-Ferrous Gluconate®; Novo-
Ferrogluc
Therapeutic Category Iron Salt; Mineral, Oral
Generic Availability (U.S.) Yes
Use Prevention and treatment of iron deficiency anemias
(OTC: FDA approved in adults); has also been used as
supplemental therapy for patients receiving epoetin alfa

Pregnancy Considerations It is recommended that pregnant women meet the dietary requirements of iron with diet and/or supplements in order to prevent adverse events associated with iron deficiency anemia in pregnancy. Treatment of iron deficiency anemia in pregnant women is the same as in nonpregnant women and in most cases, oral iron preparations may be used. Except in severe cases of maternal anemia, the fetus achieves normal iron stores regardless of maternal concentrations.

Breast-Feeding Considerations Iron is normally found in breast milk. Breast milk or iron fortified formulas generally provide enough iron to meet the recommended dietary requirements of infants. The amount of iron in breast milk is generally not influenced by maternal iron status.

Contraindications Hypersensitivity to iron salts or any component; hemochromatosis, hemolytic anemia

Warnings Accidental iron overdose is a leading cause of fatal poisoning in children under 6 years of age **[U.S. Boxed Warning]**; in case of accidental overdose, contact poison control center immediately; ingestions of ≥40 mg/kg elemental iron or who have persistent symptoms should seek immediate care. Consider all iron sources when evaluating the dose of iron, including combination products, infant formulas, and liquid nutritional supplements; store out of children's reach and in child-resistant containers. Some products contain sulfites which may cause allergic reactions in susceptible individuals.

Precautions Use for longer than 6 months is not recommended; some patients may require prolonged therapy (eg, continuous bleeding or menorrhagia). Avoid use in patients with peptic ulcer, enteritis, or ulcerative colitis. Avoid in patients receiving frequent blood transfusions; patient already prone to chronic iron overload.

Adverse Reactions
Gastrointestinal: Constipation, dark stools, diarrhea, heartburn, nausea, staining of teeth, stomach cramping, vomiting
Genitourinary: Discoloration of urine
Rare but important or life-threatening: Contact irritation

Drug Interactions
Metabolism/Transport Effects None known.
Avoid Concomitant Use
Avoid concomitant use of Ferrous Gluconate with any of the following: Dimercaprol
Increased Effect/Toxicity
The levels/effects of Ferrous Gluconate may be increased by: Dimercaprol
Decreased Effect
Ferrous Gluconate may decrease the levels/effects of: Bisphosphonate Derivatives; Cefdinir; Deferiprone; Dolutegravir; Eltrombopag; Levodopa; Levothyroxine; Methyldopa; PenicillAMINE; Phosphate Supplements; Quinolone Antibiotics; Tetracycline Derivatives; Trientine

The levels/effects of Ferrous Gluconate may be decreased by: Antacids; H2-Antagonists; Pancrelipase; Proton Pump Inhibitors; Trientine

Food Interactions Cereals, dietary fiber, tea, coffee, eggs, and milk may decrease absorption.

Stability Store at 20°C to 25°C (68°F to 77°F) in child-resistant container and out of reach of children.

Mechanism of Action Replaces iron found in hemoglobin, myoglobin, and enzymes; allows the transportation of oxygen via hemoglobin

Pharmacodynamics
Onset of action: Hematologic response: Red blood cells form within 3-10 days; similar onset as parenteral iron salts
Maximum effect: Peak reticulocytosis occurs in 5-10 days, and hemoglobin values increase within 2-4 weeks

Pharmacokinetics (Adult data unless noted)
Absorption: Oral: Iron is absorbed in the duodenum and upper jejunum; in persons with normal iron stores 10% of an oral dose is absorbed, this is increased to 20% to 30% in persons with inadequate iron stores; food and achlorhydria will decrease absorption
Protein binding: To transferrin
Elimination: Excreted in the urine, sweat, sloughing of intestinal mucosa, and by menses

Dosing: Usual Note: Doses expressed as **elemental** iron.
Children and Adolescents:
Recommended daily allowance (RDA): Oral:
Children 4-8 years: 10 mg /day
Children and Adolescents 9-13 years: 8 mg /day
Adolescents 14-18 years:
Male: 11 mg /day
Female: 15 mg /day
Iron deficiency, prevention: Oral:
Note: Tablet dosage form may not be suitable for all pediatric doses. When appropriate, consider rounding to nearest whole tablet size.
Children ≥5 years in areas where anemia prevalence is >40%: 30 mg/day with folic acid (WHO, 2001)
Adolescents in areas where anemia prevalence is >40%: 60 mg/day with folic acid (WHO, 2001)
Iron deficiency, treatment of iron deficiency: Oral:
Severe iron deficiency anemia: 4-6 mg/kg/day in 3 divided doses (Carney, 2010)
Mild to moderate iron deficiency anemia: 3 mg/kg/day in 1-2 divided doses (CDC, 1998; IOM, 1993)
Adults:
Recommended daily allowance (RDA): Oral
19-50 years:
Males: 8 mg iron/day
Females 18 mg iron/day
>50 years: 8 mg iron/day
Iron deficiency, prevention: Oral: 60 mg iron/day
Iron deficiency, treatment: Oral: 60 mg iron twice daily; up to 60 mL iron 4 times/day

Administration Oral: Do not chew or crush sustained release preparations; administer with water or juice between meals for maximum absorption; may administer with food if GI upset occurs; do not administer with milk or milk products

Monitoring Parameters Serum iron, total iron binding capacity, reticulocyte count, hemoglobin, ferritin

Reference Range
Serum iron: 22-184 mcg/dL
Total iron binding capacity:
Infants: 100-400 mcg/dL
Children and Adults: 250-400 mcg/dL

Test Interactions False-positive for blood in stool by the guaiac test

Additional Information When treating iron deficiency anemias, treat for 3-4 months after hemoglobin/hematocrit return to normal in order to replenish total body stores

Elemental Iron Content of Iron Salts

Iron Salt	Elemental Iron Content (% of salt form)	Approximate Equivalent Doses (mg of iron salt)
Ferrous fumarate	33	197
Ferrous gluconate	11.6	560
Ferrous sulfate	20	324
Ferrous sulfate, exsiccated	30	217

Dosage Forms Excipient information presented when available (limited, particularly for generics); consult specific product labeling. [DSC] = Discontinued product ▶

Tablet, Oral:
Fergon: 240 (27 Fe) mg [contains tartrazine (fd&c yellow #5)]
Generic: 240 (27 Fe) mg, 324 (37.5 Fe) mg, 324 (38 Fe) mg, 325 (36 Fe) mg
Tablet, Oral [preservative free]:
Ferate: 240 (27 Fe) mg [corn free, dairy free, egg free, fragrance free, gluten free, no artificial flavor(s), sodium free, soy free, starch free, sugar free, wheat free, yeast free; contains fd&c blue #1 aluminum lake, fd&c yellow #6 aluminum lake]
Ferate: 256 (28 Fe) mg [DSC] [gluten free, lactose free, milk free, no artificial color(s), no artificial flavor(s), sodium free, soy free, sugar free, wheat free, yeast free]

References

Carney LN, Nepa A, Cohen SS, et al, "Parenteral and Enteral Nutrition Support: Determining the Best Way to Feed," In: Corkins MR, Balint J, Bobo E, et al, eds, The A.S.P.E.N Pediatric Nutrition Support Core Curriculum, Silver Spring: MD: American Society of Parenteral and Enteral Nutrition, 2010, 440-1.

Centers for Disease Control and Prevention (CDC), "Recommendations to Prevent and Control Iron Deficiency in the United States," MMWR REcomm Rep, 1998, 47(RR-3):1-36.

World Health Organization (WHO), "Iron Deficiency Anaemia: Assessment, Prevention, and Control. A Guide for Programme Managers," 2001.

Ferrous Sulfate (FER us SUL fate)

Medication Safety Issues
Sound-alike/look-alike issues:
Feosol® may be confused with Fer-In-Sol®
Fer-In-Sol® may be confused with Feosol®
Slow FE® may be confused with Slow-K®

Administration issues:
Multiple concentrations of liquid iron preparations exist. Fer-In-Sol® drops (manufactured by Mead Johnson) and a limited number of generic products are available at a concentration of 15 mg/mL. However, a suspension product, MyKidz Iron 10™ drops, is available at a concentration of 15 mg/1.5 mL. Check concentration closely prior to dispensing. Prescriptions written in milliliters (mL) should be clarified.

Related Information
Oral Medications That Should Not Be Crushed or Altered on page 2438

Brand Names: U.S. BProtected Pedia Iron [OTC]; Fer-In-Sol [OTC]; Fer-Iron [OTC]; FeroSul [OTC]; Ferro-Bob [OTC]; FerrouSul [OTC]; Iron Supplement Childrens [OTC]; Slow Fe [OTC]; Slow Iron [OTC]; Slow Release Iron [OTC] [DSC]

Brand Names: Canada Apo-Ferrous Sulfate®; Fer-In-Sol®; Ferodan™

Therapeutic Category Iron Salt; Mineral, Oral

Generic Availability (U.S.) Yes

Use Prevention and treatment of iron deficiency anemias (OTC: FDA approved in all ages); has also been used as supplemental therapy for patients receiving epoetin alfa

Pregnancy Considerations Iron crosses the placenta and fetal stores are obtained from the mother (McArdle, 2011). Iron requirements are increased in pregnant women compared to nonpregnant females (IOM, 2001). All pregnant women should be tested for iron deficiency anemia and treated with supplemental iron if needed (ACOG, 2008; CDC, 1998). Untreated iron deficiency anemia during pregnancy may be associated with an increased risk of low birth weight, preterm delivery, and perinatal mortality, as well as postpartum depression in the mother and decreased mental functioning in the offspring (ACOG, 2008; CDC, 1998; IOM, 2001). Treatment improves maternal hematologic status and neonatal birth weight (Haider, 2013).

Breast-Feeding Considerations Iron is normally found in breast milk. Breast milk has a higher concentration of bioavailable iron than cows' milk or goats' milk. Breast milk or iron-fortified formulas generally provide enough iron to meet the recommended dietary requirements of infants up to 6 months of age (CDC, 1998; IOM, 2001). Maternal iron requirements are increased in breast-feeding women (IOM, 2001). The amount of iron in breast milk is generally not influenced by maternal iron status (IOM, 1991).

Contraindications Hypersensitivity to iron salts or any component; hemochromatosis, hemolytic anemia

Warnings Avoid use in premature infants until the vitamin E stores, deficient at birth, are replenished. Accidental iron overdose is a leading cause of fatal poisoning in children under 6 years of age **[U.S. Boxed Warning]**; in case of accidental overdose, contact poison control center immediately; ingestions of ≥40 mg/kg elemental iron or who have persistent symptoms should seek immediate care; consider all iron sources when evaluating the dose of iron including combination products, infant formulas, and liquid nutritional supplements; store out of children's reach and in child-resistant containers. Some products may contain sulfites, ethanol, or polysorbate 80 (Tween 80) which may cause allergic reactions in susceptible individuals; consult product specific labeling. Some products (eg, MyKidz Iron 10) contain propylene glycol; toxicities have been reported with use of products containing propylene glycol, including hyperosmolality, lactic acidosis, seizures, and respiratory depression; in neonates large amounts of propylene glycol delivered orally, intravenously (eg, >3000 mg/day), or topically have been associated with potentially fatal toxicities which can include metabolic acidosis, seizures, renal failure, and CNS depression; use products containing propylene glycol with caution (AAP, 1997; Shehab, 2009).

Precautions Routine use for longer than 6 months is not recommended; some patients may require prolonged therapy (eg, continuous bleeding or menorrhagia). Avoid in patients with peptic ulcer, enteritis, or ulcerative colitis. Avoid in patients receiving frequent blood transfusions; patients already prone to chronic iron overload. Some liquid preparations may temporarily stain the teeth.

Adverse Reactions
Gastrointestinal: Constipation, dark stools, diarrhea, epigastric pain, GI irritation, heartburn, nausea, stomach cramping, vomiting
Genitourinary: Discoloration of urine
Miscellaneous: Liquid preparations may temporarily stain the teeth
Rare but important or life-threatening: Contact irritation

Drug Interactions
Metabolism/Transport Effects None known.
Avoid Concomitant Use
Avoid concomitant use of Ferrous Sulfate with any of the following: Dimercaprol
Increased Effect/Toxicity
The levels/effects of Ferrous Sulfate may be increased by: Dimercaprol
Decreased Effect
Ferrous Sulfate may decrease the levels/effects of: Bisphosphonate Derivatives; Cefdinir; Deferiprone; Dolutegravir; Eltrombopag; Levodopa; Levothyroxine; Methyldopa; PenicillAMINE; Phosphate Supplements; Quinolone Antibiotics; Tetracycline Derivatives; Trientine

The levels/effects of Ferrous Sulfate may be decreased by: Antacids; H2-Antagonists; Pancrelipase; Proton Pump Inhibitors; Trientine

Food Interactions Cereals, dietary fiber, tea, coffee, eggs, and milk may decrease absorption.

Stability Store at controlled room temperature in child-resistant container and out of reach of children; consult product-specific labeling for additional details.

Mechanism of Action Replaces iron, found in hemoglobin, myoglobin, and other enzymes; allows the transportation of oxygen via hemoglobin

Pharmacodynamics

Onset of action: Hematologic response: Red blood cells form within 3-10 days; similar onset as parenteral iron salts

Maximum effect: Peak reticulocytosis occurs in 5-10 days, and hemoglobin values increase within 2-4 weeks

Pharmacokinetics (Adult data unless noted)

Absorption: Oral: Iron is absorbed in the duodenum and upper jejunum; in persons with normal iron stores 10% of an oral dose is absorbed, this is increased to 20% to 30% in persons with inadequate iron stores; food and achlorhydria will decrease absorption

Protein binding: To transferrin

Elimination: Excreted in the urine, sweat, sloughing of intestinal mucosa, and by menses

Dosing: Neonatal Note: Multiple concentrations of ferrous sulfate oral liquid exist; close attention must be paid to the concentration when ordering and administering ferrous sulfate; incorrect selection or substitution of one ferrous sulfate liquid for another without proper dosage volume adjustment may result in serious over- or underdosing.

Note: Many infant formulas are fortified with iron; it is important to consider the amount delivered via formula when calculating oral iron doses.

Note: Neonatal dosages expressed in terms of **elemental** iron.

Adequate Intake (AI): Oral: 0.27 mg/day

Iron deficiency; prevention in neonates fed human milk: Oral:

Preterm (<37 weeks gestational age): 2 mg/kg/day divided every 12-24 hours; begin at 4-8 weeks PNA (maximum dose: 15 mg/day) (Baker, 2010; WHO, 2001)

Full-term: In healthy, term infants, that are full or partially breast-fed, AAP does not recommend routine additional supplementation of iron be considered until at least 4-6 months of age, if at all (Baker, 2010; Schanler, 2011)

Iron deficiency anemia; treatment: Oral:

Treatment, severe iron deficiency anemia: 4-6 mg/kg/day in 3 divided doses (Carney, 2010; Rao, 2009)

Treatment, mild to moderate iron deficiency anemia: 3 mg/kg/day in 1-2 divided doses (CDC, 1998; IOM, 1993)

Supplementation during epoetin use: Limited data available; dosing regimens variable: Usual dose: 6 mg /kg/day in 2-3 divided doses; usual range: 3-8 mg/kg/day although higher doses (up to 12 mg/kg/day) have been used in some protocols (Kleinman, 2009; Meyer, 1996; Rao, 2009)

Dosing: Usual Note: Multiple concentrations of ferrous sulfate oral liquid exist; close attention must be paid to the concentration when ordering and administering ferrous sulfate; incorrect selection or substitution of one ferrous sulfate liquid for another without proper dosage volume adjustment may result in serious over- or underdosing.

Infants, Children, and Adolescents: **Note:** Pediatric dosages expressed in terms of **elemental** iron.

Adequate intake (AI): Oral: 1-6 months: 0.27 mg iron/day

Recommended daily allowance (RDA): Oral:

Infants 7-12 months: 11 mg iron/day

Children 1-3 years: 7 mg iron/day

Children 4-8 years: 10 mg iron/day

Children and Adolescents 9-13 years: 8 mg iron/day

Adolescents 14-18 years:

Male: 11 mg iron/day

Female: 15 mg iron/day

Iron deficiency anemia; prevention: Oral:

Infants ≥4 months (receiving human milk as only nutritional source or >50% as source of nutrition without iron fortified food): 1 mg iron/kg/day (Baker, 2010);

Note: In healthy, term infants, AAP does not recommend routine additional supplementation of iron be considered until at least 4-6 months of age if breast-fed (full or partial) (Baker, 2010; Schanler, 2011)

Infants and Children 6 months to <2 years in areas where anemia prevalence is >40% and iron fortified foods not available: 2 mg/kg/day (WHO, 2001)

Children 2 years to <5 years in areas where anemia prevalence is >40%: 2 mg/kg/day (WHO, 2001)

Children ≥5 years in areas where anemia prevalence is >40%: 30 mg/day with folic acid (WHO, 2001)

Adolescent in areas where anemia prevalence is >40%: 60 mg/day with folic acid (WHO, 2001)

Treatment of iron deficiency: Infants, Children, and Adolescents:

Severe iron deficiency anemia: 4-6 mg iron/kg/day in 3 divided doses (Carney, 2010)

Mild to moderate iron deficiency anemia: 3 mg iron/kg/day in 1-2 divided doses (CDC, 1998)

Adults:

Recommended daily allowance (RDA): Oral:

19-50 years:

Males: 8 mg elemental iron/day

Females 18 mg elemental iron/day

>50 years: 8 mg elemental iron/day

Pregnancy: 27 mg elemental iron/day

Lactation: 9-10 mg elemental iron/day

Note: Adult doses expressed in terms of ferrous sulfate.

Iron deficiency anemia; prevention: Oral: 300 mg/day

Iron deficiency anemia; treatment: Oral: Immediate release: 300 mg twice daily up to 300 mg 4 times/day; Extended release: 250 mg once or twice daily

Administration Oral: Do not chew or crush extended release preparations; administer with water or juice between meals for maximum absorption; may administer with food if GI upset occurs; do not administer with milk or milk products

Monitoring Parameters Serum iron, total iron binding capacity, reticulocyte count, hemoglobin, ferritin

Reference Range

Serum iron: 22-184 mcg/dL

Total iron binding capacity:

Infants: 100-400 mcg/dL

Children and Adults: 250-400 mcg/dL

Test Interactions False-positive for blood in stool by the guaiac test

Additional Information When treating iron deficiency anemias, treat for 3-4 months after hemoglobin/hematocrit return to normal in order to replenish total body stores.

Elemental Iron Content of Iron Salts

Iron Salt	Elemental Iron Content (% of salt form)	Approximate Equivalent Doses (mg of iron salt)
Ferrous fumarate	33	197
Ferrous gluconate	11.6	560
Ferrous sulfate	20	324
Ferrous sulfate, exsiccated	30	217

Dosage Forms Excipient information presented when available (limited, particularly for generics); consult specific product labeling. [DSC] = Discontinued product

Elixir:

FeroSul: 220 (44 Fe) mg/5 mL (473 mL) [contains alcohol, usp, fd&c yellow #6 (sunset yellow), propylene

glycol, saccharin sodium, sodium benzoate; lemon flavor]
Generic: 220 (44 Fe) mg/5 mL (5 mL, 473 mL)
Liquid, Oral:
Generic: 220 (44 Fe) mg/5 mL (473 mL)
Solution, Oral:
BProtected Pedia Iron: 75 (15 Fe) mg/mL (50 mL) [alcohol free, gluten free; contains sodium metabisulfite; citrus flavor]
Fer-In-Sol: 75 (15 Fe) mg/mL (50 mL) [contains alcohol, usp, sodium bisulfite]
Fer-Iron: 75 (15 Fe) mg/mL (50 mL) [contains sodium metabisulfite; lemon flavor]
Iron Supplement Childrens: 75 (15 Fe) mg/mL (50 mL) [alcohol free, dye free, gluten free, lactose free; contains sodium bisulfite]
Generic: 75 (15 Fe) mg/mL (50 mL)
Syrup, Oral:
Generic: 300 (60 Fe) mg/5mL (5 mL)
Tablet, Oral:
Ferro-Bob: 325 (65 Fe) mg
Generic: 325 (65 Fe) mg
Tablet, Oral [preservative free]:
FerrouSul: 325 (65 Fe) mg [sodium free, starch free]
Generic: 325 (65 Fe) mg
Tablet Delayed Release, Oral:
Generic: 324 (65 Fe) mg, 325 (65 Fe) mg
Tablet Extended Release, Oral:
Slow Fe: 160 (50 Fe) mg
Slow Fe: 142 (45 Fe) mg [contains fd&c blue #1 aluminum lake, fd&c red #40 aluminum lake, fd&c yellow #6 aluminum lake]
Slow Release Iron: 140 (45 Fe) mg [DSC] [contains brilliant blue fcf (fd&c blue #1), fd&c red #40 aluminum lake, fd&c yellow #6 aluminum lake]
Tablet Extended Release, Oral [preservative free]:
Slow Iron: 160 (50 Fe) mg [gluten free]
Generic: 140 (45 Fe) mg

References

American Academy of Pediatrics Committee on Drugs. "Inactive" ingredients in pharmaceutical products: update (subject review). *Pediatrics.* 1997;99(2):268-278.
American Academy of Pediatrics, Committee on Nutrition, "Nutritional Needs of the Premature Infant," In: Kleinman RE, ed, *Pediatric Nutrition Handbook*, 6th ed, Elk Grove Village, IL: American Academy of Pediatrics; 2008, 79-112.
American College of Obstetricians and Gynecologists, "ACOG Practice Bulletin No. 95: Anemia in Pregnancy," *Obstet Gynecol*, 2008, 112 (1):201-7.
Baker RD, Greer FR, and Committee on Nutrition American Academy of Pediatrics, "Diagnosis and Prevention of Iron Deficiency and Iron-Deficiency Anemia in Infants and Young Children (0-3 Years of Age)," *Pediatrics*, 2010, 126(5):1040-50.
Carney LN, Nepa A, Cohen SS, et al, "Parenteral and Enteral Nutrition Support: Determining the Best Way to Feed," In: Corkins MR, Balint J, Bobo E, et al, eds, *The A.S.P.E.N Pediatric Nutrition Support Core Curriculum*, Silver Spring: MD: American Society of Parenteral and Enteral Nutrition, 2010, 440-1.
Centers for Disease Control and Prevention (CDC), "Recommendations to Prevent and Control Iron Deficiency in the United States," *MMWR Recomm Rep*, 1998, 47(RR-3):1-29.
Haider BA, Olofin I, Wang M, et al, "Anaemia, Prenatal Iron Use, and Risk of Adverse Pregnancy Outcomes: Systematic Review and Meta-analysis," *BMJ*, 2013, 346:f3443.
Institute of Medicine (IOM), *Dietary Reference Intakes for Vitamin A, Vitamin K, Arsenic, Boron, Chromium, Copper, Iodine, Iron, Manganese, Molybdenum, Nickel, Silicon, Vanadium, and Zinc*, Washington, DC: National Academy Press, 2001.
Institute of Medicine (IOM), "Iron Deficiency Anemia: Recommended Guidelines for the Prevention, Detection, and Management Among U.S. Children and Women of Childbearing Age," Washington, D.C.: The National Academies Press, 1993.
Institute of Medicine (IOM), "Nutrition During Lactation." Washington, DC: National Academy Press, 1991. Available at http://www.nap.edu
McArdle HJ, Lang C, Hayes H, et al, "Role of the Placenta in Regulation of Fetal Iron Status," *Nutr Rev*, 2011, 69(Suppl 1):17-22.
Meyer MP, Haworth C, Meyer JH, et al, "A Comparison of Oral and Intravenous Iron Supplementation in Preterm Infants Receiving Recombinant Erythropoietin," *J Pediatr*, 1996, 129(2):258-63.
Rao R and Georgieff MK, "Iron Therapy for Preterm Infants," *Clin Perinatol*, 2009, 36(1):27-42.
Schanler RJ, Feldman-Winter L, Landers S, et al, "Concerns With Early Universal Iron Supplementation of Breastfeeding Infants," *Pediatrics*, 2011, 127(4):e1097.
Shehab N, Lewis CL, Streetman DD, Donn SM. Exposure to the pharmaceutical excipients benzyl alcohol and propylene glycol among critically ill neonates. *Pediatr Crit Care Med*. 2009;10 (2):256-259.
World Health Organization (WHO), "Iron Deficiency Anaemia: Assessment, Prevention, and Control. A Guide for Programme Managers," 2001.

♦ **FerrouSul [OTC]** *see* Ferrous Sulfate *on page 868*

♦ **FerUS [OTC] [DSC]** *see* Polysaccharide-Iron Complex *on page 1701*

♦ **FeSO₄** *see* Ferrous Sulfate *on page 868*

♦ **Feverall [OTC]** *see* Acetaminophen *on page 47*

♦ **Fexmid** *see* Cyclobenzaprine *on page 558*

Fexofenadine (feks oh FEN a deen)

Medication Safety Issues
Sound-alike/look-alike issues:
Fexofenadine may be confused with fesoterodine
Allegra® may be confused with Viagra®
International issues:
Allegra [U.S, Canada, and multiple international markets] may be confused with Allegro brand name for fluticasone [Israel] and frovatriptan [Germany]
Brand Names: U.S. Allegra Allergy Childrens [OTC]; Allegra Allergy [OTC]; Mucinex Allergy [OTC]
Brand Names: Canada Allegra®
Therapeutic Category Antihistamine
Generic Availability (U.S.) May be product dependent
Use Symptomatic relief of seasonal allergic rhinitis (FDA approved in ages ≥2 years and adults); treatment of uncomplicated skin manifestations of chronic idiopathic urticaria (FDA approved in ages ≥6 months and adults); relief of symptoms due to hayfever or upper respiratory allergies [OTC products: Oral suspension: FDA approved in ages ≥2 years and adults; Meltable tablets: FDA approved in ages ≥6 years and adults; Tablets (12 or 24 hours): FDA approved in ages ≥12 years and adults]
Pregnancy Risk Factor C
Pregnancy Considerations Adverse events have been observed in animal reproduction studies; therefore, the manufacturer classifies fexofenadine as pregnancy category C. The use of antihistamines for the treatment of rhinitis during pregnancy is generally considered to be safe at recommended doses. Information related to the use of fexofenadine during pregnancy is limited; therefore, other agents are preferred.
Breast-Feeding Considerations It is not known if fexofenadine is excreted in breast milk. The manufacturer recommends that caution be exercised when administering fexofenadine to nursing women.
Contraindications Hypersensitivity to fexofenadine or any component
Warnings Rare hypersensitivity reactions have been reported; manifestations have been described as angioedema, chest tightness, dyspnea, flushing, and systemic anaphylaxis.
Precautions Use with caution in patients with renal impairment; dosage adjustment required. Use cautiously in patients who are also taking ketoconazole and erythromycin; although increased plasma levels of fexofenadine have been observed, no adverse effects with concomitant administration have been reported including QT prolongation which occurred when terfenadine was combined with these agents; while less sedating than other antihistamines, fexofenadine may cause drowsiness and impair ability to perform hazardous activities requiring mental

alertness. The orally disintegrating tablets and OTC meltable tablets contain aspartame which is metabolized to phenylalanine and must be used with caution in patients with phenylketonuria.

Adverse Reactions
Central nervous system: Dizziness, drowsiness, fatigue, fever, headache, pain, somnolence

Endocrine & metabolic: Dysmenorrhea

Gastrointestinal: Diarrhea, dyspepsia, nausea, vomiting

Neuromuscular & skeletal: Back pain, myalgia, pain in extremities

Otic: Otitis media

Respiratory: Cough, rhinorrhea, sinusitis, upper respiratory tract infection

Miscellaneous: Viral infection

Rare but important or life-threatening: Hypersensitivity reactions (anaphylaxis, angioedema, chest tightness, dyspnea, flushing, pruritus, rash, urticaria); insomnia, nervousness, sleep disorders, paroniria (terrifying dreams)

Drug Interactions
Metabolism/Transport Effects Substrate of CYP3A4 (minor), P-glycoprotein, SLCO1B1; **Note:** Assignment of Major/Minor substrate status based on clinically relevant drug interaction potential; **Inhibits** CYP2D6 (weak)

Avoid Concomitant Use
Avoid concomitant use of Fexofenadine with any of the following: Aclidinium; Azelastine (Nasal); Ipratropium (Oral Inhalation); Paraldehyde; Potassium Chloride; Thalidomide; Tiotropium; Umeclidinium

Increased Effect/Toxicity
Fexofenadine may increase the levels/effects of: AbobotulinumtoxinA; Alcohol (Ethyl); Analgesics (Opioid); Anticholinergic Agents; ARIPiprazole; Azelastine (Nasal); Buprenorphine; Cannabinoid-Containing Products; CNS Depressants; Hydrocodone; Methotrimeprazine; Metyrosine; Mirabegron; Mirtazapine; OnabotulinumtoxinA; Paraldehyde; Potassium Chloride; Pramipexole; RimabotulinumtoxinB; ROPINIRole; Rotigotine; Selective Serotonin Reuptake Inhibitors; Thalidomide; Thiazide Diuretics; Tiotropium; Topiramate; Zolpidem

The levels/effects of Fexofenadine may be increased by: Aclidinium; Brimonidine (Topical); Cannabis; Doxylamine; Dronabinol; Droperidol; Eltrombopag; Erythromycin (Systemic); HydrOXYzine; Ipratropium (Oral Inhalation); Itraconazole; Kava Kava; Ketoconazole (Systemic); Magnesium Sulfate; Methotrimeprazine; Nabilone; Perampanel; P-glycoprotein/ABCB1 Inhibitors; Pramlintide; Rifampin; Rufinamide; Sodium Oxybate; Tapentadol; Tetrahydrocannabinol; Umeclidinium; Verapamil

Decreased Effect
Fexofenadine may decrease the levels/effects of: Acetylcholinesterase Inhibitors (Central); Benzylpenicilloyl Polylysine; Betahistine; Hyaluronidase; Secretin

The levels/effects of Fexofenadine may be decreased by: Acetylcholinesterase Inhibitors (Central); Amphetamines; Antacids; Grapefruit Juice; P-glycoprotein/ABCB1 Inducers; Rifampin

Food Interactions High-fat meals decrease the bioavailability of fexofenadine by ~50%. Fruit juice (apple, grapefruit, orange) may decrease bioavailability of fexofenadine by ~36%. Management: Administer with water only, avoid fruit juice.

Stability Store at 20°C to 25°C (68°F to 77°F); protect from excessive moisture.

Mechanism of Action Fexofenadine is an active metabolite of terfenadine and like terfenadine it competes with histamine for H_1-receptor sites on effector cells in the gastrointestinal tract, blood vessels and respiratory tract; it appears that fexofenadine does not cross the blood-brain barrier to any appreciable degree, resulting in a reduced potential for sedation

Pharmacodynamics
Onset of action: 1 hour

Maximum effect: 2-3 hours

Duration: ≥12 hours

Pharmacokinetics (Adult data unless noted)
Absorption: Rapid

Distribution: V_d: Children: 5.4-5.8 L/kg

Protein binding: 60% to 70%

Metabolism: 5% in liver; 3.5% transformed into methylester metabolite found only in feces (possibly transformed by gut microflora)

Half-life: 14-18 hours

Time to peak serum concentration: ODT: 2 hours (4 hours with high-fat meal); Tablets: 2.6 hours; Suspension: 1 hour

Elimination: 11% excreted unchanged in urine; 80% excreted unchanged in feces

Clearance: Children: 14-18 mL/minute/kg

Dialysis: Not effectively removed by hemodialysis

Dosing: Usual Hayfever, upper respiratory allergies (OTC use): Oral:
Children 2-11 years: 30 mg twice daily

Children ≥12 years, Adolescents, and Adults: 60 mg twice daily or 180 mg once daily

Chronic idiopathic urticaria: Oral:
Infants ≥6 months to Children <2 years: 15 mg twice daily

Children 2-11 years: 30 mg twice daily

Children ≥12 years, Adolescents, and Adults: 60 mg twice daily or 180 mg once daily

Seasonal allergic rhinitis: Oral:
Children 2-11 years: 30 mg twice daily

Children ≥12 years, Adolescents, and Adults: 60 mg twice daily or 180 mg once daily

Dosing adjustment in renal impairment:
CrCl <80 mL/minute:

Infants ≥6 months to Children <2 years: 15 mg once daily

Children 2-11 years: 30 mg once daily

Children ≥12 years, Adolescents, and Adults: 60 mg once daily

Hemodialysis: Not effectively removed by hemodialysis

Administration
Suspension, tablet: May administer without respect to food. Take with water; avoid administration with fruit juices; shake suspension well before use

Orally disintegrating tablet: Take on an empty stomach. Do not remove from blister pack until ready to administer. Using dry hands, place immediately on tongue. Tablet will dissolve within seconds, and may be swallowed with or without liquid; avoid taking with fruit juices. Do not split or chew.

Monitoring Parameters Improvement in signs and symptoms of allergic rhinitis and chronic idiopathic urticaria

Test Interactions May suppress the wheal and flare reactions to skin test antigens.

Dosage Forms Excipient information presented when available (limited, particularly for generics); consult specific product labeling.

Suspension, Oral, as hydrochloride:
Allegra Allergy Childrens: 30 mg/5 mL (120 mL) [alcohol free, dye free; contains butylparaben, edetate disodium, propylene glycol, propylparaben; raspberry creme flavor]

Tablet, Oral, as hydrochloride:
Allegra Allergy: 60 mg, 180 mg

Allegra Allergy Childrens: 30 mg

Mucinex Allergy: 180 mg [contains fd&c red #40]

Generic: 60 mg, 180 mg

Tablet Dispersible, Oral, as hydrochloride:
Allegra Allergy Childrens: 30 mg [contains aspartame; orange cream flavor]

◆ **Fexofenadine Hydrochloride** *see* Fexofenadine *on page 870*

◆ **Fiber Therapy [OTC]** *see* Psyllium *on page 1773*

Filgrastim (fil GRA stim)

Medication Safety Issues
Sound-alike/look-alike issues:
Neupogen may be confused with Epogen, Neulasta, Neumega, Nutramigen
International issues:
Neupogen [U.S., Canada, and multiple international markets] may be confused with Neupro brand name for rotigotine [multiple international markets]

Brand Names: U.S. Granix; Neupogen

Brand Names: Canada Neupogen

Therapeutic Category Colony-Stimulating Factor; Hematopoietic Agent

Generic Availability (U.S.) No

Use

Cancer patients (nonmyeloid malignancies) receiving myelosuppressive chemotherapy to decrease the incidence of infection (febrile neutropenia) in regimens associated with a high incidence of neutropenia with fever [FDA approved in pediatric patients (age not specified) and adults]

Acute myelogenous leukemia (AML) following induction or consolidation chemotherapy to shorten time to neutrophil recovery and reduce the duration of fever (FDA approved in adults)

Cancer patients (nonmyeloid malignancies) receiving bone marrow transplant to shorten the duration of neutropenia and neutropenia-related events (eg, neutropenic fever) (FDA approved in adults)

Peripheral stem cell transplantation to mobilize hematopoietic progenitor cells for apheresis collection (FDA approved in adults)

Severe chronic neutropenia (SCN; chronic administration) to reduce the incidence and duration of neutropenic complications (fever, infections, oropharyngeal ulcers) in symptomatic patients with congenital, cyclic, or idiopathic neutropenia (FDA approved in ages ≥1 month and adults)

Has also been used for AIDS patients receiving zidovudine; neonatal neutropenia

Pregnancy Risk Factor C

Pregnancy Considerations Adverse events have been observed in animal reproduction studies. Filgrastim has been shown to cross the placenta in humans.

Women who become pregnant during Neupogen treatment are encouraged to enroll in the manufacturer's Pregnancy Surveillance Program (1-800-772-6436).

Breast-Feeding Considerations It is not known if filgrastim or tbo-filgrastim is excreted in breast milk. The manufacturers recommend that caution be exercised when administering filgrastim or tbo-filgrastim to nursing women.

Women who are nursing during Neupogen treatment are encouraged to enroll in the manufacturer's Lactation Surveillance program (1-800-772-6436).

Contraindications Hypersensitivity to *E. coli*-derived proteins, G-CSF, or any component

Warnings Hypersensitivity reactions characterized by rash, urticaria, facial edema, wheezing, dyspnea, tachycardia, and/or hypotension have occurred with first or subsequent doses; reactions tended to involve two or more body systems and occur more frequently with intravenous administration and generally within 30 minutes of administration. Symptoms recurred in >50% of patients when rechallenged. Rare cases of splenic rupture have been reported (may be fatal); patients must be instructed to report left upper quadrant pain or shoulder tip pain. May

precipitate severe sickle cell crises, sometimes resulting in fatalities, in patients with sickle cell disorders; carefully evaluate potential risks and benefits. Filgrastim use prior to appropriate diagnosis of severe congenital neutropenia (SCN) may impair proper evaluation and treatment for neutropenia not due to SCN. Cytogenetic abnormalities, transformation to myelodysplastic syndrome (MDS) and acute myeloid leukemia (AML) have been observed in patients treated with filgrastim for congenital neutropenia; a longer duration of treatment and poorer ANC response appear to increase the risk. Carefully consider the risk of continuing filgrastim in patients who develop abnormal cytogenetics or MDS.

Rare cases of acute respiratory distress syndrome (ARDS) have been reported (possibly due to influx of neutrophils to sites of lung inflammation); withhold or discontinue filgrastim if ARDS occurs; patients must be instructed to report respiratory distress; monitor for fever, infiltrates, or respiratory distress. Alveolar hemorrhage has been reported, manifested as pulmonary infiltrates and hemoptysis, and occurred in healthy donors undergoing PBPC collection (not FDA approved for use in healthy donors); hemoptysis resolved upon discontinuation.

Cutaneous vasculitis has been reported, generally occurring in patients with severe chronic neutropenia on long-term therapy; symptoms generally developed with increasing absolute neutrophil count (ANC) and subsided when the ANC decreased; dose reductions may improve symptoms to allow for continued therapy.

Injection contains polysorbate 80 (Tween 80®) which may cause allergic reactions in susceptible individuals. In premature neonates, thrombocytopenia, ascites, pulmonary deterioration, and renal and hepatic failure have been reported after receiving parenteral products containing polysorbate 80 (Alade, 1986; CDC, 1984). Infusion of polysorbate 80-containing solutions through polyvinyl chloride tubing may cause DEHP to leach into the solution; in immature animals, exposure to DEHP may adversely affect the development of the male reproductive tract. The packaging of some dosage forms may contain latex which may cause allergic reactions in susceptible individuals.

Precautions Do not administer 24 hours prior to or within 24 hours following the administration of chemotherapy; use with caution in any malignancy with myeloid characteristics due to G-CSF's potential to act as a growth factor; avoid concurrent radiation therapy with filgrastim; safety and efficacy have not been established with patients receiving radiation therapy.

Leukocytosis (white blood cell counts ≥100,000/mm^3) has been observed in ~2% of patients receiving G-CSF at doses >5 mcg/kg/day. Premature discontinuation of G-CSF therapy prior to the time of recovery from the expected neutrophil nadir is generally not recommended. A transient increase in neutrophil counts is typically seen 1 to 2 days after initiation of therapy. For a sustained therapeutic response, G-CSF should be continued until the post nadir absolute neutrophil count (ANC) reaches:
10,000/mm^3 in chemotherapy treated patients, or
>1000/mm^3 for 3 consecutive days in bone marrow transplant patients

Most patients experience a 30% to 50% decrease in circulating leukocytes within 1 to 2 days following discontinuation of G-CSF

Adverse Reactions
Cardiovascular: Cardiac arrhythmia, hypertension, myocardial infarction
Central nervous system: Headache
Dermatologic: Skin rash
Endocrine & metabolic: Increased lactate dehydrogenase, increased uric acid

Gastrointestinal: Nausea, peritonitis, vomiting

Hematologic & oncologic: Leukocytosis, petechiae, splenomegaly, thrombocytopenia

Hepatic: Increased serum alkaline phosphatase

Neuromuscular & skeletal: Ostealgia (commonly in the lower back, posterior iliac crest, and sternum)

Respiratory: Epistaxis

Hypersensitivity: Transfusion reaction

Miscellaneous: Fever

Rare but important or life-threatening: Alopecia, capillary leak syndrome, cerebral hemorrhage, decreased bone mineral density, erythema nodosum, exacerbation of psoriasis, hematuria, hepatomegaly, hemoptysis, hypersensitivity angiitis, hypersensitivity reaction, osteoporosis, pericarditis, proteinuria, pulmonary hemorrhage, pulmonary infiltrates, renal insufficiency, respiratory distress syndrome, severe sickle cell crisis, splenic rupture, supraventricular cardiac arrhythmia, Sweet's syndrome, tachycardia, thrombophlebitis

Drug Interactions

Metabolism/Transport Effects None known.

Avoid Concomitant Use There are no known interactions where it is recommended to avoid concomitant use.

Increased Effect/Toxicity

Filgrastim may increase the levels/effects of: Bleomycin; Cyclophosphamide; Topotecan

Decreased Effect There are no known significant interactions involving a decrease in effect.

Stability Store at 2°C to 8°C (36°F to 46°F); do not freeze; protect from direct sunlight; avoid shaking; stable for 24 hours at room temperature; solutions with concentration ≥15 mcg/mL in D₅W are stable for 24 hours; incompatible with salt solutions

Mechanism of Action Filgrastim and tbo-filgrastim are granulocyte colony stimulating factors (G-CSF) produced by recombinant DNA technology. G-CSFs stimulate the production, maturation, and activation of neutrophils to increase both their migration and cytotoxicity.

Pharmacodynamics

Onset of action: Immediate transient leukopenia with the nadir occurring 5 to 15 minutes after an I.V. dose or 30 to 60 minutes after a SubQ dose followed by a sustained elevation in neutrophil levels within the first 24 hours reaching a plateau in 3 to 5 days

Duration: Upon discontinuation of G-CSF, ANC decreases by 50% within 2 days and returns to pretreatment levels within 1 week; WBC counts return to normal range in 4 to 7 days

Pharmacokinetics (Adult data unless noted)

Distribution: V_d: 150 mL/kg

Bioavailability: Not bioavailable after oral administration

Half-life: Neonates: 4.4 hours; Adults: 1.8 to 3.5 hours

Time to peak serum concentration: SubQ: Within 2 to 6 hours

Dosing: Neonatal

Neutropenia with sepsis: I.V., SubQ: 10 mcg/kg/day divided every 12 to 24 hours for 3 to 14 days; most trials have used once daily dosing for 3 days (Carr, 2009)

Neutropenia, prophylaxis of infection: I.V., SubQ: 5 to 10 mcg/kg/day for 3 to 5 days (Carr, 2009)

Neutropenia, congenital: SubQ: Initial: 5 mcg/kg/day, followed by 10 mcg/kg/day; then titrate to response using 10 mcg/kg/day increments every 14 days until target ANC (1000 to 1500/mm³) is reached and maintained; if ANC exceeds 5000/mm³, dosage should be reduced to lowest effective dose. Typical dose range for response of patients included in the international CN registry is 3 to 10 mcg/kg/day; maximum dose: 120 mcg/kg/day (Boztug, 2008; Welte, 2006)

Neutropenia, idiopathic or cyclic: SubQ:1 to 5 mcg/kg/day once daily (Ancliff, 2003)

Dosing: Usual

Infants, Children, and Adolescents: **Note:** Details concerning dosing in combination regimens and institution protocols should also be consulted. For larger doses (eg, adolescents), rounding doses to the nearest vial size may enhance patient convenience and reduce costs without compromising clinical response.

Bone marrow transplantation, cancer patients: Limited data available: I.V., SubQ: 5 mcg/kg/day administered ≥24 hours after cytotoxic chemotherapy and ≥24 hours after bone marrow infusion (Schaison, 1998; Wagner, 2001)

Chemotherapy-induced neutropenia: I.V., SubQ: 5 mcg/kg/day once daily beginning ≥24 hours after chemotherapy; recommendations for duration of therapy vary: Manufacturer labeling is for up to 14 days or until ANC reaches 10,000/mm³; others have suggested a lower target ANC of 5,000/mm³ (Schaison, 1998; Wagner, 2001). For subsequent chemotherapy cycles, dose may be increased by 5 mcg/kg based upon patient's previous response to therapy along with duration and severity of neutropenia; reported range: 4 to 8 mcg/kg/day.

Neutropenia, idiopathic or cyclic: SubQ: 1 to 5 mcg/kg/day once daily (Ancliff, 2003)

Neutropenia due to zidovudine for HIV treatment: SubQ: 5 to 10 mcg/kg/day once daily (Working Group, 2008)

Peripheral blood progenitor cell (PBPC) mobilization, autologous bone marrow transplant: Limited data available: I.V., SubQ: 10 mcg/kg/day given for 4 to 5 days before apheresis procedure (Diaz, 2000; Wagner, 2001)

Adults: Details concerning dosing in combination regimens and institution protocols should also be consulted. Rounding doses to the nearest vial size may enhance patient convenience and reduce costs without compromising clinical response.

Bone marrow transplantation (in patients with cancer; to shorten the duration of neutropenia and neutropenia-related events): I.V., SubQ.: 10 mcg/kg/day (administer ≥24 hours after chemotherapy and ≥24 hours after bone marrow infusion); adjust the dose according to the duration and severity of neutropenia; recommended steps based on neutrophil response:

When ANC >1000/mm³ for 3 consecutive days: Reduce filgrastim dose to 5 mcg/kg/day.

If ANC remains >1000/mm³ for 3 more consecutive days: Discontinue filgrastim.

If ANC decreases to <1000/mm³: Resume at 5 mcg/kg/day.

If ANC decreases to <1000/mm³ during the 5 mcg/kg/day dose: Increase filgrastim to 10 mcg/kg/day and follow the above step

Chemotherapy-induced neutropenia: I.V., SubQ: 5 mcg/kg/day; doses may be increased by 5 mcg/kg (for each chemotherapy cycle) according to the duration and severity of the neutropenia; continue for up to 14 days or until the ANC reaches 10,000/mm³

Peripheral blood progenitor cell (PBPC) collection: SubQ: 10 mcg/kg/dose once daily, usually for 6 to 7 days. Begin at least 4 days before the first apheresis and continue until the last apheresis; consider dose adjustment for WBC >100,000/mm³

Severe chronic neutropenia: SubQ:

Congenital: Initial: 6 mcg/kg/dose twice daily; adjust the dose based on ANC and clinical response

Idiopathic/cyclic: Initial: 5 mcg/kg/day; adjust the dose based on ANC and clinical response

Administration Parenteral: **Note:** When used for neutropenia associated with chemotherapy or BMT, do not administer in the 24 hours prior to or earlier than 24 hours after cytotoxic chemotherapy.

▶

SubQ: Administer undiluted solution as a bolus injection (preferred) (Smith, 2006; Wagner, 2001); manufacturer labeling suggests may also be given as a continuous infusion for the following indications: Chemotherapy-induced neutropenia, bone marrow transplantation, and peripheral blood progenitor cell collection. For continuous infusion, dilute dose in 10 mL D_5W and infuse at a rate of 10 mL/24 hours

I.V.: May be administered as a short infusion over 15 to 30 minutes; manufacturer labeling suggests may also be given as a continuous I.V. infusion for chemotherapy-induced neutropenia or as a 4- or 24-hour infusion for bone marrow transplantation at a final concentration of at least 15 mcg/mL in D_5W. If the final concentration of G-CSF in D_5W is 5 to <15 mcg/mL, then albumin should be added to a final concentration of 2 mg/mL to prevent drug adsorption to the I.V. tubing; albumin should be added to the D_5W prior to addition of G-CSF; final concentration of G-CSF for administration <5 mcg/mL is not recommended; do not shake solution to avoid foaming.

Monitoring Parameters Temperature, CBC with differential and platelet count, hematocrit, uric acid, urinalysis, liver function tests

Reference Range Blood samples for monitoring the hematologic effects of G-CSF should be drawn just before the next dose

Test Interactions May interfere with bone imaging studies; increased hematopoietic activity of the bone marrow may appear as transient positive bone imaging changes

Dosage Forms Considerations
Prefilled syringes: Granix, Neupogen: 300 mcg/0.5 mL (0.5 mL); 480 mcg/0.8 mL (0.8 mL)
Vials: Neupogen: 300 mcg/mL (1 mL); 480 mcg/1.6 mL (1.6 mL)

Dosage Forms Excipient information presented when available (limited, particularly for generics); consult specific product labeling.
Solution, Injection:
Neupogen: 300 mcg/mL (1 mL); 480 mcg/1.6 mL (1.6 mL) [contains polysorbate 80]
Solution, Injection [preservative free]:
Neupogen: 300 mcg/0.5 mL (0.5 mL); 480 mcg/0.8 mL (0.8 mL) [contains polysorbate 80]
Solution Prefilled Syringe, Subcutaneous [preservative free]:
Granix: 300 mcg/0.5 mL (0.5 mL); 480 mcg/0.8 mL (0.8 mL) [contains polysorbate 80]

References
Alade SL, Brown RE, Paquet A Jr. Polysorbate 80 and E-Ferol toxicity. *Pediatrics.* 1986;77(4):593-597.
Ancliff PJ. Congenital neutropenia. *Blood Rev.* 2003;17(4):209-216.
Bonilla MA, Gillio AP, Ruggeiro M, et al. Effects of recombinant human granulocyte colony-stimulating factor on neutropenia in patients with congenital agranulocytosis. *N Engl J Med.* 1989;320(24):1574-1580.
Boztug K, Welte K, Zeidler C, Klein C. Congenital neutropenia syndromes. *Immunol Allergy Clin North Am.* 2008;28(2):259-275.
Carr R, Brocklehurst P, Doré CJ, et al. Granulocyte-Macrophage colony stimulating factor administered as prophylaxis for reduction of sepsis in extremely preterm, small for gestational age neonates (the PROGRAMS trial): A single-blind, multicentre, randomised controlled trial. *Lancet.* 2009;373(9659):226-33.
Carr R, Modi N, Doré C. G-CSF and GM-CSF for treating or preventing neonatal infections. *Cochrane Database Syst Rev.* 2003;3: CD003066.
Centers for Disease Control and Prevention (CDC). Unusual syndrome with fatalities among premature infants: association with a new intravenous vitamin E product. *MMWR Morb Mortal Wkly Rep.* 1984;33 (14):198-199.
DHHS Panel on Antiretroviral Therapy and Medical Management of HIV-Infected Children. Guidelines for the use of antiretroviral agents in pediatric HIV infection. February 12, 2014. Available at http://aidsinfo.nih.gov
Díaz MA, Kanold J, Vicent MG, Halle P, Madero L, Deméocq F. Using peripheral blood progenitor cells (PBPC) for transplantation in pediatric patients: a state-of-the-art review. *Bone Marrow Transplant.* 2000;26(12):1291-1298.
Gilmore MM, Stroncek DF, Korones DN. Treatment of alloimmune neonatal neutropenia with granulocyte colony-stimulating factor. *J Pediatr.* 1994;125(6 Pt 1):948-951.
Hollingshead LM, Goa KL. Recombinant granulocyte colony-stimulating factor (rG-CSF). A review of its pharmacological properties and prospective role in neutropenic conditions. *Drugs.* 1991;42 (2):300-330.
Morstyn G, Campbell L, Lieschke G, et al. Treatment of chemotherapy-induced neutropenia by subcutaneously administered granulocyte colony-stimulating factor with optimization of dose and duration of therapy. *J Clin Oncol.* 1989;7(10):1554-1562.
Schaison G, Eden OB, Henze G, et al. Recommendations on the use of colony-stimulating factors in children: conclusions of a European panel. *Eur J Pediatr.* 1998;157(12):955-966.
Smith TJ, Khatcheressian J, Lyman GH, et al. 2006 update of recommendations for the use of white blood cell growth factors: an evidence-based clinical practice guideline. *J Clin Oncol.* 2006;24 (19):3187-3205.
Update of recommendations for the use of hematopoietic colony-stimulating factors: evidence-based clinical practice guideline. American Society of Clinical Oncology. *J Clin Oncol.* 1996;14 (6):1957-1960.
Wagner LM, Furman WL. Haemopoietic growth factors in paediatric oncology: a review of the literature. *Paediatr Drugs.* 2001;3 (3):195-217.
Welte K, Zeidler C, Dale DC. Severe congenital neutropenia. *Semin Hematol.* 2006;43(3):189-195.
Wolach B. Neonatal sepsis: pathogenesis and supportive therapy. *Semin Perinatol.* 1997;21(1):28-38.

◆ **Finacea** *see* Azelaic Acid *on page 244*

◆ **Finacea® (Can)** *see* Azelaic Acid *on page 244*

◆ **First-Hydrocortisone** *see* Hydrocortisone (Topical) *on page 1038*

◆ **First-Lansoprazole** *see* Lansoprazole *on page 1206*

◆ **First-Omeprazole** *see* Omeprazole *on page 1535*

◆ **First-Testosterone** *see* Testosterone *on page 1986*

◆ **First-Testosterone MC** *see* Testosterone *on page 1986*

◆ **First-Vancomycin 25** *see* Vancomycin *on page 2110*

◆ **First-Vancomycin 50** *see* Vancomycin *on page 2110*

◆ **Fisalamine** *see* Mesalamine *on page 1347*

◆ **FK506** *see* Tacrolimus (Systemic) *on page 1963*

◆ **Flagyl** *see* MetroNIDAZOLE (Systemic) *on page 1399*

◆ **Flagyl ER** *see* MetroNIDAZOLE (Systemic) *on page 1399*

◆ **Flamazine® (Can)** *see* Silver Sulfadiazine *on page 1890*

◆ **Flanax Pain Relief [OTC]** *see* Naproxen *on page 1470*

◆ **Flarex** *see* Fluorometholone *on page 897*

◆ **Flarex® (Can)** *see* Fluorometholone *on page 897*

◆ **Flebogamma** *see* Immune Globulin *on page 1084*

◆ **Flebogamma DIF** *see* Immune Globulin *on page 1084*

Flecainide (fle KAY nide)

Medication Safety Issues
Sound-alike/look-alike issues:
Flecainide may be confused with fluconazole
Tambocor™ may be confused with Pamelor™, Temodar®, tamoxifen, Tamiflu®
BEERS Criteria medication:
This drug may be potentially inappropriate for use in geriatric patients (Quality of evidence - high; Strength of recommendation - strong).

Related Information
Medications for Which a Single Dose May Be Fatal When Ingested by a Toddler *on page 2408*

Brand Names: U.S. Tambocor [DSC]
Brand Names: Canada Apo-Flecainide®; Tambocor™
Therapeutic Category Antiarrhythmic Agent, Class I-C
Generic Availability (U.S.) Yes

Use Prevention and suppression of documented life-threatening ventricular arrhythmias (ie, sustained ventricular tachycardia); prevention of symptomatic, disabling supraventricular tachycardias in patients without structural heart disease

Pregnancy Risk Factor C

Pregnancy Considerations Adverse events have been observed in some animal reproduction studies.

Breast-Feeding Considerations Flecainide is excreted in human breast milk at concentrations as high as 4 times corresponding plasma levels.

Contraindications Hypersensitivity to flecainide or any component; preexisting second or third degree A-V block; right bundle-branch block associated with left hemiblock (bifascicular block) or trifascicular block (unless a functioning pacemaker is present); cardiogenic shock, myocardial depression

Warnings Antiarrhythmic agents should be reserved for patients with life-threatening ventricular arrhythmias **[U.S. Boxed Warning]**. In the Cardiac Arrhythmia Suppression Trial (CAST), recent (>6 days but <2 years ago) myocardial infarction patients with asymptomatic, nonlife-threatening ventricular arrhythmias did not benefit and may have been harmed by attempts to suppress the arrhythmia with flecainide or encainide. An increased mortality or nonfatal cardiac arrest rate (7.7%) was seen in the active treatment group compared with patients in the placebo group (3%). The applicability of the CAST results to other populations is unknown. The risks of class IC agents and the lack of improved survival make use in patients without life-threatening arrhythmias generally unacceptable.

Use for symptomatic nonsustained ventricular tachycardia, frequent premature ventricular complexes (PVCs), uniform and multiform PVCs and/or coupled PVCs, or chronic atrial fibrillation is not recommended. Flecainide can worsen or cause arrhythmias with an associated risk of death **[U.S. Boxed Warnings]**. Proarrhythmic effects range from an increased number of PVCs to more severe ventricular tachycardias (ie, tachycardias that are more sustained or more resistant to conversion to sinus rhythm). Risk is reduced when lower doses were initiated; monitor and adjust dose to prevent QT_c prolongation. Flecainide is not recommended for patients with chronic atrial fibrillation. When treating atrial flutter, 1:1 atrioventricular conduction may occur; pre-emptive negative chronotropic therapy (eg, digoxin, beta-blockers) may lower the risk **[U.S. Boxed Warning]**.

Precautions Use with caution in patients with pacemakers, sick sinus syndrome, CHF, myocardial dysfunction, and renal and/or hepatic impairment; use decreased doses and cautiously titrate dose according to serum concentrations and clinical effects in patients with CHF, or myocardial, liver or renal dysfunction. Flecainide may cause increases in PR, QRS, and QT intervals and new first degree or bundle branch block; use with caution and consider dosing reduction when increases in such intervals occur.

Adverse Reactions

Cardiovascular: Chest pain, edema, palpitation, proarrhythmic, sinus node dysfunction, syncope, tachycardia

Central nervous system: Anxiety, ataxia, depression, dizziness, fatigue, fever, headache, hypoesthesia, insomnia, malaise, nervousness, paresis, somnolence, tinnitus, vertigo

Dermatologic: Rash

Gastrointestinal: Abdominal pain, anorexia, constipation, diarrhea, nausea

Neuromuscular & skeletal: Paresthesias, tremor, weakness

Ocular: Blurred vision, diplopia, visual disturbances

Respiratory: Dyspnea

Rare but important or life-threatening: Alopecia, alters pacing threshold, amnesia, angina, AV block, bradycardia, bronchospasm, CHF, corneal deposits, depersonalization, euphoria, exfoliative dermatitis, granulocytopenia, heart block, increased P-R, leukopenia, metallic taste, neuropathy, paradoxical increase in ventricular rate in atrial fibrillation/flutter, paresthesia, photophobia, pneumonitis, pruritus, QRS duration, swollen lips/tongue/mouth, tardive dyskinesia, thrombocytopenia, urinary retention, urticaria, ventricular arrhythmia

Drug Interactions

Metabolism/Transport Effects Substrate of CYP1A2 (minor), CYP2D6 (major); **Note:** Assignment of Major/Minor substrate status based on clinically relevant drug interaction potential; **Inhibits** CYP2D6 (weak)

Avoid Concomitant Use

Avoid concomitant use of Flecainide with any of the following: Fosamprenavir; Highest Risk QTc-Prolonging Agents; Ivabradine; Mifepristone; Ritonavir; Saquinavir; Tipranavir

Increased Effect/Toxicity

Flecainide may increase the levels/effects of: ARIPiprazole; Digoxin; Highest Risk QTc-Prolonging Agents; Moderate Risk QTc-Prolonging Agents

The levels/effects of Flecainide may be increased by: Abiraterone Acetate; Amiodarone; Boceprevir; Carbonic Anhydrase Inhibitors; CYP2D6 Inhibitors (Moderate); CYP2D6 Inhibitors (Strong); Darunavir; Fosamprenavir; Ivabradine; Mifepristone; Mirabegron; QTc-Prolonging Agents (Indeterminate Risk and Risk Modifying); Ritonavir; Saquinavir; Sodium Bicarbonate; Sodium Lactate; Telaprevir; Tipranavir; Tromethamine; Verapamil

Decreased Effect

The levels/effects of Flecainide may be decreased by: Etravirine; Peginterferon Alfa-2b; Sodium Bicarbonate

Food Interactions Clearance may be decreased in patients following strict vegetarian diets due to urinary pH ≥8. Dairy products (milk, infant formula, yogurt) may interfere with the absorption of flecainide in infants; there is one case report of a neonate (GA 34 weeks PNA >6 days) who required extremely large doses of oral flecainide when administered every 8 hours with feedings ("milk feeds"); changing the feedings from "milk feeds" to 5% glucose feeds alone resulted in a doubling of the flecainide serum concentration and toxicity.

Mechanism of Action Class Ic antiarrhythmic; slows conduction in cardiac tissue by altering transport of ions across cell membranes; causes slight prolongation of refractory periods; decreases the rate of rise of the action potential without affecting its duration; increases electrical stimulation threshold of ventricle, His-Purkinje system; possesses local anesthetic and moderate negative inotropic effects

Pharmacokinetics (Adult data unless noted)

Absorption: Oral: Rapid and nearly complete

Distribution: V_d: Adults: 5-13.4 L/kg

Protein binding: 40% to 50% (alpha$_1$ glycoprotein)

Metabolism: In the liver

Bioavailability: 85% to 90%

Half-life, elimination: Increased half-life with CHF or renal dysfunction

Newborns: ~29 hours

Infants: 11-12 hours

Children: 8 hours

Adults: ~20 hours (range: 12-27 hours)

Time to peak serum concentration: ~3 hours (range: 1-6 hours)

Elimination: In urine as unchanged drug (10% to 50%) and metabolites

Dialysis: Not dialyzable

Dosing: Neonatal Oral: Supraventricular tachycardia: Limited data available: Initial: 2 mg/kg/day divided every 12 hours; titrate to clinical response, monitor serum concentration; mean dose required to suppress SVT: 3.35 ± 1.35 mg/kg/day in 17 neonates (n=20 treated neonates; mean PNA: 11.5 days; mean GA: 36.8 weeks; mean birthweight: 2.8 kg); study did not report resultant serum concentrations; **Note:** Acute SVT was initially controlled with I.V. flecainide (not available in U.S.) and then converted to preventative oral therapy (Ferlini, 2009). In a retrospective analysis of 39 neonates treated with digoxin and/or flecainide for SVT (median PNA at treatment: 12 days), an initial flecainide dose of 6-8 mg/kg/day divided every 12 hours was used and titrated to response and serum concentrations; final dosage range of 3.2-13.5 mg/kg/day produced successful suppression of SVT in 24 of 25 patients. The authors noted high variability in serum concentrations with initial dosing (0.23-1.14 mcg/mL) (O'Sullivan, 1995). Optimal dose not established; further studies needed.

Dosing: Usual Oral:

Children: Initial: 1-3 mg/kg/day or 50-100 mg/m^2/day in 3 divided doses; usual: 3-6 mg/kg/day or 100-150 mg/m^2/day in 3 divided doses; up to 8 mg/kg/day or 200 mg/m^2/day for uncontrolled patients with subtherapeutic levels; higher doses have been reported, however they may be associated with an increased risk of proarrhythmias; a review of world literature reports the average effective dose to be 4 mg/kg/day or 140 mg/m^2/day

Adults:

Life-threatening ventricular arrhythmias: Initial: 100 mg every 12 hours, increase by 100 mg/day (given in 2 doses/day) every 4 days; usual: ≤300 mg/day; maximum: 400 mg/day; for patients receiving 400 mg/day who are not controlled and have trough concentrations <0.6 mcg/mL, dosage may be increased to 600 mg/day

Prevention of paroxysmal supraventricular arrhythmias in patients with disabling symptoms but no structural heart disease: Initial: 50 mg every 12 hours; increase by 50 mg twice daily at 4-day intervals; maximum dose: 300 mg/day

Paroxysmal atrial fibrillation: Outpatient: "Pill-in-the-pocket" dose (for selected patients; Alboni, 2004; EHRA, 2006): 200 mg (patient weight <70 kg), 300 mg (weight ≥70 kg). May not repeat in ≤24 hours. **Note:** An initial inpatient conversion trial should have been successful before sending patient home on this approach. Patient must be taking an AV nodal-blocking agent (eg, beta-blocker, nondihydropyridine calcium channel blocker) prior to initiation of antiarrhythmic.

Dosing adjustment in renal failure:

Manufacturer recommendations: Adults: CrCl ≤35 mL/minute/1.73 m^2: Initial: 50 mg every 12 hours or 100 mg once daily; increase dose slowly at intervals >4 days; monitor plasma levels closely

Alternative adjustment: Children and Adults CrCl ≤20 mL/minute: Decrease the usual dose by 25% to 50%

Administration Oral: May be administered in children and adults without regard to food; in infants receiving milk or milk based formulas, avoid concurrent administration with feedings; monitor serum concentrations and decrease the dose when the diet changes to a decreased consumption of milk

Monitoring Parameters ECG, serum concentrations [**Note:** Obtain serum trough concentrations at steady state (after at least 3 days when doses are started or changed) or when dietary changes due to maturation or concurrent illness occur], liver enzymes, CBC with differential

Reference Range Therapeutic: 0.2-1 mcg/mL (SI: 0.4-2 micromoles/L). **Note:** Pediatric patients may respond at the lower end of the recommended therapeutic range (0.2-0.5 mcg/mL) but up to 0.8 mcg/mL may be required.

Additional Information Single oral dose flecainide for termination of PSVT in children and young adults (n=25) and combination therapy of flecainide with amiodarone for refractory tachyarrhythmias in infancy (n=9) have been reported

Dosage Forms Excipient information presented when available (limited, particularly for generics); consult specific product labeling. [DSC] = Discontinued product

Tablet, Oral, as acetate:
Tambocor: 50 mg [DSC], 100 mg [DSC], 150 mg [DSC]
Generic: 50 mg, 100 mg, 150 mg

Extemporaneous Preparations A 20 mg/mL oral liquid suspension may be made from tablets and one of three different vehicles (cherry syrup, a 1:1 mixture of Ora-Sweet® and Ora-Plus®, or a 1:1 mixture of Ora-Sweet® SF and Ora-Plus®). Crush twenty-four 100 mg tablets in a mortar and reduce to a fine powder. Add 20 mL of the chosen vehicle and mix to a uniform paste; mix while adding the vehicle in incremental proportions to **almost** 120 mL; transfer to a calibrated bottle, rinse mortar with vehicle, and add quantity of vehicle sufficient to make 120 mL. Label "shake well" and "protect from light". Stable for 60 days when stored in amber plastic prescription bottles in the dark at room temperature or refrigerated.

Allen LV and Erickson III MA, "Stability of Baclofen, Captopril, Diltiazem, Hydrochloride, Dipyridamole, and Flecainide Acetate in Extemporaneously Compounded Oral Liquids," *Am J Health Syst Pharm*, 1996, 53:2179-84.

References

Alboni P, Botto GL, Baldi N, et al, "Outpatient Treatment of Recent-Onset Atrial Fibrillation With the 'Pill-in-the-Pocket' Approach," *N Engl J Med*, 2004, 351(23):2384-91.

European Heart Rhythm Association, Heart Rhythm Society, Fuster V, et al, "ACC/AHA/ESC 2006 Guidelines for the Management of Patients With Atrial Fibrillation - Executive Summary: A Report of the American College of Cardiology/American Heart Association Task Force on Practice Guidelines and the European Society of Cardiology Committee for Practice Guidelines (Writing Committee to Revise the 2001 Guidelines for the Management of Patients With Atrial Fibrillation)," *J Am Coll Cardiol*, 2006, 48(4):854-906.

Fenrich AL Jr, Perry JC, and Friedman RA, "Flecainide and Amiodarone: Combined Therapy for Refractory Tachyarrhythmias in Infants," *J Am Coll Cardiol*, 1995, 25(5):1195-8.

Ferlini M, Colli AM, Bonanomi C, et al, "Flecainide as First-Line Treatment for Supraventricular Tachycardia in Newborns," *J Cardiovasc Med (Hagerstown)*, 2009, 10(5):372-5.

Musto B, Cavallaro C, Musto A, et al, "Flecainide Single Oral Dose for Management of Paroxysmal Supraventricular Tachycardia in Children and Young Adults," *Am Heart J*, 1992, 124(1):110-5.

O'Sullivan JJ, Gardiner HM, and Wren C, "Digoxin or Flecainide for Prophylaxis of Supraventricular Tachycardia in Infants?" *J Am Coll Cardiol*, 1995, 26(4):991-4.

Perry JC and Garson A Jr, "Flecainide Acetate for Treatment of Tachyarrhythmias in Children: Review of World Literature on Efficacy, Safety, and Dosing," *Am Heart J*, 1992, 124(6):1614-21.

Perry JC, McQuinn RL, Smith RT Jr, et al, "Flecainide Acetate for Resistant Arrhythmias in the Young: Efficacy and Pharmacokinetics," *J Am Coll Cardiol*, 1989, 14(1):185-91.

Priestley KA, Ladusans EJ, Rosenthal E, et al, "Experience With Flecainide for the Treatment of Cardiac Arrhythmias in Children," *Eur Heart J*, 1988, 9(12):1284-90.

Russell GA and Martin RP, "Flecainide Toxicity," *Arch Dis Child*, 1989, 64(6):860-2.

Zeigler V, Gillette PC, Ross BA, et al, "Flecainide for Supraventricular and Ventricular Arrhythmias in Children and Young Adults," *Am J Cardiol*, 1988, 62(10 Pt 1):818-20.

◆ **Flecainide Acetate** see Flecainide on page 874

◆ **Flector** see Diclofenac (Topical) on page 649

◆ **Fleet Bisacodyl [OTC]** see Bisacodyl on page 293

◆ **Fleet Enema [OTC]** see Sodium Phosphates on page 1913

◆ **Fleet Enema (Can)** see Sodium Phosphates on page 1913

◆ **Fleet Enema Extra [OTC]** see Sodium Phosphates on page 1913

◆ **Fleet Laxative [OTC]** see Bisacodyl on page 293

- **Fleet Liquid Glycerin Supp [OTC]** *see* Glycerin *on page 976*
- **Fleet Oil [OTC]** *see* Mineral Oil *on page 1419*
- **Fleet Pedia-Lax Enema [OTC]** *see* Sodium Phosphates *on page 1913*
- **Flexbumin** *see* Albumin *on page 82*
- **Flexeril** *see* Cyclobenzaprine *on page 558*
- **Flolan** *see* Epoprostenol *on page 770*
- **Flonase** *see* Fluticasone (Nasal) *on page 913*
- **Flonase® (Can)** *see* Fluticasone (Nasal) *on page 913*
- **Flo-Pred** *see* PrednisoLONE (Systemic) *on page 1727*
- **Floranex™ [OTC]** *see* Lactobacillus *on page 1191*
- **Flora-Q™ [OTC]** *see* Lactobacillus *on page 1191*
- **Florical [OTC]** *see* Calcium Carbonate *on page 346*
- **Florinef** *see* Fludrocortisone *on page 887*
- **Florinef® (Can)** *see* Fludrocortisone *on page 887*
- **Flovent** *see* Fluticasone (Oral Inhalation) *on page 910*
- **Flovent Diskus** *see* Fluticasone (Oral Inhalation) *on page 910*
- **Flovent HFA** *see* Fluticasone (Oral Inhalation) *on page 910*
- **Floxin Otic Singles** *see* Ofloxacin (Otic) *on page 1524*
- **Fluad (Can)** *see* Influenza Virus Vaccine (Inactivated) *on page 1103*
- **Fluarix** *see* Influenza Virus Vaccine (Inactivated) *on page 1103*
- **Fluarix Quadrivalent** *see* Influenza Virus Vaccine (Inactivated) *on page 1103*
- **Flubenisolone** *see* Betamethasone (Systemic) *on page 282*
- **Flublok** *see* Influenza Virus Vaccine (Recombinant) *on page 1112*
- **Flucelvax** *see* Influenza Virus Vaccine (Inactivated) *on page 1103*

Fluconazole (floo KOE na zole)

Medication Safety Issues
Sound-alike/look-alike issues:
Fluconazole may be confused with flecainide, FLUoxetine, furosemide, itraconazole, voriconazole
Diflucan may be confused with diclofenac, Diprivan, disulfiram
International issues:
Canesten (oral capsules) [Great Britain] may be confused with Canesten brand name for clotrimazole (various dosage forms) [multiple international markets]; Cenestin brand name estrogens (conjugated A/synthetic) [U.S., Canada]
Brand Names: U.S. Diflucan
Brand Names: Canada Apo-Fluconazole; CanesOral; CO Fluconazole; Diflucan; Dom-Fluconazole; Fluconazole Injection; Fluconazole Omega; Monicure; Mylan-Fluconazole; Novo-Fluconazole; PHL-Fluconazole; PMS-Fluconazole; PRO-Fluconazole; Riva-Fluconazole; Taro-Fluconazole; ZYM-Fluconazole
Therapeutic Category Antifungal Agent, Systemic
Generic Availability (U.S.) Yes
Use Treatment of candidiasis (vaginal, oropharyngeal, esophageal, urinary tract infections, peritonitis, pneumonia, and systemic infections); cryptococcal meningitis; antifungal prophylaxis in allogeneic bone marrow transplant recipients (All indications: FDA approved in all ages); strains of *Candida* with decreased *in vitro* susceptibility to fluconazole are being isolated with increasing frequency; fluconazole is more active against *C. albicans* than other candidal strains like *C. parapsilosis*, *C. glabrata*, and *C. tropicalis*; for some infections, an alternative to amphotericin B in patients with preexisting renal impairment or when requiring concomitant therapy with other potentially nephrotoxic drugs

Pregnancy Risk Factor C (single dose for vaginal candidiasis)/D (all other indications)

Pregnancy Considerations Adverse events have been observed in some animal reproduction studies. When used in high doses, fluconazole is teratogenic in animal studies. Following exposure during the first trimester, case reports have noted similar malformations in humans when used in higher doses (400 mg/day) over extended periods of time (Aleck, 1997). Abnormalities reported include abnormal facies, abnormal calvarial development, arthrogryposis, brachycephaly, cleft palate, congenital heart disease, femoral bowing, thin ribs and long bones. Use of lower doses (150 mg as a single dose) does not suggest an increase risk to the fetus. Most azole antifungals, including fluconazole, are recommended to be avoided during pregnancy (Pappas, 2009).

Breast-Feeding Considerations Fluconazole is excreted in breast milk. The manufacturer recommends that caution be exercised when administering fluconazole to nursing women. Fluconazole is found in breast milk at concentrations similar to maternal plasma.

Contraindications Hypersensitivity to fluconazole or any component (cross-reaction with other azole antifungal agents may occur, but has not been established; use caution); concomitant administration with other drugs known to prolong the QT interval and are metabolized via the enzyme CYP3A4 (eg, astemizole, cisapride, pimozide, quinidine)

Warnings Serious (and rarely fatal) hepatic toxicity (eg, hepatitis, cholestasis, fulminant failure) due to fluconazole has been reported; usually is reversible upon discontinuation of therapy. Patients who develop abnormal liver function tests during fluconazole therapy should be monitored closely for the development of more severe hepatic injury. Use with caution in patients with preexisting hepatic impairment; monitor liver function closely and dosage adjustment may be warranted. If clinical signs and symptoms consistent with liver disease develop that may be attributable to fluconazole, fluconazole should be discontinued. Rare cases of exfoliative skin disorders have been reported (including Stevens-Johnson syndrome and toxic epidermal necrolysis). Closely monitor patients who develop rashes during fluconazole therapy. Rare cases of anaphylaxis have been reported.

Fluconazole oral suspension contains sodium benzoate; benzoic acid (benzoate) is a metabolite of benzyl alcohol; large amounts of benzyl alcohol (≥99 mg/kg/day) have been associated with a potentially fatal toxicity ("gasping syndrome") in neonates; the "gasping syndrome" consists of metabolic acidosis, respiratory distress, gasping respirations, CNS dysfunction (including convulsions, intracranial hemorrhage), hypotension and cardiovascular collapse; use fluconazole oral suspension containing sodium benzoate with caution in neonates; *in vitro* and animal studies have shown that benzoate displaces bilirubin from protein binding sites

Precautions Use with caution and modify dosage in patients with impaired renal function. Use with caution in patients with hepatic dysfunction. The manufacturer reports rare cases of QT_c prolongation and torsade de pointes associated with fluconazole use and advises caution in patients with concomitant medications or conditions which are arrhythmogenic. Use caution in patients treated with medications having a narrow therapeutic window and which are metabolized via CYP2C9 or CYP3A4 (monitor). Use with erythromycin should be avoided (may increase risk of cardiotoxicity). May cause dizziness or seizures ▶

(rarely) which may impair physical or mental abilities; patients must be cautioned about performing tasks which require mental alertness (eg, operating machinery or driving).

Oral suspension may contain sucrose; avoid use in patients with hereditary fructose intolerance, glucose/galactose malabsorption, and sucrose-isomaltase deficiency.

Adverse Reactions

Cardiovascular: Angioedema (rare)

Central nervous system: Dizziness, headache

Dermatologic: Rash

Gastrointestinal: Abdominal pain, diarrhea, dysgeusia, dyspepsia, nausea, vomiting

Hepatic: Alkaline phosphatase increased, ALT increased, AST increased, hepatic failure (rare), hepatitis, jaundice

Miscellaneous: Anaphylactic reactions (rare)

Rare but important or life-threatening: Agranulocytosis, alopecia, cholestasis, diaphoresis, drug eruption, exanthematous pustulosis, fatigue, fever, hypercholesterolemia, hypertriglyceridemia, hypokalemia, insomnia, leukopenia, malaise, myalgia, neutropenia, paresthesia, QT prolongation, seizure, somnolence, Stevens-Johnson syndrome, thrombocytopenia, torsade de pointes, toxic epidermal necrolysis, tremor, vertigo, weakness, xerostomia

Drug Interactions

Metabolism/Transport Effects Inhibits CYP1A2 (weak), CYP2C19 (strong), CYP2C9 (moderate), CYP3A4 (moderate)

Avoid Concomitant Use

Avoid concomitant use of Fluconazole with any of the following: Bosutinib; Cisapride; Citalopram; Conivaptan; Dofetilide; Erythromycin (Systemic); Highest Risk QTc-Prolonging Agents; Ibrutinib; Ivabradine; Lomitapide; Mifepristone; Ospemifene; Pimozide; QuiNIDine; Ranolazine; Saccharomyces boulardii; Simeprevir; Tolvaptan; Ulipristal; Voriconazole

Increased Effect/Toxicity

Fluconazole may increase the levels/effects of: Alfentanil; ARIPiprazole; AtorvaSTATin; Avanafil; Benzodiazepines (metabolized by oxidation); Bosentan; Bosutinib; Budesonide (Systemic, Oral Inhalation); BusPIRone; Busulfan; Calcium Channel Blockers; Cannabis; CarBAMazepine; Carvedilol; Cilostazol; Cisapride; Citalopram; Colchicine; Conivaptan; Corticosteroids (Systemic); CycloSPORINE (Systemic); CYP2C19 Substrates; CYP2C9 Substrates; CYP3A4 Substrates; DOCEtaxel; Dofetilide; DOXOrubicin (Conventional); Dronabinol; Eletriptan; Eplerenone; Erythromycin (Systemic); Etravirine; Everolimus; FentaNYL; Fluvastatin; Fosphenytoin; Highest Risk QTc-Prolonging Agents; Ibrutinib; Imatinib; Irbesartan; Ivabradine; Ivacaftor; Lomitapide; Losartan; Lovastatin; Lurasidone; Macrolide Antibiotics; Methadone; Moderate Risk QTc-Prolonging Agents; Nevirapine; Ospemifene; OxyCODONE; Phenytoin; Pimecrolimus; Pimozide; Proton Pump Inhibitors; QuiNIDine; Ramelteon; Ranolazine; Red Yeast Rice; Rifamycin Derivatives; Rivaroxaban; Salmeterol; Saxagliptin; Sildenafil; Simeprevir; Simvastatin; Sirolimus; Solifenacin; Sulfonylureas; SUNItinib; Tacrolimus (Systemic); Tacrolimus (Topical); Tadalafil; Temsirolimus; Tetrahydrocannabinol; Tipranavir; Tofacitinib; Tolterodine; Tolvaptan; Ulipristal; Vardenafil; Vilazodone; Vitamin K Antagonists; Voriconazole; Zidovudine; Zolpidem

The levels/effects of Fluconazole may be increased by: Etravirine; Ivabradine; Macrolide Antibiotics; Mifepristone; QTc-Prolonging Agents (Indeterminate Risk and Risk Modifying)

Decreased Effect

Fluconazole may decrease the levels/effects of: Amphotericin B; Clopidogrel; Saccharomyces boulardii

The levels/effects of Fluconazole may be decreased by: Didanosine; Etravirine; Rifamycin Derivatives

Stability

Parenteral: Store solution for injection in glass at 5°C to 30°C (41°F to 86°F); store solution for injection in Viaflex® at 5°C to 25°C (41°F to 77°F). Do not freeze; do not unwrap unit until ready for use.

Oral:

Powder for oral suspension: Store dry powder at <30°C (<86°F). Following reconstitution, store at 5°C to 30°C (41°F to 86°F). Discard unused portion after 2 weeks. Do not freeze.

Tablet: Store at <30°C (<86°F).

Mechanism of Action Interferes with fungal cytochrome P450 activity (lanosterol 14-α-demethylase), decreasing ergosterol synthesis (principal sterol in fungal cell membrane) and inhibiting cell membrane formation

Pharmacokinetics (Adult data unless noted)

Absorption: Oral: Well absorbed; food does not affect extent of absorption

Distribution: ~0.6 L/kg; widely throughout body with good penetration into CSF, eye, peritoneal fluid, sputum, skin, and urine. Relative diffusion blood into CSF: Adequate with or without inflammation; CSF:blood concentration ratio: Independent of degree of meningeal inflammation: 50% to 90%

Protein binding: 11% to 12%

Bioavailability: Oral: >90%

Half-life:

Premature neonates (GA: 26-29 weeks): 73.6 hours

PNA: 6 days: 53 hours

PNA: 12 days: 47 hours

Pediatric patients (9 months to 15 years):

9 months to 13 years: Oral: 19.5-25 hours

5-15 years: I.V.: 15-18 hours

Adults: Normal renal function: ~30 hours

Time to peak serum concentration: Oral: 1-2 hours

Elimination: 80% (unchanged in urine); 11% (metabolites in urine)

Dosing: Neonatal Note: Daily dose of fluconazole is the same for oral and I.V. administration; unless otherwise specified, either dosage form may be used:

Candidiasis: I.V., Oral:

Invasive (systemic):

Prophylaxis: Dosing based on IDSA guidelines and a pharmacokinetic simulation. Duration should be guided by presence of risk factors. Further studies are needed to define optimal criteria and duration of fluconazole prophylaxis (Healy, 2009).

GA <30 weeks: Consider for neonates with a birth weight <1000 g who are in a nursery with a high rate of invasive candidiasis.

Age at initiation of therapy:

PNA <7 days: I.V.: 3 mg/kg/dose or 6 mg/kg/dose twice weekly; in ELBW, therapy initiation recommended during first 48-72 hours of life by the I.V. route and continued for 4-6 weeks or until I.V. access no longer required for care of the neonate (Pappas, 2009; *Red Book*, 2012). **Note:** Dose selection may be directed by NICU-specific *Candida* sp. susceptibility (ie, use lower dose for an organism with an MIC ≤2 mcg/mL; neither dose has been studied for organisms with an MIC >4 mcg/mL) (Pappas, 2009; Wade, 2009).

PNA ≥7-42 days: 3 mg/kg/dose once daily or 6 mg/kg/dose every 72 hours (Wade, 2009)

PNA >42 days: 6 mg/kg/dose every 48 hours (Wade, 2009)

GA 30-40 weeks: 6 mg/kg/dose every 48 hours (Wade, 2009)

Treatment:

Systemic candidiasis, invasive disease: 12 mg/kg/dose once daily for 21 days; gestational age not specified (Pappas, 2009). Others have recommended a loading dose of 25 mg/kg, followed by 12 mg/kg once daily; an evaluation of this dosing in five neonates (GA: 35-38 weeks; PNA: 16 days) showed all subjects reached target trough concentrations (>8 mcg/mL) within 24 hours (Piper, 2011; Wade, 2008; Wade, 2009). Some experts have suggested 12 mg/kg/dose every 48 hours for PNA <8 days.

Oral (thrush) (Pappas, 2009): Term neonate:

PNA ≤14 days: Initial: 6 mg/kg/dose followed by 3 mg/kg/dose every 24-72 hours for 7-14 days

PNA >14 days: Initial: 6 mg/kg/dose followed by 3 mg/kg/dose once daily for 7-14 days

Esophageal disease (Pappas, 2009): Term neonate:

PNA ≤14 days: Initial: 6 mg/kg/dose followed by 3 mg/kg/dose every 24-72 hours for a minimum of 14-21 days; duration of therapy based upon clinical response; some suggest to continue for 2 weeks after clinical resolution with a minimum of at least 3 weeks of therapy

PNA >14 days: Initial: 6 mg/kg/dose followed by 3 mg/kg/dose once daily for a minimum of 14-21 days; in some cases, doses up to 12 mg/kg may be required; duration of therapy based upon clinical response; continue for 2 weeks after clinical resolution with a minimum of at least 3 weeks of therapy

Cryptococcal, CNS disease (meningitis): I.V., Oral: PNA >14 days:

Acute treatment: 12 mg/kg/dose followed by 6-12 mg/kg/day for 10-12 weeks after CSF culture becomes negative

Prevention of relapse: 6 mg/kg/dose once daily

Dosing adjustment in renal impairment: There are no specific neonatal dosage adjustments provided in the manufacturer's labeling; some experts have used the following indication-specific dosing (Wade, 2009): Candidiasis, prophylaxis: I.V., Oral:

S_{cr} ≥1.3 mg/dL: 6 mg/kg once weekly

S_{cr} ≤1 mg/dL: Standard dosing

Dosing: Usual

Infants and Children: **Note:** Daily dose of fluconazole is the same for oral and I.V. administration; unless otherwise specified, either dosage form may be used:

General dosing, susceptible infection: I.V., Oral: Initial: 6-12 mg/kg/dose, followed by 3-12 mg/kg/dose once daily; maximum daily dose: 600 mg/**day**; duration and dosage depends on severity of infection

Candidiasis: I.V., Oral:

Prophylaxis regimens:

Chemotherapy-induced neutropenia (including stem cell transplantation): 6 mg/kg/dose once daily during induction chemotherapy and period of neutropenia risk; maximum daily dose: 400 mg/**day** (Pappas, 2009)

Postsolid organ transplant: 6 mg/kg/dose once daily for 14 days; maximum daily dose: 400 mg/**day** (Pappas, 2009)

Treatment and suppression regimens:

Esophageal infection:

Non-HIV-exposed/-positive: *Treatment:* 6 mg/kg/dose on Day 1, followed by 3 mg/kg/dose once daily for at least 21 days and at least 2 weeks following symptom resolution. In some cases, higher doses (up to 12 mg/kg/**day**) may be used; maximum daily dose: 400 mg/**day**

HIV-exposed/-positive (CDC, 2009):

Treatment: 6 mg/kg/dose on Day 1, followed by 3-6 mg/kg/dose once daily for 4-21 days; maximum daily dose: 400 mg/**day**

Relapse suppression: 3-6 mg/kg/dose once daily; maximum daily dose: 200 mg/**day**

Oropharyngeal infection:

Non-HIV-exposed/-positive: *Treatment:* 6 mg/kg/dose on Day 1, followed by 3 mg/kg/dose once daily for at least 14 days; maximum daily dose: Day 1: 200 mg/**day**; subsequent days: 100 mg/**day**

HIV-exposed/-positive: *Treatment:* 3-6 mg/kg/dose once daily for 7-14 days; maximum daily dose: 400 mg/**day** (CDC, 2009)

Systemic infection (invasive disease):

Non-HIV-exposed/-positive (neutropenic or non-neutropenic patients; reserve use for stable patients only): *Treatment:* 12 mg/kg/dose on Day 1 (maximum dose: 800 mg), followed by 12 mg/kg/dose once daily or 6 mg/kg/dose twice daily; maximum daily dose: 600 mg/**day**; treatment duration: 2 weeks after clearance from blood and symptom resolution (Filioti, 2007; Pappas, 2009; Zaoutis, 2010)

HIV-exposed/-positive: *Treatment:* 5-6 mg/kg/dose twice daily for minimum of 4 weeks; maximum daily dose: 600 mg/**day**; reserve for documented *C. albicans* or other susceptible species (CDC, 2009)

Coccidioidomycosis, meningeal infection, or in a stable patient with diffuse pulmonary or disseminated disease (HIV-exposed/-positive) (CDC, 2009): I.V., Oral:

Treatment: 5-6 mg/kg/dose twice daily; maximum daily dose: 800 mg/**day**, followed by chronic suppressive therapy

Relapse suppression: 6 mg/kg/dose once daily; maximum daily dose: 400 mg/**day**

Cryptococcal infection: I.V., Oral:

CNS disease:

Non-HIV-exposed/-positive:

Acute therapy:

Manufacturer's labeling: 12 mg/kg/dose on Day 1, followed by 6 mg/kg/dose once daily; in some cases, doses as high as 12 mg/kg/day once daily may be required dependent upon patient's response to therapy; treatment duration 10-12 weeks after CSF becomes culture negative; maximum daily dose: 800 mg/**day**

Alternate dosing: Consolidation phase: 5-6 mg/kg/dose **twice** daily; treatment duration: 8 weeks followed by maintenance therapy; maximum daily dose: 800 mg/**day** (Perfect, 2010)

Maintenance therapy: 6 mg/kg/dose once daily for 6-12 months; maximum daily dose: 200 mg/**day** (Perfect, 2010)

HIV-exposed/-positive:

Acute therapy, induction: 12 mg/kg /dose on Day 1, followed by 6-12 mg/kg/dose once daily; maximum daily dose: 800 mg/**day**; in combination with flucytosine for at least 2 weeks until significant clinical improvement and negative CSF cultures then begin consolidation therapy; reserve as alternate therapy when amphotericin (including lipid-based products) is not tolerated (CDC, 2009)

Consolidation therapy: 12 mg/kg/dose on Day 1, followed by 6-12 mg/kg/dose once daily for a minimum of 8 weeks; maximum daily dose: 800 mg/**day**; **Note:** CSF cultures should be negative prior to initiating consolidation therapy (CDC, 2009)

Relapse suppression: 6 mg/kg/dose once daily; maximum daily dose: 200 mg/**day**

Localized (non-CNS), disseminated, or pulmonary disease:

Non-HIV-exposed/-positive:

Mild-moderate pulmonary disease or localized infection: *Treatment:* 6 mg/kg once daily; maximum daily dose: 400 mg/**day**; a treatment duration of 6-12 months has been used in organ transplant recipients (Perfect, 2010)

Severe pulmonary disease, or disseminated infection; treatment:

Acute therapy: 12 mg/kg/dose on Day 1, followed by 6 mg/kg/dose once daily; in some cases, doses as high as 12 mg/kg/dose once daily may be used dependent upon patient's response to therapy; treatment duration 10-12 weeks; maximum daily dose: 800 mg/**day** (Perfect, 2010)

Maintenance therapy: 6 mg/kg/dose once daily for 6-12 months; maximum daily dose: 200 mg/**day** (Perfect, 2010)

HIV-exposed/-positive (CDC, 2009):

Treatment: 12 mg/kg/dose on Day 1, followed by 6-12 mg/kg/dose once daily; maximum daily dose: 600 mg/**day**; treatment duration variable and dependent upon infection site, severity, and clinical response; chronic suppressive therapy should be initiated upon treatment completion

Relapse suppression: 6 mg/kg/dose once daily; maximum daily dose: 200 mg/**day**

Histoplasmosis; relapse prevention (HIV-exposed/-positive): I.V., Oral: 3-6 mg/kg/dose once daily; maximum daily dose: 200 mg/**day** (CDC, 2009).

Peritonitis (Warady, 2012):

Prophylaxis during antibiotic therapy: I.V., Oral: 3-6 mg/kg/dose every 24-48 hours; maximum single dose: 200 mg

Treatment:

Peritonitis: Intraperitoneal, I.V., Oral: 6-12 mg/kg/dose every 24-48 hours; maximum single dose: 400 mg

Exit-site and tunnel infections: Oral: 6 mg/kg/dose every 24-48 hours; maximum single dose: 400 mg

Surgical prophylaxis: I.V.: 6 mg/kg as a single dose 1-2 hours prior to procedure; maximum dose: 400 mg (Bratzler, 2013)

Adolescents:

General dosing, susceptible infection: I.V., Oral: Initial: 6-12 mg/kg/dose followed by 3-12 mg/kg/dose once daily; maximum daily dose: 600 mg/**day**; duration and dosage depend on severity of infection

Blastomycosis, CNS disease (independent of HIV status): Oral: *Step-down therapy:* 800 mg once daily; initiate after 4-6 weeks of amphotericin therapy and continue for at least 12 months or until resolution of CNS abnormalities has been recommended in adult patients (Chapman, 2005)

Candidiasis: I.V., Oral:

Prophylaxis regimens:

Chemotherapy-induced neutropenia (including stem cell transplantation): 6 mg/kg/dose once daily during induction chemotherapy and period of neutropenia risk; maximum daily dose: 400 mg/**day** (Pappas, 2009)

Postsolid organ transplant: 6 mg/kg/dose once daily for 14 days; maximum daily dose: 400 mg/**day** (Pappas, 2009)

Treatment and suppression regimens:

Esophageal infection:

Non-HIV-exposed/-positive: *Treatment:* 6 mg/kg/dose on Day 1, followed by 3 mg/kg/dose once daily for at least 21 days and at least 2 weeks following symptom resolutions. In some cases, higher doses (up to 12 mg/kg/**day**) may be used; maximum daily dose: 400 mg/**day**

HIV-exposed/-positive (DHHS, 2013):

Treatment: 100 mg once daily for 14-21 days; maximum daily dose: 400 mg/**day**

Relapse suppression: 100-200 mg once daily

Oropharyngeal infection:

Non-HIV-exposed/-positive: *Treatment:* 6 mg/kg/dose on Day 1, followed by 3 mg/kg/dose once daily for at least 14 days; maximum daily dose: Day 1: 200 mg/**day**; subsequent doses: 100 mg/**day**

HIV-exposed/-positive (DHHS, 2013):

Treatment: Oral: 100 mg once daily for 7-14 days

Relapse suppression: Oral: 100 mg once daily or 3 times weekly

Systemic infection (invasive disease): Neutropenic or non-neutropenic patients (non-HIV-exposed/-positive; reserve use for stable patients only): *Treatment:* 12 mg/kg/dose on Day 1 (maximum dose: 800 mg) followed by 12 mg/kg/dose once daily or 6 mg/kg/dose twice daily (maximum daily dose: 600 mg/**day**); treatment duration: 2 weeks after clearance from blood and symptom resolution (Fioliti, 2007; Pappas, 2009; Zaoutis, 2010)

Vulvovaginal infection:

Uncomplicated (independent of HIV status): *Treatment:* Oral: 150 mg single dose (CDC, 2010; CDC, 2013)

Complicated (severe, recurrent) (HIV-exposed/-positive) (DHHS, 2013):

Treatment: 100-200 mg once daily for at least 7 days

Relapse suppression: Oral: 150 mg/dose once weekly

Coccidioidomycosis: I.V., Oral:

Non-CNS disease:

Non-HIV-exposed/-positive: *Treatment:* 400-800 mg once daily; for severe disseminated extrapulmonary infection, doses up to 2000 mg/day have been used; total therapy duration (treatment and maintenance) dependent upon site of infection; for pneumonia (diffuse) at least 12 months (if patient immunosuppressed, consider additional suppression therapy); for other disseminated (nonpulmonary infections), treatment duration based upon clinical response and may extend longer than 12 months (Galgiani, 2005)

HIV-exposed/-positive (CDC, 2013):

Prevention, first episode: Oral: 400 mg once daily

Treatment:

Mild infection or focal pneumonia: 400 mg once daily

Severe infection (eg, diffuse pulmonary infection or extrathoracic disseminated disease): 400 mg once daily in combination with amphotericin; continue fluconazole after amphotericin stopped following clinical improvement

Chronic suppressive therapy: Oral: 400 mg once daily

Meningeal infection:

Non-HIV-exposed/-positive: *Treatment:* 400-1000 mg once daily, continue indefinitely (Galgiani, 2005)

HIV-exposed/-positive (DHHS, 2013):

Treatment: 400-800 mg once daily

Suppression: Oral: 400 mg once daily

Cryptococcal infection: I.V., Oral:

CNS disease:

Non-HIV-exposed/-positive:

Treatment: Acute therapy: 12 mg/kg/dose on Day 1, followed by 6 mg/kg/dose once daily; in some cases doses as high as 12 mg/kg/dose once daily may be used dependent upon patient's response to therapy; treatment duration 10-12 weeks; maximum daily dose: 800 mg/**day**

Consolidation therapy: Oral: 10-12 mg/kg/dose once daily for 8 weeks; maximum daily dose: 800 mg/**day** (Perfect, 2010)

Maintenance therapy: Oral: 6 mg/kg/dose once daily; maximum daily dose: 200 mg/**day** (Perfect, 2010)

HIV-exposed/-positive (DHHS, 2013):

Induction: Continue therapy for at least 2 weeks

Combination therapy: 800 mg once daily with amphotericin or liposomal amphotericin; if patient unable to tolerate amphotericin (or lipid product formulations) may use 400-800 mg/dose once daily with flucytosine

Monotherapy: 1200 mg once daily

Consolidation therapy: 400 mg once daily for 8 weeks; begin after at least 2 weeks of induction therapy (ie, significant clinical improvement and negative CSF cultures)

Maintenance therapy: Oral: 200 mg once daily for at least 12 months

Localized (non-CNS), disseminated, or pulmonary disease:

Non-HIV-exposed/-positive: Cryptococcal pneumonia: Oral: *Treatment:* 6-12 mg/kg/dose once daily for 6-12 months; maximum daily dose: 800 mg/**day** (Perfect, 2010)

HIV-exposed/-positive (DHHS, 2013):

Diffuse pulmonary disease or extrapulmonary disease:

Induction: Continue therapy for at least 2 weeks

Combination therapy: 800 mg once daily with amphotericin or liposomal amphotericin; if patient unable to tolerate amphotericin (or lipid product formulations) may use 400-800 mg/dose once daily with flucytosine

Monotherapy: 1200 mg once daily

Consolidation therapy: Oral: 400 mg once daily for 8 weeks; begin after at least 2 weeks of induction therapy (ie, significant clinical improvement and negative CSF cultures)

Maintenance therapy: Oral: 200 mg once daily for at least 12 months

Focal pulmonary infiltrates or mild-moderate symptoms: Oral: 400 mg once daily for 12 months

Histoplasmosis: I.V., Oral:

Non-HIV-exposed/-positive (Wheat, 2007):

Treatment: 200-800 mg once daily

Maintenance (CNS disease): Following 8 weeks of amphotericin B, fluconazole 200-400 mg once daily for 12 months

HIV-exposed/-positive (DHHS, 2013): Duration of therapy for induction and maintenance at least 12 months

Treatment, less severe disease: Oral: 800 mg once daily

Maintenance (severe disseminated or CNS disease): Oral: 800 mg once daily

Suppression, long-term (severe disseminated or CNS disease): Oral: 400 mg once daily

Penicilliosis; prevention first episode (HIV-exposed/-positive): Oral: 400 mg once weekly (DHHS, 2013)

Peritonitis (Warady, 2012):

Prophylaxis during antibiotic therapy: I.V., Oral: 3-6 mg/kg/dose every 24-48 hours; maximum single dose: 200 mg

Treatment:

Peritonitis: Intraperitoneal, I.V., Oral: 6-12 mg/kg/dose every 24-48 hours; maximum single dose: 400 mg

Exit-site and tunnel infection: Oral: 6 mg/kg/dose every 24-48 hours; maximum single dose: 400 mg

Surgical prophylaxis: I.V.: 6 mg/kg as a single dose 1-2 hours prior to procedure; maximum dose: 400 mg (Bratzler, 2013)

Adult: **Usual dosage range:** 150 mg once **or** 200-800 mg/day; duration and dosage depend on severity of infection

Dosing adjustment in renal impairment:

Infants, Children, and Adolescents:

No adjustment for vaginal candidiasis single-dose therapy.

For multiple dosing, administer usual load then adjust daily doses as follows; based upon Schwartz calculations:

CrCl >50 mL/minute/1.73 m^2: No adjustment necessary.

CrCl 10-50 mL/minute/1.73 m^2 (no dialysis): Administer 50% of recommended dose at the normal interval.

CrCl ≤10 mL/minute/1.73 m^2: Administer 50% of recommended dose every 48 hours (Aronoff, 2007).

Intermittent hemodialysis: Dialyzable (50%): May administer 100% of daily dose (according to indication) after each dialysis session; others have suggested the following: Administer 50% of dose every 48 hours; on dialysis days administer dose after dialysis session (Aronoff, 2007)

Peritoneal dialysis: Administer 50% of recommended dose every 48 hours (Aronoff, 2007)

Continuous renal replacement (CRRT): 6 mg/kg/dose every 24 hours (Aronoff, 2007)

Adults:

No adjustment for vaginal candidiasis single-dose therapy.

For multiple dosing, administer usual load then adjust daily doses as follows: Administer loading dose of 50-400 mg, then adjust daily doses as follows:

CrCl ≤50 mL/minute (no dialysis): Administer 50% of recommended dose daily

Intermittent hemodialysis (IHD): Dialyzable (50%): May administer 100% of daily dose (according to indication) after each dialysis session. Alternatively, doses of 200-400 mg every 48-72 hours or 100-200 mg every 24 hours have been recommended (Heintz, 2009). **Note:** Dosing dependent on the assumption of 3 times/week, complete IHD sessions.

Continuous renal replacement therapy (CRRT) (Heintz, 2009; Trotman, 2005): Drug clearance is highly dependent on the method of renal replacement, filter type, and flow rate. Appropriate dosing requires close monitoring of pharmacologic response, signs of adverse reactions due to drug accumulation, as well as drug concentrations in relation to target trough (if appropriate). The following are general recommendations only (based on dialysate flow/ultrafiltration rates of 1-2 L/hour and minimal residual renal function) and should not supersede clinical judgment:

CVVH: Loading dose of 400-800 mg followed by 200-400 mg every 24 hours

CVVHD/CVVHDF: Loading dose of 400-800 mg followed by 400-800 mg every 24 hours (CVVHD or CVVHDF) or 800 mg every 24 hours (CVVHDF)

Note: Higher maintenance doses of 400 mg every 24 hours (CVVH), 800 mg every 24 hours (CVVHD), and 500-600 mg every 12 hours (CVVHDF) may be considered when treating resistant organisms and/or when employing combined ultrafiltration and dialysis flow rates of ≥2 L/hour for CVVHD/CVVHDF (Heintz, 2009; Trotman, 2005).

Dosing adjustment in hepatic impairment: There are no dosage adjustments provided in manufacturer's labeling; use with caution.

Administration

Oral: Administer without regard to meals; shake suspension well before use

Parenteral: Do not use if cloudy or precipitated. Administered by I.V. infusion over approximately 1-2 hours at a rate not to exceed 200 mg/hour; final concentration ▶

◀ 2 mg/mL; for pediatric patients receiving doses ≥6 mg/kg, administer I.V. infusion over 2 hours; pH: 4-8 (sodium chloride diluent); 3.5-6.5 (dextrose diluent)

Monitoring Parameters Periodic liver function (AST, ALT, alkaline phosphatase), renal function tests, serum potassium, CBC with differential, and platelet count

Additional Information

Dosing equivalency suggested by the manufacturer's labeling:

Pediatric patients 3 mg/kg = Adults 100 mg

Pediatric patients 6 mg/kg = Adults 200 mg

Pediatric patients 12 mg/kg = Adults 400 mg

Dosage Forms Excipient information presented when available (limited, particularly for generics); consult specific product labeling.

Solution, Intravenous:

Generic: 100 mg (50 mL); 200 mg (100 mL); 400 mg (200 mL)

Solution, Intravenous [preservative free]:

Generic: 200 mg (100 mL); 400 mg (200 mL)

Suspension Reconstituted, Oral:

Diflucan: 10 mg/mL (35 mL); 40 mg/mL (35 mL) [orange flavor]

Generic: 10 mg/mL (35 mL); 40 mg/mL (35 mL)

Tablet, Oral:

Diflucan: 50 mg, 100 mg, 150 mg, 200 mg

Generic: 50 mg, 100 mg, 150 mg, 200 mg

References

Aleck KA and Bartley DL, "Multiple Malformation Syndrome Following Fluconazole Use in Pregnancy: Report of an Additional Patient," Am J Med Genet, 1997, 72(3):253-6.

American Academy of Pediatrics (AAP). In: Pickering LK, Baker CJ, Kimberlin DW, Long SS, eds. Red Book: 2012 Report of the Committee on Infectious Diseases. 29th ed. Elk Grove Village, IL: American Academy of Pediatrics; 2012.

Aronoff GR, Bennett WM, Berns JS, et al, Drug Prescribing in Renal Failure: Dosing Guidelines for Adults and Children, 5th ed. Philadelphia, PA: American College of Physicians; 2007.

Bratzler DW, Dellinger EP, Olsen KM, et al. Clinical practice guidelines for antimicrobial prophylaxis in surgery. Am J Health Syst Pharm. 2013;70(3):195-283.

Centers for Disease Control and Prevention (CDC), "Guidelines for Prevention and Treatment of Opportunistic Infections Among HIV-Exposed and HIV-Infected Children," MMWR Recomm Rep, 2009, 58(RR-11):1-166. Available at http://aidsinfo.nih.gov/contentfiles/Pediatric_OI.pdf

Chapman SW, Dismukes WE, Proia LA. Clinical practice guidelines for the management of blastomycosis: 2008 update by the Infectious Diseases Society of America. Clin Infect Dis. 2005;41:1217-1223.

Como JA and Dismukes WE, "Oral Azole Drugs as Systemic Antifungal Therapy," N Engl J Med, 1993, 330(4):263-72.

DHHS Panel on Opportunistic Infections (OI) in HIV-Infected Adults and Adolescents, "Guidelines for Prevention and Treatment of Opportunistic Infections in HIV-Infected Adults and Adolescents: Recommendations from the Centers for Disease Control and Prevention (CDC), the National Institutes of Health (NIH), and the HIV Medicine Association (HIVMA) of the Infectious Diseases Society of America (IDSA)," May 7, 2013. Available at http://aidsinfo.nih.gov/contentfiles/lvguidelines/adult_oi.pdf

Filioti J, Spiroglou K, Panteliadis CP, et al, "Invasive Candidiasis in Pediatric Intensive Care Patients: Epidemiology, Risk Factors, Management, and Outcome," Intensive Care Med, 2007, 33(7):1272-83.

Galgiani JN, Ampel NM, Blair JE, et al. Coccidioidomycosis. Clin Infect Dis. 2005;41(9):1217-1223.

Goodman JL, Winston DJ, Greenfield RA, et al, "A Controlled Trial of Fluconazole to Prevent Fungal Infections in Patients Undergoing Bone Marrow Transplantation," N Engl J Med, 1992, 326(13):845-51.

Healy CM and Baker CJ, "Fluconazole Prophylaxis in the Neonatal Intensive Care Unit," Pediatr Infect Dis J, 2009, 28(1):49-52.

Heintz BH, Matzke GR, Dager WE, "Antimicrobial Dosing Concepts and Recommendations for Critically Ill Adult Patients Receiving Continuous Renal Replacement Therapy or Intermittent Hemodialysis," Pharmacotherapy, 2009, 29(5):562-77.

Lee JW, Seibel NL, Amantea M, et al, "Safety and Pharmacokinetics of Fluconazole in Children With Neoplastic Diseases," J Pediatr, 1992, 120(6):987-93.

Moncino MD and Gutman LT, "Severe Systemic Cryptococcal Disease in a Child: Review of Prognostic Indicators Predicting Treatment Failure and an Approach to Maintenance Therapy With Oral Fluconazole," Pediatr Infect Dis J, 1990, 9(5):363-8.

Pappas PG, Kauffman CA, Andes D, et al, "Clinical Practice Guidelines for the Management of Candidiasis: 2009 Update by the Infectious Diseases Society of America," Clin Infect Dis, 2009, 48(5):503-35.

Perfect JR, Dismukes WE, Dromer F, et al. Clinical practice guidelines for the management of cryptococcal disease: 2010 update by the Infectious Diseases Society of America. Clin Infect Dis. 2010;50 (3):291-322.

Piper L, Smith PB, Hornik CP, et al, "Fluconazole Loading Dose Pharmacokinetics and Safety in Infants," Pediatr Infect Dis J, 2011, 30(5):375-8.

Trotman RL, Williamson JC, Shoemaker DM, et al, "Antibiotic Dosing in Critically Ill Adult Patients Receiving Continuous Renal Replacement Therapy," Clin Infect Dis, 2005, 41(8):1159-66.

Viscoli C, Castagnola E, Fioredda F, et al, "Fluconazole in the Treatment of Candidiasis in Immunocompromised Children," Antimicrob Agents Chemother, 1991, 35(2):365-7.

Wade KC, Benjamin DK Jr, Kaufman DA, et al, "Fluconazole Dosing for the Prevention or Treatment of Invasive Candidiasis in Young Infants," Pediatr Infect Dis J, 2009, 28(8):717-23.

Wade KC, Wu D, Kaufman DA, et al, "Population Pharmacokinetics of Fluconazole in Young Infants," Antimicrob Agents Chemother, 2008, 52(11):4043-9.

Warady BA, Bakkaloglu S, Newland J, et al. Consensus guideline for the prevention and treatment of catheter-related infections and peritonitis in pediatric patients receiving peritoneal dialysis: 2012. Peritoneal Dialysis International. 2012;32:s32-86.

Wheat LJ, Freifeld AG, Kleiman MB, et al. Clinical practice guidelines for the management of patients with histoplasmosis: 2007 update by the Infectious Diseases Society of America. Clin Infect Dis. 2007;45 (7):807-825.

Zaoutis T, "Candidemia in Children," Curr Med Res Opin, 2010, 26 (7):1761-8.

♦ **Fluconazole Injection (Can)** see Fluconazole on page 877

♦ **Fluconazole Omega (Can)** see Fluconazole on page 877

Flucytosine (floo SYE toe seen)

Medication Safety Issues

Sound-alike/look-alike issues:

Flucytosine may be confused with fluorouracil

Ancobon® may be confused with Oncovin

High alert medication:

The Institute for Safe Medication Practices (ISMP) includes this medication among its list of drugs which have a heightened risk of causing significant patient harm when used in error.

Brand Names: U.S. Ancobon

Therapeutic Category Antifungal Agent, Systemic

Generic Availability (U.S.) Yes

Use Treatment of serious infections caused by susceptible strains of Candida (septicemia, endocarditis, pulmonary, urinary tract infections) and/or Cryptococcus (meningitis, pulmonary, septicemia, urinary tract infections) in combination with amphotericin B (FDA approved in adults)

Pregnancy Risk Factor C

Pregnancy Considerations Adverse events have been observed in some animal reproduction studies. Flucytosine is metabolized to fluorouracil which may cause adverse events if administered during pregnancy; refer to the Fluorouracil monograph for additional information.

Breast-Feeding Considerations It is not known if flucytosine is excreted in breast milk. Due to the potential for serious adverse reactions in the nursing infant, a decision should be made whether to discontinue nursing or to discontinue the drug, taking into account the importance of treatment to the mother.

Contraindications Hypersensitivity to flucytosine or any component

Warnings Use with extreme caution in patients with renal impairment **[U.S. Boxed Warning]**; renal impairment may lead to accumulation; dosage modification required in patients with impaired renal function based on serum flucytosine concentrations. Use with extreme caution in patients with bone marrow suppression, hematologic disease, patients with AIDS, patients being treated with radiation or with drugs which depress bone marrow, or a history of treatment with such drugs or radiation. Closely monitor hematologic, renal, and hepatic function of all patients receiving flucytosine **[U.S. Boxed Warning]**; bone marrow toxicity can be irreversible and is potentially fatal; hepatotoxicity and bone marrow toxicity appear to be dose related; monitor concentrations closely and adjust dose accordingly. Serum concentrations are highly variable in neonates; monitor closely (Pasqualotte, 2007); serum concentrations tended to be higher in children <12 years of age; monitor closely (Soltani, 2006).

Precautions Avoid monotherapy due to rapid emergence of resistance; more rapid emergence of fungal resistance may occur when lower doses are used.

Adverse Reactions

Cardiovascular: Cardiac arrest, myocardial toxicity, ventricular dysfunction, chest pain

Central nervous system: Ataxia, confusion, fatigue, hallucinations, headache, parkinsonism, psychosis, pyrexia, sedation, seizure, vertigo

Dermatologic: Rash, photosensitivity, pruritus, toxic epidermal necrolysis, urticaria

Endocrine & metabolic: Hypoglycemia, hypokalemia

Gastrointestinal: Abdominal pain, anorexia, diarrhea, duodenal ulcer, enterocolitis, hemorrhage, nausea, ulcerative colitis, vomiting, xerostomia

Hematologic: Agranulocytosis, anemia, aplastic anemia, bone marrow aplasia, eosinophilia, leukopenia, pancytopenia, thrombocytopenia

Hepatic: Acute hepatic injury, bilirubin increased, hepatic dysfunction, jaundice, liver enzymes increased

Neuromuscular & skeletal: Paresthesia, peripheral neuropathy, weakness

Otic: Hearing loss

Renal: Azotemia, BUN increased, crystalluria, renal failure, serum creatinine increased

Respiratory: Dyspnea, respiratory arrest

Miscellaneous: Allergic reaction

Drug Interactions

Metabolism/Transport Effects None known.

Avoid Concomitant Use

Avoid concomitant use of Flucytosine with any of the following: CloZAPine; Dipyrone; Gimeracil; Saccharomyces boulardii

Increased Effect/Toxicity

Flucytosine may increase the levels/effects of: CloZAPine

The levels/effects of Flucytosine may be increased by: Amphotericin B; Dipyrone; Gimeracil

Decreased Effect

Flucytosine may decrease the levels/effects of: Saccharomyces boulardii

The levels/effects of Flucytosine may be decreased by: Cytarabine (Conventional)

Food Interactions Food decreases the rate, but not the extent of absorption.

Stability Store at 25°C (77°F); excursions permitted between 15°C to 30°C (59°F to 86°F); protect from light.

Mechanism of Action Penetrates fungal cells and is converted to fluorouracil which competes with uracil interfering with fungal RNA and protein synthesis

Pharmacokinetics (Adult data unless noted)

Absorption: Oral: Rapid; rate of absorption is delayed in patients with renal impairment; serum concentrations are highly variable in neonates; monitor closely (Pasqualotte, 2007); serum concentrations tended to be higher in children <12 years of age; monitor closely (Soltani, 2006)

Distribution: Widely distributed into body tissues and fluids including CSF, aqueous humor, peritoneal fluid, bronchial secretions, liver, spleen, kidney, heart, and joints

V_d: Adults: 0.68 L/kg

Protein binding: 2.9% to 4%

Metabolism: Minimal hepatic metabolism; deaminated to 5-fluorouracil (probably by gut bacteria)

Bioavailability: 78% to 89%; decreased in neonates

Half-life:

Neonates: 4-34 hours (Baley, 1990)

Infants: 7.4 hours

Adults: 2.5-5 hours

Anuria: 85 hours (range: 30-250 hours)

Time to peak serum concentration: Oral:

Infants: 2.5 ± 1.3 hours

Adults: Within 2 hours

Elimination: 90% excreted unchanged in urine by glomerular filtration; small portion is excreted in the feces

Dialysis: Dialyzable (50% to 100%)

Dosing: Neonatal Note: Administer in combination with amphotericin B or another susceptible antifungal to prevent development of resistance:

General dosing, susceptible infection: Limited data available: Oral: Initial:

Body weight ≤2 kg

PNA ≤7 days: 75 mg/kg/day divided every 8 hours

PNA 8-28 days: 75 mg/kg/day divided every 6 hours

Body weight >2 kg: 75 mg/kg/day divided every 6 hours

Note: Monitoring of serum concentrations recommended; reported dosing range: 25-100 mg/kg/day in divided doses every 6-24 hours (Baley, 1990; Fernandez, 2000; Marr, 1994)

Candidal meningitis: Limited data available: Oral: 100 mg/kg/day in divided doses every 6-8 hours in combination with amphotericin B; monitoring of serum concentrations should be considered; reported range: 75-100 mg/kg/day; dosing based on a retrospective study and case reports (n=9) including premature neonates (GA: 24-28 weeks; PMA at treatment: 26-29 weeks); treatment duration in some cases was up to 6 weeks (Fernandez, 2000; Marr, 1994; Pahud, 2009)

Dosing: Usual Note: In general, administer in combination with amphotericin B or another susceptible antifungal due to development of resistance.

Infants, Children, and Adolescents:

General dosing, susceptible infections: Oral: 50-150 mg/kg/day in divided doses every 6 hours (Red Book, 2012)

Candidiasis (Pappas, 2009): Oral:

Endocarditis or implanted cardiovascular device: 25 mg/kg/dose every 6 hours in combination with amphotericin B; valve replacement or removal of hardware is strongly recommended

Endophthalmitis: 25 mg/kg/dose every 6 hours in combination with amphotericin B

Invasive (including CNS disease), treatment: 25 mg/kg/dose every 6 hours

Urinary tract infection:

Cystitis, symptomatic: 25 mg/kg/dose every 6 hours for 7-10 days

Pyelonephritis: 25 mg/kg/dose every 6 hours for 2 weeks; with or without amphotericin B; if fungal balls present, use in combination with amphotericin B and treatment duration should be until symptom resolution and clear urine culture

Cryptococcal disease; disseminated (including CNS disease); treatment (independent of HIV status): Oral: 25 mg/kg/dose every 6 hours in combination with amphotericin B or fluconazole; minimum treatment duration: ≥2 weeks; full treatment duration dependent upon: HIV status, source of infection and concomitant antifungal therapy (DHHS [adult and pediatric], 2013; Perfect, 2010; Tunkel, 2009)

Adults:

General dosing, susceptible infection: Oral: 12.5-37.5 mg/kg/dose every 6 hours

Endocarditis: Oral: 100 mg/kg/day in 3 or 4 divided doses (with amphotericin B) for at least 4-6 weeks after valve replacement (Gould, 2012; Pappas, 2009)

Meningoencephalitis, cryptococcal: Oral: Induction: 25 mg/kg/dose (with amphotericin B) every 6 hours for at least 4 weeks, or if HIV-infected at least 2 weeks; if clinical improvement, may discontinue both amphotericin and flucytosine and follow with an extended course of fluconazole (DHHS [adult], 2013; Perfect, 2010)

Dosing adjustment in renal impairment: Monitor serum concentrations.

Infants, Children, and Adolescents: There are no dosage adjustments provided in the manufacturer labeling; however, the following guidelines have been used by some clinicians:

Aronoff, 2007: Infants, Children, and non-HIV-exposed/-positive Adolescents: Based on a usual dose of 100-150 mg/kg/day divided every 6 hours

GFR 30-50 mL/minute/1.73 m^2: 25-37.5 mg/kg/dose every 8 hours

GFR 10-29 mL/minute/1.73 m^2: 25-37.5 mg/kg/dose every 12 hours

GFR <10 mL/minute/1.73 m^2: 25-37.5 mg/kg/dose every 24 hours

Hemodialysis or peritoneal dialysis: 25-37.5 mg/kg/dose every 24 hours

Continuous renal replacement therapy: 25-37.5 mg/kg/dose every 8 hours; monitor serum concentrations

DHHS [adult], 2013: HIV-exposed/-positive: Adolescents: Based on a usual dose of 25 mg/kg every 6 hours:

CrCl >40 mL/minute: No adjustment recommended

CrCl 20-40 mL/minute: 25 mg/kg every 12 hours

CrCl 10 to <20 mL/minute: 25 mg/kg every 24 hours

CrCl <10 mL/minute: 25 mg/kg every 48 hours

Hemodialysis: Administer dose after hemodialysis: 25-50 mg/kg every 48-72 hours

Adults: The manufacturer's labeling suggests using lower initial dose; the following guidelines have been used by some clinicians

Aronoff, 2007: Based on a usual dose of 37.5 mg/kg every 6 hours:

CrCl >80 mL/minute: No adjustment recommended

CrCl 50-80 mL/minute: 37.5 mg/kg every 12 hours

CrCl 10-50 mL/minute: 37.5 mg/kg every 12-24 hours

CrCl <10 mL/minute: 37.5 mg/kg every 24-48 hours, but monitor drug concentrations frequently

Hemodialysis: Administer dose after hemodialysis

Peritoneal dialysis: 500-1000 mg every 24 hours

Continuous renal replacement therapy: 37.5 mg/kg every 12-24 hours; monitor serum concentrations

DHHS [adult], 2013: Based on a usual dose of 25 mg/kg every 6 hours:

CrCl >40 mL/minute: No adjustment recommended

CrCl 20-40 mL/minute: 25 mg/kg every 12 hours

CrCl 10 to ≤20 mL/minute: 25 mg/kg every 24 hours

CrCl <10 mL/minute: 25 mg/kg every 48 hours

Hemodialysis: Administer dose after hemodialysis: 25-50 mg/kg every 48-72 hours

Dosing adjustment in hepatic impairment: There are no dosage adjustments provided in the manufacturer's labeling, but flucytosine has minimal hepatic metabolism; use caution.

Administration Oral: Administer around-the-clock to promote less variation in peak and trough serum levels; to avoid nausea and vomiting, administer a few capsules at a time over 15 minutes until full dose is taken.

Monitoring Parameters Prior to therapy: Serum electrolytes (especially potassium), CBC with differential, BUN,

and creatinine. During therapy: Serum electrolytes, creatinine, BUN, alkaline phosphatase, AST, ALT, CBC, platelet count; serum flucytosine concentrations; *in vitro* susceptibility tests to flucytosine

Reference Range

Therapeutic: Trough: 25-50 mcg/mL; peak: 50-100 mcg/mL; peak concentrations should not exceed 100 mcg/mL to avoid bone marrow toxicity and hepatotoxicity; for patients who are HIV-exposed/-positive a peak concentration of 40-60 mcg/mL is recommended (DHHS [pediatric], 2013)

Trough: Draw just prior to dose administration

Peak: Draw 2 hours after an oral dose administration

Test Interactions Flucytosine causes markedly false elevations in serum creatinine values when the Ektachem® analyzer is used. The Jaffé reaction is recommended for determining serum creatinine.

Dosage Forms Excipient information presented when available (limited, particularly for generics); consult specific product labeling.

Capsule, Oral:

Ancobon: 250 mg, 500 mg

Generic: 250 mg, 500 mg

Extemporaneous Preparations A 10 mg/mL oral suspension may be made with capsules and distilled water. Empty the contents of ten 500 mg capsules in a mortar; add small portions of distilled water and mix to a uniform paste. Mix while adding distilled water in incremental proportions to **almost** 500 mL; transfer to a 500 mL volumetric flask, rinse mortar several times with distilled water, and add sufficient quantity of distilled water to make 500 mL. Store in glass or plastic prescription bottles and label "shake well". Stable for 70 days refrigerated and 14 days at room temperature.

Wintermeyer SM and Nahata MC, "Stability of Flucytosine in an Extemporaneously Compounded Oral Liquid," *Am J Health Syst Pharm*, 1996, 53(4):407-9.

References

American Academy of Pediatrics (AAP). In: Pickering LK, Baker CJ, Kimberlin DW, Long SS, eds. Red Book: 2012 Report of the Committee on Infectious Diseases. 29th ed. Elk Grove Village, IL: American Academy of Pediatrics; 2012.

Aronoff GR, Bennett WM, Berns JS, et al, *Drug Prescribing in Renal Failure: Dosing Guidelines for Adults and Children*, 5th ed, Philadelphia, PA: American College of Physicians, 2007, 73.

Baley JE, Meyers C, Kliegman RM, et al, "Pharmacokinetics, Outcome of Treatment, and Toxic Effects of Amphotericin B and 5-Fluorocytosine in Neonates," *J Pediatr*, 1990, 116(5):791-7.

DHHS. Guidelines for the prevention and treatment of opportunistic infections among HIV-exposed and HIV-infected children: recommendations from the National Institutes of Health, Centers for Disease Control and Prevention, the HIV Medicine Association of the Infectious Diseases Society of America, the Pediatric Infectious Diseases Society, and the American Academy of Pediatrics. November 6, 2013. Available at http://aidsinfo.nih.gov

DHHS Panel on Opportunistic Infections (OI) in HIV-Infected Adults and Adolescents, "Guidelines for Prevention and Treatment of Opportunistic Infections in HIV-Infected Adults and Adolescents: Recommendations from the Centers for Disease Control and Prevention (CDC), the National Institutes of Health (NIH), and the HIV Medicine Association (HIVMA) of the Infectious Diseases Society of America (IDSA)," May 7, 2013. Available at http://aidsinfo.nih.gov/contentfiles/lvguidelines/adult_oi.pdf

Fernandez M, Moylett EH, Noyola DE, et al, "Candidal Meningitis in Neonates: A 10-Year Review," *Clin Infect Dis*, 2000, 31(2):458-63.

Gould FK, Denning DW, Elliott TS, et al, "Guidelines for the Diagnosis and Antibiotic Treatment of Endocarditis in Adults: A Report of the Working Party of the British Society for Antimicrobial Chemotherapy," *J Antimicrob Chemother*, 2012, 67(2):269-89.

Marr B, Gross S, Cunningham C, et al, "Candidal Sepsis and Meningitis in a Very-Low-Birth-Weight Infant Successfully Treated With Fluconazole and Flucytosine," *Clin Infect Dis*, 1994, 19(4):795-6.

Pahud BA, Greenhow TL, Piecuch B, et al, "Preterm Neonates With Candidal Brain Microabscesses: A Case Series," *J Perinatol*, 2009, 29(4):323-6.

Pappas PG, Kauffman CA, Andes D, et al, "Clinical Practice Guidelines for the Management of Candidiasis: 2009 Update by the Infectious Diseases Society of America," *Clin Infect Dis*, 2009, 48(5):503-35.

Pasqualotto AC, Howard SJ, Moore CB, et al, "Flucytosine Therapeutic Monitoring: 15 Years Experience From the UK," *J Antimicrob Chemother*, 2007, 59(4):791-3.

Perfect JR, Dismukes WE, Dromer F, et al, "Clinical Practice Guidelines for the Management of Cryptococcal Disease: 2010 Update by the Infectious Diseases Society of America," *Clin Infect Dis*, 2010, 50 (3):291-322.

Soltani M, Tobin CM, Bowker KE, et al, "Evidence of Excessive Concentrations of 5-Flucytosine in Children Aged Below 12 Years: A 12-Year Review of Serum Concentrations From a UK Clinical Assay Reference Laboratory," *Int J Antimicrob Agents*, 2006, 28(6):574-7.

Tunkel AR, Glaser CA, Bloch KC, et al, "The Management of Encephalitis: Clinical Practice Guidelines by the Infectious Diseases Society of America," *Clin Infect Dis*, 2008, 47(3):303-27.

◆ **Fludara** *see* Fludarabine *on page 885*

Fludarabine (floo DARE a been)

Medication Safety Issues
Sound-alike/look-alike issues:
Fludarabine may be confused with cladribine, floxuridine, Flumadine

Fludara may be confused with FUDR

High alert medication:
This medication is in a class the Institute for Safe Medication Practices (ISMP) includes among its list of drug classes which have a heightened risk of causing significant patient harm when used in error.

Related Information
Emetogenic Potential of Antineoplastic Agents in Children *on page 2327*

Safe Handling of Hazardous Drugs *on page 2419*

Brand Names: U.S. Fludara

Brand Names: Canada Fludara; Fludarabine Phosphate for Injection; Fludarabine Phosphate for Injection, USP; Fludarabine Phosphate Injection, PPC STD.

Therapeutic Category Antineoplastic Agent, Antimetabolite; Antineoplastic Agent, Antimetabolite (Purine Analog); Antineoplastic Agent, Antimetabolite (Purine Antagonist)

Generic Availability (U.S.) Yes

Use Treatment of B-cell chronic lymphocytic leukemia (CLL) unresponsive to previous therapy with an alkylating agent-containing regimen (FDA approved in ages ≥18 years); has also been used in the treatment of relapsed acute lymphocytic leukemia (ALL) or acute myeloid leukemia (AML), reduced-intensity conditioning regimens prior to allogeneic hematopoietic stem cell transplantation, non-Hodgkin's lymphomas (NHL), and AML in either refractory or in poor risk patients

Pregnancy Risk Factor D

Pregnancy Considerations Teratogenic effects were observed in animal studies. Based on the mechanism of action, fludarabine has the potential to cause fetal harm if administered during pregnancy. There are no adequate and well-controlled studies in pregnant women. Effective contraception is recommended during and for 6 months after treatment for women and men with female partners of reproductive potential.

Breast-Feeding Considerations Due to the potential for serious adverse reactions in the nursing infant, breast-feeding is not recommended.

Contraindications Hypersensitivity to fludarabine or any component

Warnings Hazardous agent; use appropriate precautions for handling and disposal (NIOSH, 2012). High doses have been associated with severe neurotoxicity **[U.S. Boxed Warning]**, including delayed blindness, coma, and death; neurotoxicity from high doses can occur 21-60 days after completing a course of fludarabine and appears to be dose related, although neurotoxicity has been reported as early as 7 days and up to 225 days. Similar neurotoxicity (agitation, coma, confusion, and seizure) has been reported with standard CLL doses; use with caution in

patients with preexisting neurologic problems; if neurotoxicity occurs, delay or discontinue therapy. Possible neurotoxic effects of chronic administration are unknown.

Severe bone marrow suppression (anemia, thrombocytopenia, and neutropenia) has been observed at therapeutic doses **[U.S. Boxed Warning]**; may be cumulative; bone marrow hypoplasia or aplasia resulting in death has been reported. Severe myelosuppression (trilineage bone marrow hypoplasia/aplasia) has been reported (rare) with a duration of significant cytopenias ranging from 2 months to 1 year. First-line combination therapy is associated with prolonged cytopenias, with anemia lasting up to 7 months, neutropenia up to 9 months, and thrombocytopenia up to 10 months (Gill, 2010). Use with caution in patients with a fever, infection, immunodeficiency, history of opportunistic infection, or preexisting hematological disorder; dosage modification may be needed in patients with bone marrow suppression. Prophylactic anti-infectives should be considered for patients with an increased risk for developing opportunistic infections.

Life-threatening and sometimes fatal autoimmune disorders, such as hemolytic anemia, autoimmune thrombocytopenia/ thrombocytopenic purpura, Evan's syndrome, and acquired hemophilia, have been reported after one or more cycles of treatment **[U.S. Boxed Warning]**. Monitor closely for hemolysis; discontinue fludarabine if hemolysis occurs; corticosteroid efficacy at controlling episodes is variable; hemolytic effects usually recur with fludarabine rechallenge in majority of patients. Concomitant therapy with pentostatin may be associated with severe and potentially fatal pulmonary toxicity **[U.S. Boxed Warning]**; concomitant use not recommended. Patients receiving blood products should only receive irradiated blood products due to the potential for transfusion-related GVHD. Fludarabine can cause fetal harm; advise women of childbearing potential to avoid becoming pregnant; contraceptive measures should be continued for 6 months post-treatment.

Precautions Use with caution in patients with renal insufficiency; clearance of the primary metabolite 2-fluoro-ara-A is reduced; dosage reductions are recommended for renal impairment; use is not recommended if CrCl <30 mL/minute; monitor closely for excessive toxicity. May cause tumor lysis syndrome characterized by hyperuricemia, hyperphosphatemia, hypocalcemia, hyperkalemia, metabolic acidosis, and renal failure; initial presentation may include flank pain and hematuria; risk is increased in patients with large tumor burden prior to treatment. Fludarabine use associated with fatigue, weakness, and visual disturbances; may impair ability to perform activities requiring mental alertness; patients should be counseled. Avoid vaccination with live vaccines during and after fludarabine treatment. Administer under the supervision of an experienced cancer chemotherapy physician **[U.S. Boxed Warning]**.

Adverse Reactions
Cardiovascular: Aneurysm, angina, arrhythmia, cerebrovascular accident, CHF, deep vein thrombosis, edema, MI, phlebitis, supraventricular tachycardia, transient ischemic attack

Central nervous system: Cerebellar syndrome, chills, depression, fatigue, fever, headache, malaise, mentation impaired, pain, sleep disorder

Dermatologic: Alopecia, pruritus, rash, seborrhea

Endocrine & metabolic: Dehydration, hyperglycemia

Gastrointestinal: Anorexia, constipation, diarrhea, dysphagia, esophagitis, gastrointestinal bleeding, mucositis, nausea/vomiting, stomatitis

Genitourinary: Dysuria, hesitancy, urinary tract infection

Hematologic: Anemia, hemorrhage, myelosuppression (nadir: 10-14 days; recovery: 5-7 weeks; dose-limiting toxicity), neutropenia (nadir: ~13 days), thrombocytopenia (nadir: ~16 days)

Hepatic: Cholelithiasis, liver failure, liver function tests abnormal

Neuromuscular & skeletal: Arthralgia, myalgia, osteoporosis, paresthesia, weakness

Ocular: Visual disturbance

Otic: Hearing loss

Renal: Hematuria, proteinuria, renal failure, renal function test abnormal

Respiratory: Allergic pneumonitis, bronchitis, cough, dyspnea, epistaxis, hemoptysis, hypoxia, pharyngitis, pneumonia, sinusitis, upper respiratory infection

Miscellaneous: Anaphylaxis, diaphoresis, infection, tumor lysis syndrome

Rare but important or life-threatening: Acute respiratory distress syndrome, blindness, bone marrow fibrosis, cerebral hemorrhage, coma, Epstein-Barr virus (EBV) associated lymphoproliferation, EBV reactivation, erythema multiforme, Evans syndrome, hemolytic anemia (autoimmune), hemophilia (acquired), hemorrhagic cystitis, herpes zoster reactivation, hyperkalemia, hyperphosphatemia, hyperuricemia, hypocalcemia, interstitial pulmonary infiltrate, metabolic acidosis, myelodysplastic syndrome/acute myeloid leukemia (usually associated with prior or concurrent treatment with other anticancer agents), opportunistic infection, optic neuritis, optic neuropathy, pancytopenia, pemphigus, pericardial effusion, peripheral neuropathy, pneumonitis, progressive multifocal leukoencephalopathy (PML), pulmonary fibrosis, pulmonary hemorrhage, respiratory distress, respiratory failure, Richter's syndrome, seizure, skin cancer (new onset or exacerbation), Stevens-Johnson syndrome, thrombocytopenia (autoimmune), thrombocytopenic purpura (autoimmune), toxic epidermal necrolysis, trilineage bone marrow aplasia, trilineage bone marrow hypoplasia, urate crystalluria, wrist drop

Also observed: Neurologic syndrome characterized by cortical blindness, coma, and paralysis (onset of neurologic symptoms may be delayed for 3-4 weeks)

Drug Interactions

Metabolism/Transport Effects None known.

Avoid Concomitant Use

Avoid concomitant use of Fludarabine with any of the following: BCG; CloZAPine; Dipyrone; Natalizumab; Pentostatin; Pimecrolimus; Tacrolimus (Topical); Tofacitinib; Vaccines (Live)

Increased Effect/Toxicity

Fludarabine may increase the levels/effects of: CloZAPine; Leflunomide; Natalizumab; Pentostatin; Tofacitinib; Vaccines (Live)

The levels/effects of Fludarabine may be increased by: Denosumab; Dipyrone; Pentostatin; Pimecrolimus; Roflumilast; Tacrolimus (Topical); Trastuzumab

Decreased Effect

Fludarabine may decrease the levels/effects of: BCG; Coccidioidin Skin Test; Sipuleucel-T; Vaccines (Inactivated); Vaccines (Live)

The levels/effects of Fludarabine may be decreased by: Echinacea; Imatinib

Stability Hazardous agent; use appropriate precautions for handling and disposal (NIOSH, 2012).

Injection: Store intact vials of powder and solution for injection at 2°C to 8°C (36°F to 46°F). Reconstituted solution at 25 mg/mL should be used within 8 hours after preparation (per manufacturer labeling). Diluted solutions of 1 mg/mL and 25 mg/mL (in D_5W or NS) are stable for 16 days at 25°C under room light; more dilution solutions (0.04 mg/mL in D_5W or NS) are stable for 48 hours at room temperature or refrigerated; discard solution if a slight haze develops.

Mechanism of Action Fludarabine inhibits DNA synthesis by inhibition of DNA polymerase and ribonucleotide reductase; also inhibits DNA primase and DNA ligase I

Pharmacokinetics (Adult data unless noted)

Distribution: V_d: 38-96 L/m^2; widely distributed with extensive tissue binding

Protein binding: 2-fluoro-ara-A: 19% to 29%

Metabolism: I.V.: Fludarabine phosphate is rapidly dephosphorylated in the plasma to 2-fluoro-ara-A (active metabolite), which subsequently enters tumor cells and is phosphorylated by deoxycytidine kinase to the active triphosphate derivative (2-fluoro-ara-ATP)

Half-life: Terminal (2-fluoro-ara-A):

Children: 12.4-19 hours

Adults: ~20 hours

Time to peak serum concentration: Oral: 1-2 hours

Elimination: Urine (60%, 23% as 2-fluoro-ara-A) within 24 hours; clearance appears to be inversely correlated with serum creatinine

Dosing: Usual

Infants, Children, and Adolescents: Refer to individual protocols; details concerning dosing in combination regimens should also be consulted.

AML: Infants, Children, and Adolescents: Limited data available: Continuous I.V. infusion: 10.5 mg/m^2 bolus followed by 30.5 mg/m^2/**day** for 48 hours in combination with cytarabine and idarubicin (Lange, 2008)

ALL or AML, relapsed: Children and Adolescents: Limited data available: I.V.:

Continuous I.V. infusion:10.5 mg/m^2 bolus followed by 30.5 mg/m^2/**day** for 48 hours in combination with cytarabine (Avramis,1998)

Intermittent I.V. dosing: 25 mg/m^2/dose once daily for 5 days in combination with cytarabine and daunorubicin was used for ALL (Parker, 2010)

Stem cell transplant (allogeneic) conditioning regimen, reduced-intensity (hematologic malignancy): Children and Adolescents: Limited data available: I.V.: 30 mg/m^2/dose once daily for 6 doses beginning 7-10 days prior to transplant (in combination with busulfan and thymoglobulin (Pulsipher, 2009)

Adults: Refer to individual protocols; details concerning dosing in combination regimens should also be consulted.

Chronic lymphocytic leukemia (CLL): I.V.: 25 mg/m^2/**day** for 5 days every 28 days

Dosing adjustment in renal impairment:

Infants, Children, and Adolescents: The following guidelines have been used by some clinicians (Aronoff, 2007): I.V.:

GFR >50 mL/minute/1.73 m^2: No adjustment required

GFR 30-50 mL/minute/1.73 m^2: Administer 80% of dose.

GFR <30 mL/minute/1.73 m^2: Not recommended.

Hemodialysis: Administer 25% of dose

Continuous ambulatory peritoneal dialysis (CAPD): Not recommended.

Continuous renal replacement therapy (CRRT): Administer 80% of dose.

Adults:

Manufacturer labeling: CLL: I.V.:

CrCl 50-79 mL/minute: Decrease dose to 20 mg/m^2

CrCl 30-49 mL/minute: Decrease dose to 15 mg/m^2

CrCl <30 mL/minute: Avoid use.

The following guidelines have been used by some clinicians (Aronoff, 2007): I.V.:

CrCl10-50 mL/minute: Administer 75% of dose.

CrCl <10 mL/minute: Administer 50% of dose.

Hemodialysis: Administer after dialysis

Continuous ambulatory peritoneal dialysis (CAPD): Administer 50% of dose.

Continuous renal replacement therapy (CRRT): Administer 75% of dose.

Dosing adjustment for toxicity:
Hematologic or nonhematologic toxicity (other than neurotoxicity): Consider treatment delay or dosage reduction.
Hemolysis: Discontinue treatment.
Neurotoxicity: Consider treatment delay or discontinuation.

Administration Hazardous agent; use appropriate precautions for handling and disposal (NIOSH, 2012).
Parenteral: Consult specific protocols.
Intermittent I.V. infusion: Infuse over 15-30 minutes; usual concentrations are: 0.25-1 mg/mL in D_5W or NS
Continuous I.V. infusion with loading dose (bolus):
Loading dose: Dilute in 20 mL D_5W and administer over 15 minutes
Continuous I.V. infusion: Dilute to 240 mL in D_5W and administer at a constant rate of 10 mL/hour

Monitoring Parameters CBC with differential, platelet count, hemoglobin, AST, ALT, creatinine, serum electrolytes, albumin, uric acid, and examination for visual changes; monitor for signs of infection and neurotoxicity

Dosage Forms Excipient information presented when available (limited, particularly for generics); consult specific product labeling.
Solution, Intravenous, as phosphate:
Generic: 50 mg/2 mL (2 mL)
Solution Reconstituted, Intravenous, as phosphate:
Fludara: 50 mg (1 ea)
Generic: 50 mg (1 ea)
Solution Reconstituted, Intravenous, as phosphate [preservative free]:
Generic: 50 mg (1 ea)

References
Aronoff GR, Bennett WM, Berns JS, et al, *Drug Prescribing in Renal Failure: Dosing Guidelines for Adults and Children*, 5th ed, Philadelphia, PA: American College of Physicians, 2007, 99, 172.
Avramis VI, Champagne J, Sato J, et al, "Pharmacology of Fludarabine Phosphate After a Phase I/II Trial by a Loading Bolus and Continuous Infusion in Pediatric Patients," *Cancer Res*, 1990, 50(22):7226-31.
Gill S, Carney D, Ritchie D, et al, "The Frequency, Manifestations, and Duration of Prolonged Cytopenias After First-Line Fludarabine Combination Chemotherapy," *Ann Oncol*, 2010, 21(2):331-4.
Lange BJ, Smith FO, Feusner J, et al, "Outcomes in CCG-2961, a Children's Oncology Group Phase 3 Trial for Untreated Pediatric Acute Myeloid Leukemia: A Report From the Children's Oncology Group," *Blood*, 2008, 111(3):1044-53.
National Institute for Occupational Safety and Health (NIOSH), "NIOSH List of Antineoplastic and Other Hazardous Drugs in Healthcare Settings 2012." Available at http://www.cdc.gov/niosh/docs/2012-150/pdfs/2012-150.pdf. Accessed January 21, 2013.
Parker C, Waters R, Leighton C, et al, "Effect of Mitoxantrone on Outcome of Children With First Relapse of Acute Lymphoblastic Leukaemia (ALL R3): An Open-Label Randomised Trial," *Lancet*, 2010, 376(9757):2009-17.
Pulsipher MA, Boucher KM, Wall D, et al, "Reduced-Intensity Allogeneic Transplantation in Pediatric Patients Ineligible for Myeloablative Therapy: Results of the Pediatric Blood and Marrow Transplant Consortium Study ONC0313," *Blood*, 2009, 114(7):1429-36.

◆ **Fludarabine Phosphate** see Fludarabine on page 885
◆ **Fludarabine Phosphate for Injection (Can)** see Fludarabine on page 885
◆ **Fludarabine Phosphate for Injection, USP (Can)** see Fludarabine on page 885
◆ **Fludarabine Phosphate Injection, PPC STD. (Can)** see Fludarabine on page 885

Fludrocortisone (floo droe KOR ti sone)

Medication Safety Issues
Sound-alike/look-alike issues:
Florinef® may be confused with Fioricet®, Fiorinal®
Related Information
Corticosteroids Systemic Equivalencies on page 2222
Brand Names: Canada Florinef®

Therapeutic Category Adrenal Corticosteroid; Corticosteroid, Systemic; Glucocorticoid; Mineralocorticoid
Generic Availability (U.S.) Yes
Use Treatment of Addison's disease; partial replacement therapy for adrenal insufficiency; treatment of salt-losing forms of congenital adrenogenital syndrome; has been used in conjunction with an increased sodium intake for the treatment of idiopathic orthostatic hypotension
Pregnancy Risk Factor C
Pregnancy Considerations Animal reproduction studies have not been conducted with fludrocortisone; adverse events have been observed with corticosteroids in animal reproduction studies. Some studies have shown an association between first trimester systemic corticosteroid use and oral clefts (Park-Wyllie, 2000; Pradat, 2003). Systemic corticosteroids may also influence fetal growth (decreased birth weight); however, information is conflicting (Lunghi, 2010). Hypoadrenalism may occur in newborns following maternal use of corticosteroids in pregnancy; monitor.

When systemic corticosteroids are needed in pregnancy, it is generally recommended to use the lowest effective dose for the shortest duration of time, avoiding high doses during the first trimester (Leachman, 2006; Lunghi, 2010). Fludrocortisone may be used to treat women during pregnancy who require therapy for congenital adrenal hyperplasia (Speiser, 2010).
Breast-Feeding Considerations Corticosteroids are excreted in human milk; information specific to fludrocortisone has not been located. The manufacturer recommends that caution be exercised when administering fludrocortisone to nursing women.
Contraindications Hypersensitivity to fludrocortisone or any component; CHF, systemic fungal infections
Precautions Dosage should be tapered gradually if therapy is discontinued; use with caution in patients with hypertension, edema, or renal dysfunction
Adverse Reactions
Cardiovascular: Cardiac enlargement, CHF, edema, hypertension
Central nervous system: Delirium, depression, emotional instability, euphoria, hallucinations, headache, insomnia, intracranial pressure increased, malaise, mood swings, nervousness, personality changes, pseudotumor cerebri, psychiatric disorders, psychoses, seizure, vertigo
Dermatologic: Acne, bruising, erythema, hirsutism, hives, hyperpigmentation, maculopapular rash, petechiae, purpura, rash, skin test reaction impaired, striae, subcutaneous fat atrophy, thin fragile skin, urticaria, wound healing (impaired)
Endocrine & metabolic: Cushing's syndrome, diabetes mellitus, glucose intolerance, growth suppression, hyperglycemia, hypokalemia, hypokalemic alkalosis, menstrual irregularities, negative nitrogen balance, pituitary-adrenal axis suppression
Gastrointestinal: Abdominal distention, esophagitis ulceration, pancreatitis, peptic ulcer
Neuromuscular & skeletal: Fractures, necrosis (femoral and humeral heads), muscle mass loss, muscle weakness, myopathy, osteoporosis, vertebral compression fractures
Ocular: Cataracts, exophthalmos, glaucoma, increased intraocular pressure
Renal: Glycosuria
Miscellaneous: Anaphylaxis (generalized), diaphoresis
Drug Interactions
Metabolism/Transport Effects None known.
Avoid Concomitant Use
Avoid concomitant use of Fludrocortisone with any of the following: Aldesleukin; BCG; Indium 111 Capromab Pendetide; Mifepristone; Natalizumab; Pimecrolimus; Tacrolimus (Topical); Tofacitinib

▶

Increased Effect/Toxicity

Fludrocortisone may increase the levels/effects of: Acetylcholinesterase Inhibitors; Amphotericin B; Androgens; Ceritinib; Deferasirox; Leflunomide; Loop Diuretics; Natalizumab; NSAID (COX-2 Inhibitor); NSAID (Nonselective); Thiazide Diuretics; Tofacitinib; Vaccines (Live); Warfarin

The levels/effects of Fludrocortisone may be increased by: Antifungal Agents (Azole Derivatives, Systemic); Aprepitant; Calcium Channel Blockers (Nondihydropyridine); Denosumab; Estrogen Derivatives; Fluconazole; Fosaprepitant; Indacaterol; Macrolide Antibiotics; Mifepristone; Neuromuscular-Blocking Agents (Nondepolarizing); Pimecrolimus; Quinolone Antibiotics; Roflumilast; Salicylates; Tacrolimus (Topical); Telaprevir; Trastuzumab

Decreased Effect

Fludrocortisone may decrease the levels/effects of: Aldesleukin; Antidiabetic Agents; BCG; Calcitriol; Coccidioidin Skin Test; Corticorelin; Hyaluronidase; Indium 111 Capromab Pendetide; Isoniazid; Salicylates; Sipuleucel-T; Telaprevir; Urea Cycle Disorder Agents; Vaccines (Inactivated)

The levels/effects of Fludrocortisone may be decreased by: Aminoglutethimide; Antacids; Barbiturates; Bile Acid Sequestrants; Echinacea; Mifepristone; Mitotane; Primidone; Rifamycin Derivatives

Mechanism of Action Very potent mineralocorticoid with high glucocorticoid activity; used primarily for its mineralocorticoid effects. Promotes increased reabsorption of sodium and loss of potassium from renal distal tubules.

Pharmacodynamics Duration: 1-2 days

Pharmacokinetics (Adult data unless noted)
Absorption: Rapid and complete from GI tract
Protein binding: 42%
Metabolism: In the liver
Half-life:
  Plasma: ~3.5 hours
  Biological: 18-36 hours

Dosing: Neonatal Oral: Congenital adrenal hyperplasia (salt losers): Maintenance: 0.05-0.2 mg/day in 1-2 divided doses (AAP, 2010; Speiser, 2010)

Dosing: Usual Oral:
Infants and Children: 0.05-0.1 mg/day
  Congenital adrenal hyperplasia (salt losers): Maintenance: 0.05-0.3 mg/day (AAP, 2000)
Adults: 0.05-0.2 mg/day

Administration Oral: May administer with food to decrease GI upset

Monitoring Parameters Serum electrolytes and glucose, blood pressure, serum renin

Additional Information In patients with salt-losing forms of congenital adrenogenital syndrome, use along with cortisone or hydrocortisone; fludrocortisone 0.1 mg has sodium retention activity equal to DOCA® 1 mg

Dosage Forms Excipient information presented when available (limited, particularly for generics); consult specific product labeling.
Tablet, Oral, as acetate:
  Generic: 0.1 mg

References

American Academy of Pediatrics, "Statement of Endorsement-Congenital Adrenal Hyperplasia Due to Steroid 21-Hydroxylase Deficiency," *Pediatrics*, 2010, 126(5):151. Available at http://pediatrics.aappublications.org/content/126/5/1051.extract. Accessed May 10, 2011.

American Academy of Pediatrics, Section on Endocrinology and Committee on Genetics, "Technical Report: Congenital Adrenal Hyperplasia," *Pediatrics*, 2000, 106(6):1511-18.

Leachman SA and Reed BR, "The Use of Dermatologic Drugs in Pregnancy and Lactation," *Dermatol Clin*, 2006, 24(2):167-97, vi.

Lunghi L, Pavan B, Biondi C, et al, "Use of Glucocorticoids in Pregnancy," *Curr Pharm Des*, 2010, 16(32):3616-37.

Park-Wyllie L, Mazzotta P, Pastuszak A, et al, "Birth defects After Maternal Exposure to Corticosteroids: Prospective Cohort Study and Meta-Analysis of Epidemiological Studies," *Teratology*, 2000, 62 (6):385-92.

Pradat P, Robert-Gnansia E, Di Tanna GL, et al, "First Trimester Exposure to Corticosteroids and Oral Clefts," *Birth Defects Res A Clin Mol Teratol*, 2003, 67(12):968-70.

Speiser PW, Azziz R, Baskin LS, et al, "Congenital Adrenal Hyperplasia Due to Steroid 21-Hydroxylase Deficiency: An Endocrine Society Clinical Practice Guideline," *J Clin Endocrinol Metab*, 2010, 95 (9):4133-60.

◆ **Fludrocortisone Acetate** *see* Fludrocortisone *on page 887*

◆ **Flulaval** *see* Influenza Virus Vaccine (Inactivated) *on page 1103*

◆ **Flulaval Quadrivalent** *see* Influenza Virus Vaccine (Inactivated) *on page 1103*

◆ **Flumadine** *see* Rimantadine *on page 1830*

◆ **Flumadine® (Can)** *see* Rimantadine *on page 1830*

Flumazenil (FLOO may ze nil)

Medication Safety Issues
Sound-alike/look-alike issues:
Flumazenil may be confused with influenza virus vaccine

Brand Names: Canada Anexate; Flumazenil Injection; Flumazenil Injection, USP; Romazicon

Therapeutic Category Antidote, Benzodiazepine

Generic Availability (U.S.) Yes

Use Benzodiazepine antagonist; reverses sedative effects of benzodiazepines used in general anesthesia or conscious sedation; management of benzodiazepine overdose; **not indicated** for ethanol, barbiturate, general anesthetic or opioid overdose

Pregnancy Risk Factor C

Pregnancy Considerations Teratogenic effects were not seen in animal reproduction studies. Embryocidal effects were seen at large doses. Use during labor and delivery is not recommended.In general, medications used as antidotes should take into consideration the health and prognosis of the mother; antidotes should be administered to pregnant women if there is a clear indication for use and should not be withheld because of fears of teratogenicity (Bailey, 2003).

Breast-Feeding Considerations It is not known if flumazenil is excreted in breast milk. The manufacturer recommends that caution be used if administering to breast-feeding women.

Contraindications Hypersensitivity to flumazenil, any component, or benzodiazepines; patients given benzodiazepines for control of potentially life-threatening conditions (eg, control of intracranial pressure or status epilepticus); patients with signs of serious cyclic-antidepressant overdosage

Warnings Flumazenil may precipitate seizures in high risk patients **[U.S. Boxed Warning]**; possible risk factors for seizures include patients physically dependent on benzodiazepines, patients treated with benzodiazepines for seizure disorders or other reasons, patients who received recent repeated doses of parenteral benzodiazepines, overdose patients with seizure activity prior to flumazenil, patients with serious cyclic antidepressant or mixed drug overdoses, patients with concurrent major sedative-hypnotic drug withdrawal, and patients with severe hepatic impairment. Higher than normal doses of benzodiazepines may be required to treat these seizures. Mixed drug overdose patients who have ingested drugs that increase the likelihood of seizures (eg, cocaine, lithium, cyclosporine, cyclic antidepressants, bupropion, methylxanthines, MAO inhibitors, isoniazid, or propoxyphene) are at extremely high risk for seizures (flumazenil may be contraindicated in these patients). Flumazenil is not recommended in epileptic patients receiving chronic benzodiazepine therapy or in cases of serious cyclic antidepressant overdoses. Dosage of flumazenil should be individualized; clinicians should be prepared to manage seizure activity.

Precautions Resedation may occur with flumazenil use (due to its short half-life in comparison to some benzodiazepines); pediatric patients (especially 1-5 years of age) may experience resedation; these patients may require repeat bolus doses or continuous infusion; monitor patients for return of sedation, respiratory depression, and other residual benzodiazepine effects. Flumazenil should be used with caution in the intensive care unit because of increased risk of unrecognized benzodiazepine dependence in such settings. Flumazenil may provoke panic attacks in patients with panic disorder. Do not use flumazenil until effects of neuromuscular blockers have been fully reversed. Use with caution in patients with liver disease and decrease the amount or frequency of repeat doses. Use with caution in patients with head injury due to possibility of precipitating convulsions or altering blood flow in patients receiving benzodiazepines. Use with caution in patients with alcoholism and other drug dependencies; these patients may also be dependent on benzodiazepines. Clinicians should not rely on flumazenil to reverse respiratory depression/hypoventilation; flumazenil is not a substitute for evaluation of oxygenation; establishing an airway and assisting ventilation, as necessary, is always the initial step in overdose management. Safety and efficacy of flumazenil have not been established in children <1 year of age.

Adverse Reactions

Cardiovascular: Flushing, palpitation, vasodilation

Central nervous system: Abnormal crying, agitation, anxiety, ataxia, depersonalization, depression, dizziness, dysphoria, emotional lability, euphoria, fatigue, headache, insomnia, malaise, nervousness, paranoia, vertigo

Endocrine & metabolic: Hot flashes

Gastrointestinal: Nausea, vomiting, xerostomia

Local: Injection site reaction, pain at injection site, rash, skin abnormality, thrombophlebitis

Neuromuscular & skeletal: Hypoesthesia, paresthesia, weakness, tremor

Ocular: Abnormal vision, blurred vision, lacrimation

Respiratory: Dyspnea, hyperventilation

Miscellaneous: Diaphoresis

Rare but important or life-threatening: Abnormal hearing, altered blood pressure increased/decreased, arrhythmia, bradycardia, chest pain, confusion, coldness sensation, delirium, difficulty concentrating, dysphonia, fear, generalized seizure, hiccups, hyperacusis, hypertension, junctional tachycardia, panic attacks, rigors, seizure, shivering, somnolence, stupor, tachycardia, thick tongue, tinnitus, transient hearing impairment, ventricular tachycardia, withdrawal syndrome

Drug Interactions

Metabolism/Transport Effects None known.

Avoid Concomitant Use There are no known interactions where it is recommended to avoid concomitant use.

Increased Effect/Toxicity There are no known significant interactions involving an increase in effect.

Decreased Effect

Flumazenil may decrease the levels/effects of: Hypnotics (Nonbenzodiazepine)

Stability Store at 25°C (77°F); compatible with D₅W, LR, or NS for 24 hours; discard any unused solution after 24 hours

Mechanism of Action Competitively inhibits the activity at the benzodiazepine receptor site on the GABA/benzodiazepine receptor complex. Flumazenil does not antagonize the CNS effect of drugs affecting GABA-ergic neurons by means other than the benzodiazepine receptor (ethanol, barbiturates, general anesthetics) and does not reverse the effects of opioids

Pharmacodynamics

Onset of action: Benzodiazepine reversal: Within 1-3 minutes

Maximum effect: 6-10 minutes

Duration: Usually <1 hour; duration is related to dose given and benzodiazepine plasma concentrations; reversal effects of flumazenil may wear off before effects of benzodiazepine and resedation may occur

Pharmacokinetics (Adult data unless noted) Follows a two compartment open model; Note: Clearance and V_d per kg are similar for children and adults, but children display more variability

Distribution: Distributes extensively in the extravascular space; Adults:

Initial V_d: 0.5 L/kg

V_dss: 0.9-1.1 L/kg

Protein binding: ~50%; primarily to albumin

Metabolism: In the liver to the de-ethylated free acid and its glucuronide conjugate

Half-life:

Children: Terminal: 20-75 minutes (mean: 40 minutes)

Adults:

Alpha: 4-11 minutes

Terminal: 40-80 minutes

Elimination: 99% hepatically eliminated; <1% excreted unchanged in urine

Clearance: Dependent upon hepatic blood flow; Adults: 0.8-1 L/hour/kg

Dosing: Neonatal

Benzodiazepine reversal:

I.V.: Note: Minimal information available; dosing is extrapolated from experiences in pediatric patients 1-17 years; Initial dose: 0.01 mg/kg given over 15 seconds; may repeat 0.01 mg/kg after 45 seconds, and then every minute to a maximum total cumulative dose of 0.05 mg/kg

Continuous I.V. infusion (as an alternative to repeat bolus doses): 0.005-0.01 mg/kg/**hour**; dose based on a case report of premature neonate (GA: 32 weeks) exposed to high doses of diazepam intrapartum (Dixon, 1998)

Myoclonus, benzodiazepine-induced: I.V.: 0.0078 mg/kg as a single dose was effective in one full-term neonate who was receiving continuous infusion midazolam (Zaw, 2001)

Dosing: Usual I.V.:

Infants and Children:

Benzodiazepine reversal when used in conscious sedation or general anesthesia: Initial dose: 0.01 mg/kg (maximum dose: 0.2 mg) given over 15 seconds; may repeat 0.01 mg/kg (maximum dose: 0.2 mg) after 45 seconds, and then every minute to a maximum total cumulative dose of 0.05 mg/kg or 1 mg, whichever is lower; usual total dose: 0.08-1 mg (mean: 0.65 mg)

Management of benzodiazepine overdose: Minimal information available; initial dose: 0.01 mg/kg (maximum dose: 0.2 mg) with repeat doses of 0.01 mg/kg (maximum dose: 0.2 mg) given every minute to a maximum total cumulative dose of 1 mg; as an alternative to repeat bolus doses, follow up continuous infusions of 0.005-0.01 mg/kg/**hour** have been used; further studies are needed

Adults:

Benzodiazepine reversal when used in conscious sedation or general anesthesia: 0.2 mg given over 15 seconds; may repeat 0.2 mg after 45 seconds and then every 60 seconds up to a total of 1 mg, usual total dose: 0.6-1 mg. In event of resedation, may repeat doses at 20-minute intervals with maximum of 1 mg/dose (given at 0.2 mg/minute); maximum dose: 3 mg in 1 hour.

Management of benzodiazepine overdose: 0.2 mg given over 30 seconds; may give 0.3 mg dose after 30 seconds if desired level of consciousness is not obtained; additional doses of 0.5 mg can be given over 30 seconds at

1-minute intervals up to a cumulative dose of 3 mg; usual cumulative dose: 1-3 mg; rarely, patients with partial response at 3 mg may require additional titration up to total dose of 5 mg; if patient has not responded 5 minutes after cumulative dose of 5 mg, the major cause of sedation is not likely due to benzodiazepines. In the event of resedation, may repeat doses at 20-minute intervals with maximum of 1 mg/dose (given at 0.5 mg/minute); maximum dose: 3 mg in 1 hour.

Dosing adjustment in hepatic impairment: Initial dose: Use normal dose; repeat doses should be decreased in size or frequency

Administration Parenteral: For I.V. use only; administer by rapid I.V. injection over 15-30 seconds via a freely running I.V. infusion into larger vein (to decrease chance of pain, phlebitis). Children: Do not exceed 0.2 mg/minute. Adults: Repeat doses: Do not exceed 0.2 mg/minute for reversal of general anesthesia and do not exceed 0.5 mg/minute for reversal of benzodiazepine overdose.

Monitoring Parameters Level of consciousness and resedation, blood pressure, heart rate, respiratory rate, continuous pulse oximetry; monitor for resedation for 1-2 hours after reversal of sedation in patients who receive benzodiazepine sedation

Additional Information Flumazenil is a weak lipophilic base. In one study of conscious sedation reversal in 107 pediatric patients (1-17 years of age), resedation occurred between 19-50 minutes after the start of flumazenil. Flumazenil has been used to successfully treat paradoxical reactions in children associated with midazolam use (eg, agitation, restlessness, combativeness) (Massanari, 1997).

Dosage Forms Excipient information presented when available (limited, particularly for generics); consult specific product labeling.
Solution, Intravenous:
Generic: 0.5 mg/5 mL (5 mL); 1 mg/10 mL (10 mL)

References

Bailey B, "Are There Teratogenic Risks Associated With Antidotes Used in the Acute Management of Poisoned Pregnant Women?" *Birth Defects Res A Clin Mol Teratol*, 2003, 67(2):133-40.

Baktai G, Szekely E, Marialigeti T, et al, "Use of Midazolam (Dormicum) and Flumazenil (Anexate) in Paediatric Bronchology," *Curr Med Res Opin*, 1992, 12(9):552-9.

Clark RF, Sage TA, Tunget C, et al, "Delayed Onset Lorazepam Poisoning Successfully Reversed By Flumazenil in a Child: Case Report and Review of the Literature," *Pediatr Emerg Care*, 1995, 11 (1):32-4.

Dixon JC, Speidel BD, and Dixon JJ, "Neonatal Flumazenil Therapy Reverses Maternal Diazepam," *Acta Paediatr*, 1998, 87(2):225-6.

Jones RD, Lawson AD, Andrew LJ, et al, "Antagonism of the Hypnotic Effect of Midazolam in Children: A Randomized, Double Blind Study of Placebo and Flumazenil Administered After Midazolam-Induced Anaesthesia," *Br J Anaesth*, 1991, 66(6):660-6.

Massanari M, Novitsky J, and Reinstein LJ, "Paradoxical Reactions in Children Associated With Midazolam Use During Endoscopy," *Clin Pediatr*, 1997, 36(12):681-4.

Richard P, Autret E, Bardol J, et al, "The Use of Flumazenil in a Neonate," *J Toxicol Clin Toxicol*, 1991, 29(1):137-40.

Roald OK and Dahl V, "Flunitrazepam Intoxication in a Child Successfully Treated With the Benzodiazepine Antagonist Flumazenil," *Crit Care Med*, 1989, 17(12):1355-6.

Shannon M, Albers G, Burkhart K, et al, "Safety and Efficacy of Flumazenil in the Reversal of Benzodiazepine-Induced Conscious Sedation. The Flumazenil Pediatric Study Group," *J Pediatr*, 1997, 131(4):582-6.

Sugarman JM and Paul RI, "Flumazenil: A Review," *Pediatr Emerg Care*, 1994, 10(1):37-43.

Zaw W, Knoppert DC, and da Silva O, "Flumazenil's Reversal of Myoclonic-Like Movements Associated With Midazolam in Term Newborns," *Pharmacotherapy*, 2001, 21(5):642-6.

◆ **Flumazenil Injection (Can)** *see* Flumazenil *on page 888*

◆ **Flumazenil Injection, USP (Can)** *see* Flumazenil *on page 888*

◆ **FluMist** *see* Influenza Virus Vaccine (Live/Attenuated) *on page 1109*

◆ **FluMist Quadrivalent** *see* Influenza Virus Vaccine (Live/Attenuated) *on page 1109*

Flunisolide (Nasal) (floo NISS oh lide)

Medication Safety Issues
Sound-alike/look-alike issues:
Flunisolide may be confused with Flumadine®, fluocinonide

Brand Names: Canada Apo-Flunisolide®; Nasalide®; Rhinalar®

Therapeutic Category Corticosteroid, Intranasal

Generic Availability (U.S.) Yes

Use Management of nasal symptoms associated with seasonal or perennial rhinitis (FDA approved in ages ≥6 years and adults)

Intranasal corticosteroids have also been used as an adjunct to antibiotics in empiric treatment of acute bacterial rhinosinusitis primarily in patients with history of allergic rhinitis (Chow, 2012) and in pediatric patients with mild obstructive sleep apnea syndrome who cannot undergo adenotonsillectomy or who still have symptoms after surgery (Marcus, 2012).

Pregnancy Risk Factor C

Pregnancy Considerations Adverse effects were observed in some animal reproduction studies. Intranasal corticosteroids are recommended for the treatment of rhinitis during pregnancy; the lowest effective dose should be used (NAEPP, 2005; Wallace, 2008).

Breast-Feeding Considerations Other corticosteroids have been found in breast milk. It is not known if sufficient quantities of flunisolide are absorbed following inhalation to produce detectable amounts in breast milk. The use of inhaled corticosteroids is not considered a contraindication to breast-feeding (NAEPP, 2005). The manufacturer recommends caution be used if administered to a nursing woman.

Contraindications Hypersensitivity to flunisolide or any component; untreated nasal mucosa infection

Warnings HPA suppression or hypercorticism (Cushing's syndrome) may occur with use of higher than recommended doses or at typical doses in susceptible patients. Acute adrenal insufficiency may occur with abrupt withdrawal after long-term use, with stress, or when converting from systemic to topical corticosteroid therapy; withdrawal or discontinuation of corticosteroids should be done carefully; patients with HPA axis suppression may require doses of systemic glucocorticosteroids prior to, during, and after unusual stress (eg, surgery). Immunosuppression may occur; patients may be more susceptible to infections; avoid exposure to chickenpox and measles.

Precautions Avoid using higher than recommended dosages; suppression of HPA function, suppression of linear growth (ie, reduction of growth velocity), reduced bone mineral density, or hypercorticism (Cushing's syndrome) may occur; titrate to lowest effective dose. Reduction in growth velocity may occur when corticosteroids are administered to pediatric patients, even at recommended doses via intranasal route (monitor growth). Use flunisolide with extreme caution in patients with respiratory tuberculosis; untreated bacterial, fungal, systemic viral or parasitic infections; or ocular herpes simplex. Localized *Candida* infections of the nose and pharynx have been reported rarely; interruption of therapy may be necessary while antifungal therapy is employed. Corticosteroids impair wound healing; avoid use in patients with recent nasal ulcers, nasal surgery, or nasal trauma; allow healing to occur before use. Glaucoma, increased intraocular pressure and cataracts have been reported following the intranasal application of corticosteroids; monitor patients who have change in vision and in patients with a history of increased ocular pressure, glaucoma, or cataracts. Use of nasal flunisolide in place of systemic corticosteroids may unmask allergies (eg, eczema, rhinitis) that were previously controlled by the systemic corticosteroids. Rare cases of immediate hypersensitivity reactions or nasal septum perforation may occur with intranasal corticosteroids.

Adverse Reactions
Respiratory: Nasal burning/stinging, nasal congestion, nasal dryness, nasal irritation, rhinitis, sneezing
Miscellaneous: Loss of smell

Drug Interactions
Metabolism/Transport Effects Substrate of CYP3A4 (minor); **Note:** Assignment of Major/Minor substrate status based on clinically relevant drug interaction potential
Avoid Concomitant Use There are no known interactions where it is recommended to avoid concomitant use.
Increased Effect/Toxicity
Flunisolide (Nasal) may increase the levels/effects of: Ceritinib
Decreased Effect There are no known significant interactions involving a decrease in effect.

Stability Store at 15°C to 25°C (59°F to 77°F).

Mechanism of Action Decreases inflammation by suppression of migration of polymorphonuclear leukocytes and reversal of increased capillary permeability; does not depress hypothalamus

Pharmacodynamics Clinical effects are due to a direct local effect rather than systemic absorption
Onset of action: Within a few days
Maximum effect:1-2 weeks

Pharmacokinetics (Adult data unless noted)
Absorption: Rapid
Bioavailability: Intranasal 50%, oral 20% (due to first-pass metabolism)
Half-life: 1-2 hours
Elimination: Urine (50%, 65% to 70% as metabolite) and feces (50%)

Dosing: Usual Note: Once symptoms are controlled, the dose should be reduced to the lowest effective amount.
Children and Adolescents: **Seasonal and perennial rhinitis:** Intranasal:
Children and Adolescents 6-14 years: Initial: 100 mcg twice daily delivered as 50 mcg (2 sprays) **per nostril** twice daily **or** 50 mcg 3 times daily delivered as 25 mcg (1 spray) **per nostril** 3 times daily; maximum daily dose: 200 mcg/**day** (4 sprays **per nostril/day**); some patients may have efficacy at a lower maintenance dose as low as 50 mcg once daily delivered as 25 mcg (1 spray) **per nostril** once daily
Adolescents ≥15 years: Initial: 100 mcg twice daily delivered as 50 mcg (2 sprays) **per nostril** twice daily; if needed, increase to 100 mcg 3 times daily delivered as 50 mcg (2 sprays) **per nostril** 3 times daily; maximum daily dose: 400 mcg/**day** (8 sprays **per nostril/day**); some patients may have efficacy at a lower maintenance dose as low as 50 mcg once daily delivered as 25 mcg (1 spray) **per nostril** once daily
Adults: **Seasonal and perennial rhinitis:** Intranasal: 100 mcg twice daily delivered as 50 mcg (2 sprays) **per nostril** twice daily; if needed, increase to 100 mcg 3 times daily delivered as 50 mcg (2 sprays) **per nostril** 3 times daily; maximum daily dose: 400 mcg/**day** (8 sprays **per nostril/day**)

Dosing adjustment in renal impairment: There are no dosage adjustments provided in the manufacturer's labeling.

Dosing adjustment in hepatic impairment: There are no dosage adjustments provided in the manufacturer's labeling.

Administration Shake well prior to each use. Before first use, prime by pressing pump 5-6 times or until a fine spray appears. Repeat priming if ≥5 days between use or if dissembled for cleaning. Administer at regular intervals.

Blow nose to clear nostrils. Insert applicator into nostril, keeping bottle upright, and close off the other nostril. Breathe in through nose. While inhaling, press pump to release spray. Do not spray into eyes. Discard after labeled number of doses has been used, even if bottle is not completely empty.

Monitoring Parameters Mucous membranes for signs of fungal infection, growth (pediatric patients), signs/symptoms of HPA axis suppression/adrenal insufficiency; ocular changes

Additional Information When used short term as adjunctive therapy in acute bacterial rhinosinusitis (ABRS), intranasal steroids show modest symptomatic improvement and few adverse effects; improvement is primarily due to increased sinus drainage. Use should be considered optional in ABRS; however, intranasal corticosteroids should be routinely prescribed to ABRS patients who have a history of or concurrent allergic rhinitis (Chow, 2012).

Dosage Forms Excipient information presented when available (limited, particularly for generics); consult specific product labeling. [DSC] = Discontinued product
Solution, Nasal:
Generic: 25 mcg/actuation (0.025%) (25 mL); 29 mcg/actuation (0.025%) (25 mL [DSC])

References
Chow AW, Benninger MS, Brook I, et al, "IDSA Clinical Practice Guideline for Acute Bacterial Rhinosinusitis in Children and Adults," *Clin Infect Dis*, 2012, 54(8):e72-e112.
Marcus CL, Brooks LJ, Draper KA, et al, "Diagnosis and Management of Childhood Obstructive Sleep Apnea Syndrome," *Pediatrics*, 2012, 130(3):576-84.
NAEPP Working Group Report on "Managing Asthma During Pregnancy: Recommendations for Pharmacologic Treatment," National Institutes of Health, National Heart, Lung, and Blood Institute, NIH Publication No. 05-5236, March 2005. Available at http://www.nhlbi.nih.gov/health/prof/lung/asthma/astpreg/astpreg_full.pdf
Wallace DV, Dykewicz MS, Bernstein DI, et al, "The Diagnosis and Management of Rhinitis: An Updated Practice Parameter," *J Allergy Clin Immunol*, 2008, 122(2 Suppl):S1-84.

Fluocinolone (Ophthalmic) (floo oh SIN oh lone)

Medication Safety Issues
Sound-alike/look-alike issues:
Fluocinolone may be confused with fluocinonide

Brand Names: U.S. Retisert
Brand Names: Canada Retisert®
Therapeutic Category Corticosteroid, Ophthalmic
Generic Availability (U.S.) No

Use Treatment of chronic, noninfectious uveitis affecting the posterior segment of the eye (FDA approved in adults)

Pregnancy Considerations Animal studies have not been conducted with this product; however, adverse events have been observed with corticosteroids in animal reproduction studies.

Breast-Feeding Considerations Systemic corticosteroids are excreted in human milk. It is not known if sufficient quantities of fluocinolone are absorbed following ocular administration to produce detectable amounts in breast milk.

Contraindications Hypersensitivity to fluocinolone or any component; viral, fungal, and mycobacterial ocular infections; hypersensitivity to other corticosteroids

Warnings Transient decrease in visual acuity of 1-4 weeks duration following implantation may occur. Increased IOP or glaucoma may occur; use with caution in glaucoma patients; routine monitoring of IOP is recommended; patients may require use of medications or other treatments to lower IOP. Prolonged use of ocular corticosteroids may also increase the risk of secondary ocular infections, cataract formation, delayed wound healing, perforation of globe (if thinning of sclera occurs), or optic nerve damage. Unilateral implantation is recommended to minimize risk of postoperative infections in both eyes. ▶

◀ Procedural complications with implantation may occur (eg, cataract formation, choroidal detachment, endophthalmitis, hypotony, retinal detachment, vitreous loss, or hemorrhage).

Precautions Safety and efficacy have not been established in children <12 years of age.

Adverse Reactions

Central nervous system: Dizziness, fever, headache, pain, pyrexia

Dermatologic: Rash

Gastrointestinal: Nausea, vomiting

Neuromuscular & skeletal: Arthralgia, back pain, limb pain

Ocular: Abnormal sensation, blepharitis, blurred vision, cataract, choroidal detachment, conjunctival edema/chemosis, conjunctival hemorrhage, conjunctival hyperemia, corneal edema, dry eye, eye discharge, eye irritation/inflammation, eyelid edema, eye swelling, glaucoma, hypotony, intraocular pressure increased, eye pain, macular edema, maculopathy, photophobia, photopsia; procedural complications (eg, cataract fragments, implant migration, wound complications); pruritus, ptosis, retinal hemorrhage, tearing, visual acuity decreased, visual disturbance, vitreous floaters, vitreous hemorrhage, vitreous opacities

Respiratory: Cough, influenza, nasopharyngitis, sinusitis, upper respiratory infection

Miscellaneous: Secondary infection (bacterial, viral, or fungal)

Drug Interactions

Metabolism/Transport Effects None known.

Avoid Concomitant Use There are no known interactions where it is recommended to avoid concomitant use.

Increased Effect/Toxicity

Fluocinolone (Ophthalmic) may increase the levels/effects of: Ceritinib

Decreased Effect There are no known significant interactions involving a decrease in effect.

Stability Store in original container at 15°C to 25°C (59°F to 77°F); protect from freezing.

Pharmacokinetics (Adult data unless noted)

Absorption: Systemic absorption is negligible

Duration: Releases fluocinolone acetonide at a rate of 0.6 mcg/day, decreasing over 30 days to a steady-state release rate of 0.3-0.4 mcg/day for 30 months

Distribution: Aqueous and vitreous humor

Dosing: Usual Chronic uveitis: One silicone-encased tablet (0.59 mg) surgically implanted into the posterior segment of the eye is designed to release 0.6 mcg/day, decreasing over 30 days to a steady-state release rate of 0.3-0.4 mcg/day for 30 months. Recurrence of uveitis denotes depletion of tablet, requiring reimplantation.

Administration Handle only by suture tab to avoid damaging the tablet integrity and adversely affecting release characteristics. Maintain strict adherence to aseptic handling of product; do not resterilize.

Dosage Forms Excipient information presented when available (limited, particularly for generics); consult specific product labeling.

Implant, Intraocular, as acetonide:

Retisert: 0.59 mg (1 ea)

Fluocinolone (Otic) (floo oh SIN oh lone)

Medication Safety Issues

Sound-alike/look-alike issues:

Fluocinolone may be confused with fluocinonide

Brand Names: U.S. DermOtic

Therapeutic Category Adrenal Corticosteroid; Anti-inflammatory Agent

Generic Availability (U.S.) Yes

Use Relief of chronic eczematous external otitis

Pregnancy Risk Factor C

Pregnancy Considerations Adverse events have been observed with corticosteroids in animal reproduction studies. In general, the use of topical corticosteroids during pregnancy is not considered to have significant risk; however, intrauterine growth retardation in the infant has been reported (rare). The use of large amounts or for prolonged periods of time should be avoided.

Breast-Feeding Considerations Systemic corticosteroids are excreted in human milk. It is not known if sufficient quantities of fluocinolone are absorbed following topical administration to produce detectable amounts in breast milk.

Contraindications Hypersensitivity to fluocinolone or any component; **Note:** Contains peanut oil.

Warnings Infants and small children may be more susceptible to adrenal axis suppression from topical corticosteroid therapy; systemic effects may occur when used on large areas of the body, denuded areas, for prolonged periods of time, or with an occlusive dressing. Hypothalamic pituitary adrenal (HPA) axis suppression may occur; acute adrenal insufficiency may occur with abrupt withdrawal after long-term use or with stress; withdrawal or discontinuation should be done carefully; patients with HPA axis suppression may require doses of systemic glucocorticosteroids prior to, during, and after unusual stress (eg, surgery). Contains refined peanut oil; use with caution in patients with peanut hypersensitivity.

Adverse Reactions

Dermatologic: Acneiform eruptions, allergic contact dermatitis, burning, dryness, erythema, folliculitis, irritation, itching, hypopigmentation, keratosis pilaris, miliaria, skin atrophy, striae

Otic: Ear infection

Drug Interactions

Metabolism/Transport Effects None known.

Avoid Concomitant Use There are no known interactions where it is recommended to avoid concomitant use.

Increased Effect/Toxicity There are no known significant interactions involving an increase in effect.

Decreased Effect There are no known significant interactions involving a decrease in effect.

Mechanism of Action A synthetic fluorinated corticosteroid of low-to-moderate potency. The mechanism of action for all topical corticosteroids is not well defined, however, is believed to be a combination of anti-inflammatory, antipruritic, and vasoconstrictive properties.

Dosing: Usual Children ≥2 years and Adults: 5 drops into the affected ear twice daily for 1-2 weeks

Additional Information DermOtic® is made with 48% refined peanut oil, NF (peanut protein is below 0.5 ppm)

Dosage Forms Excipient information presented when available (limited, particularly for generics); consult specific product labeling.

Oil, Otic, as acetonide:

DermOtic: 0.01% (20 mL) [contains isopropyl alcohol, peanut oil]

Generic: 0.01% (20 mL)

Fluocinolone (Topical) (floo oh SIN oh lone)

Medication Safety Issues

Sound-alike/look-alike issues:

Fluocinolone may be confused with fluocinonide

Related Information

Topical Corticosteroids *on page 2224*

Brand Names: U.S. Capex; Derma-Smoothe/FS Body; Derma-Smoothe/FS Scalp; Fluocinolone Acetonide Body; Fluocinolone Acetonide Scalp; Synalar; Synalar (Cream); Synalar (Ointment); Synalar TS

Brand Names: Canada Capex®; Derma-Smoothe/FS®; Synalar®

Therapeutic Category Adrenal Corticosteroid; Anti-inflammatory Agent; Corticosteroid, Topical; Glucocorticoid

Generic Availability (U.S.) May be product dependent

Use Relief of susceptible inflammatory dermatosis

Capex™ shampoo: Adults: Treatment of seborrheic dermatitis of the scalp

Derma-Smoothe/FS®: Children ≤2 years: Moderate to severe atopic dermatitis (for use ≤4 weeks); Adults: Atopic dermatitis or psoriasis of the scalp

Pregnancy Risk Factor C

Pregnancy Considerations Adverse events have been observed with corticosteroids in animal reproduction studies. In general, the use of topical corticosteroids during pregnancy is not considered to have significant risk; however, intrauterine growth retardation in the infant has been reported (rare). The use of large amounts or for prolonged periods of time should be avoided.

Breast-Feeding Considerations Systemic corticosteroids are excreted in human milk. It is not known if sufficient quantities of fluocinolone are absorbed following topical administration to produce detectable amounts in breast milk. Hypertension in the nursing infant has been reported following corticosteroid ointment applied to the nipples. Use with caution.

Contraindications Hypersensitivity to fluocinolone or any component; TB of skin; herpes (including varicella); **Note:** Contains peanut oil.

Warnings Infants and small children may be more susceptible to adrenal axis suppression from topical corticosteroid therapy; systemic effects may occur when used on large areas of the body, denuded areas, for prolonged periods of time, or with an occlusive dressing. Derma-Smoothe/FS® contains refined peanut oil; use with caution in patients with peanut hypersensitivity. Hypothalamic pituitary adrenal (HPA) axis suppression may occur; acute adrenal insufficiency may occur with abrupt withdrawal after long-term use or with stress; withdrawal or discontinuation should be done carefully; patients with HPA axis suppression may require doses of systemic glucocorticosteroids prior to, during, and after unusual stress (eg, surgery).

Adverse Reactions

Cardiovascular: Intracranial hypertension (rare)

Central nervous system: Telangiectasia

Dermatologic: Acneiform eruptions, allergic contact dermatitis, burning, dryness, folliculitis, irritation, itching, hypertrichosis, hypopigmentation, miliaria, perioral dermatitis, skin atrophy, striae

Endocrine & metabolic: Cushing's syndrome, HPA axis suppression

Otic: Ear infection

Miscellaneous: Herpes simplex, secondary infection

Drug Interactions

Metabolism/Transport Effects None known.

Avoid Concomitant Use

Avoid concomitant use of Fluocinolone (Topical) with any of the following: Aldesleukin

Increased Effect/Toxicity

Fluocinolone (Topical) may increase the levels/effects of: Ceritinib; Deferasirox

The levels/effects of Fluocinolone (Topical) may be increased by: Telaprevir

Decreased Effect

Fluocinolone (Topical) may decrease the levels/effects of: Aldesleukin; Corticorelin; Hyaluronidase; Telaprevir

Stability Store at controlled room temperature in tightly closed container.

Mechanism of Action A synthetic fluorinated corticosteroid of low-to-moderate potency. The mechanism of action for all topical corticosteroids is not well defined, however, is believed to be a combination of anti-inflammatory, antipruritic, and vasoconstrictive properties.

Pharmacokinetics (Adult data unless noted)

Absorption: Dependent on strength of preparation, amount applied, nature of skin at application site, vehicle, and use of occlusive dressing; increased in areas of skin damage, inflammation, or occlusion

Distribution: Throughout local skin; absorbed drug is distributed rapidly into muscle, liver, skin, intestines, and kidneys

Metabolism: Primarily in skin; small amount absorbed into systemic circulation is primarily hepatic to inactive compounds

Excretion: Urine (primarily as glucuronide and sulfate, also as unconjugated products); feces (small amounts)

Dosing: Usual Children and Adults: Topical: Apply thin layer 2-4 times/day

Capex™ shampoo: Adults: Thoroughly wet hair and scalp; apply ≤1 ounce to scalp area; massage well; work into lather; allow to remain on scalp for 5 minutes; then rinse hair and scalp thoroughly; repeat daily until symptoms subside; **Note:** Once patient is symptom-free, once-weekly use usually keeps itching and flaking of dandruff from returning.

Derma-Smoothe/FS®:

Children ≥2 years: Atopic dermatitis: Apply in a thin layer to moistened skin of affected area twice daily for ≤4 weeks

Adults:

Atopic dermatitis: Apply a thin layer to affected area 3 times/day

Scalp psoriasis: Thoroughly wet or dampen hair and scalp; apply to scalp in a thin layer, massage well; cover scalp with shower cap (supplied); leave for a minimum of 4 hours or overnight, then wash hair and rinse thoroughly

Administration Apply sparingly in a thin film; rub in lightly

Capex™ shampoo: Shake well before use; do not bandage, wrap, or cover treated scalp area unless directed by physician; discard shampoo after 3 months (**Note:** Pharmacist must empty the contents of the 12 mg fluocinolone acetonide capsule into the shampoo base before dispensing to patient)

Derma-Smoothe/FS®: Do not apply to face or diaper area; avoid application to intertriginous areas (may increase local adverse effects)

Additional Information Considered a moderate-potency steroid (Derma-Smoothe/FS® and Capex™ shampoo are considered to be low to medium potency); Derma-Smoothe/FS® is made with 48% refined peanut oil, NF (peanut protein is <0.5 ppm)

Dosage Forms Excipient information presented when available (limited, particularly for generics); consult specific product labeling.

Cream, External, as acetonide:

Synalar: 0.025% (120 g) [contains cetyl alcohol, edetate disodium, methylparaben, propylene glycol, propylparaben]

Generic: 0.01% (15 g, 60 g); 0.025% (15 g, 60 g)

Kit, External, as acetonide:

Synalar (Cream): 0.025% [contains cetyl alcohol, edetate disodium, methylparaben, propylene glycol, propylparaben]

Synalar (Ointment): 0.025%

Synalar TS: 0.01% [contains propylene glycol]

Oil, External, as acetonide:

Derma-Smoothe/FS Body: 0.01% (118.28 mL) [contains isopropyl alcohol, peanut oil]

Derma-Smoothe/FS Scalp: 0.01% (118.28 mL) [contains isopropyl alcohol, peanut oil]

Fluocinolone Acetonide Body: 0.01% (118.28 mL) [contains isopropyl alcohol, peanut oil]

Fluocinolone Acetonide Scalp: 0.01% (118.28 mL) [contains isopropyl alcohol, peanut oil]

◀ Ointment, External, as acetonide:
Synalar: 0.025% (120 g)
Generic: 0.025% (15 g, 60 g)
Shampoo, External, as acetonide:
Capex: 0.01% (120 mL)
Solution, External, as acetonide:
Synalar: 0.01% (60 mL, 90 mL) [contains propylene glycol]
Generic: 0.01% (60 mL)

◆ **Fluocinolone Acetonide** see Fluocinolone (Ophthalmic) on page 891

◆ **Fluocinolone Acetonide** see Fluocinolone (Otic) on page 892

◆ **Fluocinolone Acetonide** see Fluocinolone (Topical) on page 892

◆ **Fluocinolone Acetonide Body** see Fluocinolone (Topical) on page 892

◆ **Fluocinolone Acetonide Scalp** see Fluocinolone (Topical) on page 892

Fluocinonide (floo oh SIN oh nide)

Medication Safety Issues
Sound-alike/look-alike issues:
Fluocinonide may be confused with flunisolide, fluocinolone
Lidex® may be confused with Lasix®, Videx®
Related Information
Topical Corticosteroids on page 2224
Brand Names: U.S. Vanos
Brand Names: Canada Lidemol®; Lidex®; Lyderm®; Tiamol®; Topactin®; Topsyn®
Therapeutic Category Adrenal Corticosteroid; Anti-inflammatory Agent; Corticosteroid, Topical; Glucocorticoid
Generic Availability (U.S.) Yes
Use Inflammation of corticosteroid-responsive dermatoses
Pregnancy Risk Factor C
Pregnancy Considerations Teratogenic effects have been observed in animals administered potent topical corticosteroids. Topical products are not recommended for extensive use, in large quantities, or for long periods of time in pregnant women.
Breast-Feeding Considerations It is not known if topical application will result in detectable quantities in breast milk.
Contraindications Hypersensitivity to fluocinonide or any component; viral, fungal, or tubercular skin lesions; herpes (including varicella)
Warnings Infants and small children may be more susceptible to adrenal axis suppression from topical corticosteroid therapy; systemic effects may occur when used on large areas of the body, denuded areas, for prolonged periods of time, or with occlusive dressings
Adverse Reactions
Cardiovascular: Intracranial hypertension
Dermatologic: Acne, allergic dermatitis, contact dermatitis, dry skin, folliculitis, hypertrichosis, hypopigmentation, maceration of the skin, miliaria, perioral dermatitis, pruritus, skin atrophy, striae, telangiectasia
Endocrine & metabolic: Cushing's syndrome, growth retardation, HPA axis suppression, hyperglycemia
Local: Burning, irritation
Renal: Glycosuria
Miscellaneous: Secondary infection
Drug Interactions
Metabolism/Transport Effects None known.
Avoid Concomitant Use
Avoid concomitant use of Fluocinonide with any of the following: Aldesleukin

Increased Effect/Toxicity
Fluocinonide may increase the levels/effects of: Ceritinib; Deferasirox

The levels/effects of Fluocinonide may be increased by: Telaprevir
Decreased Effect
Fluocinonide may decrease the levels/effects of: Aldesleukin; Corticorelin; Hyaluronidase; Telaprevir
Mechanism of Action Fluorinated topical corticosteroid considered to be of high potency. The mechanism of action for all topical corticosteroids is not well defined, however, is felt to be a combination of three important properties: anti-inflammatory activity, immunosuppressive properties, and antiproliferative actions.
Dosing: Usual Children and Adults: Topical: Apply thin layer to affected area 2-4 times/day depending on the severity of the condition
Administration Topical: Apply sparingly in a thin film; rub in lightly
Additional Information Considered to be a high potency steroid
Dosage Forms Excipient information presented when available (limited, particularly for generics); consult specific product labeling.
Cream, External:
Vanos: 0.1% (30 g, 60 g, 120 g)
Generic: 0.05% (15 g, 30 g, 60 g, 120 g); 0.1% (30 g, 60 g, 120 g)
Gel, External:
Generic: 0.05% (15 g, 30 g, 60 g)
Ointment, External:
Generic: 0.05% (15 g, 30 g, 60 g)
Solution, External:
Generic: 0.05% (20 mL, 60 mL)

◆ **Fluohydrisone Acetate** see Fludrocortisone on page 887

◆ **Fluohydrocortisone Acetate** see Fludrocortisone on page 887

◆ **Fluorabon** see Fluoride on page 894

◆ **Fluor-A-Day** see Fluoride on page 894

Fluoride (FLOR ide)

Medication Safety Issues
Sound-alike/look-alike issues:
Phos-Flur may be confused with PhosLo
International issues:
Fluorex [France] may be confused with Flarex brand name for fluorometholone [U.S., Canada, and multiple international markets] and Fluarix brand name for influenza virus vaccine (inactivated) [U.S., and multiple international markets]
Brand Names: U.S. Act Kids [OTC]; Act Restoring [OTC]; Act Total Care [OTC]; Act [OTC]; CaviRinse; Clinpro 5000; ControlRx; ControlRx Multi; Denta 5000 Plus; DentaGel; Fluor-A-Day; Fluorabon; Fluorinse; Fluoritab; Flura-Drops; Gel-Kam Rinse; Gel-Kam [OTC]; Just For Kids [OTC]; Lozi-Flur; NeutraCare; NeutraGard Advanced; Omni Gel [OTC]; OrthoWash; PerioMed; Phos-Flur; Phos-Flur Rinse [OTC]; PreviDent; PreviDent 5000 Booster; PreviDent 5000 Booster Plus; PreviDent 5000 Dry Mouth; PreviDent 5000 Plus; StanGard Perio; Stop
Brand Names: Canada Fluor-A-Day
Therapeutic Category Mineral, Oral; Mineral, Oral Topical
Generic Availability (U.S.) Yes: Excludes lozenge, gel drops
Use Prevention of dental caries
Pregnancy Risk Factor B

Pregnancy Considerations Fluoride crosses the placenta and can be found in the fetal circulation (IOM, 1997). Adverse events have not been observed in animal reproduction studies; epidemiological studies in areas with high levels of fluorinated water have not shown an increase in adverse effects. Heavy exposure *in utero* may be linked to skeletal fluorosis seen later in childhood.

Breast-Feeding Considerations Low concentrations of fluoride can be found in breast milk and the amount is not significantly affected by supplementation or concentrations in drinking water (IOM, 1997). The manufacturer recommends that caution be exercised when administering fluoride to nursing women.

Contraindications Hypersensitivity to fluoride or any component; when fluoride content of drinking water exceeds 0.7 ppm; low sodium or sodium-free diets; do not use 1 mg tablets in children <3 years of age or when drinking water fluoride content is ≥0.3 ppm; do not use 1 mg/5 mL rinse (as supplement) in children <6 years of age

Warnings Some products may contain tartrazine which may cause allergic reactions in susceptible individuals

Precautions Prolonged ingestion with excessive doses may result in dental fluorosis and osseous changes; dosage should be adjusted in proportion to the amount of fluoride in the drinking water; do **not** exceed recommended dosage

Adverse Reactions Rare but important or life-threatening: Discoloration of teeth, nausea, rash, vomiting

Drug Interactions

Metabolism/Transport Effects None known.

Avoid Concomitant Use There are no known interactions where it is recommended to avoid concomitant use.

Increased Effect/Toxicity There are no known significant interactions involving an increase in effect.

Decreased Effect There are no known significant interactions involving a decrease in effect.

Stability Sodium fluoride solutions decompose in glass containers; store only in tightly closed plastic containers; aqueous solutions of stannous fluoride decompose within hours of preparation; prepare solutions immediately before use

Mechanism of Action Promotes remineralization of decalcified enamel; inhibits the cariogenic microbial process in dental plaque; increases tooth resistance to acid dissolution

Pharmacokinetics (Adult data unless noted)
Absorption: Via GI tract, lungs, and skin
Distribution: 50% of fluoride is deposited in teeth and bone after ingestion; crosses placenta; appears in breast milk; topical application works superficially on enamel and plaque
Elimination: In urine and feces

Dosing: Neonatal Adequate Intake (AI): 0.01 mg/day; supplementation is not recommended in neonates

Dosing: Usual Oral:
Adequate Intake (AI):
Infants, Children, and Adolescents:
0-6 months: 0.01 mg/day; additional supplementation is not recommended in infants <6 months of age
7-12 months: 0.5 mg/day
1-3 years: 0.7 mg/day
4-8 years: 1 mg/day
9-13 years: 2 mg/day
14-18 years: 3 mg/day
Adults:
Males: 4 mg/day
Females: 3 mg/day
The recommended daily fluoride intake is adjusted in proportion to the fluoride content of available drinking water; see **Recommended Daily Fluoride Dose** table

Recommended Daily Fluoride Dose

Fluoride Content of Drinking Water	Daily Dose, Oral Fluoride (mg)
<0.3 ppm	
Birth - 6 mo	0
6 mo to 3 y	0.25
3-6 y	0.5
6-16 y	1
0.3-0.6 ppm	
Birth - 3 y	0
3-6 y	0.25
6-16 y	0.5
>0.6 ppm	
All ages	0

Adapted from *AAP News*, 1995, 11(2):18.

Dental rinse: See **Sodium Fluoride Dental Rinse Dosing** table
Sodium fluoride (dosage based upon concentration of solution):
Note: 2% concentrations are administered by dental personnel only

Sodium Fluoride Dental Rinse Dosing

Age	% Solution	Dosage
6 y	0.05%	10 mL daily
6-12 y	0.02%	10 mL twice daily
	0.2%	5 mL once weekly
>12 y	0.02%	10 mL twice daily
	0.2%	10 mL once weekly

Acidulated phosphate fluoride rinse: Children 6 years and Adults: 5-10 mL of 0.02% daily at bedtime

Gel:
Acidulated phosphate fluoride: Adults: 4-8 drops of 0.5% gel daily or for desensitizing exposed root surfaces, use a few drops of 0.5% to 1.2% gel applied and brushed onto affected area each night
Stannous fluoride: Children >6 years and Adults: Apply 0.4% gel to teeth once daily

Administration Oral:
Dental gel: Do **not** swallow; gel drops are placed in trough of applicator; applicator is applied over upper and lower teeth at same time; bite down for 6 minutes
Dental rinse: Swish or rinse in mouth then expectorate; do not swallow
Tablet: Dissolve in mouth, chew, swallow whole, or add to drinking water or fruit juice; administer with food (but not milk) to eliminate GI upset

Reference Range Total plasma fluoride: 0.14-0.19 mcg/mL

Dosage Forms Excipient information presented when available (limited, particularly for generics); consult specific product labeling.
Cream, oral, as sodium [toothpaste]: 1.1% (51 g) [equivalent to fluoride 2.5 mg/dose]
Denta 5000 Plus: 1.1% (51 g) [spearmint flavor; equivalent to fluoride 2.5 mg/dose]
PreviDent 5000 Plus: 1.1% (51 g) [contains sodium benzoate; fruitastic flavor; equivalent to fluoride 2.5 mg/dose]

◀ PreviDent 5000 Plus: 1.1% (51 g) [contains sodium benzoate; spearmint flavor; equivalent to fluoride 2.5 mg/dose]

Gel, topical, as acidulated phosphate:
Phos-Flur: 1.1% (51 g) [contains propylene glycol, sodium benzoate; mint flavor; equivalent to fluoride 0.5%]

Gel, oral, as sodium [toothpaste]:
PreviDent 5000 Booster: 1.1% (100 mL, 106 mL) [contains sodium benzoate; fruitastic flavor; equivalent to fluoride 2.5 mg/dose]
PreviDent 5000 Booster: 1.1% (100 mL, 106 mL) [contains sodium benzoate; spearmint flavor; equivalent to fluoride 2.5 mg/dose]
PreviDent 5000 Booster Plus: 1.1% (100 mL) [contains sodium benzoate; fruitastic flavor; equivalent to fluoride 2.5 mg/dose]
PreviDent 5000 Booster Plus: 1.1% (100 mL) [contains sodium benzoate; spearmint flavor; equivalent to fluoride 2.5 mg/dose]
PreviDent 5000 Dry Mouth: 1.1% (100 mL) [mint flavor; equivalent to fluoride 2.5 mg/dose]

Gel, topical, as sodium: 1.1% (56 g) [equivalent to fluoride 2 mg/dose]
DentaGel: 1.1% (56 g) [fresh mint flavor; neutral pH; equivalent to fluoride 2 mg/dose]
NeutraCare: 1.1% (60 g) [grape flavor; neutral pH]
NeutraCare: 1.1% (60 g) [mint flavor; neutral pH]
NeutraGard Advanced: 1.1% (60 g) [mint flavor; neutral pH]
NeutraGard Advanced: 1.1% (60 g) [mixed berry flavor; neutral pH]
PreviDent: 1.1% (56 g) [mint flavor; equivalent to fluoride 2 mg/dose]
PreviDent: 1.1% (56 g) [very berry flavor; equivalent to fluoride 2 mg/dose]

Gel, topical, as stannous fluoride:
Gel-Kam: 0.4% (129 g) [cinnamon flavor]
Gel-Kam: 0.4% (129 g) [fruit & berry flavor]
Gel-Kam: 0.4% (129 g) [mint flavor]
Just For Kids: 0.4% (122 g) [bubblegum flavor]
Just For Kids: 0.4% (122 g) [fruit-punch flavor]
Just For Kids: 0.4% (122 g) [grapey grape flavor]
Omni Gel: 0.4% (122 g) [cinnamon flavor]
Omni Gel: 0.4% (122 g) [grape flavor]
Omni Gel: 0.4% (122 g) [mint flavor]
Omni Gel: 0.4% (122 g) [natural flavor]
Omni Gel: 0.4% (122 g) [raspberry flavor]
Stop: 0.4% (120 g) [bubblegum flavor]
Stop: 0.4% (120 g) [mint flavor]

Liquid, oral, as base:
Fluoritab: 0.125 mg/drop [dye free]

Lozenge, oral, as sodium:
Lozi-Flur: 2.21 mg (90s) [sugar free; cherry flavor; equivalent to fluoride 1 mg]

Paste, oral, as sodium [toothpaste]:
Clinpro 5000: 1.1% (113 g) [vanilla-mint flavor]
ControlRx: 1.1% (57 g) [berry flavor]
ControlRx: 1.1% (57 g) [vanilla-mint flavor]
ControlRx Multi: 1.1% (57 g) [vanilla-mint flavor]

Solution, oral, as fluoride [rinse]:
Act Total Care: 0.02% (1000 mL) [ethanol free; contains menthol, propylene glycol, sodium benzoate, tartrazine; fresh mint flavor; equivalent to fluoride 0.009%]

Solution, oral, as sodium [drops]: 1.1 mg/mL (50 mL) [equivalent to fluoride 0.5 mg/mL]
Fluor-A-Day: 0.278 mg/drop (30 mL) [equivalent to fluoride 0.125 mg/drop]
Fluorabon: 0.55 mg/0.6 mL (60 mL) [dye free, sugar free; equivalent to fluoride 0.25 mg/0.6 mL]
Flura-Drops: 0.55 mg/drop (24 mL) [dye free, sugar free; contains natural rubber/natural latex in packaging; equivalent to fluoride 0.25 mg/drop]

Solution, oral, as sodium [rinse]: 0.2% (473 mL)
Act: 0.05% (532 mL) [contains benzyl alcohol, propylene glycol, sodium benzoate, tartrazine; cinnamon flavor; equivalent to fluoride 0.02%]
Act: 0.05% (532 mL) [contains propylene glycol, sodium benzoate, tartrazine; mint flavor; equivalent to fluoride 0.02%]
Act Kids: 0.05% (532 mL) [ethanol free; contains benzyl alcohol, propylene glycol, sodium benzoate; bubblegum flavor; equivalent to fluoride 0.02%]
Act Kids: 0.05% (500 mL) [ethanol free; contains benzyl alcohol, propylene glycol, sodium benzoate; ocean berry flavor; equivalent to fluoride 0.02%]
Act Restoring: 0.02% (1000 mL) [contains ethanol 11%, propylene glycol, sodium benzoate; Cool Splash mint flavor; equivalent to fluoride 0.009%]
Act Restoring: 0.02% (1000 mL) [contains ethanol 11%, propylene glycol, sodium benzoate; Cool Splash spearmint flavor; equivalent to fluoride 0.009%]
Act Restoring: 0.05% (532 mL) [contains ethanol 11%, propylene glycol, sodium benzoate; Cool Splash mint flavor; equivalent to fluoride 0.02%]
Act Restoring: 0.05% (532 mL) [contains ethanol 11%, propylene glycol, sodium benzoate; Cool Splash spearmint flavor; equivalent to fluoride 0.02%]
Act Restoring: 0.05% (532 mL) [contains ethanol 11%, propylene glycol, sodium benzoate; Cool Splash vanilla-mint flavor; equivalent to fluoride 0.02%]
Act Total Care: 0.02% (1000 mL) [contains ethanol 11%, propylene glycol, sodium benzoate; icy clean mint flavor; equivalent to fluoride 0.009%]
Act Total Care: 0.05% (88 mL, 532 mL) [contains ethanol 11%, propylene glycol, sodium benzoate; icy clean mint flavor; equivalent to fluoride 0.02%]
Act Total Care: 0.05% (88 mL, 532 mL) [ethanol free; contains menthol, propylene glycol, sodium benzoate, tartrazine; fresh mint flavor; equivalent to fluoride 0.02%]
CaviRinse: 0.2% (240 mL) [mint flavor]
Fluorinse: 0.2% (480 mL) [ethanol free; cinnamon flavor]
Fluorinse: 0.2% (480 mL) [ethanol free; mint flavor]
OrthoWash: 0.044% (480 mL) [contains sodium benzoate; grape flavor]
OrthoWash: 0.044% (480 mL) [contains sodium benzoate; strawberry flavor]
Phos-Flur Rinse: 0.044% (473 mL) [ethanol free, sugar free; bubblegum flavor]
Phos-Flur Rinse: 0.044% (473 mL) [ethanol free, sugar free; gushing grape flavor]
Phos-Flur Rinse: 0.044% (500 mL) [sugar free; cool mint flavor]
PreviDent: 0.2% (473 mL) [contains benzoic acid, ethanol 6%, sodium benzoate; cool mint flavor]

Solution, oral, as stannous fluoride [concentrated rinse]: 0.63% (300 mL) [equivalent to fluoride 7 mg/30 mL dose]
Gel-Kam Rinse: 0.63% (300 mL) [mint flavor; equivalent to fluoride 7 mg/30 mL dose]
PerioMed: 0.63% (284 mL) [ethanol free; cinnamon flavor; equivalent to fluoride 7 mg/30 mL dose]
PerioMed: 0.63% (284 mL) [ethanol free; mint flavor; equivalent to fluoride 7 mg/30 mL dose]
PerioMed: 0.63% (284 mL) [ethanol free; tropical fruit flavor; equivalent to fluoride 7 mg/30 mL dose]
StanGard Perio: 0.63% (284 mL) [mint flavor]

Tablet, chewable, oral, as sodium: 0.55 mg [equivalent to fluoride 0.25 mg], 1.1 mg [equivalent to fluoride 0.5 mg], 2.2 mg [equivalent to fluoride 1 mg]
Fluor-A-Day: 0.55 mg [raspberry flavor; equivalent to fluoride 0.25 mg]
Fluor-A-Day: 1.1 mg [raspberry flavor; equivalent to fluoride 0.5 mg]
Fluor-A-Day: 2.2 mg [raspberry flavor; equivalent to fluoride 1 mg]

Fluoritab: 2.2 mg [cherry flavor; equivalent to fluoride 1 mg]

Fluoritab: 1.1 mg [dye free; cherry flavor; equivalent to fluoride 0.5 mg]

References

Centers for Disease Control and Prevention, "Recommendations for Using Fluoride to Prevent and Control Dental Caries in the United States," *MMWR Recomm Rep*, 2001, 50(RR-14):1-42. Available at http://www.cdc.gov/mmwr/preview/mmwrhtml/rr5014a1.htm.

"Dietary Reference Intakes for Calcium, Phosphorus, Magnesium, Vitamin D, and Fluoride. Standing Committee on the Scientific Evaluation of Dietary Reference Intakes, Food and Nutrition Board, Institute of Medicine," National Academy of Sciences, Washington, DC: National Academy Press, 1997.

◆ **Fluorinse** *see* Fluoride *on page* 894

◆ **Fluoritab** *see* Fluoride *on page* 894

◆ **5-Fluorocytosine** *see* Flucytosine *on page* 882

◆ **9α-Fluorohydrocortisone Acetate** *see* Fludrocortisone *on page* 887

Fluorometholone (flure oh METH oh lone)

Medication Safety Issues
International issues:
Flarex [U.S., Canada, and multiple international markets] may be confused with Fluarix brand name for influenza virus vaccine (inactivated) [U.S. and multiple international markets] and Fluorex brand name for fluoride [France]

Brand Names: U.S. Flarex; FML; FML Forte; FML Liquifilm

Brand Names: Canada Flarex®; FML Forte®; FML®; PMS-Fluorometholone

Therapeutic Category Adrenal Corticosteroid; Anti-inflammatory Agent, Ophthalmic; Corticosteroid, Ophthalmic; Glucocorticoid

Generic Availability (U.S.) May be product dependent

Use Inflammatory conditions of the eye, including keratitis, iritis, cyclitis, and conjunctivitis

Pregnancy Risk Factor C

Pregnancy Considerations Teratogenic effects were observed in animal reproduction studies following use of ophthalmic fluorometholone. The extent of systemic absorption following topical application of the ophthalmic drops is not known.

Breast-Feeding Considerations Systemic corticosteroids are excreted in human milk. The extent of systemic absorption following topical application of the ophthalmic drops is not known.

Contraindications Hypersensitivity to fluorometholone, other corticosteroids, or any component; herpes simplex keratitis, fungal diseases of ocular structures, mycobacterial infections of the eye, and most viral diseases of cornea and conjunctiva

Warnings Not recommended for children <2 years of age

Precautions Prolonged use may result in glaucoma, increased intraocular pressure, or other ocular damage

Adverse Reactions
Dermatologic: Skin rash
Endocrine & metabolic: Hypercorticoidism (rare)
Gastrointestinal: Dysgeusia
Hypersensitivity: Hypersensitivity reaction
Ophthalmic: Bacterial eye infection (secondary), blurred vision, burning sensation of eyes, cataract, decreased visual acuity, erythema of eyelid, eye discharge, eye irritation, eyelid edema, eye pain, eye pruritus, foreign body sensation of eye, fungal eye infection (secondary), glaucoma, increased intraocular pressure, increased lacrimation, optic nerve damage, stinging of eyes, swelling of eye, viral eye infection (secondary), visual field defect, wound healing impairment

Drug Interactions
Metabolism/Transport Effects None known.

Avoid Concomitant Use
Avoid concomitant use of Fluorometholone with any of the following: Aldesleukin

Increased Effect/Toxicity
Fluorometholone may increase the levels/effects of: Ceritinib; Deferasirox

The levels/effects of Fluorometholone may be increased by: Telaprevir

Decreased Effect
Fluorometholone may decrease the levels/effects of: Aldesleukin; Corticorelin; Hyaluronidase; Telaprevir

Mechanism of Action Corticosteroids inhibit the inflammatory response including edema, capillary dilation, leukocyte migration, and scar formation. Fluorometholone penetrates cells readily to induce the production of lipocortins. These proteins modulate the activity of prostaglandins and leukotrienes.

Pharmacokinetics (Adult data unless noted) Absorption: Into aqueous humor with slight systemic absorption

Dosing: Usual Children >2 years and Adults: Ophthalmic:
Ointment: May be applied every 4 hours in severe cases or 1-3 times/day in mild to moderate cases.

Drops: Instill 1-2 drops into conjunctival sac every hour during day, every 2 hours at night until favorable response is obtained, then use 1 drop every 4 hours; in mild or moderate inflammation: 1-2 drops into conjunctival sac 2-4 times/day.

Administration Ophthalmic: Avoid contact of medication tube or bottle tip with skin or eye; suspension: Shake well before use; apply finger pressure to lacrimal sac during and for 1-2 minutes after instillation to decrease risk of absorption and systemic effects; the preservative (benzalkonium chloride) may be absorbed by soft contact lenses; wait at least 15 minutes after administration of suspension before inserting soft contact lenses

Monitoring Parameters Intraocular pressure (if used ≥10 days)

Dosage Forms Excipient information presented when available (limited, particularly for generics); consult specific product labeling.
Ointment, Ophthalmic, as base:
FML: 0.1% (3.5 g) [contains phenylmercuric acetate]
Suspension, Ophthalmic, as acetate:
Flarex: 0.1% (5 mL)
Suspension, Ophthalmic, as base:
FML Forte: 0.25% (5 mL, 10 mL)
FML Liquifilm: 0.1% (5 mL, 10 mL)
Generic: 0.1% (5 mL, 10 mL, 15 mL)

◆ **Fluoroplex** *see* Fluorouracil (Topical) *on page* 900

◆ **Fluoroplex® (Can)** *see* Fluorouracil (Topical) *on page* 900

◆ **Fluoro Uracil** *see* Fluorouracil (Systemic) *on page* 897

◆ **5-Fluorouracil** *see* Fluorouracil (Systemic) *on page* 897

◆ **5-Fluorouracil** *see* Fluorouracil (Topical) *on page* 900

Fluorouracil (Systemic) (flure oh YOOR a sil)

Medication Safety Issues
Sound-alike/look-alike issues:
Fluorouracil may be confused with floxuridine, flucytosine

High alert medication:
This medication is in a class the Institute for Safe Medication Practices (ISMP) includes among its list of drug classes which have a heightened risk of causing significant patient harm when used in error.

Related Information

Emetogenic Potential of Antineoplastic Agents in Children *on page 2327*

Management of Drug Extravasations *on page 2255*

Safe Handling of Hazardous Drugs *on page 2419*

Brand Names: U.S. Adrucil

Brand Names: Canada Fluorouracil Injection

Therapeutic Category Antineoplastic Agent, Antimetabolite

Generic Availability (U.S.) Yes

Use Treatment of carcinoma of stomach (gastric), colon, rectum, breast, and pancreas (FDA approved in adults); has also been used for the treatment of hepatoblastoma, nasopharyngeal carcinoma, head and neck cancer, bladder cancer, and cervical cancer

Pregnancy Risk Factor D

Pregnancy Considerations Adverse effects (increased resorptions, embryolethality, and teratogenicity) have been observed in animal reproduction studies. Based on the mechanism of action, fluorouracil may cause fetal harm if administered during pregnancy (according to the manufacturer's labeling). The National Comprehensive Cancer Network (NCCN) breast cancer guidelines (v.3.2012) state that chemotherapy, if indicated, may be administered to pregnant women with breast cancer as part of a combination chemotherapy regimen (common regimens administered during pregnancy include doxorubicin, cyclophosphamide, and fluorouracil); chemotherapy should not be administered during the first trimester, after 35 weeks gestation, or within 3 weeks of planned delivery.

Breast-Feeding Considerations Based on the mechanism of action, the manufacturer's labeling recommends against breast-feeding if receiving fluorouracil.

Contraindications Hypersensitivity to fluorouracil or any component; patients with poor nutritional status, bone marrow suppression, or potentially serious infections

Warnings Hazardous agent; use appropriate precautions for handling and disposal (NIOSH, 2012). Discontinue if intractable vomiting, diarrhea, stomatitis, esophagopharyngitis, GI ulceration/bleeding, hemorrhage, or precipitous falls in leukocyte or platelet counts occur.

Absence of the dihydropyrimidine dehydrogenase (DPD) enzyme may result in prolonged fluorouracil clearance. Administration to patients with genetic DPD enzyme deficiency has been associated with increased toxicity (diarrhea, stomatitis, neutropenia, and neurotoxicity) following administration. Discontinue if symptoms of DPD enzyme deficiency occur; rechallenge is not recommended since it has resulted in recurrent toxicity (despite dose reduction).

Precautions Use with caution in patients with renal or hepatic impairment. Use with caution in patients who have had high-dose pelvic radiation, previous use of alkylating agents, or with widespread metastatic marrow involvement. Palmar-plantar erythrodysesthesia (hand-foot) syndrome has been associated with use; symptoms include a tingling sensation, which may progress to pain, and then to symmetrical swelling and erythema with tenderness; desquamation may occur; generally resolves over 5-7 days with treatment interruption. Should be administered under the supervision of a physician experienced in cancer chemotherapy **[U.S. Boxed Warning]**. Due to risk of severe toxic reactions, patients should be hospitalized during the initial course of therapy **[U.S. Boxed Warning]**.

Adverse Reactions Toxicity depends on duration of treatment and/or rate of administration

Cardiovascular: Angina, arrhythmia, heart failure, MI, myocardial ischemia, vasospasm, ventricular ectopy

Central nervous system: Acute cerebellar syndrome, confusion, disorientation, euphoria, headache, nystagmus, stroke

Dermatologic: Alopecia, dermatitis, dry skin, fissuring, nail changes (nail loss), palmar-plantar erythrodysesthesia

syndrome, pruritic maculopapular rash, photosensitivity, Stevens-Johnson syndrome, toxic epidermal necrolysis, vein pigmentation

Gastrointestinal: Anorexia, bleeding, diarrhea, esophagopharyngitis, mesenteric ischemia (acute), nausea, sloughing, stomatitis, ulceration, vomiting

Hematologic: Agranulocytosis, anemia, leukopenia (nadir: days 9-14; recovery by day 30), pancytopenia, thrombocytopenia

Local: Thrombophlebitis

Ocular: Lacrimation, lacrimal duct stenosis, photophobia, visual changes

Respiratory: Epistaxis

Miscellaneous: Anaphylaxis, generalized allergic reactions

Drug Interactions

Metabolism/Transport Effects Inhibits CYP2C9 (strong)

Avoid Concomitant Use

Avoid concomitant use of Fluorouracil (Systemic) with any of the following: BCG; CloZAPine; Dipyrone; Gimeracil; Natalizumab; Pimecrolimus; Tacrolimus (Topical); Tofacitinib; Vaccines (Live)

Increased Effect/Toxicity

Fluorouracil (Systemic) may increase the levels/effects of: Bosentan; Carvedilol; CloZAPine; CYP2C9 Substrates; Diclofenac (Systemic); Dronabinol; Fosphenytoin; Lacosamide; Leflunomide; Natalizumab; Ospemifene; Phenytoin; Tetrahydrocannabinol; Tofacitinib; Vaccines (Live); Vitamin K Antagonists

The levels/effects of Fluorouracil (Systemic) may be increased by: Cannabis; Cimetidine; Denosumab; Dipyrone; Gemcitabine; Gimeracil; Leucovorin Calcium-Levoleucovorin; MetroNIDAZOLE (Systemic); Pimecrolimus; Roflumilast; SORAfenib; Tacrolimus (Topical); Trastuzumab

Decreased Effect

Fluorouracil (Systemic) may decrease the levels/effects of: BCG; Coccidioidin Skin Test; Sipuleucel-T; Vaccines (Inactivated); Vaccines (Live)

The levels/effects of Fluorouracil (Systemic) may be decreased by: Echinacea; SORAfenib

Stability Store intact vials at room temperature; protect from light; retain in carton until time of use. Slight discoloration of injection may occur during storage; does not usually denote decomposition. If exposed to cold temperatures, a precipitate may form; vigorous shaking and gentle heating to 60°C (140°F) will dissolve the precipitate without impairing the potency; allow to cool to body temperature before administration.

According to the manufacturer, pharmacy bulk vials should be used within 4 hours of initial entry. Solutions for infusion should be used promptly. Fluorouracil 50 mg/mL in NS was stable in polypropylene infusion pump syringes for 7 days when stored at 30°C (86°F) (Stiles, 1996). Stability of fluorouracil 1 mg/mL or 10 mg/mL in NS or D$_5$W in PVC bags was demonstrated for up to 14 days at 4°C (39.2°F) and 21°C (69.8°F) (Martel, 1996). Stability of undiluted fluorouracil (50 mg/mL) in ethylene-vinyl acetate ambulatory pump reservoirs was demonstrated for 3 days at 4°C (39.2°F) (precipitate formed after 3 days) and for 14 days at 33°C (91.4°F) (Martel, 1996). Stability of undiluted fluorouracil (50 mg/mL) in PVC ambulatory pump reservoirs was demonstrated for 5 days at 4°C (39.2°F) (precipitate formed after 5 days) and for 14 days at 33°C (91.4°F) (Martel, 1996).

Mechanism of Action A pyrimidine analog antimetabolite that interferes with DNA and RNA synthesis; after activation, F-UMP (an active metabolite) is incorporated into RNA to replace uracil and inhibit cell growth; the active metabolite F-dUMP, inhibits thymidylate synthetase, depleting thymidine triphosphate (a necessary component of DNA synthesis).

Pharmacokinetics (Adult data unless noted)

Distribution: Penetrates tumors, intestinal mucosa, liver, bone marrow, ascitic fluid, brain tissue, and CSF

Metabolism: Hepatic (90%); via a dehydrogenase enzyme; FU must be metabolized to be active metabolites, 5-fluoroxyuridine monophosphate (F-UMP) and 5-5-fluoro-2'-deoxyuridine-5'-O-monophosphate (F-dUMP)

Half-life: 16 minutes (range: 8-20 minutes); two metabolites, F-dUMP and F-UMP, have prolonged half-lives depending on the type of tissue

Elimination: Urine (7% to 20% as unchanged drug within 6 hours; also as metabolites within 9-10 hours); lung (as expired CO_2)

Dosing: Usual

Pediatric: **Note:** Dose, frequency, number of doses, and/or start date may vary by protocol and treatment phase. Refer to individual protocols.

Hepatoblastoma: Limited data available: Infants, Children, and Adolescents: I.V.: 600 mg/m²/dose every 3 weeks on day 2 or 3 (in combination with cisplatin, vincristine ± doxorubicin) (Douglas, 1993; Ortega, 2000; Watanabe, 2013)

Nasopharyngeal carcinoma: Limited data available: Children ≥8 years and Adolescents: Continuous I.V. infusion: 1000 mg/m²/day for 3-5 days every 3-4 weeks for 3-4 cycles (in combination with other chemotherapy agents) (Buehrlen, 2012; Casanova, 2012; Mertens, 2005; Rodriguez-Galindo, 2005)

Adult: **Note:** Utilize patient's actual body weight (full weight) for calculation of body surface area- or weight-based dosing, particularly when the intent of therapy is curative; manage regimen-related toxicities in the same manner as for nonobese patients; if a dose reduction is utilized due to toxicity, consider resumption of full weight-based dosing with subsequent cycles, especially if cause of toxicity (eg, hepatic or renal impairment) is resolved (Griggs, 2012). Details concerning dosing in combination regimens should be consulted:

Breast cancer: I.V.:

CEF regimen: 500 mg/m² on days 1 and 8 every 28 days (in combination with cyclophosphamide and epirubicin) for 6 cycles (Levine, 1998)

CMF regimen: 600 mg/m² on days 1 and 8 every 28 days (in combination with cyclophosphamide and methotrexate) for 6 cycles (Goldhirsch, 1998; Levine, 1998)

FAC regimen: 500 mg/m² on days 1 and 8 every 21-28 days (in combination with cyclophosphamide and doxorubicin) for 6 cycles (Assikis, 2003)

Colorectal cancer: I.V.:

FLOX regimen: 500 mg/m² bolus on days 1, 8, 15, 22, 29, and 36 (1 hour after leucovorin) every 8 weeks (in combination with leucovorin and oxaliplatin) for 3 cycles (Kuebler, 2007)

FOLFOX6 and mFOLFOX6 regimen: 400 mg/m² bolus on day 1, followed by 1200 mg/m²/day continuous infusion for 2 days (over 46 hours) every 2 weeks (in combination with leucovorin and oxaliplatin) until disease progression or unacceptable toxicity (Cheeseman, 2002)

FOLFIRI regimen: 400 mg/m² bolus on day 1, followed by 1200 mg/m²/day continuous infusion for 2 days (over 46 hours) every 2 weeks (in combination with leucovorin and irinotecan) until disease progression or unacceptable toxicity; after 2 cycles, may increase continuous infusion fluorouracil dose to 1500 mg/m²/day (over 46 hours) (André, 1999)

Roswell Park regimen: 500 mg/m² (bolus) on days 1, 8, 15, 22, 29, and 36 (1 hour after leucovorin) every 8 weeks (in combination with leucovorin) for 4 cycles (Haller, 2005)

Gastric cancer: I.V.:

CF regimen: 750-1000 mg/m²/day continuous infusion days 1-4 and 29-32 of a 35-day treatment cycle (preoperative chemoradiation; in combination with cisplatin) (NCCN Gastric Cancer Guidelines v2.2012; Tepper, 2008)

ECF regimen (resectable disease): 200 mg/m²/day continuous infusion days 1-21 every 3 weeks (in combination with epirubicin and cisplatin) for 6 cycles (3 cycles preoperatively and 3 cycles postoperatively) (Cunningham, 2006)

ECF or EOF regimen (advanced disease): 200 mg/m²/day continuous infusion days 1-21 every 3 weeks (in combination with epirubicin and either cisplatin or oxaliplatin) for a planned duration of 24 weeks (Sumpter, 2005)

TCF or DCF regimen: 750 mg/m²/day continuous infusion days 1-5 every 3 weeks or 1000 mg/m²/day continuous infusion days 1-5 every 4 weeks (in combination with docetaxel and cisplatin) until disease progression or unacceptable toxicity (Ajani, 2007; NCCN Gastric Cancer Guidelines v2.2012; Van Cutsem, 2006)

ToGA regimen (HER2-positive): 800 mg/m²/day continuous infusion days 1-5 every 3 weeks (in combination with cisplatin and trastuzumab) until disease progression or unacceptable toxicity (Bang, 2010)

Pancreatic cancer: I.V.:

Chemoradiation therapy: 250 mg/m²/day continuous infusion for 3 weeks prior to and then throughout radiation therapy (Regine, 2008)

Fluorouracil-Leucovorin: 425 mg/m²/day (bolus) days 1-5 every 28 days (in combination with leucovorin) for 6 cycles (Neoptolemos, 2010)

FOLFIRINOX regimen: 400 mg/m² bolus on day 1, followed by 1200 mg/m²/day continuous infusion for 2 days (over 46 hours) every 14 days (in combination with leucovorin, irinotecan, and oxaliplatin) until disease progression or unacceptable toxicity for a recommended 12 cycles (Conroy, 2011)

Dosing adjustment in renal impairment: Adult: There are no dosage adjustments provided in the manufacturer's labeling; however, extreme caution should be used in patients with renal impairment. The following adjustments have been recommended:

CrCl <50 mL/minute and continuous renal replacement therapy (CRRT): No dosage adjustment necessary (Aronoff, 2007).

Hemodialysis:

Administer standard dose following hemodialysis on dialysis days (Janus, 2010).

Administer 50% of standard dose following hemodialysis (Aronoff, 2007).

Dosing adjustment in hepatic impairment: Adult: There are no dosage adjustments provided in the manufacturer's labeling; however, extreme caution should be used in patients with hepatic impairment. The following adjustments have been recommended:

Hepatic impairment (degree not specified): Administer <50% of dose, then increase if toxicity does not occur (Koren, 1992)

Bilirubin >5 mg/dL: Avoid use (Floyd, 2006)

Administration Hazardous agent; use appropriate precautions for handling and disposal (NIOSH, 2012). Administration rate varies by protocol; refer to specific reference for protocol. May be administered undiluted by I.V. push, or further diluted in appropriate fluids and administered by I.V. bolus, or as a continuous infusion. Avoid extravasation (may be an irritant).

Vesicant/Extravasation Risk May be an irritant

Monitoring Parameters CBC with differential and platelet count, renal function tests, liver function tests; signs of palmar-plantar erythrodysesthesia syndrome, stomatitis,

◄ diarrhea, hemorrhage, or gastrointestinal ulcers or bleeding

Dosage Forms Excipient information presented when available (limited, particularly for generics); consult specific product labeling.

Solution, Intravenous:

Adrucil: 500 mg/10 mL (10 mL); 2.5 g/50 mL (50 mL); 5 g/100 mL (100 mL)

Generic: 500 mg/10 mL (10 mL); 1 g/20 mL (20 mL); 2.5 g/50 mL (50 mL); 5 g/100 mL (100 mL)

References

Adrucil (fluouracil) [prescribing information]. Irvine, CA: Teva Parenteral Medicines, Inc; July 2007.

Ajani JA, Moiseyenko VM, Tjulandin S, et al, "Quality of Life With Docetaxel Plus Cisplatin and Fluorouracil Compared With Cisplatin and Fluorouracil From a Phase III Trial for Advanced Gastric or Gastroesophageal Adenocarcinoma: The V-325 Study Group," J Clin Oncol, 2007, 25(22):3210-6.

André T, Louvet C, Maindrault-Goebel F, et al, "CPT-11 (Irinotecan) Addition to Bimonthly, High-Dose Leucovorin and Bolus and Continuous-Infusion 5-Fluorouracil (FOLFIRI) for Pretreated Metastatic Colorectal Cancer. GERCOR," Eur J Cancer, 1999, 35(9):1343-7.

Aronoff GR, Bennett WM, Berns JS, et al, Drug Prescribing in Renal Failure: Dosing Guidelines for Adults and Children, 5th ed. Philadelphia, PA: American College of Physicians; 2007.

Assikis V, Buzdar A, Yang Y, et al, "A Phase III Trial of Sequential Adjuvant Chemotherapy for Operable Breast Carcinoma: Final Analysis With 10-Year Follow-Up," Cancer, 2003, 97(11):2716-23.

Balis FM, Holcenberg JS and Bleyer WA, "Clinical Pharmacokinetics of Commonly Used Anticancer Drugs," Clin Pharmacokinet, 1983, 8 (3):202-32.

Bang YJ, Van Cutsem E, Feyereisiova A, et al, "Trastuzumab in Combination With Chemotherapy Versus Chemotherapy Alone for Treatment of HER2-Positive Advanced Gastric or Gastro-Oesophageal Junction Cancer (ToGA): A Phase 3, Open-Label, Randomised Controlled Trial," Lancet, 2010, 376(9742):687-97.

Buehrlen M, Zwaan CM, Granzen B, et al. Multimodal treatment, including interferon beta, of nasopharyngeal carcinoma in children and young adults: preliminary results from the prospective, multicenter study NPC-2003-GPOH/DCOG. Cancer. 2012;118 (19):4892-4900.

Casanova M, Bisogno G, Gandola L, et al. A prospective protocol for nasopharyngeal carcinoma in children and adolescents: the Italian Rare Tumors in Pediatric Age (TREP) project. Cancer. 2012;118 (10):2718-2725.

Cheeseman SL, Joel SP, Chester JD, et al, "A 'Modified de Gramont' Regimen of Fluorouracil, Alone and With Oxaliplatin, for Advanced Colorectal Cancer," Br J Cancer, 2002, 87(4):393-9.

Conroy T, Desseigne F, Ychou M, et al, "FOLFIRINOX Versus Gemcitabine for Metastatic Pancreatic Cancer," N Engl J Med, 2011, 364 (19):1817-25.

Cunningham D, Allum WH, Stenning SP, et al, "Perioperative Chemotherapy Versus Surgery Alone for Resectable Gastroesophageal Cancer," N Engl J Med, 2006, 355(1):11-20.

Douglass EC, Reynolds M, Finegold M, Cantor AB, Glicksman A. Cisplatin, vincristine, and fluorouracil therapy for hepatoblastoma: a Pediatric Oncology Group study. J Clin Oncol. 1993;11(1):96-99.

Fluouracil [prescribing information]. Ahmedabad, Gujurat, India: Intas Pharmaceuticals Ltd; March 2007.

Floyd J, Mirza I, Sachs B, et al, "Hepatotoxicity of Chemotherapy," Semin Oncol, 2006, 33(1):50-67.

Goldhirsch A, Colleoni M, Coates AS, et al, "Adding Adjuvant CMF Chemotherapy to Either Radiotherapy or Tamoxifen: Are All CMFs Alike? The International Breast Cancer Study Group (IBCSG)," Ann Oncol, 1998, 9(5):489-93.

Griggs JJ, Mangu PB, Anderson H, et al, "Appropriate Chemotherapy Dosing For Obese Adult Patients With Cancer: American Society of Clinical Oncology Clinical Practice Guideline," J Clin Oncol, 2012, 30 (13):1553-61.

Haller DG, Catalano PJ, Macdonald JS, et al, "Phase III Study of Fluorouracil, Leucovorin, and Levamisole in High-Risk Stage II and III Colon Cancer: Final Report of Intergroup 0089," J Clin Oncol, 2005, 23(34):8671-8.

Janus N, Thariat J, Boulanger H, et al, "Proposal for Dosage Adjustment and Timing of Chemotherapy in Hemodialyzed Patients," Ann Oncol, 2010, 21(7):1395-403.

Koren G, Beatty K, Seto A, et al, "The Effects of Impaired Liver Function on the Elimination of Antineoplastic Agents," Ann Pharmacother, 1992, 26(3):363-71.

Kuebler JP, Wieand HS, O'Connell MJ, et al, "Oxaliplatin Combined With Weekly Bolus Fluorouracil and Leucovorin as Surgical Adjuvant Chemotherapy for Stage II and III Colon Cancer: Results From NSABP C-07," J Clin Oncol, 2007, 25(16):2198-204.

Levine MN, Bramwell VH, Pritchard KI, et al, "Randomized Trial of Intensive Cyclophosphamide, Epirubicin, and Fluorouracil Chemotherapy Compared With Cyclophosphamide, Methotrexate, and Fluorouracil in Premenopausal Women With Node-Positive Breast Cancer, National Cancer Institute of Canada Clinical Trials Group," J Clin Oncol, 1998, 16(8):2651-8.

Martel P, Petit I, Pinguet F, Poujol S, Astre C, Fabbro M. Long-term stability of 5-fluorouracil stored in PVC bags and in ambulatory pump reservoirs. J Pharm Biomed Anal. 1996;14(4):395-399.

Mertens R, Granzen B, Lassay L, et al. Treatment of nasopharyngeal carcinoma in children and adolescents: definitive results of a multicenter study (NPC-91-GPOH). Cancer. 2005;104(5):1083-1089.

National Comprehensive Cancer Network® (NCCN), "Clinical Practice Guidelines in Oncology™: Gastric Cancer," Version 2.2012. Available at http://www.nccn.org/professionals/physician_gls/PDF/gastric.pdf

National Institute for Occupational Safety and Health (NIOSH), "NIOSH List of Antineoplastic and Other Hazardous Drugs in Healthcare Settings 2012." Available at http://www.cdc.gov/niosh/docs/2012-150/pdfs/2012-150.pdf. Accessed January 21, 2013.

Neoptolemos JP, Stocken DD, Bassi C, et al, "Adjuvant Chemotherapy With Fluorouracil Plus Folinic Acid Vs Gemcitabine Following Pancreatic Cancer Resection: A Randomized Controlled Trial," JAMA, 2010, 304(10):1073-81.

Ortega JA, Douglass EC, Feusner JH, et al, "Randomized Comparison of Cisplatin/Vincristine/Fluorouracil and Cisplatin/Continuous Infusion Doxorubicin for Treatment of Pediatric Hepatoblastoma: A Report From the Children's Cancer Group and the Pediatric Oncology Group," J Clin Oncol, 2000, 18(14):2665-75.

Regine WF, Winter KA, Abrams RA, et al, "Fluorouracil vs Gemcitabine Chemotherapy Before and After Fluorouracil-Based Chemoradiation Following Resection of Pancreatic Adenocarcinoma: A Randomized Controlled Trial," JAMA, 2008, 299(9):1019-26.

Rodriguez-Galindo C, Wofford M, Castleberry RP, et al, "Preradiation Chemotherapy With Methotrexate, Cisplatin, 5-Fluorouracil, and Leucovorin for Pediatric Nasopharyngeal Carcinoma," Cancer, 2005, 103 (4):850-7.

Sumpter K, Harper-Wynne C, Cunningham D, et al, "Report of Two Protocol Planned Interim Analyses in a Randomized Multicenter Phase III Study Comparing Capecitabine With Fluorouracil and Oxaliplatin With Cisplatin in Patients With Advanced Oesophagogastric Cancer Receiving ECF," Br J Cancer, 2005, 92(11):1976-83.

Tepper J, Krasna MJ, Niedzwiecki D, et al, "Phase III Trial of Trimodality Therapy With Cisplatin, Fluorouracil, Radiotherapy, and Surgery Compared With Surgery Alone for Esophageal Cancer: CALGB 9781," J Clin Oncol, 2008, 26(7):1086-92.

Van Cutsem E, Moiseyenko VM, Tjulandin S, et al, "Phase III Study of Docetaxel and Cisplatin Plus Fluorouracil Compared With Cisplatin and Fluorouracil As First-Line Therapy for Advanced Gastric Cancer: A Report of the V325 Study Group," J Clin Oncol, 2006, 24 (31):4991-7.

Watanabe K. Current chemotherapeutic approaches for hepatoblastoma. Int J Clin Oncol. 2013;18(6):955-961.

Fluorouracil (Topical) (flure oh YOOR a sil)

Medication Safety Issues

Sound-alike/look-alike issues:

Fluorouracil may be confused with flucytosine

High alert medication:

The Institute for Safe Medication Practices (ISMP) includes this medication among its list of drugs which have a heightened risk of causing significant patient harm when used in error.

Related Information

Safe Handling of Hazardous Drugs on page 2419

Brand Names: U.S. Carac; Efudex; Fluoroplex

Brand Names: Canada Efudex®; Fluoroplex®

Therapeutic Category Antineoplastic Agent, Antimetabolite

Generic Availability (U.S.) Yes

Use Management of multiple actinic or solar keratoses and superficial basal cell carcinomas (FDA approved in adults)

Pregnancy Risk Factor X

Pregnancy Considerations Teratogenic effects have been observed with parenteral administration in animal studies; fetal defects and miscarriages have been reported following use of topical products in humans. Use is contraindicated during pregnancy.

Breast-Feeding Considerations It is not known if fluorouracil (topical) is excreted in breast milk. Due to the potential for serious adverse reactions in the nursing infant, a decision should be made whether to discontinue nursing or to discontinue the drug, taking into account the importance of treatment to the mother.

Contraindications Hypersensitivity to fluorouracil or any component

Warnings Hazardous agent; use appropriate precautions for handling and disposal (NIOSH, 2012).

Administration to patients with genetic dihydropyrimidine dehydrogenase (DPD) enzyme deficiency has been associated with increased toxicity following administration (diarrhea, stomatitis, neutropenia, and neurotoxicity). Absence of the DPD enzyme may result in prolonged fluorouracil clearance. Systemic toxicity normally associated with parenteral administration has also been associated with topical use, particularly in patients with DPD enzyme deficiency; discontinue if symptoms of DPD enzyme deficiency occur.

Avoid topical application to mucous membranes due to potential for local inflammation and ulceration. The use of occlusive dressings with topical preparations may increase the severity of inflammation in nearby skin areas. Avoid exposure to ultraviolet rays during and immediately following therapy.

Adverse Reactions Note: Systemic toxicity normally associated with parenteral administration (including neutropenia, neurotoxicity, and gastrointestinal toxicity) has been associated with topical use particularly in patients with a genetic deficiency of dihydropyrimidine dehydrogenase (DPD).

Central nervous system: Headache, insomnia, irritability
Dermatologic: Alopecia, photosensitivity, pruritus, rash, scarring, telangiectasia
Gastrointestinal: Medicinal taste, stomatitis
Hematologic: Leukocytosis, thrombocytopenia
Local: Application site reactions: Allergic contact dermatitis, burning, crusting, dryness, edema, erosion, erythema, hyperpigmentation, irritation, pain, soreness, ulceration
Ocular: Eye irritation (burning, watering, sensitivity, stinging, itching)
Miscellaneous: Birth defects, herpes simplex, miscarriage

Drug Interactions
Metabolism/Transport Effects Inhibits CYP2C9 (weak)
Avoid Concomitant Use
Avoid concomitant use of Fluorouracil (Topical) with any of the following: BCG; Natalizumab; Pimecrolimus; Tacrolimus (Topical); Tofacitinib; Vaccines (Live)
Increased Effect/Toxicity
Fluorouracil (Topical) may increase the levels/effects of: Fosphenytoin; Leflunomide; Natalizumab; Phenytoin; Tofacitinib; Vaccines (Live); Vitamin K Antagonists

The levels/effects of Fluorouracil (Topical) may be increased by: Denosumab; Gemcitabine; Leucovorin Calcium-Levoleucovorin; Pimecrolimus; Roflumilast; SORAfenib; Tacrolimus (Topical); Trastuzumab
Decreased Effect
Fluorouracil (Topical) may decrease the levels/effects of: BCG; Coccidioidin Skin Test; Sipuleucel-T; Vaccines (Inactivated); Vaccines (Live)

The levels/effects of Fluorouracil (Topical) may be decreased by: Echinacea; SORAfenib
Stability Hazardous agent; use appropriate precautions for handling and disposal (NIOSH, 2012). Store at controlled room temperature 15°C to 30°C (59°F to 86°F).
Mechanism of Action A pyrimidine antimetabolite that interferes with DNA synthesis by blocking the methylation of deoxyuridylic acid; fluorouracil inhibits thymidylate synthetase (TS), or is incorporated into RNA. The reduced

folate cofactor is required for tight binding to occur between the 5-FdUMP and TS.
Dosing: Usual Children and Adults:
Actinic keratoses:
Efudex® or Fluoroplex®: Apply twice daily
Carac™: Apply once daily
Basal cell carcinoma: Efudex®: Apply twice daily
Administration Hazardous agent; use appropriate precautions for handling and disposal (NIOSH, 2012). For external use only. Not for ophthalmic or intravaginal use. Cleanse affected area thoroughly and wait 10 minutes before applying. Apply with a nonmetallic applicator or gloved fingers in a sufficient amount to cover affected area. Avoid contact with eyes, eyelids, nostrils, and mouth. Do not cover area with an occlusive dressing. Wash hands after application.
1% or 2%: Apply to lesions on the head and neck for the treatment of multiple actinic keratoses.
5%: Use on lesions in areas other than the head and neck for multiple actinic keratoses; only 5% preparations are used for the treatment of superficial basal cell carcinoma
Dosage Forms Excipient information presented when available (limited, particularly for generics); consult specific product labeling.
Cream, External:
Carac: 0.5% (30 g) [contains methylparaben, polysorbate 80, propylene glycol, propylparaben, trolamine (triethanolamine)]
Efudex: 5% (40 g)
Fluoroplex: 1% (30 g) [contains benzyl alcohol]
Generic: 5% (40 g)
Solution, External:
Generic: 2% (10 mL); 5% (10 mL)
References
National Institute for Occupational Safety and Health (NIOSH), "NIOSH List of Antineoplastic and Other Hazardous Drugs in Healthcare Settings 2012." Available at http://www.cdc.gov/niosh/docs/2012-150/pdfs/2012-150.pdf. Accessed January 21, 2013.

◆ **Fluorouracil Injection (Can)** *see* Fluorouracil (Systemic) *on page 897*
◆ **Fluouracil** *see* Fluorouracil (Systemic) *on page 897*

FLUoxetine (floo OKS e teen)

Medication Safety Issues
Sound-alike/look-alike issues:
FLUoxetine may be confused with DULoxetine, famotidine, Feldene, fluconazole, fluvastatin, fluvoxaMINE, fosinopril, furosemide, PARoxetine, thiothixene, vortioxetine
PROzac may be confused with Paxil, Prelone, PriLOSEC, Prograf, Proscar, ProSom, Provera
Sarafem may be confused with Serophene
BEERS Criteria medication:
This drug may be potentially inappropriate for use in geriatric patients (Quality of evidence - moderate; Strength of recommendation - strong).
International issues:
Reneuron [Spain] may be confused with Remeron brand name for mirtazapine [U.S., Canada, and multiple international markets]
Related Information
Antidepressant Agents *on page 2219*
Oral Medications That Should Not Be Crushed or Altered *on page 2438*
Brand Names: U.S. PROzac; PROzac Weekly; Sarafem
Brand Names: Canada Apo-Fluoxetine; Ava-Fluoxetine; CO Fluoxetine; Dom-Fluoxetine; Fluoxetine Capsules BP; FXT 40; Gen-Fluoxetine; JAMP-Fluoxetine; Mint-Fluoxetine; Mylan-Fluoxetine; Novo-Fluoxetine; Nu-Fluoxetine; PHL-Fluoxetine; PMS-Fluoxetine; PRO-Fluoxetine;

Prozac; Q-Fluoxetine; ratio-Fluoxetine; Riva-Fluoxetine; Sandoz-Fluoxetine; Teva-Fluoxetine; ZYM-Fluoxetine

Therapeutic Category Antidepressant, Selective Serotonin Reuptake Inhibitor (SSRI)

Generic Availability (U.S.) Yes

Use Treatment (acute and maintenance) of major depressive disorder (FDA approved in ages ≥8 years and adults); treatment (acute and maintenance) of obsessive-compulsive disorder (FDA approved in ages ≥7 years and adults); treatment of bulimia nervosa (FDA approved in adults); treatment of panic disorder with or without agoraphobia (FDA approved in adults); treatment of premenstrual dysphoric disorder (PMDD) (Sarafem®: FDA approved in adults); has also been used for anxiety and/or selective mutism and repetitive behavior associated with an autism spectrum disorder (eg, autism, Asperger's syndrome, pervasive developmental disorders)

Medication Guide Available Yes

Pregnancy Risk Factor C

Pregnancy Considerations Adverse events have been observed in animal reproduction studies. Fluoxetine and its metabolite cross the human placenta. An increased risk of teratogenic effects, including cardiovascular defects, may be associated with maternal use of fluoxetine or other SSRIs; however, available information is conflicting. Nonteratogenic effects in the newborn following SSRI/SNRI exposure late in the third trimester include respiratory distress, cyanosis, apnea, seizures, temperature instability, feeding difficulty, vomiting, hypoglycemia, hypo- or hypertonia, hyper-reflexia, jitteriness, irritability, constant crying, and tremor. Symptoms may be due to the toxicity of the SSRIs/SNRIs or a discontinuation syndrome and may be consistent with serotonin syndrome associated with SSRI treatment. Persistent pulmonary hypertension of the newborn (PPHN) has also been reported with SSRI exposure. The long-term effects of in utero SSRI exposure on infant development and behavior are not known.

Due to pregnancy-induced physiologic changes, women who are pregnant may require dose adjustments of fluoxetine to achieve euthymia. The ACOG recommends that therapy with SSRIs or SNRIs during pregnancy be individualized; treatment of depression during pregnancy should incorporate the clinical expertise of the mental health clinician, obstetrician, primary healthcare provider, and pediatrician. According to the American Psychiatric Association (APA), the risks of medication treatment should be weighed against other treatment options and untreated depression. For women who discontinue antidepressant medications during pregnancy and who may be at high risk for postpartum depression, the medications can be restarted following delivery. Treatment algorithms have been developed by the ACOG and the APA for the management of depression in women prior to conception and during pregnancy.

Breast-Feeding Considerations Fluoxetine and its metabolite are excreted into breast milk and can be detected in the serum of breast-feeding infants. Concentrations in breast milk are variable. In comparison to other SSRIs, fluoxetine concentrations in breast milk are higher and adverse events have been observed in nursing infants. Maternal use of an SSRI during pregnancy may cause delayed milk secretion. Breast-feeding is not recommended by the manufacturer. Long-term effects on development and behavior have not been studied.

Contraindications Hypersensitivity to fluoxetine or any component; use of MAO inhibitors within 14 days (potentially fatal reactions may occur; do not use MAO inhibitors for at least 5 weeks after fluoxetine is discontinued); concurrent use of thioridazine or use within 5 weeks after fluoxetine is discontinued; concurrent use of pimozide

Warnings Clinical worsening of depression or suicidal ideation and behavior may occur in children and adults with major depressive disorder **[U.S. Boxed Warning]**. In clinical trials, antidepressants increased the risk of suicidal thinking and behavior (suicidality) in children, adolescents, and young adults (18-24 years of age) with major depressive disorder and other psychiatric disorders. This risk must be considered before prescribing antidepressants for any clinical use. Short-term studies did **not** show an increased risk of suicidality with antidepressant use in patients >24 years of age and showed a decreased risk in patients ≥65 years.

Patients of all ages who are treated with antidepressants for any indication require appropriate monitoring and close observation for clinical worsening of depression, suicidality, and unusual changes in behavior, especially during the first few months after antidepressant initiation or when the dose is adjusted. Family members and caregivers should be instructed to closely observe the patient (ie, daily) and communicate condition with healthcare provider. Patients should also be monitored for associated behaviors (eg, anxiety, agitation, panic attacks, insomnia, irritability, hostility, aggressiveness, impulsivity, akathisia, hypomania, mania) which may increase the risk for worsening depression or suicidality. Worsening depression or emergence of suicidality (or associated behaviors listed above) that is abrupt in onset, severe, or not part of the presenting symptoms, may require discontinuation or modification of drug therapy. SSRI-associated behavioral activation (ie, restlessness, hyperkinesis, hyperactivity, agitation) is two- to threefold more prevalent in children compared to adolescents; it is more prevalent in adolescents compared to adults. Somnolence (including sedation and drowsiness) is more common in adults compared to children and adolescents (Safer, 2006).

Avoid abrupt discontinuation; discontinuation symptoms (including agitation, dysphoria, anxiety, confusion, dizziness, hypomania, nightmares, and other symptoms) may occur if therapy is abruptly discontinued or dose reduced; taper the dose to minimize risks of discontinuation symptoms; if intolerable symptoms occur following a decrease in dosage or upon discontinuation of therapy, consider resuming the previous dose with a more gradual taper. To reduce risk of intentional overdose, write prescriptions for the smallest quantity consistent with good patient care. Screen individuals for bipolar disorder prior to treatment (using antidepressants alone may induce manic episodes in patients with this condition). Potentially fatal serotonin syndrome may occur when SSRIs are used in combination with serotonergic drugs (eg, triptans) or drugs that impair the metabolism of serotonin (eg, MAO inhibitors).

Rash or urticaria may occur along with leukocytosis, fever, edema, arthralgia, lymphadenopathy, respiratory distress, and other symptoms; rare cases of vasculitis and lupus-like syndrome have been reported; anaphylactoid reactions including laryngospasm, bronchospasm, angioedema, and urticaria may occur; discontinue use if rash or other allergic reaction occurs.

Persistent pulmonary hypertension of the newborn (PPHN) has been reported with use during pregnancy; the FDA has reviewed further studies and data evaluating this risk which have shown conflicting results. The FDA has concluded that based on available data, it is unclear whether SSRI use during pregnancy causes PPHN. Neonates born to women receiving SSRIs later during the third trimester may experience respiratory distress, apnea, cyanosis, temperature instability, vomiting, feeding difficulty, hypoglycemia, constant crying, irritability, hypotonia, hypertonia, hyper-reflexia, tremor, jitteriness, and seizures; these symptoms may be due to a direct toxic effect, withdrawal syndrome, or (in some cases) serotonin syndrome. Withdrawal symptoms occur in 30% of neonates exposed to SSRIs in utero; monitor newborns for at least 48 hours after birth; long-term effects of *in utero* exposure to SSRIs are unknown (Levinson-Castiel, 2006). Use with caution during third trimester of pregnancy.

Oral solution contains benzoic acid; benzoic acid (benzoate) is a metabolite of benzyl alcohol; large amounts of benzyl alcohol (≥99 mg/kg/day) have been associated with a potentially fatal toxicity ("gasping syndrome") in neonates; avoid use of fluoxetine products containing benzoic acid in neonates; *in vitro* and animal studies have shown that benzoate displaces bilirubin from protein binding sites

Precautions May cause abnormal bleeding (eg, ecchymosis, purpura, upper GI bleeding); use with caution in patients with impaired platelet aggregation and with concurrent use of aspirin, NSAIDs, or other drugs that affect coagulation. A recent report describes five children (age: 8-15 years) who developed epistaxis (n=4) or bruising (n=1) while receiving SSRI therapy (sertraline) (Lake, 2000). May cause insomnia, anxiety, or nervousness. May impair cognitive or motor performance. Use with caution in patients with hepatic impairment; dosage reduction required. Use with caution in renal impairment, seizure disorders, cardiac dysfunction, diabetes mellitus. Use with caution in patients receiving diuretics or those who are volume-depleted (may cause hyponatremia or SIADH). May cause mydriasis; use with caution in patients at risk of acute narrow-angle glaucoma or with increased intraocular pressure.

May cause anorexia or weight loss; use with caution in patients where weight loss is undesirable. Fluoxetine may cause decreased growth (smaller increases in weight and height) in children and adolescent patients; currently, no studies directly evaluate fluoxetine's long-term effects on growth, development, and maturation of pediatric patients; periodic monitoring of height and weight in pediatric patients is recommended. Case reports of decreased growth in children receiving fluoxetine or fluvoxamine (n=4; age: 11.6-13.7 years) for 6 months to 5 years suggest a suppression of growth hormone secretion during SSRI therapy (Weintrob, 2002). Further studies are needed. SSRI-associated vomiting is two- to threefold more prevalent in children compared to adolescents and is more prevalent in adolescents compared to adults (Safer, 2006).

Significant toxicities have been observed after exposure to fluoxetine in juvenile animals (some occurring at clinically relevant doses). Toxicities included myotoxicity (eg, skeletal muscle damage and necrosis, elevated serum CPK), impaired bone development, and long-term neurobehavioral and reproductive toxicity. The clinical significance of these findings is uncertain.

Adverse Reactions

Cardiovascular: Chest pain, hemorrhage, hypertension, palpitation, vasodilation

Central nervous system: Abnormal dreams, abnormal thinking, agitation, amnesia, anxiety, chills, confusion, dizziness, emotional lability, headache, insomnia, nervousness, sleep disorder, somnolence

Dermatologic: Pruritus, rash

Endocrine & metabolic: Ejaculation abnormal, impotence, libido decreased, menorrhagia

Gastrointestinal: Anorexia, appetite decreased, constipation, diarrhea, dyspepsia, flatulence, nausea, taste perversion, thirst, vomiting, weight gain, weight loss, xerostomia

Genitourinary: Urinary frequency

Neuromuscular & skeletal: Hyperkinesia, tremor, weakness

Ocular: Vision abnormal

Otic: Ear pain, tinnitus

Respiratory: Pharyngitis, sinusitis, yawn

Miscellaneous: Diaphoresis, epistaxis, flu-like syndrome

Rare but important or life-threatening: Acne, acute abdominal syndrome, akathisia, albuminuria, allergies, alopecia, amenorrhea, anaphylactoid reactions, anemia, angina, aphthous stomatitis, aplastic anemia, arrhythmia, arthritis, asthma, ataxia, atrial fibrillation, balance disorder, bone pain, bruising, bruxism, bursitis, cardiac arrest, cataract, cerebrovascular accident, CHF, cholelithiasis, cholestatic jaundice, colitis, dehydration, delusions, depersonalization, dyskinesia, dysphagia, dysuria, ecchymosis, edema, eosinophilic pneumonia, erythema multiforme, erythema nodosum, esophagitis, euphoria, exfoliative dermatitis, extrapyramidal symptoms (rare), gastritis, gastroenteritis, GI ulcer, glossitis, gout, gynecological bleeding, gynecomastia, hallucinations, hepatic failure/necrosis, hepatitis, hiccup, hostility, hypercholesteremia, hyperprolactinemia, hypertonia, hyperventilation, hypoglycemia, hypokalemia, hyponatremia (possibly in association with SIADH), hypotension, hypothyroidism, immune-related hemolytic anemia, kidney failure, laryngospasm, laryngeal edema, leg cramps, liver function test abnormalities, lupus-like syndrome, malaise, melena, migraine, misuse/abuse, MI, mydriasis, myoclonus, neuroleptic malignant syndrome (NMS), optic neuritis, orthostatic hypotension, pancreatitis, pancytopenia, paranoid reaction, petechia, photosensitivity reaction, priapism, pulmonary embolism, pulmonary fibrosis, pulmonary hypertension, purpuric rash, QT prolongation, serotonin syndrome, Stevens-Johnson syndrome, suicidal ideation, syncope, tachycardia, thrombocytopenia, thrombocytopenic purpura, toxic epidermal necrolysis, vasculitis, ventricular tachycardia (including torsade de pointes), violent behavior

Drug Interactions

Metabolism/Transport Effects Substrate of CYP1A2 (minor), CYP2B6 (minor), CYP2C19 (minor), CYP2C9 (major), CYP2D6 (major), CYP2E1 (minor), CYP3A4 (minor); **Note:** Assignment of Major/Minor substrate status based on clinically relevant drug interaction potential; **Inhibits** CYP1A2 (weak), CYP2B6 (weak), CYP2C19 (moderate), CYP2C9 (weak), CYP2D6 (strong)

Avoid Concomitant Use

Avoid concomitant use of FLUoxetine with any of the following: Dosulepin; Haloperidol; Highest Risk QTc-Prolonging Agents; Iobenguane I 123; Ivabradine; Linezolid; MAO Inhibitors; Methylene Blue; Mifepristone; Moderate Risk QTc-Prolonging Agents; Pimozide; Propafenone; Tamoxifen; Thioridazine; Tryptophan; Urokinase; Ziprasidone

Increased Effect/Toxicity

FLUoxetine may increase the levels/effects of: Agents with Antiplatelet Properties; Anticoagulants; Antidepressants (Serotonin Reuptake Inhibitor/Antagonist); Antipsychotics; Apixaban; ARIPiprazole; Aspirin; AtoMOXetine; Benzodiazepines (metabolized by oxidation); Beta-Blockers; BusPIRone; CarBAMazepine; Collagenase (Systemic); CYP2C19 Substrates; CYP2D6 Substrates; Dabigatran Etexilate; Desmopressin; Dextromethorphan; Dosulepin; DOXOrubicin (Conventional); Fesoterodine; Fosphenytoin; Haloperidol; Highest Risk QTc-Prolonging Agents; Hypoglycemic Agents; Ibritumomab; Methylene Blue; Metoprolol; Mexiletine; Nebivolol; NIFEdipine; NiMODipine; NSAID (COX-2 Inhibitor); NSAID (Nonselective); Phenytoin; Pimozide; Propafenone; Rivaroxaban; Salicylates; Serotonin Modulators; Thiazide Diuretics; Thioridazine; Thrombolytic Agents; Tositumomab and Iodine I 131 Tositumomab; TraMADol; Tricyclic Antidepressants; Urokinase; Vitamin K Antagonists; Vortioxetine; Ziprasidone

The levels/effects of FLUoxetine may be increased by: Abiraterone Acetate; Alcohol (Ethyl); Analgesics (Opioid); Antiemetics (5HT3 Antagonists); Antipsychotics; ARIPiprazole; BuPROPion; BusPIRone; Cimetidine; CNS

Depressants; Cobicistat; CYP2C9 Inhibitors (Moderate); CYP2C9 Inhibitors (Strong); CYP2D6 Inhibitors (Moderate); CYP2D6 Inhibitors (Strong); Darunavir; Fosphenytoin; Glucosamine; Herbs (Anticoagulant/Antiplatelet Properties); Ibrutinib; Ivabradine; Linezolid; Lithium; MAO Inhibitors; Metoclopramide; Metyrosine; Mifepristone; Moderate Risk QTc-Prolonging Agents; Multivitamins/Fluoride (with ADE); Multivitamins/Minerals (with ADEK, Folate, Iron); Multivitamins/Minerals (with AE, No Iron); Nonsteroidal Anti-Inflammatory Agents; Omega-3 Fatty Acids; Pentosan Polysulfate Sodium; Pentoxifylline; Propafenone; Prostacyclin Analogues; QTc-Prolonging Agents (Indeterminate Risk and Risk Modifying); TraMADol; Tryptophan; Vitamin E; Ziprasidone

Decreased Effect

FLUoxetine may decrease the levels/effects of: Clopidogrel; Codeine; Iobenguane I 123; Ioflupane I 123; Tamoxifen; Thyroid Products

The levels/effects of FLUoxetine may be decreased by: CarBAMazepine; CYP2C9 Inducers (Strong); Cyproheptadine; Dabrafenib; Nonsteroidal Anti-Inflammatory Agents; NSAID (COX-2 Inhibitor); NSAID (Nonselective); Peginterferon Alfa-2b

Stability All dosage forms should be stored at controlled room temperature; protect from light.

Mechanism of Action Inhibits CNS neuron serotonin reuptake; minimal or no effect on reuptake of norepinephrine or dopamine; does not significantly bind to alpha-adrenergic, histamine, or cholinergic receptors

Pharmacodynamics Maximum effect: Antidepressant: Usually occur after >4 weeks; due to long half-life, resolution of adverse reactions after discontinuation may be slow

Pharmacokinetics (Adult data unless noted) Note: Average steady-state fluoxetine serum concentrations in children (n=10; 6 to <13 years of age) were 2-fold higher than in adolescents (n=11; 13 to <18 years of age); all patients received 20 mg/day; average steady-state norfluoxetine serum concentrations were 1.5-fold higher in the children compared with adolescents; differences in weight almost entirely explained the differences in serum concentrations

Absorption: Oral: Well absorbed; enteric-coated pellets contained in Prozac® Weekly™ resist dissolution until GI pH >5.5 and therefore delay onset of absorption 1-2 hours compared to immediate release formulations

Distribution: V_d: 12-43 L/kg; widely distributed

Protein binding: ~95% (albumin and alpha$_1$-glycoprotein)

Metabolism: Hepatic, via CYP2C19 and 2D6, to norfluoxetine (activity equal to fluoxetine) and other metabolites

Bioavailability: Capsules, tablets, solution, and weekly capsules are bioequivalent

Half-life:

Fluoxetine: Acute dosing: 1-3 days; chronic dosing: 4-6 days; cirrhosis: 7.6 days

Norfluoxetine: Acute and chronic dosing: 4-16 days; cirrhosis: 12 days

Time to peak serum concentration: Immediate release formulation: After 6-8 hours

Elimination: Urine (10% as norfluoxetine, 2.5% to 5% as fluoxetine)

Dialysis: Not removed by hemodialysis

Note: Weekly formulation results in greater fluctuations between peak and trough concentrations of fluoxetine and norfluoxetine compared to once-daily dosing (24% daily/164% weekly; 17% daily/43% weekly, respectively). Trough concentrations are 76% lower for fluoxetine and 47% lower for norfluoxetine than the concentrations maintained by 20 mg once-daily dosing. Steady-state fluoxetine concentrations are ~50% lower following the once-weekly regimen compared to 20 mg once daily.

Dosing: Usual Note: Upon discontinuation of fluoxetine therapy, gradually taper dose. If intolerable symptoms occur following a dose reduction, consider resuming the previously prescribed dose and/or decrease dose at a more gradual rate. If used for an extended period of time, long-term usefulness of fluoxetine should be periodically re-evaluated for the individual patient.

Children and Adolescents:

Anxiety with associated phobias and panic attacks: Very limited data available: Children 2-6 years: Oral: 5 mg/dose or 0.25 mg/kg/dose once daily; adequate trial is considered to be 8-10 weeks; continuation of therapy should be evaluated at 6-9 months after initiation; dosing based on case report in a 2.5-year old child and expert recommendations (Gleason, 2007)

Bulimia nervosa adjunct therapy with cognitive behavioral therapy: Limited data available: Children ≥12 years and Adolescents: Oral: Initial: 20 mg once daily for 3 days, then 40 mg once daily for 3 days, then 60 mg once daily; dosing based on an open-label study of 10 pediatric patients (age: 12-18 years) which showed significant decrease in number of weekly purges; other reports describe use in adolescents (Gable, 2005; Kotler, 2003; Rosen, 2010)

Depression:

Manufacturer's labeling: Children ≥8 years and Adolescents:

Lower weight Children: Oral: Initial: 10 mg once daily; usual daily dose: 10 mg/**day**; if needed, may increase dose to 20 mg once daily after several weeks; maximum daily dose: 20 mg/**day**

Higher weight Children and Adolescents: Oral: Initial: 10-20 mg once daily; in patients started at 10 mg once daily, may increase dose to 20 mg after 1 week; maximum daily dose: 20 mg/**day**

Alternate dosing: Limited data available: Lower initial dosing has been recommended by some experts (Dopheide, 2006; Gleason, 2007):

Children ≤11 years: Oral: Initial: 5 mg once daily; clinically, doses have been titrated up to 40 mg once daily in pediatric patients

Children ≥12 years and Adolescents: Oral: Initial: 10 mg once daily; clinically, doses have been titrated up to 40 mg once daily in pediatric patients

Obsessive-compulsive disorder:

Children <7 years: Limited data available: Oral: Initial: 5 mg once daily (Gleason, 2007)

Children ≥7 years and Adolescents: Oral:

Lower weight Children: Initial: 10 mg once daily; if needed, may increase dose after several weeks; usual daily dose: 20-30 mg/**day**; minimal experience with doses >20 mg/**day**; no experience with doses >60 mg/**day**

Higher weight Children and Adolescents: Initial: 10 mg once daily; increase dose to 20 mg once daily after 2 weeks; may increase dose after several more weeks, if needed; usual daily dose: 20-60 mg/**day**

Repetitive behavior associated with autism spectrum disorders (ASD): Limited data available: Children ≥5 years and Adolescents: Oral: Initial: 2.5 mg once daily for 7 days; then may titrate at weekly intervals using weight-based dosing: 0.3 mg/kg/**day** during week 2; followed by 0.5 mg/kg/**day** during week 3, up to a maximum of 0.8 mg/kg/**day**; dosing based on a double-blind, crossover, placebo-controlled trial in 39 pediatric patients (age: 5-16 years) which showed statistically significant improvement in behavior scores compared to placebo; mean final dose: 9.9 mg/**day** (range: 2.4-20 mg/**day**) or 0.36 ± 0.116 mg/kg/**day** (Hollander, 2005)

Selective mutism: Limited data available: Children ≥5 years and Adolescents: Oral: Initial: 5 mg once daily for 7 days, then increase to 10 mg daily for 7 days, and then increase to 20 mg daily; may further titrate in 20 mg/**day** increments if needed every 2 weeks; maximum daily dose: 60 mg/**day**. Dosing is based on an open-label study of 21 pediatric patients (age: 5-14 years); positive responses were reported in 76% of patients and required a dose of at least 20 mg/**day**; mean final dose: 28.1 mg/**day** (1.1 mg/kg/**day**) (Dummitt, 1996). Weight-based dosing has been reported in a double-blind placebo-controlled trial (treatment group: n=6; placebo: n=9; age: 6-12 years) using the following titration: 0.2 mg/kg/**day** for 1 week, then 0.4 mg/kg/**day** for 1 week, then 0.6 mg/kg/**day** for 10 weeks; mean final dose: 21.4 mg/**day** (Black,1994). To fully assess therapeutic response, a therapeutic trial of at least 9-12 weeks or longer has been suggested (Black, 1994; Dummitt; 1996; Kaakeh, 2008).

Adults: **Depression, obsessive-compulsive disorder, premenstrual dysphoric disorder, bulimia:** Oral: Initial: 20 mg once daily in the morning; may increase after several weeks by 20 mg/**day** increments; maximum daily dose: 80 mg/**day**; doses >20 mg may be given once daily or divided twice daily. **Note:** Lower doses of 5-10 mg/**day** have been used for initial treatment.

Bulimia nervosa: Oral: 60 mg once daily

Depression: Oral: Initial: 20 mg once daily; may increase after several weeks if inadequate response (maximum: 80 mg/**day**). Patients maintained on Prozac® 20 mg/day may be changed to Prozac® Weekly™ 90 mg/week, starting dose 7 days after the last 20 mg/day dose

Depression associated with bipolar disorder (in combination with olanzapine): Oral: Initial: 20 mg in the evening; adjust as tolerated to usual range of 20-50 mg/**day**. See **"Note"** below.

Obsessive-compulsive disorder: Oral: Initial: 20 mg once daily; may increase after several weeks if inadequate response; recommended range: 20-60 mg/**day** (maximum daily dose: 80 mg/**day**)

Panic disorder: Oral: Initial: 10 mg once daily; after 1 week, increase to 20 mg/**day**; may increase after several weeks; doses >60 mg/**day** have not been evaluated

Premenstrual dysphoric disorder (Sarafem®): Oral: 20 mg once daily continuously **or** 20 mg once daily starting 14 days prior to menstruation and through first full day of menses (repeat with each cycle)

Treatment-resistant depression (in combination with olanzapine): Oral: Initial: 20 mg in the evening; adjust as tolerated to usual range of 20-50 mg/**day**. See **"Note"**.

Note: When using individual components of fluoxetine with olanzapine rather than fixed dose combination product (Symbyax®), approximate dosage correspondence is as follows:

Olanzapine 2.5 mg + fluoxetine 20 mg = Symbyax® 3/25

Olanzapine 5 mg + fluoxetine 20 mg = Symbyax® 6/25

Olanzapine 12.5 mg + fluoxetine 20 mg = Symbyax® 12/25

Olanzapine 5 mg + fluoxetine 50 mg = Symbyax® 6/50

Olanzapine 12.5 mg + fluoxetine 50 mg = Symbyax® 12/50

Dosage adjustment in renal impairment: Children, Adolescents, and Adults: Adjustment not routinely needed

Single dose studies: Adults: Pharmacokinetics of fluoxetine and norfluoxetine were similar among subjects with all levels of impaired renal function, including anephric patients on chronic hemodialysis.

Chronic administration: Additional accumulation of fluoxetine or norfluoxetine may occur in patients with severely impaired renal function.

Dosage adjustment in hepatic impairment:

Children and Adolescents: Elimination half-life of fluoxetine is prolonged in patients with hepatic impairment; lower doses or less frequent administration are recommended

Adults: Elimination half-life of fluoxetine is prolonged in patients with hepatic impairment; lower doses or less frequent administration are recommended

Cirrhosis patient: Administer a lower dose or less frequent dosing interval

Compensated cirrhosis without ascites: Administer 50% of normal dose

Administration Oral: May be administered without regard to food

Indication specific:

Major depressive disorder and obsessive compulsive disorder: Take in the morning; if twice daily dosing, take at morning and noon

Bipolar I disorder and treatment-resistant depression (with concurrent olanzapine): Take in the evening

Bulimia: Take in the morning

Monitoring Parameters Liver function, weight, serum glucose; serum sodium (in volume depleted patients); monitor for rash and signs or symptoms of anaphylactoid reactions; monitor height and weight in pediatric patients periodically. Monitor patient periodically for symptom resolution; monitor for worsening depression, suicidality, and associated behaviors (especially at the beginning of therapy or when doses are increased or decreased)

Reference Range Therapeutic levels have not been well established:

Therapeutic: Fluoxetine 100-800 ng/mL (SI: 289-2314 nmol/L); norfluoxetine 100-600 ng/mL (SI: 289-1735 nmol/L)

Toxic: (Fluoxetine plus norfluoxetine): >2000 ng/mL (SI: >5784 nmol/L)

Dosage Forms Excipient information presented when available (limited, particularly for generics); consult specific product labeling.

Capsule, Oral:
PROzac: 10 mg, 20 mg, 40 mg
Generic: 10 mg, 20 mg, 40 mg

Capsule Delayed Release, Oral:
PROzac Weekly: 90 mg
Generic: 90 mg

Solution, Oral:
Generic: 20 mg/5 mL (5 mL, 120 mL)

Tablet, Oral:
Sarafem: 10 mg, 20 mg [contains fd&c yellow #10 aluminum lake, fd&c yellow #6 aluminum lake]
Generic: 10 mg, 20 mg, 60 mg

Extemporaneous Preparations Note: Commercial oral solution is available (4 mg/mL)

A 1 mg/mL fluoxetine oral solution may be prepared using the commercially available preparation (4 mg/mL). In separate graduated cylinders, measure 5 mL of the commercially available fluoxetine preparation and 15 mL of Simple Syrup, NF. Mix thoroughly in incremental proportions. For a 2 mg/mL solution, mix equal proportions of both the commercially available fluoxetine preparation and Simple Syrup, NF. Label "refrigerate". Both concentrations are stable for up to 56 days.

Nahata MC, Pai VB, and Hipple TF, *Pediatric Drug Formulations*, 5th ed, Cincinnati, OH: Harvey Whitney Books Co, 2004.

References

Black B and Uhde TW, "Treatment of Elective Mutism With Fluoxetine: A Double Blind, Placebo-Controlled Study," *J Am Acad Child Adolesc Psychiatry*, 1994, 33(7):1000-6.

Chambers CD, Hernandez-Diaz S, Van Marter LJ, et al, "Selective Serotonin-Reuptake Inhibitors and Risk of Persistent Pulmonary Hypertension of the Newborn," *N Engl J Med*, 2006, 354(6):579-87.

DeSilva KE, Le Flore DB, Marston BJ, et al, "Serotonin Syndrome in HIV-Infected Individuals Receiving Antiretroviral Therapy and Fluoxetine," *AIDS*, 2001, 15(10):1281-5.

Dopheide JA, "Recognizing and Treating Depression in Children and Adolescents," *Am J Health Syst Pharm*, 2006, 63(3):233-43.

Dow SP, Sonies BC, Scheib D, et al, "Practical Guidelines for the Assessment and Treatment of Selective Mutism," *J Am Acad Child Adolesc Psychiatry*, 1995, 34(7):836-46.

Dummit ES 3rd, Klein RG, Tancer NK, et al, "Fluoxetine Treatment of Children With Selective Mutism: An Open Trial," *J Am Acad Child Adolesc Psychiatry*, 1996, 35(5):615-21.

Gable KN and Dopheide JA, "Psychotropic Medication Use at a Private Eating Disorders Treatment Facility: A Retrospective Chart Review and Descriptive Data Analysis," *Curr Ther Res Clin Exp*, 2005, 66:572-88.

Gleason MM, Egger HL, Emslie GJ, et al, "Psychopharmacological Treatment for Very Young Children: Contexts and Guidelines," *J Am Acad Child Adolesc Psychiatry*, 2007, 46(12):1532-72.

Hollander E, Phillips A, Chaplin W, et al, "A Placebo Controlled Crossover Trial of Liquid Fluoxetine on Repetitive Behaviors in Childhood and Adolescent Autism," *Neuropsychopharmacology*, 2005, 30 (3):582-9.

Kaakeh Y and Stumpf JL, "Treatment of Selective Mutism: Focus on Selective Serotonin Reuptake Inhibitors," *Pharmacotherapy*, 2008, 28 (2):214-24.

Kotler LA, Devlin MJ, Davies M, et al, "An Open Trial of Fluoxetine for Adolescents With Bulimia Nervosa," *J Child Adolesc Psychopharmacol*, 2003, 13(3):329-35.

Lake MB, Birmaher B, Wassick S, et al, "Bleeding and Selective Serotonin Reuptake Inhibitors in Childhood and Adolescence," *J Child Adolesc Psychopharmacol*, 2000, 10(1):35-8.

Levinson-Castiel R, Merlob P, Linder N, et al, "Neonatal Abstinence Syndrome After *in utero* Exposure to Selective Serotonin Reuptake Inhibitors in Term Infants," *Arch Pediatr Adolesc Med*, 2006, 160 (2):173-6.

McPheeters ML, Warren Z, Sathe N, et al, "A Systematic Review of Medical Treatments for Children With Autism Spectrum Disorders," *Pediatrics*, 2011, 127(5):e1312-21.

Rosen DS and American Academy of Pediatrics Committee on Adolescence, "Identification and Management of Eating Disorders in Children and Adolescents," *Pediatrics*, 2010, 126(6):1240-53.

Safer DJ and Zito JM, "Treatment Emergent Adverse Effects of Selective Serotonin Reuptake Inhibitors by Age Group: Children vs. Adolescents," *J Child Adolesc Psychopharmacol*, 2006, 16 (1/2):159-69.

Weintrob N, Cohen D, Klipper-Aurbach Y, et al, "Decreased Growth During Therapy With Selective Serotonin Reuptake Inhibitors," *Arch Pediatr Adolesc Med*, 2002, 156(7):696-701.

◆ **Fluoxetine Capsules BP (Can)** *see* FLUoxetine *on page 901*

◆ **Fluoxetine Hydrochloride** *see* FLUoxetine *on page 901*

Fluoxymesterone (floo oks i MES te rone)

Medication Safety Issues
International issues:
Halotestin [Great Britain] may be confused with Haldol brand name for haloperidol [U.S. and multiple international markets]

Related Information
Safe Handling of Hazardous Drugs *on page 2419*

Brand Names: U.S. Androxy

Therapeutic Category Androgen

Generic Availability (U.S.) May be product dependent

Use Replacement of endogenous testicular hormone; in females used as palliative treatment of breast cancer, postpartum breast engorgement

Pregnancy Risk Factor X

Pregnancy Considerations Use is contraindicated in women who are or may become pregnant. May cause androgenic effects to the female fetus; clitoral hypertrophy, labial fusion, urogenital sinus defect, vaginal atresia, and ambiguous genitalia have been reported.

Breast-Feeding Considerations It is not known if fluoxymesterone is excreted in breast milk. Due to the potential for serious adverse reactions in the nursing infant, a decision should be made whether to discontinue nursing or to discontinue the drug, taking into account the importance of treatment to the mother.

Contraindications Hypersensitivity to fluoxymesterone or any component; serious cardiac disease, liver or kidney disease

Warnings Hazardous agent; use appropriate precautions for handling and disposal (NIOSH, 2012). Some tablets (brand name) contain tartrazine which may cause allergic reactions in susceptible individuals.

Precautions May accelerate bone maturation without producing compensatory gain in linear growth; in prepubertal children perform radiographic examination of the hand and wrist every 6 months to determine the rate of bone maturation and to assess the effect of treatment on the epiphyseal centers

Adverse Reactions
Male: Gynecomastia, oligospermia (at higher doses), priapism, prostatic carcinoma, prostatic hypertrophy, testicular atrophy

Female: Menstrual irregularities (including amenorrhea), virilism (including deepening of the voice, clitoris hypertrophy)

Cardiovascular: Edema

Central nervous system: Anxiety, depression, headache

Dermatologic: Acne, hirsutism, "male pattern" baldness

Endocrine & metabolic: Electrolyte abnormalities (sodium, chloride, calcium, potassium, and inorganic phosphate retention), hypercholesterolemia, libido changes (increased or decreased), water retention

Gastrointestinal: GI irritation, nausea, vomiting

Genitourinary: Prostatic hyperplasia

Hematologic: Clotting factor suppression, polycythemia

Hepatic: Cholestatic jaundice, hepatic coma (rare), hepatic dysfunction, hepatocellular neoplasms (rare), liver function tests abnormal, peliosis hepatitis (rare)

Neuromuscular & skeletal: Paresthesia

Miscellaneous: Hypersensitivity, nonimmunologic anaphylaxis (formerly known as anaphylactoid reaction)

Drug Interactions
Metabolism/Transport Effects None known.

Avoid Concomitant Use There are no known interactions where it is recommended to avoid concomitant use.

Increased Effect/Toxicity
Fluoxymesterone may increase the levels/effects of: Antidiabetic Agents; CycloSPORINE (Systemic); Vitamin K Antagonists

The levels/effects of Fluoxymesterone may be increased by: Corticosteroids (Systemic)

Decreased Effect There are no known significant interactions involving a decrease in effect.

Stability Hazardous agent; use appropriate precautions for handling and disposal (NIOSH, 2012).

Mechanism of Action Synthetic derivative of testosterone; responsible for the normal growth and development of male sex hormones, male sex organs, and maintenance of secondary sex characteristics; large doses suppress endogenous testosterone release

Pharmacokinetics (Adult data unless noted)
Absorption: Oral: Rapid

Protein binding: 98%

Metabolism: In the liver

Half-life: 10-100 minutes

Elimination: Enterohepatic circulation and urinary excretion (90%)

Halogenated derivative of testosterone with up to 5 times the activity of methyltestosterone

Dosing: Usual Adults: Oral:

Male:

Hypogonadism: 5-20 mg/day

Delayed puberty: 2.5-20 mg/day for 4-6 months

Female:
Inoperable breast carcinoma: 10-40 mg/day in divided doses for 1-3 months
Breast engorgement: 2.5 mg after delivery, 5-10 mg/day in divided doses for 4-5 days

Administration Hazardous agent; use appropriate precautions for handling and disposal (NIOSH, 2012).

Monitoring Parameters Periodic radiographic exams of hand and wrist (when used in children); hemoglobin, hematocrit (if receiving high dosages or long-term therapy)

Test Interactions Decreased levels of thyroxine-binding globulin; decreased total T_4 serum levels; increased resin uptake of T_3 and T_4

Controlled Substance C-III

Dosage Forms Excipient information presented when available (limited, particularly for generics); consult specific product labeling.
Tablet, Oral:
Androxy: 10 mg [scored]

References
National Institute for Occupational Safety and Health (NIOSH), "NIOSH List of Antineoplastic and Other Hazardous Drugs in Healthcare Settings 2012." Available at http://www.cdc.gov/niosh/docs/2012-150/pdfs/2012-150.pdf. Accessed January 21, 2013.

♦ **5-Fluracil** see Fluorouracil (Systemic) on page 897
♦ **Flura-Drops** see Fluoride on page 894

Flurazepam (flure AZ e pam)

Medication Safety Issues
Sound-alike/look-alike issues:
Flurazepam may be confused with temazepam
Dalmane® may be confused with Demulen®
BEERS Criteria medication:
This drug may be potentially inappropriate for use in geriatric patients (Quality of evidence - high; Strength of recommendation - strong).

Brand Names: Canada Apo-Flurazepam®; Dalmane®; Som Pam

Therapeutic Category Benzodiazepine; Hypnotic; Sedative

Generic Availability (U.S.) Yes

Use Short-term treatment of insomnia (FDA approved in ages ≥15 years)

Medication Guide Available Yes

Pregnancy Considerations All benzodiazepines are assumed to cross the placenta. Teratogenic effects have been observed with some benzodiazepines; however, additional studies are needed. The incidence of premature birth and low birth weights may be increased following maternal use of benzodiazepines; hypoglycemia and respiratory problems in the neonate may occur following exposure late in pregnancy. Neonatal withdrawal symptoms may occur within days to weeks after birth and "floppy infant syndrome" (which also includes withdrawal symptoms) has been reported with some benzodiazepines (Bergman, 1992; Iqbal, 2002; Wikner, 2007). Neonatal depression has been observed, specifically following exposure to flurazepam when used maternally for 10 consecutive days prior to delivery. Serum levels of N-desalkylflurazepam were measurable in the infant during the first 4 days of life. Use of flurazepam during pregnancy is contraindicated.

Breast-Feeding Considerations Although information specific to flurazepam has not been located, all benzodiazepines are expected to be excreted into breast milk. Drowsiness, lethargy, or weight loss in nursing infants have been observed in case reports following maternal use of some benzodiazepines (Iqbal, 2002).

Contraindications Hypersensitivity to flurazepam or any component (there may be cross-sensitivity with other benzodiazepines), pregnancy, preexisting CNS depression, respiratory depression, narrow-angle glaucoma

Warnings Evaluate patient carefully for medical or psychiatric causes of insomnia prior to initiation of drug treatment; failure of flurazepam to treat insomnia (after 7-10 days of therapy), a worsening of insomnia, the emergence of behavioral changes, or thinking abnormalities may indicate a medical or psychiatric illness requiring evaluation; these effects also have been reported with flurazepam use. Due to possible adverse effects, use lowest effective dose. Abrupt discontinuation after prolonged use may result in withdrawal symptoms or rebound insomnia.

Hypersensitivity reactions including anaphylaxis and angioedema may occur. Hazardous sleep-related activities, such as sleep-driving (driving while not fully awake without any recollection of driving), preparing and eating food, and making phone calls while asleep have also been reported. Effects with other sedative drugs or ethanol may be potentiated.

Precautions Use with caution in patients with depression, chronic pulmonary insufficiency, impaired renal or hepatic function, or low albumin. May cause CNS depression impairing physical and mental capabilities; patients should be cautioned about performing tasks which require mental alertness (operating machinery or driving). Use with caution in patients receiving other CNS depressants or in patients with a history of drug dependence.

Adverse Reactions
Cardiovascular: Chest pain, flushing, hypotension, palpitation
Central nervous system: Apprehension, ataxia, confusion, depression, dizziness, drowsiness, euphoria, faintness, falling, hallucinations, hangover effect, headache, irritability, lightheadedness, memory impairment, nervousness, paradoxical reactions, restlessness, slurred speech, staggering, talkativeness
Dermatologic: Pruritus, rash
Gastrointestinal: Appetite increased/decreased, bitter taste, constipation, diarrhea, GI pain, heartburn, nausea, salivation increased/excessive, upset stomach, vomiting, weight gain/loss, xerostomia
Hematologic: Granulocytopenia, leukopenia
Hepatic: Alkaline phosphatase increased, ALT increased, AST increased, cholestatic jaundice, total bilirubin increased
Neuromuscular & skeletal: Body/joint pain, dysarthria, reflex slowing, weakness
Ocular: Blurred vision, burning eyes, difficulty focusing
Respiratory: Apnea, dyspnea
Miscellaneous: Diaphoresis, drug dependence
Postmarketing and/or case reports: Anaphylaxis, angioedema, complex sleep-related behavior (sleep-driving, cooking or eating food, making phone calls)

Drug Interactions
Metabolism/Transport Effects Substrate of CYP3A4 (major); **Note:** Assignment of Major/Minor substrate status based on clinically relevant drug interaction potential; **Inhibits** CYP2E1 (weak)

Avoid Concomitant Use
Avoid concomitant use of Flurazepam with any of the following: Azelastine (Nasal); Conivaptan; Fusidic Acid (Systemic); Methadone; OLANZapine; Paraldehyde; Sodium Oxybate; Thalidomide

Increased Effect/Toxicity
Flurazepam may increase the levels/effects of: Alcohol (Ethyl); Azelastine (Nasal); Buprenorphine; CloZAPine; CNS Depressants; Hydrocodone; Methadone; Methotrimeprazine; Metyrosine; Mirtazapine; Paraldehyde; Pramipexole; ROPINIRole; Rotigotine; Selective Serotonin Reuptake Inhibitors; Sodium Oxybate; Thalidomide; Zolpidem

◀

The levels/effects of Flurazepam may be increased by: Antifungal Agents (Azole Derivatives, Systemic); Aprepitant; Brimonidine (Topical); Calcium Channel Blockers (Nondihydropyridine); Cannabis; Ceritinib; Cimetidine; Conivaptan; Contraceptives (Estrogens); Contraceptives (Progestins); CYP3A4 Inhibitors (Moderate); CYP3A4 Inhibitors (Strong); Dasatinib; Doxylamine; Dronabinol; Droperidol; Fosamprenavir; Fosaprepitant; Fusidic Acid (Systemic); Grapefruit Juice; HydrOXYzine; Isoniazid; Ivacaftor; Kava Kava; Luliconazole; Magnesium Sulfate; Methotrimeprazine; Mifepristone; Nabilone; OLANZapine; Perampanel; Proton Pump Inhibitors; Ritonavir; Rufinamide; Saquinavir; Selective Serotonin Reuptake Inhibitors; Simeprevir; Stiripentol; Tapentadol; Tetrahydrocannabinol

Decreased Effect

The levels/effects of Flurazepam may be decreased by: Bosentan; CarBAMazepine; CYP3A4 Inducers (Strong); Dabrafenib; Deferasirox; Mitotane; Rifamycin Derivatives; Siltuximab; St Johns Wort; Theophylline Derivatives; Tocilizumab; Yohimbine

Food Interactions Serum levels and response to flurazepam may be increased by grapefruit juice, but unlikely because of flurazepam's high oral bioavailability. Management: Keep grapefruit consumption consistent.

Stability

Dalmane®: Store at controlled room temperature at 25°C (77°F); excursions permitted to 15°C to 30°C (59°F to 86°F)

Generic: Store at controlled room temperature at 20°C to 25°C (68°F to 77°F); protect from light and moisture; dispense in tightly closed, light-resistant container

Mechanism of Action Binds to stereospecific benzodiazepine receptors on the postsynaptic GABA neuron at several sites within the central nervous system, including the limbic system, reticular formation. Enhancement of the inhibitory effect of GABA on neuronal excitability results by increased neuronal membrane permeability to chloride ions. This shift in chloride ions results in hyperpolarization (a less excitable state) and stabilization.

Pharmacodynamics Hypnotic effects:

Onset of action: 15-20 minutes

Maximum effect: 3-6 hours

Duration: 7-8 hours

Pharmacokinetics (Adult data unless noted)

Absorption: Rapid

Distribution: V_d: Adults: 3.4 L/kg

Protein binding: ~97%

Metabolism: Hepatic to N-desalkylflurazepam (active) and N-hydroxyethylflurazepam

Half-life: Adults:

Flurazepam: Mean: 2.3 hours

N-desalkylflurazepam: Single dose: 74-90 hours; multiple doses: 111-113 hours

Time to peak serum concentration:

Flurazepam: 30–60 minutes

N-desalkylflurazepam: 10.6 hours (range: 7.6-13.6 hours)

N-hydroxyethylflurazepam: ~1 hour

Elimination: Urine: N-hydroxyethylflurazepam (22% to 55%); N-desalkylflurazepam (<1%)

Dosing: Usual Oral:

Children:

<15 years: Dose not established; use not recommended by manufacturer

≥15 years: 15 mg at bedtime

Adults: 15-30 mg at bedtime

Administration May be administered without regard to meals; administer dose at bedtime

Controlled Substance C-IV

Dosage Forms Excipient information presented when available (limited, particularly for generics); consult specific product labeling.

Capsule, Oral, as hydrochloride:

Generic: 15 mg, 30 mg

References

Bergman U, Rosa FW, Baum C, et al, "Effects of Exposure to Benzodiazepine During Fetal Life," *Lancet*, 1992, 340(8821):694-6.

Cooper SF and Drolet D, "Protein Binding of Flurazepam and Its Major Metabolites in Plasma," *Curr Ther Res*, 1982, 32(5):757-60.

Greenblatt DJ, Harmatz JS, Engelhardt N, et al, "Pharmacokinetic Determinants of Dynamic Differences Among Three Benzodiazepine Hypnotics. Flurazepam, Temazepam, and Triazolam," *Arch Gen Psychiatry*, 1989, 46(4):326-32.

Iqbal MM, Sobhan T, Ryals T, et al, "Effects of Commonly Used Benzodiazepines on the Fetus, the Neonate, and the Nursing Infant," *Psychiatr Serv*, 2002, 53(1):39-49.

Vozeh S, Schmidlin O, and Taeschner W, "Pharmacokinetic Drug Data," *Clin Pharmacokinet*, 1988, 15(4):254-82.

Wikner BN, Stiller CO, Bergman U, et al, "Use of Benzodiazepines and Benzodiazepine Receptor Agonists During Pregnancy: Neonatal Outcome and Congenital Malformations," *Pharmacoepidemiol Drug Saf*, 2007, 16(11):1203-10.

◆ **Flurazepam Hydrochloride** see Flurazepam on page 907

Flurbiprofen (Systemic) (flure BI proe fen)

Medication Safety Issues

Sound-alike/look-alike issues:

Flurbiprofen may be confused with fenoprofen

Ansaid may be confused with Asacol, Axid

Brand Names: Canada Alti-Flurbiprofen; Ansaid; Apo-Flurbiprofen; Froben; Froben-SR; Novo-Flurprofen; Nu-Flurprofen

Therapeutic Category Analgesic, Non-narcotic; Anti-inflammatory Agent; Nonsteroidal Anti-inflammatory Drug (NSAID), Oral

Generic Availability (U.S.) Yes

Use Management of inflammatory disease and rheumatoid disorders, dysmenorrhea, pain

Medication Guide Available Yes

Pregnancy Risk Factor C

Pregnancy Considerations Adverse events were not observed in the initial animal reproduction studies; therefore, the manufacturer classifies flurbiprofen as pregnancy category C. NSAID exposure during the first trimester is not strongly associated with congenital malformations; however, cardiovascular anomalies and cleft palate have been observed following NSAID exposure in some studies. The use of an NSAID close to conception may be associated with an increased risk of miscarriage. Nonteratogenic effects have been observed following NSAID administration during the third trimester including myocardial degenerative changes, prenatal constriction of the ductus arteriosus, fetal tricuspid regurgitation, failure of the ductus arteriosus to close postnatally; renal dysfunction or failure, oligohydramnios; gastrointestinal bleeding or perforation, increased risk of necrotizing enterocolitis; intracranial bleeding (including intraventricular hemorrhage), platelet dysfunction with resultant bleeding; pulmonary hypertension. Because they may cause premature closure of the ductus arteriosus, use of NSAIDs late in pregnancy should be avoided (use after 31 or 32 weeks gestation is not recommended by some clinicians). The chronic use of NSAIDs in women of reproductive age may be associated with infertility that is reversible upon discontinuation of the medication.

Breast-Feeding Considerations Low levels of flurbiprofen are found in breast milk. Breast-feeding is not recommended by the manufacturer. The pharmacokinetics of flurbiprofen immediately postpartum are similar to healthy volunteers.

Contraindications Hypersensitivity to flurbiprofen or any component; history of asthma, urticaria, or allergic-type reaction to aspirin or other NSAIDs; patients with the "aspirin triad" [asthma, rhinitis (with or without nasal polyps), and aspirin intolerance] (fatal asthmatic and ana-phylactoid reactions may occur in these patients); perioperative pain in the setting of coronary artery bypass graft (CABG)

Warnings NSAIDs are associated with an increased risk of adverse cardiovascular thrombotic events, including potentially fatal MI and stroke **[U.S. Boxed Warning]**; risk may be increased with duration of use or preexisting cardiovascular risk factors or disease; carefully evaluate cardiovascular risk profile prior to prescribing; use the lowest effective dose for the shortest duration of time, taking into consideration individual patient treatment goals; alternate therapies should be considered for patients at high risk. Use is contraindicated for treatment of perioperative pain in the setting of CABG surgery **[U.S. Boxed Warning]**; an increased incidence of MI and stroke was found in patients receiving COX-2 selective NSAIDs for the treatment of pain within the first 10-14 days after CABG surgery. NSAIDs may cause fluid retention, edema, and new-onset or worsening of preexisting hypertension; use with caution in patients with hypertension, CHF, or fluid retention. Concurrent administration of ibuprofen, and potentially other nonselective NSAIDs, may interfere with aspirin's cardioprotective effect.

NSAIDs may increase the risk of gastrointestinal inflammation, ulceration, bleeding, and perforation **[U.S. Boxed Warning]**. These events, which can be potentially fatal, may occur at any time during therapy, and without warning. Avoid the use of NSAIDs in patients with active GI bleeding or ulcer disease. Use NSAIDs with extreme caution in patients with a history of GI bleeding or ulcers (these patients have a 10-fold increased risk for developing a GI bleed). Use NSAIDs with caution in patients with other risk factors which may increase GI bleeding (eg, concurrent therapy with aspirin, anticoagulants, and/or corticosteroids, longer duration of NSAID use, smoking, use of alcohol, and poor general health). Use the lowest effective dose for the shortest duration of time, taking into consideration individual patient treatment goals; alternate therapies should be considered for patients at high risk.

NSAIDs may compromise existing renal function. Renal toxicity may occur in patients with impaired renal function, dehydration, heart failure, liver dysfunction, those taking diuretics and ACE inhibitors; use with caution in these patients; monitor renal function closely. NSAIDs are not recommended for use in patients with advanced renal disease. Long-term use of NSAIDs may cause renal papillary necrosis and other renal injury.

Fatal asthmatic and anaphylactoid reactions may occur in patients with the "aspirin triad" who receive NSAIDs. NSAIDs may cause serious dermatologic adverse reactions including exfoliative dermatitis, Stevens-Johnson syndrome, and toxic epidermal necrolysis. Avoid use of NSAIDs in late pregnancy as they may cause premature closure of the ductus arteriosus.

Precautions Use with caution in renal or hepatic impairment, GI disease, cardiac disease, and patients receiving anticoagulants.

Adverse Reactions

Cardiovascular: Edema

Central nervous system: Amnesia, anxiety, depression, dizziness, headache, insomnia, malaise, nervousness, somnolence, vertigo

Dermatologic: Rash

Gastrointestinal: Abdominal pain, constipation, diarrhea, dyspepsia, flatulence, GI bleeding, nausea, vomiting, weight changes

Hepatic: Liver enzymes increased

Neuromuscular & skeletal: Reflexes increased, tremor, weakness

Ocular: Vision changes

Otic: Tinnitus

Respiratory: Rhinitis

Rare but important or life-threatening: Anaphylactic reaction, anemia, angioedema, asthma, bruising, cerebrovascular ischemia, CHF, confusion, eczema, eosinophilia, epistaxis, exfoliative dermatitis, fever, gastric/peptic ulcer, hematocrit increased, hematuria, hemoglobin decreased, hepatitis, hypertension, hyperuricemia, interstitial nephritis, jaundice, leukopenia, paresthesia, parosmia, photosensitivity, pruritus, purpura, renal failure, stomatitis, thrombocytopenia, toxic epidermal necrolysis, urticaria, vasodilation

Drug Interactions

Metabolism/Transport Effects Substrate of CYP2C9 (minor); **Note:** Assignment of Major/Minor substrate status based on clinically relevant drug interaction potential; **Inhibits** CYP2C9 (weak)

Avoid Concomitant Use

Avoid concomitant use of Flurbiprofen (Systemic) with any of the following: Floctafenine; Ketorolac (Nasal); Ketorolac (Systemic); NSAID (COX-2 Inhibitor); Omacetaxine; Urokinase

Increased Effect/Toxicity

Flurbiprofen (Systemic) may increase the levels/effects of: 5-ASA Derivatives; Agents with Antiplatelet Properties; Aliskiren; Aminoglycosides; Anticoagulants; Apixaban; Bisphosphonate Derivatives; Collagenase (Systemic); CycloSPORINE (Systemic); Dabigatran Etexilate; Deferasirox; Desmopressin; Digoxin; Eplerenone; Haloperidol; Ibrutinomab; Lithium; Methotrexate; Nonsteroidal Anti-Inflammatory Agents; NSAID (COX-2 Inhibitor); Omacetaxine; PEMEtrexed; Porfimer; Potassium-Sparing Diuretics; PRALAtrexate; Quinolone Antibiotics; Rivaroxaban; Salicylates; Tenofovir; Thrombolytic Agents; Tositumomab and Iodine I 131 Tositumomab; Urokinase; Vancomycin; Vitamin K Antagonists

The levels/effects of Flurbiprofen (Systemic) may be increased by: ACE Inhibitors; Angiotensin II Receptor Blockers; Antidepressants (Tricyclic, Tertiary Amine); Corticosteroids (Systemic); CycloSPORINE (Systemic); Dasatinib; Floctafenine; Glucosamine; Herbs (Anticoagulant/Antiplatelet Properties); Ibrutinib; Ketorolac (Nasal); Ketorolac (Systemic); Multivitamins/Fluoride (with ADE); Multivitamins/Minerals (with ADEK, Folate, Iron); Multivitamins/Minerals (with AE, No Iron); Nonsteroidal Anti-Inflammatory Agents; Omega-3 Fatty Acids; Pentosan Polysulfate Sodium; Pentoxifylline; Probenecid; Prostacyclin Analogues; Selective Serotonin Reuptake Inhibitors; Serotonin/Norepinephrine Reuptake Inhibitors; Sodium Phosphates; Tipranavir; Treprostinil; Vitamin E

Decreased Effect

Flurbiprofen (Systemic) may decrease the levels/effects of: ACE Inhibitors; Agents with Antiplatelet Properties; Aliskiren; Angiotensin II Receptor Blockers; Beta-Blockers; Eplerenone; HydrALAZINE; Loop Diuretics; Potassium-Sparing Diuretics; Prostaglandins (Ophthalmic); Salicylates; Selective Serotonin Reuptake Inhibitors; Thiazide Diuretics

The levels/effects of Flurbiprofen (Systemic) may be decreased by: Bile Acid Sequestrants; Nonsteroidal Anti-Inflammatory Agents; Salicylates

Food Interactions Food may decrease the rate but not the extent of absorption. Management: May administer with food, milk, or antacid to decrease GI effects.

Mechanism of Action Reversibly inhibits cyclooxygenase-1 and 2 (COX-1 and 2) enzymes, which results in decreased formation of prostaglandin precursors; has antipyretic, analgesic, and anti-inflammatory properties

Other proposed mechanisms not fully elucidated (and possibly contributing to the anti-inflammatory effect to varying degrees), include inhibiting chemotaxis, altering lymphocyte activity, inhibiting neutrophil aggregation/activation, and decreasing proinflammatory cytokine levels.

Pharmacokinetics (Adult data unless noted)
Time to peak serum concentration: Within 1.5-2 hours
Elimination: 95% in urine

Dosing: Usual Adults: Oral:
Arthritis: 200-300 mg/day in 2-4 divided doses; maximum dose: 100 mg/dose; maximum: 300 mg/day
Dysmenorrhea: 50 mg 4 times/day

Administration Administer with food, milk, or antacid to decrease GI effects.

Monitoring Parameters CBC, platelets, BUN, serum creatinine, liver enzymes, occult blood loss

Dosage Forms Excipient information presented when available (limited, particularly for generics); consult specific product labeling.
Tablet, Oral:
Generic: 50 mg, 100 mg

Flurbiprofen (Ophthalmic) (flure BI proe fen)

Medication Safety Issues
Sound-alike/look-alike issues:
Flurbiprofen may be confused with fenoprofen
Ocufen® may be confused with Ocuflox®
International issues:
Ocufen [U.S., Canada, and multiple international markets] may be confused with Ocupres brand name for timolol [India]; Ocupress brand name for dorzolamide [Brazil]

Brand Names: U.S. Ocufen

Therapeutic Category Anti-inflammatory Agent, Ophthalmic; Nonsteroidal Anti-inflammatory Drug (NSAID), Ophthalmic

Generic Availability (U.S.) Yes

Use For inhibition of intraoperative trauma-induced miosis; the value of flurbiprofen for the prevention and management of postoperative ocular inflammation and postoperative cystoid macular edema remains to be determined

Pregnancy Risk Factor C

Pregnancy Considerations Adverse events were observed following systemic administration of flurbiprofen in animal reproduction studies; therefore, flurbiprofen ophthalmic is classified as pregnancy category C. Information related to systemic absorption following topical application of the eye drops has not been located. Systemic absorption would be required in order for flurbiprofen to cross the placenta and reach the fetus. Refer to the Flurbiprofen (Systemic) monograph for additional information.

Breast-Feeding Considerations When administered orally, flurbiprofen enters breast milk. Refer to the Flurbiprofen (Systemic) monograph for details. Information related to systemic absorption following topical application of the eye drops has not been located. Systemic absorption would be required in order for flurbiprofen to enter breast milk. Breast-feeding is not recommended by the manufacturer.

Contraindications Hypersensitivity to flurbiprofen or any component

Warnings An increased risk of bleeding in ocular tissues may occur in conjunction with ocular surgery. Use with caution in patients with sensitivity to acetylsalicylic acid or other nonsteroidal anti-inflammatory agents.

Precautions Use with caution in patients with known bleeding tendencies or those receiving anticoagulants. Wound healing time may be slowed or delayed.

Adverse Reactions Ocular: Bleeding tendency increased in ocular tissue (in conjunction with ocular surgery), burning (transient), fibrosis, hyperemia, hyphema, irritation, miosis, mydriasis, stinging (transient)

Drug Interactions
Metabolism/Transport Effects None known.

Avoid Concomitant Use There are no known interactions where it is recommended to avoid concomitant use.

Increased Effect/Toxicity There are no known significant interactions involving an increase in effect.

Decreased Effect There are no known significant interactions involving a decrease in effect.

Mechanism of Action Reversibly inhibits cyclooxygenase-1 and 2 (COX-1 and 2) enzymes, which results in decreased formation of prostaglandin precursors; has antipyretic, analgesic, and anti-inflammatory properties

Other proposed mechanisms not fully elucidated (and possibly contributing to the anti-inflammatory effect to varying degrees), include inhibiting chemotaxis, altering lymphocyte activity, inhibiting neutrophil aggregation/activation, and decreasing proinflammatory cytokine levels.

Dosing: Usual Children and Adults: Instill 1 drop every 30 minutes starting 2 hours prior to surgery (total of 4 drops to each affected eye)

Administration Instill drops into affected eye(s); avoid contact of container tip with skin or eye; apply finger pressure to lacrimal sac during and for 1-2 minutes after instillation to decrease risk of absorption and systemic effects

Monitoring Parameters Periodic eye exams

Dosage Forms Excipient information presented when available (limited, particularly for generics); consult specific product labeling.
Solution, Ophthalmic, as sodium:
Ocufen: 0.03% (2.5 mL) [contains edetate disodium, thimerosal]
Generic: 0.03% (2.5 mL)

◆ **Flurbiprofen Sodium** see Flurbiprofen (Ophthalmic) on page 910

◆ **Flurbiprofen Sodium** see Flurbiprofen (Systemic) on page 908

◆ **5-Flurocytosine** see Flucytosine on page 882

Fluticasone (Oral Inhalation) (floo TIK a sone)

Medication Safety Issues
Sound-alike/look-alike issues:
Flovent may be confused with Flonase
International issues:
Allegro: Brand name for fluticasone [Israel], but also the brand name for frovatriptan [Germany]
Allegro [Israel] may be confused with Allegra and Allegra-D brand names for fexofenadine and fexofenadine/pseudoephedrine, respectively [U.S., Canada, and multiple international markets]
Flovent [U.S., Canada] may be confused with Flogen brand name for naproxen [Mexico]; Flogene brand name for piroxicam [Brazil]

Related Information
Inhaled Corticosteroids on page 2223

Brand Names: U.S. Flovent Diskus; Flovent HFA

Brand Names: Canada Flovent Diskus; Flovent HFA

Therapeutic Category Adrenal Corticosteroid; Anti-inflammatory Agent; Antiasthmatic; Corticosteroid, Inhalant (Oral); Glucocorticoid

Generic Availability (U.S.) No

Use Oral inhalation: Long-term (chronic) control of persistent bronchial asthma; **not** indicated for the relief of acute bronchospasm. Also used to help reduce or discontinue oral corticosteroid therapy for asthma (FDA approved in ages ≥4 years and adults)
Oral (swallowed; using metered dose inhaler): Has been used for eosinophilic esophagitis

Pregnancy Risk Factor C

Pregnancy Considerations Adverse events were observed in some animal reproduction studies.

Hypoadrenalism may occur in infants born to mothers receiving corticosteroids during pregnancy. Based on available data, an overall increased risk of congenital malformations or a decrease in fetal growth has not been associated with maternal use of inhaled corticosteroids during pregnancy (Bakhireva, 2005; NAEPP, 2005; Namazy, 2004). Uncontrolled asthma is associated with adverse events in pregnancy (increased risk of perinatal mortality, pre-eclampsia, preterm birth, low birth weight infants). Inhaled corticosteroids are recommended for the treatment of asthma during pregnancy (most information available using budesonide) (ACOG, 2008; NAEPP, 2005).

Breast-Feeding Considerations Systemic corticosteroids are excreted in human milk. It is not known if sufficient quantities of fluticasone are absorbed following inhalation to produce detectable amounts in breast milk. The manufacturer recommends that caution be exercised when administering fluticasone to nursing women. The use of inhaled corticosteroids is not considered a contraindication to breast-feeding (NAEPP, 2005).

Contraindications Hypersensitivity to fluticasone or any component; primary treatment of status asthmaticus

Warnings Fatalities have occurred due to adrenal insufficiency in asthmatic patients during and after switching from systemic corticosteroids to aerosol steroids; several months may be required for full recovery of hypothalamic-pituitary-adrenal (HPA) axis function; patients receiving higher doses of systemic corticosteroids (eg, adults receiving ≥20 mg of prednisone per day) may be at greater risk; during this period of HPA axis suppression, aerosol steroids do **not** provide the systemic glucocorticoid or mineralocorticoid activity needed to treat patients requiring stress doses (ie, patients with major stress such as trauma, surgery, infections, or other conditions associated with severe electrolyte loss). When used at high doses or for a prolonged time, hypercorticism and HPA axis suppression (including adrenal crisis) may occur; use with inhaled or systemic corticosteroids (even alternate-day dosing) may increase risk of HPA axis suppression. Acute adrenal insufficiency may occur with abrupt withdrawal after long-term use or with stress; withdrawal and discontinuation of corticosteroids should be done carefully; patients with HPA axis suppression may require doses of systemic glucocorticosteroids prior to, during, and after unusual stress (eg, surgery). Immunosuppression may occur; patients may be more susceptible to infections; avoid exposure to chickenpox and measles. Switching patients from systemic corticosteroids to aerosol steroids may unmask allergic conditions previously treated by the systemic steroid. Bronchospasm may occur after use of inhaled asthma medications.

Potent inhibitors of cytochrome P450 isoenzyme CYP3A4 (eg, ritonavir) may significantly increase fluticasone serum concentrations and result in systemic corticosteroid effects. Powder for oral inhalation (Flovent® Diskus®) contains lactose (milk proteins) which may cause allergic reactions in patients with severe milk protein allergy.

Precautions Avoid using higher than recommended doses; suppression of HPA function, suppression of linear growth (ie, reduction of growth velocity), reduced bone mineral density, hypercorticism (Cushing's syndrome), hyperglycemia, or glucosuria may occur; these adverse effects (as well as intracranial hypertension) may occur with topical use and have been reported in pediatric patients. Use with extreme caution in patients with respiratory tuberculosis, untreated systemic infections, or ocular herpes simplex. Use with caution and monitor patients closely with hepatic dysfunction. Eosinophilic conditions (eosinophilia, vasculitic rash, cardiac complications, worsening pulmonary symptoms, and/or neuropathy) may occur and are usually associated with withdrawal or decrease of oral corticosteroids after the initiation of

fluticasone (oral inhalation); a causal relationship by fluticasone has not been established. Increased IOP, glaucoma, and cataracts may occur with long-term use of inhaled corticosteroids.

Adverse Reactions

Central nervous system: Fatigue, fever, headache, malaise, pain

Dermatologic: Pruritus, rash

Gastrointestinal: Gastrointestinal infection (including viral), gastrointestinal discomfort/pain, nausea, oral candidiasis, vomiting

Neuromuscular & skeletal: Arthralgia, articular rheumatism, muscle injury, musculoskeletal pain

Respiratory: Bronchitis, cough, hoarseness/dysphonia, nasal congestion, rhinitis, sinusitis/sinus infection, throat irritation, upper respiratory tract inflammation/infection, viral respiratory infection

Miscellaneous: Viral infection

Rare but important or life-threatening: Aggression, agitation, anaphylactic reaction (rare with both products; Diskus® - some patients with severe milk allergy), angioedema, anxiety, aphonia, asthma exacerbation, behavioral changes (eg, hyperactivity and irritability in children; rare), bone mineral density decreased, bronchospasm (immediate and delayed), cataracts, chest tightness, Churg-Strauss syndrome, contusion, Cushingoid features, cutaneous hypersensitivity, depression, dyspnea, ecchymoses, eosinophilia, facial edema, growth velocity reduction in children/adolescents, HPA axis suppression, hyperglycemia, hypersensitivity reactions (immediate and delayed), laryngitis, migraine, muscle rigidity/stiffness/tightness, oropharyngeal edema, osteoporosis, paradoxical bronchospasm, pneumonia, restlessness, throat soreness, tooth discoloration, urticaria, vasculitis, wheeze

Drug Interactions

Metabolism/Transport Effects Substrate of CYP3A4 (major); **Note:** Assignment of Major/Minor substrate status based on clinically relevant drug interaction potential

Avoid Concomitant Use

Avoid concomitant use of Fluticasone (Oral Inhalation) with any of the following: Aldesleukin; BCG; Cobicistat; Conivaptan; Fusidic Acid (Systemic); Natalizumab; Pimecrolimus; Tacrolimus (Topical); Tofacitinib

Increased Effect/Toxicity

Fluticasone (Oral Inhalation) may increase the levels/effects of: Amphotericin B; Ceritinib; Deferasirox; Leflunomide; Loop Diuretics; Natalizumab; Thiazide Diuretics; Tofacitinib

The levels/effects of Fluticasone (Oral Inhalation) may be increased by: Ceritinib; Cobicistat; Conivaptan; CYP3A4 Inhibitors (Moderate); CYP3A4 Inhibitors (Strong); Dasatinib; Denosumab; Fusidic Acid (Systemic); Ivacaftor; Luliconazole; Mifepristone; Pimecrolimus; Simeprevir; Stiripentol; Tacrolimus (Topical); Telaprevir; Trastuzumab

Decreased Effect

Fluticasone (Oral Inhalation) may decrease the levels/effects of: Aldesleukin; Antidiabetic Agents; BCG; Coccidioidin Skin Test; Corticorelin; Hyaluronidase; Sipuleucel-T; Telaprevir; Vaccines (Inactivated)

The levels/effects of Fluticasone (Oral Inhalation) may be decreased by: Echinacea

Stability

Flovent® HFA: Store at controlled room temperature of 25°C (77°F) with mouthpiece down. Do not use or store near heat or open flame. Do not expose to temperatures >120°F. Do not puncture or incinerate. Discard device when the dose counter reads "000."

Diskus®: Store at controlled room temperature; keep dry; protect from direct heat or sunlight; discard Diskus® 6 weeks (for 50 mcg strength) or 2 months (for 100 mcg and 250 mcg strengths) after opening moistureproof foil overwrap or when dose indicator reads "0" (whichever comes first); **Note:** Diskus® device is not reusable.

Mechanism of Action Fluticasone belongs to a group of corticosteroids which utilizes a fluorocarbothioate ester linkage at the 17 carbon position; extremely potent vasoconstrictive and anti-inflammatory activity. The effectiveness of inhaled fluticasone is due to its direct local effect.

Pharmacodynamics Oral inhalation: Clinical effects are due to direct local effect rather than systemic absorption
Onset of action: Variable; may occur within 24 hours
Maximum effect: 1-2 weeks or more
Duration after discontinuation: Several days or more

Pharmacokinetics (Adult data unless noted)
Distribution: V_d: 4.2 L/kg
Protein binding: 91% to 99%
Metabolism: Via cytochrome P450 3A4 pathway to 17β-carboxylic acid (inactive)
Bioavailability: Oral inhalation: Flovent®: 30% of dose delivered from actuator; Flovent® HFA: 30% lower than Flovent®; Diskus®: 18%
Half-life: 7.8 hours

Dosing: Neonatal Inhalation: Bronchopulmonary dysplasia, treatment: See **Dosing: Usual** for dosing in infants (PNA in clinical trials >28 days)

Dosing: Usual
Oral inhalation:
Asthma: If adequate response is not seen after 2 weeks of initial dosage, increase dosage; doses should be titrated to the lowest effective dose once asthma is controlled:
Inhalation aerosol (Flovent® HFA): Manufacturer's recommendations:
Children 4-11 years: Initial: 88 mcg twice daily; maximum dose: 88 mcg twice daily
Children ≥12 years and Adults:
Patients previously treated with bronchodilators only: Initial: 88 mcg twice daily; maximum dose: 440 mcg twice daily
Patients treated with an inhaled corticosteroid: Initial: 88-220 mcg twice daily; maximum dose: 440 mcg twice daily; may start doses above 88 mcg twice daily in poorly controlled patients or in those who previously required higher doses of inhaled corticosteroids
Patients previously treated with oral corticosteroids: 440 mcg twice daily; maximum dose: 880 mcg twice daily
NIH Asthma Guidelines (NAEPP, 2007) (give in divided doses twice daily):
Children <12 years:
"Low" dose: 88-176 mcg/day (44 mcg/puff: 2-4 puffs/day)
"Medium" dose: >176-352 mcg/day (44 mcg/puff: 4-8 puffs/day or 110 mcg/puff: 2-3 puffs/day)
"High" dose: >352 mcg/day (110 mcg/puff: >3 puffs/day or 220 mcg/puff: >1 puff/day)
Children ≥12 years and Adults:
"Low" dose: 88-264 mcg/day (44 mcg/puff: 2-6 puffs/day or 110 mcg/puff: 2 puffs/day)
"Medium" dose: >264-440 mcg/day (110 mcg/puff: 2-4 puffs/day)
"High" dose: >440 mcg/day (110 mcg/puff: >4 puffs/day or 220 mcg/puff: >2 puffs/day)
Bronchopulmonary dysplasia, treatment: Infants: Some centers have used 2-4 puffs (44 mcg/puff) every 12 hours via a face mask and a spacer. One trial used fixed doses administered via a spacer and neonatal anesthesia bag (into ventilator, directly into nasopharyngeal endotracheal tube, or with a face mask) in 16 former preterm neonates (GA: ≤32 weeks; PNA: 28-60 days); chest radiograph score was improved compared to placebo; the treatment group had increased blood pressure compared to baseline; the authors conclude that the trial results do not support the use of fluticasone in oxygen-dependent patients with moderate BPD; exact dosing cannot be replicated in the U.S. with available products (Dugas, 2005)
Body weight:
0.5-1.2 kg: 125 mcg every 12 hours for 3 weeks, followed by 125 mcg once daily for the 4th week
≥1.2 kg: 250 mcg every 12 hours for 3 weeks, followed by 250 mcg once daily for the 4th week

Inhalation powder (Flovent® Diskus®): Manufacturer's recommendations:
Children 4-11 years: Patients previously treated with bronchodilators alone or inhaled corticosteroids: Initial: 50 mcg twice daily; maximum dose: 100 mcg twice daily; may start higher initial dose in poorly controlled patients or in those who previously required higher doses of inhaled corticosteroids
Adolescents and Adults:
Patients previously treated with bronchodilators alone: Initial: 100 mcg twice daily; maximum dose: 500 mcg twice daily
Patients previously treated with inhaled corticosteroids: Initial: 100-250 mcg twice daily; maximum dose: 500 mcg twice daily; may start doses above 100 mcg twice daily in poorly controlled patients or in those who previously required higher doses of inhaled corticosteroids
Patients previously treated with oral corticosteroids: Initial: 500-1000 mcg twice daily (select dose based on assessment of individual patient); maximum dose: 1000 mcg twice daily; **Note:** Inability to reduce oral corticosteroid therapy may indicate need for maximum fluticasone dose.
NIH Asthma Guidelines (NAEPP, 2007) (give in divided doses twice daily):
Children 5-11 years:
"Low" dose: 100-200 mcg/day (50 mcg/puff: 2-4 puffs/day or 100 mcg/puff: 1-2 puffs/day)
"Medium" dose: >200-400 mcg/day (50 mcg/puff: 4-8 puffs/day or 100 mcg/puff: 2-4 puffs/day)
"High" dose: >400 mcg/day (50 mcg/puff: >8 puffs/day or 100 mcg/puff: >4 puffs/day)
Children ≥12 years and Adults:
"Low" dose: 100-300 mcg/day (50 mcg/puff: 2-6 puffs/day or 100 mcg/puff: 1-3 puffs/day)
"Medium" dose: >300-500 mcg/day (50 mcg/puff: 6-10 puffs/day or 100 mcg/puff: 3-5 puffs/day)
"High" dose: >500 mcg/day (50 mcg/puff: >10 puffs/day or 100 mcg/puff: >5 puffs/day)

Oral (swallowed): Note: Patients use an oral inhaler without a spacer and swallow the medication.
Children: Eosinophilic esophagitis: Optimal dose and dosing regimen are not established. Dosing from two more recent studies is presented.
A randomized, double-blind, placebo-controlled trial (n=31) demonstrated efficacy by assessment of histologic remission (Konikoff, 2006): Children: 3-16 years: 440 mcg twice daily for 3 months
A prospective, randomized trial (n=80) compared swallowed fluticasone to oral prednisone; a greater degree of improvement in histologic response was seen in the prednisone group; however, no difference in clinical response was observed between the two groups (Schaffer, 2008):
Children: 1-10 years: 220 mcg 4 times daily for 4 weeks, 220 mcg 3 times daily for 3 weeks, 220 mcg twice daily for 3 weeks, 220 mcg daily for 2 weeks
Children and Adolescents: 11-18 years: 440 mcg 4 times daily for 4 weeks, 440 mcg 3 times daily for 3 weeks, 440 mcg twice daily for 3 weeks, 440 mcg daily for 2 weeks

Dosage adjustment in hepatic impairment: Use with caution; monitor patients closely; **Note:** Fluticasone is primarily eliminated via hepatic metabolism and serum concentrations may be elevated in patients with hepatic disease.

Administration

Oral inhalation: Rinse mouth with water (without swallowing) after inhalation to decrease chance of oral candidiasis.

Aerosol inhalation: Shake canister well for 5 seconds before each spray; use at room temperature. Inhaler must be primed before first use with four test sprays (spray into air away from face, shake well for 5 seconds between sprays) and primed again with one test spray if not used for >7 days or if dropped. Use a spacer device for children <8 years of age. Patient should contact pharmacy for refill when the dose counter reads "020." Discard device when the dose counter reads "000." Do not try to alter numbers on counter or remove the counter from the metal canister. Do not immerse canister into water (ie, do not use "float test" to determine contents).

Powder for oral inhalation: Flovent® Diskus®: Do not use with spacer device; do not exhale into Diskus®; do not wash or take apart; activate and use Diskus® in horizontal position

Oral (swallowed): **Note:** This method of administration is for treatment of eosinophilic esophagitis only. Use metered dose inhaler. Do not use a spacer. Shake canister well for 5 seconds before each spray. Prime inhaler as outlined above. Actuate inhaler and spray medication into pharynx; swallow the medication (rather than inhale). Do not eat, drink, or rinse mouth for 30 minutes following administration (Konikoff, 2006; Schaefer, 2008).

Monitoring Parameters Check mucus membranes for signs of fungal infection; monitor growth in pediatric patients; monitor IOP with therapy >6 weeks. Monitor for symptoms of asthma, FEV_1, peak flow, and/or other pulmonary function tests. Assess HPA suppression in patients using potent topical steroids applied to a large surface area or to areas under occlusion.

Additional Information Flovent® HFA does **not** contain CFCs as the propellant; Flovent® HFA is packaged in a plastic-coated, moisture-protective foil pouch that also contains a desiccant; the desiccant should be discarded when the pouch is opened

When using fluticasone oral inhalation to help reduce or discontinue oral corticosteroid therapy, begin prednisone taper after at least 1 week of fluticasone inhalation therapy; do not decrease prednisone faster than 2.5 mg/day on a weekly basis; monitor patients for signs of asthma instability and adrenal insufficiency; decrease fluticasone to lowest effective dose **after** prednisone reduction is complete. If bronchospasm with wheezing occurs after oral inhalation use, a fast-acting bronchodilator may be used; discontinue orally inhaled corticosteroid and initiate alternative chronic therapy.

Oral (swallowed) use: In the study by Schaffer that compared swallowed fluticasone to oral prednisone, systemic adverse effects occurred more frequently in the oral prednisone group; esophageal candidiasis occurred in 15% of patients using swallowed fluticasone (Schaffer, 2008).

Dosage Forms Considerations

Flovent HFA 10.6 g and 12 g canisters contain 120 inhalations.

Dosage Forms Excipient information presented when available (limited, particularly for generics); consult specific product labeling.

Aerosol, Inhalation, as propionate:
Flovent HFA: 44 mcg/actuation (10.6 g); 110 mcg/actuation (12 g); 220 mcg/actuation (12 g)

Aerosol Powder Breath Activated, Inhalation, as propionate:
Flovent Diskus: 50 mcg/blister (60 ea); 100 mcg/blister (28 ea, 60 ea); 250 mcg/blister (28 ea, 60 ea) [contains lactose]

References

ACOG Committee on Practice Bulletins-Obstetrics, "ACOG Practice Bulletin: Clinical Management Guidelines for Obstetrician-Gynecologists Number 90, February 2008: Asthma in Pregnancy," Obstet Gynecol, 2008, 111(2 Pt 1):457-64.

Bakhireva LN, Jones KL, Schatz M, et al, "Asthma Medication Use in Pregnancy and Fetal Growth," J Allergy Clin Immunol, 2005, 116 (3):503-9.

Dugas MA, Nguyen D, Frenette L, et al, "Fluticasone Inhalation in Moderate Cases of Bronchopulmonary Dysplasia," Pediatrics, 2005, 115(5):566-72.

Fok TF, Lam K, Dolovich M, et al, "Randomised Controlled Study of Early Use of Inhaled Corticosteroid in Preterm Infants With Respiratory Distress Syndrome," Arch Dis Child Fetal Neonatal Ed, 1999, 80 (3):203-8.

Konikoff MR, Noel RJ, Blanchard C, et al, "A Randomized, Double-Blind, Placebo-Controlled Trial of Fluticasone Propionate for Pediatric Eosinophilic Esophagitis," Gastroenterology, 2006, 131(5):1381-91.

Namazy J, Schatz M, Long L, et al, "Use of Inhaled Steroids by Pregnant Asthmatic Women Does Not Reduce Intrauterine Growth," J Allergy Clin Immunol, 2004, 113(3):427-32.

National Asthma Education and Prevention Program (NAEPP), "Expert Panel Report 3 (EPR-3): Guidelines for the Diagnosis and Management of Asthma," Clinical Practice Guidelines, National Institutes of Health, National Heart, Lung, and Blood Institute, NIH Publication No. 08-4051, prepublication 2007. Available at http://www.nhlbi.nih.gov/guidelines/asthma/asthgdln.htm.

National Asthma Education and Prevention Program (NAEPP) Working Group Report on "Managing Asthma During Pregnancy: Recommendations for Pharmacologic Treatment," National Institutes of Health, National Heart, Lung, and Blood Institute, NIH Publication No. 05-5236, March 2005. Available at http://www.nhlbi.nih.gov/health/prof/lung/asthma/astpreg/astpreg_full.pdf

Ng PC, Fok TF, Liu F, et al, "Effects of Inhaled Corticosteroids on Systemic Blood Pressure in Preterm Infants," Biol Neonate, 2004, 86(3):201-6.

Schaffer ET, Fitzgerald JF, Molleston JP, et al, "Comparison of Oral Prednisone and Topical Fluticasone in the Treatment of Eosinophilic Esophagitis: A Randomized Trial in Children," Clin Gastroenterol Hepatol, 2008, 6(2):165-73.

Fluticasone (Nasal) (floo TIK a sone)

Medication Safety Issues

Sound-alike/look-alike issues:
Flonase® may be confused with Flovent®

International issues:
Allegro: Brand name for fluticasone [Israel], but also the brand name for frovatriptan [Germany]

Allegro [Israel] may be confused with Allegra and Allegra-D brand names for fexofenadine and fexofenadine/pseudoephedrine, respectively, [U.S., Canada, and multiple international markets]

Brand Names: U.S. Flonase; Veramyst

Brand Names: Canada Apo-Fluticasone®; Avamys®; Flonase®; ratio-Fluticasone

Therapeutic Category Corticosteroid, Intranasal

Generic Availability (U.S.) Yes

Use

Flonase®: Management of nasal symptoms associated with seasonal and perennial allergic rhinitis and nonallergic rhinitis (FDA approved in ages ≥4 years and adults)

Veramyst®: Management of nasal symptoms associated with seasonal and perennial allergic rhinitis (FDA approved in ages ≥2 years and adults)

Intranasal corticosteroids have also been used as an adjunct to antibiotics in empiric treatment of acute bacterial rhinosinusitis primarily in patients with history of allergic rhinitis (Chow, 2012) and in pediatric patients with mild obstructive sleep apnea syndrome who cannot undergo adenotonsillectomy or who still have symptoms after surgery (Marcus, 2012).

◄ **Pregnancy Risk Factor** C

Pregnancy Considerations Adverse events were observed in some animal reproduction studies. Hypoadrenalism may occur in newborns following maternal use of corticosteroids in pregnancy; monitor. Intranasal corticosteroids are recommended for the treatment of rhinitis during pregnancy; the lowest effective dose should be used (NAEPP, 2005; Wallace, 2008).

Breast-Feeding Considerations Systemic corticosteroids are excreted in human milk. It is not known if sufficient quantities of fluticasone are absorbed following inhalation to produce detectable amounts in breast milk. The manufacturer recommends caution be used if administered to nursing women. The use of inhaled corticosteroids is not considered a contraindication to breast-feeding (NAEPP, 2005).

Contraindications Hypersensitivity to fluticasone or any component

Warnings HPA suppression or hypercorticism (Cushing's syndrome) may occur with use of higher than recommended doses or at typical doses in susceptible patients. Acute adrenal insufficiency may occur with abrupt withdrawal after long-term use, with stress, or when converting from systemic to topical corticosteroid therapy; withdrawal or discontinuation of corticosteroids should be done carefully; patients with HPA axis suppression may require doses of systemic glucocorticosteroids prior to, during, and after unusual stress (eg, surgery). Immunosuppression may occur; patients may be more susceptible to infections; avoid exposure to chickenpox and measles. Epistaxis may occur.

Potent inhibitors of cytochrome P450 isoenzyme CYP3A4 (eg, ritonavir, ketoconazole) may significantly increase fluticasone serum concentrations and result in systemic corticosteroid effects.

Fluticasone is available in furoate and propionate salt formulations which are not interchangeable on a mcg-per-mcg basis.

Precautions Avoid using higher than recommended dosages; suppression of HPA function, suppression of linear growth (ie, reduction of growth velocity), reduced bone mineral density, or hypercorticism (Cushing's syndrome) may occur; titrate to lowest effective dose. Reduction in growth velocity may occur when corticosteroids are administered to pediatric patients, even at recommended doses via intranasal route (monitor growth). In a small pediatric study conducted over 1 year, no statistically significant effect on growth velocity or clinically relevant changes in bone mineral density or HPA axis function were observed in children 3-9 years of age receiving fluticasone propionate nasal spray (200 mcg/day; n=56) versus placebo (n=52); effects at higher doses or in susceptible pediatric patients cannot be ruled out. Use fluticasone with extreme caution in patients with respiratory tuberculosis; untreated bacterial, fungal, systemic viral or parasitic infections; or ocular herpes simplex. Localized *Candida* infections of the nose and pharynx have been reported rarely; interruption of therapy may be necessary while antifungal therapy is employed. Corticosteroids impair wound healing; avoid use in patients with recent nasal ulcers, nasal surgery, or nasal trauma; allow healing to occur before use. Glaucoma, increased intraocular pressure and cataracts have been reported following the intranasal application of corticosteroids; monitor patients who have change in vision and in patients with a history of increased ocular pressure, glaucoma, or cataracts. Use of nasal fluticasone in place of systemic corticosteroids may unmask allergies (eg, eczema, rhinitis) that were previously controlled by the systemic corticosteroids. Rare cases of immediate hypersensitivity reactions or nasal septum perforation may occur with intranasal corticosteroids.

Adverse Reactions

Central nervous system: Dizziness, fever, headache

Gastrointestinal: Abdominal pain, diarrhea, nausea, vomiting

Neuromuscular & skeletal: Back pain

Respiratory: Asthma symptoms, blood in nasal mucous, bronchitis, cough, epistaxis, nasal ulcer, pharyngitis, pharyngolaryngeal pain, runny nose

Miscellaneous: Aches and pains, flu-like syndrome

Rare but important or life-threatening: Alteration or loss of sense of taste and/or smell, anaphylaxis/anaphylactoid reactions, angioedema, AST increased, AV block (second degree), cataracts, conjunctivitis, glaucoma, hypersensitivity reactions, increased intraocular pressure, nasal candidiasis, nasal septal perforation (rare), psychomotor hyperactivity, skin rash, tremor, vaginal candidiasis

Drug Interactions

Metabolism/Transport Effects Substrate of CYP3A4 (minor); **Note:** Assignment of Major/Minor substrate status based on clinically relevant drug interaction potential

Avoid Concomitant Use

Avoid concomitant use of Fluticasone (Nasal) with any of the following: Ritonavir

Increased Effect/Toxicity

Fluticasone (Nasal) may increase the levels/effects of: Ceritinib

The levels/effects of Fluticasone (Nasal) may be increased by: Cobicistat; CYP3A4 Inhibitors (Strong); Ritonavir; Telaprevir

Decreased Effect There are no known significant interactions involving a decrease in effect.

Stability

Flonase®: Store between 4°C to 30°C (39°F to 86°F)

Veramyst®: Store between 15°C to 30°C (59°F to 86°F) in upright position. Do not refrigerate or freeze.

Mechanism of Action Fluticasone belongs to a group of corticosteroids which utilizes a fluorocarbothioate ester linkage at the 17 carbon position; extremely potent vasoconstrictive and anti-inflammatory activity

Pharmacodynamics Onset of action: Variable; may occur within 24 hours

Pharmacokinetics (Adult data unless noted) Bioavailability: ≤2%

Dosing: Usual Note: Product formulations are not interchangeable: Flonase®: One spray delivers 50 mcg; Veramyst®: One spray delivers 27.5 mcg

Children and Adolescents: **Seasonal and perennial rhinitis:** Intranasal: **Note:** For optimal effects, nasal spray should be used at regular intervals (eg, once or twice daily); however, some patients ≥12 years of age with seasonal allergic rhinitis may have effective control of symptoms with prn (as needed) use.

Flonase® (fluticasone propionate): Children ≥4 years and Adolescents: Initial: 100 mcg once daily delivered as 50 mcg (1 spray) **per nostril** once daily. If response is inadequate, increase to 200 mcg once daily given as 100 mcg (2 sprays) **per nostril** once daily. Once symptoms are controlled, reduce dose to 100 mcg once daily delivered as 50 mcg (1 spray) **per nostril** once daily.

Veramyst® (fluticasone furoate):

Children 2-11 years: Initial: 55 mcg once daily delivered as 27.5 mcg (1 spray) **per nostril** once daily; if response is inadequate, increase to 110 mcg once daily delivered as 55 mcg (2 sprays) **per nostril** once daily; once symptoms have been controlled, the dosage may be reduced to 55 mcg once daily delivered as 27.5 mcg (1 spray) **per nostril** once daily

Children ≥12 years and Adolescents: Initial: 110 mcg once daily delivered as 55 mcg (2 sprays) **per nostril** once daily; once symptoms are controlled, dosage may be reduced to 55 mcg once daily delivered as 27.5 mcg (1 spray) **per nostril** once daily

Adults: **Seasonal and perennial rhinitis:** Intranasal: **Note:** For optimal effects, nasal spray should be used at regular intervals (eg, once or twice daily); however, some adult patients with seasonal allergic rhinitis may have effective control of symptoms with prn (as needed) use.

Flonase® (fluticasone propionate): Initial: 200 mcg once daily delivered as 100 mcg (2 sprays) **per nostril** once daily; alternatively, the same total daily dosage may be divided and given as 100 mcg twice daily administered as 50 mcg (1 spray) **per nostril** twice daily. After the first few days, dosage may be reduced to 100 mcg once daily delivered as 50 mcg (1 spray) **per nostril** once daily for maintenance therapy.

Veramyst® (fluticasone furoate): Initial: 110 mcg once daily delivered as 55 mcg (2 sprays) **per nostril** once daily; once symptoms are controlled, may reduce dosage to 55 mcg once daily delivered as 27.5 mcg (1 spray) **per nostril** for maintenance therapy.

Dosing adjustment in renal impairment: No adjustment required.

Dosing adjustment in hepatic impairment: There are no dosage adjustments provided in the manufacturer's labeling. Use with caution in patients with severe hepatic impairment; systemic availability of fluticasone may be increased in patients with hepatic impairment.

Administration Shake well prior to each use. Blow nose to clear nostrils before each use. Insert applicator into nostril, keeping bottle upright, and close off the other nostril. Breathe in through nose. While inhaling, press pump to release spray. Do not spray into eyes. Discard after labeled number of doses has been used, even if bottle is not completely empty.

Flonase®: Prime pump (press 6 times until fine spray appears) prior to first use or if spray unused for ≥7 days.

Veramyst®: Prime pump (press 6 times until fine spray appears) prior to first use, if spray unused for >30 days, or if cap left off bottle for ≥5 days.

Monitoring Parameters Mucous membranes for signs of fungal infection, growth (pediatric patients), signs/symptoms of HPA axis suppression/adrenal insufficiency; ocular changes

Additional Information When used short term as adjunctive therapy in acute bacterial rhinosinusitis (ABRS), intranasal steroids show modest symptomatic improvement and few adverse effects, improvement is primarily due to increased sinus drainage. Use should be considered optional in ABRS; however, intranasal corticosteroids should be routinely prescribed to ABRS patients who have a history of or concurrent allergic rhinitis (Chow, 2012).

Dosage Forms Considerations

Flonase 16 g bottles and Veramyst 10 g bottles contain 120 sprays each.

Dosage Forms Excipient information presented when available (limited, particularly for generics); consult specific product labeling.

Suspension, Nasal, as furoate:

Veramyst: 27.5 mcg/spray (10 g) [contains benzalkonium chloride]

Suspension, Nasal, as propionate:

Flonase: 50 mcg/actuation (16 g) [contains benzalkonium chloride, polysorbate 80]

Generic: 50 mcg/actuation (16 g); 50 mcg/actuation (16 g)

References

Bakhireva LN, Jones KL, Schatz M, et al, "Asthma Medication Use in Pregnancy and Fetal Growth," *J Allergy Clin Immunol*, 2005, 116 (3):503-9.

Chow AW, Benninger MS, Brook I, et al, "IDSA Clinical Practice Guideline For Acute Bacterial Rhinosinusitis in Children and Adults," *Clin Infect Dis*, 2012, 54(8):e72-e112.

Marcus CL, Brooks LJ, Draper KA, et al, "Diagnosis and Management of Childhood Obstructive Sleep Apnea Syndrome," *Pediatrics*, 2012, 130(3):576-84.

NAEPP Working Group Report on "Managing Asthma During Pregnancy: Recommendations for Pharmacologic Treatment," National Institutes of Health, National Heart, Lung, and Blood Institute, NIH Publication No. 05-5236, March 2005. Available at http://www.nhlbi. nih.gov/health/prof/lung/asthma/astpreg_full.pdf

Namazy J, Schatz M, Long L, et al, "Use of Inhaled Steroids by Pregnant Asthmatic Women Does Not Reduce Intrauterine Growth," *J Allergy Clin Immunol*, 2004, 113(3):427-32.

Wallace DV, Dykewicz MS, Bernstein DI, et al, "The Diagnosis and Management of Rhinitis: An Updated Practice Parameter," *J Allergy Clin Immunol*, 2008, 122(2 Suppl):S1-84.

Fluticasone (Topical) (floo TIK a sone)

Medication Safety Issues

Sound-alike/look-alike issues:

Cutivate® may be confused with Ultravate®

International issues:

Allegro: Brand name for fluticasone [Israel], but also the brand name for frovatriptan [Germany]

Allegro [Israel] may be confused with Allegra and Allegra-D brand names for fexofenadine and fexofenadine/pseudoephedrine, respectively, [U.S., Canada, and multiple international markets]

Related Information

Topical Corticosteroids *on page 2224*

Brand Names: U.S. Cutivate

Brand Names: Canada Cutivate™

Therapeutic Category Corticosteroid, Topical

Generic Availability (U.S.) Yes

Use

Cream: Relief of inflammation and pruritus associated with corticosteroid-responsive dermatoses (eg, atopic dermatitis) (medium potency topical corticosteroid) (FDA approved in ages ≥3 months and adults)

Lotion: Relief of inflammation and pruritus associated with atopic dermatitis (FDA approved in ages ≥1 year and adults)

Ointment: Relief of inflammation and pruritus associated with corticosteroid-responsive dermatoses (medium potency topical corticosteroid) (FDA approved in adults)

Pregnancy Risk Factor C

Pregnancy Considerations Adverse events have been observed with systemic corticosteroids in animal reproduction studies. In general, the use of topical corticosteroids during pregnancy is not considered to have significant risk; however, intrauterine growth retardation in the infant has been reported (rare). The use of large amounts or for prolonged periods of time should be avoided.

Breast-Feeding Considerations Systemic corticosteroids are excreted in human milk. It is not known if sufficient quantities of fluticasone are absorbed following topical administration to produce detectable amounts in breast milk. Hypertension in the nursing infant has been reported following corticosteroid ointment applied to the nipples. Use with caution.

Contraindications Hypersensitivity to fluticasone or any component

Warnings Adverse systemic effects may occur when topical steroids are used on large areas of the body, denuded areas, for prolonged periods of time, with an occlusive dressing, and/or in infants or small children; infants and small children may be more susceptible to HPA axis suppression or other systemic toxicities due to a larger skin surface area to body mass ratio; use with caution in pediatric patients. HPA axis suppression occurred in two children (2 and 5 years old) of 43 pediatric patients treated topically with fluticasone cream for 4 weeks; application covered at least 35% of body surface area. HPA axis ▶

suppression was not reported with use of fluticasone lotion for at least 3-4 weeks in young pediatric patients (4 months to <6 years) during clinical trials; however, it cannot be ruled out when topical fluticasone is used in any patient and especially with longer use.

Do not use for the treatment of rosacea, perioral dermatitis, or in the presence of skin atrophy or infection at treatment site. Cutivate® lotion and cream contain imidurea, an excipient; imidurea releases trace amounts of formaldehyde which may cause allergic sensitization, irritation, or may prevent healing or worsen dermatitis; avoid use in patients with sensitivity to formaldehyde; discontinue if irritation occurs and institute appropriate therapy.

Precautions Avoid using higher than recommended doses; suppression of HPA function, suppression of linear growth (ie, reduction of growth velocity), reduced bone mineral density, hypercorticism (Cushing's syndrome), hyperglycemia, or glucosuria may occur; these adverse effects (as well as intracranial hypertension) may occur with topical use and have been reported in pediatric patients.

Enhanced tumor growth has been reported in mice exposed concurrently to low-level ultraviolet (UV) radiation and topical fluticasone lotion and lotion vehicle alone; clinical applicability of these results to humans is unknown; enhanced tumor growth in humans has not been reported; however, patients should minimize UV light exposure when using fluticasone topical products; avoid excessive or unnecessary exposure to natural and artificial sunlight, including sunbathing, tanning booths, sun lamps, etc.

Adverse Reactions

Dermatologic: Dryness, eczema infection, exacerbation of eczema, pruritus, rash (erythematous; children), skin irritation, telangiectasia (children)

Neuromuscular & skeletal: Numbness of fingers

Rare but important or life-threatening: Acneiform eruptions, atrophy, blurred vision, Cushing syndrome, dermatitis, edema, folliculitis, hemorrhage, hyperglycemia, immunosuppression, leukopenia, secondary infection, sepsis, skin discoloration, thrombocytopenia, urticaria, viral warts

Reported with other topical corticosteroids (in decreasing order of occurrence): Hypopigmentation, perioral dermatitis, allergic contact dermatitis, skin atrophy, striae, hypertrichosis, miliaria, pustular psoriasis from chronic plaque psoriasis

Drug Interactions

Metabolism/Transport Effects Substrate of CYP3A4 (minor); **Note:** Assignment of Major/Minor substrate status based on clinically relevant drug interaction potential

Avoid Concomitant Use

Avoid concomitant use of Fluticasone (Topical) with any of the following: Aldesleukin

Increased Effect/Toxicity

Fluticasone (Topical) may increase the levels/effects of: Ceritinib; Deferasirox

The levels/effects of Fluticasone (Topical) may be increased by: Telaprevir

Decreased Effect

Fluticasone (Topical) may decrease the levels/effects of: Aldesleukin; Corticorelin; Hyaluronidase; Telaprevir

Stability

Cream, ointment: Store at 2°C to 30°C (36°F to 86°F).

Lotion: Store at 15°C to 30°C (59°F to 86°F). Do not refrigerate; keep tightly closed.

Mechanism of Action Fluticasone belongs to a group of corticosteroids which utilizes a fluorocarbothioate ester linkage at the 17 carbon position; extremely potent vasoconstrictive and anti-inflammatory activity; has a weak HPA inhibitory potency when applied topically, which gives the drug a high therapeutic index. The mechanism of action for all topical corticosteroids is believed to be a combination of three important properties: anti-inflammatory activity, immunosuppressive properties, and antiproliferative actions.

Dosing: Usual Topical: **Note:** If no improvement is seen within 2 weeks, reassessment of diagnosis may be necessary.

Infants, Children, and Adolescents: **Note:** Safety and efficacy of use >4 weeks in pediatric patients have not been established.

Atopic dermatitis:

Infants ≥3 months, Children, and Adolescents: Cream: Apply sparingly to affected area once or twice daily

Children ≥1 year and Adolescents: Lotion: Apply sparingly to affected area once daily

Corticosteroid-responsive dermatoses: Infants ≥3 months, Children, and Adolescents: Cream: Apply sparingly to affected area twice daily

Adults:

Atopic dermatitis: Cream, lotion: Apply sparingly to affected area once or twice daily

Corticosteroid-responsive dermatoses: Cream, lotion, ointment: Apply sparingly to affected area twice daily

Administration Apply sparingly to affected area, gently rub in until disappears; do not use on open skin; avoid application on face, underarms, or groin area unless directed by physician; avoid contact with eyes; do not occlude area unless directed; do not apply to diaper area

Dosage Forms Excipient information presented when available (limited, particularly for generics); consult specific product labeling.

Cream, External, as propionate:

Cutivate: 0.05% (30 g, 60 g) [contains cetyl alcohol, propylene glycol]

Generic: 0.05% (15 g, 30 g, 60 g)

Lotion, External, as propionate:

Cutivate: 0.05% (120 mL) [contains cetostearyl alcohol, methylparaben, propylene glycol, propylparaben]

Generic: 0.05% (60 mL, 120 mL)

Ointment, External, as propionate:

Cutivate: 0.005% (30 g, 60 g)

Generic: 0.005% (15 g, 30 g, 60 g)

References

Schaffer ET, Fitzgerald JF, Molleston JP, et al, "Comparison of Oral Prednisone and Topical Fluticasone in the Treatment of Eosinophilic Esophagitis: A Randomized Trial in Children," Clin Gastroenterol Hepatol, 2008, 6(2):165-73.

Fluticasone and Salmeterol

(floo TIK a sone & sal ME te role)

Medication Safety Issues

Sound-alike/look-alike issues:

Advair may be confused with Adcirca, Advicor

Brand Names: U.S. Advair Diskus; Advair HFA

Brand Names: Canada Advair; Advair Diskus

Therapeutic Category Adrenal Corticosteroid; Adrenergic Agonist Agent; Anti-inflammatory Agent; Antiasthmatic; Beta₂-Adrenergic Agonist; Bronchodilator; Corticosteroid, Inhalant (Oral); Glucocorticoid

Generic Availability (U.S.) No

Use

Advair Diskus®, Advair® HFA: Maintenance treatment of asthma (Advair Diskus®: FDA approved in ages ≥4 years and adults; Advair® HFA: FDA approved in ages ≥12 years and adults); **NOT** indicated for the relief of acute bronchospasm

Advair Diskus®: Maintenance treatment of airflow obstruction in patients with COPD associated with chronic bronchitis and emphysema (FDA approved in adults); **NOT** indicated for the relief of acute bronchospasm

Medication Guide Available Yes

Pregnancy Risk Factor C

Pregnancy Considerations Adverse events were observed in animal reproduction studies using this combination. Refer to individual agents.

Breast-Feeding Considerations It is not known if fluticasone or salmeterol are excreted into breast milk. The manufacturer recommends that caution be used if administering this combination to breast-feeding women. Refer to individual agents.

Contraindications Hypersensitivity to salmeterol, adrenergic amines, fluticasone, or any component; severe hypersensitivity to milk proteins (Advair Diskus®); primary treatment of status asthmaticus or other acute episodes of asthma or COPD

Warnings Long-acting beta$_2$-adrenergic agents (LABAs), including salmeterol, increase the risk of asthma-related deaths **[U.S. Boxed Warning]**. Fluticasone and salmeterol should only be prescribed in patients not adequately controlled on long-term asthma-controller medications (ie, inhaled corticosteroid) or disease severity requires initiation with two maintenance therapies. In a large clinical trial, LABA (salmeterol) use was associated with an increase in asthma-related deaths compared to placebo (when added to usual asthma therapy); risk is considered a class effect among all LABAs. Data are not available to determine if the addition of an inhaled corticosteroid lessens this increased risk of death associated with LABA use or if LABA use also increases the risk of death in patients with COPD. Assess patients at regular intervals once asthma control is maintained on combination therapy to determine if step down therapy is appropriate (without loss of asthma control), and if the patient can be maintained on an inhaled corticosteroid alone. LABAs are not appropriate in patients whose asthma is adequately controlled on low- or medium-dose inhaled corticosteroids. LABAs may increase the risk of asthma-related hospitalization in pediatric and adolescent patients **[U.S. Boxed Warning]**; when addition of a LABA is clinically indicated in patients <18 years of age, a combination product containing a LABA and an inhaled corticosteroid is preferred to ensure compliance.

Fluticasone and salmeterol should not be used to relieve acute asthmatic or COPD symptoms, rapidly deteriorating or potentially life-threatening episodes of asthma or COPD; acute episodes should be treated with short-acting beta$_2$-agonist. Routine use of inhaled, short-acting beta$_2$-agonists should be discontinued prior to initiation of fluticasone and salmeterol. Fluticasone and salmeterol should not be used more frequently than recommended (twice daily), at higher doses or with any additional long-acting beta$_2$-adrenergic agonist; adverse cardiovascular effects (possibly fatal) have been reported with excessive beta$_2$-adrenergic overstimulation.

Fatalities have occurred due to adrenal insufficiency in asthmatic patients during and after switching from systemic corticosteroids to inhaled steroids; several months may be required for full recovery of hypothalamic-pituitary-adrenal (HPA) function; patients receiving higher doses of systemic corticosteroids (eg, adults receiving ≥20 mg of prednisone per day) may be at greater risk; during this period of adrenal suppression, inhaled steroids do not provide the systemic glucocorticoid or mineralocorticoid activity needed to treat patients requiring stress doses (ie, patients with major stress such as trauma, surgery, infections, or other conditions associated with severe electrolyte loss); when used at high doses HPA suppression may occur; use of inhaled or systemic corticosteroids (even alternate-day dosing) may increase risk of HPA suppression. Acute adrenal insufficiency may occur with abrupt withdrawal after long-term use or with stress; withdrawal and discontinuation of corticosteroid therapy should be done carefully; patients with HPA axis suppression may require doses of systemic glucocorticosteroids prior to, during, and after unusual stress (eg, surgery). Switching

patients from systemic corticosteroids to inhaled steroids may unmask allergic conditions (eg, rhinitis, conjunctivitis, eczema, arthritis, eosinophilic conditions) previously suppressed by the systemic steroid. Immunosuppression may occur; patients may be more susceptible to infections; avoid exposure to chickenpox and measles. Lower respiratory tract infections, including pneumonia, have been reported in patients with COPD using the oral inhalation with an even higher incidence in the elderly.

C. albicans infections of the mouth and pharynx may occur with orally inhaled corticosteroid use, mostly mild to moderate; interruption of therapy may be necessary at times while antifungal therapy is employed; advise patients to rinse mouth after use. Hypersensitivity reactions with angioedema and swelling of the lips, tongue, and pharynx have been reported rarely.

Not recommended for use with strong CYP3A4 inhibitors (eg, ketoconazole, ritonavir, atazanavir, clarithromycin, indinavir, itraconazole, nefazodone, nelfinavir, saquinavir, telithromycin) due to potential for an increased risk of cardiovascular events and may also increase mometasone serum concentrations and result in systemic corticosteroids effects.

Precautions Use with caution in patients with cardiovascular disorders (especially coronary insufficiency, arrhythmias, hypertension, heart failure); although uncommon at recommended doses, beta-agonists may cause elevation in BP and HR and result in CNS stimulation and excitation. Caution should also be used in patients with thyrotoxicosis, seizure disorders, or conditions that are unusually sensitive to the effects of sympathomimetic amines. Transient hypokalemia from intracellular shunting may occur and produce adverse cardiovascular effects. Use with caution in patients with diabetes mellitus (DM); beta$_2$-agonists can increase serum glucose aggravating preexisting DM and ketoacidosis. Use caution in patients with hepatic impairment. Immediate hypersensitivity reactions (urticaria, angioedema, rash, bronchospasm) have been reported. Powder for oral inhalation (Advair Diskus®) contains lactose; very rare anaphylactic reactions have been reported in patients with severe milk protein allergy.

Suppression of HPA function, suppression of linear growth (ie, reduction of growth velocity), reduced bone mineral density or hypercorticism (Cushing's syndrome) may occur; titrate to lowest effective dose. Reduction in growth velocity [mean: 1 cm/year (range: 0.3-1.8 cm)] may occur when corticosteroids are administered to pediatric patients, even at recommended doses via inhaled route; related to dose and duration of exposure; monitor growth. Use with extreme caution in patients with respiratory tuberculosis, untreated systemic infections, or ocular herpes simplex. Rare cases of increased IOP, glaucoma, or cataracts have been reported with inhaled corticosteroids, including fluticasone. Pneumonia and other lower respiratory tract infections have been reported in patients with COPD following the use of inhaled corticosteroids; monitor COPD patients closely since pneumonia symptoms may overlap symptoms of exacerbations.

Adverse Reactions

Cardiovascular: Arrhythmia, chest symptoms, fluid retention, MI, palpitation, syncope, tachycardia

Central nervous system: Compressed nerve syndromes, dizziness, headache, hypnagogic effects, migraine, pain, sleep disorders, tremor

Dermatologic: Dermatitis, dermatosis, eczema, hives, skin flakiness, urticaria, viral skin infection

Endocrine & metabolic: Hypothyroidism, menstruation symptoms

Gastrointestinal: Constipation, dental discomfort/pain, diarrhea, gastrointestinal infection, GI pain/discomfort, hemorrhoids, nausea, oral candidiasis, oral discomfort/pain, oral erythema/rash, oral ulcerations, unusual taste, viral GI infection, vomiting, weight gain

Genitourinary: Urinary tract infection

Hematologic: Contusions/hematomas

Hepatic: Abnormal liver function test

Neuromuscular & skeletal: Arthralgia, articular rheumatism, bone/cartilage disorders, bone pain, cramps, fractures, muscle injuries, muscle pain, muscle spasm, muscle stiffness, musculoskeletal pain, tightness/rigidity

Ocular: Conjunctivitis, edema, eye redness, keratitis, xerophthalmia

Respiratory: Blood in nasal mucosa, bronchitis, congestion, cough, dysphonia, ear/nose/throat infection, epistaxis, hoarseness, laryngitis, lower respiratory hemorrhage, lower respiratory tract infection, nasal irritation, pneumonia, rhinitis, rhinorrhea/postnasal drip, sinusitis, sneezing, throat irritation, upper respiratory tract infection, upper respiratory tract inflammation, viral respiratory tract infection

Miscellaneous: Allergies/allergic reactions, bacterial infection, burns, candidiasis, diaphoresis, sweat/sebum disorders, viral infection, wounds and lacerations

Rare but important or life-threatening: Asthma exacerbation (serious and some fatal), abdominal pain, agitation, aggression, anaphylactic reaction (some in patients with severe milk allergy [Diskus®]), angioedema, aphonia, atrial fibrillation, bronchospasm, cataracts, chest congestion, chest tightness, choking, contact dermatitis, Cushing syndrome, Cushingoid features, depression, dysmenorrhea, dyspepsia, dyspnea, earache, ecchymoses, edema (facial, oropharyngeal), eosinophilic conditions, glaucoma, growth velocity reduction in children/adolescents, hyperactivity, hypercorticism, hyperglycemia, hypersensitivity reaction (immediate and delayed), hypertension, hypokalemia, hypothyroidism, influenza, intraocular pressure increased, irritability, laryngeal spasm/irritation, irregular menstruation, myositis, osteoporosis, pallor, paresthesia, paradoxical tracheitis, paranasal sinus pain, photodermatitis, PID, rash, restlessness, stridor, supraventricular tachycardia, syncope, vaginal candidiasis, vaginitis, vulvovaginitis, rare cases of vasculitis (Churg-Strauss syndrome), ventricular tachycardia, wheezing, xerostomia

Drug Interactions

Metabolism/Transport Effects Refer to individual components.

Avoid Concomitant Use

Avoid concomitant use of Fluticasone and Salmeterol with any of the following: Aldesleukin; BCG; Beta-Blockers (Nonselective); Cobicistat; Conivaptan; CYP3A4 Inhibitors (Strong); Fusidic Acid (Systemic); Iobenguane I 123; Long-Acting Beta2-Agonists; Natalizumab; Pimecrolimus; Tacrolimus (Topical); Telaprevir; Tipranavir; Tofacitinib

Increased Effect/Toxicity

Fluticasone and Salmeterol may increase the levels/effects of: Amphotericin B; Atosiban; Ceritinib; Deferasirox; Highest Risk QTc-Prolonging Agents; Leflunomide; Long-Acting Beta2-Agonists; Loop Diuretics; Moderate Risk QTc-Prolonging Agents; Natalizumab; Sympathomimetics; Thiazide Diuretics; Tofacitinib

The levels/effects of Fluticasone and Salmeterol may be increased by: AtoMOXetine; Cannabinoid-Containing Products; Ceritinib; Cobicistat; Conivaptan; CYP3A4 Inhibitors (Moderate); CYP3A4 Inhibitors (Strong); Dasatinib; Denosumab; Fusidic Acid (Systemic); Ivacaftor; Linezolid; Luliconazole; MAO Inhibitors; Mifepristone; Pimecrolimus; Simeprevir; Tacrolimus (Topical); Telaprevir; Tipranavir; Trastuzumab; Tricyclic Antidepressants

Decreased Effect

Fluticasone and Salmeterol may decrease the levels/effects of: Aldesleukin; Antidiabetic Agents; BCG; Coccidioidin Skin Test; Corticorelin; Hyaluronidase; Iobenguane I 123; Sipuleucel-T; Vaccines (Inactivated)

The levels/effects of Fluticasone and Salmeterol may be decreased by: Beta-Blockers (Beta1 Selective); Beta-Blockers (Nonselective); Betahistine; Echinacea

Stability

Advair Diskus®: Store at 20°C to 25°C (68°F to 77°F). Store in a dry place out of direct heat or sunlight. Discard device 1 month after removal from foil pouch or when the dose indicator reads "0" (whichever comes first); device is not reusable.

Advair® HFA: Store at controlled room temperature of 25°C (77°F); excursions permitted to 15°C to 30°C (59°F to 86°F). Do not expose to temperatures >120°F; do not puncture or incinerate. Store with mouthpiece down. When the counter reads "000," discard device.

Mechanism of Action Combination of fluticasone (corticosteroid) and salmeterol (long-acting beta$_2$-agonist) designed to improve pulmonary function and control over what is produced by either agent when used alone. Because fluticasone and salmeterol act locally in the lung, plasma levels do not predict therapeutic effect.

Fluticasone: The mechanism of action for all topical corticosteroids is believed to be a combination of three important properties: Anti-inflammatory activity, immunosuppressive properties, and antiproliferative actions. Fluticasone has extremely potent vasoconstrictive and anti-inflammatory activity.

Salmeterol: Relaxes bronchial smooth muscle by selective action on beta$_2$-receptors with little effect on heart rate

Pharmacodynamics See individual agents.

Pharmacokinetics (Adult data unless noted) See individual agents.

Dosing: Usual

Asthma, maintenance treatment: Note: Titrate dosage to the lowest effective strength which maintains control of asthma. Dose may be increased after 2 weeks if patient does not respond adequately.

Oral powder for inhalation: Advair Diskus®:

Children 4-11 years without prior inhaled corticosteroid: Fluticasone 100 mcg/salmeterol 50 mcg (Advair™ Diskus® 100/50) 1 inhalation twice daily

Children ≥12 years and Adults without prior inhaled corticosteroid: Fluticasone 100 mcg/salmeterol 50 mcg (Advair™ Diskus® 100/50) 1 inhalation twice daily

Children ≥12 years and Adults currently receiving an inhaled corticosteroid: The starting dose is dependent upon the current steroid therapy, see table on next page.

Oral inhalation: Metered dose inhaler: Advair® HFA:

Children ≥12 years and Adults without prior inhaled corticosteroid: 2 inhalations twice daily of either fluticasone 45 mcg/salmeterol 21 mcg (Advair® HFA 45/21) or fluticasone 115 mcg/salmeterol 21 mcg (Advair® HFA 115/21); not to exceed 2 inhalations twice daily of fluticasone 230 mcg/salmeterol 21 mcg (Advair® HFA 230/21)

Children ≥12 years and Adults currently receiving an inhaled corticosteroid: The starting dose is dependent upon the current steroid therapy; see table. Not to exceed 2 inhalations twice daily of fluticasone 230 mcg/salmeterol 21 mcg (Advair® HFA 230/21)

COPD, maintenance treatment: Oral powder for inhalation: Advair Diskus®: Adults: Fluticasone 250 mcg/salmeterol 50 mcg (Advair Diskus® 250/50) 1 inhalation twice daily

Recommended Starting Dose of Fluticasone / Salmeterol (Advair® Diskus®) for Patients Currently Taking Inhaled Corticosteroids

Current Daily Dose of Inhaled Corticosteroid[1]		Advair Diskus® 1 inhalation twice daily
Beclomethasone dipropionate HFA inhalation aerosol	160 mcg	100/50
	320 mcg	250/50
	640 mcg	500/50
Budesonide inhalation aerosol	≤400 mcg	100/50
	800-1200 mcg	250/50
	1600 mcg	500/50
Flunisolide inhalation aerosol	≤1000 mcg	100/50
	1250-2000 mcg	250/50
Flunisolide HFA inhalation aerosol	≤320 mcg	100/50
	640 mcg	250/50
Fluticasone propionate HFA inhalation aerosol	≤176 mcg	100/50
	440 mcg	250/50
	660-880 mcg	500/50
Fluticasone propionate inhalation powder	≤200 mcg	100/50
	500 mcg	250/50
	1000 mcg	500/50
Mometasone furoate inhalation powder	220 mcg	100/50
	440 mcg	250/50
	880 mcg	500/50
Triamcinolone acetate inhalation aerosol	≤1000 mcg	100/50
	1100-1600 mcg	250/50

[1]Not for use in patients transferring from systemic corticosteroid therapy

Recommended Starting Dose of Fluticasone / Salmeterol (Advair® HFA) for Patients Currently Taking Inhaled Corticosteroids

Current Daily Dose of Inhaled Corticosteroid[1]		Advair® HFA 2 inhalations twice daily
Beclomethasone dipropionate HFA inhalation aerosol	≤160 mcg	45/21
	320 mcg	115/21
	640 mcg	230/21
Budesonide inhalation powder	≤400 mcg	45/21
	800-1200 mcg	115/21
	1600 mcg	230/21
Flunisolide CFC inhalation aerosol	≤1000 mcg	45/21
	1250-2000 mcg	115/21
Flunisolide HFA inhalation aerosol	≤320 mcg	45/21
	640 mcg	115/21
Fluticasone propionate HFA inhalation aerosol	≤176 mcg	45/21
	440 mcg	115/21
	660-880 mcg	230/21

(continued)

Current Daily Dose of Inhaled Corticosteroid[1]		Advair® HFA 2 inhalations twice daily
Fluticasone propionate inhalation powder	≤200 mcg	45/21
	500 mcg	115/21
	1000 mcg	230/21
Mometasone furoate inhalation powder	220 mcg	45/21
	440 mcg	115/21
	880 mcg	230/21
Triamcinolone acetonide inhalation aerosol	≤1000 mcg	45/21
	1100-1600 mcg	115/21

[1]Not for use in patients transferring from systemic corticosteroid therapy

Administration Oral inhalation:

Advair Diskus®, powder for oral inhalation: A device containing a double-foil blister of a powder formulation for oral inhalation; each blister contains 1 complete dose of both medications; the medication is opened by activating the device, dispersed into the airstream created by the patient inhaling through the mouthpiece; it may not be used with a spacer. Follow the patient directions for use which are provided with each device; do not exhale into the Diskus® or attempt to take it apart. Always activate and use the Diskus® in a level, horizontal position. Do not wash the mouthpiece or any part of the Diskus®; it must be kept dry.

Advair® HFA, metered dose inhalation: Prime before using the first time by releasing 4 test sprays into the air away from the face, shaking well for 5 seconds before each spray. Reprime with 2 test sprays if the inhaler has been dropped or not used for more than 4 weeks; discard after 120 actuations. Never immerse canister into water. Shake well for 5 seconds before using.

Monitoring Parameters Pulmonary function tests, vital signs, CNS stimulation, serum glucose, serum potassium; check mucous membranes for signs of fungal infection; monitor growth in pediatric patients

Additional Information When fluticasone/salmeterol is initiated in patients previously receiving a short-acting beta agonist, instruct the patient to discontinue regular use of the short-acting beta agonist and to utilize the shorter-acting agent for symptomatic acute episodes only.

Dosage Forms Excipient information presented when available (limited, particularly for generics); consult specific product labeling. [DSC] = Discontinued product

Aerosol, for oral inhalation:

Advair HFA:

45/21: Fluticasone propionate 45 mcg and salmeterol 21 mcg per inhalation (8 g) [chlorofluorocarbon free; 60 metered actuations]

45/21: Fluticasone propionate 45 mcg and salmeterol 21 mcg per inhalation (12 g) [chlorofluorocarbon free; 120 metered actuations]

115/21: Fluticasone propionate 115 mcg and salmeterol 21 mcg per inhalation (8 g) [chlorofluorocarbon free; 60 metered actuations]

115/21: Fluticasone propionate 115 mcg and salmeterol 21 mcg per inhalation (12 g) [chlorofluorocarbon free; 120 metered actuations]

230/21: Fluticasone propionate 230 mcg and salmeterol 21 mcg per inhalation (8 g) [chlorofluorocarbon free; 60 metered actuations]

230/21: Fluticasone propionate 230 mcg and salmeterol 21 mcg per inhalation (12 g) [chlorofluorocarbon free; 120 metered actuations]

◄ Powder, for oral inhalation:
Advair Diskus:
100/50: Fluticasone propionate 100 mcg and salmeterol 50 mcg (14s, 60s) [contains lactose]
250/50: Fluticasone propionate 250 mcg and salmeterol 50 mcg (14s, 60s) [contains lactose]
500/50: Fluticasone propionate 500 mcg and salmeterol 50 mcg (14s, 60s) [contains lactose]

References

National Asthma Education and Prevention Program (NAEPP), "Expert Panel Report 3 (EPR-3): Guidelines for the Diagnosis and Management of Asthma," *Clinical Practice Guidelines*, National Institutes of Health, National Heart, Lung, and Blood Institute, NIH Publication No. 08-4051, prepublication 2007; available at http://www.nhlbi.nih.gov/guidelines/asthma/asthgdln.htm.

◆ **Fluticasone Furoate** see Fluticasone (Nasal) on page 913

◆ **Fluticasone Propionate** see Fluticasone (Nasal) on page 913

◆ **Fluticasone Propionate** see Fluticasone (Oral Inhalation) on page 910

◆ **Fluticasone Propionate** see Fluticasone (Topical) on page 915

◆ **Fluticasone Propionate and Salmeterol Xinafoate** see Fluticasone and Salmeterol on page 916

Fluvastatin (FLOO va sta tin)

Medication Safety Issues

Sound-alike/look-alike issues:
Fluvastatin may be confused with fluoxetine, nystatin, pitavastatin

Related Information

Oral Medications That Should Not Be Crushed or Altered on page 2438

Brand Names: U.S. Lescol; Lescol XL

Brand Names: Canada Lescol; Lescol XL; Teva-Fluvastatin

Therapeutic Category Antilipemic Agent; HMG-CoA Reductase Inhibitor

Generic Availability (U.S.) May be product dependent

Use Adjunct to dietary therapy to reduce elevated total-C, LDL-C, and apo-B levels in patients with heterozygous familial hypercholesterolemia (HFH) and if LDC-C remains ≥190 mg/dL or if ≥160 mg/dL with family history of premature cardiovascular disease or presence of ≥2 cardiovascular risk factors [FDA approved in ages 10-16 years (girls ≥1 year postmenarche)]. Adjunct to dietary therapy to reduce elevated total cholesterol (total-C), LDL-C, triglyceride, and apolipoprotein B (apo-B) levels and to increase HDL-C in primary hypercholesterolemia, and mixed dyslipidemia (Fredrickson types IIa and IIb) (FDA approved in adults); to slow the progression of coronary atherosclerosis in patients with coronary heart disease (FDA approved in adults); to reduce risk of coronary revascularization procedures in patients with coronary heart disease (FDA approved in adults)

Pregnancy Risk Factor X

Pregnancy Considerations Adverse events were not observed in animal reproduction studies. There are reports of congenital anomalies following maternal use of HMG-CoA reductase inhibitors in pregnancy; however, maternal disease, differences in specific agents used, and the low rates of exposure limit the interpretation of the available data (Godfrey, 2012; Lecarpentier, 2012). Cholesterol biosynthesis may be important in fetal development; serum cholesterol and triglycerides increase normally during pregnancy. The discontinuation of lipid lowering medications temporarily during pregnancy is not expected to have significant impact on the long term outcomes of primary hypercholesterolemia treatment.

Use of fluvastatin is contraindicated in pregnancy. HMG-CoA reductase inhibitors should be discontinued prior to pregnancy (ADA, 2013). If treatment of dyslipidemias is needed in pregnant women or in women of reproductive age, other agents are preferred (Berglund, 2012; Stone, 2013). The manufacturer recommends administration to women of childbearing potential only when conception is highly unlikely and patients have been informed of potential hazards.

Breast-Feeding Considerations It is not known if fluvastatin is excreted into breast milk. Due to the potential for serious adverse reactions in a nursing infant, use while breast-feeding is contraindicated by the manufacturer.

Contraindications Hypersensitivity to fluvastatin or any component; active liver disease; unexplained persistent elevations of serum transaminases; pregnancy; breast-feeding

Warnings Patients receiving HMG-CoA reductase inhibitors have developed rhabdomyolysis with or without acute renal failure and/or myopathy; patients should be monitored closely; risk is dose related and is increased with concurrent use of other lipid-lowering medications (eg, fibric acid derivatives or niacin at doses >1 g/day). With concurrent use of cyclosporine and fluconazole; dosage reductions of fluvastatin recommended. Ensure patient is on the lowest effective fluvastatin dose in all circumstances. Discontinue in any patient in which CPK levels are markedly elevated (>10 times ULN) or if myopathy is suspected/diagnosed; monitoring of CPK may be warranted, but may not prevent severe myopathy. The manufacturer recommends temporary discontinuation for elective major surgery, acute medical or surgical conditions, or in any patient experiencing an acute or serious condition predisposing to renal failure (eg, sepsis, hypotension, trauma, uncontrolled seizures). However, based upon current evidence, HMG-CoA reductase inhibitor therapy should be continued in the perioperative period unless risk outweighs cardioprotective benefit. Use caution in patients with renal impairment, inadequately treated hypothyroidism, and those taking other drugs associated with myopathy (eg, colchicine); these patients are predisposed to myopathy. Patients should be instructed to report unexplained muscle pain, tenderness, weakness, or brown urine.

Autoimmune-mediated myopathy (IMNM), has been reported (rarely) with HMG-CoA reductase inhibitor therapy; presents as proximal muscle weakness with elevated CPK levels, which persists despite discontinuation of HMG-CoA reductase inhibitor therapy; additionally, muscle biopsy may show necrotizing myopathy with limited inflammation; immunosuppressive therapy (eg, corticosteroids, azathioprine) may be used for treatment.

Postmarketing reports of fatal and nonfatal hepatic failure are rare; if serious hepatotoxicity with clinical symptoms and/or hyperbilirubinemia or jaundice occurs during treatment, interrupt therapy. If an alternate etiology is not identified, do not restart fluvastatin. Liver enzyme tests should be obtained at baseline and as clinically indicated; routine periodic monitoring of liver enzymes is not necessary. Use with caution in patients with history of heavy alcohol use or a previous history of liver disease; active liver disease and unexplained persistent elevations of serum transaminases are contraindications for use.

Precautions Use caution in patients with conditions or on medications that reduce steroidogenesis (eg, ketoconazole, spironolactone, cimetidine). Increases in Hb A_{1c} and fasting blood glucose have been reported with HMG-CoA reductase inhibitors; however, the benefits of statin therapy far outweigh the risk of dysglycemia. Secondary causes of hyperlipidemia should be ruled out prior to therapy; has not been studied in conditions where the major abnormality is elevation of chylomicrons, VLDL, or IDL (hyperlipoproteinemia Types I, III, IV, or V).

Although rare, reversible cognitive impairment (including confusion, forgetfulness, amnesia, and memory loss) can occur with HMG-CoA reductase inhibitors. These cognitive symptoms have been reported at variable times during therapy (1 day to years after initiation) and are reversible with discontinuation; resolution usually occurs within ~3 weeks. Cases have not been associated with fixed or progressive dementia; nor have they been associated with age, specific HMG CoA reductase inhibitor, dose, or concomitant medication use

Adverse Reactions As reported with fluvastatin capsules; in general, adverse reactions reported with fluvastatin extended release tablet were similar, but the incidence was less.

Central nervous system: Fatigue, headache, insomnia
Gastrointestinal: Abdominal pain, diarrhea, dyspepsia, nausea
Genitourinary: Urinary tract infection
Neuromuscular & skeletal: Myalgia
Respiratory: Bronchitis, sinusitis
Rare but important or life-threatening (including additional class-related events - not necessarily reported with fluvastatin therapy): Alopecia, amnesia (reversible), anaphylaxis, angioedema, arthralgia, arthritis, blood glucose increased, cataracts, cholestatic jaundice, cirrhosis, cognitive impairment (reversible), confusion (reversible), CPK increased (>10x normal), depression, dermatomyositis, dyspnea, eosinophilia, erectile dysfunction, erythema multiforme, ESR increased, facial paresis, fatty liver, fever, fulminant hepatic necrosis, glycosylated hemoglobin (Hb A$_{1c}$) increased, gynecomastia, hemolytic anemia, hepatitis, hepatoma, hypersensitivity reaction, immune-mediated necrotizing myopathy (IMNM), impotence, interstitial lung disease, leukopenia, memory disturbance (reversible), memory impairment (reversible), muscle cramps, myopathy, nodules, ophthalmoplegia, pancreatitis, paresthesia, peripheral nerve palsy, peripheral neuropathy, photosensitivity, polymyalgia rheumatica, positive ANA, pruritus, psychic disturbance, purpura, rash, renal failure (secondary to rhabdomyolysis), rhabdomyolysis, skin discoloration, Stevens-Johnson syndrome, systemic lupus erythematosus-like syndrome, taste alteration, thrombocytopenia, thyroid dysfunction, toxic epidermal necrolysis, transaminases increased, tremor, urticaria, vasculitis, vertigo

Drug Interactions

Metabolism/Transport Effects Substrate of CYP2C9 (minor), CYP2D6 (minor), CYP3A4 (minor), SLCO1B1; **Note:** Assignment of Major/Minor substrate status based on clinically relevant drug interaction potential; **Inhibits** CYP1A2 (weak), CYP2C8 (weak), CYP2C9 (moderate), CYP2D6 (weak), CYP3A4 (weak)

Avoid Concomitant Use

Avoid concomitant use of Fluvastatin with any of the following: Fusidic Acid (Systemic); Gemfibrozil; Pimozide; Red Yeast Rice

Increased Effect/Toxicity

Fluvastatin may increase the levels/effects of: ARIPiprazole; Bosentan; Cannabis; Carvedilol; CYP2C9 Substrates; DAPTOmycin; Dofetilide; Dronabinol; Lomitapide; PAZOPanib; Pimozide; Tetrahydrocannabinol; Trabectedin; Vitamin K Antagonists

The levels/effects of Fluvastatin may be increased by: Amiodarone; Bezafibrate; Boceprevir; Colchicine; CycloSPORINE (Systemic); Cyproterone; Eltrombopag; Fenofibrate and Derivatives; Fluconazole; Fusidic Acid (Systemic); Gemfibrozil; Mifepristone; Niacin; Niacinamide; Raltegravir; Red Yeast Rice; Telaprevir

Decreased Effect

Fluvastatin may decrease the levels/effects of: Lanthanum

The levels/effects of Fluvastatin may be decreased by: Antacids; Cholestyramine Resin; Etravirine; Fosphenytoin; Peginterferon Alfa-2b; Phenytoin; Rifamycin Derivatives

Food Interactions Food reduces rate but not the extent of absorption. Management: Administer without regard to meals.

Stability Store at 25°C (77°F), excursions permitted to 15°C to 30°C (59°F to 86°F); protect from light; dispense in a tightly closed container.

Mechanism of Action Acts by competitively inhibiting 3-hydroxyl-3-methylglutaryl-coenzyme A (HMG-CoA) reductase, the enzyme that catalyzes the reduction of HMG-CoA to mevalonate; this is an early rate-limiting step in cholesterol biosynthesis. HDL is increased while total, LDL, and VLDL cholesterols; apolipoprotein B; and plasma triglycerides are decreased.

Pharmacodynamics

Maximum effect: LDL-C reduction: Achieved within 4 weeks

Pharmacokinetics (Adult data unless noted)

Distribution: Adults: V_d: 0.35 L/kg
Protein binding: >98%
Metabolism: To inactive and active metabolites (oxidative metabolism via CYP2C9 [75%], 2C8 [~5%], and 3A4 [~20%] isoenzymes); active forms do not circulate systemically; extensive (saturable) first-pass hepatic extraction
Bioavailability: Absolute: Capsule: 24%; Extended release tablet: 29%
Half-life: Capsule: <3 hours; Extended release tablet: 9 hours
Time to peak serum concentration: Capsule: 1 hour; Extended release tablet: 3 hours
Elimination: Feces (90%); urine (5%)

Dosing: Usual

Children and Adolescents: **Hyperlipidemia or heterozygous familial and nonfamilial hypercholesterolemia: Note:** Begin treatment if after adequate trial of diet the following are present: LDL-C ≥190 mg/dL or LDL-C remains ≥160 mg/dL and positive family history of premature cardiovascular disease or meets NCEP classification (NHLBI, 2011). Therapy may be considered for children 8-9 years of age meeting the above criteria or for children with diabetes mellitus and LDL-C ≥130 mg/dL (Daniels, 2008).

Children and Adolescents (10-16 years): Oral:
Immediate release capsule: Initial: 20 mg once daily; may titrate dose or frequency (twice daily dosing) at 6-week intervals; maximum dose: 40 mg twice daily
Extended release tablet: Should not be used to initiate therapy; may convert patient if total daily dose is 80 mg/day

Adults: **Dyslipidemia or delay in progression of CAD:** Oral:
Patients requiring ≥25% decrease in LDL-C: 40 mg capsule once daily in the evening, 80 mg extended release tablet once daily (anytime), or 40 mg capsule twice daily
Patients requiring <25% decrease in LDL-C: Initial: 20 mg capsule once daily in the evening; may increase based on tolerability and response to a maximum daily dose: 80 mg/**day**, given in 2 divided doses (immediate release capsule) or as a single daily dose (extended release tablet)

Dosing adjustment for fluvastatin with concomitant medications: Children, Adolescents, and Adults:
Cyclosporine, fluconazole: Do not exceed 20 mg twice daily

Dosing adjustment in renal impairment: Adults:
Mild to moderate renal impairment: No dosage adjustment needed.
Severe renal impairment: Use with caution (doses >40 mg/day have not been studied).

Dosing adjustment in hepatic impairment: There are no dosage adjustments provided in the manufacturer labeling; systemic exposure may be increased in patients with liver disease; use is contraindicated in patients with active liver disease or unexplained transaminase elevations.

Administration Fluvastatin may be taken without regard to meals.
Immediate release capsules: Do not open capsules; do not use two 40 mg capsules for an 80 mg once daily dose; extended release formulation should be used.
Extended release tablet: Do not break, chew, or crush; swallow whole.

Monitoring Parameters
Pediatric patients: Baseline: ALT, AST, and creatine phosphokinase levels (CPK); fasting lipid panel (FLP) and repeat ALT and AST should be checked after 4 weeks of therapy; if no myopathy symptoms or laboratory abnormalities, then monitor FLP, ALT, and AST every 3-4 months during the first year and then every 6 months thereafter (NHLBI, 2011).
Adults: Baseline CPK (recheck CPK in any patient with symptoms suggestive of myopathy; discontinue therapy if markedly elevated); baseline liver function tests (LFTs) and repeat when clinically indicated thereafter. Patients with elevated transaminase levels should have a second (confirmatory) test and frequent monitoring until values normalize; discontinue if increase in ALT/AST is persistently >3 times ULN (NCEP, 2002).
Lipid panel (total cholesterol, HDL, LDL, triglycerides): ATP III recommendations (NCEP, 2002): Baseline; 6-8 weeks after initiation of drug therapy; if dose increased, then at 6-8 weeks until final dose determined. Once treatment goal achieved, follow-up intervals may be reduced to every 4-6 months. Lipid panel should be assessed at least annually, and preferably at each clinic visit.
Manufacturer's recommendation: Analyze lipid panel at initiation and 4 weeks after each titration

Dosage Forms Excipient information presented when available (limited, particularly for generics); consult specific product labeling.
Capsule, Oral:
Lescol: 20 mg, 40 mg
Generic: 20 mg, 40 mg
Tablet Extended Release 24 Hour, Oral:
Lescol XL: 80 mg

References

American Diabetes Association, "Standards of Medical Care in Diabetes-2013," *Diabetes Care*, 2013, 36(Suppl 1):S11-66.
Berglund L, Brunzell JD, Goldberg AC, et al, "Evaluation and Treatment of Hypertriglyceridemia: An Endocrine Society Clinical Practice Guideline," *J Clin Endocrinol Metab*, 2012, 97(9):2969-89.
Daniels SR, Greer FR, and Committee on Nutrition, "Lipid Screening and Cardiovascular Health in Childhood," *Pediatrics*, 2008, 122 (1):198-208.
"Executive Summary of the Third Report of the National Cholesterol Education Program (NCEP) Expert Panel on Detection, Evaluation, and Treatment of High Blood Cholesterol in Adults (Adult Treatment Panel III)," *JAMA*, 2001, 285(19):2486-97.
Godfrey LM, Erramouspe J, and Cleveland KW, "Teratogenic Risk of Statins in Pregnancy," *Ann Pharmacother*, 2012, 46(10):1419-24.
Lecarpentier E, Morel O, Fournier T, et al, "Statins and Pregnancy: Between Supposed Risks and Theoretical Benefits," *Drugs*, 2012, 72 (6):773-88.
McCrindle BW, Urbina EM, Dennison BA, et al, "Drug Therapy of High-Risk Lipid Abnormalities in Children and Adolescents: A Scientific Statement from the American Heart Association Atherosclerosis, Hypertension, and Obesity in Youth Committee, Council of Cardiovascular Disease in the Young, With the Council on Cardiovascular Nursing," *Circulation*, 2007, 115(14):1948-67.
National Heart, Lung, and Blood Institute, "Expert Panel on Integrated Guidelines for Cardiovascular Health and Risk Reduction in Children and Adolescents," Clinical Practice Guidelines, 2011, National Institutes of Health. Available at http://www.nhlbi.nih.gov/guidelines/cvd_ped/peds_guidelines_full.pdf
van der Graaf A, Nierman MC, Firth JC, et al, "Efficacy and Safety of Fluvastatin in Children and Adolescents With Heterozygous Familial Hypercholesterolaemia," *Acta Paediatr*, 2006, 95(11):1461-6

◆ **Fluviral (Can)** *see* Influenza Virus Vaccine (Inactivated) *on page 1103*

◆ **Fluvirin** *see* Influenza Virus Vaccine (Inactivated) *on page 1103*

◆ **Fluvirin Preservative Free** *see* Influenza Virus Vaccine (Inactivated) *on page 1103*

FluvoxaMINE (floo VOKS a meen)

Medication Safety Issues
Sound-alike/look-alike issues:
FluvoxaMINE may be confused with flavoxATE, FLUoxetine, fluPHENAZine
Luvox may be confused with Lasix, Levoxyl, Lovenox
BEERS Criteria medication:
This drug may be potentially inappropriate for use in geriatric patients (Quality of evidence - moderate; Strength of recommendation - strong).

Related Information
Antidepressant Agents *on page 2219*
Oral Medications That Should Not Be Crushed or Altered *on page 2438*

Brand Names: U.S. Luvox CR
Brand Names: Canada Apo-Fluvoxamine; Ava-Fluvoxamine; CO Fluvoxamine; Dom-Fluvoxamine; Luvox; Novo-Fluvoxamine; PHL-Fluvoxamine; PMS-Fluvoxamine; ratio-Fluvoxamine; Riva-Fluvox; Sandoz-Fluvoxamine
Therapeutic Category Antidepressant, Selective Serotonin Reuptake Inhibitor (SSRI)
Generic Availability (U.S.) Yes
Use
Tablets: Treatment of obsessive-compulsive disorder (OCD) (FDA approved in ages ≥8 years and adults)
Extended-release capsules: Treatment of obsessive-compulsive disorder (OCD) (FDA approved in adults)
Medication Guide Available Yes
Pregnancy Risk Factor C
Pregnancy Considerations Adverse events have been observed in animal reproduction studies. Fluvoxamine crosses the human placenta. An increased risk of teratogenic effects, including cardiovascular defects, may be associated with maternal use of fluvoxamine or other SSRIs; however, available information is conflicting. Nonteratogenic effects in the newborn following SSRI/SNRI exposure late in the third trimester include respiratory distress, cyanosis, apnea, seizures, temperature instability, feeding difficulty, vomiting, hypoglycemia, hypo- or hypertonia, hyper-reflexia, jitteriness, constant crying, and tremor. Symptoms may be due to the toxicity of the SSRIs/SNRIs or a discontinuation syndrome and may be consistent with serotonin syndrome associated with SSRI treatment. Persistent pulmonary hypertension of the newborn (PPHN) has also been reported with SSRI exposure. The long-term effects of *in utero* SSRI exposure on infant development and behavior are not known.

The ACOG recommends that therapy with SSRIs or SNRIs during pregnancy be individualized; treatment of depression during pregnancy should incorporate the clinical expertise of the mental health clinician, obstetrician, primary healthcare provider, and pediatrician. According to the American Psychiatric Association (APA), the risks of medication treatment should be weighed against other treatment options and untreated depression. For women who discontinue antidepressant medications during pregnancy and who may be at high risk for postpartum depression, the medications can be restarted following delivery. Treatment algorithms have been developed by the ACOG and the APA for the management of depression in women prior to conception and during pregnancy.

Breast-Feeding Considerations Fluvoxamine is excreted in breast milk. Based on case reports, the dose the infant receives is relatively small and adverse events have not been observed. Adverse events have been reported in nursing infants exposed to some SSRIs. According to the manufacturer, the decision to continue or discontinue breast-feeding during therapy should take into account the risk of exposure to the infant and the benefits of treatment to the mother.

The long-term effects on development and behavior have not been studied; therefore, fluvoxamine should be prescribed to a mother who is breast-feeding only when the benefits outweigh the potential risks. Maternal use of an SSRI during pregnancy may cause delayed milk secretion.

Contraindications Hypersensitivity to fluvoxamine or any component; concurrent use with alosetron, pimozide, ramelteon, thioridazine, or tizanidine; use of MAO inhibitors within 14 days (potentially fatal reactions may occur)

Warnings Clinical worsening of depression or suicidal ideation and behavior may occur in children and adults with major depressive disorder **[U.S. Boxed Warning]**. In clinical trials, antidepressants increased the risk of suicidal thinking and behavior (suicidality) in children, adolescents, and young adults (18-24 years of age) with major depressive disorder and other psychiatric disorders. This risk must be considered before prescribing antidepressants for any clinical use. Short-term studies did **not** show an increased risk of suicidality with antidepressant use in patients >24 years of age and showed a decreased risk in patients ≥65 years.

Patients of all ages who are treated with antidepressants for any indication require appropriate monitoring and close observation for clinical worsening of depression, suicidality, and unusual changes in behavior, especially during the first few months after antidepressant initiation or when the dose is adjusted. Family members and caregivers should be instructed to closely observe the patient (ie, daily) and communicate condition with healthcare provider. Patients should also be monitored for associated behaviors (eg, anxiety, agitation, panic attacks, insomnia, irritability, hostility, aggressiveness, impulsivity, akathisia, hypomania, mania) which may increase the risk for worsening depression or suicidality. Worsening depression or emergence of suicidality (or associated behaviors listed above) that is abrupt in onset, severe, or not part of the presenting symptoms, may require discontinuation or modification of drug therapy. SSRI-associated behavioral activation (ie, restlessness, hyperkinesis, hyperactivity, agitation) is two- to threefold more prevalent in children compared to adolescents; it is more prevalent in adolescents compared to adults. Somnolence (including sedation and drowsiness) is more common in adults compared to children and adolescents (Safer, 2006).

Avoid abrupt discontinuation; withdrawal syndrome with discontinuation symptoms (including agitation, dysphoria, anxiety, confusion, dizziness, hypomania, nightmares, irritability, sensory disturbances, headache, lethargy, emotional lability, insomnia, tinnitus, and seizures) may occur if therapy is abruptly discontinued or dose reduced; taper the dose to minimize risks of discontinuation symptoms. If intolerable symptoms occur following a decrease in dosage or upon discontinuation of therapy, consider resuming the previous dose with a more gradual taper. To reduce risk of intentional overdose, write prescriptions for the smallest quantity consistent with good patient care.

May worsen psychosis in some patients or precipitate a shift to mania or hypomania in patients with bipolar disorder. Monotherapy in patients with bipolar disorder should be avoided. Patients presenting with depressive symptoms should be screened for bipolar disorder. Fluvoxamine is not FDA approved for the treatment of bipolar depression.

Potentially fatal serotonin syndrome (SS) or neuroleptic malignant syndrome (NMS)-like reactions have occurred with selective serotonin reuptake inhibitors (SSRIs) and serotonin/norepinephrine reuptake inhibitors (SNRIs) when used alone, and particularly when used in combination with serotonergic drugs (eg, triptans), drugs that impair the metabolism of serotonin (eg, MAO inhibitors), or antidopaminergic agents (eg, antipsychotics). Identification and differentiation of SS (eg, tremor, myoclonus, agitation) and more severe NMS-like reactions (eg, hyperthermia, muscle rigidity, autonomic instability, mental status changes) can be complex; monitor patients closely for either syndrome. Discontinue treatment (and any concomitant serotonergic and/or antidopaminergic agents) immediately if signs or symptoms arise and initiate supportive symptomatic therapy. Tryptophan (which can be metabolized to serotonin) and the herbal medicine St John's wort (*Hypericum perforatum*) may increase serious side effects (concomitant use of these agents with fluvoxamine is not recommended).

Precautions Fluvoxamine may cause abnormal bleeding (eg, ecchymosis, purpura, upper GI bleeding); use with caution in patients with impaired platelet aggregation and with concurrent use of aspirin, NSAIDs, or other drugs that affect coagulation. May impair cognitive or motor performance. SSRI-associated vomiting is two- to threefold more prevalent in children compared to adolescents and is more prevalent in adolescents compared to adults (Safer, 2006). Use with caution in patients with seizure disorders (monitor closely; avoid use in patients with unstable epilepsy), concomitant illnesses that may affect hepatic metabolism or hemodynamic responses (eg, unstable cardiac disease, recent MI), and in suicidal patients; use with caution and decrease dose in patients with hepatic dysfunction; use with caution in patients with severe renal impairment. Use with caution in patients receiving diuretics or those who are volume depleted (may cause hyponatremia or SIADH). No clinical studies have assessed the combined use of fluvoxamine and electroconvulsive therapy; however, use with caution in patients receiving electroconvulsive therapy; may increase the risks associated with electroconvulsive therapy, consider discontinuing, when possible, prior to electroconvulsive therapy treatment.

Use with caution during third trimester of pregnancy [newborns may experience adverse effects or withdrawal symptoms (consider risk and benefits); exposure to SSRIs late in pregnancy may also be associated with an increased risk for persistent pulmonary hypertension of the newborn (Chambers, 2006)].

Adverse Reactions

Cardiovascular: Chest pain, edema, hyper-/hypotension, palpitation, syncope, tachycardia, vasodilation

Central nervous system: Abnormal dreams, abnormal thinking, agitation, amnesia, anxiety, apathy, chills, CNS stimulation, depression, dizziness, headache, insomnia, malaise, manic reaction, nervousness, neurosis, pain, psychotic reaction, somnolence

Dermatologic: Acne, bruising

Endocrine & metabolic: Anorgasmia, libido decreased, menorrhagia, sexual function abnormal

Gastrointestinal: Abdominal pain, anorexia, constipation, diarrhea, dyspepsia, dysphagia, flatulence, gingivitis, nausea, taste perversion, toothache and dental caries, vomiting, weight gain/loss, xerostomia

Genitourinary: Ejaculation abnormal, impotence, polyuria, urinary tract infection, urinary retention

Hepatic: Liver function tests abnormal

Neuromuscular & skeletal: Hyper-/hypokinesia, hypertonia, myalgia, myoclonus, paresthesia, tremor, twitching, weakness

Ocular: Amblyopia

Respiratory: Bronchitis, cough increased, dyspnea, epistaxis, laryngitis, pharyngitis, sinusitis, upper respiratory infection, yawn

Miscellaneous: Diaphoresis, flu-like syndrome, viral infection

Rare but important or life-threatening: Acute renal failure, agranulocytosis, akinesia, allergic reaction, anaphylactic reaction, anemia, angina, angioedema, anuria, aplastic anemia, apnea, asthma, ataxia, AV block, bradycardia, bullous eruption, cardiomyopathy, cardiorespiratory arrest, cerebrovascular accident, cholecystitis, cholelithiasis, colitis, conduction delay, coronary artery disease, diplopia, dyskinesia, dystonia, extrapyramidal syndrome, embolus, GI bleeding, goiter, hallucinations, heart failure, hematemesis, hematuria, Henoch-Schönlein purpura (IgA vasculitis), hepatitis, hemoptysis, homicidal ideation, hypercholesterolemia, hyper-/hypoglycemia, hypokalemia, hyponatremia, hypothyroidism, ileus, interstitial lung disease, intestinal obstruction, jaundice, leukopenia, leukocytosis, loss of consciousness, lymphadenopathy, MI, myasthenia, myopathy, neuralgia, neuroleptic malignant syndrome, neuropathy, pancreatitis, paralysis, pericarditis, porphyria, purpura, QT prolongation, retinal detachment, rhabdomyolysis, serotonin syndrome, ST segment changes, seizure, Stevens-Johnson syndrome, suicidal tendencies, supraventricular extrasystoles, tardive dyskinesia, thrombocytopenia, toxic epidermal necrolysis, vasculitis, ventricular arrhythmia, ventricular tachycardia (including torsade de pointes), white blood cells decreased

Drug Interactions

Metabolism/Transport Effects Substrate of CYP1A2 (major), CYP2D6 (major); **Note:** Assignment of Major/Minor substrate status based on clinically relevant drug interaction potential; **Inhibits** CYP1A2 (strong), CYP2B6 (weak), CYP2C19 (strong), CYP2C9 (weak), CYP2D6 (weak), CYP3A4 (weak)

Avoid Concomitant Use

Avoid concomitant use of FluvoxaMINE with any of the following: Agomelatine; Alosetron; Dosulepin; Iobenguane I 123; Linezolid; MAO Inhibitors; Methylene Blue; Pimozide; Pirfenidone; Pomalidomide; Ramelteon; Tasimelteon; Thioridazine; TiZANidine; Tryptophan; Urokinase

Increased Effect/Toxicity

FluvoxaMINE may increase the levels/effects of: Agents with Antiplatelet Properties; Agomelatine; Alosetron; Anticoagulants; Antidepressants (Serotonin Reuptake Inhibitor/Antagonist); Antipsychotics; Apixaban; ARIPiprazole; Asenapine; Aspirin; Bendamustine; Benzodiazepines (metabolized by oxidation); Bromazepam; BusPIRone; CarBAMazepine; Citalopram; CloZAPine; Collagenase (Systemic); CYP1A2 Substrates; CYP2C19 Substrates; Dabigatran Etexilate; Desmopressin; Dofetilide; Dosulepin; DULoxetine; Erlotinib; Fosphenytoin; Haloperidol; Hypoglycemic Agents; Ibritumomab; Lomitapide; Methadone; Methylene Blue; Mexiletine; NSAID (COX-2 Inhibitor); NSAID (Nonselective); OLANZapine; Phenytoin; Pimozide; Pirfenidone; Pomalidomide; Propafenone; Propranolol; QuiNIDine; Ramelteon; Rivaroxaban; Roflumilast; Ropivacaine; Salicylates; Serotonin Modulators; Tasimelteon; Theophylline Derivatives; Thiazide Diuretics; Thioridazine; Thrombolytic Agents; TiZANidine; Tositumomab and Iodine I 131 Tositumomab; TraMADol; Tricyclic Antidepressants; Urokinase; Vitamin K Antagonists; Zolpidem

The levels/effects of FluvoxaMINE may be increased by: Abiraterone Acetate; Alcohol (Ethyl); Analgesics (Opioid); Antiemetics (5HT3 Antagonists); Antipsychotics; BuPROPion; BusPIRone; Cimetidine; CNS Depressants; Cobicistat; CYP1A2 Inhibitors (Moderate); CYP1A2 Inhibitors (Strong); CYP2D6 Inhibitors (Moderate); CYP2D6 Inhibitors (Strong); Darunavir; Dasatinib; Deferasirox; DULoxetine; Glucosamine; Grapefruit Juice; Herbs (Anticoagulant/Antiplatelet Properties); Ibrutinib; Linezolid; Lithium; MAO Inhibitors; Metoclopramide; Metyrosine; Multivitamins/Fluoride (with ADE); Multivitamins/Minerals (with ADEK, Folate, Iron); Multivitamins/Minerals (with AE, No Iron); Nonsteroidal Anti-Inflammatory Agents; Omega-3 Fatty Acids; Pentosan Polysulfate Sodium; Pentoxifylline; Prostacyclin Analogues; TraMADol; Tryptophan; Vemurafenib; Vitamin E

Decreased Effect

FluvoxaMINE may decrease the levels/effects of: Clopidogrel; Iobenguane I 123; Ioflupane I 123; Thyroid Products

The levels/effects of FluvoxaMINE may be decreased by: Cannabis; CarBAMazepine; CYP1A2 Inducers (Strong); Cyproheptadine; Cyproterone; Nonsteroidal Anti-Inflammatory Agents; NSAID (COX-2 Inhibitor); NSAID (Nonselective); Peginterferon Alfa-2b

Stability Protect from high humidity and store at controlled room temperature of 25°C (77°F). Dispense in tight containers. Avoid exposing extended-release capsules to temperatures >30°C (86°F).

Mechanism of Action Inhibits CNS neuron serotonin uptake; minimal or no effect on reuptake of norepinephrine or dopamine; does not significantly bind to alpha-adrenergic, histamine or cholinergic receptors

Pharmacodynamics

Onset of action: 1-2 weeks

Maximum effect: 8-12 weeks

Duration: 1-2 days

Pharmacokinetics (Adult data unless noted) Note: Steady-state plasma concentrations (following administration of the immediate-release product) have been noted to be 2-3 times higher in children than those in adolescents; female children demonstrated a significantly higher AUC and peak concentration than males.

Distribution: V_d, apparent: Adults: ~25 L/kg

Protein binding: ~80%, primarily to albumin

Metabolism: Extensive via the liver; major metabolic routes are oxidative demethylation and deamination; dose-dependent (nonlinear) pharmacokinetics

Bioavailability: Immediate release: 53%; extended release: 84% (compared to immediate release); bioavailability is not significantly affected by food for either formulation

Half-life: Adults: 15.6 hours

Time to peak serum concentration: 3-8 hours

Elimination: 94% of the dose is excreted in the urine, primarily as metabolites; 2% as unchanged drug

Clearance: Hepatic dysfunction: Decreased by 30%

Dosing: Usual Oral:

Obsessive compulsive disorder:

Children 8-17 years: Immediate release: Initial: 25 mg once daily at bedtime; adjust in 25 mg increments at 7- to 14-day intervals, as tolerated, to maximum therapeutic benefit; usual dosage range: 50-200 mg/day; daily doses >50 mg should be divided into 2 doses; administer larger portion at bedtime

Maximum: Children: 8-11 years: 200 mg/day; Adolescents: 300 mg/day; lower doses may be effective in female versus male patients

Note: Slower titration of dose every 2-4 weeks may minimize the risk of behavioral activation; behavioral activation associated with SSRI use increases the risk of suicidal behavior. Higher mg/kg doses are needed in children compared to adolescents.

Adults:

Immediate release: Initial: 50 mg once daily at bedtime; adjust in 50 mg increments at 4- to 7-day intervals; usual dosage range: 100-300 mg/day; daily doses >100 mg should be divided into 2 doses; administer larger portion at bedtime; maximum dose: 300 mg/day

Extended release: Initial: 100 mg once daily at bedtime; may be increased in 50 mg increments at intervals of at least 1 week; usual dosage range: 100-300 mg/day; maximum dose: 300 mg/day

Dosage adjustment in hepatic impairment: Decrease initial dose and dose titration; titrate slowly

Administration May be administered without regard to meals. Do not chew or crush extended-release capsule; swallow whole.

Monitoring Parameters Monitor patient periodically for symptom resolution; monitor for worsening depression, suicidality, and associated behaviors (especially at the beginning of therapy or when doses are increased or decreased. Monitor for anxiety, social functioning, mania, panic attacks; akathisia, weight gain or loss, nutritional intake, sleep. Monitor for signs and symptoms of serotonin syndrome or neuroleptic malignant syndrome-like reactions.

Additional Information A recent report (Lake, 2000) describes 5 children (age 8-15 years) who developed epistaxis (n=4) or bruising (n=1) while receiving sertraline therapy. Another recent report describes the SSRI discontinuation syndrome in 6 children; the syndrome was similar to that reported in adults (Diler, 2002). Due to limited long-term studies, the clinical usefulness of fluvoxamine should be periodically re-evaluated in patients receiving the drug for extended intervals; effects of long term use of fluvoxamine on pediatric growth, development, and maturation have not been directly assessed. **Note:** Case reports of decreased growth in children receiving fluoxetine or fluvoxamine (n=4; age: 11.6-13.7 years) for 6 months to 5 years suggest a suppression of growth hormone secretion during SSRI therapy (Weintrob, 2002). Further studies are needed.

Neonates born to women receiving SSRIs late during the third trimester may experience respiratory distress, apnea, cyanosis, temperature instability, vomiting, feeding difficulty, hypoglycemia, constant crying, irritability, hypotonia, hypertonia, hyper-reflexia, tremor, jitteriness, and seizures; these symptoms may be due to a direct toxic effect, withdrawal syndrome, or (in some cases) serotonin syndrome. Withdrawal symptoms occur in 30% of neonates exposed to SSRIs *in utero*; monitor newborns for at least 48 hours after birth; long-term effects of *in utero* exposure to SSRIs are unknown (Levinson-Castiel, 2006).

Dosage Forms Excipient information presented when available (limited, particularly for generics); consult specific product labeling.

Capsule Extended Release 24 Hour, Oral, as maleate:
Luvox CR: 100 mg, 150 mg [gluten free; contains fd&c blue #2 (indigotine)]
Generic: 100 mg, 150 mg
Tablet, Oral, as maleate:
Generic: 25 mg, 50 mg, 100 mg

References

Chambers CD, Hernandez-Diaz S, Van Marter LJ, et al, "Selective Serotonin-Reuptake Inhibitors and Risk of Persistent Pulmonary Hypertension of the Newborn," *N Engl J Med*, 2006, 354(6):579-87.
Cheer SM and Figgitt DP, "Fluvoxamine: A Review of Its Therapeutic Potential in the Management of Anxiety Disorders in Children and Adolescents," *Paediatr Drugs*, 2001, 3(10):763-81.
Cheer SM and Figgitt DP, "Spotlight on Fluvoxamine in Anxiety Disorders in Children and Adolescents," *CNS Drugs*, 2002, 16(2):139-44.
de Vries MH, Raghoebar M, Mathlener IS, et al, "Single and Multiple Oral Dose Fluvoxamine Kinetics in Young and Elderly Subjects," *Ther Drug Monit*, 1992, 14(6):493-8.
Diler R and Avci A, "Selective Serotonin Reuptake Inhibitor Discontinuation Syndrome in Children: Six Case Reports," *Current Therapeutic Research*, 2002, 63(3):188-97.
Dopheide JA, "Recognizing and Treating Depression in Children and Adolescents," *Am J of Health Syst Pharm*, 2006, 63(3):233-43.
"Fluvoxamine for the Treatment of Anxiety Disorders in Children and Adolescents. The Research Unit on Pediatric Psychopharmacology Anxiety Study Group," *N Engl J Med*, 2001, 344(17):1279-85.
Grimsley SR and Jann MW, "Paroxetine, Sertraline, and Fluvoxamine: New Selective Serotonin Reuptake Inhibitors," *Clin Pharm*, 1992, 11 (11):930-57.
Lake MB, Birmaher B, Wassick S, et al, "Bleeding and Selective Serotonin Reuptake Inhibitors in Childhood and Adolescence," *J Child Adolesc Psychopharmacol*, 2000, 10(1):35-8.
Levinson-Castiel R, Merlob P, Linder N, et al, "Neonatal Abstinence Syndrome After *in utero* Exposure to Selective Serotonin Reuptake Inhibitors in Term Infants," *Arch Pediatr Adolesc Med*, 2006, 160 (2):173-6.
Pass SE and Simpson RW, "Discontinuation and Reinstitution of Medications During the Perioperative Period," *Am J Health Syst Pharm*, 2004, 61(9):899-912.
Reinblatt SP and Riddle MA, "Selective Serotonin Reuptake Inhibitor-Induced Apathy: A Pediatric Case Series," *J Child Adolesc Psychopharmacol*, 2006, 16(1/2):227-33.
Riddle MA, Reeve EA, Yaryura-Tobias JA, et al, "Fluvoxamine for Children and Adolescents With Obsessive-Compulsive Disorder: A Randomized, Controlled, Multicenter Trial," *J Am Acad Child Adolesc Psychiatry*, 2001, 40(2):222-9.
Roose SP, Glassman AH, Attia E, et al, "Comparative Efficacy of Selective Serotonin Reuptake Inhibitors and Tricyclics in the Treatment of Melancholia," *Am J Psychiatry*, 1994, 151(12):1735-9.
Safer DJ and Zito JM, "Treatment Emergent Adverse Effects of Selective Serotonin Reuptake Inhibitors by Age Group: Children vs. Adolescents," *J Child Adolesc Psychopharmacol*, 2006, 16 (1/2):159-69.
Weintrob N, Cohen D, Klipper-Aurbach Y, et al, "Decreased Growth During Therapy With Selective Serotonin Reuptake Inhibitors," *Arch Pediatr Adolesc Med*, 2002, 156(7):696-701.

◆ **Fluzone** *see* Influenza Virus Vaccine (Inactivated) *on page 1103*

◆ **Fluzone High-Dose** *see* Influenza Virus Vaccine (Inactivated) *on page 1103*

◆ **Fluzone Pediatric PF** *see* Influenza Virus Vaccine (Inactivated) *on page 1103*

◆ **Fluzone Preservative Free** *see* Influenza Virus Vaccine (Inactivated) *on page 1103*

◆ **Fluzone Quadrivalent** *see* Influenza Virus Vaccine (Inactivated) *on page 1103*

◆ **FML** *see* Fluorometholone *on page 897*

◆ **FML® (Can)** *see* Fluorometholone *on page 897*

◆ **FML Forte** *see* Fluorometholone *on page 897*

◆ **FML Forte® (Can)** *see* Fluorometholone *on page 897*

◆ **FML Liquifilm** *see* Fluorometholone *on page 897*

◆ **Focalin** *see* Dexmethylphenidate *on page 623*

◆ **Focalin XR** *see* Dexmethylphenidate *on page 623*

◆ **Foille [OTC]** *see* Benzocaine *on page 273*

◆ **Folacin** *see* Folic Acid *on page 925*

◆ **Folate** *see* Folic Acid *on page 925*

Folic Acid (FOE lik AS id)

Medication Safety Issues
Sound-alike/look-alike issues:
Folic acid may be confused with folinic acid
Brand Names: U.S. FA-8 [OTC]
Brand Names: Canada Apo-Folic®
Therapeutic Category Nutritional Supplement; Vitamin, Water Soluble
Generic Availability (U.S.) Yes
Use Treatment of megaloblastic and macrocytic anemias due to folate deficiency (FDA approved in all ages); has also been used as a dietary supplement to prevent neural tube defects and prevention of gingival hyperplasia due to phenytoin

◀ **Pregnancy Risk Factor** A

Pregnancy Considerations Water soluble vitamins cross the placenta. Folate requirements increase during pregnancy. Folate supplementation during the periconceptual period decreases the risk of neural tube defects. Folate supplementation (doses larger than the RDA) is recommended for women who may become pregnant (IOM, 1998).

Breast-Feeding Considerations Folate is found in breast milk; concentrations are not affected by dietary intake unless the mother has a severe deficiency (IOM, 1998).

Contraindications Hypersensitivity to folic acid or any component

Warnings Folic acid doses >0.1 mg may mask the hematologic effects of B_{12} deficiency, thus obscuring the diagnosis of pernicious anemia while allowing the neurologic complications due to B_{12} deficiency to progress; folic acid is not appropriate for monotherapy for treatment of pernicious, aplastic, or normocytic anemias when anemia is present with vitamin B_{12} deficiency.

Folic acid injection contains benzyl alcohol (1.5%) as preservative, which may cause allergic reactions in susceptible individuals; large amounts of benzyl alcohol (≥99 mg/kg/day) have been associated with a potentially fatal toxicity ("gasping syndrome") in neonates; the "gasping syndrome" consists of metabolic acidosis, respiratory distress, gasping respirations, CNS dysfunction (including convulsions, intracranial hemorrhage), hypotension and cardiovascular collapse; use caution with injection in neonates; *in vitro* and animal studies have shown that benzoate, a metabolite of benzyl alcohol, displaces bilirubin from protein-binding sites

Precautions Use with caution in patients with depressed hematopoiesis, alcoholism, and deficiencies of other vitamins; resistance to treatment with folic acid may occur.

The parenteral product contains aluminum; toxic aluminum concentrations may be seen with high doses, prolonged use, or renal dysfunction. Premature neonates are at higher risk due to immature renal function and aluminum intake from other parenteral sources. Parenteral aluminum exposure of >4-5 mcg/kg/day is associated with CNS and bone toxicity and tissue loading may occur at lower doses.

Adverse Reactions
Cardiovascular: Flushing (slight)
Central nervous system: Malaise (general)
Dermatologic: Erythema, pruritus, rash
Respiratory: Bronchospasm
Miscellaneous: Allergic reaction

Drug Interactions
Metabolism/Transport Effects None known.
Avoid Concomitant Use
Avoid concomitant use of Folic Acid with any of the following: Raltitrexed
Increased Effect/Toxicity There are no known significant interactions involving an increase in effect.
Decreased Effect
Folic Acid may decrease the levels/effects of: Fosphenytoin; PHENobarbital; Phenytoin; Primidone; Raltitrexed

The levels/effects of Folic Acid may be decreased by: Green Tea; SulfaSALAzine

Stability Store at 20°C to 25°C (68°F to 77°F); protect from light.

Mechanism of Action Folic acid is necessary for formation of a number of coenzymes in many metabolic systems, particularly for purine and pyrimidine synthesis; required for nucleoprotein synthesis and maintenance in erythropoiesis; stimulates WBC and platelet production in folate deficiency anemia. Folic acid enhances the metabolism of formic acid, the toxic metabolite of methanol, to nontoxic metabolites (unlabeled use).

Pharmacodynamics Maximum effect: Oral: Within 30-60 minutes

Pharmacokinetics (Adult data unless noted)
Absorption: In the proximal part of the small intestine
Bioavailability: Oral: Folic acid supplement: ~100%; in presence of food: 85%; Dietary folate: 50% (IOM, 1999)
Metabolism: Hepatic
Time to peak serum concentration: Oral: 1 hour
Elimination: Trace amounts of unchanged drug in urine; 90% of dose as metabolites

Dosing: Neonatal
Enteral daily recommendations; adequate intake (Vanek, 2012): Oral:
Premature neonates: 25-50 mcg/kg/day
Full-term neonates: 65 mcg/day
Parenteral nutrition, maintenance requirement of folic acid (Vanek, 2012): I.V.:
Premature neonates: 56 mcg/kg/day
Full-term neonates: 140 mcg/day

Dosing: Usual
Infants, Children, and Adolescents:
Adequate intake (AI): Oral: **Note:** Dosing presented as dietary folate equivalents (DFE) to adjust for ~50% decreased bioavailability of food folate compared with that of folic acid supplement.
1-6 months: 65 mcg/day
7-12 months: 80 mcg/day
Recommended daily allowance (RDA): Oral: **Note:** Dosing presented as dietary folate equivalents (DFE) to adjust for ~50% decreased bioavailability of food folate compared with that of folic acid supplement.
1-3 years: 150 mcg/day
4-8 years: 200 mcg/day
9-13 years: 300 mcg/day
Adolescents ≥14 years: 400 mcg/day
Anemia (folic acid deficiency); treatment: Oral, I.M., I.V., SubQ:
Infants: 0.1 mg/day
Children <4 years: Up to 0.3 mg/day
Children >4 years and Adolescents: 0.4 mg/day
Parenteral nutrition, maintenance requirement of folic acid (Vanek, 2012): I.V.:
Infants: 56 mcg/kg/day
Children and Adolescents ≤13 years: 140 mcg/day
Adolescents ≥14 years: 400 mcg/day
Gingival hyperplasia due to phenytoin, prevention: Limited data available: Oral: Children ≥6 years and Adolescents: 0.5 mg/day was used in a double-blind, randomized, placebo-controlled trial of 120 pediatric patients (treatment arm, n=62; age range: 6-15 years) who were started on phenytoin therapy within the last month for a seizure disorder; results showed a statistically significant difference in development of hyperplasia (treatment arm: 21% vs placebo: 88%); severity of cases less in treatment arm than placebo; study duration: 6 months (Arya, 2011)
Adults:
Recommended daily allowance (RDA): Expressed as dietary folate equivalents: Oral: 400 mcg/day
Pregnancy: 600 mcg/day
Lactation: 500 mcg/day
Anemia (folic acid deficiency); treatment: Oral, I.M., I.V., SubQ:
Nonpregnant and nonlactating adults: 0.4 mg/day
Pregnant and lactating women: 0.8 mg/day
Prevention of neural tube defects: Oral:
Females of childbearing potential: 400-800 mcg/day (USPSTF, 2009)
Females at high-risk or with family history of neural tube defects: 4 mg/day (ACOG, 2003)

Administration
Oral: May be administered without regard to meals

Parenteral:

I.M., SubQ: May administer undiluted deep I.M. or SubQ

I.V.: May administer doses ≤5 mg undiluted over ≥1 minute **or** may dilute ≤5 mg in 50 mL of NS or D₅W (maximum concentration: 0.1 mg/mL) and infuse over 30 minutes. May also be added to I.V. maintenance solutions and given as an infusion.

Monitoring Parameters CBC with differential

Reference Range Total folate: Normal: 5-15 ng/mL; folate deficiency: <5 ng/mL; megaloblastic anemia: <2 ng/mL

Test Interactions Falsely low serum concentrations may occur with the *Lactobacillus casei* assay method in patients on anti-infectives (eg, tetracycline)

Additional Information Dietary folate equivalents (DFE) is used to adjust for ~50% decreased bioavailability of food folate compared with that of folic acid supplement:

1 mcg DFE = 0.6 mcg folic acid from fortified food or as a supplement taken with meals, or

1 mcg DFE of food folate = 0.5 mcg of a supplement taken on an empty stomach

As of January 1998, the FDA has required manufacturers of enriched flour, bread, corn meal, pasta, rice, and other grain products to add folic acid to their products. The intent is to help decrease the risk of neural tube defects by increasing folic acid intake. Other foods which contain folic acid include dark green leafy vegetables, citrus fruits and juices, and lentils.

Dosage Forms Excipient information presented when available (limited, particularly for generics); consult specific product labeling.

Capsule, Oral [preservative free]:
  FA-8: 0.8 mg [dye free, sugar free, yeast free]
  Generic: 5 mg, 20 mg
Solution, Injection, as sodium folate:
  Generic: 5 mg/mL (10 mL)
Tablet, Oral:
  Generic: 400 mcg, 800 mcg, 1 mg
Tablet, Oral [preservative free]:
  FA-8: 800 mcg [dye free]
  Generic: 400 mcg, 800 mcg

Extemporaneous Preparations A 1 mg/mL folic acid oral solution may be made with tablets. Heat 90 mL of purified water almost to boiling. Dissolve parabens (methylparaben 200 mg and propylparaben 20 mg) in the heated water; cool to room temperature. Crush one-hundred 1 mg tablets, then dissolve folic acid in the solution. Adjust pH to 8-8.5 with sodium hydroxide 10%; add sufficient quantity of purified water to make 100 mL; mix well. Stable for 30 days at room temperature (Allen, 2007).

A 0.05 mg/mL folic acid oral solution may be prepared using the injectable formulation (5 mg/mL). Mix 1 mL of injectable folic acid with 90 mL of purified water. Adjust pH to 8-8.5 with sodium hydroxide 10%; add sufficient quantity of purified water to make 100 mL; mix well. Stable for 30 days at room temperature (Nahata, 2004).

Allen LV Jr, "Folic Acid 1-mg/mL Oral Liquid," *Int J Pharm Compound*, 2007, 11(3):244.

Nahata MC, Pai VB, and Hipple TF, *Pediatric Drug Formulations*, 5th ed, Cincinnati, OH: Harvey Whitney Books Co, 2004.

References

ACOG Committee on Practice Bulletins, "Clinical Management Guidelines for Obstetrician-Gynecologists. Number 44, July 2003 (Replaces Committee Opinion Number 252, March 2001)," *Obstet Gynecol*, 2003, 102(1):203-13.

Arya R, Gulati S, Kabra M, et al, "Folic Acid Supplementation Prevents Phenytoin-Induced Gingival Overgrowth in Children," *Neurology*, 2011, 76(15):1338-43.

Department Health & Human Services, Food Drug Administration, "Aluminum in Large and Small Volume Parenterals Used in Total Parenteral Nutrition," *Federal Register*, 2000, 65(17):4103-11.

IOM (Institute of Medicine), *Dietary Reference Intakes for Thiamin, Riboflavin, Niacin, Vitamin B6, Folate, Vitamin B₁₂, Pantothenic Acid, Biotin and Choline*, Washington, DC: National Academy Press, 1998.

U.S. Preventive Services Task Force (USPSTF), "Folic Acid for the Prevention of Neural Tube Defects: U.S. Preventive Services Task Force Recommendation Statement," *Ann Intern Med*, 2009, 150(9):626-31.

Vanek VW, Borum P, Buchman A, et al, "A.S.P.E.N. Position Paper: Recommendations for Changes in Commercially Available Parenteral Multivitamin and Multi-trace Element Products," *Nutr Clin Pract*, 2012, 27(4):440-91.

◆ **Folinate Calcium** *see* Leucovorin Calcium *on page 1213*

◆ **Folinic Acid (error prone synonym)** *see* Leucovorin Calcium *on page 1213*

Fomepizole (foe ME pi zole)

Medication Safety Issues
Sound-alike/look-alike issues:
  Fomepizole may be confused with omeprazole
Brand Names: U.S. Antizol
Brand Names: Canada Antizol
Therapeutic Category Antidote, Ethylene Glycol Toxicity; Antidote, Methanol Toxicity
Generic Availability (U.S.) Yes
Use Antidote for ethylene glycol (antifreeze) or methanol toxicity; may be useful in propylene glycol toxicity; FDA approved in ages ≥18 years
Pregnancy Risk Factor C
Pregnancy Considerations Animal reproduction studies have not been conducted. In general, medications used as antidotes should take into consideration the health and prognosis of the mother; antidotes should be administered to pregnant women if there is a clear indication for use and should not be withheld because of fears of teratogenicity (Bailey, 2003).
Breast-Feeding Considerations It is not known if fomepizole is excreted in breast milk. The manufacturer recommends that caution be exercised when administering fomepizole to nursing women.
Contraindications Hypersensitivity to fomepizole, other pyrazoles, or any component
Warnings By inhibiting the action of alcohol dehydrogenase, fomepizole reduces the elimination of alcohol; this must be considered when using fomepizole, as alcohol is often ingested concomitantly by patients with ethylene glycol intoxication; likewise, alcohol may reduce the elimination of fomepizole by the same mechanism. Pediatric administration is not FDA approved; however, safe and efficacious use in this patient population for ethylene glycol and methanol intoxication has been reported (Baum, 2000; Benitez, 2000; Boyer, 2001; Brown, 2001; De Brabander, 2005; Detaille, 2004; Fisher, 1998). Consider consultation with a clinical toxicologist or poison control center.
Precautions Management of ethylene glycol ingestion may require treatment of metabolic acidosis, acute renal failure, adult respiratory distress syndrome, and hypocalcemia; dialysis should be considered, in addition to fomepizole therapy, in patients with acute renal failure, severe metabolic acidosis, or a serum ethylene glycol concentration >50 mg/dL; adjust dosage for renal dysfunction
Adverse Reactions
Cardiovascular: Bradycardia, facial flush, hypotension, shock, tachycardia
Central nervous system: Agitation, anxiety, dizziness, drowsiness increased, fever, headache, lightheadedness, seizure, vertigo
Dermatologic: Rash
Endocrine & metabolic: Liver function tests increased
Gastrointestinal: Abdominal pain, appetite decreased, bad/metallic taste, diarrhea, heartburn, nausea, vomiting
Hematologic: Anemia, disseminated intravascular coagulation (DIC), eosinophilia, lymphangitis
Local: Application site reaction, injection site inflammation, pain during injection, phlebitis

◀ Neuromuscular & skeletal: Backache
Ocular: Nystagmus, transient blurred vision, visual disturbances
Renal: Anuria
Respiratory: Abnormal smell, hiccups, pharyngitis
Miscellaneous: Multiorgan failure, speech disturbances
Rare but important or life-threatening: Mild allergic reactions (mild rash, eosinophilia)

Drug Interactions

Metabolism/Transport Effects None known.

Avoid Concomitant Use There are no known interactions where it is recommended to avoid concomitant use.

Increased Effect/Toxicity There are no known significant interactions involving an increase in effect.

Decreased Effect There are no known significant interactions involving a decrease in effect.

Food Interactions Ethanol decreases the rate of fomepizole elimination by ~50%; conversely, fomepizole decreases the rate of elimination of ethanol by ~40%.

Stability Store at room temperature; fomepizole solidifies at temperatures <25°C (77°F); if solidification occurs, liquefy by running the vial under warm water or by holding in the hand; solidification does not affect the efficacy, safety, or stability of fomepizole; stabile diluted in NS or D_5W for 48 hours; does not contain a preservative; use within 24 hours of dilution

Mechanism of Action Fomepizole competitively inhibits alcohol dehydrogenase, an enzyme which catalyzes the metabolism of ethanol, ethylene glycol, and methanol to their toxic metabolites. Ethylene glycol is metabolized to glycoaldehyde, then oxidized to glycolate, glyoxylate, and oxalate. Glycolate and oxalate are responsible for metabolic acidosis and renal damage. Methanol is metabolized to formaldehyde, then oxidized to formic acid. Formic acid is responsible for metabolic acidosis and visual disturbances.

Pharmacokinetics (Adult data unless noted)

Distribution: V_d: 0.6-1.02 L/kg; rapidly distributes into total body water

Protein binding: Negligible

Metabolism: Liver; primarily to 4-carboxypyrazole; after single doses, exhibits saturable, Michaelis-Menton kinetics; with multiple dosing, fomepizole induces its own metabolism via the cytochrome P450 system; after enzyme induction elimination follows first order kinetics

Elimination: 1% to 3.5% excreted unchanged in the urine

Dialysis: Dialyzable

Dosing: Usual I.V.:

Children and Adults **not requiring** hemodialysis: Initial: 15 mg/kg loading dose; followed by 10 mg/kg every 12 hours for 4 doses; then 15 mg/kg every 12 hours until ethylene glycol or methanol levels have been reduced to <20 mg/dL

Children and Adults **requiring** hemodialysis: Since fomepizole is dialyzable, follow the above dose recommendations at intervals related to institution of hemodialysis and its duration:

Dose at the beginning of hemodialysis:

If <6 hours since last fomepizole dose: Do **not** administer dose

If ≥6 hours since last fomepizole dose: Administer next scheduled dose

Dose during hemodialysis: Administer every 4 hours or as continuous infusion 1-1.5 mg/kg/hour

Dose at the time hemodialysis is completed (dependent upon the time between the last dose and the end of hemodialysis):

<1 hour: Do **not** administer at the end of hemodialysis

1-3 hours: Administer 1/2 of the next scheduled dose

>3 hours: Administer the next scheduled dose

Maintenance dose off hemodialysis: Give next scheduled dose 12 hours from last dose administered

Dosage adjustment in renal impairment: Fomepizole is substantially excreted by the kidney and the risk of toxic reactions to this drug may be increased in patients with impaired renal function; no dosage recommendations for patients with impaired renal function have been established

Administration Parenteral: I.V. Dilute in at least 100 mL NS or D_5W (<25 mg/mL); infuse over 30 minutes; rapid infusion of concentrations ≥25 mg/mL has been associated with vein irritation and phlebosclerosis

Monitoring Parameters Vital signs, arterial blood gases, acid-base status, urinary oxalate, anion and osmolar gaps, clinical signs and symptoms of toxicity (arrhythmias, seizures, coma); serum and urinary ethylene glycol or serum methanol level depending upon the agent ingested; formic acid level (methanol ingestion)

Reference Range Ethylene glycol or methanol serum concentration: Goal: <20 mg/dL; therapeutic plasma fomepizole level: 0.8 mcg/mL

Additional Information If ethylene glycol poisoning is left untreated, the natural progression of the poisoning leads to accumulation of toxic metabolites, including glycolic and oxalic acids; these metabolites can induce metabolic acidosis, seizures, stupor, coma, calcium oxaluria, acute tubular necrosis and death; as ethylene glycol levels diminish in the blood when metabolized to glycolate, the diagnosis of this poisoning may be difficult

Dosage Forms Excipient information presented when available (limited, particularly for generics); consult specific product labeling.

Solution, Intravenous [preservative free]:

Antizol: 1 g/mL (1.5 mL)

Generic: 1 g/mL (1.5 mL); 1.5 g/1.5 mL (1.5 mL)

References

Bailey B, "Are There Teratogenic Risks Associated With Antidotes Used in the Acute Management of Poisoned Pregnant Women?" *Birth Defects Res A Clin Mol Teratol*, 2003, 67(2):133-40.

Baum CR, Langman CB, Oker EE, et al, "Fomepizole Treatment of Ethylene Glycol Poisoning in an Infant," *Pediatrics*, 2000, 106 (6):1489-91.

Benitez JG, Swanson-Biearman B, and Krenzelok EP, "Nystagmus Secondary to Fomepizole Administration in a Pediatric Patient," *J Toxicol Clin Toxicol*, 2000, 38(7):795-8.

Boyer EW, Mejia M, Woolf A, et al, "Severe Ethylene Glycol Ingestion Treated Without Hemodialysis," *Pediatrics*, 2001, 107(1):172-3.

Brown MJ, Shannon MW, Woolf A, et al, "Childhood Methanol Ingestion Treated With Fomepizole and Hemodialysis," *Pediatrics*, 2001, 108 (4):e77-9.

De Brabander N, Wojciechowski M, De Decker K, et al, "Fomepizole as a Therapeutic Strategy in Paediatric Methanol Poisoning: A Case Report and Review of the Literature," *Eur J Pediatr*, 2005, 164 (3):158-61.

Detaille T, Wallemacq P, Clement de Clety S, et al, "Fomepizole Alone for Severe Infant Ethylene Glycol Poisoning," *Pediatr Crit Care Med*, 2004, 5(5):490-1.

Druteika DP, Zed PJ, and Ensom MH, "Role of Fomepizole in the Management of Ethylene Glycol Toxicity," *Pharmacotherapy*, 2002, 22(3):365-72.

Fisher DM and Diaz JE, "Pediatric Methanol Poisoning Treated With Fomepizole (Antizol®)," *J Toxicol Clin Toxicol*, 1998, 36:512.

◆ **Foradil (Can)** *see* Formoterol *on page 929*

◆ **Foradil Aerolizer** *see* Formoterol *on page 929*

◆ **Forfivo XL** *see* BuPROPion *on page 327*

Formoterol (for MOH te rol)

Medication Safety Issues
Sound-alike/look-alike issues:
Foradil may be confused with Toradol
Administration issues:
Foradil capsules for inhalation are for administration via Aerolizer inhaler and are **not** for oral use.
International issues:
Foradil [U.S., Canada, and multiple international markets] may be confused with Theradol brand name for tramadol [Netherlands]

Brand Names: U.S. Foradil Aerolizer; Perforomist
Brand Names: Canada Foradil; Oxeze Turbuhaler
Therapeutic Category Adrenergic Agonist Agent; Antiasthmatic; Beta₂-Adrenergic Agonist; Bronchodilator; Sympathomimetic

Generic Availability (U.S.) No

Use
Foradil® Aerolizer™: Concomitant therapy with inhaled corticosteroids for maintenance treatment of asthma and prevention of bronchospasm in patients with reversible obstructive airway disease, including patients with nocturnal symptoms (FDA approved in ≥5 years and adults); prevention of exercise-induced bronchospasm as concomitant therapy in patients with persistent asthma and as monotherapy in those without persistent asthma (FDA approved in ≥5 years and adults); **NOT** indicated for the relief of acute bronchospasm

Foradil® Aerolizer™, Perforomist™: Maintenance treatment of bronchoconstriction in COPD (FDA approved in adults); **NOT** indicated for the relief of acute bronchospasm

Medication Guide Available Yes
Pregnancy Risk Factor C
Pregnancy Considerations Adverse events were observed in some animal reproduction studies. Formoterol has the potential to affect uterine contractility if administered during labor.

Uncontrolled asthma is associated with adverse events on pregnancy (increased risk of perinatal mortality, preeclampsia, preterm birth, low birth weight infants). Although data related to its use in pregnancy is limited, formoterol may be used as an alternative agent when a long-acting beta agonist is needed to treat moderate persistent or severe persistent asthma in pregnant women (NAEPP, 2005).

Breast-Feeding Considerations It is not known if formoterol is excreted into breast milk. The manufacturer recommends that caution be exercised when administering formoterol to nursing women. The use of beta₂-receptor agonists are not considered a contraindication to breast-feeding (NAEPP, 2005).

Contraindications Hypersensitivity to formoterol, adrenergic amines, or any component; monotherapy in the treatment of asthma (ie, use without a concomitant long-term asthma control medication, such as an inhaled corticosteroid); treatment of status asthmaticus or other acute episodes of asthma or COPD

Warnings Long-acting beta₂-adrenergic agents (LABAs), including formoterol, increase the risk of asthma-related deaths **[U.S. Boxed Warning]**. Formoterol should only be prescribed in patients not adequately controlled on long-term asthma-controller medications (ie, inhaled corticosteroid) or whose disease requires initiation of two maintenance therapies; monotherapy with a LABA is contraindicated in the treatment of asthma. In a large clinical trial, LABA (salmeterol) use was associated with an increase in asthma-related deaths compared to placebo (when added to usual asthma therapy); risk is considered a class effect among all LABAs. Data are not available to determine if the addition of an inhaled corticosteroid lessens this increased risk of death associated with LABA use or if LABA use also increases the risk of death in patients with COPD. Assess patients at regular intervals once asthma control is maintained on combination therapy to determine if step down therapy is appropriate (without loss of asthma control), and if the patient can be maintained on an inhaled corticosteroid alone. LABAs are not appropriate in patients whose asthma is adequately controlled on low- or medium-dose inhaled corticosteroids. LABAs may increase the risk of asthma-related hospitalization in pediatric and adolescent patients **[U.S. Boxed Warning]**. When addition of a LABA is clinically indicated in patients <18 years of age, a combination product containing a LABA and an inhaled corticosteroid is preferred to ensure compliance.

Formoterol should not be used to relieve acute asthmatic or COPD symptoms or rapidly deteriorating or potentially life-threatening episodes of asthma or COPD; acute episodes should be treated with short-acting beta₂-agonists. Routine use of inhaled, short-acting beta₂-agonists should be discontinued prior to initiation of formoterol. Corticosteroids should not be stopped or reduced when formeterol is initiated. Formoterol should not be used more frequently than recommended (twice daily), at higher doses, or with any additional long-acting beta₂-adrenergic agonist; adverse cardiovascular effects (possibly fatal) have been reported with excessive beta₂-adrenergic overstimulation. Use with strong CYP3A4 inhibitors (eg, ketoconazole, ritonavir, atazanavir, clarithromycin, indinavir, itraconazole, nefazodone, nelfinavir, saquinavir, telithromycin) is not recommended due to potential for an increased risk of cardiovascular events. Paroxysmal bronchospasm (which can be fatal) has been reported with formoterol and other inhaled beta₂-agonists; if this occurs, discontinue treatment; most commonly occurs with first use of a new canister or vial. Symptoms of laryngeal spasm, irritation, or swelling, such as stridor and choking, have been reported; if occurs, discontinue treatment. Because LABAs may disguise poorly controlled persistent asthma, frequent or chronic use of LABAs for exercise-induced bronchospasm is discouraged by the NAEPP Asthma Guidelines (NAEPP, 2007). Foradil® capsules should **only** be used with the Aerolizer™ inhaler and should **not** be taken orally.

Precautions Use with caution in patients with cardiovascular disorders (especially coronary insufficiency, arrhythmias, hypertension, heart failure, aneurysm), although uncommon at recommended doses, beta-agonists may cause elevation in BP and HR and result in CNS stimulation and excitation. Caution should also be used in patients with thyrotoxicosis, seizure disorders, pheochromocytoma, or conditions that are unusually sensitive to sympathomimetic amines. Transient hypokalemia from intracellular shunting may occur and produce adverse cardiovascular effects. Use with caution in patients with diabetes mellitus (DM); beta₂-agonists can increase serum glucose aggravating preexisting DM and ketoacidosis. Use caution in patients with hepatic impairment. Immediate hypersensitivity reactions (urticaria, angioedema, rash, bronchospasm) have been reported. Foradil® aerolizer contains lactose; very rare anaphylactic reactions have been reported in patients with severe milk protein allergy.

Adverse Reactions
Cardiovascular: Chest pain, palpitation
Central nervous system: Anxiety, dizziness, dysphonia, fever, headache, insomnia
Dermatologic: Pruritus, rash
Gastrointestinal: Abdominal pain, diarrhea, dyspepsia, gastroenteritis, nausea, vomiting, xerostomia
Neuromuscular & skeletal: Muscle cramps, tremor
Respiratory: Asthma exacerbation, bronchitis, dyspnea, infection, pharyngitis, sinusitis, tonsillitis

Miscellaneous: Viral infection

Rare but important or life-threatening: Acute asthma deterioration, anaphylactic reactions (severe hypotension/angioedema), agitation, angina, arrhythmia, atrial fibrillation, bronchospasm (paradoxical), cough, fatigue, hyperglycemia, hypertension, hypokalemia, glucose intolerance, malaise, metabolic acidosis, nervousness, QTc prolongation, tachycardia, ventricular extrasystoles

Drug Interactions

Metabolism/Transport Effects Substrate of CYP2C9 (minor); **Note:** Assignment of Major/Minor substrate status based on clinically relevant drug interaction potential

Avoid Concomitant Use

Avoid concomitant use of Formoterol with any of the following: Beta-Blockers (Nonselective); Highest Risk QTc-Prolonging Agents; Iobenguane I 123; Ivabradine; Long-Acting Beta2-Agonists; Mifepristone

Increased Effect/Toxicity

Formoterol may increase the levels/effects of: Atosiban; Highest Risk QTc-Prolonging Agents; Long-Acting Beta2-Agonists; Loop Diuretics; Moderate Risk QTc-Prolonging Agents; Sympathomimetics; Thiazide Diuretics

The levels/effects of Formoterol may be increased by: AtoMOXetine; Caffeine and Caffeine Containing Products; Cannabinoid-Containing Products; Inhalational Anesthetics; Ivabradine; Linezolid; MAO Inhibitors; Mifepristone; QTc-Prolonging Agents (Indeterminate Risk and Risk Modifying); Theophylline Derivatives; Tricyclic Antidepressants

Decreased Effect

Formoterol may decrease the levels/effects of: Iobenguane I 123

The levels/effects of Formoterol may be decreased by: Beta-Blockers (Beta1 Selective); Beta-Blockers (Nonselective); Betahistine

Stability

Foradil® Aerolizer™: Prior to dispensing, store in refrigerator at 2°C to 8°C (36°F to 46°F); after dispensing, store at controlled room temperature at 20°C to 25°C (68°F to 77°F); protect from heat and moisture. Capsules should always be stored in the blister pack and only removed immediately before use. Use within 4 months of purchase date or product expiration date, whichever comes first.

Performoist™: Prior to dispensing, store in refrigerator at 2°C to 8°C (36°F to 46°F); after dispensing, store at controlled room temperature at 20°C to 25°C (68°F to 77°F) for up to 3 months. Protect from heat. Unit-dose vials should always be stored in the foil pouch and only removed immediately before use.

Mechanism of Action Relaxes bronchial smooth muscle by selective action on beta$_2$ receptors with little effect on heart rate. Formoterol has a long-acting effect.

Pharmacodynamics

Onset of action: Powder for oral inhalation: 1-3 minutes

Peak effect:

Powder for oral inhalation: 80% of peak effect within 15 minutes

Solution for nebulization: Median: 2 hours

Duration: Improvement in FEV$_1$ observed for 12 hours in most patients

Pharmacokinetics (Adult data unless noted)

Absorption: Rapidly into plasma

Protein binding: 61% to 64%

Metabolism: Extensive via glucuronidation and o-demethylation; CYP2D6, CYP2C8/9, CYP2C19, CYP2A6 involved in O-demethylation

Half-life:

Powder for oral inhalation: ~10-14 hours

Solution for nebulization: ~7 hours

Time to peak serum concentration: Inhalation: 5 minutes

Elimination:

Children 5-12 years: 7% to 9% eliminated in urine as direct glucuronide metabolites, 6% as unchanged drug

Adults: 15% to 18% eliminated in urine as direct glucuronide metabolites, 2% to 10% as unchanged drug

Dosing: Usual

Asthma, maintenance treatment: Children ≥5 years, Adolescents, and Adults: Inhalation: Foradil® Aerolizer™: 12 mcg (contents of 1 capsule aerosolized) twice daily, 12 hours apart; maximum daily dose: 24 mcg; **Note:** For long-term asthma control, long-acting beta$_2$-agonists should be used in combination with inhaled corticosteroids and **not** as monotherapy

Exercise-induced asthma, prevention: Children ≥5 years, Adolescents, and Adults: Inhalation: Foradil® Aerolizer™: 12 mcg (contents of 1 capsule aerosolized) 15 minutes prior to exercise; additional doses should not be used for 12 hours; maximum daily dose: 24 mcg; patients who are using formoterol twice daily should **not** use an additional formoterol dose prior to exercise; if twice daily use is not effective during exercise, consider other appropriate therapy; **Note:** Because long-acting beta$_2$-agonists (LABAs) may disguise poorly-controlled persistent asthma, frequent or chronic use of LABAs for exercise-induced bronchospasm is discouraged by the NAEPP Asthma Guidelines (NAEPP, 2007).

COPD, maintenance treatment: Adults: Inhalation:

Foradil® Aerolizer™: 12 mcg (contents of 1 capsule aerosolized) twice daily, 12 hours apart; maximum daily dose: 24 mcg

Performoist™: 20 mcg (2 mL) twice daily by nebulization; maximum daily dose: 40 mcg

Administration

Foradil® Aerolizer™: Remove capsule from foil blister immediately before use. The contents of a capsule are aerosolized via a device called an Aerolizer™. Place the capsule into the Aerolizer™. The capsule is pierced by pressing and releasing the buttons on the side of the Aerolizer™. The formoterol formulation is dispersed into the air stream when the patient inhales rapidly and deeply through the mouthpiece. The patient should not exhale into the device. May not be used with spacer device.

Performoist™: Remove unit-dose vial from foil pouch immediately before use. Solution does not require dilution prior to administration; do not mix other medications with Performoist™ solution. Place contents of vial into the reservoir of a standard jet nebulizer connected to an air compressor; nebulize until all of the medication has been inhaled. Discard any unused medication immediately. Not for oral ingestion.

Monitoring Parameters Pulmonary function tests, vital signs, CNS stimulation, serum glucose, serum potassium

Additional Information When formoterol is initiated in patients previously receiving a short-acting beta agonist, instruct the patient to discontinue the regular use of the short-acting beta agonist and to utilize the shorter-acting agent for symptomatic or acute episodes only.

Dosage Forms Excipient information presented when available (limited, particularly for generics); consult specific product labeling.

Capsule, Inhalation, as fumarate:

Foradil Aerolizer: 12 mcg [contains milk protein]

Nebulization Solution, Inhalation, as fumarate dihydrate:

Performoist: 20 mcg/2 mL (2 mL)

References

Bisgaard H, "Long-acting Beta$_2$-Agonists in Management of Childhood Asthma: A Critical Review of the Literature," *Pediatr Pulmonol*, 2000, 29(3):221-34

National Asthma Education and Prevention Program (NAEPP), "Expert Panel Report 3 (EPR-3): Guidelines for the Diagnosis and Management of Asthma," Clinical Practice Guidelines, National Institutes of Health, National Heart, Lung, and Blood Institute, NIH Publication No. 08-4051, prepublication 2007. Available at http://www.nhlbi.nih.gov/guidelines/asthma/asthgdln.htm

National Asthma Education and Prevention Program (NAEPP) Working Group Report on "Managing Asthma During Pregnancy: Recommendations for Pharmacologic Treatment," National Institutes of Health, National Heart, Lung, and Blood Institute, NIH Publication No. 05-5236, March 2005. Available at http://www.nhlbi.nih.gov/health/prof/lung/asthma/astpreg/astpreg_full.pdf

♦ **Formoterol and Budesonide** see Budesonide and Formoterol on page 314

♦ **Formoterol and Mometasone** see Mometasone and Formoterol on page 1436

♦ **Formoterol and Mometasone Furoate** see Mometasone and Formoterol on page 1436

♦ **Formoterol Fumarate** see Formoterol on page 929

♦ **Formoterol Fumarate Dihydrate** see Formoterol on page 929

♦ **Formoterol Fumarate Dihydrate and Budesonide** see Budesonide and Formoterol on page 314

♦ **Formoterol Fumarate Dihydrate and Mometasone** see Mometasone and Formoterol on page 1436

♦ **Formula E 400 [OTC]** see Vitamin E on page 2148

♦ **Formulex (Can)** see Dicyclomine on page 652

♦ **5-Formyl Tetrahydrofolate** see Leucovorin Calcium on page 1213

♦ **Fortamet** see MetFORMIN on page 1353

♦ **Fortaz** see CefTAZidime on page 413

♦ **Fortaz in D₅W** see CefTAZidime on page 413

♦ **Fortesta** see Testosterone on page 1986

♦ **Fortical** see Calcitonin on page 340

Fosamprenavir (FOS am pren a veer)

Medication Safety Issues
Sound-alike/look-alike issues:
Lexiva® may be confused with Levitra®
Related Information
Adult and Adolescent HIV on page 2348
Pediatric HIV on page 2338
Perinatal HIV on page 2356
Brand Names: U.S. Lexiva
Brand Names: Canada Telzir®
Therapeutic Category Antiretroviral Agent; HIV Agents (Anti-HIV Agents); Protease Inhibitor
Generic Availability (U.S.) No
Use
Treatment of HIV infection in combination with other antiretroviral agents (boosted with ritonavir) in therapy-naïve patients (FDA approved in ages ≥4 weeks and adults); **Note:** Current guidelines **do not recommend** a boosted regimen in therapy-naïve patients <6 months due to low systemic exposure (DHHS [pediatric]; 2014)
Treatment of HIV infection in combination with other antiretroviral agents (boosted with ritonavir) in therapy-experienced patients (FDA approved in ages ≥6 months and adults)
Treatment of HIV infection in combination with other antiretroviral agents (unboosted; without ritonavir) (FDA approved in therapy-naïve patients ages ≥2 years and adults); **Note:** Current guidelines **do not recommend** an unboosted regimen in pediatric patients due to low systemic exposure (DHHS [pediatric]; 2014)
Note: HIV regimens consisting of **three** antiretroviral agents are strongly recommended.
Pregnancy Risk Factor C

Pregnancy Considerations Adverse events were observed in some animal reproduction studies. Fosamprenavir has a low level of transfer across the human placenta. A small increased risk of preterm birth has been associated with maternal use of protease inhibitor-based combination antiretroviral (ARV) therapy during pregnancy; however, the benefits of use generally outweigh this risk and protease inhibitors (PIs) should not be withheld if otherwise recommended. Hyperglycemia, new onset of diabetes mellitus, or diabetic ketoacidosis have been reported with PIs; it is not clear if pregnancy increases this risk. The DHHS Perinatal HIV Guidelines note there are insufficient data to recommend use during pregnancy; however, if used, they recommend that fosamprenavir be given with low-dose ritonavir boosting.

Regardless of CD4 count or HIV RNA copy number, all HIV-infected pregnant women should receive a combination antiretroviral ARV drug regimen. A combination of antepartum, intrapartum, and infant ARV prophylaxis is recommended. ARV therapy should be started as soon as possible in women with symptomatic infection. Although earlier initiation may be more effective in reducing the perinatal transmission of HIV, initiation may be delayed until after 12 weeks gestation in women who do not require immediate treatment after careful consideration of maternal conditions (eg, nausea and vomiting) and the potential risks of first trimester fetal exposure for specific agents A scheduled cesarean delivery at 38 weeks gestation is recommended for all women with HIV RNA >1000 copies/mL or unknown concentrations near delivery in order to decrease transmission. If ARV therapy must be interrupted for <24 hours during the peripartum period, stop then restart all medications simultaneously in order to decrease the chance of developing resistance. Long-term follow-up is recommended for all infants exposed to ARV medications. In couples who want to conceive, the HIV-infected partner should attain maximum viral suppression prior to conception.

Health care providers are encouraged to enroll pregnant women exposed to antiretroviral medications in the Antiretroviral Pregnancy Registry (1-800-258-4263 or www.APRegistry.com). Health care providers caring for HIV-infected women and their infants may contact the National Perinatal HIV Hotline (888-448-8765) for clinical consultation (DHHS [perinatal], 2014).

Breast-Feeding Considerations It is not known if fosamprenavir is excreted into breast milk. Maternal or infant antiretroviral therapy does not completely eliminate the risk of postnatal HIV transmission. In addition, multiclass-resistant virus has been detected in breast-feeding infants despite maternal therapy. Therefore, in the United States, where formula is accessible, affordable, safe, and sustainable, and the risk of infant mortality due to diarrhea and respiratory infections is low, complete avoidance of breast-feeding by HIV-infected women is recommended to decrease potential transmission of HIV (DHHS [perinatal], 2014).

Contraindications Hypersensitivity to fosamprenavir, amprenavir, or any component; concurrent therapy with CYP3A4 substrates with a narrow therapeutic window; concomitant therapy with alfuzosin, cisapride, delavirdine, dihydroergotamine, ergonovine, ergotamine, methylergonovine, lovastatin, midazolam, pimozide, rifampin, sildenafil [for treatment of pulmonary arterial hypertension (eg, Revatio)], simvastatin, St John's wort, and triazolam; if fosamprenavir is administered with ritonavir, flecainide and propafenone are also contraindicated.

Warnings Fosamprenavir (a prodrug of amprenavir) is a potent CYP3A4 isoenzyme inhibitor that interacts with numerous drugs. Due to potential serious and/or life-threatening drug interactions, some drugs are contraindicated and the following drugs require serum concentration monitoring if coadministered with fosamprenavir: Amiodarone, systemic lidocaine, tricyclic antidepressants, and quinidine. Concurrent use with rifampin, St John's wort, certain cholesterol-lowering agents (lovastatin, simvastatin), and delavirdine are contraindicated.

Rash may occur (incidence: ~19%); usually mild to moderate, maculopapular, some pruritic; median onset: 11 days, median duration: 13 days. Severe and life-threatening skin reactions (including Stevens-Johnson syndrome) may occur (<1% of patients); discontinue fosamprenavir in patients who develop severe or life-threatening rashes or in patients with moderate rashes and systemic symptoms. Acute hemolytic anemia has been reported. Spontaneous bleeding episodes have been reported in patients with hemophilia type A and B receiving protease inhibitors. New-onset diabetes mellitus, exacerbations of diabetes, and hyperglycemia have been reported in HIV-infected patients receiving protease inhibitors. Higher than recommended combination doses of fosamprenavir and ritonavir may result in increased risk of transaminase elevations. Cases of nephrolithiasis have been reported with fosamprenavir use; consider temporary or permanent discontinuation of therapy if symptoms develop.

Significant elevations of serum triglycerides and cholesterol may occur; obtain serum triglyceride and cholesterol prior to initiation of therapy and periodically thereafter; manage lipid elevations appropriately. Modifiable risk factors for cardiovascular disease (eg, smoking, diabetes, hypertension) should also be monitored and managed appropriately.

Precautions Use with caution in patients with diabetes mellitus, sulfonamide allergy (fosamprenavir is a sulfonamide), or hemophilia. Use with caution and decrease the dose in patients with hepatic impairment; patients coinfected with hepatitis B or C and those with baseline liver enzyme elevation may be at risk for elevated liver enzymes with fosamprenavir therapy.

Fat redistribution and accumulation [ie, central obesity, peripheral wasting, facial wasting, breast enlargement, dorsocervical fat enlargement (buffalo hump), and cushingoid appearance] have been observed in patients receiving antiretroviral agents (causal relationship not established).

Immune reconstitution syndrome (an acute inflammatory response to residual or indolent opportunistic infections) may occur in HIV patients during initial treatment with combination antiretroviral agents; this syndrome may require further patient assessment and therapy. Autoimmune disorders (eg, Graves' disease, Guillain-Barré syndrome, and polymyositis) have been reported in patients experiencing immune reconstitution; time to onset is variable and may occur many months after antiretroviral treatment is initiated.

May cause vomiting; reported in 30% of pediatric patients (regardless of causality) receiving fosamprenavir twice daily with ritonavir (compared to 10% of adults) and occurred in 56% of children 2 to 5 years of age receiving twice daily fosamprenavir without ritonavir (compared to 16% of adults).

Adverse Reactions

Central nervous system: Fatigue, headache

Dermatologic: Pruritus, rash (onset: ~11 days; duration: ~13 days)

Endocrine & metabolic: Hyperglycemia, hypertriglyceridemia

Gastrointestinal: Abdominal pain, diarrhea, nausea, serum lipase increased, vomiting

Hematologic: Neutropenia

Hepatic: Transaminases increased

Rare but important or life-threatening: Angioedema, hypercholesterolemia, myocardial infarction, nephrolithiasis, oral paresthesia, QT prolongation (with amprenavir), Stevens-Johnson syndrome, stroke

Frequency not defined: Diabetes mellitus, fat redistribution, and immune reconstitution syndrome have been associated with protease inhibitor therapy. Spontaneous bleeding has been reported in patients with hemophilia A or B following treatment with protease inhibitors. Acute hemolytic anemia has been reported in association with amprenavir use.

Drug Interactions

Metabolism/Transport Effects Substrate of CYP2C9 (minor), CYP2D6 (minor), CYP3A4 (major), P-glycoprotein; **Note:** Assignment of Major/Minor substrate status based on clinically relevant drug interaction potential; **Inhibits** CYP2C19 (weak), CYP3A4 (strong)

Avoid Concomitant Use

Avoid concomitant use of Fosamprenavir with any of the following: Ado-Trastuzumab Emtansine; Alfuzosin; Amiodarone; Apixaban; Avanafil; Axitinib; Bosutinib; Cabozantinib; Ceritinib; Cisapride; Conivaptan; Crizotinib; Delavirdine; Dronedarone; Eplerenone; Ergot Derivatives; Etravirine; Everolimus; Flecainide; Halofantrine; Ibrutinib; Ivabradine; Lapatinib; Lomitapide; Lovastatin; Lurasidone; Macitentan; Midazolam; Nilotinib; Nisoldipine; Pimozide; Propafenone; QuiNIDine; Ranolazine; Red Yeast Rice; Regorafenib; Rifampin; Rivaroxaban; Salmeterol; Silodosin; Simeprevir; Simvastatin; St Johns Wort; Tamsulosin; Telaprevir; Ticagrelor; Tipranavir; Tolvaptan; Toremifene; Triazolam; Ulipristal; Vemurafenib; VinCRIStine (Liposomal); Vorapaxar

Increased Effect/Toxicity

Fosamprenavir may increase the levels/effects of: Ado-Trastuzumab Emtansine; Alfuzosin; Almotriptan; Alosetron; ALPRAZolam; Amiodarone; Apixaban; ARIPiprazole; AtorvaSTATin; Avanafil; Axitinib; Bedaquiline; Bortezomib; Bosentan; Bosutinib; Brentuximab Vedotin; Brinzolamide; Budesonide (Nasal); Budesonide (Systemic, Oral Inhalation); Cabozantinib; Calcium Channel Blockers (Dihydropyridine); Calcium Channel Blockers (Nondihydropyridine); Cannabis; CarBAMazepine; Ceritinib; Cisapride; Clarithromycin; Clorazepate; Colchicine; Conivaptan; Corticosteroids (Orally Inhaled); Crizotinib; Cyclophosphamide; CycloSPORINE (Systemic); CYP3A4 Substrates; Diazepam; Digoxin; Dofetilide; DOXOrubicin (Conventional); Dronabinol; Dronedarone; Dutasteride; Enfuvirtide; Eplerenone; Ergot Derivatives; Everolimus; FentaNYL; Fesoterodine; Flecainide; Flurazepam; Fluticasone (Nasal); Fluticasone (Oral Inhalation); GuanFACINE; Halofantrine; Ibrutinib; Iloperidone; Imatinib; Itraconazole; Ivabradine; Ivacaftor; Ixabepilone; Ketoconazole (Systemic); Lacosamide; Lapatinib; Levomilnacipran; Lomitapide; Lovastatin; Lumefantrine; Lurasidone; Macitentan; Maraviroc; Meperidine; MethylPREDNISolone; Midazolam; Mifepristone; Nefazodone; Nilotinib; Nisoldipine; Ospemifene; OxyCODONE; Paricalcitol; PAZOPanib; Pimecrolimus; Pimozide; PONATinib; Propafenone; Protease Inhibitors; QUEtiapine; QuiNIDine; Ranolazine; Red Yeast Rice; Regorafenib; Repaglinide; Rifabutin; Rilpivirine; Riociguat; Rivaroxaban; RomiDEPsin; Rosuvastatin; Ruxolitinib; Salmeterol; Saxagliptin; Sildenafil; Silodosin; Simeprevir; Simvastatin; SORAfenib; Tacrolimus (Systemic); Tacrolimus (Topical); Tadalafil; Tamsulosin; Temsirolimus; Tetrahydrocannabinol; Ticagrelor; Tofacitinib; Tolterodine; Tolvaptan; Toremifene; TraZODone; Triazolam; Tricyclic Antidepressants; Ulipristal; Vardenafil; Vemurafenib; Vilazodone; VinCRIStine (Liposomal); Vorapaxar; Voriconazole; Warfarin; Zuclopenthixol

The levels/effects of Fosamprenavir may be increased by: Clarithromycin; CycloSPORINE (Systemic);

Delavirdine; Enfuvirtide; Etravirine; Fosphenytoin; Itraconazole; Ketoconazole (Systemic); P-glycoprotein/ABCB1 Inhibitors; Phenytoin; Posaconazole; Rifabutin; Simeprevir; Voriconazole

Decreased Effect

Fosamprenavir may decrease the levels/effects of: Abacavir; Boceprevir; Clarithromycin; Contraceptives (Estrogens); Contraceptives (Progestins); Delavirdine; Dolutegravir; Fosphenytoin; Ifosfamide; Lopinavir; Meperidine; Methadone; PARoxetine; Phenytoin; Posaconazole; Prasugrel; Raltegravir; Telaprevir; Ticagrelor; Valproic Acid and Derivatives; Zidovudine

The levels/effects of Fosamprenavir may be decreased by: Antacids; Boceprevir; Bosentan; CarBAMazepine; Contraceptives (Progestins); CYP3A4 Inducers (Strong); Dabrafenib; Deferasirox; Efavirenz; Garlic; H2-Antagonists; Methadone; Mitotane; Nevirapine; Peginterferon Alfa-2b; P-glycoprotein/ABCB1 Inducers; Raltegravir; Rifampin; Siltuximab; St Johns Wort; Telaprevir; Tipranavir; Tocilizumab

Stability

Oral suspension: Store at 5°C to 30°C (41°F to 86°F). Do not freeze. Refrigeration is not required, but it may improve the taste of the suspension for some patients.

Tablets: Store at 25°C (77°F) in tightly closed container; excursions permitted to 15°C to 30°C (59°F to 86°F)

Mechanism of Action Fosamprenavir is rapidly and almost completely converted to amprenavir by cellular phosphatases *in vivo*. Amprenavir binds to the site of HIV-1 protease activity and inhibits cleavage of viral Gag-Pol polyprotein precursors into individual functional proteins required for infectious HIV. This results in the formation of immature, noninfectious viral particles.

Pharmacokinetics (Adult data unless noted)

Protein binding: 90%; primarily to alpha$_1$ acid glycoprotein; concentration-dependent binding; protein binding is decreased in patients with hepatic impairment

Metabolism: Fosamprenavir is the prodrug of amprenavir; fosamprenavir is rapidly hydrolyzed to amprenavir and inorganic phosphate by cellular phosphatases in the gut epithelium as it is absorbed; amprenavir is metabolized in the liver via cytochrome P450 CYP3A4 isoenzyme system; glucuronide conjugation of oxidized metabolites also occurs

Bioavailability: Absolute oral bioavailability is not established. Similar amprenavir AUCs occurred in adults when single doses of the oral suspension versus tablets were administered in the fasted state; however, the suspension provided a 14.5% higher peak concentration.

Half-life: Amprenavir: Adults: 7.7 hours

Time to peak serum concentration: Amprenavir (single dose of fosamprenavir): Median: 2.5 hours; range: 1.5 to 4 hours

Elimination: Minimal excretion of unchanged drug in urine (1%) and feces; 75% of dose excreted as metabolites via biliary tract into feces and 14% excreted as metabolites in urine

Dosing: Neonatal Not approved for use; appropriate dose is unknown.

Dosing: Usual

Pediatric: **HIV infection, treatment:** Use in combination with other antiretroviral agents: Oral: **Note:** Maximum dose should not exceed adult dose. Once-daily dosing of fosamprenavir is **not** recommended in pediatric patients; data from a pediatric once-daily dosing study of fosamprenavir plus ritonavir were insufficient to support once-daily dosing in any pediatric patient population.

Antiretroviral-naive patients:

Ritonavir unboosted regimen:

Infants and Children <2 years: Not approved for use; appropriate dose is unknown

Children ≥2 years and Adolescents:

AIDS*info* guidelines: Do not use due to low systemic exposure (DHHS [pediatric], 2014)

Manufacturer's labeling: 30 mg/kg/dose twice daily; maximum dose 1400 mg/dose

Ritonavir boosted regimen:

Infants, Children, and Adolescents:

AIDS*info* guidelines: Do not use in infants <6 months due to low systemic exposure; do not use in former premature neonates (ie, born at <38 weeks gestation) (DHHS [pediatric], 2014)

Manufacturer's labeling: Use only in infants born at ≥38 weeks GA and who are at least 28 days PNA

<11 kg: Fosamprenavir 45 mg/kg/dose **plus** ritonavir 7 mg/kg/dose twice daily

11 to <15 kg: Fosamprenavir 30 mg/kg/dose **plus** ritonavir 3 mg/kg/dose twice daily

15 to <20 kg: Fosamprenavir 23 mg/kg/dose **plus** ritonavir 3 mg/kg/dose twice daily

≥20 kg: Fosamprenavir 18 mg/kg/dose (maximum dose: 700 mg) twice daily **plus** ritonavir 3 mg/kg/dose (maximum dose: 100 mg) twice daily

Note: When combined with ritonavir, fosamprenavir tablets may be administered to children who weigh ≥39 kg.

Antiretroviral therapy-experienced:

Ritonavir boosted regimen:

Infants <6 months: Not approved for use; appropriate dose is unknown

Infants ≥6 months, Children, and Adolescents:

<11 kg: Fosamprenavir 45 mg/kg/dose **plus** ritonavir 7 mg/kg/dose twice daily

11 to <15 kg: Fosamprenavir 30 mg/kg/dose **plus** ritonavir 3 mg/kg/dose twice daily

15 to <20 kg: Fosamprenavir 23 mg/kg/dose **plus** ritonavir 3 mg/kg/dose twice daily

≥20 kg: Fosamprenavir 18 mg/kg/dose (maximum dose: 700 mg) twice daily **plus** ritonavir 3 mg/kg/dose twice daily (maximum dose: 100 mg) twice daily

Note: When combined with ritonavir, fosamprenavir tablets may be administered to children who weigh ≥39 kg

Adult: **HIV infection, treatment: Note:** Use in combination with other antiretroviral agents: Oral:

Antiretroviral-naïve patients:

Unboosted regimen (ie, regimen without ritonavir): Fosamprenavir 1400 mg twice daily. **Note:** This regimen is not recommended due to inferior potency compared to other protease inhibitor based regimens and the potential for cross-resistance to darunavir (DHHS [adult], 2014).

Ritonavir boosted regimens:

Once-daily regimen: Fosamprenavir 1400 mg **plus** ritonavir 100 to 200 mg once daily

Twice-daily regimen: Fosamprenavir 700 mg **plus** ritonavir 100 mg twice daily

Protease inhibitor-experienced: Fosamprenavir 700 mg **plus** ritonavir 100 mg twice daily. **Note:** Once-daily dosing of fosamprenavir is not recommended in protease inhibitor-experienced patients.

Dosing adjustments for concomitant therapy: Adults:

Concomitant therapy with efavirenz: Note: Only ritonavir-boosted regimens should be used when efavirenz is used in combination with fosamprenavir.

Once-daily regimen: Protease inhibitor-naïve **only:** Fosamprenavir 1400 mg **plus** ritonavir 300 mg **plus** efavirenz 600 mg once daily

Twice-daily regimen: Fosamprenavir 700 mg **plus** ritonavir 100 mg twice daily with efavirenz 600 mg once daily. **Note:** No change in ritonavir dosage is required when patients receive efavirenz with twice-daily dosing of fosamprenavir with ritonavir.

Combination therapy with maraviroc: Fosamprenavir 700 mg **plus** ritonavir 100 mg **plus** maraviroc 150 mg all dosed twice daily

Dosing adjustment in renal impairment: No dosage adjustment required (DHHS [adult], 2014)

Dosing adjustment in hepatic impairment: Use with caution: Adults:

Mild impairment (Child-Pugh score 5 to 6): Reduce dosage of fosamprenavir to 700 mg twice daily without concurrent ritonavir (therapy-naïve) or fosamprenavir 700 mg twice daily plus ritonavir 100 mg once daily (therapy-naïve or PI-experienced)

Moderate impairment (Child-Pugh score 7 to 9): Reduce dosage of fosamprenavir to 700 mg twice daily without concurrent ritonavir (therapy-naïve) or fosamprenavir 450 mg twice daily plus ritonavir 100 mg once daily (therapy-naïve or PI-experienced)

Severe impairment (Child-Pugh score 10 to 15): Reduce dosage of fosamprenavir to 350 mg twice daily without concurrent ritonavir (therapy naïve) or use fosamprenavir 300 mg twice daily plus ritonavir 100 mg once daily (therapy naïve or protease inhibitor experienced).

Administration Oral: Do not administer concurrently with antacids or buffered formulations of other medications (separate administration by 1 hour).

Oral suspension: Administer **with** food to pediatric patients; administer **without** food to adults. Readminister dose of suspension if emesis occurs within 30 minutes after dosing. Shake suspension vigorously prior to use.

Tablets: Administer **with** food to pediatric patients and adult patients when coadministered with ritonavir; may be administered without regard to meals in adults if not taken with ritonavir (DHHS [adult, pediatric], 2014)

Monitoring Parameters Note: Monitor CD4 percentage (if <5 years of age) or CD4 count (if ≥5 years of age) at least every 3 to 4 months (DHHS [pediatric], 2014).

Prior to initiation of therapy: Genotypic resistance testing, CD4 and viral load (every 3 to 4 months), CBC with differential, LFTs, BUN, creatinine, electrolytes, glucose, lipid panel, urinalysis (every 6 to 12 months), and assessment of readiness for adherence with medication regimen. At initiation and with any change in treatment regimen: CBC with differential, electrolytes, calcium, phosphate, glucose, LFTs, bilirubin, urinalysis (at initiation), BUN, creatinine, albumin, total protein, lipid panel (at initiation), CD4, and viral load. After 1 to 2 weeks of therapy: Signs of medication toxicity and adherence. After 2 to 4 weeks of therapy: CBC with differential, viral load, signs of medication toxicity, and adherence; then every 3 to 4 months: CBC with differential, electrolytes, glucose, LFTs, bilirubin, BUN, creatinine, CD4, viral load, signs of medication toxicity, and adherence. Every 6 to 12 months: Lipid panel and urinalysis. CD4 monitoring frequency may be decreased to every 6 to 12 months in children who are adherent to therapy if the value is well above the threshold for opportunistic infections, viral suppression is sustained, and the clinical status is stable for more than 2 to 3 years (DHHS [pediatric], 2014). Monitor for growth and development, signs of HIV-specific physical conditions, HIV disease progression, opportunistic infections or hepatitis.

Reference Range Plasma trough concentration: Amprenavir: ≥400 ng/mL (DHHS [adult, pediatric], 2014)

Additional Information Oral suspension contains 50 mg/mL of fosamprenavir as fosamprenavir calcium and is equivalent to amprenavir 43 mg/mL. Fosamprenavir calcium 700 mg (1 tablet) is approximately equal to amprenavir 600 mg.

Dosage Forms Excipient information presented when available (limited, particularly for generics); consult specific product labeling.

Suspension, Oral, as calcium:

Lexiva: 50 mg/mL (225 mL) [contains methylparaben, polysorbate 80, propylene glycol, propylparaben; grape bubblegum peppermint flavor]

Tablet, Oral, as calcium:

Lexiva: 700 mg

References

Chapman TM, Plosker GL, Perry CM. Fosamprenavir: a review of its use in the management of antiretroviral therapy-naïve patients with HIV infection. *Drugs.* 2004;64(18):2101-2124.

DHHS Panel on Antiretroviral Guidelines for Adults and Adolescents. Guidelines for the use of antiretroviral agents in HIV-1-infected adults and adolescents, Department of Health and Human Services. May 1, 2014. Available at http://www.aidsinfo.nih.gov/ContentFiles/AdultandAdolescentGL.pdf

DHHS Panel on Antiretroviral Therapy and Medical Management of HIV-Infected Children. Guidelines for the use of antiretroviral agents in pediatric HIV infection. February 12, 2014. Available at http://aidsinfo.nih.gov

DHHS Panel on Treatment of HIV-Infected Pregnant Women and Prevention of Perinatal Transmission. Recommendations for the use of antiretroviral drugs in pregnant HIV-1-infected women for maternal health and interventions to reduce perinatal HIV-1 transmission in the United States. March 28, 2014. Available at http://aidsinfo.nih.gov

Wire MB, Shelton MJ, Studenberg S. Fosamprenavir: clinical pharmacokinetics and drug interactions of the amprenavir prodrug. *Clin Pharmacokinet.* 2006;45(2):137-168.

♦ **Fosamprenavir Calcium** see Fosamprenavir on page 931

Fosaprepitant (fos a PRE pi tant)

Medication Safety Issues

Sound-alike/look-alike issues:

Fosaprepitant may be confused with aprepitant, fosamprenavir, fospropofol

Emend® for Injection (fosaprepitant) may be confused with Emend® (aprepitant) which is an oral capsule formulation.

Brand Names: U.S. Emend

Brand Names: Canada Emend® IV

Therapeutic Category Antiemetic; Substance P/Neurokinin 1 Receptor Antagonist

Generic Availability (U.S.) No

Use Prevention of acute and delayed nausea and vomiting associated with initial and repeat courses of moderate and highly emetogenic cancer chemotherapy (MEC & HEC) in combination with other antiemetic agents (FDA approved in ages ≥18 years and adults)

Pregnancy Risk Factor B

Pregnancy Considerations Teratogenic effects were not observed in animal reproduction studies for aprepitant. Use during pregnancy only if clearly needed. Efficacy of hormonal contraceptive may be reduced; alternative or additional methods of contraception should be used both during treatment with fosaprepitant or aprepitant and for at least 1 month following the last fosaprepitant/aprepitant dose.

Breast-Feeding Considerations It is not known if fosaprepitant is excreted in breast milk. Due to the potential for serious adverse reactions in the nursing infant, a decision should be made whether to discontinue nursing or to discontinue the drug, taking into account the importance of treatment to the mother.

Contraindications Hypersensitivity to fosaprepitant, aprepitant, polysorbate 80, or any component; concurrent use with pimozide or cisapride

Warnings Immediate hypersensitivity has been reported (rarely) during infusion with fosaprepitant. Stop infusion with hypersensitivity symptoms (anaphylaxis, dyspnea, erythema, or flushing); do not reinitiate.

Fosaprepitant is rapidly converted to aprepitant. Fosaprepitant and aprepitant have the potential to significantly interact with many medications; increased serum concentrations of pimozide or cisapride could result in serious or life-threatening adverse effects. Concomitant use with warfarin may result in clinically significant decrease in INR; patients on warfarin should have INR monitored closely, particularly at 7-10 days following initiation of fosaprepitant therapy.

Efficacy of oral contraceptives may be reduced during treatment with fosaprepitant; alternative or additional methods of birth control should be used both during treatment with fosaprepitant and for at least 1 month following the last fosaprepitant dose. Contains polysorbate 80 (Tween 80®) which may cause allergic reactions in susceptible individuals. Infusion of polysorbate 80 containing solutions through polyvinyl chloride tubing may cause DEHP to leach into the solution; in immature animals, exposure to DEHP may adversely affect the development of the male reproductive tract.

Precautions Use with caution in patients with severe hepatic impairment (Child-Pugh score >9); use has not been studied. Use with caution in patients receiving medications metabolized by CYP3A4 as decreased metabolism and subsequent elevation of serum concentration may occur; the effect of aprepitant on orally administered CYP3A4 substrates may be greater than that seen with intravenously administered CYP3A4 substrates. Use with caution and monitor use closely in patients receiving docetaxel, paclitaxel, etoposide, irinotecan, ifosfamide, imatinib, vinorelbine, vinblastine, and vincristine as they are known to be metabolized by CYP3A4 isoenzymes.

Chronic continuous use for prevention of nausea and vomiting is not recommended because it has not been studied. Fosaprepitant has not been studied for the treatment of established nausea and vomiting.

Adverse Reactions Adverse reactions reported with aprepitant and fosaprepitant (as part of a combination chemotherapy regimen) occurring at a higher frequency than standard antiemetic therapy:

Central nervous system: Fatigue, headache
Gastrointestinal: Anorexia, constipation, diarrhea, dyspepsia, eructation
Hepatic: ALT increased, AST increased
Local: Injection site reactions (includes erythema, induration, pain, pruritus, or thrombophlebitis)
Neuromuscular & skeletal: Weakness
Miscellaneous: Hiccups
Rare but important or life-threatening: Abdominal pain, alkaline phosphatase increased, anaphylactic reaction, anemia, angioedema, bradycardia, candidiasis, cardiovascular disorder, chest discomfort, chills, cognitive disorder, conjunctivitis, cough, disorientation, dizziness, duodenal ulcer (perforating), dyspnea, edema, erythema, flushing, gait disturbance, hematuria (microscopic), hyperglycemia, hyperhydrosis, hypersensitivity reaction, hypertension, hyponatremia, miosis, nausea, neutropenia, neutropenic colitis, neutropenic fever, palpitation, photosensitivity, pollakiuria, polyuria, pruritus, rash, sensory disturbance, somnolence, staphylococcal infection, Stevens-Johnson syndrome, stomatitis, subileus, tinnitus, toxic epidermal necrolysis, urticaria, visual acuity decreased, vomiting, wheezing

Drug Interactions
Metabolism/Transport Effects Substrate of CYP1A2 (minor), CYP2C19 (minor), CYP3A4 (major); **Note:** Assignment of Major/Minor substrate status based on clinically relevant drug interaction potential; **Inhibits** CYP2C19 (weak), CYP2C9 (weak), CYP3A4 (moderate); **Induces** CYP2C9 (weak/moderate), CYP3A4 (weak/moderate)

Avoid Concomitant Use
Avoid concomitant use of Fosaprepitant with any of the following: Astemizole; Axitinib; Bosutinib; Cisapride; Conivaptan; Fusidic Acid (Systemic); Ibrutinib; Ivabradine; Lomitapide; Pimozide; Simeprevir; Terfenadine; Tolvaptan; Uliprista l

Increased Effect/Toxicity
Fosaprepitant may increase the levels/effects of: Astemizole; Avanafil; Benzodiazepines (metabolized by oxidation); Bosentan; Bosutinib; Budesonide (Systemic, Oral Inhalation); Cannabis; Cisapride; Colchicine; Corticosteroids (Systemic); CYP3A4 Substrates; Diltiazem; Dofetilide; DOXOrubicin (Conventional); Dronabinol; Eplerenone; Everolimus; FentaNYL; Halofantrine; Ibrutinib; Imatinib; Ivabradine; Ivacaftor; Lomitapide; Lurasidone; OxyCODONE; Pimecrolimus; Pimozide; Propafenone; Ranolazine; Rivaroxaban; Salmeterol; Saxagliptin; Simeprevir; Terfenadine; Tetrahydrocannabinol; Tolvaptan; Uliprista l; Vilazodone; Zuclopenthixol

The levels/effects of Fosaprepitant may be increased by: Ceritinib; Conivaptan; CYP3A4 Inhibitors (Moderate); CYP3A4 Inhibitors (Strong); Dasatinib; Diltiazem; Fusidic Acid (Systemic); Luliconazole; Mifepristone; Stiripentol

Decreased Effect
Fosaprepitant may decrease the levels/effects of: ARIPiprazole; Axitinib; Contraceptives (Estrogens); Contraceptives (Progestins); Ifosfamide; PARoxetine; Saxagliptin; Simeprevir; TOLBUTamide; Warfarin

The levels/effects of Fosaprepitant may be decreased by: Bosentan; CYP3A4 Inducers (Strong); Dabrafenib; Deferasirox; Mitotane; PARoxetine; Rifampin; Siltuximab; St Johns Wort; Tocilizumab

Food Interactions Aprepitant serum concentration may be increased when taken with grapefruit juice. Management: Avoid concurrent use.

Stability Store intact vials at 2°C to 8°C (36°F to 46°F). Stable for 24 hours at ≤25°C (≤77°F) after dilution in NS.

Mechanism of Action Fosaprepitant is a prodrug of aprepitant, a substance P/neurokinin 1 (NK1) receptor antagonist. It is rapidly converted to aprepitant which prevents acute and delayed vomiting by inhibiting the substance P/neurokinin 1 (NK1) receptor; augments the antiemetic activity of the 5-HT$_3$ receptor antagonist and corticosteroid activity and inhibits chemotherapy-induced emesis.

Pharmacokinetics (Adult data unless noted)
Distribution: V$_d$: Fosaprepitant: ~5 L; Aprepitant: V$_d$: ~70 L; crosses the blood-brain barrier
Protein binding: Aprepitant: >95%
Metabolism:
  Fosaprepitant: Hepatic and extrahepatic; rapidly (within 30 minutes after the end of infusion) converted to aprepitant (nearly complete conversion)
  Aprepitant: Hepatic via CYP3A4 (major); CYP1A2 and CYP2C19 (minor); forms 7 weakly-active metabolites
Half-life: Fosaprepitant: ~2 minutes; Aprepitant: ~9-13 hours
Elimination: Urine (57%); feces (45%)
Clearance: 62-90 mL/minute

Dosing: Usual Adults: I.V.: **Prevention of chemotherapy-induced nausea and vomiting:**
Single-dose regimen (for highly emetogenic chemotherapy): 150 mg over 20-30 minutes ~30 minutes prior to chemotherapy on day 1 only (in combination with a 5-HT$_3$ antagonist on day 1 and dexamethasone on days 1-4)
3-day regimen (for highly emetogenic chemotherapy): 115 mg over 15 minutes 30 minutes prior to chemotherapy on day 1, followed by aprepitant 80 mg orally on days 2 and 3 (in combination with a 5-HT$_3$ antagonist on day 1 and dexamethasone on days 1-4)

3-day regimen (for moderately emetogenic chemotherapy): 115 mg over 15 minutes 30 minutes prior to chemotherapy on day 1, followed by aprepitant 80 mg orally on days 2 and 3 (in combination with a 5-HT$_3$ antagonist and dexamethasone on day 1)

Dosage adjustment in renal impairment:
Mild, moderate, or severe impairment: No adjustment required
Dialysis-dependent end-stage renal disease (ESRD): No adjustment required

Dosage adjustment in hepatic impairment:
Mild to moderate impairment (Child-Pugh score 5-9): No adjustment necessary
Severe impairment (Child-Pugh score >9): Use caution; no data available

Administration Parenteral: Reconstitute vial with 5 mL NS; further dilute in NS to a final concentration of 1 mg/mL; administer 30 minutes prior to chemotherapy; infusion rate is dose-dependent: 150 mg over 20-30 minutes and 115 mg over 15 minutes

Monitoring Parameters Immediate hypersensitivity reactions during infusion (anaphylaxis, dyspnea, erythema, or flushing). If reaction occurs, infusion should be stopped and not reinitiated.

Dosage Forms Excipient information presented when available (limited, particularly for generics); consult specific product labeling.
Solution Reconstituted, Intravenous:
Emend: 150 mg (1 ea) [contains disodium edta, polysorbate 80]

References
Cocquyt V, Van Belle S, Reinhardt RR, et al, "Comparison of L-758,298, a Prodrug for the Selective Neurokinin-1 Antagonist, L-754,030, With Ondansetron for the Prevention of Cisplatin-Induced Emesis," *Eur J Cancer*, 2001, 37(7):835-42.
Lasseter KC, Gambelle J, Jin B, et al, "Tolerability of Fosaprepitant and Bioequivalency to Aprepitant in Healthy Subjects," *J Clin Pharmacol*, 2007,47 (7):834-40.
Marbury TC, Jin B, Panebianco D, et al, "Lack of Effect of Aprepitant or its Prodrug Fosaprepitant on QTc Intervals in Healthy Subjects," *Anesth Analg*, 2009, 109(2):418-25.
Multinational Association of Supportive Care in Cancer (MASCC), "Antiemetic Guidelines," Updated April 2010. Available at http://data.-memberclicks.com/site/mascc/MASCC_Guidelines_English_2010.pdf
National Comprehensive Cancer Network® (NCCN), "Clinical Practice Guidelines in Oncology™: Antiemesis," Version 1.2011. Available at http://www.nccn.org/professionals/physician_gls/PDF/antiemesis.pdf
Van Belle S, Lichinitser SR, Navari RM, et al, "Prevention of Cisplatin-Induced Acute and Delayed Emesis by the Selective Neurokinin-1 Antagonists, L-758,298 and MK-869," *Cancer*, 2002, 94(11):3032-41.

◆ **Fosaprepitant Dimeglumine** *see* Fosaprepitant *on page 934*

Foscarnet (fos KAR net)

Brand Names: U.S. Foscavir
Brand Names: Canada Foscavir®
Therapeutic Category Antiviral Agent, Parenteral
Generic Availability (U.S.) Yes
Use Alternative to ganciclovir for treatment of CMV infections; treatment of CMV retinitis in patients with acquired immunodeficiency syndrome (FDA approved in adults); treatment of acyclovir-resistant mucocutaneous herpes simplex virus infections in immunocompromised patients and acyclovir-resistant herpes zoster infections (FDA approved in adults)
Pregnancy Risk Factor C
Pregnancy Considerations Associated with an increase in skeletal anomalies in animal studies at approximately the equivalent of 13% to 33% of the maximal daily human dose. There are no adequate and well controlled studies in pregnant women. A single case report of use during the third trimester with normal infant outcome was observed. Monitoring of amniotic fluid volumes by ultrasound is

recommended weekly after 20 weeks of gestation to detect oligohydramnios.

Breast-Feeding Considerations The CDC recommends **not** to breast-feed if diagnosed with HIV to avoid postnatal transmission of the virus.

Contraindications Hypersensitivity to foscarnet or any component

Warnings Renal impairment occurs to some degree in the majority of patients treated with foscarnet **[U.S. Boxed Warning]**; renal impairment may occur at any time and is usually reversible within 1 week following dose adjustment or discontinuation of therapy; however, several patients have died with renal failure within 4 weeks of stopping foscarnet. To reduce the risk of nephrotoxicity and the potential to administer a relative overdose, always calculate the CrCl even if serum creatinine is within the normal range. Dosage adjustments are recommended for renal dysfunction; safety and efficacy data in adult patients with a baseline S$_{cr}$ >2.8 mg/dL or CrCl <50 mL/minute are limited. Adequate hydration may reduce the risk of nephrotoxicity and prehydration is recommended; foscarnet use is not recommended in patients with a CrCl <0.4 mL/kg/minute.

Foscarnet is deposited in teeth and bone of young, growing animals; it has adversely affected tooth enamel development in rats; deposition in human bone has also been demonstrated; safety and effectiveness in children has not been fully evaluated.

Serum electrolyte imbalance occurs in 6% to 48% of patients (hypocalcemia, low ionized calcium, hypo- or hyperphosphatemia, hypokalemia, or hypomagnesemia). Patients with a low ionized calcium may experience perioral tingling, numbness, parasthesia, tetany, and seizures.

Seizures related to electrolyte/mineral imbalance may occur **[U.S. Boxed Warning]**; incidence has been reported in up to 10% of HIV patients. Risk factors for seizures include impaired baseline renal function, low total serum calcium, and underlying CNS condition. Some patients who have experienced seizures have been able to continue or resume foscarnet treatment after their mineral or electrolyte abnormality has been corrected, their underlying disease state treated, or their dose decreased.

Precautions Use with caution in patients with renal impairment, patients with altered electrolyte levels, and patients with neurologic or cardiac abnormalities; adjust dose for patients with impaired renal function; discontinue treatment in adults if serum creatinine ≥2.9 mg/dL; therapy can be restarted if serum creatinine ≤2 mg/dL. Anemia and granulocytopenia have been reported; monitor CBC; foscarnet is a venous irritant, infuse only into veins with adequate blood flow

Adverse Reactions
Cardiovascular: Chest pain, ECG changes, edema, facial edema, flushing, hyper-/hypotension, palpitation
Central nervous system: Agitation, aggressiveness, amnesia, anxiety, aphasia, ataxia, confusion, coordination abnormal, dementia, depression, dizziness, EEG abnormal, fatigue, fever, hallucination, headache, hypoesthesia, insomnia, malaise, meningitis, nervousness, pain, seizures, somnolence, stupor
Dermatologic: Erythematous rash, maculopapular rash, pruritus, rash, seborrhea, skin discoloration, skin ulceration
Endocrine & metabolic: Acidosis, hyper-/hypophosphatemia, hypocalcemia, hypokalemia, hypomagnesemia, hyponatremia
Gastrointestinal: Abdominal pain, anorexia, cachexia, constipation, diarrhea, dysphagia, dyspepsia, flatulence, melena, nausea, pancreatitis, rectal hemorrhage, taste perversion, ulcerative stomatitis, vomiting, weight loss, xerostomia

Genitourinary: Dysuria, nocturia, urinary retention, urinary tract infection

Hematologic: Anemia, bone marrow suppression, granulocytopenia, leukopenia, lymphadenopathy, thrombocytopenia, thrombosis

Hepatic: Alkaline phosphatase increased, ALT increased, AST increased, hepatic function abnormal, LDH increased

Local: Abscess, injection site pain/inflammation

Neuromuscular & skeletal: Arthralgia, back pain, involuntary muscle contraction, leg cramps, myalgia, neuropathy (peripheral), paresthesia, rigors, tremor, weakness

Ocular: Conjunctivitis, eye pain, vision abnormalities

Renal: Abnormal renal function, acute renal failure, albuminuria, BUN increased, creatinine clearance decreased, polyuria

Respiratory: Cough, bronchospasm, dyspnea, hemoptysis, pharyngitis, pneumonia, pneumothorax, pulmonary infiltrates, respiratory failure, rhinitis, sinusitis, stridor

Miscellaneous: Diaphoresis, flu-like syndrome, infection (bacterial and fungal), malignancies (lymphoma/sarcoma), sepsis, thirst

Rare but important or life-threatening: Cardiac arrest, coma, diabetes insipidus (usually nephrogenic), erythema multiforme, hematuria, hypoproteinemia, myositis, neutropenia, pancytopenia, QT_c prolongation, renal calculus, rhabdomyolysis, Stevens-Johnson syndrome, syndrome of inappropriate antidiuretic hormone (SIADH), toxic epidermal necrolysis, ventricular arrhythmia

Drug Interactions

Metabolism/Transport Effects None known.

Avoid Concomitant Use There are no known interactions where it is recommended to avoid concomitant use.

Increased Effect/Toxicity

Foscarnet may increase the levels/effects of: Highest Risk QTc-Prolonging Agents; Moderate Risk QTc-Prolonging Agents

The levels/effects of Foscarnet may be increased by: Mifepristone; Pentamidine

Decreased Effect There are no known significant interactions involving a decrease in effect.

Stability Store unopened vials at 20°C to 25°C (68°F to 77°F); protect from temperatures >40°C and from freezing. Diluted solution is stable for 24 hours at room temperature or under refrigeration; incompatible with dextrose ≥30%, LR, TPN, vancomycin, digoxin, ganciclovir, midazolam, and I.V. solutions containing calcium or magnesium

Mechanism of Action Pyrophosphate analogue which acts as a noncompetitive inhibitor of many viral RNA and DNA polymerases as well as HIV reverse transcriptase. Similar to ganciclovir, foscarnet is a virostatic agent. Foscarnet does not require activation by thymidine kinase.

Pharmacokinetics (Adult data unless noted)

Distribution: V_d: ~0.5 L/kg; up to 28% of cumulative I.V. dose may be deposited in bone; CSF levels are ~2/3 of serum concentrations

Protein binding: 14% to 17%

Half-life, plasma: Adults: 2-4.5 hours

Elimination: 80% to 90% excreted unchanged in urine

Dosing: Usual

Infants and Children:

Cytomegalovirus (CMV) infection (HIV-exposed/-positive) (CDC, 2009):

CNS disease:

Treatment; induction: I.V.: 60 mg/kg/dose every 8 hours in combination with ganciclovir; continue until symptom improvement, followed by chronic suppressive (maintenance) therapy

Maintenance therapy: I.V.: 90-120 mg/kg/dose once daily

Retinitis, disseminated disease:

Treatment; induction: I.V.: 60 mg/kg/dose every 8 hours for 14-21 days with or without ganciclovir, followed by chronic suppressive (maintenance) therapy

Maintenance therapy: I.V.: 90-120 mg/kg/dose once daily

Herpes simplex virus (HSV) infection acyclovir-resistant; treatment (HIV-exposed/-positive) (CDC, 2009): I.V.: 40 mg/kg/dose every 8 hours or 60 mg/kg/dose every 12 hours for up to 3 weeks or until lesions heal; repeat treatment may lead to the development of resistance

Varicella zoster virus (VZ) infection (HIV-exposed/-positive) (CDC, 2009):

Chickenpox not responding to acyclovir; treatment: I.V.: 40-60 mg/kg/dose every 8 hours for 7-10 days

Zoster: Progressive outer retinal necrosis; treatment:

I.V.: 90 mg/kg/dose every 12 hours in combination with ganciclovir intravenous and intravitreal foscarnet and/or ganciclovir

Intravitreal: 1.2 mg/0.05 mL per dose twice weekly in combination with systemic foscarnet and ganciclovir and/or intravitreal ganciclovir

Adolescents:

Cytomegalovirus (CMV) retinitis (HIV-exposed/-positive) (CDC, 2009a):

Treatment; induction: I.V.: 60 mg/kg/dose every 8 hours for 14-21 days **or** 90 mg/kg every 12 hours for 14-21 days

Maintenance therapy: I.V.: 90-120 mg/kg/dose once daily

Herpes simplex virus (HSV) infection acyclovir-resistant; treatment (HIV-exposed/-positive) (CDC, 2009a): I.V.: 40 mg/kg/dose every 8-12 hours until clinical response

Varicella zoster virus (VZ) infection (HIV-exposed/-positive) (CDC, 2009a):

Chickenpox not responding to acyclovir; treatment: I.V.: 90 mg/kg/dose every 12 hours

Zoster: Progressive outer retinal necrosis; treatment:

I.V.: 90 mg/kg/dose every 12 hours in combination with systemic ganciclovir and intravitreal foscarnet and/or ganciclovir

Intravitreal: 1.2 mg/0.05 mL per dose twice weekly in combination with systemic foscarnet and ganciclovir and/or intravitreal ganciclovir

Adults:

Cytomegalovirus (CMV) retinitis: I.V.:

Treatment; induction: 60 mg/kg/dose every 8 hours for 14-21 days **or** 90 mg/kg/dose every 12 hours for 14-21 days

Maintenance therapy: 90-120 mg/kg/day as a single daily infusion

Herpes simplex virus (HSV) infection acyclovir-resistant; treatment: I.V.: 40 mg/kg/dose every 8-12 hours for 14-21 days

Dosing interval in renal impairment: Adults:

CMV Induction (equivalent to 60 mg/kg every 8 hours):

CrCl >1.4 mL/minute/kg: 60 mg/kg every 8 hours

CrCl >1-1.4 mL/minute/kg: 45 mg/kg every 8 hours

CrCl >0.8-1 mL/minute/kg: 50 mg/kg every 12 hours

CrCl >0.6-0.8 mL/minute/kg: 40 mg/kg every 12 hours

CrCl >0.5-0.6 mL/minute/kg: 60 mg/kg every 24 hours

CrCl ≥0.4-0.5 mL/minute/kg: 50 mg/kg every 24 hours

CrCl <0.4 mL/minute/kg: Not recommended

CMV Induction (equivalent to 90 mg/kg every 12 hours):

CrCl >1.4 mL/minute/kg: 90 mg/kg every 12 hours

CrCl >1-1.4 mL/minute/kg: 70 mg/kg every 12 hours

CrCl >0.8-1 mL/minute/kg: 50 mg/kg every 12 hours

CrCl >0.6-0.8 mL/minute/kg: 80 mg/kg every 24 hours

CrCl >0.5-0.6 mL/minute/kg: 60 mg/kg every 24 hours
CrCl ≥0.4-0.5 mL/minute/kg: 50 mg/kg every 24 hours
CrCl <0.4 mL/minute/kg: Not recommended

CMV Maintenance:
CrCl >1.4 mL/minute/kg: 90-120 mg/kg every 24 hours
CrCl >1-1.4 mL/minute/kg: 70-90 mg/kg every 24 hours
CrCl >0.8-1 mL/minute/kg: 50-65 mg/kg every 24 hours
CrCl >0.6-0.8 mL/minute/kg: 80-105 mg/kg every 48 hours
CrCl >0.5-0.6 mL/minute/kg: 60-80 mg/kg every 48 hours
CrCl ≥0.4-0.5 mL/minute/kg: 50-65 mg/kg every 48 hours
CrCl <0.4 mL/minute/kg: Not recommended

HSV Infection (equivalent to 40 mg/kg every 8 hours):
CrCl >1.4 mL/minute/kg: 40 mg/kg every 8 hours
CrCl >1-1.4 mL/minute/kg: 30 mg/kg every 8 hours
CrCl >0.8-1 mL/minute/kg: 35 mg/kg every 12 hours
CrCl >0.6-0.8 mL/minute/kg: 25 mg/kg every 12 hours
CrCl >0.5-0.6 mL/minute/kg: 40 mg/kg every 24 hours
CrCl ≥0.4-0.5 mL/minute/kg: 35 mg/kg every 24 hours
CrCl <0.4 mL/minute/kg: Not recommended

HSV Infection (equivalent to 40 mg/kg every 12 hours):
CrCl >1.4 mL/minute/kg: 40 mg/kg every 12 hours
CrCl >1-1.4 mL/minute/kg: 30 mg/kg every 12 hours
CrCl >0.8-1 mL/minute/kg: 20 mg/kg every 12 hours
CrCl >0.6-0.8 mL/minute/kg: 35 mg/kg every 24 hours
CrCl >0.5-0.6 mL/minute/kg: 25 mg/kg every 24 hours
CrCl ≥0.4-0.5 mL/minute/kg: 20 mg/kg every 24 hours
CrCl <0.4 mL/minute/kg: Not recommended

Administration Parenteral: For central I.V. administration, may administer undiluted 24 mg/mL solution; for peripheral I.V. administration, must be further diluted with D₅W or NS to a final concentration ≤12 mg/mL. Administer using an infusion pump at a rate **not to exceed** 60 mg/kg/dose over 1 hour or 120 mg/kg/dose over 2 hours (1 mg/kg/minute).
Hydration:
Initial: Prehydration prior to initial infusion: Children: 10-20 mL/kg (maximum: 1000 mL) of age-appropriate fluid (usually NS); adults: 750-1000 mL NS or D₅W
Subsequent foscarnet doses: Concurrent hydration: Children: 10-20 mL/kg (maximum: 1000 mL) of age-appropriate fluid; adults: 500-1000 mL NS or D₅W; concurrent hydration volume is dependent on foscarnet dose

Monitoring Parameters Serum creatinine, calcium, phosphorus, potassium, magnesium; CBC, ophthalmologic exams, clinical signs of polyuria, and polydipsia

Reference Range Therapeutic serum concentration for CMV: 150 mcg/mL

Dosage Forms Excipient information presented when available (limited, particularly for generics); consult specific product labeling.
Solution, Intravenous, as sodium:
Foscavir: 24 mg/mL (250 mL)
Generic: 24 mg/mL (500 mL)

References

Aweeka FT, Jacobson MA, Martin-Munley S, et al, "Effect of Renal Disease and Hemodialysis on Foscarnet Pharmacokinetics and Dosing Recommendations," *J Acquir Immune Defic Syndr Hum Retrovirol*, 1999, 20(4):350-7.
Butler KM, DeSmet MD, Husson RN, et al, "Treatment of Aggressive Cytomegalovirus Retinitis With Ganciclovir in Combination With Foscarnet in a Child Infected With Human Immunodeficiency Virus," *J Pediatr*, 1992, 120(3):483-6.
Centers for Disease Control and Prevention (CDC), "Guidelines for Prevention and Treatment of Opportunistic Infections in HIV-Infected Adults and Adolescents: Recommendations From CDC, the National Institutes of Health, and the HIV Medicine Association of the Infectious Diseases Society of America," *MMWR Recomm Rep*, 2009a, 58 (RR-4):1-207.
Centers for Disease Control and Prevention (CDC), "Guidelines for the Prevention and Treatment of Opportunistic Infections Among HIV-Exposed and HIV-Infected Children," *MMWR Recomm Rep*, 2009, 58(RR-11):1-166. Available at http://aidsinfo.nih.gov/contentfiles/Pediatric_OI.pdf

◆ **Foscavir** *see* Foscarnet *on page* 936
◆ **Foscavir® (Can)** *see* Foscarnet *on page* 936

Fosinopril (foe SIN oh pril)

Medication Safety Issues
Sound-alike/look-alike issues:
Fosinopril may be confused with FLUoxetine, Fosamax®, furosemide, lisinopril
Monopril may be confused with Accupril®, minoxidil, moexipril, Monoket®, Monurol®, ramipril

Brand Names: Canada Apo-Fosinopril; Ava-Fosinopril; Jamp-Fosinopril; Mylan-Fosinopril; PMS-Fosinopril; RAN-Fosinopril; Riva-Fosinopril; Teva-Fosinopril

Therapeutic Category Angiotensin-Converting Enzyme (ACE) Inhibitor; Antihypertensive Agent

Generic Availability (U.S.) Yes

Use Treatment of hypertension, either alone or in combination with other antihypertensive agents (FDA approved in ages ≥6 years and adults); adjunctive treatment of heart failure (FDA approved in adults)

Pregnancy Risk Factor D

Pregnancy Considerations [U.S. Boxed Warning]: Drugs that act on the renin-angiotensin system can cause injury and death to the developing fetus. Discontinue as soon as possible once pregnancy is detected. Drugs that act on the renin-angiotensin system are associated with oligohydramnios. Oligohydramnios, due to decreased fetal renal function, may lead to fetal lung hypoplasia and skeletal malformations. Their use in pregnancy is also associated with anuria, hypotension, renal failure, skull hypoplasia, and death in the fetus/neonate. The exposed fetus should be monitored for fetal growth, amniotic fluid volume, and organ formation. Infants exposed *in utero* should be monitored for hyperkalemia, hypotension, and oliguria (exchange transfusions or dialysis may be needed). These adverse events are generally associated with maternal use in the second and third trimesters.

Untreated chronic maternal hypertension is associated with adverse events in the fetus, infant, and mother. The use angiotensin-converting enzyme inhibitors is not recommended to treat chronic uncomplicated hypertension or heart failure in pregnant women and should generally be avoided in women of reproductive potential (ACOG, 2013; Yancy, 2013).

Breast-Feeding Considerations Fosinoprilat is excreted in breast milk. Breast-feeding is not recommended by the manufacturer.

Contraindications Hypersensitivity to fosinopril, any component, or other ACE inhibitors; patients with idiopathic or hereditary angioedema or a history of angioedema with previous ACE inhibitor use

Warnings Angioedema can occur at any time during treatment (especially following first dose). Angioedema may occur in the head, neck, extremities, or intestines; patients with angioedema of the intestines may present with abdominal pain (with or without nausea or vomiting); angioedema of the larynx, glottis, or tongue may cause airway obstruction, especially in patients with a history of airway surgery. Prolonged monitoring may be required, even in patients with swelling of only the tongue (ie, without respiratory distress) because treatment with corticosteroids and antihistamines may not be sufficient; very rare fatalities have occurred with angioedema of the larynx or tongue; appropriate treatment (eg, establishing patent airway and/or SubQ epinephrine) should be readily available for patients with angioedema of larynx, glottis, or tongue, in whom airway obstruction is likely to occur.

Anaphylactic/anaphylactoid reactions can occur with ACE inhibitors. Life-threatening anaphylactoid reactions may be seen during hemodialysis (eg, CVVHD) with high-flux dialysis membranes (eg, AN69), and rarely, during low density lipoprotein apheresis with dextran sulfate cellulose. Rare cases of anaphylactoid reactions have been reported in patients undergoing sensitization treatment with hymenoptera (bee, wasp) venom while receiving ACE inhibitors.

Fosinopril has been associated with rare but potentially fatal cases of agranulocytosis, neutropenia, or leukopenia with myeloid hypoplasia; higher risk for development of neutropenia is associated with renal impairment; risk is further increased in patients with both renal impairment and collagen vascular disease (eg, systemic lupus erythematosus). Onset of neutropenia is usually within 3 months of fosinopril initiation; closely monitor CBC with differential for the first 3 months of therapy and periodically thereafter in these patients; neutrophil count generally returns to baseline within 2 weeks of discontinuation.

ACE inhibitor use has been associated with deterioration of renal function and/or increases in serum creatinine, particularly in patients with low renal blood flow (eg, renal artery stenosis, heart failure) whose glomerular filtration rate (GFR) is dependent on efferent arteriolar vasoconstriction by angiotensin II; deterioration may result in oliguria, acute renal failure, and progressive azotemia. Small increases in serum creatinine may occur following initiation; consider discontinuation only in patients with progressive and/or significant deterioration in renal function.

A rare toxicity associated with ACE inhibitors includes cholestatic jaundice, which may progress to fulminant hepatic necrosis; discontinue if marked elevation of hepatic transaminases or jaundice occurs and intitate appropriate medical treatment.

Drugs that act on the renin-angiotensin system can cause injury and death to the developing fetus. Discontinue as soon as possible once pregnancy is detected **[U.S. Boxed Warning]**.

Concomitant use of an ARB or renin inhibitor (eg, aliskiren) is associated with an increased risk of hypotension, hyperkalemia, and renal dysfunction. Concomitant use with aliskiren should be avoided in patients with GFR <60 mL/minute and is contraindicated in patients with diabetes mellitus (regardless of GFR).

Precautions Use with caution in patients with renal impairment; dosage reduction may be necessary; avoid rapid dosage escalation which may lead to further renal impairment. Use with caution in patients with unstented unilateral/bilateral renal artery stenosis. When unstented bilateral renal artery stenosis is present, use is generally avoided due to the elevated risk of deterioration in renal function unless possible benefits outweigh risks.

Use with caution when initiating therapy and in volume-depleted patients; may cause symptomatic hypotension with or without syncope, usually with the first several doses; correct volume depletion prior to initiation; initiate lower doses in patients with sodium or volume depletion; close monitoring of patient is required, especially with initial dosing and dosing increases; blood pressure must be lowered at a rate appropriate for the patient's clinical condition. Although dose reduction may be necessary, hypotension alone is not a reason for discontinuation of future ACE inhibitor use, especially in patients with heart failure in whom a reduction in systolic blood pressure is a desirable objective. Use caution in patients with ischemic heart disease or cerebrovascular disease during therapy initiation; observe closely due to the potential consequences posed by falling blood pressure (eg, MI, stroke); fluid replacement may be required to restore blood pressure; therapy may then be resumed; discontinue therapy in patients whose hypotension recurs. Use with caution in patients with severe aortic stenosis; may reduce coronary perfusion, resulting in ischemia. Use with caution in patients with hypertrophic cardiomyopathy (HCM) and outflow tract obstruction since reduction in afterload may worsen symptoms associated with this condition.

May cause hyperkalemia; risk factors include renal dysfunction, diabetes mellitus, concomitant use of potassium-sparing diuretics, potassium supplements, and/or potassium-containing salts; use with caution, if at all, with these agents and monitor potassium closely.

Use with caution before, during, or immediately after major surgery; cardiopulmonary bypass, intraoperative blood loss or vasodilating anesthesia increases endogenous renin release; use of ACE inhibitors perioperatively will blunt angiotensin II formation and may result in hypotension.

Racial differences were identified in a multicentered, prospective, double-blind, placebo-controlled trial that investigated the dose-response of fosinopril in 253 children 6-16 years of age; this study found that black children required a higher dose of fosinopril (per kg body weight) in order to adequately control blood pressure (Menon, 2006); the findings of this study are consistent with adult studies assessing ACE inhibitors; consider dosage adjustments in these patients.

An ACE inhibitor cough is a dry, hacking, nonproductive one that usually occurs within the first few months of treatment and should generally resolve within 1-4 weeks after discontinuation of the ACE inhibitor. In pediatric patients, an isolated dry hacking cough lasting >3 weeks was reported in 7 of 42 pediatric patients (17%) receiving ACE inhibitors (von Vigier, 2000); a review of pediatric randomized-controlled ACE inhibitor trials reported a lower incidence of 3.2% (Baker-Smith, 2010). Other causes of cough should be considered (eg, pulmonary congestion in patients with heart failure) and excluded prior to discontinuation.

Adverse Reactions Higher rates of adverse reactions have generally been noted in patients with CHF. However, the frequency of adverse effects associated with placebo is also increased in this population.

Cardiovascular: Orthostatic hypotension, palpitation
Central nervous system: Dizziness, fatigue, headache
Endocrine & metabolic: Hyperkalemia
Gastrointestinal: Diarrhea, nausea, vomiting
Hepatic: Transaminases increased
Neuromuscular & skeletal: Musculoskeletal pain, noncardiac chest pain, weakness
Renal: Renal function worsening (in patients with bilateral renal artery stenosis or hypovolemia), serum creatinine increased
Respiratory: Cough
Miscellaneous: Upper respiratory infection
Rare but important or life-threatening: Anaphylactoid reaction, angina, angioedema, arthralgia, bronchospasm, cerebral infarction, cerebrovascular accident, gout, hepatitis, hepatomegaly, myalgia, MI, pancreatitis, paresthesia, photosensitivity, pleuritic chest pain, pruritus, rash, renal insufficiency, shock, sudden death, syncope, TIA, tinnitus, urticaria, vertigo. In a small number of patients, a symptom complex of cough, bronchospasm, and eosinophilia has been observed with fosinopril.
Other events reported with ACE inhibitors: Acute renal failure, agranulocytosis, anemia, aplastic anemia, bullous pemphigus, cardiac arrest, eosinophilic pneumonitis, exfoliative dermatitis, gynecomastia, hemolytic anemia, hepatic failure, jaundice, neutropenia, pancytopenia, Stevens-Johnson syndrome, symptomatic hyponatremia, thrombocytopenia. In addition, a syndrome which may include arthralgia, elevated ESR, eosinophilia and

positive ANA, fever, interstitial nephritis, myalgia, rash, and vasculitis has been reported for other ACE inhibitors.

Drug Interactions

Metabolism/Transport Effects None known.

Avoid Concomitant Use There are no known interactions where it is recommended to avoid concomitant use.

Increased Effect/Toxicity

Fosinopril may increase the levels/effects of: Allopurinol; Amifostine; Antihypertensives; AzaTHIOprine; CycloSPORINE (Systemic); DULoxetine; Ferric Gluconate; Gold Sodium Thiomalate; Grass Pollen Allergen Extract (5 Grass Extract); Hypotensive Agents; Iron Dextran Complex; Lithium; Nonsteroidal Anti-Inflammatory Agents; Obinutuzumab; RiTUXimab; Sodium Phosphates

The levels/effects of Fosinopril may be increased by: Alfuzosin; Aliskiren; Angiotensin II Receptor Blockers; Barbiturates; Brimonidine (Topical); Canagliflozin; Diazoxide; DPP-IV Inhibitors; Eplerenone; Everolimus; Heparin; Heparin (Low Molecular Weight); Herbs (Hypotensive Properties); Loop Diuretics; MAO Inhibitors; Pentoxifylline; Phosphodiesterase 5 Inhibitors; Potassium Salts; Potassium-Sparing Diuretics; Prostacyclin Analogues; Sirolimus; Temsirolimus; Thiazide Diuretics; TiZANidine; Tolvaptan; Trimethoprim

Decreased Effect

The levels/effects of Fosinopril may be decreased by: Antacids; Aprotinin; Herbs (Hypertensive Properties); Icatibant; Lanthanum; Methylphenidate; Nonsteroidal Anti-Inflammatory Agents; Salicylates; Yohimbine

Stability Store at 25°C (77°F); excursions permitted to 15°C to 30°C (59°F to 86°F). Protect from moisture; keep bottle tightly closed.

Mechanism of Action Competitive inhibitor of angiotensin-converting enzyme (ACE); prevents conversion of angiotensin I to angiotensin II, a potent vasoconstrictor; results in lower levels of angiotensin II which causes an increase in plasma renin activity and a reduction in aldosterone secretion; a CNS mechanism may also be involved in hypotensive effect as angiotensin II increases adrenergic outflow from CNS; vasoactive kallikreins may be decreased in conversion to active hormones by ACE inhibitors, thus reducing blood pressure

Pharmacodynamics

Onset of action: Antihypertensive effect: 1 hour

Maximum effect: Antihypertensive effect: 2-6 hours postdose

Duration: Antihypertensive effect: 24 hours

Pharmacokinetics (Adult data unless noted)

Absorption: Slow and incomplete

Protein binding: 95%

Metabolism: Fosinopril is a prodrug (inactive) and is hydrolyzed to fosinoprilat (active) by intestinal wall and hepatic esterases; fosinopril is also metabolized to a glucuronide conjugate and a p-hydroxy metabolite of fosinoprilat

Bioavailability: 36%

Half-life: Fosinoprilat:

Children and Adolescents 6-16 years: 11-13 hours

Adults: 12 hours

Adults with CHF: 14 hours

Time to peak serum concentration: ~3 hours

Elimination: Urine and feces (as fosinoprilat and other metabolites in roughly equal proportions, 45% to 50%)

Dosing: Usual Note: Dosage must be titrated according to patient's response; use lowest effective dose.

Children ≥6 years and Adolescents: **Hypertension:** Oral:

≤50 kg: Initial: 0.1 mg/kg/dose once daily; reported range studied: 0.1-0.6 mg/kg/day; maximum daily dose: 40 mg/**day**; some patients may require a lower initial dose (Li, 2004; NHLBI, 2011)

>50 kg: Initial: 5-10 mg once daily, as monotherapy; maximum daily dose: 40 mg/**day**

Adults:

Hypertension: Oral: Initial: 10 mg once daily; usual maintenance: 20-40 mg/day. May need to divide the dose into two if trough effect is inadequate; discontinue the diuretic, if possible 2-3 days before initiation of therapy; resume diuretic therapy carefully, if needed.

Heart failure: Oral: Initial: 10 mg once daily (5 mg once daily if renal dysfunction present or if patient has been vigorously diuresed); increase dose, as needed, to a maximum of 40 mg once daily over several weeks; usual dose: 20-40 mg/day. If hypotension, orthostasis, or azotemia occurs during titration, consider decreasing concomitant diuretic dose, if any.

Dosage adjustment in renal impairment: Children, Adolescents, and Adults: None needed since hepatobiliary elimination compensates adequately for diminished renal elimination.

Dosage adjustment in hepatic impairment: Children, Adolescents, and Adults: Decrease dose and monitor effects.

Administration Oral: May be administered without regard to food.

Monitoring Parameters Blood pressure, BUN, serum creatinine, renal function, urine dipstick for protein, serum potassium, WBC with differential, especially during first 3 months of therapy for patients with renal impairment and/or collagen vascular disease; monitor for angioedema and anaphylactoid reactions; hypovolemia and postural hypotension when beginning therapy, adjusting dosage, and on a regular basis throughout

Test Interactions May cause false low serum digoxin levels with the Digi-Tab RIA kit for digoxin.

Dosage Forms Excipient information presented when available (limited, particularly for generics); consult specific product labeling.

Tablet, Oral, as sodium:

Generic: 10 mg, 20 mg, 40 mg

References

ACOG Committee on Practice Bulletins. Practice bulletin no. 125: chronic hypertension in pregnancy. *Obstet Gynecol.* 2012;119(2 Pt 1):396.

ALLHAT Officers and Coordinators for the ALLHAT Collaborative Research Group, "Major Outcomes in High-Risk Hypertensive Patients Randomized to Angiotensin-Converting Enzyme Inhibitor or Calcium Channel Blocker vs Diuretic: The Antihypertensive and Lipid-Lowering Treatment to Prevent Heart Attack Trial (ALLHAT)," *JAMA,* 2002, 288(23):2981-97.

Antman EM, Anbe DT, Armstrong PW, et al, "ACC/AHA Guidelines for the Management of Patients With ST-Elevation Myocardial Infarction - Executive Summary: A Report of the American College of Cardiology/American Heart Association Task Force on Practice Guidelines (Writing Committee to Revise the 1999 Guidelines for the Management of Patients With Acute Myocardial Infarction)," *Circulation,* 2004, 110:588-636.

Baker-Smith CM, Benjamin DK Jr, Califf RM, et al, "Cough in Pediatric Patients Receiving Angiotensin-Converting Enzyme Inhibitor Therapy or Angiotensin Receptor Blocker Therapy in Randomized Controlled Trials," *Clin Pharmacol Ther,* 2010, 87(6):668-71.

Brown NJ, Ray WA, Snowden M, et al, "Black Americans Have an Increased Rate of Angiotensin-Converting Enzyme Inhibitor-Associated Angioedema," *Clin Pharmacol Ther,* 1996, 60(1):8-13.

Chase MP, Fiarman GS, Scholz FJ, et al, "Angioedema of the Small Bowel Due to an Angiotensin-Converting Enzyme Inhibitor," *J Clin Gastroenterol,* 2000, 31(3):254-7.

Chobanian AV, Bakris GL, Black HR, et al, "The Seventh Report of the Joint National Committee on Prevention, Detection, Evaluation, and Treatment of High Blood Pressure: The JNC 7 Report," *JAMA,* 2003, 289(19):2560-72.

"Consensus Recommendations for the Management of Chronic Heart Failure. On Behalf of the Membership of the Advisory Council to Improve Outcomes Nationwide in Heart Failure," *Am J Cardiol,* 1999, 83(2A):1A-38A.

Cooper WO, Hernandez-Diaz S, Arbogast PG, et al, "Major Congenital Malformations After First-Trimester Exposure to ACE Inhibitors," *N Engl J Med,* 2006, 354(23):2443-51.

"Guidelines for the Evaluation and Management of Heart Failure. Report of the American College of Cardiology/American Heart Association Task Force on Practice Guidelines (Committee on Evaluation and Management of Heart Failure)," *Circulation,* 1995, 92(9):2764-84.

Hunt SA, Abraham WT, Chin MH, et al, "2009 Focused Update Incorporated into the ACC/AHA 2005 Guidelines for the Diagnosis and Management of Heart Failure in Adults: A Report of the American College of Cardiology Foundation/American Heart Association Task Force on Practice Guidelines Developed in Collaboration With the International Society for Heart and Lung Transplantation," *Circulation*, 2009, 119(14):e391-479.

"K/DOQI Clinical Practice Guidelines for Chronic Kidney Disease: Evaluation, Classification, and Stratification. Kidney Disease Outcome Quality Initiative," *Am J Kidney Dis*, 2002, 39(2 Suppl 2):1-246.

Konstam MA, Dracup K, Baker DW, et al, "Heart Failure Evaluation and Care of Patients With Left Ventricular Systolic Dysfunction," *J Card Fail*, 1995, 1(2):183-7.

Li JS, Berezny K, Kilaru R, et al, "Is the Extrapolated Adult Dose of Fosinopril Safe and Effective in Treating Hypertensive Children?" *Hypertension*, 2004, 44(3):289-93.

Mastrobattista JM, "Angiotensin Converting Enzyme Inhibitors in Pregnancy," *Semin Perinatol*, 1997, 21(2):124-34.

Menon S, Berezny KY, Kilaru R, et al, "Racial Differences are Seen in Blood Pressure Response to Fosinopril in Hypertensive Children," *Am Heart J*, 2006,152(2):394-9.

National Heart, Lung, and Blood Institute, "Expert Panel on Integrated Guidelines for Cardiovascular Health and Risk Reduction in Children and Adolescents," Clinical Practice Guidelines, 2011, National Institutes of Health. Available at http://www.nhlbi.nih.gov/guidelines/cvd_ped/peds_guidelines_full.pdf. Last accessed: October 24, 2012.

National High Blood Pressure Education Program Working Group on High Blood Pressure in Children and Adolescents, "The Fourth Report on the Diagnosis, Evaluation, and Treatment of High Blood Pressure in Children and Adolescents," *Pediatrics*, 2004, 114(2 Suppl):555-76.

Packer M, Poole-Wilson PA, Armstrong PW, et al, "Comparative Effects of Low and High Doses of the Angiotensin-Converting Enzyme Inhibitor, Lisinopril, on Morbidity and Mortality in Chronic Heart Failure," *Circulation*, 1999, 100(23):2312-8.

Quan A, "Fetopathy Associated With Exposure to Angiotensin Converting Enzyme Inhibitors and Angiotensin Receptor Antagonists," *Early Hum Dev*, 2006, 82(1):23-8.

Sliwa K, Fett J, Elkayam U. Peripartum cardiomyopathy. *Lancet*. 2006;368(9536):687-693.

Smoger SH and Sayed MA, "Simultaneous Mucosal and Small Bowel Angioedema Due to Captopril," *South Med J*, 1998, 91(11):1060-3.

von Vigier RO, Mozzettini S, Truttmann AC, et al, "Cough is Common in Children Prescribed Angiotensin Converting Enzyme Inhibitors," *Nephron*, 2000, 84(1):98.

Yancy CW, Jessup M, Bozkurt B, et al; ACCF/AHA Task Force Members. 2013 ACCF/AHA Guideline for the Management of Heart Failure: A Report of the American College of Cardiology Foundation/American Heart Association Task Force on Practice Guidelines [published online ahead of print June 5, 2013]. *J Am Coll Cardiol*. 2013.

Yi Z, Li Z, Wu XC, et al, "Effect of Fosinopril in Children With Steroid-Resistant Idiopathic Nephrotic Syndrome," *Pediatr Nephrol*, 2006, 21 (7):967-72.

◆ **Fosinopril Sodium** see Fosinopril on page 938

Fosphenytoin (FOS fen i toyn)

Medication Safety Issues
Sound-alike/look-alike issues:
Cerebyx may be confused with CeleBREX®, CeleXA®, Cerezyme®, Cervarix®
Fosphenytoin may be confused with fospropofol
Administration issues:
Overdoses have occurred due to confusion between the **mg per mL concentration** of fosphenytoin (50 mg phenytoin equivalent (PE)/mL) and **total drug content per vial** (either 100 mg PE/2 mL vial or 500 mg PE/10 mL vial). ISMP recommends that the total drug content per container is identified instead of the concentration in mg per mL to avoid confusion and potential overdoses. Additionally, since most errors have occurred with overdoses in children, ISMP recommends that pediatric hospitals consider stocking only the 2 mL vial.

Related Information
Phenytoin on page 1663
Brand Names: U.S. Cerebyx
Brand Names: Canada Cerebyx®
Therapeutic Category Anticonvulsant, Hydantoin
Generic Availability (U.S.) Yes
Use Management of generalized convulsive status epilepticus; short-term (≤5 days) parenteral administration of phenytoin when other routes are not possible; prevention and treatment of seizures occurring during neurosurgery (All indications: FDA approved in adults)

Pregnancy Risk Factor D

Pregnancy Considerations Fosphenytoin is the prodrug of phenytoin. Refer to Phenytoin monograph for additional information.

Breast-Feeding Considerations Fosphenytoin is the prodrug of phenytoin. It is not known if fosphenytoin is excreted in breast milk prior to conversion to phenytoin. Refer to Phenytoin monograph for additional information.

Contraindications Hypersensitivity to fosphenytoin, phenytoin, other hydantoins, or any component; second- and third-degree AV block, sinoatrial block, sinus bradycardia, Adams-Stokes syndrome; concurrent use of delavirdine [due to loss of virologic response and possible resistance to delavirdine or other non-nucleoside reverse transcriptase inhibitors (NNRTIs)]

Warnings Doses of fosphenytoin are **always expressed as their phenytoin sodium equivalent (PE); thus phenytoin sodium: 1 mg = fosphenytoin 1 mg PE. It is NOT appropriate to convert mg of fosphenytoin to mg of phenytoin.** Dosing errors have also occurred due to misinterpretation of vial concentrations and total vial content resulting in two- or tenfold overdoses (some fatal); ensure correct volume of fosphenytoin is withdrawn from vial when preparing doses.

Fosphenytoin I.V. administration should not exceed 150 mg phenytoin equivalents (PE)/minute **[U.S. Boxed Warning]**. Hypotension and severe cardiac arrhythmias (eg, heart block, QT prolongation, ventricular tachycardia, ventricular fibrillation) may occur with rapid I.V. administration; asystole, cardiac arrest, and death may result; adverse cardiac events have been reported at or below the recommended infusion rate; use with caution in patients with hypotension and/or severe myocardial insufficiency. In the treatment of status epilepticus in adults, the rate of I.V. administration is 150 mg PE/minute. Safety and efficacy of fosphenytoin in pediatric patients has not been established; based on experience with parenteral fosphenytoin, consider a maximum I.V. infusion rate in pediatric patients of 1-3 mg PE/kg/minute (Hegenbarth, 2008). In a nonemergent situation, administer more slowly or use oral phenytoin. Cardiac monitoring is necessary during and after administration of intravenous fosphenytoin; reduction in rate of administration or discontinuation of infusion may be necessary.

Abrupt withdrawal of fosphenytoin may precipitate status epilepticus; do not discontinue abruptly; fosphenytoin should be withdrawn gradually, unless safety concerns (eg, allergic or hypersensitivity reaction) require a more rapid withdrawal.

Acute hepatotoxicity associated with a hypersensitivity syndrome characterized by fever, skin eruptions, and lymphadenopathy has been reported with phenytoin and occurs within the first 2 months of treatment; discontinue if skin rash or lymphadenopathy occur. Other reported manifestations of hepatotoxicity include jaundice, hepatomegaly, increased serum transaminase levels, leukocytosis, and eosinophilia. Serious skin reactions, including toxic epidermal necrolysis (TEN) and Stevens-Johnson syndrome (SJS), although rarely reported (with phenytoin), have resulted in fatalities; fosphenytoin should be discontinued if there are any signs of rash and patient should be evaluated for signs and symptoms of drug reaction with eosinophilia and systemic symptoms (DRESS). Preliminary data suggests that patients testing positive for the human leukocyte antigen (HLA) allele HLA-B*1502 have an increased risk of developing SJS and/or TEN. The risk appears to be highest in the early months of therapy initiation. The presence of this genetic variant exists in up to 15% of people of Asian descent in China, Thailand, Malaysia, Indonesia, Taiwan, and the Philippines, and may vary from <1% in Japanese and Koreans to 2% to 4% of South Asians and Indians. This variant is virtually absent in those of Caucasian, African-American, Hispanic, or European ancestry; consider avoiding fosphenytoin use in patients *HLA-B*1502* allele-positive if other therapeutic options are available. **Note:** Carbamazepine, another antiepileptic with a chemical structure similar to phenytoin, includes in the manufacturer labeling a recommendation to screen patients of Asian descent for the *HLA-B*1502* allele prior to initiating therapy; this is not a current recommendation in the fosphenytoin or phenytoin manufacturer labeling.

A spectrum of hematologic effects have been reported with phenytoin use (eg, agranulocytosis, neutropenia, leukopenia, thrombocytopenia, pancytopenia, and anemias); patients with a previous history of adverse hematologic reaction to any drug may be at increased risk. Early detection of hematologic change is important; advise patients of early signs and symptoms including fever, infections, easy bruising, and petechial or purpuric hemorrhage.

The "purple glove syndrome" (ie, discoloration with edema and pain of distal limb) may rarely occur following peripheral I.V. administration of fosphenytoin; incidence may be less compared to phenytoin; symptoms may resolve spontaneously; however, skin necrosis and limb ischemia may occur. In general, fosphenytoin has significantly less venous irritation and phlebitis compared with an equimolar dose of phenytoin (Jamerson, 1994).

Precautions Use with caution in patients with any condition associated with low serum albumin levels, which will increase the free fraction of phenytoin in the serum and, therefore, the pharmacologic response. Use with caution in renal impairment; serum concentrations may be difficult to interpret; consider monitoring free (unbound) concentrations; also consider the phosphate load delivered with fosphenytoin (0.0037 mmol phosphate/mg PE fosphenytoin). Use with caution in hepatic impairment; clearance may be substantially reduced in cirrhosis; frequent monitoring of free (unbound) serum concentrations should be considered. Use with caution in patients with underlying cardiac disease; use is contraindicated in bradycardia, sinoatrial block, second- and third-degree heart block, or Adam-Stokes syndrome. Use with caution in patients with porphyria; may cause exacerbations. Should not be used to treat absence seizures; phenytoin has been shown to increase frequency. May cause sedation, confusional states, or cerebellar dysfunction (loss of motor coordination) at higher total serum phenytoin concentrations, or at lower total serum concentrations when the free fraction of phenytoin is increased; possible permanent cerebellum damage may occur with chronic toxic serum concentrations; effects with other sedative drugs or ethanol may be potentiated; use with caution in patients who are debilitated. Use with caution in diabetic patients; may cause hyperglycemia. Severe burning or pruritus and/or paresthesias, mostly perineal, may occur upon administration, usually at the maximum administration rate and last from minutes to hours; occurrence and intensity may be lessened by slowing or temporarily stopping the infusion.

Pediatric patients may be at increased risk for vitamin D deficiency; with chronic therapy, phenytoin may cause catabolism of vitamin D; the daily vitamin D requirement may be increased in these patients (≥400 units/day); vitamin D status should be periodically monitored with laboratory data (Misra, 2008; Wagner, 2008).

Adverse Reactions The more important adverse clinical events caused by the I.V. use of fosphenytoin or phenytoin are cardiovascular collapse and/or central nervous system

depression. Hypotension can occur when either drug is administered rapidly by the I.V. route.

The adverse clinical events most commonly observed with the use of fosphenytoin in clinical trials were nystagmus, dizziness, pruritus, paresthesia, headache, somnolence, and ataxia. Paresthesia and pruritus were seen more often following fosphenytoin (versus phenytoin) administration and occurred more often with I.V. fosphenytoin than with I.M. administration. These events were dose and rate related (adult doses ≥15 mg/kg at a rate of 150 mg PE/minute). These sensations, generally described as itching, burning, or tingling are usually not at the infusion site. The location of the discomfort varied with the groin mentioned most frequently. The paresthesia and pruritus were transient events that occurred within several minutes of the start of infusion and generally resolved within 10 minutes after completion of infusion.

Transient pruritus, tinnitus, nystagmus, somnolence, and ataxia occurred 2-3 times more often at adult doses ≥15 mg/kg and rates ≥150 mg PE/minute.

I.V. and I.M. administration (as reported in clinical trials):
Cardiovascular: Facial edema, hypertension
Central nervous system: Chills, fever, intracranial hypertension, nervousness
Endocrine & metabolic: Hypokalemia
Neuromuscular & skeletal: Hyperreflexia, myasthenia

I.V. administration (maximum dose/rate):
Central nervous system: Ataxia, dizziness, nystagmus, somnolence
Dermatologic: Pruritus
Cardiovascular: Hypotension, tachycardia, vasodilation
Central nervous system: Agitation, brain edema, dysarthria, extrapyramidal syndrome, headache, hypoesthesia, incoordination, paresthesia, stupor, tremor, vertigo
Gastrointestinal: Dry mouth, nausea, tongue disorder, vomiting
Neuromuscular & skeletal: Back pain, muscle weakness, pelvic pain
Ocular: Amblyopia, diplopia
Otic: Deafness, tinnitus
Miscellaneous: Taste perversion

I.M. administration (substitute for oral phenytoin):
Central nervous system: Ataxia, dizziness, headache, incoordination, nystagmus, paresthesia, reflexes decreased, somnolence, tremor
Dermatologic: Pruritus
Gastrointestinal: Nausea, vomiting
Hematologic/lymphatic: Ecchymosis
Neuromuscular & skeletal: Muscle weakness

I.V. and I.M. administration: Rare but important or life-threatening: Acidosis, acute hepatic failure, acute hepatotoxicity, alkalosis, akathisia, amnesia, anemia, anorexia, aphasia, apnea, arthralgia, asthma, atrial flutter, Babinski sign positive, bundle branch block, cachexia, cardiac arrest, cardiomegaly, cerebral hemorrhage, cerebral infarct, CHF, circumoral paresthesia, CNS depression, cyanosis, dehydration, diabetes insipidus, dyskinesia, dysphagia, dyspnea, edema, emotional lability, encephalopathy, epistaxis, extrapyramidal symptoms, GI hemorrhage, hemiplegia, hemoptysis, hostility, hyperacusis, hyperesthesia, hyper-/hypokinesia, hyperkalemia, hyperventilation, hypochromic anemia, hypophosphatemia, hypotonia, hypoxia, ileus, injection site (edema, hemorrhage, inflammation), ketosis, leg cramps, leukocytosis, leukopenia, LFTs abnormal, malaise, migraine, myalgia, mydriasis, myopathy, neurosis, orthostatic hypotension, palpitation, paralysis, parosmia, petechia, photophobia, photosensitivity reaction, psychosis, pulmonary embolus, QT interval prolongation, rash (maculopapular or pustular), renal failure, sinus bradycardia, shock, subdural hematoma, syncope, Stevens-Johnson syndrome, tenesmus, thrombocytopenia, thrombophlebitis, tongue edema, toxic epidermal necrolysis, urticaria, ventricular extrasystoles, visual field defect

Drug Interactions

Metabolism/Transport Effects Substrate of CYP2C19 (major), CYP2C9 (major), CYP3A4 (minor); **Note:** Assignment of Major/Minor substrate status based on clinically relevant drug interaction potential; **Induces** CYP2B6 (strong), CYP2C19 (strong), CYP2C8 (strong), CYP2C9 (strong), CYP3A4 (strong), P-glycoprotein

Avoid Concomitant Use

Avoid concomitant use of Fosphenytoin with any of the following: Abiraterone Acetate; Apixaban; Apremilast; Artemether; Axitinib; Azelastine (Nasal); Bedaquiline; Boceprevir; Bortezomib; Bosutinib; Cabozantinib; Ceritinib; CloZAPine; Crizotinib; Dabigatran Etexilate; Darunavir; Delavirdine; Dienogest; Dolutegravir; Dronedarone; Enzalutamide; Etravirine; Everolimus; Ibrutinib; Itraconazole; Ivacaftor; Lapatinib; Lumefantrine; Lurasidone; Macitentan; Mifepristone; NIFEdipine; Nilotinib; Nisoldipine; Paraldehyde; PAZOPanib; PONATinib; Praziquantel; Ranolazine; Regorafenib; Rilpivirine; Rivaroxaban; Roflumilast; RomiDEPsin; Simeprevir; Sofosbuvir; SORAfenib; Tasimelteon; Telaprevir; Thalidomide; Ticagrelor; Tofacitinib; Tolvaptan; Toremifene; Ulipristal; Vandetanib; Vemurafenib; VinCRIStine (Liposomal); Vorapaxar

Increased Effect/Toxicity

Fosphenytoin may increase the levels/effects of: Amiodarone; Azelastine (Nasal); Buprenorphine; Ciprofloxacin (Systemic); Clarithromycin; CNS Depressants; FLUoxetine; Fosamprenavir; Highest Risk QTc-Prolonging Agents; Hydrocodone; Lithium; Methotrexate; Methotrimeprazine; Metyrosine; Moderate Risk QTc-Prolonging Agents; Neuromuscular-Blocking Agents (Nondepolarizing); Paraldehyde; PHENobarbital; Pramipexole; QuiNIDine; ROPINIRole; Rotigotine; Selective Serotonin Reuptake Inhibitors; Thalidomide; Vitamin K Antagonists; Zolpidem

The levels/effects of Fosphenytoin may be increased by: Alcohol (Ethyl); Allopurinol; Amiodarone; Antifungal Agents (Azole Derivatives, Systemic); Benzodiazepines; Brimonidine (Topical); Calcium Channel Blockers; Cannabis; Capecitabine; CarBAMazepine; Carbonic Anhydrase Inhibitors; CeFAZolin; Chloramphenicol; Cimetidine; Clarithromycin; CYP2C19 Inhibitors (Moderate); CYP2C19 Inhibitors (Strong); CYP2C9 Inhibitors (Moderate); CYP2C9 Inhibitors (Strong); Delavirdine; Dexmethylphenidate; Disopyramide; Disulfiram; Doxylamine; Dronabinol; Droperidol; Efavirenz; Eslicarbazepine; Ethosuximide; Felbamate; Floxuridine; Fluconazole; Fluorouracil (Systemic); Fluorouracil (Topical); FLUoxetine; FluvoxaMINE; Halothane; HydrOXYzine; Isoniazid; Kava Kava; Luliconazole; Magnesium Sulfate; Methotrimeprazine; Methylphenidate; MetroNIDAZOLE (Systemic); Nabilone; Omeprazole; OXcarbazepine; Rufinamide; Sertraline; Sodium Oxybate; Tacrolimus (Systemic); Tapentadol; Tegafur; Telaprevir; Tetrahydrocannabinol; Ticlopidine; Topiramate; TraZODone; Trimethoprim; Vitamin K Antagonists

Decreased Effect

Fosphenytoin may decrease the levels/effects of: Abiraterone Acetate; Acetaminophen; Afatinib; Amiodarone; Antifungal Agents (Azole Derivatives, Systemic); Apixaban; Apremilast; ARIPiprazole; Artemether; Axitinib; Bazedoxifene; Bedaquiline; Boceprevir; Bortezomib; Bosutinib; Brentuximab Vedotin; Busulfan; Cabozantinib; Canagliflozin; Cannabidiol; Cannabis; CarBAMazepine; Ceritinib; Chloramphenicol; Clarithromycin; CloZAPine; Cobicistat; Contraceptives (Estrogens); Contraceptives (Progestins); Crizotinib; CycloSPORINE (Systemic);

CYP2B6 Substrates; CYP2C19 Substrates; CYP2C8 Substrates; CYP2C9 Substrates; CYP3A4 Substrates; Dabigatran Etexilate; Darunavir; Dasatinib; Deferasirox; Delavirdine; Diclofenac (Systemic); Dienogest; Disopyramide; Dolutegravir; DOXOrubicin (Conventional); Doxycycline; Dronabinol; Dronedarone; Efavirenz; Elvitegravir; Enzalutamide; Eslicarbazepine; Ethosuximide; Etoposide; Etoposide Phosphate; Etravirine; Everolimus; Exemestane; Felbamate; FentaNYL; Flunarizine; Gefitinib; GuanFACINE; HMG-CoA Reductase Inhibitors; Ibrutinib; Imatinib; Irinotecan; Itraconazole; Ivacaftor; Ixabepilone; Lacosamide; LamoTRIgine; Lapatinib; Levodopa; Linagliptin; Loop Diuretics; Lopinavir; Lumefantrine; Lurasidone; Macitentan; Maraviroc; Mebendazole; Meperidine; Methadone; MethylPREDNISolone; MetroNIDAZOLE (Systemic); Metyrapone; Mexiletine; Mifepristone; Nelfinavir; Neuromuscular-Blocking Agents (Nondepolarizing); NIFEdipine; Nilotinib; Nisoldipine; Omeprazole; OXcarbazepine; PAZOPanib; Perampanel; P-glycoprotein/ABCB1 Substrates; PONATinib; Praziquantel; PrednisoLONE (Systemic); PredniSONE; Primidone; QUEtiapine; QuiNIDine; QuiNINE; Ranolazine; Regorafenib; Rilpivirine; Ritonavir; Rivaroxaban; Roflumilast; RomiDEPsin; Rufinamide; Saxagliptin; Sertraline; Simeprevir; Sirolimus; Sofosbuvir; SORAfenib; SUNItinib; Tacrolimus (Systemic); Tadalafil; Tasimelteon; Telaprevir; Temsirolimus; Teniposide; Tetrahydrocannabinol; Theophylline Derivatives; Thyroid Products; Ticagrelor; Tipranavir; Tofacitinib; Tolvaptan; Topiramate; Topotecan; Toremifene; TraZODone; Treprostinil; Trimethoprim; Ulipristal; Valproic Acid and Derivatives; Vandetanib; Vemurafenib; Vilazodone; VinCRIStine; VinCRIStine (Liposomal); Vorapaxar; Vortioxetine; Zonisamide

The levels/effects of Fosphenytoin may be decreased by: Alcohol (Ethyl); Antacids; CarBAMazepine; Ciprofloxacin (Systemic); CYP2C19 Inducers (Strong); CYP2C9 Inducers (Strong); Dabrafenib; Diazoxide; Enzalutamide; Folic Acid; Fosamprenavir; Ketorolac (Nasal); Ketorolac (Systemic); Leucovorin Calcium-Levoleucovorin; Levomefolate; Lopinavir; Mefloquine; Methotrexate; Methylfolate; Multivitamins/Minerals (with ADEK, Folate, Iron); Nelfinavir; Orlistat; Peginterferon Alfa-2b; PHENobarbital; Platinum Derivatives; Pyridoxine; Rifampin; Ritonavir; Theophylline Derivatives; Tipranavir; Valproic Acid and Derivatives; Vigabatrin; VinCRIStine

Food Interactions

Acute use: Ethanol inhibits metabolism of phenytoin. Management: Monitor patients.

Chronic use: Ethanol stimulates metabolism of phenytoin. Management: Monitor patients.

Stability Store intact vials at 2°C to 8°C (36°F to 46°F); do not store at room temperature for >48 hours; do not use vials containing particulate matter. Fosphenytoin at concentrations of 1, 8, and 20 mg phenytoin sodium equivalents **(PE)**/mL in D₅W or NS is stable for 30 days when stored at 25°C or 4°C in glass bottles or polyvinyl chloride infusion bags, and when frozen at -20°C in polyvinyl chloride infusion bags. After removal from the freezer, these solutions are stable for 7 days at 25°C or 4°C (Fischer, 1997).

Undiluted fosphenytoin injection (50 mg **PE**/mL) is stable in polypropylene syringes for 30 days at 25°C, 4°C, or frozen at -20°C (Fischer, 1997).

Fosphenytoin at concentrations of 1, 8, and 20 mg **PE**/mL prepared in D₅/½NS, D₅/¼NS with KCl 20 mEq/L, D₅/½NS with 40 mEq/L, LR, D₅LR, D₁₀W, amino acid 10%, mannitol 20%, hetastarch 6% in NS or Plasma-Lyte® A injection is stable in polyvinyl chloride bags for 7 days when stored at 25°C (room temperature) (Fischer, 1997).

◄ **Mechanism of Action** Diphosphate ester salt of phenytoin which acts as a water soluble prodrug of phenytoin;
after administration, plasma esterases convert fosphenytoin to phosphate, formaldehyde, and phenytoin as the
active moiety; phenytoin works by stabilizing neuronal
membranes and decreasing seizure activity by increasing
efflux or decreasing influx of sodium ions across cell
membranes in the motor cortex during generation of nerve
impulses

Pharmacokinetics (Adult data unless noted) The
pharmacokinetics of fosphenytoin-derived phenytoin are
the same as those for phenytoin. Parameters listed below
are for fosphenytoin (the prodrug) unless otherwise noted.
Note: The pharmacokinetics of intravenous fosphenytoin
in pediatric patients have been evaluated in two studies
(n=49, age range: 1 day to 16.7 years; n=8, age range:
5-18 years) and found to be similar to the pharmacokinetics observed in young adults; the conversion rate of
fosphenytoin to phenytoin was consistent throughout childhood (Fischer, 2003; Pellock, 1996).
Bioavailability: I.M., I.V.: 100%
Distribution: V_d: 4.3-10.8 L; V_d of fosphenytoin increases
with dose and rate of administration (Fischer, 2003)
Protein binding: 95% to 99% primarily to albumin; binding
of fosphenytoin to protein is saturable (the percent bound
decreases as total concentration increases); fosphenytoin displaces phenytoin from protein binding sites; during
the time fosphenytoin is being converted to phenytoin,
fosphenytoin may temporarily increase the free fraction of
phenytoin up to 30% unbound
Metabolism: Each millimole of fosphenytoin is metabolized
to 1 millimole of phenytoin, phosphate, and formaldehyde; formaldehyde is converted to formate, which is
then metabolized by a folate-dependent mechanism;
conversion of fosphenytoin to phenytoin increases with
increasing dose and infusion rate, most likely due to a
decrease in fosphenytoin protein binding
Half-life:
Conversion of fosphenytoin to phenytoin:
Pediatric patients (ages: 1 day to 16.7 years): 8.3
minutes (range: 2.5-18.5 minutes) (Fischer, 2003)
Adults: Mean range: 7-15 minutes (Fischer, 2003)
Time for complete conversion to phenytoin:
I.M.: 4 hours after injection
I.V.: 2 hours after the end of infusion
Time to peak serum concentration (phenytoin):
I.V.: Adults: 30-60 minutes from the beginning of fosphe-
nytoin infusion (Fischer, 2003)
I.M.:
Neonates and Infants ≤6 months: 1-3 hours was
reported in a case series (n=3; PNA: 15-47 days)
(Fischer, 2003)
Pediatric patients >7 months: Therapeutic concentra-
tions within 30 minutes; time to maximum serum
concentration not reported (Fischer, 2003)
Adults: 3 hours
Elimination: 0% fosphenytoin excreted in urine

Dosing: Neonatal
The dose, concentration in solutions, and infusion
rates for fosphenytoin are expressed as **PHENYTOIN
SODIUM EQUIVALENTS (PE)**

**Fosphenytoin should ALWAYS be prescribed and dis-
pensed in mg of PE**; otherwise, significant medication
errors may occur

Note: A limited number of clinical studies have been
conducted; based on pharmacokinetic studies, experts
recommend the following (Fischer, 2003): Use the neonatal I.V. phenytoin dosing guidelines to dose fosphenytoin using doses in **PE** equal to the phenytoin doses (ie,
phenytoin 1 mg = fosphenytoin 1 mg **PE**). Dosage
should be individualized based upon clinical response
and serum concentrations.

Status epilepticus; neonatal seizures: Limited data
available: Loading dose: I.M., I.V.: 15-20 mg PE/kg; then
begin maintenance therapy usually 12 hours after dose.
Note: Phenobarbital is the preferred antiepileptic agent
for treatment of neonatal seizures (Hegenbarth, 2008).
**Seizures; maintenance therapy, short-term when oral
route not available or appropriate:** Limited data available:
Not currently on phenytoin: **Note:** Assess if loading dose
is required; calculate loading dose as above for status
epilepticus.
I.M. or I.V.: Initial: 5 mg PE/kg/day in 2 divided doses;
usual range: 4-8 mg PE/kg/day in 2 divided doses;
some patients may require dosing every 8 hours; dosing based on phenytoin recommendations for this
patient population; in adult patients, treatment duration
>5 days has not been evaluated.
Substitution for oral phenytoin therapy: I.M. or I.V.: May
be substituted for oral phenytoin sodium at the same
total daily dose; due to bioavailability differences of oral
phenytoin dosage forms, serum phenytoin concentrations may increase when I.M. or I.V. fosphenytoin is
substituted for oral phenytoin sodium therapy; monitor
serum concentrations closely when converting dosage form.

Dosing: Usual
The dose, concentration in solutions, and infusion
rates for fosphenytoin are expressed as **PHENYTOIN
SODIUM EQUIVALENTS (PE)**

**Fosphenytoin should ALWAYS be prescribed and dis-
pensed in mg of PE**; otherwise significant medication
errors may occur

Infants, Children, and Adolescents: I.V.: **Note:** A limited
number of clinical studies have been conducted in pediatric patients; based on pharmacokinetic studies, experts
recommend the following (Fischer, 2003): Use the pediatric I.V. phenytoin dosing guidelines to dose fosphenytoin
using doses in **PE** equal to the phenytoin doses (ie,
phenytoin 1 mg = fosphenytoin 1 mg **PE**). Dosage
should be individualized based upon clinical response
and serum concentrations.
Status epilepticus: Limited data available: Loading
dose: I.M., I.V.: 15-20 mg PE/kg; maximum dose:
1000 mg PE; then begin maintenance therapy usually
12 hours after dose (Brophy, 2012; Hegenbarth, 2008).
An additional load of 5 mg PE/kg may be given 10
minutes after initial loading infusion completed if status
epilepticus is not resolved; however, some experts
recommend trying another agent once a total loading
dose of 20 mg PE/kg has been given (Brophy, 2012).
**Seizures; maintenance therapy, short-term when oral
route not available or appropriate:** Limited data available; dosing presented based on phenytoin recommendations for this patient population:
Not currently receiving phenytoin: **Note:** Assess if loading dose is required; calculate loading dose as above
for status epilepticus.
Maintenance therapy: I.M., I.V.: Initial 5 mg PE/kg/day
divided twice daily; usual range: 4-8 mg PE/kg/day
divided twice daily; maximum daily dose: 300 mg
PE/**day**. Some experts suggest higher maintenance
doses (8-10 mg PE/kg/day) may be necessary in
infants and young children (Guerrini, 2006). Dosing
should be based upon ideal body weight (IBW); in
adult patients, treatment duration >5 days has not
been evaluated.
Substitution for oral phenytoin therapy: I.M. or I.V.: May
be substituted for oral phenytoin sodium at the same
total daily dose; however, Dilantin® capsules are
~90% bioavailable by the oral route; phenytoin, supplied as fosphenytoin, is 100% bioavailable by both
the I.M. and I.V. routes; for this reason, plasma

phenytoin concentrations may increase when I.M. or I.V. fosphenytoin is substituted for oral phenytoin sodium therapy; in adult clinical trials, I.M. fosphenytoin was administered as a single daily dose utilizing either 1 or 2 injection sites; some patients may require more frequent dosing

Seizure prophylaxis, traumatic brain injury: Limited data available; efficacy results variable; dosing based on experience with phenytoin: I.V.: Initial: 18 mg PE/kg loading dose; followed by 6 mg PE/kg/day divided every 8 hours for 48 hours was used in a double-blind, placebo-controlled trial of 102 pediatric patients (n=46 treatment group; median age: 6.4 years) and showed no significant difference in seizure frequency between groups; however, the trial was stopped early due to a very low seizure frequency among both study groups (Young, 2004). In a retrospective trial, reduced seizure frequency with prophylactic phenytoin use was described (Lewis, 1993). **Note:** Current guidelines suggest that prophylactic phenytoin may be considered to reduce the incidence of early post-traumatic seizures in pediatric patients with severe traumatic brain injuries but it does not reduce the risk of long-term seizures or improve neurologic outcome (Kochanek, 2012). Further studies are needed.

Adults: **Note:** The dose, concentration in solutions, and infusion rates for fosphenytoin are expressed as phenytoin sodium equivalents (PE); fosphenytoin should always be prescribed and dispensed in phenytoin sodium equivalents (PE).

Status epilepticus: I.V.: Loading dose: 15-20 mg PE/kg administered at 100-150 mg PE/minute

Nonemergent loading and maintenance dosing:
Loading dose: I.M., I.V.: 10-20 mg PE/kg; for I.V. administration, infuse more slowly (eg, over 30 minutes); maximum rate: 150 mg PE/minute
Initial daily maintenance dose: I.M., I.V.: 4-6 mg PE/kg/day in divided doses

Substitution for oral phenytoin therapy: I.M. or I.V.: May be substituted for oral phenytoin sodium at the same total daily dose; however, Dilantin® capsules are ~90% bioavailable by the oral route; phenytoin, supplied as fosphenytoin, is 100% bioavailable by both the I.M. and I.V. routes; for this reason, plasma phenytoin concentrations may increase when I.M. or I.V. fosphenytoin is substituted for oral phenytoin sodium therapy; in clinical trials, I.M. fosphenytoin was administered as a single daily dose utilizing either 1 or 2 injection sites; some patients may require more frequent dosing.

Dosing adjustment in renal impairment: Adults: No initial dosage adjustment necessary. Free (unbound) phenytoin serum concentrations should be monitored closely in patients with renal disease or in those with hypoalbuminemia, free phenytoin serum concentrations may be increased; furthermore, fosphenytoinconversion to phenytoin may be increased without a similar increase in phenytoin conversion in these patients leading to increase frequency and severity of adverse events.

Dosing adjustment in hepatic impairment: Adults: No initial dosage adjustment necessary. Phenytoin clearance may be substantially reduced in cirrhosis and serum concentration monitoring with dose adjustment advisable. Free (unbound) phenytoin concentrations should be monitored closely in patients with hepatic disease or in those with hypoalbuminemia; free phenytoin concentrations may be increased; furthermore, fosphenytoin conversion to phenytoin may be increased without a similar increase in phenytoin clearance in these patients leading to increased frequency and severity of adverse events.

Administration
I.M.: May administer undiluted; the quadricep area has been recommended as an injection site; in adults, fosphenytoin has been administered as a single daily dose using 1-4 injection sites (up to 20 mL per site well tolerated in adults) (Meek, 1999; Pryor, 2001)

I.V.: Further dilute solution for injection with D_5W or NS to final concentration of 1.5-25 mg PE/mL; administer as intermittent I.V. infusion; do not administer as a continuous infusion or I.V. push

Maximum rates of infusion:
Pediatric patients: Administer at **1-3 mg PE/kg/minute up to a maximum of 150 mg PE/minute** (Brophy, 2012; Hegenbarth, 2008); slower administration reduces incidence of cardiovascular events (eg, hypotension, arrhythmia) as well as severity of paresthesias and pruritus. For nonemergent situations, may administer loading dose more slowly (eg, over 30 minutes) (Fischer, 2003). Highly sensitive patients (eg, patients with preexisting cardiovascular conditions) should receive fosphenytoin more slowly (Meek, 1999).

Adults: **Do not exceed 150 mg PE/minute.** Slower administration reduces incidence of cardiovascular events (eg, hypotension, arrhythmia) as well as severity of paresthesias and pruritus. For nonemergent situations, may administer loading dose more slowly [eg, over 30 minutes (~33 mg PE/minute for 1000 mg PE) **or** 50-100 mg PE/minute (Fischer, 2003)]. Highly sensitive patients (eg, elderly, patients with preexisting cardiovascular conditions) should receive fosphenytoin more slowly (25-50 mg PE/minute) (Meek, 1999).

Monitoring Parameters CBC with differential, platelets, serum glucose, liver function. Serum phenytoin concentrations: If available, free phenytoin concentrations should be obtained in patients with hyperbilirubinemia, renal impairment, uremia, or hypoalbuminemia; in adult patients, if free phenytoin concentrations are unavailable, the adjusted total concentration may be determined based upon equations. Trough serum concentrations are generally recommended for routine monitoring. To ensure therapeutic concentration is attained, peak serum concentrations may be measured 1 hour after the end of an I.V. infusion (particularly after a loading dose).

Additional monitoring with I.V. use: Continuous cardiac monitoring (rate, rhythm, blood pressure) and clinical observation during administration is recommended; blood pressure and pulse should be monitored every 15 minutes for 1 hour after administration with nonemergency use (Meek, 1999); emergency use may require more frequent monitoring and for a longer time after administration; infusion site reactions

Reference Range Note: Information based on experience with phenytoin.
Timing of serum samples: The apparent serum half-life varies with the dosage and the drug follows Michaelis-Menten kinetics. In adults, the average apparent half-life is about 24 hours; in pediatric patients, the apparent half-life is age-dependent (longer in neonates). Steady-state concentrations are reached in 5-10 days.

Toxicity is measured clinically and some patients may require levels outside the suggested therapeutic range.
Therapeutic range:
Total phenytoin:
Neonates: 8-15 mcg/mL
Pediatric patients ≥1 month and Adults: 10-20 mcg/mL ▶

Concentrations of 5-10 mcg/mL may be therapeutic for some patients, but concentrations <5 mcg/mL are not likely to be effective

50% of adult patients show decreased frequency of seizures at concentrations >10 mcg/mL

86% of adult patients show decreased frequency of seizures at concentrations >15 mcg/mL

Add another anticonvulsant if satisfactory therapeutic response is not achieved with a phenytoin concentration of 20 mcg/mL.

Free phenytoin: 1-2.5 mcg/mL

Total phenytoin:

Toxic: >30 mcg/mL (SI: >119 micromole/L)

Lethal: >100 mcg/mL (SI: >400 micromole/L)

After a loading dose: If rapid therapeutic serum concentrations are needed, initial concentrations may be drawn after 1 hour (after end of I.V. loading dose) to aid in determining maintenance dose or need to reload.

Rapid achievement: Early assessment of serum concentrations: Draw within 2-3 days of therapy initiation to ensure that the patient's metabolism is not remarkably different from that which would be predicted by average literature-derived pharmacokinetic parameters; early serum concentrations should be used cautiously in design of new dosing regimens.

See Phenytoin monograph for further information.

Test Interactions Falsely high plasma phenytoin concentrations (due to cross-reactivity with fosphenytoin) when measured by immunoanalytical techniques (eg, TD$_X$®, TD$_X$FL$_X$™, Emit® 2000) prior to complete conversion of fosphenytoin to phenytoin. Phenytoin may produce falsely low results for dexamethasone or metyrapone tests.

Additional Information Dosing equivalency: Fosphenytoin sodium 1.5 mg is equivalent to phenytoin sodium 1 mg which is equivalent to fosphenytoin 1 mg **PE**

Fosphenytoin is water soluble and has a lower pH (8.8) than phenytoin (12), irritation at injection site or phlebitis is reduced.

Formaldehyde production from fosphenytoin is not expected to be clinically significant in adults with short-term use (eg, 1 week); potentially harmful amounts of phosphate and formaldehyde could occur with an overdose of fosphenytoin; fosphenytoin is more water soluble than phenytoin and, therefore, the injection does not contain propylene glycol; antiarrhythmic effects should be similar to phenytoin

Overdose may result in: Lethargy, nausea, vomiting, hypotension, syncope, tachycardia, bradycardia, asystole, cardiac arrest, hypocalcemia, and metabolic acidosis; fatalities have also been reported

Dosage Forms Excipient information presented when available (limited, particularly for generics); consult specific product labeling.

Solution, Injection, as sodium:

Cerebyx: 100 mg PE/2 mL (2 mL); 500 mg PE/10 mL (10 mL)

Generic: 100 mg PE/2 mL (2 mL); 500 mg PE/10 mL (10 mL)

References

Adams BD, Buckley NH, Kim JY, et al, "Fosphenytoin May Cause Hemodynamically Unstable Bradydysrhythmias," *J Emerg Med*, 2006, 30(1):75-9.

Brophy GM, Bell R, Claassen J, et al, "Guidelines for the Evaluation and Management of Status Epilepticus," *Neurocrit Care*, 2012, 17(1):3-23.

Fischer JH, Cwik MS, Luer MS, et al, "Stability of Fosphenytoin Sodium With Intravenous Solutions in Glass Bottles, Polyvinyl Chloride Bags, and Polypropylene Syringes," *Ann Pharmacother*, 1997, 31(5):553-9.

Fischer JH, Patel TV, and Fischer PA, "Fosphenytoin: Clinical Pharmacokinetics and Comparative Advantages in the Acute Treatment of Seizures," *Clin Pharmacokinet*, 2003, 42(1):33-58.

Guerrini R, "Epilepsy in Children," *Lancet*, 2006, 367(9509):499-524.

Hegenbarth MA and American Academy of Pediatrics Committee on Drugs, "Preparing for Pediatric Emergencies: Drugs to Consider," *Pediatrics*, 2008, 121(2):433-43.

Jamerson BD, Dukes GE, Brouwer KL, et al, "Venous Irritation Related to Intravenous Administration of Phenytoin Versus Fosphenytoin," *Pharmacotherapy*, 1994, 14(1):47-52.

Kochanek PM, Carney N, Adelson PD, et al, "Guidelines for the Acute Medical Management of Severe Traumatic Brain Injury in Infants, Children, and Adolescents-Second Edition," *Pediatr Crit Care Med*, 2012, 13(Suppl 1):S1-82.

Koul R and Deleu D, "Subtherapeutic Free Phenytoin Levels Following Fosphenytoin Therapy in Status Epilepticus," *Neurology*, 2002, 58 (1):147-8.

Kriel RL and Cifuentes RF, "Fosphenytoin in Infants of Extremely Low Birth Weight," *Pediatr Neurol*, 2001, 24(3):219-21.

Lewis RJ, Yee L, Inkelis SH, et al, "Clinical Predictors of Post-Traumatic Seizures in Children With Head Trauma," *Ann Emerg Med*, 1993, 22 (7):1114-8.

McBryde KD, Wilcox J, and Kher KK, "Hyperphosphatemia Due to Fosphenytoin in a Pediatric ESRD Patient," *Pediatr Nephrol*, 2005, 20(8):1182-5.

Meek PD, Davis SN, Collins DM, et al, "Guidelines for Nonemergency Use of Parenteral Phenytoin Products: Proceedings of an Expert Panel Consensus Process. Panel on Nonemergency Use of Parenteral Phenytoin Products," *Arch Intern Med*, 1999, 159(22):2639-44.

Misra M, Pacaud D, Petryk A, Collett-Solberg PF, Kappy M, Drug and Therapeutics Committee of the Lawson Wilkins Pediatric Endocrine Society. Vitamin D deficiency in children and its management: review of current knowledge and recommendations. *Pediatrics*. 2008;122 (2):398-417.

Morton LD, "Clinical Experience With Fosphenytoin in Children," *J Child Neurol*, 1998, 13(Suppl 1):S19-22.

Ogutu BR, Newton CR, Muchohi SN, et al, "Pharmacokinetics and Clinical Effects of Phenytoin and Fosphenytoin in Children With Severe Malaria and Status Epilepticus," *Br J Clin Pharmacol*, 2003, 56(1):112-9.

Pellock JM, "Fosphenytoin Use in Children," *Neurology*, 1996, 46(6 Suppl 1):S14-6.

Pryor FM, Gidal B, Ramsay RE, et al, "Fosphenytoin: Pharmacokinetics and Tolerance of Intramuscular Loading Doses," *Epilepsia*, 2001, 42 (2):245-50.

Takeoka M, Krishnamoorthy KS, Soman TB, et al, "Fosphenytoin in Infants," *J Child Neurol*, 1998, 13(11):537-40.

Wagner CL, Greer FR, American Academy of Pediatrics Section on Breastfeeding, American Academy of Pediatrics Committee on Nutrition. Prevention of rickets and vitamin D deficiency in infants, children, and adolescents. *Pediatrics*. 2008;122(5):1142-1152.

Young KD, Okada PJ, Sokolove PE, et al, "A Randomized, Double-Blinded, Placebo-Controlled Trial of Phenytoin for the Prevention of Early Posttraumatic Seizures in Children With Moderate to Severe Blunt Head Injury," *Ann Emerg Med*, 2004, 43(4):435-46.

◆ **Fosphenytoin Sodium** *see* Fosphenytoin *on page 941*

◆ **Fresenius Propoven** *see* Propofol *on page 1755*

◆ **Frisium (Can)** *see* CloBAZam *on page 504*

◆ **Froben (Can)** *see* Flurbiprofen (Systemic) *on page 908*

◆ **Froben-SR (Can)** *see* Flurbiprofen (Systemic) *on page 908*

◆ **Fruit C [OTC]** *see* Ascorbic Acid *on page 206*

◆ **Fruit C 500 [OTC]** *see* Ascorbic Acid *on page 206*

◆ **Fruity C [OTC]** *see* Ascorbic Acid *on page 206*

◆ **Frusemide** *see* Furosemide *on page 948*

◆ **FTC** *see* Emtricitabine *on page 738*

◆ **FTC, TDF, and EFV** *see* Efavirenz, Emtricitabine, and Tenofovir *on page 735*

◆ **FU** *see* Fluorouracil (Systemic) *on page 897*

◆ **FU** *see* Fluorouracil (Topical) *on page 900*

◆ **5-FU** *see* Fluorouracil (Systemic) *on page 897*

◆ **5-FU** *see* Fluorouracil (Topical) *on page 900*

Fulvestrant (fool VES trant)

Related Information

Safe Handling of Hazardous Drugs *on page 2419*

Brand Names: U.S. Faslodex

Brand Names: Canada Faslodex®

Therapeutic Category Antineoplastic Agent, Estrogen Receptor Antagonist

Generic Availability (U.S.) No

Use Treatment of hormone receptor-positive metastatic breast cancer in postmenopausal women with disease progression following antiestrogen therapy (FDA approved in adults); has also been used in treatment of McCune-Albright Syndrome (MAS) in girls associated with progressive precocious puberty

Pregnancy Risk Factor D

Pregnancy Considerations Fetal loss and abnormalities were observed in animal studies. Approved for use only in postmenopausal women. If used prior to confirmed menopause, women of reproductive potential should be advised not to become pregnant.

Breast-Feeding Considerations Approved for use only in postmenopausal women.

Contraindications Hypersensitivity to fulvestrant or any component

Warnings Hazardous agent; use appropriate precautions for handling and disposal (NIOSH, 2012). May cause fetal harm if administered during pregnancy; women of childbearing potential should be advised to avoid becoming pregnant during therapy; if pregnancy occurs during therapy, patient should be counseled regarding potential fetal hazards. Injectable solution contains benzyl alcohol which may cause allergic reactions in susceptible individuals; may contain ethanol (10%, w/v) and castor oil.

Precautions Use with caution in patients with hepatic impairment; dosage adjustment is recommended in moderate impairment; safety and efficacy have not been established in severe impairment. Use with caution in patients with a history of bleeding disorders (including thrombocytopenia) and/or patients on anticoagulant therapy; bleeding/hematoma may occur from I.M. administration.

Adverse Reactions

Cardiovascular: Ischemic disorder

Central nervous system: Fatigue, headache

Endocrine & metabolic: Hot flushes

Gastrointestinal: Anorexia, constipation, nausea, vomiting, weight gain

Genitourinary: Urinary tract infection

Hepatic: Alkaline phosphatase increased, transaminases increased

Local: Injection site pain

Neuromuscular & skeletal: Arthralgia, back pain, bone pain, extremity pain, joint disorders, musculoskeletal pain, weakness

Respiratory: Cough, dyspnea

Rare but important or life-threatening (reported with 250 mg or 500 mg dose): Angioedema, hepatitis, hypersensitivity reactions, leukopenia, liver failure, osteoporosis, thrombosis, vaginal bleeding

Drug Interactions

Metabolism/Transport Effects Substrate of CYP3A4 (minor); **Note:** Assignment of Major/Minor substrate status based on clinically relevant drug interaction potential

Avoid Concomitant Use There are no known interactions where it is recommended to avoid concomitant use.

Increased Effect/Toxicity There are no known significant interactions involving an increase in effect.

Decreased Effect There are no known significant interactions involving a decrease in effect.

Stability Hazardous agent; use appropriate precautions for handling and disposal (NIOSH, 2012). Store in original carton at 2°C to 8°C (36°F to 46°F); protect from light.

Mechanism of Action Estrogen receptor antagonist; competitively binds to estrogen receptors on tumors and other tissue targets, producing a nuclear complex that causes a dose-related down-regulation of estrogen receptors and inhibits tumor growth.

Pharmacodynamics Duration: I.M.: Steady state concentrations reached within first month, when administered with additional dose given 2 weeks following the initial dose; plasma levels maintained for at least 1 month

Pharmacokinetics (Adult data unless noted)

Distribution: V_d: ~3-5 L/kg

Protein binding: 99%; to plasma proteins (VLDL, LDL, and HDL lipoprotein fractions)

Metabolism: Hepatic via multiple biotransformation pathways (CYP3A4 substrate involved in oxidation pathway, although relative contribution to metabolism unknown); metabolites formed are either less active or have similar activity to parent compound

Half-life:

Children 1-10 years: 70.4 days (Sims, 2012)

Adults: 250 mg: ~40 days

Excretion: Feces (~90%); urine (<1%)

Clearance: Children 1-8 years: Decreased by 32% compared to adults

Dosing: Usual

Children 1-10 years: **McCune-Albright Syndrome; progressive precocious puberty:** Limited data available: I.M.: 4 mg/kg once monthly; dosing based on a trial in 30 girls ≤10 years of age (range: 1-8.5 years) who received monthly injections for 1 year; significant decrease in vaginal bleeding and reduction in rates of skeletal maturation were reported; further studies are needed (Sims, 2012)

Adults: **Breast cancer, metastatic (postmenopausal women):** I.M.: Initial: 500 mg on days 1, 15, and 29; Maintenance: 500 mg once monthly

Dosage adjustment in renal impairment: Adults:

CrCl ≥30 mL/minute: No dosage adjustment required.

CrCl <30 mL/minute: No dosage adjustment provided in manufacturer's labeling (has not been studied); however, renal elimination of fulvestrant is negligible.

Dosage adjustment in hepatic impairment: Adults:

Mild impairment (Child-Pugh class A): No dosage adjustment required.

Moderate impairment (Child-Pugh class B): Decrease initial and maintenance doses to 250 mg.

Severe impairment (Child-Pugh class C): Use has not been evaluated.

Administration Hazardous agent; use appropriate precautions for handling and disposal (NIOSH, 2012). **For I.M. administration only; do not administer I.V., SubQ, or intra-arterially.** In adults, administer 500 mg dose as two 5 mL injections (one in each buttock) slowly over 1-2 minutes per injection; depending upon final dose volume, pediatric patients may be able to receive entire dose as one injection.

Monitoring Parameters McCune-Albright syndrome: In the pediatric clinical trial (study duration: 12 months), the following were monitored: Serum estradiol, testosterone, LH, and FSH (baseline, and at 3, 6, 12 months of therapy); liver function test (baseline and at 12 months of therapy); CBC and INR at baseline; assessments of puberty status and growth at baseline and periodically during therapy [6 and 12 months: Height, weight, Tanner stage, bone age (radiographs), vaginal bleeding data, and pelvic ultrasounds] (Sims, 2012)

Dosage Forms Excipient information presented when available (limited, particularly for generics); consult specific product labeling.

Solution, Intramuscular:

Faslodex: 250 mg/5 mL (5 mL) [contains alcohol, usp, benzyl alcohol, benzyl benzoate]

References

National Institute for Occupational Safety and Health (NIOSH), "NIOSH List of Antineoplastic and Other Hazardous Drugs in Healthcare Settings 2012." Available at http://www.cdc.gov/niosh/docs/2012-150/pdfs/2012-150.pdf. Accessed January 21, 2013.

Sims EK, Garnett S, Guzman F, et al, "Fulvestrant Treatment of Precocious Puberty in Girls With McCune-Albright Syndrome," *Int J Pediatr Endocrinol*, 2012, 2012(1):26.

◆ **Fungi-Guard [OTC]** *see* Tolnaftate *on page 2044*

◆ **Fungi-Nail® [OTC]** *see* Undecylenic Acid and Derivatives *on page 2095*

◆ **Fungizone (Can)** *see* Amphotericin B (Conventional) *on page 147*

◆ **Fungoid-D [OTC]** *see* Tolnaftate *on page 2044*

◆ **Fungoid Tincture [OTC]** *see* Miconazole (Topical) *on page 1410*

◆ **Furadantin** *see* Nitrofurantoin *on page 1502*

◆ **Furazosin** *see* Prazosin *on page 1724*

Furosemide (fyoor OH se mide)

Medication Safety Issues
Sound-alike/look-alike issues:
Furosemide may be confused with famotidine, finasteride, fluconazole, FLUoxetine, fosinopril, loperamide, torsemide

Lasix may be confused with Lanoxin, Lidex, Lomotil, Lovenox, Luvox, Luxiq

International issues:
Lasix [U.S., Canada, and multiple international markets] may be confused with Esidrex brand name for hydrochlorothiazide [multiple international markets]; Esidrix brand name for hydrochlorothiazide [Germany]

Urex [Australia, Hong Kong, Turkey] may be confused with Eurax brand name for crotamiton [U.S., Canada, and multiple international markets]

Brand Names: U.S. Lasix

Brand Names: Canada Apo-Furosemide; AVA-Furosemide; Bio-Furosemide; Dom-Furosemide; Furosemide Injection Sandoz Standard; Furosemide Injection, USP; Furosemide Special; Furosemide Special Injection; Lasix; Lasix Special; Novo-Semide; NTP-Furosemide; Nu-Furosemide; PMS-Furosemide; Teva-Furosemide

Therapeutic Category Antihypertensive Agent; Diuretic, Loop

Generic Availability (U.S.) Yes

Use Management of edema associated with heart failure and hepatic or renal disease; used alone or in combination with antihypertensives in treatment of hypertension

Pregnancy Risk Factor C

Pregnancy Considerations Animal studies have demonstrated maternal death, fetal toxicity, and fetal loss. There are no adequate and well-controlled studies in pregnant women. Crosses the placenta. Increased fetal urine production, electrolyte disturbances reported. Generally, use of diuretics during pregnancy is avoided due to risk of decreased placental perfusion. Monitor fetal growth if used during pregnancy; may increase birth weight.

Breast-Feeding Considerations Crosses into breast milk; may suppress lactation

Contraindications Hypersensitivity to furosemide or any component of the formulation; anuria

Warnings Loop diuretics are potent diuretics; excess amounts can lead to profound diuresis with fluid and electrolyte loss **[U.S. Boxed Warning]**; monitor for and correct electrolyte disturbances; adjust dose to avoid dehydration. Potassium supplementation and/or use of potassium-sparing diuretics may be necessary to prevent hypokalemia. Monitor fluid status and renal function in an attempt to prevent oliguria, azotemia, and reversible increases in BUN and creatinine; close medical supervision of aggressive diuresis required. Coadministration of antihypertensives may increase the risk of hypotension.

Ototoxicity has been demonstrated following administration of furosemide and other loop diuretics. Other possible

risk factors may include use in renal impairment, excessive doses, rapid injection, and concurrent use of other ototoxins (eg, aminoglycosides).

Oral solution may contain propylene glycol; toxicities have been reported with use of products containing propylene glycol, including hyperosmolality, lactic acidosis, seizures, and respiratory depression; in neonates large amounts of propylene glycol delivered orally, intravenously (eg, >3000 mg/day), or topically have been associated with potentially fatal toxicities which can include metabolic acidosis, seizures, renal failure, and CNS depression; use oral solution containing propylene glycol with caution (AAP, 1997; Shehab, 2009).

Precautions Use with caution in patients with cirrhosis; avoid sudden changes in fluid and electrolyte balance and acid/base status which may lead to hepatic encephalopathy. Administration with an aldosterone antagonist or potassium-sparing diuretic may provide additional diuretic efficacy and maintain normokalemia. Chemical similarities are present among sulfonamides, sulfonylureas, carbonic anhydrase inhibitors, thiazides, and loop diuretics (except ethacrynic acid). Use in patients with sulfonylurea allergy is specifically contraindicated in product labeling; a risk of cross-reaction exists in patients with allergy to any of these compounds; avoid use when previous reaction has been severe. Discontinue if signs of hypersensitivity are noted. Oral solution may contain sorbital which can cause diarrhea.

Adverse Reactions

Cardiovascular: Acute hypotension, chronic aortitis, necrotizing angiitis, orthostatic hypotension, vasculitis

Central nervous system: Dizziness, fever, headache, hepatic encephalopathy, lightheadedness, restlessness, vertigo

Dermatologic: Bullous pemphigoid, cutaneous vasculitis, drug rash with eosinophilia and systemic symptoms (DRESS), erythema multiforme, exanthematous pustulosis (generalized), exfoliative dermatitis, photosensitivity, pruritus, purpura, rash, Stevens-Johnson syndrome, toxic epidermal necrolysis, urticaria

Endocrine & metabolic: Cholesterol and triglycerides increased, glucose tolerance test altered, gout, hyperglycemia, hyperuricemia, hypocalcemia, hypochloremia, hypokalemia, hypomagnesemia, hyponatremia, metabolic alkalosis

Gastrointestinal: Anorexia, constipation, cramping, diarrhea, nausea, oral and gastric irritation, pancreatitis, vomiting

Genitourinary: Urinary bladder spasm, urinary frequency

Hematological: Agranulocytosis (rare), anemia, aplastic anemia (rare), eosinophilia, hemolytic anemia, leukopenia, thrombocytopenia

Hepatic: Intrahepatic cholestatic jaundice, ischemic hepatitis, liver enzymes increased

Local: Injection site pain (following I.M. injection), thrombophlebitis

Neuromuscular & skeletal: Muscle spasm, paresthesia, weakness

Ocular: Blurred vision, xanthopsia

Otic: Hearing impairment (reversible or permanent with rapid I.V. or I.M. administration), tinnitus

Renal: Allergic interstitial nephritis, fall in glomerular filtration rate and renal blood flow (due to overdiuresis), glycosuria, transient rise in BUN

Miscellaneous: Anaphylaxis (rare), exacerbate or activate systemic lupus erythematosus

Drug Interactions

Metabolism/Transport Effects None known.

Avoid Concomitant Use

Avoid concomitant use of Furosemide with any of the following: Chloral Hydrate; Ethacrynic Acid

Increased Effect/Toxicity

Furosemide may increase the levels/effects of: ACE Inhibitors; Allopurinol; Amifostine; Aminoglycosides; Antihypertensives; Cardiac Glycosides; Chloral Hydrate; CISplatin; Dofetilide; DULoxetine; Ethacrynic Acid; Hypotensive Agents; Ivabradine; Lithium; Methotrexate; Neuromuscular-Blocking Agents; Obinutuzumab; RisperiDONE; RiTUXimab; Salicylates; Sodium Phosphates; Topiramate

The levels/effects of Furosemide may be increased by: Alfuzosin; Analgesics (Opioid); Barbiturates; Beta2-Agonists; Brimonidine (Topical); Canagliflozin; Corticosteroids (Orally Inhaled); Corticosteroids (Systemic); CycloSPORINE (Systemic); Diazoxide; Herbs (Hypotensive Properties); Licorice; MAO Inhibitors; Methotrexate; Pentoxifylline; Phosphodiesterase 5 Inhibitors; Probenecid; Prostacyclin Analogues

Decreased Effect

Furosemide may decrease the levels/effects of: Hypoglycemic Agents; Lithium; Neuromuscular-Blocking Agents

The levels/effects of Furosemide may be decreased by: Aliskiren; Bile Acid Sequestrants; Fosphenytoin; Herbs (Hypertensive Properties); Methotrexate; Methylphenidate; Nonsteroidal Anti-Inflammatory Agents; Phenytoin; Probenecid; Salicylates; Sucralfate; Yohimbine

Food Interactions Furosemide serum levels may be decreased if taken with food. Management: Administer on an empty stomach.

Stability Furosemide injection should be stored at controlled room temperature and protected from light; exposure to light may cause discoloration; do not use furosemide solutions if they have a yellow color; refrigeration may result in precipitation or crystallization, however, resolubilization at room temperature or warming may be performed without affecting the stability; furosemide solutions are unstable in acidic media but very stable in basic media; I.V. infusion solution mixed in NS or D_5W solution is stable for 24 hours at room temperature

Tablets: Store at 25°C (77°F); excursions permitted to 15°C to 30°C (59°F to 89°F)

Mechanism of Action Inhibits reabsorption of sodium and chloride in the ascending loop of Henle and distal renal tubule, interfering with the chloride-binding cotransport system, thus causing increased excretion of water, sodium, chloride, magnesium, and calcium

Pharmacodynamics

Onset of action:
Oral: Within 30-60 minutes
I.M.: 30 minutes
I.V.: 5 minutes
Maximum effect: Oral: Within 1-2 hours
Duration:
Oral: 6-8 hours
I.V.: 2 hours

Pharmacokinetics (Adult data unless noted)

Absorption: 65% in patients with normal renal function, decreases to 45% in patients with renal failure
Protein binding: 98%
Half-life: Adults:
Normal renal function: 30 minutes
Renal failure: 9 hours
Elimination: 50% of oral dose and 80% of I.V. dose excreted unchanged in the urine within 24 hours; the remainder is eliminated by other nonrenal pathways including liver metabolism and excretion of unchanged drug in feces

Dosing: Neonatal

Edema:
Oral: Doses of 1 mg/kg/dose 1-2 times/day have been used

I.M., I.V.: **Note:** Significant absorption within ECMO circuit; avoid administration directly into circuit; high doses may be required for adequate diuretic effect (Buck, 2003):
GA <31 weeks: 1 mg/kg/dose every 24 hours; accumulation and increased risk of toxicity may be observed with doses >2 mg/kg or doses of 1 mg/kg given more frequently than every 24 hours (Mirochnick, 1988)
GA ≥31 weeks: 1-2 mg/kg/dose every 12-24 hours
Continuous I.V. infusion: 0.2 mg/kg/hour, increase in 0.1 mg/kg/hour increments every 12-24 hours to a maximum infusion rate of 0.4 mg/kg/hour (Luciani, 1997; Schoemaker, 2002)
Pulmonary edema: Inhalation: 1-2 mg/kg/dose diluted in 2 mL NS as a single dose (Brion, 2009)

Dosing: Usual

Infants and Children:
Oral: 2 mg/kg once daily; if ineffective, may increase in increments of 1-2 mg/kg/dose every 6-8 hours; not to exceed 6 mg/kg/dose. In most cases, it is not necessary to exceed individual doses of 4 mg/kg or a dosing frequency of once or twice daily
I.M., I.V.: 1-2 mg/kg/dose every 6-12 hours
Continuous infusion: 0.05 mg/kg/hour; titrate dosage to clinical effect
Adults:
Edema, heart failure:
Oral: Initial: 20-80 mg/dose with the same dose repeated or increased in increments of 20-40 mg/dose at intervals of 6-8 hours; usual maintenance dose interval is once or twice daily; may be titrated up to 600 mg/day with severe edematous states. **Note:** May also be given on 2-4 consecutive days every week
I.M., I.V.: 20-40 mg/dose; repeat in 1-2 hours as needed and increase by 20 mg/dose until the desired effect has been obtained; usual dosing interval: 6-12 hours
Continuous I.V. infusion: Initial I.V. bolus dose of 20-40 mg over 1-2 minutes, followed by continuous I.V. infusion doses of 10-40 mg/hour. If urine output is <1 mL/kg/hour, increase as necessary to a maximum of 80-160 mg/hour. The risk associated with higher infusion rates (80-160 mg/hour) must be weighed against alternative strategies. **Note:** ACC/AHA 2005 guidelines for chronic HF recommend 40 mg I.V. dose followed by 10-40 mg/hour infusion.
Acute pulmonary edema: I.V.: 40 mg over 1-2 minutes; if response not adequate within 1 hour, may increase dose to 80 mg; **Note:** ACC/AHA 2005 guidelines for chronic HF recommend a maximum single dose of 160-200 mg.
Hypertension, resistant (JNC 7): Oral: 20-80 mg/day in 2 divided doses
Refractory CHF: Oral, I.V.: Doses up to 8 g/day have been used

Dosing adjustment in renal impairment: Adults: Acute renal failure: High doses (up to 1-3 g/day - oral/I.V.) have been used to initiate desired response; avoid use in oliguric states
Dialysis: Not removed by hemo- or peritoneal dialysis; supplemental dose is not necessary

Dosing adjustment in hepatic disease: Diminished natriuretic effect with increased sensitivity to hypokalemia and volume depletion in cirrhosis; monitor effects, particularly with high doses

Usual Infusion Concentrations: Neonatal I.V. infusion: 2 mg/mL **or** undiluted as 10 mg/mL
Usual Infusion Concentrations: Pediatric I.V. infusion: 1 mg/mL **or** 2 mg/mL **or** undiluted as 10 mg/mL

Administration

Oral: May administer with food or milk to decrease GI distress
Parenteral: I.V.: May be administered undiluted direct I.V. at a maximum rate of 0.5 mg/kg/minute (not to exceed

4 mg/minute); may also be diluted for infusion 1-2 mg/mL (maximum concentration: 10 mg/mL) over 10-15 minutes (following maximum rate as above); in adults, 20-40 mg undiluted solution may be administered over 1-2 minutes

Monitoring Parameters Serum electrolytes, renal function, blood pressure, hearing (if high dosages used)

Additional Information Single dose studies utilizing nebulized furosemide at 1-2 mg/kg/dose (diluted to a final volume of 2 mL with NS) have been shown to be effective in improving pulmonary function in preterm infants with bronchopulmonary dysplasia undergoing mechanical ventilation; no diuresis or systemic side effects were noted

Dosage Forms Excipient information presented when available (limited, particularly for generics); consult specific product labeling.

Solution, Injection:
Generic: 10 mg/mL (2 mL, 4 mL, 10 mL)
Solution, Injection [preservative free]:
Generic: 10 mg/mL (2 mL, 4 mL, 10 mL)
Solution, Oral:
Generic: 8 mg/mL (5 mL, 500 mL); 10 mg/mL (60 mL, 120 mL)
Tablet, Oral:
Lasix: 20 mg
Lasix: 40 mg, 80 mg [scored]
Generic: 20 mg, 40 mg, 80 mg

References

American Academy of Pediatrics Committee on Drugs. "Inactive" ingredients in pharmaceutical products: update (subject review). Pediatrics. 1997;99(2):268-278.

Aufricht C, Votava F, Marx M, et al, "Intratracheal Furosemide in Infants After Cardiac Surgery: Its Effects on Lung Mechanics and Urinary Output, and Its Levels in Plasma and Tracheal Aspirate," Intensive Care Med, 1997, 23(9):992-7.

Brion LP, Primhak RA, and Yong W, "Aerosolized Diuretics for Preterm Infants With (or Developing) Chronic Lung Disease," Cochrane Database Syst Rev, 2006, 3:CD001694.

Buck ML, "Pharmacokinetic Changes During Extracorporeal Membrane Oxygenation: Implications for Drug Therapy of Neonates," Clin Pharmacokinet, 2003, 42(5):403-17.

Chobanian AV, Bakris GL, Black HR, et al, "The Seventh Report of the Joint National Committee on Prevention, Detection, Evaluation, and Treatment of High Blood Pressure: The JNC 7 Report," JAMA, 2003, 289(19):2560-72.

Copeland JG, Campbell DW, Plachetka JR, et al, "Diuresis With Continuous Infusion of Furosemide After Cardiac Surgery," Am J Surg, 1983, 146(6):796-9.

Engle MA, Lewy JE, Lewy PR, et al, "The Use of Furosemide in the Treatment of Edema in Infants and Children," Pediatrics, 1978, 62 (5):811-8.

Hunt SA, Abraham WT, Chin MH, et al, "ACC/AHA 2005 Guideline Update for the Diagnosis and Management of Chronic Heart Failure in the Adult-Summary Article: A Report of the American College of Cardiology/American Heart Association Task Force on Practice Guidelines (Writing Committee to Update the 2001 Guidelines for the Evaluation and Management of Heart Failure)," J Am Coll Cardiol, 2005, 46(6):1116-43.

Institute for Safe Medication Practices (ISMP), "Standard Concentrations of Neonatal Drug Infusions," ISMP, 2011.

Luciani GB, Nichani S, Chang AC, et al, "Continuous Versus Intermittent Furosemide Infusion in Critically Ill Infants After Open Heart Operations," Ann Thorac Surg, 1997, 64(4):1133-9.

Mirochnick MH, Miceli JJ, Kramer PA, et al, "Furosemide Pharmacokinetics in Very Low Birth Weight Infants," J Pediatr, 1988, 112 (4):653-7.

Pai VB and Nahata MC, "Aerosolized Furosemide in the Treatment of Acute Respiratory Distress and Possible Bronchopulmonary Dysplasia in Preterm Neonates," Ann Pharmacother, 2000, 34(3):386-92.

Prandota J, "Clinical Pharmacology of Furosemide in Children: A Supplement," Am J Ther, 2001, 8(4):275-89.

Rastogi A, Luayon M, Ajayi OA, et al, "Nebulized Furosemide in Infants With Bronchopulmonary Dysplasia," J Pediatr, 1994, 125(6 Pt 1):976-9.

Rudy DW, Voelker JR, Greene PK, et al, "Loop Diuretics for Chronic Renal Insufficiency: A Continuous Infusion Is More Efficacious Than Bolus Therapy," Ann Intern Med, 1991, 115(5):360-6.

Schoemaker RC, van dDer Vorst MM, van Heel IR, et al, "Development of an Optimal Furosemide Infusion Strategy in Infants With Modeling and Simulation," Clin Pharmacol Ther, 2002, 72(4):383-90.

Shehab N, Lewis CL, Streetman DD, Donn SM. Exposure to the pharmaceutical excipients benzyl alcohol and propylene glycol

among critically ill neonates. Pediatr Crit Care Med. 2009;10 (2):256-259.

♦ **Furosemide Injection Sandoz Standard (Can)** see Furosemide on page 948

♦ **Furosemide Injection, USP (Can)** see Furosemide on page 948

♦ **Furosemide Special (Can)** see Furosemide on page 948

♦ **Furosemide Special Injection (Can)** see Furosemide on page 948

♦ **Fuzeon** see Enfuvirtide on page 750

♦ **Fuzeon® (Can)** see Enfuvirtide on page 750

♦ **FVIII/vWF** see Antihemophilic Factor/von Willebrand Factor Complex (Human) on page 177

♦ **FXT 40 (Can)** see FLUoxetine on page 901

♦ **GAA** see Alglucosidase Alfa on page 95

Gabapentin (GA ba pen tin)

Medication Safety Issues
Sound-alike/look-alike issues:
Neurontin may be confused with Motrin, Neoral, nitrofurantoin, Noroxin, Zarontin

Related Information
Oral Medications That Should Not Be Crushed or Altered on page 2438

Brand Names: U.S. Gralise; Gralise Starter; Neurontin

Brand Names: Canada Apo-Gabapentin; Auro-Gabapentin; CO Gabapentin; Dom-Gabapentin; Gabapentin Tablets USP; GD-Gabapentin; JAMP-Gabapentin; Mylan-Gabapentin; Neurontin; PHL-Gabapentin; PMS-Gabapentin; PRO-Gabapentin; RAN-Gabapentin; ratio-Gabapentin; Riva-Gabapentin; Teva-Gabapentin

Therapeutic Category Anticonvulsant, Miscellaneous

Generic Availability (U.S.) May be product dependent

Use Adjunct for treatment of partial seizures with or without secondary generalized seizures (Neurontin®: FDA approved in ages >12 years and adults); adjunct for treatment of partial seizures (Neurontin®: FDA approved in ages 3-12 years); management of post-herpetic neuralgia (Gralise™, Neurontin®: FDA approved in adults); also used as adjunct in the treatment of neuropathic pain

Medication Guide Available Yes

Pregnancy Risk Factor C

Pregnancy Considerations Adverse events have been observed in animal reproduction studies. Gabapentin crosses the placenta. In a small study (n=6), the umbilical/maternal plasma concentration ratio was ~1.74. Neonatal concentrations declined quickly after delivery and at 24 hours of life were ~27% of the cord blood concentrations at birth (gabapentin neonatal half-life ~14 hours) (Ohman, 2005). Outcome data following maternal use of gabapentin during pregnancy is limited (Holmes, 2012).

Patients exposed to gabapentin during pregnancy are encouraged to enroll in the North American Antiepileptic Drug (NAAED) Pregnancy Registry by calling 1-888-233-2334. Additional information is available at www.aedpregnancyregistry.org.

Breast-Feeding Considerations Gabapentin is excreted in human breast milk. Per the manufacturer, a nursed infant could be exposed to ~1 mg/kg/day of gabapentin; the effect on the child is not known. Use in breast-feeding women only if the benefits to the mother outweigh the potential risk to the infant.

In a small study of breast-feeding women (n=6), the estimated exposure of gabapentin to the nursing infants was ~1% to 4% of the weight-adjusted maternal dose (sampling occurred from 12-97 days after delivery and maternal doses ranged from 600-2100 mg daily). Gabapentin was detected in the serum of 2 nursing infants 2-3 weeks after delivery and in 1 infant after 3 months of breast-feeding. Serum concentrations were <12% of the maternal plasma concentrations and <5% of those measured in the umbilical cord. Adverse events were not reported in the breast-fed infants (Ohman, 2005).

Contraindications Hypersensitivity to gabapentin or any component

Warnings Neuropsychiatric adverse events, such as emotional lability (eg, behavioral problems), hostility, aggressive behaviors, thought disorder (eg, problems with concentration and school performance) and hyperkinesia (eg, hyperactivity and restlessness), have been reported in pediatric patients. Most of these pediatric neuropsychiatric adverse events are mild to moderate in terms of intensity but discontinuation of gabapentin may be required; children with mental retardation and attention deficit disorders may be at increased risk for behavioral side effects. Anticonvulsants should not be discontinued abruptly because of the possibility of increasing seizure frequency or precipitating status epilepticus; therapy should be withdrawn gradually over at least 1 week, unless safety concerns require a more rapid withdrawal.

Potentially serious, sometimes fatal, multiorgan hypersensitivity [also known as drug reaction with eosinophilia and systemic symptoms (DRESS)] has been reported with some antiepileptic drugs, including gabapentin. Monitor for signs and symptoms of possible disparate manifestations associated with lymphatic, hepatic, renal, cardiac, and/or hematologic systems; fever, rash, and eosinophilia may also be present. Discontinue immediately if suspected. Gabapentin may cause CNS depression, which may impair physical or mental abilities; patients must be cautioned about performing tasks which require mental alertness (eg, operating machinery or driving).

Antiepileptic drugs (AEDs) increase the risk of suicidal behavior and ideation in patients receiving these medications for any indication. Pooled analyses of placebo-controlled trials involving 11 different AEDs (regardless of indication) showed a twofold increased risk of suicidal thoughts or behavior (estimated incidence rate: 0.43% in AED treated patients compared to 0.24% of patients receiving placebo); increased risk was observed as early as 1 week after initiation of AED and continued through duration of trials (most trials ≤24 weeks); risk did not vary significantly by age (age range: 5-100 years). Consider risks and benefits of AEDs before prescribing. Monitor all patients receiving an AED for emergence of suicidal thoughts or behavior, thoughts of self-harm, any unusual changes in behavior or mood, or the emergence or worsening of depressive symptoms; notify healthcare provider immediately if symptoms or concerning behavior occur. **Note:** The FDA requires a Medication Guide for all antiepileptic drugs informing patients of this risk.

The safety and efficacy of extended release gabapentin (Gralise™) has not been studied in patients with epilepsy. **Precautions** Use with caution in patients with severe renal dysfunction; dose adjustment is required. Male rat studies demonstrated an association with pancreatic acinar adenocarcinoma; the clinical significance in humans is unknown.

Gabapentin immediate release (Neurontin®) and extended release (Gralise™) products are not interchangeable with each other or with gabapentin enacarbil (Horizant™) due to differences in formulations, indications, and pharmacokinetics.

Adverse Reactions

Cardiovascular: Peripheral edema, vasodilatation
Central nervous system: Abnormal gait, abnormality in thinking, amnesia, ataxia, depression, dizziness (more common in adults), drowsiness (more common in adults), emotional lability (children), fatigue (more common in adults), headache, hostility (children), hyperesthesia, hyperkinesia (children), lethargy, nervousness, pain, tremor, twitching, vertigo
Dermatologic: Pruritus, skin rash
Endocrine & metabolic: Hyperglycemia, weight gain
Gastrointestinal: Abdominal pain, constipation, dental disease, diarrhea, dry throat, dyspepsia, flatulence, increased appetite, nausea and vomiting (more common in children), xerostomia
Genitourinary: Impotence, urinary tract infection
Hematologic & oncologic: Decreased white blood cell count, leukopenia
Infection: Infection, viral infection (children)
Neuromuscular & skeletal: Back pain, bone fracture, dysarthria, limb pain, myalgia, weakness
Ophthalmic: Blurred vision, conjunctivitis, diplopia, nystagmus
Otic: Otitis media
Respiratory: Bronchitis (children), cough, nasopharyngitis, pharyngitis, respiratory tract infection (children), rhinitis
Miscellaneous: Fever (children)
Rare but important or life-threatening: Acute renal failure, altered serum glucose, anemia, angina pectoris, angioedema, aphasia, aspiration pneumonia, blindness, blood coagulation disorder, bradycardia, brain disease, breast hypertrophy, cardiac arrhythmia (various), cardiac failure, cerebrovascular accident, CNS neoplasm, colitis, confusion, Cushingoid appearance, DRESS syndrome, drug abuse, drug dependence, erythema multiforme, facial paralysis, fecal incontinence, gastroenteritis, glaucoma, glycosuria, hearing loss, heart block, hematemesis, hematuria, hemiplegia, hemorrhage, hepatitis, hepatomegaly, herpes zoster, hyperlipidemia, hypertension, hyperthyroidism, hyperventilation, hyponatremia, hypotension, hypothyroidism, hypoventilation, increased creatine phosphokinase, increased liver enzymes, increased serum creatinine, jaundice, joint swelling, leukocytosis, lymphadenopathy, lymphocytosis, memory impairment, meningism, migraine, movement disorder, myocardial infarction, myoclonus (local), nephrolithiasis, nephrosis, nerve palsy, non-Hodgkin's lymphoma, ovarian failure, pancreatitis, peptic ulcer, pericardial effusion, pericardial rub, pericarditis, peripheral vascular disease, pneumonia, psychosis, pulmonary thromboembolism, purpura, retinopathy, rhabdomyolysis, seasonal allergy, skin necrosis, status epilepticus, Stevens-Johnson syndrome, subdural hematoma, suicidal ideation, suicidal tendencies, syncope, tachycardia, thrombocytopenia, thrombophlebitis, tumor growth, withdrawal syndrome

Drug Interactions

Metabolism/Transport Effects None known.

Avoid Concomitant Use

Avoid concomitant use of Gabapentin with any of the following: Azelastine (Nasal); Paraldehyde; Thalidomide

Increased Effect/Toxicity

Gabapentin may increase the levels/effects of: Alcohol (Ethyl); Azelastine (Nasal); Buprenorphine; CNS Depressants; Hydrocodone; Methotrimeprazine; Metyrosine; Mirtazapine; Paraldehyde; Pramipexole; ROPINIRole; Rotigotine; Selective Serotonin Reuptake Inhibitors; Thalidomide; Zolpidem

The levels/effects of Gabapentin may be increased by: Brimonidine (Topical); Cannabis; Doxylamine; Dronabinol; Droperidol; HydrOXYzine; Kava Kava; Magnesium Salts; Methotrimeprazine; Nabilone; Perampanel; Rufinamide; Sodium Oxybate; Tapentadol; Tetrahydrocannabinol

Decreased Effect

The levels/effects of Gabapentin may be decreased by:
Antacids; Ketorolac (Nasal); Ketorolac (Systemic); Magnesium Salts; Mefloquine; Orlistat

Food Interactions Tablet, solution (immediate release): No significant effect on rate or extent of absorption; tablet (extended release): Increases rate and extent of absorption. Management: Administer immediate release products without regard to food. Administer extended release products with food.

Stability

Capsules and tablets: Store at 25°C (77°F); excursions permitted to 15°C to 30°C (59°F to 86°F).
Oral solution: Store at 2°C to 8°C (36°F to 46°F).

Mechanism of Action Gabapentin is structurally related to GABA. However, it does not bind to GABA$_A$ or GABA$_B$ receptors, and it does not appear to influence synthesis or uptake of GABA. High affinity gabapentin binding sites have been located throughout the brain; these sites correspond to the presence of voltage-gated calcium channels specifically possessing the alpha-2-delta-1 subunit. This channel appears to be located presynaptically, and may modulate the release of excitatory neurotransmitters which participate in epileptogenesis and nociception.

Pharmacokinetics (Adult data unless noted)

Absorption: Variable, from proximal small bowel by L-amino transport system; saturable process; dose-dependent
Distribution: V$_d$: 58 ± 6 L; CSF concentrations are ~20% of plasma concentrations
Protein binding: <3% (not clinically significant)
Metabolism: Not metabolized
Bioavailability:
Immediate release: ~60% (300 mg dose given 3 times/day); bioavailability decreases with increasing doses; bioavailability is 27% with 1600 mg dose given 3 times/day
Extended release: Variable; increased with higher fat content meal
Time to peak serum concentration:
Immediate release:
Infants 1 month to Children 12 years: 2-3 hours
Adults: 2-4 hours
Extended release: 8 hours
Half-life, elimination:
Infants 1 month to Children 12 years: 4.7 hours
Adults, normal: 5-7 hours; increased half-life with decreased renal function; anuric adult patients: 132 hours; adults during hemodialysis: 3.8 hours
Elimination: Excreted unchanged in the urine (75% to 80%) and feces (10% to 20%)
Clearance: **Note:** Apparent oral clearance is directly proportional to CrCl: Clearance in infants is highly variable; oral clearance (per kg) in children <5 years of age is higher than in children ≥5 years of age

Dosing: Usual Note: Do not exceed 12 hours between doses with 3 times daily dosing:
Children and Adolescents:
Seizures, adjunctive treatment: Immediate release: Oral: **Note:** If gabapentin is discontinued or if another anticonvulsant is added to therapy, it should be done slowly over a minimum of 1 week.
Children 3-12 years:
Initial: 10-15 mg/kg/**day** divided into 3 doses daily; titrate dose upward over ~3 days
Maintenance usual dose:
Children 3-4 years: 40 mg/kg/**day** divided into 3 doses daily
Children ≥5 to12 years: 25-35 mg/kg/**day** divided into 3 doses daily
Note: Doses up to 50 mg/kg/**day** were well-tolerated in one long-term study.

Adolescents: Initial: 300 mg 3 times daily; titrate dose upward if needed; usual maintenance dose: 900-1800 mg/day divided into 3 doses daily; doses up to 2400 mg/day divided into 3 doses daily are well tolerated long-term; maximum daily dose: 3600 mg/**day**
Neuropathic pain: Limited data available: Immediate release: Oral: Children and Adolescents: Initial: 5 mg/kg/dose up to 300 mg at bedtime; day 2: Increase to 5 mg/kg/dose twice daily (up to 300 mg twice daily); day 3: Increase to 5 mg/kg/dose 3 times daily (up to 300 mg 3 times daily); further titrate with dosage increases (not frequency) to effect; American Pain Society (APS) recommends a lower initial dose of 2 mg/kg/**day** which may be considered if concurrent analgesics are also sedating; usual dosage range: 8-35 mg/kg/**day** divided into 3 doses daily (APS, 2008; Galloway, 2000); maximum daily dose: 3600 mg/**day**
Adults:
Anticonvulsant: Oral: Immediate release:
Initial: 300 mg 3 times daily; if necessary the dose may be gradually increased up to 1800 mg/**day**
Maintenance: 900-1800 mg/**day** administered in 3 divided doses; doses of up to 2400 mg/**day** have been tolerated in long-term clinical studies; doses up to 3600 mg/**day** have been tolerated in short-term studies
Note: If gabapentin is discontinued or if another anticonvulsant is added to therapy, it should be done slowly over a minimum of 1 week.
Post-herpetic neuralgia: Oral:
Immediate release: Day 1: 300 mg once; day 2: 300 mg twice daily; Day 3: 300 mg 3 times daily; titrate dose as needed for pain relief (range: 1800-3600 mg/**day** in divided doses; doses >1800 mg/**day** do not generally show greater benefit)
Extended release (Gralise™): Day 1: 300 mg once daily, Day 2: 600 mg once daily, Days 3-6: 900 mg once daily, Days 7-10: 1200 mg once daily, Days 11-14: 1500 mg once daily, Days ≥15: 1800 mg once daily

Dosing adjustment in renal impairment
Immediate release:
Children <12 years: There are no dosing adjustments provided in the manufacturer's labeling (has not been studied).
Children ≥12 years, Adolescents, and Adults: See table.

Gabapentin Dosing Adjustments in Renal Impairment

Creatinine Clearance (mL/min)	Total Daily Dose Range (mg/day)	Dosage Regimens (Maintenance Doses) (mg)				
≥60	900-3600	300 3 times/day	400 3 times/day	600 3 times/day	800 3 times/day	1200 tid
>30-59	400-1400	200 twice daily	300 twice daily	400 twice daily	500 twice daily	700 twice daily
>15-29	200-700	200 daily	300 daily	400 daily	500 daily	700 daily
15[1]	100-300	100 daily	125 daily	150 daily	200 daily	300 daily
Hemodialysis[2]		Posthemodialysis Supplemental Dose				
		125 mg	150 mg	200 mg	250 mg	350 mg

[1]CrCl <15 mL/minute: Reduce daily dose in proportion to creatinine clearance.

[2]Supplemental dose should be administered after each 4 hours of hemodialysis (patients on hemodialysis should also receive maintenance doses based on renal function as listed in the upper portion of the table).

Extended release (Gralise®): **Note:** Follow initial dose titration schedule if treatment-naive.

CrCl ≥60 mL/minute: 1800 mg once daily

CrCl >30-59 mL/minute: 600-1800 mg once daily; dependent on tolerability and clinical response

CrCl <30 mL/minute: Use is not recommended.

ESRD requiring hemodialysis: Use is not recommended.

Dosing adjustment in hepatic impairment: There are no dosage adjustments provided in the manufacturer's labeling; however, adjustment not necessary since gabapentin is not hepatically metabolized.

Administration

Immediate release: Capsule, tablet, solution: Administer first dose on first day at bedtime to avoid somnolence and dizziness. May be administered without regard to meals; administration with meals may decrease adverse GI effects; dose may be administered as combination of dosage forms; do not administer within 2 hours of magnesium- or aluminum-containing antacids. When given 3 times daily, the maximum time between doses should not exceed 12 hours. The 600 mg and 800 mg tablets are scored and may be split if a half-tablet is needed; manufacturer recommends that half tablets not used within several days of breaking the scored tablets should be discarded. Contents of capsule may be mixed in drinks (eg, orange juice) or food (eg, applesauce) if necessary (Khurana, 1996).

Extended release: Tablet: Take with evening meal. Swallow whole; do not chew, crush, or split.

Monitoring Parameters Seizure frequency and duration; renal function; weight; behavior in children; signs and symptoms of suicidality (eg, anxiety, depression, behavior changes)

Reference Range Minimum effective serum concentration may be 2 mcg/mL; **routine monitoring of drug levels is not required**

Test Interactions False positives have been reported with the Ames N-Multistix SG® dipstick test for urine protein

Additional Information Gabapentin is not effective for absence seizures; gabapentin does not induce liver enzymes

Dosage Forms Excipient information presented when available (limited, particularly for generics); consult specific product labeling.

Capsule, Oral:

Neurontin: 100 mg, 300 mg, 400 mg

Generic: 100 mg, 300 mg, 400 mg

Miscellaneous, Oral:

Gralise Starter: 300 & 600 mg (78 ea) [contains soybean lecithin]

Solution, Oral:

Neurontin: 250 mg/5 mL (470 mL) [strawberry anise flavor]

Generic: 250 mg/5 mL (5 mL, 6 mL, 470 mL, 473 mL)

Tablet, Oral:

Gralise: 300 mg [contains soybean lecithin]

Gralise: 600 mg

Neurontin: 600 mg, 800 mg [scored]

Generic: 600 mg, 800 mg

Extemporaneous Preparations Note: Commercial oral solution is available (50 mg/mL)

A 100 mg/mL suspension may be made with tablets (immediate release) and either a 1:1 mixture of Ora-Sweet® (100 mL) and Ora-Plus® (100 mL) or 1:1 mixture of methylcellulose 1% (100 mL) and Simple Syrup N.F. (100 mL). Crush sixty-seven 300 mg tablets in a mortar and reduce to a fine powder. Add small portions of the chosen vehicle and mix to a uniform paste; mix while adding the vehicle in incremental proportions to **almost** 200 mL; transfer to a calibrated bottle, rinse mortar with vehicle, and add sufficient quantity of vehicle to make 200 mL.

Label "shake well" and "refrigerate". Stable for 91 days refrigerated (preferred) or 56 days at room temperature.

Nahata MC, Pai VB, and Hipple TF, *Pediatric Drug Formulations*, 5th ed, Cincinnati, OH: Harvey Whitney Books Co, 2004.

References

Andrews CO and Fischer JH, "Gabapentin: A New Agent for the Management of Epilepsy," *Ann Pharmacother*, 1994, 28(10):1188-96.

Galloway KS and Yaster M, "Pain and Symptom Control in Terminally Ill Children," *Pediatr Clin North Am*, 2000, 47(3):711-46.

Holmes LB and Hernandez-Diaz S, "Newer Anticonvulsants: Lamotrigine, Topiramate, and Gabapentin," *Birth Defects Res A Clin Mol Teratol*, 2012, 94(8):599-606.

Khurana DS, Riviello J, Helmers S, et al, "Efficacy of Gabapentin Therapy in Children With Refractory Partial Seizures," *J Pediatr*, 1996, 128(6):829-33.

Laird MA and Gidal BE, "Use of Gabapentin in the Treatment of Neuropathic Pain," *Ann Pharmacother*, 2000, 34(6):802-7.

Lee DO, Steingard RJ, Cesena M, et al, "Behavioral Side Effects of Gabapentin in Children," *Epilepsia*, 1996, 37(1):87-90.

Leiderman D, Garofalo E, and LaMoreaux L, "Gabapentin Patients With Absence Seizures: Two Double-Blind, Placebo Controlled Studies," *Epilepsia*, 1993, 34(Suppl 6):45 (abstract).

Ohman I, Vitols S, and Tomson T, "Pharmacokinetics of Gabapentin During Delivery, in the Neonatal Period, and Lactation: Does a Fetal Accumulation Occur During Pregnancy?" *Epilepsia*, 2005, 46 (10):1621-4.

Pressler KL, Jabbour JT, Rose DF, et al, "Gabapentin and Aggression in Pediatric Patients: A Review of the Literature," *Journal of Pediatric Pharmacy Practice*, 1998, 3(2):100-5.

"Principles of Analgesic Use in the Treatment of Acute Pain and Cancer Pain," 6th ed, Glenview, IL: American Pain Society, 2008.

◆ **Gabapentin Tablets USP (Can)** *see* Gabapentin *on page 950*

◆ **Gabitril** *see* TiaGABine *on page 2020*

◆ **Gablofen** *see* Baclofen *on page 259*

Galsulfase (gal SUL fase)

Brand Names: U.S. Naglazyme

Therapeutic Category Enzyme

Generic Availability (U.S.) No

Use Treatment of mucopolysaccharidosis VI (MPS VI, Maroteaux-Lamy Syndrome) for improvement of walking and stair-climbing capacity [FDA approved in pediatric patients (age not specified) and adults ≤29 years]

Pregnancy Risk Factor B

Pregnancy Considerations Fetal harm was not reported in animal studies. There are no studies in pregnant women. Pregnant women are encouraged to enroll in the Clinical Surveillance Program.

Breast-Feeding Considerations Breast-feeding women are encouraged to enroll in the Clinical Surveillance Program.

Contraindications Hypersensitivity to galsulfase or any component

Warnings Severe hypersensitivity reactions, including anaphylactic reactions and anaphylactic shock, have been reported during and within 24 hours after infusion; immediate treatment for hypersensitivity reactions should be available during administration; discontinue treatment immediately if signs or symptoms occur; use caution with readministration.

Immune-mediated reactions (Type III) have been reported (including membranous glomerulonephritis); monitor patients closely and consider discontinuation of treatment if signs or symptoms occur; use caution with readministration; in some cases rechallenge with treatment has been successful.

Infusion-related reactions including angioneurotic edema, hypotension, dyspnea, bronchospasm, respiratory distress, apnea, urticaria, fever, chills, rigors, headache, rash, nausea, vomiting, increased blood pressure, retrosternal pain, abdominal pain, malaise, and joint pain have been reported and may be severe; reactions may occur as late as week 146 of treatment. Predisposing factors for infusion-related reactions have not been identified. Patients should be premedicated with antihistamines with or without antipyretics 30-60 minutes prior to start of the infusion; evaluate airway prior to therapy (due to possible effects of antihistamine use). Despite pretreatment, infusion-related reactions have been reported in up to 56% of patients (ie, 33 of 59 pretreated patients); and 70% experienced recurrent reactions during multiple infusions although not necessarily consecutive treatments. In case of reaction, decrease the rate of infusion, temporarily discontinue the infusion, and/or administer additional antihistamines, antipyretics, and possibly corticosteroids. In patients who experience an infusion-related reaction, subsequent doses may be managed by using a lower infusion rate. For severe reactions, the risks and benefits of readministering should be evaluated.

Worsening and new-onset spinal/cervical cord compression (SCC) have been reported. Monitor patients for signs and symptoms of SCC (eg, back pain, limb paralysis, urinary and fecal incontinence).

Injection contains polysorbate 80 (Tween 80®) which may cause allergic reactions in susceptible individuals. In premature neonates, thrombocytopenia, ascites, pulmonary deterioration, and renal and hepatic failure have been reported after receiving parenteral products containing polysorbate 80 (Alade, 1986; CDC, 1984). Infusion of polysorbate 80-containing solutions through polyvinyl chloride tubing may cause DEHP to leach into the solution; in immature animals, exposure to DEHP may adversely affect the development of the male reproductive tract.

Precautions Use caution in patients with compromised respiratory function or acute respiratory disease; there may be a higher risk of serious complications from infusion reactions. Use with caution in patients who are at risk of fluid overload; may cause heart failure; patients particularly at risk include those with weight <20 kg, underlying respiratory disease, or compromised cardiopulmonary function; monitor patients closely including prolonged observation times postinfusion. Use with caution in patients with sleep apnea; antihistamine pretreatment may increase the risk of apneic episodes; consider use of nonsedating antihistamine and have apneic treatment options (supplemental oxygen, CPAP) readily available. Consider delaying the galsulfase infusion in patients with febrile illness or with acute respiratory illness.

Adverse Reactions

Cardiovascular: Chest pain, hypertension

Central nervous system: Absent reflexes, chills, headache, malaise, pain

Dermatologic: Pruritus, skin rash, urticaria

Gastrointestinal: Abdominal pain, gastroenteritis, nausea, vomiting

Hypersensitivity: Angioedema

Neuromuscular & skeletal: Areflexia

Ophthalmic: Conjunctivitis, corneal opacity (increased)

Otic: Auditory impairment, otalgia

Respiratory: Apnea, dyspnea, laryngeal edema, nasal congestion, pharyngitis, respiratory distress

Miscellaneous: Antibody development, fever, infusion related reaction, umbilical hernia

Rare but important or life-threatening: Anaphylaxis, bradycardia, bronchospasm, cyanosis, erythema, hypotension, hypoxia, pallor, paresthesia, renal disease (membranous), respiratory failure, shock, spinal cord compression, tachycardia, tachypnea, thrombocytopenia

Drug Interactions

Metabolism/Transport Effects None known.

Avoid Concomitant Use There are no known interactions where it is recommended to avoid concomitant use.

Increased Effect/Toxicity There are no known significant interactions involving an increase in effect.

Decreased Effect There are no known significant interactions involving a decrease in effect.

Stability Store intact vials at 2°C to 8°C (36°F to 46°F); do not shake or freeze; protect from light. Allow vials to reach room temperature prior to dilution; however, do not keep vials at room temperature longer than 24 hours. Following dilution, administer immediately. May store diluted solution under refrigeration; storage after dilution should not exceed 48 hours from the time of preparation to completion of infusion. Room temperature storage of diluted preparation is not recommended except during infusion. Do not infuse with other medication products.

Mechanism of Action Galsulfase is a recombinant form of N-acetylgalactosamine 4-sulfatase, produced in Chinese hamster cells. A deficiency of this enzyme leads to accumulation of the glycosaminoglycan dermatan sulfate in various tissues, causing progressive disease which includes decreased growth, skeletal deformities, upper airway obstruction, clouding of the cornea, heart disease, and coarse facial features. Replacement of this enzyme has been shown to improve mobility and physical function (measured by walking and stair-climbing).

Pharmacokinetics (Adult data unless noted) Note: Data based on mixed patient population of children ≥5 years and adults <29 years.

Half-life elimination: Week 1: Median: 9 minutes (range: 6-21 minutes); Week 24: Median: 26 minutes (range: 8-40 minutes)

Dosing: Usual Note: Premedicate with antihistamines with or without antipyretics 30-60 minutes prior to infusion.

MPS VI:

Infants: Limited data available: I.V: 1 or 2 mg/kg/dose once weekly has been used in four infants (3-12 months); similar safety results to those of older patients were reported

Children, Adolescents, and Adults: I.V.: 1 mg/kg/dose once weekly

Administration Parenteral: I.V.: Without the use of a filter needle, slowly withdraw calculated dose from vial and dilute in NS to a final volume of 250 mL or 100 mL (if patient weight <20 kg or susceptible to volume overload); do not shake. Infuse via an infusion pump and PVC infusion set with in-line, low-protein-binding 0.2 micrometer filter over at least 4 hours. Infuse 250 mL solution at 6 mL/hour for the first hour; if well-tolerated, increase rate to 80 mL/hour for the remaining 3 hours. For 100 mL infusion, use a lower rate to ensure infusion over at least 4 hours. Infusion time may be extended up to 20 hours if infusion reactions occur. If hypersensitivity or infusion-related reaction occurs, discontinue immediately. pH: 5.8

Monitoring Parameters Vital signs; presence of infusion-related reactions (chills, pruritis, urticaria, dyspnea, rash, shortness of breath, nausea, abdominal pain); in clinical studies, tests of mobility and physical function were monitored at baseline and every 6 weeks.

Additional Information In order to better understand MPS VI disease progression and to monitor long-term effects of galsulfase, a voluntary Clinical Surveillance Program has been established. Monitoring also includes the effect of galsulfase on pregnant women and their offspring, and during lactation. For more information, visit www.naglazyme.com/en/clinical-resources/surveillance-program.aspx or call (800) 983-4587.

Dosage Forms Excipient information presented when available (limited, particularly for generics); consult specific product labeling.

Solution, Intravenous [preservative free]:

Naglazyme: 1 mg/mL (5 mL) [contains mouse protein (murine) (hamster), polysorbate 80]

References

Alade SL, Brown RE, and Paquet A Jr, "Polysorbate 80 and E-Ferol Toxicity," Pediatrics, 1986, 77(4):593-7.

Centers for Disease Control (CDC), "Unusual Syndrome With Fatalities Among Premature Infants: Association With a New Intravenous Vitamin E Product," *MMWR Morb Mortal Wkly Rep*, 1984, 33 (14):198-9.

European Medicines Agency, Nalgazyme Product Information. Available at http://www.ema.europa.eu/docs/en_GB/document_library/EPAR_-_Product_Information/human/000640/WC500024289.pdf. Date accessed: May 23, 2012.

Giugliani R, Harmatz P, and Wraith JE, "Management Guidelines for Mucopolysaccharidosis VI," *Pediatrics*, 2007, 120(2):405-18.

Harmatz P, Giugliani R, Schwartz IV, et al, "Long-Term Follow-Up of Endurance and Safety Outcomes During Enzyme Replacement Therapy for Mucopolysaccharidosis VI: Final Results of Three Clinical Studies of Recombinant Human N-Acetylgalactosamine 4-Sulfatase," *Mol Genet Metab*, 2008, 94(4):469-75.

Harmatz P, Ketteridge D, Giugliani R, et al, "Direct Comparison of Measures of Endurance, Mobility, and Joint Function During Enzyme-Replacement Therapy of Mucopolysaccharidosis VI (Maroteaux-Lamy Syndrome): Results After 48 Weeks in a Phase 2 Open-Label Clinical Study of Recombinant Human N-Acetylgalactosamine 4-Sulfatase," *Pediatrics*, 2005, 115(6):e681-9.

Harmatz P, Whitley CB, Waber L, et al, "Enzyme Replacement Therapy in Mucopolysaccharidosis VI (Maroteaux-Lamy Syndrome)," *J Pediatr*, 2004, 144:574-80.

Hendriksz CJ, Giugliani R, Harmatz P, et al, "Design, Baseline Characteristics, and Early Findings of the MPS VI (Mucopolysaccharidosis VI) Clinical Surveillance Program (CSP)," *J Inherit Metab Dis*, 2011.

♦ **Galzin** *see* Zinc Acetate *on page 2174*

♦ **GamaSTAN S/D** *see* Immune Globulin *on page 1084*

♦ **Gamastan S/D (Can)** *see* Immune Globulin *on page 1084*

♦ **Gamma Benzene Hexachloride** *see* Lindane *on page 1250*

♦ **Gammagard** *see* Immune Globulin *on page 1084*

♦ **Gammagard Liquid (Can)** *see* Immune Globulin *on page 1084*

♦ **Gammagard S/D** *see* Immune Globulin *on page 1084*

♦ **Gammagard S/D Less IgA** *see* Immune Globulin *on page 1084*

♦ **Gamma Globulin** *see* Immune Globulin *on page 1084*

♦ **Gammaked** *see* Immune Globulin *on page 1084*

♦ **Gammaphos** *see* Amifostine *on page 116*

♦ **Gammaplex** *see* Immune Globulin *on page 1084*

♦ **Gamunex (Can)** *see* Immune Globulin *on page 1084*

♦ **Gamunex-C** *see* Immune Globulin *on page 1084*

Ganciclovir (Systemic) (gan SYE kloe veer)

Medication Safety Issues
Sound-alike/look-alike issues:
Cytovene® may be confused with Cytosar®, Cytosar-U
Ganciclovir may be confused with acyclovir

Related Information
Safe Handling of Hazardous Drugs *on page 2419*

Brand Names: U.S. Cytovene

Brand Names: Canada Cytovene®

Therapeutic Category Antiviral Agent, Parenteral

Generic Availability (U.S.) Yes

Use Treatment of cytomegalovirus (CMV) retinitis in immunocompromised patients, including patients with AIDS (FDA approved in adults); prevention of CMV disease in transplant recipients at risk for CMV (FDA approved in adults); has also been used in CMV GI infections and pneumonitis; ganciclovir also has antiviral activity against herpes simplex virus types 1 and 2

Pregnancy Risk Factor C

Pregnancy Considerations [U.S. Boxed Warning]: Animal studies have demonstrated carcinogenic and teratogenic effects, and inhibition of spermatogenesis. Female patients should use effective contraception during therapy; male patients should use a barrier contraceptive during and for at least 90 days after therapy.

Breast-Feeding Considerations Due to the carcinogenic and teratogenic effects observed in animal studies, the possibility of adverse events in a nursing infant is considered likely. Therefore, nursing should be discontinued during therapy. In addition, the CDC recommends **not** to breast-feed if diagnosed with HIV to avoid postnatal transmission of the virus.

Contraindications Hypersensitivity to ganciclovir, acyclovir, or any component; absolute neutrophil count <500/mm^3; platelet count <25,000/mm^3

Warnings Hazardous agent; use appropriate precautions for handling and disposal (NIOSH, 2012).

Granulocytopenia (neutropenia), anemia, and thrombocytopenia may occur **[U.S. Boxed Warning]**. Dosage adjustment or interruption of therapy may be necessary in patients with neutropenia, anemia, and/or thrombocytopenia; ganciclovir should not be administered if ANC <500/mm^3 or if platelet count <25,000/mm^3.

Animal studies have demonstrated carcinogenic and teratogenic effects, and inhibition of spermatogenesis **[U.S. Boxed Warning]**; due to its mutagenic potential, contraceptive precautions for female and male patients need to be followed during and for at least 90 days after therapy with the drug; phlebitis may occur at site of infusion; infuse only into veins with adequate blood flow.

Precautions Use with caution in patients with renal impairment. Use with extreme caution in children since long-term safety has not been determined and due to ganciclovir's potential for long-term carcinogenic and adverse reproductive effects.

Adverse Reactions
Central nervous system: Chills, fever, neuropathy
Dermatologic: Pruritus
Gastrointestinal: Anorexia, diarrhea, vomiting
Hematologic: Anemia, leukopenia, neutropenia with ANC <500/mm^3, thrombocytopenia
Ocular: Retinal detachment (relationship to ganciclovir not established)
Renal: Serum creatinine increased
Miscellaneous: Diaphoresis, sepsis
Rare but important or life-threatening: Allergic reaction (including anaphylaxis), alopecia, arrhythmia, bronchospasm, cardiac arrest, cataracts, cholestasis, coma, dyspnea, edema, encephalopathy, exfoliative dermatitis, extrapyramidal symptoms, hepatitis, hepatic failure, pancreatitis, pancytopenia, pulmonary fibrosis, psychosis, rhabdomyolysis, seizure, alopecia, urticaria, eosinophilia, hemorrhage, Stevens-Johnson syndrome, torsade de pointes, renal failure, SIADH, visual loss

Drug Interactions
Metabolism/Transport Effects None known.

Avoid Concomitant Use
Avoid concomitant use of Ganciclovir (Systemic) with any of the following: Imipenem

Increased Effect/Toxicity
Ganciclovir (Systemic) may increase the levels/effects of: Imipenem; Mycophenolate; Reverse Transcriptase Inhibitors (Nucleoside); Tenofovir

The levels/effects of Ganciclovir (Systemic) may be increased by: Mycophenolate; Probenecid; Tenofovir

Decreased Effect There are no known significant interactions involving a decrease in effect.

Stability Hazardous agent; use appropriate precautions for handling and disposal (NIOSH, 2012). Intact vials should be stored at 25°C (77°F); excursions permitted to 15°C to 30°C (59°F to 86°F).

Reconstituted solution is stable for 12 hours at room temperature; do not refrigerate; diluted I.V. ganciclovir solutions in D$_5$W or NS with a concentration ≤10 mg/mL are stable for 28 days under refrigeration; however, the manufacturer recommends use within 24 hours due to SWI reconstitution.

Mechanism of Action Ganciclovir is phosphorylated to a substrate which competitively inhibits the binding of deoxyguanosine triphosphate to DNA polymerase resulting in inhibition of viral DNA synthesis

Pharmacokinetics (Adult data unless noted)

Distribution: Distributes to most body fluids, tissues, and organs, including the eyes and brain

V_d:

Children 9 months to 12 years: 0.64 ± 0.22 L/kg

Adults: 0.74 ± 0.15 L/kg

Protein binding: 1% to 2%

Half-life (prolonged with impaired renal function):

Neonates 2-49 days of age: 2.4 hours

Children 9 months to 12 years: 2.4 ± 0.7 hours

Adults: Mean: 2.5-3.6 hours (range: 1.7-5.8 hours)

Elimination: Majority (80% to 99%) excreted as unchanged drug in the urine

Dialysis: 40% to 50% removed by a 4-hour hemodialysis

Dosing: Neonatal I.V.: **Congenital CMV (symptomatic; CNS-disease); treatment (independent of HIV status):** 6 mg/kg/dose every 12 hours for 6 weeks; if neonate diagnosed as HIV-positive, a longer duration of therapy may be considered (CDC, 2009; Redbook, 2009)

Dosing: Usual I.V.:

CMV infection:

Congenital CMV (symptomatic; CNS-disease); treatment (independent of HIV status): 6 mg/kg/dose every 12 hours for 6 weeks; if neonate diagnosed as HIV-positive a longer duration of therapy may be considered (CDC, 2009; Redbook, 2009)

CNS infection, treatment (HIV-exposed/-positive): Infants and Children: 5 mg/kg/dose every 12 hours plus foscarnet; continue until symptoms improve, followed by chronic suppression (CDC, 2009)

Disseminated disease and retinitis, treatment:

Induction therapy:

Infants ≥3 months and Children: 5 mg/kg/dose every 12 hours for 14-21 days; may be increased to 7.5 mg/kg/dose every 12 hours (CDC, 2009)

Adults: Manufacturer's labeling: 5 mg/kg/dose every 12 hours for 14-21 days

Maintenance therapy:

Infants ≥3 months and Children: 5 mg/kg/dose as a single daily dose for 5-7 days/week (CDC, 2009)

Adults: Manufacturer's labeling: 5 mg/kg/dose as a single daily dose for 7 days/week or 6 mg/kg/dose for 5 days/week

Secondary prevention in HIV-exposed/-infected patients: Infants and Children: 5 mg/kg/dose once daily (CDC, 2009)

Prevention in transplant recipients: Children and Adults: Initial: 5 mg/kg/dose every 12 hours for 1-2 weeks, followed by 5 mg/kg/dose once daily 7 days/week or 6 mg/kg/dose once daily 5 days/week for 100 days

Prevention in lung/heart-lung transplant patients (CMV-positive donor with CMV-positive recipient): Children and Adults: 6 mg/kg/dose once daily for 28 days

Other CMV infections: Children and Adults: Initial: 5 mg/kg/dose every 12 hours for 14-21 days; maintenance therapy: 5 mg/kg/dose once daily for 7 days/week or 6 mg/kg/dose once daily for 5 days/week

Varicella zoster; progressive outer retinal necrosis: Infants, Children, Adolescents, and Adults: 5 mg/kg/dose every 12 hours plus systemic foscarnet and intravitreal ganciclovir or foscarnet (CDC, 2009; Kaplan, 2009)

Dosing interval in renal impairment: Adults:

Induction:

CrCl 50-69 mL/minute: Administer 2.5 mg/kg/dose every 12 hours

CrCl 25-49 mL/minute: Administer 2.5 mg/kg/dose every 24 hours

CrCl 10-24 mL/minute: Administer 1.25 mg/kg/dose every 24 hours

CrCl <10 mL/minute: Administer 1.25 mg/kg/dose 3 times/week following hemodialysis

Maintenance:

CrCl 50-69 mL/minute: Administer 2.5 mg/kg/dose every 24 hours

CrCl 25-49 mL/minute: Administer 1.25 mg/kg/dose every 24 hours

CrCl 10-24 mL/minute: Administer 0.625 mg/kg/dose every 24 hours

CrCl <10 mL/minute: Administer 0.625 mg/kg/dose 3 times/week following hemodialysis

Intermittent hemodialysis (IHD) (administer after hemodialysis on dialysis days): Dialyzable (50%): CMV Infection: I.V.: Induction: 1.25 mg/kg every 48-72 hours; Maintenance: 0.625 mg/kg every 48-72 hours. **Note:** Dosing dependent on the assumption of 3 times/week, complete IHD sessions.

Peritoneal dialysis (PD): Dose as for CrCl <10 mL/minute

Continuous renal replacement therapy (CRRT) (Heintz, 2009; Trotman, 2005): Drug clearance is highly dependent on the method of renal replacement, filter type, and flow rate. Appropriate dosing requires close monitoring of pharmacologic response, signs of adverse reactions due to drug accumulation, as well as drug concentrations in relation to target trough (if appropriate). The following are general recommendations only (based on dialysate flow/ultrafiltration rates of 1-2 L/hour and minimal residual renal function) and should not supersede clinical judgment: CMV infection:

CVVH: I.V.: Induction: 2.5 mg/kg every 24 hours; Maintenance: 1.25 mg/kg every 24 hours

CVVHD/CVVHDF: I.V.: Induction: 2.5 mg/kg every 12 hours; Maintenance: 2.5 mg/kg every 24 hours

Administration Follow same precautions utilized with antineoplastic agents when preparing and administering ganciclovir.

Parenteral: Reconstitute with SWI **not** bacteriostatic water because parabens may cause precipitation; further dilute to a final concentration not to exceed 10 mg/mL. Administer by slow I.V. infusion over at least 1 hour; too rapid infusion can cause increased toxicity and excessive plasma levels. Flush line well with NS before and after administration. Do not administer I.M. or SubQ; due to high pH, may cause severe tissue irritation.

Hazardous agent; use appropriate precautions for handling and disposal (NIOSH, 2012).

Monitoring Parameters CBC with differential and platelet count, urine output, serum creatinine, ophthalmologic exams, liver enzyme tests, blood pressure, urinalysis

Additional Information Sodium content of 1 g: 4 mEq

Dosage Forms Excipient information presented when available (limited, particularly for generics); consult specific product labeling.

Solution Reconstituted, Intravenous:

Cytovene: 500 mg (1 ea)

Generic: 500 mg (1 ea)

References

Amir J, Wolf DG, and Levy I, "Treatment of Symptomatic Congenital Cytomegalovirus Infection With Intravenous Ganciclovir Followed by Long-Term Oral Valganciclovir," *Eur J Pediatr*, 2010, 169(9):1061-7.

Centers for Disease Control and Prevention (CDC), "Guidelines for the Prevention and Treatment of Opportunistic Infections Among HIV-Exposed and HIV-Infected Children," *MMWR Recomm Rep*, 2009, 58(RR-11):1-166. Available at http://aidsinfo.nih.gov/contentfiles/Pediatric_OI.pdf

Centers for Disease Control and Prevention, "Guidelines for Prevention and Treatment of Opportunistic Infections in HIV-Infected Adults and Adolescents: Recommendations From CDC, the National Institutes of Health, and the HIV Medicine Association of the Infectious Diseases Society of America," *MMWR Recomm Rep*, 2009, 58(RR-4):1-216.

Fletcher C, Sawchuk R, Chinnock B, et al, "Human Pharmacokinetics of the Antiviral Drug DHPG," *Clin Pharmacol Ther*, 1986, 40(3):281-6.

Goodrich JM, Bowden RA, Fisher L, et al, "Ganciclovir Prophylaxis to Prevent Cytomegalovirus Disease After Allogeneic Marrow Transplant," *Ann Intern Med*, 1993, 118(3):173-8.

Gudnason T, Belani KK, and Balfour HH Jr, "Ganciclovir Treatment of Cytomegalovirus Disease in Immunocompromised Children," *Pediatr Infect Dis J*, 1989, 8(7):436-40.

Heintz BH, Matzke GR, and Dager WE, "Antimicrobial Dosing Concepts and Recommendations for Critically Ill Adult Patients Receiving Continuous Renal Replacement Therapy or Intermittent Hemodialysis," *Pharmacotherapy*, 2009, 29(5):562-77.

Merigan TC, Renlund DG, Keay S, et al, "A Controlled Trial of Ganciclovir to Prevent Cytomegalovirus Disease After Heart Transplantation," *N Engl J Med*, 1992, 326(18):1182-6.

National Institute for Occupational Safety and Health (NIOSH), "NIOSH List of Antineoplastic and Other Hazardous Drugs in Healthcare Settings 2012." Available at http://www.cdc.gov/niosh/docs/2012-150/pdfs/2012-150.pdf. Accessed January 21, 2013.

Red Book: 2009 Report of the Committee on Infectious Diseases, "Group B Streptococcal Infections," 28th ed, Pickering LK, ed, Elk Grove Village, IL: American Academy of Pediatrics, 2009.

Schleiss MR, "Antiviral Therapy of Congenital Cytomegalovirus Infection," *Semin Pediatr Infect Dis*, 2005, 16(1):50-9.

Trotman RL, Williamson JC, Shoemaker DM, et al, "Antibiotic Dosing in Critically Ill Adult Patients Receiving Continuous Renal Replacement Therapy," *Clin Infect Dis*, 2005, 41:1159-66.

Ganciclovir (Ophthalmic) (gan SYE kloe veer)

Medication Safety Issues
Sound-alike/look-alike issues:
Ganciclovir may be confused with acyclovir, valGANciclovir

Related Information
Safe Handling of Hazardous Drugs *on page 2419*

Brand Names: U.S. Zirgan

Generic Availability (U.S.) No

Use
Intravitreal implant: Treatment of CMV retinitis in patients with AIDS (FDA approved in ages ≥9 years and adults)

Ophthalmic gel: Treatment of acute herpetic keratitis (dendritic ulcers) (FDA approved in ages ≥2 years and adults)

Pregnancy Risk Factor C

Pregnancy Considerations Adverse events were observed in animal reproduction studies conducted with systemic ganciclovir. Based on animal studies, a U.S. Boxed Warning has been added to the labeling of the systemic product and effective contraception is recommended in males and females using systemic therapy. The amount of ganciclovir available systemically following topical application of the Zirgan® ophthalmic gel is significantly less in comparison I.V. doses (0.1%).

Breast-Feeding Considerations The amount of ganciclovir available systemically following ophthalmic application is not known. The manufacturer recommends that caution be used with administration of the ophthalmic gel to nursing women. Nursing mothers with herpetic lesions near or on the breast should avoid breast-feeding (AAP, 2012).

Contraindications Hypersensitivity to ganciclovir, acyclovir, or any component; intravitreal implant: Any clinical condition contraindicating intraocular surgery, such as external infection or severe thrombocytopenia

Warnings Hazardous agent; use appropriate precautions for handling and disposal (NIOSH, 2012).

Intravitreal implant: Following implantation, immediate and temporary decrease in visual acuity will be seen for 2-4 weeks; does not treat systemic CMV infection; monitor patients for signs and symptoms of systemic disease.

Gel formulation: Contact lenses should not be worn during therapy (or in any patient with herpetic keratitis); formulation is intended for topical ophthalmic use only.

Precautions Use with caution in children because long-term safety has not been determined and because of the potential long-term carcinogenic and adverse reproductive effects of ganciclovir.

Adverse Reactions Ocular: Blurred vision, conjunctival hyperemia, irritation, punctate keratitis

Drug Interactions
Metabolism/Transport Effects None known.

Avoid Concomitant Use There are no known interactions where it is recommended to avoid concomitant use.

Increased Effect/Toxicity There are no known significant interactions involving an increase in effect.

Decreased Effect There are no known significant interactions involving a decrease in effect.

Stability Hazardous agent; use appropriate precautions for handling and disposal (NIOSH, 2012).

Intravitreal implant: Store at 15°C to 30°C (59°F to 86°F); protect from freezing, excessive heat, and light.

Ophthalmic gel: Store at 15°C to 25°C (59°F to 77°F); do not freeze.

Mechanism of Action Ganciclovir is phosphorylated to a substrate which competitively inhibits the binding of deoxyguanosine triphosphate to DNA polymerase resulting in inhibition of viral DNA synthesis

Pharmacokinetics (Adult data unless noted) Absorption: Ophthalmic gel: Systemic absorption (0.1% in comparison to I.V. doses)

Dosing: Usual
CMV retinitis: Sustained release intravitreal implant:
Children ≥9 years: One implant for 5- to 8-month period; following depletion of ganciclovir, as evidenced by progression of retinitis, implant may be removed and replaced

Adults: One implant for 5- to 8-month period; following depletion of ganciclovir, as evidenced by progression of retinitis, implant may be removed and replaced

Herpetic keratitis: Ophthalmic gel: Children ≥2 years and Adults: Apply 1 drop in affected eye 5 times/day (approximately every 3 hours while awake) until corneal ulcer heals, then 1 drop 3 times/day for 7 days

Administration Ophthalmic gel: Gel is intended for topical ophthalmic use only.

Hazardous agent; use appropriate precautions for handling and disposal (NIOSH, 2012).

Dosage Forms Excipient information presented when available (limited, particularly for generics); consult specific product labeling.

Gel, Ophthalmic:
Zirgan: 0.15% (5 g) [contains benzalkonium chloride]

References
American Academy of Pediatrics (AAP) Policy Statement, "Breastfeeding and the Use of Human Milk," *Pediatrics*, 2012, 129(3):e827-41.

Centers for Disease Control and Prevention, "Guidelines for the Prevention and Treatment of Opportunistic Infections Among HIV-Exposed and HIV-Infected Children: Recommendations From CDC, the National Institutes of Health, the HIV Medicine Association of the Infectious Diseases Society of America, the Pediatric Infectious Diseases Society, and the American Academy of Pediatrics," *MMWR Recomm Rep*, 2009, 58(RR-11):1-166. Available at http://aidsinfo.nih.gov/contentfiles/Pediatric_OI.pdf

National Institute for Occupational Safety and Health (NIOSH), "NIOSH List of Antineoplastic and Other Hazardous Drugs in Healthcare Settings 2012." Available at http://www.cdc.gov/niosh/docs/2012-150/pdfs/2012-150.pdf. Accessed January 21, 2013.

◆ **GAR-936** *see* Tigecycline *on page 2025*

◆ **Garamycin** *see* Gentamicin (Ophthalmic) *on page 966*

◆ **Garamycin® (Can)** *see* Gentamicin (Ophthalmic) *on page 966*

◆ **Gardasil** *see* Papillomavirus (Types 6, 11, 16, 18) Vaccine (Human, Recombinant) *on page 1600*

◆ **Gas-X [OTC]** *see* Simethicone *on page 1891*

◆ **Gas-X Childrens [OTC]** *see* Simethicone *on page 1891*

◆ **Gas-X Extra Strength [OTC]** *see* Simethicone *on page 1891*

◆ **Gas-X Infant Drops [OTC]** *see* Simethicone *on page 1891*

◆ **Gas-X Ultra Strength [OTC]** *see* Simethicone *on page 1891*

◆ **GasAid [OTC]** *see* Simethicone *on page 1891*

◆ **Gas Free Extra Strength [OTC]** *see* Simethicone *on page 1891*

◆ **Gas Relief [OTC]** *see* Simethicone *on page 1891*

◆ **Gas Relief Extra Strength [OTC]** *see* Simethicone *on page 1891*

◆ **Gas Relief Ultra Strength [OTC]** *see* Simethicone *on page 1891*

◆ **Gastrocrom** *see* Cromolyn (Systemic, Oral Inhalation) *on page 551*

Gatifloxacin (gat i FLOKS a sin)

Brand Names: U.S. Zymaxid
Brand Names: Canada Zymar
Therapeutic Category Antibiotic, Ophthalmic; Antibiotic, Quinolone
Generic Availability (U.S.) Yes
Use Treatment of bacterial conjunctivitis caused by susceptible organisms (FDA approved in ages ≥1 year and adults).
Pregnancy Risk Factor C
Pregnancy Considerations Gatifloxacin has been shown to be fetotoxic in animal studies. Quinolone exposure during human pregnancy has been reported with other agents (refer to Ciprofloxacin (Systemic) and Ofloxacin (Systemic) monographs). Following ophthalmic administration, serum concentrations of gatifloxacin are below the limits of quantification (<5 ng/mL). Systemic absorption would be required in order for gatifloxacin to cross the placenta.
Breast-Feeding Considerations Other quinolones are known to be excreted in breast milk. The manufacturer recommends using caution if gatifloxacin is administered while nursing.
Contraindications Hypersensitivity to gatifloxacin, other quinolone antibiotics, or any component
Warnings Severe hypersensitivity reactions, including anaphylaxis, have occurred with systemic quinolone therapy, including gatifloxacin. The spectrum of these reactions can vary widely. Prompt discontinuation of drug should occur if skin rash or other symptoms arise. **Not for injection into the eye.** Eye drops should not be introduced directly into the anterior chamber of the eye.
Precautions Prolonged use may result in fungal or bacterial superinfection. Contact lenses should not be worn during therapy.
Adverse Reactions
Cardiovascular: Edema
Dermatologic: Contact dermatitis, erythema
Gastrointestinal: Taste disturbance
Ocular: Conjunctival irritation, discharge, dry eye, edema, irritation, keratitis, lacrimation increased, pain, papillary conjunctivitis, visual acuity decreased
Respiratory: Rhinorrhea
Rare but important or life-threatening: Angioedema, blepharitis (allergic), chemosis, conjunctival cyst, conjunctival hemorrhage, corneal deposits, corneal disorder, corneal ulcer, dermatitis, dizziness, endophthalmitis, eye redness, iritis, keratoconjunctivitis, macular edema, nausea, paresthesia (oral), photophobia, pruritus, subepithelial opacities, tinnitus, tremor, urticaria, uveitis, vision blurred, throat sore
Drug Interactions
Metabolism/Transport Effects None known.

Avoid Concomitant Use There are no known interactions where it is recommended to avoid concomitant use.
Increased Effect/Toxicity There are no known significant interactions involving an increase in effect.
Decreased Effect There are no known significant interactions involving a decrease in effect.
Stability Store between 15°C to 25°C (59°F to 77°F); do not freeze.
Mechanism of Action Gatifloxacin is a DNA gyrase inhibitor, and also inhibits topoisomerase IV. DNA gyrase (topoisomerase II) is an essential bacterial enzyme that maintains the superhelical structure of DNA. DNA gyrase is required for DNA replication and transcription, DNA repair, recombination, and transposition; inhibition is bactericidal.
Pharmacokinetics (Adult data unless noted) Absorption: Not measurable
Dosing: Usual Children ≥1 year and Adults:
Zymar®: Days 1 and 2: Instill 1 drop into affected eye(s) every 2 hours while awake (maximum: 8 times/day). Days 3-7: Instill 1 drop into affected eye(s) up to 4 times/day while awake.
Zymaxid™: Day 1: Instill 1 drop into affected eye(s) every 2 hours while awake (maximum: 8 times/day). Days 2-7: Instill 1 drop into affected eye(s) 2-4 times/day while awake.
Administration For topical ophthalmic use only; avoid touching tip of applicator to eye, fingers, or other surfaces. Apply finger pressure to lacrimal sac during and for 1-2 minutes after instillation to decrease risk of absorption and systemic effects.
Monitoring Parameters Signs of infection
Test Interactions Some quinolones may produce a false-positive urine screening result for opioids using commercially-available immunoassay kits. This has been demonstrated most consistently for levofloxacin and ofloxacin, but other quinolones have shown cross-reactivity in certain assay kits. Confirmation of positive opioid screens by more specific methods should be considered.
Additional Information Evidence of damage to weight-bearing joints in pediatric populations with ophthalmic administration has not been shown.
Dosage Forms Excipient information presented when available (limited, particularly for generics); consult specific product labeling.
Solution, Ophthalmic:
Zymaxid: 0.5% (2.5 mL) [contains benzalkonium chloride, edetate disodium]
Generic: 0.5% (2.5 mL)
References
Cervantes LJ and Mah FS, "Clinical Use of Gatifloxacin Ophthalmic Solution for Treatment of Bacterial Conjunctivitis," *Clin Ophthalmol*, 2011, 5:495-502.

◆ **GaviLAX [OTC]** *see* Polyethylene Glycol 3350 *on page 1696*

◆ **GaviLyte-C** *see* Polyethylene Glycol-Electrolyte Solution *on page 1697*

◆ **GaviLyte-G** *see* Polyethylene Glycol-Electrolyte Solution *on page 1697*

◆ **GaviLyte-N** *see* Polyethylene Glycol-Electrolyte Solution *on page 1697*

◆ **G-CSF** *see* Filgrastim *on page 872*

◆ **G-CSF (PEG Conjugate)** *see* Pegfilgrastim *on page 1616*

◆ **GCV Sodium** *see* Ganciclovir (Systemic) *on page 955*

◆ **GD-Amlodipine (Can)** *see* AmLODIPine *on page 135*

◆ **GD-Atorvastatin (Can)** *see* AtorvaSTATin *on page 227*

◆ **GD-Azithromycin (Can)** *see* Azithromycin (Systemic) *on page 247*

- ◆ **GD-Gabapentin (Can)** *see* Gabapentin *on page 950*
- ◆ **GD-Sertraline (Can)** *see* Sertraline *on page 1879*
- ◆ **GD-Sildenafil (Can)** *see* Sildenafil *on page 1884*
- ◆ **GD-Terbinafine (Can)** *see* Terbinafine (Systemic) *on page 1982*
- ◆ **GD-Topiramate (Can)** *see* Topiramate *on page 2046*
- ◆ **GD-Venlafaxine XR (Can)** *see* Venlafaxine *on page 2125*
- ◆ **Gel-Kam [OTC]** *see* Fluoride *on page 894*
- ◆ **Gel-Kam Rinse** *see* Fluoride *on page 894*
- ◆ **Gelnique** *see* Oxybutynin *on page 1568*
- ◆ **GelRite™ [OTC]** *see* Alcohol (Ethyl) *on page 88*
- ◆ **Gel-Stat™ [OTC]** *see* Alcohol (Ethyl) *on page 88*
- ◆ **Gelusil® Extra Strength (Can)** *see* Aluminum Hydroxide and Magnesium Hydroxide *on page 111*

Gemcitabine (jem SITE a been)

Medication Safety Issues
Sound-alike/look-alike issues:
Gemcitabine may be confused with gemtuzumab
Gemzar may be confused with Zinecard
High alert medication:
This medication is in a class the Institute for Safe Medication Practices (ISMP) includes among its list of drug classes which have a heightened risk of causing significant patient harm when used in error.
International issues:
In Canada, gemcitabine is available as a concentrated solution for injection in different strengths (38 mg/mL and 40 mg/mL), and a powder for reconstitution (final concentration of 38 mg/mL after reconstitution). Verify product concentration prior to preparation for administration.

Related Information
Emetogenic Potential of Antineoplastic Agents in Children *on page 2327*
Management of Drug Extravasations *on page 2255*
Safe Handling of Hazardous Drugs *on page 2419*

Brand Names: U.S. Gemzar

Brand Names: Canada Gemcitabine For Injection; Gemcitabine For Injection, USP; Gemcitabine Hydrochloride For Injection; Gemcitabine Sun For Injection; Gemzar

Therapeutic Category Antineoplastic Agent, Antimetabolite (Pyrimidine Antagonist)

Generic Availability (U.S.) Yes

Use Treatment of locally advanced, inoperable (stage IIIA or IIIB), or metastatic (stage IV) nonsmall cell lung cancer (NSCLC), metastatic breast cancer, and advanced relapsed ovarian cancer as part of combination therapy (FDA approved in adults); treatment of locally advanced or metastatic pancreatic cancer as a single agent (FDA approved in adults); has also been used in the treatment of refractory solid tumors (including brain tumors), refractory or relapsed Hodgkin's lymphoma, and refractory germ cell tumors

Pregnancy Risk Factor D

Pregnancy Considerations Adverse events were observed in animal reproduction studies. May cause fetal harm if administered during pregnancy; adverse effects in reproduction are anticipated based on the mechanism of action.

Breast-Feeding Considerations It is not known if gemcitabine is excreted in breast milk. Due to the potential for serious adverse reactions in the nursing infant, the decision to discontinue gemcitabine or to discontinue breast-feeding should take into account the benefits of treatment to the mother.

Contraindications Hypersensitivity to gemcitabine or any component

Warnings Hazardous agent; use appropriate precautions for handling and disposal (NIOSH, 2012). Prolongation of the infusion time >60 minutes as well as more frequent than once weekly dosing have been shown to increase toxicity. Longer infusion times allow increased accumulation of the active metabolite, gemcitabine triphosphate, optimizing the pharmacokinetics. Myelosuppression is usually the dose-limiting toxicity; monitor CBC with differential and platelet count prior to each dose; reduce or withhold dose depending on the degree of hematologic toxicity. Gemcitabine has been reported to cause hemolytic uremic syndrome and/or renal failure requiring dialysis or leading to death; monitor renal function prior to initial dose and then periodically. Hepatotoxicity, including liver failure and death, has been reported with gemcitabine use; monitor hepatic function prior to initial dose and then periodically. Pulmonary toxicity has also been reported with use. Discontinue gemcitabine if severe lung, renal, or hepatotoxicity occurs. Gemcitabine may cause fever in the absence of clinical infection.

Precautions Use with caution in patients with renal or hepatic impairment. Use with caution in patients receiving concurrent radiation therapy; radiation toxicity, including tissue injury, severe mucositis, esophagitis, or pneumonitis has been reported with concurrent and nonconcurrent administration. Gemcitabine and radiation therapy have radiosensitizing activity when given ≤7 days apart; lower gemcitabine doses with concurrent radiation therapy may produce less severe toxicity; however, an optimum regimen for combination therapy has not been determined for all tumor types; radiation recall may occur when gemcitabine and radiation therapy are given >7 days apart.

Adverse Reactions Adverse reactions reported for single-agent use of gemcitabine only; bone marrow depression is the dose-limiting toxicity.
Cardiovascular: Edema, peripheral edema
Central nervous system: Drowsiness, paresthesia
Dermatologic: Alopecia, pruritus, skin rash
Gastrointestinal: Diarrhea, nausea and vomiting, stomatitis
Genitourinary: Hematuria, increased blood urea nitrogen, proteinuria
Hematologic & oncologic: Anemia, hemorrhage, leukopenia, neutropenia, thrombocytopenia
Hepatic: Increased serum alkaline phosphatase, increased serum ALT, increased serum AST, increased serum bilirubin
Infection: Infection
Local: Injection site reaction
Renal: Increased serum creatinine
Respiratory: Bronchospasm, dyspnea
Miscellaneous: Fever, flu-like symptoms
Rare but important or life-threatening (reported with single-agent use or with combination therapy): Adult respiratory distress syndrome (acute), anaphylactoid reaction, Budd-Chiari syndrome, bullous pemphigoid, capillary leak syndrome, cardiac arrhythmia, cardiac failure, cellulitis, cerebrovascular accident, desquamation, digital vasculitis, gangrene of skin or other tissue, hemolytic-uremic syndrome, hepatic cirrhosis, hepatic necrosis, hepatic veno-occlusive disease, hepatotoxicity (rare), hypertension, hypotension, increased gamma-glutamyl transferase, interstitial pneumonitis, myocardial infarction, neuropathy, petechiae, pulmonary edema, pulmonary fibrosis, radiation recall phenomenon, renal failure, respiratory failure, reversible posterior leukoencephalopathy syndrome, sepsis, supraventricular cardiac arrhythmia, thrombotic thrombocytopenic purpura

Drug Interactions
Metabolism/Transport Effects None known.

◀ **Avoid Concomitant Use**
Avoid concomitant use of Gemcitabine with any of the following: BCG; CloZAPine; Dipyrone; Natalizumab; Pimecrolimus; Tacrolimus (Topical); Tofacitinib; Vaccines (Live)

Increased Effect/Toxicity
Gemcitabine may increase the levels/effects of: Bleomycin; CloZAPine; Fluorouracil (Systemic); Fluorouracil (Topical); Leflunomide; Natalizumab; Tofacitinib; Vaccines (Live); Vitamin K Antagonists

The levels/effects of Gemcitabine may be increased by: Denosumab; Dipyrone; Pimecrolimus; Roflumilast; Tacrolimus (Topical); Trastuzumab

Decreased Effect
Gemcitabine may decrease the levels/effects of: BCG; Coccidioidin Skin Test; Sipuleucel-T; Vaccines (Inactivated); Vaccines (Live); Vitamin K Antagonists

The levels/effects of Gemcitabine may be decreased by: Echinacea

Stability Hazardous agent; use appropriate precautions for handling and disposal (NIOSH, 2012).
Lyophilized powder: Store intact vial at 20°C to 25°C (68°F to 77°F); reconstituted vials are stable up to 24 hours at room temperature; do not refrigerate as crystallization may occur
Solution for injection: Store intact vials at 2°C to 8°C (36°F to 46°F); do not freeze. Solutions further diluted in NS are stable for 24 hours at room temperature. Do not refrigerate.

Mechanism of Action A pyrimidine antimetabolite that inhibits DNA synthesis by inhibition of DNA polymerase and ribonucleotide reductase, cell cycle-specific for the S-phase of the cycle (also blocks cellular progression at G1/S-phase). Gemcitabine is phosphorylated intracellularly by deoxycytidine kinase to gemcitabine monophosphate, which is further phosphorylated to active metabolites gemcitabine diphosphate and gemcitabine triphosphate. Gemcitabine diphosphate inhibits DNA synthesis by inhibiting ribonucleotide reductase; gemcitabine triphosphate incorporates into DNA and inhibits DNA polymerase.

Pharmacokinetics (Adult data unless noted)
Distribution: Widely distributed into tissues; present in ascitic fluid
V_d:
I.V. infusion <70 minutes: 50 L/m^2
I.V. infusion 70-285 minutes: 370 L/m^2
Protein binding: Negligible
Metabolism: Intracellularly by nucleoside kinases to active di- and triphosphate metabolites; metabolized by cytidine deaminase to an inactive metabolite
Half-life:
I.V. infusion <70 minutes: 0.7-1.6 hours
I.V. infusion 70-285 minutes: 4.1-10.6 hours
Elimination: 92% to 98% excreted in the urine as gemcitabine (<10%) and inactive uracil metabolite, difluorodeoxyuridine (dFdU)

Dosing: Usual Details concerning dosing in combination regimens should also be consulted. **Note:** Prolongation of the infusion time >60 minutes and administration more frequently than once weekly have been shown to increase toxicity. Refer to individual protocols: I.V.:
Children and Adolescents:
Hodgkin's lymphoma, refractory or relapsed:
Children ≥10 years and Adolescents: 1000 mg/m^2/dose over 100 minutes on days 1 and 8 (in combination with vinorelbine); repeat cycle every 21 days (Cole, 2009)
Adolescents ≥17 years: 1000 mg/m^2/dose over 60 minutes on days 1, 8, and 15 (in combination with vinorelbine); repeat cycle every 28 days (Suyani, 2011) **or** 800 mg/m^2/dose on days 1 and 4 (in combination with ifosfamide and vinorelbine); repeat cycle every 21 days (Santoro, 2007)

Sarcomas, refractory or relapsed (including Ewing's sarcoma, osteosarcoma): Children ≥3 years and Adolescents: 675 **or** 1000 mg/m^2/dose over 90 minutes on days 1 and 8 (in combination with docetaxel); repeat cycle every 21 days (Mora, 2009; Navid, 2008) **or** 1000 mg/m^2/dose over 30 minutes on days 1 and 8 (in combination with oxaliplatin and irinotecan); repeat cycle every 28 days (Hartmann, 2011)

Solid tumors, refractory or relapsed: Children ≥1 year and Adolescents: 1000 mg/m^2/dose over 30 minutes on days 1 and 8 (in combination with oxaliplatin and irinotecan); repeat cycle every 28 days (Hartmann, 2011) **or** 1000 mg/m^2/dose over 100 minutes on day 1 (in combination with oxaliplatin); repeat cycle every 14 days (Geoerger, 2011)
Note: Dosage reductions for toxicity (Geoerger, 2011): 800 mg/m^2/dose over 80 minutes if grade 3/4 nonhematological toxicity, grade 4 neutropenia with documented infection or lasting >7 days, grade 3/4 thrombocytopenia lasting >7 days or requiring platelets during >7 days, or delay of next cycle ≥14 days; if necessary dose could be reduced a second time to 600 mg/m^2/dose

Germ cell tumor, refractory: Adolescents ≥16 years: 1200 mg/m^2/dose over 30 minutes on days 1, 8, and 15; repeat cycle every 28 days for up to 6 cycles (Einhorn, 1999)

Adults:
Breast cancer, metastatic (AGC should be ≥1500/mm^3 and platelets ≥100,000/mm^3 prior to each cycle): 1250 mg/m^2 over 30 minutes on days 1 and 8; repeat cycle every 21 days (in combination with paclitaxel)

Nonsmall cell lung cancer, locally advanced or metastatic (in combination with cisplatin): 1000 mg/m^2 over 30 minutes on days 1, 8, and 15; repeat cycle every 28 days **or** 1250 mg/m^2 over 30 minutes on days 1 and 8; repeat cycle every 21 days

Ovarian cancer, advanced (AGC should be ≥1500/mm^3 and platelets ≥100,000/mm^3 prior to each cycle): 1000 mg/m^2 over 30 minutes days 1 and 8; repeat cycle every 21 days (in combination with carboplatin)

Pancreatic cancer, locally advanced or metastatic: Initial: 1000 mg/m^2 over 30 minutes once weekly for up to 7 weeks followed by 1 week of rest; then 1000 mg/m^2 once weekly for 3 weeks out of every 4 weeks
Dose escalation: Patients who complete an entire cycle of therapy may have the dose in subsequent cycles increased by 25% as long as the absolute granulocyte count (AGC) nadir is >1500/mm^3, platelet nadir is >100,000/mm^3, and nonhematologic toxicity is less than WHO Grade 1. If the increased dose is tolerated (with the same parameters) the dose in subsequent cycles may again be increased by 20%.

Dosing adjustment for renal impairment: Adults: The manufacturer's labeling does not contain dosing adjustment guidelines; use with caution in patients with preexisting renal dysfunction. Discontinue if severe renal toxicity or hemolytic uremic syndrome (HUS) occur during gemcitabine treatment.
The following adjustments have been made by some clinicians (Janus, 2010; Li, 2007):
Mild to severe renal impairment: No adjustment required
ESRD with hemodialysis: Hemodialysis should begin 6-12 hours after gemcitabine infusion

Dosing adjustment for hepatic impairment: Adults: The manufacturer's labeling does not contain dosing adjustment guidelines; use with caution. Discontinue if severe hepatotoxicity occurs during treatment with gemcitabine. The following guidelines have been used by some clinicians:

Transaminases elevated (with normal bilirubin): No adjustment required (Venook, 2000)

Serum bilirubin >1.6 mg/dL: Use initial dose of 800 mg/m² ; may escalate if tolerated (Ecklund, 2005; Floyd, 2006; Venook, 2000)

Dosing adjustment for hematologic toxicity: Adults:

Breast cancer: Adjustments based on granulocyte and platelet counts on day 8:

AGC ≥1200/mm³ **and** platelet count >75,000/mm³ : Administer 100% of full dose

AGC 1000-1199/mm³ **or** platelet count 50,000-75,000/mm³ : Administer 75% of full dose

AGC 700-999/mm³ **and** platelet count ≥50,000/mm³ : Administer 50% of full dose

AGC <700/mm³ **or** platelet count <50,000/mm³ : Hold dose

Severe (grades 3 or 4) nonhematologic toxicity (except alopecia, nausea, and vomiting): Hold or decrease dose by 50%. Paclitaxel dose may also need adjusted.

Nonsmall cell lung cancer: Refer to guidelines for pancreatic cancer. Cisplatin dosage may also need adjusted.

Severe (grades 3 or 4) nonhematologic toxicity (except alopecia, nausea, and vomiting): Hold or decrease dose by 50%

Ovarian cancer:

Adjustments based on granulocyte and platelet counts on day 8:

AGC ≥1500/mm³ **and** platelet count ≥100,000/mm³ : Administer 100% of full dose

AGC 1000-1499/mm³ **and/or** platelet count 75,000-99,999/mm³ : Administer 50% of full dose

AGC <1000/mm³ **and/or** platelet count <75,000/mm³ : Hold dose

Severe (grades 3 or 4) nonhematologic toxicity (except nausea and vomiting): Hold or decrease dose by 50%. Carboplatin dose may also need adjusted.

Dose adjustment for subsequent cycles:

AGC <500/mm³ for >5 days, AGC <100/mm³ for >3 days, febrile neutropenia, platelet count <25,000/mm³, cycle delay >1 week due to toxicity: Reduce gemcitabine to 800 mg/m² on days 1 and 8

For recurrence of any of the above toxicities after initial dose reduction: Administer gemcitabine 800 mg/m2 on day 1 only for the subsequent cycle

Pancreatic cancer:

AGC ≥1000/mm³ **and** platelet count ≥100,000/mm³ : Administer 100% of full dose

AGC 500-999/mm³ **or** platelet count 50,000-99,999/mm³ : Administer 75% of full dose

AGC <500/mm³ **or** platelet count <50,000/mm³ : Hold dose

Administration I.V.: Hazardous agent; use appropriate precautions for handling and disposal (NIOSH, 2012). Reconstitute lyophilized powder according to manufacturer's labeling to a final concentration of 38 mg/mL (solution must be reconstituted to ≤40 mg/mL to completely dissolve). Maximum concentration for administration: 38 mg/mL; gemcitabine can be further diluted with 50-500 mL NS to concentrations as low as 0.1 mg/mL. Infuse over 30-90 minutes based on the protocol. Prolongation of the infusion time >60 minutes has been shown to prolong gemcitabine's half-life and increase toxicity in adults; gemcitabine has been studied in adults utilizing a fixed-dose rate (FDR) of 10 mg/m²/minute (Ko, 2006;

Tempero, 2003); patients who receive gemcitabine FDR experience more grade 3/4 hematologic toxicity (Ko, 2006; Poplin, 2009). pH 2.7-3.3

Vesicant/Extravasation Risk May be an irritant

Monitoring Parameters CBC with differential and platelet count prior to each dose; monitor renal and hepatic function prior to initial dose and then periodically, bilirubin, LDH, and reticulocyte count; monitor serum electrolytes, including potassium, magnesium, and calcium (when in combination therapy with cisplatin)

Dosage Forms Excipient information presented when available (limited, particularly for generics); consult specific product labeling.

Solution, Intravenous:

Generic: 200 mg/5.26 mL (5.26 mL); 1 g/26.3 mL (26.3 mL); 2 g/52.6 mL (52.6 mL)

Solution Reconstituted, Intravenous:

Gemzar: 200 mg (1 ea); 1 g (1 ea)

Generic: 200 mg (1 ea); 1 g (1 ea); 2 g (1 ea)

Solution Reconstituted, Intravenous [preservative free]:

Generic: 200 mg (1 ea); 1 g (1 ea)

References

Cole PD, Schwartz CL, Drachtman RA, et al, "Phase II Study of Weekly Gemcitabine and Vinorelbine for Children With Recurrent or Refractory Hodgkin's Disease: A Children's Oncology Group Report," *J Clin Oncol*, 2009, 27(9):1456-61.

Eklund JW, Trifilio S, and Mulcahy MF, "Chemotherapy Dosing in the Setting of Liver Dysfunction," *Oncology (Williston Park)*, 2005, 19 (8):1057-63.

Einhorn LH, Stender MJ, and Williams SD, "Phase II Trial of Gemcitabine in Refractory Germ Cell Tumors," *J Clin Oncol*, 1999, 17 (2):509-11.

Floyd J, Mirza I, Sachs B, et al, "Hepatotoxicity of Chemotherapy," *Semin Oncol*, 2006, 33(1):50-67.

Geoerger B, Chisholm J, Le Deley MC, et al, "Phase II Study of Gemcitabine Combined With Oxaliplatin in Relapsed or Refractory Paediatric Solid Malignancies: An Innovative Therapy for Children With Cancer European Consortium Study," *Eur J Cancer*, 2011, 47 (2):230-8.

Hartmann C, Weinel P, Schmid H, et al, "Oxaliplatin, Irinotecan, and Gemcitabine: A Novel Combination in the Therapy of Progressed, Relapsed, or Refractory Tumors in Children," *J Pediatr Hematol Oncol*, 2011, 33(5):344-9.

Janus N, Thariat J, Boulanger H, et al, "Proposal for Dosage Adjustment and Timing of Chemotherapy in Hemodialyzed Patients," *Ann Oncol*, 2010, 21(7):1395-403.

Ko AH, Dito E, Schillinger B, et al, "Phase II Study of Fixed Dose Rate Gemcitabine With Cisplatin for Metastatic Adenocarcinoma of the Pancreas," *J Clin Oncol*, 2006, 24(3):379-85.

Li YF, Fu S, Hu W, et al, "Systemic Anticancer Therapy in Gynecological Cancer Patients With Renal Dysfunction," *Int J Gynecol Cancer*, 2007, 17(4):739-63.

Mora J, Cruz CO, Parareda A, et al, "Treatment of Relapsed/Refractory Pediatric Sarcomas With Gemcitabine and Docetaxel," *J Pediatr Hematol Oncol*, 2009, 31(10):723-9.

National Institute for Occupational Safety and Health (NIOSH), "NIOSH List of Antineoplastic and Other Hazardous Drugs in Healthcare Settings 2012." Available at http://www.cdc.gov/niosh/docs/2012-150/pdfs/2012-150.pdf. Accessed January 21, 2013.

Navid F, Willert JR, McCarville MB, et al, "Combination of Gemcitabine and Docetaxel in the Treatment of Children and Young Adults With Refractory Bone Sarcoma," *Cancer*, 2008, 113(2):419-25.

Ozkaynak MF and Jayabose S, "Gemcitabine and Vinorelbine as a Salvage Regimen for Relapse in Hodgkin Lymphoma After Autologous Hematopoietic Stem Cell Transplantation," *Pediatr Hematol Oncol*, 2004, 21(2):107-13.

Poplin E, Feng Y, Berlin J, et al, "Phase III, Randomized Study of Gemcitabine and Oxaliplatin Versus Gemcitabine (Fixed-Dose Rate Infusion) Compared With Gemcitabine (30-Minute Infusion) in Patients With Pancreatic Carcinoma E6201: A Trial of the Eastern Cooperative Oncology Group," *J Clin Oncol*, 2009, 27(23):3778-85.

Reid JM, Qu W, Safgren SL, et al, "Phase I Trial and Pharmacokinetics of Gemcitabine in Children With Advanced Solid Tumors," *J Clin Oncol*, 2004, 22(12):2445-51.

Santoro A, Magagnoli M, Spina M, et al, "Ifosfamide, Gemcitabine, and Vinorelbine: A New Induction Regimen for Refractory and Relapsed Hodgkin's Lymphoma," *Haematologica*, 2007, 92(1):35-41.

Suyani E, Sucak GT, Akı ŞZ, et al, "Gemcitabine and Vinorelbine Combination Is Effective in Both as a Salvage and Mobilization Regimen in Relapsed or Refractory Hodgkin Lymphoma Prior to ASCT," *Ann Hematol*, 2011, 90(6):685-91.

Tempero M, Plunkett W, Ruiz Van Haperen V, et al, "Randomized Phase II Comparison of Dose-Intense Gemcitabine: Thirty-Minute Infusion and Fixed Dose Rate Infusion in Patients With Pancreatic Adenocarcinoma," *J Clin Oncol*, 2003, 21(18):3402-8.

Venook AP, Egorin MJ, Rosner GL, et al, "Phase I and Pharmacokinetic Trial of Gemcitabine in Patients With Hepatic or Renal Dysfunction: Cancer and Leukemia Group B 9565," *J Clin Oncol*, 2000, 18 (14):2780-7.

◆ **Gemcitabine For Injection (Can)** *see* Gemcitabine *on page 959*

◆ **Gemcitabine For Injection, USP (Can)** *see* Gemcitabine *on page 959*

◆ **Gemcitabine Hydrochloride** *see* Gemcitabine *on page 959*

◆ **Gemcitabine Hydrochloride For Injection (Can)** *see* Gemcitabine *on page 959*

◆ **Gemcitabine Sun For Injection (Can)** *see* Gemcitabine *on page 959*

◆ **Gemzar** *see* Gemcitabine *on page 959*

◆ **Genahist [OTC]** *see* DiphenhydrAMINE (Systemic) *on page 673*

◆ **Genaphed [OTC]** *see* Pseudoephedrine *on page 1770*

◆ **Gen-Clozapine (Can)** *see* CloZAPine *on page 527*

◆ **Gene-Activated Human Acid-Beta-Glucosidase** *see* Velaglucerase Alfa *on page 2124*

◆ **Generlac** *see* Lactulose *on page 1193*

◆ **Gen-Fluoxetine (Can)** *see* FLUoxetine *on page 901*

◆ **Gengraf** *see* CycloSPORINE (Systemic) *on page 564*

◆ **Gen-Hydroxychloroquine (Can)** *see* Hydroxychloroquine *on page 1048*

◆ **Gen-Hydroxyurea (Can)** *see* Hydroxyurea *on page 1051*

◆ **Gen-Ipratropium (Can)** *see* Ipratropium (Oral Inhalation) *on page 1144*

◆ **Gen-Medroxy (Can)** *see* MedroxyPROGESTERone *on page 1318*

◆ **Gen-Nizatidine (Can)** *see* Nizatidine *on page 1508*

◆ **Genotropin** *see* Somatropin *on page 1920*

◆ **Genotropin MiniQuick** *see* Somatropin *on page 1920*

◆ **Genpril [OTC]** *see* Ibuprofen *on page 1059*

◆ **Gentak** *see* Gentamicin (Ophthalmic) *on page 966*

◆ **Gentak® (Can)** *see* Gentamicin (Ophthalmic) *on page 966*

Gentamicin (Systemic) (jen ta MYE sin)

Medication Safety Issues

Sound-alike/look-alike issues:
Gentamicin may be confused with gentian violet, kanamycin, vancomycin

High alert medication:
The Institute for Safe Medication Practices (ISMP) includes this medication (intrathecal administration) among its list of drug classes which have a heightened risk of causing significant patient harm when used in error.

Brand Names: Canada Gentamicin Injection, USP

Therapeutic Category Antibiotic, Aminoglycoside

Generic Availability (U.S.) Yes

Use Treatment of documented or suspected infections caused by susceptible gram-negative bacilli, including *Pseudomonas*, *E. coli*, *Proteus*, *Serratia*, and gram-positive *Staphylococcus* (FDA approved in all ages); treatment of bone infections, CNS infections, respiratory tract infections, skin and soft tissue infections, as well as abdominal and urinary tract infections, endocarditis, and septicemia; used in combination with ampicillin as empiric therapy for sepsis in newborns

Pregnancy Risk Factor D

Pregnancy Considerations Gentamicin crosses the placenta and produces detectable serum levels in the fetus. Renal toxicity has been described in two case reports following first trimester exposure. There are several reports of total irreversible bilateral congenital deafness in children whose mothers received streptomycin during pregnancy; therefore, the manufacturer classifies gentamicin as pregnancy category D. Although ototoxicity has not been reported following maternal use of gentamicin, a potential for harm exists. **[U.S. Boxed Warning]: Aminoglycosides may cause fetal harm if administered to a pregnant woman.**

Due to pregnancy induced physiologic changes, some pharmacokinetic parameters of gentamicin may be altered. Pregnant women have an average-to-larger volume of distribution which may result in lower serum peak levels than for the same dose in nonpregnant women. Serum half-life is also shorter.

Breast-Feeding Considerations Gentamicin is excreted into breast milk; however, it is not well absorbed when taken orally. This limited oral absorption may minimize exposure to the nursing infant. Nondose-related effects could include modification of bowel flora.

Contraindications Hypersensitivity to gentamicin, any component, or other aminoglycosides

Warnings Aminoglycosides are associated with significant nephrotoxicity **[U.S. Boxed Warning]**. Vestibular and permanent bilateral auditory ototoxicity can occur **[U.S. Boxed Warning]**; tinnitus or vertigo are indications of vestibular injury and impending bilateral irreversible deafness; early ototoxicity usually affects high-pitched sound. Risk of nephrotoxicity and ototoxicity is increased in patients with impaired renal function, dehydration, high-dose therapy, or prolonged therapy. Peak and trough serum concentrations should be monitored periodically during therapy to assure adequate concentrations are achieved and to avoid potentially toxic levels **[U.S. Boxed Warning]**. Ototoxicity is associated with high serum concentrations persisting for prolonged periods; nephrotoxicity is associated with high serum trough concentrations. Risk of nephrotoxicity increases when used concurrently with other potentially nephrotoxic drugs **[U.S. Boxed Warning]**; renal damage is usually reversible. Risk of ototoxicity increases with use of potent diuretics **[U.S. Boxed Warning]**. Prolonged use may result in fungal or bacterial superinfection, including *C. difficile*-associated diarrhea (CDAD) and pseudomembranous colitis; CDAD has been observed >2 months postantibiotic treatment. Once-daily gentamicin administration has been associated with a pyrogenic endotoxin-like reaction (fever, chills, hypotension, tachycardia); some products contain sulfites which may cause allergic reactions in susceptible individuals. Not intended for long-term therapy due to toxic hazards associated with extended administration. Aminoglycosides can cause fetal harm when administered to a pregnant woman **[U.S. Boxed Warning]**; aminoglycosides have been associated with several reports of total irreversible bilateral congenital deafness in pediatric patients exposed *in utero*. Hemodialysis can be used for overdose or toxic reactions **[U.S. Boxed Warning]** particularly if renal function decreased; peritoneal dialysis removal is less than hemodialysis; in neonates, may consider exchange transfusions.

Precautions Use with caution in patients with preexisting renal impairment; modify dosage in patients with renal impairment; monitor renal and eighth nerve function in patients with known or suspected renal impairment **[U.S. Boxed Warning]**. Use with caution in patients with auditory or vestibular impairment. Use with caution in patients with myasthenia gravis, hypocalcemia, and in conditions which depress neuromuscular transmission; may cause neuromuscular blockade and respiratory paralysis; risk increased with concomitant use of anesthesia or muscle relaxants. Use with caution in pediatric patients on extracorporeal membrane oxygenation (ECMO); pharmacokinetics of aminoglycosides may be altered; dosage adjustment and close monitoring necessary.

Avoid intramuscular administration in paralyzed patients, due to poor circulation in the atrophic muscles which may result in slower absorption and lower peak serum concentrations; use intravenous route. Oral use for the prevention of NEC in premature neonates may potentially increase risk for development of resistant bacteria; routine use is not recommended (Bury, 2001; Reber, 2004).

Adverse Reactions

Cardiovascular: Edema, hyper/hypotension

Central nervous system: Ataxia, confusion, depression, dizziness, drowsiness, encephalopathy, fever, headache, lethargy, pseudomotor cerebri, seizures, vertigo

Dermatologic: Alopecia, erythema, itching, purpura, rash, urticaria

Endocrine & metabolic: Hypocalcemia, hypokalemia, hypomagnesemia, hyponatremia

Gastrointestinal: Anorexia, appetite decreased, *C. difficile*-associated diarrhea, enterocolitis, nausea, salivation increased, splenomegaly, stomatitis, vomiting, weight loss

Hematologic: Agranulocytosis, anemia, eosinophilia, granulocytopenia, leukopenia, reticulocytes increased/decreased, thrombocytopenia

Hepatic: Hepatomegaly, LFTs increased

Local: Injection site reactions, pain at injection site, phlebitis/thrombophlebitis

Neuromuscular & skeletal: Arthralgia, gait instability, muscle cramps, muscle twitching, muscle weakness, myasthenia gravis-like syndrome, numbness, paresthesia, peripheral neuropathy, tremor, weakness

Ocular: Visual disturbances

Otic: Hearing impairment, hearing loss (associated with persistently increased serum concentrations; early toxicity usually affects high-pitched sound), tinnitus

Renal: BUN increased, casts (hyaline, granular) in urine, creatinine clearance decreased, distal tubular dysfunction, Fanconi-like syndrome (high dose, prolonged course) (infants and adults), oliguria, renal failure (high trough serum concentrations), polyuria, proteinuria, serum creatinine increased, tubular necrosis, urine specific gravity decreased

Respiratory: Dyspnea, laryngeal edema, pulmonary fibrosis, respiratory depression

Miscellaneous: Allergic reaction, anaphylaxis, anaphylactoid reactions

Drug Interactions

Metabolism/Transport Effects None known.

Avoid Concomitant Use

Avoid concomitant use of Gentamicin (Systemic) with any of the following: Agalsidase Alfa; Agalsidase Beta; BCG; Mannitol

Increased Effect/Toxicity

Gentamicin (Systemic) may increase the levels/effects of: AbobotulinumtoxinA; Bisphosphonate Derivatives; CARBOplatin; Colistimethate; CycloSPORINE (Systemic); Neuromuscular-Blocking Agents; OnabotulinumtoxinA; RimabotulinumtoxinB; Tenofovir

The levels/effects of Gentamicin (Systemic) may be increased by: Amphotericin B; Capreomycin; Cephalosporins (2nd Generation); Cephalosporins (3rd Generation); Cephalosporins (4th Generation); CISplatin; Loop Diuretics; Mannitol; Nonsteroidal Anti-Inflammatory Agents; Tenofovir; Vancomycin

Decreased Effect

Gentamicin (Systemic) may decrease the levels/effects of: Agalsidase Alfa; Agalsidase Beta; BCG; Sodium Picosulfate; Typhoid Vaccine

The levels/effects of Gentamicin (Systemic) may be decreased by: Penicillins

Stability Store at 20°C to 25°C (68°F to 77°F).

Premix solution: Do not freeze.

Mechanism of Action Interferes with bacterial protein synthesis by binding to 30S and 50S ribosomal subunits resulting in a defective bacterial cell membrane

Pharmacodynamics Displays concentration-dependent killing; bacteriocidal

Pharmacokinetics (Adult data unless noted)

Absorption:

Oral: Poorly absorbed (<2%)

Intramuscular: Rapid and complete

Distribution: Primarily in the extracellular fluid volume and in most tissues; poor penetration into CSF; drug accumulates in the renal cortex; small amounts distribute into bile, sputum, saliva, and tears

V_d: Higher in neonates than older pediatric patients; also increased in patients with edema, ascites, fluid overload; decreased in patients with dehydration:

Neonates: 0.45 ± 0.1 L/kg

Infants: 0.4 ± 0.1 L/kg

Children: 0.35 ± 0.15 L/kg

Adolescents: 0.3 ± 0.1 L/kg

Adults: 0.2-0.3 L/kg

Protein binding: <30%

Half-life:

Neonates:

<1 week: 3-11.5 hours

1 week to 1 month: 3-6 hours

Infants: 4 ± 1 hour

Children: 2 ± 1 hour

Adolescents: 1.5 ± 1 hour

Adults with normal renal function: 1.5-3 hours

Anuria: 36-70 hours

Time to peak serum concentration:

I.M.: Within 30-90 minutes

I.V.: 30 minutes after 30-minute infusion; **Note:** Distribution may be prolonged after larger doses. One study reported a 1.7-hour distribution period after a 60-minute, high-dose aminoglycoside infusion (Demczar, 1997).

Elimination: Clearance is directly related to renal function; eliminated almost completely by glomerular filtration of unchanged drug with excretion into urine

Clearance:

Neonates: 0.045 ± 0.01 L/hour/kg

Infants: 0.1 ± 0.05 L/hour/kg

Children: 0.1 ± 0.03 L/hour/kg

Adolescents: 0.09 ± 0.03 L/hour/kg

Dialyzable (50% to 100%)

Dosing: Neonatal Note: Dosage should be based on actual weight unless the patient has hydrops fetalis. Dosage should be individualized based upon serum concentration monitoring.

General dosing; susceptible infection: I.V.: Extended-interval dosing strategies may vary by institution as a wide variety of dosing regimens have been studied. Consider single-dose administration with serum concentration monitoring in patients with urine output <1 mL/kg/hour or serum creatinine >1.3 mg/dL rather than scheduled dosing. Consider prolongation of dosing interval when coadministered with ibuprofen or indomethacin or in neonates with history of the following: Birth depression, birth hypoxia/asphyxia, or cyanotic congenital heart disease. Some dosing based on tobramycin studies.

Age-directed dosing (de Hoog, 2002; DiCenzo, 2003; Hagen, 2009; Hansen, 2003; Ohler, 2000; Serane, 2009):
GA <32 weeks: 4-5 mg/kg/dose every 48 hours
GA 32-36 weeks: 4-5 mg/kg/dose every 36 hours
GA ≥37 weeks: 4-5 mg/kg/dose every 24 hours
Note: In some trials, a fixed interval of every 24 hours was used with dosages ranging from 2.5-4 mg/kg/dose based on GA (ie, lower doses were used for younger GA).

Weight-directed dosing (*Red Book* 2012): I.M., I.V.:
Body weight <1 kg:
PNA ≤14 days: 5 mg/kg/dose every 48 hours
PNA 15-28 days: 4-5 mg/kg/dose every 24-48 hours
Body weight 1-2 kg:
PNA ≤7 days: 5 mg/kg/dose every 48 hours
PNA 8-28 days: 4-5 mg/kg/dose every 24-48 hours
Body weight >2 kg:
PNA ≤7 days: 4 mg/kg/dose every 24 hours
PNA 8-28 days: 4 mg/kg/dose every 12-24 hours

ECMO, initial dosing in full-term neonates: I.V.: Initial dose: 2.5-3 mg/kg/dose every 18-24 hours; some experts recommend a higher initial dose of 5 mg/kg/dose; subsequent doses should be individualized by monitoring serum drug concentrations; when ECMO is discontinued, dosage may require readjustment due to large shifts in body water (Buck, 2003; Southgate, 1989)

CNS infection (VP-shunt infection, ventriculitis): Limited information available: Intraventricular/intrathecal **(use a preservative free preparation):** 1 mg/**day** (Tunkel, 2004)

NEC, prevention: Limited data available; efficacy results variable: Oral: 2.5 mg/kg/dose every 6 hours beginning at birth and continued for 1 week was used in 22 neonates at high risk for the development of NEC (including prematurity, asphyxia, use of a UAC); results showed significant decrease in incidence of NEC with treatment group compared to placebo (Bury, 2001; Grylack, 1978); due to risk of resistant bacteria development, clinical benefits and risk with use should be evaluated prior to use. Further studies are needed.

Surgical prophylaxis: I.V.: 2.5-3 mg/kg as a single dose (*Red Book*, 2012)

Dosing: Usual Note: Dosage should be based on an estimate of ideal body weight. In morbidly obese children, adolescents, and adults, dosage requirement may best be estimated using a dosing weight of IBW + 0.4 (TBW - IBW). Dosage should be individualized based upon serum concentration monitoring.

Infants, Children, and Adolescents: **Note:** Some dosing is based on tobramycin studies:
General dosing:
Conventional dosing: I.M., I.V.: 2.5 mg/kg/dose every 8 hours; some pediatric patients may require larger doses (ie, patients undergoing continuous hemofiltration, patients with major burns, febrile granulocytopenic patients); modify dose based on individual patient requirements as determined by renal function, serum drug concentrations, and patient-specific clinical parameters
Manufacturer's recommendations: I.M., I.V.:
Infants: 2.5 mg/kg/dose every 8 hours
Children: 2-2.5 mg/kg/dose every 8 hours
Extended-interval dosing: I.V.:
Weight-directed: 4.5-7.5 mg/kg/dose every 24 hours in patients with normal renal function (Contopoulos-Ioannidis, 2004; *Red Book*, 2012)
Age-directed: Based on data from 114 patients, the following has been suggested (McDade, 2010):
3 months to <2 years: 9.5 mg/kg/dose every 24 hours
2 to <8 years: 8.5 mg/kg/dose every 24 hours
≥8 years: 7 mg/kg/dose every 24 hours

CNS infection:
Meningitis (Tunkel, 2004):
Infants and Children: I.V. 7.5 mg/kg/**day** divided every 8 hours
Adolescents: I.V.: 5 mg/kg/**day** divided every 8 hours
VP-shunt infection, ventriculitis: Limited data available:
Intraventricular/intrathecal **(use a preservative free preparation)** (Tunkel, 2004):
Infants >3 months and Children: 1-2 mg/**day**
Adults: 4-8 mg/**day**

Cystic fibrosis, pulmonary infection:
Conventional dosing: I.M., I.V.: 3.3 mg/kg/dose every 8 hours
Extended-interval dosing: I.V.: 10-12 mg/kg/dose every 24 hours (Flume, 2009; Van Meter, 2009); **Note:** The CF Foundation recommends extended-interval dosing as preferred over conventional dosing.

Endocarditis, treatment: I.M., I.V.: 3 mg/kg/**day** divided into 1-3 doses in combination with other antibiotics dependent upon organism and source of infection (ie, valve-type) (Baddour, 2007; Liu, 2011)

Intra-abdominal infection, complicated: I.V.: 3-7.5 mg/kg/**day** divided every 8-24 hours (Solomkin, 2010)

Peritonitis (CAPD) (Warady, 2012): Intraperitoneal:
Intermittent:
Anuric: 0.6 mg/kg/dose every 24 hours in the long dwell
Nonanuric: 0.75 mg/kg/dose every 24 hours in the long dwell
Continuous: Loading dose: 8 mg per liter of dialysate; maintenance dose: 4 mg per liter

Surgical prophylaxis: I.V.:
AAP recommendations (*Red Book*, 2012): 2 mg/kg as a single dose
ASHP recommendation, endorsed by IDSA (Bratzler, 2013): Children and Adolescents: 2.5 mg/kg as a single dose

UTI: Extended-interval dosing: I.V.: Based on data from 179 patients, the following age-directed dosing has been suggested (Carapetis, 2001):
1 month to <5 years: 7.5 mg/kg/dose every 24 hours
5-10 years: 6 mg/kg/dose every 24 hours
>10 years: 4.5 mg/kg/dose every 24 hours

Adults: **General dosing, susceptible infection:**
Conventional: I.M., I.V.: 1-2.5 mg/kg/dose every 8-12 hours; to ensure adequate peak concentrations early in therapy, higher initial dosage may be considered in selected patients when extracellular water is increased (edema, septic shock, postsurgical, or trauma)
Once daily: I.V.: 4-7 mg/kg/dose once daily; some clinicians recommend this approach for all patients with normal renal function; this dose is at least as efficacious with similar, if not less, toxicity than conventional dosing

Dosing adjustment in renal impairment:
Infants, Children, and Adolescents: I.M., I.V.:
The following adjustments have been recommended (Aronoff, 2007): **Note:** Renally adjusted dose recommendations are based on doses of 2.5 mg/kg/dose every 8 hours:
GFR >50 mL/minute/1.73 m^2: No adjustment required
GFR 30-50 mL/minute/1.73 m^2: Administer every 12-18 hours
GFR 10-29 mL/minute/1.73 m^2: Administer every 18-24 hours
GFR <10 mL/minute/1.73 m^2: Administer every 48-72 hours
Intermittent hemodialysis: 2 mg/kg/dose; redose as indicated by serum concentration
Peritoneal dialysis (PD): 2 mg/kg/dose; redose as indicated by serum concentration

Continuous renal replacement therapy (CRRT): 2-2.5 mg/kg/dose every 12-24 hours, monitor serum concentrations

Adults:

Conventional dosing:
CrCl ≥60 mL/minute: Administer every 8 hours
CrCl 40-60 mL/minute: Administer every 12 hours
CrCl 20-40 mL/minute: Administer every 24 hours
CrCl <20 mL/minute: Loading dose, then monitor concentrations
High-dose therapy: Interval may be extended (eg, every 48 hours) in patients with moderate renal impairment (CrCl 30-59 mL/minute) and/or adjusted based on serum concentration determinations

Intermittent hemodialysis (IHD) (administer after hemodialysis on dialysis days) (Heintz, 2009): Dialyzable (~50%; variable; dependent on filter, duration, and type of IHD; **Note:** Dosing dependent on the assumption of 3 times/week, complete IHD sessions:
Loading dose: 2-3 mg/kg loading dose followed by:
Mild UTI or synergy: 1 mg/kg every 48-72 hours; consider redosing for pre-HD or post-HD serum concentrations <1 mcg/mL
Moderate to severe UTI: 1-1.5 mg/kg every 48-72 hours; consider redosing for pre-HD serum concentrations <1.5-2 mcg/mL or post-HD concentrations <1 mcg/mL
Systemic gram-negative rod infection: 1.5-2 mg/kg every 48-72 hours; consider redosing for pre-HD serum concentrations <3-5 mcg/mL or post-HD concentrations <2 mcg/mL

Peritoneal dialysis (PD):
Administration via PD fluid:
Gram-positive infection (eg, synergy): 3-4 mg/L (3-4 mcg/mL) of PD fluid
Gram-negative infection: 4-8 mg/L (4-8 mcg/mL) of PD fluid
Administration via I.V., I.M. route during PD: Dose as for CrCl <10 mL/minute and follow serum concentrations

Continuous renal replacement therapy (CRRT) (Heintz, 2009; Trotman, 2005): Drug clearance is highly dependent on the method of renal replacement, filter type, and flow rate. Appropriate dosing requires close monitoring of pharmacologic response, signs of adverse reactions due to drug accumulation, as well as drug concentrations in relation to target trough (if appropriate). The following are general recommendations only (based on dialysate flow/ultrafiltration rates of 1-2 L/hour and minimal residual renal function) and should not supersede clinical judgment:
CVVH/CVVHD/CVVHDF: Loading dose of 2-3 mg/kg followed by:
Mild UTI or synergy: 1 mg/kg every 24-36 hours (redose when serum concentration <1 mcg/mL)
Moderate to severe UTI: 1-1.5 mg/kg every 24-36 hours (redose when serum concentration <1.5-2 mcg/mL)
Systemic gram-negative infection: 1.5-2.5 mg/kg every 24-48 hours (redose when serum concentration <3-5 mcg/mL)

Administration

I.M.: Administer undiluted by deep I.M. route. Slower absorption and lower peak concentrations, probably due to poor circulation in the atrophic muscle, may occur following I.M. injection; in paralyzed patients, suggest I.V. route.

I.V.: Administer by slow intermittent infusion over 30-60 minutes (administer higher doses over 60 minutes) or by direct injection over 15 minutes; final concentration for I.V. administration should not exceed 10 mg/mL; administer beta-lactams at least 1 hour before or after

gentamicin; simultaneous administration may result in reduced antibacterial efficacy

Monitoring Parameters

Urinalysis, urine output, BUN, serum creatinine, peak and trough serum gentamicin concentrations, hearing test especially for those at risk for ototoxicity or who will be receiving prolonged therapy (>2 weeks), CBC with differential

With conventional dosing, typically obtain serum concentration after the third dose; exceptions for earlier monitoring may include neonates or patients with rapidly changing renal function. With extended-interval dosing, usually obtain serum concentration after first, second, or third dose.

Not all infants and children who receive aminoglycosides require monitoring of serum aminoglycoside concentrations. Indications for use of aminoglycoside serum concentration monitoring include:
Treatment course >5 days
Patients with decreased or changing renal function
Patients with poor therapeutic response
Neonates and Infants <3 months of age
Atypical body constituency (obesity, expanded extracellular fluid volume)
Clinical need for higher doses or shorter intervals (eg, cystic fibrosis, burns, endocarditis, meningitis, critically ill patients, relatively resistant organism)
Patients on hemodialysis or chronic ambulatory peritoneal dialysis
Signs of nephrotoxicity or ototoxicity
Concomitant use of other nephrotoxic agents

Reference Range

Conventional dosing: Timing of serum samples: Draw peak 30 minutes after 30-minute infusion has been completed or 1 hour following I.M. injection or beginning of infusion; draw trough immediately before next dose
Therapeutic concentrations:
Peak:
Serious infections: 6-8 mcg/mL (12-17 micromole/L)
Life-threatening infections: 8-10 mcg/mL (17-21 micromole/L)
Urinary tract infections: 4-6 mcg/mL
Synergy against gram-positive organisms: 3-5 mcg/mL
Trough:
Serious infections: 0.5-1 mcg/mL
Life-threatening infections: 1-2 mcg/mL
The American Thoracic Society (ATS) recommends trough levels of <1 mcg/mL for adult patients with hospital-acquired pneumonia.

Extended-interval: Note: Pediatric therapeutic monitoring protocols have not been standardized; peak values are 2-3 times greater with extended-interval dosing regimens compared to conventional dosing
Noncystic fibrosis patients: Consider monitoring serum concentration 18-20 hours after the start of the infusion to ensure the drug-free interval does not exceed typical postantibiotic effect (PAE) duration.
Cystic fibrosis patients: Clinically two methods are utilized. Peak: 25-35 mcg/mL (some centers use 20-30 mcg/mL); 18- to 20-hour value: Detectable but <1 mcg/mL; trough: Nondetectable
Method A: Obtain two serum concentrations at least 1 half-life apart after distribution is complete (eg, obtain a serum concentration 2 hours and 10 hours after the start of the infusion), calculate elimination rate and extrapolate C_{max} and C_{min}
Method B: Obtain a peak serum concentration 60 minutes after a 60-minute infusion and a serum concentration 18-20 hours after the start of the infusion to ensure the drug-free interval does not exceed typical postantibiotic effect (PAE) duration (4-6 hours)

Test Interactions Some penicillin derivatives may accelerate the degradation of aminoglycosides *in vitro*, leading to a potential underestimation of aminoglycoside serum concentration.

Additional Information Some penicillins (eg, carbenicillin, ticarcillin, and piperacillin) have been shown to inactivate aminoglycosides *in vitro*. This has been observed to a greater extent with tobramycin and gentamicin, while amikacin has shown greater stability against inactivation. Concurrent use of these agents may pose a risk of reduced antibacterial efficacy in vivo, particularly in the setting of profound renal impairment; however, definitive clinical evidence is lacking. If combination penicillin/aminoglycoside therapy is desired in a patient with renal dysfunction, separation of doses (if feasible), and routine monitoring of aminoglycoside levels, CBC, and clinical response should be considered.

Dosage Forms Excipient information presented when available (limited, particularly for generics); consult specific product labeling.

Solution, Injection:

Generic: 10 mg/mL (2 mL); 40 mg/mL (2 mL, 20 mL)

Solution, Injection [preservative free]:

Generic: 10 mg/mL (2 mL)

Solution, Intravenous:

Generic: 60 mg (50 mL); 70 mg (50 mL); 80 mg (50 mL, 100 mL); 90 mg (100 mL); 100 mg (50 mL, 100 mL); 120 mg (100 mL); 10 mg/mL (6 mL, 8 mL, 10 mL)

References

American Academy of Pediatrics (AAP). In: Pickering LK, Baker CJ, Kimberlin DW, Long SS, eds. *Red Book: 2012 Report of the Committee on Infectious Diseases.* 29th ed. Elk Grove Village, IL: American Academy of Pediatrics; 2012.

Aronoff GR, Bennett WM, Berns JS, et al, *Drug Prescribing in Renal Failure: Dosing Guidelines for Adults and Children*, 5th ed, Philadelphia, PA: American College of Physicians, 2007.

Baddour LM, Wilson WR, Bayer AS, et al, "Infective Endocarditis: Diagnosis, Antimicrobial Therapy, and Management of Complications: A Statement for Healthcare Professionals From the Committee on Rheumatic Fever, Endocarditis, and Kawasaki Disease, Council on Cardiovascular Disease in the Young, and the Councils on Clinical Cardiology, Stroke, and Cardiovascular Surgery and Anesthesia, American Heart Association: Endorsed by the Infectious Diseases Society of America," *Circulation*, 2005, 111(23):e394-434.

Bhatt-Mehta V, Johnson CE, and Schumacher RE, "Gentamicin Pharmacokinetics in Term Neonates Receiving Extracorporeal Membrane Oxygenation," *Pharmacotherapy*, 1992, 12(1):28-32.

Bratzler DW, Dellinger EP, Olsen KM, et al, "Clinical Practice Guidelines for Antimicrobial Prophylaxis in Surgery," *Am J Health Syst Pharm*, 2013, 70(3):195-283.

Buck ML, "Pharmacokinetic Changes During Extracorporeal Membrane Oxygenation: Implications for Drug Therapy of Neonates," *Clin Pharmacokinet*, 2003, 42(5):403-17.

Bury RG and Tudehope D, "Enteral Antibiotics for Preventing Necrotizing Enterocolitis in Low Birthweight or Preterm Infants," *Cochrane Database Syst Rev*, 2001, (1):CD000405.

Carapetis JR, Jaquiery AL, Buttery JP, et al, "Randomized, Controlled Trial Comparing Once Daily and Three Times Daily Gentamicin in Children With Urinary Tract Infections," *Pediatr Infect Dis J*, 2001, 20 (3):240-6.

Contopoulos-Ioannidis DG, Giotis ND, Baliatsa DV, et al, "Extended-Interval Aminoglycoside Administration for Children: A Meta-Analysis," *Pediatrics*, 2004, 114(1):e111-8.

de Hoog M, Mouton JW, Schoemaker RC, et al, "Extended-Interval Dosing of Tobramycin in Neonates: Implications for Therapeutic Drug Monitoring," *Clin Pharmacol Ther*, 2002, 71(5):349-58.

Demczar DJ, Nafziger AN, and Bertino JS Jr, "Pharmacokinetics of Gentamicin at Traditional Versus High Doses: Implications for Once-Daily Aminoglycoside Dosing," *Antimicrob Agents Chemother*, 1997, 41(5):1115-9.

DiCenzo R, Forrest A, Slish JC, et al, "A Gentamicin Pharmacokinetic Population Model and Once-Daily Dosing Algorithm for Neonates," *Pharmacotherapy*, 2003, 23(5):585-91.

Flume PA, Mogayzel PJ Jr, Robinson KA, et al, "Cystic Fibrosis Pulmonary Guidelines: Treatment of Pulmonary Exacerbations," *Am J Respir Crit Care Med*, 2009, 180(9):802-8.

Gilbert DN, "Once-Daily Aminoglycoside Therapy," *Antimicrob Agents Chemother*, 1991, 35(3):399-405.

Grylack LJ and Scanlon JW, "Oral Gentamicin Therapy in the Prevention of Neonatal Necrotizing Enterocolitis. A Controlled Double-Blind Trial," *Am J Dis Child*, 1978, 132(12):1192-4.

Hagen I and Øymar K, "Pharmacological Differences Between Once Daily and Twice Daily Gentamicin Dosage in Newborns With Suspected Sepsis," *Pharm World Sci*, 2009, 31(1):18-23.

Hansen A, Forbes P, Arnold A, et al, "Once-Daily Gentamicin Dosing for the Preterm and Term Newborn: Proposal for a Simple Regimen That Achieves Target Levels," *J Perinatol*, 2003, 23(8):635-9.

Heintz BH, Matzke GR, and Dager WE, "Antimicrobial Dosing Concepts and Recommendations for Critically Ill Adult Patients Receiving Continuous Renal Replacement Therapy or Intermittent Hemodialysis," *Pharmacotherapy*, 2009, 29(5):562-77.

Knoderer CA, Everett JA, and Buss WF, "Clinical Issues Surrounding Once-Daily Aminoglycoside Dosing in Children," *Pharmacotherapy*, 2003, 23(1):44-56.

Kraus DM, Pai MP, and Rodvold KA, "Efficacy and Tolerability of Extended-Interval Aminoglycoside Administration in Pediatric Patients," *Paediatr Drugs*, 2002, 4(7):469-84.

Liu C, Bayer A, Cosgrove SE, et al, "Clinical Practice Guidelines by the Infectious Diseases Society of America for the Treatment of Methicillin-Resistant *Staphylococcus aureus* Infections in Adults and Children," *Clin Infect Dis*, 2011, 52(3):e18-55.

McDade EJ, Wagner JL, Moffett BS, et al, "Once-Daily Gentamicin Dosing in Pediatric Patients Without Cystic Fibrosis," *Pharmacotherapy*, 2010, 30(3):248-53.

Ohler KH, Menke JA, and Fuller L, "Use of Higher Dose Extended Interval Aminoglycosides in a Neonatal Intensive Care Unit," *Am J Perinatol*, 2000, 17(6):285-90.

Reimche LD, Rooney ME, Hindmarsh KW, et al, "An Evaluation of Gentamicin Dosing According to Renal Function in Neonates With Suspected Sepsis," *Am J Perinatol*, 1987, 4(3):262-5.

Serane TV, Zengeya S, Penford G, et al, "Once Daily Dose Gentamicin in Neonates - Is Our Dosing Correct?" *Acta Paediatr*, 2009, 98 (7):1100-5.

Shevchuk YM and Taylor DM, "Aminoglycoside Volume of Distribution in Pediatric Patients," *DICP*, 1989, 33(6):817-9.

Solomkin JS, Mazuski JE, Bradley JS, et al, "Diagnosis and Management of Complicated Intra-abdominal Infections in Adults and Children: Guidelines by the Surgical Infection Society and the Infectious Diseases Society of America," *Clin Infect Dis*, 2010, 50(2):133-64.

Southgate WM, DiPiro JT, and Robertson AF, "Pharmacokinetics of Gentamicin in Neonates on Extracorporeal Membrane Oxygenation," *Antimicrob Agents Chemother*, 1989, 33(6):817-9.

Trotman RL, Williamson JC, Shoemaker DM, et al, "Antibiotic Dosing in Critically Ill Adult Patients Receiving Continuous Renal Replacement Therapy," *Clin Infect Dis*, 2005, 41(8):1159-66.

Tunkel AR, Hartman BJ, Kaplan SL, et al, "Practice Guidelines for the Management of Bacterial Meningitis," *Clin Infect Dis*, 2004, 39 (9):1267-84.

Van den Anker, JN, personal communication, June, 2011.

Van Meter DJ, Corriveau M, Ahern JW, et al, "A Survey of Once-Daily Dosage Tobramycin Therapy in Patients With Cystic Fibrosis," *Pediatr Pulmonol*, 2009, 44(4):325-9.

Warady BA, Bakkaloglu S, Newland J, et al, "Consensus Guidelines for the Prevention and Treatment of Catheter-Related Infections and Peritonitis in Pediatric Patients Receiving Peritoneal Dialysis: 2012 Update," *Perit Dial Int*, 2012, (32 Suppl 2):S32-86.

Gentamicin (Ophthalmic) (jen ta MYE sin)

Medication Safety Issues

Sound-alike/look-alike issues:

Gentamicin may be confused with gentian violet, kanamycin, vancomycin

Brand Names: U.S. Garamycin; Gentak

Brand Names: Canada Diogent®; Garamycin®; Gentak®; Gentocin; PMS-Gentamicin

Therapeutic Category Antibiotic, Aminoglycoside; Antibiotic, Ophthalmic

Generic Availability (U.S.) Yes

Use Topical treatment of ophthalmic infections caused by susceptible bacteria (FDA approved in ages ≥1 month and adults)

Pregnancy Risk Factor C

Pregnancy Considerations Adverse events were observed following systemic administration of gentamicin in animal reproduction studies; therefore, gentamicin ophthalmic is classified as pregnancy category C. The amount of gentamicin available systemically following application of the ophthalmic drops is below the limit of detection (<0.5 mcg/mL). Systemic absorption would be required in order for gentamicin to cross the placenta and reach the fetus. When administered I.M. or I.V., gentamicin crosses the placenta. Refer to the Gentamicin (Systemic) monograph for details.

Breast-Feeding Considerations When administered I.M., gentamicin is detected in breast milk. The portion that reaches the maternal milk would then be poorly absorbed by the infant's gastrointestinal tract. Refer to the Gentamicin (Systemic) monograph for details. The amount of gentamicin available systemically following application of the ophthalmic drops is below the limit of detection (<0.5 mcg/mL).

Contraindications Hypersensitivity to gentamicin, any component, or other aminoglycosides

Warnings Solution is not for injection into the eye, including the anterior chamber of the eye, nor for subconjunctival injection. Topical use has been associated with local sensitization (redness, irritation); discontinue if sensitization is noted. Prolonged use may result in fungal or bacterial superinfection; if purulent discharge, inflammation, or pain are increased, therapy should be reevaluated. Not intended for long-term therapy. Ointment may delay corneal healing. Ointment should not be used for routine prophylaxis for ophthalmia neonatorum due to recent reports of severe ocular reactions described as eyelid erythema and swelling, ocular discharge, and periocular blistering, typically reported within 48 hours after administration (Binenbaum, 2010; Nathawad, 2011).

Adverse Reactions

Ophthalmic: Burning, irritation

Rare but important or life-threatening: Allergic reaction, corneal ulceration, hallucinations, purpura, thrombocytopenia

Drug Interactions

Metabolism/Transport Effects None known.

Avoid Concomitant Use There are no known interactions where it is recommended to avoid concomitant use.

Increased Effect/Toxicity There are no known significant interactions involving an increase in effect.

Decreased Effect There are no known significant interactions involving a decrease in effect.

Stability

Ointment: Store at 2°C to 30°C (36°F to 86°F)

Solution: Store at 20°C to 25°C (68°F to 77°F); avoid exposure to excessive heat.

Mechanism of Action Interferes with bacterial protein synthesis by binding to 30S and 50S ribosomal subunits resulting in a defective bacterial cell membrane

Pharmacokinetics (Adult data unless noted) Absorption: Ophthalmic drops: Systemic absorption: Undetected (<0.5 mcg/mL)

Dosing: Neonatal Ophthalmic infections: Limited data available: Ophthalmic:

Ointment: Apply 2-3 times daily; **Note:** Use should be reserved for treatment of susceptible infection and not routine prophylaxis for ophthalmia neonatorum.

Solution: Instill 1-2 drops every 4 hours; up to 2 drops every hour for severe infections

Dosing: Usual

Infants, Children, and Adolescents: **Ophthalmic infections:** Ophthalmic:

Ointment: Instill ½ inch (1.25 cm) 2-3 times daily

Solution: Instill 1-2 drops every 4 hours; up to 2 drops every hour for severe infections

Adults: **Ophthalmic infections:** Ophthalmic:

Ointment: Instill ½ inch (1.25 cm) 2-3 times daily

Solution: Instill 1-2 drops every 4 hours; up to 2 drops every hour for severe infections

Dosing adjustment in renal impairment: There are no dosage adjustments provided in the manufacturer's labeling; however, dosage adjustment unlikely necessary due to low systemic absorption.

Dosing adjustment in hepatic impairment: There are no dosage adjustments provided in the manufacturer's

labeling; however, dosage adjustment unlikely necessary due to low systemic absorption.

Administration Gentamicin solution is not for subconjunctival injection. Solution may be instilled into the affected eye or a small amount of ointment may be placed into the conjunctival sac. Avoid contaminating tip of the solution bottle or ointment tube.

Solution: Apply finger pressure to lacrimal sac during and for 1-2 minutes after instillation to decrease risk of absorption and systemic effects

Dosage Forms Excipient information presented when available (limited, particularly for generics); consult specific product labeling.

Ointment, Ophthalmic:

Garamycin: 0.3% (3.5 g)

Gentak: 0.3% (3.5 g) [contains methylparaben, propylparaben]

Generic: 0.3% (3.5 g)

Solution, Ophthalmic:

Garamycin: 0.3% (5 mL) [contains benzalkonium chloride]

Generic: 0.3% (5 mL, 15 mL)

References

Binenbaum G, Bruno CJ, Forbes BJ, et al, "Periocular Ulcerative Dermatitis Associated With Gentamicin Ointment Prophylaxis in Newborns," *J Pediatr*, 2010, 156(2):320-1.

Bras JF and Coyle-Gilchrist MM, "Genticin in Conjunctivitis and Keratitis," *Br J Ophthalmol*, 1968, 52(7):560-1.

Nathawad R, Mendez H, Ahmad A, et al, "Severe Ocular Reactions After Neonatal Ocular Prophylaxis With Gentamicin Ophthalmic Ointment," *Pediatr Infect Dis J*, 2011, 30(2):175-6.

Gentamicin (Topical) (jen ta MYE sin)

Medication Safety Issues

Sound-alike/look-alike issues:

Gentamicin may be confused with gentian violet, kanamycin, vancomycin

Brand Names: Canada PMS-Gentamicin; ratio-Gentamicin

Therapeutic Category Antibiotic, Aminoglycoside; Antibiotic, Topical

Generic Availability (U.S.) Yes

Use Used to treat superficial infections of the skin including folliculitis, impetigo contagiosa, furunculosis, sycosis barbae, ecthyma, pyoderma gangrenosum, infectious eczematoid dermatitits, pustular acne, pustular psoriasis, infected seborrheic dermatitits or contact dermatitis, and infected excoriations (FDA approved for ages >1 year and adults)

Pregnancy Considerations When administered I.M. or I.V., gentamicin crosses the placenta and produces detectable serum levels in the fetus. Refer to the Gentamicin (Systemic) monograph for details. Systemic absorption following topical application would be required in order for gentamicin to cross the placenta and reach the fetus. Gentamicin is measurable in the serum following topical application to burn patients.

Breast-Feeding Considerations When administered I.M., gentamicin enters breast milk; however, it is not well absorbed when taken orally. Refer to the Gentamicin (Systemic) monograph for details.

Contraindications Hypersensitivity to gentamicin, any component, or other aminoglycosides

Warnings Prolonged use may result in fungal or bacterial superinfection; discontinue if superinfection is noted. Topical use has been associated with local sensitization (redness, irritation); discontinue if sensitization is noted. Not intended for long-term therapy.

Adverse Reactions Dermatologic: Erythema, pruritus

Drug Interactions

Metabolism/Transport Effects None known.

◀

Avoid Concomitant Use
Avoid concomitant use of Gentamicin (Topical) with any of the following: BCG

Increased Effect/Toxicity There are no known significant interactions involving an increase in effect.

Decreased Effect
Gentamicin (Topical) may decrease the levels/effects of: BCG; Sodium Picosulfate

Stability Store at room temperature.

Mechanism of Action Interferes with bacterial protein synthesis by binding to 30S and 50S ribosomal subunits resulting in a defective bacterial cell membrane

Dosing: Usual Infants, Children, and Adults: Apply 3-4 times/day

Administration Apply a small amount gently to the cleansed affected area

Test Interactions Some penicillin derivatives may accelerate the degradation of aminoglycosides *in vitro*, leading to a potential underestimation of aminoglycoside serum concentration.

Dosage Forms Excipient information presented when available (limited, particularly for generics); consult specific product labeling.

Cream, External:
  Generic: 0.1% (15 g, 30 g)
Ointment, External:
  Generic: 0.1% (15 g, 30 g)

◆ **Gentamicin and Prednisolone** *see* Prednisolone and Gentamicin *on page 1731*

◆ **Gentamicin Injection, USP (Can)** *see* Gentamicin (Systemic) *on page 962*

◆ **Gentamicin Sulfate** *see* Gentamicin (Ophthalmic) *on page 966*

◆ **Gentamicin Sulfate** *see* Gentamicin (Systemic) *on page 962*

Gentian Violet (JEN shun VYE oh let)

Medication Safety Issues
Sound-alike/look-alike issues:
Gentian violet may be confused with gentamicin

Therapeutic Category Antibacterial, Topical; Antifungal Agent, Topical

Generic Availability (U.S.) Yes

Use Treatment of cutaneous or mucocutaneous infections caused by *Candida albicans* and other superficial skin infections refractory to topical nystatin, clotrimazole, miconazole, or econazole

Breast-Feeding Considerations Due to the potential for serious adverse reactions in the nursing infant, breast-feeding is not recommended; safer alternatives for topical skin infections are available (Stoukides, 1993).

Contraindications Hypersensitivity to gentian violet; ulcerated areas; patients with porphyria

Warnings May result in staining of the skin when applied to granulation tissue; tracheitis may result from swallowing gentian violet solution, laryngeal obstruction following frequent or prolonged use

Adverse Reactions
Dermatologic: Necrotic skin reactions, staining, vesicle formation
Gastrointestinal: Esophagitis, gastrointestinal irritation, ulceration of mucous membranes
Genitourinary: Hemorrhagic cystitis
Local: Burning, irritation
Ocular: Keratoconjunctivitis
Respiratory: Epistaxis, laryngitis, laryngeal obstruction, tracheitis
Miscellaneous: Allergic contact dermatitis, sensitivity reactions

Drug Interactions
Metabolism/Transport Effects None known.
Avoid Concomitant Use
Avoid concomitant use of Gentian Violet with any of the following: BCG

Increased Effect/Toxicity There are no known significant interactions involving an increase in effect.

Decreased Effect
Gentian Violet may decrease the levels/effects of: BCG; Sodium Picosulfate

Mechanism of Action Topical antiseptic/germicide effective against some vegetative gram-positive bacteria, particularly *Staphylococcus* sp, and some yeast; it is much less effective against gram-negative bacteria and is ineffective against acid-fast bacteria

Dosing: Usual Topical: Oral candidiasis:
Infants: Apply to affected area (under tongue or on lesion) twice daily; solutions diluted to 0.25% to 0.5% may be less irritating.
Children and Adults: Apply to affected area once or twice daily; solutions diluted to 0.25% to 0.5% may be less irritating. Do not swallow.

Administration Topical: Apply to lesions with cotton; do not apply to ulcerative lesions on the face. Keep affected area dry and exposed to air.

Additional Information 0.25% or 0.5% solution is less irritating than a 1% to 2% solution and is reported to be as effective

Dosage Forms Excipient information presented when available (limited, particularly for generics); consult specific product labeling.
Solution, External:
  Generic: 1% (59 mL); 2% (59 mL)

References
Stoukides C, "Topical Medications and Breastfeeding," *J Hum Lact*, 1993, 9(3):185-7.

◆ **Gentle Laxative [OTC]** *see* Bisacodyl *on page 293*

◆ **Gentocin (Can)** *see* Gentamicin (Ophthalmic) *on page 966*

◆ **Gen-Triazolam (Can)** *see* Triazolam *on page 2080*

◆ **Geodon** *see* Ziprasidone *on page 2178*

◆ **Geri-Dryl [OTC]** *see* DiphenhydrAMINE (Systemic) *on page 673*

◆ **Geri-Hydrolac™ [OTC]** *see* Lactic Acid and Ammonium Hydroxide *on page 1191*

◆ **Geri-Hydrolac™-12 [OTC]** *see* Lactic Acid and Ammonium Hydroxide *on page 1191*

◆ **Geri-kot [OTC]** *see* Senna *on page 1877*

◆ **Geri-Mucil [OTC]** *see* Psyllium *on page 1773*

◆ **Geri-Stool [OTC]** *see* Docusate and Senna *on page 702*

◆ **Geri-Tussin [OTC]** *see* GuaiFENesin *on page 984*

◆ **GG** *see* GuaiFENesin *on page 984*

◆ **GI87084B** *see* Remifentanil *on page 1811*

◆ **Giazo** *see* Balsalazide *on page 261*

◆ **Glargine Insulin** *see* Insulin Glargine *on page 1121*

◆ **GlcCerase** *see* Velaglucerase Alfa *on page 2124*

◆ **Gleevec** *see* Imatinib *on page 1072*

◆ **Gliadel Wafer** *see* Carmustine *on page 382*

◆ **Gliadel Wafer® (Can)** *see* Carmustine *on page 382*

◆ **Glibenclamide** *see* GlyBURIDE *on page 974*

GlipiZIDE (GLIP i zide)

Medication Safety Issues
Sound-alike/look-alike issues:
GlipiZIDE may be confused with glimepiride, glyBURIDE

Glucotrol® may be confused with Glucophage®, Glucotrol® XL, glyBURIDE, GlycoTrol (dietary supplement)

High alert medication:
The Institute for Safe Medication Practices (ISMP) includes this medication among its list of drugs which have a heightened risk of causing significant patient harm when used in error.

Related Information
Medications for Which a Single Dose May Be Fatal When Ingested by a Toddler *on page 2408*
Oral Medications That Should Not Be Crushed or Altered *on page 2438*

Brand Names: U.S. GlipiZIDE XL; Glucotrol; Glucotrol XL

Therapeutic Category Antidiabetic Agent, Oral; Antidiabetic Agent, Sulfonylurea; Hypoglycemic Agent, Oral

Generic Availability (U.S.) Yes

Use Management of type II diabetes mellitus (noninsulin-dependent, NIDDM) when hyperglycemia cannot be managed by diet alone; may be used concomitantly with metformin or insulin to improve glycemic control

Pregnancy Risk Factor C

Pregnancy Considerations Adverse events have been observed in some animal reproduction studies. Glipizide was found to cross the placenta in vitro (Elliott, 1994). Severe hypoglycemia lasting 4-10 days has been noted in infants born to mothers taking a sulfonylurea at the time of delivery.

For women with diabetes, maternal hyperglycemia can be associated with adverse effects in the fetus, neonate, and mother. To prevent adverse events, prior to conception and throughout pregnancy, the maternal HbA_{1c} should be kept close to normal but without causing significant hypoglycemia. The use of most oral antihyperglycemic agents in pregnant women is not recommended for routine management of GDM or type 2 diabetes mellitus in pregnant women; insulin is the drug of choice for the control of diabetes mellitus during pregnancy (ACOG, 2005; ADA, 2013; Kitzmiller, 2008; Metzger, 2007). The manufacturer recommends if glipizide is used during pregnancy it should be discontinued at least 1 month before the expected delivery date.

Breast-Feeding Considerations Data from two mother-infant pairs note that glipizide was not detected in breast milk (Feig, 2005). Breast-feeding is encouraged for all women including those with diabetes; all types of insulin may be used while breast-feeding and some oral agents, including glipizide, may be acceptable for use as well (Metzger 2007). According to the manufacturer, due to the potential for hypoglycemia in the nursing infant, a decision should be made whether to discontinue nursing or to discontinue the drug, taking into account the importance of treatment to the mother.

Contraindications Hypersensitivity to glipizide or any component; type 1 diabetes mellitus (insulin-dependent, IDDM), diabetic ketoacidosis with or without coma

Warnings Product labeling states oral hypoglycemic drugs may be associated with an increased cardiovascular mortality as compared to treatment with diet alone or diet plus insulin; data to support this association are limited, and several studies, including a large prospective trial (UKPDS) have not supported an association.

Loss of efficacy may be observed following prolonged use as a result of the progression of type 2 diabetes mellitus which results in continued beta cell destruction. In patients who were previously responding to sulfonylurea therapy, consider additional factors which may be contributing to decreased efficacy (eg, inappropriate dose, nonadherence to diet and exercise regimen). If no contributing factors can be identified, consider discontinuing use of the sulfonylurea due to secondary failure of treatment. Additional antidiabetic therapy (eg, insulin) will be required. It may be necessary to discontinue therapy and administer insulin if the patient is exposed to stress (fever, trauma, infection, surgery).

Chemical similarities are present among sulfonamides, sulfonylureas, carbonic anhydrase inhibitors, thiazides, and loop diuretics (except ethacrynic acid); use in patients with sulfonamide allergy is not specifically contraindicated in product labeling; however, a risk of cross-reaction exists in patients with allergy to any of these compounds; avoid use when previous reaction has been severe

The extended release formulation consists of drug within a nondeformable matrix; following drug release/absorption, the matrix/shell is expelled in the stool. The use of nondeformable products in patients with known stricture/narrowing of the GI tract has been associated with symptoms of obstruction. Avoid use of extended release tablets (Glucotrol XL) in patients with severe gastrointestinal narrowing or esophageal dysmotility.

Precautions All sulfonylurea drugs are capable of producing severe hypoglycemia. Hypoglycemia is more likely to occur when caloric intake is deficient, after severe or prolonged exercise, when ethanol is ingested, or when more than one glucose-lowering drug is used. It is also more likely in elderly patients, malnourished patients, patients with adrenal or pituitary insufficiency, and in patients with impaired renal or hepatic function; use with caution. Autonomic neuropathy, advanced age, and concomitant use of beta-blockers or other sympatholytic agents may impair the patient's ability to recognize the signs and symptoms of hypoglycemia; use with caution.

Patients with G6PD deficiency may be at an increased risk of sulfonylurea-induced hemolytic anemia; however, cases have also been described in patients without G6PD deficiency during postmarketing surveillance; use with caution and consider a nonsulfonylurea alternative in patients with G6PD deficiency.

Adverse Reactions
Cardiovascular: Syncope
Central nervous system: Anxiety, depression, dizziness, drowsiness, headache, hypoesthesia, insomnia, nervousness, pain
Dermatologic: Eczema, erythema, maculopapular eruptions, morbilliform eruptions, pruritus, rash, urticaria
Endocrine & metabolic: Hypoglycemia
Gastrointestinal: Abdominal pain, constipation, diarrhea, dyspepsia, flatulence, nausea, vomiting
Hepatic: Alkaline phosphatase increased, AST increased, LDH increased
Neuromuscular & skeletal: Arthralgia, leg cramps, myalgia, paresthesia, tremor
Ocular: Blurred vision
Renal: Blood urea nitrogen increased, creatinine increased
Respiratory: Rhinitis
Miscellaneous: Diaphoresis
Rare but important or life-threatening: Agranulocytosis, anorexia, aplastic anemia, arrhythmia, blood in stool, cholestatic jaundice, conjunctivitis, disulfiram-like reaction, edema, gait instability, hemolytic anemia, hypertension, hypertonia, hyponatremia, jaundice, leukopenia, liver injury, migraine, pancytopenia, photosensitivity, porphyria, retinal hemorrhage, SIADH, thrombocytopenia, vertigo

Drug Interactions
Metabolism/Transport Effects Substrate of CYP2C9 (major); **Note:** Assignment of Major/Minor substrate status based on clinically relevant drug interaction potential

Avoid Concomitant Use There are no known interactions where it is recommended to avoid concomitant use.

Increased Effect/Toxicity

GlipiZIDE may increase the levels/effects of: Alcohol (Ethyl); Carbocisteine; Hypoglycemic Agents; Porfimer; Vitamin K Antagonists

The levels/effects of GlipiZIDE may be increased by: Androgens; Beta-Blockers; Ceritinib; Chloramphenicol; Cimetidine; Clarithromycin; Cyclic Antidepressants; CYP2C9 Inhibitors (Moderate); CYP2C9 Inhibitors (Strong); Fibric Acid Derivatives; Fluconazole; GLP-1 Agonists; Herbs (Hypoglycemic Properties); MAO Inhibitors; Metreleptin; Miconazole (Oral); Mifepristone; Pegvisomant; Posaconazole; Probenecid; Quinolone Antibiotics; Ranitidine; Salicylates; Selective Serotonin Reuptake Inhibitors; Sulfonamide Derivatives; Vitamin K Antagonists; Voriconazole

Decreased Effect

The levels/effects of GlipiZIDE may be decreased by: Colesevelam; Corticosteroids (Orally Inhaled); Corticosteroids (Systemic); CYP2C9 Inducers (Strong); Dabrafenib; Danazol; Loop Diuretics; Luteinizing Hormone-Releasing Hormone Analogs; Peginterferon Alfa-2b; Quinolone Antibiotics; Rifampin; Somatropin; Thiazide Diuretics

Food Interactions

Ethanol: May cause rare disulfiram reactions. Management: Monitor patients.

Food: A delayed release of insulin may occur if glipizide is taken with food. Management: Immediate release tablets should be administered 30 minutes before meals to avoid erratic absorption.

Stability Store at room temperature; protect from light

Mechanism of Action Stimulates insulin release from the pancreatic beta cells; reduces glucose output from the liver; insulin sensitivity is increased at peripheral target sites

Pharmacodynamics

Onset of action: Immediate release formulation: 15-30 minutes; extended release formulation: 2-3 hours

Maximum effect: Immediate release formulation: Within 2-3 hours; extended release formulation: 6-12 hours

Duration: Immediate release formulation: 12-24 hours; extended release formulation: 24 hours

Average decrease in fasting blood glucose (when used as monotherapy): 60-70 mg/dL

Pharmacokinetics (Adult data unless noted)

Absorption: Rapid and complete

Distribution: V_d: Adults: 10 L

Protein binding: 98% to 99%

Metabolism: Extensive liver metabolism to inactive metabolites

Bioavailability: 80% to 100%

Half-life: Adults: 2-5 hours

Time to peak serum concentration:

Immediate release formulation: 1-3 hours

Extended release formulation: 6-12 hours

Elimination: <10% of drug excreted into urine as unchanged drug; 90% of drug excreted as metabolites in urine and 10% excreted in feces

Dosing: Usual Adults: Oral:

Management of noninsulin-dependent diabetes mellitus in patients **previously untreated:** Initial: 5 mg/day immediate release or extended release tablets; adjust dosage in 2.5-5 mg daily increments in intervals of 3-7 days for immediate release tablets or 5 mg daily increments in intervals of at least 7 days for extended release tablets; if total daily dose for immediate release tablets is >15 mg, divide into twice daily dosage; maximum daily dose for immediate release tablets: 40 mg; maximum daily dose for extended release tablets: 20 mg

Note: Patients may be converted from immediate release tablets to extended release tablets by giving the nearest equivalent total daily dose once daily

Management of noninsulin-dependent diabetes mellitus in patients **previously maintained on insulin:**

Insulin dosage ≤20 units/day: Use recommended initial dose and abruptly discontinue insulin

Insulin dosage >20 units/day: Use recommended initial dose and reduce daily insulin dosage by 50%; continue to withdraw daily insulin dosage gradually over several days as tolerated with incremental increases of glipizide

Dosing adjustment/comments in renal impairment: CrCl <10 mL/minute: Some investigators recommend not using

Dosing adjustment in hepatic impairment: Reduce initial dosage to 2.5 mg/day

Administration Oral: Administer immediate release tablets 30 minutes before a meal; extended release tablets should be swallowed whole and administered with breakfast; do not cut, crush, or chew

Monitoring Parameters Signs and symptoms of hypoglycemia, fasting blood glucose, glycosylated hemoglobin (hemoglobin A_{1c})

Reference Range Target range:

Blood glucose: Fasting and preprandial: 80-120 mg/dL; bedtime: 100-140 mg/dL

Glycosylated hemoglobin (hemoglobin A_{1c}): <7%

Additional Information When transferring from other sulfonylurea antidiabetic agents to glyburide, with the exception of chlorpropamide, the administration of the other agent may be abruptly discontinued; due to the prolonged elimination half-life of chlorpropamide, a 2- to 3-day drug-free interval may be advisable before glipizide therapy is begun

Dosage Forms Excipient information presented when available (limited, particularly for generics); consult specific product labeling.

Tablet, Oral:

Glucotrol: 5 mg, 10 mg [scored]

Generic: 5 mg, 10 mg

Tablet Extended Release 24 Hour, Oral:

GlipiZIDE XL: 2.5 mg, 5 mg, 10 mg

Glucotrol XL: 2.5 mg, 5 mg, 10 mg

Generic: 2.5 mg, 5 mg, 10 mg

References

American College of Obstetricians and Gynecologists (ACOG) Committee on Practice Bulletins, "Clinical Management Guidelines for Obstetrician-Gynecologists. Number 60, March 2005. Progestational Diabetes Mellitus," *Obstet Gynecol*, 2005, 105(3):675-85.

American Diabetes Association, "Standards of Medical Care in Diabetes – 2013," *Diabetes Care*, 2013, 36(Suppl 1):11-66.

DeFronzo RA, "Pharmacologic Therapy for Type 2 Diabetes Mellitus," *Ann Intern Med*, 1999, 131(4):281-303.

Elliott BD, Schenker S, Langer O, et al, "Comparative Placental Transport of Oral Hypoglycemic Agents in Humans: A Model of Human Placental Drug Transfer," *Am J Obstet Gynecol*, 1994, 171(3):653-60.

Feig DS, Briggs GG, Kraemer JM, et al, "Transfer of Glyburide and Glipizide Into Breast Milk," *Diabetes Care*, 2005, 28(8):1851-5.

"Intensive Blood-Glucose Control With Sulphonylureas or Insulin Compared With Conventional Treatment and Risk of Complications in Patients With Type 2 Diabetes (UKPDS 33) UK Prospective Diabetes Study (UKPDS) Group," *Lancet*, 1998, 352(9131):837-53.

Kitzmiller JL, Block JM, Brown FM, et al, "Managing Preexisting Diabetes for Pregnancy: Summary of Evidence and Consensus Recommendations for Care," *Diabetes Care*, 2008, 31(5):1060-79.

Metzger BE, Buchanan TA, Coustan DR, et al, "Summary and Recommendations of the Fifth International Workshop-Conference on Gestational Diabetes Mellitus," *Diabetes Care*, 2007, 30(Suppl 2):S251-60.

◆ **GlipiZIDE XL** *see* GlipiZIDE *on page 968*

◆ **Glivec** *see* Imatinib *on page 1072*

◆ **GlucaGen** *see* Glucagon *on page 970*

◆ **GlucaGen HypoKit** *see* Glucagon *on page 970*

Glucagon (GLOO ka gon)

Brand Names: U.S. GlucaGen; GlucaGen HypoKit; Glucagon Emergency

Brand Names: Canada GlucaGen; GlucaGen HypoKit
Therapeutic Category Antihypoglycemic Agent
Generic Availability (U.S.) No
Use Treatment of severe hypoglycemia [FDA approved in pediatric patients (age not specified) and adults]; diagnostic aid in the radiologic examination of GI tract to temporarily inhibit GI tract movement (FDA approved in adults); has also been used for prevention of hypoglycemia during illness and management of beta-blocker or calcium channel blocker toxicity
Pregnancy Risk Factor B
Pregnancy Considerations Adverse events have not been observed in animal reproduction studies.
Breast-Feeding Considerations Glucagon is not absorbed from the GI tract and therefore, it is unlikely adverse effects would occur in a breast-feeding infant.
Contraindications Hypersensitivity to glucagon or any component including lactose; pheochromocytoma; insulinoma
Warnings Exogenous glucagon administration to patients with insulinoma will cause an initial rise in blood glucose followed by rebound hypoglycemia; use is contraindicated in these patients; use with caution in patients with a history suggestive of insulinoma or glucagonoma (existing or suggestive history). Exogenous glucagon may cause the release of catecholamines, resulting in an increase in blood pressure; use is contraindicated in patients with pheochromacytoma; use with caution in patients with a history suggestive of pheochromacytoma. Glucagon depletes glycogen stores, supplemental carbohydrates (which may include I.V. dextrose) should be administered as soon as physically possible. If a patient fails to respond to glucagon, I.V. dextrose must be given.

Hypersensitivity reactions including rash/urticaria and anaphylactic shock (respiratory distress and hypotension) have been reported; most anaphylactic reactions occurred during endoscopic examinations.
Precautions Use with caution in patients with adrenal insufficiency, chronic hypoglycemia, or prolonged starvation or fasting; levels of glucose stores in liver may be decreased leading to decreased efficacy of glucagon. Use with caution in patients with cardiac disease who receive glucagon for endoscopic or radiologic procedures.
Adverse Reactions
Cardiovascular: Hypertension, hypotension (up to 2 hours after GI procedures), tachycardia
Gastrointestinal: Nausea, vomiting (high incidence with rapid administration of high doses)
Miscellaneous: Anaphylaxis, hypersensitivity reactions
Drug Interactions
Metabolism/Transport Effects None known.
Avoid Concomitant Use There are no known interactions where it is recommended to avoid concomitant use.
Increased Effect/Toxicity
Glucagon may increase the levels/effects of: Vitamin K Antagonists
Decreased Effect
The levels/effects of Glucagon may be decreased by: Indomethacin
Food Interactions Glucagon depletes glycogen stores.
Stability Prior to reconstitution, store intact vials at 20°C to 25°C (69°F to 77°F); do not freeze. Keep in original carton to protect from light. Use reconstituted solution immediately. If solution shows any sign of gel formation or particles, it should be discarded. May be kept at 5°C for up to 48 hours if necessary.
Mechanism of Action Stimulates adenylate cyclase to produce increased cyclic AMP, which promotes hepatic glycogenolysis and gluconeogenesis, causing a raise in blood glucose levels; antihypoglycemic effect requires preexisting hepatic glycogen stores. Extra hepatic effects

of glucagon include relaxation of the smooth muscle of the stomach, duodenum, small bowel, and colon.
Pharmacodynamics
Blood glucose increase:
Onset of action: I.M.: 10 minutes; I.V.: 1 minute
Peak effect: I.M.: 26-30 minutes; SubQ: 30 minutes
Duration: I.M., I.V.: 60-90 minutes

GI tract relaxation:
Onset of action: I.M.: 4-10 minutes; I.V.: ≤1 minute
Duration: I.M.: 12-32 minutes; I.V.: 9-25 minutes
Pharmacokinetics (Adult data unless noted)
Distribution: V_d: 0.25 L/kg
Metabolism: Primarily hepatic; some inactivation occurring renally and in plasma
Half-life, plasma: I.M.: 45 minutes; I.V.: 8-18 minutes
Dosing: Neonatal
Hypoglycemia, persistent:
I.M., I.V., SubQ: 0.02-0.2 mg/kg/dose (maximum dose: 1 mg), may repeat dose in 20 minutes if needed (Hawdon, 1993; Mehta, 1987); **Note:** Wide variance in doses exists between manufacturer's labeling and published case reports.
Continuous I.V. infusion: 1 mg infused over 24 hours; doses >0.02 mg/kg/**hour** did not produce additional benefit; dosing based on a retrospective observation of 55 newborns (GA: 24-41 weeks) with hypoglycemia due to multiple causes (Miralles, 2002)
Congenital hyperinsulinism; hyperinsulinemic hypoglycemia: Continuous I.V. infusion: 0.005-0.02 mg/kg/**hour**; some centers use a lower dose (0.001 mg/kg/**hour**) in combination with octreotide (Aynsley-Green, 2000; Hussain, 2004, Kapoor, 2009)
Dosing: Usual
Pediatric:
Hypoglycemia, severe; treatment:
Weight-directed dosing:
Manufacturer's labeling: Infants, Children, or Adolescents weighing <20 kg: Glucagon: I.M., I.V., SubQ: 0.02-0.03 mg/kg; maximum dose: 0.5 mg
Alternate dosing: Infants, Children, and Adolescents:
AAP: I.M., I.V., SubQ: 0.03 mg/kg; maximum dose: 1 mg (Hegenbarth, 2008)
IDF-ISPAD: I.M., SubQ: 0.01-0.03 mg/kg; maximum dose dependent on age: <12 years: 0.5 mg; ≥12 years: 1 mg (IDF-ISPAD, 2011)
Fixed dosing; age-directed:
Manufacturer's labeling: GlucaGen: I.M., I.V., SubQ:
Infants and Children <6 years: 0.5 mg
Children and Adolescents ≥6 years: 1 mg
Alternate dosing: I.M., SubQ:
IDF-ISPAD (IDF-ISPAD, 2011):
Infants and Children <12 years: 0.5 mg
Children and Adolescents ≥12 years: 1 mg
CDA (Canadian Diabetes Association, 2013):
Infants and Children ≤5 years: 0.5 mg
Children and Adolescents >5 years: 1 mg
Fixed dosing; weight-directed: Infants, Children, and Adolescents: Manufacturer's labeling: I.M., I.V., SubQ:
Glucagon: Patient weight:
<20 kg: 0.5 mg
≥20 kg: 1 mg
GlucaGen: Patient weight:
<25 kg: 0.5 mg
≥25 kg: 1 mg
Hypoglycemia, prevention during illness (fixed dosing, mini-dose): Limited data available (Haymond, 2001; IDF-ISPAD, 2011): SubQ: **Note:** These doses are lower than hypoglycemia treatment doses and have been shown to prevent hypoglycemia for several hours during hypoglycemia-associated illness (eg, gastroenteritis, nausea/vomiting).
Infants and Children <2 years: 0.02 mg

Children and Adolescents 2-15 years: 0.01 mg per year of age

Adolescents >15 years: 0.15 mg

Beta-blocker or calcium channel blocker toxicity/overdose:

Infants and Children: Limited data available (Hegenbarth, 2008): I.V.:

Loading dose: 0.03-0.15 mg/kg

Continuous I.V. infusion: 0.07 mg/kg/hour; maximum rate: 5 mg/hour

Adolescents [Hegenbarth, 2008; PALS guidelines (Kleinman, 2010)]: I.V.:

Loading dose: 5-10 mg over several minutes

Continuous I.V. infusion: 1-5 mg/hour

Adult:

Hypoglycemia: I.M., I.V., SubQ: 1 mg; may repeat in 20 minutes as needed; **Note:** I.V. dextrose should be administered as soon as it is available; if patient fails to respond to glucagon, I.V. dextrose must be given.

Beta-blocker- or calcium channel blocker-induced myocardial depression (with or without hypotension) unresponsive to standard measures: I.V.: 3-10 mg (or 0.05-0.15 mg/kg) bolus followed by an infusion of 3-5 mg/hour (or 0.05-0.1 mg/kg/hour); titrate infusion rate to achieve adequate hemodynamic response (ACLS, 2010)

Diagnostic aid:

I.M.: 1-2 mg 10 minutes prior to gastrointestinal procedure

I.V.: 0.25-2 mg 10 minutes prior to gastrointestinal procedure

Dosing adjustments in renal impairment: There are no dosage adjustment provided in manufacturer's labeling.

Dosing adjustments in hepatic impairment: There are no dosage adjustment provided in manufacturer's labeling.

Administration Parenteral: Reconstitute powder for injection by adding 1 mL of sterile diluent to a vial containing 1 unit of the drug, to prepare a 1 mg of glucagon/mL solution. In pediatric patients, doses >2 mg should be reconstituted with SWI (Hegenbarth, 2008). Gently roll vial to dissolve. May administer I.M., I.V., or SubQ. When treating beta-blocker/calcium channel blocker toxicity, initial loading dose (bolus) should be administered over 3-5 minutes. A solution for continuous I.V. infusion may be prepared with further dilution in NS or D₅W (Love, 1998); in adults the usual I.V. infusion concentration is 0.08 mg/mL (4 mg in 50 mL D₅W).

Mini-dose: Reconstitute powder for injection to 1 mg/mL using sterile diluent provided; inject subcutaneously using an insulin syringe (U-100); 1 unit on the syringe provides 0.01 mg of glucagon (Haymond, 2001; IDF-ISPAD, 2011)

Monitoring Parameters Blood glucose, blood pressure, ECG, heart rate, mentation; in pediatric patients when used for hypoglycemia prevention (mini-doses), monitor blood glucose [every 30 minutes for the first hours and then at least hourly (or more often if appropriate)] (Haymond, 2001)

Dosage Forms Excipient information presented when available (limited, particularly for generics); consult specific product labeling.

Kit, Injection:

Glucagon Emergency: 1 mg

Solution Reconstituted, Injection, as hydrochloride:

GlucaGen: 1 mg (1 ea)

GlucaGen HypoKit: 1 mg (1 ea)

References

American Diabetes Association. Standards of medical care in diabetes-2014. *Diabetes Care.* 2014;37 Suppl 1:S14-80.

Aynsley-Green A, Hussain K, Hall J, et al, "Practical Management of Hyperinsulinism in Infancy," *Arch Dis Child Fetal Neonatal Ed,* 2000, 82(2):98-107.

Canadian Diabetes Association Clinical Practice Guidelines Expert Committee. Type 1 diabetes in children and adolescents. *Can J Diabetes* 2013;37:S153-162.

Field JM, Hazinski MF, Sayre MR, et al. Part 1: executive summary: 2010 American Heart Association Guidelines for Cardiopulmonary Resuscitation and Emergency Cardiovascular Care. *Circulation.* 2010;122(18 Suppl 3):S640-656.

Hawdon JM, Aynsley-Green A, and Ward Platt MP, "Neonatal Blood Glucose Concentrations: Metabolic Effects of Intravenous Glucagon and Intragastric Medium Chain Triglyceride," *Arch Dis Child,* 1993, 68 (3 Spec No):255-61.

Haymond MW, Schreiner B. Mini-dose glucagon rescue for hypoglycemia in children with type 1 diabetes. *Diabetes Care.* 2001;24 (4):643-645.

Hegenbarth MA, American Academy of Pediatrics Committee on Drugs. Preparing for pediatric emergencies: drugs to consider. *Pediatrics.* 2008;121(2):433-443.

Hussain K and Aynsley-Green A, "Hyperinsulinaemic Hypoglycaemia in Preterm Neonates," *Arch Dis Child Fetal Neonatal Ed,* 2004, 89 (1):65-7.

IDF/ISPAD. Global guideline for diabetes in childhood and adolescence, 2013. Available at http://www.idf.org/global-idfispad-guideline-diabetes-childhood-and-adolescence. Date accessed: April 14, 2014.

Kapoor RR, Flanagan SE, James C, et al, "Hyperinsulinaemic Hypoglycaemia," *Arch Dis Child,* 2009, 94(6):450-57.

Kleinman ME, Chameides L, Schexnayder SM, et al. Part 14: pediatric advanced life support: 2010 American Heart Association Guidelines for Cardiopulmonary Resuscitation and Emergency Cardiovascular Care.*Circulation.* 2010;122(18 Suppl 3):S876-908.

Love JN, Sachdeva DK, Bessman ES, Curtis LA, Howell JM. A potential role for glucagon in the treatment of drug-induced symptomatic bradycardia. *Chest.* 1998;114(1):323-326.

Mehta A, Wootton R, Cheng KN, et al, "Effect of Diazoxide or Glucagon on Hepatic Glucose Production Rate During Extreme Neonatal Hypoglycaemia," *Arch Dis Child,* 1987, 62(9):924-30.

Miralles RE, Lodha A, Perlman M, et al, "Experience With Intravenous Glucagon Infusions as a Treatment for Resistant Neonatal Hypoglycemia," *Arch Pediatr Adolesc Med,* 2002, 156(10):999-1004.

Vanden Hoek TL, Morrison LJ, Shuster M, et al. Part 12: cardiac arrest in special situations: 2010 American Heart Association Guidelines for Cardiopulmonary Resuscitation and Emergency Cardiovascular Care. *Circulation.* 2010;122(18 Suppl 3):S829-861.

◆ **Glucagon Emergency** see Glucagon *on page 970*

◆ **Glucagon Hydrochloride** see Glucagon *on page 970*

Glucarpidase (gloo KAR pid ase)

Brand Names: U.S. Voraxaze

Therapeutic Category Antidote; Enzyme

Generic Availability (U.S.) No

Use Treatment of toxic plasma methotrexate concentrations (>1 micromole/L) in patients with delayed clearance due to renal impairment (FDA approved in ages ≥1 month and adults); has also been used as a rescue agent to reduce methotrexate toxicity in patients with accidental intrathecal methotrexate overdose

Note: Due to the risk of subtherapeutic methotrexate exposure, glucarpidase is **not** indicated when methotrexate clearance is within expected range (plasma methotrexate concentration ≤2 standard deviations of mean methotrexate excretion curve specific for dose administered) **or** with normal renal function or mild renal impairment

Prescribing and Access Restrictions Voraxaze® is distributed through ASD Healthcare; procurement information is available (24 hours a day; 365 days a year) at 1-855-7-VORAXAZE (1-855-786-7292). Voraxaze® is also commercially available in the U.S. through certain pharmacy wholesalers on a drop-ship basis; orders will only be processed during business hours for overnight delivery. For additional information, refer to http://www.btgplc.com/products/specialty-pharmaceuticals/voraxaze.

Pregnancy Risk Factor C

Pregnancy Considerations Animal reproduction studies have not been conducted. If administered to a pregnant woman, the risk to the fetus is unknown; use only if clearly needed. In general, medications used as antidotes should take into consideration the health and prognosis of the mother.

Breast-Feeding Considerations Caution should be used if administered to a breast-feeding woman.

Contraindications Hypersensitivity to glucarpidase or any component

Warnings Hypersensitivity reactions which may be serious have been reported rarely (<1%). Methotrexate concentrations determined by immunoassays are unreliable when samples are collected within 48 hours of glucarpidase administration; DAMPA, an inactive methotrexate metabolite with a half-life of 9 hours, may interfere with immunoassay and result in the overestimation of the methotrexate serum concentration (when collected within 48 hours of glucarpidase administration). The only reliable method of measuring methotrexate serum concentrations during this time period is the chromatographic method.

Precautions Use should be accompanied with concomitant leucovorin therapy, adequate hydration, and urinary alkalinization. Use caution with leucovorin administration times; leucovorin calcium is a substrate for glucarpidase and may compete with methotrexate for binding sites; do not administer leucovorin calcium within 2 hours before or after a glucarpidase dose.

In children, upon resolution of renal dysfunction following glucarpidase therapy, rechallenge with high-dose methotrexate therapy has been successfully completed; monitor renal function and serum methotrexate concentrations closely in these patients (Christensen, 2012).

Intrathecal glucarpidase use for an intrathecal methotrexate overdose should be used in conjunction with immediate lumbar drainage (Widemann, 2004).

Adverse Reactions

Cardiovascular: Flushing, hypotension

Central nervous system: Headache

Gastrointestinal: Nausea/vomiting

Immunologic: Antibody development

Neuromuscular & skeletal: Paresthesia

Rare but important or life-threatening: Blurred vision, diarrhea, hypersensitivity reaction, hypertension, localized warm feeling, skin rash, throat irritation, tremor

Drug Interactions

Metabolism/Transport Effects None known.

Avoid Concomitant Use There are no known interactions where it is recommended to avoid concomitant use.

Increased Effect/Toxicity There are no known significant interactions involving an increase in effect.

Decreased Effect

Glucarpidase may decrease the levels/effects of: Leucovorin Calcium-Levoleucovorin

Stability Store intact vials at 2°C to 8°C (36°F to 46°F); do not freeze. Reconstituted solutions should be used immediately or may be stored for up to 4 hours under refrigeration.

Mechanism of Action Recombinant enzyme which rapidly hydrolyzes the carboxyl-terminal glutamate residue from extracellular methotrexate into inactive metabolites (DAMPA and glutamate), resulting in a rapid reduction of methotrexate concentrations independent of renal function

Pharmacodynamics

Onset of action: Methotrexate toxicity: I.V.: Within 15 minutes a ≥97% reduction of methotrexate serum concentrations

Duration: Methotrexate toxicity: Up to 8 days a >95% of methotrexate serum concentration reduction maintained

Pharmacokinetics (Adult data unless noted)

Distribution: V_d: I.V.: 3.6 L; distribution restricted to plasma volume

Half-life: I.V.: Normal renal function: 6-9 hours; impaired renal function (CrCl <30 mL/minute): 8-10 hours (Phillips, 2008)

Dosing: Usual Infants, Children, Adolescents, and Adults:

Methotrexate toxicity: I.V.: 50 units/kg as a single dose (Buchen, 2005; Widemann, 1997; Widemann, 2010)

Intrathecal methotrexate overdose: Limited data available: Children ≥5 years, Adolescents, and Adults: Intrathecal: 2000 units as soon as possible after accidental exposure (O'Marcaigh, 1996; Widemann, 2004); further studies are needed.

Dosage adjustment in renal impairment: Infants, Children, Adolescents, and Adults: No dosage adjustment necessary

Dosage adjustment in hepatic impairment: Infants, Children, Adolescents, and Adults: No dosage adjustment provided in the manufacturer's labeling; has not been studied

Administration

I.V.: Reconstitute each vial (1000 units/vial) with 1 mL NS; mix gently by rolling or tilting vial; do not shake. Prior to administration, flush I.V. line; infuse glucarpidase over 5 minutes; flush I.V. line after administration.

Intrathecal: Reconstitute 2000 units with 12 mL preservative-free NS (Widemann, 2004); typically administered over 5 minutes via lumbar route, ventriculostomy, Ommaya reservoir, or lumbar and ventriculostomy (O'Marcaigh, 1996; Widemann, 2004); others reports of lower doses (1000 units) have been administered through ventricular or lumbar catheter over 5 minutes (O'Marcaigh, 1996)

Monitoring Parameters Serum methotrexate concentrations using chromatographic method if <48 hours from glucarpidase administration (DAMPA interferes with immunoassay results until >48 hours). CBC with differential, bilirubin, ALT, AST, serum creatinine; evaluate for signs/symptoms of methotrexate toxicity

Test Interactions Methotrexate levels: During the first 48 hours following glucarpidase administration, the only reliable method of measuring methotrexate concentrations is the chromatographic method. DAMPA, an inactive methotrexate metabolite with a half-life of 9 hours, may interfere with immunoassay and result in the overestimation of the methotrexate concentration (when collected within 48 hours of glucarpidase administration).

Additional Information Leucovorin calcium administration should be continued after glucarpidase; the same dose as was given prior to glucarpidase should be continued for the first 48 hours after glucarpidase; after 48 hours, leucovorin doses should be based on methotrexate concentrations. A single methotrexate concentration should not determine when leucovorin should be discontinued; continue leucovorin until the methotrexate concentration remains below the threshold for leucovorin treatment for ≥3 days.

Dosage Forms Excipient information presented when available (limited, particularly for generics); consult specific product labeling.

Solution Reconstituted, Intravenous [preservative free]:
  Voraxaze: 1000 units (1 ea)

References

Buchen S, Ngampolo D, Melton RG, et al, "Carboxypeptidase G2 Rescue in Patients With Methotrexate Intoxication and Renal Failure," *Br J Cancer*, 2005, 92(3):480-7.

Christensen AM, Pauley JL, Molinelli AR, et al, "Resumption of High-Dose Methotrexate After Acute Kidney Injury and Glucarpidase Use in Pediatric Oncology Patients," *Cancer*, 2012.

O'Marcaigh AS, Johnson CM, Smithson WA, et al, "Successful Treatment of Intrathecal Methotrexate Overdose by Using Ventriculolumbar Perfusion and Intrathecal Instillation of Carboxypeptidase G2," *Mayo Clin Proc*, 1996, 71(2):161-5.

Phillips M, Smith W, Balan G, et al, "Pharmacokinetics of Glucarpidase in Subjects With Normal and Impaired Renal Function," *J Clin Pharmacol*, 2008, 48(3):279-84.

Widemann BC, Balis FM, Kim A, et al, "Glucarpidase, Leucovorin, and Thymidine for High-Dose Methotrexate-Induced Renal Dysfunction: Clinical and Pharmacologic Factors Affecting Outcome," *J Clin Oncol*, 2010, 28(25):3979-86.

Widemann BC, Balis FM, Murphy RF, et al, "Carboxypeptidase-G2, Thymidine, and Leucovorin Rescue in Cancer Patients With Methotrexate-Induced Renal Dysfunction," *J Clin Oncol*, 1997, 15 (5):2125-34.

Widemann BC, Balis FM, Shalabi A, et al, "Treatment of Accidental Intrathecal Methotrexate Overdose With Intrathecal Carboxypeptidase G2," *J Natl Cancer Inst*, 2004, 96(20):1557-9.

◆ **Glucobay™ (Can)** see Acarbose on page 46
◆ **Glucophage** see MetFORMIN on page 1353
◆ **Glucophage® (Can)** see MetFORMIN on page 1353
◆ **Glucophage XR** see MetFORMIN on page 1353
◆ **Glucose** see Dextrose on page 637
◆ **Glucose Monohydrate** see Dextrose on page 637
◆ **Glucose Nursette [OTC]** see Dextrose on page 637
◆ **Glucotrol** see GlipiZIDE on page 968
◆ **Glucotrol XL** see GlipiZIDE on page 968
◆ **Glulisine Insulin** see Insulin Glulisine on page 1123
◆ **Glumetza** see MetFORMIN on page 1353
◆ **Glumetza® (Can)** see MetFORMIN on page 1353
◆ **Glutol [OTC]** see Dextrose on page 637
◆ **Glutose 15 [OTC]** see Dextrose on page 637
◆ **Glutose 45 [OTC]** see Dextrose on page 637
◆ **Glybenclamide** see GlyBURIDE on page 974
◆ **Glybenzcyclamide** see GlyBURIDE on page 974

GlyBURIDE (GLYE byoor ide)

Medication Safety Issues
Sound-alike/look-alike issues:
GlyBURIDE may be confused with glipiZIDE, Glucotrol
DiaβBeta may be confused with Zebeta

High alert medication:
The Institute for Safe Medication Practices (ISMP) includes this medication among its list of drugs which have a heightened risk of causing significant patient harm when used in error.

BEERS Criteria medication:
This drug may be potentially inappropriate for use in geriatric patients (Quality of evidence - high; Strength of recommendation - strong).

Related Information
Medications for Which a Single Dose May Be Fatal When Ingested to a Toddler on page 2408

Brand Names: U.S. Diabeta; Glynase

Brand Names: Canada Apo-Glyburide; Ava-Glyburide; DiaBeta; Dom-Glyburide; Euglucon; Mylan-Glybe; PMS-Glyburide; PRO-Glyburide; ratio-Glyburide; Riva-Glyburide; Sandoz-Glyburide; Teva-Glyburide

Therapeutic Category Antidiabetic Agent, Oral; Antidiabetic Agent, Sulfonylurea; Hypoglycemic Agent, Oral

Generic Availability (U.S.) Yes

Use Adjunct to diet and exercise for the management of type II diabetes mellitus (noninsulin-dependent, NIDDM); may be used concomitantly with metformin or insulin to improve glycemic control

Pregnancy Risk Factor B/C (manufacturer dependent)

Pregnancy Considerations Outcomes of animal reproduction studies differ by manufacturer labeling. Glyburide crosses the placenta. Some pharmacokinetic properties of glyburide may change during pregnancy (Hebert, 2009).

Glyburide has been evaluated as an alternative for the treatment of GDM. The severity of GDM at diagnosis, the gestational age at diagnosis, and certain maternal characteristics may determine the appropriateness of this use. Most pregnancy outcome information is from studies evaluating glyburide in pregnant women with GDM when therapy was started after the period of organogenesis. Severe hypoglycemia lasting 4-10 days has been noted in infants born to mothers taking a sulfonylurea at the time of delivery. Additional adverse maternal and fetal events have been noted in some studies and may be influenced by maternal glycemic control and/or differences in study design (Bertini, 2005; Ekpebegh, 2007; Joy, 2012; Langer, 2000; Langer, 2005). Due to the potential for neonatal hypoglycemia, the manufacturer recommends that if glyburide is used during pregnancy, it should be discontinued at least 2 weeks before the expected delivery date

For women with diabetes, maternal hyperglycemia itself can be associated with adverse effects in the fetus, neonate, and mother. To prevent adverse events, prior to conception and throughout pregnancy, the maternal HbA_{1c} should be kept close to normal but without causing significant hypoglycemia. Glyburide may be used as an adjunct to medical nutrition therapy in carefully selected patients for the treatment of GDM; maternal glucose and fetal markers should be monitored closely. Insulin is the drug of choice for the control of type 1 or type 2 diabetes mellitus during pregnancy (ACOG, 2005; ADA, 2013; Kitzmiller, 2008; Metzger, 2007).

Breast-Feeding Considerations Data from initial studies note that glyburide was not detected in breast milk (Feig, 2005). According to the manufacturer, due to the potential for hypoglycemia in the nursing infant, a decision should be made whether to discontinue nursing or to discontinue the drug, taking into account the importance of treatment to the mother. Current guidelines note that breast-feeding is encouraged for all women, including those with diabetes; all types of insulin may be used while breast-feeding and some oral agents, including glyburide, may be acceptable for use as well (Metzger, 2007).

Contraindications Hypersensitivity to glyburide or any component; type 1 diabetes mellitus (insulin-dependent, IDDM), diabetic ketoacidosis with or without coma; concomitant use with bosentan

Documentation of allergenic cross-reactivity for sulfonylureas is limited; however, because of similarities in chemical structure and/or pharmacologic actions, the possibility of cross-sensitivity cannot be ruled out with certainty.

Warnings Chemical similarities are present among sulfonamides, sulfonylureas, carbonic anhydrase inhibitors, thiazides, and loop diuretics (except ethacrynic acid). Use in patients with sulfonamide allergy is not specifically contraindicated in product labeling; however, there is a risk of cross-reaction in patients with allergies to any of these compounds; avoid use when the previous reaction has been severe.

Product labeling states oral hypoglycemic drugs may be associated with an increased cardiovascular mortality as compared to treatment with diet alone or diet plus insulin; data to support this association are limited, and several studies, including a large prospective trial (UKPDS) have not supported an association.

Loss of efficacy may be observed following prolonged use as a result of the progression of type 2 diabetes mellitus which results in continued beta cell destruction. In patients who were previously responding to sulfonylurea therapy, consider additional factors which may be contributing to decreased efficacy (eg, inappropriate dose, nonadherence to diet and exercise regimen). If no contributing factors can be identified, consider discontinuing use of the sulfonylurea due to secondary failure of treatment. Additional antidiabetic therapy (eg, insulin) will be required. It may be necessary to discontinue therapy and administer insulin if the patient is exposed to stress (fever, trauma, infection, surgery).

Formulations of micronized glyburide (Glynase, Micronase) are **not** bioequivalent with conventional formulations (eg, DiaβBeta) and dosage should be retitrated when transferring patients from one formulation to the other or from other hypoglycemic agents.

Precautions All sulfonylurea drugs are capable of producing severe hypoglycemia. Hypoglycemia is more likely to occur when caloric intake is deficient, after severe or prolonged exercise, when ethanol is ingested, or when more than one glucose-lowering drug is used. It is also more likely in elderly patients, malnourished or debilitated patients, and in patients with severe renal or hepatic impairment, adrenal and/or pituitary insufficiency; use with caution. Patients with G6PD deficiency may be at an increased risk of sulfonylurea-induced hemolytic anemia; however, cases have also been described in patients without G6PD deficiency during postmarketing surveillance. Use with caution and consider a nonsulfonylurea alternative in patients with G6PD deficiency.

Adverse Reactions

Cardiovascular: Vasculitis

Central nervous system: Dizziness, headache

Dermatologic: Angioedema, erythema, maculopapular eruptions, morbilliform eruptions, photosensitivity reaction, pruritus, purpura, rash, urticaria

Endocrine & metabolic: Disulfiram-like reaction, hypoglycemia, hyponatremia (SIADH reported with other sulfonylureas)

Gastrointestinal: Anorexia, constipation, diarrhea, epigastric fullness, heartburn, nausea

Genitourinary: Nocturia

Hematologic: Agranulocytosis, aplastic anemia, hemolytic anemia, leukopenia, pancytopenia, porphyria cutanea tarda, thrombocytopenia

Hepatic: Cholestatic jaundice, hepatitis, liver failure, transaminase increased

Neuromuscular & skeletal: Arthralgia, myalgia, paresthesia

Ocular: Blurred vision

Renal: Diuretic effect (minor)

Miscellaneous: Allergic reaction

Drug Interactions

Metabolism/Transport Effects Substrate of CYP2C9 (major); **Note:** Assignment of Major/Minor substrate status based on clinically relevant drug interaction potential; **Inhibits** CYP2C8 (weak), CYP3A4 (weak)

Avoid Concomitant Use

Avoid concomitant use of GlyBURIDE with any of the following: Bosentan; Pimozide

Increased Effect/Toxicity

GlyBURIDE may increase the levels/effects of: Alcohol (Ethyl); ARIPiprazole; Bosentan; Carbocisteine; CycloSPORINE (Systemic); Dofetilide; Hypoglycemic Agents; Lomitapide; Pimozide; Porfimer; Vitamin K Antagonists

The levels/effects of GlyBURIDE may be increased by: Androgens; Beta-Blockers; Ceritinib; Chloramphenicol; Cimetidine; Clarithromycin; Cyclic Antidepressants; CYP2C9 Inhibitors (Moderate); CYP2C9 Inhibitors (Strong); Fibric Acid Derivatives; Fluconazole; GLP-1 Agonists; Herbs (Hypoglycemic Properties); MAO Inhibitors; Metreleptin; Miconazole (Oral); Mifepristone; Pegvisomant; Probenecid; Quinolone Antibiotics; Ranitidine; Salicylates; Selective Serotonin Reuptake Inhibitors; Sulfonamide Derivatives; Vitamin K Antagonists; Voriconazole

Decreased Effect

GlyBURIDE may decrease the levels/effects of: Bosentan

The levels/effects of GlyBURIDE may be decreased by: Bosentan; Colesevelam; Corticosteroids (Orally Inhaled); Corticosteroids (Systemic); CycloSPORINE (Systemic); CYP2C9 Inducers (Strong); Dabrafenib; Danazol; Loop Diuretics; Luteinizing Hormone-Releasing Hormone Analogs; Peginterferon Alfa-2b; Quinolone Antibiotics; Rifampin; Somatropin; Thiazide Diuretics

Food Interactions Ethanol may cause rare disulfiram reactions. Management: Monitor patients.

Mechanism of Action Stimulates insulin release from the pancreatic beta cells; reduces glucose output from the liver; insulin sensitivity is increased at peripheral target sites

Pharmacodynamics

Onset of action: 45-60 minutes

Maximum effect: 1.5-3 hours

Duration: Conventional formulations: 16-24 hours; micronized formulations: 12-24 hours

Average decrease in fasting blood glucose (when used as monotherapy): 60-70 mg/dL

Pharmacokinetics (Adult data unless noted)

Absorption: Reliably and almost completely absorbed

Distribution: V_d: 0.125 L/kg

Metabolism: Completely metabolized to one moderately active and several inactive metabolites

Protein binding: High (>99%)

Half-life: Biphasic: Terminal elimination half-life: Average: 1.4-1.8 hours (range: 0.7-3 hours); may be prolonged with renal or hepatic insufficiency

Time to peak serum concentration: Conventional formulation: 4 hours; micronized formulation: 2-3 hours

Elimination: 30% to 50% of dose excreted in the urine as metabolites in first 24 hours; the remainder of the metabolite via biliary excretion

Dialysis: Not dialyzable

Dosing: Usual Adults: Oral: Formulations of micronized glyburide (Glynase® Prestab®) are **not** bioequivalent with conventional formulations (eg, Diaβeta®) and dosage should be retitrated when transferring patients from one formulation to the other

Management of noninsulin-dependent diabetes mellitus in patients **previously untreated**:

Tablet (Diaβeta®):

Initial: 2.5-5 mg/day; in patients who are more sensitive to hypoglycemic drugs, start at 1.25 mg/day; increase in increments of no more than 2.5 mg/day at weekly intervals

Maintenance: 1.25-20 mg/day given as single or divided doses; maximum: 20 mg/day; doses >10 mg should be divided into twice daily doses

Micronized tablets (Glynase® Prestab®):

Initial: 1.5-3 mg/day; in patients who are more sensitive to hypoglycemic drugs, start at 0.75 mg/day; increase in increments of no more than 1.5 mg/day at weekly intervals

Maintenance: 0.75-12 mg/day given as a single dose or in divided doses; maximum: 12 mg/day; doses >6 mg/day should be divided into twice daily doses

Management of noninsulin-dependent diabetes mellitus in patients **previously maintained on insulin:** Initial dosage dependent upon previous insulin dosage, see table

Previous Daily Insulin Dosage (units)	Initial Glyburide Dosage (mg conventional formulation)	Initial Glyburide Dosage (mg micronized formulation)	Insulin Dosage Change (after glyburide started)
<20	2.5-5	1.5-3	Discontinue
20-40	5	3	Discontinue
>40	5 (increase in increments of 1.25-2.5 mg every 2-10 days)	3 (increase in increments of 0.75-1.5 mg every 2-10 days)	Reduce insulin dosage by 50% (gradually taper off insulin as glyburide dosage increased)

Dosing adjustment in renal impairment: CrCl <50 mL/minute: Not recommended

Dosing adjustment in hepatic impairment: Use conservative initial and maintenance doses and avoid use in severe disease

Administration Oral: May administer with food every morning 30 minutes before breakfast or the first main meal

Monitoring Parameters Signs and symptoms of hypoglycemia, fasting blood glucose, hemoglobin A$_{1c}$

Reference Range Target range:

Blood glucose: Fasting and preprandial: 80-120 mg/dL; bedtime: 100-140 mg/dL

Glycosylated hemoglobin (hemoglobin A$_{1c}$): <7%

Additional Information When transferring from other sulfonylurea antidiabetic agents to glyburide, with the exception of chlorpropamide, the administration of the other agent may be abruptly discontinued; due to the prolonged elimination half-life of chlorpropamide, a 2- to 3-day drug-free interval may be advisable before glyburide therapy is begun

Dosage Forms Considerations Micronized formulation: Glynase

Dosage Forms Excipient information presented when available (limited, particularly for generics); consult specific product labeling.

Tablet, Oral:

Diabeta: 1.25 mg, 2.5 mg, 5 mg [scored]

Glynase: 1.5 mg, 3 mg, 6 mg [scored]

Generic: 1.25 mg, 1.5 mg, 2.5 mg, 3 mg, 5 mg, 6 mg

References

Bertini AM, Silva JC, Taborda W, et al, "Perinatal Outcomes and the Use of Oral Hypoglycemic Agents," *J Perinat Med*, 2005, 33 (6):519-23.

DeFronzo RA, "Pharmacologic Therapy for Type 2 Diabetes Mellitus," *Ann Intern Med*, 1999, 131(4):281-303.

Ekpebegh CO, Coetzee EJ, van der Merwe L, et al, "A 10-Year Retrospective Analysis of Pregnancy Outcome in Pregestational Type 2 Diabetes: Comparison of Insulin and Oral Glucose-Lowering Agents," *Diabet Med*, 2007, 24(3):253-8.

Feig DS, Briggs GG, Kraemer JM, et al, "Transfer of Glyburide and Glipizide Into Breast Milk," *Diabetes Care*, 2005, 28(8):1851-5.

Hebert MF, Ma X, Naraharisetti SB, et al, "Are We Optimizing Gestational Diabetes Treatment With Glyburide? The Pharmacologic Basis For Better Clinical Practice," *Clin Pharmacol Ther*, 2009, 85 (6):607-14.

"Intensive Blood-Glucose Control With Sulphonylureas or Insulin Compared With Conventional Treatment and Risk of Complications in Patients With Type 2 Diabetes (UKPDS 33) UK Prospective Diabetes Study (UKPDS) Group," *Lancet*, 1998, 352(9131):837-53.

Joy S, Roman A, Istwan N, et al, "The Effect of Maternal Obesity on Pregnancy Outcomes of Women With Gestational Diabetes Controlled With Diet Only, Glyburide, or Insulin," *Am J Perinatol*, 2012, 29(8):643-8.

Langer O, Conway D, Berkus M, et al, "A Comparison of Glyburide and Insulin in Women With Gestational Diabetes Mellitus," *N Engl J Med*, 2000, 343(16):1134-8.

Langer O, Yogev Y, Xenakis EM, et al, "Insulin and Glyburide Therapy: Dosage, Severity Level of Gestational Diabetes, and Pregnancy Outcome," *Am J Obstet Gynecol* , 2005, 192(1):134-9.

Metzger BE, Buchanan TA, Coustan DR, et al, "Summary and Recommendations of the Fifth International Workshop-Conference on Gestational Diabetes Mellitus," *Diabetes Care*, 2007, 30(Suppl 2):S251-60.

◆ **Glycate** see Glycopyrrolate on page 977

Glycerin (GLIS er in)

Brand Names: U.S. Fleet Liquid Glycerin Supp [OTC]; Glycerin (Adult) [OTC]; Pedia-Lax [OTC]; Sani-Supp Adult [OTC]; Sani-Supp Pediatric [OTC]

Therapeutic Category Laxative, Osmotic

Generic Availability (U.S.) May be product dependent

Use

Oral: Gel: Relief of symptoms of dry mouth (OTC product: FDA approved in ages ≥2 years and adults)

Rectal: Suppository: Treatment of constipation (OTC product: FDA approved in ages ≥2 years and adults); has also been used to stimulate passage of meconium

Pregnancy Considerations Glycerin suppositories are generally considered safe to use during pregnancy (Cullen, 2007; Wald, 2003).

Contraindications Hypersensitivity to glycerin or any component; Suppository: Rectal bleeding

Warnings

Suppository: Overuse of laxatives may create dependency; avoid frequent or prolonged use.

Oral gel: Should be applied topically to the oral mucosa area; swallowing of product should be avoided during application, especially in young children; if swallowing of an excessive amount of glycerin occurs, consult prescriber or a local Poison Control Center.

Precautions Use suppository with caution in patients with abdominal pain, nausea, or vomiting; physician should be consulted prior to use. In children, if bowel movement does not occur within 1 hour of use or rectal bleeding occurs; consult a physician.

With oral gel, if sore mouth symptoms associated with dry mouth do not improve within 7 days or if sore throat is severe, persists more than 2 days, or is accompanied by fever, headache, rash, nausea, or vomiting consult a physician.

Adverse Reactions Rectal: Gastrointestinal: Cramping pain, rectal irritation, tenesmus

Drug Interactions

Metabolism/Transport Effects None known.

Avoid Concomitant Use There are no known interactions where it is recommended to avoid concomitant use.

Increased Effect/Toxicity There are no known significant interactions involving an increase in effect.

Decreased Effect There are no known significant interactions involving a decrease in effect.

Stability

Oral gel: Store at controlled room temperature.

Suppositories: Store at controlled room temperature. Protect from heat.

Mechanism of Action Osmotic dehydrating agent which increases osmotic pressure; draws fluid into colon and thus stimulates evacuation

Pharmacodynamics Onset of action: Laxative effect: Rectal: 15-30 minutes

Pharmacokinetics (Adult data unless noted) Absorption: Rectal: Poorly absorbed

Dosing: Neonatal Constipation: Rectal: Administered in single doses only at infrequent intervals:

Rectal solution (liquid suppository): 0.5 mL/kg/dose as an enema

Suppository: A tip or chip of the pediatric suppository

Dosing: Usual

Constipation: Rectal: Suppository: Administered in single doses only at infrequent intervals

Infants: 1 pediatric suppository as directed; typically not used more than once daily (NASPGHAN, 2006)

Children 2-5 years: 1 pediatric suppository once daily as needed or as directed

Children ≥6 years, Adolescents, and Adults: 1 adult suppository once daily as needed or as directed

Dry mouth: Oral: Oral gel: Children ≥2 years, Adolescents, and Adults: Apply a one-inch strip directly to tongue and oral cavity as needed

Administration

Oral: Apply oral gel topically to oral mucosa (tongue and oral cavity); do not rinse after use; avoid swallowing product.

Rectal: Insert suppository in the rectum and retain 15 minutes; suppository does not need to melt to produce response

Monitoring Parameters Evacuation of stool

Dosage Forms Excipient information presented when available (limited, particularly for generics); consult specific product labeling.

Enema, Rectal:
Fleet Liquid Glycerin Supp: 5.6 g/dose (7.5 mL)
Suppository, Rectal:
Glycerin (Adult): 2 g (12 ea, 24 ea, 50 ea); 2.1 g (25 ea)
Pedia-Lax: 1 g (12 ea); 2.8 g (4 mL) [contains edetate disodium]
Sani-Supp Adult: 2 g (10 ea, 25 ea)
Sani-Supp Pediatric: 1.2 g (10 ea, 25 ea)

References

Constipation Guideline Committee of the North American Society for Pediatric Gastroenterology, Hepatology and Nutrition, "Evaluation and Treatment of Constipation in Infants and Children: Recommendations of the North American Society for Pediatric Gastroenterology, Hepatology and Nutrition," *J Pediatr Gastroenterol Nutr*, 2006, 43(3): e1-13.

Cullen G and O'Donoghue D, "Constipation and Pregnancy," *Best Pract Res Clin Gastroenterol*, 2007, 21(5):807-18.

Wald A, "Constipation, Diarrhea, and Symptomatic Hemorrhoids During Pregnancy," *Gastroenterol Clin North Am*, 2003, 32(1):309-22.

Zenk KE, Koeppel RM, and Liem LA, "Comparative Efficacy of Glycerin Enemas and Suppository Chips in Neonates," *Clin Pharm*, 1993, 12 (11):846-8.

◆ **Glycerin (Adult) [OTC]** *see* Glycerin *on page* 976

◆ **Glycerol** *see* Glycerin *on page* 976

◆ **Glycerol Guaiacolate** *see* GuaiFENesin *on page* 984

◆ **Glyceryl Trinitrate** *see* Nitroglycerin *on page* 1504

◆ **GlycoLax [OTC]** *see* Polyethylene Glycol 3350 *on page* 1696

◆ **Glycon (Can)** *see* MetFORMIN *on page* 1353

◆ **Glycophos** *see* Sodium Glycerophosphate Pentahydrate *on page* 1907

Glycopyrrolate (glye koe PYE roe late)

Medication Safety Issues
International issues:
Robinul [U.S. and multiple international markets] may be confused with Reminyl brand name for galantamine [Canada and multiple international markets]

Brand Names: U.S. Cuvposa; Glycate; Robinul; Robinul-Forte

Brand Names: Canada Glycopyrrolate Injection, USP; Seebri Breezhaler

Therapeutic Category Anticholinergic Agent; Antispasmodic Agent, Gastrointestinal

Generic Availability (U.S.) Yes

Use
Oral: Adjunct in treatment of peptic ulcer disease (FDA approved in adults). **Note:** Indication listed in product labeling but currently has no place in management of peptic ulcer disease. Has also been used for control of upper airway secretions.

Oral solution (Cuvposa™): Treatment of severe chronic drooling in association with neurologic conditions (eg, cerebral palsy) (FDA approved in ages 3-16 years)

Parenteral: Used preoperatively to inhibit salivation and excessive secretions of the respiratory tract, reduce volume and acidity of gastric secretions, and blockade of cardiac vagal inhibitory reflexes during induction of anesthesia and intubation; used intraoperatively to counteract surgically, drug-induced, or vagal mediated bradyarrhythmias; reversal of the muscarinic effects of cholinergic agents, such as neostigmine and pyridostigmine, during reversal of neuromuscular blockade (FDA approved in ages ≥1 month and adults); adjunct in treatment of peptic ulcer (FDA approved in adults). **Note:** Indication of peptic ulcer listed in product labeling but currently has no place in management of peptic ulcer disease.

Pregnancy Risk Factor B (injection) / C (oral solution)

Pregnancy Considerations Teratogenic effects were not observed in animal studies. Small amounts of glycopyrrolate cross the human placenta.

Breast-Feeding Considerations May suppress lactation

Contraindications Hypersensitivity to glycopyrrolate or any component; medical conditions that preclude use of anticholinergic medication; narrow-angle glaucoma; acute hemorrhage; tachycardia; severe ulcerative colitis; obstructive uropathy; paralytic ileus; myasthenia gravis; intestinal atony; obstructive disease of GI tract (pyloric stenosis); intestinal atony in the elderly or debilitated patient, toxic megacolon complicating ulcerative colitis; oral solution (Cuvposa™): Concomitant use of solid oral dosage forms of potassium chloride

Warnings Infants, patients with Down syndrome, and children with spastic paralysis or brain damage may be hypersensitive to antimuscarinic effects. Paradoxical excitation may occur in infants and young children. May cause drowsiness and/or blurred vision, which may impair physical or mental abilities; patients must be cautioned about performing tasks which require mental alertness (eg, operating machinery or driving). May decrease sweating leading to heat prostration (eg, fever or heat stroke) in the presence of increased environmental temperature; use caution in hot weather and/or exercise. Slowing of GI muscular action can occur resulting in constipation or intestinal pseudo-obstruction. Constipation is a common dose-limiting adverse event; usually reported 4-5 days after therapy initiation or dose increases. Intestinal pseudo-obstruction can result in abdominal distention, pain, nausea, or vomiting.

Injection contains benzyl alcohol which may cause allergic reactions in susceptible individuals; large amounts of benzyl alcohol (≥99 mg/kg/day) have been associated with a potentially fatal toxicity ("gasping syndrome") in neonates; the "gasping syndrome" consists of metabolic acidosis, respiratory distress, gasping respirations, CNS dysfunction (including convulsions, intracranial hemorrhage), hypotension and cardiovascular collapse; use parenteral injection containing benzyl alcohol with caution in neonates; *in vitro* and animal studies have shown that benzoate, a metabolite of benzyl alcohol, displaces bilirubin from protein binding sites

Oral solution (Cuvpos) contains propylene glycol; toxicities have been reported with use of products containing propylene glycol, including hyperosmolality, lactic acidosis, seizures, and respiratory depression; in neonates large amounts of propylene glycol delivered orally, intravenously (eg, >3000 mg/day), or topically have been associated with potentially fatal toxicities which can include metabolic acidosis, seizures, renal failure, and CNS depression; use oral solution containing propylene glycol with caution (AAP, 1997; Shehab, 2009).

Precautions Use with caution in patients with renal impairment; if function severely impaired, dosage adjustment should be considered. Use with caution in patients with autonomic neuropathy, fever, hyperthyroidism, hepatic or renal disease, hypertension, coronary artery disease, CHF, tachyarrhythmias, reflux esophagitis, or hiatal hernia with reflux. Use with caution in patients with diarrhea; diarrhea may be a sign of incomplete intestinal obstruction, especially in patients with an ileostomy or colostomy. Discontinue treatment if this occurs. Use with caution in patients with ulcerative colitis as large doses suppress intestinal motility; may precipitate/exacerbate an ileus or toxic megacolon. Use with caution in individuals demonstrating decreased pigmentation (skin and iris coloration, dark vs light) since there has been some evidence that these individuals have an enhanced sensitivity to the anticholinergic response. In children treated with Cuvposa™, the following adverse reactions were reported with incidences ▶

>30%: Flushing, constipation, vomiting, xerostomia, and nasal congestion.

Adverse Reactions

Cardiovascular: Arrhythmias, cardiac arrest, flushing, heart block, hyper-/hypotension, malignant hyperthermia, pallor, palpitation, QT_c-interval prolongation, tachycardia

Central nervous system: Aggressiveness, agitation, confusion, crying (abnormal), dizziness, drowsiness, excitement, headache, insomnia, irritability, mood changes, pain, restlessness, nervousness, seizure

Dermatologic: Dry skin, pruritus, rash, urticaria

Endocrine & metabolic: Dehydration, lactation suppression

Gastrointestinal: Abdominal distention, abdominal pain, constipation, flatulence, retching, bloated feeling, intestinal obstruction, loss of taste, nausea, pseudo-obstructio, vomiting, xerostomia

Genitourinary: Impotence, urinary hesitancy, urinary retention, urinary tract infection

Local: Injection site reactions (edema, erythema, pain)

Neuromuscular & skeletal: Weakness

Ocular: Blurred vision, cycloplegia, mydriasis, nystagmus, ocular tension increased, photophobia, sensitivity to light increased

Respiratory: Bronchial secretion (thickening), nasal congestion, nasal dryness, pneumonia, respiratory depression, sinusitis, upper respiratory tract infection

Miscellaneous: Anaphylactoid reactions, diaphoresis decreased, hypersensitivity reactions

As reported with Seebri® Breezhaler® [Canadian product]:

Central nervous system: Headache

Gastrointestinal: Dyspepsia, gastroenteritis, vomiting, xerostomia

Genitourinary: Dysuria, urinary tract infection

Neuromuscular & skeletal: Musculoskeletal pain

Respiratory: Nasopharyngitis, rhinitis

Rare but important or life-threatening: Cough, cystitis, dental caries, diabetes mellitus, epistaxis, fatigue, hypoesthesia, palpitations, rash, throat irritation, urinary retention, weakness

Drug Interactions

Metabolism/Transport Effects None known.

Avoid Concomitant Use

Avoid concomitant use of Glycopyrrolate with any of the following: Aclidinium; Ipratropium (Oral Inhalation); Potassium Chloride; Tiotropium; Umeclidinium

Increased Effect/Toxicity

Glycopyrrolate may increase the levels/effects of: AbobotulinumtoxinA; Analgesics (Opioid); Anticholinergic Agents; Atenolol; Cannabinoid-Containing Products; Digoxin; MetFORMIN; Mirabegron; OnabotulinumtoxinA; Potassium Chloride; RimabotulinumtoxinB; Thiazide Diuretics; Tiotropium; Topiramate

The levels/effects of Glycopyrrolate may be increased by: Aclidinium; Amantadine; Ipratropium (Oral Inhalation); MAO Inhibitors; Pramlintide; Umeclidinium

Decreased Effect

Glycopyrrolate may decrease the levels/effects of: Acetylcholinesterase Inhibitors (Central); Haloperidol; Levodopa; Secretin

The levels/effects of Glycopyrrolate may be decreased by: Acetylcholinesterase Inhibitors (Central)

Food Interactions Administration with a high-fat meal significantly reduced absorption. Management: Administer on an empty stomach.

Stability Store at room temperature 20°C to 25°C (68°F to 77°F).

Parenteral: Unstable at pH >6; compatible in the same syringe with atropine, codeine, diphenhydramine, droperidol, fentanyl, hydromorphone, hydroxyzine, lidocaine, meperidine, promethazine, morphine, neostigmine, procaine, prochlorperazine, pyridostigmine, scopolamine, and trimethobenzamide

Mechanism of Action Blocks the action of acetylcholine at parasympathetic sites in smooth muscle, secretory glands, and the CNS; indirectly reduces the rate of salivation by preventing the stimulation of acetylcholine receptors

In COPD, competitively and reversibly inhibits the action of acetylcholine at muscarinic receptor subtypes 1-3 (greater affinity for subtypes 1 and 3) in bronchial smooth muscle thereby causing bronchodilation

Pharmacodynamics

Onset of action:

Oral: Within 1 hour

I.M.: 15-30 minutes

I.V.: 1 minute

Maximum effect: Oral: ~1 hour; I.M.: 30-45 minutes

Duration: Vagal effect: 2-3 hours; inhibition of salivation: Up to 7 hours; anticholinergic: Oral: 8-12 hours; Parenteral: 7 hours

Pharmacokinetics (Adult data unless noted)

Absorption: Oral tablets: Poor (~3%); variable and erratic; Oral solution: 23% lower compared to tablet

Distribution: V_d:

Pediatric patients (1-14 years): Mean range: 1.3-1.8 L/kg

Adults: 0.2-0.64 L/kg

Half-life:

Infants: 22-130 minutes

Children: 19-99 minutes

Adults: ~60-75 minutes; Oral solution: 3 hours

Elimination: Urine (as unchanged drug, I.M.: 80%, I.V.: 85%); bile (as unchanged drug)

Clearance:

Pediatric patients (1-14 years): Mean range: 1-1.4 L/kg/hour

Adults: Mean range: 0.4-0.68 L/kg/hour

Dosing: Neonatal I.V.: Limited data available: Endotracheal intubation, nonemergent: 4-10 mcg/kg as a single dose (acceptable, but not preferred vagolytic) (Kumar, 2010). A small study of 20 neonates used 3-5 mcg/kg as a single dose prior to intubation (Pokela, 1994)

Dosing: Usual

Infants, Children, and Adolescents:

Chronic drooling: Oral solution (Cuvposa™): Children and Adolescents 3-16 years: 20 mcg/kg/dose 3 times daily, titrate in increments of 20 mcg/kg/dose every 5-7 days as tolerated to response up to a maximum dose of 100 mcg/kg/dose 3 times daily; not to exceed 1500-3000 mcg/dose

Control of secretions (chronic):

Oral: 40-100 mcg/kg/dose 3-4 times daily

I.M., I.V.: 4-10 mcg/kg/dose every 3-4 hours

Reduction of secretions (preoperative): I.M.:

≤2 years: 4-9 mcg/kg/dose 30-60 minutes before procedure

>2 years: 4 mcg/kg/dose 30-60 minutes before procedure

Reversal of bradycardia, vagal reflexes (intraoperative): I.V.: 4 mcg/kg/dose (maximum dose: 100 mcg/dose) at 2-3 minute intervals

Reversal of muscarinic effects of cholinergic agents: I.V.: 0.2 mg for each 1 mg of neostigmine or 5 mg of pyridostigmine administered

Adults:

Reduction of secretions (preoperative): I.M.: 4 mcg/kg 30-60 minutes before procedure

Reversal of bradycardia, vagal reflexes (intraoperative): I.V.: 0.1 mg repeated as needed at 2-3 minute intervals

Reversal of neuromuscular blockade: I.V.: 0.2 mg for each 1 mg of neostigmine or 5 mg of pyridostigmine administered or 5-15 mcg/kg glycopyrrolate with 25-70 mcg/kg of neostigmine or 0.1-0.3 mg/kg of pyridostigmine (agents usually administered simultaneously, but glycopyrrolate may be administered first if bradycardia is present)

Dosage adjustment in renal impairment: Elimination is severely impaired in renal failure; dosage adjustment recommended.

Administration

Oral: Tablets: Administer without regard to meals; Oral solution: Administer on an empty stomach, 1 hour before or 2 hours after meals.

Parenteral: May be administered undiluted I.M. or direct I.V. at a maximum rate of 20 mcg/minute. May be diluted to a concentration of 2 mcg/mL (maximum concentration: 200 mcg/mL); infuse over 15-20 minutes; pH: 2.3.

Monitoring Parameters Heart rate; anticholinergic effects; bowel sounds; bowel movements; effects on drooling

Dosage Forms Excipient information presented when available (limited, particularly for generics); consult specific product labeling.

Solution, Injection:
Robinul: 0.2 mg/mL (1 mL); 0.4 mg/2 mL (2 mL); 1 mg/5 mL (5 mL); 4 mg/20 mL (20 mL) [contains benzyl alcohol]
Generic: 0.2 mg/mL (1 mL); 0.4 mg/2 mL (2 mL); 1 mg/5 mL (5 mL); 4 mg/20 mL (20 mL)

Solution, Oral:
Cuvposa: 1 mg/5 mL (473 mL) [contains methylparaben, propylene glycol, propylparaben, saccharin sodium; cherry flavor]

Tablet, Oral:
Glycate: 1.5 mg [dye free]
Robinul: 1 mg [scored]
Robinul-Forte: 2 mg [scored]
Generic: 1 mg, 2 mg

Extemporaneous Preparations A 0.5 mg/mL oral suspension may be made with 1 mg tablets and a 1:1 mixture of Ora-Plus® and either Ora-Sweet® or Ora-Sweet® SF. Crush thirty 1 mg tablets in a mortar and reduce to a fine powder. Prepare diluent by mixing 30 mL of Ora-Plus® with 30 mL of either Ora-Sweet® or Ora-Sweet® SF and stir vigorously. Add 30 mL of diluent (via geometric dilution) to powder until smooth suspension is obtained. Transfer suspension to 60 mL amber bottle. Rinse contents of mortar into bottle with sufficient quantity of remaining diluent to obtain 60 mL (final volume). Label "shake well". Stable at room temperature for 90 days. Due to bitter aftertaste, chocolate syrup may be administered prior to or mixed (1:1 v/v) with suspension immediately before administration (Cober, 2011).

A 0.5 mg/mL oral solution can be made from tablets. Crush fifty 1 mg tablets in a mortar and reduce to a fine powder. Add enough distilled water to make about 90 mL, mix well. Transfer to a bottle, rinse mortar with water, and add a quantity of water sufficient to make 100 mL. Label "shake well" and "protect from light". Stable at room temperature for 25 days (Gupta, 2001).

A 0.1 mg/mL oral solution may be made using glycopyrrolate 0.2 mg/mL injection without preservatives. Withdraw 50 mL from vials with a needle and syringe, add to 50 mL of a 1:1 mixture of Ora-Sweet® and Ora-Plus® in a bottle. Label "shake well", "protect from light," and "refrigerate". Stable refrigerated for 35 days (Landry, 2005).

Cober MP, Johnson CE, Sudekum D, et al, "Stability of Extemporaneously Prepared Glycopyrrolate Oral Suspensions," *Am J Health Syst Phar,*. 2011, 68(9):843-5.

Gupta VD, "Stability of an Oral Liquid Dosage Form of Glycopyrrolate Prepared from Tablets," *IJPC* 2001, 5(6):480-1.

Landry C, "Stability and Subjective Taste Acceptability of Four Glycopyrrolate Solutions for Oral Administration," *IJPC*, 2005, 9(5):396-98.

References

American Academy of Pediatrics Committee on Drugs. "Inactive" ingredients in pharmaceutical products: update (subject review). *Pediatrics.* 1997;99(2):268-278.

Hume-Smith H, McCormack J, Montgomery C, et al, "The Effect of Age on the Dose of Remifentanil for Tracheal Intubation in Infants and Children," *Paediatr Anaesth*, 2010, 20(1):19-27.

Kumar P, Denson SE, Mancuso TJ, et al, "Premedication for Nonemergency Endotracheal Intubation in the Neonate," *Pediatrics*, 2010, 125(3):608-15.

Nilsson E, Ingvarsson L, and Isern E, "Treacher Collins Syndrome With Choanal Atresia: One Way to Handle the Airway," *Paediatr Anaesth*, 2004, 14(8):700-1.

Pokela ML and Koivisto M, "Physiological Changes, Plasma Beta-Endorphin and Cortisol Responses to Tracheal Intubation in Neonates," *Acta Paediatr*, 1994, 83(2):151-6.

Shehab N, Lewis CL, Streetman DD, Donn SM. Exposure to the pharmaceutical excipients benzyl alcohol and propylene glycol among critically ill neonates. *Pediatr Crit Care Med.* 2009;10 (2):256-259.

♦ **Glycopyrrolate Injection, USP (Can)** *see* Glycopyrrolate *on page 977*

♦ **Glycopyrronium Bromide** *see* Glycopyrrolate *on page 977*

♦ **Glycosum** *see* Dextrose *on page 637*

♦ **Glydiazinamide** *see* GlipiZIDE *on page 968*

♦ **Glynase** *see* GlyBURIDE *on page 974*

♦ **Gly-Oxide [OTC]** *see* Carbamide Peroxide *on page 377*

♦ **GM-CSF** *see* Sargramostim *on page 1870*

♦ **GnRH Agonist** *see* Histrelin *on page 1016*

Gold Sodium Thiomalate
(gold SOW dee um thye oh MAL ate)

Brand Names: U.S. Myochrysine® [DSC]
Brand Names: Canada Myochrysine®
Therapeutic Category Gold Compound
Generic Availability (U.S.) No
Use Treatment of progressive rheumatoid arthritis
Pregnancy Risk Factor C
Pregnancy Considerations Adverse events were observed in animal reproduction studies
Breast-Feeding Considerations Injectable gold salts have been detected in breast milk and the serum of nursing infants
Contraindications Hypersensitivity to gold compounds, any component, systemic lupus erythematosus; avoid concomitant use of antimalarials, immunosuppressive agents, penicillamine, or phenylbutazone; severe toxicity from previous exposure or from other heavy metals; severe debilitation
Warnings Use may be associated with significant toxicity involving dermatologic, GI, hematologic, pulmonary, renal, and hepatic systems; patient education is required **[U.S. Boxed Warning]**. Signs of gold toxicity include decrease in hemoglobin, leukocytes, granulocytes and platelets, proteinuria, hematuria, or persistent diarrhea, rash, metallic taste; dermatitis (urticaria or eczema) and lesions of the mucous membranes are common and may be serious; pruritus may precede the early development of a skin reaction; advise patient to report any symptoms of toxicity; prior to each injection, the patient should be fully evaluated for any signs of adverse reactions.

Injection contains benzyl alcohol which may cause allergic reactions in susceptible individuals; large amounts of benzyl alcohol (≥99 mg/kg/day) have been associated with a potentially fatal toxicity ("gasping syndrome") in neonates; the "gasping syndrome" consists of metabolic acidosis, respiratory distress, gasping respirations, CNS dysfunction (including convulsions, intracranial hemorrhage), hypotension and cardiovascular collapse; *in vitro* and animal studies have shown that benzoate displaces bilirubin from protein binding sites; avoid use of gold sodium thiomalate in neonates

Precautions Frequent monitoring of patients for signs and symptoms of toxicity will prevent serious adverse reactions; NSAIDs and corticosteroids may be discontinued after initiating gold therapy; must not be injected I.V. Use with caution in patients with a history of blood dyscrasia; allergy or hypersensitivity to drugs, skin rash, history of hepatic or renal disease, marked hypertension, or compromised cerebral or cardiovascular circulation; ensure that CHF and diabetes are well controlled prior to starting therapy.

Adverse Reactions
Cardiovascular: Bradycardia, syncope
Central nervous system: Confusion, fever, Guillain-Barré syndrome, hallucinations, seizure
Dermatologic: Alopecia, angioedema, dermatitis, nail shedding, pruritus, rash, urticaria
Gastrointestinal: Anorexia, abdominal cramps, diarrhea, dysphagia, enterocolitis (ulcerative), gingivitis, glossitis, nausea, stomatitis, taste disturbance (metallic), thick tongue, vomiting
Hematologic: Agranulocytosis, aplastic anemia, eosinophilia, leukopenia, purpura, thrombocytopenia
Hepatic: Cholestasis, hepatitis, hepatotoxicity, jaundice
Neuromuscular & skeletal: Arthralgia, peripheral neuropathy
Ocular: Conjunctivitis, corneal ulcers, gold deposits in ocular tissues, iritis
Respiratory: Dyspnea, gold bronchitis, interstitial pneumonitis, pulmonary fibrosis
Renal: Glomerulitis, hematuria, nephrotic syndrome, proteinuria
Miscellaneous: Anaphylactoid reaction, anaphylaxis, nitritoid reaction

Drug Interactions
Metabolism/Transport Effects None known.
Avoid Concomitant Use There are no known interactions where it is recommended to avoid concomitant use.
Increased Effect/Toxicity
The levels/effects of Gold Sodium Thiomalate may be increased by: ACE Inhibitors
Decreased Effect There are no known significant interactions involving a decrease in effect.

Mechanism of Action Unknown, may decrease prostaglandin synthesis or may alter cellular mechanisms by inhibiting sulfhydryl systems

Pharmacodynamics
Onset of action: Delayed; may require up to 3 months of therapy

Pharmacokinetics (Adult data unless noted)
Distribution: Breast milk to plasma ratio: 0.02-0.3
Half-life: 5 days (range: 3-27 days); may lengthen with multiple doses
Time to peak serum concentration: I.M.: Within 3-6 hours
Elimination: Majority (50% to 90%) excreted in urine with smaller amounts (10% to 50%) excreted in feces (via bile)

Dosing: Usual I.M.:
Children: Initial: Test dose of 10 mg I.M. is recommended, followed by 1 mg/kg I.M. weekly for 20 weeks (maximum dose: 50 mg); maintenance: 1 mg/kg/dose at 2- to 4-week intervals thereafter for as long as therapy is clinically beneficial and toxicity does not develop. Administration for 2-4 months is usually required before clinical improvement is observed.
Adults: 10 mg first week; 25 mg second week; then 25-50 mg/week until clinical improvement or a 1 g cumulative dose has been given. If improvement occurs without adverse reactions, give 25-50 mg every 2 weeks for 2-20 weeks; if continues stable, give 25-50 mg every 3-4 weeks indefinitely.

Dosage adjustment in renal impairment:
CrCl 50-80 mL/minute: Administer 50% of dose
CrCl <50 mL/minute: Avoid use
Administration Parenteral: Administer I.M. only, preferably intragluteally; addition of 0.1 mL of 1% lidocaine to each injection may reduce the discomfort associated with I.M. administration; patients should be recumbent during injection and for 10 minutes afterwards; observe closely for 15 minutes after injection
Monitoring Parameters CBC with differential, platelets, hemoglobin, urinalysis for protein, white cells, red cells, and casts at baseline and prior to each injection. Skin and oral mucosa should be inspected for skin rash, bruising, or oral ulceration/stomatitis. Treatment should be withheld in patients with significant GI, renal, dermatologic, or hematologic effects (eg, platelets <100,000/mm^3, WBC <4000, granulocytes <1500/mm^3)
Reference Range Gold: Normal: 0-0.1 mcg/mL (SI: 0-0.0064 micromoles/L); Therapeutic: 1-3 mcg/mL (SI: 0.06-0.18 micromoles/L); Urine <0.1 mcg/24 hours
Dosage Forms Excipient information presented when available (limited, particularly for generics); consult specific product labeling. [DSC] = Discontinued product
Injection, solution:
Myochrysine®: 50 mg/mL (1 mL [DSC], 10 mL [DSC]) [contains benzyl alcohol]

◆ **GoLYTELY** *see* Polyethylene Glycol-Electrolyte Solution *on page 1697*

◆ **GoodSense Acid Reducer [OTC]** *see* Ranitidine *on page 1805*

◆ **GoodSense Mucus Relief [OTC]** *see* GuaiFENesin *on page 984*

◆ **GoodSense Senna Laxative [OTC]** *see* Senna *on page 1877*

◆ **Gordofilm** *see* Salicylic Acid *on page 1860*

◆ **Gordon Boro-Packs [OTC]** *see* Aluminum Acetate *on page 110*

◆ **Gordons-Vite A [OTC]** *see* Vitamin A *on page 2146*

◆ **Gordons-Vite E [OTC]** *see* Vitamin E *on page 2148*

◆ **GP 47680** *see* OXcarbazepine *on page 1564*

◆ **GR38032R** *see* Ondansetron *on page 1544*

◆ **Gralise** *see* Gabapentin *on page 950*

◆ **Gralise Starter** *see* Gabapentin *on page 950*

Granisetron (gra NI se tron)

Medication Safety Issues
Sound-alike/look-alike issues:
Granisetron may be confused with dolasetron, ondansetron, palonosetron
Brand Names: U.S. Granisol; Sancuso
Brand Names: Canada Granisetron Hydrochloride Injection; Kytril®
Therapeutic Category 5-HT$_3$ Receptor Antagonist; Antiemetic
Generic Availability (U.S.) May be product dependent
Use Prophylaxis and treatment of chemotherapy- and radiation-related nausea and emesis (FDA approved in ages 2-16 and adults); prophylaxis and treatment of postoperative nausea and vomiting (FDA approved in adults)

Transdermal patch: Prophylaxis of nausea and vomiting associated with moderate-to-high emetogenic chemotherapy regimens ≤5 days consecutive duration (FDA approved in adults)
Pregnancy Risk Factor B
Pregnancy Considerations There are no adequate or well-controlled studies in pregnant women. Teratogenic effects were not observed in animal studies. Injection

(1 mg/mL strength) contains benzyl alcohol which may cross the placenta. Use only if benefit exceeds the risk.

Breast-Feeding Considerations It is not known if granisetron is excreted in breast milk. The manufacturer recommends that caution be exercised when administering granisetron to nursing women.

Contraindications Hypersensitivity to granisetron or any component

Warnings Selective 5-HT$_3$ antagonists, including granisetron, have been associated with a number of dose-dependent increases in ECG intervals (eg, PR, QRS duration, QT/QT$_c$, JT), usually occurring 1-2 hours after I.V. administration. In general, these changes are not clinically relevant; however, when used in conjunction with other agents that prolong these intervals, arrhythmia may occur. When used with agents that prolong the QT interval (eg, Class I and III antiarrhythmics), clinically relevant QT interval prolongation may occur resulting in torsade de pointes. A number of trials have shown that 5-HT$_3$ antagonists produce QT interval prolongation to variable degrees. Reduction in heart rate may also occur with the 5-HT$_3$ antagonists. I.V. formulations of 5-HT$_3$ antagonists have more association with ECG interval changes compared to oral formulations.

Some injectable products contain benzyl alcohol which may cause allergic reactions in susceptible individuals; large amounts of benzyl alcohol (≥99 mg/kg/day) have been associated with a potentially fatal toxicity ("gasping syndrome") in neonates; the "gasping syndrome" consists of metabolic acidosis, respiratory distress, gasping respirations, CNS dysfunction (including convulsions, intracranial hemorrhage), hypotension and cardiovascular collapse; avoid use of products containing benzyl alcohol in neonates. *In vitro* and animal studies have shown that benzoate, a metabolite of benzyl alcohol, displaces bilirubin from protein-binding sites

Precautions Use with caution in patients with liver disease or in pregnant patients. Use with caution in patients following abdominal surgery; may mask progressive ileus or gastric distension. Application site reactions, generally mild, have occurred with transdermal patch use; if skin reaction is severe or generalized, remove patch. Cover patch application site with clothing to protect from natural or artificial sunlight while patch is applied and for 10 days following removal; granisetron may potentially be affected by natural or artificial sunlight. Do not apply patch to red, irritated, or damaged skin.

Adverse Reactions
Cardiovascular: Hypertension, QT$_c$ prolongation
Central nervous system: Anxiety, dizziness, fever, headache, insomnia, pain, somnolence
Dermatologic: Rash
Gastrointestinal: Abdominal pain, constipation, diarrhea, dyspepsia, taste perversion
Hepatic: Liver enzymes increased
Neuromuscular & skeletal: Weakness
Renal: Oliguria
Respiratory: Cough
Miscellaneous: Infection
Rare but important or life-threatening: Agitation, allergic reactions; anaphylaxis (including hypotension, dyspnea, urticaria); angina, application site reactions (transdermal patch), arrhythmias, atrial fibrillation, extrapyramidal syndrome, hot flashes, hypotension, hypersensitivity, syncope

Drug Interactions
Metabolism/Transport Effects Substrate of CYP3A4 (minor); **Note:** Assignment of Major/Minor substrate status based on clinically relevant drug interaction potential

Avoid Concomitant Use
Avoid concomitant use of Granisetron with any of the following: Apomorphine; Highest Risk QTc-Prolonging Agents; Ivabradine; Mifepristone

Increased Effect/Toxicity
Granisetron may increase the levels/effects of: Apomorphine; Highest Risk QTc-Prolonging Agents; Moderate Risk QTc-Prolonging Agents; Serotonin Modulators

The levels/effects of Granisetron may be increased by: Ivabradine; Mifepristone; QTc-Prolonging Agents (Indeterminate Risk and Risk Modifying)

Decreased Effect
Granisetron may decrease the levels/effects of: Tapentadol; TraMADol

Stability Tablets and injections: Store at room temperature, protect from light; injection stable when mixed in NS, D$_5$W for at least 24 hours; multi-use vial (with preservative) stable for 30 days after opening

Mechanism of Action Selective 5-HT$_3$-receptor antagonist, blocking serotonin, both peripherally on vagal nerve terminals and centrally in the chemoreceptor trigger zone

Pharmacodynamics
Onset of action: I.V.: 1-3 minutes
Duration: I.V.: ≤24 hours

Pharmacokinetics (Adult data unless noted)
Distribution: V$_d$: 2-3 L/kg; widely distributed throughout the body
Protein binding: 65%
Metabolism: Hepatic via N-demethylation, oxidation, and conjugation; some metabolites may have 5-HT$_3$ antagonist activity
Half-life:
Cancer patients: 10-12 hours
Healthy volunteers: 3-4 hours
Elimination: Primarily nonrenal, 8% to 15% of dose excreted unchanged in urine

Dosing: Usual
Treatment of chemotherapy-induced emesis: Initial dose given just prior to chemotherapy (15-60 minutes before)
Children ≥2 years and Adults: I.V.: Manufacturer's recommendation: 10 mcg/kg; or as an alternative based on clinical research: 20-40 mcg/kg/day divided once or twice daily; maximum: 3 mg/dose or 9 mg/day
As intervention therapy for breakthrough nausea and vomiting, during the first 24 hours following chemotherapy, 2 or 3 repeat infusions (same dose) have been administered
Adults: Oral: 2 mg once daily or 1 mg twice daily
Prevention and treatment of postoperative nausea and vomiting, before induction of surgery, immediately before reversal of anesthesia, or postoperatively: I.V.:
Children ≥4 years: 20-40 mcg/kg given as a single dose; not to exceed 1 mg
Adults: 0.1 mg given as a single dose; this dosage is not yet approved by the FDA; trends in randomized, double-blind, multicenter, dose-ranging studies have shown doses of 0.1 mg, 0.2 mg, and 0.3 mg to be more effective than placebo for postoperative nausea and vomiting (Gan, 2005; Shillington, 2005; Taylor, 1997); 1 mg is the FDA approved dosage
Transdermal patch: Adults: Prophylaxis of chemotherapy-related emesis: Apply 1 patch at least 24 hours prior to chemotherapy; do not apply ≥48 hours before chemotherapy. Remove patch a minimum of 24 hours after chemotherapy completion. Maximum duration: Patch may be worn up to 7 days, depending on chemotherapy regimen duration.

Administration
Oral: Given at least 1 hour prior to chemotherapy and then 12 hours later; shake oral suspension well before use

◄ Parenteral: I.V.: Infuse over 30 seconds undiluted **or** dilute in small volume NS or D$_5$W and administer over 5 minutes **or** dilute in 20-50 mL of NS or D$_5$W and infuse over 30 minutes to 1 hour

Transdermal (Sancuso®): Apply patch to clean, dry, intact skin on upper outer arm. Do not use on red, irritated, or damaged skin. Remove patch from pouch immediately before application. Do not cut patch.

Dosage Forms Excipient information presented when available (limited, particularly for generics); consult specific product labeling.

Patch, Transdermal:
Sancuso: 3.1 mg/24 hr (1 ea)
Solution, Intravenous:
Generic: 0.1 mg/mL (1 mL); 1 mg/mL (1 mL); 4 mg/4 mL (4 mL)
Solution, Intravenous [preservative free]:
Generic: 0.1 mg/mL (1 mL); 1 mg/mL (1 mL)
Solution, Oral:
Granisol: 2 mg/10 mL (30 mL) [contains fd&c yellow #6 (sunset yellow), sodium benzoate; orange flavor]
Tablet, Oral:
Generic: 1 mg

Extemporaneous Preparations Note: Commercial oral solution is available (0.2 mg/mL)

A 0.2 mg/mL oral suspension may be made with tablets. Crush twelve 1 mg tablets in a mortar and reduce to a fine powder. Add 30 mL distilled water, mix well, and transfer to a bottle. Rinse the mortar with 10 mL cherry syrup and add to bottle. Add sufficient quantity of cherry syrup to make a final volume of 60 mL. Label "shake well". Stable 14 days at room temperature or refrigerated (Quercia, 1997).

A 50 mcg/mL oral suspension may be made with tablets and one of three different vehicles (Ora-Sweet®, Ora-Plus®, or a mixture of methylcellulose 1% and Simple Syrup, N.F.). Crush one 1 mg tablet in a mortar and reduce to a fine powder. Add 20 mL of the chosen vehicle and mix to a uniform paste; transfer to a calibrated bottle. Label "shake well" and "refrigerate". Stable for 91 days refrigerated (Nahata, 1998).

Nahata MC, Morosco RS, and Hipple TF, "Stability of Granisetron Hydrochloride in Two Oral Suspensions," *Am J Health Syst Pharm*, 1998, 55(23):2511-3.

Quercia RA, Zhang J, Fan C, et al, "Stability of Granisetron Hydrochloride in an Extemporaneously Prepared Oral Liquid," *Am J Health Syst Pharm*, 1997, 54(12):1404-6.

References

"ASHP Therapeutic Guidelines on the Pharmacologic Management of Nausea and Vomiting in Adult and Pediatric Patients Receiving Chemotherapy or Radiation Therapy or Undergoing Surgery," *Am J Health Syst Pharm*, 1999, 56(8):729-64.

Gan TJ, Coop A, and Philip BK, "A Randomized, Double-Blind Study of Granisetron Plus Dexamethasone Versus Ondansetron Plus Dexamethasone to Prevent Postoperative Nausea and Vomiting in Patients Undergoing Abdominal Hysterectomy," *Aneth Analg*, 2005, 101(5):1323-9.

Hahlen K, Quintana E, Pinkerton CR, et al, "A Randomized Comparison of Intravenously Administered Granisetron Versus Chlorpromazine Plus Dexamethasone in the Prevention of Ifosfamide-Induced Emesis in Children," *J Pediatr*, 1995, 126(2):309-13.

Lemerle J, Amaral D, Southall DP, et al, "Efficacy and Safety of Granisetron in the Prevention of Chemotherapy-Induced Emesis in Paediatric Patients," *Eur J Cancer*, 1991, 27(9):1081-3.

Shillington A, et al, "Retrospective Cohort Study of Granisetron Administration for Postoperative Nausea and Vomiting Prophylaxis and Treatment," *Hosp Pharm*, 2005, 40(7): 592-8.

Taylor AM, Rosen M, Diemunsch PA, et al, "A Double-Blind, Parallel-Group, Placebo-Controlled, Dose-Ranging, Multicenter Study of Intravenous Granisetron in the Treatment of Postoperative Nausea and Vomiting in Patients Undergoing Surgery With General Anesthesia," *J Clin Anesth*, 1997, 9(8); 658-63.

◆ **Granisetron Hydrochloride Injection (Can)** *see* Granisetron *on page 980*

◆ **Granisol** *see* Granisetron *on page 980*

◆ **Granix** *see* Filgrastim *on page 872*

◆ **Granulocyte Colony Stimulating Factor** *see* Filgrastim *on page 872*

◆ **Granulocyte Colony Stimulating Factor (PEG Conjugate)** *see* Pegfilgrastim *on page 1616*

◆ **Granulocyte-Macrophage Colony Stimulating Factor** *see* Sargramostim *on page 1870*

◆ **Gravol® [OTC] (Can)** *see* DimenhyDRINATE *on page 670*

◆ **Gravol IM (Can)** *see* DimenhyDRINATE *on page 670*

◆ **Grifulvin V** *see* Griseofulvin *on page 982*

Griseofulvin (gri see oh FUL vin)

Brand Names: U.S. Grifulvin V; Gris-PEG

Therapeutic Category Antifungal Agent, Systemic

Generic Availability (U.S.) Yes

Use Treatment of tinea infections of the skin and hair caused by susceptible species of *Microsporum*, *Epidermophyton*, or *Trichophyton* (FDA approved in ages >2 years and adults) when lesions are unresponsive to topical antifungal therapy

Pregnancy Risk Factor X

Pregnancy Considerations Teratogenic effects have been observed in animal reproduction studies. Griseofulvin crosses the placenta (Pacifici, 2006). Because adverse events have also been observed in humans (two cases of conjoined twins), use during pregnancy is contraindicated. Effective contraception should be used during therapy and for 1 month after therapy is discontinued in women of reproductive potential. Men should avoid fathering a child for at least 6 months after therapy.

Breast-Feeding Considerations It is not known if griseofulvin is excreted in breast milk. women. Due to the potential for serious adverse reactions in the nursing infant, breast-feeding is not recommended.

Contraindications Hypersensitivity to griseofulvin or any component; liver failure, porphyria (interferes with porphyrin metabolism); pregnant women (may cause fetal harm)

Warnings Lupus erythematosus or lupus-like syndromes have been reported in patients receiving griseofulvin. Severe skin reactions (eg, Stevens-Johnson syndrome, toxic epidermal necrolysis, erythema multiforme) have been reported (may be serious or even fatal); discontinue use if severe skin reactions occur. May cause jaundice and elevated liver function tests or bilirubin (may be serious or even fatal); risk may be increased with prolonged therapy or high dose; monitor for hepatotoxicity and discontinue therapy if necessary.

Precautions Avoid exposure to intense sunlight to prevent photosensitivity reactions; use with caution in patients with penicillin hypersensitivity since cross-reactivity with griseofulvin is possible. Use for the prophylaxis of fungal infections has not been established; not effective for the treatment of tinea versicolor.

Adverse Reactions

Central nervous system: Dizziness, fatigue, headache, insomnia, mental confusion

Dermatologic: Angioneurotic edema (rare), erythema multiforme-like drug reaction, photosensitivity, rash (most common), urticaria (most common)

Gastrointestinal: Diarrhea, epigastric distress, GI bleeding, nausea, vomiting

Hematologic: Granulocytopenia, leukopenia (rare)

Hepatic: Hepatotoxicity

Neuromuscular & skeletal: Paresthesia (rare)

Renal: Nephrosis, proteinuria (rare)

Miscellaneous: Drug-induced lupus-like syndrome (rare), oral thrush

Rare but important or life-threatening: Bilirubin increased, liver transaminases increased, Stevens-Johnson syndrome, toxic epidermal necrolysis

Drug Interactions

Metabolism/Transport Effects Induces CYP1A2 (weak/moderate), CYP2C9 (weak/moderate), CYP3A4 (weak/moderate)

Avoid Concomitant Use

Avoid concomitant use of Griseofulvin with any of the following: Axitinib; Contraceptives (Progestins); Saccharomyces boulardii; Simeprevir

Increased Effect/Toxicity

Griseofulvin may increase the levels/effects of: Alcohol (Ethyl); Carbocisteine; Porfimer

Decreased Effect

Griseofulvin may decrease the levels/effects of: ARIPiprazole; Axitinib; Contraceptives (Estrogens); Contraceptives (Progestins); CycloSPORINE (Systemic); Ibrutinib; Saccharomyces boulardii; Saxagliptin; Simeprevir; Vitamin K Antagonists

The levels/effects of Griseofulvin may be decreased by: Barbiturates

Food Interactions

Ethanol: Concomitant use will cause a "disulfiram"-type reaction consisting of tachycardia, flushing, headache, nausea, and in some patients, vomiting and chest and/or abdominal pain. Management: Monitor patients for signs of reaction.

Food: Griseofulvin concentrations may be increased if taken with food, especially with high-fat meals. Management: Take with a fatty meal (peanuts or ice cream) to increase absorption, or with food or milk to avoid GI upset.

Stability

Suspension: Store between 20°C to 25°C (68°F to 77°F); protect from light.

Microsize tablets: Store between 20°C to 25°C (68°F to 77°F).

Ultramicrosize tablets: Store between 20°C to 25°C (68°F to 77°F); protect from light.

Gris-Peg® ultramicrosize tablets: Store between 15°C to 30°C (59°F to 86°F); protect from light.

Mechanism of Action Inhibits fungal cell mitosis at metaphase; binds to human keratin making it resistant to fungal invasion

Pharmacokinetics (Adult data unless noted)

Absorption: Ultramicrosize griseofulvin absorption is almost complete; absorption of microsize griseofulvin is variable (25% to 70% of an oral dose); absorbed from the duodenum

Distribution: Deposited in the keratin layer of skin, hair, and nails; concentrates in liver, fat, and skeletal muscles; crosses the placenta

V_d: ~1.5L (Vozeh, 1988)

Metabolism: Extensively hepatic

Half-life: 9-22 hours

Time to peak serum concentration: 4 hours

Elimination: <1% excreted unchanged in urine; also excreted in feces and perspiration

Dosing: Usual

Infants, Children, and Adolescents:

General dosing; susceptible infection (*Red Book*, 2012): Oral: Children >2 years and Adolescents:

Microsize: 10-20 mg/kg/day in single or 2 divided doses; maximum daily dose: 1000 mg/**day**

Ultramicrosize: 5-15 mg/kg/day once daily or in 2 divided doses; maximum daily dose: 750 mg/**day**

Tinea capitis: Oral:

Infants >1 month to Children ≤2 years: Limited data available: 10 mg/kg/day in single or divided doses (Higgins, 2000)

Children >2 years:

Microsize: 20-25 mg/kg/day once daily (maximum daily dose 1000 mg/day) for 6-8 weeks or until fungal cultures clear; in some cases, treatment up to 16 weeks may be necessary (Ali, 2007; Higgins, 2000, Kakourou, 2010, *Red Book*, 2012)

Ultramicrosize: 10-15 mg/kg/day once daily (maximum daily dose 750 mg/day) for 6-8 weeks or until fungal cultures clear; in some cases, treatment up to 16 weeks may be necessary (Ali, 2007; Higgins, 2000, Kakourou, 2010, *Red Book*, 2012)

Adults:

Tinea corporis:

Microsize: 500 mg daily in single or divided doses for 2-4 weeks

Ultramicrosize: 375 mg daily in single or divided doses for 2-4 weeks

Tinea cruris:

Microsize: 500 mg daily in single or divided doses 2-6 weeks (*Red Book*, 2012)

Ultramicrosize: 375 mg daily in single or divided doses 2-6 weeks (*Red Book*, 2012)

Tinea capitis:

Microsize: 500 mg daily in single or divided doses for 4-6 weeks

Ultramicrosize: 375 mg daily in single or divided doses for 4-6 weeks

Tinea pedis:

Microsize: 1000 mg daily in single or divided doses for 4-8 weeks

Ultramicrosize: 375 mg daily in single or divided doses for 4-8 weeks; doses up to 750 mg daily in divided doses have been used

Tinea unguium:

Microsize: 1000 mg daily in single or divided doses for 4-6 months or longer

Ultramicrosize: 375 mg daily in single or divided doses 4-6 months or longer; doses up to 750 mg daily in divided doses have been used

Administration Oral: Administer with a fatty meal (peanut butter or ice cream to increase absorption), or with food or milk to avoid GI upset; shake suspension well before use. Ultramicrosize tablets may be swallowed whole or crushed and sprinkled onto 1 tablespoonful of applesauce and taken immediately without chewing.

Monitoring Parameters Periodic renal, hepatic, and hematopoietic function tests

Test Interactions False-positive urinary VMA levels

Dosage Forms Considerations

Microsized formulations: Suspensions, Grifulvin V tablets

Ultramicrosize formulation: Gris-PEG tablets

Dosage Forms Excipient information presented when available (limited, particularly for generics); consult specific product labeling.

Suspension, Oral:

Generic: 125 mg/5 mL (118 mL, 120 mL)

Tablet, Oral:

Grifulvin V: 500 mg [scored]

Gris-PEG: 125 mg, 250 mg [scored]

Generic: 125 mg, 250 mg, 500 mg

References

Ali S, Graham TA, and Forgie SE, "The Assessment and Management of Tinea Capitis in Children," *Pediatr Emerg Care*, 2007, 23(9):662-5.

American Academy of Pediatrics (AAP). In: Pickering LK, Baker CJ, Kimberlin DW, Long SS, eds. *Red Book: 2012 Report of the Committee on Infectious Diseases*. 29th ed. Elk Grove Village, IL: American Academy of Pediatrics; 2012.

Fleece D, Gaughan JP, and Aronoff SC, "Griseofulvin Versus Terbinafine in the Treatment of Tinea Capitis: A Meta-Analysis of Randomized, Clinical Trials," *Pediatrics*, 2004, 114(5):1312-5.

Ginsburg CM, McCracken GH Jr, Petruska M, et al, "Effect of Feeding on Bioavailability of Griseofulvin in Children," *J Pediatr*, 1983, 102 (2):309-11.

Gupta AK, Adam P, Dlova N, et al, "Therapeutic Options for the Treatment of Tinea Capitis Caused by *Trichophyton* Species: Griseofulvin Versus the New Oral Antifungal Agents, Terbinafine, Itraconazole, and Fluconazole," *Pediatr Dermatol*, 2001, 18(5):433-8.

Gupta AK, Ryder JE, Nicol K, et al, "Superficial Fungal Infections: An Update on Pityriasis Versicolor, Seborrheic Dermatitis, Tinea Capitis, and Onychomycosis," *Clin Dermatol*, 2003, 21(5):417-25.

Higgins EM, Fuller LC, and Smith CH, "Guidelines for the Management of Tinea Capitis. British Association of Dermatologists," *Br J Dermatol*, 2000, 143(1):53-8.

Kakourou T and Uksal U, "Guidelines for the Management of Tinea Capitis in Children," *Pediatr Dermatol*, 2010, 27(3):226-8.

Lipozencic J, Skerlev M, Orofino-Costa R, et al, "A Randomized, Double-Blind, Parallel-Group, Duration-Finding Study of Oral Terbinafine and Open-Label, High-Dose Griseofulvin in Children With Tinea Capitis Due to *Microsporum* Species," *Br J Dermatol*, 2002, 146 (5):816-23.

Pacifici GM, "Placental Transfer of Antibiotics Administered to the Mother: A Review," *Int J Clin Pharmacol Ther*, 2006, 44(2):57-63.

Sethi A and Antaya R, "Systemic Antifungal Therapy for Cutaneous Infections in Children," *Pediatr Infect Dis J*, 2006, 25(7):643-4.

Vozeh S, Schmidlin O, and Taeschner W, "Pharmacokinetic Drug Data," *Clin Pharmacokinet*, 1988, 15(4):254-82.

◆ **Griseofulvin Microsize** *see* Griseofulvin *on page 982*

◆ **Griseofulvin Ultramicrosize** *see* Griseofulvin *on page 982*

◆ **Gris-PEG** *see* Griseofulvin *on page 982*

◆ **Growth Hormone, Human** *see* Somatropin *on page 1920*

◆ **GRX Hemorrhoidal [OTC]** *see* Phenylephrine (Topical) *on page 1662*

◆ **GRx HiCort 25** *see* Hydrocortisone (Topical) *on page 1038*

◆ **GSK-580299** *see* Papillomavirus (Types 16, 18) Vaccine (Human, Recombinant) *on page 1603*

◆ **GTN** *see* Nitroglycerin *on page 1504*

◆ **Guaiatussin AC** *see* Guaifenesin and Codeine *on page 985*

◆ **Guaicon DMS [OTC]** *see* Guaifenesin and Dextromethorphan *on page 987*

GuaiFENesin (gwye FEN e sin)

Medication Safety Issues
Sound-alike/look-alike issues:
GuaiFENesin may be confused with guanFACINE
Mucinex® may be confused with Mucomyst®

Related Information
Oral Medications That Should Not Be Crushed or Altered *on page 2438*

Brand Names: U.S. Altarussin [OTC]; Bidex [OTC]; Buckleys Chest Congestion [OTC]; Cough Syrup [OTC]; Diabetic Siltussin DAS-Na [OTC]; Diabetic Tussin Mucus Relief [OTC]; Diabetic Tussin [OTC]; Fenesin IR [OTC]; Geri-Tussin [OTC]; GoodSense Mucus Relief [OTC]; Iophen-NR [OTC]; Liquibid [OTC]; Liquituss GG [OTC]; Mucinex Chest Congestion Child [OTC]; Mucinex For Kids [OTC]; Mucinex Maximum Strength [OTC]; Mucinex [OTC]; Mucosa [OTC]; Mucus Relief Childrens [OTC]; Mucus Relief [OTC]; Mucus-ER [OTC]; Organ-I NR [OTC]; Q-Tussin [OTC]; Refenesen 400 [OTC]; Refenesen [OTC]; Robafen [OTC]; Robitussin Chest Congestion [OTC]; Robitussin Mucus+Chest Congest [OTC]; Scot-Tussin Expectorant [OTC]; Siltussin DAS [OTC]; Siltussin SA [OTC]; Tussin [OTC]; Xpect [OTC]

Brand Names: Canada Balminil Expectorant; Benylin® E Extra Strength; Koffex Expectorant; Robitussin®

Therapeutic Category Expectorant

Generic Availability (U.S.) May be product dependent

Use Expectorant used for the symptomatic treatment of coughs

Pregnancy Considerations Based on the limited available data, an increased risk of adverse birth outcomes has not been observed following maternal use of guaifenesin in pregnancy. Alcohol may be present in some liquid formulations of guaifenesin. If consumed in sufficient quantities during pregnancy, fetal alcohol syndrome may result. Guaifenesin has been investigated as an agent to improve cervical mucus and improve fertility.

Breast-Feeding Considerations It is not known if guaifensin is excreted in breast milk. The manufacturer recommends that caution be exercised when administering guaifensin to nursing women.

Contraindications Hypersensitivity to guaifenesin or any component

Warnings Safety and efficacy for the use of cough and cold products in children <2 years of age is limited. Serious adverse effects including death have been reported. The FDA notes that there are no approved OTC uses for these products in children <2 years of age. Healthcare providers are reminded to ask caregivers about the use of OTC cough and cold products in order to avoid exposure to multiple medications containing the same ingredient.

Some products contain sodium benzoate; benzoic acid (benzoate) is a metabolite of benzyl alcohol; large amounts of benzyl alcohol (≥99 mg/kg/day) have been associated with a potentially fatal toxicity ("gasping syndrome") in neonates; *in vitro* and animal studies have shown that benzoate displaces bilirubin from protein binding sites; avoid use of products containing sodium benzoate in neonates. Some forms contain propylene glycol; toxicities have been reported with use of products containing propylene glycol, including hyperosmolality, lactic acidosis, seizures, and respiratory depression; in neonates large amounts of propylene glycol delivered orally, intravenously (eg, >3000 mg/day), or topically have been associated with potentially fatal toxicities which can include metabolic acidosis, seizures, renal failure, and CNS depression; use products containing propylene glycol with caution (AAP, 1997; Shehab, 2009).

Precautions Some products contain phenylalanine which must be used with caution in patients with phenylketonuria.

Adverse Reactions
Central nervous system: Dizziness, drowsiness, headache
Dermatologic: Rash
Endocrine & metabolic: Uric acid levels decreased
Gastrointestinal: Nausea, stomach pain, vomiting
Rare but important or life-threatening: Kidney stone formation (with consumption of large quantities)

Drug Interactions
Metabolism/Transport Effects None known.
Avoid Concomitant Use There are no known interactions where it is recommended to avoid concomitant use.
Increased Effect/Toxicity There are no known significant interactions involving an increase in effect.
Decreased Effect There are no known significant interactions involving a decrease in effect.

Mechanism of Action Thought to act as an expectorant by irritating the gastric mucosa and stimulating respiratory tract secretions, thereby increasing respiratory fluid volumes and decreasing mucous viscosity

Pharmacokinetics (Adult data unless noted) Absorption: Well absorbed

Dosing: Usual Oral:
Children:
≥2 years: 12 mg/kg/day in 6 divided doses or as an alternative:
2-5 years: 50-100 mg every 4 hours, not to exceed 600 mg/day
6-11 years: 100-200 mg every 4 hours or as extended release product 600 mg every 12 hours; not to exceed 1.2 g/day
Children >12 years and Adults: 200-400 mg every 4 hours or as extended release product 600-1200 mg every 12 hours; not to exceed 2.4 g/day

Administration Oral: Administer with a large quantity of fluid to ensure proper action; do not crush or chew extended release tablet

Test Interactions Possible color interference with determination of 5-HIAA and VMA; discontinue for 48 hours prior to test

Dosage Forms Excipient information presented when available (limited, particularly for generics); consult specific product labeling. [DSC] = Discontinued product

Liquid, Oral:

Buckleys Chest Congestion: 100 mg/5 mL (118 mL) [alcohol free, sugar free; contains butylparaben, menthol, propylene glycol, propylparaben]

Diabetic Siltussin DAS-Na: 100 mg/5 mL (118 mL) [alcohol free, color free, fructose free, sodium free, sorbitol free, sugar free; contains aspartame, benzoic acid, methylparaben, propylene glycol; strawberry flavor]

Diabetic Tussin: 100 mg/5 mL (118 mL) [alcohol free, dye free, fructose free, sodium free, sorbitol free, sugar free; contains aspartame, menthol, methylparaben]

Diabetic Tussin Mucus Relief: 200 mg/5 mL (118 mL) [alcohol free, dye free, fructose free, sodium free, sorbitol free, sugar free; contains aspartame, benzoic acid, menthol, polyethylene glycol, propylene glycol]

Iophen-NR: 100 mg/5 mL (473 mL) [contains propylene glycol, saccharin sodium, sodium benzoate; raspberry flavor]

Liquituss GG: 200 mg/5 mL (118 mL, 473 mL) [alcohol free, sugar free; contains methylparaben, propylene glycol, propylparaben, saccharin sodium]

Mucinex Chest Congestion Child: 100 mg/5 mL (118 mL) [alcohol free; contains brilliant blue fcf (fd&c blue #1), edetate disodium, fd&c red #40, propylene glycol, sodium benzoate; grape flavor]

Mucinex Chest Congestion Child: 100 mg/5 mL (118 mL) [alcohol free; contains brilliant blue fcf (fd&c blue #1), fd&c red #40, propylene glycol, saccharin sodium, sodium benzoate; grape flavor]

Mucus Relief Childrens: 100 mg/5 mL (118 mL) [alcohol free; contains brilliant blue fcf (fd&c blue #1), fd&c red #40, propylene glycol, saccharin sodium, sodium benzoate]

Robitussin Mucus+Chest Congest: 100 mg/5 mL (118 mL) [alcohol free; contains fd&c red #40, menthol, propylene glycol, saccharin sodium, sodium benzoate]

Scot-Tussin Expectorant: 100 mg/5 mL (30 mL, 118 mL, 240 mL, 480 mL, 3780 mL) [alcohol free, dye free, saccharin free, sodium free, sorbitol free, sugar free]

Siltussin DAS: 100 mg/5 mL (118 mL) [alcohol free, dye free, sugar free; strawberry flavor]

Packet, Oral:

Mucinex For Kids: 50 mg (12 ea) [contains aspartame; grape flavor]

Mucinex For Kids: 100 mg (12 ea) [contains aspartame; bubble-gum flavor]

Solution, Oral:

Generic: 100 mg/5 mL (5 mL, 10 mL, 15 mL); 200 mg/10 mL (10 mL); 300 mg/15 mL (15 mL)

Syrup, Oral:

Altarussin: 100 mg/5 mL (120 mL, 236 mL, 473 mL, 3840 mL)

Altarussin: 100 mg/5 mL (120 mL, 240 mL, 480 mL, 3840 mL) [contains alcohol, usp]

Cough Syrup: 100 mg/5 mL (118 mL, 473 mL) [alcohol free; contains fd&c red #40, menthol, propylene glycol, saccharin sodium, sodium benzoate; fruit flavor]

Geri-Tussin: 100 mg/5 mL (473 mL) [alcohol free, sugar free; contains fd&c red #40, menthol, saccharin sodium, sodium benzoate]

Q-Tussin: 100 mg/5 mL (118 mL, 240 mL, 473 mL) [alcohol free; contains fd&c red #40, saccharin sodium, sodium benzoate; cherry flavor]

Robafen: 100 mg/5 mL (118 mL, 240 mL [DSC], 473 mL) [contains alcohol, usp; cherry flavor]

Robitussin Chest Congestion: 100 mg/5 mL (118 mL, 237 mL) [alcohol free; contains fd&c red #40, saccharin sodium, sodium benzoate; flavored flavor]

Siltussin SA: 100 mg/5 mL (118 mL, 237 mL, 473 mL) [strawberry flavor]

Tussin: 100 mg/5 mL (118 mL, 237 mL) [alcohol free]

Generic: 100 mg/5 mL (480 mL)

Tablet, Oral:

Bidex: 400 mg [DSC] [scored]

Bidex: 400 mg [scored; contains saccharin sodium]

Diabetic Tussin Mucus Relief: 400 mg [scored; dye free, sodium free, sugar free]

Fenesin IR: 400 mg

GoodSense Mucus Relief: 400 mg [scored]

Liquibid: 400 mg

Mucosa: 400 mg [scored]

Mucus Relief: 400 mg

Mucus Relief: 400 mg [scored; dye free]

Organ-I NR: 200 mg [scored]

Refenesen: 200 mg [scored; contains fd&c red #40 aluminum lake]

Refenesen 400: 400 mg [scored; dye free]

Xpect: 400 mg [scored; contains saccharin sodium]

Generic: 200 mg, 400 mg

Tablet Extended Release 12 Hour, Oral:

Mucinex: 600 mg [contains fd&c blue #1 aluminum lake]

Mucinex Maximum Strength: 1200 mg [contains fd&c blue #1 aluminum lake]

Mucus-ER: 600 mg [gluten free]

Generic: 600 mg

References
American Academy of Pediatrics Committee on Drugs. "Inactive" ingredients in pharmaceutical products: update (subject review). *Pediatrics*. 1997;99(2):268-278.

Shehab N, Lewis CL, Streetman DD, Donn SM. Exposure to the pharmaceutical excipients benzyl alcohol and propylene glycol among critically ill neonates. *Pediatr Crit Care Med*. 2009;10 (2):256-259.

◆ **Guaifenesin AC Liquid** *see* Guaifenesin and Codeine *on page 985*

Guaifenesin and Codeine
(gwye FEN e sin & KOE deen)

Brand Names: U.S. Allfen CD; Allfen CDX; Codar GF; Dex-Tuss; Guaiatussin AC; Guaifenesin AC Liquid; Iophen C-NR; M-Clear; M-Clear WC; Mar-Cof CG; Robafen AC; Virtussin A/C

Therapeutic Category Antitussive; Cough Preparation; Expectorant

Generic Availability (U.S.) Yes: Oral solution, syrup

Use Temporary control of cough due to minor throat and bronchial irritation and loosening and thinning of mucus and bronchial secretions (FDA approved in ages ≥6 years and adults)

Pregnancy Considerations See individual agents.

Breast-Feeding Considerations See individual agents.

Contraindications Hypersensitivity to guaifenesin, codeine, or any component

Additional contraindication for codeine: Postoperative pain management in pediatric patients who have undergone tonsillectomy and/or adenoidectomy (per codeine labeling)

Warnings Respiratory depression and death have occurred in children who received codeine following tonsillectomy and/or adenoidectomy and were found to have evidence of being ultrarapid metabolizers of codeine due to a CYP2D6 polymorphism; patients with this phenotype may have extensive conversion of codeine to morphine with resultant increased serum morphine concentrations; this may result in increased opioid-mediated effects and possible life-threatening respiratory depression or signs of overdose (eg, extreme sleepiness, confusion, shallow breathing) at usual therapeutic doses of codeine; codeine use is contraindicated in the postoperative pain management of pediatric patients who have undergone tonsillectomy and/or adenoidectomy. As a result, the FDA is requiring a black box warning be added to the manufacturer's labeling of some codeine-containing products (eg, particularly those indicated for analgesia) informing healthcare providers of this risk; guaifenesen/codeine products should be used with caution in pediatric patients. Deaths have also occurred in nursing infants after being exposed to high concentrations of morphine because the mothers were ultrarapid metabolizers of codeine. Ultrarapid metabolizers of codeine [ie, patients with more than two copies of functional alleles (CYP2D6 genotype with gene duplications denoted as *1/*1xN or *1/*2xN)] are at increased risk of opioid toxicity; avoid the use of codeine in these patients; consider alternative analgesics such as morphine or a nonopioid agent (Crews, 2012). The observed occurrence of the CYP2D6 "ultrarapid" phenotype is: North Africans, Ethiopians, and Arabs: 16% to 28%; African-Americans: 3%; Caucasians: 1% to 10%; Hispanics: 0.5% to 1%; and Chinese and Japanese: 0.5% to 1%. Codeine should be prescribed in all patients in the lowest effective dose and for the shortest period of time; patients and caregivers should be informed about risks and signs of morphine overdose. Due to the incidence of serious side effects and fatalities associated with codeine use in children, Health Canada is no longer recommending codeine use in any child <12 years of age.

Respiratory depression may occur even at therapeutic dosages in any patient; use with extreme caution in patients with respiratory diseases including asthma, emphysema, COPD, cor pulmonale, hypoxia, hypercapnia, preexisting respiratory depression, significantly decreased respiratory reserve, other obstructive pulmonary disease, kyphoscoliosis, or other skeletal disorder which may alter respiratory function.

Codeine may cause CNS depression which may impair physical or mental abilities; patients must be cautioned about performing tasks which require mental alertness (eg, operating machinery or driving). Use caution when combining with other CNS depressants (eg, centrally acting antiemetics, general anesthetics, phenothiazines, sedative-hypnotics) as there may be additive CNS effects. If combined therapy is needed, consider reducing the dose of one or both agents. Use with extreme caution in patients with head injury, intracranial lesions, or elevated intracranial pressure; exaggerated elevation of ICP may occur. May cause hypotension; use with caution in patients with circulatory shock, hypovolemia, impaired myocardial function, or those receiving drugs which may exaggerate hypotensive effects, including phenothiazines or general anesthetics. Codeine may obscure diagnosis or clinical course of patients with acute abdominal conditions.

Physical and psychological dependence may occur; abrupt discontinuation after prolonged use may result in withdrawal symptoms or seizures. Warn patients of possible impairment of alertness or physical coordination. Concurrent use of agonist/antagonist analgesics (ie, pentazocine, nalbuphine, and butorphanol) may precipitate withdrawal symptoms and/or reduce analgesic efficacy in patients following prolonged therapy with mu opioid agonists. High potential for abuse; healthcare providers should be alert to problems of abuse, misuse, and diversion. Infants born to women physically dependent on opioids will also be physically dependent and may experience respiratory difficulties or opioid withdrawal symptoms [neonatal abstinence syndrome (NAS)]. Onset, duration, and severity of NAS depend upon the drug used (maternal),

duration of use, maternal dose, and rate of drug elimination by the newborn. Symptoms of opioid withdrawal may include excessive crying, diarrhea, fever, hyper-reflexia, irritability, tremors, or vomiting or failure to gain weight. Opioid withdrawal syndrome in the neonate, unlike in adults, may be life-threatening and should be promptly treated.

Some products contain sodium benzoate; benzoic acid (benzoate) is a metabolite of benzyl alcohol; large amounts of benzyl alcohol (≥99 mg/kg/day) have been associated with a potentially fatal toxicity ("gasping syndrome") in neonates; *in vitro* and animal studies have shown that benzoate displaces bilirubin from protein binding sites; avoid use of sodium benzoate products in neonates. Capsules contain tartrazine which may cause allergic reactions in susceptible individuals.

Precautions Use with caution in patients with hypersensitivity reactions to other phenanthrene derivative opioid agonists (morphine, hydrocodone, hydromorphone, levorphanol, oxycodone, oxymorphone); discontinue immediately if symptoms of allergic or hypersensitivity reactions occur. Use with caution in patients with adrenal insufficiency (Addison's disease); biliary tract impairment; prostatic hyperplasia; urinary stricture; thyroid dysfunction; or severe liver, pulmonary, or renal insufficiency.

Not recommended for use for cough control in patients with a productive cough; not recommended as an antitussive for children <2 years of age. Debilitated patients may be particularly susceptible to adverse effects of opioids.

Some products contain phenylalanine which must be used with caution in patients with phenylketonuria.

Adverse Reactions See individual agents.

Drug Interactions

Metabolism/Transport Effects Refer to individual components.

Avoid Concomitant Use

Avoid concomitant use of Guaifenesin and Codeine with any of the following: Azelastine (Nasal); Paraldehyde; Thalidomide

Increased Effect/Toxicity

Guaifenesin and Codeine may increase the levels/effects of: Alcohol (Ethyl); Alvimopan; Azelastine (Nasal); Buprenorphine; CNS Depressants; Desmopressin; Diuretics; Hydrocodone; Methotrimeprazine; Metyrosine; Mirtazapine; Paraldehyde; Pramipexole; ROPINIRole; Rotigotine; Selective Serotonin Reuptake Inhibitors; Thalidomide; Zolpidem

The levels/effects of Guaifenesin and Codeine may be increased by: Amphetamines; Anticholinergic Agents; Antipsychotic Agents (Phenothiazines); Brimonidine (Topical); Cannabis; Doxylamine; Dronabinol; Droperidol; HydrOXYzine; Kava Kava; Magnesium Sulfate; Methotrimeprazine; Nabilone; Perampanel; Rufinamide; Sodium Oxybate; Somatostatin Analogs; Succinylcholine; Tapentadol; Tetrahydrocannabinol

Decreased Effect

Guaifenesin and Codeine may decrease the levels/effects of: Pegvisomant

The levels/effects of Guaifenesin and Codeine may be decreased by: Ammonium Chloride; CYP2D6 Inhibitors (Moderate); CYP2D6 Inhibitors (Strong); Mixed Agonist / Antagonist Opioids; Naltrexone

Mechanism of Action

Guaifenesin may act as an expectorant by irritating the gastric mucosa and stimulating respiratory tract secretions, thereby increasing respiratory fluid volumes and decreasing phlegm viscosity

Codeine is an antitussive that controls cough by depressing the medullary cough center

Dosing: Usual Note: Dosage units vary based on product (mg, mL, capsules, or tablets); use caution when verifying dose with product formulation.

Children ≥2 years and Adolescents: **Cough (antitussive/expectorant):** Oral:

Children 2 to <6 years: Limited data available: 1-1.5 mg/kg codeine/day divided into 4 doses administered every 4-6 hours as needed; maximum total dose: Codeine: 30 mg/24 hours or guaifenesin: 600 mg/24 hours, whichever is less.

Children 6-11 years:

Capsule: Guaifenesin 200 mg and codeine 9 mg: 1 capsule every 4 hours as needed; maximum daily dose: 6 capsules/**day**

Liquid:

Guaifenesin 100 mg and codeine 6.33 mg per 5 mL: 7.5 mL every 4-6 hours as needed; maximum daily dose: 45 mL/**day**

Guaifenesin 100-200 mg and codeine 8-10 mg per 5 mL: 5 mL every 4 hours as needed; maximum daily dose: 30 mL/**day**

Guaifenesin 225 mg and codeine 7.5 mg per 5 mL: 3.75 mL every 4-6 hours as needed; maximum total dose: 22.5 mL/24 hours

Guaifenesin 300 mg and codeine 10 mg per 5 mL: 2.5 mL every 4-6 hours as needed; maximum daily dose: 20 mL/**day**

Tablet: Guaifenesin 400 mg and codeine 10-20 mg: 1/2 tablet every 4-6 hours as needed; maximum daily dose: 3 tablets/**day**

Children ≥12 years and Adolescents:

Capsule: Guaifenesin 200 mg and codeine 9 mg: 2 capsules every 4 hours as needed; maximum daily dose: 12 capsules/**day**

Liquid:

Guaifenesin 100 mg and codeine 6.33 mg per 5 mL: 15 mL every 4-6 hours as needed; maximum daily dose: 90 mL/**day**

Guaifenesin 100-200 mg and codeine 8-10 mg per 5 mL: 10 mL every 4 hours as needed; maximum daily dose: 60 mL/**day**

Guaifenesin 225 mg and codeine 7.5 mg per 5 mL: 7.5 mL every 4-6 hours as needed; maximum total dose: 45 mL/24 hours

Guaifenesin 300 mg and codeine 10 mg per 5 mL: 5 mL every 4-6 hours as needed; maximum daily dose: 40 mL/**day**

Tablet: Guaifenesin 400 mg and codeine 10-20 mg: 1 tablet every 4-6 hours as needed; maximum daily dose: 6 tablets/**day**

Adults: **Cough (antitussive/expectorant):** Oral:

Capsule: Guaifenesin 200 mg and codeine 9 mg: 2 capsules every 4 hours as needed; maximum daily dose: 12 capsules/**day**

Liquid:

Guaifenesin 100 mg and codeine 6.33 mg per 5 mL: 15 mL every 4-6 hours as needed; maximum daily dose: 90 mL/**day**

Guaifenesin 100-200 mg and codeine 8-10 mg per 5 mL: 10 mL every 4 hours as needed; maximum daily dose: 60 mL/**day**

Guaifenesin 300 mg and codeine 10 mg per 5 mL: 5 mL every 4-6 hours as needed; maximum daily dose: 40 mL/**day**

Tablet: Guaifenesin 400 mg and codeine 10-20 mg: 1 tablet every 4-6 hours as needed; maximum daily dose: 6 tablets/**day**

Administration Oral: Administer with a large quantity of fluid to ensure proper action; may administer with food to decrease nausea and GI upset from codeine

Test Interactions May cause a colorimetric interference with certain laboratory determinations of 5-hydroxy indoleacetic acid (5-HIAA) and vanillylmandelic acid (VMA)

Controlled Substance Capsule: C-V; Liquid products: C-V; Tablet: C-III

Dosage Forms Excipient information presented when available (limited, particularly for generics); consult specific product labeling.

Capsule, oral:

M-Clear: Guaifenesin 200 mg and codeine phosphate 9 mg [contains tartrazine]

Liquid, oral:

Codar GF: Guaifenesin 200 mg and codeine phosphate 8 mg per 5 mL (473 mL) [contains propylene glycol; cotton candy flavor]

Dex-Tuss: Guaifenesin 300 mg and codeine phosphate 10 mg per 5 mL (473 mL) [ethanol free, gluten free, sugar free; contains propylene glycol; grape flavor]

Iophen C-NR: Guaifenesin 100 mg and codeine phosphate 10 mg per 5 mL (473 mL) [contains propylene glycol, sodium benzoate; raspberry flavor]

M-Clear WC: Guaifenesin 100 mg and codeine phosphate 6.33 mg per 5 mL (473 mL) [contains propylene glycol; cotton candy flavor]

Solution, oral: Guaifenesin 100 mg and codeine phosphate 10 mg per 5 mL (5 mL, 10 mL, 118 mL, 473 mL)

Mar-Cof CG: Guaifenesin 225 mg and codeine phosphate 7.5 mg per 5 mL (473 ml) [ethanol free, sugar free; contains propylene glycol, sodium benzoate, sodium 6 mg/5 mL]

Virtussin A/C: Guaifenesin 100 mg and codeine phosphate 10 mg per 5 mL (473 ml) [contains propylene glycol; cherry flavor]

Syrup, oral: Guaifenesin 100 mg and codeine phosphate 10 mg per 5 mL (473 mL)

Guaiatussin AC: Guaifenesin 100 mg and codeine phosphate 10 mg per 5 mL (5 mL, 10 mL, 118 mL, 473 mL) [sugar free; contains ethanol 3.5%, sodium 1 mg/5 mL, sodium benzoate; cherry flavor]

Robafen AC: Guaifenesin 100 mg and codeine phosphate 10 mg per 5 mL (120 mL, 480 mL) [contains ethanol 3.5%, sodium 4 mg/5 mL, sodium benzoate; cherry flavor]

Tablet, oral:

Allfen CD: Guaifenesin 400 mg and codeine phosphate 10 mg

Allfen CDX: Guaifenesin 400 mg and codeine phosphate 20 mg

References

American Academy of Pediatrics Committee on Drugs, "'Inactive' Ingredients in Pharmaceutical Products: Update (Subject Review)," *Pediatrics,* 1997, 99(2):268-78.

Guaifenesin and Dextromethorphan
(gwye FEN e sin & deks troe meth OR fan)

Medication Safety Issues
Sound-alike/look-alike issues:
Benylin may be confused with Benadryl, Ventolin

Related Information
Oral Medications That Should Not Be Crushed or Altered *on page 2438*

Brand Names: U.S. Cheracol D [OTC]; Cheracol Plus [OTC]; Coricidin HBP Chest Congestion and Cough [OTC]; Diabetic Siltussin-DM DAS-Na Maximum Strength [OTC]; Diabetic Siltussin-DM DAS-Na [OTC]; Diabetic Tussin DM Maximum Strength [OTC]; Diabetic Tussin DM [OTC]; Double Tussin DM [OTC]; Fenesin DM IR [OTC]; Guaicon DMS [OTC]; Iophen DM-NR [OTC]; Kolephrin GG/DM [OTC]; Mucinex DM Maximum Strength [OTC]; Mucinex DM [OTC]; Mucinex Fast-Max DM Max [OTC]; Mucinex Kid's Cough Mini-Melts [OTC]; Mucinex Kid's Cough [OTC]; Q-Tussin DM [OTC]; Refenesen DM [OTC]; Robafen DM [OTC]; Robitussin Peak Cold Cough + Chest Congestion DM [OTC]; Robitussin Peak Cold Maximum Strength Cough + Chest Congestion DM [OTC];

Robitussin Peak Cold Sugar-Free Cough + Chest Congestion DM [OTC]; Safe Tussin DM [OTC]; Scot-Tussin Senior [OTC]; Silexin [OTC]; Siltussin DM DAS [OTC]; Siltussin DM [OTC]; Vicks 44E [OTC]; Vicks DayQuil Mucus Control DM [OTC]; Vicks Nature Fusion Cough & Chest Congestion [OTC]; Vicks Pediatric Formula 44E [OTC]; Zyncof [OTC]

Brand Names: Canada Balminil DM E; Benylin DM-E

Therapeutic Category Antitussive; Cough Preparation; Expectorant

Generic Availability (U.S.) Yes: Excludes extended release tablet

Use Temporary control of cough due to minor throat and bronchial irritation

Pregnancy Considerations See individual agents.

Breast-Feeding Considerations See individual agents.

Contraindications Hypersensitivity to guaifenesin, dextromethorphan, or any component; use within 14 days of MAO inhibitor therapy

Warnings Some products contain sodium benzoate; benzoic acid (benzoate) is a metabolite of benzyl alcohol; large amounts of benzyl alcohol (≥99 mg/kg/day) have been associated with a potentially fatal toxicity ("gasping syndrome") in neonates; *in vitro* and animal studies have shown that benzoate displaces bilirubin from protein binding sites; avoid use of sodium benzoate products in neonates

Some products contain propylene glycol; toxicities have been reported with use of products containing propylene glycol, including hyperosmolality, lactic acidosis, seizures, and respiratory depression; in neonates large amounts of propylene glycol delivered orally, intravenously (eg, >3000 mg/day), or topically have been associated with potentially fatal toxicities which can include metabolic acidosis, seizures, renal failure, and CNS depression; use products containing propylene glycol with caution (AAP, 1997; Shehab, 2009).

Precautions Some products contain phenylalanine which must be used with caution in patients with phenylketonuria.

Adverse Reactions See individual agents.

Drug Interactions

Metabolism/Transport Effects Refer to individual components.

Avoid Concomitant Use

Avoid concomitant use of Guaifenesin and Dextromethorphan with any of the following: MAO Inhibitors

Increased Effect/Toxicity

Guaifenesin and Dextromethorphan may increase the levels/effects of: Antipsychotics; ARIPiprazole; Metoclopramide; Serotonin Modulators

The levels/effects of Guaifenesin and Dextromethorphan may be increased by: Abiraterone Acetate; Antiemetics (5HT3 Antagonists); Antipsychotics; CYP2D6 Inhibitors (Moderate); CYP2D6 Inhibitors (Strong); Darunavir; MAO Inhibitors; QuiNIDine; Selective Serotonin Reuptake Inhibitors

Decreased Effect

The levels/effects of Guaifenesin and Dextromethorphan may be decreased by: Peginterferon Alfa-2b

Mechanism of Action

Guaifenesin is thought to act as an expectorant by irritating the gastric mucosa and stimulating respiratory tract secretions, thereby increasing respiratory fluid volumes and decreasing phlegm viscosity

Dextromethorphan is a chemical relative of morphine lacking opioid properties except in overdose; controls cough by depressing the medullary cough center

Pharmacodynamics Onset of action: Antitussive effect: Oral (rapid release formulation): 15-30 minutes

Pharmacokinetics (Adult data unless noted) Absorption: Dextromethorphan is rapidly absorbed from the GI tract

Dosing: Usual Oral (dose expressed in mg of **dextromethorphan**):

Children: 1-2 mg/kg/day divided every 6-8 hours

Children >12 years and Adults: 60-120 mg/day divided every 6-8 hours or as extended release product 30-60 mg every 12 hours; not to exceed 120 mg/day

Administration Oral: Administer without regard to meals, with a large quantity of fluid to ensure proper effect; do not crush, chew, or break extended release tablets

Test Interactions See individual agents.

Dosage Forms Excipient information presented when available (limited, particularly for generics); consult specific product labeling.

Caplet, oral:

Fenesin DM IR: Guaifenesin 400 mg and dextromethorphan hydrobromide 15 mg

Refenesen DM: Guaifenesin 400 mg and dextromethorphan hydrobromide 20 mg

Capsule, softgel, oral:

Coricidin HBP Chest Congestion and Cough: Guaifenesin 200 mg and dextromethorphan hydrobromide 10 mg

Granules, oral:

Mucinex Kid's Cough Mini-Melts: Guaifenesin 100 mg and dextromethorphan hydrobromide 5 mg per packet (12s) [contains magnesium 6 mg/pack, phenylalanine 2 mg/packet, sodium 3 mg/packet; orange crème flavor]

Liquid, oral: Guaifenesin 100 mg and dextromethorphan hydrobromide 10 mg per 5 mL (480 mL)

Diabetic Tussin DM: Guaifenesin 100 mg and dextromethorphan hydrobromide 10 mg per 5 mL (120 mL) [dye free, ethanol free, sugar free; contains phenylalanine 8.4 mg/5 mL]

Diabetic Tussin DM Maximum Strength: Guaifenesin 200 mg and dextromethorphan hydrobromide 10 mg per 5 mL (120 mL) [dye free, ethanol free, sugar free; contains phenylalanine 8.4 mg/5 mL]

Double Tussin DM: Guaifenesin 300 mg and dextromethorphan hydrobromide 20 mg per 5 mL (120 mL, 480 mL) [dye free, ethanol free, sugar free]

Iophen DM-NR: Guaifenesin 100 mg and dextromethorphan hydrobromide 10 mg per 5 mL (480 mL) [contains propylene glycol, sodium benzoate; raspberry flavor]

Kolephrin GG/DM: Guaifenesin 150 mg and dextromethorphan hydrobromide 10 mg per 5 mL (120 mL) [ethanol free; cherry flavor]

Mucinex Fast-Max DM Max: Guaifenesin 400 mg and dextromethorphan hydrobromide 20 mg per 20 mL (180 mL) [contains propylene glycol, potassium 6 mg/20 mL, sodium 13 mg/20 mL]

Mucinex Kid's Cough: Guaifenesin 100 mg and dextromethorphan hydrobromide 5 mg per 5 mL (120 mL) [contains propylene glycol, sodium 3 mg/5 mL; cherry flavor]

Safe Tussin DM: Guaifenesin 100 mg and dextromethorphan hydrobromide 15 mg per 5 mL (120 mL) [contains benzoic acid, phenylalanine 4.2 mg/5 mL, and propylene glycol; orange and mint flavors]

Scot-Tussin Senior: Guaifenesin 200 mg and dextromethorphan hydrobromide 15 mg per 5 mL (120 mL) [ethanol free, sodium free, sugar free]

Vicks 44E: Guaifenesin 200 mg and dextromethorphan hydrobromide 20 mg per 15 mL (120 mL, 235 mL) [contains ethanol, sodium 31 mg/15 mL, sodium benzoate]

Vicks DayQuil Mucus Control DM: Guaifenesin 200 mg and dextromethorphan hydrobromide 10 mg per 15 mL (295 mL) [contains propylene glycol, sodium 25 mg/15 mL, sodium benzoate; citrus blend flavor]

Vicks Nature Fusion Cough & Chest Congestion: Guaifenesin 200 mg and dextromethorphan hydrobromide 20 mg per 30 mL (236 mL) [dye free, ethanol free, gluten free; contains propylene glycol, sodium 36 mg/30 mL; honey flavor]

Vicks Pediatric Formula 44E: Guaifenesin 100 mg and dextromethorphan hydrobromide 10 mg per 15 mL (120 mL) [ethanol free; contains sodium 30 mg/15 mL, sodium benzoate; cherry flavor]

Syrup, oral: Guaifenesin 100 mg and dextromethorphan hydrobromide 10 mg per 5 mL (5 mL, 10 mL, 120 mL, 480 mL)

Cheracol D: Guaifenesin 100 mg and dextromethorphan hydrobromide 10 mg per 5 mL (120 mL, 180 mL) [contains benzoic acid, ethanol 4.75%]

Cheracol Plus: Guaifenesin 100 mg and dextromethorphan hydrobromide 10 mg per 5 mL (120 mL) [contains benzoic acid, ethanol 4.75%]

Diabetic Siltussin-DM DAS-Na: Guaifenesin 100 mg and dextromethorphan hydrobromide 10 mg per 5 mL (118 mL) [ethanol free, sugar free; contains benzoic acid, phenylalanine 3 mg/5 mL, propylene glycol; strawberry flavor]

Diabetic Siltussin-DM DAS-Na Maximum Strength: Guaifenesin 200 mg and dextromethorphan hydrobromide 10 mg per 5 mL (118 mL) [ethanol free, sugar free; contains benzoic acid, phenylalanine 3 mg/5 mL, propylene glycol; strawberry flavor]

Guaicon DMS: Guaifenesin 100 mg and dextromethorphan hydrobromide 10 mg per 5 mL (10 mL) [ethanol free, sugar free]

Q-Tussin DM: Guaifenesin 100 mg and dextromethorphan hydrobromide 10 mg per 5 mL (118 mL, 237 mL, 473 mL) [ethanol free, contains sodium benzoate; cherry flavor]

Robafen DM: Guaifenesin 100 mg and dextromethorphan hydrobromide 10 mg per 5 mL (120 mL, 240 mL, 480 mL) [cherry flavor]

Robitussin Peak Cold Cough + Chest Congestion DM: Guaifenesin 100 mg and dextromethorphan hydrobromide 10 mg per 5 mL (120 mL, 240 mL) [contains menthol, propylene glycol, sodium 7 mg/5 mL, sodium benzoate]

Robitussin Peak Cold Sugar-Free Cough + Chest Congestion DM: Guaifenesin 100 mg and dextromethorphan hydrobromide 10 mg per 5 mL (120 mL) [sugar free; contains propylene glycol, sodium 3 mg/5 mL, sodium benzoate]

Robitussin Peak Cold Maximum Strength Cough + Chest Congestion DM: Guaifenesin 200 mg and dextromethorphan hydrobromide 10 mg per 5 mL (120 mL, 240 mL) [contains menthol, propylene glycol, sodium 5 mg/5 mL, sodium benzoate]

Silexin: Guaifenesin 100 mg and dextromethorphan hydrobromide 10 mg per 5 mL (45 mL) [ethanol free, sugar free)]

Siltussin DM: Guaifenesin 100 mg and dextromethorphan hydrobromide 10 mg per 5 mL (120 mL, 240 mL, 480 mL) [strawberry flavor]

Siltussin DM DAS: Guaifenesin 100 mg and dextromethorphan hydrobromide 10 mg per 5 mL (120 mL) [dye free, ethanol free, sugar free; strawberry flavor]

Zyncof: Guaifenesin 400 mg and dextromethorphan hydrobromide 20 mg per 5 mL (120 mL, 480 mL) [dye free, ethanol free, sugar free; contains propylen glycol; grape flavor]

Tablet, oral: Guaifenesin 1000 mg and dextromethorphan hydrobromide 60 mg; guaifenesin 1200 mg and dextromethorphan hydrobromide 60 mg

Silexin: Guaifenesin 100 mg and dextromethorphan hydrobromide 10 mg

Tablet, extended release, oral:
Mucinex DM: Guaifenesin 600 mg and dextromethorphan hydrobromide 30 mg
Mucinex DM Maximum Strength: Guaifenesin 1200 mg and dextromethorphan hydrobromide 60 mg

Tablet, timed release, oral [scored]: Guaifenesin 1200 mg and dextromethorphan hydrobromide 60 mg

References
American Academy of Pediatrics Committee on Drugs. "Inactive" ingredients in pharmaceutical products: update (subject review). Pediatrics. 1997;99(2):268-278.

Shehab N, Lewis CL, Streetman DD, Donn SM. Exposure to the pharmaceutical excipients benzyl alcohol and propylene glycol among critically ill neonates. Pediatr Crit Care Med. 2009;10 (2):256-259.

GuanFACINE (GWAHN fa seen)

Medication Safety Issues
Sound-alike/look-alike issues:
GuanFACINE may be confused with guaiFENesin, guanabenz, guanidine
Tenex® may be confused with Entex®, Xanax®
BEERS Criteria medication:
This drug may be potentially inappropriate for use in geriatric patients (Quality of evidence - low; Strength of recommendation - strong).
International issues:
Tenex [U.S., Canada] may be confused with Kinex brand name for biperiden [Mexico]

Related Information
Oral Medications That Should Not Be Crushed or Altered on page 2438

Brand Names: U.S. Intuniv; Tenex
Brand Names: Canada Intuniv XR
Therapeutic Category Alpha$_2$-Adrenergic Agonist
Generic Availability (U.S.) May be product dependent
Use
Immediate release: Management of hypertension alone or in combination with other hypertensive agents, especially thiazide-type diuretics (FDA approved ages ≥12 years and adults); has also been used in attention-deficit/hyperactivity disorder (ADHD), including ADHD with tic disorder (or Tourette's syndrome) and ADHD with autism or pervasive developmental disorders (PDD) comorbidities
Extended release: Short-term treatment (≤9 weeks) of ADHD as monotherapy or adjunctive therapy with stimulant medication (FDA approved in ages 6-17 years); has also been used for long-term treatment (24 months) of ADHD (Biederman, 2008; Sallee, 2009)

Pregnancy Risk Factor B
Pregnancy Considerations Adverse events were not observed in animal reproduction studies except in doses which also caused maternal toxicity. Information related to guanfacine use during pregnancy is limited (Philipp, 1980). Untreated chronic maternal hypertension is associated with adverse events in the fetus, infant, and mother. If treatment for hypertension during pregnancy is needed, other agents are preferred (ACOG, 2012; Chobanian, 2003).

Breast-Feeding Considerations It is not known if guanfacine is excreted in breast milk. The manufacturer recommends that caution be exercised when administering guanfacine to nursing women. Breast-fed infants of mothers taking medications for hypertension should be monitored for adverse effects (Chobanian, 2003).

Contraindications Hypersensitivity to guanfacine or any component

Warnings May cause bradycardia, hypotension, orthostatic hypotension, and syncope; these effects may be more pronounced during the first month of therapy. Modest, dose-dependent decreases in blood pressure and heart rate (typically asymptomatic) have also been reported. Use with caution in patients with a history of hypotension, heart block, bradycardia, cardiovascular disease, severe coronary insufficiency, recent MI, cerebrovascular disease, syncope, or a condition that predisposes patient to syncope. Use with caution with other agents that may reduce blood pressure or heart rate or increase risk of syncope. Do not abruptly discontinue; abrupt discontinuation can result in nervousness, anxiety, and rebound hypertension; dose should be tapered by no more than 1 mg every 3-7 days.

The American Heart Association recommends that all children diagnosed with ADHD who may be candidates for medication, such as guanfacine, should have a thorough cardiovascular assessment prior to initiation of therapy. These recommendations are based upon reports of serious cardiovascular adverse events (including sudden death) in patients (both children and adults) taking usual doses of stimulant medications. Most of these patients were found to have underlying structural heart disease (eg, hypertrophic obstructive cardiomyopathy). This assessment should include a combination of thorough medical history, family history, and physical examination. An ECG is not mandatory but should be considered. **Note:** In older clinical data, ECG abnormalities and four cases of sudden cardiac death were reported in children receiving clonidine (a less selective alpha$_2$-agonist) with methylphenidate; reduce dose of methylphenidate by 40% when used concurrently with clonidine; consider ECG monitoring. However, more recent (published after 2001) multicenter trials have not reported serious cardiovascular outcomes or events in medically screened children and adolescents receiving concomitant clonidine and psychostimulant therapy; the most frequent reported adverse effects with combination therapy were drowsiness, dizziness, and somnolence (Wilens, 2012). A double-blind, placebo-controlled trial of 461 pediatric patients (age: 6-17 years) examining the effect of the addition of extended release guanfacine to current psychostimulant therapy did not report any cardiovascular adverse events; in this trial, the most common (>10% incidence) treatment emergent adverse effects were headache, somnolence, fatigue, and dizziness (Wilens, 2012). Further studies are needed to examine the long-term safety and efficacy of guanfacine in combination with psychostimulants.

Several cases of skin rash with exfoliation have been reported; however, a clear causal relationship could not be established. Discontinue guanfacine and monitor patients who develop a rash. Formulations of guanfacine (immediate release vs extended release) are not interchangeable on a mg-per-mg basis (due to differences in bioavailability).

Potentially significant drug-drug interactions may exist, requiring dose or frequency adjustment, additional monitoring, and/or selection of alternative therapy. Consult drug interactions database for more detailed information.

Precautions Use with caution in patients with renal or hepatic impairment; dose reduction may be required if impairment is clinically significant. May cause drowsiness, sedation, and somnolence which may impair physical or mental abilities; patients must be cautioned about performing tasks which require mental alertness (eg, operating machinery or driving); sedating effects may be potentiated when used with other CNS depressant drugs (eg, phenothiazines, barbituates, benzodiazepines) or ethanol.

Adverse Reactions

Cardiovascular: Atrioventricular block, bradycardia, hypotension, hypertension, sinus arrhythmia, syncope

Central nervous system: Dizziness, drowsiness, emotional lability (children and adolescents 6-17 years), fatigue, headache, insomnia, irritability, lethargy

Dermatologic: Pallor

Endocrine & metabolic: Weight gain

Gastrointestinal: Abdominal pain, constipation, decreased appetite, diarrhea, dyspepsia, nausea, stomach pain, vomiting, xerostomia

Genitourinary: Impotence, urinary frequency, urinary incontinence

Hepatic: Increased serum ALT

Neuromuscular & skeletal: Weakness

Respiratory: Asthma

Miscellaneous: Fever (Biederman, 2008)

Rare but important or life-threatening: Alopecia, amnesia, cardiac failure, cardiac fibrillation, cerebrovascular accident, convulsions, depression, dermatitis, dysphagia, edema, exfoliative dermatitis, hallucinations (immediate release; children), hypersensitivity reaction, hypokinesia, iritis, mania (immediate release; children), myocardial infarction, nocturia, palpitations, paresis, rebound hypertension, renal failure, tachycardia, visual disturbance

Drug Interactions

Metabolism/Transport Effects Substrate of CYP3A4 (major); **Note:** Assignment of Major/Minor substrate status based on clinically relevant drug interaction potential

Avoid Concomitant Use

Avoid concomitant use of GuanFACINE with any of the following: Azelastine (Nasal); Ceritinib; Conivaptan; Fusidic Acid (Systemic); Iobenguane I 123; Paraldehyde; Thalidomide

Increased Effect/Toxicity

GuanFACINE may increase the levels/effects of: Alcohol (Ethyl); Amifostine; Antihypertensives; Azelastine (Nasal); Beta-Blockers; Bradycardia-Causing Agents; Buprenorphine; Ceritinib; CNS Depressants; DULoxetine; Hydrocodone; Hypotensive Agents; Methotrimeprazine; Metyrosine; Obinutuzumab; Paraldehyde; Pramipexole; RiTUXimab; ROPINIRole; Rotigotine; Selective Serotonin Reuptake Inhibitors; Thalidomide; Valproic Acid and Derivatives; Zolpidem

The levels/effects of GuanFACINE may be increased by: Alfuzosin; Barbiturates; Beta-Blockers; Brimonidine (Topical); Cannabis; Conivaptan; CYP3A4 Inhibitors (Moderate); CYP3A4 Inhibitors (Strong); Dasatinib; Diazoxide; Doxylamine; Dronabinol; Droperidol; Fusidic Acid (Systemic); Herbs (Hypotensive Properties); HydrOXYzine; Ivacaftor; Kava Kava; Luliconazole; Magnesium Sulfate; MAO Inhibitors; Methotrimeprazine; Mifepristone; Nabilone; Pentoxifylline; Perampanel; Phosphodiesterase 5 Inhibitors; Prostacyclin Analogues; Rufinamide; Simeprevir; Sodium Oxybate; Stiripentol; Tapentadol; Tetrahydrocannabinol

Decreased Effect

GuanFACINE may decrease the levels/effects of: Iobenguane I 123

The levels/effects of GuanFACINE may be decreased by: Bosentan; CYP3A4 Inducers (Strong); Dabrafenib; Deferasirox; Herbs (Hypertensive Properties); Methylphenidate; Mirtazapine; Mitotane; Serotonin/Norepinephrine Reuptake Inhibitors; Siltuximab; St Johns Wort; Tocilizumab; Tricyclic Antidepressants; Yohimbine

Stability

Immediate release: Store at room temperature between 20°C to 25°C (68°F to 77°F). Dispense in tightly closed, light-resistant container.

Extended release: Store at 25°C (77°F); excursions permitted to 15°C to 30°C (59°F to 86°F).

Mechanism of Action Guanfacine is a selective alpha$_{2A}$-adrenoreceptor agonist which reduces sympathetic nerve impulses, resulting in reduced sympathetic outflow and a subsequent decrease in vasomotor tone and heart rate. In addition, guanfacine preferentially binds postsynaptic alpha$_{2A}$-adrenoreceptors in the prefrontal cortex and has been theorized to improve delay-related firing of prefrontal cortex neurons. As a result, underlying working memory and behavioral inhibition are affected; thereby improving symptoms associated with ADHD. Guanfacine is not a CNS stimulant.

Pharmacodynamics Antihypertensive effect: Duration: 24 hours following single dose

Pharmacokinetics (Adult data unless noted) Note: When dosed at same mg dose, the extended-release product has a lower peak serum concentration (60% lower) and AUC (43% lower) compared to the immediate release formulation.

Distribution:

Immediate release: V_d: 6.3 L/kg

Extended release: V_d (apparent): Children: 23.7 L/kg; Adolescent: 19.9 L/kg (Boellner, 2007)

Protein binding: ~70%

Metabolism: Hepatic via CYP3A4

Bioavailability: Oral:

Immediate release: ~80%

Extended release (relative to immediate release): 58%

Half-life:

Immediate release: ~17 hours (range: 10-30 hours)

Extended release: Children: 14.4 hours; Adolescents: 18 hours (Boellner, 2007)

Time to peak serum concentration:

Immediate release: 2.6 hours (range: 1-4 hours)

Extended release: Children and Adolescents: 5 hours (Boellner, 2007); Adults: 4-8 hours

Elimination: ~50% (40% to 75% of dose) excreted as unchanged drug in urine; tubular secretion of the drug may occur

Dialysis: Not dialyzable in clinically significant amounts (2.4%)

Dosing: Usual Note: Immediate release and extended release products should not be interchanged on a mg-per-mg basis due to differences in pharmacokinetic profiles.

Children and Adolescents:

Attention-Deficit/Hyperactivity Disorder:

Immediate release product: Limited data available (Dopheide, 2009; Pliszka, 2007): Children ≥6 years and Adolescents:

≤45 kg: Oral: Initial: 0.5 mg once daily at bedtime; may titrate every 3-4 days in 0.5 mg/day increments to 0.5 mg twice daily, then 0.5 mg three times daily, then 0.5 mg four times daily; maximum daily dose: Patient weight 27-40.5 kg: 2 mg/**day**; 40.5-45 kg: 3 mg/**day**

>45 kg: Oral: Initial: 1 mg once daily at bedtime; may titrate every 3-4 days in 1 mg/day increments to 1 mg twice daily, then 1 mg three times daily, then 1 mg four times daily; maximum daily dose: 4 mg/**day**

Extended release product (Intuniv®): Children and Adolescents 6-17 years: Oral: Initial: 1 mg once daily administered at the same time of day (in the morning or evening); may titrate dose by no more than 1 mg/week increments, as tolerated. Usual maintenance dose: 1-4 mg/day; maximum daily dose: 4 mg/**day**. In clinical monotherapy trials, initial clinical response was associated with doses of 0.05-0.08 mg/kg once daily; increased efficacy was seen with increasing mg/kg doses; doses up to 0.12 mg/kg once daily have shown benefit when tolerated. In adjunctive therapy trials with stimulant medication, doses of 0.05-0.12 mg/kg/day produced optimal clinical response in the majority of patients.

Conversion from immediate release guanfacine to the extended release product: Discontinue the immediate release product; initiate the extended release product at the doses recommended above.

Missed doses of extended release: If patient misses two or more consecutive doses, repeat titration of dose should be considered.

Discontinuation of extended release: Taper dose by no more than 1 mg every 3-7 days.

Dosing adjustment for concomitant CYP3A4 inhibitors/inducers: Extended release:

Strong CYP3A4 inhibitors: If initiating guanfacine while taking a strong 3A4 inhibitor, do not exceed a maximum guanfacine dose of 2 mg/day. If continuing guanfacine and adding a strong CYP3A4 inhibitor, decrease guanfacine dose by 50%. If the strong CYP3A4 inhibitor is discontinued, double the guanfacine dose (maximum daily dose: 4 mg/**day**).

Strong CYP3A4 inducers: If initiating guanfacine while taking a strong CYP3A4 inducer, may titrate guanfacine up to 8 mg/day; consider faster titration (eg, 2 mg/week). If continuing guanfacine and adding a strong CYP3A4 inducer, consider increasing guanfacine gradually over 1-2 weeks to double the original dose, as tolerated. If the strong CYP3A4 inducer is discontinued, decrease guanfacine dose by 50% over 1-2 weeks (maximum daily dose: 4 mg/**day**).

Hypertension: Children ≥12 years and Adolescents: Immediate release product: Oral: 1 mg usually at bedtime; may increase, if needed, at 3- to 4-week intervals; usual range: 0.5-2 mg/day; maximum daily dose: 2 mg/**day**

Pervasive developmental disorders (PDD) and ADHD: Limited data available; efficacy results variable: Children and Adolescents 5-14 years: Immediate release product:

<25 kg: Oral: Initial: 0.25 mg once daily, increase dose as tolerated every 4 days in 0.25 mg/day increments in 2-3 divided doses; maximum daily dose: 3 mg/**day** (Scahill, 2006)

≥25 kg: Oral: Initial: 0.5 mg once daily, increase dose as tolerated every 4 days in 0.5 mg/day increments in 2-3 divided doses; maximum daily dose: 3 mg/**day** (Handen, 2008; Scahill, 2006)

Dosing based on a double-blind, placebo-controlled, 6-week crossover trial conducted in children with ADHD and autism or intellectual disabilities (n=11; age: 5-9 years); five of 11 patients showed improvement in hyperactivity scores; other patient assessment parameters did not show improvements (Handen, 2008). In an open-label 8-week pilot study in children with ADHD and PDD (n=25; mean age: 9 years; range: 5-14 years), patients showed improvement in parent- and teacher-rated hyperactivity subscale scores; increased irritability occurred in seven patients; the authors note that patients with PDD may be more sensitive to irritability-type adverse effects (Scahill, 2006). A retrospective chart review of pediatric autism spectrum disorders (n=80; age: 3-18 years) reported ~24% of patients responded to mean dose of 2.6 mg/day; the authors noted patients with Asperger's or PDD not otherwise specified (NOS) responded more frequently than those with autistic disorder or comorbidity of mental retardation (Posey, 2004). Further studies are needed.

Tic disorder and ADHD: Limited data available: Children and Adolescents 7-16 years: Immediate release product: Oral: Initial: 0.5 mg once daily at bedtime for 3 days, then 0.5 mg twice daily for 4 days, then 0.5 mg 3 times daily for 7 days; further upward titration based on clinical response; dosing based on a double-blind, placebo-controlled study in patients with ADHD and mild to moderate tics (n=34; mean age: 10.4 years; range: 7-14 years); reported final dose range: 1.5-3 mg/day in 3 divided doses; improvement in teacher-rated ADHD scores and tic scores after

8 weeks was reported (Scahill, 2001). A small open-label trial (n=10; age range: 8-16 years) used similar initial doses with dose titration; final dose range: 0.75-3 mg/day in divided doses; 7 of 10 patients required a final dose of 1.5 mg/day in divided doses (Chappell, 1995). Further studies are needed.

Adults: **Hypertension:** Immediate release: Oral: 1 mg usually at bedtime; may increase, if needed, at 3- to 4-week intervals; usual dose range (JNC 7): 0.5-2 mg once daily

Dosing adjustment in renal impairment:

Immediate release: Children ≥12 years and Adults: There are no dosage adjustments provided in the manufacturer's labeling; however, the lower end of the dosing range is recommended in patients with renal impairment; use with caution, as ~50% of the dose (40% to 75% of dose) is excreted as unchanged drug in urine.

Extended release (Intuniv®): Children ≥6 years and Adolescents: There are no dosage adjustments provided in manufacturer's labeling (has not been studied); however, dosage adjustments may be necessary in patients with significant renal impairment.

Hemodialysis: Immediate release or extended release: Dialysis clearance is low (~15% of total clearance).

Dosing adjustment in hepatic impairment:

Immediate release: Children ≥12 years and Adults: There are no specific dosage adjustments provided in the manufacturer's labeling; however, use with caution in chronic hepatic impairment; consider dosage reduction.

Extended release (Intuniv®): Children ≥6 years and Adolescents: There are no dosage adjustments provided in manufacturer's labeling (has not been studied); however, dosage adjustments may be necessary in patients with significant hepatic impairment.

Administration

Immediate release: Take at bedtime to minimize somnolence

Extended release: Take at the same time each day (either morning or evening); swallow tablet whole with water, milk, or other liquid; do not crush, break, or chew; do not administer with high-fat meal

Monitoring Parameters Heart rate, blood pressure, consider ECG monitoring in patients with history of heart disease or concurrent use of medications affecting cardiac conduction

ADHD: Evaluate patients for cardiac disease prior to initiation of therapy for ADHD with thorough medical history, family history, and physical exam; consider ECG; perform ECG and echocardiogram if findings suggest cardiac disease; promptly conduct cardiac evaluation in patients who develop chest pain, unexplained syncope, or any other symptom of cardiac disease during treatment.

Additional Information Guanfacine is a more selective alpha$_2$-agonist than clonidine; withdrawal effects less commonly occur due to its longer half-life.

Medications used to treat ADHD should be part of a total treatment program that may include other components, such as psychological, educational, and social measures. Long-term usefulness of guanfacine for the treatment of ADHD should be periodically re-evaluated in patients receiving the drug for extended periods of time.

Dosage Forms Excipient information presented when available (limited, particularly for generics); consult specific product labeling.

Tablet, Oral:
Tenex: 1 mg [contains fd&c red #40 aluminum lake]
Tenex: 2 mg [contains fd&c yellow #10 aluminum lake]
Generic: 1 mg, 2 mg
Tablet Extended Release 24 Hour, Oral:
Intuniv: 1 mg, 2 mg, 3 mg, 4 mg

References

American Academy of Pediatrics/American Heart Association Clarification of Statement on Cardiovascular Evaluation and Monitoring of Children and Adolescents With Heart Disease Receiving Medications for ADHD; available at: http://americanheart.mediaroom.com/index.-php?s=43&item=422.

American College of Obstetricians and Gynecologists (ACOG), "ACOG Practice Bulletin No. 125: Chronic Hypertension in Pregnancy," *Obstet Gynecol*, 2012, 119(2 Pt 1):396-407.

Biederman J, Melmed RD, Patel A, et al, "A Randomized, Double-Blind, Placebo-Controlled Study of Guanfacine Extended Release in Children and Adolescents With Attention-Deficit/Hyperactivity Disorder," *Pediatrics*, 2008, 121(1):e73-84.

Biederman J, Melmed RD, Patel A, et al, "Long-Term, Open-Label Extension Study of Guanfacine Extended Release in Children and Adolescents With ADHD," *CNS Spectr*, 2008, 13(12):1047-55.

Boellner SW, Pennick M, Fiske K, et al, "Pharmacokinetics of a Guanfacine Extended-Release Formulation in Children and Adolescents With Attention-Deficit-Hyperactivity Disorder," *Pharmacotherapy*, 2007, 27(9):1253-62.

Chappell PB, Riddle MA, Scahill L, et al, "Guanfacine Treatment of Comorbid Attention-Deficit Hyperactivity Disorder and Tourette's Syndrome: Preliminary Clinical Experience," *J Am Acad Child Adolesc Psychiatry*, 1995, 34(9):1140-6.

Chobanian AV, Bakris GL, Black HR, et al, "The Seventh Report of the Joint National Committee on Prevention, Detection, Evaluation, and Treatment of High Blood Pressure: The JNC 7 Report," *JAMA*, 2003, 289(19):2560-71.

Dopheide JA and Pliszka SR, "Attention-Deficit-Hyperactivity Disorder: An Update," *Pharmacotherapy*, 2009, 29(6):656-79.

Handen BL, Sahl R, and Hardan AY, "Guanfacine in Children With Autism and/or Intellectual Disabilities," *J Dev Behav Pediatr*, 2008, 29 (4):303-8.

Philipp E, "Guanfacine in the Treatment of Hypertension Due to Pre-eclamptic Toxaemia in Thirty Women," *Br J Clin Pharmacol*, 1980, 10 (Suppl 1):137-40.

Pliszka S and AACAP Work Group on Quality Issues, "Practice Parameter for the Assessment and Treatment of Children and Adolescents With Attention-Deficit/Hyperactivity Disorder," *Am Acad Child Adolesc Psychiatry*, 2007, 46(7):894-921.

Posey DJ, Puntney JI, Sasher TM, et al, "Guanfacine Treatment of Hyperactivity and Inattention in Pervasive Developmental Disorders: A Retrospective Analysis of 80 Cases," *J Child Adolesc Psychopharmacol*, 2004, 14(2):233-41.

Sallee FR, Lyne A, Wigal T, et al, "Long-Term Safety and Efficacy of Guanfacine Extended Release in Children and Adolescents With Attention-Deficit/Hyperactivity Disorder," *J Child Adolesc Psychopharmacol*, 2009, 19(3):215-26.

Sallee FR, McGough J, Wigal T, et al, "Guanfacine Extended Release in Children and Adolescents With Attention-Deficit/Hyperactivity Disorder: A Placebo-Controlled Trial," *J Am Acad Child Adolesc Psychiatry*, 2009, 48(2):155-65.

Scahill L, Aman MG, McDougle CJ, et al, "A Prospective Open Trial of Guanfacine in Children With Pervasive Developmental Disorders," *J Child Adolesc Psychopharmacol*, 2006, 16(5):589-98.

Scahill L, Chappell PB, Kim YS, et al, "A Placebo-Controlled Study of Guanfacine in the Treatment of Children With Tic Disorders and Attention Deficit Hyperactivity Disorder," *Am J Psychiatry*, 2001, 158 (7):1067-74.

Scahill L, "Alpha-2 Adrenergic Agonists in Attention Deficit Hyperactivity Disorder," *J Pediatr*, 2009, 154:S32-7.

Spencer TJ, Greenbaum M, Ginsberg LD, et al, "Safety and Effectiveness of Coadministration of Guanfacine Extended Release and Psychostimulants in Children and Adolescents With Attention-Deficit/Hyperactivity Disorder," *J Child Adolesc Psychopharmacol*, 2009, 19(5):501-10.

Vetter VL, Elia J, Erickson C, et al, "Cardiovascular Monitoring of Children and Adolescents With Heart Disease Receiving Medications for Attention Deficit/Hyperactivity Disorder [Corrected]: A Scientific Statement From the American Heart Association Council on Cardiovascular Disease in the Young Congenital Cardiac Defects Committee and the Council on Cardiovascular Nursing," *Circulation*, 2008, 117(18):2407-23.

Wilens TE, Bukstein O, Brams M, et al, "A Controlled Trial of Extended-Release Guanfacine and Psychostimulants for Attention-Deficit/Hyperactivity Disorder," *J Am Acad Child Adolesc Psychiatry*, 2012, 51(1):74-85.

◆ **Guanfacine Hydrochloride** *see* GuanFACINE *on page 989*

◆ **GW506U78** *see* Nelarabine *on page 1477*

◆ **GW433908G** *see* Fosamprenavir *on page 931*

◆ **Gyne-Lotrimin [OTC]** *see* Clotrimazole (Topical) *on page 527*

◆ **Gyne-Lotrimin 3 [OTC]** *see* Clotrimazole (Topical) *on page 527*

◆ **H1N1 Influenza Vaccine** *see* Influenza Virus Vaccine (Inactivated) *on page 1103*

◆ **H1N1 Influenza Vaccine** *see* Influenza Virus Vaccine (Live/Attenuated) *on page 1109*

◆ **H₂O₂** *see* Hydrogen Peroxide *on page 1040*

Haemophilus b Conjugate and Hepatitis B Vaccine

(he MOF i lus bee KON joo gate & hep a TYE tis bee vak SEEN)

Medication Safety Issues
Sound-alike/look-alike issues:
Comvax® may be confused with Recombivax [Recombivax HB®]

Related Information
Immunization Administration Recommendations *on page 2368*

Immunization Guidelines *on page 2373*

Brand Names: U.S. Comvax®

Therapeutic Category Vaccine

Generic Availability (U.S.) No

Use Immunization against invasive disease caused by *H. influenzae* type b and against infection caused by all known subtypes of hepatitis B virus in patients born of HBₛAg-negative mothers (FDA approved in ages 6 weeks to 15 months)

Infants born of HBₛAg-positive mothers or mothers of unknown HBₛAg status should receive hepatitis B immune globulin and monovalent hepatitis B vaccine (recombinant) at birth and should complete the hepatitis B vaccination series

Pregnancy Risk Factor C

Pregnancy Considerations Animal reproduction studies have not been conducted. This product is not indicated for use in women of childbearing age.

Breast-Feeding Considerations This product is not indicated for use in women of childbearing age. Inactivated virus vaccines do not affect the safety of breast-feeding for the mother or the infant (CDC, 2011). Breast-feeding also appears to reduce the incidence of infant fever associated with routine childhood immunization (Piscane, 2010). Breast-feeding infants should be vaccinated according to the recommended schedules (CDC, 2011).

Contraindications Hypersensitivity to hepatitis vaccine, *Haemophilus* b vaccine, yeast, or any component

Warnings Immediate treatment (including epinephrine 1:1000) for anaphylactic and/or hypersensitivity reactions should be available during vaccine use. Children with chronic illness associated with increased risk of *Haemophilus influenzae* type b disease may have impaired anti-PRP antibody responses to conjugate vaccination. Examples include those with HIV infection, immunoglobulin deficiency, anatomic or functional asplenia, and sickle cell disease, as well as recipients of bone marrow transplants and recipients of chemotherapy for malignancy. Syncope has been reported with use of injectable vaccines and may be accompanied by transient visual disturbances, weakness, or tonic-clonic movements. Procedures should be in place to avoid injuries from falling and to restore cerebral perfusion if syncope occurs (CDC, 57[17], 2008).

Comvax is not indicated for use as the "birth dose" of hepatitis B vaccine; hepatitis B vaccine (recombinant) is indicated for all infants at birth. This combination vaccine cannot be administered to any infant <6 weeks of age or >71 months of age. Infants born of HBₛAg-positive mothers or mothers of unknown HBₛAg status should receive hepatitis B vaccine (recombinant) at birth and should complete the hepatitis B vaccination series given

according to a particular schedule (refer to current ACIP recommendations). Infants born of HBₛAg-positive mothers should also receive hepatitis B immune globulin at birth.

Precautions The decision to administer or delay vaccination because of current or recent febrile illness depends on the severity of symptoms and the etiology of the disease. Immunization should be delayed during the course of an acute severe febrile illness; may administer to patients with mild acute illness (with or without fever). Use with caution in patients with coagulation disorders, including thrombocytopenia, due to an increased risk for bleeding following I.M. administration; if the patient receives antihemophilia or other similar therapy, I.M. injection can be scheduled shortly after such therapy is administered.

Use with caution in severely immunocompromised patients (eg, patients receiving chemo-/radiation therapy or other immunosuppressive therapy including high-dose corticosteroids); may have a reduced response to vaccination; inactivated vaccines should be administered ≥2 weeks prior to planned immunosuppression when feasible (IDSA [Rubin, 2013]). In general, household and close contacts of persons with altered immunocompetence may receive all age-appropriate vaccines. Vaccination may not result in effective immunity in all patients. Response depends upon multiple factors (eg, type of vaccine, age of patient) and may be improved by administering the vaccine at the recommended dose, route, and interval (CDC/ACIP [Kroger, 2011]). Infection may occur within the week of vaccination, prior to the onset of the vaccine.

Antipyretics have not been shown to prevent febrile seizures; antipyretics may be used to treat fever or discomfort following vaccination (CDC/ACIP [Kroger, 2011]). One study reported that routine prophylactic administration of acetaminophen to prevent fever prior to vaccination decreased the immune response of some vaccines; the clinical significance of this reduction in immune response has not been established (Prymula, 2009). Packaging contains natural latex rubber.

Adverse Reactions All serious adverse reactions must be reported to the U.S. Department of Health and Human Services (DHHS) Vaccine Adverse Event Reporting System (VAERS) at 1-800-822-7967 or online at https://vaers.hhs.gov/esub/index.

Central nervous system: Crying (unusual/high pitched), fever, irritability, somnolence

Dermatologic: Rash

Gastrointestinal: Anorexia, diarrhea, oral candidiasis, vomiting

Local: Injection site reactions: Erythema pain/soreness, swelling/induration

Otic: Otitis media

Respiratory: Cough, respiratory congestion, rhinorrhea, upper respiratory tract infection

Postmarketing and/or case reports: Anaphylaxis, angioedema, erythema multiforme, febrile seizure, seizure, thrombocytopenia, urticaria

Drug Interactions
Metabolism/Transport Effects None known.

Avoid Concomitant Use There are no known interactions where it is recommended to avoid concomitant use.

Increased Effect/Toxicity There are no known significant interactions involving an increase in effect.

Decreased Effect
The levels/effects of Haemophilus b Conjugate and Hepatitis B Vaccine may be decreased by: Belimumab; Fingolimod; Immunosuppressants

Stability Store at 2°C to 8°C (36°F to 48°F); do not freeze.

Mechanism of Action See individual agents.

Pharmacodynamics See individual agents.

▶

Dosing: Usual Pediatric:

Primary Immunization: Infants and Children 6 weeks through 15 months: I.M.: 0.5 mL per dose for a total of 3 doses administered as follows: 2, 4, and 12 to 15 months of age; **Note:** If the recommended schedule cannot be followed, the interval between the first two doses should be at least 6 weeks and the interval between the second and third doses should be as close as possible to 8 to 11 months.

Modified Schedule: Children who receive one dose of hepatitis B vaccine at or shortly after birth may receive Comvax on a schedule of 2, 4, and 12 to 15 months of age

Dosing adjustment in renal impairment: There are no dosage adjustments provided in the manufacturer's labeling.

Dosing adjustment in hepatic impairment: There are no dosage adjustments provided in the manufacturer's labeling.

Administration Shake well and administer I.M. in either the anterolateral aspect of the thigh or deltoid muscle of the arm; **not for I.V. or SubQ administration.**

Monitoring Parameters Observe for syncope for 15 minutes following administration. If seizure-like activity associated with syncope occurs, maintain patient in supine or Trendelenburg position to reestablish adequate cerebral perfusion.

Additional Information In order to maximize vaccination rates, the ACIP recommends simultaneous administration (ie, >1 vaccine on the same day at different anatomic sites) of all age-appropriate vaccines (live or inactivated) for which a person is eligible at a single visit, unless contraindications exist. If available, the use of combination vaccines is generally preferred over separate injections, taking into consideration provider assessment, patient preference, and potential adverse events. If separate vaccines being used, evaluate product information regarding same syringe compatibility of vaccines. Separate needles and syringes should be used for each injection. The ACIP prefers each dose of specific vaccine in a series come from the same manufacturer if possible (CDC/ACIP [Kroger, 2011]).

For additional information, please refer to the following website: http://www.cdc.gov/vaccines/vpd-vac/.

Dosage Forms Excipient information presented when available (limited, particularly for generics); consult specific product labeling.

Injection, suspension [preservative free]:

Comvax®: *Haemophilus* b capsular polysaccharide 7.5 mcg (bound to *Neisseria meningitides* OMPC 125 mcg) and hepatitis B surface antigen 5 mcg per 0.5 mL (0.5 mL) [contains aluminum; contains natural rubber/natural latex in packaging]

References

AAP Steering Committee on Quality Improvement and Management, Subcommittee on Febrile Seizures American Academy of Pediatrics. Febrile seizures: clinical practice guideline for the long-term management of the child with simple febrile seizures. *Pediatrics.* 2008;121 (6):1281-1286.

Akinsanya-Beysolow I; Advisory Committee on Immunization Practices (ACIP); ACIP Child/Adolescent Immunization Work Group; Centers for Disease Control and Prevention (CDC). Advisory Committee on Immunization Practices recommended immunization schedules for persons aged 0 through 18 years – United States, 2014. *MMWR Morb Mortal Wkly Rep.* 2014;63(5):108-109. Available at http://www.-cdc.gov/vaccines/schedules/downloads/child/0-18yrs-child-combined-schedule.pdf

Centers for Disease Control and Prevention (CDC). Syncope after vaccination – United States, January 2005-July 2007. *MMWR Morb Mortal Wkly Rep.* 2008;57(17):457-460.

Kroger AT, Atkinson WL, Marcuse EK, Pickering LK. General recommendations on immunization - recommendations of the Advisory Committee on Immunization Practices (ACIP). *MMWR Recomm Rep.* 2011;60(RR-2):1-64.

Pisacane A, Continisio P, Palma O, Cataldo S, De Michele F, Vairo U. Breastfeeding and risk for fever after immunization. *Pediatrics.* 2010;125(6):e1448-e1452.

Prymula R, Siegrist CA, Chlibek R, et al. Effect of prophylactic paracetamol administration at time of vaccination on febrile reactions and antibody responses in children: two open-label, randomised controlled trials. *Lancet.* 2009;374(9698):1339-1350.

◆ *Haemophilus* B **Conjugate (Hib)** *see* Diphtheria and Tetanus Toxoids, Acellular Pertussis, Poliovirus and *Haemophilus* b Conjugate Vaccine *on page 684*

Haemophilus b **Conjugate Vaccine**
(he MOF fi lus bee KON joo gate vak SEEN)

Related Information

Immunization Administration Recommendations *on page 2368*

Immunization Guidelines *on page 2373*

Brand Names: U.S. ActHIB; Hiberix; PedvaxHIB

Brand Names: Canada ActHIB; PedvaxHIB

Therapeutic Category Vaccine

Generic Availability (U.S.) No

Use

Routine, full series immunization of children 2 months to 5 years of age against invasive disease caused by *H. influenzae* (ActHIB: FDA approved in ages 2 months to 5 years; PedvaxHIB: FDA approved in ages 2 to 71 months)

Routine booster only immunization of children (FDA approval: Hiberix in ages 15 months to 4 years)

The Advisory Committee on Immunization Practices (ACIP) recommends vaccination for the following (CDC/ACIP [Akinsanya-Beysolow, 2014]; CDC/ACIP [Bridges, 2014]); CDC/ACIP [Briere, 2014]):

• Routine immunization in all infants and children through 59 months

• Unimmunized* children 12 through 59 months including chemotherapy recipients, anatomic or functional asplenia (including sickle cell disease), HIV infection, immunoglobulin deficiency, or early component complement deficiency

Efficacy data are not available for use in older children and adults with chronic conditions associated with an increased risk of Hib disease; however, may be used in certain situations:

• Unimmunized* children ≥5 years, adolescents, and adults with anatomic or functional asplenia (including sickle cell disease)

• Unimmunized* children ≥5 years and adolescents with HIV infection

• Children <5 years undergoing chemotherapy or radiation treatment

• Successful hematopoietic stem cell transplant recipients

• Children ≥15 months and adolescents undergoing elective splenectomy

* Unimmunized is defined as persons who have not received a primary series and booster dose or at least 1 dose of a Hib vaccine after 14 months of age

Pregnancy Risk Factor C

Pregnancy Considerations Animal reproduction studies have not been conducted.

Breast-Feeding Considerations Inactivated virus vaccines do not affect the safety of breast-feeding for the mother or the infant (CDC, 2011). Breast-feeding also appears to reduce the incidence of infant fever associated with routine childhood immunization (Piscane, 2010). Breast-feeding infants should be vaccinated according to the recommended schedules (CDC, 2011).

Contraindications Hypersensitivity to any component including tetanus toxoid (ActHIB®, Hiberix®)

Warnings Immediate treatment (including epinephrine 1:1000) for anaphylactic and/or hypersensitivity reactions should be available during vaccine use. The carrier proteins used in Haemophilus b polyribosylribitol phosphate-outer membrane polysaccharide conjugate (PRP-T, ActHIB, Hiberix) are chemically and immunologically related to toxoids contained in DTaP vaccine. Earlier or simultaneous vaccination with tetanus toxoids may be required to elicit an optimal anti-PRP antibody response. In contrast, the immunogenicity of PedvaxHIB is not affected by vaccination with DTaP. In infants in whom DTaP or DT vaccination is deferred, PedvaxHIB may be advantageous for *Haemophilus influenzae* type b vaccination. Immunization with ActHIB and Hiberix is not a substitute for routine tetanus immunization.

Children with chronic illness associated with increased risk of *Haemophilus influenzae* type b disease may have impaired anti-PRP antibody responses to conjugate vaccination. Examples include those with HIV infection, immunoglobulin deficiency, anatomic or functional asplenia, and sickle cell disease, as well as recipients of bone marrow transplants and recipients of chemotherapy for malignancy. Some children with immunologic impairment may benefit from more doses of conjugate vaccine than normally indicated. Apnea has occurred following intramuscular vaccine administration in premature infants; consider clinical status implications. Syncope has been reported with use of injectable vaccines and may be accompanied by transient visual disturbances, weakness, or tonic-clonic movements. Procedures should be in place to avoid injuries from falling and to restore cerebral perfusion if syncope occurs (CDC, 57[17], 2008).

Precautions The decision to administer or delay vaccination because of current or recent febrile illness depends on the severity of symptoms and the etiology of the disease. Immunization should be delayed during the course of an acute severe febrile illness; may administer to patients with mild acute illness (with or without fever). Use with caution in severely immunocompromised patients (eg, patients receiving chemo/radiation therapy or other immunosuppressive therapy, including high-dose corticosteroids); may have a reduced response to vaccination; inactive vaccines should be administered ≥2 weeks prior to planned immunosuppression when feasible (IDSA [Rubin, 2014]). In general, household and close contacts of persons with altered immunocompetence may receive all age-appropriate vaccines. Vaccination may not result in effective immunity in all patients. Response depends upon multiple factors (eg, type of vaccine, age of patient) and may be improved by administering the vaccine at the recommended dose, route, and interval (CDC/ACIP [Kroger, 2011]).

Administer with caution in patients with coagulation disorders, including thrombocytopenia, due to an increased risk for bleeding following I.M. administration; if the patient receives antihemophilia or other similar therapy, I.M. injection can be scheduled shortly after such therapy is administered. Antipyretics have not been shown to prevent febrile seizures; antipyretics may be used to treat fever or discomfort following vaccination (CDC/ACIP [Kroger, 2011]). One study reported that routine prophylactic administration of acetaminophen to prevent fever prior to vaccination decreased the immune response of some vaccines; the clinical significance of this reduction in immune response has not been established (Prymula, 2009). Use caution in patients with history of Guillain-Barré syndrome (GBS); carefully consider risks and benefits to vaccination in patients known to have experienced BGS within 6 weeks following a prior *Haemophilus* b vaccine.

Use of this vaccine for specific medical and/or other indications (eg, immunocompromising conditions, hepatic or kidney disease, diabetes) is also addressed in the ACIP Recommended Immunization Schedule (CDC/ACIP [Akinsanya-Beysolow, 2014]; CDC/ACIP [Bridges, 2014]). Specific recommendations for use of this vaccine in immunocompromised patients with asplenia, cancer, HIV infection, cerebrospinal fluid leaks, cochlear implants, hematopoietic stem cell transplant (prior to or after), sickle cell disease, solid organ transplant (prior to or after), or those receiving immunosuppressive therapy for chronic conditions as well as contacts of immunocompromised patients are available from the IDSA (Rubin, 2014). Some products may contain lactose; some packaging may contain natural latex rubber.

Adverse Reactions All serious adverse reactions must be reported to the U.S. Department of Health and Human Services (DHHS) Vaccine Adverse Event Reporting System (VAERS) 1-800-822-7967 or online at https://vaers.hhs.gov/esub/index. In Canada, adverse reactions may be reported to local provincial/territorial health agencies or to the Vaccine Safety Section at Public Health Agency of Canada (1-866-844-0018).

Central nervous system: Crying (unusual, high pitched, prolonged), drowsiness, fussiness, irritability, lethargy, pain, restlessness, seizure

Dermatologic: Skin rash, urticaria

Gastrointestinal: Anorexia, diarrhea, vomiting

Hematologic & oncologic: Thrombocytopenia

Local: Injection site: Erythema, induration, pain, soreness, swelling

Neuromuscular & skeletal: Weakness

Otic: Otitis media

Respiratory: Tracheitis, upper respiratory tract infection

Miscellaneous: Fever

Rare but important or life-threatening: Abscess at injection site (sterile), anaphylaxis, anaphylactoid reaction, angioedema, apnea, febrile seizures, Guillain-Barré syndrome, hypersensitivity reaction, hypotonic/hyporesponsive episode, lymphadenopathy, mass, peripheral edema, pneumonia, swelling of the injected limb (extensive), syncope, vasodepressor syncope

Drug Interactions

Metabolism/Transport Effects None known.

Avoid Concomitant Use There are no known interactions where it is recommended to avoid concomitant use.

Increased Effect/Toxicity There are no known significant interactions involving an increase in effect.

Decreased Effect

The levels/effects of Haemophilus b Conjugate Vaccine may be decreased by: Belimumab; Fingolimod; Immunosuppressants

Stability Store at 2°C to 8°C (36°F to 46°F); do not freeze; protect from light (Hiberix). Once reconstituted with saline, store under refrigeration and use within 24 hours. ActHIB reconstituted with Tripedia should be administered within 30 minutes. Hiberix saline diluent may be stored under refrigeration or at room temperature; do not freeze, discard diluent if frozen.

Mechanism of Action Stimulates production of anticapsular antibodies and provides active immunity to *Haemophilus influenzae* type b. Vaccination provides protective antibodies in >95% of infants who are vaccinated with a 2- or 3-dose series (CDC, 2012). An anti-PRP concentration of ≥1.0 mcg/mL predicts long-term protection.

Pharmacodynamics Efficacy: The initial unconjugated polysaccharide Hib vaccines produced 45% to 88% reduction in disease incidence among children at least 18 to 24 months of age. The initial protein-conjugated Hib vaccines produced >90% protection in infants after a multidose series. After the initial Hib conjugate vaccines were licensed, subsequent formulations were licensed based on noninferior antibody responses.

◄ Onset of action: Immunity develops progressively with each dose. Immunity can be inferred ~2 weeks after the initial series is complete.

Duration: Antibody concentrations exceeding 0.15 mcg/mL correlate with clinical protection from disease. Antibody concentrations exceeding 1 mcg/mL correlate with prolonged protection from disease, generally implying several years of protection.

Dosing: Usual

Pediatric:

Primary immunization: Note: Preterm infants should be vaccinated according to their chronological age, beginning at 2 months of age; number of doses for completion of Hib series dependent upon products including some combination formulations (3 doses: ActHIB, MenHibrix, Pentacel; 2 doses: PedvaxHIB, COMVAX) (see combination product monographs for specific dosing information)

Infants 6 weeks to 6 months: Minimum age for first dose is 6 weeks.

ActHib (PRP-T): I.M.: 0.5 mL per dose for a total of 3 doses administered as follows: 2, 4, and 6 months of age

PedvaxHIB (PRP-OMP): I.M.: 0.5 mL per dose for a total of 2 doses administered as follows: 2 and 4 months of age

Booster immunization:

ActHIB, PedvaxHIB: Children 12 to 15 months: I.M.: 0.5 mL as a single dose

Hiberix: Children 12 months to 4 years: I.M.: 0.5 mL as a single dose

Catch-up immunization: CDC (ACIP) recommendations (Akinsanya-Beysolow, 2014): **Note:** Do not restart the series. If doses have been given, begin the below schedule at the applicable dose number.

Infants and Children 4 to 59 months: I.M.: 0.5 mL per dose for a total of 1 to 4 doses administered as follows:

First dose given on the elected date.

Second dose given at least 4 weeks after the first dose (if first dose at <12 months of age) **or** 8 weeks after the first dose (if first dose at 12 to 14 months of age); this dose is not needed if the first dose was given at ≥15 months.

Third dose given at least 4 weeks after the second dose if currently <12 months of age and first dose at <7 months of age **or** 8 weeks after the first dose and 12 to 59 months of age if:

- currently <12 months of age and first dose at 7 to 11 months of age **or**

- currently 12 to 59 months of age and first dose <12 months of age **or**

- first two doses were PRP-OMP (PedvaxHIB) and given at <12 months of age

Third dose is not needed if the previous dose was given at ≥15 months of age.

Fourth dose given 8 weeks after the third dose: This dose is only needed for children 12 to 59 months who received 3 doses <12 months or for children at high risk who received 3 doses at any age

Children ≥5 years and Adolescents; unimmunized **and** are at increased risk for invasive Hib disease due to anatomic/functional asplenia or splenectomy, HIV infection, immunoglobulin deficiency, early component complement deficiency, or chemotherapy or radiation therapy: I.M.: 0.5 mL as a single dose; may use any of the Hib conjugate vaccines (CDC/ACIP [Briere, 2014]). Unimmunized defined as persons who have not received a primary series and booster dose or at least 1 dose of a Hib vaccine after 14 months of age.

Repeat immunization for high-risk conditions (CDC/ACIP [Briere, 2014]):

Invasive Hib disease: Infants and Children <24 months: Revaccinate with a second primary series beginning 4 weeks after onset of disease

Undergoing chemotherapy or radiation therapy: Infants and Children <60 months: If dose administered within 14 days of starting or given during therapy: Repeat the doses at least 3 months after therapy completion

Hematopoietic stem cell transplant recipient: Children and Adolescents: Revaccinate with a 3-dose regimen beginning 6 to 12 months after successful transplant, regardless of vaccination history. Doses should be administered ≥4 weeks apart.

Adult: **Immunization: Note:** Only indicated for those who have not received the childhood Hib series **and** are at increased risk for invasive Hib disease due to sickle cell disease, anatomic/functional asplenia or splenectomy: I.M.: 0.5 mL as a single dose; may use any of the Hib conjugate vaccines (CDC/ACIP [Briere, 2014])

Hematopoietic stem cell transplant: Revaccinate with a 3-dose regimen beginning 6 to 12 months after the transplant, regardless of vaccination history. Doses should be administered ≥4 weeks apart (CDC/ACIP [Briere, 2014]).

Dosing adjustment in renal impairment: There are no dosage adjustments provided in the manufacturer's labeling.

Dosing adjustment in hepatic impairment: There are no dosage adjustments provided in the manufacturer's labeling.

Administration Shake well; administer I.M. into midlateral aspect of the thigh in infants and small children; administer in the deltoid area to older children and adults; **not for I.V. or SubQ administration.** Adolescents and adults should be vaccinated while seated or lying down. U.S. law requires that the date of administration, the vaccine manufacturer, lot number of vaccine, and the administering person's name, title, and address be entered into the patient's permanent medical record.

Monitoring Parameters Observe for syncope for 15 minutes following administration. If seizure-like activity associated with syncope occurs, maintain patient in supine or Trendelenburg position to reestablish adequate cerebral perfusion.

Test Interactions May interfere with interpretation of urine antigen detection tests; antigenuria may occur up to 2 weeks following immunization

Additional Information If Hiberix is inadvertently administered during the primary vaccination series, the dose can be counted as a valid PRP-T dose that does not need repeated if administered according to schedule. In this case, a total of 3 doses completes the primary series.

In order to maximize vaccination rates, the ACIP recommends simultaneous administration (ie, >1 vaccine on the same day at different anatomic sites) of all age-appropriate vaccines (live or inactivated) for which a person is eligible at a single visit, unless contraindications exist. If available, the use of combination vaccines is generally preferred over separate injections, taking into consideration provider assessment, patient preference, and potential adverse events. If separate vaccines being used, evaluate product information regarding same syringe compatibility of vaccines. Separate needles and syringes should be used for each injection. The ACIP prefers each dose of specific vaccine in a series come from the same manufacturer if possible (CDC/ACIP [Kroger, 2011]).

For additional information, please refer to the following website: http://www.cdc.gov/vaccines/vpd-vac/.

Dosage Forms Excipient information presented when available (limited, particularly for generics); consult specific product labeling.

Injection, powder for reconstitution [preservative free]:

ActHIB *Haemophilus* b capsular polysaccharide 10 mcg [bound to tetanus toxoid 24 mcg] per 0.5 mL [contains sucrose; may be reconstituted with provided diluent (forms solution; contains natural rubber/natural latex in packaging)]

Hiberix: *Haemophilus* b capsular polysaccharide 10 mcg [bound to tetanus toxoid 25 mcg] per 0.5 mL (0.5 mL) [contains lactose 12.6 mg]

Injection, suspension:

PedvaxHIB: *Haemophilus* b capsular polysaccharide 7.5 mcg [bound to *Neisseria meningitidis* OMPC 125 mcg] per 0.5 mL (0.5 mL) [contains aluminum; natural rubber/natural latex in packaging]

References

AAP Steering Committee on Quality Improvement and Management, Subcommittee on Febrile Seizures American Academy of Pediatrics, "Febrile Seizures: Clinical Practice Guideline for the Long-Term Management of the Child With Simple Febrile Seizures," *Pediatrics*, 2008, 121(6):1281-6.

Akinsanya-Beysolow I; Advisory Committee on Immunization Practices (ACIP); ACIP Child/Adolescent Immunization Work Group; Centers for Disease Control and Prevention (CDC). Advisory Committee on Immunization Practices recommended immunization schedules for persons aged 0 through 18 years – United States, 2014. *MMWR Morb Mortal Wkly Rep.* 2014;63(5):108-109. Available at http://www.cdc.gov/vaccines/schedules/downloads/child/0-18yrs-child-combined-schedule.pdf

Bridges CB, Coyne-Beasley T; Advisory Committee on Immunization Practices (ACIP); ACIP Adult Immunization Work Group; Centers for Disease Control and Prevention (CDC). Advisory Committee on Immunization Practices recommended immunization schedule for adults aged 19 years or older – United States, 2014. *MMWR Morb Mortal Wkly Rep.* 2014;63(5):110-112. Available at http://www.cdc.gov/vaccines/schedules/downloads/adult/adult-combined-schedule.pdf

Briere EC, Rubin L, Moro P, et al. Prevention and control of Haemophilus influenzae Type b disease. Recommendations of the Advisory Committee on Immunization Practices (ACIP). *MMWR Recomm Rep.* 2014;63(RR-01):1-20.

Centers for Disease Control and Prevention (CDC), "Syncope After Vaccination-United States, January 2005-July 2007," *MMWR Morb Mortal Wkly Rep*, 2008, 2;57(17):457-60.

Kroger AT, Atkinson WL, Marcuse EK, Pickering LK. General recommendations on immunization - recommendations of the Advisory Committee on Immunization Practices (ACIP). *MMWR Recomm Rep.* 2011;60(RR-2):1-64.

Pisacane A, Continisio P, Palma O, et al, "Breastfeeding and Risk for Fever After Immunization," *Pediatrics*, 2010, 125(6):e1448-52.

Prymula R, Siegrist CA, Chlibek R, et al, "Effect of Prophylactic Paracetamol Administration at Time of Vaccination on Febrile Reactions and Antibody Responses in Children: Two Open-Label, Randomised Controlled Trials," *Lancet*, 2009, 374(9698):1339-50.

Rubin LG, Levin MJ, Ljungman P, et al. 2013 IDSA clinical practice guideline for vaccination of the immunocompromised host. *Clin Infect Dis.* 2014;58(3):e44-e100.

◆ *Haemophilus* b (meningococcal protein conjugate) Conjugate Vaccine *see Haemophilus* b Conjugate and Hepatitis B Vaccine *on page 993*

◆ *Haemophilus* B Polysaccharide *see* Diphtheria and Tetanus Toxoids, Acellular Pertussis, Poliovirus and *Haemophilus* b Conjugate Vaccine *on page 684*

◆ *Haemophilus influenzae* Type b *see Haemophilus* b Conjugate Vaccine *on page 994*

◆ Halcion *see* Triazolam *on page 2080*

◆ Halcion® (Can) *see* Triazolam *on page 2080*

◆ Haldol *see* Haloperidol *on page 998*

◆ Haldol Decanoate *see* Haloperidol *on page 998*

◆ Halfprin [OTC] *see* Aspirin *on page 212*

Halobetasol (hal oh BAY ta sol)

Medication Safety Issues

Sound-alike/look-alike issues:

Ultravate® may be confused with Cutivate®

Related Information

Topical Corticosteroids *on page 2224*

Brand Names: U.S. Halonate; Ultravate

Brand Names: Canada Ultravate®

Therapeutic Category Adrenal Corticosteroid; Anti-inflammatory Agent; Corticosteroid, Topical; Glucocorticoid

Generic Availability (U.S.) May be product dependent

Use Relief of inflammation and pruritus associated with corticosteroid-response dermatoses

Pregnancy Risk Factor C

Pregnancy Considerations Teratogenic effects have been observed in animal reproduction studies. Topical products are not recommended for extensive use, in large quantities, or for long periods of time in pregnant women (Reed, 1997).

Breast-Feeding Considerations Systemically administered corticosteroids appear in human milk and may cause adverse effects in a nursing infant. It is not known if the systemic absorption of topical halobetasol results in detectable quantities in human milk. Use with caution while breast-feeding; do not apply to nipples (Reed, 1997).

Contraindications Hypersensitivity to halobetasol propionate, other corticosteroids, or any component

Warnings Hypothalamic-pituitary-adrenal (HPA) axis suppression may occur with topical corticosteroid use; acute adrenal insufficiency may occur with abrupt withdrawal after long-term use or with stress; withdrawal or discontinuation should be done carefully; patients with HPA axis suppression may require increased doses of systemic glucocorticosteroids prior to, during, and after unusual stress (eg, surgery). Adverse systemic effects (including HPA axis suppression) may occur when topical steroids are used on large areas of the body, denuded areas, for prolonged periods of time, with an occlusive dressing, and/or in infants or small children; infants and small children may be more susceptible to HPA axis suppression or other systemic toxicities due to a larger skin surface area to body mass ratio; use with caution in pediatric patients; safety and efficacy have not been established in children <12 years of age (use is not recommended)

Do not use topical halobetasol for the treatment of rosacea or perioral dermatitis; do not apply to the face, groin, or axillae. Do not exceed maximum recommended dose or duration of therapy due to the potential development of HPA axis suppression.

Precautions Avoid using higher than recommended doses; suppression of HPA axis, suppression of linear growth (ie, reduction of growth velocity), reduced bone mineral, or hypercorticism (Cushing's syndrome) may occur. Discontinue treatment if local irritation develops. Use appropriate antibacterial or antifungal agents to treat concomitant skin infections; discontinue halobetasol treatment if infection does not resolve promptly.

Adverse Reactions

Central nervous system: Intracranial hypertension (systemic effect reported in children treated with topical corticosteroids)

Dermatologic: Acneiform eruptions, allergic contact dermatitis, dry skin, erythema, folliculitis, hypertrichosis, hypopigmentation, itching, leukoderma, miliaria, perioral dermatitis, pruritus, pustulation, rash, skin atrophy, skin infection (secondary), striae, telangiectasia, vesicles, urticaria

Endocrine: Glycosuria, HPA axis suppression, metabolic effects (hyperglycemia, hypokalemia)

Local: Burning, stinging

Neuromuscular & skeletal: Paresthesia

Drug Interactions

Metabolism/Transport Effects None known.

Avoid Concomitant Use

Avoid concomitant use of Halobetasol with any of the following: Aldesleukin

Increased Effect/Toxicity

Halobetasol may increase the levels/effects of: Ceritinib; Deferasirox

The levels/effects of Halobetasol may be increased by: Telaprevir

Decreased Effect

Halobetasol may decrease the levels/effects of: Aldesleukin; Corticorelin; Hyaluronidase; Telaprevir

Stability Store between 59°F to 86°F (15°C to 30°C)

Mechanism of Action Corticosteroids inhibit the initial manifestations of the inflammatory process (ie, capillary dilation and edema, fibrin deposition, and migration and diapedesis of leukocytes into the inflamed site) as well as later sequelae (angiogenesis, fibroblast proliferation)

Pharmacokinetics (Adult data unless noted)

Absorption: Percutaneous absorption varies and depends on many factors including vehicle used, integrity of epidermis, dose, and use of occlusive dressing; absorption is increased by occlusive dressings or with decreased integrity of skin (eg, inflammation or skin disease)

Cream: <6% of topically applied dose enters circulation within 96 hours following application

Metabolism: Hepatic

Elimination: Renal

Dosing: Usual

Children <12 years: Use not recommended (high risk of systemic adverse effects, eg, HPA axis suppression, Cushing's syndrome)

Children ≥12 years and Adults: Topical: Steroid-responsive dermatoses: Apply sparingly once or twice daily; maximum dose: 50 g/week; do not treat for >2 weeks. **Note:** To decrease risk of systemic effects, only treat small areas at any one time; discontinue therapy when control is achieved; reassess diagnosis if no improvement is seen in 2 weeks.

Administration Topical: Apply sparingly to affected area, gently rub in until disappears; do not use on open skin; do not apply to face, underarms, or groin area; avoid contact with eyes; do not occlude affected area.

Monitoring Parameters Assess HPA axis suppression in patients using potent topical steroids applied to a large surface area or to areas under occlusion (eg, ACTH stimulation test, morning plasma cortisol test, urinary free cortisol test)

Additional Information Considered to be a super high potency topical corticosteroid; patients with psoriasis who were treated with halobetasol cream or ointment in divided doses of 7 g/day for one week developed HPA axis suppression

Dosage Forms Excipient information presented when available (limited, particularly for generics); consult specific product labeling.

Cream, External, as propionate:
Ultravate: 0.05% (50 g) [contains cetyl alcohol]
Generic: 0.05% (15 g, 50 g)

Kit, External, as propionate:
Halonate: 0.05 & 12% (Foam) [contains cetyl alcohol, propylene glycol, trolamine (triethanolamine)]

Ointment, External, as propionate:
Ultravate: 0.05% (50 g) [contains propylene glycol]
Generic: 0.05% (15 g, 50 g)

References

Reed, BR, "Dermatologic Drugs, Pregnancy, and Lactation. A Conservative Guide," *Arch Dermatol,* 1997, 133(7):894-8.

◆ **Halobetasol Propionate** *see* Halobetasol *on page 997*

◆ **Halonate** *see* Halobetasol *on page 997*

Haloperidol (ha loe PER i dole)

Medication Safety Issues

Sound-alike/look-alike issues:
Haldol may be confused with Halcion, Halog, Stadol

BEERS Criteria medication:
This drug may be potentially inappropriate for use in geriatric patients (Quality of evidence - moderate; Strength of recommendation - strong).

International issues:
Haldol [U.S. and multiple international markets] may be confused with Halotestin brand name for fluoxymesterone [Great Britain]

Brand Names: U.S. Haldol; Haldol Decanoate

Brand Names: Canada Apo-Haloperidol; Apo-Haloperidol LA; Haloperidol Injection, USP; Haloperidol Long Acting; Haloperidol-LA; Haloperidol-LA Omega; Novo-Peridol; PMS-Haloperidol; PMS-Haloperidol LA

Therapeutic Category Antipsychotic Agent, Typical, Butyrophenone

Generic Availability (U.S.) Yes

Use

Injection, immediate release (lactate): Management of schizophrenia (FDA approved in adults); control of tics and vocal utterances of Tourette's disorder (FDA approved in adults); emergency sedation of severely agitated or delirious patients

Injection, extended release (decanoate): Management of schizophrenia in patients requiring prolonged parenteral antipsychotic treatment (FDA approved in adults)

Tablet and solution: Management of psychotic disorders (FDA approved in ages ≥3 years and adults), control of tics and vocal utterances of Tourette's disorder (FDA approved in ages ≥3 years and adults), treatment of severe behavioral problems in children displayed by combativeness and/or explosive hyperexcitable behavior and in short-term treatment of hyperactive children (FDA approved in ages 3-12 years); emergency sedation of severely agitated or delirious patients

Pregnancy Risk Factor C

Pregnancy Considerations Adverse events were observed in animal reproduction studies. Haloperidol crosses the placenta in humans (Newport, 2007). Although haloperidol has not been found to be a major human teratogen, an association with limb malformations following first trimester exposure in humans cannot be ruled out (ACOG, 2008; Diav-Citrin, 2005). Antipsychotic use during the third trimester of pregnancy has a risk for abnormal muscle movements (extrapyramidal symptoms [EPS]) and withdrawal symptoms in newborns following delivery. Symptoms in the newborn may include agitation, feeding disorder, hypertonia, hypotonia, respiratory distress, somnolence, and tremor; these effects may be selflimiting or require hospitalization. If needed, the minimum effective maternal dose should be used in order to decrease the risk of EPS (ACOG, 2008).

Breast-Feeding Considerations Haloperidol is found in breast milk and has been detected in the plasma and urine of nursing infants (Whalley, 1981; Yoshida, 1999). Breast engorgement, gynecomastia, and lactation are known side effects with the use of haloperidol. Breast-feeding is not recommended by the manufacturer.

Contraindications Hypersensitivity to haloperidol or any component; narrow-angle glaucoma, bone marrow suppression, CNS depression, coma, severe liver or cardiac disease, parkinsonism

Warnings Cases of sudden death, QT prolongation and torsade de pointes have occurred; risk of QT prolongation and torsade de pointes may be increased with the use of any formulation in amounts exceeding the recommended dose and with the use of I.V. administration of haloperidol lactate (not an FDA-approved route of administration). Use haloperidol with caution or avoid use in patients with electrolyte abnormalities (eg, hypokalemia, hypomagnesemia), hypothyroidism, familial long QT syndrome, concomitant medications which may augment QT prolongation, or any underlying cardiac abnormality which may also potentiate risk. If haloperidol lactate is administered I.V., monitor ECG closely for QT effects and arrhythmias. Do **not** administer haloperidol decanoate I.V.

May cause extrapyramidal symptoms, including pseudoparkinsonism, acute dystonic reactions, akathisia, and tardive dyskinesia (risk of these reactions is high relative to other neuroleptics, and is dose-dependent; to decrease risk of tardive dyskinesia: Use smallest dose and shortest duration possible; evaluate continued need periodically; risk of dystonia is increased with the use of high potency and higher doses of conventional antipsychotics and in males and younger patients). Use may be associated with neuroleptic malignant syndrome. May be sedating; use with caution in disorders where CNS depression is a feature; patients must be cautioned about performing tasks which require mental alertness (eg, operating machinery or driving). Impaired core body temperature regulation may occur; use with caution with strenuous exercise, heat exposure, dehydration, and concomitant medication possessing anticholinergic effects. Safety and efficacy have not been established in children <3 years of age.

Leukopenia, neutropenia, and agranulocytosis (sometimes fatal) have been reported in clinical trials and postmarketing reports with antipsychotic use; presence of risk factors (eg, preexisting low WBC or history of drug-induced leuko/neutropenia) should prompt periodic blood count assessment. Discontinue therapy at first signs of blood dyscrasias or if absolute neutrophil count <1000/mm³. Use is contraindicated in patients with bone marrow suppression.

An increased risk of death has been reported with the use of antipsychotics in elderly patients with dementia-related psychosis **[U.S. Boxed Warning]**; most deaths seemed to be cardiovascular (eg, sudden death, heart failure) or infectious (eg, pneumonia) in nature; haloperidol is not approved for this indication.

Injection as deconate contains benzyl alcohol which may cause allergic reactions in susceptible individuals; large amounts of benzyl alcohol (≥99 mg/kg/day) have been associated with a potentially fatal toxicity ("gasping syndrome") in neonates; avoid use of haloperidol products containing benzyl alcohol in neonates; *in vitro* and animal studies have shown that benzoate, a metabolite of benzyl alcohol, displaces bilirubin from protein binding sites

Precautions Use with caution in patients with renal or hepatic dysfunction, respiratory disease, thyrotoxicosis, cardiovascular disease, history of seizures, or EEG abnormalities; haloperidol may cause hypotension (particularly with parenteral administration), precipitation of anginal pain, anticholinergic effects (low incidence relative to other neuroleptics), elevation of prolactin levels

Adverse Reactions

Cardiovascular: Abnormal T waves with prolonged ventricular repolarization, arrhythmia, hyper-/hypotension, QT prolongation, sudden death, tachycardia, torsade de pointes

Central nervous system: Agitation, akathisia, altered central temperature regulation, anxiety, confusion, depression, drowsiness, dystonic reactions, euphoria, extrapyramidal reactions, headache, insomnia, lethargy, neuroleptic malignant syndrome (NMS), pseudoparkinsonian signs and symptoms, restlessness, seizure, tardive dyskinesia, tardive dystonia, vertigo

Dermatologic: Alopecia, contact dermatitis, hyperpigmentation, photosensitivity (rare), pruritus, rash

Endocrine & metabolic: Amenorrhea, breast engorgement, galactorrhea, gynecomastia, hyper-/hypoglycemia,

hyponatremia, lactation, mastalgia, menstrual irregularities, sexual dysfunction

Gastrointestinal: Anorexia, constipation, diarrhea, dyspepsia, hypersalivation, nausea, vomiting, xerostomia

Genitourinary: Priapism, urinary retention

Hematologic: Agranulocytosis (rare), leukopenia, leukocytosis, neutropenia, anemia, lymphomonocytosis

Hepatic: Cholestatic jaundice, obstructive jaundice

Ocular: Blurred vision

Respiratory: Bronchospasm, laryngospasm

Miscellaneous: Diaphoresis, heat stroke

Drug Interactions

Metabolism/Transport Effects Substrate of CYP1A2 (minor), CYP2D6 (major), CYP3A4 (major); **Note:** Assignment of Major/Minor substrate status based on clinically relevant drug interaction potential; **Inhibits** CYP2D6 (moderate), CYP3A4 (moderate)

Avoid Concomitant Use

Avoid concomitant use of Haloperidol with any of the following: Aclidinium; Amisulpride; Azelastine (Nasal); Bosutinib; Conivaptan; FLUoxetine; Fusidic Acid (Systemic); Highest Risk QTc-Prolonging Agents; Ibrutinib; Ipratropium (Oral Inhalation); Ivabradine; Lomitapide; Metoclopramide; Mifepristone; Paraldehyde; Pimozide; Potassium Chloride; QuiNIDine; Simeprevir; Sulpiride; Thalidomide; Thioridazine; Tiotropium; Tolvaptan; Ulipristal; Umeclidinium

Increased Effect/Toxicity

Haloperidol may increase the levels/effects of: AbobotulinumtoxinA; Alcohol (Ethyl); Amisulpride; Analgesics (Opioid); Anticholinergic Agents; ARIPiprazole; Avanafil; Azelastine (Nasal); Bosentan; Bosutinib; Budesonide (Systemic, Oral Inhalation); Buprenorphine; Cannabinoid-Containing Products; Cannabis; ChlorproMAZINE; CNS Depressants; Colchicine; CYP2D6 Substrates; CYP3A4 Substrates; DOXOrubicin (Conventional); Dronabinol; Eplerenone; Everolimus; FentaNYL; Fesoterodine; Highest Risk QTc-Prolonging Agents; Hydrocodone; Ibrutinib; Imatinib; Ivabradine; Ivacaftor; Lomitapide; Lurasidone; Methotrimeprazine; Methylphenidate; Metoprolol; Metyrosine; Mirabegron; Mirtazapine; Moderate Risk QTc-Prolonging Agents; Nebivolol; OnabotulinumtoxinA; OxyCODONE; Paraldehyde; Pimecrolimus; Pimozide; Potassium Chloride; QuiNIDine; Ranolazine; RimabotulinumtoxinB; Rivaroxaban; Salmeterol; Saxagliptin; Selective Serotonin Reuptake Inhibitors; Serotonin Modulators; Simeprevir; Sulpiride; Tetrahydrocannabinol; Thalidomide; Thiazide Diuretics; Thioridazine; Tiotropium; Tolvaptan; Topiramate; Ulipristal; Vilazodone; Zolpidem

The levels/effects of Haloperidol may be increased by: Abiraterone Acetate; Acetylcholinesterase Inhibitors (Central); Aclidinium; ARIPiprazole; Brimonidine (Topical); Cannabis; ChlorproMAZINE; Conivaptan; CYP2D6 Inhibitors (Moderate); CYP2D6 Inhibitors (Strong); CYP3A4 Inhibitors (Moderate); CYP3A4 Inhibitors (Strong); Dasatinib; Doxylamine; Dronabinol; Droperidol; FLUoxetine; FluvoxaMINE; Fusidic Acid (Systemic); HydrOXYzine; Ipratropium (Oral Inhalation); Ivabradine; Kava Kava; Lithium; Luliconazole; Magnesium Sulfate; Methotrimeprazine; Methylphenidate; Metoclopramide; Metyrosine; Mifepristone; Nabilone; Nonsteroidal Anti-Inflammatory Agents; Perampanel; Pramlintide; QTc-Prolonging Agents (Indeterminate Risk and Risk Modifying); QuiNIDine; Rufinamide; Serotonin Modulators; Sodium Oxybate; Stiripentol; Tapentadol; Tetrahydrocannabinol; Umeclidinium

Decreased Effect

Haloperidol may decrease the levels/effects of: Acetylcholinesterase Inhibitors (Central); Amphetamines; Anti-Parkinson's Agents (Dopamine Agonist); Codeine;

Ifosfamide; Quinagolide; Secretin; Tamoxifen; TraMADol; Urea Cycle Disorder Agents

The levels/effects of Haloperidol may be decreased by: Acetylcholinesterase Inhibitors (Central); Anti-Parkinson's Agents (Dopamine Agonist); ARIPiprazole; Bosentan; CarBAMazepine; CYP3A4 Inducers (Strong); Dabrafenib; Deferasirox; Glycopyrrolate; Lithium; Mitotane; Peginterferon Alfa-2b; Siltuximab; St Johns Wort; Tocilizumab

Stability All dosage forms: Store at controlled room temperature; protect from light

Oral concentrate and injection, as lactate: Do not freeze

Injection, as deconate: Do not refrigerate or freeze

Mechanism of Action Haloperidol is a butyrophenone antipsychotic which blocks postsynaptic mesolimbic dopaminergic D_1 and D_2 receptors in the brain; depresses the release of hypothalamic and hypophyseal hormones; believed to depress the reticular activating system thus affecting basal metabolism, body temperature, wakefulness, vasomotor tone, and emesis

Pharmacokinetics (Adult data unless noted)

Absorption: Oral: Well absorbed, undergoes first-pass metabolism in the liver

Distribution: Crosses the placenta; appears in breast milk

Protein binding: 92%

Metabolism: In the liver, hydroxy-metabolite is active

Bioavailability: Oral: 60%

Half-life: Adults: 20 hours; range: 13-35 hours

Elimination: Excreted in urine and feces as drug and metabolites

Dosing: Usual Note: Gradually decrease dose to the lowest effective maintenance dosage once a satisfactory therapeutic response is obtained

Children:

3-12 years (15-40 kg): Oral: Initial: 0.25-0.5 mg/day given in 2-3 divided doses; increase by 0.25-0.5 mg every 5-7 days; maximum dose: 0.15 mg/kg/day; usual maintenance:

Agitation or hyperkinesia: 0.01-0.03 mg/kg/day once daily

Tourette's disorder or nonpsychotic behavior disorders: 0.05-0.075 mg/kg/day in 2-3 divided doses

Psychotic disorders: 0.05-0.15 mg/kg/day in 2-3 divided doses

Note: Maximum effective dose has not been established; doses >6 mg/day have not been shown to further enhance behavior improvement. Preliminary findings of a double-blind, placebo controlled study reported the mean optimal dose in 12 schizophrenic children 5-12 years to be ~2 mg/day (range: 0.5-3.5 mg/day or 0.02-0.12 mg/kg/day) given in 3 divided doses

6-12 years: I.M. **(as lactate):** 1-3 mg/dose every 4-8 hours to a maximum of 0.15 mg/kg/day; switch to oral therapy as soon as able

Adults:

Oral: 0.5-5 mg 2-3 times/day; usual maximum dose: 30 mg/day; some patients may require 100 mg/day

I.M.:

As **lactate:** 2-5 mg every 4-8 hours as needed

As **decanoate:** Initial: 10-15 times the individual patients' stabilized oral dose, given at 3- to 4-week intervals

Administration

Oral: Administer with food or milk to decrease GI distress; prior to administration, dilute oral concentrate with ≥2 ounces of water or acidic beverage; do not mix oral concentrate with coffee or tea. Avoid skin contact with oral suspension or solution; may cause contact dermatitis.

Parenteral: **Decanoate** product is for I.M. use only, **do not administer decanoate I.V.** Although not FDA-approved,

haloperidol **lactate** has been administered I.V.; however, this may increase the risk of altered cardiac conduction.

Monitoring Parameters Blood pressure, heart rate, CBC with differential, liver enzymes with long-term use; serum glucose, sodium, magnesium; ECG (with non-FDA approved intravenous administration); mental status, abnormal involuntary movement scale (AIMS), extrapyramidal symptoms (EPS)

Dosage Forms Excipient information presented when available (limited, particularly for generics); consult specific product labeling.

Concentrate, Oral, as lactate [strength expressed as base]:

Generic: 2 mg/mL (5 mL, 15 mL, 120 mL)

Solution, Intramuscular, as decanoate [strength expressed as base]:

Haldol Decanoate: 50 mg/mL (1 mL); 100 mg/mL (1 mL) [contains benzyl alcohol, sesame oil]

Generic: 50 mg/mL (1 mL, 5 mL); 100 mg/mL (1 mL, 5 mL)

Solution, Injection, as lactate [strength expressed as base]:

Haldol: 5 mg/mL (1 mL)

Generic: 5 mg/mL (1 mL, 10 mL)

Solution, Injection, as lactate [strength expressed as base, preservative free]:

Generic: 5 mg/mL (1 mL)

Tablet, Oral:

Generic: 0.5 mg, 1 mg, 2 mg, 5 mg, 10 mg, 20 mg

References

ACOG Committee on Practice Bulletins-Obstetrics, "ACOG Practice Bulletin: Clinical Management Guidelines for Obstetrician-Gynecologists Number 92, April 2008 (Replaces Practice Bulletin Number 87, November 2007). Use of Psychiatric Medications During Pregnancy and Lactation," *Obstet Gynecol*, 2008, 111(4):1001-20.

Diav-Citrin O, Shechtman S, Ornoy S, et al, "Safety of Haloperidol and Penfluridol in Pregnancy: A Multicenter, Prospective, Controlled Study," *J Clin Psychiatry*, 2005, 66(3):317-22.

Newport DJ, Calamaras MR, DeVane CL, et al, "Atypical Antipsychotic Administration During Late Pregnancy: Placental Passage and Obstetrical Outcomes," *Am J Psychiatry*, 2007, 164(8):1214-20.

Serrano AC, "Haloperidol - Its Use in Children," *J Clin Psychiatry*, 1981, 42(4):154-6.

Spencer EK, Kafantaris V, Padron-Gayol MV, et al, "Haloperidol in Schizophrenic Children: Early Findings From a Study in Progress," *Psychopharmacol Bull*, 1992, 28(2):183-6.

Whalley LJ, Blain PG, and Prime JK, "Haloperidol Secreted in Breast Milk," *Br Med J (Clin Res Ed)*, 1981, 282(6278):1746-7.

Yoshida K, Smith B, and Kumar R, "Psychotropic Drugs in Mothers' Milk: A Comprehensive Review of Assay Methods, Pharmacokinetics and of Safety of Breast-Feeding," *J Psychopharmacol*, 1999, 13 (1):64-80.

◆ **Haloperidol Decanoate** *see* Haloperidol *on page 998*

◆ **Haloperidol Injection, USP (Can)** *see* Haloperidol *on page 998*

◆ **Haloperidol-LA (Can)** *see* Haloperidol *on page 998*

◆ **Haloperidol Lactate** *see* Haloperidol *on page 998*

◆ **Haloperidol-LA Omega (Can)** *see* Haloperidol *on page 998*

◆ **Haloperidol Long Acting (Can)** *see* Haloperidol *on page 998*

◆ **Harkoseride** *see* Lacosamide *on page 1189*

◆ **Havrix** *see* Hepatitis A Vaccine *on page 1005*

◆ **HAVRIX (Can)** *see* Hepatitis A Vaccine *on page 1005*

◆ **HBIG** *see* Hepatitis B Immune Globulin (Human) *on page 1008*

◆ **hCG** *see* Chorionic Gonadotropin (Human) *on page 460*

◆ **HCTZ (error-prone abbreviation)** *see* Hydrochlorothiazide *on page 1023*

◆ **HDCV** *see* Rabies Vaccine *on page 1801*

◆ **HealthyLax [OTC]** *see* Polyethylene Glycol 3350 *on page 1696*

♦ **Healthy Mama Move It Along [OTC]** *see* Docusate *on page 701*

♦ **Heartburn Relief [OTC]** *see* Famotidine *on page 843*

♦ **Heartburn Relief 24 Hour [OTC]** *see* Lansoprazole *on page 1206*

♦ **Heartburn Relief Max St [OTC]** *see* Famotidine *on page 843*

♦ **Heartburn Treatment 24 Hour [OTC]** *see* Lansoprazole *on page 1206*

♦ **Heather** *see* Norethindrone *on page 1511*

♦ **Heavy Mineral Oil** *see* Mineral Oil *on page 1419*

♦ **Hecoria** *see* Tacrolimus (Systemic) *on page 1963*

♦ **Helixate FS** *see* Antihemophilic Factor (Recombinant) *on page 172*

♦ **Hemangeol** *see* Propranolol *on page 1759*

♦ **Hemocyte [OTC]** *see* Ferrous Fumarate *on page 865*

♦ **Hemofil M** *see* Antihemophilic Factor (Human) *on page 170*

♦ **Hemorrhoidal [OTC]** *see* Phenylephrine (Topical) *on page 1662*

♦ **Hemorrhoidal HC** *see* Hydrocortisone (Topical) *on page 1038*

♦ **Hem-Prep [OTC]** *see* Phenylephrine (Topical) *on page 1662*

♦ **Hemril-30 [DSC]** *see* Hydrocortisone (Topical) *on page 1038*

♦ **HepA** *see* Hepatitis A Vaccine *on page 1005*

♦ **HepaGam B** *see* Hepatitis B Immune Globulin (Human) *on page 1008*

♦ **Hepalean (Can)** *see* Heparin *on page 1001*

♦ **Hepalean Leo (Can)** *see* Heparin *on page 1001*

♦ **Hepalean-LOK (Can)** *see* Heparin *on page 1001*

Heparin (HEP a rin)

Medication Safety Issues
Sound-alike/look-alike issues:
Heparin may be confused with Hespan®
High alert medication:
The Institute for Safe Medication Practices (ISMP) includes this medication among its list of drugs which have a heightened risk of causing significant patient harm when used in error.
National Patient Safety Goals:
The Joint Commission (TJC) requires healthcare organizations that provide anticoagulant therapy to have a process in place to reduce the risk of anticoagulant-associated patient harm. Patients receiving anticoagulants should receive individualized care through a defined process that includes standardized ordering, dispensing, administration, monitoring and education. This does not apply to routine short-term use of anticoagulants for prevention of venous thromboembolism when the expectation is that the patient's laboratory values will remain within or close to normal values (NPSG.03.05.01).

Administration issues:
The 100 unit/mL concentration should not be used to flush heparin locks, I.V. lines, or intra-arterial lines in neonates or infants <10 kg (systemic anticoagulation may occur). The 10 unit/mL flush concentration may inadvertently cause systemic anticoagulation in infants <1 kg who receive frequent flushes.

Other safety concerns:
Heparin sodium injection 10,000 units/mL and Hep-Lock U/P 10 units/mL have been confused with each other. Fatal medication errors have occurred between the two whose labels are both blue. **Never rely on color as a sole indicator to differentiate product identity.**
Labeling changes: Effective May 1st, 2013, heparin labeling is required to include the total amount of heparin per vial (rather than only including the amount of heparin per mL). During the transition, hospitals should consider only stocking the newly labeled heparin to avoid potential errors and confusion with the older labeling.
Heparin lock flush solution is intended only to maintain patency of I.V. devices and is **not** to be used for anticoagulant therapy.

Brand Names: U.S. Hep Flush-10
Brand Names: Canada Hepalean; Hepalean Leo; Hepalean-LOK
Therapeutic Category Anticoagulant
Generic Availability (U.S.) Yes
Use Prophylaxis and treatment of thromboembolic disorders [Injection: FDA approved in pediatric patients (age not specified) and adults]; **Note:** Heparin lock flush solution is intended only to maintain patency of I.V. devices and is not to be used for systemic anticoagulant therapy (FDA approved in adults)
Pregnancy Risk Factor C
Pregnancy Considerations Increased resorptions were observed in some animal reproduction studies. Heparin does not cross the placenta. Heparin may be used for the prevention and treatment of thromboembolism in pregnant women; however the use of low molecular weight heparin (LMWH) is preferred. Twice-daily heparin should be discontinued prior to induction of labor or a planned cesarean delivery. In pregnant women with mechanical heart valves, adjusted-dose LMWH or adjusted-dose heparin may be used throughout pregnancy or until week 13 of gestation when therapy can be changed to warfarin. LMWH or heparin should be resumed close to delivery. In women who are at a very high risk for thromboembolism (older generation prosthesis in mitral position or history of thromboembolism), warfarin can be used throughout pregnancy and replaced with LMWH or heparin near term; the use of low-dose aspirin is also recommended. When choosing therapy, fetal outcomes (ie, pregnancy loss, malformations), maternal outcomes (ie, VTE, hemorrhage), burden of therapy, and maternal preference should be considered (Guyatt, 2012).

Some products contain benzyl alcohol as a preservative; their use in pregnant women is contraindicated by some manufacturers; use of a preservative free formulation is recommended.

Breast-Feeding Considerations Heparin is not excreted into breast milk and can be used in breast-feeding women (Guyatt, 2012). Some products contain benzyl alcohol as a preservative; their use in breast-feeding women is contraindicated by some manufacturers due to the association of gasping syndrome in premature infants.
Contraindications Hypersensitivity to heparin or any component (unless a life-threatening situation necessitates use and use of an alternative anticoagulant is not possible); severe thrombocytopenia, uncontrollable active bleeding (unless secondary to disseminated intravascular coagulation); use when appropriate blood coagulation tests cannot be obtained at appropriate intervals (applies to full-dose heparin only). **Note:** Some products contain benzyl alcohol as a preservative; their use in neonates, infants, or pregnant or nursing mothers is contraindicated; use preservative-free heparin in these patients.

▶

Warnings Some products contain benzyl alcohol as a preservative; use of these products is contraindicated in neonates, infants, or pregnant or nursing mothers **[U.S. Boxed Warning]**. Large amounts of benzyl alcohol (≥99 mg/kg/day) have been associated with a potentially fatal toxicity ("gasping syndrome") in neonates; the "gasping syndrome" consists of metabolic acidosis, respiratory distress, gasping respirations, CNS dysfunction (including convulsions, intracranial hemorrhage), hypotension and cardiovascular collapse; *in vitro* and animal studies have shown that benzoate, a metabolite of benzyl alcohol, displaces bilirubin from protein binding sites. Some preparations contain sulfites which may cause allergic reactions in susceptible individuals.

May cause thrombocytopenia; monitor platelet count closely. Patients who develop heparin-induced thrombocytopenia (HIT) may be at risk of developing a new thrombus [heparin-induced thrombocytopenia and thrombosis (HITT)]. Discontinue therapy and consider alternatives if platelets are <100,000/mm^3 and/or thrombosis develops. HIT or HITT may be delayed and can occur up to several weeks after discontinuation of heparin. Thrombocytopenia may be more common with bovine lung heparin compared to porcine mucosa heparin; however, if a patient receiving bovine lung heparin experiences severe thrombocytopenia, it is not recommended to switch to porcine mucosa heparin because a similar reaction may occur.

Confirm the concentration of all heparin injection vials prior to administration; do not use heparin injection as a "catheter lock flush" as the injection is supplied in various concentrations including highly concentrated strengths. Fatal hemorrhages have occurred in pediatric patients when higher concentrations of heparin injection were confused with lower concentrations of heparin lock flush.

Precautions Use with caution as hemorrhage may occur; bleeding may occur at any site including internal sites such as GI bleeding, urinary tract bleeding, adrenal hemorrhage, ovarian (corpus luteum) hemorrhage, and retroperitoneal hemorrhage; risk factors for hemorrhage include: I.M. injections; intermittent I.V. injections (vs continuous I.V. infusion); increased capillary permeability; menstruation; recent surgery or invasive procedures; severe renal, hepatic, or biliary disease; indwelling catheters; subacute bacterial endocarditis; congenital or acquired bleeding disorders; active ulcerative or angiodysplastic GI diseases; continuous GI tube drainage; severe uncontrolled hypertension; history of hemorrhagic stroke; concomitant treatment with platelet inhibitors; recent GI bleeding; thrombocytopenia or platelet defects; hypertensive or diabetic retinopathy; and patients >60 years of age (especially women). Discontinue if bleeding occurs; severe hemorrhage or overdosage may require reversal of heparin with protamine.

High dosage requirements to maintain a therapeutic APTT (heparin resistance) may occur in patients with antithrombin deficiency, increased heparin clearance, elevations in heparin-binding proteins, and elevations in factor VIII and/or fibrinogen; heparin resistance is frequently encountered in patients with fever, thrombosis, thrombophlebitis, infections with thrombosing tendencies, MI, cancer, and in postsurgical patients; measurement of anticoagulant effects using antifactor Xa levels may be beneficial.

Heparin does not possess fibrinolytic activity and, therefore, cannot lyse established thrombi.

Adverse Reactions Note: Immunologically mediated heparin-induced thrombocytopenia (HIT) occurs in a small percentage of patients and is and is marked by a progressive fall in platelet counts and, in some cases, thromboembolic complications (skin necrosis, pulmonary embolism, gangrene of the extremities, stroke, or MI).

Cardiovascular: Allergic vasospastic reaction (possibly related to thrombosis), chest pain, hemorrhagic shock, shock, thrombosis

Central nervous system: Chills, fever, headache

Dermatologic: Alopecia (delayed, transient), bruising (unexplained), cutaneous necrosis, dysesthesia pedis, erythematous plaques (case reports), eczema, urticaria, purpura

Endocrine & metabolic: Adrenal hemorrhage, hyperkalemia (suppression of aldosterone synthesis), ovarian hemorrhage, rebound hyperlipidemia on discontinuation

Gastrointestinal: Constipation, hematemesis, nausea, tarry stools, vomiting

Genitourinary: Frequent or persistent erection

Hematologic: Bleeding from gums, epistaxis, hemorrhage, ovarian hemorrhage, retroperitoneal hemorrhage, thrombocytopenia (see Note)

Hepatic: Liver enzymes increased

Local: Irritation, erythema, pain, hematoma, and ulceration have been rarely reported with deep SubQ injections; I.M. injection (not recommended) is associated with a high incidence of these effects

Neuromuscular & skeletal: Peripheral neuropathy, osteoporosis (chronic therapy effect)

Ocular: Conjunctivitis (allergic reaction), lacrimation

Renal: Hematuria

Respiratory: Asthma, bronchospasm (case reports), hemoptysis, pulmonary hemorrhage, rhinitis

Miscellaneous: Allergic reactions, anaphylactoid reactions, heparin resistance, hypersensitivity (including chills, fever, and urticaria)

Drug Interactions

Metabolism/Transport Effects None known.

Avoid Concomitant Use

Avoid concomitant use of Heparin with any of the following: Apixaban; Corticorelin; Dabigatran Etexilate; Omacetaxine; Palifermin; Rivaroxaban; Streptokinase; Urokinase; Vorapaxar

Increased Effect/Toxicity

Heparin may increase the levels/effects of: ACE Inhibitors; Aliskiren; Angiotensin II Receptor Blockers; Anticoagulants; Canagliflozin; Collagenase (Systemic); Corticorelin; Deferasirox; Eplerenone; Ibritumomab; Omacetaxine; Palifermin; Potassium Salts; Potassium-Sparing Diuretics; Rivaroxaban; Tositumomab and Iodine I 131 Tositumomab

The levels/effects of Heparin may be increased by: 5-ASA Derivatives; Agents with Antiplatelet Properties; Apixaban; Aspirin; Dabigatran Etexilate; Dasatinib; Herbs (Anticoagulant/Antiplatelet Properties); Ibrutinib; Nonsteroidal Anti-Inflammatory Agents; Omega-3 Fatty Acids; Pentosan Polysulfate Sodium; Pentoxifylline; Prostacyclin Analogues; Salicylates; Streptokinase; Sugammadex; Thrombolytic Agents; Tibolone; Tipranavir; Urokinase; Vitamin E; Vorapaxar

Decreased Effect

The levels/effects of Heparin may be decreased by: Estrogen Derivatives; Nitroglycerin; Progestins

Mechanism of Action Potentiates the action of antithrombin III and thereby inactivates thrombin (as well as activated coagulation factors IX, X, XI, XII, and plasmin) and prevents the conversion of fibrinogen to fibrin; heparin also stimulates release of lipoprotein lipase (lipoprotein lipase hydrolyzes triglycerides to glycerol and free fatty acids)

Pharmacodynamics Anticoagulation effect: Onset of action:

SubQ: 20-60 minutes

I.V.: Immediate

Pharmacokinetics (Adult data unless noted)
Absorption: SubQ, I.M.: Erratic

Distribution: Does not cross the placenta; does not appear in breast milk

Metabolism: Believed to be partially metabolized in the reticuloendothelial system

Half-life: Mean: 90 minutes; range: 60-120 minutes; affected by obesity, renal function, malignancy, presence of pulmonary embolism, and infections; half-life has been reported to be dose-dependent: I.V. bolus: 25 units/kg: 30 minutes; 100 units/kg: 60 minutes; 400 units/kg: 150 minutes (Hirsh, 2008)

Elimination: Renal; small amount excreted unchanged in urine; **Note:** At therapeutic doses, elimination occurs rapidly via nonrenal mechanisms. With very high doses, renal elimination may play more of a role; however, dosage adjustment remains unnecessary for patients with renal impairment (Hirsh, 2008).

Dosing: Neonatal Note: Many concentrations of heparin are available and range from 1-20,000 units/mL. Carefully examine each prefilled syringe, bag, or vial prior to use to ensure that the correct concentration is chosen. Heparin lock flush solution is intended only to maintain patency of I.V. devices and is not to be used for anticoagulant therapy.

Line flushing: When using daily flushes of heparin to maintain patency of single and double lumen central catheters, 10 units/mL is the concentration used in neonates. Capped polyvinyl chloride catheters and peripheral heparin locks require flushing more frequently (eg, every 6-8 hours). Volume of heparin flush is usually similar to volume of catheter (or slightly greater) or may be standardized according to specific NICU policy (eg, 0.5-1 mL/flush). Dose of heparin flush used should not approach therapeutic unit per kg dose. Additional flushes should be given when stagnant blood is observed in catheter, after catheter is used for drug or blood administration, and after blood withdrawal from catheter.

TPN: Heparin 0.5-1 unit/mL (final concentration) may be added to TPN solutions, both central and peripheral. (Addition of heparin to peripheral TPN has been shown to increase duration of line patency. The final concentration of heparin used for TPN solutions may need to be decreased to 0.5 units/mL in small neonates receiving larger TPN volumes in order to avoid approaching therapeutic amounts.

Arterial lines: Heparinize with a usual final concentration of 1 unit/mL; range: 0.5-1 units/mL; in order to avoid large total doses and systemic effects, use 0.5 unit/mL in low birth weight/premature newborns and in other patients receiving multiple lines containing heparin

Peripheral arterial catheters *in situ*: Continuous I.V. infusion of heparin at a final concentration of 5 units/mL at 1 mL/hour (Monagle, 2008)

Umbilical artery catheter (UAC) prophylaxis: Low-dose heparin continuous I.V. infusion via the UAC with a heparin concentration of 0.25–1 unit/mL (Monagle, 2008)

Prophylaxis for cardiac catheterization via an artery: I.V.: Bolus: 100-150 units/kg; for prolonged procedures, further doses may be required (Monagle, 2008)

Systemic heparinization: I.V. infusion: Initial loading dose: 75 units/kg given over 10 minutes; then initial maintenance dose: 28 units/kg/hour; adjust dose to maintain APTT of 60-85 seconds (assuming this reflects an antifactor Xa level of 0.35-0.7 units/mL); see table

PROTOCOL FOR SYSTEMIC HEPARIN ADJUSTMENT
To be used after initial loading dose and maintenance I.V. infusion dose (see above) to maintain APTT of 60-85 seconds (assuming this reflects antifactor Xa level of 0.35-0.7 units/mL)

Obtain blood for APTT 4 hours after heparin loading dose and 4 hours after every infusion rate change

Obtain daily CBC and APTT after APTT is therapeutic

APTT* (seconds)	Dosage Adjustment	Time to Repeat APTT
<50	Give 50 units/kg bolus and increase infusion rate by 10%	4 h after rate change
50-59	Increase infusion rate by 10%	4 h after rate change
60-85	Keep rate the same	Next day
86-95	Decrease infusion rate by 10%	4 h after rate change
96-120	Hold infusion for 30 minutes and decrease infusion rate by 10%	4 h after rate change
>120	Hold infusion for 60 minutes and decrease infusion rate by 15%	4 h after rate change

*Adjust heparin rate to maintain APTT of 60-85 seconds, assuming this reflects antifactor-Xa level of 0.35-0.7 units/mL (reagent specific)

Modified from Monagle P, Chalmers E, Chan A, et al, "Antithrombotic Therapy in Neonates and Children," *Chest*, 2008, 133 (6):887S-968S.

Dosing: Usual
Note: Many concentrations of heparin are available and range from 1-20,000 units/mL. Carefully examine each prefilled syringe, bag, or vial prior to use to ensure that the correct concentration is chosen. Heparin lock flush solution is intended only to maintain patency of I.V. devices and is not to be used for anticoagulant therapy.

Line flushing: When using daily flushes of heparin to maintain patency of single and double lumen central catheters, 10 units/mL is commonly used for younger infants (eg, <10 kg) while 100 units/mL is used for older infants, children, and adults. Capped polyvinyl chloride catheters and peripheral heparin locks require flushing more frequently (eg, every 6-8 hours). Volume of heparin flush is usually similar to volume of catheter (or slightly greater) or may be standardized according to specific hospital's policy (eg, 2-5 mL/flush). Dose of heparin flush used should not approach therapeutic unit per kg dose. Additional flushes should be given when stagnant blood is observed in catheter, after catheter is used for drug or blood administration, and after blood withdrawal from catheter.

TPN: Infants and Children: Heparin 1 unit/mL (final concentration) may be added to TPN solutions, both central and peripheral. (Addition of heparin to peripheral TPN has been shown to increase duration of line patency.) The final concentration of heparin used for TPN solutions may need to be decreased to 0.5 units/mL in small infants receiving larger TPN volumes in order to avoid approaching therapeutic amounts.

Arterial lines: Infants and Children: Heparinize with a usual final concentration of 1 unit/mL; range: 0.5-2 units/mL; in order to avoid large total doses and systemic effects, use 0.5 unit/mL in patients receiving multiple lines containing heparin

Peripheral arterial catheters *in situ*: Infants and Children: Continuous I.V. infusion of heparin at a final concentration of 5 units/mL at 1 mL/hour (Monagle, 2008)

Prophylaxis for cardiac catheterization via an artery: Infants and Children: I.V.: Bolus: 100-150 units/kg; for prolonged procedures, further doses may be required (Monagle, 2008)

Systemic heparinization:
Infants <1 year: I.V. infusion: Initial loading dose: 75 units/kg given over 10 minutes; then initial maintenance dose: 28 units/kg/hour; adjust dose to maintain APTT of 60-85 seconds (assuming this reflects an antifactor Xa level of 0.35-0.7 units/mL); see table on next page. ▶

1003

Children >1 year:
  Intermittent I.V.: Initial: 50-100 units/kg, then 50-100 units/kg every 4 hours (**Note:** Continuous I.V. infusion is preferred):
  I.V. infusion: Initial loading dose: 75 units/kg given over 10 minutes, then initial maintenance dose: 20 units/kg/hour; adjust dose to maintain APTT of 60-85 seconds (assuming this reflects an antifactor Xa level of 0.35-0.7 units/mL); see table.

PROTOCOL FOR SYSTEMIC HEPARIN ADJUSTMENT

To be used after initial loading dose and maintenance I.V. infusion dose (see above) to maintain APTT of 60-85 seconds (assuming this reflects antifactor Xa level of 0.35-0.7 units/mL)

Obtain blood for APTT 4 hours after heparin loading dose and 4 hours after every infusion rate change

Obtain daily CBC and APTT after APTT is therapeutic

APTT* (seconds)	Dosage Adjustment	Time to Repeat APTT
<50	Give 50 units/kg bolus and increase infusion rate by 10%	4 h after rate change
50-59	Increase infusion rate by 10%	4 h after rate change
60-85	Keep rate the same	Next day
86-95	Decrease infusion rate by 10%	4 h after rate change
96-120	Hold infusion for 30 minutes and decrease infusion rate by 10%	4 h after rate change
>120	Hold infusion for 60 minutes and decrease infusion rate by 15%	4 h after rate change

*Adjust heparin rate to maintain APTT of 60-85 seconds, assuming this reflects antifactor-Xa level of 0.35-0.7 units/mL (reagent specific)

Modified from Monagle P, Chalmers E, Chan A, et al, "Antithrombotic Therapy in Neonates and Children," *Chest*, 2008, 133 (6):887S-968S.

Adults:
  Prophylaxis (low dose heparin): SubQ: 5000 units every 8-12 hours
  Intermittent I.V.: Initial: 10,000 units, then 50-70 units/kg/dose (5000-10,000 units) every 4-6 hours (**Note:** Continuous I.V. infusion is preferred)
  I.V. infusion: Initial loading dose: 80 units/kg; initial maintenance dose: 18 units/kg/hour with dose adjusted according to APTT; usual range: 10-30 units/kg/hour
Adults: *Chest*, 2008 Recommendations (Goodman, 2008; Harrington, 2008; Kearon, 2008):
  Prophylaxis of DVT and PE: SubQ: 5000 units every 8 or 12 hours or adjusted low-dose heparin
  Treatment of DVT and PE:
    I.V.: Initial (loading dose): I.V. bolus: 80 units/kg (or alternatively 5000 units); follow with continuous I.V. infusion of 18 units/kg/hour (or alternatively 1300 units/hour). Adjust dosage to achieve and maintain therapeutic APTT as determined by correlating APPT results with a therapeutic range of heparin levels as measured by antifactor Xa assay (0.3-0.7 units/mL).
    SubQ:
      Monitored dosing regimen: Initial: 17,500 units (or 250 units/kg) then 250 units/kg/dose every 12 hours. Adjust dosage to achieve and maintain therapeutic APTT as determined by correlating APPT results with a therapeutic range of heparin levels as measured by antifactor Xa assay (0.3-0.7 units/mL) when measured 6 hours after injection.
      Unmonitored dosing regimen: Initial: 333 units/kg; followed by 250 units/kg/dose every 12 hours
  Unstable angina or Non-ST-elevation myocardial infarction (NSTEMI): Initial loading dose: I.V. bolus: 60-70 units/kg (maximum: 5000 units), then initial

maintenance dose: I.V. infusion: 12-15 units/kg/hour (maximum: 1000 units/hour); adjust dose to maintain therapeutic APTT of 50-75s
STEMI after thrombolytic therapy (full dose alteplase, tenecteplase, or reteplase): Initial loading dose: I.V. bolus: 60 units/kg (maximum: 4000 units), then initial maintenance dose: I.V. infusion: 12 units/kg/hour (maximum: 1000 units/hour); adjust dose to maintain therapeutic APTT of 50-70s for 48 hours

Dosage adjustment in renal impairment: No dosage adjustment required; adjust therapeutic heparin according to aPTT or anti-Xa activity

Dosage adjustment in hepatic impairment: No dosage adjustment required; adjust therapeutic heparin according to aPTT or anti-Xa activity

Usual Infusion Concentrations: Neonatal I.V. infusion: Maintenance of line patency: 0.5 unit/mL

Usual Infusion Concentrations: Pediatric Note: Premixed solutions available

I.V. infusion: 100 units/mL

Administration Parenteral: Continuous I.V. infusion is preferred vs I.V. intermittent injections; I.V. bolus should be administered over 10 minutes; heparin lock solutions are intended only to maintain patency of I.V. devices and are **not** for systemic anticoagulation. Do not administer I.M. due to pain, irritation, and hematoma formation.

Monitoring Parameters Platelet counts, signs of bleeding, hemoglobin, hematocrit, APTT; for full-dose heparin (ie, nonlow dose), the dose should be titrated according to APTT (see table). For intermittent I.V. injections, APTT is measured 3.5-4 hours after I.V. injection.

Reference Range Venous thromboembolism: Heparin: 0.3-0.7 unit/mL anti-Xa activity (by chromogenic assay) or 0.2-0.4 unit/mL (by protamine titration); APTT: 1.5-2.5 times control (usually reflects an APTT of 60-85 seconds) (Hirsh, 2008; Kearon, 2008)

When used with thrombolytic therapy in patients with MI, a lower therapeutic range corresponding to an antiXa level of 0.2-0.5 units/mL by chromogenic assay; APTT: 1.5-2 times control (or approximately an APTT of 50-70 seconds) is recommended (Goodman, 2008)

Test Interactions Increased thyroxine (competitive protein binding methods); increased PT

Aprotinin significantly increases aPTT and celite Activated Clotting Time (ACT) which may not reflect the actual degree of anticoagulation by heparin. Kaolin-based ACTs are not affected by aprotinin to the same degree as celite ACTs. While institutional protocols may vary, a minimal celite ACT of 750 seconds or kaolin-ACT of 480 seconds is recommended in the presence of aprotinin. Consult the manufacturer's information on specific ACT test interpretation in the presence of aprotinin.

Additional Information To reverse the effects of heparin, use protamine. Heparin is available from bovine lung and from porcine intestinal mucosa sources

Duration of heparin therapy (pediatric):
  DVT and PE: At least 5-10 days
  Note: Oral anticoagulation should be started on day 1 of heparin; oral anticoagulation should be overlapped with heparin for 5 days (or more, if INR is not >2)

Updates to the United States Pharmacopeia (USP) heparin monograph were made in response to over 200 deaths linked to contaminated heparin products in 2007-2008. Serious adverse effects (including hypersensitivity reactions) were associated with a heparin-like contaminant (oversulfated chondroitin sulfate). At the time, the available quality assurance tests did not test for oversulfated chondroitin sulfate. Effective October 1, 2009, a new reference standard for heparin and a new test to determine potency (the chromogenic antifactor IIa test) were established by USP. The updated USP heparin monograph also harmonized the USP unit with the WHO international standard (IS) unit (ie, international unit). The new standard may result in a 10% reduction in potency for heparin marketed in the United States. The FDA has requested that all manufacturers differentiate (from "old" heparin products) heparin products manufactured by the new standards. The labels of products manufactured according to the new standard will have an "N" in the lot number or following the expiration date. Additionally, products manufactured by Hospira may be identified by the number "82" or higher (eg, 83, 84) at the beginning of their lot numbers. For therapeutic use, practitioners may or may not notice that larger doses of heparin are required to achieve "therapeutic" activity of anticoagulation. The impact of this change in potency should be less significant when heparin is administered by subcutaneous injection due to low and variable bioavailability. Heparin dosing should always be individualized according to the patient-specific clinical situation. Appropriate clinical judgment is essential in determining heparin dosage (Smythe, 2010).

Dosage Forms Excipient information presented when available (limited, particularly for generics); consult specific product labeling.

Solution, Injection, as sodium:
Generic: 1000 units (500 mL); 2000 units (1000 mL); 25,000 units (250 mL, 500 mL); 1000 units/mL (1 mL, 10 mL, 30 mL); 2500 units/mL (10 mL); 5000 units/mL (1 mL, 10 mL); 10,000 units/mL (1 mL, 4 mL, 5 mL); 20,000 units/mL (1 mL)

Solution, Injection, as sodium [preservative free]:
Generic: 1000 units/mL (2 mL); 5000 units/0.5 mL (0.5 mL)

Solution, Intravenous, as sodium:
Hep Flush-10: 10 units/mL (10 mL)
Generic: 10,000 units (250 mL); 12,500 units (250 mL); 20,000 units (500 mL); 25,000 units (250 mL, 500 mL); 1 units/mL (1 mL, 2 mL, 2.5 mL, 3 mL, 5 mL, 10 mL); 2 units/mL (3 mL); 10 units/mL (1 mL, 2 mL, 2.5 mL, 3 mL, 5 mL, 10 mL, 30 mL); 100 units/mL (1 mL, 2 mL, 2.5 mL, 3 mL, 5 mL, 10 mL, 30 mL); 2000 units/mL (5 mL)

Solution, Intravenous, as sodium [preservative free]:
Generic: 1 units/mL (3 mL); 10 units/mL (1 mL, 3 mL, 5 mL); 100 units/mL (1 mL, 3 mL, 5 mL)

References

Andrew M, Marzinotto V, Massicotte P, et al, "Heparin Therapy in Pediatric Patients: A Prospective Cohort Study," *Pediatr Res*, 1994, 35(1):78-83.

Goodman SG, Menon V, Cannon CP, et al, "Acute ST-Segment Elevation Myocardial Infarction: American College of Chest Physicians Evidence-Based Clinical Practice Guidelines (8th Edition)," *Chest*, 2008, 133(6 Suppl):708S-775S.

Guyatt GH, Akl EA, Crowther M, et al, "Executive Summary: Antithrombotic Therapy and Prevention of Thrombosis, 9th ed: American College of Chest Physicians Evidence-Based Clinical Practice Guidelines," *Chest*, 2012, 141(2 Suppl):7-47.

Harrington RA, Becker RC, Cannon CP, et al, "Antithrombotic Therapy for Non-ST-Segment Elevation Acute Coronary Syndromes: American College of Chest Physicians Evidence-Based Clinical Practice Guidelines (8th Edition)," *Chest*, 2008, 133(6 Suppl):670S-707S.

Hirsh J, Bauer KA, Donati MB, et al, "Parenteral Anticoagulants: American College of Chest Physicians Evidence-Based Clinical Practice Guidelines (8th Edition)," *Chest*, 2008, 133(6 Suppl):141S-159S.

Hirsh J, Guyatt G, Albers GW, et al, "Executive Summary: American College of Chest Physicians Evidence-Based Clinical Practice Guidelines (8th Edition)," *Chest*, 2008, 133(6 Suppl):71-109.

Institute for Safe Medication Practices (ISMP), "Standard Concentrations of Neonatal Drug Infusions," *ISMP*, 2011.

Kearon C, Kahn SR, Agnelli G, et al, "Antithrombotic Therapy for Venous Thromboembolic Disease: American College of Chest Physicians Evidence-Based Clinical Practice Guidelines (8th Edition)," *Chest*, 2008, 133(6 Suppl):454S-545S.

Monagle P, Chalmers E, Chan A, et al, "Antithrombotic Therapy in Neonates and Children: American College of Chest Physicians Evidence-Based Clinical Practice Guidelines (8th Edition)," *Chest*, 2008, 133(6 Suppl):887S-968S.

Newall F, Johnston L, Ignjatovic V, et al, "Unfractionated Heparin Therapy in Infants and Children," *Pediatrics*, 2009, 123(3):e510-8.

Phillips MS, "Standardizing I.V. Infusion Concentrations: National Survey Results," *Am J Health Syst Pharm*, 2011, 68(22):2176-82.

Smythe MA, Nutescu EA, and Wittkowsky AK, "Changes in the USP Heparin Monograph and Implications for Clinicians," *Pharmacotherapy*, 2010, 30(5):428-31.

◆ **Heparin Calcium** *see* Heparin *on page 1001*

◆ **Heparinized Saline** *see* Heparin *on page 1001*

◆ **Heparin Lock Flush** *see* Heparin *on page 1001*

◆ **Heparin Sodium** *see* Heparin *on page 1001*

Hepatitis A Vaccine (hep a TYE tis aye vak SEEN)

Medication Safety Issues
International issues:
Avaxim [Canada and multiple international markets] may be confused with Avastin brand name for bevacizumab [U.S., Canada, and multiple international markets]

Related Information
Immunization Administration Recommendations *on page 2368*
Immunization Guidelines *on page 2373*

Brand Names: U.S. Havrix; VAQTA
Brand Names: Canada Avaxim; Avaxim-Pediatric; HAVRIX; VAQTA
Therapeutic Category Vaccine
Generic Availability (U.S.) No

Use Active immunization against disease caused by hepatitis A virus (HAV) (FDA approved in ages ≥12 months and adults)

The Advisory Committee on Immunization Practices (ACIP) recommends routine vaccination for:
• All children ≥12 months of age (CDC [Fiore, 2006])
• All unvaccinated adults requesting protection from HAV infection (CDC [Fiore, 2006])
• Unvaccinated persons with any of the following conditions: Men who have sex with men; injection and noninjection illicit drug users; persons who work with HAV-infected primates or with HAV in a research laboratory setting; persons with chronic liver disease; patients who receive clotting-factor concentrates; persons traveling to or working in countries with high or intermediate levels of endemic HAV infection (CDC [Fiore, 2006])
• Vaccination can be a component of hepatitis A outbreak response or as postexposure prophylaxis, as determined by local public health authorities (CDC [Fiore, 2006]; CDC, 56[41], 2007)
• Unvaccinated persons who anticipate close personal contact with international adoptees from a country of intermediate to high endemicity of HAV, during their first 60 days of arrival into the United States (eg, household contacts, babysitters) (CDC, 58[36], 2009)

Pregnancy Risk Factor C
Pregnancy Considerations Animal reproduction studies have not been conducted. The safety of vaccination during pregnancy has not been determined, however, the theoretical risk to the infant is expected to be low. Inactivated vaccines have not been shown to cause increased risks to the fetus (CDC, 2011).

Breast-Feeding Considerations It is not known if this vaccine is excreted into breast milk. The manufacturer recommends that caution be used if administered to nursing women. Inactivated vaccines do not affect the safety of breast-feeding for the mother or the infant. Breast-feeding infants should be vaccinated according to the recommended schedules (CDC, 2011).

Contraindications Hypersensitivity to hepatitis A vaccine or any component, including neomycin

Warnings Immediate treatment (including epinephrine 1:1000) for anaphylactic and/or hypersensitivity reactions should be available during vaccine use. Primary ▶

immunization series should be completed at least 2 weeks prior to travel to an area of high endemicity. Syncope has been reported with use of injectable vaccines and may be accompanied by transient visual disturbances, weakness, or tonic-clonic movements. Procedures should be in place to avoid injuries from falling and to restore cerebral perfusion if syncope occurs (CDC, 57(17), 2008).

Precautions The decision to administer or delay vaccination because of current or recent febrile illness depends on the severity of symptoms and the etiology of the disease. Immunization should be delayed during the course of an acute severe febrile illness; may administer to patients with mild acute illness (with or without fever). Use with caution in severely immunocompromised patients (eg, patients receiving chemo/radiation therapy or other immunosuppressive therapy, including high-dose corticosteroids); may have a reduced response to vaccination and vaccination; inactivated vaccines should be administered ≥2 weeks prior to planned immunosuppression when feasible (IDSA [Rubin, 2013]). In general, household and close contacts of persons with altered immunocompetence may receive all age-appropriate vaccines. Vaccination may not result in effective immunity in all patients. Response depends upon multiple factors (eg, type of vaccine, age of patient) and may be improved by administering the vaccine at the recommended dose, route, and interval (CDC/ACIP [Kroger, 2011]). Due to the long incubation period for hepatitis A (15 to 50 days), unrecognized hepatitis A infection may be present at time of vaccination; immunization may not prevent infection in these patients. Patients with chronic liver disease may have decreased antibody response.

Use with caution in patients with coagulation disorders, including thrombocytopenia, due to an increased risk for bleeding following I.M. administration; if the patient receives antihemophilia or other similar therapy, I.M. injection can be scheduled shortly after such therapy is administered. Antipyretics have not been shown to prevent febrile seizures; antipyretics may be used to treat fever or discomfort following vaccination (CDC/ACIP [Kroger, 2011]). One study reported that routine prophylactic administration of acetaminophen to prevent fever prior to vaccination decreased the immune response of some vaccines; the clinical significance of this reduction in immune response has not been established (Prymula, 2009).

Use of this vaccine for specific medical and/or other indications (eg, immunocompromising conditions, hepatic or kidney disease, diabetes) is also addressed in the ACIP Recommended Immunization Schedule (CDC/ACIP [Akinsanya-Beysolow, 2014]; CDC/ACIP [Bridges, 2014]). Specific recommendations for use of this vaccine in immunocompromised patients with asplenia, cancer, HIV infection, cerebrospinal fluid leaks, cochlear implants, hematopoietic stem cell transplant (prior to or after), sickle cell disease, solid organ transplant (prior to or after), or those receiving immunosuppressive therapy for chronic conditions, as well as contacts of immunocompromised patients, are available from the IDSA (Rubin, 2014). Packaging may contain natural latex rubber; some products may contain neomycin.

Adverse Reactions All serious adverse reactions must be reported to the U.S. Department of Health and Human Services (DHHS) Vaccine Adverse Event Reporting System (VAERS) at 1-800-822-7967 or online at https://vaers.hhs.gov/esub/index. In Canada, adverse reactions may be reported to local provincial/territorial health agencies or to the Vaccine Safety Section at Public Health Agency of Canada (1-866-844-0018).

Central nervous system: Chills, drowsiness, fatigue, headache, insomnia, irritability, malaise

Dermatologic: Skin rash

Endocrine & metabolic: Menstrual disease

Gastrointestinal: Abdominal pain, anorexia, constipation, decreased appetite, diarrhea, gastroenteritis, nausea, vomiting

Local: Bruising at injection site, erythema at injection site, induration at injection site, injection site reaction (soreness, warmth), pain at injection site, swelling at injection site, tenderness at injection site

Neuromuscular & skeletal: Arm pain, back pain, myalgia, stiffness, weakness

Ophthalmic: Conjunctivitis

Otic: Otitis media

Respiratory: Asthma, cough, nasal congestion, nasopharyngitis, pharyngitis, rhinitis, rhinorrhea, upper respiratory tract infection

Miscellaneous: Excessive crying, fever (≥102°F [1-5 days postvaccination]; ≥100.4°F [1-5 days postvaccination]; >98.6°C [1-14 days postvaccination])

Rare but important or life-threatening: Anaphylaxis, angioedema, ataxia (cerebellar), bronchiolitis, bronchoconstriction, dehydration, dermatitis, encephalitis, erythema multiforme, Guillain-Barre syndrome, hematoma at injection site, hepatitis, hypersensitivity reaction, hypoesthesia, increased creatine kinase, increased serum transaminases (transient), injection site reaction (nodule), jaundice, lymphadenopathy, multiple sclerosis, myelitis, neuropathy, paresthesia, photophobia, pruritus, rash at injection site, seizure, serum sickness-like reaction, syncope, thrombocytopenia, vasculitis, wheezing

Drug Interactions

Metabolism/Transport Effects None known.

Avoid Concomitant Use There are no known interactions where it is recommended to avoid concomitant use.

Increased Effect/Toxicity There are no known significant interactions involving an increase in effect.

Decreased Effect

The levels/effects of Hepatitis A Vaccine may be decreased by: Belimumab; Fingolimod; Immunosuppressants

Stability Store at 2°C to 8°C (36°F to 46°F); do not freeze. The following stability information has also been reported for Havrix®: May be stored at room temperature for up to 72 hours (Cohen, 2007).

Mechanism of Action As an inactivated virus vaccine, hepatitis A vaccine induces active immunity against hepatitis A virus infection

Pharmacodynamics

Onset of action: Protective antibodies develop in 95% of adults after the first dose and in 100% of adults after the second dose of the vaccine; ≥97% of children and adolescents will be seropositive within 1 month of the first dose and 100% will develop protective antibodies after receiving two doses. The efficacy of preventing hepatitis A disease in children living in highly infected areas is 94% to 100% (CDC, 2012).

Duration: Protective antibodies induced by the vaccine may persist for ≥20 years (CDC, 2012).

Dosing: Usual Note: When used for primary immunization, the vaccine should be given at least 2 weeks prior to expected HAV exposure. When used prior to an international adoption, the vaccination series should begin when adoption is being planned, but at least ≥2 weeks prior to expected arrival of adoptee (CDC, 58[36], 2009). Vaccines are interchangeable for booster doses.

Pediatric:

Primary immunization:

CDC (ACIP) recommendations: Children ≥12 months: I.M.: 0.5 mL per dose for a total of two doses. All children should receive primary immunization with a 2-dose series. The series should be initiated at 12 to 23 months of age; the two doses should be separated by 6 to 18 months (CDC/ACIP [Fiore, 2006]).

Manufacturer's labeling:

Havrix: Children and Adolescents 12 months to 18 years: I.M.: 0.5 mL (720 ELISA units) per dose for a total of two doses given 6 to 12 months apart

VAQTA: Children and Adolescents 12 months to 18 years: I.M.: 0.5 mL (25 units) per dose for a total of two doses given 6 to 18 months of age apart; **Note:** VAQTA should be given at 6 to 12 months if following the primary dose of another inactivated hepatitis A vaccine.

Catch-up immunization: CDC (ACIP) recommendations (Akinsany-Beysolow, 2014): **Note:** Do not restart the series. If doses have been given, begin the following schedule at the applicable dose number. Children ≥2 years and Adolescents if immunity against hepatitis A virus infection is desired: I.M.: 0.5 mL per dose for a total of two doses separated by 6 to 18 months

Postexposure prophylaxis: Children and Adolescents without immunity: I.M.: 0.5 mL once as soon as possible following recent exposure to hepatitis A (during last two weeks) (CDC, 56[41], 2007)

Adult:

Primary immunization:

Havrix: I.M.: 1 mL (1440 ELISA units) per dose for a total of two doses given 6 to 12 months apart

VAQTA: I.M.: 1 mL (50 units) per dose for a total of two doses given 6 to 18 months apart; **Note:** VAQTA should be given at 6 to 12 months if following the primary dose of another inactivated hepatitis A vaccine.

Dosing adjustment in renal impairment: There are no dosage adjustments provided in the manufacturer's labeling.

Dosing adjustment in hepatic impairment: There are no dosage adjustments provided in the manufacturer's labeling; however, data suggest patients with chronic liver disease have a lower antibody response to HAVRIX than healthy subjects.

Administration Shake well and administer I.M. into mid-lateral aspect of the thigh in infants and small children; administer in the deltoid area to older children and adults; **not for I.V., intradermal, or SubQ administration.** Adolescents and adults should be vaccinated while seated or lying down. U.S. law requires that the date of administration, the vaccine manufacturer, lot number of vaccine, and the administering person's name, title, and address be entered into the patient's permanent medical record.

Monitoring Parameters Liver function tests. Observe for syncope for 15 minutes following administration. If seizure-like activity associated with syncope occurs, maintain patient in supine or Trendelenburg position to reestablish adequate cerebral perfusion.

Additional Information In order to maximize vaccination rates, the ACIP recommends simultaneous administration (ie, >1 vaccine on the same day at different anatomic sites) of all age-appropriate vaccines (live or inactivated) for which a person is eligible at a single visit, unless contraindications exist. If available, the use of combination vaccines is generally preferred over separate injections, taking into consideration provider assessment, patient preference, and potential adverse events. If separate vaccines being used, evaluate product information regarding same syringe compatibility of vaccines. Separate needles and syringes should be used for each injection. The ACIP prefers each dose of specific vaccine in a series come from the same manufacturer if possible (CDC/ACIP [Kroger, 2011]).

For additional information, please refer to the following website: http://www.cdc.gov/vaccines/vpd-vac/.

Dosage Forms Excipient information presented when available (limited, particularly for generics); consult specific product labeling. [DSC] = Discontinued product

Injection, suspension [adult, preservative free]:

Havrix: Hepatitis A virus antigen 1440 ELISA units/mL (1 mL) [contains aluminum, neomycin (may have trace amounts); may contain natural rubber/natural latex in prefilled syringe]

VAQTA: Hepatitis A virus antigen 50 units/mL (1 mL) [contains aluminum, natural rubber/natural latex in packaging]

Injection, suspension [pediatric, preservative free]:

Havrix: Hepatitis A virus antigen 720 ELISA units/0.5 mL (0.5 mL) [contains aluminum, neomycin (may have trace amounts); may contain natural rubber/natural latex in prefilled syringe]

Injection, suspension [pediatric/adolescent, preservative free]:

VAQTA: Hepatitis A virus antigen 25 units/0.5 mL (0.5 mL) [contains aluminum, natural rubber/natural latex in packaging]

References

AAP Steering Committee on Quality Improvement and Management, Subcommittee on Febrile Seizures American Academy of Pediatrics. Febrile seizures: clinical practice guideline for the long-term management of the child with simple febrile seizures. *Pediatrics.* 2008;121 (6):1281-1286.

Advisory Committee on Immunization Practices (ACIP) Centers for Disease Control and Prevention (CDC). Update: prevention of hepatitis A after exposure to hepatitis A virus and in international travelers. Updated recommendations of the Advisory Committee on Immunization Practices (ACIP). *MMWR Morb Mortal Wkly Rep.* 2007;56(41):1080-1084.

Akinsanya-Beysolow I; Advisory Committee on Immunization Practices (ACIP); ACIP Child/Adolescent Immunization Work Group; Centers for Disease Control and Prevention (CDC). Advisory Committee on Immunization Practices recommended immunization schedules for persons aged 0 through 18 years – United States, 2014. *MMWR Morb Mortal Wkly Rep.* 2014;63(5):108-109. Available at http://www.cdc.gov/vaccines/schedules/downloads/child/0-18yrs-child-combined-schedule.pdf

Bridges CB, Coyne-Beasley T; Advisory Committee on Immunization Practices (ACIP); ACIP Adult Immunization Work Group; Centers for Disease Control and Prevention (CDC). Advisory Committee on Immunization Practices recommended immunization schedule for adults aged 19 years or older – United States, 2014. *MMWR Morb Mortal Wkly Rep.* 2014;63(5):110-112. Available at http://www.cdc.gov/vaccines/schedules/downloads/adult/adult-combined-schedule.pdf

Centers for Disease Control and Prevention (CDC). *Epidemiology and Prevention of Vaccine-Preventable Diseases.* 12th ed. Atkinson W, Wolfe S, Hamborsky J, eds. Washington, DC: Public Health Foundation; 2012.

Centers for Disease Control and Prevention (CDC). Syncope after vaccination – United States, January 2005-July 2007. *MMWR Morb Mortal Wkly Rep.* 2008;57(17):457-460.

Centers for Disease Control and Prevention (CDC). Updated recommendations from the Advisory Committee on Immunization Practices (ACIP) for use of hepatitis A vaccine in close contacts of newly arriving international adoptees. Available at http://www.cdc.gov/mmwr/preview/mmwrhtml/mm5836a4.htm?s_cid=mm5836a4_e.

Cohen V, Jellinek SP, Teperikidis L, Berkovits E, Goldman WM. Room-temperature storage of medications labeled for refrigeration. *Am J Health-Syst Pharm.* 2007;64(16):1711-1715.

Fiore AE, Wasley A, Bell BP. Prevention of hepatitis A through active or passive immunization: recommendations of the Advisory Committee on Immunization Practices (ACIP). *MMWR Recomm Rep.* 2006;55 (RR-7):1-23. Available at http://www.cdc.gov/mmwr/PDF/rr/rr5507.pdf

Kroger AT, Atkinson WL, Marcuse EK, Pickering LK. General recommendations on immunization - recommendations of the Advisory Committee on Immunization Practices (ACIP). *MMWR Recomm Rep.* 2011;60(RR-2):1-64.

Niu MT, Salive M, Krueger C, Ellenberg SS. Two-year review of hepatitis A vaccine safety: data from the Vaccine Adverse Event Reporting System (VAERS). *Clin Infect Dis.* 1998;26(6):1475-1476.

Prymula R, Siegrist CA, Chlibek R, et al. Effect of prophylactic paracetamol administration at time of vaccination on febrile reactions and antibody responses in children: two open-label, randomised controlled trials. *Lancet.* 2009;374(9698):1339-1350.

Rubin LG, Levin MJ, Ljungman P, et al. 2013 IDSA clinical practice guideline for vaccination of the immunocompromised host. *Clin Infect Dis.* 2014;58(3):e44-e100.

Hepatitis B Immune Globulin (Human)
(hep a TYE tis bee i MYUN GLOB yoo lin YU man)

Medication Safety Issues
Sound-alike/look-alike issues:
HBIG may be confused with BabyBIG
Related Information
Immunization Administration Recommendations *on page 2368*
Immunization Guidelines *on page 2373*
Brand Names: U.S. HepaGam B; HyperHEP B S/D; Nabi-HB
Brand Names: Canada HepaGam B; HyperHEP B S/D
Therapeutic Category Immune Globulin
Generic Availability (U.S.) No
Use Parenteral:
I.M.: HepaGam B®, HyperHEP B™ S/D, Nabi-HB®: Provide prophylactic post-exposure passive immunity to hepatitis B following perinatal exposure of infants born to HB$_s$Ag-positive mothers (FDA approved in neonates and infants); provide prophylactic postexposure passive immunity to hepatitis B following acute exposure to blood containing hepatitis B surface antigen (HB$_s$Ag), sexual exposure to HB$_s$Ag-positive persons, or household exposure to persons with acute HBV infection (FDA approved in infants, children, and adults)
I.V.: HepaGam B®: Prevention of hepatitis B virus recurrence after liver transplantation in HB$_s$Ag-positive transplant patients
Note: Hepatitis B immune globulin is not indicated for treatment of active hepatitis B infection and is ineffective in the treatment of chronic active hepatitis B infection.
Pregnancy Risk Factor C
Pregnancy Considerations Animal reproduction studies have not been conducted. Use of HBIG is not contraindicated in pregnant women and may be used for postexposure prophylaxis when indicated (CDC, 2001). In addition, use of HBIG has been evaluated to reduce maternal to fetal transmission of hepatis B virus during pregnancy (ACOG, 2007)
Breast-Feeding Considerations It is not known if immune globulin from these preparations is excreted into breast milk. The manufacturer recommends that caution be used if administered to breast-feeding women. Endogenous immune globulins can be found in breast milk (Agarwal, 2011). Infants born to HBsAg-positive mothers may be breast fed (CDC, 2005). Use of HBIG is not contraindicated in breast-feeding women (CDC, 2001).
Contraindications Hypersensitivity to hepatitis B immune globulin or any component; severe allergy to gamma globulin or anti-immunoglobulin therapies. Additional contraindication: HepaGam B®: Postexposure prophylaxis in patients with severe thrombocytopenia or other coagulation disorders which would contraindicate I.M. injections (administer only if benefit outweighs the risk)
Warnings Product of human plasma; may potentially contain infectious agents which could transmit disease. Screening of donors, as well as testing and/or inactivation or removal of certain viruses, reduces this risk. Infections thought to be transmitted by this product should be reported to the manufacturer. Although extremely rare, severe hypersensitivity reactions including anaphylaxis may occur; epinephrine (1:1000) and other anaphylactic treatment agents should be readily available.

Injection may contain polysorbate 80 (Tween 80®) which may cause allergic reactions in susceptible individuals. In premature neonates, thrombocytopenia, ascites, pulmonary deterioration, and renal and hepatic failure have been reported after receiving parenteral products containing polysorbate 80 (Alade, 1986; *MMWR*, 1984). Infusion of polysorbate 80-containing solutions through polyvinyl chloride tubing may cause DEHP to leach into the solution; in immature animals, exposure to DEHP may adversely affect the development of the male reproductive tract.

Precautions Administer with caution to patients with thrombocytopenia or any coagulation disorder that would be compromised by I.M. injection; administer with caution in patients with IgA deficiency or a prior history of systemic allergic reactions following the administration of human immunoglobulin preparations. When administered I.V., do not exceed recommended infusion rates; may increase risk of adverse events (eg, hypotension, chills, dizziness, headache, pyrexia, cold sweat); patients should be monitored for adverse events during and after the infusion. Thrombotic events have been reported with administration of intravenous immune globulin; use with caution in patients of advanced age, with a history of atherosclerosis or cardiovascular and/or thrombotic risk factors, patients with impaired cardiac output, coagulation disorders, prolonged immobilization, or patients with known/suspected hyperviscosity. Consider a baseline assessment of blood viscosity in patients at risk for hyperviscosity.

Some products may contain maltose, which may result in falsely-elevated blood glucose readings.

Adverse Reactions Reported with postexposure prophylaxis. Adverse events reported in liver transplant patients included tremor and hypotension, were associated with a single infusion during the first week of treatment, and did not recur with additional infusions.

Cardiovascular: Hypotension
Central nervous system: Headache, malaise
Dermatologic: Ecchymoses, erythema
Gastrointestinal: Nausea, vomiting
Hematologic & oncologic: Change in WBC count
Hepatic: Increased liver enzymes, increased serum alkaline phosphatase
Local: Pain at injection site
Neuromuscular & skeletal: Joint stiffness, myalgia
Renal: Increased serum creatinine
Rare but important or life-threatening: Anaphylactic reaction (rare), angioedema, hypersensitivity, increased serum lipase, increased serum transaminases, sinus tachycardia
Drug Interactions
Metabolism/Transport Effects None known.
Avoid Concomitant Use There are no known interactions where it is recommended to avoid concomitant use.
Increased Effect/Toxicity There are no known significant interactions involving an increase in effect.
Decreased Effect
Hepatitis B Immune Globulin (Human) may decrease the levels/effects of: Vaccines (Live)
Stability Store at 2°C to 8°C (36°F to 46°F); do not freeze; use within 6 hours of puncturing the vial. HyperHEP B™ S/D: May be exposed to room temperature for a cumulative 7 days (Cohen, 2007).
Mechanism of Action Hepatitis B immune globulin (HBIG) is a nonpyrogenic sterile solution containing immunoglobulin G (IgG) specific to hepatitis B surface antigen (HBsAg). HBIG differs from immune globulin in the amount of anti-HBs. Immune globulin is prepared from plasma that is not preselected for anti-HBs content. HBIG is prepared from plasma preselected for high titer anti-HBs. In the U.S., HBIG has an anti-HBs high titer >1:100,000 by IRA.
Pharmacodynamics Duration: Postexposure prophylaxis: 3-6 months
Pharmacokinetics (Adult data unless noted)
Absorption: I.M.: Slow
Half-life: 17-25 days
Time to peak serum concentration: I.M.: 2-10 days

Dosing: Neonatal

Perinatal exposure, prophylaxis (CDC, 2005): **Note:** HBIG may be administered at the same time (but at a different site) or up to 1 month preceding hepatitis B vaccination without impairing the active immune response:

Neonates born to HB$_s$Ag-positive mothers: I.M.: 0.5 mL as soon after birth as possible (within 12 hours; efficacy decreases significantly if treatment is delayed >48 hours); hepatitis B vaccine series to begin at the same time; if this series is delayed for as long as 3 months, the HBIG dose may be repeated (Saari, 2003)

Neonates born to mothers with unknown HB$_s$Ag status at birth: I.M.:

Birth weight <2 kg: 0.5 mL within 12 hours of birth (along with hepatitis B vaccine) if unable to determine maternal HB$_s$Ag status within that time

Birth weight ≥2 kg: 0.5 mL within 7 days of birth while awaiting maternal HB$_s$Ag results; if mother is determined to be HB$_s$Ag positive, administer dose as soon as possible.

Dosing: Usual Note: For exposure prophylaxis, HBIG may be administered at the same time (but at a different site) or up to 1 month preceding hepatitis B vaccination without impairing the active immune response.

Infants, Children, and Adolescents:

Perinatal exposure, prophylaxis (CDC, 2005): Infants born to HB$_s$Ag-positive mothers: I.M.: 0.5 mL as a repeat of birth dose if the hepatitis B vaccination series is delayed for as long as 3 months (hepatitis B vaccine should also be administered at the same time/different site)

Postexposure, prophylaxis:

Infants <12 months: I.M.: 0.5 mL as soon as possible after exposure (eg, mother or primary caregiver with acute HBV infection); initiate hepatitis B vaccine series

Children ≥12 months and Adolescents: I.M.: 0.06 mL/kg as soon as possible after exposure (ie, within 24 hours of needlestick, ocular, or mucosal exposure or within 14 days of sexual exposure); repeat at 28-30 days after exposure

Adults:

Postexposure, prophylaxis: I.M.: 0.06 mL/kg as soon as possible after exposure (ie, within 24 hours of needlestick, ocular, or mucosal exposure or within 14 days of sexual exposure); repeat at 28-30 days after exposure

Prevention of hepatitis B recurrence in liver transplant patients: I.V.: HepaGam B™: 20,000 units/dose according to the following schedule:

Anhepatic phase (initial dose): One dose given with the liver transplant

Week 1 postop: One dose daily for 7 days (days 1-7)

Weeks 2-12 postop: One dose every 2 weeks starting on day 14

Month 4 onward: One dose monthly starting on month 4

Dose adjustment: Adjust dose to reach anti-HB$_s$ levels of 500 units/L within the first week after transplantation. In patients with surgical bleeding, abdominal fluid drainage >500 mL or those undergoing plasmapheresis, administer 10,000 units/dose every 6 hours until target anti-HB$_s$ levels are reached.

Dosing adjustment in renal impairment: There are no dosage adjustments provided in the manufacturer labeling.

Dosing adjustment in hepatic impairment: There are no dosing adjustments provided in the manufacturer labeling.

Administration

I.M.: Inject only in the anterolateral aspects of the upper thigh or the deltoid muscle; multiple injections may be necessary when the dosage is a large volume (postexposure prophylaxis). Do not administer hepatitis vaccine

and HBIG in same syringe (vaccine will be neutralized); hepatitis vaccine may be administered at the same time at a separate site

I.V.: HepaGam B™: Administer at 2 mL/minute. Decrease infusion to <1 mL/minute for patient discomfort or infusion-related adverse events. Actual volume of dosage is dependent upon potency labeled on each individual vial.

Nabi-HB®: Although not FDA approved for this purpose, Nabi-HB® has been administered intravenously in hepatitis B-positive liver transplant adult patients (Dickson, 2006).

Monitoring Parameters Liver transplant patients: anti-HB levels; infusion-related adverse events

Test Interactions

Glucose testing: HepaGam B™ contains maltose. Falsely-elevated blood glucose levels may occur when glucose monitoring devices and test strips utilizing the glucose dehydrogenase pyrroloquinolinequinone (GDH-PQQ) based methods are used.

Serological testing: Antibodies transferred following administration of immune globulins may provide misleading positive test results (eg, Coombs' test)

Dosage Forms Excipient information presented when available (limited, particularly for generics); consult specific product labeling.

Solution, Injection [preservative free]:

HepaGam B: (1 mL, 5 mL) [contains polysorbate 80]

Solution, Intramuscular:

HyperHEP B S/D: (0.5 mL, 1 mL, 5 mL)

Nabi-HB: (1 mL, 5 mL) [thimerosal free]

References

Alade SL, Brown RE, and Paquet A Jr, "Polysorbate 80 and E-Ferol Toxicity," Pediatrics, 1986, 77(4):593-7.

American College of Obstetricians and Gynecologists, ACOG Practice Bulletin No. 86: "Viral Hepatitis in Pregnancy," Obstet Gynecol, 2007, 110(4):941-56.

Centers for Disease Control and Prevention (CDC), "A Comprehensive Immunization Strategy to Eliminate Transmission of Hepatitis B Virus Infection in the United States: Recommendations of the Advisory Committee on Immunization Practices (ACIP) Part I: Immunization of Infants, Children, and Adolescents," MMWR Recomm Rep, 2005, 54(RR-16):1-31.

Centers for Disease Control and Prevention (CDC), "Unusual Syndrome With Fatalities Among Premature Infants: Association With a New Intravenous Vitamin E Product," MMWR Morb Mortal Wkly Rep, 1984, 33(14):198-9.

Centers for Disease Control and Prevention (CDC), U.S. Public Health Service, "Updated U.S. Public Health Service Guidelines for the Management of Occupational Exposures to HBV, HCV, and HIV and Recommendations for Postexposure Prophylaxis," MMWR Recomm Rep, 2001, 50(RR-11):1-52.

Cohen V, Jellinek SP, Teperikidis L, et al, "Room-Temperature Storage of Medications Labeled for Refrigeration," Am J Health-Syst Pharm, 2007, 64(16):1711-15.

Dickson RC, Terrault NA, Ishitani M, et al, "Protective Antibody Levels and Dose Requirements for IV 5% Nabi Hepatitis B Immune Globulin Combined With Lamivudine in Liver Transplantation for Hepatitis B-Induced End Stage Liver Disease," Liver Transpl, 2006, 12(1):124-33.

Saari TN and American Academy of Pediatrics Committee on Infectious Diseases, "Immunization of Preterm and Low Birth Weight Infants. American Academy of Pediatrics Committee on Infectious Diseases," Pediatrics, 2003, 112(1 Pt 1):193-8.

◆ **Hepatitis B Inactivated Virus Vaccine (recombinant DNA)** see Hepatitis B Vaccine (Recombinant) on page 1009

Hepatitis B Vaccine (Recombinant)
(hep a TYE tis bee vak SEEN ree KOM be nant)

Medication Safety Issues

Sound-alike/look-alike issues:

Engerix-B adult may be confused with Engerix-B pediatric/adolescent

Recombivax HB may be confused with Comvax

◄ **Related Information**

Immunization Administration Recommendations *on page 2368*

Immunization Guidelines *on page 2373*

Brand Names: U.S. Engerix-B; Recombivax HB

Brand Names: Canada Engerix-B; Recombivax HB

Therapeutic Category Vaccine

Generic Availability (U.S.) No

Use Immunization against infection caused by all known subtypes of hepatitis B virus (FDA approved in all ages).

The Advisory Committee on Immunization Practices (ACIP) recommends routine vaccination for the following (CDC/ACIP 60[50], 2011):

- All infants at birth (CDC/ACIP [Mast, 2005])
- All infants and children (CDC/ACIP [Mast, 2005]) (post-birth dose; refer to recommended vaccination schedule)
- All unvaccinated adults requesting protection from HBV infection (CDC/ACIP [Mast, 2006])
- All unvaccinated adults at risk for HBV infection such as those with:
  - Behavioral risks: Sexually active persons with >1 partner in a 6-month period; persons seeking evaluation or treatment for a sexually transmitted disease; men who have sex with men; injection drug users (CDC/ACIP [Mast, 2006])
  - Occupational risks: Healthcare and public safety workers with reasonably anticipated risk for exposure to blood or blood-contaminated body fluids (CDC/ACIP [Mast, 2006])
  - Medical risks: Persons with end-stage renal disease (including predialysis, hemodialysis, peritoneal dialysis, and home dialysis); persons with HIV infection; persons with chronic liver disease (CDC/ACIP [Mast, 2006]). Adults (19-59 years of age) with diabetes mellitus type 1 or type 2 should be vaccinated as soon as possible following diagnosis. Adults ≥60 years with diabetes mellitus may also be vaccinated at the discretion of their treating clinician (CDC/ACIP 60 [50], 2011).
  - Other risks: Household contacts and sex partners of persons with chronic HBV infection; residents and staff of facilities for developmentally disabled persons; international travelers to regions with high or intermediate levels of endemic HBV infection (CDC/ACIP [Mast, 2006])

In addition, the ACIP recommends vaccination for any persons who are wounded in bombings or similar mass casualty events who have penetrating injuries or nonintact skin exposure, or who have contact with mucous membranes (exception - superficial contact with intact skin), and who cannot confirm receipt of a hepatitis B vaccination (CDC [Chapman, 2008]).

Pregnancy Risk Factor C

Pregnancy Considerations Animal reproduction studies have not been conducted. The ACIP recommends HBsAg testing for all pregnant women. Based on limited data, there is no apparent risk to the fetus when the hepatitis B vaccine is administered during pregnancy. Pregnancy itself is not a contraindication to vaccination; vaccination should be considered if otherwise indicated (CDC/ACIP [Mast, 2006]).

Breast-Feeding Considerations It is not known if this vaccine is excreted into breast milk. The manufacturer recommends that caution be used if administered to a nursing woman. However, maternal vaccination is not a contraindication to breastfeeding (CDC [Schillie, 2013]). Inactivated virus vaccines do not affect the safety of breast-feeding for the mother or the infant. Breast-feeding infants should be vaccinated according to the recommended schedules (NCIRD/ACIP, 2011). Infants born to HBsAg-positive mothers may be breast-fed (CDC/ACIP

[Mast, 2005]). Female health care providers who are exposed to the hepatitis B virus do not need to discontinue nursing when the vaccine is administered as part of post exposure care (CDC [Schillie, 2013]).

Contraindications Hypersensitivity to hepatitis vaccine, yeast, or any component

Warnings Immediate treatment (including epinephrine 1:1000) for anaphylactic and/or hypersensitivity reactions should be available during vaccine use. Apnea has occurred following intramuscular vaccine administration in premature infants; consider clinical status implications. Syncope has been reported with use of injectable vaccines and may be accompanied by transient visual disturbances, weakness, or tonic-clonic movements. Procedures should be in place to avoid injuries from falling and to restore cerebral perfusion if syncope occurs (CDC, 57[17], 2008).

Precautions Use with caution in patients with multiple sclerosis; rare exacerbations of symptoms have been observed. The decision to administer or delay vaccination because of current or recent febrile illness depends on the severity of symptoms and the etiology of the disease. Immunization should be delayed during the course of an acute severe febrile illness; may administer to patients with mild acute illness (with or without fever). Use with caution in severely immunocompromised patients (eg, patients receiving chemo-/radiation therapy, or other immunosuppressive therapy including high-dose corticosteroids); may have a reduced response to vaccination; inactivated vaccines should be administered ≥2 weeks prior to planned immunosuppression when feasible (IDSA [Rubin, 2013]). In general, household and close contacts of persons with altered immunocompetence may receive all age-appropriate vaccines. Vaccination may not result in effective immunity in all patients. Response depends upon multiple factors (eg, type of vaccine, age of patient) and may be improved by administering the vaccine at the recommended dose, route, and interval (CDC/ACIP [Kroger, 2011]). Due to the long incubation period for hepatitis, unrecognized hepatitis B infection may be present prior to vaccination; immunization may not prevent infection in these patients.

Use with caution in patients with coagulation disorders including thrombocytopenia, due to an increased risk for bleeding following I.M. administration; if the patient receives antihemophilia or other similar therapy, I.M. injection can be scheduled shortly after such therapy is administered. Use with caution in patients with decreased cardiopulmonary function.

Antipyretics have not been shown to prevent febrile seizures; antipyretics may be used to treat fever or discomfort following vaccination (CDC/ACIP [Kroger, 2011]). One study reported that routine prophylactic administration of acetaminophen to prevent fever prior to vaccination decreased the immune response of some vaccines; the clinical significance of this reduction in immune response has not been established (Prymula, 2009).

Infants born to HBsAg negative mothers and weighing <2 kg at birth may have the initial dose deferred up to 30 days of chronological age or until hospital discharge. If the mother's HBsAg status at delivery is unknown or positive, hepatitis B vaccine and hepatitis B immune globulin should be administered within 12 hours of life and the first dose of the vaccine should not be counted as part of the vaccine series. Combination vaccines (eg, also containing DTaP, HIB) should not be used as a "birth" dose.

Use of this vaccine for specific medical and/or other indications (eg, immunocompromising conditions, hepatic or kidney disease, diabetes) is also addressed in the ACIP Recommended Immunization Schedule (CDC/ACIP [Akinsanya-Beysolow, 2014]; CDC/ACIP [Bridges, 2014]). Specific recommendations for use of this vaccine in immunocompromised patients with asplenia, cancer, HIV infection, cerebrospinal fluid leaks, cochlear implants, hematopoietic stem cell transplant (prior to or after), sickle cell disease, solid organ transplant (prior to or after), or those receiving immunosuppressive therapy for chronic conditions, as well as contacts of immunocompromised patients, are available from the IDSA (Rubin, 2014). Use with caution in patients with latex sensitivity; packaging may contain natural latex rubber.

Adverse Reactions All serious adverse reactions must be reported to the U.S. Department of Health and Human Services (DHHS) Vaccine Adverse Event Reporting System (VAERS) at 1-800-822-7967 or online at https://vaers.hhs.gov/esub/index.
Cardiovascular: Flushing, hypotension
Central nervous system: Body pain, chills, dizziness, drowsiness, fatigue, headache, insomnia, irritability, malaise, paresthesia, tingling sensation, vertigo
Dermatologic: Diaphoresis, pruritus, skin rash, urticaria
Gastrointestinal: Abdominal pain, anorexia, decreased appetite, diarrhea, dyspepsia, nausea, stomach cramps, vomiting
Genitourinary: Dysuria
Hematologic & oncologic: Lymphadenopathy
Hypersensitivity: Angioedema
Infection: Influenza
Local: Bruising at injection site, erythema at injection site, induration at injection site, injection site nodule, itching at injection site, local soreness/soreness at injection site, pain at injection site, swelling at injection site, tenderness at injection site, warm sensation at injection site
Neuromuscular & skeletal: Arthralgia, back pain, myalgia, neck pain, neck stiffness, shoulder pain, weakness
Otic: Otalgia
Respiratory: Cough, pharyngitis, rhinitis, upper respiratory tract infection
Miscellaneous: Fever (≥37.5°C/100°F)
Rare but important or life-threatening: Acute exacerbations of multiple sclerosis, anaphylaxis, apnea, Bell's palsy, encephalitis, febrile seizures, Guillain-Barre syndrome, herpes zoster, hypersensitivity reaction, hypoesthesia, increased erythrocyte sedimentation rate, increased liver enzymes, keratitis, lupus-like syndrome, migraine, multiple sclerosis, myelitis, neuropathy, optic neuritis, paralysis, paresis, periarteritis nodosa, peripheral neuropathy, purpura, radiculopathy, seizure, serum-sickness like reaction (may be delayed days to weeks), Stevens-Johnson syndrome, syncope, systemic lupus erythematosus, tachycardia, thrombocytopenia, transverse myelitis, uveitis, vasculitis, visual disturbances

Drug Interactions
Metabolism/Transport Effects None known.
Avoid Concomitant Use There are no known interactions where it is recommended to avoid concomitant use.
Increased Effect/Toxicity There are no known significant interactions involving an increase in effect.
Decreased Effect
The levels/effects of Hepatitis B Vaccine (Recombinant) may be decreased by: Belimumab; Fingolimod; Immunosuppressants
Stability Store at 2°C to 8°C (36°F to 46°F); do not freeze. The following stability information has also been reported for Engerix-B®: May be stored at room temperature for up to 72 hours (Cohen, 2007).
Mechanism of Action Recombinant hepatitis B vaccine is a noninfectious subunit viral vaccine, which confers active immunity via formation of antihepatitis B antibodies. The vaccine is derived from hepatitis B surface antigen (HBsAg) produced through recombinant DNA techniques from yeast cells. The portion of the hepatitis B gene which codes for HBsAg is cloned into yeast, which is then cultured to produce hepatitis B vaccine.
Pharmacodynamics Postvaccination seroprotection is found in ~95% of healthy infants, ~92% of health care personnel <40 years of age, and ~84% of health care personnel ≥40 years of age (CDC [Schillie, 2013]).
Duration: Following a 3-dose series in pediatric patients, up to 50% of patients will have low or undetectable anti-HB antibody 5 to 15 years postvaccination. However, anamnestic increases in anti-HB have been shown up to 23 years later, suggesting a lifelong immune memory response (CDC/ACIP [Mast, 2005]; CDC/ACIP [Mast, 2006]).
Dosing: Neonatal Although hepatitis B vaccine products differ by concentration (mcg/mL), when dosed in terms of volume (mL), the equivalent dose is the same between products (ie, 0.5 mL of Recombivax-HB is equivalent to 0.5 mL of Engerix-B). Combination vaccines (eg, also containing DTaP, HIB) should not be used for the "birth" dose but may be used to complete the immunization series after the infant is 6 weeks of age.
Primary immunization: Recombivax-HB, Engerix-B (Pediatric/Adolescent formulation): I.M.: 0.5 mL per dose for a total of 3 doses; the second and third dose should be given 1 and 6 months after the first dose; ideally first dose given at birth
CDC (ACIP) Recommendations:
*Neonates born to HBₛAg-**positive** mothers:* Administer first dose within the first 12 hours of life, even if premature and regardless of birth weight (hepatitis immune globulin should also be administered at the same time/different site); **Note:** Due to possible decreased immunogenicity, premature neonates <2 kg should receive 4 total doses at 0, 1, 2 to 3, and 6 to 7 months of chronological age.
*Neonates born to HBₛAg-**negative** mothers:* First dose should be given at hospital discharge, or at 1 to 2 months of age; **Note:** Premature neonates <2 kg may have the initial dose deferred up to 30 days of chronological age or at hospital discharge.
Neonates born to mothers with unknown HBₛAg status at birth: Administer first dose within 12 hours of birth even if premature and regardless of birth weight, second dose following 1 to 2 months later; if HBₛAg test is positive, the neonate should receive hepatitis immune globulin as soon as possible (no later than 12 hours of age if <2 kg or age 1 week if ≥2 kg). **Note:** Due to possible decreased immunogenicity, premature neonates <2 kg, who received an initial dose within 12 hours of birth, should receive 4 total doses at 0, 1, 2 to 3, and 6 to 7 months of chronological age.
Manufacturer's labeling: Neonates with recent exposure to the virus or certain travelers to high-risk areas: Engerix-B: 0.5 mL per dose for 4 doses given at 0, 1, 2, and 12 months
Dosing: Usual Although hepatitis B vaccine products differ by concentration (mcg/mL), when dosed in terms of volume (mL), the equivalent dose is the same between products (ie, 0.5 mL of Recombivax-HB is equivalent to 0.5 mL of Engerix-B). Combination vaccines may be used to complete the immunization series after the infant is 6 weeks of age. Please see combination vaccine monographs for dose and schedule details. Vaccines from different manufacturers are interchangeable during an immunization series with the exception of an adolescent (11 to 15 years) 2-dose Recombivax-HB regimen (CDC/ACIP [Mast, 2005]).

Pediatric:

Primary immunization:

CDC (ACIP) recommendations:

Infants: Recombivax-HB, Engerix-B (Pediatric/Adolescent formulation): I.M.: 0.5 mL per dose for a total of 3 doses given as follows: Ideally first dose is given at birth, the second dose is given at 1 to 2 months of age, and a final third dose at 6 months up to 18 months; minimum age for the final (third) dose is 24 weeks

Note: For infants born to HB$_s$Ag-**positive** mothers, anti-HB$_s$ and HB$_s$Ag levels should be checked at 9 to 18 months of age (ie, next well child visit after series completion). If anti-HB$_s$ and HB$_s$Ag are negative, reimmunize with 3 doses 2 months apart and reassess. Due to possible decreased immunogenicity, former premature neonates <2 kg should receive 4 total doses at 0, 1, 2 to 3, and 6 to 7 months of chronological age.

*Infants born of HB$_s$Ag-**positive** mothers:* First dose should be given within the first 12 hours of life, even if premature and regardless of birth weight (hepatitis immune globulin should also be administered at the same time/different site); the second dose is administered at 1 to 2 months of age and the third dose at 6 to 18 months of age; anti-HB$_s$ and HB$_s$Ag levels should be checked at 9 to 18 months of age (ie, next well child visit after series completion). If anti-HB$_s$ and HB$_s$Ag are negative, reimmunize with 3 doses 2 months apart and reassess. **Note:** Due to possible decreased immunogenicity, premature neonates <2 kg should receive 4 total doses at 0, 1, 2 to 3, and 6 to 7 months of chronological age.

*Infants born of HB$_s$Ag-**negative** mothers:* First dose should be given at hospital discharge, or at 1 to 2 months of age; another dose is given 1 to 2 months later and a final dose at 6 to 18 months of age; 4 total doses of vaccine may be given if a "birth dose" is administered and a combination vaccine is used to complete the series. If "birth dose" not received, then full-term neonates should begin vaccine series as soon as feasible. **Note:** Premature neonates <2 kg may have the initial dose deferred up to 30 days of chronological age or at hospital discharge.

Infants born of mothers whose HB$_s$Ag status is unknown at birth: First dose given within 12 hours of birth even if premature and regardless of birth weight, second dose following 1 to 2 months later; the third dose at 6 to 18 months of age; if the mother's blood HB$_s$Ag test is positive, the infant should receive hepatitis immune globulin as soon as possible (no later than 12 hours of age if <2 kg or age 1 week if ≥2 kg). **Note:** Due to possible decreased immunogenicity, premature neonates <2 kg who received an initial dose within 12 hours of birth, should receive 4 total doses at 0, 1, 2 to 3, and 6 to 7 months of chronological age.

Catch-up immunization:

CDC (ACIP) recommendations (CDC/ACIP [Akinsanya-Beysolow, 2014]): **Note:** Do not restart the series. If doses have been given, begin the below schedule at the applicable dose number.

Children ≥19 months and Adolescents: Recombivax-HB, Engerix-B (Pediatric/Adolescent formulation): I.M.: 0.5 mL per dose for 3 total doses

First dose given on the elected date

Second dose given at least 4 weeks after the first dose

Third dose given at least 8 weeks after the second dose and at least 16 weeks after the first dose; minimum age for the final (third) dose is 24 weeks

Alternate regimen: Adolescents 11 to 15 years: Recombivax HB (Adult formulation): I.M.: 1 mL per dose for 2 doses; first dose given on the elected date, second dose given 4 to 6 months later if patient still ≤15 years

Bombings or similar mass casualty events: I.M.: In persons without a reliable history of vaccination against hepatitis B and who have no known contraindications to the vaccine, vaccination should begin within 24 hours (but no later than 7 days) following the event (CDC [Chapman, 2008])

Adult:

Primary immunization: I.M.: 1 mL per dose (adult formulation) for 3 total doses administered at 0, 1, and 6 months

Note: Adult formulations of hepatitis B vaccine products differ by concentration (mcg/mL), but when dosed in terms of volume (mL), the dose of Engerix-B and Recombivax HB are the same (both 1 mL).

Alternate dosing schedules (selection of schedule should optimize compliance with vaccination): All regimens use the adult formulation administered as one dose at the following intervals (three schedules presented):

0, 1, and 4 months (CDC/ACIP [Mast, 2006])

0, 2, and 4 months (CDC/ACIP [Mast, 2006])

0, 12, and 24 months (CDC/ACIP [Mast, 2006])

Bombings or similar mass casualty events: I.M.: In persons without a reliable history of vaccination against HepB and who have no known contraindications to the vaccine, vaccination should begin within 24 hours (but no later than 7 days) following the event (CDC [Chapman, 2008]).

Postexposure management of health care personnel (HCP) (CDC [Schillie, 2013]): I.M.:

Documented vaccine responder: If the HCP has prior documentation of ≥3 doses of a hepatitis B vaccine and a postvaccination anti-HBs ≥10 mIU/mL, then additional hepatitis B vaccine is not needed, regardless of the patient's HB$_s$Ag status. HCP is considered seroprotected.

Unvaccinated or incompletely vaccinated: The primary vaccination series should be completed regardless of the source patient's Hb$_s$Ag status. If the source patient is HB$_s$AG positive or their status is unknown, 1 dose of hepatitis B vaccine and 1 dose of hepatitis B immunoglobulin (HBIG) should be administered as soon as possible.

Vaccinated with 3 doses of hepatitis B vaccine but postvaccination anti-HBs status is unknown: Test HCP for anti-HBs. If anti-HBs ≥10 mIU/mL, additional hepatitis B vaccine is not needed. If anti-HBs <10 mIU/mL, initiate revaccination by administering a single dose of the vaccine and retesting for anti-HBs in 1 to 2 months; if needed, 2 additional doses may be given and then retest anti-HBs level. Alternately, administer 3 consecutive doses of the vaccine and then retest anti-HBs level. Minimum dosing intervals are 4 weeks between doses 1 and 2 and 8 weeks between doses 2 and 3; maximum total of 6 doses of hepatitis B vaccine (including the original series). If the source patient is HB$_s$AG positive or their status is unknown, 1 dose of HBIG should also be administered.

Vaccinated with 6 doses of hepatitis B vaccine but documented as a nonresponder to the vaccine: No postexposure vaccination is recommended. If the source patient is HB$_s$AG positive or unknown, administer two doses of HBIG separated by 1 month.

Dosing adjustment in renal impairment: Hemodialysis patients often respond poorly to hepatitis B vaccination; higher vaccine doses or increased number of doses may be required. The anti-HBs (antibody to hepatitis B surface antigen) response of such persons should be tested after they are vaccinated, and those who have not responded should be revaccinated with 1 to 3 additional doses. Patients with chronic renal disease should be vaccinated as early as possible, ideally before they require hemodialysis.

Chronic renal impairment: Administer dose at 0, 1 to 2, and 4 to 6 months; repeat dose depending upon annual assessment of hepatitis B surface antigen (anti-HB) level; if anti-HB <10 milli-international units/mL administer an additional dose (CDC/ACIP [Mast, 2005])

<20 years: Dialysis and nondialysis patients; limited data available: I.M.: 20 **mcg**/dose; no specific ACIP recommendations; dosing based on a multicenter trial of 78 pediatric patients (age: 1 to 18 years) using Recombivax-HB (Dialysis formulation) and showed protective levels of antibody occurring in 75% to 97% of pediatric hemodialysis patients using higher dose (CDC/ACIP [Mast, 2005]; Watkins, 2002)

≥20 years:

Nondialysis patients: 10 **mcg**/dose (Recombivax-HB); 20 **mcg**/dose (Engerix-B)

Dialysis patients: 40 **mcg**/dose [Recombivax-HB (Dialysis formulation) or Engerix-B (Adult formulation)]

Dosing adjustment in hepatic impairment: There are no dosage adjustments provided in the manufacturer's labeling.

Administration Shake well; administer I.M. into midlateral aspect of the thigh in infants and small children; administer in the deltoid area to older children and adults; **Not for I.V. or SubQ administration.** Adolescents and adults should be vaccinated while seated or lying down. U.S. law requires that the date of administration; the vaccine manufacturer; lot number of vaccine; and the administering person's name, title, and address be entered into the patient's permanent medical record.

Monitoring Parameters HB$_s$Ag and antibodies to HB$_s$Ag (anti-HB$_s$) should be tested in infants born to mothers positive for HB$_s$Ag when they are 9 to 18 months of age; annual anti-HB in dialysis patients. Vaccination at the time of HBsAg testing: For persons in whom vaccination is recommended, the first dose of hepatitis B vaccine can be given after blood is drawn to test for HB$_s$Ag. Observe for syncope for 15 minutes following administration. If seizure-like activity associated with syncope occurs, maintain patient in supine or Trendelenburg position to reestablish adequate cerebral perfusion.

Additional Information With use of hepatitis B vaccine, hepatitis D should also be prevented since delta virus replicates only in presence of HBV infection.

In order to maximize vaccination rates, the ACIP recommends simultaneous administration (ie, >1 vaccine on the same day at different anatomic sites) of all age-appropriate vaccines (live or inactivated) for which a person is eligible at a single visit, unless contraindications exist. If available, the use of combination vaccines is generally preferred over separate injections, taking into consideration provider assessment, patient preference, and potential adverse events. If separate vaccines being used, evaluate product information regarding same syringe compatibility of vaccines. Separate needles and syringes should be used for each injection. The ACIP prefers each dose of specific vaccine in a series come from the same manufacturer if possible (CDC/ACIP [Kroger, 2011]).

For additional information, please refer to the following website: http://www.cdc.gov/vaccines/vpd-vac/.

Dosage Forms Excipient information presented when available (limited, particularly for generics); consult specific product labeling. [DSC] = Discontinued product

Injection, suspension [adult, preservative free]:

Engerix-B: Hepatitis B surface antigen 20 mcg/mL (1 mL) [contains aluminum, yeast protein, may contain natural rubber/natural latex in prefilled syringe]

Engerix-B: Hepatitis B surface antigen 20 mcg/mL (1 mL) [contains aluminum, yeast protein; vial]

Recombivax HB: Hepatitis B surface antigen 10 mcg/mL (1 mL) [contains aluminum, natural rubber/natural latex in packaging, yeast protein]

Injection, suspension [dialysis formulation, preservative free]:

Recombivax HB: Hepatitis B surface antigen 40 mcg/mL (1 mL) [contains aluminum, natural rubber/natural latex in packaging, yeast protein]

Injection, suspension [pediatric/adolescent, preservative free]:

Engerix-B: Hepatitis B surface antigen 10 mcg/0.5 mL (0.5 mL) [contains aluminum, yeast protein, may contain natural rubber/natural latex in prefilled syringe]

Recombivax HB: Hepatitis B surface antigen 5 mcg/0.5 mL (0.5 mL) [contains aluminum, natural rubber/natural latex in packaging, yeast protein]

References

AAP Steering Committee on Quality Improvement and Management, Subcommittee on Febrile Seizures American Academy of Pediatrics. Febrile seizures: clinical practice guideline for the long-term management of the child with simple febrile seizures. *Pediatrics.* 2008;121 (6):1281-1286.

Akinsanya-Beysolow I; Advisory Committee on Immunization Practices (ACIP); ACIP Child/Adolescent Immunization Work Group; Centers for Disease Control and Prevention (CDC). Advisory Committee on Immunization Practices recommended immunization schedules for persons aged 0 through 18 years – United States, 2014. *MMWR Morb Mortal Wkly Rep.* 2014;63(5):108-109. Available at http://www.cdc.gov/vaccines/schedules/downloads/child/0-18yrs-child-combined-schedule.pdf

Bridges CB, Coyne-Beasley T; Advisory Committee on Immunization Practices (ACIP); ACIP Adult Immunization Work Group; Centers for Disease Control and Prevention (CDC). Advisory Committee on Immunization Practices recommended immunization schedule for adults aged 19 years or older – United States, 2014. *MMWR Morb Mortal Wkly Rep.* 2014;63(5):110-112. Available at http://www.cdc.gov/vaccines/schedules/downloads/adult/adult-combined-schedule.pdf

Centers for Disease Control and Prevention (CDC). Guidelines for vaccinating kidney dialysis patients and patients with chronic kidney disease, summarized from recommendations of the Advisory Committee on Immunization Practices (ACIP). Available at http://www.cdc.gov/vaccines/pubs/downloads/dialysis-guide-2012.pdf

Centers for Disease Control and Prevention (CDC). Syncope after vaccination – United States, January 2005-July 2007. *MMWR Morb Mortal Wkly Rep.* 2008;57(17):457-460.

Centers for Disease Control and Prevention (CDC). Use of hepatitis B vaccination for adults with diabetes mellitus: recommendations of the Advisory Committee on Immunization Practices (ACIP). *MMWR Morb Mortal Wkly Rep.* 2011;60(50):1709-1711.

Chapman LE, Sullivent EE, Grohskopf LA, et al. Recommendations for postexposure interventions to prevent infection with hepatitis B virus, hepatitis C virus, or human immunodeficiency virus, and tetanus in persons wounded during bombings and other mass-casualty events – United States, 2008: recommendations of the Centers for Disease Control and Prevention (CDC). *MMWR Recomm Rep.* 2008;57(RR-6):1-21.

Cohen V, Jellinek SP, Teperikidis L, Berkovits E, Goldman WM. Room-temperature storage of medications labeled for refrigeration. *Am J Health-Syst Pharm.* 2007;64(16):1711-1715.

Kroger AT, Atkinson WL, Marcuse EK, Pickering LK. General recommendations on immunization - recommendations of the Advisory Committee on Immunization Practices (ACIP). *MMWR Recomm Rep.* 2011;60(RR-2):1-64.

Mast EE, Margolis HS, Fiore AE, et al. A comprehensive immunization strategy to eliminate transmission of hepatitis B virus infection in the United States: recommendations of the Advisory Committee on Immunization Practices (ACIP) part 1: immunization of infants, children, and adolescents. *MMWR Recomm Rep.* 2005;54(RR-16):1-31.

Mast EE, Weinbaum CM, Fiore AE, et al. A comprehensive immunization strategy to eliminate transmission of hepatitis B virus infection in the United States: recommendations of the Advisory Committee on Immunization Practices (ACIP) part II: immunization of adults. *MMWR Recomm Rep.* 2006;55(RR-16):1-25.

Prymula R, Siegrist CA, Chlibek R, et al. Effect of prophylactic paracetamol administration at time of vaccination on febrile reactions and antibody responses in children: two open-label, randomised controlled trials. *Lancet.* 2009;374(9698):1339-1350.

Rubin LG, Levin MJ, Ljungman P, et al. 2013 IDSA clinical practice guideline for vaccination of the immunocompromised host. *Clin Infect Dis.* 2014;58(3):e44-e100.

Saari TN, American Academy of Pediatrics Committee on Infectious Diseases. Immunization of preterm and low birth weight infants. American Academy of Pediatrics Committee on Infectious Diseases. *Pediatrics.* 2003;112(1 Pt 1):193-198.

Schillie S, Murphy TV, Sawyer M, et al. CDC guidance for evaluating health-care personnel for hepatitis B virus protection and for administering postexposure management. *MMWR Recomm Rep.* 2013;62 (RR-10):1-19.

Watkins SL, Alexander SR, Brewer ED, et al. Response to recombinant hepatitis B vaccine in children and adolescents with chronic renal failure. *Am J Kidney Dis.* 2002;40(2):365-372.

◆ **Hepatitis B Vaccine (Recombinant)** *see Haemophilus* b Conjugate and Hepatitis B Vaccine *on page 993*

◆ **HepB** *see* Hepatitis B Vaccine (Recombinant) *on page 1009*

◆ **Hep Flush-10** *see* Heparin *on page 1001*

◆ **Hepsera** *see* Adefovir *on page 75*

◆ **Heptovir (Can)** *see* LamiVUDine *on page 1194*

◆ **HES** *see* Hetastarch *on page 1014*

◆ **HES** *see* Tetrastarch *on page 1998*

◆ **HES 130/0.4** *see* Tetrastarch *on page 1998*

◆ **HES 450/0.7** *see* Hetastarch *on page 1014*

◆ **Hespan** *see* Hetastarch *on page 1014*

Hetastarch (HET a starch)

Medication Safety Issues
Sound-alike/look-alike issues:
Hespan may be confused with heparin
Brand Names: U.S. Hespan; Hextend
Brand Names: Canada Hextend
Therapeutic Category Plasma Volume Expander
Generic Availability (U.S.) Yes
Use Treatment of hypovolemia (Hespan® and Hextend®: FDA approved in adults); adjunctive use during leukapheresis to improve granulocyte harvesting and increase the yield of granulocytes by centrifugation (Hespan®: FDA approved in adults); **Note:** This is not a substitute for blood or plasma; does not have oxygen-carrying capacity.
Pregnancy Risk Factor C
Pregnancy Considerations Adverse events have been observed in some animal reproduction studies.
Breast-Feeding Considerations It is not known if hetastarch is excreted into breast milk. The manufacturer recommends that caution be exercised when administering hetastarch to nursing women.
Contraindications Hypersensitivity to hetastarch or any component; preexisting coagulation or bleeding disorders, renal failure with oliguria or anuria (not related to hypovolemia); and fluid overload condition (eg, congestive heart failure, pulmonary edema). Hextend® is also contraindicated in the treatment of lactic acidosis and in leukapheresis.
Warnings Anaphylaxis/anaphylactoid reactions have occurred and resulted in death (rare); however, a causal relationship has not been established; discontinue use with signs of hypersensitivity and administer appropriate therapy; hypersensitivity reactions may occur even after hetastarch has been discontinued. Infusion of large volumes of hetastarch or use over an extended period of time (days) may result in transient alterations of blood coagulation by hemodilution (decreased Hct and plasma protein values) and a direct inhibitory action on Factor VIII which can result in reversible von Willebrand's-like syndrome and/or a Factor VIII deficiency. Avoid administration of volumes >25% of total blood volume or >20 mL/kg in less than

24 hours and extended use. Consider replacement blood products if clinically indicated; if coagulopathy develops, it may take several days to resolve. In patients undergoing open heart surgery, increased bleeding has been reported; avoid use as cardiac bypass prime while patient is on bypass or in the immediate period following bypass discontinuation; bleeding risk decreases within hours. If used in other patient populations, discontinue use of HES at the first sign of coagulopathy. Avoid use in patients with subarachnoid hemorrhage; significant clinical bleeding and death have been reported with extended use of hetastarch over a period of days.

Administration may cause fluid overload; use with caution in patients at risk from overexpansion of blood volume, including the very young or aged patients and those at risk for developing CHF or pulmonary edema; use is contraindicated in heart failure or any preexisting condition in which volume overload is a potential concern. Monitor fluid status and rate of infusion periodically with use; in cases of severe dehydration, crystalloid should be administered first.

Avoid use in critically ill adult patients, including those with sepsis and those admitted to the ICU. HES solutions have been associated with an increased risk of mortality in the critically ill (Brunkhorst, 2008; Perel, 2012; Perner, 2012; Zarychanski, 2009) **[U.S. Boxed Warning (per the FDA; labeling updates pending)]**. The Society of Critical Care Medicine (SCCM) also recommends against the use of HES solutions for fluid resuscitation of severe sepsis and septic shock; crystalloids (eg, sodium chloride) are recommended instead (Dellinger, 2013). HES solutions have been associated with renal injury requiring renal replacement therapy in critically ill patients (Reinhart, 2012) **[U.S. Boxed Warning (per the FDA; labeling updates pending)]**. If used in patients who are not critically ill, avoid use in patients with preexisting renal dysfunction and discontinue use at the first sign of renal injury. Since the need for renal replacement therapy has been reported up to 90 days after HES administration, continue to monitor renal function in all patients for at least 90 days. HES use has also been associated with acute kidney injury in pediatric patients (Reinhart, 2012).

Precautions Use with caution in patients allergic to corn; may have cross allergy to hetastarch. Use with caution in patients with renal impairment; fluid status including urine output should be monitored closely; use is contraindicated with oliguria or anuria unrelated to hypovolemia. In presence of renal glomerular damage, hetastarch may leak into urine and increase specific gravity. Hextend® contains calcium, lactate, and potassium; use with caution in situations in which electrolyte and/or acid-base disturbances may be exacerbated (renal impairment, respiratory alkalosis). Use caution with hepatic impairment; transient elevations of indirect bilirubin have been reported; may also result in further reduction of coagulation factors and increase risk of bleeding. Use with caution in patients previously or concurrently receiving other anticoagulant drugs. May temporarily increase serum amylase concentrations (not associated with pancreatitis); elevation persists longer in patients with decreased renal function.

Adverse Reactions

Cardiovascular: Bradycardia, cardiac failure, circulatory overload, increased plasma volume, peripheral edema, tachycardia

Central nervous system: Chills, headache, intracranial hemorrhage

Dermatologic: Pruritus (dose dependent; may be delayed), skin rash

Endocrine & metabolic: Increased amylase (transient), metabolic acidosis

Gastrointestinal: Parotid gland enlargement, vomiting

Hematologic & oncologic: Anemia, blood coagulation disorder (Factor VIII deficiency, acquired von Willebrand's like syndrome, dilutional coagulopathy), disseminated intravascular coagulopathy (rare), hemolysis (rare), hemorrhage, prolonged bleeding time, prolonged partial thromboplastin time, prolonged prothrombin time, thrombocytopenia, wound hemorrhage

Hepatic: Increased serum bilirubin (indirect)

Hypersensitivity: Anaphylactoid reaction, hypersensitivity

Neuromuscular & skeletal: Myalgia

Respiratory: Bronchospasm, flu-like symptoms (mild), noncardiogenic pulmonary edema

Miscellaneous: Fever

Rare but important or life-threatening: Angioedema, cough, erythema multiforme, facial edema, hypotension, laryngeal edema, periorbital edema, renal insufficiency, severe hypotension, stridor, submaxillary gland enlargement, tachypnea, urticaria, ventricular fibrillation

Drug Interactions

Metabolism/Transport Effects None known.

Avoid Concomitant Use There are no known interactions where it is recommended to avoid concomitant use.

Increased Effect/Toxicity There are no known significant interactions involving an increase in effect.

Decreased Effect There are no known significant interactions involving a decrease in effect.

Stability Store at room temperature of 25°C (77°F); brief exposure up to 40°C (104°F) does not adversely affect product. Do not freeze; do not use if crystalline precipitate forms or is turbid deep brown. In leukapheresis, admixtures of 500-560 mL of Hespan® with citrate concentrations up to 2.5% are compatible for 24 hours.

Mechanism of Action Produces plasma volume expansion by virtue of its highly colloidal starch structure

Pharmacodynamics

Onset of volume expansion: I.V.: Within 30 minutes

Duration: 24-36 hours

Pharmacokinetics (Adult data unless noted)

Metabolism: Molecules >50,000 daltons require enzymatic degradation by the reticuloendothelial system or amylases in the blood prior to urinary and fecal excretion

Elimination: Smaller molecular weight molecules are readily excreted in urine; ~33% of dose excreted in first 24 hours in patients with normal renal function

Dosing: Usual Note: With severe dehydration, administer crystalloid first. Dose and rate of infusion dependent on amount of blood lost, on maintenance or restoration of hemodynamics, and on amount of hemodilution. Titrate to individual colloid needs, hemodynamics, and hydration status. Do not use in critically ill patients, those undergoing open heart surgery with cardiopulmonary bypass, or those with preexisting renal dysfunction.

Children and Adolescents: **Volume expansion:** I.V. infusion: Very limited data available: Children ≥1 year and Adolescents: 10 mL/kg/dose; dosing based on a small randomized, double-blinded study of 38 patients (age range: 1-15.5 years) compared hetastarch (n=20) and albumin (n=18) as a postoperative volume expander in the first 24 hours after congenital heart surgery; no differences in safety compared to albumin were found at hetastarch daily doses ≤20 mL/kg/day; patients receiving doses of 20-30 mL/kg/day were noted to have an increased PT; however, there was no difference in clinical bleeding; doses >30 mL/kg have not been studied (Brutacao, 1996).

Adults:

Plasma volume expansion: I.V. infusion: 500-1000 mL (up to 1500 mL/day) or 20 mL/kg/day (up to 1500 mL/day)

Leukapheresis (Hespan®): I.V. infusion: 250-700 mL; **Note:** Citrate anticoagulant is added before use.

Dosing adjustment in renal impairment: Adults: Avoid use in patients with preexisting renal dysfunction. Use is contraindicated in renal failure with oliguria or anuria (not related to hypovolemia). Discontinue use at the first sign of renal injury.

Dosing adjustment in hepatic impairment: Adults: No dosage adjustment provided in manufacturer's labeling; use with caution.

Administration Parenteral: I.V.: Administer I.V. only; may be administered via infusion pump or pressure infusion; if administered by pressure infusion, air should be withdrawn or expelled from bag prior to infusion to prevent air embolus. Administration rates vary depending upon the extent of blood loss, age, and clinical condition of patient but, in general, should not exceed 1.2 **g**/kg/**hour** (20 mL/kg/**hour**) in adults. Change I.V. tubing or flush copiously with normal saline before administering blood through the same line. Do not administer Hextend® with blood through the same administration set. Change I.V. tubing at least every 24 hours. Anaphylactoid reactions can occur; have epinephrine and resuscitative equipment available.

Monitoring Parameters

Volume expansion: Blood pressure, capillary refill time, CVP, RAP, MAP, urine output, heart rate, if pulmonary artery catheter in place, monitor cardiac index, PWCP, SVR, and PVR; hemoglobin, hematocrit, serum electrolytes, renal function (continue to monitor for at least 90 days after administration), acid-base balance, coagulation parameters, platelets

Leukapheresis, CBC, total leukocyte and platelet counts, leukocyte differential count, hemoglobin, hematocrit, prothrombin time, and partial thromboplastin time

Test Interactions

Serum amylase levels may be temporarily elevated following administration; could interfere with the diagnosis of pancreatitis.

Large hetastarch volumes may result in decreased coagulation factors, plasma proteins, and /or hematocrit due to dilutional effect.

Additional Information Hetastarch is a synthetic polymer derived from a waxy starch composed of amylopectin, average molecular weight of Hespan® is 600,000 kDa (range: 450,000-800,000 kDa), average molecular weight of Hextend® is 670,000 kDa (range: 450,000-800,000 kDa); each liter of Hespan® provides 154 mEq sodium chloride; each liter of Hextend® contains the following electrolytes: Sodium 143 mEq, chloride 124 mEq, lactate 28 mEq, calcium 5 mEq, magnesium 0.9 mEq, potassium 3 mEq, and dextrose 0.99 g

Dosage Forms Excipient information presented when available (limited, particularly for generics); consult specific product labeling.

Solution, Intravenous:

Hespan: 6% (500 mL)

Hextend: 6% (500 mL)

Generic: 6% (500 mL)

References

Brutocao D, Bratton SL, Thomas JR, et al, "Comparison of Hetastarch With Albumin for Postoperative Volume Expansion in Children After Cardiopulmonary Bypass," *J Cardiothoracic Vasc Anesth*, 1996, 10 (3):348-51.

Brunkhorst FM, Engel C, Bloos F, et al, "Intensive Insulin Therapy and Pentastarch Resuscitation in Severe Sepsis," *N Engl J Med*, 2008, 358(2):125-39.

Dellinger RP, Levy MM, Rhodes A, et al, "Surviving Sepsis Campaign: International Guidelines for Management of Severe Sepsis and Septic Shock: 2012," *Crit Care Med*, 2013, 41(2):580-637.

Perel P and Roberts I, "Colloids Versus Crystalloids for Fluid Resuscitation in Critically Ill Patients," *Cochrane Database Syst Rev*, 2012, 6: CD000567.

Perner A, Haase N, Guttormsen AB, et al, "Hydroxyethyl Starch 130/0.4 Versus Ringer's Acetate in Severe Sepsis," *N Engl J Med*, 2012, 367 (2):124-34; published erratum appears in *N Engl J Med*, 2012, 367 (5):481.

Reinhart K, Perner A, Sprung CL, et al, "Consensus Statement of the ESICM Task Force on Colloid Volume Therapy in Critically Ill Patients," *Intensive Care Med*, 2012, 38(3):368-83.

Zarychanski R, Turgeon AF, Fergusson DA, et al, "Renal Outcomes and Mortality Following Hydroxyethyl Starch Resuscitation of Critically Ill Patients: Systematic Review and Meta-Analysis of Randomized Trials" **ATTENTION:** The analysis and conclusions of this article are being revised by the authors. This is due to the journal Anesthesia and Analgesia's retraction of a paper by Dr. Joachim Boldt, an author in seven of the studies analyzed in this review. As such, the editors of Open Medicine recommend interpreting this review with extreme caution until Zarychanski et al. publish a new analysis and interpretation in Open Medicine. For more information, see Anesthesia and Analgesia's press release. Open Med, 2009, 3(4):e196-209.

◆ **Hexachlorocyclohexane** *see* Lindane *on page 1250*

Hexachlorophene (heks a KLOR oh feen)

Medication Safety Issues
Sound-alike/look-alike issues:
pHisoHex® may be confused with Fostex®, pHisoDerm®

Related Information
Safe Handling of Hazardous Drugs *on page 2419*

Brand Names: U.S. Phisohex [DSC]

Brand Names: Canada pHisoHex®

Therapeutic Category Antibacterial, Topical; Soap

Generic Availability (U.S.) No

Use Surgical scrub and as a bacteriostatic skin cleanser; to control an outbreak of gram-positive staphylococcal infection when other infection control procedures have been unsuccessful

Pregnancy Risk Factor C

Pregnancy Considerations Adverse events have been observed in animal reproduction studies. Hexachlorophene is absorbed systemically when applied topically. Following use as an antiseptic for vaginal exams during labor, hexachlorophene is detectable in the maternal serum and cord blood (Strickland, 1983). Vaginal use as a pack or tampon and application to mucous membranes is contraindicated.

Breast-Feeding Considerations It is not known if hexachlorophene is excreted in breast milk. Due to the potential for serious adverse reactions in the nursing infant, a decision should be made whether to discontinue nursing or to discontinue the drug, taking into account the importance of treatment to the mother.

Contraindications Hypersensitivity to halogenated phenol derivatives or hexachlorophene; use in premature infants; use on burned or denuded skin; use with an occlusive dressing; application to mucous membranes

Warnings Hazardous agent; use appropriate precautions for handling and disposal. Do not use for bathing infants; do not apply to mucous membranes; premature and low birth weight infants are particularly susceptible to hexachlorophene topical absorption; irritability, generalized clonic muscular contractions, decerebrate rigidity, and brain lesions in the white matter have occurred in infants following topical use of 6% hexachlorophene; exposure of preterm infants or patients with extensive burns has been associated with apnea, convulsions, agitation, and coma

Adverse Reactions
Central nervous system: CNS injury, irritability, seizure

Dermatologic: Dermatitis, dry skin, photosensitivity, redness

Drug Interactions
Metabolism/Transport Effects None known.

Avoid Concomitant Use
Avoid concomitant use of Hexachlorophene with any of the following: BCG

Increased Effect/Toxicity There are no known significant interactions involving an increase in effect.

Decreased Effect
Hexachlorophene may decrease the levels/effects of: BCG; Sodium Picosulfate

Stability Store in nonmetallic container (incompatible with many metals); protect from light

Mechanism of Action Bacteriostatic polychlorinated biphenyl which inhibits membrane-bound enzymes and disrupts the cell membrane

Pharmacokinetics (Adult data unless noted)
Absorption: Percutaneously through inflamed, excoriated and intact skin

Distribution: Crosses the placenta

Half-life, infants: 6.1-44.2 hours

Dosing: Usual Children and Adults: Topical: Apply 5 mL cleanser and water to area to be cleansed; lather and rinse thoroughly under running water; for use as a surgical scrub, a second application of 5 mL cleanser should be made and the hands and forearms scrubbed for an additional 3 minutes, rinsed thoroughly with running water and dried

Administration Topical: For external use only; rinse thoroughly after each use

Dosage Forms Excipient information presented when available (limited, particularly for generics); consult specific product labeling. [DSC] = Discontinued product
Liquid, External:
Phisohex: 3% (148 mL [DSC], 473 mL [DSC])

References
Lester RS, "Topical Formulary for the Pediatrician," *Pediatr Clin North Am*, 1983, 30(4):749-65.

Strickland DM, Leonard RG, Stavchansky S, et al, "Vaginal Absorption of Hexachlorophene During Labor," *Am J Obstet Gynecol*, 1983, 147 (7):769-72.

◆ **Hexamethylenetetramine** *see* Methenamine *on page 1361*

◆ **Hextend** *see* Hetastarch *on page 1014*

◆ **hGH** *see* Somatropin *on page 1920*

◆ **Hib** *see* Haemophilus b Conjugate Vaccine *on page 994*

◆ **Hib Conjugate Vaccine** *see* Haemophilus b Conjugate and Hepatitis B Vaccine *on page 993*

◆ **Hiberix** *see* Haemophilus b Conjugate Vaccine *on page 994*

◆ **Hib-HepB** *see* Haemophilus b Conjugate and Hepatitis B Vaccine *on page 993*

◆ **Hibiclens [OTC]** *see* Chlorhexidine Gluconate *on page 441*

◆ **Hibidil 1:2000 (Can)** *see* Chlorhexidine Gluconate *on page 441*

◆ **Hibistat [OTC]** *see* Chlorhexidine Gluconate *on page 441*

◆ **Hib-MenCY-TT** *see* Meningococcal Polysaccharide (Groups C and Y) and Haemophilus b Tetanus Toxoid Conjugate Vaccine *on page 1334*

◆ **High-Molecular-Weight Iron Dextran (DexFerrum)** *see* Iron Dextran Complex *on page 1153*

◆ **Hiprex** *see* Methenamine *on page 1361*

◆ **Hiprex® (Can)** *see* Methenamine *on page 1361*

◆ **Histantil (Can)** *see* Promethazine *on page 1748*

Histrelin (his TREL in)

Related Information
Safe Handling of Hazardous Drugs *on page 2419*

Brand Names: U.S. Supprelin LA; Vantas

Brand Names: Canada Vantas

Therapeutic Category Gonadotropin Releasing Hormone Agonist

Generic Availability (U.S.) No

Use

Supprelin® LA: Treatment of children with either neurogenic or idiopathic central precocious puberty (CPP) (FDA approved in ages ≥2 years)

Vantas®: Palliative treatment of advanced prostate cancer (FDA approved in adults)

Pregnancy Risk Factor X

Pregnancy Considerations Adverse events were observed in animal reproduction studies. May cause fetal harm or spontaneous abortion if administered during pregnancy. Histrelin is contraindicated for use during pregnancy or in women who may become pregnant.

Breast-Feeding Considerations It is not known if histrelin is excreted in breast milk. The products are not indicated for use in postpubertal women.

Contraindications Hypersensitivity to histrelin acetate, GnRH, GnRH-agonist analogs, or any component; females who are or may become pregnant

Warnings Hazardous agent; use appropriate precautions for handling and disposal (NIOSH, 2012).

When used for treatment of central precious puberty, initial agonistic action of histrelin may cause transient increases in estradiol serum levels (female) or testosterone levels (female and male); typically during first week of therapy; worsening of symptoms or onset of new symptoms may occur during this time; however, manifestations of puberty should decrease within 4 weeks. Rare cases of pituitary apoplexy have been observed, frequently secondary to pituitary adenoma; reported onset from 1 hour to usually <2 weeks; may present as sudden headache, vomiting, visual or mental status changes, and infrequently cardiovascular collapse; immediate medical attention required if occurs.

Transient increases in serum testosterone (in men with prostate cancer) occur during the first week of use and may result in a worsening of disease signs and symptoms (bone pain, neuropathy, hematuria, ureteral/bladder outlet obstruction, spinal cord compression) during the first week of treatment; closely observe patients for urinary tract obstruction or poor urine output in first few weeks of therapy. Spinal cord compression has been reported and may contribute to paralysis when used for prostate cancer; closely observe patients with metastatic vertebral lesions for weakness and paresthesias in first few weeks of therapy. Hyperglycemia has been reported with androgen deprivation therapy (in prostate cancer) and may manifest as diabetes or worsening of preexisting diabetes. Monitor blood glucose and/or Hb A_{1c}.

Precautions Use with caution in patients with hepatic impairment; safety and efficacy have not been established in prostate cancer patients with hepatic dysfunction. Use with caution in patients with cardiovascular disease; androgen deprivation therapy may increase the risk for cardiovascular disease (Levine, 2010); an increased risk of MI, sudden cardiac death, and stroke has been reported with GnRH agonist use in men; monitor for symptoms associated with cardiovascular disease.

Proper surgical insertion technique is essential to avoid complications. Patients should keep arm dry for 24 hours and avoid heavy lifting/strenuous exertion of insertion arm for 7 days after implantation. In prostate cancer studies, the implant was not recovered in a small number of patients. Serum testosterone rose above castrate level and the implant was not palpable or visualized (via ultrasound); it was believed to have been extruded. Some patients had continued testosterone levels below castration level even though the implant was not palpable. If the implant breaks during removal in children with CPP, the remaining pieces should be removed; confirm the removal of the entire implant (refer to manufacturer's instructions for removal procedure).

Adverse Reactions

CPP:

Endocrine & metabolic: Metrorrhagia

Local: Insertion site reaction (includes bruising, discomfort, itching, pain, protrusion of implant area, soreness, swelling, tingling); keloid scar, pain at the application site, post procedural pain, scar, suture-related complication

Rare but important or life-threatening: Amblyopia, breast tenderness, cold feeling, disease progression, dysmenorrhea, epistaxis, erythema, flu-like syndrome, gynecomastia, headache, infection at the implant site, menorrhagia, migraine, mood swings, pituitary adenoma, pituitary apoplexy, pruritus, seizures, weight gain

Prostate cancer:

Central nervous system: Fatigue, headache, insomnia

Endocrine & metabolic: Gynecomastia, hot flashes, libido decreased, sexual dysfunction

Gastrointestinal: Constipation, weight gain

Genitourinary: Testicular atrophy

Local: Implant site reaction (includes bruising, erythema, pain, soreness, swelling, tenderness)

Renal: Renal impairment

Rare but important or life-threatening: Abdominal discomfort, alopecia, anemia, appetite increased, arthralgia, AST increased, back pain, bone density decreased, bone pain, breast pain, breast tenderness, cold feeling, contusion, craving food, creatinine increased, depression, diaphoresis, dizziness, dyspnea (exertional), dysuria, fluid retention, flushing, genital pruritus, hematoma, hematuria, hepatic injury (severe), hypercalcemia, hypercholesterolemia, hyperglycemia, irritability, LDH increased, lethargy, limb pain, liver disorder, malaise, muscle twitching, myalgia, nausea, neck pain, night sweats, pain, palpitation, peripheral edema, prostatic acid phosphatase increased, pruritus, pituitary apoplexy, renal calculi, renal failure, stent occlusion, testosterone increased, tremor, urinary frequency, urinary retention, ventricular asystoles, weakness, weight loss

Drug Interactions

Metabolism/Transport Effects None known.

Avoid Concomitant Use

Avoid concomitant use of Histrelin with any of the following: Indium 111 Capromab Pendetide

Increased Effect/Toxicity

Histrelin may increase the levels/effects of: Vitamin K Antagonists

Decreased Effect

Histrelin may decrease the levels/effects of: Antidiabetic Agents; Cardiac Glycosides; Indium 111 Capromab Pendetide; Vitamin K Antagonists

Stability Hazardous agent; use appropriate precautions for handling and disposal (NIOSH, 2012).

Supprelin® LA, Vantas®: Upon delivery, separate contents of implant carton. Store implant at 2°C to 8°C (36°F to 46°F); excursions permitted to 25°C (77°F) for 7 days; if unused within the 7 days, may return to proper refrigeration until product expiration date. Keep implant wrapped in the amber pouch for protection from light; do not freeze. The insertion kit does not require refrigeration.

Mechanism of Action Potent inhibitor of gonadotropin secretion; continuous administration results in, after an initiation phase, the suppression of luteinizing hormone (LH), follicle-stimulating hormone (FSH), and a subsequent decrease in testosterone and dihydrotestosterone (males) and estrone and estradiol (premenopausal females). Testosterone levels are reduced to castrate levels in males (treated for prostate cancer) within 2-4 weeks. Additionally, in patients with CPP, linear growth velocity is slowed (improves chance of attaining predicted adult height).

◄ **Pharmacodynamics**
Onset of action:
CPP: Within 1 month
Prostate cancer: Within 2-4 weeks
Duration: 1 year (plus a few additional weeks of histrelin release)

Pharmacokinetics (Adult data unless noted)
Distribution: V_d: ~58 L
Protein binding: 70% ± 9%
Metabolism: Hepatic via C-terminal dealkylation and hydrolysis
Bioavailability: 92%
Half-life elimination: Terminal: ~4 hours
Time to peak serum concentration: 12 hours

Dosing: Usual
Children ≥2 years: **Central precocious puberty:** SubQ: Supprelin LA: 50 mg implant surgically inserted every 12 months; discontinue at the appropriate time for the onset of puberty
Adults: **Prostate cancer, advanced:** SubQ: Vantas: 50 mg implant surgically inserted every 12 months
Dosage adjustment in renal impairment: Children ≥2 years and Adults:
Vantas: CrCl: ≥15 mL/minute: No dosage adjustment necessary.
Supprelin LA: There are no dosage adjustments provided in manufacturer's labeling.
Dosage adjustment in hepatic impairment: There are no dosage adjustments provided in manufacturer's labeling; has not been adequately studied.
Administration SubQ: Surgical implantation within a sterile field using provided implantation device is required. The implant may be slightly curved when removed from refrigerator; may roll implant (in sterile-gloved hands) a few times between fingers and thumb. If resistance is felt when inserting implant into insertion tool cannula, remove and manually manipulate or roll as needed and reinsert into cannula. Insert into the inner portion of the upper arm; it is preferable to use the patient's nondominant arm for placement; implant should be placed halfway between the shoulder and the elbow at the crease between the tricep and the bicep. Implant removal should occur after ~12 months; a replacement implant may be inserted if therapy is to be continued. For removal, palpate area of incision to locate implant; if not readily palpated, ultrasound, CT, or MRI may be necessary to locate implant; plain films are not recommended because the implant is not radiopaque. Refer to manufacturer's labeling for full insertion and removal details.

Hazardous agent; use appropriate precautions for handling and disposal (NIOSH, 2012).

Monitoring Parameters
Central precocious puberty:
Manufacturer labeling: LH, FSH, estradiol, or testosterone serum concentration (after 1 month then every 6 months); height, bone age (every 6-12 months); Tanner staging, monitor for clinical evidence of suppression of CPP manifestations
Consensus recommendation: Tanner stage and growth (growth velocity, height) every 3-6 months and bone age periodically. Routine or random stimulated measurements of gonadotropins or sex steroids may be used, particularly if suboptimal response; however, use of FSH levels not typically used (Carel, 2009).
Prostate cancer: Serum testosterone levels, prostate specific antigen (PSA); bone mineral density; weakness, paresthesias, and urinary tract obstruction (especially during first few weeks of therapy); screen for diabetes; monitor for symptoms associated with cardiovascular disease

Test Interactions Results of diagnostic test of pituitary gonadotropic and gonadal functions may be affected during and after therapy

Dosage Forms Excipient information presented when available (limited, particularly for generics); consult specific product labeling.
Kit, Subcutaneous:
Supprelin LA: 50 mg
Vantas: 50 mg

References
Carel JC, Eugster EA, Rogol A, et al, "Consensus Statement on the Use of Gonadotropin-Releasing Hormone Analogs in Children," *Pediatrics*, 2009, 752-62.
Eugster EA, Clarke W, Kletter GB, et al, "Efficacy and Safety of Histrelin Subdermal Implant in Children With Central Precocious Puberty: A Multicenter Trial," *J Clin Endocrinol Metab*, 2007, 92(5):1697-704.
Levine GN, D'Amico AV, Berger P, et al, "Androgen-Deprivation Therapy in Prostate Cancer and Cardiovascular Risk. A Science Advisory From the American Heart Association, American Cancer Society, and American Urological Association," *Circulation*, 2010, 121:831-38.
National Institute for Occupational Safety and Health (NIOSH), "NIOSH List of Antineoplastic and Other Hazardous Drugs in Healthcare Settings 2012." Available at http://www.cdc.gov/niosh/docs/2012-150/pdfs/2012-150.pdf. Accessed January 21, 2013.
Rahhal S, Clarke WL, Kletter GB, et al, "Results of a Second Year of Therapy With the 12-Month Histrelin Implant for the Treatment of Central Precocious Puberty," *Int J Pediatr Endocrinol*, 2009, 2009:812517.

◆ **Histrelin Acetate** see Histrelin *on page 1016*
◆ **Hizentra** see Immune Globulin *on page 1084*
◆ **Hizentra 20%** see Immune Globulin *on page 1084*
◆ **HN₂** see Mechlorethamine (Systemic) *on page 1315*
◆ **Hold [OTC]** see Dextromethorphan *on page 636*
◆ **Homatropaire** see Homatropine *on page 1018*

Homatropine (hoe MA troe peen)

Medication Safety Issues
Sound-alike/look-alike issues:
Homatropine may be confused with Humatrope®, somatropin
Brand Names: U.S. Homatropaire; Isopto Homatropine
Therapeutic Category Anticholinergic Agent, Ophthalmic; Ophthalmic Agent, Mydriatic
Generic Availability (U.S.) Yes
Use Producing cycloplegia and mydriasis for refraction; treatment of acute inflammatory conditions of the uveal tract; relief of ciliary spasm; optical aid in some cases of axial lens opacities (All indications: Homatropine®: FDA approved in ages ≥3 months and adults, Isopto®-Homatropine: FDA approved in adults)
Pregnancy Risk Factor C
Pregnancy Considerations Animal reproduction studies have not been conducted.
Breast-Feeding Considerations Small amounts of homatropine are excreted into breast milk. Due to the potential for serious adverse reactions in the nursing infant, a decision should be made whether to discontinue nursing or to discontinue the drug, taking into account the importance of treatment to the mother.
Contraindications Hypersensitivity to homatropine or any component; primary glaucoma, patients anatomically predisposed to glaucoma (eg, narrow anterior chamber angle)
Warnings For topical ophthalmic use; do not inject. Excessive use may cause CNS disturbances, including confusion, delirium, agitation, and rarely, coma; risk may be increased in children, elderly, and patients with a known history of belladonna alkaloid sensitivity.
Precautions May cause ocular sensitivity to light; appropriate eye protection should be used. Patients should be cautioned about driving or engaging in hazardous tasks while pupils are dilated. Use may increase risk of narrow angle-closure glaucoma; an estimation of the depth of the

anterior chamber angle should be made prior to use; risk may be increased in patients with Down Syndrome as they are predisposed to angle-closure glaucoma. Use with caution in patients with keratoconus; may result in fixed pupil dilation. Use with caution in patients with hypertension. To avoid systemic absorption, apply pressure over the nasolacrimal sac for 1-3 minutes after use. Use with caution in children; may be at increased risk for systemic effects. Some products may contain benzalkonium chloride which may be adsorbed by contact lenses; remove contacts prior to administration and wait 15 minutes before reinserting.

Adverse Reactions

Cardiovascular: Edema

Central nervous system: Burning sensation, stinging sensation

Dermatologic: Eczema

Endocrine & metabolic: Increased thirst

Gastrointestinal: Xerostomia

Local: Local irritation

Ophthalmic: Blurred vision, follicular conjunctivitis, increased intraocular pressure, ocular exudate, photophobia, vascular congestion of the eye

Drug Interactions

Metabolism/Transport Effects None known.

Avoid Concomitant Use

Avoid concomitant use of Homatropine with any of the following: Aclidinium; Ipratropium (Oral Inhalation); Potassium Chloride; Tiotropium; Umeclidinium

Increased Effect/Toxicity

Homatropine may increase the levels/effects of: AbobotulinumtoxinA; Analgesics (Opioid); Anticholinergic Agents; Cannabinoid-Containing Products; Mirabegron; OnabotulinumtoxinA; Potassium Chloride; RimabotulinumtoxinB; Thiazide Diuretics; Tiotropium; Topiramate

The levels/effects of Homatropine may be increased by: Aclidinium; Ipratropium (Oral Inhalation); Pramlintide; Umeclidinium

Decreased Effect

Homatropine may decrease the levels/effects of: Acetylcholinesterase Inhibitors (Central); Secretin

The levels/effects of Homatropine may be decreased by: Acetylcholinesterase Inhibitors (Central)

Stability Store at 15°C to 30°C (59°F to 86°F); protect from light.

Isopto-Homatropine®: Store at 8°C to 24°C (46°F to 75°F).

Mechanism of Action Blocks response of iris sphincter muscle and the accommodative muscle of the ciliary body to cholinergic stimulation resulting in dilation (mydriasis) and paralysis of accommodation (cycloplegia)

Pharmacodynamics Ophthalmic:

Onset of accommodation and pupil action:

Maximum mydriatic effect: Within 10-30 minutes

Maximum cycloplegic effect: Within 30-90 minutes

Duration:

Mydriasis: Persists for 6 hours to 4 days

Cycloplegia: 10-48 hours

Dosing: Usual

Infants ≥3 months and Children:

Mydriasis and cycloplegia for refraction: Ophthalmic: 2% solution: Instill 1-2 drops immediately prior to procedure; repeat every 10-15 minutes as needed; maximum: 5 doses

Uveitis: Ophthalmic: 2% solution: Instill 1-2 drops 2-3 times daily

Adults: **Note:** Patients with heavily pigmented irides may require increased dose.

Refraction: Ophthalmic:

2% solution: 1-2 drops into eye(s); repeat every 10-15 minutes if necessary; maximum: 5 doses

5% solution: 1-2 drops into eye(s); repeat dose in 15 minutes

Uveitis: Ophthalmic: 2% or 5% solution: 1-2 drops 2-3 times daily (Alexander, 2004), may give up to every 3-4 hours for severe uveitis

Administration Ophthalmic: Wash hands before and after use. Do not touch tip of container to eye. Contact lenses should be removed before instillation; do not reinsert contact lenses within 15 minutes of drops. Finger pressure should be applied to lacrimal sac for 1-3 minutes after instillation to decrease risk of absorption and systemic reactions.

Dosage Forms Excipient information presented when available (limited, particularly for generics); consult specific product labeling.

Solution, Ophthalmic, as hydrobromide:

Homatropaire: 5% (5 mL)

Isopto Homatropine: 2% (5 mL); 5% (5 mL)

Generic: 5% (5 mL)

References

Alexander KL, Dul MW, Lalle PA et al, "Optometric Clinical Practice Guideline Care of the Patient with Anterior Uveitis," *American Optometric Association*, 2004. Available at http://www.aoa.org/documents/CPG-7.pdf

◆ **Homatropine and Hydrocodone** *see* Hydrocodone and Homatropine *on page 1032*

◆ **Homatropine Hydrobromide** *see* Homatropine *on page 1018*

◆ **Horse Antihuman Thymocyte Gamma Globulin** *see* Antithymocyte Globulin (Equine) *on page 182*

◆ **12 Hour Nasal Relief Spray [OTC]** *see* Oxymetazoline (Nasal) *on page 1577*

◆ **12 Hour Nasal Spray [OTC]** *see* Oxymetazoline (Nasal) *on page 1577*

◆ **HPV2** *see* Papillomavirus (Types 16, 18) Vaccine (Human, Recombinant) *on page 1603*

◆ **HPV4** *see* Papillomavirus (Types 6, 11, 16, 18) Vaccine (Human, Recombinant) *on page 1603*

◆ **HPV 16/18 L1 VLP/AS04 VAC** *see* Papillomavirus (Types 16, 18) Vaccine (Human, Recombinant) *on page 1603*

◆ **HPV Vaccine (Bivalent)** *see* Papillomavirus (Types 16, 18) Vaccine (Human, Recombinant) *on page 1603*

◆ **HPV Vaccine (Quadrivalent)** *see* Papillomavirus (Types 6, 11, 16, 18) Vaccine (Human, Recombinant) *on page 1600*

◆ **HRIG** *see* Rabies Immune Globulin (Human) *on page 1800*

◆ **HU** *see* Hydroxyurea *on page 1051*

◆ **HumaLOG** *see* Insulin Lispro *on page 1125*

◆ **Humalog® (Can)** *see* Insulin Lispro *on page 1125*

◆ **HumaLOG KwikPen** *see* Insulin Lispro *on page 1125*

◆ **Humalog® Mix 25 (Can)** *see* Insulin Lispro Protamine and Insulin Lispro *on page 1128*

◆ **HumaLOG® Mix 50/50™** *see* Insulin Lispro Protamine and Insulin Lispro *on page 1128*

◆ **HumaLOG® Mix 50/50™ KwikPen™** *see* Insulin Lispro Protamine and Insulin Lispro *on page 1128*

◆ **HumaLOG® Mix 75/25™** *see* Insulin Lispro Protamine and Insulin Lispro *on page 1128*

◆ **HumaLOG® Mix 75/25™ KwikPen™** *see* Insulin Lispro Protamine and Insulin Lispro *on page 1128*

◆ **Human Albumin Grifols** *see* Albumin *on page 82*

◆ **Human Antitumor Necrosis Factor Alpha** *see* Adalimumab *on page 70*

◆ **Human C1 Inhibitor** *see* C1 Inhibitor (Human) *on page 337*

- ◆ **Human Diploid Cell Cultures Rabies Vaccine** *see* Rabies Vaccine *on page 1801*
- ◆ **Human Growth Hormone** *see* Somatropin *on page 1920*
- ◆ **Human Normal Immunoglobulin** *see* Immune Globulin *on page 1084*
- ◆ **Human Papillomavirus Vaccine (Bivalent)** *see* Papillomavirus (Types 16, 18) Vaccine (Human, Recombinant) *on page 1603*
- ◆ **Human Papillomavirus Vaccine (Quadrivalent)** *see* Papillomavirus (Types 6, 11, 16, 18) Vaccine (Human, Recombinant) *on page 1600*
- ◆ **Human Rotavirus Vaccine, Attenuated (HRV)** *see* Rotavirus Vaccine *on page 1855*
- ◆ **Humate-P®** *see* Antihemophilic Factor/von Willebrand Factor Complex (Human) *on page 177*
- ◆ **Humatin (Can)** *see* Paromomycin *on page 1608*
- ◆ **Humatrope** *see* Somatropin *on page 1920*
- ◆ **Humira** *see* Adalimumab *on page 70*
- ◆ **Humira Pen** *see* Adalimumab *on page 70*
- ◆ **Humira Pen-Crohns Starter** *see* Adalimumab *on page 70*
- ◆ **Humira Pen-Psoriasis Starter** *see* Adalimumab *on page 70*
- ◆ **Humist [OTC]** *see* Sodium Chloride *on page 1902*
- ◆ **Humulin® 20/80 (Can)** *see* Insulin NPH and Insulin Regular *on page 1132*
- ◆ **HumuLIN® 70/30** *see* Insulin NPH and Insulin Regular *on page 1132*
- ◆ **Humulin® 70/30 (Can)** *see* Insulin NPH and Insulin Regular *on page 1132*
- ◆ **HumuLIN® 70/30 KwikPen** *see* Insulin NPH and Insulin Regular *on page 1132*
- ◆ **HumuLIN N [OTC]** *see* Insulin NPH *on page 1130*
- ◆ **Humulin® N (Can)** *see* Insulin NPH *on page 1130*
- ◆ **HumuLIN N KwikPen [OTC]** *see* Insulin NPH *on page 1130*
- ◆ **HumuLIN N Pen [OTC] [DSC]** *see* Insulin NPH *on page 1130*
- ◆ **HumuLIN R [OTC]** *see* Insulin Regular *on page 1134*
- ◆ **Humulin® R (Can)** *see* Insulin Regular *on page 1134*
- ◆ **HumuLIN R U-500 (CONCENTRATED)** *see* Insulin Regular *on page 1134*
- ◆ **Hurricaine [OTC]** *see* Benzocaine *on page 273*
- ◆ **HurriCaine One [OTC]** *see* Benzocaine *on page 273*

Hyaluronidase (hye al yoor ON i dase)

Related Information
Management of Drug Extravasations *on page 2255*
Brand Names: U.S. Amphadase; Hylenex; Vitrase
Therapeutic Category Antidote, Extravasation
Generic Availability (U.S.) No
Use Adjunct therapy to increase the dispersion and absorption of other drugs; adjunct therapy to increase rate of absorption of parenteral fluids given by hypodermoclysis for hydration; adjunct therapy in subcutaneous urography for improving resorption of radiopaque agents (all indications: FDA approved in all ages); has also been used in the management of I.V. extravasations
Pregnancy Risk Factor C
Pregnancy Considerations Adverse events were not observed in animal reproduction studies (not conducted with all products). Administration during labor did not cause any increase in blood loss or differences in cervical trauma. It is not known whether it affects the fetus if used

during labor. Hyaluronidase has been evaluated for use prior to intracytoplasmic sperm injection (ICSI) to increase male fertility (DeVos, 2008; Evison, 2009).
Breast-Feeding Considerations It is not known if hyaluronidase is excreted in breast milk. The manufacturer recommends that caution be exercised when administering hyaluronidase to nursing women.
Contraindications Hypersensitivity to hyaluronidase or any component
Warnings Do not administer intravenously (enzyme is rapidly inactivated); do not inject in or around infected or inflamed areas; may spread localized infection. Do not apply directly to the cornea. Should **not** be used for dopamine and alpha-agonist drug infiltrates or to reduce swelling of bites or stings. Injection may contain albumin, a human blood derivative which carries a small risk of transmitting infectious agents.
Precautions Hypersensitivity reactions may occur; a preliminary intradermal skin test may be considered. Avoid use if positive reaction occurs (ie, a wheal with pseudopods appears within 5 minutes and persists for 20-30 minutes accompanied by localized itching). Discontinue hyaluronidase if sensitization occurs during therapy. Use with caution in patients with reported history of bee sting allergy; hyaluronidase is an active component in bee venom (Lee, 2010).
Adverse Reactions
Cardiovascular: Edema
Local: Injection site reaction
Rare but important or life-threatening: Anaphylactic-like reactions (retrobulbar block or I.V. injections), anaphylaxis, hypersensitivity reaction
Drug Interactions
Metabolism/Transport Effects None known.
Avoid Concomitant Use
Avoid concomitant use of Hyaluronidase with any of the following: Phenylephrine (Systemic)
Increased Effect/Toxicity
Hyaluronidase may increase the levels/effects of: Alpha-/Beta-Agonists; DOPamine; Local Anesthetics; Phenylephrine (Systemic)
Decreased Effect
The levels/effects of Hyaluronidase may be decreased by: Antihistamines; Corticosteroids; Estrogen Derivatives; Salicylates
Stability
Amphadase™, Hylenex™: Store intact vial at 2°C to 8°C (36°F to 46°F); do not freeze. Hylenex™ is stable for <48 hours at room temperature ≤25°C (77°F). May return to the refrigerator if unopened and removed from the refrigerator for less than 48 hours. Vial may only be removed once.
Vitrase®: Store intact vial at 2°C to 8°C (35°F to 46°F); do not freeze. Protect from light. If adding to other injectable solutions, store admixture at 15°C to 25°C (59°F to 77°F) and use within 6 hours.
Mechanism of Action Enzymatically modifies the permeability of connective tissue through hydrolysis of hyaluronic acid, one of the chief components of tissue cement which offers resistance to diffusion of liquids through tissues; hyaluronidase increases the distribution/dispersion and absorption of locally injected or extravasated substances.
Pharmacodynamics
Onset of action by the SubQ or intradermal routes for the treatment of extravasation: Immediate; when used for extravasation, there is usually a reduction in swelling within 15-30 minutes after administration (Zenk, 1981)
Duration: 24-48 hours
Dosing: Neonatal
Dehydration: Hypodermoclysis: SubQ: 15 units added to each 100 mL of replacement fluid to be administered; dosing extrapolated from experience with larger volumes

(ie, in older patients, 150 units facilitates absorption of ≥1000 mL of solution). The volume of subcutaneous fluid administered is dependent upon the age, weight, and clinical condition of the patient, as well as laboratory determinations; maximum daily volume of clysis is 25 mL/kg/**day** and the rate of administration should not exceed 2 mL/minute

Extravasation: Limited data available: SubQ, intradermal: Use 5 separate 0.2 mL injections of a 15-150 units/mL solution into the extravasation site at the leading edge (Hurst, 2004; Kuensting, 2010; MacCara, 1983). **Note:** Some centers determine the concentration of hyaluronidase based upon the volume of extravasation, so for smaller extravasation volumes (<100 mL), a less concentrated solution (15 units/mL) has been used or by the medication risk of tissue toxicity (based on pH, osmolarity, known tissue toxicity); to prepare 15 units/mL solution, dilute 0.1 mL of the 150 unit/mL solution in 0.9 mL NS (MacCara, 1983).

Dosing: Usual

Infants, Children, and Adolescents:

Skin test: Intradermal: 0.02 mL (Amphadase 3 units, Hylenex 3 units, or Vitrase 4 units) of a 150 units/mL (Amphadase, Hylenex) or 200 units/mL (Vitrase) solution. Positive reaction consists of a wheal with pseudopods appearing within 5 minutes and persisting for 20-30 minutes with localized itching (transient erythema is not considered a positive reaction). Skin testing is not necessary prior to use for extravasation management.

Dehydration: Hypodermoclysis:

SubQ prior to infusion: SubQ: 150 units or 200 units, followed by subcutaneous isotonic fluid administration at a rate appropriate for age, weight, and clinical condition of the patient; 150 units facilitates absorption of ≥1000 mL of solution. If the infusion is continued greater than 24 hours, additional doses have been administered at 24 hour intervals up to a total of 3 doses (Allen, 2009)

Added to replacement solution: Dose dependent on volume to be infused; 150 units of hyaluronidase facilitates the absorption of ≥1000 mL of fluid; for patients (ie, neonates, young infants) who require smaller volumes for replacement fluid (≤100 mL), 15 units added for every 100 mL of replacement fluid has been used at some centers; maximum daily dose: 150 units/**day**

Maximum clysis volumes:

Infants and Children <3 years: Volume of a single clysis should not exceed 200 mL

Children ≥3 years and Adolescents: Rate and volume of a single clysis should not exceed those used for infusion of I.V. fluids

Dispersion/absorption enhancement of injected drugs: Children and Adolescents: SubQ: 50-300 units (usual dose: 150 units) either injected prior to drug administration or added to injection solution (consult compatibility reference prior to mixing)

Extravasation: Limited data available: SubQ, intradermal: Use 5 separate 0.2 mL injections of a 150 units/mL solution into the extravasation site at the leading edge as soon as possible (preferably within 1 hour) after extravasation is recognized (Hurst, 2004; Wiegand, 2010). **Note:** Some centers may determine concentration of hyaluronidase based upon the medication risk of tissue toxicity (risk determined by pH, osmolarity, known tissue toxicity) or by volume of extravasation so for smaller volumes (<100 mL), a less concentrated solution (15 units/mL) has been used (Hurst, 2004; MacCara, 1983; Sokol, 1998; Wiegand, 2010); to prepare 15 units/mL solution, dilute 0.1 mL of the 150 unit/mL solution in 0.9 mL NS (MacCara, 1983)

Urography, subcutaneous: SubQ: 75 units over each scapula followed by injection of contrast medium at the

same site; patient should be in the prone position during drug administration

Adults: **Dehydration: Hypodermoclysis:**

Dehydration: Hypodermoclysis: SubQ: 150 or 200 units followed by subcutaneous isotonic fluid administration ≥1000 mL **or** may be added to small volumes (≤200 mL) of subcutaneous replacement fluid. Rate and volume of a single clysis should not exceed those used for infusion of I.V. fluids.

Dispersion/absorption enhancement of injected drugs: SubQ: 50-300 units (usual dose: 150 units) either injected prior to drug administration or added to injection solution (consult compatibility reference prior to mixing)

Dosage adjustment in renal impairment: All patients: There are no dosage adjustments provided in the manufacturer's labeling; hyaluronidase exerts its effects locally and is rapidly inactivated in the blood; adverse effects would not be expected.

Dosage adjustment in hepatic impairment: All patients: There are no dosage adjustments provided in the manufacturer's labeling; hyaluronidase exerts its effects locally and is rapidly inactivated in the blood; adverse effects would not be expected.

Administration

Parenteral: Do not administer I.V. (enzyme is rapidly inactivated and desired effects will not be produced)

Treatment of extravasation: May administer undiluted (150 units/mL) or dilutions may be used for smaller volumes of extravasation. Infiltrate area of extravasation with 5 small injections at the leading edge; use 27- or 30-gauge needles and change needle between each skin entry to prevent bacterial contamination and minimize pain.

Monitoring Parameters Observe appearance of lesion for induration, swelling, discoloration, blanching, and blister formation every 15 minutes for ~2 hours

Dosage Forms Excipient information presented when available (limited, particularly for generics); consult specific product labeling.

Solution, Injection:

Amphadase: 150 units/mL (1 mL) [contains edetate disodium, thimerosal]

Solution, Injection [preservative free]:

Hylenex: 150 units/mL (1 mL) [contains albumin human, calcium chloride anhydrous, edetate disodium dihydrate, sodium hydroxide]

Vitrase: 200 units/mL (1.2 mL)

References

Allen CH, Etzwiler LS, Miller MK, et al, "Recombinant Human Hyaluronidase-Enabled Subcutaneous Pediatric Rehydration," *Pediatrics*, 2009, 124(5):e858-67.

De Vos A, Van Landuyt L, Van Ranst H, et al, "Randomized Sibling-Oocyte Study Using Recombinant Human Hyaluronidase versus Bovine-Derived Sigma Hyaluronidase in ICSI Patients," *Hum Reprod*, 2008, 23(8):1815-9.

Evison M, Pretty C, Taylor E, et al, "Human Recombinant Hyaluronidase (Cumulase) Improves Intracytoplasmic Sperm Injection Survival and Fertilization Rates," *Reprod Biomed Online*, 2009, 18(6):811-4.

Flemmer L and Chan JS, "A Pediatric Protocol for Management of Extravasation Injuries," *Pediatr Nurs*, 1993, 19(4):355-8, 424.

Hurst S, McMillan M. Innovative solutions in critical care units: extravasation guidelines. *Dimens Crit Care Nurs.* 2004;23(3):125-128.

Kuensting LL. Treatment of intravenous infiltration in a neonate. *J Pediatr Health Care.* 2010;24:184-188.

Lee A, Grummer SE, Kriegel D, et al, "Hyaluronidase," *Dermatol Surg*, 2010, 36(7):1071-7.

MacCara ME, "Extravasation: A Hazard of Intravenous Therapy," *Drug Intell Clin Pharm*, 1983, 17(10):713-7.

Raszka WV, Keuser TK, Smith FR, et al, "The Use of Hyaluronidase in the Treatment of Intravenous Extravasation Injuries," *J Perinatol*, 1990, 10(2):146-9.

Sokol DK, Dahlmann A, Dunn DW. Hyaluronidase treatment for intravenous phenytoin extravasation. *Journal of child neurology.* 1998;13(5):246-247.

Spandorfer PR, Mace SE, Okada PJ, et al, "A Randomized Clinical Trial of Recombinant Human Hyaluronidase-Facilitated Subcutaneous Versus Intravenous Rehydration in Mild to Moderately Dehydrated

Children in the Emergency Department," *Clin Ther*, 2012, 34 (11):2232-45.

Wiegand R, Brown J. Hyaluronidase for the management of dextrose extravasation. *Am J Emerg Med*. 2010;28(2):257.e1-2.

Zenk KE, Dungy Cl, and Greene GR, "Nafcillin Extravasation Injury: Use of Hyaluronidase as an Antidote," *Am J Dis Child*, 1981, 135 (12):1113-4.

◆ **Hycamtamine** see Topotecan *on page 2053*

◆ **Hycamtin** see Topotecan *on page 2053*

◆ **hycet®** see Hydrocodone and Acetaminophen *on page 1027*

◆ **Hycodan** see Hydrocodone and Homatropine *on page 1032*

◆ **Hycort™ (Can)** see Hydrocortisone (Topical) *on page 1038*

◆ **Hydeltra T.B.A. (Can)** see PrednisoLONE (Systemic) *on page 1727*

◆ **Hyderm (Can)** see Hydrocortisone (Topical) *on page 1038*

HydrALAZINE (hye DRAL a zeen)

Medication Safety Issues
Sound-alike/look-alike issues:
HydrALAZINE may be confused with hydrOXYzine

Brand Names: Canada Apo-Hydralazine®; Apresoline®; Novo-Hylazin; Nu-Hydral

Therapeutic Category Antihypertensive Agent; Vasodilator

Generic Availability (U.S.) Yes

Use Management of moderate to severe hypertension, CHF, hypertension secondary to pre-eclampsia/eclampsia, primary pulmonary hypertension

Pregnancy Risk Factor C

Pregnancy Considerations Adverse events were observed in some animal reproduction studies. Hydralazine crosses the placenta (Liedholm, 1982). Intravenous hydralazine is recommended for use in the management of acute onset severe hypertension in pregnancy and hypertension associated with pre-eclampsia (ACOG, 2011; ACOG, 2013). Untreated chronic maternal hypertension is associated with adverse events in the fetus, infant, and mother. If treatment for chronic hypertension in pregnancy is needed, other oral agents are preferred as initial therapy (ACOG, 2013).

Breast-Feeding Considerations Hydralazine is excreted into breast milk. In a case report, following a maternal dose of hydralazine 50 mg three times daily, exposure to the infant was calculated to be 0.013 mg per 75 mL breast milk (Liedholm, 1982). The manufacturer recommends that caution be used if administered to a nursing woman.

Contraindications Hypersensitivity to hydralazine or any component; dissecting aortic aneurysm, mitral valve rheumatic heart disease, coronary artery disease

Warnings Monitor blood pressure closely with I.V. use; modify dosage in patients with severe renal impairment

Precautions Discontinue hydralazine in patients who develop SLE-like syndrome or positive ANA; use with caution in patients with severe renal disease or cerebral vascular accidents

Adverse Reactions
Cardiovascular: Angina pectoris, flushing, orthostatic hypotension, palpitations, paradoxical hypertension, peripheral edema, tachycardia, vascular collapse

Central nervous system: Anxiety, chills, depression, disorientation, dizziness, fever, headache, increased intracranial pressure (I.V.; in patient with preexisting increased intracranial pressure), psychotic reaction

Dermatologic: Pruritus, rash, urticaria

Gastrointestinal: Anorexia, constipation, diarrhea, nausea, paralytic ileus, vomiting

Genitourinary: Dysuria, impotence

Hematologic: Agranulocytosis, eosinophilia, erythrocyte count reduced, hemoglobin decreased, hemolytic anemia, leukopenia, thrombocytopenia (rare)

Neuromuscular & skeletal: Muscle cramps, peripheral neuritis, rheumatoid arthritis, tremor, weakness

Ocular: Conjunctivitis, lacrimation

Respiratory: Dyspnea, nasal congestion

Miscellaneous: Diaphoresis, drug-induced lupus-like syndrome (dose related; fever, arthralgia, splenomegaly, lymphadenopathy, asthenia, myalgia, malaise, pleuritic chest pain, edema, positive ANA, positive LE cells, maculopapular facial rash, positive direct Coombs' test, pericarditis, pericardial tamponade)

Drug Interactions
Metabolism/Transport Effects Inhibits CYP3A4 (weak)

Avoid Concomitant Use
Avoid concomitant use of HydrALAZINE with any of the following: Pimozide

Increased Effect/Toxicity
HydrALAZINE may increase the levels/effects of: Amifostine; Antihypertensives; ARIPiprazole; Dofetilide; DULoxetine; Hypotensive Agents; Lomitapide; Obinutuzumab; Pimozide; RiTUXimab

The levels/effects of HydrALAZINE may be increased by: Alfuzosin; Barbiturates; Brimonidine (Topical); Diazoxide; Herbs (Hypotensive Properties); MAO Inhibitors; Pentoxifylline; Phosphodiesterase 5 Inhibitors; Prostacyclin Analogues

Decreased Effect
The levels/effects of HydrALAZINE may be decreased by: Herbs (Hypertensive Properties); Methylphenidate; Nonsteroidal Anti-Inflammatory Agents; Yohimbine

Food Interactions Food enhances bioavailability of hydralazine. Management: Administer without regard to food, but keep consistent.

Stability Changes color after contact with a metal filter; do not store intact ampuls in refrigerator

Mechanism of Action Direct vasodilation of arterioles (with little effect on veins) with decreased systemic resistance

Pharmacodynamics
Onset of action:
Oral: 20-30 minutes
I.V.: 5-20 minutes
Duration:
Oral: 2-4 hours
I.V.: 2-6 hours

Pharmacokinetics (Adult data unless noted)
Distribution: Crosses placenta; appears in breast milk
Protein-binding: 85% to 90%
Metabolism: Acetylated in the liver
Bioavailability: 30% to 50%; large first-pass effect orally
Half-life, adults: 2-8 hours; half-life varies with genetically determined acetylation rates
Elimination: 14% excreted unchanged in urine

Dosing: Usual
Infants and Children:
Oral: Initial: 0.75-1 mg/kg/day in 2-4 divided doses, not to exceed 25 mg/dose; increase over 3-4 weeks to maximum of 5 mg/kg/day in infants and 7.5 mg/kg/day in children, given in 2-4 divided doses; maximum daily dose: 200 mg/day
I.M., I.V.: Initial: 0.1-0.2 mg/kg/dose (not to exceed 20 mg) every 4-6 hours as needed; up to 1.7-3.5 mg/kg/day divided in 4-6 doses

Adults:

Oral: Initial: 10 mg 4 times/day, increase by 10-25 mg/dose every 2-5 days to maximum of 300 mg/day; usual dosage range for hypertension (JNC 7): 25-100 mg/day in 2 divided doses

I.M., I.V.: Hypertension: Initial: 10-20 mg/dose every 4-6 hours as needed, may increase to 40 mg/dose

I.M., I.V.: Pre-eclampsia/eclampsia: 5 mg/dose then 5-10 mg every 20-30 minutes as needed

Dosing interval in renal impairment:

CrCl 10-50 mL/minute: Administer every 8 hours

CrCl <10 mL/minute: Administer every 8-16 hours in fast acetylators and every 12-24 hours in slow acetylators

Administration

Oral: Administer with food

Parenteral: I.V.: Do not exceed rate of 0.2 mg/kg/minute; maximum concentration for I.V. use: 20 mg/mL

Monitoring Parameters Heart rate, blood pressure, ANA titer

Additional Information Slow acetylators, patients with decreased renal function and patients receiving >200 mg/day (chronically) are at higher risk for SLE. Titrate dosage to patient's response. Usually administered with diuretic and a beta-blocker to counteract hydralazine's side effects of sodium and water retention and reflex tachycardia.

Dosage Forms Excipient information presented when available (limited, particularly for generics); consult specific product labeling.

Solution, Injection, as hydrochloride:

Generic: 20 mg/mL (1 mL)

Tablet, Oral, as hydrochloride:

Generic: 10 mg, 25 mg, 50 mg, 100 mg

Extemporaneous Preparations A 4 mg/mL oral suspension may be made with tablets and a 1:1 mixture of Ora-Sweet SF and Ora-Plus. Crush four 100 mg tablets in a mortar and reduce to a fine powder. Add 15 mL of the vehicle and mix to a uniform paste; mix while adding the vehicle in incremental proportions to **almost** 100 mL; transfer to a calibrated bottle, rinse mortar with vehicle, and add quantity of vehicle sufficient to make 100 mL. Label "Shake Well", "Protect From Light", "Store in a Refrigerator". Stable for 2 days when stored in amber plastic prescription bottles in the dark and refrigerated (Allen, 1998).

Note: Stability reduced to 24 hours if Ora-Sweet is substituted for Ora-Sweet SF.

Allen LV Jr, Erickson MA 3rd. Stability of alprazolam, chloroquine phosphate, cisapride, enalapril maleate, and hydralazine hydrochloride in extemporaneously compounded oral liquids. *Am J Health-Syst Pharm.* 1998;55(18):1915-1920.

References

ACOG Committee on Obstetric Practice. Committee opinion no. 514: emergent therapy for acute-onset, severe hypertension with preeclampsia or eclampsia. *Obstet Gynecol.* 2011;118(6):1465-1468.

ACOG Committee on Practice Bulletins–Obstetrics, "ACOG Practice Bulletin. Diagnosis and Management of Preeclampsia and Eclampsia. Number 33, January 2002," *Obstet Gynecol*, 2002, 99(1):159-67.

American College of Obstetricians and Gynecologists (ACOG). ACOG practice bulletin no. 125: chronic hypertension in pregnancy. *Obstet Gynecol.* 2012;119(2 Pt 1):396-407.

Chobanian AV, Bakris GL, Black HR, et al, "The Seventh Report of the Joint National Committee on Prevention, Detection, Evaluation, and Treatment of High Blood Pressure: The JNC 7 Report," *JAMA*, 2003, 289(19):2560-71.

Liedholm H, Wåhlin-Boll E, Hanson A, et al, "Transplacental Passage and Breast Milk Concentrations of Hydralazine," *Eur J Clin Pharmacol*, 1982, 21(5):417-9.

◆ **Hydralazine Hydrochloride** see HydrALAZINE on page 1022

◆ **Hydrated Chloral** see Chloral Hydrate on page 436

◆ **Hydrea** see Hydroxyurea on page 1051

◆ **Hydrea® (Can)** see Hydroxyurea on page 1051

◆ **Hydrisalic [OTC]** see Salicylic Acid on page 1860

Hydrochlorothiazide (hye droe klor oh THYE a zide)

Medication Safety Issues

Sound-alike/look-alike issues:

HCTZ is an error-prone abbreviation (mistaken as hydrocortisone)

Hydrochlorothiazide may be confused with hydrocortisone, Viskazide

Microzide may be confused with Maxzide, Micronase

International issues:

Esidrex [multiple international markets] may be confused with Lasix brand name for furosemide [U.S., Canada, and multiple international markets]

Esidrix [Germany] may be confused with Lasix brand name for furosemide [U.S., Canada, and multiple international markets]

Brand Names: U.S. Microzide

Brand Names: Canada Apo-Hydro; Ava-Hydrochlorothiazide; Bio-Hydrochlorothiazide; PMS-Hydrochlorothiazide; Teva-Hydrochlorothiazide; Urozide

Therapeutic Category Antihypertensive Agent; Diuretic, Thiazide

Generic Availability (U.S.) Yes

Use Oral:

Capsules: Management of hypertension alone or in combination with other antihypertensive agents (FDA approved in adults); **Note:** Use in pregnancy should be reserved for those cases causing extreme discomfort and unrelieved by rest; should not be routinely used during pregnancy.

Tablets: Treatment of edema due to heart failure, hepatic cirrhosis, estrogen, or corticosteroid therapy (FDA approved in infants, children, and adults); treatment of various forms of renal dysfunction, including nephrotic syndrome, acute glomerulonephritis, and chronic renal failure (FDA approved in infants, children, and adults); management of hypertension either alone or in combination with other antihypertensive agents (FDA approved in infants, children, and adults); has also been used for bronchopulmonary dysplasia (BPD), idiopathic hypercalcuria, and congenital nephrogenic diabetes insipidus. **Note:** Use in pregnancy should be reserved for those cases causing extreme discomfort and unrelieved by rest; should not be routinely used during pregnancy.

Pregnancy Risk Factor B

Pregnancy Considerations Adverse events were not observed in animal reproduction studies. Thiazide diuretics cross the placenta and are found in cord blood. Maternal use may cause fetal or neonatal jaundice, thrombocytopenia, or other adverse events observed in adults. Use of thiazide diuretics to treat edema during normal pregnancies is not appropriate; use may be considered when edema is due to pathologic causes (as in the nonpregnant patient); monitor. Untreated chronic maternal hypertension is associated with adverse events in the fetus, infant, and mother (ACOG, 2013). Women who required thiazide diuretics for the treatment of hypertension prior to pregnancy may continue their use (ACOG, 2013).

Breast-Feeding Considerations Thiazide diuretics are found in breast milk. Following a single oral maternal dose of hydrochlorothiazide 50 mg, the mean breast milk concentration was 80 ng/mL (samples collected over 24 hours) and hydrochlorothiazide was not detected in the blood of the breast feeding infant (limit of detection 20 ng/mL) (Miller, 1982). Peak plasma concentrations reported in adults following hydrochlorothiazide 12.5-100 mg are 70-490 ng/mL. Due to the potential for serious adverse reactions in the nursing infant, the manufacturer recommends a decision be made whether to discontinue nursing or to discontinue the drug, taking into account the importance of treatment to the mother (Canadian labeling contraindicates use in nursing women). Diuretics have the potential to decrease milk volume and suppress lactation.

Contraindications Hypersensitivity to hydrochlorothiazide or any component; cross-sensitivity with other thiazides or sulfonamides-derived medications; anuria

Warnings Hypersensitivity reactions may occur with hydrochlorothiazide. Risk is increased in patients with a history of allergy or bronchial asthma. Chemical similarities are present among sulfonamides, sulfonylureas, carbonic anhydrase inhibitors, thiazides, and loop diuretics (except ethacrynic acid). Use in patients with sulfonamide allergy is specifically contraindicated in product labeling; however, a risk of cross-reaction exists in patients with allergy to any of these compounds; avoid use when previous reaction has been severe. Discontinue if signs of hypersensitivity are noted.

May cause hypokalemia; increased risk associated with aggressive diuresis (eg, concurrent loop diuretic use), severe cirrhosis, or after prolonged therapy; alterations in adequate oral potassium intake may also increase risk; monitor serum potassium concentrations at baseline and periodically; correct hypokalemia prior to initiating therapy. Other electrolyte disorders, including hyponatremia, hypomagnesemia, and hypochloremic metabolic alkalosis, may occur; monitor electrolytes. May cause acute transient myopia and acute angle-closure glaucoma possibly leading to permanent vision loss, typically occurring within hours to weeks following initiation; discontinue therapy immediately in patients with acute decreases in visual acuity or ocular pain. Risk factors may include a history of sulfonamide or penicillin allergy. May cause SLE exacerbation or activation. Photosensitization may occur; patients should be counseled.

Precautions Use with caution in patients with severe renal disease due to decreased efficacy and may precipitate azotemia. Use with caution in patients with severe hepatic dysfunction; in cirrhosis, avoid electrolyte and acid/base imbalances that might lead to hepatic encephalopathy. Use with caution in patients with prediabetes or diabetes mellitus; may alter glucose control. Use with caution in patients who have a history of gout; may cause hyperuricemia and in certain patients with a history of gout, a familial predisposition to gout, or chronic renal failure, gout can be precipitated. Use with caution in patients with moderate or high cholesterol concentrations.

Use with caution in patients with hypercalcemia or parathyroid disease; thiazide diuretics may decrease renal calcium excretion; pathologic changes in the parathyroid glands with hypercalcemia and hypophosphatemia have been observed with prolonged use.

Adverse Reactions The occurrence of adverse events are dose related, with the majority occurring with doses ≥25 mg.

Cardiovascular: Hypotension, necrotizing angiitis, orthostatic hypotension

Central nervous system: Dizziness, headache, paresthesia, restlessness, vertigo

Dermatologic: Alopecia, erythema multiforme, exfoliative dermatitis, skin photosensitivity, skin rash, Stevens-Johnson syndrome, toxic epidermal necrolysis, urticaria

Endocrine & metabolic: Glycosuria, hypercalcemia, hyperglycemia, hyperuricemia, hypochloremic alkalosis, hypokalemia, hypomagnesemia, hyponatremia

Gastrointestinal: Abdominal cramps, anorexia, constipation, diarrhea, gastric irritation, nausea, pancreatitis, sialadenitis, vomiting

Genitourinary: Impotence

Hematologic & oncologic: Agranulocytosis, aplastic anemia, hemolytic anemia, leukopenia, purpura, thrombocytopenia

Hepatic: Jaundice

Hypersensitivity: Anaphylaxis

Neuromuscular & skeletal: Muscle spasm, weakness

Ophthalmic: Blurred vision (transient), xanthopsia

Renal: Interstitial nephritis, renal failure, renal insufficiency

Respiratory: Respiratory distress, pneumonitis, pulmonary edema

Miscellaneous: Fever

Rare but important or life-threatening: Allergic myocarditis, eosinophilic pneumonitis, hepatic insufficiency, lip cancer (Friedman, 2012), systemic lupus erythematosus

Drug Interactions

Metabolism/Transport Effects None known.

Avoid Concomitant Use

Avoid concomitant use of Hydrochlorothiazide with any of the following: Dofetilide

Increased Effect/Toxicity

Hydrochlorothiazide may increase the levels/effects of: ACE Inhibitors; Allopurinol; Amifostine; Antihypertensives; Benazepril; Calcium Salts; CarBAMazepine; Cyclophosphamide; Diazoxide; Dofetilide; DULoxetine; Hypotensive Agents; Ivabradine; Lithium; Multivitamins/Minerals (with ADEK, Folate, Iron); Multivitamins/Minerals (with AE, No Iron); Obinutuzumab; OXcarbazepine; Porfimer; RiTUXimab; Sodium Phosphates; Topiramate; Toremifene; Valsartan; Vitamin D Analogs

The levels/effects of Hydrochlorothiazide may be increased by: Alcohol (Ethyl); Alfuzosin; Analgesics (Opioid); Anticholinergic Agents; Barbiturates; Beta2-Agonists; Brimonidine (Topical); Corticosteroids (Orally Inhaled); Corticosteroids (Systemic); Diazoxide; Herbs (Hypotensive Properties); Licorice; MAO Inhibitors; Multivitamins/Fluoride (with ADE); Pentoxifylline; Phosphodiesterase 5 Inhibitors; Prostacyclin Analogues; Selective Serotonin Reuptake Inhibitors; Valsartan

Decreased Effect

Hydrochlorothiazide may decrease the levels/effects of: Antidiabetic Agents

The levels/effects of Hydrochlorothiazide may be decreased by: Benazepril; Bile Acid Sequestrants; Herbs (Hypertensive Properties); Methylphenidate; Nonsteroidal Anti-Inflammatory Agents; Yohimbine

Stability

Capsules: Store at 20°C to 25°C (68°F to 77°F). Protect from light, moisture, and freezing.

Tablets: Store at 20°C to 25°C (68°F to 77°F); keep container tightly closed.

Mechanism of Action Inhibits sodium reabsorption in the distal tubules causing increased excretion of sodium and water as well as potassium and hydrogen ions

Pharmacodynamics

Onset of action: Diuresis: Oral:

Infants: 2-6 hours (Chemtob, 1989)

Adults: Within 2 hours

Maximum effect: Diuresis: Within 4-6 hours

Duration: Diuresis:

Infants: 8 hours (Chemtob, 1989)

Adults: 6-12 hours

Pharmacokinetics (Adult data unless noted)

Absorption: Oral: ~50% to 80%

Distribution: V_d: 3.6-7.8 L/kg

Protein binding: 68%

Half-life: 5.6-14.8 hours

Time to peak serum concentration: 1-2.5 hours

Elimination: Urine (as unchanged drug)

Dosing: Neonatal Bronchopulmonary dysplasia (BPD); diuresis, hypertension: Oral: 1-2 mg/kg/dose every 12 hours (Albersheim, 1989; Chemtob, 1989; Engelhardt, 1989)

Dosing: Usual

Infants, Children, and Adolescents:

Bronchopulmonary dysplasia: Infants: Oral: 3-4 mg/kg/day in 2 divided doses (Albersheim, 1989; Engelhardt, 1989)

Edema (diuresis):
Manufacturer labeling:
Infants 2-6 months: Oral: 1-3 mg/kg/day in 1-2 divided doses
Infants >6 months, Children, and Adolescents: Oral: 1-2 mg/kg/day in 1-2 divided doses
Maximum daily dose:
Infants and Children <2 years: 37.5 mg/**day**
Children 2-12 years: 100 mg/**day**
Adolescents: 200 mg/**day**
Hypertension: Oral: Initial: 1 mg/kg/day once daily; may increase to maximum 3 mg/kg/day; not to exceed 50 mg/day (NHBPEP, 2004; NHLBI, 2011)
Maximum daily dose:
Infants and Children <2 years: 37.5 mg/**day**
Children 2-12 years: 100 mg/**day**
Adolescents: 200 mg/**day**
Hypercalciuria: Limited data available: Oral: Initial: 1-2 mg/kg/day once daily; titrate until goal urinary calcium excretion goals reached and symptoms resolve; treatment usually continued for 1 year; maximum daily dose: 100 mg/**day** (Copelovitch, 2012).
Nephrogenic diabetes insipidus; congenital: Limited data available: Oral: 2-3 mg/kg/day in combination with amiloride; dosing based on a retrospective descriptive analysis (n=30, age range 1 month to 40 years) and a pediatric case-series (n=4). (Kirchlechner, 1999; Van Lieburg, 1999)
Adults:
Edema (diuresis): Oral: 25-100 mg/day in 1-2 doses; maximum: 200 mg/day
Hypertension: Oral: 12.5-50 mg/day; minimal increase in response and more electrolyte disturbances are seen with doses >50 mg/day
Dosage adjustment in renal impairment: CrCl <10 mL/minute: Avoid use.
Note: ACC/AHA 2009 Adult Heart Failure guidelines suggest that thiazides lose their efficacy when CrCl <40 mL/minute.

Administration Oral: May administer with food or milk; administer early in day to avoid nocturia; if multiple daily dosing, the last dose should not be administered later than 6 PM unless instructed otherwise.

Monitoring Parameters Serum electrolytes, BUN, creatinine, blood pressure, fluid balance, body weight, urinary electrolytes (if applicable); serum glucose levels

Test Interactions May interfere with parathyroid function tests and may decrease serum iodine (protein bound) without signs of thyroid disturbance.

Dosage Forms Excipient information presented when available (limited, particularly for generics); consult specific product labeling.
Capsule, Oral:
Microzide: 12.5 mg
Generic: 12.5 mg
Tablet, Oral:
Generic: 12.5 mg, 25 mg, 50 mg

References
Albersheim SG, Solimano AJ, Sharma AK, et al, "Randomized, Double-Blind, Controlled Trial of Long-Term Diuretic Therapy for Bronchopulmonary Dysplasia," *J Pediatr*, 1989, 115(4):615-20.
American College of Obstetricians and Gynecologists (ACOG), "ACOG Practice Bulletin No. 125: Chronic Hypertension in Pregnancy," *Obstet Gynecol*, 2012, 119(2 Pt 1):396-407.
Chemtob S, Kaplan BS, Sherbotie JR, et al, "Pharmacology of Diuretics in the Newborn," *Pediatr Clin North Am*, 1989, 36(5):1231-50.
Chobanian AV, Bakris GL, Black HR, et al, "The Seventh Report of the Joint National Committee on Prevention, Detection, Evaluation, and Treatment of High Blood Pressure: The JNC 7 Report," *JAMA*, 2003, 289(19):2560-72.
Copelovitch L, "Urolithiasis in Children: Medical Approach," *Pediatr Clin North Am*, 2012, 59(4):881-96.
Engelhardt B, Blalock WA, DonLevy S, et al, "Effect of Spironolactone-Hydrochlorothiazide on Lung Function in Infants With Chronic Bronchopulmonary Dysplasia," *J Pediatr*, 1989, 114:619-24.
Kirchlechner V, Koller DY, Seidl R, et al, "Treatment of Nephrogenic Diabetes Insipidus With Hydrochlorothiazide and Amiloride," *Arch Dis Child*, 1999, 80(6):548-52.
National Heart, Lung, and Blood Institute, "Expert Panel on Integrated Guidelines for Cardiovascular Health and Risk Reduction in Children and Adolescents," *Clinical Practice Guidelines*, 2011, National Institutes of Health. Available at http://www.nhlbi.nih.gov/guidelines/cvd_ped/peds_guidelines_full.pdf. Last accessed: June 2012.
Miller ME, Cohn RD, and Burghart PH, "Hydrochlorothiazide Disposition in a Mother and Her Breast-Fed Infant," *J Pediatr*, 1982, 101 (5):789-91.
National High Blood Pressure Education Program Working Group on High Blood Pressure in Children and Adolescents, "The Fourth Report on the Diagnosis, Evaluation, and Treatment of High Blood Pressure in Children and Adolescents," *Pediatrics*, 2004, 114(2 Suppl):555-76.
van der Vorst MM, Kist JE, van der Heijden AJ, et al, "Diuretics in Pediatrics: Current Knowledge and Future Prospects," *Paediatr Drugs*, 2006, 8(4):245-64.
van Lieburg AF, Knoers NV, and Monnens LA, "Clinical Presentation and Follow-Up of 30 Patients With Congenital Nephrogenic Diabetes Insipidus," *J Am Soc Nephrol*, 1999, 10(9):1958-64.

Hydrochlorothiazide and Spironolactone
(hye droe klor oh THYE a zide & speer on oh LAK tone)

Medication Safety Issues
Sound-alike/look-alike issues:
Aldactazide may be confused with Aldactone
Brand Names: U.S. Aldactazide
Brand Names: Canada Aldactazide 25; Aldactazide 50; Teva-Spironolactone/HCTZ
Therapeutic Category Antihypertensive Agent, Combination; Diuretic, Combination
Generic Availability (U.S.) Yes
Use Treatment of edematous conditions associated with heart failure, cirrhosis of the liver, and nephrotic syndrome when other diuretics are inappropriate (eg, hypokalemia) or lacked adequate response (FDA approved in adults); treatment of primary hypertension (FDA approved in adults). **Note:** Use in pregnancy should be reserved for those cases causing extreme discomfort and unrelieved by rest; should not be routinely used during pregnancy.
Pregnancy Risk Factor C
Pregnancy Considerations Animal reproduction studies have not been conducted with this combination product. See individual agents.
Breast-Feeding Considerations The active metabolite of spironolactone (canrenone) and thiazide diuretics are found in breast milk. Due to the potential for serious adverse reactions in the nursing infant, the manufacturer recommends a decision be made whether to discontinue nursing or to discontinue the drug, taking into account the importance of treatment to the mother. See individual agents.
Contraindications Hypersensitivity to hydrochlorothiazide, spironolactone, or any component; cross-sensitivity with other thiazides or sulfonamides; anuria, hyperkalemia, acute or significant renal impairment, acute or severe hepatic failure
Warnings This fixed combination is not indicated for initial therapy of hypertension or edema [U.S. Boxed Warning]; therapy requires titration to the individual patient; if dosage so determined represents this fixed combination, its use may be more convenient; use with caution in impaired hepatic function, electrolyte changes may precipitate hepatic encephalopathy; spironolactone has been shown to be a tumorigen in chronic toxicity animal studies [U.S. Boxed Warning].

Hypersensitivity reactions may occur with hydrochlorothiazide. Risk is increased in patients with a history of allergy or bronchial asthma. Chemical similarities are present among sulfonamides, sulfonylureas, carbonic anhydrase inhibitors, thiazides, and loop diuretics (except ethacrynic acid). Use in patients with sulfonamide allergy is specifically contraindicated in product labeling; however, a risk of cross-reaction exists in patients with allergy to any of these compounds; avoid use when previous reaction has been severe. Discontinue if signs of hypersensitivity are noted.

May cause acute transient myopia and acute angle-closure glaucoma with potential for loss of vision; typically occurring within hours to weeks following initiation; discontinue therapy immediately in patients with acute decreases in visual acuity or ocular pain. Risk factors may include a history of sulfonamide or penicillin allergy. May cause SLE exacerbation or activation. Photosensitization may occur; patients should be counseled. May cause gynecomastia; development associated with dose and duration of therapy; typically is reversible upon discontinuation.

Precautions Hyperkalemia may occur with spironolactone; risk factors include renal dysfunction, diabetes mellitus, and concomitant use of potassium-sparing diuretics, potassium supplements, and/or potassium-containing salts. Use cautiously, if at all, with these agents and monitor potassium closely. Concomitant administration of potassium-sparing diuretics (eg, amiloride and triamterene) and ACE inhibitors or NSAIDs has been associated with severe hyperkalemia; may cause transient elevation of BUN, possibly due to a concentration effect; sustained elevations should be evaluated.

Use with caution in patients with moderate or high cholesterol concentrations; increased cholesterol and triglyceride levels have been reported with thiazides. Use with caution in patients with prediabetes or diabetes mellitus; may alter glucose control. Use with caution in patients having a history of gout; thiazide diuretics may cause hyperuricemia and in certain patients with a history of gout, a familial predisposition to gout, or chronic renal failure, gout can be precipitated. Use with caution in patients with hypercalcemia or parathyroid disease; thiazide diuretics may decrease renal calcium excretion; pathologic changes in the parathyroid glands with hypercalcemia and hypophosphatemia have been observed with prolonged use.

Adverse Reactions See individual agents.

Drug Interactions

  Metabolism/Transport Effects None known.

  Avoid Concomitant Use

  Avoid concomitant use of Hydrochlorothiazide and Spironolactone with any of the following: AMILoride; CycloSPORINE (Systemic); Dofetilide; Tacrolimus (Systemic); Triamterene

  Increased Effect/Toxicity

  Hydrochlorothiazide and Spironolactone may increase the levels/effects of: ACE Inhibitors; Allopurinol; Amifostine; Ammonium Chloride; Antihypertensives; Benazepril; Calcium Salts; CarBAMazepine; Cardiac Glycosides; Cyclophosphamide; CycloSPORINE (Systemic); Diazoxide; Digoxin; Dofetilide; DULoxetine; Hypotensive Agents; Ivabradine; Lithium; Multivitamins/Minerals (with ADEK, Folate, Iron); Multivitamins/Minerals (with AE, No Iron); Neuromuscular-Blocking Agents (Nondepolarizing); Obinutuzumab; OXcarbazepine; Porfimer; RiTUXimab; Sodium Phosphates; Tacrolimus (Systemic); Topiramate; Toremifene; Valsartan; Vitamin D Analogs

  The levels/effects of Hydrochlorothiazide and Spironolactone may be increased by: Alcohol (Ethyl); Alfuzosin; AMILoride; Analgesics (Opioid); Angiotensin II Receptor Blockers; Anticholinergic Agents; AtorvaSTATin; Barbiturates; Beta2-Agonists; Brimonidine (Topical); Canagliflozin; Corticosteroids (Orally Inhaled); Corticosteroids (Systemic); Diazoxide; Drospirenone; Eplerenone; Heparin; Heparin (Low Molecular Weight); Herbs (Hypotensive Properties); Licorice; MAO Inhibitors; Multivitamins/Fluoride (with ADE); Nitrofurantoin; Nonsteroidal Anti-Inflammatory Agents; Pentoxifylline; Phosphodiesterase 5 Inhibitors; Potassium Salts; Prostacyclin Analogues;

Selective Serotonin Reuptake Inhibitors; Tolvaptan; Triamterene; Trimethoprim; Valsartan

  Decreased Effect

  Hydrochlorothiazide and Spironolactone may decrease the levels/effects of: Abiraterone Acetate; Alpha-/Beta-Agonists; Antidiabetic Agents; Cardiac Glycosides; Mitotane; QuiNIDine

  The levels/effects of Hydrochlorothiazide and Spironolactone may be decreased by: Benazepril; Bile Acid Sequestrants; Herbs (Hypertensive Properties); Methylphenidate; Nonsteroidal Anti-Inflammatory Agents; Yohimbine

Food Interactions Excessive potassium intake may cause hyperkalemia. Management: Avoid food with high potassium content and potassium-containing salt substitutes.

Stability Store below 25°C (77°F).

Pharmacokinetics (Adult data unless noted) See individual agents.

Dosing: Usual Note: Product is a fixed combination of equal **mg proportions of components**; the following dosage represents mg of each component (spironolactone and hydrochlorothiazide).

Infants, Children, and Adolescents: **Hypertension, diuresis:**

  Infants: Limited data available: Oral: 1-3 mg/kg/day in divided doses once or twice daily (Engelhardt, 1989)

  Children and Adolescents: Oral: Initial: 1 mg/kg/day in divided doses once or twice daily, may titrate up to maximum daily dose: 3-3.3 mg/kg/**day** or 100 mg/**day** of spironolactone (NHBPEP, 2004; NHLBI, 2011)

Adults: **Hypertension, edema:** Oral: 12.5-50 mg/day; manufacturer labeling states hydrochlorothiazide maximum 200 mg/day; however, usual dose in JNC-7 is 12.5-50 mg/day

Dosing adjustment in renal impairment: Adults: Efficacy of hydrochlorothiazide is limited in patients with CrCl <30 mL/minute; contraindicated in patients with anuria

Administration Oral: Administer in the morning; administer the last dose of multiple doses before 6 PM unless instructed otherwise

Monitoring Parameters Serum electrolytes, BUN, creatinine, blood pressure, fluid balance, body weight

Test Interactions See individual agents.

Dosage Forms Excipient information presented when available (limited, particularly for generics); consult specific product labeling.

  Tablet: Hydrochlorothiazide 25 mg and spironolactone 25 mg

  Aldactazide:

    25/25: Hydrochlorothiazide 25 mg and spironolactone 25 mg

    50/50: Hydrochlorothiazide 50 mg and spironolactone 50 mg

Extemporaneous Preparations An oral suspension containing hydrochlorothiazide 5 mg and spironolactone 5 mg per mL may be made with tablets. Crush twenty-four 25 mg hydrochlorothiazide and twenty-four 25 mg spironolactone tablets and reduce to a fine powder. Add small portions of a 1:1 mixture of Ora-Sweet and Ora-Plus and mix to a uniform paste; mix while adding the vehicle in equal proportions to **almost** 120 mL; transfer to a calibrated bottle, rinse mortar with vehicle, and add sufficient quantity of vehicle to make 120 mL. Label "shake well". Stable 60 days under refrigeration or at room temperature. Allen LV and Erickson MA, "Stability of Extemporaneously Prepared Pediatric Formulations Using Ora-Plus With Ora-Sweet and Ora-Sweet SF – Part II," *Secundum Artem,* Volume 6 (1). Available at: www.paddocklabs.com.

References

Chobanian AV, Bakris GL, Black HR, et al, "The Seventh Report of the Joint National Committee on Prevention, Detection, Evaluation, and Treatment of High Blood Pressure: The JNC 7 Report," *JAMA*, 2003, 289(19):2560-72.

Engelhardt B, Blalock WA, DonLevy S, et al, "Effect of Spironolactone-Hydrochlorothiazide on Lung Function in Infants With Chronic Bronchopulmonary Dysplasia," *J Pediatrics*, 1989, 114:619-24.

National Heart, Lung, and Blood Institute, "Expert Panel on Integrated Guidelines for Cardiovascular Health and Risk Reduction in Children and Adolescents," *Clinical Practice Guidelines*, 2011, National Institutes of Health. Available at http://www.nhlbi.nih.gov/guidelines/cvd_ped/peds_guidelines_full.pdf. Date accessed: June 11, 2012.

National High Blood Pressure Education Program Working Group on High Blood Pressure in Children and Adolescents, "The Fourth Report on the Diagnosis, Evaluation, and Treatment of High Blood Pressure in Children and Adolescents," *Pediatrics*, 2004, 114(2 Suppl 4th Report):555-76.

Hydrocodone and Acetaminophen
(hye droe KOE done & a seet a MIN oh fen)

Medication Safety Issues
Sound-alike/look-alike issues:
Hydrocodone and Acetaminophen may be confused with Oxycodone and Acetaminophen

Lorcet® may be confused with Fioricet®

Lortab® may be confused with Cortef®

Vicodin® may be confused with Hycodan, Indocin®

Zydone® may be confused with Vytone

High alert medication:
The Institute for Safe Medication Practices (ISMP) includes this medication among its list of drug classes which have a heightened risk of causing significant patient harm when used in error.

Other safety concerns:
Duplicate therapy issues: This product contains acetaminophen, which may be a component of other combination products. Do not exceed the maximum recommended daily dose of acetaminophen.

Related Information
Opioid Conversion Table *on page 2242*

Brand Names: U.S. hycet®; Lorcet® 10/650 [DSC]; Lorcet® Plus [DSC]; Lortab®; Maxidone® [DSC]; Norco®; Stagesic™ [DSC]; Vicodin ES®; Vicodin HP®; Vicodin®; Xodol® 10/300; Xodol® 5/300; Xodol® 7.5/300; Zamicet™; Zolvit® [DSC]; Zydone® [DSC]

Therapeutic Category Analgesic, Narcotic; Antitussive; Cough Preparation

Generic Availability (U.S.) Yes: Oral solution, tablet

Use Relief of moderate to moderately severe pain (Oral solution or oral elixir: FDA approved in ages ≥2 years and adults; Capsules and tablets: FDA approved in adults)

Pregnancy Risk Factor C

Pregnancy Considerations Animal reproduction studies have not been conducted with this combination product. See individual agents.

Breast-Feeding Considerations Acetaminophen and hydrocodone are excreted in breast milk. Due to the potential for serious adverse reactions in the nursing infant, the manufacturer recommends a decision be made whether to discontinue nursing or to discontinue the drug, taking into account the importance of treatment to the mother. See individual agents.

Contraindications Hypersensitivity to hydrocodone, acetaminophen, or any component; CNS depression; severe respiratory depression

Warnings Acetaminophen may cause severe hepatotoxicity **[U.S. Boxed Warning]**, potentially requiring liver transplant or resulting in death; hepatotoxicity is usually associated with excessive acetaminophen intake (>4 g/day in adults). Risk is increased with alcohol use, preexisting liver disease, and intake of more than one source of acetaminophen-containing medications. Chronic daily dosing in adults has also resulted in liver damage in some

patients. Do not exceed maximum daily doses; consider acetaminophen content of all products (prescription and OTC), including combination products when evaluating the total daily dose of acetaminophen; adults ingesting >4 g/day of acetaminophen should seek medical attention immediately.

Hypersensitivity and anaphylactic reactions have been reported with acetaminophen and hydrocodone; use with caution in patients with hypersensitivity reactions to other phenanthrene derivative opioid agonists (morphine, codeine, hydromorphone, oxycodone, oxymorphone, levorphanol); discontinue immediately if symptoms of allergic or hypersensitivity reactions occur. Serious and potentially fatal skin reactions, including acute generalized exanthematous pustulosis (AGEP), Stevens-Johnson syndrome (SJS), and toxic epidermal necrolysis (TEN), have occurred rarely with acetaminophen use. Discontinue therapy at the first appearance of skin rash.

Hydrocodone may cause CNS depression which may impair physical or mental abilities; patients must be cautioned about performing tasks which require mental alertness (eg, operating machinery or driving). Respiratory depression may occur even at therapeutic dosages; use with extreme caution in infants and in patients with respiratory diseases including asthma, emphysema, COPD, cor pulmonale, hypoxia, hypercapnia, preexisting respiratory depression, significantly decreased respiratory reserve, other obstructive pulmonary disease, kyphoscoliosis, or other skeletal disorder which may alter respiratory function.

Use with extreme caution in patients with head injury, intracranial lesions, or elevated intracranial pressure; exaggerated elevation of ICP may occur. May cause hypotension; use with caution in patients with circulatory shock, hypovolemia, impaired myocardial function, or those receiving drugs which may exaggerate hypotensive effects (including phenothiazines or general anesthetics). Hydrocodone may obscure diagnosis or clinical course of patients with acute abdominal conditions.

Physical and psychological dependence may occur; abrupt discontinuation after prolonged use may result in withdrawal symptoms; warn patients of possible impairment of alertness or physical coordination; concurrent use of agonist/antagonist analgesics (ie, pentazocine, nalbuphine, and butorphanol) may precipitate withdrawal symptoms and/or reduce analgesic efficacy in patients following prolonged therapy with mu opioid agonists such as hydrocodone. High potential for abuse; healthcare providers should be alert to problems of abuse, misuse, and diversion. Infants born to women physically dependent on opioids will also be physically dependent and may experience respiratory difficulties or opioid withdrawal symptoms ([neonatal abstinence syndrome NAS)]. Onset, duration, and severity of NAS depend upon the drug used (maternal), duration of use, maternal dose, and rate of drug elimination by the newborn. Symptoms of opioid withdrawal may include excessive crying, diarrhea, fever, hyper-reflexia, irritability, tremors, or vomiting or failure to gain weight. Opioid withdrawal syndrome in the neonate may be life-threatening and should be promptly treated.

Due to the role of CYP2D6 in the metabolism of hydrocodone to hydromorphone (an active metabolite with higher binding affinity to mu-opioid receptors compared to hydrocodone), patients with genetic variations of CYP2D6, including "poor metabolizers" or "extensive metabolizers," may have decreased or increased hydromorphone formation, respectively. Variable effects in positive and negative opioid effects have been reported in these patients; however, unlike codeine, limited data exists with hydrocodone to determine if clinically significant differences of analgesia and toxicity can be predicted based on

▶

CYP2D6 phenotype (Hutchinson, 2004; Otton, 1993; Zhou, 2009).

Some tablets contain tartrazine which may cause allergic reactions in susceptible individuals. Some liquid formulations contain propylene glycol and alcohol (~7%); toxicities have been reported with use of products containing propylene glycol, including hyperosmolality, lactic acidosis, seizures, and respiratory depression; in neonates large amounts of propylene glycol delivered orally, intravenously (eg, >3000 mg/day), or topically have been associated with potentially fatal toxicities which can include metabolic acidosis, seizures, renal failure, and CNS depression; use products containing propylene glycol with caution (AAP, 1997; Shehab, 2009).

Precautions Use with caution in patients with adrenal insufficiency (Addison's disease), biliary tract disease, pancreatitis, CNS depression/coma, acute alcoholism, delirium tremens, hypothyroidism (myxedema), severe liver, pulmonary or renal impairment, urinary stricture, prostatic hypertrophy, or seizures.

Use caution when combining with other CNS depressants (eg, centrally acting antiemetics, general anesthetics, phenothiazines, sedative-hypnotics) as there may be additive CNS effects. If combined therapy is needed, consider reducing the dose of one or both agents.

Although several case reports of acetaminophen-associated hemolytic anemia have been reported in patients with G-6-PD deficiency, a direct cause and effect relationship has not been well established (concurrent illnesses such as fever or infection may precipitate hemolytic anemia in patients with G-6-PD deficiency); therefore, acetaminophen is generally thought to be safe when given in therapeutic doses to patients with G-6-PD deficiency.

Adverse Reactions

Cardiovascular: Bradycardia, cardiac arrest, circulatory collapse, coma, hypotension

Central nervous system: Anxiety, dizziness, drowsiness, dysphoria, euphoria, fear, lethargy, lightheadedness, malaise, mental clouding, mental impairment, mood changes, physiological dependence, sedation, somnolence, stupor

Dermatologic: Pruritus, rash

Endocrine & metabolic: Hypoglycemic coma

Gastrointestinal: Abdominal pain, constipation, gastric distress, heartburn, nausea, peptic ulcer, vomiting, xerostomia

Genitourinary: Ureteral spasm, urinary retention, vesical sphincter spasm

Hematologic: Agranulocytosis, bleeding time prolonged, hemolytic anemia, iron deficiency anemia, occult blood loss, thrombocytopenia

Hepatic: Hepatic necrosis, hepatitis

Neuromuscular & skeletal: Skeletal muscle rigidity

Otic: Hearing impairment or loss (chronic overdose)

Renal: Renal toxicity, renal tubular necrosis

Respiratory: Acute airway obstruction, apnea, dyspnea, respiratory depression (dose related)

Miscellaneous: Allergic reactions, clamminess, diaphoresis

Drug Interactions

Metabolism/Transport Effects Refer to individual components.

Avoid Concomitant Use

Avoid concomitant use of Hydrocodone and Acetaminophen with any of the following: Alcohol (Ethyl); Azelastine (Nasal); Conivaptan; Fusidic Acid (Systemic); MAO Inhibitors; Paraldehyde; Pimozide; Thalidomide

Increased Effect/Toxicity

Hydrocodone and Acetaminophen may increase the levels/effects of: Alvimopan; Azelastine (Nasal); Buprenorphine; Busulfan; Dasatinib; Desmopressin; Diuretics;

Dofetilide; Imatinib; Lomitapide; Methotrimeprazine; Metyrosine; Mipomersen; Paraldehyde; Phenylephrine (Systemic); Pimozide; Pramipexole; Prilocaine; ROPINIRole; Rotigotine; Selective Serotonin Reuptake Inhibitors; Sodium Nitrite; SORAfenib; Thalidomide; Vitamin K Antagonists; Zolpidem

The levels/effects of Hydrocodone and Acetaminophen may be increased by: Alcohol (Ethyl); Amphetamines; Anticholinergic Agents; Brimonidine (Topical); Cannabis; Ceritinib; CNS Depressants; Conivaptan; CYP3A4 Inhibitors (Moderate); CYP3A4 Inhibitors (Strong); Dasatinib; Dronabinol; Droperidol; Fusidic Acid (Systemic); Isoniazid; Ivacaftor; Kava Kava; Luliconazole; Magnesium Sulfate; MAO Inhibitors; Methotrimeprazine; Metyrapone; Mifepristone; Nabilone; Nitric Oxide; Perampanel; Probenecid; Rufinamide; Simeprevir; Sodium Oxybate; SORAfenib; Stiripentol; Succinylcholine; Tapentadol; Tetrahydrocannabinol

Decreased Effect

Hydrocodone and Acetaminophen may decrease the levels/effects of: Pegvisomant

The levels/effects of Hydrocodone and Acetaminophen may be decreased by: Ammonium Chloride; Bosentan; Cholestyramine Resin; CYP3A4 Inducers (Strong); Dabrafenib; Deferasirox; Mitotane; Naltrexone; Peginterferon Alfa-2b; QuiNIDine; Siltuximab; St Johns Wort; Tocilizumab

Stability Store at 20°C to 25°C (68°F to 77°F); protect from light. Capsules: Protect from moisture.

Mechanism of Action Hydrocodone, as with other opioid analgesics, blocks pain perception in the cerebral cortex by binding to specific receptor molecules (opiate receptors) within the neuronal membranes of synapses. This binding results in a decreased synaptic chemical transmission throughout the CNS thus inhibiting the flow of pain sensations into the higher centers. Mu and kappa are the two subtypes of the opiate receptor which hydrocodone binds to cause analgesia.

Acetaminophen inhibits the synthesis of prostaglandins in the CNS and peripherally blocks pain impulse generation; produces antipyresis from inhibition of hypothalamic heat-regulating center.

Pharmacodynamics Opioid analgesia:

Onset of action: Within 10-20 minutes

Duration: 4-6 hours

Pharmacokinetics (Adult data unless noted) Hydrocodone:

Metabolism: Hepatic; O-demethylation via primarily CYP2D6 to hydromorphone (major, active metabolite with 10- to 33-fold higher or as much as a >100-fold higher binding affinity for the mu-opioid receptor than hydrocodone); N-demethylation via CYP3A4 to norhydrocodone (major metabolite); ~40% of metabolism/clearance occurs via non-CYP pathways, including 5-ketosteroid reduction to 6-alpha-hydrocol and 6-beta-hydrocol, and other elimination pathways (eg, fecal, biliary, intestinal, renal) (Hutchinson, 2004; Volpe, 2011; Zhou, 2009)

Half-life elimination: ~4 hours

Time to peak serum concentration: 1-1.6 hours

Elimination: Urine (26% of single dose in 72 hours, with ~12% as unchanged drug, 5% as norhydrocodone, 4% as conjugated hydrocodone, 3% as 6-hydrocodol, and 0.1% as conjugated 6-hydromorphol) (Zhou, 2009)

Dosing: Usual Note: Doses based on hydrocodone; titrate to appropriate analgesic effect.

Infants, Children, and Adolescents: Analgesic; opioid-naive patients (American Pain Society, 2008; Kleigman, 2011): Limited data available in infants and children <2 years: **Note:** Maximum daily dose of acetaminophen should be limited to ≤75 mg/kg/**day** in ≤5 divided doses and not to exceed 4000 mg/**day** (and possibly less in patients with hepatic impairment or ethanol use).

Patient weight:
<50 kg: Oral: Usual initial dose: Hydrocodone 0.1-0.2 mg/kg/dose every 4-6 hours; in infants, reduced doses and close monitoring should be considered due to possible increased sensitivity to respiratory depressant effects; use with caution in infants.

≥50 kg: Oral: Usual initial dose: Hydrocodone 5-10 mg every 4-6 hours

Adults: **Analgesic:** Oral: Average starting dose in opioid-naive patients: Hydrocodone 5-10 mg 4 times daily; maximum daily dose of acetaminophen should be limited to ≤4000 mg/day (and possibly less in patients with hepatic impairment or ethanol use).

Dosage ranges (based on specific product labeling): Hydrocodone 2.5-10 mg every 4-6 hours; maximum dose of hydrocodone may be limited by the acetaminophen content of specific product

Administration Oral: May administer with food or milk to decrease GI distress

Monitoring Parameters Pain relief; respiratory rate; mental status; blood pressure; signs of misuse, abuse, and addiction

Test Interactions Acetaminophen may cause false-positive urinary 5-hydroxyindoleacetic acid.

Controlled Substance C-III

Dosage Forms Excipient information presented when available (limited, particularly for generics); consult specific product labeling.

Capsule, oral:
Stagesic™: Hydrocodone bitartrate 5 mg and acetaminophen 500 mg [DSC]

Elixir, oral:
Lortab®: Hydrocodone bitartrate 7.5 mg and acetaminophen 500 mg per 15 mL (480 mL) [contains ethanol 7%, propylene glycol; tropical fruit punch flavor] [DSC]
Lortab®: Hydrocodone bitartrate 10 mg and acetaminophen 300 mg per 15 mL (480 mL) [contains ethanol 7%, propylene glycol; tropical fruit punch flavor]

Solution, oral: Hydrocodone bitartrate 7.5 mg and acetaminophen 325 mg per 15 mL; hydrocodone bitartrate 7.5 mg and acetaminophen 500 mg per 15 mL (5 mL [DSC], 10 mL [DSC], 15 mL [DSC], 118 mL [DSC], 473 mL [DSC])

hycet®: Hydrocodone bitartrate 7.5 mg and acetaminophen 325 mg per 15 mL (473 mL) [contains ethanol 7%, propylene glycol; tropical fruit punch flavor]
Zamicet™: Hydrocodone bitartrate 10 mg and acetaminophen 325 mg per 15 mL (473 mL) [contains ethanol 6.7%, propylene glycol; fruit flavor]
Zolvit®: Hydrocodone bitartrate 10 mg and acetaminophen 300 mg per 15 mL (480 mL) [contains ethanol 7%, propylene glycol; tropical fruit punch flavor] [DSC]

Tablet, oral:
Hydrocodone bitartrate 2.5 mg and acetaminophen 325 mg
Hydrocodone bitartrate 2.5 mg and acetaminophen 500 mg [DSC]
Hydrocodone bitartrate 5 mg and acetaminophen 300 mg
Hydrocodone bitartrate 5 mg and acetaminophen 325 mg
Hydrocodone bitartrate 5 mg and acetaminophen 500 mg [DSC]
Hydrocodone bitartrate 7.5 mg and acetaminophen 300 mg
Hydrocodone bitartrate 7.5 mg and acetaminophen 325 mg
Hydrocodone bitartrate 7.5 mg and acetaminophen 500 mg [DSC]
Hydrocodone bitartrate 7.5 mg and acetaminophen 650 mg [DSC]

Hydrocodone bitartrate 7.5 mg and acetaminophen 750 mg DSC]
Hydrocodone bitartrate 10 mg and acetaminophen 300 mg
Hydrocodone bitartrate 10 mg and acetaminophen 325 mg
Hydrocodone bitartrate 10 mg and acetaminophen 500 mg [DSC]
Hydrocodone bitartrate 10 mg and acetaminophen 650 mg DSC]
Hydrocodone bitartrate 10 mg and acetaminophen 750 mg [DSC]
Lorcet® 10/650: Hydrocodone bitartrate 10 mg and acetaminophen 650 mg [DSC]
Lorcet® Plus: Hydrocodone bitartrate 7.5 mg and acetaminophen 650 mg [DSC]
Lortab®:
5/500: Hydrocodone bitartrate 5 mg and acetaminophen 500 mg [DSC]
7.5/500: Hydrocodone bitartrate 7.5 mg and acetaminophen 500 mg [DSC]
10/500: Hydrocodone bitartrate 10 mg and acetaminophen 500 mg [DSC]
Maxidone®: Hydrocodone bitartrate 10 mg and acetaminophen 750 mg [DSC]
Norco®:
Hydrocodone bitartrate 5 mg and acetaminophen 325 mg
Hydrocodone bitartrate 7.5 mg and acetaminophen 325 mg
Hydrocodone bitartrate 10 mg and acetaminophen 325 mg
Vicodin®: Hydrocodone bitartrate 5 mg and acetaminophen 300 mg
Vicodin ES®: Hydrocodone bitartrate 7.5 mg and acetaminophen 300 mg
Vicodin HP®: Hydrocodone bitartrate 10 mg and acetaminophen 300 mg
Xodol®:
5/300: Hydrocodone bitartrate 5 mg and acetaminophen 300 mg
7.5/300: Hydrocodone bitartrate 7.5 mg and acetaminophen 300 mg
10/300: Hydrocodone bitartrate 10 mg and acetaminophen 300 mg
Zydone®:
Hydrocodone bitartrate 5 mg and acetaminophen 400 mg [DSC]
Hydrocodone bitartrate 7.5 mg and acetaminophen 400 mg [DSC]
Hydrocodone bitartrate 10 mg and acetaminophen 400 mg [DSC]

References

American Academy of Pediatrics Committee on Drugs. "Inactive" ingredients in pharmaceutical products: update (subject review). *Pediatrics.* 1997;99(2):268-278.

Bean-Lijewski JD, Kruitbosch SH, Hutchinson L, et al, "Post-Tonsillectomy Pain Management in Children: Can We Do Better?" *Otolaryngol Head Neck Surg,* 2007, 137(4):545-51.

Broussard CS, Rasmussen SA, Reefhuis J, et al. National birth defects prevention study: maternal treatment with opioid analgesics and risk for birth defects. *Am J Obstet Gynecol.* 2011;204(4):314.

Hutchinson MR, Menelaou A, Foster DJ, et al. CYP2D6 and CYP3A4 involvement in the primary oxidative metabolism of hydrocodone by human liver microsomes. *Br J of Clin Pharm.* 2004;57(3):287-297.

Kliegman RM, Stanton BF, St. Gemell JW, et al, eds. *Nelson Textbook of Pediatrics.* 19th ed. Philadelphia, PA: Saunders Elsevier;2011.

Otton SV, Schadel M, Cheung SW, et al. CYP2D6 phenotype determines the metabolic conversion of hydrocodone to hydromorphone. *Clin Pharmacol Ther.* 1993;54(5):463-472.

"Principles of Analgesic Use in the Treatment of Acute Pain and Cancer Pain," 6th ed, Glenview, IL: American Pain Society, 2008.

Sauberan JB, Anderson PO, Lane JR, et al. Breast milk hydrocodone and hydromorphone levels in mothers using hydrocodone for postpartum pain. *Obstet Gynecol.* 2011;117(3):611-617.

Shehab N, Lewis CL, Streetman DD, Donn SM. Exposure to the pharmaceutical excipients benzyl alcohol and propylene glycol

◀ among critically ill neonates. *Pediatr Crit Care Med.* 2009;10
(2):256-259.

Volpe DA, McMahon Tobin GA, Mellon RD, et al. Uniform assessment
and ranking of opioid mu receptor binding constants for selected
opioid drugs. *Regul Toxicol Pharmacol.* 2011;59(3):385-390.

Zhou S. Polymorphism of human cytochrome P450 2D6 and its clinical
significance. *Clin Pharmacokinet.* 2009;48(12):761-804.

Hydrocodone and Chlorpheniramine
(hye droe KOE done & klor fen IR a meen)

Medication Safety Issues
Sound-alike/look-alike issues:
Tussionex represents a different product in the U.S. than
it does in Canada. In the U.S., Tussionex (Pennkinetic)
contains hydrocodone and chlorpheniramine, while in
Canada the product bearing this name contains hydrocodone and phenyltoloxamine.

High alert medication:
The Institute for Safe Medication Practices (ISMP)
includes this medication among its list of drug classes
which have a heightened risk of causing significant
patient harm when used in error.

Brand Names: U.S. TussiCaps; Tussionex Pennkinetic;
Vituz

Therapeutic Category Antihistamine; Antitussive; Cough
Preparation

Generic Availability (U.S.) Yes: Extended release suspension

Use Symptomatic relief of cough and upper respiratory
symptoms associated with cold and allergy (Extended
release: Capsules, Suspension: FDA approved in ages
≥6 years and adults; Immediate release: Oral solution:
FDA approved in ages ≥18 years and adults)

Pregnancy Risk Factor C

Pregnancy Considerations Animal reproduction studies
have not been conducted with this combination product.
See individual agents.

Breast-Feeding Considerations Hydrocodone and
chlorpheniramine are excreted into breast milk. Due to
the potential for serious adverse reactions in the nursing
infant, the manufacturer recommends a decision be made
whether to discontinue nursing or to discontinue the drug,
taking into account the importance of treatment to the
mother. See individual agents.

Contraindications Hypersensitivity to hydrocodone,
chlorpheniramine, or any component
Dosage form-specific contraindications:
Extended release capsule and extended release suspension: Children <6 years of age
Immediate release oral solution: Concurrent use during
or within 14 days of MAO inhibitor therapy; narrow angle
glaucoma; urinary retention; severe hypertension;
severe coronary artery disease

Warnings Underlying cause of cough should be determined prior to prescribing. Dose should not be increased
if cough does not respond; re-evaluate within 5 days for
possible underlying pathology. Hydrocodone produces
dose-related respiratory depression which can be fatal;
use is contraindicated in infants and children <6 years
due to fatal respiratory depression. Use with caution in
children ≥6 years, patients with pulmonary disease (including asthma) or decreased ventilatory function, or postoperative patients. Hydrocodone may cause CNS
depression which may impair physical or mental abilities;
patients must be cautioned about performing tasks which
require mental alertness (eg, operating machinery or driving); use caution when combining with other CNS depressants (eg, centrally acting antiemetics, general
anesthetics, phenothiazines, sedative-hypnotics) as there
may be additive CNS effects; if combination therapy with
one of these types of agents is needed with hydrocodone,
consider reducing the dose of one or both agents. Potentially significant drug interactions may exist, requiring dose

or frequency adjustment, additional monitoring, and/or
selection of alternative therapy.

Hydrocodone may exaggerate elevated intracranial pressure (ICP); use with extreme caution in patients with head
injury, intracranial lesions, or elevated ICP. Hydrocodone
may obscure diagnosis or clinical course of patients with
acute abdominal conditions; has been shown to decrease
gastrointestinal motility; use with caution in postoperative
patients especially after intra-abdominal surgery. Concurrent use of anticholinergics may result in paralytic ileus;
use caution. Physical and psychological dependence may
occur; abrupt discontinuation after prolonged use may
result in withdrawal symptoms. Accurate measuring devices should be used to measure solution and suspension
doses. Calibrated oral syringes are most accurate. Household teaspoons and tablespoons are not recommended for
measurement.

Due to the role of CYP2D6 in the metabolism of hydrocodone to hydromorphone (an active metabolite with
higher binding affinity to mu-opioid receptors compared
to hydrocodone), patients with genetic variations of
CYP2D6, including "poor metabolizers" or "extensive
metabolizers," may have decreased or increased hydromorphone formation, respectively. Variable effects in positive and negative opioid effects have been reported in
these patients; however, unlike codeine, limited data exists
with hydrocodone to determine if clinically significant differences of analgesia and toxicity can be predicted based on
CYP2D6 phenotype (Hutchinson, 2004; Otton, 1993;
Zhou, 2009).

Tussionnex contains polysorbate 80 (Tween 80); which
may cause allergic reactions in susceptible individuals.
TussiCaps, Tussionnex, and Vituz contain propylene glycol; toxicities have been reported with use of products
containing propylene glycol, including hyperosmolality,
lactic acidosis, seizures, and respiratory depression; in
neonates large amounts of propylene glycol delivered
orally, intravenously (eg, >3000 mg/day), or topically have
been associated with potentially fatal toxicities which can
include metabolic acidosis, seizures, renal failure, and
CNS depression; use hydrocodone/chlorpheniramine
products containing propylene glycol with caution (AAP,
1997; Shehab, 2009).

Precautions Use with caution in patients with hypersensitivity to other phenanthrene derivative opioid agonists
(morphine, codeine, hydromorphone, oxycodone, oxymorphone, levorphanol); discontinue immediately if symptoms
of allergic or hypersensitivity reactions occur. Use with
caution in patients with adrenal insufficiency (Addison's
disease); biliary tract disease (may cause constriction of
sphincter of Oddi); pancreatitis; obstructive bowel disease;
CNS depression/coma; acute alcoholism; delirium tremens; hypothyroidism (myxedema); severe liver, pulmonary, or renal impairment; urethral stricture or prostatic
hypertrophy (Vituz use is contraindicated in patients with
urinary retention). Use with caution in patients with
increased intraocular pressure or glaucoma; Vituz use is
contraindicated in narrow angle glaucoma. Hydrocodone
suppresses the cough reflex; caution should be exercised
when this agent is used postoperatively and in patients
with pulmonary diseases.

Adverse Reactions Also refer to Chlorpheniramine monograph.
Cardiovascular: Chest tightness
Central nervous system: Agitation, anxiety, confusion,
decreased mental acuity, dizziness, drowsiness, drug
dependence, dysphoria, euphoria, fear, headache, irritability, lethargy, mood changes, sedation
Dermatologic: Diaphoresis, erythema, pruritus, skin rash,
urticaria

Gastrointestinal: Abdominal distension, abdominal pain, acute pancreatitis, constipation, decreased appetite, dyspepsia, epigastric distress, nausea, vomiting, xerostomia

Genitourinary: Dysuria, ureteral spasm, urinary frequency, urinary hesitancy, urinary retention

Neuromuscular & skeletal: Facial dyskinesia, tremor, vesicle sphincter spasm

Ophthalmic: Blurred vision, diplopia, visual disturbance

Respiratory: Dry throat, dyspnea, laryngismus, respiratory depression, wheezing

Drug Interactions

Metabolism/Transport Effects

Hydrocodone: **Substrate** of CYP2D6 (major)

Chlorpheniramine: **Substrate** of CYP2D6 (minor), 3A4 (major); **Inhibits** CYP2D6 (weak)

Avoid Concomitant Use

Avoid concomitant use of Hydrocodone and Chlorpheniramine with any of the following: Aclidinium; Alcohol (Ethyl); Azelastine (Nasal); Conivaptan; Fusidic Acid (Systemic); Ipratropium (Oral Inhalation); MAO Inhibitors; Paraldehyde; Potassium Chloride; Thalidomide; Tiotropium; Umeclidinium

Increased Effect/Toxicity

Based on **hydrocodone** component: Increased toxicity: CNS depressants, MAO inhibitors, general anesthetics, and tricyclic antidepressants may potentiate the effects of opiate agonists; dextroamphetamine may enhance the analgesic effect of opiate agonists

Based on **chlorpheniramine** component: CYP2D6 enzyme substrate; Increased toxicity (CNS depression): CNS depressants, MAO inhibitors, tricyclic antidepressants, phenothiazines

Decreased Effect

Hydrocodone and Chlorpheniramine may decrease the levels/effects of: Acetylcholinesterase Inhibitors (Central); Benzylpenicilloyl Polylysine; Betahistine; Hyaluronidase; Pegvisomant; Secretin

The levels/effects of Hydrocodone and Chlorpheniramine may be decreased by: Acetylcholinesterase Inhibitors (Central); Ammonium Chloride; Amphetamines; Bosentan; CYP3A4 Inducers (Strong); Dabrafenib; Deferasirox; Mitotane; Naltrexone; Peginterferon Alfa-2b; Siltuximab; St Johns Wort; Tocilizumab

Stability

Extended release:

Capsule (TussiCaps): Store at 20°C to 25°C (68°F to 77°F).

Extended release suspension (Tussionex Pennkinetic): Store at 20°C to 25°C (68°F to 77°F); excursions permitted to 15°C to 30°C (59°F to 86°F).

Immediate release oral solution (Vituz): Store at 20°C to 25°C (68°F to 77°F); protect from light.

Mechanism of Action

Hydrocodone binds to opiate receptors in the CNS, altering the perception of and response to pain; suppresses cough in medullary center; produces generalized CNS depression

Chlorpheniramine competes with histamine for H_1-receptor sites on effector cells in the gastrointestinal tract, blood vessels, and respiratory tract

Pharmacodynamics

Onset of action: Chlorpheniramine: 6 hours

Duration: Chlorpheniramine: 24 hours

Pharmacokinetics (Adult data unless noted)

Distribution: V_d: Chlorpheniramine:

Children: 3.8 L/kg

Adults: 2.5-3.2 L/kg

Protein binding: Chlorpheniramine: 69% to 72%

Metabolism:

Chlorpheniramine: Substantial metabolism in GI mucosa and on first pass through liver

Hydrocodone: O-demethylation via primarily CYP2D6 to hydromorphone (major, active metabolite with ~10- to 33-fold higher or as much as a >100-fold higher binding affinity for the mu-opioid receptor than hydrocodone); N-demethylation via CYP3A4 to norhydrocodone (major metabolite); and ~40% of metabolism/clearance occurs via other non-CYP pathways, including 6-ketosteroid reduction to 6-alpha-hydrocol and 6-beta-hydrocol, and other elimination pathways (eg, fecal, biliary, intestinal, renal) (Hutchinson, 2004; Volpe, 2011; Zhou, 2009)

Half-life elimination:

Chlorpheniramine:

Children: Average: 9.6-13.1 hours (range: 5.2-23.1 hours)

Adults: 12-43 hours

Hydrocodone: ~4 hours

Time to peak serum concentration:

Extended release suspension:

Chlorpheniramine: 6.3 hours

Hydrocodone: 3.4 hours

Immediate release oral solution:

Chlorpheniramine: 3.5 hours

Hydrocodone: 1.4 hours

Elimination:

Chlorpheniramine: 35% excreted in 48 hours

Hydrocodone: Urine (26% of single dose in 72 hours, with ~12% as unchanged drug, 5% as norhydrocodone, 4% as conjugated hydrocodone, 3% as 6-hydrocodol, and 0.21% as conjugated 6-hydromorphol) (Zhou, 2009)

Dosing: Usual Note: Dosage units vary based on product (mg, mL, capsules, or tablets); use caution when verifying dose with product formulation.

Pediatric: **Cough (antitussive/antihistamine):** Oral: **Note:** Immediate release oral solution is **NOT** indicated for patients <18 years.

Children 6 to <12 years: Extended release:

Capsules (hydrocodone 5 mg and chlorpheniramine 4 mg per capsule): One capsule every 12 hours; maximum daily dose: 2 capsules/24 hours

Suspension (hydrocodone 10 mg and chlorpheniramine 8 mg per 5 mL): 2.5 mL every 12 hours; maximum daily dose: 5 mL/24 hours

Children ≥12 years and Adolescents: Extended release:

Capsules (hydrocodone 10 mg and chlorpheniramine 8 mg per capsule): One capsule every 12 hours; maximum daily dose: 2 capsules/24 hours

Suspension: (hydrocodone 10 mg and chlorpheniramine 8 mg per 5 mL): 5 mL every 12 hours; maximum daily dose: 10 mL/24 hours

Adult: **Cough (antitussive/antihistamine):** Oral:

Immediate release: Oral solution: 5 mL every 4-6 hours as needed; maximum daily dose: 20 mL/24 hours

Extended release:

Capsules (hydrocodone 10 mg and chlorpheniramine 8 mg per capsule): One capsule every 12 hours; maximum daily dose: 2 capsules/24 hours

Suspension: 5 mL every 12 hours; maximum daily dose: 10 mL/24 hours

Dosing adjustment in renal impairment: There are no dosage adjustments provided in the manufacturer's labeling; use with caution.

Dosing adjustment in hepatic impairment: There are no dosage adjustments provided in the manufacturer's labeling; use with caution.

Administration

Extended release:

Capsules: Administer without regard to meals. Do not dilute with fluid or mix with other medications. Do not give more frequently than every 12 hours. ▶

Suspension: Shake well before using. Do not dilute with fluid or mix with other medications. Use calibrated oral syringe to measure doses. Do not give more frequently than every 12 hours.

Immediate release: Oral solution: To prevent overdose, use calibrated oral syringe to measure doses.

Test Interactions Chlorpheniramine: May suppress the wheal and flare reactions to skin test antigens.

Controlled Substance C-III

Dosage Forms Excipient information presented when available (limited, particularly for generics); consult specific product labeling.

Capsule, extended release, oral:

TussiCaps® 5/4: Hydrocodone polistirex [equivalent to hydrocodone bitartrate 5 mg] and chlorpheniramine polistirex [equivalent to chlorpheniramine maleate 4 mg]

TussiCaps® 10/8: Hydrocodone polistirex [equivalent to hydrocodone bitartrate 10 mg] and chlorpheniramine polistirex [equivalent to chlorpheniramine maleate 8 mg]

Solution, oral:

Vituz®: Hydrocodone bitartrate 5 mg and chlorpheniramine maleate 4 mg per 5 mL (480 mL) [contains propylene glycol; grape flavor]

Suspension, extended release, oral: Hydrocodone polistirex [equivalent to hydrocodone bitartrate 10 mg] and chlorpheniramine polistirex [equivalent to chlorpheniramine maleate 8 mg] per 5 mL (480 mL)

Tussionex® Pennkinetic®: Hydrocodone polistirex [equivalent to hydrocodone bitartrate 10 mg] and chlorpheniramine polistirex [equivalent to chlorpheniramine maleate 8 mg] per 5 mL (115 mL, 480 mL [DSC]) [contains propylene glycol]

References

American Academy of Pediatrics Committee on Drugs, "'Inactive' Ingredients in Pharmaceutical Products: Update (Subject Review)," *Pediatr*, 1997, 99(2):268-78.

Broussard CS, Rasmussen SA, Reefhuis J, et al, "National Birth Defects Prevention Study: Maternal Treatment With Opioid Analgesics and Risk for Birth Defects," *Am J Obstet Gynecol*, 2011, 204 (4):314.

Hutchinson MR, Menelaou A, Foster DJ, et al, "CYP2D6 and CYP3A4 Involvement in the Primary Oxidative Metabolism of Hydrocodone by Human Liver Microsomes," *Br J Clin Pharmacol*, 2004, 57(3):287-97.

Otton SV, Schadel M, Cheung SW, et al, "CYP2D6 Phenotype Determines the Metabolic Conversion of Hydrocodone to Hydromorphone," *Clin Pharmacol Ther*, 1993, 54(5):463-72.

Sauberan JB, Anderson PO, Lane JR, et al, "Breast Milk Hydrocodone and Hydromorphone Levels in Mothers Using Hydrocodone for Postpartum Pain," *Obstet Gynecol*, 2011, 117(3):611-7.

Shehab N, Lewis CL, Streetman DD, Donn SM. Exposure to the pharmaceutical excipients benzyl alcohol and propylene glycol among critically ill neonates. *Pediatr Crit Care Med*. 2009;10 (2):256-259.

TussiCaps (hydrocodone polistirex and chlorpheniramine polistirex) [prescribing information]. Richmond, VA: ECR Pharmaceuticals; June 2012.

Tussionex (hydrocodone polistirex and chlorpheniramine polistirex) [prescribing information]. Smyrna, GA: UCB, Inc.; June 2011.

Vituz (hydrocodone bitartrate and chlorpheniramine maleate) [prescribing information]. Madison, MS: Hawthorn Pharmaceuticals, Inc.; February 2013.

Volpe DA, McMahon Tobin GA, Mellon RD, et al, "Uniform Assessment and Ranking of Opioid Mu Receptor Binding Constants for Selected Opioid Drugs," *Regul Toxicol Pharmacol*, 2011, 59(3):385-90.

Zhou SF, "Polymorphism of Human Cytochrome P450 2D6 and Its Clinical Significance: Part II," *Clin Pharmacokinet*, 2009, 48 (12):761-804.

Hydrocodone and Homatropine
(hye droe KOE done & hoe MA troe peen)

Medication Safety Issues

Sound-alike/look-alike issues:

Hycodan may be confused with Vicodin®

High alert medication:

The Institute for Safe Medication Practices (ISMP) includes this medication among its list of drug classes which have a heightened risk of causing significant patient harm when used in error.

Brand Names: U.S. Hydromet®; Tussigon®

Therapeutic Category Antitussive; Cough Preparation

Generic Availability (U.S.) Yes

Use Symptomatic relief of cough (FDA approved in ages ≥6 years and adults)

Pregnancy Risk Factor C

Pregnancy Considerations Animal reproduction studies have not been conducted with this combination. See individual agents.

Breast-Feeding Considerations Hydrocodone and homatropine are excreted in breast milk. Due to the potential for serious adverse reactions in the nursing infant, the manufacturer recommends a decision be made whether to discontinue nursing or to discontinue the drug, taking into account the importance of treatment to the mother. See individual agents.

Contraindications Hypersensitivity to hydrocodone, homatropine, or any component

Warnings Underlying cause of cough should be determined prior to prescribing. Dose should not be increased if cough does not respond; re-evaluate within 5 days for possible underlying pathology. Hydrocodone produces dose-related respiratory depression which can be fatal; use with caution in children, patients with pulmonary disease (including asthma) or decreased ventilatory function, or postoperative patients. Hydrocodone may cause CNS depression which may impair physical or mental abilities; patients must be cautioned about performing tasks which require mental alertness (eg, operating machinery or driving); use caution when combining with other CNS depressants (eg, centrally acting antiemetics, general anesthetics, phenothiazines, sedative-hypnotics) as there may be additive CNS effects. If combination therapy is needed, consider reducing the dose of one or both agents. Potentially significant interactions may exist, requiring dose or frequency adjustment, additional monitoring, and/or selection of alternative therapy.

Hydrocodone may exaggerate elevated intracranial pressure (ICP); use with extreme caution in patients with head injury, intracranial lesions, or elevated ICP. Hydrocodone may obscure diagnosis or clinical course of patients with acute abdominal conditions; has been shown to decrease gastrointestinal motility; use with caution in postoperative patients especially after intra-abdominal surgery. Physical and psychological dependence may occur; abrupt discontinuation after prolonged use may result in withdrawal symptoms.

Due to the role of CYP2D6 in the metabolism of hydrocodone to hydromorphone (an active metabolite with higher binding affinity to mu-opioid receptors compared to hydrocodone), patients with genetic variations of CYP2D6, including "poor metabolizers" or "extensive metabolizers" may have decreased or increased hydromorphone formation, respectively. Variable effects in positive and negative opioid effects have been reported in these patients; however, unlike codeine, limited data exists with hydrocodone to determine if clinically significant differences of analgesia and toxicity can be predicted based on CYP2D6 phenotype (Hutchinson, 2004; Otton, 1993; Zhou, 2009).

The oral syrup may contain propylene glycol; toxicities have been reported with use of products containing propylene glycol, including hyperosmolality, lactic acidosis, seizures, and respiratory depression; in neonates large amounts of propylene glycol delivered orally, intravenously (eg, >3000 mg/day), or topically have been associated with potentially fatal toxicities which can include metabolic acidosis, seizures, renal failure, and CNS depression; use oral syrup containing propylene glycol with caution (AAP, 1997; Shehab, 2009). Hydrocodone/homatropine syrup also contains sodium benzoate; benzoic acid (benzoate) is a metabolite of benzyl alcohol; large amounts of benzyl alcohol (≥99 mg/kg/day) have been associated with a potentially fatal toxicity ("gasping syndrome") in neonates; use hydrocodone/homatropine syrup containing sodium benzoate with caution in neonates; *in vitro* and animal studies have shown that benzoate displaces bilirubin from protein binding sites.

Precautions Use with caution in patients with hypersensitivity to other phenanthrene derivative opioid agonists (morphine, codeine, hydromorphone, oxycodone, oxymorphone, levorphanol); discontinue immediately if symptoms of allergic or hypersensitivity reactions occur. Use with caution in patients with adrenal insufficiency (Addison's disease); biliary tract disease (may cause constriction of sphincter of Oddi); pancreatitis; CNS depression/coma; acute alcoholism; delirium tremens; hypothyroidism (myxedema); severe liver, pulmonary, or renal impairment; urethral stricture or prostatic hypertrophy. Use with caution in patients with increased intraocular pressure or glaucoma.

Adverse Reactions

Central nervous system: Anxiety, dizziness, drowsiness, dysphoria, fear, lethargy, mental clouding, mental impairment, mood changes, sedation

Dermatologic: Pruritus, rash

Gastrointestinal: Constipation, nausea, vomiting, xerostomia

Genitourinary: Urinary retention, urinary tract spasm

Respiratory: Respiratory depression

Miscellaneous: Physical and psychological dependence with prolonged use

Rare but important or life-threatening: Cardiorespiratory arrest

Drug Interactions

Metabolism/Transport Effects Hydrocodone: **Substrate** of CYP2D6 (major)

Avoid Concomitant Use

Avoid concomitant use of Hydrocodone and Homatropine with any of the following: Aclidinium; Alcohol (Ethyl); Azelastine (Nasal); Conivaptan; Fusidic Acid (Systemic); Ipratropium (Oral Inhalation); MAO Inhibitors; Paraldehyde; Potassium Chloride; Thalidomide; Tiotropium; Umeclidinium

Increased Effect/Toxicity

Based on **hydrocodone** component: Increased toxicity: CNS depressants, MAO inhibitors, general anesthetics, and tricyclic antidepressants may potentiate the effects of opiate agonists; dextroamphetamine may enhance the analgesic effect of opiate agonists

Based on **homatropine** component:

Phenothiazine and TCAs may increase anticholinergic effects when used concurrently.

Sympathomimetic amines may cause tachyarrhythmias; avoid concurrent use

Decreased Effect

Hydrocodone and Homatropine may decrease the levels/effects of: Acetylcholinesterase Inhibitors (Central); Pegvisomant; Secretin

The levels/effects of Hydrocodone and Homatropine may be decreased by: Acetylcholinesterase Inhibitors (Central); Ammonium Chloride; Bosentan; CYP3A4 Inducers

(Strong); Dabrafenib; Deferasirox; Mitotane; Naltrexone; QuiNIDine; Siltuximab; St Johns Wort; Tocilizumab

Stability Syrup (Hydromet); tablets (Tussigon): Store at 15°C to 30°C (59°F to 86°F); protect syrup (Hydromet) from light

Mechanism of Action

Hydrocodone binds to opiate receptors in the CNS, altering the perception of and response to pain; suppresses cough in medullary center; produces generalized CNS depression.

Homatropine is an anticholinergic agent, present in a subtherapeutic amount to discourage deliberate overdose.

Pharmacokinetics (Adult data unless noted) Hydrocodone:

Metabolism: Hepatic; O-demethylation via primarily CYP2D6 to hydromorphone (major, active metabolite with ~10- to 33-fold higher or as much as a >100-fold higher binding affinity for the mu-opioid receptor than hydrocodone); N-demethylation via CYP3A4 to norhydrocodone (major metabolite); and ~40% of metabolism/clearance occurs via other non-CYP pathways, including 6-ketosteroid reduction to 6-alpha-hydrocol and 6-beta-hydrocol, and other elimination pathways (eg, fecal, biliary, intestinal, renal) (Hutchinson, 2004; Volpe, 2011; Zhou, 2009)

Half-life elimination: ~4 hours

Time to peak serum concentration: 1.3 ± 0.3 hours

Elimination: Urine (26% of single dose in 72 hours, with ~12% as unchanged drug, 5% as norhydrocodone, 4% as conjugated hydrocodone, 3% as 6-hydrocodol, and 0.21% as conjugated 6-hydromorphol) (Zhou, 2009)

Dosing: Usual

Pediatric: **Cough (antitussive):** Oral:

Tablet (Hydrocodone 5 mg and homatropine 1.5 mg per tablet):

Children 6-12 years: One-half (1/2) tablet every 4-6 hours as needed; maximum daily dose: 3 tablets/24 hours

Adolescents: One tablet every 4-6 hours as needed; maximum daily dose: 6 tablets/24 hours

Syrup (Hydrocodone 5 mg and homatropine 1.5 mg per 5 mL):

Children 6-12 years: 2.5 mL every 4-6 hours as needed; maximum daily dose: 15 mL/24 hours

Adolescents: 5 mL every 4-6 hours as needed; maximum daily dose: 30 mL/24 hours

Adult: **Cough (antitussive):** Oral:

Tablet (Hydrocodone 5 mg and homatropine 1.5 mg): One tablet every 4-6 hours as needed; maximum daily dose: 6 tablets/24 hours

Syrup: 5 mL every 4-6 hours as needed; maximum daily dose: 30 mL/24 hours

Dosing adjustment in renal impairment: There are no dosage adjustments provided in the manufacturer's labeling.

Dosing adjustment in hepatic impairment: There are no dosage adjustments provided in the manufacturer's labeling.

Administration To prevent overdose, administer syrup with an accurate measuring device (not a household teaspoon).

Test Interactions Increased ALT, AST

Controlled Substance C-III

Dosage Forms Excipient information presented when available (limited, particularly for generics); consult specific product labeling. [DSC] = Discontinued product

Syrup:

Hydromet®: Hydrocodone bitartrate 5 mg and homatropine methylbromide 1.5 mg per 5 mL (480 mL) [cherry flavor]

Generic: Hydrocodone bitartrate 5 mg and homatropine methylbromide 1.5 mg per 5 mL (473 mL)

Tablet:
Tussigon®: Hydrocodone bitartrate 5 mg and homatropine methylbromide 1.5 mg
Generic: Hydrocodone bitartrate 5 mg and homatropine methylbromide 1.5 mg

References

American Academy of Pediatrics Committee on Drugs, "'Inactive' Ingredients in Pharmaceutical Products: Update (Subject Review)," *Pediatr*, 1997, 99(2):268-78.

Broussard CS, Rasmussen SA, Reefhuis J, et al, "National Birth Defects Prevention Study: Maternal Treatment With Opioid Analgesics and Risk for Birth Defects," *Am J Obstet Gynecol*, 2011, 204 (4):314.

Hutchinson MR, Menelaou A, Foster DJ, et al, "CYP2D6 and CYP3A4 Involvement in the Primary Oxidative Metabolism of Hydrocodone by Human Liver Microsomes," *Br J Clin Pharmacol*, 2004, 57(3):287-97.

Hydrocodone bitartrate and homotropine methylbromide syrup [prescribing information]. Morton Grove, IL: Morton Grove Pharmaceuticals; September 2009.

Hydromet (hydrocodone bitartrate and homatropine methylbromide) [prescribing information]. March 2008.

Otton SV, Schadel M, Cheung SW, et al, "CYP2D6 Phenotype Determines the Metabolic Conversion of Hydrocodone to Hydromorphone," *Clin Pharmacol Ther*, 1993, 54(5):463-72.

Sauberan JB, Anderson PO, Lane JR, et al, "Breast Milk Hydrocodone and Hydromorphone Levels in Mothers Using Hydrocodone for Postpartum Pain," *Obstet Gynecol*, 2011, 117(3):611-7.

Shehab N, Lewis CL, Streetman DD, Donn SM. Exposure to the pharmaceutical excipients benzyl alcohol and propylene glycol among critically ill neonates. *Pediatr Crit Care Med.* 2009;10 (2):256-259.

Tussigon (hydrocodone bitartrate and homatropine methylbromide) [prescribing information]. Bristol, TN: King Pharmaceuticals; October 2006.

Volpe DA, McMahon Tobin GA, Mellon RD, et al, "Uniform Assessment and Ranking of Opioid Mu Receptor Binding Constants for Selected Opioid Drugs," *Regul Toxicol Pharmacol*, 2011, 59(3):385-90.

Zhou SF, "Polymorphism of Human Cytochrome P450 2D6 and Its Clinical Significance: Part II," *Clin Pharmacokinet*, 2009, 48 (12):761-804.

◆ **Hydrocodone Bitartrate and Homatropine Methylbromide** see Hydrocodone and Homatropine *on page 1032*

◆ **Hydrocodone Polistirex and Chlorpheniramine Polistirex** see Hydrocodone and Chlorpheniramine *on page 1030*

Hydrocortisone (Systemic)
(hye droe KOR ti sone)

Medication Safety Issues
Sound-alike/look-alike issues:
Hydrocortisone may be confused with hydrocodone, hydroxychloroquine, hydrochlorothiazide
Cortef® may be confused with Coreg®, Lortab®
HCT (occasional abbreviation for hydrocortisone) is an error-prone abbreviation (mistaken as hydrochlorothiazide)
Solu-CORTEF® may be confused with Solu-MEDROL®

Related Information
Corticosteroids Systemic Equivalencies *on page 2222*
Emetogenic Potential of Antineoplastic Agents in Children *on page 2327*

Brand Names: U.S. A-Hydrocort; Cortef; Solu-CORTEF
Brand Names: Canada Cortef®; Solu-Cortef®
Therapeutic Category Adrenal Corticosteroid; Anti-inflammatory Agent; Antiasthmatic; Corticosteroid, Systemic; Glucocorticoid
Generic Availability (U.S.) May be product dependent
Use Anti-inflammatory or immunosuppressant agent in the treatment of a variety of diseases, including those of allergic, hematologic, dermatologic, gastrointestinal, ophthalmic, neoplastic, rheumatic, autoimmune, nervous system, renal, and respiratory origin [FDA approved in pediatric patients (age not specified) and adults]; primary or secondary adrenocorticoid deficiency (drug of choice) [FDA approved in pediatric patients (age not specified) and adults]; has also been used for management of septic

shock and in neonates for treatment of hypotension and prevention of bronchopulmonary dysplasia
Pregnancy Risk Factor C
Pregnancy Considerations Adverse events have been observed with corticosteroids in animal reproduction studies. Some studies have shown an association between first trimester systemic corticosteroid use and oral clefts (Park-Wyllie, 2000; Pradat, 2003). Systemic corticosteroids may also influence fetal growth (decreased birth weight); however, information is conflicting (Lunghi, 2010). Hypoadrenalism may occur in newborns following maternal use of corticosteroids in pregnancy (monitor). When systemic corticosteroids are needed in pregnancy, it is generally recommended to use the lowest effective dose for the shortest duration of time, avoiding high doses during the first trimester (Leachman, 2006; Lunghi, 2010; Makol, 2011; Østensen, 2009).
Breast-Feeding Considerations Corticosteroids are excreted in breast milk. The manufacturer notes that when used systemically, maternal use of corticosteroids have the potential to cause adverse events in a nursing infant (eg, growth suppression, interfere with endogenous corticosteroid production). If there is concern about exposure to the infant, some guidelines recommend waiting 4 hours after the maternal dose of an oral systemic corticosteroid before breast-feeding in order to decrease potential exposure to the nursing infant (based on a study using prednisolone) (Bae, 2011; Leachman, 2006; Makol, 2011; Ost, 1985).
Contraindications Hypersensitivity to hydrocortisone or any component; serious infections, except septic shock or tuberculous meningitis; viral, fungal, or tubercular skin lesions
Warnings Hypothalamic-pituitary-adrenal (HPA) suppression may occur, particularly in younger children or in patients receiving high doses for prolonged periods; acute adrenal insufficiency (adrenal crisis) may occur with abrupt withdrawal after long-term therapy or with stress; withdrawal and discontinuation of corticosteroids should be tapered slowly and carefully; patients with HPA axis suppression may require doses of systemic glucocorticosteroids prior to, during, and after unusual stress (eg, surgery).

Immunosuppression may occur; patients may be more susceptible to infections; prolonged use of corticosteroids may also increase the incidence of secondary infection, mask acute infection (including fungal infections), prolong or exacerbate viral or fungal infections, activate latent opportunistic infections, or limit response to vaccines. Exposure to chickenpox should be avoided; corticosteroids should not be used to treat ocular herpes simplex; use caution in patients with a history of ocular herpes simplex. Corticosteroids should not be used for cerebral malaria or viral hepatitis. Close observation is required in patients with latent tuberculosis and/or TB reactivity; restrict use in active TB (only in conjunction with antituberculosis treatment).

May cause osteoporosis (at any age) or inhibition of bone growth in pediatric patients. Use with caution in patients with osteoporosis. In a population-based study of children, risk of fracture was shown to be increased with >4 courses of corticosteroids; underlying clinical condition may also impact bone health and osteoporotic effect of corticosteroids (Leonard, 2006).

May cause GI bleeding or perforation. In premature neonates, reports of gastrointestinal perforation in the hydrocortisone treatment arm have resulted in the closure of two large BPD clinical trials (Peltoniemi, 2005; Watterberg, 2004); concomitant use with indomethacin or ibuprofen may increase the risk and should be avoided in this population (Seri, 2006). Use with caution in patients with

GI disease (diverticulitis, peptic ulcer disease, ulcerative colitis).

Corticosteroid use may cause psychiatric disturbances, including depression, euphoria, insomnia, mood swings, and personality changes. preexisting psychiatric conditions may be exacerbated by corticosteroid use. Acute myopathy may occur with high doses, usually in patients with neuromuscular transmission disorders; myopathy may involve ocular and/or respiratory muscles; monitor creatine kinase; recovery may be delayed. Increased IOP may occur, especially with prolonged use; in children, increased IOP has been shown to be dose-dependent and produce a greater IOP in children <6 years than older children (Lam, 2005). Rare cases of anaphylactoid reactions have been reported with corticosteroids.

Manufacturer-supplied diluents for injection (eg, Solu-Cortef®) contain benzyl alcohol which may cause allergic reactions in susceptible individuals; oral suspension contains benzoic acid; benzoic acid (benzoate) is a metabolite of benzyl alcohol; large amounts of benzyl alcohol (≥99 mg/kg/day) have been associated with a potentially fatal toxicity ("gasping syndrome") in neonates; the "gasping syndrome" consists of metabolic acidosis, respiratory distress, gasping respirations, CNS dysfunction (including convulsions, intracranial hemorrhage), hypotension and cardiovascular collapse; avoid use of hydrocortisone products containing benzoic acid, benzyl alcohol, or benzyl benzoate in neonates; in vitro and animal studies have shown that benzoate displaces bilirubin from protein binding sites

Precautions Avoid using higher than recommended doses; suppression of HPA function, suppression of linear growth (ie, reduction of growth velocity), reduced bone mineral density, hypercorticism (Cushing's syndrome), hyperglycemia, or glucosuria may occur; titrate to lowest effective dose. Reduction in growth velocity may occur when corticosteroids are administered to pediatric patients by any route (monitor growth). Use with extreme caution in patients with respiratory tuberculosis or untreated systemic infections. Use with caution in patients with hypertension, heart failure, or renal impairment; long-term use has been associated with fluid retention and hypertension. High-dose corticosteroids should not be used for management of head injury; increased mortality was observed in patients receiving high-dose I.V. methylprednisolone. Use with caution in patients with myasthenia gravis; exacerbation of symptoms has occurred, especially during initial treatment with corticosteroids. Use with caution in patients with hepatic impairment, including cirrhosis; enhanced pharmacologic effect due to decreased metabolism and long-term use has been associated with fluid retention. Use with caution following acute MI; corticosteroids have been associated with myocardial rupture. Hypertrophic cardiomyopathy has been reported in premature neonates.

Use with caution in patients with diabetes; corticosteroids may alter glucose regulation, leading to hyperglycemia. Use with caution in patients with cataracts and/or glaucoma; increased intraocular pressure, open-angle glaucoma, and cataracts have occurred with prolonged use; consider routine eye exams in chronic users. Use with caution in patients with a history of seizure disorder; seizures have been reported with adrenal crisis. Use with caution in patients with thyroid dysfunction; changes in thyroid status may necessitate dosage adjustments; metabolic clearance of corticosteroids increases in hyperthyroid patients and decreases in hypothyroid patients. Prolonged treatment with corticosteroids has been associated with the development of Kaposi's sarcoma (case reports); if noted, discontinuation of therapy should be considered. Use with caution in patients with thromboembolic tendencies or thrombophlebitis.

Adverse Reactions

Cardiovascular: Arrhythmias, bradycardia, cardiac arrest, cardiomegaly, circulatory collapse, congestive heart failure, edema, fat embolism, hypertension, hypertrophic cardiomyopathy (premature infants), myocardial rupture (post MI), syncope, tachycardia, thromboembolism, vasculitis

Central nervous system: Delirium, depression, emotional instability, euphoria, hallucinations, headache, insomnia, intracranial pressure increased, malaise, mood swings, nervousness, neuritis, neuropathy, personality changes, pseudotumor cerebri, psychic disorders, psychoses, seizure, vertigo

Dermatologic: Acne, allergic dermatitis, alopecia, bruising, burning/tingling, dry scaly skin, edema, erythema, hirsutism, hyper-/hypopigmentation, impaired wound healing, petechiae, rash, skin atrophy, skin test reaction impaired, sterile abscess, striae, urticaria

Endocrine & metabolic: Adrenal suppression, alkalosis, amenorrhea, carbohydrate intolerance increased, Cushing's syndrome, diabetes mellitus, glucose intolerance, growth suppression, hyperglycemia, hyperlipidemia, hypokalemia, hypokalemic alkalosis, menstrual irregularities, negative nitrogen balance, pituitary-adrenal axis suppression, potassium loss, protein catabolism, sodium and water retention, sperm motility increased/decreased, spermatogenesis increased/decreased

Gastrointestinal: Abdominal distention, appetite increased, bowel dysfunction (intrathecal administration), indigestion, nausea, pancreatitis, peptic ulcer, gastrointestinal perforation, ulcerative esophagitis, vomiting, weight gain

Genitourinary: Bladder dysfunction (intrathecal administration)

Hematologic: Leukocytosis (transient)

Hepatic: Hepatomegaly, transaminases increased

Local: Atrophy (at injection site), postinjection flare (intraarticular use), thrombophlebitis

Neuromuscular & skeletal: Arthralgia, necrosis (femoral and humoral heads), Charcot-like arthropathy, fractures, muscle mass loss, muscle weakness, myopathy, osteoporosis, tendon rupture, vertebral compression fractures

Ocular: Cataracts, exophthalmoses, glaucoma, intraocular pressure increased

Miscellaneous: Abnormal fat deposits, anaphylaxis, avascular necrosis, diaphoresis, hiccups, hypersensitivity reactions, infection, secondary malignancy

Drug Interactions

Metabolism/Transport Effects Substrate of CYP3A4 (minor), P-glycoprotein; **Note:** Assignment of Major/Minor substrate status based on clinically relevant drug interaction potential; **Induces** CYP3A4 (weak/moderate)

Avoid Concomitant Use

Avoid concomitant use of Hydrocortisone (Systemic) with any of the following: Aldesleukin; Axitinib; BCG; Indium 111 Capromab Pendetide; Mifepristone; Natalizumab; Pimecrolimus; Simeprevir; Tacrolimus (Topical); Tofacitinib

Increased Effect/Toxicity

Hydrocortisone (Systemic) may increase the levels/ effects of: Acetylcholinesterase Inhibitors; Amphotericin B; Androgens; Ceritinib; Deferasirox; Leflunomide; Loop Diuretics; Natalizumab; NSAID (COX-2 Inhibitor); NSAID (Nonselective); Thiazide Diuretics; Tofacitinib; Vaccines (Live); Warfarin

The levels/effects of Hydrocortisone (Systemic) may be increased by: Antifungal Agents (Azole Derivatives, Systemic); Aprepitant; Calcium Channel Blockers (Nondihydropyridine); Denosumab; Estrogen Derivatives; Fluconazole; Fosaprepitant; Indacaterol; Macrolide Antibiotics; Mifepristone; Neuromuscular-Blocking Agents (Nondepolarizing); P-glycoprotein/ABCB1 Inhibitors;

◀ Pimecrolimus; Quinolone Antibiotics; Roflumilast; Salicylates; Tacrolimus (Topical); Telaprevir; Trastuzumab

Decreased Effect

Hydrocortisone (Systemic) may decrease the levels/ effects of: Aldesleukin; Antidiabetic Agents; ARIPiprazole; Axitinib; BCG; Calcitriol; Coccidioidin Skin Test; Corticorelin; Hyaluronidase; Ibrutinib; Indium 111 Capromab Pendetide; Isoniazid; Salicylates; Saxagliptin; Simeprevir; Sipuleucel-T; Telaprevir; Urea Cycle Disorder Agents; Vaccines (Inactivated)

The levels/effects of Hydrocortisone (Systemic) may be decreased by: Aminoglutethimide; Antacids; Barbiturates; Bile Acid Sequestrants; Echinacea; Mifepristone; Mitotane; P-glycoprotein/ABCB1 Inducers; Primidone; Rifamycin Derivatives

Stability

Oral: Store at 20°C to 25°C (68°F to 77°F).

Parenteral: Store at controlled room temperature 20°C to 25°C (59°F to 86°F). Reconstituted solution is clear, light yellow and heat labile.

After initial reconstitution, hydrocortisone sodium succinate solutions are stable for 3 days at room temperature or under refrigeration when protected from light. Stability of parenteral admixture (Solu-Cortef®) at room temperature (25°C) and at refrigeration temperature (4°C) is concentration-dependent:

1 mg/mL: 24 hours

2-60 mg/mL: At least 4 hours

Mechanism of Action Decreases inflammation by suppression of migration of polymorphonuclear leukocytes and reversal of increased capillary permeability

Pharmacodynamics Anti-inflammatory effects:

Maximum effect:

Oral: 12-24 hours

I.V.: 4-6 hours

Duration: 8-12 hours

Pharmacokinetics (Adult data unless noted)

Absorption: Rapid

Metabolism: In the liver

Half-life, biologic: 8-12 hours

Elimination: Renally, mainly as 17-hydroxysteroids and 17-ketosteroids

Dosing: Neonatal Dose should be based on severity of disease and patient response.

Bronchopulmonary dysplasia, prevention (preterm neonates with prenatal inflammatory exposure): PNA ≤48 hours: I.V.: 1 mg/kg/day divided every 12 hours for 9 or 12 days followed by 0.5 mg/kg/day divided every 12 hours for 3 days; low-dose (ie, physiologic replacement) has been shown to be effective at improving survival without BPD in chorioamnionitis-exposed ELBW neonates (birth weight: 500-999 g) (Watterberg, 1999; Watterberg, 2004; Watterberg, 2010); of note, a higher incidence of gastrointestinal perforation in the treatment arm resulted in early study closure of the largest trial (Watterberg, 2004). In another trial of VLBW neonates (PNA ≤36 hours, GA <30 weeks, birth weight: 500-1250 g), higher dosages (ie, stress dose): 2 mg/kg/ day divided every 8 hours for 2 days followed by 1.5 mg/kg/day divided every 8 hours for 2 days followed by 0.75 mg/kg/day divided every 12 hours for 6 days showed a trend in the treatment arm of decreased severity of respiratory failure, shorten length of oxygen therapy and promotion of PDA closure; this trial was closed early due to higher incidence of gastrointestinal perforation in the treatment arm versus placebo (Peltoniemi, 2005). **Note:** The AAP suggests that for neonates with prenatal inflammatory exposure, low-dose hydrocortisone therapy (1 mg/kg/day) during the first 2 weeks of life may improve survival without BPD and without adverse neurodevelopmental outcomes (Watterberg, 2010).

Congenital adrenal hyperplasia: Oral [tablets (crushed)]: Initial: 10-15 mg/m²/day in 3 divided doses; higher initial doses (20 mg/m²/day) may be required to achieve initial target hormone serum concentrations. Administer morning dose as early as possible. Due to uneven distribution of the drug in the liquid, use of oral suspension is **not** recommended [AAP, 2000; Speiser (Endocrine Society), 2010]

Hypoglycemia, refractory (refractory to continuous glucose infusion of >12-15 mg/kg/minute): Oral, I.V.: 5 mg/kg/day divided every 8-12 hours or 1-2 mg/kg/**dose** every 6 hours

Hypotension, refractory; shock: I.V.: Limited data available; dosage regimens variable (Brierley, 2009; Higgins, 2010): 3 mg/kg/day divided every 8 hours for 5 days; dosing based on the largest, prospective, randomized, placebo-controlled trial of 48 hypotensive, VLBW neonates (PNA: <7 days; GA: <32 weeks; birth weight: <1500 g) who were also receiving dopamine at doses ≥10 mcg/kg/minute (Ng, 2006); other smaller trials have used 2 mg/kg/day divided every 12 hours for 1-3 days (Seri, 2001) or 2 mg/kg once, followed by 2 mg/kg/day divided every 12 hours for 4 doses (Noori, 2006)

Dosing: Usual Dose should be based on severity of disease and patient response.

Infants, Children, and Adolescents:

Adrenal insufficiency (acute): I.M., I.V.:

Infants and young Children: 1-2 mg/kg/**dose** I.V. bolus, then 25-150 mg/day in divided doses every 6-8 hours

Older Children: 1-2 mg/kg/**dose** I.V. bolus, then 150-250 mg/day in divided doses every 6-8 hours

Anti-inflammatory or immunosuppressive:

Infants and Children:

Oral: 2.5-10 mg/kg/day or 75-300 mg/m²/day divided every 6-8 hours

I.M., I.V.: 1-5 mg/kg/day or 30-150 mg/m²/day divided every 12-24 hours

Adolescents: Oral, I.M., I.V., SubQ: 15-240 mg every 12 hours

Congenital adrenal hyperplasia: Oral (tablets): AAP Recommendations: **Note:** Administer morning dose as early as possible. Tablets may result in more reliable serum concentrations than oral liquid formulation; use of oral suspension is not recommended. Individualize dose by monitoring growth, hormone levels, and bone age; mineralocorticoid (eg, fludrocortisone) and sodium supplement may be required in salt losers (AAP, 2000; AAP, 2010; Endocrine Society, 2010)

Initial: 10-15 mg/m²/day in 3 divided doses; higher initial doses (20 mg/m²/day) may be required to achieve initial target hormone serum concentrations (AAP, 2010; Endocrine Society, 2010).

Maintenance dose: Usual requirement:

Infants: 2.5-5 mg/**dose** 3 times/day

Children: 5-10 mg/**dose** 3 times/day;

Physiologic replacement: Infants and Children: Oral: 8-10 mg/m²/day divided every 8 hours; up to 12 mg/m²/ day in some patients (Ahmet, 2011; Gupta, 2008; Maguire, 2007).

Septic shock: Infants, Children, and Adolescents: I.V.: Initial: 1-2 mg/kg/day (intermittent or as continuous I.V. infusion); doses may be titrated up to 50 mg/kg/day if necessary for shock reversal (Brierley, 2009); alternative dosing suggests 50 mg/m²/day (Dellinger, 2008); **Note:** Use recommended only in catecholamine-resistant shock and suspected or proven adrenal insufficiency

Adults:

Adrenal insufficiency (acute): I.M., I.V.: 100 mg I.V. bolus, then 300 mg/day in divided doses every 8 hours or as a continuous infusion for 48 hours; once patient is stable, change to oral, 50 mg every 8 hours for 6 doses, then taper to 30-50 mg/day in divided doses

Adrenal insufficiency (chronic), physiologic replacement: Oral: 15-25 mg/day in 2-3 divided doses. **Note:** Studies suggest administering one-half to two-thirds of the daily dose in the morning in order to mimic the physiological cortisol secretion pattern. If the twice-daily regimen is utilized, the second dose should be administered 6-8 hours following the first dose (Arlt, 2003).

Anti-inflammatory or immunosuppressive: Oral, I.M., I.V.: 15-240 mg every 12 hours

Congenital adrenal hyperplasia: Oral: 15-25 mg/day in 2-3 divided doses (Speiser, 2010)

Septic shock: I.V.: 50 mg every 6 hours (Annane, 2002; Marik, 2008); not to exceed 300 mg/day (Dellinger, 2008). Practice guidelines also recommend alternative dosing of 100 mg bolus, followed by continuous infusion of 10 mg/hour (240 mg/day). Taper slowly (for total of 11 days) and do not stop abruptly. **Note:** Fludrocortisone is optional with use of hydrocortisone.

Status asthmaticus: I.V.: 1-2 mg/kg/dose every 6 hours for 24 hours, then maintenance of 0.5-1 mg/kg every 6 hours

Stress dosing (surgery) in patients known to be adrenally-suppressed or on chronic systemic steroids: I.V.:

Minor stress (ie, inguinal herniorrhaphy): 25 mg/day for 1 day

Moderate stress (ie, joint replacement, cholecystectomy): 50-75 mg/day (25 mg every 8-12 hours) for 1-2 days

Major stress (pancreatoduodenectomy, esophagogastrectomy, cardiac surgery): 100-150 mg/day (50 mg every 8-12 hours) for 2-3 days

Administration

Oral: Administer with food or milk to decrease GI upset

Parenteral: Hydrocortisone sodium succinate may be administered by I.M. or I.V. routes. Dermal and/or subdermal skin depression may occur at the site of injection. Avoid injection into deltoid muscle (high incidence of SubQ atrophy); pH 7-8

I.V. bolus: Dilute to 50 mg/mL and administer over at least 30 seconds; for large doses (≥500 mg in adults), administer over 10 minutes

Intermittent I.V. infusion: Dilute to 1 mg/mL and administer over 20-30 minutes; usual maximum concentration: 5 mg/mL

Note: In adult patients, when administration of a small volume of fluid is needed, concentrations up to 60 mg/mL (100-3000 mg in 50 mL D_5W or NS) may be administered by direct I.V. or I.V. piggyback.

Monitoring Parameters Blood pressure; weight; serum glucose; electrolytes; growth in pediatric patients; presence of infection, bone mineral density; assess HPA axis suppression (eg, ACTH stimulation test, morning plasma cortisol test, urinary free cortisol test). Monitor IOP with therapy >6 weeks.

Reference Range Hydrocortisone (normal endogenous morning levels): 4-30 mcg/mL

Test Interactions Interferes with skin tests

Additional Information Cortef® oral suspension was reformulated in July 1998; the suspending agent was changed from tragacanth to xanthan gum; this suspension was found **not** to be bioequivalent to hydrocortisone tablets in the treatment of children with congenital adrenal hyperplasia; children required higher doses of the suspension (19.6 mg/m²/day) compared to the tablets (15.2 mg/m²/day); based on these findings, Cortef® suspension was voluntarily recalled from the market on July 18, 2000 (Merke, 2001).

In premature neonates, the use of high-dose dexamethasone (approximately >0.5 mg/kg/day) for the prevention or treatment of BPD has been associated with adverse neurodevelopmental outcomes, including higher rates of cerebral palsy without additional clinical benefit over lower doses; current data does not support use of high doses, further studies are needed (Watterberg, 2010). Data specific to hydrocortisone use in this population has shown that use <7 days of therapy does not appear to be associated with adverse neurodevelopmental outcomes (Needelman, 2010).

Hydrocortisone has been studied in children with cystic fibrosis and an ongoing lower respiratory tract infection using 2.5 mg/kg/**dose** every 6 hours for 10 days in addition to standard therapies. A double-blind, placebo- controlled trial of 22 infants and children (age: <18 months; mean: 8.8-9.5 months) showed no significant difference in pulmonary function on day 10 of therapy between treatment and placebo groups; however, at 1-2 months after discharge, follow-up testing showed significant, sustained improvement of pulmonary function in the hydrocortisone group compared to placebo (Tepper, 1997). Further studies are needed and hydrocortisone is not recommended for routine use in current cystic fibrosis guidelines (Flume, 2009).

Dosage Forms Excipient information presented when available (limited, particularly for generics); consult specific product labeling.

Solution Reconstituted, Injection, as sodium succinate [strength expressed as base]:
A-Hydrocort: 100 mg (1 ea)
Solu-CORTEF: 100 mg (1 ea)

Solution Reconstituted, Injection, as sodium succinate [strength expressed as base, preservative free]:
Solu-CORTEF: 100 mg (1 ea); 250 mg (1 ea); 500 mg (1 ea); 1000 mg (1 ea)

Tablet, Oral, as base:
Cortef: 5 mg, 10 mg, 20 mg [scored]
Generic: 5 mg, 10 mg, 20 mg

Extemporaneous Preparations A 2.5 mg/mL oral suspension may be made with either tablets or powder and a vehicle containing sodium carboxymethylcellulose (1 g), syrup BP (10 mL), hydroxybenzoate 0.1% preservatives (0.1 g), polysorbate 80 (0.5 mL), citric acid (0.6 g), and water. To make the vehicle, dissolve the hydroxybenzoate, citric acid, and syrup BP in hot water. Cool solution and add the carboxymethylcellulose; leave overnight. Crush twelve-and-one-half 20 mg hydrocortisone tablets (or use 250 mg of powder) in a mortar and reduce to a fine powder while adding polysorbate 80. Add small portions of vehicle and mix to a uniform paste; mix while adding the vehicle in incremental proportions to **almost** 100 mL; transfer to a calibrated bottle, rinse mortar with vehicle, and add sufficient quantity of vehicle to make 100 mL. Label "shake well" and "refrigerate". Stable for 90 days.

Fawcett JP, Boulton DW, Jiang R, et al, "Stability of Hydrocortisone Oral Suspensions Prepared From Tablets and Powder," *Ann Pharmacother*, 1995, 29(10):987-90.

References

Ahmet A, Kim H, and Spier S, "Adrenal Suppression: A Practical Guide to the Screening and Management of this Under-Recognized Complication of Inhaled Corticosteroid Therapy," *Allergy Asthma Clin Immunol*, 2011, 7:13.

American Academy of Pediatrics, "Statement of Endorsement-Congenital Adrenal Hyperplasia Due to Steroid 21-Hydroxylase Deficiency," *Pediatrics*, 2010, 126(5):1051. Available at http://pediatrics.aappublications.org/cgi/content/extract/126/5/1051. Accessed May 10, 2011.

American Academy of Pediatrics, Section on Endocrinology and Committee on Genetics, "Technical Report: Congenital Adrenal Hyperplasia," *Pediatrics*, 2000, 106(6):1511-8.

Annane D, Sébille V, Charpentier C, et al, "Effect of Treatment With Low Doses of Hydrocortisone and Fludrocortisone on Mortality in Patients With Septic Shock," *JAMA*, 2002, 288(7):862-71.

Arlt W and Allolio B, "Adrenal Insufficiency," *Lancet*, 2003, 361 (9372):1881-93.

Bae YS, Van Voorhees AS, Hsu S, et al, "Review of Treatment Options For Psoriasis in Pregnant or Lactating Women: From the Medical Board of the National Psoriasis Foundation," *J Am Acad Dermatol*, 2012, 67(3):459-77.

Baker CF, Barks JD, Engmann C, et al, "Hydrocortisone Administration for the Treatment of Refractory Hypotension in Critically Ill Newborns," *J Perinatol*, 2008, 28(6):412-9.

Brierley J, Carcillo JA, Choong K, et al, "Clinical Practice Parameters for Hemodynamic Support of Pediatric and Neonatal Septic Shock: 2007 Update From the American College of Critical Care Medicine," *Crit Care Med*, 2009, 37(2):666-88.

Carcillo JA and Fields AI, "Clinical Practice Parameters for Hemodynamic Support of Pediatric and Neonatal Patients in Septic Shock," *Crit Care Med*, 2002, 30(6):1365-78.

Cowett RM and Loughead JL, "Neonatal Glucose Metabolism: Differential Diagnoses, Evaluation, and Treatment of Hypoglycemia," *Neonatal Netw*, 2002, 21(4):9-19.

Dellinger RP, Levy MM, Carlet JM, et al, "Surviving Sepsis Campaign: International Guidelines for Management of Severe Sepsis and Septic Shock: 2008," *Intensive Care Med*, 2008, 34(1):17-60.

Flume PA, Mogayzel PJ Jr, Robinson KA, et al, "Cystic Fibrosis Pulmonary Guidelines: Treatment of Pulmonary Exacerbations," *Am J Respir Crit Care Med*, 2009, 180(9):802-8.

Gupta P and Bhatia V, "Corticosteroid Physiology and Principles of Therapy," *Indian J Pediatr*, 2008, 75(10):1039-44.

Halamek LP and Stevenson DK, "Neonatal Hypoglycemia, Part II: Pathophysiology and Therapy," *Clin Pediatr (Phila)*, 1998, 37(1):11-6.

Han YY, Carcillo JA, Dragotta MA, et al, "Early Reversal of Pediatric-Neonatal Septic Shock by Community Physicians is Associated With Improved Outcome," *Pediatrics*, 2003, 112(4):793-9.

Higgins S, Friedlich P, and Seri I, "Hydrocortisone for Hypotension and Vasopressor Dependence in Preterm Neonates: A Meta-Analysis," *J Perinatol*, 2010, 30(6):373-8.

Jain A, Aggarwal R, Jeevasanker M, et al, "Hypoglycemia in the Newborn," *Indian J Pediatr*, 2008, 75(1):63-7.

Lam DS, Fan DS, Ng JS, et al, "Ocular Hypertensive and Anti-Inflammatory Responses to Different Dosages of Topical Dexamethasone in Children: A Randomized Trial," *Clin Experiment Ophthalmol*, 2005, 33 (3):252-8.

Leachman SA and Reed BR, "The Use of Dermatologic Drugs in Pregnancy and Lactation," *Dermatol Clin*, 2006, 24(2):167-97, vi.

Leonard MB, "Glucocorticoid-Induced Osteoporosis in Children: Impact of the Underlying Disease," *Pediatrics*, 2007, 119 Suppl 2:S166-74.

Lunghi L, Pavan B, Biondi C, et al, "Use of Glucocorticoids in Pregnancy," *Curr Pharm Des*, 2010, 16(32):3616-37.

Maguire AM, Ambler GR, Moore B, et al, "Prolonged Hypocortisolemia in Hydrocortisone Replacement Regimens in Adrenocorticotrophic Hormone Deficiency," *Pediatrics*, 2007, 120(1):164-71.

Makol A, Wright K, and Amin S, "Rheumatoid Arthritis and Pregnancy: Safety Considerations in Pharmacological Management," *Drugs*, 2011, 71(15):1973-87.

Marik PE, Pastores SM, Annane D, et al, "Recommendations for the Diagnosis and Management of Corticosteroid Insufficiency in Critically Ill Adult Patients: Consensus Statements From an International Task Force by the American College of Critical Care Medicine," *Crit Care Med*, 2008, 36(6):1937-49.

Merke DP, Cho D, Calis KA, et al, "Hydrocortisone Suspension and Hydrocortisone Tablets are not Bioequivalent in the Treatment of Children With Congenital Adrenal Hyperplasia," *J Clin Endocrinol Metab*, 2001, 86(1):441-5.

Needelman H, Hoskoppal A, Roberts H, et al, "The Effect of Hydrocortisone on Neurodevelopmental Outcome in Premature Infants Less Than 29 Weeks' Gestation," *J Child Neurol*, 2010, 25(4):448-52.

Ng PC, Lee CH, Bnur FL, et al, "A Double-Blind, Randomized, Controlled Study of a 'Stress Dose' of Hydrocortisone for Rescue Treatment of Refractory Hypotension in Preterm Infants," *Pediatrics*, 2006, 117(2):367-75.

Noori S, Friedlich P, Wong P, et al, "Hemodynamic Changes After Low-Dosage Hydrocortisone Administration in Vasopressor-Treated Preterm and Term Neonates," *Pediatrics*, 2006, 118(4):1456-66.

Østensen M and Forger F, "Management of RA Medications in Pregnant Patients," *Nat Rev Rheumatol*, 2009, 5(7):382-90.

Ost L, Wettrell G, Bjorkhem I, et al, "Prednisolone Excretion in Human Milk," *J Pediatr*, 1985, 106(6):1008-11.

Park-Wyllie L, Mazzotta P, Pastuszak A, et al, "Birth Defects After Maternal Exposure to Corticosteroids: Prospective Cohort Study and Meta-Analysis of Epidemiological Studies," *Teratology*, 2000, 62 (6):385-92.

Peltoniemi O, Kari MA, Heinonen K, et al, "Pretreatment Cortisol Values May Predict Responses to Hydrocortisone Administration for the Prevention of Bronchopulmonary Dysplasia in High-Risk Infants," *J Pediatr*, 2005, 146(5):632-7.

Pradat P, Robert-Gnansia E, Di Tanna GL, et al, "First Trimester Exposure to Corticosteroids and Oral Clefts," *Birth Defects Res A Clin Mol Teratol*, 2003, 67(12):968-70.

Seri I, "Hydrocortisone and Vasopressor-Resistant Shock in Preterm Neonates," *Pediatrics*, 2006, 117(2):516-8.

Seri I, Tan R, and Evans J, "Cardiovascular Effects of Hydrocortisone in Preterm Infants With Pressor-Resistant Hypotension," *Pediatrics*, 2001, 107(5):1070-4.

Speiser PW, Azziz R, Baskin LS, et al, "Congenital Adrenal Hyperplasia Due to Steroid 21-Hydroxylase Deficiency: An Endocrine Society Clinical Practice Guideline," *J Clin Endocrinol Metab*, 2010, 95 (9):4133-60.

Tepper RS, Eigen H, Stevens J, et al, "Lower Respiratory Illness in Infants and Young Children With Cystic Fibrosis: Evaluation of Treatment With Intravenous Hydrocortisone," *Pediatr Pulmonol*, 1997, 24 (1):48-51.

Watterberg KL and American Academy of Pediatrics Committee on Fetus and Newborn, "Policy Statement–Postnatal Corticosteroids to Prevent or Treat Bronchopulmonary Dysplasia," *Pediatrics*, 2010, 126 (4):800-8.

Watterberg KL, Gerdes JS, Cole CH, et al, "Prophylaxis of Early Adrenal Insufficiency to Prevent Bronchopulmonary Dysplasia: A Multicenter Trial," *Pediatrics*, 2004, 114(6):1649-57.

Watterberg KL, Gerdes JS, Gifford KL, et al, "Prophylaxis Against Early Adrenal Insufficiency to Prevent Chronic Lung Disease in Premature Infants," *Pediatrics*, 1999, 104(6):1258-63.

Hydrocortisone (Topical) (hye droe KOR ti sone)

Medication Safety Issues
Sound-alike/look-alike issues:
Hydrocortisone may be confused with hydrocodone, hydroxychloroquine, hydrochlorothiazide

Anusol® may be confused with Anusol-HC®, Aplisol®, Aquasol®

Cortizone® may be confused with cortisone

HCT (occasional abbreviation for hydrocortisone) is an error-prone abbreviation (mistaken as hydrochlorothiazide)

Hytone® may be confused with Vytone®

Proctocort® may be confused with ProctoCream®

International issues:
Nutracort [multiple international markets] may be confused with Nitrocor brand name of nitroglycerin [Italy, Russia, and Venezuela]

Related Information
Topical Corticosteroids *on page 2224*

Brand Names: U.S. Ala Cort; Ala Scalp; Anti-Itch Maximum Strength [OTC]; Anucort-HC; Anusol-HC; Aquanil HC [OTC]; Beta HC [OTC]; Colocort; CortAlo; Cortenema; Corticool [OTC]; Cortifoam; Dermasorb HC; First-Hydrocortisone; GRx HiCort 25; Hemril-30 [DSC]; Hydro Skin Maximum Strength [OTC]; Hydrocortisone Max St [OTC]; Hydrocortisone Max St/12 Moist [OTC]; HydroSKIN [OTC]; Instacort 10 [OTC]; Instacort 5 [OTC]; Locoid; Locoid Lipocream; Med-Derm Hydrocortisone [OTC]; Medi-First Hydrocortisone [OTC]; NuCort; NuZon; Pandel; Pediaderm HC; Preparation H Hydrocortisone [OTC]; Procto-Pak; Proctocort; Proctosol HC; Proctozone-HC; Recort Plus [OTC]; Rectacort-HC; Rederm [OTC]; Sarnol-HC [OTC]; Scalacort; Scalacort DK; Scalpicin Maximum Strength [OTC]; Texacort; TheraCort [OTC]; Westcort

Brand Names: Canada Aquacort®; Cortamed®; Cortenema®; Cortifoam™; Emo-Cort®; Hycort™; Hyderm; HydroVal®; Locoid®; Prevex® HC; Sarna® HC; Westcort®

Therapeutic Category Anti-inflammatory Agent; Anti-inflammatory Agent, Rectal; Corticosteroid, Rectal; Corticosteroid, Topical; Glucocorticoid

Generic Availability (U.S.) May be product dependent

Use Relief of inflammation and pruritus associated with corticosteroid-responsive dermatoses; adjunctive treatment of ulcerative colitis

Pregnancy Risk Factor C

Pregnancy Considerations Adverse events have been observed with corticosteroids in animal reproduction studies. Topical products are not recommended for extensive use, in large quantities, or for long periods of time in pregnant women (Reed, 1997).

Breast-Feeding Considerations Systemically administered corticosteroids are excreted in breast milk and endogenous hydrocortisone is also found in human milk. It is not known if systemic absorption following topical administration results in detectable quantities in human milk. Use with caution while breast-feeding; do not apply to nipples (Reed, 1997).

Contraindications Hypersensitivity to hydrocortisone or any component

Rectal suspension: Systemic fungal infections; ileocolostomy during the immediate or early postoperative period

Warnings Hypothalamic-pituitary-adrenal (HPA) suppression may occur; acute adrenal insufficiency (adrenal crisis) may occur with abrupt withdrawal after long-term therapy or with stress; withdrawal and discontinuation of corticosteroids should be done carefully; immunosuppression may occur; may cause inhibition of bone growth in pediatric patients

Adverse systemic effects may occur when topical steroids are used in large areas of the body, denuded areas, for prolonged periods of time, with an occlusive dressing, and/or in infants and small children; infants and small children may be more susceptible to HPA axis suppression or other systemic toxicities due to larger skin surface area to body mass ratio; use with caution in pediatric patients

Precautions Avoid using higher than recommended doses; reduction in growth velocity may occur when corticosteroids are administered to pediatric patients by any route (monitor growth)

Use hydrocortisone retention enema with caution in patients with possible impending perforation, abscess, or other pyogenic infection; fresh intestinal anastomoses; obstruction, extensive fistulas, and sinus tracts; active or latent peptic ulcer; diverticulitis; renal insufficiency; hypertension; osteoporosis; or myasthenia gravis

Adverse Reactions Local adverse events presented. Adverse events similar to those observed with systemic absorption are also observed, especially following rectal use. Refer to the Hydrocortisone (Systemic) monograph for details.

Cream, ointment: Acneiform eruptions, burning, dryness, folliculitis, hypertrichosis, hypopigmentation, irritation, itching, maceration of skin, miliaria, perioral dermatitis, secondary infection, skin atrophy, striae

Enema: Burning, pain, rectal bleeding

Suppositories: Allergic contact dermatitis, burning, dryness, folliculitis, hypopigmentation, itching, secondary infection

Drug Interactions

Metabolism/Transport Effects Substrate of CYP3A4 (minor); **Note:** Assignment of Major/Minor substrate status based on clinically relevant drug interaction potential

Avoid Concomitant Use

Avoid concomitant use of Hydrocortisone (Topical) with any of the following: Aldesleukin

Increased Effect/Toxicity

Hydrocortisone (Topical) may increase the levels/effects of: Ceritinib; Deferasirox

The levels/effects of Hydrocortisone (Topical) may be increased by: Telaprevir

Decreased Effect

Hydrocortisone (Topical) may decrease the levels/effects of: Aldesleukin; Corticorelin; Hyaluronidase; Telaprevir

Mechanism of Action Decreases inflammation by suppression of migration of polymorphonuclear leukocytes and reversal of increased capillary permeability

Pharmacokinetics (Adult data unless noted)

Absorption: Topical corticosteroids are absorbed percutaneously. The extent is dependent on several factors, including epidermal integrity (intact vs abraded skin), formulation, age of the patient, and the use of occlusive dressings. Percutaneous absorption of topical steroids is increased in neonates (especially preterm neonates), infants, and young children. Rectal absorption is more substantial than most topical preparations; therefore, systemic effects are more common.

Metabolism: In the liver

Half-life, biologic: 8-12 hours

Elimination: Renally, mainly as 17-hydroxysteroids and 17-ketosteroids

Dosing: Usual

Topical: Children and Adults: Usual: Apply 2-3 times/day (depending on severity); may be applied up to 4 times/day

Rectal: Adolescents and Adults: Insert 1 application 1-2 times/day for 2-3 weeks

Ulcerative colitis: One enema nightly for 21 days, or until remission occurs; clinical symptoms should subside within 3-5 days; discontinue use if no improvement within 2-3 weeks; some patients may require 2-3 months of therapy; if therapy lasts >21 days, discontinue slowly by decreasing use to every other night for 2-3 weeks

Administration

Rectal: Patient should lie on left side during administration and for 30 minutes after; retain enema for at least 1 hour, preferably all night

Topical: Apply a thin film to clean, dry skin and rub in gently; avoid contact with eyes. Do not apply to face, underarms, or groin unless directed by physician. Do not wrap or bandage affected area unless directed by physician. Do not apply to diaper areas because diapers or plastic pants may be occlusive.

Monitoring Parameters Growth in pediatric patients; assess HPA axis suppression in patients using topical steroids applied to a large surface area or to areas under occlusion (eg, ACTH stimulation test, morning plasma cortisol test, urinary free cortisol test).

Additional Information To facilitate retention of enema, prior antidiarrheal medication or sedation may be required (especially when beginning therapy)

Dosage Forms Excipient information presented when available (limited, particularly for generics); consult specific product labeling. [DSC] = Discontinued product

Cream, External, as acetate:

Hydrocortisone Max St: 1% (28.4 g)

Cream, External, as base:

Ala Cort: 1% (28.4 g, 85.2 g) [contains cetyl alcohol, propylene glycol]

Anti-Itch Maximum Strength: 1% (28 g) [contains cetyl alcohol, methylparaben]

Anti-Itch Maximum Strength: 1% (28 g) [contains cetyl alcohol, methylparaben, propylene glycol, propylparaben]

Hydrocortisone Max St/12 Moist: 1% (28.4 g) [contains cetearyl alcohol, methylparaben, propylene glycol, propylparaben]

HydroSKIN: 1% (28 g) [contains benzyl alcohol]

Instacort 5: 0.5% (28.4 g)

Med-Derm Hydrocortisone: 0.5% (30 g); 1% (30 g)

Medi-First Hydrocortisone: 1% (1 ea) [contains trolamine (triethanolamine)]

Preparation H Hydrocortisone: 1% (26 g)

Recort Plus: 1% (30 g)

Generic: 0.5% (15 g, 28.35 g, 28.4 g, 30 g); 1% (1 g, 1.5 g, 14.2 g, 20 g, 28 g, 28.35 g, 28.4 g, 30 g, 120 g, 453.6 g, 454 g); 2.5% (20 g, 28 g, 28.35 g, 30 g, 453.6 g)

Cream, Rectal, as base:

Anusol-HC: 2.5% (30 g)

Procto-Pak: 1% (28.4 g)

Proctocort: 1% (28.35 g) [contains cetyl alcohol, propylene glycol]

Proctosol HC: 2.5% (28.35 g)

Proctozone-HC: 2.5% (30 g)

Cream, External, as butyrate:

Locoid: 0.1% (15 g, 45 g) [contains butylparaben, propylparaben]

Locoid Lipocream: 0.1% (45 g, 60 g)
Generic: 0.1% (15 g, 45 g, 60 g)
Cream, External, as probutate:
Pandel: 0.1% (15 g, 45 g, 80 g) [contains butylparaben, methylparaben, propylene glycol]
Cream, External, as valerate:
Generic: 0.2% (15 g, 45 g, 60 g)
Enema, Rectal, as base:
Colocort: 100 mg/60 mL (60 mL)
Cortenema: 100 mg/60 mL (60 mL) [contains methylparaben, polysorbate 80]
Generic: 100 mg/60 mL (60 mL)
Foam, Rectal, as acetate:
Cortifoam: 90 mg (15 g) [contains cetyl alcohol, methylparaben, propylene glycol, propylparaben, trolamine (triethanolamine)]
Gel, External, as acetate:
CortAlo: 2% (43 g) [contains benzyl alcohol, menthol, trolamine (triethanolamine)]
NuZon: 2% (43 g) [contains menthol, trolamine (triethanolamine)]
Generic: 2% (43 g)
Gel, External, as base:
Corticool: 1% (42.53 g) [contains cremophor el, propylene glycol]
First-Hydrocortisone: 10% (60 g) [contains propylene glycol, simethicone]
Instacort 10: 1% (30 g)
Kit, External, as base:
Dermasorb HC: 2% [contains menthol, methylparaben, propylene glycol, propylparaben]
Pediaderm HC: 2% [contains benzalkonium chloride, cetyl alcohol, isopropyl alcohol, methylparaben, propylene glycol, propylparaben]
Scalacort DK: Hydrocortisone lotion 2% and Sal Acid 2% and sulfur 2% [contains benzalkonium chloride, isopropyl alcohol, methylparaben, propylene glycol, propylparaben, soybean lecithin]
Lotion, External, as acetate:
NuCort: 2% (60 g) [contains benzyl alcohol, cetyl alcohol, menthol, trolamine (triethanolamine)]
Lotion, External, as base:
Ala Scalp: 2% (29.6 mL) [contains benzalkonium chloride, isopropyl alcohol, propylene glycol]
Aquanil HC: 1% (120 mL)
Beta HC: 1% (60 mL)
Hydro Skin Maximum Strength: 1% (118 mL) [contains benzyl alcohol]
Rederm: 1% (120 mL)
Sarnol-HC: 1% (59 mL)
Scalacort: 2% (29.6 mL) [contains benzalkonium chloride, isopropyl alcohol, propylene glycol]
TheraCort: 1% (118 mL) [contains methylparaben, propylene glycol, propylparaben, trolamine (triethanolamine)]
Generic: 1% (114 g); 2.5% (59 mL, 118 mL)
Lotion, External, as butyrate:
Locoid: 0.1% (59 mL, 118 mL) [contains butylparaben, cetostearyl alcohol, propylparaben]
Ointment, External, as base:
Generic: 0.5% (28.35 g, 30 g); 1% (25 g, 28 g, 28.35 g, 28.4 g, 30 g, 110 g, 430 g, 453.6 g); 2.5% (20 g, 28.35 g, 453.6 g, 454 g)
Ointment, External, as butyrate:
Locoid: 0.1% (15 g, 45 g)
Generic: 0.1% (15 g, 45 g)
Ointment, External, as valerate:
Westcort: 0.2% (15 g, 45 g, 60 g) [contains propylene glycol]
Generic: 0.2% (15 g, 45 g, 60 g)
Solution, External, as base:
Scalpicin Maximum Strength: 1% (44 mL) [contains disodium edta, menthol, propylene glycol]

Texacort: 2.5% (30 mL) [lipid free, paraben free; contains alcohol, usp]
Solution, External, as butyrate:
Locoid: 0.1% (60 mL) [contains isopropyl alcohol]
Generic: 0.1% (20 mL, 60 mL)
Suppository, Rectal, as acetate:
Anucort-HC: 25 mg (12 ea, 24 ea, 100 ea)
Anusol-HC: 25 mg (12 ea, 24 ea)
GRx HiCort 25: 25 mg (12 ea)
Hemril-30: 30 mg (12 ea [DSC], 24 ea [DSC])
Proctocort: 30 mg (12 ea)
Rectacort-HC: 25 mg (12 ea, 24 ea)
Generic: 25 mg (12 ea, 24 ea); 30 mg (12 ea)

References

Reed, BR, "Dermatologic Drugs, Pregnancy, and Lactation. A Conservative Guide," Arch Dermatol, 1997, 133(7):894-8.

◆ **Hydrocortisone Acetate** see Hydrocortisone (Topical) on page 1038

◆ **Hydrocortisone and Acyclovir** see Acyclovir and Hydrocortisone on page 69

◆ **Hydrocortisone and Ciprofloxacin** see Ciprofloxacin and Hydrocortisone on page 477

◆ **Hydrocortisone, Bacitracin, Neomycin, and Polymyxin B** see Bacitracin, Neomycin, Polymyxin B, and Hydrocortisone on page 258

◆ **Hydrocortisone Butyrate** see Hydrocortisone (Topical) on page 1038

◆ **Hydrocortisone Max St [OTC]** see Hydrocortisone (Topical) on page 1038

◆ **Hydrocortisone Max St/12 Moist [OTC]** see Hydrocortisone (Topical) on page 1038

◆ **Hydrocortisone, Neomycin, and Polymyxin B** see Neomycin, Polymyxin B, and Hydrocortisone on page 1485

◆ **Hydrocortisone Probutate** see Hydrocortisone (Topical) on page 1038

◆ **Hydrocortisone Sodium Succinate** see Hydrocortisone (Systemic) on page 1034

◆ **Hydrocortisone Valerate** see Hydrocortisone (Topical) on page 1038

◆ **Hydrodiuril** see Hydrochlorothiazide on page 1023

◆ **Hydrogen Dioxide** see Hydrogen Peroxide on page 1040

Hydrogen Peroxide (HYE droe jen per OKS ide)

Therapeutic Category Antibacterial, Otic; Antibacterial, Topical; Antibiotic, Oral Rinse
Use Cleanse wounds, suppurating ulcers, and local infections; used in the treatment of inflammatory conditions of the external auditory canal and as a mouthwash or gargle; hydrogen peroxide concentrate (30%) has been used as a hair bleach and as a tooth bleaching agent
Contraindications Should not be used in abscesses
Warnings Hydrogen peroxide concentrate (30%) is a caustic liquid; it should not be tasted since it is strongly irritating to skin or mucous membranes
Precautions Repeat use as a mouthwash or gargle may produce irritation of the buccal mucous membrane or "hairy tongue"; bandages should not be applied too quickly after its use
Stability Protect from light and heat; decomposes upon standing, upon repeated agitation, or when in contact with oxidizing or reducing substances
Mechanism of Action Antiseptic oxidant that slowly releases oxygen and water upon contact with serum or tissue catalase
Pharmacodynamics Duration: Only while bubbling action occurs

Dosing: Usual Children and Adults:

Mouthwash or gargle: Dilute the 3% solution with an equal volume of water; swish around in the mouth over the affected area for at least 1 minute and then expel; use up to 4 times/day (after meals and at bedtime)

Topical:

1.5% to 3% solution for cleansing wounds

1.5% gel for cleansing wounds or mouth/gum irritations: Apply a small amount to the affected area for at least 1 minute, then expectorate; use up to 4 times/day (after meals and at bedtime)

Administration Topical: Do not inject or instill into closed body cavities from which released oxygen cannot escape; strong solutions (30.5%) of hydrogen peroxide should not be applied undiluted to tissues

Dosage Forms

Gel, oral: 1.5% (15 g)

Solution:

Concentrate: 30.5% (480 mL)

Topical: 3% (120 mL, 480 mL)

♦ **Hydromet®** see Hydrocodone and Homatropine on page 1032

♦ **Hydromorph Contin (Can)** see HYDROmorphone on page 1041

HYDROmorphone (hye droe MOR fone)

Medication Safety Issues

Sound-alike/look-alike issues:

Dilaudid may be confused with Demerol, Dilantin

HYDROmorphone may be confused with morphine; significant overdoses have occurred when hydromorphone products have been inadvertently administered instead of morphine sulfate. Commercially available prefilled syringes of both products looks similar and are often stored in close proximity to each other. **Note:** Hydromorphone 1 mg oral is approximately equal to morphine 4 mg oral; hydromorphone 1 mg I.V. is approximately equal to morphine 5 mg I.V.

High alert medication:

The Institute for Safe Medication Practices (ISMP) includes this medication among its list of drug classes which have a heightened risk of causing significant patient harm when used in error.

Administration issues:

Dilaudid, Dilaudid-HP: Extreme caution should be taken to avoid confusing the highly-concentrated (Dilaudid-HP) injection with the less-concentrated (Dilaudid) injectable product.

Exalgo: Extreme caution should be taken to avoid confusing the extended release Exalgo 8 mg tablets with immediate release hydromorphone 8 mg tablets.

Significant differences exist between oral and I.V. dosing. Use caution when converting from one route of administration to another.

Related Information

Opioid Conversion Table on page 2242

Oral Medications That Should Not Be Crushed or Altered on page 2438

Patient Information for Disposal of Unused Medications on page 2412

Brand Names: U.S. Dilaudid; Dilaudid-HP; Exalgo

Brand Names: Canada Dilaudid; Dilaudid-HP; Hydromorph Contin; Hydromorphone HP; Hydromorphone HP 10; Hydromorphone HP 20; Hydromorphone HP 50; Hydromorphone HP Forte; Hydromorphone Hydrochloride Injection, USP; Jurnista; PMS-Hydromorphone; Teva-Hydromorphone

Therapeutic Category Analgesic, Narcotic; Antitussive

Generic Availability (U.S.) May be product dependent

Use

Oral (immediate release): Management of moderate to severe pain (FDA approved in adults); has also been used as an antitussive at lower doses

Oral (extended release; Exalgo): For once-daily administration for the management of moderate to severe pain in **opioid-tolerant** patients who require continuous, around-the-clock analgesia for an extended period of time (FDA approved in adults). Should **NOT** be used as an as-needed analgesic or for management of acute or post-operative pain.

Parenteral: Management of moderate to severe pain (FDA approved in adults)

Parenteral (concentrated; Dilaudid-HP injection): Use in **opioid-tolerant** patients who require larger than usual doses of opioids for pain relief (FDA approved in adults)

Note: Patients are considered to be opioid-tolerant if they have been taking oral morphine ≥60 mg/day, fentanyl transdermal ≥25 mcg/hour, oral oxycodone ≥30 mg/day, oral hydromorphone ≥8 mg/day, oral oxymorphone ≥25 mg/day, or an equianalgesic dose of another opioid for ≥1 week

Prescribing and Access Restrictions Exalgo: As a requirement of the REMS program, healthcare providers who prescribe Exalgo need to receive training on the proper use and potential risks of Exalgo. For training, please refer to http://www.exalgorems.com. Prescribers will need retraining every 2 years or following any significant changes to the Exalgo REMS program.

Medication Guide Available Yes

Pregnancy Risk Factor C

Pregnancy Considerations Adverse events were observed in some animal reproduction studies. Hydromorphone crosses the placenta. Some dosage forms are specifically contraindicated for use in obstetrical analgesia.

When used for pain relief during labor, opioids may temporarily affect the heart rate of the fetus (ACOG, 2002). Monitor the neonate for respiratory depression if hydromorphone is used during labor.

If chronic opioid exposure occurs in pregnancy, adverse events in the newborn (including withdrawal) may occur; monitoring of the neonate is recommended. The minimum effective dose should be used if opioids are needed (Chou, 2009). Neonatal abstinence syndrome following opioid exposure may present with autonomic (eg, fever, temperature instability), gastrointestinal (eg, diarrhea, vomiting, poor feeding/weight gain), or neurologic (eg, high pitched crying, increased muscle tone, irritability, seizure, tremor) symptoms (Dow, 2012; Hudak, 2012).

Breast-Feeding Considerations Low concentrations of hydromorphone can be found in breast milk. Withdrawal symptoms may be observed in breast-feeding infants when opioid analgesics are discontinued. Breast-feeding is not recommended by the manufacturer. Parenteral opioids used during labor have the potential to interfere with a newborn's natural reflex to nurse within the first few hours after birth. Nursing infants exposed to large doses of opioids should be monitored for apnea and sedation (Montgomery, 2012).

Contraindications Hypersensitivity to hydromorphone or any component; significant respiratory depression (especially in settings without resuscitative equipment or without adequate respiratory monitoring); severe CNS depression; patients with severe or acute asthma, paralytic ileus (known or suspected); pregnancy (prolonged use or high doses at term). Additional product-specific contraindications: Dilaudid: Obstetrical analgesia, hypersensitivity to known sulfite-containing medications; Dilaudid-HP: Opioid-nontolerant patients, obstetrical analgesia, hypersensitivity to known sulfite-containing medications; Exalgo: Opioid-nontolerant patients; preexisting GI surgery or diseases resulting in narrowing of GI tract, loops in the GI tract, or GI

◄ obstruction; hypersensitivity to known sulfite-containing medications.

Warnings Respiratory depression may occur **[U.S. Boxed Warning]**; use with extreme caution in patients with preexisting respiratory depression, CNS depression, decreased respiratory reserve, hypoxia, hypercapnia, significant COPD, cor pulmonale, severe obesity, sleep apnea, myxedema, kyphoscoliosis or other skeletal disorders which may alter respiratory function; critical respiratory depression may occur, even at therapeutic dosages. Hypotension may occur, especially in hypovolemic patients or those receiving medications that compromise vasomotor tone (eg, general anesthetics, phenothiazines); use with extreme caution in patients with circulatory shock. Orthostatic hypotension may occur in ambulatory patients. Physical and psychological dependence may occur; abrupt discontinuation after prolonged use may result in withdrawal symptoms or seizures. Warn patient of possible impairment of alertness or physical coordination. Interactions with other CNS drugs may occur **[U.S. Boxed Warning]**. Healthcare provider should be alert to problems of abuse, misuse, addiction, and diversion **[U.S. Boxed Warning]**; risk of opioid abuse is increased in patients with a history or family history of alcohol or drug abuse or mental illness. Infants born to women physically dependent on opioids will also be physically dependent and may experience respiratory difficulties or opioid withdrawal symptoms [neonatal abstinence syndrome (NAS)]. Onset, duration, and severity of NAS depend upon the drug used (maternal), duration of use, maternal dose, and rate of drug elimination by the newborn. Symptoms of opioid withdrawal may include excessive crying, diarrhea, fever, hyper-reflexia, irritability, tremors, vomiting, or failure to gain weight. Opioid withdrawal syndrome in the neonate, unlike in adults, may be life-threatening and should be promptly treated.

Do not confuse the highly concentrated (Dilaudid-HP) injection with the less-concentrated (Dilaudid) injectable product **[U.S. Boxed Warning]**; significant overdose or death could result. Injection (4 mg/mL, 10 mg/mL, and powder for reconstitution), oral liquid, and tablets may contain sodium metabisulfite, which may cause allergic reactions in susceptible individuals. Rubber stopper of multiple dose vials contains latex which may cause allergic reactions in susceptible individuals; avoid use in patients with allergy to latex.

Exalgo extended release tablets are for use only in opioid-tolerant patients **[U.S. Boxed Warning]**; fatal respiratory depression may occur in patients who are not opioid-tolerant. Exalgo is indicated for the management of moderate to severe pain when around-the-clock pain control is needed for an extended time period; not for use as an as-needed analgesic or for the management of acute or postoperative pain. Tablets should be swallowed whole; do not crush, break, chew, dissolve, or inject **[U.S. Boxed Warning]**; doing so may lead to rapid release and absorption of a potentially fatal dose of hydromorphone. Injection of the tablet excipients may be toxic and cause lethal complications. Accidental consumption of Exalgo extended release tablets may lead to fatal overdose, especially in children **[U.S. Boxed Warning]**. Tablets may be visible on abdominal x-rays, especially when digital enhancing techniques are used.

Exalgo extended release tablets are nondeformable; do not administer to patients with preexisting severe gastrointestinal narrowing (eg, esophageal motility, small bowel inflammatory disease, short gut syndrome, history of peritonitis, cystic fibrosis, chronic intestinal pseudo-obstruction, Meckel's diverticulum); obstruction may occur. Exalgo is not recommended for use within 14 days of

MAO inhibitors; severe and unpredictable potentiation by MAO inhibitors has been reported with opioid analgesics.

Precautions Use with caution in patients with hypersensitivity reactions to other phenanthrene derivative opioid agonists (morphine, hydrocodone, levorphanol, oxycodone, oxymorphone, codeine). Use with caution and reduce the initial dose in patients with significant liver, respiratory, or renal disease; hypothyroidism or myxedema; CNS depression or coma; respiratory depression; adrenocortical insufficiency; toxic psychosis; seizures; acute abdominal conditions; post-GI surgery; biliary tract disease; pancreatitis; prostatic hypertrophy or urethral stricture; acute alcoholism; delirium tremens; kyphoscoliosis and in debilitated patients. Use with extreme caution in patients with head injury, intracranial lesions, or elevated intracranial pressure; exaggerated elevation of ICP may occur. Seizures and myoclonus have been reported in severely compromised patients receiving high doses of parenteral hydromorphone. Use with caution in patients undergoing biliary tract surgery (opioids may cause spasm of the sphincter of Oddi).

Adverse Reactions

Cardiovascular: Bradycardia, extrasystoles, flushing (facial), hypertension, hypotension, palpitations, peripheral edema, peripheral vasodilation, syncope, tachycardia

Central nervous system: Abnormal dreams, abnormal gait, abnormality in thinking, aggressive behavior, agitation, apprehension, ataxia, brain disease, burning sensation of skin (Exalgo), central nervous system depression, chills, cognitive dysfunction, confusion, decreased body temperature (Exalgo), depression, disruption of body temperature regulation (Exalgo), dizziness, drowsiness, drug dependence, dysarthria, dysphoria, equilibrium disturbance, euphoria, fatigue, hallucination, headache, hyperesthesia, hyperreflexia, hypoesthesia, hypothermia, increased intracranial pressure, insomnia, lack of concentration, lethargy, malaise, memory impairment, mood changes, myoclonus, nervousness, painful defecation, panic attack, paranoia, paresthesia, psychomotor agitation, restlessness, sedation, seizure, sleep disorder (Exalgo), suicidal ideation, uncontrolled crying, vertigo

Dermatologic: Diaphoresis, erythema (Exalgo), hyperhidrosis, pruritus, skin rash, urticaria

Endocrine & metabolic: Antidiuretic effect, decreased amylase, decreased libido, decreased plasma testosterone, dehydration, fluid retention, hyperuricemia, hypokalemia, weight loss

Gastrointestinal: Abdominal distention, anal fissure, anorexia, bezoar formation (Exalgo), biliary tract spasm, constipation, decreased appetite, decreased gastrointestinal motility (Exalgo), delayed gastric emptying, diarrhea, diverticulitis, diverticulosis, duodenitis, dysgeusia, dysphagia, eructation, flatulence, gastroenteritis, gastroesophageal reflux disease (aggravated; Exalgo), hematochezia, increased appetite, intestinal perforation (large intestine; Exalgo), nausea, paralytic ileus, stomach cramps, vomiting, xerostomia

Genitourinary: Bladder spasm, decreased urine output, difficulty in micturition, dysuria, erectile dysfunction, hypogonadism, sexual disorder, ureteral spasm, urinary frequency, urinary hesitancy, urinary retention

Hematologic & oncologic: Oxygen desaturation

Hepatic: Increased liver enzymes

Hypersensitivity: Histamine release

Local: Pain at injection site, post-injection flare

Neuromuscular & skeletal: Arthralgia, dyskinesia, laryngospasm, muscle rigidity, muscle spasm, myalgia, tremor, weakness

Ophthalmic: Blurred vision, diplopia, dry eye syndrome, miosis, nystagmus

Otic: Tinnitus

Respiratory: Apnea, bronchospasm, dyspnea, flu-like symptoms (Exalgo), hyperventilation, hypoxia, respiratory depression, respiratory distress, rhinorrhea

Rare but important or life-threatening: Angioedema, hypersensitivity

Drug Interactions

Metabolism/Transport Effects None known.

Avoid Concomitant Use

Avoid concomitant use of HYDROmorphone with any of the following: Azelastine (Nasal); MAO Inhibitors; Paraldehyde; Thalidomide

Increased Effect/Toxicity

HYDROmorphone may increase the levels/effects of: Alcohol (Ethyl); Alvimopan; Azelastine (Nasal); Buprenorphine; CNS Depressants; Desmopressin; Diuretics; Hydrocodone; Methotrimeprazine; Metyrosine; Mirtazapine; Paraldehyde; Pramipexole; ROPINIRole; Rotigotine; Selective Serotonin Reuptake Inhibitors; Thalidomide; Zolpidem

The levels/effects of HYDROmorphone may be increased by: Amphetamines; Anticholinergic Agents; Antipsychotic Agents (Phenothiazines); Brimonidine (Topical); Cannabis; Doxylamine; Dronabinol; Droperidol; HydrOXYzine; Kava Kava; Magnesium Sulfate; MAO Inhibitors; Methotrimeprazine; Nabilone; Perampanel; Rufinamide; Sodium Oxybate; Succinylcholine; Tapentadol; Tetrahydrocannabinol

Decreased Effect

HYDROmorphone may decrease the levels/effects of: Pegvisomant

The levels/effects of HYDROmorphone may be decreased by: Ammonium Chloride; Mixed Agonist / Antagonist Opioids; Naltrexone

Stability

Oral, parenteral: Store at 15°C to 30°C (59°F to 86°F); protect from light. A slight yellow discoloration of injection has not been associated with a loss of potency; injection is stable for at least 24 hours when protected from light and stored at 25°C in most common large volume parenteral solutions.

Rectal (suppository): Store in refrigerator.

Mechanism of Action Binds to opioid receptors in the CNS, causing inhibition of ascending pain pathways, altering the perception of and response to pain; causes cough supression by direct central action in the medulla; produces generalized CNS depression

Pharmacodynamics Analgesic effects:

Onset of action:

Oral: Immediate release formulations: Within 15-30 minutes

I.V.: Within 5 minutes

Maximum effect:

Oral: Immediate release formulations: Within 30-90 minutes

I.V.: 10-20 minutes

Duration: Oral: Immediate release formulations, I.V.: 4-5 hours; suppository may provide longer duration of effect

Pharmacokinetics (Adult data unless noted)

Absorption:

I.M.: Variable

Oral: Rapidly absorbed; extensive first-pass effect

Distribution: V_d: 4 L/kg

Protein binding: ~8% to 19%

Metabolism: Primarily in the liver via glucuronidation to inactive metabolites; >95% is metabolized to hydromorphone-3-glucuronide; minor amounts as 6-hydroxy reduction metabolites

Bioavailability: Oral: 62%

Half-life: 2-3 hours; Exalgo: Apparent half-life: ~11 hours

Time to peak serum concentration: Oral: Immediate release: 30-60 minutes; Exalgo: 12-16 hours

Elimination: In urine, principally as glucuronide conjugates; minimal unchanged drug is excreted in urine (~7%) and feces (1%)

Dosing: Usual

Antitussive: Oral:

Children 6-12 years: 0.5 mg every 3-4 hours as needed

Adolescents: 1 mg every 3-4 hours as needed

Pain: Doses should be titrated to appropriate analgesic effects, while minimizing adverse effects; when changing routes of administration, note that oral doses are less than one-half as effective as parenteral doses (may be only $1/5$ as effective):

Infants >6 months who weigh >10 kg (Friedrichsdorf, 2007; Zernikow, 2009):

Oral: Usual initial: 0.03 mg/kg/dose every 4 hours as needed; usual range: 0.03-0.06 mg/kg/dose

I.V.: Usual initial: 0.01 mg/kg/dose every 3-6 hours as needed

Continuous I.V. infusion: Usual initial: 0.003-0.005 mg/kg/**hour**

Children <50 kg and Adolescents <50 kg:

Oral: 0.03-0.08 mg/kg/dose every 3-4 hours as needed

Note: The American Pain Society (2008) recommends an initial oral dose of 0.06 mg/kg for severe pain in children.

I.V.: 0.015 mg/kg/dose every 3-6 hours as needed

Continuous I.V. infusion: Usual initial: 0.003-0.005 mg/kg/**hour** (maximum: 0.2 mg/**hour**) (Friedrichsdorf, 2007; Zernikow, 2009)

Patient-controlled analgesia (PCA): Opioid-naïve:

Children ≥5 years: **Note:** PCA has been used in children as young as 5 years of age; however, clinicians need to assess children 5-8 years of age to determine if they are able to use the PCA device correctly. All patients should receive an initial loading dose of an analgesic (to attain adequate control of pain) before starting PCA for maintenance. Adjust doses, lockouts, and limits based on required loading dose, age, state of health, and presence of opioid tolerance. Use lower end of dosing range for opioid-naïve. Assess patient and pain control at regular intervals and adjust settings if needed (American Pain Society, 2008):

Usual concentration: 0.2 mg/mL

Demand dose: Usual initial: 0.003-0.004 mg/kg/dose; usual range: 0.003-0.005 mg/kg/dose

Lockout: Usual initial: 5 doses/hour

Lockout interval: Range: 6-10 minutes

Usual basal rate: 0-0.004 mg/kg/**hour**

Children >50 kg and Adolescents >50 kg:

Oral: Initial: Opioid-naïve: 1-2 mg/dose every 3-4 hours as needed; patients with prior opioid exposure may tolerate higher initial doses; usual adult dose: 2-4 mg/dose; doses up to 8 mg have been used in adults

I.V.: Initial: Opioid-naïve: 0.2-0.6 mg/dose every 2-4 hours as needed; patients with prior opioid exposure may tolerate higher initial doses.

Patient-controlled analgesia (PCA): **Note:** All patients should receive an initial loading dose of an analgesic (to attain adequate control of pain) before starting PCA for maintenance. Adjust doses, lockouts, and limits based on required loading dose, age, state of health, and presence of opioid tolerance. Use lower end of dosing range for opioid-naïve. Assess patient and pain control at regular intervals and adjust settings if needed (American Pain Society, 2008):

Usual concentration: 0.2 mg/mL

Demand dose: Usual initial: 0.1-0.2 mg; usual range: 0.05-0.4 mg

Lockout interval: Usual initial: 6 minutes; usual range: 5-10 minutes

I.M., SubQ: **Note:** I.M. use may result in variable absorption and a lag time to peak effect.

Initial: Opioid-naïve: 0.8-1 mg every 4-6 hours as needed; patients with prior opioid exposure may require higher initial doses; usual dosage range: 1-2 mg every 3-6 hours as needed

Rectal: 3 mg (1 suppository) every 4-8 hours as needed

Adults:

Acute pain (moderate to severe): Note: These are guidelines and do not represent the maximum doses that may be required in all patients. Doses should be titrated to provide adequate pain relief. When changing routes of administration, oral doses and parenteral doses are **NOT** equivalent; parenteral doses are up to 5 times more potent. Therefore, when administered parenterally, one-fifth of the oral dose will provide similar analgesia.

Oral: Initial: Opioid-naïve: 2-4 mg every 3-4 hours as needed; elderly/debilitated patients may require lower doses; patients with prior opioid exposure may require higher initial doses. **Note:** In adults with severe pain, the American Pain Society recommends an initial dose of 4-8 mg.

I.V.: Initial: Opioid-naïve: 0.2-0.6 mg every 2-3 hours as needed; patients with prior opioid exposure may require higher initial doses.

Continuous I.V. infusion: Usual dosage range: 0.5-1 mg/**hour** (based on 70 kg patient) or 7-15 mcg/kg/**hour**

Patient-controlled analgesia (PCA): **Note:** Opioid-naïve: Consider lower end of dosing range:
Usual concentration: 0.2 mg/mL
Demand dose: Usual: 0.1-0.2 mg; range: 0.05-0.4 mg
Lockout interval: 5-10 minutes

Epidural PCA (de Leon-Casasola, 1996; Liu, 2010; Smith, 2009):
Bolus dose: 0.4-1 mg
Infusion rate: 0.03-0.3 mg/**hour**
Demand dose: 0.02-0.05 mg
Lockout interval: 10-15 minutes

I.M., SubQ: **Note:** I.M. use may result in variable absorption and lag time to peak effect.
Initial: Opioid-naïve: 0.8-1 mg every 4-6 hours as needed; patients with prior opioid exposure may require higher initial doses.
Usual dosage range: 1-2 mg every 4-6 hours as needed

Rectal: 3 mg every 6-8 hours as needed

Chronic pain: Note: Patients taking opioids chronically may become tolerant and require doses higher than the usual dosage range to maintain the desired effect. Tolerance can be managed by appropriate dose titration. There is no optimal or maximal dose for hydromorphone in chronic pain. The appropriate dose is one that relieves pain throughout its dosing interval without causing unmanageable side effects.

Extended release formulation (Exalgo): Oral: Dose requires individualization: Dosing range: 8-64 mg every 24 hours. For use in opioid-tolerant patients only; discontinue all other extended release opioids when starting therapy. Suggested recommendations for converting to Exalgo from other analgesics are presented, but when selecting the initial dose, other characteristics (eg, patient status, degree of opioid tolerance, concurrent medications, type of pain, risk factors for addiction or diversion, etc) should also be considered.

Individualization of dose: Pain relief and adverse events should be assessed frequently. Dose increases may occur not more often than every 3-4 days; consider titrating with increases of 25% to 50% of the current daily dose. If more than 2 doses of rescue medications are needed within 24 hours for 2 consecutive days, consider increasing

the dose of Exalgo. Do not administer more frequently than every 24 hours.

Discontinuing Exalgo: Taper by gradually decreasing the dose by 25% to 50% every 2-3 days to a dose of 8 mg every 24 hours before discontinuing therapy.

Conversion from other oral hydromorphone formulations to Exalgo: Start with the equivalent total daily dose of hydromorphone administered once daily. May titrate every 3-4 days until adequate pain relief with tolerable side effects have been achieved.

Conversion from other opioids to Exalgo: In general, start Exalgo at 50% of the calculated total daily dose every 24 hours. Titrate until adequate pain relief with tolerable side effects has been achieved. The following conversion ratios may be used to convert from **oral** opioid therapy to Exalgo.

Conversion ratios to Exalgo (see table): Select the opioid, sum the total daily dose, then multiply by the conversion ratio to calculate the approximate oral hydromorphone equivalent; start Exalgo at 50% of the calculated total daily dose every 24 hours. (**Note:** The conversion ratios and approximate equivalent doses in this conversion table are only to be used for the conversion from current opioid therapy to Exalgo).

Conversion Ratios to Exalgo[1]

Previous Opioid	Approximate Equivalent Oral Dose	Oral Conversion Ratio[2]
Hydromorphone	12 mg	1
Codeine	200 mg	0.06
Hydrocodone	30 mg	0.4
Methadone[3]	20 mg	0.6
Morphine	60 mg	0.2
Oxycodone	30 mg	0.4
Oxymorphone	20 mg	0.6

[1]*Approximate* equivalent doses for conversion from current opioid therapy to Exalgo.

[2]Ratio for converting oral opioid dose to approximate hydromorphone equivalent dose.

[3]Monitor closely; ratio between methadone and other opioid agonists may vary widely as a function of previous drug exposure. Methadone has a long half-life and may accumulate in the plasma.

Conversion from transdermal fentanyl to Exalgo: Treatment with Exalgo can be started 18 hours after the removal of the transdermal fentanyl patch. For every fentanyl 25 mcg/hour transdermal dose, the equianalgesic dose of Exalgo is 12 mg every 24 hours. An appropriate starting dose is 50% of the calculated total daily dose given every 24 hours

Dosing adjustment in renal impairment: Decrease initial dose and monitor closely; for injection, manufacturer recommends 1/4 to 1/2 initial dosage reductions. Adults: Exalgo: If moderate impairment, start with a reduced dose and monitor closely. For severe impairment, consider use of an alternate analgesic with better dosing flexibility.

Dosing adjustment in hepatic impairment: Decrease initial dose and monitor closely; for injection, manufacturer recommends 1/4 to 1/2 initial dosage reductions. Adults: Dose adjustment should be considered. Exalgo: In patients with moderate to severe hepatic impairment, start with a reduced dose and monitor closely; consider use of an alternate analgesic with better dosing flexibility.

Administration

Oral:

Immediate release: Administer with food or milk to decrease GI upset.

Extended release tablets (Exalgo): Tablets should be swallowed whole; do not crush, break, chew, dissolve, or inject. May be taken with or without food.

Parenteral: I.V.: Administer via slow I.V. injection over at least 2-3 minutes

Rectal: Insert suppository rectally and retain

Monitoring Parameters Pain relief, respiratory rate, heart rate, blood pressure

Test Interactions Some quinolones may produce a false-positive urine screening result for opioids using commercially-available immunoassay kits. This has been demonstrated most consistently for levofloxacin and ofloxacin, but other quinolones have shown cross-reactivity in certain assay kits. Confirmation of positive opioid screens by more specific methods should be considered.

Additional Information Equianalgesic doses: Morphine 10 mg I.M. = hydromorphone 1.5 mg I.M.

Controlled Substance C-II

Dosage Forms Excipient information presented when available (limited, particularly for generics); consult specific product labeling.

Liquid, Oral, as hydrochloride:

Dilaudid: 1 mg/mL (473 mL) [contains methylparaben, propylparaben, sodium metabisulfite; sweet flavor]

Generic: 1 mg/mL (473 mL)

Solution, Injection, as hydrochloride:

Dilaudid: 1 mg/mL (1 mL); 2 mg/mL (1 mL); 4 mg/mL (1 mL)

Dilaudid-HP: 10 mg/mL (1 mL, 5 mL, 50 mL)

Generic: 1 mg/mL (0.5 mL, 1 mL); 2 mg/mL (1 mL, 20 mL); 4 mg/mL (1 mL); 10 mg/mL (1 mL); 50 mg/5 mL (5 mL); 500 mg/50 mL (50 mL)

Solution, Injection, as hydrochloride [preservative free]:

Generic: 10 mg/mL (1 mL); 50 mg/5 mL (5 mL); 500 mg/ 50 mL (50 mL)

Solution Reconstituted, Injection, as hydrochloride:

Dilaudid-HP: 250 mg (1 ea)

Suppository, Rectal, as hydrochloride:

Generic: 3 mg (6 ea)

Tablet, Oral, as hydrochloride:

Dilaudid: 2 mg, 4 mg [contains fd&c yellow #10 aluminum lake, sodium metabisulfite]

Dilaudid: 8 mg [scored; contains sodium metabisulfite]

Generic: 2 mg, 4 mg, 8 mg

Tablet ER 24 Hour Abuse-Deterrent, Oral, as hydrochloride:

Exalgo: 8 mg, 12 mg, 16 mg, 32 mg [contains sodium metabisulfite]

Generic: 8 mg, 12 mg, 16 mg, 32 mg

References

ACOG Committee on Practice Bulletins-Obstetrics, "ACOG Practice Bulletin. Clinical Management Guidelines for Obstetrician-Gynecologists Number 36, July 2002. Obstetric Analgesia and Anesthesia," *Obstet Gynecol*, 2002, 100(1):177-91.

Berde CB and Sethna NF, "Analgesics for the Treatment of Pain in Children," *N Engl J Med*, 2002, 347(14):1094-103.

Carr D, Jacox A, Chapman CR, et al, "Clinical Practice Guideline Number 1: Acute Pain Management: Operative or Medical Procedures and Trauma," Rockville, Maryland: U.S. Department of Health and Human Services, Public Health Service, Agency for Health Care Policy and Research, AHCPR Publication No 92-0032, 1992.

Chou R, Fanciullo GJ, Fine PG, et al, "Clinical Guidelines For the Use of Chronic Opioid Therapy in Chronic Noncancer Pain," *J Pain*, 2009, 10 (2):113-30.

de Leon-Casasola OA and Lema MJ, "Postoperative Epidural Opioid Analgesia: What Are the Choices?" *Anesth Analg*, 1996, 83 (4):867-75.

Dow K, Ordean A, Murphy-Oikonen J, et al, "Neonatal Abstinence Syndrome Clinical Practice Guidelines For Ontario," *J Popul Ther Clin Pharmacol*, 2012, 19(3):e488-506.

Friedrichsdorf SJ and Kang TI, "The Management of Pain in Children With Life-Limiting Illnesses," *Pediatr Clin North Am*, 2007, 54 (5):645-72.

Hudak ML, Tan RC, Committee On Drugs, et al, "Neonatal Drug Withdrawal," *Pediatrics*, 2012, 129(2):e540-60.

Jacox A, Carr D, Payne R, et al, "Clinical Practice Guideline Number 9: Management of Cancer Pain," Rockville, Maryland: U.S. Department of Health and Human Services, Public Health Service, Agency for Health Care Policy and Research, AHCPR Publication No. 94-0592, 1994.

Liu SS, Bieltz M, Wukovits B, et al, "Prospective Survey of Patient-Controlled Epidural Analgesia With Bupivacaine and Hydromorphone in 3736 Postoperative Orthopedic Patients," *Reg Anesth Pain Med*, 2010, 35(4):351-4.

Montgomery A, Hale TW, and Academy of Breastfeeding Medicine, "ABM Clinical Protocol #15: Analgesia and Anesthesia For the Breastfeeding Mother, Revised 2012," *Breastfeed Med*, 2012, 7 (6):547-53.

Phillips MS, "Standardizing I.V. Infusion Concentrations: National Survey Results," *Am J Health Syst Pharm*, 2011, 68(22):2176-82.

"Principles of Analgesic Use in the Treatment of Acute Pain and Cancer Pain," 6th ed, Glenview, IL: American Pain Society, 2008.

Smith HS, *Current Therapy in Pain*, 1st ed, Philadelphia, PA: Saunders, 2009.

Zernikow B, Michel E, Craig F, et al, "Pediatric Palliative Care: Use of Opioids for the Management of Pain," *Paediatr Drugs*, 2009, 11 (2):129-51.

◆ **Hydromorphone HP (Can)** *see* HYDROmorphone *on page 1041*

◆ **Hydromorphone HP 10 (Can)** *see* HYDROmorphone *on page 1041*

◆ **Hydromorphone HP 20 (Can)** *see* HYDROmorphone *on page 1041*

◆ **Hydromorphone HP 50 (Can)** *see* HYDROmorphone *on page 1041*

◆ **Hydromorphone HP Forte (Can)** *see* HYDROmorphone *on page 1041*

◆ **Hydromorphone Hydrochloride** *see* HYDROmorphone *on page 1041*

◆ **Hydromorphone Hydrochloride Injection, USP (Can)** *see* HYDROmorphone *on page 1041*

◆ **HydroSKIN [OTC]** *see* Hydrocortisone (Topical) *on page 1038*

◆ **Hydro Skin Maximum Strength [OTC]** *see* Hydrocortisone (Topical) *on page 1038*

◆ **HydroVal® (Can)** *see* Hydrocortisone (Topical) *on page 1038*

Hydroxocobalamin (hye droks oh koe BAL a min)

Brand Names: U.S. Cyanokit

Brand Names: Canada Cyanokit

Therapeutic Category Antidote, Cyanide; Nutritional Supplement; Vitamin, Water Soluble

Generic Availability (U.S.) May be product dependent

Use

I.M. injection: Treatment of pernicious anemia and other vitamin B_{12} deficiency states; dietary supplement particularly in conditions of increased requirements (eg, pregnancy, thyrotoxicosis, hemorrhage, malignancy, liver or kidney disease) [FDA approved in pediatric patients (all ages) and adults]

I.V. infusion (Cyanokit®): Treatment of cyanide poisoning (FDA approved in adults)

Pregnancy Risk Factor C

Pregnancy Considerations Animal studies are insufficient to determine the effect, if any, on pregnancy or fetal development. There are no adequate and well-controlled studies in pregnant women. Data on the use of hydroxocobalamin in pregnancy for the treatment of cyanide poisoning and cobalamin defects are limited. In general, medications used as antidotes should take into consideration the health and prognosis of the mother; antidotes ▶

should be administered to pregnant women if there is a clear indication for use and should not be withheld because of fears of teratogenicity (Bailey, 2003).

Breast-Feeding Considerations It is not known if hydroxocobalamin is excreted in breast milk. Hydroxocobalamin may be administered in life-threatening situations; therefore, use in a breast-feeding woman is not contraindicated. Because of the unknown potential for adverse reactions in nursing infants, the patient should discontinue nursing.

Contraindications Hypersensitivity to hydroxocobalamin, cyanocobalamin, cobalt, or any component

Warnings Anaphylactic shock has occurred after parenteral vitamin B_{12} administration; intradermal skin testing may be used prior to administration in individuals sensitive to cobalt

When using Cyanokit®: Increased blood pressure (>180 mm Hg systolic or >110 mm Hg diastolic) is associated with infusion; elevations usually noted at beginning of infusion, peak toward the end of infusion, and return to baseline within 4 hours of infusion. May offset hypotension induced by nitrite administration or cyanide.

Due to the risk of serious adverse effects, use with caution in patients where the diagnosis of cyanide poisoning is uncertain. However, if clinical suspicion of cyanide poisoning is high, treatment should not be delayed. Treatment of cyanide poisoning should include decontamination and supportive therapy. Collection of pretreatment blood cyanide concentrations does not preclude administration and should not delay administration in the emergency management of highly suspected or confirmed cyanide toxicity. Pretreatment levels may be useful as postinfusion levels may be inaccurate. Fire victims may present with both cyanide and carbon monoxide poisoning. In this scenario, hydroxocobalamin is the agent of choice for cyanide intoxication. Hydroxocobalamin can discolor the skin and exudates, complicating the assessment of burn severity. Use caution with concurrent use of other cyanide antidotes; safety has not been established. Consider consultation with a poison control center at 1-800-222-1222.

Precautions When using solution for I.M. injection as treatment of severe vitamin B_{12}, megaloblastic anemia may result in thrombocytosis and severe hypokalemia, sometimes fatal, due to intracellular potassium shift upon anemia resolution. Use caution in folic acid deficient megaloblastic anemia; administration of vitamin B_{12} alone is not a substitute for folic acid and might mask true diagnosis. Blunted therapeutic response to vitamin B_{12} may occur in certain conditions (eg, infection, uremia, concurrent iron or folic acid deficiency) or in patients on medications with bone marrow suppressant properties (eg, chloramphenicol). Neurologic manifestations of vitamin B_{12} deficiency will not be prevented with folic acid unless vitamin B_{12} is also given; spinal cord degeneration might also occur when folic acid is used as a substitute for vitamin B_{12} in anemia prevention. Vitamin B_{12} deficiency masks signs of polycythemia vera; vitamin B_{12} administration may unmask this condition.

Photosensitivity is a potential concern; avoid direct sunlight while skin remains discolored. Will produce chromaturia which may last up to 5 weeks after administration. Hydroxocobalamin may interfere with and/or trip alarms in patients who use hemodialysis machines that rely on colorimetric technology.

Adverse Reactions

I.M. injection:
Dermatologic: Exanthema (transient), itching
Gastrointestinal: Diarrhea (mild, transient)
Local: Injection site pain
Miscellaneous: Anaphylaxis, feeling of swelling of the entire body

I.V. infusion (Cyanokit®):
Cardiovascular: Blood pressure increased, chest discomfort, hot flashes, peripheral edema
Central nervous system: Dizziness, headache, memory impairment, restlessness
Dermatologic: Angioneurotic edema (postmarketing reports), erythema (may last up to 2 weeks), pruritus, rash (predominantly acneiform; can appear 7-28 days after administration and usually resolves within a few weeks), urticaria
Gastrointestinal: Abdominal discomfort, diarrhea, dyspepsia, dysphagia, hematochezia, nausea, vomiting
Genitourinary: Chromaturia (may last up to 5 weeks after administration)
Hematologic: Lymphocytes decreased
Local: Infusion site reaction
Ocular: Irritation, redness, swelling
Respiratory: Dry throat, dyspnea, throat tightness
Miscellaneous: Allergic reaction (including anaphylaxis)

Drug Interactions

Metabolism/Transport Effects None known.

Avoid Concomitant Use There are no known interactions where it is recommended to avoid concomitant use.

Increased Effect/Toxicity There are no known significant interactions involving an increase in effect.

Decreased Effect There are no known significant interactions involving a decrease in effect.

Stability
Solution for I.M. injection: Store at 20°C to 25°C (68°F to 77°F). Protect from light.
I.V. infusion (Cyanokit®): Prior to reconstitution, store at 25°C (77°F); excursions permitted to 15°C to 30°C (59°F to 86°F).
Cyanokit® may be exposed at short intervals to temperatures outside of room temperature for transport of lyophilized form:
Usual transport: ≤15 days at 5°C to 40°C (41°F to 104°F)
Desert transport: ≤4 days at 5°C to 60°C (41°F to 140°F)
Freezing/defrosting cycles: ≤15 days at -20°C to 40°C (-4°F to 104°F)
Reconstituted vials (Cyanokit®) are stable for 6 hours at temperatures not exceeding 40°C (104°F).

Mechanism of Action Hydroxocobalamin (vitamin B_{12a}) is a precursor to cyanocobalamin (vitamin B_{12}). Cyanocobalamin acts as a coenzyme for various metabolic functions, including fat and carbohydrate metabolism and protein synthesis, used in cell replication and hematopoiesis. In the presence of cyanide, each hydroxocobalamin molecule can bind one cyanide ion by displacing it for the hydroxo ligand linked to the trivalent cobalt ion, forming cyanocobalamin, which is then excreted in the urine.

Pharmacodynamics Onset of action: I.M.: Megaloblastic anemia: Increased reticulocytes: 2-5 days

Pharmacokinetics (Adult data unless noted)
Distribution: Principally stored in the liver; also stored in the kidneys and adrenals
Protein binding: I.M. solution: Bound to transcobalamin II; I.V.: Cyanokit®: Significant; forms various cobalamin-(III) complexes
Half-life: I.V.: 26-31 hours
Metabolism: Converted in the tissues to active coenzymes methylcobalamin and deoxyadenosylcobalamin
Time to peak serum concentration: 2 hours
Elimination: Urine (50% to 60% within initial 72 hours)

Dosing: Neonatal I.M.:
Congenital transcobalamin deficiency: 1000 mcg twice weekly
Cobalamin C disease: 1000 mcg/dose once daily was used in a single full-term neonate in conjunction with carnitine and folinic acid (Kind, 2002)

Dosing: Usual

Infants, Children, and Adolescents: Note: Due to large difference in dose for different indications; pediatric dosage may be presented in mg or **mcg**; verify dosing units.

Cyanide poisoning: Cyanokit®: Limited data available: **Note:** If cyanide poisoning is suspected, antidotal therapy must be given immediately: I.V.: 70 mg/kg as a single infusion; maximum dose: 5000 mg; may repeat a second dose of 35 mg/kg (maximum dose: 2500 mg) depending on the severity of poisoning and clinical response (Shepherd, 2008)

Vitamin B$_{12}$ deficiency (pernicious anemia); treatment (uncomplicated disease): I.M.:

Manufacturer labeling: Initial: 100 **mcg**/day for ≥2 weeks total dose range: 1000-5000 **mcg**; maintenance: 30-50 **mcg**/month

Alternate dosing: Initial: 1000 **mcg**/day for 7 days, then 100 **mcg** once weekly for 1 month; then maintenance: 100 **mcg**/month

Adults:

Cyanide poisoning: (Cyanokit®): **Note:** If cyanide poisoning is suspected, antidotal therapy must be given immediately. I.V.: Initial: 5 g as single infusion; may repeat a second 5 g dose depending on the severity of poisoning and clinical response: maximum cumulative dose: 10 g

Vitamin B$_{12}$ deficiency (pernicious anemia); treatment: I.M.: Initial: 30 **mcg** once daily for 5-10 days; maintenance: 100-200 **mcg** once per month. **Note:** Larger doses may be required in critically ill patients or if patient has neurologic disease, an infectious disease, or hyperthyroidism.

Dosing adjustment in renal impairment: There are no dosage adjustments provided in manufacturer's labeling (has not been studied).

Dosing adjustment in hepatic impairment: There are no dosage adjustments provided in manufacturer's labeling (has not been studied).

Administration Parenteral:

I.M.: Administer 1000 mcg/mL injection I.M. only; do not administer SubQ

I.V.: Cyanokit®: Reconstitute 5 g vial with 200 mL NS using provided transfer spike; if NS unavailable, may use LR, or D$_5$W; invert or "rock" each vial for at least 60 seconds; do not shake; discard if solution is **not** dark red. Administer as I.V. infusion over 15 minutes; if second dose is needed, administer second dose over 15 minutes to 2 hours depending upon the patient's clinical state. Hydroxocobalamin is chemically incompatible with sodium thiosulfate and sodium nitrite and separate I.V. lines must be used if concomitant administration is desired **(the safety of coadministration is not established).**

Monitoring Parameters

Vitamin B$_{12}$, hematocrit, hemoglobin, reticulocyte count, red blood cell counts, folate and iron levels should be obtained prior to treatment and periodically during treatment.

Cyanide poisoning: Blood pressure and heart rate during and after infusion, serum lactate levels, venous-arterial PO$_2$gradient. Pretreatment cyanide levels may be useful as post infusion levels may be inaccurate.

Megaloblastic anemia: In addition to normal hematological parameters, serum potassium and platelet counts should be monitored during therapy, particularly in the first 48 hours of treatment.

Reference Range

Vitamin B$_{12}$: Normal: 200-900 pg/mL; vitamin B$_{12}$ deficiency: <200 pg/mL; megaloblastic anemia: <100 pg/mL

Cyanide poisoning: Blood cyanide levels may be used for diagnosis confirmation; however, reliable levels require prompt testing and proper storage conditions

Cyanide levels related to clinical symptomatology:

Tachycardia/flushing: 0.5-1 mg/L

Obtundation: 1-2.5 mg/L

Coma: 2.5-3 mg/L

Death: >3 mg/L

Test Interactions The following values may be affected, *in vitro*, following hydroxocobalamin 5 g dose. Interference following hydroxocobalamin 10 g dose can be expected to last up to an additional 24 hours. **Note:** Extent and duration of interference dependent on analyzer used and patient variability.

Falsely elevated:

Basophils, hemoglobin, MCH, and MCHC [duration: 12-16 hours]

Albumin, alkaline phosphatase, cholesterol, creatinine, glucose, total protein, and triglycerides [duration: 24 hours]

Bilirubin [duration: up to 4 days]

Urinalysis: Glucose, protein, erythrocytes, leukocytes, ketones, bilirubin, urobilinogen, nitrite [duration: 2-8 days]

Falsely decreased: ALT and amylase [duration: 24 hours]

Unpredictable:

AST, CK, CKMB, LDH, phosphate, and uric acid [duration: 24 hours]

PT (quick or INR) and aPTT [duration: 24-48 hours]

Urine pH [duration: 2-8 days]

May also interfere with colorimetric tests and cause hemodialysis machines to shut down due to false detection of a blood leak from the blood-like appearance of the solution.

Additional Information Cyanocobalamin is preferred over hydroxocobalamin as a treatment agent for anemia due to reports of antibody formation to the hydroxocobalamin-transcobalamin complex. Cyanide is a clear colorless gas or liquid with a faint bitter almond odor. Cyanide reacts with trivalent ions in cytochrome oxidase in the mitochondria leading to histotoxic hypoxia and lactic acidosis. Signs and symptoms of cyanide toxicity include headache, altered mental status, dyspnea, mydriasis, chest tightness, nausea, vomiting, tachycardia/hypertension (initially), bradycardia/hypotension (later), seizures, cardiovascular collapse, or coma. Expert advice from a regional poison control center for appropriate use may be obtained (1-800-222-1222). Guidelines suggest that at least 10 **g** be stocked. This is enough to treat 1 patient weighing 100 kg for an initial 8- to 24-hour period (Dart, 2009).

Dosage Forms Excipient information presented when available (limited, particularly for generics); consult specific product labeling.

Solution, Intramuscular:

Generic: 1000 mcg/mL (30 mL)

Solution Reconstituted, Intravenous:

Cyanokit: 5 g (1 ea)

References

Bailey B, "Are There Teratogenic Risks Associated With Antidotes Used in the Acute Management of Poisoned Pregnant Women?" *Birth Defects Res A Clin Mol Teratol*, 2003, 67(2):133-40.

Dart RC, Borron SW, Caravati EM, et al, "Expert Consensus Guidelines for Stocking of Antidotes in Hospitals That Provide Emergency Care," *Ann Emerg Med*, 2009, 54(3):386-394.

Geraci MJ, McCoy SL, and Aquino ME, "Woman With Red Uurine: Hydroxocobalamin-Induced Chromaturia," *J Emerg Med*, 2012, 43(3):e207-9.

Kind T, Levy J, Lee M, et al, "Cobalamin C Disease Presenting as Hemolytic-Uremic Syndrome in the Neonatal Period," *J Pediatr Hematol Oncol*, 2002, 24(4):327-9.

Shepherd G and Velez LI, "Role of Hydroxocobalamin in Acute Cyanide Poisoning," *Ann Pharmacother*, 2008, 42(5):661-9.

◆ **Hydroxycarbamide** see Hydroxyurea on page 1051

Hydroxychloroquine (hye droks ee KLOR oh kwin)

Medication Safety Issues
Sound-alike/look-alike issues:
Hydroxychloroquine may be confused with hydrocortisone

Plaquenil may be confused with Platinol

Related Information
Medications for Which a Single Dose May Be Fatal When Ingested by a Toddler *on page 2408*

Brand Names: U.S. Plaquenil

Brand Names: Canada Apo-Hydroxyquine; Gen-Hydroxychloroquine; Mylan-Hydroxychloroquine; Plaquenil; PRO-Hydroxyquine

Therapeutic Category Antimalarial Agent; Antirheumatic, Disease Modifying

Generic Availability (U.S.) Yes

Use Suppression or treatment of malaria caused by susceptible *P. vivax*, *P. ovale*, *P. malariae*, and some strains of *P. falciparum* (not effective against chloroquine-resistant strains of *P. falciparum*; not active against pre-erythrocytic or exoerythrocytic tissue stages of *Plasmodium*); treatment of systemic lupus erythematosus (SLE) and acute or chronic rheumatoid arthritis

Pregnancy Considerations Hydroxychloroquine can be detected in the cord blood at delivery in concentrations similar to those in the maternal serum (Costedoat-Chalumeau, 2002). In animal reproduction studies with chloroquine, accumulation in fetal ocular tissues was observed and remained for several months following drug elimination from the rest of the body. Based on available human data, an increased risk of fetal ocular toxicity has not been observed following maternal use of hydroxychloroquine, but additional studies are needed to confirm (Osadchy, 2011).

Maternal lupus is associated with adverse maternal and fetal events; however, pregnancy outcomes may be improved if conception does not occur until the disease has been inactive for ≥6 months. Hydroxychloroquine is one of the medications recommended for the management of lupus and lupus nephritis in pregnant women. If pregnancy is detected during therapy, it should not be stopped (could precipitate a flare in maternal disease and exposure to the fetus will still continue for 6-8 weeks due to tissue binding) (Baer, 2011; Bertsias, 2012; Hahn, 2012; Levy, 2001). Maternal use of hydroxychloroquine may also decrease the incidence of cardiac malformations associated with neonatal lupus (Izmirly, 2012).

Malaria infection in pregnant women may be more severe than in nonpregnant women and has a high risk of maternal and perinatal morbidity and mortality. Therefore, pregnant women and women who are likely to become pregnant are advised to avoid travel to malaria-risk areas. Hydroxychloroquine is recommended as an alternative treatment of pregnant women for uncomplicated malaria in chloroquine-sensitive regions (refer to current guidelines) (CDC, 2011).

Women exposed to hydroxychloroquine for the treatment of rheumatoid arthritis or systemic lupus erythematosus during pregnancy may be enrolled in the Organization of Teratology Information Specialists (OTIS) Autoimmune Diseases Study pregnancy registry (877-311-8972).

Breast-Feeding Considerations Hydroxychloroquine is excreted into breast milk in low concentrations (Costedoat-Chalumeau, 2002; Ostensen, 1985). In a case report, hydroxychloroquine concentrations were ~100 ng/mL in the maternal serum and 3.2 ng/mL in breast milk 15-24 hours after an initial maternal dose of 200 mg twice daily; the highest milk concentration was 10.6 ng/mL when measured 39-48 hours into the dosing regimen (Østensen, 1985)

Contraindications Hypersensitivity to hydroxychloroquine, 4-aminoquinoline derivatives, or any component; retinal or visual field changes; patients with porphyria or psoriasis

Warnings Children are especially sensitive to 4-aminoquinoline compounds; long-term use in children is contraindicated; daily dose >6-6.5 mg/kg/day in patients with abnormal hepatic or renal function may be associated with an increased risk of retinal toxicity

Precautions Use with caution in patients with hepatic disease, G-6-PD deficiency, and patients on concurrent therapy with known hepatotoxic drugs

Adverse Reactions
Cardiovascular: Cardiomyopathy (rare, relationship to hydroxychloroquine unclear)

Central nervous system: Ataxia, dizziness, emotional changes, headache, irritability, lassitude, nervousness, nightmares, psychosis, seizure, vertigo

Dermatologic: Alopecia, angioedema, bleaching of hair, pigmentation changes (skin and mucosal; black-blue color), rash (acute generalized exanthematous pustulosis, erythema annulare centrifugum, exfoliative dermatitis, lichenoid, maculopapular, morbilliform, purpuric, Stevens-Johnson syndrome, urticarial), urticaria

Gastrointestinal: Abdominal cramping, anorexia, diarrhea, nausea, vomiting, weight loss

Hematologic: Agranulocytosis, aplastic anemia, hemolysis (in patients with glucose-6-phosphate deficiency), leukopenia, thrombocytopenia

Hepatic: Abnormal liver function/hepatic failure (isolated cases)

Neuromuscular & skeletal: Myopathy, palsy, or neuromyopathy leading to progressive weakness and atrophy of proximal muscle groups (may be associated with mild sensory changes, loss of deep tendon reflexes, and abnormal nerve conduction)

Ocular: Abnormal color vision, abnormal retinal pigmentation, atrophy, attenuation of retinal arterioles, corneal changes/deposits (visual disturbances, blurred vision, photophobia [reversible on discontinuation]), decreased visual acuity, disturbance in accommodation, keratopathy, macular edema, nystagmus, optic disc pallor/atrophy, pigmentary retinopathy, retinopathy (early changes reversible [may progress despite discontinuation if advanced]), scotoma

Otic: Deafness, tinnitus

Miscellaneous: Exacerbation of porphyria and nonlight sensitive psoriasis

Respiratory: Bronchospasm, respiratory failure (myopathy-related)

Drug Interactions
Metabolism/Transport Effects None known.

Avoid Concomitant Use
Avoid concomitant use of Hydroxychloroquine with any of the following: Artemether; BCG; Lumefantrine; Mefloquine; Natalizumab; Pimecrolimus; Tacrolimus (Topical); Tofacitinib

Increased Effect/Toxicity
Hydroxychloroquine may increase the levels/effects of: Antipsychotic Agents (Phenothiazines); Beta-Blockers; Cardiac Glycosides; Dapsone (Systemic); Dapsone (Topical); Leflunomide; Lumefantrine; Mefloquine; Natalizumab; Tofacitinib; Vaccines (Live)

The levels/effects of Hydroxychloroquine may be increased by: Artemether; Dapsone (Systemic); Denosumab; Mefloquine; Pimecrolimus; Roflumilast; Tacrolimus (Topical); Trastuzumab

Decreased Effect

Hydroxychloroquine may decrease the levels/effects of: Anthelmintics; BCG; Coccidioidin Skin Test; Sipuleucel-T; Vaccines (Inactivated)

The levels/effects of Hydroxychloroquine may be decreased by: Echinacea

Stability Store tablets at room temperature; protect from light

Mechanism of Action Interferes with digestive vacuole function within sensitive malarial parasites by increasing the pH and interfering with lysosomal degradation of hemoglobin; inhibits locomotion of neutrophils and chemotaxis of eosinophils; impairs complement-dependent antigen-antibody reactions

Pharmacodynamics Onset of action for JRA: 2-4 months, up to 6 months

Pharmacokinetics (Adult data unless noted)

Absorption: Highly variable (31% to 100%)

Distribution: Extensive distribution to most body fluids and tissues; excreted into breast milk; crosses the placenta

Metabolism: In the liver

Bioavailability: Increased when administered with food

Elimination: Metabolites and unchanged drug slowly excreted in the urine

Dosing: Usual Oral:

Children:

Chemoprophylaxis of malaria: 5 mg/kg **(base)** once weekly; do not exceed the recommended adult dose; begin 2 weeks before exposure; continue for 4 weeks after leaving endemic area

Uncomplicated acute attack of malaria: 10 mg/kg **(base)** initial dose; followed by 5 mg/kg **(base)** in 6-8 hours on day 1; 5 mg/kg **(base)** as a single dose on day 2 and on day 3

JRA or SLE: 3-5 mg/kg/day **(as sulfate)** divided 1-2 times/day to a maximum of 400 mg/day **(as sulfate)**; not to exceed 7 mg/kg/day

Adults:

Chemoprophylaxis of malaria: 310 mg **(base)** once weekly on same day each week; begin 2 weeks before exposure; continue for 4 weeks after leaving endemic area

Uncomplicated acute attack of malaria: 620 mg **(base)** first dose day one; 310 mg **(base)** in 6-8 hours day one; 310 mg **(base)** as a single dose day 2; and 310 mg **(base)** as a single dose on day 3

Rheumatoid arthritis: 400-600 mg/day **(as sulfate)** once daily to start; increase dose until optimum response level is reached; usually after 4-12 weeks dose should be reduced by 50% and a maintenance dose given of 200-400 mg/day **(as sulfate)** divided 1-2 times/day

Lupus erythematosus: 400 mg/day **(as sulfate)** every day or twice daily for several weeks depending on response; 200-400 mg/day **(as sulfate)** for prolonged maintenance therapy

Administration Oral: Administer with food or milk to decrease GI distress

Monitoring Parameters Ophthalmologic examination at baseline and every 3 months with prolonged therapy (including visual acuity, slit-lamp, fundoscopic, and visual field exam), CBC with differential and platelet count; check for muscular weakness with prolonged therapy

Dosage Forms Excipient information presented when available (limited, particularly for generics); consult specific product labeling.

Tablet, Oral:

Generic: 200 mg

Tablet, Oral, as sulfate:

Plaquenil: 200 mg

Generic: 200 mg

Extemporaneous Preparations A 25 mg/mL hydroxychloroquine sulfate oral suspension may be made with tablets. With a towel moistened with alcohol, remove the coating from fifteen 200 mg hydroxychloroquine sulfate tablets. Crush tablets in a mortar and reduce to a fine powder. Add 15 mL of Ora-Plus® and mix to a uniform paste; add an additional 45 mL of vehicle and mix until uniform. Mix while adding sterile water for irrigation in incremental proportions to **almost** 120 mL; transfer to a calibrated bottle, rinse mortar with sterile water, and add sufficient quantity of sterile water to make 120 mL. Label "shake well". A 30-day expiration date is recommended, although stability testing has not been performed.

Pesko LJ, "Compounding: Hydroxychloroquine," *Am Druggist*, 1993, 207(4):57.

References

Baer AN, Witter FR, and Petri M, "Lupus and Pregnancy," *Obstet Gynecol Surv*, 2011, 66(10):639-53.

Bertsias GK, Tektonidou M, Amoura Z, et al, "Joint European League Against Rheumatism and European Renal Association-European Dialysis and Transplant Association (EULAR/ERA-EDTA) Recommendations For the Management of Adult and Paediatric Lupus Nephritis," *Ann Rheum Dis*, 2012, 71(11):1771-82.

Centers for Disease Control and Prevention, "Guidelines for the Treatment of Malaria in the United States," available at http://www.cdc.gov/malaria/diagnosis_treatment/tx_clinicians.htm and http://www.cdc.gov/malaria/resources/pdf/treatmenttable.pdf; last accessed October 2, 2007.

Costedoat-Chalumeau N, Amoura Z, Aymard G, et al, "Evidence of Transplacental Passage of Hydroxychloroquine in Humans," *Arthritis Rheum*, 2002, 46(4):1123-4.

Emery H, "Clinical Aspects of Systemic Lupus Erythematosus in Childhood," *Pediatr Clin North Am*, 1986, 33(5):1177-90.

Giannini EH and Cawkwell GD, "Drug Treatment in Children With Juvenile Rheumatoid Arthritis. Past, Present, and Future," *Pediatr Clin North Am*, 1995, 42(5):1099-125.

"Guidelines for the Management of Rheumatoid Arthritis. American College of Rheumatology Ad Hoc Committee on Clinical Guidelines," *Arthritis Rheum*, 1996, 39(5):713-22.

Hahn BH, McMahon MA, Wilkinson A, et al, "American College of Rheumatology Guidelines For Screening, Treatment, and Management of Lupus Nephritis," *Arthritis Care Res (Hoboken)*, 2012, 64 (6):797-808.

Izmirly PM, Costedoat-Chalumeau N, Pisoni CN, et al, "Maternal Use of Hydroxychloroquine Is Associated With a Reduced Risk of Recurrent Anti-SSA/Ro-Antibody-Associated Cardiac Manifestations of Neonatal Lupus," *Circulation*, 2012, 126(1):76-82.

Levy RA, Vilela VS, Cataldo MJ, et al, "Hydroxychloroquine (HCQ) in Lupus Pregnancy: Double-Blind and Placebo-Controlled Study," *Lupus*, 2001, 10(6):401-4.

Osadchy A, Ratnapalan T, and Koren G, "Ocular Toxicity in Children Exposed *in utero* to Antimalarial Drugs: Review of the Literature," *J Rheumatol*, 2011, 38(12):2504-8.

Østensen M, Brown ND, Chiang PK, et al, "Hydroxychloroquine in Human Breast Milk," *Eur J Clin Pharmacol*, 1985, 28(3):357.

◆ **Hydroxychloroquine Sulfate** *see* Hydroxychloroquine *on page 1048*

◆ **Hydroxydaunomycin Hydrochloride** *see* DOXOrubicin (Conventional) *on page 718*

◆ **Hydroxyethylcellulose** *see* Artificial Tears *on page 205*

◆ **Hydroxyethyl Starch** *see* Hetastarch *on page 1014*

◆ **Hydroxyethyl Starch** *see* Tetrastarch *on page 1998*

◆ **Hydroxyldaunorubicin Hydrochloride** *see* DOXOrubicin (Conventional) *on page 718*

Hydroxyprogesterone Caproate

(hye droks ee proe JES te rone CAP ro ate)

Medication Safety Issues

Sound-alike/look-alike issues:

Hydroxyprogesterone caproate may be confused with medroxyPROGESTERone

Related Information

Safe Handling of Hazardous Drugs *on page 2419*

Brand Names: U.S. Makena

Therapeutic Category Progestin

Generic Availability (U.S.) No

Use To reduce the risk of preterm birth in women with singleton pregnancies who have a history of spontaneous preterm birth (delivery <37 weeks gestation) with previous singleton pregnancies (FDA approved in ages ≥16 years and adults). **Note:** Not for use in women with multiple gestations or other risk factors for preterm birth; not intended to stop active preterm labor.

Prescribing and Access Restrictions The Makena Care Connection™ is a comprehensive program for patients and healthcare providers which provides administrative support (including insurance benefit investigation and prescription fulfillment); financial and co-pay assistance for eligible patients; and treatment support (including educational information, home health care service and scheduled treatment reminders). The Makena Care Connection™ is available by calling 1-800-847-3418, Monday-Friday, 8 AM to 9 PM EST.

Pregnancy Risk Factor B

Pregnancy Considerations Teratogenic events were not observed in animal reproduction studies; embryolethality was observed in some species. Teratogenic effects were not observed in human studies following second or third trimester exposure; first trimester data not available.

Maternal serum concentrations of hydroxyprogesterone caproate are widely variable and may be decreased in women with increased BMI. Hydroxyprogesterone is metabolized by the placenta and reaches the fetal circulation. In one study, the cord:maternal concentration ratio averaged 0.2. Hydroxyprogesterone caproate was detected in cord blood when delivery occurred ≥44 days after the last injection (Cartitis, 2012; Hemauer, 2008).

Breast-Feeding Considerations Progestins have been detected in milk and have not been found to adversely affect breast-feeding, health, growth, or development of the infant. Use of hydroxyprogesterone caproate is not indicated following delivery.

Contraindications Hypersensitivity to hydroxyprogesterone or any component; current or history of thrombosis or thromboembolic disorders; carcinoma of the breast (known or suspected) or other hormone sensitive cancers (or history of); undiagnosed vaginal bleeding unrelated to pregnancy; cholestatic jaundice of pregnancy, liver tumors (benign or malignant); active liver disease, uncontrolled hypertension

Warnings Hazardous agent; use appropriate precautions for handling and disposal (NIOSH, 2012).

Arterial thrombosis, DVT, or thromboembolic events may occur; discontinue use; contraindicated with current or history of thrombosis or thromboembolic disorders. If hypertension develops during therapy, monitor patients closely; consider risks and benefits of continuation of therapy; contraindicated with uncontrolled hypertension. If jaundice develops during therapy, monitor patients closely; consider risks and benefits of continuation of therapy; contraindicated in patients with cholestatic jaundice of pregnancy. Clinical benefits related to neonatal mortality and morbidity following use have not been demonstrated. Long-term effects of hydroxyprogesterone *in utero* exposure were evaluated in a follow-up safety study of 278 children (mean age: 48 months) whose mothers were part of an earlier hydroxyprogesterone-placebo efficacy trial; no significant differences in physical development, neurodevelopment, and health status were reported between the treatment and placebo groups (Northen, 2007).

Injection contains benzyl alcohol and benzoate which may cause allergic reactions in susceptible individuals. Contains castor oil which may cause allergic reactions in susceptible individuals; discontinue if allergic reactions (eg, urticaria, pruritus, angioedema) occur.

Precautions Use caution in women with diabetes; decreased glucose tolerance may occur. Use with caution in patients with depression; discontinue if depression

occurs. Use with caution in patients with diseases which may be exacerbated by fluid retention, including asthma, epilepsy, migraine, diabetes, pre-eclampsia, cardiac or renal dysfunction; specific studies have not been conducted; elimination may be decreased.

Adverse Reactions

Cardiovascular: Preeclampsia

Dermatologic: Pruritus, urticaria

Endocrine & metabolic: Gestational diabetes

Gastrointestinal: Diarrhea, nausea

Genitourinary: Oligohydramnios, preterm labor (admission), spontaneous abortion, stillborn infant

Local: Local pruritus, pain at injection site, swelling at injection site

Miscellaneous: Nodule

Rare but important or life-threatening: Angioedema, cellulitis at injection site, cervical dilation, cervical shortening, decreased glucose tolerance, depression, fluid retention, headache, hypersensitivity reaction, hypertension, hot flash, jaundice, premature rupture of membranes, pulmonary embolism, skin rash, thromboembolic complications, urinary tract infection

Drug Interactions

Metabolism/Transport Effects Substrate of CYP3A4 (major); **Note:** Assignment of Major/Minor substrate status based on clinically relevant drug interaction potential; **Induces** CYP1A2 (weak/moderate), CYP2A6 (strong), CYP2B6 (weak/moderate)

Avoid Concomitant Use

Avoid concomitant use of Hydroxyprogesterone Caproate with any of the following: Conivaptan; Fusidic Acid (Systemic); Ulipristal

Increased Effect/Toxicity

The levels/effects of Hydroxyprogesterone Caproate may be increased by: Ceritinib; Conivaptan; CYP3A4 Inhibitors (Moderate); CYP3A4 Inhibitors (Strong); Dasatinib; Fusidic Acid (Systemic); Herbs (Progestogenic Properties); Ivacaftor; Luliconazole; Mifepristone; Simeprevir; Stiripentol

Decreased Effect

Hydroxyprogesterone Caproate may decrease the levels/effects of: Anticoagulants; CYP2A6 Substrates

The levels/effects of Hydroxyprogesterone Caproate may be decreased by: Aminoglutethimide; Bosentan; CYP3A4 Inducers (Strong); Dabrafenib; Deferasirox; Mitotane; Siltuximab; St Johns Wort; Tocilizumab; Ulipristal

Stability Hazardous agent; use appropriate precautions for handling and disposal (NIOSH, 2012). Store upright at controlled room temperature of 15°C to 30°C (59°F to 86°F); protect from light; discard within 5 weeks of first use.

Pharmacokinetics (Adult data unless noted)

Distribution: Extensively bound to albumin and corticosteroid-binding globulins

Metabolism: Hepatic via CYP3A4 and 3A5; forms metabolites

Half-life elimination: ~8 days

Time to peak, serum concentration: 3-7 days

Elimination: Urine (~30%) and feces (~50%); primarily as metabolites

Dosing: Usual

Reduce the risk of preterm birth: Adolescents ≥16 years and Adults: I.M.: 250 mg every 7 days; treatment should be initiated between 16 weeks 0 days and 20 weeks 6 days of gestation, can be continued up to 37 weeks gestation (ie, 36 weeks 6 days) or until delivery, whichever occurs first.

Administration I.M.: Withdraw dose using an 18-gauge needle; inject dose using a 21-gauge 1 1/2-inch needle. Administer by slow injection (≥1 minute) into the upper outer quadrant of the gluteus maximus by a healthcare professional. Solution is viscous and oily; do not use if solution is cloudy or contains solid particles. Apply pressure to injection site to decrease bruising and swelling.

Hazardous agent; use appropriate precautions for handling and disposal (NIOSH, 2012).

Monitoring Parameters Signs and symptoms of thromboembolic disorders; signs or symptoms of depression; signs and symptoms of jaundice; glucose in patients with diabetes; or blood pressure

Dosage Forms Excipient information presented when available (limited, particularly for generics); consult specific product labeling.

Oil, Intramuscular:

Makena: 250 mg/mL (5 mL) [contains benzyl alcohol, benzyl benzoate]

References

Caritis SN, Sharma S, Venkataramanan R, et al, "Pharmacology and Placental Transport of 17-Hydroxyprogesterone Caproate in Singleton Gestation," *Am J Obstet Gynecol*, 2012, 207(5):398.

Hemauer SJ, Yan R, Patrikeeva SL, et al, "Transplacental Transfer and Metabolism of 17-alpha-Hydroxyprogesterone Caproate," *Am J Obstet Gynecol*, 2008, 199(2):169.e1-5.

National Institute for Occupational Safety and Health (NIOSH), "NIOSH List of Antineoplastic and Other Hazardous Drugs in Healthcare Settings 2012." Available at http://www.cdc.gov/niosh/docs/2012-150/pdfs/2012-150.pdf. Accessed January 21, 2013.

Northen AT, Norman GS, Anderson K, et al, "Follow-Up of Children Exposed *in utero* to 17 Alpha-Hydroxyprogesterone Caproate Compared With Placebo," *Obstet Gynecol*, 2007, 110(4):865-72.

◆ **9-hydroxy-risperidone** *see* Paliperidone *on page 1581*

Hydroxyurea (hye droks ee yoor EE a)

Medication Safety Issues

Sound-alike/look-alike issues:

Hydroxyurea may be confused with hydrOXYzine

High alert medication:

This medication is in a class the Institute for Safe Medication Practices (ISMP) includes among its list of drug classes which have a heightened risk of causing significant patient harm when used in error.

International issues:

Hydrea [U.S., Canada, and multiple international markets] may be confused with Hydra brand name for isoniazid [Japan]

Related Information

Emetogenic Potential of Antineoplastic Agents in Children *on page 2327*

Oral Medications That Should Not Be Crushed or Altered *on page 2438*

Safe Handling of Hazardous Drugs *on page 2419*

Brand Names: U.S. Droxia; Hydrea

Brand Names: Canada Apo-Hydroxyurea; Gen-Hydroxyurea; Hydrea®; Mylan-Hydroxyurea

Therapeutic Category Antineoplastic Agent, Miscellaneous

Generic Availability (U.S.) Yes

Use Treatment of refractory chronic myelocytic leukemia (CML), melanoma, and recurrent, metastatic or inoperable ovarian carcinoma (Hydrea: FDA approved in adults); treatment of primary squamous cell carcinomas of the head and neck with radiation (excluding lip cancer) (Hydrea®: FDA approved in adults); management of sickle cell anemia in patients who have had at least three painful crises in the previous 12 months (to reduce frequency of these crises and the need for blood transfusions) (Droxia: FDA approved in adults); has also been used in the treatment of hematologic conditions, such as essential thrombocythemia, polycythemia vera, and hypereosinophilic syndrome; treatment of hyperleukocytosis due to acute myeloid leukemia; treatment of meningiomas

Pregnancy Risk Factor D

Pregnancy Considerations Animal reproduction studies have demonstrated teratogenicity and embryotoxicity at

doses lower than the usual human dose (based on BSA). Hydroxyurea may cause fetal harm if administered during pregnancy. Women of childbearing potential should be advised to avoid becoming pregnant during treatment and should use effective contraception.

Breast-Feeding Considerations Hydroxyurea is excreted in breast milk. Due to the potential for serious adverse reactions in the nursing infant, the decision to discontinue hydroxyurea or to discontinue breast-feeding should take into account the importance of treatment to the mother.

Contraindications Hypersensitivity to hydroxyurea or any component

Hydrea: Marked bone marrow suppression (WBC <2500/mm^3 or platelet count <100,000/mm^3) or severe anemia

Warnings Hazardous agent; use appropriate precautions for handling and disposal (NIOSH, 2012); wear gloves when handling and wash hands before and after contact to decrease risk of exposure. Hydroxyurea is mutagenic, clastogenic, and presumed to be a human carcinogen **[U.S. Boxed Warning]**; secondary leukemia and skin cancer have been reported in patients receiving long-term hydroxyurea therapy for myeloproliferative disorders; it is unknown if this is drug-related or disease-related. Hydroxyurea impairs fertility and is embryotoxic causing fetal malformations; women of childbearing potential should be advised to avoid becoming pregnant.

Myelosuppression (severe or life-threatening) may occur; leukopenia, including neutropenia, occurs more frequently than thrombocytopenia and anemia; typically reversible with interruption of therapy or dosage reduction. Severe anemia should be corrected prior to initiating treatment. Monitor hematologic status at baseline and periodically during therapy; in patients with sickle cell anemia, do not initiate or continue ongoing treatment if neutrophil count <2000 cells/mm^3, platelet count <80,000/mm^3, hemoglobin <4.5 g/dL, reticulocyte count <80,000/mm^3 when hemoglobin <9 g/dL. Use with caution in patients with a history of prior chemotherapy or radiation therapy; myelosuppression is more common; do not administer if WBC <2500/mm^3 or platelet count <100,000/mm^3. Self-limiting megaloblastic erythropoiesis may be seen early in treatment and can resemble pernicious anemia; however, it is unrelated to a vitamin B$_{12}$ or folic acid deficiency. Plasma iron clearance may be delayed and the rate of utilization of iron by erythrocytes may be reduced. May cause macrocytosis, which can mask folic acid deficiency; prophylactic folic acid administration is recommended for sickle cell patients.

Vasculitic ulcerations and gangrene have been reported in patients who received hydroxyurea for myeloproliferative disorders with a previous or concurrent history of interferon use; discontinue and consider alternate cytoreductive therapy if cutaneous vasculitic ulcerations develop.

When treated concomitantly with hydroxyurea and antiretroviral agents (including didanosine), HIV-infected patients are at higher risk for developing fatal and nonfatal pancreatitis, hepatotoxicity, hepatic failure, and severe peripheral neuropathy; evaluate hepatic function at baseline and periodically with therapy; discontinue immediately if signs of hepatic impairment or pancreatitis develop. Most fatal hepatic events occurred in patients receiving hydroxyurea, didanosine, and stavudine; avoid this combination.

Precautions Use with caution in patients with marked renal impairment; clearance is decreased; reduce dosage in some cases. Patients with previous radiation therapy are at risk for an exacerbation of postirradiation erythema. Administer under the supervision of a physician experienced in the treatment of sickle cell anemia **[U.S. Boxed Warning]** or in cancer chemotherapy.

◀ **Adverse Reactions**
Cardiovascular: Edema
Central nervous system: Chills, disorientation, dizziness, drowsiness (dose-related), fever, hallucinations, headache, malaise, seizure
Dermatologic: Alopecia, cutaneous vasculitic toxicities, dermatomyositis-like skin changes, facial erythema, gangrene, hyperpigmentation, maculopapular rash, nail atrophy, nail discoloration, peripheral erythema, scaling, skin atrophy, skin cancer, skin ulcer, vasculitis ulcerations, violet papules
Endocrine & metabolic: Hyperuricemia
Gastrointestinal: Anorexia, constipation, diarrhea, gastrointestinal irritation and mucositis, (potentiated with radiation therapy), nausea, pancreatitis, stomatitis, vomiting
Genitourinary: Dysuria
Hematologic: Myelosuppression (anemia, leukopenia/neutropenia [common], thrombocytopenia; hematologic recovery: within 2 weeks); macrocytosis, megaloblastic erythropoiesis, secondary leukemias (long-term use)
Hepatic: Hepatic enzymes increased, hepatotoxicity
Neuromuscular & skeletal: Peripheral neuropathy, weakness
Renal: BUN increased, creatinine increased, renal tubular dysfunction
Respiratory: Acute diffuse pulmonary infiltrates (rare), dyspnea, pulmonary fibrosis (rare)

Drug Interactions
Metabolism/Transport Effects None known.
Avoid Concomitant Use
Avoid concomitant use of Hydroxyurea with any of the following: BCG; CloZAPine; Didanosine; Dipyrone; Natalizumab; Pimecrolimus; Stavudine; Tacrolimus (Topical); Tofacitinib; Vaccines (Live)
Increased Effect/Toxicity
Hydroxyurea may increase the levels/effects of: CloZAPine; Didanosine; Leflunomide; Natalizumab; Stavudine; Tofacitinib; Vaccines (Live)

The levels/effects of Hydroxyurea may be increased by: Denosumab; Didanosine; Dipyrone; Pimecrolimus; Roflumilast; Stavudine; Tacrolimus (Topical); Trastuzumab
Decreased Effect
Hydroxyurea may decrease the levels/effects of: BCG; Coccidioidin Skin Test; Sipuleucel-T; Vaccines (Inactivated); Vaccines (Live)

The levels/effects of Hydroxyurea may be decreased by: Echinacea
Stability Hazardous agent; use appropriate precautions for handling and disposal (NIOSH, 2012). Store at 25°C (77°F); excursions permitted to 15°C to 30°C (59°F to 86°F); keep tightly closed.
Mechanism of Action Antimetabolite which selectively inhibits ribonucleoside diphosphate reductase, preventing the conversion of ribonucleotides to deoxyribonucleotides, halting the cell cycle at the G1/S phase and therefore has radiation sensitizing activity by maintaining cells in the G_1 phase and interfering with DNA repair. In sickle cell anemia, hydroxyurea increases red blood cell (RBC) hemoglobin F levels, RBC water content, deformability of sickled cells, and alters adhesion of RBCs to endothelium.
Pharmacodynamics
Onset: Sickle cell anemia: Fetal hemoglobin increase: 4-12 weeks
Maximum effect: Sickle cell anemia: 6-18 months
Pharmacokinetics (Adult data unless noted) Note: In pediatric patients, large interpatient variability and phenotypic differences have been reported (Ware, 2011).
Absorption: Relatively rapid (Rodriguez, 1998)

Distribution: Distributes widely into tissues (including into the brain); concentrates in leukocytes and erythrocytes; estimated volume of distribution approximating total body water (Gwilt, 1998)
V_d:
Children: ~12 L (range: 2.5-52) (Ware, 2011)
Adults: ~20 L/m^2 (Rodriguez, 1998)
Metabolism: 60% via hepatic metabolism and urease found in intestinal bacteria
Bioavailability: ~100% (Rodriguez, 1998)
Half-life:
Children: 1.7 hours (range: 0.65-3.05 hours) (Ware, 2011)
Adults: 1.9-3.9 hours (Gwilt, 1998)
Time to peak serum concentration:
Children: "Fast" phenotype: 15-30 minutes; "Slow" phenotype: 60-120 minutes (Ware, 2011)
Adults: 1-4 hours
Elimination: Urine (sickle cell anemia: 40% of administered dose)
Clearance):
Children: ~7 L/hour (range: 1.6-22) (Ware, 2011)
Adults: ~7.5 L/hour (Gwilt, 1998)
Dosing: Usual Note: Doses should be based on ideal or actual body weight, whichever is less (per manufacturer).
Infants ≥6 months, Children, and Adolescents: **Sickle cell anemia:** Oral: 20 mg/kg/dose once daily; increase by 5 mg/kg/**day** every 2-6 months to a maximum dose of 35 mg/kg/**day** or 2500 mg/**day**, whichever is less (Strouse, 2012); dose is titrated to patient response; if bone marrow suppression occurs, hold therapy until counts recover; if recovery is prolonged (>2 weeks) or toxicity is recurrent, decrease dose by 2.5-5 mg/kg/day (Ferster, 2001; Hankins, 2005; Heeney, 2008; Thornburg, 2009; Wang, 2001; Wang, 2011; Zimmerman, 2004)
Adults:
Antineoplastic uses: Titrate dose to patient response; if WBC count falls to <2500/mm^3, or the platelet count to <100,000/mm^3, therapy should be stopped for at least 3 days and resumed when values rise toward normal.
ASCO guidelines for chemotherapy dosing in obese adults with cancer: Utilize patient's actual body weight (full weight) for calculation of body surface area- or weight-based dosing, particularly when the intent of therapy is curative; manage regimen-related toxicities in the same manner as for nonobese patients; if a dose reduction is utilized due to toxicity, consider resumption of full weight-based dosing with subsequent cycles, especially if cause of toxicity (eg, hepatic or renal impairment) is resolved (Griggs, 2012). **Note:** The manufacturer recommends dosing based on ideal or actual body weight, whichever is less.
Chronic myelocytic leukemia (resistant): Oral: Continuous therapy: 20-30 mg/kg/dose once daily
Solid tumors (head and neck cancer, melanoma, ovarian cancer): Oral:
Intermittent therapy: 80 mg/kg as a single dose every third day
Continuous therapy: 20-30 mg/kg/dose once daily
Concomitant therapy with irradiation (head and neck cancer): 80 mg/kg as a single dose every third day starting at least 7 days before initiation of irradiation
Sickle cell anemia: Oral: Initial: 15 mg/kg/dose once daily; if blood counts are in an acceptable range, may increase by 5 mg/kg every 12 weeks until the maximum tolerated dose of 35 mg/kg/day is achieved or the dose that does not produce toxic effects (do not increase dose if blood counts are between acceptable and toxic ranges). Monitor for toxicity every 2 weeks; if toxicity occurs, withhold treatment until the bone marrow recovers, then restart with a dose reduction of 2.5 mg/kg/day; if no toxicity occurs over the next 12 weeks, then the subsequent dose may be increased by 2.5 mg/kg/day

every 12 weeks to a maximum tolerated dose (dose which does not produce hematologic toxicity for 24 consecutive weeks). If hematologic toxicity recurs a second time at a specific dose, do not retry that dose.
Acceptable hematologic ranges: Neutrophils ≥2500/mm³; platelets ≥95,000/mm³; hemoglobin >5.3 g/dL, and reticulocytes ≥95,000/mm³ if the hemoglobin concentration is <9 g/dL
Toxic hematologic ranges: Neutrophils <2000/mm³; platelets <80,000/mm³; hemoglobin <4.5 g/dL; and reticulocytes <80,000/mm³ if the hemoglobin concentration is <9 g/dL

Dosing adjustment in renal impairment:
Infants, Children, and Adolescents: The following guidelines have been used by some clinicians: Reduce initial dose to 15 mg/kg/dose once daily (Heeney, 2008)
Adults:
Manufacturer labeling:
Sickle cell anemia:
CrCl ≥60 mL/minute: No adjustment (of initial dose) required
CrCl <60 mL/minute: Reduce initial dose to 7.5 mg/kg/day (Yan, 2005); titrate to response/avoidance of toxicity (refer to usual dosing)
ESRD: Reduce initial dose to 7.5 mg/kg/dose (administer after dialysis on dialysis days); titrate to response/avoidance of toxicity
Other approved indications: It is recommended to reduce the initial dose; however, no specific guidelines are available.
The following guidelines have been used by some clinicians:
Aronoff, 2007: Adults:
CrCl >50 mL/minute: No dosage adjustment necessary.
CrCl 10-50 mL/minute: Administer 50% of dose
CrCl <10 mL/minute: Administer 20% of dose
Hemodialysis: Administer dose after dialysis on dialysis days
Continuous renal replacement therapy (CRRT): Administer 50% of dose
Kintzel, 1995:
CrCl 46-60 mL/minute: Administer 85% of dose
CrCl 31-45 mL/minute: Administer 80% of dose
CrCl <30 mL/minute: Administer 75% of dose
Dosing adjustment in hepatic impairment: Adults: There are no dosage adjustments provided in the manufacturer's labeling; closely monitor for bone marrow toxicity.
Dosing adjustment for toxicity: Adults:
Cutaneous vasculitic ulcerations: Discontinue
Gastrointestinal toxicity (severe nausea, vomiting, anorexia): Temporarily interrupt treatment
Mucositis (severe): Temporarily interrupt treatment
Pancreatitis: Discontinue permanently
Hematologic toxicity:
Antineoplastic uses (CML, head and neck cancer, melanoma, ovarian cancer): WBC <2500/mm³ or platelets <100,000/mm³: Interrupt treatment (for at least 3 days), may resume when values rise toward normal
Sickle cell anemia: Neutrophils <2000/mm³, platelets <80,000/mm³, hemoglobin <4.5 g/dL, or reticulocytes <80,000/mm³ with hemoglobin <9 g/dL: Interrupt treatment; following recovery, may resume with a dose reduction of 2.5 mg/kg/day. If no toxicity occurs over the next 12 weeks, subsequent dose may be increased by 2.5 mg/kg/day every 12 weeks to a dose which does not produce hematologic toxicity for 24 consecutive weeks. If hematologic toxicity recurs a second time at a specific dose, do not retry that dose.
Administration Hazardous agent; use appropriate precautions for handling and disposal (NIOSH, 2012)

Oral: The manufacturer does not recommend opening the capsules; observe proper handling procedures (eg, wear gloves). Doses rounded to the nearest 100 mg when using capsules allows for dosing accuracy within ~2 mg/kg/day (Heeney, 2008). For patients unable to swallow capsules, an oral solution may be prepared.
Monitoring Parameters
General: CBC with differential, liver function tests and renal function should be checked at baseline and then periodically throughout therapy; serum uric acid, signs and symptoms of pancreatitis
Sickle cell anemia: Monitor hemoglobin F levels. Monitor neutrophils, hemoglobin, platelets and reticulocytes every 2 weeks throughout therapy. If neutrophil count <2000 cells/mm³, platelet count <80,000/mm³, hemoglobin <4.5 g/dL, and reticulocyte count <80,000/mm³ when hemoglobin <9 g/dL, hold therapy until counts recover. Decrease dose by 2.5 mg/kg/day before reinitiating therapy.
Antineoplastic use: Monitor hemoglobin, platelets, and WBC counts at least weekly throughout therapy. If WBC <2500/mm³ or platelets <100,000/mm³, hold therapy until counts increase significantly. If severe anemia occurs, treat without interrupting therapy.
Test Interactions False-negative triglyceride measurement by a glycerol oxidase method. An analytical interference between hydroxyurea and enzymes (lactate dehydrogenase, urease, and uricase) may result in false elevations of lactic acid, urea, and uric acid.
Dosage Forms Excipient information presented when available (limited, particularly for generics); consult specific product labeling.
Capsule, Oral:
Droxia: 200 mg, 300 mg, 400 mg
Hydrea: 500 mg
Generic: 500 mg
Extemporaneous Preparations Hazardous agent: Use appropriate precautions for handling and disposal.

A 40 mg/mL oral suspension may be prepared with capsules and either a 1:1 mixture of Ora-Sweet® and Ora-Plus® or a 1:1 mixture of methylcellulose 1% and simple syrup NF. Empty the contents of eight 500 mg capsules into a mortar. Add small portions of chosen vehicle and mix to a uniform paste; mix while incrementally adding the vehicle to **almost** 100 mL; transfer to a calibrated bottle, rinse mortar with vehicle, and add sufficient quantity of vehicle to make 100 mL. Label "shake well" and "refrigerate". Store in plastic prescription bottles. Stable for 14 days at room temperature or refrigerated (preferred) (Nahata, 2003).

A 100 mg/mL oral solution may be prepared with capsules. Mix the contents of twenty 500 mg capsules with enough room temperature sterile water (~50 mL) to initially result in a 200 mg/mL concentration. Stir vigorously using a magnetic stirrer for several hours, then filter to remove insoluble contents. Add 50 mL Syrpalta® (flavored syrup, HUMCO) to filtered solution, resulting in 100 mL of a 100 mg/mL hydroxyurea solution. Stable for 1 month at room temperature in amber plastic bottle (Heeney, 2004).

Heeney MM, Whorton MR, Howard TA, et al, "Chemical and Functional Analysis of Hydroxyurea Oral Solutions," J Pediatr Hematol Oncol, 2004, 26(3):179-84.
Nahata MC, Morosco RS, Boster EA, et al, "Stability of Hydroxyurea in Two Extemporaneously Prepared Oral Suspensions Stored at Two Temperatures," 2003, 38:P-161(E) [abstract from 2003 ASHP Midyear Clinical Meeting].
References
Aronoff GR, Bennett WM, Berns JS, et al, Drug Prescribing in Renal Failure: Dosing Guidelines for Adults and Children, 5th ed., Philadelphia, PA: American College of Physicians, 2007, 100.
Ferster A, Tahriri P, Vermylen C, et al, "Five Years of Experience With Hydroxyurea in Children and Young Adults With Sickle Cell Disease," Blood, 2001, 97(11):3628-32.

Griggs JJ, Mangu PB, Anderson H, et al. Appropriate chemotherapy dosing for obese adult patients with cancer: American Society of Clinical Oncology Clinical Practice Guideline. *J Clin Oncol*. 2012;30 (13):1553-1561.

Gwilt PR and Tracewell WG. Pharmacokinetics and pharmacodynamics of hydroxyurea. *Clin Pharmacokinet*. 1998;34(5):347-358.

Hankins JS, Ware RE, Rogers ZR, et al, "Long-Term Hydroxyurea Therapy for Infants With Sickle Cell Anemia: The HUSOFT Extension Study," *Blood*, 2005, 106(7):2269-75.

Heeney MM and Ware RE, "Hydroxyurea for Children With Sickle Cell Disease," *Pediatr Clin North Am*, 2008, 55(2):483-501.

Heeney MM, Whorton MR, Howard TA, et al, "Chemical and Functional Analysis of Hydroxyurea Oral Solutions," *J Pediatr Hematol Oncol*, 2004, 26(3):179-84.

Kintzel PE and Dorr RT, "Anticancer Drug Renal Toxicity and Elimination: Dosing Guidelines for Altered Renal Function," *Cancer Treat Rev*, 1995, 21(1):33-64.

Maier-Redelsperger M, de Montalembert M, Flahault A, et al, "Fetal Hemoglobin and F-Cell Responses to Long-Term Hydroxyurea Treatment in Young Sickle Cell Patients. The French Study Group on Sickle Cell Disease," *Blood*, 1998, 91(12):4472-9.

National Institute for Occupational Safety and Health (NIOSH), "NIOSH List of Antineoplastic and Other Hazardous Drugs in Healthcare Settings 2012." Available at http://www.cdc.gov/niosh/docs/2012-150/pdfs/2012-150.pdf. Accessed January 21, 2013.

Rodgers GP, Dover GJ, Noguchi CT, et al, "Hematologic Responses of Patients With Sickle Cell Disease to Treatment With Hydroxyurea," *N Engl J Med*, 1990, 322(15):1037-45.

Rodgers GP, Dover GJ, Uyesaka N, et al, "Augmentation by Erythropoietin of the Fetal-Hemoglobin Response to Hydroxyurea in Sickle Cell Disease," *N Engl J Med*, 1993, 328(2):73-80.

Rodriguez GI, Kuhn JG, Weiss GR, et al, "A Bioavailability and Pharmacokinetic Study of Oral and Intravenous Hydroxyurea," *Blood*, 1998, 91(5):1533-41.

Strouse JJ, Heeney MM. Hydroxyrea for the treatment of sickle cell disease: efficacy, barriers, toxicity, and management in children. *Pediatr Blood Cancer*. 2012;59(2):365-371.

Strouse JJ, Lanzkron S, Beach MC, et al, "Hydroxyurea for Sickle Cell Disease: A Systematic Review for Efficacy and Toxicity in Children," *Pediatrics*, 2008, 122(6):1332-42.

Thornburg CD, Dixon N, Burgett S, et al, "A Pilot Study of Hydroxyurea to Prevent Chronic Organ Damage in Young Children With Sickle Cell Anemia," *Pediatr Blood Cancer*, 2009, 52(5):609-15.

Wang WC, Ware RE, Miller ST, et al, "Hydroxycarbamide in Very Young Children With Sickle-Cell Anaemia: A Multicentre, Randomised, Controlled Trial (BABY HUG)," *Lancet*, 2011, 377(9778):1663-72.

Wang WC, Wynn LW, Rogers ZR, et al, "A Two-Year Pilot Trial of Hydroxyurea in Very Young Children With Sickle Cell Anemia," *J Pediatr*, 2001, 139(6):790-6.

Ware RE, Despotovic JM, Mortier NA, et al, "Pharmacokinetics, Pharmacodynamics, and Pharmacogenetics of Hydroxyurea Treatment for Children With Sickle Cell Anemia," *Blood*, 2011, 118(18):4985-91.

Yan JH, Ataga K, Kaul S, et al. The influence of renal function on hydroxyurea pharmacokinetics in adults with sickle cell disease. *J Clin Pharmacol*. 2005;45(4):434-445.

Zimmerman SA, Schultz WH, Davis JS, et al, "Sustained Long-Term Hematologic Efficacy of Hydroxyurea at Maximum Tolerated Dose in Children With Sickle Cell Disease," *Blood*, 2004, 103(6):2039-45.

HydrOXYzine (hye DROKS i zeen)

Medication Safety Issues

Sound-alike/look-alike issues:

HydrOXYzine may be confused with hydrALAZINE, hydroxyurea

Atarax may be confused with Ativan

Vistaril may be confused with Restoril, Versed, Zestril®

BEERS Criteria medication:

This drug may be potentially inappropriate for use in geriatric patients (Quality of evidence - high; Strength of recommendation - strong).

International issues:

Vistaril [U.S. and Turkey] may be confused with Vastarel brand name for trimetazidine [multiple international markets]

Related Information

Management of Drug Extravasations *on page 2255*

Brand Names: U.S. Vistaril

Brand Names: Canada Apo-Hydroxyzine; Atarax; Hydroxyzine Hydrochloride Injection, USP; Novo-Hydroxyzin; Nu-Hydroxyzine; PMS-Hydroxyzine; Riva-Hydroxyzine

Therapeutic Category Antianxiety Agent; Antiemetic; Antihistamine; Sedative

Generic Availability (U.S.) Yes

Use

Oral: Treatment of anxiety and pruritus; preoperative sedation [FDA approved in pediatric patients (age not specified) and adults]

Parenteral: Treatment of anxiety and pruritus; perioperative sedation; antiemetic [FDA approved in infants, children, adolescents, and adults]

Pregnancy Considerations Adverse events were observed in animal reproduction studies. Hydroxyzine crosses the placenta. Maternal hydroxyzine use has generally not resulted in an increased risk of birth defects. Use of hydroxyzine early in pregnancy is contraindicated but hydroxyzine is approved for pre- and postpartum adjunctive therapy to reduce opioid dosage, treat anxiety, and control emesis. Antihistamines are recommended for the treatment pruritus with rash in pregnant women (although second generation antihistamines may be preferred). Antihistamines are not recommended for treatment of pruritus associated with intrahepatic cholestasis in pregnancy. Possible withdrawal symptoms have been observed in neonates following chronic maternal use of hydroxyzine during pregnancy.

Breast-Feeding Considerations It is not known if hydroxyzine is excreted in breast milk. Breast-feeding is not recommended by the manufacturer. Antihistamines may decrease maternal serum prolactin concentrations when administered prior to the establishment of nursing.

Contraindications Hypersensitivity to hydroxyzine or any component; subcutaneous, intravenous, or intra-arterial administration; early pregnancy

Warnings Subcutaneous, intra-arterial, and I.V. administration are contraindicated and **not** recommended under any circumstances; intravascular hemolysis, thrombosis, and digital gangrene can occur; extravasation can result in sterile abscess and marked tissue induration. May cause CNS depression, which may impair physical or mental abilities; patients must be cautioned about performing tasks which require mental alertness (eg, operating machinery or driving). Effects may be potentiated when used with other sedative drugs or ethanol; consider dosage reduction of other sedatives.

Tablets may contain FD&C Yellow No. 5 (tartrazine) which may cause allergic reactions in susceptible individuals. Injection may contain benzyl alcohol which may cause allergic reactions in susceptible individuals; syrup may contain sodium benzoate; benzoic acid (benzoate) is a metabolite of benzyl alcohol; large amounts of benzyl alcohol (≥99 mg/kg/day) have been associated with a potentially fatal toxicity ("gasping syndrome") in neonates; avoid use of hydroxyzine products containing benzyl alcohol or sodium benzoate in neonates; *in vitro* and animal studies have shown that benzoate displaces bilirubin from protein binding sites.

Precautions Use with caution in patients with narrow-angle glaucoma, prostatic hypertrophy, bladder neck obstruction, asthma, or COPD; hydroxyzine exhibits cholinergic blockade which may exacerbate these conditions; screening for glaucoma is recommended. Neonatal withdrawal symptoms, including seizures, have been reported following long-term maternal use or the use of large doses near term (Serreau, 2005). Long-term effectiveness (>4 months) for treatment of anxiety has not been assessed; use and effectiveness should be periodically re-evaluated in patients receiving the drug for extended periods of time.

Adverse Reactions

Central nervous system: Dizziness, drowsiness, fatigue, hallucination, headache, nervousness, seizure

Dermatologic: Pruritus, rash, urticaria
Gastrointestinal: Xerostomia
Neuromuscular & skeletal: Involuntary movements, paresthesia, tremor
Ocular: Blurred vision
Respiratory: Respiratory depression (at higher than recommended doses)
Miscellaneous: Allergic reaction

Drug Interactions

Metabolism/Transport Effects Inhibits CYP2D6 (weak)

Avoid Concomitant Use
Avoid concomitant use of HydrOXYzine with any of the following: Aclidinium; Azelastine (Nasal); Ipratropium (Oral Inhalation); Paraldehyde; Potassium Chloride; Thalidomide; Tiotropium; Umeclidinium

Increased Effect/Toxicity
HydrOXYzine may increase the levels/effects of: Abobotulinumtoxin A; Alcohol (Ethyl); Anticholinergic Agents; ARIPiprazole; Azelastine (Nasal); Barbiturates; Buprenorphine; Cannabinoid-Containing Products; CNS Depressants; Hydrocodone; Meperidine; Methotrimeprazine; Metyrosine; Mirabegron; Mirtazapine; OnabotulinumtoxinA; Paraldehyde; Potassium Chloride; Pramipexole; RimabotulinumtoxinB; ROPINIRole; Rotigotine; Selective Serotonin Reuptake Inhibitors; Thalidomide; Thiazide Diuretics; Tiotropium; Topiramate; Zolpidem

The levels/effects of HydrOXYzine may be increased by: Aclidinium; Brimonidine (Topical); Cannabis; Doxylamine; Dronabinol; Droperidol; Ipratropium (Oral Inhalation); Kava Kava; Magnesium Sulfate; Methotrimeprazine; Nabilone; Perampanel; Pramlintide; Rufinamide; Sodium Oxybate; Tapentadol; Tetrahydrocannabinol; Umeclidinium

Decreased Effect
HydrOXYzine may decrease the levels/effects of: Acetylcholinesterase Inhibitors (Central); Benzylpenicilloyl Polylysine; Betahistine; Hyaluronidase; Secretin

The levels/effects of HydrOXYzine may be decreased by: Acetylcholinesterase Inhibitors (Central); Amphetamines

Stability
Injection: Store at 20°C to 25°C (68°F to 77°F), excursions permitted to 15°C to 30°C (59°F to 89°F); protect from light. Discard unused portion of single-dose vial.
Oral:
Capsules: Store below 30°C (86°F); protect from light; dispense is tightly closed container.
Solution (hydrochloride salt): Store at 15°C to 30°C (59°F to 86°F); protect from light.
Tablets: Store at 20°C to 25°C (68°F to 77°F); dispense in tightly closed container.

Mechanism of Action Competes with histamine for H_1-receptor sites on effector cells in the gastrointestinal tract, blood vessels, and respiratory tract. Possesses skeletal muscle relaxing, bronchodilator, antihistamine, antiemetic, and analgesic properties.

Pharmacodynamics
Onset of action: Oral: Within 15-30 minutes; I.M.: Rapid
Maximum effect: Suppression of antihistamine-induced wheal and flare: 6-12 hours (Simons, 1984a)
Duration: Decreased histamine-induced wheal and flare areas: 2 to ≥36 hours; Suppression of pruritus: 1-12 hours (Simons, 1984a)

Pharmacokinetics (Adult data unless noted)
Absorption: Oral: Well absorbed
Distribution: V_d, apparent:
Children and Adolescents 1-14 years: 18.5 ± 8.6 L/kg (Simons, 1984)
Adults: 16 ± 3 L/kg (Simons, 1984a)

Metabolism: Hepatic to multiple metabolites, including cetirizine (active) (Simons, 1989)
Half-life:
Children and Adolescents 1-14 years (mean age: 6.1 ± 4.6 years): 7.1 ± 2.3 hours; **Note:** Half-life increased with increasing age and was 4 hours in patients 1-year old and 11 hours in a 14-year old patient (Simons, 1984)
Adults: 3 hours; one study reported a terminal half-life of 20 hours (Simons, 1984a)
Time to peak serum concentration: Oral: 2 hours
Elimination: Active metabolite (cetirizine) is renally eliminated (Simons, 1994)

Dosing: Usual
Infants, Children, and Adolescents:
Antiemetic: I.M.: 1.1 mg/kg/dose; maximum single dose: 100 mg
Anxiety:
Manufacturer's labeling: Oral:
Children <6 years: 50 mg/day in 4 divided doses
Children and Adolescents ≥6 years: 50-100 mg/day in 4 divided doses
Alternate dosing:
Oral: Children and Adolescents: 2 mg/kg/day divided every 6-8 hours as needed; **Note:** Some experts have recommended lower initial doses. Maximum single dose is age-dependent: Age <6 years: 12.5 mg; age 6-12 years: 25 mg; age >12 years: 100 mg
I.M.: Children and Adolescents: 0.5-1 mg/kg/**dose** every 4-6 hours as needed; maximum single dose: 100 mg
Pruritus; associated with allergic conditions or chronic urticaria: Oral:
Manufacturer's labeling:
Children <6 years: 50 mg/day in 4 divided doses as needed
Children and Adolescents ≥6 years: 50-100 mg/day in 4 divided doses as needed
Alternate dosing: Children and Adolescents: Oral:
Patient weight ≤40 kg: 2 mg/kg/day divided every 6-8 hours as needed (Simons, 1994); **Note:** Some experts have recommended lower doses; maximum single dose: 25 mg
Patient weight >40 kg: 25-50 mg once daily at bedtime or twice daily (Simons, 1994)
Pruritus; associated with opioid use: Children and Adolescents: Limited data available: I.M., Oral: 0.5 mg/kg/dose every 6 hours as needed; maximum single dose: 50 mg (Berde, 1990)
Sedation; procedural, pre-/postoperative:
Manufacturer's labeling:
Oral: Children and Adolescents: 0.6 mg/kg/**dose**; maximum single dose: 100 mg
I.M.: Infants, Children, and Adolescents: 1.1 mg/kg/**dose**; maximum single dose: 100 mg
Alternate dosing: Oral: Children 2-5 years: 1 mg/kg/**dose** as a single dose 30-45 minutes prior to procedure in combination with other sedatives (eg, midazolam, chloral hydrate) has been used in preschool children prior to dental procedures or echocardiograms (Chowdhury, 2005; Roach, 2010)
Adults:
Antiemetic: I.M.: 25-100 mg/dose
Anxiety:
Oral: 50-100 mg 4 times daily
I.M.: 50–100 mg every 4-6 hours as needed
Preoperative sedation:
Oral: 50-100 mg
I.M.: 25-100 mg
Pruritus: Oral: 25 mg 3-4 times daily
Psychiatric emergency: I.M.: 50-100 mg immediately; repeat every 4-6 hours as needed

Dosing adjustment in renal impairment: There are no dosage adjustments provided in the manufacturer's labeling; active metabolite (cetirizine) is renally eliminated (Simons, 1994)

Dosing adjustment in hepatic impairment: Adults: In patients with primary biliary cirrhosis, change dosing interval to every 24 hours (Simons, 1989)

Administration

Oral: May be administered without regard to food

Parenteral: Subcutaneous, intra-arterial, and I.V. administration are contraindicated and **not** recommended under any circumstances; intravascular hemolysis, thrombosis, and digital gangrene can occur; extravasation can result in sterile abscess and marked tissue induration. Administer I.M. deep in large muscle. For I.M. administration in children, injections should be made into the midlateral muscles of the thigh. In the very rare instance that I.V. administration may be necessary, slow I.V. injection through a central venous line has been used in pediatric oncology patients (Berde, 1990).

Vesicant/Extravasation Risk Vesicant (I.V. administration is contraindicated)

Monitoring Parameters Relief of symptoms, mental status, blood pressure

Test Interactions May cause false-positive serum TCA screen.

Dosage Forms Excipient information presented when available (limited, particularly for generics); consult specific product labeling.

Capsule, Oral, as pamoate:
Vistaril: 25 mg, 50 mg
Generic: 25 mg, 50 mg, 100 mg

Solution, Intramuscular, as hydrochloride:
Generic: 25 mg/mL (1 mL); 50 mg/mL (1 mL, 2 mL, 10 mL)

Solution, Oral, as hydrochloride:
Generic: 10 mg/5 mL (473 mL)

Syrup, Oral, as hydrochloride:
Generic: 10 mg/5 mL (118 mL, 473 mL)

Tablet, Oral, as hydrochloride:
Generic: 10 mg, 25 mg, 50 mg

References

Baumgartner TG, "Administration of Hydroxyzine Injection," *Am J Hosp Pharm*, 1979, 36(12):1660.

Berde C, Ablin A, Glazer J, et al, "American Academy of Pediatrics Report of the Subcommittee on Disease-Related Pain in Childhood Cancer," *Pediatrics*, 1990, 86(5 Pt 2):818-25.

Chowdhury J and Vargas KG, "Comparison of Chloral Hydrate, Meperidine, and Hydroxyzine to Midazolam Regimens for Oral Sedation of Pediatric Dental Patients," *Pediatr Dent*, 2005, 27(3):191-7.

Roach CL, Husain N, Zabinsky J, et al, "Moderate Sedation for Echocardiography of Preschoolers," *Pediatr Cardiol*, 2010, 31 (4):469-73.

Serreau R, Komiha M, Blanc F, et al, "Neonatal Seizures Associated With Maternal Hydroxyzine Hydrochloride in Late Pregnancy," *Reprod Toxicol*, 2005, 20(4):573-4.

Simons FE and Simons KJ, "The Pharmacology and Use of H1-Receptor-Antagonist Drugs," *N Engl J Med*, 1994, 330(23):1663-70.

Simons FE, Simons KJ, and Frith EM, "The Pharmacokinetics and Antihistaminic of the H₁ Receptor Antagonist Hydroxyzine," *J Allergy Clin Immunol*, 1984a, 73(1 Pt 1):69-75.

Simons FE, Simons KJ, Becker AB, et al, "Pharmacokinetics and Antipruritic Effects of Hydroxyzine in Children With Atopic Dermatitis," *J Pediatr*, 1984, 104(1):123-7.

Simons FE, Watson WT, Chen XY, et al, "The Pharmacokinetics and Pharmacodynamics of Hydroxyzine in Patients With Primary Biliary Cirrhosis," *J Clin Pharmacol*, 1989, 29(9):809-15.

Wong AR and Rasool AH, "Hydroxyzine-Induced Supraventricular Tachycardia in a Nine-Year-Old Child," *Singapore Med J*, 2004, 45 (2):90-2.

◆ **Hydroxyzine Hydrochloride** *see* HydrOXYzine *on page 1054*

◆ **Hydroxyzine Hydrochloride Injection, USP (Can)** *see* HydrOXYzine *on page 1054*

◆ **Hydroxyzine Pamoate** *see* HydrOXYzine *on page 1054*

◆ **Hydurea** *see* Hydroxyurea *on page 1051*

◆ **Hygroton** *see* Chlorthalidone *on page 453*

◆ **Hylenex** *see* Hyaluronidase *on page 1020*

◆ **HyoMax-SL** *see* Hyoscyamine *on page 1056*

◆ **Hyonatol** *see* Hyoscyamine, Atropine, Scopolamine, and Phenobarbital *on page 1058*

◆ **Hyoscine Butylbromide** *see* Scopolamine (Systemic) *on page 1872*

◆ **Hyoscine Hydrobromide** *see* Scopolamine (Ophthalmic) *on page 1874*

Hyoscyamine (hye oh SYE a meen)

Medication Safety Issues

Sound-alike/look-alike issues:
Anaspaz may be confused with Anaprox, Antispas
Levbid may be confused with Enbrel, Lithobid, Lopid, Lorabid
Levsin/SL maybe confused with Levaquin

BEERS Criteria medication:
This drug may be potentially inappropriate for use in geriatric patients (Quality of evidence - moderate; Strength of recommendation - strong).

Related Information
Oral Medications That Should Not Be Crushed or Altered *on page 2438*

Brand Names: U.S. Anaspaz; Ed-Spaz; HyoMax-SL; Hyosyne; Levbid; Levsin; Levsin/SL; NuLev; Oscimin; Oscimin SR; Symax Duotab; Symax FasTabs; Symax-SL; Symax-SR

Brand Names: Canada Levsin

Therapeutic Category Anticholinergic Agent; Antispasmodic Agent, Gastrointestinal

Generic Availability (U.S.) May be product dependent

Use Treatment of GI tract disorders caused by spasm; adjunctive therapy for peptic ulcers and hypermotility disorders of lower urinary tract; infant colic

Pregnancy Risk Factor C

Pregnancy Considerations Crosses the placenta, effects to the fetus not known; use during pregnancy only if clearly needed.

Breast-Feeding Considerations Excreted in breast milk in trace amounts. May also suppress lactation. Breast-feeding is not recommended.

Contraindications Hypersensitivity to hyoscyamine or any component; narrow-angle glaucoma, GI and GU obstruction, paralytic ileus, severe ulcerative colitis, myasthenia gravis

Warnings Low doses may cause a paradoxical decrease in heart rate; heat prostration may occur in hot weather. Some oral liquids contain sodium benzoate; benzoic acid (benzoate) is a metabolite of benzyl alcohol; large amounts of benzyl alcohol (≥99 mg/kg/day) have been associated with a potentially fatal toxicity ("gasping syndrome") in neonates; *in vitro* and animal studies have shown that benzoate displaces bilirubin from protein binding sites; avoid using products containing sodium benzoate in neonates

Precautions Use with caution in patients with hyperthyroidism, CHF, cardiac arrhythmias, prostatic hypertrophy, autonomic neuropathy, chronic lung disease, biliary tract disease, children with spastic paralysis. Disintegrating tablet (NuLev™) contains aspartame which is metabolized to phenylalanine and must be used with caution in patients with phenylketonuria.

Adverse Reactions
Cardiovascular: Flushing, palpitations, tachycardia
Central nervous system: Amnesia (short-term), ataxia, confusion (more common in elderly), dizziness, drowsiness, excitement (more common in elderly), fatigue, hallucination, headache, insomnia, nervousness, psychosis, speech disturbance

Dermatologic: Hypohidrosis, urticaria

Gastrointestinal: Abdominal pain, ageusia, bloating, constipation, diarrhea, dysgeusia, dysphagia, heartburn, nausea, vomiting, xerostomia

Genitourinary: Decreased lactation, impotence, urinary hesitancy, urinary retention

Hypersensitivity: Hypersensitivity reaction

Neuromuscular & skeletal: Weakness

Ophthalmic: Blurred vision, cycloplegia, increased intraocular pressure, mydriasis

Miscellaneous: Fever

Drug Interactions

Metabolism/Transport Effects None known.

Avoid Concomitant Use

Avoid concomitant use of Hyoscyamine with any of the following: Aclidinium; Ipratropium (Oral Inhalation); Potassium Chloride; Tiotropium; Umeclidinium

Increased Effect/Toxicity

Hyoscyamine may increase the levels/effects of: AbobotulinumtoxinA; Analgesics (Opioid); Anticholinergic Agents; Cannabinoid-Containing Products; Mirabegron; OnabotulinumtoxinA; Potassium Chloride; RimabotulinumtoxinB; Thiazide Diuretics; Tiotropium; Topiramate

The levels/effects of Hyoscyamine may be increased by: Aclidinium; Ipratropium (Oral Inhalation); Pramlintide; Umeclidinium

Decreased Effect

Hyoscyamine may decrease the levels/effects of: Acetylcholinesterase Inhibitors (Central); Secretin

The levels/effects of Hyoscyamine may be decreased by: Acetylcholinesterase Inhibitors (Central); Antacids

Mechanism of Action Blocks the action of acetylcholine at parasympathetic sites in smooth muscle, secretory glands, and the CNS; increases cardiac output, dries secretions, antagonizes histamine and serotonin

Pharmacodynamics

Onset of action:

Oral: 20-30 minutes

Sublingual: 5-20 minutes

I.V.: 2-3 minutes

Duration: 4-6 hours

Pharmacokinetics (Adult data unless noted)

Absorption: Well absorbed from the GI tract

Distribution: Crosses the placenta; small amounts appear in breast milk

Protein binding: 50%

Metabolism: In the liver

Half-life: 3.5 hours

Elimination: 30% to 50% eliminated unchanged in urine within 12 hours

Dosing: Usual

GI tract disorders:

Infants and Children <2 years: Oral: The following table lists the hyoscyamine dosage using the drop formulation; hyoscyamine drops are dosed every 4 hours as needed

Hyoscyamine Drops Dosage

Weight (kg)	Dose (drops)	Maximum Daily Dose (drops)
2.3	3	18
3.4	4	24
5	5	30
7	6	36
10	8	48
15	11	66

Oral, S.L.:

Children 2-12 years: 0.0625-0.125 mg every 4 hours as needed; maximum daily dosage 0.75 mg **or** timed release 0.375 mg every 12 hours; maximum daily dosage 0.75 mg

Children >12 years to Adults: 0.125-0.25 mg every 4 hours as needed; maximum daily dosage 1.5 mg **or** timed release 0.375-0.75 mg every 12 hours; maximum daily dosage 1.5 mg

I.V., I.M., SubQ: Children >12 years to Adults: 0.25-0.5 mg at 4-hour intervals for 1-4 doses

Adjunct to anesthesia: I.M., I.V., SubQ: Children >2 years to Adults: 5 mcg/kg given 30-60 minutes prior to induction of anesthesia

Hypermotility of lower urinary tract: Oral, S.L.: Adults: 0.15-0.3 mg four times daily; timed release: 0.375 mg every 12 hours

Reversal of neuromuscular blockage: I.V., I.M., SubQ: 0.2 mg for every 1 mg neostigmine

Administration

Oral: Administer before meals; timed release tablets are scored and may be cut for easier dosage titration; S.L.: Place under the tongue

Parenteral: May be administered I.M., I.V., and SubQ; no information is available for I.V. administration rate or dilution

Monitoring Parameters Pulse, anticholinergic effects, urine output, GI symptoms

Dosage Forms Excipient information presented when available (limited, particularly for generics); consult specific product labeling.

Elixir, Oral, as sulfate:

Hyosyne: 0.125 mg/5 mL (473 mL) [contains alcohol, usp; lemon flavor]

Generic: 0.125 mg/5 mL (473 mL)

Solution, Injection, as sulfate:

Levsin: 0.5 mg/mL (1 mL) [contains benzyl alcohol]

Solution, Oral, as sulfate:

Hyosyne: 0.125 mg/mL (15 mL) [lemon flavor]

Generic: 0.125 mg/mL (15 mL)

Tablet, Oral, as sulfate:

Levsin: 0.125 mg

Oscimin: 0.125 mg [peppermint flavor]

Generic: 0.125 mg

Tablet Dispersible, Oral, as sulfate:

Anaspaz: 0.125 mg [scored]

Ed-Spaz: 0.125 mg [scored]

NuLev: 0.125 mg [peppermint flavor]

Oscimin: 0.125 mg [peppermint flavor]

Symax FasTabs: 0.125 mg [mint flavor]

Generic: 0.125 mg

Tablet Extended Release, Oral, as sulfate:

Symax Duotab: 0.375 mg [contains brilliant blue fcf (fd&c blue #1)]

Tablet Extended Release 12 Hour, Oral, as sulfate:

Levbid: 0.375 mg

Oscimin SR: 0.375 mg

Symax-SR: 0.375 mg [scored]

Generic: 0.375 mg

Tablet Sublingual, Sublingual, as sulfate:

HyoMax-SL: 0.125 mg

Levsin/SL: 0.125 mg

Oscimin: 0.125 mg [peppermint flavor]

Symax-SL: 0.125 mg [mint flavor]

Generic: 0.125 mg

Hyoscyamine, Atropine, Scopolamine, and Phenobarbital

(hye oh SYE a meen, A troe peen, skoe POL a meen, & fee noe BAR bi tal)

Medication Safety Issues

Sound-alike/look-alike issues:
Donnatal® may be confused with Donnagel, Donnatal Extentabs®

BEERS Criteria medication:
This drug may be potentially inappropriate for use in geriatric patients (Quality of evidence - moderate; Strength of recommendation - strong).

Related Information

Oral Medications That Should Not Be Crushed or Altered on page 2438

Brand Names: U.S. Donnatal Extentabs®; Donnatal®; Hyonatol

Therapeutic Category Anticholinergic Agent; Antispasmodic Agent, Gastrointestinal

Generic Availability (U.S.) No

Use Adjunct in treatment of peptic ulcer disease, irritable bowel, spastic colitis, spastic bladder, and renal colic

Pregnancy Risk Factor C

Pregnancy Considerations Reproduction studies with this combination have not been done; refer to individual monographs.

Breast-Feeding Considerations Refer to individual monographs.

Contraindications Hypersensitivity to hyoscyamine, atropine, scopolamine, phenobarbital, or any component of the formulation; narrow-angle glaucoma; tachycardia; GI and GU obstruction; myasthenia gravis; paralytic ileus; intestinal atony; unstable cardiovascular status in acute hemorrhage; severe ulcerative colitis; hiatal hernia associated with reflux esophagitis; acute intermittent porphyria

Warnings May cause drowsiness and/or blurred vision, which may impair physical or mental abilities; patients must be cautioned about performing tasks which require mental alertness (eg, operating machinery or driving). Heat prostration can occur in the presence of high environmental temperature; use caution in hot weather and/or exercise. If diarrhea occurs, may be a sign of incomplete intestinal obstruction; treatment should be discontinued if this occurs. Low doses may cause a paradoxical decrease in heart rate due to atropine. Elixir contains ethanol (up to 23.8%).

Precautions Use with caution in patients with hepatic or renal impairment, hyperthyroidism, CAD, CHF, cardiac arrhythmias, tachycardia, hypertension, autonomic neuropathy. Use with caution in patients with a history of drug abuse or acute alcoholism; potential for drug dependency exists. Tolerance and psychological and physical dependence may occur with prolonged use; due to the phenobarbital component, should not be discontinued abruptly because of the possibility of increasing seizure frequency; therapy should be withdrawn gradually to minimize the potential of increased seizure frequency, unless safety concerns require a more rapid withdrawal. Use of anticholinergics in gastric ulcer treatment may cause a delay in gastric emptying due to antral statis.

Adverse Reactions

Cardiovascular: Palpitation, tachycardia

Central nervous system: Dizziness, drowsiness, excitement, headache, insomnia, nervousness

Dermatologic: Urticaria

Endocrine & metabolic: Lactation suppressed

Gastrointestinal: Bloating, constipation, nausea, taste loss, vomiting, xerostomia

Genitourinary: Impotence, urinary hesitancy, urinary retention

Neuromuscular & skeletal: Musculoskeletal pain, weakness

Ocular: Blurred vision, cycloplegia, mydriasis, ocular tension increased

Miscellaneous: Allergic reaction (may be severe), anaphylaxis, sweating decreased

Drug Interactions

Metabolism/Transport Effects Refer to individual components.

Avoid Concomitant Use
Avoid concomitant use of Hyoscyamine, Atropine, Scopolamine, and Phenobarbital with any of the following: Abiraterone Acetate; Aclidinium; Apixaban; Apremilast; Artemether; Axitinib; Azelastine (Nasal); Bedaquiline; Boceprevir; Bortezomib; Bosutinib; Cabozantinib; Ceritinib; CloZAPine; Crizotinib; Dabigatran Etexilate; Darunavir; Dienogest; Dolutegravir; Dronedarone; Enzalutamide; Etravirine; Everolimus; Ibrutinib; Ipratropium (Oral Inhalation); Itraconazole; Ivacaftor; Lapatinib; Lumefantrine; Lurasidone; Macitentan; Mifepristone; NIFEdipine; Nilotinib; Nisoldipine; Paraldehyde; PAZOPanib; Perampanel; Pirfenidone; Pomalidomide; PONATinib; Potassium Chloride; Praziquantel; Ranolazine; Regorafenib; Rilpivirine; Rivaroxaban; Roflumilast; RomiDEPsin; Simeprevir; Sofosbuvir; Somatostatin Acetate; SORAfenib; Stiripentol; Tasimelteon; Telaprevir; Thalidomide; Ticagrelor; Tiotropium; Tofacitinib; Tolvaptan; Toremifene; Ulipristal; Umeclidinium; Vandetanib; Vemurafenib; VinCRIStine (Liposomal); Vorapaxar; Voriconazole

Increased Effect/Toxicity
Hyoscyamine, Atropine, Scopolamine, and Phenobarbital may increase the levels/effects of: AbobotulinumtoxinA; Alcohol (Ethyl); Analgesics (Opioid); Anticholinergic Agents; Azelastine (Nasal); Buprenorphine; Clarithromycin; CNS Depressants; Hydrocodone; Hypotensive Agents; Meperidine; Methotrimeprazine; Metyrosine; Mirabegron; OnabotulinumtoxinA; Paraldehyde; Potassium Chloride; Pramipexole; Prilocaine; QuiNIDine; RimabotulinumtoxinB; Rotigotine; Selective Serotonin Reuptake Inhibitors; Sodium Nitrite; Thalidomide; Thiazide Diuretics; Tiotropium; Topiramate; Zolpidem

The levels/effects of Hyoscyamine, Atropine, Scopolamine, and Phenobarbital may be increased by: Aclidinium; Brimonidine (Topical); Cannabis; Carbonic Anhydrase Inhibitors; Chloramphenicol; Clarithromycin; Cosyntropin; CYP2C19 Inhibitors (Moderate); CYP2C19 Inhibitors (Strong); Dexmethylphenidate; Doxylamine; Dronabinol; Droperidol; Felbamate; Fosphenytoin; HydrOXYzine; Ipratropium (Oral Inhalation); Kava Kava; Luliconazole; Magnesium Sulfate; Methotrimeprazine; Methylphenidate; Nabilone; Nitric Oxide; OXcarbazepine; Phenytoin; Pramlintide; Primidone; QuiNINE; Rufinamide; Sodium Oxybate; Somatostatin Acetate; Tapentadol; Tetrahydrocannabinol; Umeclidinium; Valproic Acid and Derivatives

Decreased Effect
Hyoscyamine, Atropine, Scopolamine, and Phenobarbital may decrease the levels/effects of: Abiraterone Acetate; Acetaminophen; Acetylcholinesterase Inhibitors (Central); Afatinib; Albendazole; Apixaban; Apremilast; ARIPiprazole; Artemether; Axitinib; Bazedoxifene; Bedaquiline; Bendamustine; Beta-Blockers; Boceprevir; Bortezomib; Bosutinib; Brentuximab Vedotin; Cabozantinib; Calcium Channel Blockers; Canagliflozin; Cannabidiol; Cannabis; Ceritinib; Chloramphenicol; Clarithromycin; CloZAPine; Cobicistat; Contraceptives (Estrogens); Contraceptives (Progestins); Corticosteroids (Systemic); Crizotinib; CycloSPORINE (Systemic); CYP1A2 Substrates; CYP2A6 Substrates; CYP2B6 Substrates; CYP2C8 Substrates; CYP2C9 Substrates; CYP3A4 Substrates; Dabigatran Etexilate; Darunavir; Dasatinib; Deferasirox; Diclofenac (Systemic); Dienogest; Disopyramide;

Dolutegravir; DOXOrubicin (Conventional); Doxycycline; Dronabinol; Dronedarone; Elvitegravir; Enzalutamide; Eslicarbazepine; Etoposide; Etravirine; Everolimus; Exemestane; Felbamate; FentaNYL; Fosphenytoin; Gefitinib; Griseofulvin; GuanFACINE; Ibrutinib; Imatinib; Irinotecan; Itraconazole; Ivacaftor; Ixabepilone; Lacosamide; LamoTRIgine; Lapatinib; Linagliptin; Lopinavir; Lumefantrine; Lurasidone; Macitentan; Maraviroc; Methadone; MetroNIDAZOLE (Systemic); Mifepristone; NIFEdipine; Nilotinib; Nisoldipine; OXcarbazepine; PAZOPanib; Perampanel; P-glycoprotein/ABCB1 Substrates; Phenytoin; Pirfenidone; Pomalidomide; PONATinib; Praziquantel; Propafenone; QUEtiapine; QuiNIDine; QuiNINE; Ranolazine; Regorafenib; Rilpivirine; Rivaroxaban; Roflumilast; RomiDEPsin; Rufinamide; Saxagliptin; Secretin; Simeprevir; Sofosbuvir; SORAfenib; Stiripentol; SUNItinib; Tadalafil; Tasimelteon; Telaprevir; Teniposide; Tetrahydrocannabinol; Ticagrelor; Tipranavir; Tofacitinib; Tolvaptan; Toremifene; Treprostinil; Tricyclic Antidepressants; Uliprstal; Valproic Acid and Derivatives; Vandetanib; Vemurafenib; Vilazodone; VinCRIStine (Liposomal); Vitamin K Antagonists; Vorapaxar; Voriconazole; Vortioxetine; Zonisamide; Zuclopenthixol

The levels/effects of Hyoscyamine, Atropine, Scopolamine, and Phenobarbital may be decreased by: Acetylcholinesterase Inhibitors (Central); Amphetamines; Antacids; Cholestyramine Resin; CYP2C19 Inducers (Strong); Dabrafenib; Folic Acid; Ketorolac (Nasal); Ketorolac (Systemic); Leucovorin Calcium-Levoleucovorin; Levomefolate; Mefloquine; Methylfolate; Multivitamins/Minerals (with ADEK, Folate, Iron); Orlistat; Pyridoxine; Rifamycin Derivatives; Tipranavir

Mechanism of Action Anticholinergic agents (hyoscyamine, atropine, and scopolamine) inhibit the muscarinic actions of acetylcholine at the postganglionic parasympathetic neuroeffector sites including smooth muscle, secretory glands, and CNS sites; specific anticholinergic responses are dose-related.

Pharmacokinetics (Adult data unless noted) Absorption: Well absorbed from the GI tract

Dosing: Usual Oral:

Children: Donnatal®: 0.1 mL/kg/dose every 4 hours; maximum dose: 5 mL or see table for alternative.

Donnatal® Dosage

Weight (kg)	Dose (mL)	
	Every 4 Hours	Every 6 Hours
4.5	0.5	0.75
10	1	1.5
14	1.5	2
23	2.5	3.8
34	3.8	5
≥45	5	7.5

Adults: Donnatal®: 1-2 tablets or capsules 3-4 times/day or 5-10 mL 3-4 times/day or 1 extended release tablet every 12 hours (may increase to every 8 hours if needed)

Administration Oral: Administer 30-60 minutes before meals; do not crush or chew extended release tablets

Dosage Forms Excipient information presented when available (limited, particularly for generics); consult specific product labeling. [DSC] = Discontinued product

Elixir:
Donnatal®: Hyoscyamine sulfate 0.1037 mg, atropine sulfate 0.0194 mg, scopolamine hydrobromide 0.0065 mg, and phenobarbital 16.2 mg per 5 mL (120 mL, 480 mL) [contains ethanol <23.8%; citrus flavor] [DSC]

Donnatal®: Hyoscyamine sulfate 0.1037 mg, atropine sulfate 0.0194 mg, scopolamine hydrobromide

0.0065 mg, and phenobarbital 16.2 mg per 5 mL (120 mL, 480 mL) [contains ethanol <23.8%; grape flavor]

Tablet:
Donnatal®: Hyoscyamine sulfate 0.1037 mg, atropine sulfate 0.0194 mg, scopolamine hydrobromide 0.0065 mg, and phenobarbital 16.2 mg

Hyonatol: Hyoscyamine sulfate 0.1037 mg, atropine sulfate 0.0194 mg, scopolamine hydrobromide 0.0065 mg, and phenobarbital 16.2 mg

Tablet, extended release:
Donnatal Extentabs®: Hyoscyamine sulfate 0.3111 mg, atropine sulfate 0.0582 mg, scopolamine hydrobromide 0.0195 mg, and phenobarbital 48.6 mg

◆ **Hyoscyamine Sulfate** see Hyoscyamine on page 1056

◆ **Hyosyne** see Hyoscyamine on page 1056

◆ **HyperHEP B S/D** see Hepatitis B Immune Globulin (Human) on page 1008

◆ **HyperRAB S/D** see Rabies Immune Globulin (Human) on page 1800

◆ **HyperRHO S/D** see Rho(D) Immune Globulin on page 1815

◆ **HyperSal** see Sodium Chloride on page 1902

◆ **HyperTET S/D** see Tetanus Immune Globulin (Human) on page 1991

◆ **HyperTET™ S/D (Can)** see Tetanus Immune Globulin (Human) on page 1991

◆ **Hypertonic Saline** see Sodium Chloride on page 1902

◆ **HypoTears [OTC]** see Artificial Tears on page 205

◆ **Hytrin** see Terazosin on page 1981

◆ **Hytrin® (Can)** see Terazosin on page 1981

◆ **Ibenzmethyzin** see Procarbazine on page 1743

◆ **Ibidomide Hydrochloride** see Labetalol on page 1186

◆ **IBU-200 [OTC]** see Ibuprofen on page 1059

Ibuprofen (eye byoo PROE fen)

Medication Safety Issues
Sound-alike/look-alike issues:
Haltran may be confused with Halfprin
Motrin may be confused with Neurontin

BEERS Criteria medication:
This drug may be potentially inappropriate for use in geriatric patients (Quality of evidence - moderate; Strength of recommendation - strong).

Administration issues:
Injectable formulations: Both ibuprofen and ibuprofen lysine are available for parenteral use. Ibuprofen lysine is only indicated for closure of a clinically-significant patent ductus arteriosus.

Related Information
Oral Medications That Should Not Be Crushed or Altered on page 2438

Brand Names: U.S. Addaprin [OTC]; Advil Junior Strength [OTC]; Advil Migraine [OTC]; Advil [OTC]; Caldolor; Childrens Advil [OTC]; Childrens Ibuprofen [OTC]; Childrens Motrin Jr Strength [OTC]; Childrens Motrin [OTC]; Dyspel [OTC]; EnovaRX-Ibuprofen; Genpril [OTC]; I-Prin [OTC]; IBU-200 [OTC]; Ibuprofen Childrens [OTC]; Ibuprofen Comfort Pac; Ibuprofen Junior Strength [OTC]; Infants Advil [OTC]; Infants Ibuprofen [OTC]; KS Ibuprofen [OTC]; Motrin IB [OTC]; Motrin Infants Drops [OTC]; Motrin Junior Strength [OTC]; Motrin [OTC]; Neo-Profen; Provil [OTC]

Brand Names: Canada Advil; Advil Pediatric Drops; Apo-Ibuprofen; Caldolor; Children's Advil; Children's Europrofen; Ibuprofen Muscle and Joint; Jamp-Ibuprofen; Motrin; Motrin (Children's); Motrin IB; Novo-Profen; Pamprin

Ibuprofen Formula; PMS-Ibuprofen; Super Strength Motrin IB Liquid Gel Capsules

Therapeutic Category Analgesic, Non-narcotic; Anti-inflammatory Agent; Antipyretic; Nonsteroidal Anti-inflammatory Drug (NSAID), Oral; Nonsteroidal Anti-inflammatory Drug (NSAID), Parenteral

Generic Availability (U.S.) May be product dependent

Use

Oral:

OTC products:

Infant drops, suspension, and chewable tablets: Relief of minor aches and pains due to the common cold, flu, sore throat, headaches, and toothaches; reduction of fever (All indications: OTC products: FDA approved in ages 6 months to 11 years; consult specific product formulation for appropriate age group)

Capsule/Tablet: Relief of minor aches and pains due to the common cold, headaches, minor pain of arthritis, backache, menstrual cramps, muscle aches, and toothaches (All indications: OTC products: FDA approved in ages ≥12 years and adults)

Capsule (Advil Migraine): Treatment of migraines (OTC products: FDA approved in adults)

Prescription strength (400, 600, and 800 mg tablets): Relief of mild to moderate pain; relief of signs and symptoms of osteoarthritis and rheumatoid arthritis; treatment of primary dysmenorrhea (All indications: FDA approved in adults)

Oral ibuprofen has also been used for juvenile idiopathic arthritis (JIA), cystic fibrosis, migraine pain, gout, and for PDA closure.

Parenteral:

Ibuprofen injection (Caldolor): Management of mild to moderate pain, management of moderate to severe pain when used concurrently with an opioid analgesic, reduction of fever (All indications: FDA approved in ages ≥17 years and adults)

Ibuprofen lysine injection (NeoProfen): Treatment (ie, closure) of a clinically significant PDA when usual treatments are ineffective (FDA approved in premature neonates ≤32 weeks gestational age and weighing 500-1500 g). **Note:** The prophylactic use of ibuprofen is not currently indicated nor recommended (Ohlsson, 2011).

Medication Guide Available Yes

Pregnancy Risk Factor C/D ≥30 weeks gestation

Pregnancy Considerations Adverse events were not observed in the initial animal reproduction studies; therefore, the manufacturer classifies ibuprofen as pregnancy category C (category D: ≥30 weeks gestation). NSAID exposure during the first trimester is not strongly associated with congenital malformations; however, cardiovascular anomalies and cleft palate have been observed following NSAID exposure in some studies. The use of a NSAID close to conception may be associated with an increased risk of miscarriage. Nonteratogenic effects have been observed following NSAID administration during the third trimester including: Myocardial degenerative changes, prenatal constriction of the ductus arteriosus, fetal tricuspid regurgitation, failure of the ductus arteriosus to close postnatally; renal dysfunction or failure, oligohydramnios; gastrointestinal bleeding or perforation, increased risk of necrotizing enterocolitis; intracranial bleeding (including intraventricular hemorrhage), platelet dysfunction with resultant bleeding; pulmonary hypertension. Because they may cause premature closure of the ductus arteriosus, use of NSAIDs late in pregnancy should be avoided (use after 31 or 32 weeks gestation is not recommended by some clinicians). Product labeling for Caldolor® specifically notes that use at ≥30 weeks gestation should be avoided and therefore classifies ibuprofen as pregnancy category D at this time. The chronic use of NSAIDs in women of reproductive age may be associated with infertility that is reversible upon discontinuation of the medication. A registry is available for pregnant women exposed to autoimmune medications including ibuprofen. For additional information contact the Organization of Teratology Information Specialists, OTIS Autoimmune Diseases Study, at 877-311-8972.

Breast-Feeding Considerations Based on limited data, only very small amounts of ibuprofen are excreted into breast milk. Adverse events have not been reported in nursing infants. Because there is a potential for adverse events to occur in nursing infants, the manufacturer does not recommend the use of ibuprofen while breast-feeding. Use with caution in nursing women with hypertensive disorders of pregnancy or preexisting renal disease.

Contraindications Hypersensitivity to ibuprofen or any component; history of asthma, urticaria, or allergic-type reaction to aspirin, or other NSAIDs; patients with the "aspirin triad" [asthma, rhinitis (with or without nasal polyps), and aspirin intolerance] (fatal asthmatic and anaphylactoid reactions may occur in these patients); perioperative pain in the setting of coronary artery bypass graft (CABG)

Ibuprofen lysine injection (NeoProfen): Preterm neonates with untreated proven or suspected infection; congenital heart disease where patency of the PDA is necessary for pulmonary or systemic blood flow (eg, pulmonary atresia, severe tetralogy of Fallot, severe coarctation of aorta); bleeding (especially with active intracranial hemorrhage or GI bleed); thrombocytopenia; coagulation defects; proven or suspected necrotizing enterocolitis (NEC); significant renal dysfunction

When used for self-medication (OTC), do not use if previous allergic reaction to any other pain reliever/fever reducer; prior to or following cardiac surgery.

Warnings NSAIDs are associated with an increased risk of adverse cardiovascular thrombotic events, including potentially fatal MI and stroke **[U.S. Boxed Warning]**; risk may be increased with duration of use or preexisting cardiovascular risk factors or disease; carefully evaluate cardiovascular risk profile prior to prescribing; use the lowest effective dose for the shortest duration of time, taking into consideration individual patient treatment goals; alternate therapies should be considered for patients at high risk. Use is contraindicated for treatment of perioperative pain in the setting of CABG surgery **[U.S. Boxed Warning]**; an increased incidence of MI and stroke was found in patients receiving COX-2 selective NSAIDs for the treatment of pain within the first 10-14 days after CABG surgery. NSAIDs may cause fluid retention, edema, and new onset or worsening of preexisting hypertension; use with caution in patients with hypertension, CHF, or fluid retention. Response to ACE inhibitors, thiazides, or loop diuretics may be impaired with concurrent use of NSAIDs. Concurrent administration of ibuprofen, and potentially other nonselective NSAIDs, may interfere with aspirin's cardioprotective effect.

NSAIDs may increase the risk of gastrointestinal irritation, ulceration, bleeding, and perforation **[U.S. Boxed Warning]**. These events, which can be potentially fatal, may occur at any time during therapy, and without warning. Avoid the use of NSAIDs in patients with active GI bleeding or ulcer disease. Use NSAIDs with extreme caution in patients with a history of GI bleeding or ulcers (these patients have a 10-fold increased risk for developing a GI bleed). Use NSAIDs with caution in patients with other risk factors which may increase GI bleeding (eg, concurrent therapy with aspirin, anticoagulants, and/or corticosteroids, longer duration of NSAID use, smoking, use of alcohol, and poor general health). Use the lowest effective dose for the shortest duration of time, taking into consideration individual patient treatment goals; alternate therapies should be considered for patients at high risk.

NSAIDs may compromise existing renal function; dose-dependent decreases in prostaglandin synthesis may result from NSAID use, reducing renal blood flow which may cause renal decompensation. A single-center, 10-year, retrospective review of pediatric patients diagnosed with acute kidney injury (AKI) (n=1015; ages: ≤18 years) reported NSAIDS as a potential cause in 2.7% of patients (n=27); a higher incidence (6.6%) was reported when additional exclusion factors were included in the data analysis. Dosing information was available for 74% of the NSAID-associated AKI cases (n=20); dosing was within the recommended range in 75% (n=15) of these cases. The median age of children with NSAID-associated AKI was 14.7 years (range: 0.5-17.7 years); 15% of patients were <5 years and more likely to require dialysis than the older patients. Some experts suggest the incidence of NSAID-associated AKI found in this study is conservative due to aggressive exclusion criteria (eg, concurrent amino-glycoside or other nephrotoxic therapy) and the actual incidence may be higher (Brophy, 2013; Misurac, 2013). Patients with impaired renal function, dehydration, heart failure, liver dysfunction, and those taking diuretics and ACE inhibitors are at greater risk of renal toxicity; use with caution in these patients; rehydrate patient before starting therapy; monitor renal function closely. NSAIDs are not recommended for use in patients with advanced renal disease. Long-term use of NSAIDs may cause renal papillary necrosis and other renal injury.

In neonates, pulmonary hypertension has occurred following use; ten cases have been reported; three following early (prophylactic) administration of tromethamine ibuprofen (not available in U.S.) and seven cases following L-lysine ibuprofen for treatment of PDA (Bellini, 2006; Gournay, 2002; Ohlsson, 2013).

Anaphylactoid reactions may occur, even in patients without prior exposure; patients with "aspirin triad" [bronchial asthma, aspirin intolerance, and rhinitis (with or without nasal polyps)] are at increased risk; use is contraindicated in these patients. Do not use in patients who experience bronchospasm, asthma, rhinitis, or urticaria with NSAID or aspirin therapy. NSAIDs may cause serious and potentially fatal dermatologic adverse reactions including exfoliative dermatitis, Stevens-Johnson syndrome, and toxic epidermal necrolysis; discontinue use at first sign of skin rash or any other sign of hypersensitivity reaction. NSAIDs may mask fever and inflammation and thus decrease the ability of these signs to help diagnose infectious conditions. Avoid use of NSAIDs in late pregnancy (≥30 weeks gestation) as they may cause premature closure of the ductus arteriosus.

Some products contain sodium benzoate; benzoate is a metabolite of benzyl alcohol; large amounts of benzyl alcohol (≥99 mg/kg/day) have been associated with a potentially fatal toxicity ("gasping syndrome") in neonates; the "gasping syndrome" consists of metabolic acidosis, respiratory distress, gasping respirations, CNS dysfunction (including convulsions, intracranial hemorrhage), hypotension, and cardiovascular collapse; avoid use of ibuprofen products containing benzyl alcohol or sodium benzoate in neonates; *in vitro* and animal studies have shown that benzoate displaces bilirubin from protein binding sites. Some oral suspensions contain polysorbate 80 (Tween 80) which may cause allergic reactions in susceptible individuals. In premature neonates, thrombocytopenia, ascites, pulmonary deterioration, and renal and hepatic failure have been reported after receiving parenteral products containing polysorbate 80 (Alade, 1986; CDC, 1984). Some oral suspensions also contain propylene glycol; toxicities have been reported with use of products

containing propylene glycol, including hyperosmolality, lactic acidosis, seizures, and respiratory depression; in neonates large amounts of propylene glycol delivered orally, intravenously (eg, >3000 mg/day), or topically have been associated with potentially fatal toxicities which can include metabolic acidosis, seizures, renal failure, and CNS depression; use oral suspensions containing propylene glycol with caution (AAP, 1997; Shehab, 2009).

Precautions Use with caution in patients with decreased hepatic function; closely monitor patients with abnormal LFTs; severe hepatic reactions [eg, fulminant hepatitis, jaundice, liver failure (some cases fatal)] have occurred with NSAID use, rarely; discontinue if signs or symptoms of liver disease develop, or if systemic manifestations (eg, eosinophilia, rash, abdominal pain, diarrhea, dark urine) occur. Use with caution in patients with asthma; asthmatic patients may have aspirin-sensitive asthma which may be associated with severe and potentially fatal bronchospasm when aspirin or NSAIDs are administered. Anemia (due to occult or gross blood loss from the GI tract, fluid retention, or other effect on erythropoiesis) may occur; monitor hemoglobin and hematocrit in patients receiving long-term therapy. Use with caution and monitor carefully in patients with coagulation disorders or those receiving anticoagulants; NSAIDs inhibit platelet aggregation and may prolong bleeding time. May increase the risk of aseptic meningitis, especially in patients with systemic lupus erythematosus (SLE) and related connective tissue disorders. May cause vision changes (blurred or diminished vision, changes in color vision, scotomata); discontinue ibuprofen if such effects occur and obtain ophthalmologic examination with central visual fields and color vision testing.

Ibuprofen injection (Caldolor): Additional precautions: Product must be diluted prior to administration; hemolysis can occur if not diluted. Patients must be well hydrated before administration to reduce risk of adverse effects on the kidneys.

Ibuprofen lysine injection (NeoProfen): Avoid extravasation; I.V. solution may be irritating to tissues. Use with caution in neonates with controlled infection or those at risk for infection; ibuprofen may alter the usual signs of infection. May inhibit platelet aggregation; monitor for signs of bleeding. Use with caution in neonates when total bilirubin is elevated; ibuprofen may displace bilirubin from albumin-binding sites. Intraventricular hemorrhage has been reported; overall incidence: 29%; grade 3/4: 15%. Long-term evaluations of neurodevelopmental outcome, growth, or diseases associated with prematurity (eg, chronic lung disease, retinopathy of prematurity) following treatment have not been conducted.

OTC labeling: Prior to self-medication, patients should contact healthcare provider if they have or had recurring stomach pain or upset, ulcers, bleeding problems, high blood pressure, heart or kidney disease, other serious medical problems, or are currently taking a diuretic, aspirin, anticoagulant, or steroid drug. Recommended dosages should not be exceeded, due to an increased risk of GI bleeding. Consuming ≥3 alcoholic beverages/day or taking this medication longer than recommended may also increase the risk of GI bleeding. Stop use and consult a healthcare provider if symptoms do not improve within first 24 hours of use (children), symptoms get worse or newly appear (children and adults), fever lasts for >3 days (children and adults), or pain lasts >3 days (children) and >10 days (adults). Do not give for >10 days unless instructed by healthcare provider (children and adults). For children with severe or persistent sore throat or sore throat with symptoms such as high fever, headache, nausea, and vomiting, consult healthcare provider immediately; do not use for treatment of sore throat for >2 days or use in children <3 years of age with sore throat, unless directed by physician.

Chewable tablets contain aspartame (phenylalanine) which must be avoided (or used with caution) in patients with phenylketonuria.

Adverse Reactions

Oral:

Cardiovascular: Edema

Central nervous system: Dizziness, headache, nervousness

Dermatologic: Itching, rash

Endocrine & metabolic: Fluid retention

Gastrointestinal: Abdominal pain/cramps/distress, appetite decreased, constipation, diarrhea, dyspepsia, epigastric pain, flatulence, heartburn, nausea, vomiting

Otic: Tinnitus

Rare but important or life-threatening: Acute renal failure, agranulocytosis, anaphylaxis, aplastic anemia, azotemia, blurred vision, bone marrow suppression, confusion, creatinine clearance decreased, duodenal ulcer, edema, eosinophilia, epistaxis, erythema multiforme, gastric ulcer, GI bleed, GI hemorrhage, GI ulceration, hallucinations, hearing decreased, hematuria, hematocrit decreased, hemoglobin decreased, hemolytic anemia, hepatitis, hypertension, inhibition of platelet aggregation, jaundice, liver function tests abnormal, leukopenia, melena, neutropenia, pancreatitis, photosensitivity, Stevens-Johnson syndrome, thrombocytopenia, toxic amblyopia, toxic epidermal necrolysis, urticaria, vesiculobullous eruptions, vision changes

Injection: Ibuprofen (Caldolor®):

Cardiovascular: Edema, hypertension

Central nervous system: Dizziness, headache

Dermatologic: Pruritus

Endocrine & metabolic: Hypernatremia, hypokalemia

Gastrointestinal: Abdominal pain, dyspepsia, flatulence, nausea, vomiting

Genitourinary: Urinary retention

Hematologic: Anemia, hemorrhage, neutropenia

Renal: BUN increased

Respiratory: Cough

Injection: Ibuprofen lysine (NeoProfen®):

Cardiovascular: Edema, heart failure, intraventricular hemorrhage, hypotension, tachycardia

Central nervous system: Seizure

Dermatologic: Skin irritation

Endocrine & metabolic: Adrenal insufficiency, hypernatremia, hypocalcemia, hyper-/hypoglycemia

Gastrointestinal: Abdominal distension, feeding problems, gastritis, GI disorders, GI reflux, ileus, non NEC

Genitourinary: Urinary tract infection

Hematologic: Anemia, neutropenia, thrombocytopenia

Hepatic: Cholestasis, jaundice

Local: Injection-site reaction

Respiratory: Apnea, respiratory infection

Renal: Urea increased, renal impairment, creatinine increased, renal failure, urine output decreased (small decrease reported on days 2-6 with compensatory increase in output on day 9)

Respiratory: Respiratory failure, atelectasis

Miscellaneous: Infection, inguinal hernia, sepsis

Rare but important or life-threatening: GI perforation, necrotizing enterocolitis

Drug Interactions

Metabolism/Transport Effects Substrate of CYP2C19 (minor), CYP2C9 (minor); **Note:** Assignment of Major/Minor substrate status based on clinically relevant drug interaction potential; **Inhibits** CYP2C9 (weak)

Avoid Concomitant Use

Avoid concomitant use of Ibuprofen with any of the following: Floctafenine; Ketorolac (Nasal); Ketorolac (Systemic); NSAID (COX-2 Inhibitor); Omacetaxine; Urokinase

Increased Effect/Toxicity

Ibuprofen may increase the levels/effects of: 5-ASA Derivatives; Agents with Antiplatelet Properties; Aliskiren; Aminoglycosides; Anticoagulants; Apixaban; Bisphosphonate Derivatives; Collagenase (Systemic); CycloSPORINE (Systemic); Dabigatran Etexilate; Deferasirox; Desmopressin; Digoxin; Eplerenone; Haloperidol; Ibritumomab; Lithium; Methotrexate; Nonsteroidal Anti-Inflammatory Agents; NSAID (COX-2 Inhibitor); Omacetaxine; PEMEtrexed; Porfimer; Potassium-Sparing Diuretics; PRALAtrexate; Quinolone Antibiotics; Rivaroxaban; Salicylates; Tenofovir; Thrombolytic Agents; Tositumomab and Iodine I 131 Tositumomab; Urokinase; Vancomycin; Vitamin K Antagonists

The levels/effects of Ibuprofen may be increased by: ACE Inhibitors; Angiotensin II Receptor Blockers; Antidepressants (Tricyclic, Tertiary Amine); Corticosteroids (Systemic); CycloSPORINE (Systemic); Dasatinib; Floctafenine; Glucosamine; Herbs (Anticoagulant/Antiplatelet Properties); Ibrutinib; Ketorolac (Nasal); Ketorolac (Systemic); Multivitamins/Fluoride (with ADE); Multivitamins/Minerals (with ADEK, Folate, Iron); Multivitamins/Minerals (with AE, No Iron); Nonsteroidal Anti-Inflammatory Agents; Omega-3 Fatty Acids; Pentosan Polysulfate Sodium; Pentoxifylline; Probenecid; Prostacyclin Analogues; Selective Serotonin Reuptake Inhibitors; Serotonin/Norepinephrine Reuptake Inhibitors; Sodium Phosphates; Tipranavir; Treprostinil; Vitamin E; Voriconazole

Decreased Effect

Ibuprofen may decrease the levels/effects of: ACE Inhibitors; Agents with Antiplatelet Properties; Aliskiren; Angiotensin II Receptor Blockers; Beta-Blockers; Eplerenone; HydrALAZINE; Imatinib; Loop Diuretics; Potassium-Sparing Diuretics; Prostaglandins (Ophthalmic); Salicylates; Selective Serotonin Reuptake Inhibitors; Thiazide Diuretics

The levels/effects of Ibuprofen may be decreased by: Bile Acid Sequestrants; Nonsteroidal Anti-Inflammatory Agents; Salicylates

Food Interactions Ibuprofen peak serum levels may be decreased if taken with food. Management: Administer with food.

Stability

Oral:

Capsule: Store at 20°C to 25°C (68°F to 77°F). Avoid excessive heat >40°C (>104°F).

Oral suspension, drops, chewable tablets, tablet: Store at 20°C to 25°C (68°F to 77°F).

Parenteral:

Ibuprofen injection (Caldolor): Store intact vials at 20°C to 25°C (68°F to 77°F). Must be diluted prior to use. Dilute with D₅W, NS, or LR to a final concentration ≤4 mg/mL. Diluted solutions are stable for 24 hours at room temperature and room lighting.

Ibuprofen lysine injection (NeoProfen): Store at 20°C to 25°C (68°F to 77°F). Protect from light; store injection vials in carton until ready to use. Stable in I.V. dextrose or saline solutions. Following dilution, administer within 30 minutes of preparation. Discard unused portion of vial (vial does not contain preservative).

Mechanism of Action Reversibly inhibits cyclooxygenase-1 and 2 (COX-1 and 2) enzymes, which results in decreased formation of prostaglandin precursors; has antipyretic, analgesic, and anti-inflammatory properties

Other proposed mechanisms not fully elucidated (and possibly contributing to the anti-inflammatory effect to varying degrees), include inhibiting chemotaxis, altering lymphocyte activity, inhibiting neutrophil aggregation/activation, and decreasing proinflammatory cytokine levels.

Pharmacodynamics

Fever reduction:

Onset of action (single oral dose 8 mg/kg) (Kauffman, 1992):

Infants ≤1 year: 69 ± 22 minutes

Children ≥6 years: 109 ± 64 minutes

Maximum effect: 2-4 hours

Duration: 6-8 hours (dose-related)

Pharmacokinetics (Adult data unless noted)

Absorption: Oral: Rapid (85%)

Distribution: V_d:

Oral:

Febrile children <11 years: 0.2 L/kg

Adults: 0.12 L/kg

I.V.: Ibuprofen lysine: Premature neonates, GA <32 weeks: Variable results observed: 0.32 L/kg, others have reported: a central compartment V_d that decreases with increasing PNA and ductal closure (Van Overmeire, 2001) and a V_d, apparent: 0.062 L/kg in 21 premature neonates (GA <32 weeks, PNA: <1 day) (Aranda, 1997); a 2-compartment open model was observed

Protein binding: 90% to 99%

Metabolism: Oxidized in the liver; **Note:** Ibuprofen is a racemic mixture of R and S isomers; the R isomer (thought to be inactive) is slowly and incompletely (~60%) converted to the S isomer (active) in adults; the amount of conversion in children is not known, but it is thought to be similar to adults; a study in preterm neonates estimated the conversion to be 61% after prophylactic ibuprofen use and 86% after curative treatment (Gregoire, 2004).

Half-life:

Oral:

Infants and Children 3 months to 10 years: Oral suspension: 1.6 ± 0.7 hours (Kauffman, 1992)

Adults: 1.8-2 hours; end-stage renal disease: Unchanged

I.V.:

Ibuprofen (Caldor): 2.22-2.44 hours

Ibuprofen lysine (Neoprofen):

Premature neonates, GA <32 weeks: Reported data highly variable.

R-enantiomer: 10 hours; S-enantiomer: 25.5 hours (Gregoire, 2004)

Age-based observations:

PNA <1 day: 30.5 ± 4.2 hours (Aranda, 1997)

PNA 3 days: 43.1 ± 26.1 hours (Van Overmeire, 2001)

PNA 5 days: 26.8 ± 23.6 hours (Van Overmeire, 2001)

Time to peak serum concentration: Tablets: 1-2 hours; suspension: 1 hour

Children with cystic fibrosis (Scott, 1999):

Suspension (n=22): 0.74 ± 0.43 hours (median: 30 minutes)

Chewable tablet (n=4): 1.5 ± 0.58 hours (median: 1.5 hours)

Tablet (n=12): 1.33 ± 0.95 hours (median: 1 hour)

Elimination: Urine [primarily as metabolites (45% to 80%); ~1% as unchanged drug and 14% as conjugated]; some biliary excretion

Dosing: Neonatal PDA closure: Note: Use birth weight to calculate all doses; monitor urine output; a decrease in urine output may require dose adjustment or holding of therapy.

I.V.:

Manufacturer's labeling: Ibuprofen lysine (NeoProfen): GA ≤32 weeks weighing 500-1500 g at birth: Initial dose: 10 mg/kg, followed by two doses of 5 mg/kg/dose at 24 and 48 hours after the initial dose. A second course of treatment, alternative pharmacologic therapy, or surgery may be needed if the ductus arteriosus fails to close or reopens following the initial course of therapy.

Alternate dosing: Ibuprofen lysine: Reported dosing approach variable (standard or high-dose therapy):

Standard-dose therapy: Limited data available: GA >32 weeks: Initial dose: 10 mg/kg, followed by two doses of 5 mg/kg/dose administered at 24 hour intervals (Hirt, 2008; Meißner, 2012)

High-dose therapy: Limited data available: GA 24 to <40 weeks: Initial dose: 20 mg/kg, followed by two doses of 10 mg/kg/dose administered at 24-hour intervals has been evaluated in a total of 58 neonates in two studies (GA: 24-39 weeks, PNA ≤5 days for majority of patients). In comparison to the standard dose, these studies found a higher rate of PDA closure using high dose therapy without an increase in adverse effects (Dani, 2012; Meißner, 2012); further studies are needed. Pharmacokinetic data suggest that clearance increases with postnatal age; therefore, doses at the higher end of the dosage range may be necessary in older neonates (Hirt, 2008; Van Overmeire, 2001). Further studies are needed.

Oral suspension: Limited data available: GA <34 weeks weighing <1500 g at birth: Initial dose: 10 mg/kg, followed by two doses of 5 mg/kg/dose at 24 and 48 hours after the initial dose; doses were administered undiluted through a feeding tube and immediately followed with a flush (~1 mL) of distilled water; this dosing regimen has been used in several trials and has been shown to be safe and as effective as I.V. ibuprofen and I.V. indomethacin (Erdeve, 2012; Heyman, 2003; Lee, 2012); in one retrospective study, oral ibuprofen (n=52) was associated with lower rates of elevated serum creatinine compared to I.V. indomethacin (n=88) (Lee, 2012).

Dosing adjustment in renal impairment: I.V.: Ibuprofen lysine (Neoprofen): If anuria or marked oliguria (urinary output <0.6 mL/kg/hour) is evident at the scheduled time of the second or third dose, hold dose until renal function returns to normal. Use is contraindicated in preterm infants with significant renal impairment.

Dosing: Usual Note: To reduce the risk of adverse cardiovascular and GI effects, use the lowest effective dose for the shortest period of time:

Pediatric:

Analgesic:

I.V.: Ibuprofen injection (Caldolor): Adolescents ≥17 years: 400-800 mg every 6 hours as needed; maximum daily dose: 3200 mg/**day. Note:** Patients should be well hydrated prior to administration.

Oral:

Weight-directed dosing: Infants and Children <50 kg: Limited data available in infants <6 months: 4-10 mg/kg/dose every 6-8 hours; maximum single dose: 400 mg; maximum daily dose: 40 mg/kg/**day** (APS, 2008; Berde, 1990; Berde, 2002; Klieg-man, 2011)

Fixed dosing:

Infants and Children 6 months to 11 years: See table based upon manufacturer's labeling; use of weight to select dose is preferred; if weight is not available, then use age; doses may be repeated every 6-8 hours; maximum: 4 doses/day; treatment of sore throat for >2 days or use in infants and children <3 years of age with sore throat is not recommended, unless directed by healthcare provider.

Ibuprofen Dosing

Weight (preferred)[1]		Age	Dosage (mg)
lbs	kg		
12-17	5.4-8.1	6-11 months	50
18-23	8.2-10.8	12-23 months	75
24-35	10.9-16.3	2-3 years	100
36-47	16.4-21.7	4-5 years	150
48-59	21.8-27.2	6-8 years	200
60-71	27.3-32.6	9-10 years	250
72-95	32.7-43.2	11 years	300

[1]Manufacturer's recommendations are based on weight in pounds (OTC labeling); weight in kg listed here is derived from pounds and rounded; kg weight listed also is adjusted to allow for continuous weight ranges in kg.

Children ≥12 years and Adolescents: Oral: 200 mg every 4-6 hours as needed; if pain does not respond may increase to 400 mg; maximum daily dose: 1200 mg/**day**; treatment of pain for >10 days is not recommended, unless directed by healthcare provider

Antipyretic:

I.V.: Ibuprofen injection (Caldolor): Adolescents ≥17 years: Initial: 400 mg, then 400 mg every 4-6 hours or 100-200 mg every 4 hours as needed; maximum daily dose: 3200 mg/**day**. **Note:** Patients should be well hydrated prior to administration.

Oral:

Weight-directed dosing: Infants ≥6 months, Children, and Adolescents: 5-10 mg/kg/dose every 6-8 hours; maximum single dose: 400 mg; maximum daily dose: 40 mg/kg/**day** up to 1200 mg, unless directed by physician; under physician supervision daily doses ≤2400 mg may be used (Kliegman, 2011; Litalien, 2001; Sullivan, 2011)

Fixed dosing:

Infants and Children 6 months to 11 years: Oral: See table based upon manufacturer's labeling; use of weight to select dose is preferred; if weight is not available, then use age; doses may be repeated every 6-8 hours; maximum: 4 doses/day; treatment for >3 days is not recommended unless directed by healthcare provider

Weight (preferred)[1]		Age	Dosage (mg)
lbs	kg		
12-17	5.4-8.1	6-11 mo	50
18-23	8.2-10.8	12-23 mo	75
24-35	10.9-16.3	2-3 y	100
36-47	16.4-21.7	4-5 y	150
48-59	21.8-27.2	6-8 y	200
60-71	27.3-32.6	9-10 y	250
72-95	32.7-43.2	11 y	300

[1]Manufacturer's recommendations are based on weight in pounds (OTC labeling); weight in kg listed here is derived from pounds and rounded; kg weight listed also is adjusted to allow for continuous weight ranges in kg.

Cystic fibrosis, mild disease (to slow lung disease progression): Limited data available: Children and Adolescents 6-17 years with FEV_1 >60% predicted (Mogayzel, 2013): Oral: Initial: 20-30 mg/kg/dose twice daily; titrate to achieve peak plasma concentrations of 50-100 mcg/mL; should not eat or take pancreatic enzymes for 2 hours after the ibuprofen dose. Dosing based on a study of 41 patients (ages: 5-39 years); mean required dose: ~25 mg/kg/dose twice daily, reported range: 16.2-31.6 mg/kg/dose every 12 hours

required to achieve target concentration; results showed that chronic ibuprofen use (over 4 years) slowed the rate of decline in FEV_1; patients 5-13 years old with mild lung disease were observed to have greatest benefit; (Konstan, 1995). A follow up observational study (n=1365; ages: 6-17 years) under noncontrolled conditions (real world) showed significant improvement in the rate of decline of lung disease progression with chronic ibuprofen therapy (Konstan, 2007). **Note:** Timing of blood sampling postdose is based on dosage form: Oral suspension: Obtain blood samples at 30, 45, and 60 minutes postdose; tablets: Obtain blood samples at 1, 2, and 3 hours postdose (Litalien, 2001; Scott, 1999).

Juvenile idiopathic arthritis (JIA): Children and Adolescents: Usual range: 30-40 mg/kg/**day** in 3-4 divided doses; start at lower end of dosing range and titrate; patients with milder disease may be treated with 20 mg/kg/**day**; patients with more severe disease may require up to 50 mg/kg/**day**; maximum single dose: 800 mg; maximum daily dose: 2400 mg/**day** (Giannini, 1990; Kliegman, 2011; Litalien, 2001)

Adult:

Inflammatory disease: Oral: 400-800 mg/dose 3-4 times daily; maximum daily dose: 3200 mg/**day**

Analgesia/pain/fever/dysmenorrhea: Oral: 200-400 mg/dose every 4-6 hours; maximum daily dose: 1200 mg/**day**, unless directed by physician; under physician supervision daily doses ≤2400 mg may be used

Analgesic: I.V. (Caldolor): 400-800 mg every 6 hours as needed; maximum daily dose: 3200 mg/**day**. **Note:** Patients should be well hydrated prior to administration.

Antipyretic: I.V. (Caldolor): Initial: 400 mg, then 400 mg every 4-6 hours or 100-200 mg every 4 hours as needed; maximum daily dose: 3200 mg/**day**. **Note:** Patients should be well hydrated prior to administration.

OTC labeling:

Analgesia/Antipyretic: Oral: 200 mg every 4-6 hours as needed; maximum daily dose: 1200 mg/24 hours; treatment for >10 days is not recommended unless directed by healthcare provider

Migraine: Oral: 400 mg at onset of symptoms; maximum daily dose: 400 mg/24 hours unless directed by healthcare provider

Dosing adjustment in renal impairment:

Infants, Children, and Adolescents: Oral: There are no dosage adjustments provided in the manufacturer's labeling; however, the 2012 KDIGO guidelines provide the following recommendations for NSAIDs:

eGFR 30 to <60 mL/minute/1.73 m^2: Avoid use in patients with intercurrent disease that increases risk of acute kidney injury

eGFR <30 mL/minute/1.73 m^2: Avoid use

Adults: Oral, I.V.: There are no dosage adjustments provided in the manufacturer's labeling; however, the 2012 KDIGO guidelines provide the following recommendations for NSAIDs:

eGFR 30 to <60 mL/minute/1.73 m^2: Avoid use in patients with intercurrent disease that increases risk of acute kidney injury

eGFR <30 mL/minute/1.73 m^2: Avoid use

Dosing adjustment in hepatic impairment: Adults: Oral, I.V.: There are no dosage adjustments provided in the manufacturer's labeling; use caution and discontinue if hepatic function worsens.

Administration

Oral: Administer with food or milk to decrease GI upset; shake suspension well before use

I.V.:

Ibuprofen injection (Caldolor): For I.V. administration only; must be diluted to a final concentration of ≤4 mg/mL prior to administration; infuse over at least 30 minutes

Ibuprofen lysine injection (NeoProfen): For I.V. administration only; administration via umbilical arterial line has not been evaluated. Dilute with dextrose or saline to an appropriate volume. Infuse over 15 minutes through I.V. port closest to insertion site. Avoid extravasation. Do not administer simultaneously via same line with TPN. If needed, interrupt TPN for 15 minutes prior to and after ibuprofen administration, keeping line open with dextrose or saline.

Monitoring Parameters CBC, serum electrolytes, occult blood loss, liver enzymes; urine output, serum BUN, and creatinine in patients receiving I.V. ibuprofen, concurrent diuretics, those with decreased renal function, or in patients on chronic therapy. Monitor preterm neonates for signs of bleeding and infection; serum electrolytes, glucose, calcium and bilirubin; vital signs; monitor I.V. site for signs of extravasation. Patients receiving long-term therapy for JIA should receive periodic ophthalmological exams.

Reference Range Plasma concentrations >200 mcg/mL may be associated with severe toxicity; cystic fibrosis: therapeutic peak plasma concentration: 50-100 mcg/mL

Test Interactions May interfere with urine detection of phencyclidine, cannabinoids, and barbiturates (false-positives)

Additional Information Motrin suspension contains sucrose 0.3 g/mL and 1.6 calories/mL. Due to its effects on platelet function, ibuprofen should be withheld for at least 4-6 half-lives prior to surgical or dental procedures.

There is currently no scientific evidence to support alternating acetaminophen with ibuprofen in the treatment of fever (Mayoral, 2000)

I.V. ibuprofen is as effective as I.V. indomethacin for the treatment of PDA in preterm neonates, but is less likely to cause adverse effects on renal function (eg, oliguria, increased serum creatinine) (Aranda, 2006; Lago, 2002; Ohlsson, 2013; Van Overmeire, 2000). Ibuprofen (compared to indomethacin) also has been shown to decrease the risk of developing NEC (Ohlsson, 2013).

Dosage Forms Considerations
EnovaRX-Ibuprofen is a compounding kit. Refer to manufacturer's package insert for compounding instructions.

Dosage Forms Excipient information presented when available (limited, particularly for generics); consult specific product labeling.

Capsule, Oral:

Advil: 200 mg

Advil Migraine: 200 mg

KS Ibuprofen: 200 mg [contains fd&c blue #2 (indigotine)]

Generic: 200 mg

Cream, External:

EnovaRX-Ibuprofen: 10% (60 g, 120 g) [contains cetearyl alcohol]

Kit, Combination:

Ibuprofen Comfort Pac: 800 mg [contains methylparaben, trolamine (triethanolamine)]

Solution, Intravenous:

Caldolor: 400 mg/4 mL (4 mL); 800 mg/8 mL (8 mL)

Solution, Intravenous, as lysine [preservative free]:

NeoProfen: 10 mg/mL (2 mL)

Suspension, Oral:

Childrens Advil: 100 mg/5 mL (120 mL) [fruit flavor]

Childrens Advil: 100 mg/5 mL (120 mL) [alcohol free; grape flavor]

Childrens Advil: 100 mg/5 mL (120 mL) [alcohol free; contains brilliant blue fcf (fd&c blue #1), edetate disodium, fd&c red #40, polysorbate 80, propylene glycol, sodium benzoate; grape flavor]

Childrens Advil: 100 mg/5 mL (120 mL) [alcohol free; contains brilliant blue fcf (fd&c blue #1), propylene glycol, sodium benzoate; blue raspberry flavor]

Childrens Advil: 100 mg/5 mL (30 mL, 120 mL) [alcohol free, dye free; contains edetate disodium, polysorbate 80, propylene glycol, sodium benzoate; white grape flavor]

Childrens Advil: 50 mg/1.25 mL (15 mL) [dye free; contains propylene glycol, sodium benzoate; white grape flavor]

Childrens Ibuprofen: 100 mg/5 mL (118 mL) [alcohol free; contains brilliant blue fcf (fd&c blue #1), fd&c red #40, polysorbate 80, sodium benzoate; grape flavor]

Childrens Ibuprofen: 100 mg/5 mL (120 mL) [alcohol free; contains butylparaben, fd&c red #40, polysorbate 80, propylene glycol, sodium benzoate; bubble-gum flavor]

Childrens Ibuprofen: 100 mg/5 mL (118 mL, 237 mL, 240 mL) [alcohol free; contains fd&c red #40, fd&c yellow #10 (quinoline yellow), polysorbate 80, sodium benzoate; berry flavor]

Childrens Ibuprofen: 100 mg/5 mL (118 mL) [alcohol free; contains fd&c red #40, polysorbate 80, sodium benzoate]

Childrens Ibuprofen: 40 mg/mL (15 mL) [alcohol free; berry flavor]

Childrens Ibuprofen: 100 mg/5 mL (118 mL) [alcohol free, dye free; contains polysorbate 80, sodium benzoate]

Childrens Ibuprofen: 100 mg/5 mL (118 mL) [alcohol free, gluten free; contains brilliant blue fcf (fd&c blue #1), fd&c red #40, polysorbate 80, sodium benzoate; grape flavor]

Childrens Motrin: 40 mg/mL (15 mL) [berry flavor]

Childrens Motrin: 100 mg/5 mL (120 mL) [alcohol free]

Childrens Motrin: 100 mg/5 mL (60 mL, 120 mL) [alcohol free; contains fd&c red #40, fd&c yellow #10 (quinoline yellow), polysorbate 80, sodium benzoate; berry flavor]

Childrens Motrin: 100 mg/5 mL (120 mL) [alcohol free; contains fd&c red #40, fd&c yellow #10 (quinoline yellow), sodium benzoate; berry flavor]

Childrens Motrin: 100 mg/5 mL (120 mL) [alcohol free; contains fd&c red #40, sodium benzoate]

Childrens Motrin: 100 mg/5 mL (120 mL) [alcohol free; contains fd&c red #40, sodium benzoate]

Childrens Motrin: 100 mg/5 mL (120 mL) [alcohol free; contains fd&c red #40, sodium benzoate; bubble-gum flavor]

Childrens Motrin: 100 mg/5 mL (120 mL) [alcohol free; contains fd&c red #40, sodium benzoate; tropical punch flavor]

Childrens Motrin: 100 mg/5 mL (120 mL) [alcohol free; dye free; contains polysorbate 80, sodium benzoate]

Childrens Motrin: 100 mg/5 mL (120 mL) [alcohol free; dye free; contains sodium benzoate; berry flavor]

Ibuprofen Childrens: 100 mg/5 mL (120 mL) [alcohol free; contains butylparaben, fd&c red #40, fd&c yellow #6 (sunset yellow), polysorbate 80, propylene glycol, sodium benzoate; fruit flavor]

Ibuprofen Childrens: 100 mg/5 mL (120 mL, 240 mL) [alcohol free; contains butylparaben, fd&c yellow #6 (sunset yellow), polysorbate 80, propylene glycol, sodium benzoate; berry flavor]

Ibuprofen Childrens: 100 mg/5 mL (120 mL) [alcohol free, gluten free; contains brilliant blue fcf (fd&c blue #1), fd&c red #40, polysorbate 80, sodium benzoate; grape flavor]

Ibuprofen Childrens: 100 mg/5 mL (118 mL) [alcohol free, gluten free; contains fd&c red #40, polysorbate 80, sodium benzoate; bubble-gum flavor]

Infants Advil: 50 mg/1.25 mL (15 mL) [alcohol free, dye free; contains edetate disodium, polysorbate 80, propylene glycol, sodium benzoate; white grape flavor]

Infants Ibuprofen: 50 mg/1.25 mL (15 mL) [alcohol free; contains butylparaben, fd&c red #40, polysorbate 80, propylene glycol, sodium benzoate; berry flavor]

Infants Ibuprofen: 50 mg/1.25 mL (15 mL, 30 mL) [alcohol free, dye free; contains polysorbate 80, sodium benzoate; berry flavor]

Infants Ibuprofen: 50 mg/1.25 mL (15 mL) [alcohol free, gluten free; contains butylparaben, fd&c red #40, polysorbate 80, propylene glycol, sodium benzoate; berry flavor]

Motrin: 40 mg/mL (15 mL) [alcohol free, dye free; berry flavor]

Motrin Infants Drops: 50 mg/1.25 mL (15 mL) [alcohol free; contains fd&c red #40, polysorbate 80, sodium benzoate; berry flavor]

Motrin Infants Drops: 50 mg/1.25 mL (15 mL, 30 mL) [alcohol free, dye free; contains polysorbate 80, sodium benzoate]

Generic: 100 mg/5 mL (5 mL, 118 mL, 120 mL, 473 mL)

Tablet, Oral:

Addaprin: 200 mg

Advil: 200 mg

Advil Junior Strength: 100 mg

Dyspel: 200 mg

Genpril: 200 mg

I-Prin: 200 mg

IBU-200: 200 mg

Motrin IB: 200 mg

Motrin IB: 200 mg [contains fd&c yellow #6 (sunset yellow)]

Motrin Junior Strength: 100 mg [scored]

Provil: 200 mg

Generic: 200 mg, 400 mg, 600 mg, 800 mg

Tablet Chewable, Oral:

Advil Junior Strength: 100 mg [scored; contains aspartame, fd&c blue #2 aluminum lake; grape flavor]

Childrens Motrin: 50 mg [scored; contains aspartame, fd&c yellow #6 (sunset yellow); orange flavor]

Childrens Motrin Jr Strength: 100 mg [scored; contains aspartame, brilliant blue fcf (fd&c blue #1); grape flavor]

Ibuprofen Junior Strength: 100 mg [contains aspartame, fd&c yellow #6 (sunset yellow), soybean oil, whey protein]

Motrin Junior Strength: 100 mg [contains aspartame, brilliant blue fcf (fd&c blue #1)]

Motrin Junior Strength: 100 mg [scored; contains aspartame, fd&c yellow #6 (sunset yellow); orange flavor]

References

Alade SL, Brown RE, Paquet A. Polysorbate 80 and e-ferol toxicity. Pediatrics. 1986;77(4):593-597.

American Academy of Pediatrics Committee on Drugs. "Inactive" ingredients in pharmaceutical products: update (subject review). Pediatr. 1997;99(2):268-278.

Amoozgar H, Ghodstehrani M, and Pishva N, "Oral Ibuprofen and Ductus Arteriosus Closure in Full-Term Neonates: A Prospective Case-Control Study," Pediatr Cardiol, 2009 [Epub ahead of print].

Aranda JV and Thomas R, "Systematic Review: Intravenous Ibuprofen in Preterm Newborns," Semin Perinatol, 2006, 30(3):114-20.

Aranda JV, Varvarigou A, Beharry K, et al, "Pharmacokinetics and Protein Binding of Intravenous Ibuprofen in the Premature Newborn Infant," Acta Paediatr, 1997, 86(3):289-93.

Bellini C, Campone F, and Serra G, "Pulmonary Hypertension Following L-lysine Ibuprofen Therapy in a Preterm Infant With Patent Ductus Arteriosus," CMAJ, 2006, 174(13):1843-4.

Berde C, Ablin A, Glazer J, et al, "American Academy of Pediatrics Report of the Subcommittee on Disease-Related Pain in Childhood Cancer," Pediatrics, 1990, 86(5 Pt 2):818-25.

Berde CB, Sethna NF. Analgesics for the treatment of pain in children. N Engl J Med. 2002;347(14):1094-1103.

Brophy PD. Changing the paradigm in pediatric acute kidney injury. J Pediatr. 2013;162(6):1094-1096.

Capparelli EV, "Pharmacologic, Pharmacodynamic, and Pharmacokinetic Considerations With Intravenous Ibuprofen Lysine," J Pediatr Pharmacol Ther, 2007, 12:158-70.

Catella-Lawson F, Reilly MP, Kapoor SC, et al. "Cyclooxygenase Inhibitors and the Antiplatelet Effects of Aspirin," N Engl J Med, 2001, 345(25):1809-17.

Center for Disease Control and Prevention (CDC). Unusual syndrome with fatalities among premature infants: association with a new intravenous vitamin E product. MMWR. 1984;33(14):198-199.

Cryer B, Berlin RG, Cooper SA, et al. "Double-Blind, Randomized, Parallel, Placebo-Controlled Study Of Ibuprofen Effects On Thromboxane B2 Concentrations In Aspirin-Treated Healthy Adult Volunteers," Clin Ther, 2005, 27(2):185-191.

Dani C, Vangi V, Bertini G, et al. High-dose ibuprofen for patent ductus arteriosus in extremely preterm infants: a randomized controlled study. Clin Pharmacol Ther. 2012;91(4):590-596.

Desfrere L, Zohar S, Morville P, et al. Dose-finding study of ibuprofen in patent ductus arteriosus using the continual reassessment method. J Clin Pharm Ther. 2005;30(2):121-132.

Erdeve O, Gokmen T, Altug N, et al, "Oral Versus Intravenous Ibuprofen: Which Is Better in Closure of Patent Ductus Arteriosus?" Pediatrics, 2009, 123(4):e763.

Erdeve O, Yurttutan S, Altug N, et al. Oral versus intravenous ibuprofen for patent ductus arteriosus closure: a randomised controlled trial in extremely low birthweight infants. Arch Dis Child Fetal Neonatal Ed. 2012;97(4):F279-283.

Gal P, Ransom JL, and Davis SA, "Possible Ibuprofen-Induced Kernicterus in a Near-Term Infant With Moderate Hyperbilirubinemia," J Pediatr Pharmacol Ther, 2006, 11:245-50.

Giannini EH, Brewer EJ, Miller ML, et al. Ibuprofen suspension in the treatment of juvenile rheumatoid arthritis. Pediatric Rheumatology Collaborative Study Group. J Pediatr. 1990;117(4):645-652.

Gournay V, Savagner C, Thiriez G, et al, "Pulmonary Hypertension After Ibuprofen Prophylaxis in Very Preterm Infants," Lancet, 2002, 359 (9316):1486-8.

Gregoire N, Gualano V, Geneteau A, et al, "Population Pharmacokinetics of Ibuprofen Enantiomers in Very Premature Neonates," J Clin Pharmacol, 2004, 44(10):1114-24.

Heyman E, Morag I, Batash D, et al. Closure of patent ductus arteriosus with oral ibuprofen suspension in premature newborns: a pilot study. Pediatrics. 2003;112(5):e354.

Hirt D, Van Overmeire B, Treluyer JM, et al. An optimized ibuprofen dosing scheme for preterm neonates with patent ductus arteriosus, based on a population pharmacokinetic and pharmacodynamic study. Br J Clin Pharmacol. 2008;65(5):629-636.

Kauffman RE and Nelson MV, "Effect of Age on Ibuprofen Pharmacokinetics and Antipyretic Response," J Pediatr, 1992, 121(6):969-73.

Kidney Disease: Improving Global Outcomes (KDIGO) CKD Work Group. KDIGO 2012 clinical practice guideline for the evaluation and management of chronic kidney disease. Kidney Inter Suppl. 2013;3:1-150.

Kliegman RM, Stanton BF, St. Gemell JW, et al, eds. Nelson Textbook of Pediatrics. 19th ed. Philadelphia, PA: Saunders Elsevier;2011.

Konstan MW, Byard PJ, Hoppel CL, et al, "Effect of High-Dose Ibuprofen in Patients With Cystic Fibrosis," N Engl J Med, 1995, 332(13):848-54.

Konstan MW, Schluchter MD, Xue W, et al. Clinical use of Ibuprofen is associated with slower FEV$_1$ decline in children with cystic fibrosis. Am J Respir Crit Care Med. 2007;176(11):1084-1089.

Lago P, Bettiol T, Salvadori S, et al, "Safety and Efficacy of Ibuprofen Versus Indomethacin in Preterm Infants Treated for Patent Ductus Arteriosus: A Randomised Controlled Trial," Eur J Pediatr, 2002, 161 (4):202-7.

Lee CH, Chen HN, Tsao LY, et al. Oral ibuprofen versus intravenous indomethacin for closure of patent ductus arteriosus in very low birth weight infants. Pediatr Neonatol. 2012;53(6):346-353.

Lesko SM and Mitchell AA, "An Assessment of the Safety of Pediatric Ibuprofen. A Practitioner-Based Randomized Clinical Trial," JAMA, 1995, 273(12):929-33.

Lesko SM and Mitchell AA, "The Safety of Acetaminophen and Ibuprofen Among Children Younger Than Two Years Old," Pediatrics, 1999, 104 (4), http://www.pediatrics.org/cgi/content/full/104/4/e39.

Litalien C, Jacqz-Aigrain E. Risks and benefits of nonsteroidal anti-inflammatory drugs in children: a comparison with paracetamol. Paediatr Drugs. 2001;3(11):817-858.

Mayoral CE, Marino RV, Rosenfeld, W, et al, "Alternating Antipyretics: Is This an Alternative?" Pediatrics, 2000, 105(5):1009-12.

Meißner U, Chakrabarty R, Topf HG, et al. Improved closure of patent ductus arteriosus with high doses of ibuprofen. Pediatr Cardiol. 2012;33(4):586-590.

Misurac JM, Knoderer CA, Leiser JD, et al. Nonsteroidal anti-inflammatory drugs are an important cause of acute kidney injury in children. J Pediatr. 2013;162(6):1153-1159.

Mogayzel PJ Jr, Naureckas ET, Robinson KA, et al. Cystic fibrosis pulmonary guidelines. Chronic medications for maintenance of lung health. Am J Respir Crit Care Med. 2013;187(7):680-689.

Ohlsson A and Shah SS, "Ibuprofen for the Prevention of Patent Ductus Arteriosus in Preterm and/or Low Birth Weight Infants (Review)," Cochrane Database Syst Rev, 2011;7:CD00421.

Ohlsson A, Walia R, and Shah S, "Ibuprofen for the Treatment of Patent Ductus Arteriosus in Preterm and/or Low Birth Weight Infants," *Cochrane Database Syst Rev*, 2013, (4):CD003481.

Pai VB, Sakadjian A, and Puthoff TD, "Ibuprofen Lysine for the Prevention and Treatment of Patent Ductus Arteriosus," *Pharmacotherapy*, 2008, 28(9):1162-82.

"Principles of Analgesic Use in the Treatment of Acute Pain and Cancer Pain," 6th ed, Glenview, IL: American Pain Society, 2008.

Scott CS, Retsch-Bogart GZ, Kustra RP, et al, "The Pharmacokinetics of Ibuprofen Suspension, Chewable Tablets, and Tablets in Children With Cystic Fibrosis," *J Pediatr*, 1999, 134(1):58-63.

Shehab N, Lewis CL, Streetman DD, Donn SM. Exposure to the pharmaceutical excipients benzyl alcohol and propylene glycol among critically ill neonates. *Pediatr Crit Care Med*. 2009;10 (2):256-259.

Sullivan JE, Farrar HC, et al. Fever and antipyretic use in children. *Pediatrics*. 2011;127(3):580-587.

Van Overmeire B, "Common Clinical and Practical Questions on the Use of Intravenous Ibuprofen Lysine for the Treatment of Patent Ductus Arteriosus," *J Pediatr Pharmacol Ther*, 2007, 12:194-206.

Van Overmeire B, Smets K, Lecoutere D, et al, "A Comparison of Ibuprofen and Indomethacin for Closure of Patent Ductus Arteriosus," *N Engl J Med*, 2000, 343(10):674-81.

Van Overmeire B, Touw D, Schepens PJ, et al, "Ibuprofen Pharmacokinetics in Preterm Infants With Patent Ductus Arteriosus," *Clin Pharmacol Ther*, 2001, 70(4):336-43.

◆ **Ibuprofen and Pseudoephedrine** *see* Pseudoephedrine and Ibuprofen *on page 1772*

◆ **Ibuprofen Childrens [OTC]** *see* Ibuprofen *on page 1059*

◆ **Ibuprofen Comfort Pac** *see* Ibuprofen *on page 1059*

◆ **Ibuprofen Junior Strength [OTC]** *see* Ibuprofen *on page 1059*

◆ **Ibuprofen Lysine** *see* Ibuprofen *on page 1059*

◆ **Ibuprofen Muscle and Joint (Can)** *see* Ibuprofen *on page 1059*

◆ **IC51** *see* Japanese Encephalitis Virus Vaccine (Inactivated) *on page 1173*

◆ **ICI-182,780** *see* Fulvestrant *on page 946*

◆ **ICI-204,219** *see* Zafirlukast *on page 2164*

◆ **ICI-46474** *see* Tamoxifen *on page 1968*

◆ **ICL670** *see* Deferasirox *on page 601*

◆ **ICRF-187** *see* Dexrazoxane *on page 626*

◆ **Idamycin PFS** *see* IDArubicin *on page 1067*

IDArubicin (eye da ROO bi sin)

Medication Safety Issues
Sound-alike/look-alike issues:
IDArubicin may be confused with DOXOrubicin, DAUNOrubicin, epirubicin
Idamycin PFS® may be confused with Adriamycin

High alert medication:
The Institute for Safe Medication Practices (ISMP) includes this medication among its list of drugs which have a heightened risk of causing significant patient harm when used in error.

Related Information
Emetogenic Potential of Antineoplastic Agents in Children *on page 2327*
Management of Drug Extravasations *on page 2255*
Safe Handling of Hazardous Drugs *on page 2419*

Brand Names: U.S. Idamycin PFS

Brand Names: Canada Idamycin PFS; Idarubicin Hydrochloride Injection

Therapeutic Category Antineoplastic Agent, Anthracycline; Antineoplastic Agent, Topoisomerase II Inhibitor

Generic Availability (U.S.) Yes

Use Used in combination with other antineoplastic agents for treatment of acute myeloid leukemia (AML) (FDA approved in adults); has also been used for the treatment of acute lymphocytic leukemia (ALL)

Pregnancy Risk Factor D

Pregnancy Considerations Adverse events were observed in animal studies. Fetal fatality was noted in a case report following use in a pregnant woman during the second trimester. The manufacturer recommends that women of childbearing potential avoid pregnancy.

Breast-Feeding Considerations It is not known if idarubicin is excreted in breast milk. Breast-feeding is not recommended by the manufacturer.

Contraindications Hypersensitivity to idarubicin or any component; patients with preexisting bone marrow suppression unless the benefit warrants the risk; severe CHF, cardiomyopathy, or arrhythmias; pregnancy

Warnings Hazardous agent; use appropriate precautions for handling and disposal (NIOSH, 2012); I.V. use only, severe local tissue necrosis will result if extravasation occurs **[U.S. Boxed Warning]**. May cause myocardial toxicity (CHF, arrhythmias or cardiomyopathies) **[U.S. Boxed Warning]**; myocardial toxicity is more common in patients who have previously received anthracyclines or have preexisting cardiac disease; the risk of myocardial toxicity is also increased in patients with concomitant or prior mediastinal/pericardial irradiation, patients with anemia, bone marrow depression, infections, leukemic pericarditis, or myocarditis. Monitor cardiac function during treatment; the maximum lifetime anthracycline dose for idarubicin is approximately 137.5 mg/m²; may cause severe myelosuppression **[U.S. Boxed Warning]**; myelosuppression occurs in all patients given a therapeutic dose and is the dose-limiting adverse effect associated with idarubicin.

Precautions Use with caution and reduce dose in patients with impaired hepatic or renal function **[U.S. Boxed Warning]** and patients receiving concurrent radiation therapy. Should be administered under the supervision of an experienced cancer chemotherapy physician **[U.S. Boxed Warning]**.

Adverse Reactions
Cardiovascular: CHF (dose related), transient ECG abnormalities (supraventricular tachycardia, S-T wave changes, atrial or ventricular extrasystoles) are generally asymptomatic and self-limiting. The relative cardiotoxicity of idarubicin compared to doxorubicin is unclear. Some investigators report no increase in cardiac toxicity for adults at cumulative oral idarubicin doses up to 540 mg/m²; other reports suggest a maximum cumulative intravenous dose of 150 mg/m².

Central nervous system: Headache, seizure

Dermatologic: Alopecia, radiation recall, skin rash, urticaria

Gastrointestinal: Diarrhea, GI hemorrhage, nausea, vomiting, stomatitis

Emetic potential: Moderate (30% to 60%)

Genitourinary: Discoloration of urine (darker yellow)

Hematologic: Myelosuppression (nadir: 10-15 days; recovery: 21-28 days), primarily leukopenia; thrombocytopenia and anemia. Effects are generally less severe with oral dosing.

Hepatic: Bilirubin increased, transaminases increased

Neuromuscular & skeletal: Peripheral neuropathy

Local: Tissue necrosis upon extravasation, erythematous streaking

Rare but important or life-threatening: Cardiomyopathy, hyperuricemia, myocarditis, neutropenic typhlitis

Drug Interactions
Metabolism/Transport Effects Substrate of P-glycoprotein

Avoid Concomitant Use
Avoid concomitant use of IDArubicin with any of the following: BCG; CloZAPine; Dipyrone; Natalizumab; Pimecrolimus; Tacrolimus (Topical); Tofacitinib; Vaccines (Live)

Increased Effect/Toxicity

IDArubicin may increase the levels/effects of: CloZAPine; Leflunomide; Natalizumab; Tofacitinib; Vaccines (Live)

The levels/effects of IDArubicin may be increased by: Bevacizumab; Cyclophosphamide; Denosumab; Dipyrone; P-glycoprotein/ABCB1 Inhibitors; Pimecrolimus; Roflumilast; Tacrolimus (Topical); Taxane Derivatives; Trastuzumab

Decreased Effect

IDArubicin may decrease the levels/effects of: BCG; Cardiac Glycosides; Coccidioidin Skin Test; Sipuleucel-T; Vaccines (Inactivated); Vaccines (Live)

The levels/effects of IDArubicin may be decreased by: Cardiac Glycosides; Echinacea; P-glycoprotein/ABCB1 Inducers

Stability Hazardous agent; use appropriate precautions for handling and disposal (NIOSH, 2012). Store vials under refrigeration and protect from light; incompatible with acyclovir, ceftazidime, furosemide, hydrocortisone, sodium bicarbonate and heparin; inactivated by alkaline solutions.

Mechanism of Action Similar to doxorubicin and daunorubicin; inhibition of DNA and RNA synthesis by intercalation between DNA base pairs

Pharmacokinetics (Adult data unless noted)

Distribution:

V_d: Large volume of distribution due to extensive tissue binding; distributes into CSF

V_{dss}: 1700 L/m^2

Protein binding:

Idarubicin: 97%

Idarubicinol: 94%

Metabolism: In the liver to idarubicinol (active metabolite)

Half-life:

Children: 18.7 hours (range: 2.5-22.4 hours)

Adults: 19 hours (range: 10.5-34.7 hours)

Idarubicinol: 45-56.8 hours

Elimination: Primarily by biliary excretion; 2.3% to 6.5% of a dose is eliminated renally

Dosing: Usual AML: I.V. (refer to individual protocols):

Children: 10-12 mg/m^2 once daily for 3 days of treatment course

Adults:

Induction: 12 mg/m^2/day for 3 days

Consolidation: 10-12 mg/m^2/day for 2 days

Dosing adjustment in hepatic and/or renal impairment:

Serum creatinine ≥2 mg/dL: Reduce dose by 25%

Bilirubin >2.5 mg/dL: Reduce dose by 50%

Bilirubin >5 mg/dL: **Do not administer**

Administration Hazardous agent; use appropriate precautions for handling and disposal (NIOSH, 2012).

Do not administer I.M. or SubQ

Parenteral: I.V.: Administer by I.V. intermittent infusion over 10-30 minutes into a free flowing I.V. solution of NS or D$_5$W; administer at a final concentration of 1 mg/mL

Vesicant/Extravasation Risk Vesicant

Monitoring Parameters CBC with differential, platelet count, ECHO, ECG, serum electrolytes, creatinine, uric acid, ALT, AST, bilirubin, signs of extravasation

Dosage Forms Excipient information presented when available (limited, particularly for generics); consult specific product labeling.

Solution, Intravenous, as hydrochloride [preservative free]:

Idamycin PFS: 5 mg/5 mL (5 mL); 10 mg/10 mL (10 mL); 20 mg/20 mL (20 mL)

Generic: 5 mg/5 mL (5 mL); 10 mg/10 mL (10 mL); 20 mg/20 mL (20 mL)

References

Dinndorf PA, Avramis VI, Wiersma S, et al, "Phase I/II Study of Idarubicin Given With Continuous Infusion Fludarabine Followed by Continuous Infusion Cytarabine in Children With Acute Leukemia: A Report From the Children's Cancer Group," *J Clin Oncol*, 1997, 15 (8):2780-5.

Leahey A, Kelly K, Rorke LB, et al, "A Phase I/II Study of Idarubicin (Ida) With Continuous Infusion Fludarabine (F-ara-A) and Cytarabine (ara-C) for Refractory or Recurrent Pediatric Acute Myeloid Leukemia (AML)," *J Pediatr Hematol Oncol*, 1997, 19(4):304-8.

National Institute for Occupational Safety and Health (NIOSH), "NIOSH List of Antineoplastic and Other Hazardous Drugs in Healthcare Settings 2012." Available at http://www.cdc.gov/niosh/docs/ 2012-150/pdfs/2012-150.pdf. Accessed January 21, 2013.

Reid JM, Pendergrass TW, Krailo MD, et al, "Plasma Pharmacokinetics and Cerebrospinal Fluid Concentrations of Idarubicin and Idarubicinol in Pediatric Leukemia Patients: A Children's Cancer Study Group Report," *Cancer Res*, 1990, 50(20):6525-8.

◆ **Idarubicin Hydrochloride** *see* IDArubicin *on page 1067*

◆ **Idarubicin Hydrochloride Injection (Can)** *see* IDArubicin *on page 1067*

◆ **IDEC-C2B8** *see* RiTUXimab *on page 1841*

◆ **IDR** *see* IDArubicin *on page 1067*

◆ **IDV** *see* Indinavir *on page 1093*

◆ **iFerex 150 [OTC]** *see* Polysaccharide-Iron Complex *on page 1701*

◆ **Ifex** *see* Ifosfamide *on page 1068*

Ifosfamide (eye FOSS fa mide)

Medication Safety Issues

Sound-alike/look-alike issues:

Ifosfamide may be confused with cyclophosphamide

High alert medication:

This medication is in a class the Institute for Safe Medication Practices (ISMP) includes its list of drug classes which have a heightened risk of causing significant patient harm when used in error.

Related Information

Emetogenic Potential of Antineoplastic Agents in Children *on page 2327*

Management of Drug Extravasations *on page 2255*

Safe Handling of Hazardous Drugs *on page 2419*

Brand Names: U.S. Ifex

Brand Names: Canada Ifex

Therapeutic Category Antineoplastic Agent, Alkylating Agent

Generic Availability (U.S.) Yes

Use Treatment of germ cell testicular cancer in combination with other antineoplastic agents (FDA approved in adults); **Note:** Should be used in combination with mesna for prophylaxis of hemorrhagic cystitis; has also been used in the treatment of Hodgkin and non-Hodgkin's lymphoma, Ewing sarcoma, osteosarcoma, and soft tissue sarcomas

Pregnancy Risk Factor D

Pregnancy Considerations Embryotoxic and teratogenic effects have been observed in animal reproduction studies. Fetal growth retardation and neonatal anemia have been reported with exposure to ifosfamide-containing regimens during human pregnancy. Male and female fertility may be affected (dose and duration dependent). Ifosfamide interferes with oogenesis and spermatogenesis; amenorrhea, azoospermia, and sterility have been reported and may be irreversible. Avoid pregnancy during treatment; male patients should not father a child for at least 6 months after completion of therapy.

Breast-Feeding Considerations Breast-feeding should be avoided during ifosfamide treatment. According to the manufacturer, the decision to discontinue ifosfamide or discontinue breast-feeding should take into account the risk of exposure to the infant and the benefits of treatment to the mother.

Contraindications Hypersensitivity to ifosfamide or any component; urinary outflow obstruction

Warnings Hazardous agent; use appropriate precautions for handling and disposal (NIOSH, 2012). Severe bone marrow suppression may occur (dose-limiting toxicity) and lead to fatal infections **[U.S. Boxed Warning]**; monitor blood counts before and after each cycle; leukopenia, neutropenia, thrombocytopenia, and anemia are associated with ifosfamide; myelosuppression is dose dependent, increased with single high doses (compared to fractionated doses) and increased withrenal dysfunction. Severe myelosuppression may occur when administered in combination with other chemotherapy agents or radiation therapy. Use with caution in patients with compromised bone marrow reserve; unless clinically necessary, avoid administering to patients with WBC <2000/mm³ and platelets <50,000/mm³. Antimicrobial prophylaxis may be necessary in some neutropenic patients; administer antibiotics and/or antifungal agents for neutropenic fever. May cause significant suppression of the immune responses; may lead to serious infection, sepsis or septic shock; reported infections have included bacterial, viral, fungal, and parasitic; latent infections may be reactivated. Use with caution with other immunosuppressants or in patients with infection.

Ifosfamide may cause CNS toxicity which may be severe, resulting in encephalopathy and death **[U.S. Boxed Warning]**; monitor for CNS toxicity; discontinue for encephalopathy. Symptoms of CNS toxicity may include somnolence, confusion, dizziness, disorientation, hallucinations, cranial nerve dysfunction, blurred vision, psychotic behavior, extrapyramidal symptoms, incontinence, seizures, and/or coma and have been observed within a few hours to a few days after initial dose, and generally resolves within 2-3 days of treatment discontinuation (although may persist longer); maintain supportive care until complete resolution. Risk factors may include hypoalbuminemia, renal dysfunction, and prior history of ifosfamide-induced encephalopathy. Concomitant centrally acting medications may result in additive CNS effects. CNS effects may impair physical or mental abilities; patients must be cautioned about performing tasks which require mental alertness (eg, operating machinery or driving). Peripheral neuropathy has been reported.

Hemorrhagic cystitis may occur **[U.S. Boxed Warning]**; concomitant mesna reduces the risk of hemorrhagic cystitis. Hydration (at least 2 L/day in adults), dose fractionation, and/or mesna administration will reduce the incidence of hematuria and protect against hemorrhagic cystitis. Obtain urinalysis prior to each dose; if microscopic hematuria is detected, withhold until complete resolution. Exclude or correct urinary tract obstructions prior to treatment. Use with caution (if at all) in patients with active urinary tract infection, Hemorrhagic cystitis is dose-dependent and is increased with high single doses (compared with fractionated doses); past or concomitant bladder radiation or busulfan treatment may increase the risk for hemorrhagic cystitis. Ifosfamide may cause severe nephrotoxicity, resulting in renal failure **[U.S. Boxed Warning]**; acute and chronic renal failure, as well as renal parenchymal and tubular necrosis (including acute), have been reported; tubular damage may be delayed and may persist. Renal manifestations include decreased glomerular rate, increased creatinine, proteinuria, enzymuria, cylindruria, aminoaciduria, phosphaturia, and glycosuria. Syndrome of inappropriate antidiuretic hormone (SIADH), renal rickets, and Fanconi syndrome have been reported. Evaluate renal function prior to and during treatment; monitor urine for erythrocytes and signs of urotoxicity.

Cardiotoxicity, possibly fatal, has been reported with ifosfamide use; manifestations include arrhythmias, ST-segment or T-wave changes, cardiomyopathy, pericardial effusion, pericarditis, and epicardial fibrosis. The risk for cardiotoxicity is dose-dependent; concomitant cardiotoxic agents (eg, anthracyclines), irradiation of the cardiac region, and renal impairment may also increase the risk.

Interstitial pneumonitis, pulmonary fibrosis, and pulmonary toxicity leading to respiratory failure have been reported; monitor for signs and symptoms of pulmonary toxicity. Hepatic sinusoidal obstruction syndrome (SOS), formerly called veno-occlusive disease (VOD), has been reported with ifosfamide-containing regimens. Secondary malignancies may occur; the risk for myelodysplastic syndrome (which may progress to acute leukemia) is increased with treatment. Ifosfamide can cause fetal harm; advise women of childbearing potential to avoid becoming pregnant and men to avoid fathering a child for 6 months post-treatment. Anaphylactic/anaphylactoid reactions have been associated with ifosfamide; cross-sensitivity with similar agents may occur.

Precautions Use with caution in patients with impaired renal function, bone marrow suppression, and prior radiation therapy; risk increased for toxicity development. Ifosfamide may interfere with wound healing.

Adverse Reactions

Central nervous system: CNS toxicity or encephalopathy, fever

Dermatologic: Alopecia

Endocrine & metabolic: Metabolic acidosis

Gastrointestinal: Anorexia, nausea/vomiting

Hematologic: Anemia, leukopenia, neutropenic fever, thrombocytopenia

Hepatic: Bilirubin increased, liver dysfunction, transaminases increased

Local: Phlebitis

Renal: Hematuria (reduced with mesna), renal impairment

Miscellaneous: Infection

Rare but important or life-threatening: Acute respiratory distress syndrome, acute tubular necrosis, agranulocytosis, alkaline phosphatase increased, allergic reaction, alveolitis (allergic), amenorrhea, aminoaciduria, amnesia, anaphylactic reaction, angina, angioedema, anuria, arrhythmia, arthralgia, asterixis, atrial ectopy, atrial fibrillation/flutter, azoospermia, bladder irritation, bleeding, blurred vision, bone marrow failure, bradycardia, bradyphrenia, bronchospasm, bundle branch block, BUN increased, capillary leak syndrome, cardiac arrest, cardiogenic shock, cardiomyopathy, cardiotoxicity, catatonia, cecitis, chest pain, cholestasis, coagulopathy, colitis, conjunctivitis, creatinine clearance decreased/increased, creatinine increased, cylindruria, cytolytic hepatitis, delirium, delusion, dermatitis, diarrhea, DIC, DVT, dysesthesia, dyspnea, dysuria, echolalia, edema, ejection fraction decreased, enterocolitis, enuresis, enzymuria, erythema, extrapyramidal disorder, facial swelling, Fanconi syndrome, fatigue, gait disturbance, GGT increased, GI hemorrhage, glycosuria, gonadotropin increased, granulocytopenia, growth retardation (children), hemolytic anemia, hemolytic uremic syndrome, hemorrhagic cystitis, hepatic failure, hepatic sinusoidal obstruction syndrome (SOS; formerly veno-occlusive disease [VOD]), hepatitis fulminant, hepatitis (viral), hepatorenal syndrome, herpes zoster, hyperglycemia, hyper-/hypotension, hypersensitivity reactions, hypocalcemia, hypokalemia, hyponatremia, hypophosphatemia, hypoxia, ileus, immunosuppression, infertility, infusion site reactions (erythema, inflammation, pain, pruritus, swelling, tenderness), interstitial lung disease, jaundice, LDH increased, leukoencephalopathy, lymphopenia, malaise, mania, mental status change, methemoglobinemia, MI, mucosal inflammation/ulceration, multiorgan failure, mutism, myocardial hemorrhage, myocarditis, nephrogenic diabetes insipidus, neuralgia, neutropenia, oligospermia, oliguria, osteomalacia (adults), ovarian failure, ovulation disorder, palmar-plantar erythrodysesthesia syndrome, pancreatitis, pancytopenia, panic attack, paranoia, paresthesia, pericardial effusion, pericarditis, peripheral neuropathy, petechiae, phosphaturia, pleural effusion, *Pneumocystis jiroveci* pneumonia, pneumonia, pneumonitis, pollakiuria, polydipsia, polyneuropathy, polyuria, portal vein thrombosis, premature atrial contractions, premature menopause, progressive multifocal leukoencephalopathy, proteinuria, pruritus, pulmonary edema, pulmonary embolism, pulmonary fibrosis, pulmonary hypertension, QRS complex abnormal, radiation recall dermatitis, rash (including macular and papular), renal failure, renal parenchymal damage, renal tubular acidosis, respiratory failure, reversible posterior leukoencephalopathy syndrome (RPLS), rhabdomyolysis, rickets, salivation, secondary malignancy, seizure, sepsis, septic shock, SIADH, skin necrosis, spermatogenesis impaired, status epilepticus, sterility, Stevens-Johnson syndrome, stomatitis, ST segment abnormal, supraventricular extrasystoles, tachycardia, tinnitus, toxic epidermal necrolysis, tubulointerstitial nephritis, tumor lysis syndrome, T-wave inversion, uremia, urticaria, vasculitis, ventricular extrasystoles/fibrillation/tachycardia, ventricular failure, vertigo, visual impairment, wound healing impairment

Drug Interactions
Metabolism/Transport Effects **Substrate** of CYP2A6 (major), CYP2B6 (minor), CYP2C19 (major), CYP2C8 (minor), CYP2C9 (minor), CYP3A4 (minor); **Note:** Assignment of Major/Minor substrate status based on clinically relevant drug interaction potential; **Inhibits** CYP3A4 (weak); **Induces** CYP2C9 (weak/moderate)

Avoid Concomitant Use
Avoid concomitant use of Ifosfamide with any of the following: BCG; CloZAPine; Dipyrone; Natalizumab; Pimecrolimus; Pimozide; Tacrolimus (Topical); Tofacitinib; Vaccines (Live)

Increased Effect/Toxicity
Ifosfamide may increase the levels/effects of: ARIPiprazole; CloZAPine; Dofetilide; Leflunomide; Lomitapide; Natalizumab; Pimozide; Tofacitinib; Vaccines (Live); Vitamin K Antagonists

The levels/effects of Ifosfamide may be increased by: Busulfan; CYP2A6 Inhibitors (Moderate); CYP2A6 Inhibitors (Strong); CYP2C19 Inhibitors (Moderate); CYP2C19 Inhibitors (Strong); CYP3A4 Inducers (Strong); Denosumab; Dipyrone; Luliconazole; Pimecrolimus; Roflumilast; Tacrolimus (Topical); Trastuzumab

Decreased Effect
Ifosfamide may decrease the levels/effects of: BCG; Coccidioidin Skin Test; Sipuleucel-T; Vaccines (Inactivated); Vaccines (Live)

The levels/effects of Ifosfamide may be decreased by: CYP2A6 Inducers (Strong); CYP2C19 Inducers (Strong); CYP3A4 Inhibitors (Moderate); CYP3A4 Inhibitors (Strong); Dabrafenib; Echinacea

Stability Hazardous agent; use appropriate precautions for handling and disposal (NIOSH, 2012).
Powder for injection: Store intact vials at 20°C to 25°C (68°F to 77°F); avoid temperatures >30°C (86°F). Reconstituted solutions and diluted solutions for administration may be stored for 24 hours under refrigeration.
Solution for injection: Store intact vials at 2°C to 8°C (36°F to 46°F). Solutions diluted for administration are stable for 24 hours under refrigeration.

Mechanism of Action Causes cross-linking of strands of DNA by binding with nucleic acids and other intracellular structures; inhibits protein synthesis and DNA synthesis

Pharmacokinetics (Adult data unless noted) **Note:** Pharmacokinetics are dose-dependent.
Distribution: Approximates total body water; unchanged ifosfamide penetrates CNS but not in therapeutic concentrations
Protein binding: Negligble
Metabolism: Hepatic to active metabolites isofosforamide mustard, 4-hydroxy-ifosfamide, acrolein, and inactive dichloroethylated and carboxy metabolites; acrolein is

the agent implicated in development of hemorrhagic cystitis
Half-life: Terminal:
Low dose (1600-2400 mg/m^2): ~7 hours
High dose (3800-5000 mg/m^2): ~15 hours
Elimination:
Low dose (1600-2400 mg/m^2): Urine (12% to 18% as unchanged drug)
High dose (5000 mg/m^2): Urine (70% to 86%; 61% as unchanged drug)

Dosing: Usual Refer to individual protocols; details concerning dosing in combination regimens should also be consulted. **Note:** To prevent bladder toxicity, combination therapy with mesna (urinary protectant) and hydration, in adults: At least 2 L/day of oral or I.V. fluid; specific protocols should be consulted for hydration recommendation in pediatric patients; some centers have used 2 times maintenance.

Infants, Children, and Adolescents:
Ewing sarcoma: Limited data available; dosing regimens and combinations variable: Children and Adolescents: I.V.:
IE regimen: 1800 mg/m^2/day for 5 days in combination with mesna and etoposide every 3 weeks for 12 cycles; or may alternate with VAC (vincristine, doxorubicin, and cyclophosphamide) every 3 weeks for a total of 17 courses (Grier, 2003; Miser, 1987)
ICE regimen: 1800 mg/m^2/day for 5 days every 3-4 weeks for up to 12 cycles in combination with carboplatin, etoposide, and mesna; or may follow with 2 courses of CAV (cyclophosphamide, doxorubicin, and vincristine) (Milano, 2006; van Winkle, 2005)
VAIA regimen: 3000 mg/m^2/day on days 1, 2, 22, 23, 43, and 44 for 4 courses in combination with vincristine, doxorubicin, dactinomycin, and mesna (Paulussen, 2001) **or** 2000 mg/m^2/day for 3 days every 3 weeks for 14 courses in combination with vincristine, doxorubicin and dactinomycin (Paulussen, 2008)
VIDE regimen: 3000 mg/m^2/day over 1-3 hours for 3 days every 3 weeks for 6 courses in combination with vincristine, doxorubicin, etoposide, and mesna (Juergens, 2006)

Lymphoma, Hodgkin (HL) and Non-Hodgkin's (NHL), recurrent/refractory: Limited data available; dosing regimens and combinations variable: I.V.:
IE regimen: 1800 mg/m^2/day for 5 days alternating in combination with etoposide and mesna; alternate at 3-week intervals with DECAL [dexamethasone, etoposide, cisplatin, cytarabine (high-dose ara-C)], and L-asparaginase for 4 cycles (Kobrinsky, 2001)
ICE regimen: 1800 mg/m^2/day for 5 days every 3 weeks for 6 courses in combination with etoposide, carboplatin, and mesna (Cairo, 2004)
MIED regimen: 2000 mg/m^2/day over 2 hours on days 2-4 in combination with high dose methotrexate, etoposide and dexamethasone (and mesna); patients with NHL also received intrathecal methotrexate, hydrocortisone, and cytarabine (Sandlund, 2011)
Griffin, 2009: 3000 mg/m^2/day over 2 hours on days 3-5 in combination with rituximab and ICE (carboplatin, etoposide, and mensa) every 23 days for up to 3 courses has been used in NHL patients

Osteosarcoma: Limited data available; dosing regimens and combinations variable: Children and Adolescents: I.V.:
IE regimen: 3000 mg/m^2/day over 3 hours for 4 days every 3-4 weeks in combination with etoposide and mesna has been used in children and adolescents 7-19 years of age (Gentet, 1997)
ICE regimen: 1800 mg/m^2/day for 5 days every 3 weeks for up to 12 cycles in combination with carboplatin, etoposide, and mesna (van Winkle, 2005)

Bacci, 2003: 3000 mg/m²/day continuous infusion for 5 days (total dose: 15 g/m²) during weeks 4 and 10 (preop) and during weeks 16, 25, and 34 (postop) in combination with cisplatin, doxorubicin, methotrexate (high-dose), and mesna has been used in patients 6-39 years (median: 18.1 years) with newly diagnosed high-grade osteosarcoma of the extremity with metastases

Basaran, 2007: Adolescents: 2000 mg/m²/day over 4 hours for 3 days (days 2, 3, and 4) every 3 weeks for 3 cycles (preop) and every 4 weeks for 3 cycles (postop) in combination with cisplatin, epirubicin, and mesna has been used in patients 15-41 years (median: 22 years) (Basaran, 2007)

Le Deley, 2007: 3000 mg/m²/day over 4 hours for 4 days during weeks 4 and 9 (three additional postop courses were administered in good responders) in combination with methotrexate (high-dose), etoposide, and mesna has been used in patients 5-19 years (median: 13.3 years) (Le Deley, 2007)

Adults: **Testicular cancer:** I.V.: 1200 mg/m²/day for 5 days in combination with other chemotherapy agents and mesna every 3 weeks or after hematologic recovery

Dosage adjustments in renal impairment:
Infants, Children, and Adolescents: The following adjustments have been recommended (Aronoff, 2007):
GFR ≥10 mL/minute/1.73 m²: No dosage adjustment necessary
GFR <10 mL/minute/1.73 m²: Administer 75% of dose
Hemodialysis: 1 g/m² followed by hemodialysis 6-8 hours later
Continuous renal replacement therapy (CRRT): No dosage adjustment necessary
Adults: Manufacturer's labeling: There are no dosage adjustments provided in the manufacturer's labeling (has not been studied); ifosfamide (and metabolites) are excreted renally and may accumulate in patients with renal dysfunction. Dose reductions may be necessary.
The following adjustments have been recommended:
Aronoff, 2007:
CrCl ≥10 mL/minute: No dosage adjustment necessary
CrCl <10 mL/minute: Administer 75% of dose
Hemodialysis: No supplemental dose needed
Kintzel, 1995:
CrCl >60 mL/minute: No dosage adjustment necessary
CrCl 46-60 mL/minute: Administer 80% of dose
CrCl 31-45 mL/minute: Administer 75% of dose
CrCl ≤30 mL/minute: Administer 70% of dose

Dosage adjustments in hepatic impairment: Adults: There are no dosage adjustments provided in the manufacturer's labeling; however, ifosfamide is extensively metabolized in the liver to both active and inactive metabolites; use with caution. The following adjustments have been recommended (Floyd, 2006): Bilirubin >3 mg/dL: Administer 25% of dose.

Administration Hazardous agent; use appropriate precautions for handling and disposal (NIOSH, 2012)
I.V.: Reconstitute powder with SWI or bacteriostatic SWI to a concentration of 50 mg/mL. Further dilute with D₅W, NS, or lactated Ringer's to a final concentration not to exceed 80 mg/mL (manufacturer recommends 0.6-20 mg/mL). Administer as a slow I.V. intermittent infusion or continuous infusion; infusion times may vary by protocol; usually over at least 30 minutes; in most pediatric trials, usual infusion time was 2 hours or administer as a 24-hour infusion

Vesicant/Extravasation Risk May be an irritant

Monitoring Parameters CBC with differential (prior to each dose), urine output, urinalysis (prior to each dose), liver and renal function tests, serum electrolytes, CNS changes, signs and symptoms of pulmonary toxicity, signs and symptoms of hemorrhagic cystitis

Dosage Forms Excipient information presented when available (limited, particularly for generics); consult specific product labeling.
Kit, Intravenous:
Generic: 1-1 GM
Solution, Intravenous:
Generic: 1 g/20 mL (20 mL); 3 g/60 mL (60 mL)
Solution, Intravenous [preservative free]:
Generic: 1 g/20 mL (20 mL); 3 g/60 mL (60 mL)
Solution Reconstituted, Intravenous:
Ifex: 1 g (1 ea); 3 g (1 ea)
Generic: 1 g (1 ea); 3 g (1 ea)

References
Aronoff GR, Bennett WM, Berns JS, et al, *Drug Prescribing in Renal Failure: Dosing Guidelines for Adults and Children*, 5th ed, Philadelphia, PA: American College of Physicians, 2007.
Bacci G, Briccoli A, Rocca M, et al, "Neoadjuvant Chemotherapy for Osteosarcoma of the Extremities With Metastases at Presentation: Recent Experience at the Rizzoli Institute in 57 Patients Treated With Cisplatin, Doxorubicin, and a High Dose of Methotrexate and Ifosfamide," *Ann Oncol*, 2003, 14(7):1126-34.
Basaran M, Bavbek ES, Saglam S, et al, "A Phase II Study of Cisplatin, Ifosfamide and Epirubicin Combination Chemotherapy in Adults With Nonmetastatic and Extremity Osteosarcomas," *Oncology*, 2007, 72 (3-4):255-60.
Cairo MS, Davenport V, Bessmertny O, et al, "Phase I/II Dose Escalation Study of Recombinant Human Interleukin-11 Following Ifosfamide, Carboplatin and Etoposide in Children, Adolescents and Young Adults With Solid Tumours or Lymphoma: A Clinical, Haematological and Biological Study," *Br J Haematol*, 2005, 128(1):49-58.
Floyd J, Mirza I, Sachs B, et al, "Hepatotoxicity of Chemotherapy," *Semin Oncol*, 2006, 33(1):50-67.
Gentet JC, Brunat-Mentigny M, Demaille MC, et al, "Ifosfamide and Etoposide in Childhood Osteosarcoma. A Phase II Study of the French Society of Paediatric Oncology," *Eur J Cancer*, 1997, 33 (2):232-7.
Grier HE, Krailo MD, Tarbell NJ, et al, "Addition of Ifosfamide and Etoposide to Standard Chemotherapy for Ewing's Sarcoma and Primitive Neuroectodermal Tumor of Bone," *N Engl J Med*, 2003, 348(8):694-701.
Griffin TC, Weitzman S, Weinstein H, et al, "A Study of Rituximab and Ifosfamide, Carboplatin, and Etoposide Chemotherapy in Children With Recurrent/Refractory B-Cell (CD20+) Non-Hodgkin Lymphoma and Mature B-Cell Acute Lymphoblastic Leukemia: A Report From the Children's Oncology Group," *Pediatr Blood Cancer*, 2009, 52 (2):177-81.
Juergens C, Weston C, Lewis I, et al, "Safety Assessment of Intensive Induction With Vincristine, Ifosfamide, Doxorubicin, and Etoposide (VIDE) in the Treatment of Ewing Tumors in the EURO-E.W.I.N.G. 99 Clinical Trial," *Pediatr Blood Cancer*, 2006, 47(1):22-9.
Kintzel PE and Dorr RT, "Anticancer Drug Renal Toxicity and Elimination: Dosing Guidelines for Altered Renal Function," *Cancer Treat Rev*, 1995, 21(1):33-64.
Kobrinsky NL, Sposto R, Shah NR, et al, "Outcomes of Treatment of Children and Adolescents With Recurrent Non-Hodgkin's Lymphoma and Hodgkin's Disease With Dexamethasone, Etoposide, Cisplatin, Cytarabine, and l-Asparaginase, Maintenance Chemotherapy, and Transplantation: Children's Cancer Group Study CCG-5912," *J Clin Oncol*, 2001, 19(9):2390-6.
Le Deley MC, Guinebretière JM, Gentet JC, et al, "SFOP OS94: A Randomised Trial Comparing Preoperative High-Dose Methotrexate Plus Doxorubicin to High-Dose Methotrexate Plus Etoposide and Ifosfamide in Osteosarcoma Patients," *Eur J Cancer*, 2007, 43 (4):752-61.
Milano GM, Cozza R, Ilari I, et al, "High Histologic and Overall Response to Dose Intensification of Ifosfamide, Carboplatin, and Etoposide With Cyclophosphamide, Doxorubicin, and Vincristine in Patients With High-Risk Ewing Sarcoma Family Tumors: The Bambino Gesù Children's Hospital Experience," *Cancer*, 2006, 106 (8):1838-45.
Miser JS, Kinsella TJ, Triche TJ, et al, "Ifosfamide With Mesna Uroprotection and Etoposide: An Effective Regimen in the Treatment of Recurrent Sarcomas and Other Tumors of Children and Young Adults," *J Clin Oncol*, 1987, 5(8):1191-8.
National Institute for Occupational Safety and Health (NIOSH), "NIOSH List of Antineoplastic and Other Hazardous Drugs in Healthcare Settings 2012." Available at http://www.cdc.gov/niosh/docs/2012-150/pdfs/2012-150.pdf. Accessed January 21, 2013.
Oberlin O, Fawaz O, Rey A, et al, "Long-Term Evaluation of Ifosfamide-Related Nephrotoxicity in Children," *J Clin Oncol*, 2009, 27 (32):5350-5.

Paulussen M, Ahrens S, Dunst J, et al, "Localized Ewing Tumor of Bone: Final Results of the Cooperative Ewing's Sarcoma Study CESS 86," *J Clin Oncol*, 2001, 19(6):1818-29.

Paulussen M, Craft AW, Lewis I, et al, "Results of the EICESS-92 Study: Two Randomized Trials of Ewing's Sarcoma Treatment - Cyclophosphamide Compared With Ifosfamide in Standard-Risk Patients and Assessment of Benefit of Etoposide Added to Standard Treatment in High-Risk Patients," *J Clin Oncol*, 2008, 26(27):4385-93.

Sandlund JT, Pui CH, Mahmoud H, et al, "Efficacy of High-Dose Methotrexate, Ifosfamide, Etoposide and Dexamethasone Salvage Therapy for Recurrent or Refractory Childhood Malignant Lymphoma," *Ann Oncol*, 2011, 22(2):468-71.

Van Winkle P, Angiolillo A, Krailo M, et al, "Ifosfamide, Carboplatin, and Etoposide (ICE) Reinduction Chemotherapy in a Large Cohort of Children and Adolescents With Recurrent/Refractory Sarcoma: The Children's Cancer Group (CCG) Experience," *Pediatr Blood Cancer*, 2005, 44(4):338-47.

◆ **IG** *see* Immune Globulin *on page 1084*

◆ **IGIM** *see* Immune Globulin *on page 1084*

◆ **IGIV** *see* Immune Globulin *on page 1084*

◆ **IGIVnex (Can)** *see* Immune Globulin *on page 1084*

◆ **IGSC** *see* Immune Globulin *on page 1084*

◆ **IIV** *see* Influenza Virus Vaccine (Inactivated) *on page 1103*

◆ **IIV3** *see* Influenza Virus Vaccine (Inactivated) *on page 1103*

◆ **IIV4** *see* Influenza Virus Vaccine (Inactivated) *on page 1103*

◆ **IL-1Ra** *see* Anakinra *on page 168*

◆ **IL-2** *see* Aldesleukin *on page 90*

◆ **IL-11** *see* Oprelvekin *on page 1549*

◆ **Ilaris** *see* Canakinumab *on page 361*

◆ **Ilotycin** *see* Erythromycin (Ophthalmic) *on page 784*

Imatinib (eye MAT eh nib)

Medication Safety Issues
Sound-alike/look-alike issues:
Imatinib may be confused with axitinib, dasatinib, erlotinib, gefitinib, ibrutinib, nilotinib, PONATinib, SORAfenib, SUNItinib, vandetanib

High alert medication:
This medication is in a class the Institute for Safe Medication Practices (ISMP) includes among its list of drug classes which have a heightened risk of causing significant patient harm when used in error.

Related Information
Emetogenic Potential of Antineoplastic Agents in Children *on page 2327*
Oral Medications That Should Not Be Crushed or Altered *on page 2438*
Safe Handling of Hazardous Drugs *on page 2419*

Brand Names: U.S. Gleevec

Brand Names: Canada Apo-Imatinib; Gleevec; Teva-Imatinib

Therapeutic Category Antineoplastic Agent, BCR-ABL Tyrosine Kinase Inhibitor; Antineoplastic Agent, Tyrosine Kinase Inhibitor

Generic Availability (U.S.) No

Use
Treatment of newly diagnosed Philadelphia chromosome-positive (Ph+) acute lymphoblastic leukemia (ALL) in combination with chemotherapy (FDA approved in ages ≥1 year); treatment of newly diagnosed Ph+ chronic myeloid leukemia (CML) in chronic phase (FDA approved in ages ≥1 year and adults)

Treatment of (the following indications: FDA approved in adults): Ph+ acute lymphoblastic leukemia (ALL) (relapsed or refractory), gastrointestinal stromal tumors (GIST) kit-positive (CD117), including unresectable and/or metastatic malignant and adjuvant treatment following complete resection, aggressive systemic mastocytosis (ASM) without D816V c-Kit mutation (or c-Kit mutation status unknown), dermatofibrosarcoma protuberans (DFSP) (unresectable, recurrent, and/or metastatic), hypereosinophilic syndrome (HES) and/or chronic eosinophilic leukemia (CEL), myelodysplastic/myeloproliferative disease (MDS/MPD) associated with platelet-derived growth factor receptor (PDGFR) gene rearrangements

Has also been used in the treatment of desmoid tumors (soft tissue sarcoma); poststem cell transplant (allogeneic) follow-up treatment in CML

Pregnancy Risk Factor D

Pregnancy Considerations Animal reproduction studies have demonstrated teratogenic effects and fetal loss. Women of childbearing potential are advised not to become pregnant (female patients and female partners of male patients); highly effective contraception is recommended. Case reports of pregnancies while on therapy (both males and females) include reports of spontaneous abortion, minor abnormalities (hypospadias, pyloric stenosis, and small intestine rotation) at or shortly after birth, and other congenital abnormalities including skeletal malformations, hypoplastic lungs, exomphalos, kidney abnormalities, hydrocephalus, cerebellar hypoplasia, and cardiac defects.

Retrospective case reports of women with CML in complete hematologic response (CHR) with cytogenic response (partial or complete) who interrupted imatinib therapy due to pregnancy, demonstrated a loss of response in some patients while off treatment. At 18 months after treatment reinitiation following delivery, CHR was again achieved in all patients and cytogenic response was achieved in some patients. Cytogenetic response rates may not be at as high as compared to patients with 18 months of uninterrupted therapy (Ault, 2006; Pye, 2008).

Breast-Feeding Considerations Imatinib and its active metabolite are found in human breast milk; the milk/plasma ratio is 0.5 for imatinib and 0.9 for the active metabolite. Based on body weight, up to 10% of a therapeutic maternal dose could potentially be received by a breastfed infant, the decision to discontinue breast-feeding during therapy or to discontinue imatinib should take into account the benefits of treatment to the mother.

Contraindications Hypersensitivity to imatinib or any component

Warnings Hazardous agent; use appropriate precautions for handling and disposal (NIOSH, 2012).

May cause fluid retention, weight gain, and edema which may lead to significant complications, including pleural effusion, pericardial effusion, pulmonary edema, and ascites; risk increases with higher doses and age >65 years. Use with caution in patients where fluid accumulation may be poorly tolerated, such as cardiovascular disease (HF or hypertension) and pulmonary disease; monitor regularly for rapid weight gain or other signs/symptoms of fluid retention. Severe HF and left ventricular dysfunction (LVD) have been reported (rare), usually in patients with comorbidities and/or risk factors. Carefully monitor patients with preexisting cardiac disease or risk factors for heart failure or history of renal failure. With initiation of imatinib treatment, cardiogenic shock and/or LVD have been reported in patients with hypereosinophilic syndrome and cardiac involvement (reversible with systemic steroids, circulatory support, and temporary cessation of imatinib). Patients with high eosinophil levels and an abnormal echocardiogram or abnormal serum troponin level may benefit from prophylactic systemic steroids with the initiation of imatinib.

Severe bullous dermatologic reactions including erythema multiforme and Stevens-Johnson syndrome have been reported; recurrence has been described with rechallenge. Successful resumption at a lower dose with concomitant corticosteroids and/or antihistamine has been described; however, some patients may experience recurrent reactions.

Hepatotoxicity may occur; fatal hepatic failure and severe hepatic injury requiring liver transplantation have been reported with both short- and long-term use; monitor liver function prior to initiation and monthly or as needed thereafter; therapy interruption or dose reduction may be necessary. Transaminase and bilirubin elevations, and acute liver failure have been observed with imatinib in combination with chemotherapy.

May cause bone marrow suppression (anemia, neutropenia, and thrombocytopenia), usually occurring within the first several months of treatment. Median duration of neutropenia is 2-3 weeks; median duration of thrombocytopenia is 3-4 weeks. Monitor blood counts weekly for the first month, biweekly for the second month, and as clinically necessary thereafter. In CML, cytopenias are more common in accelerated or blast phase than in chronic phase. Severe hemorrhage (grades 3 and 4) has been reported with use, including gastrointestinal hemorrhage and/or tumor hemorrhage. The incidence of hemorrhage is higher in patients with GIST (gastrointestinal tumors may have been hemorrhage source); monitor for symptoms with treatment initiation. Opportunistic infections may be associated with use.

Tumor lysis syndrome (TLS), including fatalities, has been reported in patients with ALL, CML eosinophilic leukemias, and GIST. Risk for TLS is higher in patients with a high tumor burden or high proliferation rate; monitor closely. Correct clinically significant dehydration and treat high uric acid levels prior to initiation of imatinib.

Precautions Use with caution in hepatic and/or renal impairment; may require dosage adjustment. Use caution in thyroidectomy patients; hypothyroidism has been reported in thyroidectomy patients who were receiving thyroid hormone replacement therapy prior to initiation of imatinib; monitor thyroid function; the average onset for imatinib-induced hypothyroidism is 2 weeks; consider doubling levothyroxine doses upon initiation of imatinib (Hamnvik, 2011).

May cause GI irritation; take with food and water to minimize irritation; there have been rare reports (including fatalities) of GI perforation. Use with caution in patients who have had gastric surgery (eg, bypass, major gastrectomy, or resection); imatinib exposure may be reduced; monitor imatinib serum trough concentrations (Liu, 2011; Pavlovsky, 2009; Yoo, 2010).

Growth retardation has been reported in prepubescent children receiving imatinib for the treatment of CML (Bansal, 2012; Rastogi, 2012; Shima, 2011); the majority of the preliminary data reported statistically significant decreases in height-SD (standard deviation) scores; less commonly reported are decreases in weight-SD scores or decreased BMI; incidence and extent of growth retardation as well as other related risk factors have not been fully characterized; reported incidence from reports is highly variable (48% to 71%), with onset during the first year of therapy and persisting with treatment. One report suggests that growth velocity was restored as pubertal age was reached; however, in other reports, patients did not have improvement in height velocity and genetically predicted adult heights were not achieved. Monitor growth closely.

Potentially significant drug interactions may exist, requiring dose or frequency adjustment, additional monitoring, and/ or selection of alternative therapy. Consult drug interactions database for more detailed information. Caution is recommended while driving or operating motor vehicles and heavy machinery when taking imatinib; advise patients regarding side effects such as dizziness, blurred vision, or somnolence; reports of accidents have been received, but it is unclear if imatinib has been the direct cause in any case.

Adverse Reactions

Cardiovascular: Chest pain; edema/fluid retention (includes aggravated edema, anasarca, ascites, palpitation, pericardial effusion, peripheral edema, pulmonary edema, and superficial edema); facial edema, flushing, hypotension (children and adolescents), pleural effusion (children and adolescents)

Central nervous system: Anxiety, chills, CNS/cerebral hemorrhage, depression, dizziness, fatigue, fever, headache, hypoesthesia, insomnia, pain

Dermatologic: Alopecia, dermatitis, dry skin, erythema, photosensitivity reaction, pruritus, rash

Endocrine & metabolic: Albumin decreased, hyperglycemia, hypocalcemia, hypokalemia (more common in children and adolescents), hypoproteinemia, LDH increased

Gastrointestinal: Abdominal distension, abdominal pain, anorexia, appetite decreased, constipation, diarrhea, dyspepsia, flatulence, gastritis, gastroesophageal reflux, gastrointestinal hemorrhage, nausea, stomatitis/mucositis, taste disturbance, vomiting, weight gain/loss, xerostomia

Hematologic: Anemia, hemorrhage, leukopenia, lymphopenia, neutropenia, neutropenic fever, pancytopenia, thrombocytopenia

Hepatic: Alkaline phosphatase increased, ALT increased, AST increased, bilirubin increased, transaminases increased (children and adolescents)

Neuromuscular & skeletal: Arthralgia, back pain, bone pain, joint swelling, limb pain, muscle cramps, musculoskeletal pain, myalgia, paresthesia, peripheral neuropathy, rigors, weakness

Ocular: Blurred vision, conjunctival hemorrhage, conjunctivitis, dry eyes, lacrimation increased, periorbital edema

Renal: Serum creatinine increased

Respiratory: Cough, dyspnea, epistaxis, hypoxia, nasopharyngitis, pharyngitis, pharyngolaryngeal pain, pneumonia, pneumonitis (children and adolescents), rhinitis, upper respiratory tract infection

Miscellaneous: Diaphoresis, flu-like syndrome, infection (more common in children and adolescents), night sweats

Rare but important or life-threatening: Acute febrile neutropenic dermatosis (Sweet's syndrome), anaphylactic shock, angina, angioedema, aplastic anemia, arrhythmia, arthritis, ascites, atrial fibrillation, avascular necrosis, bullous eruption, cardiac arrest, cardiac tamponade, cardiogenic shock, cataract, cellulitis, cerebral edema, diverticulitis, embolism, eosinophilia, erythema multiforme, exanthematous pustulosis (acute generalized), exfoliative dermatitis, fungal infection, gastric ulcer, gastrointestinal obstruction, gastrointestinal perforation, glaucoma, gout, growth retardation (children), hearing loss, heart failure (severe), hematoma, hematemesis, hematuria, hemolytic anemia, hemorrhagic corpus luteum, hemorrhagic ovarian cyst, hepatic failure, hepatic necrosis, hepatitis, hepatotoxicity, herpes simplex, herpes zoster, hip osteonecrosis, hypercalcemia, hyperkalemia, hyperuricemia, hypertension, hypomagnesemia, hyponatremia, hypophosphatemia, hypothyroidism, ileus, inflammatory bowel disease, interstitial lung disease, interstitial pneumonitis, intracranial pressure increased, left ventricular dysfunction, leukocytoclastic vasculitis, lichen planus, lichenoid keratosis, lymphadenopathy, macular edema, melena, memory impairment, menorrhagia, MI, migraine, myopathy, optic neuritis, ovarian cyst (hemorrhagic), palmar-plantar erythrodysesthesia syndrome, pancreatitis, papilledema, pericarditis, psoriasis, pulmonary fibrosis, pulmonary hemorrhage, pulmonary hypertension, Raynaud's phenomenon, renal failure, respiratory failure, respiratory tract (lower) infection, restless leg syndrome, retinal hemorrhage, rhabdomyolysis, sciatica, scleral hemorrhage, seizure, sepsis, skin pigment changes, Stevens-Johnson syndrome, subdural hematoma, syncope, tachycardia, thrombocythemia, thrombosis, toxic epidermal necrolysis, tumor hemorrhage (GIST), tumor lysis syndrome, tumor necrosis, urinary tract infection, vitreous hemorrhage

Drug Interactions

Metabolism/Transport Effects Substrate of CYP1A2 (minor), CYP2C19 (minor), CYP2C8 (minor), CYP2C9 (minor), CYP2D6 (minor), CYP3A4 (major), P-glycoprotein; **Note:** Assignment of Major/Minor substrate status based on clinically relevant drug interaction potential; **Inhibits** BCRP, CYP2C9 (weak), CYP2D6 (weak), CYP3A4 (moderate), P-glycoprotein

Avoid Concomitant Use

Avoid concomitant use of Imatinib with any of the following: BCG; Bosutinib; CloZAPine; Dipyrone; Ibrutinib; Ivabradine; Lomitapide; Natalizumab; PAZOPanib; Pimecrolimus; Pimozide; Simeprevir; Tacrolimus (Topical); Tofacitinib; Tolvaptan; Ulipristal; Vaccines (Live)

Increased Effect/Toxicity

Imatinib may increase the levels/effects of: ARIPiprazole; Avanafil; Bosentan; Bosutinib; Budesonide (Systemic, Oral Inhalation); Cannabis; CloZAPine; Colchicine; CycloSPORINE (Systemic); CYP3A4 Substrates; Dofetilide; DOXOrubicin (Conventional); Dronabinol; Eplerenone; Everolimus; FentaNYL; Halofantrine; Ibrutinib; Ivabradine; Ivacaftor; Leflunomide; Lomitapide; Lurasidone; Natalizumab; OxyCODONE; PAZOPanib; Pimozide; Propafenone; Ranolazine; Rivaroxaban; Salmeterol; Saxagliptin; Simeprevir; Simvastatin; Tetrahydrocannabinol; Tofacitinib; Tolvaptan; Topotecan; Ulipristal; Vaccines (Live); Vilazodone; Vitamin K Antagonists; Warfarin; Zuclopenthixol

The levels/effects of Imatinib may be increased by: Acetaminophen; CYP3A4 Inhibitors (Moderate); CYP3A4 Inhibitors (Strong); Denosumab; Dipyrone; Lansoprazole; P-glycoprotein/ABCB1 Inhibitors; Pimecrolimus; Roflumilast; Tacrolimus (Topical); Trastuzumab

Decreased Effect

Imatinib may decrease the levels/effects of: BCG; Cardiac Glycosides; Coccidioidin Skin Test; Fludarabine; Ifosfamide; Sipuleucel-T; Vaccines (Inactivated); Vaccines (Live); Vitamin K Antagonists

The levels/effects of Imatinib may be decreased by: Bosentan; CYP3A4 Inducers (Strong); Dabrafenib; Deferasirox; Echinacea; Gemfibrozil; Ibuprofen; Mitotane; Peginterferon Alfa-2b; P-glycoprotein/ABCB1 Inducers; Rifamycin Derivatives; Siltuximab; St Johns Wort; Tocilizumab

Food Interactions Food may reduce GI irritation. Grapefruit juice may increase imatinib plasma concentration. Management: Take with a meal and a large glass of water. Avoid grapefruit juice. Maintain adequate hydration, unless instructed to restrict fluid intake.

Stability Hazardous agent; use appropriate precautions for handling and disposal (NIOSH, 2012). Store at 25°C (77°F); excursions permitted to 15°C to 30°C (59°F to 86°F); protect from moisture.

Mechanism of Action Inhibits Bcr-Abl tyrosine kinase, the constitutive abnormal gene product of the Philadelphia chromosome in chronic myeloid leukemia (CML). Inhibition of this enzyme blocks proliferation and induces apoptosis in Bcr-Abl positive cell lines as well as in fresh leukemic cells in Philadelphia chromosome positive CML. Also inhibits tyrosine kinase for platelet-derived growth factor (PDGF), stem cell factor (SCF), c-Kit, and cellular events mediated by PDGF and SCF.

Pharmacokinetics (Adult data unless noted)

Absorption: Rapid

Protein binding: ~95% to albumin and alpha$_1$-acid glycoprotein (parent drug and metabolite)

Metabolism: Hepatic via CYP3A4 (minor metabolism via CYP1A2, CYP2D6, CYP2C9, CYP2C19); primary metabolite (active): N-demethylated piperazine derivative (CGP74588); severe hepatic impairment (bilirubin >3-10 times ULN) increases AUC by 45% to 55% for imatinib and its active metabolite, respectively

Bioavailability: 98%; may be decreased in patients who have had gastric surgery (eg, bypass, total or partial resection)

Half-life elimination:

Children: Parent drug: ~15 hours

Adults: Parent drug: ~18 hours; N-desmethyl metabolite: ~40 hours

Time to peak serum concentration: 2-4 hours (adults and children)

Elimination: Feces (68% primarily as metabolites, 20% as unchanged drug); urine (≤13% primarily as metabolites, 5% as unchanged drug)

Dosing: Usual Note: Treatment may be continued until disease progression or unacceptable toxicity. The optimal duration of therapy for CML in complete remission is not yet determined. Discontinuing CML treatment is not recommended unless part of a clinical trial (Baccarani, 2009; NCCN CML guidelines v.3.2013).

Children and Adolescents:

Ph+ ALL (newly diagnosed): Oral: 340 mg/m^2/day administered once daily; in combination with chemotherapy; maximum daily dose: 600 mg/**day**

Ph+ CML (chronic phase, newly diagnosed): Oral: 340 mg/m^2/day; may administer once daily or in 2 divided doses; maximum daily dose: 600 mg/**day**

Adults: **Note:** Doses ≤600 mg should be administered once daily; 800 mg doses should be administered as 400 mg/dose twice a day

ASM with eosinophilia: Oral: Initiate at 100 mg once daily; titrate up to a maximum of 400 mg once daily (if tolerated) for insufficient response to lower dose

ASM without D816V c-Kit mutation or c-Kit mutation status unknown: Oral: 400 mg once daily

GIST (adjuvant treatment following complete resection): Oral: 400 mg once daily; recommended treatment duration: 3 years

GIST (unresectable and/or metastatic malignant): Oral: 400 mg/day; may be increased up to 800 mg/day (400 mg/dose twice daily), if tolerated, for disease progression; **Note:** Significant improvement (progression-free survival, objective response rate) was demonstrated in patients with KIT exon 9 mutation with 800 mg (versus 400 mg), although overall survival (OS) was not impacted. The higher dose did not demonstrate a difference in time to progression or OS patients with Kit exon 11 mutation or wild-type status (Debiec-Rychter, 2006; Heinrich, 2008).

DFSP: Oral: 400 mg twice daily

HES/CEL: Oral: 400 mg once daily

HES/CEL with FIP1L1-PDGFRα fusion kinase: Oral: Initiate at 100 mg once daily; titrate up to a maximum of 400 mg once daily (if tolerated) if insufficient response to lower dose

MDS/MPD: Oral: 400 mg once daily

Ph+ ALL (relapsed or refractory): Oral: 600 mg once daily

Ph+ CML: Oral

Chronic phase: 400 mg once daily; may be increased to 600 mg daily, if tolerated, for disease progression, lack of hematologic response after 3 months, lack of cytogenetic response after 6-12 months, or loss of previous hematologic or cytogenetic response; ranges up to 800 mg/day (400 mg twice daily) are included in the NCCN CML guidelines (v.3.2013)

Accelerated phase or blast crisis: 600 mg once daily; may be increased to 800 mg daily (400 mg/dose twice daily), if tolerated, for disease progression, lack of hematologic response after 3 months, lack of cytogenetic response after 6-12 months, or loss of previous hematologic or cytogenetic response

Dosing adjustment with concomitant strong CYP3A4 inducers: Children, Adolescents, and Adults: Avoid concomitant use of strong CYP3A4 inducers (eg, dexamethasone, carbamazepine, phenobarbital, phenytoin, rifabutin, rifampin); if concomitant use cannot be avoided, increase imatinib dose by at least 50% with careful monitoring.

Dosing adjustment for renal impairment:

Mild impairment (CrCl 40-59 mL/minute): Adults: Maximum recommended dose: 600 mg/day

Moderate impairment (CrCl 20-39 mL/minute): Children, Adolescents, and Adults: Decrease recommended starting dose by 50%; dose may be increased as tolerated; maximum recommended dose: 400 mg/day

Severe impairment (CrCl <20 mL/minute): Use caution; in adults with severe impairment, a dose of 100 mg/day has been tolerated (Gibbons, 2008)

Dosing adjustment for hepatic impairment: Children, Adolescents, and Adults:

Baseline:

Mild to moderate impairment: No adjustment necessary

Severe impairment: Reduce dose by 25%

During therapy (hepatotoxicity): Withhold treatment until toxicity resolves; may resume if appropriate (depending on initial severity of adverse event)

If elevations of bilirubin >3 times ULN or liver transaminases >5 times ULN occur, withhold treatment until bilirubin <1.5 times ULN and transaminases <2.5 times ULN. Resume treatment at a reduced dose as follows:

Children, Adolescents, and Adults: If current dose 340 mg/m^2/day, reduce dose to 260 mg/m^2/day; maximum dose range: 300-400 mg

Adults:

If initial dose 400 mg, reduce dose to 300 mg

If initial dose 600 mg, reduce dose to 400 mg

If initial dose 800 mg, reduce dose to 600 mg

Dosing adjustment for other nonhematologic adverse reactions: Withhold treatment until toxicity resolves; may resume if appropriate (depending on initial severity of adverse event)

Dosing adjustment for hematologic adverse reactions:

Chronic phase CML (Initial dose: Children: 340 mg/m^2/ day or Adults: 400 mg/day), ASM, MDS/MPD, and HES/CEL (initial dose: 400 mg/day), or GIST (initial dose: 400 mg): If ANC <1 x 10^9/L and/or platelets <50 x 10^9/L: Withhold until ANC ≥1.5 x 10^9/L and platelets ≥75 x 10^9/L; resume treatment at previous dose. For recurrent neutropenia and/or thrombocytopenia, withhold until recovery and reinstitute treatment at a reduced dose as follows:

Children and Adolescents: If initial dose 340 mg/m^2/ day, reduce dose to 260 mg/m^2/day

Adults: If initial dose 400 mg/day, reduce dose to 300 mg/day

CML (accelerated phase or blast crisis) and PH+ ALL: Adults (initial dose: 600 mg): If ANC <0.5 x 10^9/L and/or platelets <10 x 10^9/L, establish whether cytopenia is related to leukemia (bone marrow aspirate or biopsy). If unrelated to leukemia, reduce dose to 400 mg/day. If cytopenia persists for an additional 2 weeks, further reduce dose to 300 mg/day. If cytopenia persists for 4 weeks and is still unrelated to leukemia, withhold treatment until ANC ≥1 x 10^9/L and platelets ≥20 x 10^9/L, then resume treatment at 300 mg/day.

ASM-associated with eosinophilia and HES/CEL with FIP1L1-PDGFRα fusion kinase (starting dose: 100 mg/day): Adults: If ANC <1 x 10^9/L and/or platelets <50 x 10^9/L: Withhold until ANC ≥1.5 x 10^9/L and platelets ≥75 x 10^9/L; resume treatment at previous dose.

DFSP (initial dose: 800 mg/day): Adults: If ANC <1 x 10^9/L and/or platelets <50 x 10^9/L, withhold until ANC ≥1.5 x 10^9/L and platelets ≥75 x 10^9/L; resume treatment at reduced dose of 600 mg/day. For recurrent neutropenia and/or thrombocytopenia, withhold until recovery and reinstitute treatment with a further dose reduction to 400 mg/day.

Administration Hazardous agent; use appropriate precautions for handling and disposal (NIOSH, 2012). Should be administered orally with a meal and a large glass of water. Do not crush tablets; tablets may be dispersed in water or apple juice (using ~50 mL for 100 mg tablet, ~200 mL for 400 mg tablet); stir until tablet dissolves and administer immediately. Dosing in children may be once or twice daily when treating CML and once daily for Ph+ ALL. In adults, doses ≤600 mg may be given once daily; 800 mg dose should be administered as 400 mg twice daily. For daily dosing ≥800 mg, the 400 mg tablets should be used to reduce iron exposure (tablets are coated with ferric oxide).

Monitoring Parameters CBC (weekly for first month, biweekly for second month, then periodically thereafter), liver function tests [at baseline and monthly or as clinically indicated; more frequently (at least weekly) in patients with moderate to severe hepatic impairment (Ramanathan, 2008)], renal function, serum electrolytes (including calcium, phosphorus, potassium, and sodium levels); bone marrow cytogenetics (in CML; at 6, 12, and 18 months); fatigue, weight, and edema/fluid status; consider echocardiogram and serum troponin levels in patients with HES/CEL, and in patients with MDS/MPD or ASM with high eosinophil levels; in pediatric patients, also monitor serum glucose, albumin, and growth parameters (height, weight, BMI)

Gastric surgery (eg, bypass, major gastrectomy, or resection) patients: Monitor imatinib trough concentrations (Liu, 2011; Pavlovsky, 2009, Yoo, 2010)

Thyroid function testing (Hamnvik, 2011):

preexisting levothyroxine therapy: Obtain baseline TSH levels, then monitor every 4 weeks until levels and levothyroxine dose are stable, then monitor every 2 months

Without preexisting thyroid hormone replacement: TSH at baseline, then every 4 weeks for 4 months, then every 2-3 months

Monitor for signs/symptoms of CHF in patients at risk for cardiac failure or patients with preexisting cardiac disease; some suggest a baseline evaluation of left ventricular ejection fraction prior to initiation of imatinib therapy in all patients with known underlying heart disease or in elderly patients. Monitor for signs/symptoms of gastrointestinal irritation or perforation and dermatologic toxicities.

Dosage Forms Excipient information presented when available (limited, particularly for generics); consult specific product labeling.

▶

Tablet, Oral:
  Gleevec: 100 mg, 400 mg [scored]
Extemporaneous Preparations Hazardous agent: Use appropriate precautions for handling and disposal.

An oral suspension may be prepared by placing tablets (whole, do not crush) in a glass of water or apple juice. Use ~50 mL for 100 mg tablet, or ~200 mL for 400 mg tablet. Stir until tablets are disintegrated, then administer immediately. To ensure the full dose is administered, rinse the glass and administer residue.

Gleevec® prescribing information, Novartis Pharmaceuticals Corporation, East Hanover, NJ, 2012.

References

Ault P, Kantarjian H, O'Brien S, et al, "Pregnancy Among Patients With Chronic Myeloid Leukemia Treated With Imatinib," *J Clin Oncol*, 2006, 24(7):1204-8.

Baccarani M, Cortes J, Pane F, et al, "Chronic Myeloid Leukemia: An Update of Concepts and Management Recommendations of European LeukemiaNet," *J Clin Oncol*, 2009, 27(35):6041-51.

Bansal D, Shava U, Varma N, et al, "Imatinib Has Adverse Effect on Growth in Children With Chronic Myeloid Leukemia," *Pediatr Blood Cancer*, 2012, 59(3):481-4.

Carpenter PA, Snyder DS, Flowers ME, et al, "Prophylactic Administration of Imatinib After Hematopoietic Cell Transplantation for High-Risk Philadelphia Chromosome-Positive Leukemia," *Blood*, 2007, 109(7):2791-3.

Debiec-Rychter M, Sciot R, Le Cesne A, et al, "KIT Mutations and Dose Selection for Imatinib in Patients With Advanced Gastrointestinal Stromal Tumours," *Eur J Cancer*, 2006, 42(8):1093-103.

Gibbons J, Egorin MJ, Ramanathan RK, et al, "Phase I and Pharmacokinetic Study of Imatinib Mesylate in Patients With Advanced Malignancies and Varying Degrees of Renal Dysfunction: A Study by the National Cancer Institute Organ Dysfunction Working Group," *J Clin Oncol*, 2008, 26(4):570-6.

Hamnvik OP, Larsen PR, and Marqusee E, "Thyroid Dysfunction From Antineoplastic Agents," *J Natl Cancer Inst*, 2011, 103(21):1572-87.

Heinrich MC, Owzar K, Corless CL, et al, "Correlation of Kinase Genotype and Clinical Outcome in the North American Intergroup Phase III Trial of Imatinib Mesylate for Treatment of Advanced Gastrointestinal Stromal Tumor: CALGB 150105 Study by Cancer and Leukemia Group B and Southwest Oncology Group," *J Clin Oncol*, 2008, 26(33):5360-7.

Liu H and Artz AS, "Reduction of Imatinib Absorption After Gastric Bypass Surgery," *Leuk Lymphoma*, 2011, 52(2):310-3.

National Comprehensive Cancer Network® (NCCN) "Practice Guidelines in Oncology™: Chronic Myelogenous Leukemia Version 3.2013." Available at http://www.nccn.org/professionals/physician_gls/PDF/cml.pdf

National Institute for Occupational Safety and Health (NIOSH), "NIOSH List of Antineoplastic and Other Hazardous Drugs in Healthcare Settings 2012." Available at http://www.cdc.gov/niosh/docs/2012-150/pdfs/2012-150.pdf. Accessed January 21, 2013.

Pavlovsky C, Egorin MJ, Shah DD, et al, "Imatinib Mesylate Pharmacokinetics Before and After Sleeve Gastrectomy in a Morbidly Obese Patient With Chronic Myeloid Leukemia," *Pharmacotherapy*, 2009, 29 (9):1152-6.

Pye SM, Cortes J, Ault P, et al, "The Effects of Imatinib on Pregnancy Outcome," *Blood*, 2008, 111(12):5505-8.

Ramanathan RK, Egorin MJ, Takimoto CH, et al, "Phase I and Pharmacokinetic Study of Imatinib Mesylate in Patients With Advanced Malignancies and Varying Degrees of Liver Dysfunction: A Study by the National Cancer Institute Organ Dysfunction Working Group," *J Clin Oncol*, 2008, 26(4):563-9.

Rastogi MV, Stork L, Druker B, et al, "Imatinib Mesylate Causes Growth Deceleration in Pediatric Patients With Chronic Myelogenous Leukemia," *Pediatr Blood Cancer*, 2012, 59(5):840-5.

Shima H, Tokuyama M, Tanizawa A, et al, "Distinct Impact of Imatinib on Growth at Prepubertal and Pubertal Ages of Children With Chronic Myeloid Leukemia," *J Pediatr*, 2011, 159(4):676-81.

Yoo C, Ryu MH, Kang BW, et al, "Cross-Sectional Study of Imatinib Plasma Trough Levels in Patients With Advanced Gastrointestinal Stromal Tumors: Impact of Gastrointestinal Resection on Exposure to Imatinib," *J Clin Oncol*, 2010, 28(9):1554-9.

◆ **Imatinib Mesylate** *see* Imatinib *on page 1072*

◆ **Imferon** *see* Iron Dextran Complex *on page 1153*

◆ **IMI 30** *see* IDArubicin *on page 1067*

◆ **Imidazole Carboxamide** *see* Dacarbazine *on page 578*

◆ **Imidazole Carboxamide Dimethyltriazene** *see* Dacarbazine *on page 578*

◆ **IMIG** *see* Immune Globulin *on page 1084*

Imiglucerase (i mi GLOO ser ace)

Medication Safety Issues
Sound-alike/look-alike issues:
  Cerezyme may be confused with Cerebyx, Ceredase

Brand Names: U.S. Cerezyme

Brand Names: Canada Cerezyme

Therapeutic Category Enzyme, Glucocerebrosidase; Gaucher's Disease, Treatment Agent

Generic Availability (U.S.) No

Use Long-term enzyme replacement therapy for patients with Type 1 Gaucher's disease

Pregnancy Risk Factor C

Pregnancy Considerations Animal reproduction studies have not been conducted; however, imiglucerase has been used safely during pregnancy based on available data (Sherer, 2003; Zimran, 2009). Doses of imiglucerase should be based on prepregnancy weight and adjusted as clinically indicated (Granovsky-Grisaru, 2011).

Breast-Feeding Considerations It is not known if imiglucerase is excreted in breast milk. The manufacturer recommends that caution be exercised when administering imiglucerase to nursing women. A case report described a small amount of imiglucerase excreted into breast milk. The maximum amount of enzyme activity was obtained in the first milk at the end of the imiglucerase infusion; enzyme activity rapidly declined to preinfusion levels (Sekijima, 2010). Enzyme ingested by a nursing infant would likely degrade in their digestive system (Zimran, 2009). The benefits of nursing to the infant should be weighed against the potential for additional bone loss in the mother (Granovsky-Grisaru, 2011; Zimran, 2009).

Contraindications Hypersensitivity to imiglucerase or any component

Warnings During clinical trials, 16% of patients developed IgG antibodies reactive with imiglucerase; <1% of patients experienced anaphylactoid reactions; most patients may continue therapy after a reduction in the infusion rate and pretreatment with an antihistamine and/or corticosteroid; close observation for hypersensitivity reactions is recommended. Injection contains polysorbate 80 (Tween 80®) which may cause allergic reactions in susceptible individuals. In premature neonates, thrombocytopenia, ascites, pulmonary deterioration, and renal and hepatic failure have been reported after receiving parenteral products containing polysorbate 80 (Alade, 1986; *MMWR*, 1984). Infusion of polysorbate 80-containing solutions through polyvinyl chloride tubing may cause DEHP to leach into the solution; in immature animals, exposure to DEHP may adversely affect the development of the male reproductive tract.

Precautions Patients experiencing respiratory symptoms during treatment should be evaluated for potential pulmonary hypertension

Adverse Reactions
Cardiovascular: Tachycardia

Central nervous system: Chills, dizziness, fatigue, fever, headache

Dermatologic: Pruritus, rash

Gastrointestinal: Abdominal discomfort, diarrhea, nausea, vomiting

Neuromuscular & skeletal: Backache

Miscellaneous: Hypersensitivity reaction (symptoms may include pruritus, flushing, urticaria, angioedema, chest discomfort, dyspnea, coughing, cyanosis, hypotension, paresthesia)

Rare but important or life-threatening: Anaphylactoid reactions; cyanosis, injection site burning, swelling, or sterile abscess; peripheral edema, pneumonia, pulmonary hypertension, rigors

Drug Interactions

Metabolism/Transport Effects None known.

Avoid Concomitant Use There are no known interactions where it is recommended to avoid concomitant use.

Increased Effect/Toxicity There are no known significant interactions involving an increase in effect.

Decreased Effect There are no known significant interactions involving a decrease in effect.

Stability Store in refrigerator 2°C to 8°C (36°F to 46°F); after reconstitution, stable for 12 hours refrigerated or at room temperature; after dilution in NS, 40 units/mL solution is stable for 24 hours refrigerated; do not use if opaque particles or solution discoloration are seen

Mechanism of Action Imiglucerase is an analogue of glucocerebrosidase; it is produced by recombinant DNA technology using mammalian cell culture. Glucocerebrosidase is an enzyme deficient in Gaucher's disease. It is needed to catalyze the hydrolysis of glucocerebroside to glucose and ceramide.

Pharmacodynamics
Onset of significant improvement in symptoms:
Hepatosplenomegaly and hematologic abnormalities: Within 6 months
Improvement in bone mineralization: Noted at 80-104 weeks of therapy

Pharmacokinetics (Adult data unless noted)
Distribution: V_d: 0.09-0.15 L/kg
Half-life, elimination: 3.6-10.4 minutes
Clearance: 9.8-20.3 mL/minute/kg

Dosing: Usual I.V.: Children and Adults: 30-60 units/kg every 2 weeks; range in dosage: 2.5 units/kg 3 times/week to 60 units/kg once weekly to every 4 weeks. Initial dose should be based on disease severity and rate of progression. Children at high risk for complications from Gaucher's disease (one or more of the following: symptomatic disease including manifestations of abdominal or bone pain, fatigue, exertional limitations, weakness, and cachexia; growth failure; evidence of skeletal involvement; platelet count ≤60,000 mm³ and/or documented abnormal bleeding episode(s); Hgb ≥2.0 g/dL below lower limit for age and sex; impaired quality of life) should receive an initial dose of 60 units/kg; failure to respond to treatment within 6 months indicates the need for a higher dosage.
Maintenance: After patient response is well established a reduction in dosage may be attempted; progressive reductions may be made at intervals of 3-6 months; assess dosage frequently to maintain consistent dosage per kg body weight

Administration Parenteral: Visually inspect the powder in the vial for particulate matter prior to reconstitution. Reconstitute 200 unit vial with 5.1 mL SWI or 400 unit vial with 10.2 mL SWI resulting in a 40 units/mL concentration; visually inspect the solution following reconstitution for particulate matter; further dilute in 100-200 mL NS; infuse over 1-2 hours; may filter diluted solution through an in-line low protein-binding 0.2 micron filter during administration; do not administer products with visualized particulate matter.

Monitoring Parameters CBC, platelets, liver function tests, MRI or CT scan (spleen and liver volume), skeletal x-rays

Dosage Forms Excipient information presented when available (limited, particularly for generics); consult specific product labeling.
Solution Reconstituted, Intravenous:
Cerezyme: 200 units (1 ea); 400 units (1 ea)

References
Alade SL, Brown RE, and Paquet A Jr, "Polysorbate 80 and E-Ferol Toxicity," *Pediatrics*, 1986, 77(4):593-7.

Centers for Disease Control (CDC), "Unusual Syndrome With Fatalities Among Premature Infants: Association With a New Intravenous Vitamin E Product," *MMWR Morb Mortal Wkly Rep*, 1984, 33 (14):198-9.

Charrow J, Andersson HC, Kaplan P, et al, "Enzyme Replacement Therapy and Monitoring for Children With Type 1 Gaucher Disease: Consensus Recommendations," *J Pediatr*, 2004, 144(1):112-20.

Granovsky-Grisaru S, Belmatoug N, vom Dahl S, et al, "The Management of Pregnancy in Gaucher Disease," *Eur J Obstet Gynecol Reprod Biol*, 2011, 156(1): 3-8.

Sekijima Y, Ohashi T, Ohira S, et al, "Successful Pregnancy and Lactation Outcome in a Patient With Gaucher Disease Receiving Enzyme Replacement Therapy, and the Subsequent Distribution and Excretion of Imiglucerase in Human Breast Milk," *Clin Ther*, 2010, 32(12):2048-52.

Sherer Y, Dulitzki M, Levy Y, et al, "Successful Pregnancy Outcome in a Patient With Gaucher's Disease and Antiphospholipid Syndrome," *Ann Hematol*, 2002, 81(3):161-3.

Zimran A, Morris E, Mengel E, et al, "The Female Gaucher Patient: The Impact of Enzyme Replacement Therapy Around Key Reproductive Events (Menstruation, Pregnancy and Menopause)," *Blood Cells Mol Dis*, 2009, 43(3):264-88.

♦ **Imipemide** see Imipenem and Cilastatin on page 1077

Imipenem and Cilastatin
(i mi PEN em & sye la STAT in)

Medication Safety Issues
Sound-alike/look-alike issues:
Imipenem may be confused with ertapenem, meropenem
Primaxin® may be confused with Premarin, Primacor

Brand Names: U.S. Primaxin® I.V.

Brand Names: Canada Imipenem and Cilastatin for Injection; Primaxin I.V. Infusion; RAN-Imipenem-Cilastatin

Therapeutic Category Antibiotic, Carbapenem

Generic Availability (U.S.) Yes

Use Treatment of documented multidrug-resistant gram-negative infection of the lower respiratory tract, urinary tract, intra-abdominal, gynecologic, bone and joint, septicemias, endocarditis, and skin and skin structure due to organisms proven or suspected to be susceptible to imipenem/cilastatin (FDA approved in all ages); treatment of multiple organism infection in which other agents have an insufficient spectrum of activity or are contraindicated due to toxic potential; therapeutic alternative for treatment of gram-negative sepsis in immunocompromised patients

Pregnancy Risk Factor C

Pregnancy Considerations Teratogenic events have not been observed in animal reproduction studies. Due to pregnancy induced physiologic changes, some pharmacokinetic parameters of imipenem/cilastatin may be altered. Pregnant women have a larger volume of distribution resulting in lower serum peak levels than for the same dose in nonpregnant women. Clearance is also increased.

Breast-Feeding Considerations Imipenem is excreted in human milk. The low concentrations and low oral bioavailability suggest minimal exposure risk to the infant. The manufacturer recommends that caution be exercised when administering imipenem/cilastatin to nursing women. Nondose-related effects could include modification of bowel flora.

Contraindications Hypersensitivity to imipenem/cilastatin or any component

Warnings Serious and occasionally fatal hypersensitivity reactions have been reported in patients receiving beta-lactam therapy; careful inquiry should be made concerning previous hypersensitivity reactions to penicillins, cephalosporins, or other beta-lactams before initiating imipenem. Pseudomembranous colitis has been reported in patients receiving imipenem; prolonged use may result in superinfection.

Valproic acid (VPA) serum concentrations may be significantly decreased by concurrent carbapenem use leading to breakthrough seizures. VPA/divalproex sodium dosage adjustment may not adequately overcome this interaction; concurrent use with valproic acid/divalproex sodium is not recommended. Alternative antimicrobial agents should be considered, but if a concurrent carbapenem is necessary, consider additional antiseizure medications. Carbapenems have been associated with CNS adverse effects, including confusional states and seizures (myoclonic); use caution with CNS disorders (eg, brain lesions and history of seizures) and adjust dose in renal impairment to avoid drug accumulation, which may increase seizure risk. Seizures have been reported with imipenem therapy in children with meningitis; imipenem is not recommended in pediatric patients with CNS infections.

Precautions Use with caution in patients with history of CNS disorders including seizures or who are predisposed and in patients with a history of hypersensitivity to penicillins, cephalosporins, or other beta-lactams; use with caution and adjust dose in patients with impaired renal function.

Adverse Reactions

Cardiovascular: Tachycardia

Central nervous system: Seizure

Dermatologic: Rash

Gastrointestinal: Diarrhea, nausea, vomiting

Genitourinary: Oliguria/anuria

Local: Phlebitis/thrombophlebitis

Rare but important or life-threatening: Abdominal pain, abnormal urinalysis, acute renal failure, alkaline phosphatase increased, anaphylaxis, anemia, angioneurotic edema, asthenia, bilirubin increased, bone marrow depression, BUN/creatinine increased, candidiasis, confusion, cyanosis, dizziness, drug fever, dyspnea, encephalopathy, eosinophilia, erythema multiforme, fever, flushing, gastroenteritis, glossitis, hallucinations, hearing loss, hematocrit decreased, hemoglobin decreased, hemolytic anemia, hemorrhagic colitis, hepatitis (including fulminant onset), hepatic failure, hyperchloremia, hyperhidrosis, hyperkalemia, hypersensitivity, hyperventilation, hyponatremia, hypotension, jaundice, lactate dehydrogenase increased, leukocytosis, leukopenia, myoclonus, neutropenia (including agranulocytosis), palpitation, pancytopenia, paresthesia, pharyngeal pain, polyarthralgia, polyuria, positive Coombs' test, prothrombin time increased, pruritus vulvae, pseudomembranous colitis, psychic disturbances, rash, resistant *P. aeruginosa*, somnolence, Stevens-Johnson syndrome, thoracic spine pain, thrombocythemia, thrombocytopenia, tinnitus, tongue papillar hypertrophy, toxic epidermal necrolysis, transaminases increased, tremor, urticaria, vertigo

Drug Interactions

Metabolism/Transport Effects None known.

Avoid Concomitant Use

Avoid concomitant use of Imipenem and Cilastatin with any of the following: BCG; Ganciclovir-Valganciclovir

Increased Effect/Toxicity

Imipenem and Cilastatin may increase the levels/effects of: CycloSPORINE (Systemic)

The levels/effects of Imipenem and Cilastatin may be increased by: CycloSPORINE (Systemic); Ganciclovir-Valganciclovir; Probenecid

Decreased Effect

Imipenem and Cilastatin may decrease the levels/effects of: BCG; CycloSPORINE (Systemic); Sodium Picosulfate; Typhoid Vaccine; Valproic Acid and Derivatives

Stability Store intact vial of powder for injection below 25°C (77°F).

Per the manufacturer, solutions further diluted with D_5W, $D_{10}W$, D_5NS, $D_5^{1/4}NS$ or NS are stable for 4 hours at room temperature and 24 hours under refrigeration; additional stability data suggests solutions further diluted with NS are stable for 11 hours at room temperature (25°C) or 72 hours under refrigeration (4°C) and when further diluted with D_5W are stable for 36 hours under refrigeration (4°C).

Mechanism of Action Inhibits bacterial cell wall synthesis by binding to one or more of the penicillin-binding proteins (PBPs); which in turn inhibits the final transpeptidation step of peptidoglycan synthesis in bacterial cell walls, thus inhibiting cell wall biosynthesis. Bacteria eventually lyse due to ongoing activity of cell wall autolytic enzymes (autolysins and murein hydrolases) while cell wall assembly is arrested. Cilastatin prevents renal metabolism of imipenem by competitive inhibition of dehydropeptidase along the brush border of the renal tubules.

Pharmacokinetics (Adult data unless noted)

Distribution: Rapidly and widely to most tissues and fluids including sputum, pleural fluid, peritoneal fluid, interstitial fluid, bile, aqueous humor, and bone; highest concentrations in pleural fluid, interstitial fluid, and peritoneal fluid; only low concentrations penetrate into CSF

Protein binding:

Imipenem: 20%

Cilastatin: 40%

Metabolism: Imipenem is metabolized in the kidney by dehydropeptidase; cilastatin prevents imipenem metabolism by this enzyme; cilastatin is partially metabolized in the kidneys

Half-life, both drugs: Prolonged with renal insufficiency

Neonates (Freij, 1985):

Imipenem: 1.7-2.4 hours

Cilastatin: 3.9-6.3 hours

Infants and Children: Imipenem: 1.2 hours (Blumer, 1996)

Adults, both drugs: 1 hour

Elimination: When imipenem is given with cilastatin, urinary excretion of unchanged imipenem increases to 70%; 70% to 80% of a cilastatin dose is excreted unchanged in the urine

Dosing: Neonatal Note: Dosage recommendations are based on **imipenem** component; not the preferred carbapenem for preterm infants due to cilastatin accumulation and possible seizures (Blumer, 1996; Freij, 1985; *Red Book*, 2012; Reed, 1990); not recommended for CNS infections

General dosing, susceptible infection (*Red Book*, 2012): I.V.:

Body weight <1 kg:

PNA ≤14 days: 20 mg/kg/dose every 12 hours

PNA 15-28 days: 25 mg/kg/dose every 12 hours

Body weight 1-2 kg:

PNA ≤7 days: 20 mg/kg/dose every 12 hours

PNA 8-28 days: 25 mg/kg/dose every 12 hours

Body weight >2 kg:

PNA ≤7 days: 25 mg/kg/dose every 12 hours

PNA 8-28 days: 25 mg/kg/dose every 8 hours

Dosing: Usual Note: Dosage recommendations are based on **imipenem** component.

Infants, Children, and Adolescents:

General dosing, susceptible infection (*Red Book*, 2012): I.V.: Serious infections: 60-100 mg/kg/**day** divided every 6 hours; maximum daily dose: 4000 mg/**day**

***Burkholderia pseudomallei* (melioidosis):** I.V.: Initial: 60-100 mg/kg/**day** divided every 6-8 hours for at least 10 days; maximum daily dose: 4000 mg/**day**; continue parenteral therapy until clinical improvement, then switch to oral therapy if tolerated and/or appropriate (Currie, 2003; White, 2003)

Intra-abdominal infection, complicated: I.V.: 60-100 mg/kg/**day** divided every 6 hours; maximum dose: 500 mg (Solomkin, 2010)

Peritonitis (CAPD): Intraperitoneal: Continuous: Loading dose: 250 mg per liter of dialysate; maintenance dose: 50 mg per liter (Warady, 2012)

Pulmonary exacerbation, cystic fibrosis: I.V.: 100 mg/kg/**day** divided every 6 hours; maximum daily dose: 4000 mg/**day**; efficacy may be limited due to rapid development of resistance (Doring, 2009; Zobell, 2012)

Adults:

Usual dosage range: Weight ≥70 kg: I.V.: 250-1000 mg every 6-8 hours; maximum: 4000 mg/day. **Note:** For adults weighing <70 kg, refer to Dosing Adjustment in Renal Impairment.

Indication-specific dosing:

Mild infections: Note: Rarely a suitable option in mild infections; normally reserved for moderate-severe cases: I.V.:

Fully susceptible organisms: 250 mg every 6 hours
Moderately susceptible organisms: 500 mg every 6 hours

Moderate infections: I.V.:

Fully susceptible organisms: 500 mg every 6-8 hours
Moderately susceptible organisms: 500 mg every 6 hours or 1000 mg every 8 hours

Severe infections: I.V.:

Fully susceptible organisms: 500 mg every 6 hours
Moderately susceptible organisms: 1000 mg every 6-8 hours

Maximum daily dose should not exceed 50 mg/kg or 4000 mg/day, whichever is lower

***Pseudomonas* infections:** I.V.: 500 mg every 6 hours; **Note:** Higher doses may be required based on organism sensitivity.

Urinary tract infection, uncomplicated: I.V.: 250 mg every 6 hours

Urinary tract infection, complicated: I.V.: 500 mg every 6 hours

Dosing adjustment in renal impairment:

Infants, Children, and Adolescents: I.V.:

Manufacturer's labeling: Patient weight <30 kg and impaired renal function (not defined): Use not recommended

The following adjustments have been recommended (Aronoff, 2007): **Note:** Renally adjusted dose recommendations are based on doses of 60-100 mg/kg/day divided every 6 hours.

GFR 30-50 mL/minute/1.73 m²: Administer 7-13 mg/kg/dose every 8 hours

GFR 10-29 mL/minute/1.73 m²: Administer 7.5-12.5 mg/kg/dose every 12 hours

GFR <10 mL/minute/1.73 m²: Administer 7.5-12.5 mg/kg/dose every 24 hours

Intermittent hemodialysis (IHD): Dialysis: Moderately dialyzable (20% to 50%): 7.5-12.5 mg/kg/dose every 24 hours (administer after hemodialysis on dialysis days)

Peritoneal dialysis (PD): 7.5-12.5 mg/kg/dose every 24 hours

Continuous renal replacement therapy (CRRT): 7-13 mg/kg/dose every 8 hours

Adults: Manufacturer's labeling: Reduce dose based on creatinine clearance and/or body weight:

Imipenem and Cilastatin Dosage in Renal Impairment

Reduced I.V. Dosage Regimen Based on Creatinine Clearance (mL/minute/1.73 m²) and/or Body Weight <70 kg				
Body Weight (kg)				
≥70	**60**	**50**	**40**	**30**
Total daily dose for normal renal function: 1000 mg/day				
CrCl ≥71 250 mg q6h	250 mg q8h	125 mg q6h	125 mg q6h	125 mg q8h
CrCl 41-70 250 mg q8h	125 mg q6h	125 mg q6h	125 mg q8h	125 mg q8h
CrCl 21-40 250 mg q12h	250 mg q12h	125 mg q8h	125 mg q12h	125 mg q12h
CrCl 6-20 250 mg q12h	125 mg q12h	125 mg q12h	125 mg q12h	125 mg q12h
Total daily dose for normal renal function: 1500 mg/day				
CrCl ≥71 500 mg q8h	250 mg q6h	250 mg q6h	250 mg q8h	125 mg q6h
CrCl 41-70 250 mg q6h	250 mg q8h	250 mg q8h	125 mg q6h	125 mg q8h
CrCl 21-40 250 mg q8h	250 mg q8h	250 mg q12h	125 mg q8h	125 mg q8h
CrCl 6-20 250 mg q12h	250 mg q12h	250 mg q12h	125 mg q12h	125 mg q12h
Total daily dose for normal renal function: 2000 mg/day				
CrCl ≥71 500 mg q6h	500 mg q8h	250 mg q6h	250 mg q6h	250 mg q8h
CrCl 41-70 500 mg q8h	250 mg q6h	250 mg q6h	250 mg q8h	125 mg q6h
CrCl 21-40 250 mg q6h	250 mg q8h	250 mg q8h	250 mg q12h	125 mg q8h
CrCl 6-20 250 mg q12h	250 mg q12h	250 mg q12h	250 mg q12h	125 mg q12h
Total daily dose for normal renal function: 3000 mg/day				
CrCl ≥71 1000 mg q8h	750 mg q8h	500 mg q6h	500 mg q8h	250 mg q6h
CrCl 41-70 500 mg q6h	500 mg q8h	500 mg q8h	250 mg q6h	250 mg q8h
CrCl 21-40 500 mg q8h	500 mg q8h	250 mg q6h	250 mg q8h	250 mg q8h
CrCl 6-20 500 mg q12h	500 mg q12h	250 mg q12h	250 mg q12h	250 mg q12h
Total daily dose for normal renal function: 4000 mg/day				
CrCl ≥71 1000 mg q6h	1000 mg q8h	750 mg q8h	500 mg q6h	500 mg q8h
CrCl 41-70 750 mg q8h	750 mg q8h	500 mg q6h	500 mg q8h	250 mg q6h
CrCl 21-40 500 mg q6h	500 mg q8h	500 mg q8h	250 mg q6h	250 mg q8h
CrCl 6-20 500 mg q12h	500 mg q12h	500 mg q12h	250 mg q12h	250 mg q12h

Patients with a CrCl ≤5 mL/minute/1.73 m² should not receive imipenem/cilastatin unless hemodialysis is instituted within 48 hours.

Patients weighing <30 kg with impaired renal function should not receive imipenem/cilastatin.

Intermittent hemodialysis (IHD) (administer after hemodialysis on dialysis days): Dialysis: Moderately dialyzable (20% to 50%): Use the dosing recommendation for patients with a CrCl 6-20 mL/minute; administer dose after dialysis session and every 12 hours thereafter **or** 250-500 mg every 12 hours (Heintz, 2009). **Note:** Dosing dependent on the assumption of 3 times/week, complete IHD sessions.

Peritoneal dialysis: Dose as for CrCl 6-20 mL/minute (Somani, 1988)

Continuous renal replacement therapy (CRRT) (Heintz, 2009; Trotman, 2005): Drug clearance is highly dependent on the method of renal replacement, filter type, and flow rate. Appropriate dosing requires close monitoring of pharmacologic response, signs of adverse reactions due to drug accumulation, as well as drug concentrations in relation to target trough (if appropriate). The following are general recommendations only (based on dialysate flow/ultrafiltration rates of 1-2 L/hour and minimal residual renal function) and should not supersede clinical judgment:

CVVH: Loading dose of 1000 mg followed by either 250 mg every 6 hours **or** 500 mg every 8 hours

CVVHD: Loading dose of 1000 mg followed by either 250 mg every 6 hours **or** 500 mg every 6-8 hours

CVVHDF: Loading dose of 1000 mg followed by either 250 mg every 6 hours **or** 500 mg every 6 hours

Note: Data suggest that 500 mg every 8-12 hours may provide sufficient time above MIC to cover organisms with MIC values ≤2 mg/L; however, a higher dose of 500 mg every 6 hours is recommended for resistant organisms (particularly *Pseudomonas* spp) with MIC ≥4 mg/L or deep-seated infections (Fish, 2005).

Dosing adjustment in hepatic impairment: There are no dosage adjustments provided in the manufacturer's labeling.

Administration I.V.: Administer by I.V. intermittent infusion; final concentration should not exceed 5 mg/mL; in fluid-restricted patients, a final concentration of 7 mg/mL has been administered at some institutions (Taketomo, 2009); doses ≤500 mg may be infused over 15-30 minutes; doses >500 mg should be infused over 40-60 minutes. If nausea and/or vomiting occur during administration, decrease the rate of I.V. infusion.

Monitoring Parameters Periodic renal, hepatic, and hematologic function tests; bowel movement frequency

Test Interactions Interferes with urinary glucose determination using Clinitest®; positive Coombs' [direct]

Additional Information Sodium content: 250 mg vial contains 0.8 mEq; 500 mg vial contains 1.6 mEq

Dosage Forms Excipient information presented when available (limited, particularly for generics); consult specific product labeling.

Injection, powder for reconstitution: Imipenem 250 mg and cilastatin 250 mg; imipenem 500 mg and cilastatin 500 mg

Primaxin® I.V.: Imipenem 250 mg and cilastatin 250 mg [contains sodium 18.8 mg (0.8 mEq)]; imipenem 500 mg and cilastatin 500 mg [contains sodium 37.5 mg (1.6 mEq)]

References

Ahonkhai VI, Cyhan GM, Wilson SE, et al, "Imipenem-Cilastatin in Pediatric Patients: An Overview of Safety and Efficacy in Studies Conducted in the United States," *Pediatr Infect Dis J*, 1989, 8 (11):740-4.

American Academy of Pediatrics (AAP). In: Pickering LK, Baker CJ, Kimberlin DW, Long SS, eds. *Red Book: 2012 Report of the Committee on Infectious Diseases*. 29th ed. Elk Grove Village, IL: American Academy of Pediatrics; 2012.

Aronoff GR, Bennett WM, Berns JS, et al, *Drug Prescribing in Renal Failure: Dosing Guidelines for Adults and Children*, 5th ed, Philadelphia, PA: American College of Physicians, 2007.

Blumer JL, "Pharmacokinetic Determinants of Carbapenem Therapy in Neonates and Children," *Pediatr Infect Dis J*, 1996, 15(8):733-7.

Currie BJ, "Melioidosis: An Important Cause of Pneumonia in Residents of and Travellers Returned from Endemic Regions," *Eur Respir J*, 2003, 22(3):542-50.

Döring G, Conway SP, Heijerman HG, et al, "Antibiotic Therapy Against *Pseudomonas aeruginosa* in Cystic Fibrosis: A European Consensus," *Eur Respir J*, 2000, 16(4):749-67.

Fish DN, Teitelbaum I, and Abraham E, "Pharmacokinetics and Pharmacodynamics of Imipenem During Continuous Renal Replacement Therapy in Critically Ill Patients," *Antimicrob Agents Chemother*, 2005, 49(6):2421-8.

Freij BJ, McCracken GH Jr, Olsen KD, et al, "Pharmacokinetics of Imipenem-Cilastatin in Neonates," *Antimicrob Agents Chemother*, 1985, 27(4):431-5.

Heintz BH, Matzke GR, Dager WE, "Antimicrobial Dosing Concepts and Recommendations for Critically Ill Adult Patients Receiving Continuous Renal Replacement Therapy or Intermittent Hemodialysis," *Pharmacotherapy*, 2009, 29(5):562-77.

Overturf GD, "Use of Imipenem-Cilastatin in Pediatrics," *Pediatr Infect Dis J*, 1989, 8(11):792-4.

Reed MD, Kliegman RM, Yamashita TS, et al, "Clinical Pharmacology of Imipenem and Cilastatin in Premature Infants During the First Week of Life," *Antimicrob Agents Chemother*, 1990, 34(6):1172-7.

Solomkin JS, Mazuski JE, Bradley JS, et al, "Diagnosis and Management of Complicated Intra-Abdominal Infections in Adults and Children: Guidelines by the Surgical Infection Society and the Infectious Diseases Society of America," *Clin Infect Dis*, 2010, 50(2):133-64.

Somani P, Freimer EH, Gross ML, et al, "Pharmacokinetics of Imipenem-Cilastatin in Patients With Renal Insufficiency Undergoing Continuous Ambulatory Peritoneal Dialysis," *Antimicrob Agents Chemother*, 1988, 32(4):530-4.

Taketomo CK, personal communication, September 2009.

Trissel LA, Gilbert DL, and Wolkin AC, "Compatibility of Docetaxel With Selected Drugs During Simulated Y-Site Administration," *Int J Pharmaceut Compound*, 1999, 3(3):241-4.

Trotman RL, Williamson JC, Shoemaker DM, et al, "Antibiotic Dosing in Critically Ill Adult Patients Receiving Continuous Renal Replacement Therapy," *Clin Infect Dis*, 2005, 41(8):1159-66.

Warady BA, Bakkaloglu S, Newland J, et al, "Consensus Guidelines for the Prevention and Treatment of Catheter-Related Infections and Peritonitis in Pediatric Patients Receiving Peritoneal Dialysis: 2012 Update," *Perit Dial Int*, 2012, 32(Suppl 20):32-86.

White NJ, "Melioidosis," *Lancet*, 2003, 361(9370):1715-22.

Wong VK, Wright HT Jr, Ross LA, et al, "Imipenem/Cilastatin Treatment of Bacterial Meningitis in Children," *Pediatr Infect Dis J*, 1991, 10 (2):122-5.

♦ **Imipenem and Cilastatin for Injection (Can)** *see* Imipenem and Cilastatin *on page 1077*

Imipramine (im IP ra meen)

Medication Safety Issues

Sound-alike/look-alike issues:
Imipramine may be confused with amitriptyline, desipramine, Norpramin®

BEERS Criteria medication:
This drug may be potentially inappropriate for use in geriatric patients (Quality of evidence - high [moderate for SIADH]; Strength of recommendation - strong).

Related Information

Antidepressant Agents *on page 2219*

Medications for Which a Single Dose May Be Fatal When Ingested by a Toddler *on page 2408*

Brand Names: U.S. Tofranil; Tofranil-PM

Brand Names: Canada Impril; Novo-Pramine; PMS Imipramine

Therapeutic Category Antidepressant, Tricyclic (Tertiary Amine)

Generic Availability (U.S.) Yes

Use Treatment of childhood enuresis (Tofranil®: FDA approved in ages ≥6 years); treatment of depression (Tofranil®: FDA approved in adolescents and adults, Tofranil-PM®: FDA approved in adults); has also been used for attention-deficit/hyperactivity disorder (ADHD) and as analgesic for certain chronic and neuropathic pain

Medication Guide Available Yes

Pregnancy Considerations Animal reproduction studies are inconclusive. Congenital abnormalities have been reported in humans; however, a causal relationship has not been established. Tricyclic antidepressants may be associated with irritability, jitteriness, and convulsions (rare) in the neonate (Yonkers, 2009). Due to pregnancy-induced physiologic changes, women who are pregnant may require dose adjustments late in pregnancy to achieve euthymia (Altshuler, 1996).

The ACOG recommends that therapy for depression during pregnancy be individualized; treatment should incorporate the clinical expertise of the mental health clinician, obstetrician, primary healthcare provider, and pediatrician (ACOG, 2008). According to the American Psychiatric

Association (APA), the risks of medication treatment should be weighed against other treatment options and untreated depression. For women who discontinue antidepressant medications during pregnancy and who may be at high risk for postpartum depression, the medications can be restarted following delivery (APA, 2010). Treatment algorithms have been developed by the ACOG and the APA for the management of depression in women prior to conception and during pregnancy (Yonkers, 2009).

Breast-Feeding Considerations Imipramine and its active metabolite (desipramine) are excreted into breast milk (Sovner, 1979). Concentrations of imipramine may be similar to those in the maternal plasma. Based on information from five mother/infant pairs, following maternal use of imipramine 75-200 mg/day, the estimated exposure to the breast-feeding infant would be 0.1% to 7.5% of the weight-adjusted maternal dose. Although adverse events were not reported, infants should be monitored for signs of adverse events (Fortinguerra, 2009). Imipramine can also be detected in the urine of nursing infants (Yoshida, 1997). Breast-feeding is not recommended by the manufacturer.

Contraindications Hypersensitivity to imipramine (cross-sensitivity with other tricyclics may occur) or any component; use during acute recovery phase after MI; use of MAO inhibitors intended to treat psychiatric disorders (concurrently or within 14 days of discontinuing either imipramine or the MAO inhibitor); initiation of imipramine in a patient receiving linezolid or intravenous methylene blue

Warnings Clinical worsening of depression or suicidal ideation and behavior may occur in children and adults with major depressive disorder **[U.S. Boxed Warning]**. In clinical trials, antidepressants increased the risk of suicidal thinking and behavior (suicidality) in children, adolescents, and young adults (18-24 years of age) with major depressive disorder and other psychiatric disorders. This risk must be considered before prescribing antidepressants for any clinical use. Short-term studies did **not** show an increased risk of suicidality with antidepressant use in patients >24 years of age and showed a decreased risk in patients ≥65 years.

Patients of all ages who are treated with antidepressants for any indication require appropriate monitoring and close observation for clinical worsening of depression, suicidality, and unusual changes in behavior, especially during the first few months after antidepressant initiation or when the dose is adjusted. Family members and caregivers should be instructed to closely observe the patient (ie, daily) and communicate condition with healthcare provider. Patients should also be monitored for associated behaviors (eg, anxiety, agitation, panic attacks, insomnia, irritability, hostility, aggressiveness, impulsivity, akathisia, hypomania, mania) which may increase the risk for worsening depression or suicidality. Worsening depression or emergence of suicidality (or associated behaviors listed above) that is abrupt in onset, severe, or not part of the presenting symptoms, may require discontinuation or modification of drug therapy.

Do not discontinue abruptly in patients receiving high doses chronically (withdrawal symptoms may occur). To reduce risk of intentional overdose, write prescriptions for the smallest quantity consistent with good patient care. May worsen psychosis in some patients or precipitate a shift to mania or hypomania in patients with bipolar disorder. Antidepressant monotherapy in patients with bipolar disorder should be avoided. Patients presenting with depressive symptoms should be screened for bipolar disorder. Imipramine causes a high degree of sedation relative to other antidepressants; may impair physical or mental abilities; patients must be cautioned about performing tasks which require mental alertness (eg, operating machinery or driving).

The American Heart Association recommends that all children diagnosed with ADHD who may be candidates for medication, such as imipramine, should have a thorough cardiovascular assessment prior to initiation of therapy. These recommendations are based upon reports of serious cardiovascular adverse events (including sudden death) in patients (both children and adults) taking usual doses of stimulant medications. Most of these patients were found to have underlying structural heart disease (eg, hypertrophic obstructive cardiomyopathy). This assessment should include a combination of thorough medical history, family history, and physical examination. An ECG is not mandatory but should be considered. The manufacturer recommends not to exceed a dose of 2.5 mg/kg/day in children; ECG changes (of unknown significance) have been reported in pediatric patients who received twice this amount. Use with caution in patients with a history of cardiovascular disease (including previous MI, stroke, tachycardia, or conduction abnormalities); the risk of conduction abnormalities with this agent is high relative to other antidepressants. Baseline and periodic ECG assessment is recommended with use of higher dosages; should also be considered in elderly patients and/or patients with preexisting cardiovascular disease.

Potentially life-threatening serotonin syndrome (SS) has occurred with serotonergic agents (eg, SSRIs, SNRIs), particularly when used in combination with other serotonergic agents (eg, triptans, TCAs, fentanyl, lithium, tramadol, buspirone, St John's wort, tryptophan) or agents that impair metabolism of serotonin [eg, MAO inhibitors intended to treat psychiatric disorders, other MAO inhibitors (ie, linezolid and intravenous methylene blue)]. Monitor patients closely for signs of SS such as mental status changes (eg, agitation, hallucinations, delirium, coma); autonomic instability (eg, tachycardia, labile blood pressure, diaphoresis, dizziness, flushing, hyperthermia); neuromuscular changes (eg, tremor, rigidity, myoclonus, hyper-reflexia, incoordination); GI symptoms (eg, nausea, vomiting, diarrhea); and/or seizures. Discontinue treatment (and any concomitant serotonergic agent) immediately if signs/symptoms arise.

Concurrent use of MOA inhibitors including reversible MAO inhibitors (eg, linezolid, methylene blue) is contraindicated; however, if urgent treatment with linezolid or I.V. methylene blue is required in a patient already receiving imipramine and potential benefits outweigh potential risks, discontinue imipramine promptly and administer linezolid or I.V. methylene blue. Monitor for increased risk of hypertensive reactions for 2 weeks or until 24 hours after the last dose of linezolid or I.V. methylene blue, whichever comes first. May resume imipramine 24 hours after the last dose of linezolid or I.V. methylene blue.

Recommended to discontinue prior to elective surgery requiring general anesthesia. TCAs may rarely cause bone marrow suppression; monitor for any signs of infection and obtain CBC if symptoms (eg, fever, sore throat) evident.

Precautions Use with caution in patients with significant renal or hepatic impairment. May cause orthostatic hypotension; risk is very high relative to other antidepressants; use with caution in patients at risk of this effect or in those who would not tolerate transient hypotensive episodes (eg, cerebrovascular disease, cardiovascular disease, hypovolemia, or concurrent medication use which may predispose to hypotension/bradycardia). Use with caution in patients with respiratory compromise or sleep apnea; use is generally not recommended in patients with severe sleep apnea. Use with caution in patients at risk of seizures, including those with a history of seizures, head trauma, brain damage, alcoholism, or concurrent therapy with medications which may lower seizure threshold. Use with caution in patients with diabetes mellitus; may alter glucose regulation. Use with caution in patients with hyperthyroidism or those receiving thyroid supplementation due to concerns of pro-arrhythmogenesis.

May cause anticholinergic effects (constipation, xerostomia, blurred vision, urinary retention); use with caution in patients with decreased gastrointestinal motility, paralytic ileus, urinary retention, BPH, xerostomia, or visual problems. The degree of anticholinergic blockade produced by this agent is high relative to other antidepressants. May increase the risks associated with electroconvulsive therapy (ECT); consider discontinuing, when possible, prior to ECT treatment. Imipramine has been associated with photosensitization; avoid excessive exposure to sunlight.

Use of capsules is generally **not** recommended in children due to high mg strength and increased potential for acute overdose. Safety of imipramine for long-term chronic use in the treatment of enuresis has not been established; long-term usefulness should be periodically re-evaluated for the individual patient; medication should be tapered off gradually to achieve drug-free period for reassessment; children who relapse with enuresis during drug-free period do not always respond to subsequent courses of therapy.

Adverse Reactions Reported for tricyclic antidepressants in general.

Cardiovascular: Arrhythmia, CHF, ECG changes, heart block, hypertension, MI, orthostatic hypotension, palpitation, stroke, tachycardia

Central nervous system: Agitation, anxiety, confusion, delusions, disorientation, dizziness, drowsiness, fatigue, hallucination, headache, hypomania, insomnia, nightmares, psychosis, restlessness, seizure

Dermatologic: Alopecia, itching, petechiae, photosensitivity, purpura, rash, urticaria

Endocrine & metabolic: Breast enlargement, galactorrhea, gynecomastia, increase or decrease in blood sugar, increase or decrease in libido, SIADH

Gastrointestinal: Abdominal cramps, anorexia, black tongue, constipation, diarrhea, epigastric disorders, ileus, nausea, stomatitis, taste disturbance, vomiting, weight gain/loss, xerostomia

Genitourinary: Impotence, testicular swelling, urinary retention

Hematologic: Agranulocytosis, eosinophilia, thrombocytopenia

Hepatic: Cholestatic jaundice, transaminases increased

Neuromuscular & skeletal: Ataxia, extrapyramidal symptoms, incoordination, numbness, paresthesia, peripheral neuropathy, tingling, tremor, weakness

Ocular: Blurred vision, disturbances of accommodation, mydriasis

Otic: Tinnitus

Miscellaneous: Diaphoresis, falling, hypersensitivity (eg, drug fever, edema)

Drug Interactions

Metabolism/Transport Effects Substrate of CYP1A2 (minor), CYP2B6 (minor), CYP2C19 (major), CYP2D6 (major), CYP3A4 (minor); **Note:** Assignment of Major/Minor substrate status based on clinically relevant drug interaction potential; **Inhibits** CYP1A2 (weak), CYP2C19 (weak), CYP2D6 (moderate), CYP2E1 (weak)

Avoid Concomitant Use

Avoid concomitant use of Imipramine with any of the following: Aclidinium; Azelastine (Nasal); Iobenguane I 123; Ipratropium (Oral Inhalation); Linezolid; MAO Inhibitors; Methylene Blue; Moxonidine; Paraldehyde; Potassium Chloride; Thalidomide; Thioridazine; Tiotropium; Umeclidinium

Increased Effect/Toxicity

Imipramine may increase the levels/effects of: AbobotulinumtoxinA; Alcohol (Ethyl); Alpha-/Beta-Agonists (Direct-Acting); Alpha1-Agonists; Amphetamines; Analgesics (Opioid); Anticholinergic Agents; Antipsychotics;

ARIPiprazole; Aspirin; Azelastine (Nasal); Beta2-Agonists; Buprenorphine; Cannabinoid-Containing Products; Citalopram; CNS Depressants; CYP2D6 Substrates; Desmopressin; DOXOrubicin (Conventional); Escitalopram; Fesoterodine; Highest Risk QTc-Prolonging Agents; Hydrocodone; Methotrimeprazine; Methylene Blue; Metoprolol; Metyrosine; Mirabegron; Moderate Risk QTc-Prolonging Agents; Nebivolol; NSAID (COX-2 Inhibitor); NSAID (Nonselective); OnabotulinumtoxinA; Paraldehyde; Potassium Chloride; Pramipexole; QuiNIDine; RimabotulinumtoxinB; ROPINIRole; Rotigotine; Serotonin Modulators; Sodium Phosphates; Sulfonylureas; Thalidomide; Thiazide Diuretics; Thioridazine; Tiotropium; Topiramate; TraMADol; Vitamin K Antagonists; Yohimbine; Zolpidem

The levels/effects of Imipramine may be increased by: Abiraterone Acetate; Aclidinium; Altretamine; Antiemetics (5HT3 Antagonists); Antipsychotics; Brimonidine (Topical); BuPROPion; Cannabis; Cimetidine; Cinacalcet; Citalopram; Cobicistat; CYP2C19 Inhibitors (Moderate); CYP2C19 Inhibitors (Strong); CYP2D6 Inhibitors (Moderate); CYP2D6 Inhibitors (Strong); Darunavir; Dexmethylphenidate; Doxylamine; Dronabinol; Droperidol; DULoxetine; Escitalopram; FLUoxetine; FluvoxaMINE; HydrOXYzine; Ipratropium (Oral Inhalation); Kava Kava; Linezolid; Lithium; Luliconazole; Magnesium Sulfate; MAO Inhibitors; Methotrimeprazine; Methylphenidate; Metoclopramide; Metyrosine; Mifepristone; Nabilone; PARoxetine; Perampanel; Pramlintide; Propafenone; Protease Inhibitors; QuiNIDine; Rufinamide; Sertraline; Sodium Oxybate; Tapentadol; Terbinafine (Systemic); Tetrahydrocannabinol; Thyroid Products; TraMADol; Umeclidinium; Valproic Acid and Derivatives

Decreased Effect

Imipramine may decrease the levels/effects of: Acetylcholinesterase Inhibitors (Central); Alpha2-Agonists; Alpha2-Agonists (Ophthalmic); Codeine; Iobenguane I 123; Moxonidine; Secretin; Tamoxifen

The levels/effects of Imipramine may be decreased by: Acetylcholinesterase Inhibitors (Central); Barbiturates; CYP2C19 Inducers (Strong); Dabrafenib; Peginterferon Alfa-2b; St Johns Wort

Stability Store at 20°C to 25°C (68°F to 77°F); dispense in tightly closed container

Mechanism of Action Traditionally believed to increase the synaptic concentration of serotonin and/or norepinephrine in the central nervous system by inhibition of their reuptake by the presynaptic neuronal membrane. However, additional receptor effects have been found including desensitization of adenyl cyclase, down regulation of beta-adrenergic receptors, and down regulation of serotonin receptors.

Pharmacodynamics Maximum antidepressant effects usually occur after ≥2 weeks

Pharmacokinetics (Adult data unless noted)

Absorption: Oral: Well absorbed

Distribution:

V_d: Children: 14.5 L/kg; Adults: ~17 L/kg

Protein binding: >90% (primarily to alpha$_1$ acid glycoprotein and lipoproteins; to a lesser extent albumin)

Metabolism: Hepatic, primarily via CYP2D6 to desipramine (active) and other metabolites; significant first-pass effect

Bioavailability: 20% to 80%

Half-life: Range: 6-18 hours

Mean: Children: 11 hours; Adults: 16-17 hours

Desipramine (active metabolite): 22-28 hours

Time to peak serum concentration: Within 1-2 hours

Elimination: Urine

Dosing: Usual

Children and Adolescents: **Note:** Dosing presented is based on hydrochloride salt.

Attention-deficit/hyperactivity disorder: Children ≥6 years and Adolescents: Oral: Limited data available: Initial: 1 mg/kg/day in 1-3 divided doses; titrate as needed; maximum daily dose: 4 mg/kg/**day** or 200 mg/**day**; for doses >2 mg/kg/day, monitor serum concentrations (target: ≤200 ng/mL) (Himpel, 2005; Pliszka, 2007). **Note:** Manufacturer's labeling warns against use of doses >2.5 mg/kg/day in pediatric patients; ECG changes (of unknown significance) have been reported in pediatric patients who received twice this amount.

Depression: Oral: Limited data available: **Note:** Controlled clinical trials have not shown tricyclic antidepressants to be superior to placebo for the treatment of depression in children and adolescents; not recommended as first line medication; may be beneficial for patient with comorbid conditions (ADHD, enuresis) (Birmaher, 2007; Dopheide, 2006; Wagner, 2005).

Children: 1.5 mg/kg/day in 2-3 divided doses; titrate as needed in increments of 1 mg/kg every 3-4 days; maximum daily doses of 5 mg/kg/**day** has been used by some centers; monitor carefully especially with doses ≥3.5 mg/kg/day; manufacturer's labeling warns against use of doses >2.5 mg/kg/day in pediatric patients; ECG changes (of unknown significance) have been reported in pediatric patients who received twice this amount

Adolescents: Initial: 25-50 mg/day; increase gradually; maximum daily dose: 100 mg/**day** in single or divided doses

Enuresis: Children ≥4 years and Adolescents: Oral: Initial: 10-25 mg at bedtime, if inadequate response still seen after 1 week of therapy, increase by 25 mg/day; maximum daily dose: The lesser of: 2.5 mg/kg/**day** or 50 mg/**day** if 6 to <12 years old; and 75 mg/**day** if ≥12 years old; for early night bedwetters, drug has been shown to be more effective if given earlier and in divided amounts (eg, 25 mg in midafternoon and repeated at bedtime). **Note:** Due to the risk of serious side effects (eg, arrhythmias, heart block, seizures), imipramine is considered third-line treatment for enuresis (Deshpande, 2012).

Neuropathic pain: Note: Not the preferred TCA; amitriptyline or nortriptyline recommended as first-line TCAs. Limited data available: Initial: 0.2-0.4 mg/kg at bedtime; dose may be increased by 50% every 2-3 days up to 1-3 mg/kg/dose at bedtime (Berde, 1990). **Note:** Manufacturer labeling warns against use of doses >2.5 mg/kg/**day** in pediatric patients; ECG changes (of unknown significance) have been reported in pediatric patients who received twice this amount.

Adults: **Depression:** Oral:

Outpatients: Initial: 75 mg/day; may increase gradually to 150 mg/day. May be given in divided doses or as a single bedtime dose; maximum daily dose: 200 mg/**day**

Inpatients: Initial: 100-150 mg/day; may increase gradually to 200 mg/day; if no response after 2 weeks, may further increase to 250-300 mg/day. May be given in divided doses or as a single bedtime dose; maximum daily dose: 300 mg/**day**

Note: Maximum antidepressant effect may not be seen for 2 or more weeks after initiation of therapy.

Dosing adjustment in renal impairment: There are no dosage adjustments provided in manufacturer's labeling; use with caution.

Dosing adjustment in hepatic impairment: There are no dosage adjustments provided in manufacturer's labeling; use with caution.

Administration Oral: May administer with food to decrease GI distress. For treatment of enuresis, administer dose 1 hour before bedtime; for early night bedwetters, drug has been shown to be more effective if given earlier and in divided amounts (eg, 25 mg in midafternoon and repeated at bedtime)

Monitoring Parameters Heart rate, ECG, supine and standing blood pressure (especially in children), liver enzymes, CBC, serum drug concentrations. Obtain ECG before initiation of therapy and at appropriate intervals in patients with any evidence of cardiovascular disease and in all patients who will receive doses that are larger than usual. Monitor patient periodically for symptom resolution; monitor for worsening depression, suicidality, and associated behaviors (especially at the beginning of therapy or when doses are increased or decreased). Monitor for signs/symptoms of serotonin syndrome.

ADHD: Evaluate patients for cardiac disease prior to initiation of therapy for ADHD with thorough medical history, family history, and physical exam; consider ECG; perform ECG and echocardiogram if findings suggest cardiac disease; promptly conduct cardiac evaluation in patients who develop chest pain, unexplained syncope, or any other symptom of cardiac disease during treatment.

Reference Range Note: Utility of serum concentration monitoring controversial.

Therapeutic: Imipramine and desipramine 150-250 ng/mL (SI: 530-890 nmol/L); desipramine 150-300 ng/mL (SI: 560-1125 nmol/L)

Potentially toxic: >300 ng/mL (SI: >1070 nmol/L)

Toxic: >1000 ng/mL (SI: >3570 nmol/L)

Dosage Forms Excipient information presented when available (limited, particularly for generics); consult specific product labeling.

Capsule, Oral, as pamoate:

Tofranil-PM: 75 mg, 100 mg, 125 mg, 150 mg

Generic: 75 mg, 100 mg, 125 mg, 150 mg

Tablet, Oral, as hydrochloride:

Tofranil: 10 mg, 25 mg, 50 mg

Generic: 10 mg, 25 mg, 50 mg

References

ACOG Committee on Practice Bulletins-Obstetrics. ACOG practice bulletin: clinical management guidelines for obstetrician-gynecologists number 92, April 2008 (replaces practice bulletin number 87, November 2007). Use of psychiatric medications during pregnancy and lactation. *Obstet Gynecol.* 2008;111(4):1001-1020.

Altshuler LL, Hendrick VC. Pregnancy and psychotropic medication: changes in blood levels. *J Clin Psychopharmacol.* 1996;16(1):78-80.

American Academy of Pediatrics/American Heart Association Clarification of Statement on Cardiovascular Evaluation and Monitoring of Children and Adolescents With Heart Disease Receiving Medications for ADHD; available at: http://americanheart.mediaroom.com/index.php?s=43&item=422.

"American Academy of Pediatrics Subcommittee on Attention-Deficit/ Hyperactivity Disorder and Committee on Quality Improvement. Clinical Practice Guidelines: Treatment of the School-Aged Child With Attention-Deficit/Hyperactivity Disorder," *Pediatrics,* 2001, 108 (4):1033-44.

American Psychiatric Association (APA). Treatment recommendations for patients with major depressive disorder. 3rd ed, May 2010. Available at http://www.psychiatryonline.com/pracGuide/pracGuideTopic_7.aspx

Berde C, Ablin A, Glazer J, et al, "American Academy of Pediatrics Report of the Subcommittee on Disease-Related Pain in Childhood Cancer," *Pediatrics,* 1990, 86(5 Pt 2):818-25.

Birmaher B, Brent D, AACAP Work Group on Quality Issues, et al, "Practice Parameter for the Assessment and Treatment of Children and Adolescents With Depressive Disorders," *J Am Acad Child Adolesc Psychiatry,* 2007, 46(11):1503-26.

Deshpande AV and Caldwell PH, "Medical Management of Nocturnal Enuresis," *Paediatr Drugs,* 2012, 14(2):71-7.

Dopheide JA, "Recognizing and Treating Depression in Children and Adolescents," *Am J Health Syst Pharm,* 2006, 63(3):233-43.

Fortinguerra F, Clavenna A, and Bonati M, "Psychotropic Drug Use During Breastfeeding: A Review of the Evidence," *Pediatrics,* 2009, 124(4):e547-56.

Himpel S, Banaschewski T, Heise CA, et al, "The Safety of Nonstimulant Agents for the Treatment of Attention-Deficit Hyperactivity Disorder," *Expert Opin Drug Saf,* 2005, 4(2):311-21.

Levy HB, Harper CR, and Weinberg WA, "A Practical Approach to Children Failing in School," *Pediatr Clin North Am,* 1992, 39 (4):895-928.

Pliszka S and AACAP Work Group on Quality Issues, "Practice Parameter for the Assessment and Treatment of Children and Adolescents With Attention-Deficit/Hyperactivity Disorder," *J Am Acad Child Adolesc Psychiatry*, 2007, 46(7):894-921.

Sovner R and Orsulak PJ, "Excretion of Imipramine and Desipramine in Human Breast Milk," *Am J Psychiatry*, 1979, 136(4A):451-2.

Vetter VL, Elia J, Erickson C, et al, "Cardiovascular Monitoring of Children and Adolescents With Heart Disease Receiving Stimulant Drugs: A Scientific Statement From the American Heart Association Council on Cardiovascular Disease in the Young Congenital Cardiac Defects Committee and the Council on Cardiovascular Nursing," *Circulation*, 2008, 117(18):2407-23.

Wagner KD, "Pharmacotherapy for Major Depression in Children and Adolescents," *Prog Neuropsychopharmacol Biol Psychiatry*, 2005, 29 (5):819-26.

Yonkers KA, Wisner KL, Stewart DE, et al. The management of depression during pregnancy: a report from the American Psychiatric Association and the American College of Obstetricians and Gynecologists. *Obstet Gynecol*. 2009;114(3):703-713.

Yoshida K, Smith B, Craggs M, et al. Investigation of pharmacokinetics and of possible adverse effects in infants exposed to tricyclic antidepressants in breast-milk. *J Affect Disord*. 1997;43(3):225-237.

◆ **Imipramine Hydrochloride** see Imipramine on page 1080

◆ **Imipramine Pamoate** see Imipramine on page 1080

◆ **Imitrex** see SUMAtriptan on page 1958

◆ **Imitrex DF (Can)** see SUMAtriptan on page 1958

◆ **Imitrex Injection (Can)** see SUMAtriptan on page 1958

◆ **Imitrex Nasal Spray (Can)** see SUMAtriptan on page 1958

◆ **Imitrex STATdose Refill** see SUMAtriptan on page 1958

◆ **Imitrex STATdose System** see SUMAtriptan on page 1958

Immune Globulin (i MYUN GLOB yoo lin)

Medication Safety Issues
Sound-alike/look-alike issues:
Gamimune N may be confused with CytoGam

Immune globulin (intravenous) may be confused with hepatitis B immune globulin

Related Information
Immune Globulin Product Comparison on page 2226

Immunization Administration Recommendations on page 2368

Brand Names: U.S. Bivigam; Carimune NF; Flebogamma; Flebogamma DIF; GamaSTAN S/D; Gammagard; Gammagard S/D; Gammagard S/D Less IgA; Gammaked; Gammaplex; Gamunex-C; Hizentra; Hizentra 20%; Octagam; Privigen

Brand Names: Canada Gamastan S/D; Gammagard Liquid; Gammagard S/D; Gamunex; Hizentra; IGIVnex; Octagam 10%; Privigen

Therapeutic Category Blood Product Derivative; Immune Globulin

Generic Availability (U.S.) No

Use Treatment of primary humoral immunodeficiency syndromes (may include but not limited to: Congenital agammaglobulinemia, severe combined immunodeficiency syndromes [SCIDS], common variable immunodeficiency, X-linked immunodeficiency, Wiskott-Aldrich syndrome); acute and chronic immune thrombocytopenia (ITP); chronic inflammatory demyelinating polyneuropathy (CIDP); and multifocal motor neuropathy. Prevention of coronary artery aneurysms associated with Kawasaki syndrome (in combination with aspirin).

Adjunctive treatment of bacterial infection in patients with hypogammaglobulinemia and/or recurrent bacterial infections with B-cell chronic lymphocytic leukemia (CLL); and serious infection in immunoglobulin deficiency (select agammaglobulinemias).

To provide passive immunity for prophylaxis in the following susceptible individuals: Hepatitis A (pre-exposure and postexposure [within 14 days and prior to manifestation of disease]); measles (postexposure [within 6 days] in an unvaccinated or nonimmune person); rubella (postexposure during early pregnancy); and varicella zoster (immunosuppressed patients when varicella zoster immune globulin is unavailable).

See table for product specific indications, FDA approved age ranges, and routes of administration.

Product	Indication	FDA Approval Ages	Route(s)
Bivigam	Primary immunodeficiency (treatment)	≥6 years and adults	Intravenous
Carimune NF	Primary immunodeficiency (treatment)	Pediatric patients (age not specified) and adults	Intravenous
	Acute and chronic ITP (treatment)		
Flebogamma 5% DIF	Primary immunodeficiency (treatment)	Adults	Intravenous
Flebogamma 10% DIF	Primary immunodeficiency (treatment)	Adults	Intravenous
GamaSTAN S/D	Passive immunity - Hepatitis A	Pediatric patients (age not specified) and adults	Intramuscular
	Passive immunity - Measles		
	Passive immunity - Rubella	Adults	
	Passive immunity - Varicella	Pediatric patients (age not specified) and adults	
Gammagard Liquid	Primary immunodeficiency (treatment)	≥2 years and adults	Intravenous, Subcutaneous
	Multifocal motor neuropathy (MMN)	Adults	Intravenous
Gammagard S/D	Primary immunodeficiency (treatment)	≥2 years and adults	Intravenous
	B-cell chronic lymphocytic leukemia (CLL)	Adults	
	Chronic ITP (treatment)	Adults	
	Kawasaki syndrome	Pediatric patients (age not specified)	

(continued)

Product	Indication	FDA Approval Ages	Route(s)
Gammaked	Primary immunodeficiency (treatment)	0 to 16 years	Intravenous
		Adults	Intravenous, Subcutaneous
	Acute ITP (treatment)	Pediatric patients (age not specified) and adults	Intravenous
	Chronic inflammatory demyelinating polyneuropathy (CIDP)	Adults	Intravenous
Gammaplex	Primary immunodeficiency (treatment)	Adults	Intravenous
	Chronic ITP (treatment)	Adults	
Gamunex-C	Primary immunodeficiency (treatment)	0 to 16 years	Intravenous
		Adults	Intravenous, Subcutaneous
	Acute and chronic ITP (treatment)	Pediatric patients (age not specified) and adults	Intravenous
	Chronic inflammatory demyelinating polyneuropathy (CIDP)	Adults	Intravenous
Hizentra	Primary immunodeficiency (treatment)	≥2 years and adults	Subcutaneous
Octagam	Primary immunodeficiency (treatment)	6 to 16 years and adults	Intravenous
Privigen	Primary immunodeficiency (treatment)	≥3 years and adults	Intravenous
	Chronic ITP (treatment)	≥15 years and adults	Intravenous

Has also been used for acute disseminated encephalomyelitis (ADEM), acute myocarditis, chronic *Clostridium difficile* colitis, Guillain-Barré syndrome, hematopoietic stem cell transplantation with hypogammaglobulinemia, isoimmune hemolytic disease (Rh-incompatibility), multiple sclerosis, myasthenia gravis, neonatal sepsis, pediatric HIV infection and associated thrombocytopenia, refractory dermatomyositis, Stevens-Johnson syndrome (SJS)/toxic epidermal necrolysis (TEN), and refractory polymyositis.

Pregnancy Risk Factor C

Pregnancy Considerations Animal reproduction studies have not been conducted. Immune globulins cross the placenta in increased amounts after 30 weeks gestation. Intravenous immune globulin has been recommended for use in fetal-neonatal alloimmune thrombocytopenia and pregnancy-associated ITP (Anderson, 2007). Intravenous immune globulin is recommended to prevent measles in nonimmune women exposed during pregnancy (CDC, 2013). May also be used in postexposure prophylaxis for rubella to reduce the risk of infection and fetal damage in exposed pregnant women who will not consider therapeutic abortion (per GamaSTAN S/D product labeling; use for postexposure rubella prophylaxis is not currently recommended [CDC, 2013]).

Breast-Feeding Considerations It is not known if immune globulin from these preparations is excreted in breast milk. The manufacturer recommends that caution be exercised when administering immune globulin to nursing women.

Contraindications Hypersensitivity to immune globulin or any component; IgA deficiency (with anti-IgA antibodies and history of hypersensitivity)

Additional product specific contraindications:

GamaSTAN S/D: Isolated IgA deficiency; severe thrombocytopenia or coagulation disorders where IM injections are contraindicated

Gammaplex: Hereditary intolerance to fructose; infants/neonates for whom sucrose or fructose tolerance has not been established

Hizentra, Privigen: Hyperprolinemia

Octagam: Hypersensitivity to corn

Warnings Product of human plasma; may potentially contain infectious agents which could transmit disease. Screening of donors, as well as testing and/or inactivation or removal of certain viruses, reduces the risk. Infections thought to be transmitted by this product should be reported to the manufacturer.

Acute renal dysfunction (increased serum creatinine, oliguria, acute renal failure, osmotic nephrosis) can rarely occur with intravenous immune globulin administration and has been associated with fatalities **[U.S. Boxed Warning]**; most cases usually occur within 7 days of use (more likely with products stabilized with sucrose). Due to risk of renal dysfunction, use caution in patients with renal disease, diabetes mellitus, volume depletion, sepsis, paraproteinemia, the elderly, and concomitant use of nephrotoxic medications; the rate of infusion and concentration of solution should be minimized; discontinue if renal function deteriorates.

Thrombosis may occur following treatment with immune globulin products **[U.S. Boxed Warning]**; even in the absence of risk factors for thrombosis. For patients at risk of thrombosis (eg, advanced age, prolonged immobilization, hypercoagulable conditions, history of venous or arterial thrombosis, use of estrogens, indwelling central vascular catheters, hyperviscosity, and cardiovascular risk factors), administer at the minimum dose and lowest infusion rate practicable. Ensure adequate hydration before administration. Monitor for signs and symptoms of thrombosis and assess blood viscosity in patients at risk for hyperviscosity such as those with cryoglobulins, fasting chylomicronemia/severe hypertriglyceridemia, or monoclonal gammopathies. Do not administer as SubQ infusion in patients with ITP due to the risk of hematoma formation.

Intravenous immune globulin has been associated with antiglobulin hemolysis (acute or delayed); monitor for signs of hemolytic anemia. Cases of hemolysis-related renal dysfunction/failure or disseminated intravascular coagulation (DIC) have been reported. Risk factors associated with hemolysis include high doses (≥2000 mg/kg) given either as a single administration or divided over several days, underlying associated inflammatory conditions, and non-O blood type (FDA, 2012). High-dose regimens (1000 mg/kg for 1 to 2 days) are not recommended for individuals with fluid overload or where fluid volume may be of concern. In chronic ITP assess risk versus benefit of high dose regimen in patients with increased risk of thrombosis, hemolysis, acute kidney injury, or volume overload.

Infusion-related reactions may occur, characterized by fever, chills, nausea, vomiting, and rarely shock; risk may be increased with initial treatment, when switching brands of immune globulin, and with treatment interruptions of >8 weeks. Stop administration for any signs of infusion reaction.

Noncardiogenic pulmonary edema has been reported with immune globulin use. Transfusion-related acute lung injury (TRALI) is characterized by severe respiratory distress, pulmonary edema, hypoxemia, and fever in the presence of normal left ventricular function and usually occurs within 1 to 6 hours after the infusion. Monitor for TRALI.

Hyperproteinemia, increased serum viscosity, and hyponatremia may occur; distinguish true hyponatremia from pseudohyponatremia to prevent volume depletion, a further increase in serum viscosity and a higher risk of thrombotic events.

Hypersensitivity and anaphylactic reactions can occur; a severe decrease in blood pressure may rarely occur with anaphylactic reactions; immediate treatment (including epinephrine 1:1000) should be available. Skin testing should not be performed with GamaSTAN S/D as local irritation can occur and be misinterpreted as a positive reaction.

Aseptic meningitis syndrome has been rarely reported with intravenous and subcutaneous administration of immune globulin; usually appears within several hours to 2 days of initiation of immune globulin therapy and resolves within several days after product discontinuation. Symptoms include severe headache, nuchal rigidity, drowsiness, fever, photophobia, painful eye movements, nausea, and vomiting. Aseptic meningitis syndrome may occur more frequently with high doses (≥1000 mg/kg) and/or rapid infusion. Patients with a migraine history may be at higher risk for aseptic meningitis syndrome.

Some products contain polysorbate 80 (Tween 80) which may cause allergic reactions in susceptible individuals. In premature neonates, thrombocytopenia, ascites, pulmonary deterioration, and renal and hepatic failure have been reported after receiving parenteral products containing polysorbate 80 (Alade, 1986; CDC, 1984). Infusion of polysorbate 80 containing solutions through polyvinyl chloride tubing may cause DEHP to leach into the solution; in immature animals, exposure to DEHP may adversely affect the development of the male reproductive tract.

Precautions Not all products are interchangeable; consult manufacturer's labeling for additional information related to route of administration. Use with caution in patients with a history of cardiovascular disease or thrombotic episodes. Rapid IVIG infusion may be a possible risk factor for vascular occlusive events associated with IVIG. Do not exceed manufacturer's recommended initial infusion rate, use a lower IVIG concentration, and advance slowly in patients at risk. Monitor for adverse events during and after the infusion. Discontinue administration with signs of infusion reaction (fever, chills, nausea, vomiting, and rarely shock). Risk of adverse events may be increased with initial treatment, when switching brands of immune globulin, and with treatment interruptions of >8 weeks. Assure that patients are not volume depleted prior to the initiation of an IVIG infusion.

IgA deficiency increases the risk of hypersensitivity, especially in patients with anti-IgA antibodies present; use is contraindicated in IgA-deficient patients with antibodies against IgA and history of hypersensitivity or isolated IgA deficiency (GamaSTAN S/D).

Some clinicians may administer intravenous immune globulin products as a subcutaneous infusion based on patient tolerability and clinical judgment. SubQ infusion should begin 1 to 2 weeks after the last I.V. dose; dose should be individualized based on clinical response and serum IgG trough concentrations; for Hizentra, it is recommended that patients receive 3 months of I.V. immune globulin before initiating SubQ infusion. Consider premedicating with acetaminophen and diphenhydramine.

Response to live vaccines may be reduced following immune globulin treatment, refer to package insert or current practice guidelines for recommendations on separation intervals.

Hizentra and Privigen contain the stabilizer L-proline and are contraindicated in patients with hyperprolinemia. Some products may contain maltose, which may result in falsely elevated blood glucose readings. Maltose-containing products are contraindicated in patients with corn allergy. Some products may contain sorbitol; do not use in patients with fructose intolerance. Some products may contain sucrose or have packaging that contains natural latex/natural rubber; consult manufacturers' labeling for additional product-specific information.

Adverse Reactions

Cardiovascular: Chest tightness, edema, facial flushing, hypertension, hypotension, palpitations, tachycardia

Central nervous system: Anxiety, aseptic meningitis, chills, dizziness, drowsiness, fatigue, headache, irritability, lethargy, malaise, migraine, pain, rigors

Dermatologic: Contact dermatitis, diaphoresis, eczema, erythema, hyperhidrosis, pruritus, skin rash, urticaria

Endocrine & metabolic: Dehydration, hyperglycemia (neuromuscular disease), increased lactate dehydrogenase

Gastrointestinal: Abdominal cramps, abdominal pain, anorexia (neuromuscular disease), diarrhea, dyspepsia, gastroenteritis, gastrointestinal distress, nausea, sore throat, toothache, vomiting

Genitourinary: Anuria, oliguria, osmotic nephrosis, proximal tubular nephropathy

Hematologic & oncologic: Anemia, autoimmune hemolytic anemia, bruise, decreased hematocrit, hematoma, hemolysis (mild), hemorrhage, petechia, purpura, thrombocytopenia

Hepatic: Increased liver enzymes, increased serum bilirubin

Hypersensitivity: Anaphylaxis, angioedema, hypersensitivity reaction

Local: Infusion site reaction (swelling, erythema, warm sensation, pain, itching, or irritation), muscle rigidity at injection site (I.M.)

Neuromuscular & skeletal: Arthralgia, back pain, hip pain, leg cramps, limb pain, muscle cramps, muscle spasm, myalgia, neck pain, weakness

Ophthalmic: Conjunctivitis

Otic: Otalgia

Renal: Acute renal failure, increased blood urea nitrogen, increased serum creatinine, renal tubular necrosis

Respiratory: Bronchitis, cough, dyspnea, epistaxis, exacerbation of asthma, flu-like symptoms, nasal congestion, oropharyngeal pain, pharyngitis, rhinitis, rhinorrhea, sinus headache, sinusitis, upper respiratory tract infection, wheezing

Miscellaneous: Fever, infusion related reaction, thermal injury

Rare but important or life-threatening: Adult respiratory distress syndrome, apnea, bronchopneumonia, bullous dermatitis, cardiac arrest, cardiac failure, cerebrovascular accident, circulatory shock, coma, cyanosis, disseminated intravascular coagulation, epidermolysis, erythema multiforme, exacerbation of autoimmune pure red cell aplasia, hepatic insufficiency, hypoxemia, leukopenia, loss of consciousness, myocardial infarction, pancytopenia, phlebitis, positive direct Coombs test, pulmonary edema, pulmonary embolism, renal insufficiency, seizure, Stevens-Johnson syndrome, thromboembolism, thrombosis, transfusion-related acute lung injury

Drug Interactions

Metabolism/Transport Effects None known.

Avoid Concomitant Use There are no known interactions where it is recommended to avoid concomitant use.

Increased Effect/Toxicity There are no known significant interactions involving an increase in effect.

Decreased Effect

Immune Globulin may decrease the levels/effects of: Vaccines (Live)

Stability Stability and dilution information are product-specific. Do not freeze or heat; do not use if previously frozen or heated. Gently swirl; do not shake; avoid foaming. Discard unused portion of vials. Do not mix products from different manufacturers or with other drugs or I.V. infusion fluids.

Bivigam: Store at 2°C to 8°C (36°F to 46°F). Dilution is not recommended.

Carimune NF: Prior to reconstitution, store at ≤30°C (≤86°F). Reconstitute with NS, D₅W, or SWI. Following reconstitution in a sterile laminar air flow environment, store under refrigeration. Begin infusion within 24 hours. If reconstituted outside of a laminar flow hood, use immediately.

Flebogamma DIF: Store at 2°C to 25°C (36°F to 77°F); protect from light. Dilution is not recommended.

GamaSTAN S/D: Store at 2°C to 8°C (36°F to 46°F).

Gammagard Liquid: Store at 2°C to 8°C (36°F to 46°F) for up to 36 months or at 25°C (77°F) for up to 24 months. Dilute only with D₅W.

Gammagard S/D: Store at ≤25°C (≤77°F). Reconstitute with SWI; store reconstituted solution under refrigeration at 2°C to 8°C (36°F to 46°F) for up to 24 hours if originally prepared in a sterile laminar air flow environment.

Gamma...
month...
only w...

Gamma...
from li...

Gamun...
36 mo...
only w...

Hizentr...
protec...

Octaga...

Privige...
further...

(handwritten note overlapping text:)
- keep at room temp
- swirl, do not shake, Ø foaming.
- throw away unused.
- store at 36–46°/3 yrs
  or 125–25 77F/2 yr.
  Dilute w/DSW.

Mechanism of Action Replacement therapy for primary and secondary immunodeficiencies, and IgG antibodies against bacteria, viral, parasitic and mycoplasma antigens; interference with F_c receptors on the cells of the reticuloendothelial system for autoimmune cytopenias and ITP; provides passive immunity by increasing the antibody titer and antigen-antibody reaction potential

Pharmacodynamics

Onset of action: I.V.: Provides immediate antibody levels

Duration: I.M., I.V.: Immune effect: 3 to 4 weeks (variable)

Pharmacokinetics (Adult data unless noted) Note:

Consult manufacturers' labeling for additional product-specific information.

Half-life...
Healtl...
humo...
half-li...
infect...

Time t...
SubC...

Dosing

able w...
ufactu...
osmol...
infuse...
"Immu...

dix for details). Dosage expressed as mg/kg or mL/kg dependent upon route of administration; use extra precaution to ensure accuracy.

(handwritten note overlapping text:)
14–40 day ½ life
↓ ½ life w/ fever
onset – immediate
duration – 3–4 wks

Immune thrombocytopenia (ITP): I.V.: 400 to 1000 mg/kg/day for 2 to 5 consecutive days (total dose: 2000 mg/kg); maintenance dose: 400 to 1000 mg/kg/dose every 3 to 6 weeks based on clinical response and platelet count

Isoimmune hemolytic disease (Rh-incompatibility): I.V.: GA ≥35 weeks: 500 to 1000 mg/kg/dose once over 2 hours; if needed, dose may be repeated in 12 hours; most effective when administered as soon as possible after diagnosis (AAP Subcommittee on Hyperbilirubinemia, 2004; Girish, 2008; Gottstein, 2003; Miqdad, 2004)

Measles, prophylaxis (CDC, 2013):
Pre-exposure prophylaxis (eg, during an outbreak, travel to endemic area): Immunocompromised patients: I.V.: ≥400 mg/kg/dose within 3 weeks before anticipated exposure

Postexposure prophylaxis: Any neonate without evidence of measles immunity:
I.M.: 0.5 **mL**/kg/dose within 6 days of exposure; **Note:** Not all immune globulin preparations may be administered by the I.M. route; of the products currently available on the market, GamaSTAN S/D may be given I.M.; consult product labeling for additional information as market availability may change.
I.V.: 400 mg/kg/dose within 6 days of exposure

Myasthenia gravis (severe exacerbation): I.V.: 400 to 1000 mg/kg/dose once daily over 2 to 5 days for a total dose of 2000 mg/kg; if additional therapy required, dose should be based on clinical response and titrated to minimum effective dose (Bassan, 1998; Feasby, 2007)

Myocarditis, acute: I.V.: 2000 mg/kg as a single dose. A cohort study of 21 young patients, including neonates, showed improvement in LVF recovery and survival at 1 year as compared to untreated historical cohort (Drucker, 1994); efficacy results are variable (English, 2004; Hia, 2004; Klugman, 2010); the largest data analysis did not show clear clinical benefit nor positive impact on survival; further studies are needed (Klugman, 2010).

Sepsis, adjunctive treatment: I.V.: Limited data available; efficacy results variable: Usual dose: 500 to 1000 mg/kg/dose once daily for 1 to 3 days (Jenson, 1997; Ohlsson, 2010). The largest trial, INIS (n=3493), reported no difference in outcomes (including incidence of subsequent sepsis, death, or major disability at 2 years) between treatment and control groups using 500 mg/kg/day for 2 days (INIS Collaborative Group, 2011).

Dosing: Usual Note: Not all products are interchangeable with regards to route of administration; consult manufacturers' labeling for additional information. Product-specific dosing provided where applicable; some clinicians use ideal body weight or an adjusted ideal body weight in morbidly-obese patients to calculate an IVIG dose (Siegel, 2010, Wimperis, 2011). Dosage expressed as mg/kg or mL/kg dependent upon route of administration; use extra precaution to ensure accuracy.

Pediatric and Adult:

Acute disseminated encephalomyelitis (ADEM): I.V.: Children: 1000 mg/kg/dose once daily for 2 days (Feasby, 2007)

B-cell chronic lymphocytic leukemia (CLL): Gammagard S/D: I.V.: Adults: 400 mg/kg/dose every 3 to 4 weeks

Chronic inflammatory demyelinating polyneuropathy (CIDP): Gammaked, Gammunex-C: I.V.: Adults: Initial: 400 to 1000 mg/kg/dose once daily for 2 to 5 days for a total dose of 2000 mg/kg
Maintenance therapy: 500 to 1000 mg/kg/dose for 1 to 2 days for a total dose of 1000 mg/kg every 3 weeks; some have recommended a maximum dose of 2000 mg/kg per treatment course (Feasby, 2007)

Colitis due to *Clostridium difficile*, chronic: I.V.: Limited data available: Infants and Children: 400 mg/kg/dose every 3 weeks resulted in resolution of colitis symptoms during treatment; duration of therapy was unclear (n=5; age range: 6 to 37 months) (Abougergi, 2011; Leung, 1991; McFarland, 2000); further studies are needed

Dermatomyositis, refractory (Feasby, 2007): I.V.:

Children: 1000 mg/kg/dose once daily for 2 days

Adults: 400 to 1000 mg/kg/dose once daily over 2 to 5 days for a total dose of 2000 mg/kg

Note: If maintenance therapy is required, the dose and frequency should be based on clinical response and doses should not exceed 2000 mg/kg per treatment course.

Guillain-Barré syndrome: I.V.: Various regimens have been used:

Children: 1000 mg/kg/dose once daily for 2 days (Feasby, 2007) **or** 400 mg/kg/dose once daily for 6 days (Patwa, 2012)

Adults: 400 mg/kg/day for 6 days (Patwa, 2012) **or** 400 to 1000 mg/kg/dose once daily over 2 to 5 days for a total cumulative dose of 2000 mg/kg (Feasby, 2007)

Hematopoietic cell transplantation (HCT) with hypogammaglobulinemia (IgG <400 mg/dL), prevention of bacterial infection (Tomblyn, 2009): I.V.:

Within first 100 days after HCT:

Children (Allogeneic HCT recipients): 400 mg/kg/dose once monthly; increase dose or frequency to maintain IgG concentration >400 mg/dL

Adolescents and Adults: 500 mg/kg/dose once weekly; increase dose or frequency to maintain IgG concentration >400 mg/dL

>100 days after HCT: Children, Adolescents and Adults: 500 mg/kg/dose every 3 to 4 weeks; increase dose or frequency to maintain IgG concentration >400 mg/dL

Hepatitis A, prophylaxis: Infants, Children, Adolescents, and Adults: **Note:** Hepatitis A vaccine preferred for patients 12 months to 40 years (CDC, 2007):

I.M.: GamaSTAN S/D: **Note:** In adults, injections >10 mL should be split into multiple injections given at different sites; in pediatric patients, consider splitting doses <10 mL based on patient size

Pre-exposure prophylaxis upon travel into endemic areas:

Anticipated duration of risk <3 months: 0.02 **mL**/kg/dose as a single dose

Anticipated duration of risk ≥3 months: 0.06 **mL**/kg/dose once every 4 to 6 months if exposure continues

Postexposure prophylaxis: 0.02 **mL**/kg/dose as a single dose given within 14 days of exposure and prior to manifestation of disease; not needed if at least 1 dose of hepatitis A vaccine was given at ≥1 month before exposure (CDC, 2006)

HIV infection, pediatric (DHHS [pediatric], 2013): I.V.: Infants and Children:

Primary prophylaxis for serious bacterial infection in patients with hypogammaglobulinemia (IgG <400 mg/dL): 400 mg/kg/dose every 2 to 4 weeks

Secondary prophylaxis for invasive bacterial infections: Should only be used if subsequent infections are frequent severe infections (>2 infections during a 1-year period): 400 mg/kg/dose every 2 to 4 weeks

Immune thrombocytopenia (ITP): Infants, Children, Adolescents, and Adults: I.V.:

General dosing: **Note:** Dosing regimens variable, consult product specific information if available:

Acute therapy: 400 to 1000 mg/kg/dose once daily for 2 to 5 consecutive days for a total cumulative dose of 2000 mg/kg; in some cases, cumulative doses up to 3000 mg/kg have been used

Chronic therapy: 400 to 1000 mg/kg/dose every 3 to 6 weeks based on clinical response and platelet count

Carimune NF:

Acute therapy: 400 mg/kg/dose once daily for 2 to 5 days to maintain platelet count ≥30,000/mm^3 and/or to control significant bleeding

Chronic therapy: 400 mg/kg/dose as a single infusion; may increase to 800 to 1000 mg/kg/dose to maintain platelet count ≥30,000/mm^3 and/or to control significant bleeding

Gammagard S/D: Chronic therapy: Adults: 1000 mg/kg/dose on alternate days for up to 3 doses based on patient response and/or platelet count

Gammaked: Acute therapy: 400 to 1000 mg/kg/dose once daily for 2 to 5 consecutive days for a total cumulative dose of 2000 mg/kg; if an adequate platelet response is observed after the initial 1000 mg/kg/dose, then the subsequent dose may be held

Gammaplex: Chronic therapy: Adults: 1000 mg/kg/dose once daily for 2 days

Gamunex-C: Acute or chronic therapy: 1000 mg/kg/dose once daily for 1 to 2 days based on patient response and/or platelet response **or** for fluid-restricted patients or other conditions sensitive to volume: 400 mg/kg once daily for 5 days

Privigen: Chronic therapy: Adolescents ≥15 years and Adults: 1000 mg/kg/dose once daily for 2 days

Kawasaki disease: Infants and Children: I.V.: 2000 mg/kg as a single dose within 10 days of disease onset; must be used in combination with aspirin; if signs and symptoms persist ≥36 hours after completion of the infusion, retreatment with a second 2000 mg/kg infusion should be considered (Newburger, 2004)

Measles, prophylaxis:

Pre-exposure prophylaxis (eg, during an outbreak, travel to endemic area):

Manufacturer's labeling: Patients with primary humoral immunodeficiency:

I.V. (Gammaked, Gamunex-C, Octagam): Infants, Children, Adolescents, and Adults: ≥400 mg/kg/dose immediately before expected exposure; **Note:** Should only administer to patients whose routine dose is <400 mg/kg/dose

SubQ infusion (Hizentra): Children ≥2 years, Adolescents, and Adults:

Weekly dosing: ≥200 mg/kg/dose once weekly for 2 consecutive weeks

Biweekly dosing: ≥400 mg/kg for 1 dose

Alternate dosing: ACIP recommendations (CDC, 2013): Immunocompromised patients: Infants, Children, Adolescents, and Adults:

I.V.: ≥400 mg/kg/dose within 3 weeks before anticipated exposure

SubQ: 200 mg/kg/dose once weekly for 2 consecutive weeks prior to anticipated exposure (CDC, 2013); **Note:** Not all immune globulin preparations may be administered by the SubQ route; Hizentra is the only product currently approved for this indication that may be given SubQ; consult product labeling for additional information as market availability may change

Postexposure prophylaxis:

Manufacturer's labeling: Patients with primary humoral immunodeficiency:

I.V. (Gammaked, Gamunex-C, Octagam): Infants, Children, and Adults: 400 mg/kg/dose administered as soon as possible after exposure

SubQ infusion (Hizentra): Children ≥2 years, Adolescents, and Adults:

Weekly dosing: ≥200 mg/kg/dose as soon as possible following exposure

Biweekly dosing: ≥400 mg/kg as soon as possible following exposure

Alternate dosing: ACIP guidelines (CDC, 2013): Any person without evidence of measles immunity: Infants, Children, Adolescents, and Adults:

I.M.: 0.5 **mL**/kg/dose; maximum dose: 15 mL within 6 days of exposure; in adults, doses >10 mL should be split into multiple injections and administered at different sites; in pediatric patients, may also split doses <10 mL based on patient size. **Note:** Not all immune globulin preparations may be administered by the I.M. route; of the products currently available on the market, GamaSTAN S/D may be given I.M.; consult product labeling for additional information as market availability may change. GamaSTAN S/D manufacturer labeling suggests a lower I.M. dose of 0.25 mL/kg; however, this dosing was based on previous immune globulin potency concentrations; recent data indicates that potency from current donor populations has decreased (ie, measles immunity now from vaccinations instead of immunity from disease) requiring a higher I.M. immune globulin dose (0.5 mL/kg) in all patients without evidence of measles immunity to ensure adequate serum titers.

I.V.: 400 mg/kg/dose within 6 days of exposure

Multifocal motor neuropathy: Gammagard Liquid: I.V.: Adults: 500 to 2400 mg/kg/month based upon response

Multiple sclerosis (relapsing-remitting, when other therapies cannot be used): Children and Adults: I.V.: Dosage regimen variable; optimal dose not established: 1000 mg/kg/dose once monthly, with or without an induction of 400 mg/kg/day for 5 days (Feasby, 2007)

Myasthenia gravis (Juvenile and Adult, severe exacerbation): Children and Adults: I.V.: 400 to 1000 mg/kg/dose once daily over 2 to 5 days for a total dose of 2000 mg/kg; if additional therapy required, dose should be based on clinical response and titrated to minimum effective dose (Feasby, 2007)

Myocarditis, acute: I.V.: Infants and Children: 2000 mg/kg as a single dose. A cohort study of 21 children showed improvement in LVF recovery and survival at 1 year as compared to untreated historical cohort (Drucker, 1994); efficacy results are variable (English, 2004; Hia, 2004; Klugman, 2010); the largest data analysis did not show clear clinical benefit nor positive impact on survival; further studies are needed (Klugman, 2010)

Polymyositis, refractory: I.V.: Adults: 400 to 1000 mg/kg/dose once daily over 2 to 5 days for a total dose of 2000 mg/kg per treatment course. If maintenance therapy is required, the dose and frequency should be based on clinical response and doses should not exceed 2000 mg/kg per treatment course (Feasby, 2007).

Primary immunodeficiency disorders: Infants, Children, Adolescents, and Adults: Adjust dose/frequency based on desired IgG concentration and clinical response; a trough IgG concentration of ≥500 mg/dL has been recommended by some experts (Bonilla, 2005); consult product specific labeling for appropriate age groups.

I.V.: General dosing: 200 to 800 mg/kg/dose every 3 to 4 weeks

Carimune NF: 400 to 800 mg/kg/dose every 3 to 4 weeks

Flebogamma DIF, Gammagard Liquid, Gammagard S/D, Gammaked, Gamunex-C, Octagam: 300 to 600 mg/kg/dose every 3 to 4 weeks

Bivigam, Gammaplex: 300 to 800 mg/kg/dose every 3 to 4 weeks

Privigen: 200 to 800 mg/kg/dose every 3 to 4 weeks

SubQ infusion: Children, Adolescents, and Adults: Gammagard Liquid, Gammaked, Gamunex-C: Begin 1 week after last I.V. dose. Use the following equation to calculate initial dose:

Initial weekly dose: Dose (grams) = [1.37 x I.V. dose (grams)] divided by [I.V. dose interval (weeks)]; **Note:** For subsequent doses, refer to product labeling

Hizentra: For weekly dosing, begin 1 week after last I.V. infusion. For biweekly dosing, begin 1 or 2 weeks after last I.V. infusion or 1 week after the last Hizentra weekly infusion. **Note:** Patient should have received an I.V. immune globulin routinely for at least 3 months before switching to SubQ. Use the following equation to calculate initial dose:

Initial **weekly** dose: Dose (grams) = [Previous I.V. dose (grams)] divided by [I.V. dose interval (weeks)] then multiply by 1.53; **Note:** To convert the dose (in grams) to mL, multiply the calculated dose (in grams) by 5.

Initial **biweekly** dose: Dose (grams) = Multiply the calculated weekly dose by 2

Note: For subsequent doses refer to product labeling

Rubella, prophylaxis during pregnancy: I.M.: GamaSTAN S/D: Postexposure: 0.55 **mL**/kg/dose as a single dose within 72 hours of exposure (Watson, 1998); **Note:** Not recommended for routine use; may reduce, but not eliminate, risk for rubella. In adults, injections >10 mL should be split into multiple injections given at different sites.

Stevens-Johnson syndrome (SJS)/toxic epidermal necrolysis (TEN): I.V.: Infants, Children, and Adolescents: Limited data available: Usual dose: 1500 to 2000 mg/kg total dose as a single dose or divided over 2 to 4 days; dosing based on retrospective reviews and case reports; efficacy results are variable, further studies needed (Koh, 2010; Morci 2000; Tristani-Firouzi, 2002)

Varicella-zoster, postexposure prophylaxis (independent of HIV-status): Note: Use only if varicella-zoster immune globulin is unavailable.

I.V.: 400 mg/kg as a single infusion as soon as possible and within 10 days of exposure; ideally within 96 hours of exposure (DHHS [pediatric], 2013; *Red Book*, 2012)

I.M.: GamaSTAN S/D: 0.6 to 1.2 **mL**/kg/dose as a single dose within 72 hours of exposure; **Note:** In adults, injections >10 mL should be split into multiple injections given at different sites; in pediatric patients, consider splitting doses <10 mL based on patient size

Dosing adjustment in renal impairment: Infants, Children, Adolescents, and Adults:

I.V.: Use with caution due to risk of immune globulin-induced renal dysfunction; the rate of infusion and concentration of solution should be minimized.

I.M., SubQ infusion: There are no dosage adjustments provided in the manufacturer's labeling; risk of immune globulin-induced renal dysfunction has not been identified with I.M. and SubQ infusion administration.

Dosing adjustment in hepatic impairment: Infants, Children, Adolescents, and Adults: I.V., I.M., SubQ: There are no dosage adjustments provided in the manufacturer's labeling.

Administration Note: If plasmapheresis employed for treatment of condition, administer immune globulin **after** completion of plasmapheresis session.

I.V.: Infuse over 2 to 24 hours with initial infusion administered slowly and titrated as tolerated; administer in separate infusion line from other medications; if using primary line, flush with NS or D_5W (product specific; consult product prescribing information) prior to administration. Decrease dose, rate, and/or concentration of infusion in patients who may be at risk of renal failure. Decreasing the rate or stopping the infusion may help relieve some adverse effects (flushing, changes in pulse rate, changes in blood pressure). Epinephrine should be available during administration.

For initial treatment or in the elderly, a lower concentration and/or a slower rate of infusion should be used. Initial rate of administration and titration is specific to each IVIG product. Refrigerated product should be warmed to room temperature prior to infusion. Some products require filtration; refer to individual product labeling. Antecubital veins should be used, especially with concentrations ≥10% to prevent injection site discomfort.

Bivigam 10%: Primary humoral immunodeficiency: Initial (first 10 minutes): 0.5 mg/kg/minute (0.3 **mL**/kg/**hour**); Maintenance: Increase every 20 minutes (if tolerated) by 0.8 mg/kg/minute (0.48 **mL**/kg/**hour**) up to 6 mg/kg/minute (3.6 **mL**/kg/**hour**)

Carimune NF: Initial: 0.5 mg/kg/minute; Maintenance: Increase in 30 minutes (if tolerated) to 1 mg/kg/minute, if tolerated after 30 minutes, may increase gradually up to 3 mg/kg/minute; rate in mL/kg/hour varies based on concentration; refer to product labeling

Flebogamma DIF 10%: Primary humoral immunodeficiency: Initial: 1 mg/kg/minute (0.6 **mL**/kg/**hour**); Maintenance: Increase slowly (if tolerated) up to 8 mg/kg/minute (4.8 **mL**/kg/**hour**)

Gammagard Liquid 10%:

Multifocal motor neuropathy (MMN): Initial: 0.8 mg/kg/minute (0.5 **mL**/kg/**hour**); Maintenance: Increase gradually (if tolerated) up to 9 mg/kg/minute (5.4 **mL**/kg/**hour**)

Primary humoral immunodeficiency: Initial (first 30 minutes): 0.8 mg/kg/minute (0.5 **mL**/kg/**hour**); Maintenance: Increase every 30 minutes (if tolerated) up to 8 mg/kg/minute (5 **mL**/kg/**hour**)

Gammagard S/D: 5% solution: Initial: 0.5 **mL**/kg/**hour**; may increase (if tolerated) to a maximum rate of 4 **mL**/kg/**hour**. If 5% solution is tolerated at maximum rate, may administer 10% solution with an initial rate of 0.5 **mL**/kg/**hour**; may increase (if tolerated) to a maximum rate of 8 **mL**/kg/**hour**.

[handwritten annotation:] RN: start w/ 0.5 ml/kg/hr maintain up to 8 mL/kg/HR

g/minute (1.2 gradually (if L/kg/hour) P: Initial (first mL/kg/hour); lerated) up to

odeficiency or g/minute (0.6 se every 15 nute (4.8 **mL**/

CIDP: Initial (first 30 minutes): 2 mg/kg/minute (1.2 **mL**/kg/**hour**); Maintenance: Increase gradually (if tolerated) up to 8 mg/kg/minute (4.8 **mL**/kg/**hour**)

Primary humoral immunodeficiency or ITP: Initial (first 30 minutes): 1 mg/kg/minute (0.6 **mL**/kg/**hour**); Maintenance: Increase gradually (if tolerated) up to 8 mg/kg/minute (4.8 **mL**/kg/**hour**)

Octagam 5%: Primary humoral immunodeficiency: Initial (first 30 minutes): 0.5 mg/kg/minute (0.6 **mL**/kg/**hour**); Maintenance: Double infusion rate (if tolerated) every 30 minutes up to a maximum rate of <3.33 mg/kg/minute (4.2 **mL**/kg/**hour**)

Privigen 10%:

ITP: Initial: 0.5 mg/kg/minute (0.3 **mL**/kg/**hour**); Maintenance: Increase gradually (if tolerated) up to 4 mg/kg/minute (2.4 **mL**/kg/**hour**)

Primary humoral immunodeficiency: Initial: 0.5 mg/kg/minute (0.3 **mL**/kg/**hour**); Maintenance: Increase

gradually (if tolerated) up to 8 mg/kg/minute (4.8 **mL**/kg/**hour**)

I.M.: Administer I.M. in the anterolateral aspects of the upper thigh or deltoid muscle of the upper arm. Avoid gluteal region due to risk of injury to sciatic nerve. Divide doses >10 mL (adult) and inject in multiple sites; in pediatric patients, consider splitting doses <10 mL based on patient size.

SubQ infusion: Initial dose should be administered in a healthcare setting capable of providing monitoring and treatment in the event of hypersensitivity. Using aseptic technique, follow the infusion device manufacturer's instructions for filling the reservoir and preparing the pump. Remove air from administration set and needle by priming. Appropriate injection sites include the abdomen, thigh, upper arm, lateral hip, and/or lower back; dose may be infused into multiple sites (spaced ≥2 inches apart) simultaneously. After administration sites are clean and dry, attach infusion device (eg, primed needle and administration set); ensure blood vessel has not been inadvertently accessed; if blood is present, remove and discard needle and tubing; repeat process using a new needle and tubing and different injection site. Repeat for each administration site; deliver the dose following instructions for the infusion device. Rotate the site(s) weekly. Treatment may be transitioned to the home/home care setting in the absence of adverse reactions.

Gammagard Liquid:

Injection sites: ≤8 simultaneous injection sites

Recommended infusion rate:

<40 kg (<88 lbs): Initial infusion: 15 mL/hour per injection site; subsequent infusions: 15 to 20 mL/hour per injection site; maximum: 160 mL/hour for all simultaneous sites combined

≥40 kg (≥88 lbs): Initial infusion: 20 mL/hour per injection site; subsequent infusions: 20 to 30 mL/hour per injection site; maximum: 240 mL/hour for all simultaneous sites combined

Maximum infusion volume:

<40 kg (<88 lbs): 20 mL per injection site

≥40 kg (≥88 lbs): 30 mL per injection site

Gammaked, Gamunex-C:

Injection sites: ≤8 simultaneous injection sites

Recommended infusion rate: 20 mL/hour per injection site

Hizentra:

Injection sites:

Weekly dosing: ≤4 simultaneous injection sites **or** ≤12 sites consecutively per infusion

Biweekly dosing: Increase the number of injection sites as needed

Maximum infusion rate: First infusion: 15 mL/hour per injection site; subsequent infusions: 25 mL/hour per injection site

Maximum infusion volume: First 4 infusions: 15 mL per injection site; subsequent infusions: 20 mL per injection site; maximum: 25 mL per site as tolerated

Monitoring Parameters Renal function, urine output, IgG concentrations, hemoglobin and hematocrit, platelets (in patients with ITP); infusion- or injection-related adverse reactions, anaphylaxis, signs and symptoms of hemolysis; blood viscosity (in patients at risk for hyperviscosity); presence of antineutrophil antibodies (if TRALI is suspected); volume status; neurologic symptoms (if aseptic meningitis syndrome suspected); clinical response (as defined by disease state)

For patients at high risk of hemolysis (dose ≥2000 mg/kg, given as a single dose or divided over several days, and non-O blood type): Hemoglobin or hematocrit prior to and 36 to 96 hours postinfusion

SubQ infusion: Monitor IgG trough levels every 2 to 3 months before/after conversion from I.V.; subcutaneous infusions provide more constant IgG levels than usual I.V. immune globulin treatments

Test Interactions Octagam contains maltose. Falsely-elevated blood glucose levels may occur when glucose monitoring devices and test strips utilizing the glucose dehydrogenase pyrroloquinolinequinone (GDH-PQQ) based methods are used. Glucose monitoring devices and test strips which utilize the glucose-specific method are recommended. Passively-transferred antibodies may yield false-positive serologic testing results; may yield false-positive direct and indirect Coombs' test. Skin testing should not be performed with GamaSTAN S/D as local chemical irritation can occur and be misinterpreted as a positive reaction.

Additional Information

I.M.: When administering immune globulin for hepatitis A prophylaxis, use should be considered for the following close contacts of persons with confirmed hepatitis A: Unvaccinated household and sexual contacts, persons who have shared illicit drugs, regular babysitters, staff and attendees of child care centers, food handlers within the same establishment (CDC, 2006).

DIF: Dual inactivation plus nanofiltration

NF: Nanofiltered

S/D: Solvent detergent treated

Octagam contains sodium 30 mmol/L.

IgA content:

Bivigam: ≤200 mcg/mL

Carimune NF: Manufacturer's labeling: Trace amounts; others have reported 1000-2000 mcg/mL in a 6% solution (Siegel, 2011)

Flebogamma 5% DIF: <50 mcg/mL

Flebogamma 10% DIF: <100 mcg/mL

Gammagard Liquid: 37 mcg/mL

Gammagard S/D 5% solution: <1 mcg/mL or <2.2 mcg/mL (product dependent) (see **Note**)

Gammaked: 46 mcg/mL

Gammaplex: <10 mcg/mL

Gamunex-C: 46 mcg/mL

Hizentra: ≤50 mcg/mL

Octagam: ≤200 mcg/mL

Privigen: ≤25 mcg/mL

Note: Manufacturer has discontinued Gammagard S/D 5% solution; however, the lower IgA product will remain available by special request for patients with known reaction to IgA or IgA deficiency with antibodies.

Dosage Forms Excipient information presented when available (limited, particularly for generics); consult specific product labeling.

Injectable, Intramuscular [preservative free]:

GamaSTAN S/D: 15% to 18% [150 to 180 mg/mL] (2 mL, 10 mL)

Solution, Injection:

Gamunex-C: 1 g/10 mL (10 mL); 2.5 g/25 mL (25 mL); 5 g/50 mL (50 mL); 10 g/100 mL (100 mL); 20 g/200 mL (200 mL) [latex free]

Solution, Injection [preservative free]:

Gammagard: 1 g/10 mL (10 mL); 2.5 g/25 mL (25 mL); 5 g/50 mL (50 mL); 10 g/100 mL (100 mL); 20 g/200 mL (200 mL); 30 g/300 mL (300 mL) [latex free]

Gammaked: 1 g/10 mL (10 mL); 2.5 g/25 mL (25 mL); 5 g/50 mL (50 mL); 10 g/100 mL (100 mL); 20 g/200 mL (200 mL) [latex free]

Solution, Intravenous:

Flebogamma: 0.5 g/10 mL (10 mL)

Flebogamma DIF: 0.5 g/10 mL (10 mL); 2.5 g/50 mL (50 mL); 5 g/100 mL (100 mL)

Flebogamma DIF: 5 g/50 mL (50 mL) [contains polyethylene glycol]

Flebogamma DIF: 10 g/200 mL (200 mL)

Flebogamma DIF: 10 g/100 mL (100 mL) [contains polyethylene glycol]

Flebogamma DIF: 20 g/400 mL (400 mL)

Flebogamma DIF: 20 g/200 mL (200 mL) [contains polyethylene glycol]

Octagam: 1 g/20 mL (20 mL); 2.5 g/50 mL (50 mL); 5 g/100 mL (100 mL); 10 g/200 mL (200 mL); 25 g/500 mL (500 mL)

Octagam: 1 g/20 mL (20 mL); 5 g/100 mL (100 mL); 10 g/200 mL (200 mL) [sucrose free]

Solution, Intravenous [preservative free]:

Bivigam: 5 g/50 mL (50 mL); 10 g/100 mL (100 mL) [sugar free; contains polysorbate 80]

Gammaplex: 2.5 g/50 mL (50 mL, 400 mL); 5 g/100 mL (100 mL); 10 g/200 mL (200 mL); 20 g/400 mL (400 mL) [contains polysorbate 80]

Privigen: 5 g/50 mL (50 mL); 10 g/100 mL (100 mL); 20 g/200 mL (200 mL); 40 g/400 mL (400 mL)

Solution, Subcutaneous [preservative free]:

Hizentra: 10 g/50 mL (50 mL) [contains polysorbate 80]

Hizentra 20%: 1 g/5 mL (5 mL); 2 g/10 mL (10 mL); 4 g/20 mL (20 mL) [contains polysorbate 80]

Solution Reconstituted, Intravenous:

Carimune NF: 3 g (1 ea); 6 g (1 ea); 12 g (1 ea)

Gammagard S/D: 2.5 g (1 ea); 5 g (1 ea); 10 g (1 ea)

Solution Reconstituted, Intravenous [preservative free]:

Gammagard S/D Less IgA: 5 g (1 ea); 10 g (1 ea)

[handwritten annotation: 5g/10g reconstituted]

References

Abougergi MS [...] Treatment of [...] 2011, 56(1):1[...]

Advisory Comm[...] Wasley A, et a[...] Immunization [...] Immunization [...] (RR-7):1-23.

Alade SL, Brov[...] Toxicity," Ped[...]

American Acad[...] Kimberlin DW [...] tee on Infecti[...] Academy of [...]

American Acad[...] "Management[...] Weeks of Gestation," Pediatrics, 2004, 114(1):297-316.

Anderson D, Ali K, Blanchette V, et al, "Guidelines on the Use of Intravenous Immune Globulin for Hematologic Conditions," Transfus Med Rev, 2007, 21(2 Suppl 1):9-56.

ASHP Commission on Therapeutics, "ASHP Therapeutic Guidelines for Intravenous Immune Globulin," Am J Hosp Pharm, 1992, 49(3):652-4.

Bassan H and Spirer Z, "Intravenous Immunoglobulin in Neonatal Myasthenia Gravis," J Pediatr, 1999, 135(6):790.

Bassan H, Muhlbaur B, Tomer A, et al, "High-Dose Intravenous Immunoglobulin in Transient Neonatal Myasthenia Gravis," Pediatr Neurol, 1998, 18(2):181-3.

Bivigam (immune globulin intravenous human]) [prescribing information]. Boca Raton, FL: Biotest Pharmaceuticals Corp; June 2013.

Blanchette VS, Luke B, Andrew M, et al, "A Prospective Randomized Trial of High-Dose Intravenous Immune Globulin G Therapy, Oral Prednisone Therapy, and No Therapy in Childhood Acute Immune Thrombocytopenic Purpura," J Pediatr, 1993, 123(6):989-95.

Bonilla FA, Bernstein IL, Khan DA, et al. Practice parameter for the diagnosis and management of primary immunodeficiency. Ann Allergy Asthma Immunol. 2005;94(5 Suppl 1):S1-63.

British Committee for Standards in Haematology General Haematology Task Force, "Guidelines for the Investigation and Management of Idiopathic Thrombocytopenic Purpura in Adults, Children and in Pregnancy," Br J Haematol, 2003, 120(4):574-96.

Carimune (immune globulin intravenous [human]) [prescribing information]. Kankakee, IL: CSL Behring AG; September 2013.

Centers for Disease Control and Prevention (CDC). Prevention of hepatitis A through active or passive immunization: recommendations of the Advisory Committee on Immunization Practices (ACIP). MMWR Recomm Rep. 2006;55(RR-7):1-23.

Centers for Disease Control and Prevention (CDC), "Prevention of Measles, Rubella, Congenital Rubella Syndrome, and Mumps, 2013: Summary Recommendations of the Advisory Committee on Immunization Practices (ACIP)," MMWR Recomm Rep, 2013;62(RR-04):1-34.

Centers for Disease Control and Prevention. Unusual syndrome with fatalities among premature infants: association with a new intravenous vitamin E product. MMWR. 1984;33(14):198-199.

Centers for Disease Control and Prevention (CDC), "Update: Prevention of Hepatitis A After Exposure to Hepatitis A Virus and in International Travelers. Updated Recommendations of the Advisory

Committee on Immunization Practices (ACIP)," *MMWR Morb Mortal Wkly Rep*, 2007, 56(41):1080-4.

Cherin P and Herson S, "Indications for Intravenous Gammaglobulin Therapy in Inflammatory Myopathies," *J Neurol Neurosurg Psychiatry*, 1994, (57): 50-4.

Dalakas MC and Hohlfeld R, "Polymyositis and Dermatomyositis," *Lancet*, 2003, 362(9388):971-82.

Dalakas MC, Illa I, Dambrosia JM, et al, "A Controlled Trial of High-Dose Intravenous Immune Globulin Infusions as Treatment for Dermatomyositis," *N Engl J Med*, 1993, 329(27):1993-2000.

Dalakas MC, "Intravenous Immunoglobulin In Autoimmune Neuromuscular Diseases," *JAMA*, 2004, 291(19):2367-75.

DHHS. Guidelines for the prevention and treatment of opportunistic infections among HIV-exposed and HIV-infected children: recommendations from the National Institutes of Health, Centers for Disease Control and Prevention, the HIV Medicine Association of the Infectious Diseases Society of America, the Pediatric Infectious Diseases Society, and the American Academy of Pediatrics. November 6, 2013. Available at http://aidsinfo.nih.gov

Drucker NA, Colan SD, Lewis AB, et al, "Gamma-Globulin Treatment of Acute Myocarditis in the Pediatric Population," *Circulation*, 1994, 89 (1):252-7.

Eijkhout HW, van Der Meer JW, Kallenberg CG, et al, "The Effect of Two Different Dosages of Intravenous Immunoglobulin on the Incidence of Recurrent Infections In Patients With Primary Hypogammaglobulinemia. A Randomized, Double-Blind, Multicenter Crossover Trial," *Ann Intern Med*, 2001, 135(3):165-74.

English RF, Janosky JE, Ettedgui JA, et al, "Outcomes for Children With Acute Myocarditis," *Cardiol Young*, 2004, 14(5):488-93.

FDA Safety Communication: updated information on the risks of thrombosis and hemolysis potentially related to administration of intravenous, subcutaneous and intramuscular human immune globulin products. November, 13, 2012. Available at http://www.fda.gov/BiologicsBloodVaccines/SafetyAvailability/ucm327934.htm?source=govdelivery ljb

Feasby T, Banwell B, Benstead T, et al, "Guidelines on the Use of Intravenous Immune Globulin for Neurologic Conditions," *Transfus Med Rev*, 2007, 21(2 Suppl 1):57-107.

Flebogamma 5% DIF (immune globulin intravenous [human]) [prescribing information]. Los Angeles, CA: Grifols Biologicals Inc; September 2013.

Flebogamma 10% DIF (immune globulin intravenous [human]) [prescribing information]. Los Angeles, CA: Grifols Biologicals Inc; September 2013.

GamaSTAN S/D (immune globulin intravenous [human]) [prescribing information]. Research Triangle Park, NC: Grifols Therapeutics Inc; September 2013.

Gammagard Liquid (immune globulin intravenous [human]) [prescribing information]. Westlake Village, CA: Baxter Healthcare Corporation; September 2013.

Gammagard S/D 1 mcg (immune globulin intravenous [human]) [prescribing information]. Deerfield, IL: Baxter Healthcare Corp; September 2013.

Gammagard S/D 2.2 mcg (immune globulin intravenous [human]) [prescribing information]. Deerfield, IL: Baxter Healthcare Corp; September 2013.

Gammaked (immune globulin intravenous [human]) [prescribing information]. Fort Lee, NJ: Kedrion Biopharma, Inc; September 2013.

Gammaplex (immune globulin intravenous [human]) [prescribing information]. Raleigh, NC: BPL, Inc; September 2013.

Gamunex-C (immune globulin intravenous [human]) [prescribing information]. Research Triangle Park, NC: Grifols Therapeutics Inc; September 2013.

Girish G, Chawla D, Agarwal R, et al, "Efficacy of Two Dose Regimes of Intravenous Immunoglobulin in Rh Hemolytic Disease of Newborn--a Randomized Controlled Trial," *Indian Pediatr*, 2008, 45(8):653-9.

Gottstein R and Cooke RW, "Systematic Review of Intravenous Immunoglobulin in Haemolytic Disease of the Newborn," *Arch Dis Child Fetal Neonatal Ed*, 2003, 88(1):F6-10.

Gurcan HM and Ahmed AR, "Efficacy of Various Intravenous Immunoglobulin Therapy Protocols in Autoimmune and Chronic Inflammatory Disorders," *Ann Pharmacother*, 2007, 41(5):812-23.

Hia CP, Yip WC, Tai BC, et al, "Immunosuppressive Therapy in Acute Myocarditis: An 18 Year Systematic Review," *Arch Dis Child*, 2004, 89 (6):580-4.

Hizentra (immune globulin intravenous [human]) [prescribing information]. Kankakee, IL: CSL Behring AG; September 2013.

Hughes RA, Raphael JC, Swan AV, et al, "Intravenous Immunoglobulin for Guillain-Barre Syndrome," *Cochrane Database of Systematic Reviews*, 2008, issue 2.

Hughes RA, Wijdicks EF, Barohn R, et al, "Practice Parameter: Immunotherapy for Guillain-Barré Syndrome: Report of the Quality Standards Subcommittee of the American Academy of Neurology," *Neurology*, 2003, 61(6):736-40.

INIS Collaborative Group, Brocklehurst P, Farrell B, et al, "Treatment of Neonatal Sepsis With Intravenous Immune Globulin," *N Engl J Med*, 2011, 365(13):1201-11.

Jenson HB and Pollock BH, "Meta-Analyses of the Effectiveness of Intravenous Immune Globulin for Prevention and Treatment of Neonatal Sepsis," *Pediatrics*, 1997, 99(2):E2.

Klugman D, Berger JT, Sable CA, et al, "Pediatric Patients Hospitalized With Myocarditis: A Multi-institutional Analysis," *Pediatr Cardiol*, 2010, 31(2):222-8.

Koh MJ and Tay YK, "Stevens-Johnson Syndrome and Toxic Epidermal Necrolysis in Asian Children," *J Am Acad Dermatol*, 2010, 62 (1):54-60.

Kuwabara S, "Guillain-Barré Syndrome: Epidemiology, Pathophysiology and Management," *Drugs*, 2004, 64(6):597-610.

Leung DY, Kelly CP, Boguniewicz M, et al, "Treatment With Intravenously Administered Gamma Globulin of Chronic Relapsing Colitis Induced by *Clostridium difficile* Toxin," *J Pediatr*, 1991, 118(4 Pt 1):633-7.

McFarland LV, Brandmarker SA, and Guandalini S, "Pediatric *Clostridium difficile*: A Phantom Menace or Clinical Reality?" *J Pediatr Gastroenterol Nutr*, 2000, 31(3):220-31.

Miqdad AM, Abdelbasit OB, Shaheed MM, et al, "Intravenous Immunoglobulin G (IVIG) Therapy for Significant Hyperbilirubinemia in ABO Hemolytic Disease of the Newborn," *J Matern Fetal Neonatal Med*, 2004, 16(3):163-6.

Morici MV, Galen WK, Shetty AK, et al, "Intravenous Immunoglobulin Therapy for Children With Stevens-Johnson Syndrome," *J Rheumatol*, 2000, 27(10):2494-7.

Newburger JW, Takahashi M, Gerber MA, et al, "Diagnosis, Treatment, and Long-Term Management of Kawasaki Disease: A Statement for Health Professionals From the Committee on Rheumatic Fever, Endocarditis, and Kawasaki Disease, Council on Cardiovascular Disease in the Young, American Heart Association," *Pediatrics*, 2004, 114(6):1708-33.

NIH Consensus Conference, "Intravenous Immunoglobulin, Prevention and Treatment of Disease," *JAMA*, 1990, 264(24):3189-93.

Octagam (immune globulin intravenous [human]) [prescribing information]. Hoboken, NJ: Octapharma USA Inc; September 2013.

Ohlsson A and Lacy J, "Intravenous Immunoglobulin for Suspected or Subsequently Proven Infection in Neonates," *Cochrane Database Syst Rev*, 2010, (3):CD001239.

Patwa HS, Chaudhry V, Katzberg H, et al, "Evidence-Based Guideline: Intravenous Immunoglobulin in the Treatment of Neuromuscular Disorders: Report of the Therapeutics and Technology Assessment Subcommittee of the American Academy of Neurology," *Neurology*, 2012, 78(13):1009-15.

Privigen (immune globulin intravenous [human]) [prescribing information]. Kankakee, IL: CSL Behring AG; September 2013.

Sansome A and Dubowitz V, "Intravenous Immunoglobulin in Juvenile Dermatomyositis--Four Year Review of Nine Cases," *Arch Dis Child*, 1995, 72(1):25-8.

Siegel J, "Immune Globulins: Therapeutic, Pharmaceutical, Cost and Administration Considerations," *Pharmacy Practice News*, 2011, 20-7.

Siegel J, "Immunoglobulins and Obesity," *Pharmacy Practice News*, 2010, 37:1.

Tagher RJ, Baumann R, and Desai N, "Failure of Intravenously Administered Immunoglobulin in the Treatment of Neonatal Myasthenia Gravis," *J Pediatr*, 1999, 134(2):233-5.

Tomblyn M, Chiller T, Einsele H, et al, "Guidelines for Preventing Infectious Complications Among Hematopoietic Cell Transplantation Recipients: A Global Perspective," *Biol Blood Marrow Transplant*, 2009, 15(10):1143-238.

Tristani-Firouzi P, Petersen MJ, Saffle JR, et al, "Treatment of Toxic Epidermal Necrolysis With Intravenous Immunoglobulin in Children," *J Am Acad Dermatol*, 2002, 47(4):548-52.

"University Hospital Consortium Expert Panel for Off-Label Use of Polyvalent Intravenously Administered Immunoglobulin Preparations Consensus Statement," *JAMA*, 1995, 273(23):1865-70.

Watson JC, Hadler SC, Dykewicz CA, et al, "Measles, Mumps, and Rubella – Vaccine Use and Strategies for Elimination of Measles, Rubella, and Congenital Rubella Syndrome and Control of Mumps: Recommendations of the Advisory Committee on Immunization Practices (ACIP)," *MMWR Recomm Rep*, 1998, 47(RR-8):1-57.

Wimperis J, Lunn M, Jones A, et al, "National Health Service. Clinical Guidelines for the Use of Immunoglobulin Use: Second Edition Update, July 2011.

◆ **Immune Globulin Subcutaneous (Human)** *see* Immune Globulin *on page 1084*

◆ **Immune Serum Globulin** *see* Immune Globulin *on page 1084*

◆ **Immunine® VH (Can)** *see* Factor IX (Human) *on page 835*

◆ **Imodium® (Can)** *see* Loperamide *on page 1270*

◆ **Imodium A-D [OTC]** *see* Loperamide *on page 1270*

- ◆ **Imogam Rabies-HT** *see* Rabies Immune Globulin (Human) *on page 1800*
- ◆ **Imogam Rabies Pasteurized (Can)** *see* Rabies Immune Globulin (Human) *on page 1800*
- ◆ **Imovax® Polio (Can)** *see* Poliovirus Vaccine (Inactivated) *on page 1694*
- ◆ **Imovax Rabies** *see* Rabies Vaccine *on page 1801*
- ◆ **Impril (Can)** *see* Imipramine *on page 1080*
- ◆ **Imuran** *see* AzaTHIOprine *on page 241*
- ◆ **Inactivated Influenza Vaccine, Quadrivalent** *see* Influenza Virus Vaccine (Inactivated) *on page 1103*
- ◆ **Inactivated Influenza Vaccine, Trivalent** *see* Influenza Virus Vaccine (Inactivated) *on page 1103*
- ◆ **Increlex** *see* Mecasermin *on page 1313*
- ◆ **Inderal (Can)** *see* Propranolol *on page 1759*
- ◆ **Inderal XL** *see* Propranolol *on page 1759*
- ◆ **Inderal LA** *see* Propranolol *on page 1759*

Indinavir (in DIN a veer)

Medication Safety Issues
Sound-alike/look-alike issues:
Indinavir may be confused with Denavir®
Related Information
Adult and Adolescent HIV *on page 2348*
Oral Medications That Should Not Be Crushed or Altered *on page 2438*
Pediatric HIV *on page 2338*
Perinatal HIV *on page 2356*
Brand Names: U.S. Crixivan
Brand Names: Canada Crixivan®
Therapeutic Category Antiretroviral Agent; HIV Agents (Anti-HIV Agents); Protease Inhibitor
Generic Availability (U.S.) No
Use Treatment of HIV infection in combination with other antiretroviral agents; **Note:** HIV regimens consisting of **three** antiretroviral agents are strongly recommended (FDA approved in adults)
Pregnancy Risk Factor C
Pregnancy Considerations Adverse events were observed in some animal reproduction studies. Placental passage in humans is minimal. No increased risk of overall birth defects has been observed according to data collected by the antiretroviral pregnancy registry. A small increased risk of preterm birth has been associated with maternal use of protease inhibitor-based combination antiretroviral (ARV) therapy during pregnancy; however, the benefits of use generally outweigh this risk and protease inhibitors (PIs) should not be withheld if otherwise recommended. Hyperglycemia, new onset of diabetes mellitus, or diabetic ketoacidosis have been reported with PIs; it is not clear if pregnancy increases this risk. Hyperbilirubinemia may occur in neonates following *in utero* exposure to indinavir. Plasma concentrations of unboosted indinavir are decreased during pregnancy. Until optimal dosing during pregnancy has been established, the manufacturer does not recommend indinavir use in pregnant patients. The DHHS Perinatal HIV Guidelines do not recommend indinavir for initial therapy in antiretroviral-naïve pregnant women due to concerns regarding maternal kidney stones or neonatal hyperbilirubinemia; if needed, must be used in combination with low-dose ritonavir boosting during pregnancy.

Regardless of CD4 count or HIV RNA copy number, all HIV-infected pregnant women should receive a combination antiretroviral ARV drug regimen. A combination of antepartum, intrapartum, and infant ARV prophylaxis is recommended. ARV therapy should be started as soon as possible in women with symptomatic infection. Although earlier initiation may be more effective in reducing the perinatal transmission of HIV, initiation may be delayed until after 12 weeks gestation in women who do not require immediate treatment after careful consideration of maternal conditions (eg, nausea and vomiting) and the potential risks of first trimester fetal exposure for specific agents. A scheduled cesarean delivery at 38 weeks gestation is recommended for all women with HIV RNA >1000 copies/mL or unknown concentrations near delivery in order to decrease transmission. If ARV therapy must be interrupted for <24 hours during the peripartum period, stop then restart all medications simultaneously in order to decrease the chance of developing resistance. Long-term follow-up is recommended for all infants exposed to ARV medications. In couples who want to conceive, the HIV-infected partner should attain maximum viral suppression prior to conception.

Healthcare providers are encouraged to enroll pregnant women exposed to antiretroviral medications in the Antiretroviral Pregnancy Registry (1-800-258-4263 or www.APRegistry.com). Healthcare providers caring for HIV-infected women and their infants may contact the National Perinatal HIV Hotline (888-448-8765) for clinical consultation (DHHS [perinatal], 2014).
Breast-Feeding Considerations It is not known if indinavir is excreted into breast milk. Maternal or infant antiretroviral therapy does not completely eliminate the risk of postnatal HIV transmission. In addition, multiclass-resistant virus has been detected in breast-feeding infants despite maternal therapy. Therefore, in the United States, where formula is accessible, affordable, safe, and sustainable, and the risk of infant mortality due to diarrhea and respiratory infections is low, complete avoidance of breast-feeding by HIV-infected women is recommended to decrease potential transmission of HIV (DHHS [perinatal], 2014).
Contraindications Hypersensitivity to indinavir or any component; concurrent therapy with alfuzosin, alprazolam, amiodarone, cisapride, dihydroergotamine, ergonovine, ergotamine, methylergonovine, lovastatin, oral midazolam, pimozide, simvastatin, sildenafil [for treatment of pulmonary arterial hypertension (eg, Revatio)], triazolam
Warnings Indinavir is a CYP3A4 isoenzyme inhibitor that interacts with numerous drugs. Due to potential serious and/or life-threatening drug interactions, some drugs are contraindicated. Concurrent use with atazanavir, rifampin, or St John's wort is **not** recommended. Alteration of dose or serum concentration monitoring may be required with other medications.

Cases of nephrolithiasis, urolithiasis (children: 29%; adults: 12.4%), and nephrolithiasis associated with renal insufficiency, acute renal failure, or pyelonephritis with or without bacteremia have been reported. In pediatric patients, sterile leukocyturia (with possible elevations in serum creatinine) has been reported without clinical symptoms of nephrolithiasis. Maintain adequate hydration in all patients to minimize risk. If signs and symptoms of nephrolithiasis occur (flank pain with or without hematuria or microscopic hematuria), temporarily interrupt or discontinue therapy. Tubulointerstitial nephritis with medullary calcification and cortical atrophy has been reported in patients with asymptomatic severe leukocyturia; consider discontinuation of indinavir in patients with severe leukocyturia.

Hepatitis, including hepatic failure and death, has been reported (causal relationship not established). Spontaneous bleeding episodes have been reported in patients with hemophilia A and B. New onset diabetes mellitus, exacerbation of diabetes and hyperglycemia have been reported in HIV-infected patients receiving protease inhibitors. ▶

Acute hemolytic anemia has been reported. Indirect hyperbilirubinemia (incidence: ~14%) and elevated serum transaminases may occur. Not recommended for use in neonates due to risk of hyperbilirubinemia and kernicterus (DHHS [pediatric], 2014).

Precautions Use with caution in patients with hepatic impairment; modify dose in patients with impaired liver function. Use of indinavir in HIV-infected pregnant patients is **not** recommended; significantly lower serum concentrations were observed in these patients receiving standard adult doses; optimal dose is not currently known.

Immune reconstitution syndrome (an acute inflammatory response to residual or indolent opportunistic infections) may occur in HIV patients during initial treatment with combination antiretroviral agents; this syndrome may require further patient assessment and therapy. Autoimmune disorders (eg, Graves' disease, Guillain-Barré syndrome, and polymyositis) have been reported in patients experiencing immune reconstitution; time to onset is variable and may occur many months after antiretroviral treatment is initiated.

Fat redistribution and accumulation [ie, central obesity, peripheral wasting, facial wasting, breast enlargement, dorsocervical fat enlargement (buffalo hump), and cushingoid appearance] have been observed in patients receiving antiretroviral agents (causal relationship not established).

Adverse Reactions
Central nervous system: Dizziness, fatigue, fever, headache, malaise, somnolence
Dermatologic: Pruritus, rash
Endocrine & metabolic: Hyperglycemia
Gastrointestinal: Abdominal pain, acid reflux, anorexia, appetite increased, diarrhea, dyspepsia, nausea, serum amylase increased, taste perversion, vomiting
Hematologic: Anemia, neutropenia, thrombocytopenia
Hepatic: Hyperbilirubinemia (dose dependent), jaundice, transaminases increased
Neuromuscular & skeletal: Back pain, weakness
Renal: Dysuria, nephrolithiasis/urolithiasis, including flank pain with/without hematuria (dose dependent)
Respiratory: Cough
Rare but important or life-threatening: Abdominal distention, acute renal failure, alopecia, anaphylactoid reactions, angina, arthralgia, bleeding (spontaneous in patients with hemophilia A or B), cerebrovascular disorder, cholesterol increased, crystalluria, depression, dry skin, erythema multiforme, fat redistribution, hemolytic anemia, hepatic failure, hepatitis, hydronephrosis, hyperpigmentation, immune reconstitution syndrome, interstitial nephritis (with medullary calcification and cortical atrophy), leukocyturia (severe and asymptomatic), MI, new-onset diabetes, pancreatitis, paresthesia (oral), paronychia, pharyngitis, pyelonephritis, QT prolongation, renal insufficiency, renal failure, Stevens-Johnson syndrome, torsade de pointes, triglycerides increased, upper respiratory infection, urticaria, vasculitis

Drug Interactions
Metabolism/Transport Effects Substrate of CYP2D6 (minor), CYP3A4 (major), P-glycoprotein; **Note:** Assignment of Major/Minor substrate status based on clinically relevant drug interaction potential; **Inhibits** CYP2C19 (weak), CYP2C9 (weak), CYP2D6 (weak), CYP3A4 (strong)

Avoid Concomitant Use
Avoid concomitant use of Indinavir with any of the following: Ado-Trastuzumab Emtansine; Alfuzosin; ALPRAZolam; Amiodarone; Apixaban; Atazanavir; Avanafil; Axitinib; Bosutinib; Cabozantinib; Ceritinib; Cisapride; Conivaptan; Crizotinib; Dronedarone; Eplerenone; Ergot Derivatives; Everolimus; Halofantrine; Ibrutinib; Ivabradine; Lapatinib; Lomitapide; Lovastatin; Lurasidone;

Macitentan; Midazolam; Nilotinib; Nisoldipine; Pimozide; QuiNIDine; Ranolazine; Red Yeast Rice; Regorafenib; Rifampin; Rivaroxaban; Salmeterol; Silodosin; Simeprevir; Simvastatin; St Johns Wort; Tamsulosin; Ticagrelor; Tipranavir; Tolvaptan; Toremifene; Triazolam; Ulipristal; Vemurafenib; VinCRIStine (Liposomal); Vorapaxar

Increased Effect/Toxicity
Indinavir may increase the levels/effects of: Ado-Trastuzumab Emtansine; Alfuzosin; Almotriptan; Alosetron; ALPRAZolam; Amiodarone; Apixaban; ARIPiprazole; Atazanavir; AtorvaSTATin; Avanafil; Axitinib; Bedaquiline; Bortezomib; Bosentan; Bosutinib; Brentuximab Vedotin; Brinzolamide; Budesonide (Nasal); Budesonide (Systemic, Oral Inhalation); Cabozantinib; Calcium Channel Blockers (Dihydropyridine); Calcium Channel Blockers (Nondihydropyridine); Cannabis; CarBAMazepine; Ceritinib; Cisapride; Clarithromycin; Colchicine; Conivaptan; Corticosteroids (Orally Inhaled); Crizotinib; Cyclophosphamide; CycloSPORINE (Systemic); CYP3A4 Substrates; Dienogest; Digoxin; Dofetilide; DOXOrubicin (Conventional); Dronabinol; Dronedarone; Dutasteride; Enfuvirtide; Eplerenone; Ergot Derivatives; Everolimus; FentaNYL; Fesoterodine; Fluticasone (Nasal); Fluticasone (Oral Inhalation); GuanFACINE; Halofantrine; Ibrutinib; Iloperidone; Imatinib; Itraconazole; Ivabradine; Ivacaftor; Ixabepilone; Ketoconazole (Systemic); Lacosamide; Lapatinib; Levomilnacipran; Lomitapide; Lovastatin; Lumefantrine; Lurasidone; Macitentan; Maraviroc; Meperidine; MethylPREDNISolone; Midazolam; Mifepristone; Nefazodone; Nilotinib; Nisoldipine; Ospemifene; OxyCODONE; Paricalcitol; PAZOPanib; Pimecrolimus; Pimozide; PONATinib; Propafenone; Protease Inhibitors; QUEtiapine; QuiNIDine; Ranolazine; Red Yeast Rice; Regorafenib; Repaglinide; Rifabutin; Rilpivirine; Riociguat; Rivaroxaban; RomiDEPsin; Rosuvastatin; Ruxolitinib; Salmeterol; Saxagliptin; Sildenafil; Silodosin; Simeprevir; Simvastatin; SORAfenib; Tacrolimus (Systemic); Tacrolimus (Topical); Tadalafil; Tamsulosin; Temsirolimus; Tetrahydrocannabinol; Ticagrelor; Tofacitinib; Tolterodine; Tolvaptan; Toremifene; TraZODone; Triazolam; Tricyclic Antidepressants; Ulipristal; Vardenafil; Vemurafenib; Vilazodone; VinCRIStine (Liposomal); Vorapaxar; Zuclopenthixol

The levels/effects of Indinavir may be increased by: Atazanavir; Clarithromycin; CycloSPORINE (Systemic); Delavirdine; Enfuvirtide; Etravirine; Itraconazole; Ketoconazole (Systemic); P-glycoprotein/ABCB1 Inhibitors; Simeprevir

Decreased Effect
Indinavir may decrease the levels/effects of: Abacavir; Boceprevir; Clarithromycin; Delavirdine; Etravirine; Ifosfamide; Meperidine; Prasugrel; Ticagrelor; Valproic Acid and Derivatives; Zidovudine

The levels/effects of Indinavir may be decreased by: Antacids; Atovaquone; Boceprevir; Bosentan; CarBAMazepine; CYP3A4 Inducers (Strong); Dabrafenib; Deferasirox; Didanosine; Efavirenz; Garlic; H2-Antagonists; Mitotane; Nevirapine; Peginterferon Alfa-2b; P-glycoprotein/ABCB1 Inducers; Proton Pump Inhibitors; Rifabutin; Rifampin; Siltuximab; St Johns Wort; Tipranavir; Tocilizumab; Venlafaxine

Food Interactions Indinavir bioavailability may be decreased if taken with food. Meals high in calories, fat, and protein result in a significant decrease in drug levels. Management: Administer with water 1 hour before or 2 hours after a meal. May also be administered with other liquids (eg, skim milk, juice, coffee, tea) or a light meal (eg, toast, corn flakes). Administer around-the-clock to avoid significant fluctuation in serum levels. Drink at least 48 oz of water daily. May be taken with food when administered in combination with ritonavir.

Stability Store at 15°C to 30°C (59°F to 86°F) in original container with desiccant (capsules are sensitive to moisture).

Mechanism of Action Binds to the site of HIV-1 protease activity and inhibits cleavage of viral Gag-Pol polyprotein precursors into individual functional proteins required for infectious HIV. This results in the formation of immature, noninfectious viral particles.

Pharmacokinetics (Adult data unless noted)
Absorption: Rapid (in the fasted state); presence of food high in calories, fat, and protein significantly decreases the extent of absorption
Protein binding: 60%
Metabolism: Hepatic via CYP3A4 to inactive metabolites; 6 oxidative and 1 glucuronide conjugate metabolites have been identified
Bioavailability: Wide interpatient variability in children: 15% to 50%
Half-life:
Children 4 to 17 years (n=18): 1.1 hours
Adults: 1.8 ± 0.4 hours
Adults with mild to moderate hepatic dysfunction: 2.8 ± 0.5 hours
Time to peak serum concentration: 0.8 ± 0.3 hours
Elimination: 83% in feces as unabsorbed drug and metabolites; ~10% excreted in urine as unchanged drug

Dosing: Usual
Pediatric: **HIV infection, treatment:** Oral: Use in combination with other antiretroviral agents:
Children: Limited data available; optimal dose not established: Ritonavir-boosted: Indinavir 400 mg/m^2/dose (maximum: 800 mg) every 12 hour **plus** ritonavir 100 to 125 mg/m^2/dose (maximum 100 mg) every 12 hours; in clinical trials, this dose produced AUCs similar to adult exposure of indinavir 800 mg/ritonavir 100 mg twice daily; however, studies report high rates of inter-individual variability and toxicity in pediatric patients; several other ritonavir-boosted dosing regimens have been evaluated with supratherapeutic (indinavir 500 mg/m^2/dose every 12 hours) and subtherapeutic (indinavir 234 to 250 mg/m^2/dose every 12 hours) indinavir serum concentrations reported (DHHS [pediatric], 2014).
Adolescents:
Unboosted: 800 mg/dose every 8 hours (DHHS [adult, 2014])
Ritonavir-boosted: Indinavir 800 mg **plus** ritonavir 100 to 200 mg twice daily (DHHS [adult, pediatric] 2014)
Adult: **HIV infection, treatment:** Oral: **Note:** Use in combination with other antiretroviral agents (DHHS [adult], 2014):
Unboosted: 800 mg/dose every 8 hours
Ritonavir-boosted: Indinavir 800 mg **plus** ritonavir 100 to 200 mg twice daily

Dosing adjustment for concomitant therapy: Adolescents and Adults: The following are manufacturer labeling recommendations for adults and should also be considered in adolescent patients receiving adult dose (DHHS [adult], 2014)

Concomitant therapy with delavirdine, itraconazole, or ketoconazole: Adolescents and Adults: Reduce indinavir dose to 600 mg every 8 hours

Concomitant therapy with efavirenz or nevirapine: Adolescents and Adults: Increase indinavir dose to 1000 mg every 8 hours

Concomitant therapy with lopinavir and ritonavir (Kaletra): Adolescents and Adults: Reduce indinavir dose to 600 mg twice daily

Concomitant therapy with nelfinavir: Adolescents and Adults: Increase indinavir dose to 1200 mg twice daily

Concomitant therapy with rifabutin: Adolescents and Adults: Increase dose of indinavir to 1000 mg every 8 hours and reduce dose of rifabutin to ½ the standard dose

Dosing adjustment in renal impairment: There are no dosage adjustments provided in the manufacturer's labeling; has not been studied.

Dosing adjustment in hepatic impairment:
Children: No dosing information is available (DHHS [pediatric], 2014)
Adults:
Mild to moderate hepatic impairment: Decrease to 600 mg every 8 hours
Severe hepatic impairment: There are no dosage adjustments provided in the manufacturer's labeling; has not been studied.

Administration Administer with water on an empty stomach or with a light snack 1 hour before or 2 hours after a meal; may administer with other liquids (ie, skim milk, coffee, tea, juice) or a light snack (ie, dry toast with jelly or cornflakes with skim milk). May administer with food if taken in combination with ritonavir (ie, meal restrictions are not required). If coadministered with didanosine, give at least 1 hour apart on an empty stomach. Administer every 8 hours around-the-clock to avoid significant fluctuation in serum levels.

Monitoring Parameters Note: Monitor CD4 percentage (if <5 years of age) or CD4 count (if ≥5 years of age) at least every 3 to 4 months (DHHS [pediatric], 2014).

Prior to initiation of therapy: Genotypic resistance testing, CD4 and viral load (every 3 to 4 months), CBC with differential, LFTs, BUN, creatinine, electrolytes, glucose, urinalysis (every 6 to 12 months), and assessment of readiness for adherence with medication regimen. At initiation and with any change in treatment regimen: CBC with differential, electrolytes, calcium, phosphate, glucose, LFTs, bilirubin, urinalysis (at initiation), BUN, creatinine, albumin, total protein, lipid panel (at initiation), CD4, and viral load. After 1 to 2 weeks of therapy: Signs of medication toxicity and adherence. After 2 to 4 weeks of therapy: CBC with differential, viral load, signs of medication toxicity, and adherence; then every 3 to 4 months: CBC with differential, electrolytes, glucose, LFTs, bilirubin, BUN, creatinine, CD4, viral load, medication toxicity, and adherence. Every 6 to 12 months: Lipid panel and urinalysis. CD4 monitoring frequency may be decreased to every 6 to 12 months in children who are adherent to therapy if the value is well above the threshold for opportunistic infections, viral suppression is sustained, and the clinical status is stable for more than 2 to 3 years (DHHS [pediatric], 2014). Monitor for growth and development, signs of HIV-specific physical conditions, HIV disease progression, opportunistic infections, kidney stones, or pancreatitis.

Reference Range Trough concentration: ≥0.1 mg/L (DHHS [adult, pediatric], 2014)

Additional Information One study in children 4 to 17 years of age (n=18), adjusted the indinavir dose and dosing interval to maintain trough plasma concentrations. A mean daily dose of 2043 mg/m^2 was required with 9 of 18 children requiring doses every 6 hours (Fletcher, 2000). Other pediatric studies have also suggested that every 6 hour dosing may be needed in some children (Gatti, 2000) and that a wide range of doses (1250 to 2450 mg/m^2/day) may be required (van Rossum, 2000a). However, it should be noted that the higher incidence of renal toxicity observed in children versus adults, may preclude studying higher doses of unboosted indinavir.

Two small studies assessed the use of indinavir in combination with ritonavir. One study used doses of indinavir 500 mg/m^2/dose **plus** ritonavir 100 mg/m^2/dose twice daily (n=4; 1 to 10 years of age); one patient attained high concentrations of both drugs and developed renal toxicity (van Rossum, 2000). Another study used doses of indinavir 400 mg/m^2/dose **plus** ritonavir 125 mg/m^2/dose twice daily in children (n=14); AUC and trough concentrations were similar to adults receiving ritonavir boosted doses; however, peak concentrations were slightly decreased (Bergshoeff, 2004). A pediatric clinical trial that used these same doses demonstrated good virologic efficacy; however, 4 of 21 patients developed nephrolithiasis; a high rate of overall side effects and intolerance to the dosing regimen was observed (Fraaij, 2007). Further studies are needed.

Dosage Forms Excipient information presented when available (limited, particularly for generics); consult specific product labeling.

Capsule, Oral:
Crixivan: 200 mg, 400 mg

Extemporaneous Preparations A 10 mg/mL oral solution may be prepared using capsules. First, prepare a 100 mg/mL indinavir concentrate by adding the contents of fifteen 400 mg capsules and 60 mL purified water to a 100 mL amber glass bottle. Place bottle in an ultrasonic bath filled with water at 37°C for 60 minutes, stirring the solution every 10 minutes. Filter solution; wash bottle and filter with 6 mL purified water; cool solution to room temperature. Add 50 mL of 100 mg/mL indinavir concentrate to 360 mL viscous sweet base, 90 mL simple syrup, 1.8 g citric acid, 45 mg azorubine, 0.1M sodium hydroxide solution to pH 3, and 12 drops of lemon oil, to make a final volume of 500 mL. Mix to a uniform solution. Label "refrigerate". Stable for 2 weeks refrigerated.

Hugen PW, Burger DM, ter Hofstede HJ, et al, "Development of an Indinavir Oral Liquid for Children," *Am J Health Syst Pharm*, 2000, 57 (14):1332-9.

References

Bergshoeff AS, Fraaij PL, van Rossum AM, et al. Pharmacokinetics of indinavir combined with low-dose ritonavir in human immunodeficiency virus type 1-infected children. *Antimicrob Agents Chemother.* 2004;48(5):1904-1907.

Curras V, Hocht C, Mangano A, et al. Pharmacokinetic study of the variability of indinavir drug levels when boosted with ritonavir in HIV-infected children. *Pharmacology.* 2009;83:59-66.

DHHS Panel on Antiretroviral Guidelines for Adults and Adolescents. Guidelines for the use of antiretroviral agents in HIV-1-infected adults and adolescents, Department of Health and Human Services. May 1, 2014. Available at http://www.aidsinfo.nih.gov/ContentFiles/AdultandAdolescentGL.pdf

DHHS Panel on Antiretroviral Therapy and Medical Management of HIV-Infected Children. Guidelines for the use of antiretroviral agents in pediatric HIV infection. February 12, 2014. Available at http://aidsinfo.nih.gov

DHHS Panel on Treatment of HIV-Infected Pregnant Women and Prevention of Perinatal Transmission. Recommendations for the use of antiretroviral drugs in pregnant HIV-1-infected women for maternal health and interventions to reduce perinatal HIV-1 transmission in the United States. March 28, 2014. Available at http://aidsinfo.nih.gov

Fletcher CV, Brundage RC, Remmel RP, et al. Pharmacologic characteristics of indinavir, didanosine, and stavudine in human immunodeficiency virus-infected children receiving combination therapy. *Antimicrob Agents Chemother.* 2000;44(4):1029-1034.

Fraaij PL, Verweel G, van Rossum AM, Hartwig NG, Burger DM, de Groot R. Indinavir/low-dose ritonavir containing HAART in HIV-1 infected children has potent antiretroviral activity, but is associated with side effects and frequent discontinuation of treatment. *Infection.* 2007;35(3):186-189.

Gatti G, Vigano' A, Sala N, et al. Indinavir pharmacokinetics and pharmacodynamics in children with human immunodeficiency virus infection. *Antimicrob Agents Chemother.* 2000;44(3):752-755.

Mueller BU, Smith S, Sleasman J, et al. A phase I/II study of the protease inhibitor indinavir (MK-0639) in children with HIV infection. *Eleventh International Conference on AIDS.* Vancouver, Canada; 1996.

Piscitelli SC, Burstein AH, Chaitt D, Alfaro RM, Falloon J. Indinavir concentrations and St John's wort. *Lancet.* 2000;355(9203):547-548.

Stein DS, Fish DG, Bilello JA, Preston SL, Martineau GL, Drusano GL. A 24-week open-label phase I/II evaluation of the HIV protease inhibitor MK-639 (indinavir). *AIDS.* 1996;10(5):485-492.

van Rossum AM, de Groot R, Hartwig NG, Weemaes CM, Head S, Burger DM. Pharmacokinetics of indinavir and low-dose ritonavir in children with HIV-1 infection. *AIDS.* 2000;14(14):2209-2210.

van Rossum AM, Niesters HG, Geelen SP, et al. Clinical and virologic response to combination treatment with indinavir, zidovudine, and lamivudine in children with human immunodeficiency virus-1 infection: a multicenter study in the Netherlands. On behalf of the Dutch Study Group for Children with HIV-1 Infections. *J Pediatr.* 2000;136 (6):780-788.

◆ **Indinavir Sulfate** *see* Indinavir *on page 1093*

◆ **Indocin** *see* Indomethacin *on page 1096*

◆ **Indometacin** *see* Indomethacin *on page 1096*

Indomethacin (in doe METH a sin)

Medication Safety Issues
Sound-alike/look-alike issues:
Indocin may be confused with Imodium, Lincocin, Minocin, Vicodin

BEERS Criteria medication:
This drug may be potentially inappropriate for use in geriatric patients (Quality of evidence - moderate; Strength of recommendation - strong).

Related Information
Oral Medications That Should Not Be Crushed or Altered *on page 2438*

Brand Names: U.S. Indocin

Brand Names: Canada Apo-Indomethacin; Novo-Methacin; Pro-Indo; ratio-Indomethacin; Sandoz-Indomethacin

Therapeutic Category Analgesic, Non-narcotic; Anti-inflammatory Agent; Antipyretic; Nonsteroidal Anti-inflammatory Drug (NSAID), Oral; Nonsteroidal Anti-inflammatory Drug (NSAID), Parenteral

Generic Availability (U.S.) May be product dependent

Use Management of inflammatory diseases and rheumatoid disorders; moderate pain; acute gouty arthritis; I.V. form used as alternative to surgery for closure of patent ductus arteriosus (PDA) in neonates; has also been used for prophylaxis of PDA in VLBW neonates

Medication Guide Available Yes

Pregnancy Risk Factor C (<30 weeks gestation); C/D (≥30 weeks gestation [manufacturer specific])

Pregnancy Considerations Adverse events have been observed in animal reproduction studies; studies in pregnant women have demonstrated risk to the fetus if administered at ≥30 weeks gestation. Indomethacin crosses the placenta and can be detected in fetal plasma and amniotic fluid. Indomethacin exposure during the first trimester is not strongly associated with congenital malformations; however, cardiovascular anomalies and cleft palate have been observed following NSAID exposure in some studies. The use of an NSAID close to conception may be associated with an increased risk of miscarriage. Nonteratogenic effects have been observed following NSAID administration during the third trimester, including myocardial degenerative changes, prenatal constriction of the ductus arteriosus, failure of the ductus arteriosus to close postnatally, and fetal tricuspid regurgitation; renal dysfunction or failure, oligohydramnios; gastrointestinal bleeding or perforation, increased risk of necrotizing enterocolitis; intracranial bleeding (including intraventricular hemorrhage), platelet dysfunction with resultant bleeding; and pulmonary hypertension. The risk of fetal ductal constriction following maternal use of indomethacin is increased with gestational age and duration of therapy. Because they may cause premature closure of the ductus arteriosus, use of NSAIDs late in pregnancy should be avoided (use after 31 or 32 weeks gestation is not recommended by some clinicians). Indomethacin has been used for a short duration (eg, ≤48 hours) in the management of preterm labor.

Indomethacin should be used with caution in pregnant women with hypertension. The chronic use of NSAIDs in women of reproductive age may be associated with infertility that is reversible upon discontinuation of the medication.

Breast-Feeding Considerations Indomethacin is excreted into breast milk and low amounts have been measured in the plasma of nursing infants. Seizures in a nursing infant were observed in one case report, although adverse events have not been noted in other cases. Breast-feeding is not recommended by most manufacturers; Tivorbex may be used with caution during breast-feeding. (The therapeutic use of indomethacin is contraindicated in neonates with significant renal failure.) Hypertensive crisis and psychiatric side effects have been noted in case reports following use of indomethacin for analgesia in postpartum women. Use with caution in nursing women with hypertensive disorders of pregnancy or preexisting renal disease.

Contraindications Hypersensitivity to indomethacin or any component; history of asthma, urticaria, or allergic-type reaction to aspirin, or other NSAIDs; patients with the "aspirin triad" [asthma, rhinitis (with or without nasal polyps), and aspirin intolerance] (fatal asthmatic and anaphylactoid reactions may occur in these patients); perioperative pain in the setting of coronary artery bypass graft (CABG)

Injection is contraindicated in preterm infants with untreated proven or suspected infection; congenital heart disease where patency of the PDA is necessary for pulmonary or systemic blood flow (eg, pulmonary atresia, severe tetralogy of Fallot, severe coarctation of aorta); bleeding (especially with active intracranial hemorrhage or GI bleed); thrombocytopenia; coagulation defects; proven or suspected necrotizing enterocolitis (NEC); significant renal dysfunction

Suppositories are contraindicated for use in patients with a history of proctitis or recent rectal bleeding.

Warnings NSAIDs are associated with an increased risk of adverse cardiovascular thrombotic events, including potentially fatal MI and stroke **[U.S. Boxed Warning]**; risk may be increased with duration of use or preexisting cardiovascular risk factors or disease; carefully evaluate cardiovascular risk profile prior to prescribing; use the lowest effective dose for the shortest duration of time, taking into consideration individual patient treatment goals; alternate therapies should be considered for patients at high risk. Use is contraindicated for treatment of perioperative pain in the setting of CABG surgery **[U.S. Boxed Warning]**; an increased incidence of MI and stroke was found in patients receiving COX-2 selective NSAIDs for the treatment of pain within the first 10-14 days after CABG surgery. NSAIDs may cause fluid retention, edema, and new-onset or worsening of preexisting hypertension; use with caution in patients with hypertension, CHF, or fluid retention. Concurrent administration of ibuprofen, and potentially other nonselective NSAIDs, may interfere with aspirin's cardioprotective effect.

NSAIDs may increase the risk of gastrointestinal inflammation, ulceration, bleeding, and perforation **[U.S. Boxed Warning]**. These events, which can be potentially fatal, may occur at any time during therapy, and without warning. Avoid the use of NSAIDs in patients with active GI bleeding or ulcer disease. Use NSAIDs with extreme caution in patients with a history of GI bleeding or ulcers (these patients have a 10-fold increased risk for developing a GI bleed). Use NSAIDs with caution in patients with other risk factors which may increase GI bleeding (eg, concurrent therapy with aspirin, anticoagulants, and/or corticosteroids, longer duration of NSAID use, smoking, use of alcohol, and poor general health). Use the lowest effective dose for the shortest duration of time, taking into consideration individual patient treatment goals; alternate therapies should be considered for patients at high risk.

NSAIDs may compromise existing renal function. Renal toxicity may occur in patients with impaired renal function, dehydration, heart failure, liver dysfunction, and those taking diuretics and ACE inhibitors; use with caution in these patients; monitor renal function closely. NSAIDs are not recommended for use in patients with advanced renal disease. Long-term use of NSAIDs may cause renal papillary necrosis and other renal injury.

Fatal asthmatic and anaphylactoid reactions may occur in patients with the "aspirin triad" who receive NSAIDs. NSAIDs may cause serious dermatologic adverse reactions including exfoliative dermatitis, Stevens-Johnson syndrome, and toxic epidermal necrolysis. Avoid use of NSAIDs in late pregnancy as they may cause premature closure of the ductus arteriosus.

Precautions Use with caution in patients with cardiac dysfunction, hypertension, renal or hepatic impairment, epilepsy, patients receiving anticoagulants and for treatment of JRA in children (fatal hepatitis has been reported; monitor children closely; assess liver function periodically)

Adverse Reactions

Cardiovascular: Presyncope, syncope

Central nervous system: Depression, dizziness, drowsiness, fatigue, headache, malaise, vertigo

Dermatologic: Hyperhidrosis, pruritus, skin rash

Endocrine & metabolic: Hot flash

Gastrointestinal: Abdominal pain, constipation, decreased appetite, diarrhea, dyspepsia, epigastric pain, heartburn, nausea, rectal irritation (suppository), tenesmus (suppository), vomiting

Hematologic & oncologic: Postoperative hemorrhage

Otic: Tinnitus

Miscellaneous: Swelling (postprocedural)

Rare but important or life-threatening: Acute respiratory distress, agranulocytosis, anaphylaxis, anemia, angioedema, aphthous stomatitis, aplastic anemia, aseptic meningitis, asthma, bone marrow depression, cardiac arrhythmia, cardiac failure, cerebrovascular accident, chest pain, cholestatic jaundice, coma, confusion, convulsions, corneal deposits, depersonalization, depression, diplopia, disseminated intravascular coagulation, dysarthria, edema, erythema multiforme, erythema nodosum, exacerbation of epilepsy, exacerbation of Parkinson's disease, exfoliative dermatitis, fluid retention, gastritis, gastroenteritis, gastrointestinal hemorrhage, gastrointestinal perforation (rare), gastrointestinal ulcer, glycosuria, gynecomastia, hearing loss, hematuria, hemodynamic deterioration (patients with severe heart failure and hyponatremia), hemolytic anemia, hepatic failure, hepatic necrosis, hepatitis (including fatal cases), hyperglycemia, hyperkalemia, hypersensitivity reaction, hypertension, hypotension, immune thrombocytopenia, interstitial nephritis, intestinal obstruction, intestinal stenosis, involuntary muscle movements, jaundice, leukopenia, maculopathy, myocardial infarction, necrotizing fasciitis, nephrotic syndrome, oliguria, peripheral neuropathy, proctitis, psychosis, pulmonary edema, purpura, rectal hemorrhage, regional ileitis, renal failure, renal insufficiency, retinal disturbance, shock, significant cardiovascular event, Stevens-Johnson syndrome, stomatitis, syncope, thrombocytopenia, thrombophlebitis, toxic amblyopia, toxic epidermal necrolysis, ulcerative colitis, vaginal hemorrhage

Drug Interactions

Metabolism/Transport Effects Substrate of CYP2C19 (minor), CYP2C9 (minor); **Note:** Assignment of Major/Minor substrate status based on clinically relevant drug interaction potential; **Inhibits** CYP2C19 (weak), CYP2C9 (weak)

◀ ## Avoid Concomitant Use

Avoid concomitant use of Indomethacin with any of the following: Floctafenine; Ketorolac (Nasal); Ketorolac (Systemic); NSAID (COX-2 Inhibitor); Omacetaxine; Urokinase

Increased Effect/Toxicity

Indomethacin may increase the levels/effects of: 5-ASA Derivatives; Agents with Antiplatelet Properties; Aliskiren; Aminoglycosides; Anticoagulants; Apixaban; Bisphosphonate Derivatives; Collagenase (Systemic); CycloSPORINE (Systemic); Dabigatran Etexilate; Deferasirox; Desmopressin; Digoxin; Eplerenone; Haloperidol; Ibritumomab; Lithium; Methotrexate; Nonsteroidal Anti-Inflammatory Agents; NSAID (COX-2 Inhibitor); Omacetaxine; PEMEtrexed; Porfimer; Potassium-Sparing Diuretics; PRALAtrexate; Quinolone Antibiotics; Rivaroxaban; Salicylates; Tenofovir; Thrombolytic Agents; Tiludronate; Tositumomab and Iodine I 131 Tositumomab; Triamterene; Urokinase; Vancomycin; Vitamin K Antagonists

The levels/effects of Indomethacin may be increased by: ACE Inhibitors; Angiotensin II Receptor Blockers; Antidepressants (Tricyclic, Tertiary Amine); Corticosteroids (Systemic); CycloSPORINE (Systemic); Dasatinib; Floctafenine; Glucosamine; Herbs (Anticoagulant/Antiplatelet Properties); Ibrutinib; Ketorolac (Nasal); Ketorolac (Systemic); Multivitamins/Fluoride (with ADE); Multivitamins/Minerals (with ADEK, Folate, Iron); Multivitamins/Minerals (with AE, No Iron); Nonsteroidal Anti-Inflammatory Agents; Omega-3 Fatty Acids; Pentosan Polysulfate Sodium; Pentoxifylline; Probenecid; Prostacyclin Analogues; Selective Serotonin Reuptake Inhibitors; Serotonin/Norepinephrine Reuptake Inhibitors; Sodium Phosphates; Tipranavir; Treprostinil; Vitamin E

Decreased Effect

Indomethacin may decrease the levels/effects of: ACE Inhibitors; Agents with Antiplatelet Properties; Aliskiren; Angiotensin II Receptor Blockers; Beta-Blockers; Eplerenone; Glucagon; HydrALAZINE; Loop Diuretics; Potassium-Sparing Diuretics; Prostaglandins (Ophthalmic); Salicylates; Selective Serotonin Reuptake Inhibitors; Thiazide Diuretics

The levels/effects of Indomethacin may be decreased by: Bile Acid Sequestrants; Nonsteroidal Anti-Inflammatory Agents; Salicylates

Food Interactions Food may decrease the rate but not the extent of absorption. Indomethacin peak serum levels may be delayed if taken with food. Management: Administer with food or milk to minimize GI upset.

Stability

Oral suspension: Store below 86°F; do not freeze

I.V. product: Protect from light; not stable in alkaline solution; reconstitute just prior to administration; discard any unused portion; do not use preservative-containing diluents for reconstitution; will precipitate if reconstituted with solutions at pH <6 (product is not buffered)

Mechanism of Action Reversibly inhibits cyclooxygenase-1 and 2 (COX-1 and 2) enzymes, which results in decreased formation of prostaglandin precursors; has antipyretic, analgesic, and anti-inflammatory properties

Other proposed mechanisms not fully elucidated (and possibly contributing to the anti-inflammatory effect to varying degrees), include inhibiting chemotaxis, altering lymphocyte activity, inhibiting neutrophil aggregation/activation, and decreasing proinflammatory cytokine levels.

Pharmacokinetics (Adult data unless noted)

Absorption: Oral:

Immediate Release:

Neonates: Formulation specific

Adults: Rapid and well absorbed

Extended Release: Adults: 90% over 12 hours (**Note:** 75 mg product is designed to initially release 25 mg and then 50 mg over an extended period of time)

Distribution:

Neonates: PDA: 0.36 L/kg

Post-PDA closure: 0.26 L/kg

Adults: 0.34-1.57 L/kg

Protein binding: 99%

Metabolism: In the liver via glucuronide conjugation and other pathways

Bioavailability: Oral:

Neonates, premature: Percent bioavailability reported in the literature is highly variable and may be influenced by formulation components and indomethacin physicochemical properties (Scanlon, 1982); some have suggested that aqueous formulations are less bioavailable compared to ethanol based formulations (Mrongovious, 1982; Scanlon, 1982); aqueous suspension (in saline): 13% to 20% (Mrongovious, 1982; Sharma, 2003); ethanol based (96% v/v) suspension: 98.6% (Al Za'abi, 2007)

Adults: ~100%

Half-life:

Neonates:

Postnatal age (PNA) <2 weeks: ~20 hours

PNA >2 weeks: ~11 hours

Adults: 2.6-11.2 hours

Elimination: Significant enterohepatic recycling; 33% excreted in feces as demethylated metabolites with 1.5% as unchanged drug; 60% eliminated in urine as drug and metabolites

Clearance: Preterm neonates: ~19 mL/hour/kg (range: 4.7-45.5 mL/hour/kg) (Al Za'abi, 2007)

Dosing: Neonatal I.V.:

Patent ductus arteriosus, treatment: Initial: 0.2 mg/kg/dose, followed by 2 doses depending on postnatal age (PNA):

PNA **at time of first dose** <48 hours: 0.1 mg/kg at 12- to 24-hour intervals

PNA **at time of first dose** 2-7 days: 0.2 mg/kg at 12- to 24-hour intervals

PNA **at time of first dose** >7 days: 0.25 mg/kg at 12- to 24-hour intervals

Note: In general, may use 12-hour dosing interval if urine output >1 mL/kg/hour after prior dose; use 24-hour dosing interval if urine output is <1 mL/kg/hour but >0.6 mL/kg/hour; doses should be withheld if patient has oliguria (urine output <0.6 mL/kg/hour) or anuria

Patent ductus arteriosus, prophylaxis: Preterm neonates: Various regimens have been evaluated in VLBW neonates with first dose administered within the first 12-24 hours of life. Typical dosing: Initial: 0.1-0.2 mg/kg/dose followed by 0.1 mg/kg/dose every 12-24 hours for 2 additional doses (Fowlie, 2010)

Dosing: Usual

Inflammatory/rheumatoid disorders: **Note:** Use lowest effective dose: Oral:

Children ≥2 years: 1-2 mg/kg/day in 2-4 divided doses; maximum dose: 4 mg/kg/day; do not exceed 150-200 mg/day

Adults: 25-50 mg/dose 2-3 times/day; maximum dose: 200 mg/day; extended release capsule should be given on a 1-2 times/day schedule

Administration

Oral: Administer with food, milk, or antacids to decrease GI adverse effects; extended release capsules must be swallowed whole, do not crush or chew

Parenteral: I.V.: Administer over 20-30 minutes at a concentration of 0.5-1 mg/mL in preservative free SWI or preservative free NS

Note: Do **not** administer via I.V. bolus or I.V. infusion via an umbilical catheter into vessels near the superior mesenteric artery, as these may cause vasoconstriction and can compromise blood flow to the intestines. Do not administer intra-arterially.

Monitoring Parameters BUN, serum creatinine, potassium, liver enzymes, CBC with differential; in addition, in neonates treated for PDA: heart rate, heart murmur, blood pressure, urine output, echocardiogram, serum sodium and glucose, platelet count, and serum concentrations of concomitantly administered drugs which are renally eliminated (eg, aminoglycosides, digoxin); periodic ophthalmic exams with chronic use

Test Interactions False-negative dexamethasone suppression test

Additional Information Indomethacin may mask signs and symptoms of infections; fatalities in children have been reported, due to unrecognized overwhelming sepsis; drowsiness, lethargy, nausea, vomiting, seizures, paresthesia, headache, dizziness, tinnitus, GI bleeding, cerebral edema, and cardiac arrest have been reported with overdoses

Product Availability Tivorbex: FDA approved February 2014; anticipated availability currently unknown. Refer to the prescribing information for additional information.

Dosage Forms Excipient information presented when available (limited, particularly for generics); consult specific product labeling.

Capsule, Oral:
Generic: 25 mg, 50 mg
Capsule Extended Release, Oral:
Generic: 75 mg
Solution Reconstituted, Intravenous:
Indocin: 1 mg (1 ea)
Generic: 1 mg (1 ea)
Solution Reconstituted, Intravenous [preservative free]:
Generic: 1 mg (1 ea)
Suppository, Rectal:
Indocin: 50 mg (30 ea)
Suspension, Oral:
Indocin: 25 mg/5 mL (237 mL) [contains alcohol, usp; pineapple-coconut-mint flavor]

References

Al Za'abi M, Donovan T, Tudehope D, et al, "Orogastric and Intravenous Indomethacin Administration to Very Premature Neonates With Patent Ductus Arteriosus: Population Pharmacokinetics, Absolute Bioavailability, and Treatment Outcome," *Ther Drug Monit*, 2007, 29 (6):807-14.

Coombs RC, Morgan ME, Durbin GM, et al, "Gut Blood Flow Velocities in the Newborn: Effects of Patent Ductus Arteriosus and Parenteral Indomethacin," *Arch Dis Child*, 1990, 65(10 Spec No):1067-71.

Fowlie PW, Davis PG, and McGuire W, "Prophylactic Intravenous Indomethacin for Preventing Mortality and Morbidity in Preterm Infants," *Cochrane Database Syst Rev*, 2010, (7):CD000174.

Gersony WM, Peckham GJ, Ellison RC, et al, "Effects of Indomethacin in Premature Infants With Patent Ductus Arteriosus: Results of a National Collaborative Study," *J Pediatr*, 1983, 102(6):895-906.

Kraus DM and Pham JT, "Neonatal Therapy," *Applied Therapeutics: The Clinical Use of Drugs*, 9th ed, Koda-Kimble MA, Young LY, Kradjan WA, et al, eds, Baltimore, MD: Lippincott Williams & Wilkins, 2009.

Mrongovius R, Imbeck H, Wille L, et al, "Variability of Serum Indomethacin Concentrations After Oral and Intravenous Administration to Preterm Infants," *Eur J Pediatr*, 1982, 138(2):151-3.

Scanlon JW, "Oral Aqueous Suspension of Indomethacin Should be Abandoned," *Pediatrics*, 1982, 69(4):507.

Sharma PK, Garg SK, and Narang A, "A Preliminary Study on Pharmacokinetics of Oral Indomethacin in Premature Infants in North India," *Indian J Med Res*, 2003, 117:164-9.

◆ **Indomethacin Sodium Trihydrate** *see* Indomethacin *on page 1096*

◆ **INF-alpha 2** *see* Interferon Alfa-2b *on page 1138*

◆ **Infanrix** *see* Diphtheria and Tetanus Toxoids, and Acellular Pertussis Vaccine *on page 686*

◆ **Infants Advil [OTC]** *see* Ibuprofen *on page 1059*

◆ **Infants Gas Relief [OTC]** *see* Simethicone *on page 1891*

◆ **Infants Ibuprofen [OTC]** *see* Ibuprofen *on page 1059*

◆ **Infants Simethicone [OTC]** *see* Simethicone *on page 1891*

◆ **Infasurf** *see* Calfactant *on page 360*

◆ **Infed** *see* Iron Dextran Complex *on page 1153*

InFLIXimab (in FLIKS e mab)

Medication Safety Issues
Sound-alike/look-alike issues:
InFLIXimab may be confused with riTUXimab
Remicade® may be confused with Renacidin®, Rituxan®

Brand Names: U.S. Remicade

Brand Names: Canada Remicade®

Therapeutic Category Antirheumatic, Disease Modifying; Gastrointestinal Agent, Miscellaneous; Immunosuppressant Agent; Monoclonal Antibody; Tumor Necrosis Factor (TNF) Blocking Agent

Generic Availability (U.S.) No

Use Reduction of signs and symptoms of Crohn's disease in patients with moderate to severely active disease who have had an inadequate response to conventional therapy (FDA approved in children ≥6 years and adults); reduction of signs and symptoms of ulcerative colitis in patients with moderate to severely active disease who have had an inadequate response to conventional therapy (FDA approved in children ≥6 years and adults); in combination with methotrexate for reducing signs and symptoms, inhibiting progression of structural damage, and improving physical function in patients with moderate to severe rheumatoid arthritis (FDA approved in adults); reduction of signs and symptoms of ankylosing spondylitis (FDA approved in adults); treatment of psoriatic arthritis (to reduce signs/symptoms of active arthritis and inhibit progression of structural damage and improve physical function) (FDA approved in adults); treatment of chronic severe plaque psoriasis (FDA approved in adults)

Medication Guide Available Yes

Pregnancy Risk Factor B

Pregnancy Considerations Animal reproduction studies have not been conducted. Infliximab crosses the placenta and can be detected in the serum of infants for up to 6 months following *in utero* exposure. The safety of administering live or live-attenuated vaccines to exposed infants is not known. If a biologic agent such as infliximab is needed to treat inflammatory bowel disease during pregnancy, it is recommended to hold therapy after 30 weeks gestation (Habal, 2012).

Healthcare providers are also encouraged to enroll women exposed to infliximab during pregnancy in the Mother-ToBaby Autoimmune Diseases Study by contacting the Organization of Teratology Information Specialists (OTIS) (877-311-8972).

Breast-Feeding Considerations Small amounts of infliximab have been detected in breast milk. Information is available from three postpartum women who were administered infliximab 5 mg/kg 1-24 weeks after delivery. Infliximab was detected within 12 hours and the highest milk concentrations (0.09-0.105 mcg/mL) were seen 2-3 days after the dose. Corresponding maternal serum concentrations were 18-64 mcg/mL (Ben-Horin, 2011). Due to the potential for serious adverse reactions in the nursing infant, the manufacturer recommends a decision be made whether to discontinue nursing or to discontinue the drug, taking into account the importance of treatment to the mother.

Contraindications Hypersensitivity to infliximab, murine proteins, or any component; patients with moderate or severe (NYHA class III/IV) congestive heart failure

◄ **Warnings** Patients receiving infliximab are at increased risk for serious infections which may result in hospitalization and/or fatality **[U.S. Boxed Warning]**; infections usually developed in patients receiving concomitant immunosuppressive agents (eg, methotrexate or corticosteroids) and may present as disseminated (rather than local) disease. Active tuberculosis (or reactivation of latent tuberculosis), invasive fungal (including aspergillosis, blastomycosis, candidiasis, coccidioidomycosis, histoplasmosis, and pneumocystosis) and bacterial, viral, or other opportunistic infections (including legionellosis and listeriosis) have been reported in patients receiving TNF-blocking agents, including infliximab. Monitor closely for signs/symptoms of infection; discontinue for serious infection or sepsis. Consider risks versus benefits prior to use in patients with a history of chronic or recurrent infection. Consider empiric antifungal therapy in patients who are at risk for invasive fungal infection and develop severe systemic illness. Caution should be exercised when considering use in the elderly or in patients with conditions that predispose them to infections (eg, diabetes) or residence/travel from areas of endemic mycoses (blastomycosis, coccidioidomycosis, histoplasmosis), or with latent or localized infections. Do not initiate infliximab therapy with an active infections, including clinically important localized infection. Patients who develop a new infection while undergoing treatment should be monitored closely. Serious infections were reported when used in combination with anakinra, abatacept, or etanercept; combination with infliximab is not recommended; similar reactions may potentially occur with concurrent use of infliximab and other biological therapeutics or DMARDS used to treat similar conditions as infliximab; use caution with combination therapy. Other potentially significant interactions may exist, requiring dose or frequency adjustment, additional monitoring, and/or selection of alternative therapy. Consult drug interactions database for more detailed information.

Infliximab use has been associated with reports of leukopenia, neutropenia, thrombocytopenia, and pancytopenia (some fatal); use with caution in patients with a history of significant hematologic abnormalities; discontinue therapy if significant hematologic abnormalities develop.

Infliximab treatment has been associated with active tuberculosis (may be disseminated or extrapulmonary) or reactivation of latent infections **[U.S. Boxed Warning]**. Evaluate patients for tuberculosis risk factors and latent tuberculosis infection (with a tuberculin skin test) prior to and during therapy. Treatment of latent tuberculosis should be initiated before use. Patients with initial negative tuberculin skin tests should receive continued monitoring for tuberculosis throughout treatment. Most cases of reactivation have been reported within the first 3-6 months of treatment. Caution should be exercised when considering the use in patients who have been exposed to tuberculosis.

Rare reactivation of hepatitis B virus (HBV) has occurred in chronic carriers of the virus, usually in patients receiving concomitant immunosuppressants; evaluate for HBV prior to initiation in all patients. Monitor during and for several months following discontinuation of treatment in HBV carriers; interrupt therapy if reactivation occurs and treat appropriately with antiviral therapy; if resumption of therapy is deemed necessary, exercise caution and monitor patient closely. Severe hepatic reactions (including hepatitis, jaundice, acute hepatic failure, and cholestasis) have been reported during treatment; discontinue with jaundice or marked increase in liver enzymes (≥5 times ULN).

Hepatosplenic T-cell lymphoma has been reported in patients with Crohn's disease or ulcerative colitis treated with infliximab and concurrent or prior azathioprine or mercaptopurine use, usually reported in adolescent and young adult males **[U.S. Boxed Warning]**. Infliximab use has been associated with reports of leukopenia, neutropenia, thrombocytopenia, and pancytopenia (some fatal). Use with caution in patients with a history of significant hematologic abnormalities; discontinue therapy if significant hematologic abnormalities develop.

In children and adolescents, lymphomas and other malignancies, some fatal, have been reported with use of TNF blockers including infliximab **[U.S. Boxed Warning]**. Use may affect defenses against malignancies; impact on the development and course of malignancies is not fully defined, but may be dose dependent. In an analysis of children and adolescents who had received TNF blockers (etanercept and infliximab), the FDA identified 48 cases of malignancy. Of the 48 cases, ~50% were lymphomas (eg, Hodgkin's and non-Hodgkin's lymphoma). Other malignancies, such as leukemia, melanoma, Merkel cell carcinoma, and solid organ tumors, were reported; malignancies rarely seen in children (eg, leiomyosarcoma, hepatic malignancies, and renal cell carcinoma) were also observed. Of note, most of these cases (88%) were receiving other immunosuppressive medications (eg, azathioprine and methotrexate). As compared to the general population, an increased risk of lymphoma has been noted in clinical trials; however, rheumatoid arthritis has been previously associated with an increased rate of lymphoma. The role of TNF blockers in the development of malignancies in children cannot be excluded. The FDA also reviewed 147 postmarketing reports of leukemia (including acute myeloid leukemia, chronic lymphocytic leukemia, and chronic myeloid leukemia) in patients (children and adults) using TNF blockers. Average onset time to development of leukemia was within the first 1-2 years of TNF blocker initiation. Although most patients were receiving other immunosuppressive agents, the role of TNF blockers in the development of leukemia could not be excluded. The FDA concluded that there is a possible association with the development of leukemia and the use of TNF blockers. Patients should be monitored closely for signs and symptoms suggestive of malignancy, including periodic skin examinations; any evidence suggestive of malignancy should result in prompt discontinuation of the medication and appropriate diagnostic evaluation. Use caution in patients with a history of COPD; higher rates of malignancy were reported in COPD patients treated with infliximab. In patients with psoriasis, nonmelanoma skin cancers have been reported, particularly in those with previous phototherapy.

May also cause new-onset psoriasis; improvement was seen when the TNF blocker was discontinued; monitor closely for signs and symptoms suggestive of new-onset psoriasis, evidence of which should result in prompt discontinuation of the medication and appropriate diagnostic evaluation.

Acute infusion reactions may occur. Hypersensitivity reaction may occur within 2 hours of infusion. Medication and equipment for management of hypersensitivity reaction should be available for immediate use. Interruptions and/or reinstitution at a slower rate may be required. Pretreatment may be considered, and may be warranted in all patients with prior infusion reactions. Serum sickness-like reactions have occurred; may be associated with a decreased response to treatment. The development of antibodies to infliximab may increase the risk of hypersensitivity and/or infusion reactions; concomitant use of immunosuppressants may lessen the development of anti-infliximab antibodies. The risk of infusion reactions may be increased with retreatment after an interruption or discontinuation of prior maintenance therapy. A retrospective study of 57 children receiving 361 infliximab infusions reported that the rate of infusion-related reactions in children was similar to that in adults (9.7% incidence shown). Female gender, immunosuppressive use for <4 months, and prior infusion reactions were risk factors for subsequent infusion reactions in children (Crandall, 2003). Retreatment in psoriasis patients should be resumed as a scheduled maintenance regimen without any induction doses; use of an induction regimen should be used cautiously for retreatment of all other patients.

Rare cases of optic neuritis and demyelinating disease including multiple sclerosis, Guillain-Barré syndrome, and systemic vasculitis have been reported with infliximab therapy; use with caution in patients with preexisting or recent onset CNS demyelinating disorders or history of seizure disorder; consider discontinuation of therapy if patients develop significant CNS reactions.

Injection contains polysorbate 80 (Tween 80®) which may cause allergic reactions in susceptible individuals. Infusion of polysorbate 80-containing solutions through polyvinyl chloride tubing may cause DEHP to leach into the solution; in immature animals, exposure to DEHP may adversely affect the development of the male reproductive tract.

Precautions Use with caution in patients with mild HF (NYHA Class I, II) or decreased left ventricular function; worsening and new-onset HF has been reported; doses >5 mg/kg should not be administered in patients with moderate to severe heart failure (NYHA Class III/IV); discontinue therapy with onset of new or worsening symptoms. Positive antinuclear antibody titers have been detected in patients (with negative baselines); rare cases of autoimmune disorder, including lupus-like syndrome, have been reported; monitor and discontinue if symptoms develop. Patients should be brought up to date with all immunizations before initiating therapy. Live vaccines should not be given concurrently; there is no data available concerning secondary transmission of live vaccines in patients receiving therapy. Use caution when administering live vaccines to infants born to female patients who received infliximab therapy while pregnant; infliximab crosses the placenta and has been detected in infants' serum for up to 6 months.

Adverse Reactions

Reported in adults with rheumatoid arthritis:

Cardiovascular: Bradycardia, cardiac arrest, cardiac arrhythmia, cardiac failure, cerebral infarction, circulatory shock, edema, hypertension, hypotension, myocardial infarction, pulmonary embolism, syncope, tachycardia, thrombophlebitis (deep)

Central nervous system: Confusion, dizziness, fatigue, headache, meningitis, neuritis, pain, peripheral neuropathy, seizure, suicidal tendencies

Dermatologic: Cellulitis, diaphoresis, pruritus, skin rash

Endocrine & metabolic: Dehydration, menstrual disease

Gastrointestinal: Abdominal pain (more common in Crohn's patients), biliary colic, cholecystitis, cholelithiasis, constipation, diarrhea, dyspepsia, gastrointestinal hemorrhage, intestinal obstruction, intestinal perforation, intestinal stenosis, nausea, pancreatitis, peritonitis, rectal pain

Genitourinary: Urinary tract infection

Hematologic & oncologic: Anemia, basal cell carcinoma, hemolytic anemia, leukopenia, lymphadenopathy, malignant lymphoma, malignant neoplasm, malignant neoplasm of breast, pancytopenia, sarcoidosis, thrombocytopenia

Hepatic: Hepatitis, increased serum ALT (risk increased with concomitant methotrexate)

Hypersensitivity: Delayed hypersensitivity (plaque psoriasis), hypersensitivity reaction, serum sickness

Immunologic: Antibody development (anti-infliximab; Mayer, 2006), antibody development (double-stranded DNA), increased ANA titer

Infection: Abscess (including Crohn's patients with fistulizing disease), candidiasis, infection, sepsis

Neuromuscular & skeletal: Arthralgia, back pain, herniated disk, lupus-like syndrome, myalgia, tendon disease

Renal: Nephrolithiasis, renal failure

Respiratory: Adult respiratory distress syndrome, bronchitis, cough, dyspnea, pharyngitis, pleural effusion, pleurisy, pulmonary edema, respiratory insufficiency, rhinitis, sinusitis, upper respiratory tract infection

Miscellaneous: Fever, ulcer

The following adverse events were reported in children with Crohn's disease and were more common in children than adults:

Cardiovascular: Flushing

Gastrointestinal: Bloody stools

Hepatic: Increased liver enzymes

Hematologic & oncologic: Anemia, leukopenia, neutropenia

Hypersensitivity: Hypersensitivity reaction (respiratory)

Immunologic: Antibody development (anti-infliximab)

Infection: Bacterial infection, infection (more common with every 8-week vs every 12-week infusions), viral infection

Neuromuscular & skeletal: Bone fracture

Rare but important or life-threatening (adults or children):

Agranulocytosis, anaphylactic shock, anaphylaxis, angina pectoris, angioedema, autoimmune hepatitis, cardiac failure (worsening), cholestasis, demyelinating disease of the central nervous system (eg, multiple sclerosis, optic neuritis), demyelinating disease (peripheral; eg, Guillain-Barré syndrome, chronic inflammatory demyelinating polyneuropathy, multifocal motor neuropathy), dysgeusia, erythema multiforme, hepatic carcinoma, hepatic failure, hepatic injury, hepatitis B (reactivation), Hodgkin's lymphoma, immune thrombocytopenia, interstitial fibrosis, interstitial pneumonitis, jaundice, leukemia, liver function tests increased, lupus-like syndrome (drug-induced), malignant lymphoma (hepatosplenic T-cell [HSTCL]), malignant melanoma, malignant neoplasm (leiomyosarcoma), Merkel cell carcinoma, neuropathy, opportunistic infection, pericardial effusion, pneumonia, psoriasis (including new onset, palmoplantar, pustular, or exacerbation), reactivated tuberculosis, renal cell carcinoma, seizure, Stevens-Johnson syndrome, thrombotic thrombocytopenia purpura, toxic epidermal necrolysis, transverse myelitis, tuberculosis, vasculitis (systemic and cutaneous)

Drug Interactions

Metabolism/Transport Effects None known.

Avoid Concomitant Use

Avoid concomitant use of InFLIXimab with any of the following: Abatacept; Adalimumab; Anakinra; BCG; Belimumab; Canakinumab; Certolizumab Pegol; Etanercept; Golimumab; Natalizumab; Pimecrolimus; Rilonacept; Tacrolimus (Topical); Tocilizumab; Tofacitinib; Ustekinumab; Vaccines (Live); Vedolizumab

Increased Effect/Toxicity

InFLIXimab may increase the levels/effects of: Abatacept; Anakinra; Belimumab; Canakinumab; Certolizumab Pegol; Leflunomide; Natalizumab; Rilonacept; Tofacitinib; Vaccines (Live); Vedolizumab

The levels/effects of InFLIXimab may be increased by: Abciximab; Adalimumab; Denosumab; Etanercept; Golimumab; Pimecrolimus; Roflumilast; Tacrolimus (Topical); Tocilizumab; Trastuzumab; Ustekinumab

Decreased Effect

InFLIXimab may decrease the levels/effects of: BCG; Coccidioidin Skin Test; Sipuleucel-T; Vaccines (Inactivated); Vaccines (Live)

The levels/effects of InFLIXimab may be decreased by: Echinacea

Stability Store intact vial at 2°C to 8°C (36°F to 46°F); do not freeze; infliximab should begin within 3 hours of preparation.

Mechanism of Action Infliximab is a chimeric monoclonal antibody that binds to human tumor necrosis factor alpha (TNFα), thereby interfering with endogenous TNFα activity. Elevated TNFα levels have been found in involved tissues/fluids of patients with rheumatoid arthritis, ankylosing spondylitis, psoriatic arthritis, plaque psoriasis, Crohn disease and ulcerative colitis. Biological activities of TNFα include the induction of proinflammatory cytokines (interleukins), enhancement of leukocyte migration, activation of neutrophils and eosinophils, and the induction of acute phase reactants and tissue degrading enzymes. Animal models have shown TNFα expression causes polyarthritis, and infliximab can prevent disease as well as allow diseased joints to heal.

Pharmacodynamics

Onset:
Crohn's disease: 1-2 weeks
Rheumatoid arthritis: 3-7 days

Duration:
Crohn's disease: 8-48 weeks
Rheumatoid arthritis: 6-12 weeks

Pharmacokinetics (Adult data unless noted) Note: Pharmacokinetic data in pediatric patients (6-17 years) reported to be similar to adult values.

Distribution: Within the vascular compartment
V_d: 3-6 L (Klotz, 2007)
Half-life, terminal: 7-12 days (Klotz, 2007)

Dosing: Usual Note: Premedication with antihistamines (H_1-antagonist and/or H_2-antagonist), acetaminophen and/or corticosteroids may be considered to prevent and/or manage infusion-related reactions:

Children and Adolescents:

Crohn's disease: Children ≥6 years and Adolescents: I.V.: Initial: 5 mg/kg/dose at 0, 2, and 6 weeks, followed by maintenance: 5 mg/kg/dose every 8 weeks thereafter. **Note:** If the response is incomplete, dose has been increased up to 10 mg/kg (Rufo, 2012; Stephens, 2003); in adult patients with Crohn's disease, it has been observed that patients who do not respond by week 14 are unlikely to respond with continued dosing; consider therapy discontinuation in these patients.

Juvenile idiopathic arthritis; refractory to conventional disease modifying drugs: Limited data available: Children ≥4 years and Adolescents: I.V.: Initial: 3 mg/kg at 0, 2, and 6 weeks; then 3-6 mg/kg/dose every 8 weeks thereafter, in combination with methotrexate during induction and maintenance (Ruperto, 2010). Alternatively, some studies used 6 mg/kg/dose starting at week 14 of a methotrexate induction regimen (weeks 0-13); repeat dose (6 mg/kg/dose) at week 16 and 20, then every 8 weeks thereafter (Ruperto, 2007; Ruperto, 2010; Visvanathan, 2012).

Ulcerative colitis: Children ≥6 years and Adolescents: I.V.: Initial: 5 mg/kg/dose at 0, 2, and 6 weeks, followed by maintenance: 5 mg/kg/dose every 8 weeks thereafter. **Note:** If the response is incomplete, dose has been increased up to 10 mg/kg (Rufo, 2012; Stephens, 2003)

Adults:

Crohn's disease: I.V.: 5 mg/kg at 0, 2, and 6 weeks, followed by 5 mg/kg every 8 weeks thereafter; dose may be increased to 10 mg/kg in patients who respond but then lose their response. If no response by week 14, consider discontinuing therapy.

Rheumatoid arthritis (in combination with methotrexate): I.V.: Initial: 3 mg/kg at 0, 2, and 6 weeks, followed by 3 mg/kg every 8 weeks thereafter; doses have ranged from 3-10 mg/kg repeated at 4- to 8-week intervals

Ankylosing spondylitis: I.V.: Initial: 5 mg/kg; repeat 5 mg/kg/dose at 2 and 6 weeks after the first infusion, then every 6 weeks thereafter

Plaque psoriasis: I.V.: Initial: 5 mg/kg at 0, 2, and 6 weeks, then every 8 weeks thereafter

Psoriatic arthritis (with or without methotrexate): I.V.: Initial: 5 mg/kg at 0, 2, and 6 weeks, followed by 5 mg/kg every 8 weeks thereafter

Ulcerative colitis: I.V.: Initial: 5 mg/kg at 0, 2, and 6 weeks, then every 8 weeks thereafter

Dosage adjustment with heart failure (HF): Adults: Weigh risk versus benefits for individual patient: Moderate to severe (NYHA Class III or IV): ≤5 mg/kg

Dosing adjustment in renal impairment: There are no dosage adjustments provided in manufacturer's labeling.

Dosing adjustment in hepatic impairment: There are no dosage adjustments provided in manufacturer's labeling.

Administration Parenteral: Reconstitute vials with 10 mL SWI; swirl vial gently to dissolve powder; do not shake. Allow solution to stand for 5 minutes. Total dose of reconstituted product should be further diluted in NS to a final concentration between 0.4-4 mg/mL (usually dose added to 250 mL NS); infusion of dose should begin within 3 hours of preparation. Administer by I.V. infusion over ≥2 hours; a rate titration schedule may be used to prevent acute infusion reactions. Administer through an in-line, sterile, nonpyrogenic, low-protein-binding filter with pore size of ≤1.2 micrometers; do not infuse in the same I.V. line as other agents.

Adults: Guidelines for the treatment and prophylaxis of infusion reactions: Data limited to adult patients and dosages used in Crohn's; prospective data for other populations (pediatrics, other indications/dosing) are not available. A protocol for the treatment of infusion reactions, as well as prophylactic therapy for repeat infusions, has been published (Mayer, 2006).

Treatment of infusion reactions: Medications for the treatment of hypersensitivity reactions should be available for immediate use. For mild reactions, the rate of infusion should be decreased to 10 mL/hour. Initiate a NS infusion (500-1000 mL/hour) and appropriate symptomatic treatment (eg, acetaminophen and diphenhydramine); monitor vital signs every 10 minutes until normal. After 20 minutes, the infliximab infusion may be increased at 15-minute intervals, as tolerated, to completion [initial increase to 20 mL/hour, then 40 mL/hour, then 80 mL/hour, etc (maximum of 125 mL/hour)]. For moderate reactions, the infusion should be stopped or slowed. Initiate a NS (500-1000 mL/hour) and appropriate symptomatic treatment. Monitor vital signs every 5 minutes until normal. After 20 minutes, the infliximab infusion may be reinstituted at 10 mL/hour; then increased at 15-minute intervals, as tolerated, to completion [initial increase 20 mL/hour, then 40 mL/hour, then 80 mL/hour, etc (maximum of 125 mL/hour)]. For severe reactions, the infusion should be stopped with administration of appropriate symptomatic treatment (eg, hydrocortisone/methylprednisolone, diphenhydramine and epinephrine) and frequent monitoring of vitals. Retreatment after a severe reaction should only be done if the benefits outweigh the risks and with appropriate prophylaxis. Delayed infusion reactions typically occur 1-7 days after an infusion. Treatment should consist of appropriate symptomatic treatment (eg, acetaminophen, antihistamine, methylprednisolone).

Prophylaxis of infusion reactions: Premedication with acetaminophen and diphenhydramine 90 minutes prior to infusion may be considered in all patients with prior infusion reactions, and in patients with severe reactions corticosteroid administration is recommended. Steroid dosing may be oral (prednisone 50 mg orally every 12 hours for 3 doses prior to infusion) or intravenous (a single dose of hydrocortisone 100 mg or methylprednisolone 20-40 mg administered 20 minutes prior to the infusion). On initiation of the infusion, begin with a test dose at 10 mL/hour of infliximab for 15 minutes. Thereafter, the infusion may be increased at 15-minute intervals, as tolerated, to completion (initial increase 20 mL/hour, then 40 mL/hour, then 80 mL/hour, etc). A maximum rate of 125 mL/hour is recommended in patients who experienced prior mild-moderate reactions and 100 mL/hour is recommended in patients who experienced prior severe reactions. In patients with cutaneous flushing, aspirin may be considered (Becker, 2004). For delayed infusion reactions, premedicate with acetaminophen and diphenhydramine 90 minutes prior to infusion. On initiation of the infusion, begin with a test dose at 10 mL/hour for 15 minutes. Thereafter, the infusion may be increased to infuse over 3 hours. Postinfusion therapy with acetaminophen for 3 days and an antihistamine for 7 days is recommended. **Note:** In a trial of pediatric patients, premedication with acetaminophen (20 mg/kg; maximum single dose: 1000 mg) and cetirizine (0.3 mg/kg if <5 years, 10 mg if ≥5 years) did not significantly impact incidence of infusion-related reactions; patients should be monitored closely (Lahdenne, 2010).

Monitoring Parameters Monitor improvement of symptoms and physical function assessments. During infusion, if reaction is noted, monitor vital signs every 2-10 minutes, depending on reaction severity, until normal. Latent TB screening prior to initiating and during therapy; signs/symptoms of infection (prior to, during, and following therapy); CBC with differential; signs/symptoms/worsening of heart failure; HBV screening prior to initiating (all patients), HBV carriers (during and for several months following therapy); signs and symptoms of hypersensitivity reaction; symptoms of lupus-like syndrome; LFTs (discontinue if >5 times ULN); signs and symptoms of malignancy (eg, splenomegaly, hepatomegaly, abdominal pain, persistent fever, night sweats, weight loss).

Dosage Forms Excipient information presented when available (limited, particularly for generics); consult specific product labeling.

Solution Reconstituted, Intravenous [preservative free]:
  Remicade: 100 mg (1 ea)

References

Becker M, Rosé CD, and McIlvain-Simpson G, "Niacin-Like Reaction to Infliximab Infusion in Systemic Juvenile Rheumatoid Arthritis," *J Rheumatol*, 2004, 31(12):2529-30.

Ben-Horin S, Yavzori M, Kopylov U, et al. Detection of infliximab in breast milk of nursing mothers with inflammatory bowel disease. *J Crohns Colitis*. 2011;5(6):555-558.

Crandall WV and Mackner LM, "Infusion Reactions to Infliximab in Children and Adolescents: Frequency, Outcome and a Predictive Model," *Aliment Pharmacol Ther*, 2003, 17(1):75-84.

Habal FM, Huang VW. Review article: a decision-making algorithm for the management of pregnancy in the inflammatory bowel disease patient. *Aliment Pharmacol Ther*. 2012;35(5):501-515.

Klotz U, Teml A, and Schwab M, "Clinical Pharmacokinetics and Use of Infliximab," *Clin Pharmacokinet*, 2007, 46(8):645-60.

Lahdenne P, Wikström AM, Aalto K, et al, "Prevention of Acute Adverse Events Related to Infliximab Infusions in Pediatric Patients," *Arthritis Care Res (Hoboken)*, 2010, 62(6):785-90.

Mayer L and Young Y, "Infusion Reactions and Their Management," *Gastroenterol Clin North Am*, 2006, 35(4):857-66.

Rufo PA, Denson LA, Sylvester FA, et al, "Health Supervision in the Management of Children and Adolescents With IBD: NASPGHAN Recommendations," *J Pediatr Gastroenterol Nutr*, 2012, 55(1):93-108.

Ruperto N,,Lovell DJ, Cuttica R, et al, "A Randomized, Placebo-Controlled Trial of Infliximab Plus Methotrexate for the Treatment of Polyarticular-Course Juvenile Rheumatoid Arthritis," *Arthritis Rheum*, 2007, 56(9):3096-106.

Ruperto N, Lovell DJ, Cuttica R, et al, "Long-Term Efficacy and Safety of Infliximab Plus Methotrexate for the Treatment of Polyarticular Course Juvenile Rheumatoid Arthritis: Findings From an Open-Label Treatment Extension," *Ann Rheum Dis*, 2009 [Epub ahead of print].

Stephens MC, Shepanski MA, Mamula P, et al, "Safety and Steroid-Sparing Experience Using Infliximab for Crohn's Disease at a Pediatric Inflammatory Bowel Disease Center," *Am J Gastroenterol*, 2003, 98(1):104-11.

Thayu M, Markowitz JE, Mamula P, et al, "Hepatosplenic T-Cell Lymphoma in an Adolescent Patient After Immunomodulator and Biologic Therapy for Crohn Disease," *J Pediatr Gastroenterol Nutr*, 2005, 40(2):220-2.

Visvanathan S, Wagner C, Marini JC, et al, "The Effect of Infliximab Plus Methotrexate on the Modulation of Inflammatory Disease Markers in Juvenile Idiopathic Arthritis: Analyses From a Randomized, Placebo-Controlled Trial," *Pediatr Rheumatol Online J*, 2010, 8:24.

Wilkinson N, Jackson G, and Gardner-Medwin J, "Biologic Therapies for Juvenile Arthritis," *Arch Dis Child*, 2003, 88(3):186-91.

◆ **Infliximab, Recombinant** *see* InFLIXimab *on page 1099*

◆ **Influenza Vaccine** *see* Influenza Virus Vaccine (Inactivated) *on page 1103*

◆ **Influenza Vaccine** *see* Influenza Virus Vaccine (Live/Attenuated) *on page 1109*

Influenza Virus Vaccine (Inactivated)
(in floo EN za VYE rus vak SEEN, in ak ti VAY ted)

Medication Safety Issues
Sound-alike/look-alike issues:
  Fluarix may be confused with Flarex
  Influenza virus vaccine may be confused with flumazenil
  Influenza virus vaccine may be confused with tetanus toxoid and tuberculin products. Medication errors have occurred when tuberculin skin tests (PPD) have been inadvertently administered instead of tetanus toxoid products and influenza virus vaccine. These products are refrigerated and often stored in close proximity to each other.

International issues:
  Fluarix [U.S., Canada, and multiple international markets] may be confused with Flarex brand name for fluorometholone [U.S. and multiple international markets] and Fluorex brand name for fluoride [France]

Related Information
Immunization Administration Recommendations *on page 2368*

Immunization Guidelines *on page 2373*

Brand Names: U.S. Afluria; Afluria Preservative Free; Fluarix; Fluarix Quadrivalent; Flucelvax; Flulaval; Flulaval Quadrivalent; Fluvirin; Fluvirin Preservative Free; Fluzone; Fluzone High-Dose; Fluzone Pediatric PF; Fluzone Preservative Free; Fluzone Quadrivalent; Medical Provider EZ Flu PF; Physicians EZ Use Flu

Brand Names: Canada Agriflu; Fluad; Fluviral; Influvac; Intanza; Vaxigrip

Therapeutic Category Vaccine; Vaccine, Inactivated Virus

Generic Availability (U.S.) May be product dependent

Use For active immunization against influenza disease caused by influenza virus subtypes A and type B contained in the vaccine

Trade Name	Manufacturer	Approval age
Fluzone, Fluzone Quadrivalent	Sanofi Pasteur	≥6 months
Fluarix, Fluarix Quadrivalent	GlaxoSmithKline	≥3 years
FluLaval, FluLaval Quadrivalent	ID Biomedical Corporation of Quebec	≥3 years
Fluvirin	Novartis vaccine	≥4 years
Afluria	CSL Biotherapies	≥5 years*
Flucelvax	Novartis vaccine	≥18 years
Fluzone Intradermal	Sanofi Pasteur	18 to 64 years
Fluzone High-Dose	Sanofi Pasteur	≥65 years

*Note: Due to an increased incidence of fever and febrile seizures in infants and children <5 years of age observed with the use of the 2010 Southern Hemisphere formulation of Afluria®, the Advisory Committee on Immunization Practices (ACIP) recommends that Afluria® should not be used in infants and children 6 months through 8 years of age, although use in 5 to 8 years of age is reserved for patients if no other age-appropriate vaccine is available (AAP, 2013).

Recommendations for annual seasonal influenza vaccination: The Advisory Committee on Immunization Practices (ACIP) recommends routine annual vaccination with the seasonal influenza vaccine for all persons ≥6 months of age who do not otherwise have contraindications to the vaccine (CDC/ACIP [Grohskopf, 2013]).

The ACIP recommends use of any age and risk factor appropriate product and does not have a preferential recommendation for use of the trivalent inactivated influenza vaccine (IIV3) or the quadrivalent inactivated influenza vaccine (IIV4). In addition to the IIV products, other alternative products are available for certain patient populations: Healthy nonpregnant persons aged 2 to 49 years may receive vaccination with the live attenuated influenza vaccine (LAIV), and persons 18 to 49 years may receive vaccination with the recombinant influenza vaccine (RIV) (CDC/ACIP [Grohskopf, 2013]).

When vaccine supply is limited, target groups for vaccination (those at higher risk of complications from influenza infection and their close contacts) include the following:

- All infants ≥6 months and children 12 to 59 months of age
- Persons ≥50 years of age
- Residents of nursing homes and other long-term care facilities
- Adults and children with chronic pulmonary disorders (including asthma) or cardiovascular system disorders (except hypertension), renal, hepatic, neurologic, or metabolic disorders (including diabetes mellitus)
- Persons who have immunosuppression (including immunosuppression caused by medications or HIV)
- Infants, children, and adolescents (6 months to 18 years of age) who are receiving long-term aspirin therapy and therefore, may be at risk for developing Reye's syndrome after influenza
- Women who are or will be pregnant during influenza season

- Healthy household contacts (including children) and caregivers of neonates, infants, and children aged 0 to 59 months (particularly neonates and infants <6 months) and adults ≥50 years
- Household contacts (including children) and caregivers of persons with medical conditions which put them at high risk of complications from influenza infection
- Healthcare personnel
- American Indians/Alaska Natives
- Morbidly obese (BMI ≥40)

Pregnancy Risk Factor B/C (manufacturer specific)

Pregnancy Considerations Adverse events were not observed in animal reproduction studies. Inactivated influenza vaccine has not been shown to cause fetal harm when given to pregnant women, although information related to use in the first trimester is limited (CDC, 2013). Following maternal immunization with the inactivated influenza virus vaccine, vaccine specific antibodies are observed in the newborn (Englund, 1993; Steinhoff, 2010; Zaman, 2008; Zuccotti, 2010). Vaccination of pregnant women protects infants from influenza infection, including infants <6 months of age who are not able to be vaccinated (CDC, 2013).

Pregnant women are at an increased risk of complications from influenza infection (Rasmussen, 2008). Influenza vaccination with the inactivated influenza vaccine (IIV) is recommended for all women who are or will become pregnant during the influenza season and who do not otherwise have contraindications to the vaccine (CDC, 2013). Pregnant women should observe the same precautions as nonpregnant women to reduce the risk of exposure to influenza and other respiratory infections (CDC, 2010). When vaccine supply is limited, focus on delivering the vaccine should be given to women who are pregnant or will be pregnant during the flu season, as well as mothers of newborns and contacts or caregivers of children <5 years of age (CDC, 2013).

Healthcare providers are encouraged to refer women exposed to the influenza vaccine during pregnancy to the Vaccines and Medications in Pregnancy Surveillance System (VAMPSS) by contacting The Organization of Teratology Information Specialists (OTIS) at (877) 311-8972.

Women exposed to Flulaval, Flulaval Quadrivalent, Fluarix, or Fluarix Quadrivalent vaccine during pregnancy or their healthcare provider may also contact the GlaxoSmithKline registry at 888-452-9622.

Healthcare providers may enroll women exposed to Fluzone Intradermal or Fluzone Quadrivalent during pregnancy in the Sanofi Pasteur vaccination registry at 800-822-2463.

Breast-Feeding Considerations It is not known if inactivated influenza vaccine is excreted into breast milk. The manufacturers recommend that caution be used if administered to nursing women. Anti-influenza IgA antibodies can be detected in breast milk following maternal vaccination with the trivalent IIV vaccine (Schlaudecker, 2013). Inactivated vaccines do not affect the safety of breast-feeding for the mother or the infant (CDC, 2011). Postpartum women may be vaccinated with either IIV or LAIV (CDC, 2013). When vaccine supply is limited, focus on delivering the vaccine should be given to women who are pregnant or will be pregnant during the flu season, as well as mothers of newborns and contacts or caregivers of children <5 years of age (CDC, 2013). Breast-feeding infants should be vaccinated according to the recommended schedules (CDC, 2011a).

Contraindications Severe allergic reaction (eg, anaphylaxis) to a previous influenza vaccination; hypersensitivity to any component

Additional manufacturer contraindications for Afluria, Fluarix, Fluarix Quadrivalent, FluLaval, FluLaval Quadrivalent, Fluvirin, Fluzone, Fluzone High-Dose, Fluzone Intradermal, Fluzone Quadrivalent: History of severe allergic reaction (eg, anaphylaxis) to egg protein

Warnings Immediate treatment (including epinephrine 1:1000) for anaphylactic and/or hypersensitivity reactions should be available during vaccine use.

Postmarketing reports of increased incidence of fever and febrile seizures in children <5 years of age has been observed with the use of the 2010 Southern Hemisphere formulation of the Afluria vaccine. Febrile events have also been reported in children 5 to 9 years of age. The ACIP does not recommend use of Afluria in children <9 years of age (CDC/ACIP [Bridges, 2014]). Based on information from the CDC, an increased rate of febrile seizures has been reported in infants and young children 6 months to 4 years who received vaccination with inactivated influenza vaccine (IIV) and the 13-valent pneumococcal conjugate vaccine (PCV13) simultaneously. However, due to the risks associated with delaying either vaccine, administering them at separate visits or deviating from the recommended vaccine schedule is not currently recommended.

Oculorespiratory syndrome (ORS) is an acute, self-limiting reaction to IIV with one or more of the following symptoms appearing within 2 to 24 hours after the dose: Chest tightness, cough, difficulty breathing, facial swelling, red eyes, sore throat, or wheezing. Symptoms resolve within 48 hours of onset. The cause of ORS has not been established, but studies have suggested that it is not IgE-mediated. However, because ORS symptoms may be similar to those of an IgE-mediated hypersensitivity reaction, healthcare providers unsure of etiology of symptoms should seek advice from an allergist/immunologist when determining whether a patient may be revaccinated in subsequent seasons (CDC/ACIP [Grohskopf, 2013]).

Syncope has been reported with use of injectable vaccines and may be accompanied by transient visual disturbances, weakness, or tonic-clonic movements. Procedures should be in place to avoid injuries from falling and to restore cerebral perfusion if syncope occurs (CDC, 57[17], 2008).

Some products may contain polysorbate 80 (Tween 80) which may cause allergic reactions in susceptible individuals. Products may contain gentamicin, kanamycin, neomycin, or polymyxin; use caution in patients with known sensitivity to these agents.

Precautions The decision to administer or delay vaccination because of current or recent febrile illness depends on the severity of symptoms and the etiology of the disease. Immunization should be delayed during the course of an acute severe febrile illness; may administer to patients with mild acute illness (with or without fever). Use with caution in severely immunocompromised patients (eg, patients receiving chemo-/radiation therapy or other immunosuppressive therapy including high-dose corticosteroids); may have a reduced response to vaccination and vaccination may not result in effective immunity in all patients. Inactivated vaccine (IIV or RIV) is preferred over live virus vaccine for household members, health care workers, and others coming in close contact with severely immunosuppressed persons requiring care in a protected environment (CDC/ACIP [Grohskopf, 2013]; CDC/ACIP [Kroger, 2011]). In general, inactivated vaccines should be administered ≥2 weeks prior to planned immunosuppression when feasible (IDSA [Rubin, 2014]).

Antigenic response may not be as great as expected in HIV-infected patients with CD4 cells <100/mm^3 and viral copies of HIV type 1 >30,000/mL and a second dose does not improve immune response in these persons (CDC/ACIP [Grohskopf, 2013]). Vaccination may not result in effective immunity in all patients. Response depends upon multiple factors (eg, type of vaccine, age of patient) and may be improved by administering the vaccine at the recommended dose, route, and interval (CDC/ACIP [Kroger, 2011]). In general, household and close contacts of persons with altered immunocompetence may receive all age-appropriate vaccines. Inactivated influenza virus vaccine (IIV or RIV) is preferred over live virus vaccine for household members, healthcare workers, and others coming in close contact with severely immunosuppressed persons requiring care in a protected environment (CDC/ACIP [Grohskopf, 2013]; CDC/ACIP [Kroger, 2011]). Influenza vaccines from previous seasons must not be used (CDC/ACIP [Grohskopf, 2013]).

Use with caution in patients with history of febrile convulsions. Antipyretics have not been shown to prevent febrile seizures; antipyretics may be used to treat fever or discomfort following vaccination (CDC/ACIP [Kroger, 2011]). One study reported that routine prophylactic administration of acetaminophen to prevent fever prior to vaccination decreased the immune response of some vaccines; the clinical significance of this reduction in immune response has not been established (Prymula, 2009).

Use with caution in patients with history of Guillain-Barré syndrome (GBS); patients with history of GBS have a greater likelihood of developing GBS than those without. As a precaution, the ACIP recommends that patients with a history of GBS and who are at low risk for severe influenza complications, and patients known to have experienced GBS within 6 weeks following previous vaccination should generally not be vaccinated (consider influenza antiviral chemoprophylaxis in these patients). The benefits of vaccination may outweigh the potential risks in persons with a history of GBS who are also at high risk for complications of influenza (CDC/ACIP [Bridges, 2014]). Recent studies of patients who received the trivalent inactivated influenza vaccine or the monovalent H1N1 influenza vaccine have shown the risk of GBS is lower with vaccination than with influenza infection (Baxter, 2013; Greene, 2013; Kwong, 2013).

Use caution in patients with coagulation disorders, including thrombocytopenia, due to an increased risk for bleeding following I.M. administration; if the patient received antihemophilia or other similar therapy, I.M. injection can be scheduled shortly after such therapy is administered.

Most products are manufactured with chicken egg protein (expressed as ovalbumin content when disclosed in prescribing information). The ovalbumin content may vary from season to season and lot to lot of vaccine. Allergy to eggs must be distinguished from allergy to the vaccine. Recommendations are available from the ACIP regarding influenza vaccination to persons who report egg allergies; however, ACIP states a prior severe allergic reaction to influenza vaccine, regardless of the component suspected, is a contraindication to vaccination. Patients with a history of egg allergy who have experienced only hives following egg exposure should receive influenza vaccine using IIV (egg- or cell-culture based) or RIV, if otherwise appropriate; however, the vaccine should only be administered by a healthcare provider familiar with the manifestations of egg allergy and patients be monitored for at least 30 minutes after vaccination (CDC/ACIP [Grohskopf, 2013]). Flucelvax (ccIV3) is an inactivated influenza vaccine manufactured using cell culture technology and provides an alternative to vaccines cultured with chicken egg protein but should not be considered egg free. It may be used in persons with a mild egg allergy if age appropriate and there are no other contraindications; appropriate precautions should be observed (CDC/ACIP [Grohskopf, 2013]).

Use of this vaccine for specific medical and/or other indications (eg, immunocompromising conditions, hepatic or kidney disease, diabetes) is also addressed in the ACIP Recommended Immunization Schedule (CDC/ACIP [Akinsanya-Beysolow, 2014]; CDC/ACIP [Bridges, 2014]). Specific recommendations for use of this vaccine in immunocompromised patients with asplenia, cancer, HIV infection, cerebrospinal fluid leaks, cochlear implants, hematopoietic stem cell transplant (prior to or after), sickle cell disease, solid organ transplant (prior to or after), or those receiving immunosuppressive therapy for chronic conditions as well as contacts of immunocompromised patients are available from the IDSA (Rubin, 2014). Some products may contain polysorbate 80 (Tween 80) which may cause allergic reactions in susceptible individuals. Products may contain thimerosal; packaging may contain natural latex rubber; use caution in patients with known sensitivity to these agents.

Adverse Reactions All serious adverse reactions must be reported to the U.S. Department of Health and Human Services (DHHS) Vaccine Adverse Event Reporting System (VAERS) 1-800-822-7967 or online at https://vaers.hhs.gov/esub/index. In Canada, adverse reactions may be reported to local provincial/territorial health agencies or to the Vaccine Safety Section at Public Health Agency of Canada (1-866-844-0018).

Adverse reactions in adults ≥65 years of age may be greater using the high-dose vaccine, but are typically mild and transient.

Cardiovascular: Chest tightness, facial edema
Central nervous system: Chills, drowsiness, fatigue, fever, headache, irritability, malaise, migraine, shivering
Endocrine & metabolic: Dysmenorrhea
Gastrointestinal: Appetite decreased, diarrhea, nausea, sore throat, upper abdominal pain, vomiting
Local: Injection site reactions (including bruising, erythema, induration, inflammation, pain, soreness [≤64%; may last up to 2 days], pruritus, swelling, tenderness)
Neuromuscular & skeletal: Arthralgia, back pain, myalgia (may start within 6-12 hours and last 1-2 days; incidence generally equal to placebo in adults; occurs more frequently than placebo in children)
Ocular: Red eyes
Otic: Earache
Respiratory: Cough, nasal congestion, nasopharyngitis, pharyngolaryngeal pain, rhinitis, upper respiratory tract infection, wheezing
Miscellaneous: Diaphoresis
Rare but important or life-threatening: Allergic reactions, anaphylaxis, angioedema, convulsions, erythema multiforme, facial palsy (Bell's palsy), Guillain-Barré syndrome (GBS), Henoch-Schönlein purpura (IgA vasculitis), hypersensitivity reaction, limb paralysis, lymphadenopathy, myelitis (including encephalomyelitis and transverse myelitis), neuralgia, oculorespiratory syndrome (ORS; acute, self-limited reaction with ocular and respiratory symptoms), optic neuritis/neuropathy, paralysis, photophobia, serum sickness, Stevens-Johnson syndrome, syncope, tachycardia, thrombocytopenia, urticaria, vasculitis, vertigo

Drug Interactions
Metabolism/Transport Effects None known.
Avoid Concomitant Use There are no known interactions where it is recommended to avoid concomitant use.
Increased Effect/Toxicity There are no known significant interactions involving an increase in effect.
Decreased Effect
Influenza Virus Vaccine (Inactivated) may decrease the levels/effects of: Pneumococcal Conjugate Vaccine (13-Valent)

The levels/effects of Influenza Virus Vaccine (Inactivated) may be decreased by: Belimumab; Fingolimod;

Immunosuppressants; Pneumococcal Conjugate Vaccine (13-Valent)

Stability Store all products between 2°C to 8°C (36°F to 46°F). Potency is destroyed by freezing; do not use if product has been frozen.
Fluarix, Fluarix Quadrivalent, Flucelvax: Protect from light.
Afluria, FluLaval: Discard multiple-dose vials 28 days after initial entry. Protect from light.
Fluvirin, Fluzone, FluLaval Quadrivalent: Between uses, the multiple dose vial should be stored at 2°C to 8°C (36°F to 46°F). Protect from light.

Mechanism of Action Promotes immunity to seasonal influenza virus by inducing specific antibody production. Each year the formulation is standardized according to the U.S. Public Health Service. Preparations from previous seasons must not be used.

Pharmacodynamics
Onset of action: Most adults have antibody protection within 2 weeks of vaccination (CDC/ACIP [Grohskopf, 2013])
Duration: ≥6-8 months when vaccine is antigenically similar to circulating virus; response may be diminished in persons ≥65 years and limited evidence suggests titers may decline significantly 6 months following vaccination in this population (CDC/ACIP [Grohskopf, 2013])

Dosing: Usual Influenza seasons vary in their timing and duration from year to year. In general, vaccination should begin soon after the vaccine becomes available (and, if possible, by October) and prior to onset of influenza activity in the community; however, vaccination should continue throughout the influenza season as long as vaccine is available. Unless noted, the ACIP does not have a preference for any given IIV formulation when used within their specified age indications.
Pediatric:
Immunization: Dose frequency is per flu season.
Note: In infants and children <9 years, the number of doses needed per flu season is dependent upon vaccination history:
A single dose for the 2013-2014 season: If patient received a total of ≥2 doses of seasonal influenza vaccine since July 1, 2010
Two doses for the 2013-1014 needed (separated by ≥4 weeks) if any of the following:
• Total of ≤1 dose of seasonal vaccine since July 1, 2010 (including no previous vaccination)
• Vaccination status cannot be determined
Additional dosing considerations are provided when vaccination history is available prior to the 2010-2011 season
Fluzone, Fluzone Quadrivalent: I.M.:
Infants and Children 6 to 35 months: 0.25 mL per dose for a total of 1 or 2 doses, dependent upon vaccination history (see **Note**)
Children 3 to 8 years: 0.5 mL per dose for a total of 1 or 2 doses, dependent upon vaccination history (see **Note**)
Children ≥9 years and Adolescents: 0.5 mL per dose as a single dose
Fluarix, Fluarix Quadrivalent, FluLaval, FluLaval Quadrivalent: I.M.:
Children 3 to 8 years: 0.5 mL per dose for a total of 1 or 2 doses, dependent upon vaccination history (see **Note**)
Children ≥9 years and Adolescents: 0.5 mL per dose as a single dose
Fluvirin: I.M.:
Children 4 to 8 years: 0.5 mL per dose for a total of 1 or 2 doses, dependent upon vaccination history (see **Note**)
Children ≥9 years and Adolescents: 0.5 mL per dose as a single dose

Afluria: I.M.: **Note:** Although approved for use in children ≥5 years of age, the ACIP does not recommend use of Afluria in infants or children <9 years of age due to an increased incidence of fever and febrile seizures noted during the 2010-2011 influenza season. However, if other age appropriate vaccines are not available, children 5 to 8 years of age who are also considered at risk for influenza complications may be given Afluria after benefits and risks are discussed with parents or caregivers (AAP, 2013; CDC/ACIP [Grohskopf, 2013]).

Children 5 to 8 years: 0.5 mL per dose for a total of 1 or 2 doses, dependent upon vaccination history (see **Note**)

Children ≥9 years and Adolescents: 0.5 mL per dose as a single dose

Fluzone Intradermal: Intradermal: Adolescents ≥18 years 0.1 mL per dose as a single dose

Flucelvax: I.M.: Adolescents ≥18 years: 0.5 mL per dose as a single dose

Adult:

Immunization:

Afluria, Fluarix, Fluarix Quadrivalent, Flucelvax, Flu-Laval, FluLaval Quadrivalent, Fluvirin, Fluzone, Fluzone Quadrivalent: I.M.: 0.5 mL per dose as a single dose

Fluzone Intradermal: Age ≤64 years: Intradermal: 0.1 mL per dose as a single dose

Fluzone High-Dose: I.M.: Adults ≥65 years: 0.5 mL per dose as a single dose

Dosing adjustment in renal impairment: There are no dosage adjustments provided in manufacturer's labeling.

Dosing adjustment in hepatic impairment: There are no dosage adjustments provided in manufacturer's labeling.

Administration Adolescents and adults should be vaccinated while seated or lying down. U.S. law requires that the date of administration; the vaccine manufacturer; lot number of vaccine; the administering person's name, title, and address; and documentation of the vaccine information statement (VIS; date on VIS and date given to patient) be entered into the patient's permanent medical record.

Intradermal: Fluzone Intradermal: For intradermal administration over the deltoid muscle only. Shake gently prior to use. Hold system using the thumb and middle finger (do not place fingers on windows). Insert needle perpendicular to the skin; inject using index finger to push on plunger. Do not aspirate.

Intramuscular: Afluria, Fluarix, Fluarix Quadrivalent, Flu-Laval, FluLaval Quadrivalent, Flucelvax, Fluvirin, Fluzone, Fluzone High-Dose, Fluzone Quadrivalent: For I.M. administration only. Inspect for particulate matter and discoloration prior to administration. Shake suspension well prior to use. Jet injectors should not be used to administer inactivated influenza vaccines unless otherwise indicated in product labeling.

Infants: I.M. injection in the anterolateral aspect of the thigh using a 1-inch needle length; do not inject into the gluteal region or areas where there may be a major nerve trunk

Children and Adults: I.M. injection in the deltoid muscle using a ≥1-inch needle length; children with adequate deltoid muscle mass should be vaccinated using a 1-inch needle, in some young children (1 to 2 years) a 5/8-inch needle may be adequate (CDC [Kroger, 2011])

Patients at risk of bleeding (eg, patient receiving antihemophilic factor): For patients at risk of hemorrhage following intramuscular injection, the ACIP recommends "it should be administered intramuscularly if, in the opinion of the physician familiar with the patient's bleeding risk, the vaccine can be administered by this route with reasonable safety. If the patient receives antihemophilia or other similar therapy, intramuscular vaccination can be

scheduled shortly after such therapy is administered. A fine needle (23-gauge or smaller) can be used for the vaccination and firm pressure applied to the site (without rubbing) for at least 2 minutes. The patient should be instructed concerning the risk of hematoma from the injection." Patients on anticoagulant therapy should be considered to have the same bleeding risks and treated as those with clotting factor disorders (CDC [Kroger, 2011]).

If a pediatric vaccine (0.25 mL) is inadvertently administered to an adult an additional 0.25 mL should be administered to provide the full adult dose (0.5 mL). If the error is discovered after the patient has left, an adult dose should be given as soon as the patient can return. If an adult vaccine (0.5 mL) is inadvertently given to a child, no action needs to be taken.

Monitoring Parameters Observe for syncope for 15 minutes following administration. If seizure-like activity associated with syncope occurs, maintain patient in supine or Trendelenburg position to re-establish adequate cerebral perfusion (CDC/ACIP [Kroger, 2011]). For those individuals who report a history of egg allergy but it is determined that the inactivated vaccine can be used, observe vaccine recipient for at least 30 minutes after receipt of vaccine (CDC/ACIP [Grohskopf, 2013]).

Additional Information Pharmacies will stock the formulations(s) standardized according to the USPHS requirements for the season. Influenza vaccines from previous seasons must not be used. It is important to note that influenza seasons vary in their timing and duration from year to year. In general, vaccination should begin soon after the vaccine becomes available and prior to onset of influenza activity in the community; however, vaccination should continue throughout the influenza season as long as vaccine is available. Seasonal quadrivalent influenza vaccines contain two subtype A strains and two subtype B strains; trivalent influenza vaccines contain two subtype A strains and one subtype B strain.

When vaccine supply is not limited, either IIV or LAIV can be used in healthy, nonpregnant persons aged 2 to 49 years of age. RIV can be used in persons 18 to 49 years of age.

When vaccine supply is limited, administration should focus on the ACIP target groups. When IIV vaccine is in short supply, administering LAIV to eligible persons is encouraged to increase available IIV to those patients in whom LAIV cannot be used. During periods of inactivated influenza vaccine (IIV) shortage, the CDC and ACIP have recommended vaccination be prioritized based on the following three tiers. The grouping is based on influenza associated mortality and hospitalization rates. Those listed in group 1 should be vaccinated first, followed by persons in group 2, and then group 3. If the vaccine supply is extremely limited, group 1 has also been subdivided in three tiers, where those in group 1A should be vaccinated first, followed by 1B, then 1C.

Priority groups for vaccination with inactivated seasonal influenza vaccine during periods of vaccine shortage (CDC, 2005):

Tier 1:

Tier 1A:

Persons ≥65 years with comorbid conditions

Residents of long-term care facilities

Tier 1B:

Persons 2 to 64 years with comorbid conditions

Persons ≥65 years without comorbid conditions

Infants and Children 6 to 23 months

Pregnant women

Tier 1C:
Health care personnel
Household contacts and out-of-home caregivers of infants <6 months
Tier 2:
Household contacts of children and adults at increased risk of influenza-associated complications
Healthy persons 50 to 64 years
Tier 3: Persons 2 to 49 years without high-risk conditions

Further information available at http://www.cdc.gov/mmwr/preview/mmwrhtml/mm5430a4.htm.

In order to maximize vaccination rates, the ACIP recommends simultaneous administration (ie, >1 vaccine on the same day at different anatomic sites) of all age-appropriate vaccines (live or inactivated) for which a person is eligible at a single visit, unless contraindications exist (CDC/ACIP [Kroger, 2011]). If available, the use of combination vaccines is generally preferred over separate injections, taking into consideration provider assessment, patient preference, and potential adverse events. If separate vaccines being used, evaluate product information regarding same syringe compatibility of vaccines. Separate needles and syringes should be used for each injection. The ACIP prefers each dose of specific vaccine in a series come from the same manufacturer if possible (CDC/ACIP [Kroger, 2011]).

For additional information, please refer to the following website: http://www.cdc.gov/vaccines/vpd-vac/.

Dosage Forms Excipient information presented when available (limited, particularly for generics); consult specific product labeling.
Device, Intradermal [preservative free]:
Fluzone: 9 mcg/strain (0.1 mL); 9 mcg/strain (0.1 mL) [contains egg white (egg protein)]
Injectable, Intramuscular:
Flulaval: (5 mL) [contains egg white (egg protein), thimerosal]
Fluvirin: (5 mL) [contains egg white (egg protein), neomycin, thimerosal]
Fluzone: (5 mL) [contains egg white (egg protein), gelatin (pork), thimerosal]
Kit, Intramuscular:
Physicians EZ Use Flu: [contains egg white (egg protein), neomycin, thimerosal]
Kit, Intramuscular [preservative free]:
Medical Provider EZ Flu PF: [contains egg white (egg protein), neomycin]
Suspension, Intramuscular:
Afluria: (5 mL) [contains egg white (egg protein), neomycin sulfate, thimerosal]
Flulaval Quadrivalent: (5 mL) [contains egg white (egg protein), polysorbate 80, thimerosal]
Fluzone Quadrivalent: 0.5 mL (5 mL) [contains egg white (egg protein), thimerosal]
Suspension, Intramuscular [preservative free]:
Afluria Preservative Free: (0.5 mL) [contains egg white (egg protein), neomycin sulfate]
Fluarix: (0.5 mL) [contains egg white (egg protein), polysorbate 80]
Fluarix Quadrivalent: 0.5 mL (0.5 mL) [contains egg white (egg protein)]
Flucelvax: (0.5 mL) [contains polysorbate 80]
Fluvirin Preservative Free: (0.5 mL) [contains egg white (egg protein), neomycin]
Fluzone High-Dose: (0.5 mL) [contains egg white (egg protein)]
Fluzone Pediatric PF: (0.25 mL, 0.5 mL) [contains egg white (egg protein), gelatin (pork)]
Fluzone Preservative Free: (0.5 mL) [contains egg white (egg protein), gelatin (pork)]
Fluzone Quadrivalent: 0.25 mL (0.25 mL); 0.5 mL (0.5 mL) [contains egg white (egg protein)]

References

AAP Steering Committee on Quality Improvement and Management, Subcommittee on Febrile Seizures American Academy of Pediatrics, "Febrile Seizures: Clinical Practice Guideline for the Long-Term Management of the Child With Simple Febrile Seizures," *Pediatrics*, 2008, 121(6):1281-6.

Akinsanya-Beysolow I, Advisory Committee on Immunization Practices (ACIP), ACIP Child/Adolescent Immunization Work Group, et al. Advisory committee on immunization practices recommended immunization schedules for persons aged 0 through 18 years - United States, 2014. *MMWR Morb Mortal Wkly Rep*. 2014; 63(5):108-109. Full schedule available at http://www.cdc.gov/vaccines/schedules/downloads/child/0-18yrs-child-combined-schedule.pdf

American Academy of Pediatrics, Committee on Infectious Diseases, "Policy Statement - Recommendations for Prevention and Control of Influenza in Children, 2013-2014," *Pediatrics*, 132;e1089.

Baxter R, Bakshi N, Fireman B, et al. Lack of association of Guillain-Barre syndrome with vaccinations. *Clin Infect Dis*. 2013;57(2):197-204.

Bridges CB, Coyne-Beasley T, Advisory Committee on Immunization Practices (ACIP), ACIP Adult Immunization Work Group; Centers for Disease Control and Prevention (CDC). Advisory committee on immunization practices recommended immunization schedule for adults aged 19 years or older - United States, 2014. *MMWR Morb Mortal Wkly Rep*. 2014; 63(5):108-109. Available at: http://www.cdc.gov/vaccines/schedules/downloads/adult/adult-combined-schedule.pdf

Centers for Disease Control and Prevention (CDC), "Note to Providers: Febrile Seizures Associated With TIV & PCV13." Available at http://www.cdc.gov/vaccines/pubs/vis/tiv-pcv-note.htm

Centers for Disease Control and Prevention (CDC), "Pregnant Women & Influenza (Flu)," Atlanta: U.S. Department of Health and Human Services, Public Health Service, December 15, 2010. Available at http://www.cdc.gov/flu/protect/vaccine/pregnant.htm.

Centers for Disease Control and Prevention (CDC), "Syncope After Vaccination-United States, January 2005-July 2007," *MMWR Morb Mortal Wkly Rep*, 2008, 2;57(17):457-60.

Centers for Disease Control and Prevention (CDC). Tiered use of inactivated influenza vaccine in the event of a vaccine shortage. *MMWR Morb Mortal Wkly Rep*. 2005;54(30):749-750.

Centers for Disease Control and Prevention (CDC), "Update on Febrile Seizures in Children Following Vaccination With Influenza Vaccines and Pneumococcal Vaccines." Last updated October 2011. Available at http://www.cdc.gov/vaccinesafety/Concerns/FebrileSeizures.html

Englund JA, Mbawuike IN, Hammill H, et al. Maternal immunization with influenza or tetanus toxoid vaccine for passive antibody protection in young infants. *J Infect Dis*. 1993;168(3):647-656.

Greene SK, Rett MD, Vellozzi C, et al. Guillain-Barré syndrome, influenza vaccination, and antecedent respiratory and gastrointestinal infections: a case-centered analysis in the Vaccine Safety Datalink, 2009-2011. *PLoS One*. 2013;8(6):e67185.

Grohskopf LA, Shay D, Shimabukuro TT, et.al. Prevention and control of seasonal influenza with vaccines. *MMWR Recomm Rep*. 2013;62(RR-07):1-43.

Kroger AT, Atkinson WL, Marcuse EK, Pickering LK. General recommendations on immunization - recommendations of the Advisory Committee on Immunization Practices (ACIP). *MMWR Recomm Rep*. 2011;60(RR-2):1-64.

Kwong JC, Vasa PP, Campetelli MA, et al. Risk of Guillain-Barré syndrome after seasonal influenza vaccination and influenza health-care encounters: a self-controlled study. *Lancet Infecti Dis*. 2013;13(9):769-776.

Prymula R, Siegrist CA, Chlibek R, et al, "Effect of Prophylactic Paracetamol Administration at Time of Vaccination on Febrile Reactions and Antibody Responses in Children: Two Open-Label, Randomised Controlled Trials," *Lancet*, 2009, 374(9698):1339-50.

Rasmussen SA, Jamieson DJ, and Bresee JS, "Pandemic Influenza and Pregnant Women," *Emerg Infect Dis*, 2008, 14(1):95-100.

Rubin LG, Levin MJ, Ljungman P, et al. 2013 IDSA clinical practice guideline for vaccination of the immunocompromised host. *Clin Infect Dis*. 2014;58(3):e44-e100.

Schlaudecker EP, Steinhoff MC, Omer SB, et al. IgA and neutralizing antibodies to influenza a virus in human milk: a randomized trial of antenatal influenza immunization. *PLoS One*, 2013;8(8):e70867.

Steinhoff MC, Omer SB, Roy E, et al. Influenza immunization in pregnancy - antibody responses in mothers and infants. *N Engl J Med*. 2010;362(17):1644-1646.

U.S. Food and Drug Administration, "FDA Updated Communication on Use of Jet Injectors With Inactivated Influenza Vaccines." Last updated October 2011. Available at http://www.fda.gov/BiologicsBloodVaccines/Vaccines/QuestionsaboutVaccines/ucm276773.htm

Zaman K, Roy E, Arifeen SE, Rahman M, et al, "Effectiveness of Maternal Influenza Immunization in Mothers and Infants," *N Engl J Med*, 2008, 359(15):1555-64.

Zuccotti G, Pogliani L, Pariani E, et al. Transplacental antibody transfer following maternal immunization with a pandemic 2009 influenza A (H1N1) MF59-adjuvanted vaccine. *JAMA.* 2010;304(21):2360-2361.

Influenza Virus Vaccine (Live/Attenuated)

(in floo EN za VYE rus vak SEEN live ah TEN yoo aye ted)

Medication Safety Issues

Sound-alike/look-alike issues:

Influenza virus vaccine may be confused with flumazenil

Related Information

Immunization Administration Recommendations *on page 2368*

Immunization Guidelines *on page 2373*

Brand Names: U.S. FluMist; FluMist Quadrivalent

Brand Names: Canada FluMist

Therapeutic Category Vaccine; Vaccine, Live/Attenuated

Generic Availability (U.S.) No

Use For the active immunization against influenza disease caused by influenza virus subtypes A and type B contained in the vaccine (FDA approved in ages 2 to 49 years)

The Advisory Committee on Immunization Practices (ACIP) recommends routine annual vaccination with seasonal influenza vaccine for all persons who do not otherwise have contraindications to the vaccine. ACIP recommends use of any age- and risk factor-appropriate product. Healthy, nonpregnant persons aged 2 to 49 years may receive vaccination with the seasonal live, attenuated influenza vaccine (LAIV) (nasal spray). In addition, other alternative products are available for certain patient populations: Persons ≥6 months of age may receive the trivalent inactivated influenza vaccine (IIV3) or the quadrivalent inactivated influenza vaccine (IIV4). Persons 18 to 49 years may also receive vaccination with the recombinant influenza vaccine (RIV) (CDC/ACIP [Grohskopf, 2013]).

Pregnancy Risk Factor B

Pregnancy Considerations Adverse events were not observed in animal reproduction studies. LAIV is not recommended for use during pregnancy. Influenza vaccination with the inactivated influenza vaccine (IIV) is recommended for all women who are or will become pregnant during the influenza season and who do not otherwise have contraindications to the vaccine (CDC, 2013c).

Healthy pregnant women do not need to avoid contact with persons vaccinated with LAIV (CDC, 2013). The nasal vaccine contains the same strains of influenza A and B found in the injection. Information specific to the use of LAIV in pregnancy has not been located. Refer to the Influenza Virus Vaccine (Inactivated) monograph for additional information.

Healthcare providers are encouraged to refer women exposed to the influenza vaccine during pregnancy to the Vaccines and Medications in Pregnancy Surveillance System (VAMPSS) by contacting The Organization of Teratology Information Specialists (OTIS) at (877) 311-8972.

Breast-Feeding Considerations It is not known if the vaccine is excreted into breast milk. LAIV should be used with caution in breast-feeding women (per manufacturer) due to the possibility of virus excretion into breast milk; however, LAIV may be administered to breast-feeding women unless contraindicated due to other reasons (per CDC). Postpartum women may be vaccinated with either IIV or LAIV. When vaccine supply is limited, focus on delivering the vaccine should be given to mothers of newborns and contacts or caregivers of children <5 years of age (CDC, 2013).

Contraindications Severe allergic reaction (eg, anaphylaxis) to any component, including egg protein, gentamicin, gelatin, and arginine or after previous influenza virus

vaccination; children or adolescents receiving aspirin or aspirin-containing therapy

Warnings Immediate treatment (including epinephrine 1:1000) for anaphylactoid and/or hypersensitivity reactions should be available during vaccine use.

The nasal spray should not be used in patients with asthma or children <5 years of age with recurrent wheezing; risk of wheezing following vaccination is increased. Patients with severe asthma or active wheezing were not included in clinical trials. Children <2 years of age had increased wheezing and hospitalizations following administration in clinical trials; use of the nasal spray is not approved in this age group. ACIP does not recommend the use of LAIV in patients with chronic pulmonary disorders including asthma and children 2 to 4 years of age who have had asthma or wheezing episodes within the past year (CDC/ACIP [Grohskopf, 2013]). Due to association of Reye's syndrome with aspirin, use is of LAIV is contraindicated in pediatric patients on concurrent aspirin therapy and aspirin-containing products should be avoided for 4 weeks following vaccination in children and adolescents ≤17 years of age.

Data on the use of the nasal spray in immunocompromised patients is limited. ACIP does not recommend the use of LAIV in immunosuppressed patients (CDC/ACIP [Grohskopf, 2013]). ACIP does not recommend the use of LAIV for persons who care for severely immunocompromised individuals who require a protective environment due to the theoretical risk of transmitting the live virus from the vaccine. Persons who care for the severely immunocompromised should receive either IIV or RIV. Persons who have received LAIV should avoid contact with severely immunocompromised individuals for at least 7 days following vaccination (CDC/ACIP [Grohskopf, 2013]). In general, live vaccines should be administered ≥4 weeks **prior to** planned immunosuppression and avoided within 2 weeks of immunosuppression when feasible (Rubin, 2014).

Because safety and efficacy information is limited, the ACIP does not recommend the use of LAIV in patients with chronic disorders of the cardiovascular system (except isolated hypertension), chronic metabolic diseases (including diabetes mellitus), hematologic disorders and hemoglobinopathies, hepatic disease, HIV, neurologic/neuromuscular disorders, renal disease, and pregnancy.

Precautions The decision to administer or delay vaccination because of current or recent febrile illness depends on the severity of symptoms and the etiology of the disease. Immunization should be delayed during the course of an acute severe febrile illness; may administer to patients with mild acute illness (with or without fever) (CDC/ACIP [Kroger, 2011]). Presence of nasal congestion may decrease delivery of the vaccine to the nasopharyngeal mucosa; postpone administration until illness resolves or use the inactivated vaccine if appropriate.

Use with caution in patients with history of Guillain-Barré syndrome (GBS); patients with history of GBS have a greater likelihood of developing GBS than those without. As a precaution, the ACIP recommends that patients with a history of GBS and who are at low risk for severe influenza complications, and patients known to have experienced GBS within 6 weeks following previous vaccination should generally not be vaccinated (consider influenza antiviral chemoprophylaxis in these patients). Based on limited data, the benefits of vaccinating persons with a history of GBS who are also at high risk for complications of influenza may outweigh the risks (CDC/ACIP [Grohskopf, 2013]). Recent studies of patients who received the trivalent inactivated influenza vaccine or the monovalent H1N1 influenza vaccine have shown the risk of GBS is lower with vaccination than with influenza infection (Baxter, 2013; Greene, 2013; Kwong, 2013).

Vaccination may not result in effective immunity in all patients. Response depends upon multiple factors (eg, type of vaccine, age of patient) and may be improved by administering the vaccine at the recommended dose, route, and interval. Vaccines may not be effective if administered during periods of altered immune competence (CDC/ACIP [Kroger, 2011]). Influenza vaccines from previous seasons must not be used. Studies conducted in children comparing the trivalent inactivated influenza vaccine (IIV) and LAIV have shown significantly greater efficacy of LAIV in younger children. Information is not yet available for the quadrivalent LAIV vaccine (CDC/ACIP [Grohskopf, 2013]).

Antipyretics have not been shown to prevent febrile seizures; antipyretics may be used to treat fever or discomfort following vaccination (CDC/ACIP [Kroger, 2011]). One study reported that routine prophylactic administration of acetaminophen to prevent fever prior to vaccination decreased the immune response of some vaccines; the clinical significance of this reduction in immune response has not been established (Prymula, 2009).

Manufactured with chicken egg protein. Allergy to eggs must be distinguished from allergy to the vaccine. Recommendations are available from the CDC regarding influenza vaccination to persons who report egg allergies; however, a prior severe allergic reaction to influenza vaccine, regardless of the component suspected, is a contraindication to vaccination. Use of TIV (trivalent inactivated influenza virus) is preferred over LAIV when considering vaccination in persons reporting an egg allergy (CDC/ACIP [Grohskopf, 2013]).

Live influenza virus vaccine (LAIV) should not be given until 48 hours after the completion of influenza antiviral therapy (influenza A and B). Influenza antiviral therapy (influenza A and B) should not be administered for 2 weeks after receiving LAIV. If influenza antiviral therapy (influenza A and B) and LAIV are administered concomitantly, revaccination should be considered.

The safety of LAIV has not been established in individuals with underlying medical conditions that may predispose them to complications following wild-type influenza infection. Use of this vaccine for specific medical and/or other indications (eg, immunocompromising conditions, hepatic or kidney disease, diabetes) is also addressed in the ACIP Recommended Immunization Schedule (CDC/ACIP [Akinsanya-Beysolow, 2014]; CDC/ACIP [Bridges, 2014]). Specific recommendations for use of this vaccine in immunocompromised patients with asplenia, cancer, HIV infection, cerebrospinal fluid leaks, cochlear implants, hematopoietic stem cell transplant (prior to or after), sickle cell disease, solid organ transplant (prior to or after), or those receiving immunosuppressive therapy for chronic conditions as well as contacts of immunocompromised patients are available from the IDSA (Rubin, 2014).

Adverse Reactions All serious adverse reactions must be reported to the U.S. Department of Health and Human Services (DHHS) Vaccine Adverse Event Reporting System (VAERS) 1-800-822-7967 or online at https://vaers.hhs.gov/esub/index. In Canada, adverse reactions may be reported to local provincial/territorial health agencies or to the Vaccine Safety Section at Public Health Agency of Canada (1-866-844-0018).

Central nervous system: Chills, fever, headache, irritability, lethargy

Gastrointestinal: Abdominal pain, appetite decreased

Neuromuscular & skeletal: Muscle aches, tiredness/weakness

Otic: Otitis media

Respiratory: Sinusitis, sneezing

Respiratory: Cough, nasal congestion/ runny nose, wheezing

Rare but important or life-threatening: Anaphylactic reactions, asthma exacerbations, Bell's palsy, encephalitis (vaccine associated), epistaxis, Guillain-Barré syndrome, hypersensitivity reaction, meningitis (including eosinophilic meningitis), mitochondrial encephalomyopathy (Leigh syndrome) exacerbation, pericarditis

Drug Interactions

Metabolism/Transport Effects None known.

Avoid Concomitant Use

Avoid concomitant use of Influenza Virus Vaccine (Live/Attenuated) with any of the following: Belimumab; Fingolimod; Immunosuppressants; Salicylates

Increased Effect/Toxicity

Influenza Virus Vaccine (Live/Attenuated) may increase the levels/effects of: Salicylates

The levels/effects of Influenza Virus Vaccine (Live/Attenuated) may be increased by: Belimumab; Corticosteroids (Systemic); Dimethyl Fumarate; Fingolimod; Hydroxychloroquine; Immunosuppressants; Leflunomide; Mercaptopurine; Methotrexate

Decreased Effect

Influenza Virus Vaccine (Live/Attenuated) may decrease the levels/effects of: Tuberculin Tests

The levels/effects of Influenza Virus Vaccine (Live/Attenuated) may be decreased by: Antiviral Agents (Influenza A and B); Dimethyl Fumarate; Fingolimod; Immune Globulins; Immunosuppressants

Stability Store in refrigerator at 2°C to 8°C (36°F to 46°F); do not freeze. The vaccine may be exposed to temperatures of up to 25°C for up to 12 hours without adverse impact; return to refrigerator as soon as possible; only a single excursion outside of the recommended storage conditions is permitted.

Mechanism of Action The vaccine contains live attenuated viruses which infect and replicate within the cells lining the nasopharynx. Promotes immunity to seasonal influenza virus by inducing specific antibody production. Each year the formulation is standardized according to the U.S. Public Health Service. Preparations from previous seasons must not be used.

Pharmacodynamics

Onset of action: Adults: Most adults have antibody protection within 2 weeks of vaccination (CDC/ACIP [Grohskopf, 2013])

Duration: ≥6 to 8 months when vaccine is antigenically similar to circulating virus; response may be diminished in persons ≥65 years and limited evidence suggests titers may decline significantly 6 months following vaccination in this population (CDC/ACIP [Grohskopf, 2013])

Pharmacokinetics (Adult data unless noted) Distribution: Following nasal administration, vaccine is distributed in the nasal cavity (~90%), stomach (~3%), brain (~2%), and lung (0.4%)

Dosing: Usual Administer vaccine prior to exposure to influenza. It is important to note that influenza seasons vary in their timing and duration from year to year. In general, vaccination should begin soon after the vaccine becomes available (and, if possible, by October) and prior to onset of influenza activity in the community; however, vaccination should continue throughout the influenza season as long as vaccine is available (CDC/ACIP [Grohskopf, 2013]).

Pediatric: **Immunization:** Dose frequency is per season.

Children 2 to 8 years: Intranasal: 0.2 mL per dose (half dose per nostril); 1 or 2 doses, dependent upon vaccination history

A single dose for the 2013-2014 season: If patient received a total of ≥2 doses of seasonal influenza vaccine since July 1, 2010

Two doses for the 2013-2014 season needed (separated by ≥4 weeks) if any of the following:
- Total of ≤1 dose of seasonal vaccine since July 1, 2010 (including no previous vaccination)
- Vaccination status cannot be determined

Additional dosing considerations are provided when vaccination history is available prior to the 2010-2011 season; see current guidelines for additional information

Children and Adolescents 9 to 18 years: Intranasal: 0.2 mL per dose (half dose per nostril) (1 dose)

Adult: **Immunization:** Adults ≤49 years: Intranasal: 0.2 mL per dose (half dose per nostril) (1 dose); dose frequency is per season

Dosing adjustment in renal impairment: There are no dosage adjustments provided in manufacturer's labeling.

Dosing adjustment in hepatic impairment: There are no dosage adjustments provided in manufacturer's labeling.

Administration Intranasal: For intranasal administration only; do not inject. Administer 0.1 mL (half of the dose from a single sprayer) into each nostril while the recipient is in an upright position. Place the tip of the sprayer inside the nostril and depress plunger as rapidly as possible to deliver the dose. Remove dose divider clip and repeat into opposite nostril. The patient does not need to inhale during administration (may breath normally).

U.S. law requires that the date of administration, name of the vaccine manufacturer, lot number of vaccine, and the administering person's name, title, and address be entered into the patient's permanent medical record.

Test Interactions Administration of the intranasal influenza virus vaccine (live, LAIV) may cause a positive result on the rapid influenza diagnostic test for the 7 days after vaccine administration; for a person with influenza-like illness during this time, the positive test could be caused by either the live attenuated vaccine or wild-type influenza virus (Aly, 2004).

Additional Information Pharmacies will stock the formulations(s) standardized according to the USPHS requirements for the season. Influenza vaccines from previous seasons must not be used.

It is important to note that influenza seasons vary in their timing and duration from year to year. In general, vaccination should begin soon after the vaccine becomes available and prior to onset of influenza activity in the community. However, vaccination should continue throughout the influenza season as long as vaccine is available.

Seasonal quadrivalent influenza vaccines contain two subtype A strains and two subtype B strains; trivalent influenza vaccines contain two subtype A strains and one subtype B strain.

When vaccine supply is not limited, either IIV or LAIV can be used in healthy, nonpregnant persons aged 2 to 49 years of age. RIV can be used in persons 18 to 49 years of age.

When vaccine supply is limited, administration should focus on the ACIP target groups. When IIV vaccine is in short supply, administering LAIV to eligible persons is encouraged to increase available IIV to those patients in whom LAIV cannot be used. During periods of inactivated influenza vaccine (IIV) shortage, the CDC and ACIP have recommended vaccination be prioritized based on the following three tiers. The grouping is based on influenza-associated mortality and hospitalization rates. Those listed in group 1 should be vaccinated first, followed by persons in group 2, and then group 3. If the vaccine supply is extremely limited, group 1 has also been subdivided in three tiers, where those in group 1A should be vaccinated first, followed by 1B, then 1C.

Priority groups for vaccination with inactivated seasonal influenza vaccine during periods of vaccine shortage (CDC, 2005):

Tier 1:
Tier 1A:
Persons ≥65 years with comorbid conditions
Residents of long-term care facilities
Tier 1B:
Persons 2 to 64 years with comorbid conditions
Persons ≥65 years without comorbid conditions
Infants and Children 6 to 23 months
Pregnant women
Tier 1C:
Healthcare personnel
Household contacts and out-of-home caregivers of infants <6 months
Tier 2:
Household contacts of children and adults at increased risk of influenza-associated complications
Healthy persons 50 to 64 years
Tier 3: Persons 2 to 49 years without high-risk conditions

Further information available at http://www.cdc.gov/mmwr/preview/mmwrhtml/mm5430a4.htm

In order to maximize vaccination rates, the ACIP recommends simultaneous administration of all age-appropriate vaccines (live or inactivated) for which a person is eligible at a single visit, unless contraindications exist. The use of combination vaccines is generally preferred over separate injections, taking into consideration provider assessment, patient preference, and potential adverse events.

For additional information, please refer to the following website: http://www.cdc.gov/vaccines/vpd-vac/

Dosage Forms Excipient information presented when available (limited, particularly for generics); consult specific product labeling.

Liquid, Nasal [preservative free]:
FluMist: (1 ea) [contains egg white (egg protein), gelatin (pork)]

Suspension, Nasal [preservative free]:
FluMist Quadrivalent: (1 ea) [latex free; contains egg white (egg protein), gelatin (pork)]

References
Akinsanya-Beysolow I, Advisory Committee on Immunization Practices (ACIP), ACIP Child/Adolescent Immunization Work Group, et al. Advisory committee on immunization practices recommended immunization schedule for persons aged 0 through 18 years - United States, 2014. *MMWR Morb Mortal Wkly Rep.* 2014; 63(5):108-109. Full schedule available at http://www.cdc.gov/vaccines/schedules/downloads/child/0-18yrs-child-combined-schedule.pdf

Ali T, Scott N, Kallas W, et al. Detection of influenza antigen with rapid antibody-based tests after intranasal influenza vaccination (FluMist). *Clin Infect Dis.* 2004;38(5):760-762.

American Academy of Pediatrics, Committee on Infectious Diseases. Policy statement - recommendations for prevention and control of influenza in children, 2013-2014. *Pediatrics.* 132;e1089.

Ashkenazi S, Vertruyen A, Arisegui J, et al. Superior relative efficacy of live attenuated influenza vaccine compared with inactivated influenza vaccine in young children with recurrent respiratory tract infections. *Pediatr Infect Dis J.* 2006;25(10):870-879.

Baxter R, Bakshi N, Fireman B, et al. Lack of association of Guillain-Barre syndrome with vaccinations. *Clin Infect Dis.* 2013;57(2):197-204.

Belshe RB, Mendelman PM, Treanor J, et al, "The Efficacy of Live Attenuated, Cold-Adapted, Trivalent, Intranasal Influenza Virus Vaccine in Children," *N Engl J Med,* 1998, 338(20):1405-12.

Bridges CB, Coyne-Beasley T, Advisory Committee on Immunization Practices (ACIP), ACIP Adult Immunization Work Group; Centers for Disease Control and Prevention (CDC). Advisory committee on immunization practices recommended immunization schedule for adults aged 19 years or older - United States, 2014. *MMWR Morb Mortal Wkly Rep.* 2014; 63(5):108-109. Available at: http://www.cdc.gov/vaccines/schedules/downloads/adult/adult-combined-schedule.pdf

Centers for Disease Control and Prevention (CDC). Tiered use of inactivated influenza vaccine in the event of a vaccine shortage. *MMWR Morb Mortal Wkly Rep.* 2005;54(30):749-750.

Greene SK, Rett MD, Vellozzi C, et al. Guillain-Barré syndrome, influenza vaccination, and antecedent respiratory and gastrointestinal infections: a case-centered analysis in the Vaccine Safety Datalink, 2009-2011. *PLoS One.* 2013;8(6):e67185.

Grohskopf LA, Shay D, Shimabukuro TT, et.al. Prevention and control of seasonal influenza with vaccines. *MMWR Recomm Rep.* 2013c;62 (RR-07):1-43.

Kroger AT, Atkinson WL, Marcuse EK, Pickering LK. General recommendations on immunization - recommendations of the Advisory Committee on Immunization Practices (ACIP). *MMWR Recomm Rep.* 2011;60(RR-2):1-64.

Kwong JC, Vasa PP, Campetelli MA, et al. Risk of Guillain-Barré syndrome after seasonal influenza vaccination and influenza healthcare encounters: a self-controlled study. *Lancet Infecti Dis.* 2013;13 (9):769-776.

Piedra PA, Gaglani MJ, Riggs M, et al. Live attenuated influenza vaccine, trivalent, is safe in healthy children 18 months to 4 years, 5 to 9 years, and 10 to 18 years of age in a community-based, nonrandomized, open-label trial. *Pediatrics.* 2005;116(3):e397-407.

Piedra PA, Yan L, Kotloff K, et al. Safety of the trivalent, cold-adapted influenza vaccine in preschool-aged children. *Pediatrics.* 2002;110 (4):662-672.

Prymula R, Siegrist CA, Chlibek R, et al, "Effect of Prophylactic Paracetamol Administration at Time of Vaccination on Febrile Reactions and Antibody Responses in Children: Two Open-Label, Randomised Controlled Trials," *Lancet*, 2009, 374(9698):1339-50.

Rasmussen SA, Jamieson DJ, and Bresee JS, "Pandemic Influenza and Pregnant Women," *Emerg Infect Dis,* 2008, 14(1):95-100.

Rubin LG, Levin MJ, Ljungman P, et al. 2013 IDSA clinical practice guideline for vaccination of the immunocompromised host. *Clin Infect Dis.* 2014;58(3):e44-e100.

Zaman K, Roy E, Arifeen SE, et al. Effectiveness of maternal influenza immunization in mothers and infants. *N Engl J Med.* 2008;9 (15):1555-1564.

◆ **Influenza Virus Vaccine (Purified Surface Antigen)** *see* Influenza Virus Vaccine (Inactivated) *on page 1103*

Influenza Virus Vaccine (Recombinant)
(in floo EN za VYE rus vak SEEN ree KOM be nant)

Medication Safety Issues
Sound-alike/look-alike issues:
Influenza virus vaccine may be confused with tetanus toxoid and tuberculin products. Medication errors have occurred when tuberculin skin tests (PPD) have been inadvertently administered instead of tetanus toxoid products and influenza virus vaccine. These products are refrigerated and often stored in close proximity to each other.

Related Information
Immunization Administration Recommendations *on page 2368*

Immunization Guidelines *on page 2373*

Brand Names: U.S. Flublok

Therapeutic Category Vaccine, Recombinant

Generic Availability (U.S.) No

Use For active immunization against influenza disease caused by influenza virus subtypes A and type B contained in the vaccine (FDA approved in ages 18 to 48 years)

The Advisory Committee on Immunization Practices (ACIP) recommends routine annual vaccination with seasonal influenza vaccine for all persons who do not otherwise have contraindications to the vaccine. ACIP recommends use of any age- and risk factor-appropriate product. Persons 18 to 49 years may receive vaccination with the recombinant influenza vaccine (RIV). In addition to RIV, other products are available for certain patient populations: Healthy nonpregnant persons aged 2 to 49 years may receive vaccination with the live attenuated influenza vaccine (LAIV). Persons ≥6 months of age may receive the trivalent inactivated influenza vaccine (IIV3) or the quadrivalent inactivated influenza vaccine (IIV4) (CDC/ACIP [Grohskopf, 2013]).

Pregnancy Risk Factor B

Pregnancy Considerations Adverse events were not observed in animal reproduction studies.

Pregnant women are at an increased risk of complications from influenza infection (Rasmussen, 2008). Influenza vaccination with the inactivated influenza vaccine (IIV) is recommended for all women who are or will become pregnant during the influenza season and who do not otherwise have contraindications to the vaccine (CDC, 2013). Pregnant women should observe the same precautions as nonpregnant women to reduce the risk of exposure to influenza and other respiratory infections (CDC, 2010). When vaccine supply is limited, focus on delivering the vaccine should be given to women who are pregnant or will be pregnant during the flu season, as well as mothers of newborns and contacts or caregivers of children <5 years of age (CDC, 2013).

Information specific to the use of RIV in pregnancy has not been located; refer to the Influenza Virus Vaccine, Inactivated monograph for additional information.

Healthcare providers are encouraged to refer women exposed to the influenza vaccine during pregnancy to the *Vaccines and Medications in Pregnancy Surveillance System* (VAMPSS) by contacting The Organization of Teratology Information Specialists (OTIS) at (877) 311-8972.

Breast-Feeding Considerations It is not known if this vaccine is excreted into breast milk. The manufacturer recommends that caution be used if administered to breast-feeding women. Recombinant vaccines do not affect the safety of breast-feeding for the mother or the infant. Breast-feeding infants should be vaccinated according to the recommended schedules (CDC, 2011). When vaccine supply is limited, focus on delivering the vaccine should be given to women who are pregnant or will be pregnant during the flu season, as well as mothers of newborns and contacts or caregivers of children <5 years of age (CDC, 2013).

Contraindications Severe allergic reaction (eg, anaphylaxis) to recombinant influenza virus vaccine or any component

Warnings Immediate treatment for anaphylactic and/or hypersensitivity reactions should be available during vaccine use. Syncope has been reported with use of injectable vaccines and may be accompanied by transient visual disturbances, weakness, or tonic-clonic movements. Procedures should be in place to avoid injuries from falling and to restore cerebral perfusion if syncope occurs (CDC 57(17), 2008).

In a clinical trial of infants and children 6 months through 3 years of age, a decreased response to Flublok was reported compared to currently licensed U.S. influenza vaccine for this population suggesting that it would not be effective in children ≤3 years; safety and efficacy in older pediatric patients have not been established; use has not been studied.

Precautions Use with caution in patients with history of Guillain-Barré syndrome (GBS); patients with history of GBS have a greater likelihood of developing GBS than those without. As a precaution, the ACIP recommends that patients with a history of GBS and who are at low risk for severe influenza complications, and patients known to have experienced GBS within 6 weeks following previous vaccination should generally not be vaccinated (consider influenza antiviral chemoprophylaxis in these patients). The benefits of vaccination may outweigh the potential risks in persons with a history of GBS who are also at high risk for complications of influenza. Influenza infection itself may cause Guillain-Barré syndrome (CDC/ACIP [Grohskopf, 2013]). Recent studies of patients who received the trivalent inactivated influenza vaccine or the monovalent H1N1 influenza vaccine have shown the risk of GBS is lower with vaccination than with influenza infection (Baxter, 2013; Greene, 2013; Kwong, 2013).

Antipyretics have not been shown to prevent febrile seizures; antipyretics may be used to treat fever or discomfort following vaccination (CDC/ACIP [Kroger, 2011]). One study reported that routine prophylactic administration of acetaminophen to prevent fever prior to vaccination decreased the immune response of some vaccines; the clinical significance of this reduction in immune response has not been established (Prymula, 2008).

The decision to administer or delay vaccination because of current or recent febrile illness depends on the severity of symptoms and the etiology of the disease. Immunization should be delayed during the course of an acute severe febrile illness; may administer to patients with mild acute illness (with or without fever). Use with caution in severely immunocompromised patients (eg, patients receiving chemo-/radiation therapy or other immunosuppressive therapy including high-dose corticosteroids); may have a reduced response to vaccination. Inactivated vaccine (IIV or RIV) is preferred over live virus vaccine for household members, health care workers, and others coming in close contact with severely immunosuppressed persons requiring care in a protected environment (CDC/ACIP [Grohskopf, 2013]; CDC/ACIP [Kroger, 2011]). Vaccination may not result in effective immunity in all patients. Response depends upon multiple factors (eg, type of vaccine, age of patient) and may be improved by administering the vaccine at the recommended dose, route, and interval (CDC/ACIP [Kroger, 2011]).

Use with caution in patients with coagulation disorders, including thrombocytopenia, due to an increased risk for bleeding following I.M. administration; if patient received antihemophilia or similar therapy, I.M. injection can be scheduled shortly after such therapy is administered.

Flublok is a trivalent influenza vaccine produced using continuous insect cell lines. It is a recombinant hemagglutinin (rHA) vaccine; it does not use the influenza virus or eggs in its production process. ACIP states it may be used in persons with an egg allergy of any severity if otherwise appropriate (CDC/ACIP [Grohskopf, 2013]). Previous season vaccines: Influenza vaccines from previous seasons must not be used (CDC/ACIP [Grohskopf, 2013]).

Use of this vaccine for specific medical and/or other indications (eg, immunocompromising conditions, hepatic or kidney disease, diabetes) is also addressed in the ACIP Recommended Immunization Schedule (CDC/ACIP [Akinsanya-Beysolow, 2014]; CDC/ACIP [Bridges, 2014]).

Adverse Reactions All serious adverse reactions must be reported to the U.S. Department of Health and Human Services (DHHS) Vaccine Adverse Event Reporting System (VAERS) 1-800-822-7967 or online at https://vaers.hhs.gov/esub/index. In Canada, adverse reactions may be reported to local provincial/territorial health agencies or to the Vaccine Safety Section at Public Health Agency of Canada (1-866-844-0018).

Central nervous system: Fatigue, headache
Gastrointestinal: Nausea
Local: Injection site reactions: Pain, redness, swelling
Neuromuscular & skeletal: Muscle pain
Respiratory: Cough, nasal congestion, nasopharyngitis, pharyngolaryngeal pain, rhinorrhea, upper respiratory tract infection
Stability Store at 2°C to 8°C (36°F to 46°F); protect from light. Discard if frozen.
Mechanism of Action Promotes immunity to seasonal influenza virus by inducing specific antibody production. Each year the formulation is standardized according to the U.S. Public Health Service. Preparations from previous seasons must not be used.

Pharmacodynamics
Onset of action: Most adults have antibody protection within 2 weeks of vaccination (CDC/ACIP [Grohskopf, 2013])
Duration: ≥6-8 months when vaccine is antigenically similar to circulating virus; response may be diminished in persons ≥65 years and limited evidence suggests titers may decline significantly 6 months following vaccination in this population (CDC/ACIP [Grohskopf, 2013])
Dosing: Usual Influenza seasons vary in their timing and duration from year to year. In general, vaccination should begin soon after the vaccine becomes available (if possible, by October) and prior to onset of influenza activity in the community; however, vaccination should continue throughout the influenza season as long as vaccine is available (CDC/ACIP [Grohskopf, 2013]).
Immunization: Adolescents ≥18 years and Adults ≤49 years: I.M.: 0.5 mL per dose as a single dose per season.
Dosing adjustment in renal impairment: There are no dosage adjustments provided in manufacturer's labeling.
Dosing adjustment in hepatic impairment: There are no dosage adjustments provided in manufacturer's labeling.
Administration For I.M. administration only. Shake gently prior to use; inspect for particulate matter and discoloration prior to administration; avoid use if visible particles are present in the solution after shaking. Administer I.M. in the deltoid muscle; do not inject into the gluteal region or areas where there may be a major nerve trunk.

Unless otherwise indicated in product labeling, jet injectors should **not** be used to administer influenza vaccines (USFDA, 2011). Currently there are no influenza vaccines in the U.S. that can be given by a jet-injector device (CDC/ACIP [Grohskopf, 2013]). Adolescents and adults should be vaccinated while seated or lying down. U.S. law requires that the date of administration; the vaccine manufacturer; lot number of vaccine; the administering person's name, title, and address; and documentation of the vaccine information statement (VIS; date on VIS and date given to patient) be entered into the patient's permanent medical record.
Monitoring Parameters Monitor for syncope for 15 minutes following administration. If seizure-like activity associated with syncope occurs, maintain patient in supine or Trendelenburg position to re-establish adequate cerebral perfusion (CDC, 2011).
Additional Information Pharmacies will stock the formulation(s) standardized according to the USPHS requirements for the season. Influenza vaccines from previous seasons must not be used. Influenza is highly contagious. Incubation period is 1 to 3 days. Patients are most contagious during the 24 hours before the onset of symptoms and during their most symptomatic period.

It is important to note that influenza seasons vary in their timing and duration from year to year. In general, vaccination should begin soon after the vaccine becomes available and prior to onset of influenza activity in the community; however, vaccination should continue throughout the influenza season as long as vaccine is available.

Seasonal quadrivalent influenza vaccines contain two subtype A strains and two subtype B strains; trivalent influenza vaccines contain two subtype A strains and one subtype B strain.

When vaccine supply is not limited, either IIV or LAIV can be used in healthy, nonpregnant persons aged 2 to 49 years of age. RIV can be used in persons 18 to 49 years of age.

In order to maximize vaccination rates, the ACIP recommends simultaneous administration (ie, >1 vaccine on the same day at different anatomic sites) of all age-appropriate vaccines (live or inactivated) for which a person is eligible ▶

at a single visit, unless contraindications exist. If available, the use of combination vaccines is generally preferred over separate injections, taking into consideration provider assessment, patient preference, and potential adverse events. If separate vaccines are being used, evaluate product information regarding same syringe compatibility of vaccines. Separate needles and syringes should be used for each injection. The ACIP prefers each dose of specific vaccine in a series come from the same manufacturer if possible (CDC/ACIP [Kroger, 2011]).

For additional information, please refer to the following website: http://www.cdc.gov/vaccines/vpd-vac/

Dosage Forms Excipient information presented when available (limited, particularly for generics); consult specific product labeling.

Solution, Intramuscular [preservative free]:
Flublok: (0.5 mL)

References

Akinsanya-Beysolow I, Advisory Committee on Immunization Practices (ACIP), ACIP Child/Adolescent Immunization Work Group, et al. Advisory committee on immunization practices recommended immunization schedule for adults aged 19 years or older - United States, 2014. *MMWR Morb Mortal Wkly Rep.* 2014; 63(5):108-109. Full schedule available at http://www.cdc.gov/vaccines/schedules/downloads/child/0-18yrs-child-combined-schedule.pdf

American College of Obstetricians and Gynecologists Committee on Obstetric Practice. ACOG committee opinion no. 468: influenza vaccination during pregnancy. *Obstet Gynecol.* 2010;116 (4):1006-1007.

Baxter R, Bakshi N, Fireman B, et al. Lack of association of Guillain-Barre syndrome with vaccinations. *Clin Infect Dis.* 2013;57 (2):197-204.

Bridges CB, Coyne-Beasley T, Advisory Committee on Immunization Practices (ACIP), ACIP Adult Immunization Work Group; Centers for Disease Control and Prevention (CDC). Advisory committee on immunization practices recommended immunization schedule for adults aged 19 years or older - United States, 2014. *MMWR Morb Mortal Wkly Rep.* 2014; 63(5):108-109. Available at: http://www.cdc.gov/vaccines/schedules/downloads/adult/adult-combined-schedule.pdf

Centers for Disease Control and Prevention (CDC). Pregnant women & influenza (flu). Atlanta: U.S. Department of Health and Human Services, Public Health Service, December 15, 2010. Available at http://www.cdc.gov/flu/protect/vaccine/pregnant.htm

Centers for Disease Control and Prevention (CDC). Syncope after vaccination-United States, January 2005-July 2007. *MMWR Morb Mortal Wkly Rep.* 2008;2;57(17):457-460.

Cox MM, Patriarca PA, and Treanor J, "FluBlok, a Recombinant Hemagglutinin Influenza Vaccine," *Influenza Other Respi Viruses,* 2008, 2(6):211-9.

Greene SK, Rett MD, Vellozzi C, et al. Guillain-Barré syndrome, influenza vaccination, and antecedent respiratory and gastrointestinal infections: a case-centered analysis in the Vaccine Safety Datalink, 2009-2011. *PLoS One.* 2013;8(6):e67185.

Grohskopf LA, Shay D, Shimabukuro TT, et al. Prevention and control of seasonal influenza with vaccines. *MMWR Recomm Rep.* 2013c;62 (RR-07):1-43.

Kroger AT, Atkinson WL, Marcuse EK, Pickering LK. General recommendations on immunization - recommendations of the Advisory Committee on Immunization Practices (ACIP). *MMWR Recomm Rep.* 2011;60(RR-2):1-64.

Kwong JC, Vasa PP, Campetelli MA, et al. Risk of Guillain-Barré syndrome after seasonal influenza vaccination and influenza healthcare encounters: a self-controlled study. *Lancet Infecti Dis.* 2013;13 (9):769-776.

McPherson CE, "Development of a Novel Recombinant Influenza Vaccine In Insect Cells," *Biologicals,* 2008, 36(6):350-3.

Prymula R, Siegrist CA, Chlibek R, et al, "Effect of Prophylactic Paracetamol Administration at Time of Vaccination on Febrile Reactions and Antibody Responses in Children: Two Open-Label, Randomised Controlled Trials," *Lancet,* 2009, 374(9698):1339-50.

Rasmussen SA, Jamieson DJ, and Bresee JS, "Pandemic Influenza and Pregnant Women," *Emerg Infect Dis,* 2008, 14(1):95-100.

Steering Committee on Quality Improvement and Management, Subcommittee on Febrile Seizures American Academy of Pediatrics, "Febrile Seizures: Clinical Practice Guideline for the Long-Term Management of the Child With Simple Febrile Seizures," *Pediatrics,* 2008, 121(6):1281-6.

Treanor JJ, El Sahly H, King J, et al, "Protective Efficacy of a Trivalent Recombinant Hemagglutinin Protein Vaccine (Flublok®) Against Influenza in Healthy Adults: A Randomized, Placebo-Controlled Trial," *Vaccine,* 2011, 29(44):7733-9.

U.S. Food and Drug Administration, "FDA Updated Communication on Use of Jet Injectors With Inactivated Influenza Vaccines", October 26, 2011. Available at http://www.fda.gov/BiologicsBloodVaccines/Vaccines/QuestionsaboutVaccines/ucm276773.htm

◆ **Influenza Virus Vaccine (Split-Virus)** *see* Influenza Virus Vaccine (Inactivated) *on page 1103*

◆ **Influenza Virus Vaccine (Trivalent, Live)** *see* Influenza Virus Vaccine (Live/Attenuated) *on page 1109*

◆ **Influvac (Can)** *see* Influenza Virus Vaccine (Inactivated) *on page 1103*

◆ **Infufer (Can)** *see* Iron Dextran Complex *on page 1153*

◆ **Infumorph 200** *see* Morphine (Systemic) *on page 1440*

◆ **Infumorph 500** *see* Morphine (Systemic) *on page 1440*

◆ **INH** *see* Isoniazid *on page 1158*

◆ **InnoPran XL** *see* Propranolol *on page 1759*

◆ **Inova** *see* Benzoyl Peroxide *on page 275*

◆ **Instacort 5 [OTC]** *see* Hydrocortisone (Topical) *on page 1038*

◆ **Instacort 10 [OTC]** *see* Hydrocortisone (Topical) *on page 1038*

◆ **Insta-Glucose [OTC]** *see* Dextrose *on page 637*

Insulin Aspart (IN soo lin AS part)

Medication Safety Issues

Sound-alike/look-alike issues:
NovoLOG® may be confused with HumaLOG®, HumuLIN® R, Nimbex®, NovoLIN® N, NovoLIN® R, NovoLOG® Mix 70/30

High alert medication:
The Institute for Safe Medication Practices (ISMP) includes this medication among its list of drugs which have a heightened risk of causing significant patient harm when used in error. *Due to the number of insulin preparations, it is essential to identify/clarify the type of insulin to be used.*

Other safety concerns:
Cross-contamination may occur if insulin pens are shared among multiple patients. Steps should be taken to prohibit sharing of insulin pens.

Brand Names: U.S. NovoLOG; NovoLOG FlexPen; NovoLOG PenFill

Brand Names: Canada NovoRapid®

Therapeutic Category Antidiabetic Agent, Parenteral; Insulin, Rapid-Acting

Generic Availability (U.S.) No

Use Treatment of type 1 diabetes mellitus (insulin dependent, IDDM); type 2 diabetes mellitus (noninsulin dependent, NIDDM) to control hyperglycemia

Pregnancy Risk Factor B

Pregnancy Considerations Adverse events have not been observed in animal reproduction studies. Maternal hyperglycemia can be associated with adverse effects in the fetus, including macrosomia, neonatal hyperglycemia, and hyperbilirubinemia; the risk of congenital malformations is increased when the HbA_{1c} is >1% above the normal range.

Insulin requirements tend to fall during the first trimester of pregnancy and increase in the later trimesters, peaking at 28-32 weeks of gestation. Following delivery, insulin requirements decrease rapidly. Diabetes can also be associated with adverse effects in the mother. Poorly-treated diabetes may cause end-organ damage that may in turn negatively affect obstetric outcomes. Physiologic glucose levels should be maintained prior to and during pregnancy to decrease the risk of adverse events in the fetus and the mother. Insulin is the drug of choice for the control of diabetes mellitus during pregnancy. Insulin aspart has been demonstrated to be as safe and effective as regular human insulin when used during pregnancy and may have advantages over regular insulin during pregnancy.

Breast-Feeding Considerations It is not known if insulin aspart distributes into breast milk. Endogenous insulin can be found in breast milk. Plasma glucose concentrations in the mother affect glucose concentrations in breast milk. The gastrointestinal tract destroys insulin when administered orally; therefore, insulin is not expected to be absorbed intact by the breast-feeding infant. All types of insulin are safe for use while breast-feeding. Due to increased calorie expenditure, women with diabetes may require less insulin while nursing.

Contraindications Hypersensitivity insulin aspart or any component

Warnings Hypoglycemia is the most common adverse effect of insulin. The timing of hypoglycemia differs among various insulin formulations. Any change of insulin should be made cautiously; changing manufacturers, type, and/or method of manufacture may result in the need for a change of dosage. Hypoglycemia may result from increased work or exercise without eating.

Precautions Use with caution and adjust dosage in patients with renal impairment; use with caution and monitor closely in patient with hepatic impairment. While regular insulin is the preferred formulation for I.V. administration, both insulin aspart and insulin glulisine have been approved for I.V. use in selected clinical situations with close medical supervision and monitoring of serum potassium.

Adverse Reactions Primarily symptoms of hypoglycemia
Cardiovascular: Pallor, palpitation, tachycardia
Central nervous system: Fatigue, headache, hypothermia, loss of consciousness, mental confusion
Dermatologic: Redness, urticaria
Endocrine & metabolic: Hypoglycemia, hypokalemia
Gastrointestinal: Hunger, nausea, numbness of mouth
Local: Atrophy or hypertrophy of SubQ fat tissue; edema, itching, pain or warmth at injection site; stinging
Neuromuscular & skeletal: Muscle weakness, paresthesia, tremor
Ocular: Transient presbyopia or blurred vision
Miscellaneous: Anaphylaxis, diaphoresis, local and/or systemic hypersensitivity reactions

Drug Interactions

Metabolism/Transport Effects None known.

Avoid Concomitant Use There are no known interactions where it is recommended to avoid concomitant use.

Increased Effect/Toxicity
Insulin Aspart may increase the levels/effects of: Antidiabetic Agents (Thiazolidinedione); Hypoglycemic Agents; Quinolone Antibiotics

The levels/effects of Insulin Aspart may be increased by: Androgens; Beta-Blockers; Edetate CALCIUM Disodium; Edetate Disodium; GLP-1 Agonists; Herbs (Hypoglycemic Properties); MAO Inhibitors; Metreleptin; Pegvisomant; Salicylates; Selective Serotonin Reuptake Inhibitors

Decreased Effect
The levels/effects of Insulin Aspart may be decreased by: Corticosteroids (Orally Inhaled); Corticosteroids (Systemic); Danazol; Loop Diuretics; Luteinizing Hormone-Releasing Hormone Analogs; Somatropin; Thiazide Diuretics

Stability Store unopened container in refrigerator; do not freeze; protect from heat and light. Once opened (in use) vials may be stored in refrigerator or at room temperature for up to 28 days. Cartridges that are in use should be stored at room temperature and used within 28 days; do not refrigerate. Insulin in reservoir should be replaced every 48 hours. Discard if exposed to temperatures ≥37°C (98.6°F). May be mixed in the same syringe with NPH insulin.

Mechanism of Action Insulin acts via specific membrane-bound receptors on target tissues to regulate metabolism of carbohydrate, protein, and fats. Target organs for insulin include the liver, skeletal muscle, and adipose tissue.

Within the liver, insulin stimulates hepatic glycogen synthesis. Insulin promotes hepatic synthesis of fatty acids, which are released into the circulation as lipoproteins. Skeletal muscle effects of insulin include increased protein synthesis and increased glycogen synthesis. Within adipose tissue, insulin stimulates the processing of circulating lipoproteins to provide free fatty acids, facilitating triglyceride synthesis and storage by adipocytes; it also directly inhibits the hydrolysis of triglycerides. In addition, insulin stimulates the cellular uptake of amino acids and increases cellular permeability to several ions, including potassium, magnesium, and phosphate. By activating sodium-potassium ATPases, insulin promotes the intracellular movement of potassium.

Normally secreted by the pancreas, insulin products are manufactured for pharmacologic use through recombinant DNA technology using either *E. coli* or *Saccharomyces cerevisiae*. Insulins are categorized based on the onset, peak, and duration of effect (eg, rapid-, short-, intermediate-, and long-acting insulin). Insulin aspart is a rapid-acting insulin analog.

Pharmacodynamics Onset and duration of hypoglycemic effects depend upon the route of administration (adsorption and onset of action are more rapid after deeper I.M. injections than after SubQ), site of injection (onset and duration are progressively slower with SubQ injection into the abdomen, arm, buttock, or thigh respectively), volume and concentration of injection, and the preparation administered; local heat and massage also increase the rate of absorption.
Onset of action: 0.17-0.33 hours
Maximum effect: 1-3 hours
Duration: 3-5 hours

Pharmacokinetics (Adult data unless noted)
Protein binding: 0% to 9%
Half-life: Adults: 81 minutes
Time to peak serum concentration: 40-50 minutes
Elimination: Urine
Clearance: Adults: 1.22 L/hour/kg

Dosing: Usual Insulin aspart is a rapid-acting insulin analog which is normally administered SubQ as a premeal component of the insulin regimen or as a continuous SubQ infusion and should be used with intermediate- or long-acting insulin. When compared to insulin regular, insulin aspart has a more rapid onset and shorter duration of activity. In carefully controlled clinical settings with close medical supervision and monitoring of blood glucose and potassium, insulin aspart may also be administered I.V. Insulin requirements vary dramatically between patients and dictate frequent monitoring and close medical supervision. See Insulin Regular for additional information.

General insulin dosing:
Type 1 diabetes mellitus: Children, Adolescents, and Adults: **Note:** Multiple daily doses or continuous subcutaneous infusions guided by blood glucose monitoring are the standard of diabetes care. Combinations of insulin formulations are commonly used. The daily doses presented below are expressed as the **total units/kg/day of all insulin formulations combined**.
Initial total insulin dose: SubQ: 0.2-0.6 units/kg/day in divided doses. Conservative initial doses of 0.2-0.4 units/kg/day are often recommended to avoid the potential for hypoglycemia. A rapidly acting insulin may be the only insulin formulation used initially.

Usual maintenance range: SubQ: 0.5-1 unit/kg/day in divided doses. An estimate of anticipated needs may be based on body weight and/or activity factors as follows:

Nonobese: 0.4-0.6 units/kg/day

Obese: 0.8-1.2 units/kg/day

Pubescent Children and Adolescents: During puberty, requirements may substantially increase to >1 unit/kg/day and in some cases up to 2 units/kg/day (IDF/ISPAD, 2011)

Adjustment of dose: Dosage must be titrated to achieve glucose control and avoid hypoglycemia. Adjust dose to maintain premeal and bedtime glucose in target range. Since combinations of agents are frequently used, dosage adjustment must address the individual component of the insulin regimen which most directly influences the blood glucose value in question, based on the known onset and duration of the insulin component.

Continuous SubQ insulin infusion (insulin pump): A combination of a "basal" continuous insulin infusion rate with preprogrammed, premeal bolus doses which are patient controlled. When converting from multiple daily SubQ doses of maintenance insulin, it is advisable to reduce the basal rate to less than the equivalent of the total daily units of longer acting insulin (eg, NPH); divide the total number of units by 24 to get the basal rate in units/hour. Do not include the total units of regular insulin or other rapid-acting insulin formulations in this calculation. The same premeal regular insulin dosage may be used.

Type 2 diabetes mellitus: Augmentation therapy (patients for which diet, exercise, weight reduction, and oral hypoglycemic agents have not been adequate): Adults: SubQ: Initial dosage of 0.2 units/kg/day or 10 units/day of an intermediate-acting (eg, NPH) or long-acting insulin administered at bedtime has been recommended. As an alternative, regular insulin or rapid-acting insulin formulations administered before meals have also been used. Dosage must be carefully adjusted.

Dosing adjustment in renal impairment: There are no dosage adjustments provided in manufacturer's labeling; insulin requirements are reduced due to changes in insulin clearance or metabolism; monitor blood glucose closely.

Dosing adjustment in hepatic impairment: There are no dosage adjustments provided in manufacturer's labeling; insulin requirements may be reduced due to changes in insulin clearance or metabolism; monitor blood glucose closely.

Administration Parenteral:

SubQ: Administration is usually made into the subcutaneous fat of the thighs, arms, buttocks, or abdomen, with sites rotated; cold injections should be avoided. May be mixed in the same syringe with NPH insulin. When mixing insulin aspart with NPH insulin, aspart should be drawn into the syringe first. Administer immediately before meals (within 5-10 minutes of the start of a meal). Can be infused SubQ by external insulin pump; however, when used in an external pump, it is not recommended to be diluted with other insulin.

I.V.: Insulin aspart may be administered I.V. in selected clinical situations to control hyperglycemia. Appropriate medical supervision is required. May be diluted to a concentration between 0.05 and 1 unit/mL with NS, D_5W, or $D_{10}W$

Monitoring Parameters Urine sugar and acetone, serum glucose, electrolytes, Hb A_{1c}, lipid profile; when used intravenously, close monitoring of serum glucose and potassium are required to avoid hypoglycemia and/or hypokalemia

Reference Range

Plasma Blood Glucose and Hgb A_{1c} Goals for Type 1 Diabetes (ADA, 2013): Note: Goals should be individualized based on individual needs/circumstances (eg, patients who experience severe hypoglycemia, patients with hypoglycemic unawareness); lower goals may be reasonable if they can be achieved without excessive hypoglycemia. **Note:** Postprandial blood glucose should be measured when there is a discrepancy between preprandial blood glucose concentrations and Hb A_{1c} values and to help assess glycemia for patients who receive basal/bolus regimens. It is usually drawn 1-2 hours after starting meal and is considered to be the "peak."

Toddlers/Preschoolers (0-6 years):

Preprandial glucose: 100-180 mg/dL

Bedtime/overnight glucose: 110-200 mg/dL

Hb A_{1c}: <8.5%

School age (6-12 years):

Preprandial glucose: 90-180 mg/dL

Bedtime/overnight glucose: 100-180 mg/dL

Hb A_{1c}: <8%

Adolescents/Young Adults (13-19 years):

Preprandial glucose: 90-130 mg/dL

Bedtime/overnight glucose: 90-150 mg/dL

Hb A_{1c}: <7.5%

Adults, nonpregnant:

Preprandial glucose: 70-130 mg/dL

Postprandial glucose: <180 mg/dL

Hb A_{1c}: <7%

Criteria for diagnosis of DKA:

Serum glucose:

Children: >200 mg/dL

Adults: >250 mg/dL

Arterial pH:

Children: <7.3

Adults: <7-7.24

Bicarbonate:

Children: <15 mEq/L

Adults: <10-15 mEq/L

Moderate ketonuria or ketonemia

Additional Information

Division of daily insulin requirement ("conventional therapy"): Generally, 50% to 75% of the daily insulin dose is given as an intermediate- or long-acting form of insulin (in 1-2 daily injections). The remaining portion of the 24-hour insulin requirement is divided and administered as either regular insulin or a rapid-acting form (eg, insulin aspart) of insulin at the same time before breakfast and dinner.

Division of daily insulin requirement ("intensive therapy"): Basal insulin delivery with 1 or 2 doses of intermediate- or long-acting insulin formulations superimposed with doses of rapid- or very rapid-acting insulin (eg, insulin aspart) formulations 3 or more times daily.

Dosage Forms Excipient information presented when available (limited, particularly for generics); consult specific product labeling.

Solution, Subcutaneous:

NovoLOG: 100 units/mL (10 mL) [contains metacresol, phenol]

Solution Cartridge, Subcutaneous:

NovoLOG PenFill: 100 units/mL (3 mL) [contains metacresol, phenol]

Solution Pen-injector, Subcutaneous:

NovoLOG FlexPen: 100 units/mL (3 mL) [contains metacresol, phenol]

References

American Diabetes Association (ADA), "Standards of Medical Care in Diabetes-2013," *Diabetes Care*, 2013, (36 Suppl 1):S11-66.

International Diabetes Federation, International Society for Pediatric and Adolescent Diabetes. Global IDF/ISPAD guideline for diabetes in childhood and adolescence. 2011. Available at: http://www.idf.org/global-idfispad-guideline-diabetes-childhood-and-adolescence. Date accessed: October 21, 2013.

◆ **Insulin Aspart and Insulin Aspart Protamine** see Insulin Aspart Protamine and Insulin Aspart on page 1117

Insulin Aspart Protamine and Insulin Aspart (IN soo lin AS part PROE ta meen & IN soo lin AS part)

Medication Safety Issues
Sound-alike/look-alike issues:
NovoLOG® Mix 70/30 may be confused with HumaLOG® Mix 75/25™, HumuLIN® 70/30, NovoLIN® 70/30, NovoLOG®

High alert medication:
The Institute for Safe Medication Practices (ISMP) includes this medication among its list of drugs which have a heightened risk of causing significant patient harm when used in error. *Due to the number of insulin preparations, it is essential to identify/clarify the type of insulin to be used.*

Other safety concerns:
Cross-contamination may occur if insulin pens are shared among multiple patients. Steps should be taken to prohibit sharing of insulin pens.

Brand Names: U.S. NovoLOG® Mix 70/30; NovoLOG® Mix 70/30 FlexPen®

Brand Names: Canada NovoMix® 30

Therapeutic Category Antidiabetic Agent, Parenteral; Insulin, Combination

Generic Availability (U.S.) No

Use Treatment of type 1 diabetes mellitus (insulin dependent, IDDM); type 2 diabetes mellitus (noninsulin dependent, NIDDM) to control hyperglycemia (FDA approved in adults)

Pregnancy Risk Factor B

Pregnancy Considerations Biphasic insulin aspart (insulin aspart protamine suspension 70% [intermediate acting] and insulin aspart solution 30% [rapid acting]) was found to be comparable to biphasic human insulin (Insulin NPH suspension 70% [intermediate acting] and insulin regular solution 30% [short acting]) in a pilot study of women with gestational diabetes mellitus. All pregnancies have a background risk of adverse outcome; this risk is increased in pregnancies complicated by hyperglycemia and may be decreased with good metabolic control. Most available information for use of insulin aspart in pregnancy is from studies using the rapid action solution. Refer to Insulin Aspart monograph for additional information.

Breast-Feeding Considerations It is not known if insulin aspart distributes into breast milk. Endogenous insulin can be found in breast milk. Plasma glucose concentrations in the mother affect glucose concentrations in breast milk. The gastrointestinal tract destroys insulin when administered orally; therefore, insulin is not expected to be absorbed intact by the breast-feeding infant. All types of insulin are safe for use while breast-feeding. Due to increased calorie expenditure, women with diabetes may require less insulin while nursing.

Contraindications Hypersensitivity insulin aspart, insulin aspart protamine, or to any component; hypoglycemia

Warnings Hypoglycemia is the most common adverse effect of insulin. The timing of hypoglycemia differs among various insulin formulations. Any change of insulin should be made cautiously; changing manufacturers, type, and/or method of manufacture may result in the need for a change of dosage. Hypoglycemia may result from increased work or exercise without eating. Not for I.V. infusion or use in insulin infusion pumps.

Precautions Use with caution and adjust dosage in patients with renal impairment; use with caution and monitor closely in patient with hepatic impairment.

Adverse Reactions
Cardiovascular: Palpitation, pallor, peripheral edema, tachycardia

Central nervous system: Fatigue, headache, hypothermia, loss of consciousness, mental confusion

Dermatologic: Pruritus, rash, redness, urticaria

Endocrine & metabolic: Hypoglycemia, hypokalemia

Gastrointestinal: Hunger, nausea, numbness of mouth, weight gain

Local: Injection site reaction (including edema, itching, pain or warmth, stinging), lipoatrophy, lipodystrophy

Neuromuscular & skeletal: Muscle weakness, paresthesia, tremor

Ocular: Transient presbyopia or blurred vision

Miscellaneous: Anaphylaxis, antibodies to insulin (no change in efficacy), diaphoresis, local allergy, systemic allergic symptoms

Drug Interactions
Metabolism/Transport Effects None known.

Avoid Concomitant Use There are no known interactions where it is recommended to avoid concomitant use.

Increased Effect/Toxicity
Insulin Aspart Protamine and Insulin Aspart may increase the levels/effects of: Antidiabetic Agents (Thiazolidinedione); Hypoglycemic Agents; Quinolone Antibiotics

The levels/effects of Insulin Aspart Protamine and Insulin Aspart may be increased by: Androgens; Beta-Blockers; Edetate CALCIUM Disodium; Edetate Disodium; GLP-1 Agonists; Herbs (Hypoglycemic Properties); MAO Inhibitors; Metreleptin; Pegvisomant; Salicylates; Selective Serotonin Reuptake Inhibitors

Decreased Effect
The levels/effects of Insulin Aspart Protamine and Insulin Aspart may be decreased by: Corticosteroids (Orally Inhaled); Corticosteroids (Systemic); Danazol; Loop Diuretics; Luteinizing Hormone-Releasing Hormone Analogs; Somatropin; Thiazide Diuretics

Stability Store unopened container in refrigerator; do not freeze; protect from light. If refrigeration is not possible, vial (in use) may be stored at room temperature for up to 28 days. The pen (in use) should not be refrigerated; store below 30°C (86°F) away from direct heat or light; discard after 14 days. Do not mix or dilute with other insulins.

Mechanism of Action Insulin aspart protamine and insulin aspart is an intermediate-acting combination insulin product with a more rapid onset and similar duration of action as compared to that of insulin NPH and insulin regular combination products. Insulin acts via specific membrane-bound receptors on target tissues to regulate metabolism of carbohydrate, protein, and fats. Target organs for insulin include the liver, skeletal muscle, and adipose tissue.

Within the liver, insulin stimulates hepatic glycogen synthesis. Insulin promotes hepatic synthesis of fatty acids, which are released into the circulation as lipoproteins. Skeletal muscle effects of insulin include increased protein synthesis and increased glycogen synthesis. Within adipose tissue, insulin stimulates the processing of circulating lipoproteins to provide free fatty acids, facilitating triglyceride synthesis and storage by adipocytes; also directly inhibits the hydrolysis of triglycerides. In addition, insulin stimulates the cellular uptake of amino acids and increases cellular permeability to several ions, including potassium, magnesium, and phosphate. By activating sodium-potassium ATPases, insulin promotes the intracellular movement of potassium.

Normally secreted by the pancreas, insulin products are manufactured for pharmacologic use through recombinant ▶

DNA technology using either *E. coli* or *Saccharomyces cerevisiae*. Insulins are categorized based on the onset, peak, and duration of effect (eg, rapid-, short-, intermediate-, and long-acting insulin).

Pharmacodynamics
Onset of action: 10-20 minutes
Maximum effect: 1-4 hours
Duration: 18-24 hours

Pharmacokinetics (Adult data unless noted)
Protein binding: ≤9%
Half-life: 8-9 hours (mean)
Time to peak serum concentration: 1-1.5 hours
Elimination: Urine

Dosing: Usual Insulin aspart protamine is an intermediate-acting insulin and insulin aspart is a rapid-acting insulin administered by SubQ injection. Insulin aspart protamine and insulin aspart combination products are approximately equipotent to insulin NPH and insulin regular combination products with a similar duration of activity, but with a more rapid onset. With combination insulin products, the proportion of rapid-acting to long-acting insulin is fixed; basal vs prandial dose adjustments cannot be made. Fixed ratio insulins (such as insulin aspart protamine and insulin aspart combination) are typically administered as 2 daily doses with each dose intended to cover two meals and a snack. Because of variability in the peak effect and individual patient variability in activities, meals, etc, it may be more difficult to achieve complete glycemic control using fixed combinations of insulins; frequent monitoring and close medical supervision may be necessary. See Insulin Regular for additional information.

General insulin dosing:
Type 1 diabetes mellitus: Children, Adolescents, and Adults: **Note:** Multiple daily doses are utilized and guided by blood glucose monitoring. Combinations of different insulin formulations are commonly used. The daily doses presented below are expressed as the **total units/kg/day of all insulin formulations combined.** Insulin aspart protamine and insulin aspart combination product is **not** intended for initial therapy; basal insulin requirements should be established **first** to direct dosing of combination insulin products.
Usual maintenance range: SubQ: 0.5-1 unit/kg/day in divided doses. An estimate of anticipated needs may be based on body weight and/or activity factors as follows:
Nonobese: 0.4-0.6 units/kg/day
Obese: 0.8-1.2 units/kg/day
Pubescent Children and Adolescents: During puberty, requirements may substantially increase to >1 unit/kg/day and in some cases up to 2 units/kg/day (IDF/ISPAD, 2011)
Adjustment of dose: Dosage must be titrated to achieve glucose control and avoid hypoglycemia. Adjust dose to maintain premeal and bedtime glucose in target range. Since combinations of agents are frequently used, dosage adjustment must address the individual component of the insulin regimen which most directly influences the blood glucose value in question, based on the known onset and duration of the insulin component.
Type 2 diabetes mellitus: Augmentation therapy (patients for which diet, exercise, weight reduction, and oral hypoglycemic agents have not been adequate): Adults: SubQ: **Note:** Insulin aspart protamine and insulin aspart combination product is **not** intended for initial therapy; basal insulin requirements should be established **first** to direct dosing of combination insulin products. Dosage must be carefully adjusted.
Dosing adjustment in renal impairment: There are no dosage adjustments provided in manufacturer's labeling; insulin requirements are reduced due to changes in insulin clearance or metabolism; monitor blood glucose closely.
Dosing adjustment in hepatic impairment: There are no dosage adjustments provided in manufacturer's labeling; insulin requirements may be reduced due to changes in insulin clearance or metabolism; monitor blood glucose closely.
Administration Parenteral: SubQ: Gently roll vial or pen in the palms of the hands to resuspend before use; administer into the subcutaneous fat of the thighs, arms, buttocks, or abdomen, with sites rotated. Cold injections should be avoided. Administer within 15 minutes before a meal (type 1 diabetes) or 15 minutes before or after a meal (type 2 diabetes) (eg, before breakfast and supper). Do not mix or dilute with other insulins. **Not for I.V. administration** or use in an insulin infusion pump.
Monitoring Parameters Urine sugar and acetone, serum glucose, electrolytes, Hb A$_{1c}$, lipid profile

Reference Range
Plasma Blood Glucose and Hgb A$_{1c}$ Goals for Type 1 Diabetes (ADA, 2013): Note: Goals should be individualized based on individual needs/circumstances (eg, patients who experience severe hypoglycemia, patients with hypoglycemic unawareness); lower goals may be reasonable if they can be achieved without excessive hypoglycemia. **Note:** Postprandial blood glucose should be measured when there is a discrepancy between preprandial blood glucose concentrations and Hb A$_{1c}$ values and to help assess glycemia for patients who receive basal/bolus regimens. It is usually drawn 1-2 hours after starting meal and is considered to be the "peak."
Toddlers/Preschoolers (0-6 years):
Preprandial glucose: 100-180 mg/dL
Bedtime/overnight glucose: 110-200 mg/dL
Hb A$_{1c}$: <8.5%
School age (6-12 years):
Preprandial glucose: 90-180 mg/dL
Bedtime/overnight glucose: 100-180 mg/dL
Hb A$_{1c}$: <8%
Adolescents/Young Adults (13-19 years):
Preprandial glucose: 90-130 mg/dL
Bedtime/overnight glucose: 90-150 mg/dL
Hb A$_{1c}$: <7.5%
Adults, nonpregnant:
Preprandial glucose: 70-130 mg/dL
Postprandial glucose: <180 mg/dL
Hb A$_{1c}$: <7%
Criteria for diagnosis of DKA:
Serum glucose:
Children: >200 mg/dL
Adults: >250 mg/dL
Arterial pH:
Children: <7.3
Adults: <7-7.24
Bicarbonate:
Children: <15 mEq/L
Adults: <10-15 mEq/L
Moderate ketonuria or ketonemia

Additional Information
Division of daily insulin requirement ("conventional therapy"): Generally, 50% to 75% of the daily insulin dose is given as an intermediate- or long-acting form of insulin (in 1-2 daily injections). The remaining portion of the 24-hour insulin requirement is divided and administered as either regular insulin or a rapid-acting form of insulin at the same time before breakfast and dinner.
Division of daily insulin requirement ("intensive therapy"): Basal insulin delivery with 1 or 2 doses of intermediate- or long-acting insulin formulations superimposed with doses of rapid- or very rapid-acting insulin formulations 3 or more times daily.

Dosage Forms Excipient information presented when available (limited, particularly for generics); consult specific product labeling.

Injection, suspension:

NovoLOG® Mix 70/30: Insulin aspart protamine suspension 70% [intermediate acting] and insulin aspart solution 30% [rapid acting]: 100 units/mL (10 mL)

NovoLOG® Mix 70/30 FlexPen®: Insulin aspart protamine suspension 70% [intermediate acting] and insulin aspart solution 30% [rapid acting]: 100 units/mL (3 mL)

References

American Diabetes Association (ADA), "Standards of Medical Care in Diabetes-2013," *Diabetes Care*, 2013, (36 Suppl 1):S11-66.

International Diabetes Federation, International Society for Pediatric and Adolescent Diabetes. Global IDF/ISPAD guideline for diabetes in childhood and adolescence. 2011. Available at: http://www.idf.org/global-idfispad-guideline-diabetes-childhood-and-adolescence. Date accessed: October 21, 2013.

Insulin Detemir (IN soo lin DE te mir)

Medication Safety Issues

High alert medication:

The Institute for Safe Medication Practices (ISMP) includes this medication among its list of drugs which have a heightened risk of causing significant patient harm when used in error. *Due to the number of insulin preparations, it is essential to identify/clarify the type of insulin to be used.*

Administration issues:

Insulin detemir is a clear solution, but it is NOT intended for I.V. or I.M. administration.

Other safety concerns:

Cross-contamination may occur if insulin pens are shared among multiple patients. Steps should be taken to prohibit sharing of insulin pens.

Brand Names: U.S. Levemir; Levemir FlexPen; Levemir FlexTouch

Brand Names: Canada Levemir®

Therapeutic Category Antidiabetic Agent, Parenteral; Insulin, Intermediate-Acting

Generic Availability (U.S.) No

Use Treatment of type 1 diabetes mellitus (insulin dependent, IDDM) to improve glycemic control (FDA approved in ages ≥2 years and adults); treatment of type 2 diabetes mellitus (noninsulin dependent, NIDDM) to improve glycemic control (FDA approved in adults)

Pregnancy Risk Factor B

Pregnancy Considerations Dose-related adverse events were observed in animal reproduction studies. Limited information is available related to the use of insulin detemir in pregnancy. Maternal hyperglycemia can be associated with adverse effects in the fetus, including macrosomia, neonatal hyperglycemia, and hyperbilirubinemia; the risk of congenital malformations is increased when the HbA$_{1c}$ is >1% above the normal range. Insulin requirements tend to fall during the first trimester of pregnancy and increase in the later trimesters, peaking at 28-32 weeks of gestation. Following delivery, insulin requirements decrease rapidly. Diabetes can also be associated with adverse effects in the mother. Poorly treated diabetes may cause end-organ damage that may in turn negatively affect obstetric outcomes. Physiologic glucose levels should be maintained prior to and during pregnancy to decrease the risk of adverse events in the fetus and the mother. Insulin is the drug of choice for the control of diabetes mellitus during pregnancy.

Breast-Feeding Considerations It is not known if insulin detemir distributes into breast milk. Endogenous insulin can be found in breast milk. Plasma glucose concentrations in the mother affect glucose concentrations in breast milk. The gastrointestinal tract destroys insulin when administered orally; therefore, insulin is not expected to be absorbed intact by the breast-feeding infant. All types of insulin are safe for use while breast-feeding. Although use of insulin detemir is compatible with breast-feeding, the manufacturer recommends that caution be used when insulin detemir is used by nursing women. Due to increased calorie expenditure, women with diabetes may require less insulin while nursing.

Contraindications Hypersensitivity to insulin detemir or any component; hypoglycemia

Warnings Insulin detemir should not be used for management of diabetic ketoacidosis; a short-acting insulin is recommended. Hypoglycemia is the most common adverse effect of insulin. The timing of hypoglycemia differs among various insulin formulations. Hypoglycemia may result from increased work or exercise without eating; use of long-acting insulin preparations (eg, insulin detemir) may delay recovery from hypoglycemia. Profound and prolonged episodes of hypoglycemia may result in convulsions, unconsciousness, temporary or permanent brain damage, or even death. Insulin requirements may be altered during illness, emotional disturbances, or other stressors. Any change of insulin should be made cautiously; changing manufacturers, type, and/or method of manufacture may result in the need for a change of dosage. Although insulin detemir is a clear solution; it is NOT intended for I.V. or I.M. administration or for use in insulin infusion pumps. Severe allergic reactions, including anaphylaxis, may occur with insulin products.

Precautions Use with caution in patients with renal impairment; monitor closely; dosage adjustment may be required. Use with caution in patient with hepatic impairment; monitor closely; dosage adjustment may be required. Use with caution in patients at risk for hypokalemia (eg, concurrent loop diuretic); insulin causes a shift of potassium from the extracellular space to the intracellular space possibly causing hypokalemia; higher risk with intravenous insulin use. Untreated hypokalemia may result in respiratory paralysis, ventricular arrhythmia, and even death; monitor serum potassium and supplement potassium when necessary.

Adverse Reactions Primarily symptoms of hypoglycemia

Cardiovascular: Pallor, palpitation, tachycardia

Central nervous system: Fatigue, headache, hypothermia, loss of consciousness, mental confusion

Dermatologic: Redness, urticaria

Endocrine & metabolic: Hypoglycemia, hypokalemia

Gastrointestinal: Hunger, nausea, numbness of mouth

Local: Atrophy or hypertrophy of SubQ fat tissue; edema, itching, pain or warmth at injection site; stinging

Neuromuscular & skeletal: Muscle weakness, paresthesia, tremor

Ocular: Transient presbyopia or blurred vision

Miscellaneous: Anaphylaxis, diaphoresis, local and/or systemic hypersensitivity reactions

Drug Interactions

Metabolism/Transport Effects None known.

Avoid Concomitant Use There are no known interactions where it is recommended to avoid concomitant use.

Increased Effect/Toxicity

Insulin Detemir may increase the levels/effects of: Antidiabetic Agents (Thiazolidinedione); Hypoglycemic Agents; Quinolone Antibiotics

The levels/effects of Insulin Detemir may be increased by: Androgens; Beta-Blockers; Edetate CALCIUM Disodium; Edetate Disodium; GLP-1 Agonists; Herbs (Hypoglycemic Properties); MAO Inhibitors; Metreleptin; Pegvisomant; Salicylates; Selective Serotonin Reuptake Inhibitors

Decreased Effect

The levels/effects of Insulin Detemir may be decreased by: Corticosteroids (Orally Inhaled); Corticosteroids (Systemic); Danazol; Loop Diuretics; Luteinizing Hormone-Releasing Hormone Analogs; Somatropin; Thiazide Diuretics

Stability Store unopened vials and prefilled pens between 2°C and 8°C (36°F to 46°F) until the expiration date or at room temperature <30°C (<86°F) for 42 days; do not freeze; keep away from heat and sunlight. Once punctured (in use), vials may be stored in refrigerator or at room temperature <30°C (<86°F); use within 42 days (includes days stored at room temperature for unopened vials, if applicable). Prefilled pens that have been punctured (in use) should be stored at temperatures <30°C (<86°F) and used within 42 days (includes days stored at room temperature for unused pens, if applicable); do not freeze or refrigerate. Do not store with needle in place. Do not dilute or mix with other insulins or solutions.

Mechanism of Action Insulin acts via specific membrane-bound receptors on target tissues to regulate metabolism of carbohydrate, protein, and fats. Target organs for insulin include the liver, skeletal muscle, and adipose tissue.

Within the liver, insulin stimulates hepatic glycogen synthesis. Insulin promotes hepatic synthesis of fatty acids, which are released into the circulation as lipoproteins. Skeletal muscle effects of insulin include increased protein synthesis and increased glycogen synthesis. Within adipose tissue, insulin stimulates the processing of circulating lipoproteins to provide free fatty acids, facilitating triglyceride synthesis and storage by adipocytes; also directly inhibits the hydrolysis of triglycerides. In addition, insulin stimulates the cellular uptake of amino acids and increases cellular permeability to several ions, including potassium, magnesium, and phosphate. By activating sodium-potassium ATPases, insulin promotes the intracellular movement of potassium.

Normally secreted by the pancreas, insulin products are manufactured for pharmacologic use through recombinant DNA technology using either *E. coli* or *Saccharomyces cerevisiae*. Insulins are categorized based on the onset, peak, and duration of effect (eg, rapid-, short-, intermediate-, and long-acting insulin). Insulin detemir is an intermediate- to long-acting insulin analog.

Pharmacodynamics

Onset of action: 3-4 hours

Maximum effect: 3-9 hours (Plank, 2005)

Duration: 6-23 hours (dose dependent); **Note:** Duration is dose-dependent. At lower dosages (0.1-0.2 units/kg), mean duration is variable (5.7-12.1 hours). At 0.4 units/kg, the mean duration was 19.9 hours. At high dosages (≥0.8 units/kg) the duration is longer and less variable (mean: 22-23 hours) (Plank, 2005).

Pharmacokinetics (Adult data unless noted)

Distribution: V_d: 0.1 L/kg

Protein binding: >98% (albumin)

Bioavailability: 60%

Half-life: SubQ: 5-7 hours (dose dependent)

Time to peak serum concentration: 6-8 hours

Elimination: Urine

Dosing: Usual Insulin detemir is an intermediate-acting insulin administered by SubQ injection. When compared to insulin NPH, insulin detemir has slower, more prolonged absorption; duration of activity is dose-dependent. Insulin detemir may be given once or twice daily when used as the basal insulin component of therapy. Changing the basal insulin component from another insulin to insulin detemir can be done on a unit-to-unit basis. Insulin requirements vary dramatically between patients and dictate frequent monitoring and close medical supervision. See Insulin Regular for additional information.

General insulin dosing: Type 1 diabetes mellitus: Children, Adolescents, and Adults: **Note:** Multiple daily doses are utilized and guided by blood glucose monitoring. Combinations of insulin formulations are commonly used. The daily doses presented below are expressed as the **total units/kg/day of all insulin formulations combined.**

Usual maintenance range: SubQ: 0.5-1 unit/kg/day in divided doses. An estimate of anticipated needs may be based on body weight and/or activity factors as follows:

Nonobese: 0.4-0.6 units/kg/day

Obese: 0.8-1.2 units/kg/day

Pubescent Children and Adolescents: During puberty, requirements may substantially increase to >1 unit/kg/day and in some cases up to 2 units/kg/day (IDF/ISPAD, 2011)

Adjustment of dose: Dosage must be titrated to achieve glucose control and avoid hypoglycemia. Adjust dose to maintain premeal and bedtime glucose in target range. Since combinations of agents are frequently used, dosage adjustment must address the individual component of the insulin regimen which most directly influences the blood glucose value in question, based on the known onset and duration of the insulin component.

Insulin detemir-specific dosing:

Type 1 diabetes mellitus: Children ≥2 years, Adolescents, and Adults: SubQ: Initial dose: Approximately one-third of the total daily insulin requirement; a rapid-acting or short-acting insulin should also be used. If administered once daily, doses are generally administered with evening meals or at bedtime.

Conversion from insulin glargine or NPH insulin: Children ≥2 years, Adolescents, and Adults: SubQ: May be substituted on an equivalent unit-per-unit basis; in one Type 2 diabetes clinical trial, higher doses of insulin detemir were required than insulin NPH.

Type 2 diabetes mellitus: Adults: SubQ: Initial basal insulin dose: 10 units (**or** 0.1-0.2 units/kg) once daily in the evening; may also administer total daily dose in 2 divided doses

Conversion from insulin glargine or NPH insulin: Children ≥2 years, Adolescents, and Adults: SubQ: May be substituted on an equivalent unit-per-unit basis; in one Type 2 diabetes clinical trial, higher doses of insulin detemir were required than insulin NPH

Dosing adjustment in renal impairment: There are no dosage adjustments provided in manufacturer's labeling; insulin requirements are reduced due to changes in insulin clearance or metabolism; monitor blood glucose closely.

Dosing adjustment in hepatic impairment: There are no dosage adjustments provided in manufacturer's labeling; insulin requirements may be reduced due to changes in insulin clearance or metabolism; monitor blood glucose closely.

Administration Parenteral: SubQ: Administer into the thighs, deltoids, or abdomen, with sites rotated. Cold injections should be avoided. **Not for I.V. infusion** or use in insulin infusion pumps. Do not use if solution is viscous or cloudy; use only if clear and colorless with no visible particles. May not be diluted or mixed with other insulins or solutions. When treated once daily, administer with evening meal or at bedtime. When treated twice daily, administer evening dose with evening meal, at bedtime, or 12 hours following the morning dose.

Monitoring Parameters Urine sugar and acetone, serum glucose, electrolytes, Hb A_{1c}, lipid profile

Reference Range

Plasma Blood Glucose and Hgb A_{1c} Goals for Type 1 Diabetes (ADA, 2013): Note: Goals should be individualized based on individual needs/circumstances (eg, patients who experience severe hypoglycemia, patients with hypoglycemic unawareness); lower goals may be reasonable if they can be achieved without excessive hypoglycemia. **Note:** Postprandial blood glucose should be measured when there is a discrepancy between preprandial blood glucose concentrations and Hb A_{1c} values and to help assess glycemia for patients who receive basal/bolus regimens. It is usually drawn 1-2 hours after starting meal and is considered to be the "peak."

Toddlers/Preschoolers (0-6 years):
  Preprandial glucose: 100-180 mg/dL
  Bedtime/overnight glucose: 110-200 mg/dL
  Hb A_{1c}: <8.5%
School age (6-12 years):
  Preprandial glucose: 90-180 mg/dL
  Bedtime/overnight glucose: 100-180 mg/dL
  Hb A_{1c}: <8%
Adolescents/Young adults (13-19 years):
  Preprandial glucose: 90-130 mg/dL
  Bedtime/overnight glucose: 90-150 mg/dL
  Hb A_{1c}: <7.5%
Adults, nonpregnant:
  Preprandial glucose: 70-130 mg/dL
  Postprandial glucose: <180 mg/dL
  Hb A_{1c}: <7%

Additional Information
Division of daily insulin requirement ("conventional therapy"): Generally, 50% to 75% of the daily insulin dose is given as an intermediate-acting (eg, insulin detemir) or a long-acting form of insulin (in 1-2 daily injections). The remaining portion of the 24-hour insulin requirement is divided and administered as either regular insulin or a rapid-acting form of insulin at the same time before breakfast and dinner.

Division of daily insulin requirement ("intensive therapy"): Basal insulin delivery with 1 or 2 doses of intermediate-acting (eg, insulin detemir) or long-acting insulin formulations superimposed with doses of rapid- or very rapid-acting insulin formulations 3 or more times daily.

Dosage Forms Excipient information presented when available (limited, particularly for generics); consult specific product labeling.

Solution, Subcutaneous:
  Levemir: 100 units/mL (10 mL) [contains metacresol, phenol]
Solution Pen-injector, Subcutaneous:
  Levemir FlexPen: 100 units/mL (3 mL) [contains metacresol, phenol]
  Levemir FlexTouch: 100 units/mL (3 mL) [contains metacresol, phenol]

References
International Diabetes Federation, International Society for Pediatric and Adolescent Diabetes. Global IDF/ISPAD guideline for diabetes in childhood and adolescence. 2011. Available at: http://www.idf.org/global-idfispad-guideline-diabetes-childhood-and-adolescence. Date accessed: October 21, 2013.

Insulin Glargine (IN soo lin GLAR jeen)

Medication Safety Issues
  Sound-alike/look-alike issues:
    Insulin glargine may be confused with insulin glulisine
    Lantus® may be confused with latanoprost, Latuda®, Xalatan®
  High alert medication:
    The Institute for Safe Medication Practices (ISMP) includes this medication among its list of drugs which have a heightened risk of causing significant patient harm when used in error. *Due to the number of insulin*

preparations, it is essential to identify/clarify the type of insulin to be used.

Administration issues:
  Insulin glargine is a clear solution, but it is NOT intended for I.V. or I.M. administration.

Other safety concerns:
  Cross-contamination may occur if insulin pens are shared among multiple patients. Steps should be taken to prohibit sharing of insulin pens.

International issues:
  Lantus [U.S., Canada, and multiple international markets] may be confused with Lanvis brand name for thioguanine [Canada and multiple international markets]

Brand Names: U.S. Lantus; Lantus SoloStar
Brand Names: Canada Lantus®; Lantus® OptiSet®
Therapeutic Category Antidiabetic Agent, Parenteral; Insulin, Long-Acting
Generic Availability (U.S.) No
Use Treatment of type 1 diabetes mellitus (insulin dependent, IDDM); type 2 diabetes mellitus (noninsulin dependent, NIDDM) requiring basal (long-acting) insulin to control hyperglycemia
Pregnancy Risk Factor C
Pregnancy Considerations Adverse events have been shown in some animal studies. Maternal hyperglycemia can be associated with adverse effects in the fetus, including macrosomia, neonatal hyperglycemia, and hyperbilirubinemia; the risk of congenital malformations is increased when HbA_{1c} is >1% above the normal range.

Insulin requirements tend to fall during the first trimester of pregnancy and increase in the later trimesters, peaking at 28-32 weeks of gestation. Following delivery, insulin requirements decrease rapidly. Diabetes can also be associated with adverse effects in the mother. Poorly-treated diabetes may cause end-organ damage that may in turn negatively affect obstetric outcomes. Physiologic glucose levels should be maintained prior to and during pregnancy to decrease the risk of adverse events in the fetus and the mother. Insulin is the drug of choice for the control of diabetes mellitus during pregnancy. When compared to NPH insulin, insulin glargine has not been found to increase the risk of adverse events during pregnancy.

Breast-Feeding Considerations It is not known if significant amounts of insulin glargine distributes into breast milk. Endogenous insulin can be found in breast milk. Plasma glucose concentrations in the mother affect glucose concentrations in breast milk. The gastrointestinal tract destroys insulin when administered orally; therefore, insulin is not expected to be absorbed intact by the breast-feeding infant. All types of insulin are safe for use while breast-feeding. Due to increased calorie expenditure, women with diabetes may require less insulin while nursing.

Contraindications Hypersensitivity insulin glargine or any component

Warnings Hypoglycemia is the most common adverse effect of insulin. The timing of hypoglycemia differs among various insulin formulations. Any change of insulin should be made cautiously; changing manufacturers, type, and/or method of manufacture may result in the need for a change of dosage. Hypoglycemia may result from increased work or exercise without eating; use of long-acting insulin preparations (insulin glargine, Ultralente®) with regular insulin may delay recovery from hypoglycemia. **Not for I.V. administration** or use in insulin infusion pumps.

Precautions Use with caution and adjust dosage in patients with renal impairment; use with caution and monitor closely in patient with hepatic impairment.

Adverse Reactions Primarily symptoms of hypoglycemia
  Cardiovascular: Pallor, palpitation, tachycardia
  Central nervous system: Fatigue, headache, hypothermia, loss of consciousness, mental confusion

Dermatologic: Redness, urticaria

Endocrine & metabolic: Hypoglycemia, hypokalemia

Gastrointestinal: Hunger, nausea, numbness of mouth

Local: Atrophy or hypertrophy of SubQ fat tissue; edema, itching, pain or warmth at injection site; stinging

Neuromuscular & skeletal: Muscle weakness, paresthesia, tremor

Ocular: Transient presbyopia or blurred vision

Miscellaneous: Anaphylaxis, diaphoresis, local and/or systemic hypersensitivity reactions

Drug Interactions

Metabolism/Transport Effects None known.

Avoid Concomitant Use There are no known interactions where it is recommended to avoid concomitant use.

Increased Effect/Toxicity

Insulin Glargine may increase the levels/effects of: Antidiabetic Agents (Thiazolidinedione); Hypoglycemic Agents; Quinolone Antibiotics

The levels/effects of Insulin Glargine may be increased by: Androgens; Beta-Blockers; Edetate CALCIUM Disodium; Edetate Disodium; GLP-1 Agonists; Herbs (Hypoglycemic Properties); MAO Inhibitors; Metreleptin; Pegvisomant; Salicylates; Selective Serotonin Reuptake Inhibitors

Decreased Effect

The levels/effects of Insulin Glargine may be decreased by: Corticosteroids (Orally Inhaled); Corticosteroids (Systemic); Danazol; Loop Diuretics; Luteinizing Hormone-Releasing Hormone Analogs; Somatropin; Thiazide Diuretics

Stability Store unopened containers or cartridges in refrigerator at 2°C to 8°C (36°F to 46°F); do not freeze; protect from direct heat or light. Once opened (in use), vials may be stored in refrigerator or at room temperature for up to 28 days. Cartridges (in use; inserted into OptiClik™ delivery system) should **not** be refrigerated; store below 30°C (86°F) away from direct heat or light; discard after 28 days. May **not** be mixed with any other insulin or solution.

Mechanism of Action Insulin acts via specific membrane-bound receptors on target tissues to regulate metabolism of carbohydrate, protein, and fats. Target organs for insulin include the liver, skeletal muscle, and adipose tissue.

Within the liver, insulin stimulates hepatic glycogen synthesis. Insulin promotes hepatic synthesis of fatty acids, which are released into the circulation as lipoproteins. Skeletal muscle effects of insulin include increased protein synthesis and increased glycogen synthesis. Within adipose tissue, insulin stimulates the processing of circulating lipoproteins to provide free fatty acids, facilitating triglyceride synthesis and storage by adipocytes; also directly inhibits the hydrolysis of triglycerides. In addition, insulin stimulates the cellular uptake of amino acids and increases cellular permeability to several ions, including potassium, magnesium, and phosphate. By activating sodium-potassium ATPases, insulin promotes the intracellular movement of potassium.

Normally secreted by the pancreas, insulin products are manufactured for pharmacologic use through recombinant DNA technology using either *E. coli* or *Saccharomyces cerevisiae*. Insulins are categorized based on the onset, peak, and duration of effect (eg, rapid-, short-, intermediate-, and long-acting insulin). Insulin glargine is a long-acting insulin analog.

Pharmacodynamics

Onset of action: 3-4 hours

Duration: 24 hours

Pharmacokinetics (Adult data unless noted)

Absorption: Slow; after injection it forms microprecipitates in the skin which allow small amounts to release over time

Metabolism: Partially metabolized in the skin to form two active metabolites

Time to peak serum concentration: No pronounced peak

Elimination: Urine

Dosing: Usual Insulin glargine is a long-acting insulin administered by SubQ injection. Insulin glargine is approximately equipotent to human insulin, but has a slower onset, no pronounced peak, and a longer duration of activity. Changing the basal insulin component from another insulin to insulin glargine can be done on a unit-to-unit basis. Insulin requirements vary dramatically between patients and dictates frequent monitoring and close medical supervision. See Insulin Regular for additional information.

General insulin dosing:

Type 1 diabetes mellitus: Children, Adolescents, and Adults: **Note:** Multiple daily doses are utilized and guided by blood glucose monitoring. Combinations of insulin formulations are commonly used. The daily doses presented below are expressed as the **total units/kg/day of all insulin formulations** used. Insulin glargine must be used in combination with a short-acting insulin.

Usual maintenance range: SubQ: 0.5-1 unit/kg/day in divided doses. An estimate of anticipated needs may be based on body weight and/or activity factors as follows:

Nonobese: 0.4-0.6 units/kg/day

Obese: 0.8-1.2 units/kg/day

Pubescent Children and Adolescents: During puberty, requirements may substantially increase to >1 unit/kg/day and in some cases up to 2 units/kg/day (IDF/ISPAD, 2011)

Adjustment of dose: Dosage must be titrated to achieve glucose control and avoid hypoglycemia. Adjust dose to maintain premeal and bedtime glucose in target range. Since combinations of agents are frequently used, dosage adjustment must address the individual component of the insulin regimen which most directly influences the blood glucose value in question, based on the known onset and duration of the insulin component.

Insulin glargine-specific dosing:

Type 1 diabetes mellitus: Children ≥6 years, Adolescents, and Adults: SubQ: Initial dose: Approximately one-third of the total daily insulin requirement; a rapid-acting or short-acting insulin should also be used.

Type 2 diabetes mellitus: Adults: SubQ: Initial insulin dose: 10 units (**or** 0.2 units/kg) once daily in the evening; may also administer total daily dose in 2 divided doses

Type 1 or type 2 diabetes; previously receiving basal insulin plus bolus insulin (eg, NPH + regular insulin):

Children <6 years: SubQ: Limited data available: 40% of the established total daily insulin requirement; this resulted in a reduction in hypoglycemic episodes in 35 nonobese preschool-aged children (age range: 2.6-6.3 years) when used in conjunction with a rapid-acting insulin prior to meals (Alemzadeh, 2005).

Children ≥6 years and Adults: SubQ:

Converting from once-daily NPH insulin: May be substituted on an equivalent unit-per-unit basis

Converting from twice-daily NPH insulin: Initial dose: Use 80% of the total daily dose of NPH (eg, 20% reduction); administer once daily; adjust dosage according to patient response

Dosing adjustment in renal impairment: There are no dosage adjustments provided in manufacturer's labeling; insulin requirements are reduced due to changes in insulin clearance or metabolism; monitor blood glucose closely.

Dosing adjustment in hepatic impairment: There are no dosage adjustments provided in manufacturer's labeling; insulin requirements may be reduced due to changes in insulin clearance or metabolism; monitor blood glucose closely.

Administration Parenteral: SubQ: Administer into the subcutaneous fat of the thighs, arms, buttocks, or abdomen, with sites rotated. Cold injections should be avoided. Administer once daily, at any time of day, but at the same time each day. Do not mix with any other insulin or solution.

Monitoring Parameters Urine sugar and acetone, serum glucose, electrolytes, Hb A_{1c}, lipid profile

Reference Range

Plasma Blood Glucose and Hgb A_{1c} Goals for Type 1 Diabetes (ADA, 2013): Note: Goals should be individualized based on individual needs/circumstances (eg, patients who experience severe hypoglycemia, patients with hypoglycemic unawareness); lower goals may be reasonable if they can be achieved without excessive hypoglycemia. **Note:** Postprandial blood glucose should be measured when there is a discrepancy between preprandial blood glucose concentrations and Hb A_{1c} values and to help assess glycemia for patients who receive basal/bolus regimens. It is usually drawn 1-2 hours after starting meal and is considered to be the "peak."

Toddlers/Preschoolers (0-6 years):
Preprandial glucose: 100-180 mg/dL
Bedtime/overnight glucose: 110-200 mg/dL
Hb A_{1c}: <8.5%

School age (6-12 years):
Preprandial glucose: 90-180 mg/dL
Bedtime/overnight glucose: 100-180 mg/dL
Hb A_{1c}: <8%

Adolescents/Young Adults (13-19 years):
Preprandial glucose: 90-130 mg/dL
Bedtime/overnight glucose: 90-150 mg/dL
Hb A_{1c}: <7.5%

Adults, nonpregnant:
Preprandial glucose: 70-130 mg/dL
Postprandial glucose: <180 mg/dL
Hb A_{1c}: <7%

Criteria for diagnosis of DKA:

Serum glucose:
Children: >200 mg/dL
Adults: >250 mg/dL

Arterial pH:
Children: <7.3
Adults: <7-7.24

Bicarbonate:
Children: <15 mEq/L
Adults: <10-15 mEq/L

Moderate ketonuria or ketonemia

Additional Information

Division of daily insulin requirement ("conventional therapy"): Generally, 50% to 75% of the daily insulin dose is given as an intermediate- or long-acting form (eg, insulin glargine) of insulin (in 1-2 daily injections). The remaining portion of the 24-hour insulin requirement is divided and administered as either regular insulin or a rapid-acting form of insulin at the same time before breakfast and dinner.

Division of daily insulin requirement ("intensive therapy"): Basal insulin delivery with 1 or 2 doses of intermediate- or long-acting insulin (eg, insulin glargine) formulations superimposed with doses of rapid- or very rapid-acting insulin formulations 3 or more times daily.

Dosage Forms Excipient information presented when available (limited, particularly for generics); consult specific product labeling.

Solution, Subcutaneous:
Lantus: 100 units/mL (10 mL) [contains metacresol]

Solution Pen-injector, Subcutaneous:
Lantus SoloStar: 100 units/mL (3 mL)

References

Alemzadeh R, Berhe T, and Wyatt DT, "Flexible Insulin Therapy With Glargine Insulin Improved Glycemic Control and Reduced Severe Hypoglycemia Among Preschool-Aged Children With Type 1 Diabetes Mellitus," *Pediatrics*, 2005, 115(5):1320-4.

American Diabetes Association (ADA), "Standards of Medical Care in Diabetes-2013," *Diabetes Care*, 2013, (36 Suppl 1):S11-66.

International Diabetes Federation, International Society for Pediatric and Adolescent Diabetes. Global IDF/ISPAD guideline for diabetes in childhood and adolescence. 2011. Available at: http://www.idf.org/global-idfispad-guideline-diabetes-childhood-and-adolescence. Date accessed: October 21, 2013.

Insulin Glulisine (IN soo lin gloo LIS een)

Medication Safety Issues

Sound-alike/look-alike issues:
Insulin glulisine may be confused with insulin glargine

High alert medication:
The Institute for Safe Medication Practices (ISMP) includes this medication among its list of drugs which have a heightened risk of causing significant patient harm when used in error. *Due to the number of insulin preparations, it is essential to identify/clarify the type of insulin to be used.*

Other safety concerns:
Cross-contamination may occur if insulin pens are shared among multiple patients. Steps should be taken to prohibit sharing of insulin pens.

Brand Names: U.S. Apidra; Apidra SoloStar

Brand Names: Canada Apidra®

Therapeutic Category Insulin, Rapid-Acting

Generic Availability (U.S.) No

Use Treatment of type 1 diabetes mellitus (insulin dependent, IDDM); type 2 diabetes mellitus (noninsulin dependent, NIDDM) to control hyperglycemia

Pregnancy Risk Factor C

Pregnancy Considerations Adverse events were observed in some animal reproduction studies. Maternal hyperglycemia can be associated with adverse effects in the fetus, including macrosomia, neonatal hyperglycemia, and hyperbilirubinemia; the risk of congenital malformations is increased when the HbA$_{1c}$ is >1% above the normal range.

Insulin requirements tend to fall during the first trimester of pregnancy and increase in the later trimesters, peaking at 28-32 weeks of gestation. Following delivery, insulin requirements decrease rapidly. Diabetes can also be associated with adverse effects in the mother. Poorly-treated diabetes may cause end-organ damage that may in turn negatively affect obstetric outcomes. Physiologic glucose levels should be maintained prior to and during pregnancy to decrease the risk of adverse events in the fetus and mother. Insulin is the drug of choice for the control of diabetes mellitus during pregnancy. Due to lack of clinical studies with insulin glulisine in pregnant women, the manufacturer recommends use during pregnancy only if the potential benefit to the mother justifies any potential risk to the fetus.

Breast-Feeding Considerations It is not known if insulin glulisine distributes into breast milk. Endogenous insulin can be found in breast milk. Plasma glucose concentrations in the mother affect glucose concentrations in breast milk. The gastrointestinal tract destroys insulin when administered orally; therefore, insulin is not expected to be absorbed intact by the breast-feeding infant. All types of insulin are safe for use while breast-feeding. Although use of insulin glulisine is compatible with breast-feeding, the manufacturer recommends that caution be used when insulin glulisine is used by nursing women. Due to

◄ increased calorie expenditure, women with diabetes may require less insulin while nursing.

Contraindications Hypersensitivity to insulin glulisine or any component; do not use during episodes of hypoglycemia

Warnings Hypoglycemia is the most common adverse effect of insulin. The timing of hypoglycemia differs among various insulin formulations. Any change of insulin should be made cautiously; changing manufacturers, type, and/or method of manufacture may result in the need for a change of dosage. Hypoglycemia may result from increased work or exercise without eating.

Precautions Use with caution and adjust dosage in patients with renal impairment; use with caution and monitor closely in patient with hepatic impairment. While regular insulin is the preferred formulation for I.V. administration, both insulin aspart and insulin glulisine have been approved for I.V. use in selected clinical situations with close medical supervision and monitoring of serum potassium.

Adverse Reactions Primarily symptoms of hypoglycemia
Cardiovascular: Pallor, palpitation, tachycardia
Central nervous system: Fatigue, headache, hypothermia, loss of consciousness, mental confusion
Dermatologic: Redness, urticaria
Endocrine & metabolic: Hypoglycemia, hypokalemia
Gastrointestinal: Hunger, nausea, numbness of mouth
Local: Atrophy or hypertrophy of SubQ fat tissue; edema, itching, pain or warmth at injection site; stinging
Neuromuscular & skeletal: Muscle weakness, paresthesia, tremor
Ocular: Transient presbyopia or blurred vision
Miscellaneous: Anaphylaxis, diaphoresis, local and/or systemic hypersensitivity reactions

Drug Interactions
Metabolism/Transport Effects None known.
Avoid Concomitant Use There are no known interactions where it is recommended to avoid concomitant use.
Increased Effect/Toxicity
Insulin Glulisine may increase the levels/effects of: Antidiabetic Agents (Thiazolidinedione); Hypoglycemic Agents; Quinolone Antibiotics

The levels/effects of Insulin Glulisine may be increased by: Androgens; Beta-Blockers; Edetate CALCIUM Disodium; Edetate Disodium; GLP-1 Agonists; Herbs (Hypoglycemic Properties); MAO Inhibitors; Metreleptin; Pegvisomant; Salicylates; Selective Serotonin Reuptake Inhibitors

Decreased Effect
The levels/effects of Insulin Glulisine may be decreased by: Corticosteroids (Orally Inhaled); Corticosteroids (Systemic); Danazol; Loop Diuretics; Luteinizing Hormone-Releasing Hormone Analogs; Somatropin; Thiazide Diuretics

Stability Store unopened container in refrigerator; do not freeze; protect from heat and light. Once opened (in use) vials may be stored in refrigerator or at room temperature for up to 28 days. Cartridges that are in use should be stored at room temperature and used within 28 days; do not refrigerate. Insulin glulisine in reservoir should be replaced every 48 hours. Discard if exposed to temperatures ≥37°C (98.6°F). May be mixed in the same syringe with NPH insulin.

Mechanism of Action Insulin acts via specific membrane-bound receptors on target tissues to regulate metabolism of carbohydrate, protein, and fats. Target organs for insulin include the liver, skeletal muscle, and adipose tissue.

Within the liver, insulin stimulates hepatic glycogen synthesis. Insulin promotes hepatic synthesis of fatty acids, which are released into the circulation as lipoproteins. Skeletal muscle effects of insulin include increased protein synthesis and increased glycogen synthesis. Within adipose tissue, insulin stimulates the processing of circulating lipoproteins to provide free fatty acids, facilitating triglyceride synthesis and storage by adipocytes; also directly inhibits the hydrolysis of triglycerides. In addition, insulin stimulates the cellular uptake of amino acids and increases cellular permeability to several ions, including potassium, magnesium, and phosphate. By activating sodium-potassium ATPases, insulin promotes the intracellular movement of potassium.

Normally secreted by the pancreas, insulin products are manufactured for pharmacologic use through recombinant DNA technology using either *E. coli* or *Saccharomyces cerevisiae*. Insulins are categorized based on the onset, peak, and duration of effect (eg, rapid-, short-, intermediate-, and long-acting insulin). Insulin glulisine is a rapid-acting insulin analog.

Pharmacodynamics Onset and duration of hypoglycemic effects depend upon the route of administration (adsorption and onset of action are more rapid after deeper I.M. injections than after SubQ), site of injection (onset and duration are progressively slower with SubQ injection into the abdomen, arm, buttock, or thigh respectively), volume and concentration of injection, and the preparation administered; local heat and massage also increase the rate of absorption.
Onset of action: 5-15 minutes
Maximum effect: 45-75 minutes
Duration: 2-4 hours

Pharmacokinetics (Adult data unless noted)
Distribution: V_d: Adults: 13 L
Bioavailability: SubQ: ~70%
Half-life:
  SubQ: 42 minutes
  I.V.: 13 minutes
Time to peak serum concentration: SubQ: 60 minutes (range: 40-120 minutes)
Elimination: Urine

Dosing: Usual Insulin glulisine is a rapid-acting insulin analog which is normally administered SubQ as a premeal component of the insulin regimen or as a continuous SubQ infusion and should be used with an intermediate- or long-acting insulin. Insulin glulisine is equipotent to insulin regular, but has a more rapid onset and shorter duration of activity. In carefully controlled clinical settings with close medical supervision and monitoring of blood glucose and potassium, insulin glulisine may be administered I.V. Insulin requirements vary dramatically between patients and dictate frequent monitoring and close medical supervision. See Insulin Regular for additional information.
General insulin dosing:
  Type 1 diabetes mellitus: Children, Adolescents, and Adults: **Note:** Multiple daily doses or continuous subcutaneous infusions guided by blood glucose monitoring are utilized. Combinations of insulin formulations are commonly used. The daily doses presented below are expressed as the **total units/kg/day of all insulin formulations combined**.
  Initial dose: SubQ: 0.2-0.6 units/kg/day in divided doses. Conservative initial doses of 0.2-0.4 units/kg/day are often recommended to avoid the potential for hypoglycemia. A rapidly acting insulin may be the only insulin formulation used initially.
  Usual maintenance range: SubQ: 0.5-1 unit/kg/day in divided doses. An estimate of anticipated needs may be based on body weight and/or activity factors as follows:
  Nonobese: 0.4-0.6 units/kg/day
  Obese: 0.8-1.2 units/kg/day

Pubescent Children and Adolescents: During puberty, requirements may substantially increase to >1 unit/kg/day and in some cases up to 2 units/kg/day (IDF/ISPAD, 2011)

Adjustment of dose: Dosage must be titrated to achieve glucose control and avoid hypoglycemia. Adjust dose to maintain premeal and bedtime glucose in target range. Since combinations of agents are frequently used, dosage adjustment must address the individual component of the insulin regimen which most directly influences the blood glucose value in question, based on the known onset and duration of the insulin component.

Continuous SubQ insulin infusion (insulin pump): A combination of a "basal" continuous insulin infusion rate with preprogrammed premeal bolus doses which are patient controlled. When converting from multiple daily SubQ doses of maintenance insulin, it is advisable to reduce the basal rate to less than the equivalent of the total daily units of longer-acting insulin (eg, NPH); divide the total number of units by 24 to get the basal rate in units/hour. Do not include the total units of regular insulin or other rapid-acting insulin formulations in this calculation. The same premeal regular insulin dosage may be used.

Type 2 diabetes mellitus: Augmentation therapy (patients for which diet, exercise, weight reduction, and oral hypoglycemic agents have not been adequate): Adults: SubQ: Initial dosage of 0.2 units/kg/day or 10 units/day of an intermediate- or long-acting insulin administered at bedtime has been recommended. As an alternative, regular insulin or rapid-acting insulin (eg, insulin glulisine) formulations administered before meals have also been used. Dosage must be carefully adjusted.

Dosing adjustment in renal impairment: There are no dosage adjustments provided in manufacturer's labeling; insulin requirements are reduced due to changes in insulin clearance or metabolism; monitor blood glucose closely.

Dosing adjustment in hepatic impairment: There are no dosage adjustments provided in manufacturer's labeling; insulin requirements may be reduced due to changes in insulin clearance or metabolism; monitor blood glucose closely.

Administration Parenteral:

SubQ: Administration is usually made into the subcutaneous fat of the thighs, arms, buttocks, or abdomen, with sites rotated; cold injections should be avoided. May be mixed in the same syringe with NPH insulin. When mixing insulin glulisine with NPH insulin, glulisine should be drawn into the syringe first. Administer 15 minutes before meals or within 20 minutes after starting a meal. Can be infused SubQ by external insulin pump; however, when used in an external pump, it is not recommended to be diluted with other insulins.

I.V.: Dilute with NS to a final concentration of 0.05-1 unit/mL and administer using polyvinyl chloride infusion bags into a dedicated infusion line (the use of other bags and tubing has not been studied).

Monitoring Parameters Urine sugar and acetone, serum glucose, electrolytes, Hb A$_{1c}$, lipid profile

Reference Range

Plasma Blood Glucose and Hgb A$_{1c}$ Goals for Type 1 Diabetes (ADA, 2013): Note: Goals should be individualized based on individual needs/circumstances (eg, patients who experience severe hypoglycemia, patients with hypoglycemic unawareness); lower goals may be reasonable if they can be achieved without excessive hypoglycemia. **Note:** Postprandial blood glucose should be measured when there is a discrepancy between preprandial blood glucose concentrations and Hb A$_{1c}$ values and to help assess glycemia for patients who receive basal/bolus regimens. It is usually drawn 1-2 hours after starting meal and is considered to be the "peak."

Toddlers/Preschoolers (0-6 years):
Preprandial glucose: 100-180 mg/dL
Bedtime/overnight glucose: 110-200 mg/dL
Hb A$_{1c}$: <8.5%

School age (6-12 years):
Preprandial glucose: 90-180 mg/dL
Bedtime/overnight glucose: 100-180 mg/dL
Hb A$_{1c}$: <8%

Adolescents/Young Adults (13-19 years):
Preprandial glucose: 90-130 mg/dL
Bedtime/overnight glucose: 90-150 mg/dL
Hb A$_{1c}$: <7.5%

Adults, nonpregnant:
Preprandial glucose: 70-130 mg/dL
Postprandial glucose: <180 mg/dL
Hb A$_{1c}$: <7%

Criteria for diagnosis of DKA:
Serum glucose:
Children: >200 mg/dL
Adults: >250 mg/dL
Arterial pH:
Children: <7.3
Adults: <7-7.24
Bicarbonate:
Children: <15 mEq/L
Adults: <10-15 mEq/L
Moderate ketonuria or ketonemia

Additional Information

Division of daily insulin requirement ("conventional therapy"): Generally, 50% to 75% of the daily insulin dose is given as an intermediate- or long-acting form of insulin (in 1-2 daily injections). The remaining portion of the 24-hour insulin requirement is divided and administered as either regular insulin or a rapid-acting (eg, insulin glulisine) form of insulin at the same time before breakfast and dinner.

Division of daily insulin requirement ("intensive therapy"): Basal insulin delivery with 1 or 2 doses of intermediate- or long-acting insulin formulations superimposed with doses of rapid- or very rapid-acting insulin (eg, insulin glulisine) formulations 3 or more times daily.

Dosage Forms Excipient information presented when available (limited, particularly for generics); consult specific product labeling.

Solution, Injection:
Apidra: 100 units/mL (10 mL) [contains metacresol]
Solution Pen-injector, Subcutaneous:
Apidra SoloStar: 100 units/mL (3 mL) [contains metacresol]

References

American Diabetes Association (ADA), "Standards of Medical Care in Diabetes-2013," *Diabetes Care*, 2013, (36 Suppl 1):S11-66.

International Diabetes Federation, International Society for Pediatric and Adolescent Diabetes. Global IDF/ISPAD guideline for diabetes in childhood and adolescence. 2011. Available at: http://www.idf.org/global-idfispad-guideline-diabetes-childhood-and-adolescence. Date accessed: October 21, 2013.

Insulin Lispro (IN soo lin LYE sproe)

Medication Safety Issues

Sound-alike/look-alike issues:

HumaLOG® may be confused with HumaLOG® Mix 50/50, Humira®, HumuLIN® N, HumuLIN® R, Novo-LOG®

High alert medication:
The Institute for Safe Medication Practices (ISMP) includes this medication among its list of drugs which have a heightened risk of causing significant patient harm when used in error. *Due to the number of insulin preparations, it is essential to identify/clarify the type of insulin to be used.*

Other safety concerns:
Cross-contamination may occur if insulin pens are shared among multiple patients. Steps should be taken to prohibit sharing of insulin pens.

Brand Names: U.S. HumaLOG; HumaLOG KwikPen

Brand Names: Canada Humalog®

Therapeutic Category Antidiabetic Agent, Parenteral; Insulin, Rapid-Acting

Generic Availability (U.S.) No

Use Treatment of type 1 diabetes mellitus (insulin dependent, IDDM); type 2 diabetes mellitus (noninsulin dependent, NIDDM) to control hyperglycemia

Pregnancy Risk Factor B

Pregnancy Considerations Adverse events have not been observed in animal reproduction studies. Insulin lispro has not been shown to cross the placenta at standard clinical doses. Although congenital anomalies have been noted in case reports, when compared to regular insulin, insulin lispro has not been found to increase the risk of adverse events to the fetus in larger studies. Maternal hyperglycemia can be associated with adverse effects in the fetus, including macrosomia, neonatal hyperglycemia, and hyperbilirubinemia; the risk of congenital malformations is increased when HbA_{1c} is >1% above the normal range.

Insulin requirements tend to fall during the first trimester of pregnancy and increase in the later trimesters, peaking at 28-32 weeks of gestation. Following delivery, insulin requirements decrease rapidly. Diabetes can also be associated with adverse effects in the mother. Poorly-treated diabetes may cause end-organ damage that may in turn negatively affect obstetric outcomes. Physiologic glucose levels should be maintained prior to and during pregnancy to decrease the risk of adverse events in the fetus and mother. Insulin is the drug of choice for the control of diabetes mellitus during pregnancy. The use of insulin lispro has been shown to be as effective as regular insulin to treat diabetes in pregnancy and may have advantages over regular insulin during pregnancy.

Breast-Feeding Considerations It is not known if insulin lispro distributes into breast milk. Endogenous insulin can be found in breast milk. Plasma glucose concentrations in the mother affect glucose concentrations in breast milk. The gastrointestinal tract destroys insulin when administered orally; therefore, insulin is not expected to be absorbed intact by the breast-feeding infant. All types of insulin are safe for use while breast-feeding. Due to increased calorie expenditure, women with diabetes may require less insulin while nursing.

Contraindications Hypersensitivity lispro insulin or any component; hypoglycemia

Warnings Hypoglycemia is the most common adverse effect of insulin. The timing of hypoglycemia differs among various insulin formulations. Any change of insulin should be made cautiously; changing manufacturers, type, and/or method of manufacture may result in the need for a change of dosage. Hypoglycemia may result from increased work or exercise without eating.

Precautions Use with caution and adjust dosage in patients with renal impairment; use with caution and monitor closely in patient with hepatic impairment.

Adverse Reactions Primarily symptoms of hypoglycemia
Cardiovascular: Pallor, palpitation, tachycardia
Central nervous system: Fatigue, headache, hypothermia, loss of consciousness, mental confusion

Dermatologic: Redness, urticaria
Endocrine & metabolic: Hypoglycemia, hypokalemia
Gastrointestinal: Hunger, nausea, numbness of mouth
Local: Atrophy or hypertrophy of SubQ fat tissue; edema, itching, pain or warmth at injection site; stinging
Neuromuscular & skeletal: Muscle weakness, paresthesia, tremor
Ocular: Transient presbyopia or blurred vision
Miscellaneous: Anaphylaxis, diaphoresis, local and/or systemic hypersensitivity reactions

Drug Interactions

Metabolism/Transport Effects None known.

Avoid Concomitant Use There are no known interactions where it is recommended to avoid concomitant use.

Increased Effect/Toxicity
Insulin Lispro may increase the levels/effects of: Antidiabetic Agents (Thiazolidinedione); Hypoglycemic Agents; Quinolone Antibiotics

The levels/effects of Insulin Lispro may be increased by: Androgens; Beta-Blockers; Edetate CALCIUM Disodium; Edetate Disodium; GLP-1 Agonists; Herbs (Hypoglycemic Properties); MAO Inhibitors; Metreleptin; Pegvisomant; Salicylates; Selective Serotonin Reuptake Inhibitors

Decreased Effect
The levels/effects of Insulin Lispro may be decreased by: Corticosteroids (Orally Inhaled); Corticosteroids (Systemic); Danazol; Loop Diuretics; Luteinizing Hormone-Releasing Hormone Analogs; Somatropin; Thiazide Diuretics

Stability Store unopened vials, pens, and cartridges in the refrigerator at 2°C to 8°C (36°F to 46°F); do not freeze; protect from heat and light. Once opened (in use) vials may be stored in refrigerator or at room temperature for up to 28 days. Cartridges and pens that are in use should be stored at room temperature and used within 28 days; do not refrigerate. Insulin lispro in an insulin pump reservoir should be replaced every 7 days. Discard if exposed to temperatures ≥37°C (98.6°F).

May be mixed in the same syringe with NPH insulin; insulin lispro should be drawn into the syringe first. A sterile diluent is available from the manufacturer for preparing dilutions of Humalog®. Diluted Humalog® may be stored at 5°C (41°F) for 28 days or 30°C (86°F) for 14 days. Do not dilute insulin in cartridges or used in insulin pumps.

Mechanism of Action Insulin acts via specific membrane-bound receptors on target tissues to regulate metabolism of carbohydrate, protein, and fats. Target organs for insulin include the liver, skeletal muscle, and adipose tissue.

Within the liver, insulin stimulates hepatic glycogen synthesis. Insulin promotes hepatic synthesis of fatty acids, which are released into the circulation as lipoproteins. Skeletal muscle effects of insulin include increased protein synthesis and increased glycogen synthesis. Within adipose tissue, insulin stimulates the processing of circulating lipoproteins to provide free fatty acids, facilitating triglyceride synthesis and storage by adipocytes; also directly inhibits the hydrolysis of triglycerides. In addition, insulin stimulates the cellular uptake of amino acids and increases cellular permeability to several ions, including potassium, magnesium, and phosphate. By activating sodium-potassium ATPases, insulin promotes the intracellular movement of potassium.

Normally secreted by the pancreas, insulin products are manufactured for pharmacologic use through recombinant DNA technology using either *E. coli* or *Saccharomyces cerevisiae*. Insulins are categorized based on the onset, peak, and duration of effect (eg, rapid-, short-, intermediate-, and long-acting insulin). Insulin lispro is a rapid-acting insulin analog.

Pharmacodynamics Onset and duration of hypoglycemic effects depend upon the route of administration (adsorption and onset of action are more rapid after deeper I.M. injections than after SubQ), site of injection (onset and duration are progressively slower with SubQ injection into the abdomen, arm, buttock, or thigh respectively), volume and concentration of injection, and the preparation administered; local heat, and massage also increase the rate of absorption.

Onset of action: 15-30 minutes
Maximum effect: 0.5-2.5 hours
Duration: 3-6.5 hours

Pharmacokinetics (Adult data unless noted)
Distribution: V_d: 0.26-0.36 L/kg
Bioavailability: 55% to 77%
Half-life: SubQ: 1 hour
Excretion: Urine

Dosing: Usual Insulin lispro is a rapid-acting insulin analog which is normally administered SubQ as a premeal component of the insulin regimen or as a continuous SubQ infusion and should be used with intermediate- or long-acting insulin. When compared to insulin regular, insulin lispro has a more rapid onset and shorter duration of activity. Insulin requirements vary dramatically between patients and dictate frequent monitoring and close medical supervision. See Insulin Regular for additional information.

General insulin dosing:

Type 1 diabetes mellitus: Children, Adolescents, and Adults: **Note:** Multiple daily doses or continuous subcutaneous infusions guided by blood glucose monitoring are the standard of diabetes care. Combinations of insulin formulations are commonly used. The daily doses presented below are expressed as the **total units/kg/day of all insulin formulations combined.**

Initial dose: SubQ: 0.2-0.6 units/kg/day in divided doses. Conservative initial doses of 0.2-0.4 units/kg/day are often recommended to avoid the potential for hypoglycemia. Regular insulin may be the only insulin formulation used initially.

Usual maintenance range: SubQ: 0.5-1 unit/kg/day in divided doses. An estimate of anticipated needs may be based on body weight and/or activity factors as follows:

Nonobese: 0.4-0.6 units/kg/day
Obese: 0.8-1.2 units/kg/day

Pubescent Children and Adolescents: During puberty, requirements may substantially increase to >1 unit/kg/day and in some cases up to 2 units/kg/day (IDF/ISPAD, 2011)

Adjustment of dose: Dosage must be titrated to achieve glucose control and avoid hypoglycemia. Adjust dose to maintain premeal and bedtime glucose in target range. Since combinations of agents are frequently used, dosage adjustment must address the individual component of the insulin regimen which most directly influences the blood glucose value in question, based on the known onset and duration of the insulin component.

Continuous SubQ insulin infusion (insulin pump): A combination of a "basal" continuous insulin infusion rate with preprogrammed, premeal bolus doses which are patient controlled. When converting from multiple daily SubQ doses of maintenance insulin, it is advisable to reduce the basal rate to less than the equivalent of the total daily units of longer-acting insulin (eg, NPH); divide the total number of units by 24 to get the basal rate in units/hour. Do not include the total units of regular insulin or other rapid-acting insulin formulations in this calculation. The same premeal regular insulin dosage may be used.

Type 2 diabetes mellitus: Augmentation therapy (patients for which diet, exercise, weight reduction, and oral hypoglycemic agents have not been

adequate): Adults: SubQ: Initial dosage of 00.2 units/kg/day or 10 units/day of an intermediate- or long-acting insulin administered at bedtime has been recommended. As an alternative, regular insulin or rapid-acting insulin (eg, insulin lispro) formulations administered before meals have also been used. Dosage must be carefully adjusted.

Dosing adjustment in renal impairment: Insulin requirements are reduced due to changes in insulin clearance or metabolism; monitor blood glucose closely. There are no dosage adjustments provided in manufacturer's labeling; however, the following adjustments have been used by some clinicians (Aronoff, 2007): Adults:

CrCl >50 mL/minute: No adjustment necessary
CrCl 10-50 mL/minute: Administer at 75% of recommended dose
CrCl <10 mL/minute: Administer at 50% of recommended dose and monitor glucose closely

Hemodialysis: Because of a large molecular weight (6000 daltons), insulin is not significantly removed by either peritoneal or hemodialysis; supplemental dose is not necessary

Peritoneal dialysis: Supplemental dose is not necessary
Continuous renal replacement therapy: Administer at 75% of recommended dose

Dosing adjustment in hepatic impairment: There are no dosage adjustments provided in manufacturer's labeling; insulin requirements may be reduced due to changes in insulin clearance or metabolism; monitor blood glucose closely.

Administration Parenteral: SubQ: Administration is usually made into the subcutaneous fat of the thighs, arms, buttocks, or abdomen, with sites rotated; cold injections should be avoided. Administer 15 minutes before meals or immediately after. May be mixed in the same syringe with NPH insulin. When mixing insulin lispro with NPH insulin, lispro should be drawn into the syringe first; administer immediately after mixing. Insulin lispro can be infused SubQ by external insulin pump; however, when used in an external pump, it is not recommended to be diluted or mixed with other insulins. Insulin in the reservoir of an external pump should be changed every 7 days; infusion sets and insertion sites should be changed every 3 days; rotate infusion sites.

Monitoring Parameters Urine sugar and acetone, serum glucose, electrolytes, Hb A_{1c}, lipid profile

Reference Range

Plasma Blood Glucose and Hgb A_{1c} Goals for Type 1 Diabetes (ADA, 2013): Note: Goals should be individualized based on individual needs/circumstances (eg, patients who experience severe hypoglycemia, patients with hypoglycemic unawareness; lower goals may be reasonable if they can be achieved without excessive hypoglycemia. **Note:** Postprandial blood glucose should be measured when there is a discrepancy between prepranial blood glucose concentrations and Hb A_{1c} values and to help assess glycemia for patients who receive basal/bolus regimens. It is usually drawn 1-2 hours after starting meal and is considered to be the "peak."

Toddlers/Preschoolers (0-6 years):
 Preprandial glucose: 100-180 mg/dL
 Bedtime/overnight glucose: 110-200 mg/dL
 Hb A_{1c}: <8.5%
School age (6-12 years):
 Preprandial glucose: 90-180 mg/dL
 Bedtime/overnight glucose: 100-180 mg/dL
 Hb A_{1c}: <8%
Adolescents/Young Adults (13-19 years):
 Preprandial glucose: 90-130 mg/dL
 Bedtime/overnight glucose: 90-150 mg/dL
 Hb A_{1c}: <7.5%

Adults, nonpregnant:
Preprandial glucose: 70-130 mg/dL
Postprandial glucose: <180 mg/dL
Hb A$_{1c}$: <7%

Criteria for diagnosis of DKA:
Serum glucose:
Children: >200 mg/dL
Adults: >250 mg/dL
Arterial pH:
Children: <7.3
Adults: <7-7.24
Bicarbonate:
Children: <15 mEq/L
Adults: <10-15 mEq/L
Moderate ketonuria or ketonemia

Additional Information
Division of daily insulin requirement ("conventional therapy"): Generally, 50% to 75% of the daily insulin dose is given as an intermediate- or long-acting form of insulin (in 1-2 daily injections). The remaining portion of the 24-hour insulin requirement is divided and administered as either regular insulin or a rapid-acting form of insulin (eg, insulin lispro) at the same time before breakfast and dinner.
Division of daily insulin requirement ("intensive therapy"): Basal insulin delivery with 1 or 2 doses of intermediate- or long-acting insulin formulations superimposed with doses of rapid- or very rapid-acting insulin (eg, insulin lispro) formulations 3 or more times daily.

Dosage Forms Excipient information presented when available (limited, particularly for generics); consult specific product labeling.
Solution, Subcutaneous:
HumaLOG: 100 units/mL (3 mL, 10 mL) [contains metacresol, phenol]
HumaLOG KwikPen: 100 units/mL (3 mL) [contains metacresol, phenol]
Solution Pen-injector, Subcutaneous:
HumaLOG KwikPen: 100 units/mL (3 mL) [contains metacresol, phenol]

References
American Diabetes Association (ADA), "Standards of Medical Care in Diabetes-2013," *Diabetes Care*, 2013, (36 Suppl 1):S11-66.
International Diabetes Federation, International Society for Pediatric and Adolescent Diabetes. Global IDF/ISPAD guideline for diabetes in childhood and adolescence. 2011. Available at: http://www.idf.org/global-idfispad-guideline-diabetes-childhood-and-adolescence. Date accessed: October 21, 2013.

◆ **Insulin Lispro and Insulin Lispro Protamine** *see* Insulin Lispro Protamine and Insulin Lispro *on page 1128*

Insulin Lispro Protamine and Insulin Lispro

(IN soo lin LYE sproe PROE ta meen & IN soo lin LYE sproe)

Medication Safety Issues
Sound-alike/look-alike issues:
HumaLOG® Mix 50/50™ may be confused with HumaLOG®
HumaLOG® Mix 75/25™ may be confused with HumuLIN® 70/30, NovoLIN® 70/30, and NovoLOG® Mix 70/30

High alert medication:
The Institute for Safe Medication Practices (ISMP) includes this medication among its list of drugs which have a heightened risk of causing significant patient harm when used in error. *Due to the number of insulin preparations, it is essential to identify/clarify the type of insulin to be used.*
Other safety concerns:
Cross-contamination may occur if insulin pens are shared among multiple patients. Steps should be taken to prohibit sharing of insulin pens.

Brand Names: U.S. HumaLOG® Mix 50/50™; HumaLOG® Mix 50/50™ KwikPen™; HumaLOG® Mix 75/25™; HumaLOG® Mix 75/25™ KwikPen™
Brand Names: Canada Humalog® Mix 25
Therapeutic Category Antidiabetic Agent, Parenteral; Insulin, Combination
Generic Availability (U.S.) No
Use Treatment of type 1 diabetes mellitus (insulin dependent, IDDM); type 2 diabetes mellitus (noninsulin dependent, NIDDM) to control hyperglycemia
Pregnancy Risk Factor B
Pregnancy Considerations Adverse events have not been observed in animal reproduction studies. Insulin lispro has not been shown to cross the placenta at standard clinical doses. Although congenital anomalies have been noted in case reports, when compared to regular insulin, insulin lispro has not been found to increase the risk of adverse events to the fetus in larger studies. Maternal hyperglycemia can be associated with adverse effects in the fetus, including macrosomia, neonatal hyperglycemia, and hyperbilirubinemia; the risk of congenital malformations is increased when HbA$_{1c}$ is >1% above the normal range.

Insulin requirements tend to fall during the first trimester of pregnancy and increase in the later trimesters, peaking at 28-32 weeks of gestation. Following delivery, insulin requirements decrease rapidly. Diabetes can also be associated with adverse effects in the mother. Poorly-treated diabetes may cause end-organ damage that may in turn negatively affect obstetric outcomes. Physiologic glucose levels should be maintained prior to and during pregnancy to decrease the risk of adverse events in the fetus and mother. Insulin is the drug of choice for the control of diabetes mellitus during pregnancy. The use of insulin lispro has been shown to be as effective as regular insulin to treat diabetes in pregnancy and may have advantages over regular insulin during pregnancy.
Breast-Feeding Considerations It is not known if significant amounts of insulin lispro distribute into breast milk. Endogenous insulin can be found in breast milk. Plasma glucose concentrations in the mother affect glucose concentrations in breast milk. The gastrointestinal tract destroys insulin when administered orally; therefore, insulin is not expected to be absorbed intact by the breast-feeding infant. All types of insulin are safe for use while breast-feeding. Due to increased calorie expenditure, women with diabetes may require less insulin while nursing.
Contraindications Hypersensitivity to insulin lispro, insulin lispro protamine, or any component; hypoglycemia
Warnings Hypoglycemia is the most common adverse effect of insulin. The timing of hypoglycemia differs among various insulin formulations. Any change of insulin should be made cautiously; changing manufacturers, type, and/or method of manufacture may result in the need for a change of dosage. Hypoglycemia may result from increased work or exercise without eating. Not for I.V. infusion or use in insulin infusion pumps
Precautions Use with caution and adjust dosage in patients with renal impairment; use with caution and monitor closely in patient with hepatic impairment.
Adverse Reactions Primarily symptoms of hypoglycemia
Cardiovascular: Pallor, palpitation, tachycardia
Central nervous system: Fatigue, headache, hypothermia, loss of consciousness, mental confusion
Dermatologic: Redness, urticaria

Endocrine & metabolic: Hypoglycemia, hypokalemia
Gastrointestinal: Hunger, nausea, numbness of mouth
Local: Atrophy or hypertrophy of SubQ fat tissue; edema, itching, pain or warmth at injection site; stinging
Neuromuscular & skeletal: Muscle weakness, paresthesia, tremor
Ocular: Transient presbyopia or blurred vision
Miscellaneous: Anaphylaxis, diaphoresis, local and/or systemic hypersensitivity reactions

Drug Interactions

Metabolism/Transport Effects None known.

Avoid Concomitant Use There are no known interactions where it is recommended to avoid concomitant use.

Increased Effect/Toxicity

Insulin Lispro Protamine and Insulin Lispro may increase the levels/effects of: Antidiabetic Agents (Thiazolidinedione); Hypoglycemic Agents; Quinolone Antibiotics

The levels/effects of Insulin Lispro Protamine and Insulin Lispro may be increased by: Androgens; Beta-Blockers; Edetate CALCIUM Disodium; Edetate Disodium; GLP-1 Agonists; Herbs (Hypoglycemic Properties); MAO Inhibitors; Metreleptin; Pegvisomant; Salicylates; Selective Serotonin Reuptake Inhibitors

Decreased Effect

The levels/effects of Insulin Lispro Protamine and Insulin Lispro may be decreased by: Corticosteroids (Orally Inhaled); Corticosteroids (Systemic); Danazol; Loop Diuretics; Luteinizing Hormone-Releasing Hormone Analogs; Somatropin; Thiazide Diuretics

Stability Store unopened container or pen in refrigerator; do not freeze; protect from light. If refrigeration is not possible, vial (in use) may be stored at room temperature for up to 28 days. The pen (in use) should **not** be refrigerated; store below 30°C (86°F) away from direct heat or light; discard after 10 days. Do not mix or dilute with other insulins.

Mechanism of Action Insulin acts via specific membrane-bound receptors on target tissues to regulate metabolism of carbohydrate, protein, and fats. Target organs for insulin include the liver, skeletal muscle, and adipose tissue.

Within the liver, insulin stimulates hepatic glycogen synthesis. Insulin promotes hepatic synthesis of fatty acids, which are released into the circulation as lipoproteins. Skeletal muscle effects of insulin include increased protein synthesis and increased glycogen synthesis. Within adipose tissue, insulin stimulates the processing of circulating lipoproteins to provide free fatty acids, facilitating triglyceride synthesis and storage by adipocytes; also directly inhibits the hydrolysis of triglycerides. In addition, insulin stimulates the cellular uptake of amino acids and increases cellular permeability to several ions, including potassium, magnesium, and phosphate. By activating sodium-potassium ATPases, insulin promotes the intracellular movement of potassium.

Normally secreted by the pancreas, insulin products are manufactured for pharmacologic use through recombinant DNA technology using either *E. coli* or *Saccharomyces cerevisiae*. Insulins are categorized based on the onset, peak, and duration of effect (eg, rapid-, short-, intermediate-, and long-acting insulin). Insulin lispro protamine and insulin lispro is an intermediate-acting combination product with a more rapid onset and similar duration of action as compared to that of insulin NPH and insulin regular combination products.

Pharmacodynamics

Onset of action: 0.25-0.5 hours
Maximum effect: 2 hours
Duration: 18-24 hours

Pharmacokinetics (Adult data unless noted)

Time to peak serum concentration: 1 hour (median; range: 0.5-4 hours)

Elimination: Urine

Dosing: Usual Lispro protamine is an intermediate-acting insulin and lispro is a rapid-acting insulin administered by SubQ injection. Insulin lispro protamine and insulin lispro combination products are approximately equipotent to insulin NPH and insulin regular combination products with a similar duration of activity but a more rapid onset. With combination insulin products, the proportion of rapid-acting to long-acting insulin is fixed; basal vs prandial dose adjustments cannot be made. Fixed ratio insulins (such as insulin lispro protamine and insulin lispro combination) are typically administered as 2 daily doses with each dose intended to cover two meals and a snack. Because of variability in the peak effect and individual patient variability in activities, meals, etc, it may be more difficult to achieve complete glycemic control using fixed combinations of insulins; frequent monitoring and close medical supervision may be necessary. See Insulin Regular for additional information.

General insulin dosing:

Type 1 diabetes mellitus: Children, Adolescents, and Adults: **Note:** Multiple daily doses are utilized and guided by blood glucose monitoring. Combinations of insulin formulations are commonly used. The daily doses presented below are expressed as the **total units/kg/day of all insulin formulations combined**. Insulin lispro protamine and insulin lispro combination product is **not** intended for initial therapy; basal insulin requirements should be established **first** to direct dosing.

Usual maintenance range: SubQ: 0.5-1 unit/kg/day in divided doses. An estimate of anticipated needs may be based on body weight and/or activity factors as follows:
Nonobese: 0.4-0.6 units/kg/day
Obese: 0.8-1.2 units/kg/day
Pubescent Children and Adolescents: During puberty, requirements may substantially increase to >1 unit/kg/day and in some cases up to 2 units/kg/day (IDF/ISPAD, 2011)

Adjustment of dose: Dosage must be titrated to achieve glucose control and avoid hypoglycemia. Adjust dose to maintain premeal and bedtime glucose in target range. Since combinations of agents are frequently used, dosage adjustment must address the individual component of the insulin regimen which most directly influences the blood glucose value in question, based on the known onset and duration of the insulin component.

Type 2 diabetes mellitus: Augmentation therapy (patients for which diet, exercise, weight reduction, and oral hypoglycemic agents have not been adequate): Adults: SubQ: **Note:** Insulin lispro protamine and insulin lispro combination product is **not** intended for initial therapy; basal insulin requirements should be established **first** to direct dosing. Dosage must be carefully adjusted.

Dosing adjustment in renal impairment: There are no dosage adjustments provided in manufacturer's labeling; insulin requirements are reduced due to changes in insulin clearance or metabolism; monitor blood glucose closely.

Dosing adjustment in hepatic impairment: There are no dosage adjustments provided in manufacturer's labeling; insulin requirements may be reduced due to changes in insulin clearance or metabolism; monitor blood glucose closely.

Administration Parenteral: SubQ: Gently roll vial or pen in the palms of the hands to resuspend before use; administer into the subcutaneous fat of the thighs, arms, buttocks, or abdomen, with sites rotated. Cold injections should be avoided. Administer within 15 minutes before a meal (breakfast and supper). Do not mix or dilute with other insulins. **Not for I.V. administration** or use in an insulin infusion pump.

Monitoring Parameters Urine sugar and acetone, serum glucose, electrolytes, Hb A$_{1c}$, lipid profile

Reference Range

Plasma Blood Glucose and Hgb A$_{1c}$ Goals for Type 1 Diabetes (ADA, 2013): Note: Goals should be individualized based on individual needs/circumstances (eg, patients who experience severe hypoglycemia, patients with hypoglycemic unawareness); lower goals may be reasonable if they can be achieved without excessive hypoglycemia. **Note:** Postprandial blood glucose should be measured when there is a discrepancy between preprandial blood glucose concentrations and Hb A$_{1c}$ values and to help assess glycemia for patients who receive basal/bolus regimens. It is usually drawn 1-2 hours after starting meal and is considered to be the "peak."

Toddlers/Preschoolers (0-6 years):
Preprandial glucose: 100-180 mg/dL
Bedtime/overnight glucose: 110-200 mg/dL
Hb A$_{1c}$: <8.5%

School age (6-12 years):
Preprandial glucose: 90-180 mg/dL
Bedtime/overnight glucose: 100-180 mg/dL
Hb A$_{1c}$: <8%

Adolescents/Young Adults (13-19 years):
Preprandial glucose: 90-130 mg/dL
Bedtime/overnight glucose: 90-150 mg/dL
Hb A$_{1c}$: <7.5%

Adults, nonpregnant:
Preprandial glucose: 70-130 mg/dL
Postprandial glucose: <180 mg/dL
Hb A$_{1c}$: <7%

Criteria for diagnosis of DKA:
Serum glucose:
Children: >200 mg/dL
Adults: >250 mg/dL
Arterial pH:
Children: <7.3
Adults: <7-7.24
Bicarbonate:
Children: <15 mEq/L
Adults: <10-15 mEq/L
Moderate ketonuria or ketonemia

Additional Information

Division of daily insulin requirement ("conventional therapy"): Generally, 50% to 75% of the daily insulin dose is given as an intermediate- or long-acting form of insulin (in 1-2 daily injections). The remaining portion of the 24-hour insulin requirement is divided and administered as either regular insulin or a rapid-acting form of insulin at the same time before breakfast and dinner.

Division of daily insulin requirement ("intensive therapy"): Basal insulin delivery with 1 or 2 doses of intermediate- or long-acting insulin formulations superimposed with doses of rapid- or very rapid-acting insulin formulations 3 or more times daily.

Dosage Forms Excipient information presented when available (limited, particularly for generics); consult specific product labeling.

Injection, suspension:
HumaLOG® Mix 50/50™: Insulin lispro protamine suspension 50% [intermediate acting] and insulin lispro solution 50% [rapid acting]: 100 units/mL (10 mL)
HumaLOG® Mix 50/50™ KwikPen™: Insulin lispro protamine suspension 50% [intermediate acting] and insulin lispro solution 50% [rapid acting]: 100 units/mL (3 mL)
HumaLOG® Mix 75/25™: Insulin lispro protamine suspension 75% [intermediate acting] and insulin lispro solution 25% [rapid acting]: 100 units/mL (10 mL)
HumaLOG® Mix 75/25™ KwikPen™: Insulin lispro protamine suspension 75% [intermediate acting] and insulin lispro solution 25% [rapid acting]: 100 units/mL (3 mL)

References

American Diabetes Association (ADA), "Standards of Medical Care in Diabetes-2013," *Diabetes Care*, 2013, (36 Suppl 1):S11-66.
International Diabetes Federation, International Society for Pediatric and Adolescent Diabetes. Global IDF/ISPAD guideline for diabetes in childhood and adolescence. 2011. Available at: http://www.idf.org/global-idfispad-guideline-diabetes-childhood-and-adolescence. Date accessed: October 21, 2013.

Insulin NPH (IN soo lin N P H)

Medication Safety Issues

Sound-alike/look-alike issues:
HumuLIN® N may be confused with HumuLIN® R, HumaLOG®, Humira®
NovoLIN® N may be confused with NovoLIN® R, NovoLOG®

High alert medication:
The Institute for Safe Medication Practices (ISMP) includes this medication among its list of drugs which have a heightened risk of causing significant patient harm when used in error. *Due to the number of insulin preparations, it is essential to identify/clarify the type of insulin to be used.*

Other safety concerns:
Cross-contamination may occur if insulin pens are shared among multiple patients. Steps should be taken to prohibit sharing of insulin pens.

Brand Names: U.S. HumuLIN N KwikPen [OTC]; HumuLIN N Pen [OTC] [DSC]; HumuLIN N [OTC]; NovoLIN N ReliOn [OTC]; NovoLIN N [OTC]

Brand Names: Canada Humulin® N; Novolin® ge NPH

Therapeutic Category Antidiabetic Agent, Insulin; Insulin, Intermediate-Acting

Generic Availability (U.S.) No

Use Treatment of type 1 diabetes mellitus (insulin dependent, IDDM); type 2 diabetes mellitus (noninsulin dependent, NIDDM) to control hyperglycemia

Pregnancy Considerations Maternal hyperglycemia can be associated with adverse effects in the fetus, including macrosomia, neonatal hyperglycemia, and hyperbilirubinemia; the risk of congenital malformations is increased when the HbA$_{1c}$ is >1% above the normal range. Insulin requirements tend to fall during the first trimester of pregnancy and increase in the later trimesters, peaking at 28-32 weeks of gestation. Following delivery, insulin requirements decrease rapidly. Diabetes can also be associated with adverse effects in the mother. Poorly-treated diabetes may cause end-organ damage that may in turn negatively affect obstetric outcomes. Physiologic glucose levels should be maintained prior to and during pregnancy to decrease the risk of adverse events in the fetus and the mother. Insulin is the drug of choice for the control of diabetes mellitus during pregnancy.

Breast-Feeding Considerations Endogenous insulin distributes into breast milk. Plasma glucose concentrations in the mother affect glucose concentrations in breast milk. The gastrointestinal tract destroys insulin when administered orally; therefore, insulin is not expected to be absorbed intact by the breast-feeding infant. All types of insulin are safe for use while breast-feeding. Due to increased calorie expenditure, women with diabetes may require less insulin while nursing.

Contraindications Hypersensitivity to NPH insulin or any component

Warnings Hypoglycemia is the most common adverse effect of insulin. The timing of hypoglycemia differs among various insulin formulations. Any change of insulin should be made cautiously; changing manufacturers, type, and/or method of manufacture may result in the need for a change of dosage. Hypoglycemia may result from increased work or exercise without eating.

Precautions Use with caution and adjust dosage in patients with renal impairment; use with caution and monitor closely in patient with hepatic impairment.

Adverse Reactions Primarily symptoms of hypoglycemia

Cardiovascular: Pallor, palpitation, tachycardia

Central nervous system: Fatigue, headache, hypothermia, loss of consciousness, mental confusion

Dermatologic: Redness, urticaria

Endocrine & metabolic: Hypoglycemia, hypokalemia

Gastrointestinal: Hunger, nausea, numbness of mouth

Local: Atrophy or hypertrophy of SubQ fat tissue; edema, itching, pain or warmth at injection site; stinging

Neuromuscular & skeletal: Muscle weakness, paresthesia, tremor

Ocular: Transient presbyopia or blurred vision

Miscellaneous: Anaphylaxis, diaphoresis, local and/or systemic hypersensitivity reactions

Drug Interactions

Metabolism/Transport Effects None known.

Avoid Concomitant Use There are no known interactions where it is recommended to avoid concomitant use.

Increased Effect/Toxicity

Insulin NPH may increase the levels/effects of: Antidiabetic Agents (Thiazolidinedione); Hypoglycemic Agents; Quinolone Antibiotics

The levels/effects of Insulin NPH may be increased by: Androgens; Beta-Blockers; Edetate CALCIUM Disodium; Edetate Disodium; GLP-1 Agonists; Herbs (Hypoglycemic Properties); MAO Inhibitors; Metreleptin; Pegvisomant; Salicylates; Selective Serotonin Reuptake Inhibitors

Decreased Effect

The levels/effects of Insulin NPH may be decreased by: Corticosteroids (Orally Inhaled); Corticosteroids (Systemic); Danazol; Loop Diuretics; Luteinizing Hormone-Releasing Hormone Analogs; Somatropin; Thiazide Diuretics

Stability May be mixed with regular insulin, insulin lispro, insulin aspart, and insulin glulisine (always add the NPH insulin to the mixture last). A sterile diluent is available from the manufacturer for preparing dilutions of Humulin® N.

Humulin® N vials: Store unopened vials in refrigerator at 2°C to 8°C (36°F to 46°F); do not freeze; keep away from heat and sunlight. Once punctured (in use), vials may be stored for up to 31 days in the refrigerator between 2°C and 8°C (36°F to 46°F) or at room temperature ≤30°C (≤86°F).

Humulin® N pens: Store unopened pens in the refrigerator at 2°C to 8°C (36°F to 46°F); do not freeze; keep away from heat and sunlight. Once punctured (in use), cartridge/pen should be stored at room temperature 15°C to 30°C (59°F to 86°F) for up to 14 days.

Novolin® N: Store unopened vials in refrigerator at 2°C to 8°C (36°F to 46°F) until product expiration date or at room temperature ≤25°C (≤77°F) for up to 42 days; do not freeze; keep away from heat and sunlight. Once punctured (in use), store vials at room temperature ≤25°C (≤77°F) for up to 42 days (includes days stored at room temperature for unopened vials, if applicable); refrigeration of in use vials is not recommended.

Mechanism of Action Insulin acts via specific membrane-bound receptors on target tissues to regulate metabolism of carbohydrate, protein, and fats. Target organs for insulin include the liver, skeletal muscle, and adipose tissue.

Within the liver, insulin stimulates hepatic glycogen synthesis. Insulin promotes hepatic synthesis of fatty acids, which are released into the circulation as lipoproteins. Skeletal muscle effects of insulin include increased protein synthesis and increased glycogen synthesis. Within adipose tissue, insulin stimulates the processing of circulating lipoproteins to provide free fatty acids, facilitating triglyceride synthesis and storage by adipocytes; also directly inhibits the hydrolysis of triglycerides. In addition, insulin stimulates the cellular uptake of amino acids and increases cellular permeability to several ions, including potassium, magnesium, and phosphate. By activating sodium-potassium ATPases, insulin promotes the intracellular movement of potassium.

Normally secreted by the pancreas, insulin products are manufactured for pharmacologic use through recombinant DNA technology using either *E. coli* or *Saccharomyces cerevisiae*. Insulins are categorized based on the onset, peak, and duration of effect (eg, rapid-, short-, intermediate-, and long-acting human insulin). Insulin NPH, an isophane suspension of human insulin, is an intermediate-acting insulin.

Pharmacodynamics

Onset of action: 1-2 hours

Maximum effect: 6-14 hours

Duration: 18 to >24 hours

Pharmacokinetics (Adult data unless noted) Elimination: Urine

Dosing: Usual Insulin NPH is an intermediate-acting insulin formulation which is usually administered subcutaneously once or twice daily. When compared to insulin regular, insulin NPH has a slower onset and longer duration of activity. Insulin requirements vary dramatically between patients and dictate frequent monitoring and close medical supervision. See Insulin Regular for additional information.

Type 1 diabetes mellitus: Children, Adolescents, and Adults: **Note:** Multiple daily doses are utilized and guided by blood glucose monitoring. Combinations of insulin formulations are commonly used. The daily doses presented below are expressed as the **total units/kg/day of all insulin formulations combined.** Insulin NPH is **not** intended for initial therapy; basal insulin requirements should be established **first** to direct dosing.

Usual maintenance range: SubQ: 0.5-1 unit/kg/day in divided doses. An estimate of anticipated needs may be based on body weight and/or activity factors as follows:

Nonobese: 0.4-0.6 units/kg/day

Obese: 0.8-1.2 units/kg/day

Pubescent Children and Adolescents: During puberty, requirements may substantially increase to >1 unit/kg/day and in some cases up to 2 units/kg/day (IDF/ISPAD, 2011)

Adjustment of dose: Dosage must be titrated to achieve glucose control and avoid hypoglycemia. Adjust dose to maintain premeal and bedtime glucose in target range. Since combinations of agents are frequently used, dosage adjustment must address the individual component of the insulin regimen which most directly influences the blood glucose value in question, based on the known onset and duration of the insulin component.

Type 2 diabetes mellitus: Augmentation therapy (patients for which diet, exercise, weight reduction, and oral hypoglycemic agents have not been adequate): Adults: SubQ: Initial dosage of 0.2 units/kg/day or 10 units/day of an intermediate-acting (eg, NPH) or long-acting insulin administered at bedtime has been recommended. As an alternative, regular insulin or rapid-acting insulin formulations administered before meals have also been used. Dosage must be carefully adjusted.

Dosing adjustment in renal impairment: There are no dosage adjustments provided in manufacturer's labeling; insulin requirements are reduced due to changes in insulin clearance or metabolism; monitor blood glucose closely.

Dosing adjustment in hepatic impairment: There are no dosage adjustments provided in manufacturer's labeling; insulin requirements may be reduced due to changes in

▶

insulin clearance or metabolism; monitor blood glucose closely.

Administration Parenteral: SubQ: Gently roll vial or pen in the palms of the hands to resuspend before use; administer into the subcutaneous fat of the thighs, arms, buttocks, or abdomen, with sites rotated. Cold injections should be avoided. Administer within 15 minutes before a meal (before breakfast and supper). May be mixed with regular insulin, insulin aspart, insulin lispro, and insulin glulisine; always add NPH insulin last. **Not for I.V. administration** or use in insulin infusion pumps.

Monitoring Parameters Urine sugar and acetone, serum glucose, electrolytes, Hb A$_{1c}$, lipid profile

Reference Range

Plasma Blood Glucose and Hgb A$_{1c}$ Goals for Type 1 Diabetes (ADA, 2013): Note: Goals should be individualized based on individual needs/circumstances (eg, patients who experience severe hypoglycemia, patients with hypoglycemic unawareness); lower goals may be reasonable if they can be achieved without excessive hypoglycemia. **Note:** Postprandial blood glucose should be measured when there is a discrepancy between preprandial blood glucose concentrations and Hb A$_{1c}$ values and to help assess glycemia for patients who receive basal/bolus regimens. It is usually drawn 1-2 hours after starting meal and is considered to be the "peak."

Toddlers/Preschoolers (0-6 years):
Preprandial glucose: 100-180 mg/dL
Bedtime/overnight glucose: 110-200 mg/dL
Hb A$_{1c}$: <8.5%

School age (6-12 years):
Preprandial glucose: 90-180 mg/dL
Bedtime/overnight glucose: 100-180 mg/dL
Hb A$_{1c}$: <8%

Adolescents/Young Adults (13-19 years):
Preprandial glucose: 90-130 mg/dL
Bedtime/overnight glucose: 90-150 mg/dL
Hb A$_{1c}$: <7.5%

Adults, nonpregnant:
Preprandial glucose: 70-130 mg/dL
Postprandial glucose: <180 mg/dL
Hb A$_{1c}$: <7%

Criteria for diagnosis of DKA:
Serum glucose:
Children: >200 mg/dL
Adults: >250 mg/dL
Arterial pH:
Children: <7.3
Adults: <7-7.24
Bicarbonate:
Children: <15 mEq/L
Adults: <10-15 mEq/L
Moderate ketonuria or ketonemia

Additional Information

Division of daily insulin requirement ("conventional therapy"): Generally, 50% to 75% of the daily insulin dose is given as an intermediate-acting (eg, NPH) or long-acting form of insulin (in 1-2 daily injections). The remaining portion of the 24-hour insulin requirement is divided and administered as either regular insulin or a rapid-acting form of insulin at the same time before breakfast and dinner.

Division of daily insulin requirement ("intensive therapy"): Basal insulin delivery with 1 or 2 doses of intermediate-acting (eg, NPH) or long-acting insulin formulations superimposed with doses of rapid- or very rapid-acting insulin formulations 3 or more times daily.

Dosage Forms Excipient information presented when available (limited, particularly for generics); consult specific product labeling. [DSC] = Discontinued product

Suspension, Subcutaneous:
HumuLIN N: 100 units/mL (3 mL, 10 mL) [contains metacresol, phenol]
NovoLIN N: 100 units/mL (10 mL) [contains metacresol, phenol]
NovoLIN N ReliOn: 100 units/mL (10 mL) [contains metacresol, phenol]
Suspension Pen-injector, Subcutaneous:
HumuLIN N KwikPen: 100 units/mL (3 mL) [contains metacresol, phenol]
HumuLIN N Pen: 100 units/mL (3 mL [DSC]) [contains metacresol, phenol]

References

American Diabetes Association (ADA), "Standards of Medical Care in Diabetes-2013," *Diabetes Care*, 2013, (36 Suppl 1):S11-66.

International Diabetes Federation, International Society for Pediatric and Adolescent Diabetes. Global IDF/ISPAD guideline for diabetes in childhood and adolescence. 2011. Available at: http://www.idf.org/global-idfispad-guideline-diabetes-childhood-and-adolescence. Date accessed: October 21, 2013.

Insulin NPH and Insulin Regular
(IN soo lin N P H & IN soo lin REG yoo ler)

Medication Safety Issues
Sound-alike/look-alike issues:
HumuLIN® 70/30 may be confused with HumaLOG® Mix 75/25, HumuLIN® R, NovoLIN® 70/30, NovoLOG® Mix 70/30
NovoLIN® 70/30 may be confused with HumaLOG® Mix 75/25, HumuLIN® 70/30, HumuLIN® R, NovoLIN® R, and NovoLOG® Mix 70/30

High alert medication:
The Institute for Safe Medication Practices (ISMP) includes this medication among its list of drugs which have a heightened risk of causing significant patient harm when used in error. *Due to the number of insulin preparations, it is essential to identify/clarify the type of insulin to be used.*

Other safety concerns:
Cross-contamination may occur if insulin pens are shared among multiple patients. Steps should be taken to prohibit sharing of insulin pens.

Brand Names: U.S. HumuLIN® 70/30; HumuLIN® 70/30 KwikPen; NovoLIN® 70/30

Brand Names: Canada Humulin® 20/80; Humulin® 70/30; Novolin® ge 30/70; Novolin® ge 40/60; Novolin® ge 50/50

Therapeutic Category Antidiabetic Agent, Parenteral; Insulin, Combination

Generic Availability (U.S.) No

Use Treatment of type 1 diabetes mellitus (insulin dependent, IDDM); type 2 diabetes mellitus (noninsulin dependent, NIDDM) to control hyperglycemia

Pregnancy Considerations See individual agents.

Breast-Feeding Considerations See individual agents.

Contraindications Hypersensitivity to regular insulin, NPH insulin, or any component; hypoglycemia

Warnings Hypoglycemia is the most common adverse effect of insulin. The timing of hypoglycemia differs among various insulin formulations. Any change of insulin should be made cautiously; changing manufacturers, type, and/or method of manufacture may result in the need for a change of dosage. Hypoglycemia may result from increased work or exercise without eating. Not for I.V. infusion or use in insulin infusion pumps.

Precautions Use with caution and adjust dosage in patients with renal impairment; use with caution and monitor closely in patient with hepatic impairment.

Adverse Reactions Primarily symptoms of hypoglycemia
Cardiovascular: Pallor, palpitation, tachycardia
Central nervous system: Fatigue, headache, hypothermia, loss of consciousness, mental confusion

Dermatologic: Redness, urticaria

Endocrine & metabolic: Hypoglycemia, hypokalemia

Gastrointestinal: Hunger, nausea, numbness of mouth

Local: Atrophy or hypertrophy of SubQ fat tissue; edema, itching, pain or warmth at injection site; stinging

Neuromuscular & skeletal: Muscle weakness, paresthesia, tremor

Ocular: Transient presbyopia or blurred vision

Miscellaneous: Anaphylaxis, diaphoresis, local and/or systemic hypersensitivity reactions

Drug Interactions

Metabolism/Transport Effects None known.

Avoid Concomitant Use There are no known interactions where it is recommended to avoid concomitant use.

Increased Effect/Toxicity

Insulin NPH and Insulin Regular may increase the levels/effects of: Antidiabetic Agents (Thiazolidinedione); Hypoglycemic Agents; Quinolone Antibiotics

The levels/effects of Insulin NPH and Insulin Regular may be increased by: Androgens; Beta-Blockers; Edetate CALCIUM Disodium; Edetate Disodium; GLP-1 Agonists; Herbs (Hypoglycemic Properties); MAO Inhibitors; Metreleptin; Pegvisomant; Salicylates; Selective Serotonin Reuptake Inhibitors

Decreased Effect

The levels/effects of Insulin NPH and Insulin Regular may be decreased by: Corticosteroids (Orally Inhaled); Corticosteroids (Systemic); Danazol; Loop Diuretics; Luteinizing Hormone-Releasing Hormone Analogs; Somatropin; Thiazide Diuretics

Stability Do not mix or dilute with other insulins.

Humulin® 70/30 vials: Store unopened vials in refrigerator at 2°C to 8°C (36°F to 46°F); do not freeze; keep away from heat and sunlight. Once punctured (in use), vials may be stored for up to 31 days in the refrigerator between 2°C and 8°C (36°F to 46°F) or at room temperature ≤30°C (≤86°F).

Humulin® 70/30 pens: Store unopened pen in refrigerator at 2°C to 8°C (36°F to 46°F); do not freeze; keep away from heat and sunlight. Once punctured (in use), pen should be stored at room temperature 15°C to 30°C (59°F to 86°F) for up to 10 days.

Novolin® 70/30 vials: Store unopened vials in refrigerator at 2°C to 8°C (36°F to 46°F) until product expiration date or at room temperature ≤25°C (≤77°F) for up to 42 days; do not freeze; keep away from heat and sunlight. Once punctured (in use), store vials at room temperature ≤25°C (≤77°F) for up to 42 days (this includes any days stored at room temperature prior to opening vial); refrigeration of in use vials is not recommended.

Mechanism of Action Insulin acts via specific membrane-bound receptors on target tissues to regulate metabolism of carbohydrate, protein, and fats. Target organs for insulin include the liver, skeletal muscle, and adipose tissue.

Within the liver, insulin stimulates hepatic glycogen synthesis. Insulin promotes hepatic synthesis of fatty acids, which are released into the circulation as lipoproteins. Skeletal muscle effects of insulin include increased protein synthesis and increased glycogen synthesis. Within adipose tissue, insulin stimulates the processing of circulating lipoproteins to provide free fatty acids, facilitating triglyceride synthesis and storage by adipocytes; also directly inhibits the hydrolysis of triglycerides. In addition, insulin stimulates the cellular uptake of amino acids and increases cellular permeability to several ions, including potassium, magnesium, and phosphate. By activating sodium-potassium ATPases, insulin promotes the intracellular movement of potassium.

Normally secreted by the pancreas, insulin products are manufactured for pharmacologic use through recombinant DNA technology using either *E. coli* or *Saccharomyces*

cerevisiae. Insulins are categorized based on the onset, peak, and duration of effect (eg, rapid-, short-, intermediate-, and long-acting insulin). Insulin NPH and insulin regular is an intermediate-acting combination insulin product with a more rapid onset than that of insulin NPH alone.

Pharmacodynamics

Onset of action: Novolin® 70/30, Humulin® 70/30: 0.5 hours

Maximum effect: Novolin® 70/30, Humulin® 70/30: 1.5-12 hours

Duration: Novolin® 70/30, Humulin® 70/30: Up to 24 hours

Pharmacokinetics (Adult data unless noted)

Elimination: Urine

Dosing: Usual Insulin NPH is an intermediate-acting insulin and regular insulin is a short-acting insulin administered by SubQ injection. When compared to insulin NPH, the combination product (insulin NPH and insulin regular) has a shorter onset of action and a similar duration of action. With combination insulin products, the proportion of short-acting to long-acting insulin is fixed in the combination products; basal vs prandial dose adjustments cannot be made. Fixed ratio insulins (such as insulin NPH and insulin regular combination) are typically administered as 2 daily doses with each dose intended to cover two meals and a snack. Because of variability in the peak effect and individual patient variability in activities, meals, etc, it may be more difficult to achieve complete glycemic control using fixed combinations of insulins; frequent monitoring and close medical supervision may be necessary. See Insulin Regular for additional information.

General insulin dosing:

Type 1 diabetes mellitus: Children, Adolescents, and Adults: **Note:** Multiple daily doses are utilized and guided by blood glucose monitoring. Combinations of insulin formulations are commonly used. The daily doses presented below are expressed as the **total units/kg/day of all insulin formulations combined**. Insulin NPH and insulin regular combination product is **not** intended for initial therapy; basal insulin requirements should be established **first** to direct dosing.

Usual maintenance range: SubQ: 0.5-1 unit/kg/day in divided doses. An estimate of anticipated needs may be based on body weight and/or activity factors as follows:

Nonobese: 0.4-0.6 units/kg/day

Obese: 0.8-1.2 units/kg/day

Pubescent Children and Adolescents: During puberty, requirements may substantially increase to >1 unit/kg/day and in some cases up to 2 units/kg/day (IDF/ISPAD, 2011)

Adjustment of dose: Dosage must be titrated to achieve glucose control and avoid hypoglycemia. Adjust dose to maintain premeal and bedtime glucose in target range. Since combinations of agents are frequently used, dosage adjustment must address the individual component of the insulin regimen which most directly influences the blood glucose value in question, based on the known onset and duration of the insulin component.

Type 2 diabetes mellitus: Augmentation therapy (patients for which diet, exercise, weight reduction, and oral hypoglycemic agents have not been adequate): Adults: SubQ: **Note:** Insulin NPH and insulin regular combination product is **not** intended for initial therapy; basal insulin requirements should be established **first** to direct dosing. Dosage must be carefully adjusted.

Dosing adjustment in renal impairment: There are no dosage adjustments provided in manufacturer's labeling; insulin requirements are reduced due to changes in insulin clearance or metabolism; monitor blood glucose closely.

Dosing adjustment in hepatic impairment: There are no dosage adjustments provided in manufacturer's labeling; insulin requirements may be reduced due to changes in insulin clearance or metabolism; monitor blood glucose closely.

Administration Parenteral: SubQ: Gently roll vial or pen in the palms of the hands to resuspend before use; administer into the subcutaneous fat of the thighs, arms, buttocks, or abdomen, with sites rotated. Cold injections should be avoided. Administer within 15 minutes before a meal (before breakfast and supper). Do not mix or dilute with other insulins. **Not for I.V. administration** or use in an insulin infusion pump.

Monitoring Parameters Urine sugar and acetone, serum glucose, electrolytes, Hb A$_{1c}$, lipid profile

Reference Range

Plasma Blood Glucose and Hgb A$_{1c}$ Goals for Type 1 Diabetes (ADA, 2013): Note: Goals should be individualized based on individual needs/circumstances (eg, patients who experience severe hypoglycemia, patients with hypoglycemic unawareness); lower goals may be reasonable if they can be achieved without excessive hypoglycemia. **Note:** Postprandial blood glucose should be measured when there is a discrepancy between preprandial blood glucose concentrations and Hb A$_{1c}$ values and to help assess glycemia for patients who receive basal/bolus regimens. It is usually drawn 1-2 hours after starting meal and is considered to be the "peak."

Toddlers/Preschoolers (0-6 years):
Preprandial glucose: 100-180 mg/dL
Bedtime/overnight glucose: 110-200 mg/dL
Hb A$_{1c}$: <8.5%
School age (6-12 years):
Preprandial glucose: 90-180 mg/dL
Bedtime/overnight glucose: 100-180 mg/dL
Hb A$_{1c}$: <8%
Adolescents/Young Adults (13-19 years):
Preprandial glucose: 90-130 mg/dL
Bedtime/overnight glucose: 90-150 mg/dL
Hb A$_{1c}$: <7.5%
Adults, nonpregnant:
Preprandial glucose: 70-130 mg/dL
Postprandial glucose: <180 mg/dL
Hb A$_{1c}$: <7%

Criteria for diagnosis of DKA:
Serum glucose:
Children: >200 mg/dL
Adults: >250 mg/dL
Arterial pH:
Children: <7.3
Adults: <7-7.24
Bicarbonate:
Children: <15 mEq/L
Adults: <10-15 mEq/L
Moderate ketonuria or ketonemia

Additional Information

Division of daily insulin requirement ("conventional therapy"): Generally, 50% to 75% of the daily insulin dose is given as an intermediate-acting or long-acting form of insulin (in 1-2 daily injections). The remaining portion of the 24-hour insulin requirement is divided and administered as either regular insulin or a rapid-acting form of insulin at the same time before breakfast and dinner.

Division of daily insulin requirement ("intensive therapy"): Basal insulin delivery with 1 or 2 doses of intermediate-acting or long-acting insulin formulations superimposed with doses of rapid- or very rapid-acting insulin formulations 3 or more times daily.

Dosage Forms Excipient information presented when available (limited, particularly for generics); consult specific product labeling.

Injection, suspension:
HumuLIN® 70/30: Insulin NPH suspension 70% [intermediate acting] and insulin regular solution 30% [short acting]: 100 units/mL (3 mL, 10 mL) [vial]
HumuLIN® 70/30 KwikPen: Insulin NPH suspension 70% [intermediate acting] and insulin regular solution 30% [short acting]: 100 units/mL (3 mL)
NovoLIN® 70/30: Insulin NPH suspension 70% [intermediate acting] and insulin regular solution 30% [short acting]: 100 units/mL (10 mL) [vial]

References

American Diabetes Association (ADA), "Standards of Medical Care in Diabetes-2013," *Diabetes Care*, 2013, (36 Suppl 1):S11-66.

International Diabetes Federation, International Society for Pediatric and Adolescent Diabetes. Global IDF/ISPAD guideline for diabetes in childhood and adolescence. 2011. Available at: http://www.idf.org/global-idfispad-guideline-diabetes-childhood-and-adolescence. Date accessed: October 21, 2013.

Insulin Regular (IN soo lin REG yoo ler)

Medication Safety Issues

Sound-alike/look-alike issues:
HumuLIN R may be confused with HumaLOG, Humira, HumuLIN 70/30, HumuLIN N, NovoLIN 70/30, NovoLIN R, NovoLOG
NovoLIN R may be confused with HumuLIN R, NovoLIN 70/30, NovoLIN N, NovoLOG

High alert medication:
The Institute for Safe Medication Practices (ISMP) includes this medication among its list of drugs which have a heightened risk of causing significant patient harm when used in error. *Due to the number of insulin preparations, it is essential to identify/clarify the type of insulin to be used.*

BEERS Criteria medication:
This drug may be potentially inappropriate for use in geriatric patients (Quality of evidence - moderate; Strength of recommendation - strong).

Administration issues:
Concentrated solutions (eg, U-500) should not be available in patient care areas. U-500 regular insulin should be stored, dispensed, and administered separately from U-100 regular insulin. For patients who receive U-500 insulin in the hospital setting, highlighting the strength prominently on the patient's medical chart and medication record may help to reduce dispensing errors.

Other safety concerns:
Cross-contamination may occur if insulin pens are shared among multiple patients. Steps should be taken to prohibit sharing of insulin pens.

Brand Names: U.S. HumuLIN R U-500 (CONCENTRATED); HumuLIN R [OTC]; NovoLIN R ReliOn [OTC]; NovoLIN R [OTC]

Brand Names: Canada Humulin® R; Novolin® ge Toronto

Therapeutic Category Antidiabetic Agent, Parenteral; Antidote; Hyperkalemia, Adjunctive Treatment Agent; Insulin, Short-Acting

Generic Availability (U.S.) No

Use Treatment of insulin-dependent diabetes mellitus, also noninsulin-dependent diabetes mellitus unresponsive to treatment with diet and/or oral hypoglycemics; to assure proper utilization of glucose and reduce glucosuria in nondiabetic patients receiving parenteral nutrition (glucosuria cannot be adequately controlled with infusion rate adjustments or requires assistance in achieving optimal caloric intakes); treatment of hyperkalemia (use with glucose to shift potassium into cells to lower serum potassium levels)

Pregnancy Risk Factor B

Pregnancy Considerations Minimal amounts of endogenous insulin cross the placenta. Exogenous insulin bound to anti-insulin antibodies has been detected in cord blood.

Maternal hyperglycemia can be associated with adverse effects in the fetus, including macrosomia, neonatal hyperglycemia, and hyperbilirubinemia; the risk of congenital malformations is increased when the HbA_{1c} is >1% above the normal range. Insulin requirements tend to fall during the first trimester of pregnancy and increase in the later trimesters, peaking at 28-32 weeks of gestation. Following delivery, insulin requirements decrease rapidly. Diabetes can also be associated with adverse effects in the mother. Poorly treated diabetes may cause end-organ damage that may in turn negatively affect obstetric outcomes. Physiologic glucose levels should be maintained prior to and during pregnancy to decrease the risk of adverse events in the fetus and the mother. Insulin is the drug of choice for the control of diabetes mellitus during pregnancy.

Breast-Feeding Considerations Endogenous insulin can be found in breast milk. Plasma glucose concentrations in the mother affect glucose concentrations in breast milk. The gastrointestinal tract destroys insulin when administered orally; therefore, insulin is not expected to be absorbed intact by the breast-feeding infant. All types of insulin are safe for use while breast-feeding. Due to increased calorie expenditure, women with diabetes may require less insulin while nursing.

Contraindications Hypersensitivity to regular insulin or any component; hypoglycemia

Warnings Hypoglycemia is the most common adverse effect of insulin. The timing of hypoglycemia differs among various insulin formulations. Any change of insulin should be made cautiously; changing manufacturers, type, and/or method of manufacture may result in the need for a change of dosage. Hypoglycemia may result from increased work or exercise without eating; use of long-acting insulin preparations (insulin glargine, Ultralente®) with regular insulin may delay recovery from hypoglycemia.

Precautions Use with caution and adjust dosage in patients with renal impairment; use with caution and monitor closely in patient with hepatic impairment. While regular insulin is the preferred formulation for I.V. administration, both insulin aspart and insulin glulisine have been approved for I.V. use in selected clinical situations with close medical supervision and monitoring of serum potassium.

Adverse Reactions Primarily symptoms of hypoglycemia

Cardiovascular: Pallor, palpitation, tachycardia

Central nervous system: Fatigue, headache, hypothermia, loss of consciousness, mental confusion

Dermatologic: Redness, urticaria

Endocrine & metabolic: Hypoglycemia, hypokalemia

Gastrointestinal: Hunger, nausea, numbness of mouth

Local: Atrophy or hypertrophy of SubQ fat tissue; edema, itching, pain or warmth at injection site; stinging

Neuromuscular & skeletal: Muscle weakness, paresthesia, tremor

Ocular: Transient presbyopia or blurred vision

Miscellaneous: Anaphylaxis, diaphoresis, local and/or systemic hypersensitivity reactions

Drug Interactions

Metabolism/Transport Effects None known.

Avoid Concomitant Use There are no known interactions where it is recommended to avoid concomitant use.

Increased Effect/Toxicity

Insulin Regular may increase the levels/effects of: Antidiabetic Agents (Thiazolidinedione); Hypoglycemic Agents; Quinolone Antibiotics

The levels/effects of Insulin Regular may be increased by: Androgens; Beta-Blockers; Edetate CALCIUM Disodium; Edetate Disodium; GLP-1 Agonists; Herbs (Hypoglycemic Properties); MAO Inhibitors; Metreleptin; Pegvisomant; Salicylates; Selective Serotonin Reuptake Inhibitors

Decreased Effect

The levels/effects of Insulin Regular may be decreased by: Corticosteroids (Orally Inhaled); Corticosteroids (Systemic); Danazol; Loop Diuretics; Luteinizing Hormone-Releasing Hormone Analogs; Somatropin; Thiazide Diuretics

Stability Regular insulin should only be used if clear. May be mixed in the same syringe with NPH insulin; draw regular insulin into syringe first.

Humulin® R, Humulin® R U-500: Store unopened vials in refrigerator at 2°C to 8°C (36°F to 46°F); do not freeze; keep away from heat and sunlight. Once punctured (in use), vials may be stored in refrigerator between 2°C and 8°C (36°F to 46°F) or at room temperature ≤30°C (≤86°F) for up to 31 days.

Novolin® R: Store unopened vials in refrigerator at 2°C to 8°C (36°F to 46°F) until product expiration date or at room temperature ≤25°C (≤77°F) for up to 42 days; do not freeze; keep away from heat and sunlight. Once punctured (in use), store vials at room temperature ≤25°C (≤77°F) for up to 42 days (includes days stored at room temperature for unopened vials, if applicable); refrigeration of in use vials is not recommended.

Continuous I.V. infusion: May be diluted in NS, $^{1}/_{2}$NS, D_5W, or D_{10}W; tubing should be flushed 30 minutes prior to administration to allow adsorption as time permits.

Humulin® R: Stable for 48 hours at room temperature or for 48 hours under refrigeration followed by 48 hours at room temperature when diluted in NS at a final concentration of 0.1-1 unit/mL.

Novolin® R: Stable for 24 hours at room temperature when diluted in NS, D_5W or D_{10}W at a final concentration of 0.05-1 unit/mL.

Mechanism of Action Insulin acts via specific membrane-bound receptors on target tissues to regulate metabolism of carbohydrate, protein, and fats. Target organs for insulin include the liver, skeletal muscle, and adipose tissue.

Within the liver, insulin stimulates hepatic glycogen synthesis. Insulin promotes hepatic synthesis of fatty acids, which are released into the circulation as lipoproteins. Skeletal muscle effects of insulin include increased protein synthesis and increased glycogen synthesis. Within adipose tissue, insulin stimulates the processing of circulating lipoproteins to provide free fatty acids, facilitating triglyceride synthesis and storage by adipocytes; also directly inhibits the hydrolysis of triglycerides. In addition, insulin stimulates the cellular uptake of amino acids and increases cellular permeability to several ions, including potassium, magnesium, and phosphate. By activating sodium-potassium ATPases, insulin promotes the intracellular movement of potassium.

Normally secreted by the pancreas, insulin products are manufactured for pharmacologic use through recombinant DNA technology using either *E. coli* or *Saccharomyces cerevisiae*. Insulins are categorized based on the onset, peak, and duration of effect (eg, rapid-, short-, intermediate-, and long-acting insulin).

Pharmacodynamics Onset and duration of hypoglycemic effects depend upon the route of administration (adsorption and onset of action are more rapid after deeper I.M. injections than after SubQ), site of injection (onset and duration are progressively slower with SubQ injection into the abdomen, arm, buttock, or thigh respectively), volume and concentration of injection, and the preparation administered; local heat and massage also increase the rate of absorption.

Onset of action: Approximately 30-60 minutes

Maximum effect: 1-5 hours

Duration: 6-10 hours (may increase with dose)

Pharmacokinetics (Adult data unless noted)

Distribution: V_d: 0.26-0.36 L/kg

Half-life: SubQ: 1.5 hours

◄ Excretion: Urine

Dosing: Neonatal Note: Neonates are extremely sensitive to the effects of insulin; initiate therapy at the lower end of infusion rate and monitor closely.

Optimization of caloric intake while on parenteral nutrition: Continuous I.V. infusion: 0.01-0.1 units/kg/**hour**

Hyperkalemia: Continuous I.V. infusion: 0.05-0.1 units/kg/**hour** in conjunction with a dextrose infusion has been used in seven neonates (<28 weeks GA) (Malone, 1991).

Dosing: Usual The general objective of insulin replacement therapy is to approximate the physiologic pattern of insulin secretion. This requires a basal level of insulin throughout the day, supplemented by additional insulin at mealtimes. Since combinations using different types of insulins are frequently used, dosage adjustment must address the individual component of the insulin regimen which most directly influences the blood glucose value in question, based on the known onset and duration of the insulin component. The frequency of doses and monitoring must be individualized in consideration of the patient's ability to manage therapy.

Type 1 diabetes mellitus: Infants, Children, Adolescents, and Adults: **Note:** Multiple daily doses or continuous subcutaneous infusion guided by blood glucose monitoring are the standard of diabetes care. The daily doses presented are expressed as the **total units/kg/day of all insulin formulations combined.**

Initial dose: SubQ: 0.2-0.6 units/kg/day in divided doses. Conservative initial doses of 0.2-0.4 units/kg/day are often recommended to avoid the potential for hypoglycemia. Regular insulin may be the only insulin formulation used initially.

Division of daily insulin requirement ("conventional therapy"): Generally, 50% to 75% of the daily insulin dose is given as an intermediate- or long-acting form of insulin (in 1-2 daily injections). The remaining portion of the 24-hour insulin requirement is divided and administered as either regular insulin or a rapid-acting form of insulin at the same time before breakfast and dinner.

Division of daily insulin requirement ("intensive therapy"): Basal insulin delivery with 1 or 2 doses of intermediate- or long-acting insulin formulations superimposed with doses of rapid- or very rapid-acting insulin formulations 3 or more times daily.

Adjustment of dose: Dosage must be titrated to achieve glucose control and avoid hypoglycemia. Adjust dose to maintain premeal and bedtime glucose in target range. Since combinations of agents are frequently used, dosage adjustment must address the individual component of the insulin regimen which most directly influences the blood glucose value in question, based on the known onset and duration of the insulin component.

Usual maintenance range: 0.5-1 unit/kg/day in divided doses. An estimate of anticipated needs may be based on body weight and/or activity factors as follows:

Nonobese: 0.4-0.6 units/kg/day

Obese: 0.8-1.2 units/kg/day

Pubescent Children and Adolescents: During puberty, requirements may substantially increase to >1 unit/kg/day and in some cases up to 2 units/kg/day (IDF/ISPAD, 2011)

Continuous SubQ insulin infusion (insulin pump): A combination of a "basal" continuous insulin infusion rate with preprogrammed, premeal bolus doses which are patient controlled. When converting from multiple daily SubQ doses of maintenance insulin, it is advisable to reduce the basal rate to less than the equivalent of the total daily units of longer acting insulin (eg, NPH). Divide the total number of units by 24 to get the basal rate in units/hour. Do not include the total units of regular insulin or other rapid-acting insulin formulations in this calculation. The same premeal regular insulin dosage may be used.

Type 2 diabetes mellitus: Augmentation therapy (patients for which diet, exercise, weight reduction, and oral hypoglycemic agents have not been adequate): Adults: SubQ: Initial dosage of 0.2 units/kg/day or 10 units/day of an intermediate- or long-acting insulin administered at bedtime has been recommended. As an alternative, regular insulin or rapid-acting insulin formulations administered before meals have also been used. Dosage must be carefully adjusted.

Diabetic ketoacidosis: Note: Patients newly diagnosed with IDDM presenting in DKA or patients with blood glucose levels <800 mg/dL may be relatively "sensitive" to insulin and should receive loading and initial maintenance doses ~50% of those indicated.

Children: Continuous I.V. infusion: 0.05-0.1 units/kg/**hour** (range: 0.05-0.2 units/kg/**hour**) depending upon the rate of decrease of serum glucose (decreasing the serum glucose level too rapidly may lead to cerebral edema; optimum rate of decrease of serum glucose 80-100 mg/dL/hour). Continue infusion until acidosis clears (pH >7.3 and HCO_3 >25 mEq/L), not when the blood glucose normalizes. SubQ therapy may begin when the HCO_3 >16 mEq/L, pH >7.3, and/or anion gap <16 mEq/L. Continue I.V. insulin infusion until the onset of the SubQ insulin dose (for regular insulin: 30-60 minutes).

Adults: I.V.: Regular insulin 0.15 units/kg (~15-20 units) initially followed by an infusion of 0.1 units/kg/**hour** (~7 units/hour); increase infusion rate achieve glucose serum reduction of 50-70 mg/dL/hour. Decrease dose to 0.05-0.1 units/kg/**hour** once serum glucose reaches 250 mg/dL and ketoacidosis/acid-base abnormalities have resolved.

Hyperkalemia (after treatment with calcium and sodium bicarbonate): I.V.:

Children: Dextrose 0.5-1 g/kg (using $D_{25}W$ or $D_{50}W$) combined with regular insulin 1 unit for every 4-5 g dextrose; infuse over 2 hours **OR** as an alternative, dextrose 0.5-1 g/kg infused over 15-30 minutes followed by 0.1 unit/kg insulin SubQ or I.V.

Adults: 10 units regular insulin mixed with 25 g dextrose (50 mL $D_{50}W$) given over 15-30 minutes (ACLS, 2005); alternatively, 50 mL $D_{50}W$ over 5 minutes followed by 10 units regular insulin I.V. push over seconds may be administered in the setting of imminent cardiac arrest. In patients with ongoing cardiac arrest (eg, PEA with presumed hyperkalemia), administration of $D_{50}W$ over <5 minutes is routine. Effects on potassium are temporary. As appropriate, consider methods of enhancing potassium removal/excretion.

Dosing adjustment in renal impairment: Insulin requirements are reduced due to changes in insulin clearance or metabolism; there are no dosage adjustments provided in manufacturer's labeling; however, the following adjustments have been used by some clinicians (Aronoff, 2007): Adults:

CrCl >50 mL/minute: No adjustment necessary

CrCl 10-50 mL/minute: Administer at 75% of recommended dose

CrCl <10 mL/minute: Administer at 50% of recommended dose and monitor glucose closely

Hemodialysis: Because of a large molecular weight (6000 daltons), insulin is not significantly removed by either peritoneal or hemodialysis; supplemental dose is not necessary

Peritoneal dialysis: Supplemental dose is not necessary

Continuous renal replacement therapy: Administer at 75% of recommended dose

Dosing adjustment in hepatic impairment: There are no dosage adjustments provided in manufacturer's labeling; insulin requirements may be reduced due to changes in insulin clearance or metabolism; monitor blood glucose closely.

Usual Infusion Concentrations: Neonatal I.V. Infusion: 0.1 unit/mL **or** 0.5 unit/mL

Usual Infusion Concentrations: Pediatric I.V. infusion: 0.1 unit/mL, 0.5 unit/mL, **or** 1 unit/mL

Administration Parenteral:

SubQ, I.M.: Administration is usually made into the subcutaneous fat of the thighs, arms, buttocks, or abdomen, with sites rotated; may be administered I.M. however, SubQ is the preferred route. When mixing regular insulin with other insulin preparations, regular insulin should be drawn into the syringe first; administer 30-60 minutes before meals. May be infused SubQ by external insulin pump; however, when used in an external pump, it is not recommended to be diluted with other solutions.

I.V.: Regular insulin is the preferred insulin formulation approved for I.V. administration (insulin aspart and insulin glulisine have been approved for I.V. administration in carefully controlled clinical settings with medical supervision and close monitoring of blood glucose as well as serum potassium); to minimize absorption of insulin to I.V. solution bag or tubing:

If new tubing is **not** needed: Wait a minimum of 30 minutes between the preparation of the solution and the initiation of the infusion.

If new tubing is needed: After receiving the insulin continuous infusion solution, the administration set should be attached to the I.V. container and the line should be flushed with the insulin solution, wait 30 minutes, then flush the line again with the insulin solution prior to initiating the infusion.

Because of adsorption, the actual amount of insulin being administered could be substantially less than the apparent amount. Therefore, adjustment of the insulin drip rate should be based on the effect and not solely on the apparent insulin dose. Furthermore, the apparent I.V. infusion dose should not be used as the basis for determining the subsequent insulin dose upon discontinuing the insulin drip. Dosage adjustment requires continuous medical supervision.

Monitoring Parameters Urine sugar and acetone, serum glucose, electrolytes, Hb A$_{1c}$, lipid profile

DKA: Arterial blood gases (initial), venous pH, CBC with differential, urinalysis, serum glucose (baseline and every hour until reaches 250 mg/dL), BUN, creatinine, electrolytes, anion gap, I&O

Hyperkalemia: Serum potassium and glucose must be closely monitored to avoid hypoglycemia and/or hypokalemia.

Reference Range

Plasma Blood Glucose and Hgb A$_{1c}$ Goals for Type 1 Diabetes (ADA, 2013): Note: Goals should be individualized based on individual needs/circumstances (eg, patients who experience severe hypoglycemia, patients with hypoglycemic unawareness); lower goals may be reasonable if they can be achieved without excessive hypoglycemia. **Note:** Postprandial blood glucose should be measured when there is a discrepancy between preprandial blood glucose concentrations and Hb A$_{1c}$ values and to help assess glycemia for patients who receive basal/bolus regimens. It is usually drawn 1-2 hours after starting meal and is considered to be the "peak."

Toddlers/Preschoolers (0-6 years):
Preprandial glucose: 100-180 mg/dL
Bedtime/overnight glucose: 110-200 mg/dL
Hb A$_{1c}$: <8.5%

School age (6-12 years):
Preprandial glucose: 90-180 mg/dL
Bedtime/overnight glucose: 100-180 mg/dL
Hb A$_{1c}$: <8%

Adolescents/Young Adults (13-19 years):
Preprandial glucose: 90-130 mg/dL
Bedtime/overnight glucose: 90-150 mg/dL
Hb A$_{1c}$: <7.5%

Adults, nonpregnant:
Preprandial glucose: 70-130 mg/dL
Postprandial glucose: <180 mg/dL
Hb A$_{1c}$: <7%

Criteria for diagnosis of DKA:
Serum glucose:
Children: >200 mg/dL
Adults: >250 mg/dL

Arterial pH:
Children: <7.3
Adults: <7-7.24

Bicarbonate:
Children: <15 mEq/L
Adults: <10-15 mEq/L

Moderate ketonuria or ketonemia

Additional Information In mild diabetic ketoacidosis or unusual circumstances, for patients without I.V. access, SubQ or I.M. regular insulin has been used. Doses are similar to the doses recommended for bolus and the hourly infusion (total dose administered once per hour). If volume depletion and secondary sympathetic activation decrease local perfusion, insulin absorption may be inconsistent. For this reason, many clinicians do not recommend this approach.

Product Availability

Afrezza: FDA approved June 2014; anticipated availability currently undetermined

Afrezza is a rapid acting inhaled insulin (human insulin produced by recombinant DNA technology) indicated to improve glycemic control in adult patients with diabetes mellitus.

Dosage Forms Excipient information presented when available (limited, particularly for generics); consult specific product labeling.

Solution, Injection:
HumuLIN R: 100 units/mL (3 mL, 10 mL) [contains metacresol, phenol]
NovoLIN R: 100 units/mL (10 mL) [contains metacresol]
NovoLIN R ReliOn: 100 units/mL (10 mL) [contains metacresol]

Solution, Subcutaneous:
HumuLIN R U-500 (CONCENTRATED): 500 units/mL (20 mL) [contains metacresol]

References

"2005 American Heart Association Guidelines for Cardiopulmonary Resuscitation and Emergency Cardiovascular Care," *Circulation*, 2005, 112(24 Suppl): 1-211.

American Diabetes Association (ADA), "Standards of Medical Care in Diabetes-2013," *Diabetes Care*, 2013, (36 Suppl 1):S11-66.

American Diabetes Association, "Standards of Medical Care in Diabetes," *Diabetes Care*, 2007, 30(Suppl 1):4-41.

Institute for Safe Medication Practices (ISMP), "Standard Concentrations of Neonatal Drug Infusions," *ISMP*, 2011.

International Diabetes Federation, International Society for Pediatric and Adolescent Diabetes. Global IDF/ISPAD guideline for diabetes in childhood and adolescence. 2011. Available at: http://www.idf.org/global-idfispad-guideline-diabetes-childhood-and-adolescence. Date accessed: October 21, 2013.

Malone TA, "Glucose and Insulin Versus Cation-Exchange Resin for the Treatment of Hyperkalemia in Very Low Birth Weight Infants," *J Pediatr*, 1991, 118(1):121-3.

Phillips MS, "Standardizing I.V. Infusion Concentrations: National Survey Results," *Am J Health Syst Pharm*, 2011, 68(22):2176-82.

Simeon PS, Geffner ME, Levin SR, et al, "Continuous Insulin Infusions in Neonates: Pharmacologic Availability of Insulin in Intravenous Solutions," *J Pediatr*, 1994, 124(5 Pt 1):818-20.

◆ **Insulin Regular and Insulin NPH** *see* Insulin NPH and Insulin Regular *on page 1132*

◆ **Intanza (Can)** *see* Influenza Virus Vaccine (Inactivated) *on page 1103*

◆ **Intelence** *see* Etravirine *on page 819*

◆ **Intelence® (Can)** *see* Etravirine *on page 819*

◆ **α-2-interferon** *see* Interferon Alfa-2b *on page 1138*

◆ **Interferon Alfa-2a (PEG Conjugate)** *see* Peginterferon Alfa-2a *on page 1617*

◆ **Interferon Alfa-2b (PEG Conjugate)** *see* Peginterferon Alfa-2b *on page 1621*

Interferon Alfa-2b (in ter FEER on AL fa too bee)

Medication Safety Issues
Sound-alike/look-alike issues:
Interferon alfa-2b may be confused with interferon alfa-2a, interferon alfa-n3, pegylated interferon alfa-2b
Intron A may be confused with PEG-Intron

International issues:
Interferon alfa-2b may be confused with interferon alpha multi-subtype which is available in international markets

Related Information
Emetogenic Potential of Antineoplastic Agents in Children *on page 2327*

Brand Names: U.S. Intron-A

Brand Names: Canada Intron A

Therapeutic Category Antineoplastic Agent, Biologic Response Modulator; Biological Response Modulator; Immunomodulator, Systemic; Interferon

Generic Availability (U.S.) No

Use Treatment of chronic hepatitis B (FDA approved in ages ≥1 year and adults); chronic hepatitis C (in combination with ribavirin) (FDA approved in ages ≥3 years and adults); chronic hepatitis C (without ribavirin) (FDA approved in adults); hairy cell leukemia (FDA approved in adults); treatment of AIDS-related Kaposi's sarcoma (FDA approved in adults); condylomata acuminata (FDA approved in adults); adjuvant therapy of malignant melanoma following surgical excision (FDA approved in adults); and follicular non-Hodgkin's lymphoma (FDA approved in adults)

Other uses include hemangiomas of infancy, cutaneous ulcerations of Behçet's disease, neuroendocrine tumors (including carcinoid syndrome and islet cell tumor), cutaneous T-cell lymphoma, desmoid tumor, hepatitis D, chronic myelogenous leukemia (CML), non-Hodgkin's lymphomas (other than follicular lymphoma, see approved use), multiple myeloma, renal cell carcinoma, West Nile virus

Medication Guide Available Yes

Pregnancy Risk Factor C / X in combination with ribavirin

Pregnancy Considerations Animal reproduction studies have demonstrated abortifacient effects. Disruption of the normal menstrual cycle was also observed in animal studies; therefore, the manufacturer recommends that reliable contraception is used in women of childbearing potential. Alfa interferon is endogenous to normal amniotic fluid. *In vitro* administration studies have reported that when administered to the mother, it does not cross the placenta. Case reports of use in pregnant women are limited. The Perinatal HIV Guidelines Working Group does not recommend that interferon-alfa be used during pregnancy. Interferon alfa-2b monotherapy should only be used in pregnancy when the potential benefit to the mother justifies the possible risk to the fetus. Combination therapy with ribavirin is contraindicated in pregnancy (refer to Ribavirin monograph); two forms of contraception should be used during combination therapy and patients should have monthly pregnancy tests. A pregnancy registry has been established for women inadvertently exposed to ribavirin while pregnant (800-593-2214).

Breast-Feeding Considerations Breast milk samples obtained from a lactating mother prior to and after administration of interferon alfa-2b showed that interferon alfa is present in breast milk and administration of the medication did not significantly affect endogenous levels. Breast-feeding is not linked to the spread of hepatitis C virus; however, if nipples are cracked or bleeding, breast-feeding is not recommended. Mothers coinfected with HIV are discouraged from breast-feeding to decrease potential transmission of HIV.

Contraindications Hypersensitivity to interferon alfa or any component; autoimmune hepatitis, hepatic decompensation

Warnings Hazardous agent; use appropriate precautions for handling and disposal. Alpha interferons suppress bone marrow function which may result in severe cytopenias or aplastic anemia. Alpha interferons may cause or aggravate fatal or life-threatening neuropsychiatric, autoimmune, ischemic, and infectious disorders **[U.S. Boxed Warning]**.

May cause or aggravate severe neuropsychiatric adverse events **[U.S. Boxed Warning]**; monitor closely with clinical evaluations (periodic); discontinue treatment for severe persistent or worsening symptoms; some cases may resolve with discontinuation. Psychiatric events may include depression, psychosis, mania, suicidal behavior/ideation, and homicidal ideation, and may occur in patients with or without previous psychiatric symptoms. Careful neuropsychiatric monitoring is recommended during and for 6 months after treatment in patients who develop psychiatric disorders (including clinical depression). New or exacerbated neuropsychiatric or substance abuse disorders are best managed with early intervention. Use with caution in patients with a history of psychiatric disorders. Drug screening and periodic health evaluation (including monitoring of psychiatric symptoms) is recommended if initiating treatment in patients with coexisting psychiatric condition or substance abuse disorders, Suicidal ideation or attempts may occur more frequently in pediatric patients when compared to adults. Higher doses in elderly patients, or diseases other than hairy cell leukemia, may result in increased CNS toxicity.

Ophthalmologic disorders including vision decrease or loss, retinopathy, optic neuritis, and papilledema have occurred; close monitoring is advised. Development of autoimmune diseases including vasculitis, ITP, rheumatoid arthritis, SLE, and hepatitis have been reported in patients on alfa interferon. Patients being treated for chronic hepatitis B or C with a history of autoimmune disease or who are immunosuppressed transplant recipients should not receive interferon alfa-2b. Do not treat patients with visceral AIDS-related Kaposi's sarcoma associated with rapidly progressing or life-threatening disease.

May cause hepatotoxicity; monitor closely if abnormal liver function tests develop. A transient increase in ALT (≥2 times baseline) may occur in patients treated with interferon alfa-2b for chronic hepatitis B. Worsening and potentially fatal liver disease, including jaundice, hepatic encephalopathy, and hepatic failure have been reported in patients receiving interferon alfa for chronic hepatitis B and C with decompensated liver disease, autoimmune hepatitis, history of autoimmune disease, and immunosuppressed transplant recipients; avoid interferon treatment in these patients. Discontinue treatment in any patient developing signs or symptoms of liver failure.

Pulmonary infiltrates, pneumonitis, and pneumonia have been reported with interferon alfa therapy; occurs more frequently in patients being treated for chronic hepatitis C. Patients with fever, cough, dyspnea, or other respiratory symptoms should be evaluated with a chest x-ray; monitor closely and consider discontinuing treatment with evidence of impaired pulmonary function.

Diluent for interferon alfa-2b injection may contain benzyl alcohol which can cause allergic reactions in susceptible individuals; large amounts of benzyl alcohol (≥99 mg/kg/day) have been associated with a potentially fatal toxicity ("gasping syndrome") in neonates; the "gasping syndrome" consists of metabolic acidosis, respiratory distress, gasping respirations, CNS dysfunction (including convulsions, intracranial hemorrhage), hypotension and cardiovascular collapse; avoid use of interferon alfa-2b products containing benzyl alcohol in neonates; *in vitro* and animal studies have shown that benzoate, a metabolite of benzyl alcohol, displaces bilirubin from protein binding sites.

Injection may also contain polysorbate 80 (Tween 80®) which may cause allergic reactions in susceptible individuals. In premature neonates, thrombocytopenia, ascites, pulmonary deterioration, and renal and hepatic failure have been reported after receiving parenteral products containing polysorbate 80 (Alade, 1986; *MMWR*, 1984). Infusion of polysorbate 80-containing solutions through polyvinyl chloride tubing may cause DEHP to leach into the solution; in immature animals, exposure to DEHP may adversely affect the development of the male reproductive tract.

Precautions Use with caution in patients with pulmonary function impairment, seizure disorders, brain metastases, compromised CNS, multiple sclerosis, arrhythmias, and patients with preexisting cardiac disease, severe renal dysfunction (CrCl <50 mL/minute), hepatic impairment, or myelosuppression. Use caution in patients with diabetes, preexisting thyroid disease, coagulopathy, hypertension, or in patients receiving drugs that may cause lactic acidosis. Product of human plasma; may potentially contain infectious agents which could transmit disease. Screening of donors, as well as testing and/or inactivation or removal of certain viruses, reduces the risk. Due to differences in dosage, patients should not change brands of interferons without the concurrence of their healthcare provider.

Adverse Reactions Note: In a majority of patients, a flu-like symptom (fever, chills, tachycardia, malaise, myalgia, headache), occurs within 1-2 hours of administration; may last up to 24 hours and may be dose limiting.

Cardiovascular: Chest pain, edema, hypertension

Central nervous system: Agitation, amnesia, anxiety, chills, confusion, depression, dizziness, drowsiness, fatigue, headache, hypoesthesia, insomnia, irritability, lack of concentration, malaise, pain, paresthesia, right upper quadrant pain, rigors, vertigo

Dermatologic: Alopecia, dermatitis, diaphoresis, pruritus, skin rash, xeroderma

Endocrine & metabolic: Amenorrhea, decreased libido, weight loss

Gastrointestinal: Abdominal pain, anorexia, constipation, diarrhea, dysgeusia, dyspepsia, gingivitis, loose stools, nausea, vomiting (more common in children), xerostomia

Genitourinary: Urinary tract infection

Hematologic & oncologic: Anemia, leukopenia, neutropenia, purpura, thrombocytopenia

Hepatic: Increased serum alkaline phosphatase, increased serum ALT, increased serum AST

Infection: Candidiasis, infection, herpes virus infection

Local: Injection site reaction

Neuromuscular & skeletal: Arthralgia, back pain, myalgia, skeletal pain, weakness

Renal: Increased blood urea nitrogen, increased serum creatinine, polyuria

Respiratory: Bronchitis, cough, dyspnea, epistaxis, flu-like symptoms, nasal congestion, pharyngitis, sinusitis

Miscellaneous: Fever (more common in children)

Rare but important or life-threatening: Abnormal hepatic function tests, aggressive behavior, albuminuria, alcohol intolerance, amyotrophy, anaphylaxis, angina pectoris, angioedema, aphasia, aplastic anemia (rarely), ascites,

asthma, atrial fibrillation, Bell's palsy, bradycardia, bronchiolitis obliterans, bronchoconstriction, bronchospasm, cardiac arrhythmia, cardiac failure, cardiomegaly, cardiomyopathy, cellulitis, cerebrovascular accident, colitis, coma, conjunctivitis, coronary artery disease, cyanosis, cystitis, dehydration, diabetes mellitus, dysphasia, dysuria, eczema, epidermal cyst, erythema, erythema multiforme, erythematous rash, exacerbation of psoriasis, exacerbation of sarcoidosis, extrapyramidal reaction, extrasystoles, gastrointestinal hemorrhage, granulocytopenia, hallucination, hearing loss, heart valve disease, hematuria, hemolytic anemia, hemoptysis, hepatic encephalopathy, hepatic failure, hepatitis, hepatotoxicity, hot flash, homicidal ideation, hyperbilirubinemia, hypercalcemia, hyperglycemia, hypermenorrhea, hypersensitivity reaction (acute), hypertriglyceridemia, hyperthyroidism, hypochromic anemia, hypotension, hypothermia, hypothyroidism, hypoventilation, immune thrombocytopenia, impotence, increased lactate dehydrogenase, interstitial pneumonitis, jaundice, leukorrhea, lupus erythematosus, lymphadenitis, lymphadenopathy, lymphocytopenia, lymphocytosis, macular edema, maculopapular rash, migraine, myocardial infarction, myositis, nephrotic syndrome, neuralgia, neuropathy, nystagmus, optic neuritis, palpitations, pancreatitis, pancytopenia, papilledema, paranoia, peripheral ischemia, peripheral neuropathy, photophobia, pituitary insufficiency, pleural effusion, pneumonia, psychoneurosis, pneumothorax, proteinuria, psychosis, pulmonary embolism, pulmonary fibrosis, pulmonary hypertension, pulmonary infiltrates, pure red cell aplasia, Raynaud's phenomenon, reduced ejection fraction, renal failure, renal insufficiency, respiratory insufficiency, retinal detachment (serous), retinal thrombosis, retinal cotton-wool spot, retinal vein occlusion, rhabdomyolysis, seizure, sepsis, sexual disorder, skin photosensitivity, Stevens-Johnson syndrome, stomatitis, suicidal ideation, syncope, systemic lupus erythematosus, tachycardia, tendonitis, tissue necrosis at injection site, thrombotic thrombocytopenic purpura, thrombosis, toxic epidermal necrolysis, upper respiratory tract infection, urinary incontinence, urticaria, uterine hemorrhage, vasculitis, Vogt-Koyanagi-Harada syndrome, wheezing

Drug Interactions

Metabolism/Transport Effects Inhibits CYP1A2 (weak)

Avoid Concomitant Use

Avoid concomitant use of Interferon Alfa-2b with any of the following: CloZAPine; Dipyrone; Telbivudine

Increased Effect/Toxicity

Interferon Alfa-2b may increase the levels/effects of: Aldesleukin; CloZAPine; Methadone; Ribavirin; Telbivudine; Theophylline Derivatives; Zidovudine

The levels/effects of Interferon Alfa-2b may be increased by: Dipyrone

Decreased Effect There are no known significant interactions involving a decrease in effect.

Stability Store powder and solution for injection (vials and pens) under refrigeration at 2°C to 8°C (36°F to 46°F); do not freeze.

Powder for injection: Following reconstitution, should be used immediately, but may be stored under refrigeration for up to 24 hours.

Prefilled pens: After first use, discard unused portion after 4 weeks.

Mechanism of Action Binds to a specific receptor on the cell wall to initiate intracellular activity; multiple effects can be detected including induction of gene transcription. Inhibits cellular growth, alters the state of cellular differentiation, interferes with oncogene expression, alters cell surface antigen expression, increases phagocytic activity of macrophages, and augments cytotoxicity of lymphocytes for target cells

Pharmacokinetics (Adult data unless noted)
Metabolism: Majority of dose is thought to be metabolized in the kidney, filtered and absorbed at the renal tubule

Bioavailability:
I.M.: 83%
SubQ: 90%

Half-life, elimination:
I.M., I.V.: 2 hours
SubQ: 3 hours

Time to peak serum concentration: I.M., SubQ: ~3-8 hours

Dosing: Usual Note: Consider premedication with acetaminophen to reduce the incidence of some adverse reactions. Not all dosage forms and strengths are appropriate for all indications; refer to product labeling for details.

Infants, Children, and Adolescents:

Hemangiomas: Limited data available: SubQ: 3 million units/m²/dose once daily (Garmendia, 2001)

Hepatitis B, chronic: Children and Adolescents: SubQ: 3 million units/m²/dose 3 times/week for 1 week; then 6 million units/m²/dose 3 times/week; maximum dose: 10 million units/dose 3 times/week; total duration of therapy is 24 weeks. Higher doses may be used for retreatment or failed lower-dose therapy: 10 million units/m²/dose 3 times/week for 6 months; dosing may also be used in infants in the setting of HIV-exposure/-infection (CDC, 2009).

Hepatitis C, chronic: Children ≥3 years and Adolescents: SubQ: 3-5 million units/m²/dose 3 times/week

Hepatitis C, chronic with HIV coinfection: I.M., SubQ: 3-5 million units/m²/dose 3 times/week (maximum: 3 million units/dose) for 48 weeks, regardless of HCV genotype; with concurrent ribavirin therapy (unless contraindicated); generally treatment in children <3 years is not recommended (CDC, 2009)

Adults:

AIDS-related Kaposi's sarcoma: I.M., SubQ: 30 million units/m²/dose 3 times/week; continue until disease progression or until maximal response has been achieved after 16 weeks

Condylomata acuminata: Intralesionally: 1 million units/lesion 3 times/week (on alternate days) for 3 weeks; not to exceed 5 million units per treatment (maximum dose: 5 lesions at one time) (use only the 10 million units vial); may administer a second course at 12-16 weeks

Hairy cell leukemia: I.M., SubQ: 2 million units/m²/dose 3 times/week for up to 6 months (may continue treatment with sustained treatment response); discontinue for disease progression or failure to respond after 6 months

Hepatitis B, chronic: I.M., SubQ: 5 million units/dose given once daily **or** 10 million units/dose given 3 times/week for 4 months

Hepatitis C, chronic: I.M., SubQ: 3 million units/dose 3 times/week for 16 weeks. In patients with normalization of ALT at 16 weeks, continue treatment for 18-24 months; consider discontinuation if normalization does not occur at 16 weeks. **Note:** May be used in combination therapy with ribavirin in previously untreated patients or in patients who relapse following alpha interferon therapy.

Lymphoma (follicular): SubQ: 5 million units/dose 3 times/week for ≤18 months

Malignant melanoma adjuvant therapy:
Induction: I.V.: 20 million units/m²/dose 5 days/week for 4 weeks
Maintenance: SubQ: 10 million units/m²/dose 3 days/week for 48 weeks

Dosage adjustment for toxicity:

Hematologic toxicity (also refer to indication specified adjustments below): ANC <500/mm³ or platelets <25,000/mm³: Discontinue treatment.

Hypersensitivity reaction (acute, serious), ophthalmic disorders (new or worsening), thyroid abnormality development (which cannot be normalized with medication), signs or symptoms of liver failure: Discontinue treatment.

Liver function abnormality, pulmonary infiltrate development, evidence of pulmonary function impairment, or autoimmune disorder development, triglycerides >1000 mg/dL in adults: Monitor closely and discontinue if appropriate.

Neuropsychiatric disorders (during treatment): Children, Adolescents, and Adults:
Clinical depression or other psychiatric problem: Monitor closely during and for 6 months after treatment.
Severe depression or other psychiatric disorder: Discontinue treatment.
Persistent or worsening psychiatric symptoms, suicidal ideation, aggression towards others: Discontinue treatment and follow with appropriate psychiatric intervention.

Indication-specific, manufacturer-recommended adjustments:

Lymphoma (follicular): Adults:
Neutrophils >1000/mm³ to <1500/mm³: Reduce dose by 50%; may re-escalate to starting dose when neutrophils return to >1500/mm³
Severe toxicity (neutrophils <1000/mm³ or platelets <50,000/mm³): Temporarily withhold.
AST >5 times ULN or serum creatinine >2 mg/dL: Permanently discontinue.

Hairy cell leukemia: Adults:
Platelet count <50,000/mm³: Do not administer intramuscularly (administer SubQ instead).
Severe toxicity: Reduce dose by 50% or temporarily withhold and resume with 50% dose reduction; permanently discontinue if persistent or recurrent severe toxicity is noted.

Chronic hepatitis B: Children, Adolescents, and Adults:
WBC <1500/mm³, granulocytes <750/mm³, or platelet count <50,000/mm³, or other laboratory abnormality or severe adverse reaction: Reduce dose by 50%; may re-escalate to starting dose upon resolution of hematologic toxicity. Discontinue for persistent intolerance.
WBC <1000/mm³, granulocytes <500/mm³, or platelet count <25,000/mm³: Permanently discontinue.

Hepatitis C, chronic: Children, Adolescents, and Adults:
Severe toxicity: Reduce dose by 50% or temporarily withhold until subsides; permanently discontinue for persistent toxicities after dosage reduction.

AIDS-related Kaposi's sarcoma: Adults: Severe toxicity: Reduce dose by 50% or temporarily withhold; may resume at reduced dose with toxicity resolution; permanently discontinue for persistent/recurrent toxicities.

Malignant melanoma (induction and maintenance): Adults:
Severe toxicity, including neutrophils >250/mm³ to <500/mm³ or ALT/AST >5-10 times ULN: Temporarily withhold; resume with a 50% dose reduction when adverse reaction abates.
Neutrophils <250/mm³, ALT/AST >10 times ULN, or severe/persistent adverse reactions: Permanently discontinue.

Administration

Parenteral: Not all dosage forms are recommended for all administration routes; refer to manufacturer's labeling

Reconstitution: Powder for injection: The manufacturer recommends reconstituting vial with the diluent provided (SWI). When reconstituted with 1 mL SWI, the 10 million unit vial concentration is 10 million units/mL, the 18 million unit vial concentration is 18 million units/mL, and the 50 million unit vial concentration is 50 million units/mL. Swirl gently to mix. pH: 6.9-7.5

I.M.: Administer dose in the evening (if possible) to enhance tolerability. Rotate injection sites. Some patients may be appropriate for self-administration with appropriate training. Allow to reach room temperature prior to injection. In hairy cell leukemia treatment, if platelets are <50,000/mm³, do not administer intramuscularly (administer SubQ instead).

I.V.: To prepare solution for infusion, further dilute appropriate dose in NS 100 mL; final concentration should be ≥10 million units/100 mL. Infuse over ~20 minutes. Administer dose in the evening (if possible) to enhance tolerability.

SubQ: Suggested for those who are at risk for bleeding or are thrombocytopenic. Rotate SubQ injection site. Administer dose in the evening (if possible) to enhance tolerability. Patient should be well hydrated. Some patients may be appropriate for self-administration with appropriate training. Allow to reach room temperature prior to injection.

Intralesional: Reconstitute the 10 million unit vial with 1 mL SWI; resulting concentration is 10 million units/mL; inject dose at an angle nearly parallel to the plane of the skin, directing the needle to center of the base of the wart to infiltrate the lesion core and cause a small wheal. Only infiltrate the keratinized layer; avoid administration which is too deep or shallow. Allow to reach room temperature prior to injection.

Monitoring Parameters CBC with differential (baseline and periodic during treatment), liver function tests (baseline and periodic), electrolytes (baseline and periodic), serum creatinine (baseline), albumin, prothrombin time, triglycerides, thyroid-stimulating hormone (TSH) baseline and periodically during treatment (in patients with preexisting thyroid disorders, repeat TSH at 3 months and 6 months); chest x-ray (baseline), weight; ophthalmic exam (baseline and periodic, or with new ocular symptoms); ECG (baseline and during treatment; in patients with preexisting cardiac abnormalities or in advanced stages of cancer); neuropsychiatric changes during and for 6 months after therapy

Hepatitis B, chronic: CBC with differential and platelets and liver function tests: Baseline, weeks 1, 2, 4, 8, 12, and 16, at the end of treatment, and then 3 and 6 months post-treatment

Hepatitis C, chronic:
CBC with differential and platelets: Baseline, weeks 1 and 2, then monthly
Liver function: Every 3 months
TSH: Baseline and periodically during treatment; in patients with preexisting thyroid disorders also repeat at 3 months and 6 months

Malignant melanoma: CBC with differential and platelets and liver function tests: Weekly during induction phase, then monthly during maintenance

Oncology patients: Thyroid function monitoring (Hamnvik, 2011): TSH and anti-TPO antibodies at baseline; if TPO antibody positive, monitor TSH every 2 months; if TPO antibody negative, monitor TSH every 6 months

Dosage Forms Excipient information presented when available (limited, particularly for generics); consult specific product labeling.
Solution, Injection:
Intron-A: 6,000,000 units/mL (3.8 mL); 10,000,000 units/mL (3.2 mL)
Solution Reconstituted, Injection:
Intron-A: 10,000,000 units (1 ea) [contains benzyl alcohol]
Intron-A: 18,000,000 units (1 ea)
Intron-A: 50,000,000 units (1 ea) [contains benzyl alcohol]

References
Alade SL, Brown RE, and Paquet A Jr, "Polysorbate 80 and E-Ferol Toxicity," *Pediatrics*, 1986, 77(4):593-7.

Centers for Disease Control and Prevention (CDC), "Guidelines for the Prevention and Treatment of Opportunistic Infections Among HIV-Exposed and HIV-Infected Children," *MMWR Recomm Rep*, 2009, 58(RR-11):1-166. Available at http://aidsinfo.nih.gov/contentfiles/Pediatric_OI.pdf
Centers for Disease Control (CDC), "Unusual Syndrome With Fatalities Among Premature Infants: Association With a New Intravenous Vitamin E Product," *MMWR Morb Mortal Wkly Rep*, 1984, 33 (14):198-9.
Davis GL, Balart LA, Schiff ER, et al, "Treatment of Chronic Hepatitis C With Recombinant Interferon Alfa. A Multicenter Randomized, Controlled Trial. Hepatitis Interventional Therapy Group," *N Engl J Med*, 1989, 321(22):1501-6.
DHHS Panel on Treatment of HIV-Infected Pregnant Women and Prevention of Perinatal Transmission, "Recommendations for Use of Antiretroviral Drugs in Pregnant HIV-1-Infected Women for Maternal Health and Interventions to Reduce Perinatal HIV Transmission in the United States," July 31, 2012. Available at http://aidsinfo.nih.gov/contentfiles/lvguidelines/perinatalgl.pdf
Garmendia G, Miranda N, Borroso S, et al, "Regression of Infancy Hemangiomas With Recombinant IFN-Alpha 2b," *J Interferon Cytokine Res*, 2001, 21(1):31-8.
Gurakan F, Kocak N, Ozen H, et al, "Comparison of Standard and High Dosage Recombinant Interferon Alpha 2b for Treatment of Children With Chronic Hepatitis B Infection," *Pediatr Infect Dis J*, 2000, 19 (1):52-6.
Hamnvik OP, Larsen PR, and Marqusee E, "Thyroid Dysfunction From Antineoplastic Agents," *J Natl Cancer Inst*, 2011, 103(21):1572-87.
Kirkwood JM, Ibrahim JG, Sondak VK, et al, "High- and Low-Dose Interferon Alfa-2b in High-Risk Melanoma: First Analysis of Intergroup Trial E1690/S9111/C9190," *J Clin Oncol*, 2000, 18(12):2444-58.
Zwiener RJ, Fielman BA, Cochran C, et al, "Interferon-Alpha-2b Treatment of Chronic Hepatitis C in Children With Hemophilia," *Pediatr Infect Dis J*, 1996, 15(10):906-8.

◆ **Interferon Alpha-2b** see Interferon Alfa-2b *on page 1138*

◆ **Interleukin-1 Receptor Antagonist** see Anakinra *on page 168*

◆ **Interleukin 2** see Aldesleukin *on page 90*

◆ **Interleukin-11** see Oprelvekin *on page 1549*

◆ **Intermezzo** see Zolpidem *on page 2182*

◆ **Intralipid** see Fat Emulsion (Plant Based) *on page 846*

◆ **Intravenous Fat Emulsion** see Fat Emulsion (Plant Based) *on page 846*

◆ **Intron-A** see Interferon Alfa-2b *on page 1138*

◆ **Intron A (Can)** see Interferon Alfa-2b *on page 1138*

◆ **Intropin** see DOPamine *on page 708*

◆ **Intuniv** see GuanFACINE *on page 989*

◆ **Intuniv XR (Can)** see GuanFACINE *on page 989*

◆ **INVanz** see Ertapenem *on page 778*

◆ **Invanz (Can)** see Ertapenem *on page 778*

◆ **Invega** see Paliperidone *on page 1581*

◆ **Invega Sustenna** see Paliperidone *on page 1581*

◆ **Invirase** see Saquinavir *on page 1867*

◆ **Invirase® (Can)** see Saquinavir *on page 1867*

Iodine (EYE oh dyne)

Medication Safety Issues
Sound-alike/look-alike issues:
Iodine may be confused with codeine, Iopidine®, Lodine
Therapeutic Category Topical Skin Product
Generic Availability (U.S.) Yes
Use Used topically as an antiseptic in the management of minor, superficial skin wounds and has been used to disinfect the skin preoperatively
Pregnancy Considerations An adequate amount of iodine intake is essential for thyroid function. Iodine crosses the placenta and requirements are increased during pregnancy. Iodine deficiency in pregnancy can lead to neurologic damage in the newborn; an extreme form, cretinism, is characterized by gross mental retardation, short stature, deaf mutism, and spasticity. Large amounts ▶

of iodine during pregnancy can cause fetal goiter or hyperthyroidism. Transient hypothyroidism in the newborn has also been reported following topical or vaginal use prior to delivery.

Breast-Feeding Considerations Iodine is excreted in breast milk and is a source of iodine for the nursing infant. Actual levels are variable, but have been reported as 113-270 mcg/L in American women. Application of topical iodine antiseptic solutions can be absorbed in amounts which may affect levels in breast milk. Exposure to excess iodine may cause thyrotoxicosis. Skin rash in the nursing infant has been reported with maternal intake of potassium iodide.

Contraindications Hypersensitivity to iodine preparations or any component; neonates; Hashimoto thyroiditis, history of Grave's disease, or nontoxic nodular goiter

Warnings May be highly toxic if ingested; iodine may be absorbed systemically, especially when large wounds are treated or when used in neonates. Not for application to large areas of the body or for use with tight or air-excluding bandages. When used for self medication (OTC), do not use on deep wounds, puncture wounds, animal bites, or serious burns without consulting with healthcare provider. Notify healthcare provider if condition does not improve within 7 days. Iodosorb® is for use as topical application to wet wounds only.

Precautions Use with caution in patients with renal dysfunction; since iodine may be absorbed systemically, thyroid function may need to be monitored when used chronically or over a large area.

Adverse Reactions

Reactions reported following topical application:

Endocrine & metabolic: TSH increased

Local: Eczema, edema, irritation, pain, redness

Miscellaneous: Allergic reaction

Reactions reported more likely observed following large doses or chronic iodine intoxication; frequency not defined:

Central nervous system: Fever, headache

Dermatologic: Skin rash, angioedema, urticaria, acne

Endocrine & metabolic: Hypothyroidism

Gastrointestinal: Metallic taste, diarrhea

Hematologic: Eosinophilia, hemorrhage (mucosal)

Neuromuscular & skeletal: Arthralgia

Ocular: Swelling of eyelids

Respiratory: Pulmonary edema

Miscellaneous: Ioderma, lymph node enlargement

Drug Interactions

Metabolism/Transport Effects None known.

Avoid Concomitant Use There are no known interactions where it is recommended to avoid concomitant use.

Increased Effect/Toxicity There are no known significant interactions involving an increase in effect.

Decreased Effect There are no known significant interactions involving a decrease in effect.

Stability Store at room temperature.

Mechanism of Action Iodine is required for thyroid hormone synthesis. Iodine is also known to be a powerful broad spectrum germicidal agent effective against a wide range of bacteria, viruses, fungi, protozoa, and spores. Iodosorb® and Iodoflex™ contain iodine in hydrophilic beads of cadexomer which allows a slow release of iodine into the wound and absorption of fluid, bacteria, and other substances from the wound

Pharmacokinetics (Adult data unless noted)

Absorption: Topical: Amount absorbed systemically depends upon the iodine concentration and skin characteristics

Metabolism: Degraded by amylases normally present in wound fluid

Excretion: Urine (>90%)

Dosing: Usual Children and Adults:

Antiseptic for minor cuts, scrapes: Apply small amount to affected area 1-3 times/day

Cleaning wet ulcers and wounds (Iodosorb®, Iodoflex™): Apply to clean wound; maximum: 50 g/application and 150 g/week. Change dressing ~3 times/week; reduce applications as exudate decreases. Do not use for >3 months; discontinue when wound is free of exudate.

Administration Topical: Apply to affected areas; avoid tight bandages because iodine may cause burns on occluded skin.

Iodosorb®: Apply 1/8" to 1/4" thickness to dry sterile gauze, then place prepared gauze onto clean wound. Change dressing when gel changes color from brown to yellow/gray (~3 times/week). Remove with sterile water, saline, or wound cleanser; gently blot fluid from surface leaving wound slightly moist before reapplying gel.

Test Interactions Large amounts from excessive absorption may alter thyroid function tests.

Additional Information Sodium thiosulfate inactivates iodine and is an effective chemical antidote for iodine poisoning; solutions of sodium thiosulfate may be used to remove iodine stains from skin and clothing

Dosage Forms Excipient information presented when available (limited, particularly for generics); consult specific product labeling.

Tincture, External:

Generic: 2% (30 mL, 20000 mL); 7% (30 mL, 59 mL, 480 mL); (30 mL, 473 mL)

◆ **Iodine and Potassium Iodide** see Potassium Iodide and Iodine on page 1713

Iodixanol (EYE oh dix an ole)

Medication Safety Issues

High alert medication:

The Institute for Safe Medication Practices (ISMP) includes this medication among its list of drugs which have a heightened risk of causing significant patient harm when used in error.

Administration issues:

Not for intrathecal use.

Brand Names: U.S. Visipaque

Brand Names: Canada Visipaque™

Therapeutic Category Radiological/Contrast Media, Nonionic

Generic Availability (U.S.) No

Use Nonionic contrast media for radiological use intraarterially: Digital subtraction angiography; angiocardiography (left ventriculography and selective coronary arteriography), peripheral arteriography, visceral arteriography, and cerebralarteriography. Intravenously: Contrast enhanced computed tomography (CECT) imaging of the head and body, excretory urography, and peripheral venography

Pregnancy Risk Factor B

Pregnancy Considerations Fetal harm was not observed in animal studies. There are no adequate and well-controlled studies in pregnant women. In general, iodinated contrast media agents are avoided during pregnancy unless essential for diagnosis.

Breast-Feeding Considerations Due to the potential for adverse reactions, temporary discontinuation of breast-feeding should be considered.

Contraindications Hypersensitivity to iodixanol or any component; intrathecal administration; administration to children who have experienced prolonged fasting or received recent laxative dose(s)

Warnings For I.V. or intra-arterial use only; **may be fatal if given intrathecally [U.S. Boxed Warning]**; intrathecal injection has also resulted in serious reactions (seizures, cerebral hemorrhage, coma, paralysis, arachnoiditis, ARF, cardiac arrest, rhabdomyolysis, hyperthermia, and brain edema). May cause rare but serious thromboembolic events including MI and stroke. Iodinated contrast media has been associated with severe hypersensitivity reactions including anaphylaxis; immediate treatment for anaphylactic reactions should be available during administration of iodixanol. Use with extreme caution in patients with or suspected of having pheochromocytoma; the amount of iodixanol used should be kept to an absolute minimum and blood pressure should be closely monitored throughout the procedure in these patients. Contrast media when administered intravascularly may promote sickling in patients who are homozygous for sickle cell disease. May worsen renal insufficiency in patients with multiple myeloma. Avoid use in patients with homocystinuria due to the risk of inducing thrombosis and embolism. Avoid extravasation.

Precautions Use with caution in pediatric patients with asthma, hypersensitivity to other medication and/or allergens, cyanotic and acyanotic heart disease, CHF, serum creatinine >1.5 mg/dL, and neonates (immature renal function) due to an increased risk of adverse effects with iodixanol. Dehydration, particularly in children, may also increase the risk of adverse effects. Patients should be adequately hydrated both prior to and after iodixanol administration. In pediatric patients, apnea, arrhythmias (AV block, bundle branch block), cardiac failure, disseminated intravascular coagulation, and taste perversion have been reported. Use caution in thyroid disease; thyroid storm has been reported in patients with history of hyperthyroidism.

Adverse Reactions

Cardiovascular: Angina/chest pain

Central nervous system: Headache/migraine, vertigo

Dermatologic: Nonurticarial rash/erythema, pruritus

Gastrointestinal: Nausea, taste perversion,

Local: Injection site reactions (discomfort/pain/warmth)

Neuromuscular & skeletal: Paresthesia

Respiratory: Parosoma

Rare but important or life-threatening: Acute renal failure, anaphylactoid reaction, anaphylaxis, apnea (children only), arrhythmia (children only), asthma, AV block (children only), back pain, bundle branch block (children only), cardiac arrest, cardiac failure (children only), cerebral vascular disorder, disseminated intravascular coagulation (children only), hematoma, hemorrhage, hypersensitivity, hypertension, hypoglycemia, hypotensive collapse, peripheral ischemia, pharyngeal edema, pulmonary edema, pulmonary embolism, respiratory depression, seizure, shock

Drug Interactions

Metabolism/Transport Effects None known.

Avoid Concomitant Use There are no known interactions where it is recommended to avoid concomitant use.

Increased Effect/Toxicity

Iodixanol may increase the levels/effects of: MetFORMIN

The levels/effects of Iodixanol may be increased by: Aldesleukin

Decreased Effect There are no known significant interactions involving a decrease in effect.

Stability Store at room temperature; do not mix with or inject in I.V. lines with other medications, solutions, or TPN solutions

Mechanism of Action Opacifies vessels in the path of flow permitting radiographic imaging of internal structures.

Pharmacodynamics Following administration, the increase in tissue density is related to blood flow, the concentration of the iodixanol solution used, and the extraction of iodixanol by various interstitial tissues. The degree of enhancement is directly related to the iodine content in an administered dose.

Kidney:

Visualization: Renal parenchyma: 30-60 seconds; calyces and pelves (normal renal function): 1-3 minutes

Optimum contrast: 5-15 minutes

Pharmacokinetics (Adult data unless noted)

Distribution: V_d: Adults: 0.26 L/kg

Metabolism: Metabolites have not been identified.

Time to peak level: I.V.: Children: 0.75-1.25 hours

Half-life:

Newborns to Infants <2 months: 4.1 ± 1.4 hours

Infants 2-6 months: 2.8 ± 0.6 hours

Infants 6-12 months: 2.4 ± 0.4 hours

Children 1 to <3 years: 2.2 ± 0.5 hours

Children 3 to <12 years: 2.3 ± 0.5 hours

Adults: 2.1 ± 0.1 hours

Elimination: 97% excreted unchanged in the urine within 24 hours; <2% excreted in feces

Clearance: Adults: 110 mL/minute

Dialysis: Dialyzable (36% to 49% depending upon the membrane)

Dosing: Usual The concentration and volume of iodixanol to be used should be individualized depending upon age, weight, size of vessel, and rate of blood flow within the vessel.

Children >1 year:

Intra-arterial: Cerebral, cardiac chambers and related major arteries, and visceral studies: **320 mg iodine/mL**: 1-2 mL/kg; not to exceed 4 mL/kg

I.V.: Contrast-enhanced computerized tomography or excretory urography: **270 mg iodine/mL**: 1-2 mL/kg; not to exceed 2 mL/kg

Children >12 years and Adults: Maximum recommended total dose of iodine: 80 g

Intra-arterial: Iodixanol **320 mg iodine/mL**: Dose individualized based on injection site and study type; refer to product labeling

I.V.: Iodixanol **270 mg and 320 mg iodine/mL**: concentration and dose vary based on study type; refer to product labeling.

Dosage adjustment in renal impairment: Not studied; use caution

Administration I.V. or intra-arterial: Administer without further dilution. **Not for intrathecal administration** . Avoid extravasation.

Vesicant/Extravasation Risk Vesicant

Monitoring Parameters Monitor signs and symptoms of hypersensitivity reactions

Test Interactions Thyroid function tests (protein bound and radioactive iodine uptake studies) may be inaccurate for up to 16 days after administration; may cause false positive urine protein test using Multistix®; may affect urine specific gravity

Dosage Forms Excipient information presented when available (limited, particularly for generics); consult specific product labeling.

Solution, Intravenous:

Visipaque: 320 mg/mL (50 mL, 100 mL, 150 mL, 200 mL, 500 mL) [contains edetate calcium disodium]

Visipaque: 270 mg/mL (50 mL, 100 mL, 150 mL, 200 mL) [pyrogen free; contains edetate calcium disodium, trolamine (triethanolamine)]

Solution, Intravenous [preservative free]:
Visipaque: 320 mg/mL (50 mL) [pyrogen free; contains edetate calcium disodium]

References

Johnson WH, Lloyd TR, Victorica BE, et al, "Iodixanol Pharmacokinetics in Children," *Pediatr Cardiol*, 2001, 22(3):223-7.

Iodoquinol (eye oh doe KWIN ole)

Brand Names: U.S. Yodoxin
Brand Names: Canada Diodoquin®
Therapeutic Category Amebicide
Generic Availability (U.S.) No
Use Treatment of acute and chronic intestinal amebiasis due to *Entamoeba histolytica*; asymptomatic cyst passers; *Blastocystis hominis* infections; iodoquinol alone is ineffective for amebic hepatitis or hepatic abscess
Pregnancy Considerations There is very limited data on the use of iodoquinol during pregnancy and safety has not been established.
Breast-Feeding Considerations It is unknown if iodoquinol is excreted in human milk and safety during lactation has not been established.
Contraindications Hypersensitivity to iodine, iodoquinol, or any component; hepatic or renal damage; preexisting optic neuropathy
Precautions Use with caution in patients with thyroid disease or neurological disorders
Adverse Reactions
Central nervous system: Chills, fever, headache, vertigo
Dermatologic: Pruritus, rash, skin eruptions, urticaria
Endocrine & metabolic: Thyroid gland enlargement
Gastrointestinal: Abdominal cramps, anal itching, diarrhea, nausea, vomiting
Neuromuscular & skeletal: Peripheral neuropathy
Ocular: Optic atrophy, optic neuritis
Drug Interactions
Metabolism/Transport Effects None known.
Avoid Concomitant Use There are no known interactions where it is recommended to avoid concomitant use.
Increased Effect/Toxicity There are no known significant interactions involving an increase in effect.
Decreased Effect There are no known significant interactions involving a decrease in effect.
Mechanism of Action Contact amebicide that works in the lumen of the intestine by an unknown mechanism
Pharmacokinetics (Adult data unless noted)
Absorption: Oral: Poor and irregular
Metabolism: In the liver
Elimination: In feces; metabolites appear in urine
Dosing: Usual Oral:
Children: 30-40 mg/kg/day in 3 divided doses for 20 days; not to exceed 1.95 g/day
Adults: 650 mg 3 times/day after meals for 20 days; not to exceed 2 g/day
Administration Oral: Administer medication after meals; tablets may be crushed and mixed with applesauce or chocolate syrup
Monitoring Parameters Ophthalmologic exam
Test Interactions May increase protein-bound serum iodine concentrations reflecting a decrease in[131]I uptake; false-positive ferric chloride test for phenylketonuria
Dosage Forms Excipient information presented when available (limited, particularly for generics); consult specific product labeling.
Tablet, Oral:
Yodoxin: 210 mg, 650 mg

◆ **Ionil [OTC]** *see* Salicylic Acid *on page 1860*

◆ **Ionil-T [OTC]** *see* Coal Tar *on page 532*

◆ **Iophen C-NR** *see* Guaifenesin and Codeine *on page 985*

◆ **Iophen DM-NR [OTC]** *see* Guaifenesin and Dextromethorphan *on page 987*

◆ **Iophen-NR [OTC]** *see* GuaiFENesin *on page 984*

◆ **IPOL®** *see* Poliovirus Vaccine (Inactivated) *on page 1694*

Ipratropium (Oral Inhalation)
(i pra TROE pee um)

Medication Safety Issues
Sound-alike/look-alike issues:
Atrovent® may be confused with Alupent, Serevent®
Ipratropium may be confused with tiotropium
Brand Names: U.S. Atrovent HFA
Brand Names: Canada Atrovent HFA; Gen-Ipratropium; Mylan-Ipratropium Sterinebs; Novo-Ipramide; Nu-Ipratropium; PMS-Ipratropium; ratio-Ipratropium UDV; Teva-Ipratropium Sterinebs
Therapeutic Category Antiasthmatic; Anticholinergic Agent; Bronchodilator
Generic Availability (U.S.) May be product dependent
Use
Nebulization: Maintenance treatment of bronchospasm associated with chronic obstructive pulmonary disease (COPD), including chronic bronchitis and emphysema alone or in combination with bronchodilators (FDA approved in ages ≥12 years and adults); has also been used to treat bronchospasm associated with asthma and as a bronchodilating agent in bronchopulmonary dysplasia and neonatal respiratory distress syndrome
Oral inhalation: Atrovent HFA: Maintenance treatment of bronchospasm associated with chronic obstructive pulmonary disease (COPD), including chronic bronchitis and emphysema (FDA approved in adults); has also been used to treat bronchospasm associated with asthma and as a bronchodilating agent in bronchopulmonary dysplasia and neonatal respiratory distress syndrome
Pregnancy Risk Factor B
Pregnancy Considerations Teratogenic effects were not observed in animal studies. Inhaled ipratropium is recommended for use as additional therapy for pregnant women with severe asthma exacerbations.
Breast-Feeding Considerations It is not known if ipratropium (oral inhalation) is excreted in breast milk. The manufacturer recommends that caution be exercised when administering ipratropium (oral inhalation) to nursing women.
Contraindications Hypersensitivity to ipratropium, atropine and its derivatives, or any component
Warnings Ipratropium (both oral inhalation and nebulizer) is not indicated for the initial (first-line) treatment of acute episodes of bronchospasm where rescue therapy is required for rapid response. Ipratropium should be added to short acting beta-agonists (SABA) therapy for severe exacerbations (NIH Guidelines, 2007). Rarely, paradoxical bronchospasm may occur with use of inhaled bronchodilating agents; this should be distinguished from inadequate response. Immediate hypersensitivity reactions including urticaria, angioedema, rash, and bronchospasm have been reported.
Precautions Use with caution in patients with narrow-angle glaucoma or myasthenia gravis; ipratropium may exert systemic anticholinergic activity. May cause urinary retention; use with caution in patients with bladder neck obstruction or prostatic hypertrophy. Ipratropium is poorly absorbed from the lung; systemic effects are rare. Use with caution in patients with renal or hepatic impairment; has not been studied in these patients.

Adverse Reactions

Central nervous system: Dizziness, headache

Gastrointestinal: Dyspepsia, nausea, taste perversion, xerostomia

Genitourinary: Urinary tract infection

Neuromuscular & skeletal: Back pain

Respiratory: Bronchitis, COPD exacerbation, cough, dyspnea, rhinitis, sinusitis, upper respiratory infection

Miscellaneous: Flu-like syndrome

Rare but important or life-threatening: Accommodation disorder, anaphylactic reaction, angioedema, bronchospasm, corneal edema, eye pain (acute), glaucoma, hypersensitivity reactions, hypotension, intraocular pressure increased, laryngospasm, palpitations, stomatitis, tachycardia, urinary retention

Drug Interactions

Metabolism/Transport Effects None known.

Avoid Concomitant Use

Avoid concomitant use of Ipratropium (Oral Inhalation) with any of the following: Aclidinium; Anticholinergic Agents; Potassium Chloride; Tiotropium; Umeclidinium

Increased Effect/Toxicity

Ipratropium (Oral Inhalation) may increase the levels/effects of: AbobotulinumtoxinA; Analgesics (Opioid); Anticholinergic Agents; Cannabinoid-Containing Products; Mirabegron; OnabotulinumtoxinA; Potassium Chloride; RimabotulinumtoxinB; Thiazide Diuretics; Tiotropium; Topiramate

The levels/effects of Ipratropium (Oral Inhalation) may be increased by: Aclidinium; Pramlintide; Umeclidinium

Decreased Effect

Ipratropium (Oral Inhalation) may decrease the levels/effects of: Acetylcholinesterase Inhibitors (Central); Secretin

The levels/effects of Ipratropium (Oral Inhalation) may be decreased by: Acetylcholinesterase Inhibitors (Central)

Stability

Nebulization: Store at 15°C to 30°C (59°F to 86°F); protect from light. Compatible for 1 hour when mixed with albuterol or metaproterenol in a nebulizer.

Oral inhalation: Atrovent HFA: Store at 25°C (77°F), excursions permitted to 15°C to 30°C (59°F to 86°F). Do not puncture; do not use or store near heat or open flame.

Mechanism of Action

Blocks the action of acetylcholine at parasympathetic sites in bronchial smooth muscle causing bronchodilation; local application to nasal mucosa inhibits serous and seromucous gland secretions.

Pharmacodynamics

Bronchodilation:

Onset of action: Within 15-30 minutes

Maximum effect: Within 1-2 hours

Duration: Oral inhalation: 2-4 hours; Nebulization: 4-5 hours, up to 7-8 hours in some patients

Pharmacokinetics (Adult data unless noted)

Absorption: Not readily absorbed into the systemic circulation from the surface of the lung or from the GI tract; ~7% absorbed after nebulization of a 2 mg dose

Distribution: Following inhalation, 15% of dose reaches the lower airways

Metabolism: Partially metabolized to inactive ester hydrolysis products

Half-life: 1.6-2 hours

Elimination: Urine (50%)

Dosing: Neonatal

Bronchopulmonary dysplasia/Respiratory distress syndrome (RDS), ventilated patients: Very limited data available; optimal dose not established.

Nebulization:

Weight-based dosing: 25 mcg/kg/dose 3 times daily. Dosing based on a placebo controlled, comparative trial in 17 preterm infants (ipratropium group, n=5; EGA 25-29 weeks; PNA 19-103 days) with BPD and reported a significant decrease in respiratory resistance (Wilkie, 1987).

Fixed-dosing: Some centers have used 175 mcg/dose 3 times daily administered through the ventilator circuit; dosing based on a dose range study of 10 preterm infants with BPD (EGA 24-28 weeks, PNA 18-34 days) which showed significant reduction in respiratory resistance; additional benefit observed when administered after albuterol (Brundage, 1990).

Inhalation, MDI: 4 puffs/dose every 6-8 hours delivered as either a single dose or 2 puffs every 20 minutes for 2 inhalations. In a randomized, placebo-controlled trial in preterm neonates (PNA: 1 week; EGA: 26-34 weeks) with RDS which evaluated a single 72 mcg dose [4 puffs (18 mcg/puff product used; not currently available in the U.S.)] and reported beneficial effects on blood gases and ventilator efficiency. In another trial, which was a crossover, randomized, controlled, double-blind trial of preterm neonates (n=21, PNA: 20 ± 9 days; EGA: 27.3 ± 1.6 weeks) with RDS, a significant reduction in respiratory resistance was reported in 38% of patients after a total dose of 80 mcg [40 mcg every 20 minutes for 2 doses (20 mcg/puff product used; not currently available in the U.S.)]; higher doses [120 mcg (6 puffs)] were not shown to have additional benefit (Fayon, 2007; Lee, 1994).

Dosing: Usual

Infants, Children, and Adolescents:

Bronchospasm, wheezing: Limited data available; efficacy results variable: Infants: Nebulization: 0.125-0.25 mg (125-250 mcg) every 4 hours has been found helpful in some infants with chronic or recurrent wheezing, and some patients with bronchiolitis; however, most bronchiolitis data suggests ipratropium is not effective (Hodges, 1981; Prendiville, 1987; Schuh, 1992; Stokes, 1983; Wang, 1992).

Asthma, acute exacerbation: Limited data available: **Note:** Ipratropium has not been shown to provide further benefit once the patient is hospitalized (NIH guidelines, 2007):

Children:

Nebulization: 0.25-0.5 mg (250-500 mcg) every 20 minutes for 3 doses, then as needed

Metered-dose inhaler: 4-8 puffs every 20 minutes as needed for up to 3 hours

Adolescents:

Nebulization: 0.5 mg (500 mcg) every 20 minutes for 3 doses, then as needed

Metered-dose inhaler: 8 puffs every 20 minutes as needed for up to 3 hours

Asthma, maintenance (nonacute): Limited data available: **Note:** Evidence is lacking that ipratropium provides added benefit to beta$_2$-agonists in long-term control asthma therapy (GINA; 2012; NIH Guidelines, 2007):

Children <12 years:

Nebulization: 0.25-0.5 mg (250-500 mcg) every 6-8 hours

Metered-dose inhaler: 1-2 inhalations every 6 hours; not to exceed 12 inhalations/day

Children ≥12 years and Adolescents:

Nebulization: 0.25 mg (250 mcg) every 6 hours

Metered-dose inhaler: 2-3 inhalations every 6 hours; maximum daily dose: 12 inhalations/**day**

Bronchospasm associated with chronic pulmonary conditions: Children ≥12 years and Adolescents: Nebulization: 0.5 mg (500 mcg, one unit-dose vial) 3-4 times daily with doses 6-8 hours apart

Adults:

Asthma exacerbation, acute (NIH Asthma Guidelines, 2007):

Nebulization: 0.5 mg (500 mcg, 1 unit dose vial) every 20 minutes for 3 doses, then as needed. **Note:** Should be given in combination with a short acting beta-adrenergic agonist.

Metered-dose inhaler: 8 inhalations every 20 minutes as needed for up to 3 hours. **Note:** Should be given in combination with a short acting beta-adrenergic agonist.

Bronchospasm associated with COPD:

Nebulization: 0.5 mg (500 mcg, one unit-dose vial) 3-4 times daily, with doses 6-8 hours apart

Metered-dose inhaler: 2 inhalations 4 times daily; maximum daily dose: 12 inhalations/**day**

Dosing adjustment in renal impairment: There are no dosage adjustments provided in the manufacturer's labeling (not studied); however, dosage adjustment unlikely necessary due to low systemic absorption.

Dosing adjustment in hepatic impairment: There are no dosage adjustments provided in the manufacturer's labeling (not studied); however, dosage adjustment unlikely necessary due to low systemic absorption.

Administration

Nebulization: May be administered with or without dilution in NS; use of a nebulizer with a mouth piece, rather than a face mask, may be preferred to prevent contact with eyes

Oral Inhalation (metered-dose inhaler): Atrovent HFA: Prior to initial use, prime inhaler by releasing 2 test sprays into the air. If the inhaler has not been used for >3 days, reprime. Avoid spraying into the eyes. Use spacer device in children <8 years; use spacer device and face mask for children ≤4 years.

Additional Information Atrovent® HFA does not contain soya lecithin or any soy ingredients like the previous formulation did. Atrovent HFA supplies 21 mcg/puff from the valve and 17 mcg/puff from the mouthpiece.

Dosage Forms Considerations

Atrovent HFA 12.9 g canister contains 200 inhalations.

Dosage Forms Excipient information presented when available (limited, particularly for generics); consult specific product labeling.

Aerosol Solution, Inhalation, as bromide:

Atrovent HFA: 17 mcg/actuation (12.9 g) [contains alcohol, usp]

Solution, Inhalation, as bromide:

Generic: 0.02% (2.5 mL)

Solution, Inhalation, as bromide [preservative free]:

Generic: 0.02% (2.5 mL)

References

Brundage KL Mohsini KG, Froese AB, et al. Bronchodilator response to ipratropium bromide in infants with bronchopulmonary dysplasia. *Am Rev Respir Dis.* 1990;142:1137-1142.

Fayon M, Tayara N, Germain C, et al. Efficacy and tolerance of high-dose inhaled ipratropium bromide vs. terbutaline in intubated premature human neonates. *Neonatology.* 2007;91:167-173.

Hodges IGC, Groggins RC, Milner AD, et al. Bronchodilator effect of inhaled ipratropium bromide in wheezy toddlers. *Arch Dis Child.* 1981;56(9):729-732.

Lee H, Arnon S, Silverman M. Bronchodilator aerosol administered by metered dose inhaler and spacer in subacute neonatal respiratory distress syndrome. *Archives of Disease in Childhood.* 1994;70:218-222.

National Institute of Health, "Guidelines for the Diagnosis and Management of Asthma. NAEPP Expert Panel Report 3," August 2007. Available at: http://www.nhlbi.nih.gov/guidelines/asthma/asthgdln.pdf.

Prendiville A, Green S, Silverman M. Ipratropium bromide and airways function in wheezy infants. *Archives of Disease in Childhood.* 1987;62:397-400.

Schuh S, Johnson DW, Callahan S, et al, "Efficacy of Frequent Nebulized Ipratropium Bromide Added to Frequent High-Dose Albuterol Therapy in Severe Childhood Asthma," *J Pediatr*, 1995, 126 (4):639-45.

Schuh S, Johnson DW, Canny G, et al, "Efficacy of Adding Nebulized Ipratropium Bromide to Nebulized Albuterol Therapy in Acute Bronchiolitis," *Pediatrics*, 1992, 90(6):920-3.

Stokes GM, Milner AD, Hodges IGC, et al. Nebulized therapy in acute severe bronchitis in infancy. *Archives of Disease In Childhood.* 1983;58:279-282.

Wang EE, Milner R, Allen U, et al, "Bronchodilators for Treatment of Mild Bronchiolitis: A Factorial Randomised Trial," *Arch Dis Child*, 1992, 67(3):289-93.

Wilkie RA and Bryan MH, "Effect of Bronchodilators on Airway Resistance in Ventilator-Dependent Neonates With Chronic Lung Disease," *J Pediatr*, 1987, 111(2):278-82.

Ipratropium (Nasal) (i pra TROE pee um)

Medication Safety Issues

Sound-alike/look-alike issues:

Atrovent® may be confused with Alupent, Serevent®

Ipratropium may be confused with tiotropium

Brand Names: U.S. Atrovent

Brand Names: Canada Alti-Ipratropium; Apo-Ipravent®; Atrovent®; Mylan-Ipratropium Solution

Therapeutic Category Anticholinergic Agent

Generic Availability (U.S.) Yes

Use Symptomatic relief of rhinorrhea associated with allergic and nonallergic rhinitis

Pregnancy Risk Factor B

Pregnancy Considerations Teratogenic effects were not observed in animal studies.

Breast-Feeding Considerations It is not known if ipratropium (nasal) is excreted in breast milk. The manufacturer recommends that caution be exercised when administering ipratropium (nasal) to nursing women.

Contraindications Hypersensitivity to ipratropium, atropine, or any component

Precautions Use with caution in patients with narrow-angle glaucoma, bladder neck obstruction, or prostatic hypertrophy.

Adverse Reactions

Central nervous system: Headache

Gastrointestinal: Diarrhea, nausea, taste perversion, xerostomia

Respiratory: Epistaxis, pharyngitis, nasal congestion, nasal dryness, nasal irritation, upper respiratory tract infection

Rare but important or life-threatening: Anaphylactic reaction, angioedema, blurred vision, conjunctivitis, cough, dizziness, hoarseness, laryngospasm, nasal burning, ocular irritation, palpitation, rash, tachycardia, thirst, tinnitus, urticaria

Drug Interactions

Metabolism/Transport Effects None known.

Avoid Concomitant Use

Avoid concomitant use of Ipratropium (Nasal) with any of the following: Aclidinium; Ipratropium (Oral Inhalation); Potassium Chloride; Tiotropium; Umeclidinium

Increased Effect/Toxicity

Ipratropium (Nasal) may increase the levels/effects of: AbobotulinumtoxinA; Analgesics (Opioid); Anticholinergic Agents; Cannabinoid-Containing Products; Mirabegron; OnabotulinumtoxinA; Potassium Chloride; RimabotulinumtoxinB; Thiazide Diuretics; Tiotropium; Topiramate

The levels/effects of Ipratropium (Nasal) may be increased by: Aclidinium; Ipratropium (Oral Inhalation); Pramlintide; Umeclidinium

Decreased Effect

Ipratropium (Nasal) may decrease the levels/effects of: Acetylcholinesterase Inhibitors (Central); Secretin

The levels/effects of Ipratropium (Nasal) may be decreased by: Acetylcholinesterase Inhibitors (Central)

Stability Store at room temperature.

Mechanism of Action Local application to nasal mucosa inhibits serous and seromucous gland secretions.

Dosing: Usual
Children >6 years and Adults: 0.03%: 2 sprays in each nostril 2-3 times/day
Children >5 years and Adults: 0.06%: 2 sprays in each nostril 3-4 times/day

Administration Pump must be primed before usage by 7 actuations into the air away from the face; if not used for >24 hours, pump must be reprimed with 2 actuations; if not used >7 days, reprime with 7 actuations

Dosage Forms Considerations
Atrovent 0.03% (21 mcg/spray) nasal solution 30 mL bottles contain 345 sprays, and the 0.06% (42 mcg/spray) 15 mL bottles contain 165 sprays.

Dosage Forms Excipient information presented when available (limited, particularly for generics); consult specific product labeling.
Solution, Nasal, as bromide:
Atrovent: 0.03% (30 mL); 0.06% (15 mL)
Generic: 0.03% (30 mL); 0.06% (15 mL)

◆ **Ipratropium Bromide** *see* Ipratropium (Nasal) *on page 1146*

◆ **Ipratropium Bromide** *see* Ipratropium (Oral Inhalation) *on page 1144*

◆ **I-Prin [OTC]** *see* Ibuprofen *on page 1059*

◆ **Iproveratril Hydrochloride** *see* Verapamil *on page 2129*

◆ **IPV** *see* Poliovirus Vaccine (Inactivated) *on page 1694*

Irbesartan (ir be SAR tan)

Medication Safety Issues
Sound-alike/look-alike issues:
Avapro may be confused with Anaprox

Brand Names: U.S. Avapro

Brand Names: Canada Apo-Irbesartan; Auro-Irbesartan; Ava-Irbesartan; Avapro; CO Irbesartan; Dom-Irbesartan; JAMP-Irbesartan; Mylan-Irbesartan; PMS-Irbesartan; RAN-Irbesartan; ratio-Irbesartan; Sandoz-Irbesartan; Teva-Irbesartan

Therapeutic Category Angiotensin II Receptor Blocker; Antihypertensive Agent

Generic Availability (U.S.) Yes

Use Treatment of hypertension alone or in combination with other antihypertensives (FDA approved in adults); treatment of diabetic nephropathy in patients with type 2 diabetes mellitus (noninsulin dependent, NIDDM) and hypertension (FDA approved in adults); has also been used to reduce proteinuria in children with chronic kidney disease either as monotherapy or in addition to ACE inhibitor therapy

Pregnancy Risk Factor D

Pregnancy Considerations [U.S. Boxed Warning]: Drugs that act on the renin-angiotensin system can cause injury and death to the developing fetus. Discontinue as soon as possible once pregnancy is detected. The use of drugs which act on the renin-angiotensin system are associated with oligohydramnios. Oligohydramnios, due to decreased fetal renal function, may lead to fetal lung hypoplasia and skeletal malformations. Use is also associated with anuria, hypotension, renal failure, skull hypoplasia, and death in the fetus/neonate. The exposed fetus should be monitored for fetal growth, amniotic fluid volume, and organ formation. Infants exposed *in utero* should be monitored for hyperkalemia, hypotension, and oliguria (exchange transfusions or dialysis may be needed). These adverse events are generally associated with maternal use in the second and third trimesters.

Untreated chronic maternal hypertension is also associated with adverse events in the fetus, infant, and mother. The use of angiotensin II receptor blockers is not recommended to treat chronic uncomplicated hypertension in pregnant women and should generally be avoided in women of reproductive potential (ACOG, 2013).

Breast-Feeding Considerations It is not known if irbesartan is excreted into breast milk. Due to the potential for serious adverse reactions in the nursing infant, the manufacturer recommends a decision be made whether to discontinue nursing or to discontinue the drug, taking into account the importance of treatment to the mother.

Contraindications Hypersensitivity to irbesartan, any component, or other angiotensin II receptor blockers

Warnings Drugs that act on the renin-angiotensin system can cause injury and death to the developing fetus. Discontinue as soon as possible once pregnancy is detected **[U.S. Boxed Warning]**. Symptomatic hypotension may occur, especially in patients with an activated renin-angiotensin system (eg, volume- or salt-depleted patients receiving high doses of diuretic agents); use with caution in these patients; correct depletion before starting therapy or initiate therapy at a lower dose. Concomitant use of an ACE inhibitor or renin inhibitor (eg, aliskiren) is associated with an increased risk of hypotension, hyperkalemia, and renal dysfunction. Concomitant use with aliskiren should be avoided in patients with GFR <60 mL/minute and is contraindicated in patients with diabetes mellitus (regardless of GFR).

Angioedema has been reported rarely with some angiotensin II receptor antagonists (ARBs) and may occur at any time during treatment (especially following first dose); it may involve the head and neck (potentially compromising airway) or the intestine (presenting with abdominal pain). Patients with idiopathic or hereditary angioedema or previous angioedema associated with ACE-inhibitor therapy may be at an increased risk. Prolonged frequent monitoring may be required, especially if tongue, glottis, or larynx are involved, as they are associated with airway obstruction. Patients with a history of airway surgery may have a higher risk of airway obstruction. Discontinue therapy immediately if angioedema occurs. Aggressive early management is critical. Intramuscular (I.M.) administration of epinephrine may be necessary. Do not readminister to patients who have had angioedema with ARBs.

Precautions Use with caution in patients with impaired renal function; use is associated with deterioration of renal function and/or increases in serum creatinine, particularly in patients with low renal blood flow (eg, renal artery stenosis, heart failure); deterioration may result in oliguria, acute renal failure, or progressive azotemia. Small increases in serum creatinine may occur following initiation; consider discontinuation in patients with progressive and/or significant deterioration in renal function. Hyperkalemia may occur; risk factors include renal dysfunction, diabetes mellitus, concomitant use of potassium-sparing diuretics, potassium supplements, and/or potassium-containing salts; use with caution with these agents; monitor potassium closely.

Adverse Reactions
Cardiovascular: Orthostatic hypotension
Central nervous system: Dizziness, fatigue
Endocrine & metabolic: Hyperkalemia
Gastrointestinal: Diarrhea, dyspepsia
Respiratory: Cough, upper respiratory infection
Rare but important or life-threatening: Anemia (case report; Simonetti, 2007), angina, angioedema, arrhythmia, cardiopulmonary arrest, conjunctivitis, depression, dyspnea, ecchymosis, epistaxis, gout, heart failure, hepatitis, hypotension, jaundice, libido decreased, MI, ▶

orthostatic hypotension, paresthesia, renal failure, renal function impaired, sexual dysfunction, stroke, thrombocytopenia, transaminases increased, urticaria

Drug Interactions

Metabolism/Transport Effects Substrate of CYP2C9 (minor); **Note:** Assignment of Major/Minor substrate status based on clinically relevant drug interaction potential; **Inhibits** CYP2C8 (moderate), CYP2C9 (moderate), CYP2D6 (weak), CYP3A4 (weak)

Avoid Concomitant Use

Avoid concomitant use of Irbesartan with any of the following: Pimozide

Increased Effect/Toxicity

Irbesartan may increase the levels/effects of: ACE Inhibitors; Amifostine; Antihypertensives; ARIPiprazole; Bosentan; Cannabis; Carvedilol; CycloSPORINE (Systemic); CYP2C8 Substrates; CYP2C9 Substrates; Dofetilide; Dronabinol; DULoxetine; Hypotensive Agents; Lithium; Lomitapide; Nonsteroidal Anti-Inflammatory Agents; Obinutuzumab; Pimozide; Potassium-Sparing Diuretics; RiTUXimab; Sodium Phosphates; Tetrahydrocannabinol

The levels/effects of Irbesartan may be increased by: Alfuzosin; Aliskiren; Barbiturates; Brimonidine (Topical); Canagliflozin; Diazoxide; Eplerenone; Fluconazole; Heparin; Heparin (Low Molecular Weight); Herbs (Hypotensive Properties); MAO Inhibitors; Pentoxifylline; Phosphodiesterase 5 Inhibitors; Potassium Salts; Prostacyclin Analogues; Tolvaptan; Trimethoprim

Decreased Effect

The levels/effects of Irbesartan may be decreased by: Herbs (Hypertensive Properties); Methylphenidate; Nonsteroidal Anti-Inflammatory Agents; Rifamycin Derivatives; Yohimbine

Stability Store at controlled room temperature of 25°C (77°F).

Mechanism of Action Irbesartan is an angiotensin receptor antagonist. Angiotensin II acts as a vasoconstrictor. In addition to causing direct vasoconstriction, angiotensin II also stimulates the release of aldosterone. Once aldosterone is released, sodium as well as water are reabsorbed. The end result is an elevation in blood pressure. Irbesartan binds to the AT1 angiotensin II receptor. This binding prevents angiotensin II from binding to the receptor thereby blocking the vasoconstriction and the aldosterone secreting effects of angiotensin II.

Pharmacodynamics Antihypertensive effect:

Onset of action: 1-2 hours

Maximum effect: 3-6 hours postdose; with chronic dosing maximum effect: ~2 weeks

Duration: >24 hours

Pharmacokinetics (Adult data unless noted)

Absorption: Rapid and almost complete

Distribution: V_d: Adults: 53-93 L

Protein binding: 90%, primarily to albumin and alpha$_1$ acid gylcoprotein

Metabolism: Hepatic, via glucuronide conjugation and oxidation; oxidation occurs primarily by cytochrome P450 isoenzyme CYP2C9

Bioavailability: 60% to 80%

Half-life, elimination: Adults: 11-15 hours

Time to peak serum concentration: 1.5-2 hours

Elimination: Excreted via biliary and renal routes; feces (80%); urine (20%)

Dialysis: Not removed by hemodialysis

Dosing: Usual Note: Use a lower starting dose of 50% of the recommended initial dose in volume- and salt-depleted patients.

Children and Adolescents:

Hypertension: Limited data available (NHBPEP, 2004; NHLBI, 2011; Sakarcan, 2001): Oral:

Children 6-12 years: Initial: 75 mg once daily; may be titrated to a maximum dose of 150 mg once daily

Adolescents ≥13 years: Initial: 150 mg once daily; may be titrated to a maximum dose of 300 mg once daily

Proteinuria reduction in children with chronic kidney disease: Limited data available: Oral: Children and Adolescents 4-18 years: Studies utilized a fixed dosage based on weight categories (see below); initial doses were approximately 2 mg/kg once daily; doses were increased after 3-5 weeks and after 8-12 weeks if needed, according to specific blood pressure criteria; median final dose in the largest study (n=44; median age: 10 years): 4 mg/kg once daily (Franscini, 2002; Gartenmann, 2003; von Vigier, 2000)

10-20 kg: Initial: 37.5 mg once daily

21-40 kg: Initial: 75 mg once daily

>40 kg: Initial: 150 mg once daily

Adults:

Hypertension: Oral: Initial: 150 mg once daily; may be titrated to a maximum dose of 300 mg once daily; **Note:** Use a starting dose of 75 mg once daily in volume- or salt-depleted patients.

Nephropathy with type 2 diabetes and hypertension: Oral: Target dose: 300 mg once daily

Dosing adjustment in renal impairment: No dosage adjustment necessary with mild-to-severe impairment unless the patient is also volume depleted.

Dosing adjustment in hepatic impairment: No dosage adjustment is needed.

Administration May be administered without regard to food. Capsules may be opened and mixed with small amount of applesauce prior to administration (Sakaran, 2001).

Monitoring Parameters Blood pressure, BUN, serum creatinine, renal function, baseline and periodic serum electrolytes, urinalysis

Dosage Forms Excipient information presented when available (limited, particularly for generics); consult specific product labeling.

Tablet, Oral:

Avapro: 75 mg, 150 mg, 300 mg

Generic: 75 mg, 150 mg, 300 mg

References

American College of Obstetricians and Gynecologists (ACOG), "ACOG Practice Bulletin No. 125: Chronic Hypertension in Pregnancy," *Obstet Gynecol*, 2012, 119(2 Pt 1):396-407.

Chobanian AV, Bakris GL, Black HR, et al, "The Seventh Report of the Joint National Committee on Prevention, Detection, Evaluation, and Treatment of High Blood Pressure: The JNC 7 Report," *JAMA*, 2003, 289(19):2560-72.

Franscini LM, Von Vigier RO, Pfister R, et al, "Effectiveness and Safety of the Angiotensin II Antagonist Irbesartan in Children With Chronic Kidney Diseases," *Am J Hypertens*, 2002, 15(12):1057-63.

Gartenmann AC, Fossali E, von Vigier RO, et al, "Better Renoprotective Effect of Angiotensin II Antagonist Compared to Dihydropyridine Calcium Channel Blocker in Childhood," *Kidney Int*, 2003, 64 (4):1450-4.

Hogg RJ, Portman RJ, Milliner D, et al, "Evaluation and Management of Proteinuria and Nephrotic Syndrome in Children: Recommendations From a Pediatric Nephrology Panel Established at the National Kidney Foundation Conference on Proteinuria, Albuminuria, Risk, Assessment, Detection, and Elimination (PARADE)," *Pediatrics*, 2000, 105(6):1242-9.

National High Blood Pressure Education Program Working Group on High Blood Pressure in Children and Adolescents, "The Fourth Report on the Diagnosis, Evaluation, and Treatment of High Blood Pressure in Children and Adolescents," *Pediatrics*, 2004, 114(2 Suppl):555-76.

Sakarcan A, Tenney F, Wilson JT, et al, "The Pharmacokinetics of Irbesartan in Hypertensive Children and Adolescents," *J Clin Pharmacol*, 2001, 41(7):742-9.

Simonetti GD, Bianchetti MG, Konrad M, et al, "Severe Anemia Caused by the Angiotensin Receptor Blocker Irbesartan After Renal Transplantation," *Pediatr Nephrol*, 2007, 22(5):756-7.

von Vigier RO, Zberg PM, Teuffel O, et al, "Preliminary Experience With the Angiotensin II Receptor Antagonist Irbesartan in Chronic Kidney Disease," *Eur J Pediatr*, 2000, 159(8):590-3.

Zaffanello M, Franchini M, and Fanos V, "New Therapeutic Strategies With Combined Renin-Angiotensin System Inhibitors for Pediatric Nephropathy," *Pharmacotherapy*, 2008, 28(1):125-30.

Irinotecan (eye rye no TEE kan)

Medication Safety Issues
Sound-alike/look-alike issues:
Irinotecan may be confused with topotecan
High alert medication:
This medication is in a class the Institute for Safe Medication Practices (ISMP) includes among its list of drug classes which have a heightened risk of causing significant patient harm when used in error.

Related Information
Emetogenic Potential of Antineoplastic Agents in Children *on page 2327*
Management of Drug Extravasations *on page 2255*
Safe Handling of Hazardous Drugs *on page 2419*

Brand Names: U.S. Camptosar
Brand Names: Canada Camptosar; Irinotecan Hydrochloride Trihydrate
Therapeutic Category Antineoplastic Agent, Camptothecin; Antineoplastic Agent, Topoisomerase I Inhibitor
Generic Availability (U.S.) Yes
Use Treatment of metastatic carcinoma of the colon or rectum (FDA approved in adults); has also been used in the treatment of advanced nonsmall cell lung cancer, extensive state small cell lung cancer, recurrent or metastatic cervical cancer, esophageal cancer, metastatic or locally advanced gastric cancer, recurrent ovarian cancer, advanced pancreatic cancer, brain tumors (recurrent glioblastoma), and in children to treat recurrent or progressive Ewing's sarcoma, rhabdomyosarcoma, neuroblastoma, and other refractory solid tumors (I.V. and oral)

Pregnancy Risk Factor D
Pregnancy Considerations Adverse events were observed in animal reproduction studies. May cause fetal harm if administered during pregnancy. Women of childbearing potential should avoid becoming pregnant while receiving treatment.

Breast-Feeding Considerations It is not known if irinotecan is excreted in breast milk. Due to the potential for serious adverse reactions in the nursing infant, the manufacturer recommends a decision be made whether to discontinue nursing or to discontinue the drug, taking into account the importance of treatment to the mother.

Contraindications Hypersensitivity to irinotecan or any component; concurrent use with St John's wort or ketoconazole

Warnings Hazardous agent; use appropriate precautions for handling and disposal (NIOSH, 2012). Irinotecan is potentially embryotoxic and teratogenic if administered during pregnant women.

May cause severe, dose-limiting, and potentially fatal diarrhea **[U.S. Boxed Warning]**; early-onset and late-onset forms of severe diarrhea have been reported with irinotecan administration. Early diarrhea has occurred during or shortly after infusion and may be accompanied by symptoms of rhinitis, increased salivation, miosis, lacrimation, diaphoresis, flushing, and abdominal cramping. Atropine 0.01 mg/kg I.V. (maximum dose: 0.4 mg) may be used to prevent or treat symptoms of early diarrhea. Late diarrhea has occurred >24 hours after irinotecan administration and can be prolonged leading to life-threatening dehydration and electrolyte imbalance. Late diarrhea should be promptly treated with loperamide until a normal

pattern of bowel movements returns; fluid and electrolyte replacement may be needed for dehydration. Provide antibiotic support if patient develops persistent diarrhea (grade 3 or 4), ileus, fever, sepsis, or severe neutropenia; cefixime (8 mg/kg/day, maximum dose: 400 mg) has been used in children as prophylaxis for diarrhea beginning 5 days prior to irinotecan therapy and continued throughout course (Wagner, 2008); cefpodoxime (10 mg/kg/day divided twice daily, maximum dose: 200 mg) has also been used (McNall-Knapp, 2010; Wagner, 2010). Interrupt or reduce subsequent irinotecan doses if National Cancer Institute (NCI) grade 3 (increase of 7-9 stools daily, or incontinence, or severe cramping) or grade 4 (increase ≥10 stools daily, grossly bloody stool, or need for parenteral support) late diarrhea occurs. Cases of colitis complicated by ulceration, bleeding, ileus, and infection have been reported; initiate antibiotics promptly in patients with ileus. Renal impairment and acute renal failure have been reported, possibly due to dehydration secondary to diarrhea; use with caution in patients with renal impairment; not recommended in patients on dialysis.

May cause severe myelosuppression **[U.S. Boxed Warning]**; deaths due to sepsis following severe neutropenia have been reported with irinotecan administration; complications due to neutropenia should be promptly managed with antibiotics. Therapy should be temporarily discontinued if neutropenic fever occurs or if the absolute neutrophil count is <1000/mm^3. The dose of irinotecan should be reduced if there is a clinically significant decrease in total WBC (<200/mm^3), neutrophil count (<1500/mm^3), or platelet count (<100,000/mm^3). Fatal cases of interstitial pulmonary disease (IPD)-like events have been reported with single-agent and combination therapy. Promptly evaluate changes in baseline pulmonary symptoms or any new-onset pulmonary symptoms; discontinue therapy if IPD is diagnosed. Patients homozygous for the UGT1A1*28 allele are at increased risk of neutropenia; initial one-level dose reduction should be considered for both single-agent and combination regimens. Heterozygous carriers of the UGT1A1*28 allele may also be at increased risk; however, most patients have tolerated normal starting doses. Patients with abnormal glucuronidation of bilirubin, such as Gilbert's syndrome, may also be at greater risk of myelosuppression when receiving irinotecan. Severe hypersensitivity reactions (including anaphylaxis) have occurred. Thromboembolic events have been reported. Do not use in patients with hereditary fructose intolerance (product contains sorbitol).

Precautions Use with caution and reduce initial irinotecan dose in patients with increased total serum bilirubin concentration (1-2 mg/dL) who previously received pelvic/abdominal radiation therapy. Use with caution in patients with hepatic impairment; exposure to the active metabolite (SN-38) is increased; toxicities may be increased; dosage adjustment should be considered. Patients with even modest elevations in total serum bilirubin levels (1-2 mg/dL) have a significantly greater likelihood of experiencing first-course grade 3 or 4 neutropenia than those with bilirubin levels that were <1 mg/dL. Patients with abnormal glucuronidation of bilirubin, such as those with Gilbert's syndrome, may also be at greater risk of myelosuppression when receiving therapy with irinotecan. Avoid vaccination with live vaccines during treatment (risk of infection may be increased due to immunosuppression). Although the response to vaccines may be diminished, inactivated vaccines may be administered during treatment. High potential for CYP-mediated drug interactions exists; enzyme inducers may decrease exposure to irinotecan and SN-38 (active metabolite); enzyme inhibitors may increase exposure; when used in patients with CNS tumors, selection of antiseizure medications which are not enzyme inducers is preferred. Administer under the ▶

supervision of an experienced cancer chemotherapy physician **[U.S. Boxed Warning]**. Except as part of a clinical trial, use in combination with the fluorouracil and leucovorin "Mayo Clinic" regimen is not recommended. Increased toxicity has also been noted in patients with a baseline performance status of 2 in other combination regimens containing irinotecan, leucovorin, and fluorouracil. For I.V. use only; monitor infusion site; may cause local tissue necrosis or thrombophlebitis if extravasation occurs.

Adverse Reactions

Cardiovascular: Edema, hypotension, thromboembolic events, vasodilation

Central nervous system: Chills, cholinergic toxicity (includes rhinitis, increased salivation, miosis, lacrimation, diaphoresis, flushing and intestinal hyperperistalsis); confusion, dizziness, fever, headache, insomnia, pain, somnolence

Dermatologic: Alopecia, rash

Endocrine & metabolic: Dehydration

Gastrointestinal: Abdominal fullness/pain, anorexia, constipation, cramps, diarrhea (early/late), dyspepsia, flatulence, mucositis, nausea, stomatitis, vomiting, weight loss

Hematologic: Anemia, hemorrhage, leukopenia, neutropenia, neutropenic fever/infection, thrombocytopenia

Hepatic: Alkaline phosphatase increased, ascites and/or jaundice, AST increased, bilirubin increased

Neuromuscular & skeletal: Back pain, weakness

Respiratory: Cough, dyspnea, pneumonia, rhinitis

Miscellaneous: Diaphoresis

Rare but important or life-threatening: ALT increased, amylase increased, anaphylactoid reaction, anaphylaxis, angina, arterial thrombosis, bleeding, bradycardia, cardiac arrest, cerebral infarct, cerebrovascular accident, circulatory failure, colitis, dysrhythmia, embolus, gastrointestinal bleeding, gastrointestinal obstruction, hepatomegaly, hyperglycemia, hypersensitivity, hyponatremia, ileus, interstitial pulmonary disease (IPD), intestinal perforation, ischemic colitis, lipase increased, lymphocytopenia, megacolon, MI, myocardial ischemia, neutropenic typhlitis, pancreatitis, paresthesia, peripheral vascular disorder, pulmonary embolus; pulmonary toxicity (dyspnea, fever, reticulonodular infiltrates on chest x-ray); renal failure (acute), renal impairment, thrombocytopenia (immune mediated), thrombophlebitis, thrombosis, typhlitis, ulcerative colitis

Note: In limited pediatric experience, dehydration (often associated with severe hypokalemia and hyponatremia) was among the most significant grade 3/4 adverse events.

Drug Interactions

Metabolism/Transport Effects Substrate of CYP2B6 (major), CYP3A4 (major), P-glycoprotein, SLCO1B1, UGT1A1; **Note:** Assignment of Major/Minor substrate status based on clinically relevant drug interaction potential

Avoid Concomitant Use

Avoid concomitant use of Irinotecan with any of the following: Atazanavir; BCG; CloZAPine; Conivaptan; Dipyrone; Fusidic Acid (Systemic); Grapefruit Juice; Itraconazole; Ketoconazole (Systemic); Natalizumab; Pimecrolimus; St Johns Wort; Tacrolimus (Topical); Tofacitinib; Vaccines (Live)

Increased Effect/Toxicity

Irinotecan may increase the levels/effects of: CloZAPine; Leflunomide; Natalizumab; Tofacitinib; Vaccines (Live)

The levels/effects of Irinotecan may be increased by: Atazanavir; Bevacizumab; Ceritinib; Conivaptan; CYP2B6 Inhibitors (Moderate); CYP2B6 Inhibitors (Strong); CYP3A4 Inhibitors (Moderate); CYP3A4 Inhibitors (Strong); Dasatinib; Denosumab; Dipyrone;

Eltrombopag; Fusidic Acid (Systemic); Grapefruit Juice; Itraconazole; Ivacaftor; Ketoconazole (Systemic); Luliconazole; Mifepristone; P-glycoprotein/ABCB1 Inhibitors; Pimecrolimus; Quazepam; Regorafenib; Roflumilast; Simeprevir; SORAfenib; Stiripentol; Tacrolimus (Topical); Trastuzumab

Decreased Effect

Irinotecan may decrease the levels/effects of: BCG; Coccidioidin Skin Test; Sipuleucel-T; Vaccines (Inactivated); Vaccines (Live)

The levels/effects of Irinotecan may be decreased by: Bosentan; CarBAMazepine; CYP2B6 Inducers (Strong); CYP3A4 Inducers (Strong); Dabrafenib; Deferasirox; Echinacea; Fosphenytoin; Mitotane; P-glycoprotein/ABCB1 Inducers; PHENobarbital; Phenytoin; Siltuximab; St Johns Wort; Tocilizumab

Stability Hazardous agent; use appropriate precautions for handling and disposal (NIOSH, 2012). Store intact vials at 20°C to 25°C (68°F to 77°F); store unopened Camptosar® vials at 15°C to 30°C (59°F to 86°F); protect from light. After dilution with D_5W, resulting solution is stable for 24 hours if stored at room temperature or 48 hours if stored refrigerated, although the manufacturer recommends use within 6 hours at room temperature and 24 hours if refrigerated. Due to the relatively acidic pH, irinotecan appears to be more stable in D_5W than NS. Solution prepared with NS is stable for 24 hours at room temperature; do not refrigerate NS solutions; visible particulates may develop. Undiluted commercially available injectable solution prepared in oral syringes is stable for 21 days under refrigeration (Wagner, 2010).

Mechanism of Action Irinotecan and its active metabolite (SN-38) bind reversibly to topoisomerase I-DNA complex preventing religation of the cleaved DNA strand. This results in the accumulation of cleavable complexes and double-strand DNA breaks. As mammalian cells cannot efficiently repair these breaks, cell death consistent with S-phase cell cycle specificity occurs, leading to termination of cellular replication.

Pharmacokinetics (Adult data unless noted)

Distribution:

Children and Adolescents: ~37 L/m^2 (range: 15.2-77 L/m^2) (Ma, 2000); distributes to pleural fluid, sweat, and saliva

Adults: 33-150 L/m^2

Protein binding:

Irinotecan: 30% to 68%

SN-38 (active metabolite): 95%

Bioavailability: Median: 9%; increased in presence of gefitinib (median: 42%) (Furman, 2009)

Half-life, terminal:

Children and Adolescents (Ma, 2000):

Irinotecan: 2.66 hours (range: 1.82-4.47 hours)

SN-38 (active metabolite): 1.58 hours (range: 0.29-8.28 hours)

Adults:

Irinotecan: 6-12 hours

SN-38 (active metabolite): 10-20 hours

Time to peak serum concentration:

Irinotecan: Oral: Children and Adolescents: 3 hours (Wagner, 2010a)

SN-38: I.V.: ~1 hour following a 90-minute infusion

Metabolism: Irinotecan is converted to its active metabolite SN-38 by carboxylesterase-mediated cleavage of the carbamate bond. SN-38 undergoes conjugation by the enzyme UDP-glucuronosyl transferase 1A1 (UGT1A1) to a glucuronide metabolite in the liver. Irinotecan also undergoes oxidation by cytochrome P450 3A4 to yield to 2 inactive metabolites.

Elimination: 11% to 20% of irinotecan and <1% SN-38 is excreted in the urine; clearance in children comparable to adult rates although greater interpatient variability in pediatric patients has been reported (Ma, 2000)

Dosing: Usual Note: A reduction in the starting dose by one dose level should be considered for prior pelvic/abdominal radiotherapy, performance status of 2, or known homozygosity for UGT1A1*28 allele. Consider premedication of atropine I.V. or SubQ in patients with cholinergic symptoms (eg, increased salivation, diaphoresis, abdominal cramping) or diarrhea. Details concerning dosage in combination regimens should also be consulted.

Infants, Children, and Adolescents:

Ewing's sarcoma, recurrent or progressive: Children ≥2 years and Adolescents: I.V.: 10-20 mg/m^2/dose once daily on days 1-5 (5 doses) and days 8-12 (5 doses) every 3 weeks; in combination with temozolomide (Casey, 2009; Wagner, 2007)

Neuroblastoma, refractory or palliative: I.V.:
Single-agent: 50 mg/m^2/dose once daily on days 1-5 (5 doses); repeat cycle every 21 days (Kushner, 2005)
Combination therapy: 10 mg/m^2/dose once daily on days 1-5 (5 doses) and days 8-12 (5 doses) ever 3 weeks with temozolomide; may repeat up to 6 cycles (Bagatell, 2010)

Refractory solid tumor or CNS tumor (low-dose, protracted schedule): I.V.:
Single-agent: 15-20 mg/m^2/dose once daily on days 1-5 (5 doses) and days 8-12 (5 doses) every 3 weeks; higher doses may be tolerated (30 mg/m^2/dose) with concurrent cefpodoxime therapy (Cosetti, 2002; McGregor, 2011)
Combination therapy:
With temozolomide: Irinotecan dose: 10 mg/m^2/dose once daily on days 1-5 (5 doses) and days 8-12 (5 doses) ever 3 weeks; may repeat up to 6 cycles (Bagatell, 2010)
With temozolomide and vincristine: Irinotecan dose: 15 mg/m^2/dose once daily on days 1-5 (5 doses) and days 8-12 (5 doses) of a 28-day treatment cycle; may repeat cycle if tolerated (McNall-Knapp, 2010)

Refractory solid tumor or CNS tumor: Children and Adolescents:
I.V.:
Single-agent: 50 mg/m^2/dose once daily on days 1-5 (5 doses); repeat cycle every 21 days (Kushner, 2005)
Weekly regimen (Bomgaars, 2006):
Heavily pretreated patients: 125 mg/m^2/dose once weekly for 4 weeks over 90 minutes, repeat cycle every 6 weeks
Less-heavily pretreated patients: 160 mg/m^2/dose once weekly for 4 weeks over 90 minutes, repeat cycle every 6 weeks
Oral: Combination therapy: 90 mg/m^2/dose once daily on days 1-5 (5 doses) repeat every 3 weeks; in combination with vincristine and temozolomide (Wagner, 2010a)

Rhabdomyosarcoma, refractory or metastatic: I.V.:
Single-agent (Vassal, 2007):
<10 kg: 20 mg/**kg**/dose once every 3 weeks; if dosage reduction necessary, next cycle was 17 mg/kg/dose; if further dosage reduction necessary due to toxicity, subsequent cycles were 14 mg/kg/dose
≥10 kg: 600 mg/m^2/dose once every 3 weeks; if dosage reduction necessary, next cycle was 500 mg/m^2/dose; if further dosage reduction necessary due to toxicity, subsequent cycles were 420 mg/m^2/dose

Combination therapy with vincristine:
High-dose, short schedule: 50 mg/m^2/dose once daily for 5 days on weeks 1 and 4 (Mascarenhas, 2010)
Low-dose, protracted schedule: 20 mg/m^2/dose once daily for 5 days followed by 2 days of rest then 20 mg/m^2/dose once daily for 5 days on weeks 0, 1, 3, and 4; maximum dose: 40 mg (Pappo, 2007)

Adults:

Colorectal cancer, metastatic (single-agent therapy):
I.V.:
Weekly regimen: 125 mg/m^2 over 90 minutes on days 1, 8, 15, and 22 of a 6-week treatment cycle (may adjust upward to 150 mg/m^2 if tolerated)
Adjusted dose level -1: 100 mg/m^2
Adjusted dose level -2: 75 mg/m^2
Further adjust to 50 mg/m^2 (in decrements of 25-50 mg/m^2) if needed
Once-every-3-week regimen: 350 mg/m^2 over 90 minutes, once every 3 weeks
Adjusted dose level -1: 300 mg/m^2
Adjusted dose level -2: 250 mg/m^2
Further adjust to 200 mg/m^2 (in decrements of 25-50 mg/m^2) if needed

Colorectal cancer, metastatic (in combination with fluorouracil and leucovorin): I.V.: Six-week (42-day) cycle:
Regimen 1: 125 mg/m^2 over 90 minutes on days 1, 8, 15, and 22; to be given in combination with bolus leucovorin and fluorouracil (leucovorin administered immediately following irinotecan; fluorouracil immediately following leucovorin)
Adjusted dose level -1: 100 mg/m^2
Adjusted dose level -2: 75 mg/m^2
Further adjust if needed in decrements of ~20%
Regimen 2: 180 mg/m^2 over 90 minutes on days 1, 15, and 29; to be given in combination with infusional leucovorin and bolus/infusion fluorouracil (leucovorin administered immediately following irinotecan; fluorouracil immediately following leucovorin)
Adjusted dose level -1: 150 mg/m^2
Adjusted dose level -2: 120 mg/m^2
Further adjust if needed in decrements of ~20%

Dosing adjustment in renal impairment: Adults:
Renal impairment: No dosage adjustment provided in manufacturer's labeling (has not been studied); use with caution.
Dialysis: Use in patients with dialysis is not recommended by the manufacturer; however, literature suggests reducing weekly dose from 125 mg/m^2 to 50 mg/m^2 and administering after hemodialysis or on nondialysis days (Janus, 2010).

Dosing adjustment in hepatic impairment:
Liver metastases with normal hepatic function: No adjustment required.
Bilirubin >ULN to ≤2 mg/dL: Consider reducing initial dose by one dose level.
Bilirubin >2 mg/dL: Use is not recommended.
The following guidelines have been used by some clinicians: Bilirubin 1.5-3 mg/dL: Administer 75% of dose (Floyd, 2006).

Dosing adjustment for toxicity: It is recommended that new courses begin only after the granulocyte count recovers to ≥1500/mm^3, the platelet counts recover to ≥100,000/mm^3, and treatment-related diarrhea has fully resolved. Depending on the patient's ability to tolerate therapy, adult doses should be adjusted in increments of 25-50 mg/m^2. Treatment should be delayed 1-2 weeks to allow for recovery from treatment-related toxicities. If the patient has not recovered after a 2-week delay, consider discontinuing irinotecan. See table on the next page for adult dosage recommendations.

Colorectal Cancer: Single-Agent Schedule: Recommended Adult Dosage Modifications[1]

Toxicity NCI Grade[2] (Value)	During a Cycle of Therapy	At Start of Subsequent Cycles of Therapy (After Adequate Recovery), Compared to Starting Dose in Previous Cycle[1]	
	Weekly	Weekly	Once Every 3 Weeks
No toxicity	Maintain dose level	↑ 25 mg/m² up to a maximum dose of 150 mg/m²	Maintain dose level
Neutropenia			
1 (1500-1999/mm³)	Maintain dose level	Maintain dose level	Maintain dose level
2 (1000-1499/mm³)	↓ 25 mg/m²	Maintain dose level	Maintain dose level
3 (500-999/mm³)	Omit dose until resolved to ≤grade 2, then ↓ 25 mg/m²	↓ 25 mg/m²	↓ 50 mg/m²
4 (<500/mm³)	Omit dose until resolved to ≤grade 2, then ↓ 50 mg/m²	↓ 50 mg/m²	↓ 50 mg/m²
Neutropenic Fever (grade 4 neutropenia and ≥grade 2 fever)	Omit dose until resolved, then ↓ 50 mg/m²	↓ 50 mg/m²	↓ 50 mg/m²
Other Hematologic Toxicities	Dose modifications for leukopenia, thrombocytopenia, and anemia during a course of therapy and at the start of subsequent courses of therapy are also based on NCI toxicity criteria and are the same as recommended for neutropenia above.		
Diarrhea			
1 (2-3 stools/day >pretreatment)	Maintain dose level	Maintain dose level	Maintain dose level
2 (4-6 stools/day >pretreatment)	↓ 25 mg/m²	Maintain dose level	Maintain dose level
3 (7-9 stools/day >pretreatment)	Omit dose until resolved to ≤grade 2, then ↓ 25 mg/m²	↓ 25 mg/m²	↓ 50 mg/m²
4 (≥10 stools/day >pretreatment)	Omit dose until resolved to ≤grade 2, then ↓ 50 mg/m²	↓ 50 mg/m²	↓ 50 mg/m²
Other Nonhematologic Toxicities[3]			
1	Maintain dose level	Maintain dose level	Maintain dose level
2	↓ 25 mg/m²	↓ 25 mg/m²	↓ 50 mg/m²
3	Omit dose until resolved to ≤grade 2, then ↓ 25 mg/m²	↓ 25 mg/m²	↓ 50 mg/m²
4	Omit dose until resolved to ≤grade 2, then ↓ 50 mg/m²	↓ 50 mg/m²	↓ 50 mg/m²

[1]All dose modifications should be based on the worst preceding toxicity.

[2]National Cancer Institute Common Toxicity Criteria (version 1.0).

[3]Excludes alopecia, anorexia, asthenia.

Administration Hazardous agent; use appropriate precautions for handling and disposal (NIOSH, 2012).

Oral: In clinical pediatric trials, doses were prepared using commercially available injectable solution (20 mg/mL); doses were drawn up in oral syringes and refrigerated until ready for use; for administration, dose was mixed with cranberry grape juice (Wagner, 2010; Wagner 2010a)

Parenteral: I.V. infusion: Irinotecan should be further diluted in D₅W (preferred diluent) or NS to a final concentration of 0.12-2.8 mg/mL; infuse usually over 90 minutes dependent upon specific protocol. Higher incidence of cholinergic symptoms have been reported with more rapid infusion rates; consider premedication with atropine and oral cephalosporin antibiotics; pH:3-3.8.

Vesicant/Extravasation Risk May be an irritant

Monitoring Parameters Signs of diarrhea and dehydration, serum electrolytes, serum BUN and creatinine; infusion site for signs of inflammation; CBC with differential and platelet count, hemoglobin, liver function tests, and serum bilirubin

A test is available for genotyping of UGT1A1; however, guidelines for use are not established and not recommended in patients who have experienced toxicity as a dose reduction is already recommended (NCCN Colon Cancer Guidelines v.1.2011)

Additional Information Loperamide dosing for treatment of late diarrhea: Oral:

8-10 kg: 1 mg after the first loose bowel movement followed by 0.5 mg every 3 hours until a normal pattern of bowel movement returns. Take 0.75 mg every 4 hours during the night rather than every 3 hours.

10.1-20 kg: 1 mg after the first loose bowel movement followed by 1 mg every 3 hours until a normal pattern of bowel movement returns. Take 1 mg every 4 hours during the night rather than every 3 hours.

20.1-30 kg: 2 mg after the first loose bowel movement followed by 1 mg every 3 hours until a normal pattern of bowel movement returns. Take 2 mg every 4 hours during the night rather than every 3 hours.

30.1-43 kg: 2 mg after the first loose bowel movement followed by 1 mg every 2 hours until a normal pattern of bowel movement returns. Take 2 mg every 4 hours during the night rather than every 2 hours.

>43 kg: 4 mg after the first loose bowel movement followed by 2 mg every 2 hours until the patient is diarrhea free for 12 hours. Take 4 mg every 4 hours during the night rather than every 2 hours.

Dosage Forms Excipient information presented when available (limited, particularly for generics); consult specific product labeling.

Solution, Intravenous, as hydrochloride:
Camptosar: 40 mg/2 mL (2 mL); 100 mg/5 mL (5 mL); 300 mg/15 mL (15 mL)
Generic: 40 mg/2 mL (2 mL); 100 mg/5 mL (5 mL); 500 mg/25 mL (25 mL)

Solution, Intravenous, as hydrochloride [preservative free]:
Generic: 40 mg/2 mL (2 mL); 100 mg/5 mL (5 mL)

References

Bagatell R, London WB, Wagner LM, et al, "Phase II Study of Irinotecan and Temozolomide in Children With Relapsed or Refractory Neuroblastoma: A Children's Oncology Group Study," J Clin Oncol, 2011, 29 (2):208-13.

Bomgaars L, Kerr J, Berg S, et al, "A Phase I Study of Irinotecan Administered on a Weekly Schedule in Pediatric Patients," Pediatr Blood Cancer, 2006, 46(1):50-5.

Bomgaars LR, Bernstein M, Krailo M, et al, "Phase II Trial of Irinotecan in Children With Refractory Solid Tumors: A Children's Oncology Group Study," J Clin Oncol, 2007, 25(29):4622-7.

Casey DA, Wexler LH, Merchant MS, et al, "Irinotecan and Temozolomide for Ewing Sarcoma: The Memorial Sloan-Kettering Experience," Pediatr Blood Cancer, 2009, 53(6):1029-34.

Cosetti M, Wexler LH, Calleja E, et al, "Irinotecan for Pediatric Solid Tumors: The Memorial Sloan-Kettering Experience," J Pediatr Hematol Oncol, 2002, 24(2):101-5.

Floyd J, Mirza I, Sachs B, et al, "Hepatotoxicity of Chemotherapy," Semin Oncol, 2006, 33(1):50-67.

Furman WL, Navid F, Daw NC, et al, "Tyrosine Kinase Inhibitor Enhances the Bioavailability of Oral Irinotecan in Pediatric Patients With Refractory Solid Tumors," J Clin Oncol, 2009, 27(27):4599-604.

Gajjar A, Chintagumpala MM, Bowers DC, et al, "Effect of Intrapatient Dosage Escalation of Irinotecan on Its Pharmacokinetics in Pediatric Patients Who Have High-Grade Gliomas and Receive Enzyme-Inducing Anticonvulsant Therapy," Cancer, 2003, 97(9 Suppl):2374-80.

Janus N, Thariat J, Boulanger H, et al, "Proposal for Dosage Adjustment and Timing of Chemotherapy in Hemodialyzed Patients," *Ann Oncol,* 2010, 21(7):1395-403.

Kushner BH, Kramer K, Modak S, et al, "Five-Day Courses of Irinotecan as Palliative Therapy for Patients With Neuroblastoma," *Cancer,* 2005, 103(4):858-62.

Ma MK, Zamboni WC, Radomski KM, et al, "Pharmacokinetics of Irinotecan and Its Metabolites SN-38 and APC in Children With Recurrent Solid Tumors After Protracted Low-Dose Irinotecan," *Clin Cancer Res,* 2000, 6(3):813-9.

Mascarenhas L, Lyden ER, Breitfeld PP, et al, "Randomized Phase II Window Trial of Two Schedules of Irinotecan With Vincristine in Patients With First Relapse or Progression of Rhabdomyosarcoma: A Report From the Children's Oncology Group," *J Clin Oncol,* 2010, 28(30):4658-63.

McGregor LM, Stewart CF, Crews KR, et al, "Dose Escalation of Intravenous Irinotecan Using Oral Cefpodoxime: A Phase I Study in Pediatric Patients With Refractory Solid Tumors," *Pediatr Blood Cancer,* 2012, 58(3):372-9.

McNall-Knapp RY, Williams CN, Reeves EN, et al, "Extended Phase I Evaluation of Vincristine, Irinotecan, Temozolomide, and Antibiotic in Children With Refractory Solid Tumors," *Pediatr Blood Cancer,* 2010, 54(7):909-15.

National Institute for Occupational Safety and Health (NIOSH), "NIOSH List of Antineoplastic and Other Hazardous Drugs in Healthcare Settings 2012." Available at http://www.cdc.gov/niosh/docs/2012-150/pdfs/2012-150.pdf. Accessed January 21, 2013.

Pappo AS, Lyden E, Breitfeld P, et al, "Two Consecutive Phase II Window trials of Irinotecan Alone or in Combination With Vincristine for the Treatment of Metastatic Rhabdomyosarcoma: The Children's Oncology Group," *J Clin Oncol,* 2007, 25(4):362-9.

Vassal G, Couanet D, Stockdale E, et al, "Phase II Trial of Irinotecan in Children With Relapsed or Refractory Rhabdomyosarcoma: A Joint Study of the French Society of Pediatric Oncology and the United Kingdom Children's Cancer Study Group," *J Clin Oncol,* 2007, 25 (4):356-61.

Wagner LM, Crews KR, Stewart CF, et al, "Reducing Irinotecan-Associated Diarrhea in Children," *Pediatr Blood Cancer,* 2008, 50 (2):201-7.

Wagner LM, McAllister N, Goldsby RE, et al, "Temozolomide and Intravenous Irinotecan for Treatment of Advanced Ewing Sarcoma," *Pediatr Blood Cancer,* 2007, 48(2):132-9.

Wagner LM, "Oral Irinotecan for Treatment of Pediatric Solid Tumors: Ready for Prime Time?" *Pediatr Blood Cancer,* 2010, 54(5):661-2.

Wagner LM, Perentesis JP, Reid JM, et al, "Phase I Trial of Two Schedules of Vincristine, Oral irinotecan, and Temozolomide (VOIT) for Children With Relapsed or Refractory Solid Tumors: A Children's Oncology Group Phase I Consortium Study," *Pediatr Blood Cancer,* 2010a, 54(4):538-45.

◆ **Irinotecan HCl** see Irinotecan on page 1149

◆ **Irinotecan Hydrochloride** see Irinotecan on page 1149

◆ **Irinotecan Hydrochloride Trihydrate (Can)** see Irinotecan on page 1149

◆ **Iron Dextran** see Iron Dextran Complex on page 1153

Iron Dextran Complex
(EYE ern DEKS tran KOM pleks)

Medication Safety Issues
Sound-alike/look-alike issues:
Dexferrum may be confused with Desferal
Iron dextran complex may be confused with ferumoxytol
Brand Names: U.S. Dexferrum; Infed
Brand Names: Canada Dexiron; Infufer
Therapeutic Category Iron Salt, Parenteral; Mineral, Parenteral
Generic Availability (U.S.) No
Use Treatment of iron deficiency when oral iron administration is infeasible or ineffective (FDA approved in children ≥4 months and adults)
Pregnancy Risk Factor C
Pregnancy Considerations Adverse events have been observed in animal reproduction studies. It is not known if iron dextran (as iron dextran) crosses the placenta. It is recommended that pregnant women meet the dietary requirements of iron with diet and/or supplements in order to prevent adverse events associated with iron deficiency anemia in pregnancy. Treatment of iron deficiency anemia in pregnant women is the same as in nonpregnant women

and in most cases, oral iron preparations may be used. Except in severe cases of maternal anemia, the fetus achieves normal iron stores regardless of maternal concentrations.

Breast-Feeding Considerations Trace amounts of iron dextran (as iron dextran) are found in human milk. Iron is normally found in breast milk. Breast milk or iron fortified formulas generally provide enough iron to meet the recommended dietary requirements of infants. The amount of iron in breast milk is generally not influenced by maternal iron status.

Contraindications Hypersensitivity to the iron formulation or any component; any anemia not associated with iron deficiency

Warnings Deaths associated with parenteral iron administration following anaphylactic-type reactions have been reported **[U.S. Boxed Warning]**; treatment agents for anaphylactic reactions (eg, epinephrine, steroids, diphenhydramine) should be immediately available; a test dose is recommended prior to initial therapy; however, anaphylactic and other hypersensitivity reactions have occurred after uneventful test doses. The full risk of hypersensitivity reactions, including anaphylaxis with iron dextran products, is unknown and variable among the products; a history of drug allergy or concomitant ACE inhibitor therapy has been shown to increase risk. Iron dextran products are available in two chemical formulations that are not clinically interchangeable; a high-molecular-weight formulation (DexFerrum®) and a low-molecular-weight (INFeD®). Adverse events (including life-threatening) associated with iron dextran usually occur more with the high-molecular-weight formulation (DexFerrum®) compared to the low-molecular-weight (INFeD®) (Chertow, 2006). Rapid I.V. administration is associated with flushing; fatigue; weakness; hypotension; and chest, back, groin, or flank pain. Delayed (1-2 days) infusion reaction, including sweating, urticaria, arthralgia, back pain, chills, dizziness, and fever, may occur with large doses (eg, total dose infusion) of I.V. iron dextran; usually subsides within 3-4 days. May also occur (less commonly) with I.M. administration; subsiding within 3-7 days. Use parenteral iron only in patients where the iron deficient state is not amenable to oral iron therapy; only INFeD® is approved for I.M. administration.

Precautions Use with caution in patients with histories of significant allergies, asthma, serious hepatic impairment, preexisting cardiac disease (may exacerbate cardiovascular complications), and rheumatoid arthritis (may exacerbate joint pain and swelling); avoid use during acute kidney infection. Discontinue oral iron prior to initiating parenteral iron therapy. Exogenous hemosiderosis may result from excess iron stores; patients with refractory anemias and/or hemoglobinopathies may be prone to iron overload with unwarranted iron supplementation. Intramuscular injections of iron-carbohydrate complexes may have a risk of delayed injection site tumor development. Intramuscular iron dextran use in neonates may be associated with an increased incidence of gram negative sepsis.

In patients with chronic kidney disease (CKD) requiring iron supplementation, the I.V. route is preferred for hemodialysis patients; either oral iron or I.V. iron may be used for nondialysis and peritoneal dialysis CKD patients. In patients with cancer-related anemia (either due to cancer or chemotherapy-induced) requiring iron supplementation, the I.V. route is superior to oral therapy; I.M. administration is not recommended for parenteral iron supplementation.

Adverse Reactions Adverse event risk is reported to be higher with the high-molecular-weight iron dextran formulation.

Cardiovascular: Arrhythmia, bradycardia, cardiac arrest, chest pain, chest tightness, cyanosis, flushing, hyper-/hypotension, shock, syncope, tachycardia

Central nervous system: Chills, disorientation, dizziness, fever, headache, malaise, seizure, unconsciousness, unresponsiveness

Dermatologic: Pruritus, purpura, rash, urticaria

Gastrointestinal: Abdominal pain, diarrhea, nausea, taste alteration, vomiting

Genitourinary: Discoloration of urine

Hematologic: Leukocytosis, lymphadenopathy

Local: Injection site reactions (cellulitis, inflammation, pain, phlebitis, soreness, swelling), muscle atrophy/fibrosis (with I.M. injection), skin/tissue staining (at the site of I.M. injection), sterile abscess

Neuromuscular & skeletal: Arthralgia, arthritis/arthritis exacerbation, back pain, myalgia, paresthesia, weakness

Respiratory: Bronchospasm, dyspnea, respiratory arrest, wheezing

Renal: Hematuria

Miscellaneous: Anaphylactic reactions (sudden respiratory difficulty, cardiovascular collapse), diaphoresis

Postmarketing and/or case reports: Angioedema, tumor formation (at former injection site)

Drug Interactions

Metabolism/Transport Effects None known.

Avoid Concomitant Use

Avoid concomitant use of Iron Dextran Complex with any of the following: Dimercaprol

Increased Effect/Toxicity

The levels/effects of Iron Dextran Complex may be increased by: ACE Inhibitors; Dimercaprol

Decreased Effect There are no known significant interactions involving a decrease in effect.

Stability Store at 20°C to 25°C (68°F to 77°F); excursions permitted to 15°C to 30°C (59°F to 86°F). Variable stability reported in parenteral nutrition solution. Stable for 48 hours at room temperature in neonatal parenteral nutrition solution containing at least 2% protein (Mayhew, 1997).

Mechanism of Action The released iron, from the plasma, eventually replenishes the depleted iron stores in the bone marrow where it is incorporated into hemoglobin

Pharmacodynamics

Onset of action: Hematologic response to either oral or parenteral iron salts is essentially the same; red blood cell form and color changes within 3-10 days

Maximum effect: Peak reticulocytosis occurs in 5-10 days, and hemoglobin values increase within 2-4 weeks; serum ferritin peak: 7-9 days after I.V. dose

Pharmacokinetics (Adult data unless noted)

Absorption: I.M.: 60% absorbed after 3 days; 90% after 1-3 weeks, the balance is slowly absorbed over months

Note: Following I.V. doses, the uptake of iron by the reticuloendothelial system appears to be constant at about 40-60 mg/hour

Half-life: 48 hours

Elimination: By the reticuloendothelial system and excreted in urine and feces (via bile)

Dialysis: Not dialyzable

Dosing: Neonatal I.V. (Dexferrum®, INFeD®): **Note: Multiple forms for parenteral iron exist; close attention must be paid to the specific product when ordering and administering**; incorrect selection or substitution of one form for another without proper dosage adjustment may result in serious over- or underdosing; test doses are recommended before starting therapy.

Anemia of prematurity: 0.2-1 mg/kg/day or 20 mg/kg/week with epoetin alfa therapy

Dosing: Usual

Multiple forms for parenteral iron exist; close attention must be paid to the specific product when ordering and administering; incorrect selection or substitution of one form for another without proper dosage adjustment

may result in serious over- or underdosing; test doses are recommended before starting therapy.

Iron deficiency anemia:

I.M. (INFeD®), I.V. (Dexferrum®, INFeD®): Test dose (given 1 hour prior to starting iron dextran therapy):

Infants <10 kg: 10 mg (0.2 mL)

Children 10-20 kg: 15 mg (0.3 mL)

Children >20 kg, Adolescents, and Adults: 25 mg (0.5 mL)

Total replacement dosage of iron dextran for iron deficiency anemia:

(mL) = 0.0442 x LBW (kg) x (Hb$_n$ - Hb$_o$) + [0.26 x LBW (kg)]

LBW = lean body weight

Hb$_n$ = desired hemoglobin (g/dL) = 12 if <15 kg or 14.8 if >15 kg

Hb$_o$ = measured hemoglobin (g/dL)

Acute blood loss; total iron replacement dosage:

Assumes 1 mL of normocytic, normochromic red cells = 1 mg elemental iron

Iron dextran (mL) = 0.02 x blood loss (mL) x hematocrit (expressed as a decimal fraction)

Note: Total dose infusions have been used safely and are the preferred method of administration

I.M., I.V.: Maximum daily dose: Injected in daily or less frequent increments:

Infants <5 kg: 25 mg (0.5 mL)

Children 5-10 kg: 50 mg (1 mL)

Children >10 kg and Adults: 100 mg (2 mL)

Anemia of chronic renal failure: I.V.: National Kidney Foundation DOQI Guidelines: **Note:** Initiation of iron therapy, determination of dose, and duration of therapy should be guided by results of iron status tests combined with the Hb level and the dose of the erythropoietin stimulating agent. See Reference Range for target levels. There is insufficient evidence to recommend I.V. iron if ferritin level >500 ng/mL.

Infants and Children: Predialysis or peritoneal dialysis: As a single dose repeated as often as necessary:

<10 kg: 125 mg

10-20 kg: 250 mg

>20 kg: 500 mg

Infants and Children: Hemodialysis: Given during each dialysis for 10 doses:

<10 kg: 25 mg

10-20 kg: 50 mg

>20 kg: 100 mg

Adults: Initial: 100 mg at every dialysis for 10 doses; maintenance: 25-100 mg once, twice, or three times/week for 10 weeks (should provide 250-1000 mg total dose within 12 weeks)

Cancer-associated anemia: Adults: I.V.: 25 mg slow I.V. push test dose, followed 1 hour later by 100 mg over 5 minutes; larger doses, up to total dose infusion (over several hours) may be administered

Administration

Parenteral: Avoid dilution in dextrose due to an increased incidence of local pain and phlebitis

I.M.: Use Z-track technique for I.M. administration (deep into the upper outer quadrant of buttock); alternate buttocks with subsequent injections; administer test dose at same recommended site using the same technique.

I.V.: Infuse test dose over at least 30 seconds (INFeD®) or 5 minutes (Dexferrum®); may be injected undiluted at a rate not to exceed 50 mg/minute; dilute large or total replacement doses in NS (50-100 mL), maximum concentration 50 mg/mL and infuse over 1-6 hours at a maximum rate of 50 mg/minute

Monitoring Parameters Vital signs and other symptoms of anaphylactoid reactions (during I.V. infusion); reticulocyte count, serum ferritin, hemoglobin, serum iron concentrations, and transferrin saturation (TSAT). Ferritin and

TSAT may be inaccurate if measured within 14 days of receiving a large single dose (1000 mg in adults).

Reference Range

Serum iron:

Newborns: 110-270 mcg/dL

Infants: 30-70 mcg/dL

Children: 55-120 mcg/dL

Adults: Male: 75-175 mcg/dL; female: 65-165 mcg/dL

Total iron binding capacity:

Newborns: 59-175 mcg/dL

Infants: 100-400 mcg/dL

Children and Adults: 230-430 mcg/dL

Transferrin: 204-360 mg/dL

Percent transferrin saturation (TSAT): 20% to 50%

Iron levels >300 mcg/dL may be considered toxic; should be treated as an overdosage

Ferritin: 13-300 ng/mL

Chronic kidney disease (CKD): Targets for iron therapy (KDOQI Guidelines, 2007) to maintain Hgb 11-12 g/dL:

Children: Nondialysis CKD, hemodialysis, or peritoneal dialysis: Ferritin: >100 ng/mL and TSAT >20%

Adults: Nondialysis (CKD) or peritoneal dialysis: Ferritin: >100 ng/mL and TSAT >20%

Hemodialysis: Ferritin >200 ng/mL and TSAT >20% or CHr (content of hemoglobin in reticulocytes) >29 pg/cell

Test Interactions May cause falsely elevated values of serum bilirubin and falsely decreased values of serum calcium. Residual iron dextran may remain in reticuloendothelial cells; may affect accuracy of examination of bone marrow iron stores. Bone scans with 99m Tc-labeled bone seeking agents may show reduced bony uptake, marked renal activity, and excess blood pooling and soft tissue accumulation following I.V. iron dextran infusion or with high serum ferritin levels. Following I.M. iron dextran, bone scans with 99m Tc-diphosphonate may show dense activity in the buttocks.

Additional Information Iron storage may lag behind the appearance of normal red blood cell morphology; use periodic hematologic determination to assess therapy

Dosage Forms Considerations

Strength of iron dextran complex is expressed as elemental iron.

Dosage Forms Excipient information presented when available (limited, particularly for generics); consult specific product labeling.

Solution, Injection:

Dexferrum: 50 mg/mL (1 mL, 2 mL)

Infed: 50 mg/mL (2 mL)

References

Auerbach M, Ballard H, Trout JR, et al, "Intravenous Iron Optimizes the Response to Recombinant Human Erythropoietin in Cancer Patients With Chemotherapy-Related Anemia: A Multicenter, Open-Label, Randomized Trial," *J Clin Oncol*, 2004, 22(7):1301-7.

Auerbach M, Witt D, and Toler W, "Clinical Use of the Total Dose Intravenous Infusion of Iron Dextran," *J Lab Clin Med*, 1988, 111 (5):566-70.

Benito RP and Guerrero TC, "Response to a Single Intravenous Dose Versus Multiple Intramuscular Administration of Iron Dextran Complex: A Comparative Study," *Curr Ther Res Clin Exp*, 1973, 15 (7):373-82.

Chertow GM, Mason PD, Vaage-Nilsen O, et al, "Update on Adverse Drug Events Associated With Parenteral Iron," *Nephrol Dial Transplant*, 2006, 21(2):378-82.

Friel JK, Andrews WL, Hall MS, et al, "Intravenous Iron Administration to Very-Low-Birth-Weight Newborns Receiving Total and Partial Parenteral Nutrition," *JPEN J Parenter Enteral Nutr*, 1995, 19 (2):114-8.

"KDOQI Clinical Practice Guideline and Clinical Practice Recommendations for Anemia in Chronic Kidney Disease: 2007 Update of Hemoglobin Target," *Am J Kidney Dis*, 2007, 50(3):471-530.

Mayhew SL and Quick MW, "Compatibility of Iron Dextran With Neonatal Parenteral Nutrient Solutions," *Am J Health Syst Pharm*, 1997, 54(5):570-1.

National Comprehensive Cancer Network® (NCCN), "Practice Guidelines in Oncology™: Cancer- and Chemotherapy-Induced Anemia

Version 3.2009." Available at http://www.nccn.org/professionals/physician_gls/PDF/anemia.pdf.

♦ **Iron Fumarate** *see* Ferrous Fumarate *on page 865*

♦ **Iron Gluconate** *see* Ferrous Gluconate *on page 866*

♦ **Iron-Polysaccharide Complex** *see* Polysaccharide-Iron Complex *on page 1701*

Iron Sucrose (EYE ern SOO krose)

Medication Safety Issues

Sound-alike/look-alike issues:

Iron sucrose may be confused with ferumoxytol

Brand Names: U.S. Venofer

Brand Names: Canada Venofer

Therapeutic Category Iron Salt, Parenteral; Mineral, Parenteral

Generic Availability (U.S.) No

Use Treatment of iron deficiency anemia in hemodialysis-dependent chronic kidney disease (HDD-CKD) (FDA approved in ages ≥2 years and adults); treatment of iron deficiency anemia with concurrent erythropoietin therapy in peritoneal dialysis-dependent (PDD) CKD and nondialysis-dependent (NDD) CKD (FDA approved in ages ≥2 years); treatment of iron deficiency anemia in PDD-CKD and NDD-CKD (FDA approved in adults); has also been used for treatment of nonrenal iron deficiency anemia and supplementation of iron in patients for which oral therapy is neither effective nor tolerated (eg, long-term TPN)

Pregnancy Risk Factor B

Pregnancy Considerations Teratogenic effects were not observed in animal studies. There are no adequate and well-controlled studies in pregnant women. Based on limited data, iron sucrose may be effective for the treatment of iron-deficiency anemia in pregnancy. It is recommended that pregnant women meet the dietary requirements of iron with diet and/or supplements in order to prevent adverse events associated with iron deficiency anemia in pregnancy. Treatment of iron deficiency anemia in pregnant women is the same as in nonpregnant women and in most cases, oral iron preparations may be used. Except in severe cases of maternal anemia, the fetus achieves normal iron stores regardless of maternal concentrations.

Breast-Feeding Considerations Iron is normally found in breast milk. Breast milk or iron fortified formulas generally provide enough iron to meet the recommended dietary requirements of infants. The amount of iron in breast milk is generally not influenced by maternal iron status.

Contraindications Hypersensitivity to the iron formulation or any component

Warnings Cases of hypersensitivity reactions, including rare postmarketing anaphylactic and anaphylactoid reactions (some fatal), have been reported; monitor patients during and for ≥30 minutes after administration; discontinue immediately for signs/symptoms of a hypersensitivity reaction (shock, hypotension, loss of consciousness). Equipment and medications (eg, epinephrine, steroids, diphenhydramine) for resuscitation and trained personnel experienced in handling medical emergencies should always be immediately available. Significant hypotension has been reported frequently in hemodialysis-dependent patients; may also occur in peritoneal dialysis and nondialysis patients but incidence is substantially lower. Hypotension may be related to total dose or rate of administration; avoid rapid I.V. injection and follow recommended guidelines.

Precautions Use with caution in patients with histories of significant allergies, asthma, serious hepatic impairment, preexisting cardiac disease (may exacerbate cardiovascular complications), and rheumatoid arthritis (may exacerbate joint pain and swelling). Discontinue oral iron prior to initiating parenteral iron therapy. Exogenous hemosiderosis may result from excess iron stores; patients with refractory anemias and/or hemoglobinopathies may be prone to iron overload with unwarranted iron supplementation. In patients with chronic kidney disease (CKD) requiring iron supplementation, the I.V. route is preferred for hemodialysis patients; either oral iron or I.V. iron may be used for nondialysis and peritoneal dialysis CKD patients. Use parenteral iron products with caution in premature neonates; necrotizing enterocolitis has been reported; however, no causal relationship established.

Use caution when interchanging products [ie, generic substitution with an iron sucrose similar (ISS) preparation (not currently available in U.S.)]; an observational trial in 75 adult hemodialysis patients reported destabilization of hemoglobin and serum iron indices, resulting in higher dose requirements (Rottembourg, 2011) after conversion to an ISS preparation. A case-series (n=3) described altered infusion tolerance and adverse effects after product conversion to an ISS preparation in nonhemodialysis adult patients; observed adverse events not previously reported in the patients included hypovolemic dysregulation, urticaria, headache, peripheral edema, and myalgia (Stein, 2012).

Adverse Reactions Events are associated with use in adults unless otherwise specified.

Cardiovascular: Arteriovenous fistula thrombosis (children), chest pain, hyper-/hypotension, peripheral edema

Central nervous system: Dizziness, fever, headache

Dermatologic: Pruritus

Endocrine & metabolic: Fluid overload, gout, hyper-/hypoglycemia

Gastrointestinal: Abdominal pain, diarrhea, nausea, peritonitis (children), vomiting, taste perversion

Local: Injection site reaction

Neuromuscular & skeletal: Arthralgia, back pain, extremity pain, muscle cramps, myalgia, weakness

Ocular: Conjunctivitis

Otic: Ear pain

Respiratory: Cough, dyspnea, nasal congestion, nasopharyngitis, pharyngitis, sinusitis, upper respiratory infection

Miscellaneous: Graft complication, sepsis

Rare but important or life-threatening: Anaphylactic shock, anaphylactoid reactions, angioedema, bradycardia, cardiovascular collapse, hypersensitivity (including wheezing), loss of consciousness, necrotizing enterocolitis (reported in premature infants, no causal relationship established), seizure, shock, urine discoloration

Drug Interactions

Metabolism/Transport Effects None known.

Avoid Concomitant Use

Avoid concomitant use of Iron Sucrose with any of the following: Dimercaprol

Increased Effect/Toxicity

The levels/effects of Iron Sucrose may be increased by: Dimercaprol

Decreased Effect There are no known significant interactions involving a decrease in effect.

Stability Store intact vials at 20°C to 25°C (68°F to 77°F); excursions permitted to 15°C to 30°C (59°F to 86°F); do not freeze. Iron sucrose is stable for 7 days at room temperature or under refrigeration when undiluted in a plastic syringe or following dilution in normal saline in a plastic syringe (2-10 mg/mL) or for 7 days at room temperature following dilution in normal saline in an I.V. bag (1-2 mg/mL). The manufacturer recommends not adding to parenteral nutrition solutions; however, iron sucrose at concentrations of 0.1 mg/dL and 0.25 mg/dL in 2-in-1 parenteral nutrition solutions with neonatal-range amino acid and cysteine were shown to be stable for 24 hours;

precipitation occurred at higher concentrations (ie, 1-10 mg/dL) (MacKay, 2009).

Mechanism of Action Iron sucrose is dissociated by the reticuloendothelial system into iron and sucrose. The released iron increases serum iron concentrations and is incorporated into hemoglobin.

Pharmacodynamics

Onset of action: Hematologic response to either oral or parenteral iron salts is essentially the same; red blood cell form and color changes within 3-10 days

Maximum effect: Peak reticulocytosis occurs in 5-10 days, and hemoglobin values increase within 2-4 weeks

Pharmacokinetics (Adult data unless noted) Following I.V. doses, the uptake of iron by the reticuloendothelial system appears to be constant at about 40-60 mg/hour

Distribution: V_{dss}: Healthy adults: 7.9 L

Metabolism: Dissociated into iron and sucrose by the reticuloendothelial system

Half-life: Adolescents (nondialysis-dependent): 8 hours; adults: 6 hours

Elimination: Healthy adults: Urine (5%) within 24 hours

Dialysis: Not dialyzable

Dosing: Neonatal Multiple forms for parenteral iron exist; close attention must be paid to the specific product when ordering and administering; incorrect selection or substitution of one form for another without proper dosage adjustment may result in serious over- or under-dosing. Doses are expressed as mg of **elemental iron.**

Anemia of prematurity: Limited data available: I.V.: 1 mg/kg/**day** infused over 2 hours; dosing based on results of a small comparative trial with oral iron therapy and erythropoietin which included 29 premature neonates (GA <31 weeks; treatment group, n=10) who at the time of treatment initiation had a mean age of 23.3 ± 2.9 days, and mean weight of 1266 ± 81 g; higher reticulocyte counts and fewer transfusions were observed in the parenteral iron group compared to the oral treatment arm; due to potential oxidative injury risk in smaller, less stable premature neonates, the authors suggest that lower doses should be considered (Pollock, 2001; Pollock, 2001a). Further studies are needed.

Dosing: Usual Multiple forms for parenteral iron exist; close attention must be paid to the specific product when ordering and administering; incorrect selection or substitution of one form for another without proper dosage adjustment may result in serious over- or underdosing. Doses are expressed as mg of **elemental iron. Note:** Per National Kidney Foundation DOQI Guidelines, initiation of iron therapy, determination of dose, and duration of therapy should be guided by results of iron status tests combined with the Hb level and the dose of the erythropoietin stimulating agent. See Reference Range for target levels. There is insufficient evidence to recommend I.V. iron if ferritin level >500 ng/mL.

Infants, Children, and Adolescents:

Iron deficiency anemia in CKD:

Repletion treatment: Limited data available: Children ≥2 years and Adolescents <15 years: I.V.: 1 mg/kg/dialysis; dosing based on a dose-finding trial in 14 pediatric patients and successfully increased ferritin therapeutic levels; iron overload (serum ferritin >400 ng/mL) was reported with the higher dose used in the study (3 mg/kg/dialysis) (Leijn, 2004)

Maintenance therapy: Children ≥2 years and Adolescents: I.V.:

Hemodialysis-dependent CKD: 0.5 mg/kg/dose (maximum dose: 100 mg) every 2 weeks for 12 weeks (6 doses); may repeat if clinically indicated

Peritoneal dialysis-dependent CKD; concurrent erythropoietin therapy: 0.5 mg/kg/dose (maximum dose: 100 mg) every 4 weeks for 12 weeks (3 doses); may repeat if clinically indicated

Nondialysis-dependent CKD; concurrent erythropoietin therapy: 0.5 mg/kg/dose (maximum dose: 100 mg) every 4 weeks for 12 weeks (3 doses); may repeat if clinically indicated

Nonrenal iron deficiency anemia; treatment in patients refractory to oral therapy (eg, long-term TPN, GI malabsorption): Limited data available (Norman, 2011; Pinsk, 2008):

Calculate Iron Deficit: Total replacement dose (mg of iron) = 0.6 x weight (kg) x [100 - (actual Hgb /12 x 100)]; **Note:** In this equation, 12 is the desired target Hgb concentration; in some patients, a different target may be required.

Initial dose: I.V.: 5-7 mg/kg; maximum dose: 100 mg

Maintenance dose: I.V.: 5-7 mg/kg every 1-7 days until total replacement dose achieved; maximum single dose: 300 mg

Adults: **Iron deficiency anemia in CKD:** I.V.:

Hemodialysis-dependent CKD: 100 mg administered during consecutive dialysis sessions to a cumulative total dose of 1000 mg (10 doses); may repeat treatment if clinically indicated

Peritoneal dialysis-dependent CKD: Two infusions of 300 mg administered 14 days apart, followed by a single 400 mg infusion 14 days later (total cumulative dose of 1000 mg in 3 divided doses); may repeat treatment if clinically indicated

Nonhemodialysis-dependent CKD: 200 mg administered on 5 different occasions within a 14-day period; cumulative total dose: 1000 mg in 14-day period. **Note:** Dosage has also been administered as two infusions of 500 mg in a maximum of 250 mL normal saline infused over 3.5-4 hours on day 1 and day 14 (limited experience); may repeat treatment if clinically indicated

Administration Parenteral: May administer I.V.; avoid dilution of solution for infusion in dextrose due to an increased incidence of local pain and phlebitis; not for I.M. use.

Pediatric patients:

Premature neonates: Infusion: Dilute dose to 2 mg/mL in NS; infuse over at least 2 hours (Pollak, 2001)

Infants, Children, and Adolescents: Dependent upon indication:

CKD treatment of iron deficiency anemia:

Slow I.V. injection: Administer undiluted over 5 minutes

Infusion: Dilute dose in 25 mL of NS; infuse over 5-60 minutes

Nonrenal treatment of iron deficiency anemia: One trial reported dilution of iron dose to a final concentration of 1 mg/mL in NS and infused at 1-1.3 mL/minute (Pinsk, 2008)

Others suggest the following recommendations (Norman, 2011):

For doses ≤100 mg, dilute dose in 100 mL NS and infuse over at least 30 minutes

For doses >100 mg and ≤200 mg, dilute dose in 200 mL NS and infuse over at least 60 minutes

For doses >200 mg and ≤300 mg, dilute dose in 250 mL NS and infuse over at least 90 minutes

Adults:

Slow I.V. injection: May administer doses ≤200 mg undiluted by slow I.V. injection over 2-5 minutes; when administering to hemodialysis-dependent patients, give iron sucrose early during the dialysis session

Infusion: Dilute doses ≤200 mg in maximum of 100 mL NS and infuse over at least 15 minutes; dilute 300 mg in a maximum of 250 mL NS and infuse over 1.5 hours; dilute 400 mg in a maximum of 250 mL NS and infuse over 2.5 hours; dilute 500 mg in a maximum of 250 mL NS and infuse over 3.5-4 hours (limited experience). When administering to hemodialysis-dependent

patients, give iron sucrose early during the dialysis session. Do not dilute to concentrations <1 mg/mL.

Monitoring Parameters Hematocrit, hemoglobin, serum ferritin, transferrin, percent transferrin saturation, TIBC; takes about 4 weeks of treatment to see increased serum iron and ferritin, and decreased TIBC. Serum iron concentrations should be drawn ≥48 hours after last dose (due to rapid increase in values following administration); signs/symptoms of hypersensitivity reactions (during and ≥30 minutes following infusion); hypotension (following infusion).

Reference Range

Serum iron:

Newborns: 110-270 mcg/dL

Infants: 30-70 mcg/dL

Children: 55-120 mcg/dL

Adults: Male: 75-175 mcg/dL; female: 65-165 mcg/dL

Total iron binding capacity:

Newborns: 59-175 mcg/dL

Infants: 100-400 mcg/dL

Children and Adults: 230-430 mcg/dL

Transferrin: 204-360 mg/dL

Percent transferrin saturation (TSAT): 20% to 50%

Iron levels >300 mcg/dL may be considered toxic; should be treated as an overdosage

Ferritin: 13-300 ng/mL

Chronic kidney disease (CKD): Targets for iron therapy (KDOQI Guidelines, 2007) to maintain Hgb 11-12 g/dL:

Children: Nondialysis CKD, hemodialysis, or peritoneal dialysis: Ferritin: >100 ng/mL and TSAT >20%

Adults: Nondialysis (CKD) or peritoneal dialysis: Ferritin: >100 ng/mL and TSAT >20%

Hemodialysis: Ferritin >200 ng/mL and TSAT >20% or CHr (content of hemoglobin in reticulocytes) >29 pg/cell

Additional Information Contains sucrose: 300 mg/mL

Dosage Forms Considerations

Strength of iron sucrose is expressed as elemental iron.

Dosage Forms Excipient information presented when available (limited, particularly for generics); consult specific product labeling.

Solution, Intravenous [preservative free]:

Venofer: 20 mg/mL (2.5 mL, 5 mL, 10 mL)

References

Crary SE, Hall K, and Buchanan GR, "Intravenous Iron Sucrose for Children With Iron Deficiency Failing to Respond to Oral Iron Therapy," *Pediatr Blood Cancer*, 2011, 56(4):615-9.

"KDOQI Clinical Practice Guideline and Clinical Practice Recommendations for Anemia in Chronic Kidney Disease: 2007 Update of Hemoglobin Target," *Am J Kidney Dis*, 2007, 50(3):471-530.

Leijn E, Monnens LA, and Cornelissen EA, "Intravenous Iron Supplementation in Children on Hemodialysis," *J Nephrol*, 2004, 17 (3):423-6.

MacKay M, Rusho W, Jackson D, et al, "Physical and Chemical Stability of Iron Sucrose in Parenteral Nutrition," *Nutr Clin Pract*, 2009, 24 (6):733-7.

Norman JL and Crill CM, "Optimizing the Transition to Home Parenteral Nutrition in Pediatric Patients," *Nutr Clin Pract*, 2011, 26(3):273-85.

Pinsk V, Levy J, Moser A, et al, "Efficacy and Safety of Intravenous Iron Sucrose Therapy in a Group of Children With Iron Deficiency Anemia," *Isr Med Assoc J*, 2008, 10(5):335-8.

Pollak A, Hayde M, Hayn M, et al, "Effect of Intravenous Iron Supplementation on Erythropoiesis in Erythropoietin-Treated Premature Infants," *Pediatrics*, 2001, 107(1):78-85.

Pollak A, Widness JA, and Lombard KA, "Iron Supplementation During Erythropoietin Treatment," *Pediatrics*, 2001, 108(6): 1390-1.

Rottembourg J, Kadri A, Leonard E, et al, "Do Two Intravenous Iron Sucrose Preparations Have the Same Efficacy?" *Nephrol Dial Transplant*, 2011, 26(10):3262-7.

Stein J, Dignass A, and Chow KU, "Clinical Case Reports Raise Doubts About the Therapeutic Equivalence of an Iron Sucrose Similar Preparation Compared With Iron Sucrose Originator," *Curr Med Res Opin*, 2012, 28(2):241-3.

◆ **Iron Sulfate** see Ferrous Sulfate on page 868

◆ **Iron Supplement Childrens [OTC]** see Ferrous Sulfate on page 868

◆ **Isagel® [OTC]** see Alcohol (Ethyl) on page 88

◆ **Isentress** see Raltegravir on page 1802

◆ **ISG** see Immune Globulin on page 1084

◆ **Isoamyl Nitrite** see Amyl Nitrite on page 165

Isoniazid (eye soe NYE a zid)

Medication Safety Issues
International issues:
Hydra [Japan] may be confused with Hydrea brand name for hydroxyurea [U.S., Canada, and multiple international markets]

Brand Names: Canada Isotamine®; PMS-Isoniazid

Therapeutic Category Antitubercular Agent

Generic Availability (U.S.) Yes

Use Treatment of susceptible mycobacterial infection due to *M. tuberculosis* and prophylactically to those individuals exposed to tuberculosis (FDA approved in infant, children, and adults)

Pregnancy Risk Factor C

Pregnancy Considerations Isoniazid was found to be embryocidal in animal studies; teratogenic effects were not noted. Isoniazid crosses the human placenta. Due to the risk of tuberculosis to the fetus, treatment is recommended when the probability of maternal disease is moderate to high. The CDC recommends isoniazid as part of the initial treatment regimen (CDC, 2003). Pyridoxine supplementation is recommended (25 mg/day).

Breast-Feeding Considerations Small amounts of isoniazid are excreted in breast milk. However, women with tuberculosis should not be discouraged from breast-feeding. Pyridoxine supplementation is recommended for the mother and infant.

Contraindications Hypersensitivity to isoniazid or any component; acute liver disease; previous history of hepatic damage during isoniazid therapy

Warnings Severe and sometimes fatal hepatitis may occur **[U.S. Boxed Warning]**; usually occurs within the first 3 months of treatment, although may develop even after many months of treatment. The risk of developing hepatitis is age-related, although isoniazid-induced hepatotoxicity has been reported in children; daily ethanol consumption may also increase the risk. Patients must report any prodromal symptoms of hepatitis, such as fatigue, weakness, malaise, anorexia, nausea, abdominal pain, jaundice, or vomiting. Patients should be instructed to immediately inform prescriber and discontinue isoniazid therapy if any of these symptoms occur, even if clinical evaluation has yet to be conducted.

Precautions Use with caution in patients with hepatic or renal impairment. Use with caution and carefully monitor patients who ingest alcohol daily, are >35 years of age, currently use other medications that may interact with isoniazid, have/are at risk for peripheral neuropathy, are pregnant, are women belonging to minority groups, or have a history of adverse reactions to latent TB infection (LTBI) medications. Oral solutions may contain sorbitol (≥70%) which may cause diarrhea.

Adverse Reactions

Cardiovascular: Hypertension, palpitation, tachycardia, vasculitis

Central nervous system: Depression, dizziness, encephalopathy, fever, lethargy, memory impairment, psychosis, seizure, slurred speech, toxic encephalopathy

Dermatologic: Flushing, rash (morbilliform, maculopapular, pruritic, or exfoliative)

Endocrine & metabolic: Gynecomastia, hyperglycemia, metabolic acidosis, pellagra, pyridoxine deficiency

Gastrointestinal: Anorexia, epigastric distress, nausea, stomach pain, vomiting

Hematologic: Agranulocytosis, anemia (sideroblastic, hemolytic, or aplastic), eosinophilia, thrombocytopenia

Hepatic: Bilirubinuria, hepatic dysfunction, hepatitis (may involve progressive liver damage; risk increases with age), hyperbilirubinemia, jaundice, LFTs mildly increased

Neuromuscular & skeletal: Arthralgia, hyper-reflexia, paresthesia, peripheral neuropathy (dose-related incidence), weakness

Ocular: Blurred vision, loss of vision, optic neuritis/atrophy

Miscellaneous: Lupus-like syndrome, lymphadenopathy, rheumatic syndrome

Drug Interactions

Metabolism/Transport Effects Substrate of CYP2E1 (major); **Note:** Assignment of Major/Minor substrate status based on clinically relevant drug interaction potential; **Inhibits** CYP1A2 (weak), CYP2A6 (moderate), CYP2C19 (moderate), CYP2C9 (weak), CYP2D6 (moderate), CYP2E1 (moderate), CYP3A4 (weak); **Induces** CYP2E1 (weak/moderate)

Avoid Concomitant Use

Avoid concomitant use of Isoniazid with any of the following: Pimozide; Tegafur; Thioridazine

Increased Effect/Toxicity

Isoniazid may increase the levels/effects of: Acetaminophen; ARIPiprazole (metabolized by oxidation); CarBAMazepine; Chlorzoxazone; Citalopram; CycloSERINE; CYP2A6 Substrates; CYP2C19 Substrates; CYP2D6 Substrates; CYP2E1 Substrates; Dofetilide; DOXOrubicin (Conventional); Fesoterodine; Fosphenytoin; Lomitapide; Metoprolol; Nebivolol; Phenytoin; Pimozide; Theophylline Derivatives; Thioridazine

The levels/effects of Isoniazid may be increased by: Disulfiram; Ethionamide; Propafenone; Rifamycin Derivatives

Decreased Effect

Isoniazid may decrease the levels/effects of: Clopidogrel; Codeine; Itraconazole; Ketoconazole (Systemic); Tamoxifen; Tegafur; TraMADol

The levels/effects of Isoniazid may be decreased by: Antacids; Corticosteroids (Systemic); Cyproterone

Food Interactions

Bioavailability is decreased if taken with food. Isoniazid may also decrease folic acid absorption and alters pyridoxine metabolism. Management: Take on an empty stomach 1 hour before or 2 hours after a meal, increase dietary intake of folate, niacin, and magnesium.

Tyramine-containing food: Isoniazid has weak monoamine oxidase inhibiting activity and may potentially inhibit tyramine metabolism. Several case reports of mild reactions (flushing, palpitations, headache, mild increase in blood pressure, diaphoresis) after ingestion of certain types of cheese or red wine, have been reported (Self, 1999; Toutoungi, 1985). Management: Manufacturer's labeling recommends avoiding tyramine-containing foods (eg, aged or matured cheese, air-dried or cured meats including sausages and salamis; fava or broad bean pods, tap/draft beers, Marmite concentrate, sauerkraut, soy sauce, and other soybean condiments). However, the clinical relevance of the tyramine reaction for the vast majority of patients receiving isoniazid has been questioned due to isoniazid's weak MAO inhibition and the relatively few published case reports of the interaction. Although not fully investigated, it has been proposed that the reaction has a genetic component and may only be significant in poor or intermediate acetylators since isoniazid is primarily inactivated by acetylation (DiMartini, 1995; Toutoungi, 1985).

Histamine-containing food: Isoniazid may also inhibit diamine oxidase resulting in headache, sweating, palpitations, flushing, hypotension to histamine-containing foods (eg, skipjack, tuna, other tropical fish). Management: Manufacturer's labeling recommends avoiding histamine-containing foods.

Stability

Oral solution: Store at 15°C to 30°C (59°F to 86°F); protect from light.

Parenteral: Store at 20°C to 25°C (68°F to 77°F); protect from light; avoid freezing.

Tablet: Store at 20°C to 25°C (68°F to 77°F); protect from light.

Mechanism of Action Unknown, but may include the inhibition of mycolic acid synthesis resulting in disruption of the bacterial cell wall

Pharmacokinetics (Adult data unless noted)

Absorption: Oral, I.M.: Rapid and complete; food reduces rate and extent of absorption

Distribution: Crosses the placenta; distributes into most body tissues and fluids, including the CSF

Protein binding: 10% to 15%

Metabolism: By the liver to acetylisoniazid with decay rate determined genetically by acetylation phenotype; undergoes further hydrolysis to isonicotinic acid and acetylhydrazine

Half-life: May be prolonged in patients with impaired hepatic function or severe renal impairment

Fast acetylators: 30-100 minutes

Slow acetylators: 2-5 hours

Time to peak serum concentration: Oral: Within 1-2 hours

Elimination: 75% to 95% excreted in urine as unchanged drug and metabolites; small amounts excreted in feces and saliva

Dialysis: Dialyzable (50% to 100%)

Dosing: Usual Oral, I.M.; **Note:** Recommendations often change due to resistant strains and newly developed information; consult *MMWR* for current CDC recommendations. Intramuscular injection is available for patients who are unable to either take or absorb oral therapy.

Infants, Children <40 kg, and Adolescents ≤14 years and <40 kg:

Treatment of active TB infection: CDC Recommendations: 10-15 mg/kg/day once daily (maximum dose: 300 mg/day) **or** 20-30 mg/kg/dose (maximum dose: 900 mg) twice weekly as part of a multidrug regimen (*MMWR*, 2003)

Treatment of latent TB infection (LTBI): 10-20 mg/kg/day given once daily (maximum dose: 300 mg/day) **or** 20-40 mg/kg/dose (maximum dose: 900 mg) twice weekly; treatment duration: 9 months

Primary prophylaxis for TB in HIV-exposed/positive patients: 10-15 mg/kg/day once daily (maximum dose: 300 mg/day) **or** 20-30 mg/kg/dose (maximum dose: 900 mg) twice weekly; treatment duration: 9 months

Children and Adolescents >40 kg or Adolescents ≥15 years: See Adult Dosing

Adults:

Treatment of latent tuberculosis infection (LTBI): Oral, I.M.: CDC recommendations: 5 mg/kg (maximum: 300 mg/dose) once daily or 15 mg/kg (maximum: 900 mg/dose) twice weekly by directly observed therapy (DOT) for 6-9 months in patients who do not have HIV infection (9 months is optimal, 6 months may be considered to reduce costs of therapy) and 9 months in patients who have HIV infection. Extend to 12 months of therapy if interruptions in treatment occur (*MMWR*, 2000)

Treatment of active TB infection (drug susceptible): Oral, I.M.:

Daily therapy: CDC recommendations: 5 mg/kg/day once daily (usual dose: 300 mg/day) (*MMWR*, 2003)

Directly observed therapy (DOT): CDC recommendations: 15 mg/kg (maximum: 900 mg/dose) twice weekly or 3 times/week; **Note:** CDC guidelines state that once-weekly therapy (15 mg/kg/dose) may be considered, but only after the first 2 months of initial

therapy in HIV-negative patients, and only in combination with rifapentine (*MMWR*, 2003).

Note: Treatment may be defined by the number of doses administered (eg, "6-month" therapy involves 182 doses of INH and rifampin, and 56 doses of pyrazinamide). Six months is the shortest interval of time over which these doses may be administered, assuming no interruption of therapy.

Note: Concomitant administration of 10-50 mg/day pyridoxine is recommended in malnourished patients or those prone to neuropathy (eg, alcoholics, patients with diabetes).

Dosing adjustment in renal impairment: No dosage adjustment needed in patients with renal impairment.

Administration

Oral: Administer 1 hour before or 2 hours after meals with water; administration of isoniazid syrup has been associated with diarrhea

Parenteral: I.M.: Administer I.M. when oral therapy is not possible; injection solution pH: 6-7

Monitoring Parameters Periodic liver function tests; monitor for prodromal signs of hepatitis; ophthalmologic exam; chest x-ray

LTBI therapy: American Thoracic Society/Centers for Disease Control (ATS/CDC) recommendations: Monthly clinical evaluation, including brief physical exam for adverse events. Baseline serum AST or ALT and bilirubin should be considered for patients at higher risk for adverse events (eg, history of liver disease, chronic ethanol use, HIV-infected patients, women who are pregnant or postpartum ≤3 months, older adults with concomitant medications or diseases). Routine, periodic monitoring is recommended for any patient with an abnormal baseline or at increased risk for hepatoxicity.

Test Interactions False-positive urinary glucose with Clinitest®

Additional Information

Prophylactic use is recommended for patients with ≥5 mm positive tuberculin skin test reaction who are HIV-positive or persons with risk factors for HIV infection; close contacts of newly diagnosed person with infectious tuberculosis; persons with fibrotic changes on chest XR suggestive of previous tuberculosis or inadequate treatment; persons with organ transplants or receiving immunosuppressive therapy

Prophylactic use is recommended for patients with ≥10 mm positive tuberculin skin test reaction who recently arrived (<5 years) from endemic areas; substance abusers; residents/employees of healthcare, correctional, or long-term care facilities; children <4 years; children and adolescents exposed to high-risk adults; persons at high-risk due to certain medical conditions like silicosis, diabetes mellitus, leukemia, end-stage renal disease, chronic malabsorption syndrome, cancer of head and neck, intestinal bypass or gastrectomy, and low body weight

Dosage Forms Excipient information presented when available (limited, particularly for generics); consult specific product labeling.

Solution, Injection:
Generic: 100 mg/mL (10 mL)

Syrup, Oral:
Generic: 50 mg/5 mL (473 mL)

Tablet, Oral:
Generic: 100 mg, 300 mg

Extemporaneous Preparations Note: Commercial oral solution is available (50 mg/mL)

A 10 mg/mL oral suspension may be made with tablets, purified water, and sorbitol. Crush ten 100 mg tablets in a mortar and reduce to a fine powder. Add 10 mL of purified water and mix to a uniform paste. Mix while adding sorbitol in incremental proportions to **almost** 100 mL; transfer to a graduated cylinder, rinse mortar with sorbitol, and add quantity of sorbitol sufficient to make 100 mL (do not use sugar-based solutions). Label "shake well" and "refrigerate". Stable for 21 days refrigerated.

Nahata MC, Pai VB, and Hipple TF, *Pediatric Drug Formulations*, 5th ed, Cincinnati, OH: Harvey Whitney Books Co, 2004.

References

Ad Hoc Committee of the Scientific Assembly on Microbiology, Tuberculosis, and Pulmonary Infections, "Treatment of Tuberculosis and Tuberculosis Infection in Adults and Children," *Clin Infect Dis*, 1995, 21:9-27.

American Academy of Pediatrics, Committee on Infectious Diseases, "Chemotherapy for Tuberculosis in Infants and Children," *Pediatrics*, 1992, 89(1):161-5.

Centers for Disease Control and Prevention (CDC), "Guidelines for the Prevention and Treatment of Opportunistic Infections Among HIV-Exposed and HIV-Infected Children," *MMWR Recomm Rep*, 2009, 58(RR-11):1-166. Available at http://aidsinfo.nih.gov/contentfiles/Pediatric_OI.pdf

Centers for Disease Control and Prevention (CDC), "Severe Isoniazid-Associated Liver Injuries Among Persons Being Treated for Latent Tuberculosis Infection - United States, 2004-2008," *MMWR Morb Mortal Wkly Rep*, 2010, 59(8):224-9. Available at http://www.cdc.gov/mmwr/preview/mmwrhtml/mm5908a3.htm.

Centers for Disease Control and Prevention (CDC), "Treatment of Tuberculosis," *MMWR Recomm Rep*, 2003, 52(RR-11):1-77.

Centers for Disease Control and Prevention (CDC), "Update: Adverse Event Data and Revised American Thoracic Society/CDC Recommendations Against the Use of Rifampin and Pyrazinamide for Treatment of Latent Tuberculosis Infection-United States, 2003," *MMWR Morb Mortal Wkly Rep*, 2003, 52(31):735-9.

Starke JR, "Modern Approach to the Diagnosis and Treatment of Tuberculosis in Children," *Pediatr Clin North Am*, 1988, 35(3):441-64.

Starke JR, "Multidrug Therapy for Tuberculosis in Children," *Pediatr Infect Dis J*, 1990, 9(11):785-93.

Van Scoy RE and Wilkowske CJ, "Antituberculous Agents: Isoniazid, Rifampin, Streptomycin, Ethambutol, and Pyrazinamide," *Mayo Clin Proc*, 1983, 58(4):233-40.

◆ **Isonicotinic Acid Hydrazide** *see* Isoniazid *on page 1158*

◆ **Isonipecaine Hydrochloride** *see* Meperidine *on page 1337*

◆ **Isophane Insulin** *see* Insulin NPH *on page 1130*

◆ **Isophane Insulin and Regular Insulin** *see* Insulin NPH and Insulin Regular *on page 1132*

◆ **Isophosphamide** *see* Ifosfamide *on page 1068*

Isoproterenol (eye soe proe TER e nole)

Medication Safety Issues
Sound-alike/look-alike issues:
Isuprel® may be confused with Disophrol®, Isordil®

Related Information
Emergency Drip Calculations *on page 2191*

Brand Names: U.S. Isuprel

Therapeutic Category Adrenergic Agonist Agent; Antiasthmatic; Beta$_1$ & Beta$_2$-Adrenergic Agonist Agent; Bronchodilator; Sympathomimetic

Generic Availability (U.S.) No

Use Treatment of asthma or COPD (reversible airway obstruction); ventricular arrhythmias due to A-V nodal block; hemodynamically compromised bradyarrhythmias or atropine-resistant bradyarrhythmias, temporary use in third degree A-V block until pacemaker insertion; low cardiac output or vasoconstrictive shock states

Pregnancy Risk Factor C

Pregnancy Considerations Animal reproduction studies have not been conducted by the manufacturer. Use of isoproterenol may interfere with uterine contractions at term (Mahon, 1967).

Breast-Feeding Considerations It is not known if isoproterenol is excreted in breast milk. The manufacturer recommends that caution be exercised when administering isoproterenol to nursing women.

Contraindications Hypersensitivity to isoproterenol, other sympathomimetic amines, or any component; angina;

preexisting cardiac arrhythmias (ventricular); tachycardia or A-V block caused by cardiac glycoside intoxication; narrow-angle glaucoma

Warnings Tolerance may occur with prolonged use; when discontinuing an isoproterenol continuous infusion used for bronchodilation, the infusion **must** be gradually tapered over a 24- to 48-hour period to prevent rebound bronchospasm; injection contains sulfites which may cause allergic reactions in susceptible individuals

Precautions Use with caution in diabetics, renal or cardiovascular disease, hyperthyroidism, prostatic hypertrophy

Adverse Reactions
Cardiovascular: Angina, flushing, hyper-/hypotension, pallor, palpitation, paradoxical bradycardia (with tilt table testing), premature ventricular beats, Stokes-Adams attacks, tachyarrhythmia, ventricular arrhythmia

Central nervous system: Dizziness, headache, nervousness, restlessness, Stokes-Adams seizure

Endocrine & metabolic: Hypokalemia, serum glucose increased

Gastrointestinal: Nausea, vomiting

Neuromuscular & skeletal: Tremor, weakness

Ocular: Blurred vision

Respiratory: Dyspnea, pulmonary edema

Miscellaneous: Diaphoresis

Drug Interactions
Metabolism/Transport Effects Substrate of COMT

Avoid Concomitant Use
Avoid concomitant use of Isoproterenol with any of the following: Inhalational Anesthetics; Iobenguane I 123

Increased Effect/Toxicity
Isoproterenol may increase the levels/effects of: Sympathomimetics

The levels/effects of Isoproterenol may be increased by: AtoMOXetine; Cannabinoid-Containing Products; COMT Inhibitors; Inhalational Anesthetics; Linezolid

Decreased Effect
Isoproterenol may decrease the levels/effects of: Iobenguane I 123; Theophylline Derivatives

Mechanism of Action Stimulates beta$_1$- and beta$_2$-receptors resulting in relaxation of bronchial, GI, and uterine smooth muscle, increased heart rate and contractility, vasodilation of peripheral vasculature

Pharmacodynamics
Onset of action: I.V.: Immediately
Duration: I.V. (single dose): Few minutes

Pharmacokinetics (Adult data unless noted)
Metabolism: By conjugation in many tissues including the liver and lungs
Half-life: 2.5-5 minutes
Elimination: In urine principally as sulfate conjugates

Dosing: Neonatal Bradyarrhythmias: Continuous I.V. infusion: 0.05-2 mcg/kg/minute; titrate to effect

Dosing: Usual Bradyarrhythmias, AV nodal block, or refractory torsade de pointes: Continuous I.V. infusion:
Infants and Children: 0.05-2 mcg/kg/minute; titrate to effect
Adults: 2-20 mcg/minute; titrate to effect

Usual Infusion Concentrations: Pediatric I.V. infusion: 20 mcg/mL

Administration Parenteral: For continuous infusions, dilute in dextrose or NS to a maximum concentration of 20 mcg/mL; concentrations as high as 64 mcg/mL have been used safely and with efficacy in situations of extreme fluid restriction

Monitoring Parameters Heart rate, blood pressure, respiratory rate, arterial blood gases, central venous pressure, ECG

Additional Information Hypotension is more common in hypovolemic patients

Dosage Forms Excipient information presented when available (limited, particularly for generics); consult specific product labeling. [DSC] = Discontinued product

Solution, Injection, as hydrochloride:

Isuprel: 0.2 mg/mL (1 mL, 5 mL) [contains disodium edta]

Isuprel: 0.2 mg/mL (1 mL [DSC], 5 mL [DSC]) [contains sodium metabisulfite]

References

Mahon WA, Reid DW, and Day RA, "The *in vivo* Effects of Beta Adrenergic Stimulation and Blockade on the Human Uterus at Term," *J Pharmacol Exp Ther*, 1967, 156(1):178-85.

Rachelefsky GS and Siegel SC, "Asthma in Infants and Children - Treatment of Childhood Asthma: Part II," *J Allergy Clin Immunol*, 1985, 76(3):409-25.

◆ **Isoproterenol Hydrochloride** *see* Isoproterenol *on page 1160*

◆ **Isoptin SR** *see* Verapamil *on page 2129*

◆ **Isopto Atropine** *see* Atropine *on page 234*

◆ **Isopto® Atropine (Can)** *see* Atropine *on page 234*

◆ **Isopto Carpine** *see* Pilocarpine (Ophthalmic) *on page 1675*

◆ **Isopto® Carpine (Can)** *see* Pilocarpine (Ophthalmic) *on page 1675*

◆ **Isopto Homatropine** *see* Homatropine *on page 1018*

◆ **Isopto Hyoscine** *see* Scopolamine (Ophthalmic) *on page 1874*

◆ **Isotamine® (Can)** *see* Isoniazid *on page 1158*

ISOtretinoin (eye soe TRET i noyn)

Medication Safety Issues

Sound-alike/look-alike issues:

Accutane® may be confused with Accolate®, Accupril® Claravis™ may be confused with Cleviprex®

ISOtretinoin may be confused with tretinoin

Other safety concerns:

Isotretinoin may be confused with tretinoin (which is also called all-*trans* retinoic acid, or ATRA); while both products may have uses in cancer treatment, they are **not** interchangeable.

Related Information

Oral Medications That Should Not Be Crushed or Altered *on page 2438*

Safe Handling of Hazardous Drugs *on page 2419*

Brand Names: U.S. Absorica; Amnesteem; Claravis; Myorisan; Zenatane

Brand Names: Canada Accutane®; Clarus™

Therapeutic Category Acne Products; Antineoplastic Agent, Retinoic Acid Derivatives; Retinoic Acid Derivative; Vitamin A Derivative

Generic Availability (U.S.) No

Use Treatment of severe recalcitrant nodular acne unresponsive to conventional therapy, including systemic antibiotics (FDA approved in ages ≥12 years and adults); has also been used for the treatment of moderate acne and high-risk neuroblastoma

Prescribing and Access Restrictions As a requirement of the REMS program, access to this medication is restricted. All patients (male and female), prescribers, wholesalers, and dispensing pharmacists must register and be active in the iPLEDGE™ risk management program, designed to eliminate fetal exposures to isotretinoin. This program covers all isotretinoin products (brand and generic). The iPLEDGE™ program requires that all patients meet qualification criteria and monthly program requirements (eg, pregnancy testing). Healthcare providers can only prescribe a maximum 30-day supply at each monthly visit and must counsel patients on the iPLEDGE™ program requirements and confirm counseling via the iPLEDGE™ automated system. Registration,

activation, and additional information are provided at www.ipledgeprogram.com or by calling 866-495-0654.

Medication Guide Available Yes

Pregnancy Risk Factor X

Pregnancy Considerations Isotretinoin and its metabolites can be detected in fetal tissue following maternal use during pregnancy (Benifla, 1995; Kraft, 1989). **[U.S. Boxed Warnings]:** Use of isotretinoin is contraindicated in females who are or may become pregnant. Birth defects (facial, eye, ear, skull, central nervous system, cardiovascular, thymus and parathyroid gland abnormalities) have been noted following isotretinoin exposure during pregnancy and the risk for severe birth defects is high, with any dose or even with short treatment duration. Low IQ scores have also been reported. The risk for spontaneous abortion and premature births is increased. Because of the high likelihood of teratogenic effects, all patients (male and female), prescribers, wholesalers, and dispensing pharmacists must register and be active in the iPLEDGE™ risk evaluation and mitigation strategy (REMS) program; do not prescribe isotretinoin for women who are or who are likely to become pregnant while using the drug. If pregnancy occurs during therapy, isotretinoin should be discontinued immediately and the patient referred to an obstetrician-gynecologist specializing in reproductive toxicity. This medication is contraindicated in females of childbearing potential unless they are able to comply with the guidelines of the iPLEDGE™ pregnancy prevention program. Females of childbearing potential must have two negative pregnancy tests with a sensitivity of at least 25 mIU/mL prior to beginning therapy and testing should continue monthly during therapy. Females of childbearing potential should not become pregnant during therapy or for 1 month following discontinuation of isotretinoin. Upon discontinuation of treatment, females of childbearing potential should have a pregnancy test after their last dose and again one month after their last dose. Two forms of contraception should be continued during this time. Any pregnancies should be reported to the iPLEDGE™ program (www.ipledgeprogram.com or 866-495-0654) and the FDA through MedWatch (800-FDA-1088).

Breast-Feeding Considerations It is not known if isotretinoin is excreted in breast milk. A case report describes a green discharge from the breast of a nonlactating woman which was determined to be iatrogenic galactorrhea due to isotretinoin (Larsen, 1985). Due to the potential for serious adverse reactions in the nursing infant, the manufacturer recommends a decision be made whether to discontinue nursing or to discontinue the drug, taking into account the importance of treatment to the mother.

Contraindications Hypersensitivity to isotretinoin, parabens, vitamin A or other retinoids; patients who are pregnant or intend to become pregnant during treatment

Warnings Hazardous agent; use appropriate precautions for handling and disposal (meets NIOSH, 2012 criteria). Isotretinoin must not be used by female patients who are or may become pregnant **[U.S. Boxed Warning]**; birth defects [CNS (cerebral abnormalities, hydrocephalus, microcephaly, cranial nerve deficit, cerebellar malformation), skull, ear, eye, and cardiovascular systems, cleft palate, thymus and parathyroid gland abnormalities] have been noted following isotretinoin exposure during pregnancy and the risk for severe birth defects is high, with any dose or even with short treatment duration. Low IQ scores have been reported. The risk for spontaneous abortion and premature births is increased. Because of the high likelihood of teratogenic effects, all patients (male and female), prescribers, wholesalers, and dispensing pharmacists must register and be active in the iPLEDGE risk evaluation and mitigation strategy (REMS) program **[U.S. Boxed Warning]**. Prescription for isotretinoin should not be issued until a female patient has had negative results from two urine or serum pregnancy tests, one performed in the prescriber's office when the patient is qualified for therapy, the second one performed on the second day of next normal menstrual period or 11 days after the last unprotected act of sexual intercourse, whichever is later. Pregnancy testing and counseling should be repeated monthly. Two forms of effective contraception must be used for at least 1 month before beginning therapy, during therapy, and for 1 month after discontinuation of therapy. Upon discontinuation of treatment, females of childbearing potential should have a pregnancy test after their last dose and again 1 month after their last dose. If pregnancy occurs during treatment, isotretinoin should be discontinued immediately and patient should be referred to a physician experienced in reproductive toxicity. Patients should be instructed not to donate blood during therapy and for 1 month following discontinuation of therapy due to risk of donated blood being given to a pregnant female.

Isotretinoin may cause depression, psychosis, aggressive or violent behavior, and changes in mood; rarely, suicidal thoughts and actions have been reported with isotretinoin use. All patients should be observed closely for symptoms of depression or suicidal thoughts; discontinuation of treatment alone may not be sufficient; further evaluation may be necessary; use with extreme caution in patients with a history of psychiatric disorder.

Retinoids have been associated with pseudotumor cerebri (benign intracranial hypertension), especially in children. Concurrent use of other drugs associated with this effect (eg, tetracyclines) may increase risk. Early signs and symptoms include papilledema, headache, nausea, vomiting, and visual disturbances; discontinue if papilledema occurs. Rare postmarketing cases of severe skin reactions (eg, erythema multiforme, Stevens-Johnson syndrome, toxic epidermal necrolysis), including fatalities, have been reported; monitor for severe skin reactions; discontinue use if severe skin reaction occurs. Anaphylaxis and other types of allergic reactions, including cutaneous reactions and allergic vasculitis, have been reported.

Dose-related elevations of serum triglycerides (in excess of 800 mg/dL) have been reported with use; acute pancreatitis and fatal hemorrhagic pancreatitis (rare) have been reported; discontinue therapy if severe hypertriglyceridemia or symptoms of pancreatitis occur; use with caution in patients with or history of hypertriglyceridemia. Clinical hepatitis and elevated liver enzymes have been reported with use; may require interruption of therapy until etiology is determined. Inflammatory bowel disease has been reported with use; discontinue treatment if abdominal pain, rectal bleeding, or severe diarrhea occurs.

May decrease bone mineral density; osteoporosis, osteopenia, and bone fractures have been reported with long-term, high-dose, or multiple courses of therapy. Use with caution in patients with a genetic predisposition to bone disorders (ie, osteoporosis, osteomalacia), with disease states that can induce bone disorders including patients with anorexia nervosa or in patients receiving drugs that cause osteoporosis/osteomalacia or affect vitamin D metabolism (ie, corticosteroids, anticonvulsants). Patients may be at risk when participating in activities with repetitive impact (eg, sports). Skeletal hyperostosis, calcification of ligaments and tendons, and premature epiphyseal closure have also been reported with the use.

Vision impairment, corneal opacities, decreased tolerance to contact lenses (due to dry eyes), and decreased night vision have been reported with use. Hearing impairment has occurred, which may persist after therapy is discontinued; discontinue therapy if hearing impairment or tinnitus develops.

Absorica™ absorption is ~83% greater than Accutane® when administered under fasting conditions; they are bioequivalent when taken with a high-fat meal. Absorica™ is not interchangeable with other generic isotretinoin products. Some formulation may contain soybean oil. Isotretinoin and tretinoin (also known as ATRA) may be confused; while both products may be used in cancer treatment, they are **not** interchangeable; verify product prior to dispensing and administration to prevent medication errors.

Precautions Use with caution in patients with diabetes mellitus; impaired glucose control has been reported. Children may experience a higher frequency of some adverse effects including arthralgia (22%) and back pain (29%). This medication should only be prescribed by prescribers competent in treating severe recalcitrant nodular acne and experienced with the use of systemic retinoids. Safety of long-term use is not established and is not recommended.

Adverse Reactions

Cardiovascular: Chest pain, edema, flushing, palpitation, stroke, syncope, tachycardia, vascular thrombotic disease

Central nervous system: Aggressive behavior, depression, dizziness, drowsiness, emotional instability, fatigue, headache, insomnia, lethargy, malaise, nervousness, paresthesia, pseudotumor cerebri, psychosis, seizure, stroke, suicidal ideation, suicide attempts, suicide, violent behavior

Dermatologic: Abnormal wound healing acne fulminans, alopecia, bruising, cheilitis, cutaneous allergic reactions, dry nose, dry skin, eczema, eruptive xanthomas, facial erythema, fragility of skin, hair abnormalities, hirsutism, hyperpigmentation, hypopigmentation, increased sunburn susceptibility, nail dystrophy, paronychia, peeling of palms, peeling of soles, photoallergic reactions, photosensitizing reactions, pruritus, purpura, rash

Endocrine & metabolic: Abnormal menses, blood glucose increased, cholesterol increased, HDL decreased, hyperuricemia, triglycerides increased

Gastrointestinal: Bleeding and inflammation of the gums, colitis, esophagitis, esophageal ulceration, inflammatory bowel disease, nausea, nonspecific gastrointestinal symptoms, pancreatitis, weight loss, xerostomia

Genitourinary: Nonspecific urogenital findings

Hematologic: Agranulocytosis (rare), anemia, neutropenia, pyogenic granuloma, thrombocytopenia

Hepatic: Alkaline phosphatase increased, ALT increased, AST increased, GGTP increased, hepatitis, LDH increased

Neuromuscular & skeletal: Arthralgia, arthritis, back pain, bone abnormalities, bone mineral density decreased, calcification of tendons and ligaments, CPK increased, myalgia, premature epiphyseal closure, skeletal hyperostosis, tendonitis, weakness

Ocular: Blepharitis, cataracts, chalazion, color vision disorder, conjunctivitis, corneal opacities, eyelid inflammation, hordeolum, keratitis, night vision decreased, optic neuritis, photophobia, visual disturbances

Otic: Hearing impairment, tinnitus

Renal: Glomerulonephritis, hematuria, proteinuria, pyuria, vasculitis

Respiratory: Bronchospasms, epistaxis, respiratory infection, voice alteration, Wegener's granulomatosis

Miscellaneous: Allergic reactions, anaphylactic reactions, disseminated herpes simplex, diaphoresis, infection, lymphadenopathy

Rare but important or life-threatening: Abnormal meibomian gland secretion, erythema multiforme, meibomian gland atrophy, myopia, pseudotumor cerebri, rhabdomyolysis, Stevens-Johnson syndrome, toxic epidermal necrolysis, visual acuity decreased

Drug Interactions

Metabolism/Transport Effects None known.

Avoid Concomitant Use

Avoid concomitant use of ISOtretinoin with any of the following: Multivitamins/Fluoride (with ADE); Multivitamins/Minerals (with ADEK, Folate, Iron); Multivitamins/Minerals (with AE, No Iron); Tetracycline Derivatives; Vitamin A

Increased Effect/Toxicity

ISOtretinoin may increase the levels/effects of: Mipomersen; Porfimer; Vitamin A

The levels/effects of ISOtretinoin may be increased by: Alcohol (Ethyl); Multivitamins/Fluoride (with ADE); Multivitamins/Minerals (with ADEK, Folate, Iron); Multivitamins/Minerals (with AE, No Iron); Tetracycline Derivatives

Decreased Effect

ISOtretinoin may decrease the levels/effects of: Contraceptives (Estrogens); Contraceptives (Progestins)

Food Interactions Isotretinoin bioavailability increased if taken with food or milk. Management: Administer orally with a meal (except Absorica™ which may be taken without regard to meals).

Stability Hazardous agent; use appropriate precautions for handling and disposal (meets NIOSH, 2012 criteria).

Absorica®: Store at 20°C to 25°C (68°F to 77°F), excursions permitted to 15°C to 30°C (59°F to 86°F); protect from light.

Accutane®: Store at 15°C to 30°C (59°F to 86°F); protect from light.

Mechanism of Action Reduces sebaceous gland size and reduces sebum production in acne treatment; in neuroblastoma, decreases cell proliferation and induces differentiation

Pharmacokinetics (Adult data unless noted) Note: Pharmacokinetic parameters in adolescents (12-15 years) are similar to adults.

Absorption: Enhanced with a high-fat meal; Absorica™ absorption is ~83% greater than Accutane® when administered under fasting conditions; they are bioequivalent when taken with a high-fat meal

Protein binding: 99% to 100%; primarily albumin

Metabolism: Hepatic via CYP2B6, 2C8, 2C9, 2D6, 3A4; forms metabolites; major metabolite: 4-oxo-isotretinoin (active)

Half-life, terminal: Parent drug: 21 hours; Metabolite: 21-24 hours

Time to peak serum concentration: Fasting conditions: Within 3 hours

Elimination: Urine and feces (equal amounts)

Dosing: Usual

Children and Adolescents:

Acne vulgaris, severe recalcitrant nodular: Children ≥12 years and Adolescents: Oral: 0.5-1 mg/kg/day in 2 divided doses; for severe cases (involving trunk, nuchal region, lower back, buttocks, thighs) may require higher doses up to 2 mg/kg/day in 2 divided doses. Duration of therapy is typically 15-20 weeks or until the total cyst count decreases by 70%, whichever is sooner; an alternate reported approach is continuation until a total cumulative dose of 120 mg/kg (eg, 1 mg/kg/day for 120 days). An initial dose of ≤0.5 mg/kg/day may be used to minimize initial flaring (Strauss, 2007)

Acne vulgaris, moderate: Limited data available: Children ≥12 years and Adolescents: 20 mg/day (~0.3-0.5 mg/kg/day) continued for 6-12 months to cumulative dose 120 mg/kg has been shown effective (Amichai, 2006)

Neuroblastoma, maintenance: Children ≥1 year and Adolescents: Oral: 160 mg/m^2/day in 2 divided doses for 14 consecutive days in a 28-day cycle for 6 cycles;

begin after continuation chemotherapy or transplantation (Matthay, 1999)

Adults: **Acne vulgaris:** Oral: 0.5-1 mg/kg/day in 2 divided doses for 15-20 weeks or until the total cyst count decreases by 70%, whichever is sooner. Adults with very severe disease/scarring or primarily involves the trunk may require dosage adjustment up to 2 mg/kg/day. A second course of therapy may be initiated after a period of ≥2 months of therapy. An initial dose of ≤0.5 mg/kg/day may be used to minimize initial flaring (Strauss, 2007).

Dosing adjustment in renal impairment: There are no dosage adjustments provided in the manufacturer's labeling.

Dosing adjustment in hepatic impairment: Children, Adolescents, and Adults:

Hepatic impairment prior to treatment: There are no dosage adjustments provided in the manufacturer's labeling.

Hepatotoxicity during treatment: Liver enzymes may normalize with dosage reduction or with continued treatment; discontinue if normalization does not readily occur or if hepatitis is suspected.

Administration Oral: Administer orally with a meal (except Absorica™ which may be taken without regard to meals). According to the manufacturers' labeling, capsules should be swallowed whole with a full glass of liquid. For patients unable to swallow capsule whole, an oral liquid may be prepared; may irritate esophagus if contents are removed from the capsule.

Hazardous agent; use appropriate precautions for handling and disposal (meets NIOSH, 2012 criteria).

Monitoring Parameters CBC with differential and platelet count, baseline sedimentation rate, glucose, CPK; signs of depression, mood alteration, psychosis, aggression, severe skin reactions

Pregnancy test (for all female patients of childbearing potential): Two negative tests with a sensitivity of at least 25 mIU/mL prior to beginning therapy (the second performed at least 19 days after the first test and performed during the first 5 days of the menstrual period immediately preceding the start of therapy); monthly tests to rule out pregnancy prior to refilling prescription

Lipids: Prior to treatment and at weekly or biweekly intervals until response to treatment is established. Test should not be performed <36 hours after consumption of ethanol.

Liver function tests: Prior to treatment and at weekly or biweekly intervals until response to treatment is established.

Dosage Forms Excipient information presented when available (limited, particularly for generics); consult specific product labeling.

Capsule, Oral:

Absorica: 10 mg, 20 mg, 30 mg, 40 mg [contains soybean oil]

Amnesteem: 10 mg, 20 mg, 40 mg [contains soybean oil]

Claravis: 10 mg [contains fd&c yellow #6 (sunset yellow), soybean oil]

Claravis: 20 mg [contains soybean oil]

Claravis: 30 mg

Claravis: 40 mg [contains fd&c yellow #6 (sunset yellow), soybean oil]

Myorisan: 10 mg, 20 mg [contains soybean oil]

Myorisan: 40 mg [contains fd&c yellow #6 (sunset yellow), soybean oil]

Zenatane: 10 mg [contains brilliant blue fcf (fd&c blue #1), edetate disodium, fd&c yellow #10 (quinoline yellow), methylparaben, propylparaben, soybean oil]

Zenatane: 20 mg [contains edetate disodium, methylparaben, propylparaben, soybean oil]

Zenatane: 40 mg [contains brilliant blue fcf (fd&c blue #1), edetate disodium, fd&c blue #2 (indigotine), fd&c yellow #10 (quinoline yellow), methylparaben, propylparaben, soybean oil]

Extemporaneous Preparations Hazardous agent: Use appropriate precautions for handling and disposal of teratogenic capsule contents.

For patients unable to swallow the capsules whole, an oral liquid may be prepared with softgel capsules (not recommended by the manufacturers) by one of the following methods:

Place capsules (softgel formulations only) in small container and add warm (~37°C [97°F]) water or milk to cover capsule(s); wait 2-3 minutes until capsule is softened and then drink the milk or water with the softened capsule, or swallow softened capsule.

Puncture capsule (softgel formulations only) with needle or cut with scissors; squeeze capsule contents into 5-10 mL of milk or tube feed formula; draw mixture up into oral syringe and administer via feeding tube; flush feeding tube with ≥30 mL additional milk or tube feeding formula.

Puncture capsule (softgel formulations only) with needle or cut with scissors and draw contents into oral syringe; add 1-5 mL of medium chain triglyceride, soybean, or safflower oil to the oral syringe; mix gently and administer via feeding tube; flush feeding tube with ≥30 mL milk or tube feeding formula.

Lam MS, "Extemporaneous Compounding of Oral Liquid Dosage Formulations and Alternative Drug Delivery Methods for Anticancer Drugs," *Pharmacotherapy*, 2011, 31(2):164-92.

References

Amichai B, Shemer A, and Grunwald MH, "Low-Dose Isotretinoin in the Treatment of Acne Vulgaris," *J Am Acad Dermatol*, 2006, 54(4):644-6.

Benifla JL, Ville Y, Imbert MC, et al. Fetal tissue dosages of retinoids. Experimental study concerning a case of isotretinoin (Roaccutan) administration and pregnancy. Fetal Diagn Ther. 199510(3):189-91.

Brecher AR and Orlow SJ, "Oral Retinoid Therapy for Dermatologic Conditions in Children and Adolescents," *J Am Acad Dermatol*, 2003, 49(2):171-82.

DiGiovanna JJ and Peck GL, "Oral Synthetic Retinoid Treatment in Children," *Pediatr Dermatol*, 1983, 1(1):77-88.

Kraft JC, Nau H, Lammer E, et al. Embryonic retinoid concentrations after maternal intake of isotretinoin. N Engl J Med. 1989;321(4):262.

Larsen GK. Iatrogenic breast discharge with isotretinoin. *Arch Dermatol*. 1985;121(4):450-451.

Matthay KK, Villablanca JG, Seeger RC, et al, "Treatment of High-Risk Neuroblastoma With Intensive Chemotherapy, Radiotherapy, Autologous Bone Marrow Transplantation, and 13-cis-Retinoic Acid. Children's Cancer Group," *N Engl J Med*, 1999, 341:1165-73.

National Institute for Occupational Safety and Health (NIOSH), "NIOSH List of Antineoplastic and Other Hazardous Drugs in Healthcare Settings 2012." Available at http://www.cdc.gov/niosh/docs/2012-150/pdfs/2012-150.pdf. Accessed January 21, 2013.

Reynolds CP, Kane DJ, Einhorn PA, et al, "Response of Neuroblastoma to Retinoic Acid In Vitro, and In Vivo," *Prog Clin Biol Res*, 1991, 366:203-11.

Strauss JS, Krowchuk DP, Leyden JJ, et al, "Guidelines of Care for Acne Vulgaris Management," *J Am Acad Dermatol*, 2007, 56 (4):651-63.

◆ **Isotretinoinum** *see* ISOtretinoin *on page 1161*

Isradipine (iz RA di peen)

Therapeutic Category Antihypertensive Agent; Calcium Channel Blocker; Calcium Channel Blocker, Dihydropyridine

Generic Availability (U.S.) Yes

Use Treatment of hypertension alone or in combination with thiazide-type diuretics (FDA approved in adults)

Pregnancy Risk Factor C

Pregnancy Considerations Adverse events were not observed in animal reproduction studies when using doses that were not maternally toxic. Isradipine crosses the human placenta (Lunell, 1993). Untreated chronic maternal hypertension is associated with adverse events in the fetus, infant, and mother. If treatment for hypertension during pregnancy is needed, other agents are preferred (ACOG, 2013).

Breast-Feeding Considerations It is not known if isradipine is excreted into breast milk. Due to the potential for serious adverse reactions in the nursing infant, the manufacturer recommends a decision be made whether to discontinue nursing or to discontinue the drug, taking into account the importance of treatment to the mother.

Contraindications Hypersensitivity to isradipine or any component

Warnings Symptomatic hypotension may occur; syncope and severe dizziness have been rarely reported, especially after initiation of recommended doses. Increased angina and/or MI has occurred with initiation or dosage titration of dihydropyridine calcium channel blockers; reflex tachycardia may occur resulting in angina and/or MI in patients with obstructive coronary disease, especially in the absence of concurrent beta-blockade.

Precautions Use with caution in patients with hepatic impairment; may require lower starting dose. May cause peripheral edema; occurs within 5-7 weeks of starting therapy. Use with caution in patients with CHF; may cause negative inotropic effects especially when used in combination with beta-blockers. Use with extreme caution in patients with severe aortic stenosis; may reduce coronary perfusion resulting in ischemia. Use with caution in hypertrophic cardiomyopathy (HCM) with outflow tract obstruction since reduction in afterload may worsen symptoms associated with this condition.

Adverse Reactions

Cardiovascular: Chest pain, edema (dose related), flushing (dose related), palpitations (dose related), tachycardia

Central nervous system: Dizziness, fatigue (dose related), headache (dose related)

Dermatologic: Skin rash

Gastrointestinal: Abdominal distress, diarrhea, nausea, vomiting

Neuromuscular & skeletal: Weakness

Renal: Urinary frequency

Respiratory: Dyspnea

Rare but important or life-threatening: Atrial fibrillation, cardiac failure, cerebrovascular accident, cough, decreased libido, depression, foot cramps, hyperhidrosis, hypotension, impotence, increased liver enzymes, insomnia, leg cramps, leukopenia, myocardial infarction, nocturia, numbness, paresthesia, pruritus, sore throat, syncope, transient ischemic attacks, urticaria, ventricular fibrillation, visual disturbance

Drug Interactions

Metabolism/Transport Effects Substrate of CYP3A4 (major); **Note:** Assignment of Major/Minor substrate status based on clinically relevant drug interaction potential; **Inhibits** CYP3A4 (weak)

Avoid Concomitant Use

Avoid concomitant use of Isradipine with any of the following: Conivaptan; Fusidic Acid (Systemic); Pimozide

Increased Effect/Toxicity

Isradipine may increase the levels/effects of: Amifostine; Antihypertensives; ARIPiprazole; Atosiban; Beta-Blockers; Calcium Channel Blockers (Nondihydropyridine); DULoxetine; Fosphenytoin; Highest Risk QTc-Prolonging Agents; Hypotensive Agents; Lomitapide; Magnesium Salts; Moderate Risk QTc-Prolonging Agents; Neuromuscular-Blocking Agents (Nondepolarizing); Nitroprusside; Obinutuzumab; Phenytoin; Pimozide; RiTUXimab; Tacrolimus (Systemic)

The levels/effects of Isradipine may be increased by: Alfuzosin; Alpha1-Blockers; Antifungal Agents (Azole Derivatives, Systemic); Barbiturates; Brimonidine (Topical); Calcium Channel Blockers (Nondihydropyridine);

Ceritinib; Cimetidine; Conivaptan; CycloSPORINE (Systemic); CYP3A4 Inhibitors (Moderate); CYP3A4 Inhibitors (Strong); Dasatinib; Diazoxide; Fluconazole; Fusidic Acid (Systemic); Herbs (Hypotensive Properties); Ivacaftor; Luliconazole; Macrolide Antibiotics; Magnesium Salts; MAO Inhibitors; Mifepristone; Pentoxifylline; Phosphodiesterase 5 Inhibitors; Prostacyclin Analogues; Protease Inhibitors; Simeprevir; Stiripentol

Decreased Effect

Isradipine may decrease the levels/effects of: Clopidogrel

The levels/effects of Isradipine may be decreased by: Barbiturates; Bosentan; Calcium Salts; CarBAMazepine; CYP3A4 Inducers (Strong); Dabrafenib; Deferasirox; Efavirenz; Herbs (Hypotensive Properties); Melatonin; Methylphenidate; Mitotane; Nafcillin; Rifamycin Derivatives; Siltuximab; St Johns Wort; Tocilizumab; Yohimbine

Food Interactions Administration with food delays absorption, but does not affect availability. Management: Administer without regard to meals.

Stability Store at 20°C to 25°C (68°F to 77°F); dispense in a tight, light-resistant container.

Mechanism of Action Inhibits calcium ion from entering the "slow channels" or select voltage-sensitive areas of vascular smooth muscle and myocardium during depolarization, producing relaxation of vascular smooth muscle, resulting in coronary vasodilation and reduced blood pressure; increases myocardial oxygen delivery in patients with vasospastic angina

Pharmacodynamics

Onset of action: 2-3 hours; **Note:** Full hypotensive effect may not occur for 2-4 weeks.

Duration: >12 hours

Pharmacokinetics (Adult data unless noted)

Absorption: 90% to 95%, but large first-pass effect

Distribution: V_d (apparent): 3 L/kg

Protein binding: 95%

Metabolism: Extensive first-pass effect; hepatically metabolized via cytochrome P450 isoenzyme CYP3A4; major metabolic pathways include oxidation and ester cleavage; six inactive metabolites have been identified

Bioavailability: 15% to 24%

Mild renal impairment (CrCl 30-80 mL/minute): Increased by 45%

Severe renal impairment (CrCl <10 mL/minute); concurrent hemodialysis: Decreased by 20% to 50%

Hepatic impairment: Increased by 52%

Half-life: Alpha half-life: 1.5-2 hours; terminal half-life: 8 hours

Time to peak serum concentration: 1.5 hours

Elimination: Urine (60% to 65% as metabolites; no unchanged drug detected); feces: 25% to 30%

Dosing: Usual

Children and Adolescents: Limited data available: **Hypertension:** Oral: Initial: 0.15-0.2 mg/kg/day divided 3 or 4 times daily; titrate upwards at 2- to 4-week intervals; maximum daily dose: 0.8 mg/**day** or 20 mg/**day** (whichever is lower) (NHBPEP, 2004; NHLBI, 2011). Based on retrospective observations, higher initial doses (0.05-0.15 mg/kg/dose) administered 3-4 times daily have been suggested especially in patients with secondary hypertension and severe hypertension; usual daily dose: 0.3-0.4 mg/kg/day divided every 8 hours (range: 0.04-1.2 mg/kg/day) (Flynn, 2002; Flynn, 2009; Johnson, 1997; Strauser, 2000). **Note:** Most adult patients show no improvement with doses >10 mg daily and adverse reaction rate increases.

Adults: **Hypertension:** Oral: 2.5 mg twice daily; antihypertensive response occurs in 2-3 hours; maximal response in 2-4 weeks; increase dose at 2- to 4-week intervals at 2.5-5 mg increments; usual dose range (JNC 7): 2.5-10 mg daily in 2 divided doses. **Note:** Most patients show no improvement with doses >10 mg daily, except

adverse reaction rate increases; therefore, maximal dose in older adults should be 10 mg daily.

Dosing adjustment in renal impairment: There are no dosage adjustments provided in manufacturer's labeling; however, bioavailability is increased with mild renal impairment; trend is reversed with further renal function deterioration. Other sources recommend that no initial dosage adjustment is required in pediatric and adult patients (Aronoff, 2007). Isradipine is not removed by hemodialysis; therefore, supplemental doses after hemodialysis are not necessary (Schönholzer, 1992).

Dosing adjustment in hepatic impairment: Adults: There are no dosage adjustments provided in manufacturer's labeling; however, peak serum concentrations are increased by 32% and bioavailability is increased by 52%.

Administration Oral: May be administered without regard to meals.

Monitoring Parameters Blood pressure, heart rate, liver and renal function

Dosage Forms Excipient information presented when available (limited, particularly for generics); consult specific product labeling.

Capsule, Oral:

Generic: 2.5 mg, 5 mg

Extemporaneous Preparations A 1 mg/mL oral suspension may be made from isradipine capsules; glycerin, USP; and Simple Syrup, N.F. Empty the contents of ten 5 mg isradipine capsules into a glass mortar. Add a small portion of glycerin, USP and mix to a fine paste; mix while adding 15 mL of simple syrup and transfer contents to a 60 mL amber glass prescription bottle. Rinse mortar with 10 mL simple syrup, NF and transfer to the prescription bottle; repeat, and add quantity of vehicle sufficient to make 50 mL. Label "protect from light", "refrigerate", and "shake well". Stable for 35 days when stored in amber glass prescription bottles in the dark and refrigerated.

MacDonald JL, Johnson CE, and Jacobson P, "Stability of Isradipine in Extemporaneously Compounded Oral Liquids," *Am J Hosp Pharm,* 1994, 51(19):2409-11.

References

American College of Obstetricians and Gynecologists (ACOG), "ACOG Practice Bulletin No. 125: Chronic Hypertension in Pregnancy," *Obstet Gynecol,* 2012, 119(2 Pt 1):396-407.

Chobanian AV, Bakris GL, Black HR, et al, "The Seventh Report of the Joint National Committee on Prevention, Detection, Evaluation, and Treatment of High Blood Pressure: The JNC 7 Report," *JAMA,* 2003, 289(19):2560-72.

Flynn JT and Pasko DA, "Calcium Channel Blockers: Pharmacology and Place in Therapy of Pediatric Hypertension," *Pediatr Nephrol,* 2000, 15(3-4):302-16.

Flynn JT and Warnick SJ, "Isradipine Treatment of Hypertension in Children: A Single-Center Experience," *Pediatr Nephrol,* 2002, 17 (9):748-53.

Johnson CE, Jacobson PA, and Song MH, "Isradipine Therapy in Hypertensive Pediatric Patients," *Ann Pharmacother,* 1997, 31 (6):704-7.

Lunell NO, Bondesson U, Grunewald C, et al, "Transplacental Passage of Isradipine in the Treatment of Pregnancy-Induced Hypertension," *Am J Hypertens,* 1993, 6(3 Pt 2):110-11.

National Heart, Lung, and Blood Institute. Expert panel on integrated guidelines for cardiovascular health and risk reduction in children and adolescents. *Clinical Practice Guidelines.* 2011. Available at http:// www.nhlbi.nih.gov/guidelines/cvd_ped/peds_guidelines_full.pdf

National High Blood Pressure Education Program Working Group on High Blood Pressure in Children and Adolescents. The fourth report on the diagnosis, evaluation, and treatment of high blood pressure in children and adolescents. *Pediatrics.* 2004;114(2 Suppl):555-576.

Schönholzer K, Marone C. Pharmacokinetics and dialysability of isradipine in chronic haemodialysis patients. *Eur J Clin Pharmacol.* 1992;42 (2):231-233.

Strauser LM, Groshong T, and Tobias JD, "Initial Experience With Isradipine for the Treatment of Hypertension in Children," *South Med J,* 2000, 93(3):287-93.

◆ **Istalol** *see* Timolol (Ophthalmic) *on page 2028*

◆ **Isuprel** *see* Isoproterenol *on page 1160*

◆ **Itch Relief [OTC]** *see* DiphenhydrAMINE (Topical) on page 677

Itraconazole (i tra KOE na zole)

Medication Safety Issues
Sound-alike/look-alike issues:
Itraconazole may be confused with fluconazole, posaconazole, voriconazole
Sporanox may be confused with Suprax, Topamax
Brand Names: U.S. Onmel; Sporanox; Sporanox Pulsepak
Brand Names: Canada Sporanox
Therapeutic Category Antifungal Agent, Systemic
Generic Availability (U.S.) May be product dependent
Use Treatment of susceptible systemic fungal infections in immunocompromised and nonimmunocompromised patients including blastomycosis, coccidioidomycosis, paracoccidioidomycosis, histoplasmosis, and aspergillosis in patients who do not respond to or cannot tolerate amphotericin B (FDA approved in adults); treatment of oropharyngeal or esophageal candidiasis (oral solution only) (FDA approved in adults)

Pregnancy Risk Factor C
Pregnancy Considerations Dose related adverse events were observed in animal reproduction studies. Use is contraindicated for the treatment of onychomycosis during pregnancy. If used for the treatment of onychomycosis in women of reproductive potential, effective contraception should be used during treatment and for 2 months following treatment. Therapy should begin on the second or third day following menses. Congenital abnormalities have been reported during postmarketing surveillance, but a causal relationship has not been established.

Breast-Feeding Considerations Itraconazole is excreted in breast milk. According to the manufacturer, the decision to continue or discontinue breast-feeding during therapy should take into account the risk of exposure to the infant and the benefits of treatment to the mother.

Contraindications Hypersensitivity to itraconazole or any component; concurrent administration with cisapride, dofetilide, ergot derivatives, levomethadyl, lovastatin, midazolam (oral), nisoldipine, pimozide, quinidine, simvastatin, or triazolam; treatment of onychomycosis in patients with evidence of left ventricular dysfunction, CHF, a history of CHF, pregnant women, or women intending to become pregnant

Warnings Not recommended for treatment of onychomycosis in patients with left ventricular dysfunction or a history of CHF **[U.S. Boxed Warning]**. Negative inotropic effects have been observed following intravenous administration. Discontinue or reassess use if signs or symptoms of CHF occur during treatment **[U.S. Boxed Warning]**. Calcium channel blockers (CCBs) may cause additive negative inotropic effects when used concurrently with itraconazole. Itraconazole may also inhibit the metabolism of CCBs; therefore, use caution with concurrent use of itraconazole and CCBs due to an increased risk of heart failure. Coadministration of cisapride, pimozide, quinidine, dofetilide, or levacetylmethadol (levomethadyl) with itraconazole is contraindicated **[U.S. Boxed Warning]**. Rare cases of serious cardiovascular adverse events (including death), ventricular tachycardia, and torsade de pointes have been observed due to increased cisapride, pimozide, quinidine, dofetilide, or levomethadyl concentrations induced by itraconazole. Serious (and rarely fatal) hepatic toxicity (eg, hepatitis, cholestasis, fulminant failure) has been observed with azole therapy; monitor liver function closely and dosage adjustment may be warranted. Not recommended for use in patients with active liver disease, elevated liver enzymes, or prior hepatotoxic reactions to

other drugs. **Due to differences in bioavailability, itraconazole solution and capsules should not be used interchangeably.** The oral solution contains propylene glycol; toxicities have been reported with use of products containing propylene glycol, including hyperosmolality, lactic acidosis, seizures, and respiratory depression; in neonates large amounts of propylene glycol delivered orally, intravenously (eg, >3000 mg/day), or topically have been associated with potentially fatal toxicities which can include metabolic acidosis, seizures, renal failure, and CNS depression; use solution containing propylene glycol with caution (AAP, 1997; Shehab, 2009).

Precautions Use with caution in patients with hypersensitivity to other azole antifungal agents, patients with left ventricular dysfunction or a history of CHF, and in patients with hepatic impairment; discontinue if signs and symptoms of liver disease or CHF develop. Large differences in itraconazole pharmacokinetic parameters have been observed in cystic fibrosis patients receiving the solution; if a patient with cystic fibrosis does not respond to therapy, alternate therapies should be considered. Transient or permanent hearing loss has been reported. Quinidine (a contraindicated drug) was used concurrently in several of these cases. Hearing loss usually resolves after discontinuation, but may persist in some patients.

Adverse Reactions
Cardiovascular: Chest pain, edema, hypertension
Central nervous system: Anxiety, depression, dizziness, dreams abnormal, fatigue, fever, headache, malaise, pain
Dermatologic: Pruritus, rash
Endocrine & metabolic: Hypertriglyceridemia, hypokalemia
Gastrointestinal: Abdominal pain, appetite increased, constipation, dyspepsia, flatulence, gastritis, gastroenteritis, gingivitis, stomatitis (ulcerative), vomiting
Hepatic: LFTs abnormal
Neuromuscular & skeletal: Bursitis, myalgia, tremor, weakness
Renal: Cystitis, urinary tract infection
Respiratory: Cough, dyspnea, pharyngitis, pneumonia, rhinitis, sinusitis, sputum increased, upper respiratory infection
Miscellaneous: Diaphoresis increased, herpes zoster
Rare but important or life-threatening: Adrenal insufficiency, albuminuria, allergic reactions, alopecia, anaphylactoid reactions, anaphylaxis, angioedema, anorexia, arrhythmia, arthralgia, blurred vision, dehydration, diplopia, dysgeusia, dysphagia, erythema multiforme, exanthematous pustulosis, exfoliative dermatitis, gynecomastia, hearing loss, heart failure, hematuria, hepatic failure, hepatitis, hepatotoxicity, hot flashes, hypoesthesia, impotence, insomnia, leukocytoclastic dermatitis, leukopenia, libido decreased, menstrual disorders, neutropenia, pancreatitis, paresthesia, peripheral edema, photosensitivity, pollakiuria, pulmonary edema, rigors, serum sickness, somnolence, Stevens-Johnson syndrome, thrombocytopenia, taste perversion, tinnitus, toxic epidermal necrolysis, urinary incontinence, urticaria, vasculitis

Drug Interactions
Metabolism/Transport Effects Substrate of CYP3A4 (major); **Note:** Assignment of Major/Minor substrate status based on clinically relevant drug interaction potential; **Inhibits** CYP3A4 (strong), P-glycoprotein

Avoid Concomitant Use
Avoid concomitant use of Itraconazole with any of the following: Ado-Trastuzumab Emtansine; Alfuzosin; Aliskiren; ALPRAZolam; Apixaban; Avanafil; Axitinib; Bosutinib; Cabozantinib; Ceritinib; Cisapride; Conivaptan; Crizotinib; CYP3A4 Inducers (Strong); Dihydroergotamine; Disopyramide; Dofetilide; Dronedarone; Efavirenz; Eletriptan; Eplerenone; Ergoloid Mesylates; Ergonovine; Ergotamine; Estazolam; Everolimus;

Felodipine; Fusidic Acid (Systemic); Halofantrine; Ibrutinib; Irinotecan; Ivabradine; Lapatinib; Lomitapide; Lovastatin; Lurasidone; Macitentan; Methadone; Methylergonovine; Midazolam; Nevirapine; Nilotinib; Nisoldipine; PAZOPanib; Pimozide; QuiNIDine; Ranolazine; Red Yeast Rice; Regorafenib; Rivaroxaban; Saccharomyces boulardii; Salmeterol; Silodosin; Simeprevir; Simvastatin; Tamsulosin; Ticagrelor; Tolvaptan; Topotecan; Toremifene; Triazolam; Ulipristal; Vemurafenib; VinCRIStine (Liposomal); Vorapaxar

Increased Effect/Toxicity

Itraconazole may increase the levels/effects of: Ado-Trastuzumab Emtansine; Afatinib; Alfentanil; Alfuzosin; Aliskiren; Almotriptan; Alosetron; ALPRAZolam; Apixaban; ARIPiprazole; AtorvaSTATin; Avanafil; Axitinib; Bedaquiline; Benzodiazepines (metabolized by oxidation); Boceprevir; Bortezomib; Bosentan; Bosutinib; Brentuximab Vedotin; Brinzolamide; Budesonide (Nasal); Budesonide (Systemic, Oral Inhalation); BusPIRone; Busulfan; Cabozantinib; Calcium Channel Blockers; Cannabis; Cardiac Glycosides; Ceritinib; Cilostazol; Cisapride; Cobicistat; Colchicine; Conivaptan; Corticosteroids (Orally Inhaled); Corticosteroids (Systemic); Crizotinib; CycloSPORINE (Systemic); CYP3A4 Substrates; Dabigatran Etexilate; Darunavir; Dienogest; Dihydroergotamine; Disopyramide; DOCEtaxel; Dofetilide; DOXOrubicin (Conventional); Dronabinol; Dronedarone; Dutasteride; Eletriptan; Elvitegravir; Eplerenone; Ergoloid Mesylates; Ergonovine; Ergotamine; Estazolam; Etravirine; Everolimus; Felodipine; FentaNYL; Fesoterodine; Fexofenadine; Fluticasone (Nasal); Fluticasone (Oral Inhalation); Fosamprenavir; GuanFACINE; Halofantrine; Highest Risk QTc-Prolonging Agents; Ibrutinib; Iloperidone; Imatinib; Indinavir; Irinotecan; Ivabradine; Ivacaftor; Ixabepilone; Lacosamide; Lapatinib; Levomilnacipran; Lomitapide; Losartan; Lovastatin; Lurasidone; Macitentan; Macrolide Antibiotics; Maraviroc; Methadone; Methylergonovine; MethylPREDNISolone; Midazolam; Mifepristone; Moderate Risk QTc-Prolonging Agents; Nilotinib; Nisoldipine; Ospemifene; OxyCODONE; Paliperidone; Paricalcitol; PAZOPanib; P-glycoprotein/ABCB1 Substrates; Pimecrolimus; Pimozide; PONATinib; Pravastatin; Propafenone; Prucalopride; QUEtiapine; QuiNIDine; Ranolazine; Red Yeast Rice; Regorafenib; Repaglinide; Rifaximin; Rilpivirine; Riociguat; Rivaroxaban; RomiDEPsin; Rosuvastatin; Ruxolitinib; Salmeterol; Saquinavir; Saxagliptin; Sildenafil; Silodosin; Simeprevir; Simvastatin; Sirolimus; Solifenacin; SORAfenib; SUNItinib; Tacrolimus (Systemic); Tacrolimus (Topical); Tadalafil; Tamsulosin; Telaprevir; Temsirolimus; Tetrahydrocannabinol; Ticagrelor; Tofacitinib; Tolterodine; Tolvaptan; Topotecan; Toremifene; Triazolam; Ulipristal; Vardenafil; Vemurafenib; Vilazodone; VinBLAStine; VinCRIStine; VinCRIStine (Liposomal); Vinorelbine; Vitamin K Antagonists; Vorapaxar; Zolpidem; Zuclopenthixol

The levels/effects of Itraconazole may be increased by: Boceprevir; Cobicistat; Conivaptan; CYP3A4 Inhibitors (Moderate); CYP3A4 Inhibitors (Strong); Darunavir; Etravirine; Fosamprenavir; Fusidic Acid (Systemic); Grapefruit Juice; Indinavir; Lopinavir; Luliconazole; Macrolide Antibiotics; Mifepristone; Ritonavir; Saquinavir; Stiripentol; Telaprevir; Tipranavir

Decreased Effect

Itraconazole may decrease the levels/effects of: Amphotericin B; Ifosfamide; Meloxicam; Prasugrel; Saccharomyces boulardii; Ticagrelor

The levels/effects of Itraconazole may be decreased by: Antacids; Bosentan; CYP3A4 Inducers (Strong); Dabrafenib; Deferasirox; Didanosine; Efavirenz; Etravirine; Grapefruit Juice; H2-Antagonists; Isoniazid; Nevirapine;

Proton Pump Inhibitors; Siltuximab; St Johns Wort; Sucralfate; Tocilizumab

Food Interactions

Capsules: Absorption enhanced by food and possibly by gastric acidity. Cola drinks have been shown to increase the absorption of the capsules in patients with achlorhydria or those taking H_2-receptor antagonists or other gastric acid suppressors. Grapefruit/grapefruit juice may increase serum levels. Management: Take capsules immediately after meals. Avoid grapefruit juice.

Solution: Food decreases the bioavailability and increases the time to peak concentration. Management: Take solution on an empty stomach 1 hour before or 2 hours after meals.

Stability

Capsules: Store at controlled room temperature 15°C to 25°C (59°F to 77°F). Protect from light and moisture.
Oral solution: Store at or below 25°C (77°F). Do not freeze.

Mechanism of Action

Interferes with cytochrome P450 activity, decreasing ergosterol synthesis (principal sterol in fungal cell membrane) and inhibiting cell membrane formation

Pharmacokinetics (Adult data unless noted)

Absorption: Requires gastric acidity; capsule better absorbed with food; solution better absorbed on empty stomach

Distribution: V_d: 10 L/kg; highly lipophilic and tissue concentrations are higher than plasma concentrations. High affinity for tissues (liver, lung, kidney, adipose tissue, brain, vagina, dermis, epidermis); poor penetration into CSF, eye fluid, saliva; distributes into breast milk, bronchial exudate, and sputum

Protein binding: 99%; metabolite hydroxy-itraconazole: 99.5%

Metabolism: Extensively hepatic via CYP3A4 into >30 metabolites including hydroxy-itraconazole (major metabolite); appears to have *in vitro* antifungal activity. Main metabolic pathway is oxidation; may undergo saturation metabolism with multiple dosing

Bioavailability: Variable, ~55% (oral solution) in one small study; **Note:** Oral solution has a higher degree of bioavailability (149% ± 68%) relative to oral capsules; should not be interchanged

Half-life:
  Pediatric patients (6 months to 12 years): Oral solution: ~36 hours; metabolite hydroxy-itraconazole: ~18 hours
  Adults: Oral: Single dose: ~21 hours, steady state: 64 hours; cirrhosis (single dose): 37 hours (range: 20-54 hours)

Time to peak serum concentration: Capsules: 3-5 hours; Oral solution: 2-3 hours

Elimination: Urine (<0.03% active drug, 40% as inactive metabolites); feces (~3% to 18%)

Dialysis: Nondialyzable

Dosing: Neonatal Oral: **Note:** Limited data available; further studies are needed, consider alternative agents.

Tinea capitis (*Microsporum canis*): Oral solution: 5 mg/kg/dose once daily for 6 weeks was used in a single, full-term neonate as part of a larger open-label pilot study of seven infants (age: 3-46 weeks) who received therapy for 3-6 weeks (Binder, 2009)

Dosing: Usual Oral:

Infants and Children:
  General dosing: Limited data available: Usual reported range: 3-5 mg/kg/dose once daily; doses as high as 5-10 mg/kg/day divided every 12-24 hours have been used in 32 patients with chronic granulomatous disease for prophylaxis against Aspergillus infection; doses of 6-8 mg/kg/**day** have been used in the treatment of disseminated histoplasmosis

Candidiasis (HIV-exposed/-positive) (CDC, 2009):
Oropharyngeal, treatment: Oral solution: 2.5 mg/kg/dose twice daily for 7-14 days (maximum daily dose: 200 mg/**day** or 400 mg/**day** if fluconazole-refractory)
Esophageal, treatment: Oral solution: 5 mg/kg/**day** divided once or twice daily for 4-21 days

Coccidioidomycosis, disseminated, non-CNS (HIV-exposed/-positive) (CDC, 2009):
Treatment: Oral: 5-10 mg/kg/dose twice daily for 3 days followed by 2-5 mg/kg/dose twice daily (maximum daily dose: 400 mg/**day**); product formulation not specified
Relapse prevention: 2-5 mg/kg/dose twice daily (maximum daily dose: 400 mg/**day**); product formulation not specified

Crypotococcus (HIV-exposed/-positive) (CDC, 2009):
Treatment, consolidation therapy: Oral solution (preferred): Initial load: 2.5-5 mg/kg/dose 3 times daily (maximum daily dose: 600 mg/**day**) for 3 days (9 doses) followed by 5-10 mg/kg/**day** divided once or twice daily (maximum daily dose: 400 mg/**day**) for a minimum of 8 weeks
Relapse prevention: Oral solution: 5 mg/kg/dose once daily (maximum daily dose: 200 mg/**day**)

Histoplasmosis (HIV-exposed/-positive) (CDC, 2009):
Treatment, mild disseminated disease: Oral solution: 2-5 mg/kg/dose 3 times daily for 3 days (9 doses) followed by 2-5 mg/kg/dose twice daily for 12 months (maximum dose: 200 mg/dose)
Consolidation treatment for moderate-severe to severe disseminated disease, including CNS infection (following appropriate induction therapy): Oral solution: 2-5 mg/kg/dose 3 times daily for 3 days (9 doses) followed by 2-5 mg/kg/dose (maximum dose: 200 mg/dose) twice daily for 12 months for non-CNS disseminated disease or for ≥12 months for CNS infection as determined by clinical response.
Relapse prevention: Oral solution: 5 mg/kg/dose twice daily (maximum daily dose: 400 mg/**day**)

Tinea capitis (*Microsporum canis*): Oral solution or capsules: 5 mg/kg/dose once daily for 3-6 weeks was used in a small open-label pilot study of seven infants (age: 3-46 weeks); if capsules were used, they were opened and sprinkled on main meal of the day (Binder, 2009)

Adolescents:
General dosing: 100-600 mg/**day**; doses >200 mg/**day** are usually given in 2 divided doses; length of therapy varies from 1 day to >6 months depending on the condition and mycological response

Candidiasis (HIV-exposed/-positive) (CDC, 2009a):
Oropharyngeal, treatment: Oral solution: 200 mg once daily for 7-14 days
Esophageal, treatment: Oral solution: 200 mg once daily for 14-21 days
Vulvovaginal, uncomplicated: Oral solution: 200 mg once daily for 3-7 days

Coccidioidomycosis (HIV-exposed/-positive) (CDC, 2009a):
Mild infection, treatment (eg, focal pneumonia): 200 mg 3 times daily for 3 days followed by 200 mg twice daily
Meningitis:
Treatment: 200 mg 3 times daily for 3 days followed by 200 mg twice daily
Maintenance therapy: 200 mg twice daily
Prevention of first episode: 200 mg twice daily

Crypotococcus (CNS disease, meningitis) (HIV-exposed/-positive) (CDC, 2009a):
Consolidation therapy: 200 mg twice daily for 8 weeks or as determined by target CD4+ counts; may be initiated after at least 2 weeks of successful induction therapy (eg, significant clinical improvement and negative CSF culture)

Maintenance therapy: 200 mg once daily

Histoplasmosis (HIV-exposed/-positive) (CDC, 2009a): **Note:** Monitoring of serum concentrations recommended to ensure adequate absorption.
Mild disseminated disease, treatment: Oral solution (preferred): 200 mg 3 times/day for 3 days, then 200 mg twice daily for at least 12 months
Moderate to severe non-CNS disease, maintenance therapy: Oral solution (preferred): 200 mg 3 times/day for 3 days, then 200 mg twice daily following amphotericin B induction therapy
Meningitis, maintenance therapy: Oral solution (preferred): 200 mg twice daily or 3 times/day for ≥1 year following liposomal amphotericin B induction therapy
Long-term suppression therapy: Oral solution (preferred): 200 mg once daily
Prevention of first episode: Oral solution (preferred): 200 mg once daily

Microsporidiosis, treatment disseminated disease (HIV-exposed/-positive) (CDC, 2009a): 400 mg once daily in conjunction with albendazole

Penicilliosis (HIV-exposed/-positive) (CDC, 2009a):
Acute infection (severely ill), maintenance therapy: 400 mg once daily for 10 weeks; initiate after completion of 2 weeks induction therapy with amphotericin B
Mild disease, treatment: 400 mg once daily for 8 weeks
Maintenance therapy: 200 mg once daily

Adults: 100-800 mg/**day**; doses >200 mg/**day** are usually given in 2 divided doses; length of therapy varies from 1 day to >6 months depending on the condition and mycological response

Dosing adjustment in renal impairment: The FDA-approved labeling states to use with caution in patients with renal impairment. The following guidelines have been used by some clinicians: Adults (Aronoff, 2007):
CrCl >10 mL/minute: No adjustment recommended.
CrCl <10 mL/minute: Administer 50% of normal dose.
Poorly dialyzed; no supplemental dose or dosage adjustment necessary, including patients on intermittent hemodialysis, peritoneal dialysis, or continuous renal replacement therapy (eg, CVVHD).

Dosing adjustment in hepatic impairment: Use caution.

Administration Oral: Doses >200 mg/day are given in 2 divided doses; do not administer with antacids. **Capsule and oral solution formulations are not bioequivalent and thus are not interchangeable.** Capsule absorption is best if taken with food, therefore, it is best to administer itraconazole after meals; solution should be taken on an empty stomach. When treating oropharyngeal and esophageal candidiasis, solution should be swished vigorously in mouth, then swallowed.

Monitoring Parameters Liver function in patients with preexisting hepatic dysfunction, and in all patients being treated for longer than 1 month; serum concentrations particularly for oral therapy (due to erratic bioavailability with capsule formulation); renal function; serum potassium; monitor for prodromal signs of hepatitis

Reference Range Serum concentrations may be performed to assure therapeutic levels. Itraconazole plus the metabolite hydroxyitraconazole concentrations should be >1 mcg/mL (not to exceed 10 mcg/mL).
Timing of serum samples: Obtain level after ~2 weeks of therapy, level may be drawn anytime during the dosing interval.

Dosage Forms Excipient information presented when available (limited, particularly for generics); consult specific product labeling.
Capsule, Oral:
Sporanox: 100 mg [contains brilliant blue fcf (fd&c blue #1), d&c red #22 (eosine), fd&c blue #2 (indigotine)]

Sporanox Pulsepak: 100 mg [contains brilliant blue fcf (fd&c blue #1), d&c red #22 (eosine), fd&c blue #2 (indigotine)]
Generic: 100 mg
Solution, Oral:
Sporanox: 10 mg/mL (150 mL)
Tablet, Oral:
Onmel: 200 mg

Extemporaneous Preparations Note: Commercial oral solution is available (10 mg/mL)

A 20 mg/mL oral suspension may be made with capsules. Empty the contents of forty 100 mg capsules and add 15 mL of Alcohol, USP. Let stand for 5 minutes. Crush the beads in a mortar and reduce to a fine powder. Mix while adding a 1:1 mixture of Ora-Sweet and Ora-Plus in incremental proportions to **almost** 200 mL; transfer to a calibrated bottle, rinse mortar with vehicle, and add quantity of vehicle sufficient to make 200 mL. Label "shake well" and "refrigerate". Stable for 56 days refrigerated.

Nahata MC, Pai VB, and Hipple TF, *Pediatric Drug Formulations*, 5th ed, Cincinnati, OH: Harvey Whitney Books Co, 2004.

References

American Academy of Pediatrics Committee on Drugs. "Inactive" ingredients in pharmaceutical products: update (subject review). *Pediatrics*. 1997;99(2):268-278.

Aronoff GR, Bennett WM, Berns JS, et al, *Drug Prescribing in Renal Failure: Dosing Guidelines for Adults and Children*, 5th ed, Philadelphia, PA: American College of Physicians, 2007.

Bhandari V and Narang A, "Oral Itraconazole Therapy for Disseminated Candidiasis in Low Birth Weight Infants," *J Pediatr*, 1992, 120(2 Pt 1):330.

Binder B, Richtig E, Weger W, et al, "Tinea Capitis in Early Infancy Treated With Itraconazole: A Pilot Study," *J Eur Acad Dermatol Venereol*, 2009, 23(10):1161-3.

Centers for Disease Control and Prevention (CDC), "Guidelines for the Prevention and Treatment of Opportunistic Infections Among HIV-Exposed and HIV-Infected Children," *MMWR Recomm Rep*, 2009, 58(RR-11):1-166. Available at http://aidsinfo.nih.gov/contentfiles/Pediatric_OI.pdf

Centers for Disease Control and Prevention, "Guidelines for the Prevention and Treatment of Opportunistic Infections in HIV-Infected Adults and Adolescents: Recommendations From CDC, the National Institutes of Health, the HIV Medicine Association of the Infectious Diseases Society of America," *MMWR Recomm Rep*, 2009, 58(RR-4):1-216. Available at http://www.aidsinfo.nih.gov/contentfiles/adult_oi.pdf

Chapman SW, Dismukes WE, Proia LA, et al, "Clinical Practice Guidelines for the Management of Blastomycosis: 2008 Update by the Infectious Diseases Society of America," *Clin Infect Dis*, 2008, 46 (12):1801-12.

Cowie F, Meller ST, Cushing P, et al, "Chemoprophylaxis for Pulmonary Aspergillosis During Intensive Chemotherapy," *Arch Dis Child*, 1994, 70(2):136-8.

"Guidelines for Prevention and Treatment of Opportunistic Infections in HIV-Infected Adults and Adolescents," June 18, 2008. Available at http://aidsinfo.nih.gov

Heintz BH, Matzke GR, and Dager WE, "Antimicrobial Dosing Concepts and Recommendations for Critically Ill Adult Patients Receiving Continuous Renal Replacement Therapy or Intermittent Hemodialysis," *Pharmacotherapy*, 2009, 29(5):562-77.

Mouy R, Veber F, Blanche S, et al, "Long-Term Itraconazole Prophylaxis Against *Aspergillus* Infections in Thirty-Two Patients With Chronic Granulomatous Disease," *J Pediatr*, 1994, 125(6 Pt 1):998-1003.

Shehab N, Lewis CL, Streetman DD, Donn SM. Exposure to the pharmaceutical excipients benzyl alcohol and propylene glycol among critically ill neonates. *Pediatr Crit Care Med*. 2009;10 (2):256-259.

Tobon AM, Franco L, Espinal D, et al, "Disseminated Histoplasmosis in Children: The Role of Itraconazole Therapy," *Pediatr Infect Dis J*, 1996; 15:1002-8.

Wheat J, Freifeld AG, Kleiman MB, et al, "Clinical Practice Guidelines for the Management of Patients With Histoplasmosis: 2007 Update by the Infectious Diseases Society of America," *Clin Infect Dis*, 2007, 45 (7):807–25.

Ivacaftor (eye va KAF tor)

Brand Names: U.S. Kalydeco
Brand Names: Canada Kalydeco

Therapeutic Category Cystic Fibrosis Transmembrane Conductance Regulator Potentiator

Generic Availability (U.S.) No

Use Treatment of cystic fibrosis (CF) in patients who have a G551D mutation in the cystic fibrosis transmembrane conductance regulator (CFTR) gene (FDA approved in ages ≥6 years and adults); **Note:** Has not been shown effective in CF patients who are homozygous for the F508del mutation in the CFTR gene

Pregnancy Risk Factor B

Pregnancy Considerations Adverse events have not been observed in animal reproduction studies.

Breast-Feeding Considerations Although unknown, the manufacturer suggests that excretion of ivacaftor in breast milk is probable; caution is recommended when administering ivacaftor to nursing women.

Contraindications Hypersensitivity to ivacaftor or any component

Warnings May increase hepatic transaminases; monitor liver function at baseline, every 3 months during first year of therapy and then periodically thereafter; temporarily discontinue treatment if ALT or AST >5 times ULN; use with caution in hepatic impairment; dosage adjustment recommended in patients with moderate to severe (Child-Pugh class B or C) impairment.

Precautions Ivacaftor is a CYP3A substrate; strong CYP3A4 inducers (eg, rifampin, rifabutin, phenobarbital, carbamazepine, phenytoin, St John's wort) may reduce efficacy; concurrent use should be avoided. Consider dose reduction with concurrent moderate or strong CYP3A4 inhibitors (eg, erythromycin, ketoconazole, voriconazole) use; ivacaftor may inhibit CYP3A and P-gp substrates (eg, midazolam, diazepam, digoxin, cyclosporine, tacrolimus); monitor and use with caution. Not effective in CF patients who are homozygous for the CFTR gene F508del mutation; avoid use in these patients. Use with caution in patients with severe renal impairment (CrCl <30 mL/minute) or end-stage renal disease; ivacaftor use has not been studied. Cataracts have been observed in animal studies using juvenile rats exposed to ivacaftor (at doses approximately one-tenth the maximum recommended human dose); cataracts have not been observed in studies involving older animals. It is unknown if this potential concern seen in animals studies is relevant to humans.

Adverse Reactions

Central nervous system: Dizziness, headache
Dermatologic: Acne, rash
Gastrointestinal: Abdominal pain, diarrhea, nausea
Endocrine & metabolic: Hyperglycemia
Hepatic: Transaminases increased
Neuromuscular & skeletal: Arthralgia, musculoskeletal chest pain, myalgia
Respiratory: Nasal congestion, nasopharyngitis, oropharyngeal pain, pharyngeal erythema, pleuritic chest pain, rhinitis, sinus congestion, upper respiratory tract infection, wheezing
Miscellaneous: Bacteria in sputum
Rare but important or life-threatening: Hypoglycemia

Drug Interactions

Metabolism/Transport Effects Substrate of CYP3A4 (major); **Note:** Assignment of Major/Minor substrate status based on clinically relevant drug interaction potential; **Inhibits** CYP2C8 (weak), CYP2C9 (weak), CYP3A4 (weak), P-glycoprotein

Avoid Concomitant Use

Avoid concomitant use of Ivacaftor with any of the following: Bosutinib; Conivaptan; CYP3A4 Inducers (Strong); Fusidic Acid (Systemic); Grapefruit Juice; PAZOPanib; Pimozide; Silodosin; St Johns Wort; Topotecan; VinCRIStine (Liposomal)

Increased Effect/Toxicity

Ivacaftor may increase the levels/effects of: Afatinib; ARIPiprazole; Bosutinib; Brentuximab Vedotin; Colchicine; CYP3A4 Substrates; Dabigatran Etexilate; Dofetilide; DOXOrubicin (Conventional); Everolimus; Lomitapide; PAZOPanib; P-glycoprotein/ABCB1 Substrates; Pimozide; Prucalopride; Rifaximin; Rivaroxaban; Silodosin; Topotecan; VinCRIStine (Liposomal)

The levels/effects of Ivacaftor may be increased by: Conivaptan; CYP3A4 Inhibitors (Moderate); CYP3A4 Inhibitors (Strong); Dasatinib; Fusidic Acid (Systemic); Grapefruit Juice; Luliconazole; Mifepristone; Simeprevir; Stiripentol

Decreased Effect

The levels/effects of Ivacaftor may be decreased by: Bosentan; CYP3A4 Inducers (Strong); Dabrafenib; Deferasirox; Siltuximab; St Johns Wort; Tocilizumab

Food Interactions Ivacaftor serum concentrations may be increased when taken with grapefruit or Seville oranges. Management: Avoid concurrent use.

Stability Store at 20°C to 25°C (68°F to 77°F); excursions permitted to 15°C to 30°C (59°F to 86°F).

Mechanism of Action Potentiates epithelial cell chloride ion transport of defective (G551D mutant) cell-surface CFTR protein thereby improving the regulation of salt and water absorption and secretion in various tissues (eg, lung, gastrointestinal tract).

Pharmacodynamics Onset of action: FEV_1 increased, sweat chloride decreased within ~2 weeks

Pharmacokinetics (Adult data unless noted)

Absorption: Variable; increased (by two- to fourfold) with fatty foods

Distribution: V_d: 353 L ± 122 L

Protein binding: ~99%; primarily to alpha₁ acid glycoprotein, albumin

Metabolism: Hepatic; extensive via CYP3A4; forms 2 major metabolites [M1 (active; ⅙ potency) and M6 (inactive)]

Half-life: ~12 hours

Time to peak serum concentration: ~4 hours

Elimination: Feces (88%, 65% of administered dose as metabolites); urine (minimal, as unchanged drug)

Dosing: Usual Cystic Fibrosis:

Children ≥6 years and Adolescents: Oral: 150 mg every 12 hours

Coadministration with CYP3A4 strong inhibitors (eg, ketoconazole, itraconazole, posaconazole, voriconazole, clarithromycin, telithromycin): Oral: 150 mg twice **weekly**

Coadministration with CYP3A4 moderate inhibitors (eg, erythromycin, fluconazole): Oral: 150 mg once daily

Adults: Oral: 150 mg every 12 hours

Coadministration with CYP3A4 strong inhibitors (eg, ketoconazole, itraconazole, posaconazole, voriconazole, clarithromycin, telithromycin): Oral: 150 mg twice **weekly**

Coadministration with CYP3A4 moderate inhibitors (eg, erythromycin, fluconazole): Oral: 150 mg once daily

Dosage adjustment in renal impairment: Children ≥6 years, Adolescents, and Adults:

CrCl >30 mL/minute: No dosage adjustment necessary

CrCl ≤30 mL/minute: No dosage adjustment provided in manufacturer's labeling (not studied); use with caution

Dosage adjustment in hepatic impairment: Children ≥6 years, Adolescents, and Adults:

Mild impairment (Child-Pugh class A): No dosage adjustment necessary

Moderate impairment (Child-Pugh class B): Oral: 150 mg once daily

Severe impairment (Child-Pugh class C): Oral: Manufacturer recommends 150 mg once daily or less frequently; has not been studied, use with caution

Dosage adjustment in patients who develop elevations of aminotransferases: Children ≥6 years, Adolescents, and Adults: ALT or AST >5 times ULN: Oral: Hold ivacaftor; may resume if elevated transaminases resolved and after assessing benefits vs risks of continued treatment

Administration Administer with high-fat-containing foods (eg, butter, cheese pizza, eggs, peanut butter).

Monitoring Parameters CF mutation test (prior to therapy initiation if G551D mutation status unknown); ALT/AST at baseline, every 3 months for 1 year, then annually thereafter or as clinically indicated; FEV_1

Dosage Forms Excipient information presented when available (limited, particularly for generics); consult specific product labeling.

Tablet, Oral:

Kalydeco: 150 mg [contains fd&c blue #2 (indigotine)]

References

Accurso FJ, Rowe SM, Clancy JP, et al, "Effect of VX-770 in Persons With Cystic Fibrosis and the G551D-CFTR Mutation," *N Engl J Med*, 2010, 363(21):1991-2003.

Ramsey BW, Davies J, McElvaney NG, et al, "A CFTR Potentiator in Patients With Cystic Fibrosis and the G551D Mutation," *N Engl J Med*, 2011, 365(18):1663-72.

Ivermectin (Systemic) (eye ver MEK tin)

Brand Names: U.S. Stromectol

Therapeutic Category Anthelmintic; Anti-ectoparasitic Agent

Generic Availability (U.S.) No

Use Treatment of intestinal strongyloidiasis (FDA approved in pediatric patients ≥15 kg and adults); treatment of onchocerciasis due to the immature form of *Onchocerca volvulus* (FDA approved in pediatric patients ≥15 kg and adults). Has also been used for the treatment of other parasitic infections including but not limited to: *Ancylostoma braziliense*, *Ascaris lumbricoides*, *Gnathostoma spinigerum*, *Mansonella ozzardi*, *Mansonella streptocerca*, *Pediculus humanus capitis*, *Pediculus humanus corporis*, *Phthirus pubis*, *Trichuris trichiura*, *Sarcoptes scabiei*, *Wucheria bancrofti*

Pregnancy Risk Factor C

Pregnancy Considerations Teratogenic effects have been observed in animal reproduction studies; therefore, the manufacturer classifies ivermectin as pregnancy category C. Ivermectin is not recommended for use in pregnancy. Although studies during pregnancy are limited, several mass treatment programs have not identified an increased risk of adverse fetal, neonatal, or maternal outcomes following ivermectin use in the first and second trimesters.

Breast-Feeding Considerations Ivermectin is measurable in low concentrations in breast milk and is less than maternal plasma concentrations. Peak concentrations of ivermectin in breast milk may occur 4-12 hours after the oral dose. In one study, the calculated infant daily dose was 2.75 mcg/kg in a 1-month-old infant and would not be expected to cause adverse effects in the infant. The manufacturer and the CDC do not have safety data in children <15 kg and the CDC does not recommend the use of ivermectin in lactating women.

Contraindications Hypersensitivity to ivermectin or any component

Warnings May cause cutaneous and/or systemic reactions of varying severity (Mazzoti reaction) and ophthalmological reactions in patients with onchocerciasis; usually reported during the first 4 days after treatment and includes reactions such as arthralgia, edema, fever, hypotension, lymph node enlargement and tenderness, pruritus, synovitis, and urticarial rash. These reactions are probably due to allergic and inflammatory responses to the death of microfilariae. Supportive treatment of Mazzoti reaction includes oral hydration, recumbency, intravenous normal saline, and/or parenteral corticosteroids to treat postural hypotension; antihistamines, corticosteroids, and/or aspirin have been used to treat mild to moderate cases.

Serious and/or fatal encephalopathy has been reported rarely following treatment with ivermectin in patients with onchocerciasis and loiasis. In addition, back pain, conjunctival hemorrhage, dyspnea, urinary and/or fecal incontinence, difficulty standing/walking, mental status changes, confusion, lethargy, stupor, seizures, or coma has also been reported. Pretreatment assessment for *Loa loa* infection is recommended in any patient with significant exposure to endemic areas (West and Central Africa) prior to treatment with ivermectin. Safety and efficacy has not been established in children <15 kg. The American Academy of Pediatrics (AAP) cautions against using ivermectin in children weighing <15 kg or <2 years of age since their blood-brain barrier may be less developed than in older patients.

Precautions Use with caution in patients with hyper-reactive onchodermatitis who are more likely than others to experience severe adverse reactions such as edema and aggravation of onchodermatitis after treatment with ivermectin. Repeated courses of treatment for intestinal strongyloidiasis may be required in immunocompromised patients (eg, HIV); control of extraintestinal strongyloidiasis may necessitate suppressive (once monthly) therapy.

Adverse Reactions
Cardiovascular: Facial edema, orthostatic hypotension, peripheral edema, tachycardia
Central nervous system: Dizziness
Dermatologic: Pruritus
Gastrointestinal: Diarrhea, nausea
Hematologic: Eosinophilia, hemoglobin increased, leukocytes decreased
Hepatic: ALT increased, AST increased
Miscellaneous: Mazzotti-type reaction (with onchocerciasis): Arthralgia/synovitis, fever, lymph node enlargement/tenderness, pruritus, skin involvement (edema/urticarial rash)
Rare but important or life-threatening: Abdominal distention, abdominal pain, anemia, anorexia, anterior uveitis, asthma exacerbation, back pain, bilirubin increased, chest discomfort, chorioretinitis, choroiditis, coma, confusion, conjunctival hemorrhage (associated with onchocerciasis), conjunctivitis, constipation, dyspnea, encephalopathy (rare; associated with loiasis), eyelid edema, eye sensation abnormal, fatigue, fecal incontinence, headache, hepatitis, hypotension, INR increased (with concomitant warfarin), keratitis, lethargy, leukopenia, mental status changes, myalgia, neck pain, rash, red eye, seizure, somnolence, standing/walking difficulty, Stevens-Johnson syndrome, stupor, toxic epidermal necrolysis, tremor, urinary incontinence, urticaria, vertigo, vision loss (transient), vomiting, weakness

Drug Interactions
Metabolism/Transport Effects Substrate of CYP3A4 (minor), P-glycoprotein; **Note:** Assignment of Major/Minor substrate status based on clinically relevant drug interaction potential

Avoid Concomitant Use
Avoid concomitant use of Ivermectin (Systemic) with any of the following: BCG

Increased Effect/Toxicity
Ivermectin (Systemic) may increase the levels/effects of: Vitamin K Antagonists

The levels/effects of Ivermectin (Systemic) may be increased by: Azithromycin (Systemic); P-glycoprotein/ABCB1 Inhibitors

Decreased Effect
Ivermectin (Systemic) may decrease the levels/effects of: BCG; Sodium Picosulfate; Typhoid Vaccine

The levels/effects of Ivermectin (Systemic) may be decreased by: P-glycoprotein/ABCB1 Inducers

Food Interactions Bioavailability is increased 2.5-fold when administered following a high-fat meal. Management: Administer on an empty stomach.

Stability Store at temperatures below 30°C (86°F).

Mechanism of Action Ivermectin is a semisynthetic anthelminthic agent; it binds selectively and with strong affinity to glutamate-gated chloride ion channels which occur in invertebrate nerve and muscle cells. This leads to increased permeability of cell membranes to chloride ions then hyperpolarization of the nerve or muscle cell, and death of the parasite.

Pharmacokinetics (Adult data unless noted)
Absorption: Well absorbed
Distribution: V_d: 3.1-3.5 L/kg; High concentration in the liver and adipose tissue; excreted in breast milk in low concentrations; does not readily cross the blood-brain barrier in patients >15 kg or >2 years
Protein binding: 93% primarily to albumin
Half-life: 18 hours (range: 16-35 hours)
Time to peak serum concentration: 4 hours
Metabolism: >97% in the liver by CYP3A4; substrate of the p-glycoprotein transport system
Elimination: <1% in urine; feces

Dosing: Usual Oral: Children ≥15 kg, Adolescents, and Adults:
Onchocerciasis: 150 mcg/kg/dose as a single dose; may repeat every 3-12 months until asymptomatic
Strongyloidiasis: Manufacturer recommendations: 200 mcg/kg as a single dose; perform follow-up stool examinations; Alternative dosing: 200 mcg/kg/day once daily for 2 days (*Red Book*, 2009). In immunocompromised patients or patients with disseminated disease, may need to repeat therapy at 2-week intervals.
Ascariasis: 150-200 mcg/kg/dose as a single dose
Cutaneous larva migran due to Ancylostoma braziliense: 200 mcg/kg once daily for 1-2 days
Gnathostomiasis due to Gnathostoma spinigerum: 200 mcg/kg once daily for 2 days
Filariasis due to Mansonella streptocerca: 150 mcg/kg/dose as a single dose
Filariasis due to Mansonella ozzardi: 200 mcg/kg/dose as a single dose
Pediculosis: 400 mcg/kg/dose as a single dose on days 1 and 8 (Chosidow, 2010); alternatively, 200 mcg/kg/dose every 7 days for 3 doses (Foucault, 2006) **or** 200 mcg/kg/dose repeated once after 10 days (Jones, 2003) have been shown to be effective
Scabies due to Sarcoptes scabiei: 200 mcg/kg/dose as a single dose; may need to repeat in 10-14 days
Trichuriasis due to Trichuris trichiura: 200 mcg/kg once daily for 3 days
Filariasis due to Wucheria bancrofti: 200 mcg/kg/dose as a single dose given in combination with albendazole
Alternatively, the following weight-based dosing can be used: See tables on this page and the next page.

Weight-Based Dosage to Provide ~150 mcg/kg

Patient Weight (kg)	Single Oral Dose
15-25	3 mg
26-44	6 mg
45-64	9 mg
65-84	12 mg
≥85	150 mcg/kg

Weight-Based Dosage to Provide ~200 mcg/kg

Patient Weight (kg)	Single Oral Dose
15-24	3 mg
25-35	6 mg
36-50	9 mg
51-65	12 mg
66-79	15 mg
≥80	200 mcg/kg

Administration Oral: Administer on an empty stomach with water

Monitoring Parameters Skin and eye microfilarial counts, periodic ophthalmologic exams; follow up stool examinations

Dosage Forms Excipient information presented when available (limited, particularly for generics); consult specific product labeling.

Tablet, Oral:
  Stromectol: 3 mg

References

Chosidow O, Giraudeau B, Cottrell J, et al, "Oral Ivermectin Versus Malathion Lotion for Difficult-to-Treat Head Lice," *N Engl J Med*, 2010, 362(10):896-905.

"Drugs for Parasitic Infections," *Treatment Guidelines from the Medical Letter*, 2007, 5(Suppl):e1-15.

Foucault C, Ranque S, Badiaga S, et al, "Oral Ivermectin in the Treatment of Body Lice," *J Infect Dis*, 2006, 193(3):474-6.

Frankowski BL, Bocchini JA Jr, and Council on School Health and Committee on Infectious Diseases, "Head Lice," *Pediatrics*, 2010, 126 (2):392-403.

González Canga A, Sahagón Prieto AM, Diez Liébana MJ, et al, "The Pharmacokinetics and Interactions of Ivermectin in Humans - A Mini-Review," *AAPS J*, 2008, 10(1):42-6.

Jones KN and English JC 3rd, "Review of Common Therapeutic Options in the United States for the Treatment of Pediculosis Capitis," *Clin Infect Dis*, 2003, 36(11):1355-61.

Red Book: 2009 Report of the Committee on Infectious Diseases, 28th ed, Pickering LK, ed, Elk Grove Village, IL: American Academy of Pediatrics, 2009.

Ivermectin (Topical) (eye ver MEK tin)

Brand Names: U.S. Sklice

Therapeutic Category Antiparasitic Agent, Topical; Pediculocide

Generic Availability (U.S.) No

Use Treatment of head lice *(Pediculus capitis)* infestation (FDA approved in ages ≥6 months and adults)

Pregnancy Risk Factor C

Pregnancy Considerations Teratogenic effects have been observed in animal reproduction studies following oral administration. Refer to the Ivermectin (Systemic) monograph for additional information. Systemic absorption is less following topical application than with oral administration.

Breast-Feeding Considerations Following oral administration, ivermectin is measurable in low concentrations in breast milk. Refer to Ivermectin (Systemic) monograph for additional information. Systemic absorption is less following topical application than with oral administration.

Contraindications Hypersensitivity to ivermectin or any component

Warnings In infants <6 months, systemic absorption may be increased due to higher skin surface area to body mass ratio and immature skin barrier; risk for ivermectin toxicity potentially increased; avoid use in these patients.

Precautions For external use only on scalp and scalp hair; avoid contact with eyes. Wash hands after application.

Adverse Reactions Rare but important or life-threatening: Burning sensation on skin, conjunctivitis, dandruff, dry skin, eye irritation, ocular hyperemia

Drug Interactions

Metabolism/Transport Effects None known.

Avoid Concomitant Use There are no known interactions where it is recommended to avoid concomitant use.

Increased Effect/Toxicity There are no known significant interactions involving an increase in effect.

Decreased Effect There are no known significant interactions involving a decrease in effect.

Stability Store at 20°C to 25°C (68°F to 77°F); excursions permitted between 15°C to 30°C (59°F to 86°F); do not freeze.

Mechanism of Action Ivermectin is a semisynthetic anthelmintic agent; it binds selectively and with strong affinity to glutamate-gated chloride ion channels which occur in invertebrate nerve and muscle cells. This leads to increased permeability of cell membranes to chloride ions then hyperpolarization of the nerve or muscle cell, and death of the parasite.

Dosing: Usual Head lice: Infants ≥6 months, Children, Adolescents, and Adults: Topical: Apply sufficient amount (up to 1 tube) to completely cover dry hair and scalp; for single use only

Administration Topical: For external use only. Apply to dry scalp and hair closest to scalp first, then apply outward towards ends of hair; completely covering scalp and hair. Leave on for 10 minutes (start timing treatment after the scalp and hair have been completely covered). The hair should then be rinsed thoroughly with warm water. Avoid contact with the eyes. Nit combing is not required, although a fine-tooth comb may be used to remove treated lice and nits. Lotion is for one-time use; discard any unused portion.

Ivermectin should be a portion of a whole lice removal program, which should include washing or dry cleaning all clothing, hats, bedding, and towels recently worn or used by the patient and washing combs, brushes, and hair accessories in hot, soapy water.

Dosage Forms Excipient information presented when available (limited, particularly for generics); consult specific product labeling.

Lotion, External:
  Sklice: 0.5% (117 g) [contains methylparaben, propylparaben]

References

Frankowski BL and Bocchini JA Jr, "Head Lice," *Pediatrics*, 2010, 126 (2):392-403.

♦ **IVIG** see Immune Globulin *on page 1084*

♦ **IV Immune Globulin** see Immune Globulin *on page 1084*

♦ **Ivy-Rid [OTC]** see Benzocaine *on page 273*

♦ **Ixiaro** see Japanese Encephalitis Virus Vaccine (Inactivated) *on page 1173*

♦ **JAA-Aminophylline (Can)** see Aminophylline *on page 124*

♦ **JAMP-Allopurinol (Can)** see Allopurinol *on page 97*

♦ **JAMP-Amlodipine (Can)** see AmLODIPine *on page 135*

♦ **JAMP-Atenolol (Can)** see Atenolol *on page 222*

♦ **JAMP-Candesartan (Can)** see Candesartan *on page 363*

♦ **JAMP-Carvedilol (Can)** see Carvedilol *on page 385*

♦ **JAMP-Ciprofloxacin (Can)** see Ciprofloxacin (Systemic) *on page 471*

♦ **JAMP-Citalopram (Can)** see Citalopram *on page 484*

♦ **JAMP-Clopidogrel (Can)** see Clopidogrel *on page 521*

♦ **Jamp-Colchicine (Can)** see Colchicine *on page 537*

♦ **JAMP-Cyclobenzaprine (Can)** see Cyclobenzaprine *on page 558*

◆ **Jamp-Dicyclomine (Can)** *see* Dicyclomine *on page 652*

◆ **Jamp-Dimenhydrinate [OTC] (Can)** *see* DimenhyDRINATE *on page 670*

◆ **Jamp-Docusate [OTC] (Can)** *see* Docusate *on page 701*

◆ **JAMP-Fluoxetine (Can)** *see* FLUoxetine *on page 901*

◆ **Jamp-Fosinopril (Can)** *see* Fosinopril *on page 938*

◆ **JAMP-Gabapentin (Can)** *see* Gabapentin *on page 950*

◆ **Jamp-Ibuprofen (Can)** *see* Ibuprofen *on page 1059*

◆ **JAMP-Irbesartan (Can)** *see* Irbesartan *on page 1147*

◆ **JAMP-Letrozole (Can)** *see* Letrozole *on page 1211*

◆ **JAMP-Levetiracetam (Can)** *see* LevETIRAcetam *on page 1219*

◆ **JAMP-Lisinopril (Can)** *see* Lisinopril *on page 1262*

◆ **JAMP-Losartan (Can)** *see* Losartan *on page 1283*

◆ **JAMP-Metformin (Can)** *see* MetFORMIN *on page 1353*

◆ **JAMP-Metformin Blackberry (Can)** *see* MetFORMIN *on page 1353*

◆ **JAMP-Metoprolol-L (Can)** *see* Metoprolol *on page 1396*

◆ **Jamp-Montelukast (Can)** *see* Montelukast *on page 1438*

◆ **JAMP-Mycophenolate (Can)** *see* Mycophenolate *on page 1453*

◆ **JAMP-Omeprazole DR (Can)** *see* Omeprazole *on page 1535*

◆ **JAMP-Ondansetron (Can)** *see* Ondansetron *on page 1544*

◆ **JAMP-Pantoprazole (Can)** *see* Pantoprazole *on page 1595*

◆ **JAMP-Paroxetine (Can)** *see* PARoxetine *on page 1609*

◆ **JAMP-Pravastatin (Can)** *see* Pravastatin *on page 1720*

◆ **JAMP-Quetiapine (Can)** *see* QUEtiapine *on page 1783*

◆ **JAMP-Risperidone (Can)** *see* RisperiDONE *on page 1831*

◆ **JAMP-Rizatriptan (Can)** *see* Rizatriptan *on page 1845*

◆ **Jamp-Rosuvastatin (Can)** *see* Rosuvastatin *on page 1853*

◆ **JAMP-Sertraline (Can)** *see* Sertraline *on page 1879*

◆ **JAMP-Simvastatin (Can)** *see* Simvastatin *on page 1892*

◆ **JAMP-Terbinafine (Can)** *see* Terbinafine (Systemic) *on page 1982*

◆ **JAMP-Tobramycin (Can)** *see* Tobramycin (Systemic, Oral Inhalation) *on page 2034*

◆ **Jantoven** *see* Warfarin *on page 2156*

Japanese Encephalitis Virus Vaccine (Inactivated)

(jap a NEESE en sef a LYE tis VYE rus vak SEEN, in ak ti VAY ted)

Related Information

Immunization Administration Recommendations *on page 2368*

Immunization Guidelines *on page 2373*

Brand Names: U.S. Ixiaro

Brand Names: Canada Ixiaro

Therapeutic Category Vaccine, Inactivated Virus

Generic Availability (U.S.) No

Use Provide active immunity to Japanese encephalitis virus (Ixiaro®: FDA approved in ages ≥2 months and adults).

Japanese encephalitis vaccine is not recommended for all persons traveling to or residing in Asia. The Advisory Committee on Immunization Practices (ACIP) recommends vaccination for (CDC, 2010):

• Persons spending ≥1 month in endemic areas during transmission season.

• Research laboratory workers who may be exposed to the Japanese encephalitis virus.

Vaccination may also be considered for the following:

• Travel to areas with an ongoing outbreak

• Travelers planning to go outside of urban areas during transmission season and have an increased risk of exposure. For example, high-risk activities include extensive outdoor activity in rural areas especially at night; extensive outdoor activities such as camping, hiking, etc; staying in accommodations without air conditioning, screens or bed nets

• Travelers to endemic areas who are unsure of specific destination, activities, or duration of travel

Pregnancy Risk Factor B

Pregnancy Considerations Adverse events were not observed in animal reproduction studies. Risks of vaccine administration should be carefully considered and in general, pregnant women should only be vaccinated if they are at high risk for exposure. Infection from Japanese encephalitis during the first or second trimesters of pregnancy may increase risk of miscarriage. Intrauterine transmission of the Japanese encephalitis virus has been reported (CDC, 2010). To report inadvertent use of Ixiaro® during pregnancy, contact Novartis Vaccines (877-683-4732).

Breast-Feeding Considerations It is not known if the vaccine is excreted into breast milk; however, the ACIP does not consider breast-feeding to be a contraindication to (CDC, 2010). The manufacturer recommends that caution be used if administered to nursing women.

Contraindications Severe allergic reaction to a previous dose of the vaccine, any other Japanese encephalitis virus vaccine, or any component of the vaccine

Warnings Immediate treatment for severe hypersensitivity reactions should be available during vaccine use. Contains protamine sulfate which may cause hypersensitivity reactions in certain individuals.

Precautions Because of the potential for severe adverse reactions, Japanese encephalitis vaccine is **not** recommended for all persons traveling to or residing in Asia. Use is **not** recommended for short-term travelers (<30 days) who will not be outside of an urban area or when the visit is outside of a well-defined Japanese encephalitis virus transmission season. Risk of exposure to the Japanese encephalitis virus may vary from year to year for a particular area (CDC, 2010).

The decision to administer or delay vaccination because of current or recent febrile illness depends on the severity of symptoms and the etiology of the disease. Immunization should be delayed during the course of an acute severe febrile illness; may administer to patients with mild acute illness (with or without fever). Use with caution in severely immunocompromised patients (eg, patients receiving chemo/radiation therapy or other immunosuppressive therapy, including high-dose corticosteroids); may have a reduced response to vaccination and vaccination may not result in effective immunity in all patients. Response depends upon multiple factors (eg, type of vaccine, age of patient) and may be improved by administering the vaccine at the recommended dose, route, and interval (CDC, 2011). In general, household and close contacts of persons with altered immunocompetence may receive all age-appropriate vaccines.

Routine prophylactic administration of acetaminophen to prevent fever due to vaccines has been shown to decrease the immune response of some vaccines; the clinical ▶

significance of this reduction in immune response has not been established (Prymula, 2009).

Other means to reduce the risk of mosquito exposure (including bed nets, insect repellents, protective clothing, avoidance of travel in endemic areas, and avoidance of outdoor activity during twilight and evening periods) should be used (CDC, 2010).

Adverse Reactions Report allergic or unusual adverse reactions to the Vaccine Adverse Event Reporting System (VAERS) 1-800-822-7967 or online at https://vaers.hhs.gov/esub/index. In Canada, adverse reactions may be reported to local provincial/territorial health agencies or to the Vaccine Safety Section at Public Health Agency of Canada (1-866-844-0018).

Central nervous system: Fatigue (more common in adults), headache (more common in adults), irritability (infants, children, and adolescents; more common in infants and children <3 years)

Dermatologic: Skin rash (more common in infants and children <3 years)

Gastrointestinal: Decreased appetite (infants, children, and adolescents), diarrhea (more common in infants and children <3 years), nausea (more common in adults), vomiting (more common in infants and children <3 years)

Infection: Influenza (adults)

Local: Erythema at injection site (more common in infants and children <3 years), induration at injection site (more common in adults), itching at injection site (more common in adults), pain at injection site (more common in adults), swelling at injection site, tenderness at injection site (more common in adults)

Neuromuscular & skeletal: Back pain (adults), myalgia (more common in adults)

Respiratory: Cough (adults), flu-like symptoms (more common in adults), nasopharyngitis (adults), pharyngolaryngeal pain (adults), rhinitis (adults), sinusitis (adults), upper respiratory tract infection (adults)

Miscellaneous: Febrile seizures (children <3 years), fever (more common in infants and children <3 years)

Rare but important or life-threatening: Appendicitis, cerebral infarction, chest pain, dermatomyositis, disseminated intravascular coagulation, encephalitis, epilepsy, herpes zoster, iritis, labyrinthitis, limb abscess, limb pain, musculoskeletal injury, neuritis, oropharyngeal spasm, ovarian torsion, paresthesia, rectal hemorrhage, rupture of ovarian cyst, seizure, syncope

Drug Interactions

Metabolism/Transport Effects None known.

Avoid Concomitant Use There are no known interactions where it is recommended to avoid concomitant use.

Increased Effect/Toxicity There are no known significant interactions involving an increase in effect.

Decreased Effect

The levels/effects of Japanese Encephalitis Virus Vaccine (Inactivated) may be decreased by: Belimumab; Fingolimod; Immunosuppressants

Stability Refrigerate at 2°C to 8°C (35°F to 46°F); protect from light; do not freeze; store in original packaging to protect from light; during storage, a white precipitant in clear liquid may be observed.

Mechanism of Action This vaccine induces antibodies to neutralize the Japanese encephalitis virus. Antibody response is measured using a 50% plaque-reduction neutralization antibody test ($PRNT_{50}$); a threshold of ≥1:10 is considered protective immunity.

Pharmacokinetics (Adult data unless noted) Onset of action: Protective immunity was observed in 96% to 100% of pediatric patients (2 months to 17 years) and ~21% of adults 10 days after the first vaccine dose and adults 28 days after the second vaccine dose

Dosing: Usual

Infants ≥2 months, Children, and Adolescents:

Primary immunization schedule:

Infants 2 months to Children <3 years: I.M.: 0.25 mL/dose on days 0 and 28 for a total of 2 doses; series should be completed at least 1 week prior to potential exposure.

Children ≥3 years and Adolescents: I.M.: 0.5 mL/dose on days 0 and 28 for a total of 2 doses; series should be completed at least 1 week prior to potential exposure.

Booster dose: Adolescents ≥17 years: 0.5 mL/dose may be given prior to potential re-exposure if the primary series was completed >1 year previously; **Note:** The safety and immunogenicity of booster doses in pediatric patients <17 years has not been evaluated.

Adults:

Primary immunization schedule: I.M.: 0.5 mL/dose; a total of 2 doses given on days 0 and 28. Series should be completed at least 1 week prior to potential exposure.

Booster dose: Booster dose may be given prior to potential re-exposure if the primary series was completed >1 year previously.

Dosage adjustment in renal impairment: There are no dosage adjustments provided in manufacturer's labeling.

Dosage adjustment in hepatic impairment: There are no dosage adjustments provided in manufacturer's labeling.

Administration For I.M. injection; do not inject I.V., SubQ, or intradermally. Shake well prior to use to form a homogeneous suspension. Do not use if discolored or if particulate matter remains.

Ixiaro® is available only in a prefilled syringe containing 0.5 mL. In order to administer a 0.25 mL dose in children 2 months to <3 years, first shake the syringe to form a homogenous suspension. Attach a sterile needle to the prefilled syringe and while holding the syringe upright, discard 0.25 mL of the suspension. Attach a new sterile needle prior to administration.

Administration site (preferred):

Infants 2 to <12 months: Anterolateral aspect of the thigh

Children 1 to <3 years: Anterolateral aspect of the thigh or deltoid muscle may be used (if mass is adequate)

Children ≥3 years, Adolescents, and Adults: Deltoid muscle

U.S. law requires that the date of administration, name of manufacturer, lot number, and administering person's name, title and address be entered into patient's permanent medical record.

Additional Information Ixiaro® is a purified Japanese encephalitis vaccine made from the SA_{14}-14-2 strain grown in Vero cells (JE-VC). It was developed due to neurologic side effects observed with Je-Vax®, a vaccine derived from mice-brain cells (JE-MB) that contains additives which may contribute to the adverse effects. Studies are currently planned to determine the need for booster doses following initial vaccination with Ixiaro®. Adults who previously received Je-Vax® vaccine and require further immunization against Japanese encephalitis should be administered a 2-dose primary series of Ixiaro® [CDC 60 (20), 2011].

Dosage Forms Excipient information presented when available (limited, particularly for generics); consult specific product labeling.

Suspension, Intramuscular:

Ixiaro: (0.5 mL) [latex free; contains albumin bovine, protamine sulfate, sodium metabisulfite]

References

Centers for Disease Control and Prevention (CDC), "General Recommendations on Immunization - Recommendations of the Advisory

Committee on Immunization Practices (ACIP)," *MMWR Recomm Rep*, 2011, 60(2):1-64.

Centers for Disease Control and Prevention (CDC), "Japanese Encephalitis Vaccines. Recommendations of the Advisory Committee on Immunization Practices (ACIP)," *MMWR Recomm Rep*, 2010, 59(RR-1):1-27.

Centers for Disease Control and Prevention (CDC), "Recommendations for Use of a Booster Dose of Inactivated Vero Cell Culture-Derived Japanese Encephalitis Vaccine: Advisory Committee on Immunization Practices, 2011," *MMWR Morb Mortal Wkly Rep*, 2011, 60 (20):661-3.

Centers for Disease Control and Prevention (CDC), "Syncope After Vaccination-United States, January 2005-July 2007," *MMWR Morb Mortal Wkly Rep*, 2008, 57(17):457-60.

Prymula R, Siegrist CA, Chlibek R, et al, "Effect of Prophylactic Paracetamol Administration at Time of Vaccination on Febrile Reactions and Antibody Responses in Children: Two Open-Label, Randomised Controlled Trials," *Lancet*, 2009, 374(9698):1339-50.

◆ **Jencycla** *see* Norethindrone *on page 1511*

◆ **JE-VC (Ixiaro)** *see* Japanese Encephalitis Virus Vaccine (Inactivated) *on page 1173*

◆ **Jock Itch Spray [OTC]** *see* Tolnaftate *on page 2044*

◆ **Jolivette** *see* Norethindrone *on page 1511*

◆ **J-Tan D PD [OTC]** *see* Brompheniramine and Pseudoephedrine *on page 306*

◆ **Jurnista (Can)** *see* HYDROmorphone *on page 1041*

◆ **Just For Kids [OTC]** *see* Fluoride *on page 894*

◆ **K-10 (Can)** *see* Potassium Chloride *on page 1708*

◆ **K-99 [OTC]** *see* Potassium Gluconate *on page 1711*

◆ **Kadian** *see* Morphine (Systemic) *on page 1440*

◆ **Kala® [OTC]** *see* Lactobacillus *on page 1191*

◆ **Kaletra** *see* Lopinavir and Ritonavir *on page 1272*

◆ **Kalexate** *see* Sodium Polystyrene Sulfonate *on page 1917*

◆ **Kalydeco** *see* Ivacaftor *on page 1169*

◆ **Kank-A Mouth Pain [OTC]** *see* Benzocaine *on page 273*

◆ **Kaopectate® [OTC] (Can)** *see* Attapulgite *on page 238*

◆ **Kaopectate® Children's [OTC] (Can)** *see* Attapulgite *on page 238*

◆ **Kaopectate® Extra Strength [OTC] (Can)** *see* Attapulgite *on page 238*

◆ **Kaote DVI** *see* Antihemophilic Factor (Human) *on page 170*

◆ **Kao-Tin [OTC]** *see* Bismuth *on page 294*

◆ **Kao-Tin [OTC]** *see* Docusate *on page 701*

◆ **Kapvay** *see* CloNIDine *on page 516*

◆ **Karbinal™ ER** *see* Carbinoxamine *on page 377*

◆ **Karbinal ER** *see* Carbinoxamine *on page 377*

◆ **Kayexalate** *see* Sodium Polystyrene Sulfonate *on page 1917*

◆ **Kayexalate® (Can)** *see* Sodium Polystyrene Sulfonate *on page 1917*

◆ **K-Bicarb [OTC]** *see* Potassium Bicarbonate *on page 1707*

◆ **KCl** *see* Potassium Chloride *on page 1708*

◆ **Kdur** *see* Potassium Chloride *on page 1708*

◆ **K-Dur (Can)** *see* Potassium Chloride *on page 1708*

◆ **Kedbumin** *see* Albumin *on page 82*

◆ **K-Effervescent** *see* Potassium Bicarbonate *on page 1707*

◆ **Keflex** *see* Cephalexin *on page 429*

◆ **Kefzol** *see* CeFAZolin *on page 393*

◆ **Kenalog** *see* Triamcinolone (Systemic) *on page 2072*

◆ **Kenalog** *see* Triamcinolone (Topical) *on page 2078*

◆ **Kenalog® (Can)** *see* Triamcinolone (Topical) *on page 2078*

◆ **Keppra** *see* LevETIRAcetam *on page 1219*

◆ **Keppra XR** *see* LevETIRAcetam *on page 1219*

◆ **Keralyt** *see* Salicylic Acid *on page 1860*

◆ **Keralyt Scalp** *see* Salicylic Acid *on page 1860*

◆ **Kerr Insta-Char [OTC]** *see* Charcoal, Activated *on page 432*

◆ **Kerr Insta-Char in Sorbitol [OTC]** *see* Charcoal, Activated *on page 432*

◆ **Ketalar** *see* Ketamine *on page 1175*

Ketamine (KEET a meen)

Medication Safety Issues

Sound-alike/look-alike issues:
Ketalar may be confused with Kenalog, ketorolac

High alert medication:
The Institute for Safe Medication Practices (ISMP) includes this medication among its list of drugs which have a heightened risk of causing significant patient harm when used in error.

Related Information
Preprocedure Sedatives in Children *on page 2402*

Brand Names: U.S. Ketalar

Brand Names: Canada Ketalar; Ketamine Hydrochloride Injection, USP

Therapeutic Category General Anesthetic

Generic Availability (U.S.) Yes

Use Anesthesia, short surgical procedures, dressing changes

Pregnancy Considerations Adverse events have not been observed in animal reproduction studies. Ketamine crosses the placenta and can be detected in fetal tissue. Ketamine produces dose dependent increases in uterine contractions; effects may vary by trimester. The plasma clearance of ketamine is reduced during pregnancy. Dose related neonatal depression and decreased APGAR scores have been reported with large doses administered at delivery (Ghoneim, 1977; Little, 1972; White, 1982).

Breast-Feeding Considerations It is not known if ketamine is excreted in breast milk.

Contraindications Hypersensitivity to ketamine or any component; patients in whom a significant elevation in blood pressure would be hazardous (eg, patients with elevated intracranial pressure, hypertension, aneurysms, thyrotoxicosis, CHF, angina, or psychotic disorders)

Warnings Use only by or under the direct supervision of physicians experienced in administering general anesthetics. Resuscitative equipment should be available for use; respiratory depression or apnea may occur with rapid administration rates or with large doses. Postanesthetic emergence reactions which can manifest as vivid dreams, hallucinations and/or frank delirium occur in 12% of patients **[U.S. Boxed Warning]**; these reactions are less common in patients <15 years of age and >65 years and when given intramuscularly. Emergence reactions may occur up to 24 hours postoperatively and may be reduced by minimization of verbal, tactile, and visual patient stimulation during recovery, or by pretreatment with a benzodiazepine (using lower recommended doses of ketamine). Severe emergent reactions may require treatment with a small hypnotic dose of a short or ultra-short acting barbiturate. Prolonged use may cause physical dependence (withdrawal symptoms on discontinuation) and tolerance. Cardiac function should be continuously monitored in patients with hypertension or cardiac decompensation. Animal data suggests that exposure of the developing brain to anesthetics like ketamine (especially during the critical time of synaptogenesis) may result in long-term impairment of cognitive function (Patel, 2009).

Precautions Use with caution in patients with gastroesophageal reflux. Use with caution and decrease the dose in patients with hepatic dysfunction. Use with caution in patients with a full stomach, patients should fast (ie, be NPO) for an appropriate time before being sedated for elective procedures. Use with caution in patients with elevated CSF pressure, chronic alcoholics, and in acutely intoxicated patients. Do not use as sole anesthetic in surgery or diagnostic procedures of the pharynx, larynx, or bronchial tree or in surgical procedures involving visceral pain pathways

Adverse Reactions

Cardiovascular: Arrhythmia, bradycardia/tachycardia, hyper-/hypotension

Central nervous system: Intracranial pressure increased

Dermatologic: Erythema (transient), morbilliform rash (transient)

Gastrointestinal: Anorexia, nausea, salivation increased, vomiting

Local: Pain at the injection site, exanthema at the injection site

Neuromuscular & skeletal: Skeletal muscle tone enhanced (tonic-clonic movements)

Ocular: Diplopia, intraocular pressure increased, nystagmus

Respiratory: Airway obstruction, apnea, bronchial secretions increased, respiratory depression, laryngospasm

Miscellaneous: Anaphylaxis, dependence with prolonged use, emergence reactions (includes confusion, delirium, dreamlike state, excitement, hallucinations, irrational behavior, vivid imagery)

Drug Interactions

Metabolism/Transport Effects Substrate of CYP2B6 (major), CYP2C9 (major), CYP3A4 (major); **Note:** Assignment of Major/Minor substrate status based on clinically relevant drug interaction potential

Avoid Concomitant Use

Avoid concomitant use of Ketamine with any of the following: Azelastine (Nasal); Conivaptan; Fusidic Acid (Systemic); Paraldehyde; Thalidomide

Increased Effect/Toxicity

Ketamine may increase the levels/effects of: Alcohol (Ethyl); Azelastine (Nasal); Buprenorphine; CNS Depressants; Hydrocodone; Methotrimeprazine; Metyrosine; Mirtazapine; Paraldehyde; Pramipexole; ROPINIRole; Rotigotine; Selective Serotonin Reuptake Inhibitors; Thalidomide; Thiopental; Zolpidem

The levels/effects of Ketamine may be increased by: Brimonidine (Topical); Cannabis; Ceritinib; Conivaptan; CYP2B6 Inhibitors (Moderate); CYP2B6 Inhibitors (Strong); CYP2C9 Inhibitors (Moderate); CYP2C9 Inhibitors (Strong); CYP3A4 Inhibitors (Moderate); CYP3A4 Inhibitors (Strong); Dasatinib; Doxylamine; Dronabinol; Droperidol; Fusidic Acid (Systemic); HydrOXYzine; Ivacaftor; Kava Kava; Luliconazole; Magnesium Sulfate; Methotrimeprazine; Mifepristone; Nabilone; Perampanel; Quazepam; Rufinamide; Simeprevir; Sodium Oxybate; Stiripentol; Tapentadol; Tetrahydrocannabinol

Decreased Effect

The levels/effects of Ketamine may be decreased by: CYP2C9 Inducers (Strong); Dabrafenib; Peginterferon Alfa-2b

Stability Protect from light; do not mix with barbiturates or diazepam as precipitation may occur

Mechanism of Action Produces a cataleptic-like state in which the patient is dissociated from the surrounding environment by direct action on the cortex and limbic system. Ketamine is a noncompetitive NMDA receptor antagonist that blocks glutamate. Low (subanesthetic) doses produce analgesia, and modulate central sensitization, hyperalgesia and opioid tolerance. Reduces polysynaptic spinal reflexes.

Pharmacodynamics

Onset of action:
Anesthesia:
I.M.: 3-4 minutes
I.V.: Within 30 seconds
Analgesia:
Oral: Within 30 minutes
I.M.: Within 10-15 minutes
Duration: Following single dose:
Anesthesia:
I.M.: 12-25 minutes
I.V.: 5-10 minutes
Analgesia: I.M.: 15-30 minutes
Recovery:
I.M.: 3-4 hours
I.V.: 1-2 hours

Pharmacokinetics (Adult data unless noted)

Metabolism: In the liver via N-dealkylation, hydroxylation of cyclohexone ring, glucuronide conjugation, and dehydration of hydroxylated metabolites

Half-life:
Alpha: 10-15 minutes
Terminal: 2.5 hours

Dosing: Neonatal Note: Some neonatal experts do not recommend the use of ketamine in neonates; an increase in neuronal apoptosis has been observed in neonatal animal studies (Patel, 2009).

I.V.: Limited data available; dose not established; titrate dose to effect; further studies needed:

Adjunct to anesthesia: 0.5-2 mg/kg/dose has been reported. A study of 23 patients [mean age: 3.2 years (9 days to 7 years)] undergoing MRI received a fixed dose of 0.5 mg/kg of ketamine prior to propofol bolus and infusion. A single case report describes ketamine (1-2 mg/kg) adjunct use with sevoflurane in a one-day old neonate (GA: 33 weeks) undergoing pacemaker placement (Castilla, 2004; Tomatir, 2004).

Procedural sedation/analgesia: Full-term neonates: 0.2-1 mg/kg/dose; may repeat 0.5 mg/kg/dose as needed; use most frequently reported in cardiac catheterization and ROP corrective procedures (Jobeir, 2003; Lyon, 2008; Pees, 2003)

Dosing: Usual Note: Titrate dose to effect.

Children:
Oral: 6-10 mg/kg for 1 dose (mixed in cola or other beverage) given 30 minutes before the procedure

I.M.: 3-7 mg/kg

I.V.: Range: 0.5-2 mg/kg, use smaller doses (0.5-1 mg/kg) for sedation for minor procedures; usual induction dosage: 1-2 mg/kg

Continuous I.V. infusion: Sedation: 5-20 mcg/kg/minute; start at lower dosage listed and titrate to effect

Adults:
I.M.: 3-8 mg/kg

I.V.: Range: 1-4.5 mg/kg; usual induction dosage: 1-2 mg/kg

Children and Adults: Maintenance: Supplemental doses of $^1/_3$ to $^1/_2$ of initial dose

Administration

Oral: Use 100 mg/mL I.V. solution and mix the appropriate dose in 0.2-0.3 mL/kg of cola or other beverage

Parenteral: I.V.: Administer slowly, do not exceed 0.5 mg/kg/minute; do not administer faster than 60 seconds; maximum concentration for slow I.V. push: 50 mg/mL; **Note:** Do not inject 100 mg/mL concentration I.V. without proper dilution; dilute with an equal volume of SWI, NS, or D_5W to produce 50 mg/mL concentration for slow I.V. push. Maximum concentration for intermittent or continuous infusion: 2 mg/mL

Monitoring Parameters Cardiovascular effects, heart rate, blood pressure, respiratory rate, transcutaneous O_2 saturation

Test Interactions May interfere with urine detection of phencyclidine (false-positive).

Additional Information Used in combination with anticholinergic agents to decrease hypersalivation; should not be used for sedation for procedures that require a total lack of movement (eg, MRI, radiation therapy) due to association with purposeless movements

Controlled Substance C-III

Dosage Forms Excipient information presented when available (limited, particularly for generics); consult specific product labeling.

Solution, Injection:

Ketalar: 10 mg/mL (20 mL); 50 mg/mL (10 mL); 100 mg/mL (5 mL)

Generic: 10 mg/mL (20 mL); 50 mg/mL (10 mL); 100 mg/mL (5 mL, 10 mL)

References

Castilla M, Jerez M, Llácer M, et al, "Anaesthetic Management in a Neonate With Congenital Complete Heart Block," *Paediatr Anaesth*, 2004, 14(2):172-5.

Cote CJ, "Sedation for the Pediatric Patient: A Review," *Pediatr Clin North Am*, 1994, 41(1):31-58.

Ghoneim MM and Korttila K, "Pharmacokinetics of Intravenous Anaesthetics: Implications for Clinical Use," *Clin Pharmacokinet*, 1977, 2 (5):344-72.

Gutstein HB, Johnson KL, Heard MN, et al, "Oral Ketamine Premedication in Children," *Anesthesiology*, 1992, 76(1):28-33.

Jobeir A, Galal MO, Bulbul ZR, et al, "Use of Low-Dose Ketamine and/or Midazolam for Pediatric Cardiac Catheterization," *Pediatr Cardiol*, 2003, 24(3):236-43.

Little B, Chang T, Chucot L, et al, "Study of Ketamine as an Obstetric Anesthetic Agent," *Am J Obstet Gynecol* , 1972, 15:113(2):247-60.

Lyon F, Dabbs T, and O'Meara M, "Ketamine Sedation During the Treatment of Retinopathy of Prematurity," *Eye (Lond)*, 2008, 22 (5):684-6.

Patel P and Sun L, "Update on Neonatal Anesthetic Neurotoxicity: Insight Into Molecular Mechanisms and Relevance to Humans," *Anesthesiology*, 2009, 110(4):703-8.

Pees C, Haas NA, Ewert P, et al, "Comparison of Analgesic/Sedative Effect of Racemic Ketamine and S(+)-Ketamine During Cardiac Catheterization in Newborns and Children," *Pediatr Cardiol*, 2003, 24(5):424-9.

Saarenmaa E, Neuvonen PJ, Huttunen P, et al, "Ketamine for Procedural Pain Relief in Newborn Infants," *Arch Dis Child Fetal Neonatal Ed*, 2001, 85(1):F53-6.

Tobias JD, Phipps S, Smith B, et al, "Oral Ketamine Premedication to Alleviate the Distress of Invasive Procedures in Pediatric Oncology Patients," *Pediatrics*, 1992, 90(4):537-41.

Tobias JD and Rasmussen GE, "Pain Management and Sedation in the Pediatric Intensive Care Unit," *Pediatr Clin North Am*, 1994, 41 (6):1269-92.

Tomatir E, Atalay H, Gurses E, et al, "Effects of Low Dose Ketamine Before Induction on Propofol Anesthesia for Pediatric Magnetic Resonance Imaging," *Paediatr Anaesth*, 2004, 14(10):845-50.

White PF, Way WL, and Trevor AJ, "Ketamine – Its Pharmacology and Therapeutic Uses," *Anesthesiology*, 1982, 56(2):119-36.

◆ **Ketamine Hydrochloride** *see* Ketamine *on page 1175*

◆ **Ketamine Hydrochloride Injection, USP (Can)** *see* Ketamine *on page 1175*

Ketoconazole (Systemic) (kee toe KOE na zole)

Medication Safety Issues

Sound-alike/look-alike issues:

Nizoral may be confused with Nasarel, Neoral, Nitrol

Brand Names: Canada Apo-Ketoconazole; Teva-Ketoconazole

Therapeutic Category Antifungal Agent, Systemic

Generic Availability (U.S.) Yes

Use Treatment of susceptible fungal infections, including blastomycosis, coccidioidomycosis, histoplasmosis, paracoccidioidomycosis, and chromomycosis in patients who have failed or who are intolerant to other antifungal therapies (FDA approved in ages ≥2 years of age and adults).

Note: Due to serious adverse effects (hepatotoxicity) and significant drug interactions, ketoconazole is seldom used in pediatric patients (*Red Book* [AAP], 2012); use should be reserved for patients who have failed or are intolerant to other antifungal therapies.

Medication Guide Available Yes

Pregnancy Risk Factor C

Pregnancy Considerations Adverse effects were noted in animal reproduction studies.

Breast-Feeding Considerations In a case report, ketoconazole in concentrations of ≤0.22 mcg/mL were detected in the breast milk of a woman 1 month postpartum. She had been taking oral ketoconazole 200 mg/day for 5 days at the time of sampling. The maximum milk concentration occurred 3.25 hours after the dose and concentrations were undetectable 24 hours after the dose. Based on the highest milk concentration, the estimated dose to the nursing infant was 1.4% of the maternal dose. Breast-feeding is not recommended by the manufacturer.

Contraindications Hypersensitivity to ketoconazole or any component; acute or chronic liver disease; coadministration with alprazolam, cisapride, colchicine, disopyramide, dofetilide, dronedarone, eplerenone, ergot alkaloids (eg, dihydroergotamine, ergometrine, ergotamine, methylergometrine), felodipine, HMG-CoA reductase inhibitors (eg, lovastatin, simvastatin), irinotecan, lurasidone, methadone, oral midazolam, nisoldipine, pimozide, quinidine, ranolazine, tolvaptan, triazolam

Warnings Has been associated with hepatotoxicity, including some fatal cases and cases requiring liver transplantation **[U.S. Boxed Warning]**; some patients had no apparent risk factors for hepatic disease. Toxicity was observed after a median duration of therapy of ~4 weeks, but has also been noted after as little as 3 days; may occur when patients receive high doses for short durations or low doses for long durations. Most cases have been observed in the treatment of onychomycosis. Use with caution in patients with preexisting hepatic impairment, those on prolonged therapy and/or taking other hepatotoxic drugs concurrently. Hepatic dysfunction is typically (but not always) reversible upon discontinuation. Obtain liver function tests at baseline and frequently throughout therapy; serum ALT should be monitored weekly throughout therapy. Discontinue therapy for elevated hepatic enzymes that persist or worsen or if accompanied by signs/symptoms (eg, jaundice, nausea/vomiting, dark urine) of hepatic injury.

Use only when other effective antifungal therapy is unavailable or not tolerated and the benefits of ketoconazole treatment are considered to outweigh the risks **[U.S. Boxed Warning]**. Ketoconazole has poor penetration into cerebral-spinal fluid and should not be used to treat fungal meningitis.

Hypersensitivity reactions (including rare cases of anaphylaxis) have been reported; some reactions occurred after the initial dose. High doses of ketoconazole may depress adrenocortical function; returns to baseline upon discontinuation of therapy; recommended maximum dosing should not be exceeded. Monitor adrenal function as clinically necessary, particularly in patients with adrenal insufficiency and in patients under prolonged stress (eg, intensive care, major surgery).

Concomitant use with cisapride, disopyramide, dofetilide, dronedarone, methadone, pimozide, quinidine, and ranolazine is contraindicated due to the possible occurrence of life-threatening ventricular arrhythmias such as torsade de pointes **[U.S. Boxed Warning]**. Coadministration with HMG-CoA reductase inhibitors (eg, lovastatin, simvastatin) may increase the risk of myopathy. Concomitant use is contraindicated. Coadministration with midazolam, triazolam, and alprazolam may result in elevated plasma concentrations of the benzodiazepines, leading to prolonged hypnotic and sedative effects. Concomitant use is contraindicated. Potentially significant interactions may exist, requiring dose or frequency adjustment, additional monitoring, and/or selection of alternative therapy. Consult drug interactions database for more detailed information.

Precautions Gastric acidity is necessary for the dissolution and absorption of ketoconazole; absorption is reduced in patients with achlorhydria; administer with acidic liquids (eg, soda pop). Avoid concomitant use of drugs that decrease gastric acidity (eg, proton pump inhibitors, antacids, H₂-blockers). In animal studies, increased long bone fragility with cases of fracture has been observed with high-dose ketoconazole; careful dose selection may be advisable for patients susceptible to bone fragility (eg, postmenopausal women, elderly).

Adverse Reactions

Cardiovascular: Orthostatic hypotension, peripheral edema

Central nervous system: Fatigue, insomnia, malaise, nervousness, paresthesia

Dermatologic: Alopecia, dermatitis, erythema, erythema multiforme, pruritus, skin rash, urticaria, xeroderma

Endocrine & metabolic: Hot flash, hyperlipidemia, menstrual disease

Gastrointestinal: Abdominal pain, anorexia, constipation, dysgeusia, dyspepsia, flatulence, increased appetite, nausea, tongue discoloration, upper abdominal pain, vomiting, xerostomia

Hematologic & oncologic: Decreased platelet count

Hepatic: Jaundice

Hypersensitivity: Anaphylactoid reaction

Neuromuscular & skeletal: Myalgia, weakness

Respiratory: Epistaxis

Miscellaneous: Alcohol intolerance

Rare but important or life-threatening: Acute generalized exanthematous pustulosis, adrenocortical insufficiency (≥400 mg/day), anaphylactic shock, anaphylaxis, angioedema, azoospermia, bulging fontanel (infants), cholestatic hepatitis, cirrhosis, decreased plasma testosterone (impaired at 800 mg/day), depression, erectile dysfunction (doses >200-400 mg/day), gynecomastia, hemolytic anemia, hepatic failure, hepatic necrosis, hepatitis, hepatotoxicity, hypertriglyceridemia, hypersensitivity reaction, impotence, increased intracranial pressure (reversible), leukopenia, myopathy, papilledema, photophobia, prolonged Q-T interval on ECG, skin photosensitivity, suicidal tendencies, thrombocytopenia

Drug Interactions

Metabolism/Transport Effects Substrate of CYP3A4 (major); **Note:** Assignment of Major/Minor substrate status based on clinically relevant drug interaction potential; **Inhibits** CYP1A2 (weak), CYP2A6 (moderate), CYP2B6 (weak), CYP2C19 (moderate), CYP2C8 (weak), CYP2C9 (moderate), CYP2D6 (moderate), CYP3A4 (strong), P-glycoprotein

Avoid Concomitant Use

Avoid concomitant use of Ketoconazole (Systemic) with any of the following: Ado-Trastuzumab Emtansine; Alfuzosin; ALPRAZolam; Apixaban; Astemizole; Avanafil; Axitinib; Bosutinib; Cabozantinib; Ceritinib; Cisapride; Conivaptan; Crizotinib; Dihydroergotamine; Disopyramide; Dofetilide; Domperidone; Dronedarone; Efavirenz; Eletriptan; Eplerenone; Ergoloid Mesylates; Ergonovine; Ergotamine; Estazolam; Everolimus; Felodipine; Halofantrine; Ibrutinib; Indium 111 Capromab Pendetide; Irinotecan; Ivabradine; Lapatinib; Lomitapide; Lovastatin; Lurasidone; Macitentan; Methadone; Methylergonovine; Midazolam; Nevirapine; Nilotinib; Nisoldipine; PAZOPanib; Pimozide; QuiNIDine; Ranolazine; Red Yeast Rice; Regorafenib; Rivaroxaban; Saccharomyces boulardii; Salmeterol; Silodosin; Simeprevir; Simvastatin; Tamsulosin; Tegafur; Terfenadine; Thioridazine; Ticagrelor; Tolvaptan; Topotecan; Toremifene; Triazolam; Ulipristal; Vemurafenib; VinCRIStine (Liposomal); Vorapaxar

Increased Effect/Toxicity

Ketoconazole (Systemic) may increase the levels/effects of: Ado-Trastuzumab Emtansine; Afatinib; Alcohol (Ethyl); Alfentanil; Alfuzosin; Aliskiren; Almotriptan; Alosetron; ALPRAZolam; Apixaban; ARIPiprazole; Astemizole; AtorvaSTATin; Avanafil; Axitinib; Bedaquiline; Benzodiazepines (metabolized by oxidation); Boceprevir; Bortezomib; Bosentan; Bosutinib; Brentuximab Vedotin; Brinzolamide; Budesonide (Nasal); Budesonide (Systemic, Oral Inhalation); BusPIRone; Busulfan; Cabozantinib; Calcium Channel Blockers; Cannabis; Carbocisteine; Carvedilol; Ceritinib; Cilostazol; Cisapride; Citalopram; Cobicistat; Colchicine; Conivaptan; Corticosteroids (Orally Inhaled); Corticosteroids (Systemic); Crizotinib; CycloSPORINE (Systemic); CYP2A6 Substrates; CYP2C19 Substrates; CYP2C9 Substrates; CYP2D6 Substrates; CYP3A4 Substrates; Dabigatran Etexilate; Darunavir; Dienogest; Dihydroergotamine; Disopyramide; DOCEtaxel; Dofetilide; Domperidone; DOXOrubicin (Conventional); Dronabinol; Dronedarone; Dutasteride; Eletriptan; Elvitegravir; Eplerenone; Ergoloid Mesylates; Ergonovine; Ergotamine; Estazolam; Etravirine; Everolimus; Felodipine; FentaNYL; Fesoterodine; Fexofenadine; Fingolimod; Fluticasone (Nasal); Fluticasone (Oral Inhalation); Fosamprenavir; Fosphenytoin; GuanFACINE; Halofantrine; Highest Risk QTc-Prolonging Agents; Ibrutinib; Iloperidone; Imatinib; Indinavir; Irinotecan; Ivabradine; Ivacaftor; Ixabepilone; Lacosamide; Lapatinib; Levomilnacipran; Lomitapide; Lopinavir; Losartan; Lovastatin; Lurasidone; Macitentan; Macrolide Antibiotics; Maraviroc; Methadone; Methylergonovine; MethylPREDNISolone; Metoprolol; Midazolam; Mifepristone; Mirabegron; Moderate Risk QTc-Prolonging Agents; Nebivolol; Nilotinib; Nisoldipine; Ospemifene; OxyCODONE; Paricalcitol; PAZOPanib; P-glycoprotein/ABCB1 Substrates; Phenytoin; Pimecrolimus; Pimozide; PONATinib; Praziquantel; Propafenone; Proton Pump Inhibitors; Prucalopride; QUEtiapine; QuiNIDine; Ramelteon; Ranolazine; Red Yeast Rice; Regorafenib; Repaglinide; Rifamycin Derivatives; Rifaximin; Rilpivirine; Riociguat; Rivaroxaban; RomiDEPsin; Ruxolitinib; Salmeterol; Saquinavir; Saxagliptin; Sildenafil; Silodosin; Simeprevir; Simvastatin; Sirolimus; Solifenacin; SORAfenib; SUNItinib; Tacrolimus (Systemic); Tacrolimus (Topical); Tadalafil; Tamsulosin; Telaprevir; Temsirolimus; Terfenadine; Tetrahydrocannabinol; Thioridazine; Ticagrelor; Tofacitinib; Tolterodine; Tolvaptan; Topotecan; Toremifene; Triazolam; Ulipristal; Vardenafil; Vemurafenib; Vilazodone; VinCRIStine (Liposomal); Vitamin K Antagonists; Vorapaxar; Zolpidem; Zuclopenthixol

The levels/effects of Ketoconazole (Systemic) may be increased by: AtorvaSTATin; Boceprevir; Cobicistat; Darunavir; Domperidone; Etravirine; Fosamprenavir; Indinavir; Lopinavir; Macrolide Antibiotics; Mifepristone; Propafenone; Ritonavir; Saquinavir; Telaprevir; Tipranavir

Decreased Effect

Ketoconazole (Systemic) may decrease the levels/effects of: Amphotericin B; Clopidogrel; Codeine; Ifosfamide; Indium 111 Capromab Pendetide; Prasugrel; Saccharomyces boulardii; Tamoxifen; Tegafur; Ticagrelor

The levels/effects of Ketoconazole (Systemic) may be decreased by: Antacids; Bosentan; CYP3A4 Inducers (Strong); Dabrafenib; Deferasirox; Didanosine; Efavirenz; Etravirine; Fosphenytoin; H2-Antagonists; Isoniazid; Mitotane; Nevirapine; Phenytoin; Proton Pump Inhibitors; Rifamycin Derivatives; Rilpivirine; Siltuximab; St Johns Wort; Sucralfate; Tocilizumab

Food Interactions Ketoconazole peak serum levels may be prolonged if taken with food. Management: May administer with food or milk to decrease GI adverse effects.

Mechanism of Action Alters the permeability of the cell wall by blocking fungal cytochrome P450; inhibits biosynthesis of triglycerides and phospholipids by fungi; inhibits several fungal enzymes that results in a build-up of toxic concentrations of hydrogen peroxide; for management of prostate cancer, ketoconazole inhibits androgen synthesis

Pharmacokinetics (Adult data unless noted)

Distribution: Well into inflamed joint fluid, saliva, bile, urine, sebum, cerumen, feces, tendons, skin and soft tissue, and testes; crosses blood-brain barrier poorly; only negligible amounts reach CSF

Protein binding: ~99% (mainly albumin)

Metabolism: Partially hepatic via CYP3A4 to inactive metabolites

Bioavailability: Decreases as pH of the gastric contents increases

Half-life, biphasic:

Initial: 2 hours

Terminal: 8 hours

Time to peak serum concentration: Within 1-2 hours

Elimination: Primarily in feces (57%) with smaller amounts excreted in urine (~13%)

Dosing: Usual

Pediatric: **Fungal infections:** Children ≥2 years and Adolescents: Oral: 3.3 to 6.6 mg/kg/day once daily; maximum daily dose: 400 mg/**day**; duration of therapy variable; continue therapy until active fungal infection has resolved (based on clinical and laboratory parameters); some infections may require at least 6 months of therapy. **Note:** Due to serious adverse effects (hepatotoxicity) and significant drug interactions, ketoconazole is seldom used in pediatric patients (*Red Book* [AAP], 2012); use should be reserved for patients who have failed or are intolerant to other antifungal therapies.

Adult: **Fungal infections:** Oral: 200 to 400 mg once daily; continue therapy until active fungal infection has resolved (based on clinical and laboratory parameters); some infections may require at least 6 months of therapy

Dosing adjustment in renal impairment: No dosage adjustment provided in manufacturer's labeling. Some clinicians suggest that no dosage adjustment is necessary in mild to severe impairment (Aronoff, 2007). Not dialyzable.

Dosing adjustment in hepatic impairment: Children ≥2 years, Adolescents, and Adults:

Baseline hepatic impairment: No dosage adjustment provided in manufacturer's labeling; use with extreme caution due to risks of hepatotoxicity; use is contraindicated with acute or chronic liver disease.

Hepatotoxicity during treatment: If ALT >ULN or 30% above baseline (or if patient is symptomatic), interrupt therapy and obtain full hepatic function panel. Upon normalization of liver function, may consider resuming therapy if benefit outweighs risk (hepatotoxicity has been reported on rechallenge).

Administration Administer oral tablets 2 hours prior to antacids to prevent decreased absorption due to the high pH of gastric contents. Patients with achlorhydria should administer with acidic liquid (eg, soda pop).

Monitoring Parameters Hepatic function tests (baseline and frequently during therapy), including weekly ALT for the duration of treatment, adrenal function (as clinically necessary)

Dosage Forms Excipient information presented when available (limited, particularly for generics); consult specific product labeling.

Tablet, Oral:

Generic: 200 mg

Extemporaneous Preparations A 20 mg/mL oral suspension may be made with tablets and one of three different vehicles (a 1:1 mixture of Ora-Sweet® and Ora-Plus®, a 1:1 mixture of Ora-Sweet® SF and Ora-Plus®, or a 1:4 mixture of cherry syrup and Simple Syrup, NF). Crush twelve 200 mg tablets in a mortar and reduce to a fine powder. Add 20 mL of chosen vehicle and mix to a uniform paste; mix while adding the vehicle in incremental proportions to **almost** 120 mL; transfer to a calibrated bottle, rinse mortar with vehicle, and add quantity of vehicle sufficient to make 120 mL. Label "shake well" and "refrigerate". Stable for 60 days.

Nahata MC, Pai VB, and Hipple TF, *Pediatric Drug Formulations*, 5th ed, Cincinnati, OH: Harvey Whitney Books Co, 2004.

References

American Academy of Pediatrics (AAP). In: Pickering LK, Baker CJ, Kimberlin DW, Long SS, eds. *Red Book: 2012 Report of the Committee on Infectious Diseases*. 29th ed. Elk Grove Village, IL: American Academy of Pediatrics; 2012.

Ketoconazole (Topical) (kee toe KOE na zole)

Medication Safety Issues

Sound-alike/look-alike issues:

Nizoral may be confused with Nasarel, Neoral, Nitrol

Brand Names: U.S. Extina; Ketodan; Nizoral; Nizoral A-D [OTC]; Xolegel

Brand Names: Canada Ketoderm; Nizoral

Therapeutic Category Antifungal Agent, Topical

Generic Availability (U.S.) May be product dependent

Use

Cream: Topical treatment of tinea corporis, tinea cruris, tinea pedis, tinea versicolor, and cutaneous candidiasis (FDA approved in adults)

Foam (Extina®); gel (Xolegel®): Topical treatment of seborrheic dermatitis in immunocompetent patients (FDA approved in ages ≥12 years and adults)

Shampoo:

1% shampoo (Nizoral® A-D): Control flaking, scaling, and itching associated with dandruff (OTC product; FDA approved in ages ≥12 years and adults)

2% shampoo (Nizoral®): Topical treatment of tinea versicolor (FDA approved in adults)

Pregnancy Risk Factor C

Pregnancy Considerations Adverse effects were noted in animal reproduction studies with oral ketoconazole. Ketoconazole is not detectable in the plasma following chronic use of the shampoo.

Breast-Feeding Considerations Ketoconazole has been detected in breast milk following oral dosing. Although it is not detected in the plasma following chronic use of the shampoo, and concentrations in the plasma following application of the gel are <250 times those observed with oral dosing, the manufacturers recommend that caution be used when administering to a nursing woman.

Contraindications Hypersensitivity to ketoconazole or any component

Warnings Hypersensitivity reactions (including rare cases of anaphylaxis) have been reported. Local irritation at application site may occur; if allergic reaction or irritation occurs or disease worsens, discontinue and contact healthcare provider. Cream contains sulfites which may cause allergic reactions in susceptible individuals.

Precautions

Foam: Formulation contains alcohol and propane/butane; do not expose to open flame or smoking during or immediately after application. Do not puncture or incinerate container.

Gel: Avoid exposure of gel to open flames or smoking during or immediately after application.

Shampoo: Severe allergic reactions (including anaphylaxis) have occurred. Use may remove curl from permanently wavy hair or cause hair discoloration and changes in hair texture. Avoid contact with eyes.

Adverse Reactions

Topical cream/gel: Acne, allergic reaction, contact dermatitis (possibly related to sulfites or propylene glycol), discharge, dizziness, dryness, erythema, facial swelling, headache, impetigo, keratoconjunctivitis sicca, local burning, nail discoloration, ocular irritation/swelling, pain, paresthesia, pruritus, pustules, pyogenic granuloma, severe irritation, stinging

Topical foam: Application site burning, application site reaction, contact sensitization, dryness, erythema, pruritus, rash

Shampoo: Abnormal hair texture, alopecia, anaphylaxis, angioedema, application site reaction, burning sensation, contact dermatitis, dry skin, hair discoloration, hair loss increased, hypersensitivity, irritation, itching, oiliness/dryness of hair, pruritus, rash, scalp pustules, urticaria

Drug Interactions

Metabolism/Transport Effects None known.

Avoid Concomitant Use There are no known interactions where it is recommended to avoid concomitant use.

Increased Effect/Toxicity There are no known significant interactions involving an increase in effect.

Decreased Effect There are no known significant interactions involving a decrease in effect.

Stability

Cream: Store at 20°C to 25°C (68°F to 77°F).

Foam: Store at 20°C to 25°C (68°F to 77°F). Do not refrigerate. Do not expose to heat and/or store at >49°C (120°F). Do not store in direct sunlight. Contents are flammable.

Gel: Store at 25°C (77°F); excursions permitted to 15°C to 30°C (59°F to 86°F). Contents are flammable; do not expose to heat or flame.

Shampoo:

Nizoral®: Store at ≤25°C (≤77°F); protect from light.

Nizoral® A-D: Store between 2°C to 30°C (35°F to 86°F); protect from freezing. Protect from light.

Mechanism of Action Alters the permeability of the cell wall by blocking fungal cytochrome P450; inhibits biosynthesis of triglycerides and phospholipids by fungi; inhibits several fungal enzymes that results in a build-up of toxic concentrations of hydrogen peroxide; also inhibits androgen synthesis

Dosing: Usual

Children and Adolescents:

Dandruff (flaking, scaling, and itching; OTC labeling): Children ≥12 years and Adolescents: Topical: Shampoo (ketoconazole 1%): Shampoo every 3-4 days for up to 8 weeks; then use only as needed to control dandruff

Seborrheic dermatitis: Children ≥12 years and Adolescents: Topical:

Foam: Apply to affected area twice daily for 4 weeks

Gel: Apply to affected area once daily for 2 weeks

Adults:

Fungal infections: Topical:

Cream: Rub gently into the affected and immediate surrounding area once daily. Duration of treatment: Candidial infection or tinea corporis, cruris, or vesicolor: 2 weeks; tinea pedis: 6 weeks

Shampoo (ketoconazole 2%): Tinea versicolor: Apply to damp skin of the affected area and a wide margin surrounding this area, lather, leave on 5 minutes, and rinse (one application should be sufficient)

Seborrheic dermatitis: Topical:

Foam: Apply to affected area twice daily for 4 weeks

Gel: Apply to affected area once daily for 2 weeks

Shampoo (ketoconazole 1%; OTC labeling): Shampoo every 3-4 days for up to 8 weeks; then use only as needed to control dandruff

Dosing adjustment in renal impairment: There are no dosage adjustments provided in manufacturer's labeling;

however, dosage adjustment unlikely necessary due to low systemic absorption.

Administration For external use only; not for ophthalmic, oral, or intravaginal use. Avoid contact with eyes and other mucous membranes.

Cream: Apply to cover the affected and immediate surrounding area.

Foam (Extina®): Hold the container upright and dispense foam into cap or other cool surface; do not dispense into hands as foam will begin to melt immediately upon contact with warm skin. If fingers are warm, rinse in cold water and dry thoroughly; pick up small amounts of foam with the fingers, and gently massage into the affected area(s) until foam disappears. For hair-bearing areas, part the hair, so foam may be applied directly to skin (rather than on the hair). Avoid fire, flame, and/or smoking during and immediately following application.

Gel (Xolegel®): Apply thin layer on affected skin; wait at least 3 hours after application before washing area(s). Avoid fire, flame, and/or smoking during and immediately following application.

Shampoo:

1%: Apply to wet hair, lather and rinse hair thoroughly; repeat

2%: Apply to damp skin, covering affected area and a wide margin surrounding the area, lather, leave on 5 minutes, and rinse

Dosage Forms Excipient information presented when available (limited, particularly for generics); consult specific product labeling. [DSC] = Discontinued product

Cream, External:

Generic: 2% (15 g, 30 g, 60 g)

Foam, External:

Extina: 2% (50 g, 100 g) [contains alcohol, usp, cetyl alcohol, propylene glycol]

Ketodan: 2% (100 g) [contains alcohol, usp, cetyl alcohol, propylene glycol]

Generic: 2% (50 g [DSC], 100 g [DSC])

Gel, External:

Xolegel: 2% (45 g) [contains alcohol, usp, fd&c yellow #10 (quinoline yellow), fd&c yellow #6 (sunset yellow), propylene glycol]

Kit, External:

Ketodan: 2% [contains cetyl alcohol, edetate disodium, propylene glycol]

Shampoo, External:

Nizoral: 2% (120 mL) [contains fd&c red #40]

Nizoral A-D: 1% (125 mL, 200 mL)

Generic: 2% (120 mL)

◆ **Ketodan** see Ketoconazole (Topical) on page 1179

◆ **Ketoderm (Can)** see Ketoconazole (Topical) on page 1179

Ketorolac (Systemic) (KEE toe role ak)

Medication Safety Issues

Sound-alike/look-alike issues:

Ketorolac may be confused with Ketalar®

Toradol® may be confused with Foradil®, Inderal®, TEGretol®, traMADol, tromethamine

BEERS Criteria medication:

This drug may be potentially inappropriate for use in geriatric patients (Quality of evidence - high; Strength of recommendation - strong).

International issues:

Toradol [Canada and multiple international markets] may be confused with Theradol brand name for tramadol [Netherlands]

Brand Names: Canada Apo-Ketorolac Injectable®; Apo-Ketorolac®; Ketorolac Tromethamine Injection, USP; Novo-Ketorolac; Toradol®; Toradol® IM

Therapeutic Category Analgesic, Non-narcotic; Anti-inflammatory Agent; Antipyretic; Nonsteroidal Anti-inflammatory Drug (NSAID), Oral; Nonsteroidal Anti-inflammatory Drug (NSAID), Parenteral

Generic Availability (U.S.) Yes

Use

I.M., I.V.: Single-dose administration for moderately severe acute pain (FDA approved in ages ≥2 years and adults). Short-term (≤5 days) management of moderate to severe pain, usually postoperative pain (FDA approved in adults); has also been used to treat visceral pain associated with cancer, pain associated with trauma

Oral: Short-term (≤5 days) management of moderate to severe pain, usually postoperative pain, and only as continuation therapy of I.M. or I.V. ketorolac (FDA approved in adults); the combined duration of oral and parenteral ketorolac should not be >5 days due to the increased risk of serious adverse effects

Medication Guide Available Yes

Pregnancy Risk Factor C

Pregnancy Considerations Adverse events were observed in some animal reproduction studies. Ketorolac crosses the placenta (Walker, 1988). NSAID exposure during the first trimester is not strongly associated with congenital malformations; however, cardiovascular anomalies and cleft palate have been observed following NSAID exposure in some studies (Ericson, 2001). The use of an NSAID close to conception may be associated with an increased risk of miscarriage (Li, 2003; Nielsen, 2001). Nonteratogenic effects have been observed following NSAID administration during the third trimester, including myocardial degenerative changes, prenatal constriction of the ductus arteriosus, fetal tricuspid regurgitation, failure of the ductus arteriosus to close postnatally; renal dysfunction or failure, oligohydramnios; gastrointestinal bleeding or perforation, increased risk of necrotizing enterocolitis; intracranial bleeding (including intraventricular hemorrhage), platelet dysfunction with resultant bleeding; pulmonary hypertension (Van den Veyver, 1993). Because they may cause premature closure of the ductus arteriosus, use of NSAIDs late in pregnancy should be avoided (use after 31 or 32 weeks gestation is not recommended by some clinicians) (Moise, 1993). **[U.S. Boxed Warning]: Ketorolac is contraindicated during labor and delivery (may inhibit uterine contractions and adversely affect fetal circulation).** The chronic use of NSAIDs in women of reproductive age may be associated with infertility that is reversible upon discontinuation of the medication.

Breast-Feeding Considerations Low concentrations of ketorolac are found in breast milk (milk concentrations were <1% of the weight-adjusted maternal dose in one study [Wischnik, 1989]). The manufacturer recommends that caution be used if administered to nursing women.

Contraindications Hypersensitivity to ketorolac or any component; history of asthma, urticaria, or allergic-type reaction to aspirin or other NSAIDs; patients with the "aspirin triad" [asthma, rhinitis (with or without nasal polyps), and aspirin intolerance] (fatal asthmatic and anaphylactoid reactions may occur in these patients); patients with active peptic ulcer disease (PUD), recent GI bleeding or perforation, or history of PUD or GI bleeding; advanced renal dysfunction; patients at risk for renal failure due to hypovolemia; women in late pregnancy; women in labor and delivery or breast-feeding; preoperative prophylactic analgesia; perioperative pain in the setting of coronary artery bypass graft (CABG); patients with cerebrovascular bleeding, incomplete hemostasis, hemorrhagic diathesis, or at high risk of bleeding; contraindicated for epidural or intrathecal use due to alcohol content; concomitant use of probenecid or pentoxifylline; do not administer with aspirin or other NSAIDs

Warnings NSAIDs are associated with an increased risk of adverse cardiovascular thrombotic events, including

potentially fatal MI and stroke **[U.S. Boxed Warning]**; risk may be increased with duration of use or preexisting cardiovascular risk factors or disease; carefully evaluate cardiovascular risk profile prior to prescribing; use the lowest effective dose for the shortest duration of time, taking into consideration individual patient treatment goals; alternate therapies should be considered for patients at high risk. NSAIDs may cause fluid retention, edema, and new onset or worsening of preexisting hypertension; use with caution in patients with hypertension, CHF, or fluid retention. Concurrent administration of ibuprofen, and potentially other nonselective NSAIDs, may interfere with aspirin's cardioprotective effect. Due the effects of platelets, use is contraindicated in patients with suspected or confirmed cerebrovascular bleeding, patients with hemorrhagic diathesis, incomplete hemostasis, those at high risk for bleeding, for use as prophylactic before any major surgery, or intraoperatively when hemostasis is critical due to increased risk of bleeding **[U.S. Boxed Warning]**.

NSAIDs may increase the risk of gastrointestinal inflammation, ulceration, bleeding, and perforation **[U.S. Boxed Warning]**. These events, which can be potentially fatal, may occur at any time during therapy and without warning. Avoid the use of NSAIDs in patients with active GI bleeding or ulcer disease. Ketorolac is contraindicated in patients with active peptic ulcer disease or patients with recent or history of GI bleeding or perforation. Use NSAIDs with caution in patients with other risk factors which may increase GI bleeding (eg, concurrent therapy with aspirin, anticoagulants, and/or corticosteroids, longer duration of NSAID use, smoking, use of alcohol, and poor general health). Use the lowest effective dose for the shortest duration of time, taking into consideration individual patient treatment goals; alternate therapies should be considered for patients at high risk.

NSAIDs may compromise existing renal function. Renal toxicity may occur in patients with impaired renal function, dehydration, heart failure, liver dysfunction, and those taking diuretics and ACE inhibitors; use with caution in these patients; monitor renal function closely. Ketorolac is contraindicated in patients with advanced renal disease **[U.S. Boxed Warning]**. Long-term use of NSAIDs may cause renal papillary necrosis and other renal injury.

Hypersensitivity reactions have been reported **[U.S. Boxed Warning]**; use is contraindicated in patients with a history of hypersensitivity to ketorolac or other NSAIDs; patients with the "aspirin triad" who receive NSAIDs may be at higher risk. NSAIDs may cause serious dermatologic adverse reactions, including exfoliative dermatitis, Stevens-Johnson syndrome, and toxic epidermal necrolysis.

Use is contraindicated for pregnant women during labor and delivery due to potential adverse effects on fetal circulation **[U.S. Boxed Warning]**; also avoid use in late pregnancy; contraindicated in nursing mothers due to potential adverse effects in neonates **[U.S. Boxed Warning]**.

Duration of ketorolac therapy should not exceed 5 days and should not exceed recommended dose due to adverse effects **[U.S. Boxed Warning]**; if multiple dosage forms are used, total duration of combined therapy should not exceed 5 days. Dosage adjustment is required for patients ≥65 years and those who weigh <50 kg **[U.S. Boxed Warning]**. Use is contraindicated in patients currently receiving aspirin or other NSAIDs due to risk of cumulative toxicity **[U.S. Boxed Warning]**.

Precautions Use with caution in patients with decreased hepatic function; closely monitor patients with abnormal LFTs; severe hepatic reactions (eg, fulminant hepatitis, liver failure) have occurred with NSAID use, rarely; discontinue if signs or symptoms of liver disease develop or if ▶

systemic manifestations occur. Use with caution in patients with asthma; asthmatic patients may have aspirin-sensitive asthma which may be associated with severe and potentially fatal bronchospasm when aspirin or NSAIDs are administered. Anemia (due to occult or gross blood loss from the GI tract, fluid retention, or other effect on erythropoiesis) may occur; monitor hemoglobin and hematocrit in patients receiving long-term therapy. Use with caution and monitor carefully in patients with coagulation disorders or those receiving anticoagulants; NSAIDs inhibit platelet aggregation and may prolong bleeding time.

Adverse Reactions

Cardiovascular: Edema, hypertension

Central nervous system: Dizziness, drowsiness, headache

Dermatologic: Diaphoresis, pruritus, skin rash

Gastrointestinal: Constipation, diarrhea, dyspepsia, flatulence, gastrointestinal fullness, gastrointestinal hemorrhage, gastrointestinal pain, gastrointestinal perforation, gastrointestinal ulcer, heartburn, nausea, stomatitis, vomiting

Hematologic & oncologic: Anemia, prolonged bleeding time, purpura

Hepatic: Increased liver enzymes

Local: Pain at injection site

Otic: Tinnitus

Renal: Renal function abnormality

Rare but important or life-threatening: Abnormality in thinking, acute pancreatitis, acute renal failure, agranulocytosis, alopecia, anaphylactoid reaction, anaphylaxis, angioedema, aplastic anemia, aseptic meningitis, asthma, azotemia, bradycardia, bronchospasm, bruise, cardiac arrhythmia, cholestatic jaundice, coma, confusion, congestive heart failure, conjunctivitis, cough, cystitis, depression, dysuria, eosinophilia, epistaxis, eructation, erythema multiforme, euphoria, exacerbation of urinary frequency, exfoliative dermatitis, extrapyramidal reaction, flank pain, gastritis, glossitis, hallucination, hearing loss, hematemesis, hematuria, hemolytic anemia, hemolytic-uremic syndrome, hepatic failure, hepatitis, hyperglycemia, hyperkalemia, hyperkinesis, hypersensitivity reaction, hyponatremia, hypotension, increased susceptibility to infection, increased thirst, infertility, inflammatory bowel disease, insomnia, interstitial nephritis, jaundice, lack of concentration, laryngeal edema, leukopenia, lymphadenopathy, maculopapular rash, melena, myocardial infarction, nephritis, oliguria, palpitations, pancytopenia, paresthesia, pneumonia, polyuria, proteinuria, psychosis, pulmonary edema, rectal hemorrhage, renal failure, respiratory depression, rhinitis, seizure, sepsis, skin photosensitivity, Stevens-Johnson syndrome, stomatitis (ulcerative), stupor, syncope, tachycardia, thrombocytopenia, tongue edema, toxic epidermal necrolysis, urinary retention, urticaria, vasculitis, weight gain, wound hemorrhage (postoperative)

Drug Interactions

Metabolism/Transport Effects None known.

Avoid Concomitant Use

Avoid concomitant use of Ketorolac (Systemic) with any of the following: Aspirin; Floctafenine; Ketorolac (Nasal); Nonsteroidal Anti-Inflammatory Agents; Omacetaxine; Pentoxifylline; Probenecid; Urokinase

Increased Effect/Toxicity

Ketorolac (Systemic) may increase the levels/effects of: 5-ASA Derivatives; Agents with Antiplatelet Properties; Aliskiren; Aminoglycosides; Anticoagulants; Apixaban; Aspirin; Bisphosphonate Derivatives; Collagenase (Systemic); CycloSPORINE (Systemic); Dabigatran Etexilate; Deferasirox; Desmopressin; Digoxin; Eplerenone; Haloperidol; Ibritumomab; Lithium; Methotrexate; Neuromuscular-Blocking Agents (Nondepolarizing); Nonsteroidal Anti-Inflammatory Agents; Omacetaxine; PEMEtrexed; Pentoxifylline; Porfimer; Potassium-Sparing Diuretics; PRALAtrexate; Quinolone Antibiotics; Rivaroxaban;

Salicylates; Tenofovir; Thrombolytic Agents; Tositumomab and Iodine I 131 Tositumomab; Urokinase; Vancomycin; Vitamin K Antagonists

The levels/effects of Ketorolac (Systemic) may be increased by: ACE Inhibitors; Angiotensin II Receptor Blockers; Antidepressants (Tricyclic, Tertiary Amine); Corticosteroids (Systemic); CycloSPORINE (Systemic); Dasatinib; Floctafenine; Glucosamine; Herbs (Anticoagulant/Antiplatelet Properties); Ibrutinib; Ketorolac (Nasal); Multivitamins/Fluoride (with ADE); Multivitamins/Minerals (with ADEK, Folate, Iron); Multivitamins/Minerals (with AE, No Iron); Omega-3 Fatty Acids; Pentosan Polysulfate Sodium; Probenecid; Prostacyclin Analogues; Selective Serotonin Reuptake Inhibitors; Serotonin/Norepinephrine Reuptake Inhibitors; Sodium Phosphates; Tipranavir; Treprostinil; Vitamin E

Decreased Effect

Ketorolac (Systemic) may decrease the levels/effects of: ACE Inhibitors; Agents with Antiplatelet Properties; Aliskiren; Angiotensin II Receptor Blockers; Anticonvulsants; Aspirin; Beta-Blockers; Eplerenone; HydrALAZINE; Loop Diuretics; Potassium-Sparing Diuretics; Prostaglandins (Ophthalmic); Salicylates; Selective Serotonin Reuptake Inhibitors; Thiazide Diuretics

The levels/effects of Ketorolac (Systemic) may be decreased by: Bile Acid Sequestrants; Salicylates

Food Interactions High-fat meals may delay time to peak (by ~1 hour) and decrease peak concentrations. Management: Administer tablet with food or milk to decrease gastrointestinal distress.

Stability

Injection: Store at room temperature of 15°C to 30°C (59°F to 86°F). Protect from light; store in carton until use. Injection is clear and has a slight yellow color; additional color change indicates degradation; precipitation may occur at relatively low pH values; do not mix in same syringe with morphine, meperidine, promethazine, or hydroxyzine (precipitation will occur)

Tablet: Store at room temperature of 15°C to 30°C (59°F to 86°F).

Mechanism of Action Reversibly inhibits cyclooxygenase-1 and 2 (COX-1 and 2) enzymes, which results in decreased formation of prostaglandin precursors; has antipyretic, analgesic, and anti-inflammatory properties

Other proposed mechanisms not fully elucidated (and possibly contributing to the anti-inflammatory effect to varying degrees), include inhibiting chemotaxis, altering lymphocyte activity, inhibiting neutrophil aggregation/activation, and decreasing proinflammatory cytokine levels.

Pharmacodynamics Analgesia:

Onset of action:

Oral: 30-60 minutes

I.M., I.V.: ~30 minutes

Maximum effect:

Oral: 1.5-4 hours

I.M., I.V.: 2-3 hours

Duration: 4-6 hours

Pharmacokinetics (Adult data unless noted)

Absorption:

Oral: Well-absorbed; 100%

I.M.: Rapid and complete

Distribution: Crosses placenta, crosses into breast milk, poor penetration into CSF; follows two-compartment model

V_d beta:

Children 4-8 years: 0.19-0.44 L/kg (mean: 0.26 L/kg)

Adults: 0.11-0.33 L/kg (mean: 0.18 L/kg)

Protein binding: 99%

Metabolism: In the liver; undergoes hydroxylation and glucuronide conjugation; in children 4-8 years, V_{dss} and plasma clearance were twice as high as adults

Bioavailability: Oral, I.M.: 100%

Half-life, terminal:

Infants 6-18 months of age (n=25): S-enantiomer: 0.83 ± 0.7 hours; R-enantiomer: 4 ± 0.8 hours (Lynn, 2007)

Children:

1-16 years (n=36): Mean: 3 ± 1.1 hours (Dsida, 2002)

3-18 years (n=24): Mean: 3.8 ± 2.6 hours

4-8 years (n=10): Mean: 6 hours; range: 3.5-10 hours

Adults: Mean: ~5 hours; range: 2-9 hours [S-enantiomer ~2.5 hours (biologically active); R-enantiomer ~5 hours]

With renal impairment: Scr 1.9-5 mg/dL: Mean: ~11 hours; range: 4-19 hours

Renal dialysis patients: Mean: ~14 hours; range: 8-40 hours

Time to peak serum concentration:

Oral: ~45 minutes

I.M.: 30-45 minutes

I.V.: 1-3 minutes

Elimination: Renal excretion: 60% in urine as unchanged drug with 40% as metabolites; 6% of dose excreted in feces

Dosing: Neonatal Note: Due to a lack of substantial evidence, NSAIDs are **not** recommended for use in neonates as an adjunct to postoperative analgesia (AAP, 2006).

Full-term neonates: Multiple-dose treatment: I.V.: Dose not established; limited data available; one retrospective study (n=10; mean PNA: 3 ± 4 weeks) recommends 0.5 mg/kg/dose every 8 hours for up to 1-2 days postoperatively; do not exceed 48 hours of treatment (Burd, 2002); **Note:** To reduce the risk of adverse cardiovascular and GI effects, use the lowest effective dose for the shortest period of time.

Dosing: Usual Note: To reduce the risk of adverse cardiovascular and GI effects, use the lowest effective dose for the shortest period of time.

Infants ≥1 month and Children <2 years: Multiple-dose treatment: I.V.: 0.5 mg/kg every 6-8 hours, not to exceed 48-72 hours of treatment (Burd, 2002; Dawkins, 2009; Gupta, 2004; Moffett, 2006)

Children 2-16 years and Children >16 years who are <50 kg: Do not exceed adult doses

Single-dose treatment:

Manufacturer's recommendations:

I.M.: 1 mg/kg as a single dose; maximum dose: 30 mg

I.V.: 0.5 mg/kg as a single dose; maximum dose: 15 mg

Alternative dosing:

I.M., I.V.: 0.4-1 mg/kg as a single dose; **Note:** Limited information exists. Single I.V. doses of 0.5-1 mg/kg have been studied in children 2-16 years of age for postoperative analgesia. In one study (Maunuksela, 1992), the median required single I.V. dose was 0.4 mg/kg.

Oral: One study used 1 mg/kg as a single dose for analgesia in 30 children (mean ± SD age: 3 ± 2.5 years) undergoing bilateral myringotomy.

Multiple-dose treatment:

I.M., I.V.: 0.5 mg/kg every 6 hours, not to exceed 5 days of treatment (Buck, 1994; Dsida, 2002; Gupta, 2004; Gupta, 2005)

Oral: No pediatric studies exist.

Children >16 years and >50 kg and Adults <65 years:

Single-dose treatment:

I.M.: 60 mg as a single dose

I.V.: 30 mg as a single dose

Multiple-dose treatment:

I.M., I.V.: 30 mg every 6 hours; maximum dose: 120 mg/day

Oral: Initial: 20 mg, then 10 mg every 4-6 hours; maximum dose: 40 mg/day

Adults ≥65 years, renally impaired, or <50 kg:

Single-dose treatment:

I.M.: 30 mg as a single dose

I.V.: 15 mg as a single dose

Multiple-dose treatment:

I.M., I.V.: 15 mg every 6 hours; maximum dose: 60 mg/day

Oral: 10 mg every 4-6 hours; maximum dose: 40 mg/day

Administration

Oral: May administer with food or milk to decrease GI upset

Parenteral:

I.M.: Administer slowly and deeply into muscle; 60 mg/2 mL vial is for I.M. use only

I.V. bolus: Administer over at least 15 seconds; maximum concentration: 30 mg/mL; **Note:** I.V. ketorolac has been infused over 1-5 minutes in children.

Monitoring Parameters Signs of pain relief (eg, increased appetite and activity); BUN, serum creatinine, liver enzymes, CBC, serum electrolytes, occult blood loss, urinalysis, urine output; signs and symptoms of GI bleeding

Reference Range Serum concentration:

Therapeutic: 0.3-5 mcg/mL

Toxic: >5 mcg/mL

Additional Information 30 mg provides analgesia comparable to 12 mg of morphine or 100 mg of meperidine; ketorolac may possess an opioid-sparing effect; diarrhea, pallor, vomiting, and labored breathing may occur with overdose

Note: A single I.V. dose of ketorolac (0.75 mg/kg) in 21 children (2.5-9 years of age) undergoing outpatient strabismus surgery was associated with less postoperative emesis than morphine plus metoclopramide (Munro, 1994). However, a single dose of I.V. ketorolac (1 mg/kg) in 25 children (2-15 years of age) undergoing tonsillectomy was associated with an increase in surgical bleeding, more patients requiring extra hemostatic measures (eg, synthetic collagen, extra Neo-Synephrine® packing), and a higher estimated blood loss compared to rectal acetaminophen (Rusy, 1995); further studies are needed.

Dosage Forms Excipient information presented when available (limited, particularly for generics); consult specific product labeling.

Solution, Injection, as tromethamine:

Generic: 15 mg/mL (1 mL); 30 mg/mL (1 mL); 60 mg/2 mL (2 mL); 300 mg/10 mL (10 mL)

Solution, Intramuscular, as tromethamine:

Generic: 30 mg/mL (1 mL); 60 mg/2 mL (2 mL)

Tablet, Oral, as tromethamine:

Generic: 10 mg

References

American Academy of Pediatrics Committee on Fetus and Newborn; American Academy of Pediatrics Section on Surgery; Canadian Paediatric Society Fetus and Newborn Committee, et al, "Prevention and Management of Pain in the Neonate: An Update," *Pediatrics*, 2006, 118(5):2231-41.

Buck ML, "Clinical Experience With Ketorolac in Children," *Ann Pharmacother*, 1994, 28(9):1009-13.

Burd RS and Tobias JD, "Ketorolac for Pain Management After Abdominal Surgical Procedures in Infants," *South Med J*, 2002, 95(3):331-3.

Dawkins TN, Barclay CA, Gardiner RL, et al, "Safety of Intravenous Use of Ketorolac in Infants Following Cardiothoracic Surgery," *Cardiol Young*, 2009, 19(1):105-8.

Dsida RM, Wheeler M, Birmingham PK, et al, "Age-Stratified Pharmacokinetics of Ketorolac Tromethamine in Pediatric Surgical Patients," *Anesth Analg*, 2002, 94(2):266-70.

Ericson A and Källén BA, "Nonsteroidal Anti-Inflammatory Drugs in Early Pregnancy," *Reprod Toxicol*, 2001, 15(4):371-5.

Gupta A, Daggett C, Drant S, et al, "Prospective Randomized Trial of Ketorolac After Congenital Heart Surgery," *J Cardiothorac Vasc Anesth*, 2004, 18(4):454-7.

Gupta A, Daggett C, Ludwick J, et al, "Ketorolac After Congenital Heart Surgery: Does It Increase the Risk of Significant Bleeding Complications?" *Paediatr Anaesth*, 2005, 15(2):139-42.

▶

◄ Kumpulainen E, Kokki H, Laisalmi M, et al, "How Readily Does Ketorolac Penetrate Cerebrospinal Fluid in Children?" *J Clin Pharmacol*, 2008, 48(4):495-501.

Li DK, Liu L, and Odouli R, "Exposure to Non-Steroidal Anti-Inflammatory Drugs During Pregnancy and Risk of Miscarriage: Population Based Cohort Study," *BMJ*, 2003, 327(7411):368.

Lynn AM, Bradford H, Kantor ED, et al, "Postoperative Ketorolac Tromethamine Use in Infants Aged 6-18 Months: The Effect on Morphine Usage, Safety Assessment, and Stereo-Specific Pharmacokinetics," *Anesth Analg*, 2007, 104(5):1040-51.

Maunuksela E, Kokki H, and Bullingham RES, "Comparison of Intravenous Ketorolac With Morphine for Postoperative Pain in Children," *Clin Pharmacol Ther*, 1992, 52(4):436-43.

Moffett BS, Wann TI, Carberry KE, et al, "Safety of Ketorolac in Neonates and Infants After Cardiac Surgery," *Paediatr Anaesth*, 2006, 16(4):424-8.

Moise KJ Jr, "Effect of Advancing Gestational Age on the Frequency of Fetal Ductal Constriction in Association With Maternal Indomethacin Use," *Am J Obstet Gynecol*, 1993, 168(5):1350-3.

Munro HM, Reigger LQ, Reynolds PI, et al, "Comparison of the Analgesic and Emetic Properties of Ketorolac and Morphine for Paediatric Outpatient Strabismus Surgery," *Br J Anaesth*, 1994, 72 (6):624-8.

Nielsen GL, Sørensen HT, Larsen H, et al, "Risk of Adverse Birth Outcome and Miscarriage in Pregnant Users of Non-Steroidal Anti-Inflammatory Drugs: Population Based Observational Study and Case-Control Study," *BMJ*, 2001, 322(7281):266-70.

Rusy LM, Houck CS, Sullivan LJ, et al, "A Double-Blind Evaluation of Ketorolac Tromethamine Versus Acetaminophen in Pediatric Tonsillectomy: Analgesia and Bleeding," *Anesth Analg*, 1995, 80(2):226-9.

Van den Veyver IB and Moise KJ Jr, "Prostaglandin Synthetase Inhibitors in Pregnancy," *Obstet Gynecol Surv*, 1993, 48(7):493-502.

Walker JJ, Johnstone J, Lloyd J, et al,"The Transfer of Ketorolac Tromethamine From Maternal to Foetal Blood," *Eur J Clin Pharmacol*, 1988, 34(5):509-11.

Watcha MF, Jones MB, Lagueruela RG, et al, "Comparison of Ketorolac and Morphine as Adjuvants During Pediatric Surgery," *Anesthesiology*, 1992, 76(3):368-72.

Wischnik A, Manth SM, Lloyd J, et al, "The Excretion of Ketorolac Tromethamine Into Breast Milk After Multiple Oral Dosing," *Eur J Clin Pharmacol*, 1989, 36(5):521-4.

Zuppa AF, Mondick JT, Davis L, et al, "Population Pharmacokinetics of Ketorolac in Neonates and Young Infants," *Am J Ther*, 2009, 16 (2):143-6.

Ketorolac (Ophthalmic) (KEE toe role ak)

Medication Safety Issues
Sound-alike/look-alike issues:
Acular® may be confused with Acthar®, Ocular
Ketorolac may be confused with Ketalar®

Brand Names: U.S. Acular; Acular LS; Acuvail

Brand Names: Canada Acular LS®; Acular®; Apo-Ketorolac® Ophthalmic; ratio-Ketorolac

Therapeutic Category Anti-inflammatory Agent; Nonsteroidal Anti-inflammatory Drug (NSAID), Ophthalmic

Generic Availability (U.S.) Yes

Use
Acular®: Treatment of ocular itch associated with seasonal allergic conjunctivitis; postoperative inflammation following cataract extraction (FDA approved in ages ≥3 years and adults)

Acular LS™: Reduction of ocular pain, burning, and stinging after corneal refractive surgery (FDA approved in ages ≥3 years and adults)

Acuvail®: Treatment of postoperative pain and inflammation following cataract surgery (FDA approved in adults)

Pregnancy Risk Factor C

Pregnancy Considerations Adverse events have been observed in animal studies; therefore, the manufacturer classifies ketorolac ophthalmic as pregnancy category C. When administered I.M., ketorolac crosses the placenta. Refer to the Ketorolac (Systemic) monograph for details. The amount of ketorolac available systemically following topical application of the ophthalmic drops is significantly less in comparison to oral doses. Because they may cause premature closure of the ductus arteriosus, the use of NSAIDs late in pregnancy (including ketorolac ophthalmic drops) should be avoided.

Breast-Feeding Considerations When administered orally, ketorolac enters breast milk. The use of systemic ketorolac is contraindicated in breast-feeding women. Refer to the Ketorolac (Systemic) monograph for details. The amount of ketorolac available systemically following topical application of the ophthalmic drops is significantly less in comparison to oral doses. The manufacturer recommends that caution be used when administering ketorolac ophthalmic to breast-feeding women.

Contraindications Hypersensitivity to ketorolac or any component

Precautions Use with caution in patients with complicated ocular surgeries, corneal denervation, epithelial defects, diabetes, rheumatoid arthritis, ocular surface diseases (eg, dry eye syndrome) or ocular surgeries repeated within short periods of time; corneal thinning, erosion, or ulceration leading to possible loss of vision have been reported; discontinue if corneal epithelial breakdown occurs. Use for >24 hours prior to or for >14 days following surgery also increases risk of corneal adverse effects. Use with caution in patients with known bleeding tendencies or those receiving anticoagulants; may increase bleeding time associated with ocular surgery.

Use with caution in patients with sensitivity to acetylsalicylic acid, phenylacetic acid derivatives, or other nonsteroidal anti-inflammatory agents; bronchospasm or exacerbation of asthma may occur.

May contain benzalkonium chloride which may be absorbed by contact lenses; contact lenses should not be worn during treatment. Allow at least 5 minutes between applications with other eye drops. To avoid contamination, do not touch tip of container to any surface. To minimize the risk of infection following surgery of both eyes, two separate bottles of eye drops (one for each eye) should be used; instruct patients not to use the same bottle for both eyes.

Adverse Reactions
Central nervous system: Headache

Ocular: Conjunctival hyperemia, corneal infiltrates, iritis, ocular edema, ocular inflammation, ocular irritation, ocular pain, superficial keratitis, superficial ocular infection, transient burning/stinging

Miscellaneous: Allergic reactions

Rare but important or life-threatening: Corneal erosion, corneal perforation, corneal thinning, corneal ulcer, dry eyes, epithelial breakdown

Drug Interactions
Metabolism/Transport Effects None known.

Avoid Concomitant Use There are no known interactions where it is recommended to avoid concomitant use.

Increased Effect/Toxicity There are no known significant interactions involving an increase in effect.

Decreased Effect There are no known significant interactions involving a decrease in effect.

Stability
Acular®, Acular LS®: Store at 15°C to 25°C (59°F to 77°F); protect from light.

Acuvail®: Store at 15°C to 30°C (59°F to 86°F) in pouch with pouch ends folded closed; protect from light; single use vials, discard after use.

Mechanism of Action
Reversibly inhibits cyclooxygenase-1 and 2 (COX-1 and 2) enzymes, which results in decreased formation of prostaglandin precursors; has anti-inflammatory properties

Other proposed mechanisms not fully elucidated (and possibly contributing to the anti-inflammatory effect to varying degrees), include inhibiting chemotaxis, altering lymphocyte activity, inhibiting neutrophil aggregation/activation, and decreasing proinflammatory cytokine levels.

Dosing: Usual

Children and Adolescents:

Seasonal allergic conjunctivitis: Acular®: Children ≥3 years, Adolescents: Ophthalmic: Instill 1 drop in eye(s) 4 times daily

Postoperative inflammation following cataract extracation: Acular®: Children ≥3 years, Adolescents: Ophthalmic: Instill 1 drop in affected eye(s) 4 times daily starting 24 hours after cataract surgery and through 14 days after surgery

Postoperative pain, burning, and stinging following corneal refractive surgery: Acular LS™: Children ≥3 years, Adolescents: Ophthalmic: Instill 1 drop in affected eye 4 times daily as needed for up to 4 days after corneal refractive surgery

Adults:

Seasonal allergic conjunctivitis (relief of ocular itching): Acular®: Ophthalmic: Instill 1 drop 4 times daily

Inflammation following cataract extraction:

Acular®: Ophthalmic: Instill 1 drop to affected eye(s) 4 times daily beginning 24 hours after surgery; continue for 2 weeks

Acuvail®: Ophthalmic: Instill 1 drop twice daily into affected eye; begin treatment 1 day prior to cataract surgery and continue on day of surgery, and for 2 weeks postoperatively

Pain following corneal refractive surgery: Acular LS®: Ophthalmic: Instill 1 drop 4 times daily as needed to affected eye for up to 4 days

Administration May contain benzalkonium chloride which may be absorbed by contact lenses; contact lenses should not be worn during treatment. Instill drops into affected eye(s); avoid contact of container tip with skin or eyes; apply finger pressure to lacrimal sac during and for 1-2 minutes after instillation to decrease risk of absorption and systemic effects; wait at least 5 minutes before administering other ophthalmic drops. To minimize the risk of infection following surgery of both eyes, two separate bottles of eye drops (one for each eye) should be used; instruct patients not to use the same bottle for both eyes.

Dosage Forms Excipient information presented when available (limited, particularly for generics); consult specific product labeling.

Solution, Ophthalmic, as tromethamine:

Acular: 0.5% (5 mL) [contains benzalkonium chloride, edetate disodium]

Acular LS: 0.4% (5 mL) [contains benzalkonium chloride, edetate disodium]

Generic: 0.4% (5 mL); 0.5% (3 mL, 5 mL, 10 mL)

Solution, Ophthalmic, as tromethamine [preservative free]:

Acuvail: 0.45% (30 ea)

◆ **Ketorolac Tromethamine** see Ketorolac (Ophthalmic) on page 1184

◆ **Ketorolac Tromethamine** see Ketorolac (Systemic) on page 1180

◆ **Ketorolac Tromethamine Injection, USP (Can)** see Ketorolac (Systemic) on page 1180

Ketotifen (Ophthalmic) (kee toe TYE fen)

Medication Safety Issues

Sound-alike/look-alike issues:

Claritin™ Eye (ketotifen) may be confused with Claritin® (loratadine)

Ketotifen may be confused with ketoprofen

ZyrTEC® Itchy Eye (ketotifen) may be confused with ZyrTEC® (cetirizine)

Brand Names: U.S. Alaway Childrens Allergy [OTC]; Alaway [OTC]; Claritin Eye [OTC]; Zaditor [OTC]; ZyrTEC Itchy Eye [OTC]

Brand Names: Canada Zaditor®

Therapeutic Category Antiallergic, Ophthalmic; Histamine H_1 Antagonist, Ophthalmic

Generic Availability (U.S.) Yes

Use Temporary relief of eye itching due to allergic conjunctivitis (FDA approved in children ≥3 years and adults)

Pregnancy Risk Factor C

Pregnancy Considerations Topical ocular administration has not been studied.

Breast-Feeding Considerations Ketotifen has been identified in rat breast milk. It is not known whether detectable levels of ketotifen would appear in human breast milk following topical ocular administration.

Contraindications Hypersensitivity to ketotifen or any component

Warnings Not indicated for use in eye irritation due to contact lenses; patients should be advised not to wear contact lens if their eye is red; solution contains benzalkonium chloride which may be absorbed by soft contact lenses; wait at least 10 minutes after administration before inserting contact lenses. When used for self-medication (OTC use), notify healthcare provider if symptoms worsen or do not improve within 3 days. Contact healthcare provider if change in vision, eye pain, or redness occur. Do not use if solution is cloudy or changes color.

Adverse Reactions

Ocular: Allergic reactions, burning or stinging, conjunctivitis, discharge, dry eyes, eye pain, eyelid disorder, itching, keratitis, lacrimation disorder, mydriasis, photophobia, rash

Respiratory: Pharyngitis

Miscellaneous: Flu syndrome

Drug Interactions

Metabolism/Transport Effects None known.

Avoid Concomitant Use

Avoid concomitant use of Ketotifen (Ophthalmic) with any of the following: Aclidinium; Azelastine (Nasal); Ipratropium (Oral Inhalation); Paraldehyde; Potassium Chloride; Thalidomide; Umeclidinium

Increased Effect/Toxicity

Ketotifen (Ophthalmic) may increase the levels/effects of: AbobotulinumtoxinA; Alcohol (Ethyl); Analgesics (Opioid); Anticholinergic Agents; Azelastine (Nasal); Buprenorphine; Cannabinoid-Containing Products; CNS Depressants; Hydrocodone; Methotrimeprazine; Metyrosine; Mirabegron; Mirtazapine; OnabotulinumtoxinA; Paraldehyde; Potassium Chloride; Pramipexole; RimabotulinumtoxinB; ROPINIRole; Rotigotine; Selective Serotonin Reuptake Inhibitors; Thalidomide; Thiazide Diuretics; Topiramate; Zolpidem

The levels/effects of Ketotifen (Ophthalmic) may be increased by: Aclidinium; Brimonidine (Topical); Cannabis; Doxylamine; Dronabinol; Droperidol; HydrOXYzine; Ipratropium (Oral Inhalation); Kava Kava; Magnesium Sulfate; Methotrimeprazine; Nabilone; Perampanel; Pramlintide; Rufinamide; Sodium Oxybate; Tapentadol; Tetrahydrocannabinol; Umeclidinium

Decreased Effect

Ketotifen (Ophthalmic) may decrease the levels/effects of: Acetylcholinesterase Inhibitors (Central); Benzylpenicilloyl Polylysine; Betahistine; Hyaluronidase; Secretin

The levels/effects of Ketotifen (Ophthalmic) may be decreased by: Acetylcholinesterase Inhibitors (Central); Amphetamines

Stability Store at controlled room temperature (68°F to 77°F).

Mechanism of Action Exhibits noncompetitive H_1-receptor antagonist and mast cell stabilizer properties. Efficacy in conjunctivitis likely results from a combination of anti-inflammatory and antihistaminergic actions including interference with chemokine-induced migration of eosinophils into inflamed conjunctiva.

◀ **Pharmacodynamics**
Onset of action: 5-15 minutes
Duration: 5-8 hours

Dosing: Usual Ophthalmic: Children ≥3 years and Adults: Instill 1 drop into lower conjunctival sac of affected eye(s) twice daily, every 8-12 hours

Administration Ophthalmic: Instill into conjunctival sac avoiding contact of bottle tip with skin or eye; apply finger pressure to lacrimal sac during and for 1-2 minutes after instillation to decrease risk of absorption and systemic effects. Administer other topical ophthalmic medications at least 5 minutes apart.

Monitoring Parameters Improvement in symptomatology (eg, reduction in itching, tearing, and hyperaemia)

Dosage Forms Excipient information presented when available (limited, particularly for generics); consult specific product labeling.

Solution, Ophthalmic:
Alaway: 0.025% (10 mL) [contains benzalkonium chloride]
Alaway Childrens Allergy: 0.025% (5 mL) [contains benzalkonium chloride]
Claritin Eye: 0.025% (5 mL) [contains benzalkonium chloride]
Zaditor: 0.025% (5 mL) [contains benzalkonium chloride]
ZyrTEC Itchy Eye: 0.025% (5 mL) [contains benzalkonium chloride]
Generic: 0.025% (5 mL)

References

Horak F, et al, "Onset and Duration of Action of Ketotifen 0.025% and Emedastine 0.05% in Seasonal Allergic Conjunctivitis," *Clin Drug Invest*, 2003, 23(5): 329-37.

◆ **Ketotifen Fumarate** see Ketotifen (Ophthalmic) on page 1185

◆ **Khloditan** see Mitotane on page 1425

◆ **KI** see Potassium Iodide on page 1711

◆ **Kidrolase (Can)** see Asparaginase (E. coli) on page 208

◆ **Kineret** see Anakinra on page 168

◆ **Kineret® (Can)** see Anakinra on page 168

◆ **Kinrix®** see Diphtheria and Tetanus Toxoids, Acellular Pertussis, and Poliovirus Vaccine on page 682

◆ **Kionex** see Sodium Polystyrene Sulfonate on page 1917

◆ **Kivexa™ (Can)** see Abacavir and Lamivudine on page 39

◆ **Klaron** see Sulfacetamide (Topical) on page 1944

◆ **Klean-Prep (Can)** see Polyethylene Glycol-Electrolyte Solution on page 1697

◆ **KlonoPIN** see ClonazePAM on page 514

◆ **Klor-Con** see Potassium Chloride on page 1708

◆ **Klor-Con 10** see Potassium Chloride on page 1708

◆ **Klor-Con M10** see Potassium Chloride on page 1708

◆ **Klor-Con M15** see Potassium Chloride on page 1708

◆ **Klor-Con M20** see Potassium Chloride on page 1708

◆ **K-Lyte/Cl** see Potassium Bicarbonate and Potassium Chloride on page 1707

◆ **Koffex Expectorant (Can)** see GuaiFENesin on page 984

◆ **Kogenate FS** see Antihemophilic Factor (Recombinant) on page 172

◆ **Kogenate FS Bio-Set** see Antihemophilic Factor (Recombinant) on page 172

◆ **Kolephrin GG/DM [OTC]** see Guaifenesin and Dextromethorphan on page 987

◆ **Konakion (Can)** see Phytonadione on page 1671

◆ **Konsyl [OTC]** see Psyllium on page 1773

◆ **Konsyl-D [OTC]** see Psyllium on page 1773

◆ **Koāte®-DVI** see Antihemophilic Factor (Human) on page 170

◆ **K-Phos® Neutral** see Potassium Phosphate and Sodium Phosphate on page 1718

◆ **K-Phos® No. 2** see Potassium Phosphate and Sodium Phosphate on page 1718

◆ **Kristalose** see Lactulose on page 1193

◆ **KS Ibuprofen [OTC]** see Ibuprofen on page 1059

◆ **KS Stool Softener [OTC]** see Docusate on page 701

◆ **K-Tab** see Potassium Chloride on page 1708

◆ **Kuvan** see Sapropterin on page 1865

◆ **K-Vescent** see Potassium Chloride on page 1708

◆ **Kwell** see Lindane on page 1250

◆ **Kwellada-P [OTC] (Can)** see Permethrin on page 1647

◆ **Kytril** see Granisetron on page 980

◆ **Kytril® (Can)** see Granisetron on page 980

◆ **L-749,345** see Ertapenem on page 778

◆ **L-758,298** see Fosaprepitant on page 934

◆ **L 754030** see Aprepitant on page 190

Labetalol (la BET a lole)

Medication Safety Issues
Sound-alike/look-alike issues:
Labetalol may be confused with betaxolol, lamoTRIgine, Lipitor
Normodyne may be confused with Norpramin
Trandate may be confused with traMADol, TRENtal

High alert medication:
The Institute for Safe Medication Practices (ISMP) includes this medication among its list of drugs which have a heightened risk of causing significant patient harm when used in error.

Administration issues:
Significant differences exist between oral and I.V. dosing. Use caution when converting from one route of administration to another.

Brand Names: U.S. Trandate

Brand Names: Canada Apo-Labetalol; Labetalol Hydrochloride Injection, USP; Normodyne; Trandate

Therapeutic Category Alpha-/Beta- Adrenergic Blocker; Antihypertensive Agent

Generic Availability (U.S.) Yes

Use
Oral: Treatment of hypertension alone or in combination (particularly with thiazide or loop diuretics) (FDA approved in adults)
Parenteral: Treatment of severe hypertension (FDA approved in adults)

Pregnancy Risk Factor C

Pregnancy Considerations Adverse events have been observed in some animal reproduction studies. Labetalol crosses the placenta and can be detected in cord blood and infant serum after delivery (Haraldsson, 1989; Rogers, 1990). Fetal/neonatal bradycardia, hypoglycemia, hypotension, and/or respiratory depression have been observed following in utero exposure to labetalol. Adequate facilities for monitoring infants at birth should be available.

Untreated chronic maternal hypertension and pre-eclampsia are also associated with adverse events in the fetus, infant, and mother. Oral labetalol is considered an appropriate agent for the treatment of chronic hypertension in pregnancy; intravenous labetalol is recommended for use in the management of acute onset severe hypertension in pregnancy and hypertension associated with pre-eclampsia (ACOG, 2011; ACOG 2013).

Breast-Feeding Considerations Low amounts of labetalol are found in breast milk and can be detected in the serum of nursing infants. The manufacturer recommends that caution be exercised when administering labetalol to nursing women.

Contraindications Hypersensitivity to labetalol or any component; asthma, obstructive airway disease, cardiogenic shock, uncompensated CHF, severe bradycardia, heart block (except in patients with a functioning artificial pacemaker); conditions associated with severe and prolonged hypotension

Warnings Symptomatic hypotension with or without syncope may occur; close monitoring of patient is required especially with initial dosing and dosage increases; blood pressure should be lowered at a rate compatible with the patient's status; cerebral and cardiac adverse effects (infarction/ischemia) may occur if blood pressure is decreased too rapidly. Initiation of therapy with a low dose and gradual up-titration may help to decrease the occurrence of hypotension or syncope; patients should be advised to avoid driving or other hazardous tasks during initiation of therapy due to the risk of syncope. Orthostatic hypotension may occur with I.V. administration; patient should remain supine during and for up to 3 hours after I.V. administration. Severe hepatic injury, including some fatalities, has been rarely reported with use; periodically monitor LFTs with prolonged use.

Tablets may contain sodium benzoate; benzoic acid (benzoate) is a metabolite of benzyl alcohol; large amounts of benzyl alcohol (≥99 mg/kg/day) have been associated with a potentially fatal toxicity ("gasping syndrome") in neonates; avoid use of labetalol products containing sodium benzoate in neonates; in vitro and animal studies have shown that benzoate displaces bilirubin from protein binding sites

Precautions Use with caution and monitor closely in patients with bronchospastic or hyper-reactive airway disease; in general, patients with bronchospastic disease should not receive beta-blockers. Use with caution in patients with diabetes mellitus; may potentiate hypoglycemia and/or mask signs and symptoms; may also reduce release of insulin in response to hyperglycemia; dosage of antidiabetic agents may need to be adjusted. May depress myocardial activity and precipitate or worsen CHF; use with extreme caution and monitor closely, especially in patients with compensated heart failure. Use with caution in patients with hepatic impairment; bioavailability is increased due to decreased first-pass metabolism. May precipitate or aggravate symptoms of arterial insufficiency in patients with PVD and Raynaud's disease; use with caution and monitor for progression of arterial obstruction. Beta-blocker use has been associated with induction or exacerbation of psoriasis, but causality has not been firmly established. Use with caution in patients with a history of psychiatric illness; may cause or exacerbate CNS depression. May mask signs of hyperthyroidism (eg, tachycardia); if hyperthyroidism is suspected, carefully manage and monitor; abrupt withdrawal may exacerbate symptoms of hyperthyroidism or precipitate thyroid storm.

A-V conduction abnormalities may occur; reported incidence less than with propranolol; consider preexisting conditions, such as sick sinus syndrome, before initiating. Use with caution in patients with myasthenia gravis. In children, two cases of reversible myopathy have been reported (Willis, 1990). Beta-blocker therapy should not be withdrawn abruptly (particularly in patients with CAD), but gradually tapered to avoid acute tachycardia, hypertension, and/or ischemia. Severe exacerbation of angina, ventricular arrhythmias, and MI have been reported following abrupt withdrawal of beta-blocker therapy. Temporary but prompt resumption of beta-blocker therapy may be indicated with worsening of angina or acute coronary insufficiency. Chronic beta-blocker therapy should not be routinely withdrawn prior to major surgery.

Labetalol has been shown to be effective in lowering blood pressure and relieving symptoms in patients with pheochromocytoma; however, some patients have experienced paradoxical hypertensive responses; use with caution in patients with pheochromocytoma. Additional alpha-blockade may be required during use of labetalol. Consider diagnostic tests for pheochromocytoma prior to use. Use caution with history of severe anaphylaxis to allergens; patients taking beta-blockers may become more sensitive to repeated challenges. Treatment of anaphylaxis (eg, epinephrine) in patients taking beta-blockers may be ineffective or promote undesirable effects.

Intraoperative floppy iris syndrome has been observed in cataract surgery patients who were on or were previously treated with alpha$_1$-blockers; causality has not been established and there appears to be no benefit in discontinuing alpha-blocker therapy prior to surgery. Instruct patients to inform ophthalmologist of labetalol use when considering eye surgery.

Adverse Reactions

Cardiovascular: Edema, flushing, hypotension, orthostatic hypotension (I.V. use), ventricular arrhythmia (I.V. use)

Central nervous system: Dizziness, fatigue, headache, somnolence, vertigo

Dermatologic: Pruritus, rash, scalp tingling

Gastrointestinal: Dyspepsia, nausea, taste disturbance, vomiting

Genitourinary: Ejaculatory failure, impotence

Hepatic: Transaminases increased

Neuromuscular & skeletal: Paresthesia, weakness

Ocular: Vision abnormal

Renal: BUN increased

Respiratory: Dyspnea, nasal congestion

Miscellaneous: Diaphoresis

Rare but important or life-threatening: Alopecia (reversible), anaphylactoid reaction, ANA positive, angioedema, bradycardia, bronchospasm, cholestatic jaundice, CHF, diabetes insipidus, heart block, hepatic necrosis, hepatitis, hypersensitivity, Peyronie's disease, psoriaform rash, Raynaud's syndrome, syncope, systemic lupus erythematosus, toxic myopathy, urinary retention, urticaria

Other adverse reactions noted with beta-adrenergic blocking agents include agranulocytosis, catatonia, emotional lability, intensification of preexisting AV block, ischemic colitis. laryngospasm, mental depression, mesenteric artery thrombosis, nonthrombocytopenic purpura, respiratory distress, short-term memory loss, and thrombocytopenic purpura.

Drug Interactions

Metabolism/Transport Effects None known.

Avoid Concomitant Use

Avoid concomitant use of Labetalol with any of the following: Beta2-Agonists; Ceritinib; Floctafenine; Methacholine

Increased Effect/Toxicity

Labetalol may increase the levels/effects of: Alpha-/Beta-Agonists (Direct-Acting); Alpha1-Blockers; Alpha2-Agonists; Amifostine; Antihypertensives; Antipsychotic Agents (Phenothiazines); Bradycardia-Causing Agents; Bupivacaine; Cardiac Glycosides; Ceritinib; Cholinergic Agonists; DULoxetine; Ergot Derivatives; Fingolimod; Grass Pollen Allergen Extract (5 Grass Extract); Hypotensive Agents; Insulin; Lidocaine (Systemic); Lidocaine (Topical); Mepivacaine; Methacholine; Midodrine; Obinutuzumab; RiTUXimab; Sulfonylureas

The levels/effects of Labetalol may be increased by: Acetylcholinesterase Inhibitors; Alpha2-Agonists; Aminoquinolines (Antimalarial); Amiodarone; Anilidopiperidine Opioids; Antipsychotic Agents (Phenothiazines);

Barbiturates; Brimonidine (Topical); Calcium Channel Blockers (Dihydropyridine); Calcium Channel Blockers (Nondihydropyridine); Diazoxide; Dipyridamole; Disopyramide; Dronedarone; Floctafenine; Herbs (Hypotensive Properties); MAO Inhibitors; Pentoxifylline; Phosphodiesterase 5 Inhibitors; Propafenone; Prostacyclin Analogues; Regorafenib; Reserpine

Decreased Effect

Labetalol may decrease the levels/effects of: Beta2-Agonists; Theophylline Derivatives

The levels/effects of Labetalol may be decreased by: Barbiturates; Herbs (Hypertensive Properties); Methylphenidate; Nonsteroidal Anti-Inflammatory Agents; Rifamycin Derivatives; Yohimbine

Food Interactions Labetalol serum concentrations may be increased if taken with food. Management: Administer with food.

Stability

Tablets: Store at room temperature (refer to manufacturer's labeling for detailed storage requirements); protect from light; protect unit dose boxes from excessive moisture

Injectable: Store at room temperature (refer to manufacturer's labeling for detailed storage requirements); do not freeze; protect from light. The solution is clear to slightly yellow.

Parenteral admixture: Stability of parenteral admixture at room temperature (25°C, 77°F) and refrigeration temperature (4°C, 39°F): 3 days

Mechanism of Action Blocks alpha-, beta$_1$-, and beta$_2$-adrenergic receptor sites; elevated renins are reduced. The ratios of alpha- to beta-blockade differ depending on the route of administration: 1:3 (oral) and 1:7 (I.V.).

Pharmacodynamics

Onset of action:

Oral: 20 minutes to 2 hours

I.V.: 2-5 minutes

Maximum effect:

Oral: 1-4 hours

I.V.: 5-15 minutes

Duration:

Oral: 8-24 hours (dose dependent)

I.V.: 2-4 hours

Pharmacokinetics (Adult data unless noted)

Distribution: Crosses the placenta; small amounts in breast milk

V_d: 3-16 L/kg; mean: 9.4 L/kg

Protein-binding: 50%

Metabolism: Hepatic via primarily glucuronide conjugation; extensive first-pass effect

Bioavailability: Oral: 25%; increased bioavailability with liver disease, elderly

Time to peak serum concentration: Oral: 1-2 hours

Half-life: 5-8 hours

Elimination: Urine (55% to 60%, primarily as glucuronide conjugates, <5% as unchanged drug); possible decreased clearance in neonates and infants

Dialysis: Not removed by hemo- or peritoneal dialysis; supplemental dose is not necessary

Dosing: Usual Note: Use care with labetalol continuous I.V. infusions; the rate of administration is different for pediatric patients (mg/kg/hour) versus adult patients (mg/minute).

Infants, Children, and Adolescents:

Hypertension: Children and Adolescents: Limited data available:

Oral: Initial: 1-3 mg/kg/**day** in 2 divided doses; maximum daily dose: 10-12 mg/kg/**day**, up to 1200 mg/day (NHLBI, 2011)

I.V. (intermittent bolus): 0.2-1 mg/kg/dose; maximum dose: 40 mg; use should be reserved for severe hypertension (NHBPEP, 2004)

Hypertensive emergency: Infants, Children, and Adolescents: Continuous I.V. infusion: 0.25-3 mg/kg/**hour**; initiate at lower end of range, and titrate up slowly (NHBPEP, 2004). One retrospective study in infants and children ≤24 months of age observed reductions in blood pressure at doses up to 0.59 mg/kg/hour with little additional benefit at higher doses (Thomas, 2011).

Adults:

Hypertension: Oral: Initial: 100 mg twice daily, may increase as needed every 2-3 days by 100 mg twice daily (titration increments not to exceed 200 mg twice daily) until desired response is obtained; usual dose: 100-400 mg twice daily (JNC 7); may require up to 2400 mg/day

Acute hypertension (hypertensive emergency/urgency):

I.V. bolus: Manufacturer's labeling: Initial: 20 mg I.V. push over 2 minutes; may administer 40-80 mg at 10-minute intervals, up to 300 mg total cumulative dose; as appropriate, follow with oral antihypertensive regimen

I.V. infusion (acute loading): Manufacturer's labeling: Initial: 2 mg/minute; titrate to response up to 300 mg total cumulative dose (eg, discontinue after 2.5 hours of 2 mg/minute); usual total dose required: 50-200 mg; as appropriate, follow with oral antihypertensive regimen

Note: There is limited documentation of prolonged continuous I.V. infusions (ie, >300 mg/day). In rare clinical situations, higher continuous I.V. infusion doses up to 6 mg/minute have been used in the critical care setting (eg, aortic dissection) and up to 8 mg/minute (eg, hypertension with ongoing acute ischemic stroke). At the other extreme, continuous infusions at relatively low doses (0.03-0.1 mg/minute) have been used in some settings (following loading infusion in patients who are unable to be converted to oral regimens or in some cases as a continuation of outpatient oral regimens). These prolonged infusions should not be confused with loading infusions. Because of wide variation in the use of infusions, an awareness of institutional policies and practices is extremely important. Careful clarification of orders and specific infusion rates/units is required to avoid confusion. Due to the prolonged duration of action, careful monitoring should be extended for the duration of the infusion and for several hours after the infusion. Excessive administration may result in prolonged hypotension and/or bradycardia.

I.V. to oral conversion: Upon discontinuation of I.V. infusion, may initiate oral dose of 200 mg followed in 6-12 hours with an additional dose of 200-400 mg. Thereafter, dose patients with 400-2400 mg/day in divided doses depending on blood pressure response.

Dosage adjustment in hepatic impairment: Dosage reduction may be necessary.

Usual Infusion Concentrations: Pediatric I.V. infusion: 1 mg/mL

Administration

Oral: May administer with food but should be administered in a consistent manner with regards to meals

Parenteral:

I.V. bolus: May administer undiluted (5 mg/mL) over 2-3 minutes; maximum: 2 mg/minute

Continuous I.V. infusion: Dilute to 1 mg/mL; undiluted labetalol injection (5 mg/mL) has been administered to a very small number of adult patients who were extremely fluid restricted

Monitoring Parameters Blood pressure, heart rate, pulse, ECG; **Note:** I.V. use: Monitor closely; due to the prolonged duration of action, careful monitoring should be extended for the duration of the infusion and for several hours after the infusion; excessive administration may result in prolonged hypotension and/or bradycardia

Test Interactions False-positive urine catecholamines, vanillylmandelic acid (VMA) if measured by fluorometric or photometric methods; use HPLC or specific catecholamine radioenzymatic technique; false-positive amphetamine if measured by thin-layer chromatography or radioenzymatic assay (gas chromatographic-mass spectrometer technique should be used)

Dosage Forms Excipient information presented when available (limited, particularly for generics); consult specific product labeling.

Solution, Intravenous, as hydrochloride:
Generic: 5 mg/mL (4 mL, 20 mL, 40 mL)
Tablet, Oral, as hydrochloride:
Trandate: 100 mg, 200 mg, 300 mg [scored]
Generic: 100 mg, 200 mg, 300 mg

Extemporaneous Preparations A 40 mg/mL labetalol hydrochloride oral suspension may be made with tablets and one of three different vehicles (cherry syrup, a 1:1 mixture of Ora-Sweet® and Ora-Plus®, or a 1:1 mixture of Ora-Sweet® SF and Ora-Plus®). Crush sixteen 300 mg tablets in a mortar and reduce to a fine powder. Add 20 mL of the chosen vehicle and mix to a uniform paste; mix while adding the vehicle in incremental proportions to **almost** 120 mL; transfer to a calibrated bottle, rinse mortar with vehicle, and add quantity of vehicle sufficient to make 120 mL. Label "shake well" and "protect from light". Stable for 60 days when stored in amber plastic prescription bottles in the dark at room temperature or refrigerated (Allen, 1996).

Extemporaneously prepared solutions of labetalol hydrochloride (approximate concentrations 7-10 mg/mL) prepared in distilled water, simple syrup, apple juice, grape juice, and orange juice were stable for 4 weeks when stored in amber glass or plastic prescription bottles at room temperature or refrigerated (Nahata, 1991).

Allen LV Jr and Erickson MA 3rd, "Stability of Labetalol Hydrochloride, Metoprolol Tartrate, Verapamil Hydrochloride, and Spironolactone with Hydrochlorothiazide in Extemporaneously Compounded Oral Liquids," *Am J Health Syst Pharm*, 1996, 53(19):2304-9.

Nahata MC, "Stability of Labetalol Hydrochloride in Distilled Water, Simple Syrup, and Three Fruit Juices," *DICP*, 1991, 25(5):465-9.

References

Chobanian AV, Bakris GL, Black HR, et al, "The Seventh Report of the Joint National Committee on Prevention, Detection, Evaluation, and Treatment of High Blood Pressure: The JNC 7 report," *JAMA*, 2003, 289(19):2560-72.

National Heart, Lung, and Blood Institute, "Expert Panel on Integrated Guidelines for Cardiovascular Health and Risk Reduction in Children and Adolescents," *Clinical Practice Guidelines*, 2011, National Institutes of Health. Available at http://www.nhlbi.nih.gov/guidelines/cvd_ped/peds_guidelines_full.pdf. Date accessed: March 16, 2012.

National High Blood Pressure Education Program (NHBPEP) Working Group on High Blood Pressure in Children and Adolescents, "The Fourth Report on the Diagnosis, Evaluation, and Treatment of High Blood Pressure in Children and Adolescents," *Pediatrics*, 2004, 114(2 Suppl 4th Report):555-76.

Phillips MS, "Standardizing I.V. Infusion Concentrations: National Survey Results," *Am J Health Syst Pharm*, 2011, 68(22):2176-82.

Thomas CA, Moffett BS, Wagner JL, et al, "Safety and Efficacy of Intravenous Labetalol for Hypertension Crisis in Infants and Small Children," *Pediatr Crit Care Med*, 2011, 12(1):28-32.

Wesley AG, Hariparsad D, Pather M, et al, "Labetalol in Tetanus. The Treatment of Sympathetic Nervous System Overactivity," *Anaesthesia*, 1983, 38(3):243-9.

Willis JK, Tilton AH, Harkin JC, et al, "Reversible Myopathy Due to Labetalol," *Pediatr Neurol*, 1990, 6(4):275-6.

◆ **Labetalol Hydrochloride** *see* Labetalol *on page 1186*

◆ **Labetalol Hydrochloride Injection, USP (Can)** *see* Labetalol *on page 1186*

◆ **Lac-Hydrin®** *see* Lactic Acid and Ammonium Hydroxide *on page 1191*

◆ **Lac-Hydrin® Five [OTC]** *see* Lactic Acid and Ammonium Hydroxide *on page 1191*

◆ **LAClotion™** *see* Lactic Acid and Ammonium Hydroxide *on page 1191*

Lacosamide (la KOE sa mide)

Medication Safety Issues
Sound-alike/look-alike issues:
Lacosamide may be confused with zonisamide
Vimpat may be confused with Vimovo

Brand Names: U.S. Vimpat

Brand Names: Canada Vimpat

Therapeutic Category Anticonvulsant, Miscellaneous

Generic Availability (U.S.) No

Use
Oral: Solution, tablets: Adjunctive therapy in the treatment of partial-onset seizures (FDA approved in ages ≥17 years and adults)
Parenteral: Short-term adjunctive therapy in the treatment of partial-onset seizures when oral therapy is not feasible (FDA approved in ages ≥17 years and adults)

Medication Guide Available Yes

Pregnancy Risk Factor C

Pregnancy Considerations Adverse events were observed in animal reproduction studies. Available information related to use in pregnancy is limited; if inadvertent exposure occurs during pregnancy, close monitoring of the mother and fetus/newborn is recommended (Hoeltzenbein, 2011). Two registries are available for women exposed to lacosamide during pregnancy:
Pregnant women may contact the North American Antiepileptic Drug (AED) Pregnancy Registry (888-233-2334 or http://www.aedpregnancyregistry.org) The healthcare provider or patient may contact the UCB AED Pregnancy Registry (888-537-7734)

Breast-Feeding Considerations It is unknown if lacosamide is excreted in human milk. The manufacturer recommends a decision be made whether to discontinue nursing or to discontinue the drug, taking into account the importance of treatment to the mother.

Contraindications Hypersensitivity to lacosamide or any component

Warnings Antiepileptic drugs (AEDs) increase the risk of suicidal behavior and ideation in patients receiving these medications for any indication. Pooled analyses of placebo-controlled trials involving 11 different AEDs (regardless of indication) showed a twofold increased risk of suicidal thoughts or behavior (estimated incidence rate: 0.43% in AED treated patients compared to 0.24% in patients receiving placebo); increased risk was observed as early as 1 week after initiation of AED and continued through duration of trials (most trials ≤24 weeks); risk did not vary significantly by age (age range: 5-100 years). Consider risks and benefits of AEDs before prescribing. Monitor all patients receiving an AED for emergence of suicidal thoughts or behavior, thoughts of self-harm, any unusual changes in behavior or mood, or the emergence or worsening of depressive symptoms; notify healthcare provider immediately if symptoms or concerning behavior occur. **Note:** The FDA requires a Medication Guide for all antiepileptic drugs informing patients of this risk.

Potentially serious (sometimes fatal, possibly delayed) multiorgan hypersensitivity reactions [drug reaction with eosinophilia and systemic symptoms (DRESS)] have been reported with some antiepileptic drugs (rare). Monitor for rash, fever, and signs and symptoms of possible disparate manifestations associated with lymphatic, hepatic, renal, and/or hematologic organ systems. Discontinuation of lacosamide and conversion to alternate therapy may be required.

Dose-dependent dizziness and ataxia may occur during therapy; reported frequency: 31%. CNS effects may impair ▶

physical and mental abilities; patients must be cautioned about performing tasks which require mental alertness (eg, operating machinery or driving). Anticonvulsants should not be discontinued abruptly because of the possibility of increasing seizure frequency; therapy should be withdrawn gradually (≥1 week) to minimize the potential of increased seizure frequency, unless safety concerns require a more rapid withdrawal.

Lacosamide oral solution contains propylene glycol; toxicities have been reported with use of products containing propylene glycol, including hyperosmolality, lactic acidosis, seizures, and respiratory depression; in neonates large amounts of propylene glycol delivered orally, intravenously (eg, >3000 mg/day), or topically have been associated with potentially fatal toxicities which can include metabolic acidosis, seizures, renal failure, and CNS depression; use oral solutions containing propylene glycol with caution (AAP, 1997; Shehab, 2009).

Precautions Use with caution in hepatic or renal impairment; dosage adjustment may be necessary; use is not recommended in patients with severe hepatic impairment. Lacosamide may prolong the PR interval (dose-dependent prolongation); AV block has been reported; use with caution in patients with conduction problems (eg, first degree, second degree or higher AV block and sick sinus syndrome without pacemaker), myocardial ischemia, heart failure, or with concurrent use with other drugs that prolong the PR interval; ECG is recommended prior to initiating therapy and when at steady state. During investigational trials, atrial fibrillation/flutter, or syncope occurred slightly more often in patients with diabetic neuropathy and/or cardiovascular disease who received lacosamide versus placebo. The oral solution contains aspartame which is metabolized to phenylalanine and must be used with caution in patients with phenylketonuria.

In vitro data has shown lacosamide interferes with CRMP-2, a protein involved with neuronal differentiation and control of axonal outgrowth; potential effect on CNS development cannot be excluded. Lacosamide administered to neonatal and juvenile rats resulted in decreased brain weights and long-term neurobehavioral changes including learning and memory deficits. Studies of the effects of lacosamide on human CNS development are needed before this medication can be recommended for routine use in pediatric patients.

Adverse Reactions
Cardiovascular: Syncope (adults; dose-related: >400 mg/day)
Central nervous system: Abnormal gait, ataxia, depression, dizziness, drowsiness, equilibrium disturbance, fatigue, headache, memory impairment, vertigo
Dermatologic: Pruritus
Gastrointestinal: Diarrhea, nausea, vomiting
Hematologic & oncologic: Bruise
Hepatic: Increased serum ALT
Local: Local irritation, pain at injection site
Neuromuscular & skeletal: Tremor, weakness
Ophthalmic: Blurred vision, diplopia, nystagmus
Miscellaneous: Laceration
Rare but important or life-threatening: Abnormal hepatic function tests, acute psychosis, aggressive behavior, agitation, agranulocytosis, anemia, angioedema, atrial fibrillation, atrial flutter, atrioventricular block, bradycardia, cerebellar syndrome, cognitive dysfunction, disturbance in attention, DRESS syndrome, euphoria, falling, hallucination, hepatitis, insomnia, nephritis, neutropenia, Stevens-Johnson syndrome, toxic epidermal necrolysis, urticaria

Drug Interactions
Metabolism/Transport Effects Substrate of CYP2C19 (minor); **Note:** Assignment of Major/Minor substrate

status based on clinically relevant drug interaction potential; **Inhibits** CYP2C19 (weak)
Avoid Concomitant Use There are no known interactions where it is recommended to avoid concomitant use.
Increased Effect/Toxicity
The levels/effects of Lacosamide may be increased by: CYP2C9 Inhibitors (Strong); CYP3A4 Inhibitors (Strong); Delavirdine; NiCARdipine
Decreased Effect
The levels/effects of Lacosamide may be decreased by: CarBAMazepine; Fosphenytoin; PHENobarbital; Phenytoin
Stability
Injection: Store at 20°C to 25°C (68°F to 77°F); excursions permitted between 15°C to 30°C (59°F to 86°F). Do not freeze. Stable when mixed with compatible diluents (D_5W, NS, LR) for ≤24 hours in glass or polyvinyl chloride bags at room temperature of 15°C to 30°C (59°F to 86°F). Any unused portion should be discarded.
Oral solution, tablets: Store at 20°C to 25°C (68°F to 77°F); excursions permitted between 15°C to 30°C (59°F to 86°F). Do not freeze. Discard any unused portion of oral solution 7 weeks after opening bottle.
Mechanism of Action *In vitro* studies have shown that lacosamide stabilizes hyperexcitable neuronal membranes and inhibits repetitive neuronal firing by enhancing the slow inactivation of sodium channels (with no effects on fast inactivation of sodium channels).
Pharmacokinetics (Adult data unless noted)
Absorption: Oral: Completely
Distribution: V_d: ~0.6 L/kg
Protein binding: <15%
Metabolism: Hepatic (CYP2C19 substrate); forms metabolite, O-desmethyl-lacosamide (inactive)
Bioavailability: ~100%
Half-life elimination: 13 hours
Time to peak plasma concentration: Oral: 1-4 hours
Excretion: Urine (95%; 40% as unchanged drug, 30% as inactive metabolite, 20% as uncharacterized metabolite); feces (<0.5%)
Dialysis: Effectively removed by hemodialysis; AUC decreased by 50% following 4-hour HD session; supplemental dose recommended
Dosing: Usual Partial onset seizure:
Children ≥3 years and Adolescents ≤16 years: Limited data available: Oral: Initial: 1 mg/kg/day divided twice daily (maximum dose: 50 mg); increased at weekly intervals by 1 mg/kg/day up to 10 mg/kg/day (mean: 6.34 mg/kg/day; range: 1.7-10 mg/kg/day); dosing based on an open-label, prospective trial of 18 patients (mean age: 10.6 years; range: 3-18 years) with refractory partial seizures (Gavatha, 2011). A retrospective study of 16 patients (mean age: 15 years; range: 8-21 years) with refractory partial seizures reported a mean initial dose of 1.3 mg/kg/day and titrated to a mean maintenance dose of 4.9 mg/kg/day; maximum daily dose: 400 mg/day (Guilhoto, 2011); further studies are needed.
Adolescents ≥17 years and Adults: Oral, I.V.:
Initial: 50 mg twice daily; may be increased at weekly intervals by 100 mg/day
Maintenance dose: 200-400 mg/day in two divided doses
Note: When switching from oral to I.V. formulations, the total daily dose and frequency should be the same; I.V. therapy should only be used temporarily.
Dosing adjustment in renal impairment: Adolescents ≥17 years and Adults: Titrate dose with caution.
Mild to moderate renal impairment: No dose adjustment necessary
Severe renal impairment (CrCl ≤30 mL/minute): Maximum dose: 300 mg/day
Hemodialysis: Removed by hemodialysis; after 4-hour HD treatment, a supplemental dose of up to 50% should be considered.

Dosing adjustment in hepatic impairment: Adolescents ≥17 years and Adults: Titrate dose with caution.
Mild to moderate hepatic impairment: Maximum dose: 300 mg/day
Severe hepatic impairment: Use is not recommended

Administration
I.V.: Administer over 30-60 minutes. Can be administered without further dilution or may be further diluted with NS, LR, or D₅W. pH: 3.5-5

Oral: Solution, tablets: May be administered with or without food. Oral solution should be administered with a calibrated measuring device (not a household teaspoon or tablespoon).

Monitoring Parameters Seizure frequency, duration, and severity; patients with conduction problems or severe cardiac disease should have ECG tracing prior to start of therapy and when at steady-state; monitor hepatic and renal function; suicidality (eg, suicidal thoughts, depression, behavioral changes)

Additional Information Twice daily I.V. infusions have been used for up to 5 days.

Controlled Substance C-V

Dosage Forms Excipient information presented when available (limited, particularly for generics); consult specific product labeling.
Solution, Intravenous:
Vimpat: 200 mg/20 mL (20 mL)
Solution, Oral:
Vimpat: 10 mg/mL (200 mL, 465 mL) [contains aspartame, methylparaben, polyethylene glycol, propylene glycol; strawberry flavor]
Tablet, Oral:
Vimpat: 50 mg [contains fd&c blue #2 aluminum lake]
Vimpat: 100 mg, 150 mg
Vimpat: 200 mg [contains fd&c blue #2 aluminum lake]

References
American Academy of Pediatrics Committee on Drugs. "Inactive" ingredients in pharmaceutical products: update (subject review). *Pediatrics.* 1997;99(2):268-278.
Gavatha M, Ioannou I, and Papavasiliou AS, "Efficacy and Tolerability of Oral Lacosamide as Adjunctive Therapy in Pediatric Patients With Pharmacoresistant Focal Epilepsy," *Epilepsy Behav,* 2011, 20 (4):691-3.
Guilhoto LM, Loddenkemper T, Gooty VD, et al, "Experience With Lacosamide in a Series of Children With Drug-Resistant Focal Epilepsy," *Pediatr Neurol,* 2011, 44(6):414-9.
Hoeltzenbein M, Supcun-Ritzler S, Langthaler M, et al "Lacosamide During pregnancy: Experience of the Berlin Institute for Clinical Teratology and Drug Risk Assessment in Pregnancy," *Reprod Toxicol,* 2011, 31(2):259.
Shehab N, Lewis CL, Streetman DD, Donn SM. Exposure to the pharmaceutical excipients benzyl alcohol and propylene glycol among critically ill neonates. *Pediatr Crit Care Med.* 2009;10 (2):256-259.
Shiloh-Malawsky Y, Fan Z, Greenwood R, et al, "Successful Treatment of Childhood Prolonged Refractory Status Epilepticus With Lacosamide," *Seizure,* 2011, 20(7):586-8.

◆ **LaCrosse Complete [OTC]** *see* Sodium Phosphates on page 1913

Lactic Acid and Ammonium Hydroxide
(LAK tik AS id & a MOE nee um hye DROKS ide)

Brand Names: U.S. AmLactin® [OTC]; Geri-Hydrolac™ [OTC]; Geri-Hydrolac™-12 [OTC]; Lac-Hydrin®; Lac-Hydrin® Five [OTC]; LAClotion™

Therapeutic Category Topical Skin Product

Generic Availability (U.S.) Yes

Use Topical humectant used in the treatment of ichthyosis vulgaris, ichthyosis xerosis, and dry skin conditions

Pregnancy Risk Factor B

Pregnancy Considerations Lactic acid is a normal component in blood and tissues. Topical application in animals has not shown fetal harm.

Breast-Feeding Considerations It is not known how this medication affects normal levels of lactic acid in human milk. Because studies have not been done in nursing women, use with caution when needed.

Contraindications Hypersensitivity to ammonium lactate, parabens, or any component

Warnings May cause photosensitivity reaction

Precautions Use with caution on face due to potential irritation, particularly in fair-skinned individuals

Adverse Reactions Dermatologic: Burning/stinging, dry skin, itching, rash (including erythema and irritation)

Drug Interactions
Metabolism/Transport Effects None known.
Avoid Concomitant Use There are no known interactions where it is recommended to avoid concomitant use.
Increased Effect/Toxicity There are no known significant interactions involving an increase in effect.
Decreased Effect There are no known significant interactions involving a decrease in effect.

Stability Store at room temperature

Mechanism of Action Exact mechanism of action unknown; lactic acid is a normal component in blood and tissues. When applied topically to the skin, acts as a humectant.

Pharmacodynamics Onset of action: Ichthyosis xerosis: 3-7 days

Pharmacokinetics (Adult data unless noted) Bioavailability: 6%

Dosing: Usual Infants, Children, and Adults: Topical: Apply twice daily

Administration Topical: Apply a small amount to the affected area(s) and rub in thoroughly; avoid contact with eyes, lips, or mucous membranes; shake lotion well before use

Monitoring Parameters Physical examination of skin condition

Dosage Forms Excipient information presented when available (limited, particularly for generics); consult specific product labeling.
Cream, topical: Lactic acid 12% with ammonium hydroxide (140 g, 280 g, 385 g)
AmLactin®: Lactic acid 12% with ammonium hydroxide (140 g)
Lac-Hydrin®: Lactic acid 12% with ammonium hydroxide (280 g, 385 g)
Lotion, topical: Lactic acid 12% with ammonium hydroxide (225 g, 400 g)
AmLactin®, Lac-Hydrin®, LAClotion™: Lactic acid 12% with ammonium hydroxide (225 g, 400 g)
Geri-Hydrolac™, Lac-Hydrin® Five: Lactic acid 5% with ammonium hydroxide (120 mL, 240 mL)
Geri-Hydrolac™-12: Lactic acid 12% with ammonium hydroxide (120 mL, 240 mL)

◆ **Lactinex™ [OTC]** *see* Lactobacillus on page 1191

Lactobacillus (lak toe ba SIL us)

Brand Names: U.S. Bacid® [OTC]; Culturelle® [OTC]; Dofus [OTC]; Flora-Q™ [OTC]; Floranex™ [OTC]; Kala® [OTC]; Lactinex™ [OTC]; Lacto-Bifidus [OTC]; Lacto-Key [OTC]; Lacto-Pectin [OTC]; Lacto-TriBlend [OTC]; Megadophilus® [OTC]; MoreDophilus® [OTC]; RisaQuad®-2 [OTC]; RisaQuad™ [OTC]; Superdophilus® [OTC]; VSL #3® [OTC]; VSL #3®-DS

Brand Names: Canada Bacid®; Fermalac

Therapeutic Category Antidiarrheal

Generic Availability (U.S.) Yes

Use Treatment of uncomplicated diarrhea particularly that caused by antibiotic therapy; re-establish normal physiologic and bacterial flora of the intestinal tract

Contraindications Allergy to milk or lactose

Warnings Discontinue if high fever present

Adverse Reactions Gastrointestinal: Bloating (intestinal), flatulence

Drug Interactions

Metabolism/Transport Effects None known.

Avoid Concomitant Use There are no known interactions where it is recommended to avoid concomitant use.

Increased Effect/Toxicity There are no known significant interactions involving an increase in effect.

Decreased Effect There are no known significant interactions involving a decrease in effect.

Stability Store in the refrigerator

Mechanism of Action Helps re-establish normal intestinal flora; suppresses the growth of potentially pathogenic microorganisms by producing lactic acid which favors the establishment of an aciduric flora.

Pharmacokinetics (Adult data unless noted)
Absorption: Not orally absorbed
Distribution: Locally, primarily in the colon
Elimination: In feces

Dosing: Usual Children and Adults: Oral:
Capsule: 1-2 capsules 2-4 times/day
Granules: 1 packet added to or taken with cereal, food, milk, fruit juice, or water 3-4 times/day
Powder: 1/4-1 teaspoon 1-3 times/day with liquid
Tablet, chewable: 4 tablets 3-4 times/day; may follow each dose with a small amount of milk, fruit juice, or water
Recontamination protocol for BMT unit: 1 packet 3 times/day for 6 doses for those patients who refuse yogurt

Administration Oral: Granules, powder, or contents of capsules may be added to or administered with cereal, food, milk, fruit juice, or water

Dosage Forms Excipient information presented when available (limited, particularly for generics); consult specific product labeling.
Capsule:
Culturelle®: *L. rhamnosus* GG 10 billion colony-forming units [contains casein and whey]
Dofus: *L. acidophilus* and *L. bifidus* 10:1 ratio [beet root powder base]
Flora-Q™: *L. acidophilus* and *L. paracasei* ≥8 billion colony-forming units [also contains *Bifidobacterium* and *S. thermophilus*]
Lacto-Key:
100: *L. acidophilus* 1 billion colony-forming units [milk, soy, and yeast free; rice derived]
600: *L. acidophilus* 6 billion colony-forming units [milk, soy, and yeast free; rice derived]
Lacto-Bifidus:
100: *L. bifidus* 1 billion colony-forming units [milk, soy, and yeast free; rice derived]
600: *L. bifidus* 6 billion colony-forming units [milk, soy, and yeast free; rice derived]
Lacto-Pectin: *L. acidophilus* and *L. casei* ≥5 billion colony-forming units [also contains *Bifidobacterium lactis* and citrus pectin cellulose complex]
Lacto-TriBlend:
100: *L. acidophilus*, *L. bifidus*, and *L. bulgaricus* 1 billion colony-forming units [milk, soy and yeast free; rice derived]
600: *L. acidophilus*, *L. bifidus*, and *L. bulgaricus* 6 billion colony-forming units [milk, soy and yeast free; rice derived]
Megadophilus®, Superdophilus®: *L. acidophilus* 2 billion units [available in dairy based or dairy free formulations]
RisaQuad™: *L. acidophilus* and *L. paracasei* 8 billion colony-forming units [also includes *Bifidobacterium* and *Streptococcus thermophilus*]
VSL #3®: *L. acidophilus*, *L. plantarum*, *L. paracasei*, *L. bulgaricus* 112 billion live cells [also contains *Bifidobacterium breve*, *B. longum*, *B. infantis*, and *Streptococcus thermophilus*]

Capsule, double strength:
RisaQuad®-2: *L. acidophilus* and *L. paracasei* 16 billion colony-forming units [gluten free; also includes *Bifidobacterium* and *Streptococcus thermophilus*]
Capsule, softgel: *L. acidophilus* 100 active units
Caplet:
Bacid®: *L. acidophilus* and *L. bulgaricus* [also contains *Bifidobacterium biffidum* and *Streptococcus thermophilus*]
Granules:
Floranex™: *L. acidophilus* and *L. bulgaricus* 100 million live cells per 1 g packet (12s) [contains milk, sodium 5 mg/packet, soy]
Lactinex™: *L. acidophilus* and *L. bulgaricus* 100 million live cells per 1 g packet (12s) [gluten free; contains calcium 5 mg/packet, lactose 380 mg/packet, potassium 20 mg/packet, sodium 5 mg/packet, sucrose 34 mg/packet, whey, evaporated milk, and soy peptone]
Powder:
Lacto-TriBlend: *L. acidophilus*, *L. bifidus*, and *L. bulgaricus* 10 billion colony-forming units per 1/4 teaspoon (60 g) [milk, soy, and yeast free; rice derived]
Megadophilus®, Superdophilus®: *L. acidophilus* 2 billion units per half-teaspoon (49 g, 70 g, 84 g, 126 g) [available in dairy based or dairy free (garbanzo bean) formulations]
MoreDophilus®: *L. acidophilus* 12.4 billion units per teaspoon (30 g, 120 g) [dairy free; yeast free; soy and carrot derived]
VSL #3®: *L. acidophilus*, *L. plantarum*, *L. paracasei*, *L. bulgaricus* 450 billion live cells per sachet (10s, 30s) [gluten free; also contains *Bifidobacterium breve*, *B. longum*, *B. infantis*, and *Streptococcus thermophilus*; lemon cream flavor and unflavored]
VSL #3®-DS: *L. acidophilus*, *L. plantarum*, *L. paracasei*, *L. bulgaricus* 900 billion live cells per packet (20s,) [gluten free; also contains *Bifidobacterium breve*, *B. longum*, *B. infantis*, and *Streptococcus thermophilus*]
Tablet: *L. acidophilus* 35 million and *L. sporogenes* 25 million
Kala®: *L. acidophilus* 200 million units [dairy free, yeast free; soy based]
Tablet, chewable: *L. reuteri* 100 million organisms
Floranex™: *L. acidophilus* and *L. bulgaricus* 1 million colony-forming units [contains lactose, nonfat dried milk, whey]
Lactinex™: *L. acidophilus* and *L. bulgaricus* 1 million live cells [gluten free; contains calcium 5.2 mg/4 tablets, lactose 960 mg/4 tablets, potassium 20 mg/4 tablets, sodium 5.6 mg/4 tablets, and sucrose 500 sucrose/4 tablets; contains whey, evaporated milk, and soy peptone]
Wafer: *L. acidophilus* 90 mg and *L. bifidus* 25 mg (100s) [provides 1 billion organisms/wafer at time of manufacture; milk free]

◆ ***Lactobacillus acidophilus*** see Lactobacillus on page *1191*

◆ ***Lactobacillus bifidus*** see Lactobacillus on page *1191*

◆ ***Lactobacillus bulgaricus*** see Lactobacillus on page *1191*

◆ ***Lactobacillus casei*** see Lactobacillus on page *1191*

◆ ***Lactobacillus paracasei*** see Lactobacillus on page *1191*

◆ ***Lactobacillus plantarum*** see Lactobacillus on page *1191*

◆ ***Lactobacillus reuteri*** see Lactobacillus on page *1191*

◆ ***Lactobacillus rhamnosus* GG** see Lactobacillus on page *1191*

◆ **Lacto-Bifidus [OTC]** see Lactobacillus on page *1191*

◆ **Lactoflavin** see Riboflavin on page *1821*

◆ **Lacto-Key [OTC]** *see Lactobacillus on page 1191*
◆ **Lacto-Pectin [OTC]** *see Lactobacillus on page 1191*
◆ **Lacto-TriBlend [OTC]** *see Lactobacillus on page 1191*

Lactulose (LAK tyoo lose)

Medication Safety Issues
Sound-alike/look-alike issues:
Lactulose may be confused with lactose
Brand Names: U.S. Constulose; Enulose; Generlac; Kristalose
Brand Names: Canada Acilac; Apo-Lactulose®; Laxilose; PMS-Lactulose
Therapeutic Category Ammonium Detoxicant; Hyperammonemia Agent; Laxative, Miscellaneous
Generic Availability (U.S.) May be product dependent
Use Prevention and treatment of portal-systemic encephalopathy (PSE) (FDA approved in infants, children, adolescents, and adults); treatment of constipation (FDA approved in adults)
Pregnancy Risk Factor B
Pregnancy Considerations Adverse events have not been observed in animal reproduction studies. Lactulose is poorly absorbed following oral administration. Use of dietary fiber or bulk-forming laxatives along with increased fluid intake is generally considered first line therapy for treating constipation in pregnant women. Short-term use of lactulose is also considered to be safe/low risk when therapy is needed; however, side effects may limit its use (Cullen, 2007; Mahadevan, 2006; Prather, 2004; Wald, 2003).
Breast-Feeding Considerations It is not known if lactulose is excreted into breast milk; however, lactulose is poorly absorbed following oral administration. The manufacturer recommends that caution be used if administered to a nursing woman.
Contraindications Hypersensitivity to lactulose or any component; patients requiring low galactose diet
Warnings During proctoscopy or colonoscopy procedures involving electrocautery, a theoretical risk of reaction between hydrogen gas accumulation and electrical spark may exist; thorough bowel cleansing with a non-fermentable solution is recommended.
Precautions Use with caution in patients with diabetes mellitus (contains galactose and lactose); do not use with other laxatives especially when initiating PSE treatment as increased loose stools may falsely suggest adequate lactulose dosage. Electrolyte imbalance may occur when lactulose is used >6 months or in patients predisposed to electrolyte abnormalities; hepatic disease may predispose patients to electrolyte imbalance; infants receiving lactulose may develop hyponatremia and dehydration.
Adverse Reactions
Endocrine & metabolic: Dehydration, hypernatremia, hypokalemia
Gastrointestinal: Abdominal discomfort, abdominal distention, belching, cramping, diarrhea (excessive dose), flatulence, nausea, vomiting
Drug Interactions
Metabolism/Transport Effects None known.
Avoid Concomitant Use There are no known interactions where it is recommended to avoid concomitant use.
Increased Effect/Toxicity There are no known significant interactions involving an increase in effect.
Decreased Effect There are no known significant interactions involving a decrease in effect.
Stability Store at room temperature. Solution: Do not freeze. Protect from light. Discard solution if cloudy or very dark. Prolonged exposure to cold temperatures will cause thickening which will return to normal upon warming to room temperature.

Mechanism of Action The bacterial degradation of lactulose resulting in an acidic pH inhibits the diffusion of NH_3 into the blood by causing the conversion of NH_3 to NH_4+; also enhances the diffusion of NH_3 from the blood into the gut where conversion to NH_4+ occurs; produces an osmotic effect in the colon with resultant distention promoting peristalsis; reduces blood ammonia concentration to reduce the degree of portal systemic encephalopathy
Pharmacodynamics Onset of action:
Constipation: Up to 24-48 hours to produce a normal bowel movement
Encephalopathy: At least 24-48 hours
Pharmacokinetics (Adult data unless noted)
Absorption: Oral: Not absorbed appreciably
Metabolism: By colonic flora to lactic acid and acetic acid
Elimination: Primarily in feces; urine (≤3%)
Dosing: Usual
Constipation: Oral:
Children: 0.7-2 g/kg/**day** (1-3 mL/kg/**day**) in divided doses, maximum daily dose: 40 g/**day** (60 mL/**day**) (NASPGHAN, 2006)
Adults: 10-20 g (15-30 mL) daily; may increase to 40 g (60 mL) daily if necessary
Portal systemic encephalopathy, acute treatment: Adults:
Oral: 20-30 g (30-45 mL) every 1 hour to induce rapid laxation; reduce to 20-30 g (30-45 mL) 3-4 times daily after laxation is achieved titrate to produce 2-3 soft stools/day
Rectal administration (retention enema): 200 g (300 mL) diluted with 700 mL of water or NS via rectal balloon catheter; retain for 30-60 minutes may be repeated every 4-6 hours; transition to oral treatment prior to discontinuing rectal administration
Portal systemic encephalopathy, prevention: Oral:
Infants: 1.7-6.7 g/**day** (2.5-10 mL/**day**) in divided doses; adjust dosage to produce 2-3 stools/day
Children: 26.7-60 g/**day** (40-90 mL/**day**) in divided doses; adjust dosage to produce 2-3 stools/day
Adults: 20-30 g (30-45 mL) 3-4 times daily; adjust dose every 1-2 days to produce 2-3 soft stools/day
Administration
Oral: Administer with juice, milk, or water; dissolve crystals in 4 ounces of water or juice
Rectal: Mix with water or normal saline; administer as retention enema using a rectal balloon catheter; retain for 30-60 minutes
Monitoring Parameters Serum ammonia, serum electrolytes, fluid status, stool output
Additional Information Upon discontinuation of therapy, allow 24-48 hours for resumption of normal bowel movements
Dosage Forms Excipient information presented when available (limited, particularly for generics); consult specific product labeling.
Packet, Oral:
Kristalose: 10 g (30 ea); 20 g (30 ea)
Solution, Oral:
Constulose: 10 g/15 mL (237 mL, 946 mL) [unflavored flavor]
Enulose: 10 g/15 mL (473 mL) [unflavored flavor]
Generlac: 10 g/15 mL (473 mL, 1892 mL) [unflavored flavor]
Generic: 10 g/15 mL (15 mL, 30 mL, 236 mL, 237 mL, 473 mL, 500 mL, 946 mL, 1892 mL); 20 g/30 mL (30 mL)
References
Constipation Guideline Committee of the North American Society for Pediatric Gastroenterology, Hepatology and Nutrition, "Evaluation and Treatment of Constipation in Infants and Children: Recommendations of the North American Society for Pediatric Gastroenterology, Hepatology and Nutrition," *J Pediatr Gastroenterol Nutr*, 2006, 43(3): e1-13.

Cullen G, O'Donoghue D. Constipation and pregnancy. *Best Pract Res Clin Gastroenterol*. 2007;21(5):807-818.

Mahadevan U, Kane S. American gastroenterological association institute technical review on the use of gastrointestinal medications in pregnancy. *Gastroenterology*. 2006;131(1):283-311.

Pijpers MA, Tabbers MM, Benninga MA, et al, "Currently Recommended Treatments of Childhood Constipation Are Not Evidence Based: A Systematic Literature Review on the Effect of Laxative Treatment and Dietary Measures," *Arch Dis Child*, 2009, 94 (2):117-31.

Prather CM. Pregnancy-related constipation. *Curr Gastroenterol Rep*. 2004;6(5):402-404.

Wald A. Constipation, diarrhea, and symptomatic hemorrhoids during pregnancy. *Gastroenterol Clin North Am*. 2003;32(1):309-322.

◆ **LAIV** *see* Influenza Virus Vaccine (Live/Attenuated) *on page 1109*

◆ **LAIV₄** *see* Influenza Virus Vaccine (Live/Attenuated) *on page 1109*

◆ **L-AmB** *see* Amphotericin B (Liposomal) *on page 155*

◆ **LaMICtal** *see* LamoTRIgine *on page 1199*

◆ **Lamictal® (Can)** *see* LamoTRIgine *on page 1199*

◆ **LaMICtal ODT** *see* LamoTRIgine *on page 1199*

◆ **LaMICtal Starter** *see* LamoTRIgine *on page 1199*

◆ **LaMICtal XR** *see* LamoTRIgine *on page 1199*

◆ **LamISIL** *see* Terbinafine (Systemic) *on page 1982*

◆ **Lamisil (Can)** *see* Terbinafine (Systemic) *on page 1982*

◆ **Lamisil (Can)** *see* Terbinafine (Topical) *on page 1984*

◆ **LamISIL Advanced [OTC]** *see* Terbinafine (Topical) *on page 1984*

◆ **LamISIL AF Defense [OTC]** *see* Tolnaftate *on page 2044*

◆ **LamISIL AT [OTC]** *see* Terbinafine (Topical) *on page 1984*

◆ **LamISIL AT Jock Itch [OTC]** *see* Terbinafine (Topical) *on page 1984*

◆ **LamISIL AT Spray [OTC]** *see* Terbinafine (Topical) *on page 1984*

◆ **LamISIL Spray** *see* Terbinafine (Topical) *on page 1984*

LamiVUDine (la MI vyoo deen)

Medication Safety Issues
Sound-alike/look-alike issues:
LamiVUDine may be confused with lamoTRIgine
Epivir may be confused with Combivir

Related Information
Adult and Adolescent HIV *on page 2348*
Pediatric HIV *on page 2338*
Perinatal HIV *on page 2356*

Brand Names: U.S. Epivir; Epivir HBV

Brand Names: Canada 3TC; Apo-Lamivudine; Apo-Lamivudine HBV; Heptovir

Therapeutic Category Antiretroviral Agent; HIV Agents (Anti-HIV Agents); Nucleoside Reverse Transcriptase Inhibitor (NRTI)

Generic Availability (U.S.) May be product dependent

Use
Epivir: Treatment of HIV-1 infection in combination with other antiretroviral agents (FDA approved in ages ≥3 months and adults); **Note:** HIV regimens consisting of three antiretroviral agents are strongly recommended; has also been used for chemoprophylaxis after occupational exposure to HIV and prevention of maternal-fetal transmission of HIV infection.

Epivir-HBV: Management of chronic hepatitis B infection associated with evidence of hepatitis B viral replication and active liver inflammation (FDA approved in ages ≥2 years and adults)

Pregnancy Risk Factor C

Pregnancy Considerations Adverse events were observed in some animal reproduction studies. Lamivudine has a high level of transfer acrosses the human placenta. No increased risk of overall birth defects has been observed following first trimester exposure according to data collected by the antiretroviral pregnancy registry. The pharmacokinetics of lamivudine during pregnancy are not significantly altered and dosage adjustment is not required. Cases of lactic acidosis/hepatic steatosis syndrome related to mitochondrial toxicity have been reported in pregnant women with prolonged use of nucleoside analogues. It is not known if pregnancy itself potentiates this known side effect; however, women may be at increased risk of lactic acidosis and liver damage. In addition, these adverse events are similar to other rare but life-threatening syndromes which occur during pregnancy (eg, HELLP syndrome). Hepatic enzymes and electrolytes should be monitored in women receiving nucleoside analogues and clinicians should watch for early signs of the syndrome. In addition, mitochondrial dysfunction may develop in infants following in utero exposure. The DHHS Perinatal HIV Guidelines consider lamivudine in combination with either abacavir, tenofovir, or zidovudine to be a preferred NRTI backbone for antiretroviral-naïve pregnant women. The DHHS Perinatal HIV Guidelines also consider lamivudine plus tenofovir a recommended dual NRTI/NtRTI backbone for HIV/HBV coinfected pregnant women. Use caution with hepatitis B coinfection; hepatitis B flare may occur if lamivudine is discontinued postpartum.

Regardless of CD4 count or HIV RNA copy number, all HIV-infected pregnant women should receive a combination antiretroviral (ARV) drug regimen. A combination of antepartum, intrapartum, and infant ARV prophylaxis is recommended. ARV therapy should be started as soon as possible in women with symptomatic infection. Although earlier initiation may be more effective in reducing the perinatal transmission of HIV, initiation may be delayed until after 12 weeks gestation in women who do not require immediate treatment after careful consideration of maternal conditions (eg, nausea and vomiting) and the potential risks of first trimester fetal exposure for specific agents. A scheduled cesarean delivery at 38 weeks gestation is recommended for all women with HIV RNA >1000 copies/mL or unknown concentrations near delivery in order to decrease transmission. If ARV therapy must be interrupted for <24 hours during the peripartum period, stop then restart all medications simultaneously in order to decrease the chance of developing resistance. Long-term follow-up is recommended for all infants exposed to ARV medications. In couples who want to conceive, the HIV-infected partner should attain maximum viral suppression prior to conception.

Health care providers are encouraged to enroll pregnant women exposed to antiretroviral medications in the Antiretroviral Pregnancy Registry (1-800-258-4263 or www.APRegistry.com). Health care providers caring for HIV-infected women and their infants may contact the National Perinatal HIV Hotline (888-448-8765) for clinical consultation (DHHS [perinatal], 2014).

Breast-Feeding Considerations Lamivudine is excreted into breast milk and can be detected in the serum of nursing infants.

Maternal or infant antiretroviral therapy does not completely eliminate the risk of postnatal HIV transmission. In addition, multiclass-resistant virus has been detected in breast-feeding infants despite maternal therapy. Therefore, in the United States, where formula is accessible, affordable, safe, and sustainable, and the risk of infant mortality due to diarrhea and respiratory infections is low, complete avoidance of breast-feeding by HIV-infected women is recommended to decrease potential transmission of HIV (DHHS [perinatal], 2014).

Contraindications Hypersensitivity to lamivudine or any component

Warnings The major clinical toxicity of lamivudine in pediatric patients is pancreatitis which has occurred in 14% of patients in one open-label, uncontrolled study; discontinue lamivudine therapy if clinical signs, symptoms, or laboratory abnormalities suggestive of pancreatitis occur. Cases of lactic acidosis, severe hepatomegaly with steatosis, and death have been reported in patients receiving nucleoside analogues **[U.S. Boxed Warning]**; most of these cases have been in women; prolonged nucleoside use, obesity, and prior liver disease may be risk factors; use with extreme caution in patients with other risk factors for liver disease; discontinue therapy in patients who develop laboratory or clinical evidence of lactic acidosis or pronounced hepatotoxicity.

Infants receiving lamivudine in combination with nelfinavir (powder no longer available in the U.S.) and zidovudine for prevention of maternal-fetal transmission experienced a higher rate of neutropenia compared to zidovudine/nevirapine combination or zidovudine alone (27.5% vs 15%). Other studies in infants reported significantly higher rates of anemia and neutropenia when lamivudine was administered in combination with zidovudine (DHHS [perinatal], 2014).

HIV-infected patients should **not** receive lamivudine products intended for the treatment of hepatitis B (Epivir-HBV tablets or oral solution); these products contain lower amounts of lamivudine compared to products intended to treat HIV (Epivir tablets and oral solution) **[U.S. Boxed Warning]**. If treatment doses used for chronic hepatitis B are administered as monotherapy to a patient with unrecognized or untreated HIV infection, rapid emergence of HIV resistance will occur; this is due to the lower lamivudine doses used to treat hepatitis B compared to HIV; thus, all patients infected with hepatitis B should receive HIV counseling and testing prior to starting lamivudine for treatment of hepatitis B and periodically during treatment **[U.S. Boxed Warning]**.

HIV-infected patients who are coinfected with hepatitis B and patients infected only with hepatitis B may experience severe acute exacerbations and clinical symptoms or laboratory evidence of hepatitis when lamivudine is discontinued **[U.S. Boxed Warning]**; most cases are self-limited, but fatalities have been reported; monitor patients closely for at least several months after discontinuation of lamivudine; initiation of antihepatitis B therapy may be required. **Note:** HIV-infected patients should be screened for hepatitis B infection prior to starting lamivudine therapy. Concomitant use of combination antiretroviral therapy with interferon alfa (with or without ribavirin) has resulted in hepatic decompensation (with some fatalities) in patients coinfected with HIV and HCV; monitor patients closely, especially for hepatic decompensation; consider discontinuation of lamivudine if needed; consider dose reduction or discontinuation of interferon alfa, ribavirin, or both if clinical toxicities, including hepatic decompensation, worsen.

Oral solutions contains propylene glycol; toxicities have been reported with use of products containing propylene glycol, including hyperosmolality, lactic acidosis, seizures, and respiratory depression; in neonates large amounts of propylene glycol delivered orally, intravenously (eg, >3000 mg/day), or topically have been associated with potentially fatal toxicities which can include metabolic acidosis, seizures, renal failure, and CNS depression; use oral solutions containing propylene glycol with caution (AAP, 1997; Shehab, 2009).

Precautions Use with extreme caution and only if there is no satisfactory alternative therapy in pediatric patients with a history of pancreatitis or other significant risk factors for the development of pancreatitis. Use with caution in patients with impaired renal function; dosage adjustment required. Fat redistribution and accumulation (ie, central obesity, peripheral wasting, facial wasting, breast enlargement, dorsocervical fat enlargement [buffalo hump], and cushingoid appearance) have been observed in patients receiving antiretroviral agents (causal relationship not established).

Immune reconstitution syndrome (an acute inflammatory response to residual or indolent opportunistic infections) may occur in HIV patients during initial treatment with combination antiretroviral agents; this syndrome may require further patient assessment and therapy. Autoimmune disorders (eg, Grave's disease, Guillain-Barré syndrome, and polymyositis) have been reported in patients experiencing immune reconstitution; time to onset is variable and may occur many months after antiretroviral treatment is initiated.

Oral solutions contain sucrose (200 mg/mL); diabetic patients should be counseled. Do not administer Epivir or Epivir-HBV with other lamivudine-containing medications (eg, Combivir, Epzicom, or Trizivir) or with medications that contain emtricitabine (eg, Atripla, Complera, Emtriva, Stribild, or Truvada).

Adverse Reactions

Central nervous system: Chills, depression, dizziness, fatigue, fever, headache, insomnia

Dermatologic: Rash

Gastrointestinal: Abdominal pain, amylase increased, anorexia, diarrhea, dyspepsia, heartburn, lipase increased, nausea, pancreatitis, vomiting

Hematologic: Hemoglobinemia, neutropenia, thrombocytopenia

Hepatic: Transaminases increased

Neuromuscular & skeletal: Arthralgia, creatine phosphokinase increased, musculoskeletal pain, myalgia, neuropathy

Miscellaneous: Infections (includes ear, nose, and throat)

Rare but important or life-threatening: Alopecia, anaphylaxis, anemia, body fat redistribution, hepatitis B exacerbation, hepatomegaly, hyperbilirubinemia, hyperglycemia, immune reconstitution syndrome, lactic acidosis, lymphadenopathy, muscle weakness, paresthesia, peripheral neuropathy, pruritus, red cell aplasia, rhabdomyolysis, splenomegaly, steatosis, stomatitis, urticaria, weakness, wheezing

Drug Interactions

Metabolism/Transport Effects None known.

Avoid Concomitant Use

Avoid concomitant use of LamiVUDine with any of the following: Emtricitabine

Increased Effect/Toxicity

LamiVUDine may increase the levels/effects of: Emtricitabine

The levels/effects of LamiVUDine may be increased by: Ganciclovir-Valganciclovir; Ribavirin; Trimethoprim

Decreased Effect There are no known significant interactions involving a decrease in effect.

Food Interactions Food decreases the rate of absorption and C_{max}; however, there is no change in the systemic AUC. Management: Administer with or without food.

Stability

Oral solution:

Epivir: Store at 25°C (77°F) in a tightly closed bottle

Epivir-HBV: Store at 20°C to 25°C (68°F to 77°F) in a tightly closed bottle

Tablets: Store at 25°C (77°F); excursions permitted to 15°C to 30°C (59°F to 86°F).

Mechanism of Action Lamivudine is a cytosine analog. *In vitro*, lamivudine is triphosphorylated, the principle mode of action is inhibition of HIV reverse transcription via viral DNA chain termination; inhibits RNA- and DNA-dependent DNA polymerase activities of reverse transcriptase. In hepatitis B, the monophosphate form of lamivudine is incorporated into the viral DNA by hepatitis B virus polymerase, resulting in DNA chain termination.

Pharmacokinetics (Adult data unless noted)

Absorption: Oral: Rapid

Distribution: Into extravascular spaces

Children (n=38): CSF concentrations were 14.2 ± 7.9% of the serum concentration

V_d: 1.3 ± 0.4 L/kg

Protein binding: <36%

Metabolism: Converted intracellularly to the active triphosphate form

Bioavailability:

Children: Oral solution: 66% ± 26%

Adolescents and Adults:

150 mg tablet: 86% ± 16%

Oral solution: 87% ± 13%

Half-life:

Intracellular: 10 to 15 hours

Elimination:

Children 4 months to 14 years: 2 ± 0.6 hours

Adults with normal renal function: 5 to 7 hours

Time to peak serum concentration:

Pediatric patients 0.5 to 17 years: Median: 1.5 hours (range: 0.5 to 4 hours) (Lewis, 1996)

Adolescents 13 to 17 years: 0.5 to 1 hour

Adults: Fasting state: 0.9 hours; Fed state: 3.2 hours

Elimination: Urine (70%, unchanged); weight-corrected oral clearance is highest at age 2 years, then declines from age 2 to 12 years, where values then remain comparable to adult values

Dosing: Neonatal

HIV infection, treatment: Use in combination with other antiretroviral agents: Oral: 2 mg/kg/dose twice daily (DHHS [pediatric], 2014)

Perinatal transmission, prevention: Note: Consider for infants of mothers who received no antiretroviral therapy prior to or during labor, infants born to mothers with only intrapartum antiretroviral therapy, infants born to mothers with suboptimal viral suppression at delivery, or infants born to mothers with known antiretroviral drug-resistant virus. However, the recommended regimen for prophylaxis in these patients is zidovudine plus nevirapine (DHHS [perinatal, pediatric], 2014).

AIDS*info* recommendation: 2 mg/kg/dose twice daily; duration typically ranges from 1 to 2 weeks and is used in combinations with a 6-week-course of zidovudine, usually in combination with a 3-dose-course of nevirapine (DHHS [perinatal, pediatric], 2014)

Dosing adjustment in renal impairment for HIV: Insufficient data exist to recommend specific dosing adjustments for renal impairment; consider reducing the dose or increasing the dosing interval; use with caution; monitor closely; drug is renally eliminated

Dosing: Usual

Pediatric:

HIV infection, treatment: Use in combination with other antiretroviral agents:

Infants 1 month to <3 months: Oral: 4 mg/kg/dose twice daily (DHHS [pediatric], 2014; Tremoulet, 2007)

Infants ≥3 months, Children, and Adolescents ≤16 years: Oral: 4 mg/kg/dose twice daily; maximum dose: 150 mg/dose

Alternate dosing for patients ≥14 kg who are able to swallow tablets (using scored 150 mg tablets):

14 to 21 kg: 75 mg (½ tablet) twice daily

>21 kg to <30 kg: 75 mg (½ tablet) in the morning and 150 mg (1 tablet) in the evening

≥30 kg: 150 mg (1 tablet) twice daily

Adolescents ≥16 years (DHHS [pediatric], 2014): Oral:

Body weight <50 kg: 4 mg/kg/dose twice daily; maximum dose: 150 mg/dose

Body weight ≥50 kg: 150 mg twice daily **or** 300 mg once daily

HIV postexposure, prophylaxis: Adolescents ≥16 years: Oral: 150 mg twice daily or 300 mg once daily in combination with zidovudine, tenofovir, stavudine, or didanosine, with or without a protease inhibitor depending on risk (CDC, 2005)

Hepatitis B, treatment (Epivir-HBV) (non-HIV-exposed/-positive): Note: Use in HBV treatment is discouraged due to rapid resistance development; consider use only if other anti-HBV antiviral regimens with more favorable resistance patterns cannot be used.

Children ≥2 years and Adolescents: Oral: 3 mg/kg/dose once daily; maximum daily dose: 100 mg/**day**

AASLD practice guidelines (Lok, 2009): Treatment duration:

Hepatitis Be antigen (HBeAg) positive chronic hepatitis: Treat ≥1 year until HBeAg confirmed seroconversion and undetectable serum HBV DNA; continue therapy for ≥6 months after HBeAg seroconversion

HBeAg negative chronic hepatitis: Treat >1 year until hepatitis B surface antigen (HBsAg) clearance

Note: Patients not achieving <2 log decrease in serum HBV DNA after at least 6 months of therapy should either receive additional treatment or be switched to an alternative therapy (Lok, 2009)

Hepatitis B/HIV coinfection, treatment of both infections: Epivir: Infants, Children, and Adolescents: Oral: 4 mg/kg/dose twice daily; maximum dose: 150 mg/dose; in combination with other antiretrovirals in a HAART regimen; **Note:** The formulation and dosage of Epivir-HBV are not appropriate to treat patients infected with both HBV and HIV (DHHS [pediatric], 2013).

Adult:

HIV infection, treatment: Use with at least two other antiretroviral agents:

Weight <50 kg: Oral: 4 mg/kg twice daily; maximum dose: 150 mg/dose (DHHS [pediatric], 2014)

Weight ≥50 kg: Oral: 150 mg twice daily **or** 300 mg once daily

HIV postexposure, prophylaxis: Oral: 150 mg twice daily or 300 mg once daily in combination with zidovudine, tenofovir, stavudine, or didanosine, with or without a protease inhibitor depending on risk (CDC, 2005).

Hepatitis B, treatment (Epivir-HBV) (non-HIV-exposed/-positive): Note: Use in HBV treatment is discouraged due to rapid resistance development; consider use only if other anti-HBV antiviral regimens with more favorable resistance patterns cannot be used. Oral: 100 mg once daily

Hepatitis B/HIV coinfection, treatment of both infections: Epivir: Oral: 150 mg twice daily or 300 mg once daily, in combination with other antiretrovirals in a HAART regimen. **Note:** The formulation and dosage of Epivir-HBV are not appropriate for patients infected with both HBV and HIV. Tenofovir and lamivudine are a preferred NRTI backbone in a fully suppressive antiretroviral regimen for the treatment of HIV/HBV coinfection (DHHS [adult], 2014).

Dosing adjustment in renal impairment for HIV:

Manufacturer labeling:

Infants, Children, and Adolescents <30 kg: There are no dosage adjustments provided in the manufacturer's labeling; consider reducing the dose or increasing the dosing interval; use with caution; monitor closely

Children and Adolescents ≥30 kg and Adults:
CrCl ≥50 mL/minute: No adjustment necessary
CrCl 30 to 49 mL/minute: 150 mg once daily
CrCl 15 to 29 mL/minute: 150 mg first dose, then 100 mg once daily
CrCl 5 to 14 mL/minute: 150 mg first dose, then 50 mg once daily
CrCl <5 mL/minute: 50 mg first dose, then 25 mg once daily
Note: On dialysis days, take dose after dialysis; additional dose of lamivudine after routine (4 hour) peritoneal or hemodialysis is not required (DHHS [adult], 2014).
Alternate dosing: The following dosage adjustments have been recommended (Aronoff, 2007):
Infants, Children, and Adolescents:
GFR 30 to 50 mL/minute/1.73 m^2: 4 mg/kg/dose once daily
GFR 10 to 29 mL/minute/1.73 m^2: 2 mg/kg/dose once daily
GFR <10 mL/minute/1.73 m^2: 1 mg/kg/dose once daily
Intermittent hemodialysis (IHD): 1 mg/kg/dose once daily
Peritoneal dialysis (PD): 1 mg/kg/dose once daily
Continuous renal replacement therapy (CRRT): 4 mg/kg/dose once daily

Dosing adjustment in renal impairment for chronic hepatitis B (Epivir-HBV):
Children ≥2 years and Adolescents: There are no dosage adjustments provided in the manufacturer's labeling; reduction in the dose should be considered; use with caution; monitor closely
Adults:
CrCl ≥50 mL/minute: No adjustment necessary
CrCl 30 to 49 mL/minute: 100 mg first dose, then 50 mg once daily
CrCl 15 to 29 mL/minute: 100 mg first dose, then 25 mg once daily
CrCl 5 to 14 mL/minute: 35 mg first dose, then 15 mg once daily
CrCl <5 mL/minute: 35 mg first dose, then 10 mg once daily
Note: Additional dose of lamivudine after routine (4 hour) peritoneal or hemodialysis is not required

Dosing adjustment in hepatic impairment: No dosage adjustments required; use with caution in patients with decompensated liver disease; safety and efficacy not established with these patients.

Administration Oral: May be administered without regard to meals

Monitoring Parameters
Hepatitis B: Screen for HIV before starting lamivudine; monitor LFTs prior to, periodically during, and for at least several months after discontinuation; monitor HBV DNA levels periodically during treatment
HIV: **Note:** Monitor CD4 percentage (if <5 years of age) or CD4 count (if ≥5 years of age) at least every 3 to 4 months (DHHS [pediatric], 2014). Screen for hepatitis B before starting lamivudine. Also prior to initiation of therapy: Genotypic resistance testing, CD4 and viral load (every 3 to 4 months), CBC with differential, LFTs, BUN, creatinine, electrolytes, glucose, urinalysis (every 6 to 12 months), and assessment of readiness for adherence with medication regimen. At initiation and with any change in treatment regimen: CBC with differential, electrolytes, calcium, phosphate, glucose, LFTs, bilirubin, urinalysis (at initiation), BUN, creatinine, albumin, total protein, lipid panel (at initiation), CD4, and viral load. After 1 to 2 weeks of therapy: Signs of medication toxicity and adherence. After 2 to 4 weeks of therapy: CBC with differential, viral load, signs of medication toxicity, and adherence; then every 3 to 4 months: CBC with differential, electrolytes, glucose, LFTs, bilirubin, BUN, creatinine, CD4, viral load, signs of medication toxicity, and adherence. Lipid panel and urinalysis every 6 to 12 months. CD4 monitoring frequency may be decreased to every 6 to 12 months in children who are adherent to therapy if the value is well above the threshold for opportunistic infections, viral suppression is sustained, and the clinical status is stable for more than 2 to 3 years (DHHS [pediatric], 2014). Monitor for growth and development, signs of HIV-specific physical conditions, HIV disease progression opportunistic infections, pancreatitis, or lactic acidosis. Infants receiving lamivudine for prevention of maternal-fetal HIV transmission: Hemoglobin and neutrophil counts at 4 weeks after initiation of prophylaxis.

Dosage Forms Excipient information presented when available (limited, particularly for generics); consult specific product labeling.
Solution, Oral:
Epivir: 10 mg/mL (240 mL) [contains methylparaben, propylene glycol, propylparaben; strawberry-banana flavor]
Epivir HBV: 5 mg/mL (240 mL) [contains methylparaben, propylene glycol, propylparaben; strawberry-banana flavor]
Tablet, Oral:
Epivir: 150 mg, 300 mg
Epivir HBV: 100 mg
Generic: 100 mg, 150 mg, 300 mg

References
American Academy of Pediatrics Committee on Drugs. "Inactive" ingredients in pharmaceutical products: update (subject review). *Pediatrics.* 1997;99(2):268-278.
Aronoff GR, Bennett WM, Berns JS, et al, *Drug Prescribing in Renal Failure: Dosing Guidelines for Adults and Children*, 5th ed, Philadelphia, PA: American College of Physicians, 2007, 161.
Center for Disease Control and Prevention (CDC), "Updated U.S. Public Health Service Guidelines for the Management of Occupational Exposures to HIV and Recommendations for Postexposure Prophylaxis," *MMWR Recomm Rep,* 2005, 54(RR-9):1-17.
DHHS. Guidelines for the prevention and treatment of opportunistic infections among HIV-exposed and HIV-infected children: recommendations from the National Institutes of Health, Centers for Disease Control and Prevention, the HIV Medicine Association of the Infectious Diseases Society of America, the Pediatric Infectious Diseases Society, and the American Academy of Pediatrics. November 6, 2013. Available at http://aidsinfo.nih.gov
DHHS Panel on Antiretroviral Guidelines for Adults and Adolescents, "Guidelines for the Use of Antiretroviral Agents in HIV-Infected Adults and Adolescents," May 1, 2014. Available at http://www.aidsinfo.nih.gov
DHHS Panel on Antiretroviral Therapy and Medical Management of HIV-Infected Children, "Guidelines for the Use of Antiretroviral Agents in Pediatric HIV Infection," February 12, 2014. Available at http://aidsinfo.nih.gov
DHHS Panel on Treatment of HIV-Infected Pregnant Women and Prevention of Perinatal Transmission, "Recommendations for the Use of Antiretroviral Drugs in Pregnant HIV-1-Infected Women for Maternal Health and Interventions to Reduce Perinatal HIV-1 Transmission in the United States," March 28, 2014. Available at http://aidsinfo.nih.gov
Lewis LL, Venzon D, Church J, et al, "Lamivudine in Children With Human Immunodeficiency Virus Infection: A Phase I/II Study," *J Infect Dis,* 1996, 174(1):16-25.
Lok AS and McMahon BJ, "Chronic Hepatitis B: Update 2009," *Hepatology,* 2009, 50(3):661-2.
Nielsen-Saines K, Watts DH, Veloso VG, et al, "Three Postpartum Antiretroviral Regimens to Prevent Intrapartum HIV Infection," *N Engl J Med,* 2012, 366(25):2368-79.
Shehab N, Lewis CL, Streetman DD, Donn SM. Exposure to the pharmaceutical excipients benzyl alcohol and propylene glycol among critically ill neonates. *Pediatr Crit Care Med.* 2009;10 (2):256-259.
Tremoulet AH, Capparelli EV, Patel P, et al, "Population Pharmacokinetics of Lamivudine in Human Immunodeficiency Virus-Exposed and -Infected Infants," *Antimicrob Agents Chemother,* 2007, 51 (12):4297-302.

◆ **Lamivudine, Abacavir, and Zidovudine** see Abacavir, Lamivudine, and Zidovudine on page 41

◆ **Lamivudine and Abacavir** *see* Abacavir and Lamivudine *on page 39*

Lamivudine and Zidovudine
(la MI vyoo deen & zye DOE vyoo deen)

Medication Safety Issues
Sound-alike/look-alike issues:
Combivir® may be confused with Combivent®, Epivir®
Other safety concerns:
AZT is an error-prone abbreviation (mistaken as aza-THIOprine, aztreonam)

Related Information
Adult and Adolescent HIV *on page 2348*
Pediatric HIV *on page 2338*
Perinatal HIV *on page 2356*

Brand Names: U.S. Combivir®

Brand Names: Canada Combivir®; Teva-Lamivudine/Zidovudine

Therapeutic Category Antiretroviral Agent; HIV Agents (Anti-HIV Agents); Nucleoside Reverse Transcriptase Inhibitor (NRTI)

Generic Availability (U.S.) Yes

Use Treatment of HIV-1 infection in combination with at least one other antiretroviral agent (FDA approved in children ≥30 kg, adolescents ≥30 kg, and adults). **Note:** HIV regimens consisting of **three** antiretroviral agents are strongly recommended.

Pregnancy Risk Factor C

Pregnancy Considerations Adverse events were observed in animal reproduction studies. See individual agents. The DHHS Perinatal HIV Guidelines consider lamivudine in combination with zidovudine as one of the preferred NRTI backbones for antiretroviral-naïve pregnant women. Although use of this combination has the most experience for in pregnant women, it has an increased potential for hematologic toxicity (DHHS [perinatal], 2014).

Breast-Feeding Considerations Lamivudine and zidovudine are both excreted into breast milk. See individual agents.

Contraindications Hypersensitivity to lamivudine, zidovudine, or any component

Warnings Hazardous agent; use appropriate precautions for handling and disposal (NIOSH, 2012). Zidovudine is associated with hematologic toxicity including granulocytopenia and severe anemia requiring transfusions **[U.S. Boxed Warning]**; use with caution in patients with ANC <1000 cells/mm³ or hemoglobin <9.5 g/dL; consider interruption of therapy for significant anemia (Hgb <7.5 g/dL or reduction >25% of baseline) or neutropenia (ANC <750 cells/mm³ or reduction >50% from baseline); use of erythropoietin, filgrastim, or reduced zidovudine dosage may be necessary in some patients. Prolonged use of zidovudine may cause myositis and myopathy **[U.S. Boxed Warning]**. Cases of lactic acidosis, severe hepatomegaly with steatosis, and death have been reported with the use of lamivudine, zidovudine and other antiretroviral agents **[U.S. Boxed Warning]**; most of these cases have been in women; prolonged nucleoside use, obesity, and prior liver disease may be risk factors; use with extreme caution in patients with other risk factors for liver disease; discontinue therapy in patients who develop laboratory or clinical evidence of lactic acidosis or pronounced hepatotoxicity.

The major clinical toxicity of lamivudine in pediatric patients is pancreatitis; discontinue therapy if clinical signs, symptoms, or laboratory abnormalities suggestive of pancreatitis occur. In HIV-infected patients who are coinfected with hepatitis B, severe acute exacerbations of HBV have occurred after discontinuation of lamivudine containing medications **[U.S. Boxed Warning]**; most cases are self-limited, but fatalities have been reported; follow hepatic function of HBV-infected patients closely (clinically and with laboratory tests) for at least several months after discontinuing lamivudine therapy; initiate antihepatitis B therapy if needed. Testing for HBV is recommended prior to the initiation of lamivudine and zidovudine therapy; treatment of HIV in patients with unrecognized/untreated HBV may lead to rapid HBV resistance. Concomitant use of combination antiretroviral therapy with interferon alfa (with or without ribavirin) has resulted in hepatic decompensation (with some fatalities) in patients coinfected with HIV and HCV; monitor patients closely, especially for hepatic decompensation, neutropenia, and anemia; consider discontinuation of lamivudine and zidovudine if needed; consider dose reduction or discontinuation of interferon alfa, ribavirin, or both if clinical toxicities, including hepatic decompensation, worsen. Concomitant use of ribavirin and zidovudine may also result in exacerbation of anemia (concurrent use is **not** recommended).

Precautions Always use lamivudine and zidovudine in combination with another antiretroviral agent. Use with extreme caution and only if there is no satisfactory alternative therapy in pediatric patients with a history of pancreatitis or other significant risk factors for pancreatitis. Use with caution in patients with bone marrow compromise or in patients with impaired renal or hepatic function. The dose of lamivudine should be reduced in patients with renal dysfunction. Zidovudine therapy should be interrupted in patients with anemia, granulocytopenia, or myopathy; the dose of zidovudine should be reduced in patients with renal or hepatic impairment, or liver cirrhosis. Use of the fixed-dose combination product is **not** recommended for patients who need a dosage reduction, including children <30 kg, patients with renal or hepatic impairment, or those patients experiencing dose-limiting adverse effects (use individual antiretroviral agents to appropriately adjust dosages).

Fat redistribution and accumulation (ie, central obesity, peripheral wasting, facial wasting, breast enlargement, dorsocervical fat enlargement [buffalo hump], and cushingoid appearance) have been observed in patients receiving antiretroviral agents (causal relationship not established).

Immune reconstitution syndrome (an acute inflammatory response to residual or indolent opportunistic infections) may occur in HIV patients during initial treatment with combination antiretroviral agents; this syndrome may require further patient assessment and therapy. Autoimmune disorders (eg, Grave's disease, Guillain-Barré syndrome, and polymyositis) have been reported in patients experiencing immune reconstitution; time to onset is variable and may occur many months after antiretroviral treatment is initiated.

Combivir contains lamivudine and zidovudine as a fixed-dose combination. Do not administer Combivir with other lamivudine or zidovudine containing medications (eg, Epivir, Epzicom, Retrovir, Trizivir) or with medications that contain emtricitabine (eg, Atripla, Complera, Emtriva, Stribild, Truvada)

Adverse Reactions See individual agents.

Drug Interactions
Metabolism/Transport Effects Refer to individual components.

Avoid Concomitant Use
Avoid concomitant use of Lamivudine and Zidovudine with any of the following: CloZAPine; Dipyrone; Emtricitabine; Stavudine

Increased Effect/Toxicity
Lamivudine and Zidovudine may increase the levels/effects of: CloZAPine; Emtricitabine; Ribavirin

The levels/effects of Lamivudine and Zidovudine may be increased by: Acyclovir-Valacyclovir; Clarithromycin;

Dipyrone; DOXOrubicin (Conventional); DOXOrubicin (Liposomal); Fluconazole; Ganciclovir-Valganciclovir; Interferons; Methadone; Probenecid; Raltegravir; Trimethoprim; Valproic Acid and Derivatives

Decreased Effect
Lamivudine and Zidovudine may decrease the levels/ effects of: Stavudine

The levels/effects of Lamivudine and Zidovudine may be decreased by: Clarithromycin; DOXOrubicin (Conventional); DOXOrubicin (Liposomal); Protease Inhibitors; Rifamycin Derivatives

Stability Store at 2°C to 30°C (36°F to 86°F).

Mechanism of Action The combination of zidovudine and lamivudine is believed to act synergistically to inhibit reverse transcriptase via DNA chain termination after incorporation of the nucleoside analogue as well as to delay the emergence of mutations conferring resistance

Pharmacokinetics (Adult data unless noted) One Combivir tablet is bioequivalent to one lamivudine 150 mg tablet plus one zidovudine 300 mg tablet; see individual agents

Dosing: Usual Note: Use in combination with at least one other antiretroviral agent.

Pediatric: **HIV Treatment:**
Children and Adolescents weighing <30 kg: Not intended for use; product is a fixed-dose combination; safety and efficacy have not been established in these patients
Children and Adolescents weighing ≥30 kg: Oral: One tablet twice daily

Adult: **HIV Treatment:** Oral: One tablet twice daily

Dosing adjustment in renal impairment: All patients: CrCl <50 mL/minute: Use not recommended; use individual agents for reduction in lamivudine and zidovudine dosage.

Dosing adjustment in hepatic impairment: Use not recommended; use individual antiretroviral agents to reduce dosage.

Administration Oral: May be administered without regard to meals

Monitoring Parameters Note: Monitor CD4 percentage (if <5 years of age) or CD4 count (if ≥5 years of age) at least every 3-4 months (DHHS [pediatric], 2014).

Screen for hepatitis B before starting. Prior to initiation of therapy: Genotypic resistance testing, CD4 and viral load (every 3 to 4 months), CBC with differential, LFTs, BUN, creatinine, electrolytes, glucose, urinalysis (every 6 to 12 months), and assessment of readiness for adherence with medication regimen. At initiation and with any change in treatment regimen: CBC with differential, electrolytes, calcium, phosphate, glucose, LFTs, bilirubin, urinalysis (at initiation), BUN, creatinine, albumin, total protein, lipid panel (at initiation), CD4, and viral load. After 1 to 2 weeks of therapy: Signs of medication toxicity and adherence. After 2 to 4 weeks of therapy: CBC with differential, viral load, signs of medication toxicity, and adherence; then every 3 to 4 months: CBC with differential, electrolytes, glucose, LFTs, bilirubin, BUN, creatinine, CD4, viral load, signs of medication toxicity, and adherence. Lipid panel and urinalysis every 6 to 12 months. CD4 monitoring frequency may be decreased to every 6 to 12 months in children who are adherent to therapy if the value is well above the threshold for opportunistic infections, viral suppression is sustained, and the clinical status is stable for more than 2 to 3 years (DHHS [pediatric], 2014). Monitor for growth and development, signs of HIV-specific physical conditions, HIV disease progression, opportunistic infections, hepatotoxicity, pancreatitis, anemia, or lactic acidosis.

Dosage Forms Excipient information presented when available (limited, particularly for generics); consult specific product labeling.
Tablet, oral: Lamivudine 150 mg and zidovudine 300 mg

Combivir®: Lamivudine 150 mg and zidovudine 300 mg [scored]

References
DHHS Panel on Antiretroviral Guidelines for Adults and Adolescents, "Guidelines for the Use of Antiretroviral Agents in HIV-Infected Adults and Adolescents," May 1, 2014. Available at http://www.aidsinfo.nih.gov
DHHS Panel on Antiretroviral Therapy and Medical Management of HIV-Infected Children, "Guidelines for the Use of Antiretroviral Agents in Pediatric HIV Infection," February 12, 2014. Available at http://aidsinfo.nih.gov
National Institute for Occupational Safety and Health (NIOSH), "NIOSH List of Antineoplastic and Other Hazardous Drugs in Healthcare Settings 2012." Available at http://www.cdc.gov/niosh/docs/2012-150/pdfs/2012-150.pdf. Accessed January 21, 2013.

LamoTRIgine (la MOE tri jeen)

Medication Safety Issues
Sound-alike/look-alike issues:
LamoTRIgine may be confused with labetalol, LamISIL®, lamiVUDine, levothyroxine, Lomotil®
LaMICtal® may be confused with LamISIL®, Lomotil®

Administration issues:
Potential exists for medication errors to occur among different formulations of LaMICtal® (tablets, extended release tablets, orally disintegrating tablets, and chewable/dispersible tablets). Patients should be instructed to visually inspect tablets dispensed to verify receiving the correct medication and formulation. The medication guide includes illustrations to aid in tablet verification.

International issues:
Lamictal [U.S., Canada, and multiple international markets] may be confused with Ludiomil brand name for maprotiline [multiple international markets]
Lamotrigine [U.S., Canada, and multiple international markets] may be confused with Ludiomil brand name for maprotiline [multiple international markets]

Related Information
Oral Medications That Should Not Be Crushed or Altered *on page 2438*

Brand Names: U.S. LaMICtal; LaMICtal ODT; LaMICtal Starter; LaMICtal XR

Brand Names: Canada Apo-Lamotrigine®; Auro-Lamotrigine; Lamictal®; Mylan-Lamotrigine; PMS-Lamotrigine; ratio-Lamotrigine; Teva-Lamotrigine

Therapeutic Category Anticonvulsant, Miscellaneous

Generic Availability (U.S.) May be product dependent

Use
Tablets, chewable dispersible tablets, and orally disintegrating tablets: Adjunctive treatment of generalized seizures of Lennox-Gastaut syndrome, primary generalized tonic-clonic seizures, and partial seizures (FDA approved in ages ≥2 years and adults); monotherapy of partial seizures in patients who are converted from valproic acid or a single enzyme-inducing AED (specifically, carbamazepine, phenytoin, phenobarbital, or primidone) (FDA approved in ages ≥16 years and adults); maintenance treatment of bipolar disorder (FDA approved in ages ≥18 years and adults); has also been used as adjunctive treatment of partial seizures in ages <24 months
Extended-release tablets: Adjunctive treatment of primary generalized tonic-clonic seizures and partial onset seizures with or without secondary generalization (FDA approved in ages ≥13 years and adults); monotherapy of partial seizures in patients who are converted from a single AED (FDA approved in ages ≥13 years and adults)
Note: Preliminary investigations have shown potential efficacy as add-on therapy for absence, atypical absence, atonic, tonic, and myoclonic seizures; and as monotherapy in adults and adolescents for idiopathic generalized tonic-clonic seizures

Medication Guide Available Yes
Pregnancy Risk Factor C

Pregnancy Considerations Although teratogenic effects were not observed in animal reproduction studies, lamotrigine has been found to decrease folate concentrations in animals. Lamotrigine crosses the human placenta and can be measured in the plasma of exposed newborns (Harden and Pennell, 2009; Ohman, 2000). An overall increase in major congenital malformations has not been observed in available studies; however, an increased risk for cleft lip or cleft palate has not been ruled out (Cunnington, 2011; Hernández-Díaz, 2012; Holmes, 2012). An increased risk of malformations following maternal lamotrigine use may be associated with larger doses (Cunnington, 2007; Tomson, 2011). Polytherapy may increase the risk of congenital malformations; monotherapy with the lowest effective dose is recommended (Harden and Meader, 2009).

Due to pregnancy-induced physiologic changes, women who are pregnant may require dose adjustments of lamotrigine in order to maintain clinical response; monitoring during pregnancy should be considered (Harden and Pennell, 2009). For women with epilepsy who are planning a pregnancy in advance, baseline serum concentrations should be measured once or twice prior to pregnancy during a period when seizure control is optimal. Monitoring can then be continued up to once a month during pregnancy and every second day during the first week postpartum (Patsalos, 2008). In women taking lamotrigine who are trying to avoid pregnancy, potentially significant interactions may exist with hormone-containing contraceptives; consult drug interactions database for more detailed information.

Pregnancy registries are available for women who have been exposed to lamotrigine. Patients may enroll themselves in the North American Antiepileptic Drug (NAAED) Pregnancy Registry by calling (888) 233-2334. Additional information is available at www.aedpregnancyregistry.org.

Breast-Feeding Considerations Lamotrigine is found in breast milk and may be as high as 50% of the maternal serum concentration. Adverse events observed in breast-feeding infants include apnea, drowsiness, and poor sucking. The manufacturer recommends that caution be used if administered to a breast-feeding woman and to monitor the nursing infant.

Contraindications Hypersensitivity to lamotrigine or any component (eg, rash, angioedema, acute urticaria, extensive pruritus, mucosal ulceration)

Warnings Skin rash may occur (10% incidence in patients with epilepsy; 14% incidence in patients with bipolar disorder). Skin rash can be serious enough to require hospitalization or discontinuation of drug **[U.S. Boxed Warning]**; serious skin rashes (including Stevens-Johnson syndrome) occur in 0.8% of pediatric epilepsy patients (2-16 years of age) and 0.3% of adult epilepsy patients and in up to 0.13% of adult patients treated for bipolar and other mood disorders; rare cases of toxic epidermal necrolysis have been reported; rash-related deaths have occurred in pediatric and adult patients. In addition to pediatric age, the risk of rash may be increased in patients receiving valproic acid, high initial doses, or with rapid dosage increases; rash usually appears in the first 2-8 weeks of therapy, but may occur after prolonged treatment (eg, 6 months). Benign rashes may occur, but one cannot predict which rashes will become serious or life-threatening; the manufacturer recommends (ordinarily) discontinuation of lamotrigine at the first sign of rash (unless rash is clearly not drug related); discontinuation of lamotrigine may not prevent rash from becoming life-threatening or permanently disfiguring or disabling. Risk of nonserious rash may also be increased when the initial recommended dose or dose escalation rate is exceeded in patients with a history of rash or allergy to other AEDs.

Increased risk of developing aseptic meningitis has been reported with lamotrigine use; symptoms (eg, headache, nuchal rigidity, fever, nausea/vomiting, rash, photophobia) have generally occurred within 1-45 days following therapy initiation. In some cases, new onset hepatic, renal, and/or other organ involvement has also occurred with symptoms, possibly suggesting aseptic meningitis is associated with a hypersensitivity reaction.

Potentially fatal hypersensitivity reactions may occur; these may include multiorgan failure or dysfunction; early symptoms of hypersensitivity reaction (eg, lymphadenopathy, fever) may occur without rash; discontinue lamotrigine if another cause for symptoms cannot be established. Blood dyscrasias may occur.

Preliminary data from the North American Antiepileptic Drug Pregnancy Registry (NAAED) suggest a possible association of lamotrigine exposure in the first trimester of pregnancy with an increased chance of cleft lip and/or cleft palate. More research and data collection is needed to confirm this possible association. Pregnant women who are currently taking lamotrigine or who are thinking about taking lamotrigine should talk with their physician first, before stopping or starting this medication.

Antiepileptic drugs (AEDs) increase the risk of suicidal behavior and ideation in patients receiving these medications for any indication. Pooled analyses of placebo-controlled trials involving 11 different AEDs (regardless of indication) showed a twofold increased risk of suicidal thoughts or behavior (estimated incidence rate: 0.43% in AED treated patients compared to 0.24% of patients receiving placebo); increased risk was observed as early as 1 week after initiation of AED and continued through duration of trials (most trials ≤24 weeks); risk did not vary significantly by age (age range: 5-100 years). Consider risks and benefits of AEDs before prescribing. Monitor all patients receiving an AED for emergence of suicidal thoughts or behavior, thoughts of self-harm, any unusual changes in behavior or mood, or the emergence or worsening of depressive symptoms; notify healthcare provider immediately if symptoms or concerning behavior occur. **Note:** The FDA requires a Medication Guide for all antiepileptic drugs informing patients of this risk.

Precautions Use with caution and decrease the dose in patients with renal or moderate to severe hepatic dysfunction. Use with caution in patients with impaired cardiac function (clinical experience is limited). Use with caution and adjust the dose in patients receiving estrogen-containing oral contraceptives; estrogen-containing oral contraceptives may decrease the serum concentration of lamotrigine; dosage adjustment of lamotrigine will be necessary in most women when starting or stopping estrogen-containing oral contraceptives. Valproic acid may cause an increase in lamotrigine serum concentrations requiring dose adjustment. Patients treated for bipolar disorder should be monitored closely for clinical worsening of depressive symptoms or suicidality, especially with initiation of therapy or dosage changes; prescriptions should be written for the smallest quantity consistent with good patient care.

Do not abruptly discontinue; when discontinuing therapy, gradually reduce the dose by ~50% per week and taper over at least 2 weeks unless safety concerns require a more rapid withdrawal. Lamotrigine should **not** be restarted in patients who discontinued therapy due to lamotrigine-associated rash, unless benefits clearly outweigh risks; if restarting lamotrigine after withholding for >5 half-lives, use the initial dosing recommendations and titrate dosage accordingly (ie, do **not** restart at the previous maintenance dose). Lamotrigine binds to melanin and may possibly accumulate in the eye and other tissues rich in melanin; long-term ophthalmologic effects are unknown. A potential for the occurrence of medication errors exists with similar-sounding medications and among the different lamotrigine formulations.

Lamotrigine is **not** approved for acute treatment of mood episodes or for use in epilepsy as initial monotherapy, conversion to monotherapy from AEDs other than carbamazepine, phenytoin, phenobarbital, primidone, or valproic acid, or for conversion to monotherapy from 2 or more AEDs. A small randomized, double-blind, placebo-controlled study in pediatric patients 1-24 months of age did **not** demonstrate safety and efficacy of immediate-release lamotrigine when used as adjunctive treatment for partial seizures; lamotrigine was associated with an increased risk for infectious and respiratory adverse reactions.

Adverse Reactions

Cardiovascular: Chest pain, edema (including peripheral)

Central nervous system: Agitation, amnesia, anxiety, ataxia, confusion, depression, dizziness, dream abnormality, emotional lability, fatigue, fever, hypoesthesia, insomnia, irritability, migraine, pain, somnolence, suicidal ideation, thought abnormality

Dermatologic: Dermatitis, dry skin, rash (nonserious)
Also observed: Rash requiring hospitalization

Endocrine & metabolic: Dysmenorrhea, libido increased

Gastrointestinal: Abdominal pain, anorexia, constipation, dyspepsia, flatulence, nausea, peptic ulcer, rectal hemorrhage, vomiting, weight gain/loss, xerostomia

Genitourinary: Urinary frequency

Neuromuscular & skeletal: Arthralgia, back pain, myalgia, neck pain, paresthesia, weakness

Ocular: Amblyopia, nystagmus, vision abnormal

Respiratory: Bronchitis, cough, dyspnea, epistaxis, pharyngitis, rhinitis, sinusitis

Miscellaneous: Diaphoresis, dyspraxia, infection, reflexes increased/decreased

Rare but important or life-threatening: Accommodation abnormality, agranulocytosis, alcohol intolerance, allergic reaction, alopecia, anemia, angina, angioedema, aphasia, aplastic anemia, apnea, appetite increased, arthritis, aseptic meningitis, atrial fibrillation, bruising, cerebellar syndrome, cerebral sinus thrombosis, cerebrovascular accident, chills, choreoathetosis, CNS depression/stimulation, conjunctivitis, deafness, deep thrombophlebitis, delirium, delusions, dermatitis (exfoliative, fungal), disseminated intravascular coagulation, dysphagia, dysphoria, dystonia, ECG abnormality, ejaculation abnormal, eructation, erythema multiforme, esophagitis, euphoria, extrapyramidal syndrome, flushing, gastritis, gingivitis, goiter, hallucinations, hematuria, hemiplegia, hemolytic anemia, hemorrhage, hepatitis, hiccup, hirsutism, hot flashes, hyperalgesia, hyperglycemia, hypersensitivity reactions, hypertension, hyperventilation, hypokinesia, hypothyroidism, hypotonia, impotence, kidney failure (acute), leg cramps, leukopenia, liver function tests abnormal, lupus-like reaction, lymphadenopathy, maculopapular rash, menorrhagia, MI, mouth ulceration, movement disorder, multiorgan failure, muscle spasm, myasthenia, neuralgia, neurosis, neutropenia, orthostatic hypotension, palpitation, pancreatitis, pancytopenia, paralysis, parkinsonian exacerbation, peripheral neuritis, photophobia, polyuria, progressive immunosuppression, pruritus, pure red cell aplasia, rhabdomyolysis, salivation increased, skin discoloration, status epilepticus, Stevens-Johnson syndrome, sudden unexplained death in epilepsy (SUDEP), suicidal behavior, suicide, syncope, tachycardia, taste loss/perversion, thrombocytopenia, tic, tinnitus, tongue edema, toxic epidermal necrolysis, twitching, urinary incontinence, urticaria, vasculitis, vasodilation, withdrawal seizures

Drug Interactions

Metabolism/Transport Effects None known.

Avoid Concomitant Use

Avoid concomitant use of LamoTRIgine with any of the following: Azelastine (Nasal); Paraldehyde; Thalidomide

Increased Effect/Toxicity

LamoTRIgine may increase the levels/effects of: Alcohol (Ethyl); Azelastine (Nasal); Buprenorphine; CarBAMazepine; CNS Depressants; Desmopressin; Hydrocodone; MetFORMIN; Methotrimeprazine; Metyrosine; Mirtazapine; OLANZapine; Paraldehyde; Pramipexole; Procainamide; ROPINIRole; Rotigotine; Selective Serotonin Reuptake Inhibitors; Thalidomide; Zolpidem

The levels/effects of LamoTRIgine may be increased by: Brimonidine (Topical); Cannabis; Doxylamine; Dronabinol; Droperidol; HydrOXYzine; Kava Kava; Magnesium Sulfate; Methotrimeprazine; Nabilone; Perampanel; Rufinamide; Sodium Oxybate; Tapentadol; Tetrahydrocannabinol; Valproic Acid and Derivatives

Decreased Effect

LamoTRIgine may decrease the levels/effects of: Contraceptives (Progestins)

The levels/effects of LamoTRIgine may be decreased by: Barbiturates; CarBAMazepine; Contraceptives (Estrogens); Ezogabine; Fosphenytoin; Ketorolac (Nasal); Ketorolac (Systemic); Mefloquine; Orlistat; Phenytoin; Primidone; Rifampin; Ritonavir

Food Interactions Food has no effect on absorption.

Stability

Lamictal® tablets and chewable dispersible tablets: Store at controlled room temperature at 25°C (77°F); excursions permitted to 15°C to 30°C (59°F to 86°F); store in a dry place; protect 100 mg, 150 mg, and 200 mg tablets from light

Lamictal® orally disintegrating tablets: Store between 20°C to 25°C (68°F to 77°F); excursions permitted to 15°C to 30°C (59°F to 86°F)

Lamictal® XR™ tablets: Store at controlled room temperature at 25°C (77°F); excursions permitted to 15°C to 30°C (59°F to 86°F)

Mechanism of Action A triazine derivative which inhibits release of glutamate (an excitatory amino acid) and inhibits voltage-sensitive sodium channels, which stabilizes neuronal membranes. Lamotrigine has weak inhibitory effect on the $5-HT_3$ receptor; *in vitro* inhibits dihydrofolate reductase.

Pharmacokinetics (Adult data unless noted)

Absorption: Oral: Immediate release: Rapid, 97.6% absorbed; **Note:** Orally disintegrating tablets (either swallowed whole with water or disintegrated in the mouth) are equivalent to regular tablets (swallowed whole with water) in terms of rate and extent of absorption.

Distribution: V_d: Adults: 1.1 L/kg; range: 0.9-1.3 L/kg; crosses into breast milk

Protein binding: 55% (primarily albumin)

Metabolism: >75% metabolized in the liver via glucuronidation; autoinduction may occur

Bioavailability: Immediate release: 98%; **Note:** AUCs were similar for immediate release and extended release preparations in patients receiving nonenzyme-inducing AEDs. In subjects receiving concomitant enzyme-inducing AEDs, bioavailability of extended release product was ~21% lower than immediate-release product; in some of these subjects, a decrease in AUC of up to 70% was observed when switching from immediate-release to extended-release tablets.

Half-life:

Infants and children:

With enzyme-inducing AEDs (ie, phenytoin, phenobarbital, carbamazepine, primidone):

Infants 10 months of age to children 5.3 years: 7.7 hours (range: 6-11 hours)

Children 5-11 years: 7 hours (range: 4-10 hours)

With enzyme-inducing AED and valproic acid (VPA): Children 5-11 years: 19 hours (range: 7-31 hours)
With VPA:
Infants 10 months of age to children 5.3 years: 45 hours (range: 30-52 hours)
Children 5-11 years: 66 hours (range: 50-74 hours)
Adults:
Normal: Single dose: 33 hours; multiple dose: ~25 hours (range: 12-62 hours)
With enzyme-inducing AEDs: 13 hours (range: 8-23 hours)
With enzyme-inducing AED and VPA: ~27 hours (range: 11-52 hours)
With VPA: 59 hours (range: 30-89 hours)
Hepatic dysfunction: Child-Pugh classification:
Mild liver impairment: 46 ± 20 hours
Moderate liver impairment: 72 ± 44 hours
Severe liver impairment without ascites: 67± 11 hours
Severe liver impairment with ascites: 100 ± 48 hours
Renal dysfunction (CrCl 13 mL/minute): ~43 hours
Severe renal dysfunction (CrCl <10 mL/minute): 57.4 hours
During dialysis: 13 hours
Time to peak serum concentration: Oral: Immediate release: ~2 hours (range: 1.4-4.8 hours); select patients may have second peak at 4-6 hours due to enterohepatic recirculation. Extended release: 4-11 hours (dependent on adjunct therapy)
Elimination: 75% to 90% excreted as glucuronide metabolites and 10% as unchanged drug
Dialysis: ~20% is removed during 4-hour hemodialysis period

Dosing: Neonatal Oral: **Note:** Dosage depends on patient's concomitant medications [ie, valproic acid; enzyme-inducing AEDs (specifically phenytoin, phenobarbital, carbamazepine, and primidone); or AEDs other than carbamazepine, phenytoin, phenobarbital, primidone, or valproic acid]. Patients receiving concomitant rifampin or other drugs that induce lamotrigine glucuronidation and increase clearance should follow the same dosing regimen as that used with anticonvulsants that have this effect (eg, phenytoin, phenobarbital, carbamazepine, and primidone). Limited data available; further studies needed.

Anticonvulsant: Adjunctive (add-on) therapy for refractory seizures: PNA 14-28 days: Initial: 2 mg/kg/dose once daily; may increase by 2 mg/kg/day at intervals of at least 7 days to a maximum dose of 10 mg/kg/day; this dosing was described in a prospective, open-label trial that included five neonates (GA not reported) in the study population; all patients had previously received enzyme-inducing agents, such as phenytoin, phenobarbital, and/or carbamazepine; patients were treated with lamotrigine for 3 months (Mikati, 2002)

Dosing: Usual Note: Dosage depends on patient's concomitant medications [ie, valproic acid; enzyme-inducing AEDs (specifically phenytoin, phenobarbital, carbamazepine, and primidone); or other AEDs not previously mentioned. Patients receiving concomitant rifampin or other drugs that induce lamotrigine glucuronidation and increase clearance should follow the same dosing regimen as that used with anticonvulsants that have similar effects (eg, phenytoin, phenobarbital, carbamazepine, and primidone).

Anticonvulsant: Adjunctive (add-on) therapy:
Oral:
Immediate release formulation:
Infants and Children <24 months (Piña-Garza, 2008; Piña-Garza, 2008a): **Note:** As reported in the trials, initial doses were administered every other day if necessary due to limited strengths of commercially available products; use of an extemporaneously compounded suspension may allow for more frequent dosing; usually, daily doses are divided into 1-2 doses per day; daily doses in these trials were divided 3 times daily once sufficiently large enough to utilize commercially available products; this was done due to the possible increased clearance of lamotrigine in this age group.
Patients receiving AED regimens **containing valproic acid or nonenzyme-inducing AEDs: Note:** Studies excluded patients <6.7 kg:
Weeks 1 and 2: 0.15 mg/kg/day
Weeks 3 and 4: 0.3 mg/kg/day
Maintenance dose: Titrate dose to effect; after week 4, increase dose every week by no more than 0.3 mg/kg/day; maximum maintenance dose: 5.1 mg/kg/day in 3 divided doses not to exceed 200 mg/day; mean final dose required in open-label phase of trial was 3.1 mg/kg/day; n=51 (Piña-Garza, 2008a)
Patients receiving **enzyme-inducing** *AED regimens (eg, carbamazepine, phenytoin, phenobarbital, or primidone)* **without valproic acid:**
Weeks 1 and 2: 0.6 mg/kg/day
Weeks 3 and 4: 1.2 mg/kg/day
Maintenance dose: Titrate dose to effect; after week 4, increase dose every week by no more than 1.2 mg/kg/day; maximum maintenance dose: 15.6 mg/kg/day in 3 divided doses not to exceed 400 mg/day; mean final dose required in open-label phase of trial was 8.9 mg/kg/day; n=126 (Piña-Garza, 2008a)
Children 2-12 years: **Note: Only whole tablets should be used for dosing**; children 2-6 years will likely require maintenance doses at the higher end of recommended range; patients weighing <30 kg may need as much as a 50% increase in maintenance dose, compared with patients weighing >30 kg; titrate dose to clinical effect
Patients receiving AEDs **other than carbamazepine, phenytoin, phenobarbital, primidone, or valproic acid:**
Weeks 1 and 2: 0.3 mg/kg/day in 1-2 divided doses; round dose down to the nearest whole tablet
Weeks 3 and 4: 0.6 mg/kg/day in 2 divided doses; round dose down to the nearest whole tablet
Maintenance dose: Titrate dose to effect; after week 4, increase dose every 1-2 weeks by a calculated increment; calculate increment as 0.6 mg/kg/day rounded down to the nearest whole tablet; add this amount to the previously administered daily dose; usual maintenance: 4.5-7.5 mg/kg/day in 2 divided doses; maximum: 300 mg/day
Patients receiving AED regimens **containing valproic acid:**
Weeks 1 and 2: 0.15 mg/kg/day in 1-2 divided doses; round dose down to the nearest whole tablet; use 2 mg every other day for patients weighing >6.7 kg and <14 kg
Weeks 3 and 4: 0.3 mg/kg/day in 1-2 divided doses; round dose down to the nearest whole tablet
Maintenance dose: Titrate dose to effect; after week 4, increase dose every 1-2 weeks by a calculated increment; calculate increment as 0.3 mg/kg/day rounded down to the nearest whole tablet; add this amount to the previously administered daily dose; usual maintenance: 1-5 mg/kg/day in 1-2 divided doses; maximum: 200 mg/day. **Note:** Usual maintenance dose in children adding lamotrigine to valproic acid **alone:** 1-3 mg/kg/day

*Patients receiving **enzyme-inducing** AED regimens (eg, carbamazepine, phenytoin, phenobarbital, or primidone) **without valproic acid**:*
Weeks 1 and 2: 0.6 mg/kg/day in 2 divided doses; round dose down to the nearest whole tablet
Weeks 3 and 4: 1.2 mg/kg/day in 2 divided doses; round dose down to the nearest whole tablet
Maintenance dose: Titrate dose to effect; after week 4, increase dose every 1-2 weeks by a calculated increment; calculate increment as 1.2 mg/kg/day rounded down to the nearest whole tablet; add this amount to the previously administered daily dose; usual maintenance: 5-15 mg/kg/day in 2 divided doses; maximum: 400 mg/day

Children >12 years, Adolescents, and Adults:
*Patients receiving AEDs **other than carbamazepine, phenytoin, phenobarbital, primidone, or valproic acid**:*
Weeks 1 and 2: 25 mg every day
Weeks 3 and 4: 50 mg every day
Maintenance dose: Titrate dose to effect; after week 4, increase dose every 1-2 weeks by 50 mg/day; usual maintenance: 225-375 mg/day in 2 divided doses
*Patients receiving AED regimens **containing valproic acid**:*
Weeks 1 and 2: 25 mg every other day
Weeks 3 and 4: 25 mg every day
Maintenance dose: Titrate dose to effect; after week 4, increase dose every 1-2 weeks by 25-50 mg/day; usual maintenance in patients receiving valproic acid and other drugs that induce glucuronidation: 100-400 mg/day in 1-2 divided doses; usual maintenance in patients adding lamotrigine to valproic acid **alone**: 100-200 mg/day
*Patients receiving **enzyme-inducing** AED regimens (eg, carbamazepine, phenytoin, phenobarbital, or primidone) **without valproic acid**:*
Weeks 1 and 2: 50 mg/day
Weeks 3 and 4: 100 mg/day in 2 divided doses
Maintenance dose: Titrate dose to effect; after week 4, increase dose every 1-2 weeks by 100 mg/day; usual maintenance: 300-500 mg/day in 2 divided doses; doses as high as 700 mg/day in 2 divided doses have been used

Extended release formulation: Adolescents ≥13 years and Adults: **Note:** Dose increases after week 8 should not exceed 100 mg/day at weekly intervals
*Regimens **not containing** carbamazepine, phenytoin, phenobarbital, primidone, or valproic acid:* Initial: Weeks 1 and 2: 25 mg once daily; Weeks 3 and 4: 50 mg once daily; Week 5: 100 mg once daily; Week 6: 150 mg once daily; Week 7: 200 mg once daily; Maintenance: 300-400 mg once daily
*Regimens **containing** valproic acid:* Initial: Weeks 1 and 2: 25 mg every other day; Weeks 3 and 4: 25 mg once daily; Week 5: 50 mg once daily; Week 6: 100 mg once daily; Week 7: 150 mg once daily; Maintenance: 200-250 mg once daily
*Regimens **containing** carbamazepine, phenytoin, phenobarbital, or primidone and **without** valproic acid:* Initial: Weeks 1 and 2: 50 mg once daily; Weeks 3 and 4: 100 mg once daily; Week 5: 200 mg once daily; Week 6: 300 mg once daily; Week 7: 400 mg once daily; Maintenance: 400-600 mg once daily
Conversion from immediate release to extended release (Lamictal® XR™): Initial dose of the extended release tablet should match the total daily dose of the immediate release formulation; monitor

for seizure control, especially in patients on AED agents. Adjust dose as needed within the recommended dosing guidelines.

Anticonvulsant: Monotherapy:
Oral:
Immediate release formulations: Adolescents ≥16 years and Adults:
*Conversion from adjunctive therapy with a **single enzyme-inducing** AED (eg, carbamazepine, phenytoin, phenobarbital, or primidone and **not valproate**) to lamotrigine immediate release monotherapy:* **Note:** First add lamotrigine and titrate it (as outlined below) to the recommended maintenance monotherapy dose (500 mg/day in 2 divided doses), while maintaining the enzyme-inducing AED at a fixed level; then gradually taper the enzyme-inducing AED by 20% decrements each week to fully withdraw over a 4-week period.
Weeks 1 and 2: 50 mg/day
Weeks 3 and 4: 100 mg/day in 2 divided doses
Maintenance dose: After week 4, increase dose every 1-2 weeks by 100 mg/day; recommended maintenance monotherapy dose: 500 mg/day in 2 divided doses
*Conversion from adjunctive therapy with **valproate** to lamotrigine immediate release monotherapy:* **Note:** This is a 4-step conversion process to achieve the lamotrigine recommended monotherapy dose (500 mg/day in 2 divided doses).
First: Add lamotrigine and titrate it to a dose of 200 mg/day as follows (if not already receiving 200 mg/day), while maintaining the valproate dose at a fixed level:
Weeks 1 and 2: 25 mg every other day
Weeks 3 and 4: 25 mg every day
Then increase dose every 1-2 weeks by 25-50 mg/day
Second: Keep lamotrigine dose at 200 mg/day; slowly taper valproate dose in decrements of ≤500 mg/day per week, to a dose of 500 mg/day; maintain this dose for one week
Third: Increase lamotrigine to 300 mg/day and decrease valproate to 250 mg/day; maintain this dose for one week
Fourth: Discontinue valproate and increase lamotrigine by 100 mg/day at weekly intervals to achieve recommended maintenance monotherapy dose of 500 mg/day in 2 divided doses
Conversion from adjunctive therapy with AEDs other than enzyme-inducing AEDs or valproate to lamotrigine immediate release monotherapy: No specific guidelines available
Extended release formulation: Adolescents ≥13 years and Adults:
*Conversion from adjunctive therapy with AEDs **other than** enzyme-inducing AEDs or valproate to lamotrigine extended release monotherapy:* First add lamotrigine and titrate it (as outlined below) to a recommended lamotrigine dose of 250-300 mg once daily, while maintaining the concomitant AED at a fixed level; then gradually taper the concomitant AED by 20% decrements each week to fully withdraw over a 4-week period.
Weeks 1 and 2: 25 mg once daily
Weeks 3 and 4: 50 mg once daily
Week 5: 100 mg once daily
Week 6: 150 mg once daily
Week 7: 200 mg once daily
Maintenance: 250-300 mg once daily
*Conversion from adjunctive therapy with **valproate** to lamotrigine extended release monotherapy:* **Note:** This is a 4-step conversion process to achieve the

lamotrigine recommended extended release mono-therapy dose (250-300 mg once daily).

First: Add lamotrigine and titrate it to a dose of 150 mg/day as follows (if not already receiving 150 mg/day), while maintaining the valproate dose at a fixed level:

Weeks 1 and 2: 25 mg every other day

Weeks 3 and 4: 25 mg once daily

Week 5: 50 mg once daily

Week 6: 100 mg once daily

Week 7: 150 mg once daily

Second: Keep lamotrigine dose at 150 mg/day; slowly taper valproate dose in decrements of ≤500 mg/day per week, to a dose of 500 mg/day; maintain this dose for 1 week

Third: Increase lamotrigine to 200 mg/day and decrease valproate to 250 mg/day; maintain this dose for 1 week

Fourth: Discontinue valproate and increase lamotrigine to a maintenance dose of 250-300 mg/day

Conversion from adjunctive therapy with a **single** **enzyme-inducing** *AED (eg, carbamazepine, pheny-toin, phenobarbital, or primidone and* **not valproate***) to lamotrigine extended release monotherapy in patients with partial seizures:* **Note:** First add lamotrigine and titrate it (as outlined below) to a recommended lamotrigine dose of 500 mg/day, while maintaining the enzyme-inducing AED at a fixed level; then gradually taper the enzyme-inducing AED by 20% decrements each week to fully withdraw over a 4-week period. Two weeks following withdrawal of the enzyme-inducing AED, the dosage of lamotrigine extended release may be tapered in decrements of ≤100 mg/day at intervals of 1 week to achieve a maintenance dosage range of 250-300 mg/day

Weeks 1 and 2: 50 mg once daily

Weeks 3 and 4: 100 mg once daily

Maintenance: After week 4, increase dose every 1 week by 100 mg/day to a lamotrigine dose of 500 mg once daily

Bipolar disorder: Oral: Immediate release formulation: Adolescents ≥18 years and Adults:

Patients **not** *receiving enzyme-inducing drugs (eg, car-bamazepine, phenytoin, phenobarbital, primidone, rifampin) or valproate:*

Weeks 1 and 2: 25 mg/day

Weeks 3 and 4: 50 mg/day

Week 5: 100 mg/day

Week 6 and thereafter: 200 mg/day

Patients receiving **valproate***:*

Weeks 1 and 2: 25 mg every other day

Weeks 3 and 4: 25 mg/day

Week 5: 50 mg/day

Week 6 and thereafter: 100 mg/day

Note: If valproate is discontinued, increase daily lamotrigine dose in 50 mg increments at weekly intervals until dosage of 200 mg/day is attained.

Patients receiving **enzyme-inducing drugs** *(eg, carba-mazepine, phenytoin, phenobarbital, primidone, rifam-pin)* **without valproate***:*

Weeks 1 and 2: 50 mg/day

Weeks 3 and 4: 100 mg/day in divided doses

Week 5: 200 mg/day in divided doses

Week 6: 300 mg/day in divided doses

Week 7 and thereafter: May increase to 400 mg/day in divided doses

Note: If carbamazepine (or other enzyme-inducing drug) is discontinued, maintain current lamotrigine dose for 1 week, then decrease daily lamotrigine dose in 100 mg increments at weekly intervals until dosage of 200 mg/day is attained.

Dosage adjustment with concomitant estrogen-con-taining oral contraceptives: Follow initial lamotrigine dosing guidelines, maintenance dose should be adjusted as follows:

Patients **taking** *concomitant carbamazepine, phenytoin, phenobarbital, primidone, or other drugs, such as rifam-pin, that induce lamotrigine glucuronidation:* No dosing adjustment required

Patients **not taking** *concomitant carbamazepine, pheny-toin, phenobarbital, primidone, or other drugs, such as rifampin, that induce lamotrigine glucuronidation:* If already taking estrogen-containing oral contraceptives, the maintenance dose of lamotrigine may need to be increased by as much as twofold over the target main-tenance dose listed above. If already taking a stable dose of lamotrigine and starting an oral contraceptive agent, the lamotrigine maintenance dose may need to be increased by as much as twofold. Dose increases should start when contraceptive agent is started and titrated to clinical response increasing no more rapidly than 50-100 mg/day every week. Gradual increases of lamotrigine plasma levels may occur during the inactive "pill-free" week and will be greater when dose increases are made the week before. If increased adverse events consistently occur during "pill-free" week, overall dose adjustments may be required. Dose adjustments during "pill-free" week are not recommended. When discontin-uing combination hormonal contraceptive, dose of lamotrigine may need decreased by as much as 50%; do not decrease by more than 25% of total daily dose over a 2-week period unless clinical response or plasma levels indicate otherwise.

Discontinuing therapy: Children and Adults: Do not abruptly discontinue; when discontinuing lamotrigine therapy, gradually decrease the dose by ~50% per week and taper over at least 2 weeks unless safety concerns require a more rapid withdrawal. **Note:** If discontinuing other anticonvulsants and maintaining lamotrigine therapy, keep in mind that discontinuing carbamazepine, phenytoin, phenobarbital, primidone, or other drugs, such as rifampin, that induce lamotrigine glucuronidation should prolong the half-life of lamotri-gine; discontinuing valproic acid should shorten the half-life of lamotrigine; monitor patient closely; dosage change may be needed

Dosage adjustment in renal impairment: Use with cau-tion; has not been adequately studied; base initial dose on patient's AED regimen; decreased maintenance dos-age may be effective in patients with significant renal impairment

Dosage adjustment in hepatic impairment: Note: Adjust escalation and maintenance doses by clinical response. Mild hepatic impairment: No dosage adjustment required Moderate and severe hepatic impairment without ascites: Reduce initial, escalation, and maintenance doses by ~25%

Severe hepatic impairment with ascites: Reduce initial, escalation, and maintenance doses by 50%

Administration Oral: May be administered without regard to food. If medication is received in blisterpack, examine blisterpack before use; do not use if blisters are broken, torn, or missing.

Regular tablet: Do not chew, as a bitter taste may result; swallow tablet whole

Chewable, dispersible tablet: Only whole tablets should be administered; may swallow whole, chew, or disperse in water or diluted fruit juice; if chewed, administer a small amount of water or diluted fruit juice to help in swallowing. To disperse, add tablets to a small amount of liquid (~5 mL or enough to cover the medication); when the tablets are completely dispersed (in about 1 minute), swirl the solution and administer the entire amount immediately.

Do not attempt to administer partial quantities of dispersed tablets.

Extended-release tablet (Lamictal® XR™): May be administered without regard to meals. Swallow tablet whole; do not chew, crush, or break.

Orally disintegrating tablet (Lamictal® ODT™): Place tablet on tongue and move around in the mouth. Tablet will dissolve rapidly and can be swallowed with or without food or water.

Monitoring Parameters All patients: Monitor for hypersensitivity reactions, especially rash; CBC with differential; liver and renal function

Epilepsy: Seizure frequency, duration, and severity; serum levels of concurrent anticonvulsants; signs and symptoms of suicidality (eg, anxiety, depression, behavior changes)

Bipolar disorder: Clinical worsening of depressive symptoms or suicidality, especially with initiation of therapy or dosage changes

Reference Range The clinical value of monitoring lamotrigine plasma concentrations has not been established. Dosing should be based on therapeutic response. Proposed therapeutic range: 1-5 mcg/mL. Lamotrigine plasma concentrations of 0.25-29.1 mcg/mL have been reported in the literature.

Additional Information Low water solubility. Does **not** induce P450 microsomal enzymes. The clinical usefulness of lamotrigine should be periodically re-evaluated in patients with bipolar disorder who are receiving the drug for extended intervals (ie, >16 weeks).

The extended-release tablets contain a modified-release eroding formulation as the core of the tablet. The clear enteric coating has an aperture drilled through it on both sides of the tablet; this allows an extended release of the medication in the acidic environment within the stomach. The design of the table controls the dissolution rate of the medication over a 12-15 hour period.

Three different lamotrigine "Starter Kits" are available for adult patients for three different dosage forms (tablets, extended release tablets, and orally disintegrating tablets); each starter kit contains a blisterpack with a certain number and mg strength of tablets that are specific for initiating doses in different patient populations.

Dosage Forms Considerations

LaMICtal Kits are available as follows:

Blue - for patients already taking valproate

LaMICtal Starter: 25 mg (35s)

LaMICtal ODT (Titration): 25 mg (21s) and 50 mg (7s)

LaMICtal XR (Titration): 25 mg (21s) and 50 mg (7s)

Green- for patients already taking carbamazepine, phenytoin, phenobarbital, or primidone, and **not** taking valproate

LaMICtal Starter: 25 mg (84s) and 100 mg (14s)

LaMICtal ODT (Titration): 50 mg (42s) and 100 mg (14s)

LaMICtal XR (Titration): 50 mg (14s) and 100 mg (14s) and 200 mg (7s)

Orange - for patients not taking carbamazepine, phenytoin, phenobarbital, primidone, or valproate

LaMICtal Starter: 25 mg (42s) and 100 mg (7s)

LaMICtal ODT (Titration): 25 mg (14s) and 50 mg (14s) and 100 mg (7s)

LaMICtal XR (Titration): 25 mg (14s) and 50 mg (14s) and 100 mg (7s)

Dosage Forms Excipient information presented when available (limited, particularly for generics); consult specific product labeling.

Kit, Oral:

LaMICtal ODT: Blue Kit: 25 mg (21s) & 50 mg (7s), Green Kit: 50 mg (42s) & 100 mg (14s), Orange Kit: 25 mg (14s) & 50 mg (14s) & 100 mg (7s)

LaMICtal Starter: Blue Kit: 25 mg (35s)

LaMICtal Starter: Green Kit: 25 mg (84s) & 100 mg (14s), Orange Kit: 25 mg (42s) & 100 mg (7s) [contains fd&c yellow #6 aluminum lake]

LaMICtal XR: Green Kit: 50 mg (14s) & 100 mg (14s) & 200 mg (7s) [contains fd&c blue #2 aluminum lake, polysorbate 80]

LaMICtal XR: Blue Kit: 25 mg (21s) & 50 mg (7s), Orange Kit: 25 mg (14s) & 50 mg (14s) & 100 mg (7s) [contains polysorbate 80]

Tablet, Oral:

LaMICtal: 25 mg, 100 mg, 150 mg, 200 mg [scored]

Generic: 25 mg, 100 mg, 150 mg, 200 mg

Tablet Chewable, Oral:

LaMICtal: 2 mg [contains saccharin sodium]

LaMICtal: 5 mg [scored; berry flavor]

LaMICtal: 25 mg [berry flavor]

Generic: 5 mg, 25 mg

Tablet Dispersible, Oral:

LaMICtal ODT: 25 mg, 50 mg, 100 mg, 200 mg

Tablet Extended Release 24 Hour, Oral:

LaMICtal XR: 25 mg, 50 mg, 100 mg [contains polysorbate 80]

LaMICtal XR: 200 mg [contains fd&c blue #2 aluminum lake, polysorbate 80]

LaMICtal XR: 250 mg [contains fd&c blue #2 aluminum lake]

LaMICtal XR: 300 mg [contains polysorbate 80]

Generic: 25 mg, 50 mg, 100 mg, 200 mg, 250 mg, 300 mg

Extemporaneous Preparations A 1 mg/mL oral suspension may be made with tablets and one of two different vehicles (a 1:1 mixture of Ora-Sweet® and Ora-Plus® or a 1:1 mixture of Ora-Sweet® SF and Ora-Plus®). Crush one 100 mg tablet in a mortar and reduce to a fine powder. Add small portions of the chosen vehicle and mix to a uniform paste; mix while adding the vehicle in incremental proportions to **almost** 100 mL; transfer to a graduated cylinder, rinse mortar with vehicle, and add quantity of vehicle sufficient to make 100 mL. Label "shake well" and "protect from light". Stable for 91 days when stored in amber plastic prescription bottles in the dark at room temperature or refrigerated.

Nahata M, Morosco R, Hipple T. "Stability of Lamotrigine in Two Extemporaneously Prepared Oral Suspensions at 4 and 25 Degrees C," *Am J Health Syst Pharm*, 1999, 56(3):240-2.

References

Barr PA, Buettiker VE, and Antony JH, "Efficacy of Lamotrigine in Refractory Neonatal Seizures," *Pediatr Neurol*, 1999, 20(2):161-3.

Battino D, Estienne M, and Avanzini G, "Clinical Pharmacokinetics of Antiepileptic Drugs in Paediatric Patients: Part II. Phenytoin, Carbamazepine, Sulthiame, Lamotrigine, Vigabatrin, Oxcarbazepine, and Felbamate," *Clin Pharmacokinet*, 1995, 29(5):341-69.

Besag FM, Wallace SJ, Dulac O, et al, "Lamotrigine for the Treatment of Epilepsy in Childhood," *J Pediatr*, 1995, 127(6):991-7.

Burstein AH, "Lamotrigine," *Pharmacotherapy*, 1995, 15(2):129-43.

Cunnington M, Ferber S, Quartey G, et al, "Effect of Dose on the Frequency of Major Birth Defects Following Fetal Exposure to Lamotrigine Monotherapy in an International Observational Study," *Epilepsia*, 2007, 48(6):1207-10.

Cunnington MC, Weil JG, Messenheimer JA, et al, "Final Results From 18 Years of the International Lamotrigine Pregnancy Registry," *Neurology*, 2011, 76(21):1817-23.

Dooley J, Camfield P, Gordon K, et al, "Lamotrigine-Induced Rash in Children," *Neurology*, 1996, 46(1):240-2.

Fitton A, and Goa KL, "Lamotrigine: An Update of its Pharmacology and Therapeutic Use in Epilepsy," *Drugs*, 1995, 50(4):691-713.

Harden CL, Meador KJ, Pennell PB, et al, "Practice Parameter Update: Management Issues for Women With Epilepsy-Focus on Pregnancy (an Evidence-Based Review): Teratogenesis and Perinatal Outcomes: Report of the Quality Standards Subcommittee and Therapeutics and Technology Assessment Subcommittee of the American Academy of Neurology and American Epilepsy Society," *Neurology*, 2009, 73(2):133-41.

Harden CL, Pennell PB, Koppel BS, et al, "Practice Parameter Update Management Issues for Women With Epilepsy-Focus on Pregnancy (an Evidence-Based Review): Vitamin K, Folic Acid, Blood Levels, and Breastfeeding: Report of the Quality Standards Subcommittee and Therapeutics and Technology Assessment Subcommittee of the

American Academy of Neurology and American Epilepsy Society," *Neurology*, 2009, 73(2):142-9.

Hernández-Díaz S, Smith CR, Shen A, et al, "Comparative Safety of Antiepileptic Drugs During Pregnancy," *Neurology*, 2012, 78 (21):1692-9.

Holmes LB and Hernández-Díaz S, "Newer Anticonvulsants: Lamotrigine, Topiramate and Gabapentin," *Birth Defects Res A Clin Mol Teratol*, 2012, 94(8):599-606.

Messenheimer JA, "Lamotrigine," *Epilepsia*, 1995, 36(Suppl 2):S87-94.

Messenheimer JA, Giorgi L, and Risner ME, "The Tolerability of Lamotrigine in Children," *Drug Saf*, 2000, 22(4):303-12.

Mikati MA, Fayad M, Koleilat M, et al, "Efficacy, Tolerability, and Kinetics of Lamotrigine in Infants," *J Pediatr*, 2002, 141(1):31-5.

Ohman I, Vitols S, and Tomson T, "Lamotrigine in Pregnancy: Pharmacokinetics During Delivery, in the Neonate, and During Lactation," *Epilepsia*, 2000, 41(6):709-13.

Patsalos PN, Berry DJ, Bourgeois BF, et al, "Antiepileptic Drugs-Best Practice Guidelines for Therapeutic Drug Monitoring: A Position Paper by the Subcommission on Therapeutic Drug Monitoring, ILAE Commission on Therapeutic Strategies," *Epilepsia*, 2008, 49 (7):1239-76.

Piña-Garza JE, Elterman RD, Ayala R, et al, "Long-Term Tolerability and Efficacy of Lamotrigine in Infants 1 to 24 Months Old," *J Child Neurol*, 2008, 23(8):853-61.

Piña-Garza JE, Levisohn P, Gucuyener K, et al, "Adjunctive Lamotrigine for Partial Seizures in Patients Aged 1 to 24 Months," *Neurology*, 2008a, 70(22 Pt 2):2099-108.

Tomson T, Battino D, Bonizzoni E, et al, "Dose-Dependent Risk of Malformations With Antiepileptic Drugs: An Analysis of Data From the EURAP Epilepsy and Pregnancy Registry," *Lancet Neurol*, 2011, 10(7):609-17.

◆ **Lanoxin** *see* Digoxin *on page 658*

◆ **Lanoxin Pediatric** *see* Digoxin *on page 658*

Lansoprazole (lan SOE pra zole)

Medication Safety Issues
Sound-alike/look-alike issues:
Lansoprazole may be confused with aripiprazole, dexlansoprazole

Prevacid® may be confused with Pravachol®, Prevpac®, PriLOSEC®, Prinivil®

Related Information
Oral Medications That Should Not Be Crushed or Altered *on page 2438*

Brand Names: U.S. First-Lansoprazole; Heartburn Relief 24 Hour [OTC]; Heartburn Treatment 24 Hour [OTC]; Prevacid; Prevacid 24HR [OTC]; Prevacid SoluTab

Brand Names: Canada Apo-Lansoprazole®; Mylan-Lansoprazole; Prevacid®; Prevacid® FasTab; Teva-Lansoprazole

Therapeutic Category Gastric Acid Secretion Inhibitor; Gastrointestinal Agent, Gastric or Duodenal Ulcer Treatment; Proton Pump Inhibitor

Generic Availability (U.S.) May be product dependent

Use Short-term treatment of symptomatic gastroesophageal reflux disease (GERD) (FDA approved in ages ≥1 year and adults); short-term treatment (up to 8 weeks) for healing and symptomatic relief of all grades of erosive esophagitis (FDA approved in ages ≥1 year and adults); maintenance of healed erosive esophagitis (FDA approved in adults); short-term treatment (up to 8 weeks) of active benign gastric ulcer (FDA approved in adults); short-term treatment (≤4 weeks) for healing and symptomatic relief of active duodenal ulcer (FDA approved in adults); maintenance treatment of healed duodenal ulcers (FDA approved in adults); treatment of pathological hypersecretory conditions, including Zollinger-Ellison syndrome (FDA approved in adults); adjuvant therapy in the treatment of duodenal ulcers associated with *Helicobacter pylori* (FDA approved in adults); prevention (for patients at high risk) and treatment of NSAID-associated gastric ulcers (FDA approved in adults); relief of frequent heartburn (≥2 days/week) (OTC product: FDA approved in adults)

Medication Guide Available Yes

Pregnancy Risk Factor B

Pregnancy Considerations Adverse events were not observed in animal reproduction studies. An increased risk of hypospadias was reported following maternal use of proton pump inhibitors (PPIs) during pregnancy (Anderka, 2012), but this was based on a small number of exposures and the same association was not found in another study (Erichsen, 2012). Most available studies have not shown an increased risk of major birth defects following maternal use of PPIs during pregnancy (Diav-Citrin, 2005; Matok, 2012; Pasternak, 2010). When treating GERD in pregnancy, PPIs may be used when clinically indicated (Katz, 2013).

Breast-Feeding Considerations It is not known if lansoprazole is excreted into breast milk. Due to the potential for serious adverse reactions in the nursing infant, the manufacturer recommends a decision be made whether to discontinue nursing or to discontinue the drug, taking into account the importance of treatment to the mother.

Contraindications Hypersensitivity to lansoprazole or any component

Warnings Long-term effects are not known; enterochromaffin (ECF)-like hyperplasia and subsequent carcinoids have developed in rats following lifetime exposure to high doses (150 mg/kg/day). No reports of enterochromaffin-like (ECL) cell carcinoids, dysplasia, or neoplasia in humans have been reported. Symptomatic response to therapy does not preclude the presence of gastric malignancy. Concomitant use of PPIs with high-dose methotrexate may lead to increased and prolonged serum concentrations of methotrexate and/or its metabolite, possibly causing methotrexate toxicities; temporary discontinuation of PPIs may be considered.

Use of gastric acid inhibitors, including proton pump inhibitors (PPIs) and H_2 blockers, has been associated with an increased risk for development of acute gastroenteritis and community-acquired pneumonia (Canani, 2006). Use of PPIs may also increase the risk of *Clostridium difficile*-associated diarrhea (CDAD), especially in hospitalized patients; consider CDAD diagnosis in patients with persistent diarrhea that does not improve. Use the lowest dose and shortest duration of PPI therapy appropriate for the condition being treated.

An increased incidence of osteoporosis-related bone fractures of the hip, spine, or wrist may occur with PPI therapy; patients on high-dose (multiple daily doses) or long-term therapy (≥1 year) should be monitored. Use the lowest effective dose for the shortest duration of time, use vitamin D and calcium supplementation, and follow appropriate guidelines to reduce risk of fractures in patients at risk. Hypomagnesemia has been reported rarely, usually with prolonged PPI use of >3 months (most cases >1 year of therapy), and may be symptomatic or asymptomatic; severe cases may cause tetany, seizures, and cardiac arrhythmias. Consider obtaining serum magnesium concentrations prior to beginning long-term therapy, especially if taking concomitant digoxin, diuretics, or other drugs known to cause hypomagnesemia; and periodically thereafter. Hypomagnesemia may be corrected by magnesium supplementation, although discontinuation of lansoprazole may be necessary; magnesium concentrations typically return to normal within 1 week of stopping.

PPIs may diminish the therapeutic effect of clopidogrel thought to be due to reduced formation of the active metabolite of clopidogrel. The manufacturer of clopidogrel recommends either avoidance of both omeprazole (even when scheduled 12 hours apart) and esomeprazole or use of a PPI with comparatively less effect on the active metabolite of clopidogrel (eg, pantoprazole). Although lansoprazole exhibits the most potent CYP2C19 inhibition *in vitro* (Li, 2004; Ogilvie, 2011), an *in vivo* study of extensive CYP2C19 metabolizers showed less reduction of the active metabolite of clopidogrel by lansoprazole/dexlansoprazole compared to esomeprazole/omeprazole (Frelinger, 2012). The manufacturer of lansoprazole states that no dosage adjustment is necessary for clopidogrel when used concurrently. In contrast to these warnings, others have recommended the continued use of PPIs, regardless of the degree of inhibition, in patients with a history of GI bleeding or multiple risk factors for GI bleeding who are also receiving clopidogrel since no evidence has established clinically meaningful differences in outcome; however, a clinically-significant interaction cannot be excluded in those who are poor metabolizers of clopidogrel (Abraham, 2010; Levine, 2011).

Do not use for self-medication (OTC) if difficulty swallowing, blood in vomit, or bloody or black stools are present. Prior to use, patients should contact healthcare provider if any of the following conditions are present: Heartburn for >3 months; heartburn with dizziness, lightheadedness, or sweating; MI symptoms; frequent chest pain; frequent wheezing (especially with heartburn); unexplained weight loss; nausea/vomiting; stomach pain; or are taking other medications (interactions are common). If heartburn continues or worsens or if need to take for >14 days or more often than every 4 months, discontinue use and contact physician. May take 1-4 days for full effect.

First®-Lansoprazole powder for oral suspension contains benzyl alcohol which may cause allergic reactions in susceptible individuals; large amounts of benzyl alcohol (≥99 mg/kg/day) have been associated with a potentially fatal toxicity ("gasping syndrome") in neonates; the "gasping syndrome" consists of metabolic acidosis, respiratory distress, gasping respirations, CNS dysfunction (including convulsions, intracranial hemorrhage), hypotension and cardiovascular collapse; use oral suspension containing benzyl alcohol with caution in neonates; *in vitro* and animal studies have shown that benzoate, a metabolite of benzyl alcohol, displaces bilirubin from protein binding sites.
Precautions Use with caution in patients with liver disease; reduce dosage with severe impairment. Prevacid® SoluTabs™ contain aspartame which is metabolized to phenylalanine and must be used with caution in patients with phenylketonuria.

Adverse Reactions

Central nervous system: Dizziness, headache
Gastrointestinal: Abdominal pain, constipation, diarrhea, nausea
Rare but important or life-threatening: Abdomen enlarged, abnormal dreams, abnormal menses, abnormal stools, abnormal vision, agitation, agranulocytosis, albuminuria, allergic reaction, alkaline phosphatase increased, ALT increased, alopecia, amblyopia, amnesia, anaphylactoid reaction, anemia, angina, anorexia, anxiety, aplastic anemia, appetite increased, arrhythmia, AST increased, arthralgia, arthritis, asthma, avitaminosis, bezoar, bilirubinemia, blepharitis, blurred vision, bradycardia, breast enlargement, breast pain, breast tenderness, bronchitis, candidiasis, carcinoma, cardiospasm, cataract, cerebrovascular accident, cerebral infarction, chest pain, chills, cholelithiasis, cholesterol increased/decreased, *Clostridium difficile*-associated diarrhea (CDAD), colitis, confusion, conjunctivitis, cough increased, creatinine increased, deafness, dehydration, dementia, depersonalization, depression, diabetes mellitus, diaphoresis, diplopia, dry eyes, dry skin, dyspepsia, dysphagia, dyspnea, dysmenorrhea, dysuria, edema, electrolyte imbalance, emotional lability, enteritis, eosinophilia, epistaxis, eructation, erythema multiforme, esophageal stenosis, esophageal ulcer, esophagitis, fecal discoloration, fever, fixed eruption, flatulence, flu-like syndrome, fracture, fundic gland polyps, gastric nodules, gastrin levels increased, gastritis, gastroenteritis, gastrointestinal anomaly, gastrointestinal hemorrhage, GGTP increased/decreased, glaucoma, glucocorticoid levels increased, glossitis, glycosuria, goiter, gout, gum hemorrhage, gynecomastia, halitosis, hallucinations, hematemesis, hematuria, hemiplegia, hemolysis, hemolytic anemia, hemoptysis, hepatotoxicity, hostility aggravated, hyper-/hypoglycemia, hyperkinesia, hyperlipemia, hypertonia, hypoesthesia, hyper-/hypotension, hypomagnesemia, hypothyroidism, impotence, infection, insomnia, interstitial nephritis, kidney calculus, laryngeal neoplasia, LDH increased, leg cramps, leukopenia, leukorrhea, libido decreased/increased, liver function test abnormal, lung fibrosis, lymphadenopathy, maculopapular rash, malaise, melena, menorrhagia, migraine, moniliasis (oral), mouth ulceration, musculoskeletal pain, myalgia, myasthenia, myositis, MI, nervousness, neurosis, neutropenia, pain, palpitation, pancreatitis, pancytopenia, paresthesia, parosmia, pelvic pain, peripheral edema, pharyngitis, photophobia, platelet abnormalities, pneumonia, polyuria, pruritus, ptosis, rash, rectal hemorrhage, retinal degeneration, rhinitis, salivation increased, seizure, shock, sinusitis, skin carcinoma, sleep disorder, somnolence, speech disorder, Stevens-Johnson syndrome, stomatitis, stridor, syncope, synovitis, tachycardia, taste loss, taste perversion, tenesmus, thirst, thrombocytopenia, thrombotic thrombocytopenic purpura, tinnitus, tremor, tongue disorder, toxic epidermal necrolysis, ulcerative colitis, ulcerative stomatitis, upper respiratory inflammation, upper respiratory infection, urethral pain, urinary frequency/urgency, urination impaired, urinary retention, urinary tract infection, urticaria, vaginitis, vasodilation, vertigo, visual field defect, vomiting, weakness, WBC abnormal, weight gain/loss, xerostomia

Drug Interactions

Metabolism/Transport Effects Substrate of CYP2C19 (major), CYP2C9 (minor), CYP3A4 (major); **Note:** Assignment of Major/Minor substrate status based on clinically relevant drug interaction potential; **Inhibits** CYP2C19 (weak), CYP2C9 (weak), CYP2D6 (weak), CYP3A4 (weak); **Induces** CYP1A2 (weak/moderate)

Avoid Concomitant Use

Avoid concomitant use of Lansoprazole with any of the following: Dasatinib; Delavirdine; Erlotinib; Nelfinavir; PAZOPanib; Pimozide; PONATinib; Rilpivirine; Risedronate

Increased Effect/Toxicity

Lansoprazole may increase the levels/effects of: Amphetamine; ARIPiprazole; Dexmethylphenidate; Dextroamphetamine; Dofetilide; Imatinib; Lomitapide; Methotrexate; Methylphenidate; Pimozide; Raltegravir; Risedronate; Saquinavir; Tacrolimus (Systemic); Vitamin K Antagonists; Voriconazole

The levels/effects of Lansoprazole may be increased by: Fluconazole; Ketoconazole (Systemic); Voriconazole

Decreased Effect

Lansoprazole may decrease the levels/effects of: Atazanavir; Bisphosphonate Derivatives; Bosutinib; Cefditoren; Clopidogrel; Dabigatran Etexilate; Dabrafenib; Dasatinib; Delavirdine; Erlotinib; Gefitinib; Indinavir; Iron Salts; Itraconazole; Ketoconazole (Systemic); Mesalamine; Multivitamins/Minerals (with ADEK, Folate, Iron); Mycophenolate; Nelfinavir; Nilotinib; PAZOPanib; PONATinib; Posaconazole; Rilpivirine; Riociguat; Risedronate; Vismodegib

The levels/effects of Lansoprazole may be decreased by: Bosentan; CYP2C19 Inducers (Strong); CYP3A4 Inducers (Strong); Dabrafenib; Deferasirox; Mitotane; Siltuximab; St Johns Wort; Tipranavir; Tocilizumab

Food Interactions Prolonged treatment (≥2 years) may lead to malabsorption of dietary vitamin B_{12} and subsequent vitamin B_{12} deficiency (Lam, 2013).

Stability

Capsules, orally disintegrating tablets: Store at 25°C (77°F); excursions permitted to 15°C to 30°C (59°F to 86°F). Protect from light and moisture.

Powder for suspension (First® compounding kit): Prior to compounding, store at 15°C to 30°C (59°F to 86°F). Once compounded, the product is stable for 30 days at room temperature and under refrigeration; manufacturer recommendation is for the compounded product to be stored under refrigeration; protect from freezing. Protect from light.

Mechanism of Action

Decreases acid secretion in gastric parietal cells through inhibition of (H+, K+)-ATPase enzyme system, blocking the final step in gastric acid production.

Pharmacodynamics

Duration of antisecretory activity: ≥24 hours

Relief of symptoms:
Gastric or duodenal ulcers: 1 week
Reflux esophagitis: 1-4 weeks

Ulcer healing:
Duodenal: 2 weeks
Gastric: 4 weeks

Pharmacokinetics (Adult data unless noted)

Absorption: Extremely acid labile and will degrade in acid pH of stomach; enteric coated granules improve bioavailability (80%)

Distribution: V_d:
Children: 0.61-0.9 L/kg
Adults: 15.7 ± 1.9 L

Protein binding: 97%

Metabolism: Hepatic via CYP2C19 and 3A4 to inactive metabolites, and in parietal cells to two active metabolites that are not present in systemic circulation

Bioavailability: 80% (reduced by 50% to 70% if given 30 minutes after food)

Half-life:
Children: 1.2-1.5 hours
Adults: 1.5 ± 1 hour

Time to peak serum concentration: 1.7 hours

Elimination: Biliary excretion is major route of elimination; feces (67%); urine (33%; 14% to 25% as metabolites and <1% as unchanged drug)

Clearance:
Children: 0.57-0.71 L/hour/kg
Adults: 11.1 ± 3.8 L/hour
Adults: Hepatic impairment: 3.2-7.2 hours

Dosing: Neonatal GERD:

Oral: 0.2-0.3 mg/kg/dose once daily; dosing based on pharmacokinetic data; clearance in patients <10 weeks of age substantially decreased compared to older patients (Zhang, 2008); higher dosages of 0.5-1 mg/kg/dose once daily have been reported (Springer, 2008)

Dosing: Usual

Infants, Children, and Adolescents:

GERD, symptomatic:
Infants: **Note:** Variable efficacy has been demonstrated in the literature when treating GERD in children <12 months (Orenstein, 2009)
<10 weeks: 0.2-0.3 mg/kg/dose once daily; dosing based on pharmacokinetic data; clearance in patients <10 weeks of age substantially decreased compared to older patients (Orenstein, 2009; Zhang, 2008); for infants >4 weeks, higher doses of 1-1.5 mg/kg/dose once daily have been reported (Springer, 2008)
≥10 weeks: 1-2 mg/kg/dose once daily (Orenstein, 2009; Springer, 2008; Zhang, 2008); 7.5 mg twice daily or 15 mg once daily was shown to provide better symptom relief compared to dietary management in 68 patients (age ≥3 months) (Khoshoo, 2008)

Manufacturer's labeling:
Children 1-11 years:
≤30 kg: 15 mg once daily for up to 12 weeks
>30 kg: 30 mg once daily for up to 12 weeks
Children ≥12 years and Adolescents: Oral: 15 mg once daily for up to 8 weeks
Alternate dosing (AAP recommendation): Infants, Children, and Adolescents: 0.7-3 mg/kg/**day** (Lightdale, 2013)

Erosive esophagitis:
Children 1-11 years:
≤30 kg: 15 mg once daily for up to 12 weeks
>30 kg: 30 mg once daily for up to 12 weeks
Children ≥12 years and Adolescents: Oral: 30 mg once daily for up to 8 weeks

Adults:
Duodenal ulcer: Oral: 15 mg once daily for 4 weeks; maintenance therapy: 15 mg once daily
Erosive esophagitis: Oral: 30 mg once daily for up to 8 weeks; additional 8 weeks may be tried in those patients who failed to respond or for a recurrence of esophagitis; maintenance: 15 mg once daily
Gastric ulcer: Oral: 30 mg once daily for up to 8 weeks
GERD, symptomatic: Oral: 15 mg once daily for up to 8 weeks
Hypersecretory conditions: Oral: Initial: 60 mg once daily; adjust dosage based upon patient response and to reduce acid secretion to <10 mEq/hour (5 mEq/hour in patients with prior gastric surgery); doses of 90 mg twice daily have been used; administer doses >120 mg/day in divided doses
***Helicobacter pylori* eradication:** Oral: 30 mg twice daily for 2 weeks (in combination with amoxicillin and clarithromycin). Alternatively, in patients allergic to or intolerant of clarithromycin or in whom resistance to clarithromycin is known or suspected, lansoprazole 30 mg every 8 hours may be given for 2 weeks (in combination with amoxicillin)
NSAID-associated gastric ulcer: Oral:
Healing: 30 mg once daily for up to 8 weeks
Prevention: 15 mg once daily for up to 12 weeks
Heartburn: OTC labeling: Oral: 15 mg once daily for 14 days; may repeat 14 days of therapy every 4 months. Do not take for >14 days or more often than every 4 months, unless instructed by healthcare provider.

Dosing adjustment in renal impairment: Children, Adolescents, and Adults: No dosage adjustments are recommended

Dosing adjustment in hepatic impairment: Children, Adolescents, and Adults: Bioavailability increased in hepatic impairment; consider dose reduction for severe impairment

Administration

Oral: Administer before eating; best if taken 30 minutes before a meal (Lightdale, 2013); intact granules should not be chewed or crushed

Capsules: Swallow whole; do not chew or crush. For patients with difficulty swallowing the capsule, capsules may be opened and the intact granules sprinkled on 1 tablespoon of applesauce, Ensure® pudding, cottage cheese, yogurt, or strained pears; the mixture should be swallowed immediately. Capsules may also be opened and emptied into ~60 mL of apple juice, orange juice, or tomato juice; mix and swallow immediately. Rinse the glass with additional juice and swallow to assure complete delivery of the dose.

For nasogastric tube ≥16 French: Capsule can be opened, the granules mixed (not crushed) with 40 mL of apple juice and then injected through the NG tube into the stomach, then flush tube with additional apple juice. Do not mix with other liquids based on manufacturer labeling; additional information may be available for NG administration; contact manufacturer to obtain current recommendations.

Tablet, orally-disintegrating: Should not be swallowed whole, broken, cut, or chewed. Place the tablet on the tongue and allow to disintegrate with or without water until the particles can be swallowed.

Administration via an oral syringe: Place the 15 mg tablet in an oral syringe and draw up ~4 mL water, or place the 30 mg tablet in an oral syringe and draw up ~10 mL water. Shake gently. After tablet has dispersed, administer within 15 minutes. Refill the syringe with water (2 mL for the 15 mg tablet; 5 mL for the 30 mg tablet), shake gently, then administer any remaining contents.

For nasogastric tube ≥8 French: Place a 15 mg tablet in a syringe and draw up ~4 mL water, or place the 30 mg tablet in a syringe and draw up ~10 mL water. Shake gently. After tablet has dispersed, administer within 15 minutes. Refill the syringe with water with ~5 mL water, shake gently, and then flush the nasogastric tube.

Monitoring Parameters Patients with Zollinger-Ellison syndrome should be monitored for gastric acid output, which should be maintained at 10 mEq/hour or less during the last hour before the next lansoprazole dose; lab monitoring should include CBC, liver function, renal function, and serum gastrin levels

Dosage Forms Excipient information presented when available (limited, particularly for generics); consult specific product labeling.

Capsule Delayed Release, Oral:
Heartburn Relief 24 Hour: 15 mg [sodium free; contains brilliant blue fcf (fd&c blue #1), fd&c red #40, fd&c yellow #10 (quinoline yellow)]

Heartburn Treatment 24 Hour: 15 mg [sodium free; contains brilliant blue fcf (fd&c blue #1), fd&c yellow #10 (quinoline yellow)]

Prevacid: 15 mg, 30 mg [contains brilliant blue fcf (fd&c blue #1), fd&c red #40]

Prevacid 24HR: 15 mg [sodium free; contains brilliant blue fcf (fd&c blue #1), fd&c red #40]

Generic: 15 mg, 30 mg

Suspension, Oral:
First-Lansoprazole: 3 mg/mL (90 mL, 150 mL, 300 mL) [contains benzyl alcohol, fd&c red #40, saccharin sodium; strawberry flavor]

Tablet Dispersible, Oral:
Prevacid SoluTab: 15 mg, 30 mg [contains aspartame]

Extemporaneous Preparations A 3 mg/mL oral solution (Simplified Lansoprazole Solution [SLS]) may be made with capsules and sodium bicarbonate. Empty the contents of ten lansoprazole 30 mg capsules into a beaker. Add 100 mL sodium bicarbonate 8.4% and gently stir until dissolved (about 15 minutes). Transfer solution to an amber-colored syringe or bottle. A prior study showed that SLS was stable for 8 hours at room temperature or for 14 days refrigerated (DiGiancinto, 2000). However, a more recent study, demonstrated SLS to be stable for 48 hours at room temperature in oral syringes and for only 7 days when refrigerated (Morrison, 2013).

Note: A more palatable lansoprazole (3 mg/mL) suspension is commercially available as a compounding kit (First-Lansoprazole).

DiGiancinto JL, Olsen KM, Bergman KL, et al, "Stability of Suspension Formulations of Lansoprazole and Omeprazole Stored in Amber-Colored Plastic Oral Syringes," *Ann Pharmacother*, 2000, 34(5):600-5

Morrison JT, Lugo RA, Thigpen JC, et al, "Stability of Extemporaneously Prepared Lansoprazole Suspension at Two Temperatures," *J Pediatr Pharmacol Ther*, 2013, 18(2):122-7.

Sharma V, "Comparison of 24-hour Intragastric pH Using Four Liquid Formulations of Lansoprazole and Omeprazole," *Am J Health Syst Pharm*, 1999, 56(Suppl 4):18-21.

Sharma VK, Vasudeva R, and Howden CW, "Simplified Lansoprazole Suspension - Liquid Formulations of Lansoprazole - Effectively Suppresses Intragastric Acidity When Administered Through a Gastrostomy," *Am J Gastroenterol*, 1999, 94(7):1813-7.

References

Abraham NS, Hlatky MA, Antman EM, et al, "ACCF/ACG/AHA 2010 Expert Consensus Document on the Concomitant Use of Proton Pump Inhibitors and Thienopyridines: A Focused Update of the ACCF/ACG/AHA 2008 Expert Consensus Document on Reducing the Gastrointestinal Risks of Antiplatelet Therapy and NSAID Use: A Report of the American College of Cardiology Foundation Task Force on Expert Consensus Documents," *Circulation*, 2010, 122 (24):2619-33.

Anderka M, Mitchell AA, Louik C, et al, "Medications Used to Treat Nausea and Vomiting of Pregnancy and the Risk of Selected Birth Defects," *Birth Defects Res A Clin Mol Teratol*, 2012, 94(1):22-30.

Canani RB, Cirillo P, Roggero P, et al, "Therapy With Gastric Acidity Inhibitors Increases the Risk of Acute Gastroenteritis and Community-Acquired Pneumonia in Children," *Pediatrics*, 2006, 117(5):e817-20.

Chun AH, Eason CJ, Shi HH, et al, "Lansoprazole: An Alternative Method of Administration of a Capsule Dosage Formulation," *Clin Ther*, 1995, 17(3):441-7.

Diav-Citrin O, Arnon J, Shechtman S, et al, "The Safety of Proton Pump Inhibitors in Pregnancy: A Multicentre Prospective Controlled Study," *Aliment Pharmacol Ther*, 2005, 21(3):269-75.

Erichsen R, Mikkelsen E, Pedersen L, et al, "Maternal Use of Proton Pump Inhibitors During Early Pregnancy and the Prevalence of Hypospadias in Male Offspring," *Am J Ther*, 2012.

Frelinger AL 3rd, Lee RD, Mulford DJ, et al, "A Randomized, 2-Period, Crossover Design Study to Assess the Effects of Dexlansoprazole, Lansoprazole, Esomeprazole, and Omeprazole on the Steady-State Pharmacokinetics and Pharmacodynamics of Clopidogrel in Healthy Volunteers," *J Am Coll Cardiol*, 2012, 59(14):1304-11.

Gibbons TE and Gold BD, "The Use of Proton Pump Inhibitors in Children: A Comprehensive Review," *Paediatr Drugs*, 2003, 5 (1):25-40.

Katz PO, Gerson LB, and Vela MF, "Guidelines for the Diagnosis and Management of Gastroesophageal Reflux Disease," *Am J Gastroenterol*, 2013, 108(3):308-28.

Khoshoo V and Dhume P, "Clinical Response to 2 Dosing Regimens of Lansoprazole in Infants With Gastroesophageal Reflux," *J Pediatr Gastroenterol Nutr*, 2008, 46(3):352-4.

Levine GN, Bates ER, Blankenship JC, et al, "2011 ACCF/AHA/SCAI Guideline for Percutaneous Coronary Intervention: A Report of the American College of Cardiology Foundation/American Heart Association Task Force on Practice Guidelines and the Society for Cardiovascular Angiography and Interventions," *Circulation*, 2011, 124(23): e574-651.

Lightdale JR, Gremse DA, and the Section on Gastroenterology, Hepatology, and Nutrition," "Gastroesophageal Reflux: Management Guidance for the Pediatrician," *Pediatrics*, 2013, 131(5):e1684-95.

Li XQ, Andersson TB, Ahlström M, et al, "Comparison of Inhibitory Effects of the Proton Pump-Inhibiting Drugs Omeprazole, Esomeprazole, Lansoprazole, Pantoprazole, and Rabeprazole on Human Cytochrome P450 Activities," *Drug Metab Dispos*, 2004, 32(8):821-7.

Matok I, Levy A, Wiznitzer A, et al, "The Safety of Fetal Exposure to Proton-Pump Inhibitors During Pregnancy," *Dig Dis Sci*, 2012, 57 (3):699-705.

Oderda G, Chiorboli E, Haitink AR, et al, "Inhibition of Gastric Acidity in Children by Lansoprazole Granules," *Gastroent*, 1998, 114(4pt2): A295.

Ogilvie BW, Yerino P, Kazmi F, et al, "The Proton Pump Inhibitor, Omeprazole, But Not Lansoprazole or Pantoprazole, Is a Metabolism-Dependent Inhibitor of CYP2C19: Implications for Coadministration With Clopidogrel," *Drug Metab Dispos*, 2011, 39(11):2020-33.

Orenstein SR, Hassall E, Furmaga-Jablonska W, et al, "Multicenter, Double-Blind, Randomized, Placebo-Controlled Trial Assessing the Efficacy and Safety of Proton Pump Inhibitor Lansoprazole in Infants With Symptoms of Gastroesophageal Reflux Disease," *J Pediatr*, 2009, 154(4):514-20.

Scott LJ, "Lansoprazole: In the Management of Gastroesophageal Reflux Disease in Children," *Paediatr Drugs*, 2003, 5(1):57-61.

Springer M, Atkinson S, North J, et al, "Safety and Pharmacodynamics of Lansoprazole in Patients With Gastroesophageal Reflux Disease Aged <1 Year," *Paediatr Drugs*, 2008, 10(4):255-63.

Tran A, et al, "Pharmacokinetics/Pharmacodynamics Study of Oral Lansoprazole in Children," *Fundam Clin Pharmacol*, 1996, 10:A221.

Zhang W, Kukulka M, Witt G, et al, "Age-Dependent Pharmacokinetics of Lansoprazole in Neonates and Infants," *Paediatr Drugs*, 2008, 10 (4):265-74.

◆ **Lantus** *see* Insulin Glargine *on page 1121*

◆ **Lantus® (Can)** *see* Insulin Glargine *on page 1121*

◆ **Lantus® OptiSet® (Can)** *see* Insulin Glargine *on page 1121*

◆ **Lantus SoloStar** *see* Insulin Glargine *on page 1121*

◆ **Lanvis® (Can)** *see* Thioguanine *on page 2010*

◆ **L-Arginine** *see* Arginine *on page 195*

♦ **L-Arginine Hydrochloride** *see* Arginine *on page 195*

Laronidase (lair OH ni days)

Brand Names: U.S. Aldurazyme
Brand Names: Canada Aldurazyme®
Therapeutic Category Enzyme; Mucopolysaccharidosis I (MPS I) Disease, Treatment Agent
Generic Availability (U.S.) No
Use Treatment of patients with mucopolysaccharidosis I (MPS I) lysosomal storage disease who have one of the following clinical syndromes: Hurler's syndrome (severe), Hurler-Scheie syndrome (intermediate), or patients with the Scheie form who have moderate to severe symptoms
Pregnancy Risk Factor B
Pregnancy Considerations Teratogenic effects were not observed in animal reproduction studies. Patients are encouraged to enroll in the MPS I registry (800-745-4447 or www.MPSIregistry.com).
Breast-Feeding Considerations It is not known if laronidase is excreted in breast milk. The manufacturer recommends that caution be exercised when administering laronidase to nursing women.
Contraindications Hypersensitivity to laronidase or any component
Warnings Hypersensitivity reactions can occur at any time during laronidase therapy. Resuscitation equipment, oxygen, diphenhydramine, and a corticosteroid should be readily available to treat hypersensitivity or anaphylactic reactions. Use epinephrine with caution in patients with MPS I due to an increased prevalence of coronary artery disease in these patients. Injection contains polysorbate 80 (Tween 80®) which may cause allergic reactions in susceptible individuals. In premature neonates, thrombocytopenia, ascites, pulmonary deterioration, and renal and hepatic failure have been reported after receiving parenteral products containing polysorbate 80 (Alade, 1986; *MMWR*, 1984). Infusion of polysorbate 80-containing solutions through polyvinyl chloride tubing may cause DEHP to leach into the solution; in immature animals, exposure to DEHP may adversely affect the development of the male reproductive tract.
Precautions The risks and benefits of administering laronidase following a severe anaphylactic or hypersensitivity reaction should be considered. If laronidase is to be readministered, use caution and have appropriate resuscitation measures available.
Adverse Reactions
Cardiovascular: Chest pain, edema, facial edema, flushing, hyper-/hypotension, pallor, poor venous access, tachycardia
Central nervous system: Chills, fever, headache
Dermatologic: Hyperhidrosis, pruritus, rash, urticaria
Gastrointestinal: Abdominal pain/discomfort, diarrhea, vomiting
Hematologic: Thrombocytopenia
Hepatic: Bilirubinemia
Immunologic: Antibody development
Local: Abscess, injection site pain, injection site reaction
Neuromuscular & skeletal: Arthralgia, back pain, hyperreflexia, musculoskeletal pain, paresthesia, tremor
Ocular: Corneal opacity
Otic: Otitis media
Respiratory: Bronchospasm, cough, crepitations, dyspnea, oxygen saturation decreased, respiratory distress, upper respiratory tract infection, wheezing
Miscellaneous: Allergic reaction, feeling warm/cold, infusion reactions
Rare but important or life-threatening: Anaphylaxis, angioedema, cardiac failure, cardiorespiratory arrest, cyanosis, erythema, extravasation, pneumonia, respiratory failure

Drug Interactions
Metabolism/Transport Effects None known.
Avoid Concomitant Use There are no known interactions where it is recommended to avoid concomitant use.
Increased Effect/Toxicity There are no known significant interactions involving an increase in effect.
Decreased Effect There are no known significant interactions involving a decrease in effect.
Stability Store vials in refrigerator at 2°C to 8°C (36°F to 46°F). Do not freeze or shake. Diluted infusion solution is stable for up to 32 hours when stored at 2°C to 8°C (36°F to 46°F). Do not mix laronidase with any other drugs. Prepare the infusion using a low protein-binding container (there is no compatability information of diluted laronidase in glass containers). Total volume of infusion is determined by body weight. For patients weighing ≤20 kg (or weighing up to 30 kg and with cardiac or respiratory compromise), dilute the required dose in 100 mL NS; for patients weighing >20 kg, dilute required dose in 250 mL NS. Determine the number of vials to dilute by calculating the required dose and rounding up to the nearest whole vial. Remove and discard a volume of NS from the infusion bag equal to the volume of the calculated dose of laronidase. Slowly withdraw from vial(s) and slowly add laronidase to the NS; avoid excessive agitation, do not use filter needle. Gently rotate infusion bag to mix (do not shake).
Mechanism of Action Laronidase is a recombinant (replacement) form of α-L-iduronidase derived from Chinese hamster cells. α-L-iduronidase is an enzyme needed to break down endogenous glycosaminoglycans (GAGs) within lysosomes. A deficiency of α-L-iduronidase leads to an accumulation of GAGs, causing cellular, tissue, and organ dysfunction as seen in MPS I. Improved pulmonary function and walking capacity have been demonstrated with the administration of laronidase to patients with Hurler, Hurler-Scheie, or Scheie (with moderate-to-severe symptoms) forms of MPS.
Pharmacokinetics (Adult data unless noted)
Distribution: V_d: 0.24 to 0.6 L/kg
Half-life: 1.5-3.6 hours
Clearance: Plasma: 1.7 to 2.7 mL/minute/kg
Dosing: Usual Children, Adolescents, and Adults: I.V. infusion: 0.58 mg/kg/dose once weekly
Administration I.V. infusion:
Determine the number of vials to be diluted. Remove vials from the refrigerator and allow them to reach room temperature. Do not use if the solution is discolored or contains particulate matter. Determine the total infusion volume based on the patient's weight [dose delivered in a total volume of 100 mL (≤20 kg) or 250 mL (>20 kg)]
From an NS infusion bag, remove and discard volume of NS equal to volume of laronidase injection solution to be added to the infusion bag. Add laronidase; do not agitate solution as it denatures the enzyme. Administer with an in-line, low protein binding 0.2 micron filter.
An initial 10 mcg/kg/hour infusion rate may be incrementally increased every 15 minutes during the first hour if tolerated; increase to a maximum infusion rate of 200 mcg/kg/hour which is maintained for the remainder of the infusion (approximately 3 hours). See the following:
Initial infusion rate: 10 mcg/kg/hour for 15 minutes: If stable, increase rate to:
20 mcg/kg/hour for 15 minutes: If stable, increase rate to:
50 mcg/kg/hour for 15 minutes: If stable, increase rate to:
100 mcg/kg/hour for 15 minutes: If stable, increase rate to:
200 mcg/kg/hour for ~3 hours (remainder of the infusion)
Monitoring Parameters Vital signs, FVC, height, weight, range of motion, serum antibodies to α-L-iduronidase, urine levels of glycosaminoglycans (GAG), change in liver size

Dosage Forms Excipient information presented when available (limited, particularly for generics); consult specific product labeling.

Solution, Intravenous:

Aldurazyme: 2.9 mg/5 mL (5 mL) [contains mouse protein (murine) (hamster), polysorbate 80]

References

Alade SL, Brown RE, and Paquet A Jr, "Polysorbate 80 and E-Ferol Toxicity," *Pediatrics*, 1986, 77(4):593-7.

Centers for Disease Control (CDC), "Unusual Syndrome With Fatalities Among Premature Infants: Association With a New Intravenous Vitamin E Product," *MMWR Morb Mortal Wkly Rep*, 1984, 33 (14):198-9.

Kakkis ED, Muenzer J, Tiller GE, et al, "Enzyme-Replacement Therapy in Mucopolysaccharidosis I," *N Engl J Med*, 2001, 344(3):182-8.

◆ **Lasix** *see* Furosemide *on page 948*

◆ **Lasix Special (Can)** *see* Furosemide *on page 948*

◆ **L-ASP** *see* Asparaginase *(E. coli) on page 208*

◆ **L-asparaginase (E. coli)** *see* Asparaginase *(E. coli) on page 208*

◆ **L-asparaginase (Erwinia)** *see* Asparaginase *(Erwinia) on page 211*

◆ **L-asparaginase with Polyethylene Glycol** *see* Pegaspargase *on page 1615*

◆ **Lassar's Zinc Paste** *see* Zinc Oxide *on page 2176*

◆ **Latrodectus Antivenin** *see* Antivenin *(Latrodectus mactans) on page 185*

◆ **Latrodectus Antivenom** *see* Antivenin *(Latrodectus mactans) on page 185*

◆ **Latrodectus mactans Antivenin** *see* Antivenin *(Latrodectus mactans) on page 185*

◆ **Latrodectus mactans Antivenom** *see* Antivenin *(Latrodectus mactans) on page 185*

◆ **Lavacol® [OTC]** *see* Alcohol (Ethyl) *on page 88*

◆ **Lavoclen-4 Acne Wash** *see* Benzoyl Peroxide *on page 275*

◆ **Lavoclen-4 Creamy Wash** *see* Benzoyl Peroxide *on page 275*

◆ **Lavoclen-8 Acne Wash** *see* Benzoyl Peroxide *on page 275*

◆ **Lavoclen-8 Creamy Wash** *see* Benzoyl Peroxide *on page 275*

◆ **Laxa Basic [OTC]** *see* Docusate *on page 701*

◆ **Laxative [OTC]** *see* Bisacodyl *on page 293*

◆ **Laxilose (Can)** *see* Lactulose *on page 1193*

◆ **Lazanda** *see* FentaNYL *on page 853*

◆ **l-Bunolol Hydrochloride** *see* Levobunolol *on page 1223*

◆ **LC-4 Lidocaine [OTC]** *see* Lidocaine (Topical) *on page 1242*

◆ **LC-5 Lidocaine [OTC]** *see* Lidocaine (Topical) *on page 1242*

◆ **L-Carnitine** *see* LevOCARNitine *on page 1224*

◆ **LCD** *see* Coal Tar *on page 532*

◆ **LCM** *see* Lacosamide *on page 1189*

◆ **Lederle Leucovorin (Can)** *see* Leucovorin Calcium *on page 1213*

◆ **Lepargylic Acid** *see* Azelaic Acid *on page 244*

◆ **Lescol** *see* Fluvastatin *on page 920*

◆ **Lescol XL** *see* Fluvastatin *on page 920*

Letrozole (LET roe zole)

Medication Safety Issues

Sound-alike/look-alike issues:

Femara may be confused with Famvir, femhrt, Provera

Letrozole may be confused with anastrozole

International issues:

Letaris, a formerly marketed Dutch brand name product for letrozole, may be confused with Letairis, a U.S. brand name for ambrisentan.

Related Information

Safe Handling of Hazardous Drugs *on page 2419*

Brand Names: U.S. Femara

Brand Names: Canada Apo-Letrozole; Auro-Letrozole; Bio-Letrozole; Femara; JAMP-Letrozole; Letrozole Tablets, USP; Mar-Letrozole; MED-Letrozole; Myl-Letrozole; PMS-Letrozole; RAN-Letrozole; Sandoz-Letrozole; Teva-Letrozole; Zinda-Letrozole

Therapeutic Category Antineoplastic Agent, Aromatase Inhibitor

Generic Availability (U.S.) Yes

Use Adjuvant treatment of hormone receptor positive early breast cancer, extended adjuvant treatment of early breast cancer after 5 years of tamoxifen, first-line treatment of hormone receptor positive or hormone receptor unknown, locally advanced or metastatic breast cancer; treatment of advanced breast cancer with disease progression following antiestrogen therapy (All indications: FDA approved in postmenopausal women); has also been used in treatment of precocious puberty associated with McCune-Albright Syndrome (MAS) in girls; constitutional delay of growth and puberty (not due to growth hormone deficiency) and idiopathic short stature in boys

Pregnancy Risk Factor X

Pregnancy Considerations Adverse events were observed in animal reproduction studies. Letrozole is FDA indicated for postmenopausal women only (no clinical benefit for breast cancer has been demonstrated in premenopausal women). Use in women who are or who may become pregnant is contraindicated. Women who are perimenopausal or recently postmenopausal should use adequate contraception until postmenopausal status is fully established.

Breast-Feeding Considerations It is not known if letrozole is excreted in breast milk. Due to the potential for serious adverse reactions in the nursing infant, a decision should be made whether to discontinue nursing or to discontinue the drug, taking into account the importance of treatment to the mother.

Contraindications Hypersensitivity to letrozole or any component of the formulation; pregnancy

Warnings Hazardous agent; use appropriate precautions for handling and disposal (NIOSH, 2012). May cause decreases in bone mineral density (BMD); a decrease in hip BMD by 3.8% from baseline in letrozole-treated patients vs 2% in placebo at 2 years has been demonstrated; however, there was no statistical difference in changes to the lumbar spine BMD scores; monitor BMD. In males treated for idiopathic short stature, trabecular bone and vertebral-body deformities were observed; consider prior to therapy initiation, and monitor patients closely (Palmert, 2012). May increase total serum cholesterol; in patients treated for breast cancer with adjuvant therapy and cholesterol levels within normal limits, an increase of >1.5 x ULN in total cholesterol has been demonstrated in 8.2% of letrozole-treated patients (25% requiring lipid-lowering medications) vs 3.2% of tamoxifen-treated patients (16% requiring medications). Monitor cholesterol panel; may require antihyperlipidemics. May cause CNS depression (eg, dizziness, fatigue, and somnolence); patients should be cautioned before performing tasks which require mental alertness (eg, operating machinery or driving).

Precautions Use with caution in patients with hepatic impairment; dose adjustment recommended in patients with cirrhosis or severe hepatic dysfunction.

Adverse Reactions

Cardiovascular: Angina; cerebrovascular accident including hemorrhagic stroke, thrombotic stroke; chest pain, hypertension, MI, peripheral edema; thromboembolic event including venous thrombosis, thrombophlebitis, portal vein thrombosis, pulmonary embolism; transient ischemic attack

Central nervous system: Anxiety, depression, dizziness, fatigue, headache, insomnia, pain, somnolence, vertigo

Dermatologic: Alopecia, pruritus, rash

Endocrine & metabolic: Breast pain, hot flashes, hypercholesterolemia, hypercalcemia

Gastrointestinal: Abdominal pain, anorexia, constipation, diarrhea, dyspepsia, nausea, vomiting, weight gain, weight loss

Genitourinary: Urinary tract infection, vaginal bleeding, vaginal dryness, vaginal hemorrhage, vaginal irritation

Neuromuscular & skeletal: Arthralgia, arthritis, back pain, bone fracture, bone mineral density decreased, bone pain, limb pain, musculoskeletal pain, myalgia, osteoporosis, weakness

Ocular: Cataract

Renal: Renal disorder

Respiratory: Cough, dyspnea, pleural effusion

Miscellaneous: Diaphoresis, infection, influenza, night sweats, secondary malignancy, viral infection

Rare but important or life-threatening: Anaphylactic reaction, angioedema, arterial thrombosis, cardiac failure, carpal tunnel syndrome, endometrial cancer, endometrial hyperplasia, endometrial proliferation, erythema multiforme, hepatitis, leukopenia, memory impairment, stomatitis, tachycardia, thrombocytopenia, toxic epidermal necrolysis, trigger finger

Drug Interactions

Metabolism/Transport Effects Substrate (minor) of CYP2A6, 3A4; **Inhibits** CYP2A6 (strong), 2C19 (weak)

Avoid Concomitant Use

Avoid concomitant use of Letrozole with any of the following: Tegafur

Increased Effect/Toxicity Letrozole may increase the levels/effects of CYP2A6 substrates; example substrates include dexmedetomidine and ifosfamide.

Decreased Effect

Letrozole may decrease the levels/effects of: Cardiac Glycosides; Tegafur; Vitamin K Antagonists

The levels/effects of Letrozole may be decreased by: Tamoxifen

Stability Store at 25°C (77°F); excursions permitted to 15°C to 30°C (59°F to 86°F).

Mechanism of Action Nonsteroidal competitive inhibitor of the aromatase enzyme system which binds to the heme group of aromatase, a cytochrome P450 enzyme which catalyzes conversion of androgens to estrogens (specifically, androstenedione to estrone and testosterone to estradiol). This leads to inhibition of the enzyme and a significant reduction in plasma estrogen (estrone, estradiol and estrone sulfate) levels. Does not affect synthesis of adrenal or thyroid hormones, aldosterone, or androgens.

Pharmacodynamics Maximum effect: Plasma estradiol, estrone and estrone sulfate suppression: 2-3 days

Pharmacokinetics (Adult data unless noted)

Absorption: Rapid and well absorbed; not affected by food

Distribution: V_d: ~1.9 L/kg

Protein binding: Weak

Metabolism: Hepatic via CYP3A4 and CYP2A6 to an inactive carbinol metabolite

Half-life elimination: Terminal: ~2 days

Time to steady state serum concentration: 2-6 weeks; steady state serum concentrations are 1.5-2 times higher than single-dose values. In girls 3-9 years, steady state concentrations were 25% to 67% that of the mean adult values (Feuillan, 2007)

Half-life elimination: Terminal: ~2 days

Elimination: Urine (90%; 6% as unchanged drug, 75% as glucuronide carbinol metabolite; 9% as unidentified metabolites)

Dosing: Usual

Pediatric:

Delayed puberty and growth [CDGP (constitutional delay of growth and puberty)] (males): Very limited data available: Adolescents ≥14 years: Oral: 2.5 mg once daily in combination with testosterone therapy; dosing from a double-blind placebo-controlled trial of 33 adolescent males (treatment group: n=11); during the 12 months of therapy, bone maturation was delayed, predicted adult height values were significantly increased and markers of puberty progressed (Palmert; 2012; Wickman, 2001); further studies are needed.

McCune-Albright syndrome; precocious puberty (females): Very limited data available: Children >2-10 years at time of treatment initiation: Oral: Initial: 0.5 mg/m^2/day divided every 12 hours for days 1-7, then 1 mg/m^2/day divided every 12 hours on days 8-14, then 1.5 mg/m^2/day divided every 12 hours beginning on day 15; if needed, may further increase to 2 mg/m^2/day if markers of precocious puberty including serum estradiol levels progress. Dosing based on a pilot study of nine girls (3-8 years at time of therapy initiation) which showed long-term therapy (up to 36 months) decreased rates of growth and bone maturation; although ovarian volume decreased during the first 6 months of treatment, the mean ovarian volume increased over 1-2 years of therapy with cyst redevelopment in some patients. During the pilot study, dosing was divided twice daily to alleviate GI discomfort; however, pharmacokinetic analysis showed once daily dosing would be appropriate for young children if tolerated (Feuillan, 2007). In a case series (n=3, age range at treatment: 3-7 years), a fixed dose of 2.5 mg once daily was used for 5-19 months duration (Bercaw-Pratt, 2012).

Short-stature; idiopathic (males): Limited data available: Children and Adolescents 9-16 years: Oral: 2.5 mg once daily; dosing based experience in a double-blind, placebo-controlled trial of 30 males (treatment group: n=16; age range: 9-14 years) and a retrospective observation (n= 24; age range: 9-16 years); the duration of letrozole therapy was up to 2 years (range: 4-24 months); bone maturation delay with increases in predicted adult height values were observed with treatment (Hero, 2005; Karmazin, 2005; Shulman, 2008)

Adults: Females: Postmenopausal:

Breast cancer, advanced (first- or second-line treatment): Oral: 2.5 mg once daily; continue until tumor progression

Breast cancer, early (adjuvant treatment): Oral: 2.5 mg once daily; optimal duration unknown, duration in clinical trial is 5 years; discontinue at relapse

Breast cancer, early (extended adjuvant treatment): Oral: 2.5 mg once daily; optimal duration unknown, duration in clinical trials is 5 years (after 5 years of tamoxifen); discontinue at relapse

Dosing adjustment in renal impairment: Adults: CrCl ≥10 mL/minute: No dosage adjustment is required.

Dosing adjustment in hepatic impairment: Adults:

Mild to moderate impairment (Child-Pugh class A or B): No adjustment recommended

Severe impairment (Child-Pugh class C) or cirrhosis: 2.5 mg every other day

Administration Hazardous agent; use appropriate precautions for handling and disposal (NIOSH, 2012). May administer without regard to meals.

Monitoring Parameters Monitor periodically during therapy: Complete blood counts, thyroid function tests; serum electrolytes, cholesterol, transaminases, and creatinine; blood pressure; bone density

Delayed puberty and short stature: In the pediatric clinical trials (study durations: 1-2 years) the following were monitored (at baseline, and then typically 2 months, 5 months, 12 months, and 18 months): Growth indices (height, adult height predictions, bone age, lumbar and femoral bone mineral density), Tanner stage and serum concentration of key hormones, and other biochemical markers (eg, 17-B estradiol, LH, FSH, testosterone), lipid profile (Hero, 2005; Shulman, 2008; Wickman, 2001)

McCune-Albright syndrome: In the pediatric clinical trial (study duration: 12-36 months), the following were monitored (baseline, every 6 months): Rates of growth and bone age advance, levels of indices of bone metabolism (eg, osteocalcin and alkaline phosphatase); and urinary markers of steroid metabolism (eg, hydroxyproline, pyridinoline, etc.), mean ovarian volume, episodes of vaginal bleeding and serum concentrations of estradiol. (Feuillan, 2007)

Dosage Forms Excipient information presented when available (limited, particularly for generics); consult specific product labeling.

Tablet, Oral:
Femara: 2.5 mg
Generic: 2.5 mg

References

Feuillan P, Calis K, Hill S, Shawker T, Robey PG, Collins MT. Letrozole treatment of precocious puberty in girls with McCune-Albright syndrome: a pilot study. *J Clin Endocrinol Metab*. 2007;92:2100-2106.

Hero M, Norjavaara E, Dunkel L. Inhibition of estrogen biosynthesis with a potent aromatase inhibitor increases predicted adult height in boys with idiopathic short stature: a randomized controlled trial. *J Clin Endocrinol Metab*. 2005;90:6396-6402.

Karmazin A, Moore WV, Popovic J, Jacobson JD. The effect of letrozole on bone age progression, predicted adult height, and adrenal gland function. *J Pediatr Endocrinol Metab*. 2005;18:285-293.

National Institute for Occupational Safety and Health (NIOSH). NIOSH list of antineoplastic and other hazardous drugs in healthcare settings 2012. Available at http://www.cdc.gov/niosh/docs/2012-150/pdfs/2012-150.pdf. Accessed January 21, 2013.

Palmert MR, Dunkel L. Clinical practice. Delayed puberty. *N Engl J Med*. 2012;366(5):443-453.

Shulman DI, Francis GL, Palmert MR, et al. Use of aromatase inhibitors in children and adolescents with disorders of growth and adolescent development. *Pediatrics*. 2008;121(4):e975-983.

Wickman S, Dunkel L. Inhibition of P450 aromatase enhances gonadotropin secretion in early and midpubertal boys: evidence for a pituitary site of action of endogenous E. *J Clin Endocrinol Metab*. 2001;86 (10):4887-4894.

Wickman S, Sipilä I, Ankarberg-Lindgren C, Norjavaara E, Dunkel L. A specific aromatase inhibitor and potential increase in adult height in boys with delayed puberty: a randomised controlled. *Lancet*. 2001;357:1743-1748.

◆ **Letrozole Tablets, USP (Can)** *see* Letrozole *on page 1211*

◆ **Leucovorin** *see* Leucovorin Calcium *on page 1213*

Leucovorin Calcium (loo koe VOR in KAL see um)

Medication Safety Issues

Sound-alike/look-alike issues:

Leucovorin may be confused with Leukeran, Leukine, LEVOleucovorin

Folinic acid may be confused with folic acid

Folinic acid is an error prone synonym and should not be used

Brand Names: Canada Lederle Leucovorin

Therapeutic Category Antidote, Methotrexate; Folic Acid Derivative

Generic Availability (U.S.) Yes

Use Reduction of toxic effects of high dose methotrexate ("leucovorin rescue"); to diminish the toxicity and counteract the effects of impaired methotrexate elimination or as

an antidote for folic acid antagonist overdosage; treatment of folate deficient megaloblastic anemias of infancy, sprue, or pregnancy; nutritional deficiency when oral folate therapy is not possible; adjunctive treatment with sulfadiazine and pyrimethamine to prevent hematologic toxicity; combined with fluorouracil to prolong survival in the palliative treatment of patients with advanced colorectal cancer (FDA approved in adults); has also been used as adjunctive cofactor therapy in methanol toxicity

Pregnancy Risk Factor C

Pregnancy Considerations Animal reproduction studies have not been conducted. Leucovorin is a biologically active form of folic acid. Adequate amounts of folic acid are recommended during pregnancy. Refer to Folic Acid monograph.

Breast-Feeding Considerations Leucovorin is a biologically active form of folic acid. Adequate amounts of folic acid are recommended in breast-feeding women. Refer to Folic Acid monograph.

Contraindications Hypersensitivity to leucovorin or any component; pernicious anemia and other megaloblastic anemias secondary to the lack of vitamin B_{12}; not to be administered by intrathecal or intraventricular route (may be harmful or fatal)

Warnings Administer promptly; when the time interval between administration of folic acid antagonists and leucovorin rescue increases, its effectiveness in treatment of toxicity diminishes. In the treatment of accidental overdosages of intrathecally administered folic acid antagonists, do not administer leucovorin intrathecally as it **may be harmful or fatal if administered intrathecally**. Leucovorin enhances the toxicity of fluorouracil; when used in combination, the dosage of fluorouracil should be reduced. Combination therapy should not be initiated or continued in patients who have symptoms of GI toxicity of any severity until the symptoms have resolved; rapid clinical deterioration including death may occur; monitor combination use closely. Concomitant use with trimethoprim/sulfamethoxazole for the acute treatment of *Pneumocystis jirovecii* pneumonia in patients with HIV infection has been associated with increased rates of treatment failure and morbidity.

Precautions Parenteral therapy is recommended over oral therapy in cases where the patient is unable to tolerate oral treatment due to vomiting. Due to saturation of oral absorption with oral doses >25 mg, I.V. administration is recommended for doses >25 mg. Methotrexate serum concentrations should be monitored closely to determine the dose and duration of leucovorin rescue. Leucovorin doses may be increased, frequencies of administration altered, and duration of therapy increased depending upon the methotrexate clearance. Ascites, pleural effusion, renal insufficiency, and inadequate hydration may prolong methotrexate clearance. Refer to individual protocols or "Leucovorin Rescue Dose" graph for leucovorin dosage adjustment recommendations.

Adverse Reactions

Dermatologic: Rash, pruritus, erythema, urticaria

Hematologic: Thrombocytosis

Respiratory: Wheezing

Miscellaneous: Allergic reactions, anaphylactoid reactions

Drug Interactions

Metabolism/Transport Effects None known.

Avoid Concomitant Use

Avoid concomitant use of Leucovorin Calcium with any of the following: Raltitrexed; Trimethoprim

Increased Effect/Toxicity

Leucovorin Calcium may increase the levels/effects of: Capecitabine; Fluorouracil (Systemic); Fluorouracil (Topical); Tegafur

Decreased Effect

Leucovorin Calcium may decrease the levels/effects of: Fosphenytoin; PHENobarbital; Phenytoin; Primidone; Raltitrexed; Trimethoprim

The levels/effects of Leucovorin Calcium may be decreased by: Glucarpidase

Stability

Powder for injection: Store at room temperature of 25°C (77°F). Protect from light. Solutions reconstituted with bacteriostatic water for injection USP must be used within 7 days. When doses >10 mg/m² are used, prepare leucovorin with preservative free SWI to decrease the amount of benzyl alcohol intake; solutions reconstituted with SWI must be used immediately. Parenteral admixture is stable for 24 hours stored at room temperature (25°C) and for 4 days when stored under refrigeration (4°C).

Solution for injection: Prior to dilution, store vials under refrigeration at 2°C to 8°C (36°F to 46°F). Protect from light.

Tablet: Store at room temperature of 15°C to 30°C (59°F to 86°F).

Mechanism of Action A reduced form of folic acid, leucovorin supplies the necessary cofactor blocked by methotrexate. Leucovorin actively competes with methotrexate for transport sites, displaces methotrexate from intracellular binding sites, and restores active folate stores required for DNA/RNA synthesis. Stabilizes the binding of 5-dUMP and thymidylate synthetase, enhancing the activity of fluorouracil. When administered with pyrimethamine for the treatment of opportunistic infections, leucovorin reduces the risk for hematologic toxicity (DHHS, 2013).

Methanol toxicity treatment: Formic acid (methanol's toxic metabolite) is normally metabolized to carbon dioxide and water by 10-formyltetrahydrofolate dehydrogenase after being bound to tetrahydrofolate. Administering a source of tetrahydrofolate may aid the body in eliminating formic acid (Barceloux, 2002).

Pharmacodynamics Onset of action:

Oral: Within 30 minutes

I.V.: Within 5 minutes

Pharmacokinetics (Adult data unless noted)

Absorption: Oral, I.M.: Rapid

Metabolism: Rapidly converted to (5MTHF) 5-methyl-tetrahydrofolate (active) in the intestinal mucosa and by the liver

Bioavailability:

Oral absorption is saturable in doses >25 mg; apparent bioavailability:

Tablet, 25 mg: 97%

Tablet, 50 mg: 75%

Tablet, 100 mg: 37%

Tablet, 200 mg: 31%

Injection solution, when administered orally, provides equivalent bioavailability

Half-life: Adults: ~4-8 hours

Time to peak serum concentration:

Oral: ~2 hours

I.V. total folates: 10 minutes

5MTHF: ~1 hour

Elimination: Primarily in urine (80% to 90%) with small losses appearing in feces (5% to 8%)

Dosing: Usual Children and Adults:

Treatment of weak folic acid antagonist overdosage (eg, pyrimethamine, trimethoprim): Oral: 5-15 mg/day for 3 days or until blood counts are normal or 5 mg every 3 days; doses of 6 mg/day are needed for patients with platelet counts <100,000/mm³

Folate deficient megaloblastic anemia: I.M.: ≤1 mg/day

Megaloblastic anemia secondary to congenital deficiency of dihydrofolate reductase: I.M.: 3-6 mg/day

Leucovorin rescue (following methotrexate dosing of 12-15 g/m²): I.V.: 10 mg/m² (15 mg in adults) to start, then 10 mg/m² (15 mg in adults) every 6 hours orally for 72 hours; if serum creatinine 24 hours after methotrexate administration is elevated ≥50% **or** the serum methotrexate concentration is >5 x 10⁻⁶ M, increase leucovorin dose to 100 mg/m²/dose (150 mg in adults) every 3 hours until serum methotrexate concentration is less than 1 x 10⁻⁸ M (see graph for further dosing recommendations as a function of plasma methotrexate concentration vs time); if methotrexate clearance is delayed, continue leucovorin therapy until methotrexate concentration is 0.05 x 10⁻⁸ M

LEUCOVORIN RESCUE DOSE
(Determined by Plasma Methotrexate Level and Time After Start of Methotrexate Infusion)

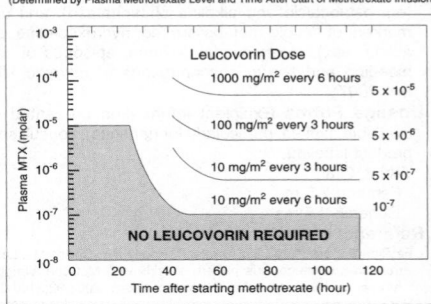

Prevention of pyrimethamine hematologic toxicity: Infants, Children, Adolescents, and Adults: Oral: Dosage varies according to specific toxoplasmosis regimen (treatment or prophylaxis), see Pyrimethamine monograph for specific regimen details (CDC, 2009)

Colorectal cancer: Adults: I.V.: 200 mg/m² in combination with fluorouracil 370 mg/m² or 20 mg/m² used in combination with fluorouracil 425 mg/m²; treatment is daily for 5 days and repeated at 4-5 week intervals; refer to individual protocols

Methotrexate overdose: **Note:** The amount of leucovorin administered should equal the amount of methotrexate inadvertently administered. I.V.: 1 mg per mg of methotrexate inadvertently administered; 100-1000 mg/m² every 3-6 hours has been used; administer until methotrexate concentrations decrease to goal concentration or longer if methotrexate concentrations are unavailable or if patient has renal dysfunction or third-space storage (ascite, pleural effusion)

An approximate nomogram for leucovorin rescue in cancer patients receiving high-dose methotrexate based upon a 48-hour methotrexate concentration may be considered (Widemann, 2006). Leucovorin dosage and frequency based on the methotrexate concentration:

≥80 micromole/L: 1000 mg/m² every 6 hours

≥8 to <80 micromole/L: 100 mg/m² every 3 hours

≥2 to <8 micromole/L: 10 mg/m² every 3 hours

≥0.1 to <2 micromole/L: 10 mg/m² every 6 hours

Use of I.T. leucovorin is not advised (Jardine, 1996; Smith, 2008).

Post I.T. methotrexate: I.V.: Post high-dose methotrexate: 100-1000 mg/m²/dose until the serum methotrexate concentration is less than 1 x 10⁻⁷ molar

Cofactor therapy in methanol toxicity: I.V.: 1 mg/kg (maximum dose: 50 mg) over 30-60 minutes every 4-6 hours. Therapy should continue until methanol and formic acid have been completely eliminated (Barceloux, 2002)

Administration

Oral: **This drug should be given parenterally instead of orally in patients with GI toxicity, nausea, vomiting, and when individual doses are >25 mg.**

Parenteral: I.M., I.V.: Reconstitute 50 mg or 100 mg powder for injection vials with 5-10 mL SWI (350 mg vial requires 17 mL diluent resulting in 20 mg/mL final concentration); for I.V. administration, infuse at a maximum rate of 160 mg/minute; **not for intrathecal or intraventricular administration.**

Monitoring Parameters

Leucovorin rescue: CBC with differential; plasma methotrexate concentrations, serum creatinine. Leucovorin is continued until the plasma methotrexate concentration is less than 1×10^{-7} molar or $<0.5 \times 10^{-7}$ molar in situations of delayed methotrexate clearance. Each dose of leucovorin is increased if the plasma methotrexate concentration is excessively high. With 4- to 6-hour high-dose methotrexate infusions, plasma drug values in excess of 5×10^{-5} and 10^{-6} molar at 24 and 48 hours after starting the infusion, respectively, are often predictive of delayed methotrexate clearance; see leucovorin rescue dose graph.

When used with fluorouracil: CBC with differential, platelets, LFTs, electrolytes

Dosage Forms

Excipient information presented when available (limited, particularly for generics); consult specific product labeling.

Solution, Injection [strength expressed as base]:
Generic: 300 mg/30 mL (30 mL)

Solution Reconstituted, Injection [strength expressed as base]:
Generic: 100 mg (1 ea); 200 mg (1 ea); 350 mg (1 ea); 500 mg (1 ea)

Solution Reconstituted, Injection [strength expressed as base, preservative free]:
Generic: 50 mg (1 ea); 100 mg (1 ea); 200 mg (1 ea); 350 mg (1 ea)

Tablet, Oral [strength expressed as base]:
Generic: 5 mg, 10 mg, 15 mg, 25 mg

Extemporaneous Preparations

A 5 mg/mL oral suspension may be prepared with tablets, Cologel, and a 2:1 mixture of simple syrup and wild cherry syrup. Crush twenty-four 25 mg tablets in a glass mortar and reduce to a fine powder; transfer powder to amber bottle. Add 30 mL Cologel and shake mixture thoroughly. Add a quantity of syrup mixture sufficient to make 120 mL. Label "shake well" and "refrigerate". Stable for 28 days refrigerated.

Lam MS. Extemporaneous Compounding of Oral Liquid Dosage Formulations and Alternative Drug Delivery Methods for Anticancer Drugs. *Pharmacotherapy.* 2011;31(2):164-192.

References

Centers for Disease Control and Prevention, "Guidelines for the Prevention and Treatment of Opportunistic Infections Among HIV-Exposed and HIV-Infected Children," *MMWR Recomm Rep,* 2009, 58(RR-11):1-164. Available at http://aidsinfo.nih.gov/contentfiles/Pediatric_OI.pdf

Barceloux DG, Bond GR, Krenzelok EP, et al, "American Academy of Clinical Toxicology Practice Guidelines on the Treatment of Methanol Poisoning," *J Toxicol Clin Toxicol,* 2002, 40(4):415-46.

Jardine LF, Ingram LC, and Bleyer WA, "Intrathecal Leucovorin After Intrathecal Methotrexate Overdose," *J Pediatr Hematol Oncol,* 1996, 18(3):302-4.

Smith SW and Nelson LS, "Case Files of the New York City Poison Control Center: Antidotal Strategies for the Management of Methotrexate Toxicity," *J Med Toxicol,* 2008, 4(2):132-40.

Widemann BC and Adamson PC, "Understanding and Managing Methotrexate Nephrotoxicity," *Oncologist,* 2006, 11(6):694-703.

◆ **Leukeran** *see* Chlorambucil *on page 437*

◆ **Leukeran® (Can)** *see* Chlorambucil *on page 437*

◆ **Leukine** *see* Sargramostim *on page 1870*

Leuprolide (loo PROE lide)

Medication Safety Issues

Sound-alike/look-alike issues:
Lupron Depot (1-month or 3-month formulation) may be confused with Lupron Depot-Ped (1-month or 3-month formulation)

Lupron Depot-Ped is available in two formulations, a 1-month formulation and a 3-month formulation. Both formulations offer an 11.25 mg strength which may further add confusion.

Related Information

Safe Handling of Hazardous Drugs *on page 2419*

Brand Names: U.S. Eligard; Lupron Depot; Lupron Depot-Ped

Brand Names: Canada Eligard; Lupron; Lupron Depot

Therapeutic Category Antineoplastic Agent, Hormone (Gonadotropin Hormone-Releasing Analog); Luteinizing Hormone-Releasing Hormone Analog

Generic Availability (U.S.) Yes

Use Treatment of precocious puberty (FDA approved in females ages <8 years and males ages <9 years); palliative treatment of advanced prostate carcinoma (FDA approved in adults); treatment of anemia caused by uterine leiomyomata (fibroids) (FDA approved in adults); management of endometriosis (FDA approved in adults); has also been used in the treatment of breast cancer, infertility, and as a gonadotropin-releasing hormone analog (GnRHa) stimulation test

Pregnancy Risk Factor X

Pregnancy Considerations Adverse events were observed in animal reproduction studies. Pregnancy must be excluded prior to the start of treatment. Although leuprolide usually inhibits ovulation and stops menstruation, contraception is not ensured and a nonhormonal contraceptive should be used. Use is contraindicated in pregnant women.

Breast-Feeding Considerations It is not known if leuprolide is excreted into breast milk; use is contraindicated in nursing women.

Contraindications Hypersensitivity to leuprolide, gonadotropin-releasing hormone (GnRH), GnRH agonist analogs, or any component; pregnancy; breast-feeding

Warnings Hazardous agent; use appropriate precautions for handling and disposal (NIOSH, 2012); gonadotropin-releasing hormone (GnRH) analog treatment of rodents has shown an increased incidence of pituitary tumors. Urinary tract obstruction, bone pain, neuropathy, hematuria, or spinal cord compression may occur upon initiation of therapy. Decreased bone density has been reported when used for ≥6 months and may not be reversible. Leuprolide may cause spontaneous abortion or fetal harm when administered to a pregnant woman. Rare cases of pituitary apoplexy (frequently secondary to pituitary adenoma) have been observed with leuprolide administration (onset from 1 hour to usually <2 weeks after the first dose); may present as sudden headache, vomiting, visual or mental status changes, and infrequently cardiovascular collapse; immediate medical attention required. Seizures have been reported in patients receiving leuprolide. An increase in pubertal signs and symptoms may occur in the first 2-4 weeks of therapy due to the initial stimulatory effect of leuprolide before suppression occurs.

Leuprolide injection for subcutaneous use contains benzyl alcohol which may cause allergic reactions in susceptible individuals; large amounts of benzyl alcohol (≥99 mg/kg/day) have been associated with a potentially fatal toxicity ("gasping syndrome") in neonates; avoid use of leuprolide products containing benzyl alcohol in neonates; *in vitro* and animal studies have shown that benzoate, a metabolite of benzyl alcohol, displaces bilirubin from protein binding sites. Depot injection formulations may contain polysorbate 80 (Tween 80®) which may cause allergic reactions in susceptible individuals.

Precautions Use with caution in patients with risk factors for decreased bone mineral density (BMD) (ie, chronic alcohol or tobacco use, strong family history of osteoporosis, or chronic use of medications that can impact BMD, such as corticosteroids or anticonvulsants). Use caution in patients with a history of psychiatric illness; alteration in mood, memory impairment, and depression have been associated with use. Females treated for precocious puberty may experience menses or spotting during the first 2 months of treatment; notify healthcare provider if bleeding continues after the second month. Vehicle used in depot injectable formulations (polylactide-co-glycolide microspheres) has rarely been associated with retinal artery occlusion in patients with abnormal arteriovenous anastomosis. Due to differences in release properties, combinations of dosage forms or fractions of dosage forms should not be interchanged.

Adverse Reactions

Children (based on 1-month and 3-month pediatric formulations combined)

Cardiovascular: Vasodilation

Central nervous system: Emotional lability, headache, mood changes, pain

Dermatologic: Acne vulgaris, seborrhea, skin rash (including erythema multiforme)

Endocrine & metabolic: Weight gain

Genitourinary: Vaginal discharge, vaginal hemorrhage, vaginitis

Local: Injection site reaction, pain at injection site

Rare but important or life-threatening: Abnormal gait, alopecia, arthralgia, asthma, body odor, bradycardia, cervix disease, decreased visual acuity, depression, dysmenorrhea, dysphagia, epistaxis, excessive crying, feminization, gingivitis, goiter, growth suppression, gynecomastia, hirsutism, hyperhidrosis, hyperkinesia, hypersensitivity reaction, hypertension, infection, leukoderma, myopathy, obesity, peripheral edema, personality disorder, precocious puberty, purpura, skin striae, syncope, urinary incontinence

Adults: Note: For prostate cancer treatment, an initial rise in serum testosterone concentrations may cause "tumor flare" or worsening of symptoms, including bone pain, neuropathy, hematuria, or ureteral or bladder outlet obstruction during the first 2 weeks. Similarly, an initial increase in estradiol levels, with a temporary worsening of symptoms, may occur in women treated with leuprolide.

Delayed release formulations:

Cardiovascular: Angina pectoris, atrial fibrillation, bradycardia, cardiac arrhythmia, cardiac failure, edema, hypertension, hypotension, palpitations, syncope, tachycardia, thrombophlebitis (deep)

Central nervous system: Anxiety, confusion, delusions, dementia, depression, dizziness, fatigue, fever, headache, insomnia, nervousness, neuropathy, ostealgia, pain, paralysis, paresthesia, seizure

Dermatologic: Acne vulgaris, allergic skin reaction, alopecia, cellulitis, diaphoresis, pruritus, rash

Endocrine & metabolic: Decreased prostatic acid phosphatase, decreased serum bicarbonate, dehydration, gynecomastia, hirsutism, hot flash, hypercholesterolemia, hyperglycemia, hyperlipidemia, hyperuricemia, hypoalbuminemia, hypocholesterolemia, hypoproteinemia, increased prostatic acid phosphatase, libido decreased, menstrual disorder, weight changes

Gastrointestinal: Anorexia, change in bowel habits, constipation, diarrhea, dysphagia, gastric ulcer, gastroenteritis, gastrointestinal hemorrhage, intestinal obstruction, nausea and vomiting

Genitourinary: Balanitis, bladder spasm, dysuria, erectile dysfunction, genitourinary complaint, hematuria, impotence, lactation, mastalgia, nocturia, penile disease, testicular atrophy, testicular disease, testicular pain, urinary incontinence, urinary retention, urinary urgency, urinary tract infection, vaginitis

Hematologic & oncologic: Anemia, bruise, change in platelet count (increased), eosinophilia, leukopenia, lymphadenopathy

Hepatic: Abnormal hepatic function tests, hepatomegaly, prolonged partial thromboplastin time, prolonged prothrombin time

Hypersensitivity: Hypersensitivity reaction

Infection: Infection

Local: Burning sensation at injection site (transient), erythema at injection site, pain at injection site

Neuromuscular & skeletal: Arthralgia, arthropathy, myalgia, pathological fracture, weakness

Renal: Decreased urine specific gravity, increased blood urea nitrogen, increased serum creatinine, increased urine specific gravity, polyuria

Respiratory: Cough, dyspnea, emphysema, epistaxis, flu-like symptoms, hemoptysis, pleural effusion, pulmonary edema

Miscellaneous: Fever

Immediate release formulation:

Cardiovascular: Angina pectoris, cardiac arrhythmia, cardiac failure, ECG changes, heart murmur, hypertension, myocardial infarction, peripheral edema, pulmonary embolism, syncope, thrombophlebitis

Central nervous system: Anxiety, depression, dizziness, headache, insomnia, fatigue, fever, nervousness, ostealgia, pain, peripheral neuropathy

Endocrine & metabolic: decreased libido, diabetes mellitus, goiter, gynecomastia, hot flash, hypercalcemia, hypoglycemia

Dermatologic: Alopecia, dermatitis, hyperpigmentation, pruritus, skin lesion

Gastrointestinal: Anorexia, constipation, diarrhea, dysphagia, diarrhea, dysphagia, gastrointestinal hemorrhage, nausea and vomiting, peptic ulcer, rectal polyps

Genitourinary: Bladder spasm, decreased testicular size, dysuria, hematuria, impotence, incontinence, mastalgia, testicular pain, urinary frequency, urinary tract infection, urinary tract obstruction

Hematologic & oncologic: Anemia, bruise

Infection: Infection

Local: Injection site reaction

Neuromuscular & skeletal: Weakness

Ophthalmic: Blurred vision

Renal: Increased blood urea nitrogen, increased serum creatinine, hematuria

Respiratory: Cough, dyspnea, pneumonia, pulmonary fibrosis

Miscellaneous: Fever, inflammation

Children and Adults: *Any formulations:* Rare but important or life-threatening: Abscess at injection site, anaphylaxis, anaphylactoid reaction, asthma, bone fracture (spine), cerebrovascular accident, convulsions, coronary artery disease, decreased white blood cell count, diabetes mellitus, fibromyalgia syndrome (arthralgia/myalgia, headaches, GI distress), hemoptysis, hepatic injury, hepatic insufficiency, hepatotoxicity, hyperuricemia, hypokalemia, hypoproteinemia, induration at injection site, interstitial pulmonary disease, leukocytosis, myocardial infarction, osteopenia, paralysis, penile swelling, peripheral neuropathy; pituitary apoplexy (cardiovascular collapse, mental status altered, ophthalmoplegia, sudden headache, visual changes, vomiting); prolonged QT interval on ECG, prostate pain, pulmonary embolism, pulmonary infiltrates, retroperitoneal fibrosis (pelvic), seizure, skin photosensitivity, suicidal ideation (rare), tenosynovitis (symptoms), thrombocytopenia, transient ischemic attacks

Drug Interactions

Metabolism/Transport Effects None known.

Avoid Concomitant Use

Avoid concomitant use of Leuprolide with any of the following: Indium 111 Capromab Pendetide

Increased Effect/Toxicity There are no known significant interactions involving an increase in effect.

Decreased Effect

Leuprolide may decrease the levels/effects of: Antidiabetic Agents; Indium 111 Capromab Pendetide

Stability Hazardous agent; use appropriate precautions for handling and disposal (NIOSH, 2012).

Parenteral:

I.M.: Lupron Depot®, Lupron Depot-Ped®: Store at room temperature of 25°C (77°F); excursions permitted to 15°C to 30°C (59°F to 86°F)

SubQ:

Leuprolide acetate 5 mg/mL solution: Store at 20°C to 25°C (68°F to 77°F); excursions permitted to 15°C to 30°C (59°F to 86°F). Protect from light and store vial in carton until use. Do not freeze.

Eligard®: Store at 2°C to 8°C (36°F to 46°F). Allow to reach room temperature prior to using; once mixed, must be administered within 30 minutes.

Mechanism of Action Leuprolide, is an agonist of luteinizing hormone-releasing hormone (LHRH). Acting as a potent inhibitor of gonadotropin secretion; continuous administration results in suppression of ovarian and testicular steroidogenesis due to decreased levels of LH and FSH with subsequent decrease in testosterone (male) and estrogen (female) levels. In males, testosterone levels are reduced to below castrate levels. Leuprolide may also have a direct inhibitory effect on the testes, and act by a different mechanism not directly related to reduction in serum testosterone.

Pharmacodynamics

Onset of action: Serum testosterone levels first increase within 3 days of therapy, then decrease after 2-4 weeks with continued therapy

Onset of therapeutic suppression for precocious puberty:

Leuprolide: 2-4 weeks

Leuprolide depot: 1 month

Pharmacokinetics (Adult data unless noted)

Absorption: Requires parenteral administration since it is rapidly destroyed within the GI tract

Protein binding: 43% to 49%

Bioavailability: SubQ: 94%

Half-life: 3 hours

Elimination: Not well defined

Dosing: Usual

Children: **Precocious puberty: Note:** Initiate for girls <8 years or boys <9 years; consider discontinuing leuprolide therapy in girls by age 11 and boys by age 12.

I.M.:

Lupron Depot-Ped® (monthly formulation):

Manufacturer's labeling: Initial:

≤25 kg: 7.5 mg every 4 weeks; titrate dose in 3.75 mg increments every 4 weeks until clinical or laboratory tests indicate adequate suppression

>25-37.5 kg: 11.25 mg every 4 weeks; titrate dose in 3.75 mg increments every 4 weeks until clinical or laboratory tests indicate adequate suppression

>37.5 kg: 15 mg every 4 weeks; titrate dose in 3.75 mg increments every 4 weeks until clinical or laboratory tests indicate adequate suppression

Alternative dosing: Initial: 0.2-0.3 mg/kg/dose every 4 weeks (Carel, 2009)

Lupron Depot-Ped® (3-month formulation): 11.25 mg or 30 mg every 12 weeks

SubQ (Leuprolide acetate 5 mg/mL solution): Initial: 50 **mcg**/kg/dose once daily; may titrate dose upward by 10 **mcg**/kg/day if suppression of ovarian or testicular steroidogenesis is not achieved. **Note:** Higher **mcg**/kg doses may be required in younger children.

Leuprolide (GNrHa) Stimulation Test (Female): SubQ (Leuprolide acetate 5 mg/mL solution): 20 **mcg**/kg once; measure LH and FSH at baseline and after administration (usually two spaced measurements ≤120 minutes [eg, 30 and 60 minutes **or** 60 and 120 minutes]) (Houk, 2008; Sathasivam, 2010; Sathasivam, 2011)

Adults:

Advanced prostate cancer:

I.M.:

Lupron Depot® 7.5 mg (monthly): 7.5 mg every month **or**

Lupron Depot® 22.5 mg (3 month): 22.5 mg every 12 weeks **or**

Lupron Depot® 30 mg (4 month): 30 mg every 16 weeks **or**

Lupron Depot® 45 mg (6 month): 45 mg every 24 weeks

SubQ:

Eligard®: 7.5 mg monthly **or** 22.5 mg every 3 months **or** 30 mg every 4 months **or** 45 mg every 6 months

Leuprolide acetate 5 mg/mL solution: 1 mg/day

Endometriosis: I.M.: Initial therapy may be with leuprolide alone or in combination with norethindrone; if retreatment for an additional 6 months is necessary, concomitant norethindrone should be used. Retreatment is not recommended for longer than one additional 6-month course.

Lupron Depot®: 3.75 mg every month for up to 6 months **or**

Lupron Depot®-3 month: 11.25 mg every 3 months for up to 2 doses (6 months total duration of treatment)

Uterine leiomyomata (fibroids): I.M. (in combination with iron):

Lupron Depot®: 3.75 mg every month for up to 3 months **or**

Lupron Depot®-3 month: 11.25 mg as a single injection

Administration Hazardous agent; use appropriate precautions for handling and disposal (NIOSH, 2012)

Parenteral: Do not administer I.V.

I.M. (Lupron Depot®, Lupron Depot-Ped®): Administer as a single injection; rotate administration site periodically. Reconstitute only with diluent provided. Upon reconstitution, a milky suspension is formed; does not contain preservatives and should be used immediately.

SubQ:

Leuprolide acetate 5 mg/mL solution: Administer undiluted into areas on the arm, thigh, or abdomen; rotate injection site. If an alternate syringe from the manufacturer-provided syringe is required, insulin syringes should be used

Eligard®: Vary injection site; choose site with adequate subcutaneous tissue (eg, upper or midabdomen, upper buttocks); avoid areas that may be compressed or rubbed (eg, belt or waistband)

Monitoring Parameters Precocious puberty: Height, weight, bone age, Tanner staging test, GnRH testing (blood LH and FSH levels), testosterone in males and estradiol in females; closely monitor patients with prostatic carcinoma for plasma testosterone, acid phosphatase, and signs of weakness, paresthesias, and urinary tract obstruction during the first few weeks of therapy

Test Interactions Interferes with pituitary gonadotropic and gonadal function tests during and up to 3 months after monthly administration of leuprolide therapy.

Dosage Forms Excipient information presented when available (limited, particularly for generics); consult specific product labeling.

◀ Kit, Injection, as acetate:
Generic: 1 mg/0.2 mL
Kit, Intramuscular, as acetate:
Lupron Depot: 7.5 mg, 45 mg [latex free; contains polysorbate 80]
Kit, Intramuscular, as acetate [preservative free]:
Lupron Depot: 3.75 mg, 11.25 mg, 22.5 mg, 30 mg [latex free; contains polysorbate 80]
Lupron Depot-Ped: 7.5 mg, 11.25 mg, 15 mg, 30 mg (Ped), 11.25 mg (Ped) [latex free; contains polysorbate 80]
Kit, Subcutaneous, as acetate:
Eligard: 7.5 mg, 22.5 mg, 30 mg, 45 mg

References

Carel JC, Eugster EA, Rogol A, et al, "Consensus Statement on the Use of Gonadotropin-Releasing Hormone Analogs in Children," *Pediatrics*, 2009, 123(4):e752-62.

Kappy MS, Stuart T, and Perelman A, "Efficacy of Leuprolide Therapy in Children With Central Precocious Puberty," *Am J Dis Child*, 1988, 142 (10):1061-4.

Lee PA and Page JG, "Effects of Leuprolide in the Treatment of Central Precocious Puberty," *J Pediatr*, 1989, 114(2):321-4.

National Institute for Occupational Safety and Health (NIOSH), "NIOSH List of Antineoplastic and Other Hazardous Drugs in Healthcare Settings 2012." Available at http://www.cdc.gov/niosh/docs/2012-150/pdfs/2012-150.pdf. Accessed January 21, 2013.

Tanaka T, Niimi H, Matsuo N, et al, "Results of Long-Term Follow-Up After Treatment of Central Precocious Puberty With Leuprorelin Acetate: Evaluation of Effectiveness of Treatment and Recovery of Gonadal Function. The TAP-144-SR Japanese Study Group on Central Precocious Puberty," *J Clin Endocrinol Metab*, 2005, 90 (3):1371-6.

◆ **Leuprolide Acetate** *see* Leuprolide *on page 1215*

◆ **Leuprorelin Acetate** *see* Leuprolide *on page 1215*

◆ **Leurocristine Sulfate** *see* VinCRIStine *on page 2138*

◆ **Leustatin** *see* Cladribine *on page 488*

Levalbuterol (leve al BYOO ter ole)

Medication Safety Issues
Sound-alike/look-alike issues:
Xopenex may be confused with Xanax

Brand Names: U.S. Xopenex; Xopenex Concentrate; Xopenex HFA

Therapeutic Category Adrenergic Agonist Agent; Antiasthmatic; Beta$_2$-Adrenergic Agonist; Bronchodilator; Sympathomimetic

Generic Availability (U.S.) May be product dependent

Use Treatment and prevention of bronchospasm in patients with reversible obstructive airway disease

Pregnancy Risk Factor C

Pregnancy Considerations Teratogenic effects were not observed in animal reproduction studies; however, racemic albuterol was teratogenic in some species. Beta-agonists may interfere with uterine contractility if administered during labor.

Uncontrolled asthma is associated with adverse events on pregnancy (increased risk of perinatal mortality, preeclampsia, preterm birth, low birth weight infants). Other beta$_2$-receptor agonists are currently preferred for the treatment of asthma during pregnancy (NAEPP, 2005).

Breast-Feeding Considerations It is not known whether levalbuterol is excreted in human milk. Although breastfeeding is not recommended by the manufacturer, the use of beta$_2$-receptor agonists are not considered a contraindication to breast-feeding (NAEPP, 2005).

Contraindications Hypersensitivity to levalbuterol, any component, albuterol, or adrenergic amine

Warnings Paradoxical bronchospasm may occur, especially with the first use. Excessive use of inhaled sympathomimetics has been associated with death possibly due to cardiac arrest. Increasing use (>2 days/week) for symptom relief generally indicates inadequate control of asthma

and the need for initiating or intensifying anti-inflammatory treatment. Regularly scheduled, daily, chronic use of short-acting beta agonists (eg, levalbuterol) is not recommended (NAEPP, 2007).

Precautions Use with caution in patients with hyperthyroidism, hypokalemia, diabetes mellitus, cardiovascular disorders including coronary insufficiency, hypertension, or history of cardiac arrhythmias; excessive or prolonged use can lead to tolerance

Adverse Reactions
Cardiovascular: Tachycardia

Central nervous system: Anxiety, dizziness, headache, migraine, nervousness, weakness

Dermatologic: Rash

Endocrine & metabolic: Serum glucose increased, serum potassium decreased

Gastrointestinal: Diarrhea, dyspepsia

Neuromuscular & skeletal: Leg cramps, tremor

Respiratory: Asthma, cough, nasal edema, pharyngitis, rhinitis, sinusitis, viral infection

Miscellaneous: Accidental injury, flu-like syndrome, viral infection,

Rare but important or life-threatening: Abnormal ECG, acne, anaphylaxis, angina, angioedema, arrhythmia, atrial fibrillation, chest pain, dysmenorrhea, epistaxis, extrasystole, gastroenteritis, gastroesophageal reflux disease, hematuria, hypertension, hypoesthesia (hand), hypokalemia, lymphadenopathy, metabolic acidosis, myalgia, nausea, oropharyngeal dryness, paresthesia, supraventricular arrhythmia, syncope, vaginal moniliasis

Note: Immediate hypersensitivity reactions have occurred (including angioedema, oropharyngeal edema, urticaria, and anaphylaxis).

Drug Interactions
Metabolism/Transport Effects None known.

Avoid Concomitant Use
Avoid concomitant use of Levalbuterol with any of the following: Beta-Blockers (Nonselective); Iobenguane I 123

Increased Effect/Toxicity
Levalbuterol may increase the levels/effects of: Atosiban; Loop Diuretics; Sympathomimetics; Thiazide Diuretics

The levels/effects of Levalbuterol may be increased by: AtoMOXetine; Cannabinoid-Containing Products; Linezolid; MAO Inhibitors; Tricyclic Antidepressants

Decreased Effect
Levalbuterol may decrease the levels/effects of: Iobenguane I 123

The levels/effects of Levalbuterol may be decreased by: Beta-Blockers (Beta1 Selective); Beta-Blockers (Nonselective); Betahistine

Stability Store all formulations at room temperature; protect from light; discard nebulized solution if it is not colorless; after the foil covering is opened, use within 2 weeks; if removed from the foil pouch, use within 1 week; vials of concentrated solution should be used immediately after removing from foil pouch; store aerosol with mouthpiece up; discard after 200 actuations

Mechanism of Action Relaxes bronchial smooth muscle by action on beta$_2$-receptors with little effect on heart rate

Pharmacodynamics
Onset of action: Nebulized: 10-17 minutes; aerosol: 5.5-10 minutes

Maximum effect: Nebulized: 1.5 hours; aerosol: 77 minutes

Duration: Nebulized: 5-6 hours; aerosol: 3-6 hours

Pharmacokinetics (Adult data unless noted) Nebulization:

Distribution: V$_d$: Adults: 1900 L

Metabolism: In the liver to an inactive sulfate

Half-life: 3.3-4.0 hours

Time to peak serum concentration: 0.2-1.8 hours

Elimination: 3% to 6% excreted unchanged in urine

Dosing: Neonatal Note: May consider using half of the albuterol dose; albuterol is a 1:1 racemic mixture and levalbuterol is the active isomer; limited data available; further studies needed.

Nebulization **(dosage expressed in terms of mg levalbuterol):** 0.31 mg/dose every 8 hours was administered to 31 VLBW neonates (mean GA: 28.1 weeks; mean birth weight: 1127 g) for >2 weeks; no untoward hemodynamic effects were noted (Mhanna, 2009)

Dosing: Usual

Acute asthma exacerbation (NAEPP, 2007) **(dosage expressed in terms of mg levalbuterol):**

Nebulization:

Children: 0.075 mg/kg (minimum dose: 1.25 mg) every 20 minutes for 3 doses then 0.075-0.15 mg/kg (not to exceed 5 mg) every 1-4 hours as needed

Adults: 1.25-2.5 mg every 20 minutes for 3 doses then 1.25-5 mg every 1-4 hours as needed

Inhalation: MDI: 45 mcg/spray:

Children: 4-8 puffs every 20 minutes for 3 doses then every 1-4 hours

Adults: 4-8 puffs every 20 minutes for up to 4 hours then every 1-4 hours as needed

Maintenance therapy (nonacute) (NAEPP, 2007): Not recommended for long-term, daily maintenance treatment; regular use exceeding 2 days/week for symptom control indicates the need for additional long-term control therapy

Nebulization:

Children 0-4 years: 0.31-1.25 mg every 4-6 hours as needed

Children ≥5 years and Adults: 0.31-0.63 mg every 8 hours as needed

Inhalation: MDI: 45 mcg/spray:

Children <5 years: Not FDA approved

Children ≥5 years and Adults: 2 inhalations every 4-6 hours as needed

Administration

Inhalation: Nebulization: dilution required for concentrated solution

Oral inhalation: Prime the inhaler (before first use or if it has not been used for more than 2 weeks) by releasing 4 test sprays into the air away from the face; shake well before use; use spacer for children <8 years of age

Monitoring Parameters Serum potassium, oxygen saturation, heart rate, pulmonary function tests, respiratory rate, use of accessory muscles during respiration, suprasternal retractions; arterial or capillary blood gases (if patient's condition warrants)

Additional Information Levalbuterol administered in ½ the mg dose of albuterol (eg, 0.63 mg levalbuterol to 1.25 mg albuterol) provides comparable efficacy and safety. Levalbuterol has not been evaluated by continuous nebulization (NIH Guidelines, 2007).

Dosage Forms Considerations Xopenex HFA 15 g canisters contain 200 inhalations and 8.4 g canisters contain 80 inhalations.

Dosage Forms Excipient information presented when available (limited, particularly for generics); consult specific product labeling.

Aerosol, Inhalation, as tartrate [strength expressed as base]:

Xopenex HFA: 45 mcg/actuation (15 g)

Nebulization Solution, Inhalation, as hydrochloride [strength expressed as base]:

Xopenex: 0.63 mg/3 mL (3 mL); 1.25 mg/3 mL (3 mL)

Generic: 0.63 mg/3 mL (3 mL)

Nebulization Solution, Inhalation, as hydrochloride [strength expressed as base, preservative free]:

Xopenex: 0.31 mg/3 mL (3 mL)

Xopenex Concentrate: 1.25 mg/0.5 mL (30 ea)

Generic: 0.31 mg/3 mL (3 mL); 0.63 mg/3 mL (3 mL); 1.25 mg/3 mL (3 mL); 1.25 mg/0.5 mL (1 ea, 30 ea)

References

Gawchik SM, Saccar CL, Noonan M, et al, "The Safety and Efficacy of Nebulized Levalbuterol Compared With Racemic Albuterol and Placebo in the Treatment of Asthma in Pediatric Patients," *J Allergy Clin Immunol*, 1999, 103(4):615-21.

Lotvall J, Palmqvist M, Arvidsson P, et al, "The Therapeutic Ratio of R-Albuterol Is Comparable With That of RS-Albuterol in Asthmatic Patients," *J Allergy Clin Immunol*, 2001, 108(5):726-31.

Mhanna MJ, Patel JS, Patel S, et al, "The Effects of Racemic Albuterol Versus Levalbuterol in Very Low Birth Weight Infants," *Pediatr Pulmonol*, 2009, 44(8):778-83.

Milgrom H, Skoner DP, Bensch G, et al, "Low-Dose Levalbuterol in Children With Asthma: Safety and Efficacy in Comparison With Placebo and Racemic Albuterol," *J Allergy Clin Immunol*, 2001, 108 (6):938-45.

"National Asthma Education and Prevention Program. Expert Panel Report: Guidelines for the Diagnosis and Management of Asthma Update on Selected Topics–2002," *J Allergy Clin Immunol*, 2002, 110 (5 Suppl):S141-219.

National Asthma Education and Prevention Program (NAEPP), "Expert Panel Report 3 (EPR-3): Guidelines for the Diagnosis and Management of Asthma," *Clinical Practice Guidelines*, National Institutes of Health, National Heart, Lung, and Blood Institute, NIH Publication No. 08-4051, prepublication 2007; available at http://www.nhlbi.nih.gov/guidelines/asthma/asthgdln.htm.

National Asthma Education and Prevention Program (NAEPP) Working Group Report on "Managing Asthma During Pregnancy: Recommendations for Pharmacologic Treatment," National Institutes of Health, National Heart, Lung, and Blood Institute, NIH Publication No. 05-5236, March 2005. Available at http://www.nhlbi.nih.gov/health/prof/lung/asthma/astpreg/astpreg_full.pdf

◆ **Levalbuterol Hydrochloride** see Levalbuterol on page 1218

◆ **Levalbuterol Tartrate** see Levalbuterol on page 1218

◆ **Levaquin** see Levofloxacin (Systemic) on page 1228

◆ **Levarterenol Bitartrate** see Norepinephrine on page 1510

◆ **Levate (Can)** see Amitriptyline on page 133

◆ **Levbid** see Hyoscyamine on page 1056

◆ **Levemir** see Insulin Detemir on page 1119

◆ **Levemir® (Can)** see Insulin Detemir on page 1119

◆ **Levemir FlexPen** see Insulin Detemir on page 1119

◆ **Levemir FlexTouch** see Insulin Detemir on page 1119

LevETIRAcetam (lee va tye RA se tam)

Medication Safety Issues

Sound-alike/look-alike issues:

Keppra may be confused with Keflex, Keppra XR

LevETIRAcetam may be confused with levOCARNitine, levofloxacin

Potential for dispensing errors between Keppra and Kaletra (lopinavir/ritonavir)

Related Information

Oral Medications That Should Not Be Crushed or Altered on page 2438

Brand Names: U.S. Keppra; Keppra XR

Brand Names: Canada Apo-Levetiracetam; Auro-Levetiracetam; Ava-Levetiracetam; CO Levetiracetam; Dom-Levetiracetam; JAMP-Levetiracetam; Keppra; PHL-Levetiracetam; PMS-Levetiracetam; PRO-Levetiracetam; RAN-Levetiracetam

Therapeutic Category Anticonvulsant, Miscellaneous

Generic Availability (U.S.) Yes

Use

Oral:

Oral solution and immediate release tablets: Adjunctive therapy in the treatment of partial onset seizures (FDA approved in ages ≥1 month and adults); adjunctive therapy in the treatment of juvenile myoclonic epilepsy (FDA approved in ages ≥12 years) and myoclonic seizures (FDA approved in adults); adjunctive therapy in the treatment of primary generalized tonic-clonic seizures (FDA approved in ages ≥6 years and adults); has also been used for treatment of neonatal seizures, as adjunctive therapy for the treatment of generalized epilepsy with photosensitivity and Lennox-Gastaut syndrome, monotherapy for the treatment of various seizures types, treatment of tics in patients with Tourette syndrome, prophylaxis in pediatric migraine, and bipolar disorder

Extended release tablets: Adjunctive therapy in the treatment of partial onset seizures (FDA approved in ages ≥16 years and adults)

I.V.: Adjunctive therapy in the treatment of partial onset seizures (FDA approved in ages ≥16 years and adults); adjunctive therapy in the treatment of myoclonic seizures in patients with juvenile myoclonic epilepsy (FDA approved in ages ≥16 years and adults); adjunctive therapy in the treatment of primary generalized tonic-clinic seizures in patients with idiopathic generalized epilepsy (FDA approved in ages ≥16 years and adults); temporary use in patients in whom oral administration is not feasible (FDA approved in ages ≥16 years and adults); has also been used for treatment of refractory status epilepticus or acute repetitive seizure activity

Medication Guide Available Yes

Pregnancy Risk Factor C

Pregnancy Considerations Developmental toxicities were observed in animal reproduction studies. Levetiracetam crosses the placenta and can be detected in the neonate at birth. Concentrations in the umbilical cord at delivery are similar to those in the maternal plasma. Serum concentrations of levetiracetam may decrease as pregnancy progresses; monitor carefully throughout pregnancy and postpartum (Tomson, 2007).

Two registries are available for women exposed to levetiracetam during pregnancy: Pregnant women may enroll themselves into the North American Antiepileptic Drug (AED) Pregnancy Registry (888-233-2334 or http://www.aedpregnancyregistry.org/). The patient or healthcare provider may contact the UCB AED Pregnancy Registry (888-537-7734).

The North American AED registry has published data collected from pregnant women taking levetiracetam monotherapy from 1997-2011 (n=450). Eleven major malformations were diagnosed within 12 weeks of birth. The relative risk of major malformations was not increased in comparison to women with epilepsy not taking AEDs (n=442; RR 2.2, 95% CI 0.8-6.4) or in comparison to women using lamotrigine monotherapy (n=1562; RR 1.2, 95% CI 0.6-2.5) (Hernández-Díaz, 2012).

Breast-Feeding Considerations Levetiracetam can be detected in breast milk. Using data from 11 women collected 4-23 days after delivery, the estimated exposure of levetiracetam to the breast-feeding infant would be ~2 mg/kg/day (relative infant dose 7.9% of the weight-adjusted maternal dose). Adverse events were not reported in the nursing infants (Tomson, 2007). Due to the potential for serious adverse reactions in the nursing infant, the manufacturer recommends a decision be made whether to discontinue nursing or to discontinue the drug, taking into account the importance of treatment to the mother.

Contraindications Hypersensitivity to levetiracetam or any component

Warnings Neuropsychiatric adverse events including somnolence, fatigue, coordination difficulties (noted in adults only), behavioral abnormalities (eg, aggression, agitation, anxiety, anger, hostility, irritability, depression) and psychotic symptoms (psychosis, hallucinations) may occur; incidence of behavioral abnormalities may be increased in children (37.6%) versus adults (13.3%); dosage reductions may be required. CNS effects may impair physical

and mental abilities; patients must be cautioned about performing tasks which require mental alertness (eg, driving or operating heavy machinery); use caution when combining with other sedating drugs or ethanol; sedative effects may be potentiated. Do not abruptly discontinue therapy; withdraw gradually to lessen chance for increased seizure frequency.

Antiepileptic drugs (AEDs) increase the risk of suicidal behavior and ideation in patients receiving these medications for any indication. Pooled analyses of placebo-controlled trials involving 11 different AEDs (regardless of indication) showed a twofold increased risk of suicidal thoughts or behavior (estimated incidence rate: 0.43% in AED treated patients compared to 0.24% of patients receiving placebo); increased risk was observed as early as 1 week after initiation of AED and continued through duration of trials (most trials ≤24 weeks); risk did not vary significantly by age (age range: 5-100 years). Consider risks and benefits of AEDs before prescribing. Monitor all patients receiving an AED for emergence of suicidal thoughts or behavior, thoughts of self-harm, any unusual changes in behavior or mood, or the emergence or worsening of depressive symptoms; notify healthcare provider immediately if symptoms or concerning behavior occur. **Note:** The FDA requires a Medication Guide for all antiepileptic drugs informing patients of this risk.

Severe dermatologic reactions, including toxic epidermal necrolysis and Stevens-Johnson syndrome, have been reported in children and adults; onset usually within ~2 weeks of treatment initiation, but may be delayed (>4 months); discontinue drug if there are any signs of a hypersensitivity reaction or unspecified rash.

Precautions Use with caution and decrease dose in patients with renal dysfunction. Hematologic abnormalities (small but statistically significant decreases in RBC count, Hgb, Hct, WBC count, and neutrophils) may occur. Eosinophilia has also been reported. Isolated elevations in diastolic blood pressure measurements have been reported in infants and children 1 month to <4 years of age receiving levetiracetam; however, no difference was noted in mean diastolic measurements of these patients vs placebo group. Similar effects have not been observed in older children and adults. In pediatric clinical trials, the most frequently reported adverse reactions in pediatric patients 4 to <16 years of age were fatigue, aggression, nasal congestion, decreased appetite, and irritability and in younger pediatric patients (1 month to <4 years of age) were somnolence and irritability; additionally, children may experience a higher frequency of certain adverse effects than adults, including the following: behavioral abnormalities (37.6% vs 13.3%), aggression/hostility (10% vs 2%), vomiting (reported in children only, 15%), and cough (9% vs 2%).

Adverse Reactions

Cardiovascular: Facial edema, increased blood pressure (diastolic; infants and children <4 years)

Central nervous system: Aggressive behavior (children and adolescents 4-16 years), agitation, amnesia, anxiety, ataxia, behavioral problems (including aggression, anger, apathy, depersonalization, hyperkinesias, neurosis); confusion, depression, dizziness, drowsiness, emotional lability, falling (children and adolescents 4-16 years), fatigue, headache, hostility, insomnia, irritability, lethargy (children and adolescents 4-16 years), nervousness, pain, paranoia (children and adolescents 4-16 years), paresthesia, personality disorder, psychotic symptoms (more common in infants and children <4 years), sedation (children), vertigo

Dermatologic: Bruise, pruritus, skin discoloration, skin rash

Endocrine & metabolic: Dehydration

Gastrointestinal: Anorexia, decreased appetite (children and adolescents 4-16 years), diarrhea, constipation (children and adolescents 4-16 years), gastroenteritis, nausea, upper abdominal pain (children and adolescents 4-16 years), vomiting (children and adolescents 4-16 years)

Genitourinary: Urine abnormality

Hematologic & oncologic: Decreased white blood cell count, eosinophilia (children and adolescents 4-16 years)

Infection: Infection, influenza, viral infection

Neuromuscular & skeletal: Arthralgia (children and adolescents 4-16 years), hyperreflexia, neck pain, sprain (children and adolescents 4-16 years), weakness

Ophthalmic: Amblyopia, conjunctivitis, diplopia

Otic: Otalgia

Renal: Albuminuria

Respiratory: Asthma, cough, flu-like symptoms, nasal congestion (children and adolescents 4-16 years), nasopharyngitis, pharyngitis, pharyngolaryngeal pain (children and adolescents 4-16 years), rhinitis, sinusitis

Miscellaneous: Accidental injury (children and adolescents 4-16 years)

Rare but important or life-threatening: Abnormal hepatic function tests, agranulocytosis, alopecia, anemia, catatonia, choreoathetosis, decreased hematocrit, decreased hemoglobin, decreased red blood cells, DRESS syndrome, dyskinesia, eczema, equilibrium disturbance, erythema multiforme, hepatic failure, hepatitis, leukopenia, myasthenia, neutropenia, pancreatitis, pancytopenia (with bone marrow suppression), panic attack, psychotic symptoms, Stevens-Johnson syndrome, suicidal ideation, suicidal tendencies, thrombocytopenia, toxic epidermal necrolysis, weight loss

Drug Interactions

Metabolism/Transport Effects None known.

Avoid Concomitant Use

Avoid concomitant use of LevETIRAcetam with any of the following: Azelastine (Nasal); Paraldehyde; Thalidomide

Increased Effect/Toxicity

LevETIRAcetam may increase the levels/effects of: Alcohol (Ethyl); Azelastine (Nasal); Buprenorphine; CNS Depressants; Hydrocodone; Methotrimeprazine; Metyrosine; Mirtazapine; Paraldehyde; Pramipexole; ROPINIRole; Rotigotine; Selective Serotonin Reuptake Inhibitors; Thalidomide; Zolpidem

The levels/effects of LevETIRAcetam may be increased by: Brimonidine (Topical); Cannabis; Doxylamine; Dronabinol; Droperidol; HydrOXYzine; Kava Kava; Magnesium Sulfate; Methotrimeprazine; Nabilone; Perampanel; Rufinamide; Sodium Oxybate; Tapentadol; Tetrahydrocannabinol

Decreased Effect

The levels/effects of LevETIRAcetam may be decreased by: Ketorolac (Nasal); Ketorolac (Systemic); Mefloquine; Orlistat

Food Interactions Food may delay, but does not affect the extent of absorption. Management: Administer without regard to meals.

Stability

Oral solution, tablets: Store at 25°C (77°F), excursion permitted to 59°F to 86°F (15°C to 30°C), keep away from heat and light

Parenteral:

Premixed solution: Store at 20°C to 25°C (68°F to 77°F)

Vials: Store intact vials at 25°C (77°F); excursions permitted to 15°C to 30°C (59°F to 86°F); upon further dilution in D_5W, NS, or LR, admixed solution is stable for at least 24 hours in polyvinyl chloride bags stored at controlled room temperature

Mechanism of Action The precise mechanism by which levetiracetam exerts its antiepileptic effect is unknown. However, several studies have suggested the mechanism may involve one or more of the following central pharmacologic effects: inhibition of voltage-dependent N-type calcium channels; facilitation of GABA-ergic inhibitory transmission through displacement of negative modulators; reduction of delayed rectifier potassium current; and/or binding to synaptic proteins which modulate neurotransmitter release.

Pharmacokinetics (Adult data unless noted)

Absorption: Oral: Rapid and complete

Distribution: V_d: Approximates volume of intracellular and extracellular water; V_d:

Infants and Children <4 years: 0.63 ± 0.08 L/kg (Glauser, 2007)

Children 6-12 years: 0.72 ± 0.12 L/kg (Pellock, 2001)

Adults: 0.5-0.7 L/kg

Protein binding: <10%

Metabolism: Not extensive; 24% of dose is metabolized by enzymatic hydrolysis of acetamide group (major metabolic pathway; hydrolysis occurs primarily in the blood; not cytochrome P450 dependent); two minor metabolites (one via hydroxylation of 2-oxo-pyrrolidine ring and one via opening of the 2-oxo-pyrrolidine ring in position 5) are also formed; metabolites are inactive and renally excreted

Bioavailability: Oral: 100%; bioavailability of extended release tablets is similar to immediate release tablets; tablets, oral solution, and injection are bioequivalent

Half-life: Increased in patients with renal dysfunction:

Infants and Children <4 years: 5.3 ± 1.3 hours (Glauser, 2007)

Children 4-12 years: 6 ± 1.1 hours (Pellock, 2001)

Adults: 6-8 hours

Time to peak serum concentration: Oral:

Oral solution: Fasting infants and children <4 years: 1.4 ± 0.9 hours

Immediate release: Fasting adults and children: 1 hour

Extended release: 4 hours; median time to peak is 2 hours longer in the fed state

Elimination: 66% excreted in urine as unchanged drug and 27% as inactive metabolites; undergoes glomerular filtration and subsequent partial tubular reabsorption

Clearance: Correlated with creatinine clearance; clearance is decreased in patients with renal dysfunction

Infants <6 months: 1.23 mL/minute/kg (Glauser, 2007)

Infants and Children 6 months-4 years: 1.57 mL/minute/kg (Glauser, 2007)

Children 6-12 years: 1.43 mL/min/kg; 30% to 40% higher than adults on a per kg basis (Pellock, 2001)

Dialysis: Hemodialysis: Standard 4-hour treatment removes ~50% of the drug from the body; supplemental doses after dialysis are recommended

Dosing: Neonatal Neonatal Seizures:

I.V.: Limited data available: 10 mg/kg/day divided twice daily; increase dosage by 10 mg/kg over 3 days to 30 mg/kg/day; additional increases up to 45-60 mg/kg/day have been used with persistent seizure activity or clinical EEG findings. Dosing based on an open-label study of 38 patients [n=19 premature neonates GA <28 weeks (birth weight: 0.41-1.33 kg); n=6 premature neonates GA: 28-36 weeks (birth weight: 1.25-1.89 kg); n=13 term neonates] which reported a decrease in seizure frequency (ie, after 1 week of therapy, 30/38 patients were seizure-free). The investigators noted that patients with extensive intracerebral hemorrhage tended to be less responsive to therapy (Ramantani, 2011). For treatment of status epilepticus, loading doses of 20-30 mg/kg/ dose have been used by some centers (Abend, 2009).

Oral: Dose not established, limited data available: Initial: 10 mg/kg/day in 1-2 divided doses; increase daily by 10 mg/kg to 30 mg/kg/day (maximum reported dose: 60 mg/kg/day). Dosing based on two prospective, open-label studies [n=38 (n=19, GA: <28 weeks; n=6, GA: 28-36 weeks, n=13 term]; n=6, GA: >30 weeks], a case series (n=3, 2 days to 3 months) which showed levetiracetam was effective at increasing seizure-free interval, and a report of pediatric neurologists' NICU experience (Fürwentsches, 2010; Ramantani, 2011; Shoemaker, 2007; Silverstein, 2008).

Dosing: Usual Note: When switching from oral to I.V. formulation, the total daily dose should be the same.

Infants, Children, and Adolescents <16 years: **Note:** Use oral solution in infants and children ≤20 kg; either oral solution or immediate release tablets may be used in children and adolescents >20 kg.

Myoclonic seizures: Children ≥12 years and Adolescents <16 years: Oral (immediate release: tablets or solution): Initial 500 mg twice daily; increase dosage every 2 weeks by 500 mg/dose twice daily, to the recommended dose of 1500 mg twice daily. Efficacy of doses other than 3000 mg/day has not been established.

Partial onset seizures:
Infants 1 to <6 months: Oral (immediate release: solution): Initial: 7 mg/kg/dose twice daily; increase dosage every 2 weeks by 7 mg/kg/dose twice daily as tolerated, to the recommended dose of 21 mg/kg/dose twice daily; effectiveness of lower doses has not been established; during clinical trials, the mean daily dose was 35 mg/kg/**day**

Infants ≥6 months and Children <4 years: Oral [immediate release: solution or tablets (patient weight >20 kg)]: Initial: 10 mg/kg/dose twice daily; increase dosage every 2 weeks by 10 mg/kg/dose twice daily, as tolerated, to the recommended dose of 25 mg/kg/dose twice daily; may reduce daily dose if not tolerated; during clinical trials, the mean daily dose was 47 mg/kg/**day**

Children ≥4 years and Adolescents <16 years: Oral (immediate release):
Oral solution: Initial: 10 mg/kg/dose twice daily; increase dosage every 2 weeks by 10 mg/kg/dose twice daily, as tolerated, to a maximum of 30 mg/kg/dose twice daily; maximum daily dose: 3000 mg/**day**; may reduce daily dose if not tolerated; during clinical trials, the mean daily dose was 44 mg/kg/**day**
Tablets: Fixed-dosing:
20-40 kg: Initial: 250 mg twice daily, increase every 2 weeks by 250 mg twice daily to the maximum recommended dose of 750 mg twice daily
>40 kg: Initial: 500 mg twice daily, increase every 2 weeks by 500 mg twice daily to the maximum recommended dose of 1500 mg twice daily

Primary generalized tonic-clonic seizures: Children 6 to <16 years: Oral [immediate release: solution or tablets (patient weight >20kg)]: Initial: 10 mg/kg/dose twice daily; increase dosage every 2 weeks by 10 mg/kg/dose given twice daily, to the recommended dose of 30 mg/kg/dose twice daily. Efficacy of doses other than 60 mg/kg/day has not been established.

Status epilepticus or acute repetitive seizure activity: Limited data available: I.V.: Loading dose: 50 mg/kg/dose (maximum dose: 2500 mg); followed by I.V. or oral maintenance dosing determined by clinical response; reported I.V. maintenance dose: 30-55 mg/kg/day divided twice daily (Kirmani, 2009; Ng, 2010). Dosing based on a prospective study (n=30, 6 months to <15 years), several retrospective observations, and case reports (n >100; youngest patient: 1 day old; reported loading dose range: 6.5-89 mg/kg) (Abend, 2009; Gallentine, 2009; Goraya, 2008; Kirmani, 2009; Ng, 2010; Reiter, 2010).

Adolescents ≥16 years and Adults:
Myoclonic seizures:
Oral: Immediate release: 500 mg twice daily; may increase every 2 weeks by 500 mg/dose to the recommended dose of 1500 mg twice daily. Efficacy of doses other than 3000 mg/**day** has not been established.

I.V.: Initial: 500 mg twice daily; increase dosage every 2 weeks by 500 mg/dose given twice daily, to the recommended dose of 1500 mg twice daily. Efficacy of doses other than 3000 mg/day has not been established.

Partial onset seizures:
Oral:
Immediate release: Initial: 500 mg twice daily; may increase every 2 weeks by 500 mg/dose given twice daily, if tolerated, to a maximum of 1500 mg twice daily. Doses >3000 mg/**day** have been used in trials; however, there is no evidence of increased benefit.
Extended release: Initial: 1000 mg once daily; may increase every 2 weeks by 1000 mg/day to a maximum of 3000 mg once daily
I.V.: Initial: 500 mg twice daily; may increase every 2 weeks by 500 mg/dose given twice daily, if tolerated, to a maximum of 1500 mg twice daily. Oral doses >3000 mg/day have been used in trials; however, there is no evidence of increased benefit.

Primary generalized tonic-clonic seizures:
Oral: Immediate release: Initial: 500 mg twice daily; increase dosage every 2 weeks by 500 mg/dose given twice daily, to the recommended dose of 1500 mg twice daily. Efficacy of doses other than 3000 mg/**day** has not been established.
I.V.: Initial: 500 mg twice daily; increase dosage every 2 weeks by 500 mg/dose given twice daily, to the recommended dose of 1500 mg twice daily. Efficacy of doses other than 3000 mg/**day** has not been established.

Dosing adjustment in renal impairment:
Infants, Children, and Adolescents <16 years (Aronoff, 2007):
GFR <50 mL/minute/1.73 m^2: Administer 50% of the dose
Hemodialysis: Administer 50% of normal dose every 24 hours; a supplemental dose after hemodialysis is recommended
CAPD: Administer 50% of normal dose
CRRT: Administer 50% of normal dose
Adolescents ≥16 years and Adults:
Immediate release and I.V. formulations:
CrCl >80 mL/minute/1.73 m^2: 500-1500 mg every 12 hours
CrCl 50-80 mL/minute/1.73 m^2: 500-1000 mg every 12 hours
CrCl 30-50 mL/minute/1.73 m^2: 250-750 mg every 12 hours
CrCl <30 mL/minute/1.73 m^2: 250-500 mg every 12 hours
End-stage renal disease patients using dialysis: 500-1000 mg every 24 hours; a supplemental dose of 250-500 mg following dialysis is recommended
Peritoneal dialysis (PD): 500-1000 mg every 24 hours (Aronoff, 2007)
Continuous renal replacement therapy (CRRT): 250-750 mg every 12 hours (Arnoff, 2007)
Extended release tablets: Adults:
CrCl >80 mL/minute/1.73 m^2: 1000-3000 mg every 24 hours
CrCl 50-80 mL/minute/1.73 m^2: 1000-2000 mg every 24 hours
CrCl 30-50 mL/minute/1.73 m^2: 500-1500 mg every 24 hours
CrCl <30 mL/minute/1.73 m^2: 500-1000 mg every 24 hours
End-stage renal disease patients using dialysis: Use immediate release product

Dosing adjustment in hepatic impairment: No dosage adjustment necessary

Administration

Oral: May be administered without regard to meals; swallow tablets (both immediate release and extended release) whole; do not break, crush, or chew. Oral solution should be administered with calibrated measuring device (not household teaspoon or tablespoon).

Parenteral: I.V.: Vials: Must be diluted prior to use. Premixed 100 mL bags: Do not dilute further prior to use. Vials and premixed bags: Do not use if solution contains particulate matter or is discolored. Discard unused portions; does not contain preservative. pH: 5.5

Pediatric patients <16 years: Dilute dose from vial in NS to final concentration 15 mg/mL; infuse over 15 minutes (Ng, 2010).

Adolescents ≥16 years and Adults: May use premix 100 mL bags or prepare dose from vials and dilute in 100 mL of D_5W, NS, or LR; infuse over 15 minutes

Others have safely used a 1:1 dilution of drug from vial with D_5W or NS infused over 5-6 minutes (with doses up to 60 mg/kg) through a peripheral site in patients 4-32 years of age (Wheless, 2009).

Monitoring Parameters Seizure frequency, duration, and severity; behavioral abnormalities and neuropsychiatric adverse events; renal function; CBC; signs and symptoms of suicidality (eg, anxiety, depression, behavior changes)

Reference Range Therapeutic range and benefit of therapeutic drug monitoring have not been established; concentrations of 6-20 mg/L (35-120 micromol/L) were attained in adult study patients receiving doses of 1000-3000 mg/day

Additional Information A recent, small, retrospective study used a rapid dosage titration of levetiracetam in 8 children, 19 months to 17 years of age (mean age: 8.6 years). Full maintenance doses of levetiracetam were achieved over a titration period of 2-14 days (mean: 10 days). The drug was effective and well-tolerated; however, one patient developed adverse behavioral effects. Further studies are needed before rapid titration of levetiracetam can be routinely recommended (Vaisleib, 2008).

In a preliminary report, levetiracetam-associated behavioral abnormalities were successfully treated with pyridoxine in 5 of 6 children, 2-10 years of age; further studies are needed before this treatment can be recommended (Miller, 2002). Levetiracetam- induced psychosis (including visual and auditory hallucinations and persecutive delusions) has been reported in pediatric patients (Kossoff, 2001).

Dosage Forms Excipient information presented when available (limited, particularly for generics); consult specific product labeling.

Solution, Intravenous:

Keppra: 500 mg/5 mL (5 mL)

Generic: 500 mg/100 mL (100 mL); 1000 mg/100 mL (100 mL); 1500 mg/100 mL (100 mL); 500 mg/5 mL (5 mL)

Solution, Intravenous [preservative free]:

Generic: 500 mg/5 mL (5 mL)

Solution, Oral:

Keppra: 100 mg/mL (473 mL) [gluten free, lactose free; contains acesulfame potassium, methylparaben, propylparaben; grape flavor]

Generic: 100 mg/mL (5 mL, 473 mL, 500 mL)

Tablet, Oral:

Keppra: 250 mg [scored; contains fd&c blue #2 (indigotine)]

Keppra: 500 mg [scored]

Keppra: 750 mg [scored; contains fd&c yellow #6 (sunset yellow)]

Keppra: 1000 mg [scored]

Generic: 250 mg, 500 mg, 750 mg, 1000 mg

Tablet Extended Release 24 Hour, Oral:

Keppra XR: 500 mg, 750 mg

Generic: 500 mg, 750 mg

References

Abend NS, Monk HM, Licht DJ, et al, "Intravenous Levetiracetam in Critically Ill Children With Status Epilepticus or Acute Repetitive Seizures," *Pediatr Crit Care Med*, 2009, 10(4):505-10.

Aronoff GR, Bennett WM, Berns JS, et al, *Drug Prescribing in Renal Failure: Dosing Guidelines for Adults and Children*, 5th ed. Philadelphia, PA: American College of Physicians, 2007, 89, 165.

Fürwentsches A, Bussmann C, Ramantani G, et al, "Levetiracetam in the Treatment of Neonatal Seizures: A Pilot Study," *Seizure*, 2010, 19 (3):185-9.

Gallentine WB, Hunnicutt AS, and Husain AM, "Levetiracetam in Children With Refractory Status Epilepticus," *Epilepsy Behav*, 2009, 14(1):215-8.

Glauser TA, Mitchell WG, Weinstock A, et al, "Pharmacokinetics of Levetiracetam in Infants and Young Children With Epilepsy," *Epilepsia*, 2007, 48(6):1117-22.

Goraya JS, Khurana DS, Valencia I, et al, "Intravenous Levetiracetam in Children With Epilepsy," *Pediatr Neurol*, 2008, 38(3):177-80.

Grosso S, Cordelli DM, Franzoni E, et al, "Efficacy and Safety of Levetiracetam in Infants and Young Children With Refractory Epilepsy," *Seizure*, 2007, 16(4):345-50.

Hernández-Díaz S, Smith CR, Shen A, et al, "Comparative Safety of Antiepileptic Drugs During Pregnancy," *Neurology*, 2012, 8 (21):1692-9.

Kirmani BF, Crisp ED, Kayani S, et al, "Role of Intravenous Levetiracetam in Acute Seizure Management of Children," *Pediatr Neurol*, 2009, 41(1):37-9.

Kossoff EH, Bergey GK, Freeman JM, et al, "Levetiracetam Psychosis in Children With Epilepsy," *Epilepsia*, 2001, 42(12):1611-3.

Mandelbaum DE, Bunch M, Kugler SL, et al, "Efficacy of Levetiracetam at 12 Months in Children Classified By Seizure Type, Cognitive Status, and Previous Anticonvulsant Drug Use," *J Child Neurol*, 2005, 20(7):590-4.

Miller GS, "Pyridoxine Ameliorates Adverse Behavioral Effects of Levetiracetam in Children," *Epilepsia*, 2002, 43(Suppl 7):S62.

Ng YT, Hastriter EV, Cardenas JF, et al, "Intravenous Levetiracetam in Children With Seizures: A Prospective Safety Study," *J Child Neurol*, 2010, 25(5):551-5.

Opp J, Tuxhorn I, May T, et al, "Levetiracetam in Children With Refractory Epilepsy: A Multicenter Open Label Study in Germany," *Seizure*, 2005, 14(7):476-84.

Pellock JM, Glauser TA, Bebin EM, et al, "Pharmacokinetic Study of Levetiracetam in Children," *Epilepsia*, 2001, 42(12):1574-9.

Perry MS and Benatar M, "Efficacy and Tolerability of Levetiracetam in Children Younger Than 4 Years: A Retrospective Review," *Epilepsia*, 2007, 48(6):1123-7.

Ramantani G, Ikonomidou C, Walter B, et al, "Levetiracetam: Safety and Efficacy in Neonatal Seizures," *Eur J Paediatr Neurol*, 2011, 15 (1):1-7.

Reiter PD, Huff AD, Knupp KG, et al, "Intravenous Levetiracetam in the Management of Acute Seizures in Children," *Pediatr Neurol*, 2010, 43 (2):117-21.

Shoemaker MT and Rotenberg JS, "Levetiracetam for the Treatment of Neonatal Seizures," *J Child Neurol*, 2007, 22(1):95-8.

Silverstein FS and Ferriero DM, "Off-Label Use of Antiepileptic Drugs for the Treatment of Neonatal Seizures," *Pediatr Neurol*, 2008, 39 (2):77-9.

Tomson T, Palm R, Källén K, et al, "Pharmacokinetics of Levetiracetam During Pregnancy, Delivery, in the Neonatal Period, and Lactation," *Epilepsia*, 2007, 48(6):1111-6.

Vaisleib II and Neft RA, "Rapid Dosage Titration of Levetiracetam in Children," *Pharmacotherapy*, 2008, 28(3):393-6.

Wheless JW, Clarke D, Hovinga CA, et al, "Rapid Infusion of a Loading Dose of Intravenous Levetiracetam With Minimal Dilution: A Safety Study," *J Child Neurol*, 2009, 24(8):946-51.

Levobunolol (lee voe BYOO noe lole)

Medication Safety Issues

Sound-alike/look-alike issues:

Levobunolol may be confused with levocabastine

Betagan® may be confused with Betadine®, Betoptic® S

Brand Names: U.S. Betagan

Brand Names: Canada Apo-Levobunolol®; Betagan®; Novo-Levobunolol; PMS-Levobunolol; Ratio-Levobunolol; Sandoz-Levobunolol

Therapeutic Category Beta-Adrenergic Blocker, Ophthalmic

Generic Availability (U.S.) Yes

Use To lower intraocular pressure in chronic open-angle glaucoma or ocular hypertension

Pregnancy Risk Factor C

Pregnancy Considerations Adverse events have been observed in some animal reproduction studies. If ophthalmic agents are needed for the treatment of glaucoma during pregnancy, the minimum effective dose should be used in combination with punctual occlusion to decrease potential exposure to the fetus (Johnson,2001; Samples, 1988)

Breast-Feeding Considerations It is not known if levobunolol is excreted in breast milk; however, systemic beta-blockers and topical timolol are excreted in breast milk. The manufacturer recommends that caution be exercised when administering levobunolol to nursing women. The minimum effective dose should be used in combination with punctual occlusion to decrease potential exposure to the nursing infant (Johnson, 2001; Samples, 1988).

Contraindications Hypersensitivity to levobunolol or any component; asthma, severe COPD, sinus bradycardia, second or third degree A-V block, cardiogenic shock

Warnings Contains metabisulfite which may cause allergic reactions in susceptible individuals; use only in combination with miotic for patients with angle closure glaucoma; products contain sulfites which may cause allergic reactions in susceptible individuals

Precautions Use with caution in patients with CHF, diabetes mellitus, hyperthyroidism, myasthenia gravis

Adverse Reactions

Cardiovascular: Arrhythmia, bradycardia, cardiac arrest cerebral ischemia, cerebrovascular accident, chest pain, congestive heart failure, heart block, hypotension, palpitation, syncope

Central nervous system: Ataxia (transient), confusion, depression, dizziness, headache, lethargy

Dermatologic: Alopecia, erythema, pruritus, rash, Stevens-Johnson syndrome, urticaria

Endocrine & metabolic: Hypoglycemia masked

Gastrointestinal: Diarrhea, nausea

Genitourinary: Impotence

Neuromuscular & skeletal: Myasthenia gravis exacerbation, paresthesia, weakness

Ocular: Blepharoconjunctivitis, blepharoptosis, conjunctivitis, corneal sensitivity decreased, diplopia, iridocyclitis, keratitis, ptosis, stinging/burning, visual disturbances

Respiratory: Bronchospasm, dyspnea, nasal congestion, respiratory failure

Miscellaneous: Hypersensitivity

Drug Interactions

Metabolism/Transport Effects None known.

Avoid Concomitant Use

Avoid concomitant use of Levobunolol with any of the following: Beta2-Agonists; Ceritinib; Floctafenine; Methacholine

Increased Effect/Toxicity

Levobunolol may increase the levels/effects of: Alpha-/Beta-Agonists (Direct-Acting); Bradycardia-Causing Agents; Bupivacaine; Ceritinib; Cholinergic Agonists; DULoxetine; Ergot Derivatives; Fingolimod; Grass Pollen Allergen Extract (5 Grass Extract); Hypotensive Agents; Lidocaine (Systemic); Lidocaine (Topical); Mepivacaine; Methacholine; Midodrine

The levels/effects of Levobunolol may be increased by: Anilidopiperidine Opioids; Barbiturates; Dronedarone; Floctafenine; MAO Inhibitors; Regorafenib; Reserpine

Decreased Effect

Levobunolol may decrease the levels/effects of: Beta2-Agonists; Theophylline Derivatives

Mechanism of Action A nonselective beta-adrenergic blocking agent that lowers intraocular pressure by reducing aqueous humor production and possibly increases the outflow of aqueous humor

Pharmacodynamics

Onset of action: Following ophthalmic instillation, decreases in intraocular pressure can be noted within 1 hour

Maximum effect: Within 2-6 hours

Maximal effectiveness: 2-3 weeks

Duration: 1-7 days

Pharmacokinetics (Adult data unless noted)

Absorption: May be absorbed systemically and produce systemic side effects

Metabolism: Extensively metabolized into several metabolites; primary metabolite (active) dihydrolevobunolol

Elimination: Not well defined

Dosing: Usual Adults: 1-2 drops of 0.5% solution in eye(s) once daily or 1-2 drops of 0.25% solution twice daily; may increase to 1 drop of 0.5% solution twice daily

Administration Intraocular: Apply drops into conjunctival sac of affected eye(s); avoid contacting bottle tip with skin; apply gentle pressure to lacrimal sac during and immediately following instillation (1-2 minutes) to decrease systemic absorption; see manufacturer's information regarding proper usage of C Cap (compliance cap)

Monitoring Parameters Intraocular pressure

Dosage Forms Excipient information presented when available (limited, particularly for generics); consult specific product labeling.

Solution, Ophthalmic, as hydrochloride:

Betagan: 0.5% (5 mL, 10 mL, 15 mL)

Generic: 0.25% (5 mL, 10 mL); 0.5% (5 mL, 10 mL, 15 mL)

References

Johnson SM, Martinez M, and Freedman S, "Management of Glaucoma in Pregnancy and Lactation," *Surv Ophthalmol*, 2001, 45(5):449-54.

Samples JR and Meyer SM, "Use of Ophthalmic Medications in Pregnant and Nursing Women," *Am J Ophthalmol*, 1988, 106 (5):616-23.

◆ **Levobunolol Hydrochloride** *see* Levobunolol *on page 1223*

LevOCARNitine (lee voe KAR ni teen)

Medication Safety Issues

Sound-alike/look-alike issues:

LevOCARNitine may be confused with levETIRAcetam, levocabastine

Brand Names: U.S. Carnitor; Carnitor SF

Brand Names: Canada Carnitor

Therapeutic Category Nutritional Supplement

Generic Availability (U.S.) Yes

Use

Oral: Solution, tablets: Treatment of primary or secondary carnitine deficiency (FDA approved infants, children, and adults); has also been used in cyclic vomiting syndrome for the prevention of episodes

Parenteral: Treatment of secondary carnitine deficiency and prevention and treatment of carnitine deficiency in patients undergoing dialysis for end-stage renal disease (ESRD) [FDA approved in pediatric patients (age not specified) and adults]; has also been used for treatment of valproic acid toxicity

Pregnancy Risk Factor B

Pregnancy Considerations Teratogenic effects were not observed in animal studies. There are no adequate and well-controlled studies in pregnant women. However, carnitine is a naturally occurring substance in mammalian metabolism.

Breast-Feeding Considerations In breast-feeding women, use must be weighed against the potential exposure of the infant to increased carnitine intake.

Contraindications Hypersensitivity to carnitine or any component

Precautions Use with caution in patients with seizure disorders or in those at risk of seizures (eg, CNS mass or medications which may lower seizure threshold); both new onset seizure activity and increased frequency of seizures have been reported. Safety and efficacy of oral carnitine has not been established in ESRD; chronic administration of high doses of oral carnitine in patients with severely compromised renal function or ESRD on dialysis may result in accumulation of potentially toxic metabolites, trimethylamine and trimethylamine-N-oxide. Routine prophylactic use of carnitine in children receiving valproic acid to avoid carnitine deficiency and hepatotoxicity is probably not indicated (Freeman, 1994). Myasthenia has been reported in uremic patients on D,L-carnitine not L-carnitine.

Adverse Reactions

Intravenous: Noted with hemodialysis patients.

Cardiovascular: Atrial fibrillation, chest pain, ECG abnormality, hypertension, palpitation, peripheral edema, tachycardia, vascular disorder

Central nervous system: Depression, dizziness, fever, headache, seizures, vertigo

Dermatologic: Rash

Endocrine & metabolic: Hypercalcemia, parathyroid disorder

Gastrointestinal: Abdominal pain, anorexia, diarrhea, gastritis, gastrointestinal disorder, melena, nausea, taste perversion, vomiting, weight gain/loss

Hematologic: Anemia, hemorrhage

Neuromuscular & skeletal: Paresthesia, weakness

Ocular: Amblyopia, eye disorder

Respiratory: Bronchitis, cough, rhinitis

Miscellaneous: Accidental injury, allergic reaction, body odor, drug dependence, infection

Oral:

Central nervous system: Seizures

Gastrointestinal: Abdominal cramps, diarrhea, nausea, vomiting

Miscellaneous: Body odor

Rare but important or life-threatening: Myasthenic syndrome (uremic patients)

Drug Interactions

Metabolism/Transport Effects None known.

Avoid Concomitant Use There are no known interactions where it is recommended to avoid concomitant use.

Increased Effect/Toxicity There are no known significant interactions involving an increase in effect.

Decreased Effect There are no known significant interactions involving a decrease in effect.

Stability Store at 25°C (77°F). Solution for I.V. infusion is stable for 24 hours when mixed in NS or LR at a concentration of 0.5-8 mg/mL and stored at 25°C (77°F) in PVC bags; stable in parenteral nutrition solutions for up to 24 hours

Mechanism of Action Carnitine is a naturally occurring metabolic compound which functions as a carrier molecule for long-chain fatty acids within the mitochondria, facilitating energy production. Carnitine deficiency is associated with accumulation of excess acyl CoA esters and disruption of intermediary metabolism. Carnitine supplementation increases carnitine plasma concentrations. The effects on specific metabolic alterations have not been evaluated. ESRD patients on maintenance hemodialysis may have low plasma carnitine levels because of reduced intake of meat and dairy products, reduced renal synthesis, and dialytic losses. Certain clinical conditions (malaise, muscle weakness, cardiomyopathy and arrhythmias) in hemodialysis patients may be related to carnitine deficiency.

In patients with valproic acid toxicity, administration of exogenous carnitine shifts the metabolism of valproic acid towards β-oxidation and away from ω-oxidation and potentially hepatotoxic metabolite production.

Pharmacokinetics (Adult data unless noted)

Protein binding: Does not bind

Metabolism: Hepatic to trimethylamine and trimethylamine-N-oxide

Bioavailability:

Tablet: 15.1% ± 5.3%

Solution: 15.9% ± 4.9%

Half-life, terminal: 17.4 hours

Time to peak serum concentration: Oral: 3.3 hours

Elimination: Urine (76%, 4% to 9% as unchanged drug); feces (<1% as unchanged drug)

Dosing: Neonatal

Carnitine deficiency, treatment: Limited data available:

Note: Dosage should be individualized based upon patient response and serum carnitine concentrations.

Primary deficiency: Oral: Initial: 50 mg/kg/**day** in divided doses every 3-4 hours; titrate slowly as needed to 50-100 mg/kg/**day** in divided doses

Secondary deficiency (other inborn errors of metabolism):

Oral: Initial: 50 mg/kg/**day** in divided doses every 3-4 hours; titrate slowly as needed to 50-100 mg/kg/**day** in divided doses; some conditions may require higher daily doses (eg, 300 mg/kg/day) (Kölker, 2011; Sutton, 2012)

I.V.: 50 mg/kg as a single dose; titrate based on patient response. In patients with severe metabolic crisis, a 50 mg/kg loading dose followed by an equivalent dose given over the next 24 hours divided every 3-6 hours may be required; some conditions may require higher daily doses (eg, 300 mg/kg/day) (Sutton, 2012)

Supplement to parenteral nutrition: Limited data available: Premature neonates GA <34 weeks: I.V.: Initial: 8-10 mg/kg/**day** in parenteral nutrition solution; may increase up to 20 mg/kg/**day** based on free and total plasma carnitine concentrations (ASPEN Pediatric Nutrition Support Core Curriculum, 2010)

Dosing: Usual

Infants, Children, and Adolescents:

Carnitine deficiency, treatment: Note: Dosage should be individualized based upon patient response and serum carnitine concentrations.

Primary deficiency: Oral: Initial: 50 mg/kg/**day** in divided doses; may titrate slowly as needed to 100 mg/kg/**day** in divided doses; maximum daily dose: 3000 mg/**day**

Dosing interval (product specific):

Oral solution: Divided doses at evenly spaced intervals with or during meals (every 3-4 hours)

Tablets: Divide daily dose into 2-3 doses

Secondary deficiency:

Oral: Initial: 50 mg/kg/**day** in divided doses; may titrate slowly as needed to 100 mg/kg/**day** in divided doses; some conditions may require higher daily doses (eg, 300 mg/kg/**day**); maximum daily dose: 3000 mg/**day** (Kölker, 2011; Sutton, 2012)

Dosing interval (product specific):

Oral solution: Divided doses at evenly spaced intervals with or during meals (every 3-4 hours)

Tablets: Divide daily dose into 2-3 doses

I.V.: 50 mg/kg as a single dose; titrate based on patient response. In patients with severe metabolic crisis, a 50 mg/kg loading dose followed by an equivalent dose given over the next 24 hours divided every 3-6 hours, may be required; maximum daily dose: 300 mg/kg/**day**

ESRD patients on hemodialysis: Limited data available: Children and Adolescents: I.V.: 10-20 mg/kg dry body weight after each dialysis session; evaluate clinical response at 3-month intervals and titrate to the lowest effective dose. Therapy should be discontinued if no improvement after 9-12 months of therapy. **Note:** Current guidelines do not support the routine use of levocarnitine in dialysis patients (KDOQI Guidelines, 2006; KDOQI Work Group, 2009); however, the National Kidney Foundation indicates levocarnitine therapy in patients with hyporesponsiveness to erythropoietin-based products, symptomatic intradialytic hypotension, NYHA functional class III-IV or ACC/AHA stage C-D heart failure or symptomatic cardiomyopathy, or muscle weakness and fatigability affecting quality of life which are unresponsive to standard medical therapy (Eknoyan, 2003).

Valproic acid toxicity, acute: Children and Adolescents: Limited data available; dosing based on level of hepatic involvement:

No hepatotoxicity: I.V.: 100 mg/kg/**day** divided every 6 hours until serum ammonia and valproic acid concentrations begin to decrease and clinical improvement is evident; maximum dose: 3000 mg (Russell, 2007)

Symptomatic hyperammonemia or hepatotoxicity: Reported dosing regimens variable: I.V.: Loading dose: 100 mg/kg, maximum loading dose: 6 **g**; followed by 50 mg/kg/dose every 8 hours or 15 mg/kg/dose every 4 hours, maximum dose: 3000 mg; continue treatment until serum ammonia concentrations begin to decrease and clinical improvement is evident; patients may require several days of therapy (Perrott, 2010; Russell, 2007)

Cyclic vomiting syndrome, prevention: Limited data available: Children and Adolescents: Oral: 50-100 mg/kg/**day** in divided doses 2-3 times daily; maximum dose: 1000 mg (Li, 2008)

Adults:

Primary carnitine deficiency:

Oral solution: Initial: 1000 mg daily in divided doses (spaced every 3-4 hours throughout the day); titrate slowly as needed to 1000-3000 mg per day in divided doses; higher doses may be needed in some patients

Tablets: Oral: 990 mg 2-3 times daily

I.V.: 50 mg/kg; titrate based on patient response. In patients with severe metabolic crisis, a 50 mg/kg loading dose followed by an equivalent dose given over the next 24 hours (divided every 3 or 4 hours, never less than every 6 hours) may be required. Maximum daily dose: 300 mg/kg/**day**

ESRD patients on hemodialysis: I.V.: 20 mg/kg after each dialysis session; evaluate clinical response at 3-month intervals and titrate to the lowest effective dose. Therapy should be discontinued if no improvement after 9-12 months of therapy. **Note:** Current guidelines do not support the routine use of levocarnitine in dialysis patients (KDOQI guidelines, 2000); however, the National Kidney Foundation indicates levocarnitine therapy in patients with hyporesponsiveness to erythropoietin-based products, symptomatic intradialytic hypotension, NYHA functional class III-IV or ACC/AHA stage C-D heart failure or symptomatic cardiomyopathy, or muscle weakness and fatigability affecting quality of life which are unresponsive to standard medical therapy (Eknoyan, 2003).

Note: Safety and efficacy of oral carnitine have not been established in ESRD. Chronic administration of high **oral** doses to patients with severely compromised renal function or ESRD patients on dialysis may result in accumulation of **potentially toxic** metabolites.

Administration

Oral solution: May be taken directly or diluted in either beverages or liquid food; consume slowly; doses should be spaced evenly throughout the day, preferably during or following meals (every 3-4 hours) to improve tolerance

Parenteral: Dependent upon use:

Carnitine deficiency: May be administered undiluted (200 mg/mL) as I.V. push over 2-3 minutes **or** further diluted in LR or NS to a final concentration of 0.5-8 mg/mL and administered as an intermittent I.V. infusion typically over 30 minutes **or** as a continuous infusion

ESRD on hemodialysis: May be administered undiluted (200 mg/mL) I.V. push over 2-3 minutes into the venous return line

Valproic acid toxicity: May be administered undiluted (200 mg/mL) I.V. push over 2-3 minutes or further diluted in LR or NS to a final concentration of 0.5-8 mg/mL and administered by intermittent infusion over 30 minutes

Monitoring Parameters

Carnitine serum concentrations should be obtained at baseline and subsequently monitored weekly to monthly. In metabolic disorders: Blood chemistry, vital signs, and plasma carnitine concentration. In ESRD patients on dialysis: National Kidney Foundation guidelines recommend basing treatment on clinical signs and symptoms; evaluate response at 3-month intervals and discontinue if no clinical improvement noted within 9-12 months (Eknoyan, 2003).

Valproic acid toxicity: Serum valproic acid concentrations (every 4-6 hours until a downward trend is observed), electrolytes, blood gases, mental status, hepatic function, serum ammonia concentration, serum lactate, and platelets

Reference Range Plasma free carnitine level: >20 micromoles/L; plasma total carnitine level 30-60 micromoles/L; to evaluate for carnitine deficiency determine the plasma acylcarnitine/free carnitine ratio (A/F ratio)

A/F ratio = [plasma total carnitine - free carnitine] divided by free carnitine

Normal plasma A/F ratio = 0.25; in carnitine deficiency A/F ratio >0.4

Dosage Forms Excipient information presented when available (limited, particularly for generics); consult specific product labeling.

Capsule, Oral:

Generic: 250 mg

Capsule, Oral [preservative free]:

Generic: 250 mg

Solution, Intravenous:

Carnitor: 200 mg/mL (5 mL)

Generic: 200 mg/mL (5 mL, 12.5 mL)

Solution, Intravenous [preservative free]:

Generic: 200 mg/mL (5 mL)

Solution, Oral:

Carnitor: 1 g/10 mL (118 mL) [contains methylparaben, propylparaben; cherry flavor]

Carnitor SF: 1 g/10 mL (118 mL) [sugar free; contains methylparaben, propylparaben, saccharin sodium; cherry flavor]

Generic: 1 g/10 mL (118 mL)

Tablet, Oral:

Carnitor: 330 mg

Generic: 250 mg, 330 mg

References

Bonner CM, De Brie KL, Hug G, et al, "Effects of Parenteral L-Carnitine Supplementation on Fat Metabolism and Nutrition in Premature Neonates," *J Pediatr*, 1995, 126(2):287-92.

Borum PR, "Carnitine in Neonatal Nutrition," *J Child Neurol*, 1995, 10 (Suppl 2):S25-31.

Eknoyan G, Latos DL, and Lindberg J, "Practice Recommendations for the Use of L-carnitine in Dialysis-Related Carnitine Disorder. National Kidney Foundation Carnitine Consensus Conference," *Am J Kidney Dis*, 2003, 41(4):868-76.

Eyer F, Felgenhauer N, Gempel K, et al, "Acute Valproate Poisoning: Pharmacokinetics, Alteration in Fatty Acid Metabolism, and Changes During Therapy," *J Clin Psychopharmacol*, 2005, 25(4):376-80.

Freeman JM, Vining EP, Cost S, et al, "Does Carnitine Administration Improve the Symptoms Attributed to Anticonvulsant Medications?: A Double-Blinded, Crossover Study," *Pediatrics*, 1994, 93(6 Pt 1):893-5.

Helms RA, Mauer EC, and Hay WW Jr, "Effect of Intravenous L-Carnitine on Growth Parameters and Fat Metabolism During Parenteral Nutrition in Neonates," *JPEN J Parenter Enteral Nutr*, 1990, 14 (5):448-53.

Katiyar A and Aaron C, "Case Files of the Children's Hospital of Michigan Regional Poison Control Center: The Use of Carnitine for the Management of Acute Valproic Acid Toxicity," *J Med Toxicol*, 2007, 3(3):129-38.

KDOQI Work Group, "KDOQI Clinical Practice Guideline for Nutrition in Children With CKD: 2008 Update. Executive Summary," *Am J Kidney Dis*, 2009, 53(3 Suppl 2):S11-104.

Li BU, Lefevre F, Chelimsky GG, et al, "North American Society for Pediatric Gastroenterology, Hepatology, and Nutrition Consensus Statement on the Diagnosis and Management of Cyclic Vomiting Syndrome," *J Pediatr Gastroenterol Nutr*, 2008, 47(3):379-93.

Mock CM and Schwetschenau KH, "Levocarnitine for Valproic Acid-Induced Hyperammonemic Encephalopathy," *Am J Health Syst Pharm*, 2012, 69(1):35-9.

National Kidney Foundation, "KDOQI Clinical Practice Guidelines and Clinical Practice Recommendations for Anemia in Chronic Kidney Disease," *Am J Kidney Dis*, 2006, 47(5 Suppl 3):S11-145.

Perrott J, Murphy NG, and Zed PJ, "L-Carnitine for Acute Valproic Acid Overdose: A Systematic Review of Published Cases," *Ann Pharmacother*, 2010, 44(7-8):1287-93.

Russell S, "Carnitine as an Antidote for Acute Valproate Toxicity in Children," *Curr Opin Pediatr*, 2007, 19(2):206-10.

Levocetirizine (LEE vo se TI ra zeen)

Medication Safety Issues
Sound-alike/look-alike issues:
Levocetirizine may be confused with cetirizine
Brand Names: U.S. Xyzal
Therapeutic Category Antihistamine
Generic Availability (U.S.) Yes
Use Relief of symptoms associated with perennial allergic rhinitis (FDA approved in ages ≥6 months and adults), seasonal allergic rhinitis (FDA approved in ages ≥2 years and adults), and treatment of the uncomplicated skin manifestations of chronic idiopathic urticaria (FDA approved in ages ≥6 months and adults)
Pregnancy Risk Factor B
Pregnancy Considerations Adverse events have not been observed in animal reproduction studies; therefore, the manufacturer classifies levocetirizine as pregnancy category B. The use of antihistamines for the treatment of rhinitis during pregnancy is generally considered to be safe at recommended doses. Information related to the use of levocitirizine during pregnancy is limited; therefore, other agents are preferred. Levocetirizine is the active enantiomer of cetirizine; refer to the Cetirizine monograph for additional information.
Breast-Feeding Considerations It is not known if levocetirizine is excreted in breast milk. Breast-feeding is not recommended by the manufacturer.
Contraindications Hypersensitivity to levocetirizine, cetirizine, hydroxyzine, or any component; end stage renal disease (CrCl <10 mL/minute); patients undergoing dialysis; infants and children 6 months to 11 years with impaired renal function
Warnings Safety and efficacy for the use of cough and cold products in children <2 years of age is limited. Serious adverse effects including death have been reported. The FDA notes that there are no approved OTC uses for these products in children <2 years of age. Healthcare providers are reminded to ask caregivers about the use of OTC cough and cold products in order to avoid exposure to multiple medications containing the same ingredient.

May cause drowsiness; patients must be cautioned about performing tasks which require mental alertness (eg, operating machinery or driving); alcohol may have additive effects; avoid concurrent use

Precautions Use with caution in patients with mild to moderate renal dysfunction and adjust dosage. Use with caution in patients at risk for genitourinary obstruction (eg, spinal cord lesion); urinary retention has been reported; discontinue if urinary retention occurs
Adverse Reactions
Central nervous system: Drowsiness, fatigue
Gastrointestinal: Constipation, diarrhea, vomiting, xerostomia
Neuromuscular & skeletal: Weakness
Otic: Otitis media
Respiratory: Cough, epistaxis, nasopharyngitis, pharyngitis
Miscellaneous: Fever (children 4%)
Rare but important or life-threatening: Aggressive behavior, agitation, anaphylaxis, angioedema, dysuria, fixed-drug eruption, hepatitis, hypersensitivity, increased serum bilirubin, increased serum transaminases, movement disorder (including dystonia and oculogyric crisis), myalgia, nausea, palpitations, paresthesia, pruritus, skin rash, seizure, suicidal ideation, syncope, urinary retention, urticaria, visual disturbances, weight gain
Drug Interactions
Metabolism/Transport Effects None known.
Avoid Concomitant Use
Avoid concomitant use of Levocetirizine with any of the following: Aclidinium; Azelastine (Nasal); Ipratropium (Oral Inhalation); Paraldehyde; Potassium Chloride; Thalidomide; Tiotropium; Umeclidinium
Increased Effect/Toxicity
Levocetirizine may increase the levels/effects of: AbobotulinumtoxinA; Alcohol (Ethyl); Analgesics (Opioid); Anticholinergic Agents; Azelastine (Nasal); Buprenorphine; Cannabinoid-Containing Products; CNS Depressants; Hydrocodone; Methotrimeprazine; Metyrosine; Mirabegron; Mirtazapine; OnabotulinumtoxinA; Paraldehyde; Potassium Chloride; Pramipexole; RimabotulinumtoxinB; ROPINIRole; Rotigotine; Selective Serotonin Reuptake Inhibitors; Thalidomide; Thiazide Diuretics; Tiotropium; Topiramate; Zolpidem

The levels/effects of Levocetirizine may be increased by: Aclidinium; Brimonidine (Topical); Cannabis; Doxylamine; Dronabinol; Droperidol; HydrOXYzine; Ipratropium (Oral Inhalation); Kava Kava; Magnesium Sulfate; Methotrimeprazine; Nabilone; Perampanel; Pramlintide; Rufinamide; Sodium Oxybate; Tapentadol; Tetrahydrocannabinol; Umeclidinium
Decreased Effect
Levocetirizine may decrease the levels/effects of: Acetylcholinesterase Inhibitors (Central); Benzylpenicilloyl Polylysine; Betahistine; Hyaluronidase; Secretin

The levels/effects of Levocetirizine may be decreased by: Acetylcholinesterase Inhibitors (Central); Amphetamines
Stability Store at 20°C to 25°C (68°F to 77°F); excursions permitted to 15°C to 30°C (59°F to 86°F).
Mechanism of Action Levocetirizine is an antihistamine which selectively competes with histamine for H_1-receptor sites on effector cells in the gastrointestinal tract, blood vessels, and respiratory tract. Levocetirizine, the active enantiomer of cetirizine, has twice the binding affinity at the H_1-receptor compared to cetirizine.
Pharmacodynamics
Duration: 24 hours
Pharmacokinetics (Adult data unless noted)
Absorption: Well absorbed from the GI tract
Distribution: V_d:
  Children: 0.4 L/kg
  Adults: 0.4 L/kg
Protein binding: 91% to 92%

Metabolism: Limited hepatic metabolism (~14% of a dose); metabolic pathways include aromatic oxidation, N- and O-dealkylation, and taurine conjugation

Half-life:
Children 1-2 years: ~4 hours
Children 6-11 years: ~6 hours (24% less than adult half-life)
Adults: 8 hours

Time to peak serum concentration:
Children: 1.2 hours
Adults: Oral solution: 0.5 hours; Tablet: 0.9 hours

Elimination: 85.4% excreted unchanged in urine; 12.9% in feces

Clearance:
Children 1-2 years: 1 mL/kg/minute
Children 6-11 years: 0.82 mL/kg/minute
Adults: 0.63 mL/kg/minute

Dialysis: <10% removed during hemodialysis

Dosing: Usual

Pediatric:

Allergic rhinitis, perennial: Oral:
Infants and Children 6 months to 5 years: 1.25 mg once daily (in the evening); maximum daily dose: 1.25 mg/**day**
Children 6-11 years: 2.5 mg once daily (in the evening); maximum: 2.5 mg/**day**
Children ≥12 years and Adolescents: 5 mg once daily (in the evening); some patients may experience relief of symptoms with 2.5 mg once daily

Allergic rhinitis, seasonal: Oral:
Children 2-5 years: 1.25 mg once daily (in the evening); maximum: 1.25 mg/**day**
Children 6-11 years: 2.5 mg once daily (in the evening); maximum: 2.5 mg/**day**
Children ≥12 years and Adolescents: 5 mg once daily (in the evening); some patients may experience relief of symptoms with 2.5 mg once daily

Urticaria, chronic: Oral:
Infants and Children 6 months to 5 years: 1.25 mg once daily (in the evening); maximum daily dose: 1.25 mg/**day**
Children 6-11 years: 2.5 mg once daily (in the evening); maximum: 2.5 mg/**day**
Children ≥12 years and Adolescents: 5 mg once daily (in the evening); some patients may experience relief of symptoms with 2.5 mg once daily

Adult: **Allergic rhinitis, chronic urticaria:** Oral: 5 mg once daily (in the evening); some patients may experience relief of symptoms with 2.5 mg once daily

Dosing adjustment in renal impairment:
Infants and Children 6 months to 11 years: Contraindicated
Children ≥12 years, Adolescents, and Adults:
CrCl 50-80 mL/minute: 2.5 mg once daily
CrCl 30-50 mL/minute: 2.5 mg once every other day
CrCl 10-30 mL/minute: 2.5 mg twice weekly (every 3 or 4 days)
CrCl <10 mL/minute or on hemodialysis: Contraindicated

Dosing adjustment in hepatic impairment: No dosage adjustment necessary.

Administration Administer without regard to food in the evening.

Dosage Forms Excipient information presented when available (limited, particularly for generics); consult specific product labeling.
Solution, Oral, as dihydrochloride:
Xyzal: 2.5 mg/5 mL (148 mL) [contains methylparaben, propylparaben, saccharin]
Generic: 2.5 mg/5 mL (148 mL)

Tablet, Oral, as dihydrochloride:
Xyzal: 5 mg [scored]
Generic: 5 mg

References
Cranswick N, Turzíkova J, Fuchs M, et al, "Levocetirizine in 1-2 Year Old Children: Pharmacokinetic and Pharmacodynamic Profile," *Int J Clin Pharmacol Ther*, 2005, 43(4):172-7.
Simons FE and Simons KJ, "Levocetirizine: Pharmacokinetics and Pharmacodynamics in Children Age 6 to 11 Years," *J Allergy Clin Immunol*, 2005, 116(2):355-61.

◆ **Levocetirizine Dihydrochloride** see Levocetirizine on page 1227

Levofloxacin (Systemic) (lee voe FLOKS a sin)

Medication Safety Issues
Sound-alike/look-alike issues:
Levaquin may be confused with Levoxyl, Levsin/SL, Lovenox
Levofloxacin may be confused with levETIRAcetam, levodopa, Levophed, levothyroxine

Brand Names: U.S. Levaquin

Brand Names: Canada APO-Levofloxacin; AVA-Levofloxacin; CO Levofloxacin; Levaquin; Mylan-Levofloxacin; Novo-Levofloxacin; PMS-Levofloxacin; Sandoz-Levofloxacin

Therapeutic Category Antibiotic, Quinolone

Generic Availability (U.S.) Yes

Use Treatment of plague and postexposure prevention of inhalational anthrax (FDA approved for ages ≥6 months and adults); treatment of acute bacterial sinusitis, pneumonia (nosocomial and community-acquired), acute bacterial exacerbation of chronic bronchitis, skin and skin structure infections (uncomplicated or complicated), chronic bacterial prostatitis, urinary tract infections (uncomplicated or complicated), and acute pyelonephritis due to multidrug-resistant organisms susceptible to levofloxacin (FDA approved in ages ≥18 years and adults). Has also been used to treat pulmonary exacerbations in cystic fibrosis and multidrug-resistant tuberculosis.

Medication Guide Available Yes

Pregnancy Risk Factor C

Pregnancy Considerations Adverse events have been observed in some animal studies; therefore, the manufacturer classifies levofloxacin as pregnancy category C. Levofloxacin crosses the placenta. Quinolone exposure during human pregnancy has been reported with other agents (see Ciprofloxacin [Systemic] and Ofloxacin [Systemic] monographs). To date, no specific teratogenic effect or increased pregnancy risk has been identified; however, because of concerns of cartilage damage in immature animals exposed to quinolones and the limited levofloxacin specific data, levofloxacin should only be used during pregnancy if a safer option is not available.

Breast-Feeding Considerations Based on data from a case report, small amounts of levofloxacin are excreted in breast milk. Breast-feeding is not recommended by the manufacturer. Levofloxacin is the L-isomer of ofloxacin. Ofloxacin has also been shown to have minimal concentrations in human milk. Nondose-related effects could include modification of bowel flora.

Contraindications Hypersensitivity to levofloxacin, any component, or other quinolones

Warnings Tendonitis and tendon rupture have been reported with fluoroquinolones in patients of all ages [U.S. Boxed Warning]; increased risk in patients taking concomitant corticosteroids; with rheumatoid arthritis; age >60 years; and with kidney, heart, or lung transplants; usually involves the Achilles, hand, or shoulder tendons and can occur during therapy or up to a few months after therapy completion. Increased osteochondrosis in immature rats and dogs was observed with levofloxacin and fluoroquinolones have caused arthropathy with erosions of the cartilage in weight-bearing joints of immature animals. In a pooled safety data analysis of more than 2500 pediatric patients (6 months to 16 years), musculoskeletal events [eg, tendinopathy (inflammation or tendon rupture), arthritis (joint inflammation with redness and/or swelling), arthralgia (pain), or gait abnormality (limping, refusal to walk) were observed more frequently at 2 months and 12 months after treatment with levofloxacin than comparative treatment; the most frequently reported event was joint pain (85%). No physical joint abnormalities were observed; however, cumulative long-term (up to 5 years) outcomes showed musculoskeletal adverse events (including ongoing arthropathy; peripheral neuropathy; abnormal bone development; scoliosis; walking difficulty; myalgia; tendon injury; hypermobility syndrome; or pain in the spine, shoulder, or hip) were slightly higher in the comparator group than levofloxacin. Safety of use in pediatric patients for >14 days of therapy has not reported; in available pediatric safety data, the typical duration of therapy was around 10 days (CAP, AOM) (Bradley, 2011).

Fluoroquinolones, including levofloxacin, may exacerbate muscle weakness associated with myasthenia gravis **[U.S. Boxed Warning]**; cases of severe exacerbations, including the need for ventilatory support and deaths, have been reported; avoid use in patients with myasthenia gravis. Peripheral neuropathy has been reported (rare); may occur soon after initiation of therapy and may be irreversible; discontinue if symptoms of sensory or sensorimotor neuropathy occur.

Toxic psychoses, tremor, restlessness, anxiety, lightheadedness, paranoia, depression, nightmares, insomnia, confusion, and very rarely hallucinations, increased intracranial pressure (including pseudotumor cerebri), or seizures may occur; use with caution in patients with known or suspected CNS disorder; discontinue in patients who experience significant CNS adverse effects (eg, dizziness, hallucinations, seizures, suicidal ideations or actions). Rare cases of polyneuropathy affecting small and/or large axons, resulting in paresthesias, hypoesthesias, dysesthesias, and weakness, have been reported in patients receiving levofloxacin. Discontinue levofloxacin if patient experiences pain, burning, tingling, numbness, or weakness or is found to have deficits in light touch, pain, temperature, position sense, vibrating sensation, or motor strength.

Serious and occasionally fatal hypersensitivity and/or anaphylactic reactions have been reported often following the first dose. Hypersensitivity reactions have been accompanied by cardiovascular collapse, hypotension/shock, seizure, loss of consciousness, tingling, angioedema, airway obstruction, dyspnea, urticaria, itching, and skin reactions. If these reactions occur, discontinue levofloxacin. Resuscitation equipment, oxygen, epinephrine, antihistamine, and a corticosteroid should be readily available to treat hypersensitivity reactions.

Idiosyncratic reactions, including toxic epidermal necrolysis, vasculitis, pneumonitis, nephritis, hepatic failure, and/or cytopenias, have usually occurred after multiple doses. Discontinue drug if these reactions occur. Unrelated to hypersensitivity, severe hepatotoxicity (including acute hepatitis and fatalities) has been reported; discontinue therapy immediately if signs and symptoms of hepatitis occur. Prolonged use may result in superinfection, including C. difficile-associated diarrhea and pseudomembranous colitis.

Oral solution contains benzyl alcohol and propylene glycol which may be toxic to newborns in high doses; benzyl alcohol may cause allergic reactions in susceptible individuals; large amounts of benzyl alcohol (≥99 mg/kg/day)

have been associated with a potentially fatal toxicity ("gasping syndrome"). Toxicities have been reported with use of products containing propylene glycol, including hyperosmolality, lactic acidosis, seizures and respiratory depression; in neonates large amounts of propylene glycol delivered orally, intravenously (eg, >3000 mg/day), or topically have been associated with potentially fatal toxicities which can include metabolic acidosis, seizures, renal failure, and CNS depression; use oral solution containing propylene glycol with caution (AAP, 1997; Shehab, 2009).

Precautions Use with caution in patients with renal impairment; dosage adjustment required. Rarely, crystalluria has occurred; urine alkalinity may increase the risk; ensure adequate hydration during therapy. Use with caution in patients with G6PD deficiency; hemolytic reactions may (rarely) occur with quinolone use in patients with latent or actual G6PD deficiency. Use with caution in individuals at risk of seizures (CNS disorders or severe cerebral arteriosclerosis), or concurrent therapy with medications which may lower seizure threshold; potential for seizures with use exists, although very rare; may be increased with concomitant NSAID therapy.

Fluoroquinolones may prolong QT_C interval and rare cases of torsade de pointes have been reported in patients taking levofloxacin; avoid use in patients with a history of QT_c prolongation, uncorrected hypokalemia or hypomagnesemia, on concurrent therapy with Class Ia or Class III antiarrhythmics or other medications known to prolong the QT interval (cisapride, erythromycin, antipsychotics, and tricyclic antidepressants), or in patients with bradycardia, cardiomyopathy, or recent myocardial ischemia.

May cause alterations in glucose regulation; fluoroquinolones have been associated with the development of serious, and sometimes fatal, hypoglycemia; most often reported in elderly patients with diabetes, but has also been reported in patients without a prior history of diabetes; prompt identification and treatment of hypoglycemia is essential. Individual quinolones may differ in their potential to cause this effect; was most evident with gatifloxacin (no longer marketed as systemic formulation). Hyperglycemia has also been associated with the use of fluoroquinolones. Patients should be monitored closely for signs/symptoms of disordered glucose regulation.

May rarely cause moderate to severe phototoxicity reactions; avoid excessive sunlight and take precautions to limit exposure (eg, loose-fitting clothing, sunscreen); discontinue use if phototoxicity occurs.

In pediatric patients, fluoroquinolones are not routinely first-line therapy, but after assessment of risks and benefits, can be considered a reasonable alternative for situations where no safe and effective substitute is available [eg, resistance (common CF pathogens, multidrug resistant-tuberculosis)] or in situations where the only alternative is parenteral therapy and levofloxacin offers an oral therapy option [eg, acute otitis media/sinusitis (S. pneumoniae, H. influenza; pneumonia (S. pneumoniae, Mycoplasma pneumonia)] (Bradley, 2011).

Adverse Reactions
Cardiovascular: Chest pain, edema
Central nervous system: Dizziness, headache, insomnia
Dermatologic: Pruritus, skin rash
Gastrointestinal: Abdominal pain, constipation, diarrhea, dyspepsia, nausea, vomiting
Genitourinary: Vaginitis
Infection: Candidiasis
Local: Injection site reaction
Respiratory: Dyspnea
Rare but important or life-threatening: Abnormal electroencephalogram, abnormal gait, acute renal failure, ageusia, agranulocytosis, anaphylactoid reaction, anemia (including aplastic and hemolytic), anorexia, anosmia,

◄ brain disease (rare), cardiac arrest, cardiac arrhythmia (including ventricular tachycardia/fibrillation and torsade de pointes), *Clostridium difficile*-associated diarrhea, confusion, convulsions, crystalluria, cylindruria, depression, elevation in serum levels of skeletal-muscle enzymes, eosinophilia, epistaxis, erythema multiforme, esophagitis, exacerbation of myasthenia gravis, gastritis (including gastroenteritis), glossitis, granulocytopenia, hallucination, hepatic failure (some fatal), hepatic insufficiency, hepatitis, hyperglycemia, hyperkalemia, hyperkinesias, hypersensitivity reaction (including anaphylaxis, angioedema, rash, pneumonitis, and serum sickness), hypertension, hypertonia, hypoacusis, hypoglycemia, hypotension, increased INR, increased intracranial pressure, increased serum alkaline phosphatase, increased serum transaminases, interstitial nephritis, intestinal obstruction, jaundice, leukocytosis, leukopenia, leukorrhea, lymphadenopathy, multiorgan failure, muscle injury, muscle spasm, pancreatitis, pancytopenia, paralysis, paranoia, peripheral neuropathy (may be irreversible), phlebitis, phototoxicity, prolonged prothrombin time, prolonged Q-T interval on ECG, pseudotumor cerebri, psychosis, renal function abnormality, rhabdomyolysis, rupture of tendon, scotoma, seizure, skeletal pain, skin photosensitivity, sleep disorder (including abnormal dreams and nightmares), Stevens-Johnson syndrome, stomatitis, suicidal ideation, syncope, tachycardia, tendonitis, toxic epidermal necrolysis, toxic psychosis, thrombocytopenia (including thrombotic thrombocytopenic purpura), uveitis, vasculitis (leukocytoclastic), vasodilatation, visual disturbances(including diplopia), voice disorder

Drug Interactions

Metabolism/Transport Effects None known.

Avoid Concomitant Use

Avoid concomitant use of Levofloxacin (Systemic) with any of the following: BCG; Highest Risk QTc-Prolonging Agents; Ivabradine; Mifepristone; Strontium Ranelate

Increased Effect/Toxicity

Levofloxacin (Systemic) may increase the levels/effects of: Corticosteroids (Systemic); Highest Risk QTc-Prolonging Agents; Moderate Risk QTc-Prolonging Agents; Porfimer; Sulfonylureas; Tacrolimus (Systemic); Varenicline; Vitamin K Antagonists

The levels/effects of Levofloxacin (Systemic) may be increased by: Insulin; Ivabradine; Mifepristone; Nonsteroidal Anti-Inflammatory Agents; Probenecid; QTc-Prolonging Agents (Indeterminate Risk and Risk Modifying)

Decreased Effect

Levofloxacin (Systemic) may decrease the levels/effects of: BCG; Didanosine; Mycophenolate; Sodium Picosulfate; Sulfonylureas; Typhoid Vaccine

The levels/effects of Levofloxacin (Systemic) may be decreased by: Antacids; Calcium Salts; Didanosine; Iron Salts; Lanthanum; Magnesium Salts; Multivitamins/Minerals (with ADEK, Folate, Iron); Multivitamins/Minerals (with AE, No Iron); Quinapril; Sevelamer; Strontium Ranelate; Sucralfate; Zinc Salts

Stability

Oral:
Solution: Store at 25°C (77°F); excursions permitted to 15°C to 30°C (59°F to 86°F).
Tablets: Store at 15°C to 30°C (59°F to 86°F).

Parenteral:
Vial: Store at room temperature; protect from light; solutions further diluted to 5 mg/mL in appropriate fluid are stable: Room temperature: 72 hours; refrigeration: 14 days; and frozen at -20°C (-4°F): 6 months. If frozen, do not thaw in microwave or by bath immersion; do not refreeze.
Premixed: Store at ≤25°C (77°F); do not freeze. Brief exposure to 40°C (104°F) does not affect product. Protect from light.

Mechanism of Action As the S(-) enantiomer of the fluoroquinolone, ofloxacin, levofloxacin, inhibits DNA-gyrase in susceptible organisms thereby inhibits relaxation of supercoiled DNA and promotes breakage of DNA strands. DNA gyrase (topoisomerase II), is an essential bacterial enzyme that maintains the superhelical structure of DNA and is required for DNA replication and transcription, DNA repair, recombination, and transposition.

Pharmacokinetics (Adult data unless noted) Levofloxacin absorption (as indicated by C_{max} and t_{max}) and distribution in children are not age-dependent and are comparable to those in adults.

Absorption: Well-absorbed; levofloxacin oral tablet and solution formulations are bioequivalent

Distribution: Widely distributed in the body, including blister fluid, skin tissue, macrophages, prostate, and lung tissue; CSF concentrations ~15% of serum concentrations

V_d: I.V. (Chien, 2005):
Infants ≥6 months, Children, and Adolescents ≤16 years: Mean range: 1.44-1.57 L/kg; reported values not statistically different between pediatric age subgroups; distribution not age-dependent
Adults: 1.27 L/kg

Protein binding: 24% to 38%, primarily to albumin

Bioavailability: Oral: 99%

Half-life:
Infants ≥6 months and Children ≤5 years: ~4 hours (Chien, 2005)
Children 5-10 years: 4.8 hours (Chien, 2005)
Children 10-12 years: 5.4 hours (Chien, 2005)
Children 12-16 years: 6 hours (Chien, 2005)
Adults: 6-8 hours

Time to peak serum concentration: Oral: Within 1-2 hours

Elimination: 87% excreted unchanged in urine over 48 hours by tubular secretion and glomerular filtration; 4% in feces

Clearance: I.V.: (Chien, 2005):
Infants and Children 6 months to 2 years: 0.35 ± 0.13 L/hour/kg
Children 2-5 years: 0.32 ± 0.08 L/hour/kg
Children 5-10 years: 0.25 ± 0.05 L/hour/kg
Children 10-12 years: 0.19 ± 0.05 L/hour/kg
Children 12-16 years: 0.18 ± 0.03 L/hour/kg
Adults: 0.15 ± 0.02 L/hour/kg

Dosing: Usual

Pediatric: **Note:** In pediatric patients, fluoroquinolones are not routinely first-line therapy, but after assessment of risks and benefits, can be considered a reasonable alternative for situations where no safe and effective substitute is available [eg, resistance (cystic fibrosis)] or in situations where the only alternative is parenteral therapy and levofloxacin offers an oral therapy option (Bradley, 2011). Use of levofloxacin in infants <6 months has not been studied.

General dosing, susceptible infection (Bradley, 2011): Infants ≥6 months, Children, and Adolescents:
Oral, I.V.:
<5 years: 8-10 mg/kg/dose twice daily
≥5 years: 10 mg/kg/dose once daily; maximum dose: 750 mg/**day**

Anthrax, postexposure (inhalation): Infants ≥6 months, Children, and Adolescents: Oral, I.V.: **Note:** Begin as soon as possible after exposure:
<50 kg: 8 mg/kg/dose every 12 hours for 60 days; maximum dose: 250 mg
≥50 kg: 500 mg every 24 hours for 60 days

Cystic fibrosis pulmonary exacerbation: Limited data available (Bradley, 2011): Infants ≥6 months, Children, and Adolescents: Oral, I.V.: Some centers have used:
<5 years: 10 mg/kg/dose twice daily
≥5 years: 10 mg/kg/dose once daily; maximum dose: 750 mg/**day**

Peritoneal dialysis; tunnel or exit site infection: Limited data available: Oral: 10 mg/kg/dose every 48 hours; maximum initial dose: 500 mg; maximum subsequent doses: 250 mg (Warady, 2012)

Plague *(Yersinia pestis),* **prophylaxis or treatment:** Infants ≥6 months, Children, and Adolescents: Oral, I.V.: **Note:** Begin as soon as possible after exposure: <50 kg: 8 mg/kg/dose every 12 hours for 10-14 days; maximum dose: 250 mg

≥50 kg: 500 mg every 24 hours for 10-14 days

Pneumonia, community-acquired (CAP) (Bradley-IDSA/PIDS, 2011a): **Note:** May consider addition of vancomycin or clindamycin to empiric therapy if community-acquired MRSA suspected. In children ≥5 years, a macrolide antibiotic should be added if atypical pneumonia cannot be ruled out.

Typical pathogens:

Haemophilus influenzae:

Mild infection/step down therapy: Oral:

Infants ≥6 months and Children <5 years: 8-10 mg/kg/dose every 12 hours; maximum daily dose: 750 mg/**day**

Children ≥5 years and Adolescents ≤16 years: 8-10 mg/kg/dose once every 24 hours; maximum daily dose: 750 mg/**day**

Severe infections: I.V.:

Infants ≥6 months and Children <5 years: 8-10 mg/kg/dose every 12 hours; maximum daily dose: 750 mg/**day**

Children ≥5 years and Adolescents ≤16 years: 8-10 mg/kg/dose once every 24 hours; maximum daily dose: 750 mg/**day**

Streptococcus pneumoniae:

Penicillin-sensitive: Mild infection/step down therapy: Oral: **Note:** Levofloxacin is not recommended for routine use for the treatment of mild to moderate infection (*Red Book*, 2012)

Infants ≥6 months and Children <5 years: 8-10 mg/kg/dose every 12 hours; maximum daily dose: 750 mg/**day**

Children ≥5 years and Adolescents ≤16 years: 8-10 mg/kg/dose once every 24 hours; maximum daily dose: 750 mg/**day**

Penicillin-resistant: Mild infection/step-down therapy: Oral: **Note:** Levofloxacin is not recommended for routine use for the treatment of mild to moderate infection (*Red Book*, 2012)

Infants ≥6 months and Children <5 years: 8-10 mg/kg/dose every 12 hours; maximum daily dose: 750 mg/**day**

Children ≥5 years and Adolescents ≤16 years: 8-10 mg/kg/dose once every 24 hours; maximum daily dose: 750 mg/**day**

Severe infections: I.V.:

Infants ≥6 months and Children <5 years: 8-10 mg/kg/dose every 12 hours; maximum daily dose: 750 mg/**day**

Children ≥5 years and Adolescents ≤16 years: 8-10 mg/kg/dose once every 24 hours; maximum daily dose: 750 mg/**day**

Atypical pathogens (*Mycoplasma pneumonia* or *Chlamydia ssp*):

Mild infection/step-down therapy: Oral: Adolescents with skeletal maturity: 500 mg/dose once daily

Severe infections: I.V.:

Infants ≥6 months and Children <5 years: 8-10 mg/kg/dose every 12 hours; maximum daily dose: 750 mg/**day**

Children ≥5 years and Adolescents ≤16 years: 8-10 mg/kg/dose once every 24 hours; maximum daily dose: 750 mg/**day**

Rhinosinusitis, acute bacterial: Note: Recommended in the following types of patients: Type I penicillin

allergy, after failure of initial therapy or in patients at risk for antibiotic resistance (eg, daycare attendance, age <2 years, recent hospitalization, antibiotic use within the past month) (Chow, 2012). Children and Adolescents: Oral, I.V.: 10-20 mg/kg/**day** divided every 12-24 hours for 10-14 days; maximum daily dose: 500 mg/**day**

Surgical prophylaxis: Children and Adolescents: I.V.: 10 mg/kg as a single dose 120 minutes prior to procedure; maximum dose: 500 mg; **Note:** While fluoroquinolones have been associated with an increased risk of tendinitis/tendon rupture in all ages, use of these agents for single-dose prophylaxis is generally safe (Bratzler, 2013).

Tuberculosis, multidrug-resistant: Limited data available: **Note:** Use in combination with at least 2-3 additional anti-TB agents (overall multidrug regimen dependent upon susceptibility profile/patterns) (Seddon, 2012): Oral:

Infants and Children <5 years: 7.5-10 mg/kg/dose every 12 hours; maximum daily dose: 750 mg/day

Children ≥5 years and Adolescents: 7.5-10 mg/kg/dose every 24 hours; maximum daily dose: 750 mg/day

Adult:

Anthrax, postexposure (inhalation): Oral, I.V.: 500 mg every 24 hours for 60 days beginning as soon as possible after exposure

Bronchitis, chronic: Oral, I.V.: 500 mg every 24 hours for at least 7 days

Chlamydia trachomatis **sexually transmitted infections:** Oral: 500 mg every 24 hours for 7 days (CDC, 2010)

Epididymitis, nongonococcal: Oral: 500 mg once daily for 10 days (CDC, 2010)

Intra-abdominal infection, complicated, community-acquired (in combination with metronidazole): I.V.: 750 mg once daily for 4-7 days (provided source controlled). **Note:** Avoid using in settings where *E. coli* susceptibility to fluoroquinolones is <90% (Solomkin, 2010).

Pelvic inflammatory disease: Oral: 500 mg once daily for 14 days with or without concomitant metronidazole; **Note:** The CDC recommends use as an alternative therapy only if standard parenteral cephalosporin therapy is not feasible and community prevalence of quinolone-resistant gonococcal organisms is low. Culture sensitivity must be confirmed (CDC, 2010).

Plague *(Yersinia pestis),* **prophylaxis or treatment:** Oral, I.V.: 500 mg every 24 hours for 10-14 days, beginning as soon as possible after exposure

Pneumonia: Oral, I.V.:

Community-acquired: 500 mg every 24 hours for 7-14 days or 750 mg every 24 hours for 5 days (efficacy of 5-day regimen for multidrug resistant *S. Pneumoniae* not established)

Nosocomial: 750 mg every 24 hours for 7-14 days

Prostatitis, chronic bacterial: Oral, I.V.: 500 mg every 24 hours for 28 days

Rhinosinusitis, acute bacterial: Oral, I.V.:

Manufacturer's recommendations: 500 mg every 24 hours for 10-14 days or 750 mg every 24 hours for 5 days

Alternate recommendations: 500 mg every 24 hours for 5-7 days (Chow, 2012)

Skin and skin structure infections: Oral, I.V.:

Complicated: 750 mg every 24 hours for 7-14 days

Uncomplicated: 500 mg every 24 hours for 7-10 days

Urethritis, nongonococcal: Oral: 500 mg every 24 hours for 7 days (CDC, 2010)

Urinary tract infection (UTI): Oral, I.V.:

Complicated or acute pyelonephritis: 250 mg every 24 hours for 10 days or 750 mg every 24 hours for 5 days

Uncomplicated: 250 mg every 24 hours for 3 days

Dosing interval in renal impairment:

Infants, Children, and Adolescents: The following adjustments have been recommended (Aronoff, 2007). **Note:** Renally adjusted dose recommendations are based on doses of 5-10 mg/kg/dose every 12 hours for children ≤5 years and 5-10 mg/kg/dose every 24 hours for children >5 years.

GFR ≥30 mL/minute/1.73 m^2: No adjustment necessary

GFR 10-29 mL/minute/1.73 m^2: 5-10 mg/kg/dose every 24 hours

GFR <10 mL/minute/1.73 m^2: 5-10 mg/kg/dose every 48 hours

Intermittent hemodialysis: 5-10 mg/kg/dose every 48 hours; not removed by hemodialysis; supplemental levofloxacin doses are not required

Peritoneal dialysis (PD): 5-10 mg/kg/dose every 48 hours; not removed by peritoneal dialysis; supplemental levofloxacin doses are not required

Continuous renal replacement therapy (CRRT): 10 mg/kg/dose every 24 hours

Adults:

Normal renal function dosing of 250 mg/day:

CrCl 20-49 mL/minute: No dosage adjustment required

CrCl 10-19 mL/minute: Administer 250 mg every 48 hours (except in uncomplicated UTI, where no dosage adjustment is required)

Hemodialysis (administer after hemodialysis on dialysis days)/peritoneal dialysis (PD): No information available

Normal renal function dosing of 500 mg/day:

CrCl 20-49 mL/minute: Administer 500 mg initial dose, followed by 250 mg every 24 hours

CrCl 10-19 mL/minute: Administer 500 mg initial dose, followed by 250 mg every 48 hours

Hemodialysis (administer after hemodialysis on dialysis days)/peritoneal dialysis (PD): Administer 500 mg initial dose, followed by 250 mg every 48 hours; not removed by hemodialysis or peritoneal dialysis; supplemental levofloxacin doses are not required

Normal renal function dosing of 750 mg/day:

CrCl 20-49 mL/minute: Administer 750 mg every 48 hours

CrCl 10-19 mL/minute: Administer 750 mg initial dose, followed by 500 mg every 48 hours

Hemodialysis (administer after hemodialysis on dialysis days)/peritoneal dialysis (PD): Administer 750 mg initial dose, followed by 500 mg every 48 hours; not removed by hemodialysis or peritoneal dialysis; supplemental levofloxacin doses are not required

Normal renal function dosing of 750 or 1000 mg daily (treatment of tuberculosis **only**) (CDC, 2003): CrCl <30 mL/minute: Administer 750 or 1000 mg 3 times per week (in hemodialysis patients administer after dialysis on dialysis days)

Continuous renal replacement therapy (CRRT) (Heintz, 2009; Trotman, 2005): Drug clearance is highly dependent on the method of renal replacement, filter type, and flow rate. Appropriate dosing requires close monitoring of pharmacologic response, signs of adverse reactions due to drug accumulation, as well as drug concentrations in relation to target trough (if appropriate). The following are general recommendations only (based on dialysate flow/ultrafiltration rates of 1-2 L/hour and minimal residual renal function) and should not supersede clinical judgment:

CVVH: Loading dose of 500-750 mg followed by 250 mg every 24 hours

CVVHD: Loading dose of 500-750 mg followed by 250-500 mg every 24 hours

CVVHDF: Loading dose of 500-750 mg followed by 250-750 mg every 24 hours

Dosing adjustment in hepatic impairment: There are no dosage adjustments provided in the manufacturer's labeling; has not been studied.

Administration

Oral: Tablets may be administered with or without food; oral solution should be administered 1 hour before or 2 hours after eating; avoid antacid use within 2 hours of administration

Parenteral: If preparing from vials, further dilute dose at a concentration not to exceed 5 mg/mL. Administer by slow I.V. infusion over 60-90 minutes (250-500 mg over 60 minutes; 750 mg over 90 minutes); avoid rapid or bolus I.V. infusion due to risk of hypotension; maintain adequate hydration to prevent crystalluria or cylinduria; not for I.M., SubQ, or intrathecal administration

Monitoring Parameters Evaluation of organ system functions (renal, hepatic, and hematopoietic) is recommended periodically during therapy; the possibility of crystalluria should be assessed; WBC and signs of infection; number and type of stools/day for diarrhea; hydration status; patients receiving concurrent levofloxacin and theophylline should have serum levels of theophylline monitored; monitor INR in patients receiving warfarin; monitor blood glucose in patients receiving antidiabetic agents or patients with a history of diabetes

Test Interactions Some quinolones may produce a false-positive urine screening result for opioids using commercially-available immunoassay kits. This has been demonstrated most consistently for levofloxacin and ofloxacin, but other quinolones have shown cross-reactivity in certain assay kits. Confirmation of positive opioid screens by more specific methods should be considered.

Additional Information A nebulized formulation is currently under investigation in clinical trials; Levofloxacin 240 mg inhalation over ~5 minutes once daily for 7 days was well tolerated in cystic fibrosis (CF) patients (n=10, age 33.6 ± 16.4 years). In another study, CF patients were given one of three doses (120 mg once daily, 240 mg once daily, 240 mg twice daily) or placebo for 28 days (n=114 treated, 37 placebo, age 28.7 ± 9 years). All three doses were well tolerated and resulted in decreased *Pseudomonas aeruginosa* density in sputum. Further studies are needed (Geller, 2011; Geller, 2011a).

Dosage Forms Excipient information presented when available (limited, particularly for generics); consult specific product labeling.

Solution, Intravenous [preservative free]:

Levaquin: 250 mg/50 mL (50 mL); 500 mg/100 mL (100 mL); 750 mg/150 mL (150 mL)

Generic: 250 mg/50 mL (50 mL); 500 mg/100 mL (100 mL); 750 mg/150 mL (150 mL); 25 mg/mL (20 mL, 30 mL)

Solution, Oral:

Levaquin: 25 mg/mL (480 mL) [contains propylene glycol]

Generic: 25 mg/mL (10 mL, 20 mL, 100 mL, 200 mL, 480 mL)

Tablet, Oral:

Levaquin: 250 mg, 500 mg, 750 mg

Generic: 250 mg, 500 mg, 750 mg

Extemporaneous Preparations Note: Commercial oral solution is available (25 mg/mL)

A 50 mg/mL oral suspension may be made with tablets and a 1:1 mixture of Ora-Plus® and strawberry syrup NF. Crush six 500 mg levofloxacin tablets in a mortar and reduce to a fine powder. Add small portions of the vehicle and mix to a uniform paste; mix while adding the vehicle in incremental proportions to **almost** 60 mL; transfer to a graduated cylinder, rinse mortar with vehicle, and add quantity of vehicle sufficient to make 60 mL. Label "shake well". Stable for 57 days when stored in amber plastic prescription bottles at room temperature or refrigerated.

VandenBussche HL, Johnson CE, and Fontana EM, et al, "Stability of Levofloxacin in an Extemporaneously Compounded Oral Liquid," *Am J Health Syst Pharm*, 1999, 56(22):2316-8.

References

American Academy of Pediatrics Committee on Drugs. "Inactive" ingredients in pharmaceutical products: update (subject review). *Pediatrics*. 1997;99(2):268-278.

Bradley JS, Byington CL, Shah SS, et al, "The Management of Community-Acquired Pneumonia in Infants and Children Older Than 3 Months of Age: Clinical Practice Guidelines by the Pediatric Infectious Diseases Society and the Infectious Diseases Society of America", *Clin Infect Dis*, 2011, 53(7):e25-76.

Bradley JS, Jackson MA, Committee on Infectious Diseases, American Academy of Pediatrics. The use of systemic and topical fluoroquinolones. *Pediatrics*. 2011a;128:e1034-1045.

Bradley JS, Nelson JD, Kimberlin DK, et al, eds. *Nelson's Pocket Book of Pediatric Antimicrobial Therapy*. 19th ed. Philadelphia, PA: Lippincott Williams & Wilkins; 2012.

Bratzler DW, Dellinger EP, Olsen KM, et al, "Clinical Practice Guidelines for Antimicrobial Prophylaxis in Surgery," *Surg Infect (Larchmt)*, 2013, 14(1):73-156.

Centers for Disease Control and Prevention (CDC), "Sexually Transmitted Diseases Treatment Guidelines, 2010," *MMWR Recomm Rep*, 2010, 59(RR-12):1-110.

Chien S, Wells TG, Blumer JL, et al, "Levofloxacin Pharmacokinetics in Children," *J Clin Pharmacol*, 2005, 45(2):153-60.

Chow AW, Benninger MS, Brook I, et al, "IDSA Clinical Practice Guideline for Acute Bacterial Rhinosinusitis in Children and Adults," *Clin Infect Dis*, 2012, 54(8):72-112.

Ernst ME, Ernst EJ, and Klepser ME, "Levofloxacin and Trovafloxacin: The Next Generation of Fluoroquinolones?" *Am J Health Syst Pharm*, 1997, 54(22):2569-84.

Geller DE, Flume PA, Staab D, et al, "Levofloxacin Inhalation Solution (MP-376) in Patients With Cystic Fibrosis With *Pseudomonas aeruginosa*," *Am J Respir Crit Care Med*, 2011, 183(11):1510-6.

Geller DE, Flume PA, Griffith DC, et al, "Pharmacokinetics and Safety of MP-376 (Levofloxacin Inhalation Solution) in Cystic Fibrosis Subjects," *Antimicrob Agents Chemother*, 2011a, 55(6):2636-40.

Heintz BH, Matzke GR, Dager WE, "Antimicrobial Dosing Concepts and Recommendations for Critically Ill Adult Patients Receiving Continuous Renal Replacement Therapy or Intermittent Hemodialysis," *Pharmacotherapy*, 2009, 29(5):562-77.

Schaad UB, "Role of the New Quinolones in Pediatric Practice," *Pediatr Infect Dis J*, 1992, 11(12):1043-6.

Shehab N, Lewis CL, Streetman DD, Donn SM. Exposure to the pharmaceutical excipients benzyl alcohol and propylene glycol among critically ill neonates. *Pediatr Crit Care Med*. 2009;10 (2):256-259.

Seddon JA, Furin JJ, Gale M, et al, "Caring for Children With Drug-Resistant Tuberculosis: Practice-Based Recommendations," *Am J Respir Crit Care Med*, 2012, 186(10):953-64.

Solomkin JS, Mazuski JE, Bradley JS, et al, "Diagnosis and Management of Complicated Intra-abdominal Infection in Adults and Children: Guidelines by the Surgical Infection Society and the Infectious Diseases Society of America," *Clin Infect Dis*, 2010, 50(2):133-64.

Trotman RL, Williamson JC, Shoemaker DM, et al, "Antibiotic Dosing in Critically Ill Adult Patients Receiving Continuous Renal Replacement Therapy," *Clin Infect Dis*, 2005, 41:1159-66.

Warady BA, Bakkaloglu S, Newland J, et al, "Consensus Guidelines for the Prevention and Treatment of Catheter-Related Infections and Peritonitis in Pediatric Patients Receiving Peritoneal Dialysis: 2012 Update," *Perit Dial Int*, 2012, (32 Suppl 2):S32-86.

Levofloxacin (Ophthalmic) (lee voe FLOKS a sin)

Medication Safety Issues

Sound-alike/look-alike issues:

Levofloxacin may be confused with levETIRAcetam, levodopa, levothyroxine

Therapeutic Category Antibiotic, Ophthalmic; Antibiotic, Quinolone

Generic Availability (U.S.) Yes

Use Used ophthalmically for treatment of bacterial conjunctivitis due to *S. aureus* (methicillin-susceptible strains), *S. epidermidis*, *S. pneumoniae*, *Streptococcus* (groups C/F), *Streptococcus* (group G), Viridans group *Streptococci*, *Corynebacterium* spp, *H. influenzae*, *Acinetobacter*

Pregnancy Risk Factor C

Pregnancy Considerations Adverse events have been observed in some animal studies; therefore, the manufacturer classifies levofloxacin ophthalmic as pregnancy category C. When administered orally or I.V., levofloxacin crosses the placenta. Refer to the Levofloxacin (Systemic) monograph for details. The amount of levofloxacin available systemically following topical application of the ophthalmic drops is significantly less in comparison to oral or I.V. doses.

Breast-Feeding Considerations When administered orally or I.V., levofloxacin enters breast milk. Refer to the Levofloxacin (Systemic) monograph for details. The amount of levofloxacin available systemically following topical application of the ophthalmic drops is significantly less in comparison to oral or I.V. doses. The manufacturer recommends that caution be exercised when administering levofloxacin eye drops to nursing women.

Contraindications Hypersensitivity to levofloxacin, any component, or other quinolones

Warnings There have been reports of tendon inflammation and/or rupture with systemic quinolone antibiotics. Exposure following ophthalmic administration is substantially lower than with systemic therapy.

Precautions Severe hypersensitivity reactions, including anaphylaxis, have occurred with quinolone therapy (primarily with systemic use). Prolonged use may result in fungal or bacterial superinfection.

Adverse Reactions

Gastrointestinal: Taste disturbance

Ocular: Decreased vision (transient), foreign body sensation, ocular pain or discomfort, photophobia, transient ocular burning

Rare but important or life-threatening: Allergic reaction, lid edema, ocular dryness, ocular itching

Drug Interactions

Metabolism/Transport Effects None known.

Avoid Concomitant Use There are no known interactions where it is recommended to avoid concomitant use.

Increased Effect/Toxicity There are no known significant interactions involving an increase in effect.

Decreased Effect There are no known significant interactions involving a decrease in effect.

Stability Store at room temperature.

Mechanism of Action As the S(-) enantiomer of the fluoroquinolone, ofloxacin, levofloxacin, inhibits DNA-gyrase in susceptible organisms thereby inhibits relaxation of supercoiled DNA and promotes breakage of DNA strands. DNA gyrase (topoisomerase II), is an essential bacterial enzyme that maintains the superhelical structure of DNA and is required for DNA replication and transcription, DNA repair, recombination, and transposition.

Pharmacokinetics (Adult data unless noted) Absorption: Only small amounts are absorbed systemically after ophthalmic instillation.

Dosing: Usual

Children ≥1 year and Adults: Bacterial conjunctivitis: 0.5% solution:

Treatment day 1 and day 2: Instill 1-2 drops into affected eye(s) every 2 hours while awake, up to 8 times/day

Treatment day 3-7: Instill 1-2 drops into affected eye(s) every 4 hours while awake, up to 4 times/day

Children ≥6 years and Adults: Bacterial corneal ulcer: 1.5% solution:

Treatment days 1-3: Instill 1-2 drops into affected eye(s) every 30 minutes to 2 hours while awake and ~4 and 6 hours after retiring

Treatment day 4 through treatment completion: Instill 1-2 drops into affected eye(s) every 1-4 hours while awake

Administration Not for subconjunctival injection or for use into anterior chamber of the eye. Contact lenses should not be worn during treatment. Instill drops into conjunctival sac of affected eye(s); apply finger pressure to lacrimal sac during and for 1-2 minutes after instillation to decrease risk of absorption and systemic effects; avoid contacting bottle tip with skin

Dosage Forms Excipient information presented when available (limited, particularly for generics); consult specific product labeling.

Solution, Ophthalmic:
Generic: 0.5% (5 mL)

◆ **Levophed** *see* Norepinephrine *on page 1510*

◆ **Levophed® (Can)** *see* Norepinephrine *on page 1510*

◆ **Levosalbutamol** *see* Levalbuterol *on page 1218*

◆ **Levothroid [DSC]** *see* Levothyroxine *on page 1234*

Levothyroxine (lee voe thye ROKS een)

Medication Safety Issues
Sound-alike/look-alike issues:
Levothyroxine may be confused with lamoTRIgine, Lanoxin, levofloxacin, liothyronine
Levoxyl may be confused with Lanoxin, Levaquin, Luvox
Synthroid may be confused with Symmetrel

Administration issues:
Significant differences exist between oral and I.V. dosing. Use caution when converting from one route of administration to another.

Other safety concerns:
To avoid errors due to misinterpretation of a decimal point, always express dosage in mcg (**not** mg).

Brand Names: U.S. Levothroid [DSC]; Levoxyl; Synthroid; Tirosint; Unithroid; Unithroid Direct

Brand Names: Canada Eltroxin; Levothyroxine Sodium; Levothyroxine Sodium for Injection; Synthroid

Therapeutic Category Thyroid Product

Generic Availability (U.S.) May be product dependent

Use
Oral:
Tablets: Replacement or supplemental therapy in congenital or acquired hypothyroidism of any etiology (FDA approved in all ages); pituitary TSH suppressant for the treatment or prevention of various types of euthyroid goiter, thyroid nodules, thyroiditis, multinodular goiter, and thyroid cancer (FDA approved in adults); **Note:** Not indicated for treatment of transient hypothyroidism associated with subacute thyroiditis

Capsules (Tirosint®): Replacement or supplemental therapy in congenital or acquired hypothyroidism of any etiology (FDA approved in older children and adults); pituitary TSH suppressant for the treatment or prevention of various types of euthyroid goiter, thyroid nodules, thyroiditis, multinodular goiter, and thyroid cancer (FDA approved in adults); **Note:** Not indicated for treatment of transient hypothyroidism associated with subacute thyroiditis

Parenteral: Treatment of myxedema coma (FDA approved in adults); has also been used for organ donor management

Pregnancy Risk Factor A

Pregnancy Considerations Endogenous thyroid hormones minimally cross the placenta; the fetal thyroid becomes active around the end of the first trimester. Levothyroxine has not been shown to increase the risk of congenital abnormalities.

Uncontrolled maternal hypothyroidism may result in adverse neonatal outcomes (eg, premature birth, low birth weight, and respiratory distress) and adverse maternal outcomes (eg, spontaneous abortion, pre-eclampsia, stillbirth, and premature delivery). To prevent adverse events, normal maternal thyroid function should be maintained prior to conception and throughout pregnancy. Levothyroxine is considered the treatment of choice for the control of hypothyroidism during pregnancy. Due to alterations of endogenous maternal thyroid hormones, the levothyroxine dose may need to be increased during pregnancy and the dose usually needs to be decreased after delivery.

Breast-Feeding Considerations Endogenous thyroid hormones are minimally found in breast milk. The amount of endogenous thyroxine found in breast milk does not influence infant plasma thyroid values. Levothyroxine was not found to cause adverse events to the infant or mother during breast-feeding. Adequate thyroid hormone concentrations are required to maintain normal lactation. Appropriate levothyroxine doses should be continued during breast-feeding.

Contraindications Hypersensitivity to levothyroxine sodium or any component;
Additionally:
Oral formulations (tablets and capsules): Acute MI; thyrotoxicosis of any etiology; uncorrected adrenal insufficiency
Capsules (Tirosint®): Inability to swallow capsule whole (eg, infants, small children)

Warnings Not for use in the treatment of obesity or for weight loss **[U.S. Boxed Warning]**; in euthyroid patients, doses within the range of daily hormonal requirements are ineffective for weight reduction; larger doses may produce serious or even life-threatening toxic effects particularly when used with some anorectic drugs (sympathomimetic amines). Should not be used for treatment of infertility without unrelated hypothyroidism.

Overtreatment may result in craniosynostosis in infants and premature closure of epiphyses in children; monitor use closely.

Levoxyl® oral tablets may rapidly swell and disintegrate, causing choking or gagging (should be administered with a full glass of water); use caution in patients with dysphagia or other swallowing disorders.

Precautions Use with extreme caution in patients with adrenal insufficiency; symptoms may be exaggerated or aggravated. Use with caution and reduce dosage in patients with angina pectoris and other cardiovascular disease; chronic hypothyroidism predisposes patients to coronary artery disease. Use with caution in patients with diabetes mellitus and insipidus; symptoms may be exaggerated or aggravated. Use with caution in patients with myxedema; symptoms may be exaggerated or aggravated.

Routine use of T_4 for TSH suppression is not recommended in patients with benign thyroid nodules and should never be fully suppressive (TSH <0.1 mIU/mL) (Cooper, 2009; Gharib, 2010). Use of T_4 for TSH suppression is often physician-dependent; may be considered in select patients, including patients who reside in iodine-deficient areas, young patients with small thyroid nodules, and patients with nonfunctioning nodular goiters (Gharib, 2010). Use of T_4 for TSH suppression should be avoided in postmenopausal women; men >60 years of age; patients with cardiovascular disease, osteoporosis, or systemic illness; and patients with large thyroid nodules, long-standing goiters, or low-normal TSH levels (Gharib, 2010).

Long-term therapy can decrease bone mineral density; postmenopausal women and women using suppressive doses should receive the lowest dose necessary for clinical response.

In neonates and infants, cardiac overload, arrhythmias, and aspiration from avid suckling may occur during initiation of therapy (eg, first 2 weeks); monitor closely.

Adverse Reactions

Cardiovascular: Angina pectoris, cardiac arrest, cardiac arrhythmia, congestive heart failure, flushing, hypertension, increased pulse, myocardial infarction, palpitations, tachycardia

Central nervous system: Anxiety, choking sensation (Levoxyl), emotional lability, fatigue, headache, heat intolerance, hyperactivity, insomnia, irritability, myasthenia, nervousness, pseudotumor cerebri (children), seizure (rare)

Dermatologic: Alopecia, diaphoresis

Endocrine & metabolic: Menstrual disease, weight loss

Gastrointestinal: Abdominal cramps, diarrhea, dysphagia (Levoxyl), gag reflex (Levoxyl), increased appetite, vomiting

Genitourinary: Infertility

Hepatic: Increased liver enzymes

Hypersensitivity: Hypersensitivity (to inactive ingredients; symptoms include urticaria, pruritus, rash, flushing, angioedema, GI symptoms, fever, arthralgia, serum sickness, wheezing)

Neuromuscular & skeletal: Decreased bone mineral density, slipped capital femoral epiphysis (children), tremor

Respiratory: Dyspnea

Miscellaneous: Fever

Drug Interactions

Metabolism/Transport Effects None known.

Avoid Concomitant Use

Avoid concomitant use of Levothyroxine with any of the following: Sodium Iodide I131; Sucroferric Oxyhydroxide

Increased Effect/Toxicity

Levothyroxine may increase the levels/effects of: Tricyclic Antidepressants; Vitamin K Antagonists

The levels/effects of Levothyroxine may be increased by: Piracetam

Decreased Effect

Levothyroxine may decrease the levels/effects of: Sodium Iodide I131; Theophylline Derivatives

The levels/effects of Levothyroxine may be decreased by: Aluminum Hydroxide; Bile Acid Sequestrants; Calcium Polystyrene Sulfonate; Calcium Salts; CarBAMazepine; Estrogen Derivatives; Fosphenytoin; Iron Salts; Lanthanum; Multivitamins/Minerals (with ADEK, Folate, Iron); Orlistat; Phenytoin; Raloxifene; Rifampin; Selective Serotonin Reuptake Inhibitors; Sevelamer; Sodium Polystyrene Sulfonate; Sucralfate; Sucroferric Oxyhydroxide

Food Interactions Taking levothyroxine with enteral nutrition may cause reduced bioavailability and may lower serum thyroxine levels leading to signs or symptoms of hypothyroidism. Soybean flour (infant formula), cottonseed meal, walnuts, and dietary fiber may decrease absorption of levothyroxine from the GI tract. Management: Take in the morning on an empty stomach at least 30 minutes before food. Consider an increase in dose if taken with enteral tube feed.

Stability

Oral:

Synthroid®, Levotroid®, Tirosint®: Store at 25°C (77°F); excursions permitted to 15°C to 30°C (59°F to 86°F). Protect from light and moisture.

Unithroid®, Levoxyl®: Store at 20°C to 25°C (68°F to 77°F); excursions permitted to 15°C to 30°C (59°F to 86°F). Protect from light and moisture.

Parenteral: Store intact vial at 20°C to 25°C (68°F to 77°F); protect from light; manufacturer recommends use immediately after preparation.

Stability in polypropylene syringes (100 mcg/mL in NS) at 5°C ± 1°C is 7 days (Gupta, 2000).

Stability in latex-free, PVC minibags stored at 25°C is dependent upon concentration and light exposure: 0.4 mcg/mL in NS is stable for 18 hours protected from light and ~17 hours when exposed to light; 2 mcg/mL in NS is stable for 12 hours protected from light and 6.5 hours when exposed to light

Mechanism of Action Levothyroxine (T_4) is a synthetic form of thyroxine, an endogenous hormone secreted by the thyroid gland. T_4 is converted to its active metabolite, L-triiodothyronine (T_3). Thyroid hormones (T_4 and T_3) then bind to thyroid receptor proteins in the cell nucleus and exert metabolic effects through control of DNA transcription and protein synthesis; involved in normal metabolism, growth, and development; promotes gluconeogenesis, increases utilization and mobilization of glycogen stores, and stimulates protein synthesis, increases basal metabolic rate

Pharmacodynamics

Onset of action: Therapeutic:

Oral: 3-5 days

I.V.: Within 6-8 hours

Maximum effect: 4-6 weeks

Pharmacokinetics (Adult data unless noted)

Absorption: Oral: Erratic (40% to 80%, per manufacturer); decreases with age

Bioavailability: Oral tablets: 64% (nonfasting state) to 79% to 81% (fasting state) (Dickerson, 2010; Fish, 1987)

Protein binding: >99%; bound to plasma proteins, including thyroxine-binding globulin, thyroxine-binding prealbumin, and albumin

Metabolism: Hepatic to triiodothyronine (T_3; active); ~80% T_4 deiodinated in kidney and periphery; glucuronidation/conjugation also occurs; undergoes enterohepatic recirculation

Half-life: Euthyroid: 6-7 days; Hypothyroid: 9-10 days; Hyperthyroid: 3-4 days

Time to peak serum concentration: 2-4 hours

Elimination: Urine (major route of elimination; decreases with age); feces (~20%)

Dosing: Neonatal Note: Doses should be adjusted based on clinical response and laboratory parameters; on a weight basis, dosing is higher in neonates, infants, and children than adults due to the higher metabolic clearance.

Congenital hypothyroidism:

Oral: 10 to 15 mcg/kg once daily; titrate as rapidly as possible (<2 weeks after initiation of therapy) to achieve target serum T_4 concentration (>10 mcg/dL); in full-size, term infants, some have suggested an initial dose of 50 mcg/day. If patient at risk for development of cardiac failure, begin with a lower dose (25 mcg/day). In severe cases of hypothyroidism (serum T_4 <5 mcg/dL), begin treatment at a higher dosage of ~50 mcg/day (12 to 17 mcg/kg/dose) (AAP, 2006; Selva, 2002).

I.V., I.M.: 50% to 75% of the oral dose

Organ donor management in brain-dead patients (hormone replacement therapy): I.V.: Initial: 5 mcg/kg bolus dose, followed by 1.4 mcg/kg/**hour** infusion (Zuppa, 2004)

Dosing: Usual Note: Doses should be adjusted based on clinical response and laboratory parameters; on a weight basis, dosing is higher in infants and children than adults due to the higher metabolic clearance.

Pediatric:

Hypothyroidism (acquired or congenital): Note: Hyperactivity in older children may be minimized by starting at one-quarter (25%) of the recommended dose and increasing each week by that amount until the full dose is achieved (4 weeks). Children with severe or chronic hypothyroidism should be started at 25 mcg/day; adjust dose by 25 mcg every 2 to 4 weeks.

Oral:

1 to 3 months: 10 to 15 mcg/kg once daily; if the infant is at risk for development of cardiac failure, use a lower starting dose of ~25 mcg/day; if the initial serum T_4 is very low (<5 mcg/dL), begin treatment at a higher dosage of ~50 mcg/day (12 to 17 mcg/kg/day) (AAP, 2006; Selva, 2002)

3 to 6 months: 8 to 10 mcg/kg once daily

6 to 12 months: 6 to 8 mcg/kg once daily

1 to 5 years: 5 to 6 mcg/kg once daily

6 to 12 years: 4 to 5 mcg/kg once daily

>12 years with incomplete growth and puberty: 2 to 3 mcg/kg once daily

Adolescents with growth and puberty complete: 1.7 mcg/kg once daily

I.V., I.M.: Infants, Children, and Adolescents: 50% to 75% of the oral dose; alternatively, some clinicians administer up to 80% of the oral dose in adults patients. **Note:** Bioavailability of the oral formulation is highly variable, but absorption has been measured to be ~80%, when the oral tablet formulation was administered in the recommended fasting state (Dickerson, 2010; Fish, 1987).

Organ donor management in brain-dead patients (hormone replacement therapy) (Nakagawa, 2008; Zuppa, 2004): I.V.:

Infants <6 months: Initial: 5 mcg/kg bolus dose, followed by 1.4 mcg/kg/**hour** infusion

Infants 6 to 12 months: Initial: 4 mcg/kg bolus dose, followed by 1.3 mcg/kg/**hour** infusion

Children 1 to 5 years: Initial: 3 mcg/kg bolus dose, followed by 1.2 mcg/kg/**hour** infusion

Children 6 to 12 years: Initial: 2.5 mcg/kg bolus dose, followed by 1 mcg/kg/**hour** infusion

Children ≥12 years and Adolescents ≤16 years: Initial: 1.5 mcg/kg bolus dose, followed by 0.8 mcg/kg/**hour** infusion

Adolescents >16 years: Initial: 0.8 mcg/kg bolus dose, followed by 0.8 mcg/kg/**hour** infusion

Adult:

Hypothyroidism: Adults <50 years of age and older adults who have been recently treated for hyperthyroidism or who have been hypothyroid for only a few months:

Oral: ~1.7 mcg/kg/day usual doses are ≤200 mcg/day [range: 100 to 125 mcg/day (70 kg adult)]; doses ≥300 mcg/day are rare (consider poor compliance, malabsorption, and/or drug interactions). Titrate dose every 6 weeks.

Note: Patients with combined hypothyroidism and cardiac disease should be monitored carefully for changes in stability.

I.V., I.M.: 50% of the oral dose; alternatively, some clinicians administer up to 80% of the oral dose. **Note:** Bioavailability of the oral formulation is highly variable, but absorption has been measured to be ~80%, when the oral tablet formulation was administered in the recommended fasting state (Dickerson, 2010; Fish, 1987).

Severe hypothyroidism: Oral: Initial: 12.5 to 25 mcg/day; adjust dose by 25 mcg/day every 2 to 4 weeks as appropriate

Subclinical hypothyroidism (if treated): Oral: 1 mcg/kg once daily

Myxedema coma or stupor: I.V.: 200 to 500 mcg one time, then 100 to 300 mcg the next day if necessary; smaller doses should be considered in patients with cardiovascular disease

TSH suppression: Oral:

Well-differentiated thyroid cancer: Highly individualized; doses >2 mcg/kg/day may be needed to suppress TSH to <0.1 mIU/L in intermediate- to high-risk tumors. Low-risk tumors may be maintained at or slightly below the lower limit of normal (0.1 to 0.5 mIU/L) (Cooper, 2009).

Benign nodules and nontoxic multinodular goiter: Routine use of T_4 for TSH suppression is not recommended in patients with benign thyroid nodules. In patients deemed appropriate candidates, treatment should never be fully suppressive (TSH <0.1 mIU/L) (Cooper, 2009; Gharib, 2010). Avoid use if TSH is already suppressed.

Administration

Oral:

Capsules: Must be swallowed whole; do not cut, crush, or attempt to dissolve capsules in water to prepare a suspension

Tablets: Administer on an empty stomach 30 to 60 minutes prior to breakfast with a full glass of water to prevent gagging. If administration on an empty stomach poses a challenge, particularly in infants and small children, it may be administered with food to improve adherence and consistency of administration. For infants, crush tablet and mix with breast-milk, non-soy-based formula, or water and use immediately (Zeitler, 2010).

Parenteral: Reconstitute vial with 5 mL NS, final concentration dependent upon vial size; administer I.V. over 2- to 3-minute period; may administer I.M.

Monitoring Parameters T_4, TSH, heart rate, blood pressure, clinical signs of hypo- and hyperthyroidism; growth, bone development (children); TSH is the most reliable guide for evaluating adequacy of thyroid replacement dosage. TSH may be elevated during the first few months of thyroid replacement despite patients being clinically euthyroid. In cases where T_4 remains low and TSH is within normal limits, an evaluation of "free" (unbound) T_4 is needed to evaluate further increase in dosage.

In congenital hypothyroidism, adequacy of replacement should be determined using both TSH and total- or free-T_4. During the first 3 years of life, total- or free-T_4 should be maintained in the upper 1/2 of the normal range; this should result in normalization of the TSH. In some patients, TSH may not normalize due to a resetting of the pituitary-thyroid feedback as a result of in utero hypothyroidism. Monitor closely for cardiac overload, arrhythmias, and aspiration from avid suckling.

Pediatric patients: Monitor closely for under/overtreatment. Undertreatment may decrease intellectual development and linear growth and lead to poor school performance due to impaired concentration and slowed mentation. Overtreatment may adversely affect brain maturation and accelerate bone age (leading to premature closure of the epiphyses and reduced adult height); craniosynostosis has been reported in infants. Perform routine clinical examinations at regular intervals (to assess mental and physical growth and development). Monitor TSH and total or free T_4 at 2 and 4 weeks after starting treatment, every 1-2 months during the first year of life, every 2-3 months between ages 1-3 years, and every 3-12 months thereafter until growth is completed; repeat tests two weeks after any change in dosage.

Adults: Monitor TSH every 6-8 weeks until normalized, 8-12 weeks after dosage changes, and every 6-12 months throughout therapy.

Reference Range

Thyroid Function Tests

Lab Parameters	Age	Normal Range
T₄ (thyroxine) serum concentration	1-7 days	10.1-20.9 mcg/dL
	8-14 days	9.8-16.6 mcg/dL
	1 month to 1 year	5.5-16.0 mcg/dL
	>1 year	4.0-12.0 mcg/dL
Free thyroxine index (FTI)	1-3 days	9.3-26.6
	1-4 weeks	7.6-20.8
	1-4 months	7.4-17.9
	4-12 months	5.1-14.5
	1-6 years	5.7-13.3
	>6 years	4.8-14.0
T₃ serum concentration	Newborns	100-470 ng/dL
	1-5 years	100-260 ng/dL
	5-10 years	90-240 ng/dL
	10 years to Adult	70-210 ng/dL
T₃ uptake		35%-45%
TSH serum concentration	Cord	3-22 micro international units/mL
	1-3 days	<40 micro international units/mL
	3-7 days	<25 micro international units/mL
	>7 days	0-10 micro international units/mL

Test Interactions Many drugs may have effects on thyroid function tests (see Additional Information). Pregnancy, infectious hepatitis, and acute intermittent porphyria may increase TBG concentrations; nephrosis, severe hypoproteinemia, severe liver disease, and acromegaly may decrease TBG concentrations.

Additional Information Equivalent doses: The following statement on relative potency of thyroid products is included in a joint statement by American Thyroid Association (ATA), American Association of Clinical Endocrinologists (AACE) and The Endocrine Society (TES): For purposes of conversion, levothyroxine sodium (T₄) 100 mcg is usually considered equivalent to desiccated thyroid 60 mg, thyroglobulin 60 mg, or liothyronine sodium (T₃) 25 mcg. However, these are rough guidelines only and do not obviate the careful re-evaluation of a patient when switching thyroid hormone preparations, including a change from one brand of levothyroxine to another. Joint position statement is available at http://www.thyroid.org/professionals/advocacy/04_12_08_thyroxine.html.

Note: Several medications have effects on thyroid production or conversion. The impact in thyroid replacement has not been specifically evaluated, but patient response should be monitored:

Methimazole: Decreases thyroid hormone secretion, while propylthiouracil decrease thyroid hormone secretion and decreases conversion of T₄ to T₃.

Beta-adrenergic antagonists: Decrease conversion of T₄ to T₃ (dose related, propranolol ≥160 mg/day); patients may be clinically euthyroid.

Iodide, iodine-containing radiographic contrast agents may decrease thyroid hormone secretion; may also increase thyroid hormone secretion, especially in patients with Graves' disease.

Other agents reported to impact on thyroid production/conversion include aminoglutethimide, amiodarone, chloral hydrate, diazepam, ethionamide, interferon-alpha, interleukin-2, lithium, lovastatin (case report), glucocorticoids (dose-related), mercaptopurine, sulfonamides, thiazide diuretics, and tolbutamide.

In addition, a number of medications have been noted to cause transient depression in TSH secretion, which may complicate interpretation of monitoring tests for levothyroxine, including corticosteroids, octreotide, and dopamine. Metoclopramide may increase TSH secretion

Dosage Forms Excipient information presented when available (limited, particularly for generics); consult specific product labeling. [DSC] = Discontinued product

Capsule, Oral, as sodium:

Tirosint: 13 mcg, 25 mcg, 50 mcg, 75 mcg, 88 mcg, 100 mcg, 112 mcg, 125 mcg, 137 mcg, 150 mcg

Solution Reconstituted, Intravenous, as sodium [preservative free]:

Generic: 100 mcg (1 ea); 200 mcg (1 ea); 500 mcg (1 ea)

Tablet, Oral, as sodium:

Levothroid: 25 mcg [DSC] [scored; contains fd&c yellow #6 aluminum lake]

Levothroid: 50 mcg [DSC] [scored]

Levothroid: 75 mcg [DSC] [scored; contains fd&c blue #2 aluminum lake, fd&c red #40 aluminum lake]

Levothroid: 88 mcg [DSC] [scored; contains fd&c blue #1 aluminum lake, fd&c yellow #10 aluminum lake, fd&c yellow #6 aluminum lake]

Levothroid: 100 mcg [DSC] [scored; contains fd&c yellow #10 aluminum lake, fd&c yellow #6 aluminum lake]

Levothroid: 112 mcg [DSC] [scored]

Levothroid: 125 mcg [DSC] [scored; contains fd&c blue #1 aluminum lake, fd&c red #40 aluminum lake, fd&c yellow #6 aluminum lake]

Levothroid: 137 mcg [DSC] [scored; contains fd&c blue #1 aluminum lake]

Levothroid: 150 mcg [DSC] [scored; contains fd&c blue #2 aluminum lake]

Levothroid: 175 mcg [DSC] [scored; contains fd&c blue #1 aluminum lake]

Levothroid: 200 mcg [DSC] [scored; contains fd&c red #40 aluminum lake]

Levothroid: 300 mcg [DSC] [scored; contains fd&c blue #1 aluminum lake, fd&c yellow #10 (quinoline yellow), fd&c yellow #6 aluminum lake]

Levoxyl: 25 mcg [scored; contains fd&c yellow #6 aluminum lake]

Levoxyl: 50 mcg [scored]

Levoxyl: 75 mcg [scored; contains fd&c blue #1 aluminum lake]

Levoxyl: 88 mcg [scored; contains fd&c blue #1 aluminum lake, fd&c yellow #10 aluminum lake, fd&c yellow #6 aluminum lake]

Levoxyl: 100 mcg [scored; contains fd&c yellow #10 aluminum lake, fd&c yellow #6 aluminum lake]

Levoxyl: 112 mcg [scored; contains fd&c red #40 aluminum lake, fd&c yellow #6 aluminum lake]

Levoxyl: 125 mcg [scored; contains fd&c red #40 aluminum lake, fd&c yellow #10 aluminum lake]

Levoxyl: 137 mcg, 150 mcg [scored; contains fd&c blue #1 aluminum lake]

Levoxyl: 175 mcg [scored; contains fd&c blue #1 aluminum lake, fd&c yellow #10 aluminum lake]

Levoxyl: 200 mcg [scored; contains fd&c yellow #10 aluminum lake]

Synthroid: 25 mcg [scored; contains fd&c yellow #6 aluminum lake]

Synthroid: 50 mcg [scored]

Synthroid: 75 mcg [scored; contains fd&c blue #2 aluminum lake, fd&c red #40 aluminum lake]

Synthroid: 88 mcg [scored; contains fd&c blue #1 aluminum lake, fd&c yellow #10 aluminum lake, fd&c yellow #6 aluminum lake]

Synthroid: 100 mcg [scored; contains fd&c yellow #10 aluminum lake, fd&c yellow #6 aluminum lake]

Synthroid: 112 mcg [scored]

Synthroid: 125 mcg [scored; contains fd&c blue #1 aluminum lake, fd&c red #40 aluminum lake, fd&c yellow #6 aluminum lake]

Synthroid: 137 mcg [scored; contains fd&c blue #1 aluminum lake]

Synthroid: 150 mcg [scored; contains fd&c blue #2 aluminum lake]

Synthroid: 175 mcg [scored; contains fd&c blue #1 aluminum lake]

Synthroid: 200 mcg [scored; contains fd&c red #40 aluminum lake]

Synthroid: 300 mcg [scored; contains fd&c blue #1 aluminum lake, fd&c yellow #10 aluminum lake, fd&c yellow #6 aluminum lake]

Unithroid: 25 mcg [contains fd&c yellow #6 aluminum lake]

Unithroid: 25 mcg [scored; contains fd&c yellow #6 aluminum lake]

Unithroid: 50 mcg

Unithroid: 50 mcg, 75 mcg [scored]

Unithroid: 75 mcg [contains fd&c blue #2 aluminum lake, fd&c red #40 aluminum lake]

Unithroid: 88 mcg [scored]

Unithroid: 88 mcg [contains fd&c blue #1 aluminum lake, fd&c yellow #10 aluminum lake, fd&c yellow #6 aluminum lake]

Unithroid: 100 mcg [contains fd&c yellow #10 aluminum lake, fd&c yellow #6 aluminum lake]

Unithroid: 100 mcg [scored; contains fd&c yellow #10 aluminum lake, fd&c yellow #6 aluminum lake]

Unithroid: 112 mcg

Unithroid: 112 mcg [scored]

Unithroid: 125 mcg [contains fd&c blue #1 aluminum lake, fd&c red #40 aluminum lake, fd&c yellow #6 aluminum lake]

Unithroid: 125 mcg [scored; contains fd&c blue #1 aluminum lake, fd&c red #40 aluminum lake, fd&c yellow #6 aluminum lake]

Unithroid: 137 mcg [contains fd&c blue #1 aluminum lake]

Unithroid: 150 mcg [contains fd&c blue #2 aluminum lake]

Unithroid: 150 mcg [scored; contains fd&c blue #2 aluminum lake]

Unithroid: 175 mcg [scored]

Unithroid: 175 mcg [contains fd&c blue #1 aluminum lake]

Unithroid: 200 mcg [scored]

Unithroid: 200 mcg [contains fd&c red #40 aluminum lake]

Unithroid: 300 mcg [contains fd&c blue #1 aluminum lake, fd&c yellow #10 (quinoline yellow), fd&c yellow #6 aluminum lake]

Unithroid: 300 mcg [scored; contains fd&c blue #1 aluminum lake, fd&c yellow #10 aluminum lake, fd&c yellow #6 aluminum lake]

Unithroid Direct: 25 mcg [scored; contains fd&c yellow #6 aluminum lake]

Unithroid Direct: 50 mcg [scored]

Unithroid Direct: 75 mcg, 88 mcg [scored; contains fd&c blue #1 aluminum lake, fd&c blue #2 aluminum lake, fd&c red #40 aluminum lake, fd&c yellow #10 aluminum lake, fd&c yellow #6 aluminum lake]

Unithroid Direct: 100 mcg [scored; contains fd&c yellow #10 aluminum lake, fd&c yellow #6 aluminum lake]

Unithroid Direct: 112 mcg [scored]

Unithroid Direct: 125 mcg [scored; contains fd&c blue #1 aluminum lake, fd&c red #40 aluminum lake, fd&c yellow #6 aluminum lake]

Unithroid Direct: 150 mcg [scored; contains fd&c blue #2 aluminum lake]

Unithroid Direct: 175 mcg [scored; contains fd&c blue #1 aluminum lake]

Unithroid Direct: 200 mcg [scored; contains fd&c red #40 aluminum lake]

Unithroid Direct: 300 mcg [scored; contains fd&c blue #1 aluminum lake, fd&c yellow #10 aluminum lake, fd&c yellow #6 aluminum lake]

Generic: 25 mcg, 50 mcg, 75 mcg, 88 mcg, 100 mcg, 112 mcg, 125 mcg, 137 mcg, 150 mcg, 175 mcg, 200 mcg, 300 mcg

Extemporaneous Preparations A 25 mcg/mL oral suspension may be made with tablets and 40 mL glycerol. Crush twenty-five 0.1 mg levothyroxine tablets in a mortar and reduce to a fine powder. Add small portions of glycerol and mix to a uniform suspension. Transfer to a calibrated 100 mL amber bottle; rinse the mortar with about 10 mL of glycerol and pour into the bottle; repeat until all 40 mL of glycerol is used. Add quantity of water sufficient to make 100 mL. Label "shake well" and "refrigerate". Stable for 8 days refrigerated.

Boulton DW, Fawcett JP, and Woods DJ, "Stability of an Extemporaneously Compounded Levothyroxine Sodium Oral Liquid," *Am J Health Syst Pharm*, 1996, 53(10):1157-61.

References

American Academy of Pediatrics, Rose SR, Section on Endocrinology and Committee on Genetics, American Thyroid Association, et al, "Update of Newborn Screening and Therapy for Congenital Hypothyroidism," *Pediatrics*, 2006, 117(6):2290-303.

Cooper DS, Kloos RT, Mazzaferri EL, et al, "Revised American Thyroid Association Management Guidelines for Patients With Thyroid Nodules and Differentiated Thyroid Cancer," *Thyroid*, 2009, 19 (11):1167-214.

de Groot JW, Zonnenberg BA, Plukker JT, et al, "Imatinib Induces Hypothyroidism in Patients Receiving Levothyroxine," *Clin Pharmacol Ther*, 2005, 78(4):433-8.

Dickerson DN, Maish GO 3rd, Minard G, et al, "Clinical Relevancy of Levothyroxine – Continuous Enteral Nutrition Interaction," *Nutr Clin Pract*, 2010, 25(6):646-52.

Fish LH, Schwartz HL, Cavenaugh J, et al, "Replacement Dose, Metabolism, and Bioavailability of Levothyroxine in the Treatment of Hypothyroidism," *N Engl J Med*, 316(13):764-70.

Gharib H, Papini E, Paschke R, et al, "American Association of Clinical Endocrinologists, Associazione Medici Endocrinologi, and European Thyroid Association Medical Guidelines for Clinical Practice for Diagnosis and Management of Thyroid Nodules," *Endocr Pract*, 2010, 16 (Supp 1):1-43.

Gupta VD, "Stability of Levothyroxine Sodium Injection in Polypropylene Syringes," *Int J Pharm Compound*, 2000, 4(6):482-3.

Nakagawa TA, "Updated Pediatric Donor Management and Dosing Guidelines," 2008. Available at http://www.natco1.org/prof_development/documents/FINALNATCOPedDonorManagementGuidelines_-Jan08.pdf. Last accessed June 2012.

Selva KA, Mandel SH, Rien L, et al, "Initial Treatment Dose of L-thyroxine in Congenital Hypothyroidism," *J Pediatr*, 2002, 141 (6):786-92.

Strong DK, Decarie D, and Ensom MHH, "Stability of Levothyroxine in Sodium Chloride for IV Administration," *Can J Hosp Pharm*, 2010, 63 (6):437-43.

Zeitler P, Solberg P, and Pharmacy and Therapeutics Committee of the Lawson Wilkins Pediatric Endocrine Society, "Food and Levothyroxine Administration in Infants and Children," *J Pediatr*, 2010, 157 (1):13-14.

Zuppa AF, Nadkarni V, Davis L, et al, "The Effect of a Thyroid Hormone Infusion on Vasopressor Support in Critically Ill Children With Cessation of Neurologic Function," *Crit Care Med*, 2004, 32(11):2318-22.

◆ **Levothyroxine and Liothyronine** see Liotrix on page 1258

◆ **Levothyroxine and Liothyronine** see Thyroid, Desiccated on page 2018

◆ **Levothyroxine Sodium** see Levothyroxine on page 1234

◆ **Levothyroxine Sodium for Injection (Can)** see Levothyroxine on page 1234

◆ **Levoxyl** see Levothyroxine on page 1234

◆ **Levsin** see Hyoscyamine on page 1056

◆ **Levsin/SL** *see* Hyoscyamine *on page 1056*

◆ **Lexapro** *see* Escitalopram *on page 788*

◆ **Lexiva** *see* Fosamprenavir *on page 931*

◆ **LH-RH Agonist** *see* Histrelin *on page 1016*

◆ *l***-Hyoscyamine Sulfate** *see* Hyoscyamine *on page 1056*

◆ **Lialda** *see* Mesalamine *on page 1347*

◆ **Lidemol® (Can)** *see* Fluocinonide *on page 894*

◆ **Lidex** *see* Fluocinonide *on page 894*

◆ **Lidex® (Can)** *see* Fluocinonide *on page 894*

Lidocaine (Systemic) (LYE doe kane)

Medication Safety Issues
High alert medication:
The Institute for Safe Medication Practices (ISMP) includes this medication (epidural administration; I.V. formulation) among its list of drugs which have a heightened risk of causing significant patient harm when used in error.
International issues:
Lidosen [Italy] may be confused with Lincocin brand name for lincomycin [U.S., Canada, and multiple international markets]; Lodosyn brand name for carbidopa [U.S.]

Brand Names: U.S. Xylocaine; Xylocaine (Cardiac); Xylocaine-MPF
Brand Names: Canada Xylocard®
Therapeutic Category Antiarrhythmic Agent, Class I-B; Local Anesthetic, Injectable
Generic Availability (U.S.) Yes
Use Treatment of ventricular arrhythmias (FDA approved in adults); local or regional anesthetic [FDA approved in pediatric patients (age not specified) and adults]
PALS guidelines recommend lidocaine when amiodarone is not available for cardiac arrest with pulseless VT or VF (unresponsive to defibrillation, CPR, and epinephrine administration); consider in patients with cocaine overdose to prevent arrhythmias secondary to MI
ACLS guidelines recommend lidocaine when amiodarone is not available for cardiac arrest with pulseless VT or VF (unresponsive to defibrillation, CPR, and vasopressor administration); it is not considered to be the drug of choice but may be considered for stable monomorphic VT (in patients with preserved ventricular function) and for polymorphic VT (with normal baseline and prolonged QT interval).

Pregnancy Risk Factor B
Pregnancy Considerations Adverse events were not observed in animal reproduction studies. Lidocaine and its metabolites cross the placenta and can be detected in the fetal circulation following injection (Cavalli, 2004; Mitani, 1987). Adverse reactions in the fetus/neonate may affect the CNS, heart, or peripheral vascular tone. Fetal heart monitoring is recommended. Lidocaine injection is approved for obstetric analgesia. Lidocaine administered by local infiltration is used to provide analgesia prior to episiotomy and during repair of obstetric lacerations (ACOG, 2002). Administration by the perineal route may result in greater absorption than administration by the epidural route (Cavalli, 2004). Cumulative exposure from all routes of administration should be considered. When used as an antiarrhythmic, ACLS guidelines recommend using the same dose that would be used in a nonpregnant woman (Vanden Hoek, 2010).
Breast-Feeding Considerations Lidocaine is excreted into breast milk. The manufacturer recommends that caution be used when administered to a nursing woman. When administered by injection for dental or obstetric analgesia, small amounts are detected in breast milk; oral bioavailability to the nursing infant is expected to be low

and the amount of lidocaine available to the nursing infant would not be expected to cause adverse events (Lebedevs, 1993; Ortega, 1999). Cumulative exposure from all routes of administration should be considered.
Contraindications Hypersensitivity to lidocaine, amide-type local anesthetics, or any component; patients with Adams-Stokes syndrome, Wolff-Parkinson-White syndrome, or with severe degree of S-A, A-V or intraventricular heart block (without a pacemaker)
Warnings Decrease dose in patients with decreased cardiac output or hepatic disease; do not use lidocaine solutions containing epinephrine for treatment of arrhythmias; do not use preservative-containing solution for epidural, spinal, or I.V. administration.

Chondroitin (necrosis and destruction of cartilage) has been reported following continuous intra-articular infusion of local anesthetics for extended periods of time (48-72 hours); patients presented as early as 2 months following the infusion with joint pain, stiffness, and loss of motion; more than 50% of patients required additional surgery, including arthroscopy or joint replacement; intra-articular administration of local anesthetics is not an FDA-approved route of administration.

Premixed infusions containing dextrose may cause hypersensitivity reactions in patients allergic to corn or corn products; some products contain benzyl alcohol or bisulfites (consult specific product information) which may cause allergic reactions in susceptible individuals; large amounts of benzyl alcohol (≥99 mg/kg/day) have been associated with a potentially fatal toxicity ("gasping syndrome") in neonates; the "gasping syndrome" consists of metabolic acidosis, respiratory distress, gasping respirations, CNS dysfunction (including convulsions, intracranial hemorrhage), hypotension, and cardiovascular collapse; avoid use of lidocaine products containing benzyl alcohol in neonates; *in vitro* and animal studies have shown that benzoate, a metabolite of benzyl alcohol, displaces bilirubin from protein-binding sites.
Precautions Use with caution in patients with hepatic disease, heart failure, marked hypoxia, severe respiratory depression, hypovolemia, or shock; incomplete heart block or bradycardia, atrial fibrillation; pseudocholinesterase deficiency
Adverse Reactions Effects vary with route of administration. Many effects are dose related.
Cardiovascular: Arrhythmia, bradycardia, arterial spasms, cardiovascular collapse, defibrillator threshold increased, edema, flushing, heart block, hypotension, sinus node supression, vascular insufficiency (periarticular injections)
Central nervous system: Agitation, anxiety, apprehension, coma, confusion, disorientation, dizziness, drowsiness, euphoria, hallucinations, headache, hyperesthesia, hypoesthesia, lethargy, lightheadedness, nervousness, psychosis, seizure, slurred speech, somnolence, unconsciousness
Gastrointestinal: Metallic taste, nausea, vomiting
Local: Thrombophlebitis
Intradermal system: Application site reactions: Bruising/burning/contusion/hemorrhage/pain, edema, erythema, petechiae, pruritus
Neuromuscular & skeletal: Paresthesia, transient radicular pain (subarachnoid administration), tremor, twitching, weakness
Otic: Tinnitus
Respiratory: Bronchospasm, dyspnea, respiratory depression or arrest
Miscellaneous: Allergic reactions, anaphylactic reaction, anaphylactoid reaction, sensitivity to temperature extremes

▶

Following spinal anesthesia: Cauda equina syndrome, double vision, hypotension, nausea, peripheral nerve symptoms, positional headache, respiratory inadequacy, shivering

Rare but important or life-threatening: Asystole, confusion, disorientation, flushing, headache, hyper-/hypoesthesia, hypersensitivity, methemoglobinemia, nervousness, skin reaction, weakness

Drug Interactions

Metabolism/Transport Effects Substrate of CYP1A2 (major), CYP2A6 (minor), CYP2B6 (minor), CYP2C9 (minor), CYP3A4 (major); **Note:** Assignment of Major/Minor substrate status based on clinically relevant drug interaction potential; **Inhibits** CYP1A2 (weak)

Avoid Concomitant Use

Avoid concomitant use of Lidocaine (Systemic) with any of the following: Conivaptan; Fusidic Acid (Systemic); Saquinavir

Increased Effect/Toxicity

Lidocaine (Systemic) may increase the levels/effects of: Prilocaine; Sodium Nitrite

The levels/effects of Lidocaine (Systemic) may be increased by: Abiraterone Acetate; Amiodarone; Beta-Blockers; Ceritinib; Conivaptan; CYP1A2 Inhibitors (Moderate); CYP1A2 Inhibitors (Strong); CYP3A4 Inhibitors (Moderate); CYP3A4 Inhibitors (Strong); Dasatinib; Deferasirox; Disopyramide; Fusidic Acid (Systemic); Hyaluronidase; Ivacaftor; Luliconazole; Mifepristone; Nitric Oxide; Saquinavir; Simeprevir; Stiripentol; Telaprevir; Vemurafenib

Decreased Effect

Lidocaine (Systemic) may decrease the levels/effects of: Technetium Tc 99m Tilmanocept

The levels/effects of Lidocaine (Systemic) may be decreased by: Bosentan; Cannabis; CYP1A2 Inducers (Strong); CYP3A4 Inducers (Strong); Cyproterone; Dabrafenib; Deferasirox; Etravirine; Mitotane; Siltuximab; St Johns Wort; Tocilizumab

Stability Store at room temperature. Stability of parenteral admixture at room temperature (25°C): Use the expiration date on premixed bag; once out of overwrap, stability is 30 days.

Mechanism of Action Class Ib antiarrhythmic; suppresses automaticity of conduction tissue, by increasing electrical stimulation threshold of ventricle, His-Purkinje system, and spontaneous depolarization of the ventricles during diastole by a direct action on the tissues; blocks both the initiation and conduction of nerve impulses by decreasing the neuronal membrane's permeability to sodium ions, which results in inhibition of depolarization with resultant blockade of conduction

Pharmacodynamics Antiarrhythmic effect:
Onset of action (single I.V. bolus dose): 45-90 seconds
Duration: 10-20 minutes

Pharmacokinetics (Adult data unless noted)

Distribution: Crosses blood-brain and placental barriers; distributes into breast milk; breast milk to plasma ratio: 0.4

V_d: 1.5 ± 0.6 L/kg; range: 0.7-2.7 L/kg; V_d alterable by many patient factors; decreased in CHF and liver disease

Protein binding: 60% to 80%; binds to alpha$_1$-acid glycoprotein

Metabolism: 90% in the liver; active metabolites monoethylglycinexylidide (MEGX) and glycinexylidide (GX) can accumulate and may cause CNS toxicity

Half-life, biphasic:
Alpha: 7-30 minutes
Beta, terminal: Infants, premature: 3.2 hours; Adults: 1.5-2 hours

CHF, liver disease, shock, severe renal disease: Prolonged half-life

Elimination: <10% excreted unchanged in urine; ~90% as metabolite

Dialysis: Dialyzable (0% to 5%)

Dosing: Neonatal Antiarrhythmic: Ventricular tachycardia, ventricular fibrillation: I.V., I.O.:

Loading dose: 1 mg/kg/dose; follow with continuous infusion; may repeat bolus; **Note:** Neonates with reduced hepatic function or decreased hepatic blood flow (eg, CHF or postcardiac surgery) should receive 1/2 the usual loading dose.

Continuous I.V. infusion: 20-50 mcg/kg/minute; use lower dose for neonates with shock, hepatic disease, cardiac arrest, or CHF

Dosing: Usual

Antiarrhythmic:

Infants, Children, and Adolescents (PALS, 2010):

I.V., I.O.: (**Note:** Use if amiodarone is not available, for pulseless VT or VF; give after defibrillation attempts, CPR, and epinephrine):

Loading dose: 1 mg/kg/dose; follow with continuous I.V. infusion (PALS, 2010); may administer second bolus of 0.5-1 mg/kg/dose if delay between bolus and start of infusion is >15 minutes (PALS, 2010); **Note:** Patients with reduced hepatic function or decreased hepatic blood flow (eg, CHF or postcardiac surgery) should receive 1/2 the usual loading dose.

Continuous I.V. infusion: 20-50 mcg/kg/minute. Per manufacturer, use a maximum of 20 mcg/kg/minute in patients with shock, hepatic disease, cardiac arrest, or CHF

E.T.: 2-3 mg/kg/dose; flush with 5 mL of NS and follow with 5 assisted manual ventilations

Adults (ACLS, 2010):

VF or pulseless VT (after defibrillation attempts, CPR, and vasopressor administration) if amiodarone is not available:

I.V., I.O.: Initial: 1-1.5 mg/kg. If refractory VF or pulseless VT, repeat 0.5-0.75 mg/kg bolus every 5-10 minutes (maximum cumulative dose: 3 mg/kg). Follow with continuous infusion (1-4 mg/minute) after return of perfusion. Reappearance of arrhythmia during constant infusion: 0.5 mg/kg bolus and reassessment of infusion (Zipes, 1999)

E.T. (loading dose only): 2-3.75 mg/kg (2-2.5 times the recommended I.V. dose); dilute in 5-10 mL NS or sterile water. **Note:** Absorption is greater with sterile water and results in less impairment of PaO$_2$.

Hemodynamically stable monomorphic VT: I.V.: 1-1.5 mg/kg; repeat with 0.5-0.75 mg/kg every 5-10 minutes as necessary (maximum cumulative dose: 3 mg/kg). Follow with continuous infusion of 1-4 mg/minute or 30-50 mcg/kg/minute

Note: Dose reduction (eg, of maintenance infusion) necessary in patients with CHF, shock, or hepatic disease.

Anesthesia, local injectable: Children and Adults: Dose varies with procedure, degree of anesthesia needed, vascularity of tissue, duration of anesthesia required, and physical condition of patient; maximum dose: 4.5 mg/kg not to exceed 300 mg.

Usual Infusion Concentrations: Pediatric Note: Premixed solutions available

I.V. infusion: 8000 **mcg**/mL

Administration

Endotracheal:

Children: Flush with 5 mL of NS after E.T. administration; follow with 5 assisted manual ventilations

Adults: Dilute in NS or sterile water prior to E.T. administration. Absorption is greater with sterile water and results in less impairment of PaO$_2$ (Hähnel, 1990).

Flush with 5 mL of NS and follow immediately with several quick insufflations and continue chest compressions.

Parenteral: I.V.: Solutions of 40-200 mg/mL must be diluted for I.V. use; final concentration not to exceed 20 mg/mL for I.V. push or 8 mg/mL for I.V. infusion. The manufacturer recommends that when given I.V. push, the rate of administration should not exceed 0.7 mg/kg/ minute or 50 mg/minute, whichever is less; however, during acute situations (eg, pulseless VT or VF), administration by rapid I.V. push has been used by some clinicians in practice. I.V. continuous infusion must be administered with a calibrated infusion device.

Monitoring Parameters Monitor ECG continuously; serum concentrations with continuous infusion; I.V. site (local thrombophlebitis may occur with prolonged infusions)

Reference Range
Therapeutic: 1.5-5 mcg/mL (SI: 6-21 micromoles/L)
Potentially toxic: >6 mcg/mL (SI: >26 micromoles/L)
Toxic: >9 mcg/mL (SI: >38 micromoles/L)

Dosage Forms Excipient information presented when available (limited, particularly for generics); consult specific product labeling.
Solution, Injection, as hydrochloride:
Xylocaine: 0.5% (50 mL); 1% (20 mL, 50 mL); 2% (10 mL, 20 mL, 50 mL) [contains methylparaben]
Xylocaine-MPF: 0.5% (50 mL); 1% (2 mL, 5 mL, 10 mL, 30 mL); 1.5% (10 mL, 20 mL); 2% (2 mL, 5 mL, 10 mL); 4% (5 mL) [methylparaben free]
Generic: 0.5% (50 mL); 1% (2 mL, 5 mL, 10 mL, 20 mL, 30 mL, 50 mL); 1.5% (20 mL); 2% (2 mL, 5 mL, 20 mL, 50 mL)
Solution, Injection, as hydrochloride [preservative free]:
Generic: 0.5% (50 mL); 1% (2 mL, 5 mL, 30 mL); 1.5% (20 mL); 2% (2 mL, 5 mL, 10 mL); 4% (5 mL)
Solution, Intravenous, as hydrochloride:
Xylocaine (Cardiac): 20 mg/mL (5 mL)
Generic: 10 mg/mL (5 mL); 20 mg/mL (5 mL); 0.4% [4 mg/mL] (250 mL, 500 mL); 0.8% [8 mg/mL] (250 mL); 2% (5 mL); 5% [50 mg/mL] (2 mL)
Solution, Intravenous, as hydrochloride [preservative free]:
Generic: 10 mg/mL (5 mL); 20 mg/mL (5 mL)

References
ACOG Committee on Practice Bulletins-Obstetrics, "ACOG Practice Bulletin. Clinical Management Guidelines for Obstetrician-Gynecologists Number 36, July 2002. Obstetric Analgesia and Anesthesia," *Obstet Gynecol*, 2002, 100(1):177-91.
Cavalli Rde C, Lanchote VL, Duarte G, et al, "Pharmacokinetics and Transplacental Transfer of Lidocaine and its Metabolite For Perineal Analgesic Assistance to Pregnant Women," *Eur J Clin Pharmacol*, 2004, 60(8):569-74.
Field JM, Hazinski MF, Sayre MR, et al, "Part 1: Executive Summary: 2010 American Heart Association Guidelines for Cardiopulmonary Resuscitation and Emergency Cardiovascular Care," *Circulation*, 2010, 122(18 Suppl 3):640-56.
Hähnel JH, Lindner KH, Schürmann C, et al, "Plasma Lidocaine Levels and PaO₂ With Endobronchial Administration: Dilution With Normal Saline or Distilled Water?" *Ann Emerg Med*, 1990, 19(11):1314-7.
Kleinman ME, Chameides L, Schexnayder SM, et al, "Part 14: Pediatric Advanced Life Support: 2010 American Heart Association Guidelines for Cardiopulmonary Resuscitation and Emergency Cardiovascular Care," *Circulation*, 2010, 122(18 Suppl 3):876-908.
Lebedevs TH, Wojnar-Horton RE, Yapp P, et al, "Excretion of Lignocaine and its Metabolite Monoethylglycinexylidide in Breast Milk Following its Use in a Dental Procedure. A Case Report," *J Clin Periodontol*, 1993, 20(8):606-8.
Mitani GM, Steinberg I, Lien EJ, et al, "The Pharmacokinetics of Antiarrhythmic Agents in Pregnancy and Lactation," *Clin Pharmacokinet*, 1987, 12(4):253-91.
Neumar RW, Otto CW, Link MS, et al, "Part 8: Adult Advanced Cardiovascular Life Support: 2010 American Heart Association Guidelines for Cardiopulmonary Resuscitation and Emergency Cardiovascular Care," *Circulation*, 2010, 122(18 Suppl 3):729-67.
Ortega D, Viviand X, Lorec AM, et al, "Excretion of Lidocaine and Bupivacaine in Breast Milk Following Epidural Anesthesia For Cesarean Delivery," *Acta Anaesthesiol Scand*, 1999, 43(4):394-7.
Phillips MS, "Standardizing I.V. Infusion Concentrations: National Survey Results," *Am J Health Syst Pharm*, 2011, 68(22):2176-82.
Vanden Hoek TL, Morrison LJ, Shuster M, et al, "Part 12: Cardiac Arrest in Special Situations: 2010 American Heart Association Guidelines for Cardiopulmonary Resuscitation and Emergency Cardiovascular Care," *Circulation*, 2010, 122(18 Suppl 3):829-61.
Zipes DP and Jalife J, "Lidocaine," *Cardiac Electrophysiology: From Cell to Bedside*, 3rd ed, Philadelphia, PA: WB Saunders Co, 1999, 896.

Lidocaine (Ophthalmic) (LYE doe kane)

Brand Names: U.S. Akten
Therapeutic Category Local Anesthetic, Ophthalmic
Generic Availability (U.S.) No
Use Local anesthetic for ophthalmic procedures (FDA approved in adults; refer to product specific information regarding FDA approval in pediatric patients)
Pregnancy Risk Factor B
Pregnancy Considerations Adverse events were not observed in animal reproduction studies. Although systemic exposure is not expected following application of the ophthalmic gel, cumulative exposure from all routes of administration should be considered.
Breast-Feeding Considerations When administered by injection for dental or obstetric analgesia, small amounts of lidocaine are detected in breast milk (Lebedevs, 1993; Ortega, 1999). Although systemic exposure is not expected following application of the ophthalmic gel, cumulative exposure from all routes of administration should be considered.
Contraindications Hypersensitivity to lidocaine, amide-type local anesthetics, or any component
Warnings For topical ophthalmic use only; not for injection; prolonged use may cause permanent corneal ulceration and/or opacification with loss of vision.
Adverse Reactions
Local: Burning
Ocular: Conjunctival hyperemia, corneal epithelial changes, diplopia, visual changes
Drug Interactions
Metabolism/Transport Effects None known.
Avoid Concomitant Use There are no known interactions where it is recommended to avoid concomitant use.
Increased Effect/Toxicity There are no known significant interactions involving an increase in effect.
Decreased Effect There are no known significant interactions involving a decrease in effect.
Stability Store at 15°C to 25°C (59°F to 77°F). Protect from light. Discard after use.
Mechanism of Action Local anesthetics block both the initiation and conduction of nerve impulses by decreasing the neuronal membrane's permeability to sodium ions, which results in inhibition of depolarization with resultant blockade of conduction.
Pharmacodynamics Local anesthetic effect:
Onset of action: 20 seconds to 5 minutes (median: 40 seconds)
Duration: 5-30 minutes (mean: 15 minutes)
Dosing: Usual Anesthesia, ocular: Ophthalmic gel (Akten®): Children and Adults: Apply 2 drops to ocular surface in area where procedure to occur; may reapply to maintain effect
Dosage Forms Excipient information presented when available (limited, particularly for generics); consult specific product labeling.
Gel, Ophthalmic [preservative free]:
Akten: 3.5% (1 mL)

References
Busbee BG, Alam A, and Reichel E, "Lidocaine Hydrochloride Gel for Ocular Anesthesia: Results of a Prospective, Randomized Study," *Ophthalmic Surg Lasers Imaging*, 2008, 39(5):386-90.
Lebedevs TH, Wojnar-Horton RE, Yapp P, et al, "Excretion of Lignocaine and its Metabolite Monoethylglycinexylidide in Breast Milk

◄ Following its Use in a Dental Procedure. A Case Report," *J Clin Periodontol*, 1993, 20(8):606-8.

Ortega D, Viviand X, Lorec AM, et al, "Excretion of Lidocaine and Bupivacaine in Breast Milk Following Epidural Anesthesia For Cesarean Delivery," *Acta Anaesthesiol Scand*, 1999, 43(4):394-7.

Lidocaine (Topical) (LYE doe kane)

Brand Names: U.S. AneCream [OTC]; AneCream5 [OTC]; EnovaRX-Lidocaine HCl; LC-4 Lidocaine [OTC]; LC-5 Lidocaine [OTC]; Lidoderm; LidoRx; LMX 4 Plus [OTC]; LMX 4 [OTC]; LMX 5 [OTC]; LTA 360 Kit; Predator [OTC]; RectiCare [OTC]; Tecnu First Aid [OTC]; Topicaine 5 [OTC]; Topicaine [OTC]; Xolido XP [OTC]; Xylocaine

Brand Names: Canada Betacaine; Lidodan; Lidoderm; Maxilene; Xylocaine

Therapeutic Category Analgesic, Topical; Local Anesthetic, Topical; Local Anesthetic, Transdermal

Generic Availability (U.S.) May be product dependent

Use In general, local anesthetic for oral mucous membrane; laser/cosmetic surgeries; minor burns, cuts, and abrasions of the skin; specific uses will vary based on product formulation (FDA approved in adults; refer to product specific information regarding FDA approval in pediatric patients)

Product-specific indications:

Topical patch (Lidoderm): Relief of allodynia (painful hypersensitivity) and postherpetic neuralgia (FDA approved in adults)

Rectal (L-M-X 5): Temporary relief of pain and itching due to anorectal disorders (FDA approved in ages ≥12 years and adults)

Oral solution (2% viscous): Topical anesthesia of irritated oral mucous membranes and pharyngeal tissue (FDA approved in infants, children, and adults); **Note:** Not approved for relief of teething pain and discomfort in infants and children; serious adverse (toxic) effects have been reported (AAP, 2011; AAPD, 2012; ISMP, 2014)

Topical solution (4%): Topical anesthesia of accessible mucous membranes of the oral and nasal cavities and proximal portions of the digestive tract. [FDA approved in children (age not specified) and adults]; **Note:** Not approved for relief of teething pain and discomfort in infants and children; serious adverse (toxic) effects have been reported (AAP, 2011; AAPD, 2012; ISMP, 2014).

Pregnancy Risk Factor B

Pregnancy Considerations Adverse events were not observed in animal reproduction studies using the injection. Lidocaine and its metabolites cross the placenta and can be detected in the fetal circulation following injection (Cavalli, 2004; Mitani, 1987). The amount of lidocaine absorbed topically (and therefore available systemically to potentially reach the fetus) varies by dose administered, duration of exposure, and site of application. Cumulative exposure from all routes of administration should be considered.

Breast-Feeding Considerations Lidocaine is excreted into breast milk. The manufacturer recommends that caution be used when administered to a nursing woman. When administered by injection for dental or obstetric analgesia, small amounts are detected in breast milk; oral bioavailability to the nursing infant is expected to be low. The amount of lidocaine available to the nursing infant would not be expected to cause adverse events (Lebedevs, 1993; Ortega, 1999). Cumulative exposure from all routes of administration should be considered.

Contraindications Hypersensitivity to lidocaine, amide-type local anesthetics, or any component

Warnings Topical anesthetic use of lidocaine oral solution [2% (viscous), 4%] can result in high systemic concentrations and lead to serious toxic effects (eg, arrhythmias,

methemoglobinemia, seizures, coma, respiratory depression, death) in pediatric patients. In infants and children, seizures (some fatal) have been reported following topical lidocaine ingestion at serum concentrations within the therapeutic range of 1 to 5 mcg/mL (Curtis, 2009); others have reported toxic effects with excessive doses or frequent application of topical oral lidocaine solution that resulted in high plasma concentrations. Multiple cases of seizures, including fatalities, have occurred in pediatric patients using viscous lidocaine for oral discomfort (eg, teething pain, herpetic gingivostomatitis) (Curtis, 2009; Giard, 1983; Gonzalez del Rey, 1994; Hess, 1988; Mofenson, 1983; Puczynski, 1985; Rothstein, 1982; Smith, 1992). After reviewing reports (n=22) of serious adverse effects including deaths, the FDA announced in June 2014 that a boxed warning will be added to lidocaine topical 2% (viscous) product labeling stating the product should not be used for treatment of teething pain in infants and children. Lidocaine oral solution is not approved for treatment of teething pain or discomfort; off-label use is strongly discouraged and should be avoided. When used for oral irritation, the solution should not be swallowed, but should be applied topically with a cotton swab to individual lesions or the excess should be expectorated (swish and spit). Toxicology data suggests that in infants and children <6 years, ingestion of as little as 5 mL of lidocaine may result in serious toxicity and emergency care should be sought (Curtis, 2009). Additionally, the FDA recommends against using topical OTC medications for teething pain as some products (eg, benzocaine) for teething pain is also discouraged by AAP, and The American Academy of Pediatric Dentistry (AAPD, 2012). The AAP recommends managing teething pain with a chilled (not frozen) teething ring or gently rubbing/massaging with the caregiver's finger.

Topical anesthetic use of lidocaine creams prior to cosmetic or other medical procedures can result in high systemic concentrations and lead to toxic effects (eg, arrhythmias, methemoglobinemia, seizures, coma, respiratory depression, death). Toxic effects may occur, particularly when topical anesthetics are applied in large amounts or to large areas of the skin; left on for long periods of time; used with materials, wraps, or dressings to cover the skin after application; or applied to broken skin, rashes, or areas of skin irritation. These practices may increase the degree of systemic absorption and should be avoided. Consumers should consult their healthcare provider for instructions on safe use prior to applying topical anesthetics for medical or cosmetic purposes. Use a product with the lowest amount of anesthetic and apply the least amount possible to relieve pain. Some topical products are not recommended for use on otic or mucous membranes; specific product labeling should be consulted.

Safety and efficacy of topical patch have not been established in pediatric patients. Topical patches (both used and unused) may cause toxicities in children; used patches still contain large amounts of lidocaine; store and dispose patches out of the reach of children. Applying the topical patch to larger areas, for longer than recommended, or to broken or inflamed skin may result in increased absorption, high serum concentrations, and serious adverse effects; apply topical patch to intact skin only. Do not expose topical patch application site to external heat sources (eg, electric blankets, heating pads, heated water beds, heat lamps, tanning lamps, hot tubs, hot baths, saunas, sunbathing); although not evaluated, temperature-dependent increases in drug released from patch may occur. Topical patch may contain conducting metal (eg, aluminum) which may cause a burn to the skin during an MRI scan; remove topical patch prior to MRI; reapply patch after scan is completed. Due to the potential for altered electrical conductivity, remove topical patch before cardioversion or defibrillation.

Lidocaine cream (AneCream, L-M-X 4, L-M-X 5), lidocaine foam (Anestafoam), and lidocaine gel (Topicaine) contain benzyl alcohol which may cause allergic reactions in susceptible individuals; large amounts of benzyl alcohol (≥99 mg/kg/day) have been associated with a potentially fatal toxicity ("gasping syndrome") in neonates; the "gasping syndrome" consists of metabolic acidosis, respiratory distress, gasping respirations, CNS dysfunction (including convulsions, intracranial hemorrhage), hypotension, and cardiovascular collapse; use lidocaine products containing benzyl alcohol with caution in neonates; *in vitro* and animal studies have shown that benzoate, a metabolite of benzyl alcohol, displaces bilirubin from protein binding sites. Lidocaine cream (AneCream, L-M-X 4, L-M-X 5), lidocaine foam (Anestafoam), lidocaine gel (Burn Jel), and lidocaine topical patch (Lidoderm) contain propylene glycol; toxicities have been reported with use of products containing propylene glycol, including hyperosmolality, lactic acidosis, seizures, and respiratory depression; in neonates large amounts of propylene glycol delivered orally, intravenously (eg, >3000 mg/day), or topically have been associated with potentially fatal toxicities which can include metabolic acidosis, seizures, renal failure, and CNS depression; use products containing propylene glycol with caution (AAP, 1997; Shehab, 2009).Some products contain polysorbate 80 or bisulfites (consult specific product information) which may cause allergic reactions in susceptible individuals.

Precautions Use with caution in patients with hepatic disease due to diminished ability to metabolize systemically absorbed lidocaine. Use with caution in severe shock, heart block, or heart failure.

Adverse Reactions Note: Adverse effects vary with formulation and extent of systemic absorption; children may be at increased risk.

Cardiovascular: Cyanosis, tachycardia

Central nervous system: Anxiety, confusion, dizziness, lethargy, lightheadedness, somnolence

Dermatologic: Angioedema, bruising (topical patch), contact dermatitis, depigmentation (topical patch), edema of the skin, itching, petechia (topical patch), pruritus, rash, urticaria

Hematologic: Methemoglobinemia

Local: Irritation (topical patch)

Neuromuscular & skeletal: Pain exacerbation (topical patch), paresthesia, weakness

Respiratory: Hypoxia

Neuromuscular & skeletal: Pain exacerbation (topical patch)

Drug Interactions

Metabolism/Transport Effects Substrate of CYP1A2 (major), CYP2A6 (minor), CYP2B6 (minor), CYP2C9 (minor), CYP3A4 (major); **Note:** Assignment of Major/Minor substrate status based on clinically relevant drug interaction potential; **Inhibits** CYP1A2 (weak)

Avoid Concomitant Use

Avoid concomitant use of Lidocaine (Topical) with any of the following: Conivaptan; Fusidic Acid (Systemic)

Increased Effect/Toxicity

Lidocaine (Topical) may increase the levels/effects of: Antiarrhythmic Agents (Class III); Prilocaine; Sodium Nitrite

The levels/effects of Lidocaine (Topical) may be increased by: Abiraterone Acetate; Antiarrhythmic Agents (Class III); Beta-Blockers; Ceritinib; Conivaptan; CYP1A2 Inhibitors (Moderate); CYP1A2 Inhibitors (Strong); CYP3A4 Inhibitors (Moderate); CYP3A4 Inhibitors (Strong); Dasatinib; Deferasirox; Disopyramide; Fusidic Acid (Systemic); Ivacaftor; Luliconazole; Mifepristone; Nitric Oxide; Simeprevir; Stiripentol; Vemurafenib

Decreased Effect

The levels/effects of Lidocaine (Topical) may be decreased by: Bosentan; Cannabis; CYP1A2 Inducers (Strong); CYP3A4 Inducers (Strong); Cyproterone; Dabrafenib; Deferasirox; Mitotane; Siltuximab; St Johns Wort; Tocilizumab

Stability All formulations: Store at controlled room temperature; see product-specific labeling for any additional storage requirements.

Mechanism of Action Blocks both the initiation and conduction of nerve impulses by decreasing the neuronal membrane's permeability to sodium ions, which results in inhibition of depolarization with resultant blockade of conduction

Pharmacodynamics Local anesthetic effect:

Onset of action:

Jelly: 3-5 minutes

Patch (5%): ~4 hours (Davies, 2004)

Pharmacokinetics (Adult data unless noted)

Absorption: Extent and rate variable; dependent upon concentration, dose, application site, and duration of exposure.

Topical patch (5%): 3% ± 2% is expected to be absorbed with recommended doses

Metabolism: 90% hepatic; active metabolites monoethylglycinexylidide (MEGX) and glycinexylidide (GX) can accumulate and may cause CNS toxicity

Time to peak serum concentration: Topical patch (5%): 11 hours (following application of 3 patches)

Elimination: Urine (<10% as unchanged drug)

Dosing: Neonatal Anesthetic for circumsion: Cream: L-M-X 4: Full-term neonates: Topical: Apply 2 g of cream (80 mg lidocaine) to foreskin and penis; occlude with plastic wrap; leave on for 20 minutes (Lehr, 2005)

Dosing: Usual

Infants, Children, and Adolescents:

Anesthetic: Topical:

Gel, ointment: Children ≥2 years and Adolescents: Apply to affected area up to 3-4 times daily as needed; maximum dose: 4.5 mg/kg; not to exceed 300 mg

Jelly: Children: Dose varies with age and weight; maximum dose: 4.5 mg/kg

Oral inflammation or irritation: Topical: **Note:** Not approved for relief of teething pain and discomfort in infants and children; serious adverse (toxic) effects have been reported; AAP, AAPD, and ISMP strongly discourage use (AAP, 2011; AAPD, 2012; ISMP, 2014).

Oral solution (2% viscous): Dose should be adjusted according to patient's age, weight, and physical condition:

Infants and Children <3 years: 25 mg/dose (1.25 mL) applied to area with a cotton-tipped applicator no more frequently than every 3 hours; maximum: 4 doses per 12-hour period; should not be swallowed

Children ≥3 years and Adolescents: Do not exceed 4.5 mg/kg/dose; maximum single dose: 300 mg; swished in the mouth and spit out no more frequently than every 3 hours; maximum: 4 doses per 12-hour period

Topical solution (4%): **Note:** For use on mucous membranes of the oral and nasal cavities and proximal portions of the digestive tract; use lowest effective dose. Children and Adolescents: Do not exceed 4.5 mg/kg/dose; maximum single dose: 300 mg; applied with cotton applicator, cotton pack, or via spray; should not be swallowed

Skin irritation: Topical: Cream:

L-M-X 4: Children ≥2 years and Adolescents: Apply up to 3-4 times daily to intact skin

L-M-X 5: Relief of anorectal pain and itching: Children ≥12 years and Adolescents: Apply to affected area up to 6 times daily

Adults: **Anesthetic, topical:**
Cream:
L-M-X 4: Skin irritation: Apply up to 3-4 times daily to intact skin
L-M-X 5: Relief of anorectal pain and itching: Apply to affected area up to 6 times/day
Gel, ointment: Apply to affected area ≤4 times/day as needed (maximum dose: 4.5 mg/kg, not to exceed 300 mg)
Jelly: Maximum dose: 30 mL (600 mg) in any 12-hour period:
Anesthesia of male urethra: 5-30 mL (100-600 mg)
Anesthesia of female urethra: 3-5 mL (60-100 mg)
Oral topical solution (2% viscous):
Anesthesia of the mouth: 15 mL swished in the mouth and spit out no more frequently than every 3 hours [maximum: 4.5 mg/kg (or 300 mg/dose); 8 doses per 24-hour period]
Anesthesia of the pharynx: 15 mL gargled no more frequently than every 3 hours [maximum: 4.5 mg/kg (or 300 mg/dose); 8 doses per 24-hour period]; may be swallowed
Topical patch:
Lidoderm: Postherpetic neuralgia: Apply patch to most painful area. Up to 3 patches may be applied in a single application. Patch(es) may remain in place for up to 12 hours in any 24-hour period.
LidoPatch: Pain (localized): Apply patch to painful area. Patch may remain in place for up to 12 hours in any 24-hour period. No more than 1 patch should be used in a 24-hour period.
Topical solution (4%): **Note:** For use in mucous membranes of oral and nasal cavities and proximal GI tract; use lowest effective dose. Apply 1-5 mL (40-200 mg) to affected area (maximum dose: 4.5 mg/kg, not to exceed 300 mg/dose)

Administration

Gel (Topicaine): Apply a moderately thick layer to affected area (~1/8" thick). Allow time for numbness to develop (~20-60 minutes after application). When used prior to laser surgery, avoid mucous membranes; remove prior to laser treatment.
Oral solution (2% viscous):
Mouth irritation or inflammation: Have patient swish medication around mouth and then spit it out. In children <3 years, apply small amount to affected area with cotton-tipped applicator.
Pharyngeal anesthesia: Adults: Patient should gargle and may swallow medication.
Topical patch:
Lidoderm: Apply to intact skin to cover most painful area immediately after removal from protective envelope. May be cut (with scissors, prior to removal of release liner) to appropriate size. Clothing may be worn over application area. After removal from skin, fold used patches so the adhesive side sticks to itself; avoid contact with eyes. Remove immediately if burning sensation occurs. Wash hands after application. Avoid exposing application site to external heat sources (eg, heating pad, electric blanket, heat lamp, hot tub). Dispose of patch properly and keep out of reach of children.
LidoPatch: Remove protective film and apply to painful area. Avoid contact with eyes or mucous membranes. Do not apply to open wounds or sensitive skin and do not bandage tightly. Wash hands after application. Avoid exposing application site to external heat sources (eg, heating pad, electric blanket, heat lamp, hot tub).

Dosage Forms Considerations

EnovaRX-Lidocaine is a compounding kit. Refer to manufacturer's package insert for compounding instructions.

Dosage Forms

Excipient information presented when available (limited, particularly for generics); consult specific product labeling.
Cream, External:
AneCream: 4% (5 g, 15 g, 30 g) [contains benzyl alcohol, polysorbate 80, propylene glycol, trolamine (triethanolamine)]
AneCream5: 5% (15 g, 30 g) [contains benzyl alcohol, polysorbate 80, propylene glycol, trolamine (triethanolamine)]
LC-4 Lidocaine: 4% (45 g) [contains cetyl alcohol]
LC-5 Lidocaine: 5% (45 g) [contains cetyl alcohol]
LMX 4: 4% (5 g, 15 g, 30 g) [contains benzyl alcohol]
LMX 5: 5% (15 g, 30 g) [contains benzyl alcohol]
RectiCare: 5% (30 g) [contains benzyl alcohol, polysorbate 80, propylene glycol, trolamine (triethanolamine)]
Cream, External, as hydrochloride:
EnovaRX-Lidocaine HCl: 5% (60 g, 120 g); 10% (60 g, 120 g) [contains cetyl alcohol]
Predator: 4% (63 g) [contains propylene glycol, trolamine (triethanolamine)]
Xolido XP: 4% (118 mL) [contains methylisothiazolinone]
Generic: 3% (28.3 g, 28.35 g, 85 g)
Gel, External:
Tecnu First Aid: 0.2-2.5% (56.7 g) [contains disodium edta]
Topicaine: 4% (10 g, 30 g, 113 g) [contains benzyl alcohol, disodium edta]
Topicaine 5: 5% (10 g, 30 g, 113 g) [contains benzyl alcohol, disodium edta]
Gel, External, as hydrochloride:
LidoRx: 3% (10 mL, 30 mL) [contains isopropyl alcohol, trolamine (triethanolamine)]
Generic: 2% (5 mL, 20 mL, 30 mL)
Gel, External, as hydrochloride [preservative free]:
Generic: 2% (5 mL, 10 mL)
Kit, External:
AneCream: 4% [contains benzyl alcohol, polysorbate 80, propylene glycol, trolamine (triethanolamine)]
LMX 4 Plus: 4% [contains benzyl alcohol]
Lotion, External, as hydrochloride:
Generic: 3% (177 mL)
Ointment, External:
Generic: 5% (30 g, 50 g)
Ointment, External, as hydrochloride:
Generic: 5% (35.44 g, 50 g)
Patch, External:
Lidoderm: 5% (1 ea, 30 ea) [contains disodium edta, methylparaben, propylene glycol, propylparaben]
Generic: 5% (1 ea, 30 ea)
Solution, External, as hydrochloride:
Xylocaine: 4% (50 mL) [contains methylparaben]
Generic: 4% (50 mL)
Solution, Mouth/Throat, as hydrochloride:
Generic: 2% (15 mL, 100 mL)
Solution, Mouth/Throat, as hydrochloride [preservative free]:
LTA 360 Kit: 4% (4 mL)
Generic: 4% (4 mL)

References

American Academy of Pediatrics Committee on Drugs. "Inactive" ingredients in pharmaceutical products: update (subject review). *Pediatrics.* 1997;99(2):268-278.
American Academy of Pediatric Dentistry. Guideline on infant oral health care. 2012. Available at http://www.aapd.org/media/Policies_-Guidelines/G_infantOralHealthCare.pdf
American Academy of Pediatrics Oral Health Initiative. A pediatric guide to children's oral health. January, 2011. Available at http://www2.aap.org/commpeds/dochs/oralhealth/docs/OralHealthFCpagesF2_2_1.pdf
Cavalli Rde C, Lanchote VL, Duarte G, et al, "Pharmacokinetics and Transplacental Transfer of Lidocaine and its Metabolite For Perineal Analgesic Assistance to Pregnant Women," *Eur J Clin Pharmacol,* 2004, 60(8):569-74.

Curtis LA, Dolan TS, Seibert HE. Are one or two dangerous? Lidocaine and topical anesthetic exposures in children. *J Emerg Med.* 2009;37 (1):32-39.

Davies PS and Galer BS, "Review of Lidocaine Patch 5% Studies in the Treatment of Postherpetic Neuralgia," *Drugs*, 2004, 64(9):937-47.

Giard MJ, Uden DL, Whitlock DJ, Watson DM. Seizures induced by oral viscous lidocaine. *Clin Pharm.* 1983;2(2):110.

Gonzalez del Rey J, Wason S, Druckenbrod RW. Lidocaine overdose: another preventable case? *Pediatr Emerg Care.* 1994;10(6): 344-346.

Hess GP, Walson PD. Seizures secondary to oral viscous lidocaine. *Ann Emerg Med.* 1988;17(7):725-727.

Institute for Safe Medication Practice (ISMP). Topical anesthetics for teething infants. ISMP Medication Safety Alert. January 14, 2014. Available at http://www.ismp.org/newsletters/acutecare/issues/20140116.pdf

Lebedevs TH, Wojnar-Horton RE, Yapp P, et al, "Excretion of Lignocaine and its Metabolite Monoethylglycinexylidide in Breast Milk Following its Use in a Dental Procedure. A Case Report," *J Clin Periodontol*, 1993, 20(8):606-8.

Lehr VT, Cepeda E, Frattarelli DA, et al, "Lidocaine 4% Cream Compared With Lidocaine 2.5% and Prilocaine 2.5% or Dorsal Penile Block for Circumcision," *Am J Perinatol*, 2005, 22(5):231-7.

Mitani GM, Steinberg I, Lien EJ, et al, "The Pharmacokinetics of Antiarrhythmic Agents in Pregnancy and Lactation," *Clin Pharmacokinet*, 1987, 12(4):253-91.

Mofenson HC, Caraccio TR, Miller H, Greensher J. Lidocaine toxicity from topical mucosal application. With a review of the clinical pharmacology of lidocaine. *Clin Pediatr (Phila)*, 1983;22(3):190-192.

Ortega D, Viviand X, Lorec AM, et al, "Excretion of Lidocaine and Bupivacaine in Breast Milk Following Epidural Anesthesia for Cesarean Delivery," *Acta Anaesthesiol Scand*, 1999, 43(4):394-7.

Puczynski MS, Ow EP, Rust C. Cardiopulmonary arrest due to misuse of viscous lidocaine. *Arch Otolaryngol.* 1985;111(11):768-769.

Rothstein P, Dornbusch J, Shaywitz BA. Prolonged seizures associated with the use of viscous lidocaine. *J Pediatr.* 101(3):461-463.

Sakai RI, Lattin JE. Lidocaine ingestion. *Am J Dis Child.* 1980;1344 (3):323.

Shehab N, Lewis CL, Streetman DD, Donn SM. Exposure to the pharmaceutical excipients benzyl alcohol and propylene glycol among critically ill neonates. *Pediatr Crit Care Med.* 2009;10 (2):256-259.

Smith M, Wolfram W, Rose R. Toxicity-seizures in an infant caused by (or related to) oral viscous lidocaine use. *J Emerg Med.* 1992;10 (5):587-590.

Lidocaine and Epinephrine

(LYE doe kane & ep i NEF rin)

Brand Names: U.S. Lignospan® Forte; Lignospan® Standard; Xylocaine® MPF With Epinephrine; Xylocaine® With Epinephrine

Brand Names: Canada Xylocaine® With Epinephrine

Therapeutic Category Local Anesthetic, Injectable

Generic Availability (U.S.) Yes

Use Local infiltration anesthesia [FDA approved in pediatric patients (age not specified) and adults]

Pregnancy Risk Factor B

Pregnancy Considerations See individual agents.

Breast-Feeding Considerations Refer to Lidocaine (Systemic) and Epinephrine (Systemic) monographs.

Contraindications Hypersensitivity to epinephrine, lidocaine, amide-type local anesthetics, or any component

Warnings Chondrolysis (necrosis and destruction of cartilage) has been reported following continuous intra-articular infusion of local anesthetics for extended periods of time (48-72 hours); patients presented as early as 2 months following the infusion with joint pain, stiffness, and loss of motion; more than 50% of patients required additional surgery, including arthroscopy or joint replacement; intra-articular administration of local anesthetics is not an FDA-approved route of administration. Some products contain sodium or potassium metabisulfite which may cause allergic reactions in susceptible individuals.

Precautions Do not use solutions in distal portions of the body (digits, nose, ears, penis); do not use large doses in patients with conduction defects (ie, heart block)

Adverse Reactions Degree of adverse effects in the central nervous system and cardiovascular system are directly related to the blood levels of lidocaine. The effects below are more likely to occur after systemic administration rather than infiltration.

Cardiovascular: Myocardial effects include a decrease in contraction force as well as a decrease in electrical excitability and myocardial conduction rate resulting in bradycardia and reduction in cardiac output.

Central nervous system: High blood levels result in anxiety, confusion, disorientation, dizziness, restlessness, seizure, and tremor. This is followed by depression of CNS resulting in somnolence, unconsciousness and possible respiratory arrest. In some cases, symptoms of CNS stimulation may be absent and the primary CNS effects are somnolence and unconsciousness.

Gastrointestinal: Nausea, vomiting

Hypersensitivity reactions: Extremely rare, but may be manifest as dermatologic reactions and edema at injection site. Asthmatic syndromes have occurred. Patients may exhibit hypersensitivity to bisulfites contained in local anesthetic solution to prevent oxidation of epinephrine. In general, patients reacting to bisulfites have a history of asthma and their airways are hyper-reactive to asthmatic syndrome.

Psychogenic reactions: It is common to misinterpret psychogenic responses to local anesthetic injection as an allergic reaction. Intraoral injections are perceived by many patients as a stressful procedure in dentistry. Common symptoms to this stress are diaphoresis, generalized pallor, fainting feeling, hyperventilation, palpitation.

Drug Interactions

Metabolism/Transport Effects Refer to individual components.

Avoid Concomitant Use

Avoid concomitant use of Lidocaine and Epinephrine with any of the following: Ergot Derivatives; Iobenguane I 123; Lurasidone

Increased Effect/Toxicity

Lidocaine and Epinephrine may increase the levels/effects of: Lurasidone; Sympathomimetics

The levels/effects of Lidocaine and Epinephrine may be increased by: AtoMOXetine; Beta-Blockers; Cannabinoid-Containing Products; COMT Inhibitors; Ergot Derivatives; Hyaluronidase; Inhalational Anesthetics; Linezolid; MAO Inhibitors; Serotonin/Norepinephrine Reuptake Inhibitors; Tricyclic Antidepressants

Decreased Effect

Lidocaine and Epinephrine may decrease the levels/effects of: Benzylpenicilloyl Polylysine; Iobenguane I 123

The levels/effects of Lidocaine and Epinephrine may be decreased by: Alpha1-Blockers; Promethazine; Spironolactone

Mechanism of Action Lidocaine blocks both the initiation and conduction of nerve impulses via decreased permeability of sodium ions; epinephrine increases the duration of action of lidocaine by causing vasoconstriction (via alpha effects) which slows the vascular absorption of lidocaine

Pharmacodynamics

Maximum effect: Within 5 minutes

Duration: 2-6 hours, dependent on dose and anesthetic procedure

Dosing: Usual Dosage varies with the anesthetic procedure

Children: Use lidocaine concentrations of 0.5% or 1% (or even more dilute) to decrease possibility of toxicity; lidocaine dose (when using combination product of lidocaine and epinephrine) should not exceed 7 mg/kg/dose; do not repeat within 2 hours

◀ **Administration** Local injection: Before injecting, withdraw syringe plunger to make sure that injection is not into vein or artery; do not administer I.V. or intra-arterially

Additional Information Use preservative free solutions for epidural or caudal use

Dosage Forms Excipient information presented when available (limited, particularly for generics); consult specific product labeling. [DSC] = Discontinued product

Injection, solution:
0.5% / 1:200,000: Lidocaine hydrochloride 0.5% [5 mg/mL] and epinephrine 1:200,000 (50 mL)

1% / 1:100,000: Lidocaine hydrochloride 1% [10 mg/mL] and epinephrine 1:100,000 (20 mL, 30 mL, 50 mL)

2% / 1:100,000: Lidocaine hydrochloride 2% [20 mg/mL] and epinephrine 1:100,000 (30 mL, 50 mL)

Xylocaine® with Epinephrine:
0.5% / 1:200,000: Lidocaine hydrochloride 0.5% [5 mg/mL] and epinephrine 1:200,000 (50 mL) [contains methylparaben]

1% / 1:100,000: Lidocaine hydrochloride 1% [10 mg/mL] and epinephrine 1:100,000 (10 mL, 20 mL, 50 mL) [contains methylparaben]

2% / 1:100,000: Lidocaine hydrochloride 2% [20 mg/mL] and epinephrine 1:100,000 (10 mL, 20 mL, 50 mL) [contains methylparaben]

Injection, solution [preservative free]:
1.5% / 1:200,000: Lidocaine hydrochloride 1.5% [15 mg/mL] and epinephrine 1:200,000 (5 mL, 30 mL)

2% / 1:200,000: Lidocaine hydrochloride 2% [20 mg/mL] and epinephrine 1:200,000 (20 mL)

Xylocaine®-MPF with Epinephrine:
1% / 1:200,000: Lidocaine hydrochloride 1% [10 mg/mL] and epinephrine 1:200,000 (5 mL, 10 mL, 30 mL) [contains sodium metabisulfite]

1.5% / 1:200,000: Lidocaine hydrochloride 1.5% [15 mg/mL] and epinephrine 1:200,000 (5 mL, 10 mL, 30 mL) [contains sodium metabisulfite]

2% / 1:200,000: Lidocaine hydrochloride 2% [20 mg/mL] and epinephrine 1:200,000 (5 mL, 10 mL, 20 mL) [contains sodium metabisulfite]

Injection, solution [for dental use]:
2% / 1:50,000: Lidocaine hydrochloride 2% [20 mg/mL] and epinephrine 1:50,000 (1.7 mL, 1.8 mL)

2% / 1:100,000: Lidocaine hydrochloride 2% [20 mg/mL] and epinephrine 1:100,000 (1.7 mL, 1.8 mL)

Lignospan® Forte: 2% / 1:50,000: Lidocaine hydrochloride 2% [20 mg/mL] and epinephrine 1:50,000 (1.7 mL) [contains edetate disodium, potassium metabisulfite]

Lignospan® Standard: 2% / 1:100,000: Lidocaine hydrochloride 2% [20 mg/mL] and epinephrine 1:100,000 (1.7 mL) [contains edetate disodium, potassium metabisulfite]

Xylocaine® Dental with Epinephrine:
2% / 1:50,000: Lidocaine hydrochloride 2% [20 mg/mL] and epinephrine 1:50,000 (1.7 mL; 1.8 mL [DSC]) [contains sodium metabisulfite]

2% / 1:100,000: Lidocaine hydrochloride 2% [20 mg/mL] and epinephrine 1:100,000 (1.7 mL; 1.8 mL [DSC]) [contains sodium metabisulfite]

Lidocaine and Prilocaine
(LYE doe kane & PRIL oh kane)

Brand Names: U.S. EMLA®; Oraqix®
Brand Names: Canada EMLA®; Oraqix®
Therapeutic Category Analgesic, Topical; Antipruritic, Topical; Local Anesthetic, Topical
Generic Availability (U.S.) Yes: Cream
Use
Cream: Topical anesthetic for use on normal intact skin to provide local analgesia for minor procedures such as I.V. cannulation or venipuncture; topical anesthetic for

superficial minor surgery of genital mucous membranes and as an adjunct for local infiltration anesthesia in genital mucous membranes [FDA approved in neonates (full-term), pediatric, and adult patients]; has also been used for painful procedures, such as lumbar puncture and skin graft harvesting

Periodontal gel: Topical anesthetic for use in periodontal pockets during scaling or root planing procedures (FDA approved in adults)

Pregnancy Risk Factor B

Pregnancy Considerations Animal reproduction studies were not conducted with this combination. Lidocaine and prilocaine cross the placenta. Their use is not contraindicated during labor and delivery. Refer to individual agents.

Breast-Feeding Considerations Lidocaine is excreted in breast milk; excretion of prilocaine in breast milk unknown; however, systemic absorption following topical application is expected to be low. The manufacturer recommends that caution be exercised when administering to nursing women. Refer to individual agents.

Contraindications Hypersensitivity to lidocaine, prilocaine, amide-type local anesthetics, or any component

Warnings Methemoglobinemia has been reported with lidocaine and prilocaine cream; methemoglobinemia is a serious and potentially fatal condition in which the amount of oxygen carried through the blood stream is greatly reduced; signs and symptoms may include pale-, gray-, or blue-colored skin, lips, and nail beds; headache; light-headedness; shortness of breath; fatigue; and rapid heart rate; symptoms may not develop until hours after exposure; many cases were associated with large doses and/or application areas; very young patients and patients with G-6-PD deficiency are more susceptible to development of methemoglobinemia; do not use in patients with congenital or idiopathic methemoglobinemia, neonates <37 weeks gestation, or in infants <12 months of age who are receiving concurrent treatment with methemoglobin-inducing agents (ie, sulfas, acetaminophen, benzocaine, chloroquine, dapsone, nitrofurantoin, nitroglycerin, nitroprusside, phenobarbital, phenytoin, primaquine, quinine).

Topical use prior to cosmetic procedures can result in high systemic levels and lead to toxic effects (eg, arrhythmias, seizures, coma, respiratory depression, and death). Toxic effects may occur particularly when topical anesthetics are applied in large amounts or to large areas of the skin; left on for long periods of time; used with materials, wraps, or dressings to cover the skin after application; or applied to broken skin, rashes, or areas of skin irritation. These practices may increase the degree of systemic absorption and should be avoided. The FDA recommends that consumers consult their healthcare provider for instructions on safe use, prior to applying topical anesthetics for medical or cosmetic purposes. Use of products with the lowest amount of anesthetic and applying the least amount possible to relieve pain is also recommended. Do not use if penetration or migration beyond the tympanic membrane is possible; animal data has shown ototoxicity with inner ear instillation.

Precautions Use with caution in patients with severe hepatic disease, patients with G-6-PD deficiency, and patients taking drugs associated with drug-induced methemoglobinemia; adjust dosage by using smaller areas for application in small children (especially infants <3 months of age) or patients with impaired renal or hepatic function. Patients who are acutely ill or debilitated may be more sensitive to the systemic effect of lidocaine/prilocaine; use with caution and reduce dosage if necessary. Use with caution in patients receiving class I and class III antiarrhythmic drugs (eg, tocainide, mexiletine, amiodarone, bretylium, sotalol, dofetilide) since systemic absorption occurs and synergistic toxicity is possible. Topical lidocaine and prilocaine cream has been shown to inhibit bacterial and viral growth; effect on intradermal administration of live vaccines has not been determined. Avoid use near the eyes; severe irritation may occur. In small infants and children, an occlusive bandage may prevent the child from placing the cream in his/her mouth or smearing the cream on the eyes. Oraqix® should only be used with the Oraqix® dispenser; do not use with standard dental syringes; do not inject Oraqix®.

Adverse Reactions

Cream/patch:

Dermatologic: Hyperpigmentation, urticaria

Genitourinary: Blistering of foreskin (rare)

Local: Burning, edema, erythema, itching, pallor, petechia, purpura, stinging

Miscellaneous: Alteration in temperature sensation (local)

Rare but important or life-threatening: Anaphylactic shock, angioedema, central nervous system depression, central nervous system stimulation, central nervous system toxicity (high dose), circulatory shock (high dose), hypersensitivity reactions, hypotension, methemoglobinemia (high dose)

Periodontal gel:

Central nervous system: Fatigue

Gastrointestinal: Bitter taste, nausea

Local: Application site reaction (includes abscess, edema, irritation, numbness, pain, ulceration, vesicles)

Respiratory: Infection

Miscellaneous: Allergic reactions, flu-like syndrome

Drug Interactions

Metabolism/Transport Effects Refer to individual components.

Avoid Concomitant Use

Avoid concomitant use of Lidocaine and Prilocaine with any of the following: Conivaptan; Fusidic Acid (Systemic)

Increased Effect/Toxicity

Lidocaine and Prilocaine may increase the levels/effects of: Antiarrhythmic Agents (Class III); Prilocaine; Sodium Nitrite

The levels/effects of Lidocaine and Prilocaine may be increased by: Abiraterone Acetate; Antiarrhythmic Agents (Class III); Beta-Blockers; Ceritinib; Conivaptan; CYP1A2 Inhibitors (Moderate); CYP1A2 Inhibitors (Strong); CYP3A4 Inhibitors (Moderate); CYP3A4 Inhibitors (Strong); Dasatinib; Deferasirox; Disopyramide; Fusidic Acid (Systemic); Hyaluronidase; Ivacaftor; Luliconazole; Methemoglobinemia Associated Agents; Mifepristone; Nitric Oxide; Simeprevir; Stiripentol; Vemurafenib

Decreased Effect

Lidocaine and Prilocaine may decrease the levels/effects of: Technetium Tc 99m Tilmanocept

The levels/effects of Lidocaine and Prilocaine may be decreased by: Bosentan; Cannabis; CYP1A2 Inducers (Strong); CYP3A4 Inducers (Strong); Cyproterone; Dabrafenib; Deferasirox; Mitotane; Siltuximab; St Johns Wort; Tocilizumab

Stability

Cream: Store at 20°C to 25°C (68°F to 77°F); keep container tightly closed when not in use

Periodontal gel: Store at 25°C (77°F); excursion permitted to 15°C to 30°C (59°F to 86°F); do not freeze. May turn opaque at temperature <5°C; opacity will disappear when warmed to room temperature

Mechanism of Action Local anesthetic action occurs by stabilization of neuronal membranes and inhibiting the ionic fluxes required for the initiation and conduction of impulses

Pharmacodynamics

Cream:

Onset of action: Dermal analgesia: 1 hour; genital mucosal analgesia: 5-10 minutes

Maximum effect: Dermal analgesia: 2-3 hours; genital mucosal analgesia: 15-20 minutes

Duration: 1-2 hours after removal of the cream

Periodontal gel:

Onset of action: 30 seconds

Duration: ~20 minutes

Pharmacokinetics (Adult data unless noted) Note: Unless specified, data refers to the topical cream product formulation.

Absorption: Related to the duration of application and to the area over which it is applied

3-hour application: 3.6% lidocaine and 6.1% prilocaine were absorbed

24-hour application: 16.2% lidocaine and 33.5% prilocaine were absorbed

Distribution: Both cross the blood-brain barrier

V_d:

Lidocaine: 1.1-2.1 L/kg

Prilocaine: 0.7-4.4 L/kg

Protein binding:

Lidocaine: 70%

Prilocaine: 55%

Metabolism:

Lidocaine: Metabolized by the liver to inactive and active metabolites

Prilocaine: Metabolized in both the liver and kidneys

Half-life:

Cream:

Lidocaine: 65-150 minutes, prolonged in cardiac or hepatic dysfunction

Prilocaine: 10-150 minutes, prolonged in hepatic or renal dysfunction

Periodontal gel:

Lidocaine: 2.2-6.5 hours, prolonged in hepatic dysfunction

Prilocaine: 2-5.7 hours, prolonged in hepatic dysfunction

Dosing: Neonatal Topical cream:

GA <37 weeks: **Topical anesthetic:** 0.5 g/dose has been most frequently reported (Weise, 2005). One study of 30 preterm neonates (GA: ≥30 weeks) showed application to the heel for 1 hour resulted in no measurable changes in methemoglobin levels; others have reported similar findings (Taddio, 1995; Weise, 2005)

GA ≥37 weeks:

Painful procedures (ie, intramuscular injections): Apply 1 g/site 60 minutes prior to procedure

Circumcision: Apply 1-2 g to prepuce and cover with occlusive dressing for 60-90 minutes prior to procedure (Weise, 2005)

Topical anesthetic: Manufacturer labeling: Maximum dose and application area (based on application to intact skin): Weight <5 kg:

Maximum total dose: 1 g

Maximum application area: 10 cm²

Maximum application time: 1 hour

◀ **Dosing: Usual**

Infants and Children: **Anesthetic:** Topical cream: Dose should be individualized based on procedure and area to be anesthetized.

Maximum Recommended Dose and Application Area for Infants and Children Based on Application to Intact Skin

Age and Body Weight Requirements	Maximum Total Dose	Maximum Application Area	Maximum Application Time
1 to <3 mo or <5 kg	1g	10 cm^2	1 h
3 to <12 mo and >5 kg	2 g	20 cm^2	4 h
1-6 y and >10 kg	10 g	100 cm^2	4 h
7-12 y and >20 kg	20 g	200 cm^2	4 h

Adult:

Anesthetic: Topical cream: Apply a thick layer to intact skin and cover with an occlusive dressing; **Note:** Dermal analgesia can be expected to increase for up to 3 hours under occlusive dressing and persist for 1-2 hours after removal of the cream.

Minor dermal procedures (eg, I.V. cannulation or venipuncture): Topical cream: Apply 2.5 g of cream 1/2 of the 5 g tube) over 20-25 cm^2 of skin surface area for at least 1 hour.

Major dermal procedures (eg, more painful dermatological procedures involving a larger skin area such as split thickness skin graft harvesting): Topical cream: Apply 2 g of cream per 10 cm^2 of skin and allow to remain in contact with the skin for at least 2 hours.

Adult male genital skin (eg, pretreatment prior to local anesthetic infiltration): Apply a thick layer of cream (1 g/10 cm^2) to the skin surface for 15 minutes. Local anesthetic infiltration should be performed immediately after removal of cream.

Adult female genital mucous membranes: Minor procedures (eg, removal of condylomata acuminata, pretreatment for local anesthetic infiltration): Apply 5-10 g (thick layer) of cream for 5-10 minutes

Periodontal gel (Oraqix®): Apply on gingival margin around selected teeth using blunt-tipped applicator included in package. Wait 30 seconds, then fill the periodontal pockets using the blunt-tipped applicator until gel becomes visible at the gingival margin. Wait another 30 seconds before starting treatment. May reapply if anesthesia starts to wear off; maximum recommended dose per treatment session: 5 cartridges (8.5 g)

Administration Topical:

Cream: Do not use on open wounds or the eyes; apply a thick layer of cream to intact skin and cover with an occlusive dressing

Periodontal gel: Oraqix® is a viscous liquid; **not for injection**; should be in the liquid form before administration; if gel forms refrigerate until becomes liquid again. Do not use dental cartridge warmers; heat will cause product to gel. Apply slowly and evenly on gingival margin around selected teeth using Oraqix® Dispenser; not intended to be used with standard dental syringes.

Dosage Forms Excipient information presented when available (limited, particularly for generics); consult specific product labeling.

Cream, topical: Lidocaine 2.5% and prilocaine 2.5% (5 g, 30 g)

EMLA®: Lidocaine 2.5% and prilocaine 2.5% (5 g, 30 g)

Gel, periodontal:

Oraqix®: Lidocaine 2.5% and prilocaine 2.5% (1.7 g)

References

Broadman LM, Soliman IE, Hannallah RS, et al, "Analgesic Efficacy of Eutectic Mixture of Local Anesthetics (EMLA®) vs Intradermal Infiltration Prior to Venous Cannulation in Children," *Am J Anaesth*, 1987, 34:S56.

Carbajal R, Biran V, Lenclen R, et al, "EMLA Cream and Nitrous Oxide to Alleviate Pain Induced by Palivizumab (Synagis) Intramuscular Injections in Infants and Young Children," *Pediatrics*, 2008, 121(6): e1591-8.

Halperin DL, Koren G, Attias D, et al, "Topical Skin Anesthesia for Venous Subcutaneous Drug Reservoir and Lumbar Puncture in Children," *Pediatrics*, 1989, 84(2):281-4.

Kaur G, Gupta P, and Kumar A, "A Randomized Trial of Eutectic Mixture of Local Anesthetics During Lumbar Puncture in Newborns," *Arch Pediatr Adolesc Med*, 2003, 157(11):1065-70.

Robieux I, Kumar R, Radhakrishnan S, et al, "Assessing Pain and Analgesia With a Lidocaine-Prilocaine Emulsion in Infants and Toddlers During Venipuncture," *J Pediatr*, 1991, 118(6):971-3.

Taddio A, Shennan AT, Stevens B, et al, "Safety of Lidocaine-Prilocaine Cream in the Treatment of Preterm Neonates," *J Pediatr*, 1995, 127 (6):1002-5.

Weise KL and Nahata MC, "EMLA for Painful Procedures in Infants," *J Pediatr Health Care*, 2005, 19(1):42-7.

Lidocaine and Tetracaine

(LYE doe kane & TET ra kane)

Medication Safety Issues

Other safety concerns:

Transdermal patch may contain conducting metal (eg, iron); remove patch prior to MRI.

Brand Names: U.S. Pliaglis; Synera

Therapeutic Category Analgesic, Topical; Local Anesthetic, Topical

Generic Availability (U.S.) No

Use Topical anesthetic for use on intact skin to provide local analgesia for superficial venous access, including venipuncture, and for superficial dermatological procedures, including excision, electrodesiccation, and shave biopsy of skin lesions.

Pregnancy Risk Factor B

Pregnancy Considerations Adverse effects have not been observed in animal reproduction studies with this combination. Systemic absorption following topical application is expected to be low. Systemic absorption would be required in order for lidocaine and tetracaine to cross the placenta and reach the fetus. Refer to Lidocaine (Systemic, Topical) and Tetracaine (Systemic) monographs.

Breast-Feeding Considerations Lidocaine is excreted in breast milk; it is not known if tetracaine is excreted in breast milk. Systemic absorption following topical application is expected to be low; according to the manufacturer, the small amount ingested by a nursing infant would not be expected to cause adverse events. The manufacturer recommends that caution be exercised if administered to nursing women. Refer to Lidocaine (Systemic, Topical) and Tetracaine (Systemic) monographs.

Contraindications Hypersensitivity to lidocaine, tetracaine, local anesthetics of the amide or ester type, para-aminobenzoic acid, or any component

Warnings Since the heating element in the patch contains iron powder, **remove patch before** magnetic resonance imaging. Do not cut patch or remove the top cover since this could result in the patch heating to temperatures that can cause thermal injury. Keeping a patch on longer than recommended or applying multiple patches simultaneously or sequentially can result in systemic absorption sufficient to cause serious adverse effects due to the local anesthetic components. Transdermal patch may contain conducting metal (eg, aluminum) which may cause a burn to the skin during an MRI scan; remove patch prior to MRI; reapply patch after scan is completed.

Topical use prior to cosmetic procedures can result in high systemic levels and lead to toxic effects (eg, arrhythmias, seizures, coma, respiratory depression, and death). Toxic effects may occur particularly when topical anesthetics are applied in large amounts or to large areas of the skin; left on for long periods of time; used with materials, wraps, or dressings to cover the skin after application; or applied to broken skin, rashes, or areas of skin irritation. These practices may increase the degree of systemic absorption and should be avoided. The FDA recommends that consumers consult their healthcare provider for instructions on safe use, prior to applying topical anesthetics for medical or cosmetic purposes. Use of products with the lowest amount of anesthetic and applying the least amount possible to relieve pain is also recommended.

Precautions Use with caution in patients who are more sensitive to the systemic effects of lidocaine and tetracaine, including acutely ill, debilitated patients. Use with caution in patients with severe liver disease, pseudocholinesterase deficiency, and patients receiving class I antiarrhythmics and/or local anesthetics (systemic toxic effects may be additive or synergistic with lidocaine and tetracaine).

Adverse Reactions Also see individual agents.

Central nervous system: Dizziness, drowsiness, headache

Dermatologic: Acne vulgaris, application site dermatitis, application site rash, ecchymosis, erythema, local discoloration, localized blanching, maculopapular rash, skin edema, xeroderma

Gastrointestinal: Nausea, vomiting

Hematologic & oncologic: Petechial rash

Rare but important or life-threatening: Anaphylactoid reaction, blepharitis, burning sensation of skin, dehydration, diaphoresis, euphoria, hyperventilation, infection, loss of consciousness, nervousness, pain, paresthesia, pharyngitis, pruritus, stupor, syncope, twitching, urticaria, vesiculobullous dermatitis

Drug Interactions

Metabolism/Transport Effects Refer to individual components.

Avoid Concomitant Use

Avoid concomitant use of Lidocaine and Tetracaine with any of the following: Conivaptan; Fusidic Acid (Systemic)

Increased Effect/Toxicity

Lidocaine and Tetracaine may increase the levels/effects of: Antiarrhythmic Agents (Class III); Prilocaine; Sodium Nitrite

The levels/effects of Lidocaine and Tetracaine may be increased by: Abiraterone Acetate; Antiarrhythmic Agents (Class III); Beta-Blockers; Ceritinib; Conivaptan; CYP1A2 Inhibitors (Moderate); CYP1A2 Inhibitors (Strong); CYP3A4 Inhibitors (Moderate); CYP3A4 Inhibitors (Strong); Dasatinib; Deferasirox; Disopyramide; Fusidic Acid (Systemic); Ivacaftor; Luliconazole; Mifepristone; Nitric Oxide; Simeprevir; Stiripentol; Vemurafenib

Decreased Effect

The levels/effects of Lidocaine and Tetracaine may be decreased by: Bosentan; Cannabis; CYP1A2 Inducers (Strong); CYP3A4 Inducers (Strong); Cyproterone; Dabrafenib; Deferasirox; Mitotane; Siltuximab; St Johns Wort; Tocilizumab

Stability Store at room temperature.

Mechanism of Action Local anesthetic action occurs by stabilization of neuronal membranes and inhibiting the sodium ion fluxes required for the initiation and conduction of impulses.

Pharmacodynamics Onset of action: 20 minutes

Pharmacokinetics (Adult data unless noted)

Distribution: Lidocaine crosses the placental and blood-brain barriers; lidocaine is excreted in breast milk

V_d: Lidocaine:

Neonates: 2.75 L/kg

Adults: 1.1 L/kg

Protein binding: Lidocaine: 70%

Metabolism:

Lidocaine: Metabolized in the liver by cytochrome P450 CYP1A2 and partially by CYP3A4 to inactive and active metabolites monoethylglycinexylidide (MEGX) and glycinexylidide (GX)

Tetracaine: Hydrolysis by plasma esterases to primary metabolites para-aminobenzoic acid and diethylaminoethanol

Half-life: Lidocaine: Adults: 1.8 hours

Elimination: Lidocaine: Excreted in urine as metabolites and parent drug

Dosing: Usual Topical: Children ≥3 years and Adults:

Venipuncture or I.V. cannulation: Apply to intact skin for 20-30 minutes before venous access

Superficial dermatologic procedures: Apply to intact skin for 30 minutes before procedure

Note: Maximum dose: Current patch removed and one additional patch applied at a new location to facilitate venous access is acceptable after a failed attempt. Otherwise, simultaneous or sequential application of multiple patches is **not recommended**.

Administration Topical: Do not use on mucous membranes or the eyes; apply to **intact skin** immediately after opening the pouch. Do **not** cut or remove the top cover of the patch as this could result in **thermal injury**. Do not cover the holes on the top of the patch as this could cause the patch to not heat up. Avoid contact with the eyes due to potential irritation or abrasion. If contact occurs, immediately wash out the eye with water or saline, and protect the eye until sensation returns. Wash hands after handling patch. The adhesive sides of a used patch should be folded together; used patch should be disposed of immediately.

Monitoring Parameters Pain assessment

Additional Information Contains CHADD® self-warming heating element which facilitates drug delivery (when used appropriately, the patch is designed to increase skin temperature by <5°C); patch is latex free. A used patch will still contain large amounts of lidocaine and tetracaine (at least 90% of the initial amount).

Dosage Forms Excipient information presented when available (limited, particularly for generics); consult specific product labeling.

Cream, external:

Pliaglis: Lidocaine 7% and tetracaine 7% (30 g, 100 g) [contains methylparaben, propylparaben]

Patch, transdermal:

Synera: Lidocaine 70 mg and tetracaine 70 mg (10s) [contains heating component, metal; each patch is ~50 cm^2]

References

Sethna NF, Verghese ST, Hannallah RS, et al, "A Randomized Controlled Trial to Evaluate S-Caine Patch for Reducing Pain Associated With Vascular Access in Children," *Anesthesiology*, 2005, 102 (2):403-8.

◆ **Lidocaine Hydrochloride** *see* Lidocaine (Ophthalmic) *on page 1241*

◆ **Lidocaine Hydrochloride** *see* Lidocaine (Systemic) *on page 1239*

◆ **Lidocaine Hydrochloride** *see* Lidocaine (Topical) *on page 1242*

◆ **Lidocaine Patch** *see* Lidocaine (Topical) *on page 1242*

◆ **Lidodan (Can)** *see* Lidocaine (Topical) *on page 1242*

◆ **Lidoderm** *see* Lidocaine (Topical) *on page 1242*

◆ **LidoRx** *see* Lidocaine (Topical) *on page 1242*

◆ **LID-Pack® (Can)** *see* Bacitracin and Polymyxin B *on page 257*

◆ **Lignocaine Hydrochloride** *see* Lidocaine (Ophthalmic) *on page 1241*

◆ **Lignocaine Hydrochloride** *see* Lidocaine (Systemic) *on page 1239*

◆ **Lignocaine Hydrochloride** *see* Lidocaine (Topical) *on page 1242*

◆ **Lignospan® Forte** *see* Lidocaine and Epinephrine *on page 1245*

◆ **Lignospan® Standard** *see* Lidocaine and Epinephrine *on page 1245*

Lindane (LIN dane)

Related Information
Safe Handling of Hazardous Drugs *on page 2419*
Therapeutic Category Antiparasitic Agent, Topical; Pediculocide; Scabicidal Agent; Shampoos
Generic Availability (U.S.) Yes
Use
Lotion: Second-line treatment of scabies (*Sarcoptes scabiei*) in patients intolerant to or who have failed other treatment options [FDA approved in pediatric patients (age not specified) and adults]
Shampoo: Second-line treatment of *Pediculus humanus capitis* (head lice), and *Pthirus pubis* (crab lice) and their ova in patients intolerant to or who have failed other treatment options [FDA approved in pediatric patients (age not specified) and adults]
Medication Guide Available Yes
Pregnancy Risk Factor C
Pregnancy Considerations Adverse events have been observed in animal reproduction studies. Animal studies suggest possible neurologic abnormalities due to the increased susceptibility of drug and the immature central nervous system of the fetus. Lindane is lipophilic and may accumulate in the placenta. Use in pregnant women is contraindicated in some guidelines (CDC, 2010).
Breast-Feeding Considerations Lindane is excreted in breast milk. Nursing mothers should interrupt breast-feeding, express and discard milk for at least 24 hours following use. In addition, skin-to-skin contact between the infant and affected area should be avoided. Use in nursing women is contraindicated in some guidelines (CDC, 2010).
Contraindications Hypersensitivity to lindane or any component; premature neonates; uncontrolled seizure disorders; crusted (Norwegian) scabies or other skin conditions which may increase systemic absorption (eg, atopic dermatitis, psoriasis)
Warnings Hazardous agent; use appropriate precautions for handling and disposal. May be associated with severe neurologic toxicities; seizures and death have been reported with lindane [U.S. Boxed Warning]; may occur with prolonged, repeated, or single use; risk may be increased in infants, children, patients <50 kg, or the elderly. Use is contraindicated in premature infants and patients with uncontrolled seizure disorders [U.S. Boxed Warning]. Premature infants may have increased systemic exposure due to increased permeability of skin, larger skin surface area to volume ratio, and immature hepatic development compared to full-term infants. Use with caution in patients with a history of seizures, head trauma, HIV infection, or with conditions which may increase risk of seizures or medications which decrease seizure threshold. When lotion is used in small infants and young children, cover hands to prevent accidental lindane ingestion from thumbsucking; consider alternative therapy for the treatment of scabies in infants and young children <2 years of age (ie, permethrin). Due to availability of other effective treatments, lindane is no longer recommended for the treatment of scabies or lice in pediatric patients (Frankowski, 2010; *Red Book*, 2012). Oil-based skin or hair products and moist warm skin may increase systemic absorption; skin and hair should be clean and dry prior to application. For external use only; avoid contact with the face, eyes, mucous membranes, and urethral meatus.

Not considered first-line therapy; use only in patients who have failed or are intolerant to other agents [U.S. Boxed Warning]. Instruct patients on proper use, including the amount to apply, how long to leave on, and to avoid

retreatment. Itching may occur as a result of killing scabies and does not necessarily indicate treatment failure or need for retreatment [U.S. Boxed Warning].
Precautions Use with caution in patients with hepatic impairment. Individuals applying on another person should wear gloves during application. Natural latex gloves are permeable to lindane; use low permeability gloves (eg, nitrile, latex with neoprene, or sheer vinyl); thoroughly clean hands after application.
Adverse Reactions
Central nervous system: Ataxia, dizziness, localized burning, neurotoxicity (risk greater in patients <110 lbs [50 kg]), restlessness, seizure, stinging sensation
Dermatologic: Contact dermatitis, eczematous rash
Hematologic & oncologic: Aplastic anemia (CDC, 2010)
Rare but important or life-threatening: Alopecia, dermatitis, headache, pain, paresthesia, pruritus, urticaria
Drug Interactions
Metabolism/Transport Effects None known.
Avoid Concomitant Use There are no known interactions where it is recommended to avoid concomitant use.
Increased Effect/Toxicity There are no known significant interactions involving an increase in effect.
Decreased Effect There are no known significant interactions involving a decrease in effect.
Stability
Store at 20°C to 25°C (68°F to 77°F).
Mechanism of Action Directly absorbed by parasites and ova through the exoskeleton; stimulates the nervous system resulting in seizures and death of parasitic arthropods
Pharmacokinetics (Adult data unless noted)
Absorption: Topical: ~10% systemically; absorption higher when applied to weeping or excoriated skin (Ginsburg, 1977)
Metabolism: Hepatic
Half-life: Infants ≥5 months and Children ≤8 years (Ginsburg, 1977):
Healthy skin: 21.4 hours
Infected skin: 17.9 hours
Time to peak serum concentration: Infants ≥5 months and Children: Topical: 6 hours
Elimination: In urine and feces
Dosing: Usual
Infants, Children, and Adolescents: **Note:** The AAP no longer recommends lindane as a treatment option for head lice or scabies in pediatric patients due to safety concerns (*Red Book*, 2012); use extreme caution in infants, children, and adolescents weighing <50 kg.
Head lice: Shampoo: Topical: Apply shampoo to dry hair and massage into hair for 4 minutes. Add small amounts of water to form lather, then immediately rinse lather away. Amount of shampoo needed is based on length and density of hair; most patients require ≤30 mL; maximum dose: 60 mL. Do not retreat.
Scabies: Lotion: Topical: Apply a thin layer of lotion and massage it on skin from the neck to the toes. Most patients require ≤30 mL; maximum dose: 60 mL. Do not retreat. Do not leave on for more than 12 hours.
Infants and Children: Wash off 6 hours after application (Pramanik, 1979)
Adults:
Head lice, crab lice: Topical: Apply shampoo to dry hair and massage into hair for 4 minutes; add small quantities of water to hair until lather forms, then rinse hair thoroughly and comb with a fine tooth comb to remove nits. Amount of shampoo needed is based on length and density of hair; most patients will require 30 mL (maximum: 60 mL). Do not retreat.
Scabies: Topical: Apply a thin layer of lotion and massage it on skin from the neck to the toes; after 8-12 hours; bathe and remove the drug; most patients will

require 30 mL; larger adults may require up to 60 mL. Do not retreat. Do not leave on for more than 12 hours.

Dosing adjustment in renal impairment: There are no dosage adjustments provided in the manufacturer's labeling.

Dosing adjustment in hepatic impairment: There are no dosage adjustments provided in the manufacturer's labeling.

Administration Shake well prior to use. For topical use only; never administer orally. Caregivers should apply with gloves (avoid natural latex, may be permeable to lindane). Rinse off with warm (not hot) water.

Lotion: Apply to dry, cool skin; do not apply to face or eyes. In infants when treating scabies, medication should be applied head to toe since those areas may also be affected (CDC, 2010; *Red Book*, 2012). Before application, wait at least 1 hour after bathing or showering (wet or warm skin increases absorption). Skin should be clean and free of any other lotions, creams, or oil prior to lindane application. Do not use on open wounds or sores. Do not use occlusive dressings (eg, diaper). Trim nails prior to use and apply under fingernails.

Shampoo: Apply to clean, dry hair. Wait at least 1 hour after washing and drying hair before applying lindane shampoo. Hair should be washed with a shampoo not containing a conditioner; hair and skin of head and neck should be free of any lotions, oils, or creams prior to lindane application. Do not cover with shower cap or towel.

Hazardous agent; use appropriate precautions for handling and disposal (EPA, U-listed).

Additional Information Excessive absorption may result in overdose with signs and symptoms which include nausea, vomiting, seizures, headaches, arrhythmias, apnea, pulmonary edema, hematuria, hepatitis, coma, and even death (Pramanik, 1979; Singal, 2006)

Dosage Forms Excipient information presented when available (limited, particularly for generics); consult specific product labeling.

Lotion, External:
Generic: 1% (60 mL)
Shampoo, External:
Generic: 1% (60 mL)

References
American Academy of Pediatrics (AAP). In: Pickering LK, Baker CJ, Kimberlin DW, Long SS, eds. *Red Book: 2012 Report of the Committee on Infectious Diseases.* 29th ed. Elk Grove Village, IL: American Academy of Pediatrics; 2012.

Centers for Disease Control and Prevention (CDC). Scabies - treatment. November 3, 2011. Available at http://www.cdc.gov/parasites/scabies/treatment.html

Centers for Disease Control and Prevention (CDC), "Sexually Transmitted Diseases Treatment Guidelines, 2010," *MMWR Recomm Rep,* 2010, 59(RR-12):1-110.

Frankowski BL, Bocchini JA Jr, and Council on School Health and Committee on Infectious Diseases, "Head Lice," *Pediatrics,* 2010, 126 (2):392-403.

Ginsburg CM, Lowry W, and Reisch JS, "Absorption of Lindane (Gamma Benzene Hexachloride) in Infants and Children," *J Pediatr,* 1977, 91(6):998-1000.

Pramanik AK and Hansen RC, "Transcutaneous Gamma Benzene Hexachloride Absorption and Toxicity in Infants and Children," *Arch Dermatol,* 1979, 115(10):1224-5.

Red Book: 2012 Report of the Committee on Infectious Diseases, "Pediculosis capitis (Head Lice)" 29th ed, Pickering LK, ed, Elk Grove Village, IL: American Academy of Pediatrics, 2012.

Red Book: 2012 Report of the Committee on Infectious Diseases, "Scabies" 29th ed, Pickering LK, ed, Elk Grove Village, IL: American Academy of Pediatrics, 2012.

Linezolid (li NE zoh lid)

Medication Safety Issues
Sound-alike/look-alike issues:
Zyvox may be confused with Zosyn, Zovirax
Brand Names: U.S. Zyvox

Brand Names: Canada Zyvoxam
Therapeutic Category Antibiotic, Oxazolidinone
Generic Availability (U.S.) No
Use Treatment of community-acquired pneumonia, hospital-acquired pneumonia, uncomplicated and complicated skin and soft tissue infections (including diabetic foot infections without concomitant osteomyelitis), and bacteremia caused by susceptible organisms, such as vancomycin-resistant *Enterococcus faecium* (VREF), *Streptococcus pneumoniae* including multidrug resistant strains, *Staphylococcus aureus* including MRSA, *Streptococcus pyogenes,* or *Streptococcus agalactiae* (FDA approved in all ages). **Note:** There have been reports of vancomycin-resistant *E. faecium* and *S. aureus* (methicillin-resistant) developing resistance to linezolid during its clinical use.

Pregnancy Risk Factor C
Pregnancy Considerations Adverse effects were observed in some animal reproduction studies at doses that were also maternally toxic. Information related to linezolid use during pregnancy is limited.

Breast-Feeding Considerations Linezolid is excreted into breast milk. The manufacturer advises caution if administering linezolid to a breast-feeding woman. Non-dose-related effects could include modification of bowel flora.

Contraindications Hypersensitivity to linezolid or any component; concurrent use or within 2 weeks of MAO inhibitors; patients with uncontrolled hypertension, pheochromocytoma, thyrotoxicosis, and/or taking sympathomimetics (eg, pseudoephedrine), vasopressive agents (eg, epinephrine, norepinephrine), or dopaminergic agents (eg, dopamine, dobutamine) unless closely monitored for increased blood pressure; patients with carcinoid syndrome and/or taking SSRIs, tricyclic antidepressants, serotonin 5-HT$_{1B, 1D}$ receptor agonists, meperidine, or buspirone unless closely monitored for sign/symptoms of serotonin syndrome

Warnings Linezolid is a reversible, nonselective MAO inhibitor with the potential to have the same interactions as other MAO inhibitors. May cause serotonin syndrome; symptoms include agitation, confusion, hallucinations, hyper-reflexia, myoclonus, shivering, and tachycardia, may occur with concomitant proserotonergic drugs (eg, SSRIs/SNRIs or triptans) or agents which reduce linezolid's metabolism; concurrent use with these medications is contraindicated unless patient is closely monitored for signs/symptoms of serotonin syndrome. Hypoglycemic episodes have been reported; use with caution and closely monitor glucose in diabetic patients; dose reductions/discontinuation of concurrent hypoglycemic agents or discontinuation of linezolid may be required. Thrombocytopenia, anemia, leukopenia, and pancytopenia have been reported in patients receiving linezolid and may be dependent on duration of therapy (generally >2 weeks of treatment); monitor patients' CBC weekly during linezolid therapy; discontinuation of therapy may be required in patients who develop or have worsening myelosuppression; use with caution in patients with preexisting myelosuppression.

C. difficile-associated colitis has been reported; fluid and electrolyte management, protein supplementation, antibiotic treatment, and surgical evaluation may be indicated. Peripheral and optic neuropathy with vision loss have been reported primarily in patients treated for longer than 28 days with linezolid. Cases of lactic acidosis in which patients experienced repeated episodes of nausea and vomiting, acidosis, and low bicarbonate levels have been reported; patients experiencing these symptoms should be evaluated immediately. Linezolid should not be used in the empiric treatment of catheter-related bloodstream infections (CRBSI) but may be appropriate for targeted therapy ▶

(eg, patient with CRBSI due to vancomycin-resistant enterococci) (Mermel, 2009).

The manufacturer does not recommend the use of linezolid for empiric treatment of pediatric CNS infections since therapeutic linezolid concentrations are not consistently achieved or maintained in the CSF of patients with ventriculoperitoneal shunts. However, limited data in the form of case reports in pediatric and adult patients suggest that linezolid may be useful in treating gram-positive CNS infections that have failed to respond to other treatment options (Cook, 2005; da Silva, 2007; Milstone, 2007; Shaikh, 2001; Villani, 2002).

Oral suspension contains sodium benzoate; benzoic acid (benzoate) is a metabolite of benzyl alcohol; large amounts of benzyl alcohol (≥99 mg/kg/day) have been associated with a potentially fatal toxicity ("gasping syndrome") in neonates; the "gasping syndrome" consists of metabolic acidosis, respiratory distress, gasping respirations, CNS dysfunction (including convulsions, intracranial hemorrhage), hypotension, and cardiovascular collapse; use caution when administering oral suspension containing sodium benzoate to neonates; in vitro and animal studies have shown that benzoate displaces bilirubin from protein binding sites.

Precautions Use with caution and monitor closely in patients with uncontrolled hypertension, untreated hyperthyroidism, carcinoid syndrome, or pheochromocytoma; linezolid has not been studied in patients with these conditions; use is contraindicated if close monitoring unavailable. Use with caution in patients with a history of or risk factors for seizures; seizures have been reported with use. Use with caution in renal impairment; while no adjustment recommended, the two primary metabolites may accumulate in patients with renal impairment; the clinical significance is unknown; risk of accumulation of metabolites versus the benefit of therapy should be weighed; monitor for hematopoietic and neuropathic adverse events when administering for extended periods in patients with renal impairment. Use with caution in severe hepatic impairment (Child-Pugh class C); use has not been adequately evaluated.

Linezolid suspension contains aspartame which is metabolized to phenylalanine and must be used with caution in patients with phenylketonuria.

Adverse Reactions

Central nervous system: Dizziness, headache, insomnia, vertigo (children)

Dermatologic: Pruritus (children), skin rash

Endocrine & metabolic: Increased amylase, increased lactate dehydrogenase

Gastrointestinal: Abdominal pain, constipation, diarrhea, dysgeusia, increased serum lipase, loose stools (children), nausea, oral candidiasis, pancreatitis, tongue discoloration, vomiting

Genitourinary: Vulvovaginal candidiasis

Hematologic & oncologic: Anemia, decreased hemoglobin, eosinophilia (children), leukopenia (more common in children), neutropenia (more common in children), thrombocytopenia

Hepatic: Abnormal hepatic function tests, increased serum alkaline phosphatase, increased serum ALT, increased serum AST (adults), increased serum bilirubin (more common in children)

Infection: Fungal infection

Renal: Increased blood urea nitrogen, increased serum creatinine

Miscellaneous: Fever

Rare but important or life-threatening: Anaphylaxis, angioedema, bullous skin disease, Clostridium difficile-associated diarrhea, convulsions, hypertension, hypoglycemia, lactic acidosis, optic neuropathy, pancytopenia, peripheral neuropathy, rhabdomyolysis, seizures, serotonin syndrome (with concurrent use of other serotonergic agents), Stevens-Johnson syndrome, vision loss

Drug Interactions

Metabolism/Transport Effects Inhibits Monoamine Oxidase

Avoid Concomitant Use

Avoid concomitant use of Linezolid with any of the following: Alcohol (Ethyl); Anilidopiperidine Opioids; Apraclonidine; AtoMOXetine; BCG; Bezafibrate; Buprenorphine; BuPROPion; BusPIRone; CarBAMazepine; CloZAPine; Cyclobenzaprine; Cyproheptadine; Dexmethylphenidate; Dextromethorphan; Diethylpropion; Dipyrone; Hydrocodone; HYDROmorphone; Isometheptene; Levonordefrin; MAO Inhibitors; Maprotiline; Meperidine; Methyldopa; Methylene Blue; Methylphenidate; Mirtazapine; Morphine (Liposomal); Morphine (Systemic); Nefazodone; Oxymorphone; Pholcodine; Pizotifen; Selective Serotonin Reuptake Inhibitors; Serotonin 5-HT1D Receptor Agonists; Serotonin/Norepinephrine Reuptake Inhibitors; Tapentadol; Tetrabenazine; Tetrahydrozoline (Nasal); TraZODone; Tricyclic Antidepressants; Tryptophan

Increased Effect/Toxicity

Linezolid may increase the levels/effects of: Antipsychotics; Apraclonidine; AtoMOXetine; Betahistine; Bezafibrate; Brimonidine (Ophthalmic); Brimonidine (Topical); BuPROPion; CloZAPine; Cyproheptadine; Dexmethylphenidate; Dextromethorphan; Diethylpropion; Domperidone; Doxylamine; Hydrocodone; HYDROmorphone; Hypoglycemic Agents; Isometheptene; Levonordefrin; Lithium; Meperidine; Methadone; Methyldopa; Methylene Blue; Methylphenidate; Metoclopramide; Mirtazapine; Morphine (Liposomal); Morphine (Systemic); Nefazodone; OxyCODONE; Pizotifen; Reserpine; Selective Serotonin Reuptake Inhibitors; Serotonin 5-HT1D Receptor Agonists; Serotonin Modulators; Serotonin/Norepinephrine Reuptake Inhibitors; Sympathomimetics; Tetrahydrozoline (Nasal); TraZODone; Tricyclic Antidepressants

The levels/effects of Linezolid may be increased by: Alcohol (Ethyl); Anilidopiperidine Opioids; Antiemetics (5HT3 Antagonists); Antipsychotics; Buprenorphine; BusPIRone; CarBAMazepine; COMT Inhibitors; Cyclobenzaprine; Dipyrone; Levodopa; MAO Inhibitors; Maprotiline; Oxymorphone; Pholcodine; Tapentadol; Tetrabenazine; TraMADol; Tryptophan

Decreased Effect

Linezolid may decrease the levels/effects of: BCG; Domperidone; Sodium Picosulfate; Typhoid Vaccine

The levels/effects of Linezolid may be decreased by: Cyproheptadine; Domperidone

Food Interactions Concurrent ingestion of foods rich in tyramine, dopamine, tyrosine, phenylalanine, tryptophan, or caffeine may cause sudden and severe high blood pressure (hypertensive crisis or serotonin syndrome). Beverages containing tyramine (eg, hearty red wine and beer) may increase toxic effects. Management: Avoid tyramine-containing foods (aged or matured cheese, air-dried or cured meats including sausages and salamis; fava or broad bean pods, tap/draft beers, Marmite concentrate, sauerkraut, soy sauce, and other soybean condiments). Food's freshness is also an important concern; improperly stored or spoiled food can create an environment in which tyramine concentrations may increase. Avoid foods containing dopamine, tyrosine, phenylalanine, tryptophan, or caffeine. Avoid beverages containing tyramine.

Stability Store at 25°C (77°F); excursions permitted to 15°C to 30°C (59°F to 86°F); protect from light.

Injection (premix infusion): Do not freeze. Store in overwrap until ready for use. The yellow color of the injectable solution may intensify over time without adversely affecting potency.

Oral suspension: Store reconstituted oral suspension at room temperature and use within 21 days.

Tablets: Protect from moisture.

Mechanism of Action Inhibits bacterial protein synthesis by binding to bacterial 23S ribosomal RNA of the 50S subunit. This prevents the formation of a functional 70S initiation complex that is essential for the bacterial translation process. Linezolid is bacteriostatic against enterococci and staphylococci and bactericidal against most strains of streptococci.

Pharmacokinetics (Adult data unless noted)

Absorption: Well absorbed orally

Distribution: Well-perfused tissues

V_d:

Preterm neonates <1 week: 0.81 L/kg

Full-term neonates <1 week: 0.78 L/kg

Full-term neonates ≥1 week to ≤28 days: 0.66 L/kg

Infants >28 days to <3 months: 0.79 L/kg

Infants and Children 3 months to 11 years: 0.69 L/kg

Adolescents: 0.61 L/kg

Adults: 0.65 L/kg

Protein binding: 31%

Metabolism: Hepatic via oxidation of the morpholine ring, resulting in two inactive metabolites (aminoethoxyacetic acid, hydroxyethyl glycine); minimally metabolized; may be mediated by cytochrome P450

Bioavailability: 100%

Half-life:

Preterm neonates <1 week: 5.6 hours

Full-term neonates <1 week: 3 hours

Full-term neonates ≥1 week to ≤28 days: 1.5 hours

Infants >28 days to <3 months: 1.8 hours

Infants and Children 3 months to 11 years: 2.9 hours

Adolescents: 4.1 hours

Adults: 4.9 hours

Time to peak serum concentration: Oral: 1-2 hours

Elimination: Urine (~30% of total dose as parent drug, ~50% of total dose as metabolites); two metabolites of linezolid may accumulate in patients with severe renal impairment; feces (~9% of total dose as metabolites); Nonrenal clearance accounts for ~65% of the total clearance

Clearance:

Preterm neonates <1 week: 2 mL/minute/kg

Full-term neonates <1 week: 3.8 mL/minute/kg

Full-term neonates ≥1 week to ≤28 days: 5.1 mL/minute/kg

Infants >28 days to <3 months: 5.4 mL/minute/kg

Infants and Children 3 months to 11 years: 3.8 mL/minute/kg

Adolescents: 2.1 mL/minute/kg

Adults: 1.7 mL/minute/kg

Dialysis: 30% removed in a 3-hour hemodialysis session (linezolid dose should be given after hemodialysis)

Dosing: Neonatal

General dosing, susceptible infection (*Red Book*, 2012): I.V.:

Body weight <1 kg:

PNA ≤14 days: 10 mg/kg/dose every 12 hours

PNA 15-28 days: 10 mg/kg/dose every 8 hours

Body weight 1-2 kg:

PNA ≤7 days: 10 mg/kg/dose every 12 hours

PNA 8-28 days: 10 mg/kg/dose every 8 hours

Body weight >2 kg: 10 mg/kg/dose every 8 hours

Bacteremia: Oral, I.V.: **Note:** Treatment should continue for 10-28 days depending on the organism

GA <34 weeks:

PNA <7 days: 10 mg/kg/dose every 12 hours

PNA ≥7 days: 10 mg/kg/dose every 8 hours

GA ≥34 weeks and PNA 0-28 days: 10 mg/kg/dose every 8 hours

Pneumonia, community- or hospital-acquired: Oral, I.V.: **Note:** Treatment should continue for 10-14 days.

GA <34 weeks:

PNA <7 days: 10 mg/kg/dose every 12 hours

PNA ≥7 days: 10 mg/kg/dose every 8 hours

GA ≥34 weeks and PNA 0-28 days: 10 mg/kg/dose every 8 hours

Skin and skin structure infections, complicated and uncomplicated: Oral, I.V.: **Note:** Treatment should continue for 10-14 days; reserve I.V. use for complicated infections only.

GA <34 weeks:

PNA <7 days: 10 mg/kg/dose every 12 hours

PNA ≥7 days: 10 mg/kg/dose every 8 hours

GA ≥34 weeks and PNA 0-28 days: 10 mg/kg/dose every 8 hours

Vancomycin-resistant *Enterococcus faecium* (VREF) infection: Oral, I.V.: **Note:** Treatment should continue for 14-28 days.

GA <34 weeks:

PNA <7 days: 10 mg/kg/dose every 12 hours

PNA ≥7 days: 10 mg/kg/dose every 8 hours

GA ≥34 weeks and PNA 0-28 days: 10 mg/kg/dose every 8 hours

Note: Case reports describe the use of higher doses up to 12-15 mg/kg/dose every 8 hours to treat VRE endocarditis and meningitis/ventriculitis in former premature neonates (n=2; GA: 26, 35 weeks; age at treatment: Term) (Ang, 2003; Kumar, 2007).

Dosing: Usual

Infants, Children, and Adolescents:

General dosing, susceptible infection (mild, moderate, or severe) (*Red Book*, 2012): Oral, I.V.:

Infants and Children <12 years: 10 mg/kg/dose every 8 hours, maximum dose: 600 mg

Children ≥12 years and Adolescents: 600 mg every 12 hours

Bacteremia: Oral, I.V.: **Note:** Treatment should continue for 10-28 days depending on the organism.

Infants and Children <12 years: 10 mg/kg/dose every 8 hours; maximum dose: 600 mg

Children ≥12 years and Adolescents: 600 mg every 12 hours

Bone and joint infection (Liu, 2011):

Osteomyelitis [*S. aureus* (methicillin-resistant)]: Oral, I.V.: **Note:** Treatment should continue for a minimum of 4-6 weeks.

Infants and Children <12 years: 10 mg/kg/dose every 8 hours; maximum dose: 600 mg

Children ≥12 years and Adolescents: 600 mg every 12 hours

Septic arthritis [*S. aureus* (methicillin-resistant)]: Oral, I.V.: **Note:** Treatment should continue for a minimum of 3-4 weeks.

Infants and Children <12 years: 10 mg/kg/dose every 8 hours; maximum dose: 600 mg

Children ≥12 years and Adolescents: 600 mg every 12 hours

Catheter-related infections, Staphylococcal (methicillin-resistant) or enterococcal (resistant) (confirmed infection): Oral, I.V.: **Note:** Not recommended use for empiric treatment (Mermel, 2009).

Infants and Children <12 years: 10 mg/kg/dose every 8 hours; maximum dose: 600 mg

Children ≥12 years and Adolescents: 10 mg/kg/dose every 12 hours; maximum dose: 600 mg

CNS infection:

Brain abscess, subdural empyema, spinal epidural abscess [*S. aureus* (methicillin-resistant)]: Oral, I.V.: **Note:** Treatment should continue for 4-6 weeks (Liu, 2011). **Note:** The manufacturer does not recommend the use of linezolid for empiric treatment of pediatric CNS infections since therapeutic linezolid ▶

concentrations are not consistently achieved or maintained in the CSF of patients with ventriculoperitoneal shunts.

Infants and Children <12 years: 10 mg/kg/dose every 8 hours; maximum dose: 600 mg

Children ≥12 years and Adolescents: 600 mg every 12 hours

Meningitis [*S. aureus* (methicillin-resistant)]: Oral, I.V.: **Note:** Treatment should continue for 2 weeks (Liu, 2011; Tunkel, 2004).

Infants and Children <12 years: 10 mg/kg/dose every 8 hours; maximum dose: 600 mg

Children ≥12 years and Adolescents: 600 mg every 12 hours

Endocarditis, treatment [*E. faecium* (vancomycin-resistant)]: Oral, I.V.: **Note:** Treatment should continue for at least 8 weeks (Baddour, 2005).

Infants and Children <12 years: 10 mg/kg/dose every 8 hours; maximum dose: 600 mg

Children ≥12 years and Adolescents: 600 mg every 12 hours

Pneumonia

Community- or hospital-acquired (non-MRSA): Oral, I.V.: **Note:** Treatment should continue for 10-14 days.

Infants and Children <12 years: 10 mg/kg/dose every 8 hours; maximum dose: 600 mg

Children ≥12 years and Adolescents: 600 mg every 12 hours

S. aureus (methicillin-resistant): Oral, I.V.: **Note:** Treatment should continue for 7-21 days depending on severity (Liu, 2011).

Infants and Children <12 years: 10 mg/kg/dose every 8 hours; maximum dose: 600 mg

Children ≥12 years and Adolescents: 600 mg every 12 hours

Septic thrombosis of cavernous or dural venous sinus [*S. aureus* (methicillin-resistant)]: Oral, I.V.: **Note:** Treatment should continue for 4-6 weeks (Liu, 2011).

Infants and Children <12 years: 10 mg/kg/dose every 8 hours; maximum dose: 600 mg

Children ≥12 years and Adolescents: 600 mg every 12 hours

Skin and skin structure infections: Note: Treatment should continue for 10-14 days.

Uncomplicated:

Infants and Children <5 years: Oral: 10 mg/kg/dose every 8 hours

Children 5-11 years: Oral: 10 mg/kg/dose every 12 hours; maximum dose: 600 mg

Children ≥12 years and Adolescents: Oral: 600 mg every 12 hours

Complicated:

Infants and Children <12 years: Oral, I.V.: 10 mg/kg/dose every 8 hours; maximum dose: 600 mg

Children ≥12 years and Adolescents: Oral, I.V.: 600 mg every 12 hours

Tuberculosis, multidrug-resistant: Limited data available: Oral: **Note:** Experience in pediatric patients reflects extrapolation of dosing approach used in adult patients which includes a lower daily dose to decrease risk of adverse effects due to the anticipated long duration of therapy and if toxicity does occur, further dosage reductions (a 25% to 50% dose decrease or increased dosing interval have been used); reported treatment duration dependent upon clinical course; reported range: 13-36 months in pediatric patients. All reports describe linezolid as part of a multidrug antimycobacterial regimen; other reported agents within the combination therapy were variable, dependent upon specific organism sensitivities, and generally included 3-5 other agents. Further studies are needed.

Infants ≥4 months and Children: 10-12 mg/kg/dose twice daily; maximum dose: 600 mg; dosing based on case reports describing successful treatment in infants and a young child (n=3; ages: 4.5 months, 11 months, and 23 months) (Pinon, 2010; Schaaf, 2009). Use has also been reported in a 10-year old child, treatment was successfully completed with dosing of 600 mg once daily (Condos, 2008).

Adolescents: 600 mg once daily was reported in a retrospective review of 30 patients (n= 4 adolescents) and a case report (patient age: 14 years) (Dauby, 2011; Schecter, 2010). In another case series, 600 mg twice daily dosing was used for the initial 2 weeks of therapy and then decreased to once daily dosing; at reduced dosage, patients seemed to have decreased hematologic toxicity while neurotoxicity remained unchanged (Park, 2006).

Vancomycin-resistant *Enterococcus faecium* (VREF) infections: Oral, I.V.: **Note:** Treatment should continue for 14-28 days.

Infants and Children <12 years: 10 mg/kg/dose every 8 hours, maximum dose: 600 mg

Children ≥12 years and Adolescents: Oral, I.V.: 600 mg every 12 hours

Adults:

Usual dosage: Oral, I.V.: 600 mg every 12 hours

Indication-specific dosing:

MRSA infections (Liu, 2011): Oral, I.V.: 600 mg every 12 hours; duration of therapy dependent upon site of infection and clinical response

Pneumonia, community- or hospital-acquired: Oral, I.V.: 600 mg every 12 hours for 10-14 days. **Note:** In contrast to the manufacturer's recommendations, current guidelines for the treatment of community-acquired, healthcare-, hospital-, and ventilator-associated pneumonia recommend that the duration of therapy be reduced to as short as 7 days (vs 10-14 days) in patients who demonstrate good clinical response (ATS/IDSA, 2005; ATS/IDSA, 2011).

Skin and skin structure infections

Complicated: Oral, I.V.: 600 mg every 12 hours for 10-14 days. **Note:** For diabetic foot infections, initial treatment duration is up to 4 weeks depending on severity of infection and response to therapy (Lipsky, 2012).

Uncomplicated: Oral: 400 mg every 12 hours for 10-14 days. **Note:** 400 mg dose is recommended in the product labeling; however, 600 mg dose is commonly employed clinically; consider 5- to 10-day treatment course as opposed to the manufacturer recommended 10-14 days (Liu, 2011; Stevens, 2005). For diabetic foot infections, may extend treatment duration up to 4 weeks if slow to resolve (Lipsky, 2012).

VREF infections, including concurrent bacteremia: Oral, I.V.: 600 mg every 12 hours for 14-28 days

Dosage adjustment in renal impairment: No adjustment is recommended. The two primary metabolites may accumulate in patients with renal impairment but the clinical significance is unknown. Weigh the risk of accumulation of metabolites versus the benefit of therapy.

Infants, Children, and Adolescents: The following adjustments have been recommended (Aronoff, 2007): **Note:** Renally adjusted dose recommendations are based on doses of 10 mg/kg/dose every 8 hours (for ages <5 years) or every 12 hours (for ages 5-11 years).

Intermittent hemodialysis: 10 mg/kg/dose every 12 hours

Peritoneal dialysis (PD): 10 mg/kg/dose every 12 hours

Continuous renal replacement therapy (CRRT): No adjustment necessary

Adults: Intermittent hemodialysis (administer after hemodialysis on dialysis days): Dialyzable (~30% removed during 3-hour dialysis session): If administration time is not immediately after dialysis session, may consider administration of a supplemental dose especially early in the treatment course to maintain levels above the MIC (Brier, 2003). Others have recommended no supplemental dose or dosage adjustment for patients on intermittent hemodialysis, peritoneal dialysis, or continuous renal replacement therapy (eg, CVVHD) (Heintz, 2009; Trotman, 2005).

Dosage adjustment in hepatic impairment:
Mild to moderate impairment (Child Pugh class A or B): No adjustment is recommended.
Severe hepatic impairment (Child Pugh Class C): Use has not been adequately evaluated.

Administration
Oral: Administer with or without food. With reconstituted suspension, gently invert bottle 3-5 times before use. Do not shake.
Parenteral: I.V.: Check infusion bag for minute leaks and solution for particulate matter prior to administration. The 2 mg/mL infusion should be administered without further dilution over 30-120 minutes. Flush line before and after infusion with a linezolid-compatible I.V. solution like D_5W, NS, or LR.

Monitoring Parameters CBC (weekly), particularly in patients at increased risk for bleeding, patients with pre-existing thrombocytopenia or myelosuppression, patients with chronic infection who have received or who are on concomitant antibiotics, or concomitant medications that decrease platelet count or function or produce bone marrow suppression, and inpatients requiring >2 weeks of therapy; number and type of stools/day for diarrhea; visual function in patients requiring ≥3 months of therapy or in patients reporting new visual symptoms

Dosage Forms Excipient information presented when available (limited, particularly for generics); consult specific product labeling.
Solution, Intravenous:
Zyvox: 2 mg/mL (100 mL, 300 mL)
Suspension Reconstituted, Oral:
Zyvox: 100 mg/5 mL (150 mL) [orange flavor]
Tablet, Oral:
Zyvox: 600 mg

References
American Academy of Pediatrics (AAP). In: Pickering LK, Baker CJ, Kimberlin DW, Long SS, eds. *Red Book: 2012 Report of the Committee on Infectious Diseases.* 29th ed. Elk Grove Village, IL: American Academy of Pediatrics; 2012.

American Thoracic Society and Infectious Diseases Society of America, "Guidelines for the Management of Adults With Hospital-Acquired, Ventilator-Associated, and Healthcare-Associated Pneumonia," *Am J Respir Crit Care Med*, 2005, 171(4):388-416.

Ang JY, Lua JL, Turner DR, et al, "Vancomycin-Resistant *Enterococcus faecium* Endocarditis in a Premature Infant Successfully Treated With Linezolid," *Pediatr Infect Dis J*, 2003, 22(12):1101-3.

Aronoff GR, Bennett WM, Berns JS, et al, *Drug Prescribing in Renal Failure: Dosing Guidelines for Adults and Children*, 5th ed. Philadelphia, PA: American College of Physicians; 2007, 167.

Baddour LM, Wilson WR, Bayer AS, et al, "Infective Endocarditis: Diagnosis, Antimicrobial Therapy, and Management of Complications: A Statement for Healthcare Professionals From the Committee on Rheumatic Fever, Endocarditis, and Kawasaki Disease, Council on Cardiovascular Disease in the Young, and the Councils on Clinical Cardiology, Stroke, and Cardiovascular Surgery and Anesthesia, American Heart Association: Endorsed by the Infectious Diseases Society of America," *Circulation*, 2005, 111(23):e394-434.

Bradley JS, Byington CL, Shah SS, et al, "The Management of Community-Acquired Pneumonia in Infants and Children Older Than 3 Months of Age: Clinical Practice Guidelines by the Pediatric Infectious Diseases Society and the Infectious Diseases Society of America", *Clin Infect Dis*, 2011, 53(7):617-30.

Brier ME, Stalker DJ, Aronoff GR, et al, "Pharmacokinetics of Linezolid in Subjects With Renal Dysfunction," *Antimicrob Agents Chemother*, 2003, 47(9):2775-80.

Clemett D and Markham A, "Linezolid," *Drugs*, 2000, 59(4):815-27.

Condos R, Hadgiangelis N, Leibert E, et al, "Case Series Report of a Linezolid-Containing Regimen for Extensively Drug-Resistant Tuberculosis," *Chest*, 2008, 134(1):187-92.

Cook AM, Ramsey CN, Martin CA, et al, "Linezolid for the Treatment of a Heteroresistant *Staphylococcus aureus* Shunt Infection," *Pediatr Neurosurg*, 2005, 41(2):102-4.

da Silva PS, Monteiro Neto H, and Sejas LM, "Successful Treatment of Vancomycin-Resistant Enterococcus Ventriculitis in a Child," *Braz J Infect Dis*, 2007, 11(2):297-9.

Dauby N, Muylle I, Mouchet F, et al, "Meropenem/Clavulanate and Linezolid Treatment for Extensively Drug-Resistant Tuberculosis," *Pediatr Infect Dis J*, 2011, 30(9):812-3.

Dotis J, Iosifidis E, Ioannidou M, et al, "Use of Linezolid in Pediatrics: A Critical Review," *Int J Infect Dis*, 2010, 14(8):e638-48.

Heintz BH, Matzke GR, Dager WE, "Antimicrobial Dosing Concepts and Recommendations for Critically Ill Adult Patients Receiving Continuous Renal Replacement Therapy or Intermittent Hemodialysis," *Pharmacotherapy*, 2009, 29(5):562-77.

Jungbluth GL, Welshman IR, and Hopkins NK, "Linezolid Pharmacokinetics in Pediatric Patients: An Overview," *Pediatr Infect Dis J*, 2003, 22(9 Suppl):153-7.

Kearns GL, Abdel-Rahman SM, Blumer JL, et al, "Single Dose Pharmacokinetics of Linezolid in Infants and Children," *Pediatr Infect Dis J*, 2000, 19(12):1178-84.

Kearns GL, Jungbluth GL, Abdel-Rahman SM, et al, "Impact of Ontogeny on Linezolid Disposition in Neonates and Infants," *Clin Pharmacol Ther*, 2003, 74(5):413-22.

Kumar S, Kohlhoff S, Valencia G, et al, "Treatment of Vancomycin-Resistant *Enterococcus faecium* Ventriculitis in a Neonate," *Int J Antimicrob Agents*, 2007, 29(6):740-1.

Lipsky BA, Berendt AR, Deery HG, et al, "Diagnosis and Treatment of Diabetic Foot Infections," *Clin Infect Dis*, 2004, 39(7):885-910.

Liu C, Bayer A, Cosgrove SE, et al, "Clinical Practice Guidelines by the Infectious Diseases Society of America for the Treatment of Methicillin-Resistant *Staphylococcus aureus* Infections in Adults and Children: Executive Summary," *Clin Infect Dis*, 2011, 52(3):285-92.

Mermel LA, Allon M, Bouza E, et al, "Clinical Practice Guidelines for the Diagnosis and Management of Intravascular Catheter-Related Infection: 2009 Update by the Infectious Diseases Society of America," *Clin Infect Dis*, 2009, 49(1):1-45.

Meyer B, Kornek GV, Nikfardjam M, et al, "Multiple-Dose Pharmacokinetics of Linezolid During Continuous Venovenous Haemofiltration," *J Antimicrob Chemother*, 2005, 56(1):172-9.

Milstone AM, Dick J, Carcon B, et al, "Cerebrospinal Fluid Penetration and Bacteriostatic Activity of Linezolid Against *Enterococcus faecalis* in a Child With a Ventriculoperitoneal Shunt Infection," *Pediatr Neurosurg*, 2007, 43(5):406-9.

Park IN, Hong SB, Oh YM, et al, "Efficacy and Tolerability of Daily-Half Dose Linezolid in Patients With Intractable Multidrug-Resistant Tuberculosis," *J Antimicrob Chemother*, 2006, 58(3):701-4.

Pinon M, Scolfaro C, Bignamini E, et al, "Two pediatric Cases of Multidrug-Resistant Tuberculosis Treated With Linezolid and Moxifloxacin," *Pediatrics*, 2010, 126(5):e1253-6.

Schaaf HS, Willemse M, and Donald PR, "Long-Term Linezolid Treatment in a Young Child With Extensively Drug-Resistant Tuberculosis," *Pediatr Infect Dis J*, 2009, 28(8):748-50.

Schecter GF, Scott C, True L, et al, "Linezolid in the Teatment of Multidrug-Resistant Tuberculosis," *Clin Infect Dis*, 2010, 50(1):49-55.

Shaikh ZH, Peloquin CA, and Ericsson CD, "Successful Treatment of Vancomycin-Resistant *Enterococcus faecium* Meningitis With Linezolid: Case Report and Literature Review," *Scand J Infect Dis*, 2001, 33(5):375-9.

Stevens DL, Bisno AL, Chambers HF, et al, "Practice Guidelines for the Diagnosis and Management of Skin and Soft-Tissue Infections," *Clin Infect Dis*, 2005, 41(10):1373-406.

Tan TQ, "Update on the Use of Linezolid: A Pediatric Perspective," *Pediatr Infect Dis J*, 2004, 23(10):955-6.

Taylor JJ, Wilson JW, and Estes LL, "Linezolid and Serotonergic Drug Interactions: A Retrospective Survey," *Clin Infect Dis*, 2006, 43 (2):180-7.

Trotman RL, Williamson JC, Shoemaker DM, et al, "Antibiotic Dosing in Critically Ill Adult Patients Receiving Continuous Renal Replacement Therapy," *Clin Infect Dis*, 2005, 41:1159-66.

Tunkel AR, Hartman BJ, Kaplan SL, et al, "Practice Guidelines for the Management of Bacterial Meningitis," *Clin Infect Dis*, 2004, 39 (9):1267-84.

Villani P, Regazzi MB, Marubbi F, et al, "Cerebrospinal Fluid Linezolid Concentrations in Postneurosurgical Central Nervous System Infections," *Antimicrob Agents Chemother*, 2002, 46(3):936-7.

◆ **Lioresal** *see* Baclofen *on page 259*

◆ **Lioresal® (Can)** *see* Baclofen *on page 259*

◆ **Lioresal® D.S. (Can)** *see* Baclofen *on page 259*

◆ **Lioresal® Intrathecal (Can)** *see* Baclofen *on page 259*

Liothyronine (lye oh THYE roe neen)

Medication Safety Issues
Sound-alike/look-alike issues:
Liothyronine may be confused with levothyroxine
Other safety concerns:
T3 is an error-prone abbreviation (mistaken as acetaminophen and codeine [ie, Tylenol® #3])
Brand Names: U.S. Cytomel; Triostat
Brand Names: Canada Cytomel®
Therapeutic Category Thyroid Product
Generic Availability (U.S.) Yes
Use Replacement or supplemental therapy in congenital or acquired hypothyroidism; treatment or prevention of euthyroid goiters including thyroid nodules and chronic lymphocytic thyroiditis; as a diagnostic aid in suppression tests to differentiate suspected mild hyperthyroidism or thyroid gland autonomy
Pregnancy Risk Factor A
Pregnancy Considerations
Endogenous thyroid hormones minimally cross the placenta; the fetal thyroid becomes active around the end of the first trimester. Liothyronine has not been found to increase the risk of teratogenic or adverse effects following maternal use during pregnancy.

Uncontrolled maternal hypothyroidism may result in adverse neonatal and maternal outcomes. To prevent adverse events, normal maternal thyroid function should be maintained prior to conception and throughout pregnancy. Levothyroxine is considered the treatment of choice for the control of hypothyroidism during pregnancy.
Breast-Feeding Considerations Endogenous thyroid hormones are minimally found in breast milk.
Contraindications Hypersensitivity to liothyronine sodium or any component; recent MI or thyrotoxicosis; uncorrected adrenal insufficiency
Warnings Not for use in the treatment of obesity or for weight loss **[U.S. Boxed Warning]**; in euthyroid patients, doses within the range of daily hormonal requirements are ineffective for weight reduction; larger doses may produce serious or even life-threatening toxic effects particularly when used with some anorectic drugs (sympathomimetic amines). Short duration of action permits more rapid assessment of dosage changes and rapid diminution of adverse effects upon discontinuation; transient partial loss of hair in pediatrics may be seen in the first few months of therapy.
Precautions Use with extreme caution in patients with cardiovascular disease, adrenal insufficiency, or coronary artery disease; use with extreme caution in patients receiving digoxin or vasopressors; use with caution in patients with diabetes mellitus and diabetes insipidus as symptoms of their disease may be exaggerated or aggravated; myxedematous patients are very sensitive to thyroid supplements; initiate therapy at very low doses and increase gradually
Adverse Reactions
Cardiovascular: Arrhythmia, cardiopulmonary arrest, hypotension, MI, tachycardia
Rare but important or life-threatening: Allergic skin reactions, angina, CHF, fever, hypertension, phlebitis, twitching
Drug Interactions
Metabolism/Transport Effects None known.
Avoid Concomitant Use
Avoid concomitant use of Liothyronine with any of the following: Sodium Iodide I131
Increased Effect/Toxicity
Liothyronine may increase the levels/effects of: Tricyclic Antidepressants; Vitamin K Antagonists

The levels/effects of Liothyronine may be increased by: Piracetam
Decreased Effect
Liothyronine may decrease the levels/effects of: Sodium Iodide I131; Theophylline Derivatives

The levels/effects of Liothyronine may be decreased by: Bile Acid Sequestrants; Calcium Polystyrene Sulfonate; Calcium Salts; CarBAMazepine; Estrogen Derivatives; Fosphenytoin; Lanthanum; Phenytoin; Rifampin; Selective Serotonin Reuptake Inhibitors; Sodium Polystyrene Sulfonate
Stability Store tablets at controlled room temperature; refrigerate parenteral solution at temperatures between 2°C and 8°C (36°F to 46°F)
Mechanism of Action Exact mechanism of action is unknown; however, it is believed the thyroid hormone exerts its many metabolic effects through control of DNA transcription and protein synthesis; involved in normal metabolism, growth, and development; promotes gluconeogenesis, increases utilization and mobilization of glycogen stores, and stimulates protein synthesis, increases basal metabolic rate
Pharmacodynamics I.V., Oral:
Onset of action: Within a few hours
Maximum effect: Within 48 hours
Duration: Up to 72 hours
Pharmacokinetics (Adult data unless noted)
Absorption: Oral: Well absorbed (~85% to 90%)
Metabolism: In the liver to inactive compounds
Half-life: 25 hours (range: 16-49 hours); hypothyroid 1.4 days; hyperthyroid 0.6 days
Elimination: 76% to 83% In urine
Dosing: Neonatal Congenital hypothyroidism: Oral: 5 mcg/day; increase by 5 mcg every 3 days to a maximum dosage of 20 mcg/day; **Note:** AAP recommends levothyroxine over liothyronine for treatment of hypothyroidism in neonates (AAP, 2006)
Postcardiac surgery replacement: Limited data available; optimal dosage not established; further studies needed: Continuous I.V. infusion: 0.05-0.15 mcg/kg/hour adjusted to maintain a serum T_3 concentration 80-200 ng/dL; dosing based on experience in five neonates who, on postoperative days 0-2, required mechanical ventilation and exhibited total serum T_3 <60 ng/dL (Chowdhury, 2001; Dimmick, 2008)
Dosing: Usual
Congenital hypothyroidism: Infants and Children <3 years: Oral: 5 mcg/day; increase by 5 mcg every 3 days to a maximum dosage of 20 mcg/day for infants, 50 mcg/day for children 1-3 years of age
Hypothyroidism:
Children: Oral: 5 mcg/day increase in 5 mcg/day increments every 3-4 days;
Usual maintenance dose:
Infants: 20 mcg/day
Children 1-3 years: 50 mcg/day
Children >3 years: Full adult dosage may be necessary
Adults: Oral: 25 mcg/day increase in 12.5-25 mcg/day increments every 1-2 weeks to a maximum of 100 mcg/day
Goiter, nontoxic:
Children: Oral: 5 mcg/day increase in 5 mcg/day increments every 1-2 weeks; usual maintenance dose 15-20 mcg/day
Adults: Oral: 5 mcg/day; increase in 5-10 mcg/day increments every 1-2 weeks; when 25 mcg is reached, increase dosage in 12.5-25 mcg increments every 1-2 weeks; usual maintenance dosage: 75 mcg/day
T_3 suppression test: Adults: Oral: 75-100 mcg/day for 7 days

Myxedema coma: Adults:

I.V.: 25-50 mcg; reduce dosage in patients with known or suspected cardiovascular disease to 10-20 mcg

Note: Normally, at least 4 hours should be allowed between I.V. doses to adequately assess therapeutic response and no more than 12 hours should elapse between doses to avoid fluctuations in hormone levels.

Oral (**Note:** Due to potential poor oral absorption in the acute phase of myxedema, oral therapy should be avoided until the clinical situation has been stabilized): 5 mcg/day; increase in 5-10 mcg/day increments every 1-2 weeks; when 25 mcg/day is reached; increase by 5-25 mcg/day increments every 1-2 weeks; usual maintenance dose: 50-100 mcg/day

Administration

Oral: Administer on an empty stomach

Parenteral: Adults: I.V.: For I.V. use only; **do not administer SubQ or I.M.** Administer at a rate of 10 mcg/minute. Administer doses at least 4 hours, and no more than 12 hours, apart. Resume oral therapy as soon as the clinical situation has been stabilized and the patient is able to take oral medication. If **levothyroxine** is used for oral therapy, there is a delay of several days in the onset of activity; therefore, discontinue I.V. therapy gradually.

Monitoring Parameters T_3, TSH, heart rate, blood pressure, clinical signs of hypo- and hyperthyroidism; TSH is the most reliable guide for evaluating adequacy of thyroid replacement dosage. TSH may be elevated during the first few months of thyroid replacement despite patients being clinically euthyroid.

Suggested frequency for monitoring thyroid function tests in children: Every 1-2 months during the first year of life, every 2-3 months between ages 1-3 years, and every 3-12 months thereafter until growth is completed; repeat tests two weeks after any change in dosage.

Reference Range

Thyroid Function Tests

Lab Parameters	Age	Normal Range
T_4 (thyroxine) serum concentration	1-7 days	10.1-20.9 mcg/dL
	8-14 days	9.8-16.6 mcg/dL
	1 month to 1 year	5.5-16.0 mcg/dL
	>1 year	4.0-12.0 mcg/dL
Free thyroxine index (FTI)	1-3 days	9.3-26.6
	1-4 weeks	7.6-20.8
	1-4 months	7.4-17.9
	4-12 months	5.1-14.5
	1-6 years	5.7-13.3
	>6 years	4.8-14.0
T_3 serum concentration	Newborns	100-470 ng/dL
	1-5 years	100-260 ng/dL
	5-10 years	90-240 ng/dL
	10 years to Adult	70-210 ng/dL
T_3 uptake		35%-45%
TSH serum concentration	Cord	3-22 micro international units/mL
	1-3 days	<40 micro international units/mL
	3-7 days	<25 micro international units/mL
	>7 days	0-10 micro international units/mL

Test Interactions Many drugs may have effects on thyroid function tests (see Additional Information). Pregnancy, infectious hepatitis, and acute intermittent porphyria may increase TBG concentrations; nephrosis, severe hypoproteinemia, severe liver disease, and acromegaly may decrease TBG concentrations.

Additional Information Equivalent doses: The following statement on relative potency of thyroid products is included in a joint statement by American Thyroid Association (ATA), American Association of Clinical Endocrinologists (AACE) and The Endocrine Society (TES): For purposes of conversion, levothyroxine sodium (T_4) 100 mcg is usually considered equivalent to desiccated thyroid 60 mg, thyroglobulin 60 mg, or liothyronine sodium (T_3) 25 mcg. However, these are rough guidelines only and do not obviate the careful re-evaluation of a patient when switching thyroid hormone preparations, including a change from one brand of levothyroxine to another. Joint position statement is available at http://www.thyroid.org/professionals/advocacy/04_12_08_thyroxine.html.

A synthetic form of L-Triiodothyronine (T_3) can be used in patients allergic to products derived from pork or beef.

Note: Several medications have effects on thyroid production or conversion. The impact in thyroid replacement has not been specifically evaluated, but patient response should be monitored:

Methimazole: Decreases thyroid hormone secretion, while propylthiouracil decrease thyroid hormone secretion and decreases conversion of T_4 to T_3.

Beta-adrenergic antagonists: Decrease conversion of T_4 to T_3 (dose related, propranolol ≥160 mg/day); patients may be clinically euthyroid.

Iodide, iodine-containing radiographic contrast agents may decrease thyroid hormone secretion; may also increase thyroid hormone secretion, especially in patients with Graves' disease.

Other agents reported to impact on thyroid production/conversion include aminoglutethimide, amiodarone, chloral hydrate, diazepam, ethionamide, interferon-alpha, interleukin-2, lithium, lovastatin (case report), glucocorticoids (dose-related), mercaptopurine, sulfonamides, thiazide diuretics, and tolbutamide.

In addition, a number of medications have been noted to cause transient depression in TSH secretion, which may complicate interpretation of monitoring tests for thyroid hormones, including corticosteroids, octreotide, and dopamine. Metoclopramide may increase TSH secretion.

Dosage Forms Excipient information presented when available (limited, particularly for generics); consult specific product labeling.

Solution, Intravenous:

Triostat: 10 mcg/mL (1 mL) [contains alcohol, usp]

Generic: 10 mcg/mL (1 mL)

Tablet, Oral:

Cytomel: 5 mcg

Cytomel: 25 mcg, 50 mcg [scored]

Generic: 5 mcg, 25 mcg, 50 mcg

References

American Academy of Pediatrics, Rose SR, Section on Endocrinology and Committee on Genetics, American Thyroid Association, et al, "Update of Newborn Screening and Therapy for Congenital Hypothyroidism," Pediatrics, 2006, 117(6):2290-303.

Chowdhury D, Ojamaa K, Parnell VA, et al, "A Prospective Randomized Clinical Study of Thyroid Hormone Treatment After Operations for Complex Congenital Heart Disease," J Thorac Cardiovasc Surg, 2001, 122(5):1023-5

Dimmick S, Badawi N, and Randell T, "Thyroid Hormone Supplementation for the Prevention of Morbidity and Mortality in Infants Undergoing Cardiac Surgery," *Cochrane Database Syst Rev*, 2004, (3): CD004220.

Gahart BL, Nazareno AR. *2014 Intravenous Medications: A Handbook for Nurses and Health Professionals*. 30th ed. St Louis, MO: Elsevier/Mosby; 2014, 745-47.

◆ **Liothyronine and Levothyroxine** *see* Liotrix *on page 1258*

◆ **Liothyronine Sodium** *see* Liothyronine *on page 1256*

Liotrix (LYE oh triks)

Medication Safety Issues
Sound-alike/look-alike issues:
Liotrix may be confused with Klotrix®
Thyrolar® may be confused with Thyrogen®
Brand Names: U.S. Thyrolar®
Brand Names: Canada Thyrolar®
Therapeutic Category Thyroid Product
Generic Availability (U.S.) No
Use Replacement or supplemental therapy in hypothyroidism of any etiology (FDA approved in all ages); pituitary TSH suppressant for the prevention or treatment of various types of euthyroid goiter, thyroid nodules, thyroiditis (Hashimoto's), multinodular goiter, and thyroid cancer (FDA approved in adults); diagnostic agent in suppression tests to diagnose suspected mild hyperthyroidism or to demonstrate thyroid gland autonomy (FDA approved in adults); **Note:** Not indicated for treatment of transient hypothyroidism associated with subacute thyroiditis
Pregnancy Risk Factor A
Pregnancy Considerations Endogenous thyroid hormones minimally cross the placenta; the fetal thyroid becomes active around the end of the first trimester. Liotrix has not been found to increase the risk of adverse effects following maternal use during pregnancy.

Uncontrolled maternal hypothyroidism may result in adverse neonatal and maternal outcomes. To prevent adverse events, normal maternal thyroid function should be maintained prior to conception and throughout pregnancy. Levothyroxine is considered the treatment of choice for the control of hypothyroidism during pregnancy.
Breast-Feeding Considerations Endogenous thyroid hormones are minimally found in breast milk and are not associated with adverse events.
Contraindications Hypersensitivity to liotrix or any component; untreated thyrotoxicosis, uncorrected adrenal insufficiency
Warnings Not for use in the treatment of obesity or for weight loss **[U.S. Boxed Warning]**; in euthyroid patients, doses within the range of daily hormonal requirements are ineffective for weight reduction; larger doses may produce serious or even life-threatening toxic effects particularly when used with some anorectic drugs (sympathomimetic amines). Should not be used for treatment of infertility without unrelated hypothyroidism.

Overtreatment may result in craniosynostosis in infants and premature closure of epiphyses in children; monitor use closely.
Precautions Use with extreme caution in patients with adrenal insufficiency; symptoms may be exaggerated or aggravated. Use with caution and reduce dosage in patients with angina pectoris or other cardiovascular disease; chronic hypothyroidism predisposes patients to coronary artery disease. Use with caution in patients with diabetes mellitus and insipidus; symptoms may be exaggerated or aggravated. Use with caution in patients with myxedema; symptoms may be exaggerated or aggravated. May cause transient alopecia in children during first

few months of therapy. In neonates and infants, cardiac overload, arrhythmias, and aspiration from avid suckling may occur during initiation of therapy (eg, first 2 weeks); monitor closely.
Adverse Reactions
Cardiovascular: Blood pressure increased, cardiac arrhythmia, chest pain, palpitation, tachycardia
Central nervous system: Anxiety, ataxia, fever, headache, insomnia, nervousness
Dermatologic: Alopecia, hyperhydrosis, pruritus, urticaria
Endocrine & metabolic: Changes in menstrual cycle, increased appetite, weight loss
Gastrointestinal: Abdominal cramps, constipation, diarrhea, nausea, vomiting
Neuromuscular & skeletal: Hand tremor, myalgia, tremor
Respiratory: Dyspnea
Miscellaneous: Allergic skin reactions (rare), diaphoresis
Drug Interactions
Metabolism/Transport Effects None known.
Avoid Concomitant Use
Avoid concomitant use of Liotrix with any of the following: Sodium Iodide I131
Increased Effect/Toxicity
Liotrix may increase the levels/effects of: Tricyclic Antidepressants; Vitamin K Antagonists

The levels/effects of Liotrix may be increased by: Piracetam
Decreased Effect
Liotrix may decrease the levels/effects of: Sodium Iodide I131; Theophylline Derivatives

The levels/effects of Liotrix may be decreased by: Bile Acid Sequestrants; Calcium Polystyrene Sulfonate; Calcium Salts; CarBAMazepine; Estrogen Derivatives; Fosphenytoin; Lanthanum; Phenytoin; Rifampin; Selective Serotonin Reuptake Inhibitors; Sodium Polystyrene Sulfonate
Stability Store at 2°C to 8°C (36°F to 46°F); protect from light.
Mechanism of Action The primary active compound is T_3 (triiodothyronine), which may be converted from T_4 (thyroxine) and then circulates throughout the body to influence growth and maturation of various tissues. Liotrix is uniform mixture of synthetic T_4 and T_3 in 4:1 ratio; exact mechanism of action is unknown; however, it is believed the thyroid hormone exerts its many metabolic effects through control of DNA transcription and protein synthesis; involved in normal metabolism, growth, and development; promotes gluconeogenesis, increases utilization and mobilization of glycogen stores and stimulates protein synthesis, increases basal metabolic rate
Pharmacodynamics Onset of action: T_3: ~3 hours
Pharmacokinetics (Adult data unless noted)
Absorption: T_4: 40% to 80%; T_3: 95%
Protein binding: T_4: >99% bound to plasma proteins including thyroxine-binding globulin, thyroxine-binding prealbumin, and albumin
Metabolism: Hepatic to triiodothyronine (active); ~80% T_4 deiodinated in kidney and periphery; glucuronidation/conjugation also occurs; undergoes enterohepatic recirculation
Half-life elimination:
T_4: Euthyroid: 6-7 days; Hyperthyroid: 3-4 days; Hypothyroid: 9-10 days
T_3: 2.5 days

Time to peak serum concentration: T_4: 2-4 hours; T_3: 2-3 days

Elimination: Urine (major route of elimination); partially feces

Dosing: Neonatal Note: Doses should be adjusted based on clinical response and laboratory parameters

Congenital hypothyroidism: Note: AAP recommends levothyroxine as the preferred treatment for hypothyroidism in neonates (AAP, 2006). Neonates should have therapy initiated at full doses. Oral: Usual daily dosage range: Liothyronine (T_3): 3.1-6.25 mcg; levothyroxine (T_4): 12.5-25 mcg once daily

Dosing: Usual Note: Doses should be adjusted based on clinical response and laboratory parameters

Infants, Children, and Adolescents:

Congenital hypothyroidism: Note: Infants should have therapy initiated at full doses. Oral: Usual daily dosage range:

Infants 1-6 months: Liothyronine (T_3): 3.1-6.25 mcg/Levothyroxine (T_4): 12.5-25 mcg once daily

Infants >6-12 months: Liothyronine (T_3): 6.25-9.35 mcg/Levothyroxine (T_4): 25-37.5 mcg once daily

Children 1-5 years: Liothyronine (T_3): 9.35-12.5 mcg/Levothyroxine (T_4): 37.5-50 mcg once daily

Children 6-12 years: Liothyronine (T_3): 12.5-18.75 mcg/Levothyroxine (T_4): 50-75 mcg once daily

Adolescents: Typical doses >Liothyronine (T_3): 18.75 mcg; levothyroxine (T_4): 75 mcg once daily

Adults:

Hypothyroidism: Oral: Initial: Liothyronine (T_3) 6.25 mcg/Levothyroxine (T_4) 25 mcg once daily; may increase by liothyronine 3.1 mcg/Levothyroxine 12.5 mcg every 2-3 weeks. A lower initial dose (liothyronine 3.1 mcg/Levothyroxine 12.5 mcg) is recommended in patients with long-standing myxedema, especially if cardiovascular impairment coexists. If angina occurs, reduce dose (usual maintenance dose: Liothyronine 12.5-25 mcg/Levothyroxine 50-100 mcg)

Monitoring Parameters T_4, TSH, heart rate, blood pressure, clinical signs of hypo- and hyperthyroidism; TSH is the most reliable guide for evaluating adequacy of thyroid replacement dosage. TSH may be elevated during the first few months of thyroid replacement despite patients being clinically euthyroid. In cases where T_4 remains low and TSH is within normal limits, an evaluation of "free" (unbound) T_4 is needed to evaluate further increase in dosage.

In congenital hypothyroidism, adequacy of replacement should be determined using both TSH and total- or free-T_4. During the first 3 years of life, total- or free-T_4 should be maintained in the upper 1/2 of the normal range; this should result in normalization of TSH. In some patients, TSH may not normalize due to a resetting of the pituitary-thyroid feedback as a result of *in utero* hypothyroidism. Monitor closely for cardiac overload, arrhythmias, and aspiration from avid suckling.

Pediatric patients: Monitor closely for under/overtreatment. Undertreatment may decrease intellectual development and linear growth, and lead to poor school performance due to impaired concentration and slowed mentation. Overtreatment may adversely affect brain maturation, accelerate bone age (leading to premature closure of the epiphyses and reduced adult height); craniosynostosis has been reported in infants. Perform routine clinical examinations at regular intervals (to assess mental and physical growth and development). Suggested frequency for monitoring thyroid function tests: Every 1-2 months during the first year of life, every 2-3 months between ages 1-3 years, and every 3-12 months thereafter until growth is completed; repeat tests 2 weeks after any change in dosage.

Reference Range

Thyroid Function Tests

Lab Parameters	Age	Normal Range
T_4 (thyroxine) serum concentration	1-7 days	10.1-20.9 mcg/dL
	8-14 days	9.8-16.6 mcg/dL
	1 month to 1 year	5.5-16.0 mcg/dL
	>1 year	4.0-12.0 mcg/dL
Free thyroxine index (FTI)	1-3 days	9.3-26.6
	1-4 weeks	7.6-20.8
	1-4 months	7.4-17.9
	4-12 months	5.1-14.5
	1-6 years	5.7-13.3
	>6 years	4.8-14.0
T_3 serum concentration	Newborns	100-470 ng/dL
	1-5 years	100-260 ng/dL
	5-10 years	90-240 ng/dL
	10 years to Adult	70-210 ng/dL
T_3 uptake		35%-45%
TSH serum concentration	Cord	3-22 micro international units/mL
	1-3 days	<40 micro international units/mL
	3-7 days	<25 micro international units/mL
	>7 days	0-10 micro international units/mL

Test Interactions Many drugs may have effects on thyroid function tests; para-aminosalicylic acid, aminoglutethimide, amiodarone, barbiturates, carbamazepine, chloral hydrate, clofibrate, colestipol, corticosteroids, danazol, diazepam, estrogens, ethionamide, fluorouracil, I.V. heparin, insulin, lithium, methadone, methimazole, mitotane, nitroprusside, oxyphenbutazone, phenylbutazone, PTU, perphenazine, phenytoin, propranolol, salicylates, sulfonylureas, and thiazides

Additional Information Equivalent doses: The following statement on relative potency of thyroid products is included in a joint statement by American Thyroid Association (ATA), American Association of Clinical Endocrinologists (AACE) and The Endocrine Society (TES): For purposes of conversion, levothyroxine sodium (T_4) 100 mcg is usually considered equivalent to desiccated thyroid 60 mg, thyroglobulin 60 mg, or liothyronine sodium (T_3) 25 mcg. However, these are rough guidelines only and do not obviate the careful re-evaluation of a patient when switching thyroid hormone preparations, including a change from one brand of levothyroxine to another. Joint position statement is available at http://www.thyroid.org/professionals/advocacy/04_12_08_thyroxine.html.

Dosage Forms Excipient information presented when available (limited, particularly for generics); consult specific product labeling.

Tablet, oral:

Thyrolar®: 1/4 [levothyroxine sodium 12.5 mcg and liothyronine sodium 3.1 mcg]

Thyrolar®: 1/2 [levothyroxine sodium 25 mcg and liothyronine sodium 6.25 mcg]

Thyrolar®: 1 [levothyroxine sodium 50 mcg and liothyronine sodium 12.5 mcg]

Thyrolar®: 2 [levothyroxine sodium 100 mcg and liothyronine sodium 25 mcg]

Thyrolar®: 3 [levothyroxine sodium 150 mcg and liothyronine sodium 37.5 mcg]

◀ **References**
American Academy of Pediatrics, Rose SR, Section on Endocrinology and Committee on Genetics, American Thyroid Association, et al, "Update of Newborn Screening and Therapy for Congenital Hypothyroidism," *Pediatrics*, 2006, 117(6):2290-303.

◆ **Lipancreatin** *see* Pancrelipase *on page 1591*

◆ **Lipase, Protease, and Amylase** *see* Pancrelipase *on page 1591*

◆ **Lipitor** *see* AtorvaSTATin *on page 227*

◆ **Liposyn III** *see* Fat Emulsion (Plant Based) *on page 846*

◆ **Liquibid [OTC]** *see* GuaiFENesin *on page 984*

◆ **Liquid Antidote** *see* Charcoal, Activated *on page 432*

◆ **Liquid Paraffin** *see* Mineral Oil *on page 1419*

◆ **Liquituss GG [OTC]** *see* GuaiFENesin *on page 984*

Lisdexamfetamine (lis dex am FET a meen)

Medication Safety Issues
Sound-alike/look-alike issues:
Vyvanse may be confused with Visanne, ViVAXIM, Vytorin, Glucovance, Vivactil
Brand Names: U.S. Vyvanse
Brand Names: Canada Vyvanse
Therapeutic Category Amphetamine; Central Nervous System Stimulant
Generic Availability (U.S.) No
Use Treatment of attention-deficit/hyperactivity disorder (ADHD) (FDA approved in ages ≥6 years and adults)
Medication Guide Available Yes
Pregnancy Risk Factor C
Pregnancy Considerations Adverse effects have not been observed in animal reproduction studies. Lisdexamfetamine is converted to dextroamphetamine. The majority of human data is based on illicit amphetamine/methamphetamine exposure and not from therapeutic maternal use (Golub, 2005). Use of amphetamines during pregnancy may lead to an increased risk of premature birth and low birth weight; newborns may experience symptoms of withdrawal. Behavioral problems may also occur later in childhood (LaGasse, 2012).
Breast-Feeding Considerations The majority of human data is based on illicit amphetamine/methamphetamine exposure and not from therapeutic maternal use (Golub, 2005). Amphetamines are excreted into breast milk and use may decrease milk production. Increased irritability, agitation, and crying have been reported in nursing infants (ACOG, 2011). According to the manufacturer, the decision to continue or discontinue breast-feeding during therapy should take into account the risk of exposure to the infant and the benefits of treatment to the mother.
Contraindications Hypersensitivity or idiosyncrasy to lisdexamfetamine, other sympathomimetic amines, or any component; concurrent use or use within 14 days of MAO inhibitors (hypertensive crisis may occur)
Warnings Serious cardiovascular events including sudden death may occur in patients with preexisting structural cardiac abnormalities or other serious heart problems. Sudden death has been reported in children and adolescents; sudden death, stroke, and MI have been reported in adults. Avoid the use of amphetamines in patients with known serious structural cardiac abnormalities, cardiomyopathy, serious heart rhythm abnormalities, coronary artery disease, or other serious cardiac problems that could place patients at an increased risk to the sympathomimetic effects of amphetamines. Patients should be carefully evaluated for cardiac disease prior to initiation of therapy. The American Heart Association recommends that all children diagnosed with ADHD who may be candidates for medication, such as lisdexamfetamine, should have a thorough cardiovascular assessment prior to

initiation of therapy. This assessment should include a combination of medical history, family history, and physical examination focusing on cardiovascular disease risk factors. An ECG is not mandatory but should be considered.

If a child displays symptoms of cardiovascular disease, including chest pain, dyspnea, or fainting, parents should seek immediate medical care for the child. In a recent retrospective study on the possible association between stimulant medication use and sudden death in children, 564 previously healthy children who died suddenly in motor vehicle accidents were compared to a group of 564 previously healthy children who died suddenly. Two of the 564 (0.4%) children in motor vehicle accidents were taking stimulant medications compared to 10 of 564 (1.8%) children who died suddenly. While the authors of this study conclude there may be an association between stimulant use and sudden death in children, there were a number of limitations to the study and the FDA cannot conclude this information impacts the overall risk:benefit profile of these medications (Gould, 2009). In a large retrospective cohort study involving 1,200,438 children and young adults (aged 2-24 years), none of the currently available stimulant medications or atomoxetine were shown to increase the risk of serious cardiovascular events (ie, acute MI, sudden cardiac death, or stroke) in current (adjusted hazard ratio: 0.75; 95% CI: 0.31-1.85) or former (adjusted hazard ratio: 1.03; 95% CI: 0.57-1.89) users compared to nonusers. It should be noted that due to the upper limit of the 95% CI, the study could not rule out a doubling of the risk, albeit low (Cooper, 2011).

Stimulant medications may increase blood pressure (average increase 2-4 mm Hg) and heart rate (average increase 3-6 bpm); some patients may experience greater increases; use stimulant medications with caution in patients with hypertension, heart failure, recent MI, advanced arteriosclerosis, ventricular arrhythmia, and other cardiovascular conditions that may be exacerbated by increases in blood pressure or heart rate.

Psychiatric adverse events may occur. Stimulants may exacerbate symptoms of behavior disturbance and thought disorder in patients with preexisting psychosis. New-onset psychosis or mania may occur with stimulant use in patients without a prior history of psychotic illness or mania, even at standard doses. Stimulants may induce mixed/manic episodes in patients with bipolar disorder; patients should be screened for bipolar disorder prior to treatment; consider discontinuation if such symptoms (eg, delusional thinking, hallucinations, or mania) occur. May be associated with aggressive behavior or hostility (monitor for development or worsening of these behaviors).

Long-term effects in pediatric patients have not been determined. Use of stimulants in children has been associated with growth suppression; in pediatric clinical trials after 4 weeks of therapy, higher lisdexamfetamine doses were associated with greater weight loss; adolescents may experience larger weight loss than children; monitor growth; treatment interruption may be needed. Appetite suppression may occur; monitor weight during therapy, particularly in children.

Stimulants may lower seizure threshold leading to new-onset or breakthrough seizure activity; use with caution in patients with a history of seizure disorder. Visual disturbances (difficulty in accommodation and blurred vision) have been reported. May exacerbate motor and phonic tics and Tourette's syndrome.

CNS stimulants, including lisdexamfetamine, possess a high potential for abuse **[U.S. Boxed Warning]**; assess for risk of abuse prior to prescribing and monitor for signs of abuse and dependence while on therapy **[U.S. Boxed Warning]**; use with caution in patients with history of ethanol or drug abuse; misuse may cause sudden death and serious cardiovascular adverse events. Prolonged administration may lead to drug dependence; abrupt discontinuation following high doses or for prolonged periods may result in symptoms of withdrawal; avoid abrupt discontinuation in patients who have received amphetamines for prolonged periods. Amphetamines may impair the ability to engage in potentially hazardous activities.

May cause hypersensitivity reactions including anaphylaxis, Stevens-Johnson syndrome, angioedema, and urticaria.

Precautions Use with caution in patients with hyperthyroidism, glaucoma, and agitated states. Prescriptions should be written for the smallest quantity consistent with good patient care to minimize possibility of overdose.

Adverse Reactions

Cardiovascular: Increased blood pressure (adults), increased heart rate (adults)

Central nervous system: Agitation (adults), akathisia (adults), anxiety (adults), dizziness (children), drowsiness (children), emotional lability (children), insomnia, irritability (children), restlessness (adults), tics (children)

Dermatologic: Hyperhidrosis (adults), skin rash (children)

Endocrine & metabolic: Weight loss (more common in children and adolescents)

Gastrointestinal: Abdominal pain (children), anorexia (adults), appetite decreased (more common in children and adolescents), diarrhea (adults), nausea, vomiting (children), xerostomia (more common in adults)

Genitourinary: Decreased libido (adults), erectile dysfunction (adults)

Neuromuscular & skeletal: Tremor (adults)

Respiratory: Dyspnea (adults)

Miscellaneous: Fever (children)

Rare but important or life-threatening: Accommodation disturbance, anaphylaxis, angioedema, cardiomyopathy, change in libido, depression, diplopia, excoriation, frequent erections, hallucination, hepatitis (eosinophilic), hostility, hypersensitivity, hypertension, mania, mydriasis, overstimulation, peripheral vascular insufficiency, prolonged erection, psychotic reaction, Raynaud's phenomenon, seizure, Stevens-Johnson syndrome, tachycardia, Tourette's syndrome

Drug Interactions

Metabolism/Transport Effects None known.

Avoid Concomitant Use

Avoid concomitant use of Lisdexamfetamine with any of the following: Iobenguane I 123; MAO Inhibitors

Increased Effect/Toxicity

Lisdexamfetamine may increase the levels/effects of: Analgesics (Opioid); Sympathomimetics

The levels/effects of Lisdexamfetamine may be increased by: Alkalinizing Agents; Antacids; AtoMOXetine; Cannabinoid-Containing Products; Carbonic Anhydrase Inhibitors; Linezolid; MAO Inhibitors; Tricyclic Antidepressants

Decreased Effect

Lisdexamfetamine may decrease the levels/effects of: Antihistamines; Ethosuximide; Iobenguane I 123; Ioflupane I 123; PHENobarbital; Phenytoin

The levels/effects of Lisdexamfetamine may be decreased by: Ammonium Chloride; Antipsychotics; Ascorbic Acid; Gastrointestinal Acidifying Agents; Lithium; Methenamine; Multivitamins/Fluoride (with ADE); Multivitamins/Minerals (with ADEK, Folate, Iron); Multivitamins/Minerals (with AE, No Iron); Urinary Acidifying Agents

Food Interactions High-fat meal prolongs T_{max} by ~1 hour. Management: Administer without regard to meals.

Stability Store at 25°C (77°F); excursions permitted to 15°C to 30°C (59°F to 86°F); protect from light; dispense in tightly-closed container.

Mechanism of Action Lisdexamfetamine dimesylate is a prodrug that is converted to the active component dextroamphetamine (a noncatecholamine, sympathomimetic amine). Amphetamines are noncatecholamine, sympathomimetic amines that cause release of catecholamines (primarily dopamine and norepinephrine) from their storage sites in the presynaptic nerve terminals. A less significant mechanism may include their ability to block the reuptake of catecholamines by competitive inhibition.

Pharmacodynamics

Onset of action: 1 hour (AAP, 2011)

Duration of action: 10-12 hours (AAP, 2011)

Pharmacokinetics (Adult data unless noted)

Absorption: Rapid

Distribution: Dextroamphetamine: V_d: 3.5-4.6 L/kg; distributes into CNS; mean CSF concentrations are 80% of plasma

Metabolism: Metabolized in the blood by hydrolytic activity of red blood cells to dextroamphetamine and l-lysine; not metabolized by CYP P450

Half-life elimination: Lisdexamfetamine: <1 hour; dextroamphetamine: 10-13 hours

Time to peak serum concentration:

Lisdexamfetamine: Children 6-12 years: 1 hour (fasting)

Dextroamphetamine:

Children 6-12 years: 3.5 hours (fasting)

Adults: 3.8 hours (fasting), 4.7 hours (after a high-fat meal)

Elimination: Urine (96%; 42% of dose as amphetamine, 2% as lisdexamfetamine, 25% as hippuric acid); feces (minimal)

Dosing: Usual

Children ≥6 years and Adolescents: **Attention-deficit/hyperactivity disorder: Note:** Individualize dosage based on patient need and response to therapy. Administer at the lowest effective dose.

Manufacturer's labeling: Oral: Initial: 30 mg once daily in the morning; may increase in increments of 10 mg or 20 mg/day at weekly intervals until optimal response is obtained; maximum daily dose: 70 mg/**day**

Alternate dosing: Oral: Initial: 20 mg once daily; may increase in increments of 10 or 20 mg/day at 3-7 day intervals until optimal response is obtained; maximum daily dose: 70 mg/**day** (AAP, 2011)

Adults: **Attention-deficit/hyperactivity disorder: Note:** Individualize dosage based on patient need and response to therapy. Administer at the lowest effective dose. Oral: Initial: 30 mg once daily in the morning; may increase in increments of 10 mg or 20 mg/day at weekly intervals until optimal response is obtained; maximum daily dose: 70 mg/**day**

Administration Administer in the morning with or without food; avoid afternoon doses to prevent insomnia. Swallow capsule whole, do not chew; capsule may be opened and the entire contents dissolved in glass of water; stir until dispersed completely and consume the resulting solution immediately; do not store solution; do not divide capsule; do not take less than 1 capsule daily.

Monitoring Parameters Evaluate patients for cardiac disease prior to initiation of therapy with thorough medical history, family history, and physical exam; consider ECG; perform ECG and echocardiogram if findings suggest cardiac disease; promptly conduct cardiac evaluation in patients who develop chest pain, unexplained syncope, or any other symptom of cardiac disease during treatment. Monitor CNS activity; blood pressure and heart rate (baseline, following dose increases, and periodically during treatment), sleep, appetite, abnormal movements, height, weight, BMI, growth in children. Patients should be re-evaluated at appropriate intervals to assess continued need of the medication. Observe for signs/symptoms of aggression or hostility, or depression. Monitor for visual disturbances. Monitor for signs of misuse, abuse, and addiction.

Test Interactions Amphetamines may elevate plasma corticosteroid levels; may interfere with urinary steroid determinations.

Additional Information Treatment for ADHD should include "drug holiday" or periodic discontinuation in order to assess the patient's requirements, decrease tolerance, and limit suppression of linear growth and weight. Medications used to treat ADHD should be part of a total treatment program that may include other components such as psychological, educational, and social measures.

Controlled Substance C-II

Dosage Forms Excipient information presented when available (limited, particularly for generics); consult specific product labeling.

Capsule, Oral, as dimesylate:

Vyvanse: 20 mg, 30 mg, 40 mg, 50 mg, 60 mg, 70 mg [contains brilliant blue fcf (fd&c blue #1), fd&c red #40, fd&c yellow #10 (quinoline yellow)]

References

American Academy of Pediatrics, "ADHD: Clinical Practice Guideline for the Diagnosis, Evaluation, and Treatment of Attention-Deficit/Hyperactivity Disorder in Children and Adolescents," *Pediatrics*, 2011,128(5):1007-22.

American Academy of Pediatrics/American Heart Association Clarification of Statement on Cardiovascular Evaluation and Monitoring of Children and Adolescents With Heart Disease Receiving Medications for ADHD; available at: http://americanheart.mediaroom.com/index.php?s=43&item=422.

American College of Obstetricians and Gynecologists (ACOG) Committee Opinion: No. 479, "Methamphetamine Abuse in Women of Reproductive Age," *Obstet Gynecol*, 2011, 117(3):751-5.

Biederman J, Krishnan S, Zhang Y, et al, "Efficacy and Tolerability of Lisdexamfetamine Dimesylate (NRP-104) in Children With Attention-Deficit/Hyperactivity Disorder: A Phase III, Multicenter, Randomized, Double-Blind, Forced-Dose, Parallel-Group Study," *Clin Ther*, 2007, 29(3):450-63.

Cooper WO, Habel LA, Sox CM, et al, "ADHD Drugs and Serious Cardiovascular Events in Children and Young Adults," *N Engl J Med*, 2011, 365(20):1896-904.

Golub M, Costa L, Crofton K, et al, "NTP-CERHR Expert Panel Report on the Reproductive and Developmental Toxicity of Amphetamine and Methamphetamine," *Birth Defects Res B Dev Reprod Toxicol*, 2005, 74(6):471-584.

Gould MS, Walsh BT, Munfakh JL, et al, "Sudden Death and Use of Stimulant Medications in Youths," *Am J Psychiatry*, 2009, 166 (9):992-1001.

LaGasse LL, Derauf C, Smith LM, et al, "Prenatal Methamphetamine Exposure and Childhood Behavior Problems at 3 and 5 Years of Age," *Pediatrics*, 2012, 129(4):681-8.

Nissen SE, "ADHD and Cardiovascular Risk," *N Engl J Med*, 2006, 354:1445-8.

Pliszka S and AACAP Work Group on Quality Issues, "Practice Parameter for the Assessment and Treatment of Children and Adolescents With Attention-Deficit/Hyperactivity Disorder," *J Am Acad Child Adolesc Psychiatry*, 2007, 46(7):894-921.

Vetter VL, Elia J, Erickson CH, et al, "Cardiovascular Monitoring of Children and Adolescents With Heart Disease Receiving Stimulant Drugs. A Scientific Statement from the American Heart Association Council on Cardiovascular Disease in the Young Congenital Cardiac Defects Committee and the Council on Cardiovascular Nursing," *Circulation*, 2008, 117:2407-23.

◆ **Lisdexamfetamine Dimesylate** see Lisdexamfetamine on page *1260*

◆ **Lisdexamphetamine** see Lisdexamfetamine on page *1260*

Lisinopril (lyse IN oh pril)

Medication Safety Issues

Sound-alike/look-alike issues:

Lisinopril may be confused with fosinopril, Lioresal, Lipitor, RisperDAL

Prinivil® may be confused with Plendil, Pravachol, Prevacid, PriLOSEC, Proventil

Zestril® may be confused with Desyrel, Restoril, Vistaril, Zegerid, Zerit, Zetia, Zostrix, ZyPREXA

International issues:

Acepril [Malaysia] may be confused with Accupril which is a brand name for quinapril [U.S.]

Acepril: Brand name for lisinopril [Malaysia], but also the brand name for captopril [Great Britain]; enalapril [Hungary, Switzerland]

Brand Names: U.S. Prinivil; Zestril

Brand Names: Canada Apo-Lisinopril; Auro-Lisinopril; CO Lisinopril; Dom-Lisinopril; JAMP-Lisinopril; Mylan-Lisinopril; PMS-Lisinopril; Prinivil; PRO-Lisinopril; RAN-Lisinopril; ratio-Lisinopril P; ratio-Lisinopril Z; Riva-Lisinopril; Sandoz-Lisinopril; Teva-Lisinopril (Type P); Teva-Lisinopril (Type Z); Zestril

Therapeutic Category Angiotensin-Converting Enzyme (ACE) Inhibitor; Antihypertensive Agent

Generic Availability (U.S.) Yes

Use Treatment of hypertension, either alone or in combination with other antihypertensive agents (FDA approved in ages 6-16 years and adults); adjunctive therapy in treatment of heart failure (HF) (FDA approved in adults); treatment of acute myocardial infarction (MI) within 24 hours in hemodynamically-stable patients to improve survival (FDA approved in adults); has also been used for the treatment of proteinuria associated with IgA nephropathy and for its reno-protective effects in patients with diabetes mellitus and renal parenchymal disease

Pregnancy Risk Factor D

Pregnancy Considerations [U.S. Boxed Warning]: Drugs that act on the renin-angiotensin system can cause injury and death to the developing fetus. Discontinue as soon as possible once pregnancy is detected. Lisinopril crosses the placenta; teratogenic effects may occur following maternal use during pregnancy. Drugs that act on the renin-angiotensin system are associated with oligohydramnios. Oligohydramnios, due to decreased fetal renal function, may lead to fetal lung hypoplasia and skeletal malformations. Their use in pregnancy is also associated with anuria, hypotension, renal failure, skull hypoplasia, and death in the fetus/neonate. Chronic maternal hypertension itself is also associated with adverse events in the fetus/infant. ACE inhibitors are not recommended during pregnancy to treat maternal hypertension or heart failure. Use of an ACE inhibitor should also be avoided in any woman of reproductive age. Women who are planning a pregnancy should be considered for other medication options if an ACE inhibitor is currently prescribed or the ACE inhibitor should be discontinued as soon as possible once pregnancy is detected. The exposed fetus should be monitored for fetal growth, amniotic fluid volume, and organ formation. Infants exposed to an ACE inhibitor *in utero* should be monitored for hyperkalemia, hypotension, and oliguria (exchange transfusions or dialysis may be needed). These adverse events are generally associated with maternal use in the second and third trimesters.

Untreated chronic maternal hypertension is also associated with adverse events in the fetus, infant, and mother. The use of ACE inhibitors is not recommended to treat chronic uncomplicated hypertension in pregnant women and should generally be avoided in women of reproductive potential (ACOG, 2013).

Breast-Feeding Considerations It is not known if lisinopril is excreted in breast milk. Breast-feeding is not recommended by the manufacturer.

Contraindications Hypersensitivity to lisinopril, any component, or other ACE inhibitors; patients with idiopathic or hereditary angioedema or a history of angioedema with previous ACE inhibitor use

Warnings Angioedema can occur at any time during treatment (especially following first dose). The relative risk of angioedema with ACE inhibitors is higher within the first 30 days of use (compared to >1 year of use), for Black Americans (compared to Whites), for lisinopril or enalapril (compared to captopril), and for patients previously hospitalized within 30 days (Brown, 1996). Angioedema may occur in the head, neck, extremities, or intestines; patients with angioedema of the intestines may present with abdominal pain (with or without nausea or vomiting); angioedema of the larynx, glottis, or tongue may cause airway obstruction, especially in patients with a history of airway surgery; prolonged monitoring may be required, even in patients with swelling of only the tongue (ie, without respiratory distress) because treatment with corticosteroids and antihistamines may not be sufficient; very rare fatalities have occurred with angioedema of the larynx or tongue; appropriate treatment (eg, establishing patent airway and/or SubQ epinephrine) should be readily available for patients with angioedema of larynx, glottis, or tongue, in whom airway obstruction is likely to occur.

Anaphylactic/anaphylactoid reactions can occur with ACE inhibitors. Life-threatening anaphylactoid reactions may be seen during hemodialysis (eg, CVVHD) with high-flux dialysis membranes (eg, AN69), and rarely, during low density lipoprotein apheresis with dextran sulfate cellulose. Rare cases of anaphylactoid reactions have been reported in patients undergoing sensitization treatment with hymenoptera (eg, bee, wasp) venom while receiving ACE inhibitors.

ACE inhibitor therapy has been associated with rare but potentially fatal cases of agranulocytosis, neutropenia, or leukopenia with myeloid hypoplasia; higher risk for development of neutropenia is associated with renal impairment; risk is further increased in patients with both renal impairment and collagen vascular disease (eg, systemic lupus erythematosus). Onset of neutropenia is usually within 3 months of ACE inhibitor initiation; closely monitor CBC with differential for the first 3 months of therapy and periodically thereafter in these patients; neutrophil count generally returns to baseline within 2 weeks of discontinuation.

ACE inhibitor use has been associated with deterioration of renal function and/or increases in serum creatinine, particularly in patients with low renal blood flow (eg, renal artery stenosis, heart failure) whose glomerular filtration rate (GFR) is dependent on efferent arteriolar vasoconstriction by angiotensin II; deterioration may result in oliguria, acute renal failure, and progressive azotemia. Small increases in serum creatinine may occur following initiation; consider discontinuation only in patients with progressive and/or significant deterioration in renal function.

A rare toxicity associated with ACE inhibitors includes cholestatic jaundice, which may progress to fulminant hepatic necrosis; discontinue if marked elevation of hepatic transaminases or jaundice occurs and initiate appropriate medical treatment.

Drugs that act on the renin-angiotensin system can cause injury and death to the developing fetus. Discontinue as soon as possible once pregnancy is detected **[U.S. Boxed Warning]**.

Concomitant use of an ARB or renin inhibitor (eg, aliskiren) is associated with an increased risk of hypotension, hyperkalemia, and renal dysfunction. Concomitant use with aliskiren should be avoided in patients with GFR <60 mL/minute and is contraindicated in patients with diabetes mellitus (regardless of GFR).

Precautions Use with caution in patients with renal impairment; dosage reduction may be necessary; avoid rapid dosage escalation which may lead to further renal impairment. Use with caution in patients with unstented

unilateral/bilateral renal artery stenosis. When unstented bilateral renal artery stenosis is present, use is generally avoided due to the elevated risk of deterioration in renal function unless possible benefits outweigh risks.

Use with caution when initiating therapy and in volume-depleted patients; may cause symptomatic hypotension with or without syncope, usually with the first several doses; correct volume depletion prior to initiation; initiate lower doses in patients with sodium or volume depletion; close monitoring of patient is required especially with initial dosing and dosing increases; blood pressure must be lowered at a rate appropriate for the patient's clinical condition. Although dose reduction may be necessary, hypotension alone is not a reason for discontinuation of future ACE inhibitor use especially in patients with heart failure where a reduction in systolic blood pressure is a desirable observation. Use caution in patients with ischemic heart disease or cerebrovascular disease during therapy initiation; observe closely due to the potential consequences posed by falling blood pressure (eg, MI, stroke); fluid replacement, may be required to restore blood pressure; therapy may then be resumed; discontinue therapy in patients whose hypotension recurs. Use with caution in patients with severe aortic stenosis; may reduce coronary perfusion resulting in ischemia. Use with caution in patients with hypertrophic cardiomyopathy (HCM) and outflow tract obstruction since reduction in afterload may worsen symptoms associated with this condition.

May cause hyperkalemia; risk factors include renal dysfunction, diabetes mellitus, concomitant use of potassium-sparing diuretics, potassium supplements, and/or potassium-containing salts; use with caution, if at all, with these agents, and monitor potassium closely. Concurrent use of angiotensin receptor blockers (ARBs) may increase the risk of clinically significant adverse events (eg, renal dysfunction, hyperkalemia).

Use with caution before, during, or immediately after major surgery; cardiopulmonary bypass, intraoperative blood loss or vasodilating anesthesia increases endogenous renin release; use of ACE inhibitors perioperatively will blunt angiotensin II formation and may result in hypotension.

An ACE inhibitor cough is a dry, hacking, nonproductive one that usually occurs within the first few months of treatment and should generally resolve within 1-4 weeks after discontinuation of the ACE inhibitor. In pediatric patients, an isolated dry hacking cough lasting >3 weeks was reported in 7 of 42 pediatric patients (17%) receiving ACE inhibitors (von Vigier, 2000); a review of pediatric randomized controlled ACE inhibitor trials reported a lower incidence of 3.2% (Baker-Smith, 2010). Other causes of cough should be considered (eg, pulmonary congestion in patients with heart failure) and excluded prior to discontinuation.

Adverse Reactions Note: Higher rates of adverse reactions have generally been noted in patients with heart failure. However, the frequency of adverse effects associated with placebo is also increased in this population.

Cardiovascular: Chest pain, hypotension, orthostatic effects, syncope

Central nervous system: Dizziness, fatigue, headache

Dermatologic: Skin rash

Endocrine & metabolic: Hyperkalemia, increased nonprotein nitrogen

Gastrointestinal: Abdominal pain, diarrhea, nausea, vomiting

Genitourinary: Impotence

Hematologic & oncologic: Decreased hemoglobin (small)

Infection: Common cold

Neuromuscular & skeletal: Weakness

Renal: Increased blood urea nitrogen, increased serum creatinine (often transient), renal insufficiency (in patients with bilateral renal artery stenosis or hypovolemia)

Respiratory: Cough, upper respiratory tract infection

Rare but important or life-threatening: Acute renal failure, alopecia, anaphylactoid reactions, angioedema, anuria, arthritis, asthma, atrial fibrillation, atrial tachycardia, azotemia, bone marrow suppression, bradycardia, cardiac arrest, cardiac arrhythmia, cerebrovascular accident, diabetes mellitus, eosinophilia, eosinophilic pneumonitis, gout, hemolytic anemia, hemoptysis, hepatic necrosis, hepatitis, herpes zoster, hypersomnia, hyponatremia, increased erythrocyte sedimentation rate, interstitial nephritis, intestinal angioedema, leukopenia, malignant neoplasm of lung, memory impairment, mood changes, myocardial infarction, neutropenia, oliguria, orthostatic hypotension, pancreatitis, pemphigus, peripheral neuropathy, pleural effusion, pneumonia, positive ANA titer, pseudolymphoma (cutaneous), psoriasis, pulmonary embolism, pulmonary infarct, SIADH, skin infection, skin photosensitivity, Stevens-Johnson syndrome, systemic lupus erythematosus, thrombocytopenia, toxic epidermal necrolysis, transient ischemic attacks, tremor, urinary tract infection, vasculitis, ventricular tachycardia, viral infection, vision loss, visual hallucination (Doane, 2013)

Drug Interactions

Metabolism/Transport Effects None known.

Avoid Concomitant Use There are no known interactions where it is recommended to avoid concomitant use.

Increased Effect/Toxicity

Lisinopril may increase the levels/effects of: Allopurinol; Amifostine; Antihypertensives; AzaTHIOprine; CycloSPORINE (Systemic); DULoxetine; Ferric Gluconate; Gold Sodium Thiomalate; Grass Pollen Allergen Extract (5 Grass Extract); Hypotensive Agents; Iron Dextran Complex; Lithium; Nonsteroidal Anti-Inflammatory Agents; Obinutuzumab; RiTUXimab; Sodium Phosphates

The levels/effects of Lisinopril may be increased by: Alfuzosin; Aliskiren; Angiotensin II Receptor Blockers; Barbiturates; Brimonidine (Topical); Canagliflozin; Diazoxide; DPP-IV Inhibitors; Eplerenone; Everolimus; Heparin; Heparin (Low Molecular Weight); Herbs (Hypotensive Properties); Loop Diuretics; MAO Inhibitors; Pentoxifylline; Phosphodiesterase 5 Inhibitors; Potassium Salts; Potassium-Sparing Diuretics; Prostacyclin Analogues; Sirolimus; Temsirolimus; Thiazide Diuretics; TiZANidine; Tolvaptan; Trimethoprim

Decreased Effect

The levels/effects of Lisinopril may be decreased by: Antacids; Aprotinin; Herbs (Hypertensive Properties); Icatibant; Lanthanum; Methylphenidate; Nonsteroidal Anti-Inflammatory Agents; Salicylates; Yohimbine

Mechanism of Action Competitive inhibitor of angiotensin-converting enzyme (ACE); prevents conversion of angiotensin I to angiotensin II, a potent vasoconstrictor; results in lower levels of angiotensin II which causes an increase in plasma renin activity and a reduction in aldosterone secretion; a CNS mechanism may also be involved in hypotensive effect as angiotensin II increases adrenergic outflow from CNS; vasoactive kallikreins may be decreased in conversion to active hormones by ACE inhibitors, thus reducing blood pressure

Pharmacodynamics

Onset of action: Antihyptensive effect: 1 hour

Maximum effect: Antihypertensive effect: 6-8 hours

Duration: 24 hours

Pharmacokinetics (Adult data unless noted)

Absorption: Oral:

Pediatric patients:

2-15 years: 20% to 36% (Hogg, 2007)

6-16 years: 28%

Adults: 25% (range: 6% to 60%)

Protein binding: 25%

Half-life: 11-13 hours; half-life increases with renal dysfunction

Time to peak serum concentration:

Pediatric patients 6 months to 15 years: Median (range): 5-6 hours (Hogg, 2007)

Adults: Within 7 hours

Elimination: Primarily urine as unchanged drug

Dialysis: Removable by hemodialysis

Dosing: Usual

Infants, Children, and Adolescents:

Hypertension: Note: Dosage must be titrated according to patient's response; **reduce dose by 50% in patients with hyponatremia, hypovolemia, severe CHF, decreased renal function, or receiving diuretics.** If possible, discontinue diuretics 2-3 days prior to initiating lisinopril; restart diuretic, if needed, after blood pressure is stable:

Infants: Limited data available: Oral: Initial: 0.07-0.1 mg/kg/dose once daily; may increase at ≥2 weeks intervals; maximum daily dose: 0.5 mg/kg/**day**; dosing based on a retrospective study of pediatric patients (n=123; 59 with hypertension; age range: 2 months to 18 years) which initiated therapy in the hospital to allow for close observation; median maximum dose in patients 1 month to <2 years (n=13): 0.159 mg/kg/day; (Raes, 2007); further studies are needed.

Children <6 years: Limited data available: Oral: Initial: 0.07-0.1 mg/kg/dose once daily; maximum initial daily dose: 5 mg/**day**; increase dose at 1- to 2-week intervals; maximum daily dose: 0.6 mg/kg/**day** or 40 mg/**day** (NHBPEP, 2004; NHLBI, 2011; Raes, 2007)

Children ≥6 years and Adolescents: Oral: Initial: 0.07-0.1 mg/kg/dose once daily; maximum initial daily dose: 5 mg/**day**; increase dose at 1- to 2-week intervals; maximum daily dose: 0.6 mg/kg/**day** or 40 mg/**day**

Proteinuria (mild IgA nephropathy): Children ≥4 years and Adolescents: Limited data available: Oral: Initial: 0.2 mg/kg/dose once daily (maximum initial dose: 10 mg) for 7 days, then increase to 0.4 mg/kg/dose once daily (maximum dose: 20 mg); dosing based on a pilot study of 40 pediatric patients (mean age: 11.4 years; range: 4-15 years) who during a 2-year treatment period showed statistically significant resolution of proteinuria in 82% of patients; five patients developed dizziness during treatment period and four of them required dosage reduction (50% to 75%) (Nakanishi, 2008); further studies are needed.

Renal protection (diabetes mellitus or renal parenchymal disease): Infants, Children, and Adolescents: Limited data available: Oral: Initial: 0.1 mg/kg/dose once daily; maximum initial daily dose: 5 mg/day; dosing based on a retrospective study of pediatric patients (n=123 of which 60 had either DM or renal parenchymal disease; age range: 2 months to 18 years); the protocol included therapy initiation within the hospital to allow for close observation initially; median maximum dose: 0.135 mg/kg/day (Raes, 2007); further studies are needed.

Adults:

Heart failure: Oral: Initial: 2.5-5 mg once daily; then increase by no more than 10 mg increments at intervals no less than 2 weeks to a maximum daily dose of 40 mg. Usual maintenance: 5-40 mg/day as a single dose. Target dose: 20-40 mg once daily (ACC/AHA 2009 Heart Failure Guidelines). **Note:** If patient has hyponatremia (serum sodium <130 mEq/L) or renal impairment (CrCl <30 mL/minute or creatinine >3 mg/dL), then initial dose should be 2.5 mg/day.

Hypertension: Oral: Usual dosage range (JNC 7): 10-40 mg/day

Not maintained on diuretic: Initial: 10 mg/day

Maintained on diuretic: Initial: 5 mg/day

Note: Antihypertensive effect may diminish toward the end of the dosing interval especially with doses of 10 mg/day. An increased dose may aid in extending the duration of antihypertensive effect. Doses up to 80 mg/day have been used, but do not appear to give greater effect.

Patients taking diuretics should have them discontinued 2-3 days prior to initiating lisinopril if possible. Restart diuretic after blood pressure is stable if needed. If diuretic cannot be discontinued prior to therapy, begin with 5 mg with close supervision until stable blood pressure. In patients with hyponatremia (<130 mEq/L), start dose at 2.5 mg/day.

Acute myocardial infarction (within 24 hours in hemodynamically stable patients): Oral: 5 mg immediately, then 5 mg at 24 hours, 10 mg at 48 hours, and 10 mg every day thereafter for 6 weeks. Patients should continue to receive standard treatments such as thrombolytics, aspirin, and beta-blockers.

Dosing adjustment in renal impairment:

Infants, Children, and Adolescents:

Manufacturer labeling: Children ≥6 years and Adolescents ≤16 years: CrCl <30 mL/minute/1.73 m^2: Use is not recommended

Alternate dosing (Aronoff, 2007):

GFR >50 mL/minute/1.73 m^2: No dosage adjustment necessary

GFR 10-50 mL/minute/1.73 m^2: Administer 50% of usual dose

GFR <10 mL/minute/1.73 m^2: Administer 25% of usual dose

Intermittent hemodialysis: Administer 25% of usual dose

Peritoneal dialysis (PD): Administer 25% of usual dose

Continuous renal replacement therapy (CRRT): Administer 50% of usual dose

Adults: Manufacturer's labeling:

Heart failure: CrCl <30 mL/minute or serum creatinine >3 mg/dL: Initial: 2.5 mg/day

Hypertension: Initial doses should be modified and upward titration should be cautious, based on response (maximum: 40 mg/day)

CrCl >30 mL/minute: Initial: 10 mg/day

CrCl 10-30 mL/minute: Initial: 5 mg/day

Hemodialysis: Initial: 2.5 mg/day; dialyzable (50%)

Administration Oral: May be administered without regard to food

Monitoring Parameters Blood pressure, BUN, serum creatinine, renal function, urine dipstick for protein, serum potassium, WBC with differential, especially during first 3 months of therapy for patients with renal impairment and/or collagen vascular disease; monitor for angioedema and anaphylactoid reactions; hypovolemia and postural hypotension when beginning therapy, adjusting dosage, and on a regular basis throughout

Test Interactions May cause false-positive results in urine acetone determinations using sodium nitroprusside reagent

Dosage Forms Excipient information presented when available (limited, particularly for generics); consult specific product labeling.

Tablet, Oral:

Prinivil: 5 mg, 10 mg, 20 mg [scored]

Zestril: 2.5 mg

Zestril: 5 mg [scored]

Zestril: 10 mg, 20 mg, 30 mg, 40 mg

Generic: 2.5 mg, 5 mg, 10 mg, 20 mg, 30 mg, 40 mg

Extemporaneous Preparations A 1 mg/mL lisinopril oral suspension may be made with tablets and a 1:1 mixture of Ora-Plus® and Ora-Sweet®. Crush ten 10 mg tablets in a mortar and reduce to a fine powder. Add small portions of the vehicle and mix to a uniform paste; mix while adding the vehicle in incremental proportions to **almost** 100 mL; transfer to a graduated cylinder; rinse mortar with vehicle, and add quantity of vehicle sufficient to make 100 mL. Store in amber plastic prescription bottles; label "shake well". Stable for 13 weeks at room temperature or refrigerated (Nahata, 2004).

A 1 mg/mL lisinopril oral suspension also be made with tablets, methylcellulose 1% with parabens, and simple syrup NF. Crush ten 10 mg tablets in a mortar and reduce to a fine powder. Add 7.7 mL of methylcellulose gel and mix to a uniform paste; mix while adding the simple syrup in incremental proportions to **almost** 100 mL; transfer to a graduated cylinder; rinse mortar with vehicle, and add quantity of vehicle sufficient to make 100 mL. Store in amber plastic prescription bottles; label "shake well". Stable for 13 weeks refrigerated or 8 weeks at room temperature (Nahata, 2004).

A 2 mg/mL lisinopril syrup may be made with powder (Sigma Chemical Company, St. Louis, MO) and simple syrup. Dissolve 1 g of lisinopril powder in 30 mL of distilled water. Mix while adding simple syrup in incremental proportions in a quantity sufficient to make 500 mL. Label "shake well" and "refrigerate". Stable for 30 days when stored in amber plastic prescription bottles at room temperature or refrigerated. **Note:** Although no visual evidence of microbial growth was observed, the authors recommend refrigeration to inhibit microbial growth (Webster, 1997).

Nahata MC and Morosco RS, "Stability of Lisinopril in Two Liquid Dosage Forms," *Ann Pharmacother*, 2004, 38(3):396-9.

Prinivil® prescribing information, Merck & Co, Inc, Whitehouse Station, NJ, 2008.

Thompson KC, Zhao Z, Mazakas JM, et al, "Characterization of an Extemporaneous Liquid Formulation of Lisinopril," *Am J Health Syst Pharm*, 2003, 60(1):69-74.

Webster AA, English BA, and Rose DJ, "The Stability of Lisinopril as an Extemporaneous Syrup," *Intr J Pharmaceut Compound*, 1997, 1:352-3.

Zestril® prescribing information, AstraZeneca Pharmaceuticals, Wilmington, DE, 2007.

References

Baker-Smith CM, Benjamin DK Jr, Califf RM, et al, "Cough in Pediatric Patients Receiving Angiotensin-Converting Enzyme Inhibitor Therapy or Angiotensin Receptor Blocker Therapy in Randomized Controlled Trials," *Clin Pharmacol Ther*, 2010, 87(6):668-71.

Brown NJ, Ray WA, Snowden M, et al, "Black Americans Have an Increased Rate of Angiotensin-Converting Enzyme Inhibitor-Associated Angioedema," *Clin Pharmacol Ther*, 1996, 60(1):8-13.

Chobanian AV, Bakris GL, Black HR, et al, "The Seventh Report of the Joint National Committee on Prevention, Detection, Evaluation, and Treatment of High Blood Pressure: The JNC 7 Report," *JAMA*, 2003, 289(19):2560-72.

Hogg RJ, Delucchi A, Sakihara G, et al, "A Multicenter Study of the Pharmacokinetics of Lisinopril in Pediatric Patients With Hypertension," *Pediatr Nephrol*, 2007, 22(5):695-701.

Nakanishi K, Iijima K, Ishikura K, et al, "Efficacy and Safety of Lisinopril for Mild Childhood IgA Nephropathy: A Pilot Study," *Pediatr Nephrol*, 2009, 24(4):845-9.

National Heart, Lung, and Blood Institute, "Expert Panel on Integrated Guidelines for Cardiovascular Health and Risk Reduction in Children and Adolescents," *Clinical Practice Guidelines*, 2011, National Institutes of Health. Available at http://www.nhlbi.nih.gov/guidelines/cvd_ped/peds_guidelines_full.pdf

National High Blood Pressure Education Program Working Group on High Blood Pressure in Children and Adolescents, "The Fourth Report on the Diagnosis, Evaluation, and Treatment of High Blood Pressure in Children and Adolescents," *Pediatrics*, 2004, 114(2 Suppl):555-76.

Raes A, Malfait F, Van Aken S, et al, "Lisinopril in Paediatric Medicine: A Retrospective Chart Review of Long-Term Treatment in Children," *J Renin Angiotensin Aldosterone Syst*, 2007, 8(1):3-12.

Raia JJ Jr, Barone JA, Byerly WG, et al, "Angiotensin-Converting Enzymes Inhibitors: A Comparative Review," *DICP*, 1990, 24(5):506-25.

Soffer B, Zhang Z, Miller K, et al, "A Double-Blind, Placebo-Controlled, Dose-Response Study of the Effectiveness and Safety of Lisinopril for Children With Hypertension," *Am J Hypertens*, 2003, 16(10):795-800.

von Vigier RO, Mozzettini S, Truttmann AC, et al, "Cough is Common in Children Prescribed Converting Enzyme Inhibitors," *Nephron*, 2000, 84(1):98.

◆ **Lispro Insulin** *see* Insulin Lispro *on page 1125*

◆ **Lithane™ (Can)** *see* Lithium *on page 1266*

Lithium (LITH ee um)

Medication Safety Issues
Sound-alike/look-alike issues:
Eskalith may be confused with Estratest
Lithium may be confused with lanthanum
Lithobid® may be confused with Levbid®, Lithostat®
Other safety concerns:
Do not confuse **mEq** (milliequivalent) with **mg** (milligram). **Note:** 300 mg lithium carbonate or citrate contain 8 mEq lithium. Dosage should be written in **mg** (milligrams) to avoid confusion.
Check prescriptions for unusually high volumes of the syrup for dosing errors.

Related Information
Oral Medications That Should Not Be Crushed or Altered *on page 2438*

Brand Names: U.S. Lithobid

Brand Names: Canada Apo-Lithium® Carbonate; Apo-Lithium® Carbonate SR; Carbolith™; Duralith®; Euro-Lithium; Lithane™; Lithmax; PHL-Lithium Carbonate; PMS-Lithium Carbonate; PMS-Lithium Citrate

Therapeutic Category Antidepressant, Miscellaneous; Antimanic Agent

Generic Availability (U.S.) Yes

Use Management of acute manic episodes (FDA approved in ages ≥12 years and adults); maintenance treatment of mania in individuals with bipolar disorder (maintenance treatment decreases frequency and diminishes intensity of subsequent manic episodes) (FDA approved in ages ≥12 years and adults); has also been used as adjunct treatment for depression; used investigationally to treat severe aggression in children and adolescents with conduct disorder

Pregnancy Risk Factor D

Pregnancy Considerations Adverse events have been observed in animal reproduction studies. Lithium crosses the placenta in concentrations similar to those in the maternal plasma (Newport, 2005). Cardiac malformations in the infant, including Ebstein's anomaly, are associated with use of lithium during the first trimester of pregnancy. Other adverse events including polyhydramnios, fetal/neonatal cardiac arrhythmias, hypoglycemia, diabetes insipidus, changes in thyroid function, premature delivery, floppy infant syndrome, or neonatal lithium toxicity are associated with lithium exposure when used later in pregnancy (ACOG, 2008). The incidence of adverse events may be associated with higher maternal doses (Newport, 2005).

Due to pregnancy-induced physiologic changes, women who are pregnant may require dose adjustments of lithium to achieve euthymia and avoid toxicity (ACOG, 2008; Grandjean, 2009; Yonkers, 2011).

For planned pregnancies, use of lithium during the first trimester should be avoided if possible (Grandjean, 2009). If lithium is needed during pregnancy, the minimum effective dose should be used, maternal serum concentrations should be monitored, and consideration should be given to start therapy after the period of organogenesis; lithium should be suspended 24-48 hours prior to delivery or at the onset of labor when delivery is spontaneous, then restarted when the patient is medically stable after delivery

(ACOG, 2008; Grandjean, 2009; Newport, 2005). Fetal echocardiography should be considered if first trimester exposure occurs (ACOG, 2008).

Breast-Feeding Considerations Lithium is excreted into breast milk and serum concentrations of nursing infants may be 10% to 50% of the maternal serum concentration (Grandjean, 2009). Hypotonia, hypothermia, cyanosis, electrocardiogram changes, and lethargy have been reported in nursing infants (ACOG, 2008). It is generally recommended that breast-feeding be avoided during maternal use of lithium; however, treatment may be continued in appropriately selected patients (Grandjean, 2009; Sharma, 2009; Viguera, 2007). The hydration status of the nursing infant and maternal serum concentrations of lithium should be monitored (ACOG, 2008). In addition, monitor the infant for lethargy, growth, and feeding problems; obtain infant serum concentrations only if clinical concerns arise (Bogen, 2012; Yonkers, 2011). Long-term effects on development and behavior have not been studied (ACOG, 2008; Grandjean, 2009).

Contraindications Hypersensitivity to lithium or any component

Warnings Lithium toxicity is closely related to serum concentrations and can occur at therapeutic doses **[U.S. Boxed Warning]**; serum lithium determinations are required to monitor therapy. Lithium should generally be avoided in patients with severe cardiovascular or renal disease, severe dehydration or debilitation, sodium depletion, and in patients receiving ACE inhibitors or diuretics (these patients are at very high risk of lithium toxicity). Chronic lithium therapy may result in diminished renal concentrating ability (eg, nephrogenic diabetes insipidus) and has been associated with morphologic changes with glomerular and interstitial fibrosis and atrophy of nephrons. Renal function (including assessment of tubular and glomerular function) should be assessed before initiation of and during lithium therapy; treatment should be re-evaluated if progressive or sudden changes in renal function occur during therapy. An encephalopathic syndrome (resembling neuroleptic malignant syndrome) may occur in patients receiving lithium with haloperidol or other antipsychotic agents. Patients and caregivers should be informed of the symptoms of lithium toxicity.

Capsule may contain benzyl alcohol which may cause allergic reactions in susceptible individuals; solution may contain sodium benzoate; benzoic acid (benzoate) is a metabolite of benzyl alcohol; large amounts of benzyl alcohol (≥99 mg/kg/day) have been associated with a potentially fatal toxicity ("gasping syndrome") in neonates; avoid use of lithium products containing benzyl alcohol in neonates; *in vitro* and animal studies have shown that benzoate, a metabolite of benzyl alcohol, displaces bilirubin from protein binding sites

Precautions Use with extreme caution in patients with cardiovascular or thyroid disease, patients receiving medications that alter sodium excretion (eg, diuretics, ACE inhibitors, or NSAIDs), and in patients with significant fluid loss (protracted sweating, diarrhea, or prolonged fever); monitor lithium concentrations closely, lithium dosage reduction or temporary cessation may be required. Use with caution and modify dose in patients with renal dysfunction.

Adverse Reactions
Cardiovascular: Bradycardia, cardiac arrhythmia, edema, flattened or inverted T waves (reversible), hypotension, sinus node dysfunction, syncope
Central nervous system: Blackout spells, coma, confusion, dizziness, dystonia, fatigue, headache, lethargy, pseudotumor cerebri, psychomotor retardation, restlessness, sedation, seizure, slowed intellectual functioning, slurred speech, stupor, tics, vertigo

Dermatologic: Alopecia, dry or thinning of hair, exacerbation of psoriasis, folliculitis, rash

Endocrine & metabolic: Diabetes insipidus, euthyroid goiter and/or hypothyroidism, hyperglycemia, hyperthyroidism

Gastrointestinal: Anorexia, diarrhea, excessive salivation, metallic taste, nausea, polydipsia, salivary gland swelling, vomiting, weight gain, xerostomia

Genitourinary: Albuminuria, glycosuria, incontinence, oliguria, polyuria

Hematologic: Leukocytosis

Neuromuscular & skeletal: Ataxia, choreoathetoid movements, hyperactive deep tendon reflexes, muscle hyperirritability, myasthenia gravis (rare), tremor

Ocular: Blurred vision, nystagmus, transient scotoma

Miscellaneous: Coldness and painful discoloration of fingers and toes

Postmarketing and/or case reports: Drug-induced Brugada syndrome

Drug Interactions

Metabolism/Transport Effects None known.

Avoid Concomitant Use There are no known interactions where it is recommended to avoid concomitant use.

Increased Effect/Toxicity

Lithium may increase the levels/effects of: Antipsychotics; Highest Risk QTc-Prolonging Agents; Metoclopramide; Moderate Risk QTc-Prolonging Agents; Neuromuscular-Blocking Agents; Selective Serotonin Reuptake Inhibitors; Serotonin Modulators; Tricyclic Antidepressants

The levels/effects of Lithium may be increased by: ACE Inhibitors; Angiotensin II Receptor Blockers; Antiemetics (5HT3 Antagonists); Calcium Channel Blockers (Nondihydropyridine); CarBAMazepine; Desmopressin; Eplerenone; Fosphenytoin; Loop Diuretics; MAO Inhibitors; Methyldopa; Mifepristone; Nonsteroidal Anti-Inflammatory Agents; Phenytoin; Potassium Iodide; Thiazide Diuretics; Topiramate

Decreased Effect

Lithium may decrease the levels/effects of: Amphetamines; Antipsychotics; Desmopressin

The levels/effects of Lithium may be decreased by: Calcitonin; Calcium Polystyrene Sulfonate; Carbonic Anhydrase Inhibitors; Loop Diuretics; Sodium Bicarbonate; Sodium Chloride; Sodium Polystyrene Sulfonate; Theophylline Derivatives

Stability

Extended release tablets: Store between 15°C and 30°C (59°F to 86°F). Protect from moisture; dispense in tightly closed container.

Immediate release tablets and capsules: Store at 25°C (77°F); excursions permitted to 15°C to 30°C (59°F to 86°F). Protect from moisture; dispense in tightly closed container.

Oral solution: Store at 25°C (77°F); excursions permitted to 15°C to 30°C (59°F to 86°F). Dispense in tightly closed container.

Mechanism of Action Alters cation transport across cell membrane in nerve and muscle cells and influences reuptake of serotonin and/or norepinephrine; second messenger systems involving the phosphatidylinositol cycle are inhibited; postsynaptic D2 receptor supersensitivity is inhibited

Pharmacokinetics (Adult data unless noted)

Distribution: Crosses the placenta; appears in breast milk at 35% to 50% of the concentrations in serum

Adults:

V_d: Initial: 0.3-0.4 L/kg

V_{dss}: 0.7-1 L/kg

Half-life, terminal: Adults: 18-24 hours, can increase to more than 36 hours in patients with renal impairment

Time to peak serum concentration (immediate release product): Within 0.5-2 hours

Elimination: 90% to 98% of a dose is excreted in the urine as unchanged drug; other excretory routes include feces (1%) and sweat (4% to 5%)

Dialysis: Dialyzable (50% to 100%)

Dosing: Usual Oral: Monitor serum concentrations and clinical response (efficacy and toxicity) to determine proper dose:

Bipolar Disorder:

Children 6-12 years: 15-60 mg/kg/day in 3-4 divided doses (immediate release); dose not to exceed usual adult dosage; initiate at lower dose and adjust dose weekly based on serum concentrations

Adolescents: 600-1800 mg/day in 3-4 divided doses (immediate release) or 2 divided doses for extended release tablets

Adults: 300 mg 3-4 times/day (immediate release) or 450-900 mg of extended release tablets twice daily; usual maximum maintenance dose: 2.4 g/day

Dosing adjustment in renal impairment:

CrCl 10-50 mL/minute: Administer 50% to 75% of normal dose

CrCl <10 mL/minute: Administer 25% to 50% of normal dose

Administration Oral: Administer with meals to decrease GI upset. Do not crush or chew extended release dosage form; swallow whole

Monitoring Parameters Serum lithium concentration every 3-4 days during initial therapy; once patient is clinically stable and serum concentrations are stable, serum lithium may be obtained every 1-2 months; obtain lithium serum concentrations 8-12 hours postdose (ie, just before next dose). Monitor renal, hepatic, thyroid and cardiovascular function; CBC with differential, urinalysis, serum sodium, calcium, potassium

Reference Range

Therapeutic: Acute mania: 0.6-1.2 mEq/L (SI: 0.6-1.2 mmol/L); protection against future episodes in most patients with bipolar disorder: 0.8-1 mEq/L (SI: 0.8-1 mmol/L). A higher rate of relapse is described in subjects who are maintained <0.4 mEq/L (SI: <0.4 mmol/L)

Toxic: >2 mEq/L (SI: >2 mmol/L)

Concentration-related adverse effects:

GI complaints/tremor: 1.5-2 mEq/L

Confusion/somnolence: 2-2.5 mEq/L

Seizures/death: >2.5 mEq/L

Additional Information In terms of efficacy, the results of studies using lithium to treat severe aggression in children and adolescents with conduct disorders, are mixed. A double-blind, placebo-controlled trial in patients 10-17 years of age (n=40) demonstrated efficacy for lithium in reducing aggressive behavior in psychiatrically hospitalized patients with conduct disorder and severe aggression. Lithium was initiated at 600 mg/day and titrated upwards by 300 mg/day. Final lithium carbonate doses ranged from 900-2100 mg/day divided into 3 doses/day (mean ± SD: 1425 ± 321 mg/day); serum lithium concentrations ranged from 0.78-1.55 mmol/L (mean ± SD: 1.07 ± 0.19 mmol/L) (Malone, 2000). In an earlier double-blind, placebo-controlled study in 50 children 5-12 years of age (mean ± SD: 9.4 ± 1.8 years), lithium was also initiated at 600 mg/day in 3 divided doses. Doses were titrated upwards in 300 mg/day increments. The mean optimal lithium dose was 1248 mg/day (range: 600-1800 mg/day); serum lithium concentrations ranged from 0.53-1.79 mmol/L (mean: 1.12 mmol/L). Doses >1500 mg/day and serum concentrations >1.13 mmol/L did not provide additional benefit (Campbell, 1995). Several other studies have not demonstrated efficacy; further studies are needed.

Dosage Forms Excipient information presented when available (limited, particularly for generics); consult specific product labeling.

Capsule, Oral, as carbonate:
Generic: 150 mg, 300 mg, 600 mg
Solution, Oral, as citrate:
Generic: 8 mEq/5 mL (5 mL, 500 mL)
Tablet, Oral, as carbonate:
Generic: 300 mg
Tablet Extended Release, Oral, as carbonate:
Lithobid: 300 mg [contains fd&c blue #2 aluminum lake, fd&c red #40 aluminum lake, fd&c yellow #6 aluminum lake]
Generic: 300 mg, 450 mg

References

ACOG Committee on Practice Bulletins-Obstetrics, "ACOG Practice Bulletin: Clinical Management Guidelines for Obstetrician-Gynecologists Number 92, April 2008 (Replaces Practice Bulletin Number 87, November 2007). Use of Psychiatric Medications During Pregnancy and Lactation," Obstet Gynecol, 2008, 111(4):1001-20.

Bogen DL, Sit D, Genovese A, et al, "Three Cases of Lithium Exposure and Exclusive Breastfeeding," Arch Womens Ment Health, 2012, 15 (1):69-72.

Campbell M, Adams PB, Small AM, et al, "Lithium in Hospitalized Aggressive Children With Conduct Disorder: A Double-Blind and Placebo-Controlled Study," J Am Acad Child Adolesc Psychiatry, 1995, 34(4):445-53.

Campbell M, Kafantaris V, and Cueva JE, "An Update on the Use of Lithium Carbonate in Aggressive Children and Adolescents With Conduct Disorder," Psychopharmacol Bull, 1995a, 31(1):93-102.

Flaherty B and Krenzelok EP, "Neonatal Lithium Toxicity as a Result of Maternal Toxicity," Vet Hum Toxicol, 1997, 39(2):92-3.

Grandjean EM and Aubry JM, "Lithium: Updated Human Knowledge Using an Evidence-Based Approach: Part III: Clinical Safety," CNS Drugs, 2009, 23(5):397-418.

Levy HB, Harper CR, and Weinberg WA, "A Practical Approach to Children Failing in School," Pediatr Clin North Am, 1992, 39 (4):895-928.

Malone RP, Delaney MA, Luebbert JF, et al, "A Double-Blind Placebo-Controlled Study of Lithium in Hospitalized Aggressive Children and Adolescents With Conduct Disorder," Arch Gen Psychiatry, 2000, 57 (7):649-54.

Newport DJ, Viguera AC, Beach AJ, et al, "Lithium Placental Passage and Obstetrical Outcome: Implications for Clinical Management During Late Pregnancy," Am J Psychiatry, 2005, 162(11):2162-70.

Sharma V, Burt VK, and Ritchie HL, "Bipolar II Postpartum Depression: Detection, Diagnosis, and Treatment," Am J Psychiatry, 2009, 166 (11):1217-21.

Viguera AC, Newport DJ, Ritchie J, et al, "Lithium in Breast Milk and Nursing Infants: Clinical Implications," Am J Psychiatry, 2007, 164 (2):342-5.

Weller EB, Weller RA, and Fristad MA, "Lithium Dosage Guide for Prepubertal Children: A Preliminary Report," J Am Acad Child Psychiatry, 1986, 25(1):92-5.

Yonkers KA, Vigod S, and Ross LE, "Diagnosis, Pathophysiology, and Management of Mood Disorders in Pregnant and Postpartum Women," Obstet Gynecol, 2011, 117(4):961-77.

◆ **Lithium Carbonate** see Lithium on page 1266

◆ **Lithium Citrate** see Lithium on page 1266

◆ **Lithmax (Can)** see Lithium on page 1266

◆ **Lithobid** see Lithium on page 1266

◆ **Little Colds Cough Formula [OTC]** see Dextromethorphan on page 636

◆ **Little Colds Decongestant [OTC]** see Phenylephrine (Systemic) on page 1658

◆ **Little Fevers [OTC]** see Acetaminophen on page 47

◆ **Live Attenuated Influenza Vaccine** see Influenza Virus Vaccine (Live/Attenuated) on page 1109

◆ **Live Attenuated Influenza Vaccine (Quadrivalent)** see Influenza Virus Vaccine (Live/Attenuated) on page 1109

◆ **10% LMD** see Dextran on page 628

◆ **LMD in D₅W** see Dextran on page 628

◆ **LMD in NaCl** see Dextran on page 628

◆ **LMX 4 [OTC]** see Lidocaine (Topical) on page 1242

◆ **LMX 4 Plus [OTC]** see Lidocaine (Topical) on page 1242

◆ **LMX 5 [OTC]** see Lidocaine (Topical) on page 1242

◆ **Locoid** see Hydrocortisone (Topical) on page 1038

◆ **Locoid® (Can)** see Hydrocortisone (Topical) on page 1038

◆ **Locoid Lipocream** see Hydrocortisone (Topical) on page 1038

◆ **Lodalis (Can)** see Colesevelam on page 539

◆ **Lodine** see Etodolac on page 812

◆ **Lodrane D [OTC]** see Brompheniramine and Pseudoephedrine on page 306

◆ **LoHist PSB [OTC] [DSC]** see Brompheniramine and Pseudoephedrine on page 306

◆ **L-OHP** see Oxaliplatin on page 1557

◆ **Lomotil®** see Diphenoxylate and Atropine on page 678

Lomustine (loe MUS teen)

Medication Safety Issues

Sound-alike/look-alike issues:
Lomustine may be confused with bendamustine, carmustine

High alert medication:
This medication is in a class the Institute for Safe Medication Practices (ISMP) includes among its list of drug classes which have a heightened risk of causing significant patient harm when used in error.

Administration issues:
Lomustine should only be administered as a single dose once every 6 weeks; serious adverse events have occurred when lomustine was inadvertently administered daily.

Related Information

Emetogenic Potential of Antineoplastic Agents in Children on page 2327

Oral Medications That Should Not Be Crushed or Altered on page 2438

Safe Handling of Hazardous Drugs on page 2419

Brand Names: Canada CeeNU

Therapeutic Category Antineoplastic Agent, Alkylating Agent; Antineoplastic Agent, Alkylating Agent (Nitrosourea)

Generic Availability (U.S.) Yes

Use Treatment of primary or metastatic brain tumors (after surgery and/or radiation therapy) [FDA approved in pediatric patients (age not specified) and adults]; treatment of relapsed or refractory Hodgkin's disease (as part of a combination chemotherapy regimen) [FDA approved in pediatric patients (age not specified) and adults]; has also been used in the treatment of medulloblastoma

Pregnancy Risk Factor D

Pregnancy Considerations Adverse effects have been observed in animal reproduction studies. May cause fetal harm when administered to a pregnant woman. Women of childbearing potential should be advised to avoid pregnancy during treatment with lomustine.

Breast-Feeding Considerations It is not known if lomustine is excreted in breast milk. Due to the potential for serious adverse reactions in the nursing infant, the decision to discontinue lomustine or to discontinue breast-feeding should take into account the importance of treatment to the mother.

Contraindications Hypersensitivity to lomustine or any component

Warnings Hazardous agent; use appropriate precautions for handling and disposal (NIOSH, 2012). Cumulative and delayed bone marrow suppression, notably thrombocytopenia and leukopenia, may lead to bleeding and overwhelming infection in an already compromised patient **[U.S. Boxed Warning]**: monitor blood counts weekly for at least 6 weeks after administration. Use with caution in patients with depressed platelet, leukocyte, or erythrocyte counts. Because bone marrow toxicity is cumulative; dose adjustments should be based on nadir counts from prior dose. At FDA approved dosages, lomustine should only be administered as a single dose once every 6 weeks due to delayed myelotoxicity; serious errors have occurred when lomustine was inadvertently administered daily.

May cause pulmonary toxicity (infiltrates and/or fibrosis); usually related to cumulative doses >1100 mg/m^2. May be delayed (has been reported up to 17 years after childhood administration in combination with radiation therapy). Patients with baseline forced vital capacity (FVC) or carbon monoxide diffusing capacity (DLco) <70% of predicted levels are at increased risk. Lomustine has been found to be clastogenic, teratogenic, embryotoxic, and carcinogenic in animals. Long-term use may be associated with the development of secondary malignancies.

Precautions Use with caution in patients with hepatic impairment; reversible hepatotoxicity (transaminase, alkaline phosphatase, and bilirubin elevations) has been reported; monitor liver function tests periodically. Kidney damage has been observed; azotemia, decreased kidney size, and renal failure have been reported with long-term use; use with caution in patients with renal impairment; monitor renal function tests periodically; dosage adjustment may be required. Should be administered under the supervision of a physician experienced in the use of cancer chemotherapy agents **[U.S. Boxed Warning]**.

Adverse Reactions

Central nervous system: Ataxia, disorientation, lethargy
Dermatologic: Alopecia, skin rash
Gastrointestinal: Stomatitis; nausea and vomiting, usually within 3-6 hours after oral administration. Administration of the dose at bedtime, with an antiemetic, significantly reduces both the incidence and severity of nausea.
Hematologic: Anemia, bone marrow dysplasia, leukemia (acute)
Myelosuppression, common, dose-limiting, may be cumulative and irreversible; leukopenia (nadir: 5-6 weeks; recovery 6-8 weeks); thrombocytopenia (nadir: 4 weeks; recovery 5-6 weeks)
Hepatic: Alkaline phosphatase increased, bilirubin increased, hepatotoxicity, kidney size decreased, transaminases increased
Neuromuscular & skeletal: Dysarthria
Ocular: Blindness, optic atrophy, visual disturbances
Renal: Azotemia (progressive), renal damage, renal failure
Respiratory: Pulmonary fibrosis, pulmonary infiltrates

Drug Interactions

Metabolism/Transport Effects Substrate of CYP2D6 (minor); **Note:** Assignment of Major/Minor substrate status based on clinically relevant drug interaction potential; **Inhibits** CYP2D6 (weak), CYP3A4 (weak)

Avoid Concomitant Use

Avoid concomitant use of Lomustine with any of the following: BCG; CloZAPine; Dipyrone; Natalizumab; Pimecrolimus; Pimozide; Tacrolimus (Topical); Tofacitinib; Vaccines (Live)

Increased Effect/Toxicity

Lomustine may increase the levels/effects of: ARIPiprazole; CloZAPine; Dofetilide; Leflunomide; Lomitapide; Natalizumab; Pimozide; Tofacitinib; Vaccines (Live)

The levels/effects of Lomustine may be increased by: Denosumab; Dipyrone; Pimecrolimus; Roflumilast; Tacrolimus (Topical); Trastuzumab

Decreased Effect

Lomustine may decrease the levels/effects of: BCG; Coccidioidin Skin Test; Sipuleucel-T; Vaccines (Inactivated); Vaccines (Live)

The levels/effects of Lomustine may be decreased by: Echinacea; Peginterferon Alfa-2b

Stability Store at 25°C (77°F); excursions permitted to 15°C to 30°C (59°F to 86°F). Avoid exposure to excessive heat (>40°C; 104°F).

Mechanism of Action Inhibits DNA and RNA synthesis via carbamylation of DNA polymerase, alkylation of DNA, and alteration of RNA, proteins, and enzymes

Pharmacokinetics (Adult data unless noted)

Absorption: Rapid and complete absorption from the GI tract (30-60 minutes)
Distribution: Widely distributed; lomustine and/or its metabolites penetrate into the CNS; CSF level is ≥50% of plasma concentration
Metabolism: Rapidly hepatic via hydroxylation producing at least two active metabolites; enterohepatically recycled
Half-life (metabolites): 16-48 hours
Time to peak serum concentration (of active metabolite): Within 3 hours
Elimination: Urine (~50%, as metabolites); feces (<5%); expired air (<10%)

Dosing: Usual

Note: Repeat courses should only be administered after adequate recovery of leukocytes to >4000/mm^3 and platelets to >100,000/mm^3. Details concerning dosage in combination regimens should also be consulted; dose, frequency, number of doses, and start date may vary by protocol and treatment phase.

Pediatric:

Brain tumors:

General dosing: Manufacturer's labeling: Infants, Children, and Adolescents: Oral: 130 mg/m^2 as a single dose every 6 weeks (dosage reductions may be recommended for combination chemotherapy regimens)

Compromised marrow function: Reduce initial dose to 100 mg/m^2 as a single dose once every 6 weeks; **Note:** Subsequent doses may require adjustment after initial treatment according to platelet and leukocyte counts.

Medulloblastoma: Children ≥3 years and Adolescents: Limited data available: Oral: 75 mg/m^2 on day 0 of each chemotherapy cycle in combination with cisplatin, vincristine, and radiotherapy (Packer, 2006; Packer, 2013)

Gliomas: Infants, Children, and Adolescents: Limited data available: Oral: 110 mg/m^2 on day 3 of a 6-week cycle in combination with thioguanine, vincristine, and procarbazine for up to 8 cycles for low grade, nonoperable (usually) gliomas (including astrocytomas) (Ater, 2012; Lancaster, 2003; Levin, 2000). For treatment of high grade glioma, 90 mg/m^2 on day 1 every 4 weeks (or repeated when counts recovered) in combination with temozolamide and radiotherapy was used in a Phase I trial of children ≥4 years and adolescents (Jackaki, 2008).

Hodgkin's lymphoma: Infants, Children, and Adolescents: Initial: 130 mg/m^2 as a single dose every 6 weeks (dosage reductions may be recommended for combination chemotherapy regimens): **Note:** Subsequent doses may require adjustment after initial treatment according to platelet and leukocyte counts.

Compromised marrow function: Reduce initial dose to 100 mg/m^2 as a single dose once every 6 weeks

Adult: **Note:** Utilize patient's actual body weight (full weight) for calculation of body surface area- or weight-based dosing, particularly when the intent of therapy is curative; manage regimen-related toxicities in the same manner as for nonobese patients; if a dose reduction is utilized due to toxicity, consider resumption of full weight-based dosing with subsequent cycles, especially if cause of toxicity (eg, hepatic or renal impairment) is resolved (Griggs, 2012).

Brain tumors, Hodgkin's lymphoma: Oral: 130 mg/m^2 as a single dose once every 6 weeks (dosage reductions may be recommended for combination chemotherapy regimens)

Compromised marrow function: Reduce dose to 100 mg/m^2 as a single dose once every 6 weeks

Dosage adjustment based on hematologic response (nadir) for subsequent cycles: Pediatric and Adult patients:

Leukocytes ≥3000/mm^3, platelets ≥75,000/mm^3: No adjustment required

Leukocytes 2000-2999/mm^3, platelets 25,000-74,999/mm^3: Administer 70% of prior dose

Leukocytes <2000/mm^3, platelets <25,000/mm^3: Administer 50% of prior dose

Dosing adjustment in renal impairment: There are no dosage adjustments provided in manufacturer's labeling. The following adjustments have been recommended:

Adults:

Aronoff, 2007:

CrCl >50 mL/minute: No adjustment necessary

CrCl 10-50 mL/minute: Administer 75% of dose

CrCl <10 mL/minute: Administer 25% to 50% of dose

Hemodialysis: Supplemental dose is not necessary

Peritoneal dialysis (PD): Administer 25% to 50% of dose

Kintzel, 1995:

CrCl 46-60 mL/minute: Administer 75% of normal dose

CrCl 31-45 mL/minute: Administer 70% of normal dose

CrCl ≤30 mL/minute: Avoid use

Dosing adjustment in hepatic impairment: There are no dosage adjustments provided in manufacturer's labeling; however, lomustine is hepatically metabolized and caution should be used in patients with hepatic dysfunction.

Administration Hazardous agent; use appropriate precautions for handling and disposal (NIOSH, 2012). Do not break capsules; wear impervious gloves when handling; avoid exposure to broken capsules.

Oral: Administer with fluids on an empty stomach and at bedtime; do not administer food or drink for 2 hours after lomustine administration to decrease incidence of nausea and vomiting. Standard antiemetics may be administered prior to lomustine if needed. Varying strengths of capsules may be required to obtain necessary dose.

Monitoring Parameters CBC with differential and platelet count (for at least 6 weeks after dose), hepatic and renal function tests (periodically), pulmonary function tests (baseline and periodically)

Dosage Forms Excipient information presented when available (limited, particularly for generics); consult specific product labeling.

Capsule, Oral:

Generic: 10 mg, 40 mg, 100 mg

References

Aronoff GR, Bennett WM, Berns JS, et al, *Drug Prescribing in Renal Failure: Dosing Guidelines for Adults and Children*, 5th ed, Philadelphia, PA: American College of Physicians, 2007, 97, 177.

Ater JL, Zhou T, Holmes E, et al. Randomized study of two chemotherapy regimens for treatment of low-grade glioma in young children: a report from the Children's Oncology Group. *J Clin Oncol*. 2012;30 (21):2641-2647.

Berg SL, Grisell DL, DeLaney TF, et al, "Principles of Treatment of Pediatric Solid Tumors," *Pediatr Clin North Am*, 1991, 38(2):249-67.

Griggs JJ, Mangu PB, Anderson H, et al, "Appropriate Chemotherapy Dosing For Obese Adult Patients With Cancer: American Society of Clinical Oncology Clinical Practice Guideline," *J Clin Oncol*, 2012, 30 (13):1553-61.

Jakacki RI, Yates A, Blaney SM, et al, "A Phase I Trial of Temozolomide and Lomustine in Newly Diagnosed High-Grade Gliomas of Childhood," *Neuro Oncol*, 2008, 10(4):569-76.

Kintzel PE and Dorr RT, "Anticancer Drug Renal Toxicity and Elimination: Dosing Guidelines for Altered Renal Function," *Cancer Treat Rev*, 1995, 21(1):33-64.

Lancaster DL, Hoddes JA, Michalski A. Tolerance of nitrosurea-based multiagen chemotherapy regime for low-grade pediatric gliomas. *J Neurooncol*. 2003;63(3):289-294.

Levin VA, Lamborn K, Wara W. Phase II study of 6-thioguanine, procarbazine, dibromodulcitol, lomustine, and vincristine chemotherapy with radiotherapy for treating malignant glioma in children. *Neuro Oncol*. 2000;2(1):22-28.

National Institute for Occupational Safety and Health (NIOSH), "NIOSH List of Antineoplastic and Other Hazardous Drugs in Healthcare Settings 2012." Available at http://www.cdc.gov/niosh/docs/2012-150/pdfs/2012-150.pdf. Accessed January 21, 2013.

Packer RJ, Gajjar A, Vezina G, et al, "Phase III Study of Craniospinal Radiation Therapy Followed by Adjuvant Chemotherapy for Newly Diagnosed Average-Risk Medulloblastoma," *J Clin Oncol*, 2006, 24 (25):4202-8.

Packer RJ, Zhou T, Holmes E, Vezina G, Gajjar A. Survival and secondary tumors in children with medulloblastoma receiving radiotherapy and adjuvant chemotherapy: results of Children's Oncology Group Trial A9961. *Neuro-Oncology*. 2013,15:97-103.

◆ **Lomustinum** *see* Lomustine *on page 1268*

◆ **Longastatin** *see* Octreotide *on page 1518*

◆ **Long Lasting Nasal Spray [OTC]** *see* Oxymetazoline (Nasal) *on page 1577*

◆ **Loniten (Can)** *see* Minoxidil (Systemic) *on page 1422*

◆ **Loperacap (Can)** *see* Loperamide *on page 1270*

Loperamide (loe PER a mide)

Medication Safety Issues

Sound-alike/look-alike issues:

Imodium® A-D may be confused with Indocin®

Loperamide may be confused with furosemide, Lomotil®

International issues:

Indiaral [France] may be confused with Inderal and Inderal LA brand names for propranolol [U.S., Canada, and multiple international markets]

Lomotil: Brand name for loperamide [Mexico, Philippines], but also the brand name for diphenoxylate [U.S., Canada, and multiple international markets]

Lomotil [Mexico, Phillipines] may be confused with Ludiomil brand name for maprotiline [multiple international markets]

Brand Names: U.S. Anti-Diarrheal [OTC]; Diamode [OTC]; Imodium A-D [OTC]; Loperamide A-D [OTC]

Brand Names: Canada Apo-Loperamide®; Diarr-Eze; Dom-Loperamide; Imodium®; Loperacap; Novo-Loperamide; PMS-Loperamine; Rhoxal-loperamide; Rho®-Loperamine; Riva-Loperamide; Sandoz-Loperamide

Therapeutic Category Antidiarrheal

Generic Availability (U.S.) May be product dependent

Use Treatment of acute diarrhea including traveler's diarrhea (FDA approved in ages ≥2 years and adults; OTC use: FDA approved in ages ≥6 years and adults); treatment of chronic diarrhea associated with inflammatory bowel disease (FDA approved in adults); has also been used for chronic functional diarrhea (idiopathic), chronic diarrhea caused by short bowel syndrome or organic lesions; to decrease the volume of ileostomy discharge; management of antiretroviral-induced diarrhea and irinotecan-induced (late-onset) diarrhea

Pregnancy Risk Factor C

Pregnancy Considerations Teratogenic effects were not observed in animal reproduction studies. Information related to loperamide use in pregnancy is limited and data is conflicting (Einarson, 2000; Källén, 2008). For acute diarrhea in pregnant women, some clinicians recommend oral rehydration and dietary changes; loperamide in small amounts may be used only if symptoms are disabling (Wald, 2003).

Breast-Feeding Considerations Small amounts of loperamide are excreted in human breast milk (information is based on studies using loperamide oxide, the prodrug of loperamide [Nikodem, 1992]). The manufacturer does not recommend use in nursing women.

Contraindications Hypersensitivity to loperamide or any component; abdominal pain in the absence of diarrhea

Warnings Loperamide is for symptom-directed use and should not be the primary treatment of acute dysentery (ie, blood in stools, high fever), acute ulcerative colitis, bacterial enterocolitis caused by *Salmonella*, *Shigella*, and *Campylobacter*, or in pseudomembraneous colitis; once underlying diagnosis is made, other disease-specific treatment may be indicated. Should not be used when inhibition of peristalsis is undesirable or dangerous due to potential for ileus, megacolon and/or toxic megacolon. Discontinue therapy if constipation, abdominal distension, blood in stool, or ileus develop. Concurrent fluid and electrolyte replacement is often necessary in all age groups depending upon severity of diarrhea; young pediatric patients are particularly susceptible.

Antidiarrheal agents are not recommended as part of the management of acute gastroenteritis in infants and children because they do not address the underlying cause (ie, do not treat the infection) and have a risk of serious adverse events (CDC, 2003). A meta-analysis evaluating the use of loperamide for adjunct treatment of acute bacterial gastroenteritis in pediatric patients identified that infants and children <3 years, malnourished, moderately to severely dehydrated, or those with bloody diarrhea have a higher risk of serious adverse events (ileus, lethargy, death) even at therapeutic doses (≤0.25 mg/kg/day) and potential benefit does not outweigh risks; use should be avoided in this subset of pediatric patients (Li, 2007). The manufacturer recommends to avoid use in infants and children <2 years. Older children with milder infection and adolescents may see benefit from loperamide therapy including decreased duration of diarrhea and stool counts; monitor closely for adverse effects or worsening of infection (CDC, 2003; Li, 2007).

In HIV-positive or AIDS patients, stop therapy at first signs of abdominal distension; cases of toxic megacolon in these patients have occurred while receiving loperamide for infectious colitis due to viral or bacterial pathogens.

When used for acute diarrhea, notify healthcare provider if symptoms do not improve within 48 hours or sooner if blood appears in stools, or fever or abdominal distention develops; not recommended for self-medication in patients <6 years. Use of the lowest effective dose of loperamide for the shortest duration is recommended.

May cause hypersensitivity reactions; rare cases of anaphylaxis and anaphylactic shock have been reported. May cause drowsiness or dizziness, which may impair physical or mental abilities; patients must be cautioned about performing tasks which require mental alertness (eg, operating machinery or driving).

Some products may contain benzoic acid and sodium benzoate; benzoic acid (benzoate) is a metabolite of benzyl alcohol; large amounts of benzyl alcohol (≥99 mg/kg/day) have been associated with a potentially fatal toxicity ("gasping syndrome") in neonates; *in vitro* and animal studies have shown that benzoate displaces bilirubin from protein binding sites; avoid use in neonates. The chewable tablets may contain milk powder; may cause hypersensitivity reaction in susceptible patients.

Precautions Use with caution in hepatic impairment; first-pass metabolism of loperamide potentially decreased; monitor closely for signs of CNS toxicity

Adverse Reactions

Central nervous system: Dizziness

Gastrointestinal: Abdominal cramping, constipation, nausea

Postmarketing and/or case reports: Abdominal distention, abdominal pain, allergic reactions, anaphylactic shock, anaphylactoid reactions, angioedema, bullous eruption (rare), drowsiness, dyspepsia, erythema multiforme (rare), fatigue, flatulence, hypersensitivity, paralytic ileus, megacolon, pruritus, rash, Stevens-Johnson syndrome (rare), toxic epidermal necrolysis (rare), toxic megacolon, urinary retention, urticaria, vomiting, xerostomia

Drug Interactions

Metabolism/Transport Effects Substrate of P-glycoprotein

Avoid Concomitant Use There are no known interactions where it is recommended to avoid concomitant use.

Increased Effect/Toxicity

The levels/effects of Loperamide may be increased by: P-glycoprotein/ABCB1 Inhibitors

Decreased Effect

The levels/effects of Loperamide may be decreased by: P-glycoprotein/ABCB1 Inducers

Stability

Oral capsules: Store at 15°C to 25°C (59°F to 77°F). Other oral formulations: Store at 20°C to 25°C (68°F to 77°F).

Mechanism of Action Acts directly on circular and longitudinal intestinal muscles, through the opioid receptor, to inhibit peristalsis and prolong transit time; reduces fecal volume, increases viscosity, and diminishes fluid and electrolyte loss; demonstrates antisecretory activity. Loperamide increases tone on the anal sphincter

Pharmacodynamics Onset of action: Within 30-60 minutes

Pharmacokinetics (Adult data unless noted)

Absorption: Rapid; poor; extensive first-pass

Protein binding: 97%

Bioavailability: 0.3%

Metabolism: Hepatic via oxidative N-demethylation to inactive metabolites; primary pathways include CYP2C8, CYP2D6, and CYP3A4

Half-life: Mean range: 14-20 hours

Time to peak serum concentration: Mean range: 4-6 hours

Elimination: Feces (15% to 33%; unchanged drug); urine (1.3%; unchanged drug or metabolites)

Dosing: Usual

Infants, Children, and Adolescents:

Acute diarrhea: Oral: Children ≥2 years and Adolescents: **Note:** For patients small for chronological age, may consider dosing according to weight range and not by age group. Use lowest effective dose for shortest duration.

Children:

2-5 years weighing 13 to <21 kg: Initial: 1 mg with first loose stool followed by 1 mg/dose after each subsequent loose stool; maximum daily dose: 3 mg/**day**

6-8 years weighing 21-27 kg: Initial: 2 mg with first loose stool followed by 1 mg/dose after each subsequent loose stool; maximum daily dose: 4 mg/**day**

9-11 years weighing 27.1-43 kg: Initial: 2 mg with first loose stool followed by 1 mg/dose after each subsequent loose stool; maximum daily dose: 6 mg/**day**

Children ≥12 years and Adolescents: Initial: 4 mg with first loose stool followed by 2 mg/dose after each subsequent loose stool; maximum daily dose: 8 mg/**day**

Chronic diarrhea; secondary to intestinal failure, short-bowel syndrome, or other noninfectious causes: Limited data available; dosing regimens variable: Oral: Infants ≥2 months and Children: 0.08-0.24 mg/kg/day divided 2-3 times/day was reported in a case series of 10 pediatric patients (age range: 2-52 months) (Buts, 1975). In a case-series of six infants and young children, higher dosing was described: Initial: 1-1.5 mg/kg/day in 4 divided doses with subsequent dose decreased as stool output and diet tolerance improved and patient weight increased. Reported final dose range of 0.25-0.5 mg/kg/day in 2 divided doses was used long-term until patient achieved target weight and dietary goals; reported duration of therapy: 6 months to ~2 years (Sandhu, 1983); maximum single dose: 2 mg

Irinotecan-induced (delayed) diarrhea: Limited data available; consult individual protocols; some organizations have used the following:

Fixed dosing (Children's Oncology Group recommendation):

Children ≥2-12 years:

<13 kg: Initial: 0.5 mg after the first loose bowel movement, followed by 0.5 mg every 3 hours while awake; during the night, may administer every 4 hours; maximum daily dose: 4 mg/**day**

13 kg to <20 kg: Initial: 1 mg after the first loose bowel movement, followed by 1 mg every 4 hours; maximum daily dose: 6 mg/**day**

20 kg to <30 kg: Initial: 2 mg after the first loose bowel movement, followed by 1 mg every 3 hours while awake; during the night, may administer every 4 hours; maximum daily dose: 8 mg/**day**

30 kg to <43 kg: Initial: 2 mg after the first loose bowel movement, followed by 1 mg every 2 hours while awake; during the night, may administer every 4 hours; maximum daily dose: 12 mg/**day**

Adolescents weighing ≥43 kg: Initial: 4 mg after the first loose bowel movement, followed by 2 mg after each loose stool; maximum daily dose: 16 mg/**day**

Weight-based dosing: Children and Adolescents 2 to <15 years (Vassal, 2007):

Grade 1 or 2: 0.03 mg/kg/dose every 4 hours

Grade 3 or 4: 0.06 mg/kg/dose every 4 hours

Maximum single dose dependent upon weight

<13 kg: 0.5 mg

13 to <20 kg: 1 mg

20 to <43 kg: Initial: 2 mg; subsequent doses: 1 mg

≥43 kg: Initial: 4 mg; subsequent doses: 2 mg

Adults:

Acute diarrhea: Oral: Initial: 4 mg, followed by 2 mg after each loose stool, up to 16 mg/day

Chronic diarrhea: Oral: Initial: Follow acute diarrhea; maintenance dose should be slowly titrated downward to minimum required to control symptoms (typically, 4-8 mg/day in divided doses)

Traveler's diarrhea: Oral: Initial: 4 mg after first loose stool, followed by 2 mg after each subsequent stool (maximum dose: 8 mg/day)

Dosing adjustment in renal impairment: No adjustment required.

Dosing adjustment in hepatic impairment: There are no dosage adjustments provided in the manufacturer labeling. Due to possible effects on first-pass metabolism, use with caution and monitor closely for signs of CNS toxicity.

Administration Oral: Drink plenty of fluids to help prevent dehydration

Dosage Forms Excipient information presented when available (limited, particularly for generics); consult specific product labeling.

Capsule, Oral, as hydrochloride:

Generic: 2 mg

Liquid, Oral, as hydrochloride:

Imodium A-D: 1 mg/7.5 mL (120 mL, 240 mL) [contains brilliant blue fcf (fd&c blue #1), fd&c yellow #10 (quinoline yellow), propylene glycol, sodium benzoate]

Imodium A-D: 1 mg/7.5 mL (30 mL, 120 mL, 240 mL, 360 mL) [contains brilliant blue fcf (fd&c blue #1), fd&c yellow #10 (quinoline yellow), propylene glycol, sodium benzoate; mint flavor]

Generic: 1 mg/5 mL (5 mL, 10 mL, 118 mL)

Suspension, Oral, as hydrochloride:

Generic: 1 mg/7.5 mL (120 mL)

Tablet, Oral, as hydrochloride:

Anti-Diarrheal: 2 mg

Anti-Diarrheal: 2 mg [scored]

Anti-Diarrheal: 2 mg [contains brilliant blue fcf (fd&c blue #1), fd&c yellow #10 (quinoline yellow)]

Anti-Diarrheal: 2 mg [scored; contains brilliant blue fcf (fd&c blue #1), fd&c yellow #10 (quinoline yellow)]

Anti-Diarrheal: 2 mg [contains fd&c blue #1 aluminum lake, fd&c yellow #10 (quinoline yellow)]

Diamode: 2 mg [scored]

Imodium A-D: 2 mg [scored; contains brilliant blue fcf (fd&c blue #1), fd&c yellow #10 (quinoline yellow)]

Imodium A-D: 2 mg [scored; contains fd&c blue #1 aluminum lake, fd&c yellow #10 aluminum lake]

Loperamide A-D: 2 mg

Tablet Chewable, Oral, as hydrochloride:

Imodium A-D: 2 mg [contains fd&c blue #1 aluminum lake, fd&c yellow #10 aluminum lake; cool mint flavor]

References

Buts JP, Petit BF, and de Meyer R, "Letter: Loperamide in Treatment of Persistent Diarrhoea in Children," Br Med J, 1975, 3(5986):766-7.

Centers for Disease Control and Prevention (CDC), "Managing Acute Gastroenteritis Among Children: Oral Rehydration, Maintenance, and Nutritional Therapy," MMWR Recomm Rep, 2003, 52(RR-16):1-16.

Einarson A, Mastroiacovo P, Arnon J, et al, "Prospective, Controlled, Multicentre Study of Loperamide in Pregnancy," Can J Gastroenterol, 2000, 14(3):185-7.

Hamdi I and Dodge JA, "Toddler Diarrhoea: Observations on the Effects of Aspirin and Loperamide," J Pediatr Gastroenterol Nutr, 1985, 4 (3):362-5.

Källén B, Nilsson E, and Otterblad Olausson P, "Maternal Use of Loperamide in Early Pregnancy and Delivery Outcome," Acta Paediatr, 2008, 97(5):541-5.

Li ST, Grossman DC, and Cummings P, "Loperamide Therapy for Acute Diarrhea in Children: Systematic Review and Meta-analysis," PLoS Med, 2007, 4(3):e98.

Nikodem VC and Hofmeyr GJ, "Secretion of the Antidiarrhoeal Agent Loperamide Oxide in Breast Milk," Eur J Clin Pharmacol, 1992, 42 (6):695-6.

Sandhu BK, Tripp JH, Milla PJ, et al, "Loperamide in Severe Protracted Diarrhoea," Arch Dis Child, 1983, 58(1):39-43.

Vassal G, Couanet D, Stockdale E, et al, "Phase II Trial of Irinotecan in Children With Relapsed or Refractory Rhabdomyosarcoma: A Joint Study of the French Society of Pediatric Oncology and the United Kingdom Children's Cancer Study Group," J Clin Oncol, 2007, 25 (4):356-61.

Wald A, "Constipation, Diarrhea, and Symptomatic Hemorrhoids During Pregnancy," Gastroenterol Clin North Am, 2003, 32(1):309-22.

◆ **Loperamide A-D [OTC]** see Loperamide on page 1270

◆ **Loperamide Hydrochloride** see Loperamide on page 1270

Lopinavir and Ritonavir

(loe PIN a veer & ri TOE na vir)

Medication Safety Issues

Sound-alike/look-alike issues:

Potential for dispensing errors between Kaletra® and Keppra® (levETIRAcetam)

Administration issues:

Children's doses are based on weight and calculated by milligrams of lopinavir. Care should be taken to accurately calculate the dose. The oral solution contains lopinavir 80 mg and ritonavir 20 mg per one mL. Children <12 years of age (and ≤40 kg) who are not taking certain concomitant antiretroviral medications will receive <5 mL of solution per dose.

Related Information

Adult and Adolescent HIV on page 2348

Oral Medications That Should Not Be Crushed or Altered on page 2438

Pediatric HIV on page 2338

Perinatal HIV on page 2356

Brand Names: U.S. Kaletra

Brand Names: Canada Kaletra

Therapeutic Category Antiretroviral Agent; HIV Agents (Anti-HIV Agents); Protease Inhibitor

Generic Availability (U.S.) No

Use Treatment of HIV infection in combination with other antiretroviral agents (FDA approved in ages ≥14 days and adults); **Note:** HIV regimens consisting of three antiretroviral agents are strongly recommended.

Medication Guide Available Yes

Pregnancy Risk Factor C

Pregnancy Considerations Adverse events were not seen in animal reproduction studies, except at doses which were also maternally toxic. Lopinavir/ritonavir has a low level of transfer across the placenta. Based on information collected by the Antiretroviral Pregnancy Registry, an increased risk of teratogenic effects has not been observed in humans. The DHHS Perinatal HIV Guidelines consider lopinavir/ritonavir to be a preferred protease inhibitor for use in antiretroviral-naive pregnant women. Due to a decrease in bioavailability, a dose increase is suggested during the second and third trimesters of pregnancy, especially in PI-experienced women. Monitor virologic response (and lopinavir serum concentrations if available) if the standard dose is used. Once-daily dosing is not recommended during pregnancy. A small increased risk of preterm birth has been associated with maternal use of protease inhibitor-based combination antiretroviral (ARV) therapy during pregnancy; however, the benefits of use generally outweigh this risk and protease inhibitors (PIs) should not be withheld if otherwise recommended. Hyperglycemia, new onset of diabetes mellitus, or diabetic ketoacidosis have been reported with PIs; it is not clear if pregnancy increases this risk.

Regardless of CD4 count or HIV RNA copy number, all HIV-infected pregnant women should receive a combination antiretroviral ARV drug regimen. A combination of antepartum, intrapartum, and infant ARV prophylaxis is recommended. ARV therapy should be started as soon as possible in women with symptomatic infection. Although earlier initiation may be more effective in reducing the perinatal transmission of HIV, initiation may be delayed until after 12 weeks gestation in women who do not require immediate treatment after careful consideration of maternal conditions (eg, nausea and vomiting) and the potential risks of first trimester fetal exposure for specific agents. A scheduled cesarean delivery at 38 weeks gestation is recommended for all women with HIV RNA >1000 copies/mL or unknown concentrations near delivery in order to decrease transmission. If ARV therapy must be interrupted for <24 hours during the peripartum period, stop then restart all medications simultaneously in order to decrease the chance of developing resistance. Long-term follow-up is recommended for all infants exposed to ARV medications. In couples who want to conceive, the HIV-infected partner should attain maximum viral suppression prior to conception..

Health care providers are encouraged to enroll pregnant women exposed to antiretroviral medications in the Antiretroviral Pregnancy Registry (1-800-258-4263 or www.-APRegistry.com). Health care providers caring for HIV-infected women and their infants may contact the National Perinatal HIV Hotline (888-448-8765) for clinical consultation (DHHS [perinatal], 2014).

Breast-Feeding Considerations Lopinavir/ritonavir concentrations are very low to undetectable in breast milk and undetectable in the serum of nursing infants. Maternal or infant antiretroviral therapy does not completely eliminate the risk of postnatal HIV transmission. In addition, multiclass-resistant virus has been detected in breast-feeding infants despite maternal therapy. Therefore, in the United States, where formula is accessible, affordable, safe, and

sustainable, and the risk of infant mortality due to diarrhea and respiratory infections is low, complete avoidance of breast-feeding by HIV-infected women is recommended to decrease potential transmission of HIV (DHHS [perinatal], 2014).

Contraindications Hypersensitivity (eg, Stevens-Johnson syndrome, erythema multiforme, toxic epidermal necrolysis, urticaria, angioedema) to lopinavir, ritonavir, or any component; concurrent therapy with medications that largely rely on cytochrome P450 isoenzymes CYP3A for clearance and that have an association between increased plasma concentrations and serious or life-threatening effects [eg, alfuzosin, cisapride, dihydroergotamine, ergonovine, ergotamine, lovastatin, methylergonovine, midazolam (oral), pimozide, sildenafil (when used for pulmonary arterial hypertension), simvastatin, triazolam]; concurrent therapy with strong CYP3A4 inducers that significantly decrease lopinavir serum concentrations which may lead to treatment failure or development of resistance or cross-resistance [eg, rifampin or the herbal medicine St John's wort (*Hypericum perforatum*)]

Once-daily dosing: Adult patients with ≥3 lopinavir-resistance-associated substitutions (L10F/I/R/V, K20M/N/R, L24I, L33F, M36I, I47V, G48V, I54L/T/V, V82A/C/F/S/T, and I84V); those receiving fosamprenavir, efavirenz, nevirapine, or nelfinavir, carbamazepine, phenobarbital, phenytoin, or in children <18 years of age

Warnings Lopinavir and ritonavir are potent CYP3A isoenzyme inhibitors that interact with numerous drugs. Due to potential serious and/or life-threatening drug interactions, some drugs are contraindicated and other medications may require concentration monitoring or dosage adjustment if coadministered with lopinavir and ritonavir. Concomitant use with certain medications may require dosage adjustment of lopinavir and ritonavir.

Potentially fatal pancreatitis may occur; markedly elevated serum triglycerides is a risk factor for developing pancreatitis; advanced HIV disease or a history of pancreatitis may also place patients at increased risk; discontinue lopinavir and ritonavir therapy if clinical signs, symptoms, or laboratory abnormalities suggestive of pancreatitis occur. New onset diabetes mellitus, exacerbations of diabetes, and hyperglycemia have been reported in HIV-infected patients receiving protease inhibitors. Possible higher risk of myocardial infarction associated with the cumulative use of lopinavir/ritonavir has been reported (DHHS, [adult] 2014).

Serious cardiac, renal, CNS, or respiratory problems have been reported in preterm neonates receiving lopinavir/ritonavir oral solution. The oral solution contains 42.4% ethanol (v/v) and 15.3% propylene glycol (w/v). Ethanol competitively inhibits propylene glycol metabolism, which may lead to propylene glycol toxicity due to impaired elimination in neonates. Preterm neonates are at an increased risk of adverse events from propylene glycol toxicity, including cardiotoxicity (complete AV block, bradycardia, cardiomyopathy), lactic acidosis, CNS depression, respiratory complications, acute renal failure, and death. Do not use oral solution in neonates if the patient is either PNA <14 days old or PMA <42 weeks. Toxicities have been reported with the use of products containing propylene glycol in all ages, including hyperosmolality, lactic acidosis, seizures, and respiratory depression. Due to concentration of ethanol in oral solution, an overdose in a child may cause potentially lethal alcohol toxicity. Treatment for overdose should be supportive and include general poisoning management; activated charcoal may help remove unabsorbed medication; dialysis unlikely to be of benefit; however, dialysis can remove alcohol and propylene glycol. In pediatric patients 14 days to 6 months of age, the total amounts of ethanol and propylene glycol delivered from all medications should be considered to

◀ avoid toxicity. Neonates and young infants should be closely monitored for increases in serum osmolality, serum creatinine, and other signs of propylene glycol toxicity (eg, CNS depression, seizures, cardiac arrhythmias, hemolysis); in neonates particularly, symptoms should be distinguished from sepsis.

A fatal accidental overdose occurred in a 2.1 kg, 44-day old infant (born at 30 weeks gestational age) with HIV who received a single dose of 6.5 mL of lopinavir/ritonavir oral solution. The infant died of cardiogenic shock 9 days later. Healthcare providers are reminded that lopinavir/ritonavir oral solution is highly concentrated. To minimize the risk for medication errors, healthcare providers should pay special attention to accurate calculation of the dose, transcription of the medication order, dispensing information, dosing instructions, and proper measurement of the dose. New pediatric tablets containing lopinavir 100 mg and ritonavir 25 mg (ie, 1/2 the amount in regular tablets) are now available; caution should be taken so that dosing and dispensing errors do not occur.

Precautions Use with caution in patients with hepatic impairment (lopinavir and ritonavir are primarily metabolized by the liver); hepatitis or markedly elevated transaminases prior to therapy may increase risk for developing or worsening elevations in liver enzymes or for hepatic decompensation; hepatic dysfunction (including fatalities) have been reported; in general, these occurred in patients with advanced HIV disease who were taking multiple concomitant medications and who had underlying chronic hepatitis or cirrhosis; a causal relationship with lopinavir/ritonavir has not been established; monitor liver enzymes prior to therapy and periodically during treatment; consider more frequent monitoring of liver enzymes in patients with concurrent chronic hepatitis or cirrhosis, especially during the first few months of lopinavir/ritonavir therapy.

May alter cardiac conduction and prolong the QT_c and/or PR interval; second and third degree AV block and torsade de pointes have been observed; use with caution in patients with underlying structural heart disease, preexisting conduction system abnormalities, ischemic heart disease, or cardiomyopathies. Avoid use in combination with QT_c- or PR-interval prolonging drugs or in patients with hypokalemia or congenital long-QT syndrome. Spontaneous bleeding episodes have been reported in patients with hemophilia type A and B receiving protease inhibitors. Large increases in total cholesterol (incidence: 3% to 19%; children: 3%) and triglycerides (incidence: 4% to 36%) have been reported; patients should be monitored prior to therapy and periodically during treatment.

Immune reconstitution syndrome (an acute inflammatory response to residual or indolent opportunistic infections) may occur in HIV patients during initial treatment with combination antiretroviral agents; this syndrome may require further patient assessment and therapy. Autoimmune disorders (eg, Graves' disease, Guillain-Barré syndrome, and polymyositis) have been reported in patients experiencing immune reconstitution; time to onset is variable and may occur many months after antiretroviral treatment is initiated.

Fat redistribution and accumulation [ie, central obesity, peripheral wasting, facial wasting, breast enlargement, dorsocervical fat enlargement (buffalo hump), and cushingoid appearance] have been observed in patients receiving antiretroviral agents (causal relationship not established).

May cause diarrhea (5% to 28%; children: 12%); in one adult study, incidence of diarrhea was higher in patients receiving once-daily dosing compared to twice-daily dosing. Children may have a higher incidence of vomiting (21% vs ≤6%). May cause taste perversion in children (incidence: 22%).

Adverse Reactions Data presented for short- and long-term combination antiretroviral therapy in both protease inhibitor experienced and naïve patients.

Cardiovascular: Vasodilation

Central nervous system: Anxiety, fatigue, headache, insomnia

Dermatologic: Rash (more common in children), skin infection (including cellulitis, folliculitis, furuncle)

Endocrine & metabolic: Hypercholesterolemia, hyperglycemia, hypertriglyceridemia, hyperuricemia, sodium decreased or increased (children), triglycerides increased

Gastrointestinal: Abdominal pain, abnormal taste/taste perversion (more common in children), amylase increased diarrhea, dyspepsia, flatulence, gastroenteritis, lipase increased, nausea, vomiting (more common in children), weight loss

Hematologic: Neutropenia, platelets decreased (children)

Hepatic: ALT increased, AST increased, bilirubin increased (more common in children), GGT increased, hepatitis (including increased AST, ALT, and gamma-glutamyl transferase)

Hypersensitivity: Hypersensitivity (including urticaria and angioedema)

Neuromuscular & skeletal: Musculoskeletal pain, weakness

Respiratory: Lower respiratory tract infection, upper respiratory tract infection

Rare but important or life-threatening: Abnormal vision, acne, allergic reaction, alopecia, amenorrhea, amnesia, anemia, anorexia, asthma, ataxia, atherosclerotic disease, atrial fibrillation, atrioventricular block, AV block (second and third degree), avitaminosis, bacterial infection, benign neoplasm, body fat redistribution (including facial wasting), bone necrosis, bradyarrhythmia, breast enlargement, bronchitis, cerebral infarction, cerebrovascular accident, chest pain, cholangitis, cholecystitis, confusion, constipation, creatinine clearance decreased, Cushing's syndrome, cyst, deep vein thrombosis, dehydration, depression, diabetes mellitus, duodenitis, dyskinesia, eczema, edema, encephalopathy, enteritis, enterocolitis, erythema multiforme, esophagitis, exfoliative dermatitis, extrapyramidal symptoms, facial edema, facial paralysis, fatty deposits, fecal incontinence, gastritis, gastrointestinal hemorrhage, gastrointestinal ulcer, GERD, glucose intolerance, gynecomastia, hematuria, hemorrhagic colitis, hemorrhoids, hepatic dysfunction, hepatomegaly, hyperacusis, hyperhidrosis, hypermenorrhea, hypertension, hypertonia, hypertrophy, hypogonadism (males), hypothyroidism, immune reconstitution syndrome, impotence, inorganic phosphorus decreased, jaundice, lactic acidosis, leukopenia, liver steatosis, liver tenderness, lung edema, lymphadenopathy, maculopapular rash, MI, migraine, mouth ulceration, neoplasm, nephritis, neuropathy, obesity, orthostatic hypotension, otitis media, pancreatitis, periodontitis, peripheral edema, peripheral neuropathy, propylene glycol toxicity (preterm neonates [includes cardiomyopathy, lactic acidosis, acute renal failure, respiratory complications]), PR prolongation, QT prolongation, rectal hemorrhage, renal failure, rhabdomyolysis, seborrhea, seizure, sialadenitis, skin discoloration, skin ulcer, splenomegaly, Stevens-Johnson syndrome, stomatitis, striae, thrombophlebitis, torsade de pointes, tricuspid regurgitation, vasculitis, viral infection, weight gain

Drug Interactions

Metabolism/Transport Effects Refer to individual components.

Avoid Concomitant Use

Avoid concomitant use of Lopinavir and Ritonavir with any of the following: Ado-Trastuzumab Emtansine; Alfuzosin; Amiodarone; Apixaban; Atovaquone; Avanafil; Axitinib; Bosutinib; Cabozantinib; Ceritinib; Cisapride; Conivaptan; Crizotinib; Darunavir; Disulfiram; Dronedarone; Enzalutamide; Eplerenone; Ergot Derivatives; Etravirine; Everolimus; Flecainide; Fluticasone (Nasal); Fusidic Acid (Systemic); Halofantrine; Highest Risk QTc-Prolonging Agents; Ibrutinib; Ivabradine; Lapatinib; Lomitapide; Lovastatin; Lurasidone; Macitentan; Methadone; Midazolam; Mifepristone; Moderate Risk QTc-Prolonging Agents; Nilotinib; Nisoldipine; PAZOPanib; Pimozide; Propafenone; QuiNIDine; QuiNINE; Ranolazine; Red Yeast Rice; Regorafenib; Rifampin; Rivaroxaban; Salmeterol; Silodosin; Simeprevir; Simvastatin; St Johns Wort; Tamoxifen; Tamsulosin; Telaprevir; Thioridazine; Ticagrelor; Tipranavir; Tolvaptan; Topotecan; Toremifene; TraZODone; Triazolam; Uliprstal; Vemurafenib; VinCRIStine (Liposomal); Vorapaxar; Voriconazole

Increased Effect/Toxicity

Lopinavir and Ritonavir may increase the levels/effects of: Ado-Trastuzumab Emtansine; Afatinib; Alfuzosin; Almotriptan; Alosetron; ALPRAZolam; Amiodarone; Apixaban; ARIPiprazole; AtoMOXetine; AtorvaSTATin; Avanafil; Axitinib; Bosentan; Bosutinib; Brentuximab Vedotin; Brinzolamide; Budesonide (Nasal); Budesonide (Systemic, Oral Inhalation); Cabozantinib; Calcium Channel Blockers (Dihydropyridine); Calcium Channel Blockers (Nondihydropyridine); Cannabis; Ceritinib; Cisapride; Colchicine; Conivaptan; Contraceptives (Progestins); Corticosteroids (Orally Inhaled); Crizotinib; Cyclophosphamide; CycloSPORINE (Systemic); CYP2C8 Substrates; CYP2D6 Substrates; CYP3A4 Substrates; Dabigatran Etexilate; Digoxin; DOXOrubicin (Conventional); Dronabinol; Dronedarone; Dutasteride; Enfuvirtide; Enzalutamide; Eplerenone; Ergot Derivatives; Estazolam; Everolimus; FentaNYL; Fesoterodine; Flecainide; Fluticasone (Nasal); Fluticasone (Oral Inhalation); Fusidic Acid (Systemic); GuanFACINE; Halofantrine; Highest Risk QTc-Prolonging Agents; Ibrutinib; Imatinib; Itraconazole; Ivabradine; Ivacaftor; Ixabepilone; Ketoconazole (Systemic); Lacosamide; Lapatinib; Levomilnacipran; Linagliptin; Lomitapide; Lovastatin; Lurasidone; Macitentan; Maraviroc; Meperidine; MethylPREDNISolone; Metoprolol; Midazolam; Nebivolol; Nefazodone; Nelfinavir; Nilotinib; Nisoldipine; Ospemifene; OxyCODONE; Paricalcitol; PAZOPanib; P-glycoprotein/ABCB1 Substrates; Pimecrolimus; Pimozide; Pioglitazone; PONATinib; PrednisoLONE (Systemic); PredniSONE; Propafenone; Protease Inhibitors; Prucalopride; QuiNIDine; QuiNINE; Ranolazine; Red Yeast Rice; Regorafenib; Rifabutin; Rifaximin; Rilpivirine; Riociguat; Rivaroxaban; Rosuvastatin; Ruxolitinib; Salmeterol; Saxagliptin; Sildenafil; Silodosin; Simeprevir; Simvastatin; Tacrolimus (Systemic); Tacrolimus (Topical); Tadalafil; Tamsulosin; Temsirolimus; Tenofovir; Tetrahydrocannabinol; Thioridazine; Ticagrelor; Tofacitinib; Tolterodine; Tolvaptan; Topotecan; Toremifene; TraZODone; Treprostinil; Triamcinolone (Systemic); Triazolam; Uliprstal; Vardenafil; Vemurafenib; Vilazodone; VinBLAStine; VinCRIStine; VinCRIStine (Liposomal); Vorapaxar; Vortioxetine

The levels/effects of Lopinavir and Ritonavir may be increased by: ARIPiprazole; CycloSPORINE (Systemic); Delavirdine; Disulfiram; Enfuvirtide; Fusidic Acid (Systemic); Ivabradine; Ketoconazole (Systemic); Methadone; MetroNIDAZOLE (Topical); Mifepristone; Moderate Risk QTc-Prolonging Agents; P-glycoprotein/ABCB1 Inhibitors; QTc-Prolonging Agents (Indeterminate Risk and Risk Modifying); QuiNINE; Rifabutin; Rifampin; Simeprevir

Decreased Effect

Lopinavir and Ritonavir may decrease the levels/effects of: Abacavir; Atovaquone; Axitinib; Boceprevir; BuPROPion; Canagliflozin; Codeine; Contraceptives (Estrogens); Contraceptives (Progestins); CYP2C19 Substrates; Darunavir; Deferasirox; Delavirdine; Didanosine; Etravirine; Fosphenytoin; LamoTRIgine; Meperidine; Methadone; Phenytoin; Prasugrel; Proguanil; QuiNINE; Simeprevir; Tamoxifen; Telaprevir; Ticagrelor; Valproic Acid and Derivatives; Voriconazole; Warfarin; Zidovudine

The levels/effects of Lopinavir and Ritonavir may be decreased by: Antacids; Boceprevir; Bosentan; CarBAMazepine; CYP3A4 Inducers (Strong); Dabrafenib; Efavirenz; Fosamprenavir; Fosphenytoin; Garlic; Mitotane; Nelfinavir; Nevirapine; Peginterferon Alfa-2b; P-glycoprotein/ABCB1 Inducers; PHENobarbital; Phenytoin; Rifampin; Siltuximab; St Johns Wort; Tipranavir; Tocilizumab

Food Interactions Moderate- to high-fat meals increase the C_{max} and AUC of lopinavir/ritonavir oral solution; no significant changes observed with oral tablets. Management: Take oral solution with food; take tablet with or without food.

Stability

Oral solution: Store at 2°C to 8°C (36°F to 46°F) until dispensed; refrigerated products are stable until labeled expiration date; stability at room temperature: 2 months; avoid exposure to excessive heat.

Tablets: Store at 20°C to 25°C (68°F to 77°F). Dispense in original container or USP equivalent tight container. Do not expose to high humidity outside original container or USP equivalent tight container for >2 weeks.

Mechanism of Action A coformulation of lopinavir and ritonavir. The lopinavir component binds to the site of HIV-1 protease activity and inhibits the cleavage of viral Gag-Pol polyprotein precursors into individual functional proteins required for infectious HIV. This results in the formation of immature, noninfectious viral particles. The ritonavir component inhibits the CYP3A metabolism of lopinavir, allowing increased plasma levels of lopinavir.

Pharmacokinetics (Adult data unless noted) Information below refers to Lopinavir; see Ritonavir for additional information.

Protein binding: 98% to 99%; binds to both alpha$_1$ - acid glycoprotein and albumin; higher affinity for alpha$_1$-acid glycoprotein; decreased protein binding in patients with mild to moderate hepatic impairment

Metabolism: Primarily oxidative, via cytochrome P450 CYP3A isoenzyme; 13 oxidative metabolites identified; may induce its own metabolism

Bioavailability: Absolute bioavailability not established; AUC for oral solution was 22% lower than capsule when given under fasting conditions; concentrations were similar under nonfasting conditions

Half-life: Mean: 5 to 6 hours

Elimination: 2.2% of dose eliminated unchanged in urine; 83% of dose eliminated in feces

Clearance: (Apparent oral): 6 to 7 L/hour

Dialysis: Unlikely to remove significant amounts of drug (due to high protein binding)

Dosing: Neonatal HIV infection, treatment: Oral: Use in combination with other antiretroviral agents: **Note:** Dosage is based on patient body weight or surface area and is presented here based on lopinavir component. **Once daily dosing has not been studied in neonates, and therefore, is not recommended.**

PNA <14 days or PMA <42 weeks: Do not use due to potential toxicity from excipients; no data about appropriate dose or safety exists (DHHS [pediatric], 2014)

PNA ≥14 days and PMA ≥42 weeks:

Patients receiving concomitant antiretroviral therapy **without efavirenz, fosamprenavir, nelfinavir, or nevirapine***:*

Manufacturer's labeling: Lopinavir 16 mg/kg/dose or 300 mg/m²/dose twice daily

AIDS*Info* guidelines (DHHS [pediatric], 2014): Lopinavir 300 mg/m²/dose twice daily

Note: Neonates who receive the 300 mg/m²/dose twice daily may have lower serum trough concentrations compared to adults; evaluate neonates and adjust dose for incremental growth at frequent intervals (DHHS [pediatric], 2014).

Patients receiving concomitant antiretroviral therapy **with** *efavirenz, fosamprenavir, nelfinavir, or nevirapine:* Dosage information does not exist; lopinavir/ritonavir is not recommended in neonates who are receiving these agents.

Dosing: Usual

Pediatric: **HIV infection, treatment:** Oral: Use in combination with other antiretroviral agents: **Note:** Pediatric dosage is based on patient body weight or surface area and is presented here based on lopinavir component. **Do not exceed recommended adult dose.** Use of tablets in patients <15 kg or <0.6 m² is **not** recommended (use oral solution). **Once daily dosing in pediatric patients is not recommended**; in a study of treatment experienced children, once daily dosing resulted in a lower trough concentration and less virological control (Foissac, 2011)

Infants 1 to 6 months:

Patients receiving concomitant antiretroviral therapy **without** *efavirenz, fosamprenavir, nelfinavir, or nevirapine:* Lopinavir 16 mg/kg/dose or 300 mg/m²/dose twice daily. **Note:** Infants who receive 300 mg/m²/dose twice daily may have lower trough concentrations compared to adults; evaluate infants and adjust dose for incremental growth at frequent intervals (DHHS [pediatric], 2014).

Patients receiving concomitant antiretroviral therapy **with** *efavirenz, fosamprenavir, nelfinavir, or nevirapine:* Dosage information does not exist; lopinavir/ritonavir is not recommended in infants ≤6 months of age who are receiving these agents.

Infants >6 months, Children, and Adolescents:

Patients receiving concomitant antiretroviral therapy **without** *efavirenz, fosamprenavir, nelfinavir, or nevirapine*:

BSA-directed dosing:

Manufacturer's labeling: Lopinavir 230 mg/m²/dose twice daily; maximum dose: 400 mg/dose

Alternate fixed dosing for patients who are able to swallow tablets:

BSA ≥0.6 to <0.9 m²: Lopinavir 200 mg twice daily

BSA ≥0.9 to <1.4 m²: Lopinavir 300 mg twice daily

BSA ≥1.4 m²: Lopinavir 400 mg twice daily

AIDS*Info* guidelines (DHHS [pediatric], 2014):

Infants >6 to 12 months: Lopinavir 300 mg/m²/dose twice daily; **Note:** Infants who receive 300 mg/m²/dose twice daily may have lower trough concentrations compared to adults; evaluate infants and adjust dose for incremental growth at frequent intervals

Children and Adolescents >12 months to 18 years:

Antiretroviral-naïve: Lopinavir 230 mg/m²/dose (maximum dose: 400 mg) twice daily; others have suggested 300 mg/m²/dose twice daily if the oral solution is used. **Note:** For patients already receiving lopinavir and ritonavir, an immediate dosage reduction at 12 months of age is **not** recommended; patients are allowed

to "grow into" the 230 mg/m²/dose dosage as they gain weight over time.

Antiretroviral-experienced or suspected decreased sensitivity to lopinavir: Lopinavir 300 mg/m²/dose (maximum dose: 400 mg) twice daily

Weight-directed dosing:

<15 kg: Lopinavir 12 mg/kg/dose twice daily

≥15 to 40 kg: Lopinavir 10 mg/kg/dose twice daily

>40 kg: Lopinavir 400 mg twice daily

Fixed dosing for patients who are able to swallow tablets: AIDS*Info* guidelines (DHHS [pediatric], 2014):

Antiretroviral-naïve: Weight band dosing to give ~230 mg/m²/dose:

≥15 to 25 kg: Lopinavir 200 mg twice daily

>25 to 35 kg: Lopinavir 300 mg twice daily

>35 kg: Lopinavir 400 mg twice daily

Antiretroviral-experienced or suspected decreased sensitivity to lopinavir: Weight band dosing to give ~300 mg/m²/dose:

15 to 20 kg: 200 mg twice daily

>20 to 30 kg: 300 mg twice daily

>30 to 45 kg: 400 mg twice daily

>45 kg: 400 mg or 500 mg twice daily

Patients receiving concomitant antiretroviral therapy **with** *efavirenz, fosamprenavir, nelfinavir, or nevirapine (or treatment-experienced patients not receiving these agents who have suspected decreased susceptibility to lopinavir):*

BSA-directed dosing:

Manufacturer's labeling: Lopinavir 300 mg/m²/dose twice daily; maximum single lopinavir dose: Oral solution: 533 mg; Tablet: 500 mg

Alternative dosing for patients who are able to swallow tablets:

BSA ≥0.6 to <0.8 m²: Lopinavir 200 mg twice daily

BSA ≥0.8 to <1.2 m²: Lopinavir 300 mg twice daily

BSA ≥1.2 to <1.7 m²: Lopinavir 400 mg twice daily

BSA ≥1.7 m²: Lopinavir 500 mg twice daily; **Note:** Therapy-experienced patients in whom decreased susceptibility to lopinavir is suspected or confirmed may receive lopinavir 600 mg twice daily (DHHS [pediatric], 2014).

AIDS*Info* guidelines (DHHS [pediatric], 2014): Lopinavir 300 mg/m²/dose twice daily; maximum single lopinavir dose: Oral solution: 533 mg; Tablet: 500 mg

Weight-directed dosing:

<15 kg: Lopinavir 13 mg/kg/dose twice daily

≥15 to 45 kg: Lopinavir 11 mg/kg/dose twice daily

>45 kg:

Oral solution: Lopinavir 533 mg (6.5 mL) twice daily

Tablets: Lopinavir 500 mg twice daily

Fixed dosing for patients who are able to swallow tablets:

≥15 to 20 kg: Lopinavir 200 mg twice daily

>20 to 30 kg: Lopinavir 300 mg twice daily

>30 to 45 kg: Lopinavir 400 mg twice daily

>45 kg: Lopinavir 400 mg or 500 mg twice daily; **Note:** Therapy-experienced patients in whom decreased susceptibility to lopinavir is suspected or confirmed may receive lopinavir 600 mg twice daily (DHHS [pediatric], 2014).

Adult: **HIV infection, treatment:** Oral: Use in combination with other antiretroviral agents:

*Patients receiving concomitant antiretroviral therapy **without efavirenz, fosamprenavir, nelfinavir, or nevirapine:***

Therapy-naïve or therapy-experienced: Lopinavir 400 mg/ritonavir 100 mg twice daily.

Once-daily dosing: **Antiretroviral-naïve patients or experienced patients with <3 lopinavir resistance-associated amino acid substitutions in protease enzyme:** Lopinavir 800 mg/ritonavir 200 mg once daily

Note: Once daily dosing is **not** recommended for antiretroviral-experienced patients with ≥3 lopinavir-resistance-associated substitutions (L10F/I/R/V, K20M/N/R, L24I, L33F, M36I, I47V, G48V, I54L/T/V, V82A/C/F/S/T, and I84V), or for patients receiving efavirenz, fosamprenavir, nelfinavir, nevirapine, carbamazepine, phenobarbital, or phenytoin; once daily dosing has not been evaluated with concurrent use of indinavir or saquinavir

*Dosing adjustment for combination therapy **with efavirenz, fosamprenavir, nelfinavir, or nevirapine: Note:*** Once daily dosing is **not** recommended:

Oral solution: Lopinavir 533 mg/ritonavir 133 mg (6.5 mL) twice daily

Tablets: Lopinavir 500 mg/ritonavir 125 mg twice daily

Dosing adjustment in renal impairment: Has not been studied in patients with renal impairment; however, a decrease in clearance is not expected. Avoid once daily dosing in patients on hemodialysis (DHHS [adult], 2014).

Dosing adjustment in hepatic impairment: Lopinavir AUC may be increased ~30% in patients with mild to moderate hepatic impairment; use with caution. No data available in patients with severe impairment.

Administration Oral:

Oral solution: Administer with food to enhance bioavailability and decrease kinetic variability; use a calibrated oral dosing syringe to measure and administer the oral solution; **Note:** Dose must be accurately measured and administered to pediatric patients as oral solution is very concentrated and a fatal accidental overdose has been reported

Methods to improve poor palatability of the oral solution include numbing the taste buds with ice chips before or after drug administration, or administering the medication with sweet or tangy foods, chocolate syrup, or peanut butter to help mask the taste; flavoring the solution prior to dispensing may also help improve palatability (DHHS [pediatric], 2014).

Tablets: May be administered without regard to meals; swallow tablets whole, do not crush, break, or chew; crushing tablets was shown to decrease AUC of lopinavir and ritonavir by 45% and 47%, respectively (Best, 2011)

Monitoring Parameters Note: Monitor CD4 percentage (if <5 years of age) or CD4 count (if ≥5 years of age) at least every 3 to 4 months (DHHS [pediatric], 2014).

Prior to initiation of therapy: Genotypic resistance testing, CD4 and viral load (every 3 to 4 months), CBC with differential, LFTs, BUN, creatinine, electrolytes, glucose, urinalysis (every 6 to 12 months), and assessment of readiness for adherence with medication regimen. At initiation and with any change in treatment regimen: CBC with differential, electrolytes, calcium, phosphate, glucose, LFTs, bilirubin, urinalysis (at initiation), BUN, creatinine, albumin, total protein, lipid panel (at initiation), CD4, and viral load. After 1 to 2 weeks of therapy: Signs of medication toxicity and adherence. After 2 to 4 weeks of therapy: CBC with differential, viral load, signs of medication toxicity, and adherence; then every 3 to 4 months: CBC with differential, electrolytes, glucose, LFTs, bilirubin,

BUN, creatinine, CD4, viral load, signs of medication toxicity, and adherence. Every 6 to 12 months: Lipid panel and urinalysis. CD4 monitoring frequency may be decreased to every 6 to 12 months in children who are adherent to therapy if the value is well above the threshold for opportunistic infections, viral suppression is sustained, and the clinical status is stable for more than 2 to 3 years (DHHS [pediatric], 2014). Monitor for growth and development, signs of HIV-specific physical conditions, HIV disease progression, opportunistic infections or pancreatitis.

Due to potential toxicity from excipients in the oral solution, in pediatric patients 14 days to 6 months of age, the total amounts of ethanol and propylene glycol delivered from all medications should be monitored to avoid toxicity. Neonates and young infants should be closely monitored for increases in serum osmolality, serum creatinine, and other signs of propylene glycol toxicity (eg, CNS depression, seizures, cardiac arrhythmias, hemolysis); in neonates particularly, symptoms should be distinguished from sepsis.

Reference Range Plasma trough concentration: Lopinavir: ≥1000 ng/mL (DHHS [adult, pediatric], 2014)

Additional Information Preliminary studies have reported response rates (defined as viral loads <400 copies/mL) of 91%, 81%, and 33% for patients with 0 to 5, 6 to 7, and 8 to 10 protease mutations at baseline, respectively (Hurst, 2000).

Dosage Forms Excipient information presented when available (limited, particularly for generics); consult specific product labeling.

Solution, oral:

Kaletra: Lopinavir 80 mg and ritonavir 20 mg per 1 mL (160 mL) [contains ethanol 42.4%, menthol, propylene glycol; cotton candy flavor]]

Tablet:

Kaletra:

Lopinavir 100 mg and ritonavir 25 mg

Lopinavir 200 mg and ritonavir 50 mg

References

American Academy of Pediatrics Committee on Drugs. "Inactive" ingredients in pharmaceutical products: update (subject review). *Pediatrics.* 1997;99(2):268-278.

Best BM, Capparelli EV, Diep H, et al. Pharmacokinetics of lopinavir/ritonavir crushed versus whole tablets in children. *J Acquir Immune Defic Syndr.* 2011;58(4):385-391.

DHHS Panel on Antiretroviral Guidelines for Adults and Adolescents. Guidelines for the use of antiretroviral agents in HIV-1-infected adults and adolescents, Department of Health and Human Services. May 1, 2014. Available at http://www.aidsinfo.nih.gov/ContentFiles/AdultandAdolescentGL.pdf

DHHS Panel on Antiretroviral Therapy and Medical Management of HIV-Infected Children. Guidelines for the use of antiretroviral agents in pediatric HIV infection. February 12, 2014. Available at http://aidsinfo.nih.gov

DHHS Panel on Treatment of HIV-Infected Pregnant Women and Prevention of Perinatal Transmission. Recommendations for the use of antiretroviral drugs in pregnant HIV-1-infected women for maternal health and interventions to reduce perinatal HIV-1 transmission in the United States. March 28, 2014. Available at http://aidsinfo.nih.gov

Foissac F, Urien S, Hirt D, et al. Pharmacokinetics and virological efficacy after switch to once-daily lopinavir-ritonavir in treatment-experienced HIV-1-infected children. *Antimicrob Agents Chemother.* 2011;55(9):4320-4325.

Hurst M, Faulds D. Lopinavir. *Drugs.* 2000;60(6):1371-1379.

Mangum EM, Graham KK. Lopinavir-ritonavir: a new protease inhibitor. *Pharmacotherapy.* 2001;21(11):1352-1363.

Morris JL, Kraus DM. New antiretroviral therapies for pediatric HIV infection. *J Pediatr Pharmacol Ther.* 2005;10:215-247.

Shehab N, Lewis CL, Streetman DD, Donn SM. Exposure to the pharmaceutical excipients benzyl alcohol and propylene glycol among critically ill neonates. *Pediatr Crit Care Med.* 2009;10(2):256-259.

◆ **Lopresor (Can)** *see* Metoprolol *on page 1396*

◆ **Lopresor SR (Can)** *see* Metoprolol *on page 1396*

◆ **Lopressor** *see* Metoprolol *on page 1396*

◆ **Loprox** *see* Ciclopirox *on page 465*

◆ **Loradamed [OTC]** *see* Loratadine *on page 1278*

Loratadine (lor AT a deen)

Medication Safety Issues
Sound-alike/look-alike issues:
Claritin may be confused with clarithromycin
Claritin (loratadine) may be confused with Claritin Eye (ketotifen)
Lorcaserin hydrochloride may be confused with lorcaserin hydrochloride

BEERS Criteria medication:
This drug may be potentially inappropriate for use in geriatric patients (Quality of evidence - varies based on comorbidity; Strength of recommendation - varies based on comorbidity)

Brand Names: U.S. Alavert [OTC]; Allergy Relief For Kids [OTC]; Allergy Relief [OTC]; Allergy [OTC]; Childrens Loratadine [OTC]; Claritin Reditabs [OTC]; Claritin [OTC]; Loradamed [OTC]; Loratadine Childrens [OTC]; Loratadine Hives Relief [OTC]; Triaminic Allerchews [OTC]

Brand Names: Canada Apo-Loratadine; Claritin®; Claritin® Kids

Therapeutic Category Antihistamine

Generic Availability (U.S.) May be product dependent

Use Symptomatic relief of nasal and non-nasal symptoms of allergic rhinitis; treatment of chronic idiopathic urticaria

Pregnancy Considerations Maternal use of loratadine has not been associated with an increased risk of major malformations. The use of antihistamines for the treatment of rhinitis during pregnancy is generally considered to be safe at recommended doses. Although safety data is limited, loratadine may be the preferred second generation antihistamine for the treatment of rhinitis or urticaria during pregnancy.

Breast-Feeding Considerations Small amounts of loratadine and its active metabolite, desloratadine, are excreted into breast milk.

Contraindications Hypersensitivity to loratadine or any component

Warnings Use with caution and adjust dosage in patients with severe liver impairment or renal impairment; Claritin® syrup contains sodium benzoate; benzoic acid (benzoate) is a metabolite of benzyl alcohol; large amounts of benzyl alcohol (≥99 mg/kg/day) have been associated with a potentially fatal toxicity ("gasping syndrome") in neonates; *in vitro* and animal studies have shown that benzoate displaces bilirubin from protein binding sites; avoid use in neonates

Precautions Use cautiously in patients who are also taking ketoconazole, itraconazole, fluconazole, erythromycin, clarithromycin, or other drugs which may impair loratadine's hepatic metabolism; although increased plasma levels of loratadine have been observed, no adverse effects with concomitant administration have been reported including QT interval prolongation which has occurred when similar antihistamines, terfenadine and astemizole, were combined with these agents; while less sedating than other antihistamines, loratadine may cause drowsiness and impair ability to perform hazardous activities requiring mental alertness. Use cautiously in breast-feeding women as breast milk levels of loratadine are equivalent to serum levels. Some tablets contain phenylalanine which must be avoided (or used with caution) in patients with phenylketonuria.

Adverse Reactions
Central nervous system: Fatigue, headache, malaise, nervousness, somnolence
Dermatologic: Rash
Gastrointestinal: Abdominal pain, stomatitis, xerostomia
Neuromuscular & skeletal: Hyperkinesia
Ocular: Conjunctivitis
Respiratory: dysphonia, epistaxis, pharyngitis, upper respiratory infection, wheezing
Miscellaneous: Flu-like syndrome, viral infection
Rare but important or life-threatening: Abnormal hepatic function, agitation, alopecia, altered lacrimation, altered micturition, altered salivation, altered taste, amnesia, anaphylaxis, angioneurotic edema, anorexia, arthralgia, back pain, blepharospasm, blurred vision, breast enlargement, breast pain, bronchospasm, chest pain, confusion, depression, dizziness, dysmenorrhea, dyspnea, erythema multiforme, hemoptysis, hepatic necrosis, hepatitis, hypotension, impaired concentration, impotence, insomnia, irritability, jaundice, menorrhagia, migraine, nausea, palpitation, paresthesia, paroniria, peripheral edema, photosensitivity, pruritus, purpura, rigors, seizure, supraventricular tachyarrhythmia, syncope, tachycardia, tremor, urinary discoloration, urticaria, thrombocytopenia, vaginitis, vertigo, vomiting, weight gain

Drug Interactions
Metabolism/Transport Effects Substrate of CYP2D6 (minor), CYP3A4 (minor), P-glycoprotein; **Note:** Assignment of Major/Minor substrate status based on clinically relevant drug interaction potential; **Inhibits** CYP2C19 (weak), CYP2C8 (weak), CYP2D6 (weak)

Avoid Concomitant Use
Avoid concomitant use of Loratadine with any of the following: Aclidinium; Azelastine (Nasal); Ipratropium (Oral Inhalation); Paraldehyde; Potassium Chloride; Thalidomide; Tiotropium; Umeclidinium

Increased Effect/Toxicity
Loratadine may increase the levels/effects of: AbobotulinumtoxinA; Alcohol (Ethyl); Analgesics (Opioid); Anticholinergic Agents; ARIPiprazole; Azelastine (Nasal); Buprenorphine; Cannabinoid-Containing Products; CNS Depressants; Hydrocodone; Methotrimeprazine; Metyrosine; Mirabegron; Mirtazapine; OnabotulinumtoxinA; Paraldehyde; Potassium Chloride; Pramipexole; RimabotulinumtoxinB; ROPINIRole; Rotigotine; Selective Serotonin Reuptake Inhibitors; Thalidomide; Thiazide Diuretics; Tiotropium; Topiramate; Zolpidem

The levels/effects of Loratadine may be increased by: Aclidinium; Amiodarone; Brimonidine (Topical); Cannabis; Doxylamine; Dronabinol; Droperidol; HydrOXYzine; Ipratropium (Oral Inhalation); Kava Kava; Magnesium Sulfate; Methotrimeprazine; Nabilone; Perampanel; P-glycoprotein/ABCB1 Inhibitors; Pramlintide; Rufinamide; Sodium Oxybate; Tapentadol; Tetrahydrocannabinol; Umeclidinium

Decreased Effect
Loratadine may decrease the levels/effects of: Acetylcholinesterase Inhibitors (Central); Benzylpenicilloyl Polylysine; Betahistine; Hyaluronidase; Secretin

The levels/effects of Loratadine may be decreased by: Acetylcholinesterase Inhibitors (Central); Amphetamines; Peginterferon Alfa-2b; P-glycoprotein/ABCB1 Inducers

Food Interactions Food increases bioavailability and delays peak. Management: Administer without regard to meals.

Mechanism of Action Long-acting tricyclic antihistamine with selective peripheral histamine H_1-receptor antagonistic properties

Pharmacodynamics
Onset of action: Within 1-3 hours
Maximum effect: 8-12 hours
Duration: >24 hours

Pharmacokinetics (Adult data unless noted)
Absorption: Rapid; food increases total bioavailability (AUC) by 40%
Distribution: Binds preferentially to peripheral nervous system H_1 receptors; no appreciable entry into CNS;

loratadine and metabolite pass easily into breast milk and achieve concentrations equivalent to plasma levels; breast milk to plasma ratio: 1.17

Protein binding: 97% (loratadine), 73% to 77% (metabolite)

Metabolism: Extensive first-pass metabolism by cytochrome P450 system to an active metabolite (descarboethoxyloratadine)

Half-life: 8.4 hours (loratadine), 28 hours (metabolite)

Time to peak serum concentration: 1-2 hours

Elimination: 80% eliminated via urine & feces as metabolic products

Dosing: Usual Oral:

Children 2-5 years: 5 mg once daily

Children ≥6 years and Adults: 10 mg once daily

Dosing interval in renal (GFR <30 mL/minute) or hepatic impairment: Administer dosage every other day

Administration Oral: Administer without regard to meals; place Claritin® RediTab® (rapidly disintegrating tablet) on the tongue; tablet disintegration occurs rapidly; may administer with or without water

Monitoring Parameters Improvement in signs and symptoms of allergic rhinitis or chronic idiopathic urticaria

Reference Range Therapeutic serum levels (not used clinically): Loratadine: 2.5-100 ng/mL; active metabolite: 0.5-100 ng/mL

Test Interactions May suppress the wheal and flare reactions to skin test antigens

Dosage Forms Excipient information presented when available (limited, particularly for generics); consult specific product labeling.

Capsule, Oral:

Claritin: 10 mg [contains brilliant blue fcf (fd&c blue #1)]

Solution, Oral:

Childrens Loratadine: 5 mg/5 mL (120 mL) [alcohol free, dye free, sugar free; contains propylene glycol, sodium benzoate; grape flavor]

Loratadine Childrens: 5 mg/5 mL (120 mL) [alcohol free, dye free, sugar free; contains propylene glycol, sodium benzoate; fruit flavor]

Loratadine Hives Relief: 5 mg/5 mL (120 mL) [alcohol free, dye free, sugar free; contains propylene glycol, sodium benzoate; grape flavor]

Syrup, Oral:

Allergy Relief: 5 mg/5 mL (236 mL) [alcohol free; contains propylene glycol, sodium benzoate]

Allergy Relief For Kids: 5 mg/5 mL (120 mL) [contains propylene glycol, sodium benzoate; fruit flavor]

Childrens Loratadine: 5 mg/5 mL (120 mL) [fruit flavor]

Childrens Loratadine: 5 mg/5 mL (120 mL) [alcohol free, dye free; contains propylene glycol, sodium benzoate, sodium metabisulfite; grape flavor]

Claritin: 5 mg/5 mL (60 mL, 120 mL, 150 mL) [alcohol free, color free, dye free, sugar free; contains edetate disodium, propylene glycol, sodium benzoate; grape flavor]

Loratadine Childrens: 5 mg/5 mL (120 mL) [sugar free; contains polyethylene glycol, propylene glycol, sodium benzoate, sodium metabisulfite; grape flavor]

Tablet, Oral:

Alavert: 10 mg

Allergy: 10 mg

Allergy Relief: 10 mg

Claritin: 10 mg

Loradamed: 10 mg

Generic: 10 mg

Tablet Chewable, Oral:

Claritin: 5 mg [contains aspartame, fd&c blue #2 aluminum lake; grape flavor]

Tablet Dispersible, Oral:

Alavert: 10 mg [contains aspartame]

Alavert: 10 mg [contains aspartame; bubble-gum flavor]

Alavert: 10 mg [contains aspartame; citrus flavor]

Allergy: 10 mg [contains aspartame]

Allergy Relief: 10 mg [contains aspartame]

Allergy Relief: 10 mg [contains aspartame; fruit flavor]

Claritin Reditabs: 5 mg, 10 mg

Triaminic Allerchews: 10 mg

References

Lin CC, Radwanski E, Affrime M, et al, "Pharmacokinetics of Loratadine in Pediatric Subjects," *Am J Therapeut*, 1995, 2:504-8.

Luck JC and Evrard HM, "Atrial Fibrillation Associated With Loratadine Use," *J Allergy Clin Immunol*, 1995, 95(2):282.

Lutsky BN, Klose P, Melon J, et al, "A Comparative Study of the Efficacy and Safety of Loratadine Syrup and Terfenadine Suspension in the Treatment of 3 to 6 Year Old Children With Seasonal Allergic Rhinitis," *Clin Ther*, 1993, 15(5):855-65.

Salmun LM, Herron JM, Banfield C, et al, "The Pharmacokinetics, Electrocardiographic Effects, and Tolerability of Loratadine Syrup in Children Aged 2 to 5 Years," *Clin Ther*, 2000, 22(5):613-21.

◆ **Loratadine-D 12 Hour [OTC]** *see* Loratadine and Pseudoephedrine *on page 1279*

Loratadine and Pseudoephedrine
(lor AT a deen & soo doe e FED rin)

Medication Safety Issues

Sound-alike/look-alike issues:

Claritin-D® may be confused with Claritin-D® 24

Claritin-D® 24 may be confused with Claritin-D®

Related Information

Oral Medications That Should Not Be Crushed or Altered *on page 2438*

Brand Names: U.S. Alavert™ Allergy and Sinus [OTC]; Claritin-D® 12 Hour Allergy & Congestion [OTC]; Claritin-D® 24 Hour Allergy & Congestion [OTC]; Loratadine-D 12 Hour [OTC]

Brand Names: Canada Chlor-Tripolon ND®; Claritin® Extra; Claritin® Liberator

Therapeutic Category Antihistamine/Decongestant Combination

Generic Availability (U.S.) Yes

Use Symptomatic relief of symptoms of seasonal allergic rhinitis and nasal congestion

Contraindications Hypersensitivity to loratadine, pseudoephedrine, or any component; MAO inhibitor therapy; severe hypertension; severe coronary artery disease; narrow-angle glaucoma

Precautions Use with caution and adjust dosage in patients with renal impairment; use with caution in patients with hyperthyroidism, diabetes mellitus, prostatic hypertrophy, mild to moderate hypertension, arrhythmias; use cautiously in patients who are also taking ketoconazole, itraconazole, fluconazole, erythromycin, clarithromycin, or other drugs which may impair loratadine's hepatic metabolism; although increased plasma levels of loratadine have been observed, no adverse effects with concomitant administration have been reported including QT interval prolongation which has occurred when similar antihistamines, terfenadine and astemizole, were combined with these agents; while less sedating than other antihistamines, loratadine may cause drowsiness and impair ability to perform hazardous activities requiring mental alertness, the CNS stimulant properties of pseudoephedrine may counteract this effect. Use cautiously in breast-feeding women as breast milk levels of loratadine are equivalent to serum levels.

Adverse Reactions See individual agents.

Drug Interactions

Metabolism/Transport Effects Refer to individual components.

Avoid Concomitant Use

Avoid concomitant use of Loratadine and Pseudoephedrine with any of the following: Aclidinium; Azelastine (Nasal); Ergot Derivatives; Iobenguane I 123; Ipratropium (Oral Inhalation); MAO Inhibitors; Paraldehyde; Potassium Chloride; Thalidomide; Tiotropium; Umeclidinium

◀ **Increased Effect/Toxicity**

Loratadine and Pseudoephedrine may increase the levels/effects of: AbobotulinumtoxinA; Alcohol (Ethyl); Analgesics (Opioid); Anticholinergic Agents; ARIPiprazole; Azelastine (Nasal); Buprenorphine; Cannabinoid-Containing Products; CNS Depressants; Hydrocodone; Methotrimeprazine; Metyrosine; Mirabegron; Mirtazapine; OnabotulinumtoxinA; Paraldehyde; Potassium Chloride; Pramipexole; RimabotulinumtoxinB; ROPINIRole; Rotigotine; Selective Serotonin Reuptake Inhibitors; Sympathomimetics; Thalidomide; Thiazide Diuretics; Tiotropium; Topiramate; Zolpidem

The levels/effects of Loratadine and Pseudoephedrine may be increased by: Aclidinium; Alkalinizing Agents; Amiodarone; AtoMOXetine; Brimonidine (Topical); Cannabinoid-Containing Products; Cannabis; Carbonic Anhydrase Inhibitors; Doxylamine; Dronabinol; Droperidol; Ergot Derivatives; HydrOXYzine; Ipratropium (Oral Inhalation); Kava Kava; Linezolid; Magnesium Sulfate; MAO Inhibitors; Methotrimeprazine; Nabilone; Perampanel; P-glycoprotein/ABCB1 Inhibitors; Pramlintide; Rufinamide; Serotonin/Norepinephrine Reuptake Inhibitors; Sodium Oxybate; Tapentadol; Tetrahydrocannabinol; Umeclidinium

Decreased Effect

Loratadine and Pseudoephedrine may decrease the levels/effects of: Acetylcholinesterase Inhibitors (Central); Benzylpenicilloyl Polylysine; Betahistine; FentaNYL; Hyaluronidase; Iobenguane I 123; Secretin

The levels/effects of Loratadine and Pseudoephedrine may be decreased by: Acetylcholinesterase Inhibitors (Central); Alpha1-Blockers; Amphetamines; Peginterferon Alfa-2b; P-glycoprotein/ABCB1 Inducers; Spironolactone; Urinary Acidifying Agents

Food Interactions See individual agents.

Pharmacokinetics (Adult data unless noted) See individual agents.

Dosing: Usual Oral: Children ≥12 years and Adults:

Alavert™ Allergy and Sinus, Claritin-D® 12-Hour, Loratadine-D 12 Hour: 1 tablet every 12 hours

Claritin-D® 24-Hour: 1 tablet every 24 hours

Dosage adjustment in renal impairment: CrCl <30 mL/minute:

Alavert™ Allergy and Sinus, Claritin-D® 12-Hour, Loratadine-D 12 Hour: 1 tablet every 24 hours

Claritin-D® 24-Hour: 1 tablet every other day

Administration Oral: Administer on an empty stomach or before meals; swallow extended release tablets whole, do not chew or crush

Monitoring Parameters Improvement in signs and symptoms of allergic rhinitis or nasal congestion

Reference Range Therapeutic serum levels (not used clinically): Loratadine: 2.5-100 ng/mL; active metabolite: 0.5-100 ng/mL

Test Interactions See individual agents.

Dosage Forms Excipient information presented when available (limited, particularly for generics); consult specific product labeling.

Tablet, extended release: Loratadine 10 mg and pseudoephedrine sulfate 240 mg

Alavert™ Allergy and Sinus: Loratadine 5 mg and pseudoephedrine sulfate 120 mg

Claritin-D® 12 Hour Allergy & Congestion: Loratadine 5 mg and pseudoephedrine sulfate 120 mg [contains calcium 30 mg/tablet]

Claritin-D® 24 Hour Allergy & Congestion: Loratadine 10 mg and pseudoephedrine sulfate 240 mg [contains calcium 25 mg/tablet]

Loratadine-D 12 Hour: Loratadine 5 mg and pseudoephedrine sulfate 120 mg

◆ **Loratadine Childrens [OTC]** *see* Loratadine *on page 1278*

◆ **Loratadine Hives Relief [OTC]** *see* Loratadine *on page 1278*

LORazepam (lor A ze pam)

Medication Safety Issues

Sound-alike/look-alike issues:

LORazepam may be confused with ALPRAZolam, clonazePAM, diazepam, KlonoPIN, Lovaza, temazepam, zolpidem

Ativan may be confused with Ambien, Atarax, Atgam, Avitene

BEERS Criteria medication:

This drug may be potentially inappropriate for use in geriatric patients (Quality of evidence - high; Strength of recommendation - strong).

Administration issues:

Injection dosage form contains propylene glycol. Monitor for toxicity when administering continuous lorazepam infusions.

Related Information

Preprocedure Sedatives in Children *on page 2402*

Brand Names: U.S. Ativan; LORazepam Intensol

Brand Names: Canada Apo-Lorazepam; Ativan; Dom-Lorazepam; Lorazepam Injection, USP; PHL-Lorazepam; PMS-Lorazepam; PRO-Lorazepam; Teva-Lorazepam

Therapeutic Category Antianxiety Agent; Anticonvulsant; Benzodiazepine; Antiemetic; Benzodiazepine; Hypnotic; Sedative

Generic Availability (U.S.) Yes

Use Management of anxiety; status epilepticus; preoperative sedation and amnesia; adjunct to antiemetic therapy

Pregnancy Risk Factor D

Pregnancy Considerations Teratogenic effects have been observed in some animal reproduction studies. Lorazepam and its metabolite cross the human placenta. Teratogenic effects in humans have been observed with some benzodiazepines (including lorazepam); however, additional studies are needed. The incidence of premature birth and low birth weights may be increased following maternal use of benzodiazepines; hypoglycemia and respiratory problems in the neonate may occur following exposure late in pregnancy. Neonatal withdrawal symptoms may occur within days to weeks after birth and "floppy infant syndrome" (which also includes withdrawal symptoms) have been reported with some benzodiazepines (including lorazepam). Elimination of lorazepam in the newborn infant is slow; following *in utero* exposure, term infants may excrete lorazepam for up to 8 days (Bergman, 1992; Iqbal, 2002; Wikner, 2007).

Breast-Feeding Considerations Lorazepam can be detected in breast milk. Drowsiness, lethargy, or weight loss in nursing infants have been observed in case reports following maternal use of some benzodiazepines (Iqbal, 2002). Breast-feeding is not recommended by the manufacturer.

Contraindications Hypersensitivity to lorazepam or any component; there may be a cross-sensitivity with other benzodiazepines; do not use in a comatose patient, those with preexisting CNS depression, narrow-angle glaucoma, severe uncontrolled pain, severe hypotension

Warnings Benzodiazepines may cause significant and potentially fatal respiratory depression, both if used alone and if used in combination with other CNS depressants. May cause CNS depression, which may impair physical or mental abilities; patients must be cautioned about performing tasks which require mental alertness (eg, operating machinery or driving). May cause emergent or worsening of preexisting depression; not recommended for use in patients with a primary depressive disorder or psychosis, particularly if suicidal risk may be present; do not use without adequate antidepressant therapy.

May cause physical and psychological dependence with prolonged use; do not abruptly discontinue; rebound or withdrawal symptoms (including seizures) may occur following abrupt discontinuation or large decreases in dose. Use caution when reducing dose or withdrawing therapy; decrease slowly and monitor for withdrawal symptoms. Flumazenil may cause acute withdrawal in patients receiving long-term benzodiazepine therapy. Potential for drug dependency exists; use benzodiazepines with caution in patients with a history of drug abuse, alcoholism, or significant personality disorders; risk of dependence increases with higher dosage and longer duration of therapy.

Dilute injection prior to I.V. use with equal volume of compatible diluent (D$_5$W, NS, SWI); do not inject intra-arterially, arteriospasm and gangrene may occur. Injection contains 2% benzyl alcohol and polyethylene glycol, which may be toxic to newborns in high doses; benzyl alcohol may cause allergic reactions in susceptible individuals; large amounts of benzyl alcohol (≥99 mg/kg/day) have been associated with a potentially fatal toxicity ("gasping syndrome") in neonates; the "gasping syndrome" consists of metabolic acidosis, respiratory distress, gasping respirations, CNS dysfunction (including convulsions, intracranial hemorrhage), hypotension and cardiovascular collapse; use lorazepam products containing benzyl alcohol with caution in neonates; *in vitro* and animal studies have shown that benzoate, a metabolite of benzyl alcohol, displaces bilirubin from protein binding sites.

Concentrated oral solution and injection contain propylene glycol; toxicities have been reported with use of products containing propylene glycol, including hyperosmolality, lactic acidosis, seizures, and respiratory depression; in neonates large amounts of propylene glycol delivered orally, intravenously (eg, >3000 mg/day), or topically have been associated with potentially fatal toxicities which can include metabolic acidosis, seizures, renal failure, and CNS depression; use products containing propylene glycol with caution (AAP, 1997; Shehab, 2009).

Precautions Use with caution in neonates, especially in preterm infants; several cases of neurotoxicity and myoclonus (rhythmic myoclonic jerking) have been reported. Use with caution in patients with renal or hepatic impairment; benzodiazepines may worsen hepatic encephalopathy; decrease dosage in patients with severe hepatic insufficiency. Use with caution in patients with compromised pulmonary function (including those with COPD or sleep apnea), CNS depression, or those receiving other CNS depressants. Debilitated patients may be more susceptible to the sedative effects of benzodiazepines; monitor closely; titrate dosage carefully according to patient response.

Benzodiazepines have been associated with anterograde amnesia; they do not have analgesic, antidepressant, or antipsychotic properties. Paradoxical reactions, including hyperactive or aggressive behavior, have been reported with benzodiazepines, particularly in pediatric/adolescent or psychiatric patients; discontinue drug if this occurs. As a hypnotic, should be used only after evaluation of potential causes of sleep disturbance. Failure of sleep disturbance to resolve after 7-10 days may indicate psychiatric or medical illness. A worsening of insomnia or the emergence of new abnormalities of thought or behavior may represent unrecognized psychiatric or medical illness and require immediate and careful evaluation.

Safety and efficacy of long-term use (>4 months) have not been established; long-term usefulness should be periodically re-evaluated for the individual patient. Safety and efficacy of oral lorazepam in children <12 years and safety of injectable lorazepam in children <18 years have not been established.

Adverse Reactions

Cardiovascular: Hypotension

Central nervous system: Aggressive behavior, agitation, akathisia, amnesia, anxiety, central nervous system stimulation, coma, disinhibition, disorientation, dizziness, drowsiness, dysarthria, euphoria, excitement, extrapyramidal reaction, fatigue, headache, hostility, hypothermia, irritability, mania, memory impairment, outbursts of anger, psychosis, sedation, seizures, sleep apnea (exacerbation), sleep disturbances, slurred speech, stupor, suicidal behavior, suicidal ideation, unsteadiness, vertigo

Dermatologic: Alopecia, skin rash

Gastrointestinal: Changes in appetite, constipation

Endocrine & metabolic: Change in libido, hyponatremia, SIADH

Genitourinary: Impotence, orgasm disturbance

Hematologic & oncologic: Agranulocytosis, pancytopenia, thrombocytopenia

Hepatic: Increased serum alkaline phosphatase, increased serum bilirubin, increased serum transaminases, jaundice

Hypersensitivity: Anaphylaxis, anaphylactoid reaction, hypersensitivity reaction

Local: Erythema at injection site, pain at injection site

Neuromuscular & skeletal: Weakness

Ophthalmic: Visual disturbances (including diplopia and blurred vision)

Respiratory: Apnea, exacerbation of obstructive pulmonary disease, hypoventilation, nasal congestion, respiratory depression, respiratory failure, worsening of sleep apnea

Rare but important or life-threatening: Abnormal gait, abnormal hepatic function tests, abnormality in thinking, acidosis, cardiac arrhythmia, ataxia, blood coagulation disorder, bradycardia, cardiac arrest, cardiac failure, cerebral edema, confusion, convulsions, cystitis, decreased mental acuity, delirium, depression, drug dependence (with prolonged use), drug toxicity (polyethylene glycol or propylene glycol poisoning [prolonged I.V. infusion]), excessive crying, gastrointestinal hemorrhage, hallucinations, hearing loss, heart block, hematologic abnormality, hepatotoxicity, hypertension, hyperventilation, hyporeflexia, infection, injection site reaction, myoclonus, neuroleptic malignant syndrome, paralysis, pericardial effusion, pheochromocytoma (aggravation), pneumothorax, pulmonary edema, pulmonary hemorrhage, pulmonary hypertension, seizure, tachycardia, urinary incontinence, ventricular arrhythmia, withdrawal syndrome

Drug Interactions

Metabolism/Transport Effects None known.

Avoid Concomitant Use

Avoid concomitant use of LORazepam with any of the following: Azelastine (Nasal); Methadone; OLANZapine; Paraldehyde; Sodium Oxybate; Thalidomide

Increased Effect/Toxicity

LORazepam may increase the levels/effects of: Alcohol (Ethyl); Azelastine (Nasal); Buprenorphine; CloZAPine; CNS Depressants; Fosphenytoin; Hydrocodone; Methadone; Methotrimeprazine; Metyrosine; Mirtazapine; Paraldehyde; Phenytoin; Pramipexole; ROPINIRole; Rotigotine; Selective Serotonin Reuptake Inhibitors; Sodium Oxybate; Thalidomide; Zolpidem

The levels/effects of LORazepam may be increased by: Brimonidine (Topical); Cannabis; Doxylamine; Dronabinol; Droperidol; HydrOXYzine; Kava Kava; Loxapine; Magnesium Sulfate; Methotrimeprazine; Nabilone; OLANZapine; Perampanel; Probenecid; Rufinamide; Tapentadol; Tetrahydrocannabinol; Valproic Acid and Derivatives

◄ **Decreased Effect**
The levels/effects of LORazepam may be decreased by:
Theophylline Derivatives; Yohimbine

Stability
I.V.: Store intact vials in the refrigerator; room temperature storage information may be available; contact product manufacturer to obtain current recommendations; protect from light. Do not use if injection is discolored or contains precipitate.

Oral solution: Store at 2°C to 8°C (36°F to 46°F); dispense only in the original bottle and with the calibrated dropper provided. Discard open bottle after 90 days.

Tablets: Store at 25°C (77°F); excursions permitted to 15°C to 30°C (59°F to 86°F); dispense in tightly closed container.

Mechanism of Action Binds to stereospecific benzodiazepine receptors on the postsynaptic GABA neuron at several sites within the central nervous system, including the limbic system, reticular formation. Enhancement of the inhibitory effect of GABA on neuronal excitability results by increased neuronal membrane permeability to chloride ions. This shift in chloride ions results in hyperpolarization (a less excitable state) and stabilization.

Pharmacodynamics Sedation:
Onset of action:
Oral: Within 60 minutes
I.M.: 30-60 minutes
I.V.: 15-30 minutes
Duration: 8-12 hours

Pharmacokinetics (Adult data unless noted)
Absorption: Oral, I.M.: Rapid, complete
Distribution: Crosses into placenta; crosses into breast milk
V_d:
Neonates: 0.76 L/kg
Adults: 1.3 L/kg
Protein binding: ~85%
Metabolism: Primarily by glucuronide conjugation in the liver to an inactive metabolite (lorazepam glucuronide)
Bioavailability: Oral: 90% to 93%
Half-life:
Full-term neonates: 40.2 hours; range: 18-73 hours
Older Children: 10.5 hours; range: 6-17 hours
Adults: 12.9 hours; range: 10-16 hours
Time to peak serum concentration: Oral: 2 hours
Elimination: In urine primarily as the glucuronide conjugate
Dialysis: Lorazepam: Poorly dialyzable; lorazepam glucuronide: May be highly dialyzable

Dosing: Neonatal Status epilepticus: I.V.: 0.05 mg/kg slow I.V. over 2-5 minutes; may repeat in 10-15 minutes (see warning regarding benzyl alcohol)

Dosing: Usual
Adjunct to antiemetic therapy:
Children: I.V.: Limited information exists in the literature, especially for multiple doses:
Single dose: 0.04-0.08 mg/kg/dose prior to chemotherapy (maximum dose: 4 mg)
Multiple doses: Some centers use 0.02-0.05 mg/kg/dose (maximum dose: 2 mg) every 6 hours as needed
Adults: Oral, I.V.: 0.5-2 mg every 4-6 hours as needed
Anxiety/sedation:
Infants and Children: Oral, I.V.: Usual: 0.05 mg/kg/dose (maximum dose: 2 mg/dose) every 4-8 hours; range: 0.02-0.1 mg/kg
Adults: Oral: 1-10 mg/day in 2-3 divided doses; usual dose: 2-6 mg/day in divided doses
Insomnia: Adults: Oral: 2-4 mg at bedtime
Operative amnesia: Adults: I.V.: Up to 0.05 mg/kg; maximum dose: 4 mg/dose
Preoperative: Adults: I.M.: 0.05 mg/kg administered 2 hours before surgery; maximum dose: 4 mg/dose; I.V.: 0.044 mg/kg 15-20 minutes before surgery; usual maximum dose: 2 mg/dose

Sedation (preprocedure): Infants and Children:
Oral, I.M., I.V.: Usual: 0.05 mg/kg; range: 0.02-0.09 mg/kg
I.V.: May use smaller doses (eg, 0.01-0.03 mg/kg) and repeat every 20 minutes, as needed to titrate to effect
Status epilepticus: I.V.:
Infants and Children: 0.05-0.1 mg/kg (maximum: 4 mg/dose) slow I.V. over 2-5 minutes (maximum rate: 2 mg/minute); may repeat every 10-15 minutes if needed (Hegenbarth, 2008; Sabo-Graham, 1998)
Adolescents: 0.07 mg/kg (maximum: 4 mg/dose) slow I.V. over 2-5 minutes (maximum rate: 2 mg/minute); may repeat in 10-15 minutes if needed; usual total maximum dose: 8 mg (Crawford, 1987)
Adults: 4 mg/dose slow I.V. over 2-5 minutes (maximum rate: 2 mg/minute); may repeat in 10-15 minutes; usual total maximum dose: 8 mg

Dosage adjustment in renal impairment: I.V.: Risk of propylene glycol toxicity. Monitor closely if using for prolonged periods of time or at high doses.

Dosage adjustment in hepatic impairment: Use with caution; benzodiazepines may worsen hepatic encephalopathy; decrease dosage in patients with severe hepatic insufficiency.

Administration
Oral: May administer with food to decrease GI distress; dilute oral solution in water, juice, soda, or semisolid food (eg, applesauce, pudding). Single oral doses >0.09 mg/kg produced increased ataxia without increasing sedative benefit vs lower doses. Since both strengths of injection contain 2% benzyl alcohol, some experts recommend using the 4 mg/mL strength for dilution with **preservative free** SWI to make a 0.4 mg/mL dilution for I.V. use in neonates (in order to decrease the amount of benzyl alcohol delivered to the neonate); however, the stability of this dilution has not been studied.
Parenteral:
I.V.: Do not exceed 2 mg/minute or 0.05 mg/kg over 2-5 minutes; dilute I.V. dose with equal volume of compatible diluent (D_5W, NS, SWI); administer I.V. using repeated aspiration with slow I.V. injection, to make sure the injection is not intra-arterial and that perivascular extravasation has not occurred
I.M.: Administer undiluted by deep injection into muscle mass

Monitoring Parameters Respiratory rate, blood pressure, heart rate; CBC with differential and liver function with long-term use

Additional Information Diarrhea in a 9-month old infant receiving high-dose oral lorazepam was attributed to the lorazepam oral solution that contains polyethylene glycol and propylene glycol (both are osmotically active); diarrhea resolved when crushed tablets were substituted for the oral solution (Marshall, 1995). To avoid the adverse effects of polyethylene glycol and propylene glycol that are found in the commercially available oral solution, a 1 mg/mL oral suspension can also be made from tablets.

Lorazepam crosses the placenta. Neonatal withdrawal symptoms (or symptoms of toxicity) may occur in infants of mothers who receive benzodiazepines during the late phase of pregnancy or at delivery. Reported symptoms include: Hypoactivity, hypotonia, feeding problems, respiratory depression, apnea, hypothermia, and impaired metabolic response to cold stress. Lorazepam enters breast milk. Sedation, irritability, and inability to suckle may occur in infants exposed to lorazepam from breast milk.

Controlled Substance C-IV

Dosage Forms Excipient information presented when available (limited, particularly for generics); consult specific product labeling.

Concentrate, Oral:
LORazepam Intensol: 2 mg/mL (30 mL) [alcohol free, dye free, sugar free; unflavored flavor]
Generic: 2 mg/mL (30 mL)
Solution, Injection:
Ativan: 2 mg/mL (1 mL, 10 mL); 4 mg/mL (1 mL, 10 mL) [contains benzyl alcohol, polyethylene glycol, propylene glycol]
Generic: 2 mg/mL (1 mL, 10 mL); 4 mg/mL (1 mL, 10 mL)
Tablet, Oral:
Ativan: 0.5 mg
Ativan: 1 mg, 2 mg [scored]
Generic: 0.5 mg, 1 mg, 2 mg

Extemporaneous Preparations Note: Commercial oral solution is available (2 mg/mL)

Two different 1 mg/mL oral suspensions may be made from different generic lorazepam tablets (Mylan Pharmaceuticals or Watson Laboratories), sterile water, Ora-Sweet, and Ora-Plus.

Mylan tablets: Place one-hundred-eighty 2 mg tablets in a 12-ounce amber glass bottle; add 144 mL of sterile water to disperse the tablets; shake until slurry is formed. Add 108 mL Ora-Plus in incremental proportions; then add a quantity of Ora-Sweet sufficient to make 360 mL. Label "shake well" and "refrigerate". Stable for 91 days when stored in amber glass prescription bottles at room temperature or refrigerated (preferred).

Watson tablets: Place one-hundred-eighty 2 mg tablets in a 12-ounce amber glass bottle; add 48 mL sterile water to disperse the tablets; shake until slurry is formed. Add 156 mL of Ora-Plus in incremental proportions; then add a quantity of Ora-Sweet sufficient to make 360 mL. Label "shake well" and "refrigerate". Store in amber glass prescription bottles. Stable for 63 days at room temperature or 91 days refrigerated.

Lee ME, Lugo RA, Rusho WJ, et al, "Chemical Stability of Extemporaneously Prepared Lorazepam Suspension at Two Temperatures," *J Pediatr Pharmacol Ther*, 2004, 9(4):254-58.

References

American Academy of Pediatrics Committee on Drugs. "Inactive" ingredients in pharmaceutical products: update (subject review). *Pediatrics*. 1997;99(2):268-278.

Bergman U, Rosa FW, Baum C, et al, "Effects of Exposure to Benzodiazepine During Fetal Life," *Lancet*, 1992, 340(8821):694-6.

Crawford TO, Mitchell WG, and Snodgrass SR, "Lorazepam in Childhood Status Epilepticus and Serial Seizures: Effectiveness and Tachyphylaxis," *Neurology*, 1987, 37(2):190-5.

Deshmukh A, Wittert W, Schnitzler E, et al, "Lorazepam in the Treatment of Refractory Neonatal Seizures: A Pilot Study," *Am J Dis Child*, 1986, 140(10):1042-4.

Hegenbarth MA and American Academy of Pediatrics Committee on Drugs, "Preparing for Pediatric Emergencies: Drugs to Consider," *Pediatrics*, 2008, 121(2):433-43.

Henry DW, Burwinkle JW, and Klutman NE, "Determination of Sedative and Amnestic Doses of Lorazepam in Children," *Clin Pharm*, 1991, 10 (8):625-9.

Iqbal MM, Sobhan T, Ryals T, et al, "Effects of Commonly Used Benzodiazepines on the Fetus, the Neonate, and the Nursing Infant," *Psychiatr Serv*, 2002, 53(1):39-49.

Lee DS, Wong HA, and Knoppert DC, "Myoclonus Associated With Lorazepam Therapy in Very-Low-Birth-Weight Infants," *Biol Neonate*, 1994, 66(6):311-5.

Marshall JD, Farrar HC, and Kearns GL, "Diarrhea Associated With Enteral Benzodiazepine Solutions," *J Pediatr*, 1995, 126(4):657-9.

McDermott CA, Kowalczyk AL, Schnitzler ER, et al, "Pharmacokinetics of Lorazepam in Critically Ill Neonates With Seizures," *J Pediatr*, 1992, 120(3):479-83.

Sabo-Graham T and Seay AR, "Management of Status Epilepticus in Children," *Pediatr Rev*, 1998, 19(9):306-9.

Shehab N, Lewis CL, Streetman DD, Donn SM. Exposure to the pharmaceutical excipients benzyl alcohol and propylene glycol among critically ill neonates. *Pediatr Crit Care Med*. 2009;10 (2):256-259.

Wikner BN, Stiller CO, Bergman U, et al, "Use of Benzodiazepines and Benzodiazepine Receptor Agonists During Pregnancy: Neonatal Outcome and Congenital Malformations," *Pharmacoepidemiol Drug Saf*, 2007, 16(11):1203-10.

◆ **Lorazepam Injection, USP (Can)** see LORazepam on page 1280

◆ **LORazepam Intensol** see LORazepam on page 1280

◆ **Lorcet® 10/650 [DSC]** see Hydrocodone and Acetaminophen on page 1027

◆ **Lorcet® Plus [DSC]** see Hydrocodone and Acetaminophen on page 1027

◆ **Lortab®** see Hydrocodone and Acetaminophen on page 1027

◆ **Lorzone** see Chlorzoxazone on page 454

Losartan (loe SAR tan)

Medication Safety Issues
Sound-alike/look-alike issues:
Cozaar may be confused with Colace, Coreg, Hyzaar, Zocor
Losartan may be confused with locaserin, valsartan

Brand Names: U.S. Cozaar

Brand Names: Canada Apo-Losartan; Auro-Losartan; CO Losartan; Cozaar; JAMP-Losartan; Mint-Losartan; Mylan-Losartan; PMS-Losartan; RAN-Losartan; Sandoz Losartan; Teva-Losartan

Therapeutic Category Angiotensin II Receptor Blocker; Antihypertensive Agent

Generic Availability (U.S.) Yes

Use Treatment of hypertension alone or in combination with other antihypertensive agents (FDA approved in ages 6-16 years and adults); treatment of diabetic nephropathy in patients with type 2 diabetes mellitus (noninsulin dependent, NIDDM) and hypertension (FDA approved in adults); reduction of the risk of stroke in patients with hypertension and left ventricular hypertrophy (FDA approved in adults); has also been used to reduce proteinuria in children with chronic kidney disease, either as monotherapy or in addition to ACE inhibitor therapy, and in Marfan's Syndrome to slow the rate of progression of aortic-root dilation

Pregnancy Risk Factor D

Pregnancy Considerations [U.S. Boxed Warning]: Drugs that act on the renin-angiotensin system can cause injury and death to the developing fetus. Discontinue as soon as possible once pregnancy is detected. The use of drugs which act on the renin-angiotensin system are associated with oligohydramnios. Oligohydramnios, due to decreased fetal renal function, may lead to fetal lung hypoplasia and skeletal malformations. Use is also associated with anuria, hypotension, renal failure, skull hypoplasia, and death in the fetus/neonate. The exposed fetus should be monitored for fetal growth, amniotic fluid volume, and organ formation. Infants exposed *in utero* should be monitored for hyperkalemia, hypotension, and oliguria (exchange transfusions or dialysis may be needed). These adverse events are generally associated with maternal use in the second and third trimesters.

Untreated chronic maternal hypertension is also associated with adverse events in the fetus, infant, and mother. The use of angiotensin II receptor blockers is not recommended to treat chronic uncomplicated hypertension in pregnant women and should generally be avoided in women of reproductive potential (ACOG, 2013).

Breast-Feeding Considerations It is not known if losartan is found in breast milk. Due to the potential for serious adverse reactions in the nursing infant, the manufacturer recommends a decision be made whether to discontinue nursing or to discontinue the drug, taking into account the importance of treatment to the mother.

Contraindications Hypersensitivity to losartan, any component, or other angiotensin II receptor blockers

◄ **Warnings** Drugs that act on the renin-angiotensin system can cause injury and death to the developing fetus. Discontinue as soon as possible once pregnancy is detected **[U.S. Boxed Warning]**. Use with caution in volume-depleted patients (eg, those on thiazide diuretics); correct depletion first or use a lower starting dose. Symptomatic hypotension may occur, especially in patients with an activated renin-angiotensin system (eg, volume- or salt-depleted patients receiving high doses of diuretic agents); use with caution in these patients; correct depletion before starting therapy or initiate therapy at a lower dose. Concomitant use of an ACE inhibitor or renin inhibitor (eg, aliskiren) is associated with an increased risk of hypotension, hyperkalemia, and renal dysfunction. Concomitant use with aliskiren should be avoided in patients with GFR <60 mL/minute and is contraindicated in patients with diabetes mellitus (regardless of GFR).

Angioedema has been reported rarely with some angiotensin II receptor antagonists (ARBs) and may occur at any time during treatment (especially following first dose); it may involve the head and neck (potentially compromising airway) or the intestine (presenting with abdominal pain). Patients with idiopathic or hereditary angioedema or previous angioedema associated with ACE-inhibitor therapy may be at an increased risk. Prolonged frequent monitoring may be required, especially if tongue, glottis, or larynx are involved, as they are associated with airway obstruction. Patients with a history of airway surgery may have a higher risk of airway obstruction. Discontinue therapy immediately if angioedema occurs. Aggressive early management is critical. Intramuscular (I.M.) administration of epinephrine may be necessary. Do not readminister to patients who have had angioedema with ARBs.

Precautions Use with caution and reduce dosage in patients with hepatic impairment (clearance of losartan is reduced in these patients). Use with caution in patients with impaired renal function; use is associated with deterioration of renal function and/or increases in serum creatinine, particularly in patients with low renal blood flow (eg, renal artery stenosis, heart failure); deterioration may result in oliguria, acute renal failure, or progressive azotemia. Small increases in serum creatinine may occur following initiation; consider discontinuation in patients with progressive and/or significant deterioration in renal function. Hyperkalemia may occur; risk factors include renal dysfunction, diabetes mellitus, concomitant use of potassium-sparing diuretics, potassium supplements, and/or potassium-containing salts; use with caution in these patients and with these agents; monitor potassium closely. Not recommended for use in children <6 years of age or in children with GFR <30 mL/minute/1.73m² (no data exists).

Adverse Reactions
Cardiovascular: Chest pain, hypotension, orthostatic hypotension, first-dose hypotension (dose related)
Central nervous system: Dizziness, fatigue, fever, hypoesthesia, insomnia
Dermatology: Cellulitis
Endocrine: Hyperkalemia, hypoglycemia
Gastrointestinal: Abdominal pain, diarrhea, dyspepsia, gastritis, nausea, weight gain
Genitourinary: Urinary tract infection
Hematologic: Anemia
Neuromuscular & skeletal: Back pain, knee pain, leg pain, muscle cramps, muscular weakness, myalgia, weakness
Respiratory: Bronchitis, cough, nasal congestion, sinusitis, upper respiratory infection
Miscellaneous: Flu-like syndrome, infection
Frequency ≤placebo: Abdominal pain, edema, headache, nausea, pharyngitis
Rare but important or life-threatening: Acute psychosis with paranoid delusions, ageusia, allergic reaction, alopecia, anaphylactic reactions, anemia, angina,

angioedema, anorexia, anxiety, arrhythmia, arthralgia, arthritis, ataxia, AV block (second degree), bilirubin increased, blurred vision, bradycardia, bronchitis, BUN increased, confusion, conjunctivitis, constipation, CVA, depression, dermatitis, dysgeusia, dyspnea, ecchymosis, epistaxis, erythroderma, erythema, facial edema, fever, flatulence, flushing, gastritis, gout, hematocrit decreased, hemoglobin decreased, Henoch-Schönlein purpura (IgA vasculitis), hepatitis, hyponatremia, hypotension, impotence, joint swelling, maculopapular rash, malaise, memory impairment, MI, migraine, muscle weakness, myositis, neoplasm, nervousness, orthostatic effects, pancreatitis, paresthesia, peripheral neuropathy, pharyngitis, photosensitivity, pruritus, rash, rhabdomyolysis, rhinitis, serum creatinine increased, sleep disorder, somnolence, syncope, tachycardia, taste perversion, thrombocytopenia, tinnitus, transaminases increased, tremor, urinary frequency, urticaria, vasculitis, ventricular arrhythmia, vertigo, visual acuity decreased, vomiting, xerostomia

Drug Interactions
Metabolism/Transport Effects Substrate of CYP2C9 (major), CYP3A4 (major); **Note:** Assignment of Major/Minor substrate status based on clinically relevant drug interaction potential; **Inhibits** CYP1A2 (weak), CYP2C19 (weak), CYP2C8 (moderate), CYP2C9 (moderate), CYP3A4 (weak)

Avoid Concomitant Use
Avoid concomitant use of Losartan with any of the following: Pimozide

Increased Effect/Toxicity
Losartan may increase the levels/effects of: ACE Inhibitors; Amifostine; Antihypertensives; ARIPiprazole; Bosentan; Cannabis; Carvedilol; CycloSPORINE (Systemic); CYP2C8 Substrates; CYP2C9 Substrates; Dofetilide; Dronabinol; DULoxetine; Hypotensive Agents; Lithium; Lomitapide; Nonsteroidal Anti-Inflammatory Agents; Obinutuzumab; Pimozide; Potassium-Sparing Diuretics; RiTUXimab; Sodium Phosphates; Tetrahydrocannabinol

The levels/effects of Losartan may be increased by: Alfuzosin; Aliskiren; Antifungal Agents (Azole Derivatives, Systemic); Barbiturates; Brimonidine (Topical); Canagliflozin; Ceritinib; CYP2C9 Inhibitors (Moderate); CYP2C9 Inhibitors (Strong); Diazoxide; Eplerenone; Fluconazole; Heparin; Heparin (Low Molecular Weight); Herbs (Hypotensive Properties); MAO Inhibitors; Mifepristone; Milk Thistle; Pentoxifylline; Phosphodiesterase 5 Inhibitors; Potassium Salts; Prostacyclin Analogues; Tolvaptan; Trimethoprim

Decreased Effect
The levels/effects of Losartan may be decreased by: Bosentan; CYP2C9 Inducers (Strong); CYP3A4 Inducers (Strong); Dabrafenib; Deferasirox; Herbs (Hypertensive Properties); Methylphenidate; Mitotane; Nonsteroidal Anti-Inflammatory Agents; Peginterferon Alfa-2b; Siltuximab; St Johns Wort; Tocilizumab; Yohimbine

Stability Store at controlled room temperature at 25°C (77°F) in tightly closed container. Protect from light.

Mechanism of Action As a selective and competitive, nonpeptide angiotensin II receptor antagonist, losartan blocks the vasoconstrictor and aldosterone-secreting effects of angiotensin II; losartan interacts reversibly at the AT1 and AT2 receptors of many tissues and has slow dissociation kinetics; its affinity for the AT1 receptor is 1000 times greater than the AT2 receptor. Angiotensin II receptor antagonists may induce a more complete inhibition of the renin-angiotensin system than ACE inhibitors, they do not affect the response to bradykinin, and are less likely to be associated with nonrenin-angiotensin effects (eg, cough and angioedema). Losartan increases urinary flow rate and in addition to being natriuretic and kaliuretic, increases excretion of chloride, magnesium, uric acid, calcium, and phosphate.

Pharmacodynamics Antihypertensive effect:
Maximum effect: 6 hours postdose; with chronic dosing, substantial hypotensive effects are seen within 1 week; maximum effect: 3-6 weeks
Duration: 24 hours

Pharmacokinetics (Adult data unless noted) Note: No significant differences in pharmacokinetic parameters have been identified across studied pediatric age groups (6-16 years) and adult population.
Absorption: Oral: Well-absorbed
Distribution: V_d: Adults:
Losartan: ~34 L
E-3174: ~12 L
Protein binding: Highly bound, >98%; primarily to albumin
Metabolism: Extensive first-pass effect; metabolized in the liver via CYP2C9 and 3A4 to active carboxylic metabolite, E-3174 (14% of dose; 40 times more potent than losartan) and several inactive metabolites
Bioavailability: Oral: 33%; AUC of E-3174 is four times greater than that of losartan; extemporaneously prepared suspension and tablet have similar bioavailability of losartan and E-3174
Half-life elimination:
Losartan:
Children 6-16 years: 2.3 ± 0.8 hours
Adults: 2.1 ± 0.7 hours
E-3174:
Children 6-16 years: 5.6 ± 1.2 hours
Adults: 7.4 ± 2.4 hours
Time to peak serum concentration:
Losartan:
Children: 2 hours
Adults: 1 hour
E-3174:
Children: 4 hours
Adults: 3.5 hours
Excretion: Biliary excretion plays a role in the elimination of parent drug and metabolites; 35% of an oral dose is eliminated in the urine and 60% in the feces; 4% of dose is eliminated as unchanged drug in the urine; 6% as E-3174
Clearance: Adults:
Plasma:
Losartan: 600 mL/minute
E-3174: 50 mL/minute
Renal:
Losartan: 75 mL/minute
E-3174: 25 mL/minute
Dialysis: Losartan and E-3174: Not removed by hemodialysis

Dosing: Usual
Children:
Hypertension:
Children and Adolescents 6-16 years: Oral: Initial: 0.7 mg/kg once daily (maximum dose: 50 mg); titrate to desired effect up to a maximum dose of 1.4 mg/kg/day or 100 mg/day; may be administered once daily or divided twice daily (NHBPEP, 2004; NHLBI, 2011); **Note:** Doses >1.4 mg/kg/day (or >100 mg/day) have not been studied (Shahinfar, 2005).
Adolescents ≥17 years: Oral: Initial: 50 mg once daily; increase dose to achieve desired effect; total daily dosage range: 25-100 mg/day; can be administered once or twice daily; **Note:** Patients receiving diuretics or with intravascular volume depletion: Initial dose: 25 mg once daily
Proteinuria reduction in children with chronic kidney disease: Limited data available: Children ≥4 years and Adolescents: Oral: Initial: 0.4-0.8 mg/kg/day; increase dose if no adverse effects occur and blood pressure remains >90th percentile or proteinuria does not fall

<50% of baseline excretion; doses can be increased slowly up to 1 mg/kg/day (maximum: 50 mg/day); dosing based on experience from three retrospective clinical trials (Chandar, 2007; Ellis, 2003; Ellis, 2004)
Marfan's syndrome aortic-root dilation: Limited data available: Children and Adolescents 14 months to 16 years: Oral: Initial: 0.6 mg/kg/day for 3 weeks (while assessing for adverse events); then gradually increase dose to 1.4 mg/kg/day (maximum: 100 mg/day); dosing based on preliminary results of a small (n=18), nonrandomized, retrospective, clinical study (Brooke, 2008); further studies are needed
Adults:
Hypertension: Oral: Initial: 50 mg once daily; can be administered once or twice daily; increase dose to achieve desired effect; total daily dosage range: 25-100 mg/day; **Note:** Patients receiving diuretics or with intravascular volume depletion: Initial dose: 25 mg once daily
Nephropathy in patients with type 2 diabetes and hypertension: Oral: Initial: 50 mg once daily; can be increased to 100 mg once daily based on blood pressure response
Stroke reduction (HTN with LVH): Oral: Initial: 50 mg once daily (maximum daily dose: 100 mg); may be used in combination with a thiazide diuretic
Dosing adjustment in renal impairment:
Children: Use is not recommended if CrCl <30 mL/minute/1.73 m^2
Adults: No initial dosage adjustment necessary
Dosing adjustment in hepatic impairment:
Children: No specific dosing recommendations provided by manufacturer; however, it is advisable to initiate at a reduced dosage.
Adults: Reduce initial dose to 25 mg/day

Administration May be administered with or without food.

Monitoring Parameters Blood pressure, BUN, serum creatinine, renal function, baseline and periodic serum electrolytes, urinalysis

Additional Information Potassium content: 25 mg tablets: 2.12 mg (0.054 mEq); 50 mg tablets: 4.24 mg (0.108 mEq); 100 mg tablets: 8.48 mg (0.216 mEq)

Evidence from the LIFE study (Dahlöf, 2002) suggests that when used to reduce the risk of stroke in patients with HTN and LVH, losartan may not be effective in the African-American population.

Dosage Forms Excipient information presented when available (limited, particularly for generics); consult specific product labeling.
Tablet, Oral, as potassium:
Cozaar: 25 mg
Cozaar: 50 mg [scored]
Cozaar: 100 mg
Generic: 25 mg, 50 mg, 100 mg

Extemporaneous Preparations A 2.5 mg/mL losartan oral suspension may be made with tablets and a 1:1 mixture of Ora-Plus® and Ora-Sweet® SF. Combine 10 mL of purified water and ten losartan 50 mg tablets in an 8-ounce amber polyethylene terephthalate bottle. Shake well for at least 2 minutes. Allow concentrate to stand for 1 hour, then shake for 1 minute. Separately, prepare 190 mL of a 1:1 mixture of Ora-Plus® and Ora-Sweet® SF; add to tablet and water mixture in the bottle and shake for 1 minute. Label "shake well" and "refrigerate". Return promptly to refrigerator after each use. Stable for 4 weeks when stored in amber polyethylene terephthalate prescription bottles and refrigerated (Cozaar prescribing information, 2014).

Cozaar prescribing information, Merck & Co, Inc, Whitehouse Station, NJ, 2014.

References
American College of Obstetricians and Gynecologists (ACOG), "ACOG Practice Bulletin No. 125: Chronic Hypertension in Pregnancy," *Obstet Gynecol*, 2012, 119(2 Pt 1):396-407.

Brooke BS, Habashi JP, Judge DP, et al, "Angiotensin II Blockade and Aortic-Root Dilation in Marfan's Syndrome," *N Engl J Med*, 2008, 358 (26):2787-95.

Butani L, "Angiotensin Blockade in Children With Chronic Glomerulonephritis and Heavy Proteinuria," *Pediatr Nephrol*, 2005, 20 (11):1651-4.

Chandar J, Abitbol C, Montané B, et al, "Angiotensin Blockade as Sole Treatment for Proteinuric Kidney Disease in Children," *Nephrol Dial Transplant*, 2007, 22(5):1332-7.

Chobanian AV, Bakris GL, Black HR, et al, "The Seventh Report of the Joint National Committee on Prevention, Detection, Evaluation, and Treatment of High Blood Pressure: The JNC 7 Report," *JAMA*, 2003, 289(19):2560-71.

Dahlöf B, Devereux RB, Kjeldsen SE, et al, "Cardiovascular Morbidity and Mortality in the Losartan Intervention For Endpoint Reduction in Hypertension Study (LIFE): A Randomised Trial Against Atenolol," *Lancet*, 2002, 359(9311):995-1003.

Ellis D, Moritz ML, Vats A, et al, "Antihypertensive and Renoprotective Efficacy and Safety of Losartan. A Long-Term Study in Children With Renal Disorders," *Am J Hypertens*, 2004, 17(10):928-35.

Ellis D, Vats A, Moritz ML, et al, "Long-Term Antiproteinuric and Renoprotective Efficacy and Safety of Losartan in Children With Proteinuria," *J Pediatr*, 2003, 143(1):89-97.

Hogg RJ, Portman RJ, Milliner D, et al, "Evaluation and Management of Proteinuria and Nephrotic Syndrome in Children: Recommendations From a Pediatric Nephrology Panel Established at the National Kidney Foundation Conference on Proteinuria, Albuminuria, Risk, Assessment, Detection, and Elimination (PARADE)," *Pediatrics*, 2000, 105(6):1242-9.

Litwin M, Grenda R, Sladowska J, et al, "Add-On Therapy With Angiotensin II Receptor 1 Blocker in Children With Chronic Kidney Disease Already Treated With Angiotensin-Converting Enzyme Inhibitors," *Pediatr Nephrol*, 2006, 21(11):1716-22.

National Heart, Lung, and Blood Institute, "Expert Panel on Integrated Guidelines for Cardiovascular Health and Risk Reduction in Children and Adolescents," Clinical Practice Guidelines, 2011, National Institutes of Health. Available at http://www.nhlbi.nih.gov/guidelines/cvd_ped/peds_guidelines_full.pdf

National High Blood Pressure Education Program Working Group on High Blood Pressure in Children and Adolescents, "The Fourth Report on the Diagnosis, Evaluation, and Treatment of High Blood Pressure in Children and Adolescents," *Pediatrics*, 2004, 114(2 Suppl):555-76.

Shahinfar S, Cano F, Soffer BA, et al, "A Double-Blind, Dose-Response Study of Losartan in Hypertensive Children," *Am J Hypertens*, 2005, 18(2 Pt 1):183-90.

White CT, Macpherson CF, Hurley RM, et al, "Antiproteinuric Effects of Enalapril and Losartan: A Pilot Study," *Pediatr Nephrol*, 2003, 18 (10):1038-43.

Zaffanello M, Franchini M, and Fanos V, "New Therapeutic Strategies With Combined Renin-Angiotensin System Inhibitors for Pediatric Nephropathy," *Pharmacotherapy*, 2008, 28(1):125-30.

◆ **Losartan Potassium** *see* Losartan *on page 1283*

◆ **Losec (Can)** *see* Omeprazole *on page 1535*

◆ **Lotensin** *see* Benazepril *on page 270*

◆ **Lotrimin AF [OTC]** *see* Clotrimazole (Topical) *on page 527*

◆ **Lotrimin AF [OTC]** *see* Miconazole (Topical) *on page 1410*

◆ **Lotrimin AF Deodorant Powder [OTC]** *see* Miconazole (Topical) *on page 1410*

◆ **Lotrimin AF For Her [OTC]** *see* Clotrimazole (Topical) *on page 527*

◆ **Lotrimin AF Jock Itch Powder [OTC]** *see* Miconazole (Topical) *on page 1410*

◆ **Lotrimin AF Powder [OTC]** *see* Miconazole (Topical) *on page 1410*

Lovastatin (LOE va sta tin)

Medication Safety Issues
Sound-alike/look-alike issues:

Lovastatin may be confused with atorvaSTATin, Leustatin, Livostin, Lotensin, nystatin, pitavastatin

Mevacor may be confused with Benicar, Lipitor

International issues:

Lovacol [Chile and Finland] may be confused with Levatol brand name for penbutolol [U.S.]

Lovastin [Malaysia, Poland, and Singapore] may be confused with Livostin brand name for levocabastine [multiple international markets]

Mevacor [U.S., Canada, and multiple international markets] may be confused with Mivacron brand name for mivacurium [multiple international markets]

Related Information
Oral Medications That Should Not Be Crushed or Altered *on page 2438*

Brand Names: U.S. Altoprev; Mevacor

Brand Names: Canada Apo-Lovastatin; Ava-Lovastatin; CO Lovastatin; Dom-Lovastatin; Mevacor; Mylan-Lovastatin; PHL-Lovastatin; PMS-Lovastatin; PRO-Lovastatin; Riva-Lovastatin; Sandoz-Lovastatin; Teva-Lovastatin

Therapeutic Category Antilipemic Agent; HMG-CoA Reductase Inhibitor

Generic Availability (U.S.) May be product dependent

Use Treatment of heterozygous familial hypercholesterolemia as adjunct to dietary therapy to decrease elevated serum total and low density lipoprotein and apolipoprotein B levels [immediate release tablets: FDA approved in males and postmenarcheal (>1 year) females ages 10-17 years]

Treatment of primary hypercholesterolemia as adjunct to dietary therapy to decrease elevated serum total and low density lipoprotein cholesterol (LDL-C) (immediate and extended release tablets: FDA approved in adults); to reduce the risk of myocardial infarction, unstable angina, and coronary revascularization procedures in patients without symptomatic disease with average to moderately elevated total and LDL-C and below average HDL-cholesterol (primary prevention) and slow progression of coronary atherosclerosis in patients with coronary heart disease (immediate and extended release tablets: FDA approved in adults)

Pregnancy Risk Factor X

Pregnancy Considerations Adverse events were observed in animal reproduction studies. There are reports of congenital anomalies following maternal use of HMG-CoA reductase inhibitors in pregnancy; however, maternal disease, differences in specific agents used, and the low rates of exposure limit the interpretation of the available data (Godfrey, 2012; Lecarpentier, 2012). Cholesterol biosynthesis may be important in fetal development; serum cholesterol and triglycerides increase normally during pregnancy. The discontinuation of lipid lowering medications temporarily during pregnancy is not expected to have significant impact on the long term outcomes of primary hypercholesterolemia treatment.

Use of lovastatin is contraindicated in pregnancy. HMG-CoA reductase inhibitors should be discontinued prior to pregnancy (ADA, 2013). If treatment of dyslipidemias is needed in pregnant women or in women of reproductive age, other agents are preferred (Berglund, 2012; Stone, 2013). The manufacturer recommends administration to women of childbearing potential only when conception is highly unlikely and patients have been informed of potential hazards.

Breast-Feeding Considerations It is not known if lovastatin is excreted into breast milk. Due to the potential for serious adverse reactions in a nursing infant, use while breast-feeding is contraindicated by the manufacturer.

Contraindications Hypersensitivity to lovastatin or any component; active liver disease; unexplained persistent elevations of serum transaminases; concomitant use of strong CYP3A4 inhibitors [eg, clarithromycin, erythromycin, itraconazole, ketoconazole, nefazodone, posaconazole, protease inhibitors (including boceprevir and telaprevir), telithromycin, cobicistat-containing products]; pregnancy; breast-feeding

Warnings Patients receiving HMG-CoA reductase inhibitors have developed rhabdomyolysis with or without acute renal failure and/or myopathy; patients should be monitored closely; risk is dose-related and is increased with concurrent use of other lipid-lowering medications (eg, fibric acid derivatives or niacin at doses ≥1 g/day) or during concurrent use with potent CYP3A4 inhibitor (contraindication) and large quantities of grapefruit juice (>1 quart/day). The manufacturer recommends temporary discontinuation for elective major surgery, acute medical or surgical conditions, or in any patient experiencing an acute or serious condition predisposing to renal failure (eg, sepsis, hypotension, trauma, uncontrolled seizures). However, based upon current evidence, HMG-CoA reductase inhibitor therapy should be continued in the perioperative period unless risk outweighs cardioprotective benefit. Immune-mediated necrotizing myopathy (IMNM), an autoimmune-mediated myopathy, has been reported (rarely) with HMG-CoA reductase inhibitor therapy. IMNM presents as proximal muscle weakness with elevated CPK levels, which persists despite discontinuation of HMG-CoA reductase inhibitor therapy; additionally, muscle biopsy may show necrotizing myopathy with limited inflammation; immunosuppressive therapy (eg, corticosteroids, azathioprine) may be used for treatment.

Postmarketing reports of fatal and nonfatal hepatic failure are rare; if serious hepatotoxicity with clinical symptoms and/or hyperbilirubinemia or jaundice occurs during treatment, interrupt therapy. If an alternate etiology is not identified, do not restart lovastatin. Liver enzyme tests should be obtained at baseline and as clinically indicated; routine periodic monitoring of liver enzymes is not necessary. Use with caution in patients with history of heavy alcohol use or a previous history of liver disease.

Precautions Use with caution and modify dose in patients with renal impairment. HMG-CoA reductase inhibitors have a high potential for drug interactions; concomitant use of lovastatin with some drugs may require cautious use, may not be recommended, may require dosage adjustments, or may be contraindicated. Increases in Hb A_{1c} and fasting blood glucose have been reported with HMG-CoA reductase inhibitors; however, the benefits of statin therapy far outweigh the risk of dysglycemia. Lovastatin is less effective in patients with rare **homozygous** familial hypercholesterolemia and may be more likely to elevate serum transaminases.

Adverse Reactions

Central nervous system: Dizziness, headache

Dermatologic: Rash

Gastrointestinal: Abdominal pain, constipation, diarrhea, dyspepsia, flatulence, nausea

Neuromuscular & skeletal: Increased CPK (>2x normal), muscle cramps, myalgia, weakness

Ocular: Blurred vision

Rare but important or life-threatening: Acid regurgitation, alopecia, amnesia (reversible), arthralgia, blood glucose increased, chest pain, cognitive impairment (reversible), confusion (reversible), dermatomyositis, diabetes mellitus (new onset), eye irritation, glycosylated hemoglobin (Hb A_{1c}) increased, insomnia, leg pain, memory disturbance (reversible), memory impairment (reversible), paresthesia, pruritus, vomiting, xerostomia

Additional class-related events or case reports (not necessarily reported with lovastatin therapy): Alkaline phosphatase increased, alteration in taste, anaphylaxis, angioedema, anorexia, anxiety, arthritis, cataracts, chills, cholestatic jaundice, cirrhosis, depression, dryness of skin/mucous membranes, dyspnea, eosinophilia, erectile dysfunction, erythema multiforme, ESR increased, facial paresis, fatty liver, fever, flushing, fulminant hepatic necrosis, GGT increased, gynecomastia, hemolytic anemia, hepatic failure (fatal and nonfatal), hepatitis, hepatoma, hyperbilirubinemia, hypersensitivity reaction, immune-mediated necrotizing myopathy (IMNM), impaired extraocular muscle movement, impotence, interstitial lung disease, leukopenia, libido decreased, malaise, myopathy, nail changes, nodules, ophthalmoplegia, pancreatitis, peripheral nerve palsy, peripheral neuropathy, photosensitivity, polymyalgia rheumatica, positive ANA, psychic disturbance, purpura, renal failure (secondary to rhabdomyolysis), rhabdomyolysis, skin discoloration, Stevens-Johnson syndrome, systemic lupus erythematosus-like syndrome, thrombocytopenia, thyroid dysfunction, toxic epidermal necrolysis, transaminases increased, tremor, urticaria, vasculitis, vertigo

Drug Interactions

Metabolism/Transport Effects Substrate of CYP3A4 (major), P-glycoprotein; **Note:** Assignment of Major/Minor substrate status based on clinically relevant drug interaction potential; **Inhibits** CYP2C9 (weak), CYP3A4 (weak)

Avoid Concomitant Use

Avoid concomitant use of Lovastatin with any of the following: Boceprevir; Clarithromycin; Conivaptan; CycloSPORINE (Systemic); CYP3A4 Inhibitors (Strong); Erythromycin (Systemic); Fusidic Acid (Systemic); Gemfibrozil; Lomitapide; Mifepristone; Pimozide; Protease Inhibitors; Red Yeast Rice; Telaprevir; Telithromycin

Increased Effect/Toxicity

Lovastatin may increase the levels/effects of: ARIPiprazole; DAPTOmycin; Diltiazem; Dofetilide; PAZOPanib; Pimozide; Trabectedin; Vitamin K Antagonists

The levels/effects of Lovastatin may be increased by: Amiodarone; Azithromycin (Systemic); Bezafibrate; Boceprevir; Ceritinib; Clarithromycin; Colchicine; Conivaptan; CycloSPORINE (Systemic); CYP3A4 Inhibitors (Moderate); CYP3A4 Inhibitors (Strong); Cyproterone; Danazol; Dasatinib; Diltiazem; Dronedarone; Erythromycin (Systemic); Fenofibrate and Derivatives; Fluconazole; Fusidic Acid (Systemic); Gemfibrozil; Grapefruit Juice; Ivacaftor; Lomitapide; Luliconazole; Mifepristone; Niacin; Niacinamide; P-glycoprotein/ABCB1 Inhibitors; Protease Inhibitors; QuiNINE; Raltegravir; Ranolazine; Red Yeast Rice; Sildenafil; Simeprevir; Telaprevir; Telithromycin; Ticagrelor; Verapamil

Decreased Effect

Lovastatin may decrease the levels/effects of: Lanthanum

The levels/effects of Lovastatin may be decreased by: Antacids; Bosentan; CYP3A4 Inducers (Strong); Dabrafenib; Deferasirox; Efavirenz; Etravirine; Fosphenytoin; Mitotane; P-glycoprotein/ABCB1 Inducers; Phenytoin; Rifamycin Derivatives; Siltuximab; St Johns Wort; Tocilizumab

Food Interactions Food decreases the bioavailability of lovastatin extended release tablets and increases the bioavailability of lovastatin immediate release tablets. Lovastatin serum concentrations may be increased if taken with grapefruit juice. Management: Avoid concurrent intake of large quantities (>1 quart/day) of grapefruit juice.

Stability

Immediate release tablets: Store at 20°C to 25°C (68°F to 77°F); protect from light.

Extended release tablets: Store at 20°C to 25°C (68°F to 77°F); excursions permitted to 15°C to 30°C (59°F to 86°F); avoid excessive heat and humidity.

Mechanism of Action Lovastatin acts by competitively inhibiting 3-hydroxyl-3-methylglutaryl-coenzyme A (HMG-CoA) reductase, the enzyme that catalyzes the rate-limiting step in cholesterol biosynthesis

◀ **Pharmacodynamics**
Onset of action: LDL-cholesterol reduction: 3 days
Maximum effect: LDL-cholesterol reduction: 4-6 weeks
LDL-C reduction: 40 mg/day: 31% (for each doubling of this dose, LDL-C is lowered by ~6%)
Average HDL-C increase: 5% to 15%
Average triglyceride reduction: 7% to 30%

Pharmacokinetics (Adult data unless noted)
Absorption: Oral: 30% absorbed but less than 5% reaches the systemic circulation due to an extensive first-pass effect; absorption increased with extended release tablets
Protein binding: 95%
Half-life: 1.1-1.7 hours
Time to peak serum concentration:
Immediate release: 2-4 hours
Extended release: 12-14 hours
Elimination: ~80% to 85% of dose excreted in feces and 10% in urine

Dosing: Usual
Children and Adolescents:
Heterozygous familial hypercholesterolemia: Note: Begin treatment if after adequate trial of diet the following are present: LDL-C >189 mg/dL or LDL-C remains >160 mg/dL and positive family history of premature cardiovascular disease or meets NCEP classification. Females must be ≥1 year postmenarche.
Children and Adolescents 10-17 years: Oral: Immediate release tablet:
LDL reduction <20%: Initial: 10 mg once daily with evening meal
LDL reduction ≥20%: Initial: 20 mg once daily with evening meal
Usual range: 10-40 mg once daily with evening meal; may titrate at 4-week intervals; maximum daily dose: 40 mg/**day**

Adults: **Dyslipidemia and primary prevention of CAD: Note:** Doses should be individualized according to the baseline LDL-cholesterol levels, the recommended goal of therapy, and patient response. For patients requiring smaller reductions in cholesterol, the use of the extended release tablet is not recommended; consider use of immediate release formulation.
Immediate release tablet: Oral: Initial: 20 mg once daily with evening meal; adjust dosage at 4-week intervals; maximum daily dose: 80 mg/**day**
Extended release tablet: Oral: Initial: 20, 40, or 60 mg once daily at bedtime; adjust dosage at 4-week intervals; maximum daily dose: 60 mg/**day**

Dosage adjustment in patients who are concomitantly receiving amiodarone: Adults: Dose should not exceed 40 mg/day

Dosage adjustment in patients who are concomitantly receiving danazol, diltiazem, or verapamil: Adults: Initial: 10 mg once daily, not to exceed 20 mg/day

Dosage adjustment in renal impairment: CrCl <30 mL/minute:
Immediate release: Children ≥10 years, Adolescents, and Adults: Doses exceeding 20 mg/day should be carefully considered and implemented cautiously
Extended release: Adults: Initial: 20 mg once daily at bedtime; doses exceeding 20 mg/day should be carefully considered and implemented cautiously

Dosage adjustment in hepatic impairment: There are no dosage adjustment provided in manufacturer's labeling (has not been studied); use is contraindicated in active liver disease or unexplained transaminase elevations.

Administration Oral:
Immediate release tablets: Take with the evening meal.
Extended release tablets: Take at bedtime; do not crush or chew.

Monitoring Parameters
Pediatric patients: Baseline: ALT, AST, and creatine phosphokinase levels (CPK); fasting lipid panel (FLP) and repeat ALT and AST should be checked after 4 weeks of therapy; if no myopathy symptoms or laboratory abnormalities, then monitor FLP, ALT, and AST every 3-4 months during the first year and then every 6 months thereafter (NHLBI, 2011).
Adults: Baseline CPK (recheck CPK in any patient with symptoms suggestive of myopathy; discontinue therapy if markedly elevated); baseline liver function tests (LFTs) and repeat when clinically indicated thereafter. Patients with elevated transaminase levels should have a second (confirmatory) test and frequent monitoring until values normalize; discontinue if increase in ALT/AST is persistently >3 times ULN (NCEP, 2002).
Lipid panel (total cholesterol, HDL, LDL, triglycerides):
ATP III recommendations (NCEP, 2002): Baseline; 6-8 weeks after initiation of drug therapy; if dose increased, then at 6-8 weeks until final dose determined. Once treatment goal achieved, follow-up intervals may be reduced to every 4-6 months. Lipid panel should be assessed at least annually, and preferably at each clinic visit.
Manufacturer recommendation: Analyze lipid panel at intervals of 4 weeks or more.

Dosage Forms Excipient information presented when available (limited, particularly for generics); consult specific product labeling.
Tablet, Oral:
Mevacor: 20 mg, 40 mg
Generic: 10 mg, 20 mg, 40 mg
Tablet Extended Release 24 Hour, Oral:
Altoprev: 20 mg, 40 mg, 60 mg [contains fd&c yellow #6 (sunset yellow)]

References
American Academy of Pediatrics Committee on Nutrition, "Cholesterol in Childhood," *Pediatrics*, 1998, 101(1 Pt 1):141-7.
American Academy of Pediatrics, "National Cholesterol Education Program: Report of the Expert Panel on Blood Cholesterol Levels in Children and Adolescents," *Pediatrics*, 1992, 89(3 Pt 2):525-84.
American Diabetes Association, "Standards of Medical Care in Diabetes-2013," *Diabetes Care*, 2013, 36(Suppl 1):S11-66.
Berglund L, Brunzell JD, Goldberg AC, et al, "Evaluation and Treatment of Hypertriglyceridemia: An Endocrine Society Clinical Practice Guideline," *J Clin Endocrinol Metab*, 2012, 97(9):2969-89.
Daniels SR, Greer FR, and Committee on Nutrition, "Lipid Screening and Cardiovascular Health in Childhood," *Pediatrics*, 2008, 122 (1):198-208.
Duplaga BA, "Treatment of Childhood Hypercholesterolemia With HMG-CoA Reductase Inhibitors," *Ann Pharmacother*, 1999, 33 (11):1224-7.
"Executive Summary of The Third Report of The National Cholesterol Education Program (NCEP) Expert Panel on Detection, Evaluation, and Treatment of High Blood Cholesterol in Adults (Adult Treatment Panel III)," *JAMA*, 2001, 285(19):2486-97.
Godfrey LM, Erramouspe J, and Cleveland KW, "Teratogenic Risk of Statins in Pregnancy," *Ann Pharmacother*, 2012, 46(10):1419-24.
Grundy SM, Cleeman JI, Merz CN, et al, "Implications of Recent Clinical Trials for the National Cholesterol Education Program Adult Treatment Panel III Guidelines," *Circulation*, 2004, 110(2):227-39.
Lambert M, Lupien PJ, Gagne C, et al, "Treatment of Familial Hypercholesterolemia in Children and Adolescents: Effect of Lovastatin. Canadian Lovastatin in Children Study Group," *Pediatrics*, 1996, 97 (5):619-28.
Lecarpentier E, Morel O, Fournier T, et al, "Statins and Pregnancy: Between Supposed Risks and Theoretical Benefits," *Drugs*, 2012, 72 (6):773-88.
McCrindle BW, Urbina EM, Dennison BA, et al, "Drug Therapy of High-Risk Lipid Abnormalities in Children and Adolescents: A Scientific Statement from the American Heart Association Atherosclerosis, Hypertension, and Obesity in Youth Committee, Council of Cardiovascular Disease in the Young, With the Council on Cardiovascular Nursing," *Circulation*, 2007, 115(14):1948-67.
National Heart, Lung, and Blood Institute, "Expert Panel on Integrated Guidelines for Cardiovascular Health and Risk Reduction in Children and Adolescents," *Clinical Practice Guidelines*, 2011, National Institutes of Health. Available at http://www.nhlbi.nih.gov/guidelines/cvd_ped/peds_guidelines_full.pdf

Stein EA, Illingworth DR, Kwiterovich PO Jr, et al, "Efficacy and Safety of Lovastatin in Adolescent Males With Heterozygous Familial Hypercholesterolemia: A Randomized Controlled Trial," *JAMA*, 1999, 281 (2):137-44.

"Third Report of the National Cholesterol Education Program Expert Panel on Detection, Evaluation, and Treatment of High Blood Cholesterol in Adults (Adult Treatment Panel III)," May 2001, www.nhlbi. nih.gov/guidelines/cholesterol.

◆ **Lovenox** see Enoxaparin on page 752

◆ **Lovenox HP (Can)** see Enoxaparin on page 752

◆ **Low-Molecular-Weight Iron Dextran (INFeD)** see Iron Dextran Complex on page 1153

◆ **Lozi-Flur** see Fluoride on page 894

◆ **L-PAM** see Melphalan on page 1328

◆ **L-Phenylalanine Mustard** see Melphalan on page 1328

◆ **L-Sarcolysin** see Melphalan on page 1328

◆ **LTA 360 Kit** see Lidocaine (Topical) on page 1242

◆ **LTG** see LamoTRIgine on page 1199

◆ **L-Thyroxine Sodium** see Levothyroxine on page 1234

◆ **Lu-26-054** see Escitalopram on page 788

Lucinactant (loo sin AK tant)

Brand Names: U.S. Surfaxin
Therapeutic Category Lung Surfactant
Generic Availability (U.S.) No
Use Prevention of respiratory distress syndrome (RDS) in premature neonates at high risk for RDS (FDA approved in neonates)
Contraindications Hypersensitivity to lucinactant or any component
Warnings Lucinactant should only be administered by clinicians experienced in resuscitation, intubation, stabilization, and ventilatory management of premature neonates in a critical care setting. Lucinactant rapidly affects oxygenation and lung compliance; the neonate may require frequent adjustments to oxygen delivery and ventilator settings. Transient episodes of bradycardia, decreased oxygen saturation, endotracheal tube blockage, or reflux of lucinactant into endotracheal tube may occur; interrupt dosing procedure and initiate measures to alleviate the problem and stabilize neonate's condition; may reinstitute therapy after the patient is stable. In clinical trials of lucinactant in adults with acute respiratory distress syndrome (ARDS), an increased incidence of sepsis, pneumothorax, pulmonary embolism, hypotension, sepsis, and death was observed; use for the treatment of ARDS in adults is not appropriate.
Precautions For endotracheal administration only.
Adverse Reactions Events observed during the dosing procedure:
Cardiovascular: Bradycardia
Local: Endotracheal tube obstruction, endotracheal tube reflux
Respiratory: Oxygen desaturation
Drug Interactions
Metabolism/Transport Effects None known.
Avoid Concomitant Use
Avoid concomitant use of Lucinactant with any of the following: Ceritinib
Increased Effect/Toxicity
Lucinactant may increase the levels/effects of: Bradycardia-Causing Agents; Ceritinib
Decreased Effect There are no known significant interactions involving a decrease in effect.
Stability Store intact vials at 2°C to 8°C (36°F to 46°F); do not freeze. Protect from light.
Mechanism of Action Surfactant administration replaces deficient or ineffective endogenous lung surfactant in neonates at risk of developing RDS. Surfactant prevents the alveoli from collapsing during expiration by lowering surface tension between air and alveolar surfaces. Lucinactant, a synthetic surfactant containing phospholipids, also contains sinapultide (KL4 peptide) which resembles and is believed to mimic the action of one of the human surfactant proteins (SPs), namely SP-B.

Dosing: Neonatal
Respiratory distress syndrome, prophylaxis: Premature neonates: Endotracheal: 5.8 mL/kg/dose; may repeat for up to 3 subsequent doses (total of 4 doses) at ≥6 hour intervals within the first 48 hours of life. **Note:** Use in neonates with birthweight >1250 g has not been evaluated.

Administration For endotracheal administration only.

Prior to administration, verify that the suspension has been properly warmed; shake vial vigorously; visually inspect to ensure the suspension is uniform, free-flowing, and opaque white to off-white. Vials are for single use only; discard any unused portion. If not used immediately after warming, may store protected from light for up to 2 hours at room temperature; do not return to refrigerator after warming. Discard warmed vial if not used within 2 hours.

Slowly draw up the appropriate amount of lucinactant into a single, appropriately sized syringe (depending on total dose volume) using a 16- or 18-gauge needle. Neonate may be suctioned prior to administration; allow neonate to stabilize prior to administration. Administer endotracheally by instilling through a 5-French end-hole catheter inserted into the endotracheal tube. Administer in four aliquots of 1.45 mL/kg each (¼ of total volume) alternating positions between right and left lateral decubitus. Each aliquot is instilled as a bolus with continued positive pressure ventilation; evaluate neonate's respiratory status and allow for stabilization between aliquots; oxygen saturation and heart rate should be ≥90% and >120 bpm, respectively, prior to administering the next aliquot. Following administration of one full dose (four aliquots), withhold suctioning for 1 hour unless signs of significant airway obstruction occur and keep the neonate's bed elevated ≥10° for at least 1-2 hours.
Monitoring Parameters Continuous heart rate and transcutaneous O_2 saturation; ventilator settings; frequent ABG sampling is necessary to prevent postdosing hyperoxia and hypocarbia.
Additional Information Each mL contains 30 mg phospholipids (22.5 mg dipalmitoylphosphatidylcholine and 7.5 mg palmitoyloleoyl-phosphatidylglycerol, sodium salt), 4.05 mg palmitic acid, and 0.862 mg sinapultide.
References

Moya FR, Gadzinowski J, Bancalari E, et al, "A Multicenter, Randomized, Masked, Comparison Trial of Lucinactant, Colfosceril Palmitate, and Beractant for the Prevention of Respiratory Distress Syndrome Among Very Preterm Infants," *Pediatrics*, 2005, 115(4):1018-29.

Moya FR, Sinha S, Gadzinowski J, et al, "One-Year Follow-up of Very Preterm Infants Who Received Lucinactant for Prevention of Respiratory Distress Syndrome: Results From 2 Multicenter Randomized, Controlled Trials," *Pediatrics*, 2007, 119(6): e1361-70.

Sinha SK, Lacaze-Masmonteil T, Valls i Soler A, et al, "A Multicenter, Randomized, Controlled Trial of Lucinactant Versus Poractant Alfa Among Very Premature Infants at High Risk for Respiratory Distress Syndrome," *Pediatrics*, 2005, 115(4):1030-8.

◆ **Lugol's Solution** see Potassium Iodide and Iodine on page 1713

◆ **Lumefantrine and Artemether** see Artemether and Lumefantrine on page 203

◆ **Luminal Sodium** see PHENobarbital on page 1651

◆ **Lumizyme** see Alglucosidase Alfa on page 95

◆ **Lupron (Can)** see Leuprolide on page 1215

◆ **Lupron Depot** see Leuprolide on page 1215

◆ **Lupron Depot-Ped** see Leuprolide on page 1215

◆ **Luvox** see FluvoxaMINE on page 922

- ◆ **Luvox CR** *see* FluvoxaMINE *on page 922*
- ◆ **Luxiq** *see* Betamethasone (Topical) *on page 285*
- ◆ **LY139603** *see* AtoMOXetine *on page 224*
- ◆ **LY146032** *see* DAPTOmycin *on page 589*
- ◆ **LY170053** *see* OLANZapine *on page 1525*
- ◆ **LY-188011** *see* Gemcitabine *on page 959*
- ◆ **Lyderm® (Can)** *see* Fluocinonide *on page 894*
- ◆ **Lymphocyte Immune Globulin** *see* Antithymocyte Globulin (Equine) *on page 182*
- ◆ **Lymphocyte Mitogenic Factor** *see* Aldesleukin *on page 90*
- ◆ **Lysodren** *see* Mitotane *on page 1425*
- ◆ **Lysteda** *see* Tranexamic Acid *on page 2063*
- ◆ **Lyza** *see* Norethindrone *on page 1511*
- ◆ **Maalox [OTC]** *see* Calcium Carbonate *on page 346*
- ◆ **Maalox Childrens [OTC]** *see* Calcium Carbonate *on page 346*
- ◆ **Macrobid** *see* Nitrofurantoin *on page 1502*
- ◆ **Macrodantin** *see* Nitrofurantoin *on page 1502*
- ◆ **Macrogol** *see* Polyethylene Glycol 3350 *on page 1696*

Mafenide (MA fe nide)

Brand Names: U.S. Sulfamylon
Therapeutic Category Antibiotic, Topical
Generic Availability (U.S.) May be product dependent
Use Adjunct in the treatment of second and third degree burns to prevent septicemia caused by susceptible organisms such as *Pseudomonas aeruginosa*

Pregnancy Risk Factor C
Pregnancy Considerations Adverse events were not observed in animal reproduction studies using an oral preparation. Safety and efficacy have not been established in pregnant women. The manufacturer does not recommended use in women of childbearing potential unless the burn area covers >20% of the total body surface or when benefits of treatment outweigh possible risks to the fetus.

Breast-Feeding Considerations It is not known if mafenide is excreted in breast milk. Due to the potential for serious adverse reactions in the nursing infant, a decision should be made whether to discontinue nursing or to discontinue the drug, taking into account the importance of treatment to the mother.

Contraindications Hypersensitivity to mafenide or any component
Warnings Superinfection with nonsusceptible organisms has occurred in burn wounds treated with mafenide; some products contain sulfites which may cause allergic reactions in susceptible individuals
Precautions Use with caution in patients with renal impairment and in patients with G-6-PD deficiency

Adverse Reactions
Cardiovascular: Edema, facial edema
Dermatologic: Erythema, maceration, pruritus, rash, urticaria
Endocrine & metabolic: Hyperchloremia, metabolic acidosis
Gastrointestinal: Diarrhea (following accidental ingestion)
Hematologic: Bleeding, bone marrow suppression, DIC, eosinophilia, hemolytic anemia, porphyria
Local: Blisters, burning sensation, excoriation, pain
Respiratory: Dyspnea, hyperventilation, pCO_2 decreased, tachypnea
Miscellaneous: Hypersensitivity

Drug Interactions
Metabolism/Transport Effects None known.

Avoid Concomitant Use
Avoid concomitant use of Mafenide with any of the following: BCG
Increased Effect/Toxicity
Mafenide may increase the levels/effects of: Prilocaine; Sodium Nitrite

The levels/effects of Mafenide may be increased by: Nitric Oxide
Decreased Effect
Mafenide may decrease the levels/effects of: BCG; Sodium Picosulfate

Stability Prepared topical solution is stable for 48 hours at room temperature
Mechanism of Action As a sulfonamide, mafenide interferes with bacterial folic acid synthesis through competitive inhibition of para-aminobenzoic acid. Spectrum of activity encompasses both gram positive and negative organisms, including *Pseudomonas* and some anaerobes.

Pharmacokinetics (Adult data unless noted)
Absorption: Diffuses through devascularized areas and is rapidly absorbed from burned surface
Metabolism: To para-carboxybenzene sulfonamide which is a carbonic anhydrase inhibitor
Time to peak serum concentration: Topical: 2-4 hours
Elimination: In urine as metabolites

Dosing: Usual Children ≥3 months and Adults: Topical
Cream: Apply once or twice daily; apply to a thickness of approximately 16 mm; the burned area should be covered with cream at all times
Solution: Irrigate dressing every 4 hours or as needed to keep gauze moistened

Administration Topical:
Cream: Apply to cleansed, debrided, burned area with a sterile-gloved hand
Solution: Reconstitute 50 g powder by adding to 1 liter sterile water or 1 liter NS for irrigation; mix until completely dissolved; filter solution through a 0.22 micron filter before use; cover area with gauze and the dressing wetted with mafenide solution; wound dressing may be left undisturbed for up to 5 days

Monitoring Parameters Acid base balance, improvement of wound healing
Dosage Forms Excipient information presented when available (limited, particularly for generics); consult specific product labeling.
Cream, External, as acetate [strength expressed as base]:
Sulfamylon: 85 mg/g (56.7 g, 113.4 g, 453.6 g) [contains methylparaben, propylparaben, sodium metabisulfite]
Packet, External, as acetate:
Sulfamylon: 50 g (1 ea, 5 ea)
Generic: 50 g (1 ea, 5 ea)

- ◆ **Mafenide Acetate** *see* Mafenide *on page 1290*
- ◆ **Mag-200 [OTC]** *see* Magnesium Oxide *on page 1296*
- ◆ **Mag-Al [OTC]** *see* Aluminum Hydroxide and Magnesium Hydroxide *on page 111*
- ◆ **Mag-Al Ultimate [OTC]** *see* Aluminum Hydroxide and Magnesium Hydroxide *on page 111*
- ◆ **Mag Citrate** *see* Magnesium Citrate *on page 1292*
- ◆ **Mag-Delay [OTC]** *see* Magnesium Chloride *on page 1291*
- ◆ **Mag-G [OTC]** *see* Magnesium Gluconate *on page 1293*
- ◆ **Magic Bullets [OTC]** *see* Bisacodyl *on page 293*
- ◆ **Maginex™ [OTC]** *see* Magnesium L-aspartate Hydrochloride *on page 1295*
- ◆ **Maginex™ DS [OTC]** *see* Magnesium L-aspartate Hydrochloride *on page 1295*
- ◆ **Magnesia Magma** *see* Magnesium Hydroxide *on page 1294*

Magnesium Chloride (mag NEE zhum KLOR ide)

Related Information
Oral Medications That Should Not Be Crushed or Altered on page 2438

Brand Names: U.S. Chloromag; Mag-Delay [OTC]; Mag-SR Plus Calcium [OTC]; Mag-SR [OTC]; Slow Magnesium/Calcium [OTC]; Slow-Mag [OTC]

Therapeutic Category Electrolyte Supplement, Oral; Electrolyte Supplement, Parenteral; Magnesium Salt

Generic Availability (U.S.) Yes

Use Treatment and prevention of hypomagnesemia; dietary supplement

Pregnancy Risk Factor C

Pregnancy Considerations Animal reproduction studies have not been conducted. Magnesium crosses the placenta; serum levels in the fetus correlate with those in the mother (Idama, 1998; Osada, 2002).

Breast-Feeding Considerations Magnesium is found in breast milk; concentrations remain constant during the first year of lactation and are not influenced by dietary intake under normal conditions. Magnesium requirements are the same in lactating and non-lactating females (IOM, 1997).

Contraindications Hypersensitivity to magnesium salt(s) or any component; serious renal impairment, myocardial damage, heart block; patients with colostomy or ileostomy, intestinal obstruction, impaction, or perforation, appendicitis, abdominal pain

Warnings Multiple salt forms of magnesium exist; close attention must be paid to the salt form when ordering and administering magnesium; **incorrect selection or substitution of one salt for another without proper dosage adjustment may result in serious over- or under-dosing**

Magnesium chloride injection contains benzyl alcohol which may cause allergic reactions in susceptible individuals; large amounts of benzyl alcohol (≥ 99 mg/kg/day) have been associated with a potentially fatal toxicity ("gasping syndrome") in neonates; the "gasping syndrome" consists of metabolic acidosis, respiratory distress, gasping respirations, CNS dysfunction (including convulsions, intracranial hemorrhage), hypotension and cardiovascular collapse; avoid or use magnesium chloride injection with caution in neonates

Precautions Use with caution in patients with impaired renal function (accumulation of magnesium may lead to magnesium intoxication); use with caution in digitalized patients (may alter cardiac conduction leading to heart block). The parenteral product may contain aluminum; toxic aluminum concentrations may be seen with high doses, prolonged use, or renal dysfunction. Premature neonates are at higher risk due to immature renal function and aluminum intake from other parenteral sources. Parenteral aluminum exposure of >4-5 mcg/kg/day is associated with CNS and bone toxicity and tissue loading may occur at lower doses.

Adverse Reactions Gastrointestinal: Diarrhea (excessive oral doses)

Drug Interactions
Metabolism/Transport Effects None known.

Avoid Concomitant Use

Avoid concomitant use of Magnesium Chloride with any of the following: Raltegravir

Increased Effect/Toxicity

Magnesium Chloride may increase the levels/effects of: Calcium Channel Blockers; Gabapentin; Neuromuscular-Blocking Agents

The levels/effects of Magnesium Chloride may be increased by: Alfacalcidol; Calcitriol; Calcium Channel Blockers

Decreased Effect

Magnesium Chloride may decrease the levels/effects of: Bisphosphonate Derivatives; Deferiprone; Dolutegravir; Eltrombopag; Gabapentin; Multivitamins/Fluoride (with ADE); Mycophenolate; Phosphate Supplements; Quinolone Antibiotics; Raltegravir; Tetracycline Derivatives; Trientine

The levels/effects of Magnesium Chloride may be decreased by: Trientine

Mechanism of Action Magnesium is important as a cofactor in many enzymatic reactions in the body involving protein synthesis and carbohydrate metabolism (at least 300 enzymatic reactions require magnesium). Actions on lipoprotein lipase have been found to be important in reducing serum cholesterol and on sodium/potassium ATPase in promoting polarization (eg, neuromuscular functioning).

Pharmacokinetics (Adult data unless noted)
Absorption: Oral: Up to 30%
Elimination: Renal with unabsorbed drug excreted in feces

Dosing: Neonatal
Hypomagnesemia: I.V.: Magnesium chloride: 0.2-0.4 mEq/kg/dose every 8-12 hours for 2-3 doses
Daily maintenance magnesium: I.V.: 0.25-0.5 mEq magnesium/kg/day (**Note:** mEq denotes amount of magnesium ion only not the total salt form.)

Dosing: Usual
Hypomagnesemia: Children:
I.M., I.V.: Magnesium chloride: 0.2-0.4 mEq/kg/dose every 4-6 hours for 3-4 doses; maximum single dose: 16 mEq
Oral: **Note:** Achieving optimal magnesium levels using oral therapy may be difficult due to the propensity for magnesium to cause diarrhea; I.V. replacement may be more appropriate particularly in situations of severe deficit: **Magnesium chloride:** 10-20 mg/kg elemental magnesium per dose up to 4 times/day
Dietary supplement: Adults: Oral: (Mag 64®, Mag Delay™, Slow-Mag®): 2 tablets once daily
Daily maintenance magnesium: I.V.: Magnesium chloride: Infants and Children ≤45 kg: 0.25-0.5 mEq/kg/day
Adolescents >45 kg and Adults: 0.2-0.5 mEq/kg/day or 3-10 mEq/1000 kcal/day (maximum: 8-20 mEq/day)

Dosing adjustment in renal impairment: Patients in severe renal failure should not receive magnesium due to toxicity from accumulation. Patients with a CrCl <25 mL/minute receiving magnesium should have serum magnesium levels monitored.

Administration
Oral: Tablet: Take with full glass of water; do not chew or crush sustained release formulations
Parenteral: Intermittent infusion: Dilute to a concentration of 0.5 mEq/mL (maximum concentration: 1.6 mEq/mL, and infuse over 2-4 hours; do not exceed 1 mEq/kg/hour; in severe circumstances, half of the dosage to be administered may be infused over the first 15-20 minutes

Monitoring Parameters Serum magnesium, deep tendon reflexes, respiratory rate, renal function, blood pressure, stool output (laxative use)

Reference Range
Neonates and Infants: 1.5-2.3 mEq/L
Children: 1.5-2.0 mEq/L
Adults: 1.4-2.0 mEq/L

Additional Information Magnesium chloride 500 mg = 59 mg **elemental** magnesium = 4.9 mEq magnesium

Elemental Magnesium Content of Magnesium Salts

Magnesium Salt	Elemental Magnesium (mg/500 mg salt)	Magnesium (mEq/500 mg salt)
Magnesium chloride	59	4.9
Magnesium gluconate	27	2.4
Magnesium L-aspartate	49.6	4.1
Magnesium oxide	302	25
Magnesium sulfate	49.3	4.1

Adverse effects associated with elevated serum magnesium concentrations may include:

>3 mg/dL: Blocked peripheral neuromuscular transmission leading to anticonvulsant effects, depressed CNS

>5 mg/dL: Depressed deep tendon reflexes, flushing, somnolence

>12 mg/dL: Complete heart block, respiratory paralysis

Dosage Forms Considerations

1 g magnesium chloride = elemental magnesium 120 mg = magnesium 9.85 mEq = magnesium 4.93 mmol

Elemental magnesium 64 mg = magnesium 5.26 mEq = magnesium 2.62 mmol

Dosage Forms Excipient information presented when available (limited, particularly for generics); consult specific product labeling.

Solution, Injection, as hexahydrate:

Chloromag: 200 mg/mL (50 mL) [contains benzyl alcohol]

Generic: 200 mg/mL (50 mL)

Tablet Delayed Release, Oral:

Mag-SR Plus Calcium: 64-106 mg [starch free, sugar free]

Slow Magnesium/Calcium: 64-106 mg

Slow-Mag: 71.5-119 mg [contains fd&c blue #2 aluminum lake]

Tablet Extended Release, Oral:

Mag-Delay: 535 (64 mg) mg

Mag-SR: 535 (64 mg) mg [starch free, sugar free]

References

Department Health & Human Services, Food Drug Administration, "Aluminum in Large and Small Volume Parenterals Used in Total Parenteral Nutrition," *Federal Register*, 2000, 65(17):4103-11.

Idama TO and Lindow SW, "Magnesium Sulphate: A Review of Clinical Pharmacology Applied to Obstetrics," *Br J Obstet Gynaecol*, 1998, 105(3):260-8.

IOM (Institute of Medicine), *Dietary Reference Intakes for Calcium, Phosphorus, Magnesium, Vitamin D, and Fluoride*, National Academy of Sciences, Washington, DC, 1997.

Osada H, Watanabe Y, Nishimura Y, at al, "Profile of Trace Element Concentrations in the Feto-Placental Unit in Relation to Fetal Growth," *Acta Obstet Gynecol Scand*, 2002, 81(10):931-7.

Magnesium Citrate (mag NEE zhum SIT rate)

Brand Names: U.S. Citroma [OTC]

Brand Names: Canada Citro-Mag

Therapeutic Category Laxative, Osmotic; Magnesium Salt

Generic Availability (U.S.) Yes

Use Short-term treatment of constipation

Pregnancy Considerations Magnesium crosses the placenta; serum concentrations in the fetus are similar to those in the mother (Idama, 1998; Osada, 2002). The American Gastroenterological Association considers the use of magnesium citrate as a laxative to be low risk in pregnancy, but long term use should be avoided (not the preferred treatment of chronic constipation) (Mahadevan, 2006).

Breast-Feeding Considerations Magnesium is found in breast milk; concentrations remain constant during the first year of lactation and are not influenced by dietary intake under normal conditions (IOM, 1997).

Contraindications Hypersensitivity to magnesium salt(s) or any component; serious renal impairment, myocardial damage, heart block; patients with colostomy or ileostomy, intestinal obstruction, impaction, or perforation, appendicitis, abdominal pain

Warnings Multiple salt forms of magnesium exist; close attention must be paid to the salt form when ordering and administering magnesium; **incorrect selection or substitution of one salt for another without proper dosage adjustment may result in serious over- or under-dosing.**

Precautions Use with caution in patients with impaired renal function (accumulation of magnesium may lead to magnesium intoxication)

Adverse Reactions Gastrointestinal: Abdominal pain, diarrhea, gas formation, nausea, vomiting

Drug Interactions

Metabolism/Transport Effects None known.

Avoid Concomitant Use

Avoid concomitant use of Magnesium Citrate with any of the following: Calcium Polystyrene Sulfonate; Raltegravir; Sodium Polystyrene Sulfonate

Increased Effect/Toxicity

Magnesium Citrate may increase the levels/effects of: Aluminum Hydroxide; Calcium Channel Blockers; Calcium Polystyrene Sulfonate; Gabapentin; Neuromuscular-Blocking Agents; Sodium Polystyrene Sulfonate

The levels/effects of Magnesium Citrate may be increased by: Alfacalcidol; Calcitriol; Calcium Channel Blockers

Decreased Effect

Magnesium Citrate may decrease the levels/effects of: Bisphosphonate Derivatives; Deferiprone; Dolutegravir; Eltrombopag; Gabapentin; Multivitamins/Fluoride (with ADE); Mycophenolate; Phosphate Supplements; Quinolone Antibiotics; Raltegravir; Tetracycline Derivatives; Trientine

The levels/effects of Magnesium Citrate may be decreased by: Trientine

Mechanism of Action Promotes bowel evacuation by causing osmotic retention of fluid which distends the colon with increased peristaltic activity

Pharmacodynamics Onset of action: Laxative: Oral: 4-8 hours

Pharmacokinetics (Adult data unless noted)

Absorption: Oral: Up to 30%

Elimination: Renal with unabsorbed drug excreted in feces

Dosing: Usual Cathartic: Oral:

Children <6 years: 2-4 mL/kg/dose given once or in divided doses

Children 6-12 years: 100-150 mL/dose given once or in divided doses

Children >12 years and Adults: 150-300 mL/dose given once or in divided doses

Dosing adjustment in renal impairment: Patients in severe renal failure should not receive magnesium due to toxicity from accumulation. Patients with a CrCl <25 mL/minute receiving magnesium should have serum magnesium levels monitored.

Administration Oral:

Solution: Mix with water and administer on an empty stomach.

Tablet: Take with full glass of water.

Monitoring Parameters Stool output

Test Interactions Increased magnesium; decreased protein, decreased calcium (S), decreased potassium (S)

Dosage Forms Considerations

1 g magnesium citrate ≈ elemental magnesium 160 mg = magnesium 13 mEq = magnesium 6.5 mmol

Dosage Forms Excipient information presented when available (limited, particularly for generics); consult specific product labeling.

Solution, Oral:

Citroma: 1.745 g/30 mL (296 mL) [contains polyethylene glycol, saccharin sodium; lemon flavor]

Citroma: 1.745 g/30 mL (296 mL) [low sodium; lemon flavor]

Citroma: 1.745 g/30 mL (296 mL) [low sodium; contains fd&c red #40, saccharin sodium; cherry flavor]

Generic: 1.745 g/30 mL (296 mL)

Tablet, Oral:

Generic: 100 mg

References

Idama TO and Lindow SW, "Magnesium Sulphate: A Review of Clinical Pharmacology Applied to Obstetrics," *Br J Obstet Gynaecol*, 1998, 105(3):260-8.

Institute of Medicine (IOM), *Dietary Reference Intakes for Calcium, Phosphorus, Magnesium, Vitamin D, and Fluoride*, Washington, DC: The National Academies Press, 1997.

Mahadevan U and Kane S, "American Gastroenterological Association Institute Medical Position Statement on the Use of Gastrointestinal Medications in Pregnancy," *Gastroenterology*, 2006, 131(1):278-82.

Osada H, Watanabe Y, Nishimura Y, et al, "Profile of Trace Element Concentrations in the Feto-Placental Unit in Relation to Fetal Growth," *Acta Obstet Gynecol Scand*, 2002, 81(10):931-7.

Magnesium Gluconate
(mag NEE zhum GLOO koe nate)

Brand Names: U.S. Mag-G [OTC]; Magonate [OTC]

Therapeutic Category Electrolyte Supplement, Oral; Magnesium Salt

Generic Availability (U.S.) May be product dependent

Use Treatment and prevention of hypomagnesemia; dietary supplement

Pregnancy Considerations Magnesium crosses the placenta; serum concentrations in the fetus are similar to those in the mother (Idama, 1998; Osada, 2002).

Breast-Feeding Considerations Magnesium is found in breast milk; concentrations remain constant during the first year of lactation and are not influenced by dietary intake under normal conditions. Magnesium requirements are the same in lactating and nonlactating females (IOM, 1997).

Contraindications Hypersensitivity to magnesium salt(s) or any component; serious renal impairment, myocardial damage, heart block; patients with colostomy or ileostomy, intestinal obstruction, impaction, or perforation, appendicitis, abdominal pain

Warnings Multiple salt forms of magnesium exist; close attention must be paid to the salt form when ordering and administering magnesium; **incorrect selection or substitution of one salt for another without proper dosage adjustment may result in serious over- or under-dosing**

Magonate® solution contains sodium benzoate; benzoic acid (benzoate) is a metabolite of benzyl alcohol; large amounts of benzyl alcohol (≥99 mg/kg/day) have been associated with a potentially fatal toxicity ("gasping syndrome") in neonates; *in vitro* and animal studies have shown that benzoate displaces bilirubin from protein binding sites; avoid use of Magonate® solution in neonates

Precautions Use with caution in patients with impaired renal function (accumulation of magnesium may lead to magnesium intoxication)

Adverse Reactions Gastrointestinal: Diarrhea (excessive oral doses)

Drug Interactions

Metabolism/Transport Effects None known.

Avoid Concomitant Use

Avoid concomitant use of Magnesium Gluconate with any of the following: Raltegravir

Increased Effect/Toxicity

Magnesium Gluconate may increase the levels/effects of: Calcium Channel Blockers; Gabapentin; Neuromuscular-Blocking Agents

The levels/effects of Magnesium Gluconate may be increased by: Alfacalcidol; Calcitriol; Calcium Channel Blockers

Decreased Effect

Magnesium Gluconate may decrease the levels/effects of: Bisphosphonate Derivatives; Deferiprone; Dolutegravir; Eltrombopag; Gabapentin; Multivitamins/Fluoride (with ADE); Mycophenolate; Phosphate Supplements; Quinolone Antibiotics; Raltegravir; Tetracycline Derivatives; Trientine

The levels/effects of Magnesium Gluconate may be decreased by: Trientine

Mechanism of Action Magnesium is important as a cofactor in many enzymatic reactions in the body involving protein synthesis and carbohydrate metabolism (at least 300 enzymatic reactions require magnesium). Actions on lipoprotein lipase have been found to be important in reducing serum cholesterol and on sodium/potassium ATPase in promoting polarization (eg, neuromuscular functioning).

Pharmacokinetics (Adult data unless noted)

Absorption: Oral: Up to 30%

Elimination: Renal with unabsorbed drug excreted in feces

Dosing: Neonatal Recommended daily allowance of magnesium: Oral: 40 mg/day

Dosing: Usual Oral: **Note:** Achieving optimal magnesium levels using oral therapy may be difficult due to the propensity for magnesium to cause diarrhea: I.V. replacement may be more appropriate particularly in situations of severe deficit.

Recommended daily allowance of magnesium: See table.

Magnesium – Recommended Daily Allowance (RDA) and Estimated Average Requirement (EAR) (in terms of elemental magnesium)

Age	RDA (mg/day)	EAR (mg/day)
1 to <6 mo	40	30
6 to <12 mo	60	75
1-3 y	80	65
4-8 y	130	110
Male		
9-13 y	240	200
14-18 y	410	340
Female		
9-13 y	240	200
14-18 y	360	300

Prevention and treatment of hypomagnesemia:

Children: 10-20 mg/kg **elemental** magnesium per dose up to 4 times/day

Adults: 500-1000 mg 3 times/day

Dosing adjustment in renal impairment: Patients in severe renal failure should not receive magnesium due to toxicity from accumulation. Patients with a CrCl <25 mL/minute receiving magnesium should have serum magnesium levels monitored.

Administration Oral:

Solution: Mix with water and administer on an empty stomach.

Tablet: Take with full glass of water.

◄ **Additional Information** Magnesium gluconate 500 mg = 27 mg **elemental** magnesium = 2.4 mEq magnesium

Elemental Magnesium Content of Magnesium Salts

Magnesium Salt	Elemental Magnesium (mg/500 mg salt)	Magnesium (mEq/500 mg salt)
Magnesium chloride	59	4.9
Magnesium gluconate	27	2.4
Magnesium L-aspartate	49.6	4.1
Magnesium oxide	302	25
Magnesium sulfate	49.3	4.1

Adverse effects associated with elevated serum magnesium concentrations may include:

>3 mg/dL: Blocked peripheral neuromuscular transmission leading to anticonvulsant effects, depressed CNS

>5 mg/dL: Depressed deep tendon reflexes, flushing, somnolence

>12 mg/dL: Complete heart block, respiratory paralysis

Dosage Forms Considerations

1 g magnesium gluconate = elemental magnesium 54 mg = magnesium 4.5 mEq = magnesium 2.25 mmol

Dosage Forms Excipient information presented when available (limited, particularly for generics); consult specific product labeling.

Liquid, Oral:

Magonate: Magnesium carbonate equivalent to magnesium gluconate 1000 mg (54 mg elemental magnesium) per 5 mL (355 mL) [contains sodium benzoate; mixed melon flavor]

Tablet, Oral:

Mag-G: 500 mg (27 mg elemental magnesium)

Magonate: 500 mg (27 mg elemental magnesium) [scored]

Magonate: 500 mg (27 mg elemental magnesium) [scored; contains fd&c yellow #6 aluminum lake]

Generic: Elemental magnesium 27.5 mg

Tablet, Oral [preservative free]:

Generic: 500 mg (27 mg elemental magnesium)

References

Idama TO and Lindow SW, "Magnesium Sulphate: A Review of Clinical Pharmacology Applied to Obstetrics," *Br J Obstet Gynaecol*, 1998, 105(3):260-8.

Institute of Medicine (IOM), *Dietary Reference Intakes for Calcium, Phosphorus, Magnesium, Vitamin D, and Fluoride*, National Academy of Sciences, Washington, DC, 1997.

Osada H, Watanabe Y, Nishimura Y, et al, "Profile of Trace Element Concentrations in the Feto-placental Unit in Relation to Fetal Growth," *Acta Obstet Gynecol Scand*, 2002, 81(10):931-7.

Magnesium Hydroxide
(mag NEE zhum hye DROKS ide)

Brand Names: U.S. Dulcolax Milk of Magnesia [OTC]; Milk of Magnesia Concentrate [OTC]; Milk of Magnesia [OTC]; Pedia-Lax [OTC]

Therapeutic Category Antacid; Laxative, Osmotic

Generic Availability (U.S.) May be product dependent

Use Short-term treatment of constipation; treatment of hyperacidity symptoms

Pregnancy Considerations Magnesium crosses the placenta; serum concentrations in the fetus are similar to those in the mother (Idama, 1998; Osada, 2002). The American Gastroenterological Association considers the use of magnesium containing antacids to be low risk in pregnancy (Mahadevan, 2006).

Breast-Feeding Considerations Magnesium is found in breast milk; concentrations remain constant during the first year of lactation and are not influenced by dietary intake under normal conditions (IOM, 1997).

Contraindications Hypersensitivity to magnesium salt(s) or any component; serious renal impairment, myocardial damage, heart block; patients with colostomy or ileostomy, intestinal obstruction, impaction, or perforation, appendicitis, abdominal pain

Warnings Multiple salt forms of magnesium exist; close attention must be paid to the salt form when ordering and administering magnesium; **incorrect selection or substitution of one salt for another without proper dosage adjustment may result in serious over- or under-dosing**

Precautions Use with caution in patients with impaired renal function (accumulation of magnesium may lead to magnesium intoxication)

Drug Interactions

Metabolism/Transport Effects None known.

Avoid Concomitant Use

Avoid concomitant use of Magnesium Hydroxide with any of the following: Calcium Polystyrene Sulfonate; PONATinib; QuiNINE; Raltegravir; Sodium Polystyrene Sulfonate

Increased Effect/Toxicity

Magnesium Hydroxide may increase the levels/effects of: Amphetamines; Calcium Channel Blockers; Calcium Polystyrene Sulfonate; Dexmethylphenidate; Gabapentin; Methylphenidate; Misoprostol; Neuromuscular-Blocking Agents; QuiNIDine; Sodium Polystyrene Sulfonate

The levels/effects of Magnesium Hydroxide may be increased by: Alfacalcidol; Calcitriol; Calcium Channel Blockers

Decreased Effect

Magnesium Hydroxide may decrease the levels/effects of: ACE Inhibitors; Allopurinol; Anticonvulsants (Hydantoin); Antipsychotic Agents (Phenothiazines); Atazanavir; Bisacodyl; Bisphosphonate Derivatives; Bosutinib; Cefditoren; Cefpodoxime; Cefuroxime; Chloroquine; Corticosteroids (Oral); Dabigatran Etexilate; Dabrafenib; Dasatinib; Deferiprone; Delavirdine; Dolutegravir; Eltrombopag; Elvitegravir; Erlotinib; Fexofenadine; Gabapentin; HMG-CoA Reductase Inhibitors; Hyoscyamine; Iron Salts; Isoniazid; Itraconazole; Ketoconazole (Systemic); Mesalamine; Methenamine; Multivitamins/Fluoride (with ADE); Multivitamins/Minerals (with ADEK, Folate, Iron); Mycophenolate; Nilotinib; PAZOPanib; PenicillAMINE; Phosphate Supplements; PONATinib; Potassium Acid Phosphate; Protease Inhibitors; QuiNINE; Quinolone Antibiotics; Raltegravir; Rilpivirine; Riociguat; Strontium Ranelate; Sulpiride; Tetracycline Derivatives; Trientine; Vismodegib

The levels/effects of Magnesium Hydroxide may be decreased by: Trientine

Mechanism of Action Promotes bowel evacuation by causing osmotic retention of fluid which distends the colon with increased peristaltic activity; reacts with hydrochloric acid in stomach to form magnesium chloride

Pharmacokinetics (Adult data unless noted)

Absorption: Oral: Up to 30%

Elimination: Renal with unabsorbed drug excreted in feces

Dosing: Usual Oral:

Liquid: Dosage based upon regular strength liquid (400 mg/5 mL); when using concentrated magnesium hydroxide solution, reduce recommended dose by 1/2:

Children <2 years: 0.5 mL/kg/dose

Children 2-5 years: 5-15 mL/day once before bedtime or in divided doses

Children 6-11 years: 15-30 mL/day once before bedtime or in divided doses

Children ≥12 years and Adults: 30-60 mL/day once before bedtime or in divided doses

Tablet:
Children 2-5 years: 311-622 mg (1-2 tablets) once before bedtime or in divided doses
Children 6-11 years: 933-1244 mg (3-4 tablets) once before bedtime or in divided doses
Children ≥12 years and Adults: 1866-2488 mg (6-8 tablets) once before bedtime or in divided doses

Magnesium hydroxide and mineral oil (Phillips'® M-O) (infant dosage to provide equivalent dosage of magnesium hydroxide listed above):
Children <2 years: 0.6 mL/kg/dose
Children 2-5 years: 5-15 mL/day once or in divided doses
Children 6-11 years: 15-30 mL/day once or in divided doses
Children ≥12 years and Adults: 30-60 mL once or in divided doses

Antacid: Oral:
Children:
Liquid: 2.5-5 mL/dose, up to 4 times/day
Tablet: 311 mg (1 tablet) up to 4 times/day
Adults:
Liquid: 5-15 mL/dose, up to 4 times/day
Liquid concentrate: 2.5-7.5 mL/dose, up to 4 times/day
Tablet: 622-1244 mg/dose (2-4 tablets) up to 4 times/day

Dosing adjustment in renal impairment: Patients in severe renal failure should not receive magnesium due to toxicity from accumulation. Patients with a CrCl <25 mL/minute receiving magnesium should have serum magnesium levels monitored.

Administration Oral:
Solution: Mix with water and administer on an empty stomach.
Tablet: Take with full glass of water.

Test Interactions Increased magnesium; decreased protein, calcium (S), decreased potassium (S)

Dosage Forms Excipient information presented when available (limited, particularly for generics); consult specific product labeling. [DSC] = Discontinued product
Suspension, Oral:
Dulcolax Milk of Magnesia: 400 mg/5 mL (355 mL) [sugar free; unflavored flavor]
Dulcolax Milk of Magnesia: 400 mg/5 mL (355 mL) [sugar free; contains saccharin sodium; mint flavor]
Milk of Magnesia: 400 mg/5 mL (355 mL, 480 mL); 1200 mg/15 mL (355 mL)
Milk of Magnesia: 1200 mg/15 mL (355 mL) [mint flavor]
Milk of Magnesia: 7.75% (360 mL, 473 mL [DSC], 480 mL)
Milk of Magnesia: 7.75% (355 mL, 473 mL) [mint flavor]
Milk of Magnesia: 7.75% (30 mL) [spearmint flavor]
Milk of Magnesia: 1200 mg/15 mL (355 mL) [gluten free, stimulant free, sugar free; contains saccharin sodium]
Milk of Magnesia: 400 mg/5 mL (355 mL, 473 mL) [low sodium, sugar free]
Milk of Magnesia: 400 mg/5 mL (473 mL, 769 mL); 1200 mg/15 mL (355 mL) [stimulant free, sugar free]
Milk of Magnesia: 1200 mg/15 mL (355 mL) [stimulant free, sugar free; contains saccharin sodium]
Milk of Magnesia: 400 mg/5 mL (473 mL); 1200 mg/15 mL (355 mL) [sugar free]
Milk of Magnesia Concentrate: 2400 mg/10 mL (100 mL, 400 mL) [lemon flavor]
Milk of Magnesia Concentrate: 2400 mg/10 mL (10 mL) [contains methylparaben, propylene glycol, propylparaben, saccharin sodium; lemon flavor]
Tablet Chewable, Oral:
Pedia-Lax: 400 mg [scored; stimulant free; contains fd&c red #40 aluminum lake; watermelon flavor]

References
Idama TO and Lindow SW, "Magnesium Sulphate: A Review of Clinical Pharmacology Applied to Obstetrics," *Br J Obstet Gynaecol*, 1998, 105(3):260-8.

Institute of Medicine (IOM), *Dietary Reference Intakes for Calcium, Phosphorus, Magnesium, Vitamin D, and Fluoride*, National Academy of Sciences, Washington, DC, 1997.
Mahadevan U and Kane S, "American Gastroenterological Association Institute Medical Position Statement on the Use of Gastrointestinal Medications in Pregnancy," *Gastroenterology*, 2006, 131(1):278-82.
Osada H, Watanabe Y, Nishimura Y, et al, "Profile of Trace Element Concentrations in the Feto-placental Unit in Relation to Fetal Growth," *Acta Obstet Gynecol Scand*, 2002, 81(10):931-7.

◆ **Magnesium Hydroxide and Aluminum Hydroxide** *see* Aluminum Hydroxide and Magnesium Hydroxide *on page 111*

Magnesium L-aspartate Hydrochloride
(mag NEE zhum el as PAR tate hye droe KLOR ide)

Brand Names: U.S. Maginex™ DS [OTC]; Maginex™ [OTC]
Therapeutic Category Electrolyte Supplement, Oral; Magnesium Salt
Generic Availability (U.S.) No
Use Magnesium supplement
Pregnancy Considerations Magnesium crosses the placenta; serum concentrations in the fetus are similar to those in the mother (Idama, 1998; Osada, 2002).
Breast-Feeding Considerations Magnesium is found in breast milk; concentrations remain constant during the first year of lactation and are not influenced by dietary intake under normal conditions. Magnesium requirements are the same in lactating and nonlactating females (IOM, 1997).
Contraindications Hypersensitivity to magnesium salt(s) or any component; serious renal impairment, myocardial damage, heart block; patients with colostomy or ileostomy, intestinal obstruction, impaction, or perforation, appendicitis, abdominal pain
Warnings Multiple salt forms of magnesium exist; close attention must be paid to the salt form when ordering and administering magnesium; **incorrect selection or substitution of one salt for another without proper dosage adjustment may result in serious over- or under-dosing**
Precautions Use with caution in patients with impaired renal function (accumulation of magnesium may lead to magnesium intoxication)
Adverse Reactions Gastrointestinal: Abdominal cramps, diarrhea (excessive oral doses), gas formation
Drug Interactions
Metabolism/Transport Effects None known.
Avoid Concomitant Use
Avoid concomitant use of Magnesium L-aspartate Hydrochloride with any of the following: Raltegravir
Increased Effect/Toxicity
Magnesium L-aspartate Hydrochloride may increase the levels/effects of: Calcium Channel Blockers; Gabapentin; Neuromuscular-Blocking Agents

The levels/effects of Magnesium L-aspartate Hydrochloride may be increased by: Alfacalcidol; Calcitriol; Calcium Channel Blockers
Decreased Effect
Magnesium L-aspartate Hydrochloride may decrease the levels/effects of: Bisphosphonate Derivatives; Deferiprone; Dolutegravir; Eltrombopag; Gabapentin; Multivitamins/Fluoride (with ADE); Mycophenolate; Phosphate Supplements; Quinolone Antibiotics; Raltegravir; Tetracycline Derivatives; Trientine

The levels/effects of Magnesium L-aspartate Hydrochloride may be decreased by: Trientine
Mechanism of Action Magnesium is important as a cofactor in many enzymatic reactions in the body involving protein synthesis and carbohydrate metabolism (at least 300 enzymatic reactions require magnesium). Actions on lipoprotein lipase have been found to be important in

reducing serum cholesterol and on sodium/potassium ATPase in promoting polarization (eg, neuromuscular functioning).

Pharmacokinetics (Adult data unless noted)
Absorption: Oral: Up to 30%
Elimination: Renal with unabsorbed drug excreted in feces

Dosing: Neonatal Recommended daily allowance of magnesium: Oral: 40 mg/day

Dosing: Usual Oral:
Recommended daily allowance of magnesium: See table.

Magnesium – Recommended Daily Allowance (RDA) and Estimated Average Requirement (EAR) (in terms of elemental magnesium)

Age	RDA (mg/day)	EAR (mg/day)
1 to <6 mo	40	30
6 to <12 mo	60	75
1-3 y	80	65
4-8 y	130	110
Male		
9-13 y	240	200
14-18 y	410	340
Female		
9-13 y	240	200
14-18 y	360	300

Hypomagnesemia: **Note:** Achieving optimal magnesium levels using oral therapy may be difficult due to the propensity for magnesium to cause diarrhea: I.V. replacement may be more appropriate particularly in situations of severe deficit:
Children: 10-20 mg/kg elemental magnesium per dose up to 4 times/day
Dietary supplement: Adults: 1230 mg up to 3 times/day
Dosing adjustment in renal impairment: Patients in severe renal failure should not receive magnesium due to toxicity from accumulation. Patients with a CrCl <25 mL/minute receiving magnesium should have serum magnesium levels monitored.

Administration Oral:
Granules: Mix each packet in 4 ounces water or juice prior to administration
Tablet: Take with full glass of water
Additional Information Magnesium L-aspartate 500 mg = 49.6 mg **elemental** magnesium = 4.1 mEq magnesium

Elemental Magnesium Content of Magnesium Salts

Magnesium Salt	Elemental Magnesium (mg/500 mg salt)	Magnesium (mEq/500 mg salt)
Magnesium chloride	59	4.9
Magnesium gluconate	27	2.4
Magnesium L-aspartate	49.6	4.1
Magnesium oxide	302	25
Magnesium sulfate	49.3	4.1

Dosage Forms Considerations 1 g magnesium L-aspartate Hydrochloride ≈ elemental magnesium 100 m = magnesium 8.1 mEq = magnesium 4.05 mmol
Dosage Forms Excipient information presented when available (limited, particularly for generics); consult specific product labeling.

Granules for solution, oral [preservative free]:
Maginex™ DS: 1230 mg/packet (30s) [sugar free; lemon flavor; equivalent to elemental magnesium 122 mg]

Tablet, enteric coated, oral [preservative free]:
Maginex™: 615 mg [sugar free; equivalent to elemental magnesium 61 mg]

References
Idama TO and Lindow SW, "Magnesium Sulphate: A Review of Clinical Pharmacology Applied to Obstetrics," *Br J Obstet Gynaecol*, 1998, 105(3):260-8.
IOM (Institute of Medicine), *Dietary Reference Intakes for Calcium, Phosphorus, Magnesium, Vitamin D, and Fluoride*, National Academy of Sciences, Washington, DC, 1997.
Osada H, Watanabe Y, Nishimura Y, et al, "Profile of Trace Element Concentrations in the Feto-Placental Unit in Relation to Fetal Growth," *Acta Obstet Gynecol Scand*, 2002, 81(10):931-7.

Magnesium Oxide (mag NEE zhum OKS ide)

Brand Names: U.S. Mag-200 [OTC]; Maox [OTC]; Uro-Mag [OTC]
Therapeutic Category Electrolyte Supplement, Oral; Laxative, Osmotic; Magnesium Salt
Generic Availability (U.S.) May be product dependent
Use Magnesium supplement; short-term treatment of constipation; treatment of hyperacidity symptoms
Pregnancy Considerations Magnesium crosses the placenta; serum concentrations in the fetus are similar to those in the mother (Idama, 1998; Osada, 2002)
Breast-Feeding Considerations Magnesium is found in breast milk; concentrations remain constant during the first year of lactation and are not influenced by dietary intake under normal conditions. Magnesium requirements are the same in lactating and nonlactating females (IOM,1997).
Contraindications Hypersensitivity to magnesium salt(s) or any component; serious renal impairment, myocardial damage, heart block; patients with colostomy or ileostomy, intestinal obstruction, impaction, or perforation, appendicitis, abdominal pain
Warnings Multiple salt forms of magnesium exist; close attention must be paid to the salt form when ordering and administering magnesium; **incorrect selection or substitution of one salt for another without proper dosage adjustment may result in serious over- or under-dosing**
Precautions Use with caution in patients with impaired renal function (accumulation of magnesium may lead to magnesium intoxication)
Adverse Reactions Gastrointestinal: Diarrhea (excessive oral doses)
Drug Interactions
Metabolism/Transport Effects None known.
Avoid Concomitant Use
Avoid concomitant use of Magnesium Oxide with any of the following: Calcium Polystyrene Sulfonate; Raltegravir; Sodium Polystyrene Sulfonate
Increased Effect/Toxicity
Magnesium Oxide may increase the levels/effects of: Calcium Channel Blockers; Calcium Polystyrene Sulfonate; Gabapentin; Neuromuscular-Blocking Agents; Sodium Polystyrene Sulfonate

The levels/effects of Magnesium Oxide may be increased by: Alfacalcidol; Calcitriol; Calcium Channel Blockers
Decreased Effect
Magnesium Oxide may decrease the levels/effects of: Bisphosphonate Derivatives; Deferiprone; Dolutegravir; Eltrombopag; Gabapentin; Multivitamins/Fluoride (with ADE); Mycophenolate; Phosphate Supplements; Quinolone Antibiotics; Raltegravir; Tetracycline Derivatives; Trientine

The levels/effects of Magnesium Oxide may be decreased by: Trientine
Mechanism of Action Magnesium is important as a cofactor in many enzymatic reactions in the body involving protein synthesis and carbohydrate metabolism (at least

300 enzymatic reactions require magnesium). Actions on lipoprotein lipase have been found to be important in reducing serum cholesterol and on sodium/potassium ATPase in promoting polarization (eg, neuromuscular functioning).

Pharmacokinetics (Adult data unless noted)
Absorption: Oral: Up to 30%
Elimination: Renal with unabsorbed drug excreted in feces

Dosing: Neonatal Recommended daily allowance of magnesium: Oral: 40 mg/day

Dosing: Usual Oral:
Recommended daily allowance of magnesium: See table.

Magnesium – Recommended Daily Allowance (RDA) and Estimated Average Requirement (EAR) (in terms of elemental magnesium)

Age	RDA (mg/day)	EAR (mg/day)
1 to <6 mo	40	30
6 to <12 mo	60	75
1-3 y	80	65
4-8 y	130	110
Male		
9-13 y	240	200
14-18 y	410	340
Female		
9-13 y	240	200
14-18 y	360	300

Antacid: Adults: 140 mg 3-4 times/day or 400-840 mg/day
Cathartic: Adults: 2-4 g at bedtime
Hypomagnesemia: **Note:** Achieving optimal magnesium levels using oral therapy may be difficult due to the propensity for magnesium to cause diarrhea: I.V. replacement may be more appropriate particularly in situations of severe deficit.
Children: 10-20 mg/kg elemental magnesium per dose up to 4 times/day

Dosing adjustment in renal impairment: Patients in severe renal failure should not receive magnesium due to toxicity from accumulation. Patients with a CrCl <25 mL/minute receiving magnesium should have serum magnesium levels monitored.

Administration Oral: Tablet: Take with full glass of water.

Reference Range
Neonates and Infants: 1.5-2.3 mEq/L
Children: 1.5-2.0 mEq/L
Adults: 1.4-2.0 mEq/L

Additional Information Magnesium oxide 500 mg = 302 mg **elemental** magnesium = 25 mEq magnesium

Elemental Magnesium Content of Magnesium Salts

Magnesium Salt	Elemental Magnesium (mg/500 mg salt)	Magnesium (mEq/500 mg salt)
Magnesium chloride	59	4.9
Magnesium gluconate	27	2.4
Magnesium L-aspartate	49.6	4.1
Magnesium oxide	302	25
Magnesium sulfate	49.3	4.1

Adverse effects associated with elevated serum magnesium concentrations may include:
>3 mg/dL: Blocked peripheral neuromuscular transmission leading to anticonvulsant effects, depressed CNS
>5 mg/dL: Depressed deep tendon reflexes, flushing, somnolence
>12 mg/dL: Complete heart block, respiratory paralysis

Dosage Forms Considerations
400 mg magnesium oxide = elemental magnesium 240 mg = magnesium 19.9 mEq = magnesium 9.85 mmol
Dosage Forms Excipient information presented when available (limited, particularly for generics); consult specific product labeling.
Capsule, Oral:
Uro-Mag: 140 mg
Tablet, Oral:
Mag-200: 200 mg [contains para-aminobenzoic acid]
Maox: 420 mg [contains tartrazine (fd&c yellow #5)]
Generic: 250 mg, 400 mg, 420 mg
Tablet, Oral [preservative free]:
Generic: 400 mg, 500 mg

References
Idama TO and Lindow SW, "Magnesium Sulphate: A Review of Clinical Pharmacology Applied to Obstetrics," Br J Obstet Gynaecol, 1998, 105(3):260-8.
IOM (Institute of Medicine), Dietary Reference Intakes for Calcium, Phosphorus, Magnesium, Vitamin D, and Fluoride, National Academy of Sciences, Washington, DC, 1997.
Osada H, Watanabe Y, Nishimura Y, et al, "Profile of Trace Element Concentrations in the Feto-Placental Unit in Relation to Fetal Growth," Acta Obstet Gynecol Scand, 2002, 81(10):931-7.

Magnesium Sulfate (mag NEE zhum SUL fate)

Medication Safety Issues
Sound-alike/look-alike issues:
Magnesium sulfate may be confused with manganese sulfate, morphine sulfate
MgSO$_4$ is an error-prone abbreviation (mistaken as morphine sulfate)
High alert medication:
The Institute for Safe Medication Practices (ISMP) includes this medication (I.V. formulation) among its list of drugs which have a heightened risk of causing significant patient harm when used in error.

Brand Names: U.S. Epsom Salt [OTC]

Therapeutic Category Anticonvulsant; Electrolyte Supplement, Oral; Electrolyte Supplement, Parenteral; Magnesium Salt

Generic Availability (U.S.) Yes

Use Treatment and prevention of hypomagnesemia, treatment of hypertension, torsade de pointes, and encephalopathy and seizures associated with acute nephritis; prevention and treatment of seizures in severe preeclampsia or eclampsia; prevention of premature labor; adjunctive treatment for bronchodilation in moderate to severe acute asthma

Pregnancy Risk Factor D

Pregnancy Considerations Magnesium crosses the placenta; serum concentrations in the fetus are similar to those in the mother (Idama, 1998; Osada, 2002). Continuous maternal use for >5-7 days (in doses such as those used for preterm labor, an off-label use) may cause fetal hypocalcemia and bone abnormalities, as well as fractures in the neonate. Magnesium sulfate injection is used for the prevention and treatment of seizures in pregnant or postpartum women with severe pre-eclampsia or eclampsia (ACOG, 2013). Magnesium sulfate may also be used prior to early preterm delivery to reduce the risk of cerebral palsy (ACOG, 2010; Reeves, 2011). Tocolytics may be used for the short-term (48 hour) prolongation of pregnancy to allow for the administration of antenatal steroids and should not be used prior to fetal viability or when the risks of use to the fetus or mother are greater than the risk of preterm birth; maintenance therapy with tocolytics is ineffective and not recommended. Magnesium sulfate injection may be used in conjunction with tocolytics for neuroprotection (it is not preferred for use as a tocolytic); however, an increased risk of maternal complications may be observed when used in combination with some tocolytic agents (ACOG, 2012).

Breast-Feeding Considerations Magnesium is found in breast milk; concentrations remain constant during the first year of lactation and are not influenced by dietary intake under normal conditions. Magnesium requirements are the same in lactating and nonlactating females (IOM, 1997). When magnesium sulfate is used in the intrapartum management of eclampsia, breast milk concentrations are generally increased for only ~24 hours after the end of treatment (Idama, 1998). The manufacturer recommends that caution be used if administered to nursing women.

Contraindications Hypersensitivity to magnesium salt(s) or any component; serious renal impairment, myocardial damage, heart block; patients with colostomy or ileostomy, intestinal obstruction, impaction, or perforation, appendicitis, abdominal pain; I.V. use for pre-eclampsia/eclampsia during the 2 hours prior to delivery

Warnings Multiple salt forms of magnesium exist; close attention must be paid to the salt form when ordering and administering magnesium; **incorrect selection or substitution of one salt for another without proper dosage adjustment may result in serious over- or under-dosing**

Precautions Use with caution in patients with impaired renal function (accumulation of magnesium may lead to magnesium intoxication)

Adverse Reactions Adverse effects on neuromuscular function may occur at lower concentrations in patients with neuromuscular disease (eg, myasthenia gravis).

Cardiovascular: Flushing (I.V.; dose related), hypotension (I.V.; rate related), vasodilation (I.V.; rate related)

Endocrine & metabolic: Hypermagnesemia

Drug Interactions

Metabolism/Transport Effects None known.

Avoid Concomitant Use

Avoid concomitant use of Magnesium Sulfate with any of the following: Calcium Polystyrene Sulfonate; Raltegravir; Sodium Polystyrene Sulfonate

Increased Effect/Toxicity

Magnesium Sulfate may increase the levels/effects of: Calcium Channel Blockers; Calcium Polystyrene Sulfonate; CNS Depressants; Gabapentin; Neuromuscular-Blocking Agents; Sodium Polystyrene Sulfonate

The levels/effects of Magnesium Sulfate may be increased by: Alfacalcidol; Calcitriol; Calcium Channel Blockers

Decreased Effect

Magnesium Sulfate may decrease the levels/effects of: Bisphosphonate Derivatives; Deferiprone; Dolutegravir; Eltrombopag; Gabapentin; Multivitamins/Fluoride (with ADE); Mycophenolate; Phosphate Supplements; Quinolone Antibiotics; Raltegravir; Tetracycline Derivatives; Trientine

The levels/effects of Magnesium Sulfate may be decreased by: Ketorolac (Nasal); Ketorolac (Systemic); Mefloquine; Orlistat; Trientine

Food Interactions Increased alcohol intake can deplete magnesium stores (IOM, 1997).

Mechanism of Action When taken orally, magnesium promotes bowel evacuation by causing osmotic retention of fluid which distends the colon with increased peristaltic activity; parenterally, magnesium decreases acetylcholine in motor nerve terminals and acts on myocardium by slowing rate of S-A node impulse formation and prolonging conduction time. Magnesium is necessary for the movement of calcium, sodium, and potassium in and out of cells, as well as stabilizing excitable membranes.

Intravenous magnesium may improve pulmonary function in patients with asthma; causes relaxation of bronchial smooth muscle independent of serum magnesium concentration.

Pharmacodynamics

Onset of action:
Anticonvulsant:
I.M.: 60 minutes
I.V.: Immediately
Laxative: Oral: 4-8 hours
Duration: Anticonvulsant:
I.M.: 3-4 hours
I.V.: 30 minutes

Pharmacokinetics (Adult data unless noted) Elimination: Renal with unabsorbed drug excreted in feces

Dosing: Neonatal Note: 1 g of magnesium sulfate = 98.6 mg **elemental** magnesium = 8.12 mEq magnesium; treatment depends on severity and clinical status

Hypomagnesemia: I.V.: 25-50 mg magnesium sulfate/kg/dose (equal to 0.2-0.4 mEq magnesium/kg/dose) every 8-12 hours for 2-3 doses

Daily maintenance magnesium: I.V.: 0.25-0.5 mEq magnesium/kg/day (**Note:** mEq denotes amount of magnesium ion only not the total salt form.)

Dosing: Usual

Hypomagnesemia:
Children: I.M., I.V.: 25-50 mg magnesium sulfate/kg/dose (equal to 0.2-0.4 mEq magnesium/kg/dose) every 4-6 hours for 3-4 doses; maximum single dose: 2000 mg magnesium sulfate (equal to 16 mEq magnesium)

Adults: I.M., I.V.: 1 g magnesium sulfate every 6 hours for 4 doses, or 250 mg magnesium sulfate/kg over a 4-hour period; for severe hypomagnesemia: 8-12 g magnesium sulfate/day in divided doses has been used

Daily maintenance magnesium: I.V.: **Note:** mEq denotes amount of magnesium ion only not the total salt form

Infants and Children ≤45 kg: 0.25-0.5 mEq magnesium/kg/day

Adolescents >45 kg and Adults: 0.2-0.5 mEq magnesium/kg/day or 3-10 mEq magnesium/1000 kcal/day (maximum: 8-24 mEq magnesium/day)

Management of seizures and hypertension: I.M., I.V.:
Children: 20-100 mg magnesium sulfate/kg/dose every 4-6 hours as needed; in severe cases, doses as high as 200 mg magnesium sulfate/kg/dose have been used

Adults: 1 g magnesium sulfate every 6 hours for 4 doses as needed

Prevention of premature labor: I.V.: Adolescents and Adults: Initial loading dose: 4-6 g magnesium sulfate followed by a continuous infusion of 2-3 g/hour

Treatment and prevention of seizures in severe pre-eclampsia or eclampsia: Adolescents and Adults:
Manufacturer's labeling: An initial total dose of 10-14 g administered as follows: 4 g magnesium sulfate I.V. infusion with simultaneous I.M. injections of 4 to 5 g of magnesium sulfate in each buttock. After the initial I.V./I.M. doses, may administer a 1-2 g magnesium sulfate/hour continuous infusion **or** may follow with I.M. doses of 4-5 g magnesium sulfate into alternate buttocks every 4 hours as necessary; maximum dose: 40 g/24 hours. I.V. use for pre-eclampsia/eclampsia is contraindicated during the 2 hours prior to delivery.

Alternate dosing: I.V.: 4-6 g loading dose followed by 1-2 g/hour continuous infusion for at least 24 hours (ACOG, 2013)

Treatment of torsade de pointes VT: I.V.:
Infants and Children: 25-50 mg magnesium sulfate/kg/dose; not to exceed 2 g magnesium sulfate/dose

Adults: 1-2 g magnesium sulfate/dose

Bronchodilation (adjunctive treatment in severe acute asthma for patients who have life-threatening exacerbations and in those whose exacerbations remain in the severe category after 1 hour of intensive conventional therapy, NIH Guidelines, 2007): I.V.:
Children: 25-75 mg magnesium sulfate/kg/dose (maximum dose: 2 g) as a single dose

Adults: 2 g magnesium sulfate as a single dose

Note: Literature evaluating magnesium sulfate's efficacy in the relief of bronchospasm has utilized single dosages in patients with acute symptomatology who have received aerosol β-agonist therapy with inconsistent results. A recent study (Ciarallo, 2000) showed significant improvement in pulmonary function in children who received a single dose of 40 mg/kg magnesium sulfate vs. placebo; pulmonary index scores after magnesium sulfate 75 mg/kg (maximum: 2.5 g) vs. placebo were not statistically different in 54 children between 1-18 years of age (Scarfone, 2000).

Dosing adjustment in renal impairment: Patients in severe renal failure should not receive magnesium due to toxicity from accumulation. Patients with a CrCl <25 mL/minute receiving magnesium should have serum magnesium levels monitored.

Administration Parenteral:

I.M.:

Infants and Children: Dilute to a maximum concentration of 20% (ie, 200 mg/mL magnesium sulfate or 1.6 mEq/mL) prior to injection (Phelps, 2013)

Adults: May administer as 25% or 50%

I.V.:

I.V. push: Must dilute to a concentration ≤20% (200 mg/mL of magnesium sulfate) and should generally not be given any faster than 150 mg/minute; in pediatric patients with pulseless torsades, may administer as a bolus (Hegenbarth, 2008) and in adult patients with persistent pulseless VT or VF with known hypomagnesemia may administer over 1-2 minutes (Dager, 2006). ACLS guidelines recommend administration over 15 minutes in patients with torsade de pointes (ACLS, 2010). In patients not in cardiac arrest, hypotension and asystole may occur with rapid administration.

Intermittent infusion: Dilute in an appropriate fluid to a usual concentration of 0.5 mEq/mL (60 mg/mL of **magnesium sulfate**); maximum concentration: 20% (ie,1.6 mEq/mL or 200 mg/mL of magnesium sulfate). Rate of infusion dependent upon use:

For general replacement therapy:

Pediatric patients: Infuse over 1-4 hours; do not exceed 1 mEq/kg/hour (125 mg/kg/hour of magnesium sulfate)

Adults: Up to 50% of an I.V. dose may be eliminated in the urine; therefore, slower administration may improve retention. If severely symptomatic, may administer ≤4000 mg over 4-5 minutes. For doses <6 g, infuse over 8-12 hours and for larger doses, infuse over 24 hours if patient asymptomatic (Kraft, 2005); maximum rate: 150 mg/minute

Acute/emergent therapy:

Pediatric patients (Hegenbarth, 2008):

Hypomagnesemia or torsades with pulses: 10-20 minutes

Status asthmaticus: 15-30 minutes

Adults: ≤150 mg/minute; in cases of severe eclampsia with seizures, faster rates may be necessary

Continuous infusion: Dilute in an appropriate fluid at a concentration not to exceed 20% (ie,1.6 mEq/mL or 200 mg/mL of magnesium sulfate)

Monitoring Parameters Serum magnesium, deep tendon reflexes, respiratory rate, renal function, blood pressure, stool output (laxative use)

Reference Range

Neonates and Infants: 1.5-2.3 mEq/L

Children: 1.5-2.0 mEq/L

Adults: 1.4-2.0 mEq/L

Additional Information Magnesium sulfate 500 mg = 49.3 mg **elemental** magnesium = 4.1 mEq magnesium. Nebulized magnesium sulfate in varying concentrations/dosages has been used successfully with and without beta₂-adrenergic agonists in the treatment of acute asthma (Blitz, 2006).

Note: 1 g of magnesium sulfate = 98.6 mg **elemental** magnesium = 8.12 mEq magnesium

Elemental Magnesium Content of Magnesium Salts

Magnesium Salt	Elemental Magnesium (mg/500 mg salt)	Magnesium (mEq/500 mg salt)
Magnesium chloride	59	4.9
Magnesium gluconate	27	2.4
Magnesium L-aspartate	49.6	4.1
Magnesium oxide	302	25
Magnesium sulfate	49.3	4.1

Adverse effects associated with elevated serum magnesium concentrations may include:

>3 mg/dL: Blocked peripheral neuromuscular transmission leading to anticonvulsant effects, depressed CNS

>5 mg/dL: Depressed deep tendon reflexes, flushing, somnolence

>12 mg/dL: Complete heart block, respiratory paralysis

Dosage Forms Considerations

1 g of magnesium sulfate = elemental magnesium 98.6 mg = magnesium 8.12 mEq = magnesium 4.06 mmol

Magnesium sulfate 1% [10 mg/mL] in Dextrose 5% injection is equivalent to elemental magnesium 0.081 mEq/mL.

Magnesium sulfate 2% [20 mg/mL] in Dextrose 5% injection is equivalent to elemental magnesium 0.162 mEq/mL.

Magnesium sulfate 4% [40 mg/mL] in Water injection is equivalent to elemental magnesium 0.325 mEq/mL.

Magnesium sulfate 8% [80 mg/mL] in Water injection is equivalent to elemental magnesium 0.65 mEq/mL.

Magnesium sulfate 50% injection is equivalent to elemental magnesium 4 mEq/mL.

Dosage Forms Excipient information presented when available (limited, particularly for generics); consult specific product labeling.

Capsule, Oral:

Generic: 70 mg

Granules, Oral:

Epsom Salt: (454 g, 1810 g, 1816 g)

Solution, Injection:

Generic: 40 mg/mL (50 mL, 100 mL, 500 mL, 1000 mL); 80 mg/mL (50 mL); 50% (2 mL, 10 mL, 20 mL, 50 mL)

Solution, Intravenous:

Generic: 10 mg/mL (100 mL); 20 mg/mL (500 mL)

References

"2005 American Heart Association (AHA) Guidelines for Cardiopulmonary Resuscitation (CPR) and Emergency Cardiovascular Care (ECC) of Pediatric and Neonatal Patients: Pediatric Advanced Life Support," *Pediatrics*, 2006, 117(5):1005-28.

ACOG Practice Bulletin, "Diagnosis and Management of Preeclampsia and Eclampsia. Number 33, January 2002," *Obstet Gynecol*, 2002, 99 (1):159-67.

ACOG Practice Bulletin No. 127: "Management of Preterm Labor,"*Obstet Gynecol*, 2012, 119(6):1308.

American College of Obstetricians and Gynecologists (ACOG) Committee on Obstetric Practice, "Committee Opinion No. 455: Magnesium Sulfate Before Anticipated Preterm Birth for Neuroprotection," *Obstet Gynecol*, 2010, 115(3):669-71.

American College of Obstetricians and Gynecologists (ACOG). Task Force Report on Hypertension in Pregnancy. http://www.acog.org/Resources_And_Publications/Task_Force_and_Work_Group_Reports/Hypertension_in_Pregnancy. Updated 2013. Accessed February 3, 2014.

Blitz M, Blitz S, Beasely R, et al, "Inhaled Magnesium Sulfate in the Treatment of Acute Asthma," *Cochrane Database Syst Rev*, 2005, 19 (4):CD003898.

Briggs GG and Wan SR, "Drug Therapy During Labor and Delivery, Part 2," *Am J Health Syst Pharm*, 2006, 63(12):1131-9.

Bloch H, Silverman R, Mancherje N, et al, "Intravenous Magnesium Sulfate as an Adjunct in the Treatment of Acute Asthma," *Chest*, 1995, 107(6):1576-81.

Chernow B, Smith J, Rainey TG, et al, "Hypomagnesemia: Implications for the Critical Care Specialist," *Crit Care Med*, 1982, 10(3):193-6.

Cheuk DK, Chau TC, and Lee SL, "A Meta-analysis on Intravenous Magnesium Sulphate for Treating Acute Asthma," *Arch Dis Child*, 2005, 90(1):74-7.

Ciarallo L, Brousseau D, and Reinert S, "Higher-Dose Intravenous Magnesium Therapy for Children With Moderate to Severe Acute Asthma," *Arch Pediatr Adolesc Med*, 2000, 154(10):979-83.

Ciarallo L, Sauer AH, and Shannon MW, "Intravenous Magnesium Therapy for Moderate to Severe Pediatric Asthma: Results of a Randomized, Placebo-Controlled Trial," *J Pediatr*, 1996, 129 (6):809-14.

Dager WE, Sanoski CA, Wiggins BS, et al, "Pharmacotherapy Considerations in Advanced Cardiac Life Support," *Pharmacotherapy*, 2006, 26(12):1703-29.

"Dietary Reference Intakes for Calcium, Phosphorus, Magnesium, Vitamin D, and Fluoride. Standing Committee on the Scientific Evaluation of Dietary Reference Intakes, Food and Nutrition Board, Institute of Medicine," National Academy of Sciences, Washington, DC: National Academy Press, 1997.

"Guidelines for the Diagnosis and Management of Asthma. NAEPP Expert Panel Report 3," August 2007, www.nhlbi.nih.gov/guidelines/asthma/asthgdln.pdf.

Hegenbarth MA, American Academy of Pediatrics Committee on Drugs. Preparing for pediatric emergencies: drugs to consider. *Pediatrics.* 2008;121(2):433-443.

Idama TO and Lindow SW, "Magnesium Sulphate: A Review of Clinical Pharmacology Applied to Obstetrics," *Br J Obstet Gynaecol*, 1998, 105(3):260-8.

Institute of Medicine (IOM), *Dietary Reference Intakes for Calcium, Phosphorus, Magnesium, Vitamin D, and Fluoride*, National Academy of Sciences, Washington, DC, 1997.

Kleinman ME, Chameides L, Schexnayder SM, et al, "Part 14: Pediatric Advanced Life Support (PALS): 2010 American Heart Association Guidelines for Cardiopulmonary Resuscitation and Emergency Cardiovascular Care," *Circulation*, 2010, 122(18 Suppl 3):876-908.

Kraft MD, Btaiche IF, Sacks GS, et al, "Treatment of Electrolyte Disorders in Adult Patients in the Intensive Care Unit," *Am J Health-Syst Pharm*, 2005, 62(16):1663-82.

Neumar RW, Otto CW, Link MS, et al, "Part 8: Adult Advanced Cardiovascular Life Support (ACLS): 2010 American Heart Association Guidelines for Cardiopulmonary Resuscitation and Emergency Cardiovascular Care," *Circulation*, 2010, 122(18 Suppl 3):729-67.

Osada H, Watanabe Y, Nishimura Y, et al, "Profile of Trace Element Concentrations in the Feto-placental Unit in Relation to Fetal Growth," *Acta Obstet Gynecol Scand*, 2002, 81(10):931-7.

Phelps SJ, Hak EB, Crill CM, eds. *Teddy Bear Book: Pediatric Injectable Drugs.* 10th ed. Bethesda, MD: American Society of Health-System Pharmacists;2013.

Reeves SA, Gibbs RS, and Clark SL, "Magnesium for Fetal Neuroprotection," *Am J Obstet Gynecol*, 2011, 204(3):202.1-4.

Scarfone RJ, Loiselle JM, Joffe MD, et al, "A Randomized Trial of Magnesium in the Emergency Department Treatment of Children With Asthma," *Ann Emerg Med*, 2000, 36(6):572-8.

◆ **Magonate [OTC]** *see* Magnesium Gluconate *on page 1293*

◆ **Mag Oxide** *see* Magnesium Oxide *on page 1296*

◆ **Mag-SR [OTC]** *see* Magnesium Chloride *on page 1291*

◆ **Mag-SR Plus Calcium [OTC]** *see* Magnesium Chloride *on page 1291*

◆ **MAH** *see* Magnesium L-aspartate Hydrochloride *on page 1295*

◆ **Makena** *see* Hydroxyprogesterone Caproate *on page 1049*

◆ **Malarone®** *see* Atovaquone and Proguanil *on page 231*

◆ **Malarone® Pediatric (Can)** *see* Atovaquone and Proguanil *on page 231*

Malathion (mal a THYE on)

Brand Names: U.S. Ovide

Therapeutic Category Antiparasitic Agent, Topical; Pediculocide; Scabicidal Agent

Generic Availability (U.S.) Yes

Use Treatment of *Pediculus capitis* (head lice and their ova) (FDA approved in ages ≥6 years and adults)

Pregnancy Risk Factor B

Pregnancy Considerations Adverse events have not been observed in animal reproduction studies

Breast-Feeding Considerations It is not known if the malathion 0.5% lotion formulation is excreted in breast milk. Use with caution if administered to or handled by breast-feeding mothers.

Contraindications Hypersensitivity to malathion or any component; use in neonates or infants

Warnings Lotion is flammable (78% isopropyl alcohol); do not expose lotion or hair wetted with malathion to open flames or electric heat sources (eg, hair dryer, curling iron, flat iron). Do not smoke while applying lotion or while hair is wet.

Skin irritation may occur; temporarily discontinue use; chemical burns, including second-degree burns, and stinging sensations may occur with use.

Systemic absorption may be increased in infants and neonates due to higher skin surface area to body mass ratio and immature skin barrier; risk for malathion toxicity potentially increased; use is contraindicated in these patients.

Precautions For external use only; if contact with eyes occurs, flush immediately with water; wash hands after application.

Adverse Reactions

Dermatologic: Chemical burns (including second-degree burns), skin/scalp irritation, stinging sensations

Ocular: Conjunctivitis (following contact with eyes)

Drug Interactions

Metabolism/Transport Effects None known.

Avoid Concomitant Use There are no known interactions where it is recommended to avoid concomitant use.

Increased Effect/Toxicity There are no known significant interactions involving an increase in effect.

Decreased Effect There are no known significant interactions involving a decrease in effect.

Stability Store at 20°C to 25°C (68°F to 77°F); do not expose to heat and open flames.

Mechanism of Action Organophosphate that acts as a pediculicide by inhibiting cholinesterase activity in *Pediculus humanus capitis* (head lice and their ova)

Dosing: Usual

Children ≥2 years and Adolescents:

Head lice: Children ≥6 years and Adolescents: Topical: Apply sufficient amount to cover and thoroughly moisten dry hair and scalp, leave on for 8-12 hours (typically overnight application); may shampoo upon completion; during clinical trials, a maximum dose of 2 fl oz was used. **Note:** In a blinded-comparative trial with permethrin; a shorter application time of 20 minutes was shown effective (AAP, 2010; Meinking, 2004). Further treatment is generally not necessary.

Head lice resistant to permethrin/pyrethrins or previously failed courses: Children 2-5 years: Limited data available: Topical: Apply sufficient amount to cover and thoroughly moisten dry hair and scalp, leave on for 8-12 hours (typically overnight application); may shampoo upon completion; during clinical trials, a maximum dose of 2 fl oz was used (AAP, 2010)

Adults: **Head lice:** Topical: Apply sufficient amount to cover and thoroughly moisten dry hair and scalp; shampoo after 8-12 hours. If required, repeat with second application in 7-9 days. Further treatment is generally not necessary.

Administration Topical: For external use only; avoid contact with eyes. Apply to dry hair and scalp and rub gently until thoroughly moistened; pay special attention to the back of the head and neck. Allow hair to dry naturally; do not use heat; leave hair uncovered; after 8-12 hours, wash hair with a nonmedicated shampoo; rinse and use a fine-toothed (nit) comb to remove dead lice and eggs. Wash hands immediately after use.

Malathion should be a portion of a whole lice removal program, which should include washing or dry cleaning all clothing, hats, bedding, and towels recently worn or used by the patient and washing combs, brushes, and hair accessories in hot, soapy water.

Dosage Forms Excipient information presented when available (limited, particularly for generics); consult specific product labeling.

Lotion, External:
    Ovide: 0.5% (59 mL) [contains isopropyl alcohol]
    Generic: 0.5% (59 mL)

References

Frankowski BL and Bocchini JA Jr, "American Academy of Pediatrics, Clinical Report: Head Lice," *Pediatrics*, 2010, 126(2):392-403.

Meinking TL, Vicaria M, Eyerdam DH, et al, "Efficacy of a Reduced Application Time of Ovide Lotion (0.5% Malathion) Compared to Nix Creme Rinse (1% Permethrin) for the Treatment of Head Lice," *Pediatr Dermatol*, 2004, 21(6):670-4.

◆ **Manda-Citalopram (Can)** *see* Citalopram *on page 484*

◆ **Mandelamine® (Can)** *see* Methenamine *on page 1361*

◆ **Mandrake** *see* Podophyllum Resin *on page 1693*

◆ **Manganese** *see* Trace Elements *on page 2059*

Mannitol (MAN i tole)

Medication Safety Issues
  Sound-alike/look-alike issues:
    Osmitrol® may be confused with esmolol
Related Information
  Management of Drug Extravasations *on page 2255*
Brand Names: U.S. Aridol; Osmitrol; Resectisol
Brand Names: Canada Osmitrol®
Therapeutic Category Diuretic, Osmotic
Generic Availability (U.S.) May be product dependent
Use

Injection: Reduction of increased intracranial pressure (ICP) associated with cerebral edema and increased intraocular pressure (IOP) [FDA approved in pediatric patients (age not specified) and adults]; promotion of urinary excretion of toxic substances and diuresis in the prevention and/or treatment of oliguria or anuria due to acute renal failure [FDA approved in pediatric patients (age not specified) and adults]. **Note:** Although FDA-labeled indications, the use of mannitol for the prevention of acute renal failure and/or promotion of diuresis is not routinely recommended (Kellum, 2008).

Irrigation solution, genitourinary: Irrigation in transurethral prostatic resection or other transurethral surgical procedures (FDA approved in adults)

Oral inhalation powder: Assessment of bronchial hyper-responsiveness (FDA approved in ages ≥6 years and adults)

Pregnancy Risk Factor C

Pregnancy Considerations Reproduction studies have not been conducted.

Breast-Feeding Considerations It is not known if mannitol is excreted in breast milk. The manufacturer recommends that caution be exercised when administering mannitol to nursing women.

Contraindications

Injection: Hypersensitivity to mannitol or any component; severe renal disease (anuria); severe dehydration; active intracranial bleeding except during craniotomy; severe pulmonary edema or congestion; progressive heart failure, pulmonary congestion, or renal dysfunction after mannitol administration (or history thereof)

Irrigation solution, genitourinary: Hypersensitivity to mannitol or any component; anuria; use as an injection

Powder for inhalation: Hypersensitivity to mannitol, gelatin, or any component; conditions that may be compromised by induced bronchospasm or repeated spirometry (eg, aortic or cerebral aneurysm, uncontrolled hypertension, recent MI or cerebral vascular accident)

Warnings Use of I.V. mannitol can lead to profound diuresis with fluid and electrolyte loss; close medical supervision and dose evaluation are required. Monitor and correct electrolyte disturbances; adjust dose to avoid dehydration. May cause severe osmotic nephrosis and/or renal dysfunction especially with high doses; use with caution in patients taking other nephrotoxic agents, with sepsis, or preexisting renal disease. To minimize adverse renal effects, adjust dosage to keep serum osmolality less than 320 mOsm/L; discontinue if evidence of acute tubular necrosis occurs. May cause progressive heart failure or pulmonary congestion after administration; if occurs, subsequent use is contraindicated.

Mannitol may increase cerebral blood flow, increase the risk of postoperative bleeding in neurosurgical patients, and worsen intracranial hypertension in children who develop generalized cerebral hyperemia during the first 24-48 hours after traumatic brain injury.

Powder for inhalation (Aridol™): Mannitol may cause severe bronchospasm. Bronchial challenge testing should be for diagnostic purposes only and performed by trained professionals; patients should not be left unattended during testing. Do not use in patients with clinically apparent asthma or very low baseline pulmonary function (eg, FEV_1 <1-1.5 L or <70% of the predicted values). Medications (eg, short-acting inhaled beta-agonist) and equipment for the treatment of severe bronchospasm should be readily available during use. **[U.S. Boxed Warning]**; use with caution in patients with conditions that may increase sensitivity to bronchoconstriction (eg, severe cough, ventilatory impairment, spirometry-induced bronchoconstriction, hemoptysis of unknown origin, pneumothorax; recent abdominal, thoracic, or intraocular surgery; unstable angina, active upper or lower respiratory tract infection). Patients who have ≥10% reduction in FEV_1 on administration of the 0 mg capsule, patients with a positive response to bronchial challenge testing, or patients who develop significant respiratory symptoms should be treated with a short-acting inhaled beta-agonist and monitored until full recovery to baseline; discontinue further testing. Bronchial challenge testing should not be performed in children <6 years of age as these patients are unable to provide reliable spirometric results.

Precautions Use with caution in patients with renal impairment; intravenous mannitol should not be administered until adequacy of renal function and urine flow is established; may use 1-2 test doses to assess renal response. Use with caution in patients with hyponatremia; the shift of sodium-free intracellular fluid into the extracellular space that occurs after mannitol infusion may lower serum sodium further.

In patients being treated for cerebral edema, mannitol may accumulate in the brain (causing rebound increases in intracranial pressure); this may occur if brain tissue is injured or if mannitol is used or circulating for extended periods of time (eg, as with continuous infusion); thus, intermittent boluses are preferred. If hypotension occurs, monitor cerebral perfusion pressure to ensure it is adequate. Cardiovascular status should also be evaluated; significant extracellular fluid expansion may occur and lead to fulminant congestive heart failure. Do not administer electrolyte-free mannitol solutions with blood. Mannitol is a vesicant; avoid extravasation.

◄ Irrigation solution should be used with caution in severe cardiopulmonary or renal dysfunction. Irrigating fluids used during transurethral prostatectomy may be absorbed systemically; the resultant osmotic diuresis may significantly affect cardiopulmonary and renal dynamics.

Adverse Reactions

Inhalation:
Cardiovascular: Chest discomfort

Central nervous system: Dizziness, headache

Gastrointestinal: Nausea, retching, throat irritation

Respiratory: Cough, dyspnea, pharyngolaryngeal pain, rhinorrhea, wheezing

Rare but important or life-threatening: FEV_1 decreased, gagging

Injection:
Cardiovascular: Chest pain, CHF, circulatory overload, hyper-/hypotension, peripheral edema, tachycardia

Central nervous system: Chills, convulsions, dizziness, fever, headache

Dermatologic: Bullous eruption, urticaria

Endocrine & metabolic: Fluid and electrolyte imbalance, dehydration and hypovolemia secondary to rapid diuresis, hyperglycemia, hypernatremia, hyponatremia (dilutional), hyperosmolality-induced hyperkalemia, metabolic acidosis (dilutional), osmolar gap increased, water intoxication

Gastrointestinal: Nausea, vomiting, xerostomia

Genitourinary: Dysuria, polyuria

Local: Pain, thrombophlebitis, tissue necrosis

Ocular: Blurred vision

Renal: Acute renal failure, acute tubular necrosis (adult dose >200 g/day; serum osmolality >320 mOsm/L)

Respiratory: Pulmonary edema, rhinitis

Miscellaneous: Allergic reactions

Drug Interactions

Metabolism/Transport Effects None known.

Avoid Concomitant Use
Avoid concomitant use of Mannitol with any of the following: Aminoglycosides

Increased Effect/Toxicity
Mannitol may increase the levels/effects of: Amifostine; Aminoglycosides; Antihypertensives; DULoxetine; Hypotensive Agents; Obinutuzumab; RiTUXimab; Sodium Phosphates

The levels/effects of Mannitol may be increased by: Alfuzosin; Analgesics (Opioid); Barbiturates; Brimonidine (Topical); Diazoxide; Herbs (Hypotensive Properties); MAO Inhibitors; Pentoxifylline; Phosphodiesterase 5 Inhibitors; Prostacyclin Analogues

Decreased Effect
The levels/effects of Mannitol may be decreased by: Herbs (Hypertensive Properties); Methylphenidate; Yohimbine

Stability
Injection: Store intact vials at room temperature 15°C to 30°C (59°F to 86°F); store flexible container at 25°C (77°F); excursions permitted up to 40°C (104°F); protect parenteral dosage forms from freezing; avoid excessive heat. Mannitol preparations with concentrations ≥15% may crystallize at low temperatures; do not use solutions that contain crystals; some products may be warmed in a hot water bath and shaken vigorously to resolubilize crystals (see product information for brand-specific instructions); solutions should be cooled to body temperature before using; incompatible with strongly acidic or alkaline solutions; potassium chloride or sodium chloride may cause precipitation of mannitol 20% or 25% solution. Discard unused portion.

Irrigation: Store at room temperature 25°C (77°F); excursions permitted to 40°C (104°F). Avoid excessive heat; do not warm above 66°C (150°F). Do not freeze.

Contains no antimicrobial or bacteriostatic agents; contents should be used promptly after opening to minimize the possibility of bacterial growth or pyrogen formation; discard unused portion.

Powder for inhalation: Store at <25°C (<77°F); excursions permitted to 15°C to 30°C (59°F to 86°F). Do not refrigerate or freeze.

Mechanism of Action
Produces an osmotic diuresis by increasing the osmotic pressure of glomerular filtrate, which inhibits tubular reabsorption of water and electrolytes and increases urinary output. Mechanism of action in reduction of intracranial pressure (ICP) is controversial. However, it is thought that mannitol reduces ICP by reducing blood viscosity which transiently increases cerebral blood flow and oxygen transport. This in turn reduces cerebral blood volume and ICP. Furthermore, mannitol reduces ICP by withdrawing water from the brain parenchyma and excretes water in the urine (Allen, 2009; Bratton, 2007; Miller, 2010).

Pharmacodynamics
Onset of action:
Bronchospasm, challenge: Inhalation: Within 1 minute if positive response

Diuresis: I.V.: Within 1-3 hours

ICP reduction: I.V.: Within 15 minutes

Duration: ICP reduction: I.V.: 3-6 hours

Pharmacokinetics (Adult data unless noted)
Distribution: 34.3 L; remains confined to extracellular space; does not penetrate blood-brain barrier except in very high concentrations or with acidosis

Metabolism: Minimal amounts in the liver to glycogen

Bioavailability: Inhalation: Absolute: 59% (relative to oral administration: 96%)

Half-life:
Injection: 0.25-1.7 hours; 6-36 hours in renal failure

Inhalation: 4.7 hours

Time to peak serum concentration: Inhalation: 1.5 hours

Elimination: Urine (~55% to 87% as unchanged drug by glomerular filtration)

Dosing: Neonatal
Acute renal failure: I.V.: 0.5-1 g/kg/dose (Andreoli, 2004); some experts recommend against routine use due to the risk of IVH in low birth weight neonates (solution is hypertonic) or the precipitation of CHF if a lack of response occurs (Andreoli, 2004; Chua, 2005)

Dosing: Usual
Infants, Children and Adolescents: **Note:** The manufacturer's labeling recommends a test dose prior to starting I.V. mannitol therapy in patients with marked oliguria or suspected renal insufficiency.

Acute renal failure (oliguria): I.V.: Initial: 0.5-1 g/kg/dose infused over 2-6 hours; usual range: 0.25-2 g/kg/dose; may repeat dose every 4-6 hours; do not repeat dose if oliguria persists. **Note:** Although FDA-labeled indications, the use of mannitol for the prevention of acute renal failure and/or promotion of diuresis is not routinely recommended (Kellum, 2008).

Test dose (to assess adequate renal function): I.V.: 0.2 g/kg (maximum dose: 12.5 g) over 3-5 minutes to produce a urine flow of at least 1 mL/kg/hour for 1-3 hours

Bronchial hyper-responsiveness assessment: Children ≥6 years and Adolescents: Oral inhalation: Administer in a stepwise fashion (measuring FEV_1 in duplicate at baseline and after each administration) until the patient has a positive response or 635 mg of mannitol has been administered (whichever comes first).

Positive test: 15% reduction in FEV_1 from baseline or 10% incremental reduction in FEV_1 between consecutive doses

Negative test: Administration of full dose (635 mg) without reduction in FEV_1 sufficient to meet criteria for a positive test

Administration should be as follows:

Stepwise Administration Schedule

Dose #	Dose (mg)	Cumulative Dose (mg)	Capsules/Dose
1	0	0	1
2	5	5	1
3	10	15	1
4	20	35	1
5	40	75	1
6	80	155	2 x 40 mg caps
7	160	315	4 x 40 mg caps
8	160	475	4 x 40 mg caps
9	160	635	4 x 40 mg caps

Intracranial pressure (ICP), reduction: I.V.: Usual range: 0.25-1 g/kg/dose infused over 20-30 minutes; repeat as needed to maintain serum osmolality <300-320 mOsm/kg (Bratton, 2007; Hegenbarth, 2008; Kochanek, 2012). **Note:** The manufacturer's labeling allows for higher single doses up to 2 g/kg/dose.

Intraocular pressure (IOP), reduction: I.V.: 1-2 g/kg/dose **or** 30-60 g/m^2/dose infused over 30-60 minutes administered 1-1.5 hours prior to surgery

IOP (traumatic hyphema), reduction: I.V.: 1.5 g/kg/dose infused over 45 minutes twice daily for IOP >35 mm Hg; may administer every 8 hours in patients with extremely high pressure (Crouch, 1999)

Adults:

Bronchial hyper-responsiveness, assessment: Inhalation: Administer in a stepwise fashion (measuring FEV$_1$ in duplicate at baseline and after each administration) until the patient has a positive response or 635 mg of mannitol has been administered (whichever comes first).

Positive test: 15% reduction in FEV$_1$ from baseline or 10% incremental reduction in FEV$_1$ between consecutive doses

Negative test: Administration of full dose (635 mg) without reduction in FEV$_1$ sufficient to meet criteria for a positive test

Administration should be as follows:

Stepwise Administration Schedule

Dose #	Dose (mg)	Cumulative Dose (mg)	Capsules/Dose
1	0	0	1
2	5	5	1
3	10	15	1
4	20	35	1
5	40	75	1
6	80	155	2 x 40 mg caps
7	160	315	4 x 40 mg caps
8	160	475	4 x 40 mg caps
9	160	635	4 x 40 mg caps

Increased intracranial pressure (ICP), cerebral edema: I.V.: 0.25-1 g/kg/dose; may repeat every 6-8 hours as needed (Bratton, 2007; Kochanek, 2012); maintain serum osmolality <300-320 mOsm/kg (Kochanek, 2012; Rabinstein, 2006)

Intraocular pressure (IOP), reduction: I.V.: 0.25-2 g/kg infused over 30-60 minutes administered 1-1.5 hours prior to surgery

IOP (traumatic hyphema), reduction: I.V.: 1.5 g/kg infused over 45 minutes twice daily for IOP >35 mm Hg; may administer every 8 hours in patients with extremely high pressure (Crouch, 1999)

Transurethral irrigation: Topical: Use 5% urogenital solution as required for irrigation.

Dosage adjustment for renal impairment: Contraindicated in severe renal impairment. Use with caution in patients with underlying renal disease. May be used to reduce the incidence of acute tubular necrosis when administered prior to revascularization during kidney transplantation.

Dosage adjustment for hepatic impairment: No adjustment required.

Administration

Irrigation: For irrigation only; not for injection: Administer using only the appropriate transurethral urologic instrumentation. Do not warm above 66°C (150°F).

I.V.: Do not administer I.M. or SubQ. In-line filter set (≤5 micron) should always be used for mannitol infusion with concentrations ≥20%; maximum concentration for administration: 25%. Inspect for crystals prior to administration; if crystals are present, redissolve by warming solution. Do not administer with blood; crenation and agglutination of red blood cells may occur. pH: 4.5-7. Infusion rate is dependent upon indication:

Acute renal failure: Administer over 2-6 hours

Cerebral edema or increased intracranial pressure: Administer over 20-30 minutes

Test dose (for oliguria): Administer over 3-5 minutes

Oral inhalation (Aridol™): Administer using supplied single patient use inhaler; do not puncture capsule more than once; do not swallow capsules. A nose clip may be used if preferred. The patient should exhale completely, followed by a controlled rapid deep inspiration from the device; hold breath for 5 seconds and exhale through the mouth. Measure FEV$_1$ in duplicate 60 seconds after inhalation; repeat process until positive response or full dose (635 mg) has been administered.

Vesicant/Extravasation Risk Vesicant (at concentrations >5%)

Monitoring Parameters

Renal function, daily fluid intake and output, serum electrolytes, serum and urine osmolality; for treatment of elevated intracranial pressure, maintain serum osmolality <300-320 mOsm/kg

Bronchial challenge test: Standard spirometry prior to bronchial challenge test; FEV$_1$ in duplicate 60 seconds after administration of each step of test

Additional Information Approximate osmolarity: Mannitol 20%: 1100 mOsm/L; mannitol 25%: 1375 mOsm/L

Bronchial challenge testing: The dose of inhaled mannitol which causes a 15% reduction in FEV$_1$ is expressed as PD$_{15}$

Dosage Forms Excipient information presented when available (limited, particularly for generics); consult specific product labeling.

Kit, Inhalation:
  Aridol:
Solution, Intravenous:
  Osmitrol: 5% (1000 mL); 10% (500 mL); 15% (500 mL); 20% (250 mL, 500 mL)
  Generic: 5% (1000 mL); 10% (500 mL); 15% (500 mL); 20% (250 mL, 500 mL); 25% (50 mL)
Solution, Intravenous [preservative free]:
  Generic: 25% (50 mL)
Solution, Irrigation:
  Resectisol: 5% (2000 mL)

References

Allen CH and Ward JD, "An Evidence-Based Approach to Management of Increased Intracranial Pressure," *Crit Care Clin*, 1998, 14 (3):485-95.

Andreoli SP, "Acute Renal Failure in the Newborn," *Semin Perinatol*, 2004, 28(2):112-23.

Bratton SL, Chestnut RM, Ghajar J, et al, "Guidelines for the Management of Severe Traumatic Brain Injury. II. Hyperosmolar Therapy," *J Neurotrauma*, 2007, 24(Suppl 1):14-20.

Broderick J, Connolly S, Feldmann E, et al, "Guidelines for the Management of Spontaneous Intracerebral Hemorrhage in Adults: 2007 Update: A Guideline From the American Heart Association/American Stroke Association Stroke Council, High Blood Pressure Research Council, and the Quality of Care and Outcomes in Research Interdisciplinary Working Group," *Stroke*, 2007, 38(6):2001-23.

Chua AN and Sarwal MM, "Acute Renal Failure Management in the Neonate," *NeoReviews*, 2005, 6:e369-76.

Crouch ER Jr and Crouch ER, "Management of Traumatic Hyphema: Therapeutic Options," *J Pediatr Ophthalmol Strabismus*, 1999, 36 (5):238-50.

Hegenbarth MA and American Academy of Pediatrics Committee on Drugs, "Preparing for Pediatric Emergencies: Drugs to Consider," *Pediatrics*, 2008, 121(2):433-43.

Kellum JA, Cerda J, Kaplan LJ, et al, "Fluids for Prevention and Management of Acute Kidney Injury," *Int J Artif Organs*, 2008, 31 (2):96-110.

Kochanek PM, Carney N, Adelson PD, et al, "Guidelines for the Acute Medical Management of Severe Traumatic Brain Injury in Infants, Children, and Adolescents–Second Edition," *Pediatr Crit Care Med*, 2012, 13(Suppl 1):1-82.

Miller RD, *Miller's Anesthesia*, 7th ed, Philadelphia PA: Churchill Livingstone, 2010.

National Asthma Education and Prevention Program (NAEPP), "Expert Panel Report 3 (EPR-3): Guidelines for the Diagnosis and Management of Asthma," *Clinical Practice Guidelines*, National Institutes of Health, National Heart, Lung, and Blood Institute, NIH Publication No. 08-4051, prepublication 2007; available at http://www.nhlbi.nih.gov/guidelines/asthma/asthgdln.htm.

Rabinstein AA, "Treatment of Cerebral Edema," *Neurologist*, 2006, 12 (2):59-73.

◆ **Maox [OTC]** *see* Magnesium Oxide *on page 1296*

◆ **Mapap [OTC]** *see* Acetaminophen *on page 47*

◆ **Mapap Arthritis Pain [OTC]** *see* Acetaminophen *on page 47*

◆ **Mapap Children's [OTC]** *see* Acetaminophen *on page 47*

◆ **Mapap Extra Strength [OTC]** *see* Acetaminophen *on page 47*

◆ **Mapap Infant's [OTC]** *see* Acetaminophen *on page 47*

◆ **Mapap Junior Rapid Tabs [OTC]** *see* Acetaminophen *on page 47*

◆ **Mapezine (Can)** *see* CarBAMazepine *on page 372*

◆ **Mar-Allopurinol (Can)** *see* Allopurinol *on page 97*

◆ **Mar-Amlodipine (Can)** *see* AmLODIPine *on page 135*

Maraviroc (mah RAV er rock)

Related Information
Adult and Adolescent HIV *on page 2348*
Pediatric HIV *on page 2338*
Perinatal HIV *on page 2356*
Brand Names: U.S. Selzentry
Brand Names: Canada Celsentri
Therapeutic Category Antiretroviral Agent; Antiretroviral, CCR5 Antagonist (Anti-HIV); CCR5 Antagonist; HIV Agents (Anti-HIV Agents)
Generic Availability (U.S.) No
Use Treatment of CCR5-tropic HIV-1 infection, in combination with other antiretroviral agents (FDA approved in ages ≥16 years and adults); **Note:** HIV regimens consisting of **three** antiretroviral agents are strongly recommended.
Medication Guide Available Yes
Pregnancy Risk Factor B
Pregnancy Considerations Adverse fetal effects were not observed in animal reproduction studies. Maraviroc has minimal to low transfer across the human placenta. The DHHS Perinatal HIV Guidelines note there are insufficient data to recommend use in pregnancy.

Regardless of CD4 count or HIV RNA copy number, all HIV-infected pregnant women should receive a combination antiretroviral (ARV) drug regimen. A combination of antepartum, intrapartum, and infant ARV prophylaxis is recommended. ARV therapy should be started as soon as possible in women with symptomatic infection. Although earlier initiation may be more effective in reducing the perinatal transmission of HIV, initiation may be delayed until after 12 weeks gestation in women who do not require immediate treatment after careful consideration of maternal conditions (eg, nausea and vomiting) and the potential risks of first trimester fetal exposure for specific agents. A scheduled cesarean delivery at 38 weeks gestation is recommended for all women with HIV RNA >1000 copies/mL or unknown concentrations near delivery in order to decrease transmission. If ARV therapy must be interrupted for <24 hours during the peripartum period, stop then restart all medications simultaneously in order to decrease the chance of developing resistance. Long-term follow-up is recommended for all infants exposed to ARV medications. In couples who want to conceive, the HIV-infected partner should attain maximum viral suppression prior to conception.

Health care providers are encouraged to enroll pregnant women exposed to antiretroviral medications in the Antiretroviral Pregnancy Registry (1-800-258-4263 or www.APRegistry.com). Health care providers caring for HIV-infected women and their infants may contact the National Perinatal HIV Hotline (888-448-8765) for clinical consultation (DHHS [perinatal], 2014).

Breast-Feeding Considerations It is not known if maraviroc is excreted into breast milk. Maternal or infant antiretroviral therapy does not completely eliminate the risk of postnatal HIV transmission. In addition, multiclass-resistant virus has been detected in breast-feeding infants despite maternal therapy. Therefore, in the United States, where formula is accessible, affordable, safe, and sustainable, and the risk of infant mortality due to diarrhea and respiratory infections is low, complete avoidance of breast-feeding by HIV-infected women is recommended to decrease potential transmission of HIV (DHHS [perinatal], 2014).

Contraindications Hypersensitivity to maraviroc or any component; severe renal impairment (CrCl <30 mL/minute) or end-stage renal disease (ESRD) in patients who are taking potent CYP3A4 inhibitors or inducers

Warnings Hepatotoxicity with allergic type features has been reported with use of maraviroc **[U.S. Boxed Warning]**; some cases have been life-threatening; hepatotoxicity usually develops after 1 month of treatment and may be preceded by severe rash or systemic allergic type reactions including pruritic rash, eosinophilia, fever, increased IgE, and/or hepatic adverse events (transaminase increases or signs/symptoms of hepatitis); immediately evaluate patients with signs and symptoms of allergic reaction or hepatitis (with or without allergy symptoms). Use with caution in patients with preexisting hepatic dysfunction or coinfection with hepatitis B or C; however, hepatotoxicity has occurred in the absence of preexisting hepatic conditions. Monitor hepatic function at baseline and as clinically indicated during treatment. Consider discontinuation in any patient with possible hepatitis or with elevated transaminases combined with systemic allergic events; rechallenge with maraviroc is not recommended (DHHS [pediatric], 2014).

Severe, potentially life-threatening skin and hypersensitivity reactions have been reported; most commonly when maraviroc is taken concomitantly with other drugs associated with these reactions. These include Stevens-Johnson syndrome, toxic epidermal necrolysis (TEN) and drug rash with eosinophilia and systemic symptoms (DRESS); discontinue treatment if severe rash or moderate symptoms accompanied by other systemic symptoms occur (including fever, malaise, muscle or joint aches, blisters, oral lesions, conjunctivitis, facial edema, lip swelling, eosinophilia).

Monitor closely for signs/symptoms of developing infections; use associated with a small increase of certain upper respiratory tract infections and herpes virus infections during clinical trials. May affect immune surveillance and lead to an increased risk of malignancy due to pharmacologic mechanism of action (maraviroc antagonizes the CCR5 coreceptor located on some immune cells); no increase in malignancy has been observed. Long-term follow-up needed to assess this risk.

Precautions Use with caution in patients with mild or moderate renal impairment; renal impairment may increase maraviroc serum concentrations. Symptomatic postural hypotension has occurred; use with caution in patients at risk for postural hypotension due to concomitant medication or history of condition; may cause dizziness or postural dizziness; patients should be cautioned to avoid driving or operating machinery. An increased risk of postural hypotension may occur in patients with severe renal insufficiency or in those with ESRD; reduce dose in patients with severe renal dysfunction who experience postural hypotension. Use with caution in patients with cardiovascular disease or cardiac risk factors; during trials, a small increase in cardiovascular events (myocardial ischemia and/or infarction) occurred in treated patients compared to placebo, although a contributory relationship relative to therapy is unknown. Of note, patients experiencing events generally had cardiac disease/risk factors prior to therapy. Use with caution in patients taking strong CYP3A4/P-glycoprotein inhibitors and moderate or strong CYP3A4/P-glycoprotein inducers; may require dosage adjustments. Concurrent use of these agents with maraviroc is contraindicated in patients with severe renal dysfunction (CrCl <30 mL/minute). Potentially significant interactions may exist, requiring dose or frequency adjustment, additional monitoring, and/or selection of alternative therapy. Consult drug interactions database for more detailed information.

Prior to therapy, coreceptor tropism testing should be performed for presence of CCR5-tropic only virus HIV-1 infection. Maraviroc should only be used in patients with documented CCR5-tropic only virus; efficacy has not been demonstrated in CXCR4-tropic HIV-1 or dual/mixed tropism patients (eg, CCR5-tropic and CXCR4-tropic); studies have found that in mixed tropism patients, the CCR5-tropic virus will be suppressed and the CXCR4-tropic virus will continue to proliferate. A phenotypic tropism assay is generally preferred to determine HIV-1 coreceptor usage compared to genotypic testing; a genotypic tropism assay should be considered as an alternative test (DHHS [adult], 2014).

Immune reconstitution syndrome (an acute inflammatory response to residual or indolent opportunistic infections) may occur in HIV patients during initial treatment with combination antiretroviral agents; this syndrome may require further patient assessment and therapy. Autoimmune disorders (eg, Graves' disease, Guillain-Barré syndrome, and polymyositis) have been reported in patients experiencing immune reconstitution; time to onset is variable and may occur many months after antiretroviral treatment is initiated.

Adverse Reactions
Cardiovascular: Vascular hypertensive disorder
Central nervous system: Amnesia, anxiety, depression, dizziness (including postural dizziness), fever, impaired consciousness, insomnia, pain, paresthesia, peripheral neuropathy, sensory disturbance
Dermatologic: Acne vulgaris, alopecia, erythema, folliculitis, pruritus, skin neoplasm (benign), skin rash, tinea
Endocrine & metabolic: Lipodystrophy
Gastrointestinal: Change in appetite, constipation, decreased gastrointestinal motility

Genitourinary: Genitourinary complaint (urinary tract/bladder symptoms), warts (genital)
Hematologic & oncologic: Neutropenia (grades 3/4)
Hepatic: Increased serum ALT (grades 3/4), increased serum AST (grades 3/4), increased serum bilirubin (grades 3/4)
Infection: Bacterial infection, herpes infection, *Neisseria*
Neuromuscular & skeletal: Arthralgia, myalgia
Ophthalmic: Conjunctivitis, eye infection
Otic: Otitis media
Respiratory: Bronchitis, cough, irregular breathing, lower respiratory tract infections, nasal congestion, paranasal sinus disease, sinusitis, upper respiratory tract infection
Miscellaneous: Flu-like symptoms, sweat gland disturbances
Rare but important or life-threatening: Anal cancer, angina pectoris, basal cell carcinoma, bile duct neoplasm, bone marrow depression, carcinoma *in situ* of esophagus, cardiac failure, cerebrovascular accident, cholestatic jaundice, coronary artery disease, coronary artery occlusion, endocarditis, endocrine neoplasm, hepatic cirrhosis, hepatic failure, hepatotoxicity, hypoplastic anemia, immune reconstitution syndrome, increased creatine kinase, ischemic heart disease, liver metastases, lymphoma, meningitis (viral), multiorgan hypersensitivity, myocardial infarction, myositis, osteonecrosis, pneumonia, portal vein thrombosis, rhabdomyolysis, seizure, septic shock, squamous cell carcinoma, Stevens-Johnson syndrome, syncope, T-cell lymphoma, tongue neoplasm, toxic epidermal necrolysis, tremor

Drug Interactions
Metabolism/Transport Effects Substrate of CYP3A4 (major), P-glycoprotein; **Note:** Assignment of Major/Minor substrate status based on clinically relevant drug interaction potential

Avoid Concomitant Use
Avoid concomitant use of Maraviroc with any of the following: Conivaptan; Fusidic Acid (Systemic); St Johns Wort

Increased Effect/Toxicity
The levels/effects of Maraviroc may be increased by: Ceritinib; Conivaptan; CYP3A4 Inhibitors (Moderate); CYP3A4 Inhibitors (Strong); Dasatinib; Fusidic Acid (Systemic); Ivacaftor; Luliconazole; Mifepristone; Simeprevir; Stiripentol

Decreased Effect
The levels/effects of Maraviroc may be decreased by: Bosentan; CYP3A4 Inducers (Strong); Dabrafenib; Deferasirox; Efavirenz; Etravirine; Mitotane; Siltuximab; St Johns Wort; Tocilizumab

Stability Store at 25°C (77°F); excursions permitted to 15°C to 30°C (59°F to 86°F).

Mechanism of Action Maraviroc, a CCR5 antagonist, selectively and reversibly binds to the chemokine (C-C motif receptor 5 [CCR5]) coreceptors located on human CD4 cells. CCR5 antagonism prevents interaction between the human CCR5 coreceptor and the gp120 subunit of the viral envelope glycoprotein, thereby inhibiting gp120 conformational change required for CCR5-tropic HIV-1 fusion with the CD4 cell and subsequent cell entry.

Pharmacokinetics (Adult data unless noted)
Distribution: V_d: ~194 L
Protein binding: ~76%
Metabolism: Hepatic, via CYP3A to inactive metabolites
Bioavailability: 23% to 33% (maraviroc is a substrate for the efflux transporter P-gp)
Half-life elimination: 14 to 18 hours
Time to peak, plasma: 0.5 to 4 hours
Elimination: Urine (~20%, 8% as unchanged drug); feces (76%, 25% as unchanged drug)

Dosing: Usual

Pediatric: **HIV infection, treatment:** Use in combination with other antiretroviral agents: Adolescents ≥16 years: Oral: 300 mg twice daily (DHHS [pediatric], 2014)

Adult: **HIV infection, treatment:** Use in combination with other antiretroviral agents: Oral: 300 mg twice daily (DHHS [adult], 2014)

Dosing adjustment for concomitant CYP3A4 inhibitors/inducers: Adolescents ≥16 years and Adults:

CYP3A inhibitors (with or without a CYP3A4 inducer): 150 mg twice daily; dose recommended when maraviroc administered concomitantly with strong CYP3A inhibitors including (but not limited to) protease inhibitors (excluding tipranavir/ritonavir), boceprevir, delavirdine, ketoconazole, itraconazole, clarithromycin, nefazodone, telaprevir, and telithromycin.

CYP3A inducers (without a strong CYP3A4 inhibitor): 600 mg twice daily; dose recommended when maraviroc administered concomitantly with CYP3A inducers including (but not limited to) efavirenz, etravirine, rifampin, carbamazepine, phenobarbital, and phenytoin.

Dosing adjustment in renal impairment: Adolescents ≥16 years and Adults (DHHS [adults], 2013):

CrCl ≥30 mL/minute: No adjustment required

CrCl <30 mL/minute:

CrCl <30 mL/minute or ESRD and concomitant potent CYP3A inhibitors (with or without a CYP3A4 inducer) or concomitant potent CYP3A4 inducer (without a CYP3A4 inhibitor): Use is contraindicated

CrCl <30 mL/minute or ESRD and concomitant medications (eg, tipranavir/ritonavir, nevirapine, raltegravir, all NRTIs, and enfuvirtide): 300 mg twice daily. If postural hypotension occurs, reduce dose to 150 mg twice daily.

CrCl <30 mL/minute and experiencing postural hypotension: Reduce dose to 150 mg twice daily

Hemodialysis has minimal effect on clearance

Dosing adjustment in hepatic impairment: Adolescents ≥16 years and Adults:

Mild to moderate impairment: Use with caution; maraviroc concentrations are increased although dosage adjustment is not recommended

Moderate impairment (with concomitant strong CYP3A4 inhibitor): Use with caution; monitor closely for adverse events

Severe impairment: Patient population has not been studied

Administration May administer without regards to meals.

Monitoring Parameters Note: Monitor CD4 percentage (if <5 years of age) or CD4 count (if ≥5 years of age) at least every 3 to 4 months (DHHS [pediatric], 2014).

Prior to initiation of therapy: Genotypic resistance testing, CD4 and viral load (every 3 to 4 months), CBC with differential, LFTs, BUN, creatinine, tropism testing, electrolytes, glucose, and urinalysis (every 6 to 12 months), and assessment of readiness for adherence with medication regimen. At initiation and with any change in treatment regimen: CBC with differential, electrolytes, calcium, phosphate, glucose, LFTs, bilirubin, urinalysis (at initiation), BUN, creatinine, albumin, total protein, lipid panel (at initiation), CD4, and viral load. After 1 to 2 weeks of therapy: Signs of medication toxicity and adherence. After 2 to 4 weeks of therapy: CBC with differential, viral load, signs of medication toxicity, and adherence; then every 3 to 4 months: CBC with differential, electrolytes, glucose, LFTs, bilirubin, BUN, creatinine, CD4, viral load, signs of medication toxicity, and adherence. Every 6 to 12 months: Lipid panel and urinalysis. CD4 monitoring frequency may be decreased to every 6 to 12 months in children who are adherent to therapy if the value is well above the threshold for opportunistic infections, viral suppression is sustained,

and the clinical status is stable for more than 2 to 3 years (DHHS [pediatric], 2014). Monitor for growth and development, signs of HIV-specific physical conditions, HIV disease progression, opportunistic infections, postural hypotension, or hepatitis.

Reference Range Plasma trough concentration: ≥50 ng/mL (DHHS [adult, pediatric], 2014)

Dosage Forms Excipient information presented when available (limited, particularly for generics); consult specific product labeling.

Tablet, Oral:

Selzentry: 150 mg, 300 mg [contains fd&c blue #2 aluminum lake, soybean lecithin]

References

DHHS Panel on Antiretroviral Guidelines for Adults and Adolescents. Guidelines for the use of antiretroviral agents in HIV-1-infected adults and adolescents, Department of Health and Human Services. May 1, 2014. Available at http://www.aidsinfo.nih.gov/ContentFiles/AdultandAdolescentGL.pdf

DHHS Panel on Antiretroviral Therapy and Medical Management of HIV-Infected Children. Guidelines for the use of antiretroviral agents in pediatric HIV infection. February 12, 2014. Available at http://aidsinfo.nih.gov

DHHS Panel on Treatment of HIV-Infected Pregnant Women and Prevention of Perinatal Transmission. Recommendations for the use of antiretroviral drugs in pregnant HIV-1-infected women for maternal health and interventions to reduce perinatal HIV-1 transmission in the United States. March 28, 2014. Available at http://aidsinfo.nih.gov

Dorr P, Westby M, Dobbs S, et al. Maraviroc (UK-427,857), a potent, orally bioavailable, and selective small-molecule inhibitor of chemokine receptor CCR5 with broad-spectrum anti-human immunodeficiency virus type 1 activity. Antimicrob Agents Chemother. 2005;49 (11):4721-4732.

◆ **Marcaine** see Bupivacaine on page 318

◆ **Marcaine® (Can)** see Bupivacaine on page 318

◆ **Marcaine Preservative Free** see Bupivacaine on page 318

◆ **Marcaine Spinal** see Bupivacaine on page 318

◆ **Mar-Ciprofloxacin (Can)** see Ciprofloxacin (Systemic) on page 471

◆ **Mar-Cof CG** see Guaifenesin and Codeine on page 985

◆ **Marinol** see Dronabinol on page 725

◆ **Marinol® (Can)** see Dronabinol on page 725

◆ **Mar-Letrozole (Can)** see Letrozole on page 1211

◆ **Mar-Metformin (Can)** see MetFORMIN on page 1353

◆ **Mar-Montelukast (Can)** see Montelukast on page 1438

◆ **Mar-Quetiapine (Can)** see QUEtiapine on page 1783

◆ **Mar-Risperidone (Can)** see RisperiDONE on page 1831

◆ **Mar-Rizatriptan (Can)** see Rizatriptan on page 1845

◆ **Mar-Simvastatin (Can)** see Simvastatin on page 1892

◆ **Matulane** see Procarbazine on page 1743

◆ **Matzim LA** see Diltiazem on page 667

◆ **3M Avagard [OTC]** see Chlorhexidine Gluconate on page 441

◆ **Maxair Autohaler [DSC]** see Pirbuterol on page 1683

◆ **Maxalt** see Rizatriptan on page 1845

◆ **Maxalt™ (Can)** see Rizatriptan on page 1845

◆ **Maxalt-MLT** see Rizatriptan on page 1845

◆ **Maxalt RPD™ (Can)** see Rizatriptan on page 1845

◆ **Maxidex** see Dexamethasone (Ophthalmic) on page 619

◆ **Maxidex® (Can)** see Dexamethasone (Ophthalmic) on page 619

◆ **Maxidol (Can)** see Naproxen on page 1470

◆ **Maxidone® [DSC]** see Hydrocodone and Acetaminophen on page 1027

◆ **Maxilene (Can)** see Lidocaine (Topical) on page 1242

◆ **Maxipime** see Cefepime on page 398

- **Maxitrol®** *see* Neomycin, Polymyxin B, and Dexamethasone *on page 1484*
- **May Apple** *see* Podophyllum Resin *on page 1693*
- **M-Clear** *see* Guaifenesin and Codeine *on page 985*
- **M-Clear WC** *see* Guaifenesin and Codeine *on page 985*
- **MCT** *see* Medium Chain Triglycerides *on page 1318*
- **MCT Oil [OTC]** *see* Medium Chain Triglycerides *on page 1318*
- **MCT Oil (Can)** *see* Medium Chain Triglycerides *on page 1318*
- **MCV** *see* Meningococcal (Groups A / C / Y and W-135) Diphtheria Conjugate Vaccine *on page 1330*
- **MCV4** *see* Meningococcal (Groups A / C / Y and W-135) Diphtheria Conjugate Vaccine *on page 1330*
- **MDL 73,147EF** *see* Dolasetron *on page 703*
- **ME-609** *see* Acyclovir and Hydrocortisone *on page 69*

Measles, Mumps, and Rubella Virus Vaccine (MEE zels, mumpz & roo BEL a VYE rus vak SEEN)

Medication Safety Issues
Sound-alike/look-alike issues:
MMR (measles, mumps and rubella virus vaccine) may be confused with MMRV (measles, mumps, rubella, and varicella) vaccine

Related Information
Immunization Administration Recommendations *on page 2368*

Immunization Guidelines *on page 2373*

Brand Names: U.S. M-M-R II

Brand Names: Canada M-M-R II; Priorix

Therapeutic Category Vaccine, Live Virus

Generic Availability (U.S.) No

Use Provide active immunity to measles, mumps, and rubella viruses (FDA approved in ages ≥12 months and adults)

The Advisory Committee on Immunization Practices (ACIP) recommends routine vaccination for the following (CDC/ACIP [McLean, 2013]):
- All children (first dose given at 12 to 15 months of age)
- Adults born 1957 or later (without evidence of immunity or documentation of vaccination). Vaccine may be given to adults born prior to 1957 if they do not have contraindications to the MMR vaccine.
- Adults at higher risk for exposure to and transmission of measles, mumps, and rubella should receive special consideration for vaccination, unless an acceptable evidence of immunity exists. This includes international travelers, persons attending colleges and other post high school education, and persons working in healthcare facilities.

Pregnancy Risk Factor C

Pregnancy Considerations Animal reproduction studies have not been conducted. It is not known whether this vaccine can cause fetal harm or affect reproduction capacity. Based on information collected following inadvertent administration during pregnancy, adverse events have not been observed following use of rubella vaccine. However, theoretical risks cannot be ruled out; use of this vaccine is contraindicated in pregnant females and should not be administered to women trying to conceive. The manufacturer recommends that pregnancy be avoided for 3 months after vaccine administration. The Advisory Committee on Immunization Practices (ACIP) recommends that pregnancy should be avoided for 28 days following vaccination. The risk of congenital rubella syndrome following vaccination is significantly less than the risk associated following infection therefore inadvertent administration of

MMR during pregnancy is not considered an indication to terminate pregnancy.

Adverse events have been reported following natural infection in unvaccinated pregnant women. Measles infection during pregnancy may increase the risk of premature labor, preterm delivery, spontaneous abortion and low birth weights. Rubella infection during the first trimester may lead to miscarriages, stillbirths, and congenital rubella syndrome (includes auditory, ophthalmic, cardiac and neurologic defects; intrauterine and postnatal growth retardation); fetal rubella infection can occur during any trimester of pregnancy. Maternal mumps infection during the first trimester may increase the risk of spontaneous abortion or intrauterine fetal death. Sterility in males and infertility in prepubescent females may also occur with natural mumps infection.

Prenatal screening is recommended for all pregnant women who lack evidence of rubella immunity. Women of childbearing age without documentation of rubella vaccination or serologic evidence of immunity should be vaccinated (for women of childbearing potential, birth prior to 1957 is not acceptable evidence of immunity to rubella). Women who are pregnant should be vaccinated upon completion or termination of pregnancy, prior to discharge. Household contacts of pregnant women may be vaccinated (CDC, 2013c).

Breast-Feeding Considerations Lactating women may secrete the rubella component of the vaccine into breast milk. Evidence of rubella infection has occurred in breast-fed infants following maternal immunization, most without severe disease. It is not known if the measles or mumps components of the vaccine are found in breast milk. The manufacturer recommends that caution be used if administered to nursing women. Breast-feeding is not a contraindication to vaccination. Breast-feeding infants should be vaccinated according to the recommended schedules (CDC, 2011).

Contraindications Hypersensitivity to measles, mumps, and rubella vaccine, gelatin or any component; history of anaphylactic reactions to neomycin; individuals with blood dyscrasias, leukemia, lymphomas, or other malignant neoplasms affecting the bone marrow or lymphatic systems; concurrent immunosuppressive therapy (does not include corticosteroids as replacement therapy); primary and acquired immunodeficiency states; family history of congenital or hereditary immunodeficiency (until immune competence in the vaccine recipient is demonstrated); current febrile illness or active febrile infection (per manufacturer's labeling); pregnancy

Warnings MMR vaccine is contraindicated in severely immunocompromised patients. The ACIP does **not** recommend vaccination for persons with primary or acquired immunodeficiency (including immunosuppression associated with cellular immunodeficiency, hypogammaglobulinemia, dysgammaglobulinemia and AIDs, or severe immunosuppression associated with HIV); persons with blood dyscrasia, leukemia, lymphoma, or other malignant neoplasms which affect the bone marrow or lymphatic system; persons with a family history of congenital or hereditary immunodeficiency in first degree relatives (unless immunocompetence can be established); persons taking systemic corticosteroid therapy for ≥2 weeks in doses equivalent to prednisone ≥20 mg/day (or ≥2 mg/kg in persons >10 kg). Patients with HIV infection who are asymptomatic and not severely immunosuppressed may be vaccinated (severe immunosuppression is defined as CD4+ T-lymphocyte <15% at any age or CD4 count <200 lymphocytes/mm^3 for persons >5 years) (CDC/ACIP [McLean, 2013]). Patients with leukemia who are in remission and who have not received chemotherapy for at least 3 months may be vaccinated. Defer vaccination in patients with active untreated tuberculosis. In general, households and close contacts of persons with altered immunocompetence may receive all age-appropriate vaccines (CDC/ACIP [Kroger, 2011]).

Vaccination may not result in effective immunity in all patients. Response depends upon multiple factors (eg, type of vaccine, age of patient) and may be improved by administering the vaccine at the recommended dose, route, and interval. Vaccines may not be effective if administered during periods of altered immune competence. Syncope has been reported with use of injectable vaccines and may be accompanied by transient visual disturbances, weakness, or tonic-clonic movements. Procedures should be in place to avoid injuries from falling and to restore cerebral perfusion if syncope occurs (CDC, 57[17], 2008). Use in patients with existing thrombocytopenia may result in more severe reduction in platelets; avoid use in patients with previous history of postvaccination thrombocytopenia, as rechallenge has resulted in recurrence of thrombocytopenia.

Immediate treatment (including epinephrine 1:1000) for anaphylactic/anaphylactoid reaction should be available during vaccine use. Vaccine may contain trace amounts of chick embryo antigen. Use caution in patients with history of immediate hypersensitivity/anaphylactic reactions following egg ingestion. Generally, the MMR vaccine can be safely administered to persons with an egg allergy (CDC/ACIP [Kroger, 2011]). Products may contain gelatin or neomycin; use is contraindicated in patients with a history of anaphylactic/anaphylactoid reaction to gelatin or neomycin; contact dermatitis due to neomycin is not a contraindication to the vaccine.

Precautions May consider deferring administration in patients with moderate or severe acute illness (with or without fever). Although fever is a contraindication per the manufacturer, current guidelines allow for administration to patients with mild acute illness (with or without fever) (CDC/ACIP [Kroger, 2011]; CDC/ACIP [McLean, 2013]). Use with caution in patients with history of cerebral injury, convulsions, or other conditions where stress due to fever should be avoided. Antipyretics have not been shown to prevent febrile seizures; antipyretics may be used to treat fever or discomfort following vaccination (CDC/ACIP [Kroger, 2011]). One study reported that routine prophylactic administration of acetaminophen to prevent fever prior to vaccination decreased the immune response of some vaccines; the clinical significance of this reduction in immune response has not been established (Prymula, 2009).

Defer vaccination for at least 3 months after receiving blood and plasma transfusions or immune globulin; may interfere with immune response. Exposure to measles is not a contraindication to vaccine; use within 72 hours of exposure may provide some protection; postexposure vaccination has not been shown to prevent or alter disease following mumps or rubella exposure (CDC/ACIP [McLean, 2013]). Use of this vaccine for specific medical and/or other indications (eg, immunocompromising conditions, hepatic or kidney disease, diabetes) is also addressed in the ACIP Recommended Immunization Schedule (CDC/ACIP [Akinsanya-Beysolow, 2014]; CDC/ACIP [Bridges, 2014]). Acceptable evidence of immunity is recommended for (CDC/ACIP [McLean, 2013]): Health care workers, students entering post high school educational institutions, and travelers to endemic areas.

Adverse Reactions All serious adverse reactions must be reported to the U.S. Department of Health and Human Services (DHHS) Vaccine Adverse Event Reporting System (VAERS) 1-800-822-7967 or online at https://vaers.hhs.gov/esub/index. In Canada, adverse reactions may be reported to local provincial/territorial health agencies or to the Vaccine Safety Section at Public Health Agency of Canada (1-866-844-0018).

Cardiovascular: Syncope, vasculitis

Central nervous system: Ataxia, dizziness, encephalitis, encephalopathy, febrile seizure, fever, Guillain-Barré syndrome, headache, irritability, malaise, measles inclusion body encephalitis, polyneuritis, polyneuropathy, seizure, subacute sclerosing panencephalitis,

Dermatologic: Angioneurotic edema, erythema multiforme, measles-like rash, pruritus, purpura, rash, Stevens-Johnson syndrome, urticaria

Endocrine & metabolic: Diabetes mellitus, parotitis

Gastrointestinal: Diarrhea, nausea, pancreatitis, sore throat, vomiting

Genitourinary: Epididymitis, orchitis

Hematologic: Leukocytosis, thrombocytopenia

Local: Injection site reactions which include burning, induration, redness, stinging, swelling, tenderness, wheal and flare, vesiculation

Neuromuscular & skeletal: Arthralgia/arthritis (variable; greater in women than children), myalgia, paresthesia

Ocular: Conjunctivitis, ocular palsies, optic neuritis, papillitis, retinitis, retrobulbar neuritis

Otic: Nerve deafness, otitis media

Respiratory: Bronchospasm, cough, pneumonia, pneumonitis, rhinitis

Miscellaneous: Anaphylactoid reactions, anaphylaxis, atypical measles, panniculitis, regional lymphadenopathy

Drug Interactions

Metabolism/Transport Effects None known.

Avoid Concomitant Use

Avoid concomitant use of Measles, Mumps, and Rubella Virus Vaccine with any of the following: Belimumab; Fingolimod; Immunosuppressants

Increased Effect/Toxicity

The levels/effects of Measles, Mumps, and Rubella Virus Vaccine may be increased by: Belimumab; Corticosteroids (Systemic); Dimethyl Fumarate; Fingolimod; Hydroxychloroquine; Immunosuppressants; Leflunomide; Mercaptopurine; Methotrexate

Decreased Effect

Measles, Mumps, and Rubella Virus Vaccine may decrease the levels/effects of: Tuberculin Tests

The levels/effects of Measles, Mumps, and Rubella Virus Vaccine may be decreased by: Dimethyl Fumarate; Fingolimod; Immune Globulins; Immunosuppressants

Stability To maintain potency, the lyophilized vaccine must be stored between -50°C to 8°C (-58°F to 46°F). Temperatures below -50°C (-58°F) may occur if stored in dry ice. Prior to reconstitution, store the powder at 2°C to 8°C (36°F to 46°F); protect from light. Diluent may be stored in refrigerator or at room temperature. Do not freeze diluent. After reconstitution, use as soon as possible is recommended or may be stored for 8 hours at 2°C to 8°C (36°F to 46°F) protected from light.

Mechanism of Action As a live, attenuated vaccine, MMR vaccine offers active immunity to disease caused by the measles, mumps, and rubella viruses.

Pharmacodynamics

Onset of action: The median seroconversion after 1 vaccine dose is 96% (measles), 99% (rubella), mumps (94%) (CDC/ACIP [McLean, 2013])

Duration of action: The median duration of immunity after 2 doses is ≥15 years for all components of the vaccine (CDC/ACIP [McLean, 2013])

Dosing: Usual Note: The minimum interval between two doses of MMR vaccine is 28 days (CDC/ACIP [McLean, 2013]). Refer to Additional Information for a description of acceptable evidence of immunity.

Pediatric:

Primary immunization: Children ≥12 months: SubQ: 0.5 mL per dose for a total of 2 doses given as follows: 12 to 15 months of age and the second dose at 4 to 6 years of age; the second dose is recommended prior to entering kindergarten or first grade. The second dose may be administered at any time provided at least 28 days have elapsed since the first dose (CDC/ACIP [McLean, 2013]).

Catch-up immunization: School-aged Children and Adolescents: Ensure that 2 doses have been given at least 28 days apart

Measles outbreak without acceptable evidence of immunity and at risk for exposure: Note: Should be administered within 72 hours postexposure.

Infants 6 to 11 months: SubQ: 0.5 mL per dose as a single dose (CDC/ACIP [McLean, 2013]). Children should be vaccinated at ≥12 months with standard 2-dose series

Children 1 to 4 years: Children who received 1 dose (0.5 mL I.M.) of MMR should be considered for a second dose if the outbreak involves preschool-aged children (CDC/ACIP [McLean, 2013]).

Mumps outbreak without acceptable evidence of immunity and at risk for exposure: Children 1 to 4 years: Children who received 1 dose of MMR should be considered for a second dose (0.5 mL I.M.) if the outbreak involves preschool-aged children (CDC/ACIP [McLean, 2013])

Household/close contacts of immunocompromised persons without acceptable evidence of immunity: Children ≥12 months and Adolescents: SubQ: 0.5 mL per dose for a total of 2 doses administered at least 28 days apart unless they have acceptable evidence of immunity (CDC/ACIP [McLean, 2013])

HIV infection without evidence of MMR immunity: Children ≥12 months and Adolescents: SubQ: 0.5 mL per dose. Children and adolescents with HIV infection and without evidence of severe immunosuppression should have 2 additional doses of MMR; those with perinatal HIV infection who were vaccinated prior to effective ART should have 2 additional doses of MMR once ART is established (CDC/ACIP [McLean, 2013]).

International travel, without evidence of immunity (CDC [Akinsanya-Beysolow, 2013]; CDC/ACIP [McLean, 2013]):

Infants 6 to 11 months: SubQ: 0.5 mL per dose. Administer 1 dose of MMR before departure from the United States; these infants should be revaccinated with 2 doses of MMR with the first dose between 12 to 15 months of age (and at least 28 days after the previous dose) and the second dose at least 28 days later.

Children ≥12 months and Adolescents: SubQ: 0.5 mL per dose for 1 to 2 doses. Administer 2 doses of MMR before departure from the United States with the second dose at least 28 days later.

Adult: **Primary immunization:** SubQ: 0.5 mL per dose for a total of 1 or 2 doses administered at least 28 days apart based upon the following criteria (CDC/ACIP [McLean, 2013]):

Adults born in or after 1957 should be vaccinated unless they have acceptable evidence of immunity

Adults born prior to 1957 are considered immune to measles, mumps, and rubella but may be vaccinated with 1 dose if they do not have contraindications to the vaccine. Pregnant adults born prior to 1957 are not considered immune to rubella.

Healthcare personnel: Persons born during or after 1957 should have 2 doses of vaccine unless they have acceptable evidence of immunity. Unvaccinated persons born prior to 1957 should also consider vaccination with 2 doses unless they have laboratory evidence or laboratory confirmation of disease.

HIV infection (without severe immunosuppression): 2 doses of MMR unless there is acceptable evidence of immunity

Household/close contacts of immunocompromised persons: 2 doses of MMR unless there is acceptable evidence of immunity

International travelers: 2 doses of MMR prior to travel unless there is acceptable evidence of immunity

Measles, mumps, or rubella outbreak (community): Adults who received one dose of MMR should be considered for a second dose if the outbreak involves measles or mumps in adults. Vaccination should also be considered for persons born prior to 1957 without evidence of immunity who may be exposed to mumps. A single dose of a rubella-containing vaccine is considered adequate vaccination during a rubella outbreak

Measles, mumps, or rubella outbreak (healthcare facility): Unvaccinated health care personnel without evidence of immunity regardless of birth year should receive 2 doses during a measles or mumps outbreak and one dose during a rubella outbreak

Students: Persons entering post high school educational facilities should receive 2 doses of MMR unless they have acceptable evidence of immunity prior to enrollment

Women of childbearing potential: 1 dose of MMR unless they have acceptable evidence of immunity. Vaccination should not be given during pregnancy and pregnancy should be avoided for 28 days after vaccine administration

Dosing adjustment in renal impairment: There are no dosage adjustments provided in manufacturer's labeling.

Dosing adjustment in hepatic impairment: There are no dosage adjustments provided in manufacturer's labeling.

Administration Use entire contents of the provided diluent to reconstitute vaccine. Gently agitate to mix thoroughly. Discard if powder does not dissolve. Use as soon as possible following reconstitution; administer subcutaneously into the anterolateral aspect of the thigh or arm; **not for I.V. administration**. Adolescents and adults should be vaccinated while seated or lying down. U.S. law requires that the date of administration, the vaccine manufacturer, lot number of vaccine, and the administering person's name, title, and address be entered into the patient's permanent medical record.

Monitoring Parameters Observe for syncope for 15 minutes following administration. If seizure-like activity associated with syncope occurs, maintain patient in supine or Trendelenburg position to reestablish adequate cerebral perfusion.

Test Interactions Temporary suppression of tuberculin skin test reactivity. Tuberculin test may be given prior to vaccination, simultaneously at separate sites on the same day as measles-containing vaccine, or 4-6 weeks later (CDC, 2013c).

Additional Information Using separate sites and syringes, MMR may be administered concurrently with DTaP or *Haemophilus* b conjugate vaccine (PedvaxHIB®). Varicella vaccine may be administered with MMR using separate sites and syringes; however, if not administered simultaneously, doses should be separated by at least 30 days. Unless otherwise specified, MMR should be given 1 month before or 1 month after live viral vaccines.

Acceptable presumptive evidence of immunity includes one of the following (CDC/ACIP [McLean, 2013]):

1. Documentation of adequate vaccination (for measles, mumps, and rubella). Adequate vaccination for mumps and measles is defined as 1 dose of a live virus vaccine for preschool children and adults not at high risk and 2 doses of a live virus vaccine for school-aged children and high-risk adults. Healthcare personnel (paid and unpaid workers with potential exposure), international travelers,

and students in institutions of post high school education are considered high-risk adults.

2. Laboratory evidence of immunity or laboratory confirmation of disease (for measles, mumps, and rubella)

3. Birth prior to 1957 (measles, mumps, and rubella); for women of childbearing potential, birth prior to 1957 is not acceptable evidence of immunity to rubella.

4. Documentation of physician-diagnosed disease (for measles, mumps, or rubella) is not acceptable evidence of immunity.

Previous vaccination:
Measles: Persons who received a measles vaccine of unknown type, an inactivated measles vaccine, or further attenuated measles vaccine accompanied by immune globulin or high-titer immune globulin should be considered unvaccinated (CDC/ACIP [McLean, 2013]).

Mumps: Persons vaccinated prior to 1979 with either killed mumps vaccine or a mumps vaccine of unknown type and who are at high risk for infection should be considered for revaccination with 2 doses of MMR vaccine (CDC/ACIP [McLean, 2013]).

In order to maximize vaccination rates, the ACIP recommends simultaneous administration (ie, >1 vaccine on the same day at different anatomic sites) of all age-appropriate vaccines (live or inactivated) for which a person is eligible at a single visit, unless contraindications exist. If available, the use of combination vaccines is generally preferred over separate injections, taking into consideration provider assessment, patient preference, and potential adverse events. If separate vaccines being used, evaluate product information regarding same syringe compatibility of vaccines. Separate needles and syringes should be used for each injection. The ACIP prefers each dose of specific vaccine in a series come from the same manufacturer if possible (CDC/ACIP [Kroger, 2011]).

For additional information, please refer to the following website: http://www.cdc.gov/vaccines/vpd-vac/.

Dosage Forms Excipient information presented when available (limited, particularly for generics); consult specific product labeling.

Injection, powder for reconstitution [preservative free]:
M-M-R® II: Measles virus ≥1000 $TCID_{50}$, mumps virus ≥20,000 $TCID_{50}$, and rubella virus ≥1000 $TCID_{50}$ [contains albumin (human), bovine serum, chicken egg protein, gelatin, neomycin, sorbitol, and sucrose 1.9 mg/vial; supplied with diluent]

References
AAP Steering Committee on Quality Improvement and Management, Subcommittee on Febrile Seizures American Academy of Pediatrics, "Febrile Seizures: Clinical Practice Guideline for the Long-Term Management of the Child With Simple Febrile Seizures," *Pediatrics*, 2008, 121(6):1281-6.

Akinsanya-Beysolow I, Advisory Committee on Immunization Practices (ACIP), ACIP Child/Adolescent Immunization Work Group, et al. Advisory committee on immunization practices recommended immunization schedule for adults aged 19 years and older - United States, 2014. *MMWR Morb Mortal Wkly Rep.* 2014; 63(5):108-109. Full schedule available at http://www.cdc.gov/vaccines/schedules/downloads/child/0-18yrs-child-combined-schedule.pdf

Bridges CB, Coyne-Beasley T, Advisory Committee on Immunization Practices (ACIP), ACIP Adult Immunization Work Group; Centers for Disease Control and Prevention (CDC). Advisory committee on immunization practices recommended immunization schedule for adults aged 19 years or older - United States, 2014. *MMWR Morb Mortal Wkly Rep.* 2014; 63(5):108-109. Available at: http://www.cdc.gov/vaccines/schedules/downloads/adult/adult-combined-schedule.-pdf

Centers for Disease Control and Prevention (CDC), "Syncope After Vaccination – United States, January 2005-July 2007," *MMWR Morb Mortal Wkly Rep*, 2008, 57(17):457-60.

Kroger AT, Atkinson WL, Marcuse EK, Pickering LK. General recommendations on immunization - recommendations of the Advisory Committee on Immunization Practices (ACIP). *MMWR Recomm Rep.* 2011;60(RR-2):1-64.

McLean HQ, Fiebelkorn AP, Temte JL, et al. Prevention of measles, rubella, congenital rubella syndrome, and mumps, 2013: summary recommendations of the Advisory Committee on Immunization Practices (ACIP). *MMWR Recomm Rep.* 2013;62(RR-04):1-34.

Prymula R, Siegrist CA, Chlibek R, et al, "Effect of Prophylactic Paracetamol Administration at Time of Vaccination on Febrile Reactions and Antibody Responses in Children: Two Open-Label, Randomised Controlled Trials," *Lancet*, 2009, 374(9698):1339-50.

Measles, Mumps, Rubella, and Varicella Virus Vaccine
(MEE zels, mumpz, roo BEL a, & var i SEL a VYE rus vak SEEN)

Medication Safety Issues
Sound-alike/look-alike issues:
MMRV (measles, mumps, rubella, and varicella) vaccine may be confused with MMR (measles, mumps and rubella virus) vaccine.

Related Information
Immunization Administration Recommendations *on page 2368*

Immunization Guidelines *on page 2373*

Brand Names: U.S. ProQuad

Brand Names: Canada Priorix-Tetra

Therapeutic Category Vaccine, Live Virus

Generic Availability (U.S.) No

Use To provide active immunity to measles, mumps, rubella, and varicella viruses (FDA approved in ages 12 months to 12 years)

The Advisory Committee on Immunization Practices (ACIP) recommends routine vaccination against measles, mumps, rubella, and varicella in healthy children; the first dose should be given at 12 to 15 months of age and the second dose at 4 to 6 years of age. For children receiving their first dose at 12 to 47 months of age, either the MMRV combination vaccine or separate MMR and varicella vaccines can be used. The ACIP prefers administration of separate MMR and varicella vaccines as the first dose in this age group particularly for children with a personal or family history of seizures (CDC/ACIP [Martin, 2010]) unless the parent or caregiver expresses preference for the MMRV combination. For children receiving the first dose at ≥48 months or their second dose at any age, use of MMRV is preferred.

Pregnancy Considerations Animal reproduction studies have not been conducted. Use is contraindicated in pregnant females and pregnancy should be avoided for 3 months (per manufacturer labeling) following vaccination. The ACIP recommends that pregnancy should be avoided for 1 month following vaccination with any of the individual components of this vaccine.

Refer to the Varicella Virus Vaccine monograph and the Measles, Mumps, and Rubella Virus Vaccine monograph for additional information.

Breast-Feeding Considerations Lactating women may secrete the rubella component of the vaccine into breast milk. It is not known if the measles, mumps, or varicella components of the vaccine are found in breast milk. The manufacturer recommends that caution be used if administered to nursing women. Breast-feeding is not a contraindication to vaccination. Breast-feeding infants should be vaccinated according to the recommended schedules (CDC, 2011). Refer to the Varicella Virus Vaccine monograph and the Measles, Mumps, and Rubella Virus Vaccine monograph for additional information.

Contraindications Hypersensitivity to any component of the vaccine including gelatin; known anaphylactic reaction to neomycin; individuals with blood dyscrasias, leukemia, lymphomas, or other malignant neoplasms affecting the bone marrow or lymphatic systems; concurrent immunosuppressive therapy; primary and acquired immunodeficiency states including HIV or a family history of congenital or hereditary immunodeficiency; cellular immune deficiencies; hypogammaglobulinemic and dysgammaglobulinemic states; active untreated tuberculosis; current febrile illness (>38.5°C); pregnancy

Warnings Immediate treatment (including epinephrine 1:1000) for anaphylactic and/or hypersensitivity reactions should be available during vaccine use. Vaccine contains trace amounts of chick embryo antigen. Use caution in patients with history of immediate hypersensitivity/anaphylactic reactions following egg ingestion. Generally, the vaccine can be safely administered to persons with an egg allergy (CDC/ACIP [Kroger, 2011]). Varicella virus transmission may occur; vaccinated individuals should not have close association with susceptible high-risk individuals (eg, newborns of women without positive history of varicella and all newborns <28 weeks gestation regardless of maternal immunity, pregnant women without positive history of varicella, and immunocompromised persons) for 6 weeks following vaccination. While safety and efficacy of this combination vaccine has not been established in patients with HIV infection, MMR and varicella individual vaccines have been recommended in children with HIV infection who are asymptomatic and not immunosuppressed (CDC immunologic category 1). Defer vaccination in patients with active untreated tuberculosis. Avoid use of salicylates for 6 weeks following vaccination; varicella may increase the risk of Reye's syndrome. Syncope has been reported with use of injectable vaccines and may be accompanied by transient visual disturbances, weakness, or tonic-clonic movements. Procedures should be in place to avoid injuries from falling and to restore cerebral perfusion if syncope occurs (CDC, 57[17], 2008).

Products may contain albumin. Products may contain gelatin or neomycin; use is contraindicated in patients with a history of anaphylactic/anaphylactoid reaction to gelatin or neomycin; contact dermatitis due to neomycin is not a contraindication to the vaccine.

Precautions The decision to administer or delay vaccination because of current or recent febrile illness depends on the severity of symptoms and the etiology of the disease. Immunization should be delayed during the course of an acute severe febrile illness; may administer to patients with mild acute illness (fever ≤38.5°C or without fever); use during current fever >38.5°C is contraindicated.

Use caution with history of cerebral injury, seizures, or other conditions where stress due to fever should be avoided; reported incidence of fever ≥38.9°C (≥102°F) was 20%. Children 12 to 23 months of age have been reported to have a twofold-higher risk of developing febrile seizures with the use of the combination product MMRV compared to administration of MMR and varicella separately. For children receiving their first dose at 12 to 47 months of age, either the MMRV combination vaccine or separate MMR and varicella vaccines can be used; however, the ACIP prefers administration of separate MMR and varicella vaccines as the first dose in this age group. Because it is uncommon for a child to have their first febrile seizure after 4 years of age, the ACIP recommends the use of the combination MMRV vaccine for children receiving their first dose at ≥48 months or their second dose at any age. The ACIP recommends that children with a personal or family history of seizures be vaccinated with separate MMR and varicella vaccines, as opposed to the MMRV combination vaccine. Parents and caregivers should be provided with the benefits and risks of both options (CDC/ACIP [Marin, 2010]). Antipyretics have not been shown to prevent febrile seizures. Antipyretics may be used to treat fever or discomfort following vaccination (CDC/ACIP [Kroger, 2011]). One study reported that routine prophylactic administration of acetaminophen to prevent fever due to vaccines has been shown to decrease the immune response of some vaccines; the clinical significance of this reduction in immune response has not been established (Prymula, 2009).

Vaccination may not result in effective immunity in all patients. Response depends upon multiple factors (eg, type of vaccine, age of patient) and may be improved by administering the vaccine at the recommended dose, route, and interval. Vaccines may not be effective if administered during periods of altered immune competence (CDC/ACIP [Kroger 2011]); use is contraindicated in patients with immunosuppression. In general, live vaccines should be administered ≥4 weeks prior to planned immunosuppression and avoided within 2 weeks of immunosuppression when feasible (IDSA [Rubin, 2014]). The safety and efficacy of this combination vaccine has not been established for postexposure prophylaxis. Specific recommendations for use of this vaccine in immunocompromised patients with asplenia, cancer, HIV infection, cerebrospinal fluid leaks, cochlear implants, hematopoietic stem cell transplant (prior to or after), sickle cell disease, solid organ transplant (prior to or after), or those receiving immunosuppressive therapy for chronic conditions are available from the IDSA (Rubin, 2014).

Use caution in patients with thrombocytopenia and in patients who develop thrombocytopenia after first dose; thrombocytopenia may worsen. Defer vaccination after receiving blood and plasma transfusions or immune globulin; these products may interfere with immune response. Guidelines with suggested administration intervals are available (CDC/ACIP [Kroger, 2011]).

Adverse Reactions All serious adverse reactions must be reported to the U.S. Department of Health and Human Services (DHHS) Vaccine Adverse Event Reporting System (VAERS) 1-800-822-7967 or online at https://vaers.hhs.gov/esub/index. In Canada, adverse reactions may be reported to local provincial/territorial health agencies or to the Vaccine Safety Section at Public Health Agency of Canada (1-866-844-0018).

Also refer to Measles, Mumps, and Rubella Vaccines (Combined) (M-M-R II) and Varicella Virus Vaccine (Varivax) monographs for additional adverse reactions reported with those agents. Percentages reported following one dose of ProQuad at 12-23 months of age.

Central nervous system: Drowsiness, irritability

Dermatologic: Erythema, morbilliform rash, rash at injection site, skin rash, varicella-like rash, viral exanthem

Gastrointestinal: Diarrhea, vomiting

Local: Bruising at injection site, pain at injection site (pain/tenderness/soreness), swelling at injection site

Respiratory: Rhinorrhea, upper respiratory tract infection

Miscellaneous: Fever

Rare but important or life-threatening: Acute disseminated encephalomyelitis, febrile seizures

Drug Interactions

Metabolism/Transport Effects None known.

Avoid Concomitant Use

Avoid concomitant use of Measles, Mumps, Rubella, and Varicella Virus Vaccine with any of the following: Belimumab; Fingolimod; Immunosuppressants

Increased Effect/Toxicity

The levels/effects of Measles, Mumps, Rubella, and Varicella Virus Vaccine may be increased by: 5-ASA Derivatives; Belimumab; Corticosteroids (Systemic); Dimethyl Fumarate; Fingolimod; Hydroxychloroquine; Immunosuppressants; Leflunomide; Mercaptopurine; Methotrexate; Salicylates

Decreased Effect

Measles, Mumps, Rubella, and Varicella Virus Vaccine may decrease the levels/effects of: Tuberculin Tests

◄   *The levels/effects of Measles, Mumps, Rubella, and Varicella Virus Vaccine may be decreased by:* Dimethyl Fumarate; Fingolimod; Immune Globulins; Immunosuppressants

Stability Vaccine: Stable in a freezer for up to 18 months at temperatures between -50°C to -15°C (-58°F to +5°F). Use of dry ice may subject the vaccine to temperatures colder than -50°C (-58°F). May store at 2°C to 8°C (36°F to 46°F) for up to 72 hours prior to reconstitution; discard if not used within 72 hours; do not refreeze. Protect from light; use within 30 minutes following reconstitution. Do not freeze reconstituted vaccine.

Diluent: Store at 2°C to 8°C (36°F to 46°F) or at 20°C to 25°C (68°F to 77°F).

Mechanism of Action A live, attenuated virus vaccine that induces active immunity to disease caused by the measles, mumps, rubella, and varicella-zoster viruses.

Pharmacodynamics

Onset of action: At 6 weeks postvaccination of a single dose, the antibody response rate in healthy children 12 to 23 months of age was ~91% to 99%. Following a second dose to children <3 years of age, the observed antibody response rate was ~98% to 99%.

Duration of action: Antibody levels persist 10 years or longer in most healthy recipients. Refer to the Varicella Virus Vaccine monograph and the Measles, Mumps, and Rubella Virus Vaccine monograph for details.

Dosing: Usual

Pediatric:

Primary immunization: Children 12 months to 12 years: ProQuad: SubQ: 0.5 mL per dose. A complete immunization series for measles, mumps, rubella, and varicella requires 2 doses of all components, administered as either the combination product (MMRV-Proquad) or as separate MMR and varicella vaccines. The first dose is usually administered at 12 to 15 months of age. The second dose is administered at 4 to 6 years of age; second dose may be administered before age 4 if needed, as long as ≥3 months have elapsed since the first dose.

CDC (ACIP) recommendations: For children receiving their first dose at 12 to 47 months of age, either the MMRV combination vaccine or separate MMR and varicella vaccines can be used; however, the ACIP prefers administration of separate MMR and varicella vaccines as the first dose in this age group unless the parent or caregiver expresses preference for the MMRV combination. For children receiving the first dose at ≥48 months or their second dose at any age, use of MMRV is preferred. The ACIP recommends that children with a personal or family history of seizures be vaccinated with separate MMR and varicella vaccines, as opposed to the MMRV combination vaccine.

Allow at least 1 month between administering a dose of a measles-containing vaccine (eg, M-M-R II) and ProQuad.

Allow at least 3 months between administering a varicella-containing vaccine (eg, Varivax) and ProQuad.

Administration Parenteral: Use entire contents of provided diluent to reconstitute vaccine. Gently agitate to mix thoroughly. Discard if powder does not dissolve. Use as soon as possible following reconstitution; administer by SubQ injection into the anterolateral aspect of the thigh or deltoid region of arm; **not for I.V. administration**. U.S. law requires that the date of administration, name of manufacturer, lot number, and administering person's name, title, and address be entered into patient's permanent medical record.

Monitoring Parameters Rash, fever; observe for syncope for 15 minutes following administration. If seizure-like activity associated with syncope occurs, maintain patient in supine or Trendelenburg position to re-establish adequate cerebral perfusion.

Test Interactions May interfere with sensitivity to tuberculin skin test; administer at separate sites before, simultaneously with, or at least 4-6 weeks after vaccine.

Additional Information MMR and MMRV vaccines are both associated with febrile seizures which may occur during the first 2 weeks following vaccination. Based on preliminary information, fever ≥102°F occurs more often with MMRV (21.5%) compared to separate MMR and varicella vaccines (14.9%) in children 12 to 23 months of age. Measles-like rash also occurs more often with MMRV (3%) than with separate MMR and varicella vaccines (2.1%) in this age group. Most cases resolve spontaneously. The risk of febrile seizures may be increased twofold in children receiving MMRV at age 12 to 23 months in comparison to separate MMR and varicella vaccines (risk is highest 5-12 days after first dose). This is not observed in older children (≥47 months of age). Immunization with either MMRV or separate MMR and varicella vaccines offers equivalent immunity with the first dose. Using the combination vaccine provides the child with one less injection. Parents and/or caregivers should be provided with information related to the benefits and risks of both options. The ACIP prefers administration of separate MMR and varicella vaccines as the first dose in this age group unless the parent or caregiver expresses preference for the MMRV combination. Children with a personal or family history of seizures should be vaccinated with separate MMR and varicella vaccines, as opposed to the MMRV combination vaccine (CDC/ACIP [Marin, 2010]). Results from a larger study confirm that children who were 12 to 23 months of age when receiving their first dose of MMRV vaccine were at an increased risk of fevers and seizures within 7 to 10 days after vaccination. Healthcare visits for fever and seizures were associated with both MMRV and separate MMR and varicella vaccines; however, the relative risk for seizures following vaccination was most significant with the MMRV vaccine. Seizures occurred most often 8 to 10 days following MMRV vaccination (RR 7.6, p <0.0001), 7 to 10 days following separate MMR and varicella vaccination (RR 4.0, p<0.0001), and 7 to 11 days following MMR vaccination (RR 3.7, p<0.0001); no peak in seizures was observed following varicella vaccine alone. Healthcare visits due to fever also clustered between 7 to 10 days after vaccination with any measles-containing vaccine (MMRV RR 6.1, MMR and varicella RR 4.4, MMR RR 4.3). Following a chart review for verification of seizure type, the rate of febrile seizures was 87% following both MMRV and separate MMR and varicella vaccine administration (Klein, 2010).

In order to maximize vaccination rates, the ACIP recommends simultaneous administration (ie, >1 vaccine on the same day at different anatomic sites) of all age-appropriate vaccines (live or inactivated) for which a person is eligible at a single visit, unless contraindications exist. If available, the use of combination vaccines is generally preferred over separate injections, taking into consideration provider assessment, patient preference, and potential adverse events. If separate vaccines being used, evaluate product information regarding same syringe compatibility of vaccines. Separate needles and syringes should be used for each injection. The ACIP prefers each dose of specific vaccine in a series come from the same manufacturer if possible (CDC/ACIP [Kroger, 2011]).

For additional information, please refer to the following website: http://www.cdc.gov/vaccines/vpd-vac/.

Dosage Forms Excipient information presented when available (limited, particularly for generics); consult specific product labeling.

Injection, powder for reconstitution [preservative free]:
ProQuad: Measles virus ≥3.00 $\log_{10}$ $TCID_{50}$, mumps virus ≥4.3 $\log_{10}$ $TCID_{50}$, rubella virus ≥3.00 $\log_{10}$ $TCID_{50}$, and varicella virus ≥3.99 $\log_{10}$ PFU [contains albumin (human), bovine serum, chicken egg protein, gelatin, neomycin, sorbitol, and sucrose (≤21 mg/vial)]

References

AAP Steering Committee on Quality Improvement and Management, Subcommittee on Febrile Seizures American Academy of Pediatrics, "Febrile Seizures: Clinical Practice Guideline for the Long-Term Management of the Child With Simple Febrile Seizures," *Pediatrics*, 2008, 121(6):1281-6.

Akinsanya-Beysolow I, Advisory Committee on Immunization Practices (ACIP), ACIP Child/Adolescent Immunization Work Group, et al. Advisory committee on immunization practices recommended immunization schedules for persons aged 0 through 18 years - United States, 2014. *MMWR Morb Mortal Wkly Rep*. 2014; 63(5):108-109. Full schedule available at http://www.cdc.gov/vaccines/schedules/downloads/child/0-18yrs-child-combined-schedule.pdf

Centers for Disease Control and Prevention (CDC), "Syncope After Vaccination – United States, January 2005-July 2007," *MMWR Morb Mortal Wkly Rep*, 2008, 57(17):457-60.

Marin M, Broder KR, Temte JL, Snider DE, Seward JF. Use of combination measles, mumps, rubella, and varicella vaccine: recommendations of the Advisory Committee on Immunization Practices (ACIP). *MMWR Recomm Rep*. 2010;59(RR-3):1-12.

Klein NP, Fireman B, Yih WK, et al, "Measles-Mumps-Rubella-Varicella Combination Vaccine and the Risk of Febrile Seizures," *Pediatrics*, 2010, 126(1):e1-8.

Kroger AT, Atkinson WL, Marcuse EK, Pickering LK. General recommendations on immunization - recommendations of the Advisory Committee on Immunization Practices (ACIP). *MMWR Recomm Rep*. 2011;60(RR-2):1-64.

Nolan T, Bernstein DI, Block SL, et al, "Safety and Immunogenicity of Concurrent Administration of Live Attenuated Influenza Vaccine With Measles-Mumps-Rubella and Varicella Vaccines to Infants 12 to 15 Months of Age," *Pediatrics*, 2008, 121(3):508-16.

Prymula R, Siegrist CA, Chlibek R, et al, "Effect of Prophylactic Paracetamol Administration at Time of Vaccination on Febrile Reactions and Antibody Responses in Children: Two Open-Label, Randomised Controlled Trials," *Lancet*, 2009, 374(9698):1339-50.

Rubin LG, Levin MJ, Ljungman P, et al. 2013 IDSA clinical practice guideline for vaccination of the immunocompromised host. *Clin Infect Dis*. 2014;58(3):e44-e100.

Mebendazole (me BEN da zole)

Medication Safety Issues
Sound-alike/look-alike issues:
Mebendazole may be confused with metroNIDAZOLE

Brand Names: Canada Vermox®

Therapeutic Category Anthelmintic

Generic Availability (U.S.) May be product dependent

Use Treatment of enterobiasis (pinworm infection), trichuriasis (whipworm infection), ascariasis (roundworm infection), and hookworm infections caused by *Necator americanus* or *Ancylostoma duodenale*; drug of choice in the treatment of capillariasis

Pregnancy Risk Factor C

Pregnancy Considerations Adverse events have been observed in animal reproduction studies; adverse pregnancy outcomes have not been observed following use in pregnancy (Diav-Citrin, 2003; Gyorkos, 2006). Treatment of pinworm in pregnancy may be considered; however, the CDC suggests postponing therapy until the third trimester when possible (CDC, 2010).

Breast-Feeding Considerations Since only 2% to 10% of mebendazole is absorbed, it is unlikely that it is excreted in breast milk in significant quantities (CDC, 2010)

Contraindications Hypersensitivity to mebendazole or any component

Warnings Pregnancy and children <2 years of age are relative contraindications since safety has not been established

Adverse Reactions
Central nervous system: Dizziness, drowsiness, headache, seizure

Dermatologic: Alopecia, angioedema, exanthema, itching, rash, Stevens-Johnson syndrome, toxic epidermal necrolysis, urticaria

Gastrointestinal: Abdominal pain, diarrhea, vomiting

Hematologic: Agranulocytosis, eosinophilia, hemoglobin decreased, leukopenia, neutropenia

Hepatic: Alkaline phosphatase increased, ALT increased, AST increased, GGT increased, hepatitis

Renal: BUN increased, cylindruria, glomerulonephritis, hematuria

Miscellaneous: Hypersensitivity reactions (anaphylactic, anaphylactoid)

Drug Interactions
Metabolism/Transport Effects None known.

Avoid Concomitant Use There are no known interactions where it is recommended to avoid concomitant use.

Increased Effect/Toxicity
Mebendazole may increase the levels/effects of: MetroNIDAZOLE (Systemic); MetroNIDAZOLE (Topical)

The levels/effects of Mebendazole may be increased by: Cimetidine

Decreased Effect
The levels/effects of Mebendazole may be decreased by: Aminoquinolines (Antimalarial); CarBAMazepine; Fosphenytoin; Phenytoin

Food Interactions Mebendazole serum levels may be increased if taken with food. Management: Administer without regard to meals.

Mechanism of Action Inhibits the formation of helminth microtubules; selectively and irreversibly blocks glucose uptake and other nutrients in susceptible adult intestine-dwelling helminths

Pharmacokinetics (Adult data unless noted)
Absorption: Oral: 2% to 10%

Distribution: To liver, fat, muscle, plasma, and hepatic cysts

Protein binding: 95%

Metabolism: Extensive in the liver

Half-life: 2.8-9 hours

Time to peak serum concentration: Variable (0.5-7 hours)

Elimination: Primarily in feces as inactive metabolites with 5% to 10% eliminated in urine

Dialysis: Not dialyzable

Dosing: Usual Children and Adults: Oral:
Pinworms: Single chewable tablet (100 mg); may need to repeat after 2 weeks

Whipworms, roundworms, hookworms: 100 mg twice daily, morning and evening on 3 consecutive days; if patient is not cured within 3-4 weeks, a second course of treatment may be administered

Capillariasis: 200 mg twice daily for 20 days

Administration Oral: Administer with food; tablet can be crushed and mixed with food, swallowed whole, or chewed

Monitoring Parameters For treatment of trichuriasis, ascariasis, hookworm, or mixed infections, check for helminth ova in the feces within 3-4 weeks following the initial therapy

Product Availability Not available in U.S.

References

Centers for Disease Control and Prevention (CDC), "Parasites - Enterobiasis (also known as Pinworm Infection)," 2010. Available at http://www.cdc.gov/parasites/pinworm/health_professionals/index.html

Diav-Citrin O, Shechtman S, Arnon J, et al, "Pregnancy Outcome After Gestational Exposure to Mebendazole: A Prospective Controlled Cohort Study," *Am J Obstet Gynecol*, 2003, 188(1):282-5.

Gyorkos TW, Larocque R, Casapia M, et al, "Lack of Risk of Adverse Birth Outcomes After Deworming in Pregnant Women," *Pediatr Infect Dis J*, 2006, 25(9):791-4.

Hotez PJ, "Hookworm Disease in Children," *Pediatr Infect Dis J*, 1989, 8(8):516-20.

Mecasermin (mek a SER min)

Brand Names: U.S. Increlex

Therapeutic Category Growth Hormone

Generic Availability (U.S.) No

Use Treatment of growth failure in children with severe primary insulin-like growth factor-1 deficiency (IGF-1 deficiency; primary IGFD), or with growth hormone (GH) gene deletions who have developed neutralizing antibodies to GH (FDA approved in children ≥2 years)

Pregnancy Risk Factor C

Pregnancy Considerations Teratogenic effects were not observed in animal studies

Breast-Feeding Considerations It is not known if mecasermin is excreted in breast milk. The manufacturer recommends that caution be exercised when administering mecasermin to nursing women.

Contraindications Hypersensitivity to mecasermin or any component; patients with closed epiphyses; active or suspected neoplasia; intravenous use

Warnings Mecasermin may cause insulin-like hypoglycemic effects, especially in small children (due to inconsistent oral intake); patients should avoid high-risk activities (eg, driving) within 2-3 hours after dosing until a tolerated dose is established. Do not administer on days a patient cannot or will not eat. Increlex® should be administered with a meal or a snack. Intracranial hypertension with papilledema, visual changes, headache, nausea, and/or vomiting has been reported with growth hormone products and reverses after interruption of dosing; fundoscopic examinations are recommended. Lymphoid hypertrophy has been reported and may lead to complications, such as snoring, sleep apnea, and chronic middle ear infections; periodic examinations are recommended. Hypersensitivity and allergic reactions including anaphylaxis have been reported; if a reaction occurs discontinue treatment.

Increlex® contains benzyl alcohol which may cause allergic reactions in susceptible individuals; large amounts of benzyl alcohol (≥99 mg/kg/day) have been associated with a potentially fatal toxicity ("gasping syndrome") in neonates; avoid use of benzyl alcohol containing diluents in neonates.

Precautions Use with caution in patients with diabetes or family history of diabetes; insulin dosage may require adjustment when growth hormone therapy is instituted. Progression of scoliosis and slipped capital femoral epiphyses may occur in children experiencing rapid growth; monitor and evaluate if symptoms present. Correct thyroid or nutritional deficiencies prior to therapy. Not intended for use in patients with secondary forms of IGF-1 deficiency (GH deficiency, malnutrition, hypothyroidism, chronic anti-inflammatory steroid therapy).

Adverse Reactions

Cardiovascular: Cardiac murmur

Central nervous system: Dizziness, headache, seizure

Endocrine & metabolic: Hyper-/hypoglycemia, iron-deficiency anemia, ovarian cysts, thymus hypertrophy, thyromegaly

Gastrointestinal: Vomiting

Hepatic: Liver enzymes increased

Local: Injection site reactions: Bruising, erythema, hair growth, lipohypertrophy

Neuromuscular & skeletal: Arthralgia, bone pain, extremity pain, muscular atrophy

Ocular: Papilledema

Otic: Ear pain, hypoacusis, middle ear fluid, otitis media, serous otitis media, tympanometry abnormal

Renal: Hematuria

Respiratory: Snoring, tonsillar hypertrophy

Miscellaneous: Lymphadenopathy

Rare but important or life-threatening: Alopecia, anaphylaxis, cardiomegaly, hypercholesterolemia, hypersensitivity, hypertriglyceridemia, hypoglycemic seizure, intracranial hypertension, obstructive sleep apnea, valvulopathy

Drug Interactions

Metabolism/Transport Effects None known.

Avoid Concomitant Use There are no known interactions where it is recommended to avoid concomitant use.

Increased Effect/Toxicity There are no known significant interactions involving an increase in effect.

Decreased Effect There are no known significant interactions involving a decrease in effect.

Stability Increlex®: Store intact vial at 2°C to 8°C (35°F to 46°F); do not freeze. Protect from direct light. After initial entry into vial, store at 2°C to 8°C (35°F to 46°F), protect from direct light and use within 30 days; discard any remaining drug.

Mechanism of Action Mecasermin is an insulin-like growth factor (IGF-1) produced using recombinant DNA technology to replace endogenous IGF-1. Endogenous IGF-1 circulates predominately bound to insulin-like growth factor-binding protein-3 (IGFBP-3) and a growth hormone-dependent acid-labile subunit (ALS). Acting at receptors in the liver and other tissues, endogenous growth hormone (GH) stimulates the synthesis and secretion of IGF-1. In patients with primary severe IGF-1 deficiency, growth hormone receptors in the liver are unresponsive to GH, leading to reduced endogenous IGF-I concentrations and decreased growth (skeletal, cell, and organ). Endogenous IGF-1 also suppresses liver glucose production, stimulates peripheral glucose utilization, and has an inhibitory effect on insulin secretion.

Pharmacokinetics (Adult data unless noted)

Distribution: V_d: Severe primary IGFD: 0.184-0.33 L/kg

Protein binding: >80% bound to IGFBP-3 and an acid-labile subunit (IGFBP-3 reduced with severe primary IGFD)

Metabolism: Hepatic and renal

Bioavailability: 100% (healthy subjects)

Half-life: Severe primary IGFD: 5.8 hours

Time to peak serum concentration: 2 hours

Dosing: Usual Children and Adolescents:

Primary IGFD: Increlex®: Children ≥2 years and Adolescents: SubQ: Initial: 0.04-0.08 mg/kg/dose twice daily; if tolerated for 7 days, may increase by 0.04 mg/kg/dose; maximum dose: 0.12 mg/kg given twice daily. **Note:** Must be administered within 20 minutes of a meal or snack; omit dose if patient is unable to eat. Reduce dose if hypoglycemia occurs despite adequate food intake; dose should not be increased to make up for ≥1 omitted dose.

Dosage adjustment in renal impairment: Children ≥2 years and Adolescents: No dosage adjustments are provided in the manufacturer's labeling; has not been studied.

Dosage adjustment in hepatic impairment: Children ≥2 years and Adolescents: No dosage adjustments are provided in the manufacturer's labeling; has not been studied.

Administration SubQ: Must be administered within 20 minutes of a meal or snack. May cause hypoglycemic effects; patients should avoid high-risk activities within 2-3 hours of dosing until a tolerated dose is established. If patient is unable to eat, omit dose and do not make up for omitted dose. Rotate injection site.

Monitoring Parameters Preprandial glucose during treatment initiation and dose adjustment; hypersensitivity reactions; facial features; lymphoid tissue; funduscopic examination; growth; new onset of a limp or complaints of hip or knee pain; progression of scoliosis. Monitor small children closely due to potentially erratic food intake.

Reference Range

Severe primary IGFD is defined as follows:

Height standard deviation score ≤-3.0 **and**

Basal IGF-1 standard deviation score ≤-3.0 **and**

Growth hormone: Normal or increased

Additional Information If using syringes that measure dose in units, doses in mg/kg must be converted to units using the following formula:

Weight (kg) × Dose (mg/kg) × 1 mL/10 mg × 100 units/1 mL = units/injection

Dosage Forms Excipient information presented when available (limited, particularly for generics); consult specific product labeling.

Solution, Subcutaneous:

Increlex: 40 mg/4 mL (4 mL) [contains benzyl alcohol]

References

Backeljauw PF, Underwood LE, and GHIS Collaborative Group, "Therapy for 6.5-7.5 Years With Recombinant Insulin-Like Growth Factor I in Children With Growth Hormone Insensitivity Syndrome: A Clinical Research Center Study Syndrome," *J Clin Endocrinol Metab*, 2001, 86(4):1504-10.

Metz KA, Assa'ad A, Lierl MB, et al, "Allergic Reaction to Mecasermin," *Ann Allergy Asthma Immunol*, 2009, 103(1):82-3.

Torjusen E, Calderon J, and Rivkees SA, "Anaphylactic Reaction to Recombinant Insulin-Like Growth Factor-I," *J Pediatr Endocrinol Metab*, 2008, 21(4):381-4.

◆ **Mecasermin (rDNA Origin)** *see* Mecasermin *on page 1313*

Mechlorethamine (Systemic)
(me klor ETH a meen)

Medication Safety Issues

High alert medication:

This medication is in a class the Institute for Safe Medication Practices (ISMP) includes among its list of drug classes which have a heightened risk of causing significant patient harm when used in error.

Related Information

Emetogenic Potential of Antineoplastic Agents in Children *on page 2327*

Management of Drug Extravasations *on page 2255*

Safe Handling of Hazardous Drugs *on page 2419*

Brand Names: U.S. Mustargen

Therapeutic Category Antineoplastic Agent, Alkylating Agent; Antineoplastic Agent, Alkylating Agent (Nitrogen Mustard)

Generic Availability (U.S.) No

Use Palliative treatment of Hodgkin lymphoma and of effusions from metastatic carcinomas (FDA approved in adults); treatment of lymphosarcoma, chronic myelocytic or chronic lymphocytic leukemia, polycythemia vera, mycosis, fungoides, and bronchogenic carcinoma (FDA approved in adults); **Note:** While FDA approved for several oncologic uses, use in practice is limited.

Pregnancy Risk Factor D

Pregnancy Considerations Adverse events have been observed in animal reproduction studies. Women of childbearing potential are advised not to become pregnant during treatment. **[U.S. Boxed Warning]: Avoid exposure during pregnancy.**

Breast-Feeding Considerations It is not known if mechlorethamine is excreted in human breast milk. Due to the potential for serious adverse reactions in the nursing infant, the decision to discontinue mechlorethamine or to discontinue breast-feeding should take into account the importance of treatment to the mother.

Contraindications Hypersensitivity to mechlorethamine or any component; presence of known infection

Warnings Hazardous agent; use appropriate precautions for handling and disposal (NIOSH, 2012). Mechlorethamine is a highly toxic nitrogen mustard; avoid inhalation of vapors or dust; review and follow special handling procedures **[U.S. Boxed Warning]**; avoid dust or vapor contact with skin or eyes. If accidental skin exposure occurs, wash/irrigate thoroughly with water for at least 15 minutes, followed by 2% sodium thiosulfate solution; remove and destroy any contaminated clothing. If exposure to eye(s) occurs, promptly irrigate for at least 15 minutes with copious amounts of water, normal saline, or balanced salt ophthalmic irrigating solution; obtain ophthalmology consultation. The manufacturer recommends neutralizing remaining unused mechlorethamine, empty or partial vials, gloves, tubing, glassware, etc, after mechlorethamine administration; soak in an aqueous solution containing equal volumes of sodium thiosulfate (5%) and sodium bicarbonate (5%) for 45 minutes; rinse with water; dispose of properly.

Mechlorethamine is a potent vesicant; extravasation results in painful inflammation with induration and sloughing **[U.S. Boxed Warning]**. If extravasation occurs, promptly manage by infiltrating area with 1/6 molar sodium thiosulfate solution, followed by dry cold compresses for 6 to 12 hours. Ensure proper needle or catheter placement prior to and during infusion. Avoid extravasation.

Avoid contact during pregnancy **[U.S. Boxed Warning]**. Impaired spermatogenesis, azoospermia, and total germinal aplasia may occur in male patients treated with mechlorethamine, particularly when used in combination with other chemotherapy agents. Delayed menses, oligomenorrhea, or temporary or permanent amenorrhea may be observed in female patients treated with mechlorethamine. Alkylating agents, including mechlorethamine, are associated with an increased incidence of secondary malignancies; concurrent radiation therapy or combination chemotherapy may increase the risk.

Hypersensitivity reactions, including anaphylaxis, have been reported. May cause lymphopenia, leukopenia, granulocytopenia, thrombocytopenia, and anemia. Agranulocytopenia may occur (rare); persistent pancytopenia has been reported; immunosuppression may predispose patients to infections (bacterial, viral, or fungal); monitor blood counts. Bleeding due to thrombocytopenia may occur. Use with caution in patients where neoplasm has bone marrow involvement or in those who have received prior myelosuppressive chemotherapy; marrow function may be further compromised (possibly fatal). Bone marrow function should recover after mechlorethamine administration prior to initiating radiation therapy or other chemotherapy regimens. Bone marrow failure and other toxicities are more common in chronic lymphocytic leukemia (CLL); in general, mechlorethamine is no longer used in the treatment of CLL.

Mechlorethamine is associated with a high emetic potential (Basch, 2011); antiemetics are recommended to prevent nausea and vomiting.

Precautions Hyperuricemia may occur, especially with lymphomas; ensure adequate hydration; consider antihyperuricemic therapy if appropriate.

Should be administered under the supervision of an experienced cancer chemotherapy physician **[U.S. Boxed Warning]**. Bone and nervous system tumors typically respond poorly to treatment with mechlorethamine and the routine use of mechlorethamine in widely disseminated tumors is discouraged. Potentially significant interactions may exist, requiring dose or frequency adjustment, additional monitoring, and/or selection of alternative therapy. Consult drug interactions database for more detailed information.

Adverse Reactions

Central nervous system: Drowsiness, encephalopathy (high dose), fever, headache, lethargy, sedation, vertigo

Dermatologic: Alopecia, erythema multiforme, maculopapular rash, petechiae, rash

Endocrine & metabolic: Amenorrhea, hyperuricemia, oligomenorrhea, spermatogenesis decreased

Gastrointestinal: Anorexia, diarrhea, metallic taste, mucositis, nausea, vomiting

Hepatic: Jaundice

Hematologic: Agranulocytosis, granulocytopenia (onset 6-8 days, recovery 10-21 days), hemolytic anemia, leukopenia, lymphocytopenia, pancytopenia, secondary leukemias, thrombocytopenia

Local: Thrombophlebitis, tissue necrosis (extravasation)

Neuromuscular & skeletal: Weakness

Ocular: Lacrimation

Otic: Deafness, tinnitus

Miscellaneous: Anaphylaxis, diaphoresis, herpes zoster infection, hypersensitivity reactions

Drug Interactions

Metabolism/Transport Effects None known.

Avoid Concomitant Use

Avoid concomitant use of Mechlorethamine (Systemic) with any of the following: BCG; CloZAPine; Dipyrone; Natalizumab; Pimecrolimus; Tacrolimus (Topical); Tofacitinib; Vaccines (Live)

Increased Effect/Toxicity

Mechlorethamine (Systemic) may increase the levels/effects of: CloZAPine; Leflunomide; Natalizumab; Tofacitinib; Vaccines (Live)

The levels/effects of Mechlorethamine (Systemic) may be increased by: Denosumab; Dipyrone; Pimecrolimus; Roflumilast; Tacrolimus (Topical); Trastuzumab

Decreased Effect

Mechlorethamine (Systemic) may decrease the levels/effects of: BCG; Coccidioidin Skin Test; Sipuleucel-T; Vaccines (Inactivated); Vaccines (Live)

The levels/effects of Mechlorethamine (Systemic) may be decreased by: Echinacea

Stability Store intact vials at 15°C to 30°C (59°F to 86°F); protect from light; protect from humidity. **Must be prepared immediately before use**; degradation begins shortly after dilution.

Mechanism of Action Bifunctional alkylating agent that inhibits DNA and RNA synthesis via formation of carbonium ions; produces interstrand and intrastrand cross-links in DNA resulting in miscoding, breakage, and failure of replication. Although not cell phase-specific *per se,* mechlorethamine effect is most pronounced in the S phase, and cell proliferation is arrested in the G_2 phase.

Pharmacokinetics (Adult data unless noted)

Metabolism: Rapid hydrolysis in the plasma to active metabolites (Perry, 2012)

Half-life elimination: 15 to 20 minutes (Perry, 2012)

Dosing: Usual Note: Dosing and frequency may vary by protocol and/or treatment phase; refer to specific protocol.

Pediatric: **Hodgkin lymphoma:**

MOPP regimen: **Note:** The MOPP (with or without ABVD) regimen is generally no longer used due to improved toxicity profiles with other combination regimens used in the treatment of Hodgkin lymphoma (Kelly, 2012). Children and Adolescents: I.V.: 6 mg/m^2 on days 1 and 8 of a 28-day cycle in combination with vincristine, procarbazine, and prednisone, may or may not alternate with doxorubicin, bleomycin, vinblastine, dacarbazine (MOPP/ABVD) (Kung, 2006; Longo, 1986)

Stanford V regimen: Adolescents ≥16 years: I.V.: 6 mg/m^2 as a single dose on day 1 in weeks 1, 5, and 9 (Horning, 2000; Horning, 2002; Metzger, 2012)

Adult: **Note:** Dosage should be based on ideal dry weight (evaluate the presence of edema or ascites so that dosage is based on actual weight unaugmented by edema/ascites).

Hodgkin lymphoma: I.V.:

MOPP regimen: 6 mg/m^2 on days 1 and 8 of a 28-day treatment cycle for 6 to 8 cycles (Canellos, 1992; Devita, 1970)

Stanford V regimen: 6 mg/m^2 as a single dose on day 1 in weeks 1, 5, and 9 (Horning, 2000; Horning, 2002)

Malignant effusion: Intracavitary: 0.4 mg/kg as a single dose; although 0.2 mg/kg (10 to 20 mg) as a single dose has been used by the *intrapericardial* route

Dosing adjustment in renal impairment: There are no dosage adjustments provided in manufacturer's labeling.

Dosing adjustment in hepatic impairment: There are no dosage adjustments provided in manufacturer's labeling.

Administration Hazardous agent; use appropriate precautions for handling and disposal (NIOSH, 2012).

Intracavitary: Adults: Prepare immediately prior to administration. May further dilute in 50 to 100 mL of normal saline prior to instillation; rotate patient position every 5 to 10 minutes for 1 hour after administration to obtain uniform distribution.

Parenteral: Reconstitute powder with 10 mL SWI or NS to a final concentration of 1 mg/mL; prepare immediately prior to administration. Administer I.V. push over 1 to 5 minutes into a free-flowing I.V. solution. **DO NOT ADMINISTER I.M. or SubQ**. Mechlorethamine is associated with a high emetic potential (Basch, 2011); antiemetics are recommended to prevent nausea and vomiting.

Extravasation management: If extravasation occurs, stop infusion immediately and disconnect (leave cannula/needle in place); gently aspirate extravasated solution (do **NOT** flush the line); remove needle/cannula; elevate extremity.

Sodium thiosulfate ¹/₆ M solution: Inject subcutaneously into extravasation area using 2 mL for each mg of mechlorethamine suspected to have extravasated (Pérez Fidalgo, 2012; Polovich, 2009). Apply ice for 6 to 12 hours after sodium thiosulfate administration (Mustargen prescribing information, 2013; Polovich, 2009) **or** may apply dry cold compresses for 20 minutes 4 times daily for 1 to 2 days (Pérez Fidalgo, 2012).

Vesicant/Extravasation Risk Vesicant

Monitoring Parameters CBC with differential and platelet count, renal and hepatic function; signs/symptoms of hypersensitivity reactions, infection, and extravasation

Product Availability Mustargen: Mustargen was acquired by Recordati Rare Diseases in 2013; availability information is currently unknown.

Dosage Forms Excipient information presented when available (limited, particularly for generics); consult specific product labeling.

Solution Reconstituted, Injection, as hydrochloride:
Mustargen: 10 mg (1 ea)

References

Basch E, Prestrud AA, Hesketh PJ, et al. Antiemetics: American Society of Clinical Oncology clinical practice guideline update. *J Clin Oncol.* 2011;29(31):4189-4198.

Canellos GP, Anderson JR, Propert KJ, et al. Chemotherapy of advanced Hodgkin's disease with MOPP, ABVD, or MOPP alternating with ABVD. *N Engl J Med.* 1992;327(21):1478-1484.

Devita VT Jr, Serpick AA, Carbone PP. Combination chemotherapy in the treatment of advanced Hodgkin's disease. *Ann Intern Med.* 1970;73(6):881-895.

Dorr RT, Soble M, and Alberts DS, "Efficacy of Sodium Thiosulfate as a Local Antidote to Mechlorethamine Skin Toxicity in the Mouse," *Cancer Chemother Pharmacol.* 1988, 22(4):299-302.

Horning SJ, Hoppe RT, Breslin S, Bartlett NL, Brown BW, Rosenberg SA. Stanford V and radiotherapy for locally extensive and advanced Hodgkin's disease: mature results of a prospective clinical trial. *J Clin Oncol.* 2002;20(3):630-637.

Horning SJ, Williams J, Bartlett NL, et al. Assessment of the Stanford V regimen and consolidative radiotherapy for bulky and advanced Hodgkin's disease: Eastern Cooperative Oncology Group pilot study E1492. *J Clin Oncol.* 2000;18(5):972-980.

Kelly KM. Management of children with high-risk Hodgkin lymphoma. *Br J Haematol.* 2012;157(1):3-13.

Kung FH, Schwartz CL, Ferree CR, et al. POG 8625: a randomized trial comparing chemotherapy with chemoradiotherapy for children and adolescents with Stages I, IIA, IIIA1 Hodgkin Disease: a report from the Children's Oncology Group. *J Pediatr Hematol Oncol.* 2006;28(6):362-368.

Longo DL, Young RC, Wesley M, et al. Twenty years of MOPP therapy for Hodgkin's disease. *J Clin Oncol.* 1986;4(9):1295-1306.

Metzger ML, Billett A, Link MP. The impact of drug shortages on children with cancer – the example of mechlorethamine. *N Engl J Med.* 2012;367(26):2461-2463.

Mustargen (mechlorethamine) [prescribing information]. Lebanon, NJ: Recordati Rare Diseases Inc; February 2013.

National Institute for Occupational Safety and Health (NIOSH), "NIOSH List of Antineoplastic and Other Hazardous Drugs in Healthcare Settings 2012." Available at http://www.cdc.gov/niosh/docs/2012-150/pdfs/2012-150.pdf. Accessed January 21, 2013.

Pérez Fidalgo JA, García Fabregat L, Cervantes A, et al. Management of chemotherapy extravasation: ESMO-EONS Clinical Practice Guidelines. *Ann Oncol.* 2012;23(Suppl 7):167-173.

Perry MC, ed.*Chemotherapeutic Agents: Mechlorethamine. The Chemotherapy Source Book.* 5th ed. Philadelphia, PA: 2012.

Polovich M, Whitford JN, Olsen M, eds. *Chemotherapy and Biotherapy Guidelines and Recommendations for Practice.* 3rd ed, Pittsburgh, PA: Oncology Nursing Society, 2009.

◆ **Mechlorethamine Hydrochloride** *see* Mechlorethamine (Systemic) *on page 1315*

Meclizine (MEK li zeen)

Medication Safety Issues
Sound-alike/look-alike issues:
Antivert® may be confused with Anzemet®, Axert®
BEERS Criteria medication:
This drug may be potentially inappropriate for use in geriatric patients (Quality of evidence - varies based on comorbidity; Strength of recommendation - varies based on comorbidity)
Brand Names: U.S. Dramamine Less Drowsy [OTC]; Medi-Meclizine [OTC]; Travel Sickness [OTC]; UniVert; Vertin-32 [OTC]
Therapeutic Category Antiemetic; Antihistamine
Generic Availability (U.S.) Yes
Use Prevention and treatment of motion sickness; management of vertigo
Pregnancy Risk Factor B
Pregnancy Considerations Adverse events have been observed in animal reproduction studies; however, an increased risk of fetal abnormalities has not been observed following maternal use of meclizine during pregnancy.
Breast-Feeding Considerations It is not known if meclizine is excreted into breast milk.
Contraindications Hypersensitivity to meclizine or any component
Precautions Use with caution in patients with angle-closure glaucoma or obstructive diseases of the GI or GU tract
Adverse Reactions
Central nervous system: Drowsiness, fatigue, headache
Gastrointestinal: Vomiting, xerostomia
Ocular: Blurred vision
Miscellaneous: Anaphylactoid reaction
Drug Interactions
Metabolism/Transport Effects Substrate of CYP2D6 (minor); **Note:** Assignment of Major/Minor substrate status based on clinically relevant drug interaction potential
Avoid Concomitant Use
Avoid concomitant use of Meclizine with any of the following: Aclidinium; Azelastine (Nasal); Ipratropium (Oral Inhalation); Paraldehyde; Potassium Chloride; Thalidomide; Tiotropium; Umeclidinium
Increased Effect/Toxicity
Meclizine may increase the levels/effects of: AbobotulinumtoxinA; Alcohol (Ethyl); Analgesics (Opioid); Anticholinergic Agents; Azelastine (Nasal); Buprenorphine; Cannabinoid-Containing Products; CNS Depressants; Hydrocodone; Methotrimeprazine; Metyrosine; Mirabegron; Mirtazapine; OnabotulinumtoxinA; Paraldehyde; Potassium Chloride; Pramipexole; RimabotulinumtoxinB; ROPINIRole; Rotigotine; Selective Serotonin Reuptake Inhibitors; Thalidomide; Thiazide Diuretics; Tiotropium; Topiramate; Zolpidem

The levels/effects of Meclizine may be increased by: Aclidinium; Brimonidine (Topical); Cannabis; Doxylamine; Dronabinol; Droperidol; HydrOXYzine; Ipratropium (Oral Inhalation); Kava Kava; Magnesium Sulfate; Methotrimeprazine; Nabilone; Perampanel; Pramlintide; Rufinamide; Sodium Oxybate; Tapentadol; Tetrahydrocannabinol; Umeclidinium
Decreased Effect
Meclizine may decrease the levels/effects of: Acetylcholinesterase Inhibitors (Central); Benzylpenicilloyl Polylysine; Betahistine; Hyaluronidase; Secretin

The levels/effects of Meclizine may be decreased by: Acetylcholinesterase Inhibitors (Central); Amphetamines; Peginterferon Alfa-2b
Mechanism of Action Has central anticholinergic action by blocking chemoreceptor trigger zone; decreases excitability of the middle ear labyrinth and blocks conduction in the middle ear vestibular-cerebellar pathways
Pharmacodynamics
Onset of action: Oral: 30-60 minutes
Duration: 12-24 hours
Pharmacokinetics (Adult data unless noted)
Metabolism: In the liver
Half-life: 6 hours
Elimination: As metabolites in urine and as unchanged drug in feces
Dosing: Usual Children >12 years and Adults: Oral:
Motion sickness: 25-50 mg 1 hour before travel, repeat dose every 24 hours if needed
Vertigo: 25-100 mg/day in divided doses
Administration Oral: Administer with food to decrease GI distress
Dosage Forms Excipient information presented when available (limited, particularly for generics); consult specific product labeling.
Tablet, Oral, as hydrochloride:
Dramamine Less Drowsy: 25 mg [contains fd&c yellow #10 (quinoline yellow)]
Dramamine Less Drowsy: 25 mg [contains fd&c yellow #10 aluminum lake]
Medi-Meclizine: 25 mg
UniVert: 32 mg [scored; contains brilliant blue fcf (fd&c blue #1), fd&c yellow #10 (quinoline yellow)]
Vertin-32: 32 mg [contains brilliant blue fcf (fd&c blue #1), fd&c yellow #10 (quinoline yellow)]
Generic: 12.5 mg, 25 mg
Tablet Chewable, Oral, as hydrochloride:
Travel Sickness: 25 mg [scored; contains aspartame, fd&c red #40 aluminum lake; raspberry flavor]
Generic: 25 mg

◆ **Meclizine Hydrochloride** *see* Meclizine *on page 1317*

◆ **Meclozine Hydrochloride** *see* Meclizine *on page 1317*

◆ **Med-Baclofen (Can)** *see* Baclofen *on page 259*

◆ **Med-Derm Hydrocortisone [OTC]** *see* Hydrocortisone (Topical) *on page 1038*

◆ **Medical Provider EZ Flu PF** *see* Influenza Virus Vaccine (Inactivated) *on page 1103*

◆ **Medicinal Carbon** *see* Charcoal, Activated *on page 432*

◆ **Medicinal Charcoal** *see* Charcoal, Activated *on page 432*

◆ **Medi-First Anti-Fungal [OTC]** *see* Tolnaftate *on page 2044*

◆ **Medi-First Hydrocortisone [OTC]** *see* Hydrocortisone (Topical) *on page 1038*

◆ **Medi-Meclizine [OTC]** *see* Meclizine *on page 1317*

◆ **Medi-Phenyl [OTC]** *see* Phenylephrine (Systemic) *on page 1658*

◆ **Mediplast [OTC]** *see* Salicylic Acid *on page 1860*

◆ **Mediproxen [OTC]** *see* Naproxen *on page 1470*

Medium Chain Triglycerides
(mee DEE um chane trye GLIS er ides)

Brand Names: U.S. MCT Oil [OTC]
Brand Names: Canada MCT Oil
Therapeutic Category Caloric Agent; Nutritional Supplement
Generic Availability (U.S.) No
Use Nutritional supplement for those who cannot digest long chain fats; malabsorption associated with disorders such as pancreatic insufficiency, bile salt deficiency, and bacterial overgrowth of the small bowel; induce ketosis as a prevention for seizures (akinetic, clonic, and petit mal)
Contraindications Hypersensitivity to medium chain triglycerides or any component; should not be used in patients with hepatic encephalopathy due to earlier observations which report that short chain fatty acids may have an opioid effect on the CNS and inhibit oxidative phosphorylation
Warnings Patients with cirrhosis demonstrate higher concentrations of medium chain fatty acids in the serum and CSF than normal individuals; impaired hepatic clearance of medium chain fatty acids due to parenchymal dysfunction of medium chain fatty acid oxidation, portal systemic shunt, and impaired protein binding of fatty acid enhance the passive diffusion of medium chain fatty acids into the CSF
Precautions Use with caution in patients with hepatic cirrhosis and complications such as portacaval shunts or encephalopathy
Adverse Reactions
Endocrine & metabolic: HDL serum levels decreased and triglycerides serum levels increased (>6 months daily use)
Gastrointestinal: Abdominal pain, bloating, cramping, diarrhea, nausea
Mechanism of Action MCTs are saturated fatty acids in chains of 6-12 carbon atoms. They are water soluble and can pass directly through intestinal cell membranes and blood stream. Once taken up by the liver, they are used for metabolic energy before being stored.
Pharmacodynamics Onset of action: Octanoic acid appeared in each subject by 30 minutes following ingestion; effect on seizures in children: Within 6 weeks
Pharmacokinetics (Adult data unless noted)
Absorption: Up to 30% of dose can be absorbed unchanged as a triglyceride in the mucosal cell
Metabolism: Almost entirely oxidized by the liver to acetyl CoA fragments and to carbon dioxide; little deposited in adipose tissue or elsewhere
Elimination: As much as 20% of oral dose of MCT, recovered in expired CO_2 in 50 minutes; <10% elimination of medium chain fatty acids in feces
Dosing: Neonatal Nutritional Supplement, increase caloric content: **Note:** Dose should be individualized to patient caloric needs, current nutritional/fluid status, and other clinical parameters. Initial: 0.5 mL every other feeding, then advance to every feeding, then increase in increments of 0.25-0.5 mL/feeding at intervals of 2-3 days as tolerated; lower initial doses may be used depending upon caloric needs; product formulation provides 115 calories/15 mL
Dosing: Usual Oral:
Cystic fibrosis: Children and Adults: 45 mL/day in divided doses
Malabsorption syndromes: Adults: 15 mL 3-4 times/day
Nutritional supplement: Infants: Initial: 0.5 mL every other feeding, then advance to every feeding, then increase in increments of 0.25-0.5 mL/feeding at intervals of 2-3 days as tolerated

Seizures: Children: About 40 mL with each meal or 50% to 70% (800-1120 kcal) of total calories (1600 kcal) as the oil will induce the ketosis necessary for seizure control
Administration Oral:
Dilute with at least an equal volume of water or mix with some other vehicle such as fruit juice (should not be cold; flavoring may be added); mixture should be sipped slowly; administer no more than 15-20 mL at any one time (up to 100 mL may be administered in divided doses in a 24-hour period)
Possible GI side effects from medication can be prevented if therapy is initiated with small supplements at meals and gradually increased according to patient's tolerance
Monitoring Parameters
Nutritional supplement and malabsorption: Weight gain, height, stool output
Seizure treatment: Reduction in seizures, urine ketones
Additional Information Does not provide any essential fatty acids; contains only saturated fats; supplementation with safflower, corn oil, or other polyunsaturated vegetable oil must be given to provide the patient with the essential fatty acids; caloric content: 8.3 calories/g; 115 calories/15 mL
Dosage Forms Excipient information presented when available (limited, particularly for generics); consult specific product labeling.
Oil, oral:
MCT Oil®: 14 g/15 mL (960 mL) [gluten free; contains coconut oil; 115 cal/15 mL]

◆ **MED-Letrozole (Can)** *see* Letrozole *on page 1211*
◆ **Medrol** *see* MethylPREDNISolone *on page 1386*
◆ **Medrol Dose Pack** *see* MethylPREDNISolone *on page 1386*
◆ **Medrol (Pak)** *see* MethylPREDNISolone *on page 1386*
◆ **Med-Rosuvastatin (Can)** *see* Rosuvastatin *on page 1853*
◆ **Medroxy (Can)** *see* MedroxyPROGESTERone *on page 1318*

MedroxyPROGESTERone
(me DROKS ee proe JES te rone)

Medication Safety Issues
Sound-alike/look-alike issues:
Depo-Provera® may be confused with depo-subQ provera 104™
MedroxyPROGESTERone may be confused with hydroxyprogesterone caproate, methylPREDNISolone, methylTESTOSTERone
Provera® may be confused with Covera®, Femara®, Parlodel®, Premarin®, Proscar®, PROzac®
Administration issues:
The injectable dosage form is available in different formulations. Carefully review prescriptions to assure the correct formulation and route of administration.
Related Information
Contraceptive Comparison Table *on page 2266*
Safe Handling of Hazardous Drugs *on page 2419*
Brand Names: U.S. Depo-Provera; Depo-SubQ Provera 104; Provera
Brand Names: Canada Alti-MPA; Apo-Medroxy®; Depo-Prevera®; Depo-Provera®; Dom-Medroxyprogesterone; Gen-Medroxy; Medroxy; Medroxyprogesterone Acetate Injectable Suspension USP; Novo-Medrone; PMS-Medroxyprogesterone; Provera-Pak; Provera®; Teva-Medroxyprogesterone
Therapeutic Category Contraceptive, Progestin Only; Progestin
Generic Availability (U.S.) Yes

Use Secondary amenorrhea or abnormal uterine bleeding due to hormonal imbalance; prevention of pregnancy; reduction of endometrial hyperplasia in nonhysterectomized postmenopausal women receiving conjugated estrogens; endometrial carcinoma; management of endometriosis-associated pain (FDA approved in adults)

Pregnancy Risk Factor X

Pregnancy Considerations Use is contraindicated in women who are pregnant, as a diagnostic test for pregnancy, or for missed abortion. In general, there is not an increased risk of birth defects following inadvertent use of the injectable medroxyprogesterone (MPA) contraceptives early in pregnancy. Hypospadias has been reported in male babies and clitoral enlargement and labial fusion have been reported in female babies exposed to MPA during the first trimester of pregnancy. High doses impair fertility. Ectopic pregnancies have been reported with use of the MPA contraceptive injection. Median time to conception/return to ovulation following discontinuation of MPA contraceptive injection is 10 months following the last injection.

Breast-Feeding Considerations Medroxyprogesterone (MPA) is excreted into breast milk. Composition, quality, and quantity of breast milk are not affected; adverse developmental and behavioral effects have not been noted following exposure of infant to MPA while breast-feeding. The manufacturer does not recommend the use of MPA tablets in breast-feeding mothers; however, guidelines note that the injectable MPA contraceptives can be initiated immediately postpartum in women who are nursing (CDC, 2010; CDC, 2011; CDC, 2013).

Contraindications Hypersensitivity to medroxyprogesterone or any component; history of or current thrombophlebitis or thromboembolic disorders (DVT, PE, MI), cerebral vascular disease, undiagnosed vaginal bleeding, liver dysfunction, breast cancer or other estrogen- or progesterone-dependent neoplasia, pregnancy (known or suspected), missed abortion, diagnostic test for pregnancy

Warnings Hazardous agent; use appropriate precautions for handling and disposal (NIOSH, 2012).

Discontinue if there is a sudden partial or complete loss of vision, proptosis, diplopia, migraine, if papilledema or retinal vascular lesions are present, or any other symptom of a thromboembolic event.

Prolonged use of medroxyprogesterone as a contraceptive reduces estrogen levels and has been associated with increased bone mineral density (BMD) loss **[U.S. Boxed Warning]**. Loss is related to the duration of use and not significantly different between the SubQ and I.M. dosage forms. Bone loss may not be completely reversible on discontinuation of the drug; in adolescents following 2 years of medroxyprogesterone treatment, femoral neck and hip BMD values did not fully recover to baseline at 60 months after discontinuation of therapy; age-matched cohorts' BMD increased throughout evaluation. It is not known if use during adolescence or early adulthood will decrease peak bone mass accretion or increase the risk for osteoporitic fractures later in life. The impact on peak bone mass in adolescents should be weighed against the potential for unintended pregnancies in treatment decisions. Consider alternative contraceptive methods in patients at risk for osteoporosis (eg, metabolic bone disease, family history of osteoporosis, chronic use of medications associated with osteoporosis such as corticosteroids). Use as a long-term contraceptive agent (≥2 years) should be reserved for situations when other contraceptives are not effective or contraindicated **[U.S. Boxed Warning]**. Monitor BMD if prolonged use is necessary. Inform patients that injectable contraceptives do not protect against HIV infection or other sexually transmitted diseases **[U.S. Boxed Warning]**. When used for

contraception, the possibility of ectopic pregnancy should be considered in patients with abdominal pain.

Based on data from the Women's Health Initiative (WHI) studies, an increased risk of invasive breast cancer was observed in postmenopausal women using conjugated estrogens (CE) in combination with medroxyprogesterone acetate (MPA) **[U.S. Boxed Warning]**. This risk may be associated with duration of use and declines once combined therapy is discontinued (Chlebowski, 2009). The risk of invasive breast cancer was decreased in postmenopausal women with a hysterectomy using CE only, regardless of weight. However, the risk was not significantly decreased in women at high risk for breast cancer (family history of breast cancer, personal history of benign breast disease) (Anderson, 2012). An increase in abnormal mammogram findings has also been reported with estrogen alone or in combination with progestin therapy. Use is contraindicated in patients with known or suspected breast cancer.

MPA is used to reduce the risk of endometrial hyperplasia in nonhysterectomized postmenopausal women receiving conjugated estrogens. The use of unopposed estrogen in women with an intact uterus is associated with an increased risk of endometrial cancer. The addition of a progestin to estrogen therapy may decrease the risk of endometrial hyperplasia, a precursor to endometrial cancer. Adequate diagnostic measures, including endometrial sampling if indicated, should be performed to rule out malignancy in postmenopausal women with undiagnosed abnormal vaginal bleeding. Estrogens may exacerbate endometriosis. Malignant transformation of residual endometrial implants has been reported posthysterectomy with unopposed estrogen therapy. Consider adding a progestin in women with residual endometriosis posthysterectomy. Postmenopausal estrogen therapy and combined estrogen/progesterone therapy may increase the risk of ovarian cancer; however, the absolute risk to an individual woman is small. Although results from various studies are not consistent, risk does not appear to be significantly associated with the duration, route, or dose of therapy. In one study, the risk decreased after 2 years following discontinuation of therapy (Mørch, 2009). Although the risk of ovarian cancer is rare, women who are at an increased risk (eg, family history) should be counseled about the association (NAMS, 2012).

Estrogens with or without progestin should not be used to prevent dementia **[U.S. Boxed Warning]**. In the Women's Health Initiative Memory Study (WHIMS), an increased incidence of dementia was observed in women ≥65 years of age taking CE alone or in combination with MPA. Estrogens with or without progestin should not be used to prevent cardiovascular disease **[U.S. Boxed Warning]**. Using data from the WHI studies, an increased risk of DVT and stroke has been reported with CE and an increased risk of DVT, stroke, pulmonary emboli, and MI has been reported with CE with MPA in postmenopausal women. Additional risk factors include diabetes mellitus, hypercholesterolemia, hypertension, SLE, obesity, tobacco use, and/or history of venous thromboembolism. Risk factors should be managed appropriately; discontinue use if adverse cardiovascular events occur or are suspected. If thrombosis develops with contraceptive treatment, discontinue treatment (unless no other acceptable contraceptive alternative).

Estrogens with or without progestin should be used for the shortest duration possible at the lowest effective dose consistent with treatment goals **[U.S. Boxed Warning]**. Available data related to treatment risks are from WHI studies, which evaluated oral CE 0.625 mg with or without MPA 2.5 mg relative to placebo in postmenopausal women. Other combinations and dosage forms of estrogens and progestins were not studied. Outcomes reported from clinical trials using CE with or without MPA should be assumed to be similar for other doses and other dosage forms of estrogens and progestins until comparable data becomes available.

Anaphylaxis or anaphylactoid reactions have been reported with use of the injection; medication for the treatment of hypersensitivity reactions should be available for immediate use. Injection may contain polysorbate 80 (Tween 80®) which may cause allergic reactions in susceptible individuals.

Precautions Unscheduled bleeding/spotting may occur; presentation of irregular, unresolving vaginal bleeding following previously regular cycles warrants further evaluation, including endometrial sampling, if indicated, to rule out malignancy. May cause weight gain; contraceptive therapy with medroxyprogesterone commonly results in an average weight gain of ~2.5 kg after 1 year and ~3.7 kg after 2 years of treatment. Use with caution in patients with diseases which may be exacerbated by fluid retention, including epilepsy, asthma, migraines, or renal or cardiac dysfunction. Use caution in diabetes mellitus; may adversely affect glucose tolerance. Use with caution in patients with a history of depression; discontinue therapy if depression recurrs. Estrogen plus progestin therapy may exacerbate hepatic hemangiomas, porphyria, and SLE; use caution in women with these conditions. Elevations in plasma triglycerides may occur with estrogen and progestin therapy; use caution in patients with preexisting hypertriglyceridemia as this may lead to pancreatitis and other complications. Medroxyprogesterone is extensively metabolized in the liver; discontinue if jaundice develops or if acute or chronic hepatic disturbances occur.

Adverse Reactions Adverse effects as reported with any dosage form

Cardiovascular: Edema

Central nervous system: Depression, dizziness, fatigue, headache, insomnia, nervousness

Dermatologic: Acne, alopecia, rash

Endocrine & metabolic: Breast pain, hot flashes, libido decreased, menstrual irregularities (includes bleeding, amenorrhea, or both)

Gastrointestinal: Abdominal pain/discomfort, bloating, nausea, weight gain (>10 lbs at 24 months)

Genitourinary: Cervical smear abnormal, leukorrhea, menometrorrhagia, menorrhagia, pelvic pain, urinary tract infection, vaginitis

Genitourinary: Dysmenorrhea, leukorrhea, vaginitis

Local: Injection site reaction (SubQ administration): Atrophy, induration, pain

Rare but important or life-threatening: Allergic reaction, anaphylaxis, anaphylactoid reactions, angioedema, asthma, blood dyscrasia, bone mineral density decreased, breast cancer, breast changes, cervical cancer, chest pain, chloasma, cholestatic jaundice, deep vein thrombosis, diaphoresis, dyspnea, facial palsy, galactorrhea, glucose tolerance decreased, hirsutism, hoarseness, injection site reactions, jaundice, lack of return to fertility, lactation decreased, melasma, nipple bleeding, optic neuritis, osteoporosis, osteoporotic fractures, paralysis, paresthesia, pulmonary embolus, rectal bleeding, retinal thrombosis, scleroderma, seizure, syncope, tachycardia, thrombophlebitis, urticaria

Drug Interactions

Metabolism/Transport Effects Substrate of CYP3A4 (major); **Note:** Assignment of Major/Minor substrate status based on clinically relevant drug interaction potential; **Induces** CYP3A4 (weak/moderate)

Avoid Concomitant Use

Avoid concomitant use of MedroxyPROGESTERone with any of the following: Axitinib; Griseofulvin; Indium 111

Capromab Pendetide; Simeprevir; Tranexamic Acid; Ulipristal

Increased Effect/Toxicity

MedroxyPROGESTERone may increase the levels/effects of: Benzodiazepines (metabolized by oxidation); Selegiline; Thalidomide; Tranexamic Acid; Voriconazole

The levels/effects of MedroxyPROGESTERone may be increased by: Atazanavir; Boceprevir; Cobicistat; Herbs (Progestogenic Properties); Lopinavir; Metreleptin; Mifepristone; Tipranavir; Voriconazole

Decreased Effect

MedroxyPROGESTERone may decrease the levels/effects of: Anticoagulants; ARIPiprazole; Axitinib; Fosamprenavir; Ibrutinib; Indium 111 Capromab Pendetide; Saxagliptin; Simeprevir; Vitamin K Antagonists

The levels/effects of MedroxyPROGESTERone may be decreased by: Acitretin; Aminoglutethimide; Aprepitant; Artemether; Barbiturates; Bexarotene (Systemic); Bile Acid Sequestrants; Bosentan; CarBAMazepine; CloBAZam; CYP3A4 Inducers (Strong); Dabrafenib; Darunavir; Deferasirox; Efavirenz; Eslicarbazepine; Felbamate; Fosamprenavir; Fosaprepitant; Fosphenytoin; Griseofulvin; LamoTRIgine; Lopinavir; Metreleptin; Mifepristone; Mitotane; Mycophenolate; Nelfinavir; Nevirapine; OXcarbazepine; Perampanel; Phenytoin; Primidone; Prucalopride; Retinoic Acid Derivatives; Rifamycin Derivatives; Saquinavir; Siltuximab; St Johns Wort; Sugammadex; Telaprevir; Tocilizumab; Topiramate; Uliprista

Food Interactions Bioavailability of the oral tablet is increased when taken with food; half-life is unchanged. Management: Administer without regard to food.

Stability Hazardous agent; use appropriate precautions for handling and disposal (NIOSH, 2012). Store at 20°C to 25°C (68°F to 77°F); protect oral formulation from light.

Mechanism of Action Inhibits secretion of pituitary gonadotropins, which prevents follicular maturation and ovulation; causes endometrial thinning

Pharmacodynamics Time to ovulation (after last injection): 10 months (range: 6-12 months)

Pharmacokinetics (Adult data unless noted)

Absorption: I.M.: Slow

Protein binding: 86% to 90% primarily to albumin; does not bind to sex hormone-binding globulin

Metabolism: Extensively hepatic via hydroxylation and conjugation; forms metabolites

Bioavailability: 0.6% to 10%

Half-life:

Oral: 12-17 hours

I.M. (Depo-Provera® Contraceptive): ~50 days

SubQ: ~40 days

Time to peak serum concentration:

Oral: 2-4 hours

I.M. (Depo-Provera® Contraceptive): ~3 weeks

SubQ (depo-subQ provera 104®): 1 week

Elimination: Urine

Dosing: Usual

Adolescents and Adults:

Abnormal uterine bleeding: Oral: 5-10 mg for 5-10 days starting on day 16 or day 21 of menstrual cycle

Amenorrhea: Oral: 5-10 mg/day for 5-10 days

Contraception: First dose to be given only during first 5 days of normal menstrual period; only within 5 days postpartum if not breast-feeding, or only at sixth postpartum week if exclusively breast-feeding. When switching from other contraceptive methods, depo-subQ provera 104™ should be administered within 7 days after the last day of using the last method (pill, ring, patch).

I.M. (Depo-Provera®): 150 mg every 3 months

SubQ (depo-subQ provera 104®): 104 mg every 3 months (every 12-14 weeks)

Endometriosis-associated pain: SubQ (depo-subQ provera 104™): 104 mg every 3 months; treatment longer than 2 years is not recommended due to impact of long-term use on bone mineral density

Adults:

Accompanying cyclic estrogen therapy (postmenopausal): Oral: 5-10 mg for 12-14 consecutive days each month, starting on day 1 or day 16 of cycle; lower doses may be used if given with estrogen continuously throughout the cycle

Endometrial carcinoma, recurrent or metastatic: I.M. (Depo-Provera®): 400-1000 mg/week

Dosing adjustment in hepatic impairment: Use is contraindicated with severe impairment. Discontinue with jaundice or if liver function disturbances occur. Consider lower dose or less frequent administration with mild to moderate impairment. Use of the contraceptive injection has not been studied in patients with hepatic impairment; consideration should be given to not readminister if jaundice develops.

Administration Hazardous agent; use appropriate precautions for handling and disposal (NIOSH, 2012).

Oral: Administer with food

Parenteral:

I.M.: (Depo-Provera® Contraceptive): Shake suspension vigorously; administer by deep I.M. injection in the gluteal or deltoid muscle

SubQ (depo-subQ provera 104®): Shake vigorously; administer by subQ injection over 5-7 seconds in the anterior thigh or abdomen; avoid boney areas and the umbilicus. Do not rub the injection area; not for I.M. or I.V. use.

Monitoring Parameters Before starting therapy, a physical exam with reference to the breasts and pelvis is recommended, including a Papanicolaou smear. Exam may be deferred if appropriate prior to administration of MPA contraceptive injection; pregnancy should be ruled out prior to use. Monitor patient closely for loss of vision; sudden onset of proptosis, diplopia, or migraine; signs and symptoms of thromboembolic disorders; signs and symptoms of depression; glucose in patients with diabetes; or blood pressure. BMD with long-term use.

Adequate diagnostic measures, including endometrial sampling, if indicated, should be performed to rule out malignancy in all cases of undiagnosed abnormal vaginal bleeding.

Dosage Forms Excipient information presented when available (limited, particularly for generics); consult specific product labeling.

Suspension, Intramuscular, as acetate:
Depo-Provera: 150 mg/mL (1 mL)
Depo-Provera: 150 mg/mL (1 mL) [contains methylparaben, polyethylene glycol, polysorbate 80, propylparaben]
Depo-Provera: 400 mg/mL (2.5 mL)
Generic: 150 mg/mL (1 mL)

Suspension, Subcutaneous, as acetate:
Depo-SubQ Provera 104: 104 mg/0.65 mL (0.65 mL) [contains methylparaben, propylparaben]

Tablet, Oral, as acetate:
Provera: 2.5 mg, 5 mg, 10 mg [scored]
Generic: 2.5 mg, 5 mg, 10 mg

References

American College of Obstetricians and Gynecologists Committee on Gynecologic Practice, "ACOG Committee Opinion No. 415: Depot Medroxyprogesterone Acetate and Bone Effects," *Obstet Gynecol*, 2008, 112(3):727-30.

Anderson GL, Chlebowski RT, Aragaki AK, et al, "Conjugated Equine Oestrogen and Breast Cancer Incidence and Mortality in Postmenopausal Women With Hysterectomy: Extended Follow-Up of the Women's Health Initiative Randomised Placebo-Controlled Trial," *Lancet Oncol*, 2012.

Centers for Disease Control and Prevention (CDC). U S. medical eligibility criteria for contraceptive use, 2010. *MMWR Recomm Rep.* 201018;59(RR-4):1-86.

Centers for Disease Control and Prevention (CDC). Update to CDC's U.S. medical eligibility criteria for contraceptive use, 2010: revised recommendations for the use of contraceptive methods during the postpartum period. *MMWR Morb Mortal Wkly Rep.* 2011;60 (26):878-883.

Centers for Disease Control and Prevention (CDC). U.S. selected practice recommendations for contraceptive use, 2013: adapted from the World Health Organization selected practice recommendations for contraceptive use, 2nd edition. *MMWR Recomm Rep*, 2013, 62(RR-05):1-60.

Chlebowski RT, Kuller LH, Prentice RL, et al, "Breast Cancer After Use of Estrogen Plus Progestin in Postmenopausal Women," *N Engl J Med*, 2009, 360(6):573-87.

Mørch LS, Løkkegaard E, Andreasen AH, et al, "Hormone Therapy and Ovarian Cancer," *JAMA*, 2009, 302(3):298-305.

National Institute for Occupational Safety and Health (NIOSH), "NIOSH List of Antineoplastic and Other Hazardous Drugs in Healthcare Settings 2012." Available at http://www.cdc.gov/niosh/docs/2012-150/pdfs/2012-150.pdf. Accessed January 21, 2013.

North American Menopause Society, "The 2012 Hormone Therapy Position Statement of: The North American Menopause Society," *Menopause*, 2012, 19(3):257-71.

◆ **Medroxyprogesterone Acetate** *see* MedroxyPROGESTERone *on page 1318*

◆ **Medroxyprogesterone Acetate Injectable Suspension USP (Can)** *see* MedroxyPROGESTERone *on page 1318*

◆ **Med-Sotalol (Can)** *see* Sotalol *on page 1925*

Mefloquine (ME floe kwin)

Medication Safety Issues

International issues:

Lariam [multiple international markets] may be confused with Levaquin [Argentina, Brazil, Venezuela]

Therapeutic Category Antimalarial Agent

Generic Availability (U.S.) Yes

Use Treatment of acute malarial infections due to *Plasmodium vivax* and *Plasmodium flaciparum* (including chloroquine-resistant strains) (FDA approved in ages ≥6 months and adults); prevention of malaria due to *Plasmodium vivax* and *Plasmodium falciparum* (including chloroquine-resistant strains) (FDA approved in pediatric patients weighing ≥20 kg and adults)

Medication Guide Available Yes

Pregnancy Risk Factor B

Pregnancy Considerations Adverse events have been observed in animal reproduction studies. Mefloquine crosses the placenta; however, clinical experience with mefloquine has not shown adverse effects in pregnant women. Use with caution during pregnancy if travel to endemic areas cannot be postponed. Malaria infection in pregnant women may be more severe than in nonpregnant women and may increase the risk of adverse pregnancy outcomes. Nonpregnant women of childbearing potential are advised to use contraception and avoid pregnancy during malaria prophylaxis and for 3 months thereafter. In case of an unplanned pregnancy, treatment with mefloquine is not considered a reason for pregnancy termination. CDC treatment guidelines are available for the use of mefloquine in the treatment of malaria during pregnancy (CDC, 2013b).

Breast-Feeding Considerations Mefloquine is excreted in breast milk in small quantities (~3% to 4% of a 250 mg dose). The manufacturer recommends that caution be exercised when administering mefloquine to nursing women. Exposure to small amounts of mefloquine from breast milk is considered safe for infants (CDC, 2014).

Contraindications Hypersensitivity to mefloquine-related compounds, such as quinine and quinidine, or any component; prophylactic use in patients with depression (active or recent history of), generalized anxiety disorder, psychosis, schizophrenia, or other major psychiatric disorders, or with a history of convulsions

Warnings May cause neuropsychiatric adverse effects that can persist after mefloquine has been discontinued. During prophylactic use, if symptoms occur, discontinue therapy and substitute an alternative medication **[U.S. Boxed Warning]**. Symptoms may develop early in the course of therapy. Due to the difficulty in identifying these symptoms in infants and children, monitor closely, especially in nonverbal pediatric patients. Psychiatric symptoms may include anxiety, paranoia, depression, hallucinations, and psychosis. Suicidal ideation and suicide have also been reported. Neurologic symptoms of dizziness or vertigo, tinnitus, and loss of balance may also occur and have been reported to be permanent in some cases. Do not prescribe for prophylaxis in patients with major psychiatric disorders **[U.S. Boxed Warning]** including patients with active or recent history of depression, generalized anxiety disorder, psychosis, or schizophrenia; use is contraindicated in these patients. During prophylactic use, the occurrence of psychiatric symptoms, such as acute anxiety, depression, restlessness, or confusion, may be a prodrome to more serious neuropsychiatric adverse reactions. Use with caution in activities requiring alertness and fine motor coordination (eg, driving, piloting planes, operating machinery) with neurologic symptoms.

Hypersensitivity reactions ranging from mild skin reactions to anaphylaxis have occurred. Agranulocytosis and aplastic anemia have been reported with use.

Mefloquine may cause alterations in the ECG, including sinus bradycardia, sinus arrhythmia, first-degree AV block, QT-interval prolongation, and abnormal T waves; use caution or avoid concomitant use of drugs known to cause QT-interval prolongation (eg, halofantrine, quinine, quinidine) or inhibit (potent) the metabolism of CYP3A4 substrates (eg, ketoconazole); use with caution in patients with significant cardiac disease.

In cases of life-threatening, serious, or overwhelming malaria infections due to *Plasmodium falciparum*, patients should be treated with an intravenous malarial drug. Mefloquine may be given orally to complete the course. In cases of acute *Plasmodium vivax* infection treated with mefloquine, patients should subsequently be treated with an 8-aminoquinoline derivative (eg, primaquine) to avoid relapse. Not recommended for the treatment of malaria acquired in Southeast Asia due to drug resistance.

Precautions Use with caution in patients with hepatic impairment; elimination may be prolonged; if mefloquine is to be used for prolonged period, liver function tests should be performed periodically. When using for treatment, use with caution in patients with a history of seizures; increase risk of seizures; prophylactic use is contraindicated in patients with seizure disorder; concurrent use with chloroquine may increase risk of seizure (WHO, 2010). Potentially significant interactions may exist, requiring dose or frequency adjustment, additional monitoring, and/or selection of alternative therapy. Consult drug interactions database for more detailed information.

In children, early vomiting leading to treatment failure has been reported in some studies; consider alternate therapy if a second dose is not tolerated. If mefloquine is to be used for a prolonged period, periodic ophthalmic examinations should be performed; retinal abnormalities have not been observed with mefloquine in humans; however, abnormalities have been reported with long-term administration to rats.

Adverse Reactions

Central nervous system: Chills, dizziness, fatigue, fever, headache

Dermatologic: Rash

Gastrointestinal: Abdominal pain, appetite decreased, diarrhea, nausea, vomiting

Neuromuscular & skeletal: Myalgia

Otic: Tinnitus

Rare but important or life-threatening: Abnormal dreams, abnormal T waves, ataxia, aggressive behavior, agitation, anxiety, arrhythmia, arthralgia, AV block, cardiac arrest (with concomitant use of propranolol), chest pain, conduction abnormalities (transient), confusion, depression, diaphoresis increased, dyspepsia, dyspnea, edema, encephalopathy, erythema, erythema multiforme, exanthema, flushing, forgetfulness, hallucinations, hearing impairment, hematocrit decreased, hyper-/hypotension, insomnia, irregular pulse, leukocytosis, leukopenia, liver function tests increased, loss of balance, malaise, mood changes, muscle cramps/weakness, palpitation, panic attacks, paranoia, paresthesia, pneumonitis (allergic etiology), psychosis, QT prolongation, restlessness, somnolence, Stevens-Johnson syndrome, suicidal ideation and behavior (causal relationship not established), tachycardia, thrombocytopenia, tremor, urticaria, vertigo, visual disturbances

Drug Interactions

Metabolism/Transport Effects Substrate of CYP3A4 (major); **Note:** Assignment of Major/Minor substrate status based on clinically relevant drug interaction potential; **Inhibits** CYP2D6 (weak), CYP3A4 (weak), P-glycoprotein

Avoid Concomitant Use

Avoid concomitant use of Mefloquine with any of the following: Aminoquinolines (Antimalarial); Artemether; Bosutinib; Conivaptan; Fusidic Acid (Systemic); Halofantrine; Lumefantrine; PAZOPanib; Pimozide; QuiNINDine; QuiNINE; Silodosin; Topotecan; VinCRIStine (Liposomal)

Increased Effect/Toxicity

Mefloquine may increase the levels/effects of: Afatinib; Aminoquinolines (Antimalarial); Antipsychotic Agents (Phenothiazines); ARIPiprazole; Bosutinib; Brentuximab Vedotin; Colchicine; Dabigatran Etexilate; Dapsone (Systemic); Dapsone (Topical); DOXOrubicin (Conventional); Everolimus; Halofantrine; Highest Risk QTc-Prolonging Agents; Lomitapide; Lumefantrine; Moderate Risk QTc-Prolonging Agents; PAZOPanib; P-glycoprotein/ABCB1 Substrates; Pimozide; Prucalopride; QuiNINE; Rifaximin; Rivaroxaban; Silodosin; Topotecan; VinCRIStine (Liposomal)

The levels/effects of Mefloquine may be increased by: Aminoquinolines (Antimalarial); Artemether; Ceritinib; Conivaptan; CYP3A4 Inhibitors (Moderate); CYP3A4 Inhibitors (Strong); Dapsone (Systemic); Dasatinib; Fusidic Acid (Systemic); Ivacaftor; Luliconazole; Mifepristone; QuiNIDine; QuiNINE; Simeprevir; Stiripentol

Decreased Effect

Mefloquine may decrease the levels/effects of: Anticonvulsants

The levels/effects of Mefloquine may be decreased by: Bosentan; CYP3A4 Inducers (Strong); Dabrafenib; Deferasirox; Mitotane; Siltuximab; St Johns Wort; Tocilizumab

Food Interactions Food increases bioavailability by ~40%. Management: Take with food and at least 8 ounces of water. Maintain adequate nutrition and hydration, unless instructed to restrict fluid intake.

Stability Store at 20°C to 25°C (68°F to 77°F).

Mechanism of Action Mefloquine is a quinoline-methanol compound structurally similar to quinine; mefloquine's effectiveness in the treatment and prophylaxis of malaria is due to the destruction of the asexual blood forms of the malarial pathogens that affect humans, *Plasmodium falciparum, P. vivax*.

Pharmacokinetics (Adult data unless noted)

Absorption: Well absorbed; interpatient variability with rate observed (WHO, 2010); more complete absorption when administered as a suspension compared with tablets

Distribution: Distributes into tissues, erythrocytes, blood, urine, CSF

V_d:

Children 4-10 years: Mean: ~18-19 L/kg (Price, 1999)

Adults: ~20 L/kg

Protein binding: ~98%

Metabolism: Extensively hepatic (primarily by CYP3A4) to 2,8-bis-trifluoromethyl-4-quinoline carboxylic acid (inactive) and other metabolites

Half-life:

Children 4-10 years: Mean range: 11.6-13.6 days (range: 6.5-33 days) (Price, 1999)

Adults: ~3 weeks (range: 2-4 weeks); may be decreased during infection (2 weeks) (WHO, 2010)

Time to peak serum concentration: Median: ~17 hours (range: 6-24 hours)

Elimination: Primarily bile and feces; urine (9% of total dose as unchanged drug, 4% of total dose as primary metabolite)

Dosing: Usual Note: Dose is expressed in terms of the salt, mefloquine hydrochloride.

Infants, Children, and Adolescents: **Note:** Due to limited clinical experience and dosage form availability, WHO Guidelines exclude patients weighing <5 kg from antimalarial dosage recommendations (WHO, 2010); however, other recommendations do not exclude these patients (CDC, 2009).

Malaria, treatment (independent of HIV-status), chloroquine-sensitive: Oral: Infants ≥6 months, Children, and Adolescents:

Manufacturer's labeling: 20-25 mg/kg/day in 2 divided doses, taken 6-8 hours apart (maximum total dose: 1250 mg)

Alternate dosing: CDC Guidelines (CDC, 2009; CDC, 2013): 15 mg/kg (maximum dose: 750 mg) followed in 6-12 hours with 10 mg/kg (maximum dose: 500 mg); if clinical improvement is not seen within 48-72 hours, an alternative therapy should be used for retreatment

Malaria, treatment; uncomplicated, chloroquine-resistant *P. vivax* (independent of HIV-status): Oral: Infants ≥6 months, Children, and Adolescents: 15 mg/kg (maximum dose: 750 mg) followed in 6-12 hours with 10 mg/kg/dose (maximum dose: 500 mg) with concomitant primaquine; not recommended unless other options not available (CDC, 2009; CDC, 2013)

Malaria; chemoprophylaxis: Oral: **Note:** Begin 2 weeks before arrival in endemic area, continue weekly during travel, and for 4 weeks after leaving endemic area. Prophylaxis may begin >2 weeks prior to travel to ensure tolerance (CDC, 2014).

Weight-based dosing: 5 mg/kg/dose once weekly; maximum dose: 250 mg

Fixed dosing:

≤9 kg: 5 mg/kg/dose once weekly

>9-19 kg: 62.5 mg (¼ of 250 mg tablet) once weekly

>19-30 kg: 125 mg (½of 250 mg tablet) once weekly

>30-45 kg: 187.5 mg (¾of a 250 mg tablet) once weekly

>45 kg: 250 mg once weekly

Adults:

Malaria treatment (mild to moderate infection): 1250 mg as a single dose or 750 mg followed 6-12 hours later by 500 mg (CDC, 2011). If clinical improvement is not seen within 48-72 hours, an alternative therapy should be used for retreatment.

Malaria prophylaxis: 250 mg once weekly on the same day each week, starting 1 week (CDC, 2012: ≥2 weeks) before arrival in endemic area, continuing weekly during travel, and for 4 weeks after leaving endemic area.

Note: Prophylaxis may begin 2-3 weeks prior to travel to ensure tolerance in patients on multiple medications.

Dosing adjustment in renal impairment: No dosage adjustment necessary; only a small amount of mefloquine is renally eliminated; not removed by hemodialysis.

Dosing adjustment in hepatic impairment: There are no dosage adjustment provided in manufacturer's labeling; however, half-life may be prolonged and plasma levels may be higher in patients with hepatic impairment.

Administration Oral: Administer with food and an ample amount of water, at least 8 oz of water for adults. If vomiting occurs within 30 minutes after a dose, repeat dose. If vomiting occurs within 30-60 minutes after a dose, an additional half-dose should be administered. If vomiting recurs, monitor closely and consider alternative treatment. Administering mefloquine on a full stomach may minimize nausea and vomiting. For patients unable to swallow tablets or unable to tolerate its bitter taste, crush tablets and mix with a small amount of water, milk, applesauce, chocolate syrup, jelly, or food immediately before administration. Pulverized dose of mefloquine can be enclosed in a gelatin capsule to mask bitter taste. When used for malaria prophylaxis, dose should be taken once weekly on the same day each week.

Monitoring Parameters Sequential blood smears for percent parasitemia; periodic hepatic function tests, ophthalmologic exam

Additional Information Information on recommendations for travelers can be accessed by contacting the Centers for Disease Control and Prevention (CDC) Malaria Hotline (770-488-7788) or visit the CDC website: http://www.cdc.gov/travel/diseases.htm#malaria.

Dosage Forms Excipient information presented when available (limited, particularly for generics); consult specific product labeling.

Tablet, Oral, as hydrochloride:

Generic: 250 mg

References

Centers for Disease Control and Prevention (CDC), *CDC Health Information for International Travel 2014*. New York: Oxford University Press; 2014; Chapter 3. http://wwwnc.cdc.gov/travel/page/yellow-book-home-2014

Centers for Disease Control and Prevention (CDC), "Guidelines for the Prevention and Treatment of Opportunistic Infections Among HIV-Exposed and HIV-Infected Children," *MMWR Recomm Rep*, 2009, 58(RR-11):1-166. Available at http://aidsinfo.nih.gov/contentfiles/Pediatric_OI.pdf

Centers for Disease Control and Prevention (CDC), "Guidelines for Treatment of Malaria in the United States," Treatment Table Update, July 1, 2013. Available at http://www.cdc.gov/malaria/resources/pdf/treatmenttable.pdf

Centers for Disease Control and Prevention (CDC), "Treatment of Malaria (Guidelines for Clinicians)." July 2013b. Available at http://www.cdc.gov/malaria/resources/pdf/clinicalguidance.pdf

Dubos F, Delattre P, Demer M, et al, "Safety of Mefloquine in Infants With Acute Falciparum Malaria," *Pediatr Infect Dis J*, 2004, 23 (7):679-81.

Fryauff DJ, Owusu-agyei S, Utz G, et al, "Mefloquine Treatment for Uncomplicated Falciparum Malaria in Young Children 6-24 months of Age in Northern Ghana," *Am J Trop Med Hyg*, 2007, 76 (2):224-31.

Price R, Simpson JA, Teja-Isavatharm P, et al. Pharmacokinetics of mefloquine combined with artesunate in children with acute falciparum malaria. *Antimicrob Agents Chemother*. 1999;43(2):341-346.

Red Book: 2009 Report of the Committee on Infectious Diseases, "Drugs for Parasitic Infections," 28th ed, Pickering LK, ed, Elk Grove Village, IL: American Academy of Pediatrics, 2009, 783-816.

Red Book: 2012 Report of the Committee on Infectious Diseases, 29th ed, Pickering LK, ed, Elk Grove Village, IL: American Academy of Pediatrics, 2012.

◆ **Mefloquine Hydrochloride** *see* Mefloquine *on page 1321*

◆ **Mefoxin** *see* CefOXitin *on page 408*

◆ **Mega-C/A Plus** see Ascorbic Acid on page 206
◆ **Megace ES** see Megestrol on page 1324
◆ **Megace Oral** see Megestrol on page 1324
◆ **Megace OS (Can)** see Megestrol on page 1324
◆ **Megadophilus® [OTC]** see Lactobacillus on page 1191

Megestrol (me JES trole)

Medication Safety Issues
Sound-alike/look-alike issues:
Megace may be confused with Reglan
Megestrol may be confused with mesalamine
BEERS Criteria medication:
This drug may be potentially inappropriate for use in geriatric patients (Quality of evidence - moderate; Strength of recommendation - strong).

Related Information
Safe Handling of Hazardous Drugs on page 2419
Brand Names: U.S. Megace ES; Megace Oral
Brand Names: Canada Megace OS; Megestrol
Therapeutic Category Antineoplastic Agent, Miscellaneous; Progestin
Generic Availability (U.S.) Yes
Use Appetite stimulation and promotion of weight gain in cachexia (particularly in HIV patients) which is unresponsive to nutritional supplementation; palliative treatment of breast and endometrial carcinomas
Pregnancy Risk Factor D (tablet) / X (suspension)
Pregnancy Considerations Adverse events were demonstrated in animal reproduction studies. May cause fetal harm if administered to a pregnant woman. Use during pregnancy is contraindicated (suspension) and appropriate contraception is recommended in women who may become pregnant. In clinical studies, megestrol was shown to cause breakthrough vaginal bleeding in women.
Breast-Feeding Considerations Megestrol is excreted into breast milk. Information is available from five nursing women, ~8 weeks postpartum, who were administered megestrol 4 mg in combination with ethinyl estradiol 50 mcg daily for contraception. Maternal serum and milk samples were obtained over 5 days, beginning 10 days after therapy began. The highest concentrations of megestrol were found at the samples taken 3 hours after the maternal dose. Mean concentrations of megestrol were 6.5 ng/mL (maternal serum; range: 3.7 to 10.8 ng/mL), 4.6 ng/mL (foremilk; range: 1.1 to 12.7 ng/mL), and 5.6 ng/mL (hindmilk; range: 1.2 to 18.5 ng/mL) (Nilsson, 1977). Due to the potential for adverse reaction in the newborn, the manufacturer recommends discontinuing breast-feeding while receiving megestrol. In addition, in the United States, where formula is accessible, affordable, safe, and sustainable, and the risk of infant mortality due to diarrhea and respiratory infections is low, complete avoidance of breast-feeding by HIV-infected women is recommended to decrease potential transmission of HIV (DHHS [perinatal], 2012).
Contraindications Hypersensitivity to megestrol or any component; pregnancy (known or suspected); concomitant use with dofetilide
Warnings Hazardous agent; use appropriate precautions for handling and disposal (NIOSH, 2012). May cause fetal harm when administered during pregnancy; women of childbearing age should use appropriate contraceptive measures. May suppress HPA axis during chronic administration; acute adrenal insufficiency may occur with abrupt withdrawal after long-term use or with stress; withdrawal or discontinuation of megestrol should be done carefully. Consider providing exogenous glucocorticoids during periods of stress or severe infection.

Oral suspensions contain sodium benzoate; benzoic acid (benzoate) is a metabolite of benzyl alcohol; large amounts of benzyl alcohol (≥99 mg/kg/day) have been associated with a potentially fatal toxicity ("gasping syndrome") in neonates; in vitro and animal studies have shown that benzoate, a metabolite of benzyl alcohol, displaces bilirubin from protein-binding sites; avoid use of products containing sodium benzoate in neonates. Megestrol may inhibit the elimination of dofetilide resulting in increased dofetilide plasma concentrations and potential serious ventricular arrhythmias associated with QT interval prolongation; concomitant use with dofetilide is not recommended. Megestrol may reduce indinavir serum levels resulting in a need for increase in indinavir dose.
Precautions Use with caution in patients with history of thromboembolic disease; use caution in patients with diabetes mellitus as increased insulin requirements have been reported in association with megestrol use

Adverse Reactions
Cardiovascular: Cardiac failure, cardiomyopathy, chest pain, edema, hypertension, palpitations, peripheral edema
Central nervous system: Abnormality in thinking, carpal tunnel syndrome, confusion, convulsions, depression, headache, hypoesthesia, insomnia, lethargy, malaise, mood change, neuropathy, pain (similar to placebo), paresthesia
Dermatologic: Alopecia, dermatological disease, diaphoresis, pruritus, skin rash, vesicobullous dermatitis
Endocrine & metabolic: Adrenocortical insufficiency, albuminuria, amenorrhea, Cushing's syndrome, decreased libido, diabetes mellitus, gynecomastia, hot flash, HPA-axis suppression, hypercalcemia, hyperglycemia, increased lactate dehydrogenase, weight gain (not attributed to edema or fluid retention)
Gastrointestinal: Abdominal pain, constipation, diarrhea (similar to placebo), dyspepsia, flatulence, nausea, oral moniliasis, sialorrhea, vomiting, xerostomia
Genitourinary: Breakthrough bleeding, impotence, urinary frequency, urinary incontinence, urinary tract infection
Hematologic & oncologic: Leukopenia, sarcoma, tumor flare
Hepatic: Hepatomegaly
Infection: Candidiasis, herpes virus infection, infection
Neuromuscular & skeletal: Weakness
Ophthalmic: Amblyopia
Respiratory: Cough, dyspnea, hyperventilation, pharyngitis, pneumonia, pulmonary disorder
Miscellaneous: Fever
Rare but important or life-threatening: Decreased glucose tolerance, thromboembolic phenomena (including deep vein thrombosis, pulmonary embolism, thrombophlebitis)

Drug Interactions
Metabolism/Transport Effects None known.
Avoid Concomitant Use
Avoid concomitant use of Megestrol with any of the following: Dofetilide; Indium 111 Capromab Pendetide; Ulipristal
Increased Effect/Toxicity
Megestrol may increase the levels/effects of: Dofetilide

The levels/effects of Megestrol may be increased by: Herbs (Progestogenic Properties)
Decreased Effect
Megestrol may decrease the levels/effects of: Anticoagulants; Indium 111 Capromab Pendetide

The levels/effects of Megestrol may be decreased by: Aminoglutethimide; Ulipristal

Stability Hazardous agent; use appropriate precautions for handling and disposal (NIOSH, 2012). Store tablets and oral suspension at room temperature; protect from heat.

Mechanism of Action A synthetic progestin with antiestrogenic properties which disrupt the estrogen receptor cycle. Megestrol interferes with the normal estrogen cycle and results in a lower LH titer. May also have a direct effect on the endometrium. Megestrol is an antineoplastic progestin thought to act through an antileutenizing effect mediated via the pituitary. May stimulate appetite by antagonizing the metabolic effects of catabolic cytokines.

Pharmacodynamics Onset of action:

Antineoplastic: 2 months of continuous therapy

Weight gain: 2-4 weeks

Pharmacokinetics (Adult data unless noted)

Absorption: Well absorbed

Metabolism: In the liver

Half-life: Adults: 10-120 hours

Time to peak serum concentration:

Tablet: 2-3 hours

Suspension: 3-5 hours

Elimination: In urine (57% to 78%) and feces (8% to 30%) within 10 days

Dosing: Usual Oral: **Note:** Megace® ES is not equivalent mg per mg with other megestrol formulations (625 mg Megace® ES is equivalent to 800 mg megestrol tablets or suspension).

Appetite stimulant in cachexia: Titrate dosage to response; decrease dose if weight gain is excessive:

Children: Limited data has been reported in cachectic children with cystic fibrosis, HIV, and solid tumors: Megestrol (tablets or 40 mg/mL suspension): 7.5-10 mg/kg/day in 1-4 divided doses; not to exceed 800 mg/day or 15 mg/kg/day

Adolescents and Adults:

Megestrol (tablets or 40 mg/mL suspension): 800 mg/day in 1-4 divided doses; titrate dose to response; doses between 400-800 mg/day have been clinically effective

Megace® ES: 625 mg once daily

Breast carcinoma: Female Adults: Megestrol (tablets or 40 mg/mL suspension): 40 mg 4 times/day

Endometrial carcinoma: Female Adults: Megestrol (tablets or 40 mg/mL suspension): 40-320 mg/day in divided doses; not to exceed 800 mg/day

Uterine bleeding: Female Adults: Megestrol (tablets or 40 mg/mL suspension): 40 mg 2-4 times/day

Administration Hazardous agent; use appropriate precautions for handling and disposal (NIOSH, 2012).

Oral: Shake oral suspension well before administering; administer without regard to food

Monitoring Parameters Monitor for signs of thromboembolic phenomena and adrenal axis suppression

Appetite stimulation: Weight, caloric intake, basal cortisol level

Antineoplastic: Tumor response

Dosage Forms Excipient information presented when available (limited, particularly for generics); consult specific product labeling.

Suspension, Oral, as acetate:

Megace ES: 625 mg/5 mL (150 mL) [contains alcohol, usp, sodium benzoate; lemon-lime flavor]

Megace Oral: 40 mg/mL (240 mL) [lemon-lime flavor]

Generic: 40 mg/mL (10 mL, 240 mL, 480 mL); 400 mg/10 mL (10 mL)

Tablet, Oral, as acetate:

Generic: 20 mg, 40 mg

References

DHHS Panel on Treatment of HIV-Infected Pregnant Women and Prevention of Perinatal Transmission. Recommendations for use of antiretroviral drugs in pregnant HIV-1-infected women for maternal health and interventions to reduce perinatal HIV transmission in the United States. July 31, 2012. Available at http://aidsinfo.nih.gov/contentfiles/lvguidelines/perinatalgl.pdf

Eubanks V, Koppersmith N, Wooldridge N, et al, "Effects of Megestrol Acetate on Weight Gain, Body Composition, and Pulmonary Function in Patients With Cystic Fibrosis," *J Pediatr*, 2002, 140(4):439-44.

Nasr SZ, Hurwitz ME, Brown RW, et al, "Treatment of Anorexia and Weight Loss With Megestrol Acetate in Patients With Cystic Fibrosis," *Pediatr Pulmonol*, 1999, 28(5):380-2.

National Institute for Occupational Safety and Health (NIOSH), "NIOSH List of Antineoplastic and Other Hazardous Drugs in Healthcare Settings 2012." Available at http://www.cdc.gov/niosh/docs/2012-150/pdfs/2012-150.pdf. Accessed January 21, 2013.

Nilsson S, Nygren KG, Johansson ED. Megestrol acetate concentrations in plasma and milk during administration of an oral contraceptive containing 4 mg megestrol acetate to nursing women. *Contraception*. 1977;16(6):615-24.

Stockheim JA, Daaboul JJ, Yogev R, et al, "Adrenal Suppression in Children With the Human Immunodeficiency Virus Treated With Megestrol Acetate," *J Pediatr*, 1999, 134(3):368-70.

Tchekmedyian NS, Hickman M, and Heber D, "Treatment of Anorexia and Weight Loss With Megestrol Acetate in Patients With Cancer or Acquired Immunodeficiency Syndrome," *Semin Oncol*, 1991, 18(1 Suppl 2):35-42.

◆ **Megestrol Acetate** *see* Megestrol *on page 1324*

◆ **Mellaril** *see* Thioridazine *on page 2012*

Meloxicam (mel OKS i kam)

Medication Safety Issues

BEERS Criteria medication:

This drug may be potentially inappropriate for use in geriatric patients (Quality of evidence - moderate; Strength of recommendation - strong).

Brand Names: U.S. Meloxicam Comfort Pac; Mobic

Brand Names: Canada Apo-Meloxicam; Auro-Meloxicam; Ava-Meloxicam; CO Meloxicam; Dom-Meloxicam; Mobicox; Mylan-Meloxicam; PHL-Meloxicam; PMS-Meloxicam; ratio-Meloxicam; Teva-Meloxicam

Therapeutic Category Analgesic, Non-narcotic; Anti-inflammatory Agent; Nonsteroidal Anti-inflammatory Drug (NSAID), Oral

Generic Availability (U.S.) May be product dependent

Use Relief of signs and symptoms of pauciarticular or polyarticular juvenile idiopathic arthritis (JIA) (FDA approved in ages ≥2 years); relief of signs and symptoms of osteoarthritis and rheumatoid arthritis (FDA approved in adults)

Medication Guide Available Yes

Pregnancy Risk Factor C / D ≥30 weeks gestation

Pregnancy Considerations Adverse events were not observed in the initial animal reproduction studies; therefore, the manufacturer classifies meloxicam as pregnancy category C (category D: ≥30 weeks gestation). Meloxicam crosses the placenta. NSAID exposure during the first trimester is not strongly associated with congenital malformations; however, cardiovascular anomalies and cleft palate have been observed following NSAID exposure in some studies. The use of an NSAID close to conception may be associated with an increased risk of miscarriage. Nonteratogenic effects have been observed following NSAID administration during the third trimester including myocardial degenerative changes, prenatal constriction of the ductus arteriosus, fetal tricuspid regurgitation, failure of the ductus arteriosus to close postnatally; renal dysfunction or failure, oligohydramnios; gastrointestinal bleeding or perforation, increased risk of necrotizing enterocolitis; intracranial bleeding (including intraventricular hemorrhage), platelet dysfunction with resultant bleeding; pulmonary hypertension. Because they may cause premature closure of the ductus arteriosus, use of NSAIDs late in pregnancy should be avoided (use after 31 or 32 weeks gestation is not recommended by some clinicians). Product labeling for Mobic specifically notes that use at ≥30 weeks gestation should be avoided and therefore classifies meloxicam as pregnancy category D at this time. The ▶

◀ chronic use of NSAIDs in women of reproductive age may be associated with infertility that is reversible upon discontinuation of the medication.

Breast-Feeding Considerations It is not known whether meloxicam is excreted in human milk. Breast-feeding is not recommended by the manufacturer.

Contraindications Hypersensitivity to meloxicam or any component; history of asthma, urticaria, or allergic-type reaction to aspirin or other NSAIDs; patients with the "aspirin triad" [asthma, rhinitis (with or without nasal polyps), and aspirin intolerance] (fatal asthmatic and anaphylactoid reactions may occur in these patients); perioperative pain in the setting of coronary artery bypass graft (CABG)

Warnings NSAIDs are associated with an increased risk of adverse cardiovascular thrombotic events, including potentially fatal MI and stroke **[U.S. Boxed Warning]**. Risk may be increased with duration of use or preexisting cardiovascular risk factors or disease. Carefully evaluate individual cardiovascular risk profiles prior to prescribing. To reduce the risk of cardiovascular events, use the lowest effective dose for the shortest duration of time, taking into consideration individual patient treatment goals; alternate therapies should be considered for patients at high risk. Use is contraindicated for treatment of perioperative pain in the setting of CABG surgery **[U.S. Boxed Warning]**; an increased incidence of MI and stroke was found in patients receiving COX-2 selective NSAIDs for the treatment of pain within the first 10-14 days after CABG surgery. NSAIDs may cause fluid retention, edema, and new onset or worsening of preexisting hypertension; use with caution in patients with hypertension, CHF, or fluid retention. Concurrent administration of ibuprofen, and potentially other nonselective NSAIDs, may interfere with aspirin's cardioprotective effect.

NSAIDs may increase the risk of gastrointestinal inflammation, ulceration, bleeding, and perforation **[U.S. Boxed Warning]**. These events, which can be potentially fatal, may occur at any time during therapy and without warning. Avoid the use of NSAIDs in patients with active GI bleeding or ulcer disease. Use NSAIDs with extreme caution in patients with a history of GI bleeding or ulcers (these patients have a 10-fold increased risk for developing a GI bleed). Use NSAIDs with caution in patients with other risk factors which may increase GI bleeding (eg, concurrent therapy with aspirin, anticoagulants, and/or corticosteroids, longer duration of NSAID use, smoking, use of alcohol, and poor general health). Use the lowest effective dose for the shortest duration of time, taking into consideration individual patient treatment goals; alternate therapies should be considered for patients at high risk.

NSAIDs may compromise existing renal function; dose-dependent decreases in prostaglandin synthesis may result from NSAID use, reducing renal blood flow which may cause renal decompensation. Patients with impaired renal function, dehydration, heart failure, liver dysfunction, and in those taking diuretics and ACE inhibitors are at greatest risk of renal toxicity; use with caution in these patients; monitor renal function closely. Rehydrate patient before starting therapy. NSAIDs are not recommended for use in patients with advanced renal disease. Long-term use of NSAIDs may cause renal papillary necrosis and other renal injury.

Anaphylactoid reactions may occur, even in patients without prior exposure; patients with "aspirin triad" [bronchial asthma, aspirin intolerance, and rhinitis (with or without nasal polyps)] are at increased risk; use is contraindicated in these patients. Do not use in patients who experience bronchospasm, asthma, rhinitis, or urticaria with NSAID or aspirin therapy. NSAIDs may cause serious and potentially fatal dermatologic adverse reactions including exfoliative

dermatitis, Stevens-Johnson syndrome, and toxic epidermal necrolysis; discontinue use at first sign of skin rash or hypersensitivity. Avoid use of NSAIDs in late pregnancy (beginning at 30 weeks gestation) as they may cause premature closure of the ductus arteriosus. NSAIDs may mask fever and inflammation and thus decrease the ability of these signs to help diagnose infectious conditions.

Oral suspension contains sodium benzoate; benzoic acid (benzoate) is a metabolite of benzyl alcohol; large amounts of benzyl alcohol (≥99 mg/kg/day) have been associated with a potentially fatal toxicity ("gasping syndrome") in neonates; avoid use of meloxicam products containing sodium benzoate in neonates; *in vitro* and animal studies have shown that benzoate displaces bilirubin from protein binding sites. Oral suspension formulation may contain sorbitol; concomitant use of sorbitol-containing products and sodium polystyrene sulfonate (Kayexalate®) may cause intestinal necrosis (including fatal cases); combined use should be avoided.

Precautions Use with caution in patients with decreased hepatic function; meloxicam is significantly metabolized in the liver; closely monitor patients with abnormal LFTs; severe hepatic reactions [eg, fulminant hepatitis, jaundice, liver failure (some cases fatal)] have occurred with NSAID use, rarely; discontinue if signs or symptoms of liver disease develop, or if systemic manifestations (eg, eosinophilia, rash, abdominal pain, diarrhea, dark urine) occur. Use with caution in patients with asthma; asthmatic patients may have aspirin-sensitive asthma which may be associated with severe and potentially fatal bronchospasm when aspirin or NSAIDs are administered. Anemia (due to occult or gross blood loss from the GI tract, fluid retention, or other effect on erythropoiesis) may occur; monitor hemoglobin and hematocrit in patients receiving long-term therapy. Use with caution and monitor carefully in patients with coagulation disorders or those receiving anticoagulants; NSAIDs inhibit platelet aggregation and may prolong bleeding time. Pediatric patients ≥2 years may experience a higher frequency of some adverse effects than adults, including the following: Abdominal pain, diarrhea, fever, headache, and vomiting.

Adverse Reactions

Cardiovascular: Edema

Central nervous system: Dizziness, headache

Dermatologic: Pruritus, rash

Gastrointestinal: Abdominal pain, diarrhea, dyspepsia, flatulence, nausea

Genitourinary: Micturition, urinary tract infection

Respiratory: Cough, pharyngitis, upper respiratory infection

Miscellaneous: Falls, flu-like syndrome

Rare but important or life-threatening: Abnormal dreams, abnormal vision, agranulocytosis, albuminuria, allergic reaction, alopecia, anaphylactoid reactions, angina, angioedema, anxiety, appetite increased, arrhythmia, asthma, bilirubinemia, bronchospasm, bullous eruption, BUN increased, cardiac failure, colitis, confusion, conjunctivitis, creatinine increased, dehydration, depression, diaphoresis, duodenal perforation, duodenal ulcer, dyspnea, edema (facial), eructation, erythema multiforme, esophagitis, exfoliative dermatitis, fatigue, fever, gastric perforation, gastric ulcer, gastritis, gastroesophageal reflux, gastrointestinal hemorrhage, GGT increased, hematemesis, hematuria, hepatic failure, hepatitis, hot flushes, hyper-/hypotension, interstitial nephritis, intestinal perforation, jaundice, leukopenia, malaise, melena, MI, mood alterations, nervousness, palpitation, pancreatitis, paresthesia, photosensitivity reaction, pruritus, purpura, renal failure, seizure, shock, somnolence, Stevens-Johnson syndrome, syncope, tachycardia, taste perversion, thrombocytopenia, tinnitus, toxic epidermal necrolysis, transaminases increased, tremor, ulcerative stomatitis, urinary retention (acute), urticaria, vasculitis, vertigo, xerostomia, weight gain/loss

Drug Interactions

Metabolism/Transport Effects Substrate of CYP3A4 (minor); **Note:** Assignment of Major/Minor substrate status based on clinically relevant drug interaction potential; **Inhibits** CYP2C9 (weak)

Avoid Concomitant Use

Avoid concomitant use of Meloxicam with any of the following: Calcium Polystyrene Sulfonate; Floctafenine; Ketorolac (Nasal); Ketorolac (Systemic); NSAID (COX-2 Inhibitor); Omacetaxine; Sodium Polystyrene Sulfonate; Urokinase

Increased Effect/Toxicity

Meloxicam may increase the levels/effects of: 5-ASA Derivatives; Agents with Antiplatelet Properties; Aliskiren; Aminoglycosides; Anticoagulants; Apixaban; Bisphosphonate Derivatives; Calcium Polystyrene Sulfonate; Collagenase (Systemic); CycloSPORINE (Systemic); Dabigatran Etexilate; Deferasirox; Desmopressin; Digoxin; Eplerenone; Haloperidol; Ibritumomab; Lithium; Methotrexate; Nonsteroidal Anti-Inflammatory Agents; NSAID (COX-2 Inhibitor); Omacetaxine; PEMEtrexed; Porfimer; Potassium-Sparing Diuretics; PRALAtrexate; Quinolone Antibiotics; Rivaroxaban; Salicylates; Sodium Polystyrene Sulfonate; Tenofovir; Thrombolytic Agents; Tositumomab and Iodine I 131 Tositumomab; Urokinase; Vancomycin; Vitamin K Antagonists

The levels/effects of Meloxicam may be increased by: ACE Inhibitors; Angiotensin II Receptor Blockers; Antidepressants (Tricyclic, Tertiary Amine); Corticosteroids (Systemic); CycloSPORINE (Systemic); Dasatinib; Floctafenine; Glucosamine; Herbs (Anticoagulant/Antiplatelet Properties); Ibrutinib; Ketorolac (Nasal); Ketorolac (Systemic); Multivitamins/Fluoride (with ADE); Multivitamins/Minerals (with ADEK, Folate, Iron); Multivitamins/Minerals (with AE, No Iron); Nonsteroidal Anti-Inflammatory Agents; Omega-3 Fatty Acids; Pentosan Polysulfate Sodium; Pentoxifylline; Probenecid; Prostacyclin Analogues; Selective Serotonin Reuptake Inhibitors; Serotonin/Norepinephrine Reuptake Inhibitors; Sodium Phosphates; Tipranavir; Treprostinil; Vitamin E; Voriconazole

Decreased Effect

Meloxicam may decrease the levels/effects of: ACE Inhibitors; Agents with Antiplatelet Properties; Aliskiren; Angiotensin II Receptor Blockers; Beta-Blockers; Eplerenone; HydrALAZINE; Loop Diuretics; Potassium-Sparing Diuretics; Prostaglandins (Ophthalmic); Salicylates; Selective Serotonin Reuptake Inhibitors; Thiazide Diuretics

The levels/effects of Meloxicam may be decreased by: Bile Acid Sequestrants; Itraconazole; Nonsteroidal Anti-Inflammatory Agents; Salicylates

Stability Store at 25°C (77°F) in tightly closed container; excursions permitted 15°C to 30°C (59°F to 86°F).

Mechanism of Action Reversibly inhibits cyclooxygenase-1 and 2 (COX-1 and 2) enzymes, which results in decreased formation of prostaglandin precursors; has antipyretic, analgesic, and anti-inflammatory properties

Other proposed mechanisms not fully elucidated (and possibly contributing to the anti-inflammatory effect to varying degrees), include inhibiting chemotaxis, altering lymphocyte activity, inhibiting neutrophil aggregation/activation, and decreasing proinflammatory cytokine levels.

Pharmacokinetics (Adult data unless noted)

Distribution:

Children 2-6 years (n=7): Apparent V_d: 0.19 L/kg (Burgos-Vargas, 2004)

Children and Adolescents 7-16 years (n=11): Apparent V_d: 0.13 L/kg (Burgos-Vargas, 2004)

Adults: Vd_{ss}: 10 L

Protein binding: ~99.4% bound, primarily albumin; **Note:** Free fraction was higher in adult patients with renal failure who were receiving chronic dialysis.

Metabolism: Extensive in the liver via CYP2C9 and CYP3A4 (minor); significant biliary and or enteral secretion occurs

Bioavailability: 89%; suspension is bioequivalent to tablets

Half-life elimination:

Children 2-6 years (n=7): 13.4 hours (Burgos-Vargas, 2004)

Children and Adolescents 7-16 years (n=11): 12.7 hours (Burgos-Vargas, 2004)

Adults: 15-20 hours

Time to peak serum concentration:

Children and Adolescents 2-16 years (n=18): Suspension: Initial: 1-3 hours; secondary: 6-12 hours (Burgos-Vargas, 2004)

Adults: Initial: 4-5 hours; secondary: 12-14 hours

Elimination: Urine and feces (as inactive metabolites); <1% excreted unchanged in urine

Clearance:

Children 2-6 years (n=7): 0.17 mL/minute/kg (Burgos-Vargas, 2004)

Children and Adolescents 7-16 years (n=11): 0.12 mL/minute/kg (Burgos-Vargas, 2004)

Adults: 7-9 mL/minute

Dosing: Usual Note: To reduce the risk of adverse cardiovascular and GI effects, use the lowest effective dose for the shortest period of time; adjust dose to specific patient's clinical needs.

Children ≥2 years and Adolescents: **Juvenile idiopathic arthritis (JIA):** Oral: 0.125 mg/kg once daily; maximum daily dose: 7.5 mg/**day**; higher doses (up to 0.375 mg/kg/**day**) have not demonstrated additional benefit in clinical trials.

Adults: **Osteoarthritis, rheumatoid arthritis:** Initial: 7.5 mg once daily; some patients may receive additional benefit from an increased dose of 15 mg once daily; maximum daily dose: 15 mg/**day**

Dosing adjustment in renal impairment:

Mild to moderate impairment: Children ≥2 years, Adolescents and Adults: No dosage adjustments are recommended.

Significant impairment (CrCl <20 mL/minute): Children ≥2 years, Adolescents, and Adults: Use is not recommended (has not been studied).

Hemodialysis: Not dialyzable; additional doses are not required after dialysis: Adults: Maximum daily dose: 7.5 mg/**day**

Dosing adjustment in hepatic impairment: Children ≥2 years, Adolescents, and Adults:

Mild to moderate impairment (Child-Pugh class A or B): No dosage adjustments are recommended.

Severe impairment: There are no dosage adjustments provided in the manufacturer's labeling (has not been studied); use with caution; meloxicam is significantly metabolized in the liver.

Administration May be taken with or without meals; administer with food or milk to minimize gastrointestinal irritation. Oral suspension: Shake gently prior to use.

Monitoring Parameters Periodic CBC, liver enzymes, serum BUN and creatinine, signs and symptoms of GI bleeding

Dosage Forms Considerations

Meloxicam Comfort Pac is a kit containing meloxicam oral tablets 15 mg, and Duraflex topical gel.

Dosage Forms Excipient information presented when available (limited, particularly for generics); consult specific product labeling.

Kit, Combination:

Meloxicam Comfort Pac: 15 mg [contains methylparaben, trolamine (triethanolamine)]

Suspension, Oral:
Mobic: 7.5 mg/5 mL (100 mL) [contains saccharin sodium, sodium benzoate; raspberry flavor]
Generic: 7.5 mg/5 mL (100 mL)
Tablet, Oral:
Mobic: 7.5 mg, 15 mg
Generic: 7.5 mg, 15 mg

References

Burgos-Vargas R, Foeldvari I, Thon A, et al, "Pharmacokinetics of Meloxicam in Patients With Juvenile Rheumatoid Arthritis," *J Clin Pharmacol*, 2004, 44(8):866-72.

Ruperto N, Nikishina I, Pachanov ED, et al, "A Randomized, Double-Blind Clinical Trial of Two Doses of Meloxicam Compared With Naproxen in Children With Juvenile Idiopathic Arthritis: Short- and Long-Term Efficacy and Safety Results," *Arthritis Rheum*, 2005, 52 (2):563-72.

◆ **Meloxicam Comfort Pac** *see* Meloxicam *on page 1325*

Melphalan (MEL fa lan)

Medication Safety Issues
Sound-alike/look-alike issues:
Melphalan may be confused with Mephyton®, Myleran® Alkeran® may be confused with Alferon®, Leukeran®, Myleran®

High alert medication:
This medication is in a class the Institute for Safe Medication Practices (ISMP) includes among its list of drug classes which have a heightened risk of causing significant patient harm when used in error.

Related Information
Emetogenic Potential of Antineoplastic Agents in Children *on page 2327*
Management of Drug Extravasations *on page 2255*
Safe Handling of Hazardous Drugs *on page 2419*

Brand Names: U.S. Alkeran
Brand Names: Canada Alkeran®
Therapeutic Category Antineoplastic Agent, Alkylating Agent; Antineoplastic Agent, Alkylating Agent (Nitrogen Mustard)
Generic Availability (U.S.) May be product dependent

Use
Oral: Palliative treatment of multiple myeloma and non-resectable epithelial ovarian carcinoma (FDA approved in adults)
Parenteral: Palliative treatment of multiple myeloma for whom oral therapy is not appropriate (FDA approved in adults); has also been used as part of a conditioning regimen for autologous hematopoietic stem cell transplantation

Pregnancy Risk Factor D
Pregnancy Considerations Animal studies have demonstrated embryotoxicity and teratogenicity. Therapy may suppress ovarian function leading to amenorrhea. There are no adequate and well-controlled studies in pregnant women. May cause fetal harm if administered during pregnancy. Women of childbearing potential should be advised to avoid pregnancy while on melphalan therapy.

Breast-Feeding Considerations According to the manufacturer, melphalan should not be administered if breast-feeding.

Contraindications Hypersensitivity to melphalan or any component; patients whose disease was resistant to prior melphalan therapy

Warnings Hazardous agent; use appropriate precautions for handling and disposal (NIOSH, 2012). Produces chromosomal changes; potentially mutagenic and leukemogenic **[U.S. Boxed Warning]**. Secondary malignancies (including acute myeloid leukemia, myeloproliferative disease, and carcinoma) have been reported (some patients were receiving combination chemotherapy or radiation therapy); the risk is increased with increased treatment duration and cumulative doses.

Bone marrow suppression is common; may be severe and result in infection or bleeding; has been demonstrated more with the I.V. formulation compared to oral **[U.S. Boxed Warning]**; myelosuppression is dose-related. Monitor blood counts; may require treatment delay or dose modification for thrombocytopenia or neutropenia. Use with caution in patients with prior bone marrow suppression, impaired renal function (consider dose reduction), or who have received prior (or concurrent) chemotherapy or irradiation. Myelotoxicity is generally reversible, although irreversible bone marrow failure has been reported. Signs of infection, such as fever and WBC rise, may not occur; lethargy and confusion may be more prominent signs of infection. In patients who are candidates for autologous transplantation, avoid melphalan containing regimens prior to transplant (due to the effects on stem cell reserve).

Hypersensitivity (including anaphylaxis) has been reported in ~2% of patients receiving I.V. melphalan **[U.S. Boxed Warning]**; discontinue infusion and treat symptomatically; hypersensitivity may occur after multiple treatment cycles and may also occur (rarely) with oral melphalan; do not readminister (oral or I.V.) in patients who experience hypersensitivity.

Abnormal liver function tests may occur; hepatitis and jaundice have also been reported; hepatic sinusoidal obstruction syndrome [SOS; formerly called veno-occlusive disease (VOD)] has been reported with I.V. melphalan. Pulmonary fibrosis and interstitial pneumonitis (some fatal) have been observed with treatment.

Suppresses ovarian function and produces amenorrhea; may also cause testicular suppression.

The injection contains propylene glycol and ethanol; toxicities have been reported with use of products containing propylene glycol, including hyperosmolality, lactic acidosis, seizures, and respiratory depression; in neonates large amounts of propylene glycol delivered orally, intravenously (eg, >3000 mg/day), or topically have been associated with potentially fatal toxicities which can include metabolic acidosis, seizures, renal failure, and CNS depression; use injection containing propylene glycol with caution (AAP, 1997; Shehab, 2009).

Precautions Gastrointestinal toxicities, including nausea, vomiting, diarrhea, and mucositis, are common. When administering high-dose melphalan in autologous transplantation, cryotherapy is recommended to prevent mucositis in adults (Keefe, 2007). Dosage reduction is recommended with I.V. melphalan in patients with renal impairment; reduced initial doses may also be recommended with oral melphalan. Closely monitor patients with azotemia. Avoid administration of live vaccines to immunocompromised patients. Cross-sensitivity may exist between melphalan and chlorambucil. Extravasation may cause local tissue damage; administration by slow injection into a fast running I.V. solution into an injection port or via a central line is recommended; do not administer directly into a peripheral veins. Should be administered under the supervision of a physician experienced with cancer chemotherapy **[U.S. Boxed Warning]**.

Adverse Reactions
Gastrointestinal: Nausea, diarrhea, oral ulceration, vomiting
Hematologic: Anemia, leukopenia (nadir: 14-21 days; recovery: 28-35 days), myelosuppression, thrombocytopenia (nadir: 14-21 days; recovery: 28-35 days)
Miscellaneous: Hypersensitivity (includes bronchospasm, dyspnea, edema, hypotension, pruritus, rash, tachycardia, urticaria); secondary malignancy (cumulative dose

and duration dependent, includes acute myeloid leukemia, myeloproliferative syndrome, carcinoma)

Rare by important or life-threatening: Agranulocytosis, allergic reactions, alopecia, amenorrhea, anaphylaxis (rare), bleeding (with high-dose therapy),, bone marrow failure (irreversible), BUN increased, cardiac arrest, cardiotoxicity (angina, arrhythmia, hypertension, MI; with high-dose therapy), encephalopathy, hemolytic anemia, hemorrhagic cystitis, hepatic sinusoidal obstruction syndrome (SOS; veno-occlusive disease; high-dose I.V. melphalan), hepatitis, infection, injection site reactions (ulceration, necrosis), interstitial pneumonitis, jaundice, mucositis (with high-dose therapy), ovarian suppression, paralytic ileus (with high-dose therapy), pruritus, pulmonary fibrosis, radiation myelopathy, rash (maculopapular), renal toxicity (with high-dose therapy), seizure (with high-dose therapy), sepsis, SIADH, skin hypersensitivity, sterility, stomatitis, testicular suppression, tingling sensation, transaminases increased, vasculitis, warmth sensation

Drug Interactions

Metabolism/Transport Effects None known.

Avoid Concomitant Use

Avoid concomitant use of Melphalan with any of the following: BCG; CloZAPine; Dipyrone; Nalidixic Acid; Natalizumab; Pimecrolimus; Tacrolimus (Topical); Tofacitinib; Vaccines (Live)

Increased Effect/Toxicity

Melphalan may increase the levels/effects of: Carmustine; CloZAPine; CycloSPORINE (Systemic); Leflunomide; Natalizumab; Tofacitinib; Vaccines (Live); Vitamin K Antagonists

The levels/effects of Melphalan may be increased by: Denosumab; Dipyrone; Nalidixic Acid; Pimecrolimus; Roflumilast; Tacrolimus (Topical); Trastuzumab

Decreased Effect

Melphalan may decrease the levels/effects of: BCG; Cardiac Glycosides; Coccidioidin Skin Test; Sipuleucel-T; Vaccines (Inactivated); Vaccines (Live); Vitamin K Antagonists

The levels/effects of Melphalan may be decreased by: Echinacea

Food Interactions Food interferes with oral absorption. Management: Administer on an empty stomach.

Stability Hazardous agent; use appropriate precautions for handling and disposal (NIOSH, 2012).

Tablet: Store at 2°C to 8°C (36°F to 46°F); protect from light

Injection: Store at 15°C to 30°C (59°F to 86°F); protect from light. Dose from reconstituted 5 mg/mL solution should be immediately diluted in NS to a concentration no greater than 0.45 mg/mL (manufacturer recommended concentration) and administration be completed within 60 minutes of reconstitution; do not refrigerate since it may precipitate

Mechanism of Action Alkylating agent which is a derivative of mechlorethamine that inhibits DNA and RNA synthesis via formation of carbonium ions; cross-links strands of DNA; acts on both resting and rapidly dividing tumor cells.

Pharmacokinetics (Adult data unless noted)

Absorption: Oral: Variable and incomplete

Distribution: V_{dss}: 0.5 L/kg; Low penetration into CSF

Protein binding: 53% to 92%; primarily to albumin, 40% to 60% and α_1-acid glycoprotein (20%)

Metabolism: Hepatic; chemical hydrolysis to mono- or dihydroxymelphalan

Bioavailability: Oral: Variable; ranges from 56% to 93% depending on the presence of food (exposure is reduced with a high-fat meal)

Half-life, terminal: I.V.: 75 minutes; Oral: 1 to 2 hours

Time to peak serum concentration: Oral: Within 2 hours

Elimination: Oral: Feces (20% to 50%); urine (~10% as unchanged drug)

Dosing: Usual Refer to individual protocols; details concerning dosing in combination regimens should also be consulted; adjust dose based on patient response and weekly blood counts.

Pediatric: **Hematopoietic stem cell transplantation, conditioning regimen for autologous HSCT:** Infants, Children, and Adolescents:

Cantete, 2009, Oberlin 2006: I.V.: 140 mg/m² 2 days prior to transplantation (combined with busulfan)

Pritchard, 2005: I.V.: 180 mg/m² (with pre- and posthydration) 12 to 30 hours prior to transplantation

Berthold, 2005: I.V.: 45 mg/m²/day for 4 days starting 8 days prior to transplantation (combined with busulfan or etoposide and carboplatin)

Adult:

Multiple myeloma (palliative treatment): Note: Response is gradual; may require repeated courses to realize benefit:

Oral:

6 mg (3 tablets) once daily for 2 to 3 weeks initially, followed by up to 4 weeks rest (melphalan-free period); then a maintenance dose of 2 mg once daily as hematologic recovery begins **or**

0.15 mg/kg/day for 7 days with a 2- to 6-week rest (melphalan-free period); followed by a maintenance dose of ≤0.05 mg/kg/day as hematologic recovery begins **or**

0.25 mg/kg/day for 4 days (or 0.2 mg/kg/day for 5 days); repeat at 4- to 6-week intervals as ANC and platelet counts return to normal **or**

10 mg once daily for 7 to 10 days, institute 2 mg once daily maintenance dose after WBC >4000 cells/mm³ and platelets >100,000 cells/mm³ (~4 to 8 weeks); titrate maintenance dose to hematologic response

I.V.: 16 mg/m²/dose every 2 weeks for 4 doses, then repeat at 4-week intervals after adequate hematologic recovery

Ovarian carcinoma: Oral: 0.2 mg/kg once daily for 5 days, repeat every 4 to 5 weeks

Dosing adjustment in renal impairment: Adults:

Manufacturer's labeling:

Oral: Moderate to severe renal impairment: Consider a reduced dose initially

I.V.: BUN ≥30 mg/dL: Reduce dose by 50%

The following guidelines have been used by some clinicians:

Aronoff, 2007 (based on a 6 mg once daily dose):

CrCl >50 mL/minute: No dosage adjustment required

CrCl 10 to 50 mL/minute: Administer 75% of dose

CrCl <10 mL/minute: Administer 50% of dose

Hemodialysis: Administer dose after hemodialysis.

Continuous ambulatory peritoneal dialysis (CAPD): Administer 50% of dose.

Continuous renal replacement therapy (CRRT): Administer 75% of dose.

Kintzel, 1995:

Oral: Adjust dose in the presence of hematologic toxicity

I.V.:

CrCl 46 to 60 mL/minute: Administer 85% of normal dose.

CrCl 31 to 45 mL/minute: Administer 75% of normal dose.

CrCl <30 mL/minute: Administer 70% of normal dose.

Dosing adjustment in hepatic impairment: Adults: There are no dosage adjustments provided in the manufacturer's labeling; however, dosage adjustment does not appear to be necessary (King, 2001).

Dosing adjustment for toxicity:

Oral:

WBC <3000/mm^3: Withhold treatment until recovery

Platelets <100,000/mm^3: Withhold treatment until recovery

Parenteral: I.V.: Adjust dose based on nadir blood cell counts

Administration Hazardous agent; use appropriate precautions for handling and disposal (NIOSH, 2012).

Oral: Administer on an empty stomach; 1 hour prior to or 2 hours after meals.

Parenteral: I.V.: Stability is limited; must be prepared freshly; the time between reconstitution/dilution and administration of parenteral melphalan must be kept to a minimum (manufacturer recommends completing infusion within <60 minutes) because reconstituted and diluted solutions are unstable. Reconstitute 50 mg vial for injection initially with provided 10 mL diluent to yield a 5 mg/mL solution; shake immediately and vigorously to dissolve; immediately dilute the reconstituted solution with NS to a final concentration not to exceed 0.45 mg/mL; administer by I.V. infusion typically over 15 to 30 minutes and some centers suggest at a rate not to exceed 10 mg/minute; complete administration of I.V. dose should occur within 60 minutes of reconstitution.

Extravasation may cause local tissue damage; administration by slow injection into a fast running I.V. solution into an injection port or via a central line is recommended; do not administer by direct injection into a peripheral vein.

Vesicant/Extravasation Risk May be an irritant

Monitoring Parameters CBC with differential and platelet count (at the start of therapy and prior to each subsequent dose); serum electrolytes; serum uric acid; monitor infusion site for redness and irritation

Test Interactions False-positive Coombs' test [direct]

Dosage Forms Excipient information presented when available (limited, particularly for generics); consult specific product labeling.

Solution Reconstituted, Intravenous:

Alkeran: 50 mg (1 ea) [contains alcohol, usp, propylene glycol]

Generic: 50 mg (1 ea)

Tablet, Oral:

Alkeran: 2 mg

References

Alkeran (melphalan) [prescribing information]. Research Triangle Park, NC: GlaxoSmithKline.

Alkeran (melphalan hydrochloride) [prescribing information]. Research Triangle Park, NC: GlaxoSmithKline.

American Academy of Pediatrics Committee on Drugs. "Inactive" ingredients in pharmaceutical products: update (subject review). *Pediatrics.* 1997;99(2):268-278.

Aronoff GR, Bennett WM, Berns JS, et al, *Drug Prescribing in Renal Failure: Dosing Guidelines for Adults and Children,* 5th ed. Philadelphia, PA: American College of Physicians, 2007, 97, 177.

Berthold F, Boos J, Burdach S, et al, "Myeloablative Megatherapy With Autologous Stem-Cell Rescue Versus Oral Maintenance Chemotherapy as Consolidation Treatment in Patients With High-Risk Neuroblastoma: A Randomised Controlled Trial," *Lancet Oncol,* 2005, 6 (9):649-58.

Canete A, Gerrard M, Rubie H, et al, "Poor Survival for Infants With MYCN-Amplified Metastatic Neuroblastoma Despite Intensified Treatment: The International Society of Paediatric Oncology European Neuroblastoma Experience," *Clin Oncol,* 2009, 27(7):1014-9.

Keefe DM, Schubert MM, Elting LS, et al, "Updated Clinical Practice Guidelines for the Prevention and Treatment of Mucositis," *Cancer,* 2007, 109(5):820-31.

King PD, Perry MC. Hepatotoxicity of chemotherapy. *Oncologist.* 2001;6(2):162-176.

Lazarus HM, Phillips GL, Herzig RH, et al, "High-Dose Melphalan and the Development of Hematopoietic Stem-Cell Transplantation: 25 Years Later," *J Clin Oncol,* 2008, 26(14):2240-3.

Moreau P, Facon T, Attal M, et al, "Comparison of 200 mg/m(2) Melphalan and 8 Gy Total Body Irradiation Plus 140 mg/m(2) Melphalan as Conditioning Regimens for Peripheral Blood Stem Cell Transplantation in Patients With Newly Diagnosed Multiple Myeloma: Final Analysis of the Intergroupe Francophone du Myélome 9502 Randomized Trial," *Blood,* 2002, 99(3):731-5.

Nath CE, Shaw PJ, Montgomery K, et al, "Population Pharmacokinetics of Melphalan in Paediatric Blood or Marrow Transplant Recipients," *Br J Clin Pharmacol,* 2007, 64(2):151-64.

National Institute for Occupational Safety and Health (NIOSH), "NIOSH List of Antineoplastic and Other Hazardous Drugs in Healthcare Settings 2012." Available at http://www.cdc.gov/niosh/docs/2012-150/pdfs/2012-150.pdf. Accessed January 21, 2013.

Oberlin O, Rey A, Desfachelles AS, et al, "Impact of High-Dose Busulfan Plus Melphalan as Consolidation in Metastatic Ewing Tumors: A Study by the Société Française des Cancers de l'Enfant," *J Clin Oncol,* 2006, 24(24):3997-4002.

Ozkaynak MF, Sahdev I, Gross TG, et al, "A Pilot Study of Addition of Amifostine to Melphalan, Carboplatin, Etoposide, and Cyclophosphamide With Autologous Hematopoietic Stem Cell Transplantation in Pediatric Solid Tumors - A Pediatric Blood and Marrow Transplant Consortium Study," *J Pediatr Hematol Oncol,* 2008, 30(3):204-9.

Pinguet F, Martel P, Rouanet P, et al, "Effect of Sodium Chloride Concentration and Temperature on Melphalan Stability During Storage and Use," *Am J Hosp Pharm,* 1994, 51(21):2701-4.

Pritchard J, Cotterill SJ, Germond SM, et al, "High Dose Melphalan in the Treatment of Advanced Neuroblastoma: Results of a Randomised Trial (ENSG-1) by the European Neuroblastoma Study Group," *Pediatr Blood Cancer,* 2005, 44(4):348-57.

Schuh A, Dandridge J, Haydon P, et al, "Encephalopathy Complicating High-Dose Melphalan," *Bone Marrow Transplant,* 1999, 24 (10):1141-3.

Shehab N, Lewis CL, Streetman DD, Donn SM. Exposure to the pharmaceutical excipients benzyl alcohol and propylene glycol among critically ill neonates. *Pediatr Crit Care Med.* 2009;10 (2):256-259.

◆ **Menactra** see Meningococcal (Groups A / C / Y and W-135) Diphtheria Conjugate Vaccine *on page 1330*

◆ **MenACWY** see Meningococcal (Groups A / C / Y and W-135) Diphtheria Conjugate Vaccine *on page 1330*

◆ **MenACWY-D (Menactra)** see Meningococcal (Groups A / C / Y and W-135) Diphtheria Conjugate Vaccine *on page 1330*

◆ **MenACWY-CRM (Menveo)** see Meningococcal (Groups A / C / Y and W-135) Diphtheria Conjugate Vaccine *on page 1330*

◆ **Menhibrix** see Meningococcal Polysaccharide (Groups C and Y) and *Haemophilus* b Tetanus Toxoid Conjugate Vaccine *on page 1334*

◆ **Meningococcal Conjugate Vaccine** see Meningococcal (Groups A / C / Y and W-135) Diphtheria Conjugate Vaccine *on page 1330*

Meningococcal (Groups A / C / Y and W-135) Diphtheria Conjugate Vaccine

(me NIN joe kok al groops aye, see, why & dubl yoo won thur tee fyve dif THEER ee a KON joo gate vak SEEN)

Medication Safety Issues

Administration issue:

Menactra (MCV4) should be administered by intramuscular (I.M.) injection only. Inadvertent subcutaneous (SubQ) administration has been reported; possibly due to confusion of this product with Menomune (MPSV4), also a meningococcal polysaccharide vaccine, which is administered by the SubQ route.

Related Information

Immunization Administration Recommendations *on page 2368*

Immunization Guidelines *on page 2373*

Brand Names: U.S. Menactra; Menveo

Brand Names: Canada Menactra; Menveo

Therapeutic Category Vaccine, Inactivated Bacteria

Generic Availability (U.S.) No

Use Provide active immunization against invasive meningococcal disease caused by *N. meningitidis* serogroups A, C, Y, and W-135 (Menactra: FDA approved 9 months to 55 years; Menveo: FDA approved in ages 2 months to 55 years).

The Advisory Committee on Immunization Practices (ACIP) (CDC/ACIP [Cohn, 2013]) recommends routine vaccination of:
- Children and adolescents aged 11 to 18 years of age
- Persons ≥2 months of age who are at increased risk of meningococcal disease
- Persons (in all recommended age groups) at increased risk who are part of outbreaks caused by vaccine preventable serogroups

Those at increased risk of meningococcal disease include:
- Persons ≥2 months of age with medical conditions such as anatomical or functional asplenia or persistent complement component deficiencies (eg, C5-C9, properdin, factor H, or factor D)
- Persons ≥9 months of age that travel to or reside in countries where meningococcal disease is hyperendemic or epidemic, especially if contact with the local population will be prolonged
- Unvaccinated or incompletely vaccinated first year college students living in residence halls
- Military recruits
- Microbiologists with occupational exposure

Pregnancy Risk Factor B/C (manufacturer dependent)

Pregnancy Considerations Animal reproduction studies have not been conducted with Menactra. Limited information is available following inadvertent use of Menactra during pregnancy (Zheteyeva, 2013). Patients should contact the Sanofi Pasteur Inc vaccine registry at 1-800-822-2463 if they are pregnant or become aware they were pregnant at the time of Menactra vaccination.

Adverse events were not observed in animal reproduction studies conducted with Menveo. Limited information is available following inadvertent use of Menveo during pregnancy. Patients should contact the Novartis Vaccines and Diagnostics Inc. pregnancy registry at 1-877-311-8972 if they are pregnant or become aware they were pregnant at the time of Menveo vaccination.

Inactivated bacterial vaccines have not been shown to cause increased risks to the fetus (CDC, 60[2], 2011). Pregnancy should not preclude vaccination if indicated (CDC, 62[2], 2013).

Breast-Feeding Considerations It is not known if this vaccine is found in breast milk. The manufacturer recommends that caution be used if administered to a nursing woman. Inactivated vaccines do not affect the safety of breast-feeding for the mother or the infant. Breast-feeding infants should be vaccinated according to the recommended schedules (CDC, 60[2], 2011).

Contraindications Hypersensitivity to any component, including diphtheria toxoid or CRM$_{197}$ (a diphtheria toxin carrier protein) or other meningococcal containing vaccines

Warnings Immediate treatment (including epinephrine 1:1000) for anaphylactic and/or hypersensitivity reactions should be available during vaccine use; Guillain-Barré syndrome has been reported in a temporal relationship following Menactra administration; the risk of developing Guillain-Barré syndrome may be increased following vaccination in persons previously diagnosed with Guillain-Barré syndrome. The risk of developing Guillain-Barré syndrome was evaluated in a study of healthcare claims of persons 11 to 18 years of age (n=~9,600,000; 15% were vaccinated with Menactra); 72 cases of Guillain-Barré syndrome were confirmed and none received the vaccine within 42 days prior to symptoms; 129 reported cases of Guillain-Barré syndrome could not be confirmed or excluded. Data not currently available to assess possible risk of Guillain-Barré syndrome following use of Menveo. Individuals with a previous history of GBS should only receive Menactra after an assessment of risks and benefits; data not currently available to assess possible risk of

GBS following use of Menveo. Apnea has occurred following intramuscular vaccine administration in premature infants; consider clinical status implications. Syncope has been reported with use of injectable vaccines and may be accompanied by transient visual disturbances, weakness, or tonic-clonic movements. Procedures should be in place to avoid injuries from falling and to restore cerebral perfusion if syncope occurs (CDC, 57(17), 2008).

Precautions The decision to administer or delay vaccination because of current or recent febrile illness depends on the severity of symptoms and the etiology of the disease. Immunization should be delayed during the course of an acute severe febrile illness; may administer to patients with mild acute illness (with or without fever). Use with caution in severely immunocompromised patients (eg, patients receiving chemo/radiation therapy or other immunosuppressive therapy, including high-dose corticosteroids); may have a reduced response to vaccination; inactivated vaccines should be administered ≥2 weeks prior to planned immunosuppression when feasible (IDSA [Rubin, 2013]). In general, households and close contacts of persons with altered immunocompetence may receive all age-appropriate vaccines. Vaccination may not result in effective immunity in all patients. Response depends upon multiple factors (eg, type of vaccine, age of patient) and may be improved by administering the vaccine at the recommended dose, route, and interval (CDC/ACIP [Kroger, 2011]).

Use with caution in patients with coagulation disorders including thrombocytopenia, due to an increased risk for bleeding following I.M. administration; if the patient receives antihemophilia or other similar therapy, I.M. injection can be scheduled shortly after such therapy is administered. Children may have higher incidence of local adverse effects (erythema, swelling, tenderness). Antipyretics have not been shown to prevent febrile seizures; antipyretics may be used to treat fever or discomfort following vaccination (CDC/ACIP [Kroger, 2011]). One study reported that routine prophylactic administration of acetaminophen to prevent fever prior to vaccination decreased the immune response of some vaccines; the clinical significance of this reduction in immune response has not been established (Prymula, 2009).

Use of this vaccine for specific medical and/or other indications (eg, immunocompromising conditions, hepatic or kidney disease, diabetes) is also addressed in the ACIP Recommended Immunization Schedule (CDC/ACIP [Akinsanya-Beysolow, 2014]; CDC/ACIP [Bridges, 2014]). Specific recommendations for use of this vaccine in immunocompromised patients with asplenia, cancer, HIV infection, cerebrospinal fluid leaks, cochlear implants, hematopoietic stem cell transplant (prior to or after), sickle cell disease, solid organ transplant (prior to or after), or those receiving immunosuppressive therapy for chronic conditions as well as contacts of immunocompromised patients are available from the IDSA (Rubin, 2014).

Not to be used to treat meningococcal infections or to provide immunity against *N. meningitidis* serogroup B or diphtheria. Latex is used in stopper of the vial of Menveo; patients with known hypersensitivity should avoid doses from vial formulation and use prefilled syringe for dose.

Adverse Reactions All serious adverse reactions must be reported to the U.S. Department of Health and Human Services (DHHS) Vaccine Adverse Event Reporting System (VAERS) 1-800-822-7967 or online at https://vaers.hhs.gov/esub/index. In Canada, adverse reactions may be reported to local provincial/territorial health agencies or to the Vaccine Safety Section at Public Health Agency of Canada (1-866-844-0018).

May vary by product and age group:

Central nervous system: Chills, drowsiness, excessive crying, fatigue, headache, irritability, malaise

Dermatologic: Skin rash

Gastrointestinal: Anorexia, change in appetite, diarrhea, nausea, vomiting

Local: Erythema at injection site, induration at injection site, pain at injection site, swelling at injection site, tenderness at injection site

Neuromuscular & skeletal: Arthralgia, myalgia

Miscellaneous: Fever

Rare but important or life-threatening: Acute disseminated encephalomyelitis, anaphylactoid reaction, anaphylaxis, apnea (premature infants), appendicitis, auditory impairment, Bell's palsy, blepharoptosis, convulsions (including tonic), Cushing's syndrome, dehydration, depression, equilibrium disturbance, exfoliation of skin, facial paresis, falling, febrile seizures, gastroenteritis, Guillain-Barre syndrome, hypersensitivity, hypotension, increased serum ALT, inflammation at injection site, injection site cellulitis, Kawasaki Syndrome, ostealgia, pelvic inflammatory disease, pneumonia, pruritus at injection site, seizure, simple partial seizures, staphylococcal infection, suicidal tendencies, syncope (including vasovagal), transverse myelitis, varicella, vertebral disc disease, vestibular disturbance

Drug Interactions

Metabolism/Transport Effects None known.

Avoid Concomitant Use There are no known interactions where it is recommended to avoid concomitant use.

Increased Effect/Toxicity There are no known significant interactions involving an increase in effect.

Decreased Effect

The levels/effects of Meningococcal (Groups A / C / Y and W-135) Diphtheria Conjugate Vaccine may be decreased by: Belimumab; Fingolimod; Immunosuppressants

Stability

Menactra: Store at 2°C to 8°C (35°F to 46°F); do not freeze; protect from light. Discard product exposed to freezing.

Menveo: Prior to reconstitution, store between 2°C to 8°C (36°F to 46°F); protect from light and do not freeze. Discard product exposed to freezing. Use immediately after reconstitution but may be stored at ≤25°C (77°F) for up to 8 hours.

Mechanism of Action Induces immunity against meningococcal disease via the formation of bactericidal antibodies directed toward the polysaccharide capsular components of *Neisseria meningitidis* serogroups A, C, Y and W-135.

Dosing: Usual Note: Use of the abbreviation, MenACWY, refers to either meningococcal quadrivalent polysaccharide vaccine. MenACWY-CRM refers specifically to Menveo; MenACWY-D refers specifically to Menactra.

Pediatric:

Primary immunization:

Manufacturer's labeling: General dosing:

Menactra:

Infants ≥9 months and Children <2 years: I.M.: 0.5 mL per dose for a total of 2 doses given 3 months apart

Children ≥2 years and Adolescents: I.M.: 0.5 mL per dose as a single dose

Menveo:

Infants 2 to <7 months: I.M.: 0.5 mL per dose for a total of 4 doses administered as follows: 2, 4, 6, and 12 months of age

Infants and Children 7 to 23 months: I.M.: 0.5 mL per dose for a total of 2 doses. The second dose should be given during the second year of life and at least 3 months after the first dose.

Children ≥2 to <6 years: I.M.: 0.5 mL per dose as a single dose; for children at continued high risk of meningococcal disease, may consider an additional dose given 2 months after the first dose

Children ≥6 years and Adolescents: I.M.: 0.5 mL per dose as a single dose

CDC (ACIP) recommendations (CDC/ACIP [Cohn, 2013]):

*Primary vaccination for patients **NOT** at increased risk for meningococcal disease:*

Infants and Children<11 years: Not routinely recommended; see dosing for persons at increased risk

Children 11 to 12 years: I.M.: 0.5 mL per dose as a single dose. Children not at increased risk for meningococcal disease who may have been previously vaccinated with Hib-MenCY-TT (MenHibrix) or Men-ACWY (Menactra or Menveo) prior to their 10th birthday; should receive the routinely recommended dose of MenACWY at 11 to 12 years

Adolescents: I.M.: 0.5 mL per dose as a single dose if not previously vaccinated

Primary vaccination for patients at increased risk for meningococcal disease:

Infants and Children <2 years:

Anatomic or functional asplenia:

Infants and Children <19 months: MenACWY-CRM (Menveo): I.M.: 0.5 mL per dose for a total of 4 doses administered at 2, 4, 6, and 12 to 15 months of age

Children 19 to 23 months (incomplete vaccination): MenACWY-CRM (Menveo): I.M.: 0.5 mL per dose for a total of 2 doses given at least 3 months apart

Persistent complement component deficiency:

Infants and Children <19 months: MenACWY-CRM (Menveo): I.M.: 0.5 mL per dose for a total of 4 doses administered at 2, 4, 6, and 12 to 15 months of age

Infants and Children 7 to 23 months (unvaccinated or partially vaccinated):

MenACWY-CRM (Menveo): I.M.: 0.5 mL per dose for a total of 2 doses; the second dose should be given at age ≥12 months and at least 3 months after the first dose

MenACWY-D (Menactra): I.M.: 0.5 mL per dose for a total of 2 doses; the first dose should be given at age ≥9 months and the second dose should be given at least 3 months after the first dose.

Community outbreak (due to vaccine serogroup): Infants ≥2 months to Children 23 months: Initiate or complete an age appropriate series of MenACWY-CRM (Menveo) or MenACWY-D (Menactra); see Primary immunization above for dosing.

Travel to or residence in countries with hyperendemic or epidemic meningococcal disease: Infants ≥9 months to Children 23 months: Initiate or complete an age appropriate series of MenACWY-CRM (Menveo) or MenACWY-D (Menactra); see Primary immunization above for dosing.

Children ≥2 years and Adolescents, not previously vaccinated and who have persistent complement deficiencies, functional or anatomic asplenia, or who have HIV infection and another indication for vaccination: I.M.: 0.5 mL per dose for a total or 2 doses given 8 to12 weeks apart. If using MenACWY-D (Menactra), administer ≥4 weeks after completion of all PCV doses.

Children ≥2 years and Adolescents not previously vaccinated and who are either: First year college students ≤21 years of age living in residential housing, traveling to or residents of areas where meningococcal disease is endemic/hyperendemic, at risk during a community outbreak, or microbiologists routinely exposed to *Neisseria meningitidis*: I.M.: 0.5 mL as a single dose. If using MenACWY-D (Menactra), administer ≥4 weeks after completion of all PCV doses. College students ≤21 years should have documentation of a vaccination not more than 5 years before enrollment (preferably a dose on their 16th birthday).

Booster dose:
Booster vaccination for patients NOT at increased risk for meningococcal disease: I.M.: 0.5 mL as a single dose. If primary vaccination was at 11 to 12 years, the booster dose should be given at age 16. If the primary vaccination was given at 13 to 15 years, the booster dose should be given at age 16 to 18. Minimum interval between MenACWY (Menveo or Menactra) doses is 8 weeks. A booster dose is not needed if the primary dose was given after the 16th birthday unless the person becomes at increased risk for meningococcal disease.

Booster vaccination for patients at increased risk for meningococcal disease:
If first dose received at 2 months to 6 years of age: Repeat dose 3 years after primary vaccination and every 5 years thereafter if the person remains at increased risk.
If first dose received at ≥7 years of age: Repeat dose 5 years after primary vaccination and every 5 years thereafter if the person remains at increased risk.

Adult:
Primary immunization:
Manufacturer's labeling: General dosing: Menactra, Menveo: I.M.: 0.5 mL as a single dose
CDC (ACIP) recommendations (CDC/ACIP [Cohn, 2013]):
Primary vaccination for persons NOT at increased risk for meningococcal disease:
19 to 21 years: Not routinely recommended; may receive one 0.5 mL dose as a catch-up vaccination if no dose was received after the 16th birthday
≥22 years: Not routinely recommended; see dosing for persons at increased risk
Primary vaccination for persons at increased risk for meningococcal disease:
Adults ≤55 years not previously vaccinated and who have persistent complement deficiencies, functional or anatomic asplenia, or who have HIV infection and another indication for vaccination: I.M.: 0.5 mL per dose for a total of two doses given 8 to 12 weeks apart. If using MenACWY-D (Menactra), administer ≥4 weeks after completion of all PCV doses
Adults ≤55 years not previously vaccinated and who are either: First year college students ≤21 years of age living in residential housing, traveling to or residents of areas where meningococcal disease is endemic/hyperendemic, at risk during a community outbreak, or microbiologists routinely exposed to *Neisseria meningitidis*: I.M.: 0.5 mL as a single dose. If using MenACWY-D (Menactra), administer ≥4 weeks after completion of all PCV doses. College students ≤21 years should have documentation of a vaccination not more than 5 years before enrollment (preferably a dose on their 16th birthday).
Adults ≥56 years: Meningococcal polysaccharide vaccine (MPSV4, Menomune) is preferred for meningococcal vaccine naïve persons in this age group who require a single dose. If multiple doses are anticipated, see booster dosing for persons at increased risk.

Booster dose:
Booster vaccination for persons NOT at increased risk for meningococcal disease: Adults ≤21 years: I.M.: 0.5 mL as a single dose if the first dose was given prior to the 16th birthday. A booster dose is not needed if the primary dose was given after the 16th birthday unless the person becomes at increased risk for meningococcal disease.
Booster vaccination for persons at increased risk for meningococcal disease:
Adults ≤55 years: Repeat dose 5 years if the person remains at increased risk
Adults ≥56 years: Persons previously vaccinated with MenACWY (Menveo or Menactra) and who require revaccination or for whom multiple doses are anticipated, MenACWY (Menveo or Menactra) is preferred. Otherwise, meningococcal polysaccharide vaccine (MPSV4, Menomune) is preferred for meningococcal vaccine naïve persons in this age group who require a single dose.

Dosing adjustment in renal impairment: There are no dosage adjustments provided in manufacturer's labeling.
Dosing adjustment in hepatic impairment: There are no dosage adjustments provided in manufacturer's labeling.
Administration Administer by I.M. injection into midlateral aspect of the thigh in infants and small children; administer in the deltoid area to older children and adults; **not for intradermal, subcutaneous, or I.V. administration.** Adolescents and adults should be vaccinated while seated or lying down. U.S. law requires that the date of administration, the vaccine manufacturer, lot number of vaccine, and the administering person's name, title, and address be entered into the patient's permanent medical record.
Menveo: Prior to use, remove liquid contents from vial of MenCYW-135 and inject into vial containing MenA powder. Gently invert or swirl until dissolved. The resulting solution should be clear and colorless. A small amount of liquid will remain in the vial after withdrawing the 0.5 mL dose. Use immediately after reconstitution but may be stored at ≤25°C (77°F) for up to 8 hours. Do not mix with other vaccines in the same syringe.

Monitoring Parameters Observe for syncope for 15 minutes following administration. If seizure-like activity associated with syncope occurs, maintain patient in supine or Trendelenburg position to reestablish adequate cerebral perfusion.

Additional Information Two meningococcal (Groups A/C/Y and W-135) diphtheria conjugate vaccines are available. Menveo uses oligosaccharides of the *N. meningitidis* serogroups linked to CRM_{197} (a nontoxic diphtheria toxin carrier protein) and Menactra uses polysaccharides from the serogroups linked to diphtheria toxoid.

In order to maximize vaccination rates, the ACIP recommends simultaneous administration (ie, >1 vaccine on the same day at different anatomic sites) of all age-appropriate vaccines (live or inactivated) for which a person is eligible at a single visit, unless contraindications exist. If available, the use of combination vaccines is generally preferred over separate injections, taking into consideration provider assessment, patient preference, and potential adverse events. If separate vaccines being used, evaluate product information regarding same syringe compatibility of vaccines. Separate needles and syringes should be used for each injection. The ACIP prefers each dose of specific vaccine in a series come from the same manufacturer if possible (CDC/ACIP [Kroger, 2011]).

For additional information, please refer to the following website: http://www.cdc.gov/vaccines/vpd-vac/.

Dosage Forms Excipient information presented when available (limited, particularly for generics); consult specific product labeling.

◄ Injection, solution [preservative free]:
Menactra: 4 mcg each of polysaccharide antigen groups A, C, Y, and W-135 [bound to diphtheria toxoid 48 mcg] per 0.5 mL [MCV4 or MenACWY-D]
Menveo: MenA oligosaccharide 10 mcg, MenC oligosaccharide 5 mcg, MenY oligosaccharide 5 mcg, and MenW-135 oligosaccharide 5 mcg [bound to CRM$_{197}$ protein 32.7-64.1 mcg] per 0.5 mL (0.5 mL) [MenACWY-CRM; supplied in two vials, one containing MenA powder and one containing MenCYW-135 liquid]

References

AAP Steering Committee on Quality Improvement and Management, Subcommittee on Febrile Seizures American Academy of Pediatrics, "Febrile Seizures: Clinical Practice Guideline for the Long-Term Management of the Child With Simple Febrile Seizures," *Pediatrics*, 2008, 121(6):1281-6.

Akinsanya-Beysolow I, Advisory Committee on Immunization Practices (ACIP), ACIP Child/Adolescent Immunization Work Group, et al. Advisory committee on immunization practices recommended immunization schedule for adults aged 19 years or older - United States, 2014. *MMWR Morb Mortal Wkly Rep.* 2014; 63(5):108-109. Full schedule available at http://www.cdc.gov/vaccines/schedules/downloads/child/0-18yrs-child-combined-schedule.pdf

Bridges CB, Coyne-Beasley T, Advisory Committee on Immunization Practices (ACIP), ACIP Adult Immunization Work Group; Centers for Disease Control and Prevention (CDC). Advisory committee on immunization practices recommended immunization schedule for adults aged 19 years or older - United States, 2014. *MMWR Morb Mortal Wkly Rep.* 2014; 63(5):108-109. Available at: http://www.cdc.gov/vaccines/schedules/downloads/adult/adult-combined-schedule.-pdf

Centers for Disease Control and Prevention (CDC), "Syncope After Vaccination-United States, January 2005-July 2007," *MMWR Morb Mortal Wkly Rep*, 2008, 2;57(17):457-60.

Cohn AC, MacNeil JR, Clark TA, et al. Prevention and control of meningococcal disease: recommendations of the Advisory Committee on Immunization Practices (ACIP). *MMWR Recomm Rep.* 2013;62(RR-2):1-28.

Kroger AT, Atkinson WL, Marcuse EK, Pickering LK. General recommendations on immunization - recommendations of the Advisory Committee on Immunization Practices (ACIP). *MMWR Recomm Rep.* 2011;60(RR-2):1-64.

Menactra (Meningococcal [Groups A, C, Y and W-135] Polysaccharide Diphtheria Toxoid Conjugate Vaccine [prescribing information]. Swiftwater, PA: Sanofi Pasteur Inc; October 2013.

Menveo (Meningococcal [Groups A, C, Y and W-135] Oligosaccharide Diphtheria CRM197 Conjugate Vaccine) [prescribing information]. Cambridge, MA: Novartis Vaccines and Diagnostics, Onc; August 2013.

Prymula R, Siegrist CA, Chlibek R, et al, "Effect of Prophylactic Paracetamol Administration at Time of Vaccination on Febrile Reactions and Antibody Responses in Children: Two Open-Label, Randomised Controlled Trials," *Lancet*, 2009, 374(9698):1339-50.

Rubin LG, Levin MJ, Ljungman P, et al. 2013 IDSA clinical practice guideline for vaccination of the immunocompromised host. *Clin Infect Dis.* 2014;58(3):e44-e100.

Zheteyeva Y, Moro PL, Yue X, Broder K. Safety of meningococcal polysaccharide-protein conjugate vaccine in pregnancy: a review of the Vaccine Adverse Event Reporting System. *Am J Obstet Gynecol.* 2013;208(6):478.e1-6.

Meningococcal Polysaccharide (Groups C and Y) and *Haemophilus* b Tetanus Toxoid Conjugate Vaccine

(me NIN joe kok al pol i SAK a ride groops see & why & he MOF i lus bee TET a nus TOKS oyd KON joo gate vak SEEN)

Medication Safety Issues

Sound-alike/look-alike issues:

MenHibrix® (Meningococcal Polysaccharide (Groups C and Y) and *Haemophilus* b Tetanus Toxoid Conjugate Vaccine) may be confused with Hiberix® (*Haemophilus* b Conjugate Vaccine)

Related Information

Immunization Administration Recommendations *on page 2368*

Immunization Guidelines *on page 2373*

Brand Names: U.S. Menhibrix

Therapeutic Category Vaccine, Inactivated Bacteria

Generic Availability (U.S.) No

Use Provide active immunization against *Neisseria meningitidis* serogroups C and Y and *Haemophilus influenzae* type b (FDA approved in ages 6 weeks to 18 months)

The Advisory Committee on Immunization Practices (ACIP) recommends vaccination only for infants and children 2 to 18 months of age who are at increased risk for meningococcal disease, including those with:
• Persistent complement pathway deficiencies
• Anatomic or functional asplenia, including sickle cell disease
• Living in communities with serogroups C and Y meningococcal disease outbreaks

The ACIP does not recommend routine vaccination for infants not at increased risk for meningococcal disease. In addition, infants traveling to certain areas (eg, meningitis belt of sub-Saharan Africa) will require a meningococcal vaccine with serogroups A and W135; vaccination with Hib-MenCY-TT is not adequate (CDC/ACIP [Cohn, 2013]).

Pregnancy Risk Factor C

Pregnancy Considerations Animal reproduction studies have not been conducted.

Contraindications Hypersensitivity to any component or any meningococcal-, *H. influenzae* type b-, or tetanus-containing vaccines

Warnings Immediate treatment (including epinephrine 1:1000) for anaphylactic and/or hypersensitivity reactions should be available during vaccine use. Guillain-Barré syndrome occurring within 6 weeks of vaccines containing tetanus toxoid has been reported; consider potential risks and benefits prior to use. Syncope has been reported with use of injectable vaccines and may be accompanied by transient visual disturbances, weakness, or tonic-clonic movements. Procedures should be in place to avoid injuries from falling and to restore cerebral perfusion if syncope occurs (CDC, 57[17], 2008). Apnea has occurred following intramuscular vaccine administration in premature infants; consider clinical status implications. Menhibrix is not a substitute for routine tetanus immunization. Do not coadminister with other Hib-containing vaccines (CDC/ACIP [Cohn, 2013]).

Precautions The decision to administer or delay vaccination because of current or recent febrile illness depends on the severity of symptoms and the etiology of the disease. Immunization should be delayed during the course of an acute febrile illness. Use with caution in immunocompromised patients; has not been evaluated for use in immunosuppressed children; in general, severely immunocompromised patients [eg, patients receiving chemo/radiation therapy or other immunosuppressive therapy (including high-dose corticosteroids)] may have a reduced response to vaccination; inactivated vaccines should be administered ≥2 weeks prior to planned immunosuppression when feasible (IDSA [Rubin, 2013]). In general, households and close contacts of persons with altered immune competence may receive all age-appropriate vaccines. Vaccination may not result in effective immunity in all patients; response depends upon multiple factors (eg, type of vaccine, age of patient) and is improved by administering the vaccine at the recommended dose, route, and interval (CDC/ACIP [Kroger, 2011]).

Use with caution in patients with coagulation disorders, including thrombocytopenia, due to an increased risk for bleeding following I.M. administration; if the patient receives antihemophilia or other similar therapy, I.M. injection can be scheduled shortly after such therapy is administered. Antipyretics have not been shown to prevent febrile seizures; antipyretics may be used to treat fever or discomfort following vaccination (CDC/ACIP [Kroger, 2011]). One study reported that routine prophylactic administration of acetaminophen to prevent fever prior to vaccination decreased the immune response of some vaccines; the clinical significance of this reduction in immune response has not been established (Prymula, 2009).

Adverse Reactions All serious adverse reactions must be reported to the U.S. Department of Health and Human Services (DHHS) Vaccine Adverse Event Reporting System (VAERS) 1-800-822-7967 or online at https://vaers.hhs.gov/esub/index. In Canada, adverse reactions may be reported to local provincial/territorial health agencies or to the Vaccine Safety Section at Public Health Agency of Canada (1-866-844-0018).

Central nervous system: Fever ≥100.4°F (38°C), drowsiness, irritability

Gastrointestinal: Appetite decreased

Local: Injection site reactions: Pain, redness, swelling

Rare but important or life-threatening: Allergic reactions, anaphylactic/anaphylactoid reactions, angioedema, apnea, hypotonic-hyporesponsive episode, injection site induration, rash, somnolence, seizures (with or without fever), swelling of vaccinated limb (extensive), syncope, urticaria, vasovagal response

Drug Interactions

Metabolism/Transport Effects None known.

Avoid Concomitant Use There are no known interactions where it is recommended to avoid concomitant use.

Increased Effect/Toxicity There are no known significant interactions involving an increase in effect.

Decreased Effect

The levels/effects of Meningococcal Polysaccharide (Groups C and Y) and Haemophilus b Tetanus Toxoid Conjugate Vaccine may be decreased by: Belimumab; Fingolimod; Immunosuppressants

Stability Store intact vials at 2°C to 8°C (36°F to 46°F); protect from light.

Store diluent at 2°C to 25°C (36°F to 77°F) either under refrigeration or at room temperature; do not freeze; discard if the diluent has been frozen.

Reconstituted solution: Use immediately; do not freeze, discard if has been frozen.

Mechanism of Action Provides active immunity against meningococcal disease via the formation of bactericidal antibodies directed toward the polysaccharide capsular components of *Neisseria meningitidis* serogroups C and Y; stimulates production of anticapsular antibodies and to *Haemophilus influenzae* type b

Pharmacodynamics Onset of action: Antibody response to the components of the vaccine occurs in ≥95% of infants following the third dose and ≥98% following the fourth dose

Dosing: Usual Primary Immunization: Infants and Children 6 weeks to 18 months: I.M.: 0.5 mL per dose for a total of 4 doses administered as follows: 2, 4, 6, and 12 to 15 months of age; first dose may be administered as early as 6 weeks of age and last dose in series as late as 18 months of age

Note: The ACIP recommends vaccination only for infants 2 to 18 months of age who are at increased risk for meningococcal disease. The first dose may be given as early as 6 weeks of age and the fourth dose may be given as late as 18 months of age. If an infant at increased risk is behind on Hib vaccine doses, Hib-MenCY-TT may be used to catch up using the current Hib schedule. If the first dose of Hib-MenCY-TT is given ≥12 months of age, 2 doses should be given 8 weeks apart. If infants have/will receive a different Hib vaccine, a 2-dose series of a quadrivalent meningococcal vaccine is recommended (Menactra for ages 9 to 23 months; Menactra or Menveo for ages >23 months) (CDC/ACIP [Cohn, 2013]).

Dosing adjustment in renal impairment: There are no dosage adjustments provided in the manufacturer's labeling.

Dosing adjustment in hepatic impairment: There are no dosage adjustments provided in the manufacturer's labeling.

Administration I.M.: Reconstitute vaccine with supplied diluent; shake well; administer immediately; in infants administer to the anterolateral aspect of the thigh; in children ≥12 months to ≤18 months, the deltoid muscle of the arm may be used. Do not administer I.V. or subQ. Do not coadminister with other Hib-containing vaccines (CDC/ACIP [Cohn, 2013]). U.S. law requires that the date of administration; the vaccine manufacturer; lot number of vaccine; and the administering person's name, title, and address be entered into the patient's permanent medical record.

Monitoring Parameters Observe for syncope for 15 minutes following administration. If seizure-like activity associated with syncope occurs, maintain patient in supine or Trendelenburg position to reestablish adequate cerebral perfusion.

Test Interactions *H. influenzae* type b from the vaccine may be detected in the urine; urine antigen tests may not be diagnostic for *H. influenzae* type b infection within 1-2 weeks of vaccination

Additional Information In order to maximize vaccination rates, the ACIP recommends simultaneous administration (ie, >1 vaccine on the same day at different anatomic sites) of all age-appropriate vaccines (live or inactivated) for which a person is eligible at a single visit, unless contraindications exist. If available, the use of combination vaccines is generally preferred over separate injections, taking into consideration provider assessment, patient preference, and potential adverse events. If separate vaccines being used, evaluate product information regarding same syringe compatibility of vaccines. Separate needles and syringes should be used for each injection. The ACIP prefers each dose of specific vaccine in a series come from the same manufacturer if possible (CDC, 2011).

For additional information, please refer to the following website: http://www.cdc.gov/vaccines/vpd-vac/.

Dosage Forms Excipient information presented when available (limited, particularly for generics); consult specific product labeling.

Solution Reconstituted, Intramuscular [preservative free]:

Menhibrix: 5 mcg each of polysaccharide antigen groups C and Y, and 2.5 mcg Haemophilus b capsular polysaccharide per 0.5 mL dose (1 ea) [contains tetanus toxoid]

References

AAP Steering Committee on Quality Improvement and Management, Subcommittee on Febrile Seizures American Academy of Pediatrics, "Febrile Seizures: Clinical Practice Guideline for the Long-Term Management of the Child With Simple Febrile Seizures," *Pediatrics*, 2008, 121(6):1281-6.

Advisory Committee on Immunization Practices (ACIP) Vaccines for Children Program - Vaccines to Prevent Meningococcal Disease, Resolution No. 6/11-1. Available at: http://www.cdc.gov/vaccines/programs/vfc/downloads/resolutions/06-11mening-mcv.pdf

Akinsanya-Beysolow I, Advisory Committee on Immunization Practices (ACIP), ACIP Child/Adolescent Immunization Work Group, et al. Advisory committee on immunization practices recommended immunization schedule for adults aged 19 years or older - United States, 2014. *MMWR Morb Mortal Wkly Rep*. 2014; 63(5):108-109. Full schedule available at http://www.cdc.gov/vaccines/schedules/downloads/child/0-18yrs-child-combined-schedule.pdf

Centers for Disease Control and Prevention (CDC), "Infant Meningococcal Vaccination: Advisory Committee on Immunization Practices (ACIP) Recommendations and Rationale," *MMWR Morb Mortal Wkly Rep*, 2013, 62:52-4.

Centers for Disease Control and Prevention (CDC), "Prevention and Control of Meningococcal Disease: Recommendations of the Advisory Committee on Immunization Practices (ACIP)," *MMWR Recomm Rep*, 2013, 62(RR-2):1-28.

Centers for Disease Control and Prevention (CDC), "Syncope After Vaccination-United States, January 2005-July 2007," *MMWR Morb Mortal Wkly Rep,* 2008, 57(17):457-60.

Cohn AC, MacNeil JR, Clark TA, et al. Prevention and control of meningococcal disease: recommendations of the Advisory Committee on Immunization Practices (ACIP). *MMWR Recomm Rep.* 2013;62(RR-2):1-28.

Kroger AT, Sumaya CV, Pickering LK, et al. General recommendations on immunization - recommendations of the Advisory Committee on Immunization Practices (ACIP). *MMWR Recomm Rep.* 2011; 60(RR-2):1-64.

Prymula R, Siegrist CA, Chlibek R, et al, "Effect of Prophylactic Paracetamol Administration at Time of Vaccination on Febrile Reactions and Antibody Responses in Children: Two Open-Label, Randomised Controlled Trials," *Lancet,* 2009, 374(9698):1339-50.

Rubin LG, Levin MJ, Ljungman P, et al. 2013 IDSA clinical practice guideline for vaccination of the immunocompromised host. *Clin Infect Dis.* 2014;58(3):e44-e100.

◆ **Meningococcal Polysaccharide Vaccine** *see* Meningococcal Polysaccharide Vaccine (Groups A / C / Y and W-135) *on page 1336*

Meningococcal Polysaccharide Vaccine (Groups A / C / Y and W-135)

(me NIN joe kok al pol i SAK a ride vak SEEN groops aye, see, why & dubl yoo won thur tee fyve)

Medication Safety Issues

Administration issue:

Menomune® (MPSV4) should be administered by subcutaneous (SubQ) injection. Menactra® (MCV4), also a meningococcal polysaccharide vaccine, is to be administered by intramuscular (I.M.) injection only.

Related Information

Immunization Administration Recommendations *on page 2368*

Immunization Guidelines *on page 2373*

Brand Names: U.S. Menomune®-A/C/Y/W-135

Brand Names: Canada Menomune®-A/C/Y/W-135

Therapeutic Category Vaccine

Generic Availability (U.S.) No

Use Provide active immunity to meningococcal serogroups contained in the vaccine (FDA approved in ages ≥2 years and adults).

The Advisory Committee on Immunization Practices (ACIP) recommends routine vaccination for persons at increased risk for meningococcal disease. Meningococcal quadrivalent conjugate vaccine (MenACWY) is preferred; meningococcal polysaccharide vaccine (MPSV4) is preferred in meningococcal vaccine naïve adults ≥56 years of age requiring only a single vaccination (CDC/ACIP [Cohn, 2013]).

Those at increased risk of meningococcal disease include:
- Persons ≥2 months of age with medical conditions such as anatomical or functional asplenia or persistent complement component deficiencies (eg, C5-C9, properdin, factor H, or factor D)
- Persons ≥9 months of age that travel to or reside in countries where meningococcal disease is hyperendemic or epidemic, especially if contact with the local population will be prolonged
- Unvaccinated or incompletely vaccinated first year college students living in residence halls
- Military recruits
- Microbiologists with occupational exposure
- Persons (in all recommended age groups) at risk who are part of outbreaks caused by vaccine preventable serogroups

Pregnancy Risk Factor C

Pregnancy Considerations Animal reproduction studies have not been conducted. Inactivated bacterial vaccines have not been shown to cause increased risks to the fetus (CDC, 2011). Pregnancy should not preclude vaccination if indicated (CDC, 62[2], 2013).

Breast-Feeding Considerations It is not known if this vaccine is present in breast milk. The manufacturer recommends that caution be used if administered to a nursing woman. Inactivated vaccines do not affect the safety of breast-feeding for the mother or the infant. Breast-feeding infants should be vaccinated according to the recommended schedules (CDC, 2011).

Contraindications Hypersensitivity to any component

Warnings Immediate treatment (including epinephrine 1:1000) for anaphylactic and/or hypersensitivity reactions should be available during vaccine use. Avoid administration at the same time as whole-cell pertussis or whole-cell typhoid vaccines due to the combined endotoxin content; patients receiving immunosuppressive therapy may have diminished response. Syncope has been reported with use of injectable vaccines and may be accompanied by transient visual disturbances, weakness, or tonic-clonic movements. Procedures should be in place to avoid injuries from falling and to restore cerebral perfusion if syncope occurs (CDC, 57[17], 2008).

Precautions The decision to administer or delay vaccination because of current or recent febrile illness depends on the severity of symptoms and the etiology of the disease. Immunization should be delayed during the course of an acute severe febrile illness; may administer to patients with mild acute illness (with or without fever). Use with caution in severely immunocompromised patients (eg, patients receiving chemo/radiation therapy or other immunosuppressive therapy, including high-dose corticosteroids); may have a reduced response to vaccination; inactivated vaccines should be administered ≥2 weeks prior to planned immunosuppression when feasible (Rubin, 2014). In general, households and close contacts of persons with altered immunocompetence may receive all age-appropriate vaccines. Vaccination may not result in effective immunity in all patients. Response depends upon multiple factors (eg, type of vaccine, age of patient) and may be improved by administering the vaccine at the recommended dose, route, and interval (CDC/ACIP [Kroger, 2011]).

Children may have higher incidence of local adverse effects (erythema, swelling, tenderness). Antipyretics have not been shown to prevent febrile seizures; antipyretics may be used to treat fever or discomfort following vaccination (CDC/ACIP [Kroger, 2011]). One study reported that routine prophylactic administration of acetaminophen to prevent fever prior to vaccination decreased the immune response of some vaccines; the clinical significance of this reduction in immune response has not been established (Prymula, 2009).

Use of this vaccine for specific medical and/or other indications (eg, immunocompromising conditions, hepatic or kidney disease, diabetes) is also addressed in the ACIP Recommended Immunization Schedule (CDC/ACIP [Akinsanya-Beysolow, 2014]; CDC/ACIP [Bridges, 2014]). Specific recommendations for use of this vaccine in immunocompromised patients with asplenia, cerebrospinal fluid leaks, cochlear implants, or sickle cell disease are available from the IDSA (Rubin, 2014). Some dosage forms contain thimerosal; packaging may contain natural latex rubber.

Adverse Reactions All serious adverse reactions must be reported to the U.S. Department of Health and Human Services (DHHS) Vaccine Adverse Event Reporting System (VAERS) 1-800-822-7967 or online at https://vaers.hhs.gov/esub/index. In Canada, adverse reactions may be reported to local provincial/territorial health agencies or to the Vaccine Safety Section at Public Health Agency of Canada (1-866-844-0018).

Central nervous system: Chills, drowsiness, fatigue, fever, headache, irritability, malaise

Dermatologic: Rash

Gastrointestinal: Anorexia, diarrhea, vomiting

Local: Injection site: Induration, pain, redness, swelling

Neuromuscular & skeletal: Arthralgia

Rare but important or life-threatening: Dizziness, Guillain-Barré syndrome, hypersensitivity (angioedema, dyspnea, pruritus, rash, urticaria), myalgia, nausea, paresthesia, vasovagal syncope, weakness

Drug Interactions

Metabolism/Transport Effects None known.

Avoid Concomitant Use There are no known interactions where it is recommended to avoid concomitant use.

Increased Effect/Toxicity There are no known significant interactions involving an increase in effect.

Decreased Effect

The levels/effects of Meningococcal Polysaccharide Vaccine (Groups A / C / Y and W-135) may be decreased by: Belimumab; Fingolimod; Immunosuppressants

Stability Prior to and following reconstitution, store vaccine and diluent at 2°C to 8°C (35°F to 46°F); do not freeze. Single-use vial should be used immediately after reconstitution; use multidose vial within 35 days of reconstitution

Mechanism of Action Induces the formation of bactericidal antibodies to meningococcal antigens; the presence of these antibodies is strongly correlated with immunity to meningococcal disease caused by *Neisseria meningitidis* groups A, C, Y and W-135.

Pharmacodynamics

Onset of action: Antibody levels: 7-10 days

Duration: Antibodies against group A and C polysaccharides decline markedly (to prevaccination levels) over the first 3 years following a single dose of vaccine, especially in children <4 years of age

Dosing: Usual

Pediatric: **Immunization:** Children ≥2 years and Adolescents: SubQ: 0.5 mL as a single dose. Per the CDC/ACIP, this meningococcal vaccine is not routinely recommended for use in pediatric patients.

Adult: **Immunization:** SubQ: 0.5 mL as a single dose

CDC/ACIP recommendations:

Adults <56 years: This meningococcal vaccine is not routinely recommended.

Adults ≥56 years: Meningococcal polysaccharide vaccine (MPSV4, Menomune) is preferred for meningococcal vaccine naïve persons in this age group who are at increased risk of meningococcal infection and require a single dose (eg, travelers or during a community outbreak). Persons previously vaccinated with a quadrivalent meningococcal conjugate vaccine (MenACWY, Menveo, or Menactra) and who require revaccination or for whom multiple doses are anticipated, MenACWY is preferred (eg, persons with asplenia or microbiologists).

Administration Reconstitute using provided diluent; shake well; administer by SubQ injection into the deltoid region of the upper arm; **not for intradermal, I.M., or I.V. administration.** Adolescents and adults should be vaccinated while seated or lying down. U.S. law requires that the date of administration, the vaccine manufacturer, lot number of vaccine, and the administering person's name, title and address be entered into the patient's permanent medical record.

Monitoring Parameters Observe for syncope for 15 minutes following administration. If seizure-like activity associated with syncope occurs, maintain patient in supine or Trendelenburg position to reestablish adequate cerebral perfusion.

Additional Information In order to maximize vaccination rates, the ACIP recommends simultaneous administration (ie, >1 vaccine on the same day at different anatomic sites) of all age-appropriate vaccines (live or inactivated) for which a person is eligible at a single visit, unless contraindications exist. If available, the use of combination vaccines is generally preferred over separate injections, taking into consideration provider assessment, patient preference, and potential adverse events. If separate vaccines being used, evaluate product information regarding same syringe compatibility of vaccines. Separate needles and syringes should be used for each injection. The ACIP prefers each dose of specific vaccine in a series come from the same manufacturer if possible (CDC/ACIP [Kroger, 2011]).

For additional information, please refer to the following website: http://www.cdc.gov/vaccines/vpd-vac/.

Dosage Forms Excipient information presented when available (limited, particularly for generics); consult specific product labeling.

Injection, powder for reconstitution [MPSV4]:

Menomune®-A/C/Y/W-135: 50 mcg each of polysaccharide antigen groups A, C, Y, and W-135 per 0.5 mL dose [contains lactose 2.5-5 mg/0.5 mL, natural rubber/natural latex in packaging, thimerosal in diluent for multidose vial]

References

AAP Steering Committee on Quality Improvement and Management, Subcommittee on Febrile Seizures American Academy of Pediatrics, "Febrile Seizures: Clinical Practice Guideline for the Long-Term Management of the Child With Simple Febrile Seizures," *Pediatrics*, 2008, 121(6):1281-6.

Akinsanya-Beysolow I, Advisory Committee on Immunization Practices (ACIP), ACIP Child/Adolescent Immunization Work Group, et al. Advisory committee on immunization practices recommended immunization schedule for adults aged 19 years or older - United States, 2014. *MMWR Morb Mortal Wkly Rep.* 2014; 63(5):108-109. Full schedule available at http://www.cdc.gov/vaccines/schedules/downloads/child/0-18yrs-child-combined-schedule.pdf

Cohn AC, MacNeil JR, Clark TA, et al. Prevention and control of meningococcal disease: recommendations of the Advisory Committee on Immunization Practices (ACIP). *MMWR Recomm Rep.* 2013;62(RR-2):1-28.

Centers for Disease Control and Prevention (CDC), "Syncope After Vaccination - United States, January 2005-July 2007," *MMWR Morb Mortal Wkly Rep*, 2008, 57(17):457-60.

Kroger AT, Atkinson WL, Marcuse EK, Pickering LK. General recommendations on immunization - recommendations of the Advisory Committee on Immunization Practices (ACIP). *MMWR Recomm Rep.* 2011;60(RR-2):1-64.

Prymula R, Siegrist CA, Chlibek R, et al, "Effect of Prophylactic Paracetamol Administration at Time of Vaccination on Febrile Reactions and Antibody Responses in Children: Two Open-Label, Randomised Controlled Trials," *Lancet*, 2009, 374(9698):1339-50.

Rubin LG, Levin MJ, Ljungman P, et al. 2013 IDSA clinical practice guideline for vaccination of the immunocompromised host. *Clin Infect Dis.* 2014;58(3):e44-e100.

◆ **Menomune®-A/C/Y/W-135** *see* Meningococcal Polysaccharide Vaccine (Groups A / C / Y and W-135) *on page 1336*

◆ **Menostar** *see* Estradiol (Systemic) *on page 796*

◆ **Menveo** *see* Meningococcal (Groups A / C / Y and W-135) Diphtheria Conjugate Vaccine *on page 1330*

Meperidine (me PER i deen)

Medication Safety Issues

Sound-alike/look-alike issues:

Meperidine may be confused with meprobamate

Demerol may be confused with Demulen, Desyrel, Dilaudid, Pamelor

High alert medication:

The Institute for Safe Medication Practices (ISMP) includes this medication among its list of drug classes ▶

which have a heightened risk of causing significant patient harm when used in error.

BEERS Criteria medication:

This drug may be potentially inappropriate for use in geriatric patients (Quality of evidence - high; Strength of recommendation - strong).

Other safety concerns:

Avoid the use of meperidine for pain control, especially in elderly and renally-compromised patients because of the risk of neurotoxicity (American Pain Society, 2008; Institute for Safe Medication Practices [ISMP], 2007)

Related Information

Opioid Conversion Table *on page 2242*

Patient Information for Disposal of Unused Medications *on page 2412*

Preprocedure Sedatives in Children *on page 2402*

Brand Names: U.S. Demerol; Meperitab

Brand Names: Canada Demerol

Therapeutic Category Analgesic, Narcotic

Generic Availability (U.S.) Yes

Use

Oral: Relief of moderate to severe pain [FDA approved in pediatric patients (age not specified) and adults]

Parenteral: Relief of moderate to severe pain, preoperative medication, support of anesthesia, obstetrical analgesia [FDA approved in pediatric patients (age not specified) and adults]

Has also been used to reduce postoperative shivering and to reduce rigors from conventional amphotericin B

Pregnancy Risk Factor C

Pregnancy Considerations Animal reproduction studies have not been conducted by the manufacturer. Meperidine crosses the placenta; meperidine and its active metabolite accumulate in the fetus. Respiratory or CNS depression should be expected to occur in the newborn if maternal I.M. administration occurs within a few hours of delivery (Mattingly, 2003). When used for pain relief during labor, opioids may temporarily affect the heart rate of the fetus. Due to the prolonged half-life of the active metabolite, dose-dependant sedation in the neonate may be observed for 2-3 days following delivery. Meperidine has been used for the management of pain during labor; however, due to adverse maternal and fetal effects, other opioids may be preferred. Meperidine should also be avoided following delivery when postoperative analgesia is needed (ACOG, 2002).

If chronic opioid exposure occurs in pregnancy, adverse events in the newborn (including withdrawal) may occur; monitoring of the neonate is recommended. The minimum effective dose should be used if opioids are needed (Chou, 2009). Neonatal abstinence syndrome following opioid exposure may present with autonomic (eg, fever, temperature instability), gastrointestinal (eg, diarrhea, vomiting, poor feeding/weight gain), or neurologic (eg, high-pitched crying, increased muscle tone, irritability, seizure, tremor) symptoms (Dow, 2012; Hudak, 2012).

Breast-Feeding Considerations Meperidine is excreted in breast milk and may cause CNS and/or respiratory depression in the nursing infant. Due to the potential for serious adverse reactions in the nursing infant, the manufacturer recommends a decision be made whether to discontinue nursing or to discontinue the drug, taking into account the importance of treatment to the mother.

Small concentrations of meperidine are excreted into breast milk following single doses. With multiple doses, concentrations of meperidine and the active metabolite may increase and both are slowly eliminated by a nursing infant (Spigset, 2000). Parenteral opioids used during labor have the potential to interfere with a newborns natural reflex to nurse within the first few hours after birth. Nursing infants exposed to large doses of opioids should

be monitored for apnea and sedation. If treatment for pain in nursing women is needed, other agents are preferred (Montgomery, 2012)

Contraindications Hypersensitivity to meperidine or any component; use of MAO inhibitors within 14 days (potentially fatal reactions may occur)

Additional contraindications: Oral dosage forms: Severe respiratory insufficiency

Warnings CNS and respiratory depression may occur. Neonates and young infants may be at higher risk for adverse effects, especially respiratory depression (due to decreased elimination); use with caution and in reduced doses in this age group. Use with great caution (and only if essential) in patients with head injury, increased ICP, or other intracranial lesions (potential to depress respiration and increase ICP may be greatly exaggerated in these patients, may also obscure clinical course in patient). Use with extreme caution in patients with preexisting respiratory compromise (hypoxia and/or hypercapnia), COPD, cor pulmonale, acute asthmatic attacks, hypoxia, significantly decreased respiratory reserve; respiratory depression may occur, even at therapeutic doses. Severe hypotension may occur; use with caution in postoperative patients, in patients with hypovolemia, or in those receiving drugs which may exaggerate hypotensive effects (including phenothiazines or general anesthetics). Meperidine may be given I.V., but should be administered very slowly and as a diluted solution; rapid I.V. administration may result in increased adverse effects including severe respiratory depression, apnea, hypotension, peripheral circulatory collapse, or cardiac arrest; do not administer I.V. unless an opioid antagonist and respiratory support are immediately available. May obscure diagnosis or clinical course of patients with acute abdominal conditions.

Normeperidine, an active metabolite of meperidine, is a CNS stimulant which may precipitate anxiety, tremors, myoclonus, or seizures; risk for CNS effects increases with preexisting CNS dysfunction or clinical situations where accumulation of normeperidine may occur including: Renal impairment, prolonged use of meperidine (>48 hours), and cumulative meperidine dose (>600 mg/24 hours in adults). Oral meperidine should not be used since first-pass metabolism decreases efficacy while increasing normeperidine concentrations (American Pain Society, 2008). Use with caution and decrease the dose in patients with renal or hepatic impairment; normeperidine metabolite may accumulate in these patients. If use in acute pain (in patients without renal or CNS disease) cannot be avoided, treatment should be limited to ≤48 hours and doses should not exceed 600 mg/24 hours in adults. Oral route is not recommended for treatment of acute or chronic pain. If I.V. route is required, consider a reduced dose. Patients with prior opioid exposure may require higher initial doses. **Note:** The Institute for Safe Medication Practices (ISMP) and the American Pain Society (2008) suggest that meperidine offers no advantage over other opioids as an analgesic, and possesses unique neurotoxicity, and thus, should be avoided (American Pain Society, 2008; ISMP, 2007). **Note:** Naloxone does not reverse, and may even worsen, neurotoxicity.

Physical and psychological dependence may occur; abrupt discontinuation after prolonged use may result in withdrawal symptoms or seizures. Warn patient of possible impairment of alertness or physical coordination and orthostatic hypotension; patients must be cautioned about performing tasks which require mental alertness (eg, operating machinery or driving). Interactions with other CNS drugs may occur. Healthcare provider should be alert to problems of abuse, misuse, and diversion. Infants born to women physically dependent on opioids will also be physically dependent and may experience respiratory difficulties or opioid withdrawal symptoms [neonatal abstinence syndrome (NAS)]. Onset, duration, and severity of NAS depend upon the drug used (maternal), duration of use, maternal dose, and rate of drug elimination by the newborn. Symptoms of opioid withdrawal may include excessive crying, diarrhea, fever, hyper-reflexia, irritability, tremors, vomiting, or failure to gain weight. Opioid withdrawal syndrome in the neonate, unlike in adults, may be life-threatening and should be promptly treated.

Multiple dose vial may contain sulfites which may cause allergic reactions in susceptible individuals; oral liquid may contain sodium benzoate; benzoic acid (benzoate) is a metabolite of benzyl alcohol; large amounts of benzyl alcohol (≥99 mg/kg/day) have been associated with a potentially fatal toxicity ("gasping syndrome") in neonates; use meperidine products containing benzoic acid or sodium benzoate with caution in neonates; in vitro and animal studies have shown that benzoate displaces bilirubin from protein-binding sites

Precautions Use with caution and decrease initial dose in patients with sickle cell anemia; normeperidine (active metabolite) may accumulate and induce seizures in these patients; **Note:** Meperidine is not considered a first-line agent for treatment of acute sickle cell pain (NHLBI, 2002); it is not recommended for use in sickle cell patients by the American Pain Society (APS, 2008); use of meperidine should be reserved for brief episodes of treatment in sickle cell patients who have previously benefited from meperidine therapy, or in those who have allergies or are intolerant to other opioids (NHLBI, 2002). Use with caution in patients with adrenal insufficiency, including Addison's disease; thyroid disorders, including myxedema and hypothyroidism. Use with caution in patients with urethral stricture or prostatic hypertrophy. Use with caution in pheochromocytoma; meperidine may precipitate hypertension. Use with caution in patients with supraventricular tachycardia (including atrial flutter); may increase ventricular response rate, possibly due to a vagolytic effect. Use with caution in patients with biliary tract disease or acute pancreatitis; may cause constriction of sphincter of Oddi. Use with caution in patients who are morbidly obese. Use with caution in debilitated patients; risk of respiratory depression is increased, even at therapeutic doses. Use with caution in patients with toxic psychosis or delirium tremens. Concomitant administration of mixed agonist/antagonist opioids (eg, pentazocine, butorphanol) may reduce analgesic efficacy and/or precipitate withdrawal symptoms.

Adverse Reactions

Cardiovascular: Bradycardia, cardiac arrest, circulatory depression, hypotension, palpitation, shock, syncope, tachycardia

Central nervous system: Agitation, confusion, delirium, disorientation, dizziness, drowsiness, dysphoria, euphoria, fatigue, flushing, hallucinations, headache, intracranial pressure increased, lightheadedness, malaise, mental depression, nervousness, paradoxical CNS stimulation, restlessness, sedation, seizure (associated with metabolite accumulation), serotonin syndrome

Dermatologic: Pruritus, rash, urticaria

Gastrointestinal: Abdominal cramps, anorexia, biliary spasm, constipation, nausea, paralytic ileus, sphincter of Oddi spasm, vomiting, xerostomia

Genitourinary: Ureteral spasms, urinary retention

Local: Injection site reaction (including pain, wheal, and flare)

Neuromuscular & skeletal: Muscle twitching, myoclonus, tremor, weakness

Ocular: Visual disturbances

Respiratory: Dyspnea, respiratory arrest, respiratory depression

Miscellaneous: Anaphylaxis, diaphoresis, histamine release, hypersensitivity reactions, physical and psychological dependence

Drug Interactions

Metabolism/Transport Effects None known.

Avoid Concomitant Use

Avoid concomitant use of Meperidine with any of the following: Azelastine (Nasal); MAO Inhibitors; Paraldehyde; Thalidomide

Increased Effect/Toxicity

Meperidine may increase the levels/effects of: Alcohol (Ethyl); Alvimopan; Antipsychotics; Azelastine (Nasal); Buprenorphine; CNS Depressants; Desmopressin; Diuretics; Hydrocodone; Methotrimeprazine; Metoclopramide; Metyrosine; Paraldehyde; Pramipexole; ROPINIRole; Rotigotine; Serotonin Modulators; Thalidomide; Zolpidem

The levels/effects of Meperidine may be increased by: Amphetamines; Anticholinergic Agents; Antiemetics (5HT3 Antagonists); Antipsychotic Agents (Phenothiazines); Antipsychotics; Barbiturates; Brimonidine (Topical); Cannabis; Doxylamine; Dronabinol; Droperidol; HydrOXYzine; Kava Kava; Magnesium Sulfate; MAO Inhibitors; Methotrimeprazine; Nabilone; Perampanel; Protease Inhibitors; Rufinamide; Sodium Oxybate; Succinylcholine; Tapentadol; Tetrahydrocannabinol

Decreased Effect

Meperidine may decrease the levels/effects of: Pegvisomant

The levels/effects of Meperidine may be decreased by: Ammonium Chloride; Fosphenytoin; Mixed Agonist / Antagonist Opioids; Naltrexone; Phenytoin; Protease Inhibitors

Stability

Injection: Store at 20°C to 25°C (68°F to 77°F); excursions permitted to 15°C to 30°C (59°F to 86°F).

Tablets; oral solution: Store at 25°C (77°F); excursions permitted to 15°C to 30°C (59°F to 86°F).

Mechanism of Action Binds to opioid receptors in the CNS, causing inhibition of ascending pain pathways, altering the perception of and response to pain; produces generalized CNS depression

Pharmacodynamics Analgesia:

Onset of action:

Oral, I.M., SubQ: Within 10-15 minutes

I.V.: Within 5 minutes

Maximum effect:

Oral, I.M., SubQ: Within 1 hour

I.V.: 5-7 minutes

Duration:

Oral, I.M., SubQ: 2-4 hours

I.V.: 2-3 hours

Pharmacokinetics (Adult data unless noted)

Absorption: Oral: Erratic and highly variable

Distribution:

V_{dss}:

Neonates: Preterm 1-7 days: 8.8 L/kg; term 1-7 days: 5.6 L/kg

Infants: 1 week to 2 months: 8 L/kg; 3-18 months: 5 L/kg; 5-8 years: 2.8 L/kg

Adults: 3-4 L/kg

Protein binding: (to alpha$_1$-acid glycoprotein)

Neonates: 52%

Infants: 3-18 months: 85%

Adults: ~60% to 80%

Metabolism: Hepatic via hydrolysis and N-demethylation to meperidinic acid (inactive); also undergoes N-demethylation to normeperidine (active, has $1/2$ the analgesic effect and 2-3 times the CNS effect of meperidine)

Bioavailability: ~50% to 60%, increased bioavailability with liver disease

Half-life, terminal:
Preterm infants 3.6-65 days of age: 11.9 hours (range: 3.3-59.4 hours)
Term infants:
0.3-4 days of age: 10.7 hours (range: 4.9-16.8 hours)
26-73 days of age: 8.2 hours (range: 5.7-31.7 hours)
Neonates: 23 hours (range: 12-39 hours)
Infants 3-18 months: 2.3 hours
Children 5-8 years: 3 hours
Adults: 2.5-4 hours
Adults with liver disease: 7-11 hours
Normeperidine (active metabolite): Neonates: 30-85 hours; Adults: 8-16 hours; normeperidine half-life is dependent on renal function and can accumulate with high doses or in patients with decreased renal function; normeperidine may precipitate tremors or seizures
Elimination: ~5% meperidine eliminated unchanged in urine

Dosing: Usual Doses should be titrated to appropriate analgesic effect; when changing route of administration, note that oral doses are about half as effective as parenteral dose.

Note: The American Pain Society (2008) and ISMP (2007) do not recommend meperidine use as an analgesic. If use for acute pain (in patients without renal or CNS disease) cannot be avoided, treatment should be limited to ≤48 hours and doses should not exceed 600 mg/24 hours in adults. Oral route is not recommended for treatment of acute or chronic pain. If I.V. route is required, consider a reduced dose. Patients with prior opioid exposure may require higher initial doses.

Infants, Children, and Adolescents:
Acute pain (analgesic) (Berde, 2002): Initial:
Infants ≤6 months:
I.M., I.V., SubQ: 0.2-0.25 mg/kg/dose every 2-3 hours
Oral: 0.5-0.75 mg/kg/dose every 3-4 hours
Infants >6 months, Children, and Adolescents:
I.M., I.V., or SubQ; intermittent dosing:
Patient weight <50 kg: 0.8-1 mg/kg/dose every 2-3 hours as needed; maximum dose: 75 mg
Patient weight ≥50 kg: 50-75 mg every 2-3 hours as needed
Oral:
Patient weight <50 kg: 2-3 mg/kg/dose every 3-4 hours as needed; maximum dose: 150 mg
Patient weight ≥50 kg: 100-150 mg every 3-4 hours as needed
Analgesia for minor procedures/sedation; preoperative:
I.M., I.V., SubQ: 0.5-1 mg/kg given 30-90 minutes before the beginning of anesthesia; maximum dose: 2 mg/kg or 150 mg/dose (Zeltzer, 1990)
Oral: 2-4 mg/kg given 30-90 minutes before the beginning of anesthesia; maximum dose: 150 mg/dose
Sickle cell disease, acute crisis (NHLBI, 2002): Note: Not recommended for first-line use; reserve for brief treatment episodes in patients who have previously benefited from meperidine therapy, or in patients who have allergies or are intolerant to other opioids (eg, morphine, hydromorphone): Initial:
Patient weight <50 kg:
I.V.: 0.75-1 mg/kg every 3-4 hours as needed; maximum dose: 1.75 mg/kg/dose or 100 mg
Oral: 1.1-1.75 mg/kg every 3-4 hours as needed; maximum dose: 1.75 mg/kg/dose or 150 mg
Patient weight ≥50 kg:
I.V.: 50-150 mg every 3 hours as needed
Oral: 50-150 mg every 3-4 hours as needed
Adults: **Pain (analgesic):** Oral, I.M., SubQ: 50-150 mg every 3-4 hours as needed
Preoperatively: I.M., SubQ: 50-150 mg given 30-90 minutes before the beginning of anesthesia

Obstetrical analgesia: I.M., SubQ: 50-100 mg when pain becomes regular; may repeat at every 1-3 hours
Dosing adjustment in renal impairment: The manufacturer recommends to use with caution and reduce dose; accumulation of meperidine and its active metabolite (normeperidine) may occur. The American Pain Society and ISMP recommend to avoid use in renal impairment. (American Pain Society, 2008; ISMP, 2007).
Dosing adjustment in hepatic impairment: Use with caution and reduce dose; accumulation of meperidine and its active metabolite (normeperidine) may occur.

Administration
Oral: Administer with water; dilute oral liquid in water prior to use (use 4 oz water for adults); undiluted solution may cause topical anesthetic effect on mucous membranes
Parenteral:
Intramuscular: Preferred route; inject into a large muscle
SubQ: Suitable for occasional use; when repeated doses are required, the I.M. route of administration is preferred
Slow I.V. push: Do not administer rapid I.V., administer over at least 5 minutes and dilute to ≤10 mg/mL
Intermittent I.V. infusion: Dilute to 1 mg/mL and administer over 15-30 minutes

Monitoring Parameters Respiratory rate; oxygen saturation; mental status; blood pressure; relief of pain, level of sedation

Test Interactions Increased amylase (S), increased BSP retention, increased CPK (I.M. injections)

Additional Information Equianalgesic doses: morphine 10 mg I.M. = meperidine 75-100 mg I.M.. **Note:** Although meperidine has been used in combination with chlorpromazine and promethazine as a premedication ("Lytic Cocktail"), this combination may have a higher rate of adverse effects compared to alternative sedatives and analgesics (AAP Committee on Drugs, 1995)

Controlled Substance C-II

Dosage Forms Excipient information presented when available (limited, particularly for generics); consult specific product labeling.
Solution, Injection, as hydrochloride:
Demerol: 25 mg/mL (1 mL); 25 mg/0.5 mL (0.5 mL); 50 mg/mL (1 mL, 30 mL); 75 mg/1.5 mL (1.5 mL); 100 mg/2 mL (2 mL); 75 mg/mL (1 mL); 100 mg/mL (1 mL, 20 mL)
Generic: 10 mg/mL (30 mL); 25 mg/mL (1 mL); 50 mg/mL (1 mL); 100 mg/mL (1 mL)
Solution, Oral, as hydrochloride:
Generic: 50 mg/5 mL (500 mL)
Tablet, Oral, as hydrochloride:
Demerol: 50 mg [scored]
Demerol: 100 mg
Meperitab: 50 mg [scored]
Meperitab: 100 mg
Generic: 50 mg, 100 mg

References
ACOG Committee on Practice Bulletins-Obstetrics, "ACOG Practice Bulletin. Clinical Management Guidelines for Obstetrician-Gynecologists Number 36, July 2002. Obstetric Analgesia and Anesthesia," *Obstet Gynecol*, 2002, 100(1):177-91.
American Academy of Pediatrics (AAP) Committee on Drugs, "Reappraisal of Lytic Cocktail/Demerol®, Phenergan®, and Thorazine® (DPT) for the Sedation of Children," *Pediatrics*, 1995, 95(4):598-602.
Berde CB and Sethna NF, "Analgesics for the Treatment of Pain in Children," *N Engl J Med*, 2002, 347(14):1094-103.
Chou R, Fanciullo GJ, Fine PG, et al, "Clinical Guidelines for the Use of Chronic Opioid Therapy in Chronic Noncancer Pain," *J Pain*, 2009, 10 (2):113-30.
Dow K, Ordean A, Murphy-Oikonen J, et al, "Neonatal Abstinence Syndrome Clinical Practice Guidelines for Ontario," *J Popul Ther Clin Pharmacol*, 2012, 19(3):e488-506.
Hudak ML, Tan RC, Committee On Drugs, et al, "Neonatal Drug Withdrawal," *Pediatrics*, 2012, 129(2):e540-60.
Mattingly JE, D'Alessio J, and Ramanathan J, "Effects of Obstetric Analgesics and Anesthetics on the Neonate: A Review," *Paediatr Drugs*, 2003, 5(9):615-27.

Montgomery A, Hale TW, and Academy of Breastfeeding Medicine, "ABM Clinical Protocol #15: Analgesia and Anesthesia for the Breastfeeding Mother, Revised 2012," *Breastfeed Med*, 2012, 7(6):547-53.

National Institutes of Health, "The Management of Sickle Cell Disease," Clinical Practice Guidelines, National Institutes of Health, National Heart, Lung, and Blood Institute, Division of Blood Diseases and Resources, NIH Publication No. 02-2117, 2002. Available at http://www.nhlbi.nih.gov/health/prof/blood/sickle/sc_mngt.pdf

Institute for Safe Medication Practice, "High Alert Medication Feature: Reducing Patient Harm From Opiates," ISMP Medication Safety Alert, February 22, 2007. Available at http://www.ismp.org/Newsletters/acutecare/articles/20070222.asp.

Olkkola KT, Hamunen K, and Maunuksela EL, "Clinical Pharmacokinetics and Pharmacodynamics of Opioid Analgesics in Infants and Children," *Clin Pharmacokinet*, 1995, 28(5):385-404.

Pokela ML, Olkkola KT, Koivisto ME, et al, "Pharmacokinetics and Pharmacodynamics of Intravenous Meperidine in Neonates and Infants," *Clin Pharmacol Ther*, 1992, 52(4):342-9.

"Principles of Analgesic Use in the Treatment of Acute Pain and Cancer Pain," 6th ed, Glenview, IL: American Pain Society, 2008.

Spigset O and Hagg S, "Analgesics and Breast-Feeding: Safety Considerations," *Paediatr Drugs*, 2000, 2(3):223-38.

Zeltzer LK, Altman A, Cohen D, et al, "American Academy of Pediatrics Report of the Subcommittee on the Management of Pain Associated With Procedures in Children With Cancer," *Pediatrics*, 1990, 86(5 Pt 2):826-31.

◆ **Meperidine Hydrochloride** *see* Meperidine *on page 1337*

◆ **Meperitab** *see* Meperidine *on page 1337*

◆ **Mephyton®** *see* Phytonadione *on page 1671*

Mepivacaine (me PIV a kane)

Medication Safety Issues
Sound-alike/look-alike issues:
Mepivacaine may be confused with bupivacaine
Polocaine® may be confused with prilocaine

High alert medication:
The Institute for Safe Medication Practices (ISMP) includes this medication (epidural administration) among its list of drug classes which have a heightened risk of causing significant patient harm when used in error.

Brand Names: U.S. Carbocaine; Carbocaine Preservative-Free; Polocaine; Polocaine-MPF

Brand Names: Canada Carbocaine®; Polocaine®

Therapeutic Category Local Anesthetic, Injectable

Generic Availability (U.S.) Yes

Use Local or regional analgesia; anesthesia by local infiltration, peripheral and central neural techniques including epidural and caudal blocks; **not** for use in spinal anesthesia

Pregnancy Risk Factor C

Pregnancy Considerations Animal reproduction studies have not been conducted. Mepivacaine has been used in obstetrical analgesia.

Breast-Feeding Considerations It is not known if mepivacaine is excreted in breast milk. The manufacturer recommends that caution be exercised when administering mepivacaine to nursing women.

Contraindications Hypersensitivity to mepivacaine, other amide-type local anesthetics, or any component

Warnings Local anesthetics have been associated with rare occurrences of sudden respiratory arrest; convulsions due to systemic toxicity leading to cardiac arrest have been reported presumably due to intravascular injection. Degree of adverse effects in the CNS and cardiovascular system is directly related to the blood levels of mepivacaine, route of administration (less observed with infiltration than systemic administration), and physical status of the patient. A test dose is recommended prior to epidural administration and all reinforcing doses with continuous catheter technique. Do not use solutions containing preservatives for caudal or epidural block. Chondrolysis has been reported following continuous intra-articular infusion; intra-articular administration of local anesthetics is not an FDA-approved route of administration.

Precautions Use with extreme caution as lumbar or caudal anesthesia in patients with existing neurologic disease, spinal deformities, or severe hypertension. Use with caution in patients with cardiac disease, hepatic or renal disease. Use caution in debilitated, elderly, or acutely-ill patients; dose reduction may be required.

Adverse Reactions
Cardiovascular: Bradycardia, cardiac arrest, cardiac output decreased, heart block, hyper-/hypotension, myocardial depression, syncope, tachycardia, ventricular arrhythmias

Central nervous system: Anxiety, chills, convulsions, depression, dizziness, excitation, restlessness, tremors

Dermatologic: Angioneurotic edema, diaphoresis, erythema, pruritus, urticaria

Gastrointestinal: Fecal incontinence, nausea, vomiting

Genitourinary: Incontinence, urinary retention

Neuromuscular & skeletal: Chondrolysis (continuous intra-articular administration), paralysis

Ocular: Blurred vision, pupil constriction

Otic: Tinnitus

Respiratory: Apnea, hypoventilation, sneezing

Miscellaneous: Allergic reaction, anaphylactoid reaction

Drug Interactions

Metabolism/Transport Effects None known.

Avoid Concomitant Use There are no known interactions where it is recommended to avoid concomitant use.

Increased Effect/Toxicity
The levels/effects of Mepivacaine may be increased by: Beta-Blockers; Hyaluronidase

Decreased Effect
Mepivacaine may decrease the levels/effects of: Technetium Tc 99m Tilmanocept

Stability Store at controlled room temperature of 15°C to 30°C (59°F to 86°F). Brief exposure up to 40°C (104°F) does not adversely affect the product. Solutions may be sterilized.

Mechanism of Action Mepivacaine is an amide local anesthetic similar to lidocaine; like all local anesthetics, mepivacaine acts by preventing the generation and conduction of nerve impulses

Pharmacodynamics Route and dose dependent:
Onset of action: Range: 3-20 minutes
Duration: 2-2.5 hours

Pharmacokinetics (Adult data unless noted)
Protein binding: ~75%
Metabolism: Primarily hepatic via N-demethylation, hydroxylation, and glucuronidation
Half-life:
Neonates: 8.7-9 hours
Adults: 1.9-3 hours
Elimination: Urine (95% as metabolites)

Dosing: Usual Injectable local anesthetic: Dose varies with procedure, degree of anesthesia needed, vascularity of tissue, duration of anesthesia required, and physical condition of patient. The smaller dose/concentration (0.5%) will produce more superficial blockade, a higher dose (1%) will block sensory and sympathetic conduction without loss of motor function, a higher dose (1.5%) will provide extensive and often complete motor blockade, and 2% will produce complete sensory and motor blockade. The smallest dose and concentration required to produce the desired effect should be used.

Children: Maximum dose: 5-6 mg/kg; only concentrations <2% should be used in children <3 years or <14 kg (30 lbs)

Adults: Maximum dose: 400 mg; do not exceed 1000 mg/24 hours

Cervical, brachial, intercostal, pudendal nerve block: 5-40 mL of a 1% solution (maximum: 400 mg) **or** 5-20 mL of a 2% solution (maximum: 400 mg). For pudendal block: Inject $^1/_2$ the total dose each side.

Transvaginal block (paracervical plus pudendal): Up to 30 mL (both sides) of a 1% solution (maximum: 300 mg). Inject $^1/_2$ the total dose into each side.

Paracervical block: Up to 20 mL (both sides) of a 1% solution (maximum: 200 mg). Inject $^1/_2$ the total dose into each side. This is the maximum recommended dose per 90-minute procedure; inject slowly with 5 minutes between sides.

Caudal and epidural block (**preservative free solutions only**): 15-30 mL of a 1% solution (maximum: 300 mg) **or** 10-25 mL of a 1.5% solution (maximum: 375 mg) **or** 10-20 mL of a 2% solution (maximum: 400 mg)

Infiltration: Up to 40 mL of a 1% solution (maximum: 400 mg)

Therapeutic block (pain management): 1-5 mL of a 1% solution (maximum: 50 mg) **or** 1-5 mL of a 2% solution (maximum: 100 mg)

Administration Parenteral: Administer in small incremental doses; when using continuous intermittent catheter techniques, use frequent aspirations before and during the injection to avoid intravascular injection

Monitoring Parameters Blood pressure, heart rate, respiration, signs of CNS toxicity (lightheadedness, dizziness, tinnitus, restlessness, tremors, twitching, drowsiness, circumoral paresthesia)

Dosage Forms Excipient information presented when available (limited, particularly for generics); consult specific product labeling.

Solution, Injection, as hydrochloride:
Carbocaine: 1% (50 mL); 2% (50 mL) [contains methylparaben]
Polocaine: 1% (50 mL); 2% (50 mL) [contains methylparaben]
Generic: 3% (1.8 mL)

Solution, Injection, as hydrochloride [preservative free]:
Carbocaine Preservative-Free: 1% (30 mL); 1.5% (30 mL); 2% (20 mL)
Polocaine-MPF: 1% (30 mL); 1.5% (30 mL); 2% (20 mL) [methylparaben free]

References

Dodson WE, Hillman RE, and Hillman LS, "Brain Tissue Levels in a Fatal Case of Neonatal Mepivacaine (Carbocaine®) Poisoning," *J Pediatr*, 1975, 86(4):624-7.

Torres MJ, Garcia JJ, del Cano Moratinos AM, et al, "Fixed Drug Eruption Induced by Mepivacaine," *J Allergy Clin Immunol*, 1995, 96 (1):130-1.

◆ **Mepivacaine Hydrochloride** see Mepivacaine on page 1341

◆ **Mepron** see Atovaquone on page 229

◆ **Mepron® (Can)** see Atovaquone on page 229

◆ **Mercaptoethane Sulfonate** see Mesna on page 1350

Mercaptopurine (mer kap toe PURE een)

Medication Safety Issues
Sound-alike/look-alike issues:
Mercaptopurine may be confused with methotrexate
Purinethol may be confused with propylthiouracil
High alert medication:
This medication is in a class the Institute for Safe Medication Practices (ISMP) includes among its list of drug classes which have a heightened risk of causing significant patient harm when used in error.
Other safety concerns:
To avoid potentially serious dosage errors, the terms "6-mercaptopurine" or "6-MP" should be avoided; use of these terms has been associated with sixfold overdosages.

Azathioprine is metabolized to mercaptopurine; concurrent use of these commercially-available products has resulted in profound myelosuppression.

Related Information
Emetogenic Potential of Antineoplastic Agents in Children on page 2327
Oral Medications That Should Not Be Crushed or Altered on page 2438
Safe Handling of Hazardous Drugs on page 2419
Brand Names: U.S. Purinethol; Purixan
Brand Names: Canada Purinethol
Therapeutic Category Antineoplastic Agent, Antimetabolite; Antineoplastic Agent, Purine
Generic Availability (U.S.) May be product dependent
Use Maintenance treatment of acute lymphoblastic leukemia (ALL) in combination with other agents (eg, methotrexate) [FDA approved in pediatric patients (age not specified) and adults]; has also been used to treat inflammatory bowel disease, autoimmune hepatitis, and maintenance treatment in acute promyelocytic leukemia (APL)
Prescribing and Access Restrictions Distribution of Purixan is provided by the specialty pharmacy, AnovoRx. For ordering information, call 888-470-0904.
Pregnancy Risk Factor D
Pregnancy Considerations May cause fetal harm if administered during pregnancy. Case reports of fetal loss have been noted with mercaptopurine administration during the first trimester; adverse effects have also been noted with second and third trimester use. Women of child bearing potential should avoid becoming pregnant during treatment.
Breast-Feeding Considerations Mercaptopurine is the active metabolite of azathioprine. Following administration of azathioprine, mercaptopurine can be detected in breast milk (Gardiner, 2006). It is not known if/how much mercaptopurine is found in breast milk following oral administration. According to the manufacturer, the decision to discontinue mercaptopurine or discontinue breast-feeding during therapy should take into account the benefits of treatment to the mother.
Contraindications Hypersensitivity to mercaptopurine or any component; patients whose disease showed prior resistance to mercaptopurine or thioguanine
Warnings Hazardous agent; use appropriate precautions for handling and disposal (NIOSH, 2012). Dose-related hematologic toxicities (leukopenia, thrombocytopenia, anemias, including macrocytic anemia or pancytopenia) may occur; however, these may also be indicative of disease progression. Hematologic toxicity may be delayed; bone marrow may appear hypoplastic (could also appear normal); monitor for bleeding (due to thrombocytopenia) or infection (due to neutropenia). Patients with intermediate TPMT activity (heterozygous) may be at risk for increased myelosuppression, although will generally tolerate normal mercaptopurine doses; those with low or absent TPMT activity (homozygous) are at risk for developing severe and life-threatening hematologic toxicity and will likely require significant dose reductions. TPMT genotyping or phenotyping may assist in identifying patients at risk for developing toxicity. Monitor hematologic function closely; may require dosage reduction or temporary discontinuation of mercaptopurine if there is a rapid decrease or persistently low leukocyte counts. Patients on concurrent therapy with drugs which may inhibit TPMT (eg, olsalazine) or xanthine oxidase (eg, allopurinol) may be at higher risk for myelosuppressive effects. Reduced dosage of mercaptopurine may be recommended when used concurrently with allopurinol. Mercaptopurine is immunosuppressive; the risk for infection is increased; common signs of infection, such as fever and leukocytosis may not occur; lethargy and confusion may be more prominent signs of infection. Because azathioprine is metabolized to

mercaptopurine, concomitant use with azathioprine may result in profound myelosuppression and should be avoided. Immune response to vaccines may be diminished.

The development of secondary hemophagocytic lymphohistiocytosis (HLH), a rare and frequently fatal activation of macrophages which causes phagocytosis of all bone marrow blood cell lines, is increased (100-fold) in pediatric patients diagnosed with inflammatory bowel disease; this risk is further increased with concomitant thiopurine (ie, azathioprine or mercaptopurine) therapy, Epstein-Barr virus, or other possible infections; if patient presents with fever (at least 5 days), cervical lymphadenopathy and lymphopenia, discontinue immunosuppressive therapy and further diagnostic evaluation for HLH should be performed; diagnostic delay associated with increased mortality (Biank, 2011).

Hepatotoxicity has been reported, including jaundice, ascites, hepatic necrosis (may be fatal), intrahepatic cholestasis, parenchymal cell necrosis, and/or hepatic encephalopathy; may be due to direct hepatic cell damage or hypersensitivity. While hepatotoxicity or hepatic injury may occur at any dose, dosages >2.5 mg/kg/day are associated with a higher incidence. Signs of jaundice generally appear early in treatment, after ~1-2 months (range: 1 week to 8 years) and may resolve following discontinuation; recurrence with rechallenge has been noted. Monitor liver function tests; more frequent monitoring recommended when used in combination with other hepatotoxic drugs or in patients with preexisting hepatic impairment. Consider a reduced dose in patients with hepatic impairment. Withhold treatment for clinical signs of jaundice (hepatomegaly, anorexia, tenderness), deterioration in liver function tests, toxic hepatitis, or biliary stasis until hepatotoxicity is ruled out.

Mutagenicity reported in humans; may cause birth defects. Immunosuppressive agents, including mercaptopurine, are associated with the development of lymphoma and other malignancies. In an analysis of T-cell lymphomas associated with TNF blockers (with or without thiopurines) for the treatment of rheumatoid arthritis, Crohn's disease, ulcerative colitis, or ankylosing spondylitis, an increase in the incidence of T-cell lymphomas, most commonly mycosis fungoides/Sezary syndrome and hepatosplenic T-cell lymphoma (HSTCL) was reported (Deepak, 2013). HSTCL is a rare white blood cell cancer that is usually fatal. Most HSTCL cases occurred in patients treated with a combination of TNF blockers and thiopurines, although cases of HSTCL also occurred in patients receiving azathioprine or mercaptopurine monotherapy.

To avoid potentially serious dosage errors, the terms "6-mercaptopurine" or "6-MP" should be avoided; use of these terms has been associated with sixfold overdosages.

Precautions Use with caution in renal impairment; consider dosage adjustment; some renal adverse effects may be minimized with hydration and prophylactic antihyperuricemic therapy. Should only be used by experienced physician.

Adverse Reactions

Central nervous system: Drug fever, malaise

Dermatologic: Alopecia, hyperpigmentation, skin rash, urticaria

Endocrine & metabolic: Hyperuricemia

Gastrointestinal: Anorexia, cholestasis, diarrhea, mucositis, oral lesion, nausea (minimal), pancreatitis, sprue-like symptoms, stomach pain, ulcerative bowel lesion, vomiting (minimal)

Genitourinary: Oligospermia, renal toxicity, uricosuria

Hematologic: Anemia, bone marrow depression (onset 7-10 days; nadir 14 days; recovery: 21 days), granulocytopenia, hemorrhage, hepatosplenic T-cell lymphomas, leukopenia, lymphocytopenia, metastases, neutropenia, thrombocytopenia

Hepatic: Ascites, hepatic encephalopathy, hepatic fibrosis, hepatic injury, hepatic necrosis, hepatomegaly, hepatotoxicity, hyperbilirubinemia, increased serum transaminases, intrahepatic cholestasis, jaundice, toxic hepatitis

Immunologic: Immunosuppression

Infection: Infection

Respiratory: Pulmonary fibrosis

Drug Interactions

Metabolism/Transport Effects None known.

Avoid Concomitant Use

Avoid concomitant use of Mercaptopurine with any of the following: AzaTHIOprine; BCG; CloZAPine; Dipyrone; Febuxostat; Natalizumab; Pimecrolimus; Tacrolimus (Topical); Tofacitinib

Increased Effect/Toxicity

Mercaptopurine may increase the levels/effects of: CloZAPine; Leflunomide; Natalizumab; Tofacitinib; Vaccines (Live)

The levels/effects of Mercaptopurine may be increased by: 5-ASA Derivatives; Allopurinol; AzaTHIOprine; Denosumab; Dipyrone; DOXOrubicin (Conventional); Febuxostat; Pimecrolimus; Roflumilast; Sulfamethoxazole; Tacrolimus (Topical); Trastuzumab; Trimethoprim

Decreased Effect

Mercaptopurine may decrease the levels/effects of: BCG; Coccidioidin Skin Test; Sipuleucel-T; Vaccines (Inactivated); Vitamin K Antagonists

The levels/effects of Mercaptopurine may be decreased by: Echinacea

Food Interactions Absorption is variable with food. Management: Take on an empty stomach at the same time each day 1 hour before or 2 hours after a meal. Maintain adequate hydration, unless instructed to restrict fluid intake.

Stability Hazardous agent; use appropriate precautions for handling and disposal (NIOSH, 2012). Store at 15°C to 25°C (59°F to 77°F); protect from moisture.

Mechanism of Action Mercaptopurine is a purine antagonist which inhibits DNA and RNA synthesis; acts as false metabolite and is incorporated into DNA and RNA, eventually inhibiting their synthesis; specific for the S phase of the cell cycle

Pharmacokinetics (Adult data unless noted)

Absorption: Variable and incomplete (~50%)

Distribution: V_d >total body water; CNS penetration is negligible

Protein binding: ~19%

Metabolism: Hepatic and in GI mucosa; hepatically via xanthine oxidase and methylation via TPMT to sulfate conjugates, 6-thiouric acid, and other inactive compounds; first-pass effect

Half-life:

Children: 21 minutes

Adults: 47 minutes

Time to peak serum concentration: Within 2 hours

Elimination: Urine (46% as mercaptopurine and metabolites)

Dosing: Usual

Children and Adolescents:

Acute lymphoblastic leukemia (ALL): Refer to individual protocols.

Manufacturer's labeling: Maintenance therapy: Oral: 1.5-2.5 mg/kg/dose once daily, combined with other agents

Alternate dosing: Adolescents ≥15 years: Multiple dosage regimens reported:

Consolidation phase: Oral: 60 mg/m²/day days 0-27 days (5-week course) or 60 mg/m²/day days 0-13 and days 28-41 (9-week course) (Stock, 2008)

Early intensification (two 4-week courses): Oral: 60 mg/m²/day on days 1-14 (Larson, 1995; Larson, 1998; Stock, 2008)

Interim maintenance: Oral: 60 mg/m²/day on days 0-41 (8-week course) or 60 mg/m²/day days 1-70 (12-week course) (Larson, 1995; Larson, 1998; Stock, 2008)

Maintenance (prolonged): Oral: 50 mg 3 times daily for 2 years (Kantarjian, 2000; Thomas, 2004) or 60 mg/m²/day for 2 years from diagnosis (Larson, 1995; Larson, 1998; Stock, 2008) or 75 mg/m²/day for 2 years (girls) or 3 years (boys) from first interim maintenance (Stock, 2008)

Acute promyelocytic leukemia (APL): Limited data available: Adolescents ≥15 years: Oral: 60 mg/m²/day for 1 year; in combination with tretinoin and methotrexate (Powell, 2010)

Autoimmune hepatitis: Very limited data available: Oral: 1.5 mg/kg/day in combination with prednisone; not considered first-line, typically used for patient who do not tolerate azathioprine (Manns, 2010)

Inflammatory bowel disease (eg, Crohn's disease, ulcerative colitis): Limited data available: 1-1.5 mg/kg/day (Markowitz, 2000; Punati, 2011; Sandhu, 2010). Some data suggest that pediatric patients ≤6 years may require higher doses to achieve remission; a median dose of 1.68 mg/kg/day (maximum daily dose: 2.4 mg/kg/day) was reported to induce remission in 62% of patients vs 17% of those receiving lower doses (<1.5 mg/kg/day study group; median dose: 1.18 mg/kg/day) (Grossman, 2008; Sandborn, 2001)

Adults: **Acute lymphoblastic leukemia (ALL):** Maintenance: Oral: 1.5-2.5 mg/kg/dose once daily; also consult guidelines for details on combination regimens

Dosing adjustment with concurrent allopurinol: Children, Adolescents, and Adults: Reduce mercaptopurine dosage to 25% to 33% of the usual dose

Dosing adjustment in TPMT-deficiency: Children, Adolescents, and Adults: Dosing not established; substantial reductions are generally required only in homozygous deficiency; however, some experts also recommend dosage reduction with intermediate activity or heterozygous phenotype (Sandborn, 2001)

Dosing adjustment in renal impairment: Children and Adolescents: The manufacturer's labeling recommends starting with reduced doses in patients with renal impairment to avoid accumulation; however, no specific dosage adjustment is provided. The following adjustments have been used by some clinicians (Aronoff, 2007):

GFR >50 mL/minute/1.73m²: No adjustment required

GFR ≤50 mL/minute/1.73m²: Administer every 48 hours

Hemodialysis: Administer every 48 hours

Continuous ambulatory peritoneal dialysis (CAPD): Administer every 48 hours

Continuous renal replacement therapy (CRRT): Administer every 48 hours

Dosing adjustment in hepatic impairment: Children, Adolescents, and Adults: The manufacturer's labeling recommends considering a reduced dose in patients with hepatic impairment; however, no specific dosage adjustment is provided.

Administration Hazardous agent; use appropriate precautions for handling and disposal (NIOSH, 2012). Preferably on an empty stomach (1 hour before or 2 hours after meals). For the treatment of ALL in children: Administration in the evening has demonstration superior outcome;

administration with food did not significantly affect outcome (Schmiegelow, 1997)

Monitoring Parameters CBC with differential (weekly initially, although clinical status may require increased frequency), bone marrow exam (to evaluate marrow status), liver function tests (weekly initially, then monthly; monitor more frequently if on concomitant hepatotoxic agents), renal function, urinalysis; consider TPMT genotyping to identify TPMT defect (if severe toxicity occurs)

For use in inflammatory bowel disease, monitor CBC with differential weekly for 1 month, then biweekly for 1 month, followed by monitoring every 1-2 months throughout the course of therapy. LFTs should be assessed every 3 months. Monitor for signs/symptoms of malignancy (eg, splenomegaly, hepatomegaly, abdominal pain, persistent fever, night sweats, weight loss) (Sandhu, 2010).

Test Interactions TPMT testing: Recent transfusions may result in a misinterpretation of the actual TPMT activity. Concomitant drugs may influence TPMT activity in the blood.

Dosage Forms Excipient information presented when available (limited, particularly for generics); consult specific product labeling.

Suspension, Oral:
Purixan: 2000 mg/100 mL (100 mL) [contains aspartame, methylparaben, propylparaben]

Tablet, Oral:
Purinethol: 50 mg [scored]
Generic: 50 mg

Extemporaneous Preparations Hazardous agent: Use appropriate precautions for handling and disposal.

A 50 mg/mL oral suspension may be prepared in a vertical flow hood with tablets and a mixture of sterile water for injection (SWFI), simple syrup, and cherry syrup. Crush thirty 50 mg tablets in a mortar and reduce to a fine powder. Add ~5 mL SWFI and mix to a uniform paste; then add ~10 mL simple syrup; mix while continuing to add cherry syrup to make a final volume of 30 mL; transfer to a calibrated bottle. Label "shake well" and "caution chemotherapy". Stable for 35 days at room temperature.

Aliabadi HM, Romanick M, Desai, S, et al, "Effect of Buffer and Antioxidant on Stability of a Mercaptopurine Suspension," *Am J Health Syst Pharm*, 2008, 65(5):441-7.

References

Aronoff GR, Bennett WM, Berns JS, et al, *Drug Prescribing in Renal Failure: Dosing Guidelines for Adults and Children*, 5th ed. Philadelphia, PA: American College of Physicians; 2007, 173.

Biank VF, Sheth MK, Talano J, et al, "Association of Crohn's disease, Thiopurines, and Primary Epstein-Barr Virus Infection With Hemophagocytic Lymphohistiocytosis," *J Pediatr*, 2011, 159(5):808-12.

Deepak P, Sifuentes H, Sherid M, et al, "T-Cell Non-Hodgkin's Lymphomas Reported to the FDA AERS With Tumor Necrosis Factor-Alpha (TNF-α) Inhibitors: Results of the REFURBISH Study," *Am J Gastroenterol*, 2013, 108(1):99-105.

Gardiner SJ, Gearry RB, Roberts RL, et al, "Exposure to Thiopurine Drugs Through Breast Milk is Low Based on Metabolite Concentrations in Mother-Infant Pairs," *Br J Clin Pharmacol*, 2006, 62(4):453-6.

Gremse DA and Crissinger KD, "Ulcerative Colitis in Children: Medical Management," *Paediatr Drugs*, 2002, 4(12):807-15.

Grossman AB, Noble AJ, Mamula P, et al, "Increased Dosing Requirements for 6-Mercaptopurine and Azathioprine in Inflammatory Bowel Disease Patients Six Years and Younger," *Inflamm Bowel Dis*, 2008, 14(6):750-5.

Kantarjian HM, O'Brien S, Smith TL, et al, "Results of Treatment With Hyper-CVAD, A Dose-Intensive Regimen, in Adult Acute Lymphocytic Leukemia," *J Clin Oncol*, 2000, 18(3): 547-61.

Larson RA, Dodge RK, Burns CP, et al, "A Five-Drug Remission Induction Regimen With Intensive Consolidation for Adults With Acute Lymphoblastic Leukemia: Cancer and Leukemia Group B Study 8811," *Blood*, 1995, 85(8):2025-37.

Larson RA, Dodge RK, Linker CA, et al, "A Randomized Controlled Trial of Filgrastim During Remission Induction and Consolidation Chemotherapy for Adults With Acute Lymphoblastic Leukemia: CALGB Study 9111," *Blood*, 1998, 92(5):1556-64.

Manns MP, Czaja AJ, Gorham JD, et al, "Diagnosis and Management of Autoimmune Hepatitis," *Hepatology*, 2010, 51(6):2193-213.

Markowitz J, Grancher K, Kohn N, et al, "A Multicenter Trial of 6-Mercaptopurine and Prednisone in Children With Newly Diagnosed Crohn's Disease," *Gastroenterology*, 2000, 119(4):895-902.

Mosesso P and Palitti F, "The Genetic Toxicology of 6-Mercaptopurine," *Mutat Res*, 1993, 296(3):279-94.

National Institute for Occupational Safety and Health (NIOSH), "NIOSH List of Antineoplastic and Other Hazardous Drugs in Healthcare Settings 2012." Available at http://www.cdc.gov/niosh/docs/2012-150/pdfs/2012-150.pdf. Accessed January 21, 2013.

Parakkal D, Sifuentes H, Semer R, et al, "Hepatosplenic T-Cell Lymphoma in Patients Receiving TNF-α Inhibitor Therapy: Expanding the Groups at Risk," *Eur J Gastroenterol Hepatol*, 2011, 23(12):1150-6.

Powell BL, Moser B, Stock W, et al, "Arsenic Trioxide Improves Event-Free and Over-All Survival for Adults With Acute Promyelocytic Leukemia: North American Leukemia Intergroup Study C9710," *Blood*, 2010, 116(19):3751-7.

Punati J, Markowitz J, Lerer T, et al, "Effect of Early Immunomodulator Use in Moderate to Severe Pediatric Crohn Disease," *Inflamm Bowel Dis*, 2008, 14(7):949-54.

Sandborn WJ, "A Review of Immune Modifier Therapy for Inflammatory Bowel Disease: Azathioprine, 6-mercaptopurine, Cyclosporine, and Methotrexate," *Am J Gastroenterol*, 1996, 91(3):423-33.

Sandhu BK, Fell JME, Beattie RM, et al, "Guidelines for the Management of Inflammatory Bowel Disease in Children in the United Kingdom." *JPGN*, 2010, 50:1-13.

Schmiegelow K, Glomstein A, Kristinsson J, et al, "Impact of Morning versus Evening Schedule for Oral Methotrexate and 6-Mercaptopurine on Relapse Risk for Children With Acute Lymphoblastic Leukemia. Nordic Society for Pediatric Hematology and Oncology (NOPHO)," *J Pediatr Hematol Oncol*, 1997, 19(2):102-9.

Stock W, La M, Sanford B, et al, "What Determines the Outcomes for Adolescents and Young Adults With Acute Lymphoblastic Leukemia Treated on Cooperative Group Protocols? A Comparison of Children's Cancer Group and Cancer and Leukemia Group B Studies," *Blood*, 2008, 112(5):1646-54.

◆ **6-Mercaptopurine (error-prone abbreviation)** *see* Mercaptopurine *on page 1342*

◆ **Mercapturic Acid** *see* Acetylcysteine *on page 60*

Meropenem (mer oh PEN em)

Medication Safety Issues
Sound-alike/look-alike issues:
Meropenem may be confused with ertapenem, imipenem, metroNIDAZOLE

Brand Names: U.S. Merrem

Brand Names: Canada Meropenem For Injection; Merrem

Therapeutic Category Antibiotic, Carbapenem

Generic Availability (U.S.) Yes

Use Treatment of multidrug-resistant infection caused by gram-negative and gram-positive aerobic and anaerobic pathogens documented or suspected to be susceptible to meropenem; used in treatment of meningitis (FDA approved in pediatric patients ages ≥3 months), intra-abdominal infections and complicated skin and skin structure infections caused by susceptible *S. aureus*, *S. pyogenes*, *S. agalactiae*, *S. pneumoniae*, *H. influenzae*, *N. meningitidis*, *M. catarrhalis*, *E. coli*, *Klebsiella*, *Enterobacter*, *Serratia*, *P. aeruginosa*, *B. cepacia*, and *B. fragilis* (FDA approved in ages ≥3 months and adults); has been used for treatment of lower respiratory tract infections, acute pulmonary exacerbations in cystic fibrosis, urinary tract infections, empiric treatment of febrile neutropenia, and sepsis

Pregnancy Risk Factor B

Pregnancy Considerations Adverse events were not observed in animal reproduction studies. Incomplete transplacental transfer of meropenem was found using an *ex vivo* human perfusion model.

Breast-Feeding Considerations Small amounts of meropenem are excreted into breast milk (case report). The manufacturer recommends that caution be exercised when administering meropenem to breast-feeding women. Non-dose-related effects could include modification of bowel flora.

Contraindications Hypersensitivity to meropenem, any component, other carbapenems, or in patients who have experienced anaphylactic reactions to beta-lactams

Warnings Serious and occasionally fatal hypersensitivity reactions have been reported in patients receiving beta-lactam therapy; careful inquiry should be made concerning previous hypersensitivity reactions to penicillins, cephalosporins, or other beta-lactams before initiating meropenem. Prolonged use may result in fungal or bacterial superinfection, including *C. difficile*-associated diarrhea (CDAD) and pseudomembranous colitis; CDAD has been observed >2 months postantibiotic treatment; use with caution in patients with a history of colitis. Seizures and other CNS adverse events have been reported, most commonly in patients with renal impairment and/or underlying neurologic disorders. Valproic acid (VPA) serum concentrations may be significantly decreased by concurrent carbapenem use leading to breakthrough seizures; serum VPA concentrations should be closely monitored after initiation of meropenem. VPA dosage adjustment may not adequately compensate for this interaction. Thrombocytopenia has been reported in patients with renal dysfunction who are receiving meropenem.

Precautions Use with caution in patients with a history of seizures, CNS disease, CNS infection, and/or compromised renal function; dosage adjustment required in patients with renal impairment

Adverse Reactions
Central nervous system: Headache, pain

Dermatologic: Pruritus, rash (includes diaper-area moniliasis in infants)

Endocrine & metabolic: Hypoglycemia

Gastrointestinal: Constipation, diarrhea, glossitis, nausea, oral moniliasis, vomiting

Hematologic: Anemia

Local: Inflammation at the injection site, injection site reaction, phlebitis/thrombophlebitis

Respiratory: Apnea, pharyngitis, pneumonia

Miscellaneous: Sepsis, shock

Rare but important or life-threatening: Abdominal enlargement, abdominal pain, agitation/delirium, agranulocytosis, alkaline phosphatase increased, ALT increased, AST increased, anemia (hypochromic), angioedema, anorexia, anxiety, aPTT decreased, asthma, back pain, bilirubin increased, bradycardia, BUN increased, cardiac arrest, chest pain, chills, cholestatic jaundice/jaundice, confusion, cough, creatinine increased, depression, diaphoresis, dizziness, dyspepsia, dyspnea, dysuria, eosinophilia, epistaxis, erythema multiforme, fever, flatulence, gastrointestinal hemorrhage, hallucinations, heart failure, hematuria, hemoglobin/hematocrit decreased, hemolytic anemia, hemoperitoneum, hepatic failure, hyper-/hypotension, hypervolemia, hypokalemia, hypoxia, ileus, injection site edema, injection site pain, insomnia, intestinal obstruction, LDH increased, leukocytosis, leukopenia, melena, MI, nervousness, neutropenia, paresthesia, pelvic pain, peripheral edema, platelets decreased/increased, pleural effusion, PT decreased, pulmonary edema, positive Coombs test, pulmonary embolism, renal failure, respiratory disorder, seizure, skin ulcer, somnolence, Stevens-Johnson syndrome, syncope, tachycardia, toxic epidermal necrolysis, urinary incontinence, urticaria, vaginal moniliasis, weakness, WBC decreased, whole body pain

Drug Interactions
Metabolism/Transport Effects None known.

Avoid Concomitant Use
Avoid concomitant use of Meropenem with any of the following: BCG; Probenecid

Increased Effect/Toxicity
The levels/effects of Meropenem may be increased by: Probenecid

▶

Decreased Effect
Meropenem may decrease the levels/effects of: BCG; Sodium Picosulfate; Typhoid Vaccine; Valproic Acid and Derivatives

Stability Store intact vials at 20°C to 25°C (68°F to 77°F); meropenem reconstituted with SWI is stable for up to 2 hours at room temperature or for up to 12 hours when refrigerated; when diluted with NS to a final concentration between 2.5-50 mg/mL, the solution is stable for up to 2 hours at room temperature or 18 hours when refrigerated; when diluted with D_5W to a final concentration between 1-50 mg/mL, the solution is stable for up to 1 hour at room temperature or 8 hours when refrigerated; solutions prepared for infusion in plastic I.V. bags with NS at concentrations ranging from 1-20 mg/mL are stable for 4 hours at room temperature or 24 hours when refrigerated

Mechanism of Action Inhibits bacterial cell wall synthesis by binding to several of the penicillin-binding proteins, which in turn inhibit the final transpeptidation step of peptidoglycan synthesis in bacterial cell walls, thus inhibiting cell wall biosynthesis; bacteria eventually lyse due to ongoing activity of cell wall autolytic enzymes (autolysins and murein hydrolases) while cell wall assembly is arrested

Pharmacokinetics (Adult data unless noted)
Distribution: Penetrates into most tissues and body fluids including urinary tract, peritoneal fluid, bone, bile, lung, bronchial mucosa, muscle tissue, heart valves, and CSF (CSF penetration: Neonates and Infants ≤3 months: 70%)

V_d:
Neonates and Infants ≤3 months: Median: ~0.47 L/kg (Smith, 2011)
Children: 0.3-0.4 L/kg (Blumer, 1995)
Adults: 15-20 L
Protein binding: 2%
Metabolism: 20% is hydrolyzed in plasma to an inactive metabolite
Half-life:
Neonates and Infants ≤3 months: Median: 2.7 hours; range: 1.6- 3.8 hours (Smith, 2011)
Infants and Children 3 months to 2 years: 1.5 hours
Children 2-12 years and Adults: 1 hour
Time to peak tissue and fluid concentrations: 1 hour after the start of infusion except in bile, lung, muscle, and CSF which peak at 2-3 hours
Elimination: Cleared by the kidney with 70% excreted unchanged in urine
Clearance:
Neonates and Infants ≤3 months: 0.12 L/hour/kg (Smith, 2011)
Infants and Children: 0.26-0.37 L/hour/kg (Blumer, 1995)

Dosing: Neonatal
General dosing:
General dosing, susceptible infection (non-CNS), treatment: Limited data available: For organisms highly susceptible to meropenem, MIC <4 mcg/mL:
Age-directed dosing (Smith, 2011):
GA <32 weeks:
PNA <14 days: 20 mg/kg/dose every 12 hours
PNA ≥14 days: 20 mg/kg/dose every 8 hours
GA ≥32 weeks:
PNA <14 days: 20 mg/kg/dose every 8 hours
PNA ≥14 days: 30 mg/kg/dose every 8 hours
Weight-directed dosing (*Red Book*, 2012):
Body weight <1 kg:
PNA ≤14 days: 20 mg/kg/dose every 12 hours
PNA 15-28 days: 20 mg/kg/dose every 8 hours
Body weight 1-2 kg:
PNA ≤7 days: 20 mg/kg/dose every 12 hours
PNA 8-28 days: 20 mg/kg/dose every 8 hours
Body weight >2 kg: 20 mg/kg/dose every 8 hours

Moderately resistant infection (non-CNS), treatment: For organisms with MIC 4-8 mcg/mL: Limited data available; further studies needed: GA >30 weeks, PNA >7 days: 40 mg/kg/dose every 8 hours, some suggest as a 4-hour infusion; dosing based on a single-dose pharmacokinetic study (n=38) (van den Anker, 2009)
Meningitis: Limited data available; dose not established; further studies are needed. An evaluation of CSF concentrations in six patients using the dosing for susceptible infection [see Susceptible infection (non-CNS) dosing] reported levels to be above the target of 4 mcg/mL and highly variable (4.1-34.6 mcg/mL) at 0.3-7.9 hours (Smith, 2011); other suggest using the upper end of the dosing range (van den Anker, 2009); recommended duration of therapy dependent upon pathogen: *N. meningitides, H. influenza:* 7 days; *S. pneumoniae:* 10-14 days; *Listeria monocytogenes:* ≥21 days; aerobic gram-negative bacilli: Either 2 weeks beyond the first sterile CSF culture or >3 weeks, whichever is longer (Tunkel, 2004)

Dosing: Usual
Infants, Children, and Adolescents:
General dosing, susceptible infection (*Red Book*, 2012): I.V.:
Severe infections (non-CNS): 10-20 mg/kg/dose every 8 hours; maximum single dose: 2000 mg
Alternate dosing for infants <3 months (non-CNS): For organisms highly susceptible to meropenem, MIC <4 mcg/mL: 20-30 mg/kg/dose every 8 hours (Smith, 2011); maximum single dose: 200 mg
Cystic fibrosis, pulmonary exacerbation: Limited data available: I.V.: 40 mg/kg/dose every 8 hours; maximum single dose: 2000 mg (Zobell, 2012)
Fever/neutropenia empiric treatment: I.V.: 20 mg/kg/dose every 8 hours; maximum single dose: 1000 mg
Intra-abdominal infection, complicated: I.V.: 20 mg/kg/dose every 8 hours for 4-7 days; maximum single dose: 1000 mg (Solomkin, 2010)
Meningitis: I.V.: 40 mg/kg/dose every 8 hours; maximum single dose: 2000 mg; duration of therapy dependent upon pathogen: *N. meningitidis, H. influenza:* 7 days; *S. pneumoniae:* 10-14 days; aerobic gram-negative bacilli: 21 days (Tunkel, 2004)
Skin and skin structure infection, complicated: Infants ≥3 months, Children, and Adolescents: I.V.: 10 mg/kg/dose every 8 hours; maximum dose: 500 mg
Adults:
General dosing, susceptible infection: I.V.: 500-2000 mg every 8 hours
Intra-abdominal infection: I.V.: 1000 mg every 8 hours
Meningitis: I.V.: 2000 mg every 8 hours; duration of therapy dependent upon pathogen: *N. meningitides, H. influenza:* 7 days; *S. pneumoniae:* 10-14 days; aerobic gram-negative bacilli: 21 days (Tunkel, 2004)
Skin and skin structure infection, complicated: I.V.: 500 mg every 8 hours
Dosing adjustment in renal impairment:
Infants, Children, and Adolescents: There are no dosage adjustments provided in the manufacturer's labeling. Some clinicians have used the following (Aronoff, 2007): **Note:** Renally adjusted dose recommendations are based on doses of 20-40 mg/kg/dose every 8 hours:
GFR >50 mL/minute/1.73 m^2: No adjustment required.
GFR 30-50 mL/minute/1.73 m^2: Administer 20-40 mg/kg/dose every 12 hours
GFR 10-29 mL/minute/1.73 m^2: Administer 10-20 mg/kg/dose every 12 hours
GFR <10 mL/minute/1.73 m^2: Administer 10-20 mg/kg/dose every 24 hours
Intermittent hemodialysis (IHD): Meropenem and metabolite are readily dialyzable: 10-20 mg/kg/dose

every 24 hours; on dialysis days give dose **after** hemodialysis

Peritoneal dialysis (PD): 10-20 mg/kg/dose every 24 hours

Continuous renal replacement therapy (CRRT): 20-40 mg/kg/dose every 12 hours

Adults:

CrCl >50 mL/minute: No adjustment required.

CrCl 26-50 mL/minute: Standard dose every 12 hours

CrCl 10-25 mL/minute: One-half dose every 12 hours

CrCl <10 mL/minute: One-half dose every 24 hours

Intermittent hemodialysis (IHD) (administer after hemodialysis on dialysis days): Meropenem and its metabolites are readily dialyzable: 500 mg every 24 hours. **Note:** Dosing dependent on the assumption of 3 times weekly, complete IHD sessions (Heintz, 2009).

Peritoneal dialysis: Administer recommended dose (based on indication) every 24 hours (Aronoff, 2007).

Continuous renal replacement therapy (CRRT) (Heintz, 2009; Trotman, 2005): Drug clearance is highly dependent on the method of renal replacement, filter type, and flow rate. Appropriate dosing requires close monitoring of pharmacologic response, signs of adverse reactions due to drug accumulation, as well as drug concentrations in relation to target trough (if appropriate). The following are general recommendations only (based on dialysate flow/ultrafiltration rates of 1-2 L/hour and minimal residual renal function) and should not supersede clinical judgment:

CVVH: Loading dose of 1000 mg followed by either 500 mg every 8 hours or 1000 mg every 12 hours

CVVHD/CVVHDF: Loading dose of 1000 mg followed by either 500 mg every 6-8 hours or 1000 mg every 8-12 hours

Note: Consider giving patients receiving CVVHDF dosages of 750 mg every 8 hours or 1500 mg every 12 hours (Heintz, 2009). Substantial variability exists in various published recommendations, ranging from 1000-3000 mg/**day** in 2-3 divided doses. One gram every 12 hours achieves a target trough of ~4 mg/L.

Dosing adjustment in hepatic impairment: There are no dosage adjustments provided in the manufacturer's labeling; pharmacokinetics of meropenem are not altered in hepatic impairment so adjustment should not be necessary; use with caution.

Administration Administer by I.V. push or I.V. intermittent infusion; infuse I.V. push injection over 3-5 minutes at a final concentration not to exceed 50 mg/mL; intermittent infusion dose should be administered over 15-30 minutes at a final concentration ranging from 1-50 mg/mL in D₅W or NS; some studies have demonstrated enhanced pharmacodynamic effects when extending intermittent infusions to 4 hours (van den Anker, 2009)

Monitoring Parameters Periodic renal, hepatic, and hematologic function tests. Observe for changes in bowel frequency. Monitor for signs of anaphylaxis during first dose.

Test Interactions Positive Coombs' [direct]

Dosage Forms Excipient information presented when available (limited, particularly for generics); consult specific product labeling.

Solution Reconstituted, Intravenous:

Merrem: 500 mg (1 ea); 1 g (1 ea)

Generic: 500 mg (1 ea); 1 g (1 ea)

References

Aronoff GR, Bennett WM, Berns JS, et al, *Drug Prescribing in Renal Failure: Dosing Guidelines for Adults and Children*, 5th ed, Philadelphia, PA: American College of Physicians, 2007.

Blumer JL, Saiman L, Konstan MW, et al, "The Efficacy and Safety of Meropenem and Tobramycin Vs Ceftazidime and Tobramycin in the Treatment of Acute Pulmonary Exacerbations in Patients With Cystic Fibrosis," *Chest*, 2005, 128(4):2336-46.

Blummer JL, "Pharmacokinetic Determinants of Carbapenem Therapy in Neonates and Children," *Pediatr Infect Dis J*, 1996, 15(8):733-7.

Blummer JL, Reed MD, Kearns GL, et al, "Sequential, Single-Dose Pharmacokinetic Evaluation of Meropenem in Hospitalized Infants and Children," *Antimicrob Agents Chemother*, 1995, 39(8):1721-5.

Bradley, JS, "Meropenem: A New, Extremely Broad Spectrum Beta-lactam Antibiotic for Serious Infections in Pediatrics," *Pediatr Infect Dis J*, 1997, 16:263-8.

Bradley JS, Sauberan JB, Ambrose PG, et al, "Meropenem Pharmacokinetics, Pharmacodynamics, and Monte Carlo Simulation in the Neonate," *Pediatr Infect Dis J*, 2008, 27(9):794-9.

Craig WA, "The Pharmacology of Meropenem, a New Carbapenem Antibiotic," *Clin Infect Dis*, 1997, 24(Suppl 2):266-75.

Heintz BH, Matzke GR, and Dager WE, "Antimicrobial Dosing Concepts and Recommendations for Critically Ill Adult Patients Receiving Continuous Renal Replacement Therapy or Intermittent Hemodialysis," *Pharmacotherapy*, 2009, 29(5):562-77.

Latzin P, Fehling M, Bauernfeind A, et al, "Efficacy and Safety of Intravenous Meropenem and Tobramycin Versus Ceftazidime and Tobramycin in Cystic Fibrosis," *J Cyst Fibros*, 2008, 7(2):142-6.

Odio CM, Puig JR, Feris JM, et al, "Prospective, Randomized, Investigator-Blinded Study of the Efficacy and Safety of Meropenem vs. Cefotaxime Therapy in Bacterial Meningitis in Children. Meropenem Meningitis Study Group," *Pediatr Infect Dis J*, 1999, 18(7):581-90.

Smith PB, Cohen-Wolkowiez M, Castro LM, et al, "Populations Pharmacokinetics of Meropenem in Plasma and Cerebrospinal Fluid of Infants With Suspected or Complicated Intra-abdominal Infections, "Pediatr Infect Dis J," 2011, 30(10):844-9.

Solomkin JS, Mazuski JE, Bradley JS, et al, "Diagnosis and Management of Complicated Intra-Abdominal Infection in Adults and Children: Guidelines by the Surgical Infection Society and the Infectious Diseases Society of America," *Clin Infect Dis*, 2010, 50(2):133-64.

Trotman RL, Williamson JC, Shoemaker DM, et al, "Antibiotic Dosing in Critically Ill Adult Patients Receiving Continuous Renal Replacement Therapy," *Clin Infect Dis*, 2005, 41(8):1159-66.

Tunkel AR, Hartman BJ, Kaplan SL, et al, "Practice Guidelines for the Management of Bacterial Meningitis," *Clin Infect Dis*, 2004, 39 (9):1267-84.

van den Anker JN, Pokorna P, Kinzig-Schippers M, et al, "Meropenem Pharmacokinetics in the Newborn," *Antimicrob Agents Chemother*, 2009, 53(9):3871-9.

Ververs TF, van Dijk A, Vinks SA, et al, "Pharmacokinetics and Dosing Regimen of Meropenem in Critically Ill Patients Receiving Continuous Venovenous Hemofiltration," *Crit Care Med*, 2000, 28(10):3412-6.

Wiseman LR, Wagstaff AJ, Brogden RN, et al, "Meropenem. A Review of its Antibacterial Activity, Pharmacokinetic Properties and Clinical Efficacy," *Drugs*, 1995, 50(1):73-101.

Yildirim I, Aytac S, Ceyhan M, et al, "Piperacillin/Tazobactam Plus Amikacin Versus Carbapenem Monotherapy as Empirical Treatment of Febrile Neutropenia in Childhood Hematological Malignancies," *Pediatr Hematol Oncol*, 2008, 25(4):291-9.

Zobell JT, Young DC, Waters CD, et al, "Optimization of Anti-pseudomonal Antibiotics for Cystic Fibrosis Pulmonary Exacerbations: I. Aztreonam and Carbapenems," *Pediatr Pulmonol*, 2012, 47 (12):1147-58.

◆ **Meropenem For Injection (Can)** see Meropenem on page 1345

◆ **Merrem** see Meropenem on page 1345

Mesalamine (me SAL a meen)

Medication Safety Issues

Sound-alike/look-alike issues:

Mesalamine may be confused with mecamylamine, megestrol, memantine, metaxalone, methenamine

Apriso may be confused with Apri

Asacol may be confused with Ansaid, Os-Cal

Lialda may be confused with Aldara

Pentasa may be confused with Pancrease, Pangestyme

Related Information

Oral Medications That Should Not Be Crushed or Altered on page 2438

Brand Names: U.S. Apriso; Asacol HD; Canasa; Delzicol; Lialda; Pentasa; Rowasa; SfRowasa

Brand Names: Canada Asacol; Asacol 800; Mesasal; Mezavant; Novo-5 ASA; Pentasa; Salofalk

Therapeutic Category 5-Aminosalicylic Acid Derivative; Anti-inflammatory Agent; Anti-inflammatory Agent, Rectal

Generic Availability (U.S.) May be product dependent

Use Treatment and maintenance of remission of ulcerative colitis (UC); treatment of proctosigmoiditis and proctitis (FDA approved in adults; see manufacturer's labeling for ▶

specific indications); has also been used for Crohn's disease

Pregnancy Risk Factor B/C (product specific)

Pregnancy Considerations Adverse events were not observed in animal reproduction studies. Dibutyl phthalate (DBP) is an inactive ingredient in the enteric coating of Asacol and Asacol HD; adverse effects in male rats were noted at doses greater than the recommended human dose. Mesalamine is known to cross the placenta. An increased rate of congenital malformations has not been observed in human studies. Preterm birth, still birth and decreased birth weight have been observed; however, these events may also be due to maternal disease. When treatment for inflammatory bowel disease is needed during pregnancy, mesalamine may be used, although products with DBP should be avoided (Habal, 2012; Mottet, 2009).

Breast-Feeding Considerations Low concentrations of the parent drug (undetectable to 0.11 mg/L) and higher concentrations of the N-acetyl metabolite of the parent drug (5-18 mg/L) have been detected in human breast milk following oral or rectal maternal doses of 500 mg to 3 g daily. Adverse effects (diarrhea) in a nursing infant have been reported while the mother received rectal administration of mesalamine within 12 hours after the first dose (Nelis, 1989). The manufacturer recommends that caution be used if administered to a nursing woman. Other sources consider use of mesalamine to be safe while breastfeeding (Habal, 2012; Mottet, 2009).

Contraindications Hypersensitivity to mesalamine, aminosalicylates, salicylates, or any component including saturated vegetable fatty acid esters (Canasa™ suppositories)

Warnings Myocarditis and pericarditis should be considered in patients with chest pain; this cardiac hypersensitivity reaction has occurred rarely with mesalamine-containing products; pancreatitis should be considered in any patient with new abdominal complaints; has been implicated in the production of an acute intolerance syndrome or exacerbation of colitis (<3%), prompt discontinuation is required if this develops.

Some products may contain sulfites which may cause allergic reactions in susceptible individuals. Rowasa® and sfRowasa™ suspensions contain sodium benzoate; benzoic acid (benzoate) is a metabolite of benzyl alcohol; large amounts of benzyl alcohol (≥99 mg/kg/day) have been associated with a potentially fatal toxicity ("gasping syndrome") in neonates; *in vitro* and animal studies have shown that benzoate displaces bilirubin from protein binding sites; avoid use of Rowasa® and sfRowasa™ suspensions in neonates.

Precautions Use with caution in patients with renal impairment or a history of renal disease; renal disease, including minimal change nephropathy, acute/chronic interstitial nephritis, nephrotic syndrome, and rarely renal failure has been reported. Use with caution with other medications converted to mesalamine; evaluate renal function prior to initiation of mesalamine products and periodically during treatment. Use with caution in patients with hypersensitivity to sulfasalazine, patients with hepatic impairment, and patients with conditions predisposing to the development of myocarditis or pericarditis. Oral products are formulated to slowly release therapeutic quantities of drug; capsules have an ethylcellulose coating or enteric coating in a polymer matrix creating a controlled/extended release throughout the GI tract; tablets are coated with an acrylic-based resin and release drug after reaching the terminal ileum; use delayed release formulations with caution in patients with pyloric stenosis due to prolonged gastric retention. Apriso™ contains phenylalanine which must be avoided in patients with phenylketonuria.

Adverse Reactions Adverse effects vary depending upon dosage form.

Cardiovascular: Chest pain, hypertension, peripheral edema, vasodilation

Central nervous system: Anxiety, chills, dizziness, fatigue, headache, insomnia, malaise, migraine, nervousness, pain, paresthesia, vertigo

Dermatologic: Acne vulgaris, alopecia, diaphoresis, pruritus, skin rash

Endocrine & metabolic: Increased serum triglycerides

Gastrointestinal: Abdominal distention, abdominal pain, abnormal stools, anorectal pain (on insertion of enema tip), constipation, diarrhea, dyspepsia, eructation, exacerbation of ulcerative colitis, flatulence, gastroenteritis, gastrointestinal hemorrhage, hemorrhoids, intolerance syndrome, nausea, rectal hemorrhage, rectal pain, tenesmus, vomiting

Genitourinary: Polyuria

Hematologic & oncologic: Hematocrit/hemoglobin decreased

Hepatic: Abnormal hepatic function tests, cholestatic hepatitis, increased serum ALT increased, increased serum transaminases

Infection: Infection

Neuromuscular & skeletal: Arthralgia, arthritis, back pain, hypertonia, musculoskeletal pain (leg/joint), myalgia, weakness

Ophthalmic: Conjunctivitis, visual disturbance

Otic: Otalgia, tinnitus

Renal: Decreased creatinine clearance, hematuria

Respiratory: Bronchitis, cough, dyspnea, flu-like symptoms, nasopharyngitis, pharyngitis, sinusitis

Miscellaneous: Fever

Rare but important or life-threatening: Abdominal distention, abnormal T waves on ECG, agranulocytosis, albuminuria, alopecia, anaphylaxis, anemia, angioedema, aplastic anemia, bloody diarrhea, cholestatic jaundice, cholecystitis, constipation, DRESS syndrome, drug fever, dysuria, edema, eosinophilia, eosinophilic pneumonitis, erythema nodosum, exacerbation of asthma, fecal discoloration, frequent bowel movements, granulocytopenia, Guillain-Barré syndrome, hepatic failure, hepatic injury, hepatic necrosis, hepatitis, hepatotoxicity, hypersensitivity pneumonitis, hypersensitivity reactions, idiopathic nephrotic syndrome, increased blood urea nitrogen, increased serum bilirubin, increased serum creatinine, interstitial nephritis, interstitial pneumonitis, irregular menses, jaundice, Kawasaki-like syndrome, leukopenia, lupus-like syndrome, lymphadenopathy, mucus stools, myocarditis, nephrotoxicity, neutropenia, oligospermia, painful defecation, palpitations, pancreatitis, pancytopenia, paresthesia, perforated peptic ulcer, perianal skin irritation, pericardial effusion, pericarditis, peripheral neuropathy, pharyngolaryngeal pain, pleurisy, pneumonitis, pruritus, pulmonary interstitial fibrosis, pyoderma gangrenosum, rectal discharge, rectal polyp, renal disease, renal failure, skin photosensitivity, Stevens-Johnson syndrome, systemic lupus erythematosus, tachycardia, tenesmus, thrombocythemia, thrombocytopenia, transverse myelitis, vasodilation

Drug Interactions

Metabolism/Transport Effects None known.

Avoid Concomitant Use There are no known interactions where it is recommended to avoid concomitant use.

Increased Effect/Toxicity

Mesalamine may increase the levels/effects of: Heparin; Heparin (Low Molecular Weight); Thiopurine Analogs; Varicella Virus-Containing Vaccines

The levels/effects of Mesalamine may be increased by: Nonsteroidal Anti-Inflammatory Agents

Decreased Effect

Mesalamine may decrease the levels/effects of: Cardiac Glycosides

The levels/effects of Mesalamine may be decreased by:
Antacids; H2-Antagonists; Proton Pump Inhibitors

Stability

Oral: Store at controlled room temperature.
Apriso™, capsules: 20°C to 25°C (68°F to 77°F); excursions permitted to 15°C to 30°C (59°F to 86°F)
Asacol® HD, tablets: 20°C to 25°C (68°F to 77°F)
Lialda®, tablets: 15°C to 25°C (59°F to 77°F); excursions permitted to 30°C (86°F)
Pentasa®, capsules: Store at 25°C (77°F); excursions permitted to 15°C to 30°C (59°F to 86°F)
Rectal:
Enema: Store at 20°C to 25°C (68°F to 77°F). Once foil wrap is open, any bottles remaining after 14 days should be discarded. Contents may darken with time (do not use if dark brown).
Suppository: Store below 25°C (below 77°F). May store under refrigeration; do not freeze. Protect from direct heat, light, and humidity.

Mechanism of Action

Mesalamine (5-aminosalicylic acid) is the active component of sulfasalazine; the specific mechanism of action of mesalamine is unknown; however, it is thought that it modulates local chemical mediators of the inflammatory response, especially leukotrienes, and is also postulated to be a free radical scavenger or an inhibitor of tumor necrosis factor (TNF); action appears topical rather than systemic

Pharmacokinetics (Adult data unless noted)

Absorption:
Oral: Capsule: ~20% to 40%; Tablet: 20% to 28%
Rectal: Variable and dependent upon retention time, underlying GI disease, and colonic pH
Protein binding: Mesalamine (5-ASA): ~43%; N-acetyl-5-ASA: ~78%
Metabolism: Hepatic and via GI tract to N-acetyl-5-aminosalicylic acid
Half-life:
5-ASA: 0.5-15 hours
N-acetyl-5-ASA: 2-15 hours
Time to peak serum concentration:
Oral: Capsule: Apriso™: ~4 hours; Pentasa®: 3 hours; Tablet: Asacol® HD: 10-16 hours; Lialda®: 9-12 hours
Rectal: 4-7 hours
Elimination: Most metabolites are excreted in urine (<8% as unchanged drug); feces (<2%)

Dosing: Usual

Children and Adolescents:
Crohn's disease; treatment (mild to moderate disease); maintenance of remission: Limited data available: Oral: 50-100 mg/kg/day divided every 6-12 hours (Fish, 2004); maximum dose: 1 g/dose
Ulcerative colitis (including proctitis); treatment (mild to moderate disease); induction and maintenance of remission: Limited data available: Usual course of therapy is 3-8 weeks: Oral: 30-60 mg/kg/day divided every 6-12 hours; doses as high as 100 mg/kg/day have been used; maximum daily dose: 4 g/day (Baldassano, 1999; Fish, 2004; Leichtner, 1995; Tomomasa, 2004)
Older Children and Adolescents: Rectal:
Enema (Rowasa): 4 g once daily at bedtime (Baldassano, 1999)
Suppository (Rowasa): 500 mg once daily at bedtime; some have used twice daily (Baldassano, 1999; Heyman, 2010)
Adults:
Ulcerative colitis:
Treatment: Oral: Usual course of therapy is 3-8 weeks:
Capsule (Pentasa®): 1 g 4 times daily; **Note:** Apriso™ capsules are approved for maintenance of remission only.
Tablet: Initial:
Asacol® HD: 1.6 g 3 times daily for 6 weeks

Lialda®: 2.4-4.8 g once daily for up to 8 weeks
Maintenance of remissions: Oral:
Capsule:
Apriso™: 1.5 g once daily in the morning
Pentasa®: 1 g 4 times daily
Tablet: Lialda®: 2.4 g once daily
Note: Asacol® HD tablets are approved for treatment only.
Distal ulcerative colitis, proctosigmoiditis, or proctitis (mild to moderate), treatment: Retention enema: Adults: 60 mL (4 g) at bedtime, retained overnight, ~8 hours
Ulcerative proctitis, treatment: Rectal suppository (Canasa®): Adults: Insert 1 suppository (1000 mg) in rectum once daily at bedtime; retained for at least 1-3 hours to achieve maximum benefit
Note: Duration of rectal therapy is 3-6 weeks; some patients may require rectal and oral therapy concurrently.

Administration

Oral: Swallow tablets or capsules whole; do not break, chew, or crush
Capsule:
Apriso™: Administer with or without food; do not administer with antacids. The capsule should be swallowed whole per the manufacturer's labeling; however, opening the capsule and placing the contents (delayed release granules) on food with a pH <6 is not expected to affect the release of mesalamine once ingested (data on file, Salix Pharmaceuticals Medical Information). There is no safety/efficacy information regarding this practice. The contents of the capsules should not be chewed or crushed.
Pentasa®: If a patient is unable to swallow the capsule, some clinicians support opening the capsules and placing the contents (controlled release beads) on yogurt or peanut butter (Crohn's & Colitis Foundation of America). There are currently no published data evaluating the safety/efficacy of this practice. The contents of the capsules should not be chewed or crushed.
Tablet: Do not break outer coating of Asacol® HD or Lialda® tablets; Lialda®: Should be administered with a meal.
Rectal:
Enema: Shake well before use; retain enema for 8 hours or as long as practical
Suppository: Avoid excessive handling; retain suppository for at least 1-3 hours for maximum benefit

Test Interactions

May cause falsely-elevated urinary normetanephrine levels when measured by liquid chromatography with electrochemical detection (due to similarity in the chromatograms of normetanephrine and mesalamine's main metabolite, N-acetylaminosalicylic acid).

Dosage Forms

Excipient information presented when available (limited, particularly for generics); consult specific product labeling.
Capsule Delayed Release, Oral:
Delzicol: 400 mg
Capsule Extended Release, Oral:
Pentasa: 250 mg [contains brilliant blue fcf (fd&c blue #1), fd&c yellow #10 (quinoline yellow)]
Pentasa: 500 mg [contains brilliant blue fcf (fd&c blue #1)]
Capsule Extended Release 24 Hour, Oral:
Apriso: 0.375 g [contains aspartame]
Enema, Rectal:
SfRowasa: 4 g/60 mL (60 mL) [sulfite free; contains edetate disodium, sodium benzoate]
Generic: 4 g (60 mL)
Kit, Rectal:
Rowasa: 4 g [contains edetate disodium, potassium metabisulfite, sodium benzoate]

Generic: 4 g
Suppository, Rectal:
Canasa: 1000 mg (30 ea, 42 ea)
Tablet Delayed Release, Oral:
Asacol HD: 800 mg
Lialda: 1.2 g

References

Baldassano RN and Piccoli DA, "Inflammatory Bowel Disease in Pediatric and Adolescent Patients," *Gastroenterol Clin North Am*, 1999, 28(2):445-58.

Fish D and Kugathasan S, "Inflammatory Bowel Disease," *Adolesc Med Clin*, 2004, 15(1):67-90.

Grand RJ, Ramakrishna J, and Calenda KA, "Inflammatory Bowel Disease in the Pediatric Patient," *Gastroenterol Clin North Am*, 1995, 24(3):613-32.

Habal FM and Huang VW, "Review Article: A Decision-Making Algorithm for the Management of Pregnancy in the Inflammatory Bowel Disease Patient," *Aliment Pharmacol Ther*, 2012, 35(5):501-15.

Leichtner AM, "Aminosalicylates for the Treatment of Inflammatory Bowel Disease," *J Pediatr Gastroenterol Nutr*, 1995, 21(3):245-52.

Mottet C, Vader JP, Felley C, et al, "Appropriate Management of Special Situations in Crohn's Disease (Upper Gastro-Intestinal; Extra-Intestinal Manifestations; Drug Safety During Pregnancy and Breastfeeding): Results of a Multidisciplinary International Expert Panel-EPACT II," *J Crohns Colitis*, 2009, 3(4):257-63.

Nelis GF, "Diarrhoea Due to 5-Aminosalicylic Acid in Breast Milk," *Lancet*, 1989, 1(8634):383.

Tomomasa T, Kobayashi A, Ushijima K, et al, "Guidelines for Treatment of Ulcerative Colitis in Children," *Pediatr Int*, 2004, 46(4):494-6.

◆ **Mesalazine** *see* Mesalamine *on page 1347*

◆ **Mesasal (Can)** *see* Mesalamine *on page 1347*

◆ **M-Eslon (Can)** *see* Morphine (Systemic) *on page 1440*

Mesna (MES na)

Brand Names: U.S. Mesnex

Brand Names: Canada Mesna for injection; Uromitexan

Therapeutic Category Antidote; Antidote, Cyclophosphamide-induced Hemorrhagic Cystitis; Antidote, Ifosfamide-induced Hemorrhagic Cystitis; Chemoprotectant Agent

Generic Availability (U.S.) May be product dependent

Use Detoxifying agent used as a protectant against hemorrhagic cystitis induced by ifosfamide and cyclophosphamide [FDA approved in pediatrics (age not specified) and adults]

Pregnancy Risk Factor B

Pregnancy Considerations Adverse effects were not observed in animal reproduction studies. Use during pregnancy only if clearly needed.

Breast-Feeding Considerations It is not known if mesna is excreted in breast milk. Benzyl alcohol, a component in some formulations, does enter breast milk and may be absorbed by a nursing infant. Due to the potential for adverse reactions in the nursing infant, a decision should be made to discontinue breast-feeding or to discontinue mesna, taking into account the importance of treatment to the mother.

Contraindications Hypersensitivity to mesna, other thiol compounds, or any component

Warnings Mesna injection contains benzyl alcohol which may cause allergic reactions in susceptible individuals; large amounts of benzyl alcohol (≥99 mg/kg/day) have been associated with a potentially fatal toxicity ("gasping syndrome") in neonates; the "gasping syndrome" consists of metabolic acidosis, respiratory distress, gasping respirations, CNS dysfunction (including convulsions, intracranial hemorrhage), hypotension and cardiovascular collapse; avoid use of mesna products containing benzyl alcohol in children <2 years of age; *in vitro* and animal studies have shown that benzoate, a metabolite of benzyl alcohol, displaces bilirubin from protein binding sites. Allergic reactions have been reported; symptoms ranged from mild hypersensitivity to systemic anaphylactic reactions and may include fever, hypotension, and/or tachycardia; patients with autoimmune disorders receiving cyclophosphamide and mesna may be at increased risk.

Precautions Examine morning urine specimen for hematuria prior to ifosfamide or cyclophosphamide treatment; if hematuria develops, reduce the ifosfamide/cyclophosphamide dose or discontinue the drug and consider increasing the mesna dosage. Mesna will not prevent or alleviate other toxicities associated with ifosfamide or cyclophosphamide and will not prevent hemorrhagic cystitis in all patients. Mesna will not reduce the risk of thrombocytopenia-related hematuria. Patients should receive adequate hydration during treatment.

Adverse Reactions

Mesna alone (frequency not defined):
Cardiovascular: Flushing
Central nervous system: Dizziness, fever, headache, hyperesthesia, somnolence
Dermatologic: Rash
Gastrointestinal: Anorexia, constipation, diarrhea, flatulence, nausea, taste alteration/bad taste (with oral administration), vomiting
Local: Injection site reactions
Neuromuscular: Arthralgia, back pain, rigors
Ocular: Conjunctivitis
Respiratory: Cough, pharyngitis, rhinitis
Miscellaneous: Flu-like syndrome
Mesna alone or in combination: Rare but important or life-threatening: Allergic reaction, anaphylactic reaction, hypersensitivity, hyper-/hypotension, injection site erythema, injection site pain, limb pain, malaise, myalgia, platelets decreased, ST-segment increased, tachycardia, tachypnea, transaminases increased

Drug Interactions

Metabolism/Transport Effects None known.

Avoid Concomitant Use There are no known interactions where it is recommended to avoid concomitant use.

Increased Effect/Toxicity There are no known significant interactions involving an increase in effect.

Decreased Effect There are no known significant interactions involving a decrease in effect.

Stability Store intact vials and tablets at room temperature of 20°C to 25°C (68°F to 77°F). Opened multidose vials may be stored and used for up to 8 days after opening. Diluted solutions in D$_5$W, D$_5$NS, NS, or LR are chemically and physically stable for 48 hours at room temperature (the manufacturer recommends a final concentration of 20 mg/mL); compatible with solutions containing ifosfamide or cyclophosphamide (variable based on concentration, pH, and storage temperature); incompatible with cisplatin. Solutions of mesna (0.5-3.2 mg/mL) and cyclophosphamide (1.8-10.8 mg/mL) in D$_5$W are stable for 48 hours refrigerated or 6 hours at room temperature (Menard, 2003).

Mechanism of Action In blood, mesna is oxidized to dimesna which in turn is reduced in the kidney back to mesna, supplying a free thiol group which binds to and inactivates acrolein, the urotoxic metabolite of ifosfamide and cyclophosphamide

Pharmacokinetics (Adult data unless noted)

Distribution: No tissue penetration; following glomerular filtration, mesna disulfide is reduced in the renal tubules back to mesna and delivered to the bladder in the active form
Protein binding: 69% to 75%
Bioavailability: Oral: 50%
Half-life: 22 minutes (mesna); after I.V. administration, mesna is rapidly oxidized intravascularly to mesna disulfide (half-life: 70 minutes). I.V. followed by oral therapy has a half-life of 1-8 hours.
Elimination: Unchanged drug and metabolite are excreted primarily in the urine; time for maximum urinary mesna

excretion: 1 hour after I.V. and 2-3 hours after an oral mesna dose

Dosing: Usual Note: Mesna dosing schedule should be repeated each day ifosfamide is received. If ifosfamide dose is adjusted, the mesna dose should also be modified to maintain the mesna-to-ifosfamide ratio. Children and Adults (refer to individual protocols): **Mesna dose depends on dose of antineoplastic agent used:**

Short infusion standard-dose ifosfamide (<2.5 g/m²/day): Mesna dose is equal to 60% of the ifosfamide dose given in 3 divided doses (0, 4, and 8 hours after the start of ifosfamide)

Continuous infusion standard-dose ifosfamide (<2.5 g/m²/day): ASCO Guidelines: Mesna dose (as an I.V. bolus) is equal to 20% of the ifosfamide dose, followed by a continuous infusion of mesna at 40% of the ifosfamide dose; continue mesna infusion for 12-24 hours after completion of ifosfamide infusion (Hensley, 2009)

High-dose ifosfamide (>2.5 g/m²/day): ASCO Guidelines: Evidence for use is inadequate; more frequent and prolonged mesna administration regimens may be required

I.V. followed by Oral (for ifosfamide doses ≤2 g/m²/day): Mesna dose is equal to 100% of the ifosfamide dose, given as 20% of the ifosfamide dose I.V. at hour 0, followed by 40% of the ifosfamide dose given orally 2 and 6 hours after start of ifosfamide

When used with ifosfamide: I.V.: Mesna dose is 20% w/w of ifosfamide dose 15 minutes before and 4 and 8 hours later or combined with ifosfamide administration; for high-dose ifosfamide, mesna has been administered at a dose of 20% w/w 15 minutes before and every 3 hours for 3-6 doses or combined with ifosfamide administration; (**Note:** In clinical protocols, total daily mesna dose ranged between 60% to 160% w/w of the daily ifosfamide dose)

When used with cyclophosphamide: I.V.: Mesna dose is 20% w/w of cyclophosphamide dose 15 minutes before and every 3 hours for 3-4 doses or combined with cyclophosphamide administration; (**Note:** In clinical protocols, total daily mesna dose ranged between 60% to 160% w/w of the daily cyclophosphamide dose)

I.V. continuous infusion: Mesna doses equivalent to 60% to 100% of the ifosfamide or cyclophosphamide dose have been used

Oral: Mesna dose is 40% w/w of the antineoplastic agent dose in 3 doses at 4-hour intervals or 20 mg/kg/dose every 4 hours x 3 (oral mesna is not recommended for the first dose before ifosfamide or cyclophosphamide)

Administration

Oral: Administer orally in tablet form or dilute mesna injection solution for oral use before oral administration to decrease sulfur odor; mesna can be diluted 1:1 to 1:10 in carbonated cola drinks, fruit juices (grape, apple, tomato, and orange juice), or in plain or chocolate milk (most palatable in chilled grape juice). Patients who vomit within 2 hours after taking oral mesna should repeat the dose or receive I.V. mesna.

Parenteral: Administer by I.V. infusion over 15-30 minutes, or by continuous I.V. infusion (maintain continuous infusion for 12-24 after completion of ifosfamide infusion), or per protocol; mesna may be diluted in D_5W or NS to a final concentration of 1-20 mg/mL; may be added to solutions containing ifosfamide or cyclophosphamide

Monitoring Parameters Urinalysis

Test Interactions

Urinary ketones: False-positive tests for urinary ketones may occur in patients receiving mesna with the use of nitroprusside-based urine tests, including dipstick tests.

CPK activity: Mesna may interfere with enzymatic creatine kinase (CPK) activity tests which use a thiol compound (eg, N-acetylcysteine) for CPK reactivation; may result in a falsely low CPK level.

Ascorbic acid: Mesna may result in false-positive reactions in Tillman's reagent-based urine screening tests for ascorbic acid.

Additional Information pH of the commercial 100 mg/mL solution: 6.5-8.5. A preservative free formulation of Mesnex® injection may be obtained directly from the manufacturer. It is restricted for use in children <2 years and others who are sensitive to benzyl alcohol. Contact Bristol-Myers Squibb Company at 800-437-0994 for additional information.

Dosage Forms Excipient information presented when available (limited, particularly for generics); consult specific product labeling.

Solution, Intravenous:
Mesnex: 100 mg/mL (10 mL) [contains benzyl alcohol, edetate disodium]
Generic: 100 mg/mL (10 mL)
Tablet, Oral:
Mesnex: 400 mg [scored]

Extemporaneous Preparations An oral solution may be prepared from mesna solution for injection. Dilute solution for injection to 20 mg/mL or 50 mg/mL with orange or grape syrup. Prior to administration, syrup-diluted solutions may be diluted to a final concentration of 1, 10, or 50 mg/mL with any of the following: carbonated beverages, apple juice, orange juice, or milk. Mesna injection prepared for oral administration is stable for at least 9 days undiluted in polypropylene syringes and stored at 5°C, 24°C, 35°C; for 7 days when diluted 1:2 or 1:5 with syrups and stored at 24°C in capped tubes; or for 24 hours at 5°C when diluted to 1:2, 1:10, and 1:100 in orange or apple juice, milk, or carbonated beverages. Dilution of mesna with diet or sugar-free preparations has not been evaluated.

Goren MP, Lyman BA, Li JT. The stability of mesna in beverages and syrup for oral administration. *Cancer Chemother Pharmacol.* 1991;28 (4):298-301.

References

Ben Yehuda A, Heyman A and Steiner Salz D, "False Positive Reaction for Urinary Ketones With Mesna," *Drug Intell Clin Pharm,* 1987, 21(6): 547-8.

Brock N and Pohl J, "The Development of Mesna for Regional Detoxification," *Cancer Treat Rev,* 1983, 10(Suppl A):33-43.

"Cancer Chemotherapy," *Med Lett Drugs Ther,* 1989, 31(793):49-56.

Hensley ML, Hagerty KL, Kewalramani T, et al, "American Society of Clinical Oncology 2008 Clinical Practice Guideline Update: Use of Chemotherapy and Radiation Therapy Protectants," *J Clin Oncol,* 2009, 27(1):127-45.

Khaw SL, Downie PA, Waters KD, et al, "Adverse Hypersensitivity Reactions to Mesna as Adjunctive Therapy for Cyclophosphamide," *Pediatr Blood Cancer,* 2007, 49(3):341-3.

Menard C, Bourguignon C, Schlatter J, et al, "Stability of Cyclophosphamide and Mesna Admixtures in Polyethylene Infusion Bags," *Ann Pharmacother,* 2003, 37(12):1789-92.

Schoenike SE and Dana WJ, "Ifosfamide and Mesna," *Clin Pharm,* 1990, 9(3):179-91.

Schuchter LM, Hensley ML, Meropol NJ, et al, "2002 Update of Recommendations for the Use of Chemotherapy and Radiotherapy Protectants: Clinical Practice Guidelines of the American Society of Clinical Oncology," *J Clin Oncol,* 2002, 20(12):2895-903.

◆ **Mesna for injection (Can)** see Mesna on page 1350
◆ **Mesnex** see Mesna on page 1350
◆ **Mestinon** see Pyridostigmine on page 1776
◆ **Mestinon® (Can)** see Pyridostigmine on page 1776
◆ **Mestinon®-SR (Can)** see Pyridostigmine on page 1776
◆ **Metadate CD** see Methylphenidate on page 1379
◆ **Metadate ER** see Methylphenidate on page 1379
◆ **Metadol (Can)** see Methadone on page 1355
◆ **Metadol-D (Can)** see Methadone on page 1355
◆ **Metamucil® (Can)** see Psyllium on page 1773
◆ **Metamucil MultiHealth Fiber [OTC]** see Psyllium on page 1773

Metaproterenol (met a proe TER e nol)

Medication Safety Issues

Sound-alike/look-alike issues:

Metaproterenol may be confused with metipranolol, metoprolol

Alupent may be confused with Atrovent®

Brand Names: Canada Apo-Orciprenaline®; ratio-Orciprenaline®; Tanta-Orciprenaline®

Therapeutic Category Adrenergic Agonist Agent; Antiasthmatic; Beta$_2$-Adrenergic Agonist; Bronchodilator; Sympathomimetic

Generic Availability (U.S.) Yes

Use Bronchodilator in reversible airway obstruction due to asthma or COPD (FDA approved in ages ≥6 years and adults)

Pregnancy Risk Factor C

Pregnancy Considerations Adverse events were observed in some animal reproduction studies. Beta agonists, including metaproterenol, may interfere with uterine contractility if administered during labor; maternal and fetal tachycardia have been observed (Baillie, 1970; Tyack, 1971).

Uncontrolled asthma is associated with adverse events on pregnancy (increased risk of perinatal mortality, preeclampsia, preterm birth, low birth weight infants). Oral beta$_2$-receptor agonists are not recommended to treat asthma during pregnancy (NAEPP, 2005).

Breast-Feeding Considerations It is not known if metaproterenol is excreted into breast milk. Although breastfeeding is not recommended by the manufacturer, the use of beta$_2$-receptor agonists are not considered a contraindication to breast-feeding (NAEPP, 2005).

Contraindications Hypersensitivity to metaproterenol or any component; preexisting cardiac arrhythmias associated with tachycardia

Warnings Beta-agonists may cause elevation in blood pressure, heart rate, and result in CNS stimulation/excitation. Beta$_2$-agonists may increase risk of arrhythmia, increase serum glucose, or decrease serum potassium. Excessive use may result in cardiac arrest and death; do not use concurrently with other sympathomimetic bronchodilators. Immediate hypersensitivity reactions (urticaria, angioedema, rash, bronchospasm) have been reported. Syrup contains sodium benzoate; benzoic acid (benzoate) is a metabolite of benzyl alcohol; large amounts of benzyl alcohol (≥99 mg/kg/day) have been associated with a potentially fatal toxicity ("gasping syndrome") in neonates; in vitro and animal studies have shown that benzoate displaces bilirubin from protein binding sites; avoid use of sodium benzoate containing products in neonates.

Precautions Use with caution in patients with ischemic heart disease, hypertension, hyperthyroidism, seizure disorders, CHF, cardiac arrhythmias, glaucoma, hypokalemia, and diabetes mellitus. Metaproterenol (a less selective beta$_2$-agonist) is not recommended in the management of asthma due to potential for excessive cardiac stimulation (NAEPP, 2007). Oral systemic agents (eg, tablets, syrup) should be avoided due to increased risk of adverse effects (eg, excessive cardiac stimulation). Inhaled bronchodilators are preferred therapy for COPD exacerbations; oral systemic agents (eg, tablets, syrup) should be avoided due to increased risk of adverse effects (eg, excessive cardiac stimulation).

Adverse Reactions

Cardiovascular: Palpitation, tachycardia

Central nervous system: Dizziness, fatigue, headache, insomnia, nervousness

Neuromuscular & skeletal: Tremor

Gastrointestinal: Diarrhea, nausea

Respiratory: Asthma exacerbation

Rare but important or life-threatening: Chest pain, diaphoresis, edema, facial/finger edema, hives, hypertension, laryngeal changes, spasms, syncope, vomiting, weakness

Drug Interactions

Metabolism/Transport Effects None known.

Avoid Concomitant Use

Avoid concomitant use of Metaproterenol with any of the following: Beta-Blockers (Nonselective); Iobenguane I 123

Increased Effect/Toxicity

Metaproterenol may increase the levels/effects of: Atosiban; Loop Diuretics; Sympathomimetics; Thiazide Diuretics

The levels/effects of Metaproterenol may be increased by: AtoMOXetine; Cannabinoid-Containing Products; Linezolid; MAO Inhibitors; Tricyclic Antidepressants

Decreased Effect

Metaproterenol may decrease the levels/effects of: Iobenguane I 123

The levels/effects of Metaproterenol may be decreased by: Beta-Blockers (Beta1 Selective); Beta-Blockers (Nonselective); Betahistine

Stability

Tablets: Store at 15°C to 30°C (59°F to 86°F); protect from light and moisture.

Syrup: Store below 30°C (86°F); protect from light.

Mechanism of Action Stimulates beta$_2$-receptors which increases the conversion of adenosine triphosphate (ATP) to 3'-5'-cyclic adenosine monophosphate (cAMP), resulting in bronchial smooth muscle relaxation

Pharmacodynamics

Onset of bronchodilation: Within 30 minutes

Maximum effect: Within 1 hour

Duration: (~1-5 hours) regardless of route administered

Pharmacokinetics (Adult data unless noted)

Absorption: Oral: Well absorbed

Metabolism: Extensive first-pass in the liver (~40% of oral dose is available)

Elimination: Mainly as glucuronic acid conjugates

Dosing: Usual

Oral:

Infants and Children:

<2 years: 0.4 mg/kg/dose 3-4 times daily; in infants, the dose can be given every 8-12 hours

2-5 years: 1.3-2.6 mg/kg/**day** divided every 6-8 hours; maximum: 10 mg/dose

Children ≥6 years and Adolescents:

<27 kg: 10 mg 3-4 times daily

≥27 kg: 20 mg 3-4 times daily

Adults: 20 mg 3-4 times daily

Administration Administer with food to decrease GI distress

Monitoring Parameters Heart rate, respiratory rate, blood pressure, arterial or capillary blood gases if applicable, pulmonary function tests

Dosage Forms Excipient information presented when available (limited, particularly for generics); consult specific product labeling.

Syrup, Oral, as sulfate:

Generic: 10 mg/5 mL (473 mL)

Tablet, Oral, as sulfate:

Generic: 10 mg, 20 mg

References

Baillie P, Meehan FP, and Tyack AJ, "Treatment of Premature Labour With Orciprenaline," Br Med J, 1970, 4(5728):154-5.

Global Initiative for Chronic Obstructive Lung Disease: Global Strategy for the Diagnosis, Management, and Prevention of COPD, 2009.

National Asthma Education and Prevention Program (NAEPP), "Expert Panel Report 3 (EPR-3): Guidelines for the Diagnosis and Management of Asthma," *Clinical Practice Guidelines*, National Institutes of Health, National Heart, Lung, and Blood Institute, NIH Publication No. 08-4051, prepublication 2007; available at http://www.nhlbi.nih.gov/guidelines/asthma/asthgdln.htm

National Asthma Education and Prevention Program (NAEPP) Working Group Report on "Managing Asthma During Pregnancy: Recommendations for Pharmacologic Treatment," National Institutes of Health, National Heart, Lung, and Blood Institute, NIH Publication No. 05-5236, March 2005. Available at http://www.nhlbi.nih.gov/health/prof/lung/asthma/astpreg/astpreg_full.pdf

Tyack AJ, Baillie P, and Meehan FP, "*In-vivo* Response of the Human Uterus to Orciprenaline in Early Labour," *Br Med J*, 1971, 2 (5764):741-3.

♦ **Metaproterenol Sulfate** see Metaproterenol
on page 1352

MetFORMIN (met FOR min)

Medication Safety Issues
Sound-alike/look-alike issues:
MetFORMIN may be confused with metroNIDAZOLE
Glucophage® may be confused with Glucotrol®, Glutofac®
High alert medication:
The Institute for Safe Medication Practices (ISMP) includes this medication among its list of drug classes which have a heightened risk of causing significant patient harm when used in error.
International issues:
Dianben [Spain] may be confused with Diovan brand name for valsartan [U.S., Canada, and multiple international markets].

Glucon brand name for metformin [Malaysia, Singapore] is also the brand name for glucosamine [Singapore]
Related Information
Oral Medications That Should Not Be Crushed or Altered
on page 2438
Brand Names: U.S. Fortamet; Glucophage; Glucophage XR; Glumetza; Riomet
Brand Names: Canada Apo-Metformin®; Ava-Metformin; CO Metformin; Dom-Metformin; Glucophage®; Glumetza®; Glycon; JAMP-Metformin; JAMP-Metformin Blackberry; Mar-Metformin; Metformin FC; Mint-Metformin; Mylan-Metformin; Novo-Metformin; PHL-Metformin; PMS-Metformin; PRO-Metformin; Q-Metformin; RAN™-Metformin; ratio-Metformin; Riva-Metformin; Sandoz-Metformin FC; Septa-Metformin; Teva-Metformin
Therapeutic Category Antidiabetic Agent, Biguanide; Antidiabetic Agent, Oral; Hypoglycemic Agent, Oral
Generic Availability (U.S.) May be product dependent
Use Management of type II diabetes mellitus (noninsulin-dependent, NIDDM) as monotherapy when hyperglycemia cannot be managed with diet and exercise alone; may be used concomitantly with a sulfonylurea or insulin to improve glycemic control
Pregnancy Risk Factor B
Pregnancy Considerations Adverse events have not been observed in animal reproduction studies. Metformin has been found to cross the placenta in concentrations which may be comparable to those found in the maternal plasma. Pharmacokinetic studies suggest that clearance of metformin may increase during pregnancy and dosing may need adjusted in some women when used during the third trimester (Charles, 2006; de Oliveira Baraldi, 2011; Eyal, 2010; Gardiner, 2003; Hughes, 2006; Vanky, 2005).

An increased risk of birth defects or adverse fetal/neonatal outcomes has not been observed following maternal use of metformin for GDM or type 2 diabetes when glycemic control is maintained (Balani, 2009; Coetzee, 1979; Coetzee, 1984; Ekpebegh, 2007; Niromanesh, 2012; Rowan, 2008; Rowan, 2010; Tertti, 2008). For women with diabetes, maternal hyperglycemia itself can be associated with adverse effects in the fetus, neonate, and mother. To prevent adverse events, prior to conception and throughout pregnancy, the maternal Hb A_{1c} should be kept close to normal but without causing significant hypoglycemia. The use of metformin in pregnant women with type 2 diabetes or GDM is under study. Until additional safety and efficacy data are obtained, use is generally not recommended for routine management of GDM or type 2 diabetes mellitus during pregnancy; insulin is the drug of choice for the control of diabetes mellitus in pregnant women (ACOG, 2005; ADA, 2013; Kitzmiller, 2008; Metzger, 2007).

Metformin is recommended to treat insulin resistance associated with PCOS; however, its use may also restore spontaneous ovulation. Women with PCOS who do not desire to become pregnant should use effective contraception. Although studied for use in women with anovulatory PCOS, there is no evidence that it improves live birth rates or decreases pregnancy complications. Routine use to treat infertility related to PCOS is not currently recommended (ACOG, 2009; ASRM, 2008; Fauser, 2012).
Breast-Feeding Considerations Low amounts of metformin (generally ≤1% of the weight-adjusted maternal dose) are excreted into breast milk. Because breast milk concentrations of metformin stay relatively constant, avoiding nursing around peak plasma concentrations in the mother would not be helpful in reducing metformin exposure to the infant (Briggs, 2005; Eyal, 2010; Gardiner, 2003; Hale, 2002). Growth and development were not affected in infants born to mothers with PCOS and who took metformin while breast-feeding (Glueck, 2006).

Breast-feeding is encouraged for all women, including those with diabetes; however, the safety of metformin during breast-feeding has not yet been established (Metzger, 2007). According to the manufacturer, due to the potential for hypoglycemia in the nursing infant, a decision should be made whether to discontinue nursing or to discontinue the drug, taking into account the importance of treatment to the mother.
Contraindications Hypersensitivity to metformin or any component; renal disease or renal dysfunction (S_{cr} ≥1.5 mg/dL in males or ≥1.4 mg/dL in females) or abnormal creatinine clearance which may result from clinical conditions such as cardiovascular collapse, respiratory failure, acute MI, acute CHF, and septicemia; acute or chronic metabolic acidosis with or without coma (including diabetic ketoacidosis)
Warnings Lactic acidosis is a rare, but potentially severe consequence of therapy with metformin **[U.S. Boxed Warning]**; withhold therapy in clinical conditions which may predispose to the development of lactic acidosis (eg, hypoxemia, dehydration, hypoperfusion, sepsis) or in any patient with CHF requiring pharmacologic management; the risk of accumulation and lactic acidosis increases with the degree of impairment of renal function and age; avoid use in patients with renal function below the limit of normal for their age; measure baseline renal function and monitor annually; more frequent monitoring may be necessary depending upon the patient's clinical condition; therapy should be suspended for any surgical procedures (resume only after normal intake resumed and normal renal function is verified); temporarily discontinue therapy for 48 hours in patients undergoing radiologic studies involving the intravascular administration of iodinated contrast materials (potential for acute alteration in renal function); avoid use in patients with impaired liver function; avoid excessive acute or chronic alcohol use (alcohol potentiates the effect of metformin on lactate metabolism); lactic acidosis should be suspected in any diabetic patient receiving metformin who has evidence of acidosis when evidence of ketoacidosis is lacking ▶

◄ **Precautions** Use with caution in patients receiving medications that may affect renal function, particularly tubular secretion, as they may also affect metformin disposition; hypoglycemia (rare with metformin) may occur with inadequate caloric intake, strenuous exercise, or concurrent use with other hypoglycemic drugs

Adverse Reactions

Cardiovascular: Chest discomfort, flushing, palpitation

Central nervous system: Chills, dizziness, headache, lightheadedness

Dermatologic: Rash

Endocrine & metabolic: Hypoglycemia

Gastrointestinal: Abdominal discomfort, abdominal distention, abnormal stools, constipation, diarrhea, dyspepsia, flatulence, heartburn, indigestion, nausea, taste disorder, vomiting

Neuromuscular & skeletal: Myalgia, weakness

Respiratory: Dyspnea, upper respiratory tract infection

Miscellaneous: Decreased vitamin B_{12} levels, flu-like syndrome, increased diaphoresis, nail disorder

Rare but important or life-threatening: Lactic acidosis, leukocytoclastic vasculitis, megaloblastic anemia, pneumonitis

Drug Interactions

Metabolism/Transport Effects None known.

Avoid Concomitant Use

Avoid concomitant use of MetFORMIN with any of the following: Alcohol (Ethyl)

Increased Effect/Toxicity

MetFORMIN may increase the levels/effects of: Dalfampridine; Dofetilide

The levels/effects of MetFORMIN may be increased by: Alcohol (Ethyl); Androgens; Carbonic Anhydrase Inhibitors; Cephalexin; Cimetidine; Dalfampridine; Dolutegravir; Glycopyrrolate; Iodinated Contrast Agents; LamoTRIgine; Pegvisomant; Ranolazine; Topiramate; Trimethoprim; Vandetanib

Decreased Effect

MetFORMIN may decrease the levels/effects of: Trospium

The levels/effects of MetFORMIN may be decreased by: Corticosteroids (Orally Inhaled); Corticosteroids (Systemic); Danazol; Luteinizing Hormone-Releasing Hormone Analogs; Somatropin; Thiazide Diuretics

Food Interactions Food decreases the extent and slightly delays the absorption. Management: Administer with a meal.

Stability Tablets and oral solution: Store at 20°C to 25°C (68°F to 77°F); protect from light

Mechanism of Action Decreases hepatic glucose production, decreasing intestinal absorption of glucose and improves insulin sensitivity (increases peripheral glucose uptake and utilization)

Pharmacodynamics

Onset of action: Within days, maximum effects up to 2 weeks

Average decrease in fasting blood glucose: Children >10 years and Adults: 60-70 mg/dL

Pharmacokinetics (Adult data unless noted)

Absorption: Oral: Slowly and incompletely absorbed

Distribution: Adults: V_d: 654 ± 358 L

Protein binding, plasma: Negligible

Bioavailability: Oral: 50% to 60% (under fasting conditions)

Half-life, plasma elimination: 3-6 hours

Time to peak serum concentration: Immediate release formulation: 2-4 hours; extended release formulation: 4-8 hours (median: 7 hours)

Elimination: Renal; tubular secretion is major route; excretion: 90% in urine as unchanged drug

Dialysis: Removed by hemodialysis; clearance up to 170 mL/minute

Dosing: Usual Oral: **Note:** While significant responses may not be seen at doses <1500 mg daily, a lower recommended starting dose and gradual increase in dosage is recommended to minimize GI symptoms

Treatment of type 2 diabetes mellitus (noninsulin-dependent) in previously untreated patients or patients currently receiving sulfonylurea oral antidiabetic agents:

Children 10-16 years: Initial: 500 mg twice daily; dosage increases should be made weekly, in increments of 500 mg/day in divided doses, up to a maximum of 2000 mg/day.

Children ≥17 years and Adults:

Initial: 500 mg twice daily; dosage increases should be made weekly, in increments of 500 mg/day in 2 divided doses, up to a maximum of 2500 mg/day; doses >2000 mg/day may be better tolerated divided 3 times/day

Alternative dose: Initial: 850 mg once daily; dosage increases should be made in increments of 850 mg every 2 weeks, given in divided doses, up to a maximum of 2550 mg/day

Glucophage® XR (extended release tablets): Initial: 500 mg once daily; dosage may be increased by 500 mg weekly; maximum dose: 2000 mg once daily. If glycemic control is not achieved at maximum dose, may divide dose to 1000 mg twice daily; if doses >2000 mg/day are needed, switch to regular release tablets and titrate to maximum dose of 2550 mg/day

Glumetza™ (extended release tablet): Initial: 1000 mg once daily; may increase weekly as needed in 500 mg increments; not to exceed 2000 mg/day; if 2000 mg/day is ineffective, may consider using 1000 mg twice daily

Adjunctive agent to diabetic patient receiving insulin: Children ≥17 years and Adults: Initial: 500 mg metformin or metformin extended release once daily, continue current insulin dose; increase by 500 mg every week; maximum dose: 2500 mg metformin or 2000 mg metformin extended release; decrease insulin dose by 10% to 25% when fasting blood glucose <120 mg/dL

Dosing adjustment in renal impairment: Metformin is contraindicated in the presence of renal dysfunction

Dosing adjustment in hepatic impairment: Avoid metformin; liver disease is a risk factor for the development of lactic acidosis during metformin therapy.

Administration Oral:

Glucophage®, Riomet™: Administer in divided doses with meals

Glucophage® XR, Glumetza™: Administer with evening meal; extended release tablets should be swallowed whole; do not cut, crush, or chew

Monitoring Parameters Fasting blood glucose, hemoglobin A_{1c}, initial and periodic monitoring of hemoglobin, hematocrit, and red blood cell indices; renal function (baseline and annually)

Reference Range Target range:

Blood glucose: Fasting and preprandial: 80-120 mg/dL; bedtime: 100-140 mg/dL

Glycosylated hemoglobin (hemoglobin A_{1c}): <7%

Additional Information When transferring therapy from chlorpropamide to metformin, monitor the patient closely during the first 2 weeks due to the prolonged retention of chlorpropamide in the body, leading to overlapping drug effects and possible hypoglycemia; if the patient has not responded to 4 weeks at the maximum metformin dosage, consider a gradual addition of a sulfonylurea antidiabetic agent, even if prior primary or secondary failure to a sulfonylurea has occurred; continue metformin at the maximum dose

Dosage Forms Excipient information presented when available (limited, particularly for generics); consult specific product labeling.

Solution, Oral, as hydrochloride:
Riomet: 500 mg/5 mL (118 mL, 473 mL) [contains saccharin calcium; cherry flavor]
Tablet, Oral, as hydrochloride:
Glucophage: 500 mg, 850 mg
Glucophage: 1000 mg [scored]
Generic: 500 mg, 850 mg, 1000 mg
Tablet Extended Release 24 Hour, Oral, as hydrochloride:
Fortamet: 500 mg, 1000 mg
Glucophage XR: 500 mg, 750 mg
Glumetza: 500 mg, 1000 mg
Generic: 500 mg, 750 mg, 1000 mg

References

ACOG Committee on Practice Bulletins-Gynecology, "ACOG Practice Bulletin No. 108: Polycystic Ovary Syndrome," *Obstet Gynecol*, 2009, 114(4):936-49.

American College of Obstetricians and Gynecologists, "ACOG Practice Bulletin. Clinical Management Guidelines for Obstetrician-Gynecologists. Number 60, March 2005. Pregestational Diabetes Mellitus," *Obstet Gynecol*, 2005, 105(3):675-85.

American Diabetes Association, "Standards of Medical Care in Diabetes-2013," *Diabetes Care*, 2013, (36 Suppl 1):S11-66.

Balani J, Hyer SL, Rodin DA, et al, "Pregnancy Outcomes in Women With Gestational Diabetes Treated With Metformin or Insulin: A Case-Control Study," *Diabet Med*, 2009, 26(8):798-802.

Briggs GG, Ambrose PJ, Nageotte MP, et al, "Excretion of Metformin Into Breast Milk and the Effect on Nursing Infants," *Obstet Gynecol*, 2005, 105(6):1437-41.

Charles B, Norris R, Xiao X, et al, "Population Pharmacokinetics of Metformin in Late Pregnancy," *Ther Drug Monit*, 2006, 28(1):67-72.

Coetzee EJ and Jackson WP, "Metformin in Management of Pregnant Insulin-Independent Diabetics," *Diabetologia*, 1979, 16(4):241-5.

Coetzee EJ and Jackson WP, "Oral Hypoglycaemics in the First Trimester and Fetal Outcome," *S Afr Med J*, 1984, 65(16):635-7.

DeFronzo RA, "Pharmacologic Therapy for Type 2 Diabetes Mellitus," *Ann Intern Med*, 1999, 131(4):281-303.

de Oliveira Baraldi C, Lanchote VL, de Jesus Antunes N, et al, "Metformin Pharmacokinetics in Nondiabetic Pregnant Women With Polycystic Ovary Syndrome," *Eur J Clin Pharmacol*, 2011, 67 (10):1027-33.

Ekpebegh CO, Coetzee EJ, van der Merwe L, et al, "A 10-Year Retrospective Analysis of Pregnancy Outcome in Pregestational Type 2 Diabetes: Comparison of Insulin and Oral Glucose-Lowering Agents," *Diabet Med*, 2007, 24(3):253-8.

Eyal S, Easterling TR, Carr D, et al, "Pharmacokinetics of Metformin During Pregnancy," *Drug Metab Dispos*, 2010, 38(5):833-40.

Fauser BC, Tarlatzis BC, Rebar RW, et al, "Consensus on Women's Health Aspects of Polycystic Ovary Syndrome (PCOS): The Amsterdam ESHRE/ASRM-Sponsored 3rd PCOS Consensus Workshop Group," *Fertil Steril*, 2012, 97(1):28-38.

Gardiner SJ, Kirkpatrick CM, Begg EJ, et al, "Transfer of Metformin Into Human Milk," *Clin Pharmacol Ther*, 2003, 73(1):71-7.

Glueck CJ, Goldenberg N, Pranikoff J, et al, "Effects of Metformin-Diet Intervention Before and Throughout Pregnancy on Obstetric and Neonatal Outcomes in Patients With Polycystic Ovary Syndrome," *Curr Med Res Opin*, 2013, 29(1):55-62.

Hale TW, Kristensen JH, Hackett LP, et al, "Transfer of Metformin Into Human Milk," *Diabetologia*, 2002, 45(11):1509-14.

Hughes RC and Rowan JA, "Pregnancy in Women With Type 2 Diabetes: Who Takes Metformin and What Is the Outcome?" *Diabet Med*, 2006, 23(3):318-22.

Jones K, Arlanian S, McVie R, et al, "Metformin Improves Glycemic Control in Children With Type 2 Diabetes," *Diabetes*, 2000, 49(Suppl 1):A75.

Kitzmiller JL, Block JM, Brown FM, et al, "Managing Preexisting Diabetes for Pregnancy: Summary of Evidence and Consensus Recommendations for Care," *Diabetes Care*, 2008, 31(5):1060-79.

Metzger BE, Buchanan TA, Coustan DR, et al, "Summary and Recommendations of the Fifth International Workshop-Conference on Gestational Diabetes Mellitus," *Diabetes Care*, 2007, 30(Suppl 2):S251-60.

Niromanesh S, Alavi A, Sharbaf FR, et al, "Metformin Compared With Insulin in the Management of Gestational Diabetes Mellitus: A Randomized Clinical Trial," *Diabetes Res Clin Pract*, 2012, 98 (3):422-9.

Practice Committee of American Society for Reproductive Medicine (ASRM), "Use of Insulin-Sensitizing Agents in the Treatment of Polycystic Ovary Syndrome," *Fertil Steril*, 2008, 90(5 Suppl):S69-73.

Rowan JA, Gao W, Hague WM, et al, "Glycemia and Its Relationship to Outcomes in the Metformin in Gestational Diabetes Trial," *Diabetes Care*, 2010, 33(1):9-16.

Rowan JA, Hague WM, Gao W, et al, "Metformin Versus Insulin for the Treatment of Gestational Diabetes," *N Engl J Med*, 2008, 358 (19):2003-15.

Tertti K, Ekblad U, Vahlberg T, et al, "Comparison of Metformin and Insulin in the Treatment of Gestational Diabetes: A Retrospective, Case-Control Study," *Rev Diabet Stud*, 2008, 5(2):95-101.

"Type 2 Diabetes in Children and Adolescents. American Diabetes Association," *Diabetes Care*, 2000, 23(3):381-9.

Vanky E, Zahlsen K, Spigset O, et al, "Placental Passage of Metformin in Women With Polycystic Ovary Syndrome," *Fertil Steril*, 2005, 83 (5):1575-8.

- ♦ **Metformin FC (Can)** *see* MetFORMIN *on page 1353*
- ♦ **Metformin Hydrochloride** *see* MetFORMIN *on page 1353*

Methadone (METH a done)

Medication Safety Issues
Sound-alike/look-alike issues:
Methadone may be confused with dexmethylphenidate, Mephyton, methylphenidate, Metadate CD, Metadate ER, metolazone, morphine
High alert medication:
The Institute for Safe Medication Practices (ISMP) includes this medication among its list of drug classes which have a heightened risk of causing significant patient harm when used in error.

Related Information
Medications for Which a Single Dose May Be Fatal When Ingested by a Toddler *on page 2408*
Opioid Conversion Table *on page 2242*
Patient Information for Disposal of Unused Medications *on page 2412*

Brand Names: U.S. Dolophine; Methadone HCl Intensol; Methadose; Methadose Sugar-Free
Brand Names: Canada Metadol; Metadol-D; Methadose
Therapeutic Category Analgesic, Narcotic
Generic Availability (U.S.) Yes
Use Management of moderate to severe pain unresponsive to nonopioids; used in opioid detoxification maintenance programs and for the treatment of iatrogenic opioid dependency

Prescribing and Access Restrictions When used for treatment of opioid addiction: May only be dispensed in accordance to guidelines established by the Substance Abuse and Mental Health Services Administration's (SAMHSA) Center for Substance Abuse Treatment (CSAT). Regulations regarding methadone use may vary by state and/or country. Obtain advice from appropriate regulatory agencies and/or consult with pain management/palliative care specialists.

Note: Regulatory Exceptions to the General Requirement to Provide Opioid Agonist Treatment (per manufacturer's labeling):
1. During inpatient care, when the patient was admitted for any condition other than concurrent opioid addiction, to facilitate the treatment of the primary admitting diagnosis.
2. During an emergency period of no longer than 3 days while definitive care for the addiction is being sought in an appropriately licensed facility.

Medication Guide Available Yes
Pregnancy Risk Factor C
Pregnancy Considerations Adverse events were observed in animal reproduction studies. Methadone crosses the placenta and can be detected in cord blood, amniotic fluid, and newborn urine.

Methadone is considered the standard of care when treating opioid addition in pregnant women. Women receiving methadone for the treatment of addiction should be maintained on their daily dose of methadone in addition to receiving the same pain management options during labor and delivery as opioid-naïve women; maintenance doses of methadone will not provide adequate pain relief. ▶

Narcotic agonist-antagonists should be avoided for the treatment of labor pain in women maintained on methadone due to the risk of precipitating acute withdrawal (ACOG, 2012; Dow, 2012).

Data is available related to fetal/neonatal outcomes following maternal use of methadone during pregnancy. Information collected by the Teratogen Information System is complicated by maternal use of illicit drugs, nutrition, infection, and psychosocial circumstances. However, pregnant women in methadone treatment programs are reported to have improved fetal outcomes compared to pregnant women using illicit drugs. Fetal growth, birth weight, length, and/or head circumference may be decreased in infants born to opioid-addicted mothers treated with methadone during pregnancy. Growth deficits do not appear to persist; however, decreased performance on psychometric and behavioral tests has been found to continue into childhood. Abnormal fetal nonstress tests have also been reported. Withdrawal symptoms in the neonate may be observed up to 2-4 weeks after delivery and should be expected (ACOG, 2012). Neonatal abstinence syndrome following opioid exposure may present with autonomic (eg, fever, temperature instability), gastrointestinal (eg, diarrhea, vomiting, poor feeding/weight gain), or neurologic (eg, high-pitched crying, increased muscle tone, irritability, seizure, tremor) symptoms (Dow, 2012; Hudak, 2012).

Methadone clearance in pregnant women is increased and half-life is decreased during the 2nd and 3rd trimesters of pregnancy; the dosage of methadone may need increased or dosing interval decreased during pregnancy to avoid withdrawal symptoms in the mother. Dosage may need decreased following delivery (ACOG, 2012).

Amenorrhea may develop secondary to substance abuse; pregnancy may occur following the initiation of buprenorphine maintenance treatment. Contraception counseling is recommended to prevent unplanned pregnancies (Dow, 2012).

Breast-Feeding Considerations Methadone is excreted into breast milk; the dose to a nursing infant has been calculated to be 2% to 3% of the maternal dose (following oral doses of 10-80 mg/day). Peak methadone levels appear in breast milk 4-5 hours after an oral dose. Methadone has been detected in the plasma of some breast-fed infants whose mothers are taking methadone. Sedation and respiratory depression have been reported in nursing infants. The manufacturer recommends that women monitor their nursing infants for sedation and that they should be instructed as to when to contact their healthcare provider for emergency care. In addition, the manufacturer recommends slowly weaning to prevent withdrawal symptoms in the nursing infant.

When methadone is used to treat opioid addiction in nursing women, guidelines do not contraindicate breast-feeding as long as the infant is tolerant to the dose and other contraindications do not exist (ACOG, 2012). If additional illicit substances are being abused, women treated with methadone should pump and discard breast milk until sobriety is established (ACOG, 2012; Dow, 2012).

Contraindications Hypersensitivity to methadone or any component; severe respiratory depression (in absence of resuscitative equipment or ventilatory support); acute or severe asthma; hypercarbia; known or suspected ileus

Warnings Death and life-threatening adverse events (eg, respiratory depression, cardiac arrhythmias) in patients receiving methadone for pain control have been reported **[U.S. Boxed Warning]**. These events may be the result of unintentional overdoses, drug interactions, and cardiac toxicities associated with methadone (QT prolongation, torsade de pointes). Particular vigilance and patient monitoring is necessary during treatment initiation (including

conversion from another opioid) and dose titration. Incomplete cross-tolerance between methadone and other opioids may occur; fatalities have been reported when converting patients from chronic, high dose treatment with other opioids to methadone; knowledge of the pharmacokinetics of methadone is essential for appropriate conversion from other opioids (see package insert for conversion tables). Methadone's elimination half-life is significantly longer than its duration of analgesic action. The respiratory depressant effects of methadone occur later and persist longer than its peak analgesic effects. Carefully select initial methadone dose for pain control and slowly titrate to analgesic effect in all patients, including those who are opioid-tolerant. Instruct patients to take methadone as prescribed; do not take more methadone than prescribed without first talking with physician.

Methadone may cause prolongation of the QT interval or torsade de pointes (especially at higher doses, eg, in adults with doses >200 mg/day) **[U.S. Boxed Warning]**; use with caution in patients at risk for QT prolongation (eg, patients with cardiac hypertrophy, hypokalemia, hypomagnesemia, concomitant diuretic use), with medications known to prolong the QT interval, or with history of conduction abnormalities. Monitoring of the QT_c interval prior to and during therapy has been recommended by the Center for Substance Abuse and Treatment (CSAT).

May cause respiratory depression **[U.S. Boxed Warning]**; use with extreme caution in patients with respiratory disease or preexisting respiratory depression; methadone's effect on respiration lasts longer than analgesic effects. Use with extreme caution (and only if essential) in patients with head injury, increased ICP, or other intracranial lesions. May cause severe hypotension; use with caution in patients with severe volume depletion or circulatory shock. Tablets are to be used only for oral administration and **must not** be used for injection. Abrupt discontinuation after prolonged use may result in withdrawal symptoms or seizures.

Concentrated oral solution may contain sodium benzoate; benzoic acid (benzoate) is a metabolite of benzyl alcohol; large amounts of benzyl alcohol (≥99 mg/kg/day) have been associated with a potentially fatal toxicity ("gasping syndrome") in neonates; the "gasping syndrome" consists of metabolic acidosis, respiratory distress, gasping respirations, CNS dysfunction (including convulsions, intracranial hemorrhage), hypotension, and cardiovascular collapse; avoid use of methadone products containing sodium benzoate in neonates; in vitro and animal studies have shown that benzoate displaces bilirubin from protein binding sites. Concentrated oral solution may contain propylene glycol; toxicities have been reported with use of products containing propylene glycol, including hyperosmolality, lactic acidosis, seizures, and respiratory depression; in neonates large amounts of propylene glycol delivered orally, intravenously (eg, >3000 mg/day), or topically have been associated with potentially fatal toxicities which can include metabolic acidosis, seizures, renal failure, and CNS depression; use solution containing propylene glycol with caution (AAP, 1997; Shehab, 2009).

Precautions Due to the cumulative effects of methadone, the dose and frequency of administration need to be reduced with repeated use; use with caution in patients with hepatic, renal, pulmonary, or cardiovascular disease; use with caution and decrease dose in patients who are debilitated and those with severe renal or hepatic dysfunction, hypothyroidism, Addison's disease, urethral stricture, or prostatic hypertrophy.

Adverse Reactions During prolonged administration, adverse effects may decrease over several weeks; however, constipation and sweating may persist.

Cardiovascular: Arrhythmia, bigeminal rhythms, bradycardia, cardiac arrest, cardiomyopathy, ECG changes, edema, extrasystoles, faintness, flushing, heart failure, hypotension, palpitation, peripheral vasodilation, phlebitis, orthostatic hypotension, QT interval prolonged, shock, syncope, tachycardia, torsade de pointes, T-wave inversion, ventricular fibrillation, ventricular tachycardia

Central nervous system: Agitation, confusion, disorientation, dizziness, drowsiness, dysphoria, euphoria, hallucination, headache, insomnia, lightheadedness, sedation, seizure

Dermatologic: Hemorrhagic urticaria, pruritus, rash, urticaria

Endocrine & metabolic: Antidiuretic effect, amenorrhea, hypokalemia, hypomagnesemia, libido decreased

Gastrointestinal: Abdominal pain, anorexia, biliary tract spasm, constipation, glossitis, nausea, stomach cramps, vomiting, weight gain, xerostomia

Genitourinary: Impotence, urinary retention or hesitancy

Hematologic: Thrombocytopenia (reversible, reported in patients with chronic hepatitis)

Neuromuscular & skeletal: Weakness

Local: I.M./SubQ injection: Erythema, pain, swelling; I.V. injection: Hemorrhagic urticaria (rare), pruritus, urticaria, rash

Ocular: Miosis, visual disturbances

Respiratory: Pulmonary edema, respiratory depression, respiratory arrest

Miscellaneous: Death, diaphoresis, physical and psychological dependence

Drug Interactions

Metabolism/Transport Effects Substrate of CYP2B6 (major), CYP2C19 (minor), CYP2C9 (minor), CYP2D6 (minor), CYP3A4 (major); **Note:** Assignment of Major/Minor substrate status based on clinically relevant drug interaction potential; **Inhibits** CYP2D6 (moderate), CYP3A4 (weak)

Avoid Concomitant Use

Avoid concomitant use of Methadone with any of the following: Alcohol (Ethyl); Azelastine (Nasal); Benzodiazepines; Conivaptan; Fusidic Acid (Systemic); Highest Risk QTc-Prolonging Agents; Itraconazole; Ivabradine; Ketoconazole (Systemic); Lopinavir; Mifepristone; Paraldehyde; Pimozide; Posaconazole; Thalidomide; Thioridazine

Increased Effect/Toxicity

Methadone may increase the levels/effects of: Alvimopan; Azelastine (Nasal); Buprenorphine; CNS Depressants; CYP2D6 Substrates; Desmopressin; Diuretics; DOXOrubicin (Conventional); Fesoterodine; Highest Risk QTc-Prolonging Agents; Hydrocodone; Lomitapide; Lopinavir; Methotrimeprazine; Metoprolol; Metyrosine; Mirtazapine; Moderate Risk QTc-Prolonging Agents; Nebivolol; Paraldehyde; Pimozide; Pramipexole; ROPINIRole; Rotigotine; Saquinavir; Thalidomide; Thioridazine; Zidovudine; Zolpidem

The levels/effects of Methadone may be increased by: Alcohol (Ethyl); Amphetamines; Anticholinergic Agents; Antipsychotic Agents (Phenothiazines); Aromatase Inhibitors; Benzodiazepines; Boceprevir; Brimonidine (Topical); Cannabis; Conivaptan; CYP2B6 Inhibitors (Moderate); CYP2B6 Inhibitors (Strong); CYP3A4 Inhibitors (Moderate); CYP3A4 Inhibitors (Strong); Dasatinib; Doxylamine; Dronabinol; Droperidol; Fluconazole; Fusidic Acid (Systemic); HydrOXYzine; Interferons (Alfa); Itraconazole; Ivabradine; Ivacaftor; Kava Kava; Ketoconazole (Systemic); Luliconazole; Magnesium Sulfate; MAO Inhibitors; Methotrimeprazine; Mifepristone; Nabilone; Perampanel; Posaconazole; QTc-Prolonging Agents (Indeterminate Risk and Risk Modifying); Rufinamide; Selective Serotonin Reuptake Inhibitors;

Simeprevir; Sodium Oxybate; Stiripentol; Succinylcholine; Tapentadol; Tetrahydrocannabinol; Voriconazole

Decreased Effect

Methadone may decrease the levels/effects of: Codeine; Didanosine; Fosamprenavir; Lubiprostone; Pegvisomant; Tamoxifen; TraMADol

The levels/effects of Methadone may be decreased by: Ammonium Chloride; Boceprevir; Bosentan; CarBAMazepine; CYP3A4 Inducers (Strong); Dabrafenib; Darunavir; Deferasirox; Etravirine; Fosamprenavir; Fosphenytoin; Lopinavir; Mitotane; Mixed Agonist / Antagonist Opioids; Naltrexone; Nelfinavir; Peginterferon Alfa-2b; PHENobarbital; Phenytoin; Primidone; Reverse Transcriptase Inhibitors (Non-Nucleoside); Rifamycin Derivatives; Ritonavir; Saquinavir; Siltuximab; St Johns Wort; Telaprevir; Tipranavir; Tocilizumab

Food Interactions Grapefruit/grapefruit juice may increase levels of methadone. Management: Avoid concurrent use of grapefruit juice.

Stability Store at controlled room temperature; protect from light

Tablets: Protect from moisture

Mechanism of Action Binds to opiate receptors in the CNS, causing inhibition of ascending pain pathways, altering the perception of and response to pain; produces generalized CNS depression. Methadone has also been shown to have weak N-methyl-D-aspartate (NMDA) receptor antagonism (Callahan, 2004).

Pharmacodynamics Analgesia:

Onset of action:
Oral: Within 30-60 minutes
Parenteral: Within 10-20 minutes

Maximum effect: Parenteral: 1-2 hours

Duration: Oral: 6-8 hours; after repeated doses, duration increases to 22-48 hours

Pharmacokinetics (Adult data unless noted)

Distribution: Crosses the placenta; appears in breast milk
V_d: (Mean ± SD):
Children: 7.1 ± 2.5 L/kg
Adults: 6.1 ± 2.4 L/kg
V_{dss}: Adults: 2-6 L/kg

Protein binding: 85% to 90% (primarily to alpha$_1$-acid glycoprotein)

Metabolism: N-demethylated in the liver to an inactive metabolite

Half-life: May be prolonged with alkaline pH
Children: 19 ± 14 hours (range: 4-62 hours)
Adults: 35 ± 22 hours (range: 9-87 hours)

Elimination: In urine (<10% as unchanged drug); increased renal excretion with urine pH <6; **Note:** Methadone may persist in the liver and other tissues; slow release from tissues may prolong the pharmacologic effect despite low serum concentrations

Dialysis: Hemodialysis, peritoneal dialysis: Not established as effective for increasing the elimination of methadone (or metabolite)

Dosing: Neonatal Note: Doses should be titrated to appropriate effects.

Neonatal abstinence syndrome (opioid withdrawal): Oral, I.V.: Initial: 0.05-0.2 mg/kg/dose given every 12-24 hours or 0.5 mg/kg/day divided every 8 hours; individualize dose and tapering schedule to control symptoms of withdrawal; usually taper dose by 10% to 20% per week over 1 to 1½ months (AAP, 1998). **Note:** Due to long elimination half-life, tapering is difficult; consider alternate agent.

Dosing: Usual Note: Doses should be titrated to appropriate effects.

Children:

Analgesia: Note: Dosing interval may range from 4-12 hours during initial therapy; decrease in dose or frequency may be required (~2-5 days after initiation of therapy or dosage increase) due to accumulation with repeated doses.

I.V.: Initial: 0.1 mg/kg/dose every 4 hours for 2-3 doses, then every 6-12 hours as needed; maximum dose: 10 mg/dose

Oral, I.M., SubQ: Initial: 0.1 mg/kg/dose every 4 hours for 2-3 doses, then every 6-12 hours as needed or 0.7 mg/kg/24 hours divided every 4-6 hours as needed; maximum dose: 10 mg/dose

Iatrogenic opioid dependency: Oral: Controlled studies have not been conducted; several clinically used dosing regimens have been reported. Methadone dose **must be individualized** and will depend upon patient's previous opioid dose and severity of opioid withdrawal; patients who have received higher doses of opioids will require higher methadone doses.

General guidelines: Initial: 0.05-0.1 mg/kg/dose every 6 hours; increase by 0.05 mg/kg/dose until withdrawal symptoms are controlled; after 24-48 hours, the dosing interval can be lengthened to every 12-24 hours; to taper dose, wean by 0.05 mg/kg/day; if withdrawal symptoms recur, taper at a slower rate

Adults:

Analgesia:

Oral: Initial 5-10 mg; dosing interval may range from 4-12 hours during initial therapy; decrease in dose or frequency may be required (~2-5 days after initiation of therapy or dosage increase) due to accumulation with repeated doses

Manufacturer's recommendations: 2.5-10 mg every 3-4 hours as needed

I.V.: Manufacturer's recommendations: Opioid-naive patients: Initial: 2.5-10 mg every 8-12 hours; titrate slowly to effect; may also be administered by SubQ or I.M. injection

Detoxification: Oral: 15-40 mg/day

Maintenance of opioid dependence: Oral: 20-120 mg/day

Dosing adjustment in renal impairment: Children and Adults:

CrCl <10 mL/minute: Administer 50% to 75% of normal dose

Administration Oral: Administer with juice or water; dispersible tablet should be completely dissolved before administration; oral dose for detoxification and maintenance may be administered in Tang®, Kool-Aid®, apple juice, grape Crystal Light®

Monitoring Parameters Respiratory, cardiovascular, and mental status, pain relief (if used for analgesia), abstinence scoring system (if used for neonatal abstinence syndrome); ECG for monitoring QT_c interval prior to and during therapy.

Test Interactions Some quinolones may produce a false-positive urine screening result for opioids using commercially-available immunoassay kits. This has been demonstrated most consistently for levofloxacin and ofloxacin, but other quinolones have shown cross-reactivity in certain assay kits. Confirmation of positive opioid screens by more specific methods should be considered.

Additional Information Methadone accumulates with repeated doses and dosage may need to be adjusted downward after 3-5 days to prevent toxic effects. Some patients may benefit from every 8- to 12-hour dosing interval (pain control).

Methadone 10 mg I.M. = morphine 10 mg I.M.

The Center for Substance Abuse and Treatment (CSAT) of the Substance Abuse and Mental Health Services Administration has developed a consensus guideline statement outlining recommendations regarding ECG monitoring in patients being considered for and being treated with methadone regardless of indication. Of note, these recommendations should not supersede clinical judgment or patient preferences and may not apply to patients with terminal, intractable cancer pain. Five recommendations have been developed:

Recommendation 1: Disclosure: Clinicians should inform patients of arrhythmia risk when methadone is prescribed.

Recommendation 2: Clinical History: Clinicians should inquire about any history of structural heart disease, arrhythmia, and syncope.

Recommendation 3: Screening: Clinicians should obtain pretreatment ECG for all patients to measure QT_c interval, follow up ECG within 30 days, then annually (monitor more frequently if patient receiving >100 mg/day or if unexplained syncope or seizure occurs while on methadone).

Recommendation 4: Risk Stratification: If before or at anytime during therapy the QT_c >450-499 msecs: Discuss potential risks and benefits; monitor QT_c more frequently. If before or anytime during therapy the QT_c ≥500 msecs: Consider discontinuation or reducing methadone dose or eliminate factors promoting QT_c prolongation (eg, potassium-wasting drugs) or use alternative therapy (eg, buprenorphine).

Recommendation 5: Drug Interactions: Clinicians should be aware of interactions between methadone and other drugs that either prolong the QT interval or reduce methadone elimination.

The panel also concluded that the arrhythmia risk is directly associated with methadone's ability to block the delayed rectifier potassium channel (Ikr) and prolong repolarization. The guideline further states that the use of the Bazett formula is adequate even though it is likely to overcorrect with high heart rates. The patient should remain supine for at least 5 minutes prior to obtaining ECG. In addition, screening for QT_c prolongation using automated readings does not require a specialist (eg, cardiologist) and may be performed in a primary care setting. However, in cases when uncertainty exists about whether or not clinically significant QT_c prolongation is present, the ECG should be repeated or interpreted by a cardiologist. For more information, Krantz, 2009.

Controlled Substance C-II

Dosage Forms Excipient information presented when available (limited, particularly for generics); consult specific product labeling.

Concentrate, Oral, as hydrochloride:
Methadone HCl Intensol: 10 mg/mL (30 mL) [unflavored flavor]
Methadose: 10 mg/mL (1000 mL) [cherry flavor]
Methadose Sugar-Free: 10 mg/mL (1000 mL) [dye free, sugar free; unflavored flavor]
Generic: 10 mg/mL (30 mL, 1000 mL)
Solution, Injection, as hydrochloride:
Generic: 10 mg/mL (20 mL)
Solution, Oral, as hydrochloride:
Generic: 5 mg/5 mL (500 mL); 10 mg/5 mL (500 mL)
Tablet, Oral, as hydrochloride:
Dolophine: 5 mg, 10 mg [scored]
Methadose: 10 mg [scored]
Generic: 5 mg, 10 mg
Tablet Soluble, Oral, as hydrochloride:
Methadose: 40 mg [scored]
Generic: 40 mg

References

ACOG Committee on Health Care for Underserved Women and American Society of Addiction Medicine, "ACOG Committee Opinion No. 524: Opioid Abuse, Dependence, and Addiction in Pregnancy," *Obstet Gynecol*, 2012, 119(5):1070-6.

American Academy of Pediatrics Committee on Drugs. "Inactive" ingredients in pharmaceutical products: update (subject review). *Pediatrics*. 1997;99(2):268-278.

American Academy of Pediatrics Committee on Drugs, "Neonatal Drug Withdrawal," *Pediatrics*, 1998, 101(6):1079-88.

Anand KJ and Arnold JH, "Opioid Tolerance and Dependence in Infants and Children," *Crit Care Med*, 1994, 22(2):334-42.

Berde C, Ablin A, Glazer J, et al, "American Academy of Pediatrics Report of the Subcommittee on Disease-Related Pain in Childhood Cancer," *Pediatrics*, 1990, 86(5 Pt 2):818-25.

Dow K, Ordean A, Murphy-Oikonen J, et al, "Neonatal Abstinence Syndrome Clinical Practice Guidelines For Ontario," *J Popul Ther Clin Pharmacol*, 2012, 19(3):e488-506.

Hudak ML, Tan RC, Committee On Drugs, et al, "Neonatal Drug Withdrawal," *Pediatrics*, 2012, 129(2):e540-60.

Krantz MJ, Lewkowiez L, Hays H, et al, "Torsade de Pointes Associated With Very-High-Dose Methadone," *Ann Intern Med*, 2002, 137(6):501-4.

Krantz MJ, Martin J, Stimmel B, et al, "QT$_c$ Interval Screening in Methadone Treatment," *Ann Intern Med*, 2009, 150(6):387-95.

Lauriault G, LeBelle MJ, Lodge BA, et al, "Stability of Methadone in Four Vehicles for Oral Administration," *Am J Hosp Pharm*, 1991, 48(6):1252-6.

Olkkola KT, Hamunen K, and Maunuksela EL, "Clinical Pharmacokinetics and Pharmacodynamics of Opioid Analgesics in Infants and Children," *Clin Pharmacokinet*, 1995, 28(5):385-404.

Shehab N, Lewis CL, Streetman DD, Donn SM. Exposure to the pharmaceutical excipients benzyl alcohol and propylene glycol among critically ill neonates. *Pediatr Crit Care Med*. 2009;10(2):256-259.

- ◆ **Methadone HCl Intensol** *see* Methadone *on page 1355*
- ◆ **Methadone Hydrochloride** *see* Methadone *on page 1355*
- ◆ **Methadose** *see* Methadone *on page 1355*
- ◆ **Methadose Sugar-Free** *see* Methadone *on page 1355*

Methamphetamine (meth am FET a meen)

Medication Safety Issues
Sound-alike/look-alike issues:
Desoxyn® may be confused with digoxin

Brand Names: U.S. Desoxyn

Brand Names: Canada Desoxyn

Therapeutic Category Amphetamine; Anorexiant; Central Nervous System Stimulant

Generic Availability (U.S.) Yes

Use Treatment of attention-deficit/hyperactivity disorder (ADHD) (FDA approved in ages ≥6 years and adults); short-term (eg, few weeks) adjunct therapy to treat exogenous obesity refractory to alternative therapy (eg, repeat diets, group programs, and other drugs) (FDA approved in ages ≥12 years and adults)

Medication Guide Available Yes

Pregnancy Risk Factor C

Pregnancy Considerations Adverse effects have been observed in animal reproduction studies. Methamphetamine and amphetamine were detected in newborn tissues following intermittent maternal use of Desoxyn during pregnancy (Garriott, 1973). The majority of human data is based on illicit amphetamine/methamphetamine exposure and not from therapeutic maternal use (Golub, 2005). Use of amphetamines during pregnancy may lead to an increased risk of premature birth and low birth weight; newborns may experience symptoms of withdrawal. Behavioral problems may also occur later in childhood (LaGasse, 2012).

Breast-Feeding Considerations Methamphetamine is excreted in breast milk. The majority of human data is based on illicit amphetamine/methamphetamine exposure and not from therapeutic maternal use (Golub, 2005). Amphetamines may decrease milk production. Increased irritability, agitation, and crying have been reported in nursing infants (ACOG, 2011). Due to the potential for serious adverse reactions in the nursing infant, breast-feeding is not recommended by the manufacturer.

Contraindications Hypersensitivity or idiosyncrasy to methamphetamine, amphetamines, other sympathomimetic amines, or any component; advanced arteriosclerosis, symptomatic cardiovascular disease, moderate to severe hypertension, hyperthyroidism, glaucoma, agitated states; history of drug abuse; concurrent use or use within 14 days of MAO inhibitors (hypertensive crisis may occur)

Documentation of allergenic cross-reactivity for amphetamines is limited; however, because of similarities in chemical structure and/or pharmacologic actions, the possibility of cross-sensitivity cannot be ruled out with certainty.

Warnings Serious cardiovascular events, including sudden death, may occur in patients with preexisting structural cardiac abnormalities or other serious heart problems. Sudden death has been reported in children and adolescents; sudden death, stroke, and MI have been reported in adults. Avoid the use of amphetamines in patients with known serious structural cardiac abnormalities, cardiomyopathy, serious heart rhythm abnormalities, coronary artery disease, or other serious cardiac problems that could place patients at an increased risk to the sympathomimetic effects of amphetamines. Patients should be carefully evaluated for cardiac disease prior to initiation of therapy. If a child displays symptoms of cardiovascular disease, including chest pain, dyspnea, or fainting, parents should seek immediate medical care for the child. In a recent retrospective study on the possible association between stimulant medication use and sudden death in children, 564 previously healthy children who died suddenly in motor vehicle accidents were compared to a group of 564 previously healthy children who died suddenly. Two of the 564 (0.4%) children in motor vehicle accidents were taking stimulant medications compared to 10 of 564 (1.8%) children who died suddenly. While the authors of this study conclude there may be an association between stimulant use and sudden death in children, there were a number of limitations to the study and the FDA cannot conclude this information impacts the overall risk:benefit profile of these medications (Gould, 2009). In a large retrospective cohort study involving 1,200,438 children and young adults (aged 2-24 years), none of the currently available stimulant medications or atomoxetine were shown to increase the risk of serious cardiovascular events (ie, acute MI, sudden cardiac death, or stroke) in current (adjusted hazard ratio: 0.75; 95% CI: 0.31-1.85) or former (adjusted hazard ratio: 1.03; 95% CI: 0.57-1.89) users compared to nonusers (Cooper, 2011). **Note:** The American Heart Association recommends that all children diagnosed with ADHD who may be candidates for medication, such as methamphetamine, should have a thorough cardiovascular assessment prior to initiation of therapy. This assessment should include a combination of medical history, family history, and physical examination focusing on cardiovascular disease risk factors. An ECG is not mandatory but should be considered.

Stimulant medications may increase blood pressure (average increase: 2-4 mm Hg) and heart rate (average increase: 3-6 bpm); some patients may experience greater increases; use stimulant medications with caution in patients with hypertension and other cardiovascular conditions that may be exacerbated by increases in blood pressure or heart rate. Stimulants are associated with peripheral vasculopathy, including Raynaud's phenomenon; signs/symptoms are usually mild and intermittent and generally improve with dose reduction or discontinuation. Digital ulceration and/or soft tissue breakdown have been observed rarely; monitor for digital changes during therapy and seek further evaluation (eg, rheumatology referral) if necessary.

Psychiatric adverse events may occur. Stimulants may exacerbate symptoms of behavior disturbance and thought disorder in patients with preexisting psychosis. New-onset psychosis or mania may occur with stimulant use in patients without a prior history of psychotic illness or mania, even at standard doses. Stimulants may induce mixed/manic episode in patients with bipolar disorder; patients should be screened for bipolar disorder prior to treatment; consider discontinuation if such symptoms (eg, delusional thinking, hallucinations, or mania) occur. May be associated with aggressive behavior or hostility; monitor for development or worsening of these behaviors.

Use of stimulants in children has been associated with growth suppression; monitor growth; treatment interruption may be needed. Appetite suppression may occur; monitor weight during therapy, particularly in children. Stimulants may lower seizure threshold leading to new onset or breakthrough seizure activity; use with caution in patients with a history of seizure disorder. Visual disturbances (eg, difficulty in accommodation and blurred vision) have been reported.

Amphetamines possess a high potential for abuse **[U.S. Boxed Warning]**; misuse may cause sudden death and serious cardiovascular adverse events **[U.S. Boxed Warning]**; limit use to weight reduction programs where alternative therapy has been ineffective **[U.S. Boxed Warning]**; prolonged administration may lead to drug dependence; abrupt discontinuation following high doses or for prolonged periods may result in symptoms of withdrawal; avoid abrupt discontinuation in patients who have received amphetamines for prolonged periods; once tolerance to anorectic effects occurs (within few weeks) therapy should be discontinued. Amphetamines may impair the ability to engage in potentially hazardous activities. May exacerbate motor and phonic tics and Tourette's syndrome.

Precautions Use with caution in patients with mild hypertension and in those receiving other sympathomimetic agents; use is contraindicated in patients with moderate to severe hypertension. Use with caution in patients with diabetes mellitus; antidiabetic agent requirements may be altered with anorexigens and concomitant dietary restrictions. Prescribe or dispense least amount feasible to minimize chance of overdose.

Adverse Reactions
Cardiovascular: Cardiorespiratory arrest, hypertension, palpitations, tachycardia
Central nervous system: Dizziness, drug dependence (prolonged use), drug withdrawal, dysphoria, euphoria, exacerbation of tics (motor, phonic, and Tourette's syndrome), headache, insomnia, overstimulation, psychosis, restlessness
Dermatologic: Skin rash, urticaria
Endocrine & metabolic: Change in libido, growth suppression (children), weight loss
Gastrointestinal: Anorexia, constipation, diarrhea, unpleasant taste, xerostomia
Genitourinary: Frequent erections, impotence, prolonged erection
Neuromuscular & skeletal: Tremor
Miscellaneous: Drug tolerance (prolonged use)

Drug Interactions
Metabolism/Transport Effects Substrate of CYP2D6 (major); **Note:** Assignment of Major/Minor substrate status based on clinically relevant drug interaction potential
Avoid Concomitant Use
Avoid concomitant use of Methamphetamine with any of the following: Iobenguane I 123; MAO Inhibitors

Increased Effect/Toxicity
Methamphetamine may increase the levels/effects of: Analgesics (Opioid); Sympathomimetics

The levels/effects of Methamphetamine may be increased by: Abiraterone Acetate; Alkalinizing Agents; Antacids; AtoMOXetine; Cannabinoid-Containing Products; Carbonic Anhydrase Inhibitors; CYP2D6 Inhibitors (Moderate); CYP2D6 Inhibitors (Strong); Darunavir; Linezolid; MAO Inhibitors; Tricyclic Antidepressants
Decreased Effect
Methamphetamine may decrease the levels/effects of: Antihistamines; Ethosuximide; Iobenguane I 123; Ioflupane I 123; PHENobarbital; Phenytoin

The levels/effects of Methamphetamine may be decreased by: Ammonium Chloride; Antipsychotics; Ascorbic Acid; Gastrointestinal Acidifying Agents; Lithium; Methenamine; Multivitamins/Fluoride (with ADE); Multivitamins/Minerals (with ADEK, Folate, Iron); Multivitamins/Minerals (with AE, No Iron); Peginterferon Alfa-2b; Urinary Acidifying Agents
Food Interactions Amphetamine serum levels may be altered if taken with acidic food, juices, or vitamin C. Management: Administer 30 minutes before a meal.
Stability Store below 30°C (86°F); protect from light.
Mechanism of Action A sympathomimetic amine related to ephedrine and amphetamine with CNS stimulant activity; causes release of catecholamines (primarily dopamine and other catecholamines) from their storage sites in the presynaptic nerve terminals. Inhibits reuptake and metabolism of catecholamines through inhibition of monoamine transporters and oxidase.
Pharmacokinetics (Adult data unless noted)
Absorption: Rapid from GI tract
Metabolism: Hepatic via aromatic hydroxylation, N-dealkylation and deamination to several metabolites
Half-life: 4-5 hours
Elimination: Urine primarily (dependent on urine pH; alkaline urine increases the half-life); 62% of dose eliminated in urine within first 24 hours with ~33% as unchanged drug and remainder as metabolites
Dosing: Usual
Children and Adolescents:
Attention-deficit/hyperactivity disorder: Note: Use lowest effective individualized dose; administer first dose in early morning: Children ≥6 years and Adolescents: Oral: Initial: 5 mg once or twice daily; may increase by 5 mg increments weekly until optimum response is achieved; usual effective dose: 20-25 mg/day; dose may be divided twice daily
Exogenous obesity: Children and Adolescents ≥12 years: Oral: 5 mg administered 30 minutes before each meal; treatment duration should not exceed a few weeks
Adults:
Attention-deficit/hyperactivity disorder: Oral: Initial: 5 mg once or twice daily, may increase by 5 mg increments weekly until optimum response is achieved, usually 20-25 mg/day
Exogenous obesity: Oral: Initial: 5 mg administered 30 minutes before each meal; treatment duration should not exceed a few weeks
Administration Avoid late evening doses due to resultant insomnia.
Monitoring Parameters Evaluate patients for cardiac disease prior to initiation of therapy with thorough medical history, family history, and physical exam; consider ECG; perform ECG and echocardiogram if findings suggest cardiac disease; promptly conduct cardiac evaluation in patients who develop chest pain, unexplained syncope, or any other symptom of cardiac disease during treatment. Monitor CNS activity; blood pressure and heart rate

(baseline, following dose increases, and periodically during treatment); sleep, appetite, abnormal movements, height, body weight (BMI), growth rate in children. Patients should be re-evaluated at appropriate intervals to assess continued need for the medication. Observe for signs/symptoms of aggression, hostility, or depression. Monitor for visual disturbances.

Test Interactions Amphetamines may elevate plasma corticosteroid levels; may interfere with urinary steroid determinations.

Additional Information Treatment with methamphetamine for ADHD should include "drug holidays" or periodic discontinuation in order to assess the patient's requirements, decrease tolerance, and limit suppression of linear growth and weight. Medications used to treat ADHD should be part of a total treatment program that may include other components such as psychological, educational, and social measures.

Controlled Substance C-II

Dosage Forms Excipient information presented when available (limited, particularly for generics); consult specific product labeling.

Tablet, Oral, as hydrochloride:
Desoxyn: 5 mg [contains sodium aminobenzoate]
Generic: 5 mg

References

American Academy of Pediatrics, "ADHD: Clinical Practice Guideline for the Diagnosis, Evaluation, and Treatment of Attention-Deficit/Hyperactivity Disorder in Children and Adolescents," *Pediatrics*, 2011, 128(5):1007-22.

American Academy of Pediatrics/American Heart Association Clarification of Statement on Cardiovascular Evaluation and Monitoring of Children and Adolescents With Heart Disease Receiving Medications for ADHD; available at http://americanheart.mediaroom.com/index.-php?s=43&item=422

American College of Obstetricians and Gynecologists (ACOG) Committee on Health Care for Underserved Women, "Committee Opinion No. 479: Methamphetamine Abuse in Women of Reproductive Age," *Obstet Gynecol*, 2011, 117(3):751-5.

Cooper WO, Habel LA, Sox CM, et al, "ADHD Drugs and Serious Cardiovascular Events in Children and Young Adults," *N Engl J Med*, 2011, 365(20):1896-904.

Garriott JC and Spruill FG, "Detection of Methamphetamine in a Newborn Infant," *J Forensic Sci*, 1973, 18(4):434-6.

Golub M, Costa L, Crofton K, et al, "NTP-CERHR Expert Panel Report on the Reproductive and Developmental Toxicity of Amphetamine and Methamphetamine," *Birth Defects Res B Dev Reprod Toxicol*, 2005, 74(6):471-584.

Gould MS, Walsh BT, Munfakh JL, et al, "Sudden Death and Use of Stimulant Medications in Youths," *Am J Psychiatry*, 2009, 166 (9):992-1001.

LaGasse LL, Derauf C, Smith LM, et al, "Prenatal Methamphetamine Exposure and Childhood Behavior Problems at 3 and 5 Years of Age," *Pediatrics*, 2012, 129(4):681-8.

Pliszka S and AACAP Work Group on Quality Issues, "Practice Parameter for the Assessment and Treatment of Children and Adolescents With Attention-Deficit/Hyperactivity Disorder," *J Am Acad Child Adolesc Psychiatry*, 2007,;46(7):894-921.

Vetter VL, Elia J, Erickson C, et al, "Cardiovascular Monitoring of Children and Adolescents With Heart Disease Receiving Medications for Attention Deficit/Hyperactivity Disorder [Corrected]: A Scientific Statement From the American Heart Association Council on Cardiovascular Disease in the Young Congenital Cardiac Defects Committee and the Council on Cardiovascular Nursing," *Circulation*, 2008, 117(18):2407-23.

◆ **Methamphetamine Hydrochloride** *see* Methamphetamine *on page 1359*

Methenamine (meth EN a meen)

Medication Safety Issues
Sound-alike/look-alike issues:
Hiprex® may be confused with Mirapex®
Methenamine may be confused with mesalamine, methazolamide, methionine

Urex may be confused with Eurax®, Serax
International issues:
Urex: Brand name for methenamine [U.S. (discontinued)], but also the brand name for furosemide [Australia, China, Turkey]
Urex [U.S. (discontinued)] may be confused with Eurax brand name for crotamiton [U.S., Canada, and multiple international markets]

Brand Names: U.S. Hiprex; Urex

Brand Names: Canada Dehydral®; Hiprex®; Mandelamine®; Urasal®

Therapeutic Category Antibiotic, Miscellaneous

Generic Availability (U.S.) Yes

Use Prophylaxis or suppression of recurrent urinary tract infections

Pregnancy Risk Factor C (methenamine mandelate)

Pregnancy Considerations Methenamine hippurate did not cause adverse fetal effects in animals; animal reproduction studies have not been conducted with methenamine mandelate. Methenamine crosses the placenta and distributes to amniotic fluid. Adverse fetal effects were not observed in two human trials. Methenamine use has been shown to interfere with urine estriol concentrations if measured via acid hydrolysis. Use of enzyme hydrolysis prevents this lab interference.

Breast-Feeding Considerations Small amounts of methenamine are secreted in human milk.

Contraindications Hypersensitivity to methenamine or any component; severe dehydration, renal insufficiency (methenamine is ineffective in patients with renal impairment), hepatic insufficiency in patients receiving hippurate salt; concurrent therapy with sulfonamides

Warnings Dosage of 8 g/day for 3-4 weeks has been associated with bladder irritation, albuminuria, and hematuria; Hiprex® tablets contain tartrazine which may cause allergic reactions in susceptible individuals

Precautions Use with caution in patients with hepatic impairment. Use care to maintain an acidic pH of the urine when treating infections due to urea-splitting organisms such as *Proteus* and *Pseudomonas*.

Adverse Reactions
Dermatologic: Pruritus, rash
Gastrointestinal: Dyspepsia, nausea, vomiting
Hepatic: ALT increased (reversible; rare), AST increased (reversible; rare)
Note: Large doses (higher than recommended) have resulted in bladder irritation, frequent/painful micturition, albuminuria, and hematuria.

Drug Interactions
Metabolism/Transport Effects None known.
Avoid Concomitant Use
Avoid concomitant use of Methenamine with any of the following: BCG; Sulfonamide Derivatives
Increased Effect/Toxicity
Methenamine may increase the levels/effects of: Sulfonamide Derivatives
Decreased Effect
Methenamine may decrease the levels/effects of: Alpha-/Beta-Agonists (Indirect-Acting); Amphetamines; BCG; Sodium Picosulfate; Typhoid Vaccine

The levels/effects of Methenamine may be decreased by: Antacids; Carbonic Anhydrase Inhibitors

Food Interactions Foods/diets which alkalinize urine (pH >5.5) decrease therapeutic effect of methenamine.

Stability Protect from excessive heat

Mechanism of Action Methenamine is hydrolyzed to formaldehyde and ammonia in acidic urine; formaldehyde has nonspecific bactericidal action. Other components, hippuric acid or mandelic acid, aid in maintaining urine acidity and may aid in suppressing bacteria.

◄ **Pharmacokinetics (Adult data unless noted)**
Absorption: Readily from the GI tract; 10% to 30% of the drug will be hydrolyzed by gastric juices unless it is protected by an enteric coating
Distribution: Distributes into breast milk; crosses the placenta
Metabolism: ~10% to 25% in the liver
Half-life: 3-6 hours
Elimination: Excretion occurs via glomerular filtration and tubular secretion with ~70% to 90% of dose excreted unchanged in urine within 24 hours

Dosing: Usual Oral:
Children >2 years to 12 years: Mandelate: 50-75 mg/kg/day divided every 6-8 hours; maximum dose: 4 g/day
Children 6-12 years: Hippurate: 0.5-1 g twice daily
Children >12 years and Adults:
Hippurate: 1 g twice daily
Mandelate: 1 g 4 times/day after meals and at bedtime

Administration Oral: Administer with food to minimize GI upset; shake suspension well before use; patient should drink plenty of fluids to ensure adequate urine flow; administer with cranberry juice, ascorbic acid, or ammonium chloride to acidify urine; avoid intake of alkalinizing agents (sodium bicarbonate, antacids)

Monitoring Parameters Urinary pH, urinalysis, urine cultures, periodic liver function tests in patients receiving hippurate salt

Test Interactions Increased urinary catecholamines, 17-hydroxycorticosteroid and vanillylmandelic acid (VMA) levels; decreased urinary 5-hydroxyindoleacetic acid (5HIAA) and estriol levels

Additional Information Should not be used to treat infections outside of the lower urinary tract (ie, pyelonephritis)

Dosage Forms Excipient information presented when available (limited, particularly for generics); consult specific product labeling.
Tablet, Oral, as hippurate:
Hiprex: 1 g [scored; contains tartrazine (fd&c yellow #5)]
Urex: 1 g [scored]
Generic: 1 g
Tablet, Oral, as mandelate:
Generic: 0.5 g, 1 g

References
"Practice Parameter: The Diagnosis, Treatment, and Evaluation of the Initial Urinary Tract Infection in Febrile Infants and Young Children. American Academy of Pediatrics. Committee on Quality Improvement. Subcommittee on Urinary Tract Infection," *Pediatrics*, 1999, 103(4 Pt 1):843-52.

♦ **Methenamine Hippurate** see Methenamine on page 1361

♦ **Methenamine Mandelate** see Methenamine on page 1361

Methimazole (meth IM a zole)

Medication Safety Issues
Sound-alike/look-alike issues:
Methimazole may be confused with metolazone
Brand Names: U.S. Tapazole
Brand Names: Canada Dom-Methimazole; PHL-Methimazole; Tapazole®
Therapeutic Category Antithyroid Agent
Generic Availability (U.S.) Yes
Use Treatment of hyperthyroidism, including amelioration of hyperthyroid symptoms, prior to thyroidectomy or radioactive iodine therapy [FDA approved in pediatric patients (age not specified) and adults]
Pregnancy Risk Factor D
Pregnancy Considerations Methimazole has been found to readily cross the placenta. Congenital anomalies, including esophageal atresia, choanal atresia, aplasia

cutis, and iridic and retinal coloboma, have been observed in neonates born to mothers taking methimazole during pregnancy. Nonteratogenic adverse events, including fetal and neonatal hypothyroidism, have been observed following maternal methimazole use. The transfer of thyroid-stimulating immunoglobulins can stimulate the fetal thyroid *in utero* and transiently after delivery and may increase the risk of fetal or neonatal hyperthyroidism.

Uncontrolled maternal hyperthyroidism may result in adverse neonatal outcomes (eg, prematurity, low birth weight, infants born small for gestational age) and adverse maternal outcomes (eg, pre-eclampsia, congestive heart failure). To prevent adverse fetal and maternal events, normal maternal thyroid function should be maintained prior to conception and throughout pregnancy. Antithyroid treatment is recommended for the control of hyperthyroidism during pregnancy. Due to an increased risk of congenital anomalies with methimazole, propylthiouracil is considered first-line therapy, especially during the first trimester of pregnancy. The use of methimazole is an option during the second and third trimesters of pregnancy. If drug therapy is changed, maternal thyroid function should be monitored after 2 weeks and then every 2-4 weeks.

The severity of hyperthyroidism may fluctuate throughout pregnancy and may result in decreased dose requirements or discontinuation of methimazole 2-3 weeks prior to delivery.

Breast-Feeding Considerations Methimazole is excreted into human breast milk. The thyroid function and intellectual development of breast-fed infants are not affected by exposure to maternal methimazole during breast-feeding. The American Thyroid Association considers doses of methimazole <30 mg/day to be safe during breast-feeding. Methimazole should be administered after nursing and in divided doses (Stagnaro-Green, 2011).

Contraindications Hypersensitivity to methimazole or any component, breast-feeding (per manufacturer); however, expert analysis reports methimazole may be used with caution in nursing mothers (Mandel, 2002)

Warnings May cause significant bone marrow depression; the most severe manifestation is agranulocytosis. Aplastic anemia, thrombocytopenia, and leukopenia may also occur; use with caution in patients >40 years of age or with doses ≥40 mg/day and with extreme caution in patients receiving other drugs known to cause myelosuppression, particularly agranulocytosis. Discontinue if significant bone marrow suppression occurs, particularly agranulocytosis or aplastic anemia. The lowest effective dose should be used; monitor thyroid function tests closely. Rare, severe hepatic reactions (fulminant hepatitis, hepatic necrosis, encephalopathy) may occur; possibly fatal. Symptoms suggestive of hepatic dysfunction (eg, anorexia, pruritus, right upper quadrant pain) should be promptly evaluated; discontinue if evidence of liver abnormality develops including transaminase >3 times ULN. May cause hypoprothrombinemia and bleeding; monitor PT.

Precautions Antithyroid agents have been associated with rare but severe dermatologic reactions; rash and urticaria are more common and may not require discontinuation in all cases; discontinue in the presence of exfoliative dermatitis. Discontinue in the presence of unexplained fever. Antithyroid agents have been associated with a variety of autoimmune reactions, including a lupus-like syndrome; discontinuation may be warranted. Antithyroid agents have been associated (rarely) with the development of ANCA-positive vasculitis or leukocytoclastic vasculitis; prompt discontinuation is warranted in patients who develop vasculitis during therapy.

Adverse Reactions

Cardiovascular: ANCA-positive vasculitis, edema, leukocytoclastic vasculitis, periarteritis

Central nervous system: Drowsiness, fever, headache, neuritis, vertigo

Dermatologic: Alopecia, exfoliative dermatitis, pruritus, skin pigmentation, skin rash, urticaria

Endocrine & metabolic: Goiter, hypoglycemic coma

Gastrointestinal: Constipation, epigastric distress, loss of taste perception, nausea, salivary gland swelling, vomiting, weight gain

Hematologic: Agranulocytosis, aplastic anemia, granulocytopenia, hypoprothrombinemia, leukopenia, thrombocytopenia

Hepatic: Hepatic necrosis, hepatitis, jaundice

Neuromuscular & skeletal: Arthralgia, myalgia, paresthesia

Renal: Nephritis

Miscellaneous: Insulin autoimmune syndrome, lymphadenopathy, SLE-like syndrome

Drug Interactions

Metabolism/Transport Effects Inhibits CYP1A2 (weak), CYP2A6 (weak), CYP2B6 (weak), CYP2C19 (weak), CYP2C9 (weak), CYP2D6 (weak), CYP2E1 (weak), CYP3A4 (weak)

Avoid Concomitant Use

Avoid concomitant use of Methimazole with any of the following: CloZAPine; Dipyrone; Pimozide; Sodium Iodide I131

Increased Effect/Toxicity

Methimazole may increase the levels/effects of: ARIPiprazole; Cardiac Glycosides; CloZAPine; Dofetilide; Lomitapide; Pimozide; Theophylline Derivatives

The levels/effects of Methimazole may be increased by: Dipyrone

Decreased Effect

Methimazole may decrease the levels/effects of: Sodium Iodide I131; Vitamin K Antagonists

Stability Store at 20°C to 25°C (68°F to 77°F); excursion permitted to 15°C to 30°C (59°F to 86°F); protect from light.

Mechanism of Action Inhibits the synthesis of thyroid hormones by blocking the oxidation of iodine in the thyroid gland. As a result, methimazole inhibits the ability of iodine to combine with tyrosine to form thyroxine and triiodothyronine (T_3); does not inactivate circulating T_4 and T_3

Pharmacodynamics

Onset of action: 12-18 hours

Duration: 36-72 hours (Clark, 2006)

Pharmacokinetics (Adult data unless noted)

Absorption: Almost complete (Clark, 2006)

Distribution: Concentrated in thyroid gland

Bioavailability: ~93% (Clark, 2006)

Metabolism: Hepatic

Half-life: 4-6 hours (Clark, 2006)

Time to peak serum concentration: 1-2 hours (Clark, 2006)

Elimination: Urine

Dosing: Neonatal Congenital Hyperthyroidism: Oral: Initial: 0.25-1 mg/kg/day in 2-3 divided doses; once patient euthyroid, reduce dose (usually by ≥50%) to maintain euthyroid state

Dosing: Usual

Infants, Children, and Adolescent:

Hyperthyroidism: Oral:

Manufacturer's labeling: Initial: 0.4 mg/kg/**day** in 3 divided doses (approximately every 8 hours); maintenance: 0.2 mg/kg/**day** in 3 divided doses

Alternate dosing: Initial: 0.25-1 mg/kg/**day** in 1-3 divided doses; consider doses on low-end of range for younger children; once patient euthyroid, reduce dose (usually by ≥50%) to maintain euthyroid state

Graves' disease (Bahn, 2011): Oral: **Note:** In severe cases, higher doses may be required (50% to 100% higher); once patient euthyroid, reduce dose by ≥50% to

maintain euthyroid; duration of therapy usually 1-2 years

Weight-based dosing: Initial: 0.2-0.5 mg/kg/dose once daily (range: 0.1-1 mg/kg/dose)

Fixed dosing (using ¼, ½, or whole tablets):

Infants: 1.25 mg/day

Children 1-5 years: 2.5-5 mg/day

Children 5-10 years: 5-10 mg/day

Children 10-18 years: 10-20 mg/day

Adults

Hyperthyroidism: Oral: Initial: 15 mg/day in 3 divided doses (approximately every 8 hours) for mild hyperthyroidism; 30-40 mg/day in moderately severe hyperthyroidism; 60 mg/day in severe hyperthyroidism; maintenance: 5-15 mg/day (may be given as a single daily dose in many cases)

Adjust dosage as required to achieve and maintain serum T_3, T_4, and TSH levels in the normal range. An elevated T_3 may be the sole indicator of inadequate treatment. An elevated TSH indicates excessive antithyroid treatment.

Graves' disease: Oral: Initial: 10-20 mg once daily to restore euthyroidism; maintenance: 5-10 mg once daily for a total of 12-18 months, then tapered or discontinued if TSH is normal at that time (Bahn, 2011)

Iodine-induced thyrotoxicosis: Oral: 20-40 mg/day given either once or twice daily (Bahn, 2011)

Thyrotoxic crisis: Oral: **Note:** Recommendations vary; use in combination with other specific agents. Dosages of 20-25 mg every 6 hours have been used; once stable, dosing frequency may be reduced to once or twice daily (Nayak, 2006). The American Thyroid Association and the American Association of Clinical Endocrinologists recommend 60-80 mg/day (Bahn, 2011). Rectal administration has also been described (Nabil, 1982).

Thyrotoxicosis (type I amiodarone-induced): Oral: 40 mg once daily to restore euthyroidism (generally 3-6 months). **Note:** If high doses continue to be required, dividing the dose may be more effective (Bahn, 2011).

Dosage adjustment in renal impairment: No adjustment necessary

Administration Oral: Administer consistently in relation to meals every day

Monitoring Parameters Signs of hyper- or hypothyroidism, CBC with differential, liver function (baseline and as needed); serum thyroxine, free thyroxine index, prothrombin time

Dosage Forms Excipient information presented when available (limited, particularly for generics); consult specific product labeling.

Tablet, Oral:

Tapazole: 5 mg, 10 mg [scored]

Generic: 5 mg, 10 mg

Extemporaneous Preparations Suppositories can be made from methimazole tablets; dissolve 1200 mg methimazole in 12 mL of water and add to 52 mL cocoa butter containing 2 drops of Span 80. Stir the resulting mixture to form a water-oil emulsion and pour into 2.6 mL suppository molds to cool.

Nabil N, Miner DJ, and Amatruda JM, "Methimazole: An Alternative Route of Administration," *J Clin Endo Metab*, 1982, 54(1):180-1.

References

American College of Obstetricians and Gynecologists, "ACOG Practice Bulletin. Clinical Management Guidelines for Obstetrician-Gynecologists. Number 37, August 2002. (Replaces Practice Bulletin Number 32, November 2001). Thyroid Disease in Pregnancy," *Obstet Gynecol*, 2002, 100(2):387-96.

Bahn RS (Chair), Burch HB, Cooper DS, et al, "Hyperthyroidism and Other Causes of Thyrotoxicosis: Management Guidelines of the American Thyroid Association and American Association of Clinical Endocrinologists," *Thyroid*, 2011, 21(6):593-646.

Clark SM, Saade GR, Snodgrass WR, et al, "Pharmacokinetics and Pharmacotherapy of Thionamides in Pregnancy," *Ther Drug Monit*, 2006, 28(4):477-83.

Cooper DS, "Antithyroid Drugs," *N Engl J Med*, 2005, 352(9):905-17.

Diav-Citrin O and Ornoy A, "Teratogen Update: Antithyroid Drugs-Methimazole, Carbimazole, and Propylthiouracil," *Teratology*, 2002, 65(1):38-44.

Johansen K, Andersen AN, Kampmann JP, et al, "Excretion of Methimazole in Human Milk," *Eur J Clin Pharmacol*, 1982, 23(4):339-41.

Koren G and Soldin O, "Therapeutic Drug Monitoring of Antithyroid Drugs in Pregnancy: The Knowledge Gaps," *Ther Drug Monit*, 2006, 28(1):12-3.

Mandel SJ and Cooper DS, "The Use of Antithyroid Drugs in Pregnancy and Lactation," *J Clin Endocrinol Metab*, 2001, 86(6):2354-9.

Nabil N, Miner DJ, and Amatruda JM, "Methimazole: An Alternative Route of Administration," *J Clin Endocrinol Metab*, 1982, 54(1):180-1.

Nayak B and Burman K, "Thyrotoxicosis and Thyroid Storm," *Endocrinol Metab Clin North Am*, 2006, 35(4):663-86.

Raby C, Lagorce JF, Jambut-Absil AC, et al, "The Mechanism of Action of Synthetic Antithyroid Drugs: Iodine Complexation During Oxidation of Iodide," *Endocrinology*, 1990, 126(3):1683-91.

Stagnaro-Green A, Abalovich M, Alexander E, et al, "Guidelines of the American Thyroid Association for the Diagnosis and Management of Thyroid Disease During Pregnancy and Postpartum," *Thyroid*, 2011, 21(10):1081-125.

Methocarbamol (meth oh KAR ba mole)

Medication Safety Issues
Sound-alike/look-alike issues:
Methocarbamol may be confused with mephobarbital
Robaxin® may be confused with ribavirin, Skelaxin®
BEERS Criteria medication:
This drug may be potentially inappropriate for use in geriatric patients (Quality of evidence - moderate; Strength of recommendation - strong).
International issues:
Robaxin [U.S., Canada, Great Britain, Greece, Spain] may be confused with Rubex brand name for ascorbic acid [Ireland]; doxorubicin [Brazil]

Brand Names: U.S. Robaxin; Robaxin-750

Brand Names: Canada Robaxin®

Therapeutic Category Skeletal Muscle Relaxant, Non-paralytic

Generic Availability (U.S.) May be product dependent

Use Adjunctive treatment of muscle spasm associated with acute painful musculoskeletal conditions (eg, tetanus) (FDA approved in ages ≥16 years and adults)

Pregnancy Risk Factor C

Pregnancy Considerations Animal reproduction studies have not been conducted. The manufacturer notes that fetal and congenital abnormalities have been rarely reported following *in utero* exposure. Use during pregnancy only if clearly needed.

Breast-Feeding Considerations It is not known if methocarbamol is excreted in breast milk. The manufacturer recommends that caution be exercised when administering methocarbamol to nursing women.

Contraindications Hypersensitivity to methocarbamol or any component; renal impairment (injectable formulation)

Warnings Parenteral solution for injection is hypertonic, avoid extravasation. Use of injection in patients with impaired renal function is contraindicated due to the polyethylene glycol vehicle which, in large amounts, may be irritating to the kidneys by increasing preexisting acidosis and urea retention in patients with renal impairment

Precautions Use injectable form cautiously in patients with suspected or known seizure disorders; use with caution in myasthenia gravis patients receiving pyridostigmine; use oral formulation with caution in patients with renal or hepatic impairment; monitor these patients closely; may cause CNS depression which may impair physical or mental abilities; use with caution when used with other sedative drugs or ethanol.

Adverse Reactions
Cardiovascular: Bradycardia, flushing, hypotension, syncope

Central nervous system: Amnesia, confusion, coordination impaired (mild), dizziness, drowsiness, fever, headache, insomnia, lightheadedness, sedation, seizures, vertigo

Dermatologic: Angioneurotic edema, pruritus, rash, urticaria

Gastrointestinal: Dyspepsia, metallic taste, nausea, vomiting

Hematologic: Leukopenia

Hepatic: Jaundice

Local: Pain at injection site, thrombophlebitis

Ocular: Blurred vision, conjunctivitis, diplopia, nystagmus

Respiratory: Nasal congestion

Miscellaneous: Hypersensitivity reactions including anaphylaxis

Drug Interactions
Metabolism/Transport Effects None known.

Avoid Concomitant Use
Avoid concomitant use of Methocarbamol with any of the following: Azelastine (Nasal); Paraldehyde; Thalidomide

Increased Effect/Toxicity
Methocarbamol may increase the levels/effects of: Alcohol (Ethyl); Azelastine (Nasal); Buprenorphine; CNS Depressants; Hydrocodone; Methotrimeprazine; Metyrosine; Mirtazapine; Paraldehyde; Pramipexole; ROPINIRole; Rotigotine; Selective Serotonin Reuptake Inhibitors; Thalidomide; Zolpidem

The levels/effects of Methocarbamol may be increased by: Brimonidine (Topical); Cannabis; Doxylamine; Dronabinol; Droperidol; HydrOXYzine; Kava Kava; Magnesium Sulfate; Methotrimeprazine; Nabilone; Perampanel; Rufinamide; Sodium Oxybate; Tapentadol; Tetrahydrocannabinol

Decreased Effect
Methocarbamol may decrease the levels/effects of: Pyridostigmine

Stability
Injection: Prior to dilution, store at controlled room temperature of 20°C to 25°C (68°F to 77°F); excursions permitted to 15°C to 30°C (59°F to 86°F).

Tablet: Store at controlled room temperature of 20°C to 25°C (68°F to 77°F).

Mechanism of Action Causes skeletal muscle relaxation by general CNS depression

Pharmacodynamics Onset of action: 30 minutes

Pharmacokinetics (Adult data unless noted) Oral:
Protein binding: 46% to 50%

Metabolism: Extensive in the liver via dealkylation and hydroxylation

Half-life: 1-2 hours

Time to peak serum concentration: Within ~1-2 hours

Elimination: Clearance: Adults: 0.2-0.8 L/hour/kg

Dosing: Usual
Tetanus: I.V.:
Children (recommended **only** for use in tetanus): 15 mg/kg/dose or 500 mg/m^2/dose, may repeat every 6 hours if needed; maximum dose: 1.8 g/m^2/day for 3 days only

Adults: 1-2 g by direct I.V. injection, which may be followed by an additional 1-2 g by infusion (maximum dose: 3 g total); followed by 1-2 g every 6 hours until NG tube or oral therapy possible; total daily dose of up to 24 g may be needed; injection should not be used for more than 3 consecutive days

Muscle spasm:

Oral: Adolescents ≥16 years and Adults: 1.5 g 4 times/day for 2-3 days (up to 8 g/day may be used for severe conditions); decrease dose to 4-4.5 g/day as 1 g 4 times/day or 750 mg every 4 hours or 1.5 g 3 times/day

I.M., I.V.: Adults: Initial: 1 g; may repeat every 8 hours if oral administration not possible; maximum dose: 3 g/day for 3 consecutive days (except when treating tetanus); may be reinstituted after 2 drug-free days

Dosing adjustment in renal impairment: Clearance is reduced by as much as 40% in patients with renal failure on hemodialysis; avoid use or reduce dosage and monitor closely; do not administer parenteral formulation to patients with renal dysfunction

Dosing adjustment in hepatic impairment: Specific dosing guidelines are not available; clearance may be reduced by as much as 70% in cirrhotic patients

Administration

Parenteral: I.V.: May be injected directly I.V. without dilution at a maximum rate of >3 mL/minute; may also be diluted in NS or D$_5$W to a concentration of 4 mg/mL and infused more slowly; patient should be in the recumbent position during and for 10-15 minutes after I.V. administration. Monitor closely for extravasation; pH: 3.5-6

I.M.: Adults: Maximum of 5 mL can be administered into each gluteal region; not recommended for SubQ administration

Tablet: May be crushed and mixed with food or liquid if needed.

Monitoring Parameters Monitor closely for extravasation (I.V. administration).

Test Interactions May cause color interference in certain screening tests for 5-HIAA using nitrosonaphthol reagent and in screening tests for urinary VMA using the Gitlow method.

Dosage Forms Excipient information presented when available (limited, particularly for generics); consult specific product labeling.

Solution, Injection:
Robaxin: 100 mg/mL (10 mL)
Tablet, Oral:
Robaxin: 500 mg [scored; contains fd&c yellow #6 (sunset yellow), saccharin sodium]
Robaxin-750: 750 mg [contains fd&c yellow #10 (quinoline yellow), fd&c yellow #6 (sunset yellow), saccharin sodium]
Generic: 500 mg, 750 mg

Methohexital (meth oh HEKS i tal)

Medication Safety Issues

Sound-alike/look-alike issues:
Brevital® may be confused with Brevibloc®

High alert medication:
The Institute for Safe Medication Practices (ISMP) includes this medication among its list of drugs which have a heightened risk of causing significant patient harm when used in error.

Related Information

Preprocedure Sedatives in Children *on page 2402*

Brand Names: U.S. Brevital Sodium

Brand Names: Canada Brevital®

Therapeutic Category Barbiturate; General Anesthetic; Sedative

Generic Availability (U.S.) No

Use Induction of anesthesia prior to the use of other general anesthetic agents (I.M., rectal: FDA approved in ages >1 month; I.V.: FDA approved in adults); adjunct to subpotent inhalational anesthetic agents for short surgical procedures (I.M., rectal: FDA approved in ages >1 month; I.V.: FDA approved in adults); anesthesia for short surgical, diagnostic, or therapeutic procedures associated with minimal painful stimuli (I.M., rectal: FDA approved in ages >1 month; I.V.: FDA approved in adults); anesthesia for use with other parenteral agents, usually opioid analgesics, to supplement subpotent inhalational anesthetic agents for longer surgical procedures (FDA approved in adults); induction of hypnotic state (FDA approved in adults)

Pregnancy Risk Factor B

Pregnancy Considerations Animal studies have not shown fetal or maternal harm. There are no adequate and well-controlled studies in pregnant women. Methohexital crosses the placenta. Use only if potential benefit outweighs risk to fetus.

Breast-Feeding Considerations Methohexital is minimally excreted in breast milk and levels decline rapidly after administration. Interruption of breast-feeding is unnecessary.

Contraindications Hypersensitivity to methohexital, barbiturates, or any component; porphyria; patients in whom general anesthesia is contraindicated

Warnings Continuously monitor respiratory function, pulse oximetry, and cardiac function. Resuscitative drugs, ventilation and intubation equipment, and trained personnel should be immediately available **[U.S. Boxed Warning]**. For deep sedation, a designated individual (other than the person performing the procedure) should be present to continuously monitor the patient. Prior to I.V. administration, ensure patient has adequate I.V. access; extravasation or intra-arterial injection causes necrosis.

Precautions Use with extreme caution in patients with liver impairment, asthma, cardiovascular instability; may precipitate seizures in patients with history of convulsions, especially partial seizure disorders; prolonged administration may result in increased CNS, respiratory, and cardiovascular effects; use with caution in patients with obstructive pulmonary disease, severe hypertension or hypotension, myocardial disease, CHF, severe anemia, extreme obesity, renal impairment, or endocrine disorders. Safety and efficacy of I.V. administration in pediatric patients have not been established.

Adverse Reactions

Cardiovascular: Cardiorespiratory arrest, circulatory depression, hypotension, peripheral vascular collapse, tachycardia

Central nervous system: Anxiety, emergence delirium, headache, restlessness, seizure

Dermatologic: Erythema, pruritus, urticaria

Gastrointestinal: Abdominal pain, nausea, salivation, vomiting

Hepatic: Transaminases increased

Local: Injection site pain, nerve injury adjacent to injection site, thrombophlebitis

Neuromuscular & skeletal: Involuntary muscle movement, radial nerve palsy, rigidity, tremor, twitching

Respiratory: Apnea, bronchospasm, cough, dyspnea, hiccups, laryngospasm, respiratory depression, rhinitis

Miscellaneous: Anaphylaxis (rare)

Drug Interactions

Metabolism/Transport Effects None known.

Avoid Concomitant Use
Avoid concomitant use of Methohexital with any of the following: Azelastine (Nasal); Paraldehyde; Somatostatin Acetate; Thalidomide

Increased Effect/Toxicity
Methohexital may increase the levels/effects of: Alcohol (Ethyl); Azelastine (Nasal); Buprenorphine; CNS Depressants; Hydrocodone; Hypotensive Agents; Meperidine; Methotrimeprazine; Metyrosine; Mirtazapine; Paraldehyde; Pramipexole; ROPINIRole; Rotigotine; Selective Serotonin Reuptake Inhibitors; Thalidomide; Thiazide Diuretics; Zolpidem

The levels/effects of Methohexital may be increased by:
Brimonidine (Topical); Cannabis; Chloramphenicol; Doxylamine; Dronabinol; Droperidol; Felbamate; HydrOXYzine; Kava Kava; Magnesium Sulfate; Methotrimeprazine; Nabilone; Perampanel; Primidone; Rufinamide; Sodium Oxybate; Somatostatin Acetate; Tapentadol; Tetrahydrocannabinol; Valproic Acid and Derivatives

Decreased Effect

Methohexital may decrease the levels/effects of: Acetaminophen; Beta-Blockers; Calcium Channel Blockers; Chloramphenicol; Contraceptives (Estrogens); Contraceptives (Progestins); Corticosteroids (Systemic); CycloSPORINE (Systemic); Doxycycline; Etoposide; Etoposide Phosphate; Felbamate; LamoTRIgine; Propafenone; Teniposide; Theophylline Derivatives; Tricyclic Antidepressants; Valproic Acid and Derivatives; Vitamin K Antagonists

The levels/effects of Methohexital may be decreased by:
Multivitamins/Minerals (with ADEK, Folate, Iron); Pyridoxine; Rifamycin Derivatives

Stability Store vials at controlled room temperature of 20°C to 25°C (68°F to 77°F). Solutions should be freshly prepared and used promptly. Reconstituted solutions are chemically stable at room temperature for 24 hours; 0.2% (2 mg/mL) solutions in D_5W or NS are stable at room temperature for 24 hours.

Do not dilute with solutions containing bacteriostatic agents; acceptable diluents: D_5W, NS, SWI, or accompanying diluent (for 500 mg vial to make a 1% solution); SWI is the preferred diluent except for making the 0.2% solution for I.V. continuous infusion (use of SWI to make the 0.2% solution will result in extreme hypotonicity; D_5W or NS should be used); dilute with D_5W for I.V. or rectal administration only (not for I.M. use). Do not use I.V./I.M. solutions if not clear and colorless. Solutions are alkaline (pH 9.5-11) and incompatible with acids (eg, atropine sulfate, succinylcholine chloride); incompatible with phenol-containing solutions, silicone, and LR

Mechanism of Action Ultra short-acting I.V. barbiturate anesthetic

Pharmacodynamics
Onset of action:
I.M. (pediatric patients): 2-10 minutes
I.V.: 1 minute
Rectal (pediatric patients): 5-15 minutes
Duration:
I.M.: 1-1.5 hours
I.V.: 7-10 minutes
Rectal: 1-1.5 hours

Pharmacokinetics (Adult data unless noted)
Metabolism: In the liver via demethylation and oxidation
Bioavailability: Rectal: 17%
Elimination: Through the kidney via glomerular filtration

Dosing: Usual Doses must be titrated to effect
Manufacturer's recommendations: Infants ≥1 month and Children:
I.M.: Induction: 6.6-10 mg/kg of a 5% solution
Rectal: Induction: Usual: 25 mg/kg of a 1% solution
Alternative pediatric dosing:
Children:
I.M.: Preoperative: 5-10 mg/kg/dose of a 5% solution
I.V.:
Induction: 1-2 mg/kg/dose of a 1% solution (Björkman, 1987)
Procedural sedation: Initial: 0.5 mg/kg of a 1% solution given immediately prior to procedure; titrate dose to achieve level of sedation as needed, in increments of 0.5 mg/kg to a maximum dose of 2 mg/kg; **Note:** In the prospective phase of a study, 20 children (mean age: 26 months) undergoing emergency CT scans

required a mean dose of 1 ± 0.5 mg/kg/dose with a mean total dose of 14 ± 7.5 mg/kg (Sedik, 2001).
Rectal: Preoperative, anesthesia induction, or preprocedural: Usual: 25 mg/kg/dose; range: 20-35 mg/kg/dose; maximum dose: 500 mg/dose; give as 10% (100 mg/mL) aqueous solution 5-15 minutes prior to procedure (Bjorkman, 1987; Pomeranz, 2000)
Adults: I.V.:
Induction: Range: 1-1.5 mg/kg or 50-120 mg/dose
Maintenance: Intermittent I.V. bolus injection: 20-40 mg (2-4 mL of a 1% solution) every 4-7 minutes

Administration
Parenteral:
I.M.: Reconstitute with NS to a maximum concentration of 50 mg/mL (5% solution)
I.V.: Adults:
Bolus: Dilute with SWI (preferred), NS, or D_5W to a maximum concentration of 10 mg/mL (1% solution); for induction, infuse a 1% solution at a rate of 1 mL/5 seconds
Continuous infusion: Dilute with D_5W or NS to prepare a 0.2% solution
Rectal: Dilute with acceptable diluent to a recommended concentration of 10 mg/mL (1% solution); **Note:** 10% solution has been given rectally (Bjorkman, 1987; Pomeranz, 2000).

Monitoring Parameters Blood pressure, heart rate, respiratory rate, oxygen saturation, pulse oximetry

Additional Information Does not possess analgesic properties; Brevital® has FDA-approved labeling for I.V. use in adults, and for rectal and I.M. use only in pediatric patients >1 month of age; 100 pediatric patients (3 months to 5 years of age) received rectal methohexital (25 mg/kg) for sedation prior to computed tomography (CT) scan; sedation was adequate in 95% of patients; mean time for full sedation = 8.2 ± 3.9 minutes; mean duration of action = 79.3 ± 30.9 minutes; 10% of patients had transient side effects (Pomeranz, 2000)

Controlled Substance C-IV

Dosage Forms Excipient information presented when available (limited, particularly for generics); consult specific product labeling.
Solution Reconstituted, Injection, as sodium:
Brevital Sodium: 200 mg (1 ea); 500 mg (1 ea); 2.5 g (1 ea)

References
Björkman S, Gabrielsson J, Quaynor H, et al, "Pharmacokinetics of I.V. and Rectal Methohexitone in Children," *Br J Anaesth*, 1987, 59 (12):1541-7.

Coté CJ, "Sedation for the Pediatric Patient," *Pediatr Clin North Am*, 1994, 41(1):31-58.

Elman DS and Denson JS, "Preanesthetic Sedation of Children With Intramuscular Methohexital Sodium," *Anesth Analg*, 1965, 44 (5):494-8.

Miller JR, Grayson M, and Stoelting VK, "Sedation With Intramuscular Methohexital Sodium for Office and Clinic Ophthalmic Procedures in Children," *Am J Ophthalmol*, 1966, 62(1):38-43.

Pomeranz ES, Chudnofsky CR, Deegan TJ, et al, "Rectal Methohexital Sedation for Computed Tomography Imaging of Stable Pediatric Emergency Department Patients," *Pediatrics*, 2000, 105(5):1110-4.

Sedik H, "Use of Intravenous Methohexital as a Sedative in Pediatric Emergency Departments," *Arch Pediatr Adolesc Med*, 2001, 155 (6):665-8.

◆ **Methohexital Sodium** *see* Methohexital *on page 1365*

Methotrexate (meth oh TREKS ate)

Medication Safety Issues

Sound-alike/look-alike issues:

Methotrexate may be confused with mercaptopurine, methylPREDNISolone sodium succinate, metolazone, metroNIDAZOLE, mitoXANtrone, PRALAtrexate

High alert medication:

The Institute for Safe Medication Practices (ISMP) includes this medication among its list of drugs which have a heightened risk of causing significant patient harm when used in error.

Administration issues:

Errors have occurred (resulting in death) when methotrexate was administered as "daily" dose instead of "weekly" dose recommended for some indications. The ISMP recommends hospitals use a weekly dosage regimen default for oral methotrexate orders, with a hard stop override requiring verification of appropriate oncology indication; manual systems should require verification of an oncology indication prior to dispensing oral methotrexate for daily administration. Pharmacists should provide patient education for patients discharged on weekly oral methotrexate (ISMP, 2014).

Intrathecal medication safety: The American Society of Clinical Oncology (ASCO)/Oncology Nursing Society (ONS) chemotherapy administration safety standards (Jacobson, 2009) encourage the following safety measures for intrathecal chemotherapy:

- Intrathecal medication should not be prepared during the preparation of any other agents
- After preparation, keep in an isolated location or container clearly marked with a label identifying as "intrathecal" use only
- Delivery to the patient should only be with other medications also intended for administration into the central nervous system

Other safety concerns:

MTX is an error-prone abbreviation (mistaken as mitoxantrone or multivitamin)

International issues:

Trexall [U.S.] may be confused with Trexol brand name for tramadol [Mexico]; Truxal brand name for chlorprothixene [multiple international markets]

Related Information

Emetogenic Potential of Antineoplastic Agents in Children *on page 2327*

Safe Handling of Hazardous Drugs *on page 2419*

Brand Names: U.S. Otrexup; Rheumatrex; Trexall

Brand Names: Canada Apo-Methotrexate; Methotrexate Injection USP; Methotrexate Injection, BP; Metoject; ratio-Methotrexate Sodium

Therapeutic Category Antineoplastic Agent, Antimetabolite; Antirheumatic, Disease Modifying

Generic Availability (U.S.) May be product dependent

Use Treatment of trophoblastic neoplasms (gestational choriocarcinoma, chorioadenoma destruens, and hydatidiform mole), acute lymphocytic leukemia, osteosarcoma, breast cancer, head and neck cancer (epidermoid), cutaneous T-Cell lymphoma (advanced mycosis fungoides), lung cancer (squamous cell and small cell) [oral, parenteral: FDA approved in pediatric patients (age not specified) and adults]; treatment of meningeal leukemia [parenteral: FDA approved in pediatric patients (age not specified) and adults]; treatment of active polyarticular juvenile idiopathic arthritis (JIA) in patients who have failed to respond to other agents [oral, parenteral (Otrexup): FDA approved in ages 2-16 years]; treatment of psoriasis (severe, recalcitrant, disabling) and severe, active rheumatoid arthritis [oral, parenteral (Otrexup): FDA approved in adults]. Has also been used for the treatment and maintenance of remission in Crohn's disease, dermatomyositis, uveitis, scleroderma, ectopic pregnancy, central nervous system tumors (including nonleukemic meningeal cancers), acute promyelocytic leukemia (maintenance treatment), soft tissue sarcoma (desmoid tumors)

Pregnancy Risk Factor X (psoriasis, rheumatoid arthritis)

Pregnancy Considerations [U.S. Boxed Warning]: Methotrexate may cause fetal death and/or congenital abnormalities. Studies in animals and pregnant women have shown evidence of fetal abnormalities; therefore, the manufacturer classifies methotrexate as pregnancy category X (for psoriasis or RA). A pattern of congenital malformations associated with maternal methotrexate use is referred to as the aminopterin/methotrexate syndrome. Features of the syndrome include CNS, skeletal, and cardiac abnormalities. Low birth weight and developmental delay have also been reported. The use of methotrexate may impair fertility and cause menstrual irregularities or oligospermia during treatment and following therapy. Methotrexate is approved for the treatment of trophoblastic neoplasms (gestational choriocarcinoma, chorioadenoma destruens, and hydatidiform mole) and has been used for the medical management of ectopic pregnancy and the medical management of abortion. **[U.S. Boxed Warning]: Use is contraindicated for the treatment of psoriasis or RA in pregnant women.** Pregnancy should be excluded prior to therapy in women of childbearing potential. Use for the treatment of neoplastic diseases only when the potential benefit to the mother outweighs the possible risk to the fetus. Pregnancy should be avoided for ≥3 months following treatment in male patients and ≥1 ovulatory cycle in female patients. A registry is available for pregnant women exposed to autoimmune medications including methotrexate. For additional information contact the Organization of Teratology Information Specialists, OTIS Autoimmune Diseases Study, at 877-311-8972.

Breast-Feeding Considerations Low amounts of methotrexate are excreted into breast milk. Due to the potential for serious adverse reactions in a breast-feeding infant, use is contraindicated in nursing mothers.

Contraindications Hypersensitivity to methotrexate or any component; breast-feeding

Additional contraindications for patients with psoriasis or rheumatoid arthritis: Pregnancy, alcoholism, alcoholic liver disease or other chronic liver disease, immunodeficiency syndrome (overt or laboratory evidence); preexisting blood dyscrasias (eg, bone marrow hypoplasia, leukopenia, thrombocytopenia, significant anemia)

Warnings Hazardous agent; use appropriate precautions for handling and disposal (NIOSH, 2012). Methotrexate has been reported to cause fetal death and/or congenital anomalies; do not use for psoriasis or RA treatment in pregnant women **[U.S. Boxed Warning]**. May cause impairment of fertility, oligospermia, and menstrual dysfunction.

Bone marrow suppression may occur (sometimes fatal), aplastic anemia has been reported **[U.S. Boxed Warning]**; anemia, pancytopenia, leukopenia, neutropenia, and/or thrombocytopenia may occur. Use caution in patients with preexisting bone marrow suppression. Discontinue therapy (immediately) in JIA, RA, or psoriasis if a significant decrease in hematologic components is noted. Immune suppression may lead to potentially fatal opportunistic infections including *Pneumocystis jirovecii* pneumonia (PCP) **[U.S. Boxed Warning]**. Use methotrexate with extreme caution in patients with an active infection; contraindicated in patients with immunodeficiency syndrome. Immunization may be ineffective during methotrexate treatment. Immunization with live vaccines is not recommended; cases of disseminated vaccinia infections due to live vaccines have been reported.

Use of low-dose methotrexate has been associated with the development of malignant lymphomas **[U.S. Boxed Warning]**; may regress upon discontinuation of therapy; treat lymphoma appropriately if regression is not induced by cessation of methotrexate. Other secondary tumors have been reported.

Methotrexate has been associated with acute (elevated transaminases) and potentially fatal chronic (fibrosis, cirrhosis) hepatotoxicity **[U.S. Boxed Warning]**. Risk is related to cumulative dose (total dose: ≥1.5 g) and prolonged exposure (duration: ≥2 years). Monitor closely (with liver function tests, including serum albumin) for liver toxicities. Liver enzyme elevations may be noted, but may not be predictive of hepatic disease in long-term treatment for psoriasis [but generally is predictive in rheumatoid arthritis (RA) treatment]. With long-term use, liver biopsy may show histologic changes, fibrosis, or cirrhosis; periodic liver biopsy is recommended with long-term use for psoriasis patients with risk factors for hepatotoxicity and for persistent abnormal liver function tests in psoriasis patients without risk factors for hepatotoxicity and in all JIA and RA patients; discontinue methotrexate with moderate-to-severe change in liver biopsy. Risk factors for hepatotoxicity include history of above moderate ethanol consumption, persistent abnormal liver chemistries, history of chronic liver disease (including hepatitis B or C), family history of inheritable liver disease, diabetes, obesity, hyperlipidemia, lack of folate supplementation during methotrexate therapy, cumulative methotrexate dose exceeding 1.5 g, continuous daily methotrexate dosing, and history of significant exposure to hepatotoxic drugs. Use caution with preexisting liver impairment; may require dosage reduction. Use caution when used with other hepatotoxic agents (azathioprine, retinoids, sulfasalazine).

May cause renal damage leading to acute renal failure, especially with high-dose methotrexate; monitor renal function and methotrexate concentrations closely, maintain adequate hydration and urinary alkalinization. Use caution in osteosarcoma patients treated with high-dose methotrexate in combination with nephrotoxic chemotherapy (eg, cisplatin). Methotrexate elimination is reduced in patients with renal impairment **[U.S. Boxed Warning]**; may require dose reduction or discontinuation; monitor closely for toxicity. Elimination is reduced in patients with ascites and/or pleural effusions **[U.S. Boxed Warning]**; resulting in prolonged half-life and toxicity; may require dose reduction or discontinuation. Monitor closely for toxicity.

May cause potentially life-threatening pneumonitis (acute or chronic); may require treatment interruption; may be irreversible **[U.S. Boxed Warning]**; pulmonary symptoms may occur at any time during therapy and at any dosage); monitor closely for pulmonary symptoms, particularly dry, nonproductive cough. Other potential symptoms include fever, dyspnea, hypoxemia, or pulmonary infiltrate.

May cause neurotoxicity manifested as generalized or focal seizures; usually occurs in pediatric ALL patients receiving intermediate-dose methotrexate (1 g/m²), associated symptoms often include leukoencephalopathy (usually with concurrent cranial irradiation) and stroke-like encephalopathy (usually with high-dose regimens). Chemical arachnoiditis (headache, back pain, nuchal rigidity, fever) and myelopathy may result from intrathecal administration. Chronic leukoencephalopathy has been reported with high-dose and with intrathecal methotrexate; may be progressive and fatal. May cause dizziness and fatigue; may affect the ability to drive or operate heavy machinery.

Any dose level or route of administration may cause severe and potentially fatal dermatologic reactions, including toxic epidermal necrolysis, Stevens-Johnson syndrome, exfoliative dermatitis, skin necrosis, and erythema multiforme **[U.S. Boxed Warning]**. Recovery has been reported with treatment discontinuation. Radiation dermatitis and sunburn may be precipitated by methotrexate administration. Psoriatic lesions may be worsened by concomitant exposure to ultraviolet radiation.

Tumor lysis syndrome may occur in patients with high tumor burden **[U.S. Boxed Warning]**; use appropriate prevention and treatment.

Concurrent administration with NSAIDs may cause severe bone marrow suppression, aplastic anemia, and GI toxicity **[U.S. Boxed Warning]**. Do not administer NSAIDs prior to or during high-dose methotrexate therapy; may increase and prolong serum methotrexate concentrations. Doses used for psoriasis may still lead to unexpected toxicities; use caution when administering NSAIDs or salicylates with lower doses of methotrexate for RA. Methotrexate may increase the concentrations and effects of mercaptopurine; may require dosage adjustments. Vitamins containing folate may decrease response to systemic methotrexate; folate deficiency may increase methotrexate toxicity. Concomitant use of proton pump inhibitors with methotrexate (primarily high-dose methotrexate) may elevate and prolong serum methotrexate levels and metabolite (hydroxymethotrexate) levels (based on case reports and pharmacokinetic studies); may lead to toxicities; use with caution. Potentially significant interactions may exist, requiring dose or frequency adjustment, additional monitoring, and/or selection of alternative therapy. Consult drug interactions database for more detailed information. Concomitant methotrexate administration with radiotherapy may increase the risk of soft tissue necrosis and osteonecrosis **[U.S. Boxed Warning]**.

Gastrointestinal toxicity may occur; diarrhea and ulcerative stomatitis may require treatment interruption **[U.S. Boxed Warning]**; death from hemorrhagic enteritis or intestinal perforation has been reported. Use with caution in patients with peptic ulcer disease, ulcerative colitis. Doses ≥250 mg/m² (I.V.) are associated with moderate emetic potential; antiemetics are recommended to prevent nausea and vomiting.

When used for intrathecal administration, should not be prepared during the preparation of any other agents; after preparation, store intrathecal medications in an isolated location or container clearly marked with a label identifying as "intrathecal" use only. Delivery of intrathecal medications to the patient should only be with other medications intended for administration into the central nervous system (Jacobson, 2009).

Some injections contain benzyl alcohol which may cause allergic reactions in susceptible individuals; large amounts of benzyl alcohol (≥99 mg/kg/day) have been associated with a potentially fatal toxicity ("gasping syndrome") in neonates; the "gasping syndrome" consists of metabolic acidosis, respiratory distress, gasping respirations, CNS dysfunction (including convulsions, intracranial hemorrhage), hypotension and cardiovascular collapse; avoid use of methotrexate products containing benzyl alcohol in neonates; in vitro and animal studies have shown that benzoate, a metabolite of benzyl alcohol, displaces bilirubin from protein binding sites. Methotrexate formulations and/or diluents containing preservatives should not be used for intrathecal or high-dose therapy **[U.S. Boxed Warning]**.

Precautions Should be administered under the supervision of a physician experienced in the use of antimetabolite therapy **[U.S. Boxed Warning]**; serious and fatal toxicities have occurred at all dose levels; monitor closely. Errors have occurred (some resulting in death) when methotrexate was administered as "daily" dose instead of a "weekly" dose as intended for some indications; check orders carefully for frequency and communicate frequency to patients. For RA and psoriasis, immunosuppressive therapy should only be used when disease is active, severe, recalcitrant, and disabling; and where less toxic, traditional therapy is ineffective.

Adverse Reactions Note: Adverse reactions vary by route and dosage. Hematologic and/or gastrointestinal toxicities may be common at dosages used in chemotherapy; these reactions are much less frequent when used at typical dosages for rheumatic diseases.

Cardiovascular: Vasculitis
Central nervous system: Chills, dizziness, malaise
Central nervous system (with intrathecal administration or very high-dose therapy):
  Arachnoiditis: Acute reaction manifested as severe headache, nuchal rigidity, vomiting, and fever; may be alleviated by reducing the dose
  Central nervous system toxicity (subacute): Patients treated with 12-15 mg of intrathecal methotrexate may develop this in the second or third week of therapy; consists of motor paralysis of extremities, cranial nerve palsy, seizure, or coma. This has also been seen in pediatric cases receiving very high-dose I.V. methotrexate.
  Demyelinating disease of the central nervous system: Seen months or years after receiving methotrexate; usually in association with cranial irradiation or other systemic chemotherapy
Dermatologic: Alopecia, burning sensation of skin (psoriasis), dermatitis, erythema, hyperpigmentation, hypopigmentation, pruritus, skin photosensitivity, skin rash
Endocrine & metabolic: Diabetes mellitus, hyperuricemia
Gastrointestinal: Anorexia, aphthous stomatitis, diarrhea, gingivitis, glossitis, intestinal perforation, mucositis (dose dependent; appears in 3-7 days after therapy, resolving within 2 weeks), nausea, periportal fibrosis (chronic therapy), stomatitis, vomiting
Genitourinary: Azotemia, cystitis, oligospermia
Hematologic & oncologic: Bone marrow depression (nadir: 7-10 days), hemorrhage, leukopenia, pancytopenia, thrombocytopenia
Hepatic: Cirrhosis (chronic therapy), increased liver enzymes (chronic therapy)
Immunologic: Immunosuppression
Infection: Infection
Neuromuscular & skeletal: Arthralgia
Ophthalmic: Blurred vision
Renal: Nephropathy, renal failure; renal insufficiency: Manifested by an abrupt rise in serum creatinine and BUN and a fall in urine output; more common with high-dose methotrexate, and may be due to precipitation of the drug.
Respiratory: Pharyngitis; pneumonitis: Associated with cough, fever, and interstitial pulmonary infiltrates; treatment is to withhold methotrexate during the acute reaction
Rare but important or life-threatening: Adult respiratory distress syndrome, agranulocytosis, anaphylactoid reaction, anaphylaxis, anorexia, arterial thrombosis, bone fracture, cardiac arrhythmia, cerebral thrombosis, cerebrovascular accident, chronic obstructive pulmonary disease (interstitial), cognitive dysfunction (has been reported at low dosage), convulsions, cryptococcosis, cytomegalovirus disease (including cytomegaloviral pneumonia, sepsis, nocardiosis), deep vein thrombosis, dysarthria, enteritis, eosinophilia, erythema multiforme, exfoliative dermatitis, gastric ulcer, gastrointestinal hemorrhage, gynecomastia, hepatic failure, hepatitis, herpes simplex infection, herpes zoster, histoplasmosis, hypogammaglobulinemia, hypotension, impotence, infertility, intestinal perforation, ischemic bowel disease (mesenteric, acute), ischemic heart disease,

leukoencephalopathy (especially following craniospinal irradiation or repeated high-dose therapy; may be chronic), lymphadenopathy, lymphoma (may regress with discontinuation), lymphoproliferative disorder, myocardial infarction, nasal septum perforation, neurological signs and symptoms (at high dosages; symptoms include confusion, hemiparesis, transient blindness, and coma), neutropenia, nodule, occlusive arterial disease (acute), osteonecrosis and soft tissue necrosis (with radiotherapy), osteoporosis (with radiotherapy), pancreatitis, pericardial effusion, pericarditis, plaque erosion (psoriasis), pneumonia, pneumonia due to *Pneumocystis carinii*, proteinuria, pulmonary alveolitis, pulmonary embolism, pulmonary fibrosis, respiratory failure, retinal thrombosis, reversible posterior leukoencephalopathy syndrome, seizure (more frequent in pediatric patients with ALL), skin abnormalities related to radiation recall, skin necrosis, skin ulceration, Stevens-Johnson syndrome, supraventricular cardiac arrhythmia, syncope, telangiectasia, thromboembolism, thrombophlebitis, tissue necrosis (with radiotherapy), toxic epidermal necrolysis, tumor lysis syndrome, upper respiratory tract infection, vaccinia (disseminated; following smallpox immunization), ventricular arrhythmia

Drug Interactions

Metabolism/Transport Effects Substrate of P-glycoprotein, SLCO1B1

Avoid Concomitant Use
Avoid concomitant use of Methotrexate with any of the following: Acitretin; BCG; CloZAPine; Dipyrone; Natalizumab; Pimecrolimus; Tacrolimus (Topical); Tofacitinib

Increased Effect/Toxicity
Methotrexate may increase the levels/effects of: CloZAPine; CycloSPORINE (Systemic); Dipyrone; Leflunomide; Loop Diuretics; Natalizumab; Tegafur; Theophylline Derivatives; Tofacitinib; Vaccines (Live); Vitamin K Antagonists

The levels/effects of Methotrexate may be increased by: Acitretin; Alitretinoin (Systemic); Ciprofloxacin (Systemic); CycloSPORINE (Systemic); Denosumab; Dipyrone; Eltrombopag; Fosphenytoin-Phenytoin; Loop Diuretics; Mipomersen; Nonsteroidal Anti-Inflammatory Agents; Penicillins; P-glycoprotein/ABCB1 Inhibitors; Pimecrolimus; Probenecid; Proton Pump Inhibitors; Roflumilast; Salicylates; SulfaSALAzine; Sulfonamide Derivatives; Tacrolimus (Topical); Trastuzumab; Trimethoprim

Decreased Effect
Methotrexate may decrease the levels/effects of: BCG; Cardiac Glycosides; Coccidioidin Skin Test; Fosphenytoin-Phenytoin; Loop Diuretics; Sapropterin; Sipuleucel-T; Vaccines (Inactivated); Vitamin K Antagonists

The levels/effects of Methotrexate may be decreased by: Bile Acid Sequestrants; Echinacea; P-glycoprotein/ABCB1 Inducers

Food Interactions Methotrexate peak serum levels may be decreased if taken with food. Milk-rich foods may decrease methotrexate absorption. Management: Administer without regard to food.

Stability
Oral: Tablets: Store at room temperature of 20°C to 25°C (68°F to 77°F); excursions are permitted between 15°C and 30°C (59°F and 86°F). Protect from light.
Parenteral: Store intact vials and autoinjectors at room temperature 20°C to 25°C (68°F to 77°F); excursions may be permitted between 15°C and 30°C (59°F and 86°F). Protect from light.
  I.V.: Solution further diluted in D_5W or NS is stable for 24 hours at room temperature (21°C to 25°C).
Intrathecal: Intrathecal dilutions are preservative free and should be used as soon as possible after preparation. After preparation, store intrathecal medications (until

use) in an isolated location or container clearly marked with a label identifying as "intrathecal" use only.

Mechanism of Action Methotrexate is a folate antimetabolite that inhibits DNA synthesis, repair, and cellular replication. Methotrexate irreversibly binds to and inhibits dihydrofolate reductase, inhibiting the formation of reduced folates, and thymidylate synthetase, resulting in inhibition of purine and thymidylic acid synthesis, thus interfering with DNA synthesis, repair, and cellular replication. Methotrexate is cell cycle specific for the S phase of the cycle. Actively proliferative tissues are more susceptible to the effects of methotrexate.

The MOA in the treatment of rheumatoid arthritis is unknown, but may affect immune function. In psoriasis, methotrexate is thought to target rapidly proliferating epithelial cells in the skin.

In Crohn disease, it may have immune modulator and anti-inflammatory activity.

Pharmacodynamics Onset of action: Antirheumatic: 3-6 weeks; additional improvement may continue longer than 12 weeks

Pharmacokinetics (Adult data unless noted)
Absorption:
  Oral: Pediatric and adult patients: Highly variable; dose-dependent; decreased absorption at higher doses (pediatric patients: >40 mg/m^2; adult patients: >80 mg/m^2); possibly due to saturation effect
  I.M.: Complete
Distribution: Penetrates slowly into 3rd space fluids (eg, pleural effusions, ascites), exits slowly from these compartments (slower than from plasma); sustained concentrations retained in kidney and liver
V_d: I.V.: ~0.18 L/kg (initial); 0.4-0.8 L/kg (steady state)
Protein binding: ~50%
Metabolism: Partially metabolized by intestinal flora (after oral administration) to DAMPA by carboxypeptidase; hepatic aldehyde oxidase converts methotrexate to 7-hydroxy methotrexate; polyglutamates are produced intracellularly and are just as potent as methotrexate; their production is dose- and duration-dependent and they are slowly eliminated by the cell once formed. Polyglutamated forms can be converted back to methotrexate.
Bioavailability: Oral: In general, bioavailability is dose dependent and decreases as the dose increases
  Pediatric patients: Highly variable: 23% to 95%
  Adults: Low doses (≤30 mg/m^2): 60%
Half-life (terminal):
  Pediatric patients:
    ALL: 0.7-5.8 hours (dose range: 6.3-30 mg/m^2)
    JIA: 0.9-2.3 hours (dose range: 3.75-26.2 mg/m^2)
  Adults: Low dose: 3-10 hours; high dose: 8-15 hours
Time to peak serum concentration:
  Oral:
    Pediatric patients: 0.67-4 hours (reported for a 15 mg/m^2 dose)
    Adults: 1-2 hours
  I.M.: Pediatric and adult patients: 30-60 minutes
Elimination: Dose and route dependent; I.V.: Urine (80% to 90% as unchanged drug; 5% to 7% as 7-hydroxy methotrexate); feces (<10%)

Dosing: Usual Note: Methotrexate doses between 100-500 mg/m^2 **may require** leucovorin calcium rescue. Methotrexate doses >500 mg/m^2 **require** leucovorin calcium rescue.
Infants, Children and Adolescents: **Note:** Dosing may be presented as mg/m^2 or mg/kg; verify dosage unit for calculations; extra precautions should be taken. Frequency of dosing is indication specific (generally weekly or daily); patient harm may occur if administered incorrectly; extra precautions should be taken to verify appropriate frequency.

Acute lymphoblastic leukemia (ALL): Note: Intrathecal therapy is also administered (refer to specific reference for intrathecal dosing used within protocol):
  Consolidation/intensification phases (as part of a combination regimen): I.V.: 1000 mg/m^2 infuse over 24 hours in week 1 of intensification and 20 mg/m^2 I.M. (use 50% dose reduction if on same day as intrathecal methotrexate) on day 1 of week 2 of intensification phase; Intensification repeats every 2 weeks for a total of 12 courses (Mahoney, 2000) **or** 5000 mg/m^2 I.V. over 24 hours days 8, 22, 36, and 50 of consolidation phase (Schrappe, 2000) with leucovorin rescue
  Interim maintenance (as part of a combination regimen) (Seibel, 2008):
    I.V.: 100 mg/m^2 (escalate dose by 50 mg/m^2 each dose) on days 0, 10, 20, 30, and 40 of increased intensity interim maintenance phase
    Oral: 15 mg/m^2 on days 0, 7, 14, 21, 28, and 35 of interim maintenance phase
  Maintenance (as part of a combination regimen):
    I.M: 20 mg/m^2 weekly on day 1 of weeks 25 to 130 (Mahoney, 2000)
    Oral: 20 mg/m^2 on days 7, 14, 21, 28, 35, 42, 49, 56, 63, 70, and 77 (Seibel, 2008)
ALL, T-cell (Asselin, 2011): Children and Adolescents: **Note:** Triple intrathecal therapy is also administered (refer to specific reference for intrathecal dosing used within protocol):
  Induction (weeks 1-6; as part of a combination regimen): I.V.:
    Low dose: 40 mg/m^2 on day 2
    High dose: 500 mg/m^2 over 30 minutes followed by 4500 mg/m^2 over 23.5 hours (to complete a total dose of 5000 mg/m^2 over 24 hours) on day 22 (with leucovorin rescue)
  Consolidation (weeks 7-33; combination chemotherapy): I.V.: High dose: 500 mg/m^2/dose over 30 minutes followed by 4500 mg/m^2/dose over 23.5 hours (to complete a total dose of 5000 mg/m^2 over 24 hours) (with leucovorin rescue) in weeks 7, 10, and 13
  Continuation (weeks 34-108; combination chemotherapy): I.V., I.M.: 30 mg/m^2 weekly until 2 years after documented complete remission
ALL, CNS prophylaxis triple intrathecal therapy: Children <10 years: Intrathecal: Age-based dosing (in combination with cytarabine and hydrocortisone): Days of administration vary based on risk status and protocol; refer to institutional protocols or reference for details (Matloub, 2006):
  <2 years: 8 mg
  2 to <3 years: 10 mg
  3 to ≤8 years: 12 mg
  >8 years: 15 mg
Crohn's disease: Limited data available: Children and Adolescents: Oral, SubQ: **Note:** Should be used in patients intolerant or unresponsive to purine analog therapy (eg, azathioprine, mercaptopurine); use in combination with folic acid supplementation
  BSA-directed dosing: 15 mg/m^2 once weekly; maximum dose: 25 mg (Mack, 1998; Rufo, 2012; Sandhu, 2010; Turner, 2007)
  Fixed-dosing (Kliegman, 2011; Mack, 1998; Turner, 2007; Weiss, 2009)
    20-29 kg: 10 mg once weekly
    30-39 kg: 15 mg once weekly
    40-49 kg: 20 mg once weekly
    ≥50 kg: 25 mg once weekly
Dermatomyositis: Limited data available: Children and Adolescents: Oral, SubQ (preferred): Initial: 15 mg/m^2 **or** 1 mg/kg (whichever is less) once weekly; maximum dose: 40 mg; used in combination with corticosteroids (Huber, 2010; Ramanan, 2005)

Graft-versus-host disease, acute (aGVHD) prophylaxis: Limited data available: Children and Adolescents: I.V.: 15 mg/m^2/dose on day 1 and 10 mg/m^2/dose on days 3 and 6 after allogeneic transplant (in combination with cyclosporine and prednisone) (Chao, 1993; Chao, 2000; Ross, 1999) or 15 mg/m^2/dose on day 1 and 10 mg/m^2/dose on days 3, 6, and 11 after allogeneic transplant (in combination with cyclosporine) (Chao, 2000)

Juvenile idiopathic arthritis (JIA); polyarticular:
BSA-directed dosing: Children and Adolescents 2-16 years: Oral, I.M., SubQ: Initial: 10 mg/m^2 once weekly, adjust gradually up to 20-30 mg/m^2 once weekly; usual maximum dose: 25 mg; to reduce GI side effects, consider parenteral administration (I.M., SubQ) of higher doses (20-30 mg/m^2)
Weight-directed dosing: Children and Adolescents: Oral, SubQ: Initial: 0.5 mg/kg once weekly; maximum initial dose: 15 mg; if symptoms worsen or unchanged after 4 weeks, may increase to SubQ: 1 mg/kg; maximum dose: 30 mg; (Dewitt, 2012)

Meningeal leukemia, prophylaxis or treatment: Intrathecal: 6-12 mg/dose (based on age) every 2-7 days; continue for 1 dose beyond CSF cell count normalization. **Note:** Optimal intrathecal chemotherapy dosing should be based on age rather than on body surface area (BSA); CSF volume correlates with age and not to BSA (Bleyer, 1983; Kerr, 2001):
<1 year: 6 mg/dose
1 year: 8 mg/dose
2 years: 10 mg/dose
≥3 years: 12 mg/dose

Osteosarcoma: Limited data available: I.V.: MAP regimen (High-dose methotrexate): 12 **g**/m^2 (maximum dose: 20 **g**) over 4 hours (followed by leucovorin rescue) for 4 doses during induction (before surgery) at weeks 3, 4, 8, and 9, and for 8 doses during maintenance (after surgery) at weeks 15, 16, 20, 21, 25, 26, 30, and 31 (in combination with doxorubicin and cisplatin) (Meyers, 2005); other combinations, intervals, and doses (8-14 **g**/m^2/dose) have been described (with leucovorin rescue), refer to specific reference for details (Bacci, 2000; Bacci, 2003; Goorin, 2003; Le Deley, 2007; Meyers, 1992; Weiner, 1986; Winkler, 1988)

Psoriasis, severe; recalcitrant to topical therapy: Limited data available: Children and Adolescents: Oral, SubQ: Usual reported range: 0.2-0.4 mg/kg once weekly; reported treatment duration is highly variable: 6-178 weeks (Dadlani, 2005; deJager, 2010)

Scleroderma, localized (juvenile): Limited data available: Oral, SubQ (preferred): 1 mg/kg once weekly; maximum dose: 25 mg; alone or in combinations with corticosteroids; duration of therapy: 12 months (Li, 2012)

Uveitis, recalcitrant: Limited data available: Children and Adolescents:
BSA-directed dosing: Oral, SubQ: Most frequently reported: 15 mg/m^2 once weekly, usual range: 10-25 mg/m^2 (Foeldvari, 2005; Simonini, 2013); the SubQ route may be preferred for patients with GI symptoms, poor bioavailability or doses >15 mg/m^2 (Simonini, 2010)
Weight-directed dosing: SubQ: 0.5-1 mg/kg once weekly; maximum dose: 25 mg (Weiss, 1998)

Adults: **Note:** For oncologic uses in obese patients, utilize patient's actual body weight (full weight) for calculation of body surface area- or weight-based dosing, particularly when the intent of therapy is curative; manage regimen-related toxicities in the same manner as for nonobese patients; if a dose reduction is utilized due to toxicity, consider resumption of full weight-based dosing with subsequent cycles, especially if cause of toxicity (eg, hepatic or renal impairment) is resolved (Griggs, 2012).

Acute lymphoblastic leukemia (ALL):
Meningeal leukemia prophylaxis or treatment: Intrathecal: Manufacturer's labeling: 12 mg (maximum 15 mg/dose) every 2-7 days; continue for 1 dose beyond CSF cell count normalization. **Note:** Optimal intrathecal chemotherapy dosing should be based on age rather than on body surface area (BSA); CSF volume correlates with age and not to BSA (Bleyer, 1983; Kerr, 2001).
CALGB 8811 regimen (Larson, 1995; combination therapy):
Early intensification: Intrathecal: 15 mg day 1 of early intensification phase, repeat in 4 weeks
CNS prophylaxis/interim maintenance phase:
Intrathecal: 15 mg day 1, 8, 15, 22, and 29
Oral: 20 mg/m^2 days 36, 43, 50, 57, and 64
Prolonged maintenance: Oral: 20 mg/m^2 days 1, 8, 15, and 22 every 4 weeks for 24 months from diagnosis
Dose-intensive regimen (Kantarjian, 2000; combination therapy): I.V.: 200 mg/m^2 over 2 hours, followed by 800 mg/m^2 over 24 hours beginning day 1 (followed by leucovorin rescue) of even numbered cycles (in combination with cytarabine; alternates with Hyper-CVAD)
CNS prophylaxis: Intrathecal: 12 mg on day 2 of each cycle; duration depends on risk
Maintenance: I.V.: 10 mg/m^2/day for 5 days every month for 2 years (in combination with prednisone, vincristine, and mercaptopurine)

Breast cancer: I.V.: CMF regimen: 40 mg/m^2 days 1 and 8 every 4 weeks (in combination with cyclophosphamide and fluorouracil) for 6-12 cycles (Bonadonna, 1995; Levine, 1998)

Choriocarcinoma, chorioadenoma, gestational trophoblastic diseases: 15-30 mg oral or I.M. daily for a 5 day course; may repeat for 3-5 courses (manufacturer's labeling) **or** 100 mg/m^2 I.V. over 30 minutes followed by 200 mg/m^2 I.V. over 12 hours (with leucovorin 24 hours after the start of methotrexate), administer a second course if hCG levels plateau for 3 consecutive weeks (Garrett, 2002)

Head and neck cancer, advanced: I.V.: 40 mg/m^2 once weekly until disease progression or unacceptable toxicity (Forastiere, 1992; Guardiola, 2004; Stewart, 2009)

Lymphoma, non-Hodgkin: I.V.:
CODOX-M/IVAC regimen (Mead, 2008): Cycles 1 and 3 of CODOX-M (CODOX-M alternates with IVAC): Adults ≤65 years: I.V.: 300 mg/m^2 over 1 hour (on day 10) followed by 2700 mg/m^2 over 23 hours (with leucovorin rescue)
Hyper-CVAD alternating with high-dose methotrexate/cytarabine regimen: I.V.: 1000 mg/m^2 over 24 hours on day 1 during even courses (2, 4, 6, and 8) of 21-day treatment cycles (Thomas, 2006) or 200 mg/m^2 bolus day 1 followed by 800 mg/m^2 over 24 hours during even courses (2, 4, 6, and 8) of 21-day treatment cycles (Khouri, 1998) with leucovorin rescue

Ectopic pregnancy: Limited data available: I.M.:
Single-dose regimen: Methotrexate 50 mg/m^2 on day 1; Measure serum hCG levels on days 4 and 7; if needed, repeat dose on day 7 (Barnhart, 2009)
Two-dose regimen: Methotrexate 50 mg/m^2 on day 1; Measure serum hCG levels on day 4 and administer a second dose of methotrexate 50 mg/m^2; Measure serum hCG levels on day 7 and if needed, administer a third dose of 50 mg/m^2 (Barnhart, 2009)

Multidose regimen: Methotrexate 1 mg/kg on day 1; measure serum hCG on day 2; methotrexate 1 mg/kg on day 3;alternate days of therapy with leucovorin (ie, day 2 and day 4); measure serum hCG on day 4; continue up to a total of 4 courses based on hCG concentrations (Barnhart, 2009)

Mycosis fungoides (cutaneous T-cell lymphoma): I.M., Oral: 5-50 mg once weekly or 15-37.5 mg twice weekly for early stages (manufacturer's labeling) **or** 25 mg orally once weekly, may increase to 50 mg once weekly (Zackheim, 2003)

Osteosarcoma: Adults ≤30 years: I.V.: MAP regimen: 12 g/m^2 (maximum dose: 20 **g**) over 4 hours (followed by leucovorin rescue) for 4 doses during induction (before surgery) at weeks 3, 4, 8, and 9, and for 8 doses during maintenance (after surgery) at weeks 15, 16, 20, 21, 25, 26, 30, and 31 (in combination with doxorubicin and cisplatin) (Meyers, 2005); other combinations, intervals, age ranges, and doses (8-14 **g**/m^2/dose) have been described (with leucovorin rescue), refer to specific reference for details (Bacci, 2000; Bacci, 2003; Goorin, 2003; Le Deley, 2007; Meyers, 1992; Weiner, 1986; Winkler, 1988)

Psoriasis: Note: Some experts recommend concomitant daily folic acid (except the day of methotrexate) to reduce hematologic, gastrointestinal, and hepatic adverse events related to methotrexate.

Oral: 2.5-5 mg/dose every 12 hours for 3 doses given weekly **or**

Oral, I.M., SubQ: 10-25 mg/dose given once weekly; titrate to lowest effective dose

Note: An initial test dose of 2.5-5 mg is recommended in patients with risk factors for hematologic toxicity or renal impairment (Kalb, 2009).

Rheumatoid arthritis: Note: Some experts recommend concomitant daily folic acid (except the day of methotrexate) to reduce hematologic, gastrointestinal, and hepatic adverse events related to methotrexate.

Oral (manufacturer's labeling): 7.5 mg once weekly or 2.5 mg every 12 hours for 3 doses per week (dosage exceeding 20 mg per week may cause a higher incidence and severity of adverse events); *alternatively,* 10-15 mg once weekly, increased by 5 mg every 2-4 weeks to a maximum of 20-30 mg once weekly has been recommended by some experts (Visser, 2009)

I.M., SubQ: 10-25 mg once weekly (dosage varies, similar to oral) or 15 mg once weekly (Braun, 2008)

Dosing adjustment for toxicity: All patients:

Nonhematologic toxicity: Diarrhea, stomatitis, or vomiting which may lead to dehydration: Discontinue until recovery

Hematologic toxicity:

Psoriasis, arthritis (JIA, RA): Significant blood count decrease: Discontinue immediately.

Oncologic uses: Profound granulocytopenia and fever: Evaluate immediately; consider broad-spectrum parenteral antimicrobial coverage

Dosing adjustment in renal impairment: There are no dosage adjustments provided in the manufacturer's labeling. The following adjustments have been recommended:

Infants, Children, and Adolescents (Aronoff, 2007):

CrCl >50 mL/minute/1.73 m^2: No adjustment necessary

CrCl 10-50 mL/minute/1.73 m^2: Administer 50% of dose

CrCl <10 mL/minute/1.73 m^2: Administer 30% of dose

Hemodialysis: Administer 30% of dose

Peritoneal dialysis (PD): Administer 30% of dose

Continuous renal replacement therapy (CRRT): Administer 50% of dose

Adults:

Aronoff, 2007:

CrCl >50 mL/minute/1.73 m^2: No adjustment necessary

CrCl 10-50 mL/minute: Administer 50% of dose

CrCl <10 mL/minute: Avoid use

Hemodialysis: Administer 50% of dose

Continuous renal replacement therapy (CRRT): Administer 50% of dose

Kintzel, 1995:

CrCl 46-60 mL/minute: Administer 65% of normal dose

CrCl 31-45 mL/minute: Administer 50% of normal dose

CrCl <30 mL/minute: Avoid use

Hemodialysis patients with cancer (Janus, 2010): Administer 25% of dose after hemodialysis; monitor closely for toxicity

High-dose methotrexate, dose-intensive regimen for ALL (200 mg/m^2 over 2 hours, followed by 800 mg/m^2 over 24 hours with leucovorin rescue (Kantarjian, 2000):

Serum creatinine <1.5 mg/dL: No dosage adjustment necessary

Serum creatinine 1.5-2 mg/dL: Administer 75% of dose

Serum creatinine >2 mg/dL: Administer 50% of dose

Dosing adjustment in hepatic impairment: All patients: There are no dosage adjustment provided in the manufacturer's labeling; use with caution in patients with impaired hepatic function or preexisting hepatic dysfunction. The following adjustments have been recommended (Floyd, 2006):

Bilirubin 3.1-5 mg/dL **or** transaminases >3 times ULN: Administer 75% of dose

Bilirubin >5 mg/dL: Avoid use

Administration Hazardous agent; use appropriate precautions for handling and disposal (NIOSH, 2012).

Oral: Often preferred when low doses are being administered; administer on an empty stomach.

Parenteral:

I.M.: May be administered at concentration ≤25 mg/mL; autoinjectors should not be used for I.M. administration.

I.V.: May further dilute in D$_5$W or NS; I.V. administration may be as slow push, bolus infusion, or 24-hour continuous infusion at a concentration not to exceed 25 mg/mL (route and rate of administration depend upon indication and/or protocol; refer to specific references) (Phelps, 2013). For high-dose infusion, preservative-free formulation must be used **[U.S. Boxed Warning]**. Specific dosing schemes vary, but high dose should be followed by leucovorin calcium to prevent toxicity

SubQ:

Solution for injection: May be administered at concentration ≤25 mg/mL

Autoinjector (Otrexup): Concentration varies based on autoinjector size; patient may self-administer after appropriate training on preparation and administration and with appropriate follow-up monitoring.

Intrathecal: Prepare intrathecal solutions with preservative-free NS, or lactated Ringer's **[U.S. Boxed Warning]** to a final volume not to exceed 12 mL (volume generally based on protocol or practitioner preference). Intrathecal methotrexate concentrations may be institution specific or based on practitioner preference, generally ranging from a final concentration of 1 mg/mL (per prescribing information; Grossman, 1993; Lin, 2008) up to ~2-4 mg/mL (de Lemos, 2009; Glantz, 1999). For triple intrathecal therapy (methotrexate 12 mg/hydrocortisone 24 mg/cytarabine 36 mg), preparation to final volume of 12 mL is reported (Lin, 2008). Intrathecal medications should **NOT** be prepared during the preparation of any other agents.

Monitoring Parameters Laboratory tests should be performed on day 5 or day 6 of the weekly methotrexate cycle (eg, psoriasis, RA, JIA) to detect the leukopenia nadir and to avoid elevated LFTs 1-2 days after taking dose.

Indication-specific recommendations: **Note:** Additional recommendations may vary based upon patient age and specific protocols (refer to specific references); for all pediatric patients receiving long-term therapy (ie, chronic disease), growth parameters should also be monitored.

Psoriasis: CBC with differential and platelets (baseline, 7-14 days after initiating therapy or dosage increase, every 2-4 weeks for first few months, then every 1-3 months); BUN and serum creatinine (baseline and every 2-3 months); consider PPD for latent TB screening (baseline); LFTs (baseline, monthly for first 6 months, then every 1-2 months); chest x-ray (baseline if underlying lung disease); pulmonary function test (if methotrexate-induced lung disease suspected)

Liver biopsy:

Patients **with** risk factors for hepatotoxicity: Baseline or after 2-6 months of therapy and with each 1-1.5 g cumulative dose interval in adults

Patients **without** risk factors for hepatotoxicity: If persistent elevations in 5 of 9 AST levels during a 12-month period, or decline of serum albumin below the normal range with normal nutritional status. In adults, consider biopsy after cumulative dose of 3.5-4 g and after each additional 1.5 g.

Juvenile idiopathic arthritis: Children and Adolescents: PPD screening (baseline and annually); CBC with differential and platelets, C-reactive protein, ESR, ferritin, and LDH [baseline, at follow-up visits (1-2 weeks, 1, 2, 6, and 9 months] and with any treatment change (DeWitt, 2012). Also based on adult recommendations in RA, consider serum creatinine and LFTs (baseline then every 2-4 weeks for initial 3 months of therapy, then every 8-12 weeks for 3-6 months of therapy and then every 12 weeks after 6 months of therapy) and liver biopsy: Baseline (if persistent abnormal baseline LFTs, history of alcoholism, or chronic hepatitis B or C) or during treatment if persistent LFT elevations (6 of 12 tests abnormal over 1 year or 5 of 9 results when LFTs performed at 6-week intervals)

Rheumatoid arthritis:

CBC with differential and platelets, serum creatinine and LFTs (baseline, then every 2-4 weeks for initial 3 months of therapy, then every 8-12 weeks for 3-6 months of therapy and then every 12 weeks after 6 months of therapy); chest x-ray (baseline); pulmonary function test (if methotrexate-induced lung disease suspected); hepatitis B or C testing (baseline)

Liver biopsy: Baseline (if persistent abnormal baseline LFTs, history of alcoholism, or chronic hepatitis B or C) or during treatment if persistent LFT elevations (6 of 12 tests abnormal over 1 year or 5 of 9 results when LFTs performed at 6-week intervals)

Cancer: Baseline and frequently during treatment: CBC with differential and platelets, serum creatinine, BUN, LFTs; chest x-ray (baseline); serum methotrexate concentrations and urine pH (with high-dose therapy); pulmonary function test (if methotrexate-induced lung disease suspected)

Crohn's disease:

Children and Adolescents: In pediatric trials, frequency of monitoring varied with study protocol and duration; may vary based on clinical status and concurrent medication; consider the following: CBC with differential and platelets, LFTs, C-reactive protein, and ESR (baseline, then every 2-4 weeks during initial 8-12 weeks of therapy, then every 4-12 weeks while on therapy); chest x-ray and PFTs (annually) (Mack, 1998; Sandhu, 2010, Turner, 2007; Weiss 2009). Also, based on adult recommendations for Crohn's disease,

consider serum creatinine (baseline, then every 2-4 weeks for initial 3 months of therapy, then every 8-12 weeks for 3-6 months of therapy and then every 12 weeks after 6 months of therapy), hepatitis B or C testing (baseline) and liver biopsy: Baseline (if persistent abnormal baseline LFTs, history of alcoholism, or chronic hepatitis B or C) or during treatment if persistent LFT elevations (6 of 12 tests abnormal over 1 year or 5 of 9 results when LFTs performed at 6-week intervals).

Adults: CBC with differential and platelets, serum creatinine and LFTs (baseline then every 2-4 weeks for initial 3 months of therapy, then every 8-12 weeks for 3-6 months of therapy and then every 12 weeks after 6 months of therapy); chest x-ray (baseline); pulmonary function test (if methotrexate-induced lung disease suspected); hepatitis B or C testing (baseline) and liver biopsy: Baseline (if persistent abnormal baseline LFTs, history of alcoholism, or chronic hepatitis B or C) or during treatment if persistent LFT elevations (6 of 12 tests abnormal over 1 year or 5 of 9 results when LFTs performed at 6-week intervals)

Ectopic pregnancy: Prior to therapy, measure serum hCG, CBC with differential, liver function tests, serum creatinine. Serum hCG concentrations should decrease between treatment days 4 and 7. If hCG decreases by >15%, additional courses are not needed; however, continue to measure hCG weekly until no longer detectable. If <15% decrease is observed, repeat dose per regimen (Barnhart, 2009).

Reference Range

Therapeutic levels: Variable; toxic concentration: Variable; therapeutic range is dependent upon therapeutic approach

High-dose regimens produce drug levels that are between 0.1-1 micromole/L 24-72 hours after drug infusion.

Toxic: Low-dose therapy: >0.2 micromole/L; high-dose therapy: >1 micromole/L

Dosage Forms

Excipient information presented when available (limited, particularly for generics); consult specific product labeling.

Solution, Injection:

Generic: 25 mg/mL (2 mL, 10 mL)

Solution, Injection [preservative free]:

Generic: 25 mg/mL (2 mL, 4 mL, 8 mL, 10 mL, 40 mL); 50 mg/2 mL (2 mL); 100 mg/4 mL (4 mL); 200 mg/8 mL (8 mL); 250 mg/10 mL (10 mL); 1 g/40 mL (40 mL)

Solution Auto-injector, Subcutaneous [preservative free]:

Otrexup: 10 mg/0.4 mL (0.4 mL); 15 mg/0.4 mL (0.4 mL); 20 mg/0.4 mL (0.4 mL); 25 mg/0.4 mL (0.4 mL)

Solution Reconstituted, Injection [preservative free]:

Generic: 1 g (1 ea)

Tablet, Oral:

Rheumatrex: 2.5 mg [scored]

Trexall: 5 mg, 7.5 mg, 10 mg, 15 mg [scored]

Generic: 2.5 mg

References

ACOG Practice Bulletin. Clinical Management Guidelines of Obstetrician-Gynecologists. Number 67, October 2005. "Medical Management of Abortion," *Obstet Gynecol*, 2005, 106(4):871-82.

Aronoff GR, Bennett WM, Berns JS, et al, *Drug Prescribing in Renal Failure: Dosing Guidelines for Adults and Children*, 5th ed. Philadelphia, PA: American College of Physicians; 2007.

Asselin BL, Devidas M, Wang C, et al. Effectiveness of high-dose methotrexate in T-cell lymphoblastic leukemia and advanced-stage lymphoblastic lymphoma: a randomized study by the Children's Oncology Group (POG 9404). *Blood*. 2011;118(4):874-883.

Bacci G, Briccoli A, Rocca M, et al. Neoadjuvant chemotherapy for osteosarcoma of the extremities with metastases at presentation: recent experience at the Rizzoli Institute in 57 patients treated with cisplatin, doxorubicin, and a high dose of methotrexate and ifosfamide. *Ann Oncol*. 2003;14(7):1126-1134.

Bacci G, Ferrari S, Bertoni F, et al. Long-term outcome for patients with nonmetastatic osteosarcoma of the extremity treated at the istituto ortopedico rizzoli according to the istituto ortopedico rizzoli/osteosarcoma-2 protocol: an updated report. J Clin Oncol. 2000;18 (24):4016-4027.

Barnhart KT, "Clinical Practice. Ectopic Pregnancy," N Engl J Med, 2009, 361(4):379-87.

Bezabeh S, Mackey AC, Kluetz P, Jappar D, Korvick J. Accumulating evidence for a drug-drug interaction between methotrexate and proton pump inhibitors. Oncologist. 2012;17(4):550-554.

Bleyer WA, Coccia PF, Sather HN, et al, "Reduction in Central Nervous System Leukemia With a Pharmacokinetically Derived Intrathecal Methotrexate Dosage Regimen," J Clin Oncol. 1983;1(5):317-325.

Bonadonna G, Valagussa P, Moliterni A, et al. Adjuvant cyclophosphamide, methotrexate, and fluorouracil in node-positive breast cancer: the results of 20 years of follow-up. N Engl J Med. 1995;332 (14):901-906.

Braun J, Kästner P, Flaxenberg P, et al, "Comparison of the Clinical Efficacy and Safety of Subcutaneous Versus Oral Administration of Methotrexate in Patients With Active Rheumatoid Arthritis: Results of a Six-Month, Multicenter, Randomized, Double-Blind, Controlled, Phase IV Trial," Arthritis Rheum, 2008, 58(1):73-81.

Chao NJ, Schmidt GM, Niland JC, et al, "Cyclosporine, Methotrexate, and Prednisone Compared with Cyclosporine and Prednisone for Prophylaxis of Acute Graft-versus-Host Disease," N Engl J Med, 1993, 329(17):1225-30.

Chao NJ, Snyder DS, Jain M, et al, "Equivalence of 2 Effective Graft-Versus-Host Disease Prophylaxis Regimens: Results of a Prospective Double-Blind Randomized Trial," Biol Blood Marrow Transplant, 2000, 6(3):254-61.

Dadlani C, Orlow SJ. Treatment of children and adolescents with methotrexate, cyclosporine, and etanercept: review of the dermatologic and rheumatologic literature. J Am Acad Dermatol. 2005;52:316-340.

deJager MEA, deJong EMGJ, van de Kerkhof PCM, et al. Efficacy and safety of treatments for childhood psoriasis: a systematic literature review. J Am Acad Dermatol . 2010;62:1013-1030.

deLemos ML, Monfared S, Denyssevych T, et al. "Evaluation of Osmolality and pH of Various Concentrations of Methotrexate, Cytarabine, and Thiotepa Prepared in Normal Saline, Sterile Water for Injection, and Lactated Ringer's Solution for Intrathecal Administration," J Oncol Pharm Pract, 2009, 15(1):45-52.

DeWitt EM, Kimura Y, Beukelman T, et al. Consensus treatment plans for new-onset systemic juvenile idiopathic arthritis. Arthritis Care Res (Hoboken). 2012;64(7):1001-1010.

Feldman BM, Rider LG, Reed AM, et al. Juvenile Dermatomyositis and other idiopathic inflammatory myopathies of childhood. Lancet. 2008;371(9631):2201-2212.

Floyd J, Mirza I, Sachs B, et al, "Hepatotoxicity of Chemotherapy," Semin Oncol, 2006, 33(1):50-67.

Foeldvari I, Wierk A. Methotrexate is an effective treatment for chronic uveitis associated with juvenile idiopathic arthritis. J Rheumatol. 2005;32(2):362-365.

Forastiere AA, Metch B, Schuller DE, et al. Randomized comparison of cisplatin plus fluorouracil and carboplatin plus fluorouracil versus methotrexate in advanced squamous-cell carcinoma of the head and neck: a Southwest Oncology Group study. J Clin Oncol. 1992;10(8):1245-1251.

Garrett AP, Garner EO, Goldstein DP, Berkowitz RS. Methotrexate infusion and folinic acid as primary therapy for nonmetastatic and low-risk metastatic gestational trophoblastic tumors. 15 years of experience. J Reprod Med. 2002;47(5):355-362.

Glantz MJ, Jaeckle KA, Chamberlain MC, et al, "A Randomized Controlled Trial Comparing Intrathecal Sustained-Release Cytarabine (DepoCyt) to Intrathecal Methotrexate in Patients With Neoplastic Meningitis From Solid Tumors," Clin Cancer Res, 1999, 5 (11):3394-402.

Goorin AM, Schwartzentruber DJ, Devidas M, et al. Presurgical Chemotherapy Compared With Immediate Surgery and Adjuvant Chemotherapy for Nonmetastatic Osteosarcoma: Pediatric Oncology Group Study POG-8651. J Clin Oncol. 2003;21(8):1574-1580.

Griggs JJ, Mangu PB, Anderson H, et al, "Appropriate Chemotherapy Dosing For Obese Adult Patients With Cancer: American Society of Clinical Oncology Clinical Practice Guideline," J Clin Oncol, 2012, 30 (13):1553-61.

Grossman SA, Finkelstein DM, Ruckeschel JC, et al, "Randomized Prospective Comparison of Intraventricular Methotrexate and Thiotepa in Patients With Previously Untreated Neoplastic Meningitis. Eastern Cooperative Oncology Group," J Clin Oncol, 1993, 11 (3):561-9.

Guardiola E, Peyrade F, Chaigneau L, et al. Results of a randomised phase II study comparing docetaxel with methotrexate in patients with recurrent head and neck cancer. Eur J Cancer. 2004;40 (14):2071-2076.

Huber AM, Giannini EH, Bowyer SL, et al. Protocols for the initial treatment of moderately severe juvenile dermatomyositis: results of a Children's Arthritis and Rheumatology Research Alliance Consensus Conference. Arthritis Care Res (Hoboken). 2010;62(2):219-225.

Jacobson JO, Polovich M, McNiff KK, et al, "American Society of Clinical Oncology/Oncology Nursing Society Chemotherapy Administration Safety Standards," J Clin Oncol, 2009, 27(32):5469-75.

Janus N, Thariat J, Boulanger H, et al. Proposal for Dosage Adjustment and Timing of Chemotherapy in Hemodialyzed Patients. Ann Oncol. 2010;21(7):1395-1403.

Kalb RE, Strober B, Weinstein G, et al. "Methotrexate and Psoriasis: 2009 National Psoriasis Foundation Consensus Conference," J Am Acad Dermatol, 2009, 60(5):824-37.

Kantarjian HM, O'Brien S, Smith TL, et al. Results of Treatment With Hyper-CVAD, A Dose-Intensive Regimen, in Adult Acute Lymphocytic Leukemia. J Clin Oncol. 2000;18(3): 547-561.

Kerr JZ, Berg S, and Blaney SM, "Intrathecal Chemotherapy," Crit Rev Oncol Hematol, 2001, 37(3):227-36.

Khouri IF, Romaguera J, Kantarjian H, et al. Hyper-CVAD and High-Dose Methotrexate/Cytarabine Followed by Stem-Cell Transplantation: An Active Regimen for Aggressive Mantle-Cell Lymphoma. J Clin Oncol. 1998;16(12):3803-3809.

Kintzel PE and Dorr RT, "Anticancer Drug Renal Toxicity and Elimination: Dosing Guidelines for Altered Renal Function," Cancer Treat Rev, 1995, 21(1):33-64.

Kliegman RM, Stanton BF, St. Gemell JW, et al, eds. Nelson Textbook of Pediatrics. 19th ed. Philadelphia, PA: Saunders Elsevier;2011.

Larson RA, Dodge RK, Burns CP, et al, "A Five-Drug Remission Induction Regimen With Intensive Consolidation for Adults With Acute Lymphoblastic Leukemia: Cancer and Leukemia Group B Study 8811," Blood, 1995, 85(8):2025-37.

Le Deley MC, Guinebretière JM, Gentet JC, et al. SFOP OS94: a randomised trial comparing preoperative high-dose methotrexate plus doxorubicin to high-dose methotrexate plus etoposide and ifosfamide in osteosarcoma patients. Eur J Cancer. 2007;43(4):752-761.

Levine MN, Bramwell VH, Pritchard KI, et al. Randomized Trial of Intensive Cyclophosphamide, Epirubicin, and Fluorouracil Chemotherapy Compared With Cyclophosphamide, Methotrexate, and Fluorouracil in Premenopausal Women With Node-Positive Breast Cancer. National Cancer Institute of Canada Clinical Trials Group. J Clin Oncol. 1998;16(8):2651-2658.

Li SC, Torok KS, Pope E, et al. Development of consensus treatment plans for juvenile localized scleroderma: a roadmap toward comparative effectiveness studies in juvenile localized scleroderma. Arthrit Care Res. 2012;64(8):1175-1185.

Lin WY, Liu HC, Yeh TC, et al, "Triple Intrathecal Therapy Without Cranial Irradiation for Central Nervous System Preventive Therapy in Childhood Acute Lymphoblastic Leukemia," Pediatr Blood Cancer, 2008, 50(3):523-7.

Mack DR, Young R, Kaufman SS, et al. Methotrexate in patients with Crohn's disease after –mercaptopurine. J Pediatr. 1998;132:830-835.

Mahoney DH Jr, Shuster JJ, Nitschke R, et al. Intensification with intermediate-dose intravenous methotrexate is effective therapy for children with lower-risk B-precursor acute lymphoblastic leukemia: A Pediatric Oncology Group study. J Clin Oncol. 2000;18(6):1285-1294.

Matloub Y, Lindemulder S, Gaynon PS, et al. Intrathecal triple therapy decreases central nervous system relapse but fails to improve event-free survival when compared with intrathecal methotrexate: results of the Children's Cancer Group (CCG) 1952 study for standard-risk acute lymphoblastic leukemia, reported by the Children's Oncology Group. Blood. 2006;108(4):1165-1173.

Mead GM, Barrans SL, Qian W, et al. A Prospective Clinicopathologic Study of Dose-Modified CODOX-M/IVAC in Patients With Sporadic Burkitt Lymphoma Defined Using Cytogenetic and Immunophenotypic Criteria (MRC/NCRI LY10 Trial). Blood.2008;112(6):2248-2260.

Menter A, Korman NJ, Elmets CA, et al, "Guidelines of Care for the Management of Psoriasis and Psoriatic Arthritis: Section 4. Guidelines of Care for the Management and Treatment of Psoriasis With Traditional Systemic Agents," J Am Acad Dermatol, 2009, 61 (3):451-85.

Meyers PA, Heller G, Healey J, et al. Chemotherapy for nonmetastatic osteogenic sarcoma: the Memorial Sloan-Kettering experience. J Clin Oncol. 1992;10(1):5-15.

Meyers PA, Schwartz CL, Krailo M, et al. Osteosarcoma: a randomized, prospective trial of the addition of ifosfamide and/or muramyl tripeptide to cisplatin, doxorubicin, and high-dose methotrexate. J Clin Oncol. 2005;23(9):2004-2011.

Meyers PA, Schwartz CL, Krailo MD, et al. Osteosarcoma: the addition of muramyl tripeptide to chemotherapy improves overall survival–a report from the Children's Oncology Group. J Clin Oncol. 2008;26 (4):633-638.

Nash R, Antin J, Karanes C, et al. Phase 3 study comparing methotrexate and tacrolimus with methotrexate and cyclosporine for prophylaxis of acute graft-vs-host disease after marrow transplantation from unrelated donors. Blood. 2000;96(6):2062-2068.

National Comprehensive Cancer Network (NCCN)®, "Clinical Practice Guidelines in Oncology™: Central Nervous System Cancers," Version 2.2009. Available at: http://www.nccn.org/professionals/physician_gls/PDF/cns.pdf.

National Institute for Occupational Safety and Health (NIOSH), "NIOSH List of Antineoplastic and Other Hazardous Drugs in Healthcare Settings 2012." Available at http://www.cdc.gov/niosh/docs/2012-150/pdfs/2012-150.pdf. Accessed January 21, 2013.

Ramanan AV, Campbell-Webster N, Ota S, et al. The effectiveness of treating juvenile dermatomyositis with methotrexate and aggressively tapered corticosteroids. *Arthritis Rheum.* 2005;52(11):3570-3578.

Reiter A, Schrappe M, Tiemann M, et al. Improved treatment results in childhood B-cell neoplasms with tailored intensification of therapy: A report of the Berlin-Frankfurt-Münster Group Trial NHL-BFM 90. *Blood.* 1999;94(10):3294-3306.

Ross M, Schmidt GM, Niland JC, et al, "Cyclosporine, Methotrexate, and Prednisone Compared With Cyclosporine and Prednisone for Prevention of Acute Graft-vs.-Host Disease: Effect on Chronic Graft-vs.-Host Disease and Long-Term Survival," *Biol Blood Marrow Transplant,* 1999, 5(5):285-291.

Rufo PA, Denson LA, Sylvester FA, et al. Health supervision in the management of children and adolescents with IBD: NASPGHAN recommendations. *J Pediatr Gastroenterol Nutr.* 2012;55(1):93-108.

Sandhu BK, Fell JME, Beattie RM, et al. Guidelines for the management of inflammatory bowel disease in children in the United Kingdom. *JPGN.* 2010;50:S1-S13.

Schrappe M, Reiter A, Ludwig WD, et al. Improved outcome in childhood acute lymphoblastic leukemia despite reduced use of anthracyclines and cranial radiotherapy: results of trial ALL-BFM 90. German-Austrian-Swiss ALL-BFM Study Group. *Blood.* 2000;95(11):3310-3322.

Seibel NL, Steinherz PG, Sather HN, et al. Early postinduction intensification therapy improves survival for children and adolescents with high-risk acute lymphoblastic leukemia: a report from the Children's Oncology Group. *Blood.* 2008;111(5):2548-2555.

Simonini G, Cantarini L, Bresci C, Lorusso M, Galeazzi M, Cimaz R. Current therapeutic approaches to autoimmune chronic uveitis in children. *Autoimmun Rev.* 2010;9(10):674-683.

Simonini G, Paudyal P, Jones GT, et al. Current evidence of methotrexate efficacy in childhood chronic uveitis: a systematic review and meta-analysis approach. *Rheumatol .* 2013;52:825-831.

Stewart JS, Cohen EE, Licitra L, et al. Phase III study of gefitinib compared with intravenous methotrexate for recurrent squamous cell carcinoma of the head and neck. *J Clin Oncol.* 2009;27(11):1864-1871.

Stringer E, Bohnsack J, Bowyer SL, et al. Treatment approaches to juvenile dermatomyositis (JDM) across North America: The Childhood Arthritis and Rheumatology Research Alliance (CARRA) JDM Treatment Survey. *J Rheumatol.* 2010;37(9):1953-1961.

Thomas DA, Faderl S, O'Brien S, et al. Chemoimmunotherapy with hyper-CVAD plus rituximab for the treatment of adult Burkitt and Burkitt-type lymphoma or acute lymphoblastic leukemia. *Cancer.* 2006;106(7):1569-1580.

Turner D, Levine A, Escher J, et al. Management of pediatric ulcerative colitis: joint ECCO and ESPGHAN evidence-based consensus guidelines. *J Pediatr Gastroenterol Nutrit..* 2012;55(3):340-361.

Visser K, Katchamart W, Loza E, et al, "Multinational Evidence-Based Recommendations for the Use of Methotrexate in Rheumatic Disorders With a Focus on Rheumatoid Arthritis: Integrating Systematic Literature Research and Expert Opinion of a Broad International Panel of Rheumatologists in the 3E Initiative," *Ann Rheum Dis,* 2009, 68(7):1086-93.

Weiner MA, Harris MB, Lewis M, et al. Neoadjuvant high-dose methotrexate, cisplatin, and doxorubicin for the management of patients with nonmetastatic osteosarcoma. *Cancer Treat Rep.* 1986; 70(12):1431-1432.

Weiss B, Lerner A, Shapiro R, et al. Methotrexate treatment in pediatric Crohn disease patients intolerant or resistant to purine analogues. *J Pediatr Gastroenterol Nutr.* 2009;48:526-530.

Widemann BC, Balis FM, Murphy RF, et al, "Carboxypeptidase-G2, Thymidine, and Leucovorin Rescue in Cancer Patients With Methotrexate-Induced Renal Dysfunction," *J Clin Oncol,* 1997, 15(5):2125-34.

Widemann BC, Balis FM, Shalabi A, et al, "Treatment of Accidental Intrathecal Methotrexate Overdose With Intrathecal Carboxypeptidase G2," *J Natl Cancer Inst,* 2004, 96(20):1557-9.

Winkler K, Beron G, Delling G, et al. Neoadjuvant chemotherapy of osteosarcoma: results of a randomized cooperative trial (COSS-82) with salvage chemotherapy based on histological tumor response. *J Clin Oncol.* 1988;6(2):329-337.

◆ **Methotrexate Injection, BP (Can)** *see* Methotrexate *on page 1367*

◆ **Methotrexate Injection USP (Can)** *see* Methotrexate *on page 1367*

◆ **Methotrexate Sodium** *see* Methotrexate *on page 1367*

◆ **Methotrexatum** *see* Methotrexate *on page 1367*

Methsuximide (meth SUKS i mide)

Medication Safety Issues
Sound-alike/look-alike issues:
Methsuximide may be confused with ethosuximide

Brand Names: U.S. Celontin

Brand Names: Canada Celontin®

Therapeutic Category Anticonvulsant, Succinimide

Generic Availability (U.S.) No

Use Control of refractory absence (petit mal) seizures (FDA approved in children and adults); useful adjunct in refractory, partial complex (psychomotor) seizures

Medication Guide Available Yes

Pregnancy Considerations Patients exposed to methsuximide during pregnancy are encouraged to enroll themselves into the NAAED Pregnancy Registry by calling 1-888-233-2334. Additional information is available at www.aedpregnancyregistry.org.

Contraindications Hypersensitivity to methsuximide, other succinimides, or any component

Warnings Blood dyscrasias (sometimes fatal) have been reported (monitor hematologic function periodically or if signs/symptoms of infection develop); SLE has been reported with the use of succinimides

Antiepileptic drugs (AEDs) increase the risk of suicidal behavior and ideation in patients receiving these medications for any indication. Pooled analyses of placebo-controlled trials involving 11 different AEDs (regardless of indication) showed a twofold increased risk of suicidal thoughts or behavior (estimated incidence rate: 0.43% in AED-treated patients compared to 0.24% in patients receiving placebo); increased risk was observed as early as one week after initiation of AED and continued through duration of trials (most trials ≤24 weeks); risk did not vary significantly by age (age range: 5–100 years). Consider risks and benefits of AEDs before prescribing. Monitor all patients receiving an AED for emergence of suicidal thoughts or behavior, thoughts of self-harm, any unusual changes in behavior or mood, or the emergence or worsening of depressive symptoms; notify healthcare provider immediately if symptoms or concerning behavior occur. **Note:** The FDA is requiring that a Medication Guide be developed for all antiepileptic drugs, informing patients of this risk.

Precautions Use with caution in patients with hepatic or renal disease. Avoid abrupt withdrawal (may precipitate absence status). When used alone, methsuximide may increase tonic-clonic seizures in patients with mixed seizure disorders; methsuximide must be used in combination with other anticonvulsants in patients with both absence and tonic-clonic seizures. May cause CNS depression, which may impair physical or mental abilities; patients must be cautioned about performing tasks which require mental alertness.

Adverse Reactions
Cardiovascular: Hyperemia

Central nervous system: Aggressiveness, ataxia, confusion, depression, dizziness, drowsiness, hallucinations (auditory), headache, hypochondriacal behavior, insomnia, irritability, mental instability, mental slowness, nervousness, psychosis, suicidal behavior

Dermatologic: Pruritus, rash, Stevens-Johnson syndrome, urticaria

Gastrointestinal: Abdominal pain, anorexia, constipation, diarrhea, epigastric pain, nausea, vomiting, weight loss

Genitourinary: Hematuria (microscopic), proteinuria

Hematologic: Eosinophilia, leukopenia, monocytosis, pancytopenia

Ocular: Blurred vision, periorbital edema, photophobia

Miscellaneous: Hiccups, systemic lupus erythematosus

◀ **Drug Interactions**
Metabolism/Transport Effects Substrate of CYP2C19 (major); **Note:** Assignment of Major/Minor substrate status based on clinically relevant drug interaction potential; **Inhibits** CYP2C19 (weak)
Avoid Concomitant Use
Avoid concomitant use of Methsuximide with any of the following: Azelastine (Nasal); Paraldehyde; Thalidomide
Increased Effect/Toxicity
Methsuximide may increase the levels/effects of: Alcohol (Ethyl); Azelastine (Nasal); Buprenorphine; CNS Depressants; Hydrocodone; Methotrimeprazine; Metyrosine; Mirtazapine; Paraldehyde; Pramipexole; ROPINIRole; Rotigotine; Selective Serotonin Reuptake Inhibitors; Thalidomide; Zolpidem

The levels/effects of Methsuximide may be increased by: Brimonidine (Topical); Cannabis; CYP2C19 Inhibitors (Moderate); CYP2C19 Inhibitors (Strong); Doxylamine; Dronabinol; Droperidol; HydrOXYzine; Kava Kava; Luliconazole; Magnesium Sulfate; Methotrimeprazine; Nabilone; Perampanel; Rufinamide; Sodium Oxybate; Tapentadol; Tetrahydrocannabinol
Decreased Effect
The levels/effects of Methsuximide may be decreased by: CYP2C19 Inducers (Strong); Dabrafenib; Ketorolac (Nasal); Ketorolac (Systemic); Mefloquine; Orlistat
Stability Store at 25°C (77°F); protect from light, moisture, and excessive heat 40°C (104°F); **Note:** Methsuximide has a relatively low melting temperature (124°F); do not store in conditions that promote high temperatures (eg, in a closed vehicle)
Mechanism of Action Increases the seizure threshold and suppresses paroxysmal spike-and-wave pattern in absence seizures; depresses nerve transmission in the motor cortex
Pharmacokinetics (Adult data unless noted)
Metabolism: Rapidly demethylated in the liver to N-desmethylmethsuximide (active metabolite)
Half-life: 2-4 hours
N-desmethylmethsuximide:
  Children: 26 hours
  Adults: 28-80 hours
Time to peak serum concentration: Within 1-3 hours
Elimination: <1% in urine as unchanged drug
Dosing: Usual Oral:
Children: Initial: 10-15 mg/kg/day in 3-4 divided doses; increase weekly up to maximum of 30 mg/kg/day; mean dose required:
  <30 kg: 20 mg/kg/day
  >30 kg: 14 mg/kg/day
Adults: 300 mg/day for the first week; may increase by 300 mg/day at weekly intervals up to 1.2 g in 2-4 divided doses/day
Administration Oral: Administer with food
Monitoring Parameters CBC with differential, liver enzymes, urinalysis; measure trough serum levels for efficacy and 3-hour postdose concentrations for toxicity; signs and symptoms of suicidality (eg, anxiety, depression, behavior changes)
Reference Range Measure N-desmethylmethsuximide concentrations:
Therapeutic: 10-40 mcg/mL (SI: 53-212 micromoles/L)
Toxic: >40 mcg/mL (SI: >212 micromoles/L)
Dosage Forms Excipient information presented when available (limited, particularly for generics); consult specific product labeling.
Capsule, Oral:
  Celontin: 300 mg
References

Miles MV, Tennison MB, and Greenwood RS, "Pharmacokinetics of N-desmethylmethsuximide in Pediatric Patients," *J Pediatr*, 1989, 114(4 Pt 1):647-50.

Tennison MB, Greenwood RS, Miles MV, "Methsuximide for Intractable Childhood Seizures," *Pediatrics*, 1991, 87(2):186-9.

◆ **Methylacetoxyprogesterone** *see* MedroxyPROGESTERone *on page 1318*

Methyldopa (meth il DOE pa)

Medication Safety Issues
Sound-alike/look-alike issues:
Methyldopa may be confused with L-dopa, levodopa
BEERS Criteria medication:
This drug may be potentially inappropriate for use in geriatric patients (Quality of evidence - low; Strength of recommendation - strong).
Brand Names: Canada Methyldopa; Novo-Medopa
Therapeutic Category Alpha-Adrenergic Inhibitors, Central; Antihypertensive Agent
Generic Availability (U.S.) Yes
Use Management of moderate to severe hypertension
Pregnancy Risk Factor B/C (injectable)
Pregnancy Considerations Adverse events have not been observed in animal reproduction studies. Methyldopa crosses the placenta and appears in cord blood. Available data show use during pregnancy does not cause fetal harm and improves fetal outcomes. Untreated chronic maternal hypertension is associated with adverse events in the fetus, infant, and mother. If treatment for chronic hypertension during pregnancy is needed, methyldopa is one of the preferred agents. If an injectable agent is needed for the urgent control of acute hypertension in pregnancy, other agents are preferred (ACOG, 2013).
Breast-Feeding Considerations Methyldopa is excreted into breast milk in concentrations <1% of the weight-adjusted maternal dose (Jones, 1978; White, 1985). The manufacturer recommends that caution be exercised when administering methyldopa to nursing women.
Contraindications Hypersensitivity to methyldopa or any component; liver disease, pheochromocytoma
Warnings Injection contains sodium bisulfite which may cause allergic reactions in susceptible individuals
Precautions Use with caution and adjust dose in patients with renal dysfunction; active metabolite may accumulate in uremia
Adverse Reactions
Cardiovascular: Angina pectoris aggravation, bradycardia, carotid sinus hypersensitivity prolonged, heart failure, myocarditis, orthostatic hypotension, paradoxical pressor response (I.V. use), pericarditis, peripheral edema, symptoms of cerebrovascular insufficiency, vasculitis
Central nervous system: Bell's palsy, dizziness, drug fever, headache, lightheadedness, mental acuity decreased, mental depression, nightmares, parkinsonism, sedation
Dermatologic: Rash, toxic epidermal necrolysis
Endocrine & metabolic: Amenorrhea, breast enlargement, gynecomastia, hyperprolactinemia, lactation, libido decreased
Gastrointestinal: Abdominal distension, colitis, constipation, diarrhea, flatulence, nausea, pancreatitis, sialadenitis, sore or "black" tongue, vomiting, weight gain, xerostomia
Genitourinary: Impotence
Hematologic: Bone marrow suppression, eosinophilia, granulocytopenia, hemolytic anemia; positive tests for ANA, LE cells, rheumatoid factor, Coombs test (positive); leukopenia, thrombocytopenia
Hepatic: Abnormal LFTs, liver disorders (hepatitis), jaundice
Neuromuscular & skeletal: Arthralgia, choreoathetosis, myalgia, paresthesias, weakness
Renal: BUN increased
Respiratory: Nasal congestion
Miscellaneous: SLE-like syndrome

Drug Interactions

Metabolism/Transport Effects Substrate of COMT

Avoid Concomitant Use

Avoid concomitant use of Methyldopa with any of the following: Ceritinib; Iobenguane I 123; MAO Inhibitors

Increased Effect/Toxicity

Methyldopa may increase the levels/effects of: Amifostine; Antihypertensives; Beta-Blockers; Bradycardia-Causing Agents; Ceritinib; DULoxetine; Hypotensive Agents; Lithium; Obinutuzumab; RiTUXimab

The levels/effects of Methyldopa may be increased by: Alfuzosin; Barbiturates; Beta-Blockers; Brimonidine (Topical); COMT Inhibitors; Diazoxide; Herbs (Hypotensive Properties); MAO Inhibitors; Pentoxifylline; Phosphodiesterase 5 Inhibitors; Prostacyclin Analogues

Decreased Effect

Methyldopa may decrease the levels/effects of: Iobenguane I 123

The levels/effects of Methyldopa may be decreased by: Herbs (Hypertensive Properties); Iron Salts; Methylphenidate; Mirtazapine; Multivitamins/Minerals (with ADEK, Folate, Iron); Serotonin/Norepinephrine Reuptake Inhibitors; Tricyclic Antidepressants; Yohimbine

Mechanism of Action Stimulation of central alpha-adrenergic receptors by a false neurotransmitter (alpha-methylnorepinephrine) that results in a decreased sympathetic outflow to the heart, kidneys, and peripheral vasculature

Pharmacodynamics Hypotensive effects:

Maximum effect: Oral, I.V.: Single-dose: Within 3-6 hours; multiple-dose: 2-3 days

Duration:

Oral: Single-dose: 12-24 hours; multiple-dose: 1-2 days

I.V.: 10-16 hours

Pharmacokinetics (Adult data unless noted)

Absorption: Oral: ~50%

Distribution: Crosses placenta; appears in breast milk

Protein binding: <15%

Metabolism: In the intestine and the liver

Half-life: Elimination:

Neonates: 10-20 hours

Adults: 1-3 hours

Elimination: ~70% of systemic dose eliminated in urine as drug and metabolites

Dialysis: Slightly dialyzable (5% to 20%)

Dosing: Usual

Children:

Oral: Initial: 10 mg/kg/day in 2-4 divided doses; increase every 2 days as needed to maximum dose of 65 mg/kg/day; do not exceed 3 g/day

I.V.: Initial: 2-4 mg/kg/dose; if response is not seen within 4-6 hours, may increase to 5-10 mg/kg/dose; administer doses every 6-8 hours; maximum daily dose: 65 mg/kg or 3 g, whichever is less

Adults:

Oral: Initial: 250 mg 2-3 times/day; increase every 2 days as needed; usual dose 500 mg to 2 g daily in 2-4 divided doses; maximum dose: 3 g/day; usual dosage range (JNC 7): 250-1000 mg/day in 2 divided doses

I.V.: 250-1000 mg every 6-8 hours; maximum dose: 4 g/day

Dosing interval in renal impairment: Children and Adults:

CrCl >50 mL/minute: Administer normal dose every 8 hours

CrCl 10-50 mL/minute: Administer normal dose every 8-12 hours

CrCl <10 mL/minute: Administer normal dose every 12-24 hours

Administration

Oral: May be administered without regard to food; administer new dosage increases in the evening to minimize sedation

Parenteral: I.V.: Infuse I.V. dose slowly over 30-60 minutes at a concentration ≤10 mg/mL

Monitoring Parameters Blood pressure, CBC with differential, hemoglobin, hematocrit, Coombs' test [direct], liver enzymes

Test Interactions Methyldopa interferes with the following laboratory tests: urinary uric acid, serum creatinine (alkaline picrate method), AST (colorimetric method), and urinary catecholamines (falsely high levels)

Additional Information Most effective if used with diuretic; titrate dose to optimal blood pressure control with minimal side effects

Dosage Forms Excipient information presented when available (limited, particularly for generics); consult specific product labeling.

Solution, Intravenous, as hydrochloride:

Generic: 250 mg/5 mL (5 mL)

Tablet, Oral:

Generic: 250 mg, 500 mg

Extemporaneous Preparations A 50 mg/mL oral suspension may be made with tablets and either unpreserved Simple Syrup, N.F. or a 1:1 mixture of simple syrup (containing 0.5% citric acid) and hydrochloric acid 0.2 N. Crush ten 250 mg tablets in a glass mortar and reduce to a fine powder. To make formulation with unpreserved simple syrup, add small portions of vehicle and mix to a uniform paste; mix while adding the vehicle in incremental proportions to almost 50 mL; transfer to a calibrated bottle; rinse the mortar and pestle several times with vehicle, and add quantity of vehicle sufficient to make 50 mL. To make formulation with the second vehicle, mix powdered tablets with 25 mL of hydrochloric acid 0.2 N (0.73% w/v); dilute this mixture to 50 mL with simple syrup containing 0.5% citric acid by the method described above. Label "shake well" and "protect from light." Stable for 14 days when stored in glass prescription bottles in the dark at room temperature or refrigerated.

Newton DW, Rogers AG, Becker CH, et al, "Extemporaneous Preparation of Methyldopa in Two Syrup Vehicles," *Am J Hosp Pharm,* 1975, 32(8):817-21.

References

American College of Obstetricians and Gynecologists, "ACOG Practice Bulletin No. 125: Chronic Hypertension in Pregnancy," *Obstet Gynecol,* 2012, 119(2 Pt 1):396-407.

Chobanian AV, Bakris GL, Black HR, et al, "The Seventh Report of the Joint National Committee on Prevention, Detection, Evaluation, and Treatment of High Blood Pressure: The JNC 7 report," *JAMA,* 2003, 289(19):2560-72.

Jones HM and Cummings AJ, "A Study of the Transfer of Alpha-Methyldopa to the Human Foetus and Newborn Infant," *Br J Clin Pharmacol,* 1978, 6(5):432-4.

White WB, Andreoli JW, and Cohn RD, "Alpha-Methyldopa Disposition in Mothers With Hypertension and in Their Breast-Fed Infants," *Clin Pharmacol Ther,* 1985, 37(4):387-90.

◆ **Methyldopate Hydrochloride** *see* Methyldopa *on page 1376*

Methylene Blue (METH i leen bloo)

Medication Safety Issues

Other safety concerns:

Due to the potential for dosing errors between mg and mL of methylene blue, prescribing and dosing should only be expressed in terms of mg of methylene blue (and not as mL)

Due to potential toxicity (hemolytic anemia), do not use methylene blue to color enteral feedings to detect aspiration.

Therapeutic Category Antidote, Cyanide; Antidote, Drug-induced Methemoglobinemia

Generic Availability (U.S.) Yes

Use Antidote for cyanide poisoning and drug-induced methemoglobinemia (FDA approved use), indicator dye, bacteriostatic genitourinary antiseptic; other uses include treatment/prevention of ifosfamide-induced encephalopathy; topically, in conjunction with polychromatic light to photoinactivate viruses such as herpes simplex; alone or in combination with vitamin C for the management of chronic urolithiasis

Pregnancy Risk Factor X

Pregnancy Considerations Use during amniocentesis has shown evidence of fetal abnormalities (atresia of the ileum and jejunum, ileal occlusions, and other adverse effects); has been used orally without similar adverse events; use, however, is contraindicated in women who are or may become pregnant. In general, medications used as antidotes should take into consideration the health and prognosis of the mother.

Contraindications Hypersensitivity to methylene blue or any component; renal insufficiency; intraspinal injection

Warnings Do not inject subcutaneously or intrathecally as necrotic abscesses (SubQ) and neural damage (I.T.) including paraplegia have occurred. Methylene blue should not be added to enteral feeding products (Wessel, 2005); safety and efficacy has not been established. Serotonin syndrome has been reported with concomitant administration of methylene blue and serotonin reuptake inhibitors (eg, SSRIs, SNRIs, tricyclic antidepressants); avoid concomitant use and allow a washout period of at least 4-5 half-lives of the serotonin reuptake inhibitor prior to intravenous methylene blue use.

Precautions Use with caution in young patients (eg, infants, neonates) and in patients with severe renal insufficiency or G-6-PD deficiency; at high doses or in patients with G-6-PD-deficiency and infants, methylene blue may catalyze the oxidation of ferrous iron in hemoglobin to ferric iron causing paradoxical methemoglobinemia; monitor methemoglobin concentrations regularly during administration. Inject slowly to avoid high local concentrations and the production of methemoglobin; large I.V. doses have been associated with precordial pain and hypotension.

Adverse Reactions

Cardiovascular: Angina, arrhythmia, hypertension, precordial pain

Central nervous system: Dizziness, headache, fever, mental confusion

Dermatologic: Staining of skin

Gastrointestinal: Abdominal pain, diarrhea, fecal discoloration (blue-green), nausea, vomiting

Genitourinary: Bladder irritation, discoloration of urine (blue-green)

Hematologic: Anemia, paradoxical methemoglobinemia (high doses), transient reduction in oxygen saturation as read by pulse oximetry

Respiratory: Dyspnea

Miscellaneous: Diaphoresis

Postmarketing and/or case reports: Serotonin syndrome

Drug Interactions

Metabolism/Transport Effects Inhibits Monoamine Oxidase

Avoid Concomitant Use

Avoid concomitant use of Methylene Blue with any of the following: Aclidinium; Alcohol (Ethyl); Alpha-/Beta-Agonists (Indirect-Acting); Alpha1-Agonists; Amphetamines; Anilidopiperidine Opioids; Apraclonidine; AtoMOXetine; Bezafibrate; Buprenorphine; BuPROPion; BusPIRone; CarBAMazepine; Cyclobenzaprine; Cyproheptadine; Dexmethylphenidate; Dextromethorphan; Diethylpropion; Hydrocodone; HYDROmorphone; Ipratropium (Oral Inhalation); Isometheptene; Levonordefrin; Linezolid; MAO Inhibitors; Maprotiline; Meperidine; Methyldopa; Methylphenidate; Mirtazapine; Morphine (Liposomal); Morphine (Systemic); Nefazodone; Oxymorphone; Pholcodine; Pizotifen; Potassium Chloride; Selective Serotonin Reuptake Inhibitors; Serotonin 5-HT1D Receptor Agonists; Serotonin/Norepinephrine Reuptake Inhibitors; Tapentadol; Tetrabenazine; Tetrahydrozoline (Nasal); Tiotropium; TraZODone; Tricyclic Antidepressants; Tryptophan; Umeclidinium

Increased Effect/Toxicity

Methylene Blue may increase the levels/effects of: Abobotulinumtoxin A; Alpha-/Beta-Agonists (Indirect-Acting); Alpha1-Agonists; Amphetamines; Analgesics (Opioid); Anticholinergic Agents; Antihypertensives; Antipsychotics; Apraclonidine; AtoMOXetine; Beta2-Agonists; Betahistine; Bezafibrate; Brimonidine (Ophthalmic); Brimonidine (Topical); BuPROPion; Cannabinoid-Containing Products; Cyproheptadine; Dexmethylphenidate; Dextromethorphan; Diethylpropion; Domperidone; Doxapram; Doxylamine; EPINEPHrine (Nasal); Epinephrine (Racemic); EPINEPHrine (Systemic, Oral Inhalation); Hydrocodone; HYDROmorphone; Hypoglycemic Agents; Isometheptene; Levonordefrin; Linezolid; Lithium; Meperidine; Methadone; Methyldopa; Methylphenidate; Metoclopramide; Mirabegron; Morphine (Liposomal); Morphine (Systemic); Norepinephrine; Onabotulinumtoxin A; Orthostatic Hypotension Producing Agents; OxyCODONE; Pizotifen; Potassium Chloride; Reserpine; RimabotulinumtoxinB; Serotonin 5-HT1D Receptor Agonists; Serotonin Modulators; Tetrahydrozoline (Nasal); Thiazide Diuretics; Tiotropium; Topiramate

The levels/effects of Methylene Blue may be increased by: Aclidinium; Alcohol (Ethyl); Altretamine; Anilidopiperidine Opioids; Antiemetics (5HT3 Antagonists); Antipsychotics; Buprenorphine; BusPIRone; CarBAMazepine; COMT Inhibitors; Cyclobenzaprine; Ipratropium (Oral Inhalation); Levodopa; MAO Inhibitors; Maprotiline; Mirtazapine; Nefazodone; Oxymorphone; Pholcodine; Pramlintide; Selective Serotonin Reuptake Inhibitors; Serotonin/Norepinephrine Reuptake Inhibitors; Tapentadol; Tetrabenazine; TraMADol; TraZODone; Tricyclic Antidepressants; Tryptophan; Umeclidinium

Decreased Effect

Methylene Blue may decrease the levels/effects of: Acetylcholinesterase Inhibitors (Central); Domperidone; Secretin

The levels/effects of Methylene Blue may be decreased by: Acetylcholinesterase Inhibitors (Central); Cyproheptadine; Domperidone

Stability Store at 20°C to 25°C (68°F to 77°F); excursions permitted to 15°C to 30°C (59°F to 86°F)

Mechanism of Action Weak germicide in low concentrations, hastens the conversion of methemoglobin to hemoglobin; has opposite effect at high concentrations by converting ferrous ion of reduced hemoglobin to ferric ion to form methemoglobin; in cyanide toxicity, it combines with cyanide to form cyanmethemoglobin preventing the interference of cyanide with the cytochrome system

In the treatment of vasoplegia syndrome, methylene blue may be able to restore vascular tone by a direct inhibitory effect on endothelial nitric oxide synthase (eNOS), and probably inducible NOS (iNOS), by oxidation of enzyme-bound ferrous iron. Methylene blue also blocks the formation of cyclic guanosine monophosphate (cGMP) by inhibiting the guanylate cyclase enzyme through binding to iron in the heme complex and subsequently reducing vasorelaxation (Lenglet, 2011).

Pharmacokinetics (Adult data unless noted)

Absorption: Well-absorbed from GI tract

Bioavailability, oral: 50% to 100%

Time to peak effect: 30 minutes

Metabolism: Peripheral reduction to leukomethylene blue

Elimination: In bile, feces, and urine as leukomethylene blue

Dosing: Neonatal Note: Systemic doses as low as 2 mg/kg have been associated with hemolytic anemia and skin desquamation.

Methemoglobinemia: I.V.: 1-2 mg/kg (0.1-0.2 mL/kg of 1% solution) (Clifton, 2003)

Shock (vasodilatory) with hypotension unresponsive to fluid resuscitation, exogenous catecholamines and corticosteroids: Limited data available; further studies needed: I.V.: 1 mg/kg/dose; dosing based on a case series of five neonates (preterm: n=4; GA: 23-30 weeks) with presumed septic shock (Driscoll, 1996)

Dosing: Usual

Methemoglobinemia: Infants, Children, and Adults: I.V.: 1-2 mg/kg or 25-50 mg/m^2; may be repeated after 1 hour if necessary

Chronic methemoglobinemia: Adults: Oral: 100-300 mg/day

NADPH-methemoglobin reductase deficiency: Children: Oral: 1-1.5 mg/kg/day (maximum dose: 300 mg/day) given with 5-8 mg/kg/day ascorbic acid

Genitourinary antiseptic: Adults: Oral: 65-130 mg 3 times/day; maximum dose: 390 mg/day

Chronic urolithiasis: Adults: Oral: 65 mg 3 times/day

Ifosfamide-induced encephalopathy: Adults: Oral, I.V.:

Note: Treatment may not be necessary; encephalopathy may improve spontaneously

Prevention: 50 mg every 6-8 hours

Treatment: 50 mg as a single dose or every 4-8 hours until symptoms resolve

Administration

Oral: Administer after meals with a full glass of water; may be mixed with fruit juice to mask unpleasant taste

Parenteral: Administer undiluted by direct I.V. injection over several minutes; when administered for the treatment of ifosfamide-induced encephalopathy, may be administered either undiluted as a slow I.V. push over at least 5 minutes or diluted in 50 mL NS or D$_5$W and infused over at least 5 minutes; may be administered intraosseously

Monitoring Parameters CBC; of note, pulse oximetry is not reliable as methylene blue interferes with light emission, resulting in falsely depressed readings

Additional Information Has been used topically (0.1% solutions) in conjunction with polychromatic light to photoinactivate viruses such as herpes simplex; has been used alone or in combination with vitamin C for the management of chronic urolithiasis; skin stains may be removed using a hypochlorite solution

Dosage Forms Excipient information presented when available (limited, particularly for generics); consult specific product labeling.

Solution, Injection:
Generic: 1% (1 mL, 10 mL)

References

Albert M, Lessin MS, and Gilchrist BF, "Methylene Blue: Dangerous Dye for Neonates," *J Pediatr Surg*, 2003, 38(8):1244-5.

Clifton J 2nd and Leikin JB, "Methylene Blue," *Am J Ther*, 2003, 10 (4):289-91.

David KA and Picus J, "Evaluating Risk Factors for the Development of Ifosfamide Encephalopathy," *Am J Clin Oncol*, 2005, 28(3):277-80.

Driscoll W, Thurin S, Carrion V, et al, "Effect of Methylene Blue on Refractory Neonatal Hypotension," *J Pediatr*, 1996, 129(6):904-8.

Lenglet S, Mach F, and Montecucco F, Methylene blue: potential use of an antique molecule in vasoplegic syndrome during cardiac surgery. *Expert Rev Cardiovas Ther*. 2011;9(12):1519-25.

Maloney JP, Ryan TA, Brasel KJ, et al, "Food Dye Use in Enteral Feedings: A Review and a Call for a Moratorium," *Nutr Clin Pract*, 2002, 17(3):169-81.

Ofoegbu BN, Agarwal RP, and Lewis MA, "Methylene Blue Irrigation-Treatment of Renal Fungal Balls Causing Acute Renal Failure in a Preterm Infant," *Acta Paediatr*, 2007, 96(6):939-40.

Patel PN, "Methylene Blue for Management of Ifosfamide-Induced Encephalopathy," *Ann Pharmacother*, 2006, 40(2):299-303.

Pelgrims J, DeVos F, Van den Brande J, et al, "Methylene Blue in the Treatment and Prevention of Ifosfamide-Induced Encephalopathy: Report of 12 Cases and a Review of the Literature," *Br J Cancer*, 2000, 82(2) 291-4.

Sills MR and Zinkham WH, "Methylene Blue-Induced Heinz Body Hemolytic Anemia," *Arch Pediatr Adolesc Med*, 1994, 148(3):306-10.

Wessel J, Balint J, Crill C, et al, "Standards for Specialized Nutrition Support: Hospitalized Pediatric Patients," *Nutr Clin Pract*, 2005, 20 (1):103-16.

◆ **Methylin** see Methylphenidate on page 1379

◆ **Methylmorphine** see Codeine on page 534

Methylphenidate (meth il FEN i date)

Medication Safety Issues

Sound-alike/look-alike issues:

Metadate CD may be confused with Metadate ER

Metadate ER may be confused with methadone

Methylphenidate may be confused with methadone

Ritalin may be confused with Rifadin, ritodrine

Ritalin LA may be confused with Ritalin-SR

Related Information

Oral Medications That Should Not Be Crushed or Altered on page 2438

Patient Information for Disposal of Unused Medications on page 2412

Brand Names: U.S. Concerta; Daytrana; Metadate CD; Metadate ER; Methylin; Quillivant XR; Ritalin; Ritalin LA; Ritalin SR

Brand Names: Canada Apo-Methylphenidate; Apo-Methylphenidate SR; Biphentin; Concerta; PHL-Methylphenidate; PMS-Methylphenidate; ratio-Methylphenidate; Ritalin; Ritalin SR; Sandoz-Methylphenidate SR; Teva-Methylphenidate ER-C

Therapeutic Category Central Nervous System Stimulant

Generic Availability (U.S.) May be product dependent

Use

Oral:

Concerta®: Treatment of attention-deficit/hyperactivity disorder (ADHD) (FDA approved in ages 6-65 years)

Ritalin LA®, Quillivant™ XR: Treatment of ADHD (FDA approved in ages 6-12 years)

Metadate CD®: Treatment of ADHD (FDA approved in ages 6-15 years)

Metadate® ER, Methylin®, Ritalin®, Ritalin SR®: Treatment of ADHD, treatment of narcolepsy (All indications: FDA approved in ages ≥6 years and adults)

Topical Patch: Daytrana®: Treatment of ADHD (FDA approved in ages 6-17 years)

Medication Guide Available Yes

Pregnancy Risk Factor C

Pregnancy Considerations Adverse events were observed in animal reproduction studies. Information related to the use of methylphenidate in pregnant women with attention-deficit/hyperactivity disorder (Bolea-Akmanac, 2013; Dideriksen, 2013) or narcolepsy (Maurovich-Horvat, 2013; Thorpy, 2013) is limited.

Breast-Feeding Considerations Methylphenidate excretion into breast milk has been noted in case reports. In both cases, the authors calculated the relative infant dose to be ≤0.2% of the weight adjusted maternal dose. Adverse events were not noted in either infant, however, both were older (6 months of age and 11 months of age) and exposure was limited (Hackett, 2006; Spigset, 2007). The manufacturer recommends that caution be used if administered to a nursing woman.

Contraindications Hypersensitivity to methylphenidate or any component; glaucoma; motor tics; Tourette's syndrome (diagnosis or family history); patients with marked agitation, tension, and anxiety; use with or within 14 days following MAO inhibitor therapy (hypertensive crisis may occur)

◄ Metadate CD® and Metadate ER® are also contraindicated in patients with severe hypertension, heart failure, arrhythmia, hyperthyroidism, thyrotoxicosis, recent MI, or angina and concomitant use of halogenated anesthetics.

Warnings Serious cardiovascular events including sudden death may occur in patients with preexisting structural cardiac abnormalities or other serious heart problems. Sudden death has been reported in children and adolescents; sudden death, stroke, and MI have been reported in adults. Avoid the use of CNS stimulants in patients with known serious structural cardiac abnormalities, cardiomyopathy, serious heart rhythm abnormalities, coronary artery disease, or other serious cardiac problems that could place patients at an increased risk to the sympathomimetic effects of CNS stimulants. Patients should be carefully evaluated for cardiac disease prior to initiation of therapy. If symptoms of cardiovascular disease, including chest pain, dyspnea, or fainting are exhibited, immediate medical care should be sought. **Note:** The American Heart Association recommends that all children diagnosed with ADHD who may be candidates for medication, such as methylphenidate, should have a thorough cardiovascular assessment prior to initiation of therapy. This assessment should include a combination of medical history, family history, and physical examination focusing on cardiovascular disease risk factors. An ECG is not mandatory but should be considered. **Note:** In a recent retrospective study on the possible association between stimulant medication use and sudden death in children, 564 previously healthy children who died suddenly in motor vehicle accidents were compared to a group of 564 previously healthy children who died suddenly. Two of the 564 (0.4%) children in motor vehicle accidents were taking stimulant medications compared to 10 of 564 (1.8%) children who died suddenly. While the authors of this study conclude there may be an association between stimulant use and sudden death in children, there are a number of limitations to the study and the FDA cannot conclude this information impacts the overall risk:benefit profile of these medications (Gould, 2009). **Note:** In a large retrospective cohort study involving 1,200,438 children and young adults (age: 2-24 years), none of the currently available stimulant medications or atomoxetine were shown to increase the risk of serious cardiovascular events (ie, acute MI, sudden cardiac death, or stroke) in current (adjusted hazard ratio: 0.75; 95% CI: 0.31-1.85) or former (adjusted hazard ratio: 1.03; 95% CI: 0.57-1.89) users compared to nonusers (Cooper, 2011). It should be noted that due to the upper limit of the 95% CI, the study could not rule out a doubling of the risk, albeit low. **Note:** ECG abnormalities and 4 cases of sudden cardiac death have been reported in children receiving clonidine with methylphenidate; reduce dose of methylphenidate by 40% when used concurrently with clonidine; consider ECG monitoring.

Stimulant medications may increase blood pressure (average increase 2-4 mm Hg) and heart rate (average increase 3-6 bpm); some patients may experience greater increases; use stimulant medications with caution in patients with hypertension and other cardiovascular conditions that may be exacerbated by increases in blood pressure or heart rate. Metadate CD® and Metadate ER® use is contraindicated in patients with severe hypertension.

Psychiatric adverse events may occur. Stimulants may exacerbate symptoms of behavior disturbance and thought disorder in patients with preexisting psychosis. New-onset psychosis or mania may occur with stimulant use in patients without a prior history of psychotic illness or mania, even at standard doses. May induce mixed/manic episode in patients with bipolar disorder; patients should be screened for bipolar disorder prior to treatment; consider discontinuation if such symptoms (eg, delusional thinking, hallucinations, or mania) occur. May be associated with aggressive behavior or hostility (causal relationship not established); monitor for development or worsening of these behaviors).

Potential for drug dependency exists **[U.S. Boxed Warning]**; prolonged administration may lead to drug dependence; abrupt discontinuation following high doses or for prolonged periods may result in symptoms of withdrawal; avoid abrupt discontinuation in patients who have received methylphenidate for prolonged periods. Do not use for severe depression or normal fatigue states. CNS stimulants possess a high potential for abuse **[U.S. Boxed Warning]**; assess risk of abuse prior to initiating therapy and continue to monitor for signs of abuse throughout therapy; misuse may cause sudden death and serious cardiovascular adverse events; use with caution in patients with history of ethanol or drug abuse.

Prolonged and painful erections (priapism), sometimes requiring surgical intervention, have been reported with methylphenidate use in pediatric and adult patients. Priapism has been reported to develop after some time on the drug, often subsequent to an increase in dose and also during a period of drug withdrawal (drug holidays or discontinuation). Patients who develop abnormally sustained or frequent and painful erections should seek immediate medical attention.

Long-term effects in pediatric patients have not been determined. Use of stimulants in children has been associated with growth suppression (monitor growth; treatment interruption may be needed). Appetite suppression may occur; monitor weight during therapy, particularly in children. Stimulants may lower seizure threshold leading to new onset or breakthrough seizure activity (use with caution in patients with a history of seizure disorder). Visual disturbances (difficulty in accommodation and blurred vision) have been reported.

A potential for GI obstruction exists with Concerta® (tablet is nondeformable); do not ordinarily use in patients with severe GI narrowing (eg, esophageal motility disorders, small bowel inflammatory disease, short gut syndrome, history of cystic fibrosis, peritonitis, chronic intestinal pseudo-obstruction, or Meckel's diverticulum).

Transdermal system (Daytrana®) may cause allergic contact sensitization, characterized by intense local reactions (edema, vesicles, papules) that may spread beyond the patch site; remove patch and monitor application site if reaction occurs; seek further evaluation if erythema, edema, and/or papules do not significantly decrease or resolve within 24 hours of patch removal. Allergic sensitization may subsequently manifest systemically when methylphenidate is administered orally or via other routes; systemic sensitization reactions may include dermatitis, generalized skin eruptions, headache, fever, vomiting, diarrhea, arthralgia, or malaise; initiate oral methylphenidate under close medical supervision in patients who have experienced a contact sensitization to the transdermal system; some of these patients may **not** be able to take methylphenidate in any dosage form. Do not expose transdermal application site to direct external heat sources (eg, electric blankets, heating pads, heated water beds), a >2-fold increase in drug release may occur. Powder for oral suspension (Quillivant™ XR) contains benzoic acid; benzoic acid (benzoate) is a metabolite of benzyl alcohol; which may cause allergic reactions in susceptible individuals.

Precautions Use with caution in patients with heart failure, recent MI, hyperthyroidism, seizures, acute stress reactions, emotional instability, or history of substance abuse. Hematological monitoring is advised with long term use. Rare cases of neuroleptic malignant syndrome have been reported; usually in patients receiving concurrent medications associated with the syndrome; one case reported with concurrent first dose of venlafaxine.

Stimulants are associated with peripheral vasculopathy, including Raynaud's phenomenon; signs/symptoms are usually mild and intermittent and generally improve with dose reduction or discontinuation. Digital ulceration and/or soft tissue breakdown have been observed rarely; monitor for digital changes during therapy and seek further evaluation (eg, rheumatology) if necessary.

Use with caution in preschool-age children; clinical trials have shown children 3-5 years of age are more sensitive to methylphenidate adverse effects resulting in a greater discontinuation of therapy compared to school-age children (discontinuation rate from trials: 11% vs <1%) (Wigal, 2006). The moderate to severe adverse effect profiles in children are age-related; in preschool children, the most commonly reported adverse effects were crabbiness/irritability, emotional outbursts, difficulty falling asleep, repetitive behavior/thoughts, and decreased appetite; in school-age children, they were decreased appetite, delay of sleep onset, headache, and stomach ache (Wigal, 2006).

Chewable tablets contain aspartame which is metabolized to phenylalanine and must be avoided (or used with caution) in patients with phenylketonuria. Chewable tablets must be taken with adequate amount of liquid, otherwise tablet may swell and block the throat or esophagus and cause choking; do not use chewable tablets in patients who have difficulty swallowing; instruct patients to seek immediate medical attention if chest pain, vomiting, difficulty in breathing or swallowing occur after taking chewable tablet.

Metadate CD® contains sucrose; avoid use in hereditary problems of fructose intolerance, sucrase-isomaltose insufficiency, and glucose-galactose malabsorption. Metadate® ER contains lactose; avoid in hereditary problems of galactose intolerance, glucose-galactose malabsorption, and the Lapp lactase deficiency. Concomitant use of Metadate® CD or Metadate® ER with halogenated anesthetics is contraindicated; use may cause sudden elevations in blood pressure; if surgery is planned, do not administer Metadate® CD or Metadate® ER on day of surgery.

Adverse Reactions
All dosage forms:
Cardiovascular: Angina, cardiac arrhythmia, cerebral arteritis, cerebral hemorrhage, cerebral occlusion, cerebrovascular accidents, hyper-/hypotension, MI, murmur, palpitation, pulse increased/decreased, Raynaud's phenomenon, tachycardia, vasculitis

Central nervous system: Aggression, agitation, anger, anxiety, confusional state, depression, dizziness, drowsiness, emotional lability, fatigue, fever, headache, hypervigilance, insomnia, irritability, lethargy, motion sickness (children), nervousness, neuroleptic malignant syndrome (NMS) (rare), restlessness, stroke, tension, tic (children), Tourette's syndrome (rare), toxic psychosis, tremor, vertigo

Dermatologic: Alopecia, erythema multiforme, excoriation (children), exfoliative dermatitis, hyperhidrosis, rash, urticaria

Endocrine & metabolic: Dysmenorrhea, growth retardation, libido decreased

Gastrointestinal: Abdominal pain, anorexia, appetite decreased, bruxism, constipation, diarrhea, dyspepsia, nausea, vomiting, weight loss, xerostomia

Genitourinary: Erectile dysfunction

Hematologic: Anemia, leukopenia, pancytopenia, thrombocytopenia, thrombocytopenic purpura

Hepatic: Bilirubin increased, hepatic coma, liver function tests abnormal, transaminases increased

Neuromuscular & skeletal: Arthralgia, dyskinesia, muscle tightness, paresthesia

Ocular: Blurred vision, dry eyes, eye pain (children), mydriasis, visual accommodation disturbance

Renal: Necrotizing vasculitis

Respiratory: Cough increased, dyspnea, pharyngitis, pharyngolaryngeal pain, rhinitis, sinusitis, upper respiratory tract infection

Miscellaneous: Accidental injury, hypersensitivity reactions

Rare but important or life-threatening: Alkaline phosphatase increased, bradycardia, disorientation, extrasystole, hallucinations, hypersensitivity reactions (eg, angioedema, anaphylactic reactions, auricular swelling, bullous conditions, eruptions, exanthemas, exfoliative conditions, pruritus, rash, urticaria), impaired peripheral circulation, mania, migraine, obsessive-compulsive disorder, priapism, seizure, supraventricular tachycardia, ventricular extrasystole

Transdermal system:
Cardiovascular: Tachycardia

Central nervous system: Dizziness, emotional instability, headache, insomnia, irritability, tic

Gastrointestinal: Abdominal pain, anorexia, appetite decreased, nausea, vomiting, weight loss

Local: Application site reaction

Respiratory: Nasal congestion, nasopharyngitis

Miscellaneous: Viral infection

Rare but important or life-threatening: Allergic contact dermatitis/sensitization, anaphylaxis, angioedema, dyskinesia, hallucinations, seizures

Drug Interactions
Metabolism/Transport Effects Inhibits CYP2D6 (weak)

Avoid Concomitant Use
Avoid concomitant use of Methylphenidate with any of the following: Alcohol (Ethyl); Inhalational Anesthetics; Iobenguane I 123; MAO Inhibitors

Increased Effect/Toxicity
Methylphenidate may increase the levels/effects of: Anti-Parkinson's Agents (Dopamine Agonist); Antipsychotics; ARIPiprazole; CloNIDine; Fosphenytoin; Inhalational Anesthetics; PHENobarbital; Phenytoin; Primidone; Sympathomimetics; Tricyclic Antidepressants; Vitamin K Antagonists

The levels/effects of Methylphenidate may be increased by: Alcohol (Ethyl); Antacids; Antipsychotics; AtoMOXetine; Cannabinoid-Containing Products; H2-Antagonists; MAO Inhibitors; Proton Pump Inhibitors

Decreased Effect
Methylphenidate may decrease the levels/effects of: Antihypertensives; Iobenguane I 123; Ioflupane I 123

Food Interactions
Ethanol: Alcohol consumption increases the rate of methylphenidate release from Metadate CD and Ritalin LA (extended-release capsules), but not from Concerta (extended-release tablet); an *in vitro* study involving Metadate CD and Ritalin LA showed that an alcohol concentration of 40% resulted in 84% and 98% of the methylphenidate being released in the first hour, respectively. Management: Avoid consuming alcohol during therapy.

Food: Food may increase oral absorption of immediate release tablet/solution and chewable tablet. Management: Administer 30-45 minutes before meals.

Stability
Oral:
Immediate release formulations:
Chewable tablet: Store at 20°C to 25°C (68°F to 77°F); protect from moisture.
Oral solution: Chewable: Store at 20°C to 25°C (68°F to 77°F); protect from moisture.

◄ Tablet: (Ritalin®): Store at 25°C (77°F); excursions permitted to 15°C to 30°C (59°F to 86°F); protect from light.

Extended and sustained release formulations:

Capsule (Metadate CD®, Ritalin LA®): Store at 25°C (77°F); excursions permitted to 15°C to 30°C (59°F to 86°F).

Tablet:

Concerta®: Store at 25°C (77°F); excursions permitted to 15°C to 30°C (59°F to 86°F); protect from humidity.

Metadate® ER: Store at 20°C to 25°C (68°F to 77°F); excursions permitted to 15°C to 30°C (59°F to 86°F); protect from moisture.

Powder for oral suspension (Quillivant™ XR): Store at 25°C (77°F), excursions permitted to 15°C to 30°C (59°F to 86°F) before and after reconstitution. Once reconstituted, bottle must be used within 4 months; dispense in original container.

Transdermal system (Daytrana®): Store at 25°C (77°F); excursions permitted to 15°C to 30°C (59°F to 86°F). Keep patches stored in protective pouch. Once sealed tray or outer pouch is opened, use patches within 2 months; once an individual patch has been removed from the pouch and the protective liner removed, use immediately. Do not refrigerate or freeze.

Mechanism of Action Mild CNS stimulant; blocks the reuptake of norepinephrine and dopamine into presynaptic neurons; appears to stimulate the cerebral cortex and subcortical structures similar to amphetamines

Pharmacodynamics

Onset of action (AAP, 2011):

Oral:

Immediate release formulations [chewable tablet, oral solution, tablet (Methylin®, Ritalin®)]: 20-60 minutes

Extended release formulations [Capsule (Metadate CD®, Ritalin LA®), tablets (Concerta®)]: 20-60 minutes

Sustained release tablet (Ritalin-SR®): 60-180 minutes

Transdermal (Daytrana®): 60 minutes

Maximum effect: Oral:

Immediate release tablet: Within 2 hours

Sustained release tablet: Within 4-7 hours

Duration of action (AAP, 2011):

Oral:

Immediate release formulations [Chewable tablet, oral solution, immediate release tablet (Methylin®, Ritalin®)]: 3-5 hours

Extended release capsule (Metadate CD®, Ritalin LA®): 6-8 hours

Extended release tablet (Concerta®): 12 hours

Sustained release tablet (Ritalin-SR®): 2-6 hours

Transdermal (Daytrana®): 11-12 hours

Pharmacokinetics (Adult data unless noted) Note: Values reported below based on pediatric patient data or combined pediatric and adult data.

Absorption: Oral:

Immediate release products: Readily absorbed

Transdermal: Rate and extent of absorption is increased when applied to inflamed skin or exposed to heat; transdermal absorption may increase with chronic therapy

Distribution: V_d: d-methylphenidate: 2.65 ± 1.11 L/kg; l-methylphenidate: 1.80 ± 0.91 L/kg

Protein binding: 15%

Metabolism: Hepatic via hydroxylation (de-esterification by carboxylesterase CES1A1) to ritalinic acid (alpha-phenyl-2-piperidine acetic acid), which has little or no pharmacologic activity

Bioavailability:

Immediate release chewable tablets and oral solution: Bioequivalent to immediate release tablets

Extended release suspension (Quillivant™ XR): 95% (relative to immediate release oral solution)

Transdermal patch (Daytrana®): Lower first-pass effect compared to oral administration; thus, much lower doses (on a mg/kg basis) given via the transdermal route may still produce higher AUCs, compared to the oral route

Half-life:

Oral:

Immediate release formulations:

Chewable tablets, oral solution (Methylin®): 3 hours

Tablet (Ritalin®):

Children: 2.5 hours (range: 1.8-5.3 hours)

Adults: 3.5 hours (range: 1.3-7.7 hours)

Extended release formulations:

Capsule:

Metadate CD®: 6.8 hours

Ritalin LA®:

Children: 2.4 hours (range: 1.5-4 hours)

Adults: 3.3 hours (range: 3-4.2 hours)

Tablet (Concerta®): 3.5 hours

Suspension (Quillivant™ XR): Children ≥9 years, Adolescents, and Adults: ~5 hours

Transdermal patch (Daytrana®): Children and Adolescents 6-17 years: 4-5 hours

Time to peak serum concentration:

Oral:

Immediate release formulations:

Chewable tablets, oral solution (Methylin®): 1-2 hours

Tablet (Ritalin®): Children: 1.9 hours (range: 0.3-4.4 hours)

Extended release formulations:

Capsule (Metadate CD®): 1.5 hours

Tablet:

Concerta®: 6-10 hours

Metadate ER®: Children: 4.7 hours (range: 1.3-8.2 hours)

Powder for oral suspension (Quillivant™ XR):

Children (9-12 years): 4 hours

Adolescents (13-15 years): 2 hours

Adults: 4 hours

Sustained release tablets (Ritalin SR®): Children: 4.7 hours (range: 1.3-8.2 hours)

Transdermal patch (Daytrana®): Children 6-17 years: 8-10 hours

Elimination: 90% of dose is eliminated in the urine as metabolites and unchanged drug; main urinary metabolite (ritalinic acid) accounts for 80% of the dose; drug is also excreted in feces via bile

Dosing: Usual Note: Discontinue medication if no improvement is seen after appropriate dosage adjustment over a 1-month period of time:

Children and Adolescents:

Attention-deficit/hyperactivity disorder:

Oral:

Immediate release products (eg, Methylin®, Ritalin®):

Children 3-5 years, moderate to severe dysfunction: Limited data available; AAP considers first-line agent in this patient population if pharmacological treatment deemed necessary (AAP, 2011): Initial: 1.25 mg twice daily; titrate to effect at weekly intervals; usual reported daily range: 3.75-30 mg/day divided into two or three daily doses (Ghuman, 2008; Greenhill, 2006). In the largest trial, a multicenter, randomized, placebo-controlled, crossover study of 165 preschool children (age range: 3-5.5 years), statistically and clinically significant improvements in ADHD scores were reported with doses of 2.5 mg, 5 mg, and 7.5 mg 3 times daily; in some patients [n=7 (4%)], dose titration to 10 mg 3 times daily was necessary; the mean effective total daily dose: 14.2 ± 8.1 mg/**day**. Although ADHD scores were statistically and clinically improved with methylphenidate use, the effect size was smaller with this younger patient population than that seen in school-age children (Greenhill, 2006).

Children ≥6 years and Adolescents: Initial: 0.3 mg/kg/dose or 2.5-5 mg/dose given before breakfast and lunch; increase by 0.1 mg/kg/dose or by 5-10 mg/day at weekly intervals; usual dose: 0.3-1 mg/kg/day or 20-30 mg/**day** in 2-3 divided doses; maximum daily dose dependent upon patient weight: 2 mg/kg/day or if patient weight ≤50 kg: 60 mg/**day**; in patients >50 kg: 100 mg/day (Dopheide, 2009, Pliszka, 2007); some patients may require 3 doses/day (ie, additional dose at 4 PM)

Extended release, sustained release and long acting products:

Metadate® ER, Ritalin-SR®: Children ≥6 years and Adolescents: Sustained release and extended release tablets (duration of action ~8 hours) may be given in place of regular tablets, once the daily dose is titrated using the immediate release products and the titrated 8-hour dosage corresponds to sustained/extended release tablet size; Ritalin SR® may be administered once or twice daily (AAP, 2011). Maximum daily dose is dependent upon patient weight: ≤50 kg: 60 mg/**day**; >50 kg: 100 mg/**day** (Dopheide, 2009; Pliszka, 2007)

Concerta®: Children ≥6 years and Adolescents:

Methylphenidate-naive patients: Initial: 18 mg once daily

Patients currently using immediate release methylphenidate: Initial dose: Dosing based on current regimen and clinical judgment; suggested dosing listed below:

Switching from methylphenidate immediate release 5 mg 2-3 times daily: Concerta® 18 mg once daily

Switching from methylphenidate immediate release 10 mg 2-3 times daily: Concerta® 36 mg once daily

Switching from methylphenidate immediate release 15 mg 2-3 times daily: Concerta® 54 mg once daily

Switching from methylphenidate immediate release 20 mg 2-3 times daily: Concerta® 72 mg once daily

Dosage adjustment: May increase by Concerta® 18 mg/day increments at weekly intervals. **Note:** A dosage strength of 27 mg is available for situations in which a dosage between 18-36 mg is desired.

Maximum daily dose:

Children 6-12 years: 54 mg/day; for patients >50 kg, higher maximum daily doses may be considered (108 mg/day)

Adolescents:

≤50 kg: 72 mg/day; not to exceed ~2 mg/kg/day >50 kg:108 mg/day (Dopheide, 2009; Pliszka, 2007)

Metadate CD®: Children ≥6 years and Adolescents: Initial: 20 mg once daily; may increase by 10-20 mg/day increments at weekly intervals; maximum daily dose dependent upon patient weight: ≤50 kg: 60 mg/**day**; >50 kg: 100 mg/**day** (Dopheide, 2009; Pliszka, 2007)

Quillivant™ XR: Children 6-12 years: Initial: 20 mg once daily; may increase by 10-20 mg/day increments at weekly intervals; maximum daily dose: 60 mg/**day**

Ritalin LA®: Children ≥6 years and Adolescents:

Methylphenidate-naive patients: Initial: 20 mg once daily; may increase by 10 mg/day increments at weekly intervals; maximum daily dose dependent upon patient weight: ≤50 kg: 60 mg/**day**; >50 kg: 100 mg/**day** (Dopheide, 2009; Pliszka, 2007). **Note:** If a lower initial dose is desired, patients may begin with Ritalin LA® 10 mg once daily. Alternatively, patients may begin therapy with an immediate release product, and switch to Ritalin LA® once immediate release dosage is titrated to 5 mg twice daily (see below)

Patients currently receiving immediate release methylphenidate: Initial dose: Dosing based on current regimen and clinical judgment; use equivalent total daily dose administered once daily

Patients currently receiving methylphenidate sustained release (SR): The same total daily dose of Ritalin LA® should be used.

Dosage adjustment: May increase Ritalin LA®: by 10 mg/day increments at weekly intervals

Maximum daily dose: Dependent upon patient weight: ≤50 kg: 60 mg/**day**; >50 kg: 100 mg/**day** (Dopheide, 2009; Pliszka, 2007)

Topical: Transdermal patch (Daytrana®): Children and Adolescents 6-17 years: Initial: 10 mg (12.5 cm^2) patch once daily; apply to hip 2 hours before effect is needed and remove 9 hours after application; titrate dose based on response and tolerability; may increase to next transdermal patch dosage size no more frequently than every week. Patch may be removed before 9 hours if a shorter duration of action is required or if late day adverse effects appear. Plasma concentrations usually start to decline when the patch is removed but drug absorption may continue for several hours after patch removal. **Note:** The manufacturer's labeling recommends patients converting from another formulation of methylphenidate to the transdermal patch should be initiated at 10 mg regardless of their previous dose and titrated as needed due to the differences in bioavailability of the transdermal formulation. However, some clinicians have supported higher starting patch doses for patients converting from oral methylphenidate doses of >20 mg/day; for example, the 15 mg (18.75 cm^2) patch has been investigated to have the same effect as 22.5 mg daily of the immediate release preparation, 27 mg daily of the osmotic release preparation (Concerta®), or 20 mg daily of the encapsulated bead preparation (Metadate CD®) (Arnold, 2007).

Narcolepsy: Children ≥6 years and Adolescents: Oral:

Immediate release tablets and oral solution (Methylin®, Ritalin®): Initial: 5 mg twice daily given before breakfast and lunch; increase by 5-10 increments mg/day at weekly intervals; 2-3 times per day; maximum daily dose: 60 mg/**day** (in 2-3 divided doses)

Extended/sustained release tablets (Metadate® ER, Ritalin-SR®): May be given in place of immediate release products (duration of action: ~8 hours), once the immediate release formulation daily dose is titrated and the titrated 8-hour dosage corresponds to sustained or extended release tablet size; maximum daily dose: 60 mg/**day**

Adults:

Attention-deficit/hyperactivity disorder: Oral:

Immediate release (IR) products (tablets, chewable tablets, and solution): Initial: 5 mg twice daily, before breakfast and lunch; increase by 5-10 mg daily at weekly intervals; maximum dose: 60 mg daily (in 2-3 divided doses)

Extended release (ER), sustained release (SR) products (capsules, tablets, and oral suspension):

Concerta®: Adults <65 years:

Patients not currently taking methylphenidate: Initial dose: 18-36 mg once every morning

Patients currently taking methylphenidate: **Note:** Initial dose: Dosing based on current regimen and clinical judgment; suggested dosing listed below:

Switching from methylphenidate 5 mg 2-3 times daily: 18 mg once every morning

Switching from methylphenidate 10 mg 2-3 times daily: 36 mg once every morning

Switching from methylphenidate 15 mg 2-3 times daily: 54 mg once every morning

Switching from methylphenidate 20 mg 2-3 times daily: 72 mg once every morning

Dose adjustment: May increase dose in increments of 18 mg; dose may be adjusted at weekly intervals. A dosage strength of 27 mg is available for situations in which a dosage between 18-36 mg is desired; maximum dose: 72 mg/day

Metadate® ER, Ritalin-SR®: May be given in place of immediate release products, once the daily dose is titrated and the titrated 8-hour dosage corresponds to sustained or extended release tablet size; maximum: 60 mg/day

Metadate CD®, Quillivant™ XR: Initial: 20 mg once daily; may be adjusted in 10-20 mg increments at weekly intervals; maximum: 60 mg/day

Ritalin LA®: Initial: 20 mg once daily (l0 mg once daily may be considered for some patients); may be adjusted in 10 mg increments at weekly intervals; maximum: 60 mg/day

Conversion from immediate release or sustained release methylphenidate formulation to Ritalin LA®: Use equivalent total daily dose administered once daily.

Narcolepsy: Oral:

Immediate release tablets and solution (Methylin®, Ritalin®): Initial: 5 mg twice daily before breakfast and lunch; increase by 5-10 mg daily at weekly intervals; 10 mg 2-3 times per day; maximum daily dose: 60 mg/day (in 2-3 divided doses).

Extended/sustained release tablets (Metadate® ER, Ritalin-SR®): May be given in place of immediate release products (duration of action: ~8 hours), once the immediate release formulation daily dose is titrated and the titrated 8-hour dosage corresponds to sustained or extended release tablet size; maximum: 60 mg/day

Dosing adjustment for renal impairment:

Oral: No dosage adjustment provided in manufacturer's labeling (has not been studied); undergoes extensive metabolism to a renally eliminated metabolite with little or no pharmacologic activity.

Transdermal: No dosage adjustment provided in manufacturer's labeling (has not been studied).

Dosing adjustment for hepatic impairment: There are no dosage adjustments provided in manufacturer's labeling (has not been studied).

Administration

Oral: To avoid insomnia, last daily dose should be administered several hours before retiring.

Immediate release formulations:

Tablet (Ritalin®), oral solution (Methylin®): Administer on an empty stomach ~30-45 minutes before meals. Ensure last daily dose is administered before 6 PM if difficulty sleeping occurs.

Chewable tablet (Methylin®): Administer on an empty stomach ~30-45 minutes before meals with at least 8 ounces of water or other fluid; choking may occur if not enough fluids are taken. Ensure last daily dose is administered before 6 PM if difficulty sleeping occurs.

Extended/sustained release formulations:

Tablets:

Metadate ER®: May be taken with or without food. Swallow whole; do not crush, chew, or break tablets.

Ritalin SR®: Administer 30-45 minutes before a meal. Swallow whole; do not crush, chew, or break tablets.

Concerta®: May be administered without regard to food, but must be taken with water, milk, or juice; administer dose once daily in the morning; do not crush, chew, or divide tablets

Capsules:

Metadate CD®: Administer dose once daily in the morning, before breakfast, with water, milk, or juice; capsule may be swallowed whole or opened and contents sprinkled on a small amount (one tablespoonful) of applesauce; immediately consume drug/applesauce mixture; do not store for future use; swallow applesauce without chewing; do not crush or chew capsule contents; drink fluids after consuming drug/applesauce mixture to ensure complete swallowing of beads; do not crush, chew, or divide capsules or its contents

Ritalin LA®: Administer dose once daily in the morning; may be administered with or without food (but some food may delay absorption); capsule may be swallowed whole or may be opened and contents sprinkled on a small amount (one spoonful) of applesauce. **Note:** Applesauce should not be warm; immediately consume drug/applesauce mixture; do not store for future use; do not crush, chew, or divide capsule or its contents.

Powder for oral suspension (Quillivant™ XR): Administer in the morning with or without food. Shake bottle ≥10 seconds prior to administration. Use the oral dosing dispenser provided; wash after each use.

Topical: Transdermal (Daytrana®): Apply patch immediately after opening pouch and removing protective liner; do not use patch if pouch seal is broken; do not cut patch; do not use patches that are cut or damaged. If difficulty is experienced when separating the patch from the liner or if any medication (sticky substance) remains on the liner after separation, discard that patch and apply a new patch. Apply to clean, dry, healthy skin on the hip; do not apply to oily, damaged, or irritated skin; do not apply to the waistline; do not premedicate the patch site with hydrocortisone or other solutions, creams, ointments, or emollients. Apply at the same time each day, 2 hours before effect is needed. Alternate site of application daily (ie, use alternate hip). Press patch firmly for 30 seconds to ensure proper adherence. Remove patch 9 hours after application. Patch may be removed earlier if a shorter duration of action is required or if late day adverse effects occur.

Avoid exposure of application site to external heat source (eg, hair dryers, electric blankets, heating pads, heated water beds), which may significantly increase the rate and amount of drug absorbed. Exposure of patch to water during swimming, bathing, or showering may affect patch adherence. Do not reapply patch with dressings, tape, or other adhesives. If patch should become dislodged, may replace with new patch (to different site) but total wear time should not exceed 9 hours.

During removal, peel off patch slowly. If needed, patch removal may be helped by applying an oil-based product (ie, mineral oil, olive oil, or petroleum jelly) to the patch edges, gently working it underneath the patch edges. If a patch is not able to be removed, contact a physician or pharmacist. Nonmedical adhesive removers and acetone-based products, such as nail polish remover, should not be used to remove patches or adhesive. If adhesive residue remains on child's skin after patch removal, use an oil-based product and gently rub area to remove adhesive. Avoid touching the sticky side of the patch. Wash hands with soap and water after handling.

Dispose of used patch by folding adhesive side onto itself, and discard in toilet or appropriate lidded container; discard unused patches that are no longer needed in the same manner; protective pouch and liner should be discarded in an appropriate lidded container. **Note:** Used patches contain residual drug; keep all transdermal patches out of the reach of children.

Monitoring Parameters Evaluate patients for cardiac disease prior to initiation of therapy with thorough medical history, family history, and physical exam; consider ECG; perform ECG and echocardiogram if findings suggest cardiac disease; promptly conduct cardiac evaluation in patients who develop chest pain, unexplained syncope, or any other symptom of cardiac disease during treatment. Monitor CBC with differential, platelet count, liver enzymes, blood pressure, heart rate, height, weight, appetite, abnormal movements, growth in children. Patients should be re-evaluated at appropriate intervals to assess continued need of the medication. Observe for signs/symptoms of aggression or hostility, depression, delusional thinking, hallucinations, or mania. Monitor for visual disturbances. Monitor for signs of misuse, abuse, and addiction.

Transdermal system: Also monitor the application site for local adverse reactions and allergic contact sensitization.

Test Interactions May interfere with urine detection of amphetamines/methamphetamines (false-positive).

Additional Information Methylphenidate is a racemic mixture of d- and l-enantiomers; the d-enantiomer is more active than the l-enantiomer. Treatment with methylphenidate should include "drug holidays" or periodic discontinuation in order to assess the patient's requirements, decrease tolerance and limit suppression of linear growth and weight. Medications used to treat ADHD should be part of a total treatment program that may include other components such as psychological, educational, and social measures. Concerta®, Metadate CD®, and Ritalin LA® are formulated to deliver methylphenidate in a biphasic release profile; Concerta® is an osmotic controlled release formulation, with an immediate release (within 1 hour) outer coating; once daily Concerta® has been shown to be as effective as immediate release methylphenidate tablets administered 3 times/day (Pelham, 2001). Metadate CD® capsules contain both immediate release beads (30% of the dose) and extended release beads (70% of the dose). Ritalin LA® capsules contain both immediate release beads (50% of the dose) and enteric coated, delayed release beads (50% of the dose). Methylin® and Ritalin-SR® tablets are color and additive free; Methylin® oral solution is colorless. Concerta® tablets may be seen on abdominal x-ray under certain conditions (eg, when digital enhancing techniques are used). Quillivant™ XR powder for oral suspension contains a combination of uncoated and coated ion exchange resin complex and a buffering solution based on the Oral XR + platform (Wigal, 2013). Once reconstituted with water forms an extended release suspension that contains approximately 20% immediate release and 80% extended release methylphenidate.

Daytrana™ Transdermal System consists of an adhesive-based matrix containing active drug which is dispersed in acrylic adhesive that is dispersed in a silicone adhesive. The patch consists of 3 layers: A polyester/ethylene vinyl acetate laminate (outside) film backing, the adhesive layer containing methylphenidate, and a flouropolymer-coated polyester protective liner (which must be removed before application). Long-term use of the transdermal system or Concerta® >7 weeks, Metadate® CD >3 weeks, and Ritalin LA® >2 weeks have not been adequately studied; long-term usefulness should be periodically re-evaluated for the individual patient.

Controlled Substance C-II

Dosage Forms Excipient information presented when available (limited, particularly for generics); consult specific product labeling.

Capsule Extended Release, Oral, as hydrochloride:
Metadate CD: 10 mg, 20 mg, 30 mg [contains fd&c blue #2 (indigotine)]
Metadate CD: 40 mg
Metadate CD: 50 mg [contains fd&c blue #2 (indigotine)]
Metadate CD: 60 mg
Generic: 10 mg, 20 mg, 30 mg, 40 mg, 50 mg, 60 mg

Capsule Extended Release 24 Hour, Oral, as hydrochloride:
Ritalin LA: 10 mg, 20 mg, 30 mg, 40 mg
Generic: 20 mg, 30 mg, 40 mg

Patch, Transdermal:
Daytrana: 10 mg/9 hr (30 ea); 15 mg/9 hr (30 ea); 20 mg/9 hr (30 ea); 30 mg/9 hr (30 ea)

Solution, Oral, as hydrochloride:
Methylin: 5 mg/5 mL (500 mL); 10 mg/5 mL (500 mL) [contains polyethylene glycol]
Generic: 5 mg/5 mL (500 mL); 10 mg/5 mL (500 mL)

Suspension Reconstituted, Oral, as hydrochloride:
Quillivant XR: 25 mg/5 mL (60 mL, 120 mL, 150 mL, 180 mL) [contains sodium benzoate; banana flavor]

Tablet, Oral, as hydrochloride:
Ritalin: 5 mg
Ritalin: 10 mg, 20 mg [scored]
Generic: 5 mg, 10 mg, 20 mg

Tablet Chewable, Oral, as hydrochloride:
Methylin: 2.5 mg, 5 mg [contains aspartame; grape flavor]
Methylin: 10 mg [scored; contains aspartame; grape flavor]

Tablet Extended Release, Oral, as hydrochloride:
Concerta: 18 mg, 27 mg, 36 mg, 54 mg
Metadate ER: 20 mg
Ritalin SR: 20 mg
Generic: 10 mg, 18 mg, 20 mg, 27 mg, 36 mg, 54 mg

References

American Academy of Pediatrics, "ADHD: Clinical Practice Guideline for the Diagnosis, Evaluation, and Treatment of Attention-Deficit/Hyperactivity Disorder in Children and Adolescents," *Pediatrics*, 2011, 128(5):1007-22.

American Academy of Pediatrics/American Heart Association Clarification of Statement on Cardiovascular Evaluation and Monitoring of Children and Adolescents With Heart Disease Receiving Medications for ADHD; available at: http://americanheart.mediaroon.com/index.php?s=43&item=422.

American Academy of Pediatrics. Subcommittee on Attention-Deficit/Hyperactivity Disorder, "Clinical Practice Guideline: Treatment of the School-Aged Child With Attention-Deficit/Hyperactivity Disorder," *Pediatrics*, 2001, 108(4):1033-44.

Arnold LE, Lindsay RL, López FA, et al, "Treating Attention-Deficit/Hyperactivity Disorder With a Stimulant Transdermal Patch: The Clinical Art," *Pediatrics*, 2007, 120(5):1100-6.

Bolea-Alamanac BM, Green A, Verma G, et al, "Methylphenidate Use in Pregnancy and Lactation, a Systematic Review of Evidence," *Br J Clin Pharmacol*, 2013, doi: 10.1111/bcp.12138.

Cooper WO, Habel LA, Sox CM, et al, "ADHD Drugs and Serious Cardiovascular Events in Children and Young Adults," *N Engl J Med*, 2011, 365(20):1896-904.

Dideriksen D, Pottegård A, Hallas J, et al, "First Trimester *in utero* Exposure to Methylphenidate," *Basic Clin Pharmacol Toxicol*, 2013, 112(2):73-6.

Ghuman JK, Arnold LE, and Anthony BJ, "Psychopharmacological and Other Treatments in Preschool Children With Attention-Deficit/Hyperactivity Disorder: Current Evidence and Practice," *J Child Adolesc Psychopharmacol*, 2008, 18(5):413-47.

Gould MS, Walsh BT, Munfakh JL, et al, "Sudden Death and Use of Stimulant Medications in Youths," *Am J Psychiatry*, 2009, 166 (9):992-1001.

Greenhill L, Kollins S, Abikoff H, et al, "Efficacy and Safety of Immediate-Release Methylphenidate Treatment for Preschoolers With ADHD," *J Am Acad Child Adolesc Psychiatry*, 2006, 45(11):1284-93.

Greenhill LL, "Pharmacologic Treatment of Attention Deficit Hyperactivity Disorder," *Psychiatr Clin North Am*, 1992, 15(1):1-27.

Greenhill LL, Pliszka S, Dulcan MK, et al, "Practice Parameter for the Use of Stimulant Medications in the Treatment of Children,

◄

Adolescents, and Adults," *J Am Acad Child Adolesc Psychiatry*, 2002, 41(2 Suppl):26S-49S.

Hackett LP, Kristensen JH, Hale TW, et al, "Methylphenidate and Breast-Feeding," *Ann Pharmacother*, 2006, 40(10):1890-1.

Kelly DP and Aylward GP, "Attention Deficits in School-Aged Children and Adolescents," *Pediatr Clin North Am*, 1992, 39(3):487-512.

Maurovich-Horvat E, Kemlink D, Högl B, et al, "Narcolepsy and Pregnancy: A Retrospective European Evaluation of 249 Pregnancies," *J Sleep Res*, 2013, doi: 10.1111/jsr.12047.

Pelham WE, Gnagy EM, Burrows-Maclean L, et al, "Once-a-Day Concerta Methylphenidate Versus Three-Times-Daily Methylphenidate in Laboratory and Natural Settings," *Pediatrics*, 2001, 107(6), http://www.pediatrics.org/cgi/content/full/107/6/e105.

Pentikis HS, Simmons RD, Benedict MF, et al, "Methylphenidate Bioavailability in Adults When an Extended-Release Multiparticulate Formulation is Administered Sprinkled on Food or as an Intact Capsule," *J Am Acad Child Adolesc Psychiatry*, 2002, 41(4):443-9.

Spigset O, Brede WR, and Zahlsen K, "Excretion of Methylphenidate in Breast Milk," *Am J Psychiatry*, 2007, 164(2):348.

Thorpy M, Zhao CG, and Dauvilliers Y, "Management of Narcolepsy During Pregnancy," *Sleep Med*, 2013, 14(4):367-76.

Vetter VL, Elia J, Erickson C, et al, "Cardiovascular Monitoring of Children and Adolescents With Heart Disease Receiving Stimulant Drugs: A Scientific Statement From the American Heart Association Council on Cardiovascular Disease in the Young Congenital Cardiac Defects Committee and the Council on Cardiovascular Nursing," *Circulation*, 2008, 117(18):2407-23.

Wigal SB, Childress AC, Belden HW, et al, "NWP06, an Extended Release Oral Suspension of Methylphenidate, Improved Attention-Deficit/Hyperactivity Disorder Symptoms Compared With Placebo in a Laboratory Classroom Study," *J Child Adolesc Psychopharmacol*, January 5, 2013.

Wigal T, Greenhill L, Chuang S, et al, "Safety and Tolerability of Methylphenidate in Preschool Children With ADHD," *J Am Acad Child Adolesc Psychiatry*, 2006, 45(11):1294-303.

Wilens TE and Biederman J, "The Stimulants," *Psychiatr Clin North Am*, 1992, 15(1):191-222.

◆ **Methylphenidate Hydrochloride** *see* Methylphenidate *on page 1379*

◆ **Methylphenoxy-Benzene Propanamine** *see* AtoMOXetine *on page 224*

◆ **Methylphenyl Isoxazolyl Penicillin** *see* Oxacillin *on page 1555*

◆ **Methylphytyl Napthoquinone** *see* Phytonadione *on page 1671*

MethylPREDNISolone (meth il pred NIS oh lone)

Medication Safety Issues

Sound-alike/look-alike issues:

MethylPREDNISolone may be confused with medroxyPROGESTERone, methotrexate, methylTESTOSTERone, predniSONE

Depo-Medrol may be confused with Solu-Medrol

Medrol may be confused with Mebaral

Solu-MEDROL may be confused with salmeterol, Solu-CORTEF

International issues:

Medrol [U.S., Canada, and multiple international markets] may be confused with Medral brand name for omeprazole [Mexico]

Related Information

Corticosteroids Systemic Equivalencies *on page 2222*

Brand Names: U.S. A-Methapred; Depo-Medrol; Medrol; Medrol (Pak); Solu-MEDROL

Brand Names: Canada Depo-Medrol; Medrol; Methylprednisolone Acetate; Solu-Medrol

Therapeutic Category Adrenal Corticosteroid; Anti-inflammatory Agent; Antiasthmatic; Corticosteroid, Systemic; Glucocorticoid

Generic Availability (U.S.) Yes

Use

Systemic: Tablets, parenteral (I.V., I.M.): Anti-inflammatory or immunosuppressant agent in the treatment of a variety of diseases including those of hematologic, allergic, inflammatory, neoplastic, and autoimmune origin (FDA approved in ages >1 month and adults); has also been used for acute spinal cord injury, *Pneumocystis* pneumonia, and prevention and treatment of graft-versus-host disease following allogeneic bone marrow transplantation

Local: Depot formulations (Depo-Medrol®): [FDA approved in pediatric patients (age not specified) and adults]

Intra-articular (or soft tissue): Acute gouty arthritis, acute/subacute bursitis, acute nonspecific tenosynovitis, epicondylitis, rheumatoid arthritis, synovitis of osteoarthritis

Intralesional (injectable suspension): Alopecia areata; discoid lupus erythematosus; infiltrated, inflammatory lesions associated with granuloma annulare, lichen planus, neurodermatitis, and psoriatic plaques; keloids; necrobiosis lipoidica diabeticorum; possibly helpful in cystic tumors of an aponeurosis or tendon (ganglia)

Pregnancy Risk Factor C

Pregnancy Considerations Adverse events have been observed with corticosteroids in animal reproduction studies. Methylprednisolone crosses the placenta (Anderson, 1981). Some studies have shown an association between first trimester systemic corticosteroid use and oral clefts (Park-Wyllie, 2000; Pradat, 2003). Systemic corticosteroids may also influence fetal growth (decreased birth weight); however, information is conflicting (Lunghi, 2010). Hypoadrenalism may occur in newborns following maternal use of corticosteroids in pregnancy; monitor.

When systemic corticosteroids are needed in pregnancy, it is generally recommended to use the lowest effective dose for the shortest duration of time, avoiding high doses during the first trimester (Leachman, 2006; Lunghi, 2010; Makol, 2011; Østensen, 2009). Inhaled corticosteroids are preferred for the treatment of asthma during pregnancy. Systemic corticosteroids such as methylprednisolone may be used for the treatment of severe persistent asthma if needed; the lowest dose administered on alternate days (if possible) should be used (NAEPP, 2005).

Pregnant women exposed to methylprednisolone for anti-rejection therapy following a transplant may contact the National Transplantation Pregnancy Registry (NTPR) at 215-955-4820. Women exposed to methylprednisolone during pregnancy for the treatment of an autoimmune disease may contact the OTIS Autoimmune Diseases Study at 877-311-8972.

Breast-Feeding Considerations Corticosteroids are excreted in human milk. The manufacturer notes that when used systemically, maternal use of corticosteroids have the potential to cause adverse events in a nursing infant (eg, growth suppression, interfere with endogenous corticosteroid production) and therefore recommends a decision be made whether to discontinue nursing or to discontinue the drug, taking into account the importance of treatment to the mother. If there is concern about exposure to the infant, some guidelines recommend waiting 4 hours after the maternal dose of an oral systemic corticosteroid before breast-feeding in order to decrease potential exposure to the nursing infant (based on a study using prednisolone) (Bae, 2011; Leachman, 2006; Makol, 2011; Ost, 1985). Other guidelines note that maternal use of systemic corticosteroids is not a contraindication to breast-feeding (NAEPP, 2005).

Contraindications Hypersensitivity to methylprednisolone or any component; systemic fungal infections (except intra-articular injection in localized joint conditions); intrathecal administration; for immunosuppressive doses: Administration of live or live, attenuated vaccines

Additional patient-type contraindications:

Premature neonates: Formulations containing benzyl alcohol preservative

Idiopathic thrombocytopenia purpura: I.M. administration

Warnings Hypothalamic-pituitary-adrenal (HPA) suppression may occur, particularly in younger children or in patients receiving high doses for prolonged periods; acute adrenal insufficiency (adrenal crisis) may occur with abrupt withdrawal after long-term therapy or with stress; withdrawal and discontinuation of corticosteroids should be tapered slowly and carefully; patients with HPA axis suppression may require doses of systemic glucocorticosteroids prior to, during, and after unusual stress (eg, surgery).

Immunosuppression may occur; patients may be more susceptible to infections; prolonged use of corticosteroids may also increase the incidence of secondary infection, mask acute infection (including fungal infections), prolong or exacerbate viral or fungal infections, activate latent opportunistic infections, or limit response to vaccines. Exposure to chickenpox should be avoided; corticosteroids should not be used to treat ocular herpes simplex; use caution in patients with a history of ocular herpes simplex. Corticosteroids should not be used for cerebral malaria or viral hepatitis. Close observation is required in patients with latent tuberculosis and/or TB reactivity; restrict use in active TB (only in conjunction with antituberculosis treatment). Amebiasis should be ruled out in any patient with recent travel to tropical climates or unexplained diarrhea prior to initiation of corticosteroids. Use with great caution in patients with known or suspected *Strongyloides* infection.

May cause osteoporosis (at any age) or inhibition of bone growth in pediatric patients. Use with caution in patients with osteoporosis. In a population-based study of children, risk of fracture was shown to be increased with >4 courses of corticosteroids; underlying clinical condition may also impact bone health and osteoporotic effect of corticosteroids (Leonard, 2006).

Corticosteroid use may cause psychiatric disturbances, including depression, euphoria, insomnia, mood swings, and personality changes. preexisting psychiatric conditions may be exacerbated by corticosteroid use. Acute myopathy may occur with high doses, usually in patients with neuromuscular transmission disorders; myopathy may involve ocular and/or respiratory muscles; monitor creatine kinase; recovery may be delayed. Increased IOP may occur, especially with prolonged use; in children, increased IOP has been shown to be dose-dependent and produce a greater IOP in children <6 years than older children (Lam, 2005). Rare cases of anaphylactoid reactions have been reported with corticosteroids.

High-dose corticosteroids should not be used for the management of traumatic brain injury (an increase in mortality was observed in patients with cranial trauma who received high-dose I.V. methylprednisolone hemisuccinate). Depressions in the skin, due to dermal and/or subdermal atrophy, may occur at the site of methylprednisolone acetate injection; do not exceed recommended dose per injection; avoid injection or leakage into the dermis; avoid injection into deltoid muscle (high incidence of subcutaneous atrophy).

Methylprednisolone **acetate** I.M. injection (multiple-dose vial) and the diluent for methylprednisolone **sodium succinate** injection contain benzyl alcohol which may cause allergic reactions in susceptible individuals; large amounts of benzyl alcohol (≥99 mg/kg/day) have been associated with a potentially fatal toxicity ("gasping syndrome") in neonates; the "gasping syndrome" consists of metabolic acidosis, respiratory distress, gasping respirations, CNS dysfunction (including convulsions, intracranial hemorrhage), hypotension and cardiovascular collapse; avoid use of methylprednisolone products containing benzyl alcohol in neonates; *in vitro* and animal studies have shown that benzoate, a metabolite of benzyl alcohol, displaces bilirubin from protein binding sites. Benzyl alcohol is also potentially toxic to neural tissue when administered locally. Methylprednisolone **acetate** injection may also contain polysorbate 80 (Tween 80®) which may cause allergic reactions in susceptible individuals. In premature neonates, thrombocytopenia, ascites, pulmonary deterioration, and renal and hepatic failure have been reported after receiving parenteral products containing polysorbate 80 (Alade, 1986; *MMWR*, 1984). Infusion of polysorbate 80-containing solutions through polyvinyl chloride tubing may cause DEHP to leach into the solution; in immature animals, exposure to DEHP may adversely affect the development of the male reproductive tract.

Precautions Avoid using higher than recommended doses; suppression of HPA function, suppression of linear growth (ie, reduction of growth velocity), reduced bone mineral density, hypercorticism (Cushing's syndrome), hyperglycemia, or glucosuria may occur; titrate to lowest effective dose. Reduction in growth velocity may occur when corticosteroids are administered to pediatric patients by any route (monitor growth). Use with extreme caution in patients with respiratory tuberculosis or untreated systemic infections. Use with caution in patients with hypertension, heart failure, or renal impairment; long-term use has been associated with fluid retention and hypertension. Use with caution in patients with GI diseases (diverticulitis, peptic ulcer, ulcerative colitis) due to risk of GI bleeding and perforation. Use with caution in patients with myasthenia gravis; exacerbation of symptoms has occurred, especially during initial treatment with corticosteroids. Use with caution in patients with hepatic impairment, including cirrhosis; enhanced pharmacologic effect due to decreased metabolism and long-term use has been associated with fluid retention. Use with caution following acute MI; corticosteroids have been associated with myocardial rupture; hypertrophic cardiomyopathy has been reported in premature neonates.

Use with caution in patients with diabetes; corticosteroids may alter glucose regulation, leading to hyperglycemia. Use with caution in patients with cataracts and/or glaucoma; increased intraocular pressure, open-angle glaucoma, and cataracts have occurred with prolonged use; consider routine eye exams in chronic users. Use with caution in patients with a history of seizure disorder; seizures have been reported with adrenal crisis. Use with caution in patients with thyroid dysfunction; changes in thyroid status may necessitate dosage adjustments; metabolic clearance of corticosteroids increases in hyperthyroid patients and decreases in hypothyroid patients. Prolonged treatment with corticosteroids has been associated with the development of Kaposi's sarcoma (case reports); if noted, discontinuation of therapy should be considered. Use with caution in patients with thromboembolic tendencies or thrombophlebitis. Avoid injection into an infected site. Response to killed or inactivated vaccines cannot be predicted in patients receiving immunosuppressive doses of corticosteroids.

Systemic use is not recommended in the treatment of optic neuritis; an increased risk of new episodes may occur.

Adverse Reactions

Cardiovascular: Arrhythmias, bradycardia, cardiac arrest, cardiomegaly, circulatory collapse, congestive heart failure, edema, fat embolism, hypertension, hypertrophic cardiomyopathy in premature infants, myocardial rupture (post MI), syncope, tachycardia, thromboembolism, vasculitis

Central nervous system: Delirium, depression, emotional instability, euphoria, hallucinations, headache, intracranial pressure increased, insomnia, malaise, mood swings, nervousness, neuritis, personality changes, psychic disorders, pseudotumor cerebri (usually following discontinuation), seizure, vertigo

◄ Dermatologic: Acne, allergic dermatitis, alopecia, dry scaly skin, ecchymoses, edema, erythema, hirsutism, hyper-/hypopigmentation, hypertrichosis, impaired wound healing, petechiae, rash, skin atrophy, sterile abscess, skin test reaction impaired, striae, urticaria

Endocrine & metabolic: Adrenal suppression, amenorrhea, carbohydrate intolerance increased, Cushing's syndrome, diabetes mellitus, fluid retention, glucose intolerance, growth suppression (children), hyperglycemia, hyperlipidemia, hypokalemia, hypokalemic alkalosis, menstrual irregularities, negative nitrogen balance, pituitary-adrenal axis suppression, protein catabolism, sodium and water retention

Gastrointestinal: Abdominal distention, appetite increased, bowel/bladder dysfunction (after intrathecal administration), gastrointestinal hemorrhage, gastrointestinal perforation, nausea, pancreatitis, peptic ulcer, perforation of the small and large intestine, ulcerative esophagitis, vomiting, weight gain

Hematologic: Leukocytosis (transient)

Hepatic: Hepatomegaly, transaminases increased

Local: Postinjection flare (intra-articular use), thrombophlebitis

Neuromuscular & skeletal: Arthralgia, arthropathy, aseptic necrosis (femoral and humoral heads), fractures, muscle mass loss, muscle weakness, myopathy (particularly in conjunction with neuromuscular disease or neuromuscular-blocking agents), neuropathy, osteoporosis, parasthesia, tendon rupture, vertebral compression fractures, weakness

Ocular: Cataracts, exophthalmoses, glaucoma, intraocular pressure increased

Renal: Glycosuria

Respiratory: Pulmonary edema

Miscellaneous: Abnormal fat disposition, anaphylactoid reaction, anaphylaxis, angioedema, avascular necrosis, diaphoresis, hiccups, hypersensitivity reactions, infections, secondary malignancy

Rare but important or life-threatening: Venous thrombosis (Johannesdottir, 2013)

Drug Interactions

Metabolism/Transport Effects Substrate of CYP3A4 (minor); **Note:** Assignment of Major/Minor substrate status based on clinically relevant drug interaction potential; **Inhibits** CYP2C8 (weak), CYP3A4 (weak)

Avoid Concomitant Use

Avoid concomitant use of MethylPREDNISolone with any of the following: Aldesleukin; BCG; Indium 111 Capromab Pendetide; Mifepristone; Natalizumab; Pimecrolimus; Pimozide; Tacrolimus (Topical); Tofacitinib

Increased Effect/Toxicity

MethylPREDNISolone may increase the levels/effects of: Acetylcholinesterase Inhibitors; Amphotericin B; Androgens; ARIPiprazole; Ceritinib; CycloSPORINE (Systemic); Deferasirox; Dofetilide; Leflunomide; Lomitapide; Loop Diuretics; Natalizumab; NSAID (COX-2 Inhibitor); NSAID (Nonselective); Pimozide; Thiazide Diuretics; Tofacitinib; Vaccines (Live); Warfarin

The levels/effects of MethylPREDNISolone may be increased by: Aprepitant; Calcium Channel Blockers (Nondihydropyridine); CycloSPORINE (Systemic); CYP3A4 Inhibitors (Strong); Denosumab; Estrogen Derivatives; Fluconazole; Fosaprepitant; Indacaterol; Macrolide Antibiotics; Mifepristone; Neuromuscular-Blocking Agents (Nondepolarizing); Pimecrolimus; Quinolone Antibiotics; Roflumilast; Salicylates; Tacrolimus (Topical); Telaprevir; Trastuzumab

Decreased Effect

MethylPREDNISolone may decrease the levels/effects of: Aldesleukin; Antidiabetic Agents; BCG; Calcitriol; Coccidioidin Skin Test; Corticorelin; CycloSPORINE (Systemic); Hyaluronidase; Indium 111 Capromab Pendetide; Isoniazid; Salicylates; Sipuleucel-T; Telaprevir; Urea Cycle Disorder Agents; Vaccines (Inactivated)

The levels/effects of MethylPREDNISolone may be decreased by: Aminoglutethimide; Antacids; Barbiturates; Bile Acid Sequestrants; CarBAMazepine; Echinacea; Fosphenytoin; Mifepristone; Mitotane; Phenytoin; Primidone; Rifamycin Derivatives

Stability

Oral: Tablets: Store 20°C to 25°C (68°F to 77°F)

Parenteral:

Methylprednisolone sodium succinate: Store intact vials at 20°C to 25°C (68°F to 77°F). Protect from light. Store reconstituted solutions at 20°C to 25°C (68°F to 77°F); use within 48 hours. Reconstitute with accompanying diluent or bacteriostatic water for injection with benzyl alcohol. May further dilute in D_5W, NS or D_5NS. Stability of parenteral admixture at room temperature (25°C) and at refrigeration temperature (4°C) is 48 hours.

Methylprednisolone acetate: Store at 20°C to 25°C (68°F to 77°F). Do **not** dilute or mix with other solutions.

Mechanism of Action In a tissue-specific manner, corticosteroids regulate gene expression subsequent to binding specific intracellular receptors and translocation into the nucleus. Corticosteroids exert a wide array of physiologic effects including modulation of carbohydrate, protein, and lipid metabolism and maintenance of fluid and electrolyte homeostasis. Moreover cardiovascular, immunologic, musculoskeletal, endocrine, and neurologic physiology are influenced by corticosteroids. Decreases inflammation by suppression of migration of polymorphonuclear leukocytes and reversal of increased capillary permeability.

Pharmacodynamics The time of maximum effects and the duration of these effects is dependent upon the route of administration. See table.

Route	Maximum Effect	Duration
Oral	1-2 hours	30-36 hours
I.M. (acetate)	4-8 days	1-4 weeks
Intra-articular	1 week	1-5 weeks

Pharmacokinetics (Adult data unless noted)

Half-life:

Adolescents: 1.9 + 0.7 hours (n=6; patients 12-20 years of age; Rouster-Stevens, 2008)

Adults: 2.4-3.3 hours (Rohatagi, 1997)

Dosing: Usual Note: Adjust dose depending upon condition being treated and response of patient. The lowest possible dose should be used to control the condition; when dose reduction is possible, the dose should be reduced gradually. In life-threatening situations, parenteral doses larger than the oral dose may be needed. **Only sodium succinate salt may be given I.V.**

Infants, Children, and Adolescents:

Asthma, exacerbation:

Acute, short-course "burst" (NAEPP, 2007):

Infants and Children <12 years:

Oral: 1-2 mg/kg/day in divided doses once or twice daily for 3-10 days; maximum daily dose: 60 mg/day; **Note:** Burst should be continued until symptoms resolve or patient achieves peak expiratory flow 80% of personal best; usually requires 3-10 days of treatment (~5 days on average); longer treatment may be required

I.M. **(acetate):** This may be given in place of short-course "burst" of oral steroids in patients who are vomiting or if compliance is a problem.

Children ≤4 years: 7.5 mg/kg as a one-time dose; maximum dose: 240 mg

Children 5-11 years: 240 mg as a one-time dose

Children ≥12 years and Adolescents:

Oral: 40-60 mg/day in divided doses once or twice daily for 3-10 days; **Note:** Burst should be continued until symptoms resolve and peak expiratory flow is at least 80% of personal best; usually requires 3-10 days of treatment (~5 days on average); longer treatment may be required

I.M. **(acetate):** 240 mg as a one-time dose; **Note:** This may be given in place of short-course "burst" of oral steroids in patients who are vomiting or if compliance is a problem

Hospital/emergency medical care doses:

Infants and Children <12 years: Oral, I.V.: 1-2 mg/kg/day in 2 divided doses; maximum daily dose: 60 mg/**day**; continue until peak expiratory flow is 70% of predicted or personal best

Children ≥12 years and Adolescents: Oral, I.V.: 40-80 mg/day in divided doses once or twice daily until peak expiratory flow is 70% of predicted or personal best

Status asthmaticus (previous NAEPP guidelines; still used by some clinicians): Children: I.V.: Loading dose: 2 mg/kg/dose, then 0.5-1 mg/kg/dose every 6 hours; **Note:** See NAEPP 2007 guidelines for asthma exacerbations (emergency medical care or hospital doses) listed above

Asthma, long-term treatment (maintenance) (NAEPP, 2007):

Infants and Children <12 years: Oral: 0.25-2 mg/kg/day once daily in the morning or every other day as needed for asthma control; maximum daily dose: 60 mg/**day**

Children ≥12 years and Adolescents: Oral: 7.5-60 mg daily once daily in the morning or every other day as needed for asthma control

Anti-inflammatory or immunosuppressive: Oral, I.M. (acetate or succinate), I.V. (succinate): 0.5-1.7 mg/kg/day or 5-25 mg/m^2/day in divided doses every 6-12 hours

"Pulse" therapy: I.V. (succinate): 15-30 mg/kg/dose once daily for 3 days; maximum dose: 1000 mg

Lupus nephritis: Children and Adolescents: I.V. (succinate): High-dose "pulse" therapy: 30 mg/kg/dose or 600-1000 mg/m^2/dose once daily for 3 days; maximum dose: 1000 mg (Adams, 2006; Marks, 2010)

Spinal cord injury, acute: Children and Adolescents: I.V. (succinate): 30 mg/kg over 15 minutes followed in 45 minutes by a continuous infusion of 5.4 mg/kg/hour for 23 hours; **Note:** Due to insufficient evidence of clinical efficacy (ie, preserving or improving spinal cord function), the routine use of methylprednisolone in the treatment of acute spinal cord injury is no longer recommended. If used in this setting, methylprednisolone should not be initiated >8 hours after the injury; not effective in penetrating trauma (eg, gunshot) (Consortium for Spinal Cord Medicine, 2008).

***Pneumocystis* pneumonia; moderate or severe infection: Note:** Initiate therapy within 72 hours of diagnosis, if possible.

Infants and Children: I.V. (succinate): 1 mg/kg/dose every 6 hours on days 1-7, then 1 mg/kg/dose twice daily on days 8-9, then 0.5 mg/kg/dose twice daily on days 10 and 11, and 1 mg/kg/dose once daily on days 12-16 (CDC, 2009)

Adolescents: I.V. (succinate): 30 mg twice daily on days 1-5, then 30 mg once daily on days 6-10, then 15 mg once daily on days 11-21 (CDC, 2009a)

Graft-versus-host disease, acute (GVHD): I.V. (succinate): 1-2 mg/kg/dose once daily; if using low dose (1 mg/kg) and no improvement after 3 days, increase dose to 2 mg/kg. Continue therapy for 5-7 days; if improvement observed, may taper by 10% of starting dose every 4 days; if no improvement, then considered

steroid-refractory GVHD and additional agents should be considered (Carpenter, 2010)

Adults:

Allergic conditions: Oral: Tapered-dosage schedule (eg, dose-pack containing 21 x 4 mg tablets):

Day 1: 24 mg on day 1 administered as 8 mg (2 tablets) before breakfast, 4 mg (1 tablet) after lunch, 4 mg (1 tablet) after supper, and 8 mg (2 tablets) at bedtime **OR** 24 mg (6 tablets) as a single dose or divided into 2 or 3 doses upon initiation (regardless of time of day)

Day 2: 20 mg on day 2 administered as 4 mg (1 tablet) before breakfast, 4 mg (1 tablet) after lunch, 4 mg (1 tablet) after supper, and 8 mg (2 tablets) at bedtime

Day 3: 16 mg on day 3 administered as 4 mg (1 tablet) before breakfast, 4 mg (1 tablet) after lunch, 4 mg (1 tablet) after supper, and 4 mg (1 tablet) at bedtime

Day 4: 12 mg on day 4 administered as 4 mg (1 tablet) before breakfast, 4 mg (1 tablet) after lunch, and 4 mg (1 tablet) at bedtime

Day 5: 8 mg on day 5 administered as 4 mg (1 tablet) before breakfast and 4 mg (1 tablet) at bedtime

Day 6: 4 mg on day 6 administered as 4 mg (1 tablet) before breakfast

Anti-inflammatory or immunosuppressive:

Oral: 2-60 mg/day in 1-4 divided doses to start, followed by gradual reduction in dosage to the lowest possible level consistent with maintaining an adequate clinical response

I.M. (sodium succinate): 10-80 mg/day once daily

I.M. (acetate): 10-80 mg every 1-2 weeks

I.V. (sodium succinate): 10-40 mg over a period of several minutes and repeated I.V. or I.M. at intervals depending on clinical response; when high dosages are needed, give 30 mg/kg over a period ≥30 minutes and may be repeated every 4-6 hours for 48 hours

Arthritis: Intra-articular (acetate): Administer every 1-5 weeks

Large joints (eg, knee, ankle): 20-80 mg

Medium joints (eg, elbow, wrist): 10-40 mg

Small joints: 4-10 mg

Asthma exacerbations, including status asthmaticus (emergency medical care or hospital doses): Oral, I.V.: 40-80 mg/day in 1-2 divided doses until peak expiratory flow is 70% of predicted or personal best (NIH Asthma Guidelines, NAEPP, 2007)

Asthma, severe persistent, long-term control: Oral: 7.5-60 mg/day (or on alternate days) (NIH Asthma Guidelines, NAEPP, 2007)

Dermatitis, acute severe: I.M. (acetate): 80-120 mg as a single dose

Dermatitis, chronic: I.M. (acetate): 40-120 mg every 5-10 days

Dermatologic conditions (eg, keloids, lichen planus): Intralesional (acetate): 20-60 mg

Dermatomyositis/polymyositis: I.V. (sodium succinate): 1000 mg/day for 3-5 days for severe muscle weakness, followed by conversion to oral prednisone (Drake, 1996)

Lupus nephritis: High-dose "pulse" therapy: I.V. (sodium succinate): 500-1000 mg/day for 3 days (Ponticelli, 2010)

***Pneumocystis* pneumonia in AIDS patients:** I.V.: 30 mg twice daily for 5 days, then 30 mg once daily for 5 days, then 15 mg once daily for 11 days

Dosing adjustment in renal impairment: Slightly dialyzable (5% to 20%); administer dose posthemodialysis

Administration

Oral: Administer after meals or with food or milk; do not administer with grapefruit juice; if prescribed once daily, administer dose in the early morning to mimic the normal diurnal variation of endogenous cortisol

◀ Parenteral:

I.M.: **Acetate, Succinate:** Avoid injection into the deltoid muscle due to a high incidence of subcutaneous atrophy. Do not inject into areas that have evidence of acute local infection. Discard contents of single-dose vial after use.

I.V.: **Succinate:** Rate dependent upon dose; typically intermittent infusion is administered over 15-60 minutes. Do not administer moderate or high dose I.V. push; severe adverse effects, including hypotension, cardiac arrhythmia, and sudden death, have been reported in patients receiving high-dose methylprednisolone I.V. push over <20 minutes. **Do not give acetate form I.V.**

Low dose (eg, ≤1.8 mg/kg or ≤125 mg/dose): I.V. push over 3-15 minutes; maximum concentration: 125 mg/mL

Moderate dose (eg, ≥2 mg/kg or 250 mg/dose): Administer over 15-30 minutes

High dose (eg, ≥15 mg/kg or ≥500 mg/dose): Administer over 30-60 minutes; doses ≥1000 mg: Administer over 60 minutes. **Note:** In some of the adult spinal cord injury trials, bolus doses (30 mg/kg) have been administered over 15 minutes.

Monitoring Parameters Blood pressure, serum glucose, potassium, and calcium and clinical presence of adverse effects. Monitor intraocular pressure (if therapy >6 weeks), linear growth of pediatric patients (with chronic use), assess HPA suppression

Test Interactions Interferes with skin tests

Additional Information Sodium content of 1 g sodium succinate injection: 2.01 mEq; methylprednisolone sodium succinate 53 mg = methylprednisolone base 40 mg

Dosage Forms Excipient information presented when available (limited, particularly for generics); consult specific product labeling.

Solution Reconstituted, Injection, as sodium succinate [strength expressed as base]:

A-Methapred: 40 mg (1 ea); 125 mg (1 ea) [contains benzyl alcohol]

Solu-MEDROL: 500 mg (1 ea); 1000 mg (1 ea)

Solu-MEDROL: 2 g (1 ea) [contains benzyl alcohol]

Generic: 40 mg (1 ea); 125 mg (1 ea); 1000 mg (1 ea)

Solution Reconstituted, Injection, as sodium succinate [strength expressed as base, preservative free]:

Solu-MEDROL: 40 mg (1 ea); 125 mg (1 ea); 500 mg (1 ea); 1000 mg (1 ea)

Suspension, Injection, as acetate:

Depo-Medrol: 20 mg/mL (5 mL); 40 mg/mL (5 mL, 10 mL) [contains benzyl alcohol, polyethylene glycol, polysorbate 80]

Depo-Medrol: 40 mg/mL (1 mL) [contains polyethylene glycol]

Depo-Medrol: 80 mg/mL (1 mL)

Depo-Medrol: 80 mg/mL (5 mL) [contains benzyl alcohol, polyethylene glycol, polysorbate 80]

Depo-Medrol: 80 mg/mL (1 mL) [contains polyethylene glycol]

Generic: 40 mg/mL (1 mL, 5 mL, 10 mL); 80 mg/mL (1 mL, 5 mL)

Tablet, Oral:

Medrol: 2 mg, 4 mg, 8 mg, 16 mg, 32 mg [scored]

Medrol (Pak): 4 mg [scored]

Generic: 4 mg, 8 mg, 16 mg, 32 mg

References

Adams A, MacDermott EJ, and Lehman TJ, "Pharmacotherapy of Lupus Nephritis in Children: A Recommended Treatment Approach," *Drugs*, 2006, 66(9):1191-207.

Alade SL, Brown RE, and Paquet A Jr, "Polysorbate 80 and E-Ferol Toxicity," *Pediatrics*, 1986, 77(4):593-7.

Anderson GG, Rotchell Y, and Kaiser DG, "Placental Transfer of Methylprednisolone Following Maternal Intravenous Administration," *Am J Obstet Gynecol*, 1981, 140(6):699-701.

Bae YS, Van Voorhees AS, Hsu S, et al, "Review of Treatment Options For Psoriasis in Pregnant or Lactating Women: From the Medical Board of the National Psoriasis Foundation," *J Am Acad Dermatol*, 2012, 67(3):459-77.

Carpenter PA and Macmillan ML, "Management of Acute Graft-Versus-Host Disease in Children," *Pediatr Clin North Am*, 2010, 57(1):273-95.

Centers for Disease Control (CDC), "Guidelines for Prevention and Treatment of Opportunistic Infections in HIV-Infected Adults and Adolescents: Recommendations From CDC, the National Institutes of Health, and the HIV Medicine Association of the Infectious Diseases Society of America," *MMWR Recomm Rep*, 2009a, 58(RR-4):1-207.

Centers for Disease Control (CDC), "Guidelines for the Prevention and Treatment of Opportunistic Infections among HIV-Exposed and HIV-Infected Children: Recommendations From CDC, the National Institutes of Health, the HIV Medicine Association of the Infectious Diseases Society of America, the Pediatric Infectious Diseases Society, and the American Academy of Pediatrics," *MMWR Recomm Rep*, 2009, 58(RR-11):1-166.

Centers for Disease Control (CDC), "Unusual Syndrome With Fatalities Among Premature Infants: Association With a New Intravenous Vitamin E Product," *MMWR Morb Mortal Wkly Rep*, 1984, 33 (14):198-9.

Consortium for Spinal Cord Medicine, "Early Acute Management in Adults With Spinal Cord Injury: A Clinical Practice Guideline for Health-Care Professionals," *J Spinal Cord Med*, 2008, 31(4):403-79.

Lam DS, Fan DS, Ng JS, et al, "Ocular Hypertensive and Anti-Inflammatory Responses to Different Dosages of Topical Dexamethasone in Children: A Randomized Trial," *Clin Experiment Ophthalmol*, 2005, 33 (3):252-8.

Leachman SA and Reed BR, "The Use of Dermatologic Drugs in Pregnancy and Lactation," *Dermatol Clin*, 2006, 24(2):167-97, vi.

Leonard MB, "Glucocorticoid-Induced Osteoporosis in Children: Impact of the Underlying Disease," *Pediatrics*, 2007, 119 Suppl 2:S166-74.

Lunghi L, Pavan B, Biondi C, et al, "Use of Glucocorticoids in Pregnancy," *Curr Pharm Des*, 2010, 16(32):3616-37.

Makol A, Wright K, and Amin S, "Rheumatoid Arthritis and Pregnancy: Safety Considerations in Pharmacological Management," *Drugs*, 2011, 71(15):1973-87.

Marks SD and Tullus K, "Modern Therapeutic Strategies for Paediatric Systemic Lupus Erythematosus and Lupus Nephritis," *Acta Paediatr*, 2010, 99(7):967-74.

National Asthma Education and Prevention Program (NAEPP), "Expert Panel Report 3 (EPR-3): Guidelines for the Diagnosis and Management of Asthma," *Clinical Practice Guidelines*, National Institutes of Health, National Heart, Lung, and Blood Institute, NIH Publication No. 08-4051, prepublication 2007; available at http://www.nhlbi.nih.gov/guidelines/asthma/asthgdln.htm.

National Asthma Education and Prevention Program (NAEPP) Working Group Report on "Managing Asthma During Pregnancy: Recommendations For Pharmacologic Treatment," National Institutes of Health, National Heart, Lung, and Blood Institute, NIH Publication No. 05-5236, March 2005. Available at http://www.nhlbi.nih.gov/health/prof/lung/asthma/astpreg/astpreg_full.pdf

Østensen M and Forger F, "Management of RA Medications in Pregnant Patients," *Nat Rev Rheumatol*, 2009, 5(7):382-90.

Ost L, Wettrell G, Bjorkhem I, et al, "Prednisolone Excretion in Human Milk," *J Pediatr*, 1985, 106(6):1008-11.

Park-Wyllie L, Mazzotta P, Pastuszak A, et al, "Birth defects After Maternal Exposure to Corticosteroids: Prospective Cohort Study and Meta-Analysis of Epidemiological Studies," *Teratology*, 2000, 62 (6):385-92.

Ponticelli C, Glassock RJ, and Moroni G, "Induction and Maintenance Therapy in Proliferative Lupus Nephritis," *J Nephrol*, 2010, 23(1):9-16.

Pradat P, Robert-Gnansia E, Di Tanna GL, et al, "First Trimester Exposure to Corticosteroids and Oral Clefts," *Birth Defects Res A Clin Mol Teratol*, 2003, 67(12):968-70.

Rohatagi S, Barth J, Möllmann H, et al, "Pharmacokinetics of Methylprednisolone and Prednisolone After Single and Multiple Oral Administration," *J Clin Pharmacol*, 1997, 37(10):916-25.

Rouster-Stevens KA, Gursahaney A, Ngai KL, et al, "Pharmacokinetic Study of Oral Prednisolone Compared With Intravenous Methylprednisolone in Patients With Juvenile Dermatomyositis," *Arthritis Rheum*, 2008, 59(2):222-6.

◆ **6-α-Methylprednisolone** see MethylPREDNISolone on page 1386

◆ **Methylprednisolone Acetate** see MethylPREDNISolone on page 1386

◆ **Methylprednisolone Sodium Succinate** see MethylPREDNISolone on page 1386

◆ **4-Methylpyrazole** see Fomepizole on page 927

◆ **Methylrosaniline Chloride** see Gentian Violet on page 968

◆ **Methylthionine Chloride** *see* Methylene Blue
on page 1377

◆ **Methylthioninium Chloride** *see* Methylene Blue
on page 1377

Metoclopramide (met oh KLOE pra mide)

Medication Safety Issues
Sound-alike/look-alike issues:
Metoclopramide may be confused with metolazone, metoprolol, metroNIDAZOLE
Reglan may be confused with Megace, Regonol, Renagel, Regitine

BEERS Criteria medication:
This drug may be potentially inappropriate for use in geriatric patients (Quality of evidence - moderate; Strength of recommendation - strong).

Brand Names: U.S. Metozolv ODT; Reglan

Brand Names: Canada Apo-Metoclop; Metoclopramide Hydrochloride Injection; Metoclopramide Omega; Metonia; Nu-Metoclopramide; PMS-Metoclopramide

Therapeutic Category Antiemetic; Gastrointestinal Agent, Prokinetic

Generic Availability (U.S.) May be product dependent

Use
Oral (orally disintegrating tablet [Metizolv ODT], solution, tablet): Symptomatic treatment of gastroesophageal reflux; diabetic gastroparesis (All indications: FDA approved in adults)
Parenteral: Symptomatic treatment of acute and recurrent diabetic gastroparesis; prevention of nausea and vomiting associated with chemotherapy; prevention of postoperative nausea and vomiting (All indications: FDA approved in adults); facilitates intubation of the small intestine (postpyloric placement of enteral feeding tube) (FDA approved in pediatric patients [age not specified] and adults)

Medication Guide Available Yes

Pregnancy Risk Factor B

Pregnancy Considerations Adverse events were not observed in animal reproduction studies. Metoclopramide crosses the placenta and can be detected in cord blood and amniotic fluid (Arvela, 1983; Bylsma-Howell, 1983). Available evidence suggests safe use during pregnancy (Berkovitch, 2002; Matok, 2009; Sørensen, 2000). Metoclopramide may be used for the treatment of nausea and vomiting of pregnancy (ACOG, 2004; Levichek, 2002) and prophylaxis for nausea and vomiting associated with cesarean delivery (ASA, 2007; Mahadevan, 2006; Smith, 2011). Other agents are preferred for gastroesophageal reflux (Mahadevan, 2006).

Breast-Feeding Considerations Metoclopramide enters breast milk. Information is available from studies conducted in mothers nursing preterm infants (n=14; delivered at 23-34 weeks gestation) or term infants (n=18) and taking metoclopramide 10 mg 3 times daily. The median concentration of metoclopramide in breast milk was ~45 ng/mL in the preterm infants and the mean concentration was ~48 ng/mL in the full term infants. The authors of both studies calculated the relative infant dose to be 3% to 5%, based on a therapeutic infant dose of 0.5 mg/kg/day. Metoclopramide was also detected in the serum of one nursing full term infant (Hansen, 2005; Kauppila, 1983). Metoclopramide may increase prolactin concentrations and cause galactorrhea and gynecomastia, but studies which evaluated its use to increase milk production for women who want to nurse have had mixed results. In addition, due to the potential for adverse events, nonpharmacologic measure should be considered prior to the use of medications as galactagogues (ABM, 2011). The manufacturer recommends that caution be used if administered to a nursing woman.

Contraindications Hypersensitivity to metoclopramide or any component; GI obstruction, perforation or hemorrhage; pheochromocytoma, history of seizure disorder; concomitant medications likely to cause extrapyramidal reactions

Warnings May cause tardive dyskinesia, which is often irreversible **[U.S. Boxed Warning]**; duration of treatment and total cumulative dose are associated with an increased risk. Therapy durations >12 weeks should be avoided (except in rare cases following risk:benefit assessment). Risk appears to be increased in the elderly, women, and diabetics; however, it is not possible to predict which patients will develop tardive dyskinesia. Therapy should be discontinued in any patient if signs or symptoms appear.

Extrapyramidal symptoms (EPS) may occur, most frequently in children and young adults (<30 years of age); generally manifested as acute dystonic reactions within the initial 24-48 hours of use; risk of these reactions is increased with I.V. administration of higher doses.

Pseudoparkinsonism (eg, bradykinesia, tremor, rigidity) may also occur (usually within first 6 months of therapy) and is generally reversible following discontinuation. Neuroleptic malignant syndrome has been associated (rarely) with metoclopramide use; monitor for mental status changes, fever, muscle rigidity, and/or autonomic instability; discontinue use if signs/symptoms appear.

Patients with NADH-cytochrome b5 reductase deficiency are at increased risk for developing methemoglobinemia and/or sulfhemoglobinemia. Neonates have prolonged clearance of metoclopramide which may lead to increased serum concentrations. In addition, neonates may have decreased NADH-cytochrome b5 reductase activity. Both conditions increase the risk of developing methemoglobinemia.

Mental depression has occurred with metoclopramide use including in patients without a history of depression; symptoms range from mild to severe (suicidal ideation and suicide); use with caution in patients with a history of mental illness.

Some products contain sodium benzoate; benzoic acid (benzoate) is a metabolite of benzyl alcohol; large amounts of benzyl alcohol (≥99 mg/kg/day) have been associated with a potentially fatal toxicity ("gasping syndrome") in neonates; the "gasping syndrome" consists of metabolic acidosis, respiratory distress, gasping respirations, CNS dysfunction (including convulsions, intracranial hemorrhage), hypotension, and cardiovascular collapse; use products containing sodium benzoate with caution in neonates; *in vitro* and animal studies have shown that benzoate displaces bilirubin from protein binding sites.

Precautions Use with caution in patients with renal impairment; dosage adjustment may be needed. Use with caution in patients at risk of fluid overload (eg,CHF, cirrhosis); may cause transient increases in plasma aldosterone which could result in fluid retention or volume overload; use lowest recommended doses initially and discontinue therapy if signs/symptoms appear. Use with caution in patients with hypertension; metoclopramide has been shown to release catecholamines; use is contraindicated with pheochromocytoma because metoclopramide may cause hypertensive crisis. Use with caution following surgical anastomosis/closure; promotility agents may theoretically increase pressure in suture lines. Abrupt discontinuation may (rarely) result in withdrawal symptoms (dizziness, headache, nervousness).

Adverse Reactions
Cardiovascular: Atrioventricular block, bradycardia, congestive heart failure, flushing (following high I.V. doses), hypertension, hypotension, supraventricular tachycardia
Central nervous system: Akathisia, confusion, depression, dizziness, drowsiness (dose related), drug-induced ▶

Parkinson's disease, dystonic reaction (dose and age related), fatigue, hallucination (rare), headache, insomnia, lassitude, neuroleptic malignant syndrome (rare), restlessness, seizure, somnolence, suicidal ideation, tardive dyskinesia

Dermatologic: Skin rash, urticaria

Endocrine & metabolic: Amenorrhea, fluid retention, galactorrhea, gynecomastia, hyperprolactinemia, porphyria

Gastrointestinal: Diarrhea, nausea, vomiting

Genitourinary: Impotence, urinary frequency, urinary incontinence

Hematologic & oncologic: Agranulocytosis, leukopenia, methemoglobinemia, neutropenia, sulfhemoglobinemia

Hepatic: Hepatotoxicity (rare)

Hypersensitivity: Angioedema (rare), hypersensitivity reaction

Neuromuscular & skeletal: Laryngospasm (rare)

Ophthalmic: Visual disturbance

Respiratory: Bronchospasm, laryngeal edema (rare)

Drug Interactions

Metabolism/Transport Effects Substrate of CYP1A2 (minor), CYP2D6 (minor); **Note:** Assignment of Major/ Minor substrate status based on clinically relevant drug interaction potential; **Inhibits** CYP2D6 (weak)

Avoid Concomitant Use

Avoid concomitant use of Metoclopramide with any of the following: Antipsychotics; Droperidol; Promethazine; Tetrabenazine; Trimetazidine

Increased Effect/Toxicity

Metoclopramide may increase the levels/effects of: Antipsychotics; CycloSPORINE (Systemic); Prilocaine; Promethazine; Selective Serotonin Reuptake Inhibitors; Sodium Nitrite; Tetrabenazine; Tricyclic Antidepressants; Trimetazidine; Venlafaxine

The levels/effects of Metoclopramide may be increased by: Droperidol; Metyrosine; Nitric Oxide; Serotonin Modulators

Decreased Effect

Metoclopramide may decrease the levels/effects of: Anti-Parkinson's Agents (Dopamine Agonist); Atovaquone; Posaconazole; Quinagolide

The levels/effects of Metoclopramide may be decreased by: Peginterferon Alfa-2b

Stability

Oral: Store at 20°C to 25°C (68°F to 77°F); protect tablets and oral solution from light.

Parenteral: Store intact vial at 20°C to 25°C (68°F to 77°F); protect from light. Do not freeze. Dilutions may be stored unprotected from light for up to 24 hours after preparation.

Mechanism of Action Blocks dopamine receptors and (when given in higher doses) also blocks serotonin receptors in chemoreceptor trigger zone of the CNS; enhances the response to acetylcholine of tissue in upper GI tract causing enhanced motility and accelerated gastric emptying without stimulating gastric, biliary, or pancreatic secretions; increases lower esophageal sphincter tone

Pharmacodynamics

Onset of action:

Oral: Within 30-60 minutes

I.M.: Within 10-15 minutes

I.V.: Within 1-3 minutes

Duration: Therapeutic effects persist for 1-2 hours, regardless of route administered

Pharmacokinetics (Adult data unless noted)

Absorption: Oral: Rapid

Distribution: V_d:

Neonates, PMA 31 to 40 weeks: 6.94 L/kg (Kearns, 1998)

Infants: 4.4 L/kg

Children: 3 L/kg

Adults: 3.5 L/kg

Protein binding: ~30%

Bioavailability: Oral: 80 ± 15.5%

Half-life: Normal renal function:

Neonates, PMA 31 to 40 weeks: 5.4 hours (Kearns, 1998)

Infants: 4.15 hours (range: 2.23 to 10.3 hours) (Kearns, 1988)

Children: ~4 hours (range: 2 to 12.5 hours); half-life and clearance may be dose-dependent

Adults: 5 to 6 hours

Time to peak serum concentration: Oral:

Neonates, PMA 31 to 40 weeks: 2.45 hours (Kearns, 1998)

Infants: 2.2 hours

Adults: 1 to 2 hours

Elimination: Primarily in the urine (~85%) and feces

Dosing: Neonatal Gastroesophageal reflux: Limited data available: Oral, I.M., I.V.: Usual dose: 0.1 mg/kg/dose every 6 hours (Avery, 1994; Kimball, 2001); higher doses of 0.15 mg/kg/dose have been reported in a pharmacokinetic study of 10 preterm neonates (PMA: 31 to 40 weeks) (Kearns, 1998). In a small case series of previous VLBW (n=6; GA: 26 to 35 weeks; birth weight: 790 to 1040 g; mean PNA at treatment: 35 days), a lower dose of 0.033 mg/kg every 8 hours was reported effective in all patients (Sankaran, 1982). Doses >0.15 mg/kg may increase potential for adverse effects due to excessive serum concentrations (Kearns, 1998).

Dosing: Usual

Pediatric:

Postpyloric feeding tube placement (short bowel intubation): I.V.:

Patient age:

<6 years: 0.1 mg/kg as a single dose

6 to 14 years: 2.5 to 5 mg as a single dose

>14 years: 10 mg as a single dose

Gastroesophageal reflux: Limited data available; efficacy results variable (Vandenplas, 2009): **Note:** NASP-GHAN/ESPGHAN guidelines do not recommend metoclopramide for routine treatment of GERD; evaluate risk:benefit prior to use (Vandenplas, 2009): Infants, Children, and Adolescents: Oral: 0.1 to 0.2 mg/kg/dose every 6 to 8 hours; maximum dose: 10 mg (Chicella, 2005; Forbes, 1986; Rode, 1987; Tolia, 1989)

Postoperative nausea and vomiting; prevention: Limited data available; optimal dose not established; efficacy results variable: **Note:** Guidelines discourage use of metoclopramide; considered ineffective (Gan, 2007): Children and Adolescents: I.V: 0.1 to 0.5 mg/kg/dose as a single dose administered after induction or on arrival to PACU; maximum dose: 10 mg/dose (Ferrari, 1992; Furst, 1994; Henzi, 1999; Lin, 1992)

Chemotherapy-induced nausea and vomiting (CINV); prevention: Limited data available; optimal dose not established; efficacy results variable. **Note:** Doses required to prevent CINV are high and should not be used first-line due to increased risk of extrapyramidal symptoms (acute dystonic reactions); concurrent administration of diphenhydramine or benztropine is recommended to prevent drug-induced adverse effects (Dupuis, 2013; Roila, 1998).

POGO Guidelines (Dupuis, 2013): Infants, Children and Adolescents: **Note:** For use in patients in whom corticosteroids are contraindicated; use in combination with 5-HT$_3$ receptor antagonists.

Initial dose: I.V.: 1 mg/kg as a single dose prior to chemotherapy

Subsequent doses: Oral: 0.0375 mg/kg/dose every 6 hours

Alternate dosing: Children and Adolescents: I.V.: 1 to 2 mg/kg/dose prior to and then every 2 to 4 hours up to every 6 hours following chemotherapy; maximum: 5 doses/day (Roila, 1998; Terrin, 1984); another trial administered 2 mg/kg when chemotherapy was started followed by 2 mg/kg/dose 2, 6, and 12 hours later (Marshall, 1989)

Adult:

Diabetic gastroparesis:

Oral: 10 mg up to 4 times daily 30 minutes before meals and at bedtime for 2 to 8 weeks. Treatment >12 weeks is not recommended.

I.M., I.V. (for severe symptoms): 10 mg over 1 to 2 minutes; 10 days of I.V. therapy may be necessary before symptoms are controlled to allow transition to oral administration

Chemotherapy-induced emesis prophylaxis: I.V.: 1 to 2 mg/kg 30 minutes before chemotherapy and repeated every 2 hours for 2 doses, then every 3 hours for 3 doses (manufacturer's labeling); pretreatment with diphenhydramine will decrease risk of extrapyramidal reactions

Alternate dosing: **Note:** Metoclopramide is considered an antiemetic with a low therapeutic index; use is generally reserved for agents with low emetogenic potential or in patients intolerant/refractory to first-line antiemetics.

Low-risk chemotherapy: I.V., Oral: 10 to 40 mg prior to chemotherapy dose, then every 4 to 6 hours as needed (NCCN Antiemesis guidelines, v.1.2013)

Breakthrough treatment: I.V., Oral: 10 to 40 mg every 4 to 6 hours (NCCN Antiemesis guidelines, v.1.2013)

Delayed-emesis prophylaxis: Oral: 20 to 40 mg (or 0.5 mg/kg/dose) 2 to 4 times daily for 3 to 4 days (in combination with dexamethasone (ASCO guidelines [Kris, 2006])

Refractory or intolerant to antiemetics with a higher therapeutic index (Hesketh, 2008):

I.V.: 1 to 2 mg/kg/dose before chemotherapy and repeat 2 hours after chemotherapy

Oral: 0.5 mg/kg every 6 hours on days 2 to 4

Gastroesophageal reflux: Oral: 10 to 15 mg up to 4 times daily 30 minutes before meals or food and at bedtime; single doses of 20 mg are occasionally needed prior to provoking situations. Treatment >12 weeks is not recommended.

Postoperative nausea and vomiting prophylaxis: I.M., I.V.: 10 to 20 mg near end of surgery. **Note:** Guidelines discourage use of 10 mg metoclopramide as being ineffective (Gan, 2007); comparative study indicates higher dose (20 mg) may be efficacious (Quaynor, 2002).

Postpyloric feeding tube placement, radiological exam: I.V.: 10 mg as a single dose

Dosing adjustment in renal impairment:

Infants, Children, and Adolescents: The following adjustments have been recommended (Aronoff, 2007). **Note:** Renally adjusted dose recommendations are based on doses of 0.1 to 0.2 mg/kg/dose every 6 to 8 hours.

GFR 30 to 50 mL/minute/1.73 m^2: Administer 75% of dose

GFR 10 to 29 mL/minute/1.73 m^2: Administer 50% of dose

GFR <10 mL/minute/1.73 m^2: Administer 25% of dose

Intermittent hemodialysis: Administer 25% of dose

Peritoneal dialysis (PD): Administer 25% of dose

Continuous renal replacement therapy (CRRT): Administer 75% of dose

Adults:

CrCl <40 mL/minute: Administer 50% of recommended dose

Not dialyzable (0% to 5%); supplemental dose is not necessary

Dosing adjustment in hepatic impairment: There are no dosage adjustments provided in the manufacturer's labeling; however, metoclopramide has been used safely in patients with advanced liver disease with normal renal function.

Administration

Oral:

Orally disintegrating tablets: Administer on an empty stomach at least 30 minutes prior to food. Do not remove from packaging until time of administration. If tablet breaks or crumbles while handling, discard and remove new tablet. Using dry hands, place tablet on tongue and allow to dissolve. Swallow with saliva.

Oral solution, tablet: Administer 30 minutes before meals and at bedtime

Parenteral: May be given I.M., direct I.V. push, or by intermittent infusion. Doses ≤10 mg may be given undiluted (5 mg/mL) by direct I.V push over 1 to 2 minutes; higher doses (>10 mg) should be diluted in 50 mL of compatible solution (preferably NS) and administered over at least 15 minutes; rapid I.V. administration is associated with a transient but intense feeling of anxiety and restlessness, followed by drowsiness

Monitoring Parameters Blood pressure and heart rate (when rapid I.V. administration is used); dystonic reactions, agitation, and confusion

Dosage Forms Excipient information presented when available (limited, particularly for generics); consult specific product labeling.

Solution, Injection:

Generic: 5 mg/mL (2 mL)

Solution, Injection [preservative free]:

Generic: 5 mg/mL (2 mL)

Solution, Oral:

Generic: 5 mg/5 mL (10 mL, 473 mL); 10 mg/10 mL (10 mL)

Tablet, Oral:

Reglan: 5 mg [contains fd&c blue #1 aluminum lake, fd&c yellow #10 aluminum lake]

Reglan: 10 mg [dye free]

Generic: 5 mg, 10 mg

Tablet Dispersible, Oral:

Metozolv ODT: 5 mg

References

Academy of Breastfeeding Medicine Protocol Committee. ABM clinical protocol #9: use of galactogogues in initiating or augmenting the rate of maternal milk secretion (First Revision January 2011). *Breastfeed Med.* 2011;6(1):41-49.

American College of Obstetrics and Gynecology. ACOG practice bulletin: nausea and vomiting of pregnancy. *Obstet Gynecol.* 2004;103 (4):803-814.

American Society of Anesthesiologists (ASA) Task Force on Obstetric Anesthesia. Practice guidelines for obstetric anesthesia: an updated report by the American Society of Anesthesiologists Task Force on Obstetric Anesthesia. *Anesthesiology.* 2007;106(4):843-863.

Aronoff GR, Bennett WM, Berns JS, et al, *Drug Prescribing in Renal Failure: Dosing Guidelines for Adults and Children,* 5th ed. Philadelphia, PA: American College of Physicians; 2007.

Arvela P, Jouppila R, Kauppila A, et al. Placental transfer and hormonal effects of metoclopramide. *Eur J Clin Pharmacol.* 1983;24 (3):345-348.

Avery GB, Fletcher MA, MacDonald MG, eds. *Neonatology - Pathophysiology and Management of the Newborn.* 4th ed. J.B. Philadelphia, PA: Lippincott Company; 1994.

Berkovitch M, Mazzota P, Greenberg R, et al. Metoclopramide for nausea and vomiting of pregnancy: a prospective multicenter international study. *Am J Perinatol.* 2002;19(6):311-316.

Bylsma-Howell M, Riggs KW, McMorland GH, et al. Placental transport of metoclopramide: assessment of maternal and neonatal effects. *Can Anaesth Soc J.* 1983;30(5):487-492.

Chicella MF, Batres LA, Heesters MS, et al, "Prokinetic Drug Therapy in Children: A Review of Current Options," *Ann Pharmacother,* 2005, 39 (4):706-11.

Dupuis LL, Boodhan S, Holdsworth M, et al. Guideline for the prevention of acute nausea and vomiting due to antineoplastic medication in pediatric cancer patients. *Pediatr Blood Cancer.* 2013;60 (7):1073-1082.

Ferrari LR, Donlon JV. Metoclopramide reduces the incidence of vomiting after tonsillectomy in children. *Anesth Analg.* 1992;75(3):351-354.

Forbes D, Hodgson M, Hill R. The effects of gaviscon and metoclopramide in gastroesophageal reflux in children. *J Pediatr Gastroenterol Nutr.* 1986;5(4):556-559.

Furst SR1, Rodarte A. Prophylactic antiemetic treatment with ondansetron in children undergoing tonsillectomy. *Anesthesiology.* 1994;81(4):799-803.

Gan TJ, Meyer TA, Apfel CC, et al, "Society for Ambulatory Anesthesia Guidelines for the Management of Postoperative Nausea and Vomiting," *Anesth Analg,* 2007, 105(6):1615-28.

Hansen WF, McAndrew S, Harris K, Z et al. Metoclopramide effect on breastfeeding the preterm infant: a randomized trial. *Obstet Gynecol.* 2005;105(2):383-9.

Hesketh PJ. Chemotherapy-induced nausea and vomiting. *N Engl J Med.* 2008;358(23):2482-2494.

Henzi I, Walder B, Tramèr MR. Metoclopramide in the prevention of postoperative nausea and vomiting: a quantitative systematic review of randomized, placebo-controlled studies. *Br J Anaesth.* 1999;83(5):761-771.

Kauppila A, Arvela P, Koivisto M, et al. Metoclopramide and breast feeding: transfer into milk and the newborn. *Eur J Clin Pharmacol.* 1983;25(6):819-823.

Kearns GL, Butler HL, Lane JK, Carchman SH, Wright GJ. Metoclopramide pharmacokinetics and pharmacodynamics in infants with gastroesophageal reflux. *J Pediatr Gastroenterol Nutr.* 1988;7(6):823-829.

Kearns GL, van den Anker JN, Reed MD, et al, "Pharmacokinetics of Metoclopramide in Neonates," *J Clin Pharmacol,* 1998, 38(2):122-8.

Kimball AL, Carlton DP. Gastroesophageal reflux medications in the treatment of apnea in premature infants. *J Pediatr.* 2001;138(3):355-360.

Kris MG, Hesketh PJ, Somerfield MR, et al. American Society of Clinical Oncology Guideline for Antiemetics in Oncology: Update 2006. *J Clin Oncol.* 2006;24(18):2932-2946.

Levichek Z, Atanackovic G, Oepkes D, et al. Nausea and vomiting of pregnancy. Evidence-based treatment algorithm. *Can Fam Physician.* 2002;48:267-268, 277.

Lin DM, Furst SR, Rodarte A. A double-blinded comparison of metoclopramide and droperidol for prevention of emesis following strabismus surgery. *Anesthesiology.* 1992;76(3):357-361.

Mahadevan U, Kane S. American gastroenterological association institute technical review on the use of gastrointestinal medications in pregnancy. *Gastroenterology.* 2006;131(1):283-311.

Marshall G, Kerr S, Vowels M, O'Gorman-Hughes D, White L. Antiemetic therapy for chemotherapy-induced vomiting: metoclopramide, benztropine, dexamethasone, and lorazepam regimen compared with chlorpromazine alone. *J Pediatr.* 1989;115(1):156-160.

Matok I, Gorodischer R, Koren G, et al, "The Safety of Metoclopramide Use in the First Trimester of Pregnancy," *N Engl J Med,* 2009, 360(24):2528-35.

Metoclopramide hydrochloride injection [prescribing information]. Irvine, CA: Teva Parenteral Medicines, Inc; November 2012.

Metoclopramide hydrochloride solution [prescribing information].Baudette, MN: ANI Pharmaceuticals, Inc; March 2012.

Metozolv ODT (metoclopramide hydrochloride) [prescribing information]. Raleigh, NC: Salix Pharmaceuticals, Inc; 2011.

National Comprehensive Cancer Network® (NCCN). Clinical Practice Guidelines in Oncology: Antiemesis. Version 1.2013. Available at http://www.nccn.org/professionals/physician_gls/PDF/antiemesis.pdf

Quaynor H, Raeder JC. Incidence and severity of postoperative nausea and vomiting are aimilar after metoclopramide 20 mg and ondansetron 8 mg given by the end of laparoscopic cholecystectomies. *Acta Anaesthesiol Scand.* 2002;46(1):109-113.

Reglan (metoclopramide hydrochloride) [prescribing information]. Baudette, MN: ANI Pharmaceuticals, Inc; September 2011.

Rode H, Stunden RJ, Millar AJ, Cywes S. Esophageal pH assessment of gastroesophageal reflux in 18 patients and the effect of two prokinetic agents: cisapride and metoclopramide. *J Pediatr Surg.* 1987;22(10):931-934.

Roila F, Feyer P, Maranzano E, Olver I, Clark-Snow R, Warr D, Molassiotis A. Antiemetics in children receiving chemotherapy. *Support Care Cancer.* 2005;13(2):129-131.

Sankaran K, Yeboah E, Bingham WT, Ninan A. Use of metoclopramide in preterm infants. *Dev Pharmacol Ther.* 1982;5(3-4):114-119.

Smith I, Kranke P, Murat I, et al. European Society of Anaesthesiology. Perioperative fasting in adults and children: guidelines from the European Society of Anaesthesiology. *Eur J Anaesthesiol.* 2011;28(8):556-569.

Sørensen HT, Nielsen GL, Christensen K, et al. Birth outcome following maternal use of metoclopramide. The Euromap study group. *Br J Clin Pharmacol.* 2000;49(3):264-268.

Terrin BN, McWilliams NB, Maurer HM. Side effects of metoclopramide as an antiemetic in childhood cancer chemotherapy. *J Pediatr.* 1984;104(1):138-140.

Tolia V, Calhoun J, Kuhns L, Kauffman RE. Randomized, prospective double-blind trial of metoclopramide and placebo for gastroesophageal reflux in infants. *J Pediatr.* 1989;115(1):141-145.

Vandenplas Y, Rudolph CD, Di Lorenzo C, et al. Pediatric gastroesophageal reflux clinical practice guidelines: joint recommendations of the North American Society for Pediatric Gastroenterology, Hepatology, and Nutrition (NASPGHAN) and the European Society for Pediatric Gastroenterology, Hepatology, and Nutrition (ESPGHAN). *J Pediatr Gastroenterol Nutr.* 2009;49(4):498-547.

◆ **Metoclopramide Hydrochloride Injection (Can)** *see* Metoclopramide *on page 1391*

◆ **Metoclopramide Omega (Can)** *see* Metoclopramide *on page 1391*

◆ **Metoject (Can)** *see* Methotrexate *on page 1367*

Metolazone (me TOLE a zone)

Medication Safety Issues
Sound-alike/look-alike issues:
Metolazone may be confused with metaxalone, methadone, methazolamide, methimazole, methotrexate, metoclopramide, metoprolol, minoxidil

Zaroxolyn may be confused with Zarontin

Brand Names: U.S. Zaroxolyn

Brand Names: Canada Zaroxolyn

Therapeutic Category Antihypertensive Agent; Diuretic, Miscellaneous

Generic Availability (U.S.) Yes

Use Treatment of hypertension (alone or in combination with other antihypertensive agents); treatment of edema in CHF or renal diseases (including nephrotic syndrome and other states of impaired renal function) (All indications: FDA approved in adults)

Pregnancy Risk Factor B

Pregnancy Considerations Adverse events have not been observed in animal reproduction studies. Metolazone crosses the placenta and appears in cord blood. Hypoglycemia, hypokalemia, hyponatremia, jaundice, and thrombocytopenia are reported as complications to the fetus or newborn following maternal use of thiazide diuretics.

Breast-Feeding Considerations Metolazone is excreted in breast milk. Due to the potential for serious adverse reactions in the nursing infant, the manufacturer recommends a decision be made whether to discontinue nursing or to discontinue the drug, taking into account the importance of treatment to the mother.

Contraindications Hypersensitivity to metolazone or any component; anuria; patients with hepatic coma or precoma

Documentation of allergenic cross-reactivity for diuretics is limited. However, because of similarities in chemical structure and/or pharmacologic actions, the possibility of cross-sensitivity cannot be ruled out with certainty.

Warnings Chemical similarities are present among sulfonamides, sulfonylureas, carbonic anhydrase inhibitors, thiazides, and loop diuretics (except ethacrynic acid). Use with caution in patients with thiazide or sulfonamide allergy; avoid use when previous reaction has been severe. Discontinue if signs of hypersensitivity are noted. Sensitivity reactions, including angioedema and bronchospasm, may occur.

Severe hypokalemia and/or hyponatremia can occur rapidly following initial doses. Hypercalcemia, hypochloremic alkalosis, and/or hypomagnesemia can also occur. Correct hypokalemia before initiating therapy. Large or prolonged fluid and electrolyte losses may occur with concomitant furosemide administration. Orthostatic hypotension may occur.

Potentially significant drug-drug interactions may exist, requiring dose or frequency adjustment, additional monitoring, and/or selection of alternative therapy.

Precautions Use with caution in patients with severe renal disease; if azotemia and oliguria worsen during treatment in these patients, discontinue therapy. Use with caution in diabetes or prediabetes, may see a change in glucose control. Use with caution in SLE, may cause SLE activation or exacerbation. Use with caution in severe hepatic dysfunction. May cause photosensitivity.

Adverse Reactions

Cardiovascular: Chest pain/discomfort, necrotizing angiitis, orthostatic hypotension, palpitation, syncope, venous thrombosis, vertigo, volume depletion

Central nervous system: Chills, depression, dizziness, drowsiness, fatigue, headache, lightheadedness, restlessness

Dermatologic: Petechiae, photosensitivity, pruritus, purpura, rash, skin necrosis, Stevens-Johnson syndrome, toxic epidermal necrolysis, urticaria

Endocrine & metabolic: Gout attacks, hypercalcemia, hyperglycemia, hyperuricemia, hypochloremia, hypochloremic alkalosis, hypokalemia, hypomagnesemia, hyponatremia, hypophosphatemia

Gastrointestinal: Abdominal bloating, abdominal pain, anorexia, constipation, diarrhea, epigastric distress, nausea, pancreatitis, vomiting, xerostomia

Genitourinary: Impotence

Hematologic: Agranulocytosis, aplastic/hypoplastic anemia, hemoconcentration, leukopenia, thrombocytopenia

Hepatic: Cholestatic jaundice, hepatitis

Neuromuscular & skeletal: Joint pain, muscle cramps/spasm, neuropathy, paresthesia, weakness

Ocular: Blurred vision (transient)

Renal: BUN increased, glucosuria

Drug Interactions

Metabolism/Transport Effects None known.

Avoid Concomitant Use

Avoid concomitant use of Metolazone with any of the following: Dofetilide

Increased Effect/Toxicity

Metolazone may increase the levels/effects of: ACE Inhibitors; Allopurinol; Amifostine; Antihypertensives; Calcium Salts; CarBAMazepine; Cyclophosphamide; Diazoxide; Dofetilide; DULoxetine; Hypotensive Agents; Ivabradine; Lithium; Multivitamins/Minerals (with ADEK, Folate, Iron); Multivitamins/Minerals (with AE, No Iron); Obinutuzumab; OXcarbazepine; Porfimer; RiTUXimab; Sodium Phosphates; Topiramate; Toremifene; Vitamin D Analogs

The levels/effects of Metolazone may be increased by: Alcohol (Ethyl); Alfuzosin; Analgesics (Opioid); Anticholinergic Agents; Barbiturates; Beta2-Agonists; Brimonidine (Topical); Corticosteroids (Orally Inhaled); Corticosteroids (Systemic); Diazoxide; Herbs (Hypotensive Properties); Licorice; MAO Inhibitors; Multivitamins/Fluoride (with ADE); Pentoxifylline; Phosphodiesterase 5 Inhibitors; Prostacyclin Analogues; Selective Serotonin Reuptake Inhibitors

Decreased Effect

Metolazone may decrease the levels/effects of: Antidiabetic Agents

The levels/effects of Metolazone may be decreased by: Bile Acid Sequestrants; Herbs (Hypertensive Properties); Methylphenidate; Nonsteroidal Anti-Inflammatory Agents; Yohimbine

Stability Store at 25°C (77°F); excursions permitted to 15°C to 30°C (59°F to 86°F). Protect from light.

Mechanism of Action Inhibits sodium reabsorption in the distal tubules causing increased excretion of sodium and water, as well as, potassium and hydrogen ions

Pharmacodynamics

Onset of action: 1 hour

Duration: 12-24 hours

Pharmacokinetics (Adult data unless noted)

Absorption: Incomplete

Protein binding: 90% to 95%

Half-life: 6-20 hours

Elimination: Enterohepatic recycling; 70% to 95% excreted unchanged in urine

Dosing: Usual

Pediatric: **Edema, refractory:** Children and Adolescents: Oral: Usual range: 0.2-0.4 mg/kg/day divided every 12-24 hours in combination with furosemide; the usual maximum dose in adults is 20 mg (Arnold, 1984; Nelson, 1996). According to the manufacturer, a lower dose of 0.05-0.1 mg/kg once daily has also been reported to result in weight loss and increase urine output in some pediatric patients.

Adult:

Edema (renal disease): Oral: Initial: 5-20 mg once daily.

Edema (heart failure): Oral: Initial: 2.5 mg once daily; maximum daily dose: 20 mg (ACCF/AHA [Yancy, 2013]); **Note:** Dosing frequency may be adjusted based on patient-specific diuretic needs (eg, administration every other day or weekly) (HFSA [Lindenfeld, 2010]).

Hypertension: Oral: Initial: 2.5-5 mg once daily; adjust dose as necessary to achieve maximum therapeutic effect

Dosing adjustment in renal impairment: There are no dosage adjustments provided in the manufacturer's labeling; use caution in patients with severe renal impairment, as most of the drug is excreted by the renal route and accumulation may occur.

Doing adjustment in hepatic impairment: There are no dosage adjustments provided in manufacturer's labeling; contraindicated in hepatic coma or precoma.

Administration Oral: Administer with food to decrease GI distress; administer early in day to avoid nocturia

Monitoring Parameters Serum electrolytes, renal function, blood pressure, body weight, fluid balance

Additional Information Metolazone 5 mg is approximately equivalent to hydrochlorothiazide 50 mg

Dosage Forms Excipient information presented when available (limited, particularly for generics); consult specific product labeling.

Tablet, Oral:

Zaroxolyn: 2.5 mg, 5 mg

Generic: 2.5 mg, 5 mg, 10 mg

Extemporaneous Preparations A 1 mg/mL oral suspension may be made by with tablets and one of three different vehicles (cherry syrup diluted 1:4 with simple syrup; a 1:1 mixture of Ora-Sweet and Ora-Plus; or a 1:1 mixture of Ora-Sweet SF and Ora-Plus). Crush twelve 10 mg tablets in a mortar and reduce to a fine powder. Add small portions of the chosen vehicle and mix to a uniform paste; mix while adding the vehicle in incremental proportions to **almost** 120 mL; transfer to a calibrated bottle, rinse mortar with vehicle, and add quantity of vehicle sufficient to make 120 mL. Label "shake well" and "refrigerate". Stable for 60 days.

A 0.25 mg/mL oral suspension may be made with tablets and a 1:1 mixture of methylcellulose 1% and simple syrup. Crush one 2.5 mg tablet in a mortar and reduce to a fine powder. Add small portions of the vehicle and mix to a uniform paste; mix while adding the vehicle in incremental proportions to **almost** 10 mL; transfer to a calibrated bottle, rinse mortar with vehicle, and add quantity of vehicle sufficient to make 10 mL. Label "shake well" and "refrigerate". Stable for 91 days refrigerated (preferred), 28 days at room temperature in plastic, and 14 days at room temperature in glass.

Nahata, MC, Pai VB, and Hipple TF, *Pediatric Drug Formulations*, 5th ed, Cincinnati, OH: Harvey Whitney Books Co, 2004.

References

Arnold WC, "Efficacy of Metolazone and Furosemide in Children With Furosemide-Resistant Edema," *Pediatrics*, 1984, 74(5):872-5.

Chobanian AV, Bakris GL, Black HR, et al, "The Seventh Report of the Joint National Committee on Prevention, Detection, Evaluation, and Treatment of High Blood Pressure: The JNC 7 Report," *JAMA*, 2003, 289(19):2560-72.

Lindenfeld J, Albert NM, Boehmer JP, et al, "HFSA 2010 Comprehensive Heart Failure Practice Guideline," *J Card Fail*, 2010, 16(6): e1-194.

Nelson WE, Behrman RE, Kliegman RM, et al, eds. *Nelson Textbook of Pediatrics*. 15th ed. Philadelphia, PA: WB Saunders Company; 1996.

Wells TG, "The Pharmacology and Therapeutics of Diuretics in the Pediatric Patient," *Pediatr Clin North Am*, 1990, 37(2):463-504.

Yancy CW, Jessup M, Bozkurt B, et al; American College of Cardiology Foundation/American Heart Association Task Force on Practice Guidelines. 2013 ACCF/AHA guideline for the management of heart failure: a report of the American College of Cardiology Foundation/American Heart Association Task Force on practice guidelines. *Circulation*. 2013;128(16):e240-e327.

◆ **Metonia (Can)** *see* Metoclopramide *on page 1391*

◆ **Metopirone** *see* Metyrapone *on page 1405*

Metoprolol (me toe PROE lole)

Medication Safety Issues
Sound-alike/look-alike issues:
Lopressor may be confused with Lyrica

Metoprolol may be confused with metaproterenol, metoclopramide, metolazone, misoprostol

Metoprolol succinate may be confused with metoprolol tartrate

Toprol-XL may be confused with TEGretol, TEGretol-XR, Topamax

High alert medication:
The Institute for Safe Medication Practices (ISMP) includes this medication among its list of drugs which have a heightened risk of causing significant patient harm when used in error.

Administration issues:
Significant differences exist between oral and I.V. dosing. Use caution when converting from one route of administration to another.

Related Information
Oral Medications That Should Not Be Crushed or Altered *on page 2438*

Brand Names: U.S. Lopressor; Toprol XL

Brand Names: Canada Apo-Metoprolol; Apo-Metoprolol (Type L); Apo-Metoprolol SR; Ava-Metoprolol; Ava-Metoprolol (Type L); Betaloc; Dom-Metoprolol-B; Dom-Metoprolol-L; JAMP-Metoprolol-L; Lopresor; Lopresor SR; Metoprolol Tartrate Injection, USP; Metoprolol-25; Metoprolol-L; Mylan-Metoprolol (Type L); Nu-Metop; PMS-Metoprolol-B; PMS-Metoprolol-L; Riva-Metoprolol-L; Sandoz-Metoprolol (Type L); Sandoz-Metoprolol SR; Teva-Metoprolol

Therapeutic Category Antianginal Agent; Antiarrhythmic Agent, Class II; Antihypertensive Agent; Antimigraine Agent; Beta-Adrenergic Blocker

Generic Availability (U.S.) Yes

Use
Immediate release tablets and injection: Treatment of hypertension, alone or in combination with other agents (FDA approved in adults), angina pectoris (FDA approved in adults), and hemodynamically-stable acute myocardial infarction (to reduce cardiovascular mortality) (FDA approved in adults)

Extended release tablets: Treatment of hypertension, alone or in combination with other agents (FDA approved in ages ≥6 years and adults); angina pectoris (FDA approved in adults); and patients with heart failure (stable NYHA Class II or III) already receiving ACE inhibitors, diuretics, and/or digoxin (to reduce mortality/hospitalization) (FDA approved in adults)

Metoprolol has also been used for the treatment of ventricular arrhythmias, atrial ectopy; prevention and treatment of atrial fibrillation and atrial flutter; multifocal atrial tachycardia; symptomatic treatment of hypertrophic obstructive cardiomyopathy; essential tremor; and migraine headache prophylaxis

Pregnancy Risk Factor C

Pregnancy Considerations Adverse events were observed in animal studies; therefore, the manufacturer classifies metoprolol as pregnancy category C. Metoprolol crosses the placenta and can be detected in cord blood, amniotic fluid, and the serum of newborn infants. In a cohort study, an increased risk of cardiovascular defects was observed following maternal use of beta-blockers during pregnancy. Intrauterine growth restriction (IUGR), small placentas, as well as fetal/neonatal bradycardia, hypoglycemia, and/or respiratory depression have been observed following *in utero* exposure to beta-blockers as a class. Adequate facilities for monitoring infants at birth should be available. Untreated chronic maternal hypertension and pre-eclampsia are also associated with adverse events in the fetus, infant, and mother. The clearance of metoprolol is increased and serum concentrations and AUC of metoprolol are decreased during pregnancy. Metoprolol has been evaluated for the treatment of hypertension in pregnancy, but other agents may be more appropriate for use.

Breast-Feeding Considerations Small amounts of metoprolol can be detected in breast milk. The manufacturer recommends that caution be exercised when administering metoprolol to nursing women.

Contraindications Hypersensitivity to metoprolol, any component of the formulation, or other beta-blockers; **Note:** Additional contraindications are formulation and/or indication specific.

Immediate release tablets and injection:

Hypertension and angina: Sinus bradycardia; second- and third-degree heart block; cardiogenic shock; overt cardiac failure; sick sinus syndrome (except in patients with a functioning artificial pacemaker); severe peripheral arterial disease; pheochromocytoma (without alpha blockade)

Myocardial infarction: Severe sinus bradycardia (heart rate <45 beats/minute); significant first-degree heart block (P-R interval ≥0.24 seconds); second- and third-degree heart block; systolic blood pressure <100 mm Hg; moderate-to-severe cardiac failure

Extended release tablet: Severe bradycardia; second- and third-degree heart block; cardiogenic shock; decompensated heart failure; sick sinus syndrome (except in patients with a functioning artificial pacemaker)

Warnings May depress myocardial activity and precipitate or worsen heart failure; use with caution and monitor closely, especially in patients with compensated heart failure and during upwards titration of dose; if heart failure worsens, may need to increase diuretics and not advance the dose of metoprolol; a reduction in dose or discontinuation of metoprolol may be needed. Beta-blocker therapy should not be withdrawn abruptly (particularly in patients with CAD), but gradually tapered over 1-2 weeks to avoid acute tachycardia, hypertension, and/or ischemia **[U.S. Boxed Warning]**. Beta-blockers should generally be avoided in patients with bronchospastic disease; metoprolol, with relative beta$_1$ selectivity, should be used with caution and closely monitored in patients with bronchospastic disease; beta$_2$ stimulants and the lowest possible dose of metoprolol should be used in these patients. Metoprolol may block hypoglycemia-induced tachycardia and blood pressure changes; use with caution in patients with diabetes mellitus. Metoprolol decreases the ability of the heart to respond to reflex adrenergic stimuli and may increase the risk of general anesthesia and surgical procedures. May mask clinical signs of hyperthyroidism (exacerbation of symptoms of hyperthyroidism, including thyroid storm, may occur following abrupt discontinuation). Use with caution with potent inhibitors of cytochrome P450 CYP2D6 isoenzyme. Use with caution with verapamil, diltiazem, or anesthetic agents that decrease myocardial function (bradycardia or heart block may occur). Beta-blocker use has been associated with induction or exacerbation of psoriasis, but cause and effect have not been firmly established.

Precautions Use with caution in patients with hepatic dysfunction and in patients with peripheral vascular disease (beta-blockers may aggravate arterial insufficiency). Patients who have a history of severe anaphylactic hypersensitivity reactions to various substances may be more reactive while receiving beta-blockers; these patients may not be responsive to the normal doses of epinephrine used to treat hypersensitivity reactions. Contraindicated in patients with pheochromocytoma; if required, these patients should receive an alpha-blocking agent before receipt of any beta-blocking agent.

Adverse Reactions

Cardiovascular: Arterial insufficiency (usually Raynaud type), bradycardia, chest pain, CHF, edema (peripheral), first-degree heart block (P-R interval ≥0.26 sec), hypotension, palpitation, syncope

Central nervous system: Confusion, depression, dizziness, fatigue, hallucination, headache, insomnia, memory loss (short-term), nightmares, sleep disturbances, somnolence, vertigo

Dermatology: Photosensitivity, pruritus, psoriasis exacerbated, rash

Endocrine & metabolic: Diabetes exacerbated, libido decreased, Peyronie's disease

Gastrointestinal: Constipation, diarrhea, flatulence, gastrointestinal pain, heartburn, nausea, vomiting, xerostomia

Hematologic: Claudication

Neuromuscular & skeletal: Musculoskeletal pain

Ocular: Blurred vision, visual disturbances

Otic: Tinnitus

Respiratory: Dyspnea, rhinitis, shortness of breath, wheezing

Miscellaneous: Cold extremities

Rare but important or life-threatening: Agranulocytosis, alkaline phosphatase increased, alopecia (reversible), anxiety, arthralgia, arthritis, cardiogenic shock, diaphoresis increased, dry eyes, gangrene, hepatitis, HDL decreased, impotence, jaundice, lactate dehydrogenase increased, nervousness, paresthesia, retroperitoneal fibrosis, second-degree heart block, taste disturbance, third-degree heart block, thrombocytopenia, transaminases increased, triglycerides increased, urticaria, vomiting, weight gain

Other events reported with beta-blockers: Catatonia, emotional lability, fever, hypersensitivity reactions, laryngospasm, nonthrombocytopenic purpura, respiratory distress, thrombocytopenic purpura

Drug Interactions

Metabolism/Transport Effects Substrate of CYP2C19 (minor), CYP2D6 (major); **Note:** Assignment of Major/Minor substrate status based on clinically relevant drug interaction potential; **Inhibits** CYP2D6 (weak)

Avoid Concomitant Use

Avoid concomitant use of Metoprolol with any of the following: Ceritinib; Floctafenine; Methacholine

Increased Effect/Toxicity

Metoprolol may increase the levels/effects of: Alpha-/Beta-Agonists (Direct-Acting); Alpha1-Blockers; Alpha2-Agonists; Amifostine; Antihypertensives; Antipsychotic Agents (Phenothiazines); ARIPiprazole; Bradycardia-Causing Agents; Bupivacaine; Cardiac Glycosides; Ceritinib; Cholinergic Agonists; Ergot Derivatives; Fingolimod; Grass Pollen Allergen Extract (5 Grass Extract);

Hypotensive Agents; Insulin; Lidocaine (Systemic); Lidocaine (Topical); Mepivacaine; Methacholine; Midodrine; Obinutuzumab; RiTUXimab; Sulfonylureas

The levels/effects of Metoprolol may be increased by: Abiraterone Acetate; Acetylcholinesterase Inhibitors; Alpha2-Agonists; Aminoquinolines (Antimalarial); Anilidopiperidine Opioids; Antipsychotic Agents (Phenothiazines); Barbiturates; Brimonidine (Topical); Calcium Channel Blockers (Dihydropyridine); Calcium Channel Blockers (Nondihydropyridine); CYP2D6 Inhibitors; Darunavir; Diazoxide; Dipyridamole; Disopyramide; Dronedarone; Floctafenine; Herbs (Hypotensive Properties); MAO Inhibitors; Mirabegron; Pentoxifylline; Phosphodiesterase 5 Inhibitors; Propafenone; Prostacyclin Analogues; Regorafenib; Reserpine; Selective Serotonin Reuptake Inhibitors

Decreased Effect

Metoprolol may decrease the levels/effects of: Beta2-Agonists; Theophylline Derivatives

The levels/effects of Metoprolol may be decreased by: Barbiturates; Herbs (Hypertensive Properties); Methylphenidate; Mirabegron; Nonsteroidal Anti-Inflammatory Agents; Peginterferon Alfa-2b; Rifamycin Derivatives; Yohimbine

Food Interactions Food increases absorption. Metoprolol serum levels may be increased if taken with food. Management: Take immediate release tartrate tablets with food; succinate can be taken with or without food.

Stability

All formulations: Store at controlled room temperature of 25°C (77°F); excursions permitted to 15°C to 30°C (59°F to 86°F)

Tablets: Protect from moisture and dispense in tight, light-resistant container

Injection: Protect from light

Mechanism of Action Selective inhibitor of beta$_1$-adrenergic receptors; competitively blocks beta$_1$-receptors, with little or no effect on beta$_2$-receptors at doses <100 mg; does not exhibit any membrane stabilizing or intrinsic sympathomimetic activity

Pharmacodynamics

Beta blockade:

Onset of action: Oral: Metoprolol tartrate tablets: Within 1 hour

Maximum effect: I.V.: 20 minutes

Duration: Dose dependent

Antihypertensive effect:

Onset of action: Oral: Metoprolol tartrate tablets: Within 15 minutes

Maximum effect: Oral (multiple dosing): After 1 week

Duration: Oral: Metoprolol tartrate tablets (single dose): 6 hours; metoprolol succinate (extended release tablets): Up to 24 hours

Pharmacokinetics (Adult data unless noted) Note: The pharmacokinetics of metoprolol in hypertensive children 6-17 years of age were found to be similar to adults.

Absorption: Rapid and complete, with large first-pass effect

Distribution: Crosses the blood brain barrier; CSF concentrations are 78% of plasma concentrations

Protein binding: 12% bound to albumin

Metabolism: Significant first-pass metabolism; extensive metabolism in the liver via isoenzyme CYP2D6

Bioavailability: Oral: ~40% to 50% (Johnsson, 1975)

Half-Life:

Neonates: 5-10 hours

Adults: CYP2D6 poor metabolizers: 7.5 hours; CYP2D6 extensive metabolizers: 2.8 hours

Adults with chronic renal failure: Similar to normal adults

Elimination: 10% of an I.V. dose and <5% of an oral dose is excreted unchanged in the urine

Dosing: Usual

Oral: Hypertension:

Immediate release tablets: Children and Adolescents 1-17 years: Initial: 1-2 mg/kg/day, administered in 2 divided doses; adjust dose based on patient response; maximum: 6 mg/kg/day (≤200 mg/day) (National High Blood Pressure Education Program Working Group on High Blood Pressure in Children and Adolescents, 2004)

Extended release tablets: Manufacturer's recommendation: Children ≥6 years: Initial: 1 mg/kg once daily (maximum initial dose: 50 mg/day); adjust dose based on patient response (maximum: 2 mg/kg/day or 200 mg/day; higher doses have not been studied)

Adults:

Immediate release tablets: Initial: 100 mg/day in single or divided doses, increase at weekly intervals to desired effect; usual dosage range: 100-450 mg/day; doses >450 mg/day have not been studied; usual dosage range (JNC 7): 50-100 mg/day in 1-2 divided doses

Note: Lower once-daily dosing (especially 100 mg/day) may not control blood pressure for 24 hours; larger or more frequent dosing may be needed. Patients with bronchospastic diseases should receive the lowest possible daily dose; dose should initially be divided into 3 doses per day (to avoid high plasma concentrations).

Extended release tablets: Initial: 25-100 mg/day as a single dose; increase at weekly intervals to desired effect; doses >400 mg/day have not been studied; usual dosage range (JNC 7): 50-100 mg once daily

Oral: Congestive heart failure: Adults: Extended release tablets: Initial: NYHA Class II heart failure: 25 mg once daily; more severe heart failure: 12.5 mg once daily; may double the dose every 2 weeks as tolerated; maximum: 200 mg/day

Administration Oral:

Metoprolol tartrate tablets: Administer with food or immediately after meals

Metoprolol succinate extended release tablets: May be administered without regard to meals; Toprol-XL® tablets are scored and may be divided; do not chew or crush the half or whole tablets; swallow whole. Do not chew, crush, or break generic nonscored extended release tablets; swallow whole.

Monitoring Parameters
Blood pressure, heart rate, respirations, circulation in extremities

Additional Information
Do not abruptly discontinue therapy, taper dosage gradually over 1-2 weeks. Beta-blockers without intrinsic sympathomimetic activity (such as metoprolol) have been shown to decrease morbidity and mortality when initiated in the acute treatment of MI and continued long term; metoprolol injection is used for early treatment of definitive or suspected MI; consult adult reference for further information.

A limited number of studies assessing the use of metoprolol in hypertensive pediatric patients are available. A recent article examined the use of metoprolol extended release tablets in children 6-16 years of age (mean age: 12.5 ± 2.8 years). In part one (a 4-week double-blind dose ranging study), patients were randomized to receive placebo (n=23) or metoprolol 0.2 mg/kg/day (n=45), 1 mg/kg/day (n=23), or 2 mg/kg/day (n=49) given as once daily dosing. For patients in the higher dosing groups, doses were initiated at 0.5 mg/kg/day, and increased after 1 week to 1 mg/kg/day if tolerated. Doses were increased again after 1 week to 2 mg/kg/day if tolerated in the 2 mg/kg/day dosing group. At the end of 4 weeks, metoprolol significantly decreased systolic blood pressure in the 1 mg/kg/day and 2 mg/kg/day groups compared to placebo. Diastolic blood pressure was significantly reduced only in the 2 mg/kg/day group. In part two (a 52-week open-label trial), 100 patients received initial doses of 25 mg or 12.5 mg once daily; doses were increased every 2 weeks in 25 mg or 50 mg increments based on blood pressure and tolerability, to a maximum dose of 200 mg once daily. The mean doses were 37 ± 33 mg at study entry, 97 ± 64 mg at week 16, and 112 ± 69 mg at study end (Batisky, 2007). In an older study using nonsustained release tablets, 16 hypertensive adolescents (≥13 years of age) were treated with an initial metoprolol dose of 50 mg twice daily; patients were seen every 4-6 weeks and doses were increased to 100 mg twice daily if blood pressure was not controlled (Falkner, 1982).

Pediatric dosing information for metoprolol, for use in indications other than hypertension, is also limited; in one case report, oral metoprolol (2 mg/kg/day in 3 divided doses) helped control paroxysmal supraventricular tachycardia in a 6-month old infant receiving digoxin (Hepner, 1983). Low dose oral metoprolol (initial: 0.1 mg/kg/dose given twice daily, then increased slowly as needed to a maximum of 0.9 ± 0.7 mg/kg/day) was used to treat severe CHF that failed conventional therapy in four children (mean age: 7.8 years) with cardiomyopathy who were under consideration for heart transplantation (Shaddy, 1998). A follow-up report in 15 children, 2.5-15 years of age (mean: 8.6 ± 1.3 years) used low dose oral metoprolol [Initial: 0.1-0.2 mg/kg/dose given twice daily, then increased slowly as needed to a maximum of 1.1 ± 0.1 mg/kg/day (range: 0.5-2.3 mg/kg/day)] to treat dilated cardiomyopathy and CHF; all patients received ACE inhibitors, digoxin, and diuretics before starting metoprolol (Shaddy, 1999). Two studies (Muller, 1993; O'Marcaigh, 1994) assessed metoprolol for unexplained syncope in children at I.V. doses of 0.1-0.2 mg/kg for tilt table testing; in both studies, oral metoprolol was given after tilt table testing to select patients; initial oral doses of 0.8-2.8 mg/kg/day were used in 15 patients (8-20 years of age), but treatment was discontinued in three patients receiving 1.8-2.8 mg/kg/day due to adverse effects (Muller, 1993); oral doses of 1-2 mg/kg/day, rounded to the nearest 25 mg/day and divided into 2 doses daily were used in 19 patients (7-18 years of age) with unexplained syncope; the mean effective dose was 1.5 mg/kg/day (O'Marcaigh, 1994). High-dose beta-blocker therapy has been recommended to treat childhood hypertrophic cardiomyopathy (Ostman-Smith, 1999). Further pediatric studies are required before these doses can be recommended.

Dosage Forms
Excipient information presented when available (limited, particularly for generics); consult specific product labeling.

Solution, Intravenous, as tartrate:

Lopressor: 1 mg/mL (5 mL)

Generic: 1 mg/mL (5 mL); 5 mg/5 mL (5 mL)

Tablet, Oral, as tartrate:

Lopressor: 50 mg, 100 mg [scored]

Generic: 25 mg, 50 mg, 100 mg

Tablet Extended Release 24 Hour, Oral, as succinate:

Toprol XL: 25 mg, 50 mg, 100 mg, 200 mg [scored]

Generic: 25 mg, 50 mg, 100 mg, 200 mg

Extemporaneous Preparations
A 10 mg/mL oral suspension may be made with metoprolol tartrate tablets and one of three different vehicles (cherry syrup; a 1:1 mixture of Ora-Sweet® and Ora-Plus®; or a 1:1 mixture of Ora-Sweet® SF and Ora-Plus®). Crush twelve 100 mg tablets in a mortar and reduce to a fine powder. Add 20 mL of the

chosen vehicle and mix to a uniform paste; mix while adding the vehicle in incremental proportions to **almost** 120 mL; transfer to a calibrated bottle, rinse mortar with vehicle, and add quantity of vehicle sufficient to make 120 mL. Label "shake well" and "protect from light". Stable for 60 days.

Allen LV Jr and Erickson MA 3rd, "Stability of Labetalol Hydrochloride, Metoprolol Tartrate, Verapamil Hydrochloride, and Spironolactone With Hydrochlorothiazide in Extemporaneously Compounded Oral Liquids," *Am J Health Syst Pharm*, 1996, 53(19):2304-9.

References

Batisky DL, Sorof JM, Sugg J, et al, "Efficacy and Safety of Extended Release Metoprolol Succinate in Hypertensive Children 6 to 16 Years of Age: A Clinical Trial Experience," *J Pediatr*, 2007, 150(2):134-9.

Brauchli YB, Jick SS, Curtin F, et al, "Association Between Beta-Blockers, Other Antihypertensive Drugs and Psoriasis: Population-Based Case-Control Study," *Br J Dermatol*, 2008, 158(6):1299-307.

Chobanian AV, Bakris GL, Black HR, et al, "The Seventh Report of the Joint National Committee on Prevention, Detection, Evaluation, and Treatment of High Blood Pressure: The JNC 7 report," *JAMA*, 2003, 289(19):2560-72.

Falkner B, Lowenthal DT, and Affrime MB, "The Pharmacodynamic Effectiveness of Metoprolol in Adolescent Hypertension," *Pediatr Pharmacol (New York)*, 1982, 2(1):49-55.

Gold MH, Holy AK, and Roenigk HH Jr, "Beta-Blocking Drugs and Psoriasis. A Review of Cutaneous Side Effects and Retrospective Analysis of Their Effects on Psoriasis," *J Am Acad Dermatol*, 1988, 19 (5 Pt 1):837-41.

Hepner SI, and Davoli E, "Successful Treatment of Supraventricular Tachycardia With Metoprolol, a Cardioselective Beta Blocker," *Clin Pediatr (Phila)*, 1983, 22(7):522-3.

Johnsson G, Regårdh CG, Sölvell L. Combined pharmacokinetic and pharmacodynamic studies in man of the adrenergic beta1-receptor antagonist metoprolol. *Acta Pharmacol Toxicol (Copenh)*. 1975;36 (Suppl 5):31-44.

Morselli PL, Boutroy MJ, Bianchetti G, et al, "Pharmacokinetics of Antihypertensive Drugs in the Neonatal Period," *Dev Pharmacol Ther*, 1989, 13(2-4):190-8.

Muller G, Deal BJ, Strasburger JF, et al, "Usefulness of Metoprolol for Unexplained Syncope and Positive Response to Tilt Testing in Young Persons," *Am J Cardiol*, 1993, 71(7):592-5.

National High Blood Pressure Education Program Working Group on High Blood Pressure in Children and Adolescents, "The Fourth Report on the Diagnosis, Evaluation, and Treatment of High Blood Pressure in Children and Adolescents," *Pediatrics*, 2004, 114(2 Suppl 4th Report):555-76.

O'Marcaigh AS, MacLellan-Tobert SG, and Porter CJ, "Tilt-Table Testing and Oral Metoprolol Therapy in Young Patients With Unexplained Syncope," *Pediatrics*, 1994, 93(2):278-83.

Ostman-Smith I, Wettrell G, and Riesenfeld T, "A Cohort Study of Childhood Hypertrophic Cardiomyopathy: Improved Survival Following High-Dose Beta-Adrenoceptor Antagonist Treatment," *J Am Coll Cardiol*, 1999, 34(6):1813-22.

Schön MP and Boehncke WH, "Psoriasis," *N Engl J Med*, 2005, 352 (18):1899-912.

Shaddy RE, "Beta-Blocker Therapy in Young Children With Congestive Heart Failure Under Consideration for Heart Transplantation," *Am Heart J*, 1998, 136(1):19-21.

Shaddy RE, Tani LY, Gidding SS, et al, "Beta-Blocker Treatment of Dilated Cardiomyopathy With Congestive Heart Failure in Children: A Multi-Institutional Experience," *J Heart Lung Transplant*, 1999, 18 (3):269-74.

◆ **Metoprolol-25 (Can)** *see* Metoprolol *on page 1396*

◆ **Metoprolol-L (Can)** *see* Metoprolol *on page 1396*

◆ **Metoprolol Succinate** *see* Metoprolol *on page 1396*

◆ **Metoprolol Tartrate** *see* Metoprolol *on page 1396*

◆ **Metoprolol Tartrate Injection, USP (Can)** *see* Metoprolol *on page 1396*

◆ **Metozolv ODT** *see* Metoclopramide *on page 1391*

◆ **Metro** *see* MetroNIDAZOLE (Systemic) *on page 1399*

◆ **MetroCream** *see* MetroNIDAZOLE (Topical) *on page 1404*

◆ **Metrogel** *see* MetroNIDAZOLE (Topical) *on page 1404*

◆ **MetroGel-Vaginal** *see* MetroNIDAZOLE (Topical) *on page 1404*

◆ **MetroLotion** *see* MetroNIDAZOLE (Topical) *on page 1404*

MetroNIDAZOLE (Systemic)
(met roe NYE da zole)

Medication Safety Issues
Sound-alike/look-alike issues:

MetroNIDAZOLE may be confused with mebendazole, meropenem, metFORMIN, methotrexate, metoclopramide, miconazole

Related Information

H. pylori Treatment in Pediatric Patients *on page 2311*

Oral Medications That Should Not Be Crushed or Altered *on page 2438*

Brand Names: U.S. Flagyl; Flagyl ER; Metro

Brand Names: Canada Flagyl; Novo-Nidazol; PMS-Metronidazole

Therapeutic Category Amebicide; Antibiotic, Anaerobic; Antiprotozoal

Generic Availability (U.S.) May be product dependent

Use

Oral:

Immediate release formulation: Treatment of susceptible amebiasis (intestinal [dysentery] or liver abscess) (FDA approved in pediatric patients [age not specified] and adults); treatment of susceptible anaerobic bacterial and protozoal infections in the following conditions: Symptomatic and asymptomatic trichomoniasis; skin and skin structure infections, bone and joint infections, CNS infections, endocarditis, gynecological infections, intra-abdominal infections, and respiratory tract (lower) infections; septicemia (FDA approved in adults)

Extended release formulation: Treatment of bacterial vaginosis (FDA approved in nonpregnant, postmenarchal females)

Parenteral: Treatment of susceptible anaerobic bacteria in the following conditions: Skin and skin structure infections, bone and joint infections, CNS infections, endocarditis, gynecological infections, intra-abdominal infections, and respiratory tract (lower) infections; septicemia, surgical prophylaxis (colorectal) (all indications: FDA approved in adults)

Has also been used for treatment of giardiasis, pelvic inflammatory disease, tetanus, *H. pylori* and antibiotic-associated pseudomembranous colitis (AAPC) caused by *C. difficile*, and management of inflammatory bowel disease

Pregnancy Risk Factor B

Pregnancy Considerations Teratogenic effects have not been observed in animal reproduction studies. Metronidazole crosses the placenta and rapidly distributes into the fetal circulation. Although there have been a few reports of facial anomalies after *in utero* exposure, most studies have not found an increased risk of congenital abnormalities following maternal use of metronidazole during the first trimester of pregnancy. In studies that included women taking metronidazole during all trimesters of pregnancy, an increased risk of adverse fetal and neonatal outcomes has not been observed. Because metronidazole has been carcinogenic in some animal species, concern has been raised whether metronidazole should be used during pregnancy; however, a strong carcinogenic potential in humans has not been observed, including one study of prenatal exposure.

Metronidazole pharmacokinetics are similar between pregnant and nonpregnant patients. Bacterial vaginosis has been associated with adverse pregnancy outcomes (including preterm labor); metronidazole is recommended for the treatment of symptomatic bacterial vaginosis in pregnant patients. Vaginal trichomoniasis has been also associated with adverse pregnancy outcomes (including preterm labor). Treatment may relieve symptoms and prevent further sexual transmission; however, ▶

metronidazole has not resulted in reduced perinatal morbidity and should not be used solely to prevent preterm delivery. Some clinicians consider deferring therapy in asymptomatic women until >37 weeks gestation. Use of oral metronidazole is contraindicated during the first trimester (per the FDA approved labeling). Not recommended for treatment of *Clostridium difficile* infection in pregnancy (Surzwica, 2013). Consult current CDC guidelines for appropriate use in pregnant women.

Breast-Feeding Considerations Metronidazole and its active metabolite are measurable in the breast milk and infant plasma. Milk concentrations are similar to those in the maternal plasma and are highly variable. Peak concentrations of metronidazole in breast milk occur ~2-4 hours after the oral dose. In studies, the calculated relative infant doses have ranged from 0.13% to 36% of the weight-adjusted maternal dose. Use of metronidazole in a lactating patient is not recommended by the manufacturer. If metronidazole is given, breast-feeding should be withheld for 12-24 hours after the dose (CDC, 2010).). Not recommended for treatment of *Clostridium difficile* infection in breast-feeding women (Surzwica, 2013).

Contraindications Hypersensitivity to metronidazole, nitroimidazole derivatives, or any component; use of disulfiram within the past 2 weeks; use of alcohol or products containing propylene glycol during therapy or within 3 days of therapy discontinuation

Additional product-specific contraindications: Immediate release capsules and tablets: Pregnancy (first trimester)

Warnings Metronidazole has been shown to be carcinogenic in rodents **[U.S. Boxed Warning]**. Aseptic meningitis (with symptoms occurring within hours of a dose), encephalopathy (cerebellar toxicity with ataxis, dizziness, dysarthria, and/or CNS lesions), seizures, and neuropathies (peripheral and optic) have been reported, especially with increased doses and chronic treatment; monitor and consider discontinuation of therapy if signs/symptoms occur. Symptoms associated with aseptic meningitis and encephalopathy generally resolve following therapy discontinuation. Use with caution in patients with a history of seizure disorder.

Disulfiram-like reactions (abdominal cramps, nausea, vomiting, headaches, flushing) to ethanol have been reported with oral metronidazole; use of alcoholic beverages or products containing alcohol or propylene glycol during therapy and for at least 3 days after therapy is contraindicated for this reason.

Precautions Use with caution in patients with hepatic impairment due to potential accumulation; reduce dosage if hepatic impairment severe. Use with caution in patients with current or history of blood dyscrasias; leukopenia has occurred; monitor CBC with differential at baseline and after treatment with prolonged or repeat courses. Metronidazole injection contains 28 mEq of sodium/gram of metronidazole; use with caution in patients receiving corticosteroids or patients predisposed to edema (eg, heart failure or other sodium-retaining conditions). Use with caution in patients with end-stage renal disease (ESRD) due to potential accumulation; monitor for adverse effects. Accumulated metabolites may be rapidly removed by dialysis. Supplemental doses may be needed in patients on hemodialysis. If *H. pylori* is not eradicated in patients being treated with metronidazole in a regimen, it should be assumed that metronidazole resistance has occurred and it should not be used again. The Infectious Disease Society of America (IDSA) recommends the use of oral metronidazole for initial treatment of mild to moderate *C. difficile* infection and the use of oral vancomycin for initial treatment of severe *C. difficile* infection with or without I.V. metronidazole, depending on the presence of complications. May treat recurrent mild to moderate infection once with oral metronidazole; avoid use beyond first

reoccurrence due to potential cumulative neurotoxicity (Cohen, 2010). The American College of Gastroenterology (ACG) recommends oral vancomycin and I.V. metronidazole for severe and complicated CDI (Surawicz, 2013). Prolonged use may result in fungal superinfection; candidiasis infection (known or unknown) may be more prominent during metronidazole treatment; antifungal treatment required. Potentially significant interactions may exist, requiring dose or frequency adjustment, additional monitoring, and/or selection of alternative therapy. Consult drug interactions database for more detailed information.

Adverse Reactions

Cardiovascular: Flattened T-wave on ECG, flushing, local thrombophlebitis (I.V.), syncope

Central nervous system: Aseptic meningitis, ataxia, brain disease, confusion, depression, disulfiram-like reaction (with alcohol), dizziness, dysarthria, dyspareunia, headache, insomnia, irritability, metallic taste, peripheral neuropathy, seizure, vertigo

Dermatologic: Erythematous rash, pruritus, Stevens-Johnson syndrome, toxic epidermal necrolysis, urticaria

Gastrointestinal: Abdominal cramps, abdominal pain, anorexia, constipation, diarrhea, epigastric distress, glossitis, hairy tongue, nausea, pancreatitis (rare), proctitis, stomatitis, vomiting, xerostomia

Genitourinary: Cystitis, dark urine (rare), decreased libido, dysmenorrhea, dysuria, genital pruritus, sensation of pelvic pressure, urinary incontinence, urinary tract infection, urine abnormality, vaginal dryness, vaginitis, vulvovaginal candidiasis

Hematologic & oncologic: Neutropenia (reversible), thrombocytopenia (reversible, rare)

Immunologic: Serum sickness-like reaction (joint pains)

Infection: Bacterial infection, candidiasis

Neuromuscular & skeletal: Weakness

Ophthalmic: Optic neuropathy

Renal: Polyuria

Respiratory: Flu-like symptoms, nasal congestion, pharyngitis, rhinitis, sinusitis, upper respiratory tract infection

Miscellaneous: Fever, lesion (central nervous system, reversible)

Drug Interactions

Metabolism/Transport Effects Substrate of CYP2A6 (minor); **Note:** Assignment of Major/Minor substrate status based on clinically relevant drug interaction potential; **Inhibits** CYP2C9 (weak), CYP3A4 (weak)

Avoid Concomitant Use

Avoid concomitant use of MetroNIDAZOLE (Systemic) with any of the following: Alcohol (Ethyl); BCG; Carbocisteine; Disulfiram; Pimozide

Increased Effect/Toxicity

MetroNIDAZOLE (Systemic) may increase the levels/effects of: Alcohol (Ethyl); ARIPiprazole; Busulfan; Calcineurin Inhibitors; Carbocisteine; Fluorouracil (Systemic); Fosphenytoin; Highest Risk QTc-Prolonging Agents; Lomitapide; Moderate Risk QTc-Prolonging Agents; Phenytoin; Pimozide; Tegafur; Tipranavir; Vitamin K Antagonists

The levels/effects of MetroNIDAZOLE (Systemic) may be increased by: Disulfiram; Mebendazole; Mifepristone

Decreased Effect

MetroNIDAZOLE (Systemic) may decrease the levels/effects of: BCG; Mycophenolate; Sodium Picosulfate; Typhoid Vaccine

The levels/effects of MetroNIDAZOLE (Systemic) may be decreased by: Fosphenytoin; PHENobarbital; Phenytoin

Food Interactions

Ethanol: May cause disulfiram-like reaction characterized by flushing, headache, nausea, vomiting, sweating, or tachycardia when administered concurrently with ethanol. Management: The manufacturer recommends to avoid all ethanol or any ethanol-containing drugs during and for 3 days after therapy.

Food: Peak antibiotic serum concentration lowered and delayed, but total drug absorbed not affected. Management: Immediate-release tablets and capsules may be administered with food to minimize stomach upset. Extended release tablets should be administered on an empty stomach (1 hour before or 2 hours after meals).

Stability

Injection: Store at 25°C (77°F). Protect from light. Avoid excessive heat. Do not refrigerate. Do not remove unit from overwrap until ready for use. Discard unused solution.

Oral:

Immediate release:

Capsules: Store at 15°C to 25°C (59°F to 77°F).

Tablets: Store below 25°C (77°F) and protect from light.

Extended release, tablets: Store in a dry place at 25°C (77°F); excursions permitted to 15°C to 30°C (59°F to 86°F).

Mechanism of Action After diffusing into the organism, interacts with DNA to cause a loss of helical DNA structure and strand breakage resulting in inhibition of protein synthesis and cell death in susceptible organisms

Pharmacokinetics (Adult data unless noted)

Absorption: Oral: Well absorbed

Distribution: Widely distributed into body tissues, fluids (including bile), liver, liver abscesses, bone, pleural fluid, and vaginal secretions; crosses blood-brain barrier; saliva and CSF concentrations similar to those in plasma

Protein binding: <20%

Metabolism: Hepatic (30% to 60%) to several metabolites, including an active hydroxyl metabolite which maintains activity ~30% to 65% of the parent compound (Lamp, 1999)

Half-life:

Neonates <7 days (Jager-Roman, 1982): Within first week of life, more prolonged than with lower GA:

GA 28 to 30 weeks: 75.3 ± 16.9 hours

GA 32 to 35 weeks: 35.4 ± 1.5 hours

GA 36 to 40 weeks: 24.8 ± 1.6 hours

Neonates ≥7 days: ~22.5 hours (Upadhyaya, 1988)

Children and Adolescents: 6 to 10 hours (Lamp, 1999)

Adults: ~8 hours

Hepatic impairment: Prolonged

Time to peak serum concentration: Oral: Immediate release: 1 to 2 hours; extended release: ~5 hours

Elimination: Urine (60% to 80% as unchanged drug and metabolites; ~20% of total as unchanged drug); feces (6% to 15%)

Dosing: Neonatal

General dosing, susceptible infection:

Weight-directed dosing (Bradley, 2012; Red Book [AAP], 2012): Oral, I.V.:

Body weight <1 kg:

PNA ≤14 days: 15 mg/kg loading dose, then 7.5 mg/kg every 48 hours

PNA 15 to 28 days: 15 mg/kg every 24 hours

Body weight 1 to 2 kg:

PNA ≤7 days: 15 mg/kg loading dose, then 7.5 mg/kg every 24 to 48 hours

PNA 8 to 28 days: 15 mg/kg every 24 hours

Body weight >2 kg:

PNA ≤7 days: 15 mg/kg every 24 hours

PNA 8 to 28 days: 15 mg/kg every 12 hours

Age-directed dosing: Limited data available; dosing regimens variable: **Note:** Postmenstrual age (PMA) is the sum of gestational age (weeks) and postnatal age (weeks) (AAP, 2004).

Loading dose: 15 mg/kg

Maintenance dose:

Bradley, 2014:

PMA <34 weeks: 7.5 mg/kg/dose every 12 hours

PMA 34 to 40 weeks: 7.5 mg/kg/dose every 8 hours

Suyagh, 2011: Dosing based on pharmacokinetic analysis and modeling of 32 preterm neonates

PMA ≤25 weeks: 7.5 mg/kg every 24 hours

PMA 26 to 27 weeks: 10 mg/kg every 24 hours

PMA 28 to 33 weeks: 7.5 mg/kg every 12 hours

PMA 34 to 44 weeks: 10 mg/kg every 12 hours

PMA ≥45 weeks: 7.5 mg/kg every 6 hours

Surgical prophylaxis (IDSA/ASHP [Bratzler], 2013): I.V.:

<1200 g: 7.5 mg/kg as a single dose 30 to 60 minutes prior to procedure

≥1200 g: 15 mg/kg as a single dose 30 to 60 minutes prior to procedure

Dosing: Usual

Pediatric: **Note:** Some clinicians recommend using adjusted body weight in obese children. Dosing weight = IBW + 0.45 (TBW-IBW)

General dosing, susceptible infection (Red Book [AAP], 2012): Infants, Children, and Adolescents:

Oral: 30 to 50 mg/kg/day in divided doses 3 times daily; maximum daily dose: 2250 mg/**day**

Parenteral: I.V.: 22.5 to 40 mg/kg/day in divided doses 3 times daily; maximum daily dose: 1500 mg/**day**

Amebiasis: Infants, Children, and Adolescents: Oral: 35 to 50 mg/kg/day in divided doses every 8 hours for 7 to 10 days; maximum single dose: 750 mg (Red Book [AAP], 2012)

Appendicitis, perforated (divided dosing): Children and Adolescents: I.V.: 30 mg/kg/day in divided doses 3 times daily (Emil, 2003)

Appendicitis, perforated (once-daily dosing): Limited data available: Children and Adolescents: I.V.: 30 mg/kg once daily in combination with ceftriaxone; maximum reported daily dose: 1500 mg/day (Yardeni, 2013); however, other pediatric trials did not report a maximum; in adult patients, a maximum daily dose of 1500 mg/day for once-daily dosing is suggested (Solomokin, 2010); in pediatric patients, once-daily metronidazole in combination with ceftriaxone has been shown to have similar efficacy as triple-combination therapy with ampicillin, clindamycin, and gentamicin (Fraser, 2010; St Peter, 2006; St Peter, 2008)

Balantidiasis: Infants, Children, and Adolescents: Oral: 35 to 50 mg/kg/day in divided doses every 8 hours for 5 days; maximum single dose: 750 mg (Red Book [AAP], 2012)

***Clostridium difficile* diarrhea:** Infants, Children, and Adolescents: Oral: 30 mg/kg/day in divided doses 4 times daily for 7 to 14 days; maximum daily dose: 2000 mg/**day** (Red Book [AAP], 2012; Schutze, 2013)

Dientamoeba fragilis: Infants, Children, and Adolescents: Oral: 35 to 50 mg/kg/day in divided doses every 8 hours for 10 days; maximum dose: 750 mg/dose (Red Book [AAP], 2012)

Giardiasis: Infants, Children, and Adolescents: Oral: 15 mg/kg/day in divided doses every 8 hours for 5 to 7 days; maximum dose: 250 mg/dose (Red Book [AAP], 2012)

***Helicobacter pylori* infection:** Children and Adolescents: Oral: 20 mg/kg/day in 2 divided doses for 10 to 14 days in combination with amoxicillin and proton pump inhibitor with or without clarithromycin; maximum daily dose: 1000 mg/**day** (NASPGHAN/ESPGHAN [Koletzkol], 2011)

Inflammatory bowel disease:

Crohn disease, perianal disease; induction: Children and Adolescents: Oral: 7.5 mg/kg/dose 3 times daily for 6 weeks with or without ciprofloxacin; maximum dose: 500 mg/dose (Sandhu, 2010)

Ulcerative colitis, pouchitis, persistent: Children and Adolescents: Oral: 20 to 30 mg/kg/day in divided doses 3 times daily for 14 days with or without ciprofloxacin or oral budesonide; maximum dose: 500 mg/dose (Turner, 2012)

Intra-abdominal infection: Infants, Children, and Adolescents: I.V.: 30 to 40 mg/kg/day in divided doses 3 times daily as part of combination therapy; maximum dose: 500 mg/dose (IDSA [Solomkin], 2010)

Intra-abdominal infection, complicated: Infants, Children, and Adolescents: I.V.: 30 to 40 mg/kg/day in divided doses every 8 hours for 4 to 7 days; maximum daily dose: 1500 mg/**day** (IDSA [Solomkin], 2010)

Pelvic inflammatory disease: Adolescents: Oral: 500 mg twice daily for 14 days; give with doxycycline plus a cephalosporin (CDC, 2010; *Red Book* [AAP], 2012)

Surgical prophylaxis: Children and Adolescents: I.V.: 15 mg/kg as a single dose 30 to 60 minutes prior to procedure; maximum single dose: 500 mg (IDSA/ASHP [Bratzler], 2013)

Surgical prophylaxis, colorectal: Children and Adolescents: Oral: 15 mg/kg every 3 to 4 hours for 3 doses, starting after mechanical bowel preparation the afternoon and evening before the procedure, with or without additional oral antibiotics and with an appropriate I.V. antibiotic prophylaxis regimen; maximum dose: 1000 mg/dose (IDSA/ASHP [Bratzler], 2013)

Tetanus (*Clostridium tetani* infection): Infants, Children, and Adolescents: Oral, I.V.: 30 mg/kg/day in divided doses 4 times daily for 10 to 14 days; maximum daily dose: 4000 mg/**day** (*Red Book* [AAP], 2012)

Trichomoniasis; prophylaxis after sexual victimization and treatment: Oral:

Children <45 kg: 15 mg/kg/day in divided doses 3 times daily for 7 days; maximum daily dose: 2000 mg/**day** (*Red Book* [AAP], 2012)

Children ≥45 kg and Adolescents: 2000 mg as a single dose once (CDC, 2010; Red Book [AAP], 2012)

Vaginosis, bacterial:

Children <45 kg: 15 mg/kg/day in divided doses every 12 hours for 7 days; maximum daily dose: 1000 mg/**day** (*Red Book* [AAP], 2012)

Children >45 kg and Adolescents: 500 mg twice daily for 7 days (CDC, 2010; *Red Book* [AAP], 2012)

Adults:

Amebiasis: Oral: 500 to 750 mg every 8 hours for 5 to 10 days

Anaerobic infections: Oral, I.V.: 30 mg/kg/day in divided doses every 6 hours (~500 mg every 6 hours for a 70 kg adult); maximum daily dose 4000 mg/**day**; **Note:** Initial: 1000 mg I.V. loading dose may be administered

Bacterial vaginosis or vaginitis due to *Gardnerella mobiluncus* (CDC, 2010): Oral:

Regular release: 500 mg twice daily for 7 days

Extended release: 750 mg once daily for 7 days

***Clostridium difficile* diarrhea:** IDSA Guidelines (Cohen, 2010):

Mild to moderate infection: Oral: 500 mg 3 times daily for 10 to 14 days

Severe complicated infection: I.V.: 500 mg 3 times daily with oral vancomycin (recommended agent) for 10 to 14 days

Note: Due to the emergence of a new strain of *C. difficile*, some clinicians recommend converting to oral vancomycin therapy if the patient does not show a clear clinical response after 2 days of metronidazole therapy.

***Helicobacter pylori* infection:** Oral: 250 to 500 mg with meals and at bedtime (4 times daily) for 10 to 14 days; requires combination therapy with at least one other antibiotic and an acid-suppressing agent (proton pump inhibitor or H$_2$ blocker) (Chey, 2007)

Intra-abdominal infection, complicated, community-acquired, mild to moderate (in combination with cephalosporin or fluoroquinolone): I.V.: 500 mg

every 8 to 12 hours or 1500 mg every 24 hours for 4 to 7 days (provided source controlled) (Solomkin, 2010)

Surgical prophylaxis (colorectal): I.V. 15 mg/kg 1 hour prior to surgery; followed by 7.5 mg/kg 6 and 12 hours after initial dose

Trichomoniasis: Oral: 250 mg every 8 hours for 7 days or 375 mg twice daily for 7 days **or** 2000 mg as a single dose **or** 1000 mg twice daily for 2 doses (on same day)

Dosing adjustment in renal impairment:

Infants, Children, and Adolescents:

Manufacturer's labeling:

Mild, moderate, or severe impairment: There are no dosage adjustments provided in the manufacturer's labeling; however, decreased renal function does not alter the single-dose pharmacokinetics.

ESRD requiring dialysis: Metronidazole metabolites may accumulate; monitor for adverse events; accumulated metabolites may be rapidly removed by dialysis.

Intermittent hemodialysis (IHD): If administration cannot be separated from hemodialysis, consider supplemental dose following hemodialysis.

Peritoneal dialysis (PD): No dosage adjustment necessary

Alternate dosing: Others have used the following the adjustments (Aronoff, 2007). **Note:** Renally adjusted dose recommendations are based on doses of 15 to 30 mg/kg/**day** divided every 6 to 8 hours.

GFR ≥10 mL/minute/1.73 m^2: No adjustment required

GFR <10 mL/minute/1.73 m^2: 4 mg/kg/dose every 6 hours

Intermittent hemodialysis: Extensively removed by hemodialysis: 4 mg/kg/dose every 6 hours

Peritoneal dialysis (PD): Extensively removed by peritoneal dialysis: 4 mg/kg/dose every 6 hours

Continuous renal replacement therapy (CRRT): No adjustment required

Adults:

Manufacturer's labeling:

Mild, moderate, or severe impairment: There are no dosage adjustments provided in the manufacturer's labeling; however, decreased renal function does not alter the single-dose pharmacokinetics.

ESRD requiring dialysis: Metronidazole metabolites may accumulate; monitor for adverse events; accumulated metabolites may be rapidly removed by dialysis.

Intermittent hemodialysis (IHD): If administration cannot be separated from hemodialysis, consider supplemental dose following hemodialysis.

Peritoneal dialysis (PD): No dosage adjustment necessary

Alternate dosing:

Intermittent hemodialysis (IHD) (administer after hemodialysis on dialysis days): Extensively removed by hemodialysis: 500 mg every 8 to 12 hours. **Note:** Dosing regimen highly dependent on clinical indication (trichomoniasis vs *C. difficile* colitis) (Heintz, 2009). **Note:** Dosing dependent on the assumption of thrice-weekly, complete IHD sessions.

Continuous renal replacement therapy (CRRT) (Heintz, 2009; Trotman, 2005): Drug clearance is highly dependent on the method of renal replacement, filter type, and flow rate. Appropriate dosing requires close monitoring of pharmacologic response, signs of adverse reactions due to drug accumulation, as well as drug concentrations in relation to target trough (if appropriate). The following are general recommendations only (based on dialysate flow/ultrafiltration rates of 1 to 2 L/hour and minimal residual renal function) and should not supersede clinical judgment:

CVVH/CVVHD/CVVHDF: 500 mg every 6 to 12 hours (or per clinical indication; dosage reduction generally not necessary)

Dosing adjustment in hepatic impairment: Infants, Children, Adolescents, and Adults:

Manufacturer labeling:

Mild or moderate impairment (Child-Pugh class A or B): No dosage adjustment necessary; use with caution and monitor for adverse events

Severe impairment (Child-Pugh class C):

Immediate release tablets, injection: Reduce dose by 50%

Immediate release capsules:

Amebiasis: Adults: 375 mg 3 times daily

Trichomoniasis: Adults: 375 mg once daily

Extended release tablets: Use is not recommended.

Alternate dosing: The pharmacokinetics of a single oral 500 mg dose were not altered in patients with cirrhosis; initial dose reduction is therefore not necessary (Daneshmend, 1982). In one study of I.V. metronidazole, patients with alcoholic liver disease (with or without cirrhosis) demonstrated a prolonged elimination half-life (eg, ~18 hours). The authors recommended the dose be reduced accordingly (clearance was reduced by ~62%) and the frequency may be prolonged (eg, every 12 hours instead of every 6 hours) (Lau, 1987). In another single I.V. dose study using metronidazole metabolism to predict hepatic function, patients classified as Child-Pugh class C demonstrated a half-life of ~21.5 hours (Muscará, 1995).

Administration

Oral: Administer on an empty stomach

Immediate release: May administer with food if GI upset occurs.

Extended release: Should be taken on an empty stomach (1 hour before or 2 hours after meals); do not split, chew, or crush.

Parenteral: Administer I.V. by slow intermittent infusion over 30 to 60 minutes at a final concentration for administration of 5 to 8 mg/mL. Avoid contact of drug solution with equipment containing aluminum.

Monitoring Parameters Monitor CBC with differential at baseline and after prolonged or repeated courses of therapy. Closely monitor patients with severe hepatic impairment or ESRD for adverse reactions. Observe patients carefully if neurologic symptoms occur and consider discontinuation of therapy.

Test Interactions May interfere with AST, ALT, triglycerides, glucose, and LDH testing

Additional Information Sodium content of 500 mg ready-to-use single dose plastic container: 14 mEq

Dosage Forms Excipient information presented when available (limited, particularly for generics); consult specific product labeling.

Capsule, Oral:

Flagyl: 375 mg

Generic: 375 mg

Solution, Intravenous:

Metro: 500 mg (100 mL)

Generic: 500 mg (100 mL)

Solution, Intravenous [preservative free]:

Generic: 500 mg (100 mL)

Tablet, Oral:

Flagyl: 250 mg, 500 mg

Generic: 250 mg, 500 mg

Tablet Extended Release 24 Hour, Oral:

Flagyl ER: 750 mg

Extemporaneous Preparations A 50 mg/mL oral suspension may be made with tablets and a 1:1 mixture of Ora-Sweet and Ora-Plus. Crush twenty-four 250 mg tablets in a mortar and reduce to a fine powder. Add small portions of the vehicle and mix to a uniform paste; mix while adding the vehicle in incremental portions to **almost** 120 mL; transfer to a calibrated bottle, rinse mortar with vehicle, and add quantity of vehicle sufficient to make 120 mL. Label "shake well". Stable for 60 days at room temperature or refrigerated.

Allen LV Jr and Erickson MA 3rd, "Stability of Ketoconazole, Metolazone, Metronidazole, Procainamide Hydrochloride, and Spironolactone in Extemporaneously Compounded Oral Liquids," *Am J Health Syst Pharm*, 1996, 53(17):2073-8.

References

American Academy of Pediatrics (AAP). In: Pickering LK, Baker CJ, Kimberlin DW, Long SS, eds. *Red Book: 2012 Report of the Committee on Infectious Diseases.* 29th ed. Elk Grove Village, IL: American Academy of Pediatrics; 2012.

Aronoff GR, Bennett WM, Berns JS, et al. Drug prescribing in renal failure: dosing guidelines for adults and children. 5th ed. Philadelphia, PA: American College of Physicians; 2007.

Bratzler DW, Dellinger EP, Olsen KM, et al. Clinical practice guidelines for antimicrobial prophylaxis in surgery. *Am J Health Syst Pharm.* 2013;70(3):195-283.

Centers for Disease Control and Prevention (CDC). Sexually transmitted diseases treatment guidelines, 2010. *MMWR Recomm Rep.* 2010;59(RR-12):1-110.

Chey WD, Wong B. American College of Gastroenterology guideline on the management of *Helicobacter pylori* infection. *Am J Gastroenterol.* 2007;102(8):1808-1825.

Cohen SH, Gerding DN, Johnson S, et al. Clinical practice guidelines for *Clostridium difficile* infection in adults: 2010 update by the Society for Healthcare Epidemiology of American (SHEA) and the Infectious Diseases Society of America (IDSA). *Infect Control Hosp Epidemiol.* 2010;31(5):431-455.

Daneshmend TK, Homeida M, Kaye CM, Elamin AA, Roberts CJ. Disposition of oral metronidazole in hepatic cirrhosis and in hepatosplenic schistosomiasis. *Gut.* 1982;23(10):807-813.

Emil S, Laberge JM, Mikhail P, et al. Appendicitis in children: a ten-year update of therapeutic recommendations. *J Pediatr Surg.* 2003;38 (2):236-242.

Flagyl (metronidazole) [prescribing information]. New York, NY: G.D. Searle; June 2013.

Fraser JD, Aguayo P, Leys CM, et al. A complete course of intravenous antibiotics vs a combination of intravenous and oral antibiotics for perforated appendicitis in children: a prospective, randomized trial. *J Pediatr Surg.* 2010;45(6):1198-1202.

Heintz BH, Matzke GR, Dager WE. Antimicrobial dosing concepts and recommendations for critically ill adult patients receiving continuous renal replacement therapy or intermittent hemodialysis. *Pharmacotherapy.* 2009;29(5):562-577.

Jager-Roman E, Doyle PE, Baird-Lambert J, Cvejic M, Buchanan N. Pharmacokinetics and tissue distribution of metronidazole in the new born infant. *J Pediatr.* 1982;100(4):651-654.

Koletzko S, Jones NL, Goodman KJ, et al. Evidence-based guidelines from ESPGHAN and NASPGHAN for *Helicobacter pylori* infection in children. *J Pediatr Gastroenterol Nutr.* 2011;53(2):230-243.

Lamp KC, Freeman CD, Klutman NE, Lacy MK. Pharmacokinetics and pharmacodynamics of the nitroimidazole antimicrobials. *Clin Pharmacokinet.* 1999;36(5):353-373.

Lau AH, Evans R, Chang CW, Seligsohn R. Pharmacokinetics of metronidazole in patients with alcoholic liver disease. *Antimicrob Agents Chemother.* 1987;31(11):1662-1664.

Metronidazole [prescribing information]. Deerfield, IL: Baxter Healthcare Corporation; October 2013.

Muscará MN, Pedrazzoli J Jr, Miranda EL, et al. Plasma hydroxymetronidazole/metronidazole ratio in patients with liver disease and in healthy volunteers. *Br J Clin Pharmacol.* 1995;40(5):477-480.

Rufo PA, Denson LA, Sylvester FA, et al. Health supervision in the management of children and adolescents with IBD: NASPGHAN recommendations. *J Pediatr Gastroenterol Nutr.* 2012;55(1):93-108.

Sandhu BK, Fell JM, Beattie RM, et al. Guidelines for the management of inflammatory bowel disease in children in the United Kingdom. *J Pediatr Gastroenterol Nutr.* 2010;50(Suppl 1):S1-S13.

◀

Schutze GE, Willoughby RE. Committee on Infectious Diseases, American Academy of Pediatrics. *Clostridium difficile* infection in infants and children. *Pediatrics.* 2013;131(1):196-200.

Solomkin JS, Mazuski JE, Bradley JS, et al. Diagnosis and management of complicated intra-abdominal infection in adults and children: guidelines by the Surgical Infection Society and the Infectious Diseases Society of America. *Clin Infect Dis.* 2010;50(2):133-164.

St Peter SD, Little DC, Calkins CM, et al. A simple and more cost-effective antibiotic regimen for perforated appendicitis. *J Pediatr Surg.* 2006;41(5):1020-1024.

St Peter SD, Tsao K, Spilde TL, et al. Single daily dosing ceftriaxone and metronidazole vs standard triple antibiotic regimen for perforated appendicitis in children: a prospective randomized trial. *J Pediatr Surg.* 2008;43(6):981-985.

Surawicz CM, Brandt LJ, Binion DG, et al. Guidelines for diagnosis, treatment, and prevention of *Clostridium difficile* infections. *Am J Gastroenterol.* 2013 Apr;108(4):478-498.

Suyagh M, Collier PS, Millership JS, et al. Metronidazole population pharmacokinetics in preterm neonates using dried blood-spot sampling. *Pediatrics.* 2011;127(2):e367-e374.

Trotman RL, Williamson JC, Shoemaker DM, Salzer WL. Antibiotic dosing in critically ill adult patients receiving continuous renal replacement therapy. *Clin Infect Dis.* 2005;41(8):1159-1166.

Turner D, Levine A, Escher JC, et al. Management of pediatric ulcerative colitis: joint ECCO and ESPGHAN evidence-based consensus guidelines. *J Pediatr Gastroenterol Nutr.* 2012;55(3):340-361.

Upadhyaya P, Bhatnagar V, Basu N. Pharmacokinetics of intravenous metronidazole in neonates. *J Pediatr Surg.* 1988;23(3):263-265.

Yardeni D, Kawar B, Siplovich L, et al. Single daily dosing of ceftriaxone and metronidazole is as safe and effective as ampicillin, gentamicin and metronidazole for non-operative management of complicated appendicitis in children. *Pediat Therapeut.* 2013;3:5.

MetroNIDAZOLE (Topical) (met roe NYE da zole)

Brand Names: U.S. MetroCream; Metrogel; MetroGel-Vaginal; MetroLotion; Noritate; Rosadan; Vandazole

Brand Names: Canada MetroCream; Metrogel; MetroLotion; Nidagel; Noritate; Rosasol

Therapeutic Category Antibiotic, Topical

Generic Availability (U.S.) May be product dependent

Use

Topical: Treatment of inflammatory lesions (papules and pustules) of rosacea (FDA approved in adults)

Vaginal gel:

Metrogel: Treatment of bacterial vaginosis (FDA approved in adults)

Vandazole: Treatment of bacterial vaginosis (FDA approved in nonpregnant, postmenarchal females)

Pregnancy Risk Factor B

Pregnancy Considerations Adverse events have not been observed in animal reproduction studies. Metronidazole crosses the placenta and rapidly distributes into the fetal circulation rapidly following oral administration. The amount of metronidazole available systemically following topical application is less in comparison to oral doses. Metronidazole 1.3% vaginal gel and Vandazole are not indicated for use in pregnant patients. Oral metronidazole is preferred for the treatment of symptomatic bacterial vaginosis in pregnant patients (consult current guidelines) (CDC, 2010).

Breast-Feeding Considerations Metronidazole is excreted in breast milk following oral administration and can be detected in concentrations similar to the maternal serum. The amount of metronidazole available systemically following topical application is less in comparison to oral doses. According to the manufacturer, the decision to continue or discontinue breast-feeding during therapy should take into account the risk of exposure to the infant and the benefits of treatment to the mother; nursing women may consider pumping and discarding their milk during therapy and 24 hours after therapy.

Contraindications Hypersensitivity to metronidazole, nitroimidazole derivatives, or any component

Warnings Prolonged use may result in fungal or bacterial superinfection. Approximately 10% of women treated with the vaginal gel developed *Candida* vaginitis during or immediately after treatment. Disulfiram-like reaction to ethanol has been reported with systemic metronidazole and may occur with the vaginal gel; consider avoidance of alcoholic beverages during therapy with vaginal gel. Do not administer the vaginal gel to patients who have taken disulfiram within the past 2 weeks. Aseptic meningitis, encephalopathy, seizures, and neuropathies (peripheral and optic) have been reported with systemic therapy, especially with increased doses and chronic treatment; peripheral neuropathy has also been reported with topical products; monitor and consider discontinuation of therapy if signs/symptoms occur; use with caution in patients with CNS disease. Has been shown to be carcinogenic in rodents with oral dosing.

Precautions Use with caution in patients with hepatic impairment due to potential accumulation. May cause tearing of the eye; avoid contact with the eyes. In the event of accidental contact, wash eye out immediately. Irritant and allergic contact dermatitis has been reported; if symptoms occur may need to use less frequently or discontinue use. Use with caution in patients with blood dyscrasias.

Adverse Reactions

Topical:

Cardiovascular: Hypertension

Central nervous system: Headache

Dermatologic: Acne vulgaris, burning sensation of skin, contact dermatitis, erythema, pruritus, skin irritation, skin rash, xeroderma

Gastrointestinal: Metallic taste, nausea, unusual taste, xerostomia

Local: Hypersensitivity reaction

Neuromuscular & skeletal: Numbness of extremities, peripheral neuropathy, tingling of extremities

Ophthalmic: Eye irritation

Respiratory: Flu-like symptoms

Vaginal:

Central nervous system: Dizziness, headache

Gastrointestinal: Abdominal cramps, decreased appetite, diarrhea, gastrointestinal distress, metallic taste (or unusual taste), nausea and vomiting

Genitourinary: Cervical candidiasis (or vaginitis), dysmenorrhea, pelvic pain, vaginal discharge, vulvovaginal candidiasis, vulvovaginal irritation, vulvovaginal pruritus

Rare, but important or life-threatening: Bloating, dark urine, depression, skin rash, xerostomia

Drug Interactions

Metabolism/Transport Effects None known.

Avoid Concomitant Use

Avoid concomitant use of MetroNIDAZOLE (Topical) with any of the following: BCG

Increased Effect/Toxicity

MetroNIDAZOLE (Topical) may increase the levels/effects of: Alcohol (Ethyl); Disulfiram; Ritonavir; Tipranavir

The levels/effects of MetroNIDAZOLE (Topical) may be increased by: Mebendazole

Decreased Effect

MetroNIDAZOLE (Topical) may decrease the levels/effects of: BCG; Sodium Picosulfate

Stability

Topical cream, gel, lotion: Store at 20°C to 25°C (68°F to 77°F).

Vaginal gel: Store at 15°C to 30°C (59°F to 86°C); do not freeze.

Mechanism of Action After diffusing into the organism, interacts with DNA to cause a loss of helical DNA structure and strand breakage resulting in inhibition of protein synthesis and cell death in susceptible organisms

Pharmacokinetics (Adult data unless noted)

Absorption:

Topical: Concentrations achieved systemically after application of the 1 g topical gel and cream are <1% of those obtained after a 250 mg oral dose

Vaginal gel: ~50% of oral dose

Time to peak serum concentration:

Topical gel: 6 to 10 hours

Topical cream: 8 to 12 hours

Vaginal gel: 6 to 12 hours

Dosing: Usual

Infants, Children, and Adolescents:

Bacterial vaginosis: Intravaginal: One applicatorful (~5 g gel contains ~37.5 mg of metronidazole) intravaginally once daily at bedtime for 5 days (CDC, 2010; *Red Book* [AAP], 2012)

Periorifacial dermatitis: Infants ≥6 months, Children, and Adolescents: Limited data available: Topical: 0.75% gel: Apply thin film once or twice daily (Manders, 1992; Miller, 1994; Nguyen, 2006)

Adults:

Acne rosacea: Topical:

0.75%: Apply and rub a thin film twice daily, morning and evening, to entire affected areas after washing

1%: Apply thin film to affected area once daily after washing

Bacterial vaginosis: Intravaginal: One applicatorful (~5 g gel contains ~37.5 mg of metronidazole) intravaginally once or twice daily for 5 days; apply once in morning and evening if using twice daily; apply at bedtime if using once daily

Administration

Intravaginal: Use only **vaginal gel** intravaginally; fill applicator with medication; insert the applicator high into the vagina and press the plunger to release the medication; clean the applicator with warm soapy water and rinse well. Do not apply to the eye

Topical: Wash affected areas with a mild cleanser; then apply a thin film of drug to the affected area and rub in. Cosmetics may be used after application (wait at least 5 minutes after using lotion). Do not apply to the eye.

Dosage Forms

Excipient information presented when available (limited, particularly for generics); consult specific product labeling.

Cream, External:

MetroCream: 0.75% (45 g) [contains benzyl alcohol]

Noritate: 1% (60 g) [contains methylparaben, propylparaben, trolamine (triethanolamine)]

Rosadan: 0.75% (45 g) [contains benzyl alcohol]

Generic: 0.75% (45 g)

Gel, External:

Metrogel: 1% (55 g, 60 g) [contains methylparaben, propylparaben]

Rosadan: 0.75% (45 g) [contains edetate disodium, methylparaben, propylene glycol, propylparaben]

Generic: 0.75% (45 g); 1% (55 g, 60 g)

Gel, Vaginal:

MetroGel-Vaginal: 0.75% (70 g) [contains edetate disodium, methylparaben, propylene glycol, propylparaben]

Vandazole: 0.75% (70 g) [contains methylparaben, propylparaben]

Generic: 0.75% (70 g)

Kit, External:

Rosadan: 0.75% [contains benzyl alcohol]

Rosadan: 0.75% [contains edetate disodium, methylparaben, propylene glycol, propylparaben]

Lotion, External:

MetroLotion: 0.75% (59 mL) [contains benzyl alcohol]

Generic: 0.75% (59 mL)

References

American Academy of Pediatrics (AAP). In: Pickering LK, Baker CJ, Kimberlin DW, Long SS, eds. *Red Book: 2012 Report of the*

Committee on Infectious Diseases. 29th ed. Elk Grove Village, IL: American Academy of Pediatrics; 2012.

Centers for Disease Control and Prevention (CDC), "Sexually Transmitted Diseases Treatment Guidelines, 2010," *MMWR Recomm Rep,* 2010, 59(RR-12):1-110.

Manders SM, Lucky AW. Perioral dermatitis in childhood. *J Am Acad Dermatol.* 1992;27:688-692.

Miller SR, Shalita AR. Topical metronidazole gel (0.75%) for the treatment of perioral dermatitis in children. *J Am Acad Dermatol.* 1994;31:847-848.

Nguyen V, Eichenfield LE. Periorificial dermatitis in children and adolescents. *J Am Acad Dermatol.* 2006;55:781-785.

Red Book: 2012 Report of the Committee on Infectious Diseases, 29th ed, Pickering LK, ed, Elk Grove Village, IL: American Academy of Pediatrics, 2012.

◆ **Metronidazole Hydrochloride** *see* MetroNIDAZOLE (Systemic) *on page 1399*

◆ **Metronidazole Hydrochloride** *see* MetroNIDAZOLE (Topical) *on page 1404*

Metyrapone (me TEER a pone)

Medication Safety Issues

Sound-alike/look-alike issues:

Metyrapone may be confused with metyrosine

Brand Names: U.S. Metopirone

Therapeutic Category Diagnostic Agent, Hypothalamic-Pituitary ACTH Function

Generic Availability (U.S.) No

Use Diagnostic agent for testing hypothalamic-pituitary ACTH function [FDA approved in pediatric patients (age not specified) and adults]

Prescribing and Access Restrictions Metopirone® is available from HRA Pharma via special allocation only. Contact the manufacturer for additional information at 855-674-7663.

Pregnancy Risk Factor C

Pregnancy Considerations Animal reproduction studies have not been conducted. Subnormal response may occur in pregnant women and the fetal pituitary may be affected.

Breast-Feeding Considerations The excretion of metyrapone and its active metabolite into breast milk are described in a case report. The mother had been taking metyrapone 250 mg 4 times/day for 9 weeks and was 1 week postpartum when milk samples were obtained. Multiple milk samples taken 1-5 hours after the dose contained average concentrations of metyrapone 11.2 mcg/L and metyrapol 48.5 mcg/L over the dosing interval. The relative infant dose (metyrapone and metyrapol) was calculated to be 0.1% of the weight adjusted maternal dose.

Contraindications Hypersensitivity to metyrapone or any component; adrenal cortical insufficiency

Warnings All corticosteroid therapy should be discontinued prior to and during the metyrapone test; administration of metyrapone may induce acute adrenal insufficiency in patients with reduced adrenal secretory capacity; patients with suspected adrenocortical insufficiency should be observed closely over 24 hours

Precautions Response to test may be subnormal in patients with hypo- or hyperthyroidism. Prior to use of metapyrone, the ability of the patient's adrenal glands to respond to exogenous ACTH should be demonstrated. Metyrapone may cause dizziness and sedation which may impair physical or mental abilities; patients must be cautioned about performing tasks which require mental alertness (eg, operating machinery or driving).

Adverse Reactions

Cardiovascular: Hypotension

Central nervous system: Dizziness, headache, sedation

Dermatologic: Allergic rash

Gastrointestinal: Abdominal discomfort or pain, nausea, vomiting

◀ Hematologic: Bone marrow suppression (rare), white blood cell count decreased (rare)

Drug Interactions

Metabolism/Transport Effects Inhibits CYP2A6 (weak); **Induces** CYP3A4 (weak/moderate)

Avoid Concomitant Use

Avoid concomitant use of Metyrapone with any of the following: Axitinib; Simeprevir

Increased Effect/Toxicity

Metyrapone may increase the levels/effects of: Acetaminophen

Decreased Effect

Metyrapone may decrease the levels/effects of: ARIPiprazole; Axitinib; Ibrutinib; Saxagliptin; Simeprevir

The levels/effects of Metyrapone may be decreased by: Fosphenytoin; Phenytoin

Stability Store at ≤30°C (86°F); protect from heat and moisture.

Mechanism of Action Metyrapone inhibits the production of cortisol; blockade can be measured by the urinary increase of the metabolites of cortisol precursors in the urine (17-hyroxycorticosteroids [17-OHCS] and 17-ketogenic steroids [17-KGS]).

Pharmacodynamics Maximum effect: Peak excretion of steroid during the first 24 hours after administration

Pharmacokinetics (Adult data unless noted)

Absorption: Oral: Well absorbed; rapid

Metabolism: Reduced to metyrapol (active metabolite); parent drug and metabolite also undergo glucuronide conjugation

Half-life, elimination:

Metyrapone: 1.9 ± 0.7 hours

Metyrapol (active metabolite): Takes twice as long as metyrapone to be eliminated

Time to peak serum concentration: 1 hour

Elimination: Urine: ~5% as metyrapone (primarily as glucuronide conjugate) and ~38% as metyrapol (primarily as glucuronide conjugate)

Dosing: Usual ACTH function, diagnostic test: Oral:

Single-dose/overnight test: Children and Adults: 30 mg/kg as a single dose (maximum dose: 3000 mg) given at midnight the night before the test

Multiple-dose test:

Children: 15 mg/kg/dose every 4 hours for 6 doses; minimum dose: 250 mg; maximum dose: 750 mg

Adults: 750 mg every 4 hours for 6 doses

Administration Oral: May administer with food or milk to reduce GI irritation

Single-dose/overnight test: Administer dose at midnight with yogurt or milk.

Multiple-dose test: Administer with milk or snack 2 days following ACTH test.

Monitoring Parameters Urinary 17-OHCS; urinary 17-KGS; plasma 11-deoxycortisol

Single-dose/overnight test: Blood samples are taken the following morning (7:30-8:00 am).

Multiple-dose test: Urine is collected for 24 hours following the last day of administration.

Reference Range Normal 24-hour urinary excretion of 17-OHCS: 3-12 mg (increases following ACTH infusion)

Normal response to metyrapone:

Plasma ACTH: 44 pmol/L (200 ng/L)

Plasma 11-desoxycortisol: 0.2 micromoles/L (70 mcg/L)

24 hour urinary excretion of 17-OHCS: 2-4 time increase

24 hour urinary excretion of 17-KGS: 2 time increase

A subnormal response may be indicative of panhypopituitarism or partial hypopituitarism. An excessive response is suggestive of Cushing's syndrome associated with adrenal hyperplasia.

Dosage Forms Excipient information presented when available (limited, particularly for generics); consult specific product labeling.

Capsule, Oral:

Metopirone: 250 mg

♦ **Mevacor** see Lovastatin on page 1286

♦ **Mevinolin** see Lovastatin on page 1286

Mexiletine (meks IL e teen)

Brand Names: Canada Novo-Mexiletine

Therapeutic Category Antiarrhythmic Agent, Class I-B

Generic Availability (U.S.) Yes

Use Management of serious ventricular arrhythmias; suppression of premature ventricular contractions; diabetic neuropathy

Pregnancy Risk Factor C

Pregnancy Considerations Adverse events were observed in some animal reproduction studies. A few case reports have demonstrated safe use of mexiletine in pregnant women.

Breast-Feeding Considerations Mexiletine concentrations in breast milk are similar to those in the maternal plasma.

Contraindications Hypersensitivity to mexiletine or any component; cardiogenic shock; second or third degree heart block (except in patients with a functioning artificial pacemaker)

Warnings Antiarrhythmic agents should be reserved for patients with life-threatening ventricular arrhythmias **[U.S. Boxed Warning]**. In the Cardiac Arrhythmia Suppression Trial (CAST), recent (>6 days but <2 years ago) myocardial infarction patients with asymptomatic, nonlife-threatening ventricular arrhythmias did not benefit and may have been harmed by attempts to suppress the arrhythmia with flecainide or encainide. An increased mortality or nonfatal cardiac arrest rate (7.7%) was seen in the active treatment group compared with patients in the placebo group (3%). The applicability of the CAST results to other populations is unknown. Worsening of arrhythmia (including ventricular tachycardia or ventricular fibrillation) may occur.

Blood dyscrasias (including leukopenia, agranulocytosis, and thrombocytopenia) have been reported.

Precautions Use with caution in patients with seizure disorders, severe heart failure, hypotension, hepatic impairment; avoid dietary regimens or concomitant drug therapy that markedly change urine pH

Adverse Reactions

Cardiovascular: Angina, chest pain, palpitation, premature ventricular contractions, proarrhythmia

Central nervous system: Confusion, depression, dizziness, headache, incoordination, insomnia, lightheadedness, nervousness

Dermatologic: Rash

Gastrointestinal: Abdominal pain, constipation, diarrhea, GI distress, nausea, vomiting, xerostomia

Neuromuscular & skeletal: Arthralgias, ataxia, numbness of fingers or toes, paresthesia, trembling, tremor, unsteady gait, weakness

Ocular: Blurred vision, nystagmus

Otic: Tinnitus

Respiratory: Dyspnea

Rare but important or life-threatening: Agranulocytosis, alopecia, AV block, cardiogenic shock, CHF, dysphagia, exfoliative dermatitis, hallucinations, hepatic necrosis, hepatitis, hypotension, impotence, leukopenia, myelofibrosis, pancreatitis (rare), psychosis, pulmonary fibrosis, seizure, sinus arrest, SLE syndrome, Stevens-Johnson syndrome, syncope, thrombocytopenia, torsade de pointes, upper GI bleeding, urinary retention, urticaria

Drug Interactions

Metabolism/Transport Effects Substrate of CYP1A2 (major), CYP2D6 (major); **Note:** Assignment of Major/Minor substrate status based on clinically relevant drug interaction potential; **Inhibits** CYP1A2 (strong)

Avoid Concomitant Use

Avoid concomitant use of Mexiletine with any of the following: Agomelatine; Pirfenidone; Pomalidomide; Tasimelteon

Increased Effect/Toxicity

Mexiletine may increase the levels/effects of: Agomelatine; Bendamustine; CloZAPine; CYP1A2 Substrates; Pirfenidone; Pomalidomide; Tasimelteon; Theophylline Derivatives

The levels/effects of Mexiletine may be increased by: Abiraterone Acetate; CYP1A2 Inhibitors (Moderate); CYP1A2 Inhibitors (Strong); CYP2D6 Inhibitors (Moderate); CYP2D6 Inhibitors (Strong); Darunavir; Deferasirox; Selective Serotonin Reuptake Inhibitors; Vemurafenib

Decreased Effect

The levels/effects of Mexiletine may be decreased by: Cannabis; CYP1A2 Inducers (Strong); Cyproterone; Etravirine; Fosphenytoin; Peginterferon Alfa-2b; Phenytoin

Food Interactions Food may decrease the rate, but not the extent of oral absorption; diets which affect urine pH can increase or decrease excretion of mexiletine. Management: Avoid dietary changes that alter urine pH.

Mechanism of Action Class IB antiarrhythmic, structurally related to lidocaine, which inhibits inward sodium current, decreases rate of rise of phase 0, increases effective refractory period/action potential duration ratio

Pharmacodynamics Onset of action: Oral: 30-120 minutes

Pharmacokinetics (Adult data unless noted)

Distribution: V_d: 5-7 L/kg; found in breast milk in similar concentrations as plasma

Protein-binding: 50% to 70%

Metabolism: Extensive in the liver (some minor active metabolites)

Bioavailability: Oral: 88%

Half-life, adults: 10-14 hours; increase in half-life with hepatic or heart failure

Elimination: 10% to 15% excreted unchanged in urine; urinary acidification increases excretion

Dosing: Usual Oral:

Children: Range: 1.4-5 mg/kg/dose (mean: 3.3 mg/kg/dose) given every 8 hours; start with lower initial dose and increase according to effects and serum concentrations

Adults: Initial: 200 mg every 8 hours (may load with 400 mg if necessary); adjust dose every 2-3 days; usual dose: 200-300 mg every 8 hours; some patients may respond to the same daily dose divided every 12 hours; maximum dose: 1.2 g/day

Dosing adjustment in renal impairment: Children and Adults: CrCl <10 mL/minute: Administer 50% to 75% of normal dose

Dosing adjustment in hepatic disease: Children and Adults: Administer 25% to 30% of normal dose; patients with severe liver disease may require even lower doses, monitor closely

Administration Oral: Administer with food, milk, or antacids to decrease GI upset

Monitoring Parameters Liver enzymes, CBC, ECG, heart rate, serum concentrations

Reference Range

Therapeutic range: 0.5-2 mcg/mL

Potentially toxic: >2 mcg/mL

Test Interactions Abnormal liver function test, positive ANA, thrombocytopenia

Additional Information I.V. form under investigation

Dosage Forms Excipient information presented when available (limited, particularly for generics); consult specific product labeling.

Capsule, Oral, as hydrochloride:

Generic: 150 mg, 200 mg, 250 mg

Extemporaneous Preparations A 10 mg/mL oral suspension may be with made with capsules and either distilled water or sorbitol USP. Empty the contents of eight 150 mg capsules in a mortar and reduce to a fine powder if necessary. Add small portions of the chosen vehicle and mix to a uniform paste; mix while adding the vehicle in incremental proportions to **almost** 120 mL; transfer to a graduated cylinder, rinse mortar with vehicle, and add quantity of vehicle sufficient to make 120 mL. Label "shake well". Sorbitol suspension is stable in plastic prescription bottles for 2 weeks at room temperature and 4 weeks refrigerated; distilled water suspension is stable in plastic prescription bottles for 7 weeks at room temperature and 13 weeks refrigerated. Extended storage under refrigeration is recommended to minimize microbial contamination.

Nahata MC, Morosco RS, and Hipple TF, "Stability of Mexiletine in Two Extemporaneous Liquid Formulations Stored Under Refrigeration and at Room Temperature," *J Am Pharm Assoc (Wash),* 2000, 40 (2):257-9.

References

Moak JP, Smith RT, and Garson A Jr, "Mexiletine: An Effective Antiarrhythmic Drug for Treatment of Ventricular Arrhythmias in Congenital Heart Disease," *J Am Coll Cardiol,* 1987, 10(4):824-9.

◆ **Mezavant (Can)** *see* Mesalamine *on page 1347*

◆ **MgSO₄ (error-prone abbreviation)** *see* Magnesium Sulfate *on page 1297*

◆ **Miacalcin** *see* Calcitonin *on page 340*

◆ **Mi-Acid Gas Relief [OTC]** *see* Simethicone *on page 1891*

◆ **Micaderm [OTC]** *see* Miconazole (Topical) *on page 1410*

Micafungin (mi ka FUN gin)

Brand Names: U.S. Mycamine

Brand Names: Canada Mycamine

Therapeutic Category Antifungal Agent, Echinocandin; Antifungal Agent, Systemic

Generic Availability (U.S.) No

Use Treatment of patients with esophageal candidiasis; treatment of candidemia, acute disseminated candidiasis, *Candida* peritonitis and abscess; prophylaxis of *Candida* infections in patients undergoing hematopoietic stem cell transplant (All indications: FDA approved in ages ≥4 months and adults); has been used for treatment of invasive *Aspergillosis*; micafungin is ineffective against cryptococcosis, fusariosis, and zygomycosis

Pregnancy Risk Factor C

Pregnancy Considerations Adverse events have been observed in animal reproduction studies. There are no adequate and well-controlled studies in pregnant women. Use only if benefit outweighs risk.

Breast-Feeding Considerations It is not known if micafungin is excreted in breast milk. The manufacturer recommends that caution be exercised when administering micafungin to nursing women.

Contraindications Hypersensitivity to micafungin, other echinocandins, or any component

Warnings Cases of hypersensitivity reactions, including anaphylactoid reactions and anaphylaxis with shock, have been reported in patients who received micafungin; if reaction occurs, discontinue infusion and provide appropriate treatment. Rare cases of acute intravascular hemolysis, hemoglobinuria, and hemolytic anemia have been reported. New-onset or worsening hepatic impairment, including hepatitis and hepatic failure, has been reported; use with caution in patients receiving concomitant hepatotoxic drugs; monitor closely and evaluate appropriateness of continued use in patients who develop abnormal liver function tests during treatment. Increased BUN, serum creatinine, renal dysfunction, and/or acute renal failure have also been reported; use with caution in patients with renal impairment or who develop worsening renal function during treatment; monitor closely.

Precautions Use caution with administration through a peripheral line; local reactions may occur more frequently including infusion site inflammation, phlebitis and thrombophlebitis.

Adverse Reactions

Cardiovascular: Atrial fibrillation, bradycardia, cardiac arrest, edema, hypertension, hypotension, localized phlebitis, myocardial infarction, pericardial effusion, peripheral edema, tachycardia

Central nervous system: Anxiety, brain disease, convulsions, delirium, dizziness, fatigue, headache, insomnia, intracranial hemorrhage, rigors

Dermatologic: Pruritus (more common in pediatric patients ages 3 days through 16 years), skin rash, urticaria (more common in pediatric patients ages 3 days through 16 years)

Endocrine & metabolic: Hyperglycemia, hyperkalemia, hypernatremia, hypervolemia, hypocalcemia, hypoglycemia, hypokalemia, hypomagnesemia

Gastrointestinal: Abdominal distension, abdominal pain, anorexia, constipation, diarrhea, dyspepsia, mucositis, nausea, vomiting

Genitourinary: Decreased urine output, hematuria

Hematologic & oncologic: Anemia (more common in pediatric patients ages 3 days through 16 years), blood coagulation disorder, febrile neutropenia, neutropenia, pancytopenia, thrombocytopenia, thrombotic thrombocytopenic purpura

Hepatic: Abnormal hepatic function tests (more common in pediatric patients ages 3 days through 16 years), hepatic failure, hepatic injury, hepatomegaly, hyperbilirubinemia (more common in pediatric patients ages 3 days through 16 years), increased serum alkaline phosphatase, increased serum ALT (more common in pediatric patients ages 3 days through 16 years), increased serum AST, jaundice

Hypersensitivity: Anaphylaxis, hypersensivity reaction

Infection: Bacteremia, sepsis

Local: Venous thrombosis at injection site

Neuromuscular & skeletal: Back pain

Renal: Renal failure

Respiratory: Cough, dyspnea, epistaxis

Miscellaneous: Fever (more common in pediatric patients ages 3 days through 16 years), infusion related reaction (more common in pediatric patients ages 3 days through 16 years)

Rare but important or life-threatening: Acidosis, acute renal failure, anaphylactoid reaction, anuria, apnea, cardiac arrhythmia, cyanosis, decreased white blood cell count, deep vein thrombosis, disseminated intravascular coagulation, erythema multiforme, hemoglobinuria, hemolysis, hemolytic anemia, hepatic insufficiency, hepatitis, hiccups, hyponatremia, hypoxia, increased blood urea nitrogen, increased serum creatinine, infection, injection site reaction, oliguria, pneumonia, pulmonary embolism, renal insufficiency, renal tubular necrosis, seizure, shock, skin necrosis, Stevens-Johnson syndrome, thrombophlebitis, tissue necrosis at injection site, toxic epidermal necrolysis, vasodilatation

Drug Interactions

Metabolism/Transport Effects Substrate of CYP3A4 (minor); **Note:** Assignment of Major/Minor substrate status based on clinically relevant drug interaction potential; **Inhibits** CYP3A4 (weak)

Avoid Concomitant Use
Avoid concomitant use of Micafungin with any of the following: Pimozide; Saccharomyces boulardii

Increased Effect/Toxicity
Micafungin may increase the levels/effects of: ARIPiprazole; Dofetilide; Lomitapide; Pimozide

Decreased Effect
Micafungin may decrease the levels/effects of: Saccharomyces boulardii

Stability Store intact vials at 25°C (77°F); excursions permitted to 15°C to 30°C (59°F to 86°F); reconstituted solution may be stored in the original vial for up to 24 hours at room temperature; diluted infusion may be stored for up to 24 hours at room temperature; protect diluted solution from light; it is not necessary to cover the infusion drip chamber or the tubing.

Mechanism of Action Concentration-dependent inhibition of 1,3-beta-D-glucan synthase resulting in reduced formation of 1,3-beta-D-glucan, an essential polysaccharide comprising 30% to 60% of *Candida* cell walls (absent in mammalian cells); decreased glucan content leads to osmotic instability and cellular lysis

Pharmacokinetics (Adult data unless noted)

Absorption: Oral: Poor

Distribution: Distributes into lung, liver, and spleen; minimally to CNS and eyes (Caudle, 2012)

Preterm infants (ELBW): Reported data highly variable; possibly dependent on GA/weight, and PNA: V_{dss}:

PNA 0-1 day: 0.76 L/kg (Kawada, 2009)

PNA 4 days: 1.52 L/kg (Smith, 2009)

PNA >3 weeks: 0.43 L/kg (range: 0.28-0.66 L/kg) (Heresi, 2006)

Children 2-8 years: V_{dss}: 0.35 ± 0.18 L/kg (Seibel, 2005)

Children and Adolescents 9-17 years: V_{dss}: 0.28 ± 0.09 L/kg (Seibel, 2005)

Adults: V_d: 0.39 ± 0.11 L/kg

Protein binding:

Neonates: 96.7% (Yanni, 2011)

Adults: >99% to albumin

Metabolism: Hepatic to M-1, catechol form by arylsulfatase; further metabolized to M-2, methoxy form by catechol-O-methyltransferase; hydroxylation to M-5 by CYP3A

Half-life:

Preterm infants:

PNA <1 week: 6.7 hours (Kawada, 2009)

PNA >3 weeks: Mean 8.3 hours (range: 5.6-11 hours) (Heresi, 2006)

Pediatric patients 4 months to 16 years of age:

≤30 kg: 12.5 ± 4.6 hours

>30kg: 13.6 ± 8.8 hours

Healthy Adults: 11-21 hours

Adults receiving bone marrow or peripheral stem-cell transplantation: 10.7-13.5 hours (Carver, 2004)

Elimination: <1% of dose is eliminated unchanged renally (Herbert, 2005); 71% is eliminated in the feces

Clearance:

Preterm infants:

PNA 0-1 day: 1.48 mL/minute/kg (Kawada, 2009)

PNA 4 days: 0.58 mL/minute (Smith, 2009)

PNA >3 weeks: 0.64 mL/minute (Heresi, 2006)

Pediatric patients 4 months to 16 years of age:

≤30 kg: 0.328 mL/minute/kg

>30kg: 0.241 mL/minute/kg

Adults: ~0.3 mL/minute/kg

Dosing: Neonatal

Fungal infections, susceptible: Limited data available; dosing based on several pharmacokinetic studies in preterm infants (Benjamin, 2010; Caudle, 2012; Heresi, 2006; Hope, 2010; Smith, 2009): I.V.:

<1000 g: 10 mg/kg/day once daily; doses as high as 15 mg/kg/day have been used; dosages at the higher end of the dosing range should be considered for

treating CNS infections due to poor micafungin CNS penetration (Caudle, 2012)

≥1000 g: 7-10 mg/kg/day once daily; HIV-exposed/-positive neonates may require up to 10-12 mg/kg/day once daily (DHHS [pediatric], 2013)

Dosing: Usual

Infants <4 months:

Candidiasis:

Disseminated; treatment: Limited data available: I.V.:

Non-HIV-exposed/-positive: 2 mg/kg/day once daily; may increase higher doses (4-10 mg/kg/day) if no improvement in condition, or persistent positive cultures; reported range: 2-10 mg/kg/day; further studies are needed [Benjamin, 2010; Hope, 2010; Myacin prescribing information (European Medicines Agency), 2013; Queiroz-Telles, 2008]

HIV-exposed/-positive (critically ill): 5-7 mg/kg/day once daily; treatment duration variable, continue treatment for 2 weeks following last positive blood culture

Esophageal, treatment: HIV-exposed/-positive: 5-7 mg/kg/day once daily; treatment duration: ≥3 weeks and for at least 2 weeks following symptom resolution (DHHS [pediatric], 2013)

Infants ≥4 months, Children, and Adolescents:

Aspergillosis: I.V.:

Treatment; invasive disease: Limited data available:

Infants and Children: 1.5-3 mg/kg/day once daily; titration to a higher dose may be necessary for lack of clinical response or persistent positive cultures; reported usual maximum dose range: 4-8.6 mg/kg/day; in infants, initial doses at the higher end of the dosage range may be necessary due to pharmacokinetic differences (Denning, 2006, Emiroglu, 2011; Flynn, 2006; Kobayashi, 2007; Singer, 2003)

Adolescents:

HIV-exposed/-positive: 100-150 mg once daily (DHHS [adult], 2013)

Non-HIV-exposed/-positive: 1.5 mg/kg/day; increase if clinically indicated; maximum daily dose: 150 mg/day; dosing based on a noncomparative study of all ages, an abstract describing a study in pediatric patients 3 months to 16 years and single case report of a 13-year old who received 1.5 mg/kg/day for invasive aspergillosis; further studies are needed (Denning, 2006; Emiroglu, 2011; Flynn, 2006; Singer, 2003).

Prophylaxis in hematopoietic stem cell transplantation: I.V.: 1-3 mg/kg daily; maximum dose: 50 mg (Kusuki, 2009; Tomblyn, 2009; van Burik, 2004)

Candidiasis:

Treatment:

Acute disseminated infection, peritonitis, and abscesses: I.V.:

Non-HIV-exposed/-positive: 2 mg/kg once daily; maximum dose: 100 mg

HIV-exposed/-positive (DHHS [pediatric], 2013):

Infants <15 kg: 5-7 mg/kg once daily

Children 2-8 years and ≤40 kg: 3-4 mg/kg once daily

Children ≥9 years and Adolescents:

≤40 kg: 2-3 mg/kg once daily

>40 kg: 100 mg once daily

Esophageal candidiasis: I.V.:

Non-HIV-exposed/-positive:

≤30 kg: 3 mg/kg once daily

>30 kg: 2.5 mg/kg once daily; maximum dose:150 mg

HIV-exposed/-positive (DHHS [adult/pediatric], 2013):

Infants <15 kg: 5-7 mg/kg once daily

Children 2-8 years and ≤40kg: 3-4 mg/kg once daily

Children ≥9 years

≤40 kg: 2-3 mg/kg once daily

>40 kg: 100 mg once daily

Adolescents:

<40 kg: 2-3 mg/kg once daily

≥40 kg: 150 mg once daily; treatment duration: 14-21 days

Prophylaxis in hematopoietic stem cell transplantation: I.V.: 1 mg/kg daily; maximum dose: 50 mg; doses as high as 3 mg/kg/day have been used in trials (Kusuki, 2009)

Adults:

Candidemia, acute disseminated candidiasis, and *Candida* **peritonitis and abscesses:** I.V.: 100 mg daily; mean duration of therapy (from clinical trials): 15 days (range: 10-47 days)

Esophageal candidiasis: I.V.: 150 mg daily; mean duration of therapy (from clinical trials): 15 days (range: 10-30 days)

Prophylaxis of *Candida* **infection in hematopoietic stem cell transplantation:** I.V.: 50 mg daily

Dosing adjustment in renal impairment: Adults: No adjustment required; not dialyzable, supplemental dosing is not required following hemodialysis.

Dosing adjustment in hepatic impairment: Adults: No adjustment required.

Administration Parenteral: I.V.: Reconstitute vial with 5 mL of NS or D_5W by gently dissolving powder by swirling the vial; do **not** vigorously shake the vial. Further dilution is dose dependent on patient age: Pediatric patients: Dilute dose in NS or D_5W to a final concentration of 0.5-4 mg/mL; adults: Dilute dose in 100 mL of NS or D_5W. In pediatric patients, final concentrations >1.5 mg/mL should be administered via a central line to minimize risk of infusion reactions. Prior to administration, flush line with NS. Infuse over 1 hour; more rapid infusions may result in a higher incidence of histamine-mediated reactions. Do not coinfuse with other medications since precipitation may occur.

Monitoring Parameters Periodic liver function tests, renal function tests, CBC with differential

Dosage Forms Excipient information presented when available (limited, particularly for generics); consult specific product labeling.

Solution Reconstituted, Intravenous, as sodium:

Mycamine: 50 mg (1 ea); 100 mg (1 ea)

References

Ashouri N, Singh J, Arrieta A. Micafungin in pediatrics: when one size does not fit all. *Expert Opin Drug Metab Toxicol.* 2008;4(4):463-469.

Benjamin DK Jr, Smith PB, Arrieta A, et al, "Safety and Pharmacokinetics of Repeat-Dose Micafungin in Young Infants," *Clin Pharmacol Ther,* 2010, 87(1):93-9.

Carver PL. Micafungin. *Ann Pharmacother.* 2004;38(10):1707-1721.

Caudle KE, Inger AG, Butler DR, et.al. Echinocandin use in the neonatal intensive care unit. *Ann Pharmacother.* 2012;46:108-116.

Denning DW, Marr KA, Lau WM, et al, "Micafungin (FK463), Alone or in Combination With Other Systemic Antifungal Agents, for the Treatment of Acute Invasive Aspergillosis," *J Infect,* 2006, 53(5):337-49.

DHHS. Guidelines for the prevention and treatment of opportunistic infections among HIV-exposed and HIV-infected children: recommendations from the National Institutes of Health, Centers for Disease Control and Prevention, the HIV Medicine Association of the Infectious Diseases Society of America, the Pediatric Infectious Diseases Society, and the American Academy of Pediatrics. November 6, 2013. Available at: http://aidsinfo.nih.gov

DHHS Panel on Opportunistic Infections (OI) in HIV-Infected Adults and Adolescents, "Guidelines for Prevention and Treatment of Opportunistic Infections in HIV-Infected Adults and Adolescents: Recommendations from the Centers for Disease Control and Prevention (CDC), the National Institutes of Health (NIH), and the HIV Medicine Association (HIVMA) of the Infectious Diseases Society of America (IDSA)," May 7, 2013. Available at http://aidsinfo.nih.gov/contentfiles/lvguidelines/adult_oi.pdf

Emiroglu M. Micafungin use in children. *Expert Reviews Anti-infective Therapy.* 2011;9(9):821-834.

Flynn PM, Seibel N, Arrieta A, et al, "Treatment of Invasive Aspergillosis in Pediatric Patients With Micafungin Alone or in Combination with Other Systemic Antifungal Agents," Program and abstracts of the 46th Interscience Conference on Antimicrobial Agents and Chemotherapy, San Francisco, 2006, September 27-30 (abstract M-891).

Herbert MF, Smith HE, Marbury TC, et al. Pharmacokinetics of micafungin in healthy volunteers, volunteers with moderate liver disease, and volunteers with renal dysfunction. *J Clin Pharmacol.* 2005;45 (10):1145-1152.

Heresi GP, Gerstmann DR, Reed MD, et al, "The Pharmacokinetics and Safety of Micafungin, a Novel Echinocandin, in Premature Infants," *Pediatr Infect Dis J,* 2006, 25(12):1110-5.

Hope WW, Smith PB, Arrieta A, et al. Population pharmacokinetics of micafungin in neonates and young infants. *Antimicrob Agents Chemother.* 2010;54(6):2633-2637.

Kawada M, Fukuoka N, Kondo M, et al, "Pharmacokinetics of Prophylactic Micafungin in Very-Low-Birth-Weight Infants," *Pediatr Infect Dis J,* 2009, 28(9):840-2.

Kobayashi S, Murayama S, Tatsuzawa O, et al, "X-Linked Severe Combined Immunodeficiency (X-SCID) With High Blood Levels of Immunoglobulins and Aspergillus Pneumonia Successfully Treated With Micafangin Followed by Unrelated Cord Blood Stem Cell Transplantation," *Eur J Pediatr,* 2007, 166(3):207-10.

Kusuki S, Hashii Y, Yoshida H, et al, "Antifungal Prophylaxis With Micafungin in Patients Treated for Childhood Cancer," *Pediatr Blood Cancer,* 2009, 53(4):605-9.

Pappas PG, Kauffman CA, Andes D, et al, "Clinical Practice Guidelines for the Management of Candidiasis: 2009 Update by the Infectious Diseases Society of America," *Clin Infect Dis,* 2009, 48(5):503-35.

Queiroz-Telles F, Berezin E, Leverger G, et al, "Micafungin Versus Liposomal Amphotericin B for Pediatric Patients With Invasive Candidiasis: Substudy of a Randomized Double-Blind Trial," *Pediatr Infect Dis J,* 2008, 27(9):820-6.

Santos RP, Sánchez PJ, Mejias A, et al, "Successful Medical Treatment of Cutaneous Aspergillosis in a Premature Infant Using Liposomal Amphotericin B, Voriconazole and Micafungin," *Pediatr Infect Dis J,* 2007, 26(4):364-6.

Seibel NL, Schwartz C, Arrieta A, et al, "Safety, Tolerability, and Pharmacokinetics of Micafungin (FK463) in Febrile Neutropenic Pediatric Patients," *Antimicrob Agents Chemother,* 2005, 49 (8):3317-24.

Singer MS, Seibel NL, Vezina G, et al, "Successful Treatment of Invasive Aspergillosis in Two Patients With Acute Myelogenous Leukemia," *J Pediatr Hematol Oncol,* 2003, 25(3):252-6.

Smith PB, Walsh TJ, Hope W, et al, "Pharmacokinetics of an Elevated Dosage of Micafungin in Premature Neonates," *Pediatr Infect Dis J,* 2009, 28(5):412-5.

Tomblyn M, Chiller T, Einsele H, et.al. Guidelines for preventing infectious complications among hematopoietic cell transplantation recipients: a global perspective. *Biol Blood Marrow Transplant.* 2009;15:1143-1238.

van Burik JA, Ratanatharathorn V, Stepan DE, et al, "Micafungin Versus Fluconazole for Prophylaxis Against Invasive Fungal Infections During Neutropenia in Patients Undergoing Hematopoietic Stem Cell Transplantation," *Clin Infect Dis,* 2004, 39(10):1407-16.

Yanni, SB, Smith PB, Benjamin DK, et al. Higher clearance of micafungin in neonates compared to adults: rose of age-dependent micafungin serum binding. *Biopharm Drug Dispos.* 2011;32 (4):222-232.

♦ **Micafungin Sodium** *see* Micafungin *on page 1407*

♦ **Micatin [OTC]** *see* Miconazole (Topical) *on page 1410*

♦ **Micatin® (Can)** *see* Miconazole (Topical) *on page 1410*

♦ **Miconazole 3** *see* Miconazole (Topical) *on page 1410*

♦ **Miconazole 3 Combo Pack [OTC]** *see* Miconazole (Topical) *on page 1410*

♦ **Miconazole 7 [OTC]** *see* Miconazole (Topical) *on page 1410*

Miconazole (Topical) (mi KON a zole)

Medication Safety Issues
Sound-alike/look-alike issues:

Miconazole may be confused with metroNIDAZOLE, Micronase, Micronor®

Lotrimin® may be confused with Lotrisone®, Otrivin®

Micatin® may be confused with Miacalcin®

Brand Names: U.S. Aloe Vesta Antifungal [OTC]; Antifungal [OTC]; Azolen Tincture [OTC]; Baza Antifungal [OTC]; Carrington Antifungal [OTC]; Critic-Aid Clear AF [OTC]; Cruex Prescription Strength [OTC]; DermaFungal [OTC]; Desenex Jock Itch [OTC]; Desenex Spray [OTC]; Desenex [OTC]; Fungoid Tincture [OTC]; Lotrimin AF Deodorant Powder [OTC]; Lotrimin AF Jock Itch Powder [OTC]; Lotrimin AF Powder [OTC]; Lotrimin AF [OTC]; Micaderm [OTC]; Micatin [OTC]; Miconazole 3; Miconazole 3 Combo Pack [OTC]; Miconazole 7 [OTC]; Micro Guard [OTC]; Miranel AF [OTC]; Mitrazol [OTC]; Podactin [OTC]; Remedy Antifungal [OTC]; Secura Antifungal Extra Thick [OTC]; Secura Antifungal [OTC]; Soothe & Cool INZO Antifungal [OTC]; Triple Paste AF [OTC]; Vagistat-3 [OTC]; Zeasorb-AF [OTC]

Brand Names: Canada Dermazole; Micatin®; Micozole; Monistat®; Monistat® 3

Therapeutic Category Antifungal Agent, Topical; Antifungal Agent, Vaginal

Generic Availability (U.S.) May be product dependent

Use Treatment of vulvovaginal candidiasis; topical treatment of superficial fungal infections

Pregnancy Considerations Following vaginal administration, small amounts are absorbed systemically (Stevens, 2002). Adverse fetal events have not been observed (Czeizel, 2004). Vaginal products (7-day therapies) may be considered for the treatment of vulvovaginal candidiasis in pregnant women. This product may weaken latex condoms and diaphragms (CDC, 2010).

Breast-Feeding Considerations It is not known if miconazole is excreted in breast milk. The manufacturer recommends that caution be exercised when administering miconazole to nursing women.

Contraindications Hypersensitivity to miconazole or any component; vaginal preparation should not be used in the first trimester of pregnancy unless the drug is essential to patient's welfare

Warnings The safety of miconazole in infants <1 year of age has not been established

Precautions Use with caution in patients allergic to other imidazole-derivative antifungals (eg, clotrimazole, econazole, ketoconazole)

Adverse Reactions

Topical: Allergic contact dermatitis, burning, maceration

Vaginal: Abdominal cramps, burning, irritation, itching

Drug Interactions

Metabolism/Transport Effects None known.

Avoid Concomitant Use There are no known interactions where it is recommended to avoid concomitant use.

Increased Effect/Toxicity

Miconazole (Topical) may increase the levels/effects of: Vitamin K Antagonists

Decreased Effect There are no known significant interactions involving a decrease in effect.

Stability Store at room temperature

Mechanism of Action Inhibits biosynthesis of ergosterol, damaging the fungal cell wall membrane, which increases permeability causing leaking of nutrients

Pharmacokinetics (Adult data unless noted)

Absorption: Vaginal: Small amount absorbed systemically

Distribution: Into body tissues, joints, and fluids; poor penetration into sputum, saliva, urine, and CSF

Protein binding: 91% to 93%

Metabolism: In the liver

Half-life: Multiphasic degradation:

Alpha: 40 minutes

Beta: 126 minutes

Terminal: 24 hours

Elimination: ~50% excreted in feces and <1% in urine as unchanged drug

Dosing: Usual

Infants, Children, Adolescents, and Adults: Topical:

Tinea pedis and tinea corporis: Apply twice daily for 4 weeks

Tinea cruris: Apply twice daily for 2 weeks

Adolescents and Adults:

Vaginal: Insert contents of 1 applicator of 2% vaginal cream or 100 mg vaginal suppository at bedtime for 7 days; or 1 applicator of 4% vaginal cream or 200 mg vaginal suppository at bedtime for 3 days; or 1200 mg vaginal suppository one-time dose at bedtime or during the day

Note: Many products are available as a combination pack (contains a suppository for vaginal instillation and external cream which is applied twice daily for up to 7 days to relieve external symptoms)

Administration For external use only.

Topical: Apply sparingly to the cleansed, dry affected area; if intertriginous areas are involved, rub cream gently into the skin

Vaginal: Wash hands before using; gently insert tablet or full applicator of cream high into vagina at bedtime. Wash applicator with soap and water following use. Remain lying down for 30 minutes following administration.

Monitoring Parameters Hematocrit, hemoglobin, serum electrolytes and lipids

Dosage Forms Excipient information presented when available (limited, particularly for generics); consult specific product labeling.

Aerosol, External, as nitrate:
Desenex Spray: 2% (133 g)
Lotrimin AF: 2% (150 g)

Aerosol Powder, External, as nitrate:
Cruex Prescription Strength: 2% (85 g)
Desenex Jock Itch: 2% (113 g)
Desenex Spray: 2% (113 g)
Lotrimin AF Deodorant Powder: 2% (133 g)
Lotrimin AF Jock Itch Powder: 2% (133 g)
Lotrimin AF Powder: 2% (133 g)

Cream, External, as nitrate:
Antifungal: 2% (14 g, 28 g, 42.5 g) [contains benzoic acid]
Antifungal: 2% (113 g, 198 g) [contains cetyl alcohol, methylparaben, propylene glycol, propylparaben]
Baza Antifungal: 2% (4 g, 57 g, 142 g)
Carrington Antifungal: 2% (141 g) [contains disodium edta, methylparaben, propylene glycol, propylparaben]
Micaderm: 2% (30 g)
Micatin: 2% (14 g) [contains benzoic acid]
Micro Guard: 2% (57 g)
Podactin: 2% (28.35 g) [contains benzoic acid]
Remedy Antifungal: 2% (118 mL) [contains methylparaben, propylparaben, trolamine (triethanolamine)]
Secura Antifungal: 2% (57 g) [contains cetearyl alcohol, methylparaben, propylparaben]
Secura Antifungal Extra Thick: 2% (92 g) [contains cetearyl alcohol, methylparaben, propylparaben]
Soothe & Cool INZO Antifungal: 2% (56.7 g, 141.7 g)
Generic: 2% (15 g, 28.4 g, 30 g)

Cream, Vaginal, as nitrate:
Miconazole 7: 2% (45 g) [contains benzoic acid]
Generic: 2% (45 g)

Kit, External, as nitrate:
Fungoid Tincture: 2% [contains benzyl alcohol]

Kit, Vaginal, as nitrate:
Miconazole 3 Combo Pack: Cream, topical: 2% (9 g) and Suppository, vaginal: 200 mg (3s)
Miconazole 3 Combo Pack: Cream, topical: 2% (9 g) and Suppository, vaginal: 200 mg (3s) [contains benzoic acid]
Vagistat-3: Cream, topical: 2% (9 g) and Suppository, vaginal: 200 mg (3s) [contains benzoic acid]

Lotion, External, as nitrate:
Zeasorb-AF: 2% (56 g) [contains alcohol, usp]

Ointment, External, as nitrate:
Aloe Vesta Antifungal: 2% (56 g, 141 g)
Critic-Aid Clear AF: 2% (4 g, 57 g, 142 g)
DermaFungal: 2% (113 g)

Triple Paste AF: 2% (56.7 g) [contains polysorbate 80]

Powder, External, as nitrate:
Desenex: 2% (43 g, 85 g)
Lotrimin AF: 2% (90 g)
Micro Guard: 2% (85 g)
Mitrazol: 2% (30 g)
Remedy Antifungal: 2% (85 g)
Remedy Antifungal: 2% (85 g) [talc free; contains methylparaben]
Zeasorb-AF: 2% (71 g)
Zeasorb-AF: 2% (71 g) [starch free]

Solution, External, as nitrate:
Azolen Tincture: 2% (29.57 mL) [contains benzyl alcohol, isopropyl alcohol]
Fungoid Tincture: 2% (29.57 mL) [contains benzyl alcohol]
Miranel AF: 2% (28 g) [contains disodium edta, menthol, propylene glycol, sd alcohol 40b]

Suppository, Vaginal, as nitrate:
Miconazole 7: 100 mg (7 ea)
Miconazole 3: 200 mg (3 ea)
Generic: 100 mg (7 ea)

References
Centers for Disease Control and Prevention (CDC), "Sexually Transmitted Diseases Treatment Guidelines, 2010," *MMWR Recomm Rep*, 2010, 59(RR-12):1-110.
Czeizel AE, Kazy Z, and Puhó E, "Population-Based Case-Control Teratologic Study of Topical Miconazole," *Congenit Anom (Kyoto)*, 2004, 44(1):41-5.
Stevens RE, Konsil J, Verrill SS, et al, "Bioavailability Study of a 1200 mg Miconazole Nitrate Vaginal Ovule in Healthy Female Adults," *J Clin Pharmacol*, 2002, 42(1):52-60.

◆ **Miconazole Nitrate** see Miconazole (Topical) on page 1410

◆ **Micozole (Can)** see Miconazole (Topical) on page 1410

◆ **MICRhoGAM Ultra-Filtered Plus** see Rh$_o$(D) Immune Globulin on page 1815

◆ **Micro Guard [OTC]** see Miconazole (Topical) on page 1410

◆ **Micro-K** see Potassium Chloride on page 1708

◆ **Micro-K Extencaps (Can)** see Potassium Chloride on page 1708

◆ **Micronase** see GlyBURIDE on page 974

◆ **Micronefrin [OTC]** see EPINEPHrine (Systemic, Oral Inhalation) on page 761

◆ **Micronized Colestipol HCl** see Colestipol on page 540

◆ **Micronor® (Can)** see Norethindrone on page 1511

◆ **Microzide** see Hydrochlorothiazide on page 1023

◆ **Midamor (Can)** see AMILoride on page 121

Midazolam (MID aye zoe lam)

Medication Safety Issues

Sound-alike/look-alike issues:
Versed may be confused with VePesid, Vistaril

High alert medication:
The Institute for Safe Medication Practices (ISMP) includes this medication among its list of drugs which have a heightened risk of causing significant patient harm when used in error.

Related Information
Preprocedure Sedatives in Children on page 2402

Brand Names: Canada Midazolam Injection

Therapeutic Category Anticonvulsant, Benzodiazepine; Benzodiazepine; Hypnotic; Sedative

Generic Availability (U.S.) Yes

Use
Oral: Sedation, anxiolysis, amnesia prior to procedures or before induction of anesthesia (FDA approved in ages ≥6 months to <16 years)

◀ Parenteral: Preprocedure sedation, anxiolysis, amnesia for diagnostic or radiographic procedures (FDA approved in infants, children, adolescents, and adults); continuous I.V. sedation of intubated and mechanically ventilated patients (FDA approved in all ages); has also been used for status epilepticus

Buccal: Has been used for acute treatment of seizures

Intranasal: Has been used for preprocedure sedation, anxiolysis, amnesia for diagnostic or radiographic procedures; acute treatment of seizures

Rectal: Has been used for preprocedure sedation

Pregnancy Risk Factor D

Pregnancy Considerations Adverse events were not observed in animal reproduction studies. Midazolam has been found to cross the human placenta and can be detected in the serum of the umbilical vein and artery, as well as the amniotic fluid. Teratogenic effects have been observed with some benzodiazepines; however, additional studies are needed. The incidence of premature birth and low birth weights may be increased following maternal use of benzodiazepines; hypoglycemia and respiratory problems in the neonate may occur following exposure late in pregnancy. Neonatal withdrawal symptoms may occur within days to weeks after birth and "floppy infant syndrome" (which also includes withdrawal symptoms) have been reported with some benzodiazepines (Bergman, 1992; Iqbal, 2002; Wikner, 2007).

Breast-Feeding Considerations Midazolam and hydroxymidazolam can be detected in breast milk. Based on information from two women, 2-3 months postpartum, the half-life of midazolam in breast milk is ~1 hour. Milk concentrations were below the limit of detection (<5 nmol/L) 4 hours after a single maternal dose of midazolam 15 mg. Drowsiness, lethargy, or weight loss in nursing infants have been observed in case reports following maternal use of some benzodiazepines (Iqbal, 2002; Matheson, 1990). The manufacturer recommends that caution be exercised when administering midazolam to nursing women.

Contraindications Hypersensitivity to midazolam, any component, or cherries (syrup); cross-sensitivity with other benzodiazepines may occur; narrow-angle glaucoma; parenteral form is not for intrathecal or epidural injection

Warnings Midazolam may cause respiratory depression/arrest **[U.S. Boxed Warning]**; deaths and hypoxic encephalopathy have resulted when these were not promptly recognized and treated appropriately; dose must be individualized and patients must be appropriately monitored; serious respiratory adverse events occur most often when midazolam is used in combination with other CNS depressants; personnel and equipment needed for standard respiratory resuscitation should be immediately available during midazolam use; a dedicated individual (other than the one performing the procedure) should monitor the deeply sedated pediatric patient throughout the procedure; use with extreme caution, particularly in noncritical care settings. Initial I.V. dose in adults should not exceed 2.5 mg. Pediatric dosing is age, weight, procedure, and route dependant. Use lower doses in elderly or debilitated patients **[U.S. Boxed Warning]**. Do not administer by rapid I.V. injection in neonates **[U.S. Boxed Warning]**; severe hypotension and seizures have been reported; risk may be increased with concomitant fentanyl use. Paradoxical reactions, including hyperactive or aggressive behavior, have been reported in both adult and pediatric patients.

Syrup contains sodium benzoate and injection may contain benzyl alcohol which may cause allergic reactions in susceptible individuals; large amounts of benzyl alcohol (≥99 mg/kg/day) have been associated with a potentially fatal toxicity ("gasping syndrome") in neonates; the "gasping syndrome" consists of metabolic acidosis, respiratory distress, gasping respirations, CNS dysfunction (including convulsions, intracranial hemorrhage), hypotension and cardiovascular collapse; avoid use of midazolam products containing benzyl alcohol or sodium benzoate in neonates; a benzyl alcohol free (preservative free) injection is available; *in vitro* and animal studies have shown that benzoate, a metabolite of benzyl alcohol, displaces bilirubin from protein binding sites

Precautions Use with caution in patients with heart failure, renal impairment, pulmonary disease, hepatic dysfunction and in neonates (especially premature neonates); several cases of myoclonus (rhythmic myoclonic jerking) have been reported in premature infants (~8% incidence). Benzodiazepine withdrawal may occur if abruptly discontinued in patients receiving prolonged I.V. continuous infusions; doses should be tapered slowly with prolonged use; does not have analgesic, antidepressant, or antipsychotic properties. Does not protect against increases in heart rate or blood pressure during intubation. Should not be used in shock, coma, or acute alcohol intoxication. Avoid intra-arterial administration or extravasation of parenteral formulation. Use during upper airway procedures may increase risk of hypoventilation. Prolonged responses have been noted following extended administration by continuous infusion (possibly due to metabolite accumulation) or in the presence of drugs which inhibit midazolam metabolism.

Adverse Reactions

Cardiovascular: Hypotension

Central nervous system: Drowsiness, headache, oversedation, seizure-like activity

Gastrointestinal: Nausea, vomiting

Local: Pain and local reactions at injection site

Neuromuscular & skeletal: Myoclonic jerks (preterm infants)

Ocular: Nystagmus

Respiratory: Apnea, cough, decreased tidal volume and/or respiratory rate

Miscellaneous: Hiccups, paradoxical reaction, physical and psychological dependence with prolonged use

Rare but important or life-threatening: Agitation, amnesia, bigeminy, bronchospasm, emergence delirium, euphoria, hallucinations, laryngospasm, rash

Drug Interactions

Metabolism/Transport Effects Substrate of CYP2B6 (minor), CYP3A4 (major); **Note:** Assignment of Major/Minor substrate status based on clinically relevant drug interaction potential; **Inhibits** CYP2C8 (weak), CYP2C9 (weak), CYP3A4 (weak)

Avoid Concomitant Use

Avoid concomitant use of Midazolam with any of the following: Azelastine (Nasal); Boceprevir; Cobicistat; Conivaptan; Fusidic Acid (Systemic); Itraconazole; Ketoconazole (Systemic); Methadone; OLANZapine; Paraldehyde; Pimozide; Protease Inhibitors; Sodium Oxybate; Telaprevir; Thalidomide

Increased Effect/Toxicity

Midazolam may increase the levels/effects of: Alcohol (Ethyl); ARIPiprazole; Azelastine (Nasal); Buprenorphine; CloZAPine; CNS Depressants; Dofetilide; Hydrocodone; Lomitapide; Methadone; Methotrimeprazine; Metyrosine; Mirtazapine; Paraldehyde; Pimozide; Pramipexole; Propofol; ROPINIRole; Rotigotine; Selective Serotonin Reuptake Inhibitors; Sodium Oxybate; Thalidomide; Zolpidem

The levels/effects of Midazolam may be increased by: Antifungal Agents (Azole Derivatives, Systemic); Aprepitant; AtorvaSTATin; Boceprevir; Brimonidine (Topical); Calcium Channel Blockers (Nondihydropyridine); Cannabis; Ceritinib; Cimetidine; Cobicistat; Conivaptan; Contraceptives (Estrogens); Contraceptives (Progestins); CYP3A4 Inhibitors (Moderate); CYP3A4 Inhibitors

(Strong); Dasatinib; Doxylamine; Dronabinol; Droperidol; Fosaprepitant; Fusidic Acid (Systemic); Grapefruit Juice; HydrOXYzine; Isoniazid; Itraconazole; Ivacaftor; Kava Kava; Ketoconazole (Systemic); Luliconazole; Macrolide Antibiotics; Magnesium Sulfate; Methotrimeprazine; Mifepristone; Nabilone; OLANZapine; Perampanel; Propofol; Protease Inhibitors; Proton Pump Inhibitors; Rufinamide; Selective Serotonin Reuptake Inhibitors; Simeprevir; Stiripentol; Tapentadol; Telaprevir; Tetrahydrocannabinol

Decreased Effect
The levels/effects of Midazolam may be decreased by: Bosentan; CarBAMazepine; CYP3A4 Inducers (Strong); Dabrafenib; Deferasirox; Ginkgo Biloba; Mitotane; Rifamycin Derivatives; Siltuximab; St Johns Wort; Theophylline Derivatives; Tocilizumab; Yohimbine

Food Interactions Grapefruit juice may increase serum concentrations of midazolam. Management: Avoid concurrent use of grapefruit juice with oral midazolam.

Stability
Oral: Store at 25°C (77°F); excursions permitted to 15°C to 30°C (59°F to 86°F)

Parenteral: Store at 20°C to 25°C (68°F to 77°F), excursions permitted to 15°C to 30°C (59°F to 86°F); stable at a concentration of 0.5 mg/mL for 24 hours in D_5W or NS and for 4 hours in LR

Mechanism of Action Binds to stereospecific benzodiazepine receptors on the postsynaptic GABA neuron at several sites within the central nervous system, including the limbic system, reticular formation. Enhancement of the inhibitory effect of GABA on neuronal excitability results by increased neuronal membrane permeability to chloride ions. This shift in chloride ions results in hyperpolarization (a less excitable state) and stabilization.

Pharmacodynamics Sedation:

Onset of action:

Oral: Children: Within 10-20 minutes

I.M.:
Children: Within 5 minutes
Adults: Within 15 minutes

I.V.: Within 1-5 minutes

Intranasal: Within 5 minutes

Maximum effect:

I.M.:
Children: 15-30 minutes
Adults: 30-60 minutes

I.V.: 5-7 minutes

Intranasal: 10 minutes

Duration:

I.M.: Mean: 2 hours, up to 6 hours

I.V.: 20-30 minutes

Intranasal: 30-60 minutes

Note: Full recovery may take more than 24 hours

Pharmacokinetics (Adult data unless noted)

Absorption: Oral, nasal: Rapid

Distribution: V_d:

Preterm infants (n=24; GA: 26-34 weeks; PNA: 3-11 days): Median: 1.1 L/kg (range: 0.4-4.2 L/kg)

Infants and Children 6 months to 16 years: 1.24-2.02 L/kg

Adults: 1-3.1 L/kg

Increased V_d with CHF and chronic renal failure; widely distributed in body including CSF and brain; crosses placenta; enters fetal circulation; crosses into breast milk

Protein binding: Children >1 year and Adults: 97%; primarily to albumin

Metabolism: Extensive in the liver via cytochrome P450 CYP3A4 enzyme; undergoes hydroxylation and then glucuronide conjugation; primary metabolite (alpha-hydroxy-midazolam) is active and equipotent to midazolam

Bioavailability: Oral: 15% to 45% (syrup: 36%); I.M.: >90%; intranasal: ~60%; rectal: ~40% to 50%

Half-life, elimination: Increased half-life with cirrhosis, CHF, obesity, elderly, and acute renal failure

Preterm infants (n=24; GA: 26-34 weeks; PNA: 3-11 days): Median: 6.3 hours (range: 2.6-17.7 hours)

Neonates: 4-12 hours; seriously ill neonates: 6.5-12 hours

Children: I.V.: 2.9-4.5 hours; syrup: 2.2-6.8 hours

Adults: 3 hours (range: 1.8-6.4 hours)

Elimination: 63% to 80% excreted as alpha-hydroxy-midazolam glucuronide in urine; ~2% to 10% in feces, <1% eliminated as unchanged drug in the urine

Clearance:

Preterm infants (n=24; GA: 26-34 weeks; PNA: 3-11 days): Median: 1.8 mL/minute/kg (range: 0.7-6.7 mL/minute/kg)

Neonates <39 weeks GA: 1.17 mL/minute/kg

Neonates >39 weeks GA: 1.84 mL/minute/kg

Seriously ill neonates: 1.2-2 mL/minute/kg

Infants >3 months: 9.1 mL/minute/kg

Children >1 year: 3.2-13.3 mL/minute/kg

Healthy adults: 4.2-9 mL/minute/kg

Adults with acute renal failure: 1.9 mL/minute/kg

Dosing: Neonatal Dosage must be individualized and based on patient's age, underlying diseases, concurrent medications, and desired effect; decrease dose (by ~30%) if opioids or other CNS depressants are administered concomitantly. Patients receiving ECMO may require higher doses due to drug absorption in the ECMO circuit (Mulla, 2000). To minimize excipient load, preservative free preparations should be used; alternatively use the more concentrated midazolam injection (eg, 5 mg/mL) and dilute with SWI without preservatives.

Sedation, intermittent dosing or procedural (intubation): I.M., I.V.: 0.05-0.1 mg/kg/dose over 5 minutes (Kumar, 2010; VanLooy, 2008)

Sedation, mechanically ventilated patient: I.V.: **Note:** Use the lowest effective dose.

Manufacturer's labeling: Continuous I.V. infusion:

GA ≤32 weeks: Initial: 0.03 mg/kg/**hour** (0.5 **mcg**/kg/minute)

GA >32 weeks: Initial: 0.06 mg/kg/**hour** (1 **mcg**/kg/minute)

Alternative dosing:

Loading dose:

GA <34 weeks: **Note:** Some have recommended against the use of a loading or bolus dose due to associated hypotension; to rapidly achieve sedation, it has been suggested to begin the continuous infusion at a faster rate for the first several hours (Jacqz-Aigrain, 1992). Others have successfully used loading doses of 0.2 mg/kg given over 1 hour to prevent hypotension (Anand, 1999; Treluyer, 2005)

GA ≥34 weeks: 0.2 mg/kg/dose once (Anand, 1999; Jacqz-Aigrain, 1990; Treluyer, 2005)

Continuous I.V. infusion (Anand, 1999; Jacqz-Aigrain, 1994; Treluyer, 2005):

GA 24-26 weeks: Initial: 0.02-0.03 mg/kg/**hour** (0.33-0.5 **mcg**/kg/minute)

GA 27-29 weeks: Initial: 0.03-0.04 mg/kg/**hour** (0.5-0.67 **mcg**/kg/minute)

GA ≥30 weeks: Initial: 0.03-0.06 mg/kg/**hour** (0.5-1 **mcg**/kg/minute)

Note: After prolonged therapy, consider a slow wean of therapy to prevent signs and symptoms of withdrawal. The following regimen has been reported: If duration of therapy ≤4 days, wean over at least 2 days beginning with an initial dosage reduction of 30% to 50% followed by 20% to 30% dosage reductions every 6-8 hours; monitor closely for signs and symptoms of

◀ withdrawal with each reduction in dose. If duration of therapy is >4 days, decrease infusion rate by 25% to 50% every 12 hours, then convert to an intermittent dose every 4 hours and lastly, every 8 hours (Anand, 1999).

Seizures, refractory; status epilepticus: I.V.: Dosage regimens variable, reported doses are higher than sedative doses: **Note:** Consider omitting loading dose if patient has received an I.V. dose of a benzodiazepine; begin continuous I.V. infusion at lower end of range and titrate to lowest effective dose: Loading dose: 0.06-0.15 mg/kg/dose followed by a continuous infusion of 0.06-0.4 mg/kg/**hour** (1-7 **mcg**/kg/minute); maximum reported rate: 1.1 mg/kg/**hour** (18 mcg/kg/minute) (Boylan, 2004; Conde, 2005; Holmes, 1999)

Dosing: Usual Dosage must be individualized and based on patient's age, underlying diseases, concurrent medications, and desired effect; decrease dose (by ~30%) if opioids or other CNS depressants are administered concomitantly; use multiple small doses and titrate to desired sedative effect; allow 3-5 minutes between doses to decrease the chance of oversedation

Infants, Children, and Adolescents:

Sedation, anxiolysis, and amnesia prior to procedure or before induction of anesthesia:

I.M.: Usual: 0.1-0.15 mg/kg 30-60 minutes before surgery or procedure; range: 0.05-0.15 mg/kg; doses up to 0.5 mg/kg have been used in more anxious patients; maximum total dose: 10 mg

I.V.:

Infants 1-5 months: Limited information is available in nonintubated infants; dosing recommendations are unclear; infants <6 months are at higher risk for airway obstruction and hypoventilation; titrate dose with small increments to desired clinical effect; monitor carefully

Infants 6 months to Children 5 years: Initial: 0.05-0.1 mg/kg; titrate dose carefully; total dose of 0.6 mg/kg may be required; usual total dose maximum: 6 mg

Children 6-12 years: Initial: 0.025-0.05 mg/kg; titrate dose carefully; total doses of 0.4 mg/kg may be required; usual total dose maximum: 10 mg

Children 12-16 years: Dose as adults; usual total dose maximum: 10 mg

Intranasal: **Note:** Some investigators suggest premedication with intranasal lidocaine to decrease irritation and subsequent agitation (Chiaretti, 2011; Lugo, 1993):

Infants 1-5 months: **Note:** Very limited information exists; further studies are needed: 0.2 mg/kg (single dose) (Harcke, 1995; Mittal, 2006)

Infants ≥6 months, Children, and Adolescents: 0.2-0.3 mg/kg (maximum single dose: 10 mg); may repeat in 5-15 minutes to a maximum of 0.5 mg/kg (maximum total dose: 10 mg) (Acworth, 2001; Charetti, 2011; Harcke, 1995; Lane, 2008)

Oral: Infants >6 months, Children, and Adolescents ≤16 years: Single dose: 0.25-0.5 mg/kg once, depending on patient status and desired effect, usual: 0.5 mg/kg; maximum dose: 20 mg; **Note:** Younger patients (6 months to <6 years) and those less cooperative may require higher doses (up to 1 mg/kg); use lower initial doses (0.25 mg/kg) in patients with cardiac or respiratory compromise, concomitant CNS depressant, or high-risk surgical patients.

Rectal: Infants >6 months and Children: Usual: 0.25-0.5 mg/kg once (Krauss, 2006); doses up to 1 mg/kg have been used in infants and young children (7 months to 5 years of age) but may be associated with a higher incidence of postprocedural agitation (Kanegaye, 2003; Tanaka, 2000)

Sedation, mechanically ventilated patient: I.V.: Loading dose: 0.05-0.2 mg/kg given slow I.V. over 2-3 minutes, then follow with initial continuous I.V. infusion: 0.06-0.12 mg/kg/**hour** (1-2 **mcg**/kg/minute); titrate to the desired effect; range: 0.024-0.36 mg/kg/**hour** (0.4-6 **mcg**/kg/minute)

Seizures, acute treatment:

Buccal: Reserve for patients without I.V. access (Ashrafi, 2010; Kutlu, 2003; McIntyre, 2005; Mpimbaza, 2008; Talukdar, 2009):

Weight-based dosing: Infants ≥3 months, Children, and Adolescents: 0.2-0.5 mg/kg once; maximum dose: 10 mg

Age-based dosing (McIntyre, 2005):

Infants 6-11 months: 2.5 mg

Children 1-4 years: 5 mg

Children 5-9 years: 7.5 mg

Children and Adolescents ≥10 years: 10 mg

I.M.: 0.2 mg/kg/dose; repeat every 10-15 minutes; maximum dose: 6 mg (Hegenbarth, 2008)

Intranasal (Bhattachyaryya, 2006; Fişgin, 2000; Fişgin, 2002; Holsti, 2007; Holsti, 2010; Kutlu, 2000): Reserve for patients without I.V. access; divide dose between nares:

Infants 1-5 months: 0.2 mg/kg once; maximum dose: 10 mg

Infants and Children ≥6 months: 0.2 mg/kg; one study used 0.3 mg/kg (n=9); maximum dose: 10 mg; may repeat once to a total maximum of 0.4 mg/kg

Seizures, refractory; status epilepticus refractory to standard therapy: I.V. (Hayashi, 2007; Hegenbarth, 2008; Igartua, 1999; Koul, 1997; Koul, 2002; Morrison, 2006; Morrison, 2008; Ozdemir, 2005; Rivera, 1993; Singh, 2002; Yoshikawa, 2000):

Loading dose: 0.15-0.2 mg/kg; 0.5 mg/kg/dose was used in one high-dose midazolam study (n=17); consider using the lower end of the loading dose range in patients with hemodynamic instability or who have received other agents with hypotensive effects

Continuous I.V. infusion: Initial rate: 0.06-0.12 mg/kg/**hour** (1-2 **mcg**/kg/minute); increase rate every 15 minutes in increments of 0.06-0.12 mg/kg/**hour** (1-2 mcg/kg/minute) until seizure activity ceases; one high dose study increased by 0.24 mg/kg/**hour** (4 mcg/kg/minute); mean required dosage across a number of studies: 0.11-0.84 mg/kg/**hour** (1.87-14 mcg/kg/minute); the upper end of this range was used in one study; however, patients were titrated to burst suppression on EEG; maximum reported dose (n=1): 3 mg/kg/**hour** (50 mcg/kg/minute)

Seizures, status epilepticus, prehospital treatment: **Note:** Administered by paramedics when convulsions last >5 minutes or if convulsions are occurring after having intermittent seizures without regaining consciousness for >5 minutes: I.M.: Children and Adolescents (Silbergleit, 2012):

<13 kg: Not studied

13-40 kg: 5 mg once

>40 kg: 10 mg once

Adults:

Anesthesia: I.V.:

Induction:

Unpremedicated patients: 0.3-0.35 mg/kg (up to 0.6 mg/kg in resistant cases)

Premedicated patients: 0.15-0.35 mg/kg

Maintenance: 0.05-0.3 mg/kg as needed, or continuous I.V. infusion 0.25-1.5 mcg/kg/minute

Sedation, preoperative:

I.M.: 0.07-0.08 mg/kg 30-60 minutes prior to surgery/procedure; usual dose: 5 mg; **Note:** Reduce dose in patients with COPD, high-risk patients, patients ≥60 years of age, and patients receiving other opioids or CNS depressants.

I.V.: 0.02-0.04 mg/kg; repeat every 5 minutes as needed to desired effect or up to 0.1-0.2 mg/kg

Sedation, procedural (moderate): I.V.: Initial: 0.5-2 mg slow I.V. over at least 2 minutes; slowly titrate to effect by repeating doses every 2-3 minutes if needed; usual total dose: 2.5-5 mg

Healthy Adults <60 years:

Initial: Some patients respond to doses as low as 1 mg; no more than 2.5 mg should be administered over a period of 2 minutes. Additional doses of midazolam may be administered after a 2-minute waiting period and evaluation of sedation after each dose increment. A total dose >5 mg is generally not needed. If opioids or other CNS depressants are administered concomitantly, the midazolam dose should be reduced by 30%. A reduced dose is required for patients ≥60 years, debilitated, or chronically ill.

Maintenance: 25% of dose used to reach sedative effect

Sedation in mechanically ventilated patients: I.V.:

Manufacturer's labeling: Initial dose: 0.01-0.05 mg/kg (~0.5-4 mg); may repeat at 5- to 15-minute intervals until adequate sedation achieved; maintenance infusion: 0.02-0.1 mg/kg/**hour**. Titrate to reach desired level of sedation.

Alternative dosing: Initial dose: 0.02-0.08 mg/kg (~1-5 mg in 70 kg adult); may repeat at 5- to 15-minute intervals until adequate sedation achieved; maintenance infusion: 0.04-0.2 mg/kg/**hour**. Titrate to reach desired level of sedation (Jacobi, 2002).

Status epilepticus, refractory: Note: Intubation required; adjust dose based on hemodynamics, seizure activity, and EEG. I.V.: 0.15-0.3 mg/kg (usual dose: 5-15 mg); may repeat every 10-15 minutes as needed **or** 0.2 mg/kg bolus followed by a continuous infusion of 0.05-0.6 mg/kg/**hour** (Lowenstein, 2005; Meierkord, 2010)

Status epilepticus, prehospital treatment: Note: Administered by paramedics when convulsions last >5 minutes or if convulsions are occurring after having intermittent seizures without regaining consciousness for >5 minutes: I.M.: 10 mg once (Silbergleit, 2012)

Usual Infusion Concentrations: Neonatal I.V. Infusion: 0.1 mg/mL **or** 0.5 mg/mL

Usual Infusion Concentrations: Pediatric I.V. infusion: 0.5 mg/mL **or** 1 mg/mL

Administration

Buccal: A buccal formulation is not currently available in the U.S. Some trials used an injectable solution administered buccally. International studies used a 10 mg/mL commercially available buccal formulation. Administer to the buccal mucosa between the gums and the cheek using an oral syringe; gently massage cheek; dose may be divided to both sides of the mouth.

Intranasal: Administer using a needleless syringe into the nares over 15-30 seconds; use the 5 mg/mL injection; 1/2 of the dose may be administered to each nare; **Note:** The 5 mg/mL injection has also been administered as a nasal spray using a graded pump device (Ljungman, 2000) or using an atomizer such as the MAD® Nasal Drug delivery device (Holsti, 2007; Holsti, 2010).

Oral: Administer on empty stomach (feeding is usually contraindicated prior to sedation for procedures).

Parenteral:

I.V.: Administer by slow I.V. injection over at least 2-5 minutes [administer loading doses more slowly in preterm neonates (ie, over 60 minutes)] at a concentration of 1-5 mg/mL (maximum concentration: 5 mg/mL) or by continuous I.V. infusion; avoid extravasation; do not administer intra-arterially

I.M.: Administer deep I.M. into large muscle, generally into anterior-lateral aspect of thigh (vastus lateralis) in pediatric patients (Lam, 2005; Malamed, 1989)

Rectal: Clinical trials utilized parenteral midazolam for rectal administration; administer a 1-5 mg/mL solution through a small, lubricated catheter or tube inserted rectally; hold buttocks closed for ~5 minutes after administration

Monitoring Parameters Level of sedation, respiratory rate, heart rate, blood pressure, oxygen saturation (ie, pulse oximetry)

Additional Information Sodium content of injection: 0.14 mEq/mL. For neonates: Use preservative-free injection; alternatively, use the 5 mg/mL injection and dilute to 0.5 mg/mL with SWI without preservatives to decrease the amount of benzyl alcohol delivered to the neonate (since both concentrations of midazolam injection contain 1% benzyl alcohol). With continuous I.V. infusion, midazolam may accumulate in peripheral tissues; use lowest effective infusion rate to reduce accumulation effects. Midazolam is 3-4 times as potent as diazepam. Paradoxical reactions associated with midazolam use in children (eg, agitation, restlessness, combativeness) have been successfully treated with flumazenil (Massanari, 1997).

Controlled Substance C-IV

Dosage Forms Excipient information presented when available (limited, particularly for generics); consult specific product labeling.

Solution, Injection:

Generic: 2 mg/2 mL (2 mL); 5 mg/5 mL (5 mL); 10 mg/10 mL (10 mL); 5 mg/mL (1 mL, 2 mL, 5 mL, 10 mL); 10 mg/2 mL (2 mL); 25 mg/5 mL (5 mL); 50 mg/10 mL (10 mL)

Solution, Injection [preservative free]:

Generic: 2 mg/2 mL (2 mL); 5 mg/5 mL (5 mL); 5 mg/mL (1 mL); 10 mg/2 mL (2 mL)

Syrup, Oral:

Generic: 2 mg/mL (118 mL)

References
Adrian ER, "Intranasal Versed®: The Future of Pediatric Conscious Sedation," *Pediatr Nurs*, 1994, 20(3):287-92.

Acworth JP, Purdie D, and Clark RC, "Intravenous Ketamine Plus Midazolam Is Superior to Intranasal Midazolam for Emergency Paediatric Procedural Sedation," *Emerg Med J*, 2001, 18(1):39-45.

Anand KJ, Barton BA, McIntosh N, et al, "Analgesia and Sedation in Preterm Neonates Who Require Ventilatory Support: Results From the NOPAIN Trial. Neonatal Outcome and Prolonged Analgesia in Neonates," *Arch Pediatr Adolesc Med*, 1999, 153(4):331-8.

Ashrafi MR, Khosroshahi N, Karimi P, et al, "Efficacy and Usability of Buccal Midazolam in Controlling Acute Prolonged Convulsive Seizures in Children," *Eur J Paediatr Neurol*, 2010, 14(5):434-8.

Bergman U, Rosa FW, Baum C, et al, "Effects of Exposure to Benzodiazepine During Fetal Life," *Lancet*, 1992, 340(8821):694-6.

Bhattacharyya M, Kalra V, and Gulati S, "Intranasal Midazolam vs Rectal Diazepam in Acute Childhood Seizures," *Pediatr Neurol*, 2006, 34(5):355-9.

Booker PD, Beechey A, and Lloyd-Thomas AR, "Sedation of Children Requiring Artificial Ventilation Using an Infusion of Midazolam," *Br J Anaesth*, 1986, 58(10):1104-8.

Boylan GB, Rennie JM, Chorley G, et al, "Second-Line Anticonvulsant Treatment of Neonatal Seizures: A Video-EEG Monitoring Study," *Neurology*, 2004, 62(3):486-8.

Burtin P, Jacqz-Aigrain E, Girard P, et al, "Population Pharmacokinetics of Midazolam in Neonates," *Clin Pharmacol Ther*, 1994, 56(6 Pt 1):615-25.

Castro Conde JR, Hernández Borges AA, Doménech Martínez E, et al, "Midazolam in Neonatal Seizures With No Response to Phenobarbital," *Neurology*, 2005, 64(5):876-9.

Chiaretti A, Barone G, Rigante D, et al, "Intranasal Lidocaine and Midazolam for Procedural Sedation in Children," *Arch Dis Child*, 2011, 96(2):160-3.

de Wildt SN, Kearns GL, Hop WC, et al, "Pharmacokinetics and Metabolism of Intravenous Midazolam in Preterm Infants," *Clin Pharmacol Ther*, 2001, 70(6):525-31.

Fişgin T, Gürer Y, Senbil N, et al, "Nasal Midazolam Effects on Childhood Acute Seizures," *J Child Neurol*, 2000, 15(12):833-5.

Fişgin T, Gurer Y, Teziç T, et al, "Effects of Intranasal Midazolam and Rectal Diazepam on Acute Convulsions in Children: Prospective Randomized Study," *J Child Neurol*, 2002, 17(2):123-6.

Harcke HT, Grissom LE, and Meister MA, "Sedation in Pediatric Imaging Using Intranasal Midazolam," *Pediatr Radiol*, 1995, 25 (5):341-3.

Hayashi K, Osawa M, Aihara M, et al, "Efficacy of Intravenous Midazolam for Status Epilepticus in Childhood," *Pediatr Neurol*, 2007, 36 (6):366-72.

Hegenbarth MA and American Academy of Pediatrics Committee on Drugs, "Preparing for Pediatric Emergencies: Drugs to Consider," *Pediatrics*, 2008, 121(2):433-43.

Holmes GL and Riviello JJ Jr, "Midazolam and Pentobarbital for Refractory Status Epilepticus," *Pediatr Neurol*, 1999, 20(4):259-64.

Holsti M, Sill BL, Firth SD, et al, "Prehospital Intranasal Midazolam for the Treatment of Pediatric Seizures," *Pediatr Emerg Care*, 2007, 23 (3):148-53.

Holsti M, Dudley N, Schunk J, et al, "Intranasal Midazolam vs Rectal Diazepam for the Home Treatment of Acute Seizures in Pediatric Patients With Epilepsy," *Arch Pediatr Adolesc Med*, 2010, 164 (8):747-53.

Igartua J, Silver P, Maytal J, et al, "Midazolam Coma for Refractory Status Epilepticus in Children," *Crit Care Med*, 1999, 27(9):1982-5.

Institute for Safe Medication Practices (ISMP), "Standard Concentrations of Neonatal Drug Infusions," *ISMP*, 2011.

Iqbal MM, Sobhan T, Ryals T, et al, "Effects of Commonly Used Benzodiazepines on the Fetus, the Neonate, and the Nursing Infant," *Psychiatr Serv*, 2002, 53(1):39-49.

Jacobi J, Fraser GL, Coursin DB, et al, "Clinical Practice Guidelines for the Sustained Use of Sedatives and Analgesics in the Critically Ill Adult," *Crit Care Med*, 2002, 30(1):119-41.

Jacqz-Aigrain E, Daoud P, Burtin P, et al, "Pharmacokinetics of Midazolam During Continuous Infusion in Critically Ill Neonates," *Eur J Clin Pharmacol*, 1992, 42(3):329-32.

Jacqz-Aigrain E, Daoud P, Burtin P, et al, "Placebo-Controlled Trial of Midazolam Sedation in Mechanically Ventilated Newborn Babies," *Lancet*, 1994, 344(8923):646-50.

Jacqz-Aigrain E, Wood C, and Robieux I, "Pharmacokinetics of Midazolam in Critically Ill Neonates," *Eur J Clin Pharmacol*, 1990, 39 (2):191-2.

Koul R, Chacko A, Javed H, et al, "Eight-Year Study of Childhood Status Epilepticus: Midazolam Infusion in Management and Outcome," *J Child Neurol*, 2002, 17(12):908-10.

Koul R, Raj Aithala G, Chacko A, et al, "Continuous Midazolam Infusion as Treatment of Status Epilepticus," *Arch Dis Child*, 1997, 76 (5):445-8.

Kumar P, Denson SE, Mancuso TJ, et al, "Premedication for Nonemergency Endotracheal Intubation in the Neonate," *Pediatrics*, 2010, 125(3):608-15.

Kupietzky A and Houpt MI, "Midazolam: A Review of Its Use for Conscious Sedation of Children," *Pediatr Dent*, 1993, 15(4):237-41.

Kutlu NO, Yakinci C, Dogrul M, et al, "Intranasal Midazolam for Prolonged Convulsive Seizures," *Brain Dev*, 2000, 22(6):359-61.

Lam C, Udin RD, Malamed SF, et al, "Midazolam Premedication in Children: A Pilot Study Comparing Intramuscular and Intranasal Administration," *Anesth Prog*, 2005, 52(2):56-61.

Lane RD and Schunk JE, "Atomized Intranasal Midazolam Use for Minor Procedures in the Pediatric Emergency Department," *Pediatr Emerg Care*, 2008, 24(5):300-3.

Ljungman G, Kreuger A, Andreasson S, et al, "Midazolam Nasal Spray Reduces Procedural Anxiety in Children," *Pediatrics*, 2000, 105(1 Pt 1):73-8.

Lowenstein DH, "Treatment Options for Status Epilepticus," *Curr Opin Pharmacol*, 2005, 5(3):334-9.

Lugo RA, Fishbein M, Nahata MC, et al, "Complication of Intranasal Midazolam," *Pediatrics*, 1993, 92(4):638.

Magny JF, Zupan V, Dehan M, et al, "Midazolam and Myoclonus in Neonate," *Eur J Pediatr*, 1994, 153(5):389-90.

Malamed SF, Quinn CL, and Hatch HG, "Pediatric Sedation With Intramuscular and Intravenous Midazolam," *Anesth Prog*, 1989, 36 (4-5):155-7.

Malinovsky JM, Populaire C, Cozian A, et al, "Premedication With Midazolam in Children, Effect of Intranasal, Rectal and Oral Routes on Plasma Midazolam Concentrations," *Anaesthesia*, 1995, 50 (4):351-4.

Massanari M, Novitsky J, and Reinstein LJ, "Paradoxical Reactions in Children Associated With Midazolam Use During Endoscopy," *Clin Pediatr*, 1997, 36(12):681-4.

Matheson I, Lunde PK, Bredesen JE, et al, "Midazolam and Nitrazepam in the Maternity Ward: Milk Concentrations and Clinical Effects," *Br J Clin Pharmacol*, 1990, 30(6):787-93.

McIntyre J, Robertson S, Norris E, et al, "Safety and Efficacy of Buccal Midazolam Versus Rectal Diazepam for Emergency Treatment of Seizures in Children: A Randomised Controlled Trial," *Lancet*, 2005, 366(9481):205-10.

Meierkord H, Boon P, Engelsen B, et al, "EFNS Guideline on the Management of Status Epilepticus in Adults," *Eur J Neurol*, 2010, 17(3):348-55.

Mittal P, Manohar R, and Rawat AK, "Comparative Study of Intranasal Midazolam and Intravenous Diazepam Sedation for Procedures and Seizures," *Indian J Pediatr*, 2006, 73(11):975-8.

Morrison GC and Whitehouse WP, "High-Dose Midazolam in Convulsive Status Epilepticus," *Pediatr Neurol*, 2008, 39(3):221.

Morrison G, Gibbons E, and Whitehouse WP, "High-Dose Midazolam Therapy for Refractory Status Epilepticus in Children," *Intensive Care Med*, 2006, 32(12):2070-6.

Mpimbaza A, Ndeezi G, Staedke S, et al, "Comparison of Buccal Midazolam With Rectal Diazepam in the Treatment of Prolonged Seizures in Ugandan Children: A Randomized Clinical Trial," *Pediatrics*, 2008, 121(1):58-64.

Mulla H, Lawson G, Woodland ED, et al, "Effects of Neonatal Extracorporeal Membrane Oxygenation Circuits on Drug Disposition," *Curr Ther Res Clin Exp*, 2000, 61:838-48.

Ozdemir D, Gulez P, Uran N, et al, "Efficacy of Continuous Midazolam Infusion and Mortality in Childhood Refractory Generalized Convulsive Status Epilepticus," *Seizure*, 2005, 14(2):129-32.

Phillips MS, "Standardizing I.V. Infusion Concentrations: National Survey Results," *Am J Health Syst Pharm*, 2011, 68(22):2176-82.

Riva J, Lejbusiewicz G, Papa M, et al, "Oral Premedication With Midazolam in Paediatric Anaesthesia. Effects on Sedation and Gastric Contents," *Paediatr Anaesth*, 1997, 7(3):191-6.

Rivera R, Segnini M, Baltodano A, et al, "Midazolam in the Treatment of Status Epilepticus in Children," *Crit Care Med*, 1993, 21(7):991-4.

Silbergleit R, Durkalski V, Lowenstein D, et al, "Intramuscular Versus Intravenous Therapy for Prehospital Status Epilepticus," *N Engl J Med*, 2012, 366(7):591-600.

Silvasi DL, Rosen DA, and Rosen KR, "Continuous Intravenous Midazolam Infusion for Sedation in the Pediatric Intensive Care Unit," *Anesth Analg*, 1988, 67(3):286-8.

Singh N, Pandey RK, Saksena AK, et al, "A Comparative Evaluation of Oral Midazolam With Other Sedatives as Premedication in Pediatric Dentistry," *J Clin Pediatr Dent*, 2002, 26(2):161-4.

Talukdar B and Chakrabarty B, "Efficacy of Buccal Midazolam Compared to Intravenous Diazepam in Controlling Convulsions in Children: A Randomized Controlled Trial," *Brain Dev*, 2009, 31(10):744-9.

Treluyer JM, Zohar S, Rey E, et al, "Minimum Effective Dose of Midazolam for Sedation of Mechanically Ventilated Neonates," *J Clin Pharm Ther*, 2005, 30(5):479-85.

VanLooy JW, Schumacher RE, and Bhatt-Mehta V, "Efficacy of a Premedication Algorithm for Nonemergent Intubation in a Neonatal Intensive Care Unit," *Ann Pharmacother*, 2008, 42(7):947-55.

Wang Z, Gorski JC, Hamman MA, et al, "The Effects of St John's Wort (Hypericum perforatum) on Human Cytochrome P450 Activity," *Clin Pharmacol Ther*, 2001, 70(4):317-26.

Wikner BN, Stiller CO, Bergman U, et al, "Use of Benzodiazepines and Benzodiazepine Receptor Agonists During Pregnancy: Neonatal Outcome and Congenital Malformations," *Pharmacoepidemiol Drug Saf*, 2007, 16(11):1203-10.

Yoshikawa H, Yamazaki S, Abe T, et al, "Midazolam as a First-Line Agent for Status Epilepticus in Children," *Brain Dev*, 2000, 22 (4):239-42.

◆ **Midazolam Hydrochloride** see Midazolam
  on page 1411

◆ **Midazolam Injection (Can)** see Midazolam
  on page 1411

◆ **Migergot** see Ergotamine and Caffeine on page 777

◆ **Migranal** see Dihydroergotamine on page 665

◆ **Migranal® (Can)** see Dihydroergotamine on page 665

◆ **Milk of Magnesia [OTC]** see Magnesium Hydroxide
  on page 1294

◆ **Milk of Magnesia Concentrate [OTC]** see Magnesium
  Hydroxide on page 1294

◆ **Millipred** see PrednisoLONE (Systemic) on page 1727

◆ **Millipred DP** see PrednisoLONE (Systemic)
  on page 1727

◆ **Millipred DP 12-Day** see PrednisoLONE (Systemic)
  on page 1727

Milrinone (MIL ri none)

Medication Safety Issues
Sound-alike/look-alike issues:
Primacor may be confused with Primaxin
High alert medication:
The Institute for Safe Medication Practices (ISMP) includes this medication among its list of drugs which have a heightened risk of causing significant patient harm when used in error.

Brand Names: Canada Milrinone Lactate Injection; Primacor

Therapeutic Category Phosphodiesterase Enzyme Inhibitor

Generic Availability (U.S.) Yes

Use Short-term treatment of acute decompensated heart failure (FDA approved in adults)

Pregnancy Risk Factor C

Pregnancy Considerations Teratogenic effects have not been observed in animal reproduction studies; however, increased resorption was reported in some studies.

Breast-Feeding Considerations It is not known if milrinone is excreted in breast milk. The manufacturer recommends that caution be exercised when administering milrinone to nursing women.

Contraindications Hypersensitivity to milrinone, any component, or inamrinone (amrinone)

Warnings Longer treatment of heart failure (>48 hours) has not been shown to be safe and effective (there are no controlled trials using milrinone infusions for >48 hours); long-term oral use for heart failure was associated with no improvement in symptoms, increased risk of hospitalization, and increased risk of sudden death; monitor ECG continuously to promptly detect and manage ventricular arrhythmias. Long-term, regularly scheduled intermittent infusions are strongly discouraged (ACC/AHA 2005 Guidelines).

Precautions Avoid use in patients with severe obstructive aortic or pulmonic valvular disease; use in patients with hypertrophic subaortic stenosis may increase outflow tract obstruction. Use with caution in patients with a history of ventricular arrhythmias, atrial fibrillation, or atrial flutter. Use with caution and modify dosage in patients with impaired renal function. Hypotension may occur; monitor blood pressure and heart rate; infusion may require reduction in rate or temporary discontinuation if hypotension occurs; hypotension may be prolonged, especially in patients with renal dysfunction. Infusion site reactions may occur; monitor infusion site carefully. Milrinone is not recommended for use in patients with acute MI.

Adverse Reactions
Cardiovascular: Angina, hypotension, supraventricular arrhythmia, ventricular arrhythmia
Central nervous system: Headache
Rare but important or life-threatening: Anaphylaxis, atrial fibrillation, bronchospasm, hypokalemia, injection site reaction, liver function abnormalities, MI, rash, thrombocytopenia, torsade de pointes, tremor, ventricular fibrillation

Drug Interactions
Metabolism/Transport Effects None known.
Avoid Concomitant Use There are no known interactions where it is recommended to avoid concomitant use.
Increased Effect/Toxicity
Milrinone may increase the levels/effects of: Riociguat
Decreased Effect There are no known significant interactions involving a decrease in effect.

Stability
Storage:
Injection: Store at controlled room temperature 15°C to 30°C (59°F to 86°F); avoid freezing

Premixed infusion: Store at room temperature at 25°C (77°F); brief exposure up to 40°C (104°F) will not adversely affect drug; minimize exposure to heat; avoid excessive heat; protect from freezing

Mechanism of Action A selective phosphodiesterase inhibitor in cardiac and vascular tissue, resulting in vasodilation and inotropic effects with little chronotropic activity.

Pharmacodynamics Onset of action (improved hemodynamic function): Within 5-15 minutes

Pharmacokinetics (Adult data unless noted)
Distribution: V_d beta:
Infants (after cardiac surgery): 0.9 ± 0.4 L/kg
Children (after cardiac surgery): 0.7 ± 0.2 L/kg
Adults:
After cardiac surgery: 0.3 ± 0.1 L/kg
CHF (with single injection): 0.38 L/kg
CHF (with infusion): 0.45 L/kg
Protein binding: 70%
Half-life:
Infants (after cardiac surgery): 3.15 ± 2 hours
Children (after cardiac surgery): 1.86 ± 2 hours
Adults:
After cardiac surgery: 1.69 ± 0.18 hours
CHF: 2.3-2.4 hours
Renal impairment: Prolonged half-life
Elimination: Excreted in the urine as unchanged drug (83%) and glucuronide metabolite (12%)
Clearance:
Infants (after cardiac surgery): 3.8 ± 1 mL/kg/minute
Children (after cardiac surgery): 5.9 ± 2 mL/kg/minute
Children (with septic shock): 10.6 ± 5.3 mL/kg/minute
Adults:
After cardiac surgery: 2 ± 0.7 mL/kg/minute
CHF: 2.2-2.3 mL/kg/minute
Renal impairment: Decreased clearance

Dosing: Neonatal I.V.: A limited number of studies have used different dosing schemes; optimal dose not established; further studies needed.

Hemodynamic support: Full-term neonates: Loading dose: 50-75 mcg/kg administered over 15 minutes followed by a continuous infusion of 0.5 mcg/kg/minute; titrate to effect; range: 0.25-0.75 mcg/kg/minute has been used by several centers. One report used a loading dose of 50 mcg/kg administered over 15 minutes, followed by a continuous infusion of 0.5 mcg/kg/minute for 30 minutes in 10 neonates (3-27 days old, median age: 5 days) with low cardiac output after cardiac surgery; results showed improved hemodynamic parameters and milrinone was well tolerated (Chang, 1995)

Prevention of postoperative low cardiac output syndrome (CHD corrective surgery): Full-term neonates: Loading dose: 75 mcg/kg administered over 60 minutes followed by a continuous I.V. infusion of 0.75 mcg/kg/minute for 35 hours was used in a randomized, placebo-controlled trial of 227 patients (age: 2 days-6.9 years, median: 3 months) and showed 64% relative risk reduction for development of low cardiac output syndrome compared to placebo; a lower milrinone dose used in the study did not show a statistically significant relative risk reduction compared to placebo for the same endpoint (Hoffman, 2003)

Dosing: Usual

Infants and Children: I.V.: A limited number of studies have used different dosing schemes. Two pharmacokinetic studies propose per kg doses for pediatric patients with septic shock that are greater than those recommended for adults (Lindsay, 1998) and in infants and children after cardiac surgery (Ramamoorthy, 1998). Further pharmacodynamic studies are needed to define pediatric milrinone guidelines. Several centers are using the following guidelines:

Loading dose: 50 mcg/kg administered over 15 minutes followed by a continuous infusion of 0.5 mcg/kg/minute; range: 0.25-0.75 mcg/kg/minute; titrate dose to effect

PALS Guidelines, 2010: I.V., I.O.: Loading dose: 50 mcg/kg administered over 10-60 minutes followed by a continuous infusion of 0.25-0.75 mcg/kg/minute

Adults: I.V.: Loading dose: 50 mcg/kg slow I.V. over 10 minutes, followed by a continuous infusion of 0.5 mcg/kg/minute; range: 0.375-0.75 mcg/kg/minute; titrate dose to effect; maximum daily dose: 1.13 mg/kg/day

Dosing adjustment in renal impairment: Adult: Continuous I.V. infusion:

Manufacturer recommended adjustment:

CrCl 50 mL/minute/1.73 m²: Administer 0.43 mcg/kg/minute

CrCl 40 mL/minute/1.73 m²: Administer 0.38 mcg/kg/minute

CrCl 30 mL/minute/1.73 m²: Administer 0.33 mcg/kg/minute

CrCl 20 mL/minute/1.73 m²: Administer 0.28 mcg/kg/minute

CrCl 10 mL/minute/1.73 m²: Administer 0.23 mcg/kg/minute

CrCl 5 mL/minute/1.73 m²: Administer 0.2 mcg/kg/minute

Alternative Dosing Adjustments in Patients with Renal Impairment[1]

CrCl (mL/min)	Starting dose (mcg/kg/min)		
	0.375	0.5	0.75
50	0.25	0.375	0.5
40	0.125	0.25	0.375
30	0.0625	0.125	0.25
20	Consider alternative therapy	0.0625	0.125
10	Consider alternative therapy		0.0625
5	Consider alternative therapy		

[1]Based on expert opinion

Usual Infusion Concentrations: Pediatric Note: Premixed solutions available

I.V. infusion: 200 mcg/mL

Administration

Loading dose: Administer slow I.V. push over 15 minutes for pediatric patients and over 10 minutes in adults; loading dose may be given as undiluted solution, but may dilute to 10-20 mL (in adults) for ease of administration.

Continuous I.V. infusion: Dilute with ½NS, NS, or D₅W and administer via infusion pump or syringe pump; usual concentration: ≤200 mcg/mL; 250 mcg/mL in NS has been used (Barton, 1996). **Note:** Some pediatric centers use a concentration of 500 mcg/mL but only if infused via a central line.

Monitoring Parameters Blood pressure, heart rate, cardiac output, CI, SVR, PVR, CVP, ECG, CBC, platelet count, serum electrolytes (especially potassium and magnesium), liver enzymes, renal function; clinical signs and symptoms of CHF; monitor infusion site carefully (avoid extravasation)

Additional Information Dosing schemes and proposed dosing based on pharmacokinetic data:

Infants and children with septic shock: Twelve patients (9 months to 15 years of age) were administered a loading dose of 50 mcg/kg, followed by a continuous infusion of 0.5 mcg/kg/minute. At 1 hour after the loading dose, if patients did not respond (defined as a ≥20% increase in CI or an improvement in peripheral perfusion), an additional loading dose of 25 mcg/kg was given and the infusion rate was increased to 0.75 mcg/kg/minute. Nine of 12 patients required the additional loading dose and increased rate of infusion (Barton, 1996). A subsequent pharmacokinetic analysis of these patients recommended larger loading doses of 75 mcg/kg and infusion rates of 0.75-1 mcg/kg/minute. However, these doses were based on a one-compartment pharmacokinetic model and are higher then the mean infusion rate of 0.69 mcg/kg/minute used in the study (Lindsay, 1998). Further studies are needed.

Infants and Children after open heart surgery: A prospective, open-label trial compared a lower dose of milrinone (Group A) to a higher dose (Group B). Group A: Eleven patients received a loading dose of 25 mcg/kg given over 5 minutes followed by an infusion of 0.25 mcg/kg/minute; 30 minutes later, a second 25 mcg/kg loading dose was given and the infusion was increased to 0.5 mcg/kg/minute. Group B: 8 patients received a loading dose of 50 mcg/kg given over 10 minutes followed by an infusion of 0.5 mcg/kg/minute; 30 minutes later, a second loading dose of 25 mcg/kg was given and the infusion was increased to 0.75 mcg/kg/minute. Patients in both groups received a third loading dose of 25 mcg/kg if needed. A two-compartment model and NONMEM pharmacokinetic analyses were performed. Based on the NONMEM analysis, the authors propose the following doses: Infants: Loading dose: 104 mcg/kg and continuous infusion of 0.49 mcg/kg/minute; children: loading dose: 67 mcg/kg and continuous infusion of 0.61 mcg/kg/minute (Ramamoorthy, 1998). Further studies are needed before these proposed doses can routinely be used in the pediatric population.

Dosage Forms Excipient information presented when available (limited, particularly for generics); consult specific product labeling.

Solution, Intravenous:

Generic: 200 mcg/mL (100 mL, 200 mL); 10 mg/10 mL (10 mL); 20 mg/20 mL (20 mL); 50 mg/50 mL (50 mL)

Solution, Intravenous [preservative free]:

Generic: 200 mcg/mL (100 mL, 200 mL)

References

"ACC/AHA 2005 Guideline Update for the Diagnosis and Management of Chronic Heart Failure in the Adult: A Report of the American College of Cardiology/American Heart Association Task Force on Practice Guidelines (Writing Committee to Update the 2001 Guidelines for the Evaluation and Management of Heart Failure)," J Am Coll Cardiol, 2005, 46(6):e1-82.

"2005 American Heart Association (AHA) Guidelines for Cardiopulmonary Resuscitation (CPR) and Emergency Cardiovascular Care (ECC), Part 12: Pediatric Advanced Life Support, The American Heart Association Emergency Cardiovascular Care Committee," Circulation, 2005, 112(24 Suppl):IV58-77, 167-87.

Barton P, Garcia J, Kouatli A, et al, "Hemodynamic Effects of I.V. Milrinone Lactate in Pediatric Patients With Septic Shock. A Prospective Double-Blinded, Randomized, Placebo-Controlled, Interventional Study," Chest, 1996, 109(5):1302-12.

Chang AC, Atz AM, Wernovsky G, et al, "Milrinone: Systemic and Pulmonary Hemodynamic Effects in Neonates After Cardiac Surgery," Crit Care Med, 1995, 23(11):1907-14.

Cuffe MS, Califf RM, Adams KF Jr, et al, "Short-Term Intravenous Milrinone for Acute Exacerbation of Chronic Heart Failure: A Randomized Controlled Trial," JAMA, 2002, 287(12):1541-7.

Heart Failure Society of America, "HFSA 2006 Comprehensive Heart Failure Practice Guideline," J Card Fail, 2006, 12(1):e1-122.

Hoffman TM, Wernovsky G, Atz AM, et al, "Efficacy and Safety of Milrinone in Preventing Low Cardiac Output Syndrome in Infants and Children After Corrective Surgery for Congenital Heart Disease," *Circulation*, 2003, 107(7):996-1002.

Hoffman TM, Wernovsky G, Atz AM, et al, "Prophylactic Intravenous Use of Milrinone After Cardiac Operation in Pediatrics (PRIMACORP) Study," *Am Heart J*, 2002, 143(1):15-21.

Lindsay CA, Barton P, Lawless S, et al, "Pharmacokinetics and Pharmacodynamics of Milrinone in Pediatric Patients With Septic Shock," *J Pediatr*, 1998, 132(2):329-34.

Paradisis M, Evans N, Kluckow M, et al, "Pilot Study of Milrinone for Low Systemic Blood Flow in Very Preterm Infants," *J Pediatr*, 2006, 148(3):306-13.

Phillips MS, "Standardizing I.V. Infusion Concentrations: National Survey Results," *Am J Health Syst Pharm*, 2011, 68(22):2176-82.

Ramamoorthy C, Anderson GD, Williams GD, et al, "Pharmacokinetics and Side Effects of Milrinone in Infants and Children After Open Heart Surgery," *Anesth Analg*, 1998, 86(2):283-9.

◆ **Milrinone Lactate** *see* Milrinone *on page 1417*

◆ **Milrinone Lactate Injection (Can)** *see* Milrinone *on page 1417*

Mineral Oil (MIN er al oyl)

Medication Safety Issues
BEERS Criteria medication:
This drug may be potentially inappropriate for use in geriatric patients (Quality of evidence - moderate; Strength of recommendation - strong).

Brand Names: U.S. Fleet Oil [OTC]

Therapeutic Category Laxative, Lubricant

Generic Availability (U.S.) Yes

Use
Oral: Treatment of occasional constipation (OTC product: FDA approved in ≥6 years and adults)

Rectal: Treatment of occasional constipation; relief of fecal impaction; removal of barium sulfate residues following barium administration (OTC products: Fleet® Mineral Oil Enema; All indications: FDA approved in ages ≥2 years and adults); has also been used as preparation for bowel studies or surgery

Refer to product-specific information to determine FDA approved ages for additional products

Pregnancy Considerations The use of mineral oil for the treatment of constipation in pregnancy is not recommended (Mahadevan, 2006).

Breast-Feeding Considerations The use of mineral oil for the treatment of constipation is not recommended for nursing women (Mahadevan, 2006).

Contraindications Hypersensitivity to mineral oil or any component. Additional contraindications for oral products: Pregnancy, swallowing difficulties, bed-ridden, elderly or <6 years of age, appendicitis or its symptoms, undiagnosed rectal bleeding

Warnings Lipid pneumonitis results from aspiration of mineral oil; oral formulation should be avoided in patients with difficulty swallowing (including those with esophageal or gastric distention, dysphagia, or hiatal hernia) or who are bed-ridden; not recommended for use in infants due to increased risk of aspiration (NASPHAGAN, 2006).

When using for self-medication (OTC), consult physician prior to use if any of the following conditions are present: Abdominal pain, nausea or vomiting, a sudden change in bowel habits that persist over a period of 2 weeks, or if presently taking a stool softener laxative. If laxative use is needed for more than 1 week, rectal bleeding occurs, or fail to have a bowel movement after use, discontinue use and contact physician.

Adverse Reactions
Gastrointestinal: Abdominal cramps, diarrhea, nausea, vomiting

Respiratory: Lipid pneumonitis with aspiration

Miscellaneous: Large doses may cause anal leakage causing anal itching, hemorrhoids, irritation, perianal discomfort, soiling of clothes

Drug Interactions
Metabolism/Transport Effects None known.

Avoid Concomitant Use There are no known interactions where it is recommended to avoid concomitant use.

Increased Effect/Toxicity There are no known significant interactions involving an increase in effect.

Decreased Effect
Mineral Oil may decrease the levels/effects of: Multivitamins/Fluoride (with ADE); Multivitamins/Minerals (with ADEK, Folate, Iron); Multivitamins/Minerals (with AE, No Iron); Phytonadione; Vitamin D Analogs

Stability
Oral:
Plain (nonemulsified) liquid: Protect from sunlight.
Suspension (emulsion) (Kondremul®): Store at 15°C to 25°C (59°F to 77°F).
Rectal enema: Store at 20°C to 25°C (68°F to 77°F); protect from sunlight.

Mechanism of Action Eases passage of stool by decreasing water absorption and lubricating the intestine; retards colonic absorption of water

Pharmacodynamics
Onset of action:
Enema: 2-15 minutes
Oral: ~6-8 hours

Pharmacokinetics (Adult data unless noted)
Absorption: Minimal following oral and rectal administration
Distribution: Into intestinal mucosa, liver, spleen, and mesenteric lymph nodes
Elimination: In feces

Dosing: Usual
Children and Adolescents:
Constipation, occasional:
Oral:
Plain (nonemulsified) liquid:
Children 6-11 years: 5-15 mL/day in a single daily dose at bedtime or in divided doses; maximum daily dose: 15 mL/**day**
Children ≥12 years and Adolescents: 15-45 mL/day in a single daily dose at bedtime or in divided doses; maximum daily dose: 45 mL/**day**
Suspension (emulsion) (Kondremul®):
Children 6-11 years: 10-30 mL/day in a single daily dose or in up to 3 divided doses
Children ≥12 years and Adolescents: 30-90 mL/day in a single daily dose or in up to 3 divided doses
Rectal:
Children 2-11 years: Administer **one half** the contents of a 4.5 oz bottle as a single dose
Children ≥12 years and Adolescents: Administer the contents of one 4.5 oz bottle as a single dose
Constipation, chronic: Oral: 1-3 mL/kg/day divided in 1-2 doses (NASPGHAN, 2006)
Fecal impaction:
Oral:
Rapid disimpaction: 15-30 mL per year of age as a single dose; maximum daily dose: 240 mL/**day** (NASPGHAN, 2006)
Slow disimpaction: Oral: 3 mL/kg twice daily for 7 days
Rectal:
Children 2-11 years: Administer **one half** the contents of a 4.5 oz bottle as a single dose
Children ≥12 years and Adolescents: Administer the contents of one 4.5 oz bottle as a single dose
Removal of barium sulfate residues following barium administration: Rectal:
Children 2-11 years: Administer **one half** the contents of a 4.5 oz bottle as a single dose
Children ≥12 years and Adolescents: Administer the contents of one 4.5 oz bottle as a single dose

Adults:

Constipation:

Oral:

Plain (nonemulsified) liquid: 15-45 ml/day in a single daily dose at bedtime or in divided doses; maximum daily dose: 45 mL/**day**

Suspension (emulsion) (Kondremul®): 30-90 mL/day in a single daily dose or in up to 3 divided doses

Rectal: Administer the contents of one 4.5 oz bottle as a single dose

Fecal impaction or following barium studies: Rectal: Administer the contents of one 4.5 oz bottle as a single dose

Administration

Oral: Mineral oil may be more palatable if refrigerated (NASGHAN, 2006). **Note:** Due to risk of aspiration, do not administer to patient in supine position.

Plain (nonemulsified): Administer on an empty stomach. Take at least 2 hours before or after other medications.

Suspension (emulsion) (Kondremul®): Shake well before use. May be administered alone or mixed with warm or cold water, milk, or cocoa; do not take with meals.

Rectal: Administer with patient lying on left side and knees bent or with patient kneeling and head and chest leaning forward until left side of face is resting comfortably. Remove protective shield and gently insert enema tip into rectum with a slight side-to-side movement with tip pointing toward the navel; have patient bear down. Do not force the enema tip into the rectum as this may cause injury. Squeeze the bottle until correct dose is administered. It is not necessary to empty the bottle completely for a one-bottle dose. Remove enema tip from rectum.

Monitoring Parameters Evacuation of stool; anal leakage indicates dose too high or need for disimpaction

Additional Information Fleets® Mineral Oil Enema: 4.5 ounce enema delivers 118 mL

Dosage Forms Excipient information presented when available (limited, particularly for generics); consult specific product labeling.

Enema, Rectal:

Fleet Oil: (133 mL)

Generic: (135 mL)

Oil, Oral:

Generic: (473 mL, 500 mL, 1000 mL, 4000 mL)

References

Constipation Guideline Committee of the North American Society for Pediatric Gastroenterology, Hepatology and Nutrition (NASPGHAN), "Evaluation and Treatment of Constipation in Infants and Children: Recommendations of the North American Society for Pediatric Gastroenterology, Hepatology and Nutrition," *J Pediatr Gastroenterol Nutr*, 2006, 43(3):e1-13.

Mahadevan U and Kane S, "American Gastroenterological Association Institute Medical Position Statement on the Use of Gastrointestinal Medications in Pregnancy," *Gastroenterology*, 2006, 131(1):278-82.

◆ **Minims Cyclopentolate (Can)** *see* Cyclopentolate *on page 560*

◆ **Minims Prednisolone Sodium Phosphate (Can)** *see* PrednisoLONE (Ophthalmic) *on page 1730*

◆ **Minipress** *see* Prazosin *on page 1724*

◆ **Minirin® (Can)** *see* Desmopressin *on page 612*

◆ **Minitran** *see* Nitroglycerin *on page 1504*

◆ **Minivelle** *see* Estradiol (Systemic) *on page 796*

◆ **Minocin** *see* Minocycline *on page 1420*

◆ **Minocin® (Can)** *see* Minocycline *on page 1420*

Minocycline (mi noe SYE kleen)

Medication Safety Issues

Sound-alike/look-alike issues:

Dynacin® may be confused with Dyazide®, Dynapen

Minocin® may be confused with Indocin®, Lincocin®, Minizide®, niacin

Related Information

Oral Medications That Should Not Be Crushed or Altered *on page 2438*

Brand Names: U.S. Minocin; Solodyn

Brand Names: Canada Apo-Minocycline®; Arestin Microspheres; Dom-Minocycline; Minocin®; Mylan-Minocycline; Novo-Minocycline; PHL-Minocycline; PMS-Minocycline; ratio-Minocycline; Riva-Minocycline; Sandoz-Minocycline

Therapeutic Category Antibiotic, Tetracycline Derivative

Generic Availability (U.S.) May be product dependent

Use Treatment of susceptible gram-negative and gram-positive infections involving the respiratory tract, urinary tract, and skin/soft tissue; treatment of anthrax (inhalational, cutaneous, and gastrointestinal); brucellosis; asymptomatic meningococcal carrier state; rickettsial diseases (including Rocky Mountain spotted fever, typhus fever, Q fever); nongonococcal urethritis caused by *Ureaplasma urealyticum* or *C. trachomatis*, and gonorrhea; chlamydial infections (FDA approved in ages >8 years and adults); inflammatory acne vulgaris (FDA approved in ages ≥12 years); has been used to treat *Nocardia*, cutaneous (non-CNS) infections; *Mycobacterium marinum* cutaneous infections

Pregnancy Risk Factor D

Pregnancy Considerations Tetracyclines cross the placenta and accumulate in developing teeth and long tubular bones. Rare spontaneous reports of congenital anomalies, including limb reduction, have been reported following maternal minocycline use. Due to limited information, a causal association cannot be established. Tetracyclines may discolor fetal teeth following maternal use during pregnancy; the specific teeth involved and the portion of the tooth affected depends on the timing and duration of exposure relative to tooth calcification. As a class, tetracyclines are generally considered second-line antibiotics in pregnant women and their use should be avoided (Mylonas, 2011). Minocycline should not be used for the treatment of acne in pregnant women, or in males or females attempting to conceive a child.

Breast-Feeding Considerations Minocycline is excreted in breast milk (Brogden, 1975). According to the manufacturer, the decision to continue or discontinue breast-feeding during therapy should take into account the risk of exposure to the infant and the benefits of treatment to the mother. Oral absorption is not affected by dairy products; therefore, oral absorption of minocycline by the breast-feeding infant would not be expected to be diminished by the calcium in the maternal milk. Nondose-related effects could include modification of bowel flora. There have been case reports of black discoloration of breast milk in women taking minocycline (Basler, 1985; Hunt, 1996).

Contraindications Hypersensitivity to minocycline, other tetracyclines, or any component

Warnings Use of tetracyclines during tooth development may cause permanent discoloration of the teeth (yellow-gray to brown) and enamel hypoplasia; adult-onset tooth discoloration following long-term minocycline administration has also been reported. Do not administer to children <8 years of age due to permanent discoloration of teeth and retardation of skeletal development and bone growth (risk being greatest for children <4 years and in those receiving high doses). Minocycline has been associated with increases in BUN secondary to antianabolic effects. Pseudotumor cerebri has been reported rarely in infants and adolescents; use with isotretinoin has been associated with cases of pseudotumor cerebri; avoid concomitant treatment with isotretinoin. CNS effects (dizziness, lightheadedness, vertigo) may occur; patients must be cautioned about performing tasks which require mental alertness. Photosensitivity reaction may occur; avoid prolonged exposure to sunlight or tanning equipment; discontinue if skin erythema occurs. Azotemia, hyperphosphatemia, and acidosis have been reported in patients with significant renal dysfunction. Prolonged use may result in superinfection including *C. difficile*-associated diarrhea and pseudomembraneous colitis. Minocycline can cause fetal harm if used during pregnancy; avoid use during pregnancy. Severe, sometimes fatal, hepatic injury has been associated with minocycline use; discontinue therapy if liver injury is suspected. Rash, along with eosinophilia, fever, and organ failure (Drug Rash with Eosinophilia and Systemic Symptoms (DRESS) syndrome) has been reported; discontinue treatment immediately if DRESS syndrome is suspected.

Precautions Use with caution in patients with renal or hepatic impairment; consider dosage modification in patients with renal impairment

Adverse Reactions

Cardiovascular: Myocarditis, pericarditis, vasculitis

Central nervous system: Bulging fontanels, dizziness, fatigue, fever, headache, hypoesthesia, malaise, mood changes, paresthesia, pseudotumor cerebri, sedation, seizure, somnolence, vertigo

Dermatologic: Alopecia, angioedema, drug rash with eosinophilia and systemic symptoms (DRESS), erythema multiforme, erythema nodosum, erythematous rash, exfoliative dermatitis, hyperpigmentation of nails, maculopapular rash, photosensitivity, pigmentation of the skin and mucous membranes, pruritus, Stevens-Johnson syndrome, toxic epidermal necrolysis, urticaria

Endocrine & metabolic: Thyroid cancer, thyroid discoloration, thyroid dysfunction

Gastrointestinal: Anorexia, diarrhea, dyspepsia, dysphagia, enamel hypoplasia, enterocolitis, esophageal ulcerations, esophagitis, glossitis, inflammatory lesions (oral/anogenital), moniliasis, nausea, oral cavity discoloration, pancreatitis, pseudomembranous colitis, stomatitis, tooth discoloration, vomiting, xerostomia

Genitourinary: Balanitis, vulvovaginitis

Hematologic: Agranulocytosis, eosinophilia, hemolytic anemia, leukopenia, neutropenia, pancytopenia, thrombocytopenia

Hepatic: Autoimmune hepatitis, hepatic cholestasis, hepatic failure, hepatitis, hyperbilirubinemia, jaundice, liver enzyme increases

Local: Injection site reaction (I.V. administration)

Neuromuscular & skeletal: Arthralgia, arthritis, bone discoloration, joint stiffness, joint swelling, myalgia

Otic: Hearing loss, tinnitus

Renal: Acute renal failure, BUN increased, interstitial nephritis

Respiratory: Asthma, bronchospasm, cough, dyspnea, pneumonitis, pulmonary infiltrate (with eosinophilia)

Miscellaneous: Anaphylaxis, hypersensitivity, lupus erythematosus, lupus-like syndrome, serum sickness

Drug Interactions

Metabolism/Transport Effects None known.

Avoid Concomitant Use

Avoid concomitant use of Minocycline with any of the following: BCG; Retinoic Acid Derivatives; Strontium Ranelate

Increased Effect/Toxicity

Minocycline may increase the levels/effects of: Mipomersen; Neuromuscular-Blocking Agents; Porfimer; Retinoic Acid Derivatives; Vitamin K Antagonists

Decreased Effect

Minocycline may decrease the levels/effects of: Atazanavir; BCG; Penicillins; Sodium Picosulfate; Typhoid Vaccine

The levels/effects of Minocycline may be decreased by: Antacids; Bile Acid Sequestrants; Bismuth; Bismuth Subsalicylate; Calcium Salts; Iron Salts; Lanthanum; Magnesium Salts; Multivitamins/Minerals (with ADEK, Folate, Iron); Multivitamins/Minerals (with AE, No Iron); Quinapril; Strontium Ranelate; Sucralfate; Sucroferric Oxyhydroxide; Zinc Salts

Food Interactions Minocycline serum concentrations are not significantly altered if taken with food or dairy products. Management: Administer without regard to food.

Stability

Oral:

Capsule (including pellet-filled), tablet: Store at 20°C to 25°C (68°F to 77°F); protect from heat. Protect from light and moisture.

Extended release tablet (Solodyn®): Store at 15°C to 30°C (59°F to 86°F); protect from heat. Protect from light and moisture.

Injection: Store vials at 20°C to 25°C (68°F to 77°F) prior to reconstitution. Reconstituted solution should be further diluted immediately. Final dilution should be administered immediately; stable at room temperature for 24 hours. Incompatible with adrenocorticotropic hormone, aminophylline, amobarbital, amphotericin B, bicarbonate infusion mixtures, calcium, cefazolin, heparin, hydrocortisone, penicillin, pentobarbital, phenytoin, whole blood.

Mechanism of Action Inhibits bacterial protein synthesis by binding with the 30S and possibly the 50S ribosomal subunit(s) of susceptible bacteria; cell wall synthesis is not affected

Rheumatoid arthritis: The mechanism of action of minocycline in rheumatoid arthritis is not completely understood. It is thought to have antimicrobial, anti-inflammatory, immunomodulatory, and chondroprotective effects. More specifically, it is thought to be a potent inhibitor of metalloproteinases, which are active in rheumatoid arthritis joint destruction.

Pharmacokinetics (Adult data unless noted)

Absorption: Oral: Well absorbed

Distribution: Widely distributed to most body fluids, bile, and tissues; poor CNS penetration; deposits in fat for extended periods; crosses placenta; appears in breast milk

V_d: Adults: 0.14-0.7 L/kg

Protein binding: 55% to 96%

Bioavailability: 90% to 100%

Half-life: Adults: I.V.: 15-23 hours; Oral: 16 hours (range: 11-26 hours)

Time to peak serum concentration:

Capsules and pellet filled capsules: 1-4 hours

Tablet: 1-3 hours

Extended release tablet: 3.5-4 hours

Elimination: 5% to 12% excreted unchanged in urine

Dosing: Usual

Children >8 years and Adolescents:

Usual dosage range: Oral, I.V.: Initial: 4 mg/kg followed by 2 mg/kg/dose every 12 hours; maximum daily dose: 400 mg/**day**

Acne: Adolescents: Oral: 100 mg once daily, in some patients may increase to 150-200 mg/day (Goulden, 2003)

Acne, inflammatory, non-nodular, moderate to severe: Children ≥12 years and Adolescents: Oral (Solodyn®): **Note:** Higher doses do not confer greater efficacy and may be associated with more acute vestibular side effects: ~1 mg/kg/dose once daily for 12 weeks

45-49 kg: 45 mg once daily

50-59 kg: 55 mg once daily

60-71 kg: 65 mg once daily

72-84 kg: 80 mg once daily

85-96 kg: 90 mg once daily

97-110 kg: 105 mg once daily

111-125 kg: 115 mg once daily
126-136 kg: 135 mg once daily

Cellulitis (purulent) infection due to community-acquired MRSA: Oral: Initial: 4 mg/kg; maximum dose: 200 mg; maintenance: 2 mg/kg/dose every 12 hours for 5-10 days; maximum dose: 100 mg (Liu, 2011)

Adults:

General dosing: Oral, I.V.: Initial: 200 mg, followed by 100 mg every 12 hours; more frequent dosing intervals may be used (100-200 mg initially, followed by 50 mg 4 times daily)

Acne: Oral: 50-100 mg once or twice daily (see also Solodyn® dosing)

Asymptomatic meningococcal carrier state: Oral: 100 mg every 12 hours for 5 days; **Note:** CDC recommendations do not mention use of minocycline for eradicating nasopharyngeal carriage of meningococcus.

Chlamydial or _Ureaplasma urealyticum_ infection, uncomplicated (urethral, endocervical, or rectal): Oral, I.V.: 100 mg every 12 hours for at least 7 days

Gonococcal infection, uncomplicated (males): Oral, I.V.: Without urethritis or anorectal infection: Initial: 200 mg, followed by 100 mg every 12 hours for at least 4 days

Gonococcal infection, uncomplicated urethritis: Oral, I.V.: 100 mg every 12 hours for 5 days

Mycobacterium marinum cutaneous infection: Oral: 100 mg every 12 hours for 6-8 weeks (**Note:** Optimal dosing has not been established)

Nocardiosis, cutaneous (non-CNS): Oral: 100-200 mg every 12 hours

Syphilis: Oral, I.V.: Initial: 200 mg, followed by 100 mg every 12 hours for 10-15 days

Dosage adjustment in renal impairment: Consider decreasing dose or extending interval between doses; CrCl <80 mL/minute; maximum dose: 200 mg/day (minocycline serum level may need to be monitored)

Administration
I.V.: Reconstitute vial with 5 mL of SWI and further dilute in NS, D5W, D5NS, Ringer's injection, or LR to a final concentration not to exceed 0.4 mg/mL; infuse slowly; avoid rapid administration; the manufacturer's labeling does not provide a recommended administration rate; other tetracyclines are typically infused over 1-2 hours; the injectable route should be used only if the oral route is not feasible or adequate; prolonged intravenous therapy may be associated with thrombophlebitis

Oral: Administer with adequate fluid to decrease the risk of esophageal irritation and ulceration. Administer with or without food. Swallow pellet-filled capsule and extended release tablet whole; do not chew, crush, or split. Administer antacids, calcium supplements, iron supplements, magnesium-containing laxatives, and cholestyramine 2 hours before or after minocycline.

Monitoring Parameters CBC, serum BUN, creatinine, liver function tests. Observe for changes in bowel frequency.

Test Interactions May cause interference with fluorescence test for urinary catecholamines (false elevations)

Product Availability Ximino™ extended-release capsules: FDA approved July 2012; anticipated availability currently unknown. Consult prescribing information for additional information.

Dosage Forms Excipient information presented when available (limited, particularly for generics); consult specific product labeling.

Capsule, Oral:
Minocin: 50 mg, 75 mg, 100 mg [contains brilliant blue fcf (fd&c blue #1), fd&c yellow #10 (quinoline yellow)]
Generic: 50 mg, 75 mg, 100 mg

Kit, Combination:
Minocin: 50 mg, 100 mg [contains brilliant blue fcf (fd&c blue #1), disodium edta, fd&c yellow #10 (quinoline yellow), sodium benzoate]
Solution Reconstituted, Intravenous:
Minocin: 100 mg (1 ea)
Tablet, Oral:
Generic: 50 mg, 75 mg, 100 mg
Tablet Extended Release 24 Hour, Oral:
Solodyn: 55 mg [contains fd&c red #40]
Solodyn: 65 mg [contains brilliant blue fcf (fd&c blue #1), fd&c blue #2 (indigotine), fd&c yellow #10 (quinoline yellow)]
Solodyn: 80 mg [contains fd&c blue #2 (indigotine), fd&c red #40, fd&c yellow #6 (sunset yellow)]
Solodyn: 105 mg [contains brilliant blue fcf (fd&c blue #1)]
Solodyn: 115 mg [contains brilliant blue fcf (fd&c blue #1), fd&c blue #2 (indigotine), fd&c yellow #10 (quinoline yellow)]
Generic: 45 mg, 90 mg, 135 mg

References

American Academy of Dermatology/American Academy of Dermatology Association, "Guidelines of Care for Acne Vulgaris Management," _J Am Acad Dermatol_, 2007, 56(4):651-63.

Basler RS and Lynch PJ, "Black Galactorrhea as a Consequence of Minocycline and Phenothiazine Therapy," _Arch Dermatol_, 1985, 121 (3):417-8.

Brogden RN, Speight TM, and Avery GS, "Minocycline: A Review of Its Antibacterial and Pharmacokinetic Properties and Therapeutic Use," _Drugs_, 1975, 9(4):251-91.

Garner SE, Eady EA, Popescu C, et al, "Minocycline for Acne Vulgaris: Efficacy and Safety," _Cochrane Database Syst Rev_, 2003, (1): CD002086.

Goulden V, "Guidelines for the Management of Acne Vulgaris in Adolescents," _Paediatr Drugs_, 2003, 5(5):301-13.

Hunt MJ, Salisbury EL, Grace J, et al, "Black Breast Milk Due to Minocycline Therapy," _Br J Dermatol_, 1996, 134(5):943-4.

Liu C, Bayer A, Cosgrove SE, et al, "Clinical Practice Guidelines by the Infectious Diseases Society of America for the Treatment of Methicillin-Resistant _Staphylococcus aureus_ Infections in Adults and Children: Executive Summary," _Clin Infect Dis_, 2011, 52(3):285-92.

Mylonas I, "Antibiotic Chemotherapy During Pregnancy and Lactation Period: Aspects for Consideration," _Arch Gynecol Obstet_, 2011, 283 (1):7-18.

Sanchez AR, Rogers RS 3rd, and Sheridan PJ, "Tetracycline and Other Tetracycline-Derivative Staining of the Teeth and Oral Cavity," _Int J Dermatol_, 2004, 43(10):709-15.

Zhanel GG, Homenuik K, Nichol K, et al, "The Glycylcyclines: A Comparative Review with the Tetracyclines," _Drugs_, 2004, 64 (1):63-88.

Zouboulis CC and Piquero-Martin J, "Update and Future of Systemic Acne Treatment," _Dermatology_, 2003, 206(1):37-53.

◆ **Minocycline Hydrochloride** see Minocycline on page 1420

Minoxidil (Systemic) (mi NOKS i dil)

Medication Safety Issues

Sound-alike/look-alike issues:
Loniten may be confused with Lipitor
Minoxidil may be confused with metolazone, midodrine, Minipress, Minocin, Monopril, Noxafil

International issues:
Noxidil [Thailand] may be confused with Noxafil brand name for posaconazole [U.S. and multiple international markets]

Brand Names: Canada Loniten

Generic Availability (U.S.) Yes

Use Management of severe hypertension

Pregnancy Risk Factor C

Pregnancy Considerations Adverse events were observed in some animal studies.

Breast-Feeding Considerations Excretion in breast milk has been reported in one case report of a woman receiving 10 mg/day orally.

Contraindications Hypersensitivity to minoxidil or any component; pheochromocytoma

Warnings May cause pericardial effusion progressing to tamponade **[U.S. Boxed Warning]**; pericarditis, angina, and sodium and water retention may also occur; use of minoxidil should be reserved for treatment of hypertension in patients who have not adequately responded to maximum doses of a diuretic and two other antihypertensive agents **[U.S. Boxed Warning]**; minoxidil is usually used with a beta-blocker (to treat minoxidil-induced tachycardia) and a diuretic (for treatment of water retention/edema); avoid concomitant use of minoxidil with guanethidine; minoxidil may rapidly control blood pressure; too rapid control of blood pressure may lead to syncope, CVA, MI, or ischemia. Myocardial lesions and other adverse cardiac effects have been shown in experimental animals **[U.S. Boxed Warning]**; significance of these findings in humans is unclear.

Precautions Use with caution in patients with coronary artery disease or with recent MI, pulmonary hypertension, significant renal dysfunction, or heart failure; renal failure or dialysis patients may require dosage reduction. Elongations, thickening, and enhanced pigmentation of fine body hair between eyebrows and hairline, sideburns, cheek, and eventually back, arms, legs, and scalp is seen in ~80% of patients within the first 3-6 weeks; may take 1-6 months for hypertrichosis to reverse itself after discontinuation of the drug.

Adverse Reactions

Cardiovascular: Angina pectoris, ECG changes (T-wave changes), heart failure, peripheral edema, pericardial effusion with/without tamponade, pericarditis, rebound hypertension (in children after a gradual withdrawal), sodium and water retention, tachycardia

Dermatologic: Bullous eruption, hypertrichosis, rash, Stevens-Johnson syndrome

Endocrine & metabolic: Breast tenderness

Gastrointestinal: Nausea, vomiting, weight gain

Hematologic: Leukopenia, thrombocytopenia, transient decreased erythrocyte count (hemodilution), transient decreased hematocrit/hemoglobin (hemodilution)

Hepatic: Alkaline phosphatase increased

Renal: Serum BUN and creatinine increased (transient)

Respiratory: Pulmonary edema

Drug Interactions

Metabolism/Transport Effects None known.

Avoid Concomitant Use There are no known interactions where it is recommended to avoid concomitant use.

Increased Effect/Toxicity

Minoxidil (Systemic) may increase the levels/effects of: Amifostine; Antihypertensives; DULoxetine; Hypotensive Agents; Obinutuzumab; RiTUXimab

The levels/effects of Minoxidil (Systemic) may be increased by: Alfuzosin; Barbiturates; Brimonidine (Topical); CycloSPORINE (Systemic); Diazoxide; Herbs (Hypotensive Properties); MAO Inhibitors; Pentoxifylline; Phosphodiesterase 5 Inhibitors; Prostacyclin Analogues

Decreased Effect

The levels/effects of Minoxidil (Systemic) may be decreased by: Herbs (Hypertensive Properties); Methylphenidate; Yohimbine

Stability Store at controlled room temperature 20°C to 25°C (68°F to 77°F).

Mechanism of Action Produces vasodilation by directly relaxing arteriolar smooth muscle, with little effect on veins; effects may be mediated by cyclic AMP; stimulation of hair growth is secondary to vasodilation, increased cutaneous blood flow and stimulation of resting hair follicles

Pharmacodynamics Hypotensive effects:

Onset of action: Within 30 minutes

Maximum effect: Within 2-8 hours

Duration: Up to 2-5 days

Pharmacokinetics (Adult data unless noted)

Metabolism: 88% primarily via glucuronidation

Protein-binding: None

Bioavailability: 90%

Half-life, adults: 3.5-4.2 hours

Elimination: 12% excreted unchanged in urine

Dialysis: Dialyzable (50% to 100%)

Dosing: Usual Hypertension:

Children <12 years: Initial: 0.1-0.2 mg/kg once daily; maximum dose: 5 mg/day; increase gradually every 3 days; usual dosage: 0.25-1 mg/kg/day in 1-2 divided doses; maximum dose: 50 mg/day

Children >12 years and Adults: Initial: 5 mg once daily, increase gradually every 3 days; usual dose: 10-40 mg/day in 1-2 divided doses; maximum dose: 100 mg/day; **Note:** Usual dosage range for Adolescents ≥18 years and Adults (JNC 7): 2.5-80 mg/day in 1-2 divided doses

Administration May be administered without regard to food

Monitoring Parameters Fluids and electrolytes, body weight, blood pressure

Additional Information May take 1-6 months for hypertrichosis to totally reverse after oral minoxidil therapy is discontinued

Dosage Forms Excipient information presented when available (limited, particularly for generics); consult specific product labeling.

Tablet, Oral:

Generic: 2.5 mg, 10 mg

References

Chobanian AV, Bakris GL, Black HR, et al, "The Seventh Report of the Joint National Committee on Prevention, Detection, Evaluation, and Treatment of High Blood Pressure: The JNC 7 report," *JAMA*, 2003, 289(19):2560-72.

◆ **Mint-Amlodipine (Can)** *see* AmLODIPine *on page 135*

◆ **Mint-Atenolol (Can)** *see* Atenolol *on page 222*

◆ **Mint-Ciprofloxacin (Can)** *see* Ciprofloxacin (Systemic) *on page 471*

◆ **Mint-Citalopram (Can)** *see* Citalopram *on page 484*

◆ **Mint-Fluoxetine (Can)** *see* FLUoxetine *on page 901*

◆ **Mint-Losartan (Can)** *see* Losartan *on page 1283*

◆ **Mint-Metformin (Can)** *see* MetFORMIN *on page 1353*

◆ **Mint-Montelukast (Can)** *see* Montelukast *on page 1438*

◆ **Mint-Ondansetron (Can)** *see* Ondansetron *on page 1544*

◆ **Mint-Pantoprazole (Can)** *see* Pantoprazole *on page 1595*

◆ **Mint-Pravastatin (Can)** *see* Pravastatin *on page 1720*

◆ **Mint-Risperidon (Can)** *see* RisperiDONE *on page 1831*

◆ **Mint-Rosuvastatin (Can)** *see* Rosuvastatin *on page 1853*

◆ **MINT-Sertraline (Can)** *see* Sertraline *on page 1879*

◆ **Mint-Simvastatin (Can)** *see* Simvastatin *on page 1892*

◆ **Mint-Topiramate (Can)** *see* Topiramate *on page 2046*

◆ **Miochol-E** *see* Acetylcholine *on page 59*

◆ **Miochol®-E (Can)** *see* Acetylcholine *on page 59*

◆ **MiraLax [OTC]** *see* Polyethylene Glycol 3350 *on page 1696*

◆ **Miranel AF [OTC]** *see* Miconazole (Topical) *on page 1410*

Misoprostol (mye soe PROST ole)

Medication Safety Issues

Sound-alike/look-alike issues:

Cytotec may be confused with Cytoxan

Misoprostol may be confused with metoprolol, mifepristone

Brand Names: U.S. Cytotec

Brand Names: Canada Novo-Misoprostol; PMS-Misoprostol

Therapeutic Category Gastrointestinal Agent, Gastric Ulcer Treatment; Prostaglandin

Generic Availability (U.S.) Yes

Use Prevention of NSAID-induced gastric ulcers (FDA approved in adults)

Pregnancy Risk Factor X

Pregnancy Considerations Teratogenic effects were not observed in animal reproduction studies. Congenital anomalies following first trimester exposure have been reported, including skull defects, cranial nerve palsies, falcial malformations, and limb defects. Misoprostol may produce uterine contractions; fetal death, uterine perforation, and abortion may occur. **[U.S. Boxed Warning]: Use of misoprostol during pregnancy may cause abortion, birth defects, or premature birth. It is not to be used to reduce NSAID-induced ulcers in a woman of childbearing potential unless she is capable of complying with effective contraceptive measures and is at high risk of developing gastric ulcers and/or their complications.** If needed, the patient must have a negative pregnancy test within 2 weeks of starting therapy, she must use effective contraception during treatment, and therapy should begin on the second or third day of next normal menstrual period. Written and verbal warnings concerning the hazards of misoprostol should be provided.

Misoprostol is FDA approved for the medical termination of pregnancy of ≤49 days in conjunction with mifepristone.

Because misoprostol may induce or augment uterine contractions, it has been used off-label as a cervical-ripening agent for induction of labor in women who have not had a prior cesarean delivery or major uterine surgery. Hyperstimulation of the uterus, uterine rupture, or adverse events in the fetus or mother may occur with this use.

Breast-Feeding Considerations Misoprostol acid (the active metabolite of misoprostol) has been detected in breast milk. Concentrations following a single oral dose were 7.6-20.9 pg/mL after 1 hour and decreased to <1 pg/mL by 5 hours. Adverse events have not been reported in nursing infants (FIGO, 2012).

Contraindications Hypersensitivity to prostaglandins; pregnancy (when used to prevent NSAID-induced ulcers)

Warnings May cause abortion, premature labor, or birth defects if given to pregnant women **[U.S. Boxed Warning]**; not to be used for reducing the risk of NSAID-induced ulcers in pregnant women or women of childbearing potential unless the woman is capable of complying with effective contraceptive measures; women should have a negative serum pregnancy test within 2 weeks prior to initiating therapy with therapy begun on the second or third day of next menstrual period. **Due to the abortifacient property of this medication, patients must be warned not to give this drug to others [U.S. Boxed Warning].**

Precautions Use with caution in patients with inflammatory bowel disease due to potential for development of diarrhea. Use with caution in patients with cardiovascular disease. Use with caution in patients with renal impairment. For use only in patients at high risk of complications from gastric ulcers (eg, the elderly or patients with concomitant diseases) or patients at high risk for developing gastric ulcers (eg, those with a history of ulcers) taking NSAIDs. Misoprostol must be taken during the duration of NSAID therapy. It is not effective in preventing duodenal ulcers in patients taking NSAIDs.

Adverse Reactions

Central nervous system: Headache

Gastrointestinal: Abdominal pain, constipation, diarrhea, dyspepsia, flatulence, nausea, vomiting

Rare but important or life-threatening: Abnormal taste, abnormal vision, alkaline phosphatase increased, alopecia, anaphylaxis, anemia, amylase increase, anxiety, arrhythmia, arterial thrombosis, arthralgia, cardiac enzymes increased, chest pain, chills, confusion, CVA, deafness, depression, diaphoresis, dizziness, drowsiness, dysphagia, dyspnea, dysuria, edema, epistaxis, ESR increased, fatigue, fever, GI bleeding, GI inflammation, gingivitis, glycosuria, gout; gynecological disorders, hematuria, hepatobiliary function abnormal, hyper-/hypotension, impotence, loss of libido, MI, muscle cramps, myalgia, neuropathy, neurosis, nitrogen increased, pallor, phlebitis, polyuria, pulmonary embolism, purpura, rash, reflux, rigors, stiffness, syncope, thirst, thrombocytopenia, tinnitus, uterine rupture, weakness, weight changes

Drug Interactions

Metabolism/Transport Effects None known.

Avoid Concomitant Use

Avoid concomitant use of Misoprostol with any of the following: Carbetocin

Increased Effect/Toxicity

Misoprostol may increase the levels/effects of: Carbetocin; Oxytocin

The levels/effects of Misoprostol may be increased by: Antacids

Decreased Effect There are no known significant interactions involving a decrease in effect.

Food Interactions Misoprostol peak serum concentrations may be decreased if taken with food (not clinically significant).

Mechanism of Action Misoprostol is a synthetic prostaglandin E_1 analog that replaces the protective prostaglandins consumed with prostaglandin-inhibiting therapies (eg, NSAIDs); has been shown to induce uterine contractions

Pharmacodynamics Inhibition of gastric acid secretion:

Onset of action: 30 minutes

Maximum effect: 60-90 minutes

Duration: 3 hours

Pharmacokinetics (Adult data unless noted)

Absorption: Rapid and extensive

Protein binding (misoprostol acid): 80% to 90%

Metabolism: Extensive "first pass" de-esterification to misoprostol acid (active metabolite)

Bioavailability: 88%

Half-life (metabolite): Terminal: 20-40 minutes

Time to peak serum concentration (active metabolite):

Fasting: 14 ± 8 minutes

Elimination: In urine (~80%)

Dosing: Usual Oral: Prevention of NSAID-induced ulcers:

Adults: 200 mcg 4 times/day; if not tolerated, may decrease dose to 100 mcg 4 times/day; take for the duration of NSAID therapy

Dosage adjustment in renal impairment: Half-life, maximum plasma concentration, and bioavailability may be increased; however, a correlation has not been observed with degree of dysfunction. Decrease dose if recommended dose is not tolerated

Administration Oral: Administer after meals and at bedtime

Additional Information Has also been used to improve absorption in cystic fibrosis patients 8-16 years of age at doses of 100 mcg 4 times daily, in conjunction with pancreatic enzyme supplements (limited data available)

Dosage Forms Excipient information presented when available (limited, particularly for generics); consult specific product labeling.

Tablet, Oral:

Cytotec: 100 mcg

Cytotec: 200 mcg [scored]

Generic: 100 mcg, 200 mcg

References

Cleghorn GJ, Shepherd RW, and Holt TL, "The Use of a Synthetic Prostaglandin E1 Analogue (Misoprostol) as an Adjunct to Pancreatic Enzyme Replacement in Cystic Fibrosis," *Scand J Gastroenterol Suppl*, 1988, 143:142-7.

International Federation of Gynecology and Obstetrics (FIGO), "Prevention of Postpartum Hemorrhage With Misoprostol," *Int J Gynaecol Obstet*," 2012, 119(3):213-4.

International Federation of Gynecology and Obstetrics (FIGO), "Treatment of Postpartum Hemorrhage With Misoprostol," *Int J Gynaecol Obstet*, 2012, 119(3):215-6.

Robinson PJ, Smith AL, and Sly PD, "Duodenal pH in Cystic Fibrosis and Its Relationship to Fat Malabsorption," *Dig Dis Sci*, 1990, 35 (10):1299-304.

Mitotane (MYE toe tane)

Medication Safety Issues

Sound-alike/look-alike issues:

Mitotane may be confused with mitoMYcin, mitoXANtrone

High alert medication:

This medication is in a class the Institute for Safe Medication Practices (ISMP) includes among its list of drug classes which have a heightened risk of causing significant patient harm when used in error.

Related Information

Emetogenic Potential of Antineoplastic Agents in Children *on page 2327*

Oral Medications That Should Not Be Crushed or Altered *on page 2438*

Safe Handling of Hazardous Drugs *on page 2419*

Brand Names: U.S. Lysodren

Brand Names: Canada Lysodren

Therapeutic Category Antineoplastic Agent, Miscellaneous

Generic Availability (U.S.) No

Use Treatment of inoperable adrenocortical carcinoma (both functional and nonfunctional types) (FDA approved in adults)

Pregnancy Risk Factor D

Pregnancy Considerations Animal reproduction studies have not been conducted. May cause fetal harm if administered during pregnancy; adverse outcomes have been reported. Women of reproductive potential should use effective contraception during treatment and after treatment until plasma levels are no longer detected.

Breast-Feeding Considerations Mitotane has been detected in human breast milk. Due to the potential for serious adverse reactions in the nursing infant, breast-feeding should be discontinued until plasma levels are no longer detected.

Contraindications Hypersensitivity to mitotane or any component

Warnings Use appropriate precautions for handling and disposal (NIOSH, 2012). Because the primary action of mitotane is through adrenal suppression, discontinue mitotane temporarily with onset of shock or severe trauma; administer appropriate corticosteroid coverage **[U.S. Boxed Warning]**. Patients treated with mitotane may develop adrenal insufficiency; corticosteroid replacement with glucocorticoid and sometimes mineralocorticoid therapy is necessary. It has been recommended that replacement therapy be initiated at the start of therapy, rather than waiting for evidence of adrenal insufficiency. Mitotane can increase the metabolism of exogenous corticosteroids; higher than usual replacement steroid doses may be required. Mitotane increases hormone binding proteins; monitor free cortisol and corticotropin levels for optimal replacement.

Neurotoxicity has been reported with use; long-term use (>2 years) may lead to brain damage or functional impairment; observe patients for neurotoxicity (behavioral and neurological) at regular intervals; plasma concentrations >20 mcg/mL in adults are associated with an increased incidence of higher-grade neurotoxicity; neurologic impairment may reverse upon discontinuation. Growth, motor skill, and speech delays were observed during therapy in an infant treated for adenocarcinoma (DeLeon, 2002). CNS adverse effects, including lethargy, sedation, and vertigo may occur; patients must be cautioned about performing tasks which require mental alertness (eg, operating machinery or driving); concomitant use with other sedative drugs or ethanol may cause additive CNS effects; avoid use.

Precautions Use with caution in patients with hepatic impairment (other than metastatic lesions from adrenal cortex); metabolism may be decreased. Surgically remove tumor tissues from metastatic masses prior to initiation of treatment; rapid cytotoxic effect may cause tumor hemorrhage. Prolonged bleeding time may occur; consider bleeding possibility prior to any surgical intervention. Mitotane is a strong inducer of CYP3A4; potentially significant interactions may exist, requiring dose or frequency adjustment, additional monitoring, and/or selection of alternative therapy. Consult drug interactions database for more detailed information.

Mitotane is associated with a moderate emetic potential; antiemetics may be needed to prevent nausea and vomiting. The manufacturer recommends initiating treatment for adenocarcinoma within a hospital environment until a stabilized dose is achieved; continue treatment as long as clinical benefit (clinical status maintenance or slowed growth of metastatic lesion) is observed. In adults, clinical benefit is usually observed within 3 months at maximum tolerated dose, although 10% of patients may require more than 3 months for benefit; continuous treatment at the maximum tolerated dose is generally the best approach. Some adults have been treated for adenocarcinoma intermittently, restarting when severe symptoms reappear, although often response is no longer observed after 3 or 4 courses of intermittent treatment. Mitotane should be administered under the supervision of an experienced cancer chemotherapy physician **[U.S. Boxed Warning]**.

Adverse Reactions The majority of adverse events are dose-dependent.

Central nervous system: Central nervous system depression, confusion, dizziness, drowsiness, headache, lethargy, vertigo

Dermatologic: Skin rash

Gastrointestinal: Anorexia, diarrhea, nausea, vomiting

Neuromuscular & skeletal: Tremor, weakness

Rare but important or life-threatening: Abnormal thyroid function test, adrenocortical insufficiency, albuminuria, anemia, autoimmune hepatitis, blurred vision, brain damage (may be reversible), cataract, decreased protein-bound iodine, diplopia, generalized aches, growth suppression, gynecomastia, hematuria, hemorrhagic cystitis, hepatitis, hypercholesterolemia, hyperpyrexia, hypertension, hypertriglyceridemia, hypogonadism (primary), hypouricemia, increased gamma-glutamyl transferase, increased liver enzymes, increased serum transaminases, increased serum triglycerides, increased sex hormone binding globulin, leukopenia, macular edema, maculopathy, memory impairment, mental deficiency, mucositis, myalgia, neuropathy, neutropenia, orthostatic hypotension, prolonged bleeding time, psychological disturbances (neuro), retinopathy (toxic), thrombocytopenia

Drug Interactions

Metabolism/Transport Effects Induces CYP3A4 (strong)

Avoid Concomitant Use

Avoid concomitant use of Mitotane with any of the following: Abiraterone Acetate; Apixaban; Apremilast; Artemether; Axitinib; Bedaquiline; Boceprevir; Bortezomib; ▶

◄ Bosutinib; Cabozantinib; Ceritinib; CloZAPine; Crizotinib; Dienogest; Dronedarone; Enzalutamide; Everolimus; Ibrutinib; Itraconazole; Ivacaftor; Lapatinib; Lumefantrine; Lurasidone; Macitentan; Mifepristone; NIFEdipine; Niloti- nib; Nisoldipine; PAZOPanib; Perampanel; PONATinib; Praziquantel; Ranolazine; Regorafenib; Rivaroxaban; Roflumilast; RomiDEPsin; Simeprevir; SORAfenib; Tasi- melteon; Telaprevir; Ticagrelor; Tofacitinib; Tolvaptan; Toremifene; Ulipristal; Vandetanib; Vemurafenib; Vin- CRIStine (Liposomal); Vorapaxar

Increased Effect/Toxicity CNS depressants taken with mitotane may enhance CNS depression.

Decreased Effect Mitotane may enhance the clearance of barbiturates and warfarin by induction of the hepatic microsomal enzyme system resulting in a decreased effect. Coadministration of spironolactone has resulted in negation of mitotane's effect. Mitotane may increase clearance of phenytoin by microsomal enzyme stimula- tion.

Stability Store at 25°C (77°F); excursions permitted to 15°C to 30°C (59°F to 86°F).

Mechanism of Action Adrenolytic agent which causes adrenal cortical atrophy; affects mitochondria in adrenal cortical cells and decreases production of cortisol; also alters the peripheral metabolism of steroids

Pharmacodynamics Onset of action: Antitumor response: Achieved at serum concentrations ≥14 mcg/mL; Pediatric patients: In experience with treatment of adeno- carcinoma reported 1.5-12.5 months to reach 10 mcg/mL with subsequent rapid escalation of serum concentration, clinical response may be observed earlier (Rodriguez- Galindo, 2005; Zancanella, 2006); Adults: Typically within 3 months

Pharmacokinetics (Adult data unless noted)
Absorption: Oral: ~40%
Distribution: Stored mainly in fat tissue but is found in all body tissues
Metabolism: Hepatic and other tissues
Half-life, elimination: 18-159 days; serum concentrations undetectable after 6-9 weeks in majority of patients
Time to peak serum concentration: 3-5 hours
Elimination: Urine (~10%, as metabolites); feces (1% to 17%, as metabolites)

Dosing: Usual
Pediatric: **Adrenocortical carcinoma (stage III or IV):** Limited data available: Children and Adolescents: Oral: Initial: 0.5-1 g/day in 3 divided doses, titrate dose to target serum concentration range of 14-20 mcg/mL; initially, monitor serum concentrations every 2-4 weeks until serum concentration of 10 mcg/mL is achieved, then monitor every 1-2 weeks due to rapid drug accumulation and narrow therapeutic window; once target serum con- centration (14-20 mcg/mL) is reached, continue to mon- itor every 1-2 weeks and adjust dose to maintain therapeutic range (dosage reduction may be necessary in some cases); has also been used in combination with CED regimen (cisplatin, etoposide, and doxorubicin). An initial target daily dose of 4 g/m²/day was used in an open-label, prospective study (n=11; age range: 2-15 years); however, the reported range to initially achieve a serum concentration of 14 ± 2 mcg/mL was 1.6-7.3 g/ m²/day; and then further reductions to 1-5.3 g/m²/day were required to maintain therapeutic concentrations (Zancanella, 2006). In an ongoing trial at some centers, a similar target dose of 4 g/m²/day is being evaluated using a titration schedule: Initial dose: 1-2 g/m²/day in 4 divided doses with weekly titration in 1-2 g/m²/day incre- ments; maximum daily dose: 4 g/m²/day (NCT00304070, 2014); **Note:** In general, optimal treatment for pediatric adrenocortical carcinoma is unknown; further studies are needed.

Adult: **Adrenocortical carcinoma:** Oral:
Manufacturer's labeling: Initial: 2-6 g daily in 3-4 divided doses, then increase incrementally to 9-10 g daily in 3-4 divided doses (maximum tolerated range: 2-16 g daily, usually 9-10 g daily; maximum dose studied: 18-19 g daily); continue as long as clinical benefit is demon- strated
Alternate dosing: Limited data available: Initial: 1-2 g daily; increase by 1-2 g daily at 1-2 week intervals as tolerated to a maximum of 6-10 g daily; usual dose 4-5 g daily (Veytsman, 2009)

Dosing adjustment for toxicity: Adult:
Severe side effects: Reduce dose until a maximum tolerated dose is achieved
Significant neuropsychiatric adverse effects: Withhold treatment for at least 1 week and restart at a lower dose (Allolio, 2006)

Dosing adjustment in renal impairment: Adult: There are no dosage adjustments provided in manufacturer's labeling.

Dosing adjustment in hepatic impairment: Adult: There are no dosage adjustments provided in manufacturer's labeling; however, drug accumulation may occur in patients with liver disease; use with caution.

Administration Hazardous agent; use appropriate precau- tions for handling and disposal (NIOSH, 2012). Wear impervious gloves when handling; avoid exposure to crushed or broken tablets if possible.

Oral: In pediatric trials, tablets have been crushed and dissolved in MCT (medium-chain triglyceride) oil (ie, each gram mitotane in 2 mL MCT oil); then solution was mixed with a fat-containing food [eg, milk (white or chocolate) or yogurt] (Zancanella, 2006)

Monitoring Parameters
Adrenal function; neurologic assessments (including behavioral) at regular intervals with chronic (>2 years) use.
Pediatric: Monitor mitotane serum concentrations initially every 2-4 weeks until serum concentration of 10 mcg/mL is achieved, then monitor every 1-2 weeks (even after target concentration of 14-20 mcg/mL is reached) and use conservative dose adjustments due to drug accumu- lation and narrow therapeutic window (Zancanella, 2006)
Adult: Monitor mitotane serum concentrations (gas chro- matography-flame ionization assay) every 4-8 weeks until levels at 10-14 mg/L are attained, then monitor every 3 months; urinary free cortisol levels; TSH and free thyroxine every few months (Veytsman, 2009)

Dosage Forms Excipient information presented when available (limited, particularly for generics); consult specific product labeling.
Tablet, Oral:
Lysodren: 500 mg [scored]

References
Allolio B and Fassnacht M, "Clinical Review: Adrenocortical Carcinoma: Clinical Update," *J Clin Endocrinol Metab*, 2006, 91(6):2027-37.
De Leon DD, Lange BJ, Walterhouse D, et al, "Long-Term (15 years) Outcome in an Infant with Metastatic Adrenocortical Carcinoma," *J Clin Endocrinol Metab*, 2002, 87(10):4452-6.
National Institute for Occupational Safety and Health (NIOSH), "NIOSH List of Antineoplastic and Other Hazardous Drugs in Healthcare Settings 2012." Available at http://www.cdc.gov/niosh/docs/ 2012-150/pdfs/2012-150.pdf. Accessed January 21, 2013.
NCT0030470. Cisplatin-based chemotherapy and/or surgery in treating young patients with adrenocortical tumor. Unpublished data. Available at http://clinicaltrials.gov/ct2/show/NCT00304070?term=NC- T00304070&rank=1. Date accessed: March 20, 2014.
Ribeiro RC, Pinto EM, Zambetti GP, et al. The International Pediatric Adrenocortical Tumor Registry initiative: contributions to clinical, bio- logical, and treatment advances in pediatric adrenocortical tumors. *Mol Cell Endocrinol*. 2012;351(1):37-43.
Rodriguez-Galindo C, Figueiredo BC, Zambetti GP, et al, "Biology, Clinical Characteristics, and Management of Adrenocortical Tumors in Children," *Pediatr Blood Cancer*, 2005, 45(3):265-73.

Veytsman I, Nieman L, and Fojo T. Management of endocrine manifestations and the use of mitotane as a chemotherapeutic agent for adrenocortical carcinoma. *J Clin Oncol.* 2009;27(27):4619-4629.

Zancanella P, Pianovski MA, Oliveira BH, et al. Mitotane associated with cisplatin, etoposide, and doxorubicin in advanced childhood adrenocortical carcinoma: mitotane monitoring and tumor regression. *J Pediatr Hematol Oncol.* 2006; 28(8):513-524.

MitoXANtrone (mye toe ZAN trone)

Medication Safety Issues

Sound-alike/look-alike issues:

MitoXANtrone may be confused with methotrexate, mito-MYcin, mitotane, Mutamycin®

High alert medication:

This medication is in a class the Institute for Safe Medication Practices (ISMP) includes among its list of drug classes which have a heightened risk of causing significant patient harm when used in error.

Related Information

Emetogenic Potential of Antineoplastic Agents in Children *on page 2327*

Management of Drug Extravasations *on page 2255*

Safe Handling of Hazardous Drugs *on page 2419*

Brand Names: Canada Mitoxantrone Injection®

Therapeutic Category Antineoplastic Agent, Anthracenedione; Antineoplastic Agent, Antibiotic; Antineoplastic Agent, Topoisomerase II Inhibitor

Generic Availability (U.S.) Yes

Use Treatment of acute nonlymphocytic leukemias (ANLL; includes myelogenous, promyelocytic, monocytic, and erythroid leukemias); advanced hormone-refractory prostate cancer, secondary progressive, or relapsing-remitting multiple sclerosis (MS) (FDA approved in adults); has also been used for Hodgkin's lymphoma, non-Hodgkin's lymphomas (NHL), acute lymphocytic leukemia (ALL), myelodysplastic syndrome, breast cancer, pediatric acute myelogenous leukemia (AML), pediatric acute promyelocytic leukemia (APL); part of a conditioning regimen for autologous hematopoietic stem-cell transplantation (HSCT)

Medication Guide Available Yes

Pregnancy Risk Factor D

Pregnancy Considerations Adverse effects were noted in animal reproduction studies. May cause fetal harm if administered to a pregnant woman. Pregnancy should be avoided while on treatment. Women with multiple sclerosis who are of reproductive potential should have a pregnancy test prior to each dose.

Breast-Feeding Considerations Mitoxantrone is excreted in human milk and significant concentrations (18 ng/mL) have been reported for 28 days after the last administration. Because of the potential for serious adverse reactions in infants from mitoxantrone, breast-feeding should be discontinued before starting treatment.

Contraindications Hypersensitivity to mitoxantrone or any component

Warnings Hazardous agent; use appropriate precautions for handling and disposal (NIOSH, 2012). Mitoxantrone can cause severe myelosuppression; use is generally not recommended in patients with preexisting myelosuppression from prior chemotherapy unless the expected benefit outweighs the risk; do not use if baseline neutrophil count is <1500 cells/mm^3 (except for its use in the treatment of ANLL); monitor blood counts and monitor for infection due to neutropenia **[U.S. Boxed Warning]**. May cause myocardial toxicity and potentially-fatal heart failure (HF); risk increases with cumulative dosing. Effects may occur during therapy or may be delayed (months or years after completion of therapy). Predisposing factors for mitoxantrone-induced cardiotoxicity include prior anthracycline or anthracenedione therapy, prior cardiovascular disease, concomitant use of cardiotoxic drugs, and mediastinal/pericardial irradiation, although may also occur in patients without risk factors. Prior to therapy initiation, evaluate all patients for cardiac-related signs/symptoms, including history, physical exam, and ECG; and evaluate baseline left ventricular ejection fraction (LVEF) with echocardiogram or multigated radionuclide angiography (MUGA) or MRI. Not recommended for use in MS patients when LVEF <50%, or baseline LVEF below the lower limit of normal (LLN). Evaluate for cardiac signs/symptoms (by history, physical exam, and ECG) and evaluate LVEF (using same method as baseline LVEF) in MS patients prior to each dose and if signs/symptoms of HF develop. Use in MS should be limited to a cumulative dose ≤140 mg/m^2, and discontinued if LVEF falls below LLN or a significant decrease in LVEF is observed; decreases in LVEF and HF have been observed in patients with MS who have received cumulative doses <100 mg/m^2. Patients with MS should undergo annual LVEF evaluation following discontinuation of therapy to monitor for delayed cardiotoxicity **[U.S. Boxed Warning]**. For I.V. administration only, into a free-flowing I.V.; may cause severe local tissue damage if extravasation occurs **[U.S. Boxed Warning]**; extravasation resulting in burning, erythema, pain, swelling, and skin discoloration (blue) has been reported; extravasation may result in tissue necrosis and requires debridement for skin graft. Do not administer SubQ, I.M., or intra-arterial injections (have resulted in local/regional neuropathy); do not administer intrathecally; may cause serious and permanent neurologic damage **[U.S. Boxed Warning]**, including local nerve demyelination, seizures, coma, and paraplegia. Hazardous agent; use appropriate precautions for handling and disposal. Secondary acute myelogenous leukemia has been reported in patients treated with mitoxantrone (in both patients with cancer and with MS) **[U.S. Boxed Warning]**; acute promyelocytic leukemia (APL) has also been observed; symptoms of acute leukemia include excessive bruising, bleeding, and recurrent infections; the risk for secondary leukemia is increased in patients who are heavily pretreated, with higher doses, and with combination chemotherapy; monitor CBC, platelet count; signs and symptoms of infection prior to each course and after discontinuation of mitoxantrone; occurrence of secondary leukemia is more common when anthracyclines are given in combination with DNA-damaging agents, when patients have been heavily pretreated with cytotoxic drugs, or when anthracycline doses have been escalated. Rapid lysis of tumor cells may lead to hyperuricemia.

Precautions Dosage should be reduced in patients with preexisting bone marrow suppression, previous treatment with cardiotoxic agents, and patients with impaired hepatobiliary function. May cause urine, saliva, tears, and sweat to turn blue-green for 24 hours postinfusion; whites of eyes may have blue-green tinge. Should be administered under the supervision of a physician experienced in cancer chemotherapy agents **[U.S. Boxed Warning]**.

Adverse Reactions

Cardiovascular: Arrhythmia, cardiac function changes, CHF, ECG changes, edema, hypertension, ischemia, LVEF decreased

Central nervous system: Anxiety, chills, depression, fatigue, fever, headache, pain, seizure

Dermatologic: Alopecia, cutaneous mycosis, nail bed changes, petechiae/bruising, skin infection

Endocrine & metabolic: Amenorrhea, hypocalcemia, hyperglycemia, hypokalemia, hyponatremia, menorrhagia, menstrual disorder

Gastrointestinal: Abdominal pain, anorexia, aphthosis, constipation, diarrhea, dyspepsia, GI bleeding, mucositis, nausea, stomatitis, vomiting, weight gain/loss

Genitourinary: Abnormal urine, impotence, sterility, urinary tract infection

Hematologic: Anemia, granulocytopenia, hemoglobin decreased, hemorrhage, leukopenia, lymphopenia, neutropenia, neutropenic fever, secondary acute leukemias (includes AML, APL), thrombocytopenia

Hepatic: Alkaline phosphatase increased, GGT increased, jaundice, transaminases increased

Neuromuscular & skeletal: Arthralgia, back pain, myalgia, weakness

Ocular: Blurred vision, conjunctivitis

Renal: BUN increased, creatinine increased, hematuria, proteinuria, renal failure

Respiratory: Cough, dyspnea, pharyngitis, pneumonia, rhinitis, sinusitis, upper respiratory tract infection

Miscellaneous: Diaphoresis, fungal infection, infection, sepsis (ANLL), systemic infection

Rare but important or life-threatening: Allergic reaction, anaphylactoid reactions, anaphylaxis, chest pain, dehydration; extravasation at injection site (may result in burning, erythema, pain, skin discoloration, swelling, or tissue necrosis); interstitial pneumonitis (with combination chemotherapy), hyperuricemia, hypotension, phlebitis at the infusion site, rash, sclera discoloration (blue), tachycardia, urine discoloration (blue-green), urticaria

Drug Interactions

Metabolism/Transport Effects Inhibits CYP3A4 (weak)

Avoid Concomitant Use

Avoid concomitant use of MitoXANtrone with any of the following: BCG; CloZAPine; Dipyrone; Natalizumab; Pimecrolimus; Pimozide; Tacrolimus (Topical); Tofacitinib; Vaccines (Live)

Increased Effect/Toxicity

MitoXANtrone may increase the levels/effects of: ARIPiprazole; CloZAPine; Dofetilide; Leflunomide; Lomitapide; Natalizumab; Pimozide; Tofacitinib; Vaccines (Live)

The levels/effects of MitoXANtrone may be increased by: CycloSPORINE (Systemic); Denosumab; Dipyrone; Pimecrolimus; Roflumilast; Tacrolimus (Topical); Trastuzumab

Decreased Effect

MitoXANtrone may decrease the levels/effects of: BCG; Coccidioidin Skin Test; Sipuleucel-T; Vaccines (Inactivated); Vaccines (Live)

The levels/effects of MitoXANtrone may be decreased by: Echinacea

Stability Hazardous agent; use appropriate precautions for handling and disposal (NIOSH, 2012). Store intact vials at 15°C to 25°C (59°F to 77°F); do not freeze. Opened vials may be stored for 7 days at room temperature or 14 days when refrigerated; solutions diluted for administration are stable for 7 days at room temperature or under refrigeration, although the manufacturer recommends immediate use.

Mechanism of Action Related to the anthracyclines, mitoxantrone intercalates into DNA resulting in cross-links and strand breaks; binds to nucleic acids and inhibits DNA and RNA synthesis by template disordering and steric obstruction; replication is decreased by binding to DNA topoisomerase II and seems to inhibit the incorporation of uridine into RNA and thymidine into DNA; active throughout entire cell cycle (cell-cycle nonspecific)

Pharmacokinetics (Adult data unless noted)

Distribution: Distributes into thyroid, liver, pancreas, spleen, heart, bone marrow, and red blood cells; prolonged retention in tissues; excreted in breast milk
V_{dss}: >1000 L/m²

Protein binding: 78%

Half-life, terminal: 23-215 hours (median: 75 hours); may be prolonged with liver impairment

Elimination: 11% of dose excreted in urine (65% as unchanged drug) and 25% in bile as unchanged drug and metabolites

Dosing: Usual I.V. (refer to individual protocols):

Infants, Children, and Adolescents: Limited data available; further studies are needed.

Acute lymphocytic leukemia (ALL), relapsed: Children and Adolescents: Induction: 10 mg/m²/dose once daily for 2 days (in combination with other chemotherapeutic agents) (Parker, 2010)

Acute nonlymphocytic leukemias (ANLL):

AML:

Induction:

Infants <1 year:

Weight-based dosing: 0.4 mg/**kg**/dose over 1 hour once daily on days 3-6 for a total of 4 doses (in combination with cytarabine and gemtuzumab) (Aplenc, 2008)

BSA-based dosing: 9 mg/m²/dose once daily on days 1, 3, and 5 (in combination with cytarabine and etoposide) (Gibson, 2011) **or** 8 mg/m²/dose once daily for 5 days (in combination with cytarabine) (Perel, 2002)

Children <3 years:

Weight-based dosing: 0.4 mg/**kg**/dose over 1 hour once daily on days 3-6 for a total of 4 doses (in combination with cytarabine and gemtuzumab) (Aplenc, 2008)

BSA-based dosing: 12 mg/m²/dose once daily for 4-5 days (in combination with cytarabine); for incomplete response, may repeat at 12 mg/m²/dose once daily for 2 days (in combination with cytarabine) (Perel, 2002; Wells, 2003) **or** 12 mg/m²/dose once daily on days 1, 3, and 5 (in combination with cytarabine and etoposide) (Gibson, 2011)

Children ≥3 years and Adolescents: 12 mg/m²/dose once daily for 4-5 days (in combination with cytarabine); for incomplete response, may repeat at 12 mg/m²/dose once daily for 2 days (in combination with cytarabine) (Perel, 2002; Wells, 2003) **or** 12 mg/m²/dose once daily on days 1, 3, and 5 (in combination with cytarabine and etoposide) (Gibson, 2011) **or** 12 mg/m²/dose over 1 hour once daily on days 3-6 for a total of 4 doses (in combination with cytarabine and gemtuzumab) (Aplenc, 2008)

Consolidation:

Age-directed dosing (Gibson, 2011; Stevens, 1998): Infants <1 year: 7.5 mg/m²/dose once daily for 5 days

Children and Adolescents 1-14 years: 10 mg/m²/dose once daily for 5 days

BSA-directed dosing (Cooper, 2012):

BSA <0.6 m²: 0.4 mg/**kg**/dose once daily on days 3-6 (in combination with cytarabine and gemtuzumab)

BSA ≥0.6 m²: 12 mg/m²/dose once daily on days 3-6 (in combination with cytarabine and gemtuzumab)

APL: Consolidation: Children ≥2 years and Adolescents: 10 mg/m²/dose once daily for 5 days (Ortega, 2005; Sanz, 2004)

Adults:

Acute nonlymphocytic leukemias (ANLL):

AML induction: 12 mg/m²/dose once daily for 3 days (in combination with cytarabine); for incomplete response, may repeat 7-10 days later at 12 mg/m²/dose once daily for 2 days (Arlin, 1990)

AML consolidation (beginning ~6 weeks after initiation of the final induction course): 12 mg/m²/dose once daily for 2 days (in combination with cytarabine), repeat in 4 weeks (Arlin, 1990)

Multiple sclerosis: 12 mg/m²/dose every 3 months; maximum lifetime cumulative dose: 140 mg/m² (discontinue use with LVEF <50% or clinically significant reduction in LVEF)

Prostate cancer (advanced hormone-refractory): 12-14 mg/m²/dose every 3 weeks (in combination with corticosteroids)

Dosing adjustment in hepatic impairment: No dosage adjustment provided in the manufacturer's labeling. Dosage reduction of 50% in patients with serum bilirubin of 1.5-3 mg/dL and dosage reduction of 75% in patients with serum bilirubin >3 mg/dL have been recommended; **Note:** MS patients with hepatic impairment should not receive mitoxantrone.

Dosing adjustment for toxicity:

ANLL patients: Severe or life-threatening nonhematologic toxicity: Withhold treatment until toxicity resolves

MS Patients:

Neutrophils <1500/mm³: Use is not recommended

Signs/symptoms of HF: Evaluate for cardiac signs/symptoms and LVEF

LVEF <50% or baseline LVEF below the lower limit of normal (LLN): Use is not recommended

Administration Hazardous agent; use appropriate precautions for handling and disposal (NIOSH, 2012).

Parenteral: For I.V. administration only; do not administer by SubQ, I.M., intrathecal, or intra-arterial injection. Must be diluted prior to use; may administer by I.V. bolus over 5-15 minutes or I.V. intermittent infusion over 15-60 minutes. Avoid extravasation; may cause severe local tissue damage if extravasation occurs; pH: 3-4.5

Vesicant/Extravasation Risk Irritant with vesicant-like properties

Monitoring Parameters CBC with differential, platelet count, serum uric acid (for leukemia treatment), liver function tests, women with multiple sclerosis of childbearing potential must have a pregnancy test prior to each dose; injection site for signs of extravasation

Cardiac monitoring: Prior to initiation, evaluate all patients for cardiac-related signs/symptoms, including history, physical exam, and echocardiogram; evaluate baseline and periodic left ventricular ejection fraction (LVEF) with ECG or multigated radionuclide angiography (MUGA) or MRI. In patients with MS, evaluate for cardiac signs/symptoms (by history, physical exam, and ECG) and evaluate LVEF (using same method as baseline LVEF) prior to each dose and if signs/symptoms of HF develop. Patients with MS should undergo annual LVEF evaluation following discontinuation of therapy to monitor for delayed cardiotoxicity.

Additional Information Myelosuppression (leukocyte nadir: 10-14 days; recovery: 21 days); injection contains 0.14 mEq of sodium/mL

Dosage Forms Excipient information presented when available (limited, particularly for generics); consult specific product labeling.

Concentrate, Intravenous:

Generic: 20 mg/10 mL (10 mL); 25 mg/12.5 mL (12.5 mL); 30 mg/15 mL (15 mL)

References

Aplenc R, Alonzo TA, Gerbing RB, et al, "Safety and Efficacy of Gemtuzumab Ozogamicin in Combination With Chemotherapy for Pediatric Acute Myeloid Leukemia: A Report From the Children's Oncology Group," *J Clin Oncol*, 2008, 26(14):2390-3295.

Arlin Z, Case DC Jr, Moore J, et al, "Randomized Multicenter Trial of Cytosine Arabinoside With Mitoxantrone or Daunorubicin in Previously Untreated Adult Patients With Acute Nonlymphocytic Leukemia (ANLL). Lederle Cooperative Group," *Leukemia*, 1990, 4(3):177-83.

Cooper TM, Franklin J, Gerbing RB, et al, "AAML03P1, a Pilot Study of the Safety of Gemtuzumab Ozogamicin in Combination With Chemotherapy for Newly Diagnosed Childhood Acute Myeloid Leukemia: A Report From the Children's Oncology Group," *Cancer*, 2012, 118 (3):761-9.

Gibson BE, Webb DK, Howman AJ, et al, "Results of a Randomized Trial in Children With Acute Myeloid Leukaemia: Medical Research Council AML12 Trial," *Br J Haematol*, 2011, 155(3):366-76.

Koeller J and Eble M, "Mitoxantrone: A Novel Anthracycline Derivative," *Clin Pharm*, 1988, 7(8):574-81.

National Institute for Occupational Safety and Health (NIOSH), "NIOSH List of Antineoplastic and Other Hazardous Drugs in Healthcare Settings 2012." Available at http://www.cdc.gov/niosh/docs/2012-150/pdfs/2012-150.pdf. Accessed January 21, 2013.

Ortega JJ, Madero L, Martín G, et al, "Treatment With All-trans Retinoic Acid and Anthracycline Monochemotherapy for Children With Acute promyelocytic Leukemia: A Multicenter Study by the PETHEMA Group," *J Clin Oncol*, 2005, 23(30):7632-40.

Parker C, Waters R, Leighton C, et al, "Effect of Mitoxantrone on Outcome of Children With First Relapse of Acute Lymphoblastic Leukaemia (ALL R3): An Open-Label Randomised Trial," *Lancet*, 2010, 376(9757):2009-17.

Perel Y, Auvrignon A, Leblanc T, et al, "Impact of Addition of Maintenance Therapy to Intensive Induction and Consolidation Chemotherapy for Childhood Acute Myeloid Leukemia: Results of a Prospective Randomized Trial, LAME 89/91. Leucámie Aiğüe Myéloïde Enfant," *J Clin Oncol*, 2002, 20(12):2774-82.

Pratt CB, Vietti TJ, Etcubanas E, et al, "Novantrone® for Childhood Malignant Solid Tumors. A Pediatric Oncology Group Phase II Study," *Invest New Drugs*, 1986, 4(1):43-8.

Sanz MA, Martín G, González M, et al, "Risk-Adapted Treatment of Acute Promyelocytic Leukemia With All-trans-retinoic Acid and Anthracycline Monochemotherapy: A Multicenter Study by the PETHEMA Group," *Blood*, 2004, 103(4):1237-43.

Stevens RF, Hann IM, Wheatley K, et al, "Marked Improvements in Outcome With Chemotherapy Alone in Paediatric Acute Myeloid Leukemia: Results of the United Kingdom Medical Research Council's 10th AML Trial. MRC Childhood Leukaemia Working Party," *Br J Haematol*, 1998, 101(1):130-40.

Wells RJ, Adams MT, Alonzo TA, et al, "Mitoxantrone and Cytarabine Induction, High-Dose Cytarabine, and Etoposide Intensification for Pediatric Patients With Relapsed or Refractory Acute Myeloid Leukemia: Children's Cancer Group Study 2951," *J Clin Oncol*, 2003, 21 (15):2940-7.

◆ **Mitoxantrone Dihydrochloride** *see* MitoXANtrone *on page 1427*

◆ **Mitoxantrone HCl** *see* MitoXANtrone *on page 1427*

◆ **Mitoxantrone Hydrochloride** *see* MitoXANtrone *on page 1427*

◆ **Mitoxantrone Injection® (Can)** *see* MitoXANtrone *on page 1427*

◆ **Mitozantrone** *see* MitoXANtrone *on page 1427*

◆ **Mitrazol [OTC]** *see* Miconazole (Topical) *on page 1410*

◆ **MK462** *see* Rizatriptan *on page 1845*

◆ **MK 0517** *see* Fosaprepitant *on page 934*

◆ **MK-0518** *see* Raltegravir *on page 1802*

◆ **MK594** *see* Losartan *on page 1283*

◆ **MK0826** *see* Ertapenem *on page 778*

◆ **MK 869** *see* Aprepitant *on page 190*

◆ **MMF** *see* Mycophenolate *on page 1453*

◆ **MMR** *see* Measles, Mumps, and Rubella Virus Vaccine *on page 1307*

◆ **M-M-R II** *see* Measles, Mumps, and Rubella Virus Vaccine *on page 1307*

◆ **MMRV** *see* Measles, Mumps, Rubella, and Varicella Virus Vaccine *on page 1310*

◆ **Mobic** *see* Meloxicam *on page 1325*

◆ **Mobicox (Can)** *see* Meloxicam *on page 1325*

Modafinil (moe DAF i nil)

Brand Names: U.S. Provigil

Brand Names: Canada Alertec®

Therapeutic Category Central Nervous System Stimulant

Generic Availability (U.S.) Yes

Use To improve wakefulness in patients with excessive daytime sleepiness associated with narcolepsy and shift work sleep disorder (SWSD), as adjunctive therapy for obstructive sleep apnea/hypopnea syndrome (OSAHS) (FDA approved in adults); has also been used for attention-deficit/hyperactivity disorder (ADHD); treatment of fatigue in multiple sclerosis (MS) and other disorders

Medication Guide Available Yes

Pregnancy Risk Factor C

Pregnancy Considerations Adverse events were observed in some animal reproduction studies. Healthcare providers are encouraged to register pregnant patients exposed to modafinil by calling (866-404-4106).

Efficacy of steroidal contraceptives (including depot and implantable contraceptives) may be decreased; alternate means of contraception should be considered during therapy and for 1 month after modafinil is discontinued.

Breast-Feeding Considerations It is not known if modafinil is excreted into breast milk. The manufacturer recommends caution be used if administered to nursing women.

Contraindications Hypersensitivity to modafinil, armodafinil, or any component

Warnings Serious and life-threatening rashes, including Stevens-Johnson syndrome and toxic epidermal necrolysis, have been reported with modafinil. Although initially reported in children during clinical trials, postmarketing cases have occurred in both children and adults. Most cases have occurred within the first 5 weeks of therapy; however, rare cases have occurred after long-term use. No risk factors have been identified to predict occurrence or severity. Patients should be advised to discontinue at first sign of rash. The serious nature of these dermatologic adverse effects, as well reports of psychiatric events, have resulted in the FDA's Pediatric Advisory Committee unanimously recommending that a specific warning against the use of modafinil in children be added to the manufacturer's labeling.

May impair the ability to engage in potentially hazardous activities. The degree of sleepiness should be reassessed frequently; some patients may not return to a normal level of wakefulness. Produces psychoactive and euphoric effects, alterations of mood, perception, thinking, and feelings typical of other CNS stimulants. No clinical symptoms of withdrawal have been reported; patients should be monitored closely for abuse potential, particularly those with a prior history of drug and/or stimulant abuse.

Rare cases of multiorgan hypersensitivity reactions in association with modafinil use and lone cases of angioedema and anaphylactoid reactions with armodafinil have been reported. Signs and symptoms are diverse, reflecting the involvement of specific organs. Patients typically present with fever and rash associated with organ-system dysfunction. Patients should be advised to report any signs and symptoms related to these effects; discontinuation of therapy is recommended.

The American Heart Association recommends that all children diagnosed with ADHD who may be candidates for stimulant medication, such as modafinil, should have a thorough cardiovascular assessment prior to initiation of therapy. These recommendations are based upon reports of serious cardiovascular adverse events (including sudden death) in patients (both children and adults) taking usual doses of stimulant medications. Most of these patients were found to have underlying structural heart disease (eg, hypertrophic obstructive cardiomyopathy). This assessment should include a combination of thorough medical history, family history, and physical examination. An ECG is not mandatory but should be considered. Modafinil use is not recommended in patients with a history of angina, cardiac ischemia, recent history of MI, left ventricular hypertrophy, or patients with mitral valve prolapse who have developed mitral valve prolapse syndrome

with previous CNS stimulant use. Increase monitoring in patients with hypertension; additional antihypertensive therapy may be necessary.

Effectiveness of steroidal contraceptives may be reduced when administered concomitantly with modafinil; alternative or concomitant methods of contraception are recommended for patients receiving modafinil and for 1 month following discontinuation. Cyclosporine serum concentrations may be reduced with modafinil use; monitor cyclosporine concentrations.

Precautions Use with caution in patients with hepatic impairment; dosage reduction is recommended for patients with severe hepatic impairment. Use with caution in patients with preexisting psychosis or bipolar disorder (may induce mixed/manic episode). May exacerbate symptoms of behavior and thought disorder in psychotic patients; new-onset psychosis or mania may occur with stimulant use; observe for symptoms of aggression, hostility, or suicidal ideation. Use with caution in patients with renal impairment. Use with caution in patients with Tourette syndrome; stimulants may unmask tics. Children may experience a higher frequency of some adverse effects than adults including the following: insomnia (29% vs 5%), decreased appetite (16% vs 4%), weight loss, and abdominal pain. The following were reported in controlled, open label clinical studies in children: Cataplexy increased, hostility, hypnagogic hallucinations, suicidal ideation, and Tourette syndrome.

Adverse Reactions

Cardiovascular: Chest pain, edema, hypertension, palpitation, tachycardia, vasodilation

Central nervous system: Agitation, anxiety (dose related), chills, confusion, depression, dizziness, emotional lability, headache (occurs more frequently in adults; dose related), insomnia, nervousness, somnolence, vertigo

Dermatologic: Rash (includes some severe cases requiring hospitalization)

Gastrointestinal: Abdominal pain (occurs more frequently in children), anorexia, appetite decreased (occurs more frequently in children), constipation, diarrhea, dyspepsia, flatulence, mouth ulceration, nausea, taste perversion, weight loss (occurs more frequently in children), xerostomia

Genitourinary: Abnormal urine, hematuria, pyuria

Hematologic: Eosinophilia

Hepatic: LFTs abnormal

Neuromuscular & skeletal: Back pain, dyskinesia, hyperkinesia, hypertonia, neck rigidity, paresthesia, tremor

Ocular: Abnormal vision, amblyopia, eye pain

Respiratory: Asthma, epistaxis, lung disorder, pharyngitis, rhinitis

Miscellaneous: Diaphoresis, flu-like syndrome, herpes simplex infection, thirst

Postmarketing and/or case reports: Agranulocytosis, anaphylactic reaction, angioedema, DRESS syndrome, erythema multiforme, hypersensitivity syndrome (multiorgan), mania, psychosis, Stevens-Johnson syndrome, toxic epidermal necrolysis

Drug Interactions

Metabolism/Transport Effects Substrate of CYP3A4 (major); **Note:** Assignment of Major/Minor substrate status based on clinically relevant drug interaction potential; **Inhibits** CYP1A2 (weak), CYP2A6 (weak), CYP2C19 (moderate), CYP2C9 (weak), CYP2E1 (weak), CYP3A4 (weak); **Induces** CYP1A2 (weak/moderate), CYP2B6 (weak/moderate), CYP3A4 (weak/moderate)

Avoid Concomitant Use

Avoid concomitant use of Modafinil with any of the following: Axitinib; Bosutinib; Conivaptan; Fusidic Acid (Systemic); Iobenguane I 123; Pimozide; Simeprevir; Sofosbuvir

Increased Effect/Toxicity

Modafinil may increase the levels/effects of: Citalopram; CYP2C19 Substrates; Dofetilide; Lomitapide; Pimozide; Sympathomimetics

The levels/effects of Modafinil may be increased by: AtoMOXetine; Cannabinoid-Containing Products; Ceritinib; Conivaptan; CYP3A4 Inhibitors (Moderate); CYP3A4 Inhibitors (Strong); Dasatinib; Fusidic Acid (Systemic); Ivacaftor; Linezolid; Luliconazole; Mifepristone; Stiripentol

Decreased Effect

Modafinil may decrease the levels/effects of: ARIPiprazole; Axitinib; Bosutinib; Clopidogrel; Contraceptives (Estrogens); CycloSPORINE (Systemic); Ibrutinib; Iobenguane I 123; Saxagliptin; Simeprevir; Sofosbuvir

The levels/effects of Modafinil may be decreased by: Bosentan; CYP3A4 Inducers (Strong); Dabrafenib; Deferasirox; Mitotane; Siltuximab; St Johns Wort; Tocilizumab

Food Interactions Food delays absorption, but does not affect bioavailability. Management: Administer without regard to meals.

Stability Store at 68°F to 77°F (20°C to 25°C).

Mechanism of Action The exact mechanism of action is unclear, it does not appear to alter the release of dopamine or norepinephrine, it may exert its stimulant effects by decreasing GABA-mediated neurotransmission, although this theory has not yet been fully evaluated; several studies also suggest that an intact central alpha-adrenergic system is required for modafinil's activity; the drug increases high-frequency alpha waves while decreasing both delta and theta wave activity, and these effects are consistent with generalized increases in mental alertness

Pharmacokinetics (Adult data unless noted) Modafinil is a racemic compound (at steady state total exposure to the *l*-isomer is ~3 times that for the *d*-isomer) whose enantiomers have different pharmacokinetics and do not interconvert.

Distribution: V_d: 0.9 L/kg

Protein binding: ~60%, primarily to albumin

Metabolism: Hepatic; multiple pathways including CYP3A4

Half-life: Effective half-life: 15 hours

Time to peak serum concentration: 2-4 hours

Elimination: Urine (as metabolites; <10% as unchanged drug)

Dosing: Usual Oral:

Children: **ADHD: Note:** Reports of serious dermatologic adverse effects and psychiatric events has resulted in the FDA's Pediatric Advisory Committee unanimously recommending that a specific warning against the use of modafinil in children be added to the manufacturer's labeling; use only if first- and second-line treatments have failed and the benefits outweigh the risks

Children <30 kg: 200-340* mg once daily

Children >30 kg: 300-425* mg

Adults:

ADHD: 100-400 mg once daily (Taylor, 2000); **Note:** Randomized, double-blind, placebo-controlled pediatric studies have utilized an 85 mg film-coated tablet (currently not commercially available) to provide these dosages. All studies utilized a titration method but varied the length of titration (3 weeks vs 7-9 days); clinical improvement was noted earlier in the shorter titration period.

Narcolepsy, obstructive sleep apnea/hypopnea syndrome (OSAHS): Adults: Initial: 200 mg as a single daily dose in the morning; **Note:** Doses of up to 400 mg/day, given as a single dose, have been well tolerated, but there is no consistent evidence that this dose confers additional benefit.

Shift work sleep disorder (SWSD): Adults: Initial: 200 mg as a single dose taken ~1 hour prior to start of work shift; **Note:** Doses of up to 400 mg/day, given as a single dose, have been well tolerated, but there is no consistent evidence that this dose confers additional benefit.

Dosing adjustment in renal impairment: Safety and efficacy have not been established in severe renal impairment.

Dosing adjustment in hepatic impairment: Severe hepatic impairment: Dose should be reduced to one-half of that recommended for patients with normal liver function.

Administration Oral: May be administer without regard to food, as a single dose in the morning; administer 1 hour prior to the start of work shift in those patients with SWSD

Monitoring Parameters Monitor CNS activity, blood pressure (if hypertensive patient), heart rate, appetite

Controlled Substance C-IV

Dosage Forms Excipient information presented when available (limited, particularly for generics); consult specific product labeling.

Tablet, Oral:

Provigil: 100 mg

Provigil: 200 mg [scored]

Generic: 100 mg, 200 mg

References

Amiri S, Mohammadi MR, Mohammadi M, et al, "Modafinil as a Treatment for Attention-Deficit/Hyperactivity Disorder in Children and Adolescents: A Double-Blind, Randomized Clinical Trial," *Prog Neuropsychopharmacol Biol Psychiatry*, 2007, August 8 [Epub ahead of print].

Biederman J and Pliszka SR, "Modafinil Improves Symptoms of Attention-Deficit/Hyperactivity Disorder Across Subtypes in Children and Adolescents," *J Pediatr*, 2008, 152(3):394-9.

Biederman J, Swanson JM, Wigal SB, et al, "Efficacy and Safety of Modafinil Film-Coated Tablets in Children and Adolescents With Attention-Deficit/Hyperactivity Disorder: Results of a Randomized, Double-Blind, Placebo-Controlled, Flexible-Dose Study," *Pediatrics*, 2005, 116(6):e777-84.

Broughton RJ, Fleming JA, George, CF, et al, "Randomized, Double-Blind, Placebo-Controlled Crossover Trial of Modafinil in the Treatment of Excessive Daytime Sleepiness in Narcolepsy," *Neurology*, 1997, 49(2):444-51.

Greenhill LL, Biederman J, Boellner SW, etal, "A Randomized, Double-Blind, Placebo-Controlled Study of Modafinil Film-Coated Tablets in Children and Adolescents With Attention-Deficit/Hyperactivity Disorder," *J AM Acad Child Adolesc Psychiatry*, 2006, 45(5):503-11.

Grozinger M, "Interaction of Modafinil and Clomipramine as Comedication in a Narcoleptic Patient," *Clin Neuropharmacol*, 1998, 21 (2):127-9.

Kumar R, "Approved and Investigational Use of Modafinil: An Evidence-Based Review," *Drugs*, 2008, 68(13):1803-39.

Rugino TA and Copley TC, "Effects of Modafinil in Children With Attention-Deficit/Hyperactivity Disorder: An Open-Label Study," *J Am Acad Child Adolesc Psychiatry*, 2001, 40(2):230-5.

Schwartz JR, "Modafinil in the Treatment of Excessive Sleepiness," *Drug Des Devel Ther*, 2009, 2:71-85.

Swanson JM, Greenhill LL, Lopez FA, et al, "Modafinil Film-Coated Tablets in Children and Adolescents With Attention-Deficit/Hyperactivity Disorder: Results of a Randomized, Double-Blind, Placebo-Controlled, Fixed-Dose Study Followed by Abrupt Discontinuation," *J Clin Psychiatry*, 2006, 67(1):137-47.

Taylor FB and Russo J, "Efficacy of Modafinil Compared to Dextroamphetamine for the Treatment of Attention Deficit/Hyperactivity Disorder in Adults," *J Child Adolesc Psychopharmacol*, 2000, 10 (4):311-20.

U.S. Modafinil in Narcolepsy Multicenter Study Group, "Randomized Trial of Modafinil for the Treatment of Pathological Somnolence in Narcolepsy," *Ann Neurol*, 1998, 43(1):88-97.

Vetter VL, Elia J, Erickson C, et al, "Cardiovascular Monitoring of Children and Adolescents With Heart Disease Receiving Medications for Attention Deficit/Hyperactivity Disorder [Corrected]: A Scientific Statement From the American Heart Association Council on Cardiovascular Disease in the Young Congenital Cardiac Defects Committee and the Council on Cardiovascular Nursing," *Circulation*, 2008, 117(18):2407-23.

Wigal SB, Biederman J, Swanson JM, et al, "Efficacy and Safety of Modafinil Film-Coated Tablets in Children and Adolescents With or Without Prior Stimulant Treatment for Attention-Deficit/Hyperactivity Disorder: Pooled Analysis of 3 Randomized, Double-Blind, Placebo-Controlled Studies," *Prim Care Companion J Clin Psychiatry*, 2006, 8 (6):352-60.

◆ **Moderiba** see Ribavirin on page 1818

◆ **Modified Burow's Solution** *see* Aluminum Acetate *on page 110*

◆ **Modified Shohl's Solution** *see* Sodium Citrate and Citric Acid *on page 1906*

◆ **MOM** *see* Magnesium Hydroxide *on page 1294*

Mometasone (Oral Inhalation)
(moe MET a sone)

Related Information
Inhaled Corticosteroids *on page 2223*

Brand Names: U.S. Asmanex 120 Metered Doses; Asmanex 14 Metered Doses; Asmanex 30 Metered Doses; Asmanex 60 Metered Doses; Asmanex 7 Metered Doses

Brand Names: Canada Asmanex Twisthaler

Therapeutic Category Anti-inflammatory Agent; Antiasthmatic; Corticosteroid, Inhalant (Oral); Glucocorticoid

Generic Availability (U.S.) No

Use Maintenance treatment of asthma as prophylactic therapy (FDA approved in ages ≥4 years and adults); **NOT** indicated for the relief of acute bronchospasm. Also used to help reduce or discontinue oral corticosteroid therapy in patients with bronchial asthma.

Pregnancy Risk Factor C

Pregnancy Considerations Adverse events were observed in some animal reproduction studies. Hypoadrenalism may occur in infants born to mothers receiving corticosteroids during pregnancy. Based on available data, an overall increased risk of congenital malformations or a decrease in fetal growth has not been associated with maternal use of inhaled corticosteroids during pregnancy (Bakhireva, 2005; NAEPP, 2005; Namazy, 2004). Uncontrolled asthma is associated with adverse events in pregnancy (increased risk of perinatal mortality, pre-eclampsia, preterm birth, low birth weight infants). Inhaled corticosteroids are recommended for the treatment of asthma during pregnancy (most information available using budesonide) (ACOG, 2008; NAEPP, 2005).

Breast-Feeding Considerations Systemic corticosteroids are excreted in human milk. It is not known if sufficient quantities of mometasone are absorbed following oral inhalation to produce detectable amounts in breast milk; however, oral absorption is limited (<1%). The manufacturer recommends that caution be exercised when administering mometasone to nursing women. The use of inhaled corticosteroids is not considered a contraindication to breast-feeding (NAEPP, 2005).

Contraindications Hypersensitivity to mometasone or any component; hypersensitivity to milk proteins; primary treatment of status asthmaticus or acute bronchospasm

Warnings Fatalities have occurred due to adrenal insufficiency in asthmatic patients during and after switching from systemic corticosteroids to aerosol steroids; several months may be required for full recovery of hypothalamic-pituitary-adrenal (HPA) function; patients receiving higher doses of systemic corticosteroids (eg, adults receiving ≥20 mg of prednisone per day) may be at greater risk; during this period of HPA suppression, aerosol steroids do not provide the systemic glucocorticoid or mineralocorticoid activity needed to treat patients requiring stress doses (ie, patients with major stress, such as trauma, surgery, infections, or other conditions associated with severe electrolyte loss). When used at high doses or for a prolonged time, hypercorticism and HPA suppression (including adrenal crisis) may occur; use with inhaled or systemic corticosteroids (even alternate-day dosing) may increase risk of HPA suppression. Acute adrenal insufficiency may occur with abrupt withdrawal after long-term use or with stress; withdrawal and discontinuation of corticosteroids should be done carefully; patients with HPA axis suppression may require doses of systemic glucocorticosteroids prior to, during, and after unusual stress (eg, surgery). Immunosuppression may occur; patients may be more susceptible to infections; avoid exposure to chickenpox and measles. Switching patients from systemic corticosteroids to aerosol steroids may unmask allergic conditions previously treated by the systemic steroid. Bronchospasm may occur after use of inhaled asthma medications; a fast-acting bronchodilator may be used to treat; discontinue mometasone and initiate alternative chronic therapy

Allergic reactions, including anaphylaxis, angioedema, pruritus, and rash, have been reported. If these symptoms occur, discontinue use. Powder for oral inhalation (Asmanex® Twisthaler®) contains lactose (milk proteins) which may cause allergic reactions (including anaphylaxis) in patients with milk protein allergy.

Precautions Avoid using higher than recommended doses; suppression of HPA axis function, suppression of linear growth (ie, reduction of growth velocity), reduced bone mineral density, hypercorticism (Cushing's syndrome), hyperglycemia, or glucosuria may occur; titrate to lowest effective dose. Use with extreme caution in patients with respiratory tuberculosis, untreated systemic infections, or ocular herpes simplex. Rare cases of increased IOP, glaucoma, or cataracts have been reported with inhaled corticosteroids, including mometasone. Local oropharyngeal *Candida* infections have been reported; if they occur, treat appropriately while continuing mometasone therapy; however, therapy may need to be interrupted in some patients. Patients should be instructed to rinse mouth after each use.

Adverse Reactions
Central nervous system: Depression, fatigue, fever (children), headache, pain

Dermatologic: Bruising (children)

Gastrointestinal: Abdominal pain, anorexia, dry throat (oral inhalation), dyspepsia, gastroenteritis, nausea, vomiting

Genitourinary: Dysmenorrhea, urinary tract infection (children)

Neuromuscular & skeletal: Arthralgia, back pain, musculoskeletal pain, myalgia

Ocular: Cataracts, ocular pressure increased

Otic: Earache

Respiratory: Dysphonia, epistaxis, nasal irritation, pharyngitis, rhinitis, sinus congestion, sinusitis, upper respiratory tract infection

Miscellaneous: Flu-like syndrome, infection

Rare but important or life-threatening: Anaphylaxis, angioedema, asthma aggravated, bronchospasm, cough, dyspnea, growth suppression, hypersensitivity, pruritus, rash, wheezing

Drug Interactions
Metabolism/Transport Effects Substrate of CYP3A4 (minor); **Note:** Assignment of Major/Minor substrate status based on clinically relevant drug interaction potential

Avoid Concomitant Use
Avoid concomitant use of Mometasone (Oral Inhalation) with any of the following: Aldesleukin

Increased Effect/Toxicity
Mometasone (Oral Inhalation) may increase the levels/effects of: Amphotericin B; Ceritinib; Deferasirox; Loop Diuretics; Thiazide Diuretics

The levels/effects of Mometasone (Oral Inhalation) may be increased by: CYP3A4 Inhibitors (Strong); Telaprevir

Decreased Effect
Mometasone (Oral Inhalation) may decrease the levels/effects of: Aldesleukin; Antidiabetic Agents; Corticorelin; Hyaluronidase; Telaprevir

Stability Oral inhaler: Store at 25°C (77°F) in a dry place; excursions permitted to 15°C to 30°C (59°F to 86°F);

discard inhaler 45 days after opening foil pouch (or when dose counter reads "00")

Mechanism of Action May depress the formation, release, and activity of endogenous chemical mediators of inflammation (kinins, histamine, liposomal enzymes, prostaglandins). Leukocytes and macrophages may have to be present for the initiation of responses mediated by the above substances. Inhibits the margination and subsequent cell migration to the area of injury, and also reverses the dilatation and increased vessel permeability in the area resulting in decreased access of cells to the sites of injury.

Pharmacodynamics Clinical effects are due to direct local effect, rather than systemic absorption
Maximum effect: 1-2 weeks or more
Duration after discontinuation: Several days or more

Pharmacokinetics (Adult data unless noted)
Absorption: Systemic absorption: Single dose: <1%
Distribution: V_{dss}: Adults: 152 L
Protein binding: 98% to 99%
Metabolism: Extensive in the liver to multiple metabolites; no major metabolites are detectable in the plasma; *in vitro* incubation studies identified one minor metabolite, 6 Beta-hydroxymometasone furoate, formed via cytochrome P450 CYP3A4 pathway
Bioavailability: Single dose: <1%
Half-life: Mean: 5 hours
Elimination: Metabolites are excreted primarily via the bile with a limited amount via urine; after oral inhalation, 74% of the dose was excreted in the feces and 8% in the urine (none as unchanged drug)

Dosing: Usual Note: Maximum effects may not be seen until 1-2 weeks or longer; doses should be titrated to the lowest effective dose once asthma is controlled.

Children 4-11 years (regardless of prior therapy): **Note:** Use 110 mcg inhaler: Initial: 1 inhalation (110 mcg) once daily, administered in the evening. Maximum dose: 1 inhalation/day (110 mcg/day)

Children ≥12 years and Adults:
Patients previously treated with bronchodilators only or with inhaled corticosteroids: Initial: 1 inhalation (220 mcg) once daily, administered in the evening; may increase dose after 2 weeks if adequate response not obtained. Maximum dose: 2 inhalations/day (440 mcg/day); may be administered as 1 inhalation twice daily or 2 inhalations once daily in the evening
Patients previously treated with oral corticosteroids: Initial: 2 inhalations (440 mcg) twice daily. Maximum dose: 4 inhalations/day (880 mcg/day)
NIH Asthma Guidelines (NAEPP, 2007) (give in divided doses): **Note:** 220 mcg inhaler delivers 200 mcg mometasone furoate per actuation; NAEPP uses doses based on delivery, while manufacturer recommended doses are based on inhaler amount; Children ≥12 years and Adults:
"Low" dose: 200 mcg/day (200 mcg/puff: 1 puff/day)
"Medium" dose: 400 mcg/day (200 mcg/puff: 2 puffs/day)
"High" dose: >400 mcg/day (200 mcg/puff: >2 puffs/day)

Administration Remove inhaler from foil pouch; write date on cap label. Keep inhaler upright while removing cap, twisting in a counterclockwise direction; lifting the cap loads the device with the medication. Exhale fully prior to bringing the inhaler up to the mouth. Place inhaler in mouth, while holding it in a horizontal position. Close lips around the mouthpiece and inhale quickly and deeply. Remove the inhaler from your mouth and hold your breath for about 10 seconds, if possible. Do not exhale into inhaler. Wipe the mouthpiece dry and replace the cap immediately after each inhalation; rotate fully until click is heard. Rinse mouth with water (without swallowing) after inhalation to decrease chance of oral candidiasis. Avoid

contact of the inhaler with any liquids; do not wash; wipe with dry cloth or tissue if needed. Discard the inhaler 45 days after opening foil pouch or when dose counter reads "00."

Monitoring Parameters Monitor growth in pediatric patients. Check mucous membranes for signs of fungal infection. Monitor pulmonary function tests (eg, FEV_1, peak flow).

Additional Information When using mometasone oral inhalation to help reduce or discontinue oral corticosteroid therapy, begin prednisone taper after at least 1 week of mometasone inhalation therapy; do not decrease prednisone faster than 2.5 mg/day on a weekly basis; monitor patients for signs of asthma instability and adrenal insufficiency; decrease mometasone to lowest effective dose after prednisone reduction is complete.

Product Availability Asmanex HFA: FDA approved April 2014; anticipated availability is currently unknown.

Dosage Forms Excipient information presented when available (limited, particularly for generics); consult specific product labeling.
Aerosol Powder Breath Activated, Inhalation, as furoate:
Asmanex 120 Metered Doses: 220 mcg/INH (1 ea) [contains milk protein]
Asmanex 14 Metered Doses: 220 mcg/INH (1 ea) [contains milk protein]
Asmanex 30 Metered Doses: 110 mcg/INH (1 ea); 220 mcg/INH (1 ea) [contains milk protein]
Asmanex 60 Metered Doses: 220 mcg/INH (1 ea) [contains milk protein]
Asmanex 7 Metered Doses: 110 mcg/INH (1 ea) [contains milk protein]

References

ACOG Committee on Practice Bulletins-Obstetrics, "ACOG Practice Bulletin: Clinical Management Guidelines for Obstetrician-Gynecologists Number 90, February 2008: Asthma in Pregnancy," *Obstet Gynecol*, 2008, 111(2 Pt 1):457-64.
Bakhireva LN, Jones KL, Schatz M, et al, "Asthma Medication Use in Pregnancy and Fetal Growth," *J Allergy Clin Immunol*, 2005, 116 (3):503-9.
Namazy J, Schatz M, Long L, et al, "Use of Inhaled Steroids by Pregnant Asthmatic Women Does Not Reduce Intrauterine Growth," *J Allergy Clin Immunol*, 2004, 113(3):427-32.
National Asthma Education and Prevention Program (NAEPP), "Expert Panel Report 3 (EPR-3): Guidelines for the Diagnosis and Management of Asthma," *Clinical Practice Guidelines*, National Institutes of Health, National Heart, Lung, and Blood Institute, NIH Publication No. 08-4051, prepublication 2007. Available at http://www.nhlbi.nih.gov/guidelines/asthma/asthgdln.htm
National Asthma Education and Prevention Program (NAEPP) Working Group Report on "Managing Asthma During Pregnancy: Recommendations for Pharmacologic Treatment," National Institutes of Health, National Heart, Lung, and Blood Institute, NIH Publication No. 05-5236, March 2005. Available at http://www.nhlbi.nih.gov/health/prof/lung/asthma/astpreg/astpreg_full.pdf

Mometasone (Nasal) (moe MET a sone)

Brand Names: U.S. Nasonex
Brand Names: Canada Apo-Mometasone®; Nasonex®
Therapeutic Category Anti-inflammatory Agent; Corticosteroid, Intranasal; Glucocorticoid
Generic Availability (U.S.) No

Use Management of nasal symptoms associated with seasonal and perennial allergic rhinitis (FDA approved in ages ≥2 years and adults); prevention of seasonal allergic rhinitis (FDA approved in ages ≥12 years and adults); treatment of nasal polyps (FDA approved in adults); has also been used for management of nasal airway obstruction associated with adenoidal hypertrophy

Intranasal corticosteroids have also been used as an adjunct to antibiotics in empiric treatment of acute bacterial rhinosinusitis primarily in patients with history of allergic rhinitis (Chow, 2012) and in pediatric patients with mild obstructive sleep apnea syndrome who cannot undergo ▶

adenotonsillectomy or who still have symptoms after surgery (Marcus, 2012).

Pregnancy Risk Factor C

Pregnancy Considerations Adverse events were observed in some animal reproduction studies. Hypoadrenalism may occur in newborns following maternal use of corticosteroids in pregnancy; monitor. Intranasal corticosteroids are recommended for the treatment of rhinitis during pregnancy; the lowest effective dose should be used (NAEPP, 2005; Wallace, 2008).

Breast-Feeding Considerations Systemic corticosteroids are excreted in human milk. It is not known if sufficient quantities of mometasone are absorbed following nasal inhalation to produce detectable amounts in breast milk; however, systemic absorption is low (<1%). The use of inhaled corticosteroids is not considered a contraindication to breast-feeding (NAEPP, 2005). The manufacturer recommends caution be used if administered to a nursing woman.

Contraindications Hypersensitivity to mometasone or any component

Warnings HPA suppression or hypercorticism (Cushing's syndrome) may occur with use of higher than recommended doses or at typical doses in susceptible patients. Acute adrenal insufficiency may occur with abrupt withdrawal after long-term use, with stress, or when converting from systemic to topical corticosteroid therapy; withdrawal or discontinuation of corticosteroids should be done carefully; patients with HPA axis suppression may require doses of systemic glucocorticosteroids prior to, during, and after unusual stress (eg, surgery). Immunosuppression may occur; patients may be more susceptible to infections; avoid exposure to chickenpox and measles. Epistaxis may occur.

Precautions Avoid using higher than recommended dosages; suppression of HPA function, suppression of linear growth (ie, reduction of growth velocity), reduced bone mineral density, or hypercorticism (Cushing's syndrome) may occur; titrate to lowest effective dose. Reduction in growth velocity may occur when corticosteroids are administered to pediatric patients, even at recommended doses via intranasal route (monitor growth). Use mometasone with extreme caution in patients with respiratory tuberculosis, untreated bacterial, fungal, systemic viral or parasitic infections, or ocular herpes simplex. Localized *Candida* infections of the nose and pharynx have been reported rarely; interruption of therapy may be necessary while antifungal therapy is employed. Corticosteroids impair wound healing; avoid use in patients with recent nasal ulcers, nasal surgery, or nasal trauma; allow healing to occur before use. Glaucoma, increased intraocular pressure, and cataracts have been reported following the intranasal application of corticosteroids; monitor patients who have change in vision and in patients with a history of increased ocular pressure, glaucoma, or cataracts. Use of nasal mometasone in place of systemic corticosteroids may unmask allergies (eg, eczema, rhinitis) that were previously controlled by the systemic corticosteroids. Rare cases of immediate hypersensitivity reactions or nasal septum perforation may occur with intranasal corticosteroids.

Adverse Reactions

Central nervous system: Headache

Gastrointestinal: Diarrhea, dyspepsia, vomiting

Neuromuscular & skeletal: Musculoskeletal pain, myalgia

Ocular: Conjunctivitis

Otic: Otitis media

Respiratory: Asthma, bronchitis, nasal irritation, rhinitis, sinusitis, upper respiratory tract infection, wheezing

Miscellaneous: Flu-like syndrome, viral infection (nasal inhalation)

Rare but important or life-threatening: Anaphylaxis, angioedema, growth suppression, nasal burning, nasal

candidiasis, nasal septal perforation, nasal ulcers, oral candidiasis (nasal inhalation), smell disturbance (rare), taste disturbance (rare)

Drug Interactions

Metabolism/Transport Effects Substrate of CYP3A4 (minor); **Note:** Assignment of Major/Minor substrate status based on clinically relevant drug interaction potential

Avoid Concomitant Use There are no known interactions where it is recommended to avoid concomitant use.

Increased Effect/Toxicity

Mometasone (Nasal) may increase the levels/effects of: Ceritinib

Decreased Effect There are no known significant interactions involving a decrease in effect.

Stability Store at 25°C (77°F), excursions permitted to 15°C to 30°C (59°F to 86°F). Protect from light.

Mechanism of Action May depress the formation, release, and activity of endogenous chemical mediators of inflammation (kinins, histamine, liposomal enzymes, prostaglandins). Leukocytes and macrophages may have to be present for the initiation of responses mediated by the above substances. Inhibits the margination and subsequent cell migration to the area of injury, and also reverses the dilatation and increased vessel permeability in the area resulting in decreased access of cells to the sites of injury.

Pharmacodynamics Clinical effects are due to direct local effect, rather than systemic absorption.

Onset of action: Improvement in allergic rhinitis symptoms may be seen within 11 hours.

Maximum effect: Within 1-2 weeks after starting therapy

Pharmacokinetics (Adult data unless noted) Bioavailability: <1%

Dosing: Usual

Children and Adolescents:

Nasal airway obstruction/adenoidal hypertrophy: Intranasal: Limited data available: Children and Adolescents 3-15 years: Initial 100 mcg once daily delivered as 50 mcg (1 spray) **per nostril** once daily for 6 weeks, followed by the same dose given every 24 hours for the first 2 weeks of each month. Dosing based on two studies: The first was a randomized, placebo-controlled study (n=122; treatment arm: 67; age range; 3-15 years) in which patients received therapy for 6 weeks and 67.2% had a significant decrease in adenoid size compared to the control group (p<0.001) (Cengel, 2005). The second was a 2-stage, placebo-controlled, randomized study (n=60, treatment arm: 30; age range: 3-7 years) which showed that after 40 days of daily mometasone therapy, ~77.7% of patients were considered responders and able to avoid adenoidectomy; those who responded continued therapy every 24 or 48 hours for the first 2 weeks of three subsequent months (Berlucchi, 2007). Long-term analysis of children receiving the daily dose for the first 2 weeks of each month continued to show improvement after a mean followup period of 28 months and the need for surgery remained reduced (Berlucchi, 2008).

Allergic rhinitis: Intranasal:

Treatment:

Children 2-11 years: 100 mcg once daily delivered as 50 mcg (1 spray) **per nostril** once daily

Children ≥12 years and Adolescents: 200 mcg once daily delivered as 100 mcg (2 sprays) **per nostril** once daily

Prevention: Children ≥12 years and Adolescents: 200 mcg once daily delivered as 100 mcg (2 sprays) **per nostril** once daily beginning 2-4 weeks prior to pollen season

Nasal polyps, treatment: Intranasal: Adolescents ≥18 years: 200 mcg twice daily delivered as 100 mcg (2 sprays) **per nostril** twice daily; a lower dose of 200 mcg once daily delivered as 100 mcg (2 sprays) **per nostril** once daily may be effective in some patients

Adults:

Allergic rhinitis: Intranasal:

Treatment: 200 mcg once daily delivered as 100 mcg (2 sprays) **per nostril** once daily

Prevention: 200 mcg once daily delivered as 100 mcg (2 sprays) **per nostril** once daily beginning 2-4 weeks prior to pollen season

Nasal polyps, treatment: Intranasal: 200 mcg twice daily delivered as 100 mcg (2 sprays) **per nostril** twice daily; 200 mcg once daily delivered as 100 mcg (2 sprays) **per nostril** once daily may be effective in some patients

Dosing adjustment in renal impairment: There are no dosage adjustments provided in the manufacturer's labeling.

Dosing adjustment in hepatic impairment: There are no dosage adjustments provided in the manufacturer's labeling. Mometasone concentrations appear to increase with the severity of hepatic impairment; use with caution.

Administration Shake well prior to each use. Before first use, prime by pressing pump 10 times or until a fine spray appears. Repeat priming with 2 sprays or until a fine spray appears if ≥1 week between use. Blow nose to clear nostrils before each use. Insert applicator into nostril, keeping bottle upright, and close off the other nostril. Breathe in through nose. While inhaling, press pump to release spray. Do not spray into eyes or mouth. Discard after labeled number of doses has been used, even if bottle is not completely empty.

After removing nasal spray from container, avoid prolonged exposure of product to direct light; brief exposure to light (with normal use) is acceptable.

Monitoring Parameters Mucous membranes for signs of fungal infection, growth (pediatric patients), signs/symptoms of HPA axis suppression/adrenal insufficiency; ocular changes

Additional Information When used short term as adjunctive therapy in acute bacterial rhinosinusitis (ABRS), intranasal steroids show modest symptomatic improvement and few adverse effects; improvement is primarily due to increased sinus drainage. Use should be considered optional in ABRS; however, intranasal corticosteroids should be routinely prescribed to ABRS patients who have a history of or concurrent allergic rhinitis (Chow, 2012).

Dosage Forms Considerations Nasonex 17 g bottles contain 120 sprays.

Dosage Forms Excipient information presented when available (limited, particularly for generics); consult specific product labeling.

Suspension, Nasal, as furoate:

Nasonex: 50 mcg/actuation (17 g) [contains benzalkonium chloride]

References

Berlucchi M, Salsi D, Valetti L, et al, "The Role of Mometasone Furoate Aqueous Nasal Spray in the Treatment of Adenoidal Hypertrophy in the Pediatric Age Group: Preliminary Results of a Prospective, Randomized Study," Pediatrics, 2007, 119(6):e1392-7.

Berlucchi M, Valetti L, Parrinello G, et al, "Long-Term Follow-Up of Children Undergoing Topical Intranasal Steroid Therapy For Adenoidal Hypertrophy," Int J Pediatr Otorhinolaryngol, 2008, 72(8):1171-5.

Cengel S and Akyol MU, "The Role of Topical Nasal Steroids in the Treatment of Children With Otitis Media With Effusion and/or Adenoid Hypertrophy," Int J Pediatr Otorhinolaryngol, 2006, 70(4):639-45.

Chow AW, Benninger MS, Brook I, et al, "IDSA Clinical Practice Guideline For Acute Bacterial Rhinosinusitis in Children and Adults," Clin Infect Dis, 2012, 54(8):e72-e112.

Marcus CL, Brooks LJ, Draper KA, et al, "Diagnosis and Management of Childhood Obstructive Sleep Apnea Syndrome," Pediatrics, 2012, 130(3):576-84.

NAEPP Working Group Report on "Managing Asthma During Pregnancy: Recommendations for Pharmacologic Treatment," National Institutes of Health, National Heart, Lung, and Blood Institute, NIH Publication No. 05-5236, March 2005. Available at http://www.nhlbi.nih.gov/health/prof/lung/asthma/astpreg/astpreg_full.pdf

Wallace DV, Dykewicz MS, Bernstein DI, et al, "The Diagnosis and Management of Rhinitis: An Updated Practice Parameter," J Allergy Clin Immunol, 2008, 122(2 Suppl):S1-84.

Mometasone (Topical) (moe MET a sone)

Medication Safety Issues

Sound-alike/look-alike issues:

Elocon lotion may be confused with ophthalmic solutions. Manufacturer's labeling emphasizes the product is **NOT** for use in the eyes.

Related Information

Topical Corticosteroids on page 2224

Brand Names: U.S. Elocon

Brand Names: Canada Elocom; PMS-Mometasone; ratio-Mometasone; Taro-Mometasone

Therapeutic Category Anti-inflammatory Agent; Corticosteroid, Topical; Glucocorticoid

Generic Availability (U.S.) May be product dependent

Use Relief of the inflammation and pruritus associated with corticosteroid-responsive dermatoses (medium potency topical corticosteroid); **Note:** Due to lack of established safety and efficacy in specific age groups, the cream and ointment are not recommended for use in children <2 years of age and the lotion is not recommended for use in children <12 years of age

Pregnancy Risk Factor C

Pregnancy Considerations Adverse events have been observed in animal reproduction studies. When topical corticosteroids are needed during pregnancy, low to mid potency preparations are preferred; higher potency preparations should be used for the shortest time possible and fetal growth should be monitored (Chi, 2011; Chi, 2013). Topical products are not recommended for extensive use, in large quantities, or for long periods of time in pregnant women (Leachman, 2006).

Breast-Feeding Considerations Corticosteroids are excreted in human milk; information specific to mometasone has not been located. It is not known if systemic absorption following topical administration results in detectable quantities in human milk. The manufacturer notes that when used systemically, maternal use of corticosteroids have the potential to cause adverse events in a nursing infant (eg, growth suppression, interfere with endogenous corticosteroid production), therefore caution should be exercised if administered to nursing women. Do not apply topical corticosteroids to nipples; hypertension was noted in a nursing infant exposed to a topical corticosteroid while nursing (Leachman, 2006).

Contraindications Hypersensitivity to mometasone or any component

Warnings Adverse systemic effects may occur when topical steroids are used on large areas of the body, denuded areas, for prolonged periods of time, with an occlusive dressing, and/or in infants or small children; infants and small children may be more susceptible to HPA axis suppression or other systemic toxicities due to a larger skin surface area to body mass ratio; use with caution in pediatric patients and for no longer than 3 weeks

Precautions Avoid using higher than recommended doses; suppression of HPA axis function, suppression of linear growth (ie, reduction of growth velocity), reduced bone mineral density, hypercorticism (Cushing's syndrome), hyperglycemia, or glucosuria may occur; titrate to lowest effective dose; these adverse effects (as well as intracranial hypertension) may also occur with topical use and have been reported in pediatric patients. Do not

◄ use topical mometasone products for the treatment of diaper dermatitis.

Adverse Reactions

Dermatologic: Bacterial skin infection, burning, furunculosis, pruritus, skin atrophy, tingling/stinging

Rare but important or life-threatening: Decreased glucocorticoid concentrations (pediatrics), folliculitis, moniliasis, paresthesia, rosacea, skin depigmentation, skin atrophy

Cataract formation, reduction in growth velocity, and HPA axis suppression have been reported with other corticosteroids.

Drug Interactions

Metabolism/Transport Effects Substrate of CYP3A4 (minor); **Note:** Assignment of Major/Minor substrate status based on clinically relevant drug interaction potential

Avoid Concomitant Use

Avoid concomitant use of Mometasone (Topical) with any of the following: Aldesleukin

Increased Effect/Toxicity

Mometasone (Topical) may increase the levels/effects of: Ceritinib; Deferasirox

The levels/effects of Mometasone (Topical) may be increased by: Telaprevir

Decreased Effect

Mometasone (Topical) may decrease the levels/effects of: Aldesleukin; Corticorelin; Hyaluronidase; Telaprevir

Stability

Cream: Store between 2°C to 25°C (36°F to 77°F)

Lotion: Store between 2°C to 30°C (36°F to 86°F)

Ointment: Store at 25°C (77°F); excursions permitted to 15°C to 30°C (59°F to 86°F)

Mechanism of Action Mometasone furoate has anti-inflammatory, antipruritic, and vasoconstrictive properties. May depress the formation, release, and activity of endogenous chemical mediators of inflammation (kinins, histamine, liposomal enzymes, prostaglandins) through the induction of phospholipase A_2 inhibitory proteins (lipocortins) and sequential inhibition of the release of arachidonic acid.

Pharmacokinetics (Adult data unless noted) Absorption: 0.4% of the applied dose of the cream and 0.7% of the applied dose of the ointment enter the circulation after 8 hours of contact with normal skin (without occlusion); absorption is increased by occlusive dressings or with decreased integrity of skin (eg, inflammation or skin disease)

Dosing: Usual Apply sparingly, do not use occlusive dressings. Discontinue therapy when control is achieved; reassess diagnosis if no improvement is seen in 2 weeks.

Cream, ointment: Children ≥2 years and Adults: Apply a thin film to affected area once daily; do not use in pediatric patients for >3 weeks

Lotion: Children ≥12 years and Adults: Apply a few drops to affected area once daily; massage lightly into skin

Administration Apply sparingly; avoid contact with eyes. Do not apply to face, underarms, or groin, unless directed by physician. Do not wrap or bandage affected area unless directed by physician. Do not use for treatment of diaper dermatitis or in diaper area.

Lotion: Hold nozzle of bottle close to affected area and gently squeeze bottle.

Monitoring Parameters Monitor growth in pediatric patients; assess HPA axis suppression in patients using topical steroids applied to a large surface area or to areas under occlusion.

Additional Information Several studies conducted in children 6-23 months of age with atopic dermatitis demonstrated a high incidence of adrenal suppression when topical mometasone products were applied once daily for ~3 weeks over an average body surface area of about

40%. Of the patients with normal baseline adrenal function, adrenal suppression occurred in 16% of patients using the cream, 27% of patients using the ointment, and 29% of patients using the lotion. Follow-up testing 2-4 weeks after discontinuation of therapy demonstrated suppressed HPA axis function in 1 of 5 patients who used the cream, 3 of 8 patients who used the ointment, and 1 of 8 patients who used the lotion.

Dosage Forms Excipient information presented when available (limited, particularly for generics); consult specific product labeling.

Cream, External, as furoate:

Elocon: 0.1% (15 g, 45 g, 50 g) [contains soybean lecithin]

Generic: 0.1% (15 g, 45 g)

Lotion, External, as furoate:

Elocon: 0.1% (30 mL, 60 mL) [contains isopropyl alcohol, propylene glycol]

Ointment, External, as furoate:

Elocon: 0.1% (15 g, 45 g) [contains propylene glycol stearate]

Generic: 0.1% (15 g, 45 g)

Solution, External, as furoate:

Generic: 0.1% (30 mL, 60 mL)

References

Chi CC, Kirtschig G, Aberer W, et al. Evidence-based (S3) guideline on topical corticosteroids in pregnancy. *Br J Dermatol*. 2011;165 (5):943-952.

Chi CC, Wang SH, Mayon-White R, Wojnarowska F. Pregnancy outcomes after maternal exposure to topical corticosteroids: a UK population-based cohort study [[published online ahead of print September 4, 2013]. *JAMA Dermatol*. 2013.

Leachman SA, Reed BR. The use of dermatologic drugs in pregnancy and lactation. *Dermatol Clin*. 2006;24(2):167-197, vi.

Mometasone and Formoterol

(moe MET a sone & for MOH te rol)

Brand Names: U.S. Dulera®

Brand Names: Canada Zenhale™

Therapeutic Category Adrenal Corticosteroid; Adrenergic Agonist Agent; Anti-inflammatory Agent; Beta₂-Adrenergic Agonist; Bronchodilator; Corticosteroid, Inhalant (Oral); Glucocorticoid

Generic Availability (U.S.) No

Use Maintenance treatment of asthma (FDA approved in ages ≥12 years and adults); **NOT** indicated for the relief of acute bronchospasm

Medication Guide Available Yes

Pregnancy Risk Factor C

Pregnancy Considerations Animal reproduction studies have not been conducted with this combination. See individual agents.

Breast-Feeding Considerations It is not known if mometasone or formoterol are excreted into breast milk. According to the manufacturer, the decision to continue or discontinue breast-feeding during therapy should take into account the risk of exposure to the infant and the benefits to the mother.

Contraindications Hypersensitivity to mometasone, formoterol, adrenergic amines, or any component; treatment of acute asthma or status asthmaticus

Warnings Long-acting beta₂-agonists (LABAs), such as formoterol, increase the risk of asthma-related deaths **[U.S. Boxed Warning]**; mometasone and formoterol should only be used in patients not adequately controlled on a long-term asthma control medication (ie, inhaled corticosteroid) or whose disease severity requires initiation of two maintenance therapies. In a large clinical trial, LABA (salmeterol) use was associated with an increase in asthma-related deaths compared with placebo (when added to usual asthma therapy); risk is considered a class effect among all LABAs. Data are not available to determine if the addition of an inhaled corticosteroid lessens this increased risk of death associated with LABA use. Assess patients at regular intervals once asthma control is maintained on combination therapy to determine if step down therapy is appropriate (without loss of asthma control), and the patient can be maintained on an inhaled corticosteroid only. LABAs are not appropriate in patients whose asthma is adequately controlled on low- or medium-dose inhaled corticosteroids. LABAs may increase the risk of asthma-related hospitalization in pediatric and adolescent patients **[U.S. Boxed Warning]**.

Mometasone and formoterol should not be used to relieve acute asthmatic symptoms or rapidly deteriorating or potentially life-threatening episodes of asthma; acute episodes should be treated with short-acting beta$_2$-agonist. Routine use of inhaled, short-acting beta$_2$-agonists should be discontinued prior to initiation of mometasone and formoterol. Mometasone and formoterol should not be used more frequently than recommended (twice daily), at higher doses, nor with any additional long-acting beta$_2$-adrenergic agonist; adverse cardiovascular effects (possibly fatal) have been reported with excessive beta$_2$-adrenergic overstimulation. Paroxysmal bronchospasm (which can be fatal) has been reported with this and other inhaled beta$_2$-agonist agents. If this occurs, discontinue treatment; symptoms of laryngeal spasm, irritation, or swelling, such as stridor and choking, have been reported in patients receiving mometasone and formoterol; if this occurs, discontinue treatment.

Fatalities have occurred due to adrenal insufficiency in asthmatic patients during and after switching from systemic corticosteroids to inhaled steroids; several months may be required for full recovery of hypothalamic-pituitary-adrenal (HPA) function; patients receiving higher doses of systemic corticosteroids (eg, adults receiving ≥20 mg of prednisone per day) may be at greater risk; during this period of HPA suppression, inhaled steroids do not provide the systemic glucocorticoid or mineralocorticoid activity needed to treat patients requiring stress doses (ie, patients with major stress such as trauma, surgery, infections, or other conditions associated with severe electrolyte loss). When used at high doses, HPA suppression may occur; use with inhaled or systemic corticosteroids (even alternate day dosing) may increase risk of HPA suppression. Acute adrenal insufficiency may occur with abrupt withdrawal after long-term use or with stress; withdrawal or discontinuation of corticosteroids should be done carefully; patients with HPA axis suppression may require doses of systemic glucocorticoids prior to, during, and after unusual stress (eg, surgery). Switching patients from systemic corticosteroids to inhaled steroids may unmask allergic conditions (eg, rhinitis, conjunctivitis, eczema, arthritis, eosinophilic conditions) previously suppressed by the systemic steroid. Immunosuppression may occur; patients may be more susceptible to infections; avoid exposure to chickenpox and measles.

C. albicans infections of the mouth and pharynx may occur with orally inhaled corticosteroid use, mostly mild to moderate; interruption of therapy may be necessary at times while antifungal therapy is employed; advise patients to rinse mouth after use. Hypersensitivity reactions with angioedema and swelling of the lips, tongue, and pharynx have been reported rarely.

Precautions Use with caution in patients with cardiovascular disease (aneurysm, arrhythmia, hypertension, or HF), seizure disorders, diabetes, hypokalemia, liver dysfunction, thyrotoxicosis, pheochromocytoma, or others who are sensitive to the effects of sympathomimetic amines. Suppression of HPA function, suppression of linear growth (ie, reduction of growth velocity), reduced bone mineral density or hypercorticism (Cushing's syndrome) may occur; titrate to lowest effective dose.

Reduction in growth velocity [mean: 1 cm/year (range: 0.3-1.8 cm)] may occur when corticosteroids are administered to pediatric patients, even at recommended doses via inhaled route; related to dose and duration of exposure; monitor growth. Use with extreme caution in patients with respiratory tuberculosis, untreated systemic infections, or ocular herpes simplex. Rare cases of increased IOP, glaucoma, or cataracts have been reported with inhaled corticosteroids, including mometasone. Immediate hypersensitivity reactions (urticaria, angioedema, rash, bronchospasm) have been reported.

Use with caution with potent inhibitors of cytochrome P450 isoenzyme CYP3A4 (eg, ritonavir, ketoconazole); may increase mometasone serum concentrations and result in systemic corticosteroid effects.

Adverse Reactions Also see individual agents.

Central nervous system: Headache

Respiratory: Nasopharyngitis, sinusitis, voice disorder

Rare but important or life-threatening: Anaphylactoid reaction, anaphylaxis, angina pectoris, angioedema, atrial fibrillation, cardiac arrhythmia, exacerbation of asthma, hyperglycemia, hypertension, hypokalemia, hypotension (including severe), increased blood pressure, hypersensitivity reaction, oral candidiasis, prolonged Q-T interval on ECG, tachyarrhythmia, ventricular premature contractions

Drug Interactions

Metabolism/Transport Effects Refer to individual components.

Avoid Concomitant Use

Avoid concomitant use of Mometasone and Formoterol with any of the following: Aldesleukin; Beta-Blockers (Nonselective); Highest Risk QTc-Prolonging Agents; Iobenguane I 123; Ivabradine; Long-Acting Beta2-Agonists; Mifepristone

Increased Effect/Toxicity

Mometasone and Formoterol may increase the levels/effects of: Amphotericin B; Atosiban; Deferasirox; Highest Risk QTc-Prolonging Agents; Long-Acting Beta2-Agonists; Loop Diuretics; Moderate Risk QTc-Prolonging Agents; Sympathomimetics; Thiazide Diuretics

The levels/effects of Mometasone and Formoterol may be increased by: AtoMOXetine; Caffeine and Caffeine Containing Products; Cannabinoid-Containing Products; CYP3A4 Inhibitors (Strong); Inhalational Anesthetics; Ivabradine; Linezolid; MAO Inhibitors; Mifepristone; QTc-Prolonging Agents (Indeterminate Risk and Risk Modifying); Telaprevir; Theophylline Derivatives; Tricyclic Antidepressants

Decreased Effect

Mometasone and Formoterol may decrease the levels/effects of: Aldesleukin; Antidiabetic Agents; Corticorelin; Hyaluronidase; Iobenguane I 123; Telaprevir

The levels/effects of Mometasone and Formoterol may be decreased by: Beta-Blockers (Beta1 Selective); Beta-Blockers (Nonselective); Betahistine

Stability Store at room temperature of 20°C to 25°C (68°F to 77°F); excursions permitted to 15°C to 30°C (59°F to 86°F). Do not puncture, incinerate, or store near heat or open flame; exposure to temperatures above 120°F may cause bursting. Discard inhaler after the labeled number of inhalations have been used.

Mechanism of Action Formoterol relaxes bronchial smooth muscle by selective action on beta$_2$ receptors with little effect on heart rate. Formoterol has a long-acting effect.

Mometasone is a corticosteroid which controls the rate of protein synthesis, depresses the migration of polymorphonuclear leukocytes/fibroblasts, and reverses capillary permeability and lysosomal stabilization at the cellular level to prevent or control inflammation.

Pharmacokinetics (Adult data unless noted) See individual agents.

Dosing: Usual Oral inhalation: **Asthma, maintenance treatment:** Initial dose based on previous corticosteroid dosage.

Children and Adolescents ≥12 years:

Previous medium dose inhaled corticosteroids: Mometasone 100 mcg/formoterol 5 mcg (Dulera® 100 mcg/5 mcg): 2 inhalations twice daily; maximum daily dose: 4 inhalations/day. In patients not adequately controlled on the lower combination dose following 2 weeks of therapy, consider the higher dose combination.

Previous high dose inhaled corticosteroids: Mometasone 200 mcg/formoterol 5 mcg (Dulera® 200 mcg/5 mcg): 2 inhalations twice daily; maximum daily dose: 4 inhalations/day

Adults: Dulera® 100 mcg/5 mcg, Dulera® 200 mcg/5 mcg: 2 inhalations twice daily. Do not exceed 4 inhalations/day. In patients not adequately controlled on the lower combination dose following 2 weeks of therapy, consider the higher dose combination.

Dosing adjustment in hepatic impairment: Mometasone systemic exposure appears to increase with increasing extent of impairment; however, there is no dosage adjustment recommended in the manufacturer labeling.

Administration Prior to first use, inhaler must be primed by releasing 4 test sprays into the air; shake well before each spray. Inhaler must be reprimed if not used for >5 days. Shake well before each use. Rinse mouth after each use. Discard inhaler after the labeled number of inhalations have been used.

Monitoring Parameters Pulmonary function tests, check mucous membranes for signs of fungal infection; monitor growth in pediatric patients; serum glucose and serum potassium

Dosage Forms Excipient information presented when available (limited, particularly for generics); consult specific product labeling.

Aerosol, for oral inhalation:

Dulera®: Mometasone furoate 100 mcg and formoterol fumarate dihydrate 5 mcg per inhalation (8.8 g) [60 metered actuations]

Dulera®: Mometasone furoate 100 mcg and formoterol fumarate dihydrate 5 mcg per inhalation (13 g) [120 metered actuations]

Dulera®: Mometasone furoate 200 mcg and formoterol fumarate dihydrate 5 mcg per inhalation (8.8 g) [60 metered actuations]

Dulera®: Mometasone furoate 200 mcg and formoterol fumarate dihydrate 5 mcg per inhalation (13 g) [120 metered actuations]

References

National Asthma Education and Prevention Program (NAEPP), "Expert Panel Report 3, Guidelines for the Diagnosis and Management of Asthma," *Clinical Practice Guidelines,* National Institutes of Health, National Heart, Lung, and Blood Institute, NIH Publication No. 08-4051, prepublication 2007. Available at http://www.nhlbi.nih.gov/guidelines/asthma/asthgdln.htm

◆ **Mometasone Furoate** *see* Mometasone (Nasal) *on page 1433*

◆ **Mometasone Furoate** *see* Mometasone (Oral Inhalation) *on page 1432*

◆ **Mometasone Furoate** *see* Mometasone (Topical) *on page 1435*

◆ **Monacolin K** *see* Lovastatin *on page 1286*

◆ **Monicure (Can)** *see* Fluconazole *on page 877*

◆ **Monistat® (Can)** *see* Miconazole (Topical) *on page 1410*

◆ **Monistat® 3 (Can)** *see* Miconazole (Topical) *on page 1410*

◆ **Monoclate-P®** *see* Antihemophilic Factor (Human) *on page 170*

◆ **Monodox** *see* Doxycycline *on page 721*

◆ **Mononine** *see* Factor IX (Human) *on page 835*

◆ **Monopril** *see* Fosinopril *on page 938*

Montelukast (mon te LOO kast)

Medication Safety Issues

Sound-alike/look-alike issues:

Singulair® may be confused with Oralair™, SINEquan®

Brand Names: U.S. Singulair

Brand Names: Canada Apo-Montelukast; Auro-Montelukast; Auro-Montelukast Chewable Tablets; Dom-Montelukast; Dom-Montelukast FC; Jamp-Montelukast; Mar-Montelukast; Mint-Montelukast; Montelukast Sodium Tablets; Mylan-Montelukast; PMS-Montelukast; PMS-Montelukast FC; RAN-Montelukast; Sandoz-Montelukast; Sandoz-Montelukast Granules; Singulair; Teva-Montelukast

Therapeutic Category Antiasthmatic; Leukotriene Receptor Antagonist

Generic Availability (U.S.) Yes

Use Prophylaxis and chronic treatment of asthma (FDA approved in ages ≥12 months and adults); relief of symptoms of seasonal allergic rhinitis (FDA approved in ages ≥2 years and adults) and perennial allergic rhinitis (FDA approved in ages ≥6 months and adults); prevention of exercise-induced bronchoconstriction (FDA approved in ages ≥6 years and adults); has also been used as adjunct therapy for asthma exacerbation

Pregnancy Risk Factor B

Pregnancy Considerations Adverse events have not been observed in animal reproduction studies. Structural defects have been reported in neonates exposed to montelukast *in utero*; however, a specific pattern and relationship to montelukast has not been established. Based on available data, an increased risk of teratogenic effects has not been observed with montelukast use in pregnancy (Bakhireva, 2007; Nelsen, 2012; Sarkar, 2009). Uncontrolled asthma is associated with adverse events on pregnancy (increased risk of perinatal mortality, pre-eclampsia, preterm birth, low birth weight infants). Montelukast may be considered for use in women who had a favorable response prior to becoming pregnant; however, initiating a leukotriene receptor antagonist during pregnancy is an alternative (but not preferred) treatment option for mild persistent asthma (NAEPP, 2005).

Breast-Feeding Considerations It is not known if montelukast is excreted into breast milk. The manufacturer recommends that caution be exercised when administering montelukast to nursing women.

Contraindications Hypersensitivity to montelukast or any component

Warnings Montelukast is not indicated for use in the reversal of bronchospasm in acute asthma attacks, including status asthmaticus; therapy with montelukast can be continued during acute exacerbations. A gradual reduction of inhaled corticosteroid therapy may be appropriate after beginning montelukast therapy; clinical monitoring and caution are recommended as montelukast is not a substitute for inhaled corticosteroid therapy. Montelukast will not interrupt bronchoconstrictor response to aspirin or other NSAIDs in susceptible individuals; patients with known aspirin sensitivity should continue to avoid these agents. Rare cases of systemic eosinophilia, sometimes presenting with clinical features of vasculitis (consistent with Churg-Strauss syndrome), have been reported; these reactions may also be associated with a reduction in oral corticosteroid dosage; a causal association with montelukast has not been established.

Postmarketing reports of behavioral changes including agitation, aggression, anxiousness, depression, disorientation, hallucinations, inattention, insomnia, irritability, memory impairment, somnambulism, suicidal thinking and behavior, and tremor have been observed in pediatric and adult patients. In a retrospective analysis performed by the manufacturer, the incidence of serious behavior-related events was rare (Philip, 2009); monitor and assess patients for behavioral changes; if occur, consider risks and benefits of continued therapy. Patients should be instructed to notify prescriber if behavioral changes occur.

Precautions Use caution with concomitant administration of potent cytochrome P450 enzyme inducers, such as phenobarbital or rifampin. Chewable tablets contain aspartame which is metabolized to phenylalanine and must be avoided (or used with caution) in patients with phenylketonuria. Some products may contain lactose; avoid use in patient with galactose intolerance, Lapp lactase deficiency, or glucose-galactose malabsorption. Montelukast should not be used to treat exercise-induced bronchoconstriction if patient already on montelukast therapy for another indication (eg, chronic asthma).

Adverse Reactions

Children ≥15 years and Adults:
Central nervous system: Dizziness, fatigue, fever, headache
Dermatologic: Skin rash
Gastrointestinal: Dyspepsia, gastroenteritis, toothache
Hepatic: Increased serum ALT, increased serum AST
Neuromuscular & skeletal: Weakness
Respiratory: Cough, epistaxis, nasal congestion, sinusitis, upper respiratory tract infection

Children 2 to ≤14 years:
Central nervous system: Fever, headache
Dermatologic: Dermatitis, eczema, skin rash, urticaria
Gastrointestinal: Abdominal pain, dyspepsia, gastroenteritis, nausea
Infection: Influenza, varicella, viral infection
Ophthalmic: Conjunctivitis
Otic: Otalgia, otitis
Respiratory: Laryngitis, pharyngitis, pneumonia, rhinorrhea, sinusitis, upper respiratory tract infection

Children 6 to 23 months:
Respiratory: Cough, otitis media, pharyngitis, rhinitis, tonsillitis, upper respiratory tract infection, wheezing

Rare but important or life-threatening: Anaphylaxis, angioedema, Churg-Strauss syndrome, depression, disorientation, eosinophilia (systemic), eosinophilic pneumonitis, erythema multiforme, erythema nodosum, hallucination, hepatic eosinophilic infiltration, hepatitis (mixed pattern, hepatocellular, and cholestatic), hypersensitivity, insomnia, memory impairment, pancreatitis, paresthesia, seizure, somnambulism, Stevens-Johnson syndrome, suicidal ideation, suicidal tendencies, thrombocytopenia, toxic epidermal necrolysis, vasculitis

Drug Interactions

Metabolism/Transport Effects Substrate of CYP2C9 (major), CYP3A4 (major); **Note:** Assignment of Major/Minor substrate status based on clinically relevant drug interaction potential; **Inhibits** CYP2C8 (weak), CYP2C9 (weak)

Avoid Concomitant Use There are no known interactions where it is recommended to avoid concomitant use.

Increased Effect/Toxicity

The levels/effects of Montelukast may be increased by: Ceritinib; CYP2C9 Inhibitors (Moderate); CYP2C9 Inhibitors (Strong); Mifepristone

Decreased Effect

The levels/effects of Montelukast may be decreased by: Bosentan; CYP2C9 Inducers (Strong); CYP3A4 Inducers (Strong); Dabrafenib; Deferasirox; Mitotane; Peginterferon Alfa-2b; Siltuximab; St Johns Wort; Tocilizumab

Stability Store at 25°C (77°F); excursions permitted to 15°C to 30°C (59°F to 86°F). Protect from moisture and light; granules must be administered within 15 minutes of opening the packet.

Mechanism of Action Selective leukotriene receptor antagonist that inhibits the cysteinyl leukotriene receptor. Cysteinyl leukotrienes and leukotriene receptor occupation have been correlated with the pathophysiology of asthma, including airway edema, smooth muscle contraction, and altered cellular activity associated with the inflammatory process, which contribute to the signs and symptoms of asthma. Cysteinyl leukotrienes are also released from the nasal mucosa following allergen exposure leading to symptoms associated with allergic rhinitis (Jarvis, 2000).

Pharmacokinetics (Adult data unless noted)
Absorption: Rapid
Distribution: V_d: Adults: 8-11 L
Protein binding: >99%
Metabolism: Extensive by cytochrome P450 3A4 and 2C9
Bioavailability: Tablet:
  5 mg: 63% to 73%
  10 mg: 64%
Time to peak serum concentration: Tablet:
  4 mg: 2 hours
  5 mg: 2-2.5 hours
  10 mg: 3-4 hours
Elimination: Exclusively via bile; <0.2% excreted in urine

Dosing: Usual

Infants, Children, and Adolescents:
Allergic rhinitis: Oral:
  6 months to 5 years: 4 mg once daily
  6-14 years: 5 mg once daily
  ≥15 years: 10 mg once daily
Asthma, chronic treatment and prophylaxis: Oral:
  12 months to 5 years: 4 mg once daily
  6-14 years: 5 mg once daily
  ≥15 years: 10 mg once daily
Asthma, exacerbation (acute), adjunct therapy: Limited data available: Oral: Children 2-5 years: 4 mg/dose; in a double-blind, placebo-controlled trial of 52 children with acute asthma exacerbation, a single dose of montelukast (4 mg) with concomitant short-acting beta$_2$-agonist (salbutamol) showed lower respiratory rate and improved pulmonary indices compared to placebo (Harmanci, 2006)
Bronchoconstriction, exercise-induced; prevention: Oral: Administer dose at least 2 hours prior to exercise; additional doses should not be administered within 24 hours. Daily administration to prevent exercise-induced bronchospasm has not been evaluated.
  Children and Adolescents 6-14 years: Chewable tablet: 5 mg/dose
  Adolescents ≥15 years: Tablet: 10 mg/dose
Adults:
Asthma, allergic seasonal or perennial rhinitis: Oral: 10 mg once daily
Bronchoconstriction, exercise-induced (prevention): Oral: 10 mg at least 2 hours prior to exercise; additional doses should not be administered within 24 hours. Daily administration to prevent exercise-induced bronchoconstriction has not been evaluated.

Dosing adjustment in renal impairment: No adjustment necessary.

Dosing adjustment in hepatic impairment:
Mild to moderate impairment: No dosage adjustment necessary.
Severe impairment: There are no dosage adjustments provided in the manufacturer labeling; has not been studied.

Administration Oral: When treating asthma, administer dose in the evening. Patients with allergic rhinitis may individualize administration time (morning or evening).

Patients with both asthma and allergic rhinitis should take their dose in the evening.

Granules: May be administered directly into the mouth or mixed in cold or room temperature soft foods; based on stability studies, only applesauce, mashed carrots, rice, and ice cream should be used; granules are not intended to be dissolved in liquid (other than breast milk or infant formula) and must be administered within 15 minutes of opening the packet; liquids may be taken subsequent to administration.

Monitoring Parameters Pulmonary function tests (FEV-1), improvement in asthma symptoms, behavioral effects

Additional Information Recent studies of montelukast use in acute asthma and RSV bronchiolitis have shown promising results. Pulmonary function tests improved significantly in adult patients receiving a single dose (10 mg) montelukast along with I.V. prednisolone at the onset of an acute asthma exacerbation (Cylly, 2003). Pediatric patients with RSV positive bronchiolitis receiving daily montelukast demonstrated fewer symptoms when compared with placebo treated controls (Bisgaard, 2003).

Dosage Forms Excipient information presented when available (limited, particularly for generics); consult specific product labeling.

Packet, Oral:
Singulair: 4 mg (30 ea)
Generic: 4 mg (1 ea, 30 ea)
Tablet, Oral:
Singulair: 10 mg
Generic: 10 mg
Tablet Chewable, Oral:
Singulair: 4 mg [contains aspartame]
Singulair: 4 mg [contains aspartame; cherry flavor]
Singulair: 5 mg [contains aspartame]
Singulair: 5 mg [contains aspartame; cherry flavor]
Generic: 4 mg, 5 mg

References

Bakhireva LN, Jones KL, Schatz M, et al, "Organization of Teratology Information Specialists Collaborative Research Group. Safety of Leukotriene Receptor Antagonists in Pregnancy," *J Allergy Clin Immunol*, 2007, 119(3):618-25.

Bisgaard H, "A Randomized Trial of Montelukast in Respiratory Syncytial Virus Postbronchiolitis," *Am J Respir Crit Care Med*, 2003, 167 (3):379-83.

Cylly A, Kara A, Ozdemir T, et al, "Effects of Oral Montelukast on Airway Function in Acute Asthma," *Respir Med*, 2003, 97(5):533-6.

Global Strategy for Asthma Management and Prevention, Global Initiative for Asthma (GINA), 2011. Available at http://www.ginasthma.org

"Guidelines for the Diagnosis and Management of Asthma. NAEPP Expert Panel Report 3," 2007. Available at http://www.nhlbi.nih.gov/guidelines/asthma/asthgdln.pdf

Harmanci K, Bakirtas A, Turktas I, et al, "Oral Montelukast Treatment of Preschool-Aged Children With Acute Asthma," *Ann Allergy Asthma Immunol*, 2006, 96(5):731-5.

"National Asthma Education and Prevention Program. Expert Panel Report: Guidelines for the Diagnosis and Management of Asthma Update on Selected Topics – 2002," *J Allergy Clin Immunol*, 2002, 110 (5 Suppl):S141-219.

National Asthma Education and Prevention Program (NAEPP) Working Group Report on "Managing Asthma During Pregnancy: Recommendations for Pharmacologic Treatment," National Institutes of Health, National Heart, Lung, and Blood Institute, NIH Publication No. 05-5236, March 2005. Available at http://www.nhlbi.nih.gov/health/prof/lung/asthma/astpreg/astpreg_full.pdf

Nelsen LM, Shields KE, Cunningham ML, et al, "Congenital Malformations Among Infants Born to Women Receiving Montelukast, Inhaled Corticosteroids, and Other Asthma Medications," *J Allergy Clin Immunol*, 2012, 129(1):251-4.

Philip G, Hustad CM, Malice MP, et al, "Analysis of Behavior-Related Adverse Experiences in Clinical Trials of Montelukast," *J Allergy Clin Immunol*, 2009, 124(4):699-706.

Philip G, Hustad C, Noonan G, et al, "Reports of Suicidality in Clinical Trials of Montelukast," *J Allergy Clin Immunol*, 2009a, 124(4):691-6.

Sarkar M, Koren G, Kalra S, et al, "Montelukast Use During Pregnancy: A Multicentre, Prospective, Comparative Study of Infant Outcomes," *Eur J Clin Pharmacol* 2009, 65(12);1259-64.

◆ **Montelukast Sodium** *see* Montelukast *on page 1438*

◆ **Montelukast Sodium Tablets (Can)** *see* Montelukast *on page 1438*

◆ **MoreDophilus® [OTC]** *see* Lactobacillus *on page 1191*

◆ **Morgidox** *see* Doxycycline *on page 721*

Morphine (Systemic) (MOR feen)

Medication Safety Issues

Sound-alike/look-alike issues:
Morphine may be confused with HYDROmorphone, methadone
Morphine sulfate may be confused with magnesium sulfate
Kadian may be confused with Kapidex [DSC]
MS Contin may be confused with OxyCONTIN
MSO_4 and MS are error-prone abbreviations (mistaken as magnesium sulfate)
AVINza may be confused with Evista, INVanz
Roxanol may be confused with OxyFast, Roxicet, Roxicodone

High alert medication:
The Institute for Safe Medication Practices (ISMP) includes this medication (I.V. formulation) among its list of drug classes which have a heightened risk of causing significant patient harm when used in error.

Other safety concerns:
Use care when prescribing and/or administering morphine solutions. These products are available in different concentrations. Always prescribe dosage in mg; **not** by volume (mL).
Use caution when selecting a morphine formulation for use in neurologic infusion pumps (eg, Medtronic delivery systems). The product should be appropriately labeled as "preservative-free" and suitable for intraspinal use via continuous infusion. In addition, the product should be formulated in a pH range that is compatible with the device operation specifications.
Significant differences exist between oral and I.V. dosing. Use caution when converting from one route of administration to another.

Related Information

Medications for Which a Single Dose May Be Fatal When Ingested by a Toddler *on page 2408*
Opioid Conversion Table *on page 2242*
Oral Medications That Should Not Be Crushed or Altered *on page 2438*
Patient Information for Disposal of Unused Medications *on page 2412*
Preprocedure Sedatives in Children *on page 2402*

Brand Names: U.S. Astramorph; AVINza; Duramorph; Infumorph 200; Infumorph 500; Kadian; MS Contin

Brand Names: Canada Doloral; Kadian; M-Eslon; M.O.S. 10; M.O.S. 20; M.O.S. 30; M.O.S.-SR; M.O.S.-Sulfate; Morphine Extra Forte Injection; Morphine Forte Injection; Morphine HP; Morphine LP Epidural; Morphine SR; Morphine-EPD; MS Contin; MS Contin SRT; MS-IR; Novo-Morphine SR; PMS-Morphine Sulfate SR; ratio-Morphine; ratio-Morphine SR; Sandoz-Morphine SR; Statex; Teva-Morphine SR

Therapeutic Category Analgesic, Narcotic

Generic Availability (U.S.) Yes

Use

Oral:
Immediate release formulations (oral solution and tablets): Management of moderate to severe acute and chronic pain (FDA approved in ages ≥18 years and adults); has also been used for treatment of neonatal abstinence syndrome, iatrogenic opioid withdrawal, and palliative care management of dyspnea
Controlled and extended release products (eg, Avinza, Kadian, MS Contin): Management of moderate to

severe **chronic** pain when continuous, around-the-clock opioid analgesia is required for an extended amount of time (FDA approved in ages ≥18 years and adults); **Note:** Not intended for use as a PRN analgesic or for treatment of mild pain, acute pain, pain that is not expected to persist for an extended period of time, or for immediate postoperative pain (within 12-24 hours after surgery) unless the patient is already receiving chronic opioid therapy prior to surgery or if postoperative pain is expected to be moderate to severe and persist for an extended period of time

Parenteral:

Intravenous: Management of severe acute pain; preanes-thetic sedative [FDA approved in pediatric patients (age not specified) and adults]; has also been used for management of hypercyanotic spells associate with tetralogy of Fallot; and for palliative care management of dyspnea (including nebulization)

Epidural (at the lumbar level): Management of pain unresponsive to nonopioid analgesics (Astramorph/PF, Duramorph: FDA approved in adults); treatment of intractable chronic pain as an epidural infusion via microinfusion device (Infumorph: FDA approved in adults)

Intrathecal (at lumbar level): Management of pain unre-sponsive to nonopioid analgesics (Astramorph/PF, Duramorph: FDA approved in adults); treatment of intractable chronic pain as a continuous infusion via microinfusion device (Infumorph: FDA approved in adults)

Rectal: Suppositories: Management of severe acute and chronic pain (FDA approved in adults)

Medication Guide Available Yes

Pregnancy Risk Factor C

Pregnancy Considerations Adverse events have been observed in some animal reproduction studies. Morphine crosses the human placenta. The frequency of congenital malformations has not been reported to be greater than expected in children from mothers treated with morphine during pregnancy. However, following *in utero* exposure, infants may exhibit withdrawal, decreased brain volume (reversible), small size, decreased ventilatory response to CO_2, and increased risk of sudden infant death syndrome.

Morphine sulfate injection may be used for the manage-ment of pain during labor (ACOG, 2002); however, some manufacturers specifically contraindicate use of the injec-tion during labor when a premature birth is anticipated. When used for pain relief during labor, opioids may tem-porarily affect the heart rate of the fetus. Morphine injection may also be used to treat pain following delivery (ACOG, 2002).

If chronic opioid exposure occurs in pregnancy, adverse events in the newborn (including withdrawal) may occur; monitoring of the neonate is recommended. The minimum effective dose should be used if opioids are needed (Chou, 2009). Neonatal abstinence syndrome following opioid exposure may present with autonomic (eg, fever, temper-ature instability), gastrointestinal (eg, diarrhea, vomiting, poor feeding/weight gain), or neurologic (eg, high-pitched crying, increased muscle tone, irritability, seizure, tremor) symptoms (Dow, 2012; Hudak, 2012).

Breast-Feeding Considerations Morphine concentrates in breast milk, with a milk to plasma AUC ratio of 2.5:1. Detectable serum levels of morphine can be found in infants following morphine administration to nursing moth-ers.

Parenteral opioids used during labor have the potential to interfere with a newborn's natural reflex to nurse within the first few hours after birth. Morphine is recommended as an analgesic in nursing women due to the limited amounts found in breast milk and poor oral bioavailability in nursing infants. Nursing infants exposed to large doses of opioids should be monitored for apnea and sedation (Montgom-ery, 2012).

Treatment of the mother with single doses of morphine is not expected to cause detrimental effects in nursing infants. Breast-feeding following chronic use or in neo-nates with hepatic or renal dysfunction may lead to higher levels of morphine in the infant and a risk of adverse effects (Spigset, 2000).

The manufacturers of extended release products note that due to the potential for serious adverse reactions in the nursing infant, a decision should be made whether to discontinue nursing or to discontinue the drug, taking into account the importance of treatment to the mother.

Contraindications Hypersensitivity to morphine sulfate or any component; severe respiratory depression or respira-tory depression in a setting without resuscitative equip-ment or appropriate monitoring; acute or severe asthma

Additional contraindications:

Oral:

Immediate release tablets, solution: Hypercarbia; para-lytic ileus (known or suspected)

Controlled/extended release capsules or tablets (eg, Avinza, Kadian, MS Contin): Paralytic ileus (known or suspected)

Parenteral:

Injectable formulations: Heart failure due to chronic lung disease, cardiac arrhythmias, increased intracranial or cerebrospinal pressure, head injuries, brain tumor, acute alcoholism, delirium tremens; convulsive states such as those occurring with status epilepticus, teta-nus, and strychnine poisoning

Epidural/intrathecal: Astramorph/PF, Duramorph, Infu-morph: Usual contraindications related to neuraxial analgesia apply (eg, presence of infection at injection microinfusion site, concomitant anticoagulant therapy, uncontrolled bleeding diathesis); Astramorph/PF, Duramorph: Upper airway obstruction

Suppository: Severe CNS depression, heart failure due to chronic lung disease, cardiac arrhythmias, increased intracranial or cerebrospinal pressure, head injuries, brain tumor, acute alcoholism, delirium tremens, seizure disorder, postoperative use following biliary tract sur-gery, suspected surgical abdomen, surgical anastomo-sis, concurrent use or within 2 weeks of MAO inhibitors

Warnings An opioid-containing analgesic regimen should be individualized to each patient's needs and the optimal analgesic dose varies widely among patients; dose may be based upon the type of pain (acute versus chronic), route of administration, degree of patient's tolerance for opioids (naive vs chronic user), age, weight, and medical condi-tion.

Respiratory depression may occur even with therapeutic dosages with all morphine products and may be fatal if unrecognized. With controlled/extended release products, risk of respiratory depression is highest during initiation of therapy and dose titration **[Controlled/extended release products: U.S. Boxed Warning]**; should only be pre-scribed by physician experienced in management of chronic pain and patients should be monitored closely. Use any morphine product with extreme caution in elderly, cachectic, or debilitated patients and patients with respira-tory diseases, including asthma, emphysema, COPD, cor pulmonale, hypoxia, hypercapnia, preexisting respiratory depression, significantly decreased respiratory reserve, other obstructive pulmonary disease, kyphoscoliosis, or other skeletal disorder which may alter respiratory function; there is a greater potential for critical respiratory depres-sion in these patients. Neonates and infants <3 months of age, especially if premature, are more susceptible to respiratory depression and/or apnea; use with caution; ▶

lower doses are recommended in this age group compared to older pediatric patients.

Morphine may cause CNS depression which may impair physical or mental abilities; patients must be cautioned about performing tasks which require mental alertness (eg, operating machinery or driving). Effects may be potentiated when used with other sedative drugs including ethanol. Morphine may exaggerate elevated intracranial pressure (ICP); use with extreme caution in patients with head injury, increased ICP, or other intracranial lesions. Severe hypotension may occur; use with caution in patients with circulatory shock, hypovolemia, impaired myocardial function, or those receiving drugs which compromise vasomotor tone or exaggerate hypotensive effects (including phenothiazines or general anesthetics). Duramorph and Astromorph should not be used if patient's ability to maintain blood pressure is compromised. Orthostatic hypotension and syncope may occur in ambulatory patients. Morphine may obscure diagnosis or clinical course of patients with acute abdominal conditions.

Physical and psychological dependence may occur. Healthcare providers should be alert to problems of abuse, misuse, and diversion **[Controlled and extended release products: U.S. Boxed Warning]**; use with caution in patients with a history of drug abuse or acute alcoholism; potential for drug dependency exists. Abrupt discontinuation after prolonged use may result in withdrawal symptoms or seizures; concurrent use of agonist/antagonist analgesics (eg, pentazocine, nalbuphine, and butorphanol) may precipitate withdrawal symptoms and/or reduce the analgesic efficacy in patients following prolonged therapy with a mu opioid agonist such as morphine. Neonates born to women physically dependent on opioids will also be physically dependent and may experience respiratory difficulties or opioid withdrawal symptoms [neonatal abstinence syndrome (NAS)]. Onset, duration, and severity of NAS depend upon the drug used (maternal), duration of use, maternal dose, and rate of drug elimination by the newborn. Symptoms of neonatal abstinence syndrome may include excessive crying, high-pitched cry, diarrhea, fever, hyper-reflexia, irritability, tremors, vomiting, or failure to gain weight. Opioid withdrawal syndrome in the neonate, unlike in adults, may be life-threatening and should be promptly treated.

Controlled and extended release products are not interchangeable. When determining a generic equivalent or switching from one extended release product to another, a thorough understanding of the pharmacokinetic properties is important in determining the proper generic equivalent or proper dose of the other extended release product (review of the manufacturer's label may be necessary). Controlled and extended release products are indicated for the treatment of moderate to severe chronic pain and are not intended for PRN use. Controlled release tablets (eg, MS Contin) in 100 mg and 200 mg strengths and extended release capsules (Avinza, Kadian) in ≥90 mg strengths are for use in opioid-tolerant patients only (ie, adults taking ≥60 mg/day of morphine or equivalent for ≥1 week); fatal respiratory depression may occur if these products or their contents are administered to patients who are not tolerant to high-dose opioids. Patients should be warned not to let others use these products, since severe adverse effects, including death, may result. Fatal overdose of morphine can result from accidental ingestion, especially in children **[Controlled/extended release products: U.S. Boxed Warning]**.

Do not crush, break, chew, or dissolve controlled and extended release products **[U.S. Boxed Warning]**; a toxic or potentially fatal dose of morphine may be rapidly released. Do not administer Avinza with alcoholic beverages or ethanol-containing prescription or nonprescription products, which may disrupt extended release characteristics of the product **[U.S. Boxed Warning]**, causing a rapid release of morphine and potentially fatal overdose. Avinza capsules contain fumaric acid; dangerous quantities of fumaric acid may be ingested when >1600 mg/day of Avinza is used; serious renal toxicity may occur above the maximum dose.

Parenteral products are designed for administration by specific routes (I.V., intrathecal, epidural); use caution when prescribing, dispensing, or administering to ensure formulations used only by intended route(s). Only physicians experienced in the techniques and familiar with the clinical management of the adverse effects of epidural and intrathecal drug administration should administer drugs via the intraspinal route. Prior to administration, patients should be evaluated for contraindications for epidural or intrathecal injection (eg, anticoagulant therapy, bleeding, diathesis). When used as an epidural or intrathecal injection, monitor for delayed sedation and respiratory depression. Due to the risk of severe and/or sustained cardiopulmonary depressant effects of Astramorph/PF, Duramorph, and Infumorph, they must be administered in a fully equipped (ie, for resuscitation) and staffed environment **[U.S. Boxed Warning]**. Naloxone injection should be immediately available. Patient should remain in this environment for at least 24 hours following the initial dose. For patients receiving Infumorph via microinfusion device, patient may be observed, as appropriate, for the first several days after catheter implantation. Thoracic epidural administration has been shown to dramatically increase the risk of early and late respiratory depression. Infumorph should only be used in microinfusion devices; not for I.V., I.M., or SubQ administration or for single-dose administration. Improper or erroneous substitution of Infumorph for regular Duramorph is likely to result in serious overdosage, leading to seizures, respiratory depression and possibly a fatal outcome **[U.S. Boxed Warning]**. Inflammatory masses (eg, granulomas), some resulting in severe neurologic impairment have occurred when receiving Infumorph via indwelling intrathecal catheter; monitor carefully for new neurologic signs/symptoms. Some adverse effects are more common following epidural or intrathecal administration compared to other routes (eg, I.V. or oral); these may include: Headache, pruritus, urinary retention (may be prolonged up to 20 hours), and urinary tract spasm. Due to fewer potential adverse effects, the epidural route is preferred over the intrathecal route; intrathecal route is associated with a higher incidence of respiratory depression. Tolerance to morphine and increased epidural or intrathecal dosage requirements may occur; patients may require hospitalization and detoxification. Seizures may occur with high doses of intraspinal morphine. Myoclonic spasm of the lower extremities has been reported in adults receiving high doses of intrathecal morphine.

Accidental dermal exposure to Astramorph/PF, Duramorph, or Infumorph should be rinsed with water and contaminated clothing should be removed **[U.S. Boxed Warning]**. Prior to administration, inspect parenteral products for particulate matter and discoloration if possible. Do not use if color is darker than pale yellow or if discolored.

Concentrated oral solution (20 mg/mL) should only be used in opioid-tolerant patients (adults taking ≥60 mg/day of morphine or equivalent for ≥1 week). Precautions should be taken to avoid confusion between morphine solutions of different concentrations and dosing unit confusion (mg vs mL); the intended dose should be clearly represented as milligram (mg) of morphine not volume (mL) and additionally, the intended product concentration to be dispensed should be identified **[U.S. Boxed Warning]**. Keep morphine oral solutions out of the reach of children **[U.S.**

Boxed Warning]; a fatal overdose may result from accidental ingestion.

Injection may contain sodium metabisulfite which may cause allergic reactions in susceptible individuals; oral solution may contain sodium benzoate; benzoic acid (benzoate) is a metabolite of benzyl alcohol; large amounts of benzyl alcohol (≥99 mg/kg/day) have been associated with a potentially fatal toxicity ("gasping syndrome") in neonates; the "gasping syndrome" consists of metabolic acidosis, respiratory distress, gasping respirations, CNS dysfunction (including convulsions, intracranial hemorrhage), hypotension, and cardiovascular collapse; avoid use of morphine sulfate products containing sodium benzoate in neonates; *in vitro* and animal studies have shown that benzoate displaces bilirubin from protein binding sites.

Precautions Use with caution in patients with hypersensitivity reactions to other phenanthrene derivative opioid agonists (codeine, hydrocodone, hydromorphone, levorphanol, oxycodone, oxymorphone). Avoid the use of morphine in patients with CNS depression or coma as these patients are susceptible to intracranial effects of CO_2 retention. Use with caution in patients with biliary tract disease or acute pancreatitis; morphine may cause spasm of the sphincter of Oddi. Use with caution in patients with Addison's disease; toxic psychosis; seizure disorders; acute alcoholism; delirium tremens; hypothyroidism; severe liver, pulmonary, or renal impairment; urethral stricture; prostatic hypertrophy; or seizures. Use caution when combining with other CNS depressants (eg, centrally acting antiemetics, general anesthetics, phenothiazines, sedative-hypnotics) as there may be additive CNS effects. If combined therapy is needed, consider reducing the dose of one or both agents.

I.V., epidural, and intrathecal morphine readily pass into the fetal circulation and may result in respiratory depression in the newborn when administered during labor and delivery; resuscitative equipment should be available for the neonate to support ventilation if necessary.

Adverse Reactions Note: Individual patient differences are unpredictable. Reactions may be dose-, formulation-, and/or route-dependent.

Cardiovascular: Atrial fibrillation, bradycardia, chest pain, circulatory depression, edema, flushing, hyper-/hypotension, palpitation, peripheral edema, shock, syncope, tachycardia, vasodilation

Central nervous system: Amnesia, agitation, anxiety, apathy, apprehension, ataxia, chills, coma, confusion, delirium, depression, dizziness, dream abnormalities, drowsiness (tolerance usually develops to drowsiness with regular dosing for 1-2 weeks), dysphonia, euphoria, false sense of well being, fever, hallucination, headache (following epidural or intrathecal use), hypoesthesia, insomnia, lethargy, malaise, nervousness, physical and psychological dependence, restlessness, sedation, seizure, slurred speech, somnolence, vertigo

Dermatologic: Dry skin, pruritus (may be dose related), rash, urticaria

Endocrine & metabolic: Antidiuretic hormone release, gynecomastia, hypogonadism, hypokalemia, hyponatremia, libido decreased

Gastrointestinal: Abdominal distension, anorexia, abdominal pain, biliary colic, constipation (tolerance develops very slowly if at all), diarrhea, dyspepsia, dysphagia, flatulence, gastroenteritis, GERD, GI irritation, nausea (tolerance usually develops to nausea and vomiting with chronic use), paralytic ileus, rectal disorder, taste perversion, vomiting, weight loss, xerostomia

Genitourinary: Urinary retention (may be prolonged, up to 20 hours, following epidural or intrathecal use), bladder spasm, dysuria, ejaculation abnormal, impotence, urination decreased

Hematologic: Anemia (following intrathecal use), hematocrit decreased, leukopenia, thrombocytopenia

Hepatic: Liver function tests increased

Local: Pain at injection site

Neuromuscular & skeletal: Arthralgia, back pain, bone mineral density decreased, bone pain, foot drop, gait abnormalities, myoclonus, paresthesia, rigors, skeletal muscle rigidity, tremor, weakness

Ocular: Amblyopia, conjunctivitis, eye pain, vision problems/disturbance

Renal: Oliguria

Respiratory: Asthma, atelectasis, dyspnea, hiccups, hypercapnia, hypoxia, oxygen saturation decreased, pulmonary edema (noncardiogenic), respiratory depression, rhinitis

Miscellaneous: Diaphoresis, flu-like syndrome, histamine release, infection, thirst, voice alteration, withdrawal syndrome

Rare but important or life-threatening: Amenorrhea, anaphylaxis, apnea, biliary tract spasm, blurred vision, bronchospasm, cardiac arrest, cough reflex decreased, dehydration, diplopia, disorientation, hemorrhagic urticaria, intestinal obstruction, intracranial pressure increased, laryngospasm, menstrual irregularities, miosis, myoclonus, nystagmus, paradoxical CNS stimulation, respiratory arrest, sepsis, urinary tract spasm, thermal dysregulation, toxic psychoses

Drug Interactions

Metabolism/Transport Effects Substrate of CYP2D6 (minor), P-glycoprotein; **Note:** Assignment of Major/Minor substrate status based on clinically relevant drug interaction potential

Avoid Concomitant Use

Avoid concomitant use of Morphine (Systemic) with any of the following: Azelastine (Nasal); MAO Inhibitors; Paraldehyde; Thalidomide

Increased Effect/Toxicity

Morphine (Systemic) may increase the levels/effects of: Alcohol (Ethyl); Alvimopan; Azelastine (Nasal); Buprenorphine; CNS Depressants; Desmopressin; Diuretics; Hydrocodone; Methotrimeprazine; Metyrosine; Mirtazapine; Paraldehyde; Pramipexole; ROPINIRole; Rotigotine; Selective Serotonin Reuptake Inhibitors; Thalidomide; Zolpidem

The levels/effects of Morphine (Systemic) may be increased by: Amphetamines; Anticholinergic Agents; Antipsychotic Agents (Phenothiazines); Brimonidine (Topical); Cannabis; Doxylamine; Dronabinol; Droperidol; HydrOXYzine; Kava Kava; Magnesium Sulfate; MAO Inhibitors; Methotrimeprazine; Nabilone; Perampanel; P-glycoprotein/ABCB1 Inhibitors; Rufinamide; Sodium Oxybate; Succinylcholine; Tapentadol; Tetrahydrocannabinol

Decreased Effect

Morphine (Systemic) may decrease the levels/effects of: Clopidogrel; Pegvisomant

The levels/effects of Morphine (Systemic) may be decreased by: Ammonium Chloride; Mixed Agonist / Antagonist Opioids; Naltrexone; Peginterferon Alfa-2b; P-glycoprotein/ABCB1 Inducers; Rifamycin Derivatives

Food Interactions

Ethanol: Alcoholic beverages or ethanol-containing products may disrupt extended release formulation resulting in rapid release of entire morphine dose. Management: Avoid alcohol. **Do not administer Avinza with alcoholic beverages or ethanol-containing prescription or nonprescription products.**

Food: Administration of oral morphine solution with food may increase bioavailability (ie, a report of 34% increase in morphine AUC when morphine oral solution followed a high-fat meal). The bioavailability of Avinza, MS Contin, or Kadian does not appear to be affected by food. Management: Take consistently with or without meals.

Stability

Parenteral:

Injection (vials, prefilled syringes): Store at 20°C to 25°C (68°F to 77°F); protect from light. Degradation depends on pH and presence of oxygen; relatively stable in pH ≤4; darkening of solutions indicates degradation.

Astramorph/PF: Store in carton at 20°C to 25°C (65°F to 77°F); protect from light; do not freeze. Discard unused portion of vial (vial does not contain preservative. Do not heat sterilize.

Duramorph, Infumorph: Store in carton at 20°C to 25°C (65°F to 77°F); excursions permitted to 15°C to 30°C (59°F to 86°F); protect from light; do not freeze. Discard unused portion of vial (vial does not contain preservative). Do not heat sterilize.

Oral:

Capsule, extended release (Avinza, Kadian): Store at 25°C (77°F); excursions permitted to 15°C to 30°C (59°F to 86°F). Protect from light and moisture.

Oral solution: Store at 15°C to 30°C (59°F to 86°F); protect from moisture.

Tablet, controlled release (MS Contin): Store at 25°C (77°F); excursions permitted to 15°C to 30°C (59°F to 86°F). Protect from light.

Tablet, immediate release: Store at 15°C to 30°C (59°F to 86°F); protect from moisture.

Suppositories: Refrigerate; do not freeze.

Mechanism of Action Binds to opioid receptors in the CNS, causing inhibition of ascending pain pathways, altering the perception of and response to pain; produces generalized CNS depression

Pharmacodynamics See table.

Dosage Form / Route	Analgesia	
	Peak	Duration
Tablets	1 h	3-5 h
Oral solution	1 h	3-5 h
Epidural	1 h	12-20 h
Extended release tablets	3-4 h	8-12 h
Suppository	20-60 min	3-7 h
Subcutaneous injection	50-90 min	3-5 h
I.M. injection	30-60 min	3-5 h
I.V. injection	20 min	3-5 h

Pharmacokinetics (Adult data unless noted)

Absorption: Oral: Variable

Distribution: Distributes to skeletal muscle, liver, kidneys, lungs, intestinal tract, spleen and brain

V_d, apparent:

Pediatric cancer patients (age: 1.7-18.7 years): Median: 5.2 L/kg; a significantly higher V_d was observed in children <11 years (median: 7.1 L/kg) versus >11 years (median: 4.7 L/kg) (Hunt, 1999)

Adults: 1-6 L/kg

Protein binding:

Premature Infants: <20%

Adults: 20% to 35%

Metabolism: Hepatic via glucuronide conjugation to morphine-6-glucuronide (active) and morphine-3-glucuronide (inactive)

Bioavailability: Nebulization: 5.5 ± 3.2% (Masood, 1996)

Half-life:

Preterm: 10-20 hours

Neonates: 7.6 hours (range: 4.5-13.3 hours)

Infants 1-3 months: Median: 6.2 hours (range: 5-10 hours) (McRorie, 1992)

Infants 3-6 months: Median: 4.5 hours (range: 3.8-7.3 hours) (McRorie, 1992)

Infants 6 months to Children 2.5 years: Median: 2.9 hours (range: 1.4-7.8 hours) (McRorie, 1992)

Preschool Children: 1-2 hours

Pediatric patients with sickle cell disease (age: 6-19 years): ~1.3 hours (Dampier, 1995)

Adults: Immediate release: 2-4 hours; Avinza: ~24 hours; Kadian: 11-13 hours

Elimination: Excreted unchanged in urine:

Neonates: 3% to 15%

Adults: 2% to 12%

Clearance: **Note:** In pediatric patients, adult values are reached by 6 months to 2.5 years of age (McRorie, 1992)

Preterm: 0.5-3 mL/minute/kg

Neonates 1-7 days: Median: 5.5 mL/minute/kg (range: 3.2-8.4 mL/minute/kg) (McRorie, 1992)

Neonates 8-30 days: Median: 7.4 mL/minute/kg (range: 3.4-13.8 mL/minute/kg) (McRorie, 1992)

Infants 1-3 months: Median: 10.5 mL/minute/kg (range: 9.8-20.1 mL/minute/kg) (McRorie, 1992)

Infants 3-6 months: Median: 13.9 mL/minute/kg (range: 8.3-24.1 mL/minute/kg) (McRorie, 1992)

Infants 6 months to Children 2.5 years: Median: 21.7 mL/minute/kg (range: 5.8-28.6 mL/minute/kg) (McRorie, 1992)

Preschool Children: 20-40 mL/minute/kg

Pediatric cancer patients (age: 1.7-18.7 years): Median: 23.1 mL/minute/kg; a significantly higher clearance was observed in children <11 years (median: 37.4 mL/minute/kg) versus >11 years (median: 21.9 mL/minute/kg) (Hunt, 1999)

Pediatric patients with sickle cell disease (age: 6-19 years): ~36 mL/minute/kg (range: 6-59 mL/minute/kg) (Dampier, 1995)

Adults: 20-30 mL/minute/kg

Dosing: Neonatal Doses should be titrated to appropriate effect; when changing routes of administration in chronically treated patients, please note that oral doses are approximately one-half as effective as parenteral dose; **Note: Use preservative-free formulation:**

Analgesia:

Oral: Oral solution (2 mg/mL or 4 mg/mL): 0.08 mg/kg/dose every 4-6 hours (APA, 2012)

I.M., I.V. (preferred), SubQ: Initial: 0.05-0.1 mg/kg/dose; usual frequency every 4-6 hours, although some neonates may require every 8 hour dosing; titrate carefully to effect; maximum dose: 0.1 mg/kg/dose (Anand, 2001; Hegenbarth, 2008)

Continuous I.V. infusion: Initial: 0.01 mg/kg/hour (10 mcg/kg/hour); titrate carefully to effect; maximum: 0.03 mg/kg/hour (30 mcg/kg/hour) (Anand, 2001); some have suggested a lower usual maximum infusion rate of 0.015-0.02 mg/kg/hour (15-20 mcg/kg/hour) due to decreased elimination, increased CNS sensitivity, and adverse effects; **Note:** Some centers may use slightly higher doses, especially in neonates who develop tolerance.

Endotracheal intubation, nonemergent: I.M., I.V.: 0.05-0.1 mg/kg; allow at least 5 minutes for onset of analgesia (Kumar, 2010)

Neonatal abstinence syndrome: Limited data available: Oral: Oral solution (2 mg/mL or 4 mg/mL): Initial: 0.04 mg/kg/dose every 3-4 hours; increase by 0.04 mg/kg/dose if symptoms are not controlled; maximum dose: 0.2 mg/kg/dose (Hudak, 2012); dose and weaning schedule should be individualized based on signs and symptoms of withdrawal and/or withdrawal scores; once withdrawal symptoms are controlled, maintain dose for 48-72 hours; then taper dose usually by 10% to 20% every 2-7 days (Burgos, 2009; Hudak, 2012).

Dosing: Usual Doses should be titrated to appropriate effect; when changing routes of administration in chronically treated patients, please note that oral doses are approximately one-half as effective as parenteral dose.

Infants, Children, and Adolescents:

Acute pain, severe: Note: The use of I.M. injections is no longer recommended, especially for repeated administration due to painful administration, variable absorption, and lag time to peak effect; other routes are more reliable and less painful (American Pain Society, 2008).

Infants ≤6 months, nonventilated: **Note:** Infants <3 months of age are more susceptible to respiratory depression; lower doses are recommended (American Pain Society, 2008):

Oral: Oral solution (2 mg/mL or 4 mg/mL): 0.08-0.1 mg/kg/dose every 3-4 hours (American Pain Society, 2008; Berde, 2002)

I.V.: 0.025-0.03 mg/kg/dose every 2-4 hours (American Pain Society, 2008; Berde, 2002)

Infants >6 months, Children, and Adolescents:

Oral: Immediate release tablets, oral solution (2 mg/mL or 4 mg/mL):

Patient weight <50 kg: 0.2-0.5 mg/kg/dose every 3-4 hours as needed; some experts have recommended an initial dose of 0.3 mg/kg for severe pain; usual initial maximum dose: 15-20 mg (APA, 2012; American Pain Society, 2008; Berde, 2002)

Patient weight ≥50 kg: 15-20 mg every 3-4 hours as needed (American Pain Society, 2008; Berde, 2002)

I.M., I.V., or SubQ; intermittent dosing:

Patient weight <50 kg: Initial: 0.05 mg/kg/dose; usual range: 0.1-0.2 mg/kg/dose every 2-4 hours as needed; usual maximum dose: Infants: 2 mg/dose; Children 1-6 years: 4 mg/dose; Children 7-12 years: 8 mg/dose; Adolescents: 10 mg/dose

Patient weight ≥50 kg: Initial: 5-8 mg every 2-4 hours as needed (Berde, 2002)

Continuous I.V. infusion, SubQ continuous infusion:

Patient weight <50 kg: Initial: 0.01 mg/kg/hour (10 mcg/kg/hour); titrate carefully to effect; dosage range: 0.01-0.04 mg/kg/**hour** (10-40 mcg/kg/**hour**) (APA, 2012; Friedrichsdorf, 2007; Golianu, 2000)

Patient weight ≥50 kg: 1.5 mg/**hour** (Berde, 2002)

Conversion from intermittent I.V. morphine: Administer the patient's total daily I.V. morphine dose over 24 hours as a continuous infusion; titrate dose to appropriate effect

Epidural: Astramorph/PF, Duramorph: Limited data available: **Note: Must use preservative-free formulation:**

Intermittent: 0.015-0.05 mg/kg (15-50 **mcg**/kg) (APA, 2012; Henneberg, 1993); a trial evaluating pain relief in pediatric patients after abdominal surgery (n=76; age: newborn to 13 years median age: 12 months) administered epidural morphine every 8 hours in combination with bupivacaine during the immediate postop period; most children achieved good pain relief with this regimen (Henneberg, 1993). Maximum dose: 0.1 mg/kg (100 **mcg**/kg) or 5 mg/24 hours

Continuous epidural infusion: Infants >6 months, Children, and Adolescents: 0.001-0.005 mg/kg/**hour** (1-5 **mcg**/kg/**hour**) (Suresh, 2012)

Analgesia for minor procedures/sedation: I.V.: 0.05-0.1 mg/kg/dose; administer 5 minutes before the procedure; maximum dose: 4 mg; may repeat dose in 5 minutes if necessary (Cramton, 2012; Zeltzer, 1990)

Patient-controlled analgesia (PCA), opioid-naïve: Note: All patients should receive an initial loading dose of an analgesic (to attain adequate control of pain) before starting PCA for maintenance. Adjust doses, lockouts, and limits based on required loading dose, age, state of health, and presence of opioid tolerance. Use lower end of dosing range for opioid-naïve. Assess patient and pain control at regular intervals and adjust settings if needed (American Pain Society, 2008): I.V.: Children ≥5 years and Adolescents, weighing <50 kg: **Note:** PCA has been used in children as young as 5 years of age; however, clinicians need to assess children 5-8 years of age to determine if they are able to use the PCA device correctly (American Pain Society, 2008).

Usual concentration: 1 mg/mL

Demand dose: Usual initial: 0.02 mg/kg/dose; usual range: 0.01-0.03 mg/kg/dose

Lockout: Usual initial: 5 doses/hour

Lockout interval: Range: 6-8 minutes

Usual basal rate: 0-0.03 mg/kg/hour

Children and Adolescents, weighing ≥50 kg:

Usual concentration: 1 mg/mL

Demand dose: Usual initial: 1 mg; usual range: 0.5-2.5 mg

Lockout interval: Usual initial: 6 minutes; usual range: 5-10 minutes

Chronic pain: Note: Patients taking opioids chronically may become tolerant and require doses higher than the usual dosage range to maintain the desired effect. Tolerance can be managed by appropriate dose titration. There is no optimal or maximal dose for morphine in chronic pain. The appropriate dose is one that relieves pain throughout its dosing interval without causing unmanageable side effects. Consider total daily dose, potency, prior opioid use, degree of opioid experience and tolerance, conversion from previous opioid (including opioid formulation), patient's general condition, concurrent medications, and type and severity of pain during prescribing process.

Oral: Extended/controlled release preparations: A patient's morphine requirement should be established using immediate release formulations. Conversion to long-acting products may be considered when chronic, continuous treatment is required. Higher dosages should be reserved for use only in opioid-tolerant patients.

Capsules, extended release (Avinza): Adolescents ≥18 years: Daily dose administered once daily (for best results, administer at same time each day)

Opioid-naive: Initial: 30 mg once daily; adjust in increments ≤30 mg daily every 4 days

Conversion from other oral morphine formulations to Avinza: Total daily morphine dose given as once daily. The first dose of Avinza may be taken with the last dose of the immediate release morphine. Patients who experience breakthrough pain may require dose adjustment or rescue with a small dose of immediate release morphine. Maximum: 1600 mg daily due to fumaric acid content.

Capsules, extended release (Kadian): Adolescents ≥18 years: **Note:** Not intended for use as an initial opioid in the management of pain; use immediate release formulations before initiation. Total daily oral morphine dose may be either administered once daily or in 2 divided doses daily (every 12 hours). The first dose of Kadian may be taken with the last dose of the immediate release morphine.

Tablets, controlled release (MS Contin): Children and Adolescents: Usually not used as an initial opioid in the management of pain; use immediate release formulations to titrate dose. Total daily morphine dose may be administered in 2 divided doses daily (every 12 hours) or in 3 divided doses daily (every 8 hours).

Weight-directed dosing: 0.3-0.6 mg/kg/dose every 12 hours (Berde, 1990)

Alternate dosing; fixed dosing (Berde, 2002):

Patient weight 20 to <35 kg: 10-15 mg every 8-12 hours; **Note:** 10 mg strength not available in U.S.

Patient weight 35 to <50 kg: 15-30 mg every 8-12 hours

Patient weight ≥50 kg: 30-45 mg every 8-12 hours

Conversion from parenteral morphine or other opioids to controlled/extended release formulations: Substantial interpatient variability exists in relative potency. Therefore, it is safer to underestimate a patient's daily oral morphine requirement and provide breakthrough pain relief with immediate release morphine than to overestimate requirements. Consider the parenteral to oral morphine ratio or other oral or parenteral opioids to oral morphine conversions.

Continuous I.V. infusion, SubQ continuous infusion: Children and Adolescents: 0.01-0.04 mg/kg/**hour** (10-40 **mcg**/kg/**hour**) (APA, 2012; Friedrichsdorf, 2007; Golianu, 2000); opioid-tolerate patients may require higher doses; in a small study of terminal pediatric oncology patients (n=8; age range: 3-16 years), the median required dose was 0.04-0.07 mg/kg/**hour** (40-70 **mcg**/kg/**hour**); range: 0.025-2.6 mg/kg/**hour** (Miser, 1980); another study evaluating subcutaneous continuous infusion in children with cancer (n=17; age range: 22 months to 22 years) had similar findings; median dose: 0.06 mg/kg/**hour** (60 **mcg**/kg/**hour**); range: 0.025-1.79 mg/kg/**hour** (Miser, 1983)

Conversion from intermittent I.V. morphine: Administer the patient's total daily I.V. morphine dose over 24 hours as a continuous infusion; titrate dose to appropriate effect

Sickle cell disease, acute crisis (NHLBI, 2002): I.V.:

Infants ≥6 months and Children weighing ≤50 kg: Loading dose: 0.1-0.15 mg/kg once (maximum dose: 5 mg), then begin 0.05 mg-0.1 mg/kg/dose every 2-4 hours (maximum dose: 2.5 mg)

Children and Adolescents weighing >50 kg: Loading dose: 5-10 mg once, then begin 2.5-5 mg dose every 2-4 hours

Tetralogy of fallot, hypercyanotic spell (infundibular spasm): Limited data available: I.M., I.V., SubQ: 0.1 mg/kg has been used to decrease ventilatory drive and systemic venous return (Hegenbarth, 2008)

Palliative care, dyspnea management: Limited data available; further studies needed:

Inhalation (nebulization; preservative-free injection): Dose not established; dependent upon patient's previous or current systemic opioid exposure; doses not intended to provide analgesic activity; current systemic analgesia should be continued: Initial dose: Equivalent to patient's 4-hour systemic morphine requirement (eg, I.V. or oral dose); titrate to effect (Golianu, 2000); every 4-6 hour administration has been suggested (Cohen, 2002). In the only pediatric case report (end-stage CF, age: 10 years, weight: 20 kg), an initial dose of 2.5 mg was used and final dose was 10 mg every 4-6 hours (Cohen, 2002); from experience in adult patients, an initial dose of 5 mg has been used and reported range 2.5-30 mg administered up to every 4 hours (Ferraresi, 2005; Shirk, 2006)

I.V.: Initial: 25% of 4-hour intermittent dose; titrate until patient is comfortable (Golianu, 2000)

Oral: 0.1 mg/kg/dose every 4 hours as needed

Adults:

Acute pain (moderate to severe):

Oral (immediate release formulations): Opioid-naive: Initial: **Note:** Usual dosage range: 10-30 mg every 4 hours as needed. Patients with prior opioid exposure may require higher initial doses.

Solution: 10-20 mg every 4 hours as needed

Tablet: 15-30 mg every 4 hours as needed

I.M., SubQ: **Note:** Repeated SubQ administration causes local tissue irritation, pain, and induration. The use of I.M. injections is no longer recommended, especially for repeated administration due to painful administration, variable absorption, and lag time to peak effect; other routes are more reliable and less painful (American Pain Society, 2008).

Initial: Opioid-naive: 5-10 mg every 4 hours as needed; usual dosage range: 5-15 mg every 4 hours as needed. Patients with prior opioid exposure may require higher initial doses.

I.V.: Initial: Opioid-naive: 2.5-5 mg/dose every 3-4 hours as needed; patients with prior opioid exposure may require higher initial doses

Continuous I.V. infusion, SubQ continuous infusion: 0.8-10 mg/hour; may increase depending on pain relief/adverse effects; usual range up to 80 mg/hour. **Note:** May administer a loading dose (amount administered should depend on severity of pain) prior to initiating the infusion. A continuous (basal) infusion is not recommended in an opioid-naive patient (ISMP, 2009).

Rectal: 10-20 mg every 3-4 hours

Patient-controlled analgesia (PCA): Note: In opioid-naïve patients, consider lower end of dosing range:

Usual concentration: 1 mg/mL

Demand dose: Usual initial: 1 mg; usual range: 0.5-2.5 mg

Lockout interval: 5-10 minutes

Epidural: Note: Use preservative-free formulation; use lower doses and with extreme caution in debilitated patients. Vigilant monitoring is particularly important in these patients:

Single dose: **Lumbar region:** Astramorph/PF, Duramorph: 30-100 **mcg**/kg (optimal range: 2.5-3.75 mg; may depend upon patient comorbidities; Bujedo, 2012; Sultan, 2011)

Continuous infusion (may be combined with bupivacaine): 0.2-0.4 mg/hour (Bujedo, 2012)

Continuous microinfusion (Infumorph):

Opioid-naive: Initial: 3.5-7.5 mg over 24 hours

Opioid-tolerant: Initial: 4.5-10 mg over 24 hours, titrate to effect; usual maximum is ~30 mg per 24 hours

Intrathecal: Note: Must use preservative-free formulation; use lower doses and with extreme caution in debilitated patients. I.T. dose is usually 1/10 (one-tenth) that of epidural dosage.

Opioid-naive: Single dose: **Lumbar region:** Astramorph/PF, Duramorph: 0.1-0.3 mg (may provide adequate relief for up to 24 hours; APS, 2008); repeat doses **not** recommended. If pain recurs within 24 hours of administration, use of an alternate route of administration is recommended. **Note:** Although product labeling recommends doses up to 1 mg, an analgesic ceiling exists with doses >0.3 mg and the risk of respiratory depression is higher with doses >0.3 mg (Rathmell, 2005).

Continuous microinfusion (Infumorph): **Lumbar region:** After initial in-hospital evaluation of response to single-dose injections (Astramorph/PF,

Duramorph) the initial dose of Infumorph is 0.2-1 mg over 24 hours

Opioid-tolerant: Continuous microinfusion (Infumorph): **Lumbar region:** Dosage range: 1-10 mg over 24 hours, titrate to effect; usual maximum: ~20 mg over 24 hours

Chronic pain: Note: Patients taking opioids chronically may become tolerant and require doses higher than the usual dosage range to maintain the desired effect. Tolerance can be managed by appropriate dose titration. There is no optimal or maximal dose for morphine in chronic pain. The appropriate dose is one that relieves pain throughout its dosing interval without causing unmanageable side effects. Consider total daily dose, potency, prior opioid use, degree of opioid experience and tolerance, conversion from previous opioid (including opioid formulation), patient's general condition, concurrent medications, and type and severity of pain during prescribing process.

Oral (extended release formulations): A patient's morphine requirement should be established using immediate release formulations. Conversion to long-acting products may be considered when chronic, continuous treatment is required. Higher dosages should be reserved for use only in opioid-tolerant patients.

Capsules, extended release (Avinza):

Opioid-naive: Initial: 30 mg once daily; adjust in increments ≤30 mg daily every 4 days administered once daily (for best results, administer at same time each day)

Conversion from other oral morphine formulations to Avinza: Total daily morphine dose given once daily. The first dose of Avinza may be taken with the last dose of the immediate release morphine; maximum dose: 1600 mg daily due to fumaric acid content

Capsules, extended release (Kadian): **Note:** Not intended for use as an initial opioid in the management of pain; use immediate release formulations before initiation. Total daily oral morphine dose may be either administered once daily or in 2 divided doses daily (every 12 hours). The first dose of Kadian may be taken with the last dose of the immediate release morphine.

Tablets, extended release (MS Contin): Daily dose divided and administered every 8 or every 12 hours

Conversion from parenteral morphine or other opioids to extended release formulations: Substantial interpatient variability exists in relative potency. Therefore, it is safer to underestimate a patient's daily oral morphine requirement and provide breakthrough pain relief with immediate release morphine than to overestimate requirements. Consider the parenteral to oral morphine ratio or other oral or parenteral opioids to oral morphine conversions.

Dosing adjustment in renal impairment:

Infants, Children and Adolescents: I.V., Oral: Dosage adjustments are not provided in the manufacturer's labeling; however, the following adjustments have been recommended (Aronoff, 2007). **Note:** Renally adjusted dose recommendations are based on oral (immediate release) doses of 0.2-0.5 mg/kg/dose every 4-6 hours and I.V. doses of 0.05-0.2 mg/kg/dose every 2-4 hours:

GFR >50 mL/minute/1.73 m^2: No dosage adjustment necessary

GFR 10-50 mL/minute/1.73 m^2: Administer 75% of dose

GFR <10 mL/minute/1.73 m^2: Administer 50% of dose

Intermittent hemodialysis: Administer 50% of dose

Peritoneal dialysis (PD): Administer 50% of dose

Continuous renal replacement therapy (CRRT): Administer 75% of dose; titrate to effect

Adults:

CrCl 10-50 mL/minute: Administer 75% of normal dose

CrCl <10 mL/minute: Administer 50% of normal dose

Intermittent HD: No dosage adjustment necessary

Continuous renal replacement therapy (CRRT): Administer 75% of normal dose, titrate

Dosing adjustment in hepatic impairment: There are no dosage adjustments provided in manufacturer's labeling. Pharmacokinetics are unchanged in mild liver disease; substantial extrahepatic metabolism may occur. In cirrhosis, increases in half-life and AUC suggest dosage adjustment required.

Usual Infusion Concentrations: Neonatal I.V. infusion: 0.1 mg/mL

Usual Infusion Concentrations: Pediatric I.V. infusion: 0.1 mg/mL, 0.5 mg/mL, **or** 1 mg/mL

Administration

Oral: Administer with food

Immediate release: Oral solution: Available in multiple strengths, including a concentrated oral solution (20 mg/mL). Precautions should be taken to avoid confusion between the different concentrations; prescriptions should have the concentration specified as well as the dose clearly represented as milligram (mg) of morphine, not volume (mL). The enclosed calibrated oral syringe should always be used to administer the concentrated oral solution to ensure the dose is measured and administered accurately. The concentrated oral solution (20 mg/mL) should only be used in opioid-tolerant patients (adults taking ≥60 mg/day of morphine or equivalent for ≥1 week).

Extended/controlled release products: Do not chew, crush, break, or dissolve extended and controlled release products; swallow whole. Avinza and Kadian capsules may be opened and contents sprinkled on a small amount of applesauce and eaten immediately without chewing; rinse mouth with water and swallow to ensure all beads have been ingested; do not chew, crush, or dissolve beads or pellets from capsule as it can result in a rapid release and absorption of a potentially fatal dose of morphine. Kadian capsules may be opened and contents sprinkled into ~10 mL of water, then flushed while swirling through a prewetted 16-French gastrostomy tube fitted with a funnel at the port end; flush with water to transfer all pellets and flush the tube; do not attempt to administer via NG tube. Do not administer Avinza with alcohol.

Parenteral: **Note:** Solutions for injection should be visually inspected for particulate matter and discoloration prior to administration. Do not use if contains a precipitate or is darker in color than pale yellow or discolored in any other way.

I.V. push: Administer over at least 5 minutes at a final concentration of 0.5-5 mg/mL; rapid I.V. administration may increase adverse effects

Intermittent I.V. infusion: Administer over 15-30 minutes at a final concentration of 0.5-5 mg/mL

Continuous I.V. infusion: 0.1-1 mg/mL in D_5W, $D_{10}W$, or NS

Epidural and intrathecal: **Use only preservative-free injections.** Adults: Infumorph was developed for use in continuous microinfusion devices only; it may require dilution before use, as determined by the individual patient's dosage requirements and the characteristics of the continuous microinfusion device; not recommended for single dose I.V., I.M., or SubQ administration; filter through ≤5 micron microfilter before injecting into microinfusion device

Inhalation: Limited data available; utilize preservative free parenteral morphine and dilute with normal saline to a final volume of 5 mL (Cohen, 2002; Ferraresi, 2005; Shirk, 2006)

Monitoring Parameters Respiratory rate; oxygen saturation; mental status; blood pressure; heart rate; pain relief; signs of misuse, abuse, and addiction; level of sedation. **Note:** Resedation may occur following epidural administration. Monitor patients receiving Infumorph closely for ≥24 hours after initiation and as appropriate for the first several days after catheter implantation.

Test Interactions Some quinolones may produce a false-positive urine screening result for opioids using commercially-available immunoassay kits. This has been demonstrated most consistently for levofloxacin and ofloxacin, but other quinolones have shown cross-reactivity in certain assay kits. Confirmation of positive opioid screens by more specific methods should be considered.

Additional Information Equianalgesic doses: Codeine: 120 mg I.M. = morphine 10 mg I.M. = single dose oral morphine 60 mg or chronic dosing oral morphine 15-25 mg

Avinza capsules contain both immediate release and extended release beads; also contains fumaric acid (as an osmotic agent and local pH modifier); this product is intended for once daily oral administration only; not for PRN or postoperative use. Kadian capsules contain extended release pellets that are polymer-coated; this product is intended for every 12- or 24-hour dosing. Kadian capsules also contain talc; parenteral abuse may result in local tissue necrosis, infection, pulmonary granulomas, endocarditis, and valvular heart injury.

Controlled Substance C-II

Dosage Forms Excipient information presented when available (limited, particularly for generics); consult specific product labeling. [DSC] = Discontinued product

Capsule Extended Release 24 Hour, Oral, as sulfate:
AVINza: 30 mg [contains fd&c yellow #10 (quinoline yellow), fumaric acid]
AVINza: 45 mg [contains fd&c blue #2 (indigotine)]
AVINza: 60 mg [contains fumaric acid]
AVINza: 75 mg
AVINza: 90 mg [contains fd&c red #40, fumaric acid]
AVINza: 120 mg [contains brilliant blue fcf (fd&c blue #1), fumaric acid]
Kadian: 10 mg [contains brilliant blue fcf (fd&c blue #1)]
Kadian: 20 mg [contains fd&c yellow #10 (quinoline yellow)]
Kadian: 30 mg [contains brilliant blue fcf (fd&c blue #1)]
Kadian: 40 mg [contains brilliant blue fcf (fd&c blue #1), fd&c yellow #10 (quinoline yellow)]
Kadian: 50 mg, 60 mg [contains brilliant blue fcf (fd&c blue #1), fd&c red #40]
Kadian: 70 mg [DSC] [contains brilliant blue fcf (fd&c blue #1)]
Kadian: 80 mg [contains brilliant blue fcf (fd&c blue #1), fd&c red #40, fd&c yellow #6 (sunset yellow)]
Kadian: 100 mg [contains brilliant blue fcf (fd&c blue #1), fd&c yellow #10 (quinoline yellow)]
Kadian: 130 mg [DSC] [contains brilliant blue fcf (fd&c blue #1), fd&c red #40, fd&c yellow #6 (sunset yellow)]
Kadian: 150 mg [DSC] [contains brilliant blue fcf (fd&c blue #1), fd&c yellow #10 (quinoline yellow)]
Kadian: 200 mg
Generic: 10 mg, 20 mg, 30 mg, 45 mg, 50 mg, 60 mg, 75 mg, 80 mg, 90 mg, 100 mg, 120 mg
Device, Intramuscular, as sulfate:
Generic: 10 mg/0.7 mL (0.7 mL)
Solution, Injection, as sulfate:
Generic: 2 mg/mL (1 mL); 4 mg/mL (1 mL); 5 mg/mL (1 mL); 8 mg/mL (1 mL); 10 mg/mL (1 mL, 10 mL); 15 mg/mL (1 mL, 20 mL)
Solution, Injection, as sulfate [preservative free]:
Astramorph: 0.5 mg/mL (2 mL); 1 mg/mL (2 mL)
Duramorph: 0.5 mg/mL (10 mL); 1 mg/mL (10 mL)
Infumorph 200: 200 mg/20 mL (10 mg/mL) (20 mL) [antioxidant free]
Infumorph 500: 500 mg/20 mL (25 mg/mL) (20 mL) [antioxidant free]
Generic: 0.5 mg/mL (10 mL); 1 mg/mL (10 mL)

Solution, Intravenous, as sulfate:
Generic: 1 mg/mL (10 mL, 30 mL); 25 mg/mL (4 mL, 10 mL); 50 mg/mL (20 mL, 50 mL)
Solution, Intravenous, as sulfate [preservative free]:
Generic: 1 mg/mL (30 mL); 2 mg/mL (1 mL); 4 mg/mL (1 mL); 150 mg/30 mL (30 mL); 8 mg/mL (1 mL); 10 mg/mL (1 mL); 15 mg/mL (1 mL); 25 mg/mL (10 mL)
Solution, Oral, as sulfate:
Generic: 10 mg/5 mL (5 mL, 100 mL, 500 mL); 20 mg/5 mL (5 mL, 100 mL, 500 mL); 20 mg/mL (15 mL, 30 mL, 120 mL, 240 mL); 100 mg/5 mL (30 mL, 120 mL)
Suppository, Rectal, as sulfate:
Generic: 5 mg (12 ea); 10 mg (12 ea); 20 mg (12 ea); 30 mg (12 ea)
Tablet, Oral, as sulfate:
Generic: 15 mg, 30 mg
Tablet Extended Release, Oral, as sulfate:
MS Contin: 15 mg, 30 mg, 60 mg, 100 mg, 200 mg
Generic: 15 mg, 30 mg, 60 mg, 100 mg, 200 mg

References

ACOG Committee on Practice Bulletins-Obstetrics, "ACOG Practice Bulletin. Clinical Management Guidelines for Obstetrician-Gynecologists Number 36, July 2002. Obstetric Analgesia and Anesthesia," *Obstet Gynecol*, 2002, 100(1):177-91.

Anand KJ and International Evidence-Based Group for Neonatal Pain, "Consensus Statement for the Prevention and Management of Pain in the Newborn," *Arch Pediatr Adolesc Med*, 2001, 155(2):173-80.

Aronoff GR, Bennett WM, Berns JS, et al, *Drug Prescribing in Renal Failure: Dosing Guidelines for Adults and Children*, 5th ed, Philadelphia, PA: American College of Physicians, 2007.

Association of Paediatric Anaesthetists of Great Britain and Ireland (APA), "Good Practice in Postoperative and Procedural Pain Management, 2nd edition," *Paediatr Anaesth*, 2012, 22(Suppl 1):1-79.

Berde C, Ablin A, Glazer J, et al, "American Academy of Pediatrics Report of the Subcommittee on Disease-Related Pain in Childhood Cancer," *Pediatrics*, 1990, 86(5 Pt 2):818-25.

Berde CB and Sethna NF, "Analgesics for the Treatment of Pain in Children," *N Engl J Med*, 2002, 347(14):1094-103.

Bujedo BM, "A Clinical Approach to Neuroaxial Morphine for the Treatment of Postoperative Pain," *Pain Res Treat*, 2012, 8(3):177-92.

Burgos AE and Burke, Jr BL, "Neonatal Abstinence Syndrome," *Neoreviews*, 2009, 10(5):e222-9.

Chou R, Fanciullo GJ, Fine PG, et al, "Clinical Guidelines for the Use of Chronic Opioid Therapy in Chronic Noncancer Pain," *J Pain*, 2009, 10 (2):113-30.

Cohen SP and Dawson TC, "Nebulized Morphine as a Treatment for Dyspnea in a Child With Cystic Fibrosis," *Pediatrics*, 2002, 110(3): e38.

Cramton RE and Gruchala NE, "Managing Procedural Pain in Pediatric Patients," *Curr Opin Pediatr*, 2012, 24(4):530-8.

Dampier CD, Setty BN, Logan J, et al, "Intravenous Morphine Pharmacokinetics in Pediatric Patients With Sickle Cell Disease," *J Pediatr*, 1995, 126(3):461-7.

Dow K, Ordean A, Murphy-Oikonen J, et al, "Neonatal Abstinence Syndrome Clinical Practice Guidelines For Ontario," *J Popul Ther Clin Pharmacol*, 2012, 19(3):e488-506.

Ferraresi V, "Inhaled Opioids for the Treatment of Dyspnea," *Am J Health Syst Pharm*, 2005, 62(3):319-20.

Hegenbarth MA and American Academy of Pediatrics Committee on Drugs, "Preparing for Pediatric Emergencies: Drugs to Consider," *Pediatrics*, 2008, 121(2):433-43.

Henneberg SW, Hole P, Madsen de Haas I, et al, "Epidural Morphine for Postoperative Pain Relief in Children," *Acta Anaesthesiol Scand*, 1993, 37(7):664-7.

Hudak ML, Tan RC, AAP Committee on Drugs, et al, "Neonatal Drug Withdrawal," *Pediatrics*, 2012, 129(2):e540-60.

Hunt A, Joel S, Dick G, et al, "Population Pharmacokinetics of Oral Morphine and Its Glucuronides in Children Receiving Morphine as Immediate-Release Liquid or Sustained-Release Tablets for Cancer Pain," *J Pediatr*, 1999, 135(1):47-55.

Institute for Safe Medication Practice (ISMP), "Beware of Basal Opioid Infusions With PCA Therapy," 2009. Available at https://www.ismp.org/Newsletters/acutecare/articles/20090312.asp

Institute for Safe Medication Practices (ISMP), "Standard Concentrations of Neonatal Drug Infusions," *ISMP*, 2011.

Kumar P, Denson SE, Mancuso TJ, et al, "Premedication for Nonemergency Endotracheal Intubation in the Neonate," *Pediatrics*, 2010, 125(3):608-15.

Masood AR and Thomas SH, "Systemic Absorption of Nebulized Morphine Compared With Oral Morphine in Healthy Subjects," *Br J Clin Pharmacol*, 1996, 41(3):250-2.

McRorie TI, Lynn AM, Nespeca MK, et al, "The Maturation of Morphine Clearance and Metabolism," *Am J Dis Child*, 1992, 147(8):972-6.

Miser AW, Davis DM, Hughes CS, et al, "Continuous Subcutaneous Infusion of Morphine in Children With Cancer," *Am J Dis Child*, 1983, 137(4):383-5.

Miser AW, Miser JS, and Clark BS, "Continuous Intravenous Infusion of Morphine Sulfate for Control of Severe Pain in Children With Terminal Malignancy," *J Pediatr*, 1980, 96(5):930-2.

Montgomery A, Hale TW, and Academy of Breastfeeding Medicine, "ABM Clinical Protocol #15: Analgesia and Anesthesia for the Breast-feeding Mother, Revised 2012," *Breastfeed Med*, 2012, 7(6):547-53.

National Heart, Lung and Blood Institute (NHLBI), Division of Blood Diseases and Resources, "The Management of Sickle Cell Disease," June 2002. Available at http://www.nhlbi.nih.gov/health/prof/blood/sickle/sc_mngt.pdf

Olkkola KT, Hamunen K, and Maunuksela EL, "Clinical Pharmacokinetics and Pharmacodynamics of Opioid Analgesics in Infants and Children," *Clin Pharmacokinet*, 1995, 28(5):385-404.

Phillips MS, "Standardizing I.V. Infusion Concentrations: National Survey Results," *Am J Health Syst Pharm*, 2011, 68(22):2176-82.

"Principles of Analgesic Use in the Treatment of Acute Pain and Cancer Pain," 6th ed, Glenview, IL: American Pain Society, 2008.

Rathmell JP, Lair TR, and Nauman B, "The Role of Intrathecal Drugs in the Treatment of Acute Pain," *Anesth Analg*, 2005, 101(5 Suppl):30-43.

Shirk MB, Donahue KR, and Shirvani J, "Unlabeled Uses of Nebulized Medications," *Am J Health Syst Pharm*, 2006, 63(18):1704-16.

Spigset O and Hagg S, "Analgesics and Breast-feeding: Safety Considerations," *Paediatr Drugs*, 2000, 2(3):223-38.

Sultan P, Gutierrez MC, and Carvalho B, "Neuraxial Morphine and Respiratory Depression: Finding the Right Balance," *Drugs*, 2011, 71(14):1807-19.

Suresh S, Birmingham PK, and Kozlowski RJ, "Pediatric Pain Management," *Anesthesiol Clin*, 2012, 30(1):101-17.

Zeltzer LK, Altman A, Cohen D, et al, "American Academy of Pediatrics Report of the Subcommittee on the Management of Pain Associated With Procedures in Children With Cancer," *Pediatrics*, 1990, 86(5 Pt 2):826-31.

Morphine (Liposomal) (MOR feen)

Medication Safety Issues
Sound-alike/look-alike issues:
Morphine may be confused with HYDROmorphone

Morphine sulfate may be confused with magnesium sulfate

MSO$_4$ and MS are error-prone abbreviations (mistaken as magnesium sulfate)

High alert medication:
The Institute for Safe Medication Practices (ISMP) includes this medication among its list of drug classes which have a heightened risk of causing significant patient harm when used in error.

Brand Names: U.S. DepoDur

Therapeutic Category Analgesic, Narcotic

Generic Availability (U.S.) No

Use Epidural (at the lumbar level) single-dose management of surgical pain in adults; may be used in women undergoing cesarean section following clamping of the umbilical cord (FDA approved in adults) (not for use in vaginal labor and delivery)

Pregnancy Risk Factor C

Pregnancy Considerations Adverse events were observed in some animal reproduction studies. DepoDur® is administered as a single dose for acute, surgery-induced pain. It may be used in women undergoing cesarean section following clamping of the umbilical cord; not for use in vaginal labor and delivery.

Refer to the Morphine (Systemic) monograph for additional information.

Breast-Feeding Considerations Morphine is excreted into breast milk. Studies using this specific preparation have not been located. Due to the potential for serious adverse reactions in the nursing infant, the manufacturer recommends a decision should be made whether to discontinue nursing or to discontinue the drug (delay nursing for 48 hours after administration), taking into account the importance of treatment to the mother.

Refer to the Morphine, Systemic monograph for additional information.

Contraindications Hypersensitivity to morphine sulfate or any component; severe respiratory depression or respiratory depression in a setting without resuscitative equipment or appropriate monitoring; acute or severe asthma; upper airway obstruction; GI obstruction especially known or suspected paralytic ileus; suspected or known CNS injury, increased ICP, circulatory shock, or conditions that preclude an epidural injection

Warnings CNS and respiratory depression may occur. Use with extreme caution in patients with COPD, cor pulmonale, hypoxia, hypercapnia, preexisting respiratory depression, significantly decreased respiratory reserve, head injury, increased ICP, or other intracranial lesions. Severe hypotension may occur; use with caution in patients with circulatory shock, hypovolemia, impaired myocardial function, or those receiving drugs which may exaggerate hypotensive effects (including phenothiazines or general anesthetics).

Warn patient of possible impairment of alertness or physical coordination. Interactions with other CNS drugs may occur.

Prior to administration via epidural, evaluate benefits versus risks in patients with infection at injection site, bleeding diatheses, or anticoagulation therapy. Only physicians experienced in the techniques and familiar with the clinical management of the adverse effects of epidural drug administration should administer drugs via the intraspinal route. When morphine is used via the epidural route, severe adverse effects may occur, including significant respiratory depression; facilities must be properly equipped to resuscitate patients; monitor patients for delayed sedation. Patients must be closely monitored for a minimum of 48 hours (due to prolonged effects of extended release epidural preparation). Safety and efficacy have not been established in pediatric patients. Freezing may adversely affect modified-release mechanism of DepoDur®; check freeze indicator within carton prior to administration.

Precautions Use with caution in patients with hypersensitivity reactions to other phenanthrene derivative opioid agonists (codeine, hydrocodone, hydromorphone, levorphanol, oxycodone, oxymorphone). Use with caution in patients with biliary tract disease or acute pancreatitis (morphine may cause spasm of the sphincter of Oddi).

When administered to a pregnant woman, epidural morphine readily passes into the fetal circulation and may result in respiratory depression in the newborn; resuscitative equipment and naloxone should be available for the neonate.

Adverse Reactions
Cardiovascular: Bradycardia, hypertension, hypotension, tachycardia

Central nervous system: Anxiety, dizziness, fever, headache, insomnia, somnolence

Dermatologic: Pruritus

Gastrointestinal: Abdominal distension, constipation, dyspepsia, flatulence, nausea, paralytic ileus, vomiting

Genitourinary: Bladder spasm, oliguria, urinary retention (may be prolonged)

Hematologic: Anemia, hematocrit decreased

Local: Pain at injection site

Neuromuscular & skeletal: Back pain, hypoesthesia, paresthesia, rigors, weakness

Respiratory: Dyspnea, hypercapnia, hypoxia, oxygen saturation decreased, respiratory depression

Miscellaneous: Sweating increased

Rare but important or life-threatening: Cardiac arrest, confusion, lethargy, obtundation, respiratory arrest.

Apnea and prolonged respiratory depression have occurred following subarachnoid puncture.

Drug Interactions

Metabolism/Transport Effects Substrate of CYP2D6 (minor), P-glycoprotein; **Note:** Assignment of Major/Minor substrate status based on clinically relevant drug interaction potential

Avoid Concomitant Use

Avoid concomitant use of Morphine (Liposomal) with any of the following: Azelastine (Nasal); MAO Inhibitors; Paraldehyde; Thalidomide

Increased Effect/Toxicity

Morphine (Liposomal) may increase the levels/effects of: Alcohol (Ethyl); Alvimopan; Azelastine (Nasal); Buprenorphine; CNS Depressants; Desmopressin; Diuretics; Hydrocodone; Methotrimeprazine; Metyrosine; Mirtazapine; Paraldehyde; Pramipexole; ROPINIRole; Rotigotine; Selective Serotonin Reuptake Inhibitors; Thalidomide; Zolpidem

The levels/effects of Morphine (Liposomal) may be increased by: Amphetamines; Anticholinergic Agents; Antipsychotic Agents (Phenothiazines); Brimonidine (Topical); Cannabis; Doxylamine; Dronabinol; Droperidol; HydrOXYzine; Kava Kava; Magnesium Sulfate; MAO Inhibitors; Methotrimeprazine; Nabilone; Perampanel; P-glycoprotein/ABCB1 Inhibitors; Rufinamide; Sodium Oxybate; Succinylcholine; Tapentadol; Tetrahydrocannabinol

Decreased Effect

Morphine (Liposomal) may decrease the levels/effects of: Clopidogrel; Pegvisomant

The levels/effects of Morphine (Liposomal) may be decreased by: Ammonium Chloride; Mixed Agonist / Antagonist Opioids; Naltrexone; Peginterferon Alfa-2b; P-glycoprotein/ABCB1 Inducers

Stability Store in carton under refrigeration, 2°C to 8°C (36°F to 46°F). Do not freeze; do not use if product has been frozen or is suspected of having been frozen. Check freeze indicator (located on carton) before administration; do not administer if indicator bulb is pink or purple (this indicates drug may have been frozen). May store unopened vials at room temperature for up to 7 days. After withdrawal from vial, drug may be held at room temperature for ≤4 hours before use. Do not heat or gas sterilize. Discard unused portion of vial (vial does not contain preservatives). Do not mix with other medications.

Mechanism of Action Binds to opiate receptors in the CNS, causing inhibition of ascending pain pathways, altering the perception of and response to pain; produces generalized CNS depression

Pharmacodynamics

See Table.

Dosage Form / Route	Analgesia	
	Peak	Duration
Epidural	1 h	12-20 h

Pharmacokinetics (Adult data unless noted)

Distribution: Distributes to skeletal muscle, liver, kidneys, lungs, intestinal tract, spleen, brain, and into breast milk; crosses placenta

Protein binding: 30% to 35%

Metabolism: In the liver via glucuronide conjugation to morphine-6-glucuronide (active) and morphine-3-glucuronide (inactive)

Dosing: Usual Adults: Epidural: Surgical pain: Single dose:

Cesarean section: 10 mg

Lower abdominal or pelvic surgery: 10-15 mg; **Note:** Some patients may benefit from a 20 mg dose; however, the

incidence of adverse respiratory effects may be increased.

Major orthopedic surgery of the lower extremity: 15 mg

For epidural use only (at the lumbar level); do not administer I.V., I.M., or by the intrathecal route; not recommended for administration into thoracic epidural space or higher (has not been studied). Do not use if suspect vial has been frozen. Gently invert vial to resuspend particles immediately before use (avoid aggressive agitation). May administer undiluted or may dilute up to 5 mL total volume in preservative free NS. Product does not contain preservative; drug must be administered within 4 hours after withdrawal from vial. Do not use in-line filter during administration. Do not administer within 15 minutes of epidural lidocaine and epinephrine; do not administer any other medication into the epidural space for at least 48 hours after DepoDur®.

Monitoring Parameters Respiratory and cardiovascular status, oxygen saturation, pain relief (if used for analgesia), level of sedation. **Note:** Resedation may occur; monitor patients closely for ≥48 hours.

Additional Information DepoDur® is an extended release sterile suspension of multivesicular liposomes in NS; liposomes range in size from 17-23 micrometers (median diameter); the pharmacokinetics, safety, and efficacy of DepoDur® have not been studied in patients <18 years of age and use in these patients is **not** recommended

Controlled Substance C-II

Dosage Forms Excipient information presented when available (limited, particularly for generics); consult specific product labeling.

Suspension, Epidural, as sulfate:

DepoDur: 10 mg/mL (1 mL); 15 mg/1.5 mL (1.5 mL)

◆ **Morphine-EPD (Can)** *see* Morphine (Systemic) *on page 1440*

◆ **Morphine Extra Forte Injection (Can)** *see* Morphine (Systemic) *on page 1440*

◆ **Morphine Forte Injection (Can)** *see* Morphine (Systemic) *on page 1440*

◆ **Morphine HP (Can)** *see* Morphine (Systemic) *on page 1440*

◆ **Morphine LP Epidural (Can)** *see* Morphine (Systemic) *on page 1440*

◆ **Morphine SR (Can)** *see* Morphine (Systemic) *on page 1440*

◆ **M.O.S. 10 (Can)** *see* Morphine (Systemic) *on page 1440*

◆ **M.O.S. 20 (Can)** *see* Morphine (Systemic) *on page 1440*

◆ **M.O.S. 30 (Can)** *see* Morphine (Systemic) *on page 1440*

◆ **M.O.S.-SR (Can)** *see* Morphine (Systemic) *on page 1440*

◆ **M.O.S.-Sulfate (Can)** *see* Morphine (Systemic) *on page 1440*

◆ **Motion Sickness [OTC]** *see* DimenhyDRINATE *on page 670*

◆ **Motrin [OTC]** *see* Ibuprofen *on page 1059*

◆ **Motrin (Can)** *see* Ibuprofen *on page 1059*

◆ **Motrin (Children's) (Can)** *see* Ibuprofen *on page 1059*

◆ **Motrin IB [OTC]** *see* Ibuprofen *on page 1059*

◆ **Motrin IB (Can)** *see* Ibuprofen *on page 1059*

◆ **Motrin Infants Drops [OTC]** *see* Ibuprofen *on page 1059*

◆ **Motrin Junior Strength [OTC]** *see* Ibuprofen *on page 1059*

◆ **MoviPrep** *see* Polyethylene Glycol-Electrolyte Solution *on page 1697*

◆ **Moxatag** *see* Amoxicillin *on page 140*

◆ **Moxeza** *see* Moxifloxacin (Ophthalmic) *on page 1451*

Moxifloxacin (Ophthalmic) (moxs i FLOKS a sin)

Medication Safety Issues
International issues:
Vigamox [U.S., Canada, and multiple international markets] may be confused with Fisamox brand name for amoxicillin [Australia]

Brand Names: U.S. Moxeza; Vigamox

Brand Names: Canada Vigamox®

Therapeutic Category Antibiotic, Fluoroquinolone; Antibiotic, Ophthalmic

Generic Availability (U.S.) No

Use Treatment of bacterial conjunctivitis caused by susceptible organisms (Moxeza™: FDA approved in ages ≥4 months and adults; Vigamox®: FDA approved in ages ≥1 year and adults)

Pregnancy Risk Factor C

Pregnancy Considerations Adverse events have been observed in some animal studies; therefore, the manufacturer classifies moxifloxacin ophthalmic as pregnancy category C. Information related to moxifloxacin in pregnancy is limited. Refer to the Moxifloxacin (Systemic) monograph for available information. Quinolone exposure during human pregnancy has been reported with other agents (see Ciprofloxacin [Systemic] and Ofloxacin [Systemic] monographs).

Breast-Feeding Considerations It is not known if moxifloxacin is excreted into breast milk. The manufacturer recommends that caution be exercised when administering moxifloxacin eye drops to nursing women.

Contraindications Hypersensitivity to moxifloxacin, other quinolone antibiotics, or any component

Warnings Severe hypersensitivity reactions, including anaphylaxis, have occurred with systemic quinolone therapy, including moxifloxacin. The spectrum of these reactions can vary widely. Prompt discontinuation of drug should occur if skin rash or other symptoms arise. **Not for injection into the eye.** Eye drops should not be introduced directly into the anterior chamber of the eye.

Precautions Prolonged use may result in fungal or bacterial superinfection. Contact lenses should not be worn during therapy.

Adverse Reactions Ocular: Conjunctivitis, dry eye, ocular discomfort, ocular hyperemia, ocular irritation, ocular pain, ocular pruritus, subconjunctival hemorrhage, tearing, visual acuity decreased

Drug Interactions
Metabolism/Transport Effects None known.

Avoid Concomitant Use There are no known interactions where it is recommended to avoid concomitant use.

Increased Effect/Toxicity There are no known significant interactions involving an increase in effect.

Decreased Effect There are no known significant interactions involving a decrease in effect.

Stability Store at 2°C to 25°C (36°F to 77°F).

Mechanism of Action Moxifloxacin is a DNA gyrase inhibitor, and also inhibits topoisomerase IV. DNA gyrase (topoisomerase II) is an essential bacterial enzyme that maintains the superhelical structure of DNA. DNA gyrase is required for DNA replication and transcription, DNA repair, recombination, and transposition; inhibition is bactericidal.

Pharmacokinetics (Adult data unless noted) Absorption: Minimal systemic absorption; resulting serum concentration was 0.02% of that achieved with oral formulation

Dosing: Usual
Infants ≥4 months, Children, and Adults: Moxeza™: Instill 1 drop into affected eye(s) 2 times daily for 7 days

Children ≥1 year and Adults: Vigamox®: Instill 1 drop into affected eye(s) 3 times daily for 7 days

Administration For topical ophthalmic use only; avoid touching tip of applicator to eye, finger, or other surfaces. Apply finger pressure to lacrimal sac during and for 1-2 minutes after instillation to decrease risk of absorption and systemic effects.

Monitoring Parameters Signs of infection

Additional Information Evidence of damage to weight-bearing joints in pediatric populations with ophthalmic administration has not been shown.

Dosage Forms Excipient information presented when available (limited, particularly for generics); consult specific product labeling.

Solution, Ophthalmic:
Moxeza: 0.5% (3 mL)
Vigamox: 0.5% (3 mL)

References
Silver LH, Woodside AM, and Montgomery DB, "Clinical Safety of Moxifloxacin Ophthalmic Solution 0.5% (VIGAMOX) in Pediatric and Nonpediatric Patients With Bacterial Conjunctivitis," *Surv Ophthalmol*, 2005, 50(Suppl 1):55-63.

◆ **Moxifloxacin Hydrochloride** *see* Moxifloxacin (Ophthalmic) *on page 1451*

◆ **4-MP** *see* Fomepizole *on page 927*

◆ **MPA** *see* MedroxyPROGESTERone *on page 1318*

◆ **MPA** *see* Mycophenolate *on page 1453*

◆ **6-MP (error-prone abbreviation)** *see* Mercaptopurine *on page 1342*

◆ **MPSV** *see* Meningococcal Polysaccharide Vaccine (Groups A / C / Y and W-135) *on page 1336*

◆ **MPSV4** *see* Meningococcal Polysaccharide Vaccine (Groups A / C / Y and W-135) *on page 1336*

◆ **MRA** *see* Tocilizumab *on page 2040*

◆ **MS Contin** *see* Morphine (Systemic) *on page 1440*

◆ **MS Contin SRT (Can)** *see* Morphine (Systemic) *on page 1440*

◆ **MS (error-prone abbreviation and should not be used)** *see* Morphine (Liposomal) *on page 1449*

◆ **MS (error-prone abbreviation and should not be used)** *see* Morphine (Systemic) *on page 1440*

◆ **MS-IR (Can)** *see* Morphine (Systemic) *on page 1440*

◆ **MSO₄ (error-prone abbreviation and should not be used)** *see* Morphine (Liposomal) *on page 1449*

◆ **MSO₄ (error-prone abbreviation and should not be used)** *see* Morphine (Systemic) *on page 1440*

◆ **MTX (error-prone abbreviation)** *see* Methotrexate *on page 1367*

◆ **Mucinex [OTC]** *see* GuaiFENesin *on page 984*

◆ **Mucinex Allergy [OTC]** *see* Fexofenadine *on page 870*

◆ **Mucinex Chest Congestion Child [OTC]** *see* GuaiFENesin *on page 984*

◆ **Mucinex DM [OTC]** *see* Guaifenesin and Dextromethorphan *on page 987*

◆ **Mucinex DM Maximum Strength [OTC]** *see* Guaifenesin and Dextromethorphan *on page 987*

◆ **Mucinex Fast-Max DM Max [OTC]** *see* Guaifenesin and Dextromethorphan *on page 987*

◆ **Mucinex For Kids [OTC]** *see* GuaiFENesin *on page 984*

◆ **Mucinex Kid's Cough [OTC]** *see* Guaifenesin and Dextromethorphan *on page 987*

◆ **Mucinex Kid's Cough Mini-Melts [OTC]** *see* Guaifenesin and Dextromethorphan *on page 987*

◆ **Mucinex Maximum Strength [OTC]** *see* GuaiFENesin *on page 984*

◆ **Mucinex Nasal Spray Full Force [OTC]** *see* Oxymetazoline (Nasal) *on page 1577*

◆ **Mucinex Nasal Spray Moisture [OTC]** *see* Oxymetazoline (Nasal) *on page 1577*

◆ **Mucinex Sinus-Max Full Force [OTC]** *see* Oxymetazoline (Nasal) *on page 1577*

◆ **Mucinex Sinus-Max Moist Smart [OTC]** *see* Oxymetazoline (Nasal) *on page 1577*

◆ **Mucomyst** *see* Acetylcysteine *on page 60*

◆ **Mucomyst® (Can)** *see* Acetylcysteine *on page 60*

◆ **Mucosa [OTC]** *see* GuaiFENesin *on page 984*

◆ **Mucus-ER [OTC]** *see* GuaiFENesin *on page 984*

◆ **Mucus Relief [OTC]** *see* GuaiFENesin *on page 984*

◆ **Mucus Relief Childrens [OTC]** *see* GuaiFENesin *on page 984*

◆ **Multitrace-4** *see* Trace Elements *on page 2059*

◆ **Multitrace-4 Concentrate** *see* Trace Elements *on page 2059*

◆ **Multitrace-4 Neonatal** *see* Trace Elements *on page 2059*

◆ **Multitrace-4 Pediatric** *see* Trace Elements *on page 2059*

◆ **Multitrace-5** *see* Trace Elements *on page 2059*

◆ **Multitrace-5 Concentrate** *see* Trace Elements *on page 2059*

◆ **Mumps, Measles and Rubella Vaccines** *see* Measles, Mumps, and Rubella Virus Vaccine *on page 1307*

◆ **Mumps, Rubella, Varicella, and Measles Vaccine** *see* Measles, Mumps, Rubella, and Varicella Virus Vaccine *on page 1310*

Mupirocin (myoo PEER oh sin)

Medication Safety Issues
Sound-alike/look-alike issues:
Bactroban may be confused with bacitracin, baclofen, Bactrim
Brand Names: U.S. Bactroban; Bactroban Nasal; Centany; Centany AT
Brand Names: Canada Bactroban
Therapeutic Category Antibiotic, Topical
Generic Availability (U.S.) May be product dependent
Use
Intranasal ointment: Eradication of *Staphylococcus aureus* from nasal carriage sites as part of an infection control program to reduce the risk of infection among patients at high risk of MRSA infection during institutional outbreaks (FDA approved in ages ≥12 years and adults)
Topical cream: Topical treatment of secondarily-infected traumatic skin lesions due to susceptible strains of *S. aureus* and *Streptococcus pyogenes* (FDA approved in ages ≥3 months and adults); has also been used for prophylaxis at intravenous catheter exit sites
Topical ointment: Topical treatment of impetigo caused by susceptible strains of *S. aureus* and *S. pyogenes* (FDA approved in ages ≥2 months and adults)
Pregnancy Risk Factor B
Pregnancy Considerations Adverse events have not been observed in animal reproduction studies.
Breast-Feeding Considerations It is not known if mupirocin is excreted in breast milk. The manufacturer recommends that caution be exercised when administering mupirocin to nursing women.
Contraindications Hypersensitivity to mupirocin or any component
Warnings Potentially toxic amounts of polyethylene glycol (PEG) contained in the vehicle of topical ointment may be absorbed percutaneously in patients with extensive burns or open wounds; intranasal use of the topical ointment may irritate mucous membranes and increase nasal secretions.

Prolonged use of mupirocin may result in overgrowth of nonsusceptible organisms

Topical cream contains benzyl alcohol which may cause allergic reactions in susceptible individuals; large amounts of benzyl alcohol (≥99 mg/kg/day) have been associated with a potentially fatal toxicity ("gasping syndrome") in neonates; the "gasping syndrome" consists of metabolic acidosis, respiratory distress, gasping respirations, CNS dysfunction (including convulsions, intracranial hemorrhage), hypotension, and cardiovascular collapse; use topical cream containing benzyl alcohol with caution in neonates; *in vitro* and animal studies have shown that benzoate, a metabolite of benzyl alcohol, displaces bilirubin from protein binding sites
Precautions Use with caution in patients with impaired renal function and in burn patients
Adverse Reactions
Central nervous system: Dizziness, headache
Dermatologic: Cellulitis, dermatitis, dry skin, erythema, hives, pruritus, rash
Gastrointestinal: Abdominal pain, diarrhea, nausea, taste perversion, ulcerative stomatitis, xerostomia
Local: Burning, edema, pain, stinging, tenderness
Ocular: Blepharitis
Otic: Ear pain
Respiratory: Cough, pharyngitis, rhinitis, upper respiratory tract congestion
Miscellaneous: Secondary wound infection
Drug Interactions
Metabolism/Transport Effects None known.
Avoid Concomitant Use
Avoid concomitant use of Mupirocin with any of the following: BCG
Increased Effect/Toxicity There are no known significant interactions involving an increase in effect.
Decreased Effect
Mupirocin may decrease the levels/effects of: BCG; Sodium Picosulfate; Typhoid Vaccine
Stability Store at or below 20°C to 25°C (68°F to 77°F); do not refrigerate. Do not mix with Aquaphor®, coal tar solution, or salicylic acid.
Mechanism of Action Binds to bacterial isoleucyl transfer-RNA synthetase resulting in the inhibition of protein synthesis
Pharmacokinetics (Adult data unless noted)
Absorption: Following topical administration, penetrates the outer layers of the skin; systemic absorption is minimal through intact skin; following intranasal use in neonates significant systemic absorption reported
Protein binding: >97%
Metabolism: Skin: 3% to monic acid (inactive)
Half-life: 17-36 minutes
Elimination: Momic acid [inactive] is renally excreted
Dosing: Neonatal
Intranasal: **MRSA decolonization:** Intranasal ointment: Apply a small amount to both anterior nares 2-3 times/day for 5-10 days in conjunction with umbilical application of topical ointment (Bertin, 2006; Lally, 2004; Liu, 2011)
Topical:
Mild localized impetigo or MRSA skin infections: Ointment: Apply a small amount 3 times/day for 5-10 days (Liu, 2011)
MRSA decolonization: Ointment: Apply a small amount to umbilicus 2-3 times/day for 5-10 days in conjunction with intranasal application (Bertin, 2006; Lally, 2004)

Dosing: Usual

Intranasal: **Eradication of MRSA colonization:** Intranasal ointment:

Manufacturer recommendations: Children ≥12 years, Adolescents, and Adults: Apply 0.5 g (1/2 of unit-dose tube) twice daily for 5 days

Alternate dosing: Infants, Children, and Adults: Apply a small amount twice daily for 5-10 days (Lui, 2011)

Topical:

Cream: **Minor skin infections or infected lesions:** Infants, Children, and Adults: Apply small amount 3 times/day for 10 days; patients not showing clinical response after 5 days should be re-evaluated.

Ointment: **Minor skin infection, impetigo, infected lesions:** Infants, Children, and Adults: Apply a small amount 3-5 times/day for 5-14 days; patients not showing clinical response after 5 days should be re-evaluated.

Administration

Intranasal: Avoid contact with eyes; apply to anterior nares. Press sides of the nose together and gently massage for 1 minute after application to spread ointment throughout the inside of the nostrils.

Topical cream and ointment: For topical use only; not formulated for use on mucosal surfaces; do not apply into the eye or use intranasally; may cover with gauze dressing

Dosage Forms Excipient information presented when available (limited, particularly for generics); consult specific product labeling.

Cream, External, as calcium [strength expressed as base]:
Bactroban: 2% (15 g, 30 g)
Generic: 2% (15 g, 30 g)

Kit, External:
Centany AT: 2% [contains propylene glycol monostearate]

Ointment, External:
Bactroban: 2% (22 g)
Centany: 2% (30 g) [contains propylene glycol monostearate]
Generic: 2% (22 g)

Ointment, Nasal, as calcium [strength expressed as base]:
Bactroban Nasal: 2% (1 g)

References

Bertin ML, Vinski J, Schmitt S, et al, "Outbreak of Methicillin-Resistant *Staphylococcus aureus* Colonization and Infection in a Neonatal Intensive Care Unit Epidemiologically Linked to a Healthcare Worker With Chronic Otitis," *Infect Control Hosp Epidemiol*, 2006, 27 (6):581-5.

Britton JW, Fajardo JE, and Krafte-Jacobs B, "Comparison of Mupirocin and Erythromycin in the Treatment of Impetigo," *J Pediatr*, 1990, 117 (5):827-9.

Hayakawa T, Hayashidera T, Katsura S, et al, "Nasal Mupirocin Treatment of Pharynx-Colonized Methicillin Resistant *Staphylococcus aureus:* Preliminary Study With 10 Carrier Infants," *Pediatr Int*, 2000, 42 (1):67-70.

Hitomi S, Kubota M, Mori N, et al, "Control of a Methicillin-Resistant *Staphylococcus aureus* Outbreak in a Neonatal Intensive Care Unit by Unselective Use of Nasal Mupirocin Ointment," *J Hosp Infect*, 2000, 46(2):123-9.

Lally RT, Lanz E, and Schrock CG, "Rapid Control of an Outbreak of *Staphylococcus aureus* on a Neonatal Intensive Care Department Using Standard Infection Control Practices and Nasal Mupirocin," *Am J Infect Control*, 2004, 32(1):44-7.

Liu C, Bayer A, Cosgrove SE, et al, "Clinical Practice Guidelines by the Infectious Diseases Society of America for the Treatment of Methicillin-Resistant *Staphylococcus aureus* Infections in Adults and Children: Executive Summary," *Clin Infect Dis*, 2011, 52(3):285-92.

Oh J, von Baum H, Klaus G, et al, "Nasal Carriage of *Staphylococcus aureus* in Families of Children on Peritoneal Dialysis. European Pediatric Peritoneal Dialysis Study Group (EPPS)," *Adv Perit Dial*, 2000, 16:324-7.

Siegel JD, Rhinehart E, Jackson M, et al, "2007 Guideline for Isolation Precautions: Preventing Transmission of Infectious Agents in Health Care Settings," *Am J Infect Control*, 2007, 35(10 Suppl 2):65-164. Available at http://www.cdc.gov/ncidod/dhqp/pdf/isolation2007.pdf

Siegel JD, Rhinehart E, Jackson M, et al, "Management of Multidrug-Resistant Organisms in Health Care Settings, 2006," *Am J Infect Control*, 2007, 35(10 Suppl 2):165-93.

◆ **Mupirocin Calcium** *see* Mupirocin *on page 1452*
◆ **Murine Tears® [OTC]** *see* Artificial Tears *on page 205*
◆ **Muro 128 [OTC]** *see* Sodium Chloride *on page 1902*
◆ **Muse** *see* Alprostadil *on page 103*
◆ **Muse Pellet (Can)** *see* Alprostadil *on page 103*
◆ **Mustargen** *see* Mechlorethamine (Systemic) *on page 1315*
◆ **Mustine** *see* Mechlorethamine (Systemic) *on page 1315*
◆ **Myambutol** *see* Ethambutol *on page 807*
◆ **Mycamine** *see* Micafungin *on page 1407*
◆ **Mycelex** *see* Clotrimazole (Oral) *on page 526*
◆ **Mycobutin** *see* Rifabutin *on page 1822*
◆ **Mycobutin® (Can)** *see* Rifabutin *on page 1822*
◆ **Mycocide Clinical NS [OTC]** *see* Tolnaftate *on page 2044*

Mycophenolate (mye koe FEN oh late)

Related Information

Oral Medications That Should Not Be Crushed or Altered *on page 2438*

Safe Handling of Hazardous Drugs *on page 2419*

Brand Names: U.S. CellCept; CellCept Intravenous; Myfortic

Brand Names: Canada Apo-Mycophenolate; CellCept; CO Mycophenolate; JAMP-Mycophenolate; Myfortic; Mylan-Mycophenolate; Novo-Mycophenolate; Sandoz-Mycophenolate; Sandoz-Mycophenolate Mofetil

Therapeutic Category Immunosuppressant Agent

Generic Availability (U.S.) May be product dependent

Use

Oral: Immunosuppressant agent used in conjunction with other immunosuppressive therapies (eg, cyclosporine and corticosteroids with or without antithymocyte induction) for the prophylaxis of organ rejection in patients receiving allogeneic renal (CellCept: FDA approved in ages ≥3 months and adults; Myfortic: FDA approved in ages ≥5 years who are at least 6 months post-transplant and adults), hepatic, or cardiac transplants (CellCept: FDA approved in adults). Has also been used in nephrotic syndrome; intestine, small bowel, and bone marrow transplant patients; moderate to severe psoriasis; chronic graft-versus-host disease; myasthenia gravis; lupus nephritis; autoimmune lymphoproliferative syndrome juvenile localized scleroderma, uveitis and refractory immune thrombocytopenia (ITP).

Parenteral: Immunosuppressant agent used in conjunction with other immunosuppressive therapies (eg, cyclosporine and corticosteroids with or without antithymocyte induction) for the prophylaxis of organ rejection in patients receiving allogeneic renal, hepatic, or cardiac transplants (CellCept: FDA approved in adults)

Medication Guide Available Yes

Pregnancy Risk Factor D

Pregnancy Considerations [U.S. Boxed Warning]: Mycophenolate is associated with an increased risk of congenital malformations and first trimester pregnancy loss when used by pregnant women. Females of reproductive potential must be counseled about pregnancy prevention and planning. Alternative agents should be considered for women planning a pregnancy. Adverse events have been reported in animal reproduction studies. In humans, the following congenital malformations have been reported: external ear abnormalities, cleft lip and palate, anomalies of the distal limbs, heart, esophagus and kidney. Spontaneous abortions have also been noted.

Females of reproductive potential (girls who have entered puberty, women with a uterus who have not passed through clinically confirmed menopause) should have a negative pregnancy test with a sensitivity of ≥25 mIU/mL immediately before therapy and the test should be repeated 8-10 days later. Pregnancy tests should be repeated during routine follow-up visits. Acceptable forms of contraception should be used during treatment and for 6 weeks after therapy is discontinued. The effectiveness of hormonal contraceptive agents may be affected by mycophenolate. For women with lupus nephritis taking mycophenolate and who are planning a pregnancy, mycophenolate should be discontinued at least 6 weeks prior to trying to conceive (Hahn, 2012).

Healthcare providers should report female exposures to mycophenolate during pregnancy or within 6 weeks of discontinuing therapy to the Mycophenolate Pregnancy Registry (800-617-8191). The National Transplantation Pregnancy Registry (NTPR, Temple University) is a registry for pregnant women taking immunosuppressants following any solid organ transplant. The NTPR encourages reporting of all immunosuppressant exposures during pregnancy in transplant recipients at 877-955-6877.

Breast-Feeding Considerations It is unknown if mycophenolate is excreted in human milk. Due to potentially serious adverse reactions, the decision to discontinue the drug or discontinue breast-feeding should be considered. Breast-feeding is not recommended during therapy or for 6 weeks after treatment is complete.

Contraindications Hypersensitivity to mycophenolate mofetil, mycophenolate sodium, mycophenolic acid, or any component. Additional product-specific contraindications: CellCept: Parenteral formulation: Hypersensitivity to polysorbate 80.

Warnings

Hazardous agent; use appropriate precautions for handling and disposal (NIOSH, 2012). Immunosuppression with mycophenolate may result in an increased susceptibility to bacterial, viral, fungal, and protozoal infections, including opportunistic infections **[U.S. Boxed Warning]**; infections may be serious and potentially fatal. Due to the risk of oversuppression of the immune system, which may increase susceptibility to infection, combination immunosuppressant therapy should be used with caution. Polyomavirus-associated nephropathy (PVAN), JC virus-associated progressive multifocal leukoencephalopathy (PML), cytomegalovirus (CMV) infections, reactivation of hepatitis B (HBV) or hepatitis C (HCV) have been reported with use. A reduction in immunosuppression should be considered for patients with new or reactivated viral infections; however, in transplant recipients, the risk that reduced immunosuppression presents to the functioning graft should also be considered. PVAN, primarily from activation of BK virus, may lead to the deterioration of renal function and/or renal graft loss. PML, a potentially fatal condition, commonly presents with apathy, ataxia, cognitive deficiencies, confusion, and hemiparesis. Risk factors for development of PML include treatment with immunosuppressants and immune function impairment; consultation with a neurologist should be considered in any patient with neurological symptoms receiving immunosuppressants. Risk of CMV viremia or disease is increased in transplant recipients who are CMV seronegative at the time of transplant who receive a graft from a CMV seropositive donor. In patients infected with HBV or HCV, viral reactivation may occur; these patients should be monitored for signs of active HBV or HCV. Risk of developing lymphomas and other malignancies, particularly of the skin, is increased with mycophenolate use **[U.S. Boxed Warning]**; risk appears to be associated with the intensity and duration of immunosuppression; patients should be monitored and instructed to limit exposure to sunlight and ultraviolet light. Post-transplant lymphoproliferative disorder related to EBV infection has been reported in immunosuppressed organ transplant patients; risk is highest in EBV seronegative patients (including many young children).

Mycophenolate is associated with an increased risk of first trimester pregnancy loss, teratogenic effects, and congenital malformations, including external ear, facial abnormalities, cleft lip and palate, and anomalies of the distal limbs, heart, esophagus, and kidney **[U.S. Boxed Warning]**; women using mycophenolate during pregnancy should be encouraged to enroll in the National Transplantation Pregnancy Registry. Females of reproductive potential must be counseled about pregnancy prevention and planning. Alternative agents should be considered for women planning a pregnancy. Females of reproductive potential should have a negative pregnancy test with a sensitivity of ≥25 mIU/mL immediately before therapy and the test should be repeated 8-10 days later. Pregnancy tests should be repeated during routine follow-up visits. Acceptable forms of contraception must be initiated 4 weeks before starting mycophenolate therapy, maintained during therapy, and continued for 6 weeks after it has been discontinued. Because mycophenolate mofetil has demonstrated teratogenic effects in rats and rabbits, tablets should not be crushed, and capsules should not be opened or crushed. Avoid inhalation or direct contact with skin or mucous membranes of the powder contained in the capsules and the powder for oral suspension. Caution should be exercised in the handling and preparation of solutions of intravenous mycophenolate. Avoid skin contact with the intravenous solution and reconstituted suspension. If such contact occurs, wash thoroughly with soap and water, rinse eyes with plain water.

Neutropenia (including severe neutropenia) may occur, requiring dose reduction or interruption of treatment (risk greater from day 31-180 post-transplant). Pure red cell aplasia (PRCA), a type of anemia which can range from subclinical to severe has been reported in patients receiving mycophenolate concomitantly with other immunosuppressive agents (eg, tacrolimus, cyclosporine, corticosteroids). Symptoms may include fatigue, lethargy, or pallor. Although not precisely known, risk factors for the development of PRCA may include immunosuppression and treatment with immunosuppressant therapy. Dose reduction or discontinuation of immunosuppressive therapy may reverse PRCA; however, in transplant recipients, the risk of reduced immunosuppression and graft rejection should be considered.

CellCept and Myfortic products are not bioequivalent due to differences in absorption and should not be used interchangeably.

Some dosage forms (eg, oral suspension) may contain aspartame which is metabolized to phenylalanine and must be used with caution in patients with phenylketonuria. The intravenous formulation contains polysorbate 80 (Tween 80) which may cause allergic reactions in susceptible individuals. In premature neonates, thrombocytopenia, ascites, pulmonary deterioration, and renal and hepatic failure have been reported after receiving parenteral products containing polysorbate 80 (Alade, 1986; CDC, 1984). Infusion of polysorbate 80-containing solutions through polyvinyl chloride tubing may cause DEHP to leach into the solution; in immature animals, exposure to DEHP may adversely affect the development of the male reproductive tract.

Precautions Use with caution in patients with active serious digestive disease; use may rarely be associated with gastric or duodenal ulcers, GI bleeding, and/or perforation. Use with caution in patients with renal impairment as toxicity may be increased; may require dosage adjustment in severe impairment (ie, GFR <25 mL/minute/1.73 m^2 outside of the immediate post-transplant period). Avoid use in patients with rare hereditary deficiency of hypoxanthineguanine phosphoribosyl-transferase (HGPRT) such as Lesch-Nyhan and Kelley-Seegmiller syndrome. Intravenous solutions should be given over at least 2 hours; never administer intravenous solution by rapid or bolus injection. Live attenuated vaccines should be avoided during use; vaccinations may be less effective during therapy. Administer under the supervision of a physician experienced in immunosuppressive therapy and management of transplant patients **[U.S. Boxed Warning]**.

Adverse Reactions Note: In general, lower doses used in renal rejection patients had less adverse effects than higher doses. Rates of adverse effects were similar for each indication, except for those unique to the specific organ involved. The type of adverse effects observed in pediatric patients was similar to those seen in adults, with the exception of abdominal pain, anemia, diarrhea, fever, hypertension, infection, pharyngitis, respiratory tract infection, sepsis, and vomiting; lymphoproliferative disorder was the only type of malignancy observed.

As reported in adults following oral dosing of CellCept alone in renal, cardiac, and hepatic allograft rejection studies:

Cardiovascular: Chest pain, edema, hyper-/hypotension, peripheral edema, tachycardia

Central nervous system: Anxiety, dizziness, fever, headache, insomnia, pain

Dermatologic: Rash

Endocrine & metabolic: Hypercholesterolemia, hyperglycemia, hypocalcemia, hyper-/hypokalemia, hypomagnesemia

Gastrointestinal: Abdominal pain, anorexia, constipation, diarrhea, dyspepsia, nausea, vomiting

Genitourinary: Urinary tract infection

Hematologic: Anemia (including hypochromic), leukocytosis, leukopenia, thrombocytopenia

Hepatic: Ascites, liver function tests abnormal

Neuromuscular & skeletal: Back pain, paresthesia, tremor, weakness

Renal: BUN increased, creatinine increased, kidney function abnormal

Respiratory: Cough, dyspnea, lung disorder, pleural effusion, respiratory tract infection, sinusitis

Miscellaneous: *Candida*, herpes simplex, lactate dehydrogenase increased, sepsis

Use in combination with cyclosporine and corticosteroids:

Cardiovascular: Angina, arrhythmia, arterial thrombosis, atrial fibrillation, atrial flutter, bradycardia, cardiac arrest, cardiac failure, CHF, extrasystole, facial edema, hyper-/hypovolemia, orthostatic hypotension, pallor, palpitation, pericardial effusion, peripheral vascular disorder, supraventricular extrasystoles, supraventricular tachycardia, syncope, thrombosis, vasodilation, vasospasm, venous pressure increased, ventricular extrasystole, ventricular tachycardia

Central nervous system: Agitation, chills with fever, confusion, delirium, depression, emotional lability, hallucinations, hypoesthesia, malaise, nervousness, psychosis, seizure, somnolence, thinking abnormal, vertigo

Dermatologic: Acne, alopecia, bruising, cellulitis, fungal dermatitis, hirsutism, petechia, pruritus, skin carcinoma, skin hypertrophy, skin ulcer, vesiculobullous rash

Endocrine & metabolic: Acidosis, alkalosis, Cushing's syndrome, dehydration, diabetes mellitus, gout, hypercalcemia, hyper-hypophosphatemia, hyperlipemia, hyperuricemia, hypochloremia, hypoglycemia, hyponatremia, hypoproteinemia, hypothyroidism, parathyroid disorder

Gastrointestinal: Abdomen enlarged, dysphagia, esophagitis, flatulence, gastritis, gastroenteritis, gastrointestinal

hemorrhage, gastrointestinal moniliasis, gingivitis, gum hyperplasia, ileus, melena, mouth ulceration, oral moniliasis, stomach disorder, stomach ulcer, stomatitis, xerostomia, weight gain/loss

Genitourinary: Impotence, nocturia, pelvic pain, prostatic disorder, scrotal edema, urinary frequency, urinary incontinence, urinary retention, urinary tract disorder

Hematologic: Coagulation disorder, hemorrhage, neutropenia, pancytopenia, polycythemia, prothrombin time increased, thromboplastin time increased

Hepatic: Alkaline phosphatase increased, bilirubinemia, cholangitis, cholestatic jaundice, GGT increased, hepatitis, jaundice, liver damage, transaminases increased

Local: Abscess

Neuromuscular & skeletal: Arthralgia, hypertonia, joint disorder, leg cramps, myalgia, myasthenia, neck pain, neuropathy, osteoporosis

Ocular: Amblyopia, cataract, conjunctivitis, eye hemorrhage, lacrimation disorder, vision abnormal

Otic: Deafness, ear disorder, ear pain, tinnitus

Renal: Albuminuria, creatinine increased, dysuria, hematuria, hydronephrosis, oliguria, pyelonephritis, renal failure, renal tubular necrosis

Respiratory: Apnea, asthma, atelectasis, bronchitis, epistaxis, hemoptysis, hiccup, hyperventilation, hypoxia, respiratory acidosis, pharyngitis, pneumonia, pneumothorax, pulmonary edema, pulmonary hypertension, respiratory moniliasis, rhinitis, sputum increased, voice alteration

Miscellaneous: *Candida* (mucocutaneous), CMV tissue invasive disease, CMV viremia/syndrome, herpes zoster cutaneous disease, cyst, diaphoresis, flu-like syndrome, healing abnormal, hernia, ileus infection, neoplasm, peritonitis, thirst

Rare but important or life-threatening: Atypical mycobacterial infection, BK virus-associated nephropathy, colitis, gastrointestinal perforation, infectious endocarditis, interstitial lung disorder, intestinal villous atrophy, lymphoma, lymphoproliferative disease, malignancy, meningitis, pancreatitis, progressive multifocal leukoencephalopathy (sometimes fatal), pulmonary fibrosis (fatal), pure red cell aplasia, tuberculosis

Drug Interactions

Metabolism/Transport Effects None known.

Avoid Concomitant Use

Avoid concomitant use of Mycophenolate with any of the following: BCG; Bile Acid Sequestrants; Cholestyramine Resin; Natalizumab; Pimecrolimus; Rifamycin Derivatives; Tacrolimus (Topical); Tofacitinib; Vaccines (Live)

Increased Effect/Toxicity

Mycophenolate may increase the levels/effects of: Acyclovir-Valacyclovir; Ganciclovir-Valganciclovir; Leflunomide; Natalizumab; Tofacitinib; Vaccines (Live)

The levels/effects of Mycophenolate may be increased by: Acyclovir-Valacyclovir; Belatacept; Denosumab; Ganciclovir-Valganciclovir; Pimecrolimus; Probenecid; Roflumilast; Tacrolimus (Topical); Trastuzumab

Decreased Effect

Mycophenolate may decrease the levels/effects of: BCG; Coccidioidin Skin Test; Contraceptives (Estrogens); Contraceptives (Progestins); Sipuleucel-T; Vaccines (Inactivated); Vaccines (Live)

The levels/effects of Mycophenolate may be decreased by: Antacids; Bile Acid Sequestrants; Cholestyramine Resin; CycloSPORINE (Systemic); Echinacea; Magnesium Salts; MetroNIDAZOLE (Systemic); Penicillins; Proton Pump Inhibitors; Quinolone Antibiotics; Rifamycin Derivatives; Sevelamer

Food Interactions Food decreases C$_{max}$ of MPA by 40% following CellCept administration and 33% following Myfortic use; the extent of absorption is not changed.

Management: Take CellCept or Myfortic on an empty stomach to decrease variability; however, Cellcept may be taken with food if necessary in stable renal transplant patients.

Stability

Oral:

Capsules: Store at 25°C (77°F); excursions permitted to 15°C to 30°C (59°F to 86°F).

Tablets: Store at 25°C (77°F); excursions permitted to 15°C to 30°C (59°F to 86°F). Protect from moisture and light.

Oral suspension: Store powder for oral suspension at 25°C (77°F); excursions permitted to 15°C to 30°C (59°F to 86°F). Once reconstituted, the oral suspension may be stored in the refrigerator or at room temperature; stable for 60 days after reconstitution. Do not freeze.

Injection: Store intact vials and diluted solutions at 25°C (77°F); excursions permitted to 15°C to 30°C (59°F to 86°F). Manufacturer's labeling recommends that administration of the infusion solution should begin within 4 hours from reconstitution and dilution of the drug. Do not mix mycophenolate with any other drugs.

Mechanism of Action

MPA exhibits a cytostatic effect on T and B lymphocytes. It is an inhibitor of inosine monophosphate dehydrogenase (IMPDH) which inhibits *de novo* guanosine nucleotide synthesis. T and B lymphocytes are dependent on this pathway for proliferation.

Pharmacokinetics (Adult data unless noted)

Absorption: Rapid and extensive; early post-transplant period mycophenolic acid (MPA) AUC values are lower (~45% to 53%) than later post-transplant period (>3 months) MPA AUC values in both pediatric patients and adults

Distribution: Mean V_d:

Mycophenolate mofetil (CellCept): MPA: Oral: 4 L/kg; I.V. 3.6 L/kg

Mycophenolate sodium delayed release tablet (Myfortic): MPA: Oral: 54 L (at steady state)

Protein binding: Mycophenolic acid (MPA): >97%; Mycophenolic acid glucuronide (MPAG): 82%

Metabolism: Hepatic and via GI tract; undergoes hydrolysis by esterases to mycophenolic acid (MPA is the active metabolite); MPA is metabolized by glucuronyl transferase to mycophenolic acid glucuronide (MPAG is inactive). MPAG is converted to MPA via enterohepatic recirculation.

Bioavailability:

Mycophenolate mofetil (CellCept): 80.7% to 94%; enterohepatic recirculation contributes to MPA concentration (Staatz, 2007); two 500 mg tablets have been shown to be bioequivalent to four 250 mg capsules or 1000 mg of oral suspension

Mycophenolate sodium delayed release tablet (Myfortic): 72%

Half-life:

Mycophenolate mofetil (CellCept): MPA: Oral: 18 hours; I.V.: 17 hours

Mycophenolate sodium delayed release tablet (Myfortic): MPA: Oral: 8-16 hours; MPAG: 13-17 hours

Time to peak serum concentration: Oral:

Mycophenolate mofetil (CellCept): 0.5-1 hour

Mycophenolate sodium delayed release tablet (Myfortic): Median: 1.5-2.75 hours

Elimination:

Mycophenolate mofetil (CellCept): MPA: Urine (<1%); feces (6%); MPAG: Urine (87%)

Mycophenolate sodium delayed release tablet (Myfortic): MPA: Urine (3%); feces; MPAG: Urine (>60%)

Dosing: Usual

Note: May be used I.V. for up to 14 days; transition to oral therapy as soon as tolerated. Mycophenolate mofetil (CellCept) tablets, capsules, and suspension should not be interchanged with the delayed release tablet formulation (Myfortic) due to differences in the rate of absorption.

Pediatric:

Renal transplantation:

Mycophenolate mofetil (CellCept): Infants ≥3 months, Children, and Adolescents:

Oral:

Suspension: 600 mg/m²/dose twice daily; maximum daily dose: 2000 mg/**day**

Tablets or capsules:

BSA 1.25 m² to 1.5 m²: 750 mg twice daily

BSA >1.5 m²: 1000 mg twice daily

Mycophenolate sodium delayed release tablets (Myfortic): Children ≥5 years and Adolescents: 400 mg/m²/dose twice daily; maximum daily dose: 1440 mg/**day**

Alternate fixed dosing:

BSA <1.19 m²: Use of this formulation is not recommended

BSA 1.19 to 1.58 m²: 540 mg twice daily

BSA >1.58 m²: 720 mg twice daily

Note: Mycophenolate sodium delayed release 720 mg twice daily was shown to be bioequivalent to mycophenolate mofetil 1000 mg twice daily

Lupus nephritis: Limited data available: Mycophenolate mofetil (CellCept): Children and Adolescents: Oral:

BSA-based dosing:

Induction: 300-600 mg/m²/dose twice daily; maximum daily dose: 3000 mg/**day** (Aragon, 2010; Hobbs, 2010; Marks, 2010; Wong, 2009)

Maintenance: Initial: 300-600 mg/m²/dose twice daily; reported maximum daily dose range: 2000-3000 mg/**day** (Baskin, 2010; Cramer, 2007; Marks, 2010); once disease stabilized and remission maintained may consider dosage reduction.

Fixed dosing: Children ≥5 years and Adolescents: Induction or maintenance: Initial: 250-500 mg twice daily and gradually increased up to 750-1000 mg twice daily; doses based on small retrospective studies (n=52); doses equivalent to 10-12.5 mg/kg/dose twice daily (Appel, 2009; Falcini, 2009; Kazyra, 2010)

Nephrotic syndrome: Limited data available: Mycophenolate mofetil (CellCept): Children and Adolescents: Oral:

Frequently relapsing:

BSA-based dosing: 600 mg/m²/dose twice daily for at least 12 months; maximum daily dose: 2000 mg/**day** (Beck, 2013; Gipson, 2009; KDIGO, 2012)

Weight-based dosing: 12.5-18 mg/kg/dose twice daily; maximum daily dose: 2000 mg/**day** for 1-2 years with a tapering dose of prednisone (Gipson, 2009)

Steroid-dependent (for steroid sparing effect):

BSA-based dosing: 600 mg/m²/dose twice daily for at least 12 months; maximum daily dose: 2000 mg/**day** (Gipson, 2009; KDIGO, 2012)

Weight-based dosing: 12-18 mg/kg/dose twice daily; maximum daily dose: 2000 mg/**day** (Gipson, 2009)

Adult: **Note:** May be used I.V. for up to 14 days; transition to oral therapy as soon as tolerated.

Renal transplantation:

CellCept: I.V., Oral: 1000 mg twice daily. Doses >2000 mg daily are not recommended.

Myfortic: Oral: 720 mg twice daily

Cardiac transplantation: *CellCept:* I.V., Oral: 1500 mg twice daily

Hepatic transplantation: *CellCept:*

Oral: 1500 mg twice daily

I.V.: 1000 mg twice daily

Lupus nephritis: *CellCept:* Oral:

Induction: 1000 mg twice daily for 6 months in combination with a glucocorticoid (Ong, 2005) **or** 2000-3000 mg daily for 6 months in combination with glucocorticoids (Hahn, 2012)

Maintenance: 500-3000 mg daily (Contreras, 2004) **or** 1000 mg twice daily (Dooley, 2011) **or** 1000-2000 mg daily (Hahn, 2012)

Dosing adjustment in renal impairment:

Infants, Children, and Adolescents:

Mycophenolate mofetil (CellCept): Infants ≥3 months, Children, and Adolescents: Patients should be carefully observed; no dose adjustments are needed in renal transplant patients experiencing delayed graft function postoperatively. Avoid doses >1 g twice daily.

Mycophenolate delayed release tablet (Myfortic): Children ≥5 years and Adolescents: No dose adjustments are needed in renal transplant patients experiencing delayed graft function postoperatively; however, monitor carefully for potential concentration dependent adverse events.

Adults:

Renal transplant: GFR <25 mL/minute/1.73 m^2 outside the immediate post-transplant period:

Mycophenolate mofetil (CellCept): Avoid doses >1 g twice daily; patients should also be carefully observed; no dose adjustments are needed in renal transplant patients experiencing delayed graft function postoperatively

Mycophenolate delayed release tablet (Myfortic): No dose adjustments are needed in renal transplant patients experiencing delayed graft function postoperatively; however, monitor carefully for potential concentration dependent adverse events.

Cardiac or liver transplant: No data available; mycophenolate may be used in cardiac or hepatic transplant patients with severe chronic renal impairment if the potential benefit outweighs the potential risk.

Dosing adjustment in hepatic impairment: Infants ≥3 months, Children, Adolescents, and Adults: No dosage adjustment is recommended for renal patients with severe hepatic parenchymal disease; however, it is not currently known whether dosage adjustments are necessary for hepatic disease with other etiologies.

Dosing adjustment for toxicity (neutropenia): ANC <1.3 x 103/µL or anemia; Dosing should be interrupted or the dose reduced

Administration Hazardous agent: Use appropriate precautions for handling and disposal (NIOSH, 2012).

Oral (capsule, tablet, suspension): Administer on an empty stomach 1 hour before or 2 hours after food to avoid variability in absorption; CellCept may be administered with food in stable renal transplant patients when necessary. Shake suspension well before use; may be administered via a nasogastric tube (minimum: 8 French, 1.7 mm interior diameter); oral suspension should not be mixed with other medications. Delayed release tablets should be swallowed whole; do not crush, chew, or cut.

I.V.: Reconstitute vial with D$_5$W and further dilute to a final concentration of 6 mg/mL using D$_5$W. **Do not administer I.V. push** or by rapid I.V. bolus injection; administer by slow I.V. infusion over a period of no less than 2 hours.

Monitoring Parameters Complete blood count (weekly for first month, twice monthly during months 2 and 3, then monthly thereafter through the first year); renal and liver function; signs and symptoms of organ rejection; signs and symptoms of bacterial, fungal, protozoal, new or reactivated viral, or opportunistic infections; neurological symptoms (eg, hemiparesis, confusion, cognitive deficiencies, ataxia) suggestive of PML, pregnancy test (immediately prior to initiation and 8-10 days later in females of childbearing potential, followed by repeat tests during therapy); monitor skin (for lesions suspicious of skin cancer); monitor for signs of lymphoma

Additional Information A direct conversion factor from mycophenolate mofetil to mycophenolic acid (delayed release) is not available. In one study, adults on mycophenolate mofetil 1000 mg twice daily were successfully converted to mycophenolic acid (delayed release) 720 mg twice daily. In the same study, children (n=17) were converted from 440 ± 147 mg/m^2 twice daily to mycophenolic acid (delayed release) 432 ± 51 mg/m^2 twice daily (Massari, 2005).

Dosage Forms Excipient information presented when available (limited, particularly for generics); consult specific product labeling.

Capsule, Oral, as mofetil:

CellCept: 250 mg [contains fd&c blue #2 (indigotine)]

Generic: 250 mg

Solution Reconstituted, Intravenous, as mofetil hydrochloride:

CellCept Intravenous: 500 mg (1 ea)

Suspension Reconstituted, Oral, as mofetil:

CellCept: 200 mg/mL (160 mL) [contains aspartame, methylparaben, soybean lecithin; mixed fruit flavor]

Tablet, Oral, as mofetil:

CellCept: 500 mg [contains fd&c blue #2 aluminum lake]

Generic: 500 mg

Tablet Delayed Release, Oral, as mycophenolic acid:

Myfortic: 180 mg [contains fd&c blue #2 (indigotine)]

Myfortic: 360 mg

Generic: 180 mg, 360 mg

Extemporaneous Preparations Hazardous agent: Use appropriate precautions for handling and disposal.

A 50 mg/mL oral suspension may be made with mycophenolate mofetil capsules, Ora-Plus, and cherry syrup. In a vertical flow hood, empty six 250 mg capsules into a mortar; add 7.5 mL Ora-Plus and mix to a uniform paste. Mix while adding 15 mL of cherry syrup in incremental proportions; transfer to a calibrated bottle, rinse mortar with cherry syrup, and add sufficient quantity of cherry syrup to make 30 mL. Label "shake well". Stable for 210 days at 5°C, for 28 days at 25°C to 37°C, and for 11 days at 45°C.

Venkataramanan R, McCombs JR, Zuckerman S, et al, "Stability of Mycophenolate Mofetil as an Extemporaneous Suspension," *Ann Pharmacother*, 1998, 32(7-8):755-7.

References

Alade SL, Brown RE, and Paquet A Jr, "Polysorbate 80 and E-Ferol Toxicity," *Pediatrics*, 1986, 77(4):593-7.

Appel GB, Contreras G, Dooley MA, et al. Mycophenolate mofetil versus cyclophosphamide for induction treatment of lupus nephritis. *J Am Soc Nephrol*. 2009;20(5):1103-1112.

Aragon E, Chan YH, Ng KH, et al. Good outcomes with mycophenolate-cyclosporine-based induction protocol in children with severe proliferative lupus nephritis. *Lupus*. 2010;19(8):965-973.

Aronoff GR, Bennett WM, Berns JS, et al. *Drug Prescribing in Renal Failure: Dosing Guidelines for Adults and Children.* 5th ed. Philadelphia, PA: American College of Physicians; 2007.

Baskin E, Ozen S, Cakar N, et al. The use of low-dose cyclophosphamide followed by AZA/MMF treatment in childhood lupus nephritis. *Pediatr Nephrol*. 2010;25(1):111-117.

Beck L, Bomback AS, Choi MJ, et al. KDOQI US commentary on the 2012 KDIGO clinical practice guideline for glomerulonephritis. *Am J Kidney Dis*. 2013;62(3):403-441.

Centers for Disease Control (CDC), "Unusual Syndrome With Fatalities Among Premature Infants: Association With a New Intravenous Vitamin E Product," *MMWR Morb Mortal Wkly Rep*, 1984, 33 (14):198-9.

Contreras G, Pardo V, Leclercq B, et al. Sequential therapies for proliferative lupus nephritis. *N Engl J Med*. 2004;350(10):971-980.

Cramer CH 2nd, Mills M, Valentini RP, et al. Clinical presentation and outcome in a cohort of paediatric patients with membranous lupus nephritis. *Nephrol Dial Transplant*. 2007;22(12):3495-3500.

Dooley MA, Jayne D, Ginzler EM, et al. Mycophenolate versus azathioprine as maintenance therapy for lupus nephritis. *N Engl J Med*. 2011;365(20):1886-1895.

Ettenger R, Warshaw B, Menster M, et al, "Mycophenolate Mofetil in Pediatric Renal Transplantation: A Report of the Ped MMF Study Group." Abstract: 1996, Annual Meeting, ASTP.

Falcini F, Capannini S, Martini G, et al. Mycophenolate mofetil for the treatment of juvenile onset SLE: a multicenter study. *Lupus*. 2009;18 (2):139-143.

Gipson DS, Massengill SF, Yao L, et al, "Management of Childhood Onset Nephrotic Syndrome," *Pediatrics*, 2009, 124(2):747-57.

Hahn BH, McMahon MA, Wilkinson A, et al, "American College of Rheumatology Guidelines for Screening, Treatment, and

Management of Lupus Nephritis," *Arthritis Care Res (Hoboken)*, 2012, 64(6):797-808.

Hobbs DJ, Barletta GM, Rajpal JS, et al. Severe paediatric systemic lupus erythematosus nephritis-a single-centre experience. *Nephrol Dial Transplant.* 2010;25(2):457-463.

Hogg RJ, Fitzgibbons L, Bruick J, et al, "Mycophenolate Mofetil in Children With Frequently Relapsing Nephrotic Syndrome: A Report From the Southwest Pediatric Nephrology Study Group," *Clin J Am Soc Nephrol*, 2006, 1(6):1173-8.

Kazyra I, Pilkington C, Marks SD, et al. Mycophenolate mofetil treatment in children and adolescents with lupus. *Arch Dis Child.* 2010;95 (12):1059-1061.

Kidney disease: improving global outcomes (KDIGO) Glomerulonephritis Work Group. KDIGO clinical practice guideline for glomerulonephritis. *Kidney Inter.* 2012;2:139–274.

Kobashigawa JA, Renlund DG, Gerosa G, et al, "Similar Efficacy and Safety of Enteric-Coated Mycophenolate Sodium (EC-MPS, Myfortic) Compared With Mycophenolate Mofetil (MMF) in de novo Heart Transplant Recipients: Results of a 12-Month, Single-Blind, Randomized, Parallel-Group, Multicenter Study," *J Heart Lung Transplant*, 2006, 25(8):935-41.

Marks SD, Tullus K. Modern therapeutic strategies for paediatric systemic lupus erythematosus and lupus nephritis. *Acta Paediatr.* 2010;99(7):967-974.

Massari P, Duro-Garcia V, Girón F, et al, "Safety Assessment of the Conversion From Mycophenolate Mofetil to Enteric-Coated Mycophenolate Sodium in Stable Renal Transplant Recipients," *Transplant Proc*, 2005, 37(2):916-9.

National Institute for Occupational Safety and Health (NIOSH), "NIOSH List of Antineoplastic and Other Hazardous Drugs in Healthcare Settings 2012." Available at http://www.cdc.gov/niosh/docs/2012-150/pdfs/2012-150.pdf. Accessed January 21, 2013.

Ong LM, Hooi LS, Lim TO, et al. Randomized controlled trial of pulse intravenous cyclophosphamide versus mycophenolate mofetil in the induction therapy of proliferative lupus nephritis. *Nephrology (Carlton).* 2005;10(5):504-510.

Sollinger HW, "Mycophenolate Mofetil for the Prevention of Acute Rejection in Primary Cadaveric Renal Allograft Recipients. U.S. Renal Transplant Mycophenolate Mofetil Study Group," *Transplantation*, 1995, 60:225-32.

Staatz CE and Tett SE, "Clinical Pharmacokinetics and Pharmacodynamics of Mycophenolate in Solid Organ Transplant Recipients," *Clin Pharmacokinet*, 2007, 46(1):13-58.

Wong SN, Chan WK, Hui J, et al. Membranous lupus nephritis in Chinese children–a case series and review of the literature. *Pediatr Nephrol.* 2009 Oct;24(10):1989-1996.

◆ **Mycophenolate Mofetil** *see* Mycophenolate on page 1453

◆ **Mycophenolate Sodium** *see* Mycophenolate on page 1453

◆ **Mycophenolic Acid** *see* Mycophenolate on page 1453

◆ **Mydfrin [DSC]** *see* Phenylephrine (Ophthalmic) on page 1661

◆ **Mydfrin® (Can)** *see* Phenylephrine (Ophthalmic) on page 1661

◆ **Mydral** *see* Tropicamide on page 2092

◆ **Mydriacyl** *see* Tropicamide on page 2092

◆ **Mydriacyl® (Can)** *see* Tropicamide on page 2092

◆ **Myferon 150 [OTC]** *see* Polysaccharide-Iron Complex on page 1701

◆ **Myfortic** *see* Mycophenolate on page 1453

◆ **Mylan-Acyclovir (Can)** *see* Acyclovir (Systemic) on page 63

◆ **Mylan-Almotriptan (Can)** *see* Almotriptan on page 99

◆ **Mylan-Alprazolam (Can)** *see* ALPRAZolam on page 100

◆ **Mylan-Amantadine (Can)** *see* Amantadine on page 112

◆ **Mylan-Amiodarone (Can)** *see* Amiodarone on page 127

◆ **Mylan-Amlodipine (Can)** *see* AmLODIPine on page 135

◆ **Mylan-Amoxicillin (Can)** *see* Amoxicillin on page 140

◆ **Mylan-Anagrelide (Can)** *see* Anagrelide on page 166

◆ **Mylan-Atenolol (Can)** *see* Atenolol on page 222

◆ **Mylan-Atomoxetine (Can)** *see* AtoMOXetine on page 224

◆ **Mylan-Atorvastatin (Can)** *see* AtorvaSTATin on page 227

◆ **Mylan-Azathioprine (Can)** *see* AzaTHIOprine on page 241

◆ **Mylan-Azithromycin (Can)** *see* Azithromycin (Systemic) on page 247

◆ **Mylan-Baclofen (Can)** *see* Baclofen on page 259

◆ **Mylan-Beclo AQ (Can)** *see* Beclomethasone (Nasal) on page 267

◆ **Mylan-Bosentan (Can)** *see* Bosentan on page 298

◆ **Mylan-Budesonide AQ (Can)** *see* Budesonide (Nasal) on page 313

◆ **Mylan-Bupropion XL (Can)** *see* BuPROPion on page 327

◆ **Mylan-Candesartan (Can)** *see* Candesartan on page 363

◆ **Mylan-Captopril (Can)** *see* Captopril on page 368

◆ **Mylan-Carbamazepine CR (Can)** *see* CarBAMazepine on page 372

◆ **Mylan-Carvedilol (Can)** *see* Carvedilol on page 385

◆ **Mylan-Cimetidine (Can)** *see* Cimetidine on page 469

◆ **Mylan-Ciprofloxacin (Can)** *see* Ciprofloxacin (Systemic) on page 471

◆ **Mylan-Citalopram (Can)** *see* Citalopram on page 484

◆ **Mylan-Clarithromycin (Can)** *see* Clarithromycin on page 490

◆ **Mylan-Clindamycin (Can)** *see* Clindamycin (Systemic) on page 495

◆ **Mylan-Clobetasol Cream (Can)** *see* Clobetasol on page 506

◆ **Mylan-Clobetasol Ointment (Can)** *see* Clobetasol on page 506

◆ **Mylan-Clobetasol Scalp Application (Can)** *see* Clobetasol on page 506

◆ **Mylan-Clonazepam (Can)** *see* ClonazePAM on page 514

◆ **Mylan-Clopidogrel (Can)** *see* Clopidogrel on page 521

◆ **Mylan-Cyclobenzaprine (Can)** *see* Cyclobenzaprine on page 558

◆ **Mylan-Divalproex (Can)** *see* Valproic Acid and Derivatives on page 2102

◆ **Mylan-Doxazosin (Can)** *see* Doxazosin on page 712

◆ **Mylan-Efavirenz (Can)** *see* Efavirenz on page 731

◆ **Mylan-Enalapril (Can)** *see* Enalapril on page 744

◆ **Mylan-Esomeprazole (Can)** *see* Esomeprazole on page 793

◆ **Mylan-Etidronate (Can)** *see* Etidronate on page 810

◆ **Mylan-Famotidine (Can)** *see* Famotidine on page 843

◆ **Mylan-Fluconazole (Can)** *see* Fluconazole on page 877

◆ **Mylan-Fluoxetine (Can)** *see* FLUoxetine on page 901

◆ **Mylan-Fosinopril (Can)** *see* Fosinopril on page 938

◆ **Mylan-Gabapentin (Can)** *see* Gabapentin on page 950

◆ **Mylan-Glybe (Can)** *see* GlyBURIDE on page 974

◆ **Mylan-Hydroxychloroquine (Can)** *see* Hydroxychloroquine on page 1048

◆ **Mylan-Hydroxyurea (Can)** *see* Hydroxyurea on page 1051

◆ **Mylan-Ipratropium Solution (Can)** *see* Ipratropium (Nasal) on page 1146

◆ **Mylan-Ipratropium Sterinebs (Can)** *see* Ipratropium (Oral Inhalation) on page 1144

◆ **Mylan-Irbesartan (Can)** *see* Irbesartan on page 1147

◆ **Mylan-Lamotrigine (Can)** *see* LamoTRIgine *on page 1199*

◆ **Mylan-Lansoprazole (Can)** *see* Lansoprazole *on page 1206*

◆ **Mylan-Levofloxacin (Can)** *see* Levofloxacin (Systemic) *on page 1228*

◆ **Mylan-Lisinopril (Can)** *see* Lisinopril *on page 1262*

◆ **Mylan-Losartan (Can)** *see* Losartan *on page 1283*

◆ **Mylan-Lovastatin (Can)** *see* Lovastatin *on page 1286*

◆ **Mylan-Meloxicam (Can)** *see* Meloxicam *on page 1325*

◆ **Mylan-Metformin (Can)** *see* MetFORMIN *on page 1353*

◆ **Mylan-Metoprolol (Type L) (Can)** *see* Metoprolol *on page 1396*

◆ **Mylan-Minocycline (Can)** *see* Minocycline *on page 1420*

◆ **Mylan-Montelukast (Can)** *see* Montelukast *on page 1438*

◆ **Mylan-Mycophenolate (Can)** *see* Mycophenolate *on page 1453*

◆ **Mylan-Naproxen EC (Can)** *see* Naproxen *on page 1470*

◆ **Mylan-Nevirapine (Can)** *see* Nevirapine *on page 1487*

◆ **Mylan-Nifedipine Extended Release (Can)** *see* NIFEdipine *on page 1497*

◆ **Mylan-Nitro Sublingual Spray (Can)** *see* Nitroglycerin *on page 1504*

◆ **Mylan-Olanzapine (Can)** *see* OLANZapine *on page 1525*

◆ **Mylan-Omeprazole (Can)** *see* Omeprazole *on page 1535*

◆ **Mylan-Ondansetron (Can)** *see* Ondansetron *on page 1544*

◆ **Mylan-Oxybutynin (Can)** *see* Oxybutynin *on page 1568*

◆ **Mylan-Pantoprazole (Can)** *see* Pantoprazole *on page 1595*

◆ **Mylan-Paroxetine (Can)** *see* PARoxetine *on page 1609*

◆ **Mylan-Pravastatin (Can)** *see* Pravastatin *on page 1720*

◆ **Mylan-Quetiapine (Can)** *see* QUEtiapine *on page 1783*

◆ **Mylan-Ranitidine (Can)** *see* Ranitidine *on page 1805*

◆ **Mylan-Risperidone (Can)** *see* RisperiDONE *on page 1831*

◆ **Mylan-Rizatriptan ODT (Can)** *see* Rizatriptan *on page 1845*

◆ **Mylan-Rosuvastatin (Can)** *see* Rosuvastatin *on page 1853*

◆ **Mylan-Sertraline (Can)** *see* Sertraline *on page 1879*

◆ **Mylan-Simvastatin (Can)** *see* Simvastatin *on page 1892*

◆ **Mylan-Sotalol (Can)** *see* Sotalol *on page 1925*

◆ **Mylan-Sumatriptan (Can)** *see* SUMAtriptan *on page 1958*

◆ **Mylanta™ (Can)** *see* Aluminum Hydroxide and Magnesium Hydroxide *on page 111*

◆ **Mylan-Tamoxifen (Can)** *see* Tamoxifen *on page 1968*

◆ **Mylan-Terbinafine (Can)** *see* Terbinafine (Systemic) *on page 1982*

◆ **Mylan-Timolol (Can)** *see* Timolol (Ophthalmic) *on page 2028*

◆ **Mylan-Topiramate (Can)** *see* Topiramate *on page 2046*

◆ **Mylan-Trazodone (Can)** *see* TraZODone *on page 2065*

◆ **Mylan-Triazolam (Can)** *see* Triazolam *on page 2080*

◆ **Mylan-Valacyclovir (Can)** *see* ValACYclovir *on page 2097*

◆ **Mylan-Valproic (Can)** *see* Valproic Acid and Derivatives *on page 2102*

◆ **Mylan-Valsartan (Can)** *see* Valsartan *on page 2108*

◆ **Mylan-Venlafaxine XR (Can)** *see* Venlafaxine *on page 2125*

◆ **Mylan-Verapamil (Can)** *see* Verapamil *on page 2129*

◆ **Mylan-Verapamil SR (Can)** *see* Verapamil *on page 2129*

◆ **Mylan-Warfarin (Can)** *see* Warfarin *on page 2156*

◆ **Myleran** *see* Busulfan *on page 333*

◆ **Myleran® (Can)** *see* Busulfan *on page 333*

◆ **Myl-Letrozole (Can)** *see* Letrozole *on page 1211*

◆ **Myl-Ranitidine (Can)** *see* Ranitidine *on page 1805*

◆ **Myobloc** *see* RimabotulinumtoxinB *on page 1829*

◆ **Myochrysine® [DSC]** *see* Gold Sodium Thiomalate *on page 979*

◆ **Myochrysine® (Can)** *see* Gold Sodium Thiomalate *on page 979*

◆ **Myorisan** *see* ISOtretinoin *on page 1161*

◆ **Myozyme** *see* Alglucosidase Alfa *on page 95*

◆ **Myozyme® (Can)** *see* Alglucosidase Alfa *on page 95*

◆ **Mysoline** *see* Primidone *on page 1737*

◆ **Mytab Gas [OTC]** *see* Simethicone *on page 1891*

◆ **Mytab Gas Maximum Strength [OTC]** *see* Simethicone *on page 1891*

◆ **Mytotan** *see* Mitotane *on page 1425*

◆ **Nabi-HB** *see* Hepatitis B Immune Globulin (Human) *on page 1008*

Nabilone (NA bi lone)

Brand Names: U.S. Cesamet
Brand Names: Canada Cesamet®; PMS-Nabilone; RAN™-Nabilone; Teva-Nabilone
Therapeutic Category Antiemetic
Generic Availability (U.S.) No
Use Treatment of refractory nausea and vomiting associated with cancer chemotherapy
Pregnancy Risk Factor C
Pregnancy Considerations Adverse events have been observed in animal reproduction studies.
Breast-Feeding Considerations Because some cannabinoids are excreted in breast milk, use in breast-feeding is not recommended.
Contraindications Hypersensitivity to nabilone, cannabinoids, tetrahydrocannabinol, or any component
Warnings Nabilone has potential for abuse and/or dependence; use caution in patients with substance abuse history; limit antiemetic therapy availability to current cycle of chemotherapy. Safety and efficacy in children have not been established.
Precautions Use with caution in patients with cardiovascular disease (may cause tachycardia and orthostatic hypotension), history of substance abuse, and those with preexisting CNS depression; use caution with current or previous history of mental illness; cannabinoid use may reveal symptoms of psychiatric disorders. Psychiatric adverse reactions may persist for up to 3 days after discontinuing treatment.
Adverse Reactions
Cardiovascular: Hypotension
Central nervous system: Ataxia, concentration decreased, depersonalization, depression, disorientation, dizziness, drowsiness, dysphoria, euphoria, headache, sedation, sleep disturbance, vertigo
Gastrointestinal: Anorexia, appetite increased, nausea, xerostomia
Neuromuscular & skeletal: Weakness

Ocular: Visual disturbance

Rare but important or life-threatening: Abdominal pain, abnormal dreams, akathisia, allergic reaction, amblyopia, anemia, anhydrosis, anxiety, apathy, aphthous ulcer, arrhythmia, back pain, cerebral vascular accident, chest pain, chills, constipation, cough, diaphoresis, diarrhea, dyspepsia, dyspnea, dystonia, emotional disorder, emotional lability, epistaxis, equilibrium dysfunction, eye irritation, fatigue, fever, flushing, gastritis, hallucinations, hot flashes, hyperactivity, hypertension, infection, insomnia, joint pain, leukopenia, lightheadedness, malaise, memory disturbance, mood swings, mouth irritation, muscle pain, nasal congestion, neck pain, nervousness, neurosis (phobic), numbness, orthostatic hypotension, pain, palpitation, panic disorder, paranoia, paresthesia, perception disturbance, pharyngitis, photophobia, photosensitivity, polyuria, pruritus, psychosis (including toxic), pupil dilation, rash, seizure, sinus headache, speech disorder, stupor, syncope, tachycardia, taste perversion, thirst, thought disorder, tinnitus, tremor, urination decreased/increased, urinary retention, visual field defect, voice change, vomiting, wheezing, withdrawal, xerophthalmia

Drug Interactions

Metabolism/Transport Effects None known.

Avoid Concomitant Use There are no known interactions where it is recommended to avoid concomitant use.

Increased Effect/Toxicity

Nabilone may increase the levels/effects of: Alcohol (Ethyl); CNS Depressants; Sympathomimetics

The levels/effects of Nabilone may be increased by: Anticholinergic Agents; Cocaine

Decreased Effect There are no known significant interactions involving a decrease in effect.

Stability Store at room temperature between 15°C and 30°C (59°F and 86°F).

Mechanism of Action Antiemetic activity may be due to effect on cannabinoid receptors (CB1) within the central nervous system.

Pharmacokinetics (Adult data unless noted)

Absorption: Rapid and complete

Distribution: ~12.5 L/kg

Metabolism: To several active metabolites by oxidation and stereospecific enzyme reduction; CYP450 enzymes may also be involved

Half-life: Parent compound: 2 hours; Metabolites: 35 hours

Time to peak serum concentration: Within 2 hours

Elimination: Feces (~60%); renal (~24%)

Dosing: Usual

Oral:

Children >4 years:

<18 kg: 0.5 mg twice daily

18-30 kg: 1 mg twice daily

>30 kg: 1 mg 3 times/day

Adults: 1-2 mg twice daily (maximum: 6 mg divided in 3 doses daily)

Dosage adjustment in renal impairment: No adjustment required.

Administration Oral: Initial dose should be given 1-3 hours before chemotherapy; may be given 2-3 times/day during the entire chemotherapy course and for up to 48 hours after the last dose of chemotherapy; a dose the night before chemotherapy may be useful

Monitoring Parameters Blood pressure, heart rate; signs and symptoms of excessive use, abuse, or misuse

Controlled Substance C-II

Dosage Forms Excipient information presented when available (limited, particularly for generics); consult specific product labeling.

Capsule, Oral:

Cesamet: 1 mg [contains fd&c blue #2 (indigotine)]

References

Chan HS, Correia JA, and MacLeod SM, "Nabilone Versus Prochlorperazine for Control of Cancer Chemotherapy-Induced Emesis in Children: A Double-Blind, Crossover Trial," *Pediatrics*, 1987, 79 (6):946-52.

Dupuis LL and Nathan PC, "Options for the Prevention and Management of Acute Chemotherapy-Induced Nausea and Vomiting in Children," *Pediatr Drug*, 2003, 5(9):597-613.

Tramer MR, Carroll D, Campbell FA, et al, "Cannabinoids for Control of Chemotherapy Induced Nausea and Vomiting: Quantitative Systematic Review," *BMJ*, 2001, 323(7303):16-21.

Ward A and Holmes B, "Nabilone: A Preliminary Review of Its Pharmacological Properties and Therapeutic Use," *Drugs*, 1985, 30 (2):127-44.

♦ **NAC** *see* Acetylcysteine *on page 60*

♦ **N-Acetyl-L-cysteine** *see* Acetylcysteine *on page 60*

♦ **N Acetylcysteine** *see* Acetylcysteine *on page 60*

♦ **N-Acetyl-P-Aminophenol** *see* Acetaminophen *on page 47*

♦ **NaCl** *see* Sodium Chloride *on page 1902*

Nadolol (NAY doe lol)

Medication Safety Issues

Sound-alike/look-alike issues:

Corgard may be confused with Cognex, Coreg

International issues:

Nadolol may be confused with Mandol brand name for cefamandole [Belgium, Netherlands, New Zealand, Russia]

Brand Names: U.S. Corgard

Brand Names: Canada Apo-Nadol; Teva-Nadolol

Therapeutic Category Antianginal Agent; Antiarrhythmic Agent, Class II; Antihypertensive Agent; Antimigraine Agent; Beta-Adrenergic Blocker

Generic Availability (U.S.) Yes

Use Treatment of hypertension, alone or in combination with other agents (FDA approved in adults); treatment of angina pectoris (FDA approved in adults); has also been used for supraventricular tachycardia (SVT), thyrotoxicosis, prophylaxis of migraine headaches

Pregnancy Risk Factor C

Pregnancy Considerations Adverse events were observed in some animal reproduction studies; therefore, the manufacturer classifies nadolol as pregnancy category C. Nadolol crosses the placenta and is measurable in infant serum after birth. In a cohort study, an increased risk of cardiovascular defects was observed following maternal use of beta-blockers during pregnancy. Intrauterine growth restriction (IUGR), small placentas, as well as fetal/neonatal bradycardia, hypoglycemia, and/or respiratory depression have been observed following *in utero* exposure to beta-blockers as a class. Adequate facilities for monitoring infants at birth should be available. Untreated chronic maternal hypertension and pre-eclampsia are also associated with adverse events in the fetus, infant, and mother. Nadolol is indicated for the treatment of hypertension, but due to its long half-life and potential effects to the fetus, other agents may be more appropriate for use during pregnancy.

Breast-Feeding Considerations Nadolol is excreted into breast milk in concentrations higher than the maternal serum. According to the manufacturer, the decision to continue or discontinue breast-feeding during therapy should take into account the risk of exposure to the infant and the benefits of treatment to the mother. The time to peak milk concentration is 6 hours after the oral dose, the half-life of nadolol in breast milk is similar to that in the maternal serum, and nadolol can still be detected in breast milk for several days after the last maternal dose.

Contraindications Hypersensitivity to nadolol or any component; overt cardiac failure, cardiogenic shock, sinus bradycardia, greater than first degree conduction block, bronchial asthma

Warnings May depress myocardial activity and precipitate or worsen heart failure; use is contraindicated in overt heart failure; use with caution in compensated heart failure and monitor closely, especially during upwards titration of dose; if heart failure worsens, may need to increase diuretics and not advance the dose of nadolol; a reduction in dose or discontinuation of nadolol may be needed. Beta-blocker therapy should not be withdrawn abruptly (particularly in patients with CAD), but gradually tapered over 1-2 weeks to avoid acute tachycardia, hypertension, and/or ischemia **[U.S. Boxed Warning]**. Severe exacerbation of angina, ventricular arrhythmias, and MI have been reported following abrupt withdrawal of beta-blocker therapy. Temporary but prompt resumption of beta-blocker therapy may be indicated with worsening of angina or acute coronary insufficiency. Chronic beta-blocker therapy should not be routinely withdrawn prior to major surgery. Beta-blockers should generally be avoided in patients with bronchospastic disease (nonallergic bronchospasm, chronic bronchitis, emphysema), as bronchospasm may occur; nadolol is contraindicated for patients with asthma.

Nadolol may block hypoglycemia-induced tachycardia and blood pressure changes; use with caution in patients with diabetes mellitus. Nadolol decreases the ability of the heart to respond to reflex adrenergic stimuli and may increase the risk of general anesthesia and surgical procedures. May mask clinical signs of hyperthyroidism (eg, tachycardia). If hyperthyroidism is suspected, carefully manage and monitor; abrupt withdrawal may exacerbate symptoms of hyperthyroidism or precipitate thyroid storm. In patients with pheochromocytoma, adequate alpha-blockade is required prior to use of any beta-blocker. Use with caution in patients on concurrent verapamil, diltiazem, or digoxin; bradycardia or heart block can occur. Potentially significant drug interactions may exist, requiring dose or frequency adjustment, additional monitoring, and/or selection of alternative therapy. Consult drug interactions database for more detailed information. Beta-blocker use has been associated with induction or exacerbation of psoriasis, but cause and effect have not been firmly established.

Precautions Use with caution in patients with renal impairment; dosage adjustment required. Use with caution in patients with peripheral vascular disease and Raynaud's disease; may aggravate symptoms of arterial insufficiency; monitor for progression of arterial obstruction. Use with caution in patients with a history of severe anaphylaxis to allergens; patients taking beta-blockers may become more sensitive to repeated challenges. Treatment of anaphylaxis (eg, epinephrine) in patients taking beta-blockers may be ineffective or promote undesirable effects. Use with caution in patients with myasthenia gravis. Use with caution in patients with a history of psychiatric illness; may cause or exacerbate CNS depression.

Adverse Reactions

Cardiovascular: Atrioventricular block, bradycardia, cardiac conduction disturbance, cardiac failure, cold extremities, edema, hypotension, palpitations, peripheral vascular insufficiency, Raynaud's phenomenon

Central nervous system: Depression, dizziness, drowsiness, fatigue, insomnia, sedation

Rare but important or life-threatening: Anorexia, bloating, bronchospasm, cardiac arrhythmia, confusion (especially in the elderly), cough, decreased libido, diarrhea, dyspepsia, facial edema, hallucination, headache, impotence, nasal congestion, nausea, paresthesia, pruritus, sedation, skin rash, slurred speech, thrombocytopenia, transient alopecia, weight gain, xeroderma, xerophthalmia

Drug Interactions

Metabolism/Transport Effects Substrate of P-glycoprotein

Avoid Concomitant Use

Avoid concomitant use of Nadolol with any of the following: Beta2-Agonists; Ceritinib; Floctafenine; Methacholine

Increased Effect/Toxicity

Nadolol may increase the levels/effects of: Alpha-/Beta-Agonists (Direct-Acting); Alpha1-Blockers; Alpha2-Agonists; Amifostine; Antihypertensives; Bradycardia-Causing Agents; Bupivacaine; Cardiac Glycosides; Ceritinib; Cholinergic Agonists; DULoxetine; Ergot Derivatives; Fingolimod; Grass Pollen Allergen Extract (5 Grass Extract); Hypotensive Agents; Insulin; Lidocaine (Systemic); Lidocaine (Topical); Mepivacaine; Methacholine; Midodrine; Obinutuzumab; RiTUXimab; Sulfonylureas

The levels/effects of Nadolol may be increased by: Acetylcholinesterase Inhibitors; Alpha2-Agonists; Amiodarone; Anilidopiperidine Opioids; Barbiturates; Brimonidine (Topical); Calcium Channel Blockers (Dihydropyridine); Calcium Channel Blockers (Nondihydropyridine); Diazoxide; Dipyridamole; Disopyramide; Dronedarone; Floctafenine; Herbs (Hypotensive Properties); MAO Inhibitors; Pentoxifylline; P-glycoprotein/ABCB1 Inhibitors; Phosphodiesterase 5 Inhibitors; Prostacyclin Analogues; Regorafenib; Reserpine

Decreased Effect

Nadolol may decrease the levels/effects of: Beta2-Agonists; Theophylline Derivatives

The levels/effects of Nadolol may be decreased by: Green Tea; Herbs (Hypertensive Properties); Methylphenidate; Nonsteroidal Anti-Inflammatory Agents; P-glycoprotein/ABCB1 Inducers; Yohimbine

Stability Store at room temperature; avoid excessive heat; protect from light.

Mechanism of Action Competitively blocks response to $beta_1$- and $beta_2$-adrenergic stimulation; does not exhibit any membrane stabilizing or intrinsic sympathomimetic activity. Nonselective beta-adrenergic blockers (propranolol, nadolol) reduce portal pressure by producing splanchnic vasoconstriction ($beta_2$ effect) thereby reducing portal blood flow.

Pharmacodynamics Duration: 24 hours

Pharmacokinetics (Adult data unless noted)

Absorption: Oral: 30%

Distribution: V_d: ~2 L/kg

Protein-binding: 30%

Metabolism: Not hepatically metabolized

Half-life, elimination:

Increased half-life with decreased renal function

Infants 3-22 months (n=3): 3.2-4.3 hours (Mehta, 1992b)

Children 10 years (n=1): 15.7 hours (Mehta, 1992b)

Children ~15 years (n=1): 7.3 hours (Mehta, 1992b)

Adults: 20-24 hours; prolonged with renal impairment (up to 45 hours in severe impairment) (Herrera, 1979)

Time to peak serum concentration: 3-4 hours

Elimination: Urine (as unchanged drug)

Dosing: Usual

Infants, Children, and Adolescents:

Migraine, prophylaxis: Children >6 years and Adolescents: Limited data available: Oral: 0.25-1 mg/kg once or twice daily; begin at low end of range and slowly titrate upwards every 1-2 weeks (Linder, 2001)

SVT: Limited data available: Oral: Initial: 0.5-1 mg/kg once daily; increase dose gradually to a maximum of 2.5 mg/kg/day; dosing based on a trial of 26 pediatric patients (age range: 3 months to 15 years) which showed SVT was well controlled with a median dose of 1 mg/kg/day (Mehta, 1992)

Adults:

Angina: Oral: Initial: 40 mg once daily; increase dosage gradually by 40-80 mg increments at 3- to 7-day intervals until optimum clinical response is obtained; usual dose: 40-80 mg daily; maximum daily dose: 240 mg/**day**

Hypertension: Oral: Initial: 40 mg once daily; increase dosage gradually by 40-80 mg increments until optimum blood pressure reduction achieved; usual dosage range (JNC 7): 40-120 mg once daily; doses up to 240-320 mg/day in hypertension may be necessary

Thyrotoxicosis: 40-160 mg once daily (Bahn, 2011)

Dosage adjustment for renal impairment: Adults: Manufacturer's recommendation:

CrCl >50 mL/minute/1.73 m^2: Administer every 24 hours

CrCl 31-50 mL/minute/1.73 m^2: Administer every 24-36 hours

CrCl 10-30 mL/minute/1.73 m^2: Administer every 24-48 hours

CrCl <10 mL/minute/1.73 m^2: Administer every 40-60 hours

Dialysis: Moderately dialyzable (20% to 50%). There are no dosage adjustments for dialysis provided in the manufacturer's labeling; however, the following guidelines have been used by some clinicians (Aronoff, 2007):

ESRD requiring hemodialysis: Administer dose post-dialysis.

Peritoneal dialysis: Administer every 40-60 hours.

Dosage adjustment for hepatic impairment: There are no dosage adjustments provided in the manufacturer's labeling

Administration Oral: May administer without regard to meals

Monitoring Parameters Blood pressure, heart rate, fluid intake and output, weight

Dosage Forms Excipient information presented when available (limited, particularly for generics); consult specific product labeling.

Tablet, Oral:

Corgard: 20 mg, 40 mg, 80 mg [scored]

Generic: 20 mg, 40 mg, 80 mg

References

Bahn RS, Burch HB, Cooper, DS, et.al. Hyperthyroidism and other causes of thyrotoxicosis: management guidelines of the American Thyroid Association and American Association of Clinical Endocrinologists. *Endocrine Practice*. 2011;17(3):1-65.

Brauchli YB, Jick SS, Curtin F, et al, "Association Between Beta-Blockers, Other Antihypertensive Drugs and Psoriasis: Population-Based Case-Control Study," *Br J Dermatol*, 2008, 158(6):1299-307.

Chobanian AV, Bakris GL, Black HR, et al, "The Seventh Report of the Joint National Committee on Prevention, Detection, Evaluation, and Treatment of High Blood Pressure: The JNC 7 report," *JAMA*, 2003, 289(19):2560-72.

Gold MH, Holy AK, and Roenigk HH Jr, "Beta-Blocking Drugs and Psoriasis. A Review of Cutaneous Side Effects and Retrospective Analysis of Their Effects on Psoriasis," *J Am Acad Dermatol*, 1988, 19 (5 Pt 1):837-41.

Herrera J, Vukovich RA, Griffith DL. Elimination of nadolol by patients with renal impairment. *Br J Clin Pharmacol*. 1979;7(Suppl 2):227-231.

Linder SL and Winner P, "Pediatric Headache," *Med Clin North Am*, 2001, 85(4):1037-53.

Mehta AV and Chidambaram B, "Efficacy and Safety of Intravenous and Oral Nadolol for Supraventricular Tachycardia in Children," *J Am Coll Cardiol*, 1992a, 19(3):630-5.

Mehta AV, Chidambaram B, and Rice PJ, "Pharmacokinetics of Nadolol in Children With Supraventricular Tachycardia," *J Clin Pharmacol*, 1992b, 32(1):1023-7.

Schön MP and Boehncke WH, "Psoriasis," *N Engl J Med*, 2005, 352 (18):1899-912.

Nafcillin (naf SIL in)

Related Information

Management of Drug Extravasations *on page 2255*

Brand Names: U.S. Nallpen in Dextrose

Therapeutic Category Antibiotic, Penicillin (Antistaphylococcal)

Generic Availability (U.S.) May be product dependent

Use Treatment of bacterial infections such as osteomyelitis, septicemia, endocarditis, and CNS infections due to susceptible penicillinase-producing strains of *Staphylococcus* [FDA approved in pediatric patients (I.M.) and adults (I.M. and I.V.)]

Pregnancy Risk Factor B

Pregnancy Considerations Adverse events have not been observed in animal reproduction studies. Information specific to nafcillin use in pregnancy is limited. Maternal use of penicillins has generally not resulted in an increased risk of birth defects.

Breast-Feeding Considerations Penicillins are excreted into breast milk. The manufacturer recommends that caution be exercised when administering nafcillin to nursing women. Nondose-related effects could include modification of bowel flora.

Contraindications Hypersensitivity to nafcillin, any component, or penicillins; premixed solutions: Hypersensitivity to corn or corn products

Warnings Serious and occasionally fatal hypersensitivity (anaphylactoid) reactions have been reported in patients on penicillin therapy, especially with a history of beta-lactam hypersensitivity, history of sensitivity to multiple allergens, or previous IgE-mediated reactions (eg, anaphylaxis, angioedema, urticaria); administration to patients with confirmed penicillin allergies should be avoided; in patients with confirmed cephalosporin allergy, consider skin testing to rule out cross-sensitivity to penicillins. Immediate treatment for anaphylactic reaction should be available during administration. In a study of pediatric patients (5-19 years) receiving outpatient nafcillin for >3 weeks, significantly less rash was reported in the nafcillin group (10.3%) compared to oxacillin group (31.7%) (Maraqa, 2002).

In neonates, elimination rate is decreased due to immature hepatic and renal function; dosage adjustment is needed. Large I.V. or intraventricular doses have been associated with neurotoxicity; use caution, especially in patients with concomitant renal and hepatic dysfunction. Prolonged use may result in fungal or bacterial superinfection, including *C. difficile*-associated diarrhea (CDAD) and pseudomembranous colitis; CDAD has been observed >2 months postantibiotic treatment.

Precautions Extravasation of I.V. infusions should be avoided; hyaluronidase may be used for management if extravasation occurs (Zenk, 1981). Use with caution renal and hepatic impairment; dosage modification is necessary in patients with both severe renal and hepatic impairment. Use with caution in patients with history of significant allergies and/or asthma.

Adverse Reactions

Central nervous system: Neurotoxicity (high doses)

Gastrointestinal: *C. difficile*-associated diarrhea

Hematologic: Agranulocytosis, bone marrow depression, neutropenia

Local: Inflammation, pain, phlebitis, skin sloughing, swelling, and thrombophlebitis at the injection site; tissue necrosis with sloughing (SubQ extravasation)

Renal: Interstitial nephritis (rare), renal tubular damage (rare)

Miscellaneous: Anaphylaxis, hypersensitivity reactions (immediate and delayed; general incidence of 1% to 10% for penicillins), serum sickness

Rare but important or life-threatening: ALT increased, AST increased, bilirubin increased, cholestatic hepatitis, diarrhea, drug-induced lupus erythematosus, fever, hypokalemia, itching, nausea, rash (including bullous skin eruptions), vomiting

Drug Interactions

Metabolism/Transport Effects Induces CYP3A4 (strong)

Avoid Concomitant Use

Avoid concomitant use of Nafcillin with any of the following: Abiraterone Acetate; Apixaban; Apremilast; Artemether; Axitinib; BCG; Bedaquiline; Boceprevir; Bortezomib; Bosutinib; Cabozantinib; Ceritinib; CloZAPine; Crizotinib; Dienogest; Dronedarone; Enzalutamide; Everolimus; Ibrutinib; Itraconazole; Ivacaftor; Lapatinib; Lumefantrine; Lurasidone; Macitentan; Mifepristone; NIFEdipine; Nilotinib; Nisoldipine; PAZOPanib; Perampanel; PONATinib; Praziquantel; Probenecid; Ranolazine; Regorafenib; Rivaroxaban; Roflumilast; RomiDEPsin; Simeprevir; SORAfenib; Tasimelteon; Telaprevir; Ticagrelor; Tofacitinib; Tolvaptan; Toremifene; Ulipristal; Vandetanib; Vemurafenib; VinCRIStine (Liposomal); Vorapaxar

Increased Effect/Toxicity

Nafcillin may increase the levels/effects of: Clarithromycin; Ifosfamide; Methotrexate

The levels/effects of Nafcillin may be increased by: Clarithromycin; Probenecid

Decreased Effect

Nafcillin may decrease the levels/effects of: Abiraterone Acetate; Apixaban; Apremilast; ARIPiprazole; Artemether; Axitinib; BCG; Bedaquiline; Boceprevir; Bortezomib; Bosutinib; Brentuximab Vedotin; Cabozantinib; Calcium Channel Blockers; Cannabidiol; Cannabis; Ceritinib; Clarithromycin; CloZAPine; Contraceptives (Estrogens); Crizotinib; CycloSPORINE (Systemic); CYP3A4 Substrates; Dasatinib; Dienogest; DOXOrubicin (Conventional); Dronabinol; Dronedarone; Enzalutamide; Everolimus; Exemestane; FentaNYL; Gefitinib; GuanFACINE; Ibrutinib; Imatinib; Itraconazole; Ivacaftor; Ixabepilone; Lapatinib; Linagliptin; Lumefantrine; Lurasidone; Macitentan; Maraviroc; Mifepristone; Mycophenolate; NIFEdipine; Nilotinib; Nisoldipine; PAZOPanib; Perampanel; PONATinib; Praziquantel; QUEtiapine; Ranolazine; Regorafenib; Rivaroxaban; Roflumilast; RomiDEPsin; Saxagliptin; Simeprevir; Sodium Picosulfate; SORAfenib; SUNItinib; Tadalafil; Tasimelteon; Telaprevir; Tetrahydrocannabinol; Ticagrelor; Tofacitinib; Tolvaptan; Toremifene; Typhoid Vaccine; Ulipristal; Vandetanib; Vemurafenib; Vilazodone; VinCRIStine (Liposomal); Vitamin K Antagonists; Vorapaxar; Vortioxetine; Zuclopenthixol

The levels/effects of Nafcillin may be decreased by: Tetracycline Derivatives

Stability

Premixed infusions: Store in a freezer at -20°C or less (-4°F or less). Thaw at room temperature or under refrigeration only. Thawed bags are stable for 21 days under refrigeration or 72 hours at room temperature. Do not refreeze.

Vials: Store intact vial at 20°C to 25°C (68°F to 77°F); reconstituted parenteral solution (250 mg/mL) is stable for 3 days at room temperature and 7 days when refrigerated or 90 days when frozen. When further diluted for I.V. infusion in NS or D_5W, solution is stable for 24 hours at room temperature and 7 days when refrigerated. Solutions for ambulatory I.V. infusion reservoirs (eg, >24-hour supply) may be subject to inadvertent exposure to temperatures higher than recommended due to heat radiation from patient's skin; lower concentrations of preparation may be needed to prevent precipitation of solution in some circumstances (Chan, 2005).

Mechanism of Action Interferes with bacterial cell wall synthesis during active multiplication, causing cell wall destruction and resultant bactericidal activity against susceptible bacteria; resistant to inactivation by staphylococcal penicillinase

Pharmacokinetics (Adult data unless noted)

Distribution: Distributes into bile, synovial, pleural, ascitic, and pericardial fluids and into bone and liver; CSF penetration is poor unless meninges are inflamed

V_d:
Neonates: 0.24-0.53 L/kg
Children: 0.85-0.91 L/kg
Adults: 0.57-1.55 L/kg

Protein binding: ~90%; primarily albumin

Metabolism: Primarily hepatic; undergoes enterohepatic recirculation

Half-life:
Neonates and Infants <9 weeks:
<3 weeks: 2.2-5.5 hours
4-9 weeks: 1.2-2.3 hours
Infants and Children 1 month to 14 years: 0.75-1.9 hours
Adults: Normal renal and hepatic function: 30-60 minutes

Time to peak serum concentration: I.M.: Within 30-60 minutes

Elimination: Primarily bile/feces; urine (30% as unchanged drug)

Dialysis: Not dialyzable (0% to 5%)

Dosing: Neonatal

General dosing, susceptible infection (non-CNS): (*Red Book*, 2012): I.M., I.V.:
Body weight <1 kg:
PNA ≤14 days: 25 mg/kg/dose every 12 hours
PNA 15-28 days: 25 mg/kg/dose every 8 hours
Body weight 1-2 kg:
PNA ≤7 days: 25 mg/kg/dose every 12 hours
PNA 8-28 days: 25 mg/kg/dose every 8 hours
Body weight >2 kg:
PNA ≤7 days: 25 mg/kg/dose every 8 hours
PNA 8-28 days: 25 mg/kg/dose every 6 hours

Meningitis: I.V. (Tunkel, 2004):
PNA 0-7 days: 75 mg/kg/day in divided doses every 8-12 hours for 14-21 days
PNA 8-28 days: 100-150 mg/kg/day in divided doses every 6-8 hours for 14-21 days

Dosing: Usual

Infants, Children, and Adolescents:
General dosing, susceptible infection (*Red Book*, 2012): I.M., I.V.:
Mild to moderate infections: 100-150 mg/kg/day in divided doses every 6 hours; maximum daily dose: 4 g/**day**
Severe infections: 150-200 mg/kg/day in divided doses every 4-6 hours; maximum daily dose: 12 g/**day**

Endocarditis, oxacillin/methicillin-susceptible staphylococci (Baddour, 2005):
Native valve: I.V.: 200 mg/kg/day in divided doses every 4-6 hours for 6 weeks with gentamicin for the first 3-5 days of therapy
Prosthetic valve: I.V.: 200 mg/kg/day in divided doses every 4-6 hours for ≥6 weeks with rifampin (same duration as nafcillin) and with gentamicin for the first 2 weeks of therapy

Meningitis: I.V.: 200 mg/kg/day in divided doses every 6 hours; maximum daily dose: 12 g/**day** (Tunkel, 2004)

Skin and soft tissue infections: I.V.: 100-150 mg/kg/day in divided doses every 6 hours; maximum daily dose: 12 g/**day** (Stevens, 2005)

Adults:
General dosing, susceptible infections:
I.M.: 500 mg every 4-6 hours
I.V.: 500-2000 mg every 4-6 hours

Endocarditis, oxacillin/methicillin-susceptible staphylococci: (Baddour, 2005): I.V.:
Native valve: 12 g/24 hours in 4-6 divided doses for 6 weeks
Prosthetic valve: 12 g/24 hours in 6 divided dose for ≥6 weeks (use with rifampin for entire course and gentamicin for first 2 weeks)

Joint, prosthetic infections: I.V.: 1500-2000 mg every 4-6 hours for 4-6 weeks (2-6 weeks if in combination with rifampin), followed by oral antibiotic treatment and suppressive regimens (Osmon, 2013)

Skin and soft tissue infections: (Stevens, 2005): I.V.:
Methicillin-susceptible *Staphylococcus aureus*: 1000-2000 mg every 4 hours
Necrotizing infection *(Staphylococcus aureus)* of fascia, muscle, skin: 1000-2000 mg every 4 hours

Dosing adjustment in renal impairment: Not necessary unless renal impairment is in the setting of concomitant hepatic impairment; poorly dialyzed; no supplemental dose or dosage adjustment necessary, including patients on intermittent hemodialysis, peritoneal dialysis, or continuous renal replacement therapy (eg, CVVHD)

Dosing adjustment in hepatic impairment: No specific dosage adjustments provided in manufacturer's labeling; however, dosage adjustment may be necessary particularly in the setting of concomitant renal impairment; nafcillin primarily undergoes hepatic metabolism. In patients with both hepatic and renal impairment, monitoring of serum drug concentrations and modification of dosage may be necessary.

Administration Parenteral:
I.M.: Administer deep I.M. into a large muscle (ie, gluteus maximus) using a solution containing 250 mg/mL
I.V.: May be administered by direct I.V. injection over 5-10 minutes by diluting dose in 15-30 mL of NS or SWI or by intermittent I.V. infusion over 30-60 minutes at a final concentration not to exceed 40 mg/mL; in fluid-restricted patients, a higher concentration may be used depending on the diluent (D_5W: 71 mg/mL; NS: 62 mg/mL; SWI: 125 mg/mL) (Robinson, 1987)

Vesicant/Extravasation Risk Vesicant

Monitoring Parameters Baseline and periodic CBC with differential, urinalysis, BUN, serum creatinine, AST, and ALT; initial culture and susceptibility test; observe for signs and symptoms of anaphylaxis during first dose and I.V. site for extravasation

Test Interactions Positive Coombs' test (direct), false-positive urinary and serum proteins; may inactivate aminoglycosides *in vitro*

Additional Information In adults, 1000 mg given I.M. is expected to yield a peak serum concentration of 7.71 mcg/mL 30-60 minutes after dose.
Sodium content of 1 g injection: 2.9 mEq

Dosage Forms Excipient information presented when available (limited, particularly for generics); consult specific product labeling.
Solution, Intravenous:
Nallpen in Dextrose: 1 g/50 mL (50 mL); 2 g/100 mL (100 mL)
Solution Reconstituted, Injection:
Generic: 1 g (1 ea); 2 g (1 ea); 10 g (1 ea)
Solution Reconstituted, Injection [preservative free]:
Generic: 1 g (1 ea); 2 g (1 ea); 10 g (1 ea)
Solution Reconstituted, Intravenous:
Generic: 1 g (1 ea); 2 g (1 ea)

References

Baddour LM, Wilson WR, Bayer AS, et al, "Infective Endocarditis: Diagnosis, Antimicrobial Therapy, and Management of Complications: A Statement for Healthcare Professionals From the Committee on Rheumatic Fever, Endocarditis, and Kawasaki Disease, Council on Cardiovascular Disease in the Young, and the Councils on Clinical Cardiology, Stroke, and Cardiovascular Surgery and Anesthesia, American Heart Association: Endorsed by the Infectious Diseases Society of America," *Circulation*, 2005, 111(23):e394-434.

Banner W Jr, Gooch WM 3d, Burckart G, et al, "Pharmacokinetics of Nafcillin in Infants With Low Birth Weights," *Antimicrob Agents Chemother*, 1980, 17(4):691-4.

Chan V, "Influence of Temperature and Drug Concentration on Nafcillin Precipitation," *Am J Health Syst Pharm*, 2005, 62(13):1347-8.

Maraqa NF, Gomez MM, Rathore MH, et al, "Higher Occurrence of Hepatotoxicity and Rash in Patients Treated With Oxacillin,

Compared With Those Treated With Nafcillin and Other Commonly Used Antimicrobials," *Clin Infect Dis*, 2002, 34(1):50-4.

Osmon DR, Berbari EF, Berendt AR, et al, "Diagnosis and Management of Prosthetic Joint Infection: Clinical Practice Guidelines by the Infectious Diseases Society of America," *Clin Infect Dis*, 2013, 56 (1):e1-e25.

Red Book: 2012 Report of the Committee on Infectious Diseases, 29th ed, Pickering LK, ed, Elk Grove Village, IL: American Academy of Pediatrics, 2012.

Robinson DC, Cookson TL, and Grisafe JA, "Concentration Guidelines for Parenteral Antibiotics in Fluid-Restricted Patients," *Drug Intell Clin Pharm*, 1987, 21(12):985-9.

Stevens DL, Bisno AL, Chambers HF, et al, "Practice Guidelines for the Diagnosis and Management of Skin and Soft-Tissue Infections," *Clin Infect Dis*, 2005, 41(10):1373-406.

Tunkel AR, Hartman BJ, Kaplan SL, et al, "Practice Guidelines for the Management of Bacterial Meningitis," *Clin Infect Dis*, 2004, 39 (9):1267-84.

Zenk KE, Dungy CL, and Greene CR, "Nafcillin Extravasation Injury: Use of Hyaluronidase as an Antidote," *Am J Dis Child*, 1981, 135 (12):1113-4.

◆ **Nafcillin Sodium** *see* Nafcillin *on page 1462*

◆ **Naglazyme** *see* Galsulfase *on page 953*

◆ **NaHCO$_3$** *see* Sodium Bicarbonate *on page 1901*

Nalbuphine (NAL byoo feen)

Medication Safety Issues
Sound-alike/look-alike issues:
Nalbuphine may be confused with naloxone
Nubain may be confused with Navane®, Nebcin
High alert medication:
The Institute for Safe Medication Practices (ISMP) includes this medication among its list of drug classes which have a heightened risk of causing significant patient harm when used in error.

Therapeutic Category Analgesic, Narcotic; Opioid Partial Agonist

Generic Availability (U.S.) Yes

Use Relief of moderate to severe pain; supplement to balanced anesthesia [for preoperative and postoperative analgesia, and obstetrical analgesia (during labor and delivery)]; prevention or treatment of opioid-induced pruritus

Pregnancy Risk Factor C

Pregnancy Considerations Adverse events were observed in some animal reproduction studies. Nalbuphine crosses the placenta. Nalbuphine is approved for use in obstetrical analgesia during labor and delivery. When used for pain relief during labor, opioids may temporarily affect the heart rate of the fetus (ACOG, 2002) and severe fetal bradycardia has been reported following use of nalbuphine in labor/delivery. Fetal bradycardia may occur when administered earlier in pregnancy (not documented). Use only if clearly needed, with monitoring to detect and manage possible adverse fetal effects. Naloxone has been reported to reverse bradycardia. Newborn should be monitored for respiratory depression or bradycardia following nalbuphine use in labor.

If chronic opioid exposure occurs in pregnancy, adverse events in the newborn (including withdrawal) may occur; monitoring of the neonate is recommended. The minimum effective dose should be used if opioids are needed (Chou, 2009). Neonatal abstinence syndrome following opioid exposure may present with autonomic (eg, fever, temperature instability), gastrointestinal (eg, diarrhea, vomiting, poor feeding/weight gain), or neurologic (eg, high-pitched crying, increased muscle tone, irritability, seizure, tremor) symptoms (Dow, 2012; Hudak, 2012).

Breast-Feeding Considerations Small amounts (<1% of maternal dose) of nalbuphine are excreted in breast milk. The manufacturer recommends that caution be exercised when administering nalbuphine to nursing women.

Parenteral opioids used during labor have the potential to interfere with a newborns natural reflex to nurse within the first few hours after birth. If nalbuphine is administered to a nursing woman, it is recommended to monitor both the mother and baby for psychotomimetic reactions. Nursing infants exposed to large doses of opioids should also be monitored for apnea and sedation (Montgomery, 2012).

Contraindications Hypersensitivity to nalbuphine or any component

Warnings Abrupt discontinuation after prolonged use may result in opioid withdrawal; administration to patients receiving chronic opioids may precipitate opioid withdrawal

Neonatal and fetal adverse reactions have occurred after administration of nalbuphine to pregnant women during labor; these adverse reactions, which may be life-threatening, include: Bradycardia, respiratory depression, apnea, cyanosis, and hypotonia; use with caution in pregnancy; monitor neonates closely with maternal use in labor and delivery.

Precautions Reduce dose in patients with hepatic impairment; use with caution in patients with CNS depression, impaired respiration, recent MI, or biliary tract surgery; may produce respiratory depression or bradycardia; use with caution in patients with a history of drug dependence, head trauma or increased intracranial pressure, decreased hepatic or renal function, or patients suspected to be opioid dependent

Adverse Reactions

Central nervous system: Dizziness, headache, sedation
Gastrointestinal: Nausea/vomiting, xerostomia
Miscellaneous: Clamminess
Rare but important or life-threatening: Abdominal pain, agitation, allergic reaction, anaphylaxis, anaphylactoid reaction, anxiety, asthma, bitter taste, blurred vision, bradycardia, cardiac arrest, confusion, crying, delusion, depersonalization, depression, diaphoresis, dreams (abnormal), dyspepsia, dysphoria, dyspnea, euphoria, faintness, fever, floating sensation, flushing, gastrointestinal cramps, hallucinations, hostility, hypertension, hypotension, injection site reactions (pain, swelling, redness, burning); laryngeal edema, loss of consciousness, nervousness, numbness, pruritus, pulmonary edema, rash, respiratory depression, respiratory distress, restlessness, seizure, sensation of warmth/burning, somnolence, speech disorder, stridor, tachycardia, tingling, tremor, unreality, urinary urgency, urticaria

Drug Interactions

Metabolism/Transport Effects None known.

Avoid Concomitant Use

Avoid concomitant use of Nalbuphine with any of the following: Azelastine (Nasal); Paraldehyde; Thalidomide

Increased Effect/Toxicity

Nalbuphine may increase the levels/effects of: Alcohol (Ethyl); Alvimopan; Azelastine (Nasal); Buprenorphine; CNS Depressants; Desmopressin; Diuretics; Hydrocodone; Methotrimeprazine; Metyrosine; Mirtazapine; Paraldehyde; Pramipexole; ROPINIRole; Rotigotine; Selective Serotonin Reuptake Inhibitors; Thalidomide; Zolpidem

The levels/effects of Nalbuphine may be increased by: Amphetamines; Anticholinergic Agents; Antipsychotic Agents (Phenothiazines); Brimonidine (Topical); Cannabis; Doxylamine; Dronabinol; Droperidol; HydrOXYzine; Kava Kava; Magnesium Sulfate; Methotrimeprazine; Nabilone; Perampanel; Rufinamide; Sodium Oxybate; Succinylcholine; Tapentadol; Tetrahydrocannabinol

Decreased Effect

Nalbuphine may decrease the levels/effects of: Analgesics (Opioid); Pegvisomant

The levels/effects of Nalbuphine may be decreased by: Ammonium Chloride; Mixed Agonist / Antagonist Opioids; Naltrexone

Stability Store at controlled room temperature at 25°C (77°F); protect from excessive light; store product in carton until used; not physically compatible with nafcillin and ketorolac

Mechanism of Action Agonist of kappa opiate receptors and partial antagonist of mu opiate receptors in the CNS, causing inhibition of ascending pain pathways, altering the perception of and response to pain; produces generalized CNS depression

Pharmacodynamics

Onset of action:
I.M., SubQ: Within 15 minutes
I.V.: 2-3 minutes
Maximum effect:
I.M.: 30 minutes
I.V.: 1-3 minutes
Duration: 3-6 hours

Pharmacokinetics (Adult data unless noted)

Distribution: Crosses placenta; distributes into breast milk in small amounts (<1% of dose)
Metabolism: In the liver; extensive first-pass metabolism
Protein binding: ~50%
Half-life, terminal:
Children 1-8 years: 0.9 hours
Adults 23-32 years: ~2 hours; range: 3.5-5 hours
Adults 65-90 years: 2.3 hours
Time to peak serum concentration:
I.M.: 30 minutes
I.V.: 1-3 minutes
Elimination: Metabolites primarily in feces (via bile) and in urine; 4% to 7% eliminated unchanged in the urine

Dosing: Usual

Children 1-14 years: Premedication: I.M., I.V., SubQ: 0.2 mg/kg; maximum dose: 20 mg/dose
Children: Analgesia: I.M., I.V., SubQ: 0.1-0.15 mg/kg every 3-6 hours as needed; maximum single-dose: 20 mg/dose; maximum daily dose: 160 mg/day
Adults:
Analgesia: I.M., I.V., SubQ: 10 mg/70 kg every 3-6 hours as needed; maximum single-dose: 20 mg/dose; maximum daily dose: 160 mg/day
Surgical anesthesia supplement: I.V.: Induction: 0.3-3 mg/kg administered over 10-15 minutes; maintenance doses of 0.25-0.5 mg/kg may be given as required
Opioid-induced pruritus: I.V.: 2.5-5 mg; may repeat dose (Cohen, 1992)

Administration Parenteral: I.V.: Administer over 5-10 minutes; larger doses should be administered over 10-15 minutes

Monitoring Parameters Relief of pain, respiratory and mental status, blood pressure

Test Interactions May interfere with certain enzymatic methods used to detect opioids, depending on sensitivity and specificity of the test (refer to test manufacturer for details)

Additional Information Analgesic potency: 1 mg nalbuphine ~1 mg morphine

Dosage Forms Excipient information presented when available (limited, particularly for generics); consult specific product labeling.

Solution, Injection, as hydrochloride:
Generic: 10 mg/mL (1 mL, 10 mL); 20 mg/mL (1 mL, 10 mL)

References

ACOG Committee on Practice Bulletins-Obstetrics, "ACOG Practice Bulletin. Clinical Management Guidelines for Obstetrician-Gynecologists Number 36, July 2002. Obstetric Analgesia and Anesthesia," *Obstet Gynecol*, 2002, 100(1):177-91.

Chou R, Fanciullo GJ, Fine PG, et al, "Clinical Guidelines For the Use of Chronic Opioid Therapy in Chronic Noncancer Pain," *J Pain*, 2009, 10 (2):113-30.

Cohen SE, Ratner EF, Kreitzman TR, et al, "Nalbuphine is Better Than Naloxone for Treatment of Side Effects After Epidural Morphine," *Anesth Analg*, 1992, 75(5):747-52.

Dow K, Ordean A, Murphy-Oikonen J, et al, "Neonatal Abstinence Syndrome Clinical Practice Guidelines For Ontario," *J Popul Ther Clin Pharmacol*, 2012, 19(3):e488-506.

Hudak ML, Tan RC, Committee On Drugs, et al, "Neonatal Drug Withdrawal," *Pediatrics*, 2012, 129(2):e540-60.

Jaillon P, Gardin ME, Lecocq B, et al, "Pharmacokinetics of Nalbuphine in Infants, Young Healthy Volunteers, and Elderly Patients," *Clin Pharmacol Ther*, 1989, 46(2):226-33.

Kendrick WD, Woods AM, Daly MY, et al, "Naloxone Versus Nalbuphine Infusion for Prophylaxis of Epidural Morphine-Induced Pruritus," *Anesth Analg*, 1996, 82:641-7.

Kjellberg F and Tramer MR, "Pharmacological Control of Opioid-Induced Pruritus: A Quantitative Systematic Review of Randomized Trials," *Eur J Anaesthesiol*, 2001, 18(6):346-57.

Montgomery A, Hale TW, and Academy of Breastfeeding Medicine, "ABM Clinical Protocol #15: Analgesia and Anesthesia for the Breastfeeding Mother, Revised 2012," *Breastfeed Med*, 2012, 7(6):547-53.

Nakatsuka N, Minogue SC, Lim J, et al, "Intravenous Nalbuphine 50 Microg x kg(-1) is Ineffective for Opioid-Induced Pruritus in Pediatrics," *Can J Anaesth*, 2006, 53(11):1103-10.

◆ **Nalbuphine Hydrochloride** *see* Nalbuphine *on page 1464*

◆ **Nalcrom (Can)** *see* Cromolyn (Systemic, Oral Inhalation) *on page 551*

◆ **Nallpen** *see* Nafcillin *on page 1462*

◆ **Nallpen in Dextrose** *see* Nafcillin *on page 1462*

◆ **N-allylnoroxymorphine Hydrochloride** *see* Naloxone *on page 1466*

Naloxone (nal OKS one)

Medication Safety Issues
Sound-alike/look-alike issues:
Naloxone may be confused with Lanoxin®, nalbuphine, naltrexone

Narcan may be confused with Marcaine®, Norcuron®
International issues:
Narcan [multiple international markets] may be confused with Marcen brand name for ketazolam [Spain]

Brand Names: U.S. Evzio

Brand Names: Canada Naloxone Hydrochloride Injection®; Naloxone Hydrochloride Injection® USP

Therapeutic Category Antidote for Narcotic Agonists

Generic Availability (U.S.) May be product dependent

Use Complete or partial reversal of opioid drug effects, including respiratory depression induced by natural and synthetic opioids; diagnosis and management of known or suspected acute opioid overdose (FDA approved in all ages); has also been used for the prevention and treatment of opioid-induced pruritus

Pregnancy Risk Factor C

Pregnancy Considerations Adverse events were not observed in animal reproduction studies. Naloxone crosses the placenta. Consider the benefit to the mother and the risk to the fetus before administering to a pregnant woman who is known or suspected to be opioid dependent; may precipitate withdrawal in both the mother and fetus. In general, medications used as antidotes should take into consideration the health and prognosis of the mother; antidotes should be administered to pregnant women if there is a clear indication for use and should not be withheld because of fears of teratogenicity (Bailey, 2003). Use caution in pregnant women with mild-to-moderate hypertension during labor; severe hypertension may occur.

Breast-Feeding Considerations It is not known if naloxone is excreted into breast milk, however, systemic absorption following oral administration is low (Smith, 2012) and any exposure of naloxone to a nursing infant would therefore be limited. Since naloxone is used for opioid reversal, the opioid concentrations in the milk of a breast-feeding mother and potential transfer of the opioid to the infant should be considered.

Contraindications Hypersensitivity to naloxone or any component

Warnings In patients with physical dependence to opioids (including newborns of opioid-dependent mothers), naloxone may precipitate symptoms of acute withdrawal, including but not limited to agitation, body aches, fever, sweating, runny nose, sneezing, piloerection, yawning, weakness, shivering or trembling, nervousness, restlessness or irritability, diarrhea, nausea or vomiting, abdominal cramps, increased blood pressure, and tachycardia. Neonatal opioid withdrawal may also include convulsions, excessive crying, shrill cry, failure to feed, and hyperactive reflexes. Recurrence of respiratory depression may occur if the opioid involved is long-acting; observe patients until there is no reasonable risk of recurrent respiratory depression. Larger doses of naloxone may be required for the reversal of respiratory depression due to partial agonists or mixed agonists/antagonists. Naloxone is not effective in reversing respiratory depression due to nonopioid drugs.

Precautions Use with caution in patients with cardiovascular disease or in patients receiving medications with potential adverse cardiovascular effects (eg, hypotension, pulmonary edema, or arrhythmias); pulmonary edema and cardiovascular instability, including ventricular fibrillation, have been reported in association with abrupt reversal when using opioid antagonists. Administration of naloxone causes the release of catecholamines and may precipitate acute withdrawal or unmask pain in those who regularly take opioids; providing ventilation prior to the administration of naloxone may decrease these adverse effects. Following the use of opioids during surgery, naloxone may reverse analgesia and increase blood pressure; carefully titrate dose to reverse hypoventilation; do not fully awaken patient or reverse analgesic effect (postoperative patient). Intramuscular administration of naloxone may also reduce the risk of cardiovascular effects due to the slower onset of action.

Adverse Reactions Adverse reactions are related to reversing dependency and precipitating withdrawal. Withdrawal symptoms are the result of sympathetic excess. Adverse events occur secondarily to reversal (withdrawal) of opioid analgesia and sedation.

Cardiovascular: Cardiac arrest, fever, flushing, hypertension, hypotension, tachycardia, ventricular fibrillation ventricular tachycardia

Central nervous system: Agitation, coma, crying (excessive [neonates]), encephalopathy, hallucination, irritability, nervousness, restlessness, seizure (neonates), tremulousness

Gastrointestinal: Abdominal cramps, diarrhea, nausea, vomiting

Local: Injection site reaction

Neuromuscular & skeletal: Ache, hyperreflexia (neonates), paresthesia, piloerection, tremor, weakness

Respiratory: Dyspnea, hypoxia, pulmonary edema, respiratory depression, rhinorrhea, sneezing

Miscellaneous: Diaphoresis, hot flashes, shivering, yawning

Drug Interactions

Metabolism/Transport Effects None known.

Avoid Concomitant Use There are no known interactions where it is recommended to avoid concomitant use.

Increased Effect/Toxicity There are no known significant interactions involving an increase in effect.

Decreased Effect There are no known significant interactions involving a decrease in effect.

Stability Store at 20°C to 25°C (68°F to 77°F) (see product specific labeling for details); protect from light; stable in NS and D$_5$W at 4 mcg/mL for 24 hours; do not mix with alkaline solutions.

Mechanism of Action Pure opioid antagonist that competes and displaces opioids at opioid receptor sites

Pharmacodynamics

Onset of action:

E.T., I.M., SubQ: Within 2-5 minutes

Inhalation via nebulization: ~5 minutes (Mycyk, 2003)

Intranasal: ~8-13 minutes (Kelley, 2005; Robertson, 2009)

I.V.: Within 2 minutes

Duration: (20-60 minutes) is shorter than that of most opioids; therefore, repeated doses are usually needed

Pharmacokinetics (Adult data unless noted)

Metabolism: Primarily by glucuronidation in the liver

Half-life:

Neonates: 1.2-3 hours

Adults: 0.5-1.5 hours (mean: ~1 hour)

Elimination: In urine as metabolites

Dosing: Neonatal Note: Not recommended as part of initial resuscitative efforts in the delivery room for neonates with respiratory depression; support ventilation to improve oxygenation and heart rate (Kattwinkel, 2010):

Opioid intoxication (full reversal): (PALS Guidelines, 2010):

I.V. (preferred), I.O.: **Note:** May be administered I.M., SubQ, or E.T., but onset of action may be delayed, especially if patient has poor perfusion; E.T. preferred if I.V./I.O. route not available; doses may need to be repeated: 0.1 mg/kg/dose; repeat every 2-3 minutes if needed; may need to repeat doses every 20-60 minutes

E.T.: Optimal endotracheal dose unknown; current expert recommendations are 2-3 times the I.V. dose

Opioid-induced depression: I.V., I.M., SubQ: Manufacturer's labeling: Usual: 0.01 mg/kg/dose; **Note:** This dose is **one-tenth** of the dose used for neonatal opioid intoxication (full reversal); may repeat every 2-3 minutes as needed based on response; may need to repeat every 1-2 hours

Reversal of respiratory depression from therapeutic opioid dosing: PALS Guidelines, 2010: I.V.: 0.001-0.005 mg/kg/dose; titrate to effect. **Note:** AAP recommends a wider dosage range of 0.001-0.015 mg/kg/dose (Hegenbarth, 2008)

Dosing: Usual

Infants, Children, and Adolescents:

Opioid intoxication (full reversal):

PALS Guidelines, 2010:

I.V. (preferred), I.O.: **Note:** May be administered I.M., SubQ, or E.T., but onset of action may be delayed, especially if patient has poor perfusion; E.T. preferred if I.V./I.O. route not available; doses may need to be repeated.

Infants and Children ≤5 years or ≤20 kg: 0.1 mg/kg/dose; repeat every 2-3 minutes if needed; may need to repeat doses every 20-60 minutes

Children >5 years or >20 kg and Adolescents: 2 mg/dose; if no response, repeat every 2-3 minutes; may need to repeat doses every 20-60 minutes

E.T.: Optimal endotracheal dose unknown; current expert recommendations are 2-3 times the I.V. dose.

Manufacturer's labeling: I.V. (preferred), I.M., SubQ: Initial: 0.01 mg/kg/dose; if no response, a subsequent dose of 0.1 mg/kg may be given; **Note:** If using I.M. or SubQ route, dose should be given in divided doses.

Continuous I.V. infusion: Limited data available: Infants, Children, and Adolescents: 24-40 **mcg**/kg/**hour** has been reported (Gourlay, 1983; Lewis, 1984; Tenenbein, 1984). **Note:** Doses as low as 2.5 **mcg**/kg/**hour** have been reported in adults and a dose of 160 **mcg**/kg/**hour** was reported in one neonate (Tenenbein,

1984). If continuous infusion is required, calculate the initial dosage/**hour** based on the effective intermittent dose used and duration of adequate response seen (Tenebein, 1984) **or** use two-thirds (^{2}/$_3$) of the initial effective naloxone bolus given as the hourly infusion (Perry, 1996); titrate dose; **Note:** The infusion should be discontinued by reducing the infusion rate in decrements of 25%; closely monitor the patient (eg, pulse oximetry and respiratory rate) after each adjustment and after discontinuation of the infusion for recurrence of opioid-induced respiratory depression (Perry, 1996).

Opioid overdose: 1 mg/mL injection: Intranasal administration: Adolescents ≥13 years: 2 mg (1 mg per nostril); **Note:** Onset of action is slightly delayed compared to I.M. or I.V. routes (Barton, 2005, Kelly, 2005).

Reversal of respiratory depression from therapeutic opioid dosing:

PALS Guidelines, 2010: I.V.: 0.001-0.005 mg/kg/dose; titrate to effect; **Note:** AAP recommends a wider dosage range of 0.001-0.015 mg/kg/dose (Hegenbarth, 2008)

Manufacturer's labeling: Initial: 0.005- 0.01 mg; repeat every 2-3 minutes as needed based on response

Opioid-induced pruritus: Limited data available:

Prevention: Children ≥6 years and Adolescents ≤17 years: Continuous I.V. infusion: 0.25 **mcg**/kg/**hour** was used in a double-blind, prospective, randomized, placebo-controlled study (n=20) which showed lower incidence and severity of opioid-induced side effects (ie, pruritus, nausea) without a loss of pain control (Maxwell, 2005).

Treatment: Children ≥3 years and Adolescents: Continuous I.V. infusion: Initial: 2 **mcg**/kg/**hour**; if pruritus continues, may titrate by 0.5 **mcg**/kg/**hour** every few hours; dosing based on a retrospective study (n=30, age range: 3-20 years) with a reported mean (± SD) dose of 2.3 ± 0.68 **mcg**/kg/**hour**; monitor closely; doses ≥3 **mcg**/kg/**hour** may increase risk for loss of pain control and patients may require an increase in opioid dose (Vrchoticky, 2000).

Adults: **Note:** Available routes of administration include I.M., I.V. (preferred), and SubQ routes; other available routes (unlabeled) include inhalation via nebulization, intranasal, and intraosseous (I.O.). Endotracheal administration is the least desirable and is supported by only anecdotal evidence (case report) (Neumar, 2010):

Opioid overdose (with standard ACLS protocols):

I.V., I.M., SubQ: Initial: 0.4-2 mg; may need to repeat doses every 2-3 minutes; after reversal, may need to readminister dose(s) at a later interval (ie, 20-60 minutes) depending on type/duration of opioid. If no response is observed after 10 mg, consider other causes of respiratory depression. **Note:** May be given endotracheally as 2-2.5 times the initial I.V. dose (ie, 0.8-5 mg) (Neumar, 2010).

Continuous I.V. infusion: **Note:** For use with exposures to long-acting opioids (eg, methadone), sustained release product, and symptomatic body packers after initial naloxone response. Calculate dosage/hour based on effective intermittent dose used and duration of adequate response seen (Tenenbein, 1984) **or** use two-thirds (^{2}/$_3$) of the initial effective naloxone bolus on an hourly basis (typically 0.25-6.25 mg/hour); one-half (^{1}/$_2$) of the initial bolus dose should be readministered 15 minutes after initiation of the continuous infusion to prevent a drop in naloxone levels; adjust infusion rate as needed to assure adequate ventilation and prevent withdrawal symptoms (Goldfrank, 1986).

Inhalation via nebulization: 2 mg; may repeat. Switch to I.V. or I.M. administration when possible (Weber, 2012)

Intranasal administration: 2 mg (1 mg per nostril); may repeat in 5 minutes if respiratory depression persists. **Note:** Onset of action is slightly delayed compared to I.M. or I.V. routes (Kelly, 2005; Neumar, 2010; Robertson, 2009).

Reversal of respiratory depression with therapeutic opioid doses: I.V., I.M., SubQ: Initial: 0.04-0.4 mg; may repeat until desired response achieved. If desired response is not observed after 0.8 mg total, consider other causes of respiratory depression. **Note:** May be given endotracheally (unlabeled route) as 2-2.5 times the initial I.V. dose (ie, 0.08-1 mg) (Neumar, 2010).

Continuous I.V. infusion: **Note:** For use with exposures to long-acting opioids (eg, methadone) or sustained release products. Calculate dosage/hour based on effective intermittent dose used and duration of adequate response seen (Tenenbein, 1984) or use two-thirds ($^2/_3$) of the initial effective naloxone bolus on an hourly basis (typically 0.2-0.6 mg/hour); one-half ($^1/_2$) of the initial bolus dose should be readministered 15 minutes after initiation of the continuous infusion to prevent a drop in naloxone levels; adjust infusion rate as needed to assure adequate ventilation and prevent withdrawal symptoms (Goldfrank, 1986).

Opioid-dependent patients being treated for cancer pain (NCCN guidelines, v.2.2011): I.V.: 0.04-0.08 mg (40-80 **mcg**) slow I.V. push; administer every 30-60 seconds until improvement in symptoms; if no response is observed after total naloxone dose 1 mg, consider other causes of respiratory depression

Postoperative opioid reversal: I.V.: 0.1-0.2 mg every 2-3 minutes until desired response (adequate ventilation and alertness without significant pain). **Note:** Repeat doses may be needed within 1-2 hour intervals depending on type, dose, and timing of the last dose of opioid administered.

Administration

Endotracheal: Dilute to 1-2 mL with NS; follow with a flush ≥5 mL of NS and 5 consecutive positive-pressure ventilations

Inhalation via nebulization: Adults: Dilute 2 mg of naloxone with 3 mL of normal saline and administer via nebulizer face mask (Mycyk, 2003; Weber, 2012).

Intranasal: Adolescents and Adults: Administer total dose equally divided into each nostril using a mucosal atomizer device (MAD) (Kelly, 2005; Robertson, 2009; Vanden Hoek, 2010)

Parenteral:

I.V. push: Administer over 30 seconds as undiluted preparation. May administer I.V. push as diluted preparation by diluting 0.4 mg (1 mL) with 9 mL of normal saline for a total volume of 10 mL to achieve a concentration of 0.04 mg/mL (APS, 2008)

Continuous I.V. infusion: Dilute to 4 mcg/mL in D$_5$W or NS

I.M., I.O, SubQ: May administer I.M., I.O., or SubQ if unable to obtain I.V. access. **Note:** I.M. or SubQ administration in hypotensive patients or patients with peripheral vasoconstriction or hypoperfusion may result in erratic or delayed absorption.

Monitoring Parameters Respiratory rate, heart rate, blood pressure, temperature, level of consciousness, ABGs, or pulse oximetry

Additional Information For administration to neonates, it is no longer recommended to use a more dilute concentration (0.02 mg/mL) and product has been discontinued. Use of this concentration results in unacceptably high fluid volumes, especially in small neonates. The 0.4 mg/mL preservative-free preparation should be used and can be accurately dosed with appropriately sized syringes (1 mL).

To prevent overdose deaths, there are initiatives to dispense naloxone for self- or buddy-administration to patients at risk of opioid overdose (eg, recipients of high-dose opioids, suspected or confirmed history of illicit opioid use) and individuals likely to be present in an overdose situation (eg, family members of illicit drug users) (Albert, 2011; Bennett, 2011). Needleless administration via nebulization and the intranasal route by first responders and bystanders has also been described (Doe-Simkins, 2009; Weber, 2012). Needleless administration provides an alternative route of administration in patients with venous scarring due to illicit drug use (eg, heroin). There is a low incidence of death following naloxone reversal of opioid toxicity in patients who refuse transport to a healthcare facility (Wampler, 2011).

Some products contain methyl and propylparabens. Naloxone has been used to increase blood pressure in patients with septic shock; increases in blood pressure may last several hours; however, an increase in patient survival has not been demonstrated and in some studies serious adverse effects (eg, agitation, pulmonary edema, hypotension, cardiac arrhythmias, seizures) have been reported; naloxone is generally not used for septic shock, especially in patients with underlying pain or opioid tolerance; optimal dosage for this indication has not been established; one neonatal study (n=2) reported a positive blood pressure response, but one neonate developed intractable seizures and died.

Product Availability Evzio: FDA approved April 2014; availability anticipated in the summer of 2014. Evzio is an auto-injector indicated for the emergency treatment of known or suspected opioid overdose in settings where opioids may be present.

Dosage Forms Excipient information presented when available (limited, particularly for generics); consult specific product labeling.

Solution, Injection, as hydrochloride:
Generic: 0.4 mg/mL (1 mL, 10 mL)
Solution, Injection, as hydrochloride [preservative free]:
Generic: 1 mg/mL (2 mL)
Solution Auto-injector, Injection, as hydrochloride:
Evzio: 0.4 mg/0.4 mL (0.4 mL)

References

Albert S, Brason FW 2nd, Sanford CK, et al, "Project Lazarus: Community-Based Overdose Prevention in Rural North Carolina," *Pain Med*, 2011, (12 Suppl 2):S77-85.

American Academy of Pediatrics Committee on Drugs, "Naloxone Dosage and Route of Administration for Infants and Children: Addendum to Emergency Drug Doses for Infants and Children," *Pediatrics*, 1990, 86(3):484-5.

American Pain Society (APS), *Principles of Analgesic Use in the Treatment of Acute Pain and Cancer Pain*, 6th ed, Glenview, IL: 2008.

Bailey B, "Are There Teratogenic Risks Associated With Antidotes Used in the Acute Management of Poisoned Pregnant Women?" *Birth Defects Res A Clin Mol Teratol*, 2003, 67(2):133-40.

Barton ED, Colwell CB, Wilfe T, Fosnocht D, Gravitz C, Bryan T, et al. Efficacy of intranasal naloxone as a needleless alternative for treatment of opioid overdose in the prehospital setting. *J Emerg Med*. 2005;29:265-271.

Bennett AS, Bell A, Tomedi L, et al, "Characteristics of an Overdose Prevention, Response, and Naloxone Distribution Program in Pittsburgh and Allegheny County, Pennsylvania," *J Urban Health*, 2011, 88(6):1020-30.

Boyer EW, "Management of Opioid Analgesic Overdose," *N Engl J Med*, 2012, 367(2):146-55.

Chamberlain JM and Klein BL, "A Comprehensive Review of Naloxone for the Emergency Physician," *Am J Emerg Med*, 1994, 12(6):650-60.

Doe-Simkins M, Walley AY, Epstein A, et al, "Saved by the Nose: Bystander-Administered Intranasal Naloxone Hydrochloride for Opioid Overdose," *Am J Public Health*, 2009, 99(5):788-91.

Field JM, Hazinski MF, Sayre MR, et al, "Part 1: Executive Summary: 2010 American Heart Association Guidelines for Cardiopulmonary Resuscitation and Emergency Cardiovascular Care," *Circulation*, 2010, 122(18 Suppl 3):640-56.

Fischer CG and Cook DR, "The Respiratory and Narcotic Antagonistic Effects of Naloxone in Infants," *Anesth Analg*, 1974, 53(6):849-52.

Goldfrank L, Weisman RS, Errick JK, et al, "A Dosing Nomogram for Continuous Infusion Intravenous Naloxone," *Ann Emerg Med*, 1986, 15(5):566-70.

Gourlay GK and Coulthard K, "The Role of Naloxone Infusions in the Treatment of Overdoses of Long Half-Life Narcotic Agonists: Application to Nor-methadone," *Br J Clin Pharmacol*, 1983, 15(2):269-71.

Hegenbarth MA and American Academy of Pediatrics Committee on Drugs, "Preparing for Pediatric Emergencies: Drugs to Consider," *Pediatrics*, 2008, 121(2):433-43.

Kattwinkel J, Perlman JM, Aziz K, et al, "Part 15: Neonatal Resuscitation: 2010 American Heart Association Guidelines for Cardiopulmonary Resuscitation and Emergency Cardiovascular Care," *Circulation*, 2010, 122(18 Suppl 3):909-19.

Kelly AM, Kerr D, Dietze P, et al, "Randomised Trial of Intranasal Versus Intramuscular Naloxone in Prehospital Treatment for Suspected Opioid Overdose," *Med J Aust*, 2005, 182(1):24-7.

Kjellberg F and Tramer MR, "Pharmacological Control of Opioid-Induced Pruritus: A Quantitative Systematic Review of Randomized Trials," *Eur J Anaesthesiol*, 2001, 18(6):346-57.

Kleinman ME, Chameides L, Schexnayder SM, et al, "Part 14: Pediatric Advanced Life Support: 2010 American Heart Association Guidelines for Cardiopulmonary Resuscitation and Emergency Cardiovascular Care," *Circulation*, 2010, 122(18 Suppl 3):876-908.

Lewis JM, Klein-Schwartz W, Benson BE, et al, "Continuous Naloxone Infusion in Pediatric Narcotic Overdose," *Am J Dis Child*, 1984, 138 (10):944-6.

Maxwell LG, Kaufmann SC, and Bitzer S, "The Effects of a Small-Dose Naloxone Infusion on Opioid-Induced Side Effects and Analgesia in Children and Adolescents Treated With Intravenous Patient-controlled Analgesia: A Double-Blind, Prospective, Randomized, Controlled Study," *Anesth Analg*, 2005, 100(4):953-8.

Mycyk MB, Szyszko AL, and Aks SE, "Nebulized Naloxone Gently and Effectively Reverses Methadone Intoxication," *J Emerg Med*, 2003, 24 (2):185-7.

Neumar RW, Otto CW, Link MS, et al, "Part 8: Adult Advanced Cardiovascular Life Support: 2010 American Heart Association Guidelines for Cardiopulmonary Resuscitation and Emergency Cardiovascular Care," *Circulation*, 2010, 122(18 Suppl 3):729-67.

Perry HE and Shannon MW, "Diagnosis and Management of Opioid-and Benzodiazepine-Induced Comatose Overdose in Children," *Curr Opin Pediatr*, 1996, 8(3):243-7.

Robertson TM, Hendey GW, Stroh G, et al, "Intranasal Naloxone Is a Viable Alternative to Intravenous Naloxone for Prehospital Narcotic Overdose," *Prehosp Emerg Care*, 2009, 13(4):512-5.

Smith K, Hopp M, Mundin G, et al, "Low Absolute Bioavailability of Oral Naloxone in Healthy Subjects," *Int J Clin Pharmacol Ther*, 2012, 50 (5):360-7.

Tenenbein M, "Continuous Naloxone Infusion for Opiate Poisoning in Infancy," *J Pediatr*, 1984, 105(4):645-8.

Vanden Hoek TL, Morrison LJ, Shuster M, et al, "Part 12: Cardiac Arrest in Special Situations: 2010 American Heart Association Guidelines for Cardiopulmonary Resuscitation and Emergency Cardiovascular Care," *Circulation*, 2010, 122(18 Suppl 3):829-61.

van Vonderen JJ, Siew ML, Hooper SB, et al, "Effects of Naloxone on the Breathing Pattern of a Newborn Exposed to Maternal Opiates," *Acta Paediatr*, 2012, 101(7):e309-12.

Vrchoticky T, "Naloxone for the Treatment of Narcotic Indiced Pruritus," *Journal of Pediatric Pharmacy Practice*, 2000, 5(2):92-7.

Wampler DA, Molina DK, McManus J, et al, "No Deaths Associated With Patient Refusal of Transport After Naloxone-Reversed Opioid Overdose," *Prehosp Emerg Care*, 2011, 15(3):320-4.

Weber JM, Tataris KL, Hoffman JD, et al, "Can Nebulized Naloxone Be Used Safely and Effectively by Emergency Medical Services for Suspected Opioid Overdose," *Prehosp Emerg Care*, 2012, 16 (2):289-92.

◆ **Naloxone and Buprenorphine** *see* Buprenorphine and Naloxone *on page 324*

◆ **Naloxone Hydrochloride** *see* Naloxone *on page 1466*

◆ **Naloxone Hydrochloride Dihydrate and Buprenorphine Hydrochloride** *see* Buprenorphine and Naloxone *on page 324*

◆ **Naloxone Hydrochloride Injection® (Can)** *see* Naloxone *on page 1466*

◆ **Naloxone Hydrochloride Injection® USP (Can)** *see* Naloxone *on page 1466*

◆ **NAPA and NABZ** *see* Sodium Phenylacetate and Sodium Benzoate *on page 1911*

Naphazoline (Nasal) (naf AZ oh leen)

Medication Safety Issues
Other safety concerns:
Accidental ingestion: Serious adverse reactions (eg, coma, bradycardia, respiratory depression, sedation) requiring hospitalization have been reported in children ≤5 years of age who have accidentally ingested even small amounts (eg, 1-2 mL) of imidazoline-derivative (ie, tetrahydrozoline, oxymetazoline, or naphazoline) eye drops or nasal sprays. Store these products out of reach of children at all times. Contact poison control or seek medical attention if accidental ingestion occurs.

Brand Names: U.S. Privine® [OTC]

Therapeutic Category Decongestant, Nasal; Nasal Agent, Vasoconstrictor

Use Temporarily relieves nasal congestion associated with rhinitis, sinusitis, hay fever, or the common cold

Contraindications Hypersensitivity to naphazoline or any component

Precautions Rebound congestion may occur with extended use (use no longer than 3-5 days); use with caution in the presence of hypertension, diabetes mellitus, hyperthyroidism, heart disease, coronary artery disease, cerebral arteriosclerosis, or long-standing asthma

Adverse Reactions
Local: Transient stinging, nasal mucosa irritation, dryness, rebound congestion
Respiratory: Sneezing

Drug Interactions
Metabolism/Transport Effects None known.

Avoid Concomitant Use
Avoid concomitant use of Naphazoline (Nasal) with any of the following: Ergot Derivatives; Iobenguane I 123; MAO Inhibitors

Increased Effect/Toxicity
Naphazoline (Nasal) may increase the levels/effects of: Sympathomimetics

The levels/effects of Naphazoline (Nasal) may be increased by: AtoMOXetine; Cannabinoid-Containing Products; Ergot Derivatives; Linezolid; MAO Inhibitors; Tricyclic Antidepressants

Decreased Effect
Naphazoline (Nasal) may decrease the levels/effects of: FentaNYL; Iobenguane I 123

The levels/effects of Naphazoline (Nasal) may be decreased by: Alpha1-Blockers

Mechanism of Action Stimulates alpha-adrenergic receptors in the arterioles of the conjunctiva and the nasal mucosa to produce vasoconstriction

Pharmacodynamics
Onset of action: Decongestion occurs within 10 minutes
Duration: 2-6 hours

Dosing: Usual Intranasal not recommended for use in children <6 years of age (especially in infants) due to CNS depression; therapy should not exceed 3-5 days
Children 6-12 years: 0.05%, 1 drop or spray every 6 hours if needed
Children >12 years to Adults: 0.05%, 1-2 drops or sprays every 3-6 hours if needed

Administration Spray or drop medication into one nostril while gently occluding the other; then reverse procedure

Dosage Forms Excipient information presented when available (limited, particularly for generics); consult specific product labeling.
Solution, intranasal, as hydrochloride [drops]:
Privine®: 0.05% (25 mL) [contains benzalkonium chloride]

Solution, intranasal, as hydrochloride [spray]:
Privine®: 0.05% (20 mL) [contains benzalkonium chloride]

Naphazoline (Ophthalmic) (naf AZ oh leen)

Medication Safety Issues
Other safety concerns:
Accidental ingestion: Serious adverse reactions (eg, coma, bradycardia, respiratory depression, sedation) requiring hospitalization have been reported in children ≤5 years of age who have accidentally ingested even small amounts (eg, 1-2 mL) of imidazoline-derivative (ie, tetrahydrozoline, oxymetazoline, or naphazoline) eye drops or nasal sprays. Store these products out of reach of children at all times. Contact poison control or seek medical attention if accidental ingestion occurs.

Brand Names: U.S. Clear Eyes Redness Relief [OTC]; VasoClear [OTC]; VasoClear-A [OTC]

Brand Names: Canada Naphcon Forte®; Vasocon®

Therapeutic Category Adrenergic Agonist Agent, Ophthalmic; Ophthalmic Agent, Vasoconstrictor

Generic Availability (U.S.) Yes

Use Topical ocular vasoconstrictor (to soothe, refresh, moisturize, and relieve redness due to minor eye irritation)

Pregnancy Risk Factor C

Pregnancy Considerations Animal reproduction studies have not been conducted.

Breast-Feeding Considerations It is not known if naphazoline is excreted into breast milk. The manufacturer recommends that caution be used if administering to a nursing woman.

Contraindications Hypersensitivity to naphazoline or any component; narrow-angle glaucoma; prior to peripheral iridectomy (in patients susceptible to angle block)

Precautions Use with caution in the presence of hypertension, diabetes mellitus, hyperthyroidism, heart disease, coronary artery disease, cerebral arteriosclerosis, or longstanding asthma. May contain benzalkonium chloride; may be absorbed by soft contact lenses.

Adverse Reactions Ocular: Blurred vision, discomfort, intraocular pressure increased, irritation, lacrimation, mydriasis, punctuate keratitis, redness

Drug Interactions
Metabolism/Transport Effects None known.
Avoid Concomitant Use
Avoid concomitant use of Naphazoline (Ophthalmic) with any of the following: Ergot Derivatives; Iobenguane I 123; MAO Inhibitors
Increased Effect/Toxicity
Naphazoline (Ophthalmic) may increase the levels/effects of: Sympathomimetics

The levels/effects of Naphazoline (Ophthalmic) may be increased by: AtoMOXetine; Cannabinoid-Containing Products; Ergot Derivatives; Linezolid; MAO Inhibitors; Tricyclic Antidepressants
Decreased Effect
Naphazoline (Ophthalmic) may decrease the levels/effects of: Iobenguane I 123

The levels/effects of Naphazoline (Ophthalmic) may be decreased by: Alpha1-Blockers

Mechanism of Action Stimulates alpha-adrenergic receptors in the arterioles of the conjunctiva and the nasal mucosa to produce vasoconstriction

Dosing: Usual Note: Therapy should generally not exceed 3-4 days; not recommended for use in children <6 years of age due to CNS depression (especially in infants). Children >6 years and Adults (0.01% to 0.1%): Instill 1-2 drops every 3-4 hours

Administration Instill drops into conjunctival sac of affected eye; finger pressure should be applied to lacrimal sac during and for 1-2 minutes after instillation to decrease risk of absorption and systemic reactions; avoid contact of bottle tip with skin or eye

Dosage Forms Excipient information presented when available (limited, particularly for generics); consult specific product labeling.
Solution, Ophthalmic, as hydrochloride:
Clear Eyes Redness Relief: 0.012% (6 mL) [contains benzalkonium chloride]
VasoClear: 0.02% (15 mL)
VasoClear-A: 0.02% (15 mL)
Generic: 0.1% (15 mL)

♦ **Naphazoline Hydrochloride** *see* Naphazoline (Nasal) *on page 1469*

♦ **Naphazoline Hydrochloride** *see* Naphazoline (Ophthalmic) *on page 1470*

♦ **Naphcon Forte® (Can)** *see* Naphazoline (Ophthalmic) *on page 1470*

♦ **Naprelan** *see* Naproxen *on page 1470*

♦ **Naprosyn** *see* Naproxen *on page 1470*

♦ **Naprosyn E (Can)** *see* Naproxen *on page 1470*

Naproxen (na PROKS en)

Medication Safety Issues
Sound-alike/look-alike issues:
Naproxen may be confused with Natacyn, Nebcin
Anaprox may be confused with Anaspaz, Avapro
Naprelan may be confused with Naprosyn
Naprosyn may be confused with Natacyn, Nebcin
BEERS Criteria medication:
This drug may be potentially inappropriate for use in geriatric patients (Quality of evidence - moderate; Strength of recommendation - strong).
International issues:
Flogen [Mexico] may be confused with Flovent brand name for fluticasone [U.S., Canada]

Flogen [Mexico] may be confused with Floxin brand name for flunarizine [Thailand], norfloxacin [South Africa], ofloxacin [U.S., Canada], and perfloxacin [Philippines]

Related Information
Oral Medications That Should Not Be Crushed or Altered *on page 2438*

Brand Names: U.S. Aleve [OTC]; All Day Pain Relief [OTC]; All Day Relief [OTC]; Anaprox; Anaprox DS; EC-Naprosyn; EnovaRX-Naproxen; Flanax Pain Relief [OTC]; Mediproxen [OTC]; Naprelan; Naprosyn; Naproxen Comfort Pac; Naproxen DR

Brand Names: Canada Aleve; Anaprox; Anaprox DS; Apo-Napro-Na; Apo-Napro-Na DS; Apo-Naproxen; Apo-Naproxen EC; Apo-Naproxen SR; Ava-Naproxen EC; Maxidol; Mylan-Naproxen EC; Naprelan; Naprosyn; Naprosyn E; Naproxen Sodium DS; Naproxen-NA; Naproxen-NA DF; PMS-Naproxen; PMS-Naproxen EC; PRO-Naproxen EC; Teva-Naproxen; Teva-Naproxen EC; Teva-Naproxen Sodium; Teva-Naproxen Sodium DS; Teva-Naproxen SR

Therapeutic Category Analgesic, Non-narcotic; Anti-inflammatory Agent; Antipyretic; Nonsteroidal Anti-inflammatory Drug (NSAID), Oral

Generic Availability (U.S.) May be product dependent

Use Management of inflammatory disease and rheumatoid disorders [including rheumatoid arthritis, juvenile idiopathic arthritis (JIA), osteoarthritis, ankylosing spondylitis]; acute gout; mild to moderate pain; primary dysmenorrhea; fever; tendonitis, bursitis. **Note:** Due to delayed absorption, the delayed-release tablets are **not** recommended for initial treatment of pain

Medication Guide Available Yes

Pregnancy Risk Factor C

Pregnancy Considerations Adverse events were not observed in the initial animal reproduction studies; therefore, the manufacturer classifies naproxen as pregnancy category C. Naproxen crosses the placenta and can be detected in fetal tissue and the serum of newborn infants following *in utero* exposure. NSAID exposure during the first trimester is not strongly associated with congenital malformations; however, cardiovascular anomalies and cleft palate have been observed following NSAID exposure in some studies. The use of a NSAID close to conception may be associated with an increased risk of miscarriage. Nonteratogenic effects have been observed following NSAID administration during the third trimester including: Myocardial degenerative changes, prenatal constriction of the ductus arteriosus, fetal tricuspid regurgitation, failure of the ductus arteriosus to close postnatally; renal dysfunction or failure, oligohydramnios; gastrointestinal bleeding or perforation, increased risk of necrotizing enterocolitis; intracranial bleeding (including intraventricular hemorrhage), platelet dysfunction with resultant bleeding; pulmonary hypertension. Because they may cause premature closure of the ductus arteriosus, use of NSAIDs late in pregnancy should be avoided (use after 31 or 32 weeks gestation is not recommended by some clinicians). The chronic use of NSAIDs in women of reproductive age may be associated with infertility that is reversible upon discontinuation of the medication. A registry is available for pregnant women exposed to autoimmune medications including naproxen. For additional information contact the Organization of Teratology Information Specialists, OTIS Autoimmune Diseases Study, at (877) 311-8972.

Breast-Feeding Considerations Small amounts of naproxen are excreted into breast milk. Naproxen has been detected in the urine of a breast-feeding infant. Breast-feeding is not recommended by the manufacturer. In a study which included 20 mother-infant pairs, there were two cases of drowsiness and one case of vomiting in the breast-fed infants. Maternal naproxen dose, duration, and relationship to breast-feeding were not provided.

Contraindications Hypersensitivity to naproxen or any component; history of asthma, urticaria, or allergic-type reaction to aspirin, or other NSAIDs; patients with the "aspirin triad" [asthma, rhinitis (with or without nasal polyps), and aspirin intolerance] (fatal asthmatic and anaphylactoid reactions may occur in these patients); perioperative pain in the setting of coronary artery bypass graft (CABG)

Warnings NSAIDs are associated with an increased risk of adverse cardiovascular thrombotic events, including potentially fatal MI and stroke **[U.S. Boxed Warning]**; risk may be increased with duration of use or preexisting cardiovascular risk factors or disease; carefully evaluate cardiovascular risk profile prior to prescribing; use the lowest effective dose for the shortest duration of time, taking into consideration individual patient treatment goals; alternate therapies should be considered for patients at high risk. Use is contraindicated for treatment of perioperative pain in the setting of CABG surgery **[U.S. Boxed Warning]**; an increased incidence of MI and stroke was found in patients receiving COX-2 selective NSAIDs for the treatment of pain within the first 10-14 days after CABG surgery. NSAIDs may cause fluid retention, edema, and new onset or worsening of preexisting hypertension; use with caution in patients with hypertension, heart failure, or fluid retention; be aware of sodium content of sodium naproxen products in patients with sodium restriction. Concurrent administration of ibuprofen, and potentially other nonselective NSAIDs, may interfere with aspirin's cardioprotective effect.

NSAIDs may increase the risk of gastrointestinal irritation, ulceration, bleeding, and perforation **[U.S. Boxed Warning]**. These events, which can be potentially fatal, may occur at any time during therapy and without warning. Avoid the use of NSAIDs in patients with active GI bleeding or ulcer disease. Use NSAIDs with extreme caution in patients with a history of GI bleeding or ulcers (these patients have a 10-fold increased risk for developing a GI bleed). Use NSAIDs with caution in patients with other risk factors which may increase GI bleeding (eg, concurrent therapy with aspirin, anticoagulants and/or corticosteroids, longer duration of NSAID use, smoking, use of alcohol, and poor general health). Use the lowest effective dose for the shortest duration of time, taking into consideration individual patient treatment goals; alternate therapies should be considered for patients at high risk.

NSAIDs may compromise existing renal function. Renal toxicity may occur in patients with impaired renal function, dehydration, salt depletion, heart failure, liver dysfunction, those taking diuretics and ACE inhibitors; use with caution in these patients; monitor renal function closely. Naproxen is not recommended for use in patients with moderate to severe or severe renal impairment (CrCl <30 mL/minute). Long-term use of NSAIDs may cause renal papillary necrosis and other renal injury.

Fatal asthmatic and anaphylactoid reactions may occur in patients with the "aspirin triad" who receive NSAIDs. Avoid use of NSAIDs in late pregnancy as they may cause premature closure of the ductus arteriosus. NSAIDs can cause serious skin reactions including exfoliative dermatitis, Stevens-Johnson Syndrome, and toxic epidermal necrolysis; these events may occur without warning; discontinue use at risk appearance of rash or other sign of hypersensitivity. Pseudoporphyria (ie, increased skin fragility and blistering with scarring in sun-exposed skin) has been reported in naproxen-treated children with JIA (reported incidence, 12%); discontinue therapy if this occurs.

Precautions Use with caution in patients with decreased hepatic function; closely monitor patients with abnormal LFTs; severe hepatic reactions (eg, fulminant hepatitis, liver failure) have occurred with NSAID use, rarely; discontinue if signs or symptoms of liver disease develop, or if systemic manifestations occur. Use with caution in patients with asthma. Safety and efficacy have not been established in children <2 years of age.

OTC labeling: Prior to self-medication, patients should contact healthcare provider if they have had recurring stomach pain or upset, heartburn, ulcers, bleeding problems, asthma, allergy to aspirin or any other pain reliever or fever reducer, high blood pressure, heart or kidney disease, other serious medical problems, or are currently taking a diuretic, steroid, anticoagulant, aspirin, other NSAID, or any other drug. Recommended dosages and duration should not be exceeded, due to an increased risk of GI bleeding, MI, and stroke. Stop use and consult a healthcare provider if symptoms get worse, newly appear, or continue; if an allergic reaction occurs; if the patient feels faint, vomits blood, or has bloody or black stools; if the patient has difficulty swallowing or heartburn; if fever worsens or lasts >3 days; or if pain worsens or lasts >10 days in adults or >3 days in children. Consuming ≥3 alcoholic beverages/day or taking this medication longer than recommended may increase the risk of GI bleeding. Not for OTC use in children <12 years of age without consulting with physician.

Adverse Reactions

Cardiovascular: Edema, palpitations

Central nervous system: Dizziness, drowsiness, headache, lightheadedness, vertigo

Dermatologic: Ecchymosis, pruritus, purpura, rash, skin eruption

Endocrine & metabolic: Fluid retention

Gastrointestinal: Abdominal pain, constipation, diarrhea, dyspepsia, flatulence, gross bleeding/perforation, heartburn, indigestion, nausea, stomatitis, ulcers, vomiting

Genitourinary: Abnormal renal function

Hematologic: Anemia, bleeding time increased, ecchymosis, hemolysis

Hepatic: LFTs increased

Ocular: Visual disturbances

Otic: Hearing disturbances, tinnitus

Respiratory: Dyspnea

Miscellaneous: Diaphoresis, thirst

Rare but important or life-threatening: Agranulocytosis, alopecia, anaphylactic/anaphylactoid reaction, angioneurotic edema, arrhythmia, aseptic meningitis, asthma, blurred vision, cognitive dysfunction, colitis, coma, confusion, CHF, conjunctivitis, cystitis, depression, dream abnormalities, dysuria, eosinophilia, eosinophilic pneumonitis, erythema multiforme, exfoliative dermatitis, glossitis, granulocytopenia, hallucinations, hematemesis, hepatitis, hyper-/hypoglycemia, hyper-/hypotension, infection, interstitial nephritis, melena, jaundice, leukopenia, liver failure, lymphadenopathy, menstrual disorders, malaise, MI, muscle weakness, myalgia, oliguria, pancreatitis, pancytopenia, paresthesia, photosensitivity, pneumonia, polyuria, proteinuria, pyrexia, rectal bleeding, renal failure, renal papillary necrosis, respiratory depression, sepsis, Stevens-Johnson syndrome, tachycardia, seizure, syncope, thrombocytopenia, toxic epidermal necrolysis ulcerative stomatitis, vasculitis

Drug Interactions

Metabolism/Transport Effects Substrate of CYP1A2 (minor), CYP2C9 (minor); **Note:** Assignment of Major/Minor substrate status based on clinically relevant drug interaction potential

Avoid Concomitant Use

Avoid concomitant use of Naproxen with any of the following: Floctafenine; Ketorolac (Nasal); Ketorolac (Systemic); NSAID (COX-2 Inhibitor); Omacetaxine; Urokinase

Increased Effect/Toxicity

Naproxen may increase the levels/effects of: 5-ASA Derivatives; Agents with Antiplatelet Properties; Aliskiren; Aminoglycosides; Anticoagulants; Apixaban; Bisphosphonate Derivatives; Collagenase (Systemic); CycloSPORINE (Systemic); Dabigatran Etexilate; Deferasirox; Desmopressin; Digoxin; Eplerenone; Haloperidol; Ibritumomab; Lithium; Methotrexate; Nonsteroidal Anti-Inflammatory Agents; NSAID (COX-2 Inhibitor); Omacetaxine; PEMEtrexed; Porfimer; Potassium-Sparing Diuretics; PRALAtrexate; Quinolone Antibiotics; Rivaroxaban; Salicylates; Tenofovir; Thrombolytic Agents; Tositumomab and Iodine I 131 Tositumomab; Urokinase; Vancomycin; Vitamin K Antagonists

The levels/effects of Naproxen may be increased by: ACE Inhibitors; Angiotensin II Receptor Blockers; Antidepressants (Tricyclic, Tertiary Amine); Corticosteroids (Systemic); CycloSPORINE (Systemic); Dasatinib; Floctafenine; Glucosamine; Herbs (Anticoagulant/Antiplatelet Properties); Ibrutinib; Ketorolac (Nasal); Ketorolac (Systemic); Multivitamins/Fluoride (with ADE); Multivitamins/Minerals (with ADEK, Folate, Iron); Multivitamins/Minerals (with AE, No Iron); Nonsteroidal Anti-Inflammatory Agents; Omega-3 Fatty Acids; Pentosan Polysulfate Sodium; Pentoxifylline; Probenecid; Prostacyclin Analogues; Selective Serotonin Reuptake Inhibitors; Serotonin/Norepinephrine Reuptake Inhibitors; Sodium Phosphates; Tipranavir; Treprostinil; Vitamin E

Decreased Effect

Naproxen may decrease the levels/effects of: ACE Inhibitors; Agents with Antiplatelet Properties; Aliskiren; Angiotensin II Receptor Blockers; Beta-Blockers; Eplerenone; HydrALAZINE; Loop Diuretics; Potassium-Sparing Diuretics; Prostaglandins (Ophthalmic); Salicylates; Selective Serotonin Reuptake Inhibitors; Thiazide Diuretics

The levels/effects of Naproxen may be decreased by: Bile Acid Sequestrants; Nonsteroidal Anti-Inflammatory Agents; Salicylates

Food Interactions Naproxen absorption rate/levels may be decreased if taken with food. Management: Administer with food, milk, or antacids to decrease GI adverse effects.

Stability Store tablets and suspension at room temperature [15°C to 30°C (59°F to 86°F)]; avoid exposure of suspension to excessive heat >40°C (104°F); dispense naproxen tablets and suspension in light-resistant, well-closed containers

Mechanism of Action Reversibly inhibits cyclooxygenase-1 and 2 (COX-1 and 2) enzymes, which results in decreased formation of prostaglandin precursors; has antipyretic, analgesic, and anti-inflammatory properties

Other proposed mechanisms not fully elucidated (and possibly contributing to the anti-inflammatory effect to varying degrees), include inhibiting chemotaxis, altering lymphocyte activity, inhibiting neutrophil aggregation/activation, and decreasing proinflammatory cytokine levels.

Pharmacokinetics (Adult data unless noted)

Absorption: Oral: Almost 100%

Distribution: Crosses the placenta; ~1% distributed into breast milk

V_d: Adults: 0.16 L/kg

Protein binding: >99%

Metabolism: Extensively metabolized in the liver to 6-0-desmethyl naproxen; parent drug and desmethyl metabolite undergo further metabolism to their respective acyl-glucuronide conjugated metabolites

Bioavailability: 95%

Half-life, elimination: Children: Range: 8-17 hours

Children 8-14 years: 8-10 hours

Adults: 12-17 hours

Time to peak serum concentration:

Tablets, naproxen: 2-4 hours

Tablets, naproxen sodium: 1-2 hours

Tablets, delayed-release (empty stomach): 4-6 hours; range 2-12 hours

Tablets, delayed-release (with food): 12 hours; range: 4-24 hours

Suspension: 1-4 hours

Elimination: 95% excreted in urine (<1% as unchanged drug; <1% as 6-0-desmethyl naproxen; 66% to 92% as their conjugates); ≤3% excreted in feces

Dosing: Usual Note: Dosage expressed as naproxen base; 200 mg naproxen base is equivalent to 220 mg naproxen sodium

Oral:

Children >2 years:

Analgesia: 5-7 mg/kg/dose every 8-12 hours

Inflammatory disease, including JIA: Usual: 10-15 mg/kg/day in 2 divided doses; range: 7-20 mg/kg/day; maximum dose: 1000 mg/day. Manufacturer's recommendation for JIA: 10 mg/kg/day in 2 divided doses

Children >12 and Adults ≤65 years: OTC labeling for pain and fever: 200 mg every 8-12 hours; if needed may take 400 mg for the initial dose; maximum dose: 600 mg/day

Adults:

Rheumatoid arthritis, osteoarthritis, and ankylosing spondylitis: 500-1000 mg/day in 2 divided doses

Acute gout: Initial: 750 mg, followed by 250 mg every 8 hours until attack subsides. **Note:** Delayed release tablet is not recommended due to delayed absorption.

Mild to moderate pain, dysmenorrhea, acute tendonitis, or bursitis: Initial: 500 mg, then 500 mg every 12 hours or 250 mg every 6-8 hours as needed; maximum dose: 1250 mg/day initially, then 1000 mg/day thereafter. **Note:** Delayed release tablet is not recommended for treatment of acute pain, due to delayed absorption.

Dosage adjustment in renal impairment: Moderate to severe and severe renal impairment (CrCl <30 mL/minute): Not recommended for use

Administration Oral: Administer with food, milk, or antacids to decrease GI adverse effects. Shake suspension well before use. Do not chew, crush, or break delayed or controlled release tablet, swallow whole. Separate administration of naproxen and antacids, sucralfate, or cholestyramine by 2 hours.

Monitoring Parameters CBC with differential, platelets, BUN, serum creatinine, liver enzymes, occult blood loss, periodic ophthalmologic exams, hemoglobin, hematocrit, blood pressure

Test Interactions Naproxen may interfere with 5-HIAA urinary assays; due to an interaction with m-dinitrobenzene, naproxen should be discontinued 72 hours before adrenal function testing if the Porter-Silber test is used. May interfere with urine detection of cannabinoids and barbiturates (false-positives).

Additional Information In a multicenter, retrospective chart review, 19 children, 4-14 years of age (mean: 9.1 ± 2.9) with rheumatic fever (but without carditis, chorea, or rashes), were treated solely with naproxen (10-20 mg/kg/day divided in 2 doses) until ESR normalized (between 4-8 weeks); fever and arthritis resolved within a median of 1 day of starting therapy; no patient had side effects, or developed carditis over the following 6 months; comparative studies with aspirin that include patients with mild carditis are needed to confirm these findings (Uziel, 2000).

Due to its effects on platelet function, naproxen should be withheld for at least 4-6 half-lives prior to surgical or dental procedures.

Dosage Forms Considerations

EnovaRX-Naproxen is a compounding kit. Refer to manufacturer's package insert for compounding instructions.

Naproxen Comfort Pac is a combination kit containing naproxen tablets and Duraflex Comfort Gel

Dosage Forms Excipient information presented when available (limited, particularly for generics); consult specific product labeling.

Capsule, Oral, as sodium:
Aleve: 220 mg [contains brilliant blue fcf (fd&c blue #1)]
Cream, External:
EnovaRX-Naproxen: 10% (60 g, 120 g) [contains cetyl alcohol]
Kit, Combination:
Naproxen Comfort Pac: 500 mg [contains methylparaben, trolamine (triethanolamine)]
Suspension, Oral:
Naprosyn: 125 mg/5 mL (480 mL)
Generic: 125 mg/5 mL (500 mL)
Tablet, Oral:
Naprosyn: 250 mg [scored]
Naprosyn: 375 mg
Naprosyn: 500 mg [scored]
Generic: 250 mg, 375 mg, 500 mg
Tablet, Oral, as sodium:
Aleve: 220 mg [contains fd&c blue #2 aluminum lake]
All Day Pain Relief: 220 mg [contains fd&c blue #2 aluminum lake]
All Day Pain Relief: 220 mg [gluten free; contains fd&c blue #2 aluminum lake]
All Day Relief: 220 mg
All Day Relief: 220 mg [contains fd&c blue #2 aluminum lake]
Anaprox: 275 mg

Anaprox DS: 550 mg [scored]
Flanax Pain Relief: 220 mg [contains fd&c blue #2 (indigotine)]
Mediproxen: 220 mg
Generic: 220 mg, 275 mg, 550 mg
Tablet Delayed Release, Oral:
EC-Naprosyn: 375 mg, 500 mg
Naproxen DR: 375 mg, 500 mg
Tablet Extended Release 24 Hour, Oral, as sodium [strength expressed as base]:
Naprelan: 375 mg, 500 mg, 750 mg

References

Berde C, Ablin A, Glazer J, et al, "American Academy of Pediatrics Report of the Subcommittee on Disease-Related Pain in Childhood Cancer," *Pediatrics*, 1990, 86(5 Pt 2):818-25.

Lang BA and Finlayson LA, "Naproxen-Induced Pseudoporphyria in Patients With Juvenile Rheumatoid Arthritis," *J Pediatr*, 1994, 124 (4):639-42.

Uziel Y, Hashkes PJ, Kassem E, et al, "The Use of Naproxen in the Treatment of Children With Rheumatic Fever," *J Pediatr*, 2000, 137 (2):269-71.

Wells TG, Mortensen ME, Dietrich A, et al, "Comparison of the Pharmacokinetics of Naproxen Tablets and Suspension in Children," *J Clin Pharmacol*, 1994, 34(1):30-3.

◆ **Naproxen Comfort Pac** see Naproxen on page 1470

◆ **Naproxen DR** see Naproxen on page 1470

◆ **Naproxen-NA (Can)** see Naproxen on page 1470

◆ **Naproxen-NA DF (Can)** see Naproxen on page 1470

◆ **Naproxen Sodium** see Naproxen on page 1470

◆ **Naproxen Sodium DS (Can)** see Naproxen on page 1470

◆ **Narcan** see Naloxone on page 1466

◆ **Naropin** see Ropivacaine on page 1849

◆ **Naropin® (Can)** see Ropivacaine on page 1849

◆ **Nasacort Allergy 24HR [OTC]** see Triamcinolone (Nasal) on page 2076

◆ **Nasacort AQ** see Triamcinolone (Nasal) on page 2076

◆ **NasalCrom [OTC]** see Cromolyn (Nasal) on page 553

◆ **Nasal Decongestant [OTC]** see Phenylephrine (Systemic) on page 1658

◆ **Nasal Decongestant [OTC]** see Pseudoephedrine on page 1770

◆ **Nasal Decongestant PE Max St [OTC]** see Phenylephrine (Systemic) on page 1658

◆ **Nasal Decongestant Spray [OTC]** see Oxymetazoline (Nasal) on page 1577

◆ **Nasal Four [OTC]** see Phenylephrine (Nasal) on page 1660

◆ **Nasalide® (Can)** see Flunisolide (Nasal) on page 890

◆ **Nasal Moist [OTC]** see Sodium Chloride on page 1902

◆ **Nasal Spray 12 Hour [OTC]** see Oxymetazoline (Nasal) on page 1577

◆ **Nasal Spray Extra Moisturizing [OTC]** see Oxymetazoline (Nasal) on page 1577

◆ **Nascobal** see Cyanocobalamin on page 556

◆ **Nasonex** see Mometasone (Nasal) on page 1433

◆ **Nasonex® (Can)** see Mometasone (Nasal) on page 1433

◆ **Natesto** see Testosterone on page 1986

◆ **Natroba** see Spinosad on page 1930

◆ **NatrOVA** see Spinosad on page 1930

◆ **Natulan (Can)** see Procarbazine on page 1743

◆ **Natural Fiber Therapy [OTC]** see Psyllium on page 1773

◆ **Natural Lung Surfactant** see Beractant on page 280

- ◆ **Natural Psyllium Seed [OTC]** *see* Psyllium *on page 1773*
- ◆ **Natural Senna Laxative [OTC]** *see* Senna *on page 1877*
- ◆ **Natural Vegetable Fiber [OTC]** *see* Psyllium *on page 1773*
- ◆ **Natural Vitamin E [OTC]** *see* Vitamin E *on page 2148*
- ◆ **Nature-Throid** *see* Thyroid, Desiccated *on page 2018*
- ◆ **Nauseatol [OTC] (Can)** *see* DimenhyDRINATE *on page 670*
- ◆ **Navane** *see* Thiothixene *on page 2015*
- ◆ **Navelbine** *see* Vinorelbine *on page 2143*
- ◆ **Na-Zone [OTC]** *see* Sodium Chloride *on page 1902*
- ◆ **N-Carbamoyl-L-Glutamic Acid** *see* Carglumic Acid *on page 381*
- ◆ **N-Carbamylglutamate** *see* Carglumic Acid *on page 381*
- ◆ **Nebupent** *see* Pentamidine *on page 1637*
- ◆ **Nebusal** *see* Sodium Chloride *on page 1902*

Nedocromil (ne doe KROE mil)

Brand Names: U.S. Alocril
Brand Names: Canada Alocril®
Therapeutic Category Antiallergic, Ophthalmic
Generic Availability (U.S.) No
Use Treatment of itching associated with allergic conjunctivitis (FDA approved in ages ≥3 years and adults)
Pregnancy Risk Factor B
Pregnancy Considerations There are no well-controlled studies in pregnant women. Animal studies show no evidence of teratogenicity or harm to fetus. Additionally, nedocromil has minimal systemic absorption.
Breast-Feeding Considerations It is not known if nedocromil is excreted in breast milk. The manufacturer recommends that caution be exercised when administering nedocromil to nursing women.
Contraindications Hypersensitivity to nedocromil or any component
Precautions Contains benzalkonium chloride, which may be absorbed by contact lenses; users of contact lenses should not wear them during periods of symptomatic allergic conjunctivitis.
Adverse Reactions
Central nervous system: Headache
Gastrointestinal: Unpleasant taste
Ocular: Burning, conjunctivitis, eye redness, irritation, photophobia, stinging
Respiratory: Asthma, nasal congestion, rhinitis
Drug Interactions
Metabolism/Transport Effects None known.
Avoid Concomitant Use There are no known interactions where it is recommended to avoid concomitant use.
Increased Effect/Toxicity There are no known significant interactions involving an increase in effect.
Decreased Effect There are no known significant interactions involving a decrease in effect.
Stability Store at 2°C to 25°C (36°F to 77°F); the remaining contents of Alocril® unit dose solution should be discarded immediately after use
Mechanism of Action Inhibits the activation of and mediator release from a variety of inflammatory cell types associated with hypersensitivity reactions including eosinophils, neutrophils, macrophages, mast cells, monocytes, and platelets; it inhibits the release of histamine, leukotrienes, and slow-reacting substance of anaphylaxis.
Pharmacokinetics (Adult data unless noted)
Absorption: Systemic: Ophthalmic: <4%
Elimination: Excreted unchanged in urine 70%; feces 30%

Dosing: Usual Ophthalmic: Children ≥3 years and Adults: 1-2 drops in each eye twice daily throughout the period of exposure to allergen
Administration Ophthalmic: Instill drops into conjunctival sac; avoid contact of bottle tip with skin or eye
Dosage Forms Excipient information presented when available (limited, particularly for generics); consult specific product labeling.
Solution, Ophthalmic, as sodium:
Alocril: 2% (5 mL) [contains benzalkonium chloride]

- ◆ **Nedocromil Sodium** *see* Nedocromil *on page 1474*

Nefazodone (nef AY zoe done)

Medication Safety Issues
Sound-alike/look-alike issues:
Serzone® may be confused with selegiline, SEROquel®, sertraline
Related Information
Antidepressant Agents *on page 2219*
Therapeutic Category Antidepressant, Serotonin Reuptake Inhibitor/Antagonist
Generic Availability (U.S.) Yes
Use Treatment of depression (FDA approved in adults)
Note: Due to the risk of hepatic failure, other antidepressant agents are generally tried first
Medication Guide Available Yes
Pregnancy Risk Factor C
Pregnancy Considerations Adverse effects were observed in some animal reproduction studies. When nefazodone is taken during pregnancy, an increased risk of major malformations has not been observed in the limited number of pregnancies studied (Einarson, 2003; Einarson, 2009). The long-term effects of *in utero* exposure to nefazodone on infant development and behavior are not known.

The ACOG recommends that therapy with antidepressants during pregnancy be individualized; treatment of depression during pregnancy should incorporate the clinical expertise of the mental health clinician, obstetrician, primary healthcare provider, and pediatrician. According to the American Psychiatric Association (APA), the risks of medication treatment should be weighed against other treatment options and untreated depression. Consideration should be given to using agents with safety data in pregnancy. For women who discontinue antidepressant medications during pregnancy and who may be at high risk for postpartum depression, the medications can be restarted following delivery. Treatment algorithms have been developed by the ACOG and the APA for the management of depression in women prior to conception and during pregnancy (ACOG, 2008; APA, 2010; Yonkers, 2009).
Breast-Feeding Considerations Nefazodone and its metabolites are excreted in breast milk. Drowsiness, lethargy, poor feeding, and failure to maintain body temperature have been reported in a premature nursing infant. Adverse events were not observed in two case reports of older infants (Dodd, 2000; Yapp, 2000). The long-term effects on neurobehavior have not been studied. The manufacturer recommends that caution be exercised when administering nefazodone to nursing women.
Contraindications Hypersensitivity to nefazodone, related compounds (phenylpiperazine antidepressants), or any component; liver injury due to previous nefazodone treatment; concurrent use with astemizole, carbamazepine, cisapride, pimozide, or terfenadine; concurrent therapy with triazolam
Warnings Nefazodone is not approved for use in pediatric patients. Clinical worsening of depression or suicidal ideation and behavior may occur in children and adults with

major depressive disorder **[U.S. Boxed Warning]**. In clinical trials, antidepressants increased the risk of suicidal thinking and behavior (suicidality) in children, adolescents, and young adults (18-24 years of age) with major depressive disorder and other psychiatric disorders. This risk must be considered before prescribing antidepressants for any clinical use. Short-term studies did not show an increased risk of suicidality with antidepressant use in patients >24 years of age and showed a decreased risk in patients ≥65 years.

Patients of all ages who are treated with antidepressants for any indication require appropriate monitoring and close observation for clinical worsening of depression, suicidality, and unusual changes in behavior, especially during the first few months after antidepressant initiation or when the dose is adjusted. Family members and caregivers should be instructed to closely observe the patient (ie, daily) and communicate condition with healthcare provider. Patients should also be monitored for associated behaviors (eg, anxiety, agitation, panic attacks, insomnia, irritability, hostility, aggressiveness, impulsivity, akathisia, hypomania, mania) which may increase the risk for worsening depression or suicidality. Worsening depression or emergence of suicidality (or associated behaviors listed above) that is abrupt in onset, severe, or not part of the presenting symptoms, may require discontinuation or modification of drug therapy. If intolerable symptoms occur following a decrease in dosage or upon discontinuation of therapy, consider resuming the previous dose with a more gradual taper. Therapy should not be abruptly discontinued in patients receiving high doses for prolonged periods. To reduce risk of intentional overdose, write prescriptions for the smallest quantity consistent with good patient care.

Life-threatening hepatic failure has been reported in patients treated with nefazodone **[U.S. Boxed Warning]**. The estimated rate is 1 case of liver failure (resulting in liver transplant or death) per 250,000-300,000 patient-years of nefazodone treatment (3-4 times the background rate of liver failure); actual incidence may be higher due to under-reporting. Onset of liver injury has generally occurred between 2 weeks to 6 months of nefazodone therapy. Nefazodone should not routinely be started in patients with active liver disease or elevated baseline serum transaminases (baseline abnormalities may complicate patient monitoring). Nefazodone should be discontinued if clinical signs or symptoms suggestive of liver failure occur or if serum AST or ALT levels increase to ≥3 times the upper limit of normal. Do not reinitiate nefazodone in these patients.

Concurrent use with triazolam is contraindicated; nefazodone significantly increases triazolam serum concentrations; initial triazolam dosage must be reduced by 75% if drugs are used concomitantly; such reductions may not be possible with available dosage forms; thus, use with triazolam is contraindicated. Nefazodone significantly increases alprazolam serum concentrations; initial alprazolam dosage should be reduced by 50% if drugs are used concomitantly. Concurrent use of MAO inhibitors, use of MAO inhibitors within previous 14 days, and use of MAO inhibitors within 1 week of stopping nefazodone is not recommended; serious, potentially fatal reactions may occur. Nefazodone may potentially significantly increase plasma concentrations of astemizole, cisapride, pimozide, and terfenadine, resulting in QT prolongation and serious cardiovascular adverse events; concurrent use with any of these drugs is contraindicated. Carbamazepine will significantly decrease nefazodone serum concentrations; concurrent use is contraindicated.

May precipitate a shift to mania or hypomania in patients with bipolar disorder. Monotherapy in patients with bipolar disorder should be avoided. Patients presenting with depressive symptoms should be screened for bipolar disorder. Use with caution in patients with a history of mania. Nefazodone is not FDA approved for the treatment of bipolar depression.

Precautions Use with caution in patients with a history of seizures; seizures have been reported with nefazodone use. May cause orthostatic or postural hypotension; use with caution in patients with known cardiovascular or cerebrovascular disease or predisposing hypotensive conditions like dehydration, hypovolemia, or concurrent antihypertensive therapy. Priapism has been reported (rarely) during postmarketing surveillance; if condition occurs, therapy should be discontinued and physician contacted. Use with caution in patients with recent history of MI or unstable heart disease; nefazodone has not been studied in these patients; sinus bradycardia may occur with nefazodone use. Use with caution and decrease the dose in debilitated patients. May impair physical or mental abilities; patients must be cautioned about performing tasks which require mental alertness (eg, operating machinery or driving) until certain nefazodone does not adversely affect abilities. Visual disturbances, including blurred vision, scotoma, and visual trials have been reported. No clinical studies have assessed the combined use of nefazodone and electroconvulsive therapy; however, similar drugs may increase the risks associated with electroconvulsive therapy; consider discontinuing, when possible, prior to ECT treatment. Discontinue use prior to elective surgery (unknown interactions with general anesthetics may exist).

Adverse Reactions

Cardiovascular: Bradycardia, hypotension, orthostatic hypotension, peripheral edema, vasodilation

Central nervous system: Abnormal dreams, agitation, ataxia, chills, confusion, decreased concentration, dizziness, drowsiness, fever, headache, incoordination, insomnia, lightheadedness, memory impairment, psychomotor retardation, tremor

Dermatologic: Pruritus, rash

Endocrine & metabolic: Breast pain, decreased libido, impotence

Gastrointestinal: Constipation, diarrhea, dyspepsia, gastroenteritis, increased appetite, nausea, taste perversion, thirst, vomiting, xerostomia

Genitourinary: Urinary frequency, urinary retention

Hematologic: Decreased hematocrit

Neuromuscular & skeletal: Arthralgia, hypertonia, neck rigidity, paresthesia, tremor, weakness

Ocular: Abnormal vision, blurred vision, eye pain, visual field defect

Otic: Tinnitus

Respiratory: Bronchitis, cough, dyspnea, pharyngitis

Miscellaneous: Flu syndrome, infection

Rare but important or life-threatening: Allergic reaction, angioedema, AV block, galactorrhea, gynecomastia, hallucinations, hepatic failure, hepatic necrosis, hepatitis, hyponatremia, impotence, increased prolactin, leukopenia, liver function tests (abnormal), photosensitivity, priapism, rhabdomyolysis (with lovastatin/simvastatin), seizure, serotonin syndrome, Stevens-Johnson syndrome, thrombocytopenia

Drug Interactions

Metabolism/Transport Effects Substrate of CYP2D6 (major), CYP3A4 (major); **Note:** Assignment of Major/Minor substrate status based on clinically relevant drug interaction potential; **Inhibits** CYP1A2 (weak), CYP2B6 (weak), CYP2C8 (weak), CYP2D6 (weak), CYP3A4 (strong); **Induces** P-glycoprotein

Avoid Concomitant Use

Avoid concomitant use of Nefazodone with any of the following: Ado-Trastuzumab Emtansine; Alfuzosin; Apixaban; Avanafil; Axitinib; Bosutinib; Cabozantinib; CarBAMazepine; Ceritinib; Cisapride; Conivaptan; Crizotinib; Dabigatran Etexilate; Dronedarone; Eplerenone; ▶

Everolimus; Fusidic Acid (Systemic); Halofantrine; Ibrutinib; Ivabradine; Lapatinib; Linezolid; Lomitapide; Lovastatin; Lurasidone; Macitentan; MAO Inhibitors; Methylene Blue; Nilotinib; Nisoldipine; Pimozide; Ranolazine; Red Yeast Rice; Regorafenib; Rivaroxaban; Salmeterol; Silodosin; Simeprevir; Simvastatin; Sofosbuvir; Tamsulosin; Ticagrelor; Tolvaptan; Toremifene; Ulipristal; Vemurafenib; VinCRIStine (Liposomal); Vorapaxar

Increased Effect/Toxicity

Nefazodone may increase the levels/effects of: Ado-Trastuzumab Emtansine; Alfuzosin; Almotriptan; Alosetron; Antipsychotic Agents (Phenothiazines); Antipsychotics; Apixaban; ARIPiprazole; Avanafil; Axitinib; Bedaquiline; Bortezomib; Bosentan; Bosutinib; Brentuximab Vedotin; Brinzolamide; Budesonide (Nasal); Budesonide (Systemic, Oral Inhalation); Cabozantinib; Cannabis; CarBAMazepine; Ceritinib; Cisapride; CloZAPine; Colchicine; Conivaptan; Corticosteroids (Orally Inhaled); Crizotinib; CYP3A4 Substrates; Dienogest; Digoxin; Dofetilide; DOXOrubicin (Conventional); Dronabinol; Dronedarone; Dutasteride; Eplerenone; Everolimus; FentaNYL; Fesoterodine; Fluticasone (Nasal); Fluticasone (Oral Inhalation); GuanFACINE; Halofantrine; Ibrutinib; Iloperidone; Imatinib; Ivabradine; Ivacaftor; Ixabepilone; Lacosamide; Lapatinib; Levomilnacipran; Lomitapide; Lovastatin; Lumefantrine; Lurasidone; Macitentan; Maraviroc; Methylene Blue; MethylPREDNISolone; Metoclopramide; Mifepristone; Nilotinib; Nisoldipine; Ospemifene; OxyCODONE; Paricalcitol; PAZOPanib; Pimecrolimus; Pimozide; PONATinib; Propafenone; QUEtiapine; Ranolazine; Red Yeast Rice; Regorafenib; Repaglinide; Rilpivirine; Rivaroxaban; RomiDEPsin; Ruxolitinib; Salmeterol; Saxagliptin; Serotonin Modulators; Sildenafil; Silodosin; Simeprevir; Simvastatin; SORAfenib; Tacrolimus (Systemic); Tacrolimus (Topical); Tadalafil; Tamsulosin; Tetrahydrocannabinol; Ticagrelor; Tofacitinib; Tolterodine; Tolvaptan; Toremifene; Ulipristal; Vardenafil; Vemurafenib; Vilazodone; VinCRIStine (Liposomal); Vorapaxar; Zuclopenthixol

The levels/effects of Nefazodone may be increased by: Abiraterone Acetate; Antiemetics (5HT3 Antagonists); Antipsychotic Agents (Phenothiazines); Antipsychotics; BusPIRone; Conivaptan; CYP2D6 Inhibitors (Moderate); CYP2D6 Inhibitors (Strong); CYP3A4 Inhibitors (Moderate); CYP3A4 Inhibitors (Strong); Fusidic Acid (Systemic); Linezolid; Luliconazole; MAO Inhibitors; Mifepristone; Protease Inhibitors; Selective Serotonin Reuptake Inhibitors; Stiripentol

Decreased Effect

Nefazodone may decrease the levels/effects of: Afatinib; Brentuximab Vedotin; Dabigatran Etexilate; DOXOrubicin (Conventional); Ifosfamide; Linagliptin; P-glycoprotein/ABCB1 Substrates; Prasugrel; Sofosbuvir; Ticagrelor; VinCRIStine (Liposomal)

The levels/effects of Nefazodone may be decreased by: Bosentan; CarBAMazepine; CYP3A4 Inducers (Strong); Dabrafenib; Deferasirox; Mitotane; Peginterferon Alfa-2b; Siltuximab; St Johns Wort; Tocilizumab

Food Interactions Nefazodone absorption may be delayed and bioavailability may be decreased if taken with food. Management: Administering after meals may decrease lightheadedness and postural hypotension, but may also decrease absorption and therefore effectiveness.

Stability Store at controlled room temperature at 20°C to 25°C (68°F to 77°F); dispense in a tightly-closed, light-resistant container.

Mechanism of Action Inhibits neuronal reuptake of serotonin and norepinephrine; also blocks 5-HT$_2$ and alpha$_1$ receptors; has no significant affinity for alpha$_2$, beta-adrenergic, 5-HT$_{1A}$, cholinergic, dopaminergic, or benzodiazepine receptors

Pharmacodynamics Maximum antidepressant effect: Adults: 4-6 weeks

Pharmacokinetics (Adult data unless noted)

Absorption: Oral: Rapid and complete

Distribution: Distributes into CNS; V$_d$: 0.22-0.87 L/kg

Protein binding: >99%

Metabolism: Hepatic, via N-dealkylation and aliphatic and aromatic hydroxylation, to three active metabolites: A triazoledione metabolite, hydroxynefazodone, and m-chlorophenylpiperazine (mCPP); other metabolites have also been identified but not tested for activity

Bioavailability: Oral: Absolute: 20% (variable); AUC increased by 25% in patients with cirrhosis of the liver

Half-life elimination: **Note:** Active metabolites persist longer in all populations.

Children: 4.1 hours

Adolescents: 3.9 hours

Adults: 2-4 hours

Time to peak serum concentration: **Note:** Prolonged in presence of food

Children and Adolescents: 0.5 -1 hour

Adults: 1 hour

Elimination: Primarily urine, as metabolites (<1% is eliminated as unchanged drug in urine); feces

Dialysis: Not likely to be of benefit

Dosing: Usual Oral: Depression:

Children and Adolescents: **Note:** Not FDA approved. Limited information is available: Based on primary outcome measures, no randomized, placebo-controlled trial has shown nefazodone to be effective for the treatment of depression in pediatric patients (Findling, 2006; Laughren, 2004; Wagner, 2005); one study showed a positive trend toward efficacy (Emslie, 2000); two open-label trials [(n=28; age range: 7-17 years) and (n=10; adolescents)] showed nefazodone improved depressive symptom severity scores in children and adolescents (Findling, 2000; Goodnick, 2000); a small case series (n=7; age range: 9-17 years) showed improvement in depression severity scores in treatment refractory children and adolescents with multiple comorbid conditions (Wilens, 1997). Because efficacy has not been established in controlled clinical trials and due to the risk of hepatotoxicity, nefazodone is seldom prescribed in children and adolescents (Dopheide, 2006). If use is indicated, some experts recommend the following doses: Initial: 50 mg twice daily (100 mg/day) for at least 7 days; then increase to 100 mg twice daily (200 mg/day) for at least 7 days; then titrate at weekly intervals using 50 mg/day increments in children and 100 mg/day increments in adolescents; usual target range: 300-400 mg/day

Adults: Initial: 200 mg/day given in 2 divided doses; titrate in 100-200 mg/day increments at ≥1 week intervals; effective dosage: 300-600 mg/day in 2 divided doses

Administration May be administered with or without food

Monitoring Parameters Blood pressure, mental status, liver enzymes, clinical signs and symptoms of liver failure (discontinue nefazodone if clinical signs or symptoms suggestive of liver failure occur or if serum AST or ALT levels increase to ≥3 times the upper limit of normal; do not reinitiate nefazodone in these patients). Monitor patient periodically for symptom resolution; monitor for worsening depression, suicidality, and associated behaviors (especially at the beginning of therapy or when doses are increased or decreased).

Dosage Forms Excipient information presented when available (limited, particularly for generics); consult specific product labeling.

Tablet, Oral, as hydrochloride:

Generic: 50 mg, 100 mg, 150 mg, 200 mg, 250 mg

References

ACOG Committee on Practice Bulletins–Obstetrics, "ACOG Practice Bulletin: Clinical Management Guidelines for Obstetrician-Gynecologists Number 92, April 2008 (Replaces Practice Bulletin Number 87,

November 2007). Use of Psychiatric Medications During Pregnancy and Lactation," *Obstet Gynecol*, 2008, 111(4):1001-20.

American Psychiatric Association, "Treatment Recommendations for Patients With Major Depressive Disorder," 3rd ed, May 2010. Available at http://www.psychiatryonline.com/pracGuide/pracGuideTopic_7.aspx

Dodd S, Maguire KP, Burrows GD, et al, "Nefazodone in the Breast Milk of Nursing Mothers: A Report of Two Patients," *J Clin Psychopharmacol*, 2000, 20(6):717-8.

Dopheide JA, "Recognizing and Treating Depression in Children and Adolescents," *Am J Health Syst Pharm*, 2006, 63(3):233-43.

Dubitsky GM, "Review and Evaluation of Clinical Data: Placebo-Controlled Antidepressant Studies in Pediatric Patients. Available at www.fda.gov/ohrms/dockets/ac/04/briefing/20044065b1-08-TAB06-Dubitsky-Review.pdf. Accessed on April 21, 2009.

Einarson A, Bonari L, Voyer-Lavigne S, et al, "A Multicentre Prospective Controlled Study to Determine the Safety of Trazodone and Nefazodone Use During Pregnancy," *Can J Psychiatry*, 2003, 48(2):106-10.

Einarson A, Choi J, Einarson TR, et al, "Incidence of Major Malformations in Infants Following Antidepressant Exposure in Pregnancy: Results of a Large Prospective Cohort Study," *Can J Psychiatry*, 2009, 54(4):242-6.

Emslie GJ, Findling RL, Rynn MA, et al, "Efficacy and Safety of Nefazodone in the Treatment of Adolescents with Major Depressive Disorder," *J Child Adolesc Psychopharmacol*, 2000, 12(4):299.

Findling RL, McNamara NK, Stansbrey RJ, et al, "The Relevance of Pharmacokinetic Studies in Designing Efficacy Trials in Juvenile Major Depression," *J Child Adolesc Psychopharmacol*, 2006, 16 (1-2):131-45.

Findling RL, Preskorn SH, Marcus RN, et al, "Nefazodone Pharmacokinetics in Depressed Children and Adolescents," *J Am Acad Child Adolesc Psychiatry*, 2000, 39(8):1008-16.

Goodnick PJ, Jorge CA, Hunter T, et al, "Nefazodone Treatment of Adolescent Depression: An Open-Label Study of Response and Biochemistry," *Ann Clin Psychiatry*, 2000, 12(2):97-100.

Laughren TP, "Memorandum to Members of PDAC and Peds AC: Background Comments for February 2, 2004 Meeting of Psychopharmacological Advisory Committee (PDAC) and Pediatric Subcommittee of the Anti-Infective Drugs Advisory Committee (Peds AC)." Available at www.fda.gov/ohrms/dockets/ac/04/briefing/2004–4065b1–04-Tab02-Laughren-Jan5.pdf. Accessed on April 21, 2009.

Wagner KD, "Pharmacotherapy for Major Depression in Children and Adolescents," *Prog Neuropsychopharmacol Biol Psychiatry*, 2005, 29 (5):819-26.

Wilens TE, Spencer TJ, Biederman J, et al, "Case Study: Nefazodone for Juvenile Mood Disorders," *J Am Acad Child Adolesc Psychiatry*, 1997, 36(4):481-5.

Yapp P, Ilett KF, Kristensen JH, et al, "Drowsiness and Poor Feeding in a Breast-Fed Infant: Association With Nefazodone and Its Metabolites," *Ann Pharmacother*, 2000, 34(11):1269-72.

Yonkers KA, Wisner KL, Stewart DE, et al, "The Management of Depression During Pregnancy: A Report From the American Psychiatric Association and the American College of Obstetricians and Gynecologists," *Obstet Gynecol*, 2009, 114(3):703-13.

◆ **Nefazodone Hydrochloride** *see* Nefazodone
on page 1474

Nelarabine (nel AY re been)

Medication Safety Issues

Sound-alike/look-alike issues:

Nelarabine may be confused with clofarabine

High alert medication:

This medication is in a class the Institute for Safe Medication Practices (ISMP) includes among its list of drug classes which have a heightened risk of causing significant patient harm when used in error.

Related Information

Emetogenic Potential of Antineoplastic Agents in Children
on page 2327

Safe Handling of Hazardous Drugs *on page 2419*

Brand Names: U.S. Arranon

Brand Names: Canada Atriance™

Therapeutic Category Antineoplastic Agent, Antimetabolite

Generic Availability (U.S.) No

Use Treatment of relapsed or refractory T-cell acute lymphoblastic leukemia (ALL) and T-cell lymphoblastic lymphoma [FDA approved in pediatrics (age not specified) and adults]

Pregnancy Risk Factor D

Pregnancy Considerations Teratogenic effects were observed in animal reproduction studies. May cause fetal harm if administered during pregnancy. Women of child-bearing potential should be advised to use effective contraception and avoid becoming pregnant during therapy.

Breast-Feeding Considerations Due to the potential for serious adverse reactions in the nursing infant, the decision to discontinue breast-feeding or discontinue nelarabine should take into account the benefits of treatment to the mother.

Contraindications Hypersensitivity to nelarabine or any component

Warnings Hazardous agent; use appropriate precautions for handling and disposal (NIOSH, 2012). Severe neurotoxicity, including mental status changes, severe somnolence, seizures, and peripheral neuropathy (ranging from numbness to motor weakness or paralysis) has been reported **[U.S. Boxed Warning]**. Observe closely for signs and symptoms of neurotoxicity; discontinue if ≥grade 2. Adverse effects associated with demyelination or similar to Guillain-Barré syndrome (ascending peripheral neuropathies) have also been reported. Neurologic toxicities may not fully resolve and neurologic function may not return to baseline after treatment cessation. Neurologic toxicity is dose-limiting. Risk of neurotoxicity may increase in patients with concurrent or previous intrathecal chemotherapy or history of craniospinal irradiation. Tumor lysis syndrome (TLS) may occur as a consequence of leukemia treatment; may lead to life-threatening acute renal failure; institute adequate hydration and consider prophylactic allopurinol prior to nelarabine treatment to prevent hyperuricemia and TLS; monitor closely.

Precautions Use with caution in patients with hepatic impairment; monitor closely; risk of adverse reactions may be higher with hepatic dysfunction. Use with caution in patients with renal impairment; monitor closely; Ara-G (active moiety) clearance may be reduced with renal dysfunction. Bone marrow suppression, including leukopenia, thrombocytopenia, anemia, neutropenia, and febrile neutropenia are associated with treatment; monitor blood counts regularly. Avoid administration of live vaccines in immunocompromised patients on nelarabine therapy.

Adverse Reactions

Cardiovascular: Chest pain, edema, hypotension, peripheral edema, tachycardia

Central nervous system: Amnesia, aphasia, ataxia, attention disturbance, balance disorder, cerebral hemorrhage, coma, confusion, depressed level of consciousness, depression, dizziness, encephalopathy, fatigue, fever, headache, hemiparesis, hydrocephalus, hypoesthesia, insomnia, intracranial hemorrhage, lethargy, leukoencephalopathy, loss of consciousness, mental impairment, motor dysfunction, nerve paralysis, neuropathic pain, nerve palsy, pain, seizure, paralysis, sciatica, sensory disturbance, sensory loss, somnolence, speech disorder

Dermatologic: Petechiae

Endocrine & metabolic: Dehydration, hyper-/hypoglycemia, hypocalcemia, hypokalemia, hypomagnesemia

Gastrointestinal: Abdominal distension, abdominal pain, anorexia, constipation, diarrhea, nausea, stomatitis, taste perversion, vomiting

Hematologic: Anemia, leukopenia, neutropenia, neutropenic fever

Hepatic: Albumin decreased, AST increased, bilirubin increased, transaminases increased

Neuromuscular & skeletal: Abnormal gait, arthralgia, back pain, dysarthria, hypertonia, hyporeflexia, incoordination, limb pain, muscle weakness, myalgia, noncardiac chest pain, paresthesia, peripheral neuropathy, rigors, tremor, weakness

Ocular: Blurred vision, nystagmus

Renal: Creatinine increased

Respiratory: Cough, dyspnea, epistaxis, pleural effusion, pneumonia, sinus headache, sinusitis, wheezing

Miscellaneous: Infection

Rare but important or life-threatening: Craniospinal demyelination, neuropathy (peripheral) (similar to Guillain-Barré syndrome), opportunistic infection, pneumothorax, progressive multifocal leukoencephalopathy (PML), respiratory arrest, rhabdomyolysis, tumor lysis syndrome

Drug Interactions

Metabolism/Transport Effects None known.

Avoid Concomitant Use

Avoid concomitant use of Nelarabine with any of the following: BCG; CloZAPine; Dipyrone; Natalizumab; Pentostatin; Pimecrolimus; Tacrolimus (Topical); Tofacitinib; Vaccines (Live)

Increased Effect/Toxicity

Nelarabine may increase the levels/effects of: CloZAPine; Leflunomide; Natalizumab; Tofacitinib; Vaccines (Live)

The levels/effects of Nelarabine may be increased by: Denosumab; Dipyrone; Pimecrolimus; Roflumilast; Tacrolimus (Topical); Trastuzumab

Decreased Effect

Nelarabine may decrease the levels/effects of: BCG; Coccidioidin Skin Test; Sipuleucel-T; Vaccines (Inactivated); Vaccines (Live)

The levels/effects of Nelarabine may be decreased by: Echinacea; Pentostatin

Stability Store intact vials at 25°C (77°F); excursions permitted to 15°C to 30°C (59°F to 86°F). Undiluted injection solution is stable in a polyvinyl chloride infusion bag or glass container for up to 8 hours at up to 30°C (86°F).

Mechanism of Action Nelarabine, a prodrug of ara-G, is demethylated by adenosine deaminase to ara-G and then converted to ara-GTP. Ara-GTP is incorporated into the DNA of the leukemic blasts, leading to inhibition of DNA synthesis and inducing apoptosis. Ara-GTP appears to accumulate at higher levels in T-cells, which correlates to clinical response.

Pharmacokinetics (Adult data unless noted)

Distribution:

Nelarabine: V_{ss}: Pediatric patients: 213 ± 358 L/m^2; Adults: 197 ± 216 L/m^2

Ara-G: V_{ss}/F: Pediatric patients: 33 ± 9.3 L/m^2 Adults: 50 ± 24 L/m^2

Protein binding: Nelarabine and ara-G: <25%

Metabolism: Hepatic; demethylated by adenosine deaminase to form ara-G (active); also hydrolyzed to form methylguanine. Both ara-G and methylguanine metabolized to guanine. Guanine is deaminated into xanthine, which is further oxidized to form uric acid, which is then oxidized to form allantoin.

Half-life:

Pediatric patients: Nelarabine: 13 minutes; Ara-G: 2 hours

Adults: Nelarabine: 18 minutes; Ara-G: 3 hours

Time to peak serum concentration: Ara-G: 3-25 hours (of day 1)

Elimination: Urine (nelarabine 5% to 10%, ara-G 20% to 30%)

Clearance: Nelarabine clearance is ~30% higher in pediatric patients (259 ± 409 L/hour/m^2) than in adults (197 ± 189 L/hour/m^2); ara-G clearance in pediatric patients (11.3 ± 4.2 L/hour/m^2) is similar to adults (10.5 ± 4.5 L/hour/m^2)

Dosing: Usual Dosing and frequency may vary by protocol and/or treatment phase; refer to specific protocol.

Infants, Children, and Adolescents: **T-cell acute lymphoblastic leukemia (ALL), T-cell lymphoblastic lymphoma, relapsed/refractory:** I.V.: 650 mg/m^2/dose on days 1 through 5; repeat cycle every 21 days until transplant, disease progression, or unacceptable toxicity

Adults: **T-cell acute lymphoblastic leukemia (ALL), T-cell lymphoblastic lymphoma:** I.V.: 1500 mg/m^2/dose on days 1, 3, and 5; repeat cycle every 21 days until transplant, disease progression, or unacceptable toxicity.

Note: In obese adults; utilize patient's actual body weight (full weight) for calculation of body surface area- or weight-based dosing, particularly when the intent of therapy is curative; manage regimen-related toxicities in the same manner as for nonobese patients; if a dose reduction is utilized due to toxicity, consider resumption of full weight-based dosing with subsequent cycles, especially if cause of toxicity (eg, hepatic or renal impairment) is resolved (Griggs, 2012).

Dosage adjustment for toxicity: All patients:

Neurologic toxicity ≥grade 2: Discontinue treatment

Hematologic or other (non-neurologic) toxicity: Consider treatment delay

Dosage adjustment in renal impairment: All patients:

CrCl ≥50 mL/minute: No adjustment necessary

CrCl <50 mL/minute: There are no dosage adjustments provided in the manufacturer's labeling (although ARA-G clearance is decreased as renal function declines, data is insufficient for a dosing recommendation); monitor closely.

Dosage adjustment in hepatic impairment: All patients: There are no dosage adjustments provided in the manufacturer's labeling (has not been studied); closely monitor with severe impairment (total bilirubin >3 times ULN).

Administration Hazardous agent; use appropriate precautions for handling and disposal (NIOSH, 2012). Adequate I.V. hydration recommended to prevent tumor lysis syndrome; allopurinol may be used if hyperuricemia is anticipated.

I.V.: Transferred the appropriate nelarabine dose into an empty polyvinyl chloride (PVC) bag or glass container and administered undiluted.

Pediatric patients: Infuse over 1 hour daily for 5 consecutive days

Adults: Infuse over 2 hours on days 1, 3, and 5

Monitoring Parameters Monitor closely for neurologic toxicity (severe somnolence, seizure, peripheral neuropathy, confusion, ataxia, paresthesia, hypoesthesia, coma, or craniospinal demyelination); signs and symptoms of tumor lysis syndrome; hydration status; CBC with platelet counts, renal and liver function tests

Additional Information Contains 4.5 mg of sodium chloride per mL

Dosage Forms Excipient information presented when available (limited, particularly for generics); consult specific product labeling.

Solution, Intravenous:

Arranon: 5 mg/mL (50 mL)

References

Berg SL, Blaney SM, Devidas M, et al, "Phase II Study of Nelarabine (Compound 506U78) in Children and Young Adults With Refractory T-Cell Malignancies: A Report From the Children's Oncology Group," *J Clin Oncol*, 2005, 23(15):3376-82.

Commander LA, Seif AE, Insogna IG, et al. Salvage therapy with nelarabine, etoposide, and cyclophosphamide in relapsed/refractory paediatric T-cell lymphoblastic leukaemia and lymphoma. *Br J Haematol*. 2010;150(3):345-351.

Gandhi V, Plunkett W, Weller S, et al, "Evaluation of the Combination of Nelarabine and Fludarabine in Leukemias: Clinical Response, Pharmacokinetics, and Pharmacodynamics in Leukemia Cells," *J Clin Oncol*, 2001, 19(8):2142-52.

Griggs JJ, Mangu PB, Anderson H, et al. Appropriate chemotherapy dosing for obese adult patients with cancer: American Society of Clinical Oncology Clinical Practice Guideline. *J Clin Oncol*. 2012;30 (13):1553-1561.

Kisor DF, Plunkett W, Kurtzberg J, et al, "Pharmacokinetics of Nelarabine and 9-beta-D-Arabinofuranosyl Guanine in Pediatric and Adult Patients During a Phase I Study of Nelarabine for the Treatment of Refractory Hematologic Malignancies," *J Clin Oncol*, 2000, 18 (5):995-1003.

Kurtzberg J, Ernst TJ, Keating MJ, et al. Phase I study of 506U78 administered on a consecutive 5-day schedule in children and adults with refractory hematologic malignancies. *J Clin Oncol.* 2005;23 (15):3396-3403.

National Institute for Occupational Safety and Health (NIOSH), "NIOSH List of Antineoplastic and Other Hazardous Drugs in Healthcare Settings 2012." Available at http://www.cdc.gov/niosh/docs/2012-150/pdfs/2012-150.pdf. Accessed January 21, 2013.

Nelfinavir (nel FIN a veer)

Medication Safety Issues
Sound-alike/look-alike issues:
Nelfinavir may be confused with nevirapine
Viracept may be confused with Viramune, Viramune XR

Related Information
Adult and Adolescent HIV *on page 2348*
Pediatric HIV *on page 2338*
Perinatal HIV *on page 2356*

Brand Names: U.S. Viracept

Brand Names: Canada Viracept

Therapeutic Category Antiretroviral Agent; HIV Agents (Anti-HIV Agents); Protease Inhibitor

Generic Availability (U.S.) No

Use Treatment of HIV infection in combination with other antiretroviral agents (FDA approved in ages ≥2 years and adults). **Note:** HIV regimens consisting of **three** antiretroviral agents are strongly recommended.

Pregnancy Risk Factor B

Pregnancy Considerations Adverse events were not observed in animal reproduction studies. Nelfinavir has a minimal to low level of transfer across the human placenta. A modest increased risk of overall birth defects has been observed following first trimester exposure in humans according to data collected by the antiretroviral pregnancy registry. However, no pattern of defects has been detected. The DHHS Perinatal HIV Guidelines does not recommended nelfinavir for initial therapy in antiretroviral-naïve pregnant women due to lower viral suppression when compared to other regimens. A dose of 1250 mg twice daily has been shown to provide adequate plasma concentrations although lower and variable levels may occur late in pregnancy. A small increased risk of preterm birth has been associated with maternal use of protease inhibitor-based combination antiretroviral (ARV) therapy during pregnancy; however, the benefits of use generally outweigh this risk and protease inhibitors (PIs) should not be withheld if otherwise recommended. Hyperglycemia, new onset of diabetes mellitus, or diabetic ketoacidosis have been reported with PIs; it is not clear if pregnancy increases this risk.

Regardless of CD4 count or HIV RNA copy number, all HIV-infected pregnant women should receive a combination antiretroviral ARV drug regimen. A combination of antepartum, intrapartum, and infant ARV prophylaxis is recommended. ARV therapy should be started as soon as possible in women with symptomatic infection. Although earlier initiation may be more effective in reducing the perinatal transmission of HIV, initiation may be delayed until after 12 weeks gestation in women who do not require immediate treatment after careful consideration of maternal conditions (eg, nausea and vomiting) and the potential risks of first trimester fetal exposure for specific agents. A scheduled cesarean delivery at 38 weeks gestation is recommended for all women with HIV RNA >1000 copies/mL or unknown concentrations near delivery in order to decrease transmission. If ARV therapy must be interrupted for <24 hours during the peripartum period, stop then restart all medications simultaneously in order to decrease the chance of developing resistance. Long-term follow-up is recommended for all infants exposed to ARV medications. In couples who want to conceive, the HIV-infected partner should attain maximum viral suppression prior to conception.

Health care providers are encouraged to enroll pregnant women exposed to antiretroviral medications in the Antiretroviral Pregnancy Registry (1-800-258-4263 or www.APRegistry.com). Health care providers caring for HIV-infected women and their infants may contact the National Perinatal HIV Hotline (888-448-8765) for clinical consultation (DHHS [perinatal], 2014).

Breast-Feeding Considerations Minimal amounts of nelfinavir are excreted into breast milk and plasma concentrations in the nursing infant were undetectable. Maternal or infant antiretroviral therapy does not completely eliminate the risk of postnatal HIV transmission. In addition, multiclass-resistant virus has been detected in breast-feeding infants despite maternal therapy. Therefore, in the United States, where formula is accessible, affordable, safe, and sustainable, and the risk of infant mortality due to diarrhea and respiratory infections is low, complete avoidance of breast-feeding by HIV-infected women is recommended to decrease potential transmission of HIV (DHHS [perinatal], 2014).

Contraindications Hypersensitivity to nelfinavir or any component; concurrent therapy with alfuzosin, amiodarone, cisapride, dihydroergotamine, ergonovine, ergotamine, lovastatin, methylergonovine, midazolam (oral), pimozide, quinidine, rifampin, sildenafil [when used for the treatment of pulmonary arterial hypertension (Revatio®)], simvastatin, St John's wort, or triazolam

Warnings Nelfinavir inhibits cytochrome P450 isoenzyme CYP3A and interacts with numerous drugs. Due to potential serious and/or life-threatening drug interactions, some drugs are contraindicated; other drug interactions require alteration in dose or regimen; concurrent use with some anticonvulsants may significantly limit nelfinavir's effectiveness. Use with caution in patients taking strong CYP3A4 inhibitors, moderate or strong CYP3A4 inducers, and major CYP3A4 substrates and if coadministered with QT prolonging drugs that are metabolized by CYP3A. Spontaneous bleeding episodes have been reported in patients with hemophilia type A and B receiving protease inhibitors; additional factor VIII may be needed. New onset diabetes mellitus, exacerbations of diabetes, and hyperglycemia have been reported in HIV-infected patients receiving protease inhibitors.

Precautions Use with caution in patients with mild hepatic impairment; use is not recommended in patients with moderate or severe hepatic impairment; nelfinavir is metabolized in the liver and may also cause hepatitis and/or exacerbate preexisting hepatic dysfunction.

Fat redistribution and accumulation [ie, central obesity, peripheral wasting, facial wasting, breast enlargement, dorsocervical fat enlargement (buffalo hump), and cushingoid appearance] have been observed in patients receiving antiretroviral agents (causal relationship not established). Lipodystrophy was observed in 28% of children after a median of 49 months of receiving a nelfinavir-containing antiretroviral regimen (Scherpbier, 2006).

Immune reconstitution syndrome (an acute inflammatory response to residual or indolent opportunistic infections) may occur in HIV patients during initial treatment with combination antiretroviral agents, including nelfinavir; this syndrome may require further patient assessment and therapy. Autoimmune disorders (eg, Graves' disease, Guillain-Barré syndrome, and polymyositis) have been reported in patients experiencing immune reconstitution; time to onset is variable and may occur many months after antiretroviral treatment is initiated.

May cause diarrhea (children: 39% to 47%; adults: 14% to 20%); a secretory diarrhea mediated via a calcium-dependent process may also occur; calcium carbonate administered at the same time as nelfinavir has been used to treat this adverse effect in adults without affecting plasma concentrations of nelfinavir or its major metabolite.

Adverse Reactions
Dermatologic: Rash

Gastrointestinal: Diarrhea, flatulence, nausea

Hematologic: Lymphocytes decreased, neutrophils decreased

Rare but important or life-threatening: Abdominal pain, acute iritis, alkaline phosphatase increased, allergic reaction, amylase increased, anemia, anorexia, anxiety, arthralgia, arthritis, back pain, bilirubinemia, body fat redistribution/accumulation, cramps, creatine phosphokinase increased, dehydration, depression, dermatitis, diaphoresis, dizziness, dyspepsia, dyspnea, emotional lability, epigastric pain, eye disorder, fever, folliculitis, fungal dermatitis, gastrointestinal bleeding, GGTP increased, headache, hepatitis, hyperkinesia, hyper-/hypoglycemia, hyperlipemia; hypersensitivity reaction (bronchospasm, rash, edema); hyperuricemia, immune reconstitution syndrome, insomnia, jaundice, kidney calculus, lactic dehydrogenase increased, leukopenia, lipoatrophy, lipodystrophy, liver function tests abnormal, maculopapular rash, malaise, metabolic acidosis, migraine, mouth ulceration, myalgia, myasthenia, myopathy, pain, pancreatitis, paresthesia, pharyngitis, pruritus, QT_c prolongation, rhinitis, seizure, sexual dysfunction, sinusitis, sleep disorder, somnolence, suicidal ideation, thrombocytopenia, torsade de pointes, transaminases increased, urine abnormality, urticaria, vomiting, weakness

Drug Interactions
Metabolism/Transport Effects Substrate of CYP2C19 (major), CYP2C9 (minor), CYP2D6 (minor), CYP3A4 (major), P-glycoprotein; **Note:** Assignment of Major/Minor substrate status based on clinically relevant drug interaction potential; **Inhibits** CYP1A2 (weak), CYP2B6 (weak), CYP2C19 (weak), CYP2C9 (weak), CYP2D6 (weak), CYP3A4 (strong), P-glycoprotein

Avoid Concomitant Use
Avoid concomitant use of Nelfinavir with any of the following: Ado-Trastuzumab Emtansine; Alfuzosin; Amiodarone; Apixaban; Avanafil; Axitinib; Bosutinib; Cabozantinib; Ceritinib; Cisapride; Conivaptan; Crizotinib; Dronedarone; Eplerenone; Ergot Derivatives; Everolimus; Halofantrine; Ibrutinib; Ivabradine; Lapatinib; Lomitapide; Lovastatin; Lurasidone; Macitentan; Midazolam; Nilotinib; Nisoldipine; PAZOPanib; Pimozide; Proton Pump Inhibitors; QuiNIDine; Ranolazine; Red Yeast Rice; Regorafenib; Rifampin; Rivaroxaban; Salmeterol; Silodosin; Simeprevir; Simvastatin; St Johns Wort; Tamsulosin; Ticagrelor; Tipranavir; Tolvaptan; Topotecan; Toremifene; Triazolam; Ulipristal; Vemurafenib; VinCRIStine (Liposomal); Vorapaxar

Increased Effect/Toxicity
Nelfinavir may increase the levels/effects of: Ado-Trastuzumab Emtansine; Afatinib; Alfuzosin; Almotriptan; Alosetron; ALPRAZolam; Amiodarone; Apixaban; ARIPiprazole; AtorvaSTATin; Avanafil; Axitinib; Azithromycin (Systemic); Bedaquiline; Bortezomib; Bosentan; Bosutinib; Brentuximab Vedotin; Brinzolamide; Budesonide (Nasal); Budesonide (Systemic, Oral Inhalation); Cabozantinib; Calcium Channel Blockers (Dihydropyridine); Calcium Channel Blockers (Nondihydropyridine); Cannabis; CarBAMazepine; Ceritinib; Cisapride; Clarithromycin; Colchicine; Conivaptan; Corticosteroids (Orally Inhaled); Crizotinib; Cyclophosphamide; CycloSPORINE (Systemic); CYP3A4 Substrates; Dabigatran Etexilate; Digoxin; Dofetilide; DOXOrubicin (Conventional); Dronabinol; Dronedarone; Dutasteride; Enfuvirtide; Eplerenone; Ergot Derivatives; Everolimus; FentaNYL; Fesoterodine; Fluticasone (Nasal); Fluticasone (Oral Inhalation); GuanFACINE; Halofantrine;

Ibrutinib; Iloperidone; Imatinib; Ivabradine; Ivacaftor; Ixabepilone; Lacosamide; Lapatinib; Levomilnacipran; Lomitapide; Lovastatin; Lumefantrine; Lurasidone; Macitentan; Maraviroc; Meperidine; MethylPREDNISolone; Midazolam; Mifepristone; Nefazodone; Nilotinib; Nisoldipine; Ospemifene; OxyCODONE; Paricalcitol; PAZOPanib; P-glycoprotein/ABCB1 Substrates; Pimecrolimus; Pimozide; PONATinib; Propafenone; Protease Inhibitors; Prucalopride; QUEtiapine; QuiNIDine; Ranolazine; Red Yeast Rice; Regorafenib; Repaglinide; Rifabutin; Rifaximin; Rilpivirine; Riociguat; Rivaroxaban; RomiDEPsin; Rosuvastatin; Ruxolitinib; Salmeterol; Saxagliptin; Sildenafil; Silodosin; Simeprevir; Simvastatin; Sirolimus; SORAfenib; Tacrolimus (Systemic); Tacrolimus (Topical); Tadalafil; Tamsulosin; Temsirolimus; Tetrahydrocannabinol; Ticagrelor; Tofacitinib; Tolterodine; Tolvaptan; Topotecan; Toremifene; TraZODone; Triazolam; Tricyclic Antidepressants; Ulipristal; Vardenafil; Vemurafenib; Vilazodone; VinCRIStine (Liposomal); Vorapaxar; Warfarin; Zuclopenthixol

The levels/effects of Nelfinavir may be increased by: Clarithromycin; CycloSPORINE (Systemic); Delavirdine; Enfuvirtide; Etravirine; Lopinavir; P-glycoprotein/ABCB1 Inhibitors; Simeprevir; Voriconazole

Decreased Effect
Nelfinavir may decrease the levels/effects of: Abacavir; Boceprevir; Clarithromycin; Contraceptives (Estrogens); Contraceptives (Progestins); Delavirdine; Etravirine; Fosphenytoin; Ifosfamide; Lopinavir; Meperidine; Methadone; Phenytoin; Prasugrel; Pravastatin; Ticagrelor; Valproic Acid and Derivatives; Warfarin; Zidovudine

The levels/effects of Nelfinavir may be decreased by: Antacids; Boceprevir; Bosentan; CarBAMazepine; CYP2C19 Inducers (Strong); CYP3A4 Inducers (Strong); Dabrafenib; Deferasirox; Fosphenytoin; Garlic; H2-Antagonists; Mitotane; Nevirapine; Peginterferon Alfa-2b; P-glycoprotein/ABCB1 Inducers; Phenytoin; Proton Pump Inhibitors; Rifabutin; Rifampin; Siltuximab; St Johns Wort; Tipranavir; Tocilizumab

Food Interactions Nelfinavir taken with food increases plasma concentration time curve (AUC) by two- to threefold. Management: Administer with a meal. Do not administer with acidic food or juice (orange juice, apple juice, or applesauce) since the combination may have a bitter taste.

Stability Store at 15°C to 30°C (59°F to 86°F). Dispense in original container; keep container tightly closed.

Mechanism of Action Binds to the site of HIV-1 protease activity and inhibits cleavage of viral Gag-Pol polyprotein precursors into individual functional proteins required for infectious HIV. This results in the formation of immature, noninfectious viral particles.

Pharmacokinetics (Adult data unless noted)
Absorption: AUC is two- to threefold higher under fed conditions versus fasting; AUC is highly variable in pediatric patients due to increased clearance, problems with compliance, and inconsistent food intake with dosing

Distribution: V_d: 2 to 7 L/kg

Protein binding: >98%

Metabolism: Hepatic via multiple cytochrome P450 isoforms including CYP3A4 and CYP2C19; one active oxidative metabolite with comparable activity to the parent drug and several minor oxidative metabolites are formed

Bioavailability: 20% to 80%; **Note:** The 625 mg and 250 mg tablet formulations were shown to be bioequivalent in HIV-infected patients receiving multiple doses of 1250 mg twice daily (under fed conditions). In healthy volunteers, the 250 mg and 625 mg tablets were **not** bioequivalent; the AUC for the 625 mg tablets was 34% higher than the 250 mg tablets in fasted adults and 24% higher than the 250 mg tablets under fed conditions.

Half-life: 3.5 to 5 hours

Time to peak serum concentration: 2 to 4 hours

Elimination: 98% to 99% excreted in feces (78% as metabolites and 22% as unchanged nelfinavir); 1% to 2% excreted in urine (primarily as unchanged drug)

Dosing: Neonatal HIV infection, treatment: Not approved for use; a reliable, effective dose has not been established; a high interpatient variability in serum drug concentrations occurs; nelfinavir dosing is problematic in neonates, since the drug is best absorbed when taken with a high-fat meal; further studies are needed (DHHS [pediatric], 2014; Hirt, 2006).

Dosing: Usual

Pediatric: **HIV infection, treatment:** Use in combination with other antiretroviral agents: Oral:

Infants and Children <2 years: Not approved for use; a reliable, effective dose has not been established; high interpatient variability in serum drug concentrations occurs; nelfinavir dosing is problematic in young infants, since the drug is best absorbed when taken with a high-fat meal; further studies are needed (DHHS [pediatric], 2014; Hirt, 2006).

Children ≥2 years: **Note:** Pediatric guidelines recommend twice daily dosing (DHHS [pediatric], 2014).

Weight-directed dosing: Oral tablets (250 mg): 45 to 55 mg/kg/dose (maximum: 1250 mg) twice daily **or** 25 to 35 mg/kg/dose (maximum: 750 mg) 3 times daily; daily doses >2500 mg/day have not been studied in children. **Note:** Current guidelines rate nelfinavir as an acceptable protease inhibitor for initial therapy in children ≥2 years only in special circumstances (ie, when preferred and alternative drugs are not available or are not tolerated); due to the high variability of nelfinavir plasma concentrations in children, dosage adjustment utilizing measurement of plasma concentrations and pharmacokinetics may be beneficial (Crommentuyn, 2006; DHHS [pediatric], 2014; Fletcher, 2008).

Fixed dosing: Oral tablets (250 mg):

10 to 12 kg: 500 mg (2 tablets) twice daily **or** 250 mg (1 tablet) three times daily

13 to 18 kg: 750 mg (3 tablets) twice daily **or** 500 mg (2 tablets) three times daily

19 to 20 kg: 1000 mg (4 tablets) twice daily **or** 500 mg (2 tablets) three times daily

>20 kg: 1000 to 1250 mg (4 to 5 tablets) twice daily **or** 750 mg (3 tablets) three times daily

Adolescents: 1250 mg/dose twice daily **or** 750 mg three times daily (DHHS [adult, pediatric], 2014). **Note:** Some adolescent patients require doses higher than adults to achieve similar nelfinavir AUCs; consider the use of serum drug concentrations to guide optimal dosing (DHHS [pediatric], 2014).

Adult: **HIV infection, treatment:** Use in combination with other antiretroviral agents: Oral: 1250 mg/dose twice daily **or** 750 mg three times daily. **Note:** The DHHS Perinatal HIV Guidelines do not recommend the three times daily dosing in pregnant women (DHHS [perinatal], 2014).

Dosing adjustment in renal impairment: No adjustment necessary (DHHS [adult], 2014); has not been studied; however, since <2% of the drug is eliminated in the urine, renal impairment should have minimal effect on nelfinavir elimination

Dosing adjustment in hepatic impairment:

Mild hepatic impairment (Child-Pugh Class A): Use with caution; no dosage adjustment is necessary. In adults, nelfinavir AUC and C_{max} were not significantly different compared to subjects with normal hepatic function.

Moderate hepatic impairment (Child-Pugh Class B): Not recommended for use. In adults, nelfinavir AUC was increased by 62% and C_{max} was increased by 22% compared to subjects with normal hepatic function.

Severe hepatic impairment (Child-Pugh Class C): Use not recommended; has not been studied

Administration Administer with food to enhance bioavailability and decrease kinetic variability. Tablets can be readily dissolved in water and consumed or mixed with milk or chocolate milk; consume immediately; rinse glass with water and swallow to make sure total dose is consumed; tablets can also be crushed and administered with pudding. If coadministered with didanosine, nelfinavir should be administered 2 hours before or 1 hour after didanosine.

Monitoring Parameters Note: Monitor CD4 percentage (if <5 years of age) or CD4 count (if ≥5 years of age) at least every 3 to 4 months (DHHS [pediatric], 2014).

Prior to initiation of therapy: Genotypic resistance testing, CD4 and viral load (every 3 to 4 months), CBC with differential, LFTs, BUN, creatinine, electrolytes, glucose, urinalysis (every 6 to 12 months), and assessment of readiness for adherence with medication regimen. At initiation and with any change in treatment regimen: CBC with differential, electrolytes, calcium, phosphate, glucose, LFTs, bilirubin, urinalysis (at initiation), BUN, creatinine, albumin, total protein, lipid panel (at initiation), CD4, and viral load. After 1 to 2 weeks of therapy: Signs of medication toxicity and adherence. After 2 to 4 weeks of therapy: CBC with differential, viral load, signs of medication toxicity, and adherence; then every 3 to 4 months: CBC with differential, electrolytes, glucose, LFTs, bilirubin, BUN, creatinine, CD4, viral load, signs of medication toxicity, and adherence. Every 6 to 12 months: Lipid panel and urinalysis. CD4 monitoring frequency may be decreased to every 6 to 12 months in children who are adherent to therapy if the value is well above the threshold for opportunistic infections, viral suppression is sustained, and the clinical status is stable for more than 2 to 3 years (DHHS [pediatric], 2014). Monitor for growth and development, signs of HIV-specific physical conditions, HIV disease progression, opportunistic infections.

Reference Range Plasma trough concentration: ≥800 ng/mL mL (measurable active (M8) metabtolite) (DHHS [adult, pediatric], 2014)

Dosage Forms Excipient information presented when available (limited, particularly for generics); consult specific product labeling.

Tablet, Oral:

Viracept: 250 mg, 625 mg

References

Crommentuyn KM, Scherpbier HJ, Kuijpers TW, Mathôt RA, Huitema AD, Beijnen JH. Population pharmacokinetics and pharmacodynamics of nelfinavir and its active metabolite M8 in HIV-1-infected children. *Pediatr Infect Dis J.* 2006;25(6):538-543.

DHHS Panel on Antiretroviral Guidelines for Adults and Adolescents. Guidelines for the use of antiretroviral agents in HIV-1-infected adults and adolescents, Department of Health and Human Services. May 1, 2014. Available at http://www.aidsinfo.nih.gov/ContentFiles/AdultandAdolescentGL.pdf

DHHS Panel on Antiretroviral Therapy and Medical Management of HIV-Infected Children. Guidelines for the use of antiretroviral agents in pediatric HIV infection. February 12, 2014. Available at http://aidsinfo.nih.gov

DHHS Panel on Treatment of HIV-Infected Pregnant Women and Prevention of Perinatal Transmission. Recommendations for the use of antiretroviral drugs in pregnant HIV-1-infected women for maternal health and interventions to reduce perinatal HIV-1 transmission in the United States. March 28, 2014. Available at http://aidsinfo.nih.gov

Fletcher CV, Brundage RC, Fenton T, et al. Pharmacokinetics and pharmacodynamics of efavirenz and nelfinavir in HIV-infected children participating in an area-under-the-curve controlled trial. *Clin Pharmacol Ther.* 2008;83(2):300-306.

Hirt D, Urien S, Jullien V, et al. Age-related effects on nelfinavir and M8 pharmacokinetics: a population study with 182 children. *Antimicrob Agents Chemother.* 2006;50(3):910-916.

Scherpbier HJ, Bekker V, van Leth F, Jurriaans S, Lange JM, Kuijpers TW. Long-term experience with combination antiretroviral therapy that contains nelfinavir for up to 7 years in a pediatric cohort. *Pediatrics.* 2006;117(3):e528-e536.

◆ **Nembutal** see PENTobarbital on page 1641

◆ **Nembutal® Sodium (Can)** see PENTobarbital on page 1641

◆ **Neo-Fradin** see Neomycin on page 1482

◆ **Neofrin** see Phenylephrine (Ophthalmic) on page 1661

Neomycin (nee oh MYE sin)

Brand Names: U.S. Neo-Fradin

Therapeutic Category Ammonium Detoxicant; Antibiotic, Aminoglycoside; Antibiotic, Topical; Hyperammonemia Agent

Generic Availability (U.S.) Yes

Use

Oral solution: Adjunct therapy for hepatic coma (portal-systemic encephalopathy) by reducing ammonia-forming bacteria in the intestinal tract (FDA approved in ages ≥18 years and adults)

Oral tablets: Adjunct therapy (with erythromycin) for the suppression of normal bacterial flora of the bowel (eg, preoperative preparation); adjunct therapy for hepatic coma (portal-systemic encephalopathy) by reducing ammonia-forming bacteria in the intestinal tract (All indications: FDA approved in ages ≥18 years and adults)

Pregnancy Risk Factor D

Pregnancy Considerations Aminoglycosides cross the placenta; however, neomycin has limited maternal absorption. Therefore the portion of an orally administered maternal dose available to cross the placenta is very low. Teratogenic effects have not been observed following maternal use of neomycin. Because of several reports of total irreversible bilateral congenital deafness in children whose mothers received another aminoglycoside (streptomycin) during pregnancy, the manufacturer classifies neomycin as pregnancy category D.

Breast-Feeding Considerations It is not known if neomycin is excreted into breast milk; however, limited oral absorption by both the mother and infant would minimize exposure to the nursing infant. Nondose-related effects could include modification of bowel flora. Breast-feeding is not recommended by the manufacturer.

Contraindications Hypersensitivity to neomycin or any component, or other aminoglycosides; intestinal obstruction, inflammatory or ulcerative gastrointestinal disease

Warnings Systemic absorption occurs following oral administration; toxic reactions may occur [U.S. Boxed Warning]. Safety and efficacy not established in pediatric patients (age <18 years; use with caution); systemic absorption from gastrointestinal tract occurs; treatment should not exceed 3 consecutive weeks. Systemic absorption can also occur when neomycin is utilized for irrigation of wounds or surgical sites. Concurrent and/or sequential use of any form of other aminoglycosides and other potentially nephrotoxic and/or neurotoxic drugs should be avoided because toxicity may be additive [U.S. Boxed Warning]. May cause nephrotoxicity [U.S. Boxed Warning]; usual risk factors include preexisting renal impairment, concomitant nephrotoxic medications, advanced age, and dehydration. Discontinue treatment if signs of nephrotoxicity occur; renal damage is usually reversible. May cause neurotoxicity, including ototoxicity [U.S. Boxed Warning]; usual risk factors include preexisting renal impairment, concomitant neuro-/nephrotoxic medications, advanced age, and dehydration. Ototoxicity risk is proportional to the amount of drug given and the duration of treatment. Serial vestibular and audiometric testing should be performed; especially in high-risk patients. Tinnitus or vertigo may be indications of vestibular injury and impending bilateral irreversible damage. Discontinue treatment if signs of ototoxicity occur; risk of hearing loss continues after drug withdrawal. Avoid concurrent use of potent diuretics due to risk of ototoxicity [U.S. Boxed Warning]; intravenous use of diuretics may enhance neomycin toxicity by altering concentration in serum and tissue. May cause neuromuscular blockade and respiratory paralysis [U.S. Boxed Warning], especially when given soon after anesthesia or muscle relaxants. Prolonged use may result in fungal or bacterial superinfection, including C. difficile-associated diarrhea (CDAD) and pseudomembranous colitis; CDAD has been observed >2 months postantibiotic treatment.

Neo-Fradin oral solution contains benzoic acid; benzoic acid (benzoate) is a metabolite of benzyl alcohol; large amounts of benzyl alcohol (≥99 mg/kg/day) have been associated with a potentially fatal toxicity ("gasping syndrome") in neonates; the "gasping syndrome" consists of metabolic acidosis, respiratory distress, gasping respirations, CNS dysfunction (including convulsions, intracranial hemorrhage), hypotension, and cardiovascular collapse. Use oral solution products containing benzoic acid with caution in neonates; in vitro and animal studies have shown that benzoate displaces bilirubin from protein binding sites. Neomycin is more toxic than other aminoglycosides when given parenterally; **do not administer parenterally.**

Precautions Use with caution in patients with renal impairment; dosage modification or discontinuation required. Use with caution in patients with preexisting hearing impairment (including vertigo or tinnitus) or neuromuscular disorders (ie, myasthenia gravis). Oral doses of 12 **g**/day in adults may produce a malabsorption syndrome for a variety of substances (fat, nitrogen, cholesterol, carotene, glucose, xylose, lactose, sodium, calcium, cyanocobalamin, and iron).

Adverse Reactions

Gastrointestinal: Diarrhea, irritation or soreness of the mouth or rectal area, nausea, vomiting

Rare but important or life-threatening: Dyspnea, eosinophilia, nephrotoxicity, neurotoxicity, ototoxicity (auditory), ototoxicity (vestibular)

Drug Interactions

Metabolism/Transport Effects None known.

Avoid Concomitant Use

Avoid concomitant use of Neomycin with any of the following: BCG; Mannitol

Increased Effect/Toxicity

Neomycin may increase the levels/effects of: AbobotulinumtoxinA; Acarbose; Bisphosphonate Derivatives; CARBOplatin; Colistimethate; CycloSPORINE (Systemic); Neuromuscular-Blocking Agents; OnabotulinumtoxinA; RimabotulinumtoxinB; Tenofovir; Vitamin K Antagonists

The levels/effects of Neomycin may be increased by: Amphotericin B; Capreomycin; Cephalosporins (2nd Generation); Cephalosporins (3rd Generation); Cephalosporins (4th Generation); CISplatin; Loop Diuretics; Mannitol; Nonsteroidal Anti-Inflammatory Agents; Tenofovir; Vancomycin

Decreased Effect

Neomycin may decrease the levels/effects of: BCG; Cardiac Glycosides; Sodium Picosulfate; SORAfenib

The levels/effects of Neomycin may be decreased by: Penicillins

Stability Store at 20°C to 25°C (68°F to 77°F).

Mechanism of Action Interferes with bacterial protein synthesis by binding to 30S ribosomal subunits

Pharmacodynamics

Neomycin is bacteriocidal:

Onset of action: Bacterial growth suppression: Rapid

Duration of action: Bacterial growth suppression: 48-72 hours

Pharmacokinetics (Adult data unless noted)
Absorption: Poor orally (3%) or percutaneously; readily absorbed through denuded or abraded skin and body cavities

Distribution: V_d: 0.36 L/kg

Protein binding: 0% to 30%

Half-life: 2-3 hours (age and renal function dependent)

Time to peak serum concentration: 1-4 hours

Elimination: In urine (30% to 50% of absorbed drug as unchanged drug); 97% of an oral dose eliminated unchanged in feces

Dosing: Neonatal Note: Dosage expressed in terms of neomycin sulfate.

Diarrhea: Oral: 50-100 mg/kg/day divided every 6 hours (Marks, 1973; Red Book, 2009)

Dosing: Usual Note: Dosage expressed in terms of neomycin sulfate.

Infants, Children, and Adolescents:

Cholangitis, prophylaxis recurrent episodes after Kasai Portoenterostomy: Limited data available: Infants and Children ≤3 years: Oral: 25-50 mg/kg/day in 4 divided doses 4 days per week; continue until 2-3 years of age. Dosing based on a prospective, randomized, comparative trial and a small case series of patients ≤2 years of age at time of therapy initiation who had an episode of cholangitis after a Kasai Portoenterostomy (n=10). In the trial, two prophylactic regimens were compared (neomycin vs trimethoprim/sulfamethoxazole) against historic controls; the mean age at time of therapy initiation was 6.1 ± 3.6 months; both neomycin and trimethoprim/sulfamethoxazole decreased cholangitis incidence by ~60% and neomycin increased survival. In the case series, dosing was started at 25 mg/kg/day or 50 mg/kg/day for 5 days just prior to discharge then given 4 days per week (4 days on, 3 days off) (Bu, 2003; Mones, 1994).

Enteric infections: Oral: 50-100 mg/kg/day divided every 6-8 hours; maximum dose: 1000 mg (Bradley, 2012; Red Book, 2012); duration of treatment should not exceed 3 weeks due to GI absorption which may result in systemic toxicities

Hepatic encephalopathy: Limited data available: Oral: 50-100 mg/kg/day divided every 6 hours for a maximum of 7 days with or without lactulose (Debray, 2006; Lovejoy, 1975); some centers have used 2.5-7 g/m²/day divided every 4-6 hours for 5-6 days; maximum daily dose: 12 g/day

Preoperative intestinal antisepsis: Children and Adolescents: Oral: 15 mg/kg/dose for 3 doses administered over 10 hours (eg, at 1 PM, 2 PM, and 11 PM) the day before surgery; maximum dose: 1000 mg (Bratzler, 2013); some centers have used 90 mg/kg/day divided every 4 hours for 2-3 days; or 25 mg/kg at 1 PM, 2 PM, and 11 PM on the afternoon and evening preceding surgery; maximum dose: 1000 mg; used as an adjunct to mechanical cleansing of the intestine and in combination with erythromycin base

Adults:

Chronic hepatic insufficiency: Oral: 4000 mg/day for an indefinite period

Hepatic encephalopathy: Oral: 500-2000 mg every 6-8 hours or 4-12 g/day divided every 4-6 hours for 5-6 days

Preoperative intestinal antisepsis: Oral: 1000 mg each hour for 4 doses then 1000 mg every 4 hours for 5 doses; or 1000 mg at 1 PM, 2 PM, and 11 PM with oral erythromycin on day preceding surgery as an adjunct to mechanical cleansing of the bowel; or 6 g/day divided every 4 hours for 2-3 days

Dosage adjustment in renal impairment: Dialyzable; there are no specific dosing adjustments provided in the manufacuturer's labeling; however, renal impairment

increases the risk for toxicity and consideration should be given to reducing the dose or discontinuing therapy.

Dosage adjustment in hepatic impairment: There are no dosing adjustments provided in the manufacturer's labeling.

Monitoring Parameters Renal function tests (serum creatinine, BUN, creatinine clearance); urinalysis for increased excretion of protein, decreased specific gravity, casts and cells; serial vestibular and audiometric tests

Reference Range Toxic serum concentrations: ≥1.5 mcg/mL (Marks, 1973)

Additional Information Each 500 mg neomycin sulfate tablet contains 350 mg of neomycin base. Each 125 mg (5 mL) of oral neomycin sulfate solution contains 87.5 mg of neomycin base.

Dosage Forms Excipient information presented when available (limited, particularly for generics); consult specific product labeling.

Solution, Oral, as sulfate:
Neo-Fradin: 25 mg/mL (480 mL) [cherry flavor]

Tablet, Oral, as sulfate:
Generic: 500 mg

References
Bradley JS, Nelson JD, Kimberlin DK, et al, eds. *Nelson's Pocket Book of Pediatric Antimicrobial Therapy*. 19th ed. Philadelphia, PA: Lippincott Williams & Wilkins; 2012.

Bratzler DW, Dellinger EP, Olsen KM, et al, "Clinical Practice Guidelines for Antimicrobial Prophylaxis in Surgery," *Am J Health Syst Pharm*, 2013, 70(3):195-283.

Bu LN, Chen HL, Chang CJ, et al. Prophylactic oral antibiotics in prevention of recurrent cholangitis after the Kasai portoenterostomy. *J Pediatr Surg*. 2003;38(4):590-593.

Debray D, Yousef N, Durand P. New management options for end-stage chronic liver disease and acute liver failure. Potential for Pediatric Patients. *Pediatr Drugs*. 2006;8(1):1-13.

Lovejoy FH, Bresnan MJ, Lombroso CT, etal. Anticerebral oedema therapy in Reye's syndrome. *Archives of Disease in Childhood*. 1975;50:933-937.

Marks MI, Shapera M, Brazeau M. Pediatric antimicrobial therapy III. *Canadian Medical Association Journal*. 1973;109:213-214.

Mones RL, DeFelice AR, Preud'Homme D. Use of neomycin as the prophylaxis against recurrent cholangitis after Kasai portoenterostomy. *J Pediatric Surgery*. 1994;29(3):422-424.

Red Book: 2009 Report of the Committee on Infectious Diseases, 28th ed, Pickering LK, ed, Elk Grove Village, IL: American Academy of Pediatrics, 2009.

Red Book: 2012 Report of the Committee on Infectious Diseases, "Antibacterial Drugs Dosage Tables," 29th ed, Pickering LK, ed, Elk Grove Village, IL: American Academy of Pediatrics, 2012, 808-16.

Neomycin and Polymyxin B
(nee oh MYE sin & pol i MIKS in bee)

Brand Names: U.S. Neosporin® G.U. Irrigant

Brand Names: Canada Neosporin® Irrigating Solution

Therapeutic Category Antibiotic, Topical; Antibiotic, Urinary Irrigation; Genitourinary Irrigant

Generic Availability (U.S.) Yes

Use Short-term use as a continuous irrigant or rinse in the urinary bladder to prevent bacteriuria and gram-negative rod septicemia associated with the use of indwelling catheters

Pregnancy Risk Factor D

Pregnancy Considerations Animal reproduction studies have not been conducted with this combination; however, there are reports of total irreversible bilateral congenital deafness in children whose mothers received streptomycin during pregnancy. See individual agents.

Breast-Feeding Considerations It is not known if neomycin or polymyxin B are excreted into breast milk. See individual agents.

Contraindications Hypersensitivity to neomycin, polymyxin B, or any component; ophthalmic use; irrigation should be avoided in patients with defects in the bladder mucosa or wall

Warnings Topical neomycin is a contact sensitizer

Precautions Use with caution in patients with impaired renal function, dehydrated patients, burn patients, and patients receiving a high dose for prolonged treatment

Adverse Reactions

Dermatologic: Contact dermatitis, erythema, rash, urticaria

Genitourinary: Bladder irritation

Local: Burning

Neuromuscular & skeletal: Neuromuscular blockade

Otic: Ototoxicity

Renal: Nephrotoxicity

Drug Interactions

Metabolism/Transport Effects None known.

Avoid Concomitant Use

Avoid concomitant use of Neomycin and Polymyxin B with any of the following: BCG; Mannitol

Increased Effect/Toxicity

Neomycin and Polymyxin B may increase the levels/effects of: AbobotulinumtoxinA; Acarbose; Bisphosphonate Derivatives; CARBOplatin; Colistimethate; CycloSPORINE (Systemic); Neuromuscular-Blocking Agents; OnabotulinumtoxinA; RimabotulinumtoxinB; Tenofovir; Vitamin K Antagonists

The levels/effects of Neomycin and Polymyxin B may be increased by: Amphotericin B; Capreomycin; Cephalosporins (2nd Generation); Cephalosporins (3rd Generation); Cephalosporins (4th Generation); CISplatin; Loop Diuretics; Mannitol; Nonsteroidal Anti-Inflammatory Agents; Tenofovir; Vancomycin

Decreased Effect

Neomycin and Polymyxin B may decrease the levels/effects of: BCG; Cardiac Glycosides; Sodium Picosulfate; SORAfenib

The levels/effects of Neomycin and Polymyxin B may be decreased by: Penicillins

Stability Store irrigant solution in the refrigerator

Mechanism of Action See individual agents.

Pharmacokinetics (Adult data unless noted) Absorption: Not absorbed following topical application to intact skin; absorbed through denuded or abraded skin, peritoneum, wounds, or ulcers

Dosing: Usual Children and Adults: Bladder irrigation: 1 mL is added to 1 L of NS with administration rate adjusted to patient's urine output; usually administered via a 3-way catheter (approximately 40 mL/hour); continuous irrigation or rinse of the urinary bladder should not exceed 10 days

Administration Bladder irrigant: Do not inject irrigant solution; concentrated irrigant solution must be diluted in 1 liter NS before administration; connect irrigation container to the inflow lumen of a 3-way catheter to permit continuous irrigation of the urinary bladder

Monitoring Parameters Urinalysis, renal function

Additional Information GU irrigant contains methylparaben

Dosage Forms Excipient information presented when available (limited, particularly for generics); consult specific product labeling.

Solution, irrigation: Neomycin 40 mg and polymyxin B sulfate 200,000 units per 1 mL (1 mL, 20 mL)

Neosporin® G.U. Irrigant: Neomycin 40 mg and polymyxin sulfate B 200,000 units per 1 mL (1 mL, 20 mL)

◆ **Neomycin, Bacitracin, and Polymyxin B** see Bacitracin, Neomycin, and Polymyxin B on page 258

◆ **Neomycin, Bacitracin, Polymyxin B, and Hydrocortisone** see Bacitracin, Neomycin, Polymyxin B, and Hydrocortisone on page 258

Neomycin, Polymyxin B, and Dexamethasone

(nee oh MYE sin, pol i MIKS in bee, & deks a METH a sone)

Brand Names: U.S. Maxitrol®

Brand Names: Canada Dioptrol®; Maxitrol®

Therapeutic Category Antibiotic, Ophthalmic; Corticosteroid, Ophthalmic

Generic Availability (U.S.) Yes

Use Steroid-responsive inflammatory ocular conditions in which a corticosteroid is indicated and where bacterial infection or a risk of bacterial infection exists

Pregnancy Risk Factor C

Pregnancy Considerations Animal reproduction studies have not been conducted with this combination. See individual agents.

Breast-Feeding Considerations See individual agents.

Contraindications Hypersensitivity to dexamethasone, polymyxin, neomycin, or any component; viral diseases of the cornea and conjunctiva; mycobacterial infection of the eye; fungal disease of ocular structures; dendritic keratitis; use after uncomplicated removal of a corneal foreign body

Warnings Prolonged use may result in glaucoma, defects in visual acuity, posterior subcapsular cataract formation, and secondary ocular infections

Precautions Cutaneous sensitivity to neomycin may develop; discontinue if occurs. Suspension contains benzalkonium chloride which may be adsorbed by contact lenses; contact lenses should not be worn during treatment of ophthalmic infections. For ophthalmic use only. A maximum of 8 g of ointment or 20 mL of suspension should be prescribed initially; patients should be evaluated prior to additional refills.

Adverse Reactions See individual agents.

Drug Interactions

Metabolism/Transport Effects None known.

Avoid Concomitant Use There are no known interactions where it is recommended to avoid concomitant use.

Increased Effect/Toxicity

Neomycin, Polymyxin B, and Dexamethasone may increase the levels/effects of: Ceritinib

Decreased Effect There are no known significant interactions involving a decrease in effect.

Mechanism of Action See individual agents.

Dosing: Usual Children and Adults: Ophthalmic:

Ointment: Apply a small amount (~1/2") in the affected eye 3-4 times/day or apply at bedtime as an adjunct with drops

Suspension: Instill 1-2 drops into affected eye(s) every 4-6 hours; in severe disease, drops may be used hourly and tapered to discontinuation

Administration Ophthalmic: Shake suspension well before using; instill drop into affected eye; avoid contacting bottle tip with skin or eye; apply finger pressure to lacrimal sac during and for 1-2 minutes after instillation to decrease risk of absorption and systemic effects

Monitoring Parameters Intraocular pressure with use >10 days

Dosage Forms Excipient information presented when available (limited, particularly for generics); consult specific product labeling.

Ointment, ophthalmic: Neomycin 3.5 mg, polymyxin B sulfate 10,000 units, and dexamethasone 0.1% per g (3.5 g)

Maxitrol®: Neomycin 3.5 mg, polymyxin B sulfate 10,000 units, and dexamethasone 0.1% per g (3.5 g)

Suspension, ophthalmic [drops]: Neomycin 3.5 mg, polymyxin B sulfate 10,000 units, and dexamethasone 0.1% per 1 mL (5 mL)

Maxitrol®: Neomycin 3.5 mg, polymyxin B sulfate 10,000 units, and dexamethasone 0.1% per 1 mL (5 mL) [contains benzalkonium chloride]

Neomycin, Polymyxin B, and Hydrocortisone
(nee oh MYE sin, pol i MIKS in bee, & hye droe KOR ti sone)

Brand Names: U.S. Cortisporin; Cortomycin
Brand Names: Canada Cortimyxin; Cortisporin Otic
Therapeutic Category Antibacterial, Otic; Antibiotic, Ophthalmic; Antibiotic, Otic; Antibiotic, Topical; Corticosteroid, Ophthalmic; Corticosteroid, Otic; Corticosteroid, Topical
Generic Availability (U.S.) Yes: Excludes topical cream
Use Steroid-responsive inflammatory condition for which a corticosteroid is indicated and where bacterial infection or a risk of bacterial infection exists (Otic preparations: FDA approved in ages 2-16 years and adults; Topical cream, ophthalmic suspension: FDA approved in adults)
Pregnancy Risk Factor C
Pregnancy Considerations Animal reproduction studies have not been conducted with this combination. See individual agents.
Breast-Feeding Considerations See individual agents.
Contraindications Hypersensitivity to hydrocortisone, polymyxin B sulfate, neomycin sulfate, or any component; not for use in viral infections, fungal diseases, mycobacterial infections; perforated tympanic membrane
Warnings Neomycin may cause cutaneous and conjunctival sensitization presenting as itching, reddening, edema, and failure to heal; neomycin may cause permanent hearing loss; risk of ototoxicity is increased in patients with extended use; limit therapy to 10 days; do not use in tympanic perforation. Systemic absorption of hydrocortisone may cause HPA axis suppression which can lead to adrenal crisis; risk is increased when used over large surface areas, for prolonged periods, or with occlusive dressings; children are more susceptible to topical corticosteroid-induced HPA axis suppression and Cushing's syndrome; prolonged use of corticosteroids may also increase the incidence of secondary infection, mask acute infection (including fungal infections), prolong or exacerbate viral infections, or limit response to vaccines; prolonged treatment with corticosteroids has been associated with the development of Kaposi's sarcoma (case reports); if noted, discontinuation of therapy should be considered. The ophthalmic suspension should never be directly introduced into the anterior chamber; may delay corneal healing; prolonged use may result in ocular hypertension/glaucoma, optic nerve damage, cataract formation, visual field or acuity defects, and corneal and scleral thinning potentially resulting in perforation; may mask or worsen ophthalmic infection; otic solution contains potassium metabisulfate which may cause allergic reactions in susceptible individuals
Precautions Use with caution in patients with chronic otitis media; use caution in glaucoma; avoid use following ocular cataract surgery; inadvertent contamination of multiple-dose ophthalmic solutions has caused bacterial keratitis
Adverse Reactions For additional information, see individual agents.
Ophthalmic ointment:
Dermatologic: Delayed wound healing, rash
Ocular: Cataracts, corneal thinning, glaucoma, irritation, keratitis (bacterial), intraocular pressure increase, optic nerve damage, scleral thinning
Miscellaneous: Hypersensitivity (including anaphylaxis), secondary infection, sensitization to kanamycin, paromomycin, streptomycin, and gentamicin
Otic solution and suspension:
Dermatologic: Acneiform eruptions, allergic contact dermatitis, burning skin, dryness, folliculitis, hypertrichosis,

hypopigmentation, irritation, maceration of skin, miliaria, perioral dermatitis, pruritus, skin atrophy, striae
Ophthalmic: Ocular hypertension
Otic: Burning, ototoxicity, stinging
Renal: Nephrotoxicity
Miscellaneous: Hypersensitivity (including anaphylaxis), secondary infection, sensitization to karamycin, paromycin, streptomycin, and gentamicin
Drug Interactions
Metabolism/Transport Effects None known.
Avoid Concomitant Use There are no known interactions where it is recommended to avoid concomitant use.
Increased Effect/Toxicity There are no known significant interactions involving an increase in effect.
Decreased Effect There are no known significant interactions involving a decrease in effect.
Mechanism of Action See individual agents.
Dosing: Usual
Otic preparations (solution and suspension):
Children: 3 drops into affected ear 3-4 times/day for up to 10 days
Adults: 4 drops into affected ear 3-4 times/day for up to 10 days
Topical cream: Children and Adults: Apply thin layer to affected area 2-4 times/day for up to 7 days. Therapy should be discontinued when control is achieved or after a week; if no improvement is seen, reassessment of diagnosis may be necessary.
Ophthalmic suspension: Children and Adults: Instill 1-2 drops in the affected eye every 3-4 hours
Administration Shake ophthalmic and otic suspension well before use
Ophthalmic: Avoid contamination of the tip of the eye dropper; apply finger pressure to lacrimal sac during and for 1-2 minutes after instillation to decrease risk of absorption and systemic effects
Otic: Drops can be instilled directly into the affected ear, or a cotton wick may be saturated with suspension and inserted in ear canal. Keep wick moist with suspension every 4 hours; wick should be replaced every 24 hours.
Topical: Apply a thin layer to the cleansed, dry affected area
Monitoring Parameters If ophthalmic suspension is used >10 days or in patients with glaucoma, monitor intraocular pressure (IOP).
Additional Information Otic **suspension** is the preferred otic preparation; otic **suspension** can be used for the treatment of infections of mastoidectomy and fenestration cavities caused by susceptible organisms; otic **solution** is used **only** for superficial infections of the external auditory canal (ie, swimmer's ear)
Dosage Forms Excipient information presented when available (limited, particularly for generics); consult specific product labeling.
Cream, topical
Cortisporin®: Neomycin 3.5 mg, polymyxin B 10,000 units, and hydrocortisone acetate 5 mg per g (7.5 g)
Solution, otic: Neomycin 3.5 mg, polymyxin B 10,000 units, and hydrocortisone 10 mg per 1 mL (10 mL)
Cortisporin®: Neomycin 3.5 mg, polymyxin B 10,000 units, and hydrocortisone 10 mg per 1 mL (10 mL) [contains potassium metabisulfite]
Cortomycin: Neomycin 3.5 mg, polymyxin B 10,000 units, and hydrocortisone 10 mg per 1 mL (10 mL) [contains potassium metabisulfate]
Suspension, ophthalmic [drops]: Neomycin 3.5 mg, polymyxin B 10,000 units, and hydrocortisone 10 mg per 1 mL (7.5 mL)
Suspension, otic: Neomycin 3.5 mg, polymyxin B 10,000 units, and hydrocortisone 10 mg per 1 mL (10 mL)

Cortomycin: Neomycin 3.5 mg, polymyxin B 10,000 units, and hydrocortisone 10 mg per 1 mL (10 mL) [contains thimerosal]

◆ **Neomycin Sulfate** see Neomycin on page 1482
◆ **Neonatal Trace Metals** see Trace Elements on page 2059
◆ **Neo-Polycin™** see Bacitracin, Neomycin, and Polymyxin B on page 258
◆ **Neo-Polycin™ HC** see Bacitracin, Neomycin, Polymyxin B, and Hydrocortisone on page 258
◆ **NeoProfen** see Ibuprofen on page 1059
◆ **Neoral** see CycloSPORINE (Systemic) on page 564
◆ **Neosar** see Cyclophosphamide on page 561
◆ **Neosporin® G.U. Irrigant** see Neomycin and Polymyxin B on page 1483
◆ **Neosporin® Irrigating Solution (Can)** see Neomycin and Polymyxin B on page 1483
◆ **Neosporin® Neo To Go® [OTC]** see Bacitracin, Neomycin, and Polymyxin B on page 258
◆ **Neosporin® Topical [OTC]** see Bacitracin, Neomycin, and Polymyxin B on page 258

Neostigmine (nee oh STIG meen)

Medication Safety Issues
Sound-alike/look-alike issues:
Prostigmin may be confused with physostigmine
Brand Names: U.S. Bloxiverz; Prostigmin
Brand Names: Canada Prostigmin
Therapeutic Category Antidote, Neuromuscular Blocking Agent; Cholinergic Agent; Diagnostic Agent, Myasthenia Gravis
Generic Availability (U.S.) May be product dependent
Use Treatment of myasthenia gravis; prevention and treatment of postoperative bladder distention and urinary retention; reversal of the effects of nondepolarizing neuromuscular blocking agents after surgery
Pregnancy Risk Factor C
Pregnancy Considerations Animal reproduction studies have not been conducted; anticholinesterases have caused uterine irritability and induced premature labor with I.V. use in near-term pregnant women. When used as adjunct to analgesia in labor, adverse events to the fetus and mother are dose- and route-dependent (Habib, 2006). Neostigmine may be used to treat myasthenia gravis in pregnant women; however, if an acetylcholinesterase inhibitor is needed during pregnancy, another agent may be preferred (Norwood, 2013; Silvestri, 2012).
Breast-Feeding Considerations It is not known if neostigmine is excreted into breast milk. The manufacturer recommends caution be used if administered to nursing women. Babies born to women with myasthenia gravis may have feeding difficulties due to transient myasthenia gravis of the newborn (Norwood, 2013).
Contraindications Hypersensitivity to neostigmine, bromides, or any component; GI or GU obstruction, peritonitis
Warnings Does **not** antagonize, and may prolong the phase I block of depolarizing muscle relaxants (eg, succinylcholine); adequate facilities should be available for cardiopulmonary resuscitation when testing and adjusting dose for myasthenia gravis; have atropine and epinephrine ready to treat hypersensitivity reactions; anticholinesterase insensitivity can develop for brief or prolonged periods
Precautions Use with caution in patients with epilepsy, asthma, bradycardia, hyperthyroidism, cardiac arrhythmias, peptic ulcer, vagotonia, or recent coronary occlusion

Adverse Reactions
Cardiovascular: Arrhythmias (especially bradycardia), AV block, cardiac arrest, flushing, hypotension, nodal rhythm, nonspecific ECG changes, syncope, tachycardia
Central nervous system: Convulsions, dizziness, drowsiness, dysarthria, dysphonia, headache, loss of consciousness
Dermatologic: Skin rash, thrombophlebitis (I.V.), urticaria
Gastrointestinal: Diarrhea, dysphagia, flatulence, hyperperistalsis, nausea, salivation, stomach cramps, vomiting
Genitourinary: Urinary urgency
Neuromuscular & skeletal: Arthralgias, fasciculations, muscle cramps, spasms, weakness
Ocular: Lacrimation, small pupils
Respiratory: Bronchiolar constriction, bronchospasm, dyspnea, increased bronchial secretions, laryngospasm, respiratory arrest, respiratory depression, respiratory muscle paralysis
Miscellaneous: Allergic reactions, anaphylaxis, diaphoresis increased

Drug Interactions
Metabolism/Transport Effects None known.
Avoid Concomitant Use There are no known interactions where it is recommended to avoid concomitant use.
Increased Effect/Toxicity
Neostigmine may increase the levels/effects of: Beta-Blockers; Cholinergic Agonists; Succinylcholine

The levels/effects of Neostigmine may be increased by: Corticosteroids (Systemic)
Decreased Effect
Neostigmine may decrease the levels/effects of: Neuromuscular-Blocking Agents (Nondepolarizing)

The levels/effects of Neostigmine may be decreased by: Dipyridamole
Mechanism of Action Inhibits destruction of acetylcholine by acetylcholinesterase which facilitates transmission of impulses across myoneural junction; direct cholinomimetic effect on skeletal muscle and possible on autonomic ganglion cells and neurons of the CNS
Pharmacodynamics
Onset of action:
Oral: 45-75 minutes
I.M.: Within 20-30 minutes
I.V.: Within 1-20 minutes
Duration:
Oral: 2-4 hours
I.M.: 2-4 hours
I.V.: 1-2 hours
Pharmacokinetics (Adult data unless noted)
Absorption: Oral: Poor (~1% to 2%)
Metabolism: In the liver
Half-life: 0.5-2.1 hours
Elimination: 50% excreted renally as unchanged drug
Dosing: Usual
Myasthenia gravis:
Diagnosis: I.M. (all cholinesterase medications should be discontinued at least 8 hours before; atropine should be administered I.V. immediately prior to or I.M. 30 minutes before neostigmine):
Children: 0.025-0.04 mg/kg as a single dose
Adults: 0.02 mg/kg as a single dose
Treatment (dosage requirements are variable; adjust dosage so patient takes larger doses at times of greatest fatigue):
Children:
Oral: 2 mg/kg/day or 60 mg/m²/day every 3-4 hours; not to exceed 375 mg/day
I.M., I.V., SubQ: 0.01-0.04 mg/kg every 2-4 hours

Adults:

Oral: Initial: 15 mg/dose every 3-4 hours, gradually increase every 1-2 days; usual daily range: 15-375 mg

I.M., I.V., SubQ: 0.5-2.5 mg every 1-3 hours up to 10 mg/24 hours maximum

Reversal of nondepolarizing neuromuscular blockade after surgery in conjunction with atropine or glycopyrrolate: I.V.:

Infants: 0.025-0.1 mg/kg/dose

Children: 0.025-0.08 mg/kg/dose

Adults: 0.5-2.5 mg; total dose not to exceed 5 mg

Bladder atony: Adults: I.M., SubQ:

Prevention: 0.25 mg every 4-6 hours for 2-3 days

Treatment: 0.5-1 mg every 3 hours for 5 doses after bladder has emptied

Dosing adjustment in renal impairment:

CrCl 10-50 mL/minute: Administer 50% of normal dose

CrCl <10 mL/minute: Administer 25% of normal dose

Administration

Parenteral: May be administered undiluted by slow I.V. injection over several minutes; may be administered I.M. or SubQ

Oral: Divide dosages so patient receives larger doses at times of greatest fatigue; may be administered with or without food

Monitoring Parameters Muscle strength, heart rate, respiratory rate

Dosage Forms Excipient information presented when available (limited, particularly for generics); consult specific product labeling. [DSC] = Discontinued product

Solution, Injection, as methylsulfate:

Prostigmin: 0.5 mg/mL (1 mL, 10 mL)

Generic: 0.5 mg/mL (10 mL); 1 mg/mL (10 mL)

Solution, Intravenous, as methylsulfate:

Bloxiverz: 5 mg/10 mL (10 mL); 10 mg/10 mL (10 mL) [contains phenol]

Tablet, Oral, as bromide:

Prostigmin: 15 mg [DSC] [scored]

References

Habib AS and Gan TJ, "Use of Neostigmine in the Management of Acute Postoperative Pain and Labour Pain: A Review," *CNS Drugs*, 2006, 20(10):821-39.

Norwood F, Dhanjal M, Hill M, et al, "Myasthenia in Pregnancy: Best Practice Guidelines From a UK Multispecialty Working Group," *J Neurol Neurosurg Psychiatry*, 2013 [epub ahead of print].

Silvestri NJ and Wolfe GI, "Myasthenia Gravis," *Semin Neurol*, 2012, 32 (3):215-26.

◆ **Neostigmine Bromide** see Neostigmine on page 1486

◆ **Neostigmine Methylsulfate** see Neostigmine on page 1486

◆ **Neo-Synephrine [OTC]** see Phenylephrine (Nasal) on page 1660

◆ **Neo-Synephrine® (Can)** see Phenylephrine (Nasal) on page 1660

◆ **Neo-Synephrine 12 Hour Spray [OTC]** see Oxymetazoline (Nasal) on page 1577

◆ **Nesacaine** see Chloroprocaine on page 442

◆ **Nesacaine®-CE (Can)** see Chloroprocaine on page 442

◆ **Nesacaine-MPF** see Chloroprocaine on page 442

◆ **NESP** see Darbepoetin Alfa on page 592

◆ **Neulasta** see Pegfilgrastim on page 1616

◆ **Neumega** see Oprelvekin on page 1549

◆ **Neuotrogena T/Gel Therapeutic Shampoo [OTC] (Can)** see Coal Tar on page 532

◆ **Neupogen** see Filgrastim on page 872

◆ **Neuro-K-50 [OTC]** see Pyridoxine on page 1778

◆ **Neuro-K-250 T.D. [OTC]** see Pyridoxine on page 1778

◆ **Neuro-K-250 Vitamin B6 [OTC]** see Pyridoxine on page 1778

◆ **Neuro-K-500 [OTC]** see Pyridoxine on page 1778

◆ **Neurontin** see Gabapentin on page 950

◆ **Neut** see Sodium Bicarbonate on page 1901

◆ **NeutraCare** see Fluoride on page 894

◆ **NeutraGard Advanced** see Fluoride on page 894

◆ **Neutra-Phos** see Potassium Phosphate and Sodium Phosphate on page 1718

◆ **Neutra-Phos®-K [OTC] [DSC]** see Potassium Phosphate on page 1715

◆ **Neutrogena Clear Pore [OTC]** see Benzoyl Peroxide on page 275

◆ **Neutrogena Oil-Free Acne Wash [OTC]** see Salicylic Acid on page 1860

◆ **Neutrogena T/Gel Conditioner [OTC]** see Coal Tar on page 532

◆ **Neutrogena T/Gel Ex St [OTC]** see Coal Tar on page 532

Nevirapine (ne VYE ra peen)

Medication Safety Issues

Sound-alike/look-alike issues:

Nevirapine may be confused with nelfinavir

Viramune®, Viramune XR® may be confused with Viracept®

Related Information

Adult and Adolescent HIV on page 2348

Oral Medications That Should Not Be Crushed or Altered on page 2438

Pediatric HIV on page 2338

Perinatal HIV on page 2356

Brand Names: U.S. Viramune; Viramune XR

Brand Names: Canada Auro-Nevirapine; Mylan-Nevirapine; Teva-Nevirapine; Viramune XR®; Viramune®

Therapeutic Category Antiretroviral Agent; HIV Agents (Anti-HIV Agents); Non-nucleoside Reverse Transcriptase Inhibitor (NNRTI)

Generic Availability (U.S.) Yes

Use Treatment of HIV infection in combination with other antiretroviral agents (Immediate release: FDA approved in ages ≥15 days and adults; Extended release: FDA approved in ages ≥6 years and adults). **Note:** HIV regimens consisting of three antiretroviral agents are strongly recommended. Do not start nevirapine therapy in women with CD4+ counts >250 cells/mm^3 or in men with CD4+ counts >400 cells/mm^3 unless benefit of therapy outweighs the risk. Nevirapine has also been used as chemoprophylaxis in newborns to prevent perinatal HIV transmission.

Medication Guide Available Yes

Pregnancy Risk Factor B

Pregnancy Considerations Teratogenic effects were not observed in animal reproduction studies. Nevirapine has a high level of transfer across the human placenta. No increased risk of overall birth defects has been observed following first trimester exposure according to data collected by the antiretroviral pregnancy registry. Pharmacokinetics are not altered during pregnancy and dose adjustment is not needed. The DHHS Perinatal HIV Guidelines consider nevirapine to be an alternative NNRTI for use in antiretroviral-naïve pregnant patients. Nevirapine may be initiated in pregnant women with a CD4$^+$ lymphocyte count <250/mm^3 or continued in women who are virologically suppressed and tolerating therapy once pregnancy is detected (regardless of CD4+ lymphocyte count); however, **do not** initiate therapy in pregnant women with a CD4$^+$ lymphocyte count >250/mm^3 unless the benefit of therapy clearly outweighs the risk. Elevated transaminase concentrations at baseline may increase the risk of toxicity; the monitoring recommendation for transaminase levels is generally the same as in nonpregnant women. Hypersensitivity reactions (including hepatic toxicity and rash) are more common in women on NNRTI.

Regardless of CD4 count or HIV RNA copy number, all HIV-infected pregnant women should receive a combination antiretroviral (ARV) drug regimen. A combination of antepartum, intrapartum, and infant ARV prophylaxis is recommended. ARV therapy should be started as soon as possible in women with symptomatic infection. Although earlier initiation may be more effective in reducing the perinatal transmission of HIV, initiation may be delayed until after 12 weeks gestation in women who do not require immediate treatment after careful consideration of maternal conditions (eg, nausea and vomiting) and the potential risks of first trimester fetal exposure for specific agents. A scheduled cesarean delivery at 38 weeks gestation is recommended for all women with HIV RNA >1000 copies/mL or unknown concentrations near delivery in order to decrease transmission. If ARV therapy must be interrupted for <24 hours during the peripartum period, stop then restart all medications simultaneously in order to decrease the chance of developing resistance. Long-term follow-up is recommended for all infants exposed to ARV medications. In couples who want to conceive, the HIV-infected partner should attain maximum viral suppression prior to conception.

Health care providers are encouraged to enroll pregnant women exposed to antiretroviral medications in the Antiretroviral Pregnancy Registry (1-800-258-4263 or www.APRegistry.com). Health care providers caring for HIV-infected women and their infants may contact the National Perinatal HIV Hotline (888-448-8765) for clinical consultation (DHHS [perinatal], 2014).

Breast-Feeding Considerations Nevirapine is excreted into breast milk and measurable in the serum of nursing infants. Maternal or infant antiretroviral therapy does not completely eliminate the risk of postnatal HIV transmission. In addition, multiclass resistant virus has been detected in breast-feeding infants despite maternal therapy. Therefore, in the United States, where formula is accessible, affordable, safe, and sustainable, and the risk of infant mortality due to diarrhea and respiratory infections is low, complete avoidance of breast-feeding by HIV-infected women is recommended to decrease potential transmission of HIV (DHHS [perinatal], 2014).

Contraindications Hypersensitivity to nevirapine or any component; moderate or severe hepatic impairment (Child Pugh Class B or C); use in occupational or nonoccupational HIV postexposure prophylaxis (PEP) regimens

Warnings Severe, life-threatening, and fatal cases of skin reactions (eg, Stevens-Johnson syndrome, toxic epidermal necrolysis, and hypersensitivity reactions accompanied by rash, constitutional symptoms, and organ dysfunction) have occurred in patients receiving nevirapine **[U.S. Boxed Warning]**; discontinue nevirapine in patients who develop a severe rash or rash accompanied by fever, blistering, oral lesions, conjunctivitis, facial edema, muscle or joint aches, general malaise, fatigue, hepatitis, renal dysfunction, granulocytopenia, eosinophilia, or lymphadenopathy; do not restart nevirapine in these patients. Rash has been described as usually maculopapular erythematous cutaneous eruptions with or without pruritus, located on the trunk, face, and extremities; women may be at a higher risk for development of rash; 21% of pediatric patients developed rash. Initiating therapy at a lower dose for the first 14 days of therapy (lead-in dose) has been shown to reduce the frequency of rash. If nonsevere rash (in the absence of transaminase elevations) occurs, do not increase dose until rash has resolved. If rash continues beyond 28 days, use an alternative regimen. Concomitant use of prednisone during the first 6 weeks of therapy was associated with an increase in incidence and severity of rash. Use of prednisone to prevent nevirapine-associated rash is not recommended. Obtain liver function tests immediately in all patients who develop a rash within the first 18 weeks of therapy.

Severe, life-threatening, and fatal cases of hepatotoxicity have been reported with the use of nevirapine **[U.S. Boxed Warning]**. Hepatitis or hepatic failure may be associated with hypersensitivity reactions and may include severe rash, rash with fever, malaise, fatigue, blisters, oral lesions, conjunctivitis, facial edema, muscle or joint aches, eosinophilia, granulocytopenia, lymphadenopathy, and renal dysfunction. Rhabdomyolysis has occurred in some patients in conjunction with skin and/or hepatic reactions associated with nevirapine therapy.

Intensive monitoring is required during the initial 18 weeks of therapy to detect potentially life-threatening hepatotoxicity or skin reactions **[U.S. Boxed Warning]**. The greatest risk for these reactions occurs in the first 6 weeks of therapy. Patients with elevated AST or ALT levels, coinfection with hepatitis B or C, women with CD4+ counts >250 cells/mm^3, and men with CD4+ counts >400 cells/mm^3 may be at higher risk for rash-associated hepatic adverse events. Women with high CD4+ counts are at the greatest risk of hepatotoxicity including potentially fatal hepatic events. Serious hepatotoxicity (including hepatic failure requiring liver transplantation) has been reported in patients receiving multiple-dose regimens of nevirapine for postexposure prophylaxis; use of nevirapine for occupational and nonoccupational HIV postexposure prophylaxis is contraindicated. Discontinue immediately if any of the following occur: Signs or symptoms of hepatitis, increased LFTs in combination with rash or other systemic symptoms, severe skin or hypersensitivity reaction, or any rash with systemic symptoms **[U.S. Boxed Warning]**; do not restart after recovery.

Nevirapine induces hepatic cytochrome P450 3A and has the potential for interacting with numerous drugs. Due to potential serious and/or life-threatening drug interactions, certain drugs must be avoided. Other drug interactions require dosage adjustment. Use of efavirenz with nevirapine may increase the risk for adverse effects without increasing efficacy; concurrent use is **not** recommended. Concurrent use of St John's wort is **not** recommended; may decrease the therapeutic efficacy of nevirapine.

Due to rapid emergence of resistance, nevirapine should not be used as monotherapy or the only agent added to a failing regimen for the treatment of HIV. Use care when timing discontinuation of regimens containing nevirapine; serum concentrations are sustained after concentrations of other medications decrease, potentially leading to nevirapine resistance. Cross-resistance may be conferred to other non-nucleoside reverse transcriptase inhibitors (DHHS [adult], 2014).

The suspension formulation contains polysorbate 80 (Tween) which may cause allergic reactions in susceptible individuals.

Precautions Use with caution in patients with either renal or hepatic dysfunction; contraindicated in patients with moderate to severe hepatic impairment; elevated AST or ALT levels and/or a history of chronic hepatitis (B or C) infection are associated with a greater risk of hepatic adverse events; nevirapine may accumulate in patients with worsening hepatic function and ascites. Fat redistribution and accumulation [ie, central obesity, peripheral wasting, facial wasting, breast enlargement, dorsocervical fat enlargement (buffalo hump), and cushingoid appearance] have been observed in patients receiving antiretroviral agents (causal relationship not established).

Immune reconstitution syndrome (an acute inflammatory response to residual or indolent opportunistic infections) may occur in HIV patients during initial treatment with combination antiretroviral agents; this syndrome may require further patient assessment and therapy. Autoimmune disorders (eg, Grave's disease, Guillain-Barré syndrome, and polymyositis) have been reported in patients experiencing immune reconstitution; time to onset is variable and may occur many months after antiretroviral treatment is initiated.

Granulocytopenia may occur; more common in younger pediatric patients (2 weeks to <3 months of age) compared to older children and adults; also more common in pediatric patients receiving concomitant zidovudine. Anemia may occur at an incidence of 7.3%; it has been reported more commonly in children in postmarketing reports; however, effects of concomitant medications cannot be separated out.

In perinatally HIV-exposed infants, the sensitivity of diagnostic virologic assays, particularly HIV RNA assays, may be affected by infant combination antiretroviral prophylactic therapy. Thus, a negative result of a diagnostic virologic assay should be repeated 2 to 4 weeks after cessation of neonatal combination antiretroviral prophylactic therapy (DHHS [pediatric], 2014).

Adverse Reactions Note: Potentially life-threatening nevirapine-associated adverse effects may present with the following symptoms: Abrupt onset of flu-like symptoms, abdominal pain, jaundice, or fever with or without rash; may progress to hepatic failure with encephalopathy.

Central nervous system: Fatigue, fever, headache

Dermatologic: Rash

Endocrine & metabolic: Cholesterol increased, LDL increased

Gastrointestinal: Abdominal pain, amylase increased, diarrhea, nausea

Hematologic: Neutropenia

Hepatic: ALT increased, AST increased, symptomatic hepatic events (including hepatitis and hepatic failure)

Neuromuscular & skeletal: Arthralgia

Rare but important or life-threatening: Allergic reactions, anaphylaxis, anemia, angioedema, bullous eruptions, conjunctivitis, drug reaction with eosinophilia and systemic symptoms (DRESS), eosinophilia, hypersensitivity syndrome, hypophosphatemia, immune reconstitution syndrome, lymphadenopathy, oral lesions, redistribution/accumulation of body fat, renal dysfunction, rhabdomyolysis, Stevens-Johnson syndrome, toxic epidermal necrolysis, ulcerative stomatitis

Drug Interactions

Metabolism/Transport Effects Substrate of CYP2B6 (minor), CYP2D6 (minor), CYP3A4 (major); **Note:** Assignment of Major/Minor substrate status based on clinically relevant drug interaction potential; **Inhibits** CYP1A2 (weak), CYP2D6 (weak), CYP3A4 (weak); **Induces** CYP2B6 (strong), CYP3A4 (strong)

Avoid Concomitant Use

Avoid concomitant use of Nevirapine with any of the following: Abiraterone Acetate; Apixaban; Apremilast; Artemether; Atazanavir; Axitinib; Bedaquiline; Boceprevir; Bortezomib; Bosutinib; Cabozantinib; CarBAMazepine; Ceritinib; CloZAPine; Crizotinib; Dienogest; Dolutegravir; Dronedarone; Efavirenz; Enzalutamide; Etravirine; Everolimus; Ibrutinib; Itraconazole; Ivacaftor; Ketoconazole (Systemic); Lapatinib; Lumefantrine; Lurasidone; Macitentan; Mifepristone; NIFEdipine; Nilotinib; Nisoldipine; PAZOPanib; Perampanel; Pimozide; PONATinib; Praziquantel; Ranolazine; Regorafenib; Rilpivirine; Rivaroxaban; Roflumilast; RomiDEPsin; Simeprevir; SORAfenib; St Johns Wort; Tasimelteon; Telaprevir; Ticagrelor; Tofacitinib; Tolvaptan; Toremifene; Ulipristal; Vandetanib; Vemurafenib; VinCRIStine (Liposomal); Vorapaxar

Increased Effect/Toxicity

Nevirapine may increase the levels/effects of: Clarithromycin; Dofetilide; Efavirenz; Etravirine; Ifosfamide; Lomitapide; Pimozide; Rifabutin; Rilpivirine

The levels/effects of Nevirapine may be increased by: Atazanavir; Clarithromycin; Efavirenz; Fluconazole; Voriconazole

Decreased Effect

Nevirapine may decrease the levels/effects of: Abiraterone Acetate; Apixaban; Apremilast; ARIPiprazole; Artemether; Atazanavir; Axitinib; Bedaquiline; Boceprevir; Bortezomib; Bosutinib; Brentuximab Vedotin; Cabozantinib; Cannabidiol; Cannabis; CarBAMazepine; Caspofungin; Ceritinib; Clarithromycin; CloZAPine; Contraceptives (Estrogens); Contraceptives (Progestins); Crizotinib; CYP2B6 Substrates; CYP3A4 Substrates; Dasatinib; Dienogest; Dolutegravir; DOXOrubicin (Conventional); Dronabinol; Dronedarone; Efavirenz; Enzalutamide; Etravirine; Everolimus; Exemestane; FentaNYL; Fosamprenavir; Gefitinib; GuanFACINE; Ibrutinib; Imatinib; Indinavir; Itraconazole; Ivacaftor; Ixabepilone; Ketoconazole (Systemic); Lapatinib; Linagliptin; Lopinavir; Lumefantrine; Lurasidone; Macitentan; Maraviroc; Methadone; Mifepristone; Nelfinavir; NIFEdipine; Nilotinib; Nisoldipine; PAZOPanib; Perampanel; PONATinib; Praziquantel; QUEtiapine; Ranolazine; Regorafenib; Rifabutin; Rilpivirine; Rivaroxaban; Roflumilast; RomiDEPsin; Saquinavir; Saxagliptin; Simeprevir; SORAfenib; SUNItinib; Tadalafil; Tasimelteon; Telaprevir; Tetrahydrocannabinol; Ticagrelor; Tofacitinib; Tolvaptan; Toremifene; Ulipristal; Vandetanib; Vemurafenib; Vilazodone; VinCRIStine (Liposomal); Vorapaxar; Voriconazole; Vortioxetine; Zuclopenthixol

The levels/effects of Nevirapine may be decreased by: Bosentan; CarBAMazepine; CYP3A4 Inducers (Strong); Dabrafenib; Deferasirox; Mitotane; Peginterferon Alfa-2b; Rifabutin; Rifampin; Siltuximab; St Johns Wort; Tocilizumab

Stability Store at 25°C (77°F); excursions permitted to 15°C to 30°C (59°F to 86°F); dispense in tightly closed container.

Mechanism of Action As a non-nucleoside reverse transcriptase inhibitor, nevirapine has activity against HIV-1 by binding to reverse transcriptase. It consequently blocks the RNA-dependent and DNA-dependent DNA polymerase activities including HIV-1 replication. It does not require intracellular phosphorylation for antiviral activity.

Pharmacokinetics (Adult data unless noted)

Absorption: Rapid and readily absorbed; Immediate release: >90%

Distribution: V_d: 1.21 L/kg; widely distributed; 45% of the plasma concentration in CSF

Metabolism: Metabolized by cytochrome P450 isozymes from the CYP3A family to hydroxylated metabolites; autoinduction of metabolism occurs in 2-4 weeks with a 1.5-2 times increase in clearance; nevirapine is more rapidly metabolized in pediatric patients than in adults

Protein binding, plasma: 60%

Bioavailability:

Single dose: Immediate release: 93%; Extended release (relative to immediate release): 75%; Oral solution: 91%

Multiple dose: Extended release (relative to immediate release): Fasted conditions: 80%; fed conditions: 94%

Half-life: Adults: Single dose (45 hours); multiple dosing (25-30 hours)

Time to peak serum concentration: Immediate release: 4 hours; Extended release: ~24 hours

Elimination: 81.3% in urine as metabolites, 10.1% in feces; <3% of the total dose is eliminated in urine as parent drug

Clearance: Women have a 13.8% lower clearance compared to men; body size does not totally explain the gender difference

Dosing: Neonatal

HIV infection, treatment: Use in combination with other antiretroviral agents: **Note:** If patient experiences a nonsevere rash (in the absence of transaminase elevations) during the first 14 days of therapy, do not increase dose until rash has resolved. If rash continues beyond 28 days, use an alternative regimen. Discontinue nevirapine if severe rash, rash with constitutional symptoms, or rash with elevated hepatic transaminases occurs. If nevirapine therapy is interrupted for >14 days, restart at the initial recommended dose (ie, once daily for the first 14 days) before increasing to twice daily dosing (DHHS [pediatric], 2014).

PNA ≤14 days: Treatment dose is not defined.

PNA ≥15 days: Oral: Immediate release:

Manufacturer's labeling: Initial: 150 mg/m²/dose (maximum: 200 mg/dose) once daily for the first 14 days of therapy; increase to 150 mg/m²/dose twice daily if no rash or other adverse effects occur; maximum dose: 200 mg/dose every 12 hours

AIDS*Info* pediatric guidelines: Initial: 200 mg/m²/dose (maximum: 200 mg/dose) once daily for the first 14 days of therapy; increase to 200 mg/m²/dose (maximum: 200 mg/dose) twice daily if no rash or other adverse effects occur (DHHS [pediatric], 2014)

Prevention of perinatal HIV transmission: [DHHS (perinatal), 2014]; **Note:** Nevirapine is used in combination with a 6-week course of zidovudine in select situations (eg, infants born to HIV-infected mothers with no antiretroviral therapy prior to labor or during labor or infants born to mothers with only intrapartum antiretroviral therapy); and may be considered in other situations (eg, infants born to mothers with suboptimal viral suppression at delivery or infants born to mothers with known antiretroviral drug-resistant virus).

Newborn: Oral: Immediate release: Administer **three** doses of nevirapine within the first week of life; administer the first dose as soon as possible after birth, but within 48 hours (birth to 48 hours); administer the second dose 48 hours after the first dose; administer the third dose 96 hours after the second dose:

Birthweight 1.5 to 2 kg: 8 mg/dose

Birthweight >2 kg: 12 mg/dose

Dosing: Usual

Pediatric: **HIV infection, treatment:** Use in combination with other antiretroviral agents: **Note:** If patient experiences a nonsevere rash (in the absence of transaminase elevations) during the first 14 days of therapy, do not increase dose until rash has resolved. If rash continues beyond 28 days, use an alternative regimen. Discontinue nevirapine if severe rash, rash with constitutional symptoms, or rash with elevated hepatic transaminases occurs. **Note:** If nevirapine therapy is interrupted for >7 days (adults/adolescents) or >14 days (infants/children), restart at the initial recommended dose (ie, once daily for the first 14 days) before increasing to twice daily dosing (DHHS [adult, pediatric], 2014).

Manufacturer's labeling: Oral:

Immediate release: Infants, Children, and Adolescents: Initial: 150 mg/m²/dose (maximum: 200 mg/dose) once daily for the first 14 days of therapy; increase to 150 mg/m²/dose (maximum: 200 mg/dose) twice daily if no rash or other adverse effects occur

Extended release: Children ≥6 years and Adolescents (must be able to swallow tablets whole): **Note:** Maintenance therapy using the extended release tablet must follow a 14-day initial dosing period (lead-in) using the immediate release formulation, unless the patient is already maintained on a nevirapine

immediate release regimen. Extended release tablets should not be divided to achieve daily dose.

BSA 0.58 to 0.83 m²: 200 mg once daily

BSA 0.84 to 1.16 m²: 300 mg once daily

BSA ≥1.17 m²: 400 mg once daily

AIDS*Info* guidelines (DHHS [pediatric], 2014): Oral:

Immediate release:

Infants and Children <8 years: Initial (lead-in dosing): 200 mg/m²/dose (maximum: 200 mg/dose) once daily for the first 14 days of therapy; increase to 200 mg/m²/dose (maximum: 200 mg/dose) twice daily if no rash or other adverse effects occur; maximum dose: 200 mg twice daily

Children ≥8 years: Initial (lead-in dosing): 120 to 150 mg/m²/dose (maximum: 200 mg/dose) once daily for the first 14 days of therapy; increase to 120 to 150 mg/m²/dose (maximum: 200 mg/dose) twice daily if no rash or other adverse effects occur

Note: In a growing child, do not decrease the mg dose when the child reaches 8 years; leave the mg dose the same to achieve the appropriate mg/m²/dose as the child grows larger (as long as there are no adverse effects)

Adolescents: Initial: 200 mg/dose once daily for the first 14 days; increase to 200 mg every 12 hours if no rash or other adverse effects occur; if patient able to swallow tablets whole, may convert maintenance dose to the extended release formulation (400 mg once daily)

Extended release: Children >6 years and Adolescents (must be able to swallow tablets whole): For patients already on full-dose nevirapine, may initiate extended release preparation without lead-in dosing as long as viral load is undetectable. If initiating nevirapine therapy, begin with the age-appropriate once daily dose of the *immediate release* formulation for the first 14 days of therapy; at 14 days, if no rash or other adverse effects have occurred, increase dose to the age-appropriate dose administered once daily for the extended release formulation; maximum daily dose: 400 mg/**day**

BSA 0.58 to 0.83 m²: 200 mg once daily

BSA 0.84 to 1.16 m²: 300 mg once daily

BSA ≥1.17 m²: 400 mg once daily

Adult: **HIV infection, treatment:** Use in combination with other antiretroviral agents; **Note:** Therapy in antiretroviral-naive patients should not be initiated in patients with elevated CD4⁺ cell counts unless the benefit of therapy outweighs the risk of serious hepatotoxicity (adult/postpubertal females: CD4⁺ cell counts >250 cells/mm³; adult males: CD4⁺ cell counts >400 cells/mm³).

Initial: Immediate release: Oral: 200 mg once daily for the first 14 days

Maintenance:

Immediate release: Oral: 200 mg twice daily if no rash or other adverse effects occur during initial dosing period

Extended release: Oral: 400 mg once daily; **Note:** Maintenance therapy using the extended release tablet must follow a 14-day initial dosing period (lead-in) using the immediate release formulation, unless the patient is already maintained on a nevirapine immediate release regimen.

Dosing adjustment in renal impairment: Adult:

CrCl ≥20 mL/minute: No dosage adjustment required

CrCl <20 mL/minute: There are no dosage adjustments provided in the manufacturer's labeling; however, the following guidelines have been used by some clinicians: No dosage adjustment required

Hemodialysis: An additional 200 mg dose of immediate release tablet is recommended following dialysis. **Note:** Nevirapine metabolites may accumulate in patients on dialysis (clinical significance is unknown)

Dosing adjustment in hepatic impairment:

Mild impairment (Child-Pugh class A): There are no dosage adjustments provided in manufacturer's labeling; use with caution; monitor for symptoms of drug-induced toxicity (increased trough concentrations have been observed in some patients with hepatic fibrosis or cirrhosis).

Moderate to severe impairment (Child-Pugh class B or C): Use is contraindicated; permanently discontinue if symptomatic hepatic events occur.

Administration Oral:

Immediate release: May be administered with water, milk, or soda, with or without meals; may be administered with an antacid or didanosine. Shake suspension gently prior to administration; the use of an oral dosing syringe is recommended, especially if the dose is <5 mL; if using a dosing cup, after administration, rinse cup with water and also administer rinse.

Extended release: May be administered with or without food; swallow tablet whole; do not chew, crush, or divide.

Monitoring Parameters Note: Monitor CD4 percentage (if <5 years of age) or CD4 count (if ≥5 years of age) at least every 3 to 4 months (DHHS [pediatric], 2014)

Prior to initiation of therapy: Genotypic resistance testing, CD4 and viral load (every 3 to 4 months), CBC with differential, LFTs, BUN, creatinine, electrolytes, glucose, urinalysis (every 6 to 12 months), and assessment of readiness for adherence with medication regimen. At initiation and with any change in treatment regimen: CBC with differential, electrolytes, calcium, phosphate, glucose, LFTs, bilirubin, urinalysis (at initiation), BUN, creatinine, albumin, total protein, lipid panel (at initiation), CD4, and viral load. After 1 to 2 weeks of therapy: Signs of medication toxicity and adherence. After 2 to 4 weeks of therapy: CBC with differential, viral load, signs of toxicity, and adherence; then every 3 to 4 months: CBC with differential, electrolytes, glucose, LFTs, bilirubin, BUN, creatinine, CD4, viral load, signs of medication toxicity, and adherence. Every 6 to 12 months: Lipid panel and urinalysis. CD4 monitoring frequency may be decreased to every 6 to 12 months in children who are adherent to therapy if the value is well above the threshold for opportunistic infections, viral suppression is sustained, and the clinical status is stable for more than 2 to 3 years (DHHS [pediatric], 2014). Monitor for growth and development, signs of HIV-specific physical conditions, HIV disease progression, opportunistic infections, skin rash, or hypersensitivity.

Obtain liver function tests every 2 weeks for the first 4 weeks of therapy, then monthly for 3 months, and every 3 to 4 months thereafter. Also check liver function tests immediately if patient develops signs or symptoms consistent with hepatitis or hypersensitivity reactions and immediately in all patients who develop a rash within the first 18 weeks of therapy (DHHS [pediatric], 2014).

Reference Range Plasma trough concentration: ≥3000 ng/mL (DHHS [adult, pediatric], 2014)

Dosage Forms Excipient information presented when available (limited, particularly for generics); consult specific product labeling.

Suspension, Oral:
Viramune: 50 mg/5 mL (240 mL) [contains methylparaben, propylparaben]
Generic: 50 mg/5 mL (240 mL)

Tablet, Oral:
Viramune: 200 mg [scored]
Generic: 200 mg

Tablet Extended Release 24 Hour, Oral:
Viramune XR: 100 mg, 400 mg
Generic: 400 mg

References
Aronoff GR, Bennett WM, Berns JS, et al. *Drug Prescribing in Renal Failure: Dosing Guidelines for Adults and Children.* 5th ed. Philadelphia, PA: American College of Physicians; 2007;80.

DHHS Panel on Antiretroviral Guidelines for Adults and Adolescents. Guidelines for the use of antiretroviral agents in HIV-1-infected adults and adolescents, Department of Health and Human Services. May 1, 2014. Available at http://www.aidsinfo.nih.gov/ContentFiles/AdultandAdolescentGL.pdf

DHHS Panel on Antiretroviral Therapy and Medical Management of HIV-Infected Children. Guidelines for the use of antiretroviral agents in pediatric HIV infection. February 12, 2014. Available at http://aidsinfo.nih.gov

DHHS Panel on Treatment of HIV-Infected Pregnant Women and Prevention of Perinatal Transmission. Recommendations for the use of antiretroviral drugs in pregnant HIV-1-infected women for maternal health and interventions to reduce perinatal HIV-1 transmission in the United States. March 28, 2014. Available at http://aidsinfo.nih.gov

◆ **Nexafed [OTC]** *see* Pseudoephedrine *on page 1770*

◆ **NexIUM** *see* Esomeprazole *on page 793*

◆ **Nexium (Can)** *see* Esomeprazole *on page 793*

◆ **Nexium 24HR** *see* Esomeprazole *on page 793*

◆ **NexIUM I.V.** *see* Esomeprazole *on page 793*

◆ **Nexterone** *see* Amiodarone *on page 127*

◆ **NFV** *see* Nelfinavir *on page 1479*

◆ **NGX-4010** *see* Capsaicin *on page 367*

Niacin (NYE a sin)

Medication Safety Issues
Sound-alike/look-alike issues:
Niacin may be confused with Minocin, niacinamide, Niaspan

Related Information
Oral Medications That Should Not Be Crushed or Altered *on page 2438*

Brand Names: U.S. Niacin-50 [OTC]; Niacor; Niaspan; Slo-Niacin [OTC]

Brand Names: Canada Niaspan; Niaspan FCT; Niodan

Therapeutic Category Antilipemic Agent; Nutritional Supplement; Vitamin, Water Soluble

Generic Availability (U.S.) Yes

Use Adjunctive treatment of hyperlipidemias (FDA approved in adults); adjunctive treatment of hypertriglyceridemia in patients at risk of pancreatitis (FDA approved in adults); to lower the risk of recurrent MI in patients with hyperlipidemia (FDA approved in adults); in combination with a bile acid sequestrant to slow progression (or promote regression) of atherosclerotic disease in patients with CAD and hyperlipidemia (FDA approved in adults); has also been used in the treatment of pellagra; dietary supplement; **Note:** Niacin may be used in combination with lovastatin, simvastatin, or bile acid sequestrants for treatment of hyperlipidemias in patients who fail monotherapy; combination therapy is not indicated as initial therapy

Pregnancy Risk Factor C

Pregnancy Considerations Animal reproduction studies have not been conducted. Water soluble vitamins cross the placenta. When used as a dietary supplement, niacin requirements may be increased in pregnant women compared to nonpregnant women (IOM, 1998). It is not known if niacin at lipid-lowering doses is harmful to the developing fetus. If a woman becomes pregnant while receiving niacin for primary hypercholesterolemia, niacin should be discontinued. If a woman becomes pregnant while receiving niacin for hypertriglyceridemia, the benefits and risks of continuing niacin should be assessed on an individual basis.

Breast-Feeding Considerations Niacin is excreted in human breast milk. When used as a dietary supplement, niacin requirements may be increased in nursing women compared to non-nursing women (IOM, 1998). Because lipid-lowering doses of niacin may cause serious adverse reactions in nursing infants, a decision should be made whether to discontinue nursing or discontinue the drug, taking into account the importance of the drug to the mother.

Contraindications Hypersensitivity to niacin or any component; active liver disease, unexplained persistent increases in liver enzymes, significant or unexplained hepatic dysfunction, active peptic ulcer disease, arterial hemorrhaging

Warnings Hepatotoxicity may occur and may be more common if extended release product is substituted for immediate release product at same dosage; do not interchange extended or sustained release products for immediate release at same dosage. Cases of myopathy and rhabdomyolysis have occurred during concomitant use of niacin with HMG-CoA reductase inhibitors; risk may be increased in patients with diabetes, renal failure, or uncontrolled hypothyroidism; monitor all patients receiving both medications for clinical signs of rhabdomyolysis (muscle pain, tenderness, or weakness) and serum CPK and potassium.

Precautions Use with caution in patients with diabetes mellitus; niacin may increase fasting blood glucose (monitor glucose; adjustment of hypoglycemic therapy may be needed). May elevate uric acid concentrations, use with caution in patients predisposed to gout; large doses should be administered with caution to patients with gallbladder disease, jaundice, history of liver disease, diabetes, unstable angina, MI, renal dysfunction or heavy alcohol use; niacin may cause small increases in prothrombin time (use with caution in patients receiving anticoagulants; monitor closely)

Adverse Reactions

Cardiovascular: Arrhythmias, atrial fibrillation, edema, flushing, hypotension, orthostasis, palpitation, syncope (rare), tachycardia

Central nervous system: Chills, dizziness, headache, insomnia, migraine, nervousness, pain

Dermatologic: Acanthosis nigricans, burning skin, dry skin, hyperpigmentation, maculopapular rash, pruritus, rash, skin discoloration, urticaria

Endocrine & metabolic: Glucose tolerance decreased, gout, phosphorous levels decreased, hyperuricemia

Gastrointestinal: Abdominal pain, amylase increased, diarrhea, dyspepsia, eructation, flatulence, nausea, peptic ulcers, vomiting

Hematologic: Platelet counts decreased

Hepatic: Hepatic necrosis (rare), hepatitis, jaundice, transaminases increased (dose-related), prothrombin time increased, total bilirubin increased

Neuromuscular & skeletal: CPK increased, leg cramps, myalgia, myasthenia, myopathy (with concurrent HMG-CoA reductase inhibitor), paresthesia, rhabdomyolysis (with concurrent HMG-CoA reductase inhibitor; rare), weakness

Ocular: Blurred vision, cystoid macular edema, toxic amblyopia

Respiratory: Cough, dyspnea

Miscellaneous: Diaphoresis, hypersensitivity reactions (rare; includes anaphylaxis, angioedema, laryngismus, vesiculobullous rash), LDH increased

Drug Interactions

Metabolism/Transport Effects None known.

Avoid Concomitant Use There are no known interactions where it is recommended to avoid concomitant use.

Increased Effect/Toxicity
Niacin may increase the levels/effects of: HMG-CoA Reductase Inhibitors

The levels/effects of Niacin may be increased by: Alcohol (Ethyl)

Decreased Effect
The levels/effects of Niacin may be decreased by: Bile Acid Sequestrants

Mechanism of Action Niacin (nicotinic acid) is bioconverted to nicotinamide which is further converted to nicotinamide adenine dinucleotide (NAD+) and the hydride equivalent (NADH) which are coenzymes necessary for tissue metabolism, lipid metabolism, and glycogenolysis (Belenky, 2006; Suave, 2008). The mechanism by which niacin (in lipid-lowering doses) affects plasma lipoproteins is not fully understood. It may involve several actions including partial inhibition of release of free fatty acids from adipose tissue, and increased lipoprotein lipase activity, which may increase the rate of chylomicron triglyceride removal from plasma. Ultimately, niacin reduces total cholesterol, apolipoprotein (apo) B, triglycerides, VLDL, LDL, lipoprotein (a), and increases HDL and other important components and subfractions (eg, LPA-I) (Kamanna, 2000)

Pharmacodynamics Vasodilation:
Onset of action: Within 20 minutes
    Extended release: Within 1 hour
Duration: 20-60 minutes
    Extended release: 8-10 hours

Pharmacokinetics (Adult data unless noted)
Absorption: Oral: Rapid and extensive; ≥60% to 76% of dose is absorbed

Distribution: Crosses into breast milk

Metabolism: Extensive first-pass effect; niacin in smaller doses is converted to niacinamide which is metabolized in the liver; niacin undergoes conjugation with glycine to form nicotinuric acid; nicotinamide, nicotinamide adenine dinucleotide (NAD), and other niacin metabolites are formed via saturable pathways; Note: It is not clear whether nicotinamide is formed before or after the synthesis of NAD

Bioavailability: Single dose studies indicate that only certain Niaspan® tablet strengths are interchangeable (ie, two 500 mg tablets are equivalent to one 1000 mg tablet; however, three 500 mg tablets are **not** equivalent to two 750 mg tablets)

Half-life: 45 minutes

Time to peak serum concentration: Immediate release: ~45 minutes; extended release: 4-5 hours

Elimination: In urine, with ~33% as unchanged drug; with larger doses, a greater percentage is excreted unchanged in urine

Dosing: Neonatal Oral: Adequate intake: 2 mg/day

Dosing: Usual Note: Formulations of niacin (immediate release versus extended release) are not interchangeable.
Oral:
Infants, Children, and Adolescents:
    Adequate intake:
        1-5 months: 2 mg/day
        6-11 months: 3 mg/day
    Recommended daily allowances:
        1-3 years: 6 mg/day
        4-8 years: 8 mg/day
        9-13 years: 12 mg/day
        14-18 years: Female: 14 mg/day; Male: 16 mg/day
        ≥19 years: Refer to adult dosing
Children and Adolescents:
    Hyperlipidemia: Initial: **Note:** Routine use is not recommended due to limited safety and efficacy information: 100-250 mg/day (maximum dose: 10 mg/kg/day) in 3 divided doses with meals; increase weekly by 100 mg/day or increase every 2-3 weeks by 250 mg/day as tolerated; evaluate efficacy and adverse effects with laboratory tests at 20 mg/kg/day or 1000 mg/day (whichever is less); continue to increase if needed and as tolerated; re-evaluate at each 500 mg increment; doses up to 2250 mg/day have been used

Pellagra: 50-100 mg/dose 3 times/day (some experts prefer niacinamide for treatment due to a more favorable side effect profile)

Adults:

Recommended daily allowances (RDA) (National Academy of Sciences, 1998):

≥19 years: Female: 14 mg/day; Male: 16 mg/day

Pregnancy (all ages): 18 mg/day

Lactation (all ages): 17 mg/day

Dietary supplement: 50 mg twice daily or 100 mg once daily. **Note:** Many over-the-counter formulations exist.

Hyperlipidemia:

Immediate release formulation (Niacor®): Initial: 250 mg once daily (with evening meal); increase frequency and/or dose every 4-7 days to desired response or first-level therapeutic dose (1.5-2 g/day) in 2-3 divided doses); after 2 months, may increase at 2- to 4-week intervals to 3 g/day in 3 divided doses [maximum dose: 6 g/day (NCEP recommends 4.5 g/day) in 3 divided doses]. Usual daily dose after titration (NCEP, 2002): 1.5-3 g/day; **Note:** Many over-the-counter formulations exist.

Sustained release (or controlled release) formulations: Usual daily dose after titration (NCEP, 2002): 1-2 g/day; **Note:** Several over-the-counter formulations exist.

Extended release formulation (Niaspan®): Initial: 500 mg at bedtime for 4 weeks, then 1 g at bedtime for 4 weeks; adjust dose to response and tolerance; may increase dose every 4 weeks by 500 mg/day to a maximum of 2 g/day. Usual daily dose after titration (NCEP, 2002): 1-2 g once daily

If additional LDL-lowering is necessary with lovastatin or simvastatin: Recommended initial lovastatin or simvastatin dose: 20 mg/day; Maximum lovastatin or simvastatin dose: 40 mg/day; **Note:** Lovastatin prescribing information recommends a maximum dose of 20 mg/day with concurrent use of niacin (>1 g/day).

Pellagra: 50-100 mg 3-4 times/day, maximum dose: 500 mg/day (some experts prefer niacinamide for treatment due to more favorable side effect profile)

Dosage adjustment in renal impairment: Studies have not been performed; use with caution

Dosage adjustment in hepatic impairment: Contraindicated in patients with active liver disease, unexplained liver enzyme elevations, significant or unexplained hepatic dysfunction. Use with caution in patients with history of liver disease or those with suspected liver disease (eg, those who consume large quantities of alcohol).

Administration Oral: Administer with food or milk to decrease GI upset; administer Niaspan® with a low-fat snack (do not administer on an empty stomach). Swallow timed release tablet and capsule whole; do not break, chew, or crush. To minimize flushing, administer dose at bedtime, take aspirin (adults: 325 mg) 30 minutes before niacin, and avoid alcohol, hot drinks, or spicy food around the time of administration. Separate administration of bile acid sequestrants by at least 4-6 hours (bile acid sequestrants may decrease the absorption of niacin).

Monitoring Parameters Blood glucose, serum uric acid, periodic liver function tests, platelet count and prothrombin time (if on concurrent anticoagulant), serum phosphorus (if predisposed to hypophosphatemia). Treatment of hyperlipidemias: Baseline: Liver enzymes, uric acid, fasting glucose, and minimum of two fasting lipid profiles; repeat 4-6 weeks after dose is stabilized; once LDL-C goal is reached, repeat every 2-3 months for first year and then every 6-12 months if no sign of toxicity develops and dose remains stable. Monitor CPK and serum potassium (if on concurrent HMG-CoA reductase inhibitor).

Test Interactions False elevations in some fluorometric determinations of plasma or urinary catecholamines; false-positive urine glucose (Benedict's reagent)

Dosage Forms Excipient information presented when available (limited, particularly for generics); consult specific product labeling.

Capsule Extended Release, Oral:
Generic: 250 mg, 500 mg

Capsule Extended Release, Oral [preservative free]:
Generic: 250 mg, 500 mg

Tablet, Oral:
Niacin-50: 50 mg [starch free, sugar free, wheat free]
Niacor: 500 mg [scored]
Generic: 50 mg, 100 mg, 250 mg, 500 mg

Tablet, Oral [preservative free]:
Generic: 50 mg, 100 mg, 500 mg

Tablet Extended Release, Oral:
Niaspan: 500 mg, 750 mg, 1000 mg [contains fd&c yellow #6 aluminum lake]
Slo-Niacin: 250 mg [scored]
Slo-Niacin: 500 mg, 750 mg [scored; contains fd&c red #40]
Generic: 500 mg, 750 mg, 1000 mg

Tablet Extended Release, Oral [preservative free]:
Generic: 250 mg, 500 mg, 1000 mg

References

American Academy of Pediatrics Committee on Nutrition, "Cholesterol in Childhood," *Pediatrics*, 1998, 101(1 Pt 1):141-7.

"ASHP Therapeutic Position Statement on the Safe Use of Niacin in the Management of Dyslipidemias. American Society of Health-System Pharmacists," *Am J Health Syst Pharm*, 1997, 54(24):2815-9.

Colletti RB, Neufeld EJ, Roff NK, et al, "Niacin Treatment of Hypercholesterolemia in Children." *Pediatrics*, 1993, 92(1):78-82.

Daniels SR, Greer FR, and Committee on Nutrition, "Lipid Screening and Cardiovascular Health in Childhood," *Pediatrics*, 2008, 122(1):198-208.

"Dietary Reference Intakes for Thiamin, Riboflavin, Niacin, Vitamin B6, Folate, Vitamin B12, Pantothenic Acid, Biotin and Choline. Standing Committee on the Scientific Evaluation of Dietary Reference Intakes, Food and Nutrition Board, Institute of Medicine," National Academy of Sciences, Washington, DC: National Academy Press, 1998. Available at http://www.nap.edu.

Hegyi J, Schwartz RA, and Hegyi V, "Pellagra: Dermatitis, Dementia, and Diarrhea," *Int J Dermatol*, 2004, 43(1):1-5.

McCrindle BW, Urbina EM, Dennison BA, et al, "Drug Therapy of High-Risk Lipid Abnormalities in Children and Adolescents: A Scientific Statement from the American Heart Association Atherosclerosis, Hypertension, and Obesity in Youth Committee, Council of Cardiovascular Disease in the Young, With the Council on Cardiovascular Nursing," *Circulation*, 2007, 115(14):1948-67.

Schuna AA, "Safe Use of Niacin," *Am J Health Syst Pharm*, 1997, 54(24):2803.

"Third Report of The National Cholesterol Education Program (NCEP) Expert Panel on Detection, Evaluation, and Treatment of High Blood Cholesterol in Adults (Adult Treatment Panel III)," May 2001, www.nhlbi.nih.gov/guidelines/cholesterol.

◆ **Niacin-50 [OTC]** *see* Niacin *on page 1491*

◆ **Niacor** *see* Niacin *on page 1491*

◆ **Niaspan** *see* Niacin *on page 1491*

◆ **Niaspan FCT (Can)** *see* Niacin *on page 1491*

◆ **Niastase® (Can)** *see* Factor VIIa (Recombinant) *on page 831*

◆ **Niastase® RT (Can)** *see* Factor VIIa (Recombinant) *on page 831*

NiCARdipine (nye KAR de peen)

Medication Safety Issues

Sound-alike/look-alike issues:

NiCARdipine may be confused with niacinamide, NIFEdipine, niMODipine

◀ Cardene may be confused with Cardizem, Cardura, codeine

Administration issues:
Significant differences exist between oral and I.V. dosing. Use caution when converting from one route of administration to another.

International issues:
Cardene [U.S., Great Britain, Netherlands] may be confused with Cardem brand name for celiprolol [Spain]; Cardin brand name for simvastatin [Poland]

Related Information
Oral Medications That Should Not Be Crushed or Altered *on page 2438*

Brand Names: U.S. Cardene IV; Cardene SR

Therapeutic Category Antianginal Agent; Antihypertensive Agent; Calcium Channel Blocker; Calcium Channel Blocker, Dihydropyridine

Generic Availability (U.S.) May be product dependent

Use
Oral:
Immediate release product: Treatment of chronic stable angina and treatment of hypertension (FDA approved in adults)
Sustained release product: Treatment of hypertension (FDA approved in adults)
Parenteral: Short-term treatment of hypertension when oral treatment is not feasible (FDA approved in adults)

Pregnancy Risk Factor C

Pregnancy Considerations Adverse events were observed in some animal reproduction studies. Nicardipine has been used for the treatment of severe hypertension in pregnancy and preterm labor. Nicardipine crosses the placenta; changes in fetal heart rate, neonatal hypotension and neonatal acidosis have been observed following maternal use (rare; based on limited data). Adverse effects reported in pregnant women are generally similar to those reported in nonpregnant patients; however, pulmonary edema has been observed (Nij, 2010). Untreated chronic maternal hypertension is also associated with adverse events in the fetus, infant, and mother. If treatment for hypertension during pregnancy is needed, other agents are preferred (ACOG, 2013).

Breast-Feeding Considerations Nicardipine is minimally excreted into breast milk. Per the manufacturer, the possibility of infant exposure should be considered. In one study, peak milk concentrations ranged from 1.9-18.8 mcg/mL following oral maternal doses of 40-150 mg/day. The estimated exposure to the breast-feeding infant was calculated to be 0.073% of the weight-adjusted maternal oral dose or 0.14% of the weight-adjusted maternal I.V. dose. Adverse events were not noted in the infants.

Contraindications Hypersensitivity to nicardipine or any component; advanced aortic stenosis

Warnings Symptomatic hypotension with or without syncope may occur; monitor blood pressure carefully during initiation and dose titration; lowering of blood pressure should be done at a rate appropriate for the patient's condition; rapid drops in blood pressure may lead to arterial insufficiency; avoid systemic hypotension in patients following an acute cerebral infarct or hemorrhage.

Nicardipine may increase frequency, duration, or severity of angina or precipitate acute MI during initiation of therapy or dosage increase in patients with severe obstructive coronary artery disease. Titrate dosage slowly if utilizing I.V. nicardipine in patients with heart failure (HF).

Immediate release nicardipine capsules contain propylene glycol; toxicities have been reported with use of products containing propylene glycol, including hyperosmolality, lactic acidosis, seizures, and respiratory depression; in neonates large amounts of propylene glycol delivered orally, intravenously (eg, >3000 mg/day), or topically have

been associated with potentially fatal toxicities which can include metabolic acidosis, seizures, renal failure, and CNS depression; use ccapsules containing propylene glycol with caution (AAP, 1997; Shehab, 2009).

Precautions Use with caution and carefully titrate the dose in patients with heart failure or severe left ventricular dysfunction, particularly with concomitant beta-blockade; may experience worsened symptoms of heart failure due to mild negative inotropic effects of nicardipine. Use with caution in patients with hypertrophic cardiomyopathy with outflow tract obstruction; reduction in afterload may worsen symptoms. Titrate dose cautiously in patients with renal impairment due to reduced clearance. Use with caution and decrease the starting dose for patients with severe hepatic dysfunction and reduced hepatic blood flow; nicardipine is metabolized hepatically. Use with caution in patients with mild to moderate aortic stenosis; may reduce coronary perfusion resulting in ischemia. Use is contraindicated in patients with advanced aortic stenosis. Peripheral infusion sites (for I.V. therapy) should be changed every 12 hours to minimize venous irritation; central or large peripheral veins preferred. Abrupt withdrawal may cause rebound angina in patients with CAD. Use of immediate release product for treatment of hypertension may result in relatively large differences in peak and trough blood pressures (compared to sustained release product).

Adverse Reactions
Cardiovascular: Chest pain (I.V.), ECG abnormal, extrasystoles (I.V.), flushing, hemopericardium (I.V.), hyper-/hypotension (I.V.), increased angina (dose related), orthostasis, palpitation, peripheral edema (dose related), supraventricular tachycardia (I.V), syncope, tachycardia, vasodilation, ventricular extrasystoles (I.V.), ventricular tachycardia (I.V.)
Central nervous system: Dizziness, headache, hypoesthesia, intracranial hemorrhage, pain, somnolence
Dermatologic: Rash
Endocrine & metabolic: Hypokalemia (I.V.)
Gastrointestinal: Abdominal pain (I.V.), dry mouth, dyspepsia, nausea, vomiting (I.V.)
Genitourinary: Polyuria
Local: Injection site pain/reaction
Neuromuscular & skeletal: Myalgia, paresthesia, weakness
Renal: Hematuria
Respiratory: Dyspnea
Miscellaneous: Diaphoresis
Rare but important or life-threatening: Abnormal ECG, allergic reaction, constipation, deep vein thrombophlebitis; ECG effects (AV block, inverted T wave, ST segment depression); gingival hyperplasia, hypophosphatemia, insomnia, malaise, nervousness, nocturia, parotitis, thrombocytopenia, tinnitus, tremor, ventricular extrasystoles

Drug Interactions
Metabolism/Transport Effects Substrate of CYP1A2 (minor), CYP2C9 (minor), CYP2D6 (minor), CYP2E1 (minor), CYP3A4 (major), P-glycoprotein; **Note:** Assignment of Major/Minor substrate status based on clinically relevant drug interaction potential; **Inhibits** CYP2C19 (moderate), CYP2C9 (strong), CYP2D6 (moderate), CYP3A4 (strong), P-glycoprotein
Avoid Concomitant Use
Avoid concomitant use of NiCARdipine with any of the following: Ado-Trastuzumab Emtansine; Alfuzosin; Apixaban; Avanafil; Axitinib; Bosutinib; Cabozantinib; Ceritinib; Conivaptan; Crizotinib; Dronedarone; Eplerenone; Everolimus; Fusidic Acid (Systemic); Halofantrine; Ibrutinib; Ivabradine; Lapatinib; Lomitapide; Lovastatin; Lurasidone; Macitentan; Nilotinib; Nisoldipine; PAZOPanib; Pimozide; Ranolazine; Red Yeast Rice; Regorafenib; Rivaroxaban; Salmeterol; Silodosin; Simeprevir; Simvastatin; Tamsulosin; Thioridazine; Ticagrelor; Tolvaptan;

Topotecan; Toremifene; Ulipristal; Vemurafenib; VinCRIStine (Liposomal); Vorapaxar

Increased Effect/Toxicity

NiCARdipine may increase the levels/effects of: AdoTrastuzumab Emtansine; Afatinib; Alfuzosin; Almotriptan; Alosetron; Amifostine; Antihypertensives; Apixaban; ARIPiprazole; Atosiban; Avanafil; Axitinib; Bedaquiline; BetaBlockers; Bortezomib; Bosentan; Bosutinib; Brentuximab Vedotin; Brinzolamide; Budesonide (Nasal); Budesonide (Systemic, Oral Inhalation); Cabozantinib; Cannabis; Carvedilol; Ceritinib; Citalopram; Colchicine; Conivaptan; Corticosteroids (Orally Inhaled); Crizotinib; CYP2C19 Substrates; CYP2C9 Substrates; CYP2D6 Substrates; CYP3A4 Substrates; Dabigatran Etexilate; Diclofenac (Systemic); Dienogest; DOXOrubicin (Conventional); Dronabinol; Dronedarone; DULoxetine; Dutasteride; Eplerenone; Everolimus; FentaNYL; Fesoterodine; Fluticasone (Nasal); Fluticasone (Oral Inhalation); Fosphenytoin; GuanFACINE; Halofantrine; Highest Risk QTcProlonging Agents; Hypotensive Agents; Ibrutinib; Iloperidone; Imatinib; Ivabradine; Ivacaftor; Ixabepilone; Lacosamide; Lapatinib; Levomilnacipran; Lomitapide; Lovastatin; Lurasidone; Macitentan; Magnesium Salts; Maraviroc; MethylPREDNISolone; Metoprolol; Mifepristone; Moderate Risk QTc-Prolonging Agents; Nebivolol; Neuromuscular-Blocking Agents (Nondepolarizing); Nilotinib; Nisoldipine; Nitroprusside; Obinutuzumab; Ospemifene; OxyCODONE; Paricalcitol; PAZOPanib; Pglycoprotein/ABCB1 Substrates; Phenytoin; Pimecrolimus; Pimozide; PONATinib; Propafenone; Propranolol; Prucalopride; QUEtiapine; Ranolazine; Red Yeast Rice; Regorafenib; Repaglinide; Rifaximin; Rilpivirine; RiTUXimab; Rivaroxaban; RomiDEPsin; Ruxolitinib; Salmeterol; Saxagliptin; Sildenafil; Silodosin; Simeprevir; Simvastatin; SORAfenib; Tadalafil; Tamsulosin; Tetrahydrocannabinol; Thioridazine; Ticagrelor; Tofacitinib; Tolterodine; Tolvaptan; Topotecan; Toremifene; Ulipristal; Vardenafil; Vemurafenib; Vilazodone; VinCRIStine (Liposomal); Vorapaxar; Zuclopenthixol

The levels/effects of NiCARdipine may be increased by: Alpha1-Blockers; Antifungal Agents (Azole Derivatives, Systemic); Barbiturates; Brimonidine (Topical); Cannabis; Conivaptan; CYP3A4 Inhibitors (Moderate); CYP3A4 Inhibitors (Strong); Diazoxide; Fluconazole; Fusidic Acid (Systemic); Grapefruit Juice; Herbs (Hypotensive Properties); Luliconazole; Macrolide Antibiotics; Magnesium Salts; MAO Inhibitors; Mifepristone; Pentoxifylline; P-glycoprotein/ABCB1 Inhibitors; Propafenone; Prostacyclin Analogues; Protease Inhibitors; Stiripentol

Decreased Effect

NiCARdipine may decrease the levels/effects of: Clopidogrel; Codeine; Ifosfamide; Prasugrel; Tamoxifen; Ticagrelor

The levels/effects of NiCARdipine may be decreased by: Barbiturates; Bosentan; Calcium Salts; CarBAMazepine; CYP3A4 Inducers (Strong); Dabrafenib; Deferasirox; Efavirenz; Herbs (Hypertensive Properties); Melatonin; Methylphenidate; Mitotane; Nafcillin; Peginterferon Alfa-2b; P-glycoprotein/ABCB1 Inducers; Rifamycin Derivatives; Siltuximab; St Johns Wort; Tocilizumab; Yohimbine

Food Interactions Nicardipine average peak concentrations may be decreased if taken with food. Serum concentrations/toxicity of nicardipine may be increased by grapefruit juice. Management: Avoid grapefruit juice.

Stability

Capsules:
Immediate release: Store at 20°C to 25°C (68°F to 77°F); dispense in light-resistant container.
Sustained release: Store at 15°C to 30°C (59°F to 86°F); dispense in light-resistant container.

Injection:
Ampuls: Store at 20°C to 25°C (68°F to 77°F); protect from light. Store ampuls in carton before use; avoid exposure to elevated temperatures; freezing does not affect stability. Diluted solution (100 mcg/mL) is stable for 24 hours in glass or PVC containers at room temperature. Stability has also been demonstrated at room temperature at concentrations up to 0.5 mg/mL in PVC containers for 24 hours or in glass containers for up to 7 days (Baaske, 1996).
Premixed solution: Store at 20°C to 25°C (68°F to 77°F); protect from light. Store in carton until ready to use; avoid exposure to excessive heat; protect from freezing.

Mechanism of Action Inhibits calcium ion from entering the "slow channels" or select voltage-sensitive areas of vascular smooth muscle and myocardium during depolarization, producing a relaxation of coronary vascular smooth muscle and coronary vasodilation; increases myocardial oxygen delivery in patients with vasospastic angina

Pharmacodynamics Antihypertensive effects:
Onset of action:
I.V.: Within minutes
Oral: 0.5-2 hours
Maximum effect:
Immediate capsules: 1-2 hours
Sustained release capsules (at steady state): Sustained from 2-6 hours postdose
I.V. continuous infusion: 50% of the maximum effect is seen by 45 minutes
Duration:
Immediate release capsules: <8 hours
Sustained release capsules: 12 hours
I.V.: ≤8 hours
Continuous infusion: Upon discontinuation, a 50% decrease in effect is seen in ~30 minutes with gradual discontinuing antihypertensive effects for ~50 hours.

Pharmacokinetics (Adult data unless noted) Absorption: Oral: ~100%, but large first-pass effect
Distribution: V_d: Adults: 8.3 L/kg
Protein binding: >95%
Metabolism: Extensive, saturable, first-pass effect; dosedependent (nonlinear) pharmacokinetics; extensive hepatic metabolism; major pathway is via cytochrome P450 isoenzyme CYP3A4
Bioavailability: Oral: 35%
Half-life: Follows dose-dependent (nonlinear) pharmacokinetics; "apparent" or calculated half-life is dependent upon serum concentrations. Half-life over the first 8 hours after oral dosing is 2-4 hours; terminal half-life (oral): 8.6 hours. After I.V. infusion, serum concentrations decrease tri-exponentially; alpha half-life: 2.7 minutes; beta halflife: 44.8 minutes; terminal half-life: 14.4 hours (**Note:** Terminal half-life can only be seen after long-term infusions)
Time to peak serum concentration: Oral:
Immediate release capsule: 30-120 minutes (mean: 1 hour)
Sustained release capsule: 1-4 hours
Elimination: Urine (oral: 60% as metabolites; I.V.: 49% as metabolites; <1% as unchanged drug); feces (oral: 35%; I.V.: 43%)
Clearance: Decreased in patients with hepatic dysfunction; may be decreased in patients with renal impairment

Dosing: Neonatal Note: Oral and I.V. doses are **not** equivalent on a mg per mg basis; limited data available.
Hypertension: Continuous I.V. infusion: Initial: 0.5 mcg/kg/minute was used in one prospective, open-label study of 20 hypertensive neonates (15 preterm; median PNA: 15 days). Doses were titrated according to blood pressure; the mean maximal required dose was 0.74 ± 0.41 mcg/kg/minute (range: 0.5-2 mcg/kg/minute) and occurred at 12 ± 19 hours of nicardipine infusion. The ▶

median duration of treatment was 11 days (range: 2-43 days) (Milou, 2000). Similar doses were required in a smaller study of eight preterm infants and in one case report of a neonate who received ECMO therapy (Gouyon, 1997; McBride, 2003).

Dosing: Usual Note: Oral and I.V. doses are **not** equivalent on a mg per mg basis.

Infants, Children, and Adolescents: **Hypertension:**

Continuous I.V. infusion: **Note:** Use should be reserved for severe hypertension: Limited data available: Initial: 0.5-1 mcg/kg/minute; titrate dose according to blood pressure; rate of infusion may be increased every 15-30 minutes; usual dose: 1-3 mcg/kg/minute; maximum dose: 4-5 mcg/kg/minute (Flynn, 2000; Flynn, 2001; NHBPEP, 2004). In a retrospective analysis (n=29; mean age: 7.8 years; age range: 2 days to 18 years), the mean effective dose was 1.8 ± 0.3 mcg/kg/minute (range: 0.3-4 mcg/kg/minute); blood pressure was controlled within 2.7 ± 2.1 hours (range: 0.5-9 hours) after starting nicardipine continuous infusion (Flynn, 2001).

Alternate dosing (high dose): Infants and Children: Initial dose: 5 mcg/kg/minute; once blood pressure controlled, decrease to a lower maintenance dose. Mean maintenance doses reported: PICU patients (n=10): 2.4 mcg/kg/minute (range: 1-5 mcg/kg/minute); postop cardiac patients (n=9, age range: 6 days to 9 years; mean age: 3.3 years): 3 mcg/kg/minute (range: 2.1-5.5 mcg/kg/minute) (Tobias, 2001)

Oral: Adolescents: Very limited data available: dose not established: One case report used 20 mg every 8 hours in a 14-year old boy following cardiac transplant (Larsen, 1994). Another case transitioned from a continuous infusion (1-4 mcg/kg/minute) to oral dose of 30 mg every 8 hours in a 14-year old girl with renal disease (Michael, 1998).

Adults:

Angina: Immediate release: Oral: 20 mg 3 times daily; usual range: 60-120 mg/day; increase dose at 3-day intervals

Hypertension: Oral:

Immediate release: Initial: 20 mg 3 times daily; titrate to response; usual: 20-40 mg 3 times daily (allow 3 days between dose increases)

Sustained release: Initial: 30 mg twice daily, titrate up to 60 mg twice daily

Note: The total daily dose of immediate release product may not automatically be equivalent to the daily sustained release dose; use caution in converting.

Acute hypertension: I.V.: Initial: 5 mg/hour increased by 2.5 mg/hour every 5 minutes (for rapid titration) to every 15 minutes (for gradual titration) up to a maximum of 15 mg/hour; rapidly titrated patients, consider reduction to 3 mg/hour after response is achieved.

Substitution for oral nicardipine therapy (approximate equivalents):

Oral dose of 20 mg every 8 hours = 0.5 mg/hour I.V. infusion

Oral dose of 30 mg every 8 hours = 1.2 mg/hour I.V. infusion

Oral dose of 40 mg every 8 hours = 2.2 mg/hour I.V. infusion

Conversion to oral antihypertensive agent:

Oral antihypertensive other than nicardipine: Initiate at the same time that I.V. nicardipine is discontinued

Oral nicardipine: Initiate 1 hour prior to I.V. discontinuation

Dosing adjustment in renal impairment: Adults:

I.V.: There are no dosage adjustments provided in the manufacturer's labeling; titrate slowly; careful monitoring is warranted and dosing adjustment may be necessary.

Oral: Titrate dose carefully beginning with usual initial dose.

Dosing adjustment in hepatic impairment: Adults:

I.V.: There are no dosage adjustments provided in the manufacturer's labeling; however, nicardipine is extensively metabolized by the liver. Consider initiating at lower doses and titrating slowly; careful monitoring is warranted and dosing adjustment may be necessary.

Oral:

Immediate release: Initial dose: 20 mg twice daily; titrate dose carefully

Sustained release: There are no dosage adjustments provided in the manufacturer's labeling (has not been studied); however, nicardipine is extensively metabolized by the liver; use with caution; titrate dose slowly; careful monitoring is warranted and dosing adjustment may be necessary.

Usual Infusion Concentrations: Pediatric Note: Premixed solutions available

I.V. infusion: 100 mcg/mL **or** 500 mcg/mL

Administration

Oral: May be administered without regard to meals; avoid concurrent administration with high-fat meals. Swallow sustained release capsule whole; do not crush, break, or chew.

I.V.: Administer by slow I.V. continuous infusion through a central line or large peripheral vein; avoid extravasation. Peripheral infusion sites should be changed every 12 hours to minimize venous irritation.

Ampul: Must be diluted prior to administration; may dilute with D_5W, D_5W with KCl 40 mEq, D_5NS, $D_5^{1/2}NS$, NS, $^{1/2}NS$; manufacturer recommended concentration for infusion: 100 mcg/mL; one pediatric study used infusions of 500 mcg/mL in D_5W, NS, or other compatible solution (Flynn, 2001).

Premixed solution: No further dilution needed. For single use only, discard any unused portion. Use only if solution is clear; per manufacturer's labeling, do not to admix or run in the same line as other medications.

Monitoring Parameters Blood pressure, heart rate, hepatic and renal function; **Note:** Monitor blood pressure carefully during initiation of therapy and with dosage adjustments.

Immediate release product: Measure blood pressure at peak effects (1-2 hours after the dose) especially during initiation of therapy, and just prior to the next dose (to ensure control of blood pressure throughout dosing interval).

Sustained release product: Measure blood pressure 2-4 hours after the first dose or dosage increase and just prior to the next dose

I.V.: Monitor infusion site for extravasation; monitor blood pressure continuously during I.V. administration

Additional Information The sustained release capsule contains a powder component (containing 25% of the dose) and a spherical granule component (containing 75% of the dose). The I.V. product is buffered to a pH of 3.5.

Dosage Forms Excipient information presented when available (limited, particularly for generics); consult specific product labeling. [DSC] = Discontinued product

Capsule, Oral, as hydrochloride:

Generic: 20 mg, 30 mg

Capsule Extended Release 12 Hour, Oral, as hydrochloride:

Cardene SR: 30 mg [contains fd&c red #40]

Cardene SR: 60 mg [contains fd&c blue #2 (indigotine)]

Solution, Intravenous, as hydrochloride:

Cardene IV: 20 mg (200 mL); 40 mg (200 mL); 2.5 mg/mL (10 mL [DSC]); 40 mg (200 mL)

Generic: 2.5 mg/mL (10 mL)

References

American Academy of Pediatrics Committee on Drugs. "Inactive" ingredients in pharmaceutical products: update (subject review). *Pediatrics*. 1997;99(2):268-278.

American College of Obstetricians and Gynecologists (ACOG), "ACOG Practice Bulletin No. 125: Chronic Hypertension in Pregnancy," *Obstet Gynecol*, 2012, 119(2 Pt 1):396-407.

Baaske DM, DeMay JF, Latona CA, et al. Stability of nicardipine hydrochloride in intravenous solutions. *Am J Health Syst Pharm*. 1996;53(14):1701-1705.

Chobanian AV, Bakris GL, Black HR, et al, "The Seventh Report of the Joint National Committee on Prevention, Detection, Evaluation, and Treatment of High Blood Pressure: The JNC 7 Report," *JAMA*, 2003, 289(19):2560-71.

Flynn JT and Pasko DA, "Calcium Channel Blockers: Pharmacology and Place in Therapy of Pediatric Hypertension," *Pediatr Nephrol*, 2000, 15(3-4):302-16.

Flynn JT, Mottes TA, Brophy PD, et al, "Intravenous Nicardipine for Treatment of Severe Hypertension in Children," *J Pediatr*, 2001, 139 (1):38-43.

Gouyon JB, Geneste B, Semama DS, et al, "Intravenous Nicardipine in Hypertensive Preterm Infants," *Arch Dis Child Fetal Neonatal Ed*, 1997, 76(2):F126-7.

Larsen A and Tobias J, "Nicardipine for the Treatment of Hypertension Following Cardiac Transplantation in a 14-Year-Old Boy," *Clin Pediatr (Phila)*, 1994, 33(5):309-11.

McBride BF, White CM, Campbell M, et al, "Nicardipine to Control Neonatal Hypertension During Extracorporeal Membrane Oxygen Support," *Ann Pharmacother*, 2003, 37(5):667-70.

Michael J, Groshong T, and Tobias JD, "Nicardipine for Hypertensive Emergencies in Children With Renal Disease," *Pediatr Nephrol*, 1998, 12(1):40-2.

Milou C, Debuche-Benouachkou V, Semama DS, et al, "Intravenous Nicardipine as a First-Line Antihypertensive Drug in Neonates," *Intensive Care Med*, 2000, 26(7):956-8.

Nakagawa TA, Sartori SC, Morris A, et al, "Intravenous Nicardipine for Treatment of Postcoarctectomy Hypertension in Children," *Pediatr Cardiol*, 2004, 25(1):26-30.

National High Blood Pressure Education Program (NHBPEP) Working Group on High Blood Pressure in Children and Adolescents. The fourth report on the diagnosis, evaluation, and treatment of high blood pressure in children and adolescents. *Pediatrics*. 2004;114(2 Suppl 4th Report):555-576.

Nij Bijvank SW and Duvekot JJ, "Nicardipine for the Treatment of Severe Hypertension in Pregnancy: A Review of the Literature," *Obstet Gynecol Surv*, 2010, 65(5):341-7.

Shehab N, Lewis CL, Streetman DD, Donn SM. Exposure to the pharmaceutical excipients benzyl alcohol and propylene glycol among critically ill neonates. *Pediatr Crit Care Med*. 2009;10 (2):256-259.

Steele RM, Schuna AA, and Schreiber RT, "Calcium Antagonist-Induced Gingival Hyperplasia," *Ann Intern Med*, 1994, 120(8):663-4.

Tobias JD, "Nicardipine to Control Mean Arterial Pressure After Cardiothoracic Surgery in Infants and Children," *Am J Ther*, 2001, 8 (1):3-6.

Treluyer JM, Hubert P, Jouvet P, et al, "Intravenous Nicardipine in Hypertensive Children," *Eur J Pediatr*, 1993, 152(9):712-4.

◆ **Nicardipine Hydrochloride** *see* NiCARdipine *on page 1493*

◆ **NicAzelDoxy 30** *see* Doxycycline *on page 721*

◆ **NicAzelDoxy 60** *see* Doxycycline *on page 721*

◆ **Nicotinic Acid** *see* Niacin *on page 1491*

◆ **Nidagel (Can)** *see* MetroNIDAZOLE (Topical) *on page 1404*

◆ **Nifediac CC** *see* NIFEdipine *on page 1497*

◆ **Nifedical XL** *see* NIFEdipine *on page 1497*

NIFEdipine (nye FED i peen)

Medication Safety Issues

Sound-alike/look-alike issues:

NIFEdipine may be confused with niCARdipine, niMODipine, nisoldipine

Procardia XL may be confused with Cartia XT

BEERS Criteria medication:

This drug may be potentially inappropriate for use in geriatric patients (Quality of evidence - high; Strength of recommendation - strong).

International issues:

Depin [India] may be confused with Depen brand name for penicillamine [U.S.]; Depon brand name for acetaminophen [Greece]; Dipen brand name for diltiazem [Greece]

Nipin [Italy and Singapore] may be confused with Nipent brand name for pentostatin [U.S., Canada, and multiple international markets]

Related Information

Medications for Which a Single Dose May Be Fatal When Ingested by a Toddler *on page 2408*

Oral Medications That Should Not Be Crushed or Altered *on page 2438*

Brand Names: U.S. Adalat CC; Afeditab CR; Nifediac CC; Nifedical XL; Procardia; Procardia XL

Brand Names: Canada Adalat XL; Apo-Nifed PA; Mylan-Nifedipine Extended Release; PMS-Nifedipine

Therapeutic Category Antianginal Agent; Antihypertensive Agent; Calcium Channel Blocker; Calcium Channel Blocker, Dihydropyridine

Generic Availability (U.S.) Yes

Use

Immediate release: Treatment of chronic stable or vasospastic angina (FDA approved in adults); has also been used for treatment of hypertensive emergency in pediatric patients and high altitude pulmonary edema

Extended release:

Adalat® CC, Afeditab® CR, Nifediac CC®: Treatment of hypertension alone or in combinations with other hypertensive agents (FDA approved in adults)

Procardia XL®, Nifedical XL®: Treatment of chronic stable or vasospastic angina (FDA approved in adults); treatment of hypertension alone or in combination with other antihypertensive agents (FDA approved in adults)

Pregnancy Risk Factor C

Pregnancy Considerations Adverse events were observed in animal reproduction studies. Nifedipine crosses the placenta and small amounts can be detected in the urine of newborn infants (Manninen, 1991; Silberschmidt, 2008). An increase in perinatal asphyxia, cesarean delivery, prematurity, and intrauterine growth retardation have been reported following maternal use. Untreated chronic maternal hypertension is also associated with adverse events in the fetus, infant, and mother. If treatment for hypertension during pregnancy is needed, nifedipine is one of the preferred agents (ACOG, 2013; SOGC [Magee, 2008]).

Nifedipine has also been evaluated for the treatment of preterm labor. Tocolytics may be used for the short-term (48 hour) prolongation of pregnancy to allow for the administration of antenatal steroids and should not be used prior to fetal viability or when the risks of use to the fetus or mother are greater than the risk of preterm birth (ACOG, 2012). Nifedipine is ineffective for maintenance tocolytic therapy (ACOG, 2012; Roos, 2013).

Breast-Feeding Considerations Nifedipine is excreted into breast milk. Reported concentrations are low and similar to those in the maternal serum (Ehrenkranz, 1989; Manninen, 1991; Penny, 1989). Breast-feeding is not recommended by the U.S. manufacturer (Canadian labeling contraindicates use). Nifedipine has been used for the treatment of Raynaud's phenomenon of the nipple in breast-feeding mothers (Barrett, 2013; Wu, 2012).

Contraindications Hypersensitivity to nifedipine or any component; concomitant use with strong CYP3A4 inducers (eg, rifampin); cardiogenic shock; additionally in adults: Immediate release preparation for treatment of urgent or emergent hypertension (Chobanian, 2003) and acute MI (Antman, 2004)

Warnings Excessive hypotension may occur, especially during initiation of therapy or dosage increase (more common with concurrent beta-blocker therapy; monitor blood pressure closely); profound hypotension, MI, and death have been reported in adults when immediate release nifedipine has been used (orally or sublingually) for acute reduction of blood pressure (manufacturer does **not** recommend use of capsules for acute reduction of blood pressure); immediate release nifedipine is not FDA approved for long-term control of primary hypertension (appropriate studies to determine optimal dose or dosing interval have not been conducted). Mild to moderate peripheral edema may occur. Some dosage forms (eg, Adalat® CC and Nifediac CC®) tablets contain lactose; do not use with galactose intolerance, Lapp lactase deficiency, or glucose-galactose malabsorption syndromes

Precautions Use with caution in cirrhotic patients as clearance of nifedipine is reduced, leading to increased systemic exposure; monitor closely for adverse effects or toxicity and consider dose adjustments. May increase frequency, duration, and severity of angina or precipitate acute MI during initiation of therapy. Use with caution in patients with CHF or aortic stenosis (especially with concomitant beta-blocker). Use with caution in patients taking CYP3A4 inhibitors; may result in increased nifedipine concentrations; monitor for adverse effects/toxicity and consider dose adjustments. Use with strong CYP3A4 inducers (eg, rifampin, rifabutin, phenobarbital, phenytoin, carbamazepine, and St John's wort) is contraindicated due to reduced bioavailability and efficacy.

Use extended release dosage forms with caution in patients with alterations in GI anatomy (eg, severe GI narrowing, history of GI cancer, obstruction, bowel resection, gastric bypass, vertical banded gastroplasty, colostomy), hypomotility disorders (constipation, GERD, ileus, obesity, hypothyroidism, diabetes), and concomitant medications (H$_2$ blockers, NSAIDs, laxatives, anticholinergic agents, levothyroxine); use of extended release forms have led to serious GI obstruction and (in rare cases) bezoars.

Adverse Reactions

Cardiovascular: CHF, flushing, palpitation, peripheral edema (dose related), transient hypotension (dose related)

Central nervous system: Chills difficulties in balance, dizziness, fatigue, fever, giddiness, headache, jitteriness, lightheadedness, mood changes, nervousness, shakiness, sleep disturbances

Dermatologic: Dermatitis, pruritus, urticaria

Endocrine & metabolic: Sexual difficulties

Gastrointestinal: Constipation, cramps, diarrhea, flatulence, gingival hyperplasia, heartburn, nausea

Neuromuscular & skeletal: inflammation, joint stiffness, muscle cramps, tremor, weakness

Ocular: Blurred vision

Respiratory: Chest congestion, cough, dyspnea, nasal congestion, sore throat, wheezing

Miscellaneous: Diaphoresis

Rare but important or life-threatening: Agranulocytosis, allergic hepatitis, alopecia, anemia, angina, angioedema, aplastic anemia, arrhythmia, arthritis with positive ANA, bezoars (Procardia XL®), cerebral ischemia, depression, dysosmia, epistaxis, EPS, erectile dysfunction, erythema multiforme, erythromelalgia, exanthematous pustulosis, exfoliative dermatitis, facial edema, gastroesophageal reflux, gastrointestinal obstruction (Procardia XL®), gastrointestinal ulceration (Procardia XL®), gynecomastia, hematuria, ischemia, leukopenia, lip cancer (Friedman, 2012), memory dysfunction, migraine, myalgia, myoclonus, nocturia, paranoid syndrome, parotitis, periorbital edema, photosensitivity, polyuria, purpura, Stevens-Johnson syndrome, syncope, tachycardia, taste perversion, thrombocytopenia, tinnitus, toxic epidermal necrolysis, transient blindness, ventricular arrhythmia

Reported with use of sublingual short-acting nifedipine: Acute MI, cerebrovascular ischemia, ECG changes, fetal distress, heart block, severe hypotension, sinus arrest, stroke, syncope

Drug Interactions

Metabolism/Transport Effects Substrate of CYP2D6 (minor), CYP3A4 (major); **Note:** Assignment of Major/Minor substrate status based on clinically relevant drug interaction potential; **Inhibits** CYP1A2 (weak), CYP2C9 (weak), CYP2D6 (weak), CYP3A4 (weak)

Avoid Concomitant Use

Avoid concomitant use of NIFEdipine with any of the following: Conivaptan; CYP3A4 Inducers (Strong); Fusidic Acid (Systemic); Grapefruit Juice; Pimozide

Increased Effect/Toxicity

NIFEdipine may increase the levels/effects of: Amifostine; Antihypertensives; ARIPiprazole; Atosiban; Beta-Blockers; Calcium Channel Blockers (Nondihydropyridine); Digoxin; Dofetilide; DULoxetine; Hypotensive Agents; Lomitapide; Magnesium Salts; Neuromuscular-Blocking Agents (Nondepolarizing); Nitroprusside; Obinutuzumab; Pimozide; QuiNIDine; RiTUXimab; Tacrolimus (Systemic); VinCRIStine; VinCRIStine (Liposomal)

The levels/effects of NIFEdipine may be increased by: Alcohol (Ethyl); Alfuzosin; Alpha1-Blockers; Antifungal Agents (Azole Derivatives, Systemic); Barbiturates; Brimonidine (Topical); Calcium Channel Blockers (Nondihydropyridine); Ceritinib; Cimetidine; Cisapride; Conivaptan; CycloSPORINE (Systemic); CYP3A4 Inhibitors (Moderate); CYP3A4 Inhibitors (Strong); Dasatinib; Diazoxide; Fluconazole; FLUoxetine; Fusidic Acid (Systemic); Grapefruit Juice; Herbs (Hypotensive Properties); Ivacaftor; Luliconazole; Macrolide Antibiotics; Magnesium Salts; MAO Inhibitors; Mifepristone; Pentoxifylline; Phosphodiesterase 5 Inhibitors; Prostacyclin Analogues; Protease Inhibitors; QuiNIDine; Simeprevir; Stiripentol

Decreased Effect

NIFEdipine may decrease the levels/effects of: Clopidogrel; QuiNIDine

The levels/effects of NIFEdipine may be decreased by: Barbiturates; Bosentan; Calcium Salts; CYP3A4 Inducers (Strong); Dabrafenib; Deferasirox; Efavirenz; Herbs (Hypertensive Properties); Melatonin; Methylphenidate; Peginterferon Alfa-2b; Siltuximab; St Johns Wort; Tocilizumab; Yohimbine

Food Interactions Nifedipine serum levels may be decreased if taken with food. Food may decrease the rate but not the extent of absorption of Procardia XL®. Increased nifedipine concentrations resulting in therapeutic and vasodilator side effects, including severe hypotension and myocardial ischemia, may occur if nifedipine is taken by patients ingesting grapefruit. Management: Avoid grapefruit/grapefruit juice.

Stability

Adalat® CC, Afeditab® CR, Procardia XL®: Store below 30°C (86°F); protect from light and moisture.

Nifediac CC®, Nifedical XL®: Store at 25°C (77°F); excursions permitted to 15°C to 30°C (59°F to 86°F); protect from light and moisture.

Immediate release capsules (Procardia®): Store at 15°C to 25°C (59°F to 77°F); prevent capsules from freezing; protect from light and moisture.

Mechanism of Action Inhibits calcium ion from entering the "slow channels" or select voltage-sensitive areas of vascular smooth muscle and myocardium during depolarization, producing a relaxation of coronary vascular smooth muscle and coronary vasodilation; increases myocardial oxygen delivery in patients with vasospastic angina; also reduces peripheral vascular resistance, producing a reduction in arterial blood pressure.

Pharmacodynamics

Onset of action:

"Bite and swallow": Within 1-5 minutes

Oral:

Immediate release: Within 20-30 minutes

Extended release: 2.5-5 hours

Duration:

Immediate release: 4-8 hours

Extended release: 24 hours

Pharmacokinetics (Adult data unless noted)

Protein-binding: 92% to 98% (concentration-dependent); **Note:** Protein-binding may be significantly decreased in patients with renal or hepatic impairment

Metabolism: Hepatic via CYP3A4 to inactive metabolites

Bioavailability: Capsule: 40% to 77%; Extended release: 84% to 89% relative to immediate release capsules; bioavailability increased with significant hepatic disease

Half-life: Adults:

Normal: Immediate release: 2-5 hours; Extended release: 7 hours

Cirrhosis: 7 hours

Elimination: Urine (60% to 80% as inactive metabolites); feces

Dosing: Usual

Children and Adolescents: **Note:** Doses are usually titrated upward over 7-14 days; may increase over 3 days if clinically necessary:

Hypertensive urgency: Immediate release: Oral or "bite and swallow" (eg, bite capsule to release liquid contents then swallow): 0.1-0.25 mg/kg/dose; maximum single dose: 10 mg; may repeat if needed every 4-6 hours; monitor carefully; typically reserved for inpatient use; maximum daily dose: 1-2 mg/kg/**day** (Blaszak, 2001; Egger, 2002; Singh, 2012). **Note:** Current pediatric blood pressure guidelines do not recommend use (NHBPEP, 2004).

Hypertension (chronic treatment): Extended release: Oral: Initial: 0.25-0.5 mg/kg/**day** given once daily or divided in 2 doses per **day**; do not exceed initial adult dose (30-60 mg/**day**); titrate dose to effect; maximum dose: 3 mg/kg/**day** up to 120 mg/**day** (NHBPEP, 2004; NHLBI, 2011); some centers use a higher maximum dose: 3 mg/kg/**day** up to 180 mg/**day** (Flynn, 2000)

High altitude pulmonary edema (Pollard, 2001): Limited data available: Children and Adolescents: **Note:** Reserve treatment with NIFEdipine for unsatisfactory response to oxygen and/or altitude descent: Oral:

Immediate release: 0.5 mg/kg/dose every 8 hours; maximum dose: 20 mg

Extended release (preferred): 1.5 mg/kg/day given once daily or divided in 2 doses per **day**; maximum dose: 40 mg

Adults: **Note:** Dosage adjustments should occur at 7- to 14-day intervals, to allow for adequate assessment of new dose; when switching from immediate release to sustained release formulations, use same total daily dose.

Chronic stable or vasospastic angina: Oral:

Immediate release: Initial: 10 mg 3 times daily; usual dose: 10-20 mg 3 times daily; coronary artery spasm may require up to 20-30 mg 3-4 times daily; single doses >30 mg and total daily doses >120 mg are rarely needed; maximum daily dose: 180 mg/**day**; **Note:** Do not use for acute anginal episodes; may precipitate myocardial infarction.

Extended release: Initial: 30 or 60 mg once daily; maximum: 120-180 mg/day

Hypertension: Oral: Extended release: Initial: 30 or 60 mg once daily; maximum: 90-120 mg/day

High altitude pulmonary edema (Luks, 2010): Oral:

Prevention: Extended release: 30 mg every 12 hours starting the day before ascent and may be discontinued after staying at the same elevation for 5 days or if descent initiated

Treatment: Extended release: 30 mg every 12 hours

Administration Oral:

Immediate release: Administer with or without food. Liquid-filled capsule may be punctured and drug solution administered orally. When nifedipine is administered sublingually, only a small amount is absorbed sublingually; the observed effects are actually due to swallowing of the drug with subsequent rapid oral absorption. When measuring smaller doses from the liquid-filled capsules, completely empty the capsule to determine the concentration (may vary based on strength and by manufacturer) and administer the appropriate volume for the desired dose; the following concentrations are for Procardia®: 10 mg capsule = 10 mg/0.34 mL; 20 mg capsule = 20 mg/0.45 mL

Extended release: Tablets should be swallowed whole; do not crush, break, chew, or divide. Adalat® CC, Afeditab® CR, Nifediac CC®: Administer on an empty stomach (per manufacturer); other extended release products may not have this recommendation; consult product labeling.

Monitoring Parameters

CBC, platelets, periodic liver enzymes; blood pressure, heart rate, signs and symptoms of CHF, peripheral edema

Dosage Forms

Excipient information presented when available (limited, particularly for generics); consult specific product labeling.

Capsule, Oral:

Procardia: 10 mg

Generic: 10 mg, 20 mg

Tablet Extended Release 24 Hour, Oral:

Adalat CC: 30 mg, 60 mg, 90 mg

Afeditab CR: 30 mg, 60 mg

Nifediac CC: 30 mg, 60 mg

Nifediac CC: 90 mg [contains tartrazine (fd&c yellow #5)]

Nifedical XL: 30 mg, 60 mg

Procardia XL: 30 mg, 60 mg, 90 mg

Generic: 30 mg, 60 mg, 90 mg

Extemporaneous Preparations

A 4 mg/mL oral suspension may be made with liquid capsules (**Note:** Concentration inside capsule may vary depending on manufacturer. Procardia: 10 mg capsule contains a concentration of 10 mg/0.34 mL [29.4 mg/mL]). Puncture the top of twelve 10 mg liquid capsules with one needle to create a vent. Insert a second needle attached to a syringe and extract the liquid; transfer to a calibrated bottle and add sufficient quantity of a 1:1 mixture of Ora-Sweet and Ora-Plus to make 30 mL. Label "shake well". Stable 90 days under refrigeration or at room temperature.

Nahata MC, Morosco RS, and Willhite EA, "Stability of Nifedipine in Two Oral Suspensions Stored at Two Temperatures," *J Am Pharm Assoc,* 2002, 42(6):865-7.

References

American College of Obstetricians and Gynecologists (ACOG), "ACOG Practice Bulletin No. 125: Chronic Hypertension in Pregnancy," *Obstet Gynecol,* 2012, 119(2 Pt 1):396-407.

American College of Obstetricians and Gynecologists (ACOG), "ACOG Practice Bulletin No. 127: "Management of Preterm Labor,"*Obstet Gynecol,* 2012, 119(6):1308.

Adcock KG and Wilson JT, "Nifedipine Labeling Illustrates the Pediatric Dilemma for Off-Patent Drugs," *Pediatrics,* 2002, 109(2):319-21.

Antman EM, Anbe DT, Armstrong PW, et al, "ACC/AHA Guidelines for the Management of Patients With ST-Elevation Myocardial Infarction: A Report of the American College of Cardiology/American Heart Association Task Force on Practice Guidelines (Committee to Revise the 1999 Guidelines for the Management of Patients With Acute Myocardial Infarction)," *Circulation,* 2004, 110(9):e82-292.

Barrett ME, Heller MM, Stone HF, et al, "Raynaud Phenomenon of the Nipple in Breastfeeding mothers: An Underdiagnosed Cause of Nipple Pain," *JAMA Dermatol,* 2013, 149(3):300-6.

Blaszak RT, Savage JA, and Ellis EN, "The Use of Short-Acting Nifedipine in Pediatric Patients With Hypertension," *J Pediatr*, 2001, 139(1):34-7.

Chobanian AV, Bakris GL, Black HR, et al, "The Seventh Report of the Joint National Committee on Prevention, Detection, Evaluation, and Treatment of High Blood Pressure: The JNC 7 report," *JAMA*, 2003, 289(19):2560-72.

Dilmen U, Cagfülar MK, Senses A, et al, "Nifedipine in Hypertensive Emergencies of Children," *Am J Dis Child*, 1983, 137(12):1162-5.

Egger DW, Deming DD, Hamada N, et al, "Evaluation of the Safety of Short-Acting Nifedipine in Children With Hypertension," *Pediatr Nephrol*, 2002, 17(1):35-40.

Ehrenkranz RA, Ackerman BA, and Hulse JD, "Nifedipine Transfer Into Human Milk," *J Pediatr*, 1989, 114(3):478-80.

Flynn JT and Pasko DA, "Calcium Channel Blockers: Pharmacology and Place in Therapy of Pediatric Hypertension," *Pediatr Nephrol*, 2000, 15(3-4):302-16.

Friedman GD, Asgari MM, Warton EM, et al, "Antihypertensive Drugs and Lip Cancer in Non-Hispanic Whites," *Arch Intern Med*, 2012, 6:1-6.

Lopez-Herce J, Albajara L, Cagigas P, et al, "Treatment of Hypertensive Crisis in Children With Nifedipine," *Intensive Care Med*, 1988, 14 (5):519-21.

Luks AM, McIntosh SE, Grissom CK, et al, "Wilderness Medical Society Consensus Guidelines for the Prevention and Treatment of Acute Altitude Illness," *Wilderness Environ Med*, 2010, 21(2):146-55.

Manninen AK and Juhakoski A, "Nifedipine Concentrations in Maternal and Umbilical Serum, Amniotic Fluid, Breast Milk and Urine of Mothers and Offspring," *Int J Clin Pharmacol Res*, 1991, 11(5):231-6.

National Heart, Lung, and Blood Institute, "Expert Panel on Integrated Guidelines for Cardiovascular Health and Risk Reduction in Children and Adolescents," *Clinical Practice Guidelines*, 2011, National Institutes of Health. Available at http://www.nhlbi.nih.gov/guidelines/cvd_ped/peds_guidelines_full.pdf. Accessed: June 11, 2012.

National High Blood Pressure Education Program Working Group on High Blood Pressure in Children and Adolescents, "The Fourth Report on the Diagnosis, Evaluation, and Treatment of High Blood Pressure in Children and Adolescents," *Pediatrics*, 2004, 114(2 Suppl):555-76.

Penny WJ and Lewis MJ, "Nifedipine Is Excreted in Human Milk," *Eur J Clin Pharmacol*, 1989, 36(4):427-8.

Pollard AJ, Niermeyer S, Barry P, et al, "Children at High Altitude: An International Consensus Statement by an Ad Hoc Committee of the International Society for Mountain Medicine, March 12, 2001," *High Alt Med Biol*, 2001, 2(3):389-403.

Roos C, Spaanderman ME, Schuit E, et al, "Effect of Maintenance Tocolysis With Nifedipine in Threatened Preterm Labor on Perinatal Outcomes: a Randomized Controlled Trial," *JAMA*, 2013, 309(1):41-7.

Rosen WJ and Johnson CE, "Evaluation of Five Procedures for Measuring Nonstandard Doses of Nifedipine Liquid," *Am J Hosp Pharm*, 1989, 46(11):2313-7.

Silberschmidt AL, Kuhn-Velten WN, Juon AM, et al, "Nifedipine Concentration in Maternal and Umbilical Cord Blood After Nifedipine Gastrointestinal Therapeutic System for Tocolysis," *BJOG*, 2008, 115(4):480-85.

Singh D, Akingbola O, Yosypiv I, et al, "Emergency Management of Hypertension in Children," *Int J Nephrol*, 2012, 2012:420247.

Yiu V, Orrbine E, Rosychuk RJ, et al, "The Safety and Use of Short-Acting Nifedipine in Hospitalized Hypertensive Children," *Pediatr Nephrol*, 2004, 19(6):644-50.

Wu M, Chason R, and Wong M, "Raynaud's Phenomenon of the Nipple," *Obstet Gynecol*, 2012, 119(2 Pt 2):447-9.

◆ **Nighttime Sleep Aid [OTC]** *see* DiphenhydrAMINE (Systemic) *on page 673*

◆ **Nimbex** *see* Cisatracurium *on page 479*

◆ **Niodan (Can)** *see* Niacin *on page 1491*

◆ **Nipent** *see* Pentostatin *on page 1644*

◆ **Nipent® (Can)** *see* Pentostatin *on page 1644*

◆ **Nipride (Can)** *see* Nitroprusside *on page 1507*

◆ **Niravam** *see* ALPRAZolam *on page 100*

◆ **Nitalapram** *see* Citalopram *on page 484*

Nitazoxanide (nye ta ZOX a nide)

Brand Names: U.S. Alinia
Therapeutic Category Antiprotozoal
Generic Availability (U.S.) No

Use Treatment of diarrhea caused by *Giardia lamblia* (FDA approved in ages ≥1 year and adults); treatment of diarrhea caused by *Cryptosporidium parvum* in immunocompetent patients (FDA approved in ages ≥1 year and adults); has also been used for the treatment of amebiasis, dwarf tapeworm infection, fluke infections, and refractory or recurrent *Clostridium difficile*-associated diarrhea

Pregnancy Risk Factor B

Pregnancy Considerations Teratogenic effects were not observed in animal reproduction studies.

Breast-Feeding Considerations It is not known if nitazoxanide is excreted in breast milk. The manufacturer recommends that caution be exercised when administering nitazoxanide to nursing women.

Contraindications Hypersensitivity to nitazoxanide or any component

Warnings Suspension contains sodium benzoate; benzoic acid (benzoate) is a metabolite of benzyl alcohol; large amounts of benzyl alcohol (≥99 mg/kg/day) have been associated with a potentially fatal toxicity ("gasping syndrome") in neonates; avoid use of sodium benzoate containing products in neonates; *in vitro* and animal studies have shown that benzoate displaces bilirubin from protein binding sites

Precautions Use with caution in patients with renal, hepatic, or biliary disease since pharmacokinetics of nitazoxanide have not been studied in these patients. Use suspension dosage form with caution in diabetic patients due to sucrose content.

Adverse Reactions

Central nervous system: Headache

Gastrointestinal: Abdominal pain, diarrhea, nausea, vomiting

Rare but important or life-threatening: Allergic reaction, ALT increased, anemia, anorexia, appetite increased, creatinine increased, diaphoresis, dizziness, eye discoloration (pale yellow), fever, flatulence, hypertension, infection, malaise, pruritus, rhinitis, salivary glands enlarged, tachycardia, urine discoloration

Drug Interactions

Metabolism/Transport Effects None known.

Avoid Concomitant Use There are no known interactions where it is recommended to avoid concomitant use.

Increased Effect/Toxicity There are no known significant interactions involving an increase in effect.

Decreased Effect There are no known significant interactions involving a decrease in effect.

Food Interactions Food increases AUC. Management: Take with food.

Stability

Suspension: Prior to and following reconstitution, store at 25°C (77°F); excursions permitted to 15°C to 30°C (59°F to 86°F). Following reconstitution, discard unused portion of suspension after 7 days.

Tablet: Store at 25°C (77°F); excursions permitted to 15°C to 30°C (59°F to 86°F).

Mechanism of Action Nitazoxanide is rapidly metabolized to the active metabolite tizoxanide *in vivo*. Activity may be due to interference with the pyruvate:ferredoxin oxidoreductase (PFOR) enzyme-dependent electron transfer reaction which is essential to anaerobic metabolism. *In vitro*, nitazoxanide and tizoxanide inhibit the growth of sporozoites and oocysts of *Cryptosporidium parvum* and trophozoites of *Giardia lamblia*.

Pharmacokinetics (Adult data unless noted) Note: In pediatric patients (1-18 years of age), pharmacokinetic properties similar to adult when dosed equivalently.

Protein binding: Tizoxanide: >99%

Metabolism: Hepatic, to an active metabolite, tizoxanide. Tizoxanide undergoes conjugation to form tizoxanide glucuronide. Nitazoxanide is not detectable in the serum following oral administration.

Bioavailability: Relative bioavailability of the suspension to the tablet is 70%; tablet and suspension are not bioequivalent

Half-life: Tizoxanide: 1-1.6 hours

Time to peak serum concentration: Tizoxanide: 1-4 hours

Elimination: Tizoxanide is excreted in urine (<10%), bile, and feces (60%); tizoxanide glucuronide is excreted in urine and bile

Dosing: Usual Oral:

Cryptosporidium parvum or *Giardia lamblia* treatment of diarrhea (**Note:** May consider increasing duration up to 14 days in HIV-exposed/HIV-infected patients (CDC, 2009):

Children 1-3 years: 100 mg every 12 hours for 3 days

Children 4-11 years: 200 mg every 12 hours for 3 days

Adolescents ≥12 years and Adults: 500 mg every 12 hours for 3 days

Fasciola hepatica (sheep liver fluke) (*Red Book*, 2009):

Children 1-3 years: 100 mg every 12 hours for 7 days

Children 4-11years: 200 mg every 12 hours for 7 days

Adolescents ≥12 years and Adults: 500 mg every 12 hours for 7 days

Hymenolepis nana (dwarf tapeworm) (*Red Book*, 2009):

Children 1-3 years: 100 mg twice daily for 3 days

Children 4-11 years: 200 mg twice daily for 3 days

Adults: 500 mg once or twice daily for 3 days

C. difficile-associated diarrhea: Adults: 500 mg every 12 hours for 7-10 days

Dosage adjustment in renal and/or hepatic impairment: Specific recommendations are not available; use with caution

Administration Minimize gastric irritation by administering with food; shake suspension well prior to use

Monitoring Parameters Periodic liver function tests, stool frequency

Additional Information The oral suspension contains sucrose 1.48 g/5 mL.

Dosage Forms Excipient information presented when available (limited, particularly for generics); consult specific product labeling.

Suspension Reconstituted, Oral:

Alinia: 100 mg/5 mL (60 mL) [contains fd&c red #40, sodium benzoate; strawberry flavor]

Tablet, Oral:

Alinia: 500 mg [contains fd&c blue #2 aluminum lake, fd&c yellow #10 aluminum lake, fd&c yellow #6 aluminum lake, soybean lecithin]

References

Bobak DA, "Use of Nitazoxanide for Gastrointestinal Tract Infections: Treatment of Protozoan Parasitic Infection and Beyond," *Curr Infect Dis Rep*, 2006, 8(2):91-5.

Centers for Disease Control and Prevention (CDC), "Guidelines for the Prevention and Treatment of Opportunistic Infections Among HIV-Exposed and HIV-Infected Children," *MMWR Recomm Rep*, 2009, 58(RR-11):1-166. Available at http://aidsinfo.nih.gov/contentfiles/Pediatric_OI.pdf

Red Book: 2009 Report of the Committee on Infectious Diseases, "Drugs for Parasitic Infections," 28th ed, Pickering LK, ed, Elk Grove Village, IL: American Academy of Pediatrics, 2009, 783-816.

◆ **Nithiodote** *see* Sodium Nitrite and Sodium Thiosulfate on page 1909

Nitisinone (ni TIS i known)

Brand Names: U.S. Orfadin

Therapeutic Category Tyrosinemia Type 1, Treatment Agent

Generic Availability (U.S.) No

Use Adjunct to dietary restriction of tyrosine and phenylalanine in the treatment of hereditary tyrosinemia type 1 (HT-1) (FDA approved in all ages)

Prescribing and Access Restrictions Distributed by Orfadin4U comprehensive patient support program.

Information regarding acquisition of product may be obtained by calling 877-473-3179. Additional information can be found at http://www.orfadin.com

Pregnancy Risk Factor C

Pregnancy Considerations Adverse events have been observed in animal reproduction studies.

Breast-Feeding Considerations It is not known if nitisinone is excreted in breast milk. Due to the potential for serious adverse reactions in the nursing infant, the manufacturer recommends a decision be made whether to discontinue nursing or to discontinue the drug, taking into account the importance of treatment to the mother.

Contraindications Hypersensitivity to nitisinone or any component

Warnings Nitisinone therapy should be initiated by individuals experienced in the management of inborn errors of metabolism including treatment of HT-1. Dietary restriction of tyrosine and phenylalanine must be used in conjunction with nitisinone; inadequate dietary restriction can result in increased plasma tyrosine concentrations leading to toxic ophthalmic effects (corneal ulcers, corneal opacities, keratitis, conjunctivitis, eye pain, and photophobia), skin effects (painful hyperkeratotic plaques on the soles and palms), and variable degrees of mental retardation and developmental delay. Nitisinone dosage should not be adjusted in order to lower the plasma tyrosine concentration. Transient thrombocytopenia and leukopenia has been reported; platelet and WBC counts should be monitored regularly during nitisinone therapy.

Precautions Slit-lamp examination of the eyes should be performed prior to initiation of nitisinone therapy; patients who develop photophobia, eye pain or signs of inflammation such as redness, swelling, or burning of the eyes during treatment should be re-examined and a plasma tyrosine concentration measured; if the plasma tyrosine concentration is >500 micromoles/L, a more tyrosine- and phenylalanine-restrictive diet is indicated. Patients with HT-1 are at risk for developing porphyric crises, liver failure, or hepatic neoplasm; regular liver monitoring by imaging (ultrasound, CT scan, MRI), liver function tests, and measurement of serum alpha-fetoprotein concentration is recommended; an increase in serum alpha-fetoprotein or signs of nodules in the liver during treatment may be a sign of inadequate therapy or hepatic malignancy.

Adverse Reactions

Dermatologic: Alopecia, dry skin, exfoliative dermatitis, maculopapular rash, pruritus

Hematologic: Epistaxis, granulocytopenia, leukopenia, porphyria, thrombocytopenia

Hepatic: Hepatic failure, hepatic neoplasm

Ocular: Blepharitis, cataracts, conjunctivitis, corneal opacity, eye pain, keratitis, photophobia

Rare but important or life-threatening: Abdominal pain, amenorrhea, brain tumor, bronchitis, corneal ulceration, cyanosis, dehydration, diarrhea, enanthema, encephalopathy, gastritis, gastroenteritis, gastrointestinal hemorrhage, headache, hepatic dysfunction, hepatomegaly, hyperkinesias, hypoglycemia, infection, liver enzymes increased, melena, nervousness, otitis, pathologic fracture, respiratory insufficiency, seizure, septicemia, somnolence, thirst, tooth discoloration, tyrosine levels increased

Drug Interactions

Metabolism/Transport Effects None known.

Avoid Concomitant Use There are no known interactions where it is recommended to avoid concomitant use.

Increased Effect/Toxicity There are no known significant interactions involving an increase in effect.

Decreased Effect There are no known significant interactions involving a decrease in effect.

Food Interactions Effect of taking with food is unknown. Tyrosine toxicity can occur without proper dietary restriction of tyrosine and phenylalanine. Management: Administer at least 1 hour prior to, or 2 hours after a meal. Dietary restriction of tyrosine and phenylalanine is required.

Stability Store in refrigerator 2°C to 8°C (36°F to 46°F)

Mechanism of Action In patients with HT-1, tyrosine metabolism is interrupted due to a lack of the enzyme (fumarylacetoacetate hydrolase) needed in the last step of tyrosine degradation. Toxic metabolites of tyrosine accumulate and cause liver and kidney toxicity. Nitisinone competitively inhibits 4-hydroxyphenyl-pyruvate dioxygenase, an enzyme present early in the tyrosine degradation pathway, thereby preventing the build-up of the toxic metabolites.

Pharmacokinetics (Adult data unless noted) Note: Limited pharmacokinetic studies exist in HT-1 patients.
Bioavailability: >90% (animal studies)
Half-life: 54 hours (healthy volunteers)
Time to peak serum concentration: 3 hours (healthy volunteers)
Excretion: Equal amounts in urine and feces (McKiernan, 2006)

Dosing: Usual Oral: HT-1: **Note:** Must be used in conjunction with a diet restricted in tyrosine and phenylalanine.
Infants, Children, and Adults: Initial: 1 mg/kg/day in two divided doses; adjust dose if inadequate response, as defined by continued abnormal biological parameters (erythrocyte PBG-synthase activity, urine 5-ALA, and urine succinylacetone) despite treatment. If the aforementioned parameters are not available, may use urine succinylacetone, liver function tests, alpha-fetoprotein, serum tyrosine, and serum phenylalanine to evaluate response (exceptions may include during initiation of therapy and exacerbations).
Abnormal biological parameters at 1 month: Increase dose to 1.5 mg/kg/day
Abnormal biological parameters at 3 months: Increase to maximum dose of 2 mg/kg/day

Administration Oral: Administer in two divided doses in the morning and evening, at least 1 hour prior to, or 2 hours after a meal. The total daily dose does not need to be split evenly; divide the total dose to limit the total number of capsules administered at each interval. Capsules may be opened and contents suspended in a small quantity of water, formula, or applesauce; use immediately.

Monitoring Parameters
Dietary tyrosine and phenylalanine intake; platelets, WBC, plasma and urine succinylacetone concentrations, serum alpha-fetoprotein, serum phosphate (if renal dysfunction), hepatic
Function (ultrasound, computerized tomography, magnetic resonance imaging)
Ophthalmic exam (Slit-lamp examination prior to initiation of therapy and in patients who develop symptoms of ocular toxicity)
Plasma tyrosine concentrations should be kept <500 µmol/L to avoid toxicity

Reference Range Plasma tyrosine concentration <500 micromoles/L

Dosage Forms Excipient information presented when available (limited, particularly for generics); consult specific product labeling.
Capsule, Oral:
Orfadin: 2 mg, 5 mg, 10 mg

References
Hall MG, Wilks MF, Provan WM, et al, "Pharmacokinetics and Pharmacodynamics of NTBC (2-(2-Nitro-4-Fluoromethylbenzoyl)-1,3-Cyclohexanedione) and Mesotrione, Inhibitors of 4-Hydroxyphenyl Pyruvate Dioxygenase (HPPD) Following a Single Dose to Healthy Male Volunteers," Br J Clin Pharmacol, 2001, 52(2):169-77.
Holme E and Lindstedt S, "Diagnosis and Management of Tyrosinemia Type I," Curr Opin Pediatr, 1995, 7(6):726-32.
Holme E and Lindstedt S, "Nontransplant Treatment of Tyrosinemia," Clin Liver Dis, 2000, 4(4):805-14.
Lindstedt S, Holme E, Lock EA, et al, "Treatment of Hereditary Tyrosinaemia Type I by Inhibition of 4-Hydroxyphenylpyruvate Dioxygenase," Lancet, 1992, 340(8823):813-7.
McKiernan PJ, "Nitisinone in the Treatment of Hereditary Tyrosinaemia Type 1," Drugs, 2006, 66(6):743-50.

◆ **Nitro-Bid** see Nitroglycerin on page 1504
◆ **Nitro-Dur** see Nitroglycerin on page 1504

Nitrofurantoin (nye troe fyoor AN toyn)

Medication Safety Issues
Sound alike/look alike issues:
Macrobid may be confused with microK, Nitro-Bid
Nitrofurantoin may be confused with Neurontin®, nitroglycerin

BEERS Criteria medication:
This drug may be potentially inappropriate for use in geriatric patients (Quality of evidence - moderate; Strength of recommendation - strong).

Brand Names: U.S. Furadantin; Macrobid; Macrodantin
Brand Names: Canada Apo-Nitrofurantoin; Macrobid; Macrodantin; Novo-Furantoin; Teva-Nitrofurantoin
Therapeutic Category Antibiotic, Miscellaneous
Generic Availability (U.S.) Yes
Use Prevention and treatment of urinary tract infections caused by susceptible gram-negative and some gram-positive organisms including *E. coli*, *Klebsiella*, *Enterobacter*, enterococci, *S. saprophyticus*, and *S. aureus*; *Pseudomonas*, *Serratia*, and most species of *Proteus* are generally resistant to nitrofurantoin.
Macrodantin® and Furadantin® (FDA approved in ages ≥1 month)
Macrobid® (FDA approved in ages ≥12 years)

Pregnancy Risk Factor B (contraindicated at term)
Pregnancy Considerations Adverse effects have not been observed in animal reproduction studies. Nitrofurantoin crosses the placenta (Perry, 1967) and maternal serum concentrations may be lower in pregnancy (Philipson, 1979). Current studies evaluating maternal use of nitrofurantoin during pregnancy and the development of birth defects have had mixed results (ACOG, 2011). An increased risk of neonatal jaundice was observed following maternal nitrofurantoin use during the last 30 days of pregnancy (Nordeng, 2013). Nitrofurantoin may be used to treat infections in pregnant women; use during the first trimester should be limited to situations where no alternative therapies are available. Prescriptions should be written when clinically appropriate and for the shortest effective duration for confirmed infections (ACOG, 2011). Nitrofurantoin is contraindicated in pregnant patients at term (38-42 weeks gestation), during labor and delivery, or when the onset of labor is imminent due to the possibility of hemolytic anemia in the neonate. Alternative antibiotics should be considered in pregnant women with G-6-PD deficiency (Nordeng, 2013).

Breast-Feeding Considerations Trace amounts of nitrofurantoin can be detected in breast milk. Due to the potential for serious adverse reactions in the nursing infant, the manufacturer recommends a decision be made whether to discontinue nursing or to discontinue the drug, taking into account the importance of treatment to the mother. The therapeutic use of nitrofurantoin is contraindicated in neonates (<1 month of age) due to the possibility of hemolytic anemia caused by immature erythrocyte enzyme systems. In case reports, diarrhea was reported in two nursing infants and decreased milk volume was reported by one mother (dose, duration, relationship to breast-feeding not provided) (Ito, 1993).

Contraindications Hypersensitivity to nitrofurantoin or any component; anuria, oliguria, or significant renal impairment (CrCl <60 mL/minute or significant serum creatinine elevation); infants <1 month of age, pregnant patients at term (38-42 weeks gestation), during labor and delivery (due to the possibility of hemolytic anemia); in patients with a history of cholestatic jaundice or hepatic impairment with previous nitrofurantoin therapy

Warnings Nitrofurantoin should not be used to treat UTIs in febrile infants and young children in whom renal involvement is likely; not indicated for the treatment of pyelonephritis or perinephric abscesses; therapeutic concentrations of nitrofurantoin are not attained in the urine of patients with renal insufficiency (CrCl <60 mL/minute, anuria, or oliguria). Acute, subacute, or chronic (usually after 6 months of therapy) pulmonary reactions, including fatalities have been reported; monitor for dyspnea, cough, fever, malaise, radiologic evidence of diffuse interstitial pneumonitis or fibrosis; if these reactions occur, discontinue nitrofurantoin immediately. Hepatitis, cholestatic jaundice, chronic active hepatitis (onset may be insidious) and hepatic necrosis resulting in death may occur; monitor patients for changes in liver function; if hepatitis occurs, discontinue nitrofurantoin immediately. Peripheral neuropathy may occur; risk is increased by renal impairment, anemia, diabetes mellitus, electrolyte imbalance, vitamin B deficiency, and debilitating disease. Optic neuritis has been reported. Prolonged use may result in fungal or bacterial superinfection, including C. difficile-associated diarrhea (CDAD) and pseudomembranous colitis; CDAD has been observed >2 months postantibiotic treatment.

Precautions Use with caution in patients with G-6-PD deficiency (hemolytic anemia-induced by nitrofurantoin appears to be linked to G-6-PD deficiency in the red blood cells of affected patients), patients with anemia, vitamin B deficiency, diabetes mellitus, or electrolyte abnormalities

Adverse Reactions

Cardiovascular: ECG changes (nonspecific ST/T wave changes, bundle branch block)

Central nervous system: Bulging fontanel (infants), chills, confusion, depression, dizziness, drowsiness, headache, malaise, numbness, paresthesia, peripheral neuropathy, pseudotumor cerebri, psychotic reaction, vertigo

Dermatologic: Alopecia, erythema multiforme, exfoliative dermatitis, pruritus, skin rash (eczematous, erythematous, maculopapular), Stevens-Johnson syndrome, urticaria

Endocrine & metabolic: Hyperphosphatemia

Gastrointestinal: Abdominal pain, anorexia, Clostridium difficile associated diarrhea, constipation, diarrhea, dyspepsia, flatulence, nausea, pancreatitis, pseudomembranous colitis, sialadenitis, vomiting

Genitourinary: Urine discoloration (brown)

Hematologic & oncologic: Agranulocytosis, aplastic anemia, eosinophilia, glucose-6-phosphate dehydrogenase deficiency anemia, granulocytopenia, hemoglobin decreased, hemolytic anemia, leukopenia, megaloblastic anemia, thrombocytopenia

Hepatic: Cholestatic jaundice, hepatitis, hepatic necrosis, increased serum transaminases

Hypersensitivity: Anaphylaxis, angioedema, hypersensitivity (including acute pulmonary hypersensitivity)

Infection: Superinfection (eg, Pseudomonas or Candida)

Neuromuscular & skeletal: Arthralgia, lupus-like syndrome, myalgia, weakness

Ophthalmic: Amblyopia, nystagmus, optic neuritis

Respiratory: Acute pulmonary reaction (symptoms include chills, chest pain, cough, dyspnea, fever, and eosinophilia), cough, cyanosis, dyspnea, pneumonitis, pulmonary fibrosis (with long-term use), pulmonary infiltration

Miscellaneous: Fever

Drug Interactions

Metabolism/Transport Effects None known.

Avoid Concomitant Use

Avoid concomitant use of Nitrofurantoin with any of the following: BCG; Magnesium Trisilicate; Norfloxacin

Increased Effect/Toxicity

Nitrofurantoin may increase the levels/effects of: Eplerenone; Prilocaine; Sodium Nitrite; Spironolactone

The levels/effects of Nitrofurantoin may be increased by: Nitric Oxide; Probenecid

Decreased Effect

Nitrofurantoin may decrease the levels/effects of: BCG; Norfloxacin; Sodium Picosulfate; Typhoid Vaccine

The levels/effects of Nitrofurantoin may be decreased by: Magnesium Trisilicate

Food Interactions Nitrofurantoin serum concentrations may be increased if taken with food. Management: Administer with meals.

Stability Protect oral suspension from light; store capsules and suspension at room temperature (59°F to 86°F or 15°C to 30°C)

Mechanism of Action Nitrofurantoin is reduced by bacterial flavoproteins to reactive intermediates that inactivate or alter bacterial ribosomal proteins leading to inhibition of protein synthesis, aerobic energy metabolism, DNA, RNA, and cell wall synthesis. Nitrofurantoin is bactericidal in urine at therapeutic doses. The broad-based nature of this mode of action may explain the lack of acquired bacterial resistance to nitrofurantoin, as the necessary multiple and simultaneous mutations of the target macromolecules would likely be lethal to the bacteria.

Pharmacokinetics (Adult data unless noted)

Absorption: Well absorbed from the GI tract; macrocrystalline form is absorbed more slowly due to slower dissolution, but causes less GI distress than formulations containing microcrystals of the drug

Distribution: V_d: 0.8 L/kg; crosses the placenta; appears in breast milk and bile

Protein binding: ~40% to 60%

Metabolism: Partially in the liver

Bioavailability: Presence of food increases bioavailability

Half-life: 20-60 minutes and is prolonged with renal impairment

Elimination: As metabolites and unchanged drug (40%) in the urine and small amounts in the bile; renal excretion is via glomerular filtration and tubular secretion

Dialysis: Dialyzable

Dosing: Usual Oral:

Infants >1 month and Children: 5-7 mg/kg/day divided every 6 hours; maximum dose: 400 mg/day

Macrocrystal/monohydrate: Children >12 years: 100 mg every 12 hours for 7 days

Prophylaxis of UTI: 1-2 mg/kg/day as a single daily dose; maximum dose: 100 mg/day

Adults: 50-100 mg/dose every 6 hours; macrocrystal/monohydrate: 100 mg twice daily for 7 days

Prophylaxis of UTI: 50-100 mg/dose at bedtime

Dosing adjustment in renal impairment: CrCl <60 mL/minute: Avoid use

Administration Oral: Administer with food or milk; do not administer with antacid preparations containing magnesium trisilicate; suspension may be mixed with water, milk, fruit juice, or infant formula. Shake suspension well before use.

Monitoring Parameters Signs of pulmonary reaction; signs of numbness or tingling of the extremities; periodic liver and renal function tests; CBC; urine culture and in vitro susceptibility tests. Observe for change in bowel frequency.

Test Interactions False-positive urine glucose (Benedict's and Fehling's methods); no false positives with enzymatic tests

Dosage Forms Excipient information presented when available (limited, particularly for generics); consult specific product labeling.

Capsule, Oral:
 Macrobid: 100 mg [contains brilliant blue fcf (fd&c blue #1), fd&c red #40, fd&c yellow #10 (quinoline yellow)]
 Macrodantin: 25 mg
 Macrodantin: 50 mg, 100 mg [contains fd&c yellow #10 (quinoline yellow), fd&c yellow #6 (sunset yellow)]
 Generic: 50 mg, 100 mg
Suspension, Oral:
 Furadantin: 25 mg/5 mL (230 mL)
 Generic: 25 mg/5 mL (230 mL, 240 mL)

References
American College of Obstetricians and Gynecologists (ACOG) Committee on Obstetric Practice, "ACOG Committee Opinion No. 494: Sulfonamides, Nitrofurantoin, and Risk of Birth Defects," *Obstet Gynecol*, 2011, 117(6):1484-5.

Brendstrup L, Hjelt K, Petersen KE, et al, "Nitrofurantoin Versus Trimethoprim Prophylaxis in Recurrent Urinary Tract Infections in Children," *Acta Paediatr Scand*, 1990. 79(12):1225-34.

Coraggio MJ, Gross TP, and Roscelli JD, "Nitrofurantoin Toxicity in Children," *Pediatr Infect Dis J*, 1989, 8(3):163-6.

Ito S, Blajchman A, Stephenson M, et al. Prospective follow-up of adverse reactions in breast-fed infants exposed to maternal medication. *Am J Obstet Gynecol*. 1993;168(5):1393-13999.

Nordeng H, Lupattelli A, Romøren M, et al. Neonatal outcomes after gestational exposure to nitrofurantoin. *Obstet Gynecol*. 2013;121(2 Pt 1):306-313.

Perry JE and Leblanc AL, "Transfer of Nitrofurantoin Across the Human Placenta," *Tex Rep Biol Med*, 1967a, 25(2):265-9.

Philipson A. Pharmacokinetics of antibiotics in pregnancy and labour. *Clin Pharmacokinet*. 1979;4(4):297-309.

"Practice Parameter: The Diagnosis, Treatment, and Evaluation of the Initial Urinary Tract Infection in Febrile Infants and Young Children." American Academy of Pediatrics. Committee on Quality Improvement. Subcommittee on Urinary Tract Infection," *Pediatrics*, 1999, 103(4 Pt 1):843-52.

◆ **Nitrogen Mustard** *see* Mechlorethamine (Systemic) *on page 1315*

Nitroglycerin (nye troe GLI ser in)

Medication Safety Issues
Sound-alike/look-alike issues:
 Nitroglycerin may be confused with nitrofurantoin, nitroprusside
 Nitro-Bid may be confused with Macrobid
 Nitroderm may be confused with NicoDerm
 Nitrol may be confused with Nizoral
 Nitrostat may be confused with Nilstat, nystatin
Other safety concerns:
 Transdermal patch may contain conducting metal (eg, aluminum); remove patch prior to MRI.
International issues:
 Nitrocor [Italy, Russia, and Venezuela] may be confused with Natrecor brand name for nesiritide [U.S., Canada, and multiple international markets]; Nutracort brand name for hydrocortisone in the [U.S. and multiple international markets]; Nitro-Dur [U.S., Canada, and multiple international markets]

Related Information
 Management of Drug Extravasations *on page 2255*
 Oral Medications That Should Not Be Crushed or Altered *on page 2438*
 Safe Handling of Hazardous Drugs *on page 2419*
Brand Names: U.S. Minitran; Nitro-Bid; Nitro-Dur; Nitro-Time; Nitrolingual; NitroMist; Nitronal; Nitrostat; Rectiv
Brand Names: Canada Minitran; Mylan-Nitro Sublingual Spray; Nitro-Dur; Nitroglycerin Injection, USP; Nitrol; Nitrostat; Rho-Nitro Pump Spray; Transderm-Nitro; Trinipatch
Therapeutic Category Antianginal Agent; Antihypertensive Agent; Nitrate; Vasodilator; Vasodilator, Coronary
Generic Availability (U.S.) May be product dependent
Use Treatment or prevention of angina pectoris (FDA approved in adults)
 I.V. administration: Treatment or prevention of angina pectoris; acute decompensated heart failure (especially

when associated with acute myocardial infarction); perioperative hypertension (especially during cardiovascular surgery); induction of intraoperative hypotension (FDA approved in adults)
 Intra-anal administration (Rectiv™ ointment): Treatment of moderate to severe pain associated with chronic anal fissure (FDA approved in adults)
Pregnancy Risk Factor B/C (product specific)
Pregnancy Considerations Animal reproduction studies have not been conducted with all products; adverse events were not observed in animal reproduction studies conducted using the ointment. Nitroglycerin crosses the placenta (David, 2000). Concentrations following application of a transdermal patch 0.4 mg/hour were low but detectable in the fetal serum (fetal/maternal ratio: 0.23) (Bustard, 2003). Nitroglycerin may be used in pregnancy when immediate relaxation of the uterus is needed (ACOG, 2006; Axemo, 1998; Chandraharan, 2005). Intravenous nitroglycerin may be used to treat pre-eclampsia with pulmonary edema (ESG, 2011).
Breast-Feeding Considerations It is not known if nitroglycerin is excreted in breast milk. The manufacturer recommends that caution be exercised when administering nitroglycerin to nursing women. Information related to the use of nitroglycerin and breast-feeding is limited (Böttiger, 2010; O'Sullivan, 2011).
Contraindications Hypersensitivity to nitroglycerin, organic nitrates, or any component (including adhesives in transdermal patches); severe anemia; increased ICP; concurrent use with phosphodiesterase-5 (PDE-5) inhibitors (eg, sildenafil, tadalafil, or vardenafil); I.V. product is also contraindicated in hypotension, pericardial tamponade, restrictive cardiomyopathy, or constrictive pericarditis
Warnings May cause severe hypotension; use with caution in hypovolemia, hypotension, and right ventricular infarctions. Transdermal patch may contain conducting metal (eg, aluminum) which may cause a burn to the skin during an MRI scan; remove patch prior to MRI; reapply patch after scan is completed. Due to the potential for altered electrical conductivity, remove transdermal patch before cardioversion or defibrillation. Rectal ointment and some I.V. preparations contain propylene glycol; toxicities have been reported with use of products containing propylene glycol, including hyperosmolality, lactic acidosis, seizures, and respiratory depression; in neonates large amounts of propylene glycol delivered orally, intravenously (eg, >3000 mg/day), or topically have been associated with potentially fatal toxicities which can include metabolic acidosis, seizures, renal failure, and CNS depression; use products containing propylene glycol with caution (AAP, 1997; Shehab, 2009).
Precautions Intra-anal ointment: Use with caution when treating rectal anal fissures with nitroglycerin in patients with suspected or known significant cardiovascular disorders (eg, cardiomyopathies, heart failure, acute MI); intra-anal topical nitroglycerin administration may decrease systolic blood pressure and decrease arterial vascular resistance.
Adverse Reactions
 Cardiovascular: Bradycardia, flushing, hypotension, orthostatic hypotension, peripheral edema, syncope, tachycardia
 Central nervous system: Headache (common), dizziness, lightheadedness
 Gastrointestinal: Nausea, vomiting, xerostomia
 Neuromuscular & skeletal: Paresthesia, weakness
 Respiratory: Dyspnea, pharyngitis, rhinitis
 Miscellaneous: Diaphoresis
 Rare but important or life-threatening): Allergic reactions, anaphylactoid reaction, application site irritation (patch), blurred vision, cardiovascular collapse, contact dermatitis (ointment, patch), crescendo angina, exfoliative

dermatitis, fixed drug eruption (ointment, patch), methemoglobinemia (rare; overdose), pallor, palpitation, rash, rebound hypertension, restlessness, shock, vertigo

Drug Interactions

Metabolism/Transport Effects None known.

Avoid Concomitant Use

Avoid concomitant use of Nitroglycerin with any of the following: Ergot Derivatives; Phosphodiesterase 5 Inhibitors; Riociguat

Increased Effect/Toxicity

Nitroglycerin may increase the levels/effects of: DULoxetine; Ergot Derivatives; Hypotensive Agents; Prilocaine; Riociguat; Rosiglitazone; Sodium Nitrite

The levels/effects of Nitroglycerin may be increased by: Alfuzosin; Barbiturates; Nitric Oxide; Phosphodiesterase 5 Inhibitors

Decreased Effect

Nitroglycerin may decrease the levels/effects of: Alteplase; Heparin

The levels/effects of Nitroglycerin may be decreased by: Ergot Derivatives

Stability

I.V. solution: Doses should be made in glass bottles, EXCEL®, or PAB® containers. Adsorption occurs to soft plastic (eg, polyvinyl chloride tubing). Nitroglycerin diluted in D₅W or NS in glass containers is physically and chemically stable for 48 hours at room temperature and 7 days under refrigeration. In D₅W or NS in EXCEL®/PAB® containers it is physically and chemically stable for 24 hours at room temperature. Premixed bottles are stable according to the manufacturer's expiration dating. Sublingual tablets, topical ointment, rectal ointment: Store in tightly closed containers at 20°C to 25°C (68°F to 77°F); slow release capsules at 20°C to 25°C (68°F to 77°F); translingual spray and transdermal patch at 15°C to 30°C (59°F to 86°F); use rectal ointment within 8 weeks of opening.

Mechanism of Action
Nitroglycerin forms free radical nitric oxide. In smooth muscle, nitric oxide activates guanylate cyclase which increases guanosine 3'5' monophosphate (cGMP) leading to dephosphorylation of myosin light chains and smooth muscle relaxation. Produces a vasodilator effect on the peripheral veins and arteries with more prominent effects on the veins. Primarily reduces cardiac oxygen demand by decreasing preload (left ventricular end-diastolic pressure); may modestly reduce afterload; dilates coronary arteries and improves collateral flow to ischemic regions. For use in rectal fissures, intra-anal administration results in decreased sphincter tone and intra-anal pressure.

Pharmacodynamics

Onset of action: Sublingual tablet: 1-3 minutes; Translingual spray: Similar to sublingual tablet; Sustained release: ~60 minutes; Topical: 15-30 minutes; Transdermal: ~30 minutes; I.V.: Immediate

Peak effect: Sublingual tablet: 5 minutes; Translingual spray: 4-10 minutes; Sustained release: 2.5-4 hours; Topical: ~60 minutes; Transdermal: 120 minutes; I.V.: Immediate

Duration: Sublingual tablet: At least 25 minutes; Translingual spray: Similar to sublingual tablet; Sustained release: 4-8 hours; Topical: 7 hours; Transdermal: 10-12 hours; I.V.: 3-5 minutes

Pharmacokinetics (Adult data unless noted)

Distribution: V_d: ~3 L/kg

Protein binding: 60%

Metabolism: Extensive first-pass; metabolized hepatically to glycerol di- and mononitrate metabolites via liver reductase enzyme; subsequent metabolism to glycerol and organic nitrate; nonhepatic metabolism via red blood cells and vascular walls also occurs

Half-life: 1-4 minutes

Elimination: Excretion of inactive metabolites in urine

Dosing: Neonatal Note: Limited data exist; further studies needed.

Continuous I.V. infusion: Initial: 0.25-0.5 mcg/kg/minute; titrate by 0.5-1 mcg/kg/minute every 3-5 minutes as needed; usual dose: 1-3 mcg/kg/minute; usual maximum dose: 5 mcg/kg/minute. In one clinical study of 16 pediatric patients <24 months of age (median: 4.4 months, range: 3 days-23.7 months), a median dose of 1.8 mcg/kg/minute (range: 0.5-4 mcg/kg/minute) was reported following cardiac surgery with bypass (Williams, 1994); another trial describes a fixed dose of 1 mcg/kg/minute administered to 15 neonates (mean: 8 days of age) after cardiac surgery in conjunction with dopamine (Laitinen, 1999)

Dosing: Usual Tolerance to the hemodynamic and antianginal effects can develop within 24-48 hours of continuous use.

Infants and Children: Continuous I.V. infusion: Initial: 0.25-0.5 mcg/kg/minute; titrate by 0.5-1 mcg/kg/minute every 3-5 minutes as needed; usual dose: 1-3 mcg/kg/minute; usual maximum dose: 5 mcg/kg/minute; doses up to 20 mcg/kg/minute may be used

Adults:

Anal fissure, chronic: Intra-anal: 0.4% ointment: 1 inch (equals 1.5 mg of nitroglycerin) every 12 hours for up to 3 weeks

Angina/coronary artery disease:

Continuous I.V. infusion: **Note:** Do **not** dose per kg; adult dose is in units of mcg/minute; Initial: 5 mcg/minute, increase by 5 mcg/minute every 3-5 minutes to 20 mcg/minute, then increase as needed by 10-20 mcg/minute every 3-5 minutes (generally accepted maximum dose: 400 mcg/minute)

Oral: 2.5-6.5 mg 3-4 times daily (maximum dose: 26 mg)

Patch, transdermal: Initial: 0.2-0.4 mg/hour, titrate to 0.4-0.8 mg/hour; use a "patch-on" period of 12-14 hours per day and a "patch-off" period of 10-12 hours per day to minimize tolerance

Sublingual: 0.3-0.6 mg every 5 minutes for maximum of 3 doses in 15 minutes; may also use prophylactically 5-10 minutes prior to activities which may provoke an attack

Topical: 2% Ointment: Apply 0.5 inch upon rising and 0.5 inch 6 hours later; if necessary, the dose may be doubled to 1 inch and subsequently doubled again to 2 inches if response is inadequate. Doses of 0.5-2 inches were used in clinical trials. Recommended maximum: 2 doses/day; include a nitrate-free interval ~10-12 hours/day

Translingual: 1-2 sprays into mouth onto or under tongue every 3-5 minutes for maximum of 3 sprays in 15 minutes; may administer 5-10 minutes before activities that may precipitate angina

Usual Infusion Concentrations: Pediatric Note: Premixed solutions available

I.V. infusion: 100 **mcg**/mL, 200 **mcg**/mL, or 400 **mcg**/mL

Administration

Intra-anal ointment: Using a finger covering (eg, plastic wrap, surgical glove, finger cot), place finger beside 1 inch measuring guide on the box and squeeze ointment the length of the measuring line directly onto covered finger. Insert ointment into the anal canal using the covered finger up to first finger joint (do not insert further than the first finger joint) and apply ointment around the side of the anal canal. If intra-anal application is too painful, may apply the ointment to the outside of the anus. Wash hands following application.

Oral:

Capsule (sustained release): Administer with a full glass of water on an empty stomach; swallow whole, do not crush or chew

Sublingual tablet: Place under tongue and allow to dissolve, do not swallow, chew, or crush; do not eat or drink while tablet dissolves

Translingual spray: Do not shake container. Pump must be primed prior to first use by spraying 5 times (Nitrolingual®) or 10 times (Nitromist™); direct priming sprays into the air, away from patient and others; if pump is unused for 6 weeks, a single priming spray (Nitrolingual®) or 2 priming sprays (Nitromist™) should be completed. To administer dose, spray onto or under tongue with container as close to mouth as possible; close mouth after administration; do not inhale spray; avoid swallowing immediately after spray; do not expectorate or rinse mouth for 5-10 minutes after use

Parenteral: Continuous I.V. infusion: Dilute in D_5W or NS to 50-100 mcg/mL; maximum concentration not to exceed 400 mcg/mL; prepare in glass bottles, EXCEL® or PAB® containers [adsorption occurs to soft plastic (eg, PVC)]; administer via controlled infusion device; special administration sets intended for nitroglycerin (nonpolyvinyl chloride) must be used

Transdermal patch: Place on hair-free area of skin; rotate patch sites; **Note:** Some products are a membrane-controlled system (eg, Transderm-Nitro®); do **not** cut these patches to deliver partial doses; rate of drug delivery, reservoir contents, and adhesion may be affected; if partial dose is needed, surface area of patch can be blocked proportionally using adhesive bandage (Lee, 1997 and see specific product labeling)

Monitoring Parameters Blood pressure, heart rate (continuously with I.V. use)

Test Interactions I.V. formulation: Due to propylene glycol content, triglyceride assays dependent on glycerol oxidase may be falsely elevated.

Additional Information I.V. preparations contain alcohol and/or propylene glycol; may need to use nitrate-free interval (10-12 hours/day) to avoid tolerance development; tolerance may possibly be reversed with acetylcysteine; gradually decrease dose in patients receiving NTG for prolonged period to avoid withdrawal reaction; lingual spray contains 20% alcohol, do not spray toward flames

Dosage Forms Excipient information presented when available (limited, particularly for generics); consult specific product labeling.

Aerosol Solution, Translingual:
NitroMist: 400 mcg/spray (4.1 g, 8.5 g) [contains menthol]
Generic: 400 mcg/spray (4.1 g, 8.5 g)

Capsule Extended Release, Oral:
Nitro-Time: 2.5 mg [contains brilliant blue fcf (fd&c blue #1), fd&c red #40, fd&c yellow #10 (quinoline yellow)]
Nitro-Time: 6.5 mg [contains brilliant blue fcf (fd&c blue #1), fd&c yellow #10 (quinoline yellow), fd&c yellow #6 (sunset yellow)]
Nitro-Time: 9 mg [contains fd&c yellow #10 (quinoline yellow), fd&c yellow #6 (sunset yellow)]
Generic: 2.5 mg, 6.5 mg, 9 mg

Ointment, Rectal:
Rectiv: 0.4% (30 g) [contains propylene glycol]

Ointment, Transdermal:
Nitro-Bid: 2% (1 g, 30 g, 60 g)

Patch 24 Hour, Transdermal:
Minitran: 0.1 mg/hr (30 ea); 0.2 mg/hr (30 ea); 0.4 mg/hr (30 ea); 0.6 mg/hr (30 ea)
Nitro-Dur: 0.1 mg/hr (30 ea, 100 ea); 0.2 mg/hr (30 ea, 100 ea); 0.3 mg/hr (30 ea, 100 ea); 0.4 mg/hr (30 ea, 100 ea); 0.6 mg/hr (30 ea, 100 ea); 0.8 mg/hr (30 ea, 100 ea)

Generic: 0.1 mg/hr (30 ea, 4350 ea); 0.2 mg/hr (30 ea, 4350 ea); 0.4 mg/hr (30 ea, 4350 ea); 0.6 mg/hr (30 ea, 4350 ea)

Solution, Intravenous:
Nitronal: 1 mg/mL (25 mL, 50 mL)
Generic: 25 mg (250 mL); 50 mg (250 mL, 500 mL); 100 mg (250 mL); 200 mg (500 mL); 5 mg/mL (10 mL)

Solution, Translingual:
Nitrolingual: 0.4 mg/spray (4.9 g, 12 g) [contains alcohol, usp]
Generic: 0.4 mg/spray (4.9 g, 12 g)

Tablet Sublingual, Sublingual:
Nitrostat: 0.3 mg, 0.4 mg, 0.6 mg

References

American Academy of Pediatrics Committee on Drugs. "Inactive" ingredients in pharmaceutical products: update (subject review). *Pediatrics.* 1997;99(2):268-278.

American College of Obstetricians and Gynecologists (ACOG), "ACOG Practice Bulletin: Clinical Management Guidelines for Obstetrician-Gynecologists Number 76, October 2006: Postpartum Hemorrhage," *Obstet Gynecol,* 2006, 108(4):1039-47.

Axemo P, Fu X, Lindberg B, et al, "Intravenous Nitroglycerin for Rapid Uterine Relaxation," *Acta Obstet Gynecol Scand,* 1998, 77(1):50-3.

Böttiger Y, "Lack of Data on Glyceryl Trinitrate Risks in Breast Feeding," *Lakartidningen,* 2010, 107(22):1483.

Bustard MA, Ryan G, Seaward G, et al, "Human Maternal and Fetal Plasma Glyceryl Trinitrate Concentrations," *Am J Obstet Gynecol,* 2003, 189(6):1777-8.

Chandraharan E and Arulkumaran S, "Acute Tocolysis," *Curr Opin Obstet Gynecol,* 2005, 17(2):151-6.

David M, Walka MM, Schmid B, et al, "Nitroglycerin Application During Cesarean Delivery: Plasma Levels, Fetal/Maternal Ratio of Nitroglycerin, and Effects in Newborns," *Am J Obstet Gynecol,* 2000, 182(4):955-61.

Elkayam U, "Tolerance to Organic Nitrates: Evidence, Mechanisms, Clinical Relevance, and Strategies for Prevention," *Ann Intern Med,* 1991, 114(8):667-77.

European Society of Gynecology (ESG), Association for European Paediatric Cardiology (AEPC), German Society for Gender Medicine (DGesGM), et al, "ESC Guidelines on the Management of Cardiovascular Diseases During Pregnancy: The Task Force on the Management of Cardiovascular Diseases During Pregnancy of the European Society of Cardiology (ESC)," *Eur Heart J,* 2011, 32(24):3147-97.

Friedman WF and George BL, "Treatment of Congestive Heart Failure by Altering Loading Conditions of the Heart," *J Pediatr,* 1985, 106 (5):697-706.

Laitinen P, Happonen JM, Sairanen H, et al, "Amrinone Versus Dopamine-Nitroglycerin After Reconstructive Surgery for Complete Atrioventricular Septal Defect," *J Cardiothorac Vasc Anesth,* 1997, 11 (7):870-4.

Laitinen P, Happonen JM, Sairanen H, et al, "Amrinone Versus Dopamine and Nitroglycerin in Neonates After Arterial Switch Operation for Transposition of the Great Arteries," *J Cardiothorac Vasc Anesth,* 1999, 13(2):186-90.

Lee HA and Anderson PO, "Giving Partial Doses of Transdermal Patches," *Am J Health Syst Pharm,* 1997, 54(15):1759-60.

O'Sullivan S and Keith MP, "Raynaud phenomenon of the Nipple: A Rare Finding in Rheumatology Clinic," *J Clin Rheumatol,* 2011, 17 (7):371-2.

Shehab N, Lewis CL, Streetman DD, Donn SM. Exposure to the pharmaceutical excipients benzyl alcohol and propylene glycol among critically ill neonates. *Pediatr Crit Care Med.* 2009;10 (2):256-259.

Williams RS, Mickell JJ, Young ES, et al, "Methemoglobin Levels During Prolonged Combined Nitroglycerin and Sodium Nitroprusside Infusions in Infants After Cardiac Surgery," *J Cardiothorac Vasc Anesth,* 1994, 8(6):658-62.

◆ **Nitroglycerin Injection, USP (Can)** *see* Nitroglycerin *on page 1504*

◆ **Nitroglycerol** *see* Nitroglycerin *on page 1504*

◆ **Nitrol (Can)** *see* Nitroglycerin *on page 1504*

◆ **Nitrolingual** *see* Nitroglycerin *on page 1504*

◆ **NitroMist** *see* Nitroglycerin *on page 1504*

◆ **Nitronal** *see* Nitroglycerin *on page 1504*

◆ **Nitropress** *see* Nitroprusside *on page 1507*

Nitroprusside (nye troe PRUS ide)

Medication Safety Issues

Sound-alike/look-alike issues:

Nitroprusside may be confused with nitroglycerin

High alert medication:

The Institute for Safe Medication Practices (ISMP) includes this medication among its list of drugs which have a heightened risk of causing significant patient harm when used in error.

Related Information

Serotonin Syndrome *on page 2405*

Brand Names: U.S. Nitropress

Brand Names: Canada Nipride

Therapeutic Category Antihypertensive Agent; Vasodilator

Generic Availability (U.S.) No

Use Management of hypertensive crises; CHF; used for controlled hypotension during anesthesia

Pregnancy Risk Factor C

Pregnancy Considerations Animal studies have shown that nitroprusside may cross the placental barrier and result in fetal cyanide levels that are dose-related to maternal nitroprusside levels. However, information related to use in pregnancy is limited.

Breast-Feeding Considerations It is not known if nitroprusside is excreted in breast milk. Due to the potential for serious adverse reactions in the nursing infant, a decision should be made whether to discontinue nursing or to discontinue the drug, taking into account the importance of treatment to the mother.

Contraindications Hypersensitivity to nitroprusside or any component of the formulation; treatment of compensatory hypertension (aortic coarctation, arteriovenous shunting); high output failure; congenital optic atrophy or tobacco amblyopia

Warnings Use only as an infusion with D_5W **[U.S. Boxed Warning]**; continuously monitor patient's blood pressure **[U.S. Boxed Warning]**; may cause precipitous decreases in blood pressure. Except when used briefly or at low (<2 mcg/kg/minute) infusion rates, nitroprusside gives rise to large cyanide quantities **[U.S. Boxed Warning]**; cyanide or thiocyanate toxicity may occur; risk increased in patients with decreased renal or liver function or when using excessive doses. Do not use the maximum dose for more than 10 minutes; if blood pressure is not controlled, then discontinue infusion. Monitor for cyanide toxicity via acid-base balance and venous oxygen concentration.

Precautions Use with caution in patients with severe renal impairment, hepatic failure, hypothyroidism, hyponatremia, increased intracranial pressure

Adverse Reactions

Cardiovascular: Bradycardia, ECG changes, flushing, hypotension (excessive), palpitation, substernal distress, tachycardia

Central nervous system: Apprehension, dizziness, headache, intracranial pressure increased, restlessness

Dermatologic: Rash

Endocrine & metabolic: Metabolic acidosis (secondary to cyanide toxicity), hypothyroidism

Gastrointestinal: Abdominal pain, ileus, nausea, retching, vomiting

Hematologic: Methemoglobinemia, platelet aggregation decreased

Local: Injection site irritation

Neuromuscular & skeletal: Hyperreflexia (secondary to thiocyanate toxicity), muscle twitching

Ocular: Miosis (secondary to thiocyanate toxicity)

Otic: Tinnitus (secondary to thiocyanate toxicity)

Respiratory: Hyperoxemia (secondary to cyanide toxicity)

Miscellaneous: Cyanide toxicity, diaphoresis, thiocyanate toxicity

Drug Interactions

Metabolism/Transport Effects None known.

Avoid Concomitant Use There are no known interactions where it is recommended to avoid concomitant use.

Increased Effect/Toxicity

Nitroprusside may increase the levels/effects of: Amifostine; Antihypertensives; DULoxetine; Hypotensive Agents; Obinutuzumab; Prilocaine; RiTUXimab; Sodium Nitrite

The levels/effects of Nitroprusside may be increased by: Alfuzosin; Barbiturates; Brimonidine (Topical); Calcium Channel Blockers; Diazoxide; Herbs (Hypotensive Properties); MAO Inhibitors; Nitric Oxide; Pentoxifylline; Phosphodiesterase 5 Inhibitors; Prostacyclin Analogues

Decreased Effect

The levels/effects of Nitroprusside may be decreased by: Herbs (Hypertensive Properties); Methylphenidate; Yohimbine

Stability Discard solution 24 hours after reconstitution and dilution; discard highly colored solutions

Mechanism of Action Causes peripheral vasodilation by direct action on venous and arteriolar smooth muscle, thus reducing peripheral resistance; will increase cardiac output by decreasing afterload; reduces aortal and left ventricular impedance

Pharmacodynamics Hypotensive effects:

Onset of action: Within 2 minutes

Duration: 1-10 minutes

Pharmacokinetics (Adult data unless noted)

Metabolism: Converted to cyanide by erythrocyte and tissue sulfhydryl group interactions; cyanide is converted in the liver by the enzyme rhodanase to thiocyanate

Half-life: <10 minutes

Thiocyanate: 2.7-7 days

Elimination: Thiocyanate is excreted in the urine

Dosing: Neonatal Continuous I.V. infusion: Initial: 0.2 mcg/kg/minute and titrate to effect; doses up to 8 mcg/kg/minute have been reported; however, doses ≥1.8 mcg/kg/minute are associated with increased cyanide concentration in pediatric patients, including neonates (Moffett, 2008); reported duration of therapy was typically <6-7 days. Use in neonates has been described in several retrospective reports and case series; most recent and majority of patient experience is during cardiac surgery requiring cardiopulmonary bypass and postoperatively for afterload reduction (Benitz, 1985; Cachat, 2004; Furck, 2010; Kiran, 2006; Motta, 1995; Williams, 1994); use for 6 days at a maximum dose of 2.5 mcg/kg/minute produced profound lactic acidosis in one neonate (Meyer, 2005)

Dosing: Usual

Infants and Children: Continuous I.V. infusion: Start 0.3-0.5 mcg/kg/minute, titrate to effect; doses ≥1.8 mcg/kg/minute are associated with increased cyanide concentration in pediatric patients (Moffett, 2008); rarely need >4 mcg/kg/minute; maximum dose: 8-10 mcg/kg/minute

Adults: Continuous I.V. infusion: Initial: 0.3-0.5 mcg/kg/minute; increase in increments of 0.5 mcg/kg/minute, titrating to the desired hemodynamic effect or the appearance of headache or nausea; usual dose: 3 mcg/kg/minute; rarely need >4 mcg/kg/minute; maximum: 10 mcg/kg/minute. When >500 mcg/kg is administered by prolonged infusion of faster than 2 mcg/kg/minute, cyanide is generated faster than an unaided patient can handle.

Usual Infusion Concentrations: Pediatric I.V. infusion: 100 **mcg/mL or** 200 mcg/mL

Administration Parenteral: I.V. continuous infusion only via controlled infusion device. Not for direct injection; must dilute prior to administration; dilute in D_5W (preferred). Solution should be protected from light, but not necessary ▶

◄ to wrap administration set or I.V. tubing. Final concentration for administration: Usual maximum: 200 mcg/mL in D_5W; in fluid restricted patients a final maximum concentration of 1000 mcg/mL in D_5W has been used. May also dilute in LR or NS to 50 or 100 mcg/mL. Do not add other medications to nitroprusside solutions.

Monitoring Parameters Blood pressure, heart rate; monitor for cyanide and thiocyanate toxicity; monitor acid-base status as acidosis can be the earliest sign of cyanide toxicity; monitor thiocyanate levels if requiring prolonged infusion (>3 days) or dose ≥4 mcg/kg/minute or patient has renal dysfunction; monitor cyanide blood levels in patients with decreased hepatic function

Reference Range

Thiocyanate:

Toxic: 35-100 mcg/mL

Fatal: >200 mcg/mL

Cyanide:

Normal <0.2 mcg/mL

Normal (smoker): <0.4 mcg/mL

Toxic: >2 mcg/mL

Potentially lethal: >3 mcg/mL

Additional Information Thiocyanate toxicity includes psychoses, blurred vision, confusion, weakness, tinnitus, seizures; cyanide toxicity includes metabolic acidosis, tachycardia, pink skin, decreased pulse, decreased reflexes, altered consciousness, coma, almond smell on breath, methemoglobinemia, dilated pupils

Dosage Forms Excipient information presented when available (limited, particularly for generics); consult specific product labeling.

Solution, Intravenous, as sodium:

Nitropress: 25 mg/mL (2 mL)

References

Benitz WE, Malachowski N, Cohen RS, et al, "Use of Sodium Nitroprusside in Neonates: Efficacy and Safety," *J Pediatr*, 1985, 106 (1):102-10.

Cachat F, Bogaru A, Micheli JL, et al, "Severe Hypertension and Massive Proteinuria in a Newborn With Renal Artery Stenosis," *Pediatr Nephrol*, 2004, 19(5):544-6.

Cachat F and Guignard JP, "Reply to the Letter From C. von Schnakenburg and M. Krüger," *Pediatr Nephrol*, 2004, 19:1308-09.

Furck AK, Hansen JH, Uebing A, et al, "The Impact of Afterload Reduction on the Early Postoperative Course After the Norwood Operation - A 12-year Single-Centre Experience," *Eur J Cardiothorac Surg*, 2010, 37(2):289-95.

Kiran U, Zuber K, and Kakani M, "Combination of Low-Dose Phenoxybenzamine and Sodium Nitroprusside in Children Undergoing Cardiac Surgery," *J Cardiothorac Vasc Anesth*, 2006, 20(2):291-2.

Meyer S, Baghai A, Sailer NL, et al, "Lactic Acidosis Caused by Sodium Nitroprusside in a Newborn With Congenital Heart Disease," *Eur J Pediatr*, 2005, 164(4):253-4.

Moffett BS and Price JF, "Evaluation of Sodium Nitroprusside Toxicity in Pediatric Cardiac Surgical Patients," *Ann Pharmacother*, 2008, 42 (11):1600-4.

Motta P, Mossad E, Toscana D, et al, "Comparison of Phenoxybenzamine to Sodium Nitroprusside in Infants Undergoing Surgery," *J Cardiothorac Vasc Anesth*, 2005, 19(1):54-9.

Phillips MS, "Standardizing I.V. Infusion Concentrations: National Survey Results," *Am J Health Syst Pharm*, 2011, 68(22):2176-82.

von Schnakenburg C and Krüger M, "Note of Caution for the Use of Sodium Nitroprusside in Neonatal Hypertension," *Pediatr Nephrol*, 2004, 19(11):1307.

Williams RS, Mickell JJ, Young ES, et al, "Methemoglobin Levels During Prolonged Combined Nitroglycerin and Sodium Nitroprusside Infusions in Infants After Cardiac Surgery," *J Cardiothorac Vasc Anesth*, 1994, 8(6):658-62.

◆ **Nitroprusside Sodium** *see* Nitroprusside *on page 1507*

◆ **Nitrostat** *see* Nitroglycerin *on page 1504*

◆ **Nitro-Time** *see* Nitroglycerin *on page 1504*

◆ **Nix [OTC] (Can)** *see* Permethrin *on page 1647*

Nizatidine (ni ZA ti deen)

Medication Safety Issues

Sound-alike/look-alike issues:

Axid may be confused with Ansaid

International issues:

Tazac [Australia] may be confused with Tazact brand name for piperacillin/tazobactam [India]; Tiazac brand name for diltiazem [U.S., Canada]

Brand Names: U.S. Axid; Axid AR [OTC]

Brand Names: Canada Apo-Nizatidine; Axid; Gen-Nizatidine; Novo-Nizatidine; Nu-Nizatidine; PMS-Nizatidine

Therapeutic Category Gastrointestinal Agent, Gastric or Duodenal Ulcer Treatment; Histamine H_2 Antagonist

Generic Availability (U.S.) May be product dependent

Use Treatment and maintenance therapy of duodenal ulcer; treatment of active benign gastric ulcer; esophagitis; gastroesophageal reflux disease (GERD); adjunctive therapy in the treatment of *Helicobacter pylori*-associated duodenal ulcer

Pregnancy Risk Factor B

Pregnancy Considerations Adverse events have not been observed in animal reproduction studies; therefore, the nizatidine is classified as pregnancy category B. Nizatidine crosses the placenta. An increased risk of congenital malformations or adverse events in the newborn has generally not been observed following maternal use of nizatidine during pregnancy. Histamine H_2 antagonists have been evaluated for the treatment of gastroesophageal reflux disease (GERD), as well as gastric and duodenal ulcers during pregnancy. Although if needed, nizatidine is not the agent of choice. Histamine H_2 antagonists may be used for aspiration prophylaxis prior to cesarean delivery.

Breast-Feeding Considerations Following oral administration of nizatidine, 0.1% of the maternal dose is found in breast milk. The highest milk concentrations appear ~2 hours after a maternal dose. According to the manufacturer, the decision to continue or discontinue breast-feeding during therapy should take into account the risk of exposure to the infant and the benefits of treatment to the mother.

Contraindications Hypersensitivity to nizatidine, H_2 antagonists, or any component

Warnings Use of gastric acid inhibitors including proton pump inhibitors and H_2 blockers has been associated with an increased risk for development of acute gastroenteritis and community-acquired pneumonia (Canani, 2006). A large epidemiological study has suggested an increased risk for developing pneumonia in patients receiving H_2 receptor antagonists; however, a causal relationship with nizatidine has not been demonstrated.

Precautions Use with caution and modify dosage in patients with impaired renal function

Adverse Reactions

Central nervous system: Anxiety, dizziness, fever (reported in children), headache, insomnia, irritability (reported in children), nervousness, somnolence

Dermatologic: Pruritus, rash

Gastrointestinal: Abdominal pain, anorexia, constipation, diarrhea, dry mouth, flatulence, heartburn, nausea, vomiting

Respiratory: Reported in children: Cough, nasal congestion, nasopharyngitis

Rare but important or life-threatening: Alkaline phosphatase increased, ALT increased, anaphylaxis, anemia, AST increased, bronchospasm, confusion, eosinophilia, exfoliative dermatitis, gynecomastia, hepatitis, jaundice, laryngeal edema, serum-sickness like reactions, thrombocytopenia, thrombocytopenic purpura, vasculitis, ventricular tachycardia

Drug Interactions

Metabolism/Transport Effects Inhibits CYP3A4 (weak)

Avoid Concomitant Use

Avoid concomitant use of Nizatidine with any of the following: Dasatinib; Delavirdine; PAZOPanib; Pimozide; PONATinib; Risedronate

Increased Effect/Toxicity

Nizatidine may increase the levels/effects of: ARIPiprazole; Dexmethylphenidate; Dofetilide; Lomitapide; Methylphenidate; Pimozide; Risedronate; Saquinavir; Varenicline

Decreased Effect

Nizatidine may decrease the levels/effects of: Atazanavir; Bosutinib; Cefditoren; Cefpodoxime; Cefuroxime; Dabrafenib; Dasatinib; Delavirdine; Erlotinib; Fosamprenavir; Gefitinib; Indinavir; Iron Salts; Itraconazole; Ketoconazole (Systemic); Mesalamine; Multivitamins/Minerals (with ADEK, Folate, Iron); Nelfinavir; Nilotinib; PAZOPanib; PONATinib; Posaconazole; Rilpivirine; Vismodegib

Food Interactions Prolonged treatment (≥2 years) may lead to malabsorption of dietary vitamin B_{12} and subsequent vitamin B_{12} deficiency (Lam, 2013).

Stability Nizatidine is stable for 48 hours at room temperature when the contents of a capsule are mixed in Gatorade® lemon-lime, Cran-Grape® grape-cranberry drink, V8®, or aluminum- and magnesium hydroxide suspension (approximate concentration 2.5 mg/mL)

Mechanism of Action Competitive inhibition of histamine at H_2-receptors of the gastric parietal cells resulting in reduced gastric acid secretion, gastric volume and hydrogen ion concentration reduced. In healthy volunteers, nizatidine suppresses gastric acid secretion induced by pentagastrin infusion or food.

Pharmacodynamics Maximum effect: Duodenal ulcer: 4 weeks

Pharmacokinetics (Adult data unless noted)

Distribution: V_d: Adults: 0.8-1.5 L/kg; breast milk: 0.1% excreted into breast milk

Protein binding: 35%

Bioavailability: Oral: 70%

Half-life, elimination: Adults: 1-2 hours; anuric: 3.5-11 hours

Time to peak serum concentration: 0.5-3 hours

Elimination: 60% excreted unchanged in urine

Dosing: Usual Oral:

Infants 6 months to Children 11 years: Limited information available: 5-10 mg/kg/day divided twice daily

GERD, esophagitis: Children ≥12 years and Adults: 150 mg twice daily

Active duodenal and gastric ulcers: Adults: 300 mg once daily at bedtime or 150 mg twice daily

Maintenance of healed duodenal ulcer: Adults: 150 mg once daily

Helicobacter pylori-associated duodenal ulcer (limited information): Adults: 150 mg twice daily for 4 weeks (combined with clarithromycin and bismuth formulation; followed by 300 mg/day)

Dosing adjustment in renal impairment: Adults:

Active treatment:

CrCl 20-50 mL/minute: 150 mg once daily

CrCl <20 mL/minute: 150 mg every other day

Maintenance treatment:

CrCl 20-50 mL/minute: 150 every other day

CrCl <20 mL/minute: 150 mg every 3 days

Administration Oral: May administer with or without food; do not administer or mix with apple juice

Test Interactions False-positive urine protein using Multistix®, gastric acid secretion test, skin tests allergen extracts, serum creatinine and serum transaminase concentrations, urine protein test

Dosage Forms Excipient information presented when available (limited, particularly for generics); consult specific product labeling.

Capsule, Oral:

Axid: 300 mg

Generic: 150 mg, 300 mg

Solution, Oral:

Axid: 15 mg/mL (480 mL) [contains methylparaben, propylparaben, saccharin sodium; bubble-gum flavor]

Generic: 15 mg/mL (473 mL, 480 mL)

Tablet, Oral:

Axid AR: 75 mg

Extemporaneous Preparations A 2.5 mg/mL oral solution may be made with capsules and one of three different vehicles (lemon-lime Gatorade®, Ocean Spray® Cran-Grape® juice or V8® 100% vegetable juice). Empty the contents of one 300 mg capsule in a mortar. Add small portions of the chosen vehicle and mix to a uniform paste; mix while adding the vehicle in incremental proportions to **almost** 120 mL; transfer to a calibrated bottle, rinse mortar with vehicle, and add quantity of vehicle sufficient to make 120 mL. Label "shake well". Stable for 2 days refrigerated.

Nahata MC, Pai VB, and Hipple TF, *Pediatric Drug Formulations*, 5th ed, Cincinnati, OH: Harvey Whitney Books Co, 2004.

References

Canani RB, Cirillo P, Roggero P, et al, "Therapy With Gastric Acidity Inhibitors Increases the Risk of Acute Gastroenteritis and Community-Acquired Pneumonia in Children," *Pediatrics*, 2006, 117(5):e817-20.

Mikawa K, Nishina K, Maekawa N, et al, "Effects of Oral Nizatidine on Preoperative Gastric Fluid pH and Volume in Children," *Br J Anaesth*, 1994, 73(5):600-4.

Simeone D, Caria MC, Miele E, et al, "Treatment of Childhood Peptic Esophagitis: A Double-Blind Placebo-Controlled Trial of Nizatidine," *J Pediatr Gastroenterol Nur*, 1997, 25(1):51-5.

◆ **Nizoral** *see* Ketoconazole (Systemic) *on page 1177*

◆ **Nizoral** *see* Ketoconazole (Topical) *on page 1179*

◆ **Nizoral A-D [OTC]** *see* Ketoconazole (Topical) *on page 1179*

◆ **N-Methylhydrazine** *see* Procarbazine *on page 1743*

◆ **No Doz® Maximum Strength [OTC]** *see* Caffeine *on page 338*

◆ **Nolvadex** *see* Tamoxifen *on page 1968*

◆ **Nolvadex®-D (Can)** *see* Tamoxifen *on page 1968*

◆ **Non-Aspirin Pain Reliever [OTC]** *see* Acetaminophen *on page 47*

◆ **Non-Pseudo Sinus Decongestant [OTC]** *see* Phenylephrine (Systemic) *on page 1658*

◆ **Nora-BE** *see* Norethindrone *on page 1511*

◆ **Noradrenaline** *see* Norepinephrine *on page 1510*

◆ **Noradrenaline Acid Tartrate** *see* Norepinephrine *on page 1510*

◆ **Norco®** *see* Hydrocodone and Acetaminophen *on page 1027*

◆ **Norcuron** *see* Vecuronium *on page 2123*

◆ **Norcuron® (Can)** *see* Vecuronium *on page 2123*

◆ **Nordeoxyguanosine** *see* Ganciclovir (Ophthalmic) *on page 957*

◆ **Nordeoxyguanosine** *see* Ganciclovir (Systemic) *on page 955*

◆ **Norditropin FlexPro** *see* Somatropin *on page 1920*

◆ **Norditropin NordiFlex Pen** *see* Somatropin *on page 1920*

◆ **Norditropin Simplexx (Can)** *see* Somatropin *on page 1920*

Norepinephrine (nor ep i NEF rin)

Medication Safety Issues
Sound-alike/look-alike issues:
Levophed® may be confused with levofloxacin
High alert medication:
The Institute for Safe Medication Practices (ISMP) includes this medication among its list of drugs which have a heightened risk of causing significant patient harm when used in error.

Related Information
Emergency Drip Calculations *on page 2191*
Management of Drug Extravasations *on page 2255*
Serotonin Syndrome *on page 2405*

Brand Names: U.S. Levophed
Brand Names: Canada Levophed®
Therapeutic Category Adrenergic Agonist Agent; Alpha-Adrenergic Agonist; Sympathomimetic
Generic Availability (U.S.) Yes
Use Treatment of shock which persists after adequate fluid volume replacement; severe hypotension; cardiogenic shock

Pregnancy Risk Factor C
Pregnancy Considerations Animal reproduction studies have not been conducted. Norepinephrine is an endogenous catecholamine and crosses the placenta (Minzter, 2010; Wang, 1999).

Breast-Feeding Considerations It is not known if norepinephrine is excreted in breast milk. The manufacturer recommends that caution be exercised when administering norepinephrine to nursing women.

Contraindications Hypersensitivity to norepinephrine, bisulfites (contains metabisulfite), or any component of the formulation; hypotension from hypovolemia except as an emergency measure to maintain coronary and cerebral perfusion until volume could be replaced; mesenteric or peripheral vascular thrombosis unless it is a lifesaving procedure; during anesthesia with cyclopropane or halothane anesthesia (risk of ventricular arrhythmias)

Warnings Potent drug; must be diluted prior to use; monitor hemodynamic status; injection contains sodium metabisulfite which may cause allergic reactions in susceptible individuals. Extravasation may cause tissue necrosis (treat extravasation with phentolamine) **[U.S. Boxed Warning]**

Precautions Blood/volume depletion should be corrected, if possible, before norepinephrine therapy; extravasation may cause severe tissue necrosis; do **not** give to patients with peripheral or mesenteric vascular thrombosis because ischemia may be increased and the area of infarct extended; use with caution during cyclopropane or halothane anesthesia and in patients with occlusive vascular disease

Adverse Reactions
Cardiovascular: Arrhythmias, bradycardia, peripheral (digital) ischemia
Central nervous system: Anxiety, headache (transient)
Local: Skin necrosis (with extravasation)
Respiratory: Dyspnea, respiratory difficulty

Drug Interactions
Metabolism/Transport Effects Substrate of COMT
Avoid Concomitant Use
Avoid concomitant use of Norepinephrine with any of the following: Ergot Derivatives; Inhalational Anesthetics; Iobenguane I 123
Increased Effect/Toxicity
Norepinephrine may increase the levels/effects of: Droxidopa; Sympathomimetics

The levels/effects of Norepinephrine may be increased by: AtoMOXetine; Beta-Blockers; Cannabinoid-Containing Products; COMT Inhibitors; Ergot Derivatives; Hyaluronidase; Inhalational Anesthetics; Linezolid; MAO Inhibitors; Serotonin/Norepinephrine Reuptake Inhibitors; Tricyclic Antidepressants
Decreased Effect
Norepinephrine may decrease the levels/effects of: Benzylpenicilloyl Polylysine; Iobenguane I 123; Ioflupane I 123

The levels/effects of Norepinephrine may be decreased by: Alpha1-Blockers; Spironolactone

Stability Readily oxidized, do not use if brown coloration; dilute with D_5W, D_5W/NS, or NS (dilution in NS is not recommended by the manufacturer; however, stability in NS has been proven by others; Tremblay, 2008); not stable with alkaline solutions

Mechanism of Action Stimulates beta$_1$-adrenergic receptors and alpha-adrenergic receptors causing increased contractility and heart rate as well as vasoconstriction, thereby increasing systemic blood pressure and coronary blood flow; clinically, alpha effects (vasoconstriction) are greater than beta effects (inotropic and chronotropic effects)

Pharmacodynamics
Onset of action: Very rapid
Duration: Limited duration following I.V. injection
Pharmacokinetics (Adult data unless noted)
Metabolism: By catechol-o-methyltransferase (COMT) and monoamine oxidase (MAO)
Elimination: In urine (84% to 96% as inactive metabolites)

Dosing: Usual Continuous I.V. infusion: **Note:** Dose stated in terms of **norepinephrine base**:
Children: Initial: 0.05-0.1 mcg/kg/minute, titrate to desired effect; maximum dose: 1-2 mcg/kg/minute
Adults: Initial: 0.5-1 mcg/minute; titrate to desired response
Usual range: 8-30 mcg/minute as an infusion
ACLS dosage range: 0.5-30 mcg/minute

Usual Infusion Concentrations: Neonatal I.V. infusion: 10 mcg/mL **or** 16 mcg/mL
Usual Infusion Concentrations: Pediatric I.V. infusion: 8 mcg/mL **or** 16 mcg/mL

Administration Parenteral: Administer into large vein to avoid potential extravasation.
Vesicant/Extravasation Risk Vesicant
Monitoring Parameters Blood pressure, heart rate, urine output, peripheral perfusion
Additional Information Treat extravasations with local injections of phentolamine.

Dosage Forms Excipient information presented when available (limited, particularly for generics); consult specific product labeling.
Solution, Injection [strength expressed as base]:
Levophed: 1 mg/mL (4 mL) [contains sodium metabisulfite]
Generic: 1 mg/mL (4 mL)
Solution, Injection [strength expressed as base, preservative free]:
Generic: 1 mg/mL (4 mL)

References
Institute for Safe Medication Practices (ISMP), "Standard Concentrations of Neonatal Drug Infusions," *ISMP*, 2011.
Minzter BH, Johnson RF, Paschall RL, et al, "The Diverse Effects of Vasopressors on the Fetoplacental Circulation of the Dual Perfused Human Placenta," *Anesth Analg*, 2010, 110(3):857-62.
Phillips MS, "Standardizing I.V. Infusion Concentrations: National Survey Results," *Am J Health Syst Pharm*, 2011, 68(22):2176-82.
Tremblay M, Lessard MR, Trépanier CA, et al, "Stability of Norepinephrine Infusions Prepared in Dextrose and Normal Saline Solutions," *Can J Anaesth*, 2008, 55(3):163-7.
Wang L, Zhang W, and Zhao Y, "The Study of Maternal and Fetal Plasma Catecholamines Levels During Pregnancy and Delivery," *J Perinat Med*, 1999, 27(3):195-8.

◆ **Norepinephrine Bitartrate** *see* Norepinephrine *on page 1510*

Norethindrone (nor ETH in drone)

Medication Safety Issues
Sound-alike/look-alike issues:
Micronor® may be confused with miconazole, Micronase

Related Information
Contraceptive Comparison Table *on page 2266*
Safe Handling of Hazardous Drugs *on page 2419*

Brand Names: U.S. Aygestin; Camila; Errin; Heather; Jencycla; Jolivette; Lyza; Nor-QD; Nora-BE; Ortho Micronor

Brand Names: Canada Micronor®; Norlutate®

Therapeutic Category Contraceptive, Oral; Contraceptive, Progestin Only; Progestin

Generic Availability (U.S.) Yes

Use Treatment of amenorrhea, abnormal uterine bleeding, endometriosis, oral contraceptive

Pregnancy Risk Factor X

Pregnancy Considerations First trimester exposure may cause genital abnormalities including hypospadias in male infants and mild virilization of external female genitalia. Significant adverse events related to growth and development have not been observed (limited studies). Use is contraindicated during pregnancy. May be started immediately postpartum if not breast-feeding.

Breast-Feeding Considerations Small amounts of progestins are found in breast milk (1% to 6% of maternal serum concentration). Norethindrone can cause changes in milk production in the mother. When used for contraception, may start 3 weeks after delivery in women who are partially breast-feeding, or 6 weeks after delivery in women who are fully breast-feeding.

Contraindications Hypersensitivity to norethindrone or any component; thromboembolic disorders, severe hepatic disease, breast cancer, cerebral hemorrhage, undiagnosed vaginal bleeding; known or suspected pregnancy; as a diagnostic test for pregnancy

Warnings Hazardous agent; use appropriate precautions for handling and disposal (NIOSH, 2012). Discontinue if sudden partial or complete loss of vision, proptosis, diplopia, or migraine occur; **there is a higher rate of failure with progestin only contraceptives**; progestin-induced withdrawal bleeding occurs within 3-7 days after discontinuation of drug.

Precautions Use with caution in patients with asthma, diabetes mellitus, seizure disorder, migraine, cardiac or renal dysfunction, psychic depression; may affect lipid and carbohydrate metabolism; women with diabetes mellitus or hyperlipidemias should be monitored closely

Adverse Reactions
Cardiovascular: Cerebral embolism, cerebral thrombosis, DVT, edema

Central nervous system: Depression, dizziness, headache, insomnia, migraine, mood swings

Dermatologic: Acne, chloasma, hirsutism, melasma, pruritus, rash, urticaria

Endocrine & metabolic: Amenorrhea, breakthrough bleeding, breast enlargement/tenderness, menstrual flow changes, spotting

Gastrointestinal: Nausea, weight gain/loss

Genitourinary: Cervical erosion changes, cervical secretion changes

Hepatic: Cholestatic jaundice, liver function test abnormalities

Ocular: Optic neuritis (with or without vision loss), retinal vascular thrombosis

Respiratory: Pulmonary embolism

Miscellaneous: Anaphylactic/anaphylactoid reactions

Drug Interactions
Metabolism/Transport Effects Substrate of CYP3A4 (major); **Note:** Assignment of Major/Minor substrate status based on clinically relevant drug interaction potential; **Induces** CYP2C19 (weak/moderate)

Avoid Concomitant Use
Avoid concomitant use of Norethindrone with any of the following: Griseofulvin; Tranexamic Acid; Ulipristal

Increased Effect/Toxicity
Norethindrone may increase the levels/effects of: Benzodiazepines (metabolized by oxidation); Selegiline; Thalidomide; Tranexamic Acid; Voriconazole

The levels/effects of Norethindrone may be increased by: Atazanavir; Boceprevir; Cobicistat; Herbs (Progestogenic Properties); Lopinavir; Metreleptin; Mifepristone; Tipranavir; Voriconazole

Decreased Effect
Norethindrone may decrease the levels/effects of: Anticoagulants; Fosamprenavir; Vitamin K Antagonists

The levels/effects of Norethindrone may be decreased by: Acitretin; Aminoglutethimide; Aprepitant; Artemether; Barbiturates; Bexarotene (Systemic); Bile Acid Sequestrants; Bosentan; CarBAMazepine; CloBAZam; Colesevelam; CYP3A4 Inducers (Strong); Dabrafenib; Darunavir; Deferasirox; Efavirenz; Eslicarbazepine; Exenatide; Felbamate; Fosamprenavir; Fosaprepitant; Fosphenytoin; Griseofulvin; LamoTRIgine; Lopinavir; Metreleptin; Mifepristone; Mitotane; Mycophenolate; Nelfinavir; Nevirapine; OXcarbazepine; Perampanel; Phenytoin; Primidone; Prucalopride; Retinoic Acid Derivatives; Rifamycin Derivatives; Rufinamide; Saquinavir; Siltuximab; St Johns Wort; Sugammadex; Telaprevir; Tocilizumab; Topiramate; Ulipristal

Stability Hazardous agent; use appropriate precautions for handling and disposal (NIOSH, 2012).

Mechanism of Action Inhibits secretion of pituitary gonadotropin (LH) which prevents follicular maturation and ovulation

Pharmacokinetics (Adult data unless noted)
Absorption: Oral: Rapidly absorbed
Distribution: V_d: 4 L/kg
Protein binding: 61% to albumin and 36% to sex hormone-binding globulin (SHBG)
Metabolism: Hepatic via reduction and conjugation; first-pass effect
Bioavailability: ~65%
Half-life: ~8 hours
Time to peak serum concentration: 1 hour (range: 0.5-2 hours)
Elimination: Urine (>50% as metabolites); feces (20% to 40% as metabolites)

Dosing: Usual Adolescents and Adults: Female: Oral: Not indicated for use before menarche
Amenorrhea and abnormal uterine bleeding: Norethindrone acetate 2.5-10 mg/day for 5-10 days beginning during the latter half of the menstrual cycle
Endometriosis: Norethindrone acetate 5 mg/day for 14 days; increase at increments of 2.5 mg/day every 2 weeks up to 15 mg/day
Contraception: Progesterone only: Norethindrone 0.35 mg every day of the year starting on first day of menstrual period or the day after a miscarriage or abortion. If switching from a combined oral contraceptive, begin the day after finishing the last active combined tablet. If dose is missed, take as soon as remembered. An additional method of contraception should be used for 48 hours if dose is taken >3 hours late.

Administration Oral: Administer at the same time each day; may administer with food

Hazardous agent; use appropriate precautions for handling and disposal (NIOSH, 2012).

Dosage Forms Excipient information presented when available (limited, particularly for generics); consult specific product labeling.

Tablet, Oral:
Camila: 0.35 mg
Errin: 0.35 mg
Heather: 0.35 mg [contains fd&c yellow #10 aluminum lake, fd&c yellow #6 aluminum lake]
Jencycla: 0.35 mg [contains brilliant blue fcf (fd&c blue #1), fd&c yellow #10 (quinoline yellow)]
Jolivette: 0.35 mg
Lyza: 0.35 mg [contains fd&c yellow #10 (quinoline yellow)]
Nor-QD: 0.35 mg
Nora-BE: 0.35 mg
Ortho Micronor: 0.35 mg [contains fd&c yellow #10 (quinoline yellow)]
Generic: 0.35 mg
Tablet, Oral, as acetate:
Aygestin: 5 mg [scored]
Generic: 5 mg

References

American College of Obstetricians and Gynecologists, "ACOG Committee Opinion. Number 310, April 2005. Endometriosis in Adolescents," *Obstet Gynecol*, 2005, 105(4):921-7.

ACOG Committee on Practice Bulletins-Gynecology, "ACOG Practice Bulletin. No. 73: Use of Hormonal Contraception in Women With Coexisting Medical Conditions," *Obstet Gynecol*, 2006, 107 (6):1453-72.

National Institute for Occupational Safety and Health (NIOSH), "NIOSH List of Antineoplastic and Other Hazardous Drugs in Healthcare Settings 2012." Available at http://www.cdc.gov/niosh/docs/2012-150/pdfs/2012-150.pdf. Accessed January 21, 2013.

◆ **Norethindrone Acetate** see Norethindrone on page 1511

◆ **Norethisterone** see Norethindrone on page 1511

◆ **Noritate** see MetroNIDAZOLE (Topical) on page 1404

◆ **Norlutate® (Can)** see Norethindrone on page 1511

◆ **Normal Human Serum Albumin** see Albumin on page 82

◆ **Normal Immunoglobulin** see Immune Globulin on page 1084

◆ **Normal Saline** see Sodium Chloride on page 1902

◆ **Normal Serum Albumin (Human)** see Albumin on page 82

◆ **Normodyne (Can)** see Labetalol on page 1186

◆ **Norpace** see Disopyramide on page 694

◆ **Norpace® (Can)** see Disopyramide on page 694

◆ **Norpace CR** see Disopyramide on page 694

◆ **Norpramin** see Desipramine on page 608

◆ **Nor-QD** see Norethindrone on page 1511

◆ **Nortemp Children's [OTC]** see Acetaminophen on page 47

◆ **North American Antisnake-Bite Serum, FAB (Ovine)** see Crotalidae Polyvalent Immune Fab (Ovine) on page 553

Nortriptyline (nor TRIP ti leen)

Medication Safety Issues

Sound-alike/look-alike issues:
Aventyl® HCl may be confused with Bentyl®
Nortriptyline may be confused with amitriptyline, desipramine, Norpramin®
Pamelor™ may be confused with Demerol®, Tambocor™

BEERS Criteria medication:
This drug may be potentially inappropriate for use in geriatric patients (SIADH: Quality of evidence - moderate; Strength of recommendation - strong).

Related Information

Antidepressant Agents on page 2219

Brand Names: U.S. Pamelor

Brand Names: Canada Apo-Nortriptyline®; Ava-Nortriptyline; Aventyl®; Dom-Nortriptyline; Norventyl; Nu-Nortriptyline; PMS-Nortriptyline; Teva-Nortriptyline

Therapeutic Category Antidepressant, Tricyclic (Secondary Amine)

Generic Availability (U.S.) Yes

Use Treatment of various forms of depression, often in conjunction with psychotherapy; nocturnal enuresis

Medication Guide Available Yes

Pregnancy Considerations Animal reproduction studies are inconclusive. Nortriptyline and its metabolites cross the human placenta and can be detected in cord blood (Loughhead, 2006). Tricyclic antidepressants may be associated with irritability, jitteriness, and convulsions (rare) in the neonate (Yonkers, 2009).

The ACOG recommends that therapy for depression during pregnancy be individualized; treatment should incorporate the clinical expertise of the mental health clinician, obstetrician, primary healthcare provider, and pediatrician (ACOG, 2008). According to the American Psychiatric Association (APA), the risks of medication treatment should be weighed against other treatment options and untreated depression. For women who discontinue antidepressant medications during pregnancy and who may be at high risk for postpartum depression, the medications can be restarted following delivery (APA, 2010). Treatment algorithms have been developed by the ACOG and the APA for the management of depression in women prior to conception and during pregnancy (Yonkers, 2009).

Breast-Feeding Considerations Nortriptyline is excreted into breast milk and the M/P ratio ranged from 0.87 to 3.71 in one case report (Matheson, 1988). Based on available information, nortriptyline has not been detected in the serum of nursing infants; however, low levels of the active metabolite E-10-hydroxynortriptyline have been detected in the serum of newborns following breast-feeding (Wisner, 1991). Based on information from one mother-infant pair, following maternal use of nortriptyline 125 mg/day, the estimated exposure to the breast-feeding infant would be 0.6% to 3% of the weight-adjusted maternal dose. Adverse events have not been reported in nursing infants. Infants should be monitored for signs of adverse events; routine monitoring of infant serum concentrations is not recommended (Fortinguerra, 2009).

Contraindications Hypersensitivity to nortriptyline or amitriptyline (cross-sensitivity with other tricyclics may occur) or any component; use of MAO inhibitors within 14 days (potentially fatal reactions may occur); use during acute recovery period after MI

Warnings Nortriptyline is not approved for use in pediatric patients. Clinical worsening of depression or suicidal ideation and behavior may occur in children and adults with major depressive disorder **[U.S. Boxed Warning]**. In clinical trials, antidepressants increased the risk of suicidal thinking and behavior (suicidality) in children, adolescents, and young adults (18-24 years of age) with major depressive disorder and other psychiatric disorders. This risk must be considered before prescribing antidepressants for any clinical use. Short-term studies did **not** show an increased risk of suicidality with antidepressant use in patients >24 years of age and showed a decreased risk in patients ≥65 years.

Patients of all ages who are treated with antidepressants for any indication require appropriate monitoring and close observation for clinical worsening of depression, suicidality, and unusual changes in behavior, especially during the first few months after antidepressant initiation or when the dose is adjusted. Family members and caregivers should be instructed to closely observe the patient (ie, daily) and communicate condition with healthcare provider. Patients should also be monitored for associated behaviors (eg, anxiety, agitation, panic attacks, insomnia, irritability, hostility, aggressiveness, impulsivity, akathisia, hypomania, mania) which may increase the risk for worsening depression or suicidality. Worsening depression or emergence of suicidality (or associated behaviors listed above) that is abrupt in onset, severe, or not part of the presenting symptoms, may require discontinuation or modification of drug therapy.

Do not discontinue abruptly in patients receiving high doses chronically (withdrawal symptoms may occur). To reduce risk of intentional overdose, write prescriptions for the smallest quantity consistent with good patient care. Screen individuals for bipolar disorder prior to treatment (using antidepressants alone may induce manic episodes in patients with this condition). May worsen psychosis in some patients.

Use with extreme caution with renal or hepatic impairment. Capsule may contain sodium bisulfite and/or benzyl alcohol, both of which may cause allergic reactions in susceptible individuals; solution contains benzoic acid; benzoic acid (benzoate) is a metabolite of benzyl alcohol; large amounts of benzyl alcohol (≥99 mg/kg/day) have been associated with a potentially fatal toxicity ("gasping syndrome") in neonates; avoid use of nortriptyline products containing benzoic acid or benzyl alcohol in neonates; in vitro and animal studies have shown that benzoate displaces bilirubin from protein binding sites

Precautions Use with caution in patients with cardiac conduction disturbances, cardiovascular disease, seizure disorder, history of urinary retention, hyperthyroidism, or those receiving thyroid hormone replacement

Adverse Reactions

Cardiovascular: Arrhythmia, flushing, heart block, hypertension, MI, orthostatic hypotension, palpitation, tachycardia

Central nervous system: Agitation, anxiety, ataxia, confusion, delirium, delusions, disorientation, dizziness, drowsiness, EEG changes, exacerbation of psychosis, extrapyramidal symptoms, fatigue, hallucinations, headache, hypomania, incoordination, insomnia, nightmares, panic, restlessness, seizure

Dermatologic: Alopecia, itching, petechiae, photosensitivity, rash, urticaria

Endocrine & metabolic: Blood sugar increased/decreased, breast enlargement, galactorrhea, gynecomastia, libido increased/decreased, sexual dysfunction, SIADH

Gastrointestinal: Abdominal cramps, anorexia, black tongue, constipation, diarrhea, epigastric distress, nausea, paralytic ileus, stomatitis, taste disturbance, vomiting, weight gain/loss, xerostomia

Genitourinary: Delayed micturition, impotence, nocturia, polyuria, testicular edema, urinary retention

Hematologic: Agranulocytosis (rare), eosinophilia, purpura, thrombocytopenia

Hepatic: Cholestatic jaundice, transaminases increased

Neuromuscular & skeletal: Numbness, paresthesia, peripheral neuropathy, tingling, tremor, weakness

Ocular: Blurred vision, disturbances in accommodation, eye pain, mydriasis

Otic: Tinnitus

Miscellaneous: Allergic reactions (eg, general edema or of the face/tongue), diaphoresis (excessive), withdrawal symptoms

Drug Interactions

Metabolism/Transport Effects Substrate of CYP1A2 (minor), CYP2C19 (minor), CYP2D6 (major), CYP3A4 (minor); **Note:** Assignment of Major/Minor substrate status based on clinically relevant drug interaction potential; **Inhibits** CYP2D6 (weak), CYP2E1 (weak)

Avoid Concomitant Use

Avoid concomitant use of Nortriptyline with any of the following: Aclidinium; Azelastine (Nasal); Iobenguane I 123; Ipratropium (Oral Inhalation); Linezolid; MAO Inhibitors; Methylene Blue; Moxonidine; Paraldehyde; Potassium Chloride; Thalidomide; Tiotropium; Umeclidinium

Increased Effect/Toxicity

Nortriptyline may increase the levels/effects of: AbobotulinumtoxinA; Alcohol (Ethyl); Alpha-/Beta-Agonists (Direct-Acting); Alpha1-Agonists; Amphetamines; Analgesics (Opioid); Anticholinergic Agents; Antipsychotics; ARIPiprazole; Azelastine (Nasal); Beta2-Agonists; Buprenorphine; Cannabinoid-Containing Products; Citalopram; CNS Depressants; Desmopressin; Escitalopram; Highest Risk QTc-Prolonging Agents; Hydrocodone; Methotrimeprazine; Methylene Blue; Metyrosine; Mirabegron; Moderate Risk QTc-Prolonging Agents; OnabotulinumtoxinA; Paraldehyde; Potassium Chloride; Pramipexole; QuiNIDine; RimabotulinumtoxinB; ROPINIRole; Rotigotine; Serotonin Modulators; Sodium Phosphates; Sulfonylureas; Thalidomide; Thiazide Diuretics; Tiotropium; Topiramate; TraMADol; Vitamin K Antagonists; Yohimbine; Zolpidem

The levels/effects of Nortriptyline may be increased by: Abiraterone Acetate; Aclidinium; Altretamine; Antiemetics (5HT3 Antagonists); Antipsychotics; Brimonidine (Topical); BuPROPion; Cannabis; Cimetidine; Cinacalcet; Citalopram; Cobicistat; CYP2D6 Inhibitors (Moderate); CYP2D6 Inhibitors (Strong); Darunavir; Dexmethylphenidate; Doxylamine; Dronabinol; Droperidol; DULoxetine; Escitalopram; FLUoxetine; FluvoxaMINE; HydrOXYzine; Ipratropium (Oral Inhalation); Kava Kava; Linezolid; Lithium; Magnesium Sulfate; MAO Inhibitors; Methotrimeprazine; Methylphenidate; Metoclopramide; Metyrosine; Mifepristone; Nabilone; PARoxetine; Perampanel; Pramlintide; Protease Inhibitors; QuiNIDine; Rufinamide; Sertraline; Sodium Oxybate; Tapentadol; Terbinafine (Systemic); Tetrahydrocannabinol; Thyroid Products; TraMADol; Umeclidinium; Valproic Acid and Derivatives

Decreased Effect

Nortriptyline may decrease the levels/effects of: Acetylcholinesterase Inhibitors (Central); Alpha2-Agonists; Alpha2-Agonists (Ophthalmic); Iobenguane I 123; Moxonidine; Secretin

The levels/effects of Nortriptyline may be decreased by: Acetylcholinesterase Inhibitors (Central); Barbiturates; CarBAMazepine; Peginterferon Alfa-2b; St Johns Wort

Stability Protect from light

Mechanism of Action Traditionally believed to increase the synaptic concentration of serotonin and/or norepinephrine in the central nervous system by inhibition of their reuptake by the presynaptic neuronal membrane. However, additional receptor effects have been found including desensitization of adenyl cyclase, down regulation of beta-adrenergic receptors, and down regulation of serotonin receptors.

Pharmacodynamics Onset of action: Therapeutic antidepressant effects begin in 7-21 days; maximum effects may not occur for ≥2-3 weeks

Pharmacokinetics (Adult data unless noted)

Absorption: Oral: Rapid; well absorbed

Distribution: V_d: 14-22 L/kg; crosses placenta; enters breast milk

Protein binding: 93% to 95%

Metabolism: Undergoes significant first-pass metabolism; primarily detoxified in the liver via hydroxylation followed by glucuronide conjugation

Half-life:

Children (mean ± SD): 18 ± 4 hours

Adults (mean ± SD): 46 ± 24 hours

Time to peak serum concentration: Oral: Within 7-8.5 hours

Elimination: Metabolites and small amounts of unchanged drug excreted in urine; small amounts of biliary elimination occur

Dialysis: Not Dialyzable

Dosing: Usual Oral:

Nocturnal enuresis: Children: Administer dose 30 minutes before bedtime; usual treatment duration: ≤3 months:
6-7 years (20-25 kg): 10 mg/day
8-11 years (25-35 kg): 10-20 mg/day
>11 years (35-54 kg): 25-35 mg/day

Depression: **Note:** Not FDA approved for use in pediatric patients; controlled clinical trials have not shown tricyclic antidepressants to be superior to placebo for the treatment of depression in children and adolescents (Dopheide, 2006; Wagner, 2005).
Children 6-12 years: 1-3 mg/kg/day or 10-20 mg/day in 3-4 divided doses
Adolescents: 1-3 mg/kg/day or 30-50 mg/day in 3-4 divided doses; usual maximum dose: 150 mg/day
Adults: 25 mg 3-4 times/day up to 150 mg/day

Dosing adjustment in hepatic impairment: Use lower doses and slower titration; individualization of dosage is recommended

Administration Oral: May administer with food to decrease GI upset; dilute oral solution in water, milk, or fruit juice immediately before use; do not dilute in grape juice or carbonated beverages

Monitoring Parameters Heart rate, blood pressure, mental status, weight, plasma concentrations. Monitor patient periodically for symptom resolution; monitor for worsening depression, suicidality, and associated behaviors (especially at the beginning of therapy or when doses are increased or decreased).

Reference Range Therapeutic: 50-150 ng/mL (SI: 190-570 nmol/L)

Dosage Forms Excipient information presented when available (limited, particularly for generics); consult specific product labeling.

Capsule, Oral:
Pamelor: 10 mg, 25 mg [contains fd&c yellow #10 (quinoline yellow), fd&c yellow #6 (sunset yellow)]
Pamelor: 50 mg
Pamelor: 75 mg [contains fd&c yellow #10 (quinoline yellow), fd&c yellow #6 (sunset yellow)]
Generic: 10 mg, 25 mg, 50 mg, 75 mg

Solution, Oral:
Generic: 10 mg/5 mL (473 mL)

References

ACOG Committee on Practice Bulletins-Obstetrics. ACOG practice bulletin: clinical management guidelines for obstetrician-gynecologists number 92, April 2008 (replaces practice bulletin number 87, November 2007). Use of psychiatric medications during pregnancy and lactation. *Obstet Gynecol.* 2008;111(4):1001-1020.

American Psychiatric Association (APA). Treatment recommendations for patients with major depressive disorder. 3rd ed, May 2010. Available at http://www.psychiatryonline.com/pracGuide/pracGuideTopic_7.aspx

Dopheide JA, "Recognizing and Treating Depression in Children and Adolescents," *Am J Health Syst Pharm,* 2006, 63(3):233-43.

Levy HB, Harper CR, and Weinberg WA, "A Practical Approach to Children Failing in School," *Pediatr Clin North Am,* 1992, 39 (4):895-928

Loughhead AM, Stowe ZN, Newport DJ, et al, "Placental Passage of Tricyclic Antidepressants," *Biol Psychiatry,* 2006, 59(3):287-90.

Matheson I and Skjaeraasen J, "Milk Concentrations of Flupenthixol, Nortriptyline and Zuclopenthixol and Between-Breast Differences in Two Patients," *Eur J Clin Pharmacol,* 1988, 35(2):217-20.

Wagner KD, "Pharmacotherapy for Major Depression in Children and Adolescents," *Prog Neuropsychopharmacol Biol Psychiatry,* 2005, 29 (5):819-26.

Yonkers KA, wiser KL, Stewart DE, et al, "The Management of Depression During Pregnancy: A Report From the American Psychiatric Association and the American College of Obstetricians and Gynecologists," *upstate canicola,* 2009, 114(3):703-13.

◆ **Nortriptyline Hydrochloride** *see* Nortriptyline *on page 1512*

◆ **Norvasc** *see* AmLODIPine *on page 135*

◆ **Norventyl (Can)** *see* Nortriptyline *on page 1512*

◆ **Norvir** *see* Ritonavir *on page 1837*

◆ **Norvir® (Can)** *see* Ritonavir *on page 1837*

◆ **Norvir® SEC (Can)** *see* Ritonavir *on page 1837*

◆ **NovaFerrum 50 [OTC]** *see* Polysaccharide-Iron Complex *on page 1701*

◆ **NovaFerrum Pediatric Drops [OTC]** *see* Polysaccharide-Iron Complex *on page 1701*

◆ **Novamoxin® (Can)** *see* Amoxicillin *on page 140*

◆ **Novantrone** *see* MitoXANtrone *on page 1427*

◆ **Novarel** *see* Chorionic Gonadotropin (Human) *on page 460*

◆ **Novasen (Can)** *see* Aspirin *on page 212*

◆ **Novel Erythropoiesis-Stimulating Protein** *see* Darbepoetin Alfa *on page 592*

◆ **Novo-5 ASA (Can)** *see* Mesalamine *on page 1347*

◆ **Novo-Ampicillin (Can)** *see* Ampicillin *on page 159*

◆ **Novo-Atorvastatin (Can)** *see* AtorvaSTATin *on page 227*

◆ **Novo-Azithromycin (Can)** *see* Azithromycin (Systemic) *on page 247*

◆ **Novo-AZT (Can)** *see* Zidovudine *on page 2168*

◆ **Novo-Baclofen (Can)** *see* Baclofen *on page 259*

◆ **Novo-Bupropion SR (Can)** *see* BuPROPion *on page 327*

◆ **Novo-Buspirone (Can)** *see* BusPIRone *on page 332*

◆ **Novo-Carvedilol (Can)** *see* Carvedilol *on page 385*

◆ **Novo-Cefaclor (Can)** *see* Cefaclor *on page 391*

◆ **Novo-Chloroquine (Can)** *see* Chloroquine *on page 444*

◆ **Novo-Cholamine (Can)** *see* Cholestyramine Resin *on page 457*

◆ **Novo-Cholamine Light (Can)** *see* Cholestyramine Resin *on page 457*

◆ **Novo-Cimetidine (Can)** *see* Cimetidine *on page 469*

◆ **Novo-Ciprofloxacin (Can)** *see* Ciprofloxacin (Systemic) *on page 471*

◆ **Novo-Clavamoxin (Can)** *see* Amoxicillin and Clavulanate *on page 144*

◆ **Novo-Clobazam (Can)** *see* CloBAZam *on page 504*

◆ **Novo-Clobetasol (Can)** *see* Clobetasol *on page 506*

◆ **Novo-Clomipramine (Can)** *see* ClomiPRAMINE *on page 510*

◆ **Novo-Clonidine (Can)** *see* CloNIDine *on page 516*

◆ **Novo-Clopate (Can)** *see* Clorazepate *on page 524*

◆ **Novo-Cycloprine (Can)** *see* Cyclobenzaprine *on page 558*

◆ **Novo-Desipramine (Can)** *see* Desipramine *on page 608*

◆ **Novo-Desmopressin (Can)** *see* Desmopressin *on page 612*

◆ **Novo-Dimenate [OTC] (Can)** *see* DimenhyDRINATE *on page 670*

◆ **Novo-Dipam (Can)** *see* Diazepam *on page 640*

◆ **Novo-Divalproex (Can)** *see* Valproic Acid and Derivatives *on page 2102*

◆ **Novo-Docusate Calcium [OTC] (Can)** *see* Docusate *on page 701*

◆ **Novo-Docusate Sodium [OTC] (Can)** *see* Docusate *on page 701*

◆ **Novo-Doxepin (Can)** *see* Doxepin (Systemic) *on page 715*

◆ **Novoeight** *see* Antihemophilic Factor (Recombinant) *on page 172*

◆ **Novo-Famotidine (Can)** *see* Famotidine *on page 843*

◆ **Novo-Fentanyl (Can)** *see* FentaNYL *on page 853*

◆ **Novo-Ferrogluc (Can)** *see* Ferrous Gluconate *on page 866*

◆ **Novo-Fluconazole (Can)** *see* Fluconazole *on page 877*

◆ **Novo-Fluoxetine (Can)** *see* FLUoxetine *on page 901*

◆ **Novo-Flurprofen (Can)** *see* Flurbiprofen (Systemic) *on page 908*

◆ **Novo-Fluvoxamine (Can)** *see* FluvoxaMINE *on page 922*

◆ **Novo-Furantoin (Can)** *see* Nitrofurantoin *on page 1502*

◆ **Novo-Gesic (Can)** *see* Acetaminophen *on page 47*

◆ **Novo-Hydroxyzin (Can)** *see* HydrOXYzine *on page 1054*

◆ **Novo-Hylazin (Can)** *see* HydrALAZINE *on page 1022*

◆ **Novo-Ipramide (Can)** *see* Ipratropium (Oral Inhalation) *on page 1144*

◆ **Novo-Ketorolac (Can)** *see* Ketorolac (Systemic) *on page 1180*

◆ **Novo-Levobunolol (Can)** *see* Levobunolol *on page 1223*

◆ **Novo-Levofloxacin (Can)** *see* Levofloxacin (Systemic) *on page 1228*

◆ **Novo-Lexin (Can)** *see* Cephalexin *on page 429*

◆ **NovoLIN® 70/30** *see* Insulin NPH and Insulin Regular *on page 1132*

◆ **Novolin® ge 30/70 (Can)** *see* Insulin NPH and Insulin Regular *on page 1132*

◆ **Novolin® ge 40/60 (Can)** *see* Insulin NPH and Insulin Regular *on page 1132*

◆ **Novolin® ge 50/50 (Can)** *see* Insulin NPH and Insulin Regular *on page 1132*

◆ **Novolin® ge NPH (Can)** *see* Insulin NPH *on page 1130*

◆ **Novolin® ge Toronto (Can)** *see* Insulin Regular *on page 1134*

◆ **NovoLIN N [OTC]** *see* Insulin NPH *on page 1130*

◆ **NovoLIN N ReliOn [OTC]** *see* Insulin NPH *on page 1130*

◆ **NovoLIN R [OTC]** *see* Insulin Regular *on page 1134*

◆ **NovoLIN R ReliOn [OTC]** *see* Insulin Regular *on page 1134*

◆ **NovoLOG** *see* Insulin Aspart *on page 1114*

◆ **NovoLog 70/30** *see* Insulin Aspart Protamine and Insulin Aspart *on page 1117*

◆ **NovoLOG FlexPen** *see* Insulin Aspart *on page 1114*

◆ **NovoLOG® Mix 70/30** *see* Insulin Aspart Protamine and Insulin Aspart *on page 1117*

◆ **NovoLOG® Mix 70/30 FlexPen®** *see* Insulin Aspart Protamine and Insulin Aspart *on page 1117*

◆ **NovoLOG PenFill** *see* Insulin Aspart *on page 1114*

◆ **Novo-Loperamide (Can)** *see* Loperamide *on page 1270*

◆ **Novo-Medopa (Can)** *see* Methyldopa *on page 1376*

◆ **Novo-Medrone (Can)** *see* MedroxyPROGESTERone *on page 1318*

◆ **Novo-Metformin (Can)** *see* MetFORMIN *on page 1353*

◆ **Novo-Methacin (Can)** *see* Indomethacin *on page 1096*

◆ **Novo-Mexiletine (Can)** *see* Mexiletine *on page 1406*

◆ **Novo-Minocycline (Can)** *see* Minocycline *on page 1420*

◆ **Novo-Misoprostol (Can)** *see* Misoprostol *on page 1423*

◆ **NovoMix® 30 (Can)** *see* Insulin Aspart Protamine and Insulin Aspart *on page 1117*

◆ **Novo-Morphine SR (Can)** *see* Morphine (Systemic) *on page 1440*

◆ **Novo-Mycophenolate (Can)** *see* Mycophenolate *on page 1453*

◆ **Novo-Nidazol (Can)** *see* MetroNIDAZOLE (Systemic) *on page 1399*

◆ **Novo-Nizatidine (Can)** *see* Nizatidine *on page 1508*

◆ **Novo-Ofloxacin (Can)** *see* Ofloxacin (Systemic) *on page 1521*

◆ **Novo-Oxybutynin (Can)** *see* Oxybutynin *on page 1568*

◆ **Novo-Paroxetine (Can)** *see* PARoxetine *on page 1609*

◆ **Novo-Pen-VK (Can)** *see* Penicillin V Potassium *on page 1635*

◆ **Novo-Peridol (Can)** *see* Haloperidol *on page 998*

◆ **Novo-Pheniram (Can)** *see* Chlorpheniramine *on page 448*

◆ **Novo-Phenytoin (Can)** *see* Phenytoin *on page 1663*

◆ **Novo-Pramine (Can)** *see* Imipramine *on page 1080*

◆ **Novo-Pranol (Can)** *see* Propranolol *on page 1759*

◆ **Novo-Pravastatin (Can)** *see* Pravastatin *on page 1720*

◆ **Novo-Prazin (Can)** *see* Prazosin *on page 1724*

◆ **Novo-Prednisolone (Can)** *see* PrednisoLONE (Systemic) *on page 1727*

◆ **Novo-Prednisone (Can)** *see* PredniSONE *on page 1732*

◆ **Novo-Profen (Can)** *see* Ibuprofen *on page 1059*

◆ **Novo-Purol (Can)** *see* Allopurinol *on page 97*

◆ **Novo-Quinidin (Can)** *see* QuiNIDine *on page 1791*

◆ **Novo-Quinine (Can)** *see* QuiNINE *on page 1794*

◆ **NovoRapid® (Can)** *see* Insulin Aspart *on page 1114*

◆ **Novo-Rythro Estolate (Can)** *see* Erythromycin (Systemic) *on page 780*

◆ **Novo-Rythro Ethylsuccinate (Can)** *see* Erythromycin (Systemic) *on page 780*

◆ **Novo-Salbutamol HFA (Can)** *see* Albuterol *on page 84*

◆ **Novo-Semide (Can)** *see* Furosemide *on page 948*

◆ **NovoSeven RT** *see* Factor VIIa (Recombinant) *on page 831*

◆ **Novo-Sotalol (Can)** *see* Sotalol *on page 1925*

◆ **Novo-Sucralate (Can)** *see* Sucralfate *on page 1940*

◆ **Novo-Theophyl SR (Can)** *see* Theophylline *on page 2005*

◆ **Novo-Timol (Can)** *see* Timolol (Ophthalmic) *on page 2028*

◆ **Novo-Trazodone (Can)** *see* TraZODone *on page 2065*

◆ **Novo-Trifluzine (Can)** *see* Trifluoperazine *on page 2082*

◆ **Novo-Triptyn (Can)** *see* Amitriptyline *on page 133*

◆ **Novo-Veramil (Can)** *see* Verapamil *on page 2129*

◆ **Novo-Veramil SR (Can)** *see* Verapamil *on page 2129*

◆ **Novo-Warfarin (Can)** *see* Warfarin *on page 2156*

◆ **Noxafil** *see* Posaconazole *on page 1703*

◆ **NPH Insulin** *see* Insulin NPH *on page 1130*

◆ **NPH Insulin and Regular Insulin** *see* Insulin NPH and Insulin Regular *on page 1132*

◆ **NP Thyroid** *see* Thyroid, Desiccated *on page 2018*

◆ **NRP104** *see* Lisdexamfetamine *on page 1260*

◆ **NRS Nasal Relief [OTC]** *see* Oxymetazoline (Nasal) *on page 1577*

◆ **NTBC** *see* Nitisinone *on page 1501*

◆ **NTG** *see* Nitroglycerin *on page 1504*

- **NTP-Alprazolam (Can)** *see* ALPRAZolam *on page 100*
- **NTP-Amoxicillin (Can)** *see* Amoxicillin *on page 140*
- **NTP-Furosemide (Can)** *see* Furosemide *on page 948*
- **NTZ** *see* Nitazoxanide *on page 1500*
- **Nu-Acyclovir (Can)** *see* Acyclovir (Systemic) *on page 63*
- **Nu-Alpraz (Can)** *see* ALPRAZolam *on page 100*
- **Nu-Amoxi (Can)** *see* Amoxicillin *on page 140*
- **Nu-Ampi (Can)** *see* Ampicillin *on page 159*
- **Nu-Atenol (Can)** *see* Atenolol *on page 222*
- **Nu-Baclo (Can)** *see* Baclofen *on page 259*
- **Nubain** *see* Nalbuphine *on page 1464*
- **Nu-Carbamazepine (Can)** *see* CarBAMazepine *on page 372*
- **Nu-Cefaclor (Can)** *see* Cefaclor *on page 391*
- **Nu-Cephalex (Can)** *see* Cephalexin *on page 429*
- **Nu-Cimet (Can)** *see* Cimetidine *on page 469*
- **NuCort** *see* Hydrocortisone (Topical) *on page 1038*
- **Nu-Cromolyn (Can)** *see* Cromolyn (Systemic, Oral Inhalation) *on page 551*
- **Nu-Desipramine (Can)** *see* Desipramine *on page 608*
- **Nu-Diltiaz (Can)** *see* Diltiazem *on page 667*
- **Nu-Diltiaz-CD (Can)** *see* Diltiazem *on page 667*
- **Nu-Erythromycin-S (Can)** *see* Erythromycin (Systemic) *on page 780*
- **Nu-Famotidine (Can)** *see* Famotidine *on page 843*
- **Nu-Fluoxetine (Can)** *see* FLUoxetine *on page 901*
- **Nu-Flurprofen (Can)** *see* Flurbiprofen (Systemic) *on page 908*
- **Nu-Furosemide (Can)** *see* Furosemide *on page 948*
- **Nu-Hydral (Can)** *see* HydrALAZINE *on page 1022*
- **Nu-Hydroxyzine (Can)** *see* HydrOXYzine *on page 1054*
- **Nu-Ipratropium (Can)** *see* Ipratropium (Oral Inhalation) *on page 1144*
- **Nu-Iron [OTC]** *see* Polysaccharide-Iron Complex *on page 1701*
- **NuLev** *see* Hyoscyamine *on page 1056*
- **NuLYTELY** *see* Polyethylene Glycol-Electrolyte Solution *on page 1697*
- **Nu-Metoclopramide (Can)** *see* Metoclopramide *on page 1391*
- **Nu-Metop (Can)** *see* Metoprolol *on page 1396*
- **Nu-Nizatidine (Can)** *see* Nizatidine *on page 1508*
- **Nu-Nortriptyline (Can)** *see* Nortriptyline *on page 1512*
- **Nu-Oxybutyn (Can)** *see* Oxybutynin *on page 1568*
- **Nu-Pen-VK (Can)** *see* Penicillin V Potassium *on page 1635*
- **Nupercainal [OTC]** *see* Dibucaine *on page 645*
- **Nu-Pravastatin (Can)** *see* Pravastatin *on page 1720*
- **Nu-Prazo (Can)** *see* Prazosin *on page 1724*
- **Nu-Prochlor (Can)** *see* Prochlorperazine *on page 1745*
- **Nu-Propranolol (Can)** *see* Propranolol *on page 1759*
- **Nu-Ranit (Can)** *see* Ranitidine *on page 1805*
- **Nu-Simvastatin (Can)** *see* Simvastatin *on page 1892*
- **Nu-Sotalol (Can)** *see* Sotalol *on page 1925*
- **Nu-Sucralate (Can)** *see* Sucralfate *on page 1940*
- **Nu-Terazosin (Can)** *see* Terazosin *on page 1981*
- **Nu-Tetra (Can)** *see* Tetracycline *on page 1996*
- **Nu-Timolol (Can)** *see* Timolol (Systemic) *on page 2026*
- **Nutracort** *see* Hydrocortisone (Topical) *on page 1038*

- **Nu-Trazodone (Can)** *see* TraZODone *on page 2065*
- **Nu-Trazodone D (Can)** *see* TraZODone *on page 2065*
- **Nutr-E-Sol [OTC]** *see* Vitamin E *on page 2148*
- **Nutropin [DSC]** *see* Somatropin *on page 1920*
- **Nutropin (Can)** *see* Somatropin *on page 1920*
- **Nutropin AQ (Can)** *see* Somatropin *on page 1920*
- **Nutropin AQ NuSpin (Can)** *see* Somatropin *on page 1920*
- **Nutropin AQ NuSpin 5** *see* Somatropin *on page 1920*
- **Nutropin AQ NuSpin 10** *see* Somatropin *on page 1920*
- **Nutropin AQ NuSpin 20** *see* Somatropin *on page 1920*
- **Nutropin AQ Pen** *see* Somatropin *on page 1920*
- **Nu-Verap (Can)** *see* Verapamil *on page 2129*
- **Nu-Verap SR (Can)** *see* Verapamil *on page 2129*
- **NuZon** *see* Hydrocortisone (Topical) *on page 1038*
- **NVA237** *see* Glycopyrrolate *on page 977*
- **NVP** *see* Nevirapine *on page 1487*
- **Nyaderm (Can)** *see* Nystatin (Topical) *on page 1517*
- **Nyamyc** *see* Nystatin (Topical) *on page 1517*
- **Nycoff [OTC]** *see* Dextromethorphan *on page 636*

Nystatin (Oral) (nye STAT in)

Medication Safety Issues
Sound-alike/look-alike issues:
Nystatin may be confused with HMG-CoA reductase inhibitors (also known as "statins"; eg, atorvaSTATin, fluvastatin, lovastatin, pitavastatin, pravastatin, rosuvastatin, simvastatin), Nitrostat®

Brand Names: U.S. Bio-Statin

Brand Names: Canada PMS-Nystatin

Generic Availability (U.S.) Yes

Use Treatment of susceptible cutaneous, mucocutaneous, and oral cavity fungal infections normally caused by the *Candida* species

Pregnancy Risk Factor C

Pregnancy Considerations Animal reproduction studies have not been conducted. Adverse events in the fetus or newborn have not been reported following maternal use of vaginal nystatin during pregnancy. Absorption following oral use is poor.

Breast-Feeding Considerations Excretion into breast milk is not known; however, absorption following oral use is poor.

Contraindications Hypersensitivity to nystatin or any component

Adverse Reactions
Gastrointestinal: Diarrhea, nausea, stomach pain, vomiting
Rare but important or life-threatening: Hypersensitivity reactions

Drug Interactions
Metabolism/Transport Effects None known.

Avoid Concomitant Use
Avoid concomitant use of Nystatin (Oral) with any of the following: Saccharomyces boulardii

Increased Effect/Toxicity There are no known significant interactions involving an increase in effect.

Decreased Effect
Nystatin (Oral) may decrease the levels/effects of: Saccharomyces boulardii

Mechanism of Action Binds to sterols in fungal cell membrane, changing the cell wall permeability allowing for leakage of cellular contents

Pharmacodynamics Onset of action: Symptomatic relief from candidiasis: Within 24-72 hours

Pharmacokinetics (Adult data unless noted)
Absorption: Poorly absorbed from the GI tract

Elimination: In feces as unchanged drug

Dosing: Neonatal Oral candidiasis:

Prophylaxis: 100,000 units/dose 4 times/day divided as 50,000 units to each side of the mouth (Ganesan, 2009)

Treatment: 100,000-400,000 units/dose 4 times/day; one study of 14 patients (neonates and infants) found higher cure rates using 400,000 unit/dose 4 times/day (Hoppe, 1997)

Dosing: Usual

Oral candidiasis:

Infants: 200,000-400,000 units 4 times/day or 100,000 units to each side of mouth 4 times/day; one study of 14 patients (neonates and infants) found higher cure rates using 400,000 unit/dose 4 times/day (Hoppe, 1997)

Children and Adults: 400,000-600,000 units 4 times/day

Intestinal infections: Adults: Oral: 500,000-1,000,000 units every 8 hours

Administration Shake suspension well before use; suspension should be swished about the mouth and retained in the mouth for as long as possible (several minutes) before swallowing. For neonates and infants, paint nystatin suspension into recesses of the mouth.

Monitoring Parameters KOH smears or cultures should be used to confirm diagnosis of cutaneous or mucocutaneous candidiasis.

Dosage Forms Excipient information presented when available (limited, particularly for generics); consult specific product labeling.

Capsule, Oral [preservative free]:

Bio-Statin: 500,000 units, 1,000,000 units [dye free]

Powder, Oral:

Bio-Statin: (1 ea)

Generic: (1 ea)

Suspension, Mouth/Throat:

Generic: 100,000 units/mL (5 mL, 60 mL, 473 mL, 480 mL)

Tablet, Oral:

Generic: 500,000 units

References

Dismukes WE, Wade JS, Lee JY, et al, "A Randomized, Double-Blind Trial of Nystatin Therapy for the Candidiasis Hypersensitivity Syndrome," N Engl J Med, 1990, 323(25):1717-23.

Ganesan K, Harigopal S, Neal T, et al, "Prophylactic Oral Nystatin for Preterm Babies Under 33 Weeks' Gestation Decreases Fungal Colonisation and Invasive Fungaemia," Arch Dis Child Fetal Neonatal Ed, 2009, 94(4):F275-8.

Hoppe JE, "Treatment of Oropharyngeal Candidiasis and Candidal Diaper Dermatitis in Neonates and Infants: Review and Reappraisal," Pediatr Infect Dis J, 1997, 16(9):885-94.

Kaufman DA, "Challenging Issues in Neonatal Candidiasis," Curr Med Res Opin, 2010, 26(7):1769-78.

Nystatin (Topical) (nye STAT in)

Medication Safety Issues

Sound-alike/look-alike issues:

Nystatin may be confused with HMG-CoA reductase inhibitors (also known as "statins"; eg, atorvaSTATin, fluvastatin, lovastatin, pitavastatin, pravastatin, rosuvastatin, simvastatin), Nitrostat

Brand Names: U.S. Nyamyc; Nystop; Pedi-Dri; Pediaderm AF Complete

Brand Names: Canada Candistatin; Nyaderm

Therapeutic Category Antifungal Agent, Topical; Antifungal Agent, Vaginal

Generic Availability (U.S.) May be product dependent

Use Treatment of susceptible cutaneous, mucocutaneous, and vaginal fungal infections normally caused by the *Candida* species

Pregnancy Risk Factor C

Pregnancy Considerations Animal reproduction studies have not been conducted. Absorption following oral use is poor and nystatin is not absorbed following application to mucous membranes or intact skin.

Breast-Feeding Considerations Excretion into breast milk is not known; however, absorption following oral use is poor and nystatin is not absorbed following application to mucous membranes or intact skin.

Contraindications Hypersensitivity to nystatin or any component

Adverse Reactions

Dermatologic: Contact dermatitis, Stevens-Johnson syndrome

Rare but important or life-threatening: Hypersensitivity reactions

Drug Interactions

Metabolism/Transport Effects None known.

Avoid Concomitant Use There are no known interactions where it is recommended to avoid concomitant use.

Increased Effect/Toxicity There are no known significant interactions involving an increase in effect.

Decreased Effect There are no known significant interactions involving a decrease in effect.

Mechanism of Action Binds to sterols in fungal cell membrane, changing the cell wall permeability allowing for leakage of cellular contents

Pharmacodynamics Onset of action: Symptomatic relief from candidiasis: Within 24-72 hours

Pharmacokinetics (Adult data unless noted) Absorption: Not absorbed through mucous membranes or intact skin

Dosing: Neonatal Topical: Cutaneous candidal infections (candidal diaper dermatitis): Ointment, cream: Apply 2-4 times/day to affected area; most studies have used 4 times/day dosing (Hoppe, 1997)

Dosing: Usual Topical:

Cutaneous candidal infections: Children and Adults: Apply 2-4 times/day

Vaginal infections: Adolescents and Adults: Vaginal tablets: Insert 1 tablet/day at bedtime for 2 weeks

Administration

Cream or ointment: Gently massage formulation into the skin.

Intravaginal: Insert vaginal tablet high in the vagina.

Powder: Dust in shoes, in stockings, and on feet for treatment of candidal infection of the feet; also used on very moist lesions

Monitoring Parameters KOH smears or cultures should be used to confirm diagnosis of cutaneous or mucocutaneous candidiasis.

Dosage Forms Excipient information presented when available (limited, particularly for generics); consult specific product labeling.

Cream, External:

Generic: 100,000 units/g (15 g, 30 g)

Kit, External:

Pediaderm AF Complete: 100,000 units/g [contains methylparaben, propylene glycol, propylparaben]

Ointment, External:

Generic: 100,000 units/g (15 g, 30 g)

Powder, External:

Nyamyc: 100,000 units/g (15 g, 30 g, 60 g)

Nystop: 100,000 units/g (15 g, 30 g, 60 g)

Pedi-Dri: 100,000 units/g (56.7 g)

Generic: 100,000 units/g (15 g, 30 g, 60 g)

References

Hoppe JE, "Treatment of Oropharyngeal Candidiasis and Candidal Diaper Dermatitis in Neonates and Infants: Review and Reappraisal," Pediatr Infect Dis J, 1997, 16(9):885-94.

Ward DB, Fleischer AB Jr, Feldman SR, et al, "Characterization of Diaper Dermatitis in the United States," Arch Pediatr Adolesc Med, 2000, 154(9):943-6.

◆ **Nystop** see Nystatin (Topical) on page 1517

◆ **Nytol [OTC]** see DiphenhydrAMINE (Systemic) on page 673

- ◆ **Nytol® (Can)** *see* DiphenhydrAMINE (Systemic) *on page 673*
- ◆ **Nytol® Extra Strength (Can)** *see* DiphenhydrAMINE (Systemic) *on page 673*
- ◆ **Nytol Maximum Strength [OTC]** *see* DiphenhydrAMINE (Systemic) *on page 673*
- ◆ **OC8 [OTC]** *see* Benzoyl Peroxide *on page 275*
- ◆ **OCBZ** *see* OXcarbazepine *on page 1564*
- ◆ **Occlusal™-HP (Can)** *see* Salicylic Acid *on page 1860*
- ◆ **Ocean Complete Sinus Rinse [OTC]** *see* Sodium Chloride *on page 1902*
- ◆ **Ocean for Kids [OTC]** *see* Sodium Chloride *on page 1902*
- ◆ **Ocean Nasal Spray [OTC]** *see* Sodium Chloride *on page 1902*
- ◆ **Ocean Ultra Saline Mist [OTC]** *see* Sodium Chloride *on page 1902*
- ◆ **Octagam** *see* Immune Globulin *on page 1084*
- ◆ **Octagam 10% (Can)** *see* Immune Globulin *on page 1084*
- ◆ **Octostim® (Can)** *see* Desmopressin *on page 612*

Octreotide (ok TREE oh tide)

Medication Safety Issues
Sound-alike/look-alike issues:
Octreotide may be confused with pasireotide
SandoSTATIN may be confused with SandIMMUNE, SandoSTATIN LAR, sargramostim, simvastatin
Brand Names: U.S. SandoSTATIN; SandoSTATIN LAR Depot
Brand Names: Canada Octreotide Acetate Injection; Octreotide Acetate Omega; Sandostatin LAR; Sandostatin®
Therapeutic Category Antidiarrheal; Antidote; Antihemorrhagics; Antisecretory Agent; Somatostatin Analog
Generic Availability (U.S.) May be product dependent
Use Control of symptoms, including secretory diarrhea in patients with metastatic carcinoid or vasoactive intestinal peptide-secreting tumors (VIPomas) (FDA approved in adults); treatment of acromegaly (FDA approved in adults). Other uses include control of bleeding of esophageal varices, Cushing's syndrome, insulinomas, glucagonoma, small bowel fistulas, postgastrectomy dumping syndrome, chemotherapy-induced diarrhea, graft-versus-host disease (GVHD)-associated diarrhea, Zollinger-Ellison syndrome, persistent hyperinsulinemic hypoglycemia of infancy (nesidioblastosis), postoperative chylothorax, second-line treatment for thymic malignancies; islet cell tumors; treatment of malignant bowel obstruction; treatment of sulfonylurea overdosage (nondepot formulation); hypothalamic obesity

Pregnancy Risk Factor B
Pregnancy Considerations Adverse effects were not observed in animal reproduction studies. Octreotide crosses the placenta and can be detected in the newborn at delivery (Caron, 1995; Fassnacht, 2001; Maffeï, 2010); data concerning use in pregnancy is limited. In case reports of acromegalic women who received normal doses of octreotide during pregnancy, no congenital malformations were reported. Because normalization of IGF-1 and GH may restore fertility in women with acromegaly, women of childbearing potential should use adequate contraception during treatment. Long-acting formulations should be discontinued 2 to 3 months prior to a planned pregnancy when possible; however, octreotide therapy may be resumed in pregnant women with worsening symptoms if needed (Katznelson, 2011).

Breast-Feeding Considerations Octreotide is excreted in breast milk. In a case report, a woman was taking octreotide SubQ in doses up to 2400 mcg/day prior to and throughout pregnancy. Octreotide was measurable in the colostrum in concentrations similar to those in the maternal serum (Maffeï, 2010); however, oral absorption of octreotide is considered to be poor (Battershill, 1989). The manufacturer recommends that caution be exercised when administering octreotide to nursing women.

Contraindications Hypersensitivity to octreotide or any component

Warnings Dosage adjustment may be required to maintain symptomatic control; octreotide may affect glucose regulation; insulin requirements may be reduced in type I diabetic patients; symptomatic hypoglycemia which may be severe, has been reported; in nondiabetics and type II diabetics with partially intact insulin reserves, octreotide may decrease insulin levels and hyperglycemia may occur; monitor glucose tolerance and antidiabetic treatment closely; may worsen hypoglycemia in patients with insulinomas; patients must be monitored closely for biliary tract abnormalities (including biliary obstruction, cholecystitis, and cholelithiasis). The incidence of gallbladder stone or sludge increases with a duration of therapy ≥12 months; reported incidence in children is ~33%. In patients with neuroendocrine tumors, the NCCN guidelines (v.2.2009) recommend considering prophylactic cholecystectomy in patients undergoing abdominal surgery if octreotide treatment is planned. Postmarketing cases of serious and fatal events, including hypoxia and necrotizing enterocolitis, have been reported with octreotide use in children (usually with serious underlying conditions), particularly in children <2 years of age. In studies with octreotide depot, the incidence of cholelithiasis in children is higher than the reported incidences for adults.

Precautions Hypothyroidism, with or without goiter, has been reported in acromegalic patients; use with caution in patients with renal impairment and consider dosage modification in patients with severe renal failure requiring dialysis; use with caution in patients with hepatic impairment; dosage adjustment required in patients with established cirrhosis; use caution in diabetic patients with gastroparesis; chronic usage is associated with abnormal Schillings test and depressed vitamin B_{12} levels; monitor vitamin B_{12} levels in patients receiving long-term therapy; suppression of growth hormone (animal data) is of concern when used as long-term therapy in children. Use with caution in patients with heart failure or concomitant medications that alter heart rate or rhythm; bradycardia, conduction abnormalities, and arrhythmia have been observed in acromegalic and carcinoid syndrome patients; cardiovascular medication requirements may change; may enhance the adverse/toxic effects of other QT_c-prolonging agents. Vehicle used in depot injectable (polylactide-coglycolide microspheres) has rarely been associated with retinal artery occlusion in patients with abnormal arteriovenous anastomosis.

Adverse Reactions Adverse reactions vary by route of administration or dosage form.
Cardiovascular: Angina, arrhythmia, cardiac failure, chest pain (non-depot formulations), conduction abnormalities, edema, flushing, hematoma, hypertension, palpitation, peripheral edema, phlebitis, sinus bradycardia
Central nervous system: Abnormal gait, amnesia, anxiety, confusion, depression, dizziness, dysphonia, fatigue, fever, hallucinations, headache, hypoesthesia, insomnia, malaise, nervousness, neuralgia, neuropathy, pain, somnolence, tremor, vertigo
Dermatologic: Acne, alopecia, bruising, cellulitis, pruritus, rash (depot formulation)
Endocrine & metabolic: Breast pain, cachexia, goiter (non-depot formulations), gout, hyper-/hypoglycemia, hypokalemia, hypoproteinemia, hypothyroidism (non-depot formulations), impotence
Gastrointestinal: Abdominal pain, anorexia, biliary duct dilatation, biliary sludge (length of therapy dependent),

cholelithiasis (length of therapy dependent), colitis, constipation, cramping, dehydration, diarrhea, diverticulitis, dyspepsia, dysphagia, fat malabsorption, feces discoloration, flatulence, gastritis, gastroenteritis, gingivitis, glossitis, loose stools, melena, nausea, steatorrhea, stomatitis, taste perversion, tenesmus, vomiting, xerostomia

Genitourinary: Incontinence, pollakiuria (non-depot formulations), urinary tract infection

Hematologic: Anemia (more common with depot formulations)

Local: Injection site hematoma/pain (dose and formulation related)

Neuromuscular & skeletal: Arthralgia, arthropathy, back pain, hyperkinesia, hypertonia, joint pain, myalgia, neuropathy, paresthesia, rigors, tremor, weakness

Ocular: Blurred vision, visual disturbance

Otic: Earache, tinnitus

Renal: Albuminuria, renal abscess, renal calculus

Respiratory: Bronchitis, cough, dyspnea (non-depot formulations), epistaxis, pharyngitis, rhinitis, sinusitis, upper respiratory infection

Miscellaneous: Allergy, antibodies to octreotide, bacterial infection, cold symptoms, diaphoresis, flu symptoms, moniliasis

Rare but important or life-threatening: Amenorrhea, anaphylactic shock, anaphylactoid reactions, aneurysm, aphasia, appendicitis, arthritis, ascending cholangitis, ascites, atrial fibrillation, basal cell carcinoma, Bell's palsy, biliary obstruction, breast carcinoma, cardiac arrest, cerebral vascular disorder, CHF, cholecystitis, cholestatic hepatitis, CK increased, deafness, diabetes insipidus, diabetes mellitus, fatty liver, galactorrhea, gallbladder polyp, GI bleeding, GI hemorrhage, GI ulcer, glaucoma, gynecomastia, hematuria, hepatitis, hypoadrenalism, hypoxia (children), intestinal obstruction, intracranial hemorrhage, intraocular pressure increased, ischemia, joint effusion, malignant hyperpyrexia, MI, migraine, necrotizing enterocolitis (neonates), nephrolithiasis, neuritis, oligomenorrhea, orthostatic hypotension, pancreatitis, pancytopenia, paresis, pituitary apoplexy, pleural effusion, pneumonia, pneumothorax, polymenorrhea, pulmonary embolism, pulmonary hypertension, pulmonary nodule, Raynaud's syndrome, renal failure, renal insufficiency, retinal vein thrombosis, seizures, status asthmaticus, suicide attempt, syncope, tachycardia, thrombocytopenia, thrombophlebitis, thrombosis, weight loss

Drug Interactions

Metabolism/Transport Effects None known.

Avoid Concomitant Use

Avoid concomitant use of Octreotide with any of the following: Ceritinib

Increased Effect/Toxicity

Octreotide may increase the levels/effects of: Bradycardia-Causing Agents; Ceritinib; Codeine; Highest Risk QTc-Prolonging Agents; Hypoglycemic Agents; Moderate Risk QTc-Prolonging Agents; Pegvisomant

The levels/effects of Octreotide may be increased by: Herbs (Hypoglycemic Properties); MAO Inhibitors; Mifepristone; Salicylates; Selective Serotonin Reuptake Inhibitors

Decreased Effect

Octreotide may decrease the levels/effects of: CycloSPORINE (Systemic)

The levels/effects of Octreotide may be decreased by: Loop Diuretics

Food Interactions Octreotide may alter absorption of dietary fats. Management: Administer injections between meals to decrease GI effects.

Stability Store in refrigerator between 2°C and 8°C (36°F and 46°F); protect from light; Sandostatin® injection at room temperature at 20°C to 30°C (68°F and 86°F) and protected from light is stable for 14 days; parenteral admixtures are stable in NS for 4 days and D$_5$W for 24 hours at room temperature; stable for up to 7 days in a polypropylene syringe; not compatible in TPN solutions due to glycosyl octreotide conjugate which may have decreased activity. Sandostatin LAR® Depot must be used immediately after reconstitution

Mechanism of Action Mimics natural somatostatin by inhibiting serotonin release, and the secretion of gastrin, VIP, insulin, glucagon, secretin, motilin, and pancreatic polypeptide. Decreases growth hormone and IGF-1 in acromegaly. Octreotide provides more potent inhibition of growth hormone, glucagon, and insulin as compared to endogenous somatostatin. Also suppresses LH response to GnRH, secretion of thyroid-stimulating hormone and decreases splanchnic blood flow.

Pharmacodynamics Duration (immediate release formulation): SubQ: 6-12 hours

Pharmacokinetics (Adult data unless noted)

Absorption: SubQ: Rapid; I.M. (depot formulation): Released slowly (via microsphere degradation in the muscle)

Bioavailability: SubQ: 100%; I.M.: 60% to 63% of SubQ dose

Distribution: V$_d$:
Adults: 13.6 L
Adults with acromegaly: 21.6 ± 8.5 L

Protein binding: 65% primarily to lipoprotein (41% in acromegaly)

Metabolism: Extensive by the liver

Half-life: 1.7-1.9 hours; up to 3.7 hours with cirrhosis; up to 3.4 hours with fatty liver disease; up to 3.1 hours in renal impairment

Time to peak serum concentration: SubQ: 0.4 hours (0.7 hours acromegaly); I.M.: 1 hour

Elimination: 32% excreted unchanged in urine
Clearance:
Adults: 10 L/hour
Adults with acromegaly: 18 L/hour

Note: When using Sandostatin LAR® Depot formulation, steady-state levels are achieved after 3 injections (3 months of therapy)

Dosing: Neonatal

Chylothorax: Continuous I.V. infusion: 0.3-10 mcg/kg/**hour** titrated to response (median: 2.8 mcg/kg/**hour**) has been described in case reports; treatment duration is usually 1-3 weeks but may vary with the clinical response (Das, 2010; Roehr, 2006)

Persistent hyperinsulinemic hypoglycemia of infancy (Stanley, 1997):
Continuous I.V. infusion: Initial: 0.08-0.4 mcg/kg/**hour**; titrate dosage depending upon patient response; maximum dose: 1.67 mcg/kg/**hour**
SubQ: Initial: 2-10 mcg/kg/day divided 3-4 times daily; titrate dosage depending upon patient response; maximum daily dose: 40 mcg/kg/day

Dosing: Usual Dosage should be individualized according to the patient's response

Sandostatin®:
Infants and Children (data limited to small studies and case reports): **Note:** The following are effective dosing ranges for specific therapies: I.V., SubQ:
Diarrhea:
Continuous I.V. infusion: Initial: 1 mcg/kg bolus dose, followed by a continuous infusion of 1 mcg/kg/**hour** has been used successfully in several cases of severe diarrhea secondary to graft vs host disease
I.V., SubQ: Doses of 1-10 mcg/kg/dose every 12 hours have been used in children beginning at the low end of the range and increasing based upon the clinical response

Chylothorax:

Continuous I.V. infusion: 0.3-10 mcg/kg/**hour** titrated to response (median: 2.8 mcg/kg/**hour**) has been described in case reports; treatment duration is usually 1-3 weeks but may vary with the clinical response (Roehr, 2006)

SubQ: 40 mcg/kg/day; case reports of effective dosage range from 2-68 mcg/kg/day (Chan, 2006; Roehr, 2006)

Esophageal varices/GI bleed: 1-2 mcg/kg initial I.V. bolus followed by 1-2 mcg/kg/**hour** continuous infusion; titrate infusion rate to response; taper dose by 50% every 12 hours when no active bleeding occurs for 24 hours; may discontinue when dose is 25% of initial dose (Eroglu, 2004)

Hypothalamic obesity (from cranial insult): SubQ: 5 mcg/kg/day divided into 3 daily doses; dose may be increased bimonthly at 5 mcg/kg/day increments to a maximum of 15 mcg/kg/day divided into 3 daily doses (Lustig, 2003)

Persistent hyperinsulinemic hypoglycemia of infancy: SubQ: 2-10 mcg/kg/day divided 3-4 times daily; titrate dosage depending upon patient response; maximum daily dose: 40 mcg/kg/day (Stanley, 1997)

Treatment of sulfonylurea overdose: **Note:** SubQ is the preferred route of administration; repeat dosing, dose escalation, or initiation of a continuous infusion may be required in patients who experience recurrent hypoglycemia. Duration of treatment may exceed 24 hours. Optimal care decisions should be made based upon patient-specific details; SubQ: 1-1.5 mcg/kg/dose; repeat in 6-12 hours as needed based upon blood glucose concentrations

Adults:

Acromegaly:

SubQ, I.V.: Initial: 50 mcg 3 times/day; titrate to achieve growth hormone levels <5 ng/mL or IGF-I (somatomedin C) levels <1.9 units/mL in males and <2.2 units/mL in females. Usual effective dose is 100-200 mcg 3 times/day; range: 300-1500 mcg/day. **Note:** Should be withdrawn yearly for a 4-week interval (8 weeks for depot injection) in patients who have received irradiation. Resume if levels increase and signs/symptoms recur.

I.M. depot injection: Patients must be stabilized on subcutaneous octreotide for at least 2 weeks before switching to the long-acting depot. Upon switch: 20 mg I.M. intragluteally every 4 weeks for 3 months, then the dose may be modified based upon response.

Dosage adjustment: After 3 months of depot injections, the dosage may be continued or modified as follows:

GH ≤1 ng/mL, IGF-1 normal, and symptoms controlled: Reduce octreotide LAR® to 10 mg I.M. every 4 weeks

GH ≤2.5 ng/mL, IGF-1 normal, and symptoms controlled: Maintain octreotide LAR® at 20 mg I.M. every 4 weeks

GH >2.5 ng/mL, IGF-1 elevated, and/or symptoms uncontrolled: Increase octreotide LAR® to 30 mg I.M. every 4 weeks

Note: Patients not adequately controlled at a dose of 30 mg may increase dose to 40 mg every 4 weeks. Dosages >40 mg are not recommended.

Carcinoid tumors:

SubQ, I.V.: Initial 2 weeks: 100-600 mcg/day in 2-4 divided doses; usual range: 50-750 mcg/day (some patients may require up to 1500 mcg/day)

I.M. depot injection: Patients must be stabilized on subcutaneous octreotide for at least 2 weeks before switching to the long-acting depot. Upon switch: 20 mg I.M. intragluteally every 4 weeks for 2 months,

then the dose may be modified based upon response

Note: Patients should continue to receive their SubQ injections for the first 2 weeks at the same dose in order to maintain therapeutic levels (some patients may require 3-4 weeks of continued SubQ injections). Patients who experience periodic exacerbations of symptoms may require temporary SubQ injections in addition to depot injections (at their previous SubQ dosing regimen) until symptoms have resolved.

Dosage adjustment: See dosing adjustment for VIPomas.

VIPomas:

SubQ, I.V.: Initial 2 weeks: 200-300 mcg/day in 2-4 divided doses; titrate dose based on response/tolerance; range: 150-750 mcg/day (doses >450 mcg/day are rarely required)

I.M. depot injection: Patients must be stabilized on subcutaneous octreotide for at least 2 weeks before switching to the long-acting depot. Upon switch: 20 mg I.M. intragluteally every 4 weeks for 2 months, then the dose may be modified based upon response.

Note: Patients receiving depot injection should continue to receive their SubQ injections for the first 2 weeks at the same dose in order to maintain therapeutic levels (some patients may require 3-4 weeks of continued SubQ injections). Patients who experience periodic exacerbations of symptoms may require temporary SubQ injections in addition to depot injections (at their previous SubQ dosing regimen) until symptoms have resolved.

Dosage adjustment: After 2 months of depot injections, the dosage may be continued or modified as follows:

Increase to 30 mg I.M. every 4 weeks if symptoms are inadequately controlled

Decrease to 10 mg I.M. every 4 weeks, for a trial period, if initially responsive to 20 mg dose

Dosage >30 mg is not recommended

Dosage adjustment in renal impairment: Clearance is decreased by 50% in patients with severe renal failure requiring dialysis; consider dosage modification in these patients as follows:

• Nondialysis-dependent renal impairment: No dosage adjustment required

• Dialysis-dependent renal impairment: Depot injection: Initial dose: I.M.: 10 mg every 4 weeks; titrate based upon response (clearance is reduced by ~50%

Dosage adjustment in hepatic impairment: Patients with established cirrhosis of the liver: Depot injection: Initial dose: I.M.: 10 mg every 4 weeks; titrate based upon response

Administration Parenteral: Only Sandostatin® injection may be administered I.V. and SubQ; Sandostatin LAR® Depot may only be administered I.M.

SubQ: Use the concentration with smallest volume to deliver dose to reduce injection site pain; rotate injection site; may bring to room temperature prior to injection

I.V. infusion: Dilute Sandostatin® injection in 50-200 mL NS or D$_5$W and infuse over 15-30 minutes or over 24 hours as a continuous infusion; in emergency situations, may be administered undiluted by direct I.V. push over 3 minutes; allow solution to come to room temperature before administration

I.M. administration: Reconstitute with provided diluent; see detailed instruction booklet for complete instructions; use immediately after reconstitution; administer into gluteal area only (avoid deltoid injections due to significant pain and discomfort at injection site)

Monitoring Parameters Baseline and periodic ultrasound evaluations for cholelithiasis, blood sugar, baseline and periodic thyroid function tests, fluid and electrolyte balance, fecal fat, and serum carotene determinations; for carcinoid, monitor urinary 5-hydroxyindole acetic acid (5-HIAA), plasma serotonin, plasma substance P; for VIPoma, monitor VIP; vitamin B_{12} levels (chronic therapy); for acromegaly: growth hormone levels, IGF-I (somatomedin C), glycemic control, and antidiabetic regimen (patients with diabetes mellitus)

Reference Range Vasoactive intestinal peptide (VIP): <75 ng/L; levels vary considerably between laboratories; growth hormone level: <5 ng/mL; IGF-I (somatomedin C): males: <1.9 units/mL, females: <2.2 units/mL

Dosage Forms Excipient information presented when available (limited, particularly for generics); consult specific product labeling.

Kit, Intramuscular:
  SandoSTATIN LAR Depot: 10 mg, 20 mg, 30 mg

Solution, Injection:
  SandoSTATIN: 50 mcg/mL (1 mL); 100 mcg/mL (1 mL)
  SandoSTATIN: 200 mcg/mL (5 mL) [contains phenol]
  SandoSTATIN: 500 mcg/mL (1 mL)
  SandoSTATIN: 1000 mcg/mL (5 mL) [contains phenol]
  Generic: 50 mcg/mL (1 mL); 100 mcg/mL (1 mL); 200 mcg/mL (5 mL); 1000 mcg/5 mL (5 mL); 500 mcg/mL (1 mL); 1000 mcg/mL (5 mL)

Solution, Injection [preservative free]:
  Generic: 100 mcg/mL (1 mL); 500 mcg/mL (1 mL)

References

Battershill PE, Clissold SP. Octreotide. A review of its pharmacodynamic and pharmacokinetic properties, and therapeutic potential in conditions associated with excessive peptide secretion. *Drugs*. 1989;38(5):658-702.

Beckman RA, Siden R, Yanik GA, et al, "Continuous Octreotide Infusion for the Treatment of Secretory Diarrhea Caused by Acute Intestinal Graft-Versus-Host Disease in a Child," *J Pediatr Hematol Oncol*, 2000, 22(4):344-50.

Calello DP, Osterhoudt KC, Henretig FM, et al, "Octreotide for Pediatric Sulfonylurea Overdose: Review of 5 Cases," *Clin Toxicol*, 2005, 43:671.

Caron P, Gerbeau C, Pradayrol L. Maternal-fetal transfer of octreotide. *N Engl J Med*. 1995;333(9):601-602.

Chan SY, Lau W, Wong WH, et al, "Chylothorax in Children After Congenital Heart Surgery," *Ann Thorac Surg*, 2006, 82(5):1650-6.

Cheung Y, Leung MP, and Yip M, "Octreotide for Treatment of Postoperative Chylothorax," *J Pediatr*, 2001, 139(1):157-9.

Couper RT, Berzen A, Berall G, et al, "Clinical Response to the Long-Acting Somatostatin Analogue SMS 201-995 in a Child With Congenital Microvillus Atrophy," *Gut*, 1989, 30(7):1020-4.

Das A and Shah PS, "Octreotide for the Treatment of Chylothorax in Neonates," *Cochrane Database Syst Rev*, 2010, 9:CD006388.

Eroglu Y, Emerick KM, Whitongon PF, et al, "Octreotide Therapy for Control of Acute Gastrointestinal Bleeding in Children," *J Pediatr Gastroenterol Nutr*, 2004, 38(1):41-7.

Fasano CJ, O'Malley G, Dominici P, et al, "Comparison of Octreotide and Standard Therapy Versus Standard Therapy Alone for the Treatment of Sulfonylurea-Induced Hypoglycemia," *Ann Emerg Med*, 2008, 51(4):400-6.

Fassnacht M, Capeller B, Arlt W, et al. Octreotide LAR treatment throughout pregnancy in an acromegalic woman. *Clin Endocrinol (Oxf)*. 2001;55(3):411-5.

Jaros W, Biller J, Greer S, et al, "Successful Treatment of Idiopathic Secretory Diarrhea of Infancy With the Somatostatin Analogue SMS 201-995," *Gastroenterology*, 1988, 94(1):189-93.

Katz MD and Erstad BL, "Octreotide, A New Somatostatin Analogue," *Clin Pharm*, 1989, 8(4):255-73.

Katznelson L, Atkinson JL, Cook DM, et al. American Association of Clinical Endocrinologists medical guidelines for clinical practice for the diagnosis and treatment of acromegaly-2011 update. *Endocr Pract*. 2011;17 Suppl 4:1-44.

Kalomenidis I, "Octreotide and chylothorax," *Curr Opin Pulm Med*, 2006, 12(4):264-7.

Lugassy DM, Nelson LS, Hoffman RS, et al, "Failure of Standard Octreotide Dosing to Prevent Recurrent Hypoglycemia Following Sulfonylurea Exposure in a Child," *J Toxicol Clin Toxicol*, 2009, 47 (7):760.

Lustig RH, Hinds PS, Ringwald-Smith K, et al, "Octreotide Therapy of Pediatric Hypothalamic Obesity: A Double-Blind, Placebo-Controlled Trial," *J Clin Endocrinol Metab*, 2003, 88(6):2586-92.

Maffei P, Tamagno G, Nardelli GB, et al. Effects of octreotide exposure during pregnancy in acromegaly. *Clin Endocrinol (Oxf)*. 2010;72 (5):668-677.

McLaughlin SA, Crandall CS, and McKinney PE, "Octreotide: An Antidote for Sulfonylurea-Induced Hypoglycemia," *Ann Emerg Med*, 2000, 36(2):133-8.

Mordel A, Sivilotti ML, Old AC, et al, "Octreotide for Pediatric Sulfonylurea Poisoning," *J Toxicol Clin Toxicol*, 1998, 36(5):437.

Pratap U, Slavik Z, Ofoe VD, et al, "Octreotide to Treat Postoperative Chylothorax After Cardiac Operations in Children," *Ann Thorac Surg*, 2001, 72(5):1740-2.

Roehr CC, Jung A, Proquitté H, et al, "Somatostatin or Octreotide as Treatment Options for Chylothorax in Young Children: A Systematic Review," *Intensive Care Med*, 2006, 32(5):650-7.

Siafakas C, Fox VL, and Nurko S, "Use of Octreotide for the Treatment of Severe Gastrointestinal Bleeding in Children," *J Pediatr Gastroenterol Nutr*, 1998, 26(3):356-9.

Stanley CA, "Hyperinsulinism in Infants and Children," *Pediatr Clin North Am*, 1997, 44(2):363-74.

Tang J and Weiter JJ, "Branch Retinal Artery Occlusion After Injection of a Long-Acting Risperidone Preparation," *Ann Intern Med*, 2007, 147(4):283-4.

◆ **Octreotide Acetate** see Octreotide *on page 1518*

◆ **Octreotide Acetate Injection (Can)** see Octreotide *on page 1518*

◆ **Octreotide Acetate Omega (Can)** see Octreotide *on page 1518*

◆ **Ocudox** see Doxycycline *on page 721*

◆ **Ocufen** see Flurbiprofen (Ophthalmic) *on page 910*

◆ **Ocuflox** see Ofloxacin (Ophthalmic) *on page 1523*

◆ **Ocuflox® (Can)** see Ofloxacin (Ophthalmic) *on page 1523*

Ocular Lubricant (OK yoo lar LOO bri kant)

Brand Names: U.S. Akwa Tears® [OTC]; Refresh® Lacri-Lube® [OTC]; Tears Renewed® [OTC]

Therapeutic Category Lubricant, Ocular; Ophthalmic Agent, Miscellaneous

Use Ocular lubricant

Contraindications Hypersensitivity to any component

Warnings Discontinue if eye pain, vision change, redness or eye irritation occurs or if condition worsens or persists >72 hours

Stability Store away from heat

Mechanism of Action Forms an occlusive film on the surface of the eye to lubricate and protect the eye from drying

Dosing: Neonatal Note: Neonatal data are unavailable. Dose extrapolated from older patients. Ophthalmic: Apply ¼" of ointment to the inside of the lower lid as needed.

Dosing: Usual Infants, Children, Adolescents, and Adults: Ophthalmic: Apply ¼" of ointment to the inside of the lower lid as needed.

Administration Ophthalmic: Do not use with contact lenses; to avoid contamination, do not touch tip of container to any surface

Additional Information Contains petrolatum, mineral oil, chlorobutanol and lanolin alcohols

Dosage Forms Excipient information presented when available (limited, particularly for generics); consult specific product labeling. [DSC] = Discontinued product
  Ointment, ophthalmic: (1 g [DSC], 3.5 g [DSC])
    Akwa Tears®: 3.5 g (3.5 g)
  Ointment, ophthalmic [preservative free]:
    Tears Renewed®: 3.5 g (3.5 g)

◆ **Odans Liquor Carbonis Detergens [OTC] (Can)** see Coal Tar *on page 532*

◆ **Oesclim (Can)** see Estradiol (Systemic) *on page 796*

◆ **Ofirmev** see Acetaminophen *on page 47*

Ofloxacin (Systemic) (oh FLOKS a sin)

Brand Names: Canada Apo-Oflox®; Novo-Ofloxacin

▶

◄ **Therapeutic Category** Antibiotic, Quinolone

Generic Availability (U.S.) Yes

Use Treatment of acute bacterial exacerbations of chronic bronchitis, community-acquired pneumonia, uncomplicated skin and skin structure infections, urethral and cervical gonorrhea (acute, uncomplicated), urethritis and cervicitis (nongonococcal), pelvic inflammatory disease, uncomplicated cystitis, complicated urinary tract infections, and prostatitis caused by susceptible organisms including *S. pneumoniae, S. aureus, S. pyrogenes, C. koseri, E. aerogenes, E. coli, H. influenzae, K. pneumoniae, N. gonorrhoeae, P. mirabilis, C. trachomatis,* and *P. aeruginosa*

Medication Guide Available Yes

Pregnancy Risk Factor C

Pregnancy Considerations Adverse events have been observed in some animal studies; therefore, the manufacturer classifies ofloxacin as pregnancy category C. Ofloxacin crosses the placenta and produces measurable concentrations in the amniotic fluid. An increased risk of teratogenic effects has not been observed in animals or humans following ofloxacin use during pregnancy; however, because of concerns of cartilage damage in immature animals, ofloxacin should only be used during pregnancy if a safer option is not available. Serum concentrations of ofloxacin may be lower during pregnancy than in nonpregnant patients.

Breast-Feeding Considerations Ofloxacin is excreted in breast milk. Breast-feeding is not recommended by the manufacturer. Due to the low concentrations in human milk, minimal toxicity would be expected in the nursing infant. Nondose-related effects could include modification of bowel flora.

Contraindications Hypersensitivity to ofloxacin, any component, or other quinolones; not recommended for use in pregnant women or during breast-feeding

Warnings Oral formulation not recommended for use in children <18 years of age; ofloxacin has caused osteochondrosis in immature rats and dogs. Fluoroquinolones have caused arthropathy with erosions of the cartilage in weight-bearing joints of immature animals; Achilles tendonitis and tendon rupture have been reported with fluoroquinolones in patients of all ages **[U.S. Boxed Warning]**; risk increased in patients taking concomitant corticosteroids, patients >60 years of age, and in patients with kidney, heart, or lung transplants. Fluoroquinolones, including ofloxacin, may exacerbate muscle weakness associated with myasthenia gravis **[U.S. Boxed Warning]**; cases of severe exacerbations, including the need for ventilatory support and deaths have been reported; avoid use in patients with myasthenia gravis. Prolonged use may result in superinfection, including *C. difficile*-associated diarrhea and pseudomembranous colitis; CNS stimulation and increased intracranial pressure (including pseudotumor cerebi) may occur resulting in tremors, restlessness, confusion, hallucinations (rare), depression, nightmares, suicidal ideation, or convulsive seizures; serious and occasionally fatal hypersensitivity and/or anaphylactic reactions have been reported often following the first dose. Hypersensitivity reactions have been accompanied by cardiovascular collapse, hypotension/shock, seizure, loss of consciousness, tingling, angioedema, airway obstruction, dyspnea, urticaria, itching, and skin reactions. If these reactions occur, discontinue ofloxacin.

Precautions Use with caution in patients with known or suspected CNS disorders, seizure disorders, severe cerebral arteriosclerosis or renal impairment; modify dosage in patients with renal impairment. The use of quinolones has been linked to peripheral neuropathy (rare); discontinue if symptoms of sensory or sensorimotor neuropathy occur. Rare cases of torsade de pointes have been reported in patients taking ofloxacin so use with caution in patients on concurrent therapy with Class Ia or Class III antiarrhythmics or in patients with known prolongation of QT interval, bradycardia, cardiomyopathy, hypokalemia, or hypomagnesemia. Avoid excessive sunlight and take precautions to limit exposure (eg, loose-fitting clothing, sunscreen); may rarely cause moderate to severe phototoxicity reactions. Discontinue use if phototoxicity occurs.

Adverse Reactions

Cardiovascular: Chest pain

Central nervous system: dizziness, fatigue, headache, insomnia, nervousness, pyrexia, sleep disorders, somnolence

Dermatologic: Pruritus, rash

Gastrointestinal: Abdominal cramps, abnormal taste, appetite decreased, constipation, diarrhea, flatulence, GI distress, nausea, vomiting, xerostomia

Genitourinary: External genital pruritus in women, vaginitis

Ocular: Visual disturbances

Respiratory: Pharyngitis

Miscellaneous: Trunk pain

Rare but important or life-threatening: Anaphylaxis reactions, anxiety, blurred vision, chills, cognitive change, cough, depression, dream abnormality, ecchymosis, edema, erythema nodosum, euphoria, extremity pain, hallucinations, hearing acuity decreased, hepatic dysfunction, hepatic failure (some fatal), hepatitis, hyper-/hypoglycemia, hypertension, interstitial nephritis, intracranial pressure increased, lightheadedness, malaise, myasthenia gravis exacerbation, palpitation, paresthesia, peripheral neuropathy, photophobia, photosensitivity, pneumonitis, pseudotumor cerebri, psychotic reactions, rhabdomyolysis, seizure, Stevens-Johnson syndrome, syncope, tendonitis and tendon rupture, thirst, tinnitus, torsade de pointes, Tourette's syndrome, toxic epidermal necrolysis, vasculitis, vasodilation, vertigo, weakness, weight loss

Drug Interactions

Metabolism/Transport Effects Inhibits CYP1A2 (strong)

Avoid Concomitant Use

Avoid concomitant use of Ofloxacin (Systemic) with any of the following: Agomelatine; BCG; Highest Risk QTc-Prolonging Agents; Ivabradine; Mifepristone; Pirfenidone; Pomalidomide; Strontium Ranelate; Tasimelteon

Increased Effect/Toxicity

Ofloxacin (Systemic) may increase the levels/effects of: Agomelatine; Bendamustine; CloZAPine; Corticosteroids (Systemic); CYP1A2 Substrates; Highest Risk QTc-Prolonging Agents; Moderate Risk QTc-Prolonging Agents; Pirfenidone; Pomalidomide; Porfimer; Sulfonylureas; Tasimelteon; Theophylline Derivatives; Varenicline; Vitamin K Antagonists

The levels/effects of Ofloxacin (Systemic) may be increased by: Insulin; Ivabradine; Mifepristone; Nonsteroidal Anti-Inflammatory Agents; Probenecid; QTc-Prolonging Agents (Indeterminate Risk and Risk Modifying)

Decreased Effect

Ofloxacin (Systemic) may decrease the levels/effects of: BCG; Didanosine; Mycophenolate; Sodium Picosulfate; Sulfonylureas; Typhoid Vaccine

The levels/effects of Ofloxacin (Systemic) may be decreased by: Antacids; Calcium Salts; Didanosine; Iron Salts; Lanthanum; Magnesium Salts; Multivitamins/Minerals (with ADEK, Folate, Iron); Multivitamins/Minerals (with AE, No Iron); Quinapril; Sevelamer; Strontium Ranelate; Sucralfate; Zinc Salts

Food Interactions Ofloxacin average peak serum concentrations may be decreased by 20% if taken with food. Management: Do not administer within 2 hours of food or any antacids which contain zinc, magnesium, or aluminum.

Stability Store tablets at room temperature.

Mechanism of Action Ofloxacin is a DNA gyrase inhibitor. DNA gyrase is an essential bacterial enzyme that maintains the superhelical structure of DNA. DNA gyrase is required for DNA replication and transcription, DNA repair, recombination, and transposition; bactericidal

Pharmacokinetics (Adult data unless noted)

Absorption: Well-absorbed

Distribution: Widely distributed into body tissues and fluids, including blister fluid, cervix, lung, ovary, prostatic tissue, skin, and sputum; crosses the placenta; excreted into breast milk

V_d: 2.4-3.5 L/kg

Protein binding: 20% to 32%

Bioavailability: 98%

Half-life, biphasic: 4-7.4 hours and 20-25 hours; prolonged with renal impairment

Time to peak, serum concentration: 1-2 hours

Elimination: 68% to 90% is excreted unchanged in urine; 4% to 8% excreted in feces; <10% is metabolized

Dosing: Usual

Children: **Note:** Limited information regarding ofloxacin use in pediatric patients is currently available in the literature; some centers recommend doses of 15 mg/kg/day divided every 12 hours.

Adults:

Chronic bronchitis (acute exacerbation), community-acquired pneumonia, skin and skin structure infections (uncomplicated): 400 mg every 12 hours for 10 days

Urethral and cervical gonorrhea (acute, uncomplicated): 400 mg as a single dose

Cervicitis/urethritis (nongonococcal) due to *C. trachomatis* or mixed infections due to *C. trachomatis* and *N. gonorrhoeae*: 300 mg every 12 hours for 7 days

Pelvic inflammatory disease: 400 mg every 12 hours for 10-14 days

Cystitis (uncomplicated): 200 mg every 12 hours for 3-7 days

UTI (complicated): 200 mg every 12 hours for 10 days

Prostatitis: 300 mg every 12 hours for 6 weeks

Dosage adjustment in renal impairment: Adults:

CrCl 20-50 mL/minute: Administer usual dose every 24 hours

CrCl <20 mL/minute: Administer half the usual dose every 24 hours

Dosage adjustment in hepatic impairment: Severe impairment: Maximum dose: 400 mg/day

Administration May administer ofloxacin tablets with or without food; avoid antacids, vitamins with iron or minerals, sucralfate, or didanosine; use within 2 hours of administration; drink plenty of fluids to maintain proper hydration and urine output

Monitoring Parameters Patients receiving concurrent ofloxacin and theophylline should have serum levels of theophylline monitored; monitor INR in patients receiving warfarin; monitor blood glucose in patients receiving antidiabetic agents; monitor renal, hepatic, hematopoietic function, and electrolytes periodically; number and type of stools/day for diarrhea

Test Interactions Some quinolones may produce a false-positive urine screening result for opioids using commercially-available immunoassay kits. This has been demonstrated most consistently for levofloxacin and ofloxacin, but other quinolones have shown cross-reactivity in certain assay kits. Confirmation of positive opioid screens by more specific methods should be considered.

Dosage Forms Excipient information presented when available (limited, particularly for generics); consult specific product labeling. [DSC] = Discontinued product

Tablet, Oral:

Generic: 200 mg [DSC], 300 mg, 400 mg

References

Alghasham AA and Nahata MC, "Clinical Use of Fluoroquinolones in Children," *Ann Pharmacother*, 2000, 34(3):347-59.

Ofloxacin (Ophthalmic) (oh FLOKS a sin)

Medication Safety Issues

Sound-alike/look-alike issues:

Ocuflox® may be confused with Occlusal™-HP, Ocufen®

Brand Names: U.S. Ocuflox

Brand Names: Canada Ocuflox®

Therapeutic Category Antibiotic, Ophthalmic; Antibiotic, Quinolone

Generic Availability (U.S.) Yes

Use Treatment of bacterial keratitis due to susceptible organisms including *P. aeruginosa*, *Propionibacterium acnes*, *S. marcescens*, *S. aureus*, *S. epidermidis*, and *S. pneumoniae*; treatment of severe bacterial conjunctivitis due to susceptible organisms, including *Enterobacter cloacae*, *H. influenzae*, *P. mirabilis*, *P. aeruginosa*, *S. aureus*, *S. epidermidis*, or *S. pneumoniae*

Pregnancy Risk Factor C

Pregnancy Considerations Adverse events have been observed in some animal studies; therefore, the manufacturer classifies ofloxacin ophthalmic as pregnancy category C. When administered orally, ofloxacin crosses the placenta. Refer to the Ofloxacin (Systemic) monograph for details. The amount of ofloxacin available systemically following topical application of the ophthalmic drops is significantly less in comparison to oral doses.

Breast-Feeding Considerations When administered orally, ofloxacin enters breast milk. Refer to the Ofloxacin (Systemic) monograph for details. The amount of ofloxacin available systemically following topical application of the ophthalmic drops is significantly less in comparison to oral doses; however, due to the potential for adverse events in a nursing infant, breast-feeding is not recommended by the manufacturer.

Contraindications Hypersensitivity to ofloxacin, any component, or other quinolones

Warnings There have been reports of tendon inflammation and/or rupture with systemic quinolone antibiotics. Exposure following ophthalmic administration is substantially lower than with systemic therapy.

Precautions Severe hypersensitivity reactions, including anaphylaxis, have occurred with quinolone therapy (primarily with systemic use). Prolonged use may result in fungal or bacterial superinfection.

Adverse Reactions

Central nervous system: Dizziness

Dermatologic: Stevens-Johnson syndrome (rare), toxic epidermal necrolysis (rare)

Gastrointestinal: Nausea

Ocular: Blurred vision, burning, chemical conjunctivitis/keratitis, discomfort, dryness, edema, eye pain, foreign body sensation, itching, photophobia, redness, stinging, tearing

Drug Interactions

Metabolism/Transport Effects None known.

Avoid Concomitant Use There are no known interactions where it is recommended to avoid concomitant use.

Increased Effect/Toxicity There are no known significant interactions involving an increase in effect.

Decreased Effect There are no known significant interactions involving a decrease in effect.

Stability Store at room temperature.

Mechanism of Action Ofloxacin is a DNA gyrase inhibitor. DNA gyrase is an essential bacterial enzyme that maintains the superhelical structure of DNA. DNA gyrase is required for DNA replication and transcription, DNA repair, recombination, and transposition; bactericidal

Pharmacokinetics (Adult data unless noted) Absorption: Ocular: Minimal absorption unless inflammation or epithelial defect is present

Dosing: Usual Children >1 year and Adults:

Conjunctivitis: Instill 1-2 drops in affected eye(s) every 2-4 hours while awake for the first 2 days, then 4 times/day for an additional 5 days

Corneal ulcer: Instill 1-2 drops in affected eye(s) every 30 minutes while awake and every 4-6 hours at night for the first 2 days; then starting day 3, instill 1-2 drops every hour while awake for 4-6 additional days; thereafter, 1-2 drops 4 times/day until clinical cure is achieved

Administration Not for subconjunctival or direct injection into the anterior chamber of the eye. Apply gentle pressure to lacrimal sac during and immediately following instillation (1 minute) or instruct patient to gently close eyelid after administration, to decrease systemic absorption of ophthalmic drops; avoid contact of bottle tip with skin or eye. Remove contact lenses prior to administration (ophthalmic solution contains benzalkonium chloride which may adsorb to soft contact lenses); lenses may be inserted 15 minutes after administration.

Monitoring Parameters Slit-lamp biomicroscopy and fluorescein staining may be necessary

Dosage Forms Excipient information presented when available (limited, particularly for generics); consult specific product labeling.

Solution, Ophthalmic:
Ocuflox 0.3% (5 mL) [contains benzalkonium chloride]
Generic: 0.3% (5 mL, 10 mL)

Ofloxacin (Otic) (oh FLOKS a sin)

Medication Safety Issues
Sound-alike/look-alike issues:
Floxin may be confused with Flexeril®
International issues:
Floxin: Brand name for ofloxacin [U.S., Canada], but also the brand name for flunarizine [Thailand], norfloxacin [South Africa], and perfloxacin [Philippines]
Floxin [U.S., Canada] may be confused with Flexin brand name for diclofenac [Argentina], cyclobenzaprine [Chile], and orphenadrine [Israel]; Flogen brand name for naproxen [Mexico]

Therapeutic Category Antibiotic, Otic; Antibiotic, Quinolone

Generic Availability (U.S.) Yes

Use Treatment of chronic suppurative otitis media with or without perforation of the tympanic membrane; instillation into the ear canal of patients with tympanostomy tubes for treatment of acute otitis media caused by susceptible *S. aureus*, *S. pneumoniae*, *H. influenzae*, *M. catarrhalis*, or *P. aeruginosa*; otitis externa caused by susceptible *S. aureus* or *P. aeruginosa*

Pregnancy Risk Factor C

Pregnancy Considerations Adverse events have been observed in some animal studies; therefore, the manufacturer classifies ofloxacin otic as pregnancy category C. When administered orally, ofloxacin crosses the placenta. Refer to the Ofloxacin (Systemic) monograph for details. The amount of ofloxacin available systemically following topical application of the otic drops is significantly less in comparison to oral doses.

Breast-Feeding Considerations When administered orally, ofloxacin enters breast milk. Refer to the Ofloxacin (Systemic) monograph for details. The amount of ofloxacin available systemically following topical application of the otic drops is significantly less in comparison to oral doses; however, due to the potential for adverse events in a nursing infant, breast-feeding is not recommended by the manufacturer.

Contraindications Hypersensitivity to ofloxacin, any component, or other quinolones; patients with viral infections of the external ear canal

Precautions Severe hypersensitivity reactions, including anaphylaxis, have occurred with quinolone therapy (primarily with systemic use). Prolonged use may result in fungal or bacterial superinfection. There have been reports of tendon inflammation and/or rupture with systemic quinolone antibiotics.

Adverse Reactions
Central nervous system: Dizziness, vertigo
Dermatologic: Pruritus, rash
Gastrointestinal: Taste perversion
Local: Application site reaction
Neuromuscular & skeletal: Paresthesia
Rare but important or life-threatening: Diarrhea, fever, headache, hearing loss transient, hypertension, nausea, otorrhagia, tinnitus, transient neuropsychiatric disturbances, tremor, vomiting, xerostomia

Drug Interactions
Metabolism/Transport Effects None known.
Avoid Concomitant Use There are no known interactions where it is recommended to avoid concomitant use.
Increased Effect/Toxicity There are no known significant interactions involving an increase in effect.
Decreased Effect There are no known significant interactions involving a decrease in effect.

Stability Store at room temperature.

Mechanism of Action Ofloxacin is a DNA gyrase inhibitor. DNA gyrase is an essential bacterial enzyme that maintains the superhelical structure of DNA. DNA gyrase is required for DNA replication and transcription, DNA repair, recombination, and transposition; bactericidal

Pharmacokinetics (Adult data unless noted) Absorption: Minimal absorption unless tympanic membrane is perforated

Dosing: Usual
Acute otitis media with tympanostomy tubes: Children >1 year to 12 years: Instill 5 drops (0.25 mL) into the affected ear(s) twice daily for 10 days
Chronic suppurative otitis media with perforated tympanic membranes: Adolescents ≥12 years and Adults: Instill 10 drops (0.5 mL) into the affected ear(s) twice daily for 10-14 days
Otitis externa:
Children 6 months to 13 years: Instill 5 drops into the affected ear(s) once daily for 7 days
Adolescents ≥13 years and Adults: Instill 10 drops into the affected ear(s) once daily for 7 days

Administration Not for ophthalmic use or injection. Gently clean any discharge that can be easily removed from the outer ear. Warm otic solution by holding bottle in hand for 1-2 minutes prior to instillation. The tip of the bottle should not touch the fingers, ear, or any surface. Patient should lie on side with affected ear upward. For middle ear infections, gently press the tragus 4 times in a pumping motion to allow the drops to pass through the hole or tube in the eardrum and into the middle ear. For otitis externa infection, pull the outer ear upward and backward to allow the ear drops to flow down into the ear canal. Patient should remain on his/her side for at least 5 minutes. If necessary, repeat procedure for the other ear.

Monitoring Parameters Presence of otorrhea, cultures

Dosage Forms Excipient information presented when available (limited, particularly for generics); consult specific product labeling.

Solution, Otic:
Generic: 0.3% (5 mL, 10 mL)

◆ **17OHPC** *see* Hydroxyprogesterone Caproate *on page 1049*

◆ **9-OH-risperidone** *see* Paliperidone *on page 1581*

OLANZapine (oh LAN za peen)

Medication Safety Issues
Sound-alike/look-alike issues:
OLANZapine may be confused with olsalazine, QUEtiapine

ZyPREXA may be confused with CeleXA, Reprexain, Zestril, ZyrTEC

ZyPREXA Zydis may be confused with Zelapar, zolpidem

ZyPREXA Relprevv may be confused with ZyPREXA IntraMuscular

BEERS Criteria medication:
This drug may be potentially inappropriate for use in geriatric patients (Quality of evidence - moderate; Strength of recommendation - strong).

Brand Names: U.S. ZyPREXA; ZyPREXA Relprevv; ZyPREXA Zydis

Brand Names: Canada Apo-Olanzapine; Apo-Olanzapine ODT; Ava-Olanzapine; CO Olanzapine; CO Olanzapine ODT; Mylan-Olanzapine; Olanzapine ODT; PHL-Olanzapine; PHL-Olanzapine ODT; PMS-Olanzapine; PMS-Olanzapine ODT; Riva-Olanzapine; Riva-Olanzapine ODT; Sandoz-Olanzapine; Sandoz-Olanzapine ODT; Teva-Olanzapine; Teva-Olanzapine OD; Zyprexa; Zyprexa Intramuscular; Zyprexa Zydis

Therapeutic Category Antipsychotic Agent, Atypical

Generic Availability (U.S.) May be product dependent

Use

Oral: Treatment of schizophrenia (FDA approved in ages ≥13 years and adults); acute and maintenance treatment of manic or mixed episodes of bipolar I disorder (FDA approved in ages ≥13 years and adults); adjunctive therapy (to lithium or valproate) for treatment of manic or mixed episodes of bipolar I disorder (FDA approved in adults); in combination with fluoxetine for treatment-resistant depression or depressive episodes associated with bipolar I disorder (FDA approved in adults). Has also been used for anorexia nervosa, autism spectrum disorders, Tourette syndrome, and tic disorders. Therapy should only be initiated in pediatric patients after a thorough diagnostic evaluation and an assessment of potential long-term risks; adolescent patients experience a higher incidence of weight gain, and greater increases in total cholesterol, triglycerides, LDL, prolactin, and hepatic transaminase concentrations than adult patients; other agents with fewer risks may be preferred as first-line treatment.

Parenteral:
I.M. extended release (Zyprexa® Relprevv™): Treatment of schizophrenia (FDA approved in adults)

I.M. short-acting (Zyprexa® IntraMuscular): Treatment of acute agitation associated with schizophrenia and bipolar I mania (FDA approved in adults)

Prescribing and Access Restrictions As a requirement of the REMS program, only prescribers, healthcare facilities, and pharmacies registered with the Zyprexa Relprevv Patient Care Program are able to prescribe, distribute, or dispense Zyprexa Relprevv for patients who are enrolled in and meet all conditions of the program. Zyprexa Relprevv must be administered at a registered healthcare facility. Prescribers will need to be recertified every 3 years. Contact the Zyprexa Relprevv Patient Care Program at 1-877-772-9390.

Medication Guide Available Yes

Pregnancy Risk Factor C

Pregnancy Considerations Adverse events were observed in animal reproduction studies. Olanzapine crosses the placenta and can be detected in cord blood at birth (Newport, 2007). Information related to olanzapine use in pregnancy is limited (Goldstein, 2000). Antipsychotic use during the third trimester of pregnancy has a risk for abnormal muscle movements (extrapyramidal symptoms [EPS]) and/or withdrawal symptoms in newborns following delivery. Symptoms in the newborn may include agitation, feeding disorder, hypertonia, hypotonia, respiratory distress, somnolence, and tremor; these effects may be self-limiting or require hospitalization. Olanzapine may cause hyperprolactinemia, which may decrease reproductive function in both males and females.

The ACOG recommends that therapy during pregnancy be individualized; treatment with psychiatric medications during pregnancy should incorporate the clinical expertise of the mental health clinician, obstetrician, primary healthcare provider, and pediatrician. Safety data related to atypical antipsychotics during pregnancy is limited and routine use is not recommended. However, if a woman is inadvertently exposed to an atypical antipsychotic while pregnant, continuing therapy may be preferable to switching to a typical antipsychotic that the fetus has not yet been exposed to; consider risk:benefit (ACOG, 2008). Evaluate risk factors for gestational diabetes and weight gain if considering use of olanzapine in a pregnant woman (NICE, 2007).

Healthcare providers are encouraged to enroll women 18-45 years of age exposed to olanzapine during pregnancy in the Atypical Antipsychotics Pregnancy Registry (1-866-961-2388 or http://www.womensmentalhealth.org/pregnancyregistry).

Breast-Feeding Considerations Olanzapine is excreted into breast milk. At steady-state concentrations, it is estimated that a breast-fed infant may be exposed to ~2% of the maternal dose. In one study, the median time to peak milk concentration was ~5 hours after the maternal dose and serum concentrations in the nursing infants were low (<5 ng/mL; n=5) (Gardiner, 2003). An increased risk of adverse events in nursing infants has not been reported (Gardiner, 2003; Gilad, 2011). Breast-feeding is not recommended by the manufacturer.

Contraindications Hypersensitivity to olanzapine or any component

Warnings May cause neuroleptic malignant syndrome; symptoms include hyperpyrexia, altered mental status, muscle rigidity, autonomic instability, acute renal failure, rhabdomyolysis, and increased CPK. May cause extrapyramidal reactions, including pseudoparkinsonism, acute dystonic reactions, akathisia, and tardive dyskinesia. Risk of these reactions is dose-dependent. To decrease risk of tardive dyskinesia: Use smallest dose and shortest duration possible and evaluate continued need periodically. Risk of dystonia is increased with the use of high potency and higher doses of conventional antipsychotics and in males and younger patients.

May cause hyperglycemia, which may be severe and include potentially fatal ketoacidosis or hyperosmolar coma; there is a stronger association of hyperglycemia with olanzapine than other atypical antipsychotics. In clinical trials of adolescents, 14.3% of patients at 12 weeks of olanzapine exposure and 23.1% of patients at ≥24 weeks exposure had an increase in their fasting blood glucose concentration from the borderline category (100 mg/dL to <126 mg/dL) to high (≥126 mg/dL). Use with caution and monitor for symptoms of hyperglycemia in all patients treated with olanzapine; monitor glucose closely in patients with diabetes mellitus (or with risk factors such as family history or obesity) or with borderline increased blood glucose (fasting: 100-126 mg/dL or nonfasting: 140-200 mg/dL); measure fasting blood glucose at the beginning of therapy, periodically during therapy, and in any patient who develops signs or symptoms of hyperglycemia.

Leukopenia, neutropenia, and agranulocytosis (sometimes fatal) have been reported in clinical trials and postmarketing reports with antipsychotic use; presence of risk factors (eg, preexisting low WBC or history of drug-induced leuko-/neutropenia) should prompt periodic blood count assessment. Discontinue therapy at first signs of blood dyscrasia or if absolute neutrophil count <1000/mm^3.

Pediatric psychiatric disorders are frequently serious mental disorders which present with variable symptoms that do not always match adult diagnostic criteria. Conduct a thorough diagnostic evaluation and carefully consider risks of psychotropic medication before initiation in pediatric patients. Medication therapy for pediatric patients with bipolar disorder and schizophrenia is indicated as part of a total treatment program that frequently includes educational, psychological, and social interventions. The possibility of a suicide attempt is inherent in psychotic illness or bipolar disorder; use with caution in high-risk patients during initiation of therapy. Prescriptions should be written for the smallest quantity consistent with good patient care.

An increased risk of death has been reported with the use of antipsychotics in elderly patients with dementia-related psychosis [U.S. Boxed Warning]; most deaths seemed to be cardiovascular (eg, sudden death, heart failure) or infectious (eg, pneumonia) in nature. An increased incidence of cerebrovascular adverse events (eg, transient ischemic attack, stroke), including fatalities, has been reported with the use of olanzapine in elderly patients with dementia-related psychosis. Olanzapine is not approved for the treatment of patients with dementia-related psychosis.

Extended release I.M. injection (Zyprexa® Relprevv™): A postinjection delirium sedation syndrome, characterized by severe sedation (including coma) and/or delirium (including agitation, anxiety, confusion, disorientation, and other cognitive impairment), has been observed [U.S. Boxed Warning]; other symptoms including ataxia, aggression, convulsion, dizziness, dysarthria, extrapyramidal symptoms, hypertension, slurred speech, and weakness have been noted; in some patients, clinical signs and symptoms were associated with an inadvertent rapid rise in olanzapine serum concentrations; exact mechanism for introduction of drug into the bloodstream is unknown. Administer at a registered healthcare facility where patients are continuously monitored (≥3 hours) for symptoms of olanzapine overdose; symptom development is highest in first hour but may occur within or after 3 hours; risk of syndrome is cumulative with each injection; recovery expected by 72 hours. Upon determining alert status, patient should be escorted to their destination and not drive or operate heavy machinery for the remainder of the day. Diluent contains polysorbate 80 (Tween 80®) which may cause allergic reactions in susceptible individuals.

Precautions Use with caution in patients with hepatic impairment, signs and symptoms of hepatic impairment, or being treated with potentially hepatotoxic drugs; olanzapine may increase transaminases (primarily ALT); greater increases in hepatic transaminases were observed in adolescent patients compared to adults in clinical trials; dosage adjustment may be necessary.

Use with caution in patients with breast cancer, history of breast cancer, or other prolactin-dependent tumors; olanzapine increases prolactin concentrations; a higher incidence of hyperprolactinemia has been observed in adolescent patients treated with olanzapine than adults (47% vs 30%), high concentrations of prolactin may reduce pituitary gonadotropin secretion; galactorrhea, amenorrhea, gynecomastia, impotence, decreased bone density may occur. Use with caution in children and adolescents as adverse effects due to elevated serum prolactin concentrations have been observed; long-term effects on growth or sexual maturation have not been evaluated.

Olanzapine may cause increases in serum lipid concentration and weight gain (higher than normal) in adolescent and adult patients. Very high triglyceride concentrations (>500 mg/dL) have been observed along with modest increases in total cholesterol. In adolescent patients, increases in fasting total cholesterol, LDL cholesterol, and triglycerides were generally greater than in adult patients; measure fasting serum lipids at the beginning of therapy and periodically during therapy in these patients. Compared to adult patients, adolescent patients had both greater magnitude of weight gain and proportion of patients who had clinically significant weight gain (incidence: 29% to 40% vs 6%). With long-term olanzapine exposure (≥24 weeks), 89% of adolescents gained at least 7% of their baseline body weight, 55% gained at least 15% of their baseline body weight, and 29% gained at least 25% of their baseline body weight; discontinuation due to weight gain occurred in 2.2%. Monitor growth (including weight, height, BMI, and waist circumference) in pediatric and adolescent patients receiving olanzapine; compare weight gain to standard growth curves. **Note:** A prospective, nonrandomized, cohort study followed 338 antipsychotic naive pediatric patients (age: 4-19 years) for a median of 10.8 weeks (range: 10.5-11.2 weeks) and showed that olanzapine was associated with greater increases in weight, fat mass, BMI, and waist circumference than other atypical antipsychotics evaluated (ie, quetiapine, risperidone, and aripiprazole). The following significant mean increases in weight in kg (and% change from baseline) were reported: Olanzapine: 8.5 kg (15.2%), quetiapine: 6.1 kg (10.4%), risperidone: 5.3 kg (10.4%), and aripiprazole: 4.4 kg (8.1%) compared to the control cohort: 0.2 kg (0.65%). Also, compared to the other atypical antipsychotics evaluated, olanzapine showed higher increases in metabolic indices (eg, serum glucose, total cholesterol and LDL-C). Biannual monitoring of cardiometabolic indices after the first 3 months of therapy is suggested (Correll, 2009).

Use with caution in patients with seizure disorder or conditions that lower seizure threshold (seizures have been rarely reported); in suicidal patients; in patients with concomitant systemic illnesses, unstable heart disease, or a recent history of MI (these patients not adequately studied); and in patients at risk of aspiration pneumonia (esophageal dysmotility and aspiration have been associated with antipsychotic agents). May cause orthostatic hypotension with resultant dizziness, tachycardia, or syncope (especially during initial dose titration); use with caution in patients with history of cardiovascular disease, cerebrovascular disease, conditions predisposed to hypotension (eg, dehydration, hypovolemia) or concurrent drug therapy that can induce hypotension, bradycardia, respiratory or central nervous system depression. May alter cardiac conduction; life-threatening arrhythmias have occurred with therapeutic doses of antipsychotics.

Moderate to highly sedating; a higher frequency of sedation-related adverse events (defined as hypersomnia, lethargy, sedation, and somnolence) have been observed in adolescents compared to adults. Use with caution in disorders where CNS depression is a feature; patients must be cautioned about performing tasks which require mental alertness (eg, operating machinery or driving).

May cause anticholinergic effects; relative to other neuroleptics, olanzapine has a moderate potency of cholinergic blockade; use with caution in patients with decreased gastrointestinal motility, history of paralytic ileus or related condition, urinary retention, BPH, xerostomia, glaucoma, or myasthenia gravis. Olanzapine concentrations may be lower in patients who smoke, dosing adjustment not recommended by manufacturer but may be considered. Use with caution in patients exposed to temperature extremes; may cause alteration of temperature regulation.

Orally disintegrating tablets contain phenylalanine which must be used with caution in patients with phenylketonuria.

I.M. administration: Two different I.M. formulations are available (short-acting and extended release preparations) and are not interchangeable. Patients should remain recumbent if drowsy/dizzy until hypotension, bradycardia, and/or hypoventilation have been ruled out. Concurrent use of I.M./I.V. benzodiazepines is not recommended due to potential for excessive sedation and cardiorespiratory depression (fatalities have been reported, though causality not determined). Extended release product (Zyprexa® Relprevv™) may cause local skin irritation, use gloves during preparation.

Adverse Reactions

Oral: Unless otherwise noted, adverse events are reported for placebo-controlled trials in adult patients on monotherapy:

Cardiovascular: Chest pain, hypertension, orthostatic hypotension, peripheral edema, tachycardia

Central nervous system: Abnormal gait, akathisia, articulation impairment, dizziness (more common in adults), drowsiness (dose dependent; adolescents and adults), extrapyramidal reaction (dose dependent; more common in adults), falling, fatigue (dose dependent; adolescents and adults), headache (adolescents), hypertonia, insomnia, personality changes, restlessness (adolescents)

Endocrine & metabolic: Breast changes ([adolescents] discharge, enlargement, galactorrhea, gynecomastia, lactation disorder), increased gamma-glutamyl transferase (adolescents), increased serum prolactin (more common in adolescents), menstrual disease (amenorrhea, hypomenorrhea, delayed menstruation, oligomenorrhea), weight gain (adolescents and adults)

Gastrointestinal: Abdominal pain (adolescents), constipation (adolescents and adults), diarrhea (adolescents), dyspepsia (more common in adults), flatulence, increased appetite (more common in adolescents), nausea (dose dependent), vomiting, xerostomia (dose dependent; more common in adults)

Genitourinary: Incontinence, sexual disorder (anorgasmia, delayed ejaculation, erectile dysfunction, changes in libido, abnormal orgasm, sexual dysfunction), urinary tract infection

Hematologic & oncologic: Bruise

Hepatic: Decreased serum bilirubin (adolescents), increased liver enzyme (adolescents), increased serum ALT (adolescents and adults), increased serum AST (adolescents)

Neuromuscular & skeletal: Arthralgia (adolescents and adults), back pain, limb pain (adolescents and adults), muscle rigidity (adolescents), tremor (dose dependent), weakness (dose dependent)

Ophthalmic: Amblyopia

Respiratory: Cough, epistaxis (adolescents), nasopharyngitis (adolescents), pharyngitis, respiratory tract infection (adolescents), rhinitis, sinusitis (adolescents)

Miscellaneous: Accidental injury, fever

Rare but important or life-threatening: Accommodation disturbance, acidosis, agranulocytosis, akinesia, albuminuria, alopecia, anaphylactoid reaction, angioedema, apnea, arteritis, asthma, ataxia, atelectasis, atrial fibrillation, brain disease, cardiac arrest, cardiac failure, cerebrovascular accident, coma, confusion, deafness, diabetes mellitus, diabetic ketoacidosis, diabetic coma, dysarthria, dyskinesia, dysphagia, dystonia, dysuria, facial paralysis, glaucoma, heart failure, hematuria, hemoptysis, hemorrhage (eye, rectal, subarachnoid, vaginal), hepatic injury (cholestatic or mixed), hepatitis,

hypercholesterolemia, hypergylcemia, hyperkalemia, hyperlipidemia, hypernatremia, hypertriglyceridemia, hyperuricemia, hyperventilation, hypoesthesia, hypoglycemia, hypokalemia, hypokinesia, hyponatremia, hypoproteinemia, hypoventilation, hypoxia, intestinal obstruction, jaundice, ketosis, leukocytosis (eosinophilia), leukopenia, liver steatosis, lymphadenopathy, migraine, myasthenia, myopathy, neuralgia, neuroleptic malignant syndrome, neuropathy, neutropenia, osteoporosis, pancreatitis, paralysis, priapism, pruritus, pulmonary edema, pulmonary embolism, rhabdomyolysis, seizure, skin rash, stridor, suicidal tendencies, syncope, tardive dyskinesia, thrombocythemia, thrombocytopenia, tongue edema, transient ischemic attacks, urticaria, venous thrombosis, withdrawal syndrome

Injection: Unless otherwise noted, adverse events are reported for placebo-controlled trials in adult patients on extended release I.M. injection (Zyprexa Relprevv). Also refer to adverse reactions noted with oral therapy.

Cardiovascular: Hypertension, hypotension (short-acting), orthostatic hypotension (short-acting), prolonged Q-T interval on ECG

Central nervous system: Abnormal dreams, abnormality in thinking, auditory hallucination, dizziness, drowsiness, dysarthria, extrapyramidal reaction, fatigue, headache, pain, restlessness, sedation

Dermatologic: Acne vulgaris

Endocrine & metabolic: Weight gain

Gastrointestinal: Abdominal pain, diarrhea, flatulence, increased appetite, nausea, toothache, vomiting, xerostomia

Genitourinary: Vaginal discharge

Hepatic: Increased liver enzymes

Infection: Tooth infection, viral infection

Local: Pain at injection site

Neuromuscular & skeletal: Arthralgia, back pain, muscle spasm, stiffness, tremor, weakness (short-acting)

Otic: Otalgia

Respiratory: Cough, nasal congestion, nasopharyngitis, pharyngolaryngeal pain, sneezing, upper respiratory tract infection

Miscellaneous: Fever

Rare but important or life-threatening: Increased creatine phosphokinase, postinjection delirium/sedation syndrome, syncope (short-acting)

Drug Interactions

Metabolism/Transport Effects Substrate of CYP1A2 (major), CYP2D6 (minor); **Note:** Assignment of Major/Minor substrate status based on clinically relevant drug interaction potential; **Inhibits** CYP1A2 (weak), CYP2C19 (weak), CYP2C9 (weak), CYP2D6 (weak), CYP3A4 (weak)

Avoid Concomitant Use

Avoid concomitant use of OLANZapine with any of the following: Aclidinium; Amisulpride; Azelastine (Nasal); Benzodiazepines; Ipratropium (Oral Inhalation); Metoclopramide; Paraldehyde; Pimozide; Potassium Chloride; Sulpiride; Thalidomide; Tiotropium; Umeclidinium

Increased Effect/Toxicity

OLANZapine may increase the levels/effects of: AbobotulinumtoxinA; Alcohol (Ethyl); Amisulpride; Analgesics (Opioid); Anticholinergic Agents; ARIPiprazole; Azelastine (Nasal); Benzodiazepines; Buprenorphine; Cannabinoid-Containing Products; CNS Depressants; Highest Risk QTc-Prolonging Agents; Hydrocodone; Lomitapide; Methotrimeprazine; Methylphenidate; Metyrosine; Mirabegron; Mirtazapine; Moderate Risk QTc-Prolonging Agents; OnabotulinumtoxinA; Paraldehyde; Pimozide; Potassium Chloride; RimabotulinumtoxinB; Selective Serotonin Reuptake Inhibitors; Serotonin Modulators; Sulpiride; Thalidomide; Thiazide Diuretics; Tiotropium; Topiramate; Zolpidem ▶

The levels/effects of OLANZapine may be increased by: Abiraterone Acetate; Acetylcholinesterase Inhibitors (Central); Aclidinium; Brimonidine (Topical); Cannabis; CYP1A2 Inhibitors (Moderate); CYP1A2 Inhibitors (Strong); Deferasirox; Doxylamine; Dronabinol; Droperidol; FluvoxaMINE; HydrOXYzine; Ipratropium (Oral Inhalation); Kava Kava; LamoTRIgine; Lithium; Magnesium Sulfate; Methotrimeprazine; Methylphenidate; Metoclopramide; Metyrosine; Mifepristone; Nabilone; Perampanel; Pramlintide; Rufinamide; Serotonin Modulators; Sodium Oxybate; Tapentadol; Tetrahydrocannabinol; Umeclidinium; Vemurafenib

Decreased Effect

OLANZapine may decrease the levels/effects of: Acetylcholinesterase Inhibitors (Central); Amphetamines; Anti-Parkinson's Agents (Dopamine Agonist); Quinagolide; Secretin

The levels/effects of OLANZapine may be decreased by: Acetylcholinesterase Inhibitors (Central); Cannabis; CYP1A2 Inducers (Strong); Cyproterone; Lithium; Peginterferon Alfa-2b; Valproic Acid and Derivatives

Stability

Injection, extended release: Store at room temperature, not to exceed 30°C (86°F). Once suspension prepared, stable for 24 hours at room temperature.

Injection, short-acting: Store at 20°C to 25°C (68°F to 77°F); excursions permitted to 15°C to 30°C (59°F to 86°F); do not freeze. Protect from light. Use immediately (within 1 hour) following reconstitution. Discard any unused portion. Incompatible with diazepam, lorazepam, or haloperidol.

Tablet and orally disintegrating tablet: Store at 20°C to 25°C (68°F to 77°F); excursions permitted to 15°C to 30°C (59°F to 86°F). Protect from light and moisture.

Mechanism of Action

Olanzapine is a second generation thienobenzodiazepine antipsychotic which displays potent antagonism of serotonin 5-HT$_{2A}$ and 5-HT$_{2C}$, dopamine D$_{1-4}$, histamine H$_1$, and alpha$_1$-adrenergic receptors. Olanzapine shows moderate antagonism of 5-HT$_3$ and muscarinic M$_{1-5}$ receptors, and weak binding to GABA-A, BZD, and beta-adrenergic receptors. Although the precise mechanism of action in schizophrenia and bipolar disorder is not known, the efficacy of olanzapine is thought to be mediated through combined antagonism of dopamine and serotonin type 2 receptor sites.

Pharmacodynamics

Onset of action: Within 1-2 weeks for control of aggression, agitation, insomnia; 3-6 weeks for control of mania and positive psychotic symptoms. Adequate trial: Typically 6 weeks at maximum tolerated doses

Pharmacokinetics (Adult data unless noted)

Absorption:

I.M. (short-acting): Rapidly absorbed

Oral: Well absorbed; not affected by food; tablets and orally disintegrating tablets are bioequivalent

Distribution: Extensive throughout body; V$_d$: 1000 L

Protein binding: 93% primarily to albumin and alpha$_1$-glycoprotein

Metabolism: Highly metabolized via direct glucuronidation and cytochrome P450 mediated oxidation (CYP1A2, CYP2D6); 40% removed via first pass metabolism

Half-life:

Oral and I.M. (short-acting):

Pediatric patients (10-18 years; n=8): 37.2 ± 5.1 hours (Grothe, 2000)

Adults: 30 hours [21-54 hours (5th to 95th percentile)]

I.M. (extended release): 30 days (effective half-life)

Time to peak serum concentration: Maximum plasma concentrations after I.M. (short-acting product) administration are 5 times higher than maximum plasma concentrations produced by an oral dose.

I.M. (short-acting): 15-45 minutes

I.M. (extended release): ~7 days

Oral:

Pediatric patients (10-18 years; n=8): 4.7 ± 3.7 hours (Grothe, 2000)

Adults: ~6 hours

Elimination: Urine (57%; 7% as unchanged drug); feces (30%)

Clearance: Oral:

Pediatric patients (10-18 years; n=8): Apparent: 9.6 ± 2.4 L/hour (Grothe 2000)

Adult: Apparent: 25 L/hour [12-47 L/hour (5th to 95th percentile)]; 40% increase in olanzapine clearance in smokers; 30% decrease in females

Dialysis: Not removed by dialysis

Dosing: Usual

Oral:

Children and Adolescents:

Bipolar I disorder (acute manic or mixed episodes):

Children 4 to <6 years: Limited data available: Initial: 1.25 mg once daily; increase at weekly intervals according to response and tolerability to target dose: 10 mg/day. Dosing based on an open-label trial in 15 children (mean age: 5 ± 0.8 years; mean weight: 20.8 kg; mean required dose: 6.3 ± 2.3 mg/day) that showed significant improvement in manic symptoms (Biederman, 2005)

Children 6-12 years: Limited data available: Initial: 2.5 mg once daily; increase dose in 2.5 or 5 mg increments at weekly intervals to target dose of 10 mg once daily; maximum dose: 20 mg/day (Frazier, 2001; Kowatch, 2006; Wozniak, 2009)

Adolescents: Initial: 2.5-5 mg once daily; increase dose in 2.5 or 5 mg increments at weekly intervals to target dose of 10 mg once daily; maximum dose: 20 mg/day. In adolescent flexible-dosing (2.5-20 mg/day) clinical trials, the mean modal dose was 10.7 mg/day (mean dose: 8.9 mg/day) (Kowatch, 2006; Tohen, 2007)

Schizophrenia: Children ≥8 years (Limited data available) and Adolescents: Initial: 2.5-5 mg once daily; increase dose in 2.5 or 5 mg increments at weekly intervals to target dose of 10 mg once daily; maximum dose: 20 mg/day. **Note:** Doses up to 30 mg/day were used in one study of adolescents who were treatment refractory; however, some patients did not tolerate doses >20 mg/day (Kumra, 2008); safety and efficacy of doses >20 mg/day have not been fully evaluated. In adolescent flexible-dosing (2.5-20 mg/day) clinical trials, the mean modal dose was 12.5 mg/day (mean dose: 11.1 mg/day). Dosing in children is based on two double-blind comparison studies which included both children and adolescents [n=35, age: 8-19 years with seven children; n=13, age: 7-16 years (mean age: 12.8 + 2.4 years)] (Shaw, 2006; Sikich, 2008).

Anorexia nervosa: Children ≥9 years and Adolescents: Limited data available: 1.25-2.5 mg once daily has been shown in one small trial and several case reports to improve BMI and other disease-related symptoms (eg, eating attitudes, anxiety); another case series used initial doses of 2.5 mg once daily and final doses of 5 mg to 10 mg once daily; reported range: 1.25-12.5 mg/day; however, it has been suggested that higher doses (>2.5 mg once daily) may not be associated with greater efficacy. Further studies are needed (Boachie, 2003; Dunican, 2007; Legerro, 2010; Mehler, 2001; Mehler-Wex, 2007).

Tourette syndrome, tic disorder: Children ≥7 years and Adolescents: Limited data available:

Patient weight ≤40 kg: Initial: 2.5 mg every other day for 3 days, increase to 2.5 mg every day for remainder of week; increase to 5 mg/day by second week if needed; then increase in 5 mg increments at weekly intervals as tolerated; maximum dose: 20 mg/day

Patient weight >40 kg: Initial: 2.5 mg every day for 3 days; increase to 5 mg every day for remainder of week if needed, then increase in 5 mg increments at weekly intervals as tolerated; maximum dose: 20 mg/day

An open-label study of 10 pediatric patients (7-13 years of age) reported significant reductions in tic severity [Yale Global Tic Severity Scale (YGTSS)] from baseline at a mean final dose of 14.5 mg/day after 8 weeks of treatment (Stephens, 2004). An open-label trial of 12 children and adolescents (7-14 years of age) reported a significant reduction (30%) in total tic severity (YGTSS) at a final mean dose of 11.3 mg/day (range: 2.5-20 mg/day) (McCracken, 2008)

Adults:

Acute mania associated with bipolar disorder:

Monotherapy: Initial: 10-15 mg once daily; increase by 5 mg/day at intervals of not less than 24 hours. Maintenance: 5-20 mg/day; recommended maximum dose: 20 mg/day

Combination therapy (with lithium or valproate): Initial: 10 mg once daily; dosing range: 5-20 mg/day

Schizophrenia: Initial: 5-10 mg once daily (increase to 10 mg once daily within 5-7 days); thereafter, adjust by 5 mg/day at 1-week intervals, up to a recommended maximum of 20 mg/day. Maintenance: 10-20 mg once daily. Doses of 30-50 mg/day have been used; however, doses >10 mg/day have not demonstrated better efficacy, and safety and efficacy of doses >20 mg/day have not been evaluated.

I.M. (short-acting): **Agitation** (acute, associated with bipolar disorder or schizophrenia):

Pediatric patients: Limited data available: Children: 5 mg; Adolescents: 10 mg. Dosing based on a retrospective report of I.M. olanzapine use in an inpatient psychiatric setting which included 50 pediatric patients [children (n=15; mean age: 11 years); adolescents (n=35; mean age: 15 years)] and evaluated 163 doses administered; results showed a 90.2% response rate (Khan, 2006)

Adults: Initial dose: 10 mg (a lower dose of 5-7.5 mg may be considered when clinical factors warrant); additional doses (up to 10 mg) may be considered; however, 2-4 hours should be allowed between doses to evaluate response (maximum total daily dose: 30 mg)

I.M. (extended release): Adults:

Schizophrenia: Note: Establish tolerance to oral olanzapine prior to changing to extended release I.M. injection. It may take up to 3 months to re-establish steady-state when switching from oral olanzapine to long-acting I.M. injection. Maximum dose: 300 mg/2 weeks or 405 mg/4 weeks

Patients established on oral olanzapine 10 mg/day: Initial dose: 210 mg every 2 weeks for 4 doses or 405 mg every 4 weeks for 2 doses; Maintenance dose: 150 mg every 2 weeks or 300 mg every 4 weeks

Patients established on oral olanzapine 15 mg/day: Initial dose: 300 mg every 2 weeks for 4 doses; Maintenance dose: 210 mg every 2 weeks or 405 mg every 4 weeks

Patients established on oral olanzapine 20 mg/day: Initial and maintenance dose: 300 mg every 2 weeks

Patients who are debilitated, predisposed to hypotensive reactions, exhibit multiple factors that may result in slower metabolism, or may be more sensitive to olanzapine: Initial dose: 150 mg every 4 weeks; increase dose with caution and only if clinically needed

Dosage adjustment in renal impairment: No dosage adjustment required.

Dosage adjustment in hepatic impairment: Use with caution. Dosage adjustment may be necessary; however, no specific recommendations exist. Monitor closely.

Administration

Injection:

I.M. (short-acting): For I.M. administration only; do not administer I.V. or subcutaneously; inject slowly, deep into muscle mass. Reconstitute 10 mg vial with 2.1 mL SWI; resulting solution is ~5 mg/mL with a clear and yellow appearance.

I.M. (extended release): Adults: **For deep I.M. gluteal administration only**; do not administer injection intravenously. Add appropriate amount of provided diluent to proper vial size (see package labeling) and agitate vigorously to suspend drug. Do not use other diluents. If foam develops, let vial stand to allow foam to dissipate. If suspended drug is not used right away, agitate vial again vigorously to resuspend drug prior to withdrawal from vial. Once drug is withdrawn into syringe, use immediately. After needle insertion into muscle, aspirate to verify that no blood appears; inject slowly, deep into muscle. Do not massage injection site. Solution may be irritating to the skin; use of gloves recommended during preparation; flush skin with water if drug comes into contact with skin. Use diluent, syringes, and needles provided in convenience kit; obtain a new kit if aspiration of blood occurs.

Tablet: May be administered with or without food. Orally disintegrating tablet: Remove from foil blister by peeling back foil (do not push tablet through the foil); place tablet in mouth immediately upon removal; tablet dissolves rapidly in saliva and may be swallowed with or without liquid. No faster onset compared to oral solid.

Monitoring Parameters Vital signs; CBC with differential, fasting lipid profile, and fasting blood glucose/Hgb A_{1c} (prior to treatment, at 3 months, then annually or as symptoms warrant); periodic assessment of hepatic transaminases; weight, BMI, waist circumference; personal/family history of diabetes or obesity; orthostatic blood pressure; mental status, abnormal involuntary movement scale (AIMS), extrapyramidal symptoms (EPS). Weight should be assessed prior to treatment, at 4 weeks, 8 weeks, 12 weeks, and then at quarterly intervals. Consider switching to a different antipsychotic agent for a weight gain ≥5% of the initial weight. Monitor patient periodically for symptom resolution. Following I.M. administration, if dizziness and/or drowsiness are noted, patient should remain recumbent until resolved. Extended release I.M. injection (Zyprexa® Relprevv™): Monitor patients continuously for 3 hours after injection for symptoms of post-injection sedation syndrome and olanzapine overdose; once patient is alert, escort patient to their destination; patient should not drive or operate heavy machinery for the remainder of the day.

Additional Information Long-term usefulness of olanzapine should be periodically re-evaluated in patients receiving the drug for extended periods of time.

Additional detailed olanzapine dosing information for Children and Adolescents: Oral:

Autism spectrum disorders: Note: Limited information exists in the literature; dose not established; efficacy results have been variable; further studies are needed. A double-blind, placebo-controlled study (n=11, 6-14 years of age, study duration: 8 weeks) reported a response in only 3 of 6 treatment arm patients using an initial dose of: 2.5 mg every other day (patient weight: <40 kg) or 2.5 mg every day (patient weight: ≥40 kg); dose increased at weekly intervals in 2.5-5 mg increments as tolerated (maximum dose allowed: 20 mg/day); final dosage range: 7.5-12.5 mg/day; mean: 10 mg/day (Hollander, 2006). An open-label, 6-week, comparative study with haloperidol in 12 children (4.8-11.8 years of age) used a similar dosing regimen and reported responses in 5 of 6 patients in the olanzapine treatment arm; final dosage range: 5-10 mg/day (mean: 7.9 ± 2.5 mg/day) (Malone, 2001).

However, an open-label, 12-week study in 25 pediatric patients (6-16 years) reported a response in only three patients, final dosage range: 2.5-20 mg/day (mean: 10.7 mg/day) (Kemner, 2002).

Dosage Forms Excipient information presented when available (limited, particularly for generics); consult specific product labeling.

Solution Reconstituted, Intramuscular:

ZyPREXA: 10 mg (1 ea) [contains tartaric acid]

Generic: 10 mg (1 ea)

Suspension Reconstituted, Intramuscular:

ZyPREXA Relprevv: 210 mg (1 ea); 300 mg (1 ea); 405 mg (1 ea) [contains polysorbate 80]

Tablet, Oral:

ZyPREXA: 2.5 mg, 5 mg, 7.5 mg, 10 mg

ZyPREXA: 15 mg [contains fd&c blue #2 aluminum lake]

ZyPREXA: 20 mg

Generic: 2.5 mg, 5 mg, 7.5 mg, 10 mg, 15 mg, 20 mg

Tablet Dispersible, Oral:

ZyPREXA Zydis: 5 mg, 10 mg, 15 mg, 20 mg [contains aspartame, methylparaben sodium, propylparaben sodium]

Generic: 5 mg, 10 mg, 15 mg, 20 mg

References

ACOG Committee on Practice Bulletins-Obstetrics, "ACOG Practice Bulletin: Clinical Management Guidelines for Obstetrician-Gynecologists Number 92, April 2008 (Replaces Practice Bulletin Number 87, November 2007). Use of Psychiatric Medications During Pregnancy and Lactation," *Obstet Gynecol*, 2008, 111(4):1001-20.

American Diabetes Association; American Psychiatric Association; American Association of Clinical Endocrinologists; North American Association for the Study of Obesity, "Consensus Development Conference on Antipsychotic Drugs and Obesity and Diabetes," *Diabetes Care*, 2004, 27(2):596-601.

Biederman J, Mick E, Hammerness P, et al, "Open-Label, 8-Week Trial of Olanzapine and Risperidone for the Treatment of Bipolar Disorder in Preschool-Age Children," *Biol Psychiatry*, 2005, 58(7):589-94.

Boachie A, Goldfield GS, and Spettigue W, "Olanzapine Use as an Adjunctive Treatment for Hospitalized Children With Anorexia Nervosa: Case Reports," *Int J Eat Disord*, 2003, 33(1):98-103.

Carrillo JA, Herraiz AG, Ramos SI, et al, "Role of the Smoking-Induced Cytochrome P450 (CYP)1A2 and Polymorphic CYP2D6 in Steady-State Concentration of Olanzapine," *J Clin Psychopharmacol*, 2003, 23(2):119-27.

Chavez B, Chavez-Brown M, Sopko MA Jr, et al, "Atypical Antipsychotics in Children With Pervasive Developmental Disorders," *Paediatr Drugs*, 2007, 9(4):249-66.

Correll CU, Manu P, Olshanskiy V, et al, "Cardiometabolic Risk of Second-Generation Antipsychotic Medications During First-Time Use in Children and Adolescents," *JAMA*, 2009, 302(16):1765-73.

Dunican KC and DelDotto D, "The Role of Olanzapine in the Treatment of Anorexia Nervosa," *Ann Pharmacother*, 2007, 41(1):111-5.

Farwell WR, Stump TE, Wang J, et al, "Weight Gain and New Onset Diabetes Associated With Olanzapine and Risperidone," *J Gen Intern Med*, 2004, 19(12):1200-5.

Frazier JA, Biederman J, Tohen M, et al, " A Prospective Open-Label Treatment Trial of Olanzapine Monotherapy in Children and Adolescents With Bipolar Disorder," *J Child Adolesc Psychopharmacol*, 2001, 11(3):239-50.

Gardiner SJ, Kristensen JH, Begg EJ, et al, "Transfer of Olanzapine Into Breast Milk, Calculation of Infant Drug Dose, and Effect on Breast-Fed Infants," *Am J Psychiatry*, 2003, 160(8):1428-31.

Gilad O, Merlob P, Stahl B, et al, "Outcome of Infants Exposed to Olanzapine During Breastfeeding," *Breastfeed Med*, 2011, 6(2):55-8.

Goldstein DJ, Corbin LA, and Fung MC, "Olanzapine-Exposed Pregnancies and Lactation: Early Experience," *J Clin Psychopharmacol*, 2000, 20(4):399-403.

Grothe DR, Calis KA, Jacobsen L, et al, "Olanzapine Pharmacokinetics in Pediatric and Adolescent Inpatients With Childhood-Onset Schizophrenia," *J Clin Psychopharmacol*, 2000, 20(2):220-5.

Hollander E, Wasserman S, Swanson EN, et al, "A Double-Blind Placebo-Controlled Pilot Study of Olanzapine in Childhood/Adolescent Pervasive Developmental Disorder," *J Child Adolesc Psychopharmacol*, 2006, 16(5):541-8.

Kemner C, Willemsen-Swinkels SH, de Jonge M, et al, "Open-Label Study of Olanzapine in Children With Pervasive Developmental Disorder," *J Clin Psychopharmacol*, 2002, 22(5):455-60.

Khan SS and Mican LM, "A Naturalistic Evaluation of Intramuscular Ziprasidone Versus Intramuscular Olanzapine for the Management of Acute Agitation and Aggression in Children and Adolescents," *J Child Adolesc Psychopharmacol*, 2006, 16(6):671-7.

Kowatch RA, Fristad M, Birmaher B, et al, "Treatment Guidelines for Children and Adolescents With Bipolar Disorder," *J Am Acad Child Adolesc Psychiatry*, 2005, 44(3):213-35.

Kryzhanovskaya L, Schulz SC, McDougle C, et al, "Olanzapine Versus Placebo in Adolescents With Schizophrenia: A 6-Week, Randomized, Double-Blind, Placebo-Controlled Trial," *J Am Acad Child Adolesc Psychiatry*, 2009, 48(1):60-70.

Kumra S, Kranzler H, Gerbino-Rosen G, et al, "Clozapine and 'High-Dose' Olanzapine in Refractory Early-Onset Schizophrenia: A 12-Week Randomized and Double-Blind Comparison," *Biol Psychiatry*, 2008, 63(5):524-9.

Leggero C, Masi G, Brunori E, et al, "Low-Dose Olanzapine Monotherapy in Girls With Anorexia Nervosa, Restricting Subtype: Focus on Hyperactivity," *J Child Adolesc Psychopharmacol*, 2010, 20 (2):127-33.

Malone RP, Cater J, Sheikh RM, et al, "Olanzapine Versus Haloperidol in Children With Autistic Disorder: An Open Pilot Study," *J Am Acad Child Adolesc Psychiatry*, 2001, 40(8):887-94.

McCracken JT, Suddath R, Chang S, et al, "Effectiveness and Tolerability of Open Label Olanzapine in Children and Adolescents With Tourette Syndrome," *J Child Adolesc Psychopharmacol*, 2008, 18 (5):501-8.

Mehler C, Wewetzer C, Schulze U, et al, "Olanzapine in Children and Adolescents With Chronic Anorexia Nervosa. A Study of Five Cases," *Eur Child Adolesc Psychiatry*, 2001, 10(2):151-7.

Mehler-Wex C, Romanos M, Kirchheiner J, et al, "Atypical Antipsychotics in Severe Anorexia Nervosa in Children and Adolescents - Review and Case Reports," *Eur Eat Disord Rev*, 2008, 16(2):100-8.

National Institute for Health and Clinical Excellence (NICE), National Collaborating Centre for Mental Health," Antenatal and Postnatal Mental Health, National Clinical Practice Guideline Number 45," 2007. Available at http://publications.nice.org.uk/antenatal-and-post-natal-mental-health-cg45

Newport DJ, Calamaras MR, DeVane CL, et al, "Atypical Antipsychotic Administration During Late Pregnancy: Placental Passage and Obstetrical Outcomes," *Am J Psychiatry*, 2007, 164(8):1214-20.

Shaw P, Sporn A, Gogtay N, et al, "Childhood-Onset Schizophrenia: A Double-Blind, Randomized, Clozapine-Olanzapine Comparison," *Arch Gen Psych*, 2006, 63(7):721-30.

Sikich L, Frazier JA, McClellan J, et al, "Double-Blind Comparison of First- and Second-Generation Antipsychotics in Early-Onset Schizophrenia and Schizo-affective Disorder: Findings From the Treatment of Early-Onset Schizophrenia Spectrum Disorders (TEOSS) Study," *Am J Psychiatry*, 2008, 165(11):1420-31.

Stachnik JM and Nunn-Thompson C, "Use of Atypical Antipsychotics in the Treatment of Autistic Disorder," *Ann Pharmacother*, 2007, 41 (4):626-34.

Stephens RJ, Bassel C, and Sandor P, "Olanzapine in the Treatment of Aggression and Tics in Children With Tourette's Syndrome - A Pilot Study," *J Child Adolesc Psychopharmacol*, 2004, 14(2):255-66.

Tohen M, Kryzhanovskaya L, Carlson G, et al, "Olanzapine Versus Placebo in the Treatment of Adolescents With Bipolar Mania," *Am J Psychiatry*, 2007, 164(10):1547-56.

Wozniak J, Mick E, Waxmonsky J, et al, "Comparison of Open-Label, 8-Week Trials of Olanzapine Monotherapy and Topiramate Augmentation of Olanzapine for the Treatment of Pediatric Bipolar Disorder," *J Child Adolesc Psychopharmacol*, 2009, 19(5):539-45.

◆ **Olanzapine ODT (Can)** see OLANZapine on page *1525*

◆ **Olanzapine Pamoate** see OLANZapine on page *1525*

◆ **Oleovitamin A** see Vitamin A on page *2146*

◆ **Oleptro** see TraZODone on page *2065*

◆ **Olestyr (Can)** see Cholestyramine Resin on page *457*

◆ **Oleum Ricini** see Castor Oil on page *390*

Olmesartan (ole me SAR tan)

Medication Safety Issues

Sound-alike/look-alike issues:

Benicar may be confused with Mevacor

Brand Names: U.S. Benicar

Brand Names: Canada Olmetec

Therapeutic Category Angiotensin II Receptor Blocker; Antihypertensive Agent

Generic Availability (U.S.) No

Use Treatment of hypertension alone or in combination with other antihypertensive agents (FDA approved in ages 6-16 years and adults)

Pregnancy Risk Factor D

Pregnancy Considerations [U.S. Boxed Warning]: Drugs that act on the renin-angiotensin system can cause injury and death to the developing fetus. Discontinue as soon as possible once pregnancy is detected. The use of drugs which act on the renin-angiotensin system are associated with oligohydramnios. Oligohydramnios, due to decreased fetal renal function, may lead to fetal lung hypoplasia and skeletal malformations. Use is also associated with anuria, hypotension, renal failure, skull hypoplasia, and death in the fetus/neonate. The exposed fetus should be monitored for fetal growth, amniotic fluid volume, and organ formation. Infants exposed *in utero* should be monitored for hyperkalemia, hypotension, and oliguria (exchange transfusions or dialysis may be needed). These adverse events are generally associated with maternal use in the second and third trimesters.

Untreated chronic maternal hypertension is also associated with adverse events in the fetus, infant, and mother. The use of angiotensin II receptor blockers is not recommended to treat chronic uncomplicated hypertension in pregnant women and should generally be avoided in women of reproductive potential (ACOG, 2013).

Breast-Feeding Considerations It is not known if olmesartan is excreted into breast milk. Due to the potential for serious adverse reactions in the nursing infant, the manufacturer recommends a decision be made whether to discontinue nursing or to discontinue the drug, taking into account the importance of treatment to the mother.

Contraindications Hypersensitivity to olmesartan, any component, or other angiotensin II receptor blockers; concomitant use with aliskiren in patients with diabetes mellitus (regardless of GFR)

Warnings Drugs that act on the renin-angiotensin system can cause injury and death to the developing fetus. Discontinue as soon as possible once pregnancy is detected **[U.S. Boxed Warning]**. Use with caution in volume-depleted patients (eg, those on thiazide diuretics); correct depletion first or use a lower starting dose. Symptomatic hypotension may occur, especially in patients with an activated renin-angiotensin system (eg, volume- or salt-depleted patients receiving high doses of diuretic agents); use with caution in these patients; correct depletion before starting therapy or initiate therapy at a lower dose. Concomitant use of an ACE inhibitor or renin inhibitor (eg, aliskiren) is associated with an increased risk of hypotension, hyperkalemia, and renal dysfunction. Concomitant use with aliskiren should be avoided in patients with GFR <60 mL/minute.

Symptoms of sprue-like enteropathy (ie, severe, chronic diarrhea with significant weight loss) have been reported; may develop years after treatment initiation with villous atrophy commonly found on intestinal biopsy; if other etiologies have been excluded, discontinue treatment and consider alternate antihypertensive treatment; clinical and histologic improvement was noted after treatment was discontinued in a case series of 22 patients (Rubio-Tapia, 2012).

Angioedema has been reported rarely with some angiotensin II receptor antagonists (ARBs) and may occur at any time during treatment (especially following first dose); it may involve the head and neck (potentially compromising airway) or the intestine (presenting with abdominal pain). Patients with idiopathic or hereditary angioedema or previous angioedema associated with ACE-inhibitor therapy may be at an increased risk. Prolonged frequent monitoring may be required, especially if tongue, glottis, or larynx are involved, as they are associated with airway obstruction. Patients with a history of airway surgery may have a higher risk of airway obstruction. Discontinue therapy immediately if angioedema occurs. Aggressive

early management is critical. Intramuscular (I.M.) administration of epinephrine may be necessary. Do not readminister to patients who have had angioedema with ARBs.

Precautions Use with caution in patients with impaired renal function; use is associated with deterioration of renal function and/or increases in serum creatinine, particularly in patients with low renal blood flow (eg, renal artery stenosis, heart failure); deterioration may result in oliguria, acute renal failure, or progressive azotemia. Small increases in serum creatinine may occur following initiation; consider discontinuation in patients with progressive and/or significant deterioration in renal function. Hyperkalemia may occur; risk factors include renal dysfunction, diabetes mellitus, concomitant use of potassium-sparing diuretics, potassium supplements, and/or potassium-containing salts; use with caution in these patients and with these agents; monitor potassium closely.

Adverse Reactions

Central nervous system: Dizziness, headache

Endocrine & metabolic: Hyperglycemia, hypertriglyceridemia

Gastrointestinal: Diarrhea

Neuromuscular & skeletal: Back pain, CPK increased

Renal: Hematuria

Respiratory: Bronchitis, pharyngitis, rhinitis, sinusitis

Miscellaneous: Flu-like syndrome

Rare but important or life-threatening: Acute renal failure, alopecia, anaphylaxis, angioedema, arthritis, gastroenteritis, hypercholesterolemia, hyperkalemia, hyperlipidemia, hyperuricemia, liver enzymes increased, peripheral edema, rhabdomyolysis, serum creatinine increased, sprue-like symptoms, tachycardia

Drug Interactions

Metabolism/Transport Effects Substrate of SLCO1B1

Avoid Concomitant Use There are no known interactions where it is recommended to avoid concomitant use.

Increased Effect/Toxicity

Olmesartan may increase the levels/effects of: ACE Inhibitors; Amifostine; Antihypertensives; CycloSPORINE (Systemic); DULoxetine; Hypotensive Agents; Lithium; Nonsteroidal Anti-Inflammatory Agents; Obinutuzumab; Potassium-Sparing Diuretics; RiTUXimab; Sodium Phosphates

The levels/effects of Olmesartan may be increased by: Alfuzosin; Aliskiren; Barbiturates; Brimonidine (Topical); Canagliflozin; Diazoxide; Eltrombopag; Eplerenone; Heparin; Heparin (Low Molecular Weight); Herbs (Hypotensive Properties); MAO Inhibitors; Pentoxifylline; Phosphodiesterase 5 Inhibitors; Potassium Salts; Prostacyclin Analogues; Tolvaptan; Trimethoprim

Decreased Effect

The levels/effects of Olmesartan may be decreased by: Colesevelam; Herbs (Hypertensive Properties); Methylphenidate; Nonsteroidal Anti-Inflammatory Agents; Yohimbine

Food Interactions Food does not affect olmesartan bioavailability.

Stability Store at 20°C to 25°C (68°F to 77°F).

Mechanism of Action As a selective and competitive, nonpeptide angiotensin II receptor antagonist, olmesartan blocks the vasoconstrictor and aldosterone-secreting effects of angiotensin II; olmesartan interacts reversibly at the AT1 and AT2 receptors of many tissues and has slow dissociation kinetics; its affinity for the AT1 receptor is 12,500 times greater than the AT2 receptor. Angiotensin II receptor antagonists may induce a more complete inhibition of the renin-angiotensin system than ACE inhibitors, they do not affect the response to bradykinin, and are less likely to be associated with nonrenin-angiotensin effects (eg, cough and angioedema). Olmesartan increases urinary flow rate and, in addition to being natriuretic and kaliuretic, increases excretion of chloride, magnesium, uric acid, calcium, and phosphate.

Pharmacokinetics (Adult data unless noted)

Distribution: V_d: ~17 L

Protein binding: 99%

Metabolism: Olmesartan medoxomil is hydrolyzed during absorption from the GI tract to active olmesartan. Virtually no further metabolism occurs

Bioavailability: ~26%

Half-life elimination: Terminal: ~13 hours

Time to peak serum concentration: 1-2 hours

Elimination: All as unchanged drug: Feces (50% to 65%); urine (35% to 50%)

Clearance: 1.3 L/hour; similar data reported in pediatric patients (1-16 years) when adjusted by body weight

Dialysis: Effects of hemodialysis have not been studied

Dosing: Usual Note: Consider lower starting dose in patients with possible depletion of intravascular volume (eg, patients receiving diuretics).

Children and Adolescents: Hypertension: Oral:

Children 1-5 years and ≥5 kg: Limited data available: Initial: 0.3 mg/kg/dose once daily; if initial response inadequate after 2 weeks, dose may be increased to 0.6 mg/kg/dose once daily. Dosing was evaluated in a double-blind, placebo-controlled study of 59 patients and some efficacy was demonstrated; however, results were not statistically significant (NCT00151775, 2010).

Children and Adolescents 6-16 years:

20 to <35 kg: 10 mg once daily; if initial response inadequate after 2 weeks, dose may be increased (maximum: 20 mg/day)

≥35 kg: 20 mg once daily; if initial response inadequate after 2 weeks, dose may be increased (maximum: 40 mg/day)

Adolescents >16 years: Initial: 20 mg once daily; if initial response is inadequate, may be increased to 40 mg once daily after 2 weeks. May administer with other antihypertensive agents if blood pressure inadequately controlled with olmesartan.

Adults: Hypertension: Oral: Initial: 20 mg once daily; if initial response is inadequate, may be increased to 40 mg once daily after 2 weeks. May administer with other antihypertensive agents if blood pressure inadequately controlled with olmesartan.

Dosing adjustment in renal impairment: No specific guidelines for dosage adjustment; patients undergoing hemodialysis have not been studied. In patients with severe renal impairment (CrCl <20 mL/minute), the AUC was tripled after repeated dosing.

Dosing adjustment in hepatic impairment: No initial dosage adjustment necessary. **Note:** In patients with moderate hepatic impairment, an increase in AUC of ~60% was observed.

Administration May be administered with or without food.

Monitoring Parameters Blood pressure, serum creatinine, serum potassium

Additional Information The antihypertensive effects of olmesartan are smaller in black patients (usually a low-renin patient population); this effect of race is also seen with ACE inhibitors, beta-blockers, and other angiotensin receptor blockers. A pediatric study of olmesartan in patients 6-16 years of age found numerically smaller reductions in blood pressure in black patients compared to a racially-mixed cohort (Hazan, 2010).

Dosage Forms Excipient information presented when available (limited, particularly for generics); consult specific product labeling.

Tablet, Oral, as medoxomil:

Benicar: 5 mg, 20 mg, 40 mg

Extemporaneous Preparations A 2 mg/mL oral suspension may be made with olmesartan tablets. Combine 50 mL purified water and twenty 20 mg tablets in an 8-ounce amber bottle and allow to stand for ≥5 minutes. Shake well for ≥1 minute, then allow to stand for ≥1 minute. Repeat shaking and standing process four additional times. Add 100 mL Ora-Sweet® and 50 mL Ora-Plus® to the suspension and shake well for ≥1 minute. Label "shake well" and "refrigerate". Stable for 28 days refrigerated.

Benicar® prescribing information, Daiichi Sankyo, Inc, Parsippany, NJ, 2010.

References

American College of Obstetricians and Gynecologists (ACOG), "ACOG Practice Bulletin No. 125: Chronic Hypertension in Pregnancy," *Obstet Gynecol*, 2012, 119(2 Pt 1):396-407.

Chobanian AV, Bakris GL, Black HR, et al, "The Seventh Report of the Joint National Committee on Prevention, Detection, Evaluation, and Treatment of High Blood Pressure: The JNC 7 Report," *JAMA*, 2003, 289(19):2560-71.

Hazan L, Hernández Rodriguez OA, Bhorat AE, et al, "A Double-Blind, Dose-Response Study of the Efficacy and Safety of Olmesartan Medoxomil in Children and Adolescents With Hypertension," *Hypertension*, 2010, 55(6):1323-30.

NCT00151775, "Assessment of Efficacy and Safety of Olmesartan Medoxomil in Children and Adolescent Patients With High Blood Pressure," Unpublished data. Available at: http://clinicaltrials.gov/ct2/show/NCT00151775?term=olmesartan+children&rank=1. Date accessed: October 13, 2010.

Rubio-Tapia A, Herman ML, Ludvigsson JF, et al. Severe spruelike enteropathy associated with olmesartan. *Mayo Clin Proc*. 2012;87(8):732-738.

◆ **Olmesartan Medoxomil** see Olmesartan on page 1530

◆ **Olmetec (Can)** see Olmesartan on page 1530

Olsalazine (ole SAL a zeen)

Medication Safety Issues

Sound-alike/look-alike issues:

Olsalazine may be confused with OLANZapine

Dipentum® may be confused with Dilantin®

Brand Names: U.S. Dipentum

Brand Names: Canada Dipentum®

Therapeutic Category 5-Aminosalicylic Acid Derivative; Anti-inflammatory Agent

Generic Availability (U.S.) No

Use Maintenance of remission of ulcerative colitis in patients intolerant to sulfasalazine (FDA approved in adults)

Pregnancy Risk Factor C

Pregnancy Considerations Animal studies have demonstrated fetal developmental toxicities. There are no well-controlled studies in pregnant women. Use during pregnancy only if clearly necessary.

Breast-Feeding Considerations The active metabolite, 5-aminosalicylic acid may pass into breast milk. Diarrhea has been reported in breast-fed infants whose mothers took olsalazine.

Contraindications Hypersensitivity to olsalazine, salicylates, or any component

Warnings Diarrhea is a common adverse effect of olsalazine. May exacerbate symptoms of colitis.

Precautions Use with caution in patients with hypersensitivity to sulfasalazine or mesalamine. Use with caution in patients with asthma, severe allergies, hepatic impairment, or renal impairment.

Adverse Reactions

Central nervous system: Depression, dizziness, vertigo

Dermatologic: Pruritus, rash

Gastrointestinal: Abdominal pain/cramps, bloating, diarrhea (dose related), nausea, stomatitis, vomiting

Neuromuscular & skeletal: Arthralgia

Respiratory: Upper respiratory infection

Rare but important or life-threatening: Alkaline phosphatase increased, Alopecia, ALT increased, anemia, angioedema, aplastic anemia, AST increased, bilirubin increased, blood in stool, blurred vision, bronchospasm, cholestatic hepatitis, cholestatic jaundice, chest pain, chills, cirrhosis, dehydration, dry eyes, dyspnea, dysuria, eosinophilia, epigastric discomfort, erythema, erythema nodosum, fever, flare of symptoms, flatulence, GGT increased, heart block (second degree), hematuria, hemolytic anemia, hepatitis, hepatic failure, hepatic necrosis, hot flashes, hypertension, impotence, insomnia, interstitial nephritis, interstitial pneumonia, irritability, jaundice, Kawasaki-like syndrome, LDH increased, leukopenia, lymphopenia, menorrhagia, mood swings, muscle cramps, myalgia, myocarditis, nephrotic syndrome, neutropenia, orthostatic hypotension, palpitation, pancreatitis, pancytopenia, paresthesia, pericarditis, peripheral edema, peripheral neuropathy, photosensitivity, proteinuria, rectal bleeding, rectal discomfort, reticulocytosis, rigors, tachycardia, thrombocytopenia, tinnitus, tremor, urinary frequency, watery eyes, xerostomia

Drug Interactions

Metabolism/Transport Effects None known.

Avoid Concomitant Use There are no known interactions where it is recommended to avoid concomitant use.

Increased Effect/Toxicity

Olsalazine may increase the levels/effects of: Heparin; Heparin (Low Molecular Weight); Thiopurine Analogs; Varicella Virus-Containing Vaccines

The levels/effects of Olsalazine may be increased by: Nonsteroidal Anti-Inflammatory Agents

Decreased Effect

Olsalazine may decrease the levels/effects of: Cardiac Glycosides

Mechanism of Action Mesalamine (5-aminosalicylic acid) is the active component of olsalazine; the specific mechanism of action of mesalamine is unknown; however, it is thought that it modulates local chemical mediators of the inflammatory response, especially leukotrienes, and is also postulated to be a free radical scavenger or an inhibitor of tumor necrosis factor (TNF); action appears topical rather than systemic.

Pharmacokinetics (Adult data unless noted)

Absorption: <3%; very little intact olsalazine is systemically absorbed

Protein binding: >99%

Metabolism: Mostly by colonic bacteria to the active drug, 5-aminosalicylic acid

Bioavailability: 2.4%

Half-life, elimination: 54 minutes (in serum)

Elimination: Primarily in feces; <1% eliminated in urine

Dosing: Usual Adults: Oral: 1 g/day in 2 divided doses

Administration Oral: Administer with food in evenly divided doses

Dosage Forms Excipient information presented when available (limited, particularly for generics); consult specific product labeling.

Capsule, Oral, as sodium:

Dipentum: 250 mg

◆ **Olsalazine Sodium** *see* Olsalazine *on page 1532*

◆ **Olux** *see* Clobetasol *on page 506*

◆ **Olux-E** *see* Clobetasol *on page 506*

Omalizumab (oh mah lye ZOO mab)

Medication Safety Issues

Sound-alike/look-alike issues:

Omalizumab may be confused with obinutuzumab, ofatumumab

Brand Names: U.S. Xolair

Brand Names: Canada Xolair

Therapeutic Category Monoclonal Antibody, Anti-Asthmatic

Generic Availability (U.S.) No

Use Treatment of moderate to severe, persistent allergic asthma not adequately controlled with inhaled corticosteroids

Medication Guide Available Yes

Pregnancy Risk Factor B

Pregnancy Considerations Teratogenic effects were not observed in animal studies. There are no adequate and well-controlled studies in pregnant women. IgG molecules are known to cross the placenta; use during pregnancy only if clearly needed. A registry has been established to monitor outcomes of women exposed to omalizumab during pregnancy or within 8 weeks prior to pregnancy (866-496-5247).

Breast-Feeding Considerations It is not known if omalizumab is excreted in breast milk; however, IgG is excreted in human milk and excretion of omalizumab is expected. Effects to nursing infant are not known; use with caution.

Contraindications Hypersensitivity to omalizumab or any component

Warnings Not indicated for use in the control of acute asthma symptoms. Anaphylaxis, including delayed-onset anaphylaxis, has been reported following administration **[U.S. Boxed Warning]**; reactions usually occur within 2 hours of administration, but may occur up to 24 hours and in some cases >24 hours after treatment. Patients should receive treatment only under direct medical supervision and be observed for a minimum of 2 hours following administration; providers and patients should have appropriate treatment for anaphylaxis available. Hypersensitivity reactions may occur following any dose, even during chronic therapy; discontinue therapy following any severe reaction. Injection site reactions typically occur within 1 hour postinjection, last <8 days, and generally decrease in frequency after subsequent doses. Due to the risk of delayed anaphylaxis, patients should be fully prepared and trained on the appropriate emergency self-treatment of an anaphylactic reaction. Safety and efficacy in children <12 years of age has not been established.

Malignant neoplasms of varying types (breast, nonmelanoma skin, prostate, and parotid) were observed in 0.5% of patients during clinical trials (compared with 0.2% in controls); the majority of these patients received omalizumab for <1 year; risk of long-term exposure to omalizumab is not known. Systemic or inhaled corticosteroid use should not be abruptly discontinued upon initiation of omalizumab therapy; gradual tapering under medical supervision is recommended. In a one year clinical trial in Brazil, patients with increased risk of geohelminthic infections (roundworm, hookworm, whipworm, threadworm) experienced an increase in geohelminthic infections when compared with the control group (42% vs 53%).

Preliminary findings of an ongoing safety review suggest an increased risk of cardiovascular (eg, arrhythmias, cardiomyopathy, ischemic heart disease, heart failure, pulmonary hypertension), cerebrovascular, and thromboembolic adverse events in patients treated with omalizumab.

Precautions Dosage and frequency of administration are dependent upon the serum total IgE level and body weight. Total IgE level must be measured prior to beginning treatment. Total IgE levels are elevated during treatment and remain elevated for up to one year after the discontinuation of treatment. Remeasurement of IgE levels during omalizumab treatment should not be used as a guide to dosage. Remeasurement of IgE levels may be used after treatment has been discontinued for at least one year.

Adverse Reactions

Asthma:

Central nervous system: Dizziness, fatigue, pain

Dermatologic: Dermatitis, pruritus

Local: Injection site reaction (most reactions occurred within 1 hour, lasted <8 days, and decreased in frequency with additional dosing)

Neuromuscular & skeletal: Arm pain, arthralgia, bone fracture, leg pain

Otic: Otalgia

Rare but important or life-threatening: Alopecia, anaphylaxis, antibody development, arthritis, lymphadenopathy, malignant neoplasm, syncope, thrombocytopenia

Chronic idiopathic urticaria:

Cardiovascular: Peripheral edema

Central nervous system: Anxiety, headache, migraine

Dermatologic: Alopecia

Gastrointestinal: Toothache

Genitourinary: Urinary tract infection

Infection: Fungal infection

Local: Injection site reaction

Neuromuscular & skeletal: Arthralgia, limb pain, musculoskeletal pain, myalgia

Respiratory: Asthma, cough, nasopharyngitis, oropharyngeal pain, sinus headache, sinusitis, upper respiratory tract infection, viral upper respiratory tract infection

Miscellaneous: Fever

Drug Interactions

Metabolism/Transport Effects None known.

Avoid Concomitant Use

Avoid concomitant use of Omalizumab with any of the following: BCG; Belimumab; Natalizumab; Pimecrolimus; Tacrolimus (Topical); Tofacitinib; Vaccines (Live)

Increased Effect/Toxicity

Omalizumab may increase the levels/effects of: Belimumab; Leflunomide; Natalizumab; Tofacitinib; Vaccines (Live)

The levels/effects of Omalizumab may be increased by: Abciximab; Denosumab; Pimecrolimus; Roflumilast; Tacrolimus (Topical); Trastuzumab

Decreased Effect

Omalizumab may decrease the levels/effects of: BCG; Coccidioidin Skin Test; Sipuleucel-T; Vaccines (Inactivated); Vaccines (Live)

The levels/effects of Omalizumab may be decreased by: Echinacea

Stability Store in refrigerator at 2°C to 8°C (36°F to 46°F); omalizumab is provided in a single use vial with no preservatives; the reconstituted solution is stable for 4 hours at room temperature and 8 hours refrigerated

Mechanism of Action

Allergic asthma: Omalizumab is an IgG monoclonal antibody (recombinant DNA derived) which inhibits IgE binding to the high-affinity IgE receptor on mast cells and basophils. By decreasing bound IgE, the activation and release of mediators in the allergic response (early and late phase) is limited. Serum free IgE levels and the number of high-affinity IgE receptors are decreased. Long-term treatment in patients with allergic asthma showed a decrease in asthma exacerbations and corticosteroid usage.

Chronic idiopathic urticaria: Omalizumab binds to IgE and lowers free IgE levels. Subsequently, IgE receptors (FcεRI) on cells down-regulate. The mechanism by which these effects of omalizumab result in an improvement of chronic idiopathic urticaria symptoms is unknown.

Pharmacodynamics Response to therapy: ~12-16 weeks (87% of patients had measurable response in 12 weeks)

Pharmacokinetics (Adult data unless noted)

Absorption: Slow after SubQ administration

Distribution: V_d: 78 ± 32 mL/kg

Metabolism: Hepatic: IgG degradation by reticuloendothelial system and endothelial cells

Bioavailability: Absolute: 62%

Half-life: Adults: 1-4 weeks

Time to peak serum concentration: 7-8 days

Excretion: Primarily via hepatic degradation; intact IgG may be secreted in bile

Clearance: 2.4 ± 1.1 mL/kg/day

Dosing: Usual Dosage and frequency of administration are dependent upon the serum total IgE level and body weight. Measure total IgE level prior to beginning treatment. Total IgE levels are elevated during treatment and remain elevated for up to one year after the discontinuation of treatment. Remeasurement of IgE levels during omalizumab treatment should not be used as a guide to dosage.

Asthma: Children ≥12 years, Adolescents, and Adults: SubQ: 0.016 mg/kg/unit of IgE every 4 weeks.

Manufacturer's labeling:

IgE ≥30-100 units/mL:
  30-90 kg: 150 mg every 4 weeks
  >90-150 kg: 300 mg every 4 weeks

IgE >100-200 units/mL:
  30-90 kg: 300 mg every 4 weeks
  >90-150 kg: 225 mg every 2 weeks

IgE >200-300 units/mL:
  30-60 kg: 300 mg every 4 weeks
  >60-90 kg: 225 mg every 2 weeks
  >90-150 kg: 300 mg every 2 weeks

IgE >300-400 units/mL:
  30-70 kg: 225 mg every 2 weeks
  >70-90 kg: 300 mg every 2 weeks
  >90 kg: Do not use*

IgE >400-500 units/mL:
  30-70 kg: 300 mg every 2 weeks
  >70-90 kg: 375 mg every 2 weeks
  >90 kg: Do not use*

IgE >500-600 units/mL:
  30-60 kg: 300 mg every 2 weeks
  >60-70 kg: 375 mg every 2 weeks
  >70 kg: Do not use*

IgE >600-700 units/mL:
  30-60 kg: 375 mg every 2 weeks
  >60 kg: Do not use*

*Dosage has not been studied and approved for this weight and IgE level

Administration SubQ: Reconstitute 150 mg vial with 1.4 mL SWI; swirl vial for approximately 1 minute to evenly wet powder; repeat swirling for 5-10 seconds every 5 minutes in order to dissolve remaining solids; dissolution time is at least 20 minutes. Reconstituted solution will be viscous with no visible gel-like particles present in solution. Do not use if contents of vial do not dissolve within 40 minutes. Resulting concentration is 150 mg/1.2 mL (125 mg/mL). Due to viscosity, injection may take 5-10 seconds to administer. Doses >150 mg should be divided into more than one injection site.

Monitoring Parameters Baseline total serum IgE, pulmonary function tests, anaphylactic/hypersensitivity reactions

Test Interactions Total IgE levels are elevated for up to 1 year following treatment. Total serum IgE may be retested after interruption of therapy for 1 year or more.

Additional Information Omalizumab was used successfully in a double-blind, randomized, placebo-controlled study of 334 children between the ages of 6-12 years; omalizumab dosage was based on body weight and initial serum total IgE. Patients received omalizumab at either 2- or 4-week intervals with a dosage equal to 0.016 mg/kg/ IgE (units/mL) per 4 weeks. 55% of patients were able to discontinue corticosteroid use (Milgrom, 2003). A registry has been established to monitor outcomes of women exposed to omalizumab during pregnancy or within 8 weeks prior to pregnancy (866-496-5247).

Dosage Forms Excipient information presented when available (limited, particularly for generics); consult specific product labeling.

Solution Reconstituted, Subcutaneous [preservative free]:
Xolair: 150 mg (1 ea)

References

Berger W, Gupta N, McAlary M, et al, "Evaluation of Long-Term Safety of the Anti-IgE Antibody, Omalizumab, in Children with Allergic Asthma," *Ann Allergy Asthma Immunol*, 2003, 91(2):182-8.

Casale TB, Condemi J, LaForce C, et al, "Effect of Omalizumab on Symptoms of Seasonal Allergic Rhinitis: A Randomized Controlled Trial," *JAMA*, 2001, 286(23):2956-67.

Milgrom H, Berger W, Nayak A, et al, "Treatment of Childhood Asthma With Anti-Immunoglobulin E Antibody (Omalizumab)," *Pediatrics*, 2001, 108(2):E36.

Milgrom H, Fick RB Jr, Su JQ, et al, "Treatment of Allergic Asthma With Monoclonal Anti-IgE Antibody. rhuMAb-E25 Study Group," *Engl J Med*, 1999, 341(26):1966-73.

Strunk RC and Bloomberg GR, "Omalizumab for Asthma," *N Engl J Med*, 2006, 354(25):2689-95.

Omeprazole (oh MEP ra zole)

Medication Safety Issues

Sound-alike/look-alike issues:

Omeprazole may be confused with aripiprazole, esomeprazole, fomepizole

PriLOSEC may be confused with Plendil, Prevacid, predniSONE, prilocaine, Prinivil, Proventil, PROzac

International issues:

Losec [multiple international markets] may be confused with Lasix brand name for furosemide [U.S., Canada, and multiple international markets]

Medral [Mexico] may be confused with Medrol brand name for methylprednisolone [U.S., Canada, and multiple international markets]

Norpramin: Brand name for omeprazole [Spain], but also the brand name for desipramine [U.S., Canada] and enalapril/hydrochlorothiazide [Portugal]

Protonix: Brand name for omeprazole [Phillipines] but also the brand name for pantoprazole [U.S.]

Related Information

H. pylori Treatment in Pediatric Patients *on page 2311*

Oral Medications That Should Not Be Crushed or Altered *on page 2438*

Brand Names: U.S. First-Omeprazole; Omeprazole+Syrspend SF Alka; PriLOSEC; PriLOSEC OTC [OTC]

Brand Names: Canada Apo-Omeprazole; Auro-Omeprazole; Ava-Omeprazole; Dom-Omeprazole DR; JAMP-Omeprazole DR; Losec; Mylan-Omeprazole; PMS-Omeprazole; PMS-Omeprazole DR; Q-Omeprazole; RAN-Omeprazole; ratio-Omeprazole; Riva-Omeprazole DR; Sandoz-Omeprazole; Teva-Omeprazole

Therapeutic Category Gastric Acid Secretion Inhibitor; Gastrointestinal Agent; Gastric or Duodenal Ulcer Treatment; Proton Pump Inhibitor

Generic Availability (U.S.) May be product dependent

Use Short-term treatment (4-8 weeks) and maintenance of healing of severe erosive esophagitis (FDA approved in ages ≥1 year and adults); treatment of symptomatic gastroesophageal reflux disease (GERD) (FDA approved in ages ≥1 year and adults); short-term treatment (4-8 weeks) of active duodenal ulcers and active benign gastric ulcers (FDA approved in adults); adjunctive treatment of duodenal ulcers associated with *Helicobacter pylori* (FDA approved in adults); treatment of pathological hypersecretory conditions (FDA approved in adults); relief of frequent heartburn (OTC products; FDA approved in adults)

Medication Guide Available Yes

Pregnancy Risk Factor C

Pregnancy Considerations Adverse events were observed in some animal reproduction studies. An increased risk of hypospadias was reported following maternal use of proton pump inhibitors (PPIs) during pregnancy (Anderka, 2012), but this was based on a small number of exposures and the same association was not found in another study (Erichsen, 2012). Most available studies have not shown an increased risk of major birth defects following maternal use of omeprazole during pregnancy (Diav-Citrin, 2005; Källén, 2001; Lalkin, 1998; Matok, 2012; Pasternak, 2010). When treating GERD in pregnancy, PPIs may be used when clinically indicated (Katz, 2013).

Breast-Feeding Considerations Omeprazole is excreted into breast milk. Milk concentrations of omeprazole were studied in a breast-feeding woman at 3 weeks postpartum. The mother had taken omeprazole 20 mg daily starting her 29th week of gestation and continued after delivery. Following administration of omeprazole 20 mg, peak concentrations in the maternal serum occurred 240 minutes after the dose and peak concentrations in the breast milk were 180 minutes after the dose. The concentrations of omeprazole detected in the breast milk were <7% of the highest maternal serum concentration (Marshall, 1998).The manufacturer recommends caution be used if administered to a nursing woman. The acidic content of the nursing infants' stomach may potentially inactivate any ingested omeprazole (Marshall, 1998).

Contraindications Hypersensitivity to omeprazole, substituted benzimidazole proton pump inhibitors (eg, esomeprazole, lansoprazole), or any component

Warnings In long-term (2-year) studies in rats, omeprazole produced a dose-related increase in gastric carcinoid tumors. While available endoscopic evaluations and histologic examinations of biopsy specimens from human stomachs have not detected a risk from short-term exposure to omeprazole, further human data on the effect of sustained hypochlorhydria and hypergastrinemia are needed to rule out the possibility of an increased risk for the development of tumors in humans receiving long-term therapy.

An increased incidence of osteoporosis-related bone fractures of the hip, spine, or wrist may occur with proton pump inhibitor (PPI) therapy; patients on high-dose (multiple daily doses) or long-term (≥1 year) therapy should be monitored. Use the lowest effective dose for the shortest duration of time, use vitamin D and calcium supplementation, and follow appropriate guidelines to reduce risk of fractures in patients at risk. Hypomagnesemia has been reported rarely, usually with prolonged PPI use of >3 months (most cases >1 year of therapy), and may be symptomatic or asymptomatic; severe cases may cause tetany, seizures, and cardiac arrhythmias. Consider obtaining serum magnesium concentrations prior to beginning long-term therapy, especially if taking concomitant digoxin, diuretics, or other drugs known to cause hypomagnesemia; and periodically thereafter. Hypomagnesemia may be corrected by magnesium supplementation, although discontinuation of omeprazole may be necessary; magnesium concentrations typically return to normal within 1 week of stopping. Atrophic gastritis has been reported occasionally in gastric corpus biopsies from patients treated long-term with omeprazole. Symptomatic response to therapy does not preclude the presence of GI malignancy.

Use of gastric acid inhibitors, including proton pump inhibitors and H_2 blockers, has been associated with an increased risk for development of acute gastroenteritis and community-acquired pneumonia (Canani, 2006). Use of PPIs may also increase the risk of *Clostridium difficile*-associated diarrhea (CDAD), especially in hospitalized patients; consider CDAD diagnosis in patients with persistent diarrhea that does not improve. Use the lowest dose and shortest duration of PPI therapy appropriate for the condition being treated. Serum chromogranin A (CgA) levels may be falsely elevated if assessed while on omeprazole causing diagnostic misinterpretation if a neuroendocrine tumor suspected.

PPIs may diminish the therapeutic effect of clopidogrel, thought to be due to reduced formation of the active metabolite of clopidogrel. The manufacturer of clopidogrel recommends either avoidance of both omeprazole (even when scheduled 12 hours apart) and esomeprazole or use of a PPI with comparatively less effect on the active metabolite of clopidogrel (eg, pantoprazole). In contrast to these warnings, others have recommended the continued use of PPIs, regardless of the degree of inhibition, in patients with a history of GI bleeding or multiple risk factors for GI bleeding who are also receiving clopidogrel since no evidence has established clinically meaningful differences in outcome; however, a clinically-significant interaction cannot be excluded in those who are poor metabolizers of clopidogrel (Abraham, 2010; Levine, 2011). Concomitant use of PPIs with high-dose methotrexate may lead to increased and prolonged serum concentrations of methotrexate and/or its metabolite, possibly causing methotrexate toxicities; temporary discontinuation of PPIs may be considered.

Do not use for self-medication (OTC) if difficulty swallowing, blood in vomit, or bloody or black stools are present. Healthcare provider should be contacted prior to use if any of the following conditions are present: Heartburn for >3 months; heartburn with dizziness, lightheadedness, or sweating; MI symptoms; frequent chest pain; frequent wheezing (especially with heartburn); unexplained weight loss; nausea/vomiting; stomach pain; or taking other medications (interactions are common). If heartburn continues or worsens or if need to take for >14 days or more often than every 4 months, discontinue use and contact physician. May take 1-4 days for full effect to be seen.

First®-Omeprazole powder for oral suspension contains benzyl alcohol which may cause allergic reactions in susceptible individuals; large amounts of benzyl alcohol (≥99 mg/kg/day) have been associated with a potentially fatal toxicity ("gasping syndrome") in neonates; use oral suspension containing benzyl alcohol with caution in neonates; in vitro and animal studies have shown that benzoate, a metabolite of benzyl alcohol, displaces bilirubin from protein binding sites.

Precautions Bioavailability may be increased in patients with hepatic dysfunction or patients of Asian descent; consider dosage reductions, especially for maintenance healing of erosive esophagitis

Adverse Reactions

Central nervous system: Dizziness, headache

Dermatologic: Skin rash

Gastrointestinal: Abdominal pain, acid regurgitation, constipation, diarrhea, flatulence, nausea, vomiting

Neuromuscular & skeletal: Back pain, weakness

Respiratory: Cough, upper respiratory infection

Rare but important or life-threatening: Abdominal swelling, abnormal dreams, aggression, agranulocytosis, allergic reactions, alopecia, anaphylaxis, anemia, angina pectoris, angioedema, anorexia, apathy, arthralgia, atrophic gastritis, benign gastric polyps, blurred vision, bone fracture, bradycardia, bronchospasm, chest pain, cholestatic hepatitis, Clostridium difficile-associated diarrhea (CDAD), confusion, depression, dermatitis, diplopia, drowsiness, epistaxis, erythema multiforme, esophageal candidiasis, fecal discoloration, gastroduodenal carcinoids, glycosuria, gynecomastia, hallucinations, hematuria, hemolytic anemia, hepatic disease (hepatocellular, cholestatic, mixed), hepatic encephalopathy, hepatic failure, hepatic necrosis, hepatitis, hepatocellular hepatitis, hyperhidrosis, hypersensitivity, hypertension, hypocalcemia, hypoglycemia, hypokalemia, hypomagnesemia, hyponatremia, increased gamma glutamyl transferase, increased serum alkaline phosphatase, increased serum bilirubin, increased serum creatinine, increased serum transaminases, insomnia, interstitial nephritis, irritable bowel syndrome, jaundice, leg pain, leukocytosis, leukopenia, malaise, microscopic colitis, microscopic pyuria, mucosal atrophy (tongue), muscle cramps, myalgia, myasthenia, nervousness, neutropenia, ocular irritation, optic atrophy, optic neuritis, optic neuropathy (anterior ischemic), osteoporosis-related fracture, pain, palpitation, pancreatitis, pancytopenia, paresthesia, peripheral edema, petechiae, photophobia, pneumonia, proteinuria, pruritus, psychiatric disturbance, purpura, sleep disturbance, sore throat, Stevens-Johnson syndrome, stomatitis, tachycardia, testicular pain, thrombocytopenia, toxic epidermal necrolysis, tremor, urinary tract infection, urticaria, weight gain, xeroderma, xerophthalmia, xerostomia

Drug Interactions

Metabolism/Transport Effects Substrate of CYP2A6 (minor), CYP2C19 (major), CYP2C9 (minor), CYP2D6 (minor), CYP3A4 (minor); **Note:** Assignment of Major/Minor substrate status based on clinically relevant drug interaction potential; **Inhibits** CYP1A2 (weak), CYP2C19 (moderate), CYP2C9 (moderate), CYP2D6 (weak), CYP3A4 (weak); **Induces** CYP1A2 (weak/moderate)

Avoid Concomitant Use

Avoid concomitant use of Omeprazole with any of the following: Clopidogrel; Dasatinib; Delavirdine; Erlotinib; Nelfinavir; PAZOPanib; Pimozide; PONATinib; Rifampin; Rilpivirine; Risedronate; St Johns Wort

Increased Effect/Toxicity

Omeprazole may increase the levels/effects of: Amphetamine; ARIPiprazole; Benzodiazepines (metabolized by oxidation); Bosentan; Cannabis; Carvedilol; Cilostazol; Citalopram; CloZAPine; CycloSPORINE (Systemic); CYP2C19 Substrates; CYP2C9 Substrates; Dexmethylphenidate; Dextroamphetamine; Dofetilide; Dronabinol; Escitalopram; Fosphenytoin; Lomitapide; Methotrexate; Methylphenidate; Phenytoin; Pimozide; Raltegravir; Risedronate; Saquinavir; Tacrolimus (Systemic); Tetrahydrocannabinol; Vitamin K Antagonists; Voriconazole

The levels/effects of Omeprazole may be increased by: Fluconazole; Ketoconazole (Systemic); Voriconazole

Decreased Effect

Omeprazole may decrease the levels/effects of: Atazanavir; Bisphosphonate Derivatives; Bosutinib; Cefditoren; Clopidogrel; CloZAPine; Dabigatran Etexilate; Dabrafenib; Dasatinib; Delavirdine; Erlotinib; Gefitinib; Indinavir; Iron Salts; Itraconazole; Ketoconazole (Systemic); Mesalamine; Multivitamins/Minerals (with ADEK, Folate, Iron); Mycophenolate; Nelfinavir; Nilotinib; PAZOPanib; PONATinib; Posaconazole; Rilpivirine; Riociguat; Risedronate; Vismodegib

The levels/effects of Omeprazole may be decreased by: CYP2C19 Inducers (Strong); Dabrafenib; Fosphenytoin; Peginterferon Alfa-2b; Phenytoin; Rifampin; St Johns Wort; Tipranavir

Food Interactions Prolonged treatment (≥2 years) may lead to malabsorption of dietary vitamin B_{12} and subsequent vitamin B_{12} deficiency (Lam, 2013).

Stability Oral omeprazole stability is a function of pH; it is rapidly degraded in acidic media but has acceptable stability under alkaline conditions. Each capsule of omeprazole contains enteric-coated granules to prevent omeprazole degradation by gastric acidity.

Delayed release capsules: Store between 15°C to 30°C (59°F to 86°F); protect from light and moisture

Oral suspension: Store at 25°C (77°F); excursions permitted to 15°C to 30°C (59°F to 86°F)

Powder for suspension (compounding kit): Prior to compounding, store at 15°C to 30°C (59°F to 86°F). Once compounded, the product is stable for 30 days under refrigeration [2°C to 8°C (36°F to 46°F)]; protect from light; protect from freezing.

OTC capsules: Store at 20°C to 25°C (68°F to 77°F); protect from moisture.

Mechanism of Action Proton pump inhibitor; suppresses gastric basal and stimulated acid secretion by inhibiting the parietal cell H+/K+ ATP pump

Pharmacodynamics

Onset of action: 1 hour

Maximum effect: 2 hours

Duration: 72 hours; 50% of maximum effect at 24 hours; after stopping treatment, secretory activity gradually returns over 3-5 days

Maximum secretory inhibition: 4 days

Pharmacokinetics (Adult data unless noted)

Absorption: Rapid

Protein binding: 95%

Metabolism: Hepatic via CYP2C19 primarily and to a lesser extent via 3A4 to hydroxy, desmethyl, and sulfone metabolites (all inactive); saturable first pass effect

Bioavailability: 30% to 40%; improves slightly with repeated administration; hepatic dysfunction: ~100%; in Asians, the AUC increased up to fourfold compared to Caucasians

Half-life: 0.5-1 hour; chronic hepatic disease: 3 hours

Time to peak serum concentration: 0.5-3.5 hours

Elimination: Urine (~77% as metabolites; very small amount as unchanged drug); feces

Clearance: 500-600 mL/minute; chronic hepatic disease: 70 mL/minute

Note: Half-life and AUC were significantly reduced for omeprazole suspension when compared with an equivalent dose via the commercially available capsule in 7 adults (Song, 2001).

Dosing: Usual

Infants, Children, and Adolescents:

Erosive esophagitis: Oral: Children ≥1 year and Adolescents:

5 kg to <10 kg: 5 mg once daily

10 kg to <20 kg: 10 mg once daily

≥20 kg: 20 mg once daily

GERD: Oral:

Infants: 0.7 mg/kg/dose once daily reduced the percentage of time gastric and esophageal pH <4, as well as the number of reflux episodes in 10 infants [mean PMA: 36.1 weeks, (34-40 weeks)] in a double-blind, placebo-controlled trial (Omari, 2007); higher doses of 1-1.5 mg/kg/day have been reported (Gibbons, 2005)

Children ≥1 year and Adolescents:

Manufacturer labeling:

5 kg to <10 kg: 5 mg once daily

10 kg to <20 kg: 10 mg once daily

≥20 kg: 20 mg once daily

Alternate dosing: Infants, Children, and Adolescents: 0.7-3.3 mg/kg/day; maximum daily dose: 20 mg/**day**; the dose most frequently reported to provide healing of esophagitis and relief of GERD symptoms is 1 mg/kg/day (Lightdale, 2013; Zimmerman, 2001). In critically ill children to maintain gastric pH >5, administration every 6-8 hours may be necessary (1.5-2 mg/kg/day) (Kaufman, 2002)

Helicobacter pylori eradication: Oral: Children and Adolescents: **Note:** Usual duration of therapy is 7-14 days; use in combination with antimicrobials (eg, clarithromycin, metronidazole, amoxicillin).

Weight-based: 1-2 mg/kg/day divided into 2 doses; maximum single dose: 20 mg (Gold, 2000; Koletzko, 2011)

Fixed-dosing (Gottrand, 2001):

15-30 kg: 10 mg twice daily

>30 kg: 20 mg twice daily

Adults:

Active duodenal ulcer: Oral: 20 mg once daily for 4-8 weeks

Gastric ulcers: Oral: 40 mg once daily for 4-8 weeks

GERD, symptomatic: Oral: 20 mg once daily for up to 4 weeks

Erosive esophagitis: Oral: 20 mg once daily for 4-8 weeks

Helicobacter pylori eradication: Oral: Dose varies with regimen: 20 mg twice daily for 10 days (in combination with clarithromycin and amoxicillin) or 40 mg once daily for 14 days (in combination with clarithromycin)

Note: Presence of ulcer at the time of therapy initiation may necessitate an additional 14-18 days of omeprazole 20 mg daily (monotherapy) after completion of combination therapy

Pathological hypersecretory conditions: Oral: Initial: 60 mg once daily; doses up to 120 mg 3 times daily have been administered; administer daily doses >80 mg in divided doses

Frequent heartburn (OTC labeling): Oral: 20 mg once daily for 14 days; treatment may be repeated after 4 months if needed

Dosing adjustment in renal impairment: Children, Adolescents, and Adults: No dosage adjustments are recommended

Dosing adjustment in hepatic impairment: Children, Adolescents, and Adults: There are no dosage adjustments provided in the manufacturer's labeling. However, based on increased bioavailability, dosage adjustment should be considered, especially for maintenance healing of erosive esophagitis. Specific guidelines are not available.

Administration

Oral: Should be taken before meals; best if taken 30 minutes before a meal (Lightdale, 2013); may be administered with antacids

Capsule: Should be swallowed whole; do not chew or crush. Delayed release capsule may be opened and contents added to 1 tablespoon of applesauce; use immediately after adding to applesauce; do not chew. Follow with a cool glass of water. Applesauce should not be heated.

Oral suspension: Empty the contents of the 2.5 mg packet or 10 mg packet into 5 mL or 15 mL of water, respectively; stir, the suspension should be left to thicken for 2-3 minutes and administered within 30 minutes. If any material remains after administration, add more water, stir, and administer immediately.

Tablet: Should be swallowed whole; do not crush or chew.

Nasogastric tube administration:

Capsule: The manufacturer of Prilosec® does not give recommendations for extemporaneous preparation of omeprazole capsules for NG/OG administration. Consider using the packets for oral suspension. If packets are unavailable, methods of preparation of capsules for NG/OG administration have been described (Balaban, 1997; Phillips, 1996). An extemporaneously prepared suspension with extended stability may also be used (DiGiacinto, 2000; Quercia, 1997; Sharma, 1999).

Oral suspension: Add 5 mL of water to a catheter-tipped syringe and then add the contents of a 2.5 mg packet (or 15 mL of water for the 10 mg packet), shake the suspension well and leave to thicken for 2-3 minutes. Administer within 30 minutes of reconstitution. Use an NG or gastric tube that is a French size 6 or larger; refill syringe with an equal amount of water, shake, and flush remaining contents through NG or gastric tube.

Test Interactions Omeprazole may falsely elevate serum chromogranin A (CgA) levels. The increased CgA level may cause false-positive results in the diagnosis of a neuroendocrine tumor. Temporarily stop omeprazole ≥14 days prior to assessing CgA level; repeat level if initially elevated; use the same laboratory for all testing of CgA levels.

Dosage Forms Excipient information presented when available (limited, particularly for generics); consult specific product labeling.

Capsule Delayed Release, Oral:
PriLOSEC: 10 mg, 20 mg, 40 mg
Generic: 10 mg, 20 mg, 40 mg, 20 mg
Packet, Oral:
PriLOSEC: 2.5 mg (30 ea); 10 mg (30 ea)
Suspension, Oral:
First-Omeprazole: 2 mg/mL (90 mL, 150 mL, 300 mL) [contains benzyl alcohol, fd&c red #40, saccharin sodium; strawberry flavor]
Omeprazole+Syrspend SF Alka: 2 mg/mL (100 mL) [cherry flavor]
Tablet Delayed Release, Oral:
PriLOSEC OTC: 20 mg
Generic: 20 mg

Extemporaneous Preparations Note: More palatable omeprazole (2 mg/mL) suspensions are commercially available as compounding kits (First-Omeprazole, Omeprazole+Syrspend SF Alka Cherry Kit).

A 2 mg/mL oral omeprazole solution (Simplified Omeprazole Solution) may be made with five omeprazole 20 mg delayed release capsules and 50 mL sodium bicarbonate 8.4%. Empty capsules into beaker. Add sodium bicarbonate solution. Gently stir (about 15 minutes) until a white suspension forms. Transfer to amber-colored syringe or bottle. Stable for 14 days at room temperature or for 30 days refrigerated.

DiGiacinto JL, Olsen KM, Bergman KL, et al, "Stability of Suspension Formulations of Lansoprazole and Omeprazole Stored in Amber-Colored Plastic Oral Syringes," Ann Pharmacother, 2000, 34 (5):600-5.

Quercia R, Fan C, Liu X, et al, "Stability of Omeprazole in an Extemporaneously Prepared Oral Liquid," Am J Health Syst Pharm, 1997, 54(16):1833-6.

Sharma V, "Comparison of 24-hour Intragastric pH Using Four Liquid Formulations of Lansoprazole and Omeprazole," Am J Health Syst Pharm, 1999, 56(23 Suppl 4):18-21.

References

Abraham NS, Hlatky MA, Antman EM, et al, "CCF/ACG/AHA 2010 Expert Consensus Document on the Concomitant Use of Proton Pump Inhibitors and Thienopyridines: A Focused Update of the ACCF/ACG/AHA 2008 Expert Consensus Document on Reducing the Gastrointestinal Risks of Antiplatelet Therapy and NSAID Use: A Report of the American College of Cardiology Foundation Task Force on Expert Consensus Documents," Circulation, 2010, 122 (24):2619-33.

Anderka M, Mitchell AA, Louik C, et al, "Medications Used to Treat Nausea and Vomiting of Pregnancy and the Risk of Selected Birth Defects," Birth Defects Res A Clin Mol Teratol, 2012, 94(1):22-30.

Andersson T, Hassall E, Lundborg P, et al, "Pharmacokinetics of Orally Administered Omeprazole in Children. International Pediatric Omeprazole Pharmacokinetic Group," Am J Gastroenterol, 2000, 95 (11):3101-6.

Balaban DH, Duckworth CW, and Peura DA, "Nasogastric Omeprazole: Effects on Gastric pH in Critically Ill Patients," Am J Gastroenterol, 1997, 92(1):79-83.

Canani RB, Cirillo P, Roggero P, et al, "Therapy With Gastric Acidity Inhibitors Increases the Risk of Acute Gastroenteritis and Community-Acquired Pneumonia in Children," Pediatrics, 2006, 117(5):e817-20.

Diav-Citrin O, Arnon J, Shechtman S, et al, "The Safety of Proton Pump Inhibitors in Pregnancy: A Multicentre Prospective Controlled Study," Aliment Pharmacol Ther, 2005, 21(3):269-75.

Erichsen R, Mikkelsen E, Pedersen L, et al, "Maternal Use of Proton Pump Inhibitors During Early Pregnancy and the Prevalence of Hypospadias in Male Offspring," Am J Ther, 2012.

Gibbons TE and Gold BD, "The Use of Proton Pump Inhibitors in Children: A Comprehensive Review," Paediatr Drugs, 2003, 5 (1):25-40.

Gold BD, Colletti RB, Abbott M, et al, "Helicobacter pylori Infection in Children: Recommendations for Diagnosis and Treatment," J Pediatr Gastroenterol Nutr, 2000, 31(5):490-7.

Gottrand F, Kalach N, Spyckerelle C, et al, "Omeprazole Combined With Amoxicillin and Clarithromycin in the Eradication of Helicobacter pylori in Children With Gastritis: A Prospective Randomized Double-Blind Trial," J Pediatr, 2001, 139(5):664-8.

Gunasekaran TS and Hassall EG, "Efficacy and Safety of Omeprazole for Severe Gastroesophageal Reflux in Children," J Pediatr, 1993, 123(1):148-54.

Hassall E, Israel D, Shepherd R, "Omeprazole for Treatment of Chronic Erosive Esophagitis in Children: A Multicenter Study of Efficacy, Safety, Tolerability and Dose Requirements. International Pediatric Omeprazole Study Group," J Pediatr, 2000, 137(6):800-7.

Källén BA, "Use of Omeprazole During Pregnancy-No Hazard Demonstrated in 955 Infants Exposed During Pregnancy," Eur J Obstet Gynecol Reprod Biol, 2001, 96(1):63-8.

Kane DL, "Administration of Omeprazole (Prilosec™) in the Atypical Patient," Int J Pharm Compounding, 1997, 1(1):13.

Kato S, Ebina K, Fujii K, et al, "Effect of Omeprazole in the Treatment of Refractory Acid-Related Diseases in Childhood: Endoscopic Healing and Twenty-Four Hour Intragastric Acidity," J Pediatr, 1996, 128 (3):415-21.

Katz PO, Gerson LB, and Vela MF, "Guidelines for the Diagnosis and Management of Gastroesophageal Reflux Disease," Am J Gastroenterol, 2013, 108(3):308-28.

Kaufman SS, Lyden ER, Brown CR, et al, "Omeprazole Therapy in Pediatric Patients After Liver and Intestinal Transplantation," J Pediatr Gastroenterol Nutr, 2002, 34(2):194-8.

Koletzko S, Jones NL, Goodman KJ, et al, "Evidence-Based Guidelines From ESPGHAN and NASPGHAN for Helicobacter pylori Infection in Children," J Pediatr Gastroenterol Nutr, 2011, 53(2):230-43.

Lalkin A, Loebstein R, Addis A, et al, "The Safety of Omeprazole During Pregnancy: A Multicenter Prospective Controlled Study," Am J Obstet Gynecol, 1998, 179(3 Pt 1):727-30.

Levine GN, Bates ER, Blankenship JC, et al, "2011 ACCF/AHA/SCAI Guideline for Percutaneous Coronary Intervention: A Report of the American College of Cardiology Foundation/American Heart Association Task Force on Practice Guidelines and the Society for Cardiovascular Angiography and Interventions," Circulation, 2011, 124(23): e574-651.

Lightdale JR, Gremse DA, and the Section on Gastroenterology, Hepatology, and Nutrition," Gastroesophageal Reflux: Management Guidance for the Pediatrician," Pediatrics, 2013, 131(5):e1684-95.

Marshall JK, Thompson AB, and Armstrong D, "Omeprazole for Refractory Gastroesophageal Reflux Disease During Pregnancy and Lactation," Can J Gastroenterol, 1998, 12(3):225-7.

Matok I, Levy A, Wiznitzer A, et al, "The Safety of Fetal Exposure to Proton-Pump Inhibitors During Pregnancy," Dig Dis Sci, 2012, 57 (3):699-705.

Omari TI, Haslam RR, Lundborg P, et al, "Effect of Omeprazole on Acid Gastroesophageal Reflux and Gastric Acidity in Preterm Infants With Pathological Acid Reflux," J Pediatr Gastroenterol Nutr, 2007, 44 (1):41-4.

Pasternak B and Hviid A, "Use of Proton-Pump Inhibitors in Early Pregnancy and the Risk of Birth Defects," N Engl J Med, 2010, 363 (22):2114-23.

Song JC, Quercia RA, Fan C, et al, "Pharmacokinetic Comparison of Omeprazole Capsules and a Simplified Omeprazole Suspension," Am J Health Syst Pharm, 2001, 58(8):689-94.

Zimmermann AE, Walters JK, Katona BG, et al, "A Review of Omeprazole Use in the Treatment of Acid-Related Disorders in Children," Clin Ther, 2001, 23(5):660-79.

Omeprazole and Sodium Bicarbonate

(oh MEP ra zole & SOW dee um bye KAR bun ate)

Medication Safety Issues

Sound-alike/look-alike issues:
Zegerid may be confused with Zestril

Related Information

Oral Medications That Should Not Be Crushed or Altered on page 2438

Brand Names: U.S. Zegerid; Zegerid OTC [OTC]

Therapeutic Category Proton Pump Inhibitor; Substituted Benzimidazole

Generic Availability (U.S.) Yes: Capsule

Use Short-term (4-8 weeks) treatment of active duodenal ulcer disease or active benign gastric ulcer; treatment of symptomatic gastroesophageal reflux disease (GERD) treatment and maintenance healing of erosive esophagitis (Capsule, oral suspension: FDA approved in adults); reduction of risk of upper gastrointestinal bleeding in critically ill patients (Oral suspension: FDA approved in adults); relief of frequent (≥2 days/week), uncomplicated heartburn (OTC products: FDA approved in adults)

Medication Guide Available Yes

Pregnancy Risk Factor C

Pregnancy Considerations Adverse events were observed in animal reproduction studies with omeprazole. Refer to individual agents for additional information.

Breast-Feeding Considerations Omeprazole is excreted into breast milk. Due to the potential for serious adverse reactions in the nursing infant, the manufacturer recommends a decision be made whether to discontinue nursing or to discontinue the drug, taking into account the importance of treatment to the mother. Refer to individual monographs for additional information.

Contraindications Hypersensitivity to omeprazole, substituted benzimidazole proton pump inhibitors (eg, esomeprazole, lansoprazole), or any component.

Warnings In long-term (2-year) studies in rats, omeprazole produced a dose-related increase in gastric carcinoid tumors. While available endoscopic evaluations and histologic examinations of biopsy specimens from human stomachs have not detected a risk from short-term exposure to omeprazole, further human data on the effect of sustained hypochlorhydria and hypergastrinemia are needed to rule out the possibility of an increased risk for the development of tumors in humans receiving long-term therapy.

An increased incidence of osteoporosis-related bone fractures of the hip, spine, or wrist may occur with proton pump inhibitor (PPI) therapy; patients on high-dose (multiple daily doses) or long-term (≥1 year) therapy should be monitored. Use the lowest effective dose for the shortest duration of time, use vitamin D and calcium supplementation, and follow appropriate guidelines to reduce risk of fractures in patients at risk. Hypomagnesemia has been reported rarely, usually with prolonged PPI use of >3 months (most cases >1 year of therapy), and may be symptomatic or asymptomatic; severe cases may cause tetany, seizures, and cardiac arrhythmias. Consider obtaining serum magnesium concentrations prior to beginning long-term therapy, especially if taking concomitant digoxin, diuretics, or other drugs known to cause hypomagnesemia; and periodically thereafter. Hypomagnesemia may be corrected by magnesium supplementation, although discontinuation of omeprazole may be necessary; magnesium concentrations typically return to normal within 1 week of stopping. Atrophic gastritis has been reported occasionally in gastric corpus biopsies from patients treated long-term with omeprazole. Symptomatic response to therapy does not preclude the presence of GI malignancy. Serum chromogranin A (CgA) levels may be falsely elevated if assessed while on omeprazole causing diagnostic misinterpretation if a neuroendocrine tumor suspected.

Use of gastric acid inhibitors, including proton pump inhibitors and H₂ blockers, has been associated with an increased risk for development of acute gastroenteritis and community-acquired pneumonia (Canani, 2006). Use of PPIs may also increase the risk of *C. difficile*-associated diarrhea (CDAD), especially in hospitalized patients; consider CDAD diagnosis in patients with persistent diarrhea that does not improve. Use the lowest dose and shortest duration of PPI therapy appropriate for the condition being treated.

Proton pump inhibitors (PPIs) may diminish the therapeutic effect of clopidogrel, thought to be due to reduced formation of the active metabolite of clopidogrel. The manufacturer of clopidogrel recommends either avoidance of both omeprazole (even when scheduled 12 hours apart) and esomeprazole or use of a PPI with comparatively less effect on the active metabolite of clopidogrel (eg, pantoprazole). In contrast to these warnings, others have recommended the continued use of PPIs, regardless of the degree of inhibition, in patients with a history of GI bleeding or multiple risk factors for GI bleeding who are also receiving clopidogrel since no evidence has established clinically meaningful differences in outcome; however, a clinically significant interaction cannot be excluded in those who are poor metabolizers of clopidogrel (Abraham, 2010;

Levine, 2011). Concomitant use of PPIs with high-dose methotrexate may lead to increased and prolonged serum concentrations of methotrexate and/or its metabolite, possibly causing methotrexate toxicities; temporary discontinuation of PPIs may be considered.

Zegerid OTC™ contains polysorbate 80 (Tween 80®) which may cause allergic reactions in susceptible individuals. Do not use for self-medication (OTC) if difficulty swallowing, blood in vomit, or bloody or black stools are present. Prior to use, patients should contact healthcare provider if any of the following conditions are present: Heartburn for >3 months; heartburn with dizziness, lightheadedness, or sweating; MI symptoms, frequent chest pain, frequent wheezing (especially with heartburn), unexplained weight loss, nausea/vomiting, stomach pain, a sodium-restricted diet, or taking other medications (interactions are common). If heartburn continues or worsens, if need to take for >14 days or more often than every 4 months, discontinue use and contact physician. May take 1-4 days for full effect to be seen.

Precautions Use with caution in patients with Bartter's syndrome, hypokalemia, and respiratory alkalosis due to high content of sodium bicarbonate; avoid use in patients on sodium-restrictive diets; chronic use may lead to systemic alkalosis, edema, and weight gain. Bioavailability may be increased in patients with hepatic dysfunction or patients of Asian descent; consider dosage reductions, especially for maintenance healing of erosive esophagitis

Adverse Reactions

Cardiovascular: Atrial fibrillation, bradycardia, edema, hyper-/hypotension, supraventricular tachycardia, tachycardia, ventricular tachycardia

Central nervous system: Agitation, hyperpyrexia, pyrexia

Dermatological: Decubitus ulcer, rash

Endocrine & metabolic: Fluid overload, hyper-/hypoglycemia, hyper-/hypokalemia, hyper-/hyponatremia, hypocalcemia, hypomagnesemia, hypophosphatemia

Gastrointestinal: Constipation, diarrhea, hypomotility

Genitourinary: Urinary tract infection

Hematological: Anemia, anemia increased, thrombocytopenia

Hepatic: LFTs increased

Respiratory: ARDS, cough, nosocomial pneumonia, pneumothorax, respiratory failure

Miscellaneous: Candidal infection, oral candidiasis, sepsis

Rare but important or life-threatening (adverse event occurrence may vary based on formulation): Agranulocytosis, allergic reactions, alopecia, anaphylaxis, angina, angioedema, anorexia, atrophic gastritis, benign gastric polyps, bronchospasm, *Clostridium difficile*-associated diarrhea (CDAD), creatinine increased, depression, erythema multiforme, esophageal candidiasis, fracture, glycosuria, gynecomastia, hallucinations, hematuria, hemifacial dysesthesia, hemolytic anemia, hepatic encephalopathy, hepatic failure, hepatic necrosis interstitial nephritis, hypersensitivity, leukocytosis, leukopenia, liver disease (hepatocellular, cholestatic, mixed), metabolic alkalosis, microscopic pyuria, microscopic colitis, mucosal atrophy (tongue), neutropenia, optic neuritis, optic neuropathy, osteoporosis-related fracture, pancreatitis, pancytopenia, photosensitivity, pneumonia (CAP), proteinuria, psychiatric disturbance, purpura, seizure, Stevens-Johnson syndrome, taste perversion, tinnitus, toxic epidermal necrolysis, vertigo, xerostomia

Drug Interactions

Metabolism/Transport Effects Refer to individual components.

Avoid Concomitant Use

Avoid concomitant use of Omeprazole and Sodium Bicarbonate with any of the following: Clopidogrel; Dasatinib; Delavirdine; Erlotinib; Nelfinavir; PAZOPanib; Pimozide;

PONATinib; Rifampin; Rilpivirine; Risedronate; St Johns Wort

Increased Effect/Toxicity

Omeprazole and Sodium Bicarbonate may increase the levels/effects of: Alpha-/Beta-Agonists (Indirect-Acting); Amphetamines; ARIPiprazole; Benzodiazepines (metabolized by oxidation); Bosentan; Calcium Polystyrene Sulfonate; Cannabis; Carvedilol; Cilostazol; Citalopram; CloZAPine; CycloSPORINE (Systemic); CYP2C19 Substrates; CYP2C9 Substrates; Dexmethylphenidate; Dofetilide; Dronabinol; Escitalopram; Flecainide; Fosphenytoin; Lomitapide; Memantine; Methotrexate; Methylphenidate; Phenytoin; Pimozide; QuiNIDine; QuiNINE; Raltegravir; Risedronate; Saquinavir; Tacrolimus (Systemic); Tetrahydrocannabinol; Vitamin K Antagonists; Voriconazole

The levels/effects of Omeprazole and Sodium Bicarbonate may be increased by: AcetaZOLAMIDE; Fluconazole; Ketoconazole (Systemic); Voriconazole

Decreased Effect

Omeprazole and Sodium Bicarbonate may decrease the levels/effects of: ACE Inhibitors; Anticonvulsants (Hydantoin); Antipsychotic Agents (Phenothiazines); Atazanavir; Bisacodyl; Bisphosphonate Derivatives; Bosutinib; Cefditoren; Cefpodoxime; Cefuroxime; Chloroquine; Clopidogrel; CloZAPine; Corticosteroids (Oral); Dabigatran Etexilate; Dabrafenib; Dasatinib; Delavirdine; Elvitegravir; Erlotinib; Flecainide; Gabapentin; Gefitinib; HMG-CoA Reductase Inhibitors; Hyoscyamine; Indinavir; Iron Salts; Isoniazid; Itraconazole; Ketoconazole (Systemic); Lithium; Mesalamine; Methenamine; Multivitamins/Minerals (with ADEK, Folate, Iron); Mycophenolate; Nelfinavir; Nilotinib; PAZOPanib; PenicillAMINE; Phosphate Supplements; PONATinib; Posaconazole; Potassium Acid Phosphate; Protease Inhibitors; Rilpivirine; Riociguat; Risedronate; Sulpiride; Tetracycline Derivatives; Trientine; Vismodegib

The levels/effects of Omeprazole and Sodium Bicarbonate may be decreased by: CYP2C19 Inducers (Strong); Dabrafenib; Fosphenytoin; Peginterferon Alfa-2b; Phenytoin; Rifampin; St Johns Wort; Tipranavir

Food Interactions See individual agents.

Stability

Capsule, powder for oral suspension: Store at 25°C (77°F); excursions permitted to 15°C to 30°C (59°F to 86°F); protect from light and moisture.

OTC capsules: Store at 20°C to 25°C (68°F to 77°F); protect from moisture; keep out of high heat and humidity.

Mechanism of Action Suppresses gastric basal and stimulated acid secretion by inhibiting the parietal cell H+/K+ ATP pump

Pharmacodynamics

Onset of action: 1 hour

Maximum effect: 2 hours

Duration: 72 hours; 50% of maximum effect at 24 hours

Maximum secretory inhibition: 4 days

Pharmacokinetics (Adult data unless noted)

Absorption: Rapid

Protein binding: 95%

Metabolism: Hepatic via CYP2C19 primarily and to a lesser extent via 3A4 to hydroxy, desmethyl, and sulfone metabolites (all inactive); saturable first pass effect

Bioavailability: 30% to 40%; improves slightly with repeated administration; hepatic dysfunction: ~100%; increased in Asian patients; AUC increased up to fourfold compared to Caucasians

Half-life: ~1 hour (range: 0.4-3.2 hours); chronic hepatic disease: 3 hours

Time to peak serum concentration: ~30 minutes

Elimination: Urine (77% as metabolites, very small amount as unchanged drug); feces

Clearance: 500-600 mL/minute; chronic hepatic disease: 70 mL/minute

Dosing: Usual Note: Dosage listed is for omeprazole component; both strengths of Zegerid® capsule and powder for oral suspension have identical sodium bicarbonate content. Do not substitute two 20 mg capsules/packets for one 40 mg dose.

Children and Adolescents: **Note:** Recognizing that this formulation has not received FDA approval for use in children despite an approved dosage for omeprazole in children and considering that omeprazole has been used safely in children as an extemporaneous formulation with sodium bicarbonate, the following dosage is recommended:

Erosive esophagitis: Oral:

5 kg to <10 kg: 5 mg once daily

10 kg to <20 kg: 10 mg once daily

≥20 kg: 20 mg once daily

GERD, symptomatic: Oral:

5 kg to <10 kg: 5 mg once daily

10 kg to ≤20 kg: 10 mg once daily

>20 kg: 20 mg once daily

Alternate dosing: Infants, Children, and Adolescents: 0.7-3.3 mg/kg/day (Lightdale, 2013); maximum daily dose: 20 mg/day; 1 mg/kg/day is the dose reported most often to provide healing of esophagitis and relief of GERD symptoms (Zimmerman, 2001). To maintain gastric pH >5 in critically ill children, administration every 6-8 hours may be necessary (1.5-2 mg/kg/day) (Kaufman, 2002).

Adults:

Active duodenal ulcer: Oral: 20 mg once daily for 4-8 weeks

Erosive esophagitis: Oral: 20 mg once daily for 4-8 weeks; maintenance of healing: 20 mg once daily for up to 12 months total therapy (including treatment period of 4-8 weeks)

Gastric ulcers: Oral: 40 mg once daily for 4-8 weeks

GERD, symptomatic: Oral: 20 mg once daily for up to 4 weeks

Heartburn (OTC labeling): Oral: 20 mg once daily for 14 days. Do not take for >14 days or more often than every 4 months, unless instructed by healthcare provider.

Risk reduction of upper GI bleeding in critically ill patients (Zegerid® powder for oral suspension): Oral:

Loading dose: Day 1: 40 mg every 6-8 hours for two doses

Maintenance dose: 40 mg daily for up to 14 days; therapy >14 days has not been evaluated

Dosing adjustment in renal impairment: Adults: No dosage adjustments are recommended

Dosing adjustment in hepatic impairment: Adults: There are no dosage adjustments provided in the manufacturer's labeling; however, based on increased bioavailability, a dosage adjustment should be considered, especially for maintenance of healing of erosive esophagitis. Specific guidelines are not available.

Administration Note: Both strengths of capsule and Zegerid® powder for oral suspension have identical sodium bicarbonate content, respectively. Do not substitute two 20 mg capsules/packets for one 40 mg dose.

Capsule: Should be swallowed whole with water (do not use other liquids); do not chew or crush. Capsules should **not** be opened, sprinkled on food, or administered via NG. Best if taken at least 1 hour before breakfast.

Powder for oral suspension:

Oral: Administer 1 hour before a meal. Mix with 15-30 mL of water; stir well and drink immediately. Rinse cup with water and drink. Do not mix with other liquids or food, only water.

Nasogastric/orogastric tube: Mix well with 20 mL of water and administer immediately; flush tube with an additional 20 mL of water. Suspend enteral feeding for 3 hours before and 1 hour after administering. Do not mix with other liquids or food; only water.

Test Interactions Omeprazole may falsely elevate serum chromogranin A (CgA) levels. The increased CgA level may cause false-positive results in the diagnosis of a neuroendocrine tumor. Temporarily stop omeprazole ≥14 days prior to assessing CgA level; repeat test if CgA level is initially elevated; use the same laboratory for all testing of CgA levels.

Additional Information Each capsule of omeprazole-sodium bicarbonate contains 1100 mg (13 mEq) of sodium bicarbonate; total Na content is 304 mg and 303 mg for the prescription and OTC product, respectively. Each packet of omeprazole-sodium bicarbonate powder for oral suspension contains 1680 mg (20 mEq) of sodium bicarbonate; total Na content is 460 mg.

Dosage Forms Excipient information presented when available (limited, particularly for generics); consult specific product labeling.

Capsule, oral: Omeprazole 20 mg [immediate release] and sodium bicarbonate 1100 mg; omeprazole 40 mg [immediate release] and sodium bicarbonate 1100 mg

Zegerid®: Omeprazole 20 mg [immediate release] and sodium bicarbonate 1100 mg [contains sodium 304 mg (13 mEq) per capsule]

Zegerid®: Omeprazole 40 mg [immediate release] and sodium bicarbonate 1100 mg [contains sodium 304 mg (13 mEq) per capsule]

Zegerid OTC™: Omeprazole 20 mg [immediate release] and sodium bicarbonate 1100 mg [contains sodium 303 mg (13 mEq) per capsule]

Powder for suspension, oral:

Zegerid®: Omeprazole 20 mg and sodium bicarbonate 1680 mg per packet (30s) [contains sodium 460 mg (20 mEq) per packet]

Zegerid®: Omeprazole 40 mg and sodium bicarbonate 1680 mg per packet (30s) [contains sodium 460 mg (20 mEq) per packet]

Extemporaneous Preparations A 2 mg/mL oral suspension may be made with omeprazole-sodium bicarbonate powder and water. Pour the contents of six 20 mg omeprazole-sodium bicarbonate packets into a glass mortar. Add 30 mL water to the powder and mix to a uniform paste; mix while adding water in incremental proportions to **almost** 60 mL; transfer to a 60 mL bottle, rinse mortar with water, and add sufficient quantity of water to make 60 mL. Label "shake well" and "refrigerate". Stable for 45 days refrigerated.

Johnson CE, Cober MP, and Ludwig JL, "Stability of Partial Doses of Omeprazole-Sodium Bicarbonate Oral Suspension," *Ann Pharmacother*, 2007, 41(12):1954-61.

References

Abraham NS, Hlatky MA, Antman EM, et al, "ACCF/ACG/AHA 2010 Expert Consensus Document on the Concomitant Use of Proton Pump Inhibitors and Thienopyridines: A Focused Update of the ACCF/ACG/AHA 2008 Expert Consensus Document on Reducing the Gastrointestinal Risks of Antiplatelet Therapy and NSAID Use: A Report of the American College of Cardiology Foundation Task Force on Expert Consensus Documents," *Circulation*, 2010, 122 (24):2619-33.

Andersson T, Hassall E, Lundborg P, et al, "Pharmacokinetics of Orally Administered Omeprazole in Children. International Pediatric Omeprazole Pharmacokinetic Group," *Am J Gastroenterol*, 2000, 95 (11):3101-6.

Canani RB, Cirillo P, Roggero P, et al, "Therapy With Gastric Acidity Inhibitors Increases the Risk of Acute Gastroenteritis and Community-Acquired Pneumonia in Children," *Pediatrics*, 2006, 117(5):e817-20.

Gibbons TE and Gold BD, "The Use of Proton Pump Inhibitors in Children: A Comprehensive Review," *Paediatr Drugs*, 2003, 5 (1):25-40.

Gottrand F, Kalach N, Spyckerelle C, et al, "Omeprazole Combined With Amoxicillin and Clarithromycin in the Eradication of *Helicobacter pylori* in Children With Gastritis: A Prospective Randomized Double-Blind Trial," *J Pediatr*, 2001, 139(5):664-8.

Gunasekaran TS and Hassall EG, "Efficacy and Safety of Omeprazole for Severe Gastroesophageal Reflux in Children," *J Pediatr*, 1993, 123(1):148-54.

Hassall E, Israel D, Shepherd R, "Omeprazole for Treatment of Chronic Erosive Esophagitis in Children: A Multicenter Study of Efficacy, Safety, Tolerability and Dose Requirements. International Pediatric Omeprazole Study Group," *J Pediatr*, 2000, 137(6):800-7.

Johnson CE, Cober MP, and Ludwig JL, "Stability of Partial Doses of Omeprazole-Sodium Bicarbonate Oral Suspension," *Ann Pharmacother*, 2007, 41(12):1954-61.

Kane DL, "Administration of Omeprazole (Prilosec™) in the Atypical Patient," *Int J Pharm Compounding*, 1997, 1(1):13.

Kato S, Ebina K, Fujii K, et al, "Effect of Omeprazole in the Treatment of Refractory Acid-Related Diseases in Childhood: Endoscopic Healing and Twenty-Four Hour Intragastric Acidity," *J Pediatr*, 1996, 128 (3):415-21.

Kaufman SS, Lyden ER, Brown CR, et al, "Omeprazole Therapy in Pediatric Patients After Liver and Intestinal Transplantation," *J Pediatr Gastroenterol Nutr*, 2002, 34(2):194-8.

Levine GN, Bates ER, Blankenship JC, et al, "2011 ACCF/AHA/SCAI Guideline for Percutaneous Coronary Intervention: A Report of the American College of Cardiology Foundation/American Heart Association Task Force on Practice Guidelines and the Society for Cardiovascular Angiography and Interventions," *Circulation*, 2011, 124(23): e574-651.

Lightdale JR, Gremse DA, and Section on Gastroenterology, Hepatology, and Nutrition, "Gastroesophageal Reflux: Management Guidance for the Pediatrician," *Pediatrics*, 2013, 131(5):e1684-95.

Song JC, Quercia RA, Fan C, et al, "Pharmacokinetic Comparison of Omeprazole Capsules and a Simplified Omeprazole Suspension," *Am J Health Syst Pharm*, 2001, 58(8):689-94.

Zimmermann AE, Walters JK, Katona BG, et al, "A Review of Omeprazole Use in the Treatment of Acid-Related Disorders in Children," *Clin Ther*, 2001, 23(5):660-79.

◆ **Omeprazole Magnesium** see Omeprazole on page 1535

◆ **Omeprazole+Syrspend SF Alka** see Omeprazole on page 1535

◆ **Omnaris** see Ciclesonide (Nasal) on page 464

◆ **Omnaris HFA (Can)** see Ciclesonide (Nasal) on page 464

◆ **Omnicef** see Cefdinir on page 395

◆ **Omni Gel [OTC]** see Fluoride on page 894

◆ **Omnipred** see PrednisoLONE (Ophthalmic) on page 1730

◆ **Omnitrope** see Somatropin on page 1920

OnabotulinumtoxinA
(oh nuh BOT yoo lin num TOKS in aye)

Medication Safety Issues
Other safety concerns:
Botulinum products are not interchangeable; potency differences may exist between the products.

Brand Names: U.S. Botox; Botox Cosmetic

Brand Names: Canada Botox; Botox Cosmetic

Therapeutic Category Muscle Contracture, Treatment; Ophthalmic Agent, Toxin

Generic Availability (U.S.) No

Use Treatment of strabismus and blepharospasm associated with dystonia (including benign essential blepharospasm or VII nerve disorders) (FDA approved in ages >12 years and adults); treatment of dynamic muscle contracture in pediatric cerebral palsy patients (orphan drug); treatment of cervical dystonia (FDA approved in ages >16 and adults); treatment of severe primary axillary hyperhidrosis (not adequately controlled with topical treatments) (FDA approved in adults); temporary improvement in the appearance of lines and wrinkles of the face (moderate to severe glabellar lines associated with corrugator and/or procerus muscle activity) in adult patients ≤65 years of age; focal spasticity, specifically upper limb spasticity (FDA approved in adults); prophylaxis of chronic migraine headache (≥15 days/month with ≥4 hours/day headache duration) (FDA approved in adults). Other uses include treatment of sialorrhea, palmar hyperhidrosis, esophageal achalasia, chronic anal fissure.

Medication Guide Available Yes

Pregnancy Risk Factor C

Pregnancy Considerations Adverse events were observed in some animal reproduction studies.

Breast-Feeding Considerations It is not known if onabotulinumtoxinA is excreted in breast milk. The manufacturer recommends that caution be exercised when administering onabotulinumtoxinA to nursing women.

Contraindications Hypersensitivity to botulinum toxin or any component of the formulation; infection at the site of injection

Warnings The U.S. Food and Drug Administration (FDA) and Health Canada have issued respective early communications to healthcare professionals alerting them of serious adverse events (including fatalities) in association with the use of onabotulinumtoxinA (Botox®, Botox® Cosmetic) and rimabotulinumtoxinB (Myobloc®). Events reported are suggestive of botulism, indicating systemic spread of the botulinum toxin beyond the site of injection. Reactions were observed in both adult and pediatric patients treated for a variety of conditions with varying doses. However, the most serious outcomes, including respiratory failure and death, were associated with the use in children for cerebral palsy limb spasticity. The FDA has evaluated postmarketing cases and now reports that systemic and potentially fatal toxicity may result from local injection of the botulinum toxins in the treatment of other underlying conditions such as cerebral palsy associated with limb spasticity. Monitor patients closely for signs/symptoms of systemic toxic effects (possibly occurring 1 day to several weeks after treatment) and instruct patients to seek immediate medical attention with worsening symptoms or dysphagia, dyspnea, muscle weakness, or difficulty speaking.

AbobotulinumtoxinA (Dysport®) is not equivalent in potency to Botox®; the Dysport®:Botox® equivalency ratio is ~3:1 or 4:1, respectively; patients treated for cervical dystonia may experience dysphagia which rarely may result in dyspnea, aspiration, and pneumonia; weakness of hand muscles and blepharoptosis may occur in patients who also receive treatment for palmar and facial hyperhidrosis respectively

Precautions Presence of antibodies to onabotulinumtoxinA may reduce the effectiveness of therapy; to minimize the development of antibodies, keep the dose of onabotulinumtoxinA as low as possible. Reduced blinking from onabotulinumtoxinA injection of the orbicularis muscle can lead to corneal exposure, persistent epithelial defect, and corneal ulceration, especially in patients with VII nerve disorders; carefully test corneal sensation in eyes previously operated upon. Avoid injection into the lower lid area to avoid ectropion, and vigorously treat any epithelial defect (this may require protective drops, ointment, therapeutic soft contact lenses, or closure of the eye by patching). Retrobulbar hemorrhages sufficient to compromise retinal circulation have occurred from needle penetrations into the orbit; have appropriate instruments to decompress the orbit accessible; ocular (globe) penetrations by needles have also occurred (an ophthalmoscope to diagnose this condition should be available).

Use with caution in patients with peripheral motor neuropathic diseases (eg, amyotrophic lateral sclerosis or motor neuropathy) or neuromuscular junction disorders (eg, myasthenia gravis or Lambert-Eaton syndrome) as these patients may be at increased risk for development of significant systemic side effects including severe dysphagia and respiratory compromise; use cautiously if there is inflammation present at the proposed injection site or when excessive weakness or atrophy is present in the target muscles

Adverse Reactions Adverse effects usually occur in 1 week and may last up to several months.

Bladder dysfunction:
Gastrointestinal: Constipation
Genitourinary: Bacteriuria, dysuria, hematuria, residual urine volume increased (not requiring catheterization), urinary retention, urinary tract infection
Neuromuscular & skeletal: Gait disturbance, muscle spasm, muscular weakness

Cerebral palsy spasticity:
Central nervous system: Fever, lethargy, pain
Neuromuscular & skeletal: Falling, weakness

Cervical dystonia:
Central nervous system: Dizziness, drowsiness, fever, headache, malaise, pain, speech disorder
Gastrointestinal: Dysphagia, nausea, xerostomia
Local: Injection site reaction: Soreness
Neuromuscular & skeletal: Back pain, focal weakness, hypertonia, neck pain, numbness, stiffness, weakness
Ocular: Diplopia, ptosis
Respiratory: Cough, dyspnea, rhinitis, upper respiratory infection
Miscellaneous: Flu-like syndrome

Chronic migraines:
Cardiovascular: Hypertension
Central nervous system: Facial paresis, Headache, worsening migraine
Neuromuscular & skeletal: Muscle spasm, musculoskeletal pain, myalgia, neck pain, stiffness, weakness
Ocular: Eyelid ptosis
Respiratory: Bronchitis
Miscellaneous: Injection site pain

Focal spasticity:
Central nervous system: Fatigue
Gastrointestinal: Nausea
Neuromuscular & skeletal: Pain in extremity, weakness
Respiratory: Bronchitis

Other indications (blepharospasm, primary axillary hyperhidrosis, reduction of glabellar lines, strabismus):
Cardiovascular: Hypertension
Central nervous system: Anxiety, dizziness, facial paresis, fever, headache, pain
Dermatologic: Pruritus, rash, skin tightness
Gastrointestinal: Dyspepsia, nausea
Immunologic: Antibody development
Local: Injection site reaction: Hemorrhage, pain, soreness
Neuromuscular & skeletal: Back pain, facial pain, neck pain, weakness
Ocular: Diplopia, eyelid edema, eyelid ptosis, irritation/tearing (includes dry eye, lagophthalmos, photophobia); keratitis, superficial punctate keratitis
Respiratory: Pharyngitis
Miscellaneous: Flu-like syndrome, infection, nonaxillary sweating

Rare but important and life-threatening: *Any indication:* Abdominal distension, acute angle closure glaucoma, allergic reactions, alopecia, anaphylaxis, anorexia, anterior segment eye ischemia, arrhythmia, arthralgia, aspiration pneumonia, asthma, autonomic dysreflexia, brachial plexopathy, cardiovascular insufficiency, ciliary ganglion damage, circulatory collapse, colitis, corneal perforation, denervation, diarrhea, dysarthria, dysphonia, ectropion, entropion, erythema, erythema multiforme, eye edema, eye pain, focal facial paralysis, glaucoma, hearing loss, herpes zoster, hypoacusis, lymphadenopathy, madarosis, muscle atrophy, myalgia, myasthenia gravis exacerbation, myocardial infarction, neutralizing antibody formation, paresthesia, peripheral edema, peripheral neuropathy, pneumonia, psoriasiform eruption, radiculopathy, reduced blinking leading to corneal ulceration, respiratory depression, respiratory failure, retinal vein occlusion, retrobulbar hemorrhage, seizure, serum sickness, syncope, trismus, urinary incontinence, vertigo with nystagmus, visual disturbances, vitreous hemorrhage

Drug Interactions

Metabolism/Transport Effects None known.

Avoid Concomitant Use There are no known interactions where it is recommended to avoid concomitant use.

Increased Effect/Toxicity

OnabotulinumtoxinA may increase the levels/effects of: AbobotulinumtoxinA; RimabotulinumtoxinB

The levels/effects of OnabotulinumtoxinA may be increased by: Aminoglycosides; Anticholinergic Agents; Neuromuscular-Blocking Agents

Decreased Effect There are no known significant interactions involving a decrease in effect.

Stability Store lyophilized product in refrigerator at 2°C to 8°C (36°F to 46°F); administer within 24 hours after reconstitution; reconstituted solution may be stored in the refrigerator 2°C to 8°C (36°F to 46°F) until administered; do not freeze reconstituted solution

Mechanism of Action OnabotulinumtoxinA (previously known as botulinum toxin type A) is a neurotoxin produced by *Clostridium botulinum*, spore-forming anaerobic bacillus, which appears to affect only the presynaptic membrane of the neuromuscular junction in humans, where it prevents calcium-dependent release of acetylcholine and produces a state of denervation. Muscle inactivation persists until new fibrils grow from the nerve and form junction plates on new areas of the muscle-cell walls. Intradetrusor injection affects efferent pathways of detrusor activity by inhibiting release of acetylcholine. Intradermal injection results in temporary sweat gland denervation, reducing local sweating.

Pharmacodynamics

Strabismus:

Onset of action: 1-2 days after injection

Duration of paralysis: 2-6 weeks

Blepharospasm:

Onset of action: 3 days after injection

Maximum effect: 1-2 weeks

Duration of paralysis: 3 months

Spasticity associated with cerebral palsy

Onset of action: Several days

Duration of paralysis: 3-8 months

Reduction in axillary sweat production:

Duration of effect: 201 days (mean)

Dosing: Usual I.M.:

Strabismus:

Children 2 months to 12 years:

Horizontal or vertical deviations <20 prism diopters: 1.25 units into any one muscle

Horizontal or vertical deviations 20-25 prism diopters: 1-2.5 units into any one muscle

Persistent VI nerve palsy of ≥1 month duration: 1-1.25 units into the medial rectus muscle

Children ≥12 years and Adults:

Horizontal or vertical deviations <20 prism diopters: 1.25-2.5 units into any one muscle

Horizontal or vertical deviations 20-50 prism diopters: 2.5-5 units into any one muscle

Persistent VI nerve palsy of ≥1 month duration: 1.25-2.5 units into the medial rectus muscle

Note: Re-examine patient 7-14 days after each injection to assess effects; dosage may be increased up to twofold of the previously administered dose; do not exceed 25 units as a single injection for any one muscle

Spasticity associated with cerebral palsy: Children >18 months to Adolescents: Small muscle: 1-2 units/kg; large muscle: 3-6 units/kg; maximum dose per injection site: 50 units; maximum dose for any one visit: 12 units/kg, up to 400 units; no more than 400 units should be administered during a 3-month period

Blepharospasm: Adults: Initial: 1.25-2.5 units injected into the medial and lateral pretarsal orbicularis oculi of the upper lid and into the lateral pretarsal orbicularis oculi of the lower lid; dose may be increased up to 2.5-5 units at repeat treatment sessions; do not exceed 5 units per injection or cumulative dose of 200 units in a 30-day period

Cervical dystonia: Adults: Initial and sequential doses should be individualized related to the patient's head and neck position, localization of pain, muscle hypertrophy, and patient response; mean dose used in research trials: 236 units (range: 198-300 units) (maximum: ≤50 units/site) divided among affected muscles; limit total dose into sternocleidomastoid muscles to ≤100 units to decrease the occurrence of dysphagia

Severe primary axillary hyperhidrosis: Adults: Intradermal: 50 units per axilla injected in 0.1-0.2 mL aliquots

Reduction of glabellar lines: Adults ≤65 years: I.M.: An effective dose is determined by gross observation of the patient's ability to activate the superficial muscles injected. The location, size and use of muscles may vary markedly among individuals. Inject 0.1 mL dose into each of five sites, two in each corrugator muscle and one in the procerus muscle (total dose 0.5 mL).

Chronic migraine: Adults: I.M.: Administer 5 units/0.1 mL per site. Recommended total dose is 155 units once every 12 weeks. Each 155-unit dose should be equally divided and administered bilaterally, into 31 total sites as described below (refer to prescribing information for specific diagrams of recommended injection sites):

Corrugator: 5 units to each side (2 sites)

Procerus: 5 units (1 site only)

Frontalis: 10 units to each side (divided into 2 sites/side)

Temporalis: 20 units to each side (divided into 4 sites/side)

Occipitalis: 15 units to each side (divided into 3 sites/side)

Cervical paraspinal: 10 units to each side (divided into 2 sites/side)

Trapezius: 15 units to each side (divided into 3 sites/side)

Spasticity (focal): Adults: I.M.: Individualize dose based on patient size, extent, and location of muscle involvement, degree of spasticity, local muscle weakness, and response to prior treatment. In clinical trials, total doses up to 360 units were administered as separate injections typically divided among selected muscles; may repeat therapy at ≥3 months with appropriate dosage based upon the clinical condition of patient at time of retreatment.

Suggested guidelines for the treatment of upper limb spasticity. The lowest recommended starting dose should be used and ≤50 units/site should be administered. **Note:** Dose listed is total dose administered as individual or separate intramuscular injection(s):

Biceps brachii: 100-200 units (up to 4 sites)

Flexor digitorum profundus: 30-50 units (1 site)

Flexor digitorum sublimes: 30-50 units (1 site)

Flexor carpi radialis: 12.5-50 units (1 site)

Flexor carpi ulnaris: 12.5-50 units (1 site)

Administration Parenteral: For I.M. or intradermal administration only by individuals understanding the relevant neuromuscular and orbital anatomy and any alterations to the anatomy due to prior surgical procedures and standard electromyographic techniques; reconstitute vial with preservative-free NS to obtain an optimal injection volume of 0.1 mL; suggested diluent volumes and resulting concentrations: 1 mL (10 units/0.1 mL); 2 mL (5 units/0.1 mL), 4 mL (2.5 units/0.1 mL) or 8 mL (1.25 units/0.1 mL); gently swirl as onabotulinumtoxinA is denatured by violent agitation. Local site reactions may be minimized by careful injection into the target muscle, using a minimal volume, and slowing the rate of injection. Application of ice and topical anesthetics to the injection site may also be used.

Monitoring Parameters Monitor patients closely for signs/symptoms of systemic toxic effects (possibly occurring 1 day to several weeks after treatment)

Cervical dystonia: Toronto Western Spasmodic Torticollis Rating Scale (TWSTRS) which evaluates severity, disability, and pain

Cerebral palsy: Modified Ashworth Scale, Tardieu Scale, Gross Motor Function Measure; treatment goals include: Improved gait and balance, facilitation of patient care, increased comfort with therapy, improved tolerance of bracing, and prevention of musculoskeletal complications

Dosage Forms Excipient information presented when available (limited, particularly for generics); consult specific product labeling.

Solution Reconstituted, Injection:
Botox: 100 units (1 ea)
Solution Reconstituted, Injection [preservative free]:
Botox: 200 units (1 ea)
Solution Reconstituted, Intramuscular:
Botox Cosmetic: 100 units (1 ea) [contains albumin human]
Solution Reconstituted, Intramuscular [preservative free]:
Botox Cosmetic: 50 units (1 ea) [contains albumin human]

References

"Botulinum Toxin," *NIH Consens Statement*, 1990, 12-14, 8(8):1-20.

Benson J and Daugherty KK, "Botulinum Toxin A in the Treatment of Sialorrhea," *Ann Pharmacother*, 2007, 41(1):79-85.

Charles PD, "Botulinum Neurotoxin Serotype A: A Clinical Update on Non-cosmetic Uses," *Am J Health Syst Pharm*, 2004, 61(22 Suppl 6):S11-23.

Cheng CM, Chen JS, and Patel RP, "Unlabeled Uses of Botulinum Toxins: A Review, Part 1," *Am J Health Syst Pharm*, 2006, 63 (2):145-52.

Cheng CM, Chen JS, and Patel RP, "Unlabeled Uses of Botulinum Toxins: A Review, Part 2," *Am J Health Syst Pharm*, 2006, 63 (3):225-32.

Criswell SR, Crowner BE, and Racette BA, "The Use of Botulinum Toxin Therapy for Lower-Extremity Spasticity in Children With Cerebral Palsy," *Neurosurg Focus*, 2006, 21(2):e1.

Russman BS, Tilton A, and Gormley ME Jr, "Cerebral Palsy: A Rational Approach to a Treatment Protocol, and the Role of Botulinum Toxin in Treatment," *Muscle Nerve Suppl*, 1997, 6:S181-S193.

Scott AB, Magoon EH, McNeer KW, et al, "Botulinum Treatment of Childhood Strabismus," *Ophthalmology*, 1990, 97(11):1434-8.

◆ **Oncaspar** see Pegaspargase on page 1615

◆ **Oncovin** see VinCRIStine on page 2138

Ondansetron (on DAN se tron)

Medication Safety Issues
Sound-alike/look-alike issues:
Ondansetron may be confused with dolasetron, granisetron, palonosetron
Zofran® may be confused with Zantac®, Zosyn®

Brand Names: U.S. Zofran; Zofran ODT; Zuplenz

Brand Names: Canada Apo-Ondansetron; CO Ondansetron; Dom-Ondansetron; JAMP-Ondansetron; Mint-Ondansetron; Mylan-Ondansetron; Ondansetron Injection; Ondansetron Injection USP; Ondansetron-Odan; Ondansetron-Omega; PHL-Ondansetron; PMS-Ondansetron; RAN™-Ondansetron; ratio-Ondansetron; Sandoz-Ondansetron; Teva-Ondansetron; Zofran®; Zofran® ODT; ZYM-Ondansetron

Therapeutic Category 5-HT₃ Receptor Antagonist; Antiemetic

Generic Availability (U.S.) May be product dependent

Use
Oral:
Orally disintegrating tablets, oral solution, oral tablets: Prevention of nausea and vomiting associated with moderately emetogenic chemotherapy (FDA approved in ages ≥4 years and adults); prevention of nausea and vomiting associated with highly emetogenic cancer chemotherapy (including cisplatin) (FDA approved in ages ≥4 years and adults); prevention of nausea and vomiting associated with radiotherapy (FDA approved in adults); prevention of postoperative nausea and vomiting (FDA approved in adults); has also been used in the treatment of hyperemesis gravidarum

Soluble Film (Zuplenz®): Prevention of nausea and vomiting associated with moderately emetogenic cancer chemotherapy (FDA approved in ages ≥4 years and adults); prevention of nausea and vomiting associated with highly emetogenic cancer chemotherapy or radiotherapy (FDA approved in adults); prevention of postoperative nausea and vomiting (PONV) (FDA approved in adults)

Parenteral: Prevention of nausea and vomiting associated emetogenic cancer chemotherapy [including high-dose cisplatin (highly emetogenic)] (FDA approved in ages ≥6 months and adults); prevention of postoperative nausea and vomiting (FDA approved in ages ≥1 month and adults); has also been used in the treatment of hyperemesis gravidarum

Pregnancy Risk Factor B

Pregnancy Considerations Teratogenic effects were not observed in animal reproduction studies. Ondansetron readily crosses the human placenta in the first trimester of pregnancy and can be detected in fetal tissue (Siu, 2006). The use of ondansetron for the treatment of nausea and vomiting of pregnancy (NVP) has been evaluated. Although a significant increase in birth defects has not been described in case reports and some studies (Ferreira, 2012; Pasternak, 2013), other studies have shown a possible association with ondansetron exposure and adverse fetal events (Anderka, 2012; Einarson, 2004). Additional studies are needed to determine safety to the fetus, particularly during the first trimester. Based on available data, use is generally reserved for severe NVP (hyperemesis gravidarum) or when conventional treatments are not effective (ACOG, 2004; Koren, 2012; Levicheck, 2002; Tan, 2011). Because a dose-dependent QT-interval prolongation occurs with use, the manufacturer recommends ECG monitoring in patients with electrolyte abnormalities (which can be associated with some cases of NVP; Koren, 2012).

Breast-Feeding Considerations It is not known if ondansetron is excreted into breast milk. The manufacturer recommends caution be used if administered to nursing women.

Contraindications Hypersensitivity to ondansetron, other 5-HT₃ receptor antagonists, or any component; concurrent use of apomorphine

Warnings Profound hypotension and loss of consciousness have been reported with concurrent use of ondansetron and apomorphine; coadministration of these agents is contraindicated. QT interval prolongation and torsades de pointes have been reported with ondansetron; selective 5-HT₃ antagonists, including ondansetron, have been associated with a number of dose-dependent increases in ECG intervals (eg, PR, QRS duration, QT/QT_c, JT), usually occurring 1-2 hours after I.V. administration. Single doses >16 mg ondansetron I.V. are not recommended due to the potential for an increased risk of QT prolongation. When used with agents that prolong the QT interval (eg, Class I and III antiarrhythmics), clinically relevant QT interval prolongation may occur resulting in torsade de pointes. A number of trials have shown that 5-HT₃ antagonists produce QT interval prolongation to variable degrees. Avoid use in patients with congenital long QT syndrome. ECG monitoring is recommended if used concurrently with other agents that prolong the QT interval or in patients with electrolyte abnormalities (eg, hypokalemia, hypomagnesemia, CHF, or bradyarrhythmias.

Zofran® solution contains sodium benzoate; benzoic acid (benzoate) is a metabolite of benzyl alcohol; large amounts of benzyl alcohol (≥99 mg/kg/day) have been associated with a potentially fatal toxicity ("gasping syndrome") in neonates; *in vitro* and animal studies have shown that benzoate displaces bilirubin from protein binding sites; avoid use of Zofran® solution in neonates. Orally disintegrating tablets contain phenylalanine; use with caution in patients with phenylketonuria.

Precautions Use with caution in patients at risk of QT prolongation and/or ventricular arrhythmia, including patients with congenital long QT syndrome or other risk factors for QT prolongation [eg, medications known to prolong QT interval, electrolyte abnormalities (hypokalemia or hypomagnesemia), and cumulative high-dose anthracycline therapy]. Use with caution in patients allergic to other 5-HT$_3$ receptor antagonists; cross-reactivity has been reported. Use with caution in patients with hepatic impairment; clearance is decreased and half-life is increased; dose recommendations provided for patients with severe hepatic impairment (Child-Pugh C). Does not stimulate gastric or intestinal peristalsis; may mask progressive ileus and/or gastric distension. When used for chemotherapy-related emesis, administration should be used on a scheduled basis, not on an "as needed" (PRN) basis, since data support the use of this drug only in the prevention of nausea and vomiting and not in the rescue of nausea and vomiting. Should only be used in the first 24-48 hours of chemotherapy. Data does not support any increased efficacy in delayed nausea and vomiting.

Adverse Reactions

Central nervous system: Anxiety, dizziness, drowsiness, fatigue, headache, malaise, paresthesia, sensation of cold

Dermatologic: Pruritus, skin rash

Gastrointestinal: Constipation, diarrhea

Genitourinary: Gynecologic disease, urinary retention

Hepatic: Increased serum ALT (>2 times ULN), increased serum AST (>2 times ULN)

Local: Injection site reaction

Respiratory: Hypoxia

Miscellaneous: Fever

Rare but important or life-threatening: Angina pectoris, bradycardia, cardiac arrhythmia, cardiorespiratory arrest, extrapyramidal reaction, hepatic failure, hepatitis, hypersensitivity reaction, hypokalemia, hypotension, neuroleptic malignant syndrome, seizure, serotonin syndrome, shock, syncope, tachycardia, toxic epidermal necrolysis, transient blindness (following infusion; lasting ≤48 hours), transient blurred vision (following infusion), vascular occlusive events

Drug Interactions

Metabolism/Transport Effects Substrate of CYP1A2 (minor), CYP2C9 (minor), CYP2D6 (minor), CYP2E1 (minor), CYP3A4 (major), P-glycoprotein; **Note:** Assignment of Major/Minor substrate status based on clinically relevant drug interaction potential; **Inhibits** CYP1A2 (weak), CYP2C9 (weak), CYP2D6 (weak)

Avoid Concomitant Use

Avoid concomitant use of Ondansetron with any of the following: Apomorphine; Highest Risk QTc-Prolonging Agents; Ivabradine; Mifepristone

Increased Effect/Toxicity

Ondansetron may increase the levels/effects of: Apomorphine; ARIPiprazole; Highest Risk QTc-Prolonging Agents; Moderate Risk QTc-Prolonging Agents; Serotonin Modulators

The levels/effects of Ondansetron may be increased by: Ivabradine; Mifepristone; P-glycoprotein/ABCB1 Inhibitors; QTc-Prolonging Agents (Indeterminate Risk and Risk Modifying)

Decreased Effect

Ondansetron may decrease the levels/effects of: Tapentadol; TraMADol

The levels/effects of Ondansetron may be decreased by: Bosentan; CYP3A4 Inducers (Strong); Dabrafenib; Deferasirox; Mitotane; Peginterferon Alfa-2b; P-glycoprotein/ABCB1 Inducers; Siltuximab; St Johns Wort; Tocilizumab

Food Interactions Tablet: Food slightly increases the extent of absorption. Management: Administer without regard to meals.

Stability

Oral:

Orally disintegrating tablets, tablets: Store at 2°C to 30°C (36°F to 86°F); protect tablets from light.

Soluble film (Zuplenz®): Store at 20°C to 25°C (68°F to 77°F); store pouches in cartons; keep film in individual pouch until ready for use.

Solution: Store 15°C to 30°C (59°F to 86°F); protect from light; store upright.

Parenteral:

Premixed bag in D$_5$W: Store at 20°C to 25°C (68°F to 77°F), excursions allowed from 15°C to 30°C (59°F to 86°F); may refrigerate; avoid freezing and excessive heat; protect from light.

Vial: Store unopened vials at 2°C to 30°C (36°F to 86°F); protect from light; when diluted in NS or D$_5$W manufacturer recommends stability for 48 hours at room temperature and others have reported for 7 days at 4°C or 25°C; consult specific references for additional information.

Compatible; Y-site: Bleomycin, carboplatin, carmustine, chlorpromazine, cisplatin, cyclophosphamide, cytarabine, dacarbazine, dactinomycin, daunorubicin, dexamethasone, diphenhydramine, doxorubicin, droperidol, etoposide, fludarabine, ifosfamide, mechlorethamine, methotrexate, mesna, metoclopramide, mitoxantrone, prochlorperazine, promethazine, teniposide, vinblastine, and vincristine

Incompatible with acyclovir, ampicillin, aminophylline, furosemide, ganciclovir, lorazepam, methylprednisolone, and piperacillin

Mechanism of Action Selective 5-HT$_3$-receptor antagonist, blocking serotonin, both peripherally on vagal nerve terminals and centrally in the chemoreceptor trigger zone

Pharmacokinetics (Adult data unless noted)

Absorption: Oral: 100%; nonlinear absorption occurs with increasing oral doses; Zofran® ODT tablets are bioequivalent to Zofran® tablets; absorption does not occur via oral mucosa

Distribution: V$_d$:

Children: Surgical patients:

1-4 months: 3.5 L/kg

5-24 months: 2.3 L/kg

3-12 years: 1.65 L/kg

Children and Adolescents: Cancer patients: 4-18 years: 1.9 L/kg

Adults: 1.9 L/kg

Protein binding, plasma: 70% to 76%

Metabolism: Some first-pass metabolism; primarily by hydroxylation, followed by glucuronidation and sulfate conjugation; CYP1A2, CYP2D6, and CYP3A4 substrate; some demethylation occurs

Bioavailability: Oral: 50% to 70% due to some first-pass metabolism; in cancer patients (adults) 85% to 87% bioavailability possibly related to changes in metabolism

Half-life:

Infants 1-4 months: 6.7 hours

Infants and Children 5 months to 12 years: 2.9 hours

Adults: 3.5-5.5 hours

Mild to moderate hepatic impairment (Child-Pugh A-B): 12 hours

Severe hepatic impairment (Child-Pugh C): 20 hours
Elimination: In urine and feces; <5% of the parent drug is recovered unchanged in urine
Clearance:
Children: Surgical patients:
1-4 months: 0.401 L/kg/hour
5-24 months: 0.581 L/kg/hour
3-12 years: 0.439 L/kg/hour
Children and Adolescents: Cancer patients 4-18 years: 0.599 L/kg/hour
Adults (normal):
19-40 years: 0.381 L/kg/hour
61-74 years: 0.319 L/kg/hour
>75 years: 0.262 L/kg/hour

Dosing: Usual

Infants, Children, and Adolescents:

Chemotherapy- or radiotherapy-induced nausea and vomiting; prevention:

I.V.: Infants (Limited data available in infants <6 months), Children, and Adolescents:

Weight-directed dosing:

Highly emetogenic antineoplastic therapy: 0.15 mg/kg/dose; maximum dose: 16 mg; administer first dose 30 minutes before the start chemotherapy with subsequent doses administered 4 and 8 hours after the first dose for 3 doses total; others have recommended administering the doses every 8 hours after the initial dose (Dupuis, 2013); a once-daily single dose of 0.3 mg/kg or 0.45 mg/kg (maximum dose: 16 mg) dependent upon emetogenic potential of chemotherapy has also been reported (Holdsworth, 2006)

Moderately emetogenic antineoplastic therapy: 0.15 mg/kg/dose; maximum dose: 8 mg; administer first dose 30 minutes before the start of chemotherapy with subsequent doses every 12 hours (Dupuis, 2013)

Low emetogenic antineoplastic therapy: 0.3 mg/kg/dose once; maximum dose: 16 mg; administered 30 minutes before the start of chemotherapy (Dupuis, 2013)

Body surface area (BSA)-directed dosing:

Highly emetogenic antineoplastic therapy: 5 mg/m^2/dose; maximum dose: 16 mg; administer first dose 30 minutes before the start chemotherapy with subsequent doses administered every 8 hours (Dupuis, 2013)

Moderately emetogenic antineoplastic therapy: 5 mg/m^2/dose; maximum dose: 8 mg; administer first dose 30 minutes before the start of chemotherapy with subsequent doses every 12 hours (Dupuis, 2013)

Low emetogenic antineoplastic therapy: 10 mg/m^2/dose once; maximum dose: 16 mg; administered 30 minutes before the start of chemotherapy (Dupuis, 2013)

Oral: **Note:** Doses should be administered 30 minutes before chemotherapy or 1-2 hours prior to radiotherapy and repeated at 8-hour intervals:

Fixed dosing: Children ≥2 years and Adolescents:

Children 2-4 years: Limited data available (Carden, 1990; Pinkerton, 1990):
<0.3 m^2: 1 mg/dose every 8 hours
0.3-0.6 m^2: 2 mg/dose every 8 hours
0.6-1 m^2: 3 mg/dose every 8 hours
>1 m^2: 4 mg/dose every 8 hours

Children 4-11 years: 4 mg/dose every 8 hours

Children ≥12 years and Adolescents: 8 mg/dose every 8 hours or 24 mg once daily

Alternate dosing:

Weight-directed dosing: Infants, Children, and Adolescents: Limited data in infants and children <4 years:

Highly emetogenic antineoplastic therapy: 0.15 mg/kg/dose every 8 hours; maximum dose: 16 mg (Dupuis, 2013)

Moderately emetogenic antineoplastic therapy: 0.15 mg/kg/dose; maximum dose: 8 mg; administer first dose 30 minutes before the start of chemotherapy with subsequent doses every 12 hours (Dupuis, 2013)

Low emetogenic antineoplastic therapy: 0.3 mg/kg/dose once; maximum dose: 16 mg; administered 30 minutes before the start of chemotherapy (Dupuis, 2013)

Body surface area (BSA)-directed dosing: Infants, Children, and Adolescents: Limited data in infants and children <4 years:

Highly emetogenic antineoplastic therapy: 5 mg/m^2/dose; maximum dose: 16 mg; administer first dose 30 minutes before the start chemotherapy with subsequent doses administered every 8 hours (Dupuis, 2013)

Moderately emetogenic antineoplastic therapy: 5 mg/m^2/dose; maximum dose: 8 mg; administer first dose 30 minutes before the start of chemotherapy with subsequent doses every 12 hours (Dupuis, 2013)

Low emetogenic antineoplastic therapy: 10 mg/m^2/dose once; maximum dose: 16 mg; administered 30 minutes before the start of chemotherapy (Dupuis, 2013)

Cyclic vomiting syndrome (CVS); treatment of acute attack Limited data available; dosing based on case reports and clinical experience: Children >2 years and Adolescents:

Low dose: I.V.: 0.15 mg/kg every 4 hours as needed for up to 3 doses; maximum dose: 16 mg (Fleisher, 1995)

High dose: I.V.: 0.3-0.4 mg/kg/dose every 4-6 hours; maximum dose: 16 mg (Li, 2008); per manufacturer labeling, should not exceed 3 doses in a 24-hour period

Gastroenteritis, acute; treatment: Note: Routine use of ondansetron is not recommended in most cases of acute gastroenteritis (AAP, 2004; CDC, 2003)

I.V.: Infants and Children ≥1 month: 0.15 or 0.3 mg/kg/dose once; maximum dose: 16 mg (DeCamp, 2008)

Oral: Infants and Children 6 months to 10 years, ≥8 kg (Freedman, 2006):
8-15 kg: 2 mg/dose once
>15-30 kg: 4 mg/dose once
>30 kg: 8 mg/dose once

Postoperative nausea and vomiting; prevention: I.V.: Administer immediately before induction of anesthesia, or postoperatively if the patient is symptomatic:

Infants and Children 1 month to 12 years and ≤40 kg: 0.1 mg/kg/dose; maximum dose: 4 mg

Children >40 kg, Adolescents: 4 mg/dose

Note: Repeat doses given in response to inadequate control of nausea/vomiting from preoperative doses are generally ineffective.

Adults:

Chemotherapy-induced emesis, prevention:

I.V.: 0.15 mg/kg/dose (maximum dose: 16 mg) over 15 minutes for 3 doses, beginning 30 minutes prior to chemotherapy, followed by subsequent doses 4 and 8 hours after the first dose

Oral:

Highly emetogenic agents/single-day therapy: 24 mg given as three 8 mg tablets 30 minutes prior to the start of therapy

Moderately emetogenic agents: 8 mg beginning 30 minutes before chemotherapy; repeat dose 8 hours after initial dose, then 8 mg every 12 hours for 1-2 days after chemotherapy completed

Postoperative nausea and vomiting (PONV), prevention: Note: The manufacturer recommends administration immediately before induction of anesthesia; however, this has been shown not to be as effective as administration at the end of surgery (Sun, 1997). Repeat doses given in response to inadequate control of nausea/vomiting from preoperative doses are generally ineffective.

I.M., I.V.: 4 mg as a single dose ~30 minutes before the end of anesthesia or as treatment if vomiting occurs after surgery (Gan, 2007).

Oral: 16 mg given 1 hour prior to induction of anesthesia

Radiation-induced emesis, prophylaxis:

Total body irradiation: Oral: 8 mg 1-2 hours before each daily fraction of radiotherapy

Single high-dose fraction radiotherapy to abdomen: Oral: 8 mg 1-2 hours before irradiation, then 8 mg every 8 hours after first dose for 1-2 days after completion of radiotherapy

Daily fractionated radiotherapy to abdomen: Oral: 8 mg 1-2 hours before irradiation, then 8 mg 8 hours after first dose for each day of radiotherapy

Hyperemesis gravidum, treatment:

I.V.: 8 mg administered over 15 minutes every 12 hours

Oral: 8 mg every 12 hours

Dosing adjustment in renal impairment: No dosage adjustments are recommended (there is no experience for oral ondansetron beyond day 1).

Dosing adjustment in hepatic impairment: Adults: Severe impairment (Child-Pugh C):

I.V.: Day 1: Maximum dose: 8 mg (there is no experience beyond day 1)

Oral: Maximum daily dose: 8 mg/day

Administration

Oral (all dosage forms): May administer without regard to meals

Orally disintegrating tablet (Zofran® ODT): Do open until needed; peel foil back; do not push through foil backing. Place tablet on tongue; it will disintegrate immediately; may also swallow with fluids as whole tablet

Soluble film (Zuplenz®): Do not remove from pouch until immediately before use. Using dry hands, place film on top of tongue and allow to dissolve (4-20 seconds). Swallow with or without liquid. If using more than one film, allow each film to dissolve completely before administering the next film.

Parenteral:

I.V.:

IVPB infusion: For prevention of chemotherapy-related emesis, dilute to a maximum concentration of 1 mg/mL and infuse over 15 minutes; for cyclic vomiting syndrome, dilute in 50-100 mL of D_5W and infuse of 15-30 minutes (Fleischer, 1995)

I.V. push: May be administered I.V. undiluted over 2-5 minutes for prevention of PONV

I.M.: Administer as undiluted injection; use only in adults

Monitoring Parameters Closely monitor patients <4 months of age; baseline ECG (if applicable); serum electrolytes (K/Mg); emesis episodes

Dosage Forms Excipient information presented when available (limited, particularly for generics); consult specific product labeling.

Film, Oral:

Zuplenz: 4 mg (1 ea, 10 ea); 8 mg (1 ea, 10 ea)

Solution, Injection:

Zofran: 40 mg/20 mL (20 mL) [contains methylparaben, propylparaben]

Generic: 4 mg/2 mL (2 mL); 40 mg/20 mL (20 mL)

Solution, Injection [preservative free]:

Generic: 4 mg/2 mL (2 mL)

Solution, Oral:

Zofran: 4 mg/5 mL (50 mL) [strawberry flavor]

Generic: 4 mg/5 mL (50 mL)

Tablet, Oral:

Zofran: 4 mg, 8 mg

Generic: 4 mg, 8 mg, 24 mg

Tablet Dispersible, Oral:

Zofran ODT: 4 mg, 8 mg [contains aspartame, methylparaben sodium, propylparaben sodium; strawberry flavor]

Generic: 4 mg, 8 mg

Extemporaneous Preparations Note: Commercial oral solution is available (0.8 mg/mL).

If commercial oral solution is unavailable, a 0.8 mg/mL syrup may be made with ondansetron tablets, Ora-Plus® (Paddock), and any of the the following syrups: Cherry syrup USP, Syrpalta® (HUMCO), Ora-Sweet® (Paddock), or Ora-Sweet® Sugar-Free (Paddock). Crush ten 8 mg tablets in a mortar and reduce to a fine powder (flaking of the tablet coating occurs). Add 50 mL Ora-Plus® in 5 mL increments, mixing thoroughly; mix while adding the chosen syrup in incremental proportions to **almost** 100 mL; transfer to a calibrated bottle, rinse mortar with syrup, and add sufficient quantity of syrup to make 100 mL. Label "shake well" and "refrigerate". Stable for 42 days refrigerated (Trissel, 1996).

Rectal suppositories: Calibrate a suppository mold for the base being used. Determine the displacement factor (DF) for ondansetron for the base being used (Fattibase® = 1.1; Polybase® = 0.6). Weigh the ondansetron tablet(s). Divide the tablet weight by the DF; this result is the weight of base displaced by the drug. Subtract the weight of base displaced from the calculated weight of base required for each suppository. Grind the ondansetron tablets in a mortar and reduce to a fine powder. Weigh out the appropriate weight of suppository base. Melt the base over a water bath (<55°C). Add the ondansetron powder to the suppository base and mix well. Pour the mixture into the suppository mold and cool. Stable for at least 30 days refrigerated (Tenjarla, 1998).

Tenjarla SN, Ward ES, and Fox JL, "Ondansetron Suppositories: Extemporaneous Preparation, Drug Release, Stability and Flux Through Rabbit Rectal Membrane," *Int J Pharm Compound*, 1998, 2(1):83-8.

Trissel LA, *Trissel's Stability of Compounded Formulations*, Washington, DC: American Pharmaceutical Association, 1996.

References

Al-Ansari K, Alomary S, Abdulateef H, et al, "Metoclopramide Versus Ondansetron for the Treatment of Vomiting in Children With Acute Gastroenteritis," *J Pediatr Gastroenterol Nutr*, 2011, 53(2):156-60.

American College of Obstetrics and Gynecology, "ACOG (American College of Obstetrics and Gynecology) Practice Bulletin: Nausea and Vomiting of Pregnancy," *Obstet Gynecol*, 2004, 103(4):803-14.

Anderka M, Mitchell AA, Louik C, et al, "Medications Used to Treat Nausea and Vomiting of Pregnancy and the Risk of Selected Birth Defects," *Birth Defects Res A Clin Mol Teratol*, 2012, 94(1):22-30.

"ASHP Therapeutic Guidelines on the Pharmacologic Management of Nausea and Vomiting in Adult and Pediatric Patients Receiving Chemotherapy or Radiation Therapy or Undergoing Surgery," *Am J Health Syst Pharm*, 1999, 56(8):729-64.

Carden PA, Mitchell SL, Waters KD, et al, "Prevention of Cyclophosphamide/Cytarabine-Induced Emesis With Ondansetron in Children With Leukemia," *J Clin Oncol*, 1990, 8(9):1531-5.

Centers for Disease Control and Prevention, "Managing Acute Gastroenteritis Among Children: Oral Rehydration, Maintenance, and Nutritional Therapy," *MMWR Recomm Rep*, 2003, 52(RR-16):1-16.

DeCamp LR, Byerley JS, Doshi N, et al, "Use of Antiemetic Agents in Acute Gastroenteritis: A Systematic Review and Meta-analysis," *Arch Pediatr Adolesc Med*, 2008, 162(9):858-65.

Dupuis LL, Boodhan S, Holdsworth M, et al. Guideline for the prevention of acute nausea and vomiting due to antineoplastic medication in pediatric cancer patients. *Pediatr Blood Cancer*. 2013;60(7):1073-1082.

Einarson A, Maltepe C, Navioz Y, et al, "The Safety of Ondansetron for Nausea and Vomiting of Pregnancy: A Prospective Comparative Study," *BJOG*, 2004, 111(9):940-3.

Ferreira E, Gillet M, Lelièvre J, et al, "Ondansetron Use During Pregnancy: A Case Series," *J Popul Ther Clin Pharmacol*, 2012, 19 (1):e1-e10.

Fleisher DR, "Management of Cyclic Vomiting Syndrome," *J Pediatr Gastrenterol Nutr*, 1994, 21(Suppl 1):S52-6.

Freedman SB, Adler M, Seshadri R, et al, "Oral Ondansetron for Gastroenteritis in a Pediatric Emergency Department," *N Engl J Med*, 2006, 354(16):1698-705.

Gan TJ, Meyer TA, Apfel CC, et al, "Society for Ambulatory Anesthesia Guidelines for the Management of Postoperative Nausea and Vomiting," *Anesth Analg*, 2007, 105(6):1615-28.

Holdsworth MT, Raisch DW, and Frost J, "Acute and Delayed Nausea and Emesis Control in Pediatric Oncology Patients," *Cancer*, 2006, 106(4):931-40.

Koren G, "Motherisk Update. Is Ondansetron Safe for Use During Pregnancy?" *Can Fam Physician*, 2012, 58(10):1092-3.

Levichek Z, Atanackovic G, Oepkes D, et al, "Nausea and Vomiting of Pregnancy. Evidence-Based Treatment Algorithm," *Can Fam Physician*, 2002, 48:267-8, 277.

Li BU, Lefevre F, Chelimsky GG, et al, "North American Society for Pediatric Gastroenterology, Hepatology, and Nutrition Consensus Statement on the Diagnosis and Management of Cyclic Vomiting Syndrome," *J Pediatr Gastroenterol Nutr*, 2008, 47(3):379-93.

Marty M, Pouillart P, Scholl S, et al, "Comparison of the 5-hydroxytryptamine 3 (Serotonin) Antagonist Ondansetron (GR 38032F) With High-Dose Metoclopramide in the Control of Cisplatin-Induced Emesis," *N Engl J Med*, 1990, 322(12):816-21.

Mondick JT, Johnson BM, Haberer LJ, et al, "Population Pharmacokinetics of Intravenous Ondansetron in Oncology and Surgical Patients Aged 1-48 Months," *Eur J Clin Pharmacol*, 2010, 66(1):77-86.

Multinational Association of Supportive Care in Cancer (MASCC), "Antiemetic Guidelines," Updated April 2010. Available at http://data.memberclicks.com/site/mascc/MASCC_Guidelines_English_2010.pdf

National Comprehensive Cancer Network® (NCCN), "Clinical Practice Guidelines in Oncology™: Antiemesis," Version 2.2010. Available at http://www.nccn.org/professionals/physician_gls/PDF/antiemesis.pdf

Pasternak B, Svanström H, and Hviid A, "Ondansetron in Pregnancy and Risk of Adverse Fetal Outcomes," *N Engl J Med*, 2013, 368 (9):814-23.

Phillips RS, Gopaul S, Gibson F, et al, "Antiemetic Medication for Prevention and Treatment of Chemotherapy Induced Nausea and Vomiting in Childhood," *Cochrane Database Syst Rev*, 2010, (9): CD007786.

Pinkerton CR, Williams D, Wootton C, et al, "5-HT$_3$ Antagonist Ondansetron - An Effective Outpatient Antiemetic in Cancer Treatment," *Arch Dis Child*, 1990, 65(8):822-5.

Roila F and Del Favero A, "Ondansetron Clinical Pharmacokinetics," *Clin Pharmacokinet*, 1995, 29(2):95-109.

Seynaeve C, Schuller J, Buser K, et al, "Comparison of the Anti-emetic Efficacy of Different Doses of Ondansetron, Given as Either a Continuous Infusion or a Single Intravenous Dose, in Acute Cisplatin-Induced Emesis," *Br J Cancer* 1992, 66(1):192-7.

Siu SS, Chan MT, and Lau TK, "Placental Transfer of Ondansetron During Early Human Pregnancy," *Clin Pharmacokinet*, 2006, 45 (4):419-23.

Spahr-Schopfer IA, Lerman J, Sikich N, et al, "Pharmacokinetics of Intravenous Ondansetron in Healthy Children Undergoing Ear, Nose, and Throat Surgery," *Clin Pharmacol Ther*, 1995, 58(3):316-21.

Spector JI, Lester EP, Chevlen EM, et al, "A Comparison of Oral Ondansetron and Intravenous Granisetron for the Prevention of Nausea and Emesis Associated With Cisplatin-Based Chemotherapy," *Oncologist*, 1998, 3(6):432-438.

Tan PC and Omar SZ, "Contemporary Approaches to Hyperemesis During Pregnancy," *Curr Opin Obstet Gynecol*, 2011, 23(2):87-93.

♦ **Ondansetron Hydrochloride** *see* Ondansetron *on page 1544*

♦ **Ondansetron Injection (Can)** *see* Ondansetron *on page 1544*

♦ **Ondansetron Injection USP (Can)** *see* Ondansetron *on page 1544*

♦ **Ondansetron-Odan (Can)** *see* Ondansetron *on page 1544*

♦ **Ondansetron-Omega (Can)** *see* Ondansetron *on page 1544*

♦ **One Step Callus Remover [OTC]** *see* Salicylic Acid *on page 1860*

♦ **Onfi** *see* CloBAZam *on page 504*

♦ **Onmel** *see* Itraconazole *on page 1166*

♦ **Onsolis** *see* FentaNYL *on page 853*

♦ **OPC-14597** *see* ARIPiprazole *on page 196*

♦ **o,p'-DDD** *see* Mitotane *on page 1425*

♦ **Ophtho-Dipivefrin™ (Can)** *see* Dipivefrin *on page 692*

♦ **Opium and Belladonna** *see* Belladonna and Opium *on page 269*

Opium Tincture (OH pee um TING chur)

Medication Safety Issues
Sound-alike/look-alike issues:
Opium tincture may be confused with camphorated tincture of opium (paregoric)

High alert medication:
The Institute for Safe Medication Practices (ISMP) includes this medication among its list of drugs which have a heightened risk of causing significant patient harm when used in error.

Administration issues:
Use care when prescribing opium tincture; opium tincture is 25 times more concentrated than paregoric, each undiluted mL of opium tincture contains the equivalent of morphine 10 mg/mL.

If opium tincture is used in neonates, a 25-fold dilution should be prepared (final concentration: 0.4 mg/mL morphine). Of note, paregoric (which contains the equivalent of morphine 0.4 mg/mL) is **not** recommended for use in neonates due to the high alcohol content (~45%) and the presence of other additives; as an alternative to the use of diluted opium tincture or paregoric, ISMP recommends using a diluted preservative free injectable morphine solution orally.

Although historically opium tincture is dosed as mL/kg, the preferred dosing units are **mg**/kg (Levine, 2001). ISMP suggests hospitals evaluate the need for this product at their institution.

Other safety concerns:
DTO is an error-prone abbreviation and should never be used as an abbreviation for opium tincture (also known as *Deodorized* Tincture of Opium) due to potential for being mistaken as *Diluted* Tincture of Opium

Therapeutic Category Analgesic, Narcotic; Antidiarrheal

Generic Availability (U.S.) Yes

Use Treatment of diarrhea in adults; has also been used for the treatment of neonatal abstinence syndrome (opioid withdrawal) using **a 25-fold dilution with water** (final concentration 0.4 mg/mL morphine)

Pregnancy Risk Factor C

Pregnancy Considerations Animal reproduction studies have not been conducted. Opium tincture contains morphine; refer to the Morphine (Systemic) monograph for additional information. In addition, this preparation contains large amounts of alcohol (19%).

Breast-Feeding Considerations Opium tincture contains morphine, which is excreted into breast milk; refer to the Morphine (Systemic) monograph for additional information. In addition, this preparation contains large amounts of alcohol (19%). The manufacturer recommends that caution be used if administered to a nursing woman.

Contraindications Hypersensitivity to opium, morphine, or any component; diarrhea caused by poisoning until the toxic material has been removed; increased intracranial pressure, severe respiratory depression, severe liver or renal insufficiency. Manufacturer does not recommend use in children.

Warnings Do not confuse opium tincture with paregoric; opium tincture is 25 times more potent than paregoric; opium shares the toxic potential of opioid agonists, usual precautions of opioid agonist therapy should be observed; opium may mask dehydration by producing fluid retention in the bowel; monitor patients with prolonged or severe diarrhea carefully; abrupt discontinuation after prolonged use may result in withdrawal symptoms; oral solution contains 19% ethanol

Precautions Use with caution in patients with respiratory, hepatic, or renal dysfunction, severe prostatic hypertrophy, or history of opioid abuse; infants <3 months of age are more susceptible to respiratory depression, use with caution and in reduced doses in this age group

Adverse Reactions
Cardiovascular: Bradycardia, hypotension, palpitation, peripheral vasodilation
Central nervous system: CNS depression, dizziness, drowsiness, headache, insomnia, intracranial pressure increased, malaise, mental depression, restlessness
Gastrointestinal: Anorexia, biliary tract spasm, constipation, nausea, stomach cramps, vomiting
Genitourinary: Urination decreased, urinary tract spasm
Neuromuscular & skeletal: Weakness
Ocular: Miosis
Respiratory: Respiratory depression
Miscellaneous: Histamine release, physical and psychological dependence

Drug Interactions
Metabolism/Transport Effects None known.
Avoid Concomitant Use
Avoid concomitant use of Opium Tincture with any of the following: Azelastine (Nasal); Paraldehyde; Thalidomide
Increased Effect/Toxicity
Opium Tincture may increase the levels/effects of: Alcohol (Ethyl); Alvimopan; Azelastine (Nasal); Buprenorphine; CNS Depressants; Desmopressin; Diuretics; Hydrocodone; Methotrimeprazine; Metyrosine; Mirtazapine; Paraldehyde; Pramipexole; ROPINIRole; Rotigotine; Selective Serotonin Reuptake Inhibitors; Thalidomide; Zolpidem

The levels/effects of Opium Tincture may be increased by: Amphetamines; Anticholinergic Agents; Antipsychotic Agents (Phenothiazines); Brimonidine (Topical); Cannabis; Doxylamine; Dronabinol; Droperidol; HydrOXYzine; Kava Kava; Magnesium Sulfate; Methotrimeprazine; Nabilone; Perampanel; Rufinamide; Sodium Oxybate; Succinylcholine; Tapentadol; Tetrahydrocannabinol

Decreased Effect
Opium Tincture may decrease the levels/effects of: Pegvisomant

The levels/effects of Opium Tincture may be decreased by: Ammonium Chloride; Mixed Agonist / Antagonist Opioids; Naltrexone

Stability Store at 68°F to 77°F (20°C to 25°C); protect from light and excessive heat; do not refrigerate, decreased solubility and precipitation may occur

Mechanism of Action Contains many opioid alkaloids including morphine; its mechanism for gastric motility inhibition is primarily due to this morphine content; it results in a decrease in digestive secretions, an increase in GI muscle tone, and therefore a reduction in GI propulsion

Pharmacodynamics Duration: 4-5 hours
Pharmacokinetics (Adult data unless noted)
Absorption: Variable from GI tract
Metabolism: In the liver
Elimination: In urine and bile

Dosing: Neonatal Oral: **Note:** The following doses are expressed in **mg/kg** or **mg** dosing units of morphine.
Full-term neonates: Neonatal abstinence syndrome (opioid withdrawal): **Use a 25-fold dilution of opium tincture** (final concentration: 0.4 mg/mL morphine)
Initial: Give 0.04 **mg/kg**/dose of a 0.4 mg/mL solution with feedings every 3-4 hours; increase as needed by 0.04 **mg/kg**/dose of a 0.4 mg/mL solution every 3-4 hours until withdrawal symptoms are controlled

Usual dose: 0.08-0.2 **mg**/dose given every 3-4 hours; it is rare to exceed 0.28 **mg**/dose; stabilize withdrawal symptoms for 3-5 days, then gradually decrease the dosage (keeping the same dosage interval) over a 2- to 4-week period

Dosing: Usual Oral: **Note:** The following doses are expressed in **mg/kg** or **mg** dosing units of morphine.
Adults: Diarrhea: Usual: 6 **mg** of undiluted opium tincture (10 mg/mL morphine) every 6 hours

Administration Oral: May administer with food to decrease GI upset; for neonatal abstinence syndrome (opioid withdrawal), use a 25-fold dilution of opium tincture (final concentration 0.4 mg/mL morphine)

Monitoring Parameters Respiratory rate, blood pressure, heart rate, resolution of diarrhea, mental status; if using a 25-fold dilution to treat neonatal abstinence syndrome, monitor for resolution of withdrawal symptoms (such as irritability, high-pitched cry, stuffy nose, rhinorrhea, vomiting, poor feeding, diarrhea, sneezing, yawning etc), and signs of overtreatment (such as bradycardia, lethargy, hypotonia, irregular respirations, respiratory depression etc). An abstinence scoring system (eg, Finnegan abstinence scoring system) can be used to more objectively assess neonatal opioid withdrawal symptoms and the need for dosage adjustment.

Test Interactions Increased aminotransferase [ALT/AST] (S)

Additional Information Opium tincture contains 10 mg/mL morphine; for treatment of neonatal abstinence syndrome, a 25-fold dilution of opium tincture (final concentration: 0.4 mg/mL morphine) is preferred over paregoric; the 25-fold dilution of opium tincture contains the same morphine concentration as paregoric, but without the high amount of alcohol or additives of paregoric

Controlled Substance C-II
Dosage Forms Excipient information presented when available (limited, particularly for generics); consult specific product labeling.
Tincture, Oral:
Generic: 10 mg/mL (1%) (118 mL, 473 mL)

References
Dow K, Ordean A, Murphy-Oikonen J, et al, "Neonatal Abstinence Syndrome Clinical Practice Guidelines For Ontario," *J Popul Ther Clin Pharmacol*, 2012, 19(3):e488-506.
Hudak ML, Tan RC, Committee On Drugs, et al, "Neonatal Drug Withdrawal," *Pediatrics*, 2012, 129(2):e540-60.
Kraus DM and Pham JT, "Neonatal Therapy," *Applied Therapeutics: The Clinical Use of Drugs*, 9th ed, Koda-Kimble MA, Young LY, Kradjan WA, et al, eds, Baltimore, MD: Lippincott Williams & Wilkins, 2009.
Levine SR, Cohen MR, Blanchard MR, et al, "Guidelines for Preventing Medication Errors in Pediatrics," *J Pediatr Pharmacol Ther*, 2001, 6:427-43.
Levy M and Spino M, "Neonatal Withdrawal Syndrome: Associated Drugs and Pharmacologic Management," *Pharmacotherapy*, 1993, 13(3):202-11.
"Neonatal Drug Withdrawal. American Academy of Pediatrics Committee on Drugs," *Pediatrics*, 1998, 101(6):1079-88.

◆ **Opium Tincture, Deodorized** *see* Opium Tincture *on page 1548*

Oprelvekin (oh PREL ve kin)

Medication Safety Issues
Sound-alike/look-alike issues:
Oprelvekin may be confused with aldesleukin, Proleukin®
Neumega® may be confused with Neulasta®, Neupogen®
Brand Names: U.S. Neumega
Therapeutic Category Biological Response Modulator; Thrombopoietic Growth Factor
Generic Availability (U.S.) No

Use Prevention of severe thrombocytopenia and the reduction of the need for platelet transfusions following myelosuppressive chemotherapy in adult patients with nonmyeloid malignancies who are at high risk of severe thrombocytopenia (FDA approved in adults)

Pregnancy Risk Factor C

Pregnancy Considerations Animal studies have demonstrated adverse fetal effects. There are no adequate and well-controlled studies in pregnant women. Use during pregnancy only if the potential benefits outweigh the potential risk to the fetus.

Breast-Feeding Considerations Due to the potential for serious adverse reactions in the nursing infant, breast-feeding is not recommended.

Contraindications Hypersensitivity to oprelvekin or any component

Warnings Treatment has been associated with severe hypersensitivity reactions including anaphylaxis [U.S. Boxed Warning]; may occur with the first or with subsequent doses; permanently discontinue oprelvekin in any patient developing an allergic reaction. Not indicated following myeloablative chemotherapy as effectiveness was not significant vs placebo and toxicity (edema, conjunctival bleeding, hypotension, and tachycardia) was increased vs placebo in these patients. Severe hypokalemia and/or sudden death have been reported in patients receiving chronic diuretic therapy, ifosfamide, and oprelvekin. Moderate decreases in hemoglobin, hematocrit, and RBC without a decrease in red cell mass have been observed; this is predominately related to an increase in plasma volume (dilutional anemia) from renal sodium and water retention. Onset of dilutional anemia is within 3-5 days of oprelvekin therapy and is reversible over approximately 7 days following discontinuation of oprelvekin. Stroke has been reported in patients who develop atrial fibrillation/flutter while receiving oprelvekin. Animal studies were predictive of an effect of oprelvekin on developing bone in children; thickening of femoral and tibial growth plates was noted. Per the manufacturer, oprelvekin should not be used in children, particularly those <12 years of age, except as part of a controlled clinical trial; some adverse events occurred more frequently in children, such as tachycardia (84%), conjunctival injection (57%), cardiomegaly (21%), and periosteal changes (11%).

Dose-limiting papilledema, more frequently associated with use in children (16% vs 2% in adults), has occurred (usually following repeated cycles); use with caution in patients with preexisting papilledema or with tumors involving the central nervous system; may worsen preexisting papilledema. Patients experiencing oprelvekin-related papilledema may be at risk for visual acuity changes, including blurred vision or blindness.

Precautions Oprelvekin may cause serious fluid retention resulting in peripheral edema, facial edema, dyspnea on exertion, pulmonary edema, capillary leak syndrome, atrial arrhythmias, and exacerbation of preexisting pleural effusions. Use cautiously in patients with conditions where expansion of plasma volume should be avoided (eg, left ventricular dysfunction, CHF, hypertension). Use caution in patients with cardiac arrhythmias or conduction defects (ventricular arrhythmias generally occurring within 2-7 days of initiation of treatment have been reported postmarketing); use with caution in patients with respiratory disease; history of thromboembolic problems or stroke, and hepatic or renal dysfunction; modify dosage in patients with severe renal dysfunction

Adverse Reactions

Cardiovascular: Atrial arrhythmia, cardiomegaly, edema, palpitation, syncope, tachycardia, vasodilation

Central nervous system: Dizziness, fatigue, fever, headache, insomnia, neutropenic fever

Dermatologic: Rash

Endocrine & metabolic: Fluid retention

Gastrointestinal: Diarrhea, mucositis, nausea/vomiting, oral moniliasis, weight gain

Hematologic: Anemia (dilutional)

Neuromuscular & skeletal: Arthralgia, periostitis, weakness

Ocular: Conjunctival injection/redness/swelling, papilledema

Respiratory: Cough, dyspnea, rhinitis, pharyngitis, pleural effusion

Rare but important or life-threatening: Allergic reaction, amblyopia, anaphylaxis/anaphylactoid reactions, blindness, blurred vision, capillary leak syndrome, cardiac arrest, chest pain, dehydration, dysarthria, exfoliative dermatitis, eye hemorrhage, facial edema, fibrinogen increased, fluid overload, HF, hypoalbuminemia, hypocalcemia, hypokalemia, hypotension, injection site reactions (dermatitis, pain, discoloration), loss of consciousness, mental status changes, optic neuropathy, paresthesia, pericardial effusion, peripheral edema, pneumonia, pulmonary edema, renal failure, shock, skin discoloration, stroke, urticaria, ventricular arrhythmia, visual acuity changes, visual field defect, von Willebrand factor concentration increased, wheezing

Drug Interactions

Metabolism/Transport Effects None known.

Avoid Concomitant Use There are no known interactions where it is recommended to avoid concomitant use.

Increased Effect/Toxicity There are no known significant interactions involving an increase in effect.

Decreased Effect There are no known significant interactions involving a decrease in effect.

Stability Store vials under refrigeration between 2°C to 8°C (36°F to 46°F); protect from light; do not freeze. Use reconstituted oprelvekin within 3 hours of reconstitution; store reconstituted solution at either 2°C to 8°C (36°F to 46°F) or room temperature ≤25°C (70°F). Do not freeze reconstituted solution.

Mechanism of Action Oprelvekin is a thrombopoietic growth factor which stimulates multiple stages of megakaryocytopoiesis and thrombopoiesis, resulting in proliferation of megakaryocyte progenitors and megakaryocyte maturation, thereby increasing platelet production.

Pharmacodynamics

Onset of action: 5-9 days

Maximum effect: 14-19 days

Duration: Up to 7 days after discontinuation

Pharmacokinetics (Adult data unless noted)

Distribution: V_d: Adults: 112-152 mL/kg

Bioavailability: >80%

Metabolism: Uncertain

Half-life: Terminal: 6.9-8.1 hours

Time to peak serum concentration: 3.2 ± 2.4 hours

Elimination: Urine (primarily as metabolites)

Clearance: Adults: 2.2-2.7 mL/min/kg; clearance decreases with age and is about 1.2-1.6 times faster in children than in adults

Dosing: Usual SubQ: **Note:** First dose should not be administered until 6-24 hours after the end of chemotherapy. Discontinue the drug at least 48 hours before beginning the next cycle of chemotherapy.

Children: 25-50 mcg/kg once daily for 27 days was shown to be efficacious with decreased toxicities as compared to higher doses in one study with 47 pediatric patients (Cairo, 2005); dosing should continue until postnadir platelet count ≥50,000/mm³

Note: The manufacturer states that, until efficacy/toxicity parameters are established, the use of oprelvekin in pediatric patients (particularly those <12 years of age) should be restricted to use in controlled clinical trials.

Adults: 50 mcg/kg once daily for 10-21 days (until postnadir platelet count ≥50,000/mm³)

Dosage adjustment in renal failure: Adults: CrCl <30 mL/minute: 25 mcg/kg once daily for 10-21 days (until postnadir platelet count ≥50,000/mm³)

Administration SubQ: Reconstitute to a final concentration of 5 mg/mL with SWI; direct diluent down side of vial, gently swirl, do not shake. Administer subcutaneously in either the abdomen, thigh, hip, or upper arm (if not self-injected).

Monitoring Parameters Monitor electrolytes and fluid balance during therapy; obtain a CBC at regular intervals during therapy; monitor platelet counts until adequate recovery has occurred; renal function (at baseline)

Dosage Forms Excipient information presented when available (limited, particularly for generics); consult specific product labeling.

Solution Reconstituted, Subcutaneous [preservative free]:
Neumega: 5 mg (1 ea)

References
Adams VR and Brenner TL, "Oprelvekin (Neumega®)," *J Oncol Pharm Pract*, 1999, 5(3):117-24.
Cairo MS, Davenport V, Bessmertny O, et al, "Phase I/II Dose Escalation Study of Recombinant Human Interleukin-11 Following Ifosfamide, Carboplatin and Etoposide in Children, Adolescents and Young Adults With Solid Tumours or Lymphoma: A Clinical, Haematological and Biological Study," *Br J Haematol*, 2005, 128(1):49-58.
Du X and Williams DA, "Interleukin-11: Review of Molecular, Cell Biology, and Clinical Use," *Blood*, 1997, 89(11):3897-908.
Gordon MS, "Thrombopoietic Activity of Recombinant Human Interleukin 11 in Cancer Patients Receiving Chemotherapy," *Cancer Chemother Pharmacol*, 1996, 38 (Suppl):96-8.
Milman E, Berdon WE, Garvin JH, et al, "Periostitis Secondary to Interleukin-11 (Oprelvekin, Neumega®). Treatment for Thrombocytopenia in Pediatric Patients," *Pediatr Radiol*, 2003, 33(7):450-2.
Tepler I, Elias L, Smith JW 2d, et al, "A Randomized Placebo-Controlled Trial of Recombinant Human Interleukin-11 in Cancer Patients With Severe Thrombocytopenia Due to Chemotherapy," *Blood*, 1996, 87 (9):3607-14.
Teramura M, Kobayashi S, Yoshinaga K, et al, "Effect of Interleukin 11 on Normal and Pathological Thrombopoiesis," *Cancer Chemother Pharmacol*, 1996, 38 (Suppl):99-102.

◆ **Opticrom® (Can)** *see* Cromolyn (Ophthalmic) *on page 553*

◆ **Optimyxin® (Can)** *see* Bacitracin and Polymyxin B *on page 257*

◆ **Optivar** *see* Azelastine (Ophthalmic) *on page 247*

◆ **Oracea** *see* Doxycycline *on page 721*

◆ **Oracit®** *see* Sodium Citrate and Citric Acid *on page 1906*

◆ **Oracort (Can)** *see* Triamcinolone (Topical) *on page 2078*

◆ **Ora-film [OTC]** *see* Benzocaine *on page 273*

◆ **Oralone** *see* Triamcinolone (Topical) *on page 2078*

◆ **Oral Pain Relief Max St [OTC]** *see* Benzocaine *on page 273*

◆ **Orap** *see* Pimozide *on page 1677*

◆ **Orap® (Can)** *see* Pimozide *on page 1677*

◆ **Orapred [DSC]** *see* PrednisoLONE (Systemic) *on page 1727*

◆ **Orapred ODT** *see* PrednisoLONE (Systemic) *on page 1727*

◆ **Oraqix®** *see* Lidocaine and Prilocaine *on page 1246*

◆ **Orazinc [OTC]** *see* Zinc Sulfate *on page 2176*

◆ **Orciprenaline Sulfate** *see* Metaproterenol *on page 1352*

◆ **Orencia** *see* Abatacept *on page 44*

◆ **Orfadin** *see* Nitisinone *on page 1501*

◆ **ORG 9426** *see* Rocuronium *on page 1847*

◆ **Organ-I NR [OTC]** *see* GuaiFENesin *on page 984*

◆ **ORG NC 45** *see* Vecuronium *on page 2123*

◆ **ORO-Clense (Can)** *see* Chlorhexidine Gluconate *on page 441*

◆ **Ortho-CS 250** *see* Ascorbic Acid *on page 206*

◆ **Ortho Micronor** *see* Norethindrone *on page 1511*

◆ **Ortho,para-DDD** *see* Mitotane *on page 1425*

◆ **OrthoWash** *see* Fluoride *on page 894*

◆ **Oscal** *see* Calcium Carbonate *on page 346*

◆ **Os-Cal [OTC] [DSC]** *see* Calcium Carbonate *on page 346*

◆ **Os-Cal (Can)** *see* Calcium Carbonate *on page 346*

◆ **Oscimin** *see* Hyoscyamine *on page 1056*

◆ **Oscimin SR** *see* Hyoscyamine *on page 1056*

◆ **Oscion Cleanser** *see* Benzoyl Peroxide *on page 275*

Oseltamivir (oh sel TAM i vir)

Medication Safety Issues
Sound-alike/look-alike issues:
Tamiflu may be confused with Tambocor, Thera-Flu
Other safety concerns:
Oseltamivir (Tamiflu) oral suspension is available in a 6 mg/mL concentration and is packaged with an oral syringe calibrated in **milliliters** up to a total of 10 mL. **Instructions to the patient should be provided based on these units of measure (ie, mL). When providing oseltamivir suspension for children <1 year of age, use a lower calibrated (ie, <10 mL) oral syringe to ensure accurate dosing.**

When commercially-prepared oseltamivir oral suspension is not available, an extemporaneously prepared suspension may be compounded to provide a 6 mg/mL concentration.

Brand Names: U.S. Tamiflu
Brand Names: Canada Tamiflu
Therapeutic Category Antiviral Agent, Oral; Neuraminidase Inhibitor
Generic Availability (U.S.) No
Use Treatment of influenza infection in patients who have been symptomatic for no more than 2 days (FDA approved in ages ≥2 weeks and adults); prophylaxis of influenza exposures (FDA approved in ages ≥1 year and adults)

Has also been used for prophylaxis of influenza in ages <1 year and treatment of patients symptomatic for >2 days with severe illness (CDC, 2010)

The Advisory Committee on Immunization Practices (ACIP) recommends that antiviral **treatment** be considered for the following (see specific antiviral product monograph for appropriate patient selection):
• Persons with severe, complicated or progressive illness
• Hospitalized persons
• Persons at higher risk for influenza complications
 - Children <2 years of age (highest risk in children <6 months of age)
 - Adults ≥65 years of age
 - Persons with chronic disorders of the pulmonary (including asthma) or cardiovascular systems (except hypertension)
 - Persons with chronic metabolic diseases (including diabetes mellitus, hepatic disease, renal dysfunction, hematologic disorders (including sickle cell disease), or immunosuppression (including immunosuppression caused by medications or HIV)
 - Persons with neurologic/neuromuscular conditions (including conditions such as spinal cord injuries, seizure disorders, cerebral palsy, stroke, mental retardation, moderate to severe developmental delay, or muscular dystrophy) which may compromise respiratory function, the handling of respiratory secretions, or that can increase the risk of aspiration
 - Pregnant or postpartum women (≤2 weeks after delivery)

◄

- Persons <19 years of age on long-term aspirin therapy
- American Indians and Alaskan Natives
- Persons who are morbidly obese (BMI ≥40)
- Residents of nursing homes or other chronic care facilities
• Use may also be considered for previously healthy, non-high-risk outpatients with confirmed or suspected influenza based on clinical judgment when treatment can be started within 48 hours of illness onset.

The ACIP recommends that **prophylaxis** be considered for the following (**Note**: Postexposure chemoprophylaxis is generally only recommended when it can be started within 48 hours of most recent exposure) (see specific antiviral product monograph for appropriate patient selection):

• Postexposure prophylaxis may be considered for family or close contacts of suspected or confirmed cases, who are at higher risk of influenza complications, and who have not been vaccinated against the circulating strain at the time of the exposure or if exposure occurred within 2 weeks of vaccination.

• Postexposure prophylaxis may be considered for unvaccinated healthcare workers who had occupational exposure without protective equipment.

• Pre-exposure prophylaxis should only be used for persons at very high risk of influenza complications and who cannot be otherwise protected at times of high risk for exposure.

• Prophylaxis should also be administered to all eligible residents of institutions that house patients at high risk when needed to control outbreaks.

The ACIP recommends that treatment and prophylaxis be given to children <1 year of age when indicated.

Tamiflu® oral suspension: 75 mg dose delivers 2 g sorbitol

Hospitalized patients with severe 2009 H1N1 influenza infection may require longer (eg, ≥10 days) treatment courses. Some experts also recommend empirically doubling the treatment dose. Doubling the dose in adult outpatients was not associated with increased adverse events. As no double dose studies have been published in children, use caution. Initiate as early as possible in any hospitalized patient with suspected/confirmed influenza [interim recommendations (CDC, 2010)].

The absence of symptoms does not rule out viral influenza infection and clinical judgment should guide the decision for therapy. Treatment should not be delayed while waiting for the results of diagnostic tests. Treatment should be considered for high-risk patients with symptoms despite a negative rapid influenza test when the illness cannot be contributed to another cause. Use of oseltamivir is not a substitute for vaccination (when available); susceptibility to influenza infection returns once therapy is discontinued.

Pregnancy Risk Factor C

Pregnancy Considerations In animal reproduction studies, a dose-dependent increase in the rates of minor skeleton abnormalities was found in exposed offspring. The rate of each abnormality remained within the background rate of occurrence in the species studied. Oseltamivir phosphate and its active metabolite oseltamivir carboxylate cross the placenta (*in vitro* data). An increased risk of adverse neonatal outcomes has generally not been observed following maternal use of oseltamivir during pregnancy. Untreated influenza infection is associated with an increased risk of adverse events to the fetus and an increased risk of complications or death to the mother. Oseltamivir and zanamivir are currently recommended for the treatment or prophylaxis of influenza in pregnant women and women up to 2 weeks postpartum. Oseltamivir and zanamivir are currently recommended as an adjunct to vaccination and should not be used as a substitute for vaccination in pregnant women (consult current CDC guidelines).

Breast-Feeding Considerations Small amounts of oseltamivir and oseltamivir carboxylate have been detected in breast milk. Breast-feeding is not recommended by the manufacturer. According to the CDC, breast-feeding while taking oseltamivir can be continued. The CDC recommends that women infected with the influenza virus follow general precautions (eg, frequent hand washing) to decrease viral transmission to the child. Mothers with influenza-like illnesses at delivery should consider avoiding close contact with the infant until they have received 48 hours of antiviral medication, fever has resolved, and cough and secretions can be controlled. These measures may help decrease (but not eliminate) the risk of transmitting influenza to the newborn. During this time, breast milk can be expressed and bottle-fed to the infant by another person who is well. Protective measures, such as wearing a face mask, changing into a clean gown or clothing, and strict hand hygiene should be continued by the mother for ≥7 days after the onset of symptoms or until symptom-free for 24 hours. Infant care should be performed by a noninfected person when possible (consult current CDC guidelines). Influenza may cause serious illness in postpartum women and prompt evaluation for febrile respiratory illnesses is recommended.

Contraindications Hypersensitivity to oseltamivir, any component, or other sialic acid-based neuraminidase inhibitors

Warnings There have been postmarketing reports of neuropsychiatric events in children (including self-injury with fatalities, hallucination, confusion, and delirium). Closely monitor patients for signs of any unusual behavior. Rare but severe hypersensitivity reactions (anaphylaxis, severe dermatologic reactions) have been associated with use. Oral suspension contains sodium benzoate; benzoic acid (benzoate) is a metabolite of benzyl alcohol; large amounts of benzyl alcohol (≥99 mg/kg/day) have been associated with a potentially fatal toxicity ("gasping syndrome") in neonates; use oral suspension containing sodium benzoate with caution in neonates; *in vitro* and animal studies have shown that benzoate displaces bilirubin from protein binding sites.

Precautions Use with caution and modify dosage in patients with renal impairment. Use suspension with caution in patients with hereditary fructose intolerance since 75 mg oral suspension delivers 2 g sorbitol which is greater than the maximum daily limit; may cause diarrhea and dyspepsia. Oseltamivir is not a substitute for the influenza virus vaccine. As an antiviral agent, it will not prevent primary or concomitant bacterial infections that may occur with influenza virus. Antiviral treatment should begin within 48 hours of symptom onset; however, the CDC recommends that treatment may still be beneficial and should be started in hospitalized patients with severe, complicated or progressive illness if >48 hours. Treatment should not be delayed while awaiting results of laboratory tests for influenza. Nonhospitalized persons who are not at high risk for developing severe or complicated illness and who have a mild disease are not likely to benefit if treatment is started >48 hours after symptom onset. Non-hospitalized persons who are already beginning to recover do not need treatment.

Adverse Reactions

Gastrointestinal: Abdominal pain, diarrhea, nausea, vomiting

Ocular: Conjunctivitis

Respiratory: Epistaxis

Rare but important or life-threatening: Allergy, anaphylactic/anaphylactoid reaction, angina, arrhythmia, confusion, erythema multiforme, fracture, gastrointestinal bleeding, hemorrhagic colitis, hepatitis, liver function tests abnormal, neuropsychiatric events, pseudomembranous colitis, pyrexia, seizure, Stevens-Johnson syndrome, swelling of face or tongue, toxic epidermal necrolysis

Drug Interactions

Metabolism/Transport Effects None known.

Avoid Concomitant Use There are no known interactions where it is recommended to avoid concomitant use.

Increased Effect/Toxicity

The levels/effects of Oseltamivir may be increased by: Probenecid

Decreased Effect

Oseltamivir may decrease the levels/effects of: Influenza Virus Vaccine (Live/Attenuated)

Stability

Capsules: Store at 25°C (77°F); excursions permitted to 15°C to 30°C (59°F to 86°F).

Oral suspension: Store powder for suspension at 25°C (77°F); excursions permitted to 15°C to 30°C (59°F to 86°F). Once reconstituted, store suspension under refrigeration at 2°C to 8°C (36°F to 46°F); do not freeze. Use within 10 days of preparation if stored at room temperature or within 17 days of preparation if stored under refrigeration.

Mechanism of Action Oseltamivir, a prodrug, is hydrolyzed to the active form, oseltamivir carboxylate (OC). OC inhibits influenza virus neuraminidase, an enzyme known to cleave the budding viral progeny from its cellular envelope attachment point (neuraminic acid) just prior to release.

Pharmacodynamics Reduction in the median time to improvement: 1.3 days

Pharmacokinetics (Adult data unless noted)

Absorption: Well absorbed from the GI tract

Distribution: Adults: V_{dss}: 23-26 L

Protein binding: 3% (oseltamivir carboxylate); 42% (oseltamivir phosphate)

Metabolism: Prodrug oseltamivir phosphate is metabolized by hepatic esterases to oseltamivir carboxylate (active); neither oseltamivir phosphate or oseltamivir carboxylate are a substrate, inducer, or inhibitor of cytochrome P450 isoenzymes

Half-life:

Oseltamivir phosphate: 1-3 hours

Oseltamivir carboxylate: 6-10 hours

Elimination: >99% of oseltamivir carboxylate is eliminated by renal excretion via glomerular filtration and tubular secretion

Dosing: Neonatal Influenza, treatment: Note: Treatment should ideally begin within 48 hours; however, initiation after 48 hours may decrease mortality or duration of illness.

Premature neonates: Limited data available: GA: 24 to 37 weeks: Oral: 1 mg/kg/dose twice daily; duration not determined. This dose is expected to produce serum concentrations similar to treatment doses in infants and young children based on retrospective pharmacokinetic trial of 20 neonates (Acosta, 2010; Bradley, 2011; CDC, 2011).

Full-term neonates (Bautista, 2010; Bradley, 2011; CDC, 2011; WHO, 2010):

PNA 0 to 13 days: Limited data available: Oral: 3 mg/kg/dose once daily for 5 days

PNA 14 to 28 days: Oral: 3 mg/kg/dose twice daily for 5 days

Dosing: Usual

Pediatric:

Influenza, treatment: Note: Treatment should ideally begin within 48 hours; however, initiation after 48 hours may decrease mortality or duration of illness. Hospitalized patients may require longer (eg, ≥10 days) treatment courses. Initiate as early as possible in any hospitalized patient with suspected/confirmed influenza (CDC, 2011).

Infants:

Weight-based dosing (preferred):

CDC Recommendations (independent of HIV status) (CDC, 2012; DHHS [pediatric], 2013): Manufacturer's labeling: Oral: 3 mg/kg/dose twice daily for 5 days

IDSA/PIDS Recommendations (Bradley, 2011): Oral:

1 to 8 months: 3 mg/kg/dose twice daily

9 to 11 months: 3.5 mg/kg/dose twice daily

*Fixed dosing (use **only** if weight not available)* (AAP, 2010): Limited data available: Oral:

<3 months: 12 mg twice daily for 5 days

3 to 5 months: 20 mg twice daily for 5 days

6 to 11 months: 25 mg twice daily for 5 days

Children 12 to 23 months:

CDC Recommendations (independent of HIV status) (CDC, 2012; DHHS [pediatric], 2013): Oral:

≤15 kg: 30 mg twice daily for 5 days

>15 to 23 kg: 45 mg twice daily for 5 days

>23 kg: See dosage recommendations below for children ≥2 years

IDSA/PIDS Recommendations (Bradley, 2011): Oral: 3.5 mg/kg/dose twice daily; weight-dependent maximum dose: Weight ≤15 kg: 30 mg; Weight >15 to 23 kg: 45 mg

Children ≥2-12 years and Adolescents (independent of HIV status): **Note:** Manufacturer's labeling consistent with current CDC and IDSA/PIDS recommendations (Bradley, 2011; CDC, 2012; DHHS [pediatric], 2013): Oral:

≤15 kg: 30 mg twice daily for 5 days

>15 to 23 kg: 45 mg twice daily for 5 days

>23 to 40 kg: 60 mg twice daily for 5 days

>40 kg: 75 mg twice daily for 5 days

Influenza, prophylaxis: Note: Initiate treatment within 48 hours of contact with an infected individual. Duration of prophylaxis dependent upon type of exposure or outbreak (eg, household exposure vs hospital outbreak); see below for further details.

Infants: Limited data available

Weight-directed dosing (preferred):

CDC Recommendation (independent of HIV status) (CDC, 2012; DHHS [pediatric], 2013): Oral:

<3 months: Not recommended unless clinically critical

3 to 11 months: 3 mg/kg/dose once daily

IDSA/PIDS Recommendations (Bradley, 2011): Oral:

3 to 8 months: 3 mg/kg/dose once daily

9 to 11 months: 3.5 mg/kg/dose once daily

*Fixed dosing (use **only** if weight not available)* (AAP, 2010): Oral:

<3 months: Not recommended unless clinically critical

3 to 5 months: 20 mg once daily

6 to 11 months: 25 mg once daily

Children 12 to 23 months:

CDC Recommendations (independent of HIV status) (CDC, 2012; DHHS [pediatric], 2013): Oral:

≤15 kg: 30 mg once daily

>15 to 23 kg: 45 mg dose once daily

>23 kg: See dosage recommendations below for weight.

IDSA/PIDS Recommendations (Bradley, 2011): Oral: 3.5 mg/kg/dose once daily; weight-dependent maximum dose: Weight: ≤15 kg: 30 mg; Weight >15-23 kg: 45 mg

Children: 2 to 12 years and Adolescents (independent of HIV status): **Note:** Manufacturer's labeling consistent with current CDC and IDSA/PIDS recommendations (Bradley, 2011; CDC, 2012; DHHS [pediatric], 2013): Oral:

≤15 kg: 30 mg once daily

>15 kg to ≤23 kg: 45 mg once daily

>23 kg to ≤40 kg: 60 mg once daily
>40 kg: 75 mg once daily

Prophylaxis duration:
Individual/household exposure:
Manufacturer labeling: 10 days
Alternate recommendations:
Non-HIV-exposed/-positive: 7 days (CDC, 2012)
HIV-exposed/-positive: 10 days for household exposure; 7 days for other exposures (DHHS [pediatric], 2013)
Community/institutional outbreak:
Manufacturer recommendation: May be used for up to 6 weeks
Alternate recommendations: Continue for ≥2 weeks and until ~7 days after identification of illness onset in the last patient (CDC, 2012) or until influenza activity in community subsides or immunity obtained from immunization (Bradley, 2011). During community outbreaks, duration of protection lasts for length of dosing period; safety and efficacy have been demonstrated for use up to 6 weeks in immunocompetent patients and safety has been demonstrated for use up to 12 weeks in patients who are immunocompromised.

Adult:
Influenza, prophylaxis: Oral: 75 mg once daily; initiate prophylaxis within 48 hours of contact with an infected individual; duration of prophylaxis: 10 days (manufacturer recommendation) or alternatively 7 days (CDC, 2012). During community outbreaks, duration of protection lasts for length of dosing period; safety and efficacy have been demonstrated for use up to 6 weeks in immunocompetent patients and safety has been demonstrated for use up to 12 weeks in patients who are immunocompromised.
Prophylaxis (institutional outbreak; CDC, 2012): Continue for ≥2 weeks and until ~7 days after identification of illness onset in the last patient

Influenza, treatment: Oral: 75 mg twice daily initiated within 48 hours of onset of symptoms; duration of treatment: 5 days

Note: Hospitalized patients with severe influenza infection may require longer (eg, ≥10 days) treatment courses. Some experts have recommended empirically doubling the treatment dose (ie, 150 mg twice daily) (CDC, 2009). However, more recent data suggests that doubling of the dose is not necessary (Ariano, 2010). Initiate as early as possible in any hospitalized patient with suspected/confirmed influenza regardless of the time of presentation from symptom onset (CDC, 2011); may be administered via naso- or orogastric tube in mechanically ventilated patients (Taylor, 2008).

Dosing adjustment in renal impairment:
Children >1 year: **Influenza, treatment** (Schreuder, 2010):
Limited data available: Hemodialysis: Fixed dosing:
≤15 kg: 7.5 mg after each hemodialysis session
>15 kg to ≤23 kg: 10 mg after each hemodialysis session
>23 kg to ≤40 kg: 15 mg after each hemodialysis session
>40 kg: 30 mg after each hemodialysis session
Adults:
CrCl >30 mL/minute: No dosage adjustment necessary
CrCl 10 to 30 mL/minute:
Treatment of influenza: Decrease dose to 75 mg once daily for 5 days
Prophylaxis of influenza: Decrease dose to 75 mg every other day **or** 30 mg once daily
CrCl <10 mL/minute: No recommended dosage regimens are available for patients with end-stage renal disease
CAPD: Limited data available:
Treatment: 30 mg once weekly for one dose to provide a 5-day duration [AMMI Canada (Aoki, 2012); Robson, 2006]

Prophylaxis: 30 mg once weekly until outbreak is over [AMMI Canada (Aoki, 2012)]
Hemodialysis: Limited data available:
Treatment [AMMI Canada (Aoki, 2012)]:
Low-flux hemodialysis: 30 mg after each dialysis session for 5 days
High-flux hemodialysis: 75 mg after each dialysis session for 5 days
Prophylaxis [AMMI Canada (Aoki, 2012)]:
Low-flux hemodialysis: 30 mg after alternate dialysis sessions until outbreak is over
High-flux hemodialysis: No data
Continuous renal replacement therapy (CRRT) (High-flux):
Treatment: Limited data available: 30 mg once daily for 5 days **or** 75 mg every 48 hours to provide a 5-day duration [AMMI Canada (Aoki, 2012); Ariano, 2010]
Prophylaxis: No data [AMMI Canada (Aoki, 2012)]
Continuous veno-venous hemodialysis (CVVHD): **Note:** Limited data available; optimal dosing has not been established: 150 mg twice daily administered via nasogastric or postpyloric feeding tube for suspected or confirmed H1N1 influenza demonstrated supratherapeutic oseltamivir carboxylate concentrations at effluent rates of 3300 ± 919 mL/hour; the authors determined that the manufacturer's recommended dosage of 75 mg once daily for patients with CrCl 10-30 mL/minute will likely achieve concentrations necessary to inhibit viral neuraminidase activity at these effluent rates; however, doses greater than 75 mg once daily may be required when using higher effluent rates (Eyler, 2012).

Administration Oral: May administer with or without food; may decrease stomach upset if administered with food
Capsules: May be opened and mixed with sweetened liquid [eg, chocolate syrup, corn syrup, caramel topping, or light brown sugar (dissolved in water)]. May be administered via naso- or orogastric tube in mechanically ventilated patients; for a 150 mg dose (in adults), dissolve powder from two 75 mg capsules in 20 mL of sterile water and inject down the NG/OG tube; follow with a 10 mL sterile water flush (Taylor, 2008)
Oral suspension: Reconstitute powder for suspension with 55 mL of water to a final concentration of 6 mg/mL (final volume: 60 mL); shake suspension well before use; measure dose in calibrated oral syringe; the manufacturer provided oral syringe should not be used to measure the dose for infants (<1 year of age); a smaller total volume syringe (ie, <10 mL) should be used to accurately measure dose

Monitoring Parameters Renal function, serum glucose in patients with diabetes mellitus; signs or symptoms of unusual behavior, including attempts at self-injury, confusion, and/or delirium
Critically ill patients: Repeat rRT-PCR or viral culture may help to determine ongoing viral replication

Dosage Forms Excipient information presented when available (limited, particularly for generics); consult specific product labeling.
Capsule, Oral, as phosphate:
Tamiflu: 30 mg, 45 mg, 75 mg
Suspension Reconstituted, Oral, as base:
Tamiflu: 6 mg/mL (60 mL) [contains saccharin sodium, sodium benzoate; tutti-frutti flavor]

Extemporaneous Preparations
If the commercially prepared oral suspension is not available, the manufacturer provides the following compounding information to prepare a **6 mg/mL** suspension in emergency situations.

1. Place the specified amount of water into a polyethyleneterephthalate (PET) or glass bottle.

2. Carefully separate the capsule body and cap and pour the contents of the required number of 75 mg capsules into the PET or glass bottle.
3. Gently swirl the suspension to ensure adequate wetting of the powder for at least 2 minutes.
4. Slowly add the specified amount of vehicle to the bottle.
5. Close the bottle using a child-resistant cap and shake well for 30 seconds to completely dissolve the active drug.
6. Label "Shake Well Before Use."

Stable for 35 days refrigerated or 5 days at room temperature. The Canadian labeling suggests that preparations made with water containing preservative (ie, 0.05% sodium benzoate) are stable for 49 days refrigerated and 10 days at room temperature. Shake gently prior to use. Do **not** dispense with dosing device provided with commercially-available product.

Preparation of Oseltamivir 6 mg/mL Suspension

Body Weight	Total Volume per Patient[1]	# of 75 mg Capsules[2]	Required Volume of Water	Required Volume of Vehicle[2,3]	Treatment Dose (wt based)[4]	Prophylactic Dose (wt based)[4]
≤15 kg	75 mL	6	5 mL	69 mL	5 mL (30 mg) twice daily for 5 days	5 mL (30 mg) once daily for 10 days
16-23 kg	100 mL	8	7 mL	91 mL	7.5 mL (45 mg) twice daily for 5 days	7.5 mL (45 mg) once daily for 10 days
24-40 kg	125 mL	10	8 mL	115 mL	10 mL (60 mg) twice daily for 5 days	10 mL (60 mg) once daily for 10 days
≥41 kg	150 mL	12	10 mL	137 mL	12.5 mL (75 mg) twice daily for 5 days	12.5 mL (75 mg) once daily for 10 days

[1]Entire course of therapy.

[2]Based on total volume per patient.

[3]Acceptable vehicles are cherry syrup, Ora-Sweet® SF, or simple syrup.

[4]Using 6 mg/mL suspension.

References

Acosta EP, Jester P, Gal P, et al, "Oseltamivir Dosing for Influenza Infection in Premature Neonates," *J Infect Dis*, 2010, 202(4):563-6.

Aoki FY, Allen UD, Stiver HG, Evans GA. AMMI Canada Guidelines. The use of antiviral drugs for influenza: guidance for practitioners 2012/2013. *Can J Infect Dis Med Microbiol*. 2012;23(4):e79-92. Available at http://www.ammi.ca/media/48038/14791_aoki_final.pdf. pdf

Ariano RE, Sitar DS, Zelenitsky SA, Z, et al. Enteric absorption and pharmacokinetics of oseltamivir in critically ill patients with pandemic (H1N1) influenza. *CMAJ*. 182(4):357-363.

Bradley JS, Byington CL, Shah SS, et al, "The Management of Community-Acquired Pneumonia in Infants and Children Older Than 3 Months of Age: Clinical Practice Guidelines by the Pediatric Infectious Diseases Society and the Infectious Diseases Society of America", *Clin Infect Dis*, 2011, 53(7):e25-76.

Centers for Disease Control and Prevention, "Antiviral Agents For the Treatment and Prophylaxis of Influenza: Recommendations of the Advisory Committee on Immunization Practices (ACIP)," *MMWR Recomm Rep*, 2011, 60 (RR-1): 1-25.

Centers for Disease Control and Prevention (CDC), "Influenza Antiviral Medications: Summary for Clinicians." Available at http://www.cdc.

gov/flu/professionals/antivirals/summary-clinicians.htm. Accessed on November 26, 2012.

Centers for Disease Control, "Intensive-Care Patients with Severe Novel Influenza A (H1N1) Virus Infection," July, 17, 2009. Available at: http://www.cdc.gov/mmwr/preview/mmwrhtml/mm5827a4.htm.

Center for Disease Control and Prevention, "Interim Guidance on the Use of Influenza Antiviral Agents During the 2010-2011 Influenza Season, December 15, 2010." Available at http://www.cdc.gov/flu/professionals/antivirals/index.htm.

Eyler RF, Heung M, Pleva M, et al. Pharmacokinetics of oseltamivir and oseltamivir carboxylate in critically ill patients receiving continuous venovenous hemodialysis and/or extracorporeal membrane oxygenation. *Pharmacotherapy*. 2012;32(12):1061-1069.

DHHS. Guidelines for the prevention and treatment of opportunistic infections among HIV-exposed and HIV-infected children: recommendations from the National Institutes of Health, Centers for Disease Control and Prevention, the HIV Medicine Association of the Infectious Diseases Society of America, the Pediatric Infectious Diseases Society, and the American Academy of Pediatrics. November 6, 2013. Available at http://aidsinfo.nih.gov

Harper SA, Bradley JS, Englund JA, et al, "Seasonal Influenza in Adults and Children - Diagnosis, Treatment, Chemoprophylaxis, and Institutional Outbreak Management: Clinical Practice Guidelines of the Infectious Diseases Society of America," *Clin Infect Dis*, 2009, 48 (8):1003-32.

Hayden FG, Atmar RL, Schilling M, et al, "Use of the Selective Oral Neuraminidase Inhibitor Oseltamivir to Prevent Influenza," *N Engl J Med*, 1999, 341(18):1336-43.

Kimberlin DW, Shalabi M, Abzug MJ, et al, "Safety of Oseltamivir Compared With the Adamantanes in Children Less Than 12 Months of Age," *Pediatr Infect Dis J*, 2009, Nov 25.

Robson R, Buttimore A, Lynn K, et al, "The Pharmacokinetics and Tolerability of Oseltamivir Suspension in Patients on Haemodialysis and Continuous Ambulatory Peritoneal Dialysis," *Nephrol Dial Transplant*, 2006, 21(9):2556-62.

Schreuder MF, van der Flier M, Knops NB, et al, "Oseltamivir Dosing in Children Undergoing Hemodialysis," *Clin Infect Dis*, 2010, 50 (10):1427-8.

Taylor WRJ, Thinh BN, Anh GT, et al, "Oseltamivir is Adequately Absorbed Following Nasogastric Administration to Adult Patients With Severe H5N1 Influenza," *PLoS One*, 2008, 3(10):e3410.

Treanor JJ, Hayden FG, Vrooman PS, et al, "Efficacy and Safety of the Oral Neuraminidase Inhibitor Oseltamivir in Treating Acute Influenza: A Randomized Controlled Trial. US Oral Neuraminidase Study Group," *JAMA*, 2000, 283(8):1016-24.

Whitley RJ, Hayden FG, Reisinger KS, et al, "Oral Oseltamivir Treatment of Influenza in Children," *Pediatr Infect Dis J*, 2001, 20 (2):127-33.

Writing Committee of the WHO Consultation on Clinical Aspects of Pandemic (H1N1) 2009 Influenza, Bautista E, Chotpitayasunondh T, et al, "Clinical Aspects of Pandemic 2009 Influenza A (H1N1) Virus Infection," *N Engl J Med*, 2010, 362(18):1708-19.

World Health Organization, "WHO Guidelines for Pharmacological Management of Pandemic Influenza A (H1N1) 2009 and Other Influenza Viruses." Available at: http://www.who.int/csr/resources/publications/swineflu/h1n1_guidelines_pharmaceutical_mngt.pdf.

◆ **Osmitrol** *see* Mannitol *on page 1301*

◆ **Osmitrol® (Can)** *see* Mannitol *on page 1301*

◆ **OsmoPrep** *see* Sodium Phosphates *on page 1913*

◆ **Osteocit® (Can)** *see* Calcium Citrate *on page 351*

◆ **Ostoforte® (Can)** *see* Ergocalciferol *on page 774*

◆ **OTFC (Oral Transmucosal Fentanyl Citrate)** *see* FentaNYL *on page 853*

◆ **Otrexup** *see* Methotrexate *on page 1367*

◆ **Ovace Plus** *see* Sulfacetamide (Topical) *on page 1944*

◆ **Ovace Plus Wash** *see* Sulfacetamide (Topical) *on page 1944*

◆ **Ovace Wash** *see* Sulfacetamide (Topical) *on page 1944*

◆ **Ovide** *see* Malathion *on page 1300*

◆ **Ovol® (Can)** *see* Simethicone *on page 1891*

Oxacillin (oks a SIL in)

Brand Names: U.S. Bactocill in Dextrose

Therapeutic Category Antibiotic, Penicillin (Antistaphylococcal)

Generic Availability (U.S.) May be product dependent

Use Treatment of bacterial infections, such as osteomyelitis, septicemia, endocarditis, and CNS infections, due to susceptible penicillinase-producing strains of *Staphylococcus* (FDA approved in all ages)

Pregnancy Risk Factor B

Pregnancy Considerations Adverse events have not been observed in animal reproduction studies. Oxacillin is distributed into the amniotic fluid and is detected in cord blood. Maternal use of penicillins has generally not resulted in an increased risk of adverse fetal effects.

Breast-Feeding Considerations Oxacillin is excreted in breast milk. The manufacturer recommends that caution be exercised when administering oxacillin to nursing women. Nondose-related effects could include modification of bowel flora.

Contraindications Hypersensitivity to oxacillin, other penicillins, or any component; premixed solutions: Hypersensitivity to corn or corn products

Warnings Serious and occasionally fatal hypersensitivity (anaphylactoid) reactions have been reported in patients on penicillin therapy, especially with a history of beta-lactam hypersensitivity, history of sensitivity to multiple allergens, or previous IgE-mediated reactions (eg, anaphylaxis, angioedema, urticaria); administration to patients with confirmed penicillin allergies should be avoided; in patients with confirmed cephalosporin allergy, consider skin testing to rule out cross-sensitivity to penicillins. Immediate treatment for an anaphylactic reaction should be available during administration. In neonates, elimination rate is decreased due to immature renal function; dosage adjustment is needed; hematuria and azotemia have occurred in neonates and infants receiving high-dose oxacillin. In a study of pediatric patients (5-19 years) receiving outpatient oxacillin, significantly less rash was reported in the nafcillin group (10.3%) compared to the oxacillin group (31.7%) (Maraqa, 2002). Cases of acute hepatitis and reversible elevations of serum transaminases have been reported with oxacillin. In adult and pediatric patients receiving outpatient antibiotic therapy, oxacillin has been shown to have a significantly higher incidence of adverse events as compared to nafcillin and other antibiotics in comparator group; adverse events reported include rash, leukopenia, and hepatitis; onset after 2-3 weeks of therapy; patients should be monitored periodically throughout therapy (Dahlgren, 1997; Faden, 2009; Maraqa, 2002; Vial, 1997). Prolonged use may result in fungal or bacterial superinfection, including *C. difficile*-associated diarrhea (CDAD) and pseudomembranous colitis; CDAD has been observed >2 months postantibiotic treatment.

Precautions Use with caution in patients with renal impairment; dosage modification may be required

Adverse Reactions
Central nervous system: Fever
Dermatologic: Rash
Gastrointestinal: Diarrhea, nausea, vomiting
Hematologic: Agranulocytosis, eosinophilia, leukopenia, neutropenia, thrombocytopenia
Hepatic: Hepatotoxicity, AST increased
Renal: Acute interstitial nephritis, hematuria
Miscellaneous: Serum sickness-like reactions

Drug Interactions

Metabolism/Transport Effects None known.

Avoid Concomitant Use
Avoid concomitant use of Oxacillin with any of the following: BCG; Probenecid

Increased Effect/Toxicity
Oxacillin may increase the levels/effects of: Methotrexate; Vitamin K Antagonists

The levels/effects of Oxacillin may be increased by: Probenecid

Decreased Effect
Oxacillin may decrease the levels/effects of: BCG; Mycophenolate; Sodium Picosulfate; Typhoid Vaccine

The levels/effects of Oxacillin may be decreased by: Tetracycline Derivatives

Stability
Premixed infusions: Store in a freezer at -20°C or less (-4°F or less). Thaw at room temperature or under refrigeration only. Thawed bags are stable for 21 days under refrigeration or 48 hours at room temperature. Do not refreeze.
Vials: Store intact vial at 20°C to 25°C (68°F to 77°F); reconstituted parenteral solution (250 mg/1.5 mL) is stable for 3 days at room temperature and 7 days when refrigerated. For I.V. infusion in NS (10-100 mg/mL), solution is stable for 4 days at room temperature and 7 days when refrigerated; for I.V. infusion in D_5W (10-30 mg/mL), solution is stable for 4 days when refrigerated.

Mechanism of Action Inhibits bacterial cell wall synthesis by binding to one or more of the penicillin-binding proteins (PBPs); which in turn inhibits the final transpeptidation step of peptidoglycan synthesis in bacterial cell walls, thus inhibiting cell wall biosynthesis. Bacteria eventually lyse due to ongoing activity of cell wall autolytic enzymes (autolysins and murein hydrolases) while cell wall assembly is arrested.

Pharmacokinetics (Adult data unless noted)
Distribution: Distributes into bile, pleural, and amniotic fluids; insignificant concentrations in CNS and aqueous humor
Protein binding: ~94%; primarily albumin
Metabolism: Hepatic to inactive metabolites
Half-life:
  Neonates (PNA: 8 to 15 days): 1.6 hours
  Infants and Children ≤2 years: 0.9 to 1.8 hours
  Adults: 20 to 60 minutes
Time to peak serum concentration:
  I.M.: Within 30 to 60 minutes
  I.V.: Within 5 minutes
Elimination: Urine and feces/bile (unchanged drug)

Dosing: Neonatal
General dosing, susceptible infection (nonmeningitis): I.M., I.V.:
  Manufacturer labeling: Premature Infants and Neonates: 25 mg/kg/day
  Alternate dosing (*Red Book* [AAP, 2012]):
    Body weight <1 kg:
      PNA ≤14 days: 25 mg/kg/dose every 12 hours
      PNA 15-28 days: 25 mg/kg/dose every 8 hours
    Body weight 1-2 kg:
      PNA ≤7 days: 25 mg/kg/dose every 12 hours
      PNA 8-28 days: 25 mg/kg/dose every 8 hours
    Body weight >2 kg:
      PNA ≤7 days: 25 mg/kg/dose every 8 hours
      PNA 8-28 days: 25 mg/kg/dose every 6 hours
Meningitis: I.V. (Tunkel, 2004):
  PNA 0-7 days: 75 mg/kg/day in divided doses every 8-12 hours
  PNA 8-28 days: 150-200 mg/kg/day in divided doses every 6-8 hours

Dosing: Usual
Pediatric:
General dosing, susceptible infection: Infants, Children, and Adolescents: I.M., I.V.:
  Mild to moderate infections: I.M., I.V.:
    Manufacturer's labeling:
      Infants and Children <40 kg: 50 mg/kg/day in divided doses every 6 hours
      Children ≥40 kg and Adolescents: 250 to 500 mg every 4 to 6 hours

Alternate dosing: 100 to 150 mg/kg/day in divided doses every 6 hours; maximum daily dose: 4000 mg/**day** [*Red Book* (AAP), 2012]

Severe infections: I.M., I.V.:

Manufacturer's labeling:

Infants and Children <40 kg: 100 mg/kg/day in divided doses every 4 to 6 hours; maximum daily dose: 4000 mg/**day**

Children ≥40 kg and Adolescents: 1000 mg every 4 to 6 hours; maximum daily dose: 4000 mg/**day**

Alternate dosing: 150 to 200 mg/kg/day in divided doses every 4 to 6 hours; maximum daily dose: 12 g/**day**; however, recent manufacturer labeling suggests a maximum daily dose of 4000 mg/**day** in adults when treating severe infection [*Red Book* (AAP), 2012]

Endocarditis, oxacillin/methicillin-susceptible staphylococci (Baddour, 2005): Infants, Children, and Adolescents: I.V.:

Native valve: 200 mg/kg/day in divided doses every 4 to 6 hours for 6 weeks with gentamicin for the first 3 to 5 days of therapy

Prosthetic valve: 200 mg/kg/day in divided doses every 4 to 6 hours for ≥6 weeks with rifampin (same duration as oxacillin) and with gentamicin for the first 2 weeks of therapy

Meningitis: Infants, Children, and Adolescents: I.V.: 200 mg/kg/day in divided doses every 6 hours; maximum daily dose: 12 g/**day** (Tunkel, 2004)

Pneumonia, community-acquired (CAP) moderate to severe infection, S. aureus (methicillin-susceptible): Infants ≥3 months, Children, and Adolescents: I.V.: 150 to 200 mg/kg/day divided every 6 to 8 hours (Bradley, 2011),

Skin and soft tissue infections: I.V.: 100 to 150 mg/kg/day in divided doses every 6 hours; maximum daily dose: 12 g/**day** (Stevens, 2005)

Adults:

General dosing, susceptible infection:

Mild to moderate infections: I.M., I.V.: 250 to 500 mg every 4 to 6 hours

Severe infections: I.M., I.V.: 1000 mg every 4 to 6 hours

Dosing adjustment in renal impairment: Not dialyzable (0% to 5%). There are no dosage adjustments provided in the manufacturer's labeling.

Dosing adjustment in hepatic impairment: There are no dosage adjustments provided in the manufacturer's labeling.

Administration Parenteral:

I.M. injection: Reconstitute each gram of oxacillin with 5.7 mL of SWI to make a 167 mg/mL solution; shake well until a clear solution is obtained. Administer by deep I.M. injection into a large muscle mass (eg, gluteus maximus); avoid sciatic nerve injury.

I.V.: Reconstitute each gram of oxacillin with 10 mL of SWI which results in 100 mg/mL solution; shake well until a clear solution is obtained. May be administered by direct I.V. injection over 10 minutes at a maximum concentration of 100 mg/mL or by intermittent I.V. infusion over 15 to 30 minutes at a final concentration ≤40 mg/mL; for peripheral administration, some centers infuse oxacillin at a concentration of 20 mg/mL over 60 minutes (Dahlgren, 1997)

Monitoring Parameters Periodic CBC with differential, urinalysis, BUN, serum creatinine, AST and ALT; number and type of stools/day for diarrhea; observe I.V. site for extravasation

Test Interactions May interfere with urinary glucose tests using cupric sulfate (Benedict's solution, Clinitest®); may inactivate aminoglycosides *in vitro*; false-positive urinary and serum proteins

Additional Information Sodium content: 1 g injection: 2.5 mEq

Dosage Forms Excipient information presented when available (limited, particularly for generics); consult specific product labeling.

Solution, Intravenous:

Bactocill in Dextrose: 1 g/50 mL (50 mL); 2 g/50 mL (50 mL)

Solution Reconstituted, Injection:

Generic: 1 g (1 ea); 2 g (1 ea); 10 g (1 ea)

Solution Reconstituted, Injection [preservative free]:

Generic: 1 g (1 ea); 2 g (1 ea); 10 g (1 ea)

References

Baddour LM, Wilson WR, Bayer AS, et al, "Infective Endocarditis: Diagnosis, Antimicrobial Therapy, and Management of Complications: A Statement for Healthcare Professionals From the Committee on Rheumatic Fever, Endocarditis, and Kawasaki Disease, Council on Cardiovascular Disease in the Young, and the Councils on Clinical Cardiology, Stroke, and Cardiovascular Surgery and Anesthesia, American Heart Association: Endorsed by the Infectious Diseases Society of America," *Circulation*, 2005, 111(23):e394-434.

Bradley JS, Byington CL, Shah SS, et al, "The Management of Community-Acquired Pneumonia in Infants and Children Older Than 3 Months of Age: Clinical Practice Guidelines by the Pediatric Infectious Diseases Society and the Infectious Diseases Society of America," *Clin Infect Dis*, 2011, 53(7):e25-76.

Dahlgren AF, "Adverse Drug Reactions in Home Care Patients Receiving Nafcillin or Oxacillin," *Am J Health Syst Pharm*, 1997, 54 (10):1176-9.

Faden D and Faden HS, "The High Rate of Adverse Drug Events in Children Receiving Prolonged Outpatient Parenteral Antibiotic Therapy for Osteomyelitis," *Pediatr Infect Dis J*, 2009, 28(6):539-41.

Maraqa NF, Gomez MM, Rathore MH, et al, "Higher Occurrence of Hepatotoxicity and Rash in Patients Treated With Oxacillin, Compared With Those Treated With Nafcillin and Other Commonly Used Antimicrobials," *Clin Infect Dis*, 2002, 34(1):50-4.

Olans RN and Weiner LB, "Reversible Oxacillin Hepatotoxicity," *J Pediatr*, 1976, 89(5):835-8.

Red Book: 2012 Report of the Committee on Infectious Diseases, "Antibacterial Drugs Dosage Tables," 29th ed, Pickering LK, ed, Elk Grove Village, IL: American Academy of Pediatrics, 2012, 808-16.

Oxacillin for injection [prescribing information]. Dayton, NJ: AuroMedics Pharma LLC; January 2013.

Oxacillin [prescribing information]. Dayton, NJ: AuroMedics Pharma LLC; January 2013.

Robinson DC, Cookson TL, and Grisafe JA, "Concentration Guidelines for Parenteral Antibiotics in Fluid-Restricted Patients," *Drug Intell Clin Pharm*, 1987, 21(12):985-9.

Stevens DL, Bisno AL, Chambers HF, et al, "Practice Guidelines for the Diagnosis and Management of Skin and Soft-Tissue Infections," *Clin Infect Dis*, 2005, 41(10):1373-406.

Tunkel AR, Hartman BJ, Kaplan SL, et al, "Practice Guidelines for the Management of Bacterial Meningitis," *Clin Infect Dis*, 2004, 39 (9):1267-84.

Vial T, Biour M, Descotes J, et al, "Antibiotic-Associated Hepatitis: Update From 1990," *Ann Pharmacother*, 1997, 31(2):204-20.

◆ **Oxacillin Sodium** *see* Oxacillin *on page 1555*

◆ **Oxalatoplatin** *see* Oxaliplatin *on page 1557*

◆ **Oxalatoplatinum** *see* Oxaliplatin *on page 1557*

Oxaliplatin (ox AL i pla tin)

Medication Safety Issues

Sound-alike/look-alike issues:

Oxaliplatin may be confused with Aloxi®, carboplatin, cisplatin

High alert medication:

This medication is in a class the Institute for Safe Medication Practices (ISMP) includes among its list of drug classes which have a heightened risk of causing significant patient harm when used in error.

Related Information

Emetogenic Potential of Antineoplastic Agents in Children *on page 2327*

Management of Drug Extravasations *on page 2255*

Safe Handling of Hazardous Drugs *on page 2419*

Brand Names: U.S. Eloxatin

Brand Names: Canada Eloxatin

Therapeutic Category Antineoplastic Agent, Alkylating Agent

◀ **Generic Availability (U.S.)** Yes

Use Treatment of stage III colon cancer (adjuvant) and advanced colorectal carcinoma (FDA approved in adults); has also been used in the treatment of relapsed/refractory childhood solid tumors including CNS and non-CNS tumors

Pregnancy Risk Factor D

Pregnancy Considerations Adverse events were observed in animal reproduction studies at one-tenth the equivalent human dose. Women of childbearing potential should be advised to avoid pregnancy and use effective contraception during treatment.

Canadian labeling: Use in pregnant women is contraindicated in the Canadian labeling. Males should be advised not to father children during and for up to 6 months following therapy. May cause permanent infertility in males. Prior to initiating therapy, advise males desiring to father children, to seek counseling on sperm storage.

Breast-Feeding Considerations It is not known if oxaliplatin is excreted in breast milk. Due to the potential for serious adverse reactions in the nursing infant, the decision to discontinue breast-feeding or to discontinue oxaliplatin should take into account the benefits of treatment to the mother.

Contraindications Hypersensitivity to oxaliplatin, other platinum-containing compounds, or any component

Warnings Hazardous agent; use appropriate precautions for handling and disposal (NIOSH, 2012). Anaphylactic-like reactions may occur within minutes of oxaliplatin administration **[U.S. Boxed Warning]**; manage reactions with supportive therapy, epinephrine, corticosteroids, and antihistamines and discontinuation of therapy; oxygen and bronchodilators have also been used (Kim, 2009). Grade 3 or 4 hypersensitivity has been observed. Allergic reactions are similar to reactions reported with other platinum analogs, and may occur with any cycle. Reactions typically occur after multiple cycles; in retrospective reviews, reaction occurred at a median of 7-9 cycles, with an onset of 5-70 minutes (Kim, 2009; Polyzos, 2009). Symptoms may include bronchospasm (rare), erythema, hypotension (rare), pruritus, rash, and/or urticaria; previously-untreated patients have also experienced flushing, diaphoresis, diarrhea, shortness of breath, chest pain, hypotension, syncope, and disorientation. According to the manufacturer, rechallenge is contraindicated (deaths due to anaphylaxis have been associated with platinum derivatives). In patients rechallenged after mild hypersensitivity, reaction recurred at a higher level of severity; for patients with severe hypersensitivity, rechallenge (with 2-3 days of antihistamine and corticosteroid premedication, and prolongation of infusion time) allowed for 2-4 additional oxaliplatin cycles; however, rechallenge was not feasible in nearly two-thirds of patients due to the severity of the initial reaction (Polyzos, 2009).

Two different types of peripheral sensory neuropathy may occur: 1) an acute (within first 2 days), reversible (resolves within 14 days) sensory neuropathy with peripheral symptoms that are often exacerbated by cold (may include pharyngolaryngeal dysesthesia); avoid mucositis prophylaxis with ice chips during oxaliplatin infusion (may exacerbate symptoms); commonly recurs with subsequent doses; 2) persistent (>14 days) sensory neuropathy which presents with paresthesias, dysesthesias, hypoesthesias, and impaired proprioception that often interferes with daily activities (eg, writing, buttoning, swallowing); these symptoms may improve in some patients upon discontinuing treatment. Several retrospective studies as well as a small, underpowered randomized trial have suggested calcium and magnesium infusions before and after oxaliplatin administration may reduce incidence of cumulative sensory neuropathy; however, a recent abstract of an ongoing, placebo-controlled, double-blind study in

patients with colorectal cancer suggests there is no benefit of calcium and magnesium in preventing sensory neuropathy or in decreasing oxaliplatin discontinuation rates (Loprinzi, 2013).

May cause pulmonary fibrosis; withhold treatment for unexplained pulmonary symptoms (eg, crackles, dyspnea, nonproductive cough, pulmonary infiltrates) until interstitial lung disease or pulmonary fibrosis are excluded. May cause hepatotoxicity including rare cases of hepatitis and hepatic failure. Liver biopsy has revealed peliosis, nodular regenerative hyperplasia, sinusoidal alterations, perisinusoidal fibrosis, and veno-occlusive lesions. The presence of hepatic vascular disorders, including veno-occlusive disease, should be considered, especially in individuals developing portal hypertension or who present with elevated liver function tests. Posterior leukoencephalopathy syndrome (RPLS) has been reported with use. Signs/symptoms include headache, mental status changes, seizure, blurred vision, blindness and/or other vision changes; may be associated with hypertension. Diagnosis is confirmed with brain imaging.

Oxaliplatin is an irritant with vesicant-like properties; ensure proper needle or catheter placement prior to and during infusion; avoid extravasation. Oxaliplatin is associated with a moderate emetic potential; antiemetics are recommended to prevent nausea and vomiting. When administered as sequential infusions, taxane derivatives (docetaxel, paclitaxel) should be administered before platinum derivatives to limit myelosuppression and enhance efficacy. Oxaliplatin may cause fetal harm; pregnancy should be avoided during therapy. Potentially significant interactions may exist, requiring dose or frequency adjustment, additional monitoring, and/or selection of alternative therapy. Consult drug interactions database for more detailed information.

Precautions Use caution in patients with renal impairment since increased toxicity may occur; reduce initial dose in severe impairment.. Should be administered under the supervision of a physician experienced in the use of cancer chemotherapy agents.

Adverse Reactions

Cardiovascular: Chest pain, edema, flushing, peripheral edema, thromboembolism

Central nervous system: Dizziness, fatigue, fever, headache, insomnia, pain, peripheral neuropathy (may be dose limiting), rigors

Dermatologic: Alopecia, palmar-plantar erythrodysesthesia, skin rash

Endocrine & metabolic: Dehydration, hypokalemia

Gastrointestinal: Abdominal pain, anorexia, constipation, diarrhea, hiccups, palmar-plantar erythrodysesthesia, dyspepsia, dysphagia, flatulence, gastroesophageal reflux, mucositis, nausea, stomatitis, vomiting

Genitourinary: Dysuria

Hematologic & oncologic: Anemia, leukopenia, neutropenia, thrombocytopenia

Hepatic: Increased serum ALT, increased serum AST, increased serum bilirubin

Hypersensitivity: Hypersensitivity reaction (includes urticaria, pruritus, facial flushing, shortness of breath, bronchospasm, diaphoresis, hypotension, syncope)

Local: Injection site reaction (redness/swelling/pain)

Neuromuscular & skeletal: Arthralgia, back pain

Ocular: Abnormal lacrimation

Renal: Increased serum creatinine

Respiratory: Cough, dyspnea, epistaxis, pharyngitis, pharyngolaryngeal dysesthesia, rhinitis, upper respiratory tract infection

Miscellaneous: Fever

Rare but important or life-threatening (reported with mono- and combination therapy): Abnormal gait, acute renal failure, anaphylaxis, anaphylactic shock, anaphylactoid reaction, angioedema, aphonia, ataxia, blepharoptosis, cerebral hemorrhage, colitis, cranial nerve palsy, decreased deep tendon reflex, deafness, decreased visual acuity, diplopia, dysarthria, eosinophilic pneumonitis, fasciculations, febrile neutropenia,hematuria, hemolysis, hemolytic anemia (immuno-allergic), hemolytic-uremic syndrome, hemorrhage, hepatic failure, hepatic sinusoidal obstruction syndrome (SOS; venoocclusive disease), hepatitis, hepatotoxicity, hypertension, hypomagnesemia, hypoxia, idiopathic noncirrhotic portal hypertension (nodular regenerative hyperplasia), increased INR, increased serum alkaline phosphatase, infusion related reaction (extravasation [including necrosis]), interstitial nephritis (acute), interstitial pulmonary disease, intestinal obstruction, laryngospasm, Lhermitte's sign, metabolic acidosis, muscle spasm, myoclonus, neutropenic enterocolitis, neutropenic infection (sepsis), optic neuritis, pancreatitis, prolonged prothrombin time, purpura, rectal hemorrhage, renal tubular necrosis, reversible posterior leukoencephalopathy syndrome (RPLS), rhabdomyolysis, seizure, sepsis, temporary vision loss, thrombocytopenia (immuno-allergic), trigeminal neuralgia, visual field loss, voice disorder

Drug Interactions

Metabolism/Transport Effects None known.

Avoid Concomitant Use

Avoid concomitant use of Oxaliplatin with any of the following: BCG; CloZAPine; Dipyrone; Natalizumab; Pimecrolimus; Tacrolimus (Topical); Tofacitinib; Vaccines (Live)

Increased Effect/Toxicity

Oxaliplatin may increase the levels/effects of: CloZAPine; Leflunomide; Natalizumab; Taxane Derivatives; Tofacitinib; Topotecan; Vaccines (Live); Vitamin K Antagonists

The levels/effects of Oxaliplatin may be increased by: Denosumab; Dipyrone; Pimecrolimus; Roflumilast; Tacrolimus (Topical); Trastuzumab

Decreased Effect

Oxaliplatin may decrease the levels/effects of: BCG; Cardiac Glycosides; Coccidioidin Skin Test; Fosphenytoin-Phenytoin; Sipuleucel-T; Vaccines (Inactivated); Vaccines (Live); Vitamin K Antagonists

The levels/effects of Oxaliplatin may be decreased by: Echinacea

Stability Hazardous agent; use appropriate precautions for handling and disposal (NIOSH, 2012). Store intact vials at 25°C (77°F); excursions permitted to 15°C to 30°C (59°F to 86°F); do not freeze. Protect concentrated solution from light; store in original outer carton. According to the manufacturer, solutions diluted for infusion are stable up to 6 hours at room temperature or up to 24 hours under refrigeration. Oxaliplatin solution diluted with D_5W to a final concentration of 0.7 mg/mL (polyolefin container) has been shown to retain >90% of the original concentration for up to 30 days when stored at room temperature or refrigerated; artificial light did not affect the concentration (Andre, 2007). As this study did not examine sterility, refrigeration would be preferred to limit microbial growth. Solutions diluted for infusion do not require protection from light.

Mechanism of Action Oxaliplatin, a platinum derivative, is an alkylating agent. Following intracellular hydrolysis, the platinum compound binds to DNA forming cross-links which inhibit DNA replication and transcription, resulting in cell death. Cytotoxicity is cell-cycle nonspecific.

Pharmacokinetics (Adult data unless noted)

Distribution: V_d: 440 L

Protein binding: >90%

Metabolism: Nonenzymatic biotransformation (rapid and extensive), forms active and inactive derivatives

Half-life:

Children: Oxaliplatin ultrafilterable platinum (terminal): Median: 293 hours; range: 187-662 hours (Beaty, 2010)

Adults: Oxaliplatin ultrafilterable platinum:

Distribution:

Alpha phase: 0.4 hours

Beta phase: 16.8 hours

Terminal: 391 hours

Elimination: Urine (~54%); feces (~2%)

Dosing: Usual Refer to individual protocols; details concerning dosing in combination regimens should also be consulted.

Children and Adolescents: **Refractory or relapsed solid tumors:** Limited data available; efficacy results highly variable; has shown limited activity in pediatric patients (primarily some delayed tumor progression reported) and an acceptable safety profile; should not be used first-line; reserved for refractory cases. I.V.:

85 mg/m² or 100 mg/m² on day 1 of a 14 day cycle in combination with gemcitabine or fluorouracil/leucovorin (Georger, 2011; Macy, 2013); **or** 105 or 130 mg/m² on day 1 of a 21 day cycle in combination with doxorubicin or etoposide (respectively) (MacGregor, 2009; Mascarenhas, 2013).

Adults:

Advanced colorectal cancer: I.V.: 85 mg/m² every 2 weeks until disease progression or unacceptable toxicity; administer in combination with fluorouracil/leucovorin calcium

Stage III colon cancer (adjuvant): I.V.: 85 mg/m² every 2 weeks for 12 cycles; administer in combination with fluorouracil/leucovorin calcium

Dosing adjustment for obesity: Adults: ASCO Guidelines for appropriate chemotherapy dosing in obese adults with cancer: Utilize patient's actual body weight (full weight) for calculation of body surface area- or weight-based dosing, particularly when the intent of therapy is curative; manage regimen-related toxicities in the same manner as for nonobese patients; if a dose reduction is utilized due to toxicity, consider resumption of full weight-based dosing with subsequent cycles, especially if cause of toxicity (eg, hepatic or renal impairment) is resolved (Griggs, 2012).

Dosing adjustments for toxicity: Adults:

Acute toxicities: Longer infusion time (6 hours) may mitigate acute toxicities (eg, pharyngolaryngeal dysesthesia)

Neurosensory events:

Persistent (>7 days) grade 2 neurosensory events:

Adjuvant treatment of stage III colon cancer: Reduce dose to 75 mg/m²

Advanced colorectal cancer: Reduce dose to 65 mg/m²

Consider withholding oxaliplatin for grade 2 neuropathy lasting >7 days despite dose reduction.

Persistent (>7 days) grade 3 neurosensory events: Consider discontinuing oxaliplatin.

Gastrointestinal toxicity (grade 3/4):

Adjuvant treatment of stage III colon cancer: Delay next dose until recovery from toxicity, then reduce dose to 75 mg/m²

Advanced colorectal cancer: Delay next dose until recovery from toxicity, then reduce dose to 65 mg/m²

Hematologic toxicity (grade 4 neutropenia or grade 3/4 thrombocytopenia):

Adjuvant treatment of stage III colon cancer: Delay next dose until neutrophils recover to ≥1500/mm³ and platelets recover to ≥75,000/mm³, then reduce dose to 75 mg/m².

Advanced colorectal cancer: Delay next dose until neutrophils recover to ≥1500/mm³ and platelets recover to ≥75,000/mm³, then reduce dose to 65 mg/m².

◀ **Pulmonary toxicity (unexplained respiratory symptoms, including nonproductive cough, dyspnea, crackles, pulmonary infiltrates):** Discontinue until interstitial lung disease or pulmonary fibrosis have been excluded.

Dosing adjustment in renal impairment: Adults:

Mild to moderate impairment: No dosage adjustment required

Severe impairment: Reduce dose to 65 mg/m^2

Dosing adjustment in hepatic impairment: Adults: There are no dosage adjustments provided in the manufacturer's labeling; however, some have suggested that dosage adjustment is not necessary (Doroshow, 2003; Synold, 2007)

Administration Hazardous agent; use appropriate precautions for handling and disposal (NIOSH, 2012). In adults, oxaliplatin is associated with moderate emetic potential and preventative antiemetics recommended. **Do not prepare using a chloride-containing solution such as NaCl** due to rapid conversion to monochloroplatinum, dichloroplatinum, and diaquoplatinum; all highly reactive in sodium chloride (Takimoto, 2007).

Aqueous solution: Dilution with D$_5$W (250 or 500 mL) is required prior to administration.

Lyophilized powder: Use only SWFI or D$_5$W to reconstitute powder. To obtain final concentration of 5 mg/mL add 10 mL of diluent to 50 mg vial or 20 mL diluent to 100 mg vial. Gently swirl vial to dissolve powder. Dilution with D$_5$W (250 or 500 mL) is required prior to administration. Discard unused portion of vial.

I.V.: Administer as I.V. infusion over 2-6 hours. Flush infusion line with D$_5$W prior to administration of any concomitant medication. Do **not** use I.V. administration sets containing aluminum.

Extravasation management: If extravasation occurs, stop infusion immediately and disconnect (leave cannula/needle in place); gently aspirate extravasated solution (do **NOT** flush the line); remove needle/cannula; elevate extremity. Information conflicts regarding use of warm or cold compresses. Cold compresses could potentially precipitate or exacerbate peripheral neuropathy (de Lemos, 2005).

Vesicant/Extravasation Risk Irritant with vesicant-like properties

Cold compress may cause local vasoconstriction and reduce cellular injury; however, may cause or exacerbate peripheral neuropathy; warm compresses may increase local drug removal, although may also increase cellular uptake and injury (de Lemos, 2005).

Monitoring Parameters CBC with differential, hemoglobin, platelet count, blood chemistries (including serum creatinine, ALT, AST, and bilirubin) prior to each cycle; INR and prothrombin time (in patients on oral anticoagulant therapy); signs of neuropathy, hypersensitivity reaction, respiratory effects, and/or RPLS.

Dosage Forms Excipient information presented when available (limited, particularly for generics); consult specific product labeling.

Solution, Intravenous [preservative free]:

Eloxatin: 50 mg/10 mL (10 mL); 100 mg/20 mL (20 mL); 200 mg/40 mL (40 mL)

Generic: 50 mg/10 mL (10 mL); 100 mg/20 mL (20 mL)

Solution Reconstituted, Intravenous [preservative free]:

Generic: 50 mg (1 ea); 100 mg (1 ea)

References

André P, Cisternino S, Roy AL, et al, "Stability of Oxaliplatin in Infusion Bags Containing 5% Dextrose Injection," *Am J Health Syst Pharm*, 2007, 64(18):1950-4.

Beaty O, Berg S, Blaney S, et.al. A phase II trial and pharmacokinetic study of oxaliplatin in children with refractory solid tumors: a children's oncology group study. *Pediatr Blood Cancer*. 2010;55:440-445.

de Lemos ML, Walisser S, Management of extravasation of oxaliplatin. *J Oncol Pharm Pract*. 2005;11(4):159-162.

Doroshow JH, Synold TW, Gandara D, et al, "Pharmacology of Oxaliplatin in Solid Tumor Patients With Hepatic Dysfunction: A Preliminary Report of the National Cancer Institute Organ Dysfunction Working Group," *Semin Oncol*, 2003, 30(4 Suppl 15):14-9.

Geoerger B, Chisholm J, Deley ML, et al. Phase II study of gemcitabine combined with oxaliplatin in relapsed or refractory paediatric solid malignancies: an innovative therapy for children with Cancer European Consortium Study. *European Journal of Cancer*. 2011;47:230-238.

Griggs JJ, Mangu PB, Anderson H, et al. Appropriate chemotherapy dosing for obese adult patients with cancer: American Society of Clinical Oncology clinical practice guideline. *J Clin Oncol*. 2012;30 (13):1553-1561.

Kim BH, Bradley T, Tai J, et al. Hypersensitivity to oxaliplatin: an investigation of incidence and risk factors, and literature review. *Oncology*. 2009;76(4):231-238.

Loprinzi CL, Qin R, Dakhil SR, et al. Phase III randomized, placebo-controlled, double-blind study of intravenous calcium and magnesium to prevent oxaliplatin-induced sensory neurotoxicity (N08CB/Alliance). *J Clin Oncol*. 2013 Dec 2. [Epub ahead of print].

Macy ME, Duncan T, Whitlock J, et.al. A multi-center phase 1b study of oxaliplatin (NSC #266046) in combination with fluorouracil and leucovorin in pediatric patients with advanced solid tumors. *Pediatric Blood Cancer*. 2013;60:230-236.

Mascarenhas L, Malogolowkin M, Armenian SH, Sposto R, Venkatramani R. A phase I study of oxaliplatin and doxorubicin in pediatric patients with relapsed or refractory extracranial non-hematopoietic soldi tumors. *Pediatric Blood Cancer*. 2013;60:1103-1107.

McGregor LM, Spunt SL, Santana VM, et.al. Phase I study of an oxaliplatin-etoposide regimen in pediatric patients with recurrent solid tumors. *Cancer*. 2009;115(3):655-664.

National Institute for Occupational Safety and Health (NIOSH), "NIOSH List of Antineoplastic and Other Hazardous Drugs in Healthcare Settings 2012." Available at http://www.cdc.gov/niosh/docs/2012-150/pdfs/2012-150.pdf. Accessed January 21, 2013.

Polyzos A, Tsavaris N, Gogas H, et al. Clinical features of hypersensitivity reactions to oxaliplatin: a 10-year experience. *Oncology*. 2009;76(1):36-41.

Synold TW, Takimoto CH, Doroshow JH, et al, "Dose-Escalating and Pharmacologic Study of Oxaliplatin in Adult Cancer Patients With Impaired Hepatic Function: A National Cancer Institute Organ Dysfunction Working Group Study," *Clin Cancer Res*, 2007, 13 (12):3660-6.

Takimoto CH, Graham MA, Lockwood G, et al, "Oxaliplatin Pharmacokinetics and Pharmacodynamics in Adult Cancer Patients With Impaired Renal Function," *Clin Cancer Res*, 2007, 13(16):4832-9.

◆ **Oxandrin** see Oxandrolone on page 1560

Oxandrolone (oks AN droe lone)

Brand Names: U.S. Oxandrin

Therapeutic Category Androgen

Generic Availability (U.S.) Yes

Use Adjunctive therapy to promote weight gain after weight loss following extensive surgery, chronic infections, or severe trauma, and in some patients who, without definite pathophysiologic reasons, fail to gain or to maintain normal weight; to offset protein catabolism with prolonged corticosteroid administration and for the relief of bone pain associated with osteoporosis (All indications: FDA approved in children and adults); has also been used in the management of Turner syndrome in girls, constitutional delay of growth and puberty (CDGP), and for postoperative burn management to increase lean muscle mass and promote wound healing.

Pregnancy Risk Factor X

Pregnancy Considerations Use is contraindicated in women who are or may become pregnant; masculinization of the fetus has been reported.

Breast-Feeding Considerations It is not known if oxandrolone is excreted in breast milk. Due to the potential for serious adverse reactions in the nursing infant, breast-feeding is not recommended.

Contraindications Hypersensitivity to oxandrolone or any component; nephrosis; in females, carcinoma of breast with hypercalcemia; in males, prostate or breast cancer; hypercalcemia; pregnancy

Warnings Anabolic steroids may cause peliosis hepatis or liver cell tumors which may not be apparent until life-threatening liver failure or intra-abdominal hemorrhage develops **[U.S. Boxed Warning]**; discontinue if cholestatic hepatitis with jaundice or abnormal liver function tests; drug-induced jaundice is generally reversible when oxandrolone is discontinued; use with caution in patients with hepatic impairment.

May accelerate bone maturation without producing compensatory gain in linear growth in children; effect may continue for 6 months after the drug is stopped; in prepubertal children, perform radiographic examination of the left hand and wrist every 6 months to determine the rate of bone maturation and to assess the effect of treatment on the epiphyseal centers. May cause mild virilization in females; monitor for signs of virilization (deepening of the voice, hirsutism, acne, clitoromegaly); discontinue if evidence of mild virilization; discontinuation may prevent irreversible virilization.

May cause hypercalcemia in patients with breast cancer by stimulating osteolysis; discontinue if hypercalcemia occurs; use is contraindicated in patients with hypercalcemia and in patients with known or suspected carcinoma of the breast (in males) or in females with hypercalcemia and carcinoma of the breast. May cause blood lipid changes with increased risk of arteriosclerosis **[U.S. Boxed Warning]**.

May cause suppression of clotting factors II, V, VII, and X and increases in prothrombin time; use caution with concomitant warfarin therapy; warfarin dose may need to be significantly decreased.

Precautions Use with caution in patients with renal or hepatic impairment. Use with caution in patients with diabetes mellitus; may cause adverse effects on glucose tolerance; monitor carefully. Use with caution in patients with conditions influenced by edema (eg, cardiovascular disease, migraine, seizure disorder, renal impairment); may cause fluid retention. Use with caution in patients with COPD; monitor for COPD exacerbation or fluid retention. Anabolic steroids have not been shown to improve athletic ability.

Adverse Reactions

Cardiovascular: Edema

Central nervous system: Depression, excitation, insomnia

Dermatologic: Acne (females and prepubertal males)
Also reported in females: Hirsutism, male-pattern baldness

Endocrine & metabolic: Electrolyte imbalances, glucose intolerance, gonadotropin secretion inhibited, gynecomastia, HDL decreased, LDL increased, libido changes
Also reported in females: Clitoral enlargement, menstrual irregularities

Genitourinary:
Prepubertal males: Erections increased or persistent, penile enlargement
Postpubertal males: Bladder irritation, epididymitis, impotence, oligospermia, priapism (chronic), testicular atrophy, testicular function

Hematologic: Prothrombin time increased, suppression of clotting factors

Hepatic: Alkaline phosphatase increased, ALT increased, AST increased, bilirubin increased, cholestatic jaundice, hepatic necrosis (rare), hepatocellular neoplasms, peliosis hepatis (with long-term therapy)

Neuromuscular & skeletal: CPK increased, premature closure of epiphyses (in children)

Renal: Creatinine excretion increased

Miscellaneous: Bromsulfophthalein retention, habituation, voice alteration (deepening, in females)

Drug Interactions

Metabolism/Transport Effects None known.

Avoid Concomitant Use There are no known interactions where it is recommended to avoid concomitant use.

Increased Effect/Toxicity ACTH, adrenal steroids may increase risk of edema and acne. Oxandrolone enhances the hypoprothrombinemic effects of oral anticoagulants, and enhances the hypoglycemic effects of insulin and sulfonylureas (oral hypoglycemics).

Decreased Effect There are no known significant interactions involving a decrease in effect.

Stability Store at 20°C to 25°C (68°F to 77°F).

Mechanism of Action Synthetic testosterone derivative with similar androgenic and anabolic actions

Pharmacokinetics (Adult data unless noted)

Absorption: Oral: Well absorbed (Orr, 2004)

Protein binding: 95% (Orr, 2004)

Half-life elimination: 10-13 hours

Time to peak serum concentration: ~1 hour (Orr, 2004)

Elimination: Urine (28% as unchanged drug) (Orr, 2004)

Dosing: Usual

Pediatric:

Weight gain, adjunct: Children and Adolescents: Oral: Total daily dose: ≤0.1 mg/kg; may be repeated intermittently as needed; in adult patients, the daily dose is divided 2-4 times daily; typical duration of therapy: 2-4 weeks

Burn management, severe; to increase lean muscle mass and promote wound healing: Limited data available: Children and Adolescents: Oral: 0.1 mg/kg/dose twice daily for up to 12 months has been shown to increase lean body mass, bone mineral density, and muscle strength; shortened length of ICU stay and improved donor site wound healing were also observed (Hart, 2001; Jeschke, 2007; Murphy, 2004; Porro, 2012; Pzkora, 2005). Benefits have been shown to persist for up to 5 years post burn (Porro, 2012; Przkora, 2005).

Constitutional delay of growth and puberty (CDGP) (males): Limited data available: Children and Adolescents 9-16 years: Oral: 1.25-2.5 mg once daily in the evening; usual duration: 3-12 months although longer (~5 years) has been reported (Albanese, 1994; Buyukgebiz, 1990; Papadimitriou, 1991; Schroor, 1995; Stanhope, 1985; Stanhope, 1988; Tse, 1990)

Turner Syndrome (females): Limited data available: Children and Adolescents ≥8 years: Oral: Reported range: 0.03-0.06 mg/kg/day at bedtime in combination with growth hormone and/or estrogen; maximum single dose: 2.5 mg; due to risks of dose-related virilization, doses ≥0.05 mg/kg/day should generally be avoided. Typically, therapy initiated at 8-9 years of age and continued until goal height attained or further growth is unlikely (bone age ≥14 years and growth velocity <2 cm/year) [Bareille, 1997; NIH (Bondy), 2007, Freriks, 2013; Gault, 2011; Haeusler, 1995; Menke, 2010, Nilsson, 1996].

Adult: **Weight gain, adjunct:** Oral: 2.5-20 mg/day in 2-4 divided based on individual response; a course of therapy of 2-4 weeks is usually adequate. This may be repeated intermittently as needed.

Dosing adjustment in renal impairment: There are no dosage adjustments provided in the manufacturer's labeling. Caution is recommended because of the propensity of oxandrolone to cause edema and water retention.

Dosing adjustment in hepatic impairment: There are no dosage adjustments provided in the manufacturer's labeling.

Monitoring Parameters Liver function tests, lipid profile, hemoglobin/hematocrit; INR/PT in patients on anticoagulant therapy

Children: Radiographs of left wrist every 6 months to assess bone maturation

Females: Signs of virilization (deepening voice, hirsutism, acne, clitoromegaly); urine and serum calcium in women with breast cancer

◄ **Test Interactions** May suppress factors II, V, VII, and X; may increase PT; may decrease thyroxine-binding globulin and radioactive iodine uptake

Controlled Substance C-III

Dosage Forms Excipient information presented when available (limited, particularly for generics); consult specific product labeling.

Tablet, Oral:
Oxandrin: 2.5 mg [scored]
Oxandrin: 10 mg
Generic: 2.5 mg, 10 mg

Extemporaneous Preparations A 1 mg/mL oral suspension may be made with tablets and either a 1:1 mixture of Ora-Sweet® and Ora-Plus®, or a 1:1 mixture of Ora-Sweet® SF and Ora-Plus®. Crush twenty-four 2.5 mg tablets in a mortar to a fine powder. Add small portions of chosen vehicle and mix to a uniform paste; mix while adding the vehicle in incremental proportions to **almost** 60 mL; transfer to a calibrated bottle, rinse mortar with vehicle, and add quantity of vehicle sufficient to make 60 mL. Thoroughly mix the suspension by shaking. Label "shake well" and "protect from light". Stable for 90 days at room temperature (Johnson, 2011).

Johnson CE, Cober MP, Hawkins KA, et al, "Stability of Extemporaneously Prepared Oxandrolone Oral Suspensions," Am J Health-Syst Pharm, 2011, 68(6):519-21.

References

Albanese A, Kewley GD, Long A, Pearl KN, Robins DG, Stanhope R. Oral treatment for constitutional delay of growth and puberty in boys: a randomized trial of an anabolic steroid or testosterone undecanoate. Arch Dis Child. 1994;71(4):315-317.

Bareille P, Massarano AA, Stanhope R. Final height outcome in girls with Turner syndrome treated with a combination of low dose oestrogen and oxandrolone. Eur J Pediatr. 1997;156:358-362.

Bondy CA, Turner Syndrome Consensus Study Group. Care of girls and women with Turner Syndrome: a guideline of the Turner Syndrome Study Group. J Clin Endocrinol Metab. 2007;92(1):10-25.

Buuykgebiz A, Hindmarsh PC, Brook CGD. Treatment of constitutional delay of growth and puberty with oxandrolone compared with growth hormone. Arch Dis Child. 1990;65(4):448-449.

Freriks K, Sas TCJ, Traas MAF, et al. Long-term effects of previous oxandrolone treatment in adult women with Turner syndrome. Eur J Endocrinol. 2012;168(1):91-99.

Gault EJ, Perry R, Cole TJ, et al. Effect of oxandrolone and timing of pubertal induction on final height in Turner's syndrome: randomized, double blind, placebo controlled trial. BMJ. 2011;342:d1980.

Hart DW, Wolf SE, Ramzy PI, et al. Anabolic effects of oxandrolone after severe burn. Ann Surg. 2001;233(4):556-564.

Haeusler G, Frisch H, Schmitt K, et.al. Treatment of patients with Ullrich-Turner syndrome with conventional doses of growth hormone and the combination with testosterone or oxandrolone: effect on growth, IGF-I and IGFBP-3 concentrations. Eur J Pediatr. 1995;154(6):437-444.

Jeschke MG, Finnerty CC, Suman OE, Kulp G, Mlcak RP, Herndon DN. The effect of oxandrolone on the endocrinologic, inflammatory, and hypermetabolic responses during the acute phase postbrn. Ann Surg. 2007;246(3):351-360.

Menke LA, Sas TCJ, de Muinck Keizer-Schrama SMPF, et al. Efficacy and safety of oxandrolone in growth hormone-treated girls with Turner Syndrome. J Clin Endocrinol Metab. 2010;95(3):1151-1160.

Murphy KD, Thomas S, Mlcak RP, Chinkes DL, Klein GL, Herndon DN. Effects of long-term oxandrolone administration in severely burned children. Surgery. 2004;136(2):219-224.

Nilsson KA, Albertsson-Wikland K, Alm J, et al. Improved final height in girls with Turner's syndrome treated with growth hormone and oxandrolone. J Clin Endocrinol Metab. 1996;81(2):635-640.

Orr R, Fiatarone Singh M. The anabolic androgenic steroid oxandrolone in the treatment of wasting and catabolic disorders. Review of efficacy and safety. Drugs. 2004;64(7):725-750.

Papadimitriou A, Wacharasindhu S, Pearl K, Preece MA, Stanhope R. Treatment of constitutional growth delay in prepubertal boys with a prolonged course of low dose oxandrolone. Arch Dis Child. 1991;66(7):841-843.

Porro LJ, Herndon DN, Rodriguez MA, et al. Five-year outcomes after oxandrolone administration in severely burned children: a randomized clinical trial of safety and efficacy. J Am Coll Surg. 2012;214(4):489-504.

Przkora R, Jeschke MG, Barrow RE, et al. Metabolic and hormonal changes of severely burned children receiving long-term oxandrolone treatment. Ann Surg. 2005;242(3):384-389.

Schroor EJ, van Weissenbruch MM, Knibbe P, Delemarre-van de Waal HA. The effect of prolonged administration of an anabolic steroid

(oxandrolone) on growth in boys with constitutionally delayed growth and puberty. Eur J Pediatr. 1995;154(12):953-957.

Stanhope R, Brook CGD. Oxandrolone in low dose for constitutional delay of growth and puberty in boys. Arch Dis Child. 1985;60(4):379-381.

Stanhope R, Buchanan CR, Fenn GC, Preece MA. Double blind placebo controlled trial of low dose oxandrolone in the treatment of boys with constitutional delay of growth and puberty. Arch Dis Child. 1988;63(5):501-505.

Tse WY, Buyukgebiz A, Hindmarsh PC, Stanhope R, Preece MA, Brook CG. Long-term outcome of oxandrolone treatment in boys with constitutional delay of growth and puberty. J Pediatr. 1990;117(4):588-591.

Oxaprozin (oks a PROE zin)

Medication Safety Issues
Sound-alike/look-alike issues:
Oxaprozin may be confused with oxazepam

BEERS Criteria medication:
This drug may be potentially inappropriate for use in geriatric patients (Quality of evidence - moderate; Strength of recommendation - strong).

Brand Names: U.S. Daypro

Brand Names: Canada Apo-Oxaprozin

Therapeutic Category Analgesic, Non-narcotic; Anti-inflammatory Agent; Nonsteroidal Anti-inflammatory Drug (NSAID), Oral

Generic Availability (U.S.) Yes

Use Symptomatic relief of the signs and symptoms of osteoarthritis; adult and juvenile idiopathic arthritis (JIA)

Medication Guide Available Yes

Pregnancy Risk Factor C

Pregnancy Considerations Adverse events were not observed in the initial animal reproduction studies; therefore, the manufacturer classifies oxaprozin as pregnancy category C. NSAID exposure during the first trimester is not strongly associated with congenital malformations; however, cardiovascular anomalies and cleft palate have been observed following NSAID exposure in some studies. The use of an NSAID close to conception may be associated with an increased risk of miscarriage. Nonteratogenic effects have been observed following NSAID administration during the third trimester including myocardial degenerative changes, prenatal constriction of the ductus arteriosus, fetal tricuspid regurgitation, failure of the ductus arteriosus to close postnatally; renal dysfunction or failure, oligohydramnios; gastrointestinal bleeding or perforation, increased risk of necrotizing enterocolitis; intracranial bleeding (including intraventricular hemorrhage), platelet dysfunction with resultant bleeding; pulmonary hypertension. Because they may cause premature closure of the ductus arteriosus, use of NSAIDs late in pregnancy should be avoided (use after 31 or 32 weeks gestation is not recommended by some clinicians). The chronic use of NSAIDs in women of reproductive age may be associated with infertility that is reversible upon discontinuation of the medication. A registry is available for pregnant women exposed to autoimmune medications including oxaprozin. For additional information, contact the Organization of Teratology Information Specialists, OTIS Autoimmune Diseases Study, at 877-311-8972.

Breast-Feeding Considerations The amount of oxaprozin found in breast milk is not known; however, distribution into breast milk would be expected. Breast-feeding is not recommended by the manufacturer.

Contraindications Hypersensitivity to oxaprozin or any component; history of asthma, urticaria, or allergic-type reaction to aspirin, or other NSAIDs; patients with the "aspirin triad" [asthma, rhinitis (with or without nasal polyps), and aspirin intolerance] (fatal asthmatic and anaphylactoid reactions may occur in these patients); perioperative pain in the setting of coronary artery bypass graft (CABG)

Warnings NSAIDs are associated with an increased risk of adverse cardiovascular thrombotic events, including potentially fatal MI and stroke **[U.S. Boxed Warning]**; risk may be increased with duration of use or preexisting cardiovascular risk factors or disease; carefully evaluate cardiovascular risk profile prior to prescribing; use the lowest effective dose for the shortest duration of time, taking into consideration individual patient treatment goals; alternate therapies should be considered for patients at high risk. Use is contraindicated for treatment of perioperative pain in the setting of CABG surgery **[U.S. Boxed Warning]**; an increased incidence of MI and stroke was found in patients receiving COX-2 selective NSAIDs for the treatment of pain within the first 10-14 days after CABG surgery. NSAIDs may cause fluid retention, edema, and new onset or worsening of preexisting hypertension; use with caution in patients with hypertension, CHF, or fluid retention. Concurrent administration of ibuprofen, and potentially other nonselective NSAIDs, may interfere with aspirin's cardioprotective effect.

NSAIDs may increase the risk of gastrointestinal inflammation, ulceration, bleeding, and perforation **[U.S. Boxed Warning]**. These events, which can be potentially fatal, may occur at any time during therapy, and without warning. Avoid the use of NSAIDs in patients with active GI bleeding or ulcer disease. Use NSAIDs with extreme caution in patients with a history of GI bleeding or ulcers (these patients have a 10-fold increased risk for developing a GI bleed). Use NSAIDs with caution in patients with other risk factors which may increase GI bleeding (eg, concurrent therapy with aspirin, anticoagulants, and/or corticosteroids, longer duration of NSAID use, smoking, use of alcohol, and poor general health). Use the lowest effective dose for the shortest duration of time, taking into consideration individual patient treatment goals; alternate therapies should be considered for patients at high risk.

NSAIDs may compromise existing renal function. Renal toxicity may occur in patients with impaired renal function, dehydration, heart failure, liver dysfunction, and those taking diuretics and ACE inhibitors; use with caution in these patients; monitor renal function closely. NSAIDs are not recommended for use in patients with advanced renal disease. Long-term use of NSAIDs may cause renal papillary necrosis and other renal injury.

Fatal asthmatic and anaphylactoid reactions may occur in patients with the "aspirin triad" who receive NSAIDs. NSAIDs may cause serious dermatologic adverse reactions including exfoliative dermatitis, Stevens-Johnson syndrome, and toxic epidermal necrolysis. Avoid use of NSAIDs in late pregnancy as they may cause premature closure of the ductus arteriosus.

Precautions Severe hepatic reactions (rare) may occur. Use with caution in patients with, asthma, dehydration (rehydrate patient before starting therapy), mild-to-moderate renal dysfunction, hepatic dysfunction, coagulation disorders, or those receiving anticoagulants. Safety and efficacy in pediatric patients <6 years of age have not been established. Adverse reactions more frequently reported in patients being treated for JIA (45%) compared to adult rheumatoid arthritis patients (~30%). May cause photosensitivity reactions; incidence in JIA patients is 30%.

Adverse Reactions

Cardiovascular: Edema

Central nervous system: Confusion, depression, dizziness, headache, sedation, sleep disturbance, somnolence

Dermatologic: Pruritus, rash

Gastrointestinal: Abdominal distress, abdominal pain, anorexia, constipation, diarrhea, dyspepsia, flatulence, gastrointestinal ulcer, gross bleeding with perforation, heartburn, nausea, vomiting

Hematologic: Anemia, bleeding time increased

Hepatic: Liver enzymes increased

Otic: Tinnitus

Renal: Dysuria, renal function abnormal, urinary frequency

Rare but important or life-threatening (effects reported with oxaprozin or other NSAIDs): Acute interstitial nephritis, acute renal failure, agranulocytosis, alopecia, anaphylaxis, angioedema, anxiety, aplastic anemia, appetite changes, arrhythmia, asthma, blurred vision, bruising, coma, conjunctivitis, cystitis, death, diaphoresis, dream abnormalities, drowsiness, dyspnea, eosinophilia, eructation, erythema multiforme, esophagitis, exfoliative dermatitis, fever, gastritis, GI bleeding, glossitis, hallucinations, hearing decreased, heart failure, hematemesis, hematuria, hemolytic anemia, hemorrhoidal bleeding, hepatitis, hyperglycemia, hypersensitivity reaction, hyper-/hypotension, infection, insomnia, jaundice, leukopenia, liver failure, liver function abnormalities, lymphadenopathy, malaise, melena, meningitis, menstrual flow increased/decreased, myocardial infarction, nephrotic syndrome, nervousness, oliguria, palpitation, pancreatitis, pancytopenia, paresthesia, peptic ulcer, photosensitivity, pneumonia, polyuria, proteinuria, pseudoporphyria, pulmonary infection, purpura, rectal bleeding, renal insufficiency, respiratory depression, seizures, sepsis, serum sickness, sinusitis, Stevens-Johnson syndrome, stomatitis, syncope, tachycardia, taste alteration, thrombocytopenia, toxic epidermal necrolysis, tremor, upper respiratory tract infection, urticaria, vasculitis, vertigo, weakness, weight changes, xerostomia

Drug Interactions

Metabolism/Transport Effects None known.

Avoid Concomitant Use

Avoid concomitant use of Oxaprozin with any of the following: Floctafenine; Ketorolac (Nasal); Ketorolac (Systemic); NSAID (COX-2 Inhibitor); Omacetaxine; Urokinase

Increased Effect/Toxicity

Oxaprozin may increase the levels/effects of: 5-ASA Derivatives; Agents with Antiplatelet Properties; Aliskiren; Aminoglycosides; Anticoagulants; Apixaban; Bisphosphonate Derivatives; Collagenase (Systemic); CycloSPORINE (Systemic); Dabigatran Etexilate; Deferasirox; Desmopressin; Digoxin; Eplerenone; Haloperidol; Ibritumomab; Lithium; Methotrexate; Nonsteroidal Anti-Inflammatory Agents; NSAID (COX-2 Inhibitor); Omacetaxine; PEMEtrexed; Porfimer; Potassium-Sparing Diuretics; PRALAtrexate; Quinolone Antibiotics; Rivaroxaban; Salicylates; Tenofovir; Thrombolytic Agents; Tositumomab and Iodine I 131 Tositumomab; Urokinase; Vancomycin; Vitamin K Antagonists

The levels/effects of Oxaprozin may be increased by: ACE Inhibitors; Angiotensin II Receptor Blockers; Antidepressants (Tricyclic, Tertiary Amine); Corticosteroids (Systemic); CycloSPORINE (Systemic); Dasatinib; Floctafenine; Glucosamine; Herbs (Anticoagulant/Antiplatelet Properties); Ibrutinib; Ketorolac (Nasal); Ketorolac (Systemic); Multivitamins/Fluoride (with ADE); Multivitamins/Minerals (with ADEK, Folate, Iron); Multivitamins/Minerals (with AE, No Iron); Nonsteroidal Anti-Inflammatory Agents; Omega-3 Fatty Acids; Pentosan Polysulfate Sodium; Pentoxifylline; Probenecid; Prostacyclin Analogues; Selective Serotonin Reuptake Inhibitors; Serotonin/Norepinephrine Reuptake Inhibitors; Sodium Phosphates; Tipranavir; Treprostinil; Vitamin E

Decreased Effect

Oxaprozin may decrease the levels/effects of: ACE Inhibitors; Agents with Antiplatelet Properties; Aliskiren; Angiotensin II Receptor Blockers; Beta-Blockers; Eplerenone; HydrALAZINE; Loop Diuretics; Potassium-Sparing Diuretics; Prostaglandins (Ophthalmic); Salicylates; Selective Serotonin Reuptake Inhibitors; Thiazide Diuretics

◀ *The levels/effects of Oxaprozin may be decreased by:*
Bile Acid Sequestrants; Nonsteroidal Anti-Inflammatory Agents; Salicylates

Stability Store at 25°C (77°F); protect from light; keep bottle tightly closed

Mechanism of Action Reversibly inhibits cyclooxygenase-1 and 2 (COX-1 and 2) enzymes, which results in decreased formation of prostaglandin precursors; has antipyretic, analgesic, and anti-inflammatory properties.

Other proposed mechanisms not fully elucidated (and possibly contributing to the anti-inflammatory effect to varying degrees) include inhibiting chemotaxis, altering lymphocyte activity, inhibiting neutrophil aggregation/activation, and decreasing proinflammatory cytokine levels.

Pharmacodynamics Maximum effect: Due to its long half-life, several days of treatment are required for oxaprozin to reach its full effect

Pharmacokinetics (Adult data unless noted)
Absorption: Oral: 95%

Distribution: Distributes into synovial tissues at twice the concentration of plasma and 3 times the concentration of synovial fluid; expected to distribute into breast milk (exact amount not known)

V_d (apparent): Adults: 11-17 L per 70 kg

Protein binding: 99%, primarily to albumin; protein binding is saturable (nonlinear protein binding)

Metabolism: Hepatic via microsomal oxidation (65%) and conjugation with glucuronic acid (35%); major conjugated metabolites are ester and ether glucuronide (inactive); small amounts of an active phenolic metabolite is produced (<5%) but has limited contribution to overall activity

Half-life: Adults: 41-55 hours

Time to peak serum concentration: 2.4-3.1 hours

Elimination: Excreted in the urine (5% as unchanged drug, 65% as metabolites) and feces (35% as metabolites)

Clearance: After adjusting for body weight, no clinically important age-related differences in apparent clearance of unbound drug were identified between adult and pediatric patients ≥6 years of age

Dialysis: Not significantly removed by hemodialysis or CAPD due to high protein binding

Dosing: Usual Note: Use lowest effective dose; dose may be divided if patient does not tolerate once daily dosing; Oral:

Children 6-16 years: JIA: Dose according to body weight.
Note: Doses greater than 1200 mg have not been evaluated:
22-31 kg: 600 mg once daily
32-54 kg: 900 mg once daily
≥55 kg: 1200 mg once daily

Adults: Osteoarthritis or Rheumatoid arthritis: Usual: 1200 mg once daily; titrate to lowest effective dose; patients with low body weight should start with 600 mg daily; a one-time loading dose of 1200 mg to 1800 mg or 26 mg/kg (whichever is lower) may be given if needed; maximum daily dose: 1800 mg or 26 mg/kg (whichever is lower) in divided doses

Note: Chronic administration of doses >1200 mg/day should be reserved for adult patients >50 kg with severe disease, low risk for peptic ulcer disease, and normal hepatic and renal function; ensure that patient tolerates lower doses before advancing to larger dose

Dosing adjustment in renal impairment: Severe renal impairment or patients on dialysis: Initial: 600 mg once daily; may increase dose if needed to 1200 mg once daily with close monitoring

Dosing adjustment in hepatic impairment: Use with caution in patients with severe hepatic dysfunction (dosage reduction is not required in patients with well compensated cirrhosis)

Administration May be administered without regard to food; administer with food or milk to decrease GI distress

Monitoring Parameters CBC, occult blood loss, liver enzymes, renal function tests; blood pressure, signs and symptoms of GI bleeding

Test Interactions False-positive urine immunoassay screening tests for benzodiazepines have been reported and may occur several days after discontinuing oxaprozin.

Additional Information An open-label study of oxaprozin (10-20 mg/kg/dose once daily) in 59 JIA patients [3-16 years of age (mean age: 9 years)], reported adverse events in 58% of patients; GI symptoms occurred at a higher incidence than historically reported in adults; 9 of 30 patients (30%) who continued therapy for a total of 19-48 weeks, developed a vesicular rash on sun-exposed areas of skin; 5 of these 9 patients with rash discontinued the drug (Bass, 1985).

Dosage Forms Excipient information presented when available (limited, particularly for generics); consult specific product labeling.
Tablet, Oral:
Daypro: 600 mg [scored]
Generic: 600 mg

References
Bass JC, Athreya BH, Brewer EJ, et al, "A Once-Daily Anti-Inflammatory Drug, Oxaprozin, in the Treatment of Juvenile Rheumatoid Arthritis," *J Rheumatol*, 1985, 12(2):384-6.

OXcarbazepine (ox car BAZ e peen)

Medication Safety Issues
Sound-alike/look-alike issues:
OXcarbazepine may be confused with carBAMazepine, oxazepam
Trileptal® may be confused with TriLipix®

Related Information
Oral Medications That Should Not Be Crushed or Altered *on page 2438*
Safe Handling of Hazardous Drugs *on page 2419*

Brand Names: U.S. Oxtellar XR; Trileptal

Brand Names: Canada Apo-Oxcarbazepine®; Trileptal®

Therapeutic Category Anticonvulsant, Miscellaneous

Generic Availability (U.S.) May be product dependent

Use Oral:
Immediate release; suspension, tablet (Trileptal®): Treatment of partial seizures (FDA approved as monotherapy in ages ≥4 years and adults; FDA approved as adjunctive therapy in ages ≥2 years and adults)
Extended release; tablet (Oxtellar XR™): Adjunctive therapy for treatment of partial seizures (FDA approved in ages ≥6 years and adults)

Medication Guide Available Yes

Pregnancy Risk Factor C

Pregnancy Considerations Adverse events have been observed in animal reproduction studies; therefore, the manufacturer classifies oxcarbazepine as pregnancy category C. Oxcarbazepine, the active metabolite MHD and the inactive metabolite DHD, crosses the placenta and can be detected in the newborn. An increased risk in the overall rate of major congenital malformations has not been observed following maternal use of oxcarbazepine. Available studies have not been large enough to determine if there is an increased risk of specific defects. In general, the risk of teratogenic effects is higher with AED polytherapy than monotherapy. Plasma concentrations of MHD gradually decrease due to physiologic changes which occur during pregnancy; patients should be monitored during pregnancy and postpartum. Oxcarbazepine may decrease plasma concentrations of hormonal contraceptives.

Patients exposed to oxcarbazepine during pregnancy are encouraged to enroll themselves into the AED Pregnancy

Registry by calling 1-888-233-2334. Additional information is available at www.aedpregnancyregistry.org.

Breast-Feeding Considerations Oxcarbazepine and the active 10-hydroxy metabolite (MHD) are found in breast milk (small amounts). According to the manufacturer, the decision to continue or discontinue breast-feeding during therapy should take into account the risk of exposure to the infant and the benefits of treatment to the mother.

Contraindications Hypersensitivity to oxcarbazepine or any component

Warnings Hazardous agent; use appropriate precautions for handling and disposal (NIOSH, 2012).

Significant hyponatremia (ie, serum sodium <125 mEq/L) may occur; with immediate release use, usual onset within first 3 months of therapy, but has been reported in patients >1 year after initiation; reported incidence: Immediate release: 2.5%; extended release: 1.2%. Consider monitoring serum sodium especially in patients who receive other drugs that may cause hyponatremia and in patients with symptoms of hyponatremia (eg, nausea, headache, malaise, confusion, lethargy, obtundation, or an increase in seizure frequency or severity); dosage reduction or fluid restriction may be beneficial. Do not abruptly discontinue therapy, withdraw gradually to lessen chance for increased seizure frequency (unless a more rapid withdrawal is required due to safety concerns). Serious dermatologic reactions (including potentially fatal Stevens-Johnson syndrome and toxic epidermal necrolysis) have been reported (median onset 19 days); consider discontinuation of oxcarbazepine and alternative therapy in patients who develop skin reactions.

Rare cases of angioedema have been reported after the first or subsequent doses of oxcarbazepine; angioedema has occurred in the lips, eyelids, glottis, and larynx; angioedema of the larynx (laryngeal edema) can be fatal; permanently discontinue oxcarbazepine if any of these reactions occur; do not rechallenge or restart oxcarbazepine in these patients. Rare cases of anaphylaxis and multiorgan hypersensitivity reaction with rash, lymphadenopathy, fever, abnormal liver function tests, hepatitis, nephritis, oliguria, hepatorenal syndrome, hematological abnormalities, pruritus, asthenia, and/or arthralgia have also been reported; median time to detection: 13 days post-therapy initiation; permanently discontinue oxcarbazepine if any of these reactions occur; do not rechallenge or restart oxcarbazepine in these patients. Cross-hypersensitivity reactions with carbamazepine may occur (incidence: 25% to 30%). Agranulocytosis, leukopenia, and pancytopenia have been reported with use (rare); discontinuation and conversion to alternate therapy may be required.

Antiepileptic drugs (AEDs) increase the risk of suicidal behavior and ideation in patients receiving these medications for any indication. Pooled analyses of placebo-controlled trials involving 11 different AEDs (regardless of indication) showed a twofold increased risk of suicidal thoughts or behavior (estimated incidence rate: 0.43% in AED treated patients compared to 0.24% of patients receiving placebo); increased risk was observed as early as 1 week after initiation of AED and continued through duration of trials (most trials ≤24 weeks); risk did not vary significantly by age (age range: 5-100 years). Consider risks and benefits of AEDs before prescribing. Monitor all patients receiving an AED for emergence of suicidal thoughts or behavior, thoughts of self-harm, any unusual changes in behavior or mood, or the emergence or worsening of depressive symptoms; notify healthcare provider immediately if symptoms or concerning behavior occur. **Note:** The FDA requires Medication Guide for all antiepileptic drugs informing patients of this risk.

Trileptal® and Oxtellar XR™ are not bioequivalent and not interchangeable on a mg per mg basis; systemic absorption and resulting serum concentrations are lower with once daily Oxtellar XR™ compared to twice daily Trileptal® when administered at the same total daily dose; higher doses of Oxtellar XR™ may be necessary.

Precautions CNS adverse effects may occur, including somnolence (children: ~35%), fatigue, coordination abnormalities [ataxia and gait disturbances (children: 23%)], and cognitive symptoms [eg, difficulty concentrating, speech or language problems, and psychomotor slowing (5.8%)]; these effects may be more common when oxcarbazepine is used as add-on therapy versus monotherapy; caution patients about performing tasks which require mental alertness (eg, operating machinery or driving). Effects with other sedative drugs or ethanol may be potentiated. Use with caution in renal impairment; single-dose studies show that half-life of the primary active metabolite is prolonged and AUC is doubled in patients with CrCl <30 mL/minute; dose adjustment required in these patients.

Adverse Reactions Incidence in children was similar.

Cardiovascular: Hypotension, lower extremity edema

Central nervous system: Abnormal electroencephalogram, abnormality in thinking, agitation, amnesia, ataxia, confusion, dizziness, drowsiness, dysmetria, fatigue, feeling abnormal, fever, headache, insomnia, nervousness, speech disorder, vertigo

Dermatologic: Acne vulgaris, skin rash

Endocrine & metabolic: Hyponatremia

Gastrointestinal: Abdominal pain, constipation, diarrhea, dysgeusia, dyspepsia, gastritis, nausea, vomiting, weight gain, xerostomia

Genitourinary: Urinary frequency

Neuromuscular & skeletal: Abnormal gait, back pain, falling, myasthenia, sprain, tremor, weakness

Ophthalmic: Accommodation disturbance, diplopia, nystagmus, visual disturbance

Respiratory: Epistaxis, pulmonary infection, rhinitis, sinusitis, upper respiratory tract infection

Rare but important or life-threatening: Aggressive behavior, alopecia, anaphylaxis, angioedema, anxiety, aphasia, aphthous stomatitis, aplastic anemia, biliary colic, blepharoptosis, bradycardia, bruise, cardiac failure, cerebral hemorrhage, chest pain, cholelithiasis, colitis, conjunctival hemorrhage, delirium, delusion, dysphagia, dyspnea, dystonia, dysuria, emotional lability, enteritis, erythema multiforme, erythematosus rash, esophagitis, extrapyramidal reaction, gingival hemorrhage, gingival hyperplasia, hematuria, hemianopia, hemiplegia, hematemesis, hypersensitivity reaction, hypertension, hypocalcemia, hypoesthesia, hypokalemia, hypothyroidism, hysteria, impaired consciousness, increased gamma-glutamyl transferase, increased liver enzymes, increased serum amylase, increased serum lipase, laryngismus, leukopenia, leukorrhea, maculopapular rash, manic behavior, multiorgan hypersensitivity (eosinophilia, arthralgia, rash, fever, lymphadenopathy), muscle spasm, mydriasis, nephrolithiasis, neuralgia, nightmares, ocular edema, oculogyric crisis, orthostatic hypotension, palpitations, pancreatitis, pancytopenia, panic disorder, paralysis, photophobia, pleurisy, priapism, purpura, psychosis, renal pain, right hypochondrium pain, rigors, scotoma, seizure (aggravated), sialoadenitis, skin photosensitivity, Stevens-Johnson syndrome, stupor, suicidal ideation, suicidal tendencies, syncope, systemic lupus erythematosus, tachycardia, tetany, thrombocytopenia, toxic epidermal necrolysis, urinary tract pain, urticaria, vitiligo, voice disorder, weight loss, xerophthalmia

Drug Interactions

Metabolism/Transport Effects Induces CYP3A4 (strong)

◄ **Avoid Concomitant Use**

Avoid concomitant use of OXcarbazepine with any of the following: Abiraterone Acetate; Apixaban; Apremilast; Artemether; Axitinib; Bedaquiline; Boceprevir; Bortezomib; Bosutinib; Cabozantinib; Ceritinib; CloZAPine; Crizotinib; Dienogest; Dolutegravir; Dronedarone; Enzalutamide; Eslicarbazepine; Everolimus; Ibrutinib; Itraconazole; Ivacaftor; Lapatinib; Lumefantrine; Lurasidone; Macitentan; Mifepristone; NIFEdipine; Nilotinib; Nisoldipine; PAZOPanib; PONATinib; Praziquantel; Ranolazine; Regorafenib; Rilpivirine; Rivaroxaban; Roflumilast; RomiDEPsin; Selegiline; Simeprevir; Sofosbuvir; SORAfenib; Tasimelteon; Telaprevir; Ticagrelor; Tofacitinib; Tolvaptan; Toremifene; Ulipristal; Vandetanib; Vemurafenib; VinCRIStine (Liposomal); Vorapaxar

Increased Effect/Toxicity

OXcarbazepine may increase the levels/effects of: Clarithromycin; Fosphenytoin-Phenytoin; Ifosfamide; PHENobarbital; Selegiline

The levels/effects of OXcarbazepine may be increased by: Alcohol (Ethyl); Clarithromycin; Eslicarbazepine; Perampanel; Thiazide Diuretics

Decreased Effect

OXcarbazepine may decrease the levels/effects of: Abiraterone Acetate; Apixaban; Apremilast; ARIPiprazole; Artemether; Axitinib; Bedaquiline; Boceprevir; Bortezomib; Bosutinib; Brentuximab Vedotin; Cabozantinib; Cannabidiol; Cannabis; Ceritinib; Clarithromycin; CloZAPine; Cobicistat; Contraceptives (Estrogens); Contraceptives (Progestins); Crizotinib; CYP3A4 Substrates; Dasatinib; Dienogest; Dolutegravir; DOXOrubicin (Conventional); Dronabinol; Dronedarone; Elvitegravir; Enzalutamide; Everolimus; Exemestane; FentaNYL; Gefitinib; GuanFACINE; Ibrutinib; Imatinib; Itraconazole; Ivacaftor; Ixabepilone; Lapatinib; Linagliptin; Lumefantrine; Lurasidone; Macitentan; Maraviroc; Mifepristone; NIFEdipine; Nilotinib; Nisoldipine; PAZOPanib; Perampanel; PONATinib; Praziquantel; QUEtiapine; Ranolazine; Regorafenib; Rilpivirine; Rivaroxaban; Roflumilast; RomiDEPsin; Saxagliptin; Simeprevir; Sofosbuvir; SORAfenib; SUNItinib; Tadalafil; Tasimelteon; Telaprevir; Tetrahydrocannabinol; Ticagrelor; Tofacitinib; Tolvaptan; Toremifene; Ulipristal; Vandetanib; Vemurafenib; Vilazodone; VinCRIStine (Liposomal); Vorapaxar; Vortioxetine; Zuclopenthixol

The levels/effects of OXcarbazepine may be decreased by: CarBAMazepine; Fosphenytoin-Phenytoin; Ketorolac (Nasal); Ketorolac (Systemic); Mefloquine; Orlistat; PHENobarbital; Valproic Acid and Derivatives

Stability Hazardous agent; use appropriate precautions for handling and disposal (NIOSH, 2012). Store tablets (immediate and extended release) and suspension at 25°C (77°F); excursions permitted to 15°C to 30°C (59°F to 86°F); protect from moisture; dispense in tight, light-resistant container. Use suspension within 7 weeks of first opening container.

Mechanism of Action Pharmacological activity results from both oxcarbazepine and its monohydroxy metabolite (MHD). Precise mechanism of anticonvulsant effect has not been defined. Oxcarbazepine and MHD block voltage-sensitive sodium channels, stabilizing hyperexcited neuronal membranes, inhibiting repetitive firing, and decreasing the propagation of synaptic impulses. These actions are believed to prevent the spread of seizures. Oxcarbazepine and MHD also increase potassium conductance and modulate the activity of high-voltage activated calcium channels.

Pharmacokinetics (Adult data unless noted)

Absorption: Complete

Distribution: MHD: V_d (apparent): 49 L

Protein binding: Oxcarbazepine: 67%; MHD: 40%, primarily to albumin; parent drug and metabolite do not bind to alpha-1 acid glycoprotein

Metabolism: Oxcarbazepine is extensively metabolized in the liver to its active 10-monohydroxy metabolite (MHD); MHD undergoes further metabolism via glucuronide conjugation; 4% of dose is oxidized to the 10,11-dihydroxy metabolite (DHD) (inactive); 70% of serum concentration appears as MHD, 2% as unchanged oxcarbazepine, and the rest as minor metabolites; **Note:** Unlike carbamazepine, autoinduction of metabolism has not been observed and biotransformation of oxcarbazepine does not result in an epoxide metabolite

Bioavailability: Immediate release tablets and suspension have similar bioavailability (based on MDH serum concentrations). Extended release tablets and immediate release products are **not** bioequivalent.

Half-life:

Children (Rey, 2004):

2-5 years: MHD: Single dose: Mean range: 4.8-6.7 hours

6-12 years: MHD: Single dose: Mean range: 7.2-9.3 hours

Adults:

Immediate release: Oxcarbazepine: 2 hours; MHD: 9 hours

Extended release: Oxcarbazepine: 7-11 hours; MHD: 9-11 hours

Adults with renal impairment (CrCl <30 mL/minute): MHD: 19 hours

Time to peak serum concentration:

Children 2-12 years: Immediate release: Oxcarbazepine: 1 hour; MHD: 3-4 hours (Rey, 2004)

Adults:

Immediate release: MHD: Tablets: Median: 4.5 hours (range: 3-13 hours); Suspension: Median 6 hours

Extended release: MHD: 7 hours

Elimination: Urine (>95% of dose is excreted in the urine with <1% as unchanged parent drug), 27% as unchanged MHD, 49% as MHD glucuronides, 3% as DHD (inactive), and 13% as conjugate of oxcarbazepine and MHD); feces (<4%)

Clearance (per body weight):

Children 2 to <4 years: Increased by ~80% compared to adults

Children 4-12 years: Increased by ~40% compared to adults

Children ≥13 years: Values approach adult clearance

Dosing: Usual Note: Immediate release preparations (oral suspension and tablets) are interchangeable on a mg per mg basis; immediate release and extended release preparations are **not** bioequivalent and not interchangeable on a mg per mg basis.

Children and Adolescents:

Partial seizures, monotherapy: Oral: Immediate release (Trileptal®): Children and Adolescents 4-16 years:

Initiation of monotherapy:

Initial: 8-10 mg/kg/day in 2 divided doses; increase dose every third day by 5 mg/kg/day to achieve the recommended monotherapy maintenance dose by weight, as follows:

Maintenance dose:

20 to <25 kg: 600-900 mg/day in 2 divided doses

25 to <35 kg: 900-1200 mg/day in 2 divided doses

35 to <45 kg: 900-1500 mg/day in 2 divided doses

45 to <50 kg: 1200-1500 mg/day in 2 divided doses

50 to <60 kg: 1200-1800 mg/day in 2 divided doses

60 to <70 kg: 1200-2100 mg/day in 2 divided doses

≥70 kg: 1500-2100 mg/day in 2 divided doses

Conversion to monotherapy: Initial: 8-10 mg/kg/day in 2 divided doses, with a simultaneous initial reduction of the dose of concomitant antiepileptic drugs (AEDs); withdraw concomitant AEDs completely over 3-6 weeks, while increasing oxcarbazepine dose as needed by no more than 10 mg/kg/day at approximately weekly intervals; increase oxcarbazepine dose to achieve the recommended monotherapy maintenance dose.

Partial seizures, adjunctive therapy: Oral:

Immediate release (Trileptal®):

Children 2 to <4 years: Initial: 8-10 mg/kg/day in 2 divided doses (usual maximum initial daily dose: 600 mg/day); patients <20 kg may require a higher initial dose of 16-20 mg/kg/day in 2 divided doses; increase dose slowly over 2-4 weeks; maximum daily dose: 60 mg/kg/day

Children and Adolescents 4-16 years:

Initial: 8-10 mg/kg/day in 2 divided doses (usual maximum initial daily dose: 600 mg/day); increase dose slowly over 2 weeks to the target maintenance dose by weight, as follows:

Maintenance dose:

20-29 kg: 900 mg/day in 2 divided doses

29.1-39 kg: 1200 mg/day in 2 divided doses

>39 kg: 1800 mg/day in 2 divided doses

Note: Use of these pediatric target maintenance doses in one clinical trial resulted in doses ranging from 6-51 mg/kg/day (median dose: 31 mg/kg/day) in pediatric patients 4-16 years of age (Glauser, 2000). In children 2-4 years of age, 50% of patients were titrated to a final dose of at least 55 mg/kg/day with target dose of 60 mg/kg/day. Due to a higher drug clearance, children 2 to <4 years of age may require up to twice the dose per body weight compared to adults; children 4 to ≤12 years of age may require a 50% higher dose per body weight compared to adults.

Extended release (Oxtellar XR™): Children and Adolescents 6-17 years:

Initial: 8-10 mg/kg/day once daily; maximum initial daily dose: 600 mg/day during the first week of therapy; increase dose at weekly intervals in 8-10 mg/kg/day increments (maximum dosage incremental increase: 600 mg) to the target maintenance dose by weight, as follows:

Maintenance dose:

20-29 kg: 900 mg once daily

29.1-39 kg: 1200 mg once daily

>39 kg: 1800 mg once daily

Conversion from immediate release (Trileptal®) to extended release (Oxtellar XR™): Higher doses of Oxtellar XR™ may be necessary; on a mg per mg basis dosage forms are not bioequivalent.

Adults:

Partial seizures; adjunctive therapy (epilepsy): Oral:

Immediate release (Trileptal®): Initial: 600 mg daily in 2 divided doses; dose may be increased by as much as 600 mg/day increments at weekly intervals; recommended daily dose: 1200 mg daily in 2 divided doses. Although daily doses >1200 mg daily were somewhat more efficacious, most patients were unable to tolerate 2400 mg daily (due to CNS effects).

Extended release (Oxtellar XR™): Initial: 600 mg once daily; dosage may be increased by 600 mg/day increments at weekly intervals. Recommended daily dose is 1200-2400 mg once daily. Although daily doses >1200 mg daily were somewhat more efficacious, most patients were unable to tolerate 2400 mg daily (due to CNS effects).

Conversion to monotherapy, partial seizures (epilepsy): Patients receiving concomitant antiepileptic drugs (AEDs): Oral: Immediate release (Trileptal®): Initial: 600 mg daily in 2 divided doses while simultaneously reducing the dose of concomitant AEDs. Withdraw concomitant AEDs completely over 3-6 weeks, while increasing the oxcarbazepine dose in increments of 600 mg daily at weekly intervals, reaching the maximum oxcarbazepine dose (2400 mg daily in 2 divided

doses) in about 2-4 weeks (lower doses have been effective in patients in whom monotherapy has been initiated).

Partial seizures; monotherapy (epilepsy): Patients not receiving prior AEDs: Oral: Immediate release (Trileptal®): Initial: 600 mg daily in 2 divided doses. Increase dose by 300 mg daily every third day to a dose of 1200 mg daily. Higher dosages (2400 mg daily) have been shown to be effective in patients converted to monotherapy from other AEDs.

Conversion from immediate release (Trileptal®) to extended release (Oxtellar XR™): Higher doses of Oxtellar XR™ may be necessary.

Dosing adjustment with concomitant antiepileptic drugs (AEDs): Adults: Concomitant use with enzyme-inducing antiepileptic drugs (eg, carbamazepine, phenobarbital, phenytoin): Extended release (Oxtellar XR™): Consider initiating dose at 900 mg once daily.

Dosing adjustment in renal impairment: Children, Adolescents, and Adults:

Severe impairment (CrCl <30 mL/minute): Immediate release (Trileptal®), Extended release (Oxtellar XR™): Therapy should be initiated at lower starting dose [eg, one-half the usual starting dose (adults: 300 mg daily)] and increased slowly to achieve desired clinical response (eg, adults: Increase in 300-450 mg daily increments at weekly intervals).

ESRD (on dialysis): Immediate release formulations should be used instead of extended release formulation.

Dosing adjustment in hepatic impairment: Children, Adolescents, and Adults:

Mild to moderate impairment: Immediate release (Trileptal®), Extended release (Oxtellar XR™): No dosage adjustments are recommended.

Severe impairment:

Immediate release (Trileptal®): Use caution (not studied).

Extended release (Oxtellar XR™): Not recommended (not studied).

Administration Hazardous agent; use appropriate precautions for handling and disposal (NIOSH, 2012).

Oral:

Immediate release: May be taken without regard to meals

Suspension: Prior to using for the first time, firmly insert the manufacturer supplied plastic adapter into the neck of the bottle; cover the adapter with child-resistant cap when not in use; shake suspension well (for at least 10 seconds) before use; use manufacturer supplied oral syringe to withdraw appropriate dose; dose may be administered directly from syringe or mixed in a small amount of water immediately prior to use; after use, rinse oral syringe with warm water and allow to dry thoroughly; discard any unused portion 7 weeks after first opening bottle

Extended release: Administer on an empty stomach at least 1 hour before or 2 hours after food. Swallow whole; do not cut, crush, or chew the tablets.

Monitoring Parameters Seizure frequency, duration and severity; symptoms of CNS depression (dizziness, headache, somnolence); consider monitoring serum sodium (particularly during first three months of therapy) especially in patients who receive other drugs that may cause hyponatremia and in patients with symptoms of hyponatremia; signs and symptoms of suicidality (eg, anxiety, depression, behavior changes); hypersensitivity reactions

Test Interactions Thyroid function tests; may depress serum T_4 without affecting T_3 levels or TSH

Additional Information Oxcarbazepine is a keto analogue of carbamazepine; symptoms of overdose may include CNS depression (somnolence, ataxia, obtundation)

Dosage Forms Excipient information presented when available (limited, particularly for generics); consult specific product labeling.

Suspension, Oral:

Trileptal: 300 mg/5 mL (250 mL) [contains alcohol, usp, methyl hydroxybenzoate, propyl hydroxybenzoate, propylene glycol, saccharin sodium; lemon flavor]

Generic: 300 mg/5 mL (250 mL)

Tablet, Oral:

Trileptal: 150 mg, 300 mg, 600 mg [scored]

Generic: 150 mg, 300 mg, 600 mg

Tablet Extended Release 24 Hour, Oral:

Oxtellar XR: 150 mg, 300 mg, 600 mg

References

Glauser TA, Nigro M, Sachdeo R, et al, "Adjunctive Therapy With Oxcarbazepine in Children With Partial Seizures. The Oxcarbazepine Pediatric Study Group," *Neurology*, 2000, 54(12):2237-44.

National Institute for Occupational Safety and Health (NIOSH), "NIOSH List of Antineoplastic and Other Hazardous Drugs in Healthcare Settings 2012." Available at http://www.cdc.gov/niosh/docs/2012-150/pdfs/2012-150.pdf. Accessed January 21, 2013.

Rey E, Bulteau C, Motte J, et al, "Oxcarbazepine Pharmacokinetics and Tolerability in Children With Inadequately Controlled Epilepsy," *J Clin Pharmacol*, 2004, 44(11):1290-300.

Tecoma ES, "Oxcarbazepine," *Epilepsia*, 1999, 40(Suppl 5): S37-46.

◆ **Oxecta** see OxyCODONE on page 1569

◆ **Oxecta [DSC]** see OxyCODONE on page 1569

◆ **Oxeze Turbuhaler (Can)** see Formoterol on page 929

◆ **Oxpentifylline** see Pentoxifylline on page 1646

◆ **Oxtellar XR** see OXcarbazepine on page 1564

◆ **Oxybutyn (Can)** see Oxybutynin on page 1568

Oxybutynin (oks i BYOO ti nin)

Medication Safety Issues

Sound-alike/look-alike issues:

Oxybutynin may be confused with OxyCONTIN

Ditropan may be confused with Detrol, diazepam, Diprivan, dithranol

BEERS Criteria medication:

This drug may be potentially inappropriate for use in geriatric patients (Quality of evidence - varies based on comorbidity; Strength of recommendation - varies based on comorbidity)

Other safety concerns:

Transdermal patch may contain conducting metal (eg, aluminum); remove patch prior to MRI.

Related Information

Oral Medications That Should Not Be Crushed or Altered on page 2438

Brand Names: U.S. Ditropan XL; Gelnique; Oxytrol; Oxytrol For Women [OTC]

Brand Names: Canada Apo-Oxybutynin; Ditropan XL; Dom-Oxybutynin; Gelnique; Mylan-Oxybutynin; Novo-Oxybutynin; Nu-Oxybutyn; Oxybutyn; Oxybutynine; Oxytrol; PHL-Oxybutynin; PMS-Oxybutynin; Riva-Oxybutynin; Uromax

Therapeutic Category Antispasmodic Agent, Urinary

Generic Availability (U.S.) May be product dependent

Use Relief of bladder spasms associated with voiding in patients with uninhibited and reflex neurogenic bladder; treatment of overactive bladder with symptoms of urge urinary incontinence, urgency, and frequency (FDA approved in ages >5 and adults); symptoms of detrus or overactivity associated with a neurological condition (XL product FDA approved in ages >6 years)

Pregnancy Risk Factor B

Pregnancy Considerations Adverse events were not observed in animal reproduction studies.

Breast-Feeding Considerations It is not known if oxybutynin is excreted into breast milk. The manufacturer recommends that caution be used if administered to a nursing woman. Suppression of lactation has been reported.

Contraindications Hypersensitivity to oxybutynin or any component; glaucoma (angle-closure), partial or complete GI obstruction, GU obstruction; toxic megacolon

Warnings Transdermal patch may contain conducting metal (eg, aluminum); remove patch prior to MRI. The extended release formulation consists of drug within a nondeformable matrix; following drug release/absorption, the matrix/shell is expelled in the stool.

Precautions Use with caution in patients with hepatic or renal disease, myasthenia gravis, heart disease, hyperthyroidism, reflux esophagitis, hypertension, prostatic hypertrophy, autonomic neuropathy, ulcerative colitis, intestinal atony. After application of the alcohol-based gel product, avoid open fire or smoking until gel has dried. Once topical gel has dried, application site should be covered with clothing to avoid transfer of medicine to others.

Adverse Reactions

Oral:

Cardiovascular: Cardiac arrhythmia (sinus), decreased blood pressure, chest pain, edema, flushing, hypertension, palpitations, peripheral edema

Central nervous system: Confusion, depression, dizziness, drowsiness, fatigue, headache, insomnia, nervousness, pain

Dermatologic: Pruritus, xeroderma

Endocrine & metabolic: Fluid retention, hyperglycemia

Gastrointestinal: Abdominal pain, constipation, diarrhea, dry throat, dyspepsia, dysphagia, eructation, flatulence, gastroesophageal reflux disease, nausea, unpleasant taste, vomiting, xerostomia

Genitourinary: Cystitis, dysuria, pollakiuria, urinary hesitancy, urinary retention, urinary tract infection

Infection: Fungal infection

Neuromuscular & skeletal: Arthralgia, back pain, flank pain, limb pain, weakness

Ophthalmic: Blurred vision, eye irritation, keratoconjunctivitis sicca, xerophthalmia

Respiratory: Asthma, bronchitis, cough, dry nose, dry throat, hoarseness, nasal congestion, nasal dryness, nasopharyngitis, pharyngolaryngeal pain, sinus congestion, upper respiratory tract infection

Miscellaneous: Increased thirst

Rare but important or life-threatening: Anaphylaxis, anorexia, cycloplegia, decreased gastrointestinal motility, glaucoma, hallucination, hypersensitivity reaction, impotence, suppressed lactation, memory impairment, mydriasis, psychotic reaction, prolonged Q-T interval on ECG, seizure, tachycardia

Topical gel:

Central nervous system: Dizziness, fatigue, headache

Dermatologic: Pruritus

Gastrointestinal: Constipation, gastroenteritis, xerostomia

Genitourinary: Urinary tract infection

Local: Application site reaction (includes anesthesia, dermatitis, erythema, irritation, pain, papules, pruritus, rash)

Ophthalmic: Blurred vision, conjunctivitis, xerophthalmia

Respiratory: Nasopharyngitis, upper respiratory tract infection

Transdermal:

Gastrointestinal: Constipation, diarrhea, xerostomia

Genitourinary: Dysuria

Local: Erythema, localized vesiculation, macular eruption, pruritus, skin rash

Ophthalmic: Visual disturbance

Rare but important or life-threatening: Dizziness, drowsiness

Drug Interactions

Metabolism/Transport Effects Substrate of CYP3A4 (minor); **Note:** Assignment of Major/Minor substrate status based on clinically relevant drug interaction potential; **Inhibits** CYP2C8 (weak), CYP2D6 (weak), CYP3A4 (weak)

Avoid Concomitant Use

Avoid concomitant use of Oxybutynin with any of the following: Aclidinium; Ipratropium (Oral Inhalation); Pimozide; Potassium Chloride; Tiotropium; Umeclidinium

Increased Effect/Toxicity

Oxybutynin may increase the levels/effects of: AbobotulinumtoxinA; Analgesics (Opioid); Anticholinergic Agents; ARIPiprazole; Cannabinoid-Containing Products; Dofetilide; Lomitapide; Mirabegron; OnabotulinumtoxinA; Pimozide; Potassium Chloride; RimabotulinumtoxinB; Thiazide Diuretics; Tiotropium; Topiramate

The levels/effects of Oxybutynin may be increased by: Aclidinium; Alcohol (Ethyl); Ipratropium (Oral Inhalation); Pramlintide; Umeclidinium

Decreased Effect

Oxybutynin may decrease the levels/effects of: Acetylcholinesterase Inhibitors (Central); Secretin

The levels/effects of Oxybutynin may be decreased by: Acetylcholinesterase Inhibitors (Central)

Stability Store at controlled room temperature; protect syrup from light; keep transdermal patch in sealed pouch; protect from moisture or humidity; keep gel in sachet; protect from heat.

Mechanism of Action Direct antispasmodic effect on smooth muscle, also inhibits the action of acetylcholine on smooth muscle (exhibits 1/5 the anticholinergic activity of atropine, but has 4-10 times the antispasmodic activity); does not block effects at skeletal muscle or at autonomic ganglia; increases bladder capacity, decreases uninhibited contractions, and delays desire to void, therefore, decreases urgency and frequency

Pharmacodynamics

Immediate release formulation:
Onset of action: Oral: Within 30-60 minutes
Maximum effect: 3-6 hours
Duration: 6-10 hours
Extended release formulation: Maximum effects: 3 days
Transdermal formulation: Duration: 96 hours

Pharmacokinetics (Adult data unless noted)

Absorption: Oral: Rapid and well absorbed
Distribution: V_d: Adults: 193 L
Metabolism: Hepatic via cytochrome isozyme CYP3A4 found mostly in liver and gut wall; extensive first pass effect (not with I.V. or transdermal use); metabolized in the liver to active and inactive metabolites
Bioavailability: Oral: Immediate release: 6% (range: 1.6% to 10.9%)
Half-life: Adults: 2-3 hours
Time to peak serum concentration:
Immediate release: Within 60 minutes
Extended release: 4-6 hours
Transdermal: 24-48 hours
Elimination: <0.1% excreted unchanged in urine

Dosing: Usual

Children: Oral:
Immediate release:
1-5 years: 0.2 mg/kg/dose 2-3 times/day
>5 years: 5 mg twice daily, up to 5 mg 3 times/day
Extended release: ≥6 years: 5 mg once daily; increase as tolerated in 5 mg increments to a maximum of 20 mg/day
Adults:
Oral: 5 mg 2-3 times/day up to 5 mg 4 times/day maximum **or** extended release tablet (Ditropan® XL)

5-10 mg once daily; increase in 5 mg increments to a maximum of 30 mg/day
Topical gel: Apply contents of one sachet (100 mg/g) once daily
Transdermal: 3.9 mg/day system applied twice weekly (every 3-4 days)
Note: Should be discontinued periodically to determine whether the patient can manage without the drug and to minimize tolerance to the drug

Administration

Oral: May be administered with or without food; swallow extended release tablets whole; do not chew or crush.
Topical gel: For topical use only. Apply to clean, dry, intact skin on abdomen, thighs, or upper arms/shoulders. Rotate site; do not apply to same site on consecutive days. Wash hands after use. Cover treated area with clothing after gel has dried to prevent transfer of medication to others. Do not bathe, shower, or swim until 1 hour after gel applied.
Transdermal: Apply to dry intact skin on the abdomen, hip, or buttock. Rotate site of application with each administration and avoid application to the same site within 7 days

Test Interactions May suppress the wheal and flare reactions to skin test antigens.

Dosage Forms Excipient information presented when available (limited, particularly for generics); consult specific product labeling.
Gel, Transdermal:
Gelnique: 3% (92 g) [contains propylene glycol]
Gel, Transdermal, as chloride:
Gelnique: 10% (1 g) [contains alcohol, usp]
Patch Biweekly, Transdermal:
Oxytrol: 3.9 mg/24 hr (1 ea, 2 ea, 4 ea, 8 ea)
Oxytrol For Women: 3.9 mg/24 hr (8 ea); 3.9 mg/24hr (4 ea)
Syrup, Oral, as chloride:
Generic: 5 mg/5 mL (473 mL)
Tablet, Oral, as chloride:
Generic: 5 mg
Tablet Extended Release 24 Hour, Oral, as chloride:
Ditropan XL: 5 mg, 10 mg, 15 mg [contains polysorbate 80]
Generic: 5 mg, 10 mg, 15 mg

References

Humphreys MR and Reinberg YE, "Contemporary and Emerging Drug Treatments for Urinary Incontinence in Children," *Paediatr Drugs*, 2005, 7(3):151-62.

◆ **Oxybutynin Chloride** *see* Oxybutynin *on page 1568*

◆ **Oxybutynine (Can)** *see* Oxybutynin *on page 1568*

◆ **Oxycodan® (Can)** *see* Oxycodone and Aspirin *on page 1575*

OxyCODONE (oks i KOE done)

Medication Safety Issues

Sound-alike/look-alike issues:

OxyCODONE may be confused with HYDROcodone, OxyCONTIN, oxymorphone
OxyCONTIN may be confused with MS Contin, oxybutynin
OxyFast may be confused with Roxanol
Roxicodone may be confused with Roxanol

High alert medication:

The Institute for Safe Medication Practices (ISMP) includes this medication among its list of drug classes which have a heightened risk of causing significant patient harm when used in error.

Related Information

Opioid Conversion Table *on page 2242*
Oral Medications That Should Not Be Crushed or Altered *on page 2438*
Patient Information for Disposal of Unused Medications *on page 2412*

Brand Names: U.S. Oxecta [DSC]; OxyCONTIN; Roxicodone
Brand Names: Canada Apo-Oxycodone CR; CO Oxycodone CR; Oxy.IR; OxyContin; OxyNEO; PMS-Oxycodone; PMS-Oxycodone CR; Supeudol
Therapeutic Category Analgesic, Narcotic
Generic Availability (U.S.) May be product dependent

Use

Immediate release formulations (capsules, oral solution, and tablets): Management of moderate to severe pain (FDA approved in ages ≥18 years and adults)
Controlled release tablets (OxyContin®): For around-the-clock management of moderate to severe pain when an analgesic is needed for an extended period of time (FDA approved in ages ≥18 years and adults); immediate postoperative pain management in patients who received OxyContin® prior to surgery or if moderate to severe persistent pain is anticipated (FDA approved in ages ≥18 years and adults) **Note:** Not intended for use as a PRN analgesic or for treatment of mild pain, pain that is not expected to persist for an extended period of time, or for immediate postoperative pain (within 12-24 hours after surgery)

Prescribing and Access Restrictions As a requirement of the REMS program, healthcare providers who prescribe OxyContin need to receive training on the proper use and potential risks of OxyContin. For training, please refer to http://www.oxycontinrems.com. Prescribers will need retraining every 2 years or following any significant changes to the OxyContin REMS program.

Medication Guide Available Yes

Pregnancy Risk Factor B

Pregnancy Considerations Adverse events were not observed in animal reproduction studies. Opioids cross the placenta. Oxycodone should not be used immediately prior to or during labor.

If chronic opioid exposure occurs in pregnancy, adverse events in the newborn (including withdrawal) may occur; monitoring of the neonate is recommended. The minimum effective dose should be used if opioids are needed (Chou, 2009). Neonatal abstinence syndrome following opioid exposure may present with autonomic (eg, fever, temperature instability), gastrointestinal (eg, diarrhea, vomiting, poor feeding/weight gain), or neurologic (eg, high-pitched crying, increased muscle tone, irritability, seizure, tremor) symptoms (Dow, 2012; Hudak, 2012).

Breast-Feeding Considerations Oxycodone is excreted into breast milk. Breast-feeding is not recommended by the manufacturer. Sedation and/or respiratory depression may occur in the infant; symptoms of opioid withdrawal may occur following the cessation of breast-feeding. Nursing infants exposed to large doses of opioids should be monitored for apnea and sedation. Use caution in a woman who may be an ultrarapid metabolizer; oxycodone is a substrate for CYP2D6 and their nursing infants may be at higher risk for adverse events (Montgomery, 2012).

Contraindications Hypersensitivity to oxycodone or any component; significant respiratory depression (in settings without resuscitative equipment or without adequate respiratory monitoring); patients with hypercarbia, severe or acute asthma, paralytic ileus (known or suspected); GI obstruction

Warnings An opioid-containing analgesic regimen should be individualized to each patient's needs and the optimal analgesic dose varies widely among patients; dose may be based upon the type of pain (acute versus chronic), route of administration, degree of patient's tolerance for opioids (naive vs chronic user), age, weight, and medical condition.

Respiratory depression may occur even with therapeutic dosages with all oxycodone products and may be fatal if unrecognized. With controlled release tablets, risk of respiratory depression is highest during initiation of therapy and dose titration **[U.S. Boxed Warning]**; ensure proper dosing and titration; monitor for respiratory depression especially within the first 24-72 hours of initiation or dose escalation; should only be prescribed by physician experienced in management of chronic pain and patients should be monitored closely. Use any oxycodone product with extreme caution in elderly, cachectic, or debilitated patients and patients with respiratory diseases including asthma, emphysema, COPD, cor pulmonale, hypoxia, hypercapnia, preexisting respiratory depression, significantly decreased respiratory reserve, other obstructive pulmonary disease, kyphoscoliosis, or other skeletal disorder which may alter respiratory function; there is a greater potential for critical respiratory depression in these patients. Concomitant use with CYP3A4 inhibitors (eg, macrolides, azole antifungals, and protease inhibitors) may result in increased oxycodone concentrations and potentially fatal respiratory depression whereas use with CYP3A4 inducers (eg, carbamazepine, phenytoin, and rifampin) may result in decreased oxycodone concentrations, lack of pain relief and even withdrawal in patients with physical dependence to oxycodone.

Oxycodone may cause CNS depression which may impair physical or mental abilities; patients must be cautioned about performing tasks which require mental alertness (eg, operating machinery or driving). Oxycodone may exaggerate elevated intracranial pressure (ICP); use with extreme caution in patients with head injury, intracranial lesions, or elevated ICP. Hypotension may occur; use with caution in patients with circulatory shock, hypovolemia, impaired myocardial function, or those receiving medications that compromise vasomotor tone or exaggerate hypotensive effects (including phenothiazines or general anesthetics). Orthostatic hypotension may occur in ambulatory patients. Oxycodone may obscure diagnosis or clinical course of patients with acute abdominal conditions; has been shown to decrease gastrointestinal motility; use with caution in postoperative patients especially after intra-abdominal surgery.

Physical and psychological dependence may occur; abrupt discontinuation after prolonged use may result in withdrawal symptoms; concurrent use of agonist/antagonist analgesics (eg, pentazocine, nalbuphine, and butorphanol) may precipitate withdrawal symptoms and/or reduce the analgesic efficacy in patients following prolonged therapy with a mμ opioid agonist, such as oxycodone. High potential for abuse; healthcare providers should be alert to problems of abuse, misuse, and diversion. Infants born to women physically dependent on opioids will also be physically dependent and may experience respiratory difficulties or opioid withdrawal symptoms [neonatal abstinence syndrome (NAS)]. Onset, duration, and severity of NAS depend upon the drug used (maternal), duration of use, maternal dose, and rate of drug elimination by the newborn. Symptoms of opioid withdrawal may include excessive crying, diarrhea, fever, hyper-reflexia, irritability, tremors, vomiting, or failure to gain weight. Opioid withdrawal syndrome in the neonate, unlike in adults, may be life-threatening and should be promptly treated.

OxyContin is a controlled release oral formulation indicated for the management of moderate to severe pain when continuous analgesia is needed for an extended period of time; OxyContin is not intended for use as an "as needed" analgesic or for immediately postoperative pain management. Controlled release 60 mg and 80 mg strengths, a single dose >40 mg or a total dose >80 mg/day are for use only in opioid-tolerant patients (adults taking ≥30 mg/day of oxycodone or equivalent for ≥1 week); administration of these tablet strengths to opioid-naïve patients may cause fatal respiratory depression. Controlled release tablets may be difficult to swallow and could become lodged in throat; patients with swallowing difficulties may be at increased risk. Cases of intestinal obstruction or diverticulitis exacerbation have also been reported, including cases requiring medical intervention to remove the tablet; patients with an underlying GI disease (eg, esophageal cancer, colon cancer) may be at increased risk. Do not crush, break, or chew controlled release tablets **[U.S. Boxed Warning]**; use of broken, chewed, or crushed tablets may lead to rapid release and absorption of a potentially fatal dose. Accidental exposure may result in fatal overdose of oxycodone, especially in children **[U.S. Boxed Warning]**. Healthcare providers should be alert to problems of abuse, misuse, and diversion **[U.S. Boxed Warning]**. Patients should be assessed for risk of abuse or addiction prior to therapy and all patients should be monitored for signs of misuse, abuse, and addiction. Risk of opioid abuse is increased in patients with a history or family history of alcohol or drug abuse or mental illness.

Concentrated oral solution (20 mg/mL) should only be used in opioid-tolerant patients (adults taking ≥30 mg/day of oxycodone or equivalent for ≥1 week) **[U.S. Boxed Warning]**. Precautions should be taken to avoid confusion between oxycodone solutions of different concentrations and dosing unit confusion (mg vs mL); prescriptions for oxycodone oral solutions (20 mg/mL or 5 mg/5 mL) should be clearly written to include the intended dose (in mg not mL) and the intended product concentration to be dispensed to avoid potential dosing errors **[U.S. Boxed Warning]**. Keep oxycodone oral solutions out of the reach of children **[U.S. Boxed Warning]**. Concentrated oral solution contains sodium benzoate; benzoic acid (benzoate) is a metabolite of benzyl alcohol; large amounts of benzyl alcohol (≥99 mg/kg/day) have been associated with a potentially fatal toxicity ("gasping syndrome") in neonates; the "gasping syndrome" consists of metabolic acidosis, respiratory distress, gasping respirations, CNS dysfunction (including convulsions, intracranial hemorrhage), hypotension, and cardiovascular collapse; avoid use of oxycodone products containing sodium benzoate in neonates; *in vitro* and animal studies have shown that benzoate displaces bilirubin from protein binding sites.

Precautions Use with caution in patients with hypersensitivity to other phenanthrene derivative opioid agonists (morphine, codeine, hydrocodone, hydromorphone, oxymorphone, levorphanol); discontinue immediately if symptoms of allergic or hypersensitivity reactions occur. Use with caution in patients with adrenal insufficiency (Addison's disease); biliary tract disease; pancreatitis; CNS depression/coma; toxic psychosis; acute alcoholism; delirium tremens; hypothyroidism (myxedema); severe liver, pulmonary, or renal impairment; urethral stricture; prostatic hypertrophy; or seizures and in debilitated patients. Use caution when combining with other CNS depressants (eg, centrally acting antiemetics, general anesthetics, phenothiazines, sedative-hypnotics) as there may be additive CNS effects. If combined therapy is needed, consider reducing the dose of one or both agents. Use care in prescribing, dispensing, and administering the oral concentrated solution, inappropriate use may cause overdose.

Adverse Reactions

Cardiovascular: Orthostatic hypotension

Central nervous system: Abnormal dreams, anxiety, chills, confusion, dizziness, dysphoria, euphoria, fever, headache, insomnia, nervousness, somnolence, thought abnormalities

Dermatologic: Pruritus, rash

Gastrointestinal: Abdominal pain, anorexia, constipation, diarrhea, dyspepsia, gastritis, nausea, vomiting, xerostomia

Neuromuscular & skeletal: Twitching, weakness

Respiratory: Dyspnea, hiccups

Miscellaneous: Diaphoresis

Rare but important or life-threatening: Agitation, amnesia, anaphylactoid reaction, anaphylaxis, chest pain, dehydration, depression, diverticulitis exacerbation, dysphagia, dysuria, edema, emotional lability, eructation, hallucinations, hematuria, histamine release, hyperalgesia, hyperkinesia, hypoesthesia, hyponatremia, hypotonia, ileus, intestinal obstruction, intracranial pressure increased, malaise, paralytic ileus, paresthesia, seizures, SIADH, speech disorder, ST segment depression, stomatitis, stupor, syncope, tablet in stool (some controlled release dosage forms), tremor, urinary retention, vertigo, withdrawal syndrome

Drug Interactions

Metabolism/Transport Effects Substrate of CYP2D6 (minor), CYP3A4 (major); **Note:** Assignment of Major/Minor substrate status based on clinically relevant drug interaction potential

Avoid Concomitant Use

Avoid concomitant use of OxyCODONE with any of the following: Azelastine (Nasal); Conivaptan; Fusidic Acid (Systemic); Paraldehyde; Thalidomide

Increased Effect/Toxicity

OxyCODONE may increase the levels/effects of: Alcohol (Ethyl); Alvimopan; Azelastine (Nasal); Buprenorphine; CNS Depressants; Desmopressin; Diuretics; Hydrocodone; Methotrimeprazine; Metyrosine; Mirtazapine; Paraldehyde; Pramipexole; ROPINIRole; Rotigotine; Selective Serotonin Reuptake Inhibitors; Thalidomide; Zolpidem

The levels/effects of OxyCODONE may be increased by: Amphetamines; Anticholinergic Agents; Antipsychotic Agents (Phenothiazines); Brimonidine (Topical); Cannabis; Conivaptan; CYP3A4 Inhibitors (Moderate); CYP3A4 Inhibitors (Strong); Dasatinib; Doxylamine; Dronabinol; Droperidol; Fusidic Acid (Systemic); HydrOXYzine; Ivacaftor; Kava Kava; Luliconazole; Magnesium Sulfate; MAO Inhibitors; Methotrimeprazine; Mifepristone; Nabilone; Perampanel; Rufinamide; Simeprevir; Sodium Oxybate; Stiripentol; Succinylcholine; Tapentadol; Tetrahydrocannabinol; Voriconazole

Decreased Effect

OxyCODONE may decrease the levels/effects of: Pegvisomant

The levels/effects of OxyCODONE may be decreased by: Ammonium Chloride; Bosentan; CYP3A4 Inducers (Strong); Dabrafenib; Deferasirox; Mitotane; Mixed Agonist / Antagonist Opioids; Naltrexone; Rifampin; Siltuximab; St Johns Wort; Tocilizumab

Stability Store at 25°C (77°F); excursions permitted between 15°C to 30°C (59°F to 86°F); protect from light and moisture

Mechanism of Action Binds to opiate receptors in the CNS, causing inhibition of ascending pain pathways, altering the perception of and response to pain; produces generalized CNS depression

Pharmacodynamics Duration of action: Analgesia:
Immediate release: 4-5 hours
Controlled release (OxyContin): 12 hours

Pharmacokinetics (Adult data unless noted)
Distribution: Distributes into skeletal muscle, liver, intestinal tract, lungs, spleen, and brain; V_{dss}:
Children 2-10 years: 2.1 L/kg (range: 1.2-3.7 L/kg)

Adults: 2.6 L/kg

Protein binding: 38% to 45%

Metabolism: In the liver primarily to noroxycodone (via demethylation) and oxymorphone (via CYP2D6); noroxycodone is the major circulating metabolite, but has much weaker activity than oxycodone; oxymorphone is active, but present in low concentrations; <15% of the dose is metabolized to oxymorphone via CYP2D6; drug and metabolites undergo glucuronide conjugation

Bioavailability: 60% to 87%

Half-life, apparent:

Immediate release: 3.2 hours

Controlled release (OxyContin): 4.5 hours

Half-life, elimination:

Children 2-10 years: 1.8 hours (range: 1.2-3 hours)

Adults: 3.7 hours

Adults with renal dysfunction (CrCl <60 mL/minute): Half-life increases by 1 hour, but peak oxycodone concentrations increase by 50% and AUC increases by 60%

Adults with mild to moderate hepatic dysfunction: Half-life increases by 2.3 hours, peak oxycodone concentrations increase by 50%, and AUC increases by 95%

Elimination: In the urine as unchanged drug (≤19%) and metabolites: Conjugated oxycodone (≤50%), conjugated oxymorphone (≤14%), noroxycodone, and conjugated noroxycodone

Dosing: Usual Note: Doses should be titrated to appropriate effect:

Infants, Children, and Adolescents:

Analgesic, moderate to severe: Oral: Immediate release:

Infants ≤6 months: Limited data available: Initial dose: 0.025-0.05 mg/kg/dose every 4-6 hours as needed (Berde, 2002)

Infants >6 months, Children, and Adolescents:

Patient weight <50 kg: Initial dose: 0.1-0.2 mg/kg/dose every 4-6 hours as needed; for severe pain some experts have recommended an initial dose of 0.2 mg/kg; usual maximum dose range: 5-10 mg (American Pain Society, 2008; APA, 2012; Berde, 2002)

Patient weight ≥50 kg: Initial dose: 5-10 mg every 4-6 hours as needed; for severe pain an initial dose of 10 mg may be used; usual maximum dose: 20 mg/dose (American Pain Society, 2008; Berde, 2002)

Adolescents ≥18 years and Adults: **Analgesic, moderate to severe:** Oral:

Immediate release: Initial: 5-15 mg every 4-6 hours as needed; dosing range: 5-20 mg/dose (American Pain Society, 2008). For severe chronic pain, administer on a regularly scheduled basis, every 4-6 hours, at the lowest dose that will achieve adequate analgesia.

Controlled release (OxyContin): **Note:** Only opioid-tolerant patients should receive the 60 mg and 80 mg strengths, a single dose >40 mg, or a total dose of >80 mg/day.

Opioid-naïve: 10 mg every 12 hours

Concurrent CNS depressants: Reduce usual initial oxycodone dose by one-third (1/3) to one-half (1/2)

Conversion from transdermal fentanyl: For each 25 mcg/hour transdermal dose, substitute 10 mg controlled release oxycodone every 12 hours; should be initiated 18 hours after the removal of the transdermal fentanyl patch

Currently on opioids: Use standard conversion chart to convert daily opioid dose to oxycodone equivalent. Initiate controlled release oxycodone with one-half (1/2) the estimated oxycodone daily dose (mg/day) and provide rescue medication in the form of immediate release oxycodone. Divide the initial controlled release oxycodone daily dose in 2 (for twice-daily dosing, usually every 12 hours) and round down to nearest dosage form.

Dose adjustment: Doses may be adjusted by changing the total daily dose (not by changing the dosing interval). Doses may be adjusted every 1-2 days and may be increased by 25% to 50%. Dose should be gradually tapered when no longer required in order to prevent withdrawal.

Dosing adjustment in renal impairment:

Children and Adolescents: Dosage adjustments are not provided in the manufacturer's labeling; however, the following adjustments have been recommended (Aronoff, 2007):

GFR 10-50 mL/minute/1.73 m^2: Administer 75% of dose

GFR <10 mL/minute/1.73 m^2: Administer 50% of dose

Hemodialysis: Administer 50% of dose posthemodialysis

Peritoneal dialysis: Administer 50% of dose

Adults: CrCl <60 mL/minute: Initiate doses conservatively and carefully titrate dose to appropriate effect

Dosing adjustment in hepatic impairment: Adults:

Immediate release: Reduced initial doses may be necessary (use a conservative approach to initial dosing); adjust dose based on clinical situation.

Controlled release products: Initial: One-third (1/3) to one-half (1/2) of the usual starting dose; carefully titrate dose to appropriate effect

Administration May administer with food to decrease GI upset

Immediate release (capsule, oral solution, tablets):

Oral solution: Available in two strengths; 1 mg/mL and a concentrated oral solution (20 mg/mL). Precautions should be taken to avoid confusion between the different concentrations; prescriptions should have the concentration specified as well as the dose clearly represented as milligram (mg) of oxycodone, not volume (mL). The enclosed calibrated oral syringe should always be used to administer the concentrated oral solution to ensure the dose is measured and administered accurately. The concentrated oral solution (20 mg/mL) should only be used in opioid-tolerant patients (taking ≥30 mg/day of oxycodone or equivalent for ≥1 week).

Tablet (Oxecta): Swallow whole with adequate water to ensure complete swallowing immediately after placing in the mouth; the formulation uses technology designed to discourage common methods of tampering to prevent misuse/abuse. The tablet should not be wet prior to placing in the mouth. Do not crush, chew, or dissolve nor administer via feeding tubes (eg, gastric, NG) due to potential for obstruction.

Controlled release tablet (OxyContin): Swallow whole; do not moisten, dissolve, cut, crush, chew, or break as this would result in rapid release of oxycodone and absorption of a potentially fatal dose of drug. Administer one at a time and follow each with water immediately after placing in the mouth. For oral use only, do not administer rectally; increased risk of adverse events due to better rectal absorption.

Monitoring Parameters Pain relief, respiratory rate, mental status, blood pressure; signs of misuse, abuse, and addiction

Test Interactions Some quinolones may produce a false-positive urine screening result for opioids using commercially-available immunoassay kits. This has been demonstrated most consistently for levofloxacin and ofloxacin, but other quinolones have shown cross-reactivity in certain assay kits. Confirmation of positive opioid screens by more specific methods should be considered.

Additional Information OxyContin tablets deliver medication over 12 hours; release is pH independent. Equianalgesic doses: oral oxycodone 30 mg = morphine 10 mg I.M. = single oral dose morphine 60 mg **or** chronic dosing oral morphine 30 mg

Oxecta utilizes Acura Pharmaceutical's Aversion technology which may help discourage misuse and abuse potential. Reduced abuse potential of Oxecta compared to other immediate release oxycodone tablet formulations has not been proven; the FDA is requiring Pfizer to complete a post approval epidemiological study to determine whether the formulation actually results in a decrease of misuse/abuse. In one clinical trial in non-dependent recreational opioid users, the "drug-liking" responses and safety of crushed Oxecta tablets were compared to crushed immediate-release oxycodone tablets following the self-administered intranasal use. A small difference in "drug-liking" scores was observed, with lower scores reported in the crushed Oxecta group. In regards to safety, there was an increased incidence of nasopharyngeal and facial adverse events in the Oxecta group. In addition, there was decreased ability in the Oxecta group to completely administer the two crushed Oxecta tablets intranasally within a set time period. However, whether these differences translate into a significant clinical difference is unknown. Of note, pharmacokinetic studies showed that Oxecta is bioequivalent with oxycodone immediate release tablets with no differences in T_{max} and half-life when administered in the fasted state.

Controlled Substance C-II

Dosage Forms Excipient information presented when available (limited, particularly for generics); consult specific product labeling. [DSC] = Discontinued product

Capsule, Oral, as hydrochloride:
Generic: 5 mg
Concentrate, Oral, as hydrochloride:
Generic: 100 mg/5 mL (30 mL)
Solution, Oral, as hydrochloride:
Generic: 5 mg/5 mL (5 mL, 15 mL, 500 mL)
Tablet, Oral, as hydrochloride:
Roxicodone: 5 mg [scored]
Roxicodone: 15 mg [scored; contains fd&c blue #2 (indigotine), fd&c yellow #10 (quinoline yellow)]
Roxicodone: 30 mg [scored]
Generic: 5 mg, 10 mg, 15 mg, 20 mg, 30 mg
Tablet Abuse-Deterrent, Oral, as hydrochloride:
Oxecta: 5 mg [DSC], 7.5 mg [DSC]
Tablet ER 12 Hour Abuse-Deterrent, Oral, as hydrochloride:
OxyCONTIN: 10 mg, 15 mg, 20 mg, 30 mg, 40 mg, 60 mg
OxyCONTIN: 80 mg [contains fd&c blue #2 aluminum lake]

References

ACOG Committee on Practice Bulletins-Obstetrics, "ACOG Practice Bulletin. Clinical Management Guidelines for Obstetrician-Gynecologists Number 36, July 2002. Obstetric Analgesia and Anesthesia,' Obstet Gynecol, 2002, 100(1):177-91.

Association of Paediatric Anaesthetists of Great Britain and Ireland (APA). Good practice in postoperative and procedural pain management, 2nd edition. Paediatr Anaesth. 2012;22(Suppl 1):1-79.

Berde CB, Sethna NF. Analgesics for the treatment of pain in children. N Engl J Med. 2002;347(14):1094-1103.

Chou R, Fanciullo GJ, Fine PG, et al, "Clinical Guidelines for the Use of Chronic Opioid Therapy in Chronic Noncancer Pain," J Pain, 2009, 10 (2):113-30.

Dow K, Ordean A, Murphy-Oikonen J, et al, "Neonatal Abstinence Syndrome Clinical Practice Guidelines For Ontario," J Popul Ther Clin Pharmacol, 2012, 19(3):e488-506.

Hudak ML, Tan RC, Committee on Drugs, et al, "Neonatal Drug Withdrawal," Pediatrics, 2012, 129(2):e540-60.

Montgomery A, Hale TW, and Academy of Breastfeeding Medicine, "ABM Clinical Protocol #15: Analgesia and Anesthesia For the Breastfeeding Mother, Revised 2012," Breastfeed Med, 2012, 7 (6):547-53.

Olkkola KT, Hamunen K, and Maunuksela EL, "Clinical Pharmacokinetics and Pharmacodynamics of Opioid Analgesics in Infants and Children," Clin Pharmacokinet, 1995, 28(5):385-404.

Olkkola KT, Hamunen K, Seppala T, et al, "Pharmacokinetics and Ventilatory Effects of Intravenous Oxycodone in Postoperative Children," Br J Clin Pharmacol, 1994, 38(1):71-6.

"Principles of Analgesic Use in the Treatment of Acute Pain and Cancer Pain," 6th ed, Glenview, IL: American Pain Society, 2008.

Oxycodone and Acetaminophen
(oks i KOE done & a seet a MIN oh fen)

Medication Safety Issues

Sound-alike/look-alike issues:

Oxycodone and Acetaminophen may be confused with Hydrocodone and Acetaminophen

Endocet may be confused with Indocid

Percocet may be confused with Fioricet, Percodan

Roxicet may be confused with Roxanol

High alert medication:

The Institute for Safe Medication Practices (ISMP) includes this medication among its list of drug classes which have a heightened risk of causing significant patient harm when used in error.

Other safety concerns:

Duplicate therapy issues: This product contains acetaminophen, which may be a component of other combination products. Do not exceed the maximum recommended daily dose of acetaminophen.

Brand Names: U.S. Endocet; Percocet; Primlev; Roxicet; Xartemis XR; Xolox [DSC]

Brand Names: Canada Apo-Oxycodone/Acet; Endocet; Percocet; Percocet-Demi; PMS-Oxycodone-Acetaminophen; Ratio-Oxycocet; Rivacocet; Sandoz-Oxycodone/Acetaminophen

Therapeutic Category Analgesic, Narcotic

Generic Availability (U.S.) Yes: Excludes solution

Use Relief of moderate to moderately severe pain (FDA approved in adults)

Medication Guide Available Yes

Pregnancy Risk Factor C

Pregnancy Considerations [U.S. Boxed Warning]: Prolonged use of oxycodone/acetaminophen during pregnancy can result in neonatal opioid withdrawal syndrome, which may be life-threatening if not recognized and requires management according to protocols developed by neonatology experts. If opioid use is required for a prolonged period in a pregnant woman, advise the patient of the risk of neonatal opioid withdrawal syndrome. Animal reproduction studies have not been conducted with this combination. Refer to individual monographs for additional information.

Breast-Feeding Considerations Oxycodone and acetaminophen are both excreted into breast milk. Somnolence and lethargy have been reported in nursing infants following maternal use of this combination. Breast-feeding is not recommended by the manufacturer. Refer to individual monographs for additional information.

Contraindications Hypersensitivity to oxycodone, acetaminophen, or any component; severe respiratory depression (in unmonitored settings or the absence of resuscitative equipment); severe or acute bronchial asthma; hypercarbia; suspected or known paralytic ileus

Warnings Acetaminophen may cause severe hepatotoxicity **[U.S. Boxed Warning]**, potentially requiring liver transplant or resulting in death; hepatotoxicity is usually associated with excessive acetaminophen intake (>4 g/day in adults). Risk is increased with alcohol use, preexisting liver disease, and intake of more than one source of acetaminophen-containing medications. Chronic daily dosing in adults has also resulted in liver damage in some patients. Do not exceed maximum daily doses; consider acetaminophen content of all products (prescription and OTC) including combination products when evaluating the total daily dose of acetaminophen; adults ingesting >4 g/day of acetaminophen should seek medical attention immediately.

◄ Hypersensitivity and anaphylactic reactions have been reported with acetaminophen and oxycodone; use with caution in patients with hypersensitivity to other phenanthrene derivative opioid agonists (morphine, codeine, hydrocodone, hydromorphone, oxymorphone, levorphanol); discontinue immediately if symptoms of allergic or hypersensitivity reactions occur. Serious and potentially fatal skin reactions, including acute generalized exanthematous pustulosis (AGEP), Stevens-Johnson Syndrome (SJS), and toxic epidermal necrolysis (TEN), have occurred rarely with acetaminophen use. Discontinue therapy at the first appearance of skin rash.

Oxycodone may cause CNS depression which may impair physical or mental abilities; patients must be cautioned about performing tasks which require mental alertness (eg, operating machinery or driving). Respiratory depression may occur even at therapeutic dosages; use with extreme caution in patients with respiratory diseases including asthma, emphysema, COPD, cor pulmonale, hypoxia, hypercapnia, preexisting respiratory depression, significantly decreased respiratory reserve, other obstructive pulmonary disease, kyphoscoliosis, or other skeletal disorder which may alter respiratory function.

Use with extreme caution in patients with head injury, intracranial lesions, or elevated intracranial pressure; exaggerated elevation of ICP may occur. May cause hypotension; use with caution in patients with circulatory shock, hypovolemia, impaired myocardial function, or those receiving drugs which may exaggerate hypotensive effects (including phenothiazines or general anesthetics); may cause orthostatic hypotension in ambulatory patients. Oxycodone may obscure diagnosis or clinical course of patients with acute abdominal conditions; has been shown to decrease gastrointestinal motility; use with caution in postoperative patients especially after intra-abdominal surgery.

Physical and psychological dependence may occur; abrupt discontinuation after prolonged use may result in withdrawal symptoms; warn patients of possible impairment of alertness or physical coordination; concurrent use of agonist/antagonist analgesics (ie, pentazocine, nalbuphine, and butorphanol) may precipitate withdrawal symptoms and/or reduce analgesic efficacy in patients following prolonged therapy with mu opioid agonists, such as oxycodone. High potential for abuse; healthcare providers should be alert to problems of abuse, misuse, and diversion. Infants born to women physically dependent on opioids will also be physically dependent and may experience respiratory difficulties or opioid withdrawal symptoms [neonatal abstinence syndrome (NAS)]. Onset, duration, and severity of NAS depend upon the drug used (maternal), duration of use, maternal dose, and rate of drug elimination by the newborn. Symptoms of opioid withdrawal may include excessive crying, diarrhea, fever, hyper-reflexia, irritability, tremors, vomiting, or failure to gain weight. Opioid withdrawal syndrome in the neonate may be life-threatening and should be promptly treated.

Oral solution contains alcohol (<0.5%). Some preparations contain sodium metabisulfite which may cause allergic reactions in susceptible individuals; capsule may contain sodium benzoate; benzoic acid (benzoate) is a metabolite of benzyl alcohol; large amounts of benzyl alcohol (≥99 mg/kg/day) have been associated with a potentially fatal toxicity ("gasping syndrome") in neonates; avoid use of oxycodone and acetaminophen products containing sodium benzoate in neonates.

Precautions Use with caution in patients with adrenal insufficiency (Addison's disease); biliary tract disease; pancreatitis; CNS depression/coma; acute alcoholism; delirium tremens; hypothyroidism (myxedema); severe liver, pulmonary, or renal impairment; urinary stricture; prostatic hypertrophy; or seizures.

Use caution when combining with other CNS depressants (eg, centrally acting antiemetics, general anesthetics, phenothiazines, sedative-hypnotics) as there may be additive CNS effects. If combined therapy is needed, consider reducing the dose of one or both agents.

Although several case reports of acetaminophen-associated hemolytic anemia have been reported in patients with G-6-PD deficiency, a direct cause and effect relationship has not been well established (concurrent illnesses such as fever or infection may precipitate hemolytic anemia in patients with G-6-PD deficiency); therefore, acetaminophen is generally thought to be safe when given in therapeutic doses to patients with G-6-PD deficiency.

Adverse Reactions Also see individual agents.
Cardiovascular: Peripheral edema
Central nervous system: Dizziness, drowsiness, fatigue, headache, insomnia
Dermatologic: Erythema, excoriation, pruritus, skin blister, skin rash
Endocrine & metabolic: Hot flash
Gastrointestinal: Constipation, diarrhea, dyspepsia, nausea, vomiting, xerostomia
Genitourinary: Dysuria
Hepatic: Increased liver enzymes
Respiratory: Cough
Rare but important or life-threatening: Chest discomfort, cognitive dysfunction, dermatitis, dysphoria, euphoria, hypersensitivity reaction, hypertension, memory impairment, migraine, myoclonus, palpitations, respiratory depression, sedation, withdrawal syndrome

Drug Interactions

Metabolism/Transport Effects Refer to individual components.

Avoid Concomitant Use
Avoid concomitant use of Oxycodone and Acetaminophen with any of the following: Azelastine (Nasal); Conivaptan; Fusidic Acid (Systemic); Paraldehyde; Pimozide; Thalidomide

Increased Effect/Toxicity
Oxycodone and Acetaminophen may increase the levels/effects of: Alvimopan; ARIPiprazole; Azelastine (Nasal); Buprenorphine; Busulfan; CNS Depressants; Dasatinib; Desmopressin; Diuretics; Dofetilide; Hydrocodone; Lomitapide; Methotrimeprazine; Metyrosine; Mipomersen; Mirtazapine; Paraldehyde; Phenylephrine (Systemic); Pimozide; Pramipexole; Prilocaine; ROPINIRole; Rotigotine; Selective Serotonin Reuptake Inhibitors; Sodium Nitrite; SORAfenib; Thalidomide; Vitamin K Antagonists; Zolpidem

The levels/effects of Oxycodone and Acetaminophen may be increased by: Alcohol (Ethyl); Amphetamines; Anticholinergic Agents; Antipsychotic Agents (Phenothiazines); Brimonidine (Topical); Cannabis; Conivaptan; CYP3A4 Inhibitors (Moderate); CYP3A4 Inhibitors (Strong); Dasatinib; Doxylamine; Dronabinol; Droperidol; Fusidic Acid (Systemic); HydrOXYzine; Isoniazid; Ivacaftor; Kava Kava; Luliconazole; Magnesium Sulfate; MAO Inhibitors; Methotrimeprazine; Metyrapone; Mifepristone; Nabilone; Nitric Oxide; Perampanel; Probenecid; Rufinamide; Simeprevir; Sodium Oxybate; SORAfenib; Stiripentol; Succinylcholine; Tapentadol; Tetrahydrocannabinol; Voriconazole

Decreased Effect
Oxycodone and Acetaminophen may decrease the levels/effects of: Pegvisomant

The levels/effects of Oxycodone and Acetaminophen may be decreased by: Ammonium Chloride; Anticonvulsants (Hydantoin); Barbiturates; Bosentan;

Cholestyramine Resin; CYP3A4 Inducers (Strong); Dabrafenib; Deferasirox; Mitotane; Mixed Agonist / Antagonist Opioids; Naltrexone; Peginterferon Alfa-2b; Rifampin; Siltuximab; St Johns Wort; Tocilizumab

Mechanism of Action

Oxycodone, as with other opioid analgesics, blocks pain perception in the cerebral cortex by binding to specific receptor molecules (opiate receptors) within the neuronal membranes of synapses. This binding results in a decreased synaptic chemical transmission throughout the CNS thus inhibiting the flow of pain sensations into the higher centers. Mu and kappa are the two subtypes of the opiate receptor to which oxycodone binds to cause analgesia.

Acetaminophen inhibits the synthesis of prostaglandins in the CNS and peripherally blocks pain impulse generation; produces antipyresis from inhibition of hypothalamic heat-regulating center.

Pharmacodynamics

Onset of action: Within 10 to 15 minutes
Maximum effect: Within 1 hour
Duration: 3 to 6 hours

Pharmacokinetics (Adult data unless noted) See individual agents.

Dosing: Usual

Children and Adolescents: **Note:** Doses based on total oxycodone content; titrate dose to appropriate analgesic effects; maximum daily acetaminophen dose: 75 mg/kg/**day** not to exceed 4000 mg/**day**; do **not** exceed 5 doses in 24 hours

Analgesic, moderate: Oral: 0.1 to 0.2 mg/kg/dose; doses typically given every 4 to 6 hours as needed; manufacturer's labeling recommends every 6 hours; maximum initial oxycodone dose: 5 mg/dose (American Pain Society, 2008)

Analgesic, severe: Initial dose: Oral: 0.2 mg/kg/dose; doses typically given every 4 to 6 hours as needed; manufacturer's labeling recommends every 6 hours; maximum initial oxycodone dose: 10 mg (American Pain Society, 2008)

Adults: **Analgesic:** Initial dose is based on oxycodone content; however, the maximum daily dose is based on the acetaminophen content. Doses should be given every 4 to 6 hours as needed and titrated to appropriate analgesic effects.

Manufacturer's labeling: Moderate to moderately severe pain: Initial dose, based on oxycodone content: Oral: 2.5 to 10 mg every 6 hours as needed. Titrate according to pain severity and individual response. Do not exceed acetaminophen 4 **g**/day.

Alternate recommendations (American Pain Society, 2008):

Moderate pain: Initial dose, based on oxycodone content: Oral: 5 mg; doses typically given every 4 to 6 hours as needed; manufacturer's labeling recommends every 6 hours as needed. Do not exceed acetaminophen 4 **g**/day

Severe pain: Initial dose, based on oxycodone content: Oral: 10 to 20 mg; doses typically given every 4 to 6 hours as needed; manufacturer's labeling recommends every 6 hours as needed. Do not exceed acetaminophen 4 **g**/day

Administration Oral: May administer with food or milk to decrease GI upset

Monitoring Parameters Pain relief, respiratory rate, mental status, blood pressure; signs of misuse, abuse, and addiction

Test Interactions See individual agents.

Controlled Substance C-II

Dosage Forms Excipient information presented when available (limited, particularly for generics); consult specific product labeling. [DSC] = Discontinued product

Capsule, Oral: 5/500: Oxycodone hydrochloride 5 mg and acetaminophen 500 mg [DSC]

Solution, Oral:
Roxicet: Oxycodone hydrochloride 5 mg and acetaminophen 325 mg per 5 mL (5 mL, 500 mL) [contains ethanol <0.5%; mint flavor]

Tablet, Oral: 2.5/325: Oxycodone hydrochloride 2.5 mg and acetaminophen 325 mg; 5/325: Oxycodone hydrochloride 5 mg and acetaminophen 325 mg; 7.5/325: Oxycodone hydrochloride 7.5 mg and acetaminophen 325 mg; 7.5/500: Oxycodone hydrochloride 7.5 mg and acetaminophen 500 mg [DSC]; 10/325: Oxycodone hydrochloride 10 mg and acetaminophen 325 mg; 10/650: Oxycodone hydrochloride 10 mg and acetaminophen 650 mg [DSC]

Endocet 2.5/325: Oxycodone hydrochloride 2.5 mg and acetaminophen 325 mg

Endocet 5/325 [scored]: Oxycodone hydrochloride 5 mg and acetaminophen 325 mg

Endocet 7.5/325: Oxycodone hydrochloride 7.5 mg and acetaminophen 325 mg

Endocet 7.5/500: Oxycodone hydrochloride 7.5 mg and acetaminophen 500 mg [DSC]

Endocet 10/325: Oxycodone hydrochloride 10 mg and acetaminophen 325 mg

Endocet 10/650: Oxycodone hydrochloride 10 mg and acetaminophen 650 mg [DSC]

Magnacet 5/400: Oxycodone hydrochloride 5 mg and acetaminophen 400 mg [DSC]

Magnacet 7.5/400: Oxycodone hydrochloride 7.5 mg and acetaminophen 400 mg [DSC]

Magnacet 10/400: Oxycodone hydrochloride 10 mg and acetaminophen 400 mg [DSC]

Percocet 2.5/325: Oxycodone hydrochloride 2.5 mg and acetaminophen 325 mg

Percocet 5/325 [scored]: Oxycodone hydrochloride 5 mg and acetaminophen 325 mg

Percocet 7.5/325: Oxycodone hydrochloride 7.5 mg and acetaminophen 325 mg

Percocet 7.5/500: Oxycodone hydrochloride 7.5 mg and acetaminophen 500 mg [DSC]

Percocet 10/325: Oxycodone hydrochloride 10 mg and acetaminophen 325 mg

Percocet 10/650: Oxycodone hydrochloride 10 mg and acetaminophen 650 mg [DSC]

Primlev 5/300: Oxycodone hydrochloride 5 mg and acetaminophen 300 mg

Primlev 7.5/300: Oxycodone hydrochloride 7.5 mg and acetaminophen 300 mg

Primlev 10/300: Oxycodone hydrochloride 10 mg and acetaminophen 300 mg

Roxicet 5/325 [scored]: Oxycodone hydrochloride 5 mg and acetaminophen 325 mg

Tablet, Extended Release, Oral:
Xartemis XR: Oxycodone hydrochloride 7.5 mg and acetaminophen 325 mg

References

Olkkola KT, Hamunen K, and Maunuksela EL, "Clinical Pharmacokinetics and Pharmacodynamics of Opioid Analgesics in Infants and Children," Clin Pharmacokinet, 1995, 28(5):385-404.

"Principles of Analgesic Use in the Treatment of Acute Pain and Cancer Pain," 6th ed, Glenview, IL: American Pain Society, 2008.

Oxycodone and Aspirin (oks i KOE done & AS pir in)

Medication Safety Issues

Sound-alike/look-alike issues:

Percodan® may be confused with Decadron, Percocet®, Percogesic®, Periactin

High alert medication:

The Institute for Safe Medication Practices (ISMP) includes this medication among its list of drug classes

which have a heightened risk of causing significant patient harm when used in error.

Brand Names: U.S. Endodan®; Percodan®

Brand Names: Canada Endodan®; Oxycodan®; Percodan®

Therapeutic Category Analgesic, Narcotic

Generic Availability (U.S.) Yes

Use Relief of moderate to moderately severe pain (FDA approved in adults)

Pregnancy Risk Factor B (oxycodone); D (aspirin)

Pregnancy Considerations See individual agents.

Breast-Feeding Considerations See individual agents.

Contraindications Hypersensitivity to oxycodone, salicylates, other NSAIDs, or any component; severe or acute asthma, urticaria, or allergic-type reaction to aspirin or other NSAIDs; patients with the "aspirin triad" [asthma, rhinitis (with or without nasal polyps), and aspirin intolerance] (fatal asthmatic and anaphylactoid reactions may occur in these patients); inherited or acquired bleeding disorders (including factor VII and factor IX deficiency); significant respiratory depression; hypercarbia; known or suspected paralytic ileus; children and adolescents in the presence of viral infections (chickenpox or flu symptoms) with or without fever, due to a potential association with Reye's syndrome

Warnings Oxycodone may cause CNS depression which may impair physical or mental abilities; patients must be cautioned about performing tasks which require mental alertness (eg, operating machinery or driving). Respiratory depression may occur even at therapeutic doses; use with extreme caution in patients with preexisting respiratory depression, significantly decreased respiratory reserve, hypoxia, hypercapnia, respiratory diseases (including asthma, emphysema, significant COPD, or cor pulmonale), other obstructive pulmonary disease, kyphoscoliosis, or other skeletal disorder which may alter respiratory function.

Oxycodone may exaggerate elevated intracranial pressure; use with extreme caution in patients with head injury, intracranial lesions, or elevated ICP. Hypotension may occur; especially in hypovolemic patients or those receiving medications that compromise vasomotor tone or exaggerate hypotensive effects (including phenothiazines); use with extreme caution in patients with circulatory shock. Orthostatic hypotension may occur in ambulatory patients. Oxycodone may obscure diagnosis or clinical course of patients with acute abdominal conditions; has been shown to decrease gastrointestinal motility; use with caution in postoperative patients especially after intra-abdominal surgery.

Physical and psychological dependence may occur; abrupt discontinuation after prolonged use may result in withdrawal symptoms; warn patients of possible impairment of alertness or physical coordination; concurrent use of agonist/antagonist analgesics (ie, pentazocine, nalbuphine, and butorphanol) may precipitate withdrawal symptoms and/or reduce analgesic efficacy in patients following prolonged therapy with mu opioid agonists such as oxycodone. High potential for abuse; healthcare providers should be alert to problems of abuse, misuse, and diversion. Infants born to women physically dependent on opioids will also be physically dependent and may experience respiratory difficulties or opioid withdrawal symptoms [neonatal abstinence syndrome (NAS)]. Onset, duration, and severity of NAS depend upon the drug used (maternal), duration of use, maternal dose, and rate of drug elimination by the newborn. Symptoms of opioid withdrawal may include excessive crying, diarrhea, fever, hyper-reflexia, irritability, tremors, vomiting, or failure to gain weight. Opioid withdrawal syndrome in the neonate,

unlike in adults, may be life-threatening and should be promptly treated.

Precautions

Aspirin: Use with caution in patients with impaired hepatic or renal function, platelet or bleeding disorders, erosive gastritis, peptic ulcer, or heavy alcohol use.

Oxycodone: Use with caution in patients with hypersensitivity to other phenanthrene derivative opioid agonists (morphine, codeine, hydrocodone, hydromorphone, oxymorphone, levorphanol); discontinue immediately if symptoms of allergic or hypersensitivity reactions occur. Use with caution in patients with adrenal insufficiency (Addison's disease), biliary tract disease, pancreatitis, CNS depression, acute alcoholism, delirium tremens, kyphoscoliosis with respiratory depression, hypothyroidism (myxedema), severe liver, pulmonary or renal impairment, urinary stricture, prostatic hypertrophy, or seizures. Use caution when combining with other CNS depressants (eg centrally acting antiemetics, general anesthetics, phenothiazines, sedative-hypnotics) as there may be additive CNS effects. If combined therapy is needed, consider reducing the dose of one or both agents.

Adverse Reactions Note: Also see individual agents

Cardiovascular: Circulatory depression, hypotension, shock

Central nervous system: Dizziness, drowsiness, dysphoria, euphoria, lightheadedness, sedation

Dermatologic: Pruritus

Gastrointestinal: Constipation, nausea, vomiting

Respiratory: Apnea, respiratory arrest, respiratory depression

Drug Interactions

Metabolism/Transport Effects Refer to individual components.

Avoid Concomitant Use

Avoid concomitant use of Oxycodone and Aspirin with any of the following: Azelastine (Nasal); Conivaptan; Floctafenine; Fusidic Acid (Systemic); Influenza Virus Vaccine (Live/Attenuated); Ketorolac (Nasal); Ketorolac (Systemic); Omacetaxine; Paraldehyde; Thalidomide; Urokinase

Increased Effect/Toxicity

Oxycodone and Aspirin may increase the levels/effects of: Agents with Antiplatelet Properties; Alcohol (Ethyl); Alendronate; Alvimopan; Anticoagulants; Apixaban; Azelastine (Nasal); Buprenorphine; Carbonic Anhydrase Inhibitors; Carisoprodol; CNS Depressants; Collagenase (Systemic); Corticosteroids (Systemic); Dabigatran Etexilate; Desmopressin; Diuretics; Heparin; Hydrocodone; Hypoglycemic Agents; Ibritumomab; Methotrexate; Methotrimeprazine; Metyrosine; Mirtazapine; NSAID (COX-2 Inhibitor); Omacetaxine; Paraldehyde; PRALAtrexate; Pramipexole; Rivaroxaban; ROPINIRole; Rotigotine; Salicylates; Thalidomide; Thrombolytic Agents; Ticagrelor; Tositumomab and Iodine I 131 Tositumomab; Urokinase; Valproic Acid and Derivatives; Varicella Virus-Containing Vaccines; Vitamin K Antagonists; Zolpidem

The levels/effects of Oxycodone and Aspirin may be increased by: Agents with Antiplatelet Properties; Ammonium Chloride; Amphetamines; Anticholinergic Agents; Antidepressants (Tricyclic, Tertiary Amine); Antipsychotic Agents (Phenothiazines); Brimonidine (Topical); Cannabis; Conivaptan; CYP3A4 Inhibitors (Moderate); CYP3A4 Inhibitors (Strong); Dasatinib; Doxylamine; Dronabinol; Droperidol; Floctafenine; Fusidic Acid (Systemic); Ginkgo Biloba; Glucosamine; Herbs (Anticoagulant/Antiplatelet Properties); HydrOXYzine; Ibrutinib; Influenza Virus Vaccine (Live/Attenuated); Ivacaftor; Kava Kava; Ketorolac (Nasal); Ketorolac (Systemic); Loop Diuretics; Luliconazole; Magnesium Sulfate; MAO Inhibitors; Methotrimeprazine; Mifepristone; Multivitamins/Fluoride (with ADE);

Multivitamins/Minerals (with ADEK, Folate, Iron); Multivitamins/Minerals (with AE, No Iron); Nabilone; NSAID (Nonselective); Omega-3 Fatty Acids; Pentosan Polysulfate Sodium; Pentoxifylline; Perampanel; Potassium Acid Phosphate; Prostacyclin Analogues; Rufinamide; Selective Serotonin Reuptake Inhibitors; Serotonin/Norepinephrine Reuptake Inhibitors; Simeprevir; Sodium Oxybate; Stiripentol; Succinylcholine; Tapentadol; Tetrahydrocannabinol; Tipranavir; Treprostinil; Vitamin E; Voriconazole

Decreased Effect

Oxycodone and Aspirin may decrease the levels/effects of: ACE Inhibitors; Carisoprodol; Hyaluronidase; Loop Diuretics; Multivitamins/Fluoride (with ADE); Multivitamins/Minerals (with ADEK, Folate, Iron); Multivitamins/Minerals (with AE, No Iron); NSAID (Nonselective); Pegvisomant; Probenecid; Ticagrelor; Tiludronate

The levels/effects of Oxycodone and Aspirin may be decreased by: Ammonium Chloride; Bosentan; Corticosteroids (Systemic); CYP3A4 Inducers (Strong); Dabrafenib; Deferasirox; Floctafenine; Ketorolac (Nasal); Ketorolac (Systemic); Mitotane; Mixed Agonist / Antagonist Opioids; Naltrexone; NSAID (Nonselective); Rifampin; Siltuximab; St Johns Wort; Tocilizumab

Mechanism of Action

Oxycodone, as with other opioid analgesics, blocks pain perception in the cerebral cortex by binding to specific receptor molecules (opiate receptors) within the neuronal membranes of synapses. This binding results in a decreased synaptic chemical transmission throughout the CNS, thus inhibiting the flow of pain sensations into the higher centers. Mu and kappa are the two subtypes of the opiate receptor to which oxycodone binds to cause analgesia.

Aspirin inhibits prostaglandin synthesis by decreasing the activity of the enzyme, cyclooxygenase, which results in decreased formation of prostaglandin precursors, acts on the hypothalamic heat-regulating center to reduce fever, blocks thromboxane synthetase action which prevents formation of the platelet-aggregating substance thromboxane A_2

Pharmacokinetics (Adult data unless noted) See individual agents.

Dosing: Usual Oral:

Children and Adolescents: Note: Dosed based on total oxycodone content; titrate dose to appropriate analgesic effects; maximum daily aspirin dose: 4 g/day

Analgesic, moderate: 0.1-0.2 mg/kg/dose every 4-6 hours as needed; maximum oxycodone dose: 5 mg/dose (American Pain Society, 2008)

Analgesic, severe: Initial dose: 0.2 mg/kg/dose every 4-6 hours as needed (American Pain Society, 2008)

Adults:1 tablet every 6 hours as needed for pain; maximum aspirin dose should not exceed 4 g/**day**

Dosing adjustment in renal impairment:

Children and Adolescents: Note: No dosing recommendations are available for the combination product. The following guidelines have been used by some clinicians:
GFR 10-50 mL/minute/1.73m^2: Administer 75% of dose (Aronoff, 2007); **Note:** Based on the oxycodone component only
GFR <10 mL/minute/1.73m^2: No data available; avoid use due to aspirin component

Adults: CrCl <10 mL/minute: Adults: Avoid use due to aspirin component

Dosing adjustment in hepatic impairment: Adults: The FDA-approved labeling does not contain dosing adjustment guidelines; use with caution; if severe impairment, avoid use of aspirin

Administration May administer with food or milk to decrease GI upset

Monitoring Parameters Pain relief, respiratory rate, mental status, blood pressure; signs of misuse, abuse, and addiction

Test Interactions May cross-react with urine tests for cocaine or marijuana.

Additional Information One generic tablet contains ~5 mg oxycodone as combined salt

Controlled Substance C-II

Dosage Forms Excipient information presented when available (limited, particularly for generics); consult specific product labeling.
Tablet: Oxycodone hydrochloride 4.8355 mg and aspirin 325 mg
Endodan®, Percodan®: Oxycodone hydrochloride 4.8355 mg and aspirin 325 mg

References

"Principles of Analgesic Use in the Treatment of Acute Pain and Cancer Pain," 6th ed, Glenview, IL: American Pain Society, 2008.

◆ **Oxycodone Hydrochloride** *see* OxyCODONE *on page 1569*

◆ **OxyCONTIN** *see* OxyCODONE *on page 1569*

◆ **OxyContin (Can)** *see* OxyCODONE *on page 1569*

◆ **Oxyderm™ (Can)** *see* Benzoyl Peroxide *on page 275*

◆ **Oxy.IR (Can)** *see* OxyCODONE *on page 1569*

Oxymetazoline (Nasal) (oks i met AZ oh leen)

Medication Safety Issues

Sound-alike/look-alike issues:
Oxymetazoline may be confused with oxymetholone
Afrin may be confused with aspirin
Afrin (oxymetazoline) may be confused with Afrin (saline)
Neo-Synephrine (oxymetazoline) may be confused with Neo-Synephrine (phenylephrine, nasal)

Other safety concerns:
Accidental ingestion: Serious adverse reactions (eg, coma, bradycardia, respiratory depression, sedation) requiring hospitalization have been reported in children ≤5 years of age who have accidentally ingested even small amounts (eg, 1-2 mL) of imidazoline-derivative (ie, tetrahydrozoline, oxymetazoline, or naphazoline) eye drops or nasal sprays. Store these products out of reach of children at all times. Contact poison control or seek medical attention if accidental ingestion occurs.

Brand Names: U.S. 12 Hour Nasal Relief Spray [OTC]; 12 Hour Nasal Spray [OTC]; Afrin 12 Hour [OTC]; Afrin Extra Moisturizing [OTC]; Afrin Menthol Spray [OTC]; Afrin Nasal Spray [OTC]; Afrin NoDrip Original [OTC]; Afrin NoDrip Sinus [OTC]; Afrin Sinus [OTC]; Dristan Spray [OTC]; Long Lasting Nasal Spray [OTC]; Mucinex Nasal Spray Full Force [OTC]; Mucinex Nasal Spray Moisture [OTC]; Mucinex Sinus-Max Full Force [OTC]; Mucinex Sinus-Max Moist Smart [OTC]; Nasal Decongestant Spray [OTC]; Nasal Spray 12 Hour [OTC]; Nasal Spray Extra Moisturizing [OTC]; Neo-Synephrine 12 Hour Spray [OTC]; NRS Nasal Relief [OTC]; Sinus Nasal Spray [OTC]

Brand Names: Canada Claritin Allergic Decongestant; Dristan Long Lasting Nasal; Drixoral Nasal

Therapeutic Category Decongestant, Nasal; Nasal Agent, Vasoconstrictor; Vasoconstrictor, Nasal

Generic Availability (U.S.) Yes

Use Symptomatic relief of nasal mucosal congestion associated with acute or chronic rhinitis, the common cold, sinusitis, hay fever, or other allergies

Pregnancy Considerations Adverse fetal or neonatal effects have not been observed following normal maternal doses of oxymetazoline during the third trimester of pregnancy. Adverse events have been noted in case reports following large doses or extended use. Decongestants are not the preferred agents for the treatment of rhinitis during pregnancy. Short-term (<3 days) use of intranasal

◀ oxymetazoline may be beneficial to some patients although its safety during pregnancy has not been studied.

Contraindications Hypersensitivity to oxymetazoline or any component

Warnings Use for periods exceeding 3 days may result in severe rebound nasal congestion; excessive dosage in children may cause profound CNS depression. Some products contain benzyl alcohol which may cause allergic reactions in susceptible individuals; large amounts of benzyl alcohol (≥99 mg/kg/day) have been associated with a potentially fatal toxicity ("gasping syndrome") in neonates; the "gasping syndrome" consists of metabolic acidosis, respiratory distress, gasping respirations, CNS dysfunction (including convulsions, intracranial hemorrhage), hypotension and cardiovascular collapse; *in vitro* and animal studies have shown that benzoate, a metabolite of benzyl alcohol, displaces bilirubin from protein binding sites; avoid use of these products in neonates

Precautions Use with caution in patients with hyperthyroidism, heart disease, hypertension, diabetes mellitus, or prostatic hypertrophy

Adverse Reactions Respiratory: Dryness of the nasal mucosa, nasal irritation (temporary), rebound congestion (chronic use), sneezing

Drug Interactions

Metabolism/Transport Effects None known.

Avoid Concomitant Use

Avoid concomitant use of Oxymetazoline (Nasal) with any of the following: Ergot Derivatives; Iobenguane I 123; MAO Inhibitors

Increased Effect/Toxicity

Oxymetazoline (Nasal) may increase the levels/effects of: Sympathomimetics

The levels/effects of Oxymetazoline (Nasal) may be increased by: AtoMOXetine; Cannabinoid-Containing Products; Ergot Derivatives; Linezolid; MAO Inhibitors; Tricyclic Antidepressants

Decreased Effect

Oxymetazoline (Nasal) may decrease the levels/effects of: FentaNYL; Iobenguane I 123

The levels/effects of Oxymetazoline (Nasal) may be decreased by: Alpha1-Blockers

Mechanism of Action Stimulates alpha-adrenergic receptors in the arterioles of the nasal mucosa to produce vasoconstriction

Pharmacodynamics

Onset of action: Within 5-10 minutes

Duration: 5-6 hours

Dosing: Usual Note: Therapy should not exceed 3-5 days; avoid use in children <6 years of age. Children ≥6 years and Adults: 2-3 drops or 2-3 sprays or 1-2 metered sprays (Nōstrilla®) into each nostril twice daily

Administration Spray or apply drops into each nostril while gently occluding the other

Dosage Forms Excipient information presented when available (limited, particularly for generics); consult specific product labeling.

Solution, Nasal, as hydrochloride:

12 Hour Nasal Relief Spray: 0.05% (15 mL, 30 mL)

12 Hour Nasal Spray: 0.05% (30 mL) [contains benzalkonium chloride]

12 Hour Nasal Spray: 0.05% (30 mL) [contains benzalkonium chloride, benzyl alcohol, edetate disodium, polyethylene glycol]

Afrin 12 Hour: 0.05% (30 mL) [contains benzalkonium chloride, disodium edta, polyethylene glycol, propylene glycol]

Afrin Extra Moisturizing: 0.05% (30 mL)

Afrin Menthol Spray: 0.05% (15 mL)

Afrin Nasal Spray: 0.05% (15 mL)

Afrin Nasal Spray: 0.05% (15 mL, 20 mL, 30 mL) [contains benzalkonium chloride, disodium edta]

Afrin NoDrip Original: 0.05% (15 mL) [contains benzalkonium chloride]

Afrin NoDrip Sinus: 0.05% (15 mL) [contains benzalkonium chloride, menthol]

Afrin Sinus: 0.05% (15 mL)

Dristan Spray: 0.05% (15 mL) [contains benzalkonium chloride, disodium edta]

Long Lasting Nasal Spray: 0.05% (30 mL) [contains benzalkonium chloride]

Mucinex Nasal Spray Full Force: 0.05% (22 mL) [contains benzalkonium chloride, disodium edta, menthol, polysorbate 80]

Mucinex Nasal Spray Moisture: 0.05% (22 mL) [contains benzalkonium chloride, edetate disodium, propylene glycol]

Mucinex Sinus-Max Full Force: 0.05% (22 mL) [contains benzalkonium chloride, disodium edta, menthol, polysorbate 80, propylene glycol]

Mucinex Sinus-Max Moist Smart: 0.05% (22 mL) [contains benzalkonium chloride, disodium edta, propylene glycol]

Nasal Decongestant Spray: 0.05% (15 mL, 30 mL)

Nasal Decongestant Spray: 0.05% (15 mL, 30 mL) [contains benzalkonium chloride]

Nasal Spray 12 Hour: 0.05% (30 mL) [contains benzalkonium chloride, benzyl alcohol, edetate disodium, polyethylene glycol, propylene glycol]

Nasal Spray Extra Moisturizing: 0.05% (30 mL) [contains benzalkonium chloride, benzyl alcohol, edetate disodium, polyethylene glycol, propylene glycol]

Neo-Synephrine 12 Hour Spray: 0.05% (15 mL)

NRS Nasal Relief: 0.05% (15 mL) [contains benzalkonium chloride, benzyl alcohol, disodium edta, propylene glycol]

Sinus Nasal Spray: 0.05% (30 mL) [contains benzalkonium chloride, edetate disodium, menthol, polysorbate 80, propylene glycol]

Generic: 0.05% (30 mL)

Oxymetazoline (Ophthalmic)

(oks i met AZ oh leen)

Medication Safety Issues

Sound-alike/look-alike issues:

Oxymetazoline may be confused with oxymetholone

Visine® may be confused with Visken®

Other safety concerns:

Accidental ingestion: Serious adverse reactions (eg, coma, bradycardia, respiratory depression, sedation) requiring hospitalization have been reported in children ≤5 years of age who have accidentally ingested even small amounts (eg, 1-2 mL) of imidazoline-derivative (ie, tetrahydrozoline, oxymetazoline, or naphazoline) eye drops or nasal sprays. Store these products out of reach of children at all times. Contact poison control or seek medical attention if accidental ingestion occurs.

Brand Names: U.S. Visine-LR [OTC]

Therapeutic Category Adrenergic Agonist Agent, Ophthalmic; Vasoconstrictor, Ophthalmic

Generic Availability (U.S.) No

Use Relief of redness of eye due to minor eye irritations

Contraindications Hypersensitivity to oxymetazoline or any component

Precautions Use with caution in patients with increased intraocular pressure or glaucoma

Adverse Reactions Local: Transient burning, stinging

Drug Interactions

Metabolism/Transport Effects None known.

Avoid Concomitant Use There are no known interactions where it is recommended to avoid concomitant use.

Increased Effect/Toxicity There are no known significant interactions involving an increase in effect.

Decreased Effect There are no known significant interactions involving a decrease in effect.

Dosing: Usual Children ≥6 years and Adults: Instill 1-2 drops into the affected eye(s) 2-4 times/day (≥6 hours apart)

Administration Instill drops into conjunctival sac of affected eye(s); avoid contact of bottle tip with skin or eye; finger pressure should be applied to lacrimal sac during and for 1-2 minutes after instillation to decrease the risk of absorption and systemic reactions

Dosage Forms Excipient information presented when available (limited, particularly for generics); consult specific product labeling.

Solution, Ophthalmic, as hydrochloride:
Visine-LR: 0.025% (15 mL) [contains benzalkonium chloride]

◆ **Oxymetazoline Hydrochloride** see Oxymetazoline (Nasal) on page 1577

◆ **Oxymetazoline Hydrochloride** see Oxymetazoline (Ophthalmic) on page 1578

◆ **OxyNEO (Can)** see OxyCODONE on page 1569

◆ **Oxytrol** see Oxybutynin on page 1568

◆ **Oxytrol For Women [OTC]** see Oxybutynin on page 1568

◆ **Oysco 500 [OTC]** see Calcium Carbonate on page 346

◆ **Ozurdex** see Dexamethasone (Ophthalmic) on page 619

◆ **Ozurdex® (Can)** see Dexamethasone (Ophthalmic) on page 619

◆ **P-071** see Cetirizine on page 431

◆ **Pacerone** see Amiodarone on page 127

PACLitaxel (pac li TAKS el)

Medication Safety Issues
Sound-alike/look-alike issues:
PACLitaxel may be confused with cabazitaxel, DOCEtaxel, PARoxetine, Paxil®
PACLitaxel (conventional) may be confused with PACLitaxel (protein-bound)
Taxol® may be confused with Abraxane®, Paxil®, Taxotere®

High alert medication:
This medication is in a class the Institute for Safe Medication Practices (ISMP) includes among its list of drug classes which have a heightened risk of causing significant patient harm when used in error.

Related Information
Emetogenic Potential of Antineoplastic Agents in Children on page 2327
Management of Drug Extravasations on page 2255
Safe Handling of Hazardous Drugs on page 2419

Brand Names: Canada Apo-Paclitaxel®; Paclitaxel for Injection; Paclitaxel Injection USP

Therapeutic Category Antineoplastic Agent, Antimicrotubular; Antineoplastic Agent, Taxane Derivative

Generic Availability (U.S.) Yes

Use Treatment of breast cancer, advanced ovarian cancer, nonsmall cell lung cancer, and second-line treatment of AIDS-related Kaposi's sarcoma (FDA approved in adults); has also been used in head and neck cancer, bladder cancer, cervical cancer, small cell lung cancer, and unknown primary adenocarcinomas

Pregnancy Risk Factor D

Pregnancy Considerations Adverse events (embryotoxicity, fetal toxicity, and maternal toxicity) have been observed in animal reproduction studies at doses less than the recommended human dose. An ex vivo human placenta perfusion model illustrated that paclitaxel crossed the placenta at term. Placental transfer was low and affected by the presence of albumin; higher albumin concentrations resulted in lower paclitaxel placental transfer (Berveiller, 2012). Women of childbearing potential should be advised to avoid becoming pregnant. A pregnancy registry is available for all cancers diagnosed during pregnancy at Cooper Health (877-635-4499).

Breast-Feeding Considerations Paclitaxel is excreted in breast milk (case report). The mother (3 months postpartum) was treated with paclitaxel 30 mg/m^2 (56.1 mg) and carboplatin once weekly for papillary thyroid cancer. Milk samples were obtained 4-316 hours after the infusion given at the sixth and final week of therapy. The average paclitaxel milk concentration over the testing interval was 0.78 mg/L. Although maternal serum concentrations were not noted in the report, the relative infant dose to a nursing infant was calculated to be ~17% of the maternal dose. Paclitaxel continued to be detected in breast milk when sampled at 172 hours after the dose and was below the limit of detection when sampled at 316 hours after the infusion (Griffin, 2012). Due to the potential for serious adverse reactions in a nursing infant, breast-feeding is not recommended.

Contraindications Hypersensitivity to paclitaxel, Cremophor® EL (polyoxyethylated castor oil) or any component

Warnings Hazardous agent; use appropriate precautions for handling and disposal (NIOSH, 2012). Anaphylaxis and severe hypersensitivity reactions have occurred in 2% to 4% of patients receiving paclitaxel in clinical trials during first or subsequent infusions **[U.S. Boxed Warning]. All patients should be premedicated with a corticosteroid, diphenhydramine, and an H$_2$-receptor antagonist to prevent hypersensitivity reactions;** fatal reactions have occurred despite premedication. Patients who experience severe hypersensitivity reactions to paclitaxel should not be rechallenged with the drug. Be prepared to treat a severe hypersensitivity reaction with epinephrine, I.V. fluids, diphenhydramine, and a corticosteroid.

CNS toxicity has been reported in pediatric patients receiving high doses of paclitaxel (350-420 mg/m^2 as a 3-hour infusion) which may have resulted from the ethanol contained in the formulation. With use, peripheral neuropathy may occur; patients with preexisting neuropathies from chemotherapy or coexisting conditions (eg, diabetes mellitus) may be at a higher risk; reduce dose by 20% for severe neuropathy. Severe bone marrow suppression (primarily neutropenia) with resulting infection may occur **[U.S. Boxed Warning]**. In general, do not administer paclitaxel to patients with baseline neutrophil counts <1500/mm^3 (<1000 cells/mm^3 for patients with AIDS-related KS). Infusion-related hypotension, bradycardia, and/or hypertension may occur; frequent monitoring of vital signs is recommended, especially during the first hour of the infusion. Rare but severe conduction abnormalities have been reported; conduct cardiac monitoring during subsequent infusions for these patients.

Precautions Use with caution in patients with moderate or severe hepatic impairment; dosage adjustment may be necessary in patients with hepatic impairment, severe neutropenia, or peripheral neuropathy. Formulations contain dehydrated alcohol; may cause adverse CNS effects. Should be administered under the supervision of an experienced cancer chemotherapy physician **[U.S. Boxed Warning]**.

Adverse Reactions Myelosuppression is dose related, schedule related, and infusion-rate dependent (increased incidences with higher doses, more frequent doses, and longer infusion times) and, in general, rapidly reversible upon discontinuation.

▸

◄ Cardiovascular: Bradycardia, ECG abnormal, edema, flushing, hyper-/hypotension, rhythm abnormalities, syncope, tachycardia, venous thrombosis

Dermatologic: Alopecia, nail changes, rash

Gastrointestinal: Abdominal pain (with intraperitoneal paclitaxel), diarrhea, mucositis, nausea/vomiting, stomatitis

Hematologic: Anemia, bleeding, febrile neutropenia, leukopenia; neutropenia (onset 8-10 days, median nadir 11 days, recovery 15-21 days); thrombocytopenia

Hepatic: Alkaline phosphatase increased, AST increased, bilirubin increased

Local: Injection site reaction (erythema, tenderness, skin discoloration, swelling)

Neuromuscular & skeletal: Arthralgia/myalgia, peripheral neuropathy, weakness

Renal: Creatinine increased (observed in KS patients only)

Miscellaneous: Hypersensitivity reaction, infection

Rare but important or life-threatening: Anaphylaxis, arrhythmia, ataxia, atrial fibrillation, AV block, back pain, cardiac conduction abnormalities, cellulitis, CHF, chills, conjunctivitis, dehydration, enterocolitis, extravasation recall, hepatic encephalopathy, hepatic necrosis, induration, intestinal obstruction, intestinal perforation, interstitial pneumonia, ischemic colitis, lacrimation increased, maculopapular rash, malaise, MI, myocardial ischemia, necrotic changes and ulceration following extravasation, neuroencephalopathy, neutropenic enterocolitis, neutropenic typhlitis, ototoxicity (tinnitus and hearing loss), pancreatitis, paralytic ileus, phlebitis, pneumonitis, pruritus, pulmonary embolism, pulmonary fibrosis, radiation recall, radiation pneumonitis, renal insufficiency, seizure, skin exfoliation, skin fibrosis, skin necrosis, Stevens-Johnson syndrome, supraventricular tachycardia, toxic epidermal necrolysis, ventricular tachycardia (asymptomatic), visual disturbances (scintillating scotomata)

Drug Interactions

Metabolism/Transport Effects Substrate of CYP2C8 (major), CYP3A4 (major), P-glycoprotein; **Note:** Assignment of Major/Minor substrate status based on clinically relevant drug interaction potential; **Induces** CYP3A4 (weak/moderate)

Avoid Concomitant Use

Avoid concomitant use of PACLitaxel with any of the following: Axitinib; BCG; CloZAPine; Conivaptan; Dipyrone; Fusidic Acid (Systemic); Natalizumab; Pimecrolimus; Simeprevir; SORAfenib; Tacrolimus (Topical); Tofacitinib; Vaccines (Live)

Increased Effect/Toxicity

PACLitaxel may increase the levels/effects of: Antineoplastic Agents (Anthracycline, Systemic); Bexarotene (Systemic); CloZAPine; DOXOrubicin (Conventional); Leflunomide; Natalizumab; Tofacitinib; Trastuzumab; Vaccines (Live); Vinorelbine

The levels/effects of PACLitaxel may be increased by: Ceritinib; Conivaptan; CYP2C8 Inhibitors (Moderate); CYP2C8 Inhibitors (Strong); CYP3A4 Inhibitors (Moderate); CYP3A4 Inhibitors (Strong); Dasatinib; Deferasirox; Denosumab; Dipyrone; Fusidic Acid (Systemic); Ivacaftor; Luliconazole; Mifepristone; P-glycoprotein/ABCB1 Inhibitors; Pimecrolimus; Platinum Derivatives; Roflumilast; SORAfenib; Stiripentol; Tacrolimus (Topical)

Decreased Effect

PACLitaxel may decrease the levels/effects of: ARIPiprazole; Axitinib; BCG; Coccidioidin Skin Test; Ibrutinib; Saxagliptin; Simeprevir; Sipuleucel-T; Vaccines (Inactivated); Vaccines (Live)

The levels/effects of PACLitaxel may be decreased by: Bexarotene (Systemic); Bosentan; CYP2C8 Inducers (Strong); CYP3A4 Inducers (Strong); Dabrafenib; Deferasirox; Echinacea; Mitotane; P-glycoprotein/ABCB1 Inducers; Siltuximab; St Johns Wort; Tocilizumab; Trastuzumab

Stability Hazardous agent; use appropriate precautions for handling and disposal (NIOSH, 2012). Refrigerate intact vials or store at room temperature; undiluted vials of paclitaxel may precipitate upon refrigeration, but will redissolve at room temperature with no loss in potency; dilution of paclitaxel from 0.3 mg/mL to 1.2 mg/mL in NS or D_5W is stable for up to 48 hours at room temperature; incompatible with amphotericin B, chlorpromazine, hydroxyzine, methylprednisolone, and mitoxantrone.

Mechanism of Action Paclitaxel promotes microtubule assembly by enhancing the action of tubulin dimers, stabilizing existing microtubules, and inhibiting their disassembly, interfering with the late G_2 mitotic phase, and inhibiting cell replication. In addition, the drug can distort mitotic spindles, resulting in the breakage of chromosomes. Paclitaxel may also suppress cell proliferation and modulate immune response.

Pharmacokinetics (Adult data unless noted)

Distribution: Biphasic with initial rapid distribution to the peripheral compartment; later phase is a slow efflux of paclitaxel from the peripheral compartment

V_d: 227-688 L/m^2

Protein binding: 89% to 98%

Metabolism: Cytochrome P450 hepatic isoenzymes metabolize paclitaxel to 6 alpha-hydroxypaclitaxel

Half-life (varies with dose and infusion duration):

Children: 4.6-17 hours

Adults: 1.5-8.4 hours

Elimination: Urinary recovery of unchanged drug: 1.3% to 12.6%

Dialysis: No significant drug removal by hemodialysis

Dosing: Usual I.V. infusion (refer to individual protocols):

Children:

Treatment for refractory leukemia is still undergoing investigation: 250-360 mg/m^2/dose infused over 24 hours every 14 days

Recurrent Wilms' tumor: 250-350 mg/m^2/dose infused over 24 hours every 3 weeks

Adults:

Ovarian carcinoma: 135-175 mg/m^2/dose infused over 1-24 hours every 3 weeks

Metastatic breast cancer: 175 mg/m^2/dose infused over 3 hours every 3 weeks (protocols have used dosages ranging between 135-250 mg/m^2/dose over 1-24 hours every 3 weeks)

Kaposi's sarcoma: 135 mg/m^2/dose infused over 3 hours every 3 weeks, or 100 mg/m^2/dose infused over 3 hours every 2 weeks

Dosage adjustment in renal impairment: None

Dosage adjustment in hepatic impairment:

Total bilirubin ≤1.5 mg/dL and AST >2x normal limits: Total dose <135 mg/m^2

Total bilirubin 1.6-3.0 mg/dL: Total dose ≤75 mg/m^2

Total bilirubin ≥3.1 mg/dL: Total dose ≤50 mg/m^2

Administration Hazardous agent; use appropriate precautions for handling and disposal (NIOSH, 2012).

Parenteral: I.V.: Patients should be premedicated with a corticosteroid, diphenhydramine and an H_2-receptor antagonist 30-60 minutes prior to paclitaxel administration. To minimize patient exposure to the plasticizer diethylhexylphthalate (DEHP) from polyoxyl 35 castor oil-induced leaching of polyvinyl chloride-containing I.V. infusion bags and administration sets, prepare paclitaxel infusions in glass or in polypropylene or polyolefin bags and administer through polyethylene lined administration sets with a 0.22 micron in-line filter. Paclitaxel can be further diluted in D_5W, NS, D_5NS or D_5 in Ringer's injection to a final concentration of 0.3-1.2 mg/mL. Paclitaxel has been infused over short (1-3 hours) and long periods (24, 72, and 96 hours to 14 days continuous infusion)

Vesicant/Extravasation Risk Irritant with vesicant-like properties

Monitoring Parameters CBC with differential, platelet count, vital signs, ECG, liver function test; observe I.V. injection site for extravasation

Dosage Forms Excipient information presented when available (limited, particularly for generics); consult specific product labeling.

Concentrate, Intravenous:
Generic: 100 mg/16.7 mL (16.7 mL); 30 mg/5 mL (5 mL); 150 mg/25 mL (25 mL); 300 mg/50 mL (50 mL)

Concentrate, Intravenous [preservative free]:
Generic: 100 mg/16.7 mL (16.7 mL); 30 mg/5 mL (5 mL); 300 mg/50 mL (50 mL)

References

Berveiller P, Vinot C, Mir O, et al, "Comparative Transplacental Transfer of Taxanes Using the Human Perfused Cotyledon Placental Model," *Am J Obstet Gynecol*, 2012, 207(6):514.e1-514.e7.

Griffin SJ, Milla M, Baker TE, et al, "Transfer of Carboplatin and Paclitaxel into Breast Milk," *J Hum Lact*, 2012, 28(4):457-9.

National Institute for Occupational Safety and Health (NIOSH), "NIOSH List of Antineoplastic and Other Hazardous Drugs in Healthcare Settings 2012." Available at http://www.cdc.gov/niosh/docs/2012-150/pdfs/2012-150.pdf. Accessed January 21, 2013.

Woo MH, Gregornik D, Shearer PD, et al, "Pharmacokinetics of Paclitaxel in an Anephric Patient," *Cancer Chemother Pharmacol*, 1999, 43(1):92-6.

◆ **Paclitaxel (Conventional)** *see* PACLitaxel *on page 1579*

◆ **Paclitaxel for Injection (Can)** *see* PACLitaxel *on page 1579*

◆ **Paclitaxel Injection USP (Can)** *see* PACLitaxel *on page 1579*

◆ **Pain Eze [OTC]** *see* Acetaminophen *on page 47*

◆ **Pain & Fever Children's [OTC]** *see* Acetaminophen *on page 47*

◆ **Palafer® (Can)** *see* Ferrous Fumarate *on page 865*

◆ **Palgic [DSC]** *see* Carbinoxamine *on page 377*

Paliperidone (pal ee PER i done)

Medication Safety Issues
BEERS Criteria medication:
This drug may be potentially inappropriate for use in geriatric patients (Quality of evidence - moderate; Strength of recommendation - strong).

Related Information
Oral Medications That Should Not Be Crushed or Altered *on page 2438*

Brand Names: U.S. Invega; Invega Sustenna

Brand Names: Canada Invega; Invega Sustenna

Therapeutic Category Antipsychotic Agent, Atypical; Antipsychotic Agent, Benzisoxazole

Generic Availability (U.S.) No

Use
Oral: Treatment of schizophrenia (FDA approved in ages ≥12 years and adults); treatment of schizoaffective disorder as monotherapy or adjunctive therapy to mood stabilizers and/or antidepressants (FDA approved in adults); has also been used for treatment of irritability associated with autistic disorder

Parenteral: Treatment of schizophrenia (acute and maintenance) (FDA approved in adults)

Pregnancy Risk Factor C

Pregnancy Considerations Adverse events were not observed in animal reproduction studies. Antipsychotic use during the third trimester of pregnancy has a risk for extrapyramidal symptoms (EPS) and/or withdrawal symptoms in newborns following delivery. Symptoms in the newborn may include agitation, feeding disorder, hypertonia, hypotonia, respiratory distress, somnolence, and tremor. These effects may be self-limiting and allow recovery within hours or days with no specific treatment, or they may be severe requiring prolonged hospitalization.

Paliperidone may cause hyperprolactinemia, which may decrease reproductive function in both males and females. Paliperidone is the active metabolite of risperidone; refer to Risperidone monograph for additional information.

The ACOG recommends that therapy during pregnancy be individualized; treatment with psychiatric medications during pregnancy should incorporate the clinical expertise of the mental health clinician, obstetrician, primary healthcare provider, and pediatrician. Safety data related to atypical antipsychotics during pregnancy is limited and routine use is not recommended. However, if a woman is inadvertently exposed to an atypical antipsychotic while pregnant, continuing therapy may be preferable to switching to a typical antipsychotic that the fetus has not yet been exposed to; consider risk:benefit (ACOG, 2008).

Healthcare providers are encouraged to enroll women 18-45 years of age exposed to paliperidone during pregnancy in the Atypical Antipsychotics Pregnancy Registry (1-866-961-2388 or http://www.womensmentalhealth.org/pregnancyregistry).

Breast-Feeding Considerations Paliperidone is excreted into breast milk. According to the manufacturer, the decision to continue or discontinue breast-feeding during therapy should take into account the risk of exposure to the infant and the benefits of treatment to the mother.

Contraindications Hypersensitivity to paliperidone, risperidone, or any component

Warnings May cause neuroleptic malignant syndrome (symptoms include hyperpyrexia, altered mental status, muscle rigidity, autonomic instability, acute renal failure, rhabdomyolysis, and elevated CPK). May cause extrapyramidal reactions, including pseudoparkinsonism, acute dystonic reactions, akathisia, and tardive dyskinesia (risk of these reactions is low relative to other neuroleptics, and is dose-dependent; to decrease risk of tardive dyskinesia, use smallest dose and shortest duration possible; evaluate continued need periodically; risk of dystonia is increased with the use of high potency and higher doses of conventional antipsychotics and in males and younger patients; occurring in up to 18% of children). May cause hyperglycemia, which may be severe and include potentially fatal ketoacidosis or hyperosmolar coma; use with caution and monitor glucose closely in patients with diabetes mellitus (or with risk factors such as family history or obesity); measure fasting blood glucose at the beginning of therapy and periodically during therapy in these patients; monitor for symptoms of hyperglycemia in all patients treated with paliperidone; measure fasting blood glucose in patients who develop symptoms.

May alter cardiac conduction and prolong the QT_c interval; life-threatening arrhythmias have occurred with therapeutic doses of antipsychotics. Risk may be increased by conditions or concomitant medications which cause bradycardia, hypokalemia, and/or hypomagnesemia. Avoid use in combination with QT_c-prolonging drugs and in patients with congenital long QT syndrome or patients with history of cardiac arrhythmia.

Leukopenia, neutropenia, and agranulocytosis (sometimes fatal) have been reported in clinical trials and postmarketing reports with antipsychotic use; presence of risk factors (eg, preexisting low WBC or history of drug-induced leuko/neutropenia) should prompt periodic blood count assessment. Discontinue therapy at first signs of blood dyscrasias or if absolute neutrophil count <1000/mm³.

An increased risk of death has been reported with the use of antipsychotics in elderly patients with dementia-related psychosis **[U.S. Boxed Warning]**; most deaths seemed to be cardiovascular (eg, sudden death, heart failure) or infectious (eg, pneumonia) in nature. An increased incidence of cerebrovascular adverse events (eg, transient ischemic attack, stroke), including fatalities, has been reported in placebo-controlled trials of risperidone (paliperidone is the primary active metabolite of risperidone) in elderly patients with dementia-related psychosis. Paliperidone is not approved for the treatment of patients with dementia-related psychosis.

The possibility of a suicide attempt is inherent in psychotic illness or bipolar disorder; use with caution in high-risk patients during initiation of therapy. Prescriptions should be written for the smallest quantity consistent with good patient care.

Precautions Use with caution in patients with renal impairment; clearance is reduced (%) based on severity of impairment: Mild (32%), moderate (64%), and severe (71%); dosage adjustment required. Use with caution in patients with severe hepatic impairment, use has not been studied; in patients with mild to moderate hepatic impairment, no dosage adjustment is required. Use with caution in patients with breast cancer or other prolactin-dependent tumors; paliperidone elevates prolactin levels to a similar degree as risperidone, a drug known to elevate prolactin to a greater degree than other antipsychotic agents; high levels of prolactin may reduce pituitary gonadotropin secretion; galactorrhea, amenorrhea, gynecomastia, impotence, decreased bone density may occur. Use with caution in children and adolescents; adverse effects due to elevated prolactin levels have been observed; long-term effects on growth or sexual maturation have not been evaluated.

Paliperidone may cause a higher than normal weight gain in children and adolescents; monitor growth (including weight, height, BMI, and waist circumference) in pediatric patients receiving paliperidone; in adolescent trials, ≤19% of patients experienced a weight gain of ≥7%; monitor weight and compare to standard growth curves. Paliperidone may cause increases in metabolic indices (eg, serum cholesterol, triglycerides). Biannual monitoring of cardiometabolic indices after the first 3 months of therapy is suggested for atypical antipsychotics (Correll, 2009).

Use with caution in patients with seizure disorders or patients with conditions that lower seizure threshold; seizures have been rarely reported. Use with caution in patients with Parkinson's disease, in suicidal patients, and in those at risk of aspiration pneumonia (esophageal dysmotility and aspiration have been associated with antipsychotic agents). May cause orthostatic hypotension with resultant dizziness, tachycardia, or syncope (especially during initial dose titration); use with caution in patients with cardiovascular disease (heart failure, past MI, or myocardia ischemia), cerebrovascular disease, dehydration, hypovolemia, or other conditions which may predispose patients to hypotension; may cause hypotension when used with antihypertensive agents. May cause somnolence (dose-related), priapism (rarely), alteration of temperature regulation (use with caution in patients exposed to temperature extremes). Paliperidone exhibits antiemetic effects and may mask toxicity of other drugs or conditions (eg, intestinal obstruction, Reye's syndrome, brain tumor).

Adolescents may experience a higher frequency of certain adverse effects than adults, particularly akathisia (4% to 17% vs 1% to 10%; dose-dependent), somnolence (9% to 26% vs 1% to 12%), vomiting (≤11% vs 2% to 5%). Adolescents may experience some adverse effects not reported in adults, including amenorrhea, blurred vision, galactorrhea, gynecomastia, and tongue swelling.

Extended release tablets: Use is not recommended in patients with preexisting severe gastrointestinal narrowing disorders (esophageal motility disorders, small bowel inflammatory disease, "short gut" syndrome, history of peritonitis, cystic fibrosis, chronic intestinal pseudoobstruction, or Meckel's diverticulum); formulation consists of drug within a nonabsorbable shell; following drug release and absorption, the shell is expelled in the stool; patients with upper GI tract alterations in transit time may have increased or decreased bioavailability of paliperidone.

Paliperidone is an active metabolite of risperidone; concomitant use with risperidone has not been studied; pharmacokinetic data suggests additional paliperidone exposure and corresponding effects.

Adverse Reactions Unless otherwise noted, frequency of adverse effects is reported for the oral/I.M. formulation in adults.

Cardiovascular: Bundle branch block, orthostatic hypotension (dose dependent), tachycardia (adolescents and adults)

Central nervous system: Agitation, akathisia (adolescents and adults; dose dependent), anxiety (adolescents and adults), dizziness (adolescents and adults), drowsiness (more common in adolescents; dose dependent), dysarthria (dose dependent), dystonia (adolescents and adults; dose dependent), extrapyramidal reaction (more common in adolescents; dose dependent), fatigue (adolescents and adults), headache (adolescents and adults), lethargy (adolescents and adults), parkinsonian-like syndrome (adolescents and adults; dose dependent), sleep disorder

Endocrine & metabolic: Abnormal triglycerides (adolescents and adults), altered serum glucose (adolescents and adults), amenorrhea (adolescents and adults), blood cholesterol abnormal (adolescents and adults), galactorrhea (adolescents and adults), gynecomastia (adolescents and adults), weight gain (adolescents and adults; dose dependent)

Gastrointestinal: Abdominal pain, constipation, diarrhea, dyspepsia, increased appetite, nausea, sialorrhea (adolescents and adults; dose dependent), swollen tongue (adolescents and adults), toothache, vomiting (adolescents and adults), xerostomia (adolescents and adults)

Hematologic & oncologic: Change in HDL (adolescents and adults), change in LDL (adolescents and adults)

Local: I.M. formulation: Injection site reaction

Neuromuscular & skeletal: Back pain, dyskinesia (adolescents and adults), hyperkinesia (adolescents and adults; dose dependent), limb pain, myalgia (dose dependent), tongue paralysis (adolescents), tremor (adolescents and adults), weakness (adolescents and adults)

Ophthalmic: Blurred vision (adolescents and adults)

Respiratory: cough (dose dependent), nasopharyngitis (adolescents and adults; dose dependent), rhinitis (dose dependent), upper respiratory tract infection

Rare but important or life-threatening: Agranulocytosis, anaphylaxis, antiemetic effect, aspiration pneumonia, cerebrovascular accident, diabetes mellitus, ECG abnormality, edema, epistaxis, erectile dysfunction, first degree atrioventricular block, hyperprolactinemia, hypertension, hypertonia, increased serum ALT, increased serum AST, insomnia, intestinal obstruction, ischemia, leukopenia, neuroleptic malignant syndrome, neutropenia, orthostatic dizziness, postural orthostatic tachycardia, priapism, psychomotor agitation, retrograde ejaculation, seizure, suicidal ideation, syncope, tardive dyskinesia, thrombotic thrombocytopenic purpura, trismus, urinary incontinence, urinary retention

Drug Interactions

Metabolism/Transport Effects Substrate of P-glycoprotein

Avoid Concomitant Use

Avoid concomitant use of Paliperidone with any of the following: Amisulpride; Azelastine (Nasal); Highest Risk

QTc-Prolonging Agents; Ivabradine; Metoclopramide; Mifepristone; Moderate Risk QTc-Prolonging Agents; Paraldehyde; Sulpiride; Thalidomide

Increased Effect/Toxicity

Paliperidone may increase the levels/effects of: Alcohol (Ethyl); Amisulpride; Azelastine (Nasal); Buprenorphine; CNS Depressants; Highest Risk QTc-Prolonging Agents; Hydrocodone; Methotrimeprazine; Methylphenidate; Metyrosine; Paraldehyde; Selective Serotonin Reuptake Inhibitors; Serotonin Modulators; Sulpiride; Thalidomide; Zolpidem

The levels/effects of Paliperidone may be increased by: Acetylcholinesterase Inhibitors (Central); Brimonidine (Topical); Cannabis; Doxylamine; Dronabinol; HydrOXYzine; Itraconazole; Ivabradine; Kava Kava; Magnesium Sulfate; Methotrimeprazine; Methylphenidate; Metoclopramide; Metyrosine; Mifepristone; Moderate Risk QTc-Prolonging Agents; Nabilone; Perampanel; P-glycoprotein/ABCB1 Inhibitors; QTc-Prolonging Agents (Indeterminate Risk and Risk Modifying); RisperiDONE; Rufinamide; Serotonin Modulators; Sodium Oxybate; Tapentadol; Tetrahydrocannabinol; Valproic Acid and Derivatives

Decreased Effect

Paliperidone may decrease the levels/effects of: Amphetamines; Anti-Parkinson's Agents (Dopamine Agonist); Quinagolide

The levels/effects of Paliperidone may be decreased by: CarBAMazepine; P-glycoprotein/ABCB1 Inducers

Stability

Tablets: Store at ≤25°C (77°F); protect from moisture.

Injection: Store at 25°C (77°F); excursions permitted to 15°C to 30°C (59°F to 86°F).

Mechanism of Action

Paliperidone is considered a benzisoxazole atypical antipsychotic as it is the primary active metabolite of risperidone. As with other atypical antipsychotics, its therapeutic efficacy is believed to result from mixed central serotonergic and dopaminergic antagonism. The addition of serotonin antagonism to dopamine antagonism (classic neuroleptic mechanism) is thought to improve negative symptoms of psychoses and reduce the incidence of extrapyramidal side effects. Similar to risperidone, paliperidone demonstrates high affinity to α_1, D_2, H_1, and 5-HT_{2C} receptors, and low affinity for muscarinic and 5-HT_{1A} receptors. In contrast to risperidone, paliperidone displays nearly 10-fold lower affinity for α_2 and 5-HT_{2A} receptors, and nearly three- to fivefold less affinity for 5-HT_{1A} and 5-HT_{1D}, respectively.

Pharmacokinetics (Adult data unless noted)

Note: Pharmacokinetic parameters in adolescent patients weighing >51 kg were similar to adults; an increased drug exposure (23%) was observed in adolescent patient weighing <51 kg compared to adults and was not considered clinically significant.

Absorption: I.M.: Slow release (begins on day 1 and continues up to 126 days)

Distribution, apparent V_d: 391-487 L

Protein binding: 74%

Metabolism: Hepatic via CYP2D6 and 3A4 (limited role in elimination); minor metabolism (<10% each) via dealkylation, hydroxylation, dehydrogenation, and benzisoxazole scission

Bioavailability: Oral: 28%

Half-life:

Oral: 23 hours; prolonged with renal impairment (CrCl <80 mL/minute): 24-51 hours

I.M. (single dose): Range: 25-49 days

Time to peak serum concentration: Oral: ~24 hours; I.M.:13 days

Elimination: Urine (80%; 59% as unchanged drug); feces (11%)

Dosing: Usual

Children and Adolescents:

Schizophrenia: Children ≥12 and Adolescents: Oral: 3 mg once daily; titration not necessary; if after clinical assessment a dosage increase is required, may increase dose in 3 mg/day increments at least every 5 days; maximum daily dose is weight dependent: <51 kg: 6 mg/**day**; ≥51 kg: 12 mg/**day**; **Note:** During adolescent clinical trials, higher doses were not associated with greater efficacy, but increased risk of adverse effects.

Irritability associated with autistic disorder: Limited data available: Children ≥12 years and Adolescents: Oral: Initial: 3 mg once daily; titrate on a weekly basis in 3 mg/day increments until clinical response or intolerance; maximum daily dose: 12 mg/**day**. Dosing based on an open-label trial of 25 patients (mean age: 15.3 years; age range: 12-21 years); therapeutic response was reported in 84% of patients at a mean final dose: 7.1 mg/day (Stigler, 2012)

Adults:

Schizoaffective disorder, schizophrenia: Oral: Usual: 6 mg once daily in the morning; titration not required, though some may benefit from higher or lower doses. If dose exceeding 6 mg/day, increases of 3 mg/day are recommended no more frequently than every 4 days in schizoaffective disorder or every 5 days in schizophrenia, up to a maximum of 12 mg/day. Some patients may require only 3 mg/day.

Schizophrenia: I.M.: **Note:** Prior to initiation of I.M therapy, tolerability should be established with oral paliperidone or oral risperidone. Previous oral antipsychotics can be discontinued at the time of initiation of I.M. therapy. **Dosing based on paliperidone palmitate.**

Initiation of therapy:

Initial: 234 mg on treatment day 1 followed by 156 mg 1 week later. The second dose may be administered 2 days before or after the weekly timepoint.

Maintenance: Following the 1-week initiation regimen, begin a maintenance dose of 117 mg every month. Some patients may benefit from higher or lower monthly maintenance doses (monthly maintenance dosage range: 39-234 mg). The monthly maintenance dose may be administered 7 days before or after the monthly timepoint.

Conversion from oral paliperidone to I.M paliperidone: Initiate I.M. therapy as described using the 1-week initiation regimen. Patients previously stabilized on oral doses can expect similar steady state exposure during maintenance treatment with I.M. therapy using the following conversion:

Oral extended release dose of 12 mg, then I.M. maintenance dose of 234 mg

Oral extended release dose of 6 mg, then I.M. maintenance dose of 117 mg

Oral extended release dose of 3 mg, then I.M. maintenance dose of 39-78 mg

Switching from other long acting injectable antipsychotics to I.M. paliperidone: Initiate I.M. paliperidone in the place of the next scheduled injection and continue at monthly intervals. The 1-week initiation regimen is not required in these patients.

Dosage adjustments: Adjustments may be made monthly (full effect from adjustments may not be seen for several months)

Missed doses:

If <6 weeks has elapsed since the last monthly injection: Administer the missed dose as soon as possible and continue therapy at monthly intervals.

If >6 weeks and ≤6 months has elapsed since the last monthly injection:

If the maintenance dose was <234 mg: Administer the same dose the patient was previously stabilized

◄ on as soon as possible, followed by a second equivalent dose 1 week later, then resume maintenance dose at monthly intervals

If the maintenance dose was 234 mg: Administer a 156 mg dose as soon as possible, followed by a second dose of 156 mg 1 week later, then resume maintenance dose at monthly intervals.

If >6 months has elapsed since last monthly maintenance injection: Therapy must be reinitiated following dosing recommendations for initiation of therapy.

Dosing adjustment in renal impairment:

Children ≥12 years and Adolescents: There are no dosing adjustments provided in manufacturer's labeling.

Adults:

Oral:

CrCl 50-79 mL/minute: Initial: 3 mg once daily; maximum dose: 6 mg once daily

CrCl 10-49 mL/minute: Initial: 1.5 mg once daily; maximum dose: 3 mg once daily

CrCl <10 mL/minute: Use not recommended; not studied in this population

I.M.:

CrCl 50-79 mL/minute: Initiation of therapy: 156 mg on treatment day 1, followed by 117 mg 1 week later, followed by a maintenance dose of 78 mg every month

CrCl <50 mL/minute: Use not recommended

Dosing adjustment hepatic impairment: Oral, I.M.: No adjustment necessary for mild to moderate (Child-Pugh class A or B) impairment. Not studied in severe impairment.

Administration

Oral: Administer in the morning without regard to meals; swallow extended release tablets whole with liquids; do not crush, chew, or divide.

I.M. (Invega® Sustenna™): Shake prefilled syringe for at least 10 seconds to ensure a homogenous suspension; administer I.M. as a single injection (do not divide doses) injection should be slow and deep into the muscle. When initiating therapy, the deltoid muscle should be used for the first two doses to rapidly attain therapeutic concentrations (see manufacturer labeling for specific needle length/gauge). Monthly maintenance doses can be administered in either the deltoid muscle or upper, outer quadrant of gluteal muscle; may alternate injection sites. Do not administer I.V. or subQ; avoid inadvertent injection into vasculature.

Monitoring Parameters Blood pressure (including orthostatic) and heart rate, particularly during dosage titration; mental status, abnormal involuntary movement scale (AIMS), extrapyramidal symptoms; growth, BMI, waist circumference, and weight (in adults, weight should be assessed prior to treatment, at 4 weeks, 8 weeks, 12 weeks, and then at quarterly intervals; consider titrating to a different antipsychotic agent for a weight gain ≥5% of the initial weight); CBC with differential; liver enzymes in children (especially obese children or those who are rapidly gaining weight while receiving therapy); lipid profile; fasting blood glucose/Hgb A_{1c} (prior to treatment, at 3 months, then annually); prolactin serum concentrations

Additional Information Long-term usefulness of paliperidone should be periodically re-evaluated in patients receiving the drug for extended periods of time. Invega® is an extended release tablet based on the OROS® osmotic delivery system. Water from the GI tract enters through a semipermeable membrane coating the tablet, solubilizing the drug into a gelatinous form which, through hydrophilic expansion, is then expelled through laser-drilled holes in the coating.

Dosage Forms Excipient information presented when available (limited, particularly for generics); consult specific product labeling.

Suspension, Intramuscular, as palmitate:

Invega Sustenna: 39 mg/0.25 mL (0.25 mL); 78 mg/0.5 mL (0.5 mL); 117 mg/0.75 mL (0.75 mL); 156 mg/mL (1 mL); 234 mg/1.5 mL (1.5 mL) [contains polyethylene glycol]

Tablet Extended Release 24 Hour, Oral:

Invega: 1.5 mg, 3 mg, 6 mg, 9 mg

References

American College of Obstetricians and Gynecologists, ACOG Practice Bulletin: Clinical Management Guidelines for Obstetricians-Gynecologists No. 92 April 2008 (Replaces Practice Bulletin Number 87, November 2007), "Use of Psychiatric Medications During Pregnancy and Lactation," *Obstet Gynecol,* 2008, 111(4):1001-20.

Correll CU, Manu P, Olshanskiy V, et al, "Cardiometabolic Risk of Second-Generation Antipsychotic Medications During First-Time Use in Children and Adolescents," *JAMA,* 2009, 302(16):1765-73.

Singh J, Robb A, Vijapurkar U, et al, "A Randomized, Double-Blind Study of Paliperidone Extended-Release in Treatment of Acute Schizophrenia in Adolescents," *Biol Psychiatry,* 2011, 70(12):1179-87.

Stigler KA, Mullett JE, Erickson CA, et al, "Paliperidone for Irritability in Adolescents and Young Adults With Autistic Disorder," *Psychopharmacology (Berl),* 2012, 223(2):237-45

◆ **Paliperidone Palmitate** *see* Paliperidone *on page 1581*

Palivizumab (pah li VIZ u mab)

Medication Safety Issues

Sound-alike/look-alike issues:

Synagis may be confused with Synalgos-DC, Synflorix, Synvisc

Brand Names: U.S. Synagis

Brand Names: Canada Synagis

Therapeutic Category Monoclonal Antibody

Generic Availability (U.S.) No

Use Prevention of serious lower respiratory tract disease caused by respiratory syncytial virus (RSV) in infants and children at high risk for RSV disease (FDA approved ≤24 months of age); has also been used for I.V. treatment of active RSV infections in patients at high-risk for severe disease.

The American Academy of Pediatrics (*Red Book* [AAP], 2012) recommends RSV prophylaxis with palivizumab during RSV season for:

Infants <3 months of age who were born between gestational age 32 weeks 0 days and 34 weeks 6 days and have one of the following:
• Daycare attendance
• ≥1 sibling who is <5 years of age living in the same household

Infants <6 months of age who were born between gestational age 29 weeks 0 days to ≤31 weeks 6 days

Infants <12 months of age who were born gestational age ≤28 weeks 6 days

Infants <12 months of age with congenital airway abnormality or neuromuscular disorder that decreases the ability to manage airway secretions

Infants and children <24 months of age with chronic lung disease (CLD) necessitating medical therapy (eg, supplemental oxygen, bronchodilator, diuretic, or chronic steroid therapy) within 6 months prior to the beginning of RSV season

Infants and children ≤24 months with hemodynamically significant congenital heart disease and one of the following:
• Receiving medication to treat congestive heart failure
• Moderate to severe pulmonary hypertension
• Cyanotic heart disease

Pregnancy Risk Factor C

Pregnancy Considerations Not for adult use; reproduction studies have not been conducted

Contraindications Hypersensitivity to palivizumab or any component

Warnings Rare cases of anaphylaxis have been reported following re-exposure to palivizumab. Severe acute hypersensitivity reactions have also been reported following administration of palivizumab. Palivizumab should be permanently discontinued if a severe hypersensitivity reaction occurs. If anaphylaxis or severe allergic reaction occurs, administer epinephrine (1:1000) and provide supportive care as required.

Precautions Use with caution in patients with thrombocytopenia or any coagulation disorder; bleeding/hematoma may occur from I.M. administration. Interference (false-negatives) with immunological-based RSV diagnostic tests (antigen-detection) and viral culture assays has been reported; rely on reverse-transcriptase-polymerase chain reaction based assays and clinical findings. Safety and efficacy have not been demonstrated for treatment of established RSV disease.

Adverse Reactions

Central nervous system: Fever

Dermatologic: Rash

Miscellaneous: Antibody formation

Rare but important or life-threatening: Anaphylaxis (very rare - includes angioedema, dyspnea, hypotonia, pruritus, respiratory failure, unresponsiveness, urticaria); hypersensitivity reactions, injection site reactions, thrombocytopenia

Drug Interactions

Metabolism/Transport Effects None known.

Avoid Concomitant Use

Avoid concomitant use of Palivizumab with any of the following: Belimumab

Increased Effect/Toxicity

Palivizumab may increase the levels/effects of: Belimumab

The levels/effects of Palivizumab may be increased by: Abciximab

Decreased Effect There are no known significant interactions involving a decrease in effect.

Stability Store intact vial at 2°C to 8°C (35.6°F to 46.4°F) in original container; do not freeze. The single-use vial does not contain a preservative.

Mechanism of Action Exhibits neutralizing and fusion-inhibitory activity against RSV; these activities inhibit RSV replication in laboratory and clinical studies

Pharmacodynamics Protective trough concentrations (≥40 mcg/mL) are achieved following the second dose.

Pharmacokinetics (Adult data unless noted)

Half-life:

Infants and Children <24 months: 20 days

Adults: 18 days

Time to achieve adequate serum antibody titers: 48 hours

Dosing: Neonatal

RSV, prevention: I.M.: 15 mg/kg once monthly throughout RSV season; **Note:** AAP recommends a maximum of 3 doses for patients born GA 32 weeks 0 days through 34 weeks 6 days and <3 months of age without significant congenital heart disease or chronic lung disease and maximum of 5 doses for all others (*Red Book* [AAP], 2012).

Cardiopulmonary bypass patients: I.M.: Administer a dose as soon as possible after cardiopulmonary bypass procedure, even if <1 month from previous dose. (A 58% decrease in palivizumab serum concentrations has been noted after cardiopulmonary bypass.)

Dosing: Usual Pediatric:

RSV, prevention: Infants and Children: I.M.: 15 mg/kg once monthly throughout RSV season; **Note:** AAP recommends a maximum of 3 doses for patients born GA 32 weeks 0 days through 34 weeks 6 days and <3 months of age without significant congenital heart disease or chronic lung disease and maximum of 5 doses for all others (*Red Book* [AAP], 2012).

Cardiopulmonary bypass patients: I.M.: Administer a dose as soon as possible after cardiopulmonary bypass procedure, even if <1 month from previous dose. (A 58% decrease in palivizumab serum concentrations has been noted after cardiopulmonary bypass.)

RSV, treatment in patients at high-risk for severe disease: Limited data available: Infants, Children, and Adolescents: I.V.: 15 mg/kg as a single dose; in most patients, used in combination with ribavirin therapy; in two patients with disease progression, a single repeat dose at 3 to 5 days after the initial dose was reported (Chávez-Bueno, 2007). Dosing based on experience in 85 patients the majority of which are pediatric patients and mostly ≤2 years of age. Reported efficacy results variable, an initial double-blind, placebo-controlled trial (n=17 treatment group; all patients ≤2 years) showed statistically significant decreases in RSV tracheal aspirate concentrations vs placebo (Malley, 1998); in another double-blind, placebo-controlled trial (n=22 treatment group; all patients ≤2 years) a decrease in the days of RSV hospitalization, days of supplemental oxygen, and lower respiratory infection scores were reported relative to placebo (Sáez-Llorens, 2004); in an underpowered, observational study of hematopoietic stem cell patients (n=15; age range: 2 to 60 years) a decrease viral shedding and increased 30 day-survival vs ribavirin monotherapy (83.3% vs ~55%) was reported (Boeckh, 2001); further studies are needed.

Administration

I.M.: Administer undiluted solution I.M., preferably in the anterolateral aspect of the thigh; gluteal muscle should not be used routinely as an injection site because of the risk of damage to the sciatic nerve; injection volume over 1 mL should be given as a divided dose. Do **not** dilute product; do not shake or vigorously agitate the vial.

I.V.: In clinical trials in pediatric patients ≤2 years, has been administered IVP over 2 to 5 minutes or I.V. infusion through a 0.2 micron filter at a rate not to exceed 1 to 2 mL/minute at a final concentration of 10 to 20 mg/mL (Boeckh, 2001; Sáez-Llorens, 2004; Subramanian, 1998).

Monitoring Parameters Observe for anaphylactic or severe allergic reactions

Test Interactions May interfere (false negatives) with immunological-based RSV diagnostic tests (antigen detection) and viral culture assays; rely on reverse-transcriptase-polymerase chain reaction-based assays and clinical findings.

Additional Information RSV prophylaxis should be initiated no earlier than July 1st in Southeast Florida, September 15th in Northcentral and Southwest Florida, and November 1st in most other areas of the United States (*Red Book* [AAP], 2012).

If an infant or child receiving prophylaxis experiences a breakthrough RSV infection they should continue to receive the maximum number of doses based on their risk factors. Hospitalized infants who qualify for prophylaxis during RSV season should receive the first palivizumab dose 48 to 72 hours before discharge or promptly after discharge. Infants who have begun prophylaxis during RSV season and are hospitalized on the date when the next monthly dose is due should receive the dose as scheduled.

Antipalivizumab antibodies may develop after the fourth injection in some patients (~1%). This has not been associated with any risk of adverse events or altered serum concentrations.

Dosage Forms Excipient information presented when available (limited, particularly for generics); consult specific product labeling.

Solution, Intramuscular [preservative free]:
Synagis: 50 mg/0.5 mL (0.5 mL); 100 mg/mL (1 mL) [contains glycine, histidine]

References

American Academy of Pediatrics (AAP). In: Pickering LK, Baker CJ, Kimberlin DW, Long SS, eds. *Red Book: 2012 Report of the Committee on Infectious Diseases*. 29th ed. Elk Grove Village, IL: American Academy of Pediatrics; 2012.

Boeckh M, Berrey MM, Bowden RA, et al, "Phase 1 Evaluation of the Respiratory Syncytial Virus-Specific Monoclonal Antibody Palivizumab in Recipients of Hematopoietic Stem Cell Transplants," *J Infect Dis*, 2001, 184(3):350-4.

Chávez-Bueno S, Mejías A, Merryman RA, et al, "Intravenous Palivizumab and Ribavirin Combination for Respiratory Syncytial Virus Disease in High-Risk Pediatric Patients," *Pediatr Infect Dis J*, 2007, 26(12):1089-93.

Feltes TF, Cabalka AK, Meissner HC, et al, "Palivizumab Prophylaxis Reduces Hospitalization Due to Respiratory Syncytial Virus in Young Children With Hemodynamically Significant Congenital Heart Disease," *J Pediatr*, 2003, 143(4):532-40.

Giebels K, Marcotte JE, Podoba J, et al, "Prophylaxis Against Respiratory Syncytial Virus in Young Children With Cystic Fibrosis," *Pediatr Pulmonol*, 2008, 43(2):169-74.

Malley R, DeVincenzo J, Ramilo O, et al, "Reduction of Respiratory Syncytial Virus (RSV) in Tracheal Aspirates in Intubated Infants by Use of Humanized Monoclonal Antibody to RSV F Protein," *J Infect Dis*, 1998, 178(6):1555-61.

"Palivizumab, a Humanized Respiratory Syncytial Virus Monoclonal Antibody, Reduces Hospitalization From Respiratory Syncytial Virus Infection in High-Risk Infants. The Impact-RSV Study Group," *Pediatrics*, 1998, 102(3 Pt 1):531-7.

Sáez-Llorens X, Moreno MT, Ramilo O, et al, "Safety and Pharmacokinetics of Palivizumab Therapy in Children Hospitalized With Respiratory Syncytial Virus Infection," *Pediatr Infect Dis J*, 2004, 23 (8):707-12.

Subramanian KN, Weisman LE, Rhodes T, et al, "Safety, Tolerance and Pharmacokinetics of a Humanized Monoclonal Antibody to Respiratory Syncytial Virus in Premature Infants and Infants With Bronchopulmonary Dysplasia. MEDI-493 Study Group," *Pediatr Infect Dis J*, 1998, 17(2):110-5.

Palonosetron (pal oh NOE se tron)

Medication Safety Issues

Sound-alike/look-alike issues:
Aloxi may be confused with Eloxatin, oxaliplatin
Palonosetron may be confused with dolasetron, granisetron, ondansetron

Brand Names: U.S. Aloxi

Therapeutic Category 5-HT$_3$ Receptor Antagonist; Antiemetic

Generic Availability (U.S.) No

Use Prevention of acute and delayed chemotherapy-induced nausea and vomiting; prevention of postoperative nausea and vomiting (PONV) (FDA approved in adults)

Pregnancy Risk Factor B

Pregnancy Considerations Adverse events have not been observed in animal reproduction studies. Use during pregnancy only if needed.

Breast-Feeding Considerations It is not known if palonosetron is excreted in breast milk. Due to the potential for adverse reactions in the nursing infant, the manufacturer recommends a decision be made whether to discontinue nursing or to discontinue palonosetron, takinge into account the importance of treatment to the mother.

Contraindications Hypersensitivity to palonosetron or any component

Warnings Palonosetron may cause ECG interval changes (PR, QT$_c$, JT prolongation and QRS widening); interval prolongation could lead to cardiovascular consequences such as heart block or cardiac arrhythmias; hypersensitivity reactions may occur in patients who have exhibited hypersensitivity to other 5-HT$_3$ antagonists (eg, ondansetron, dolasetron)

Precautions Use with caution in patients with, or who may develop, prolongation of cardiac conduction intervals, particularly QT$_c$; conditions include hypokalemia, hypomagnesemia, or congenital QT syndrome; use with caution in

patients receiving antiarrhythmic or other medications known to prolong the QT interval (eg, class I or III antiarrhythmic agents) or medications known to reduce potassium or magnesium levels (eg, diuretics)

Adverse Reactions Adverse events may vary according to indication; frequency reported for adults unless otherwise noted.

Cardiovascular: Prolonged Q-T interval on ECG (more common in PONV), bradycardia (more common in PONV), hypotension, sinus bradycardia, tachycardia (nonsustained)

Central nervous system: Headache (more common in chemotherapy-associated nausea), anxiety, dizziness

Dermatologic: Pruritus

Endocrine & metabolic: Hyperkalemia

Gastrointestinal: Constipation, diarrhea, flatulence

Genitourinary: Urinary retention

Hepatic: Increased serum ALT (transient), increased serum AST (transient)

Neuromuscular & skeletal: Weakness

Rare but important or life-threatening: Allergic dermatitis, amblyopia, anaphylactic shock, anaphylaxis, anemia, anorexia, cardiac arrhythmia, decreased gastrointestinal motility, decreased platelet count, dyskinesia, dyspepsia, edema (generalized), electrolyte disturbance, epistaxis, erythema, extrasystoles, flattened T wave on ECG, flu-like symptoms, glycosuria, hyperglycemia, hypersensitivity (rare), hypersomnia, hypertension, hypokalemia, hypoventilation, insomnia, ischemic heart disease, jugular vein distention, laryngospasm, limb pain, metabolic acidosis, motion sickness, paresthesia, seizure, sinus arrhythmia, sinus tachycardia, skin rash, supraventricular extrasystole, vein discoloration, ventricular extrasystoles

Drug Interactions

Metabolism/Transport Effects Substrate of CYP1A2 (minor), CYP2D6 (minor), CYP3A4 (minor); **Note:** Assignment of Major/Minor substrate status based on clinically relevant drug interaction potential

Avoid Concomitant Use
Avoid concomitant use of Palonosetron with any of the following: Apomorphine

Increased Effect/Toxicity
Palonosetron may increase the levels/effects of: Apomorphine; Serotonin Modulators

Decreased Effect
Palonosetron may decrease the levels/effects of: Tapentadol; TraMADol

The levels/effects of Palonosetron may be decreased by: Peginterferon Alfa-2b

Stability Store at room temperature; protect from light. Do not freeze; do not mix with other drugs.

Mechanism of Action Selective 5-HT$_3$ receptor antagonist, blocking serotonin, both on vagal nerve terminals in the periphery and centrally in the chemoreceptor trigger zone

Pharmacokinetics (Adult data unless noted)

Distribution: Adults: 8.3 ± 2.5 L/kg

Protein binding: 62%

Metabolism: Metabolized to 2 minimally active metabolites (<1% activity of palonosetron)

Half-life:
Children: 21-37 hours
Adults: 40 hours

Elimination: Urine 80% to 93% (40% as unchanged drug); feces (5% to 8%)

Clearance: Adults: Total body: 160 mL/h/kg

Dosing: Usual

Children and Adolescents: Information based on small clinical trials: I.V.: Prevention of acute chemotherapy-induced nausea and vomiting

Kadota (2007): A multicenter, stratified, double-blind randomized trial of 60 pediatric patients >2 years [12 patients (1 month to 2 years) treated in an open-label fashion] showed 3 mcg/kg (maximum dose: 0.25 mg) and 10 mcg/kg (maximum dose: 0.75 mg) were well-tolerated and effective (no emesis, no rescue first 0-24 hours)

Sepõlveda-Vildósola (2008): A randomized comparison of palonosetron (0.25 mg single dose 30 minutes before chemotherapy) and ondansetron (8 mg/m^2 every 8 hours beginning 30 minutes before chemotherapy) in children 2-15 years, evaluated 100 chemotherapy courses in each arm and showed a statistically significant reduction in emetic events on days 0-3 in the palonosetron group and clinically significant reduction in emetic events on days 4-7 (up to 6 emetic events in the ondansetron group vs none with palonosetron)

Adults: I.V.:

Prevention of acute and delayed chemotherapy-induced nausea and vomiting: 0.25 mg as a single dose administered 30 minutes before chemotherapy

PONV: 0.075 mg immediately prior to anesthesia induction

Dosage adjustment in hepatic or renal impairment: No dosage adjustment is indicated

Administration Infuse I.V. undiluted over 30 seconds; do not mix with other medications. Solutions of 5 mcg/mL and 30 mcg/mL in NS, D$_5$W, D$_5$½NS, and D$_5$LR injection are stable for 48 hours at room temperature and 14 days under refrigeration

Monitoring Parameters Baseline ECG in high-risk patients, emesis episodes

Dosage Forms Excipient information presented when available (limited, particularly for generics); consult specific product labeling.

Solution, Intravenous:

Aloxi: 0.25 mg/5 mL (5 mL) [contains edetate disodium]

References

Eisenberg P, Figueroa-Vadillo J, Zamora R, et al, "Improved Prevention of Moderately Emetogenic Chemotherapy-Induced Nausea and Vomiting With Palonosetron, a Pharmacologically Novel 5-HT$_3$ Receptor Antagonist: Results of a Phase III, Single-Dose Trial Versus Dolasetron," *Cancer*, 2003, 98(11):2473-82.

Gralla R, Lichinitser M, Van Der Vegt S, et al, "Palonosetron Improves Prevention of Chemotherapy-Induced Nausea and Vomiting Following Moderately Emetogenic Chemotherapy: Results of a Double-Blind Randomized Phase III Trial Comparing Single Doses of Palonosetron With Ondansetron," *Ann Oncol*, 2003, 14(10):1570-7.

Kadota R, Shen V, and Messinger Y, "Safety, Pharmacokinetics, and Efficacy of Palonosetron in Pediatric Patients: A Multicenter, Stratified, Double-Blind, Phase 3, Randomized Study," *J Clin Oncol*, 2007, 25 (18S June 20 Suppl):9570.

Sepõlveda-Vildósola AC, Betanzos-Cabrera Y, Lastiri GG, et al, "Palonosetron Hydrochloride Is an Effective and Safe Option to Prevent Chemotherapy-Induced Nausea and Vomiting in Children," *Arch Med Res*, 2008, 39(6):601-6.

Siddiqui MA and Scott LJ, "Palonosetron," *Drugs*, 2004, 64 (10):1125-32.

Trissel LA and Xu QA, "Physical and Chemical Stability of Palonosetron HCl in 4 Infusion Solutions," *Ann Pharmacother*, 2004, 38 (10):1608-11.

◆ **Palonosetron Hydrochloride** *see* Palonosetron
on page 1586

◆ **2-PAM** *see* Pralidoxime *on page 1719*

◆ **Pamelor** *see* Nortriptyline *on page 1512*

Pamidronate (pa mi DROE nate)

Medication Safety Issues

Sound-alike/look-alike issues:

Aredia may be confused with Adriamycin

Pamidronate may be confused with papaverine

Brand Names: Canada Aredia; Pamidronate Disodium; Pamidronate Disodium Omega; PMS-Pamidronate

Therapeutic Category Antidote, Hypercalcemia; Bisphosphonate Derivative

Generic Availability (U.S.) Yes

Use Treatment of moderate or severe hypercalcemia associated with malignancy with or without bone metastases (in conjunction with adequate hydration); treatment of osteolytic bone lesions associated with multiple myeloma or metastatic breast cancer; treatment of moderate to severe Paget's disease of bone (All indications: FDA approved in adults); has also been used in the treatment of osteogenesis imperfecta and osteopenia in cerebral palsy patients

Pregnancy Risk Factor D

Pregnancy Considerations Adverse events were observed in animal reproduction studies. It is not known if bisphosphonates cross the placenta, but fetal exposure is expected (Djokanovic, 2008; Stathopoulos, 2011). Bisphosphonates are incorporated into the bone matrix and gradually released over time. The amount available in the systemic circulation varies by dose and duration of therapy. Theoretically, there may be a risk of fetal harm when pregnancy follows the completion of therapy; however, available data have not shown that exposure to bisphosphonates during pregnancy significantly increases the risk of adverse fetal events (Djokanovic, 2008; Levy, 2009; Stathopoulos, 2011). Until additional data is available, most sources recommend discontinuing bisphosphonate therapy in women of reproductive potential as early as possible prior to a planned pregnancy; use in premenopausal women should be reserved for special circumstances when rapid bone loss is occurring (Bhalla, 2010; Pereira, 2012; Stathopoulos, 2011). Because hypocalcemia has been described following *in utero* bisphosphonate exposure, exposed infants should be monitored for hypocalcemia after birth (Djokanovic, 2008; Stathopoulos, 2011).

Breast-Feeding Considerations It is not known if pamidronate is excreted in breast milk. Pamidronate was not detected in the milk of a nursing woman receiving pamidronate 30 mg I.V. monthly (therapy started ~6 months postpartum). Following the first infusion, milk was pumped and collected for 0-24 hours and 25-48 hours, and each day pooled for analysis. Pamidronate readings were below the limit of quantification (<0.4 micromole/L). During therapy, breast milk was pumped and discarded for the first 48 hours following each infusion prior to resuming nursing. The infant was breast-fed >80% of the time; adverse events were not observed in the nursing infant (Simonoski, 2000). Monitoring the serum calcium concentrations of nursing infants is recommended (Stathopoulos, 2011). Due to the potential for serious adverse reactions in the nursing infant, the manufacturer recommends a decision be made whether to discontinue nursing or to discontinue the drug, taking into account the importance of treatment to the mother.

Contraindications Hypersensitivity to pamidronate, other bisphosphonates, or any component

Warnings Hazardous agent; use appropriate precautions for handling and disposal (NIOSH, 2012). Osteonecrosis of the jaw (ONJ) has been reported in patients receiving bisphosphonates; risk factors include invasive dental procedures (eg, tooth extraction, dental implants, boney surgery); a diagnosis of cancer, with concomitant chemotherapy, radiotherapy, or corticosteroids; poor oral hygiene, ill-fitting dentures; and comorbid disorders (ie, anemia, coagulopathy, infection, preexisting dental disease). Most reported cases occurred after I.V. bisphosphonate therapy; however, cases have been reported following oral therapy. A dental exam and preventative dentistry should be performed prior to placing patients with risk factors on chronic bisphosphonate therapy. When dental procedures are required, there is no evidence that discontinuing therapy reduces the risk of developing ONJ (Assael, 2009). The risk:benefit must be assessed by the treating physician and/or dentist/surgeon prior to any invasive dental procedure. Patients developing ONJ while on bisphosphonates should receive care by an oral surgeon.

Infrequently, severe (and occasionally debilitating) bone, joint, and/or muscle pain have been reported during bisphosphonate treatment. The onset of pain ranged from a single day to several months. Consider discontinuing therapy in patients who experience severe symptoms; symptoms usually resolve upon discontinuation. Some patients experienced recurrence when rechallenged with the same drug or another bisphosphonate; avoid use in patients with a history of these symptoms in association with bisphosphonate therapy. Atypical femur fractures (after minimal or no trauma) have been reported. The fractures include subtrochanteric femur (bone just below the hip joint) and diaphyseal femur (long segment of the thigh bone). Some patients experience prodromal pain weeks or months before the fracture occurs. It is unclear if bisphosphonate therapy is the cause for these fractures. Patients receiving long-term therapy (>3-5 years) may be at an increased risk. Consider discontinuing bisphosphonate therapy in patients with a suspected femoral shaft fracture. Patients who present with thigh or groin pain in the absence of trauma should be evaluated.

May cause renal deterioration; single pamidronate doses should not exceed 90 mg; initial or single doses have been associated with renal deterioration, progressing to renal failure and dialysis. Glomerulosclerosis (focal segmental) with or without nephrotic syndrome, has also been reported, particularly in patients with multiple myeloma and breast cancer. Longer infusion times (>2 hours) may reduce the risk for renal toxicity, especially in patients with preexisting renal insufficiency. Monitor serum creatinine prior to each dose; withhold pamidronate treatment (until renal function returns to baseline) in patients with evidence of renal deterioration.

Precautions Use with caution in patients with renal impairment; evaluate serum creatinine prior to each treatment; for the treatment of bone metastases, use is not recommended in patients with severe renal impairment. With indications other than bone metastases, use clinical judgment to determine if benefits outweigh potential risks in patients with renal impairment; maintain adequate hydration [pediatric patients: 2-3 L/m² (Kerdudo, 2005)] and urinary output during treatment; use with caution with other potentially nephrotoxic drugs. Use has been associated with asymptomatic electrolyte abnormalities (including hypophosphatemia, hypokalemia, hypomagnesemia, and hypocalcemia). Rare cases of symptomatic hypocalcemia, including tetany have been reported. Use with caution in patients with a history of thyroid surgery; patients may have relative hypoparathyroidism, predisposing them to pamidronate-related hypocalcemia. Use with caution in patients with preexisting anemia, leukopenia, or thrombocytopenia; may cause myelosuppression; closely monitor during the first 2 weeks of treatment.

Bisphosphonate therapy may not be appropriate for patients with mild osteogenesis imperfect; risk:benefit has not been established. Potential adverse effects in growing children include infusion reactions and effects on bone growth. Influenza-like reactions are common after the first dose occurring at 12-36 hours after the infusion and may include fever, rash, and vomiting; treatment with standard antipyretic therapy is usually adequate and symptoms do not generally recur after later doses. Increased height has been reported and theoretical effects

of diminishing bone remodeling in a growing child may result in bone malformation or delayed recovery after fractures (Rauch, 2004).

According to the American Society of Clinical Oncology (ASCO) guidelines for bisphosphonates in multiple myeloma, treatment with pamidronate is not recommended for asymptomatic (smoldering) or indolent myeloma or with solitary plasmacytoma (Kyle, 2007). The National Comprehensive Cancer Network® (NCCN) multiple myeloma guidelines (v.2.2013) recommend bisphosphonates for all patients receiving treatment for symptomatic disease; the use of bisphosphonates in stage 1 or smoldering disease may be considered, although preferable as part of a clinical trial. Patients with Bence-Jones proteinuria and dehydration should be adequately hydrated prior to therapy.

Adverse Reactions

Cardiovascular: Atrial fibrillation, atrial flutter, cardiac failure, edema, hypertension, syncope, tachycardia

Central nervous system: Drowsiness, fatigue, headache, insomnia, psychosis, seizure

Endocrine & metabolic: Hypocalcemia, hypokalemia, hypomagnesemia, hypophosphatemia, hypothyroidism

Gastrointestinal: Abdominal pain, anorexia, constipation, diarrhea, dyspepsia, gastrointestinal hemorrhage, nausea, stomatitis, vomiting

Genitourinary: Uremia, urinary tract infection

Hematologic & oncologic: Anemia, granulocytopenia, leukopenia, metastases, neutropenia, thrombocytopenia

Infection: Candidiasis

Local: Infusion site reaction (includes induration, pain, redness, and swelling)

Neuromuscular & skeletal: Arthralgia, back pain, myalgia, ostealgia, osteonecrosis of the jaw, weakness

Renal: Increased serum creatinine

Respiratory: Cough, dyspnea, pleural effusion, rales, rhinitis, sinusitis, upper respiratory tract infection

Miscellaneous: Fever

Rare but important or life-threatening: Acute renal failure, adult respiratory distress syndrome, anaphylactic shock, angioedema, cardiac failure, confusion, episcleritis, femur fractures (atypical subtrochanteric, diaphyseal femoral), focal segmental glomerulosclerosis (including collapsing variant), glomerulonephritis, hallucination (visual), hematuria, herpes virus infection (reactivation), hyperkalemia, hypernatremia, hypersensitivity reaction, hypervolemia, hypotension, inflammation at injection site, injection site phlebitis, interstitial nephritis, interstitial pneumonitis, iridocyclitis, iritis, left heart failure, lymphocytopenia, nephrotic syndrome, orbital disease (inflammation), osteonecrosis (other than jaw), renal failure, renal insufficiency, renal tubular disease, scleritis, uveitis, xanthopsia

Drug Interactions

Metabolism/Transport Effects None known.

Avoid Concomitant Use There are no known interactions where it is recommended to avoid concomitant use.

Increased Effect/Toxicity

Pamidronate may increase the levels/effects of: Deferasirox; Phosphate Supplements

The levels/effects of Pamidronate may be increased by: Aminoglycosides; Nonsteroidal Anti-Inflammatory Agents; Systemic Angiogenesis Inhibitors; Thalidomide

Decreased Effect

The levels/effects of Pamidronate may be decreased by: Proton Pump Inhibitors

Stability

Powder for injection: Store at 20°C to 25°C (68°F to 77°F). The reconstituted solution is stable for 24 hours under refrigeration.

Solution for injection: Store at 20°C to 25°C (68°F to 77°F).

Pamidronate diluted for infusion is stable at room temperature for up to 24 hours. Incompatible with calcium-containing solutions, including LR.

Mechanism of Action Nitrogen-containing bisphosphonate; inhibits bone resorption and decreases mineralization by disrupting osteoclast activity (Gralow, 2009; Rogers, 2011)

Pharmacodynamics

Onset of action:

Hypercalcemia of malignancy: Reduction of albumin-corrected serum calcium: Children: ~48 hours (Kerdudo, 2005); Adults: ≤24 hours

Paget's disease: ~1 month for ≥50% decrease in serum alkaline phosphatase

Maximum effect: Hypercalcemia of malignancy: ≤7 days

Duration: Hypercalcemia of malignancy: 7-14 days; Paget's disease: 1-372 days

Pharmacokinetics (Adult data unless noted)

Absorption: Poorly from the GI tract

Metabolism: Not metabolized

Half-life, elimination: 28 ± 7 hours

Elimination: Biphasic: Urine (30% to 62% as unchanged drug; lower in patients with renal dysfunction) within 120 hours

Dosing: Neonatal Osteogenesis imperfecta: Limited data available: Full-term neonates, PNA ≥14 days: I.V.: Initial: 0.25 mg/kg once on day 1, then 0.5 mg/kg/dose daily days 2 and 3 of the first cycle, then 0.5 mg/kg/dose once daily for 3 days for subsequent cycles; cycles are repeated every 2 months for a total yearly dose of 9 mg/kg (Rauch, 2003; Zietlin, 2003)

Dosing: Usual Note: Due to increased risk of nephrotoxicity, single doses should not exceed 90 mg.

Infants, Children, and Adolescents:

Hypercalcemia: Limited data available: Children and Adolescents: Dosing based on several case reports and retrospective studies for treatment of hypercalcemia due to malignancy and/or immobility. Administer as a single infusion. Retreatment may be necessary if serum calcium does not return to normal or does not remain normal after initial treatment; reported interval for multiple doses is ≥24 hours.

Initial treatment: I.V.: 0.5-1 mg/kg; maximum dose: 90 mg (Kerdudo, 2005; Kutluk, 1999; Lteif, 1998; Young; 1998)

Severe, life-threatening: I.V.: 1.5-2 mg/kg; maximum dose: 90 mg; in one case report, a higher dose of 4 mg/kg was used to treat a serum calcium concentration of 18.9 mg/dL associated with bone metastases in a 4-year old child with non-Hodgkin lymphoma (Kerdudo, 2005; Kutluk, 1997; Kutluk, 1999)

Osteogenesis imperfecta: Limited data available: **Note:** Reported dosing regimens variable (ie, weight-directed vs BSA-directed); duration of treatment has not been established; however, the most benefit has been shown to occur in the first 2-4 years of treatment (Rauch, 2006).

Weight-directed dosing (Rauch, 2003; Zietlin, 2003):

Infants and Children <2 years: I.V.: Initial: 0.25 mg/kg once on day 1, then 0.5 mg/kg/dose daily days 2 and 3 of the first cycle, then 0.5 mg/kg/dose once daily for 3 days for subsequent cycles; cycles are repeated every 2 months for a total yearly dose of 9 mg/kg

Children 2-3 years: I.V.: Initial: 0.38 mg/kg once on day 1, then 0.75 mg/kg/dose daily days 2 and 3 of the first cycle, then 0.75 mg/kg/dose once daily for 3 days for subsequent cycles; cycles are repeated every 3 months for a total yearly dose of 9 mg/kg

Children >3 years and Adolescents: I.V.: Initial: 0.5 mg/kg once on day 1, then 1 mg/kg/dose daily days 2 and 3 of the first cycle, then 1 mg/kg/dose once daily for 3 days for subsequent cycles; cycles are

repeated every 4 months for a total yearly dose of 9 mg/kg

BSA-directed dosing: I.V.: Initial: 10 mg/m²/dose once a month for 3 months, then increase to 20 mg/m²/dose once a month for 3 months, then increase to 30 mg/m²/dose once a month for subsequent doses; maximum dose: 40 mg/m²/dose was used in six patients after 1-2 years due to skeletal pain and less bone mineral gain; improvements in mobility and vertebral height was noted in patients who received this regimen for 3-6 years (n=11, median age at initiation of therapy: 3.6 months, range: 3-13 months) (Astrom, 2007); another study used the same dosing in 14 prepubescent patients with mild disease (Heino, 2011)

Osteopenia associated with cerebral palsy (nonambulatory): Limited data available; dosing regimens variable: Children and Adolescents: I.V.: Initial: 1 mg/kg/dose daily for 3 days; administer every 3-4 months; minimum dose: 15 mg; maximum dose: 35 mg. Dosing based on two trials; the first included 14 pediatric patients (age range: 6-16 years, treatment group: n=7), and reported an increase in bone mineral density; therapy was used in combination with calcium and vitamin D supplementation (Henderson, 2002). In the other trial (n=25, age range: 3-19 years), a decreased incidence of fractures was noted after 1 year of therapy (Bachrach, 2010). A lower dose was used in a trial of 23 pediatric patients (age range: 4-17 years); the initial dose was 0.37 mg/kg on day 1, followed by 0.75 mg/kg on day 2, then 0.75 mg/kg/dose once daily for 2 days was used for subsequent cycles; cycles were repeated every 4 months for 1 year; maximum single dose: 45 mg (Plotkin, 2006); further studies are needed.

Adults:

Hypercalcemia of malignancy: I.V.:

Moderate cancer-related hypercalcemia (corrected serum calcium 12-13.5 mg/dL): 60-90 mg as a single dose over 2-24 hours

Severe cancer-related hypercalcemia (corrected serum calcium >13.5 mg/dL): 90 mg as a single dose over 2-24 hours

Retreatment in patients who show an initial complete or partial response (allow at least 7 days to elapse prior to retreatment): May retreat at the same dose if serum calcium does not return to normal or does not remain normal after initial treatment

Multiple myeloma, osteolytic bone lesions: I.V.: 90 mg over 4 hoursonce monthly

Breast cancer, osteolytic bone metastases: I.V.: 90 mg over 2 hours every 3-4 weeks

Paget's disease, moderate to severe: I.V.: 30 mg over 4 hours daily for 3 consecutive days (total dose = 90 mg); may retreat at initial dose if clinically indicated

Dosing adjustment in renal impairment: Adults:

Baseline: Patients with serum creatinine >3 mg/dL were excluded from clinical trials; there are only limited pharmacokinetic data in patients with CrCl <30 mL/minute

Manufacturer's recommendations:

Treatment of bone metastases: Use is not recommended in patients with severe renal impairment.

Renal impairment in indications other than bone metastases: Use clinical judgment to determine if benefit outweighs risks.

The following recommendations have been used by some clinicians:

Multiple myeloma: American Society of Clinical Oncology (ASCO) guidelines (Kyle, 2007):

Severe renal impairment (serum creatinine >3 mg/dL or CrCl <30 mL/minute) and extensive bone disease: 90 mg over 4-6 hours; however, a reduced initial dose should be considered if renal impairment was preexisting.

▶

Albuminuria >500 mg/24 hours (unexplained): Withhold dose until returns to baseline, then recheck every 3-4 weeks; consider reinitiating at a dose not to exceed 90 mg every 4 weeks and with a longer infusion time of at least 4 hours

During therapy: In patients with bone metastases, treatment should be withheld for deterioration in renal function (increase of serum creatinine ≥0.5 mg/dL in patients with normal baseline or ≥1 mg/dL in patients with abnormal baseline). Resumption of therapy may be considered when serum creatinine returns to within 10% of baseline.

Dosing adjustment in hepatic impairment: Adults:

Mild to moderate impairment (Child-Pugh class A or B): No adjustment recommended.

Severe hepatic impairment (Child-Pugh class C): There are no dosage adjustments provided in manufacturer's labeling; not studied.

Administration Hazardous agent; use appropriate precautions for handling and disposal (NIOSH, 2012).

Reconstitute powder for injection vial with 10 mL SWI.; further dilute solution for injection or reconstituted solution with D_5W, 1/2NS, or NS to a final concentration of 0.06-0.36 mg/mL; final concentration is determined by dose and condition being treated; refer to manufacturer's labeling for specific information for adult patients. In pediatric osteogenesis imperfecta trials, for neonates, infants and children <3 years, the dose was diluted in NS to a final concentration of ≤0.1 mg/mL; in children ≥3 years and adolescents, doses were added to 250 mL or 500 mL of NS (final concentration not specified) (Glorieaux, 1998; Plotkin, 2000).

Infusion rate varies by indication; longer infusion times (>2 hours) may reduce the risk for renal toxicity, especially in patients with preexisting renal insufficiency. In adults, the manufacturer recommends infusing over 2-24 hours for hypercalcemia of malignancy, over 2 hours for osteolytic bone lesions with metastatic breast cancer, and over 4 hours for Paget's disease and for osteolytic bone lesions with multiple myeloma. In pediatric trials, infusion times were 4 hours for osteogenesis imperfecta, 3-4 hours for osteopenia from immobility, and 4-6 hours for hypercalcemia; a 24-hour infusion has also been used (Henderson, 2002; Kerdudo, 2005; Kutluk, 1997; Lteif, 1998; Rauch, 2003; Young, 1998).

Monitoring Parameters Monitor serum creatinine prior to each dose; monitor serum calcium, phosphate, potassium, and magnesium; monitor for hypocalcemia for at least 2 weeks after therapy; patients with preexisting anemia, leukopenia, or thrombocytopenia should have hemoglobin, hematocrit, and CBC with differential monitored closely, particularly in the first 2 weeks following treatment; dental exam and preventative dentistry prior to therapy for patients at risk for osteonecrosis

Additional indication-specific monitoring:

Multiple myeloma: Urine albumin every 3-6 months

Osteogenesis imperfecta: In pediatric trials, motor milestones, ambulation assessment, total body length, sitting height, and arm span were recorded every 6 months. Bone density was measured every 6 months. Conventional x-rays were obtained once yearly (Heino, 2011). Urinary excretion of calcium, alkaline phosphatase, and other bone-related chemistries were also monitored.

Osteopenia associated with cerebral palsy: In pediatric trials, bone mineral density, number and location of fractures, conventional x-rays, serum vitamin D concentrations, alkaline phosphatase, and other bone related chemistries were monitored (Bachrach, 2010; Henderson, 2002; Plotkin, 2006)

Paget's disease: Monitor serum alkaline phosphatase and urinary hydroxyproline excretion

Test Interactions Bisphosphonates may interfere with diagnostic imaging agents such as technetium-99m-diphosphonate in bone scans.

Dosage Forms Excipient information presented when available (limited, particularly for generics); consult specific product labeling.

Solution, Intravenous, as disodium:

Generic: 30 mg/10 mL (10 mL); 90 mg/10 mL (10 mL)

Solution, Intravenous, as disodium [preservative free]:

Generic: 30 mg/10 mL (10 mL); 6 mg/mL (10 mL); 90 mg/10 mL (10 mL)

Solution Reconstituted, Intravenous, as disodium:

Generic: 30 mg (1 ea); 90 mg (1 ea)

References

Assael LA. Oral bisphosphonates as a cause of bisphosphonate-related osteonecrosis of the jaws: clinical findings, assessment of risks, and preventive strategies. J Oral Maxillofac Surg. 2009;67(5 Suppl):35-43.

Aström E, Jorulf H, Söderhäll S. Intravenous pamidronate treatment of infants with severe osteogenesis imperfecta. Arch Dis Child. 2007; 92 (4):332-3388.

Auron A, Tal L, Srivastava T, et.al. Reversal of hypercalcemic acute kidney injury by treatment with intravenous bisphosphonates. Pediatric Nephrology. 2009; 24:613-617.

Bachrach SJ, Kecskemethy HH, Harcke HT, et al. Decreased fracture incidence after 1 year of pamidronate treatment in children with spastic quadriplegic cerebral palsy. Dev Med Child Neurol. 2010;52 (9):837-842.

Bhalla AK, "Management of Osteoporosis in a Pre-menopausal Woman," Best Pract Res Clin Rheumatol, 2010, 24(3):313-27.

Djokanovic N, Klieger-Grossmann C, and Koren G, "Does Treatment With Bisphosphonates Endanger the Human Pregnancy?" J Obstet Gynaecol Can, 2008, 30(12):1146-8.

Glorieux FH, Bishop NH, Plotkin H, et al, "Cyclic Administration of Pamidronate in Children With Severe Osteogenesis Imperfecta," N Engl J Med, 1998, 339(14):947-52.

Heino T, Astrom E, Laurencikas E, et al. Intravenous pamidronate treatment improves growth in prepubertal osteogenesis imperfecta patients. Horm Res Paediatr. 2011;75:354-61.

Henderson RC, Lark RK, Kecskemethy HH, et al, "Bisphosphonates to Treat Osteopenia in Children With Quadriplegic Cerebral Palsy: A Randomized, Placebo-Controlled Clinical Trial," J Pediatr, 2002, 141 (5):644-51.

Kerdudo C, Aerts I, Fattet S, et al. Hypercalcemia and childhood cancer: a 7-year experience. J Pediatr Hematol Oncol. 2005;27 (1):23-27.

Kutluk MT, Hazar V, Akyuz C, et.al. Childhood cancer and hypercalcemia: report of a case treated with pamidronate. Journal of Pediatrics. 1997;130(5):828-831.

Kutluk MT. Use of bisphosphonates in hypercalcemia associated with childhood cancer. Journal of Clinical Oncology. 1999;17(6):1901.

Kyle RA, Yee GC, Somerfield MR, et al. American Society of Clinical Oncology 2007 clinical practice guideline update on the role of bisphosphonates in multiple myeloma. J Clin Oncol. 2007;25 (17):2464-2472.

Levy S, Fayez I, Taguchi N, et al, "Pregnancy Outcome Following in utero Exposure to Bisphosphonates," Bone, 2009, 44(3):428-30.

Lteif AN and Zimmerman D, "Bisphosphonates for Treatment of Childhood Hypercalcemia," Pediatrics, 1998, 102(4 Pt 1):990-3.

National Institute for Occupational Safety and Health (NIOSH), "NIOSH List of Antineoplastic and Other Hazardous Drugs in Healthcare Settings 2012." Available at http://www.cdc.gov/niosh/docs/2012-150/pdfs/2012-150.pdf. Accessed January 21, 2013.

Pereira RM, Carvalho JF, Paula AP, et al, "Guidelines for the Prevention and Treatment of Glucocorticoid-Induced Osteoporosis," Rev Bras Reumatol, 2012, 52(4):580-93.

Plotkin H, Coughlin S, Kreikemeier R, et al. Low doses of pamidronate to treat osteopenia in children with severe cerebral palsy: a pilot study. Dev Med Child Neurol. 2006;48(9):709-712.

Plotkin H, Rauch F, Bishop NJ, et al. Pamidronate treatment of severe osteogenesis imperfecta in children under 3 years of age. J Clin Endocrinol Metab. 2000;85:1846-1850.

Rauch F, Glorieux FH. Osteogenesis imperfecta. Lancet. 2004;363 (9418):1377-1385.

Rauch F, Plotkin H, Travers R, et al. Osteogenesis imperfecta types I, III, and IV: effect of pamidronate therapy on bone and mineral metabolism. J Clin Endocrinol Metab. 2003;88(3):986-992.

Rauch F, Travers R, Glorieux FH. Pamidronate in children with osteogenesis imperfecta: histomorphometric effects of long-term therapy. J Clin Endocrinol Metab. 2006;91(2):511-516.

Siminoski K, Fitzgerald AA, Flesch G, et al, "Intravenous Pamidronate for Treatment of Reflex Sympathetic Dystrophy During Breast Feeding,"J Bone Miner Res, 2000, 15(10):2052-5.

Stathopoulos IP, Liakou CG, Katsalira A, et al, "The Use of Bisphosphonates in Women Prior to or During Pregnancy and Lactation," *Hormones (Athens)*, 2011, 10(4):280-91.

Van Poznak CH, Temin S, Yee GC, et al. American Society of Clinical Oncology executive summary of the clinical practice guideline update on the role of bone-modifying agents in metastatic breast cancer. *J Clin Oncol.* 2011;29(9):1221-7

Young G, Shende A. Use of pamidronate in the management of acute cancer-related hypercalcemia in children. *Med Pediatr Oncol.* 1998;30(2):117-121.

Zeitlin L, Rauch F, Plotkin H, et al. Height and weight development during long-term therapy with cyclical intravenous pamidronate in children and adolescents with osteogenesis imperfect types I, III and IV. *Pediatrics.* 2003;111:1030–1036.

◆ **Pamidronate Disodium** *see* Pamidronate *on page 1587*

◆ **Pamidronate Disodium Omega (Can)** *see* Pamidronate *on page 1587*

◆ **Pamix [OTC]** *see* Pyrantel Pamoate *on page 1774*

◆ **Pamprin Ibuprofen Formula (Can)** *see* Ibuprofen *on page 1059*

◆ **Pancrease MT (Can)** *see* Pancrelipase *on page 1591*

◆ **Pancreatic Enzymes** *see* Pancrelipase *on page 1591*

◆ **Pancreaze** *see* Pancrelipase *on page 1591*

Pancrelipase (pan kre LYE pase)

Medication Safety Issues
Sound-alike/look-alike issues:
Pancrelipase may be confused with pancreatin

Related Information
Oral Medications That Should Not Be Crushed or Altered *on page 2438*

Brand Names: U.S. Creon; Pancreaze; Pancrelipase (Lip-Prot-Amyl); Pertzye; Ultresa; Viokace; Zenpep

Brand Names: Canada Cotazym; Creon; Pancrease MT; Ultrase; Ultrase MT; Viokase

Therapeutic Category Enzyme, Pancreatic; Pancreatic Enzyme

Generic Availability (U.S.) No

Use
Creon: Treatment of exocrine pancreatic insufficiency due to cystic fibrosis, chronic pancreatitis, pancreatectomy, or other conditions (FDA approved in infants, children, adolescents, and adults)

Pancrelipase, Pancreaze, Zenpep: Treatment of exocrine pancreatic insufficiency due to cystic fibrosis or other conditions (FDA approved in infants, children, adolescents, and adults)

Pertzye: Treatment of exocrine pancreatic insufficiency due to cystic fibrosis or other conditions (FDA approved in ages >12 months and weighing ≥8 kg and adults)

Ultresa: Treatment of exocrine pancreatic insufficiency due to cystic fibrosis or other conditions (FDA approved in ages >12 months and weighing ≥14 kg and adults)

Viokace: Treatment of exocrine pancreatic insufficiency due to chronic pancreatitis or pancreatectomy in combination with a proton pump inhibitor (FDA approved in adults)

Medication Guide Available Yes

Pregnancy Risk Factor C

Pregnancy Considerations Reproduction studies have not been conducted. Nutrition should be optimized in pregnancy; in cystic fibrosis patients with malabsorption, pancreatic enzyme replacement is not considered to cause a risk to the pregnancy.

Breast-Feeding Considerations Systemic absorption and concentration into the breast milk is unlikely, but unknown.

Contraindications Hypersensitivity to pancrelipase or any component

Warnings Fibrosing colonopathy and colonic strictures have been reported in pediatric patients. Development of

strictures has been associated with high lipase intake (mean: >6000 units/kg/meal) over a prolonged period of time in children <12 years. Patients receiving doses >2500 lipase units/kg/meal, 4000 lipase units/g of fat/day or >10,000 lipase units/kg/day should be re-evaluated or titrated downward to lowest effective dose; if required, doses of lipase >2500 units/kg/meal (or lipase >10,000 units/kg/day) should be used with caution and only with documentation of 3-day fecal fat measures. Transmission of porcine viruses is theoretically a risk; however, testing and/or inactivation or removal of certain viruses, reduces the risk. There have been no cases of transmission of an infectious illness reported.

Precautions Products are not bioequivalent; do not substitute without consulting a physician or pharmacist; CF guidelines do not recommend generic enzyme use. Crushing or chewing the contents of the capsules or mixing the contents with foods outside of product labeling may cause early release of the enzymes, causing irritation of the oral mucosa and/or loss of enzyme activity. When mixing the contents of capsules with food, the mixture should be swallowed immediately and followed with water or juice to ensure complete ingestion. Use caution in patients with gout, hyperuricemia, or renal impairment; products contain purines which may increase uric acid concentrations. Products are derived from porcine pancreatic glands; severe, allergic reactions (rare) have been observed; use with caution in patients hypersensitive to pork proteins. Viokace tablets contain lactose; use with caution in patients with lactose intolerance.

Adverse Reactions The following adverse reactions were reported in a short-term safety studies; actual frequency varies with different products; adverse events, particularly gastrointestinal events, were often greater with placebo:

Cardiovascular: Peripheral edema

Central nervous system: Dizziness, headache

Dermatologic: Rash

Endocrine & metabolic: Diabetes mellitus exacerbation, hyper-/hypoglycemia

Gastrointestinal: Abdominal pain, anal itching, biliary tract stones, diarrhea, dyspepsia, early satiety, feces abnormal, flatulence, upper abdominal pain, vomiting, weight loss

Hematologic: Anemia

Hepatic: Ascites, hydrocholecystis

Neuromuscular & skeletal: Neck pain

Otic: Ear pain

Renal: Renal cyst

Respiratory: Beta-hemolytic streptococcal infection, cough, epistaxis, nasopharyngitis, pharyngolaryngeal pain

Miscellaneous: Lymphadenopathy, viral infection

Rare but important or life-threatening (reported with various formulations of pancrelipase): Allergic reactions (severe), anaphylaxis, asthma, carcinoma recurrence, constipation, distal intestinal obstruction syndrome (DIOS), duodenitis, fibrosing colonopathy, gastritis, hives, hyperuricemia, muscle spasm, myalgia, nausea, neutropenia (transient), pruritus, transaminases increased (asymptomatic), urticaria, vision blurred

Drug Interactions
Metabolism/Transport Effects None known.

Avoid Concomitant Use There are no known interactions where it is recommended to avoid concomitant use.

Increased Effect/Toxicity There are no known significant interactions involving an increase in effect.

Decreased Effect
Pancrelipase may decrease the levels/effects of: Iron Salts; Multivitamins/Minerals (with ADEK, Folate, Iron)

Food Interactions Delayed release capsules: Enteric coated contents of delayed release capsules opened and sprinkled on alkaline foods may result in early release of pancrelipase followed by enzyme inactivation by gastric acid in the stomach after swallowing. Management: Avoid placing contents of opened capsules on alkaline food (soft acidic foods with a pH of ≤4.5 are recommended for patients who cannot swallow capsules).

Stability

Creon: Store at room temperature up to 25°C (77°F); excursions permitted to 25°C to 40°C (77°F to 104°F) for up to 30 days; protect from moisture; discard if exposed to temperature >40°C (104°F) and moisture conditions are >70%. Keep bottle tightly closed between uses.

Pancreaze: Store at ≤25°C (77°F). Protect from moisture; keep bottle tightly closed between uses.

Zenpap:

Original glass container: Store at 20°C to 25°C (68°F to 77°F); excursions permitted to 15°C to 40°C (59°F to 104°F). Protect from moisture; keep bottle tightly closed between uses.

Repackaged HDPE container: Store at ≤30°C (86°F) for up to 6 months; excursions permitted to 15°C to 40°C (59°F to 104°F) for ≤30 days. Protect from moisture; keep bottle tightly closed between uses.

Pancrelipase, Pertzye: Store at 20°C to 25°C (68°F to 77°F); brief excursions permitted to 15°C to 40°C (59°F to 104°F). Protect from moisture; keep bottle tightly closed between uses.

Ultresa: Store at 20°C to 25°C (68°F to 77°F); protect from moisture. Keep bottle tightly closed between uses.

Viokace: Store at 20°C to 25°C (68°F to 77°F); brief excursions permitted up to 40°C (104°F) for up to 24 hours. Protect from moisture; keep bottle tightly closed between uses.

Mechanism of Action Pancrelipase is a natural product harvested from the porcine pancreatic glands. It contains a combination of lipase, amylase, and protease. Products are formulated to dissolve in the more basic pH of the duodenum so that they may act locally to break down fats, protein, and starch.

Pharmacokinetics (Adult data unless noted)

Absorption: Not significantly absorbed, acts locally in the GI tract

Elimination: In feces

Dosing: Neonatal Pancreatic insufficiency: Limited data available: Oral: Lipase 2000-5000 units per feeding of formula, breast milk, or per breast-feeding. Adjust dose based on clinical symptoms and stool fat content up to 2500 units/kg/feeding. Allow several days between dose adjustments. Maximum daily dose: Lipase 10,000 units/kg/day (Borowitz, 2009). **Note:** A review of data from the CF Foundation Patient Registry suggests that the maximum daily dose of lipase may be insufficient in young infants with CF; however, the optimal dose is not established (Borowitz, 2013).

Dosing: Usual Note: Adjust dose based on body weight, clinical symptoms, and stool fat content. Allow several days between dose adjustments. Total daily dose reflects ~3 meals/day and 2-3 snacks/day, with half the mealtime dose given with a snack. Doses of lipase >2500 units/kg/meal should be used with caution and only with documentation of 3-day fecal fat measures. Doses of lipase >6000 units/kg/meal are associated with colonic stricture and should be decreased.

Infants, Children, and Adolescents: **Pancreatic insufficiency:**

Oral:

Infants: Lipase 2000-5000 units per feeding of formula, breast milk, or per breast-feeding. Maximum daily dose: Lipase 10,000 units/kg/day up to 2500 units/kg/feeding (Borowitz, 2009). **Note:** A review of data from the CF Foundation Patient Registry suggests that the maximum daily dose may be insufficient in young infants with CF; however, the optimal dose is not established (Borowitz, 2013).

Children 1 to <2 years: Dosage requirements may fluctuate as diet transitions to more solid foods. Initial dose: Lipase 1000 units/kg/meal. Dosage range: Lipase 1000-2500 units/kg/meal. Maximum daily dose: Lipase 10,000 units/kg/**day** or lipase 4000 units/g of fat/day. Higher dosing similar to infant dosing (Lipase: 2000-5000 units per feeding of formula, breast milk, or per breast-feeding) may be necessary in some patients (Borowitz, 2009).

Children 2 to <4 years: Initial dose: Lipase 1000 units/kg/meal. Dosage range: Lipase 1000-2500 units/kg/meal. Maximum daily dose: Lipase 10,000 units/kg/**day** or lipase 4000 units/g of fat/day.

≥4 years: Initial dose: Lipase 500 units/kg/meal. Dosage range: Lipase 500-2500 units/kg/meal. Maximum daily dose: Lipase 10,000 units/kg/**day** or lipase 4000 units per g of fat/day.

Enteral tube feedings: Limited data available: **Note:** With low-fat or elemental enteral formulas, pancreatic enzyme supplementation may not be necessary (Ferrie, 2011).

Continuous enteral feeding: Lipase 1000 units/g of fat provided by the daily amount of feeds administered in divided doses every 2-3 hours (Ferrie, 2011).

Overnight enteral feeding: Administer premeal dose at beginning of feeding; additional dose may be given if midway through or at the end of a feeding (Borowitz, 2002). Some centers recommend using 1000 units/g of fat provided by the overnight feed administered in 2 divided doses with the first dose as 50% of requirement or enough to cover 3 hours of feeds and the additional dose given if patient awakens at night or at the end of a feeding (Ferrie, 2011).

Adults:

Pancreatic insufficiency due to conditions such as cystic fibrosis: Oral: Initial: Lipase 500 units/kg/meal. Dosage range: Lipase 500-2500 units/kg/meal. Maximum single dose: Lipase ≤2500 units/kg/**meal**; maximum daily dose: Lipase ≤10,000 units/kg/**day** or lipase <4000 units/g of fat daily

Pancreatic insufficiency due to chronic pancreatitis or pancreatectomy: Oral:

Creon: Lipase 72,000 units/meal while consuming ≥100 g of fat per day; alternatively, lower initial doses of lipase 500 units/kg/meal with individualized dosage titrations have also been used.

Viokace (administer in combination with a proton pump inhibitor): Initial: Lipase 500 units/kg/meal. Dosage range: Lipase 500-2500 units/kg/meal. Maximum single dose: Lipase ≤2500 units/kg/**meal**; maximum daily dose: Lipase ≤10,000 units/kg/**day** or lipase <4000 units/g of fat daily.

Administration Administer with meals or snacks and swallow capsules or tablets whole with a generous amount of liquid, water, or juice. Do not crush or chew; retention in the mouth before swallowing may cause mucosal irritation and stomatitis.

Oral:

Capsules: If necessary, capsules may also be opened and contents added to a small amount of an acidic food (pH ≤4.5), such as applesauce. The food should be at room temperature and swallowed immediately after mixing. The contents of the capsule should not be crushed or chewed. Follow with water or juice to ensure complete ingestion and that no medication remains in the mouth. Creon capsules contain enteric coated spheres which are 0.71-1.6 mm in diameter. Pancreaze capsules contain enteric coated microtablets which are ~2 mm in diameter. Zenpep capsules contain enteric coated beads which are 1.8-2.5 mm in diameter.

Infants <1 year: Avoid mixing with breast milk or infant formula. Open capsule and place the contents directly into the mouth or mix with a small amount of acidic soft food (pH ≤4.5) such as applesauce, or other commercially prepared baby food (pears or bananas) at room temperature. Administer immediately after mixing (or within 15 minutes of mixing using Pancreaze). Follow with infant formula or breast milk to ensure complete ingestion and that no medication remains in the mouth.

Tablets: Tablets are not enteric coated and should be taken with a proton pump inhibitor.

Gastrostomy tube (GT): Capsules: An *in vitro* study demonstrated that Creon delayed release capsules sprinkled on a small amount of baby food (pH<4.5; applesauce or bananas manufacturerd by both Gerber and Beech-Nut) may be administered through the following G-tubes without significant loss of lipase activity: Kimberly-Clark MIC Bolus® size 18 Fr, Kimberly-Clark MIC-KEY size 16 Fr, Bard® Tri-Funnel size 18 Fr, and Bard® Button size 18 Fr (Shlieout, 2011). Some centers use sodium bicarbonate to dissolve the beads before administering into GT; may cause increase in serum bicarbonate, monitor closely (Ferrie, 2011; Nicolo, 2013).

Monitoring Parameters Stool fat content, abdominal symptoms, nutritional intake, weight, growth, stool character, serum bicarbonate if using bicarbonate for GT administration.

Additional Information Concomitant administration with an H_2-receptor antagonist or proton pump inhibitor has been used to decrease acid inactivation of enzyme activity; concomitant antacid administration may decrease effectiveness of enzymes.

Dosage Forms Excipient information presented when available (limited, particularly for generics); consult specific product labeling.

Capsule, delayed release, bicarbonate buffered enteric coated microspheres, oral [porcine derived]:

Pertzye: Lipase 8,000 USP units, protease 28,750 USP units, and amylase 30,250 USP units

Pertzye: Lipase 16,000 USP units, protease 57,500 USP units, and amylase 60,500 USP units

Capsule, delayed release, enteric coated beads, oral [porcine derived]:

Pancrelipase (Lip-Prot-Amyl): Lipase 5000 USP units, protease 17,000 USP units, amylase 27,000 USP units

Zenpep: Lipase 3000 USP units, protease 10,000 USP units, and amylase 16,000 USP units

Zenpep: Lipase 5000 USP units, protease 17,000 USP units, and amylase 27,000 USP units

Zenpep: Lipase 10,000 USP units, protease 34,000 USP units, and amylase 55,000 USP units

Zenpep: Lipase 15,000 USP units, protease 51,000 USP units, and amylase 82,000 USP units

Zenpep: Lipase 20,000 USP units, protease 68,000 USP units, and amylase 109,000 USP units

Zenpep: Lipase 25,000 USP units, protease 85,000 USP units, and amylase 136,000 USP units

Capsule, delayed release, enteric coated microspheres, oral [porcine derived]:

Creon: Lipase 3000 USP units, protease 9500 USP units, and amylase 15,000 USP units

Creon: Lipase 6000 USP units, protease 19,000 USP units, and amylase 30,000 USP units

Creon: Lipase 12,000 USP units, protease 38,000 USP units, and amylase 60,000 USP units

Creon: Lipase 24,000 USP units, protease 76,000 USP units, and amylase 120,000 USP units

Creon: Lipase 36,000 USP units, protease 114,000 USP units, and amylase 180,000 USP units

Capsule, delayed release, enteric coated microtablets, oral [porcine derived]:

Pancreaze: Lipase 4200 USP units, protease 10,000 USP units, and amylase 17,500 USP units

Pancreaze: Lipase 10,500 USP units, protease 25,000 USP units, and amylase 43,750 USP units

Pancreaze: Lipase 16,800 USP units, protease 40,000 USP units, and amylase 70,000 USP units

Pancreaze: Lipase 21,000 USP units, protease 37,000 USP units, and amylase 61,000 USP units

Capsule, delayed release, enteric coated minitablets, oral [porcine derived]:

Ultresa: Lipase 13,800 USP units, protease 27,600 USP units, and amylase 27,600 USP units

Ultresa: Lipase 20,700 USP units, protease 41,400 USP units, and amylase 41,400 USP units

Ultresa: Lipase 23,000 USP units, protease 46,000 USP units, and amylase 46,000 USP units

Tablet, oral [porcine derived]:

Viokace: Lipase 10,440 USP units, protease 39,150 USP units, and amylase 39,150 USP units

Viokace: Lipase 20,880 USP units, protease 78,300 USP units, and amylase 78,300 USP units

References

Borowitz D, Baker RD, Stallings V. Consensus report on nutrition for pediatric patients with cystic fibrosis. *J Pediatr Gastroenterol Nutr.* 2002;35(3): 246-259.

Borowitz D, Gelfond D, Maguinness K, et al. Maximal daily dose of pancreatic enzyme replacement therapy in infants with cystic fibrosis. *J Cyst Fibros.* 2013. Available at http://dx.doi.org/10.1016/j.jcf2013.05.011

Borowitz D, Robinson KA, Rosenfeld M, et al. Cystic fibrosis foundation evidence-based guidelines for the management of infants with cystic fibrosis. *J Pediatr.* 2009;155:73-93.

Borowitz DS, Grand RJ, and Durie PR, "Use of Pancreatic Enzyme Supplements for Patients With Cystic Fibrosis in the Context of Fibrosing Colonopathy. Consensus Committee," *J Pediatr,* 1995, 127(5):681-4.

Ferrie S, Graham C, Hoyle M. Pancreatic enzyme supplementation for patients receiving enteral feeds. *Nutr Clin Prac.* 2011;26(3): 349-351.

FitzSimmons SC, Burkhart GA, Borowitz D, et al, "High-Dose Pancreatic-Enzyme Supplements and Fibrosing Colonopathy in Children With Cystic Fibrosis," *N Engl J Med,* 1997, 336(18):1283-9.

Nicolo M, Stratton KW, Rooney W, et al. Pancreatic enzyme therapy for enterally fed patients with cystic fibrosis. *Nutr Clin Prac.* 2013;28(4): 485-489.

Pettei MJ, Leonidas JC, Levinne JJ, et al, "Pancolonic Disease in Cystic Fibrosis and High-Dose Pancreatic Enzyme Therapy," *J Pediatr,* 1994, 125(4):587-9.

Shlieout G, Koerner A, Maffert M, et al, "Administration of CREON® Pancrelipase Pellets Via Gastrostomy Tube Is Feasible With No Loss of Gastric Resistance or Lipase Activity: An *in vitro* Study," *Clin Drug Investig,* 2011, 31(7):e1-7.

Stallings VA, Stark LJ, Robinson KA, et al, "Evidence-Based Practice Recommendations for Nutrition-Related Management of Children and Adults With Cystic Fibrosis and Pancreatic Insufficiency: Results of a Systematic Review," *J Am Diet Assoc,* 2008, 108(5):832-9.

Taylor CG, "Colonic Strictures in Cystic Fibrosis," *Lancet,* 1994, 343 (8898):615-6.

◆ **Pancrelipase (Lip-Prot-Amyl)** *see* Pancrelipase *on page 1591*

Pancuronium (pan kyoo ROE nee um)

Medication Safety Issues
High alert medication:

The Institute for Safe Medication Practices (ISMP) includes this medication among its list of drugs which have a heightened risk of causing significant patient harm when used in error.

Other safety concerns:

United States Pharmacopeia (USP) 2006: The Interdisciplinary Safe Medication Use Expert Committee of the USP has recommended the following:

- Hospitals, clinics, and other practice sites should institute special safeguards in the storage, labeling, and use of these agents and should include these safeguards in staff orientation and competency training.

- Healthcare professionals should be on high alert (especially vigilant) whenever a neuromuscular-blocking agent (NMBA) is stocked, ordered, prepared, or administered.

Brand Names: Canada Pancuronium Bromide®
Therapeutic Category Neuromuscular Blocker Agent, Nondepolarizing; Skeletal Muscle Relaxant, Paralytic
Generic Availability (U.S.) Yes
Use Adjunct to anesthesia, to facilitate endotracheal intubation and provide skeletal muscle relaxation during surgery or mechanical ventilation (FDA approved in all ages)
Pregnancy Risk Factor C
Pregnancy Considerations Animal reproduction studies have not been conducted. Small amounts of pancuronium cross the placenta (Daily, 1984). May be used short-term in cesarean section; reduced doses recommended in patients also receiving magnesium sulfate due to enhanced effects.
Contraindications Hypersensitivity to pancuronium, bromide, or any component
Warnings Ventilation must be supported during neuromuscular blockade; pancuronium should only be administered by individuals who are experienced in the maintenance of an adequate airway and respiratory support **[U.S. Boxed Warning]**. Pancuronium does not alter consciousness; use in conjunction with adequate sedation or anesthesia. Severe allergic reactions have been reported with neuromuscular blocking agents, including pancuronium; cross-sensitivity with other neuromuscular-blocking agents may occur; use extreme caution in patients with previous anaphylactic reactions. Pancuronium injection contains benzyl alcohol which may cause allergic reactions in susceptible individuals; large amounts of benzyl alcohol (≥99 mg/kg/day) have been associated with a potentially fatal toxicity ("gasping syndrome") in neonates; the "gasping syndrome" consists of metabolic acidosis, respiratory distress, gasping respirations, CNS dysfunction (including convulsions, intracranial hemorrhage), hypotension, and cardiovascular collapse; *in vitro* and animal studies have shown that benzoate, a metabolite of benzyl alcohol, displaces bilirubin from protein binding sites; avoid use of benzyl alcohol containing products in neonates
Precautions Use with caution in patients with renal, hepatic, and/or biliary tract disease; some patients may experience prolonged recovery of neuromuscular function after administration (especially after prolonged use). Concurrent use of some antibiotics (eg, aminoglycosides, tetracyclines, polymixin B, bacitracin, colistin), particularly high doses, may enhance neuromuscular blocking effects. Many clinical conditions may affect the response to neuromuscular blockade; see table.

Clinical Conditions Affecting Neuromuscular Blockade

Potentiation	Antagonism
Acidosis	Alkalosis
Acute intermittent porphyria	Demyelinating lesions
Electrolyte abnormalities	Diabetes mellitus
Severe hyponatremia	Hypercalcemia
Severe hypocalcemia	Peripheral neuropathies
Severe hypokalemia	
Hypermagnesemia	
Hepatic failure	
Neuromuscular diseases	
Renal failure	

Adverse Reactions

Cardiovascular: Circulatory collapse, edema, elevated blood pressure and cardiac output, elevation in pulse rate, skin flushing, tachycardia
Dermatologic: Burning sensation along the vein, erythema, itching, rash
Gastrointestinal: Excessive salivation
Neuromuscular & skeletal: Profound muscle weakness
Respiratory: Bronchospasm, wheezing
Miscellaneous: Hypersensitivity reaction

Postmarketing and/or case reports: Acute quadriplegic myopathy syndrome (prolonged use), anaphylactoid reactions, anaphylaxis, myositis ossificans (prolonged use)
Drug Interactions
Metabolism/Transport Effects None known.
Avoid Concomitant Use
Avoid concomitant use of Pancuronium with any of the following: QuiNINE
Increased Effect/Toxicity
Pancuronium may increase the levels/effects of: Cardiac Glycosides; Corticosteroids (Systemic); OnabotulinumtoxinA; RimabotulinumtoxinB

The levels/effects of Pancuronium may be increased by: AbobotulinumtoxinA; Aminoglycosides; Calcium Channel Blockers; Capreomycin; Clindamycin (Topical); Colistimethate; CycloSPORINE (Systemic); Fosphenytoin-Phenytoin; Inhalational Anesthetics; Ketorolac (Nasal); Ketorolac (Systemic); Lincosamide Antibiotics; Lithium; Loop Diuretics; Magnesium Salts; Polymyxin B; Procainamide; QuiNIDine; QuiNINE; Spironolactone; Tetracycline Derivatives; Theophylline Derivatives; Vancomycin
Decreased Effect
The levels/effects of Pancuronium may be decreased by: Acetylcholinesterase Inhibitors; Fosphenytoin-Phenytoin; Loop Diuretics; Theophylline Derivatives
Stability Store at 2°C to 8°C (36°F to 46°F); also stable for up to 6 months at room temperature; compatible with D_5W, NS, D_5NS, and LR injections
Mechanism of Action Blocks neural transmission at the myoneural junction by binding with cholinergic receptor sites
Pharmacodynamics
Onset of action (Martin, 1999):
  Infants: 2-5 minutes
  Children: 2-4 minutes
  Adults: 3-5 minutes
Duration: Dose-dependent
  Children: 24 minutes (Martin, 1999)
  Adults: 22 minutes (Martin, 1999)
Pharmacokinetics (Adult data unless noted)
Distribution: V_d: 0.24-0.28 L/kg
Protein binding: 87%
Metabolism: Hepatic: 30% to 40%; active metabolite 3-hydroxypancuronium (1/2 the activity of parent drug)
Half-life: 89-161 minutes
Elimination: Urine (40%); bile (11%)
Clearance: ~1-2 mL/kg/minute
Dosing: Neonatal Paralysis/skeletal muscle relaxation:
I.V.: 0.05-0.1 mg/kg/dose (Kumar, 2010); may repeat dose every 30-60 minutes as needed or as continuous I.V. infusion of 0.02-0.04 mg/kg/**hour** or 0.4-0.6 **mcg**/kg/minute
Dosing: Usual Paralysis/skeletal muscle relaxation:
I.V.:
Infants: 0.1 mg/kg/dose every 30-60 minutes as needed or as continuous I.V. infusion of 0.02-0.04 mg/kg/**hour** or 0.4-0.6 **mcg**/kg/minute
Children: 0.15 mg/kg/dose every 30-60 minutes as needed or as continuous I.V. infusion 0.03-0.1 mg/kg/**hour** or 0.5-1.7 **mcg**/kg/minute
Adolescents and Adults: 0.15 mg/kg/dose every 30-60 minutes as needed or as a continuous I.V. infusion 0.02-0.04 mg/kg/**hour** or 0.4-0.6 **mcg**/kg/minute
Dosing adjustment in renal impairment:
CrCl 10-50 mL/minute: Administer 50% of normal dose
CrCl <10 mL/minute: Do not use
Administration Parenteral: May be administered undiluted by rapid I.V. injection; for continuous I.V. infusion, dilute to final concentration of 0.01-0.8 mg/mL in D_5NS, D_5W, LR, or NS.

Monitoring Parameters Heart rate, blood pressure, assisted ventilation status, peripheral nerve stimulator measuring twitch response

Additional Information Patients with hepatic and biliary disease have a larger V_d which may result in a higher total initial dose and possibly a slower onset of effect; the duration of neuromuscular blocking effects may be prolonged in patients with hepatic, biliary, or renal dysfunction

Dosage Forms Excipient information presented when available (limited, particularly for generics); consult specific product labeling.

Solution, Intravenous, as bromide:
Generic: 1 mg/mL (10 mL); 2 mg/mL (2 mL, 5 mL)

References
Kumar P, Denson SE, Mancuso TJ, et al, "Premedication for Non-emergency Endotracheal Intubation in the Neonate," *Pediatrics*, 2010, 125(3):608-15.
Martin LD, Bratton SL, and O'Rourke PP, "Clinical Uses and Controversies of Neuromuscular Blocking Agents in Infants and Children," *Crit Care Med*, 1999, 27(7):1358-68.

◆ **Pancuronium Bromide** *see* Pancuronium *on page 1593*
◆ **Pancuronium Bromide® (Can)** *see* Pancuronium *on page 1593*
◆ **Pandel** *see* Hydrocortisone (Topical) *on page 1038*
◆ **Panglobulin** *see* Immune Globulin *on page 1084*
◆ **PanOxyl [OTC]** *see* Benzoyl Peroxide *on page 275*
◆ **PanOxyl® (Can)** *see* Benzoyl Peroxide *on page 275*
◆ **PanOxyl-4 Creamy Wash [OTC]** *see* Benzoyl Peroxide *on page 275*
◆ **PanOxyl-8 Creamy Wash [OTC]** *see* Benzoyl Peroxide *on page 275*
◆ **PanOxyl Wash [OTC]** *see* Benzoyl Peroxide *on page 275*
◆ **Panto I.V. (Can)** *see* Pantoprazole *on page 1595*
◆ **Pantoloc (Can)** *see* Pantoprazole *on page 1595*

Pantoprazole (pan TOE pra zole)

Medication Safety Issues
Sound-alike/look-alike issues:
Pantoprazole may be confused with ARIPiprazole
Protonix may be confused with Lotronex, Lovenox, protamine

Administration issues:
Vials containing Protonix I.V. for injection are not recommended for use with spiked I.V. system adaptors. Nurses and pharmacists have reported breakage of the glass vials during attempts to connect spiked I.V. system adaptors, which may potentially result in injury to healthcare professionals.

International issues:
Protonix [U.S.] may be confused with Pretanix brand name for indapamide [Hungary]
Protonix: Brand name for pantoprazole [U.S.] but also the brand name for omeprazole [Phillipines]

Related Information
Oral Medications That Should Not Be Crushed or Altered *on page 2438*

Brand Names: U.S. Protonix

Brand Names: Canada Abbott-Pantoprazole; Apo-Pantoprazole; Ava-Pantoprazole; CO Pantoprazole; Dom-Pantoprazole; JAMP-Pantoprazole; Mint-Pantoprazole; Mylan-Pantoprazole; Panto I.V.; Pantoloc; Pantoprazole for Injection; Pantoprazole Sodium for Injection; PMS-Pantoprazole; Q-Pantoprazole; RAN-Pantoprazole; ratio-Pantoprazole; Riva-Pantoprazole; Sandoz-Pantoprazole; Tecta; Teva-Pantoprazole

Therapeutic Category Gastric Acid Secretion Inhibitor; Gastrointestinal Agent, Gastric or Duodenal Ulcer Treatment; Proton Pump Inhibitor

Generic Availability (U.S.) May be product dependent

Use
Oral: Short-term treatment (up to 8 weeks) of erosive esophagitis associated with gastroesophageal reflux disease (GERD) (FDA approved in ages ≥5 years and adults); maintenance of healing of erosive esophagitis (FDA approved in adults); treatment of pathological hypersecretory conditions, including Zollinger-Ellison syndrome (FDA approved in adults); has also been used as adjunctive therapy of duodenal ulcers associated with *Helicobacter pylori*

I.V.: Short-term treatment (7-10 days) of patients with GERD with a history of erosive esophagitis (FDA approved in adults); treatment of pathological hypersecretory conditions, including Zollinger-Ellison syndrome (FDA approved in adults); has also been used as an alternative to oral therapy in patients who are unable to continue taking oral pantoprazole

Medication Guide Available Yes

Pregnancy Risk Factor B

Pregnancy Considerations Adverse events were not observed in animal reproduction studies. Most available studies have not shown an increased risk of major birth defects following maternal use of proton pump inhibitors during pregnancy (Diav-Citrin, 2005; Erichsen, 2012; Matok, 2012; Pasternak, 2010). When treating GERD in pregnancy, PPIs may be used when clinically indicated (Katz, 2013).

Breast-Feeding Considerations Pantoprazole is excreted into breast milk. The excretion of pantoprazole into breast milk was studied in a nursing woman, 10 months postpartum. Following a single dose of pantoprazole 40 mg, maternal milk and serum samples were obtained over 24 hours. Peak concentrations appeared in both the plasma and milk 2 hours after the dose. Pantoprazole concentrations in breast milk were below the limits of detection during most of the study period. Based on this single dose study, the authors calculated the expected exposure to a nursing infant to be 0.14% of the weight-adjusted maternal dose (Plante, 2004). Due to the potential for serious adverse reactions in the nursing infant, the manufacturer recommends a decision be made whether to discontinue nursing or to discontinue the drug, taking into account the importance of treatment to the mother; however, the acidic content of the nursing infants' stomach may potentially inactivate any ingested pantoprazole (Plante, 2004).

Contraindications Hypersensitivity to pantoprazole, substituted benzimidazole proton pump inhibitors (eg, esomeprazole, omeprazole, lansoprazole), or any component

Warnings Benign and malignant neoplasia has been observed in long-term rodent studies using pantoprazole; while not reported in humans, the relevance of these findings in regards to tumorigenicity in humans is not known. Symptomatic response to therapy does not preclude the presence of gastric malignancy. Atrophic gastritis has been reported in gastric biopsies from patients treated long-term with pantoprazole, particularly in patients who were *H. pylori* positive.

Use of gastric acid inhibitors, including proton pump inhibitors and H2 blockers, has been associated with an increased risk for development of acute gastroenteritis and community-acquired pneumonia (Canani, 2006). Use of PPIs may also increase the risk of *Clostridium difficile*-associated diarrhea (CDAD), especially in hospitalized patients; consider CDAD diagnosis in patients with persistent diarrhea that does not improve. Use the lowest dose and shortest duration of PPI therapy appropriate for the condition being treated.

An increased incidence of osteoporosis-related bone fractures of the hip, spine, or wrist may occur with PPI therapy; ▶

patients on high-dose (multiple daily doses) or long-term therapy (≥1 year) should be monitored. Use the lowest effective dose for the shortest duration of time, use vitamin D and calcium supplementation, and follow appropriate guidelines to reduce risk of fractures in patients at risk.

Hypomagnesemia has been reported rarely, usually with prolonged PPI use of >3 months (most cases >1 year of therapy), and may be symptomatic or asymptomatic; severe cases may cause tetany, seizures, and cardiac arrhythmias. Consider obtaining serum magnesium concentrations prior to beginning long-term therapy, especially if taking concomitant digoxin, diuretics, or other drugs known to cause hypomagnesemia; and periodically thereafter. Hypomagnesemia may be corrected by magnesium supplementation, although discontinuation of pantoprazole may be necessary; magnesium concentrations typically return to normal within 1 week of stopping.

PPIs may diminish the therapeutic effect of clopidogrel, thought to be due to reduced formation of the active metabolite of clopidogrel. The manufacturer of clopidogrel recommends either avoidance of both omeprazole (even when scheduled 12 hours apart) and esomeprazole or use of a PPI with comparatively less effect on the active metabolite of clopidogrel. Of the PPIs, pantoprazole has the lowest degree of CYP2C19 inhibition *in vitro* (Li, 2004) and has been shown to have less effect on conversion of clopidogrel to its active metabolite compared to omeprazole (Angiolillo, 2011). In contrast to these warnings, others have recommended the continued use of PPIs, regardless of the degree of inhibition, in patients with a history of GI bleeding or multiple risk factors for GI bleeding who are also receiving clopidogrel since no evidence has established clinically meaningful differences in outcome; however, a clinically-significant interaction cannot be excluded in those who are poor metabolizers of clopidogrel (Abraham, 2010; Levine, 2011). Concomitant use of PPIs with high-dose methotrexate may lead to increased and prolonged serum concentrations of methotrexate and/or its metabolite, possibly causing methotrexate toxicities; temporary discontinuation of PPIs may be considered.

Thrombophlebitis and hypersensitivity reactions, including anaphylaxis, Stevens-Johnson syndrome, and toxic epidermal necrolysis, have been reported with I.V. administration. Pantoprazole delayed release tablets and delayed release oral suspension contain polysorbate 80 (Tween 80®) which may cause allergic reactions in susceptible individuals.

Precautions Long-term treatment (>3 years) may lead to malabsorption of cyanocobalamin (vitamin B_{12}) caused by hypo or achlorhydria. Injection contains edetate sodium (EDTA); EDTA is a potent chelator of metal ions, particularly zinc; use with caution in patients prone to zinc deficiency or receiving other EDTA-containing products. Zinc supplementation may be necessary.

Adverse Reactions
Cardiovascular: Facial edema, generalized edema
Central nervous system: Depression, dizziness, fever, headache, vertigo
Dermatologic: Photosensitivity, pruritus, rash, urticaria
Endocrine & metabolic: Triglycerides increased
Gastrointestinal: Abdominal pain, constipation, diarrhea, flatulence, nausea, vomiting, xerostomia
Genitourinary: Urinary frequency, UTI
Hematologic: Leukopenia, thrombocytopenia
Hepatic: Hepatitis, liver function tests abnormal
Local: Injection site reaction (thrombophlebitis)
Neuromuscular & skeletal: Arthralgia, CPK increased, myalgia
Ocular: Blurred vision
Respiratory: Upper respiratory tract infection
Miscellaneous: Allergic reaction

Rare but important or life-threatening: Ageusia, agranulocytosis, albuminuria, alkaline phosphatase increased, anaphylaxis (including anaphylactic shock), anemia, angioedema, angina pectoris, aphthous stomatitis, arrhythmia, asthma exacerbation, atrial fibrillation/flutter, atrophic gastritis, biliary pain, bone pain, breast pain, bursitis, cataract, CHF, cholecystitis, cholelithiasis, *Clostridium difficile*-associate diarrhea (CDAD), colitis, contact dermatitis, creatinine increased, cystitis, deafness, dehydration, diabetes mellitus, diplopia, duodenitis, dysmenorrhea, dysphagia, dysuria, ecchymosis, ECG abnormality, eosinophilia, epididymitis, epistaxis, erythema multiforme, extraocular palsy, fracture, fungal dermatitis, gastrointestinal carcinoma, gastrointestinal hemorrhage, gastrointestinal moniliasis, GGT increased, gingivitis, glaucoma, glossitis, glycosuria, goiter, gout, hallucinations, hematemesis, hematuria, hemorrhage, hepatic failure, hernia, hyperbilirubinemia, hyperesthesia, hyper-/hypotension, hyperkinesia, hyperuricemia, hypokinesia, hypomagnesemia, hyponatremia, impotence, interstitial nephritis, jaundice, kidney calculus, kidney pain, leukocytosis, lichenoid dermatitis, maculopapular rash, melena, mouth ulceration, myocardial infarction, myocardial ischemia, neoplasm, neuralgia, neuritis, optic neuropathy (including anterior ischemic), palpitation, pancreatitis, pancytopenia, paresthesia, periodontitis, pneumonia, pyelonephritis, rectal hemorrhage, retinal vascular disorder, rhabdomyolysis, scrotal edema, seizure, Stevens-Johnson syndrome, stomach ulcer, stomatitis, syncope, tachycardia, tenosynovitis, thrombosis, tinnitus, tongue discoloration, toxic epidermal necrolysis, urethritis, vision abnormal

Drug Interactions
Metabolism/Transport Effects Substrate of CYP2C19 (major), CYP2D6 (minor), CYP3A4 (minor); **Note:** Assignment of Major/Minor substrate status based on clinically relevant drug interaction potential; **Inhibits** BCRP, CYP2C19 (weak); **Induces** CYP1A2 (weak/moderate)

Avoid Concomitant Use
Avoid concomitant use of Pantoprazole with any of the following: Dasatinib; Delavirdine; Erlotinib; Nelfinavir; PAZOPanib; PONATinib; Rilpivirine; Risedronate

Increased Effect/Toxicity
Pantoprazole may increase the levels/effects of: Amphetamine; Dexmethylphenidate; Dextroamphetamine; Methotrexate; Methylphenidate; PAZOPanib; Raltegravir; Risedronate; Saquinavir; Topotecan; Voriconazole

The levels/effects of Pantoprazole may be increased by: Fluconazole; Ketoconazole (Systemic); Voriconazole

Decreased Effect
Pantoprazole may decrease the levels/effects of: Atazanavir; Bisphosphonate Derivatives; Bosutinib; Cefditoren; Clopidogrel; Dabigatran Etexilate; Dabrafenib; Dasatinib; Delavirdine; Erlotinib; Gefitinib; Indinavir; Iron Salts; Itraconazole; Ketoconazole (Systemic); Mesalamine; Multivitamins/Minerals (with ADEK, Folate, Iron); Mycophenolate; Nelfinavir; Nilotinib; PAZOPanib; PONATinib; Posaconazole; Rilpivirine; Riociguat; Risedronate; Vismodegib

The levels/effects of Pantoprazole may be decreased by: CYP2C19 Inducers (Strong); Dabrafenib; Peginterferon Alfa-2b; Tipranavir

Food Interactions Prolonged treatment (≥2 years) may lead to malabsorption of dietary vitamin B_{12} and subsequent vitamin B_{12} deficiency (Lam, 2013).

Stability Stability of oral pantoprazole is a function of pH; it is rapidly degraded in acidic media but has acceptable stability under alkaline conditions. Each tablet of pantoprazole is enteric coated to prevent degradation by gastric acidity.

Oral: Store tablet and oral suspension at 20°C to 25°C (68°F to 77°F); excursions permitted to 15°C to 30°C (59°F to 86°F).

I.V.: Prior to reconstitution, store intact vial at 20°C to 25°C (68°F to 77°F); excursions permitted to 15°C to 30°C (59°F to 86°F). Do not freeze. Protect from light prior to reconstitution; upon reconstitution, protection from light is not required. Per manufacturer's labeling, reconstituted solution is stable at room temperature for 6 hours; once further diluted, the admixed solution should be stored at room temperature and used within 24 hours from the time of initial reconstitution. Studies have shown that the reconstituted solution (4 mg/mL) in polypropylene syringes is stable up to 96 hours at room temperature (Johnson, 2005); once further diluted, the admixed solution should be used within 96 hours from the time of initial reconstitution. The preparation should be stored at 3°C to 5°C (37°F to 41°F) if it is stored beyond 48 hours to minimize discoloration.

Mechanism of Action Suppresses gastric acid secretion by inhibiting the parietal cell H^+/K^+ ATP pump

Pharmacodynamics Acid secretion:
Onset of action:
Oral: 2.5 hours
I.V.: 15-30 minutes
Maximum effect: I.V.: 2 hours
Duration: Oral, I.V.: 24 hours

Pharmacokinetics (Adult data unless noted)
Absorption: Rapid, well-absorbed
Distribution: V_d:
Children and Adolescents (Kearns, 2008):
I.V.: 2-16 years: 0.22 ± 0.14 L/kg
Oral: 5-16 years: 0.24 ± 0.09 L/kg
Adults: 11-23.6 L
Protein binding: 98%
Metabolism: Extensively hepatic; CYP2C19 (demethylation), CYP3A4; no evidence that metabolites have pharmacologic activity
Bioavailability: ~77%
Half-life:
Neonates (PMA: 37-44 weeks): ~3 hours (Ward, 2010)
Children and Adolescents (Kearns, 2008):
I.V.: 2-16 years: 1.22 ± 0.68 hours
Oral: 5-16 years: 1.27 ± 1.29 hours
Adults: 1 hour; prolonged half-life (3.5-10 hours) in slow metabolizers (CYP2C19 deficiency)
Time to peak serum concentration:
Children and Adolescents (Kearns, 2008):
I.V.: 2-16 years: 0.34 ± 0.12 hours
Oral: 5-16 years: 2.54 ± 0.72 hours
Adults: Oral: 2.5 hours
Elimination: Urine (71% as metabolites); feces (18%); pantoprazole clearance increased with weight and age (Peterson, 2009)

Dosing: Neonatal GERD, symptomatic: Limited data available: Preterm (PMA <44 weeks and weighing ≥1.5 kg) and Term Neonates: Oral: 2.5 mg (~1.2 mg/kg/dose) once daily administered 30 minutes prior to first feeding of the day was evaluated in a pharmacokinetic trial in 21 neonatal patients (preterm: 19; term: 2; mean GA: 28 weeks; range: 23-41 weeks); this dose produced slightly higher systemic exposure than adolescents and adults receiving 40 mg, but there was no evidence of accumulation with repeated administration noted; although there was a significant increase in gastric pH and the amount of time the pH >4, there was no significant difference in reflux episodes. A lower dose of 1.25 mg (0.6 mg/kg/dose) was also evaluated (n=19); however, this dose did not provide statistically significant improvements in pH-metry parameters (Kierkus, 2011; Ward, 2010); further studies are needed.

Dosing: Usual Parenteral therapy should be discontinued as soon as the patient tolerates oral therapy.

Infants, Children, and Adolescents:
GERD, symptomatic: Limited data available:
Infants and Children <5 years: Oral: 1.2 mg/kg/day once daily for 4 weeks was shown to reduce GERD symptoms but was not significantly different from placebo (n=128; age range: 1-11 months) (Winter, 2010); a pharmacokinetic trial showed this dose produced similar serum concentrations as adults receiving 40 mg in infants 1-11 months (mean age: 6.3 months) and slightly lower concentrations in children 1 to <6 years (mean age: 3.2 years) (Tammara, 2011)
Children 5-11 years: Oral: 20 or 40 mg once daily have been shown to reduce severity and frequency of symptoms within 1 week based on the GERD Assessment of Symptoms in Pediatric Patients Questionnaire (n=53, age range: 5-11 years); results also showed that while a lower dose of 10 mg improved symptoms, it took longer (3 weeks) for results (Tolia, 2006); a pharmacokinetic trial in patients 6-11 years old (n=24) showed that 40 mg once daily produced similar systemic exposure as adults receiving 40 mg; however, the authors suggested that 20 mg once daily may be appropriate for small children (Ward, 2011)
Children and Adolescents 12-16 years: Oral: 20 or 40 mg once daily was shown to reduce symptoms in patients with confirmed or clinically suspected diagnosis of GERD (n=136) based on the GERD Assessment of Symptoms in Pediatric Patients Questionnaire (Tsou, 2011); a pharmacokinetic trial showed that a 40 mg dose produced similar systemic exposure as adults receiving 40 mg; however, suggested that 20 mg once daily may be appropriate for smaller adolescents (<40 kg) (Ward, 2011)

Erosive esophagitis associated with GERD:
Children 1-5 years: Limited data available: Oral: 0.3, 0.6, or 1.2 mg/kg/day once daily for 8 weeks was used in a dose-finding study of 60 patients with histologic or erosive esophagitis. High-dose treatment (1.2 mg/kg/day) was administered as a fixed dose of either: 15 mg for 1-year-olds **or** 20 mg for 2- to 5-year-olds. Patients with erosive esophagitis (n=4) received either 0.6 or 1.2 mg/kg/day. All patients had symptomatic improvement and patients with erosive esophagitis were healed by week 8; no dose response relationship was demonstrated (Baker, 2010)
Children ≥5 years and Adolescents: Oral:
≥15 to <40 kg: 20 mg once daily for up to 8 weeks
≥40 kg: 40 mg once daily for up to 8 weeks

Gastric acid suppression; oral therapy not appropriate or tolerated: Limited data available; dosing regimens variable: I.V.: Dosing based on pharmacokinetic data from 39 pediatric patients (age range: 10 days to 16 years) which has shown doses within this range produce similar AUC as adult patients with comparable dosing; efficacy was not evaluated in either trial (Kearns, 2008; Petersen, 2009). Further studies are needed.

Weight-based dosing: Children ≥2 years and Adolescents: I.V.: 0.8 or 1.6 mg/kg once daily; maximum single dose: 80 mg; dosing from a single dose pharmacokinetic study in 18 patients (age range: 2-14 years) (Kearns, 2008). In the BSA-based dosing trial (Petersen, 2009), the final median dose when standardized to weight was 1.1 mg/kg/day (range: 0.5-4.6 mg/kg/day). (**Note:** The 4.6 mg/kg/day dose was a prescription error; however, the patient experienced no adverse consequences due to high dose) Additionally, some clinicians have used 1-2 mg/kg/day in single or divided doses.

Body surface area (BSA)-based dosing: Infants, Children, and Adolescents: I.V.: 40 mg/1.73 m²/day; if inadequate response (eg, continued symptoms or target gastric pH not achieved) may titrate up to a maximum dose of 80 mg/1.73 m²/day; dosing based on multidose pharmacokinetic analysis; in the final analysis, the median reported dose was 41.8 mg/1.73 m²/day (range: 19.9-140.6 mg/1.73 m²/day) (**Note:** The 140.6 mg/1.73 m²/day dose was a prescription error; however, the patient experienced no adverse consequences due to high dose) (Petersen, 2009).

Note: In a very small trial (n=8), a median dose of 1.1 mg/kg (0.9-2.5 mg/kg) produced similar AUC values as adults, but only produced a definable response (gastric pH >4) in one patient; in the remaining seven patients the mean percentage of time with intragastric pH ≥4 was 7.4% (Petersen, 2005). Further studies are needed to define the optimal AUC and dose (Petersen, 2009).

Adults:

Erosive esophagitis associated with GERD:
Oral:
  Treatment: 40 mg once daily for up to 8 weeks; an additional 8 weeks may be used in patients who have not healed after an 8-week course
  Maintenance of healing: 40 mg once daily
  I.V.: 40 mg once daily for 7-10 days

Hypersecretory conditions (including Zollinger-Ellison syndrome):
Oral: Initial: 40 mg twice daily; adjust dose based on patient response; doses up to 240 mg daily have been administered
I.V.: Initial: 80 mg every 12 hours; adjust dosage to maintain acid output; 160-240 mg daily in divided doses has been used for a limited period (up to 7 days)

Dosing adjustment in renal impairment: Adults: No dosage adjustment needed
Hemodialysis: Not appreciably removed by hemodialysis

Dosing adjustment in hepatic impairment: Adults: No dosage adjustment for doses up to 40 mg/day. Doses higher than 40 mg/day have not been studied in patients with hepatic impairment.

Administration
I.V.: Reconstitute powder for injection with 10 mL NS; further dilute in NS, D₅W, or LR to a final concentration of 0.4-0.8 mg/mL; infuse over 15 minutes at a rate not to exceed 7 mL/minute; for more rapid infusion, administer reconstituted solution (4 mg/mL) over 2 minutes; not for I.M. or SubQ use. Flush I.V. line with NS, D₅W, or LR before and after administration.

Oral:
  Tablet: Should be swallowed whole; do not chew or crush. May be taken without regard to meals; however, best if taken 30 minutes before a meal (Lightdale, 2013); may be administered with antacids.
  Delayed release oral suspension: Should only be administered in apple juice or applesauce and administered 30 minutes before a meal. Do not administer in water, other liquids, or foods. Per manufacturer's labeling, do not divide the 40 mg delayed release oral suspension packet to create a 20 mg dosage for pediatric patients who are unable to take the tablet formulation.
  Oral administration in apple juice: Empty intact granules into 5 mL of apple juice, stir for 5 seconds, and swallow immediately. Rinse container once or twice with apple juice and swallow immediately.
  Oral administration in applesauce: Sprinkle intact granules on 1 teaspoonful of applesauce; swallow within 10 minutes of preparation.
  Nasogastric tube administration: Separate the plunger from the barrel of a 60 mL catheter tip syringe and connect to a ≥16 French nasogastric tube. Holding the syringe attached to the tubing as high as possible, empty granules into barrel of syringe, add 10 mL of

apple juice, and gently tap/shake the barrel of the syringe to help empty the syringe. Add an additional 10 mL of apple juice and gently tap/shake the barrel to help rinse. Repeat rinse with at least 2-10 mL aliquots of apple juice. No granules should remain in the syringe.
  Oral administration in syringe: In neonatal trials, fixed dosage packets of 2.5 mg pantoprazole were mixed with grape flavoring and 2.5 mL of water and administered immediately (Ward, 2010).

Test Interactions False-positive urine screening tests for tetrahydrocannabinol (THC) have been noted in patients receiving proton pump inhibitors, including pantoprazole.

Dosage Forms Excipient information presented when available (limited, particularly for generics); consult specific product labeling.
Packet, Oral:
  Protonix: 40 mg (1 ea, 30 ea) [contains polysorbate 80]
Solution Reconstituted, Intravenous:
  Protonix: 40 mg (1 ea) [contains edetate disodium]
  Generic: 40 mg (1 ea)
Tablet Delayed Release, Oral:
  Protonix: 20 mg, 40 mg
  Generic: 20 mg, 40 mg

Extemporaneous Preparations A 2 mg/mL pantoprazole oral suspension may be made with pantoprazole tablets, sterile water, and sodium bicarbonate powder. Remove the Protonix® imprint from twenty 40 mg tablets with a paper towel dampened with ethanol (improves the look of product). Let tablets air dry. Crush the tablets in a mortar and reduce to a fine powder. Transfer to a 600 mL beaker, and add 340 mL sterile water. Place beaker on a magnetic stirrer. Add 16.8 g of sodium bicarbonate powder and stir for about 20 minutes until the tablet remnants have disintegrated. While stirring, add another 16.8 g of sodium bicarbonate powder and stir for about 5 minutes until powder has dissolved. Add enough sterile water for irrigation to bring the final volume to 400 mL. Mix well. Transfer to amber-colored bottle. Label "shake well" and "refrigerate". Stable for 62 days refrigerated.

Dentinger PJ, Swenson CF, and Anaizi NH, "Stability of Pantoprazole in an Extemporaneously Compounded Oral Liquid," *Am J Health Syst Pharm*, 2002, 59(10):953-6.

References
Abraham NS, Hlatky MA, Antman EM, et al, "CCF/ACG/AHA 2010 Expert Consensus Document on the Concomitant Use of Proton Pump Inhibitors and Thienopyridines: A Focused Update of the ACCF/AHA 2008 Expert Consensus Document on Reducing the Gastrointestinal Risks of Antiplatelet Therapy and NSAID Use: A Report of the American College of Cardiology Foundation Task Force on Expert Consensus Documents," *Circulation*, 2010, 122 (24):2619-33.

Angiolillo DJ, Gibson CM, Cheng S, et al, "Differential Effects of Omeprazole and Pantoprazole on the Pharmacodynamics and Pharmacokinetics of Clopidogrel in Healthy Subjects: Randomized, Placebo-Controlled, Crossover Comparison Studies," *Clin Pharmacol Ther*, 2011, 89(1):65-74.

Baker R, Tsou VM, Tung J, et al, "Clinical Results From a Randomized, Double-Blind, Dose-Ranging Study of Pantoprazole in Children Aged 1 Through 5 Years With Symptomatic Histologic or Erosive Esophagitis," *Clin Pediatr (Phila)*, 2010, 49(9):852-65.

Canani RB, Cirillo P, Roggero P, et al, "Therapy With Gastric Acidity Inhibitors Increases the Risk of Acute Gastroenteritis and Community-Acquired Pneumonia in Children," *Pediatrics*, 2006, 117(5):e817-20.

Diav-Citrin O, Arnon J, Shechtman S, et al, "The Safety of Proton Pump Inhibitors in Pregnancy: A Multicentre Prospective Controlled Study," *Aliment Pharmacol Ther*, 2005, 21(3):269-75.

Erichsen R, Mikkelsen E, Pedersen L, et al, "Maternal Use of Proton Pump Inhibitors During Early Pregnancy and the Prevalence of Hypospadias in Male Offspring," *Am J Ther*, 2012.

Johnson CE, "Stability of Pantoprazole in 0.9% Sodium Chloride Injection in Polypropylene Syringes," *Am J Health Syst Pharm*, 2005, 62(22):2410-2.

Katz PO, Gerson LB, and Vela MF, "Guidelines for the Diagnosis and Management of Gastroesophageal Reflux Disease," *Am J Gastroenterol*, 2013, 108(3):308-28.

Kearns GL, Blumer J, Schexnayder S, et al, "Single-Dose Pharmacokinetics of Oral and Intravenous Pantoprazole in Children and Adolescents," *J Clin Pharmacol*, 2008, 48(11):1356-65.

Kierkus J, Furmaga-Jablonska W, Sullivan JE, et al. Pharmacodynamics and safety of pantoprazole in neonates, preterm infants, and infants aged 1 through 11 months with a clinical diagnosis of gastroesophageal reflux disease. *Dig Dis Sci.* 2011;56:425-434.

Levine GN, Bates ER, Blankenship JC, et al, "2011 ACCF/AHA/SCAI Guideline for Percutaneous Coronary Intervention: A Report of the American College of Cardiology Foundation/American Heart Association Task Force on Practice Guidelines and the Society for Cardiovascular Angiography and Interventions," *Circulation,* 2011, 124(23): e574-651.

Lightdale JR, Gremse DA, and the Section on Gastroenterology, Hepatology, and Nutrition," Gastroesophageal Reflux: Management Guidance for the Pediatrician," *Pediatrics,* 2013, 131(5):e1684-95.

Li XQ, Andersson TB, Ahlström M, et al, "Comparison of Inhibitory Effects of the Proton Pump-Inhibiting Drugs Omeprazole, Esomeprazole, Lansoprazole, Pantoprazole, and Rabeprazole on Human Cytochrome P450 Activities," *Drug Metab Dispos,* 2004, 32(8):821-7.

Madrazo-De La Garza A, Dibildox M, Vargas A, et al, "Efficacy and Safety of Oral Pantoprazole 20 mg Given Once Daily for Reflux Esophagitis in Children," *J Pediatr Gastroenterol Nutr,* 2003, 36 (2):261-5.

Matok I, Levy A, Wiznitzer A, et al, "The Safety of Fetal Exposure to Proton-Pump Inhibitors During Pregnancy," *Dig Dis Sci,* 2012, 57 (3):699-705.

Pasternak B and Hviid A, "Use of Proton-Pump Inhibitors in Early Pregnancy and the Risk of Birth Defects," *N Engl J Med,* 2010, 363 (22):2114-23.

Petterson G, Faure C, Litalien C, et al. Therapeutic failure of a single intravenous dose of pantoprazole in young intensive care children. *Crit Care Med.* 2005;33(12): A170.

Pettersen G, Mouksassi MS, Theoret Y, et al. Population pharmacokinetics of intravenous pantoprazole in paediatric intensive care patients. *Br J Clin Pharmacol.* 2009;67(2):216-227.

Plante L, Ferron GM, Unruh M, et al, "Excretion of Pantoprazole in Human Breast," *J Reprod Med,* 2004, 49(10):825-7.

Tammara BK, Sullivan JE, Adcock KG, et al, "Randomized, Open-Label, Multicentre Pharmacokinetic Studies of Two Dose Levels of Pantoprazole Granules in Infants and Children Aged 1 Month Through <6 Years With Gastro-oesophageal Reflux Disease," *Clin Pharmacokinet,* 2011, 50(8):541-50.

Tolia V, Bishop PR, Tsou VM, et al. Multicenter, randomized, double-blind study comparing 10, 20 and 40 mg pantoprazole in children (5-11 years) with sympomatic gastroesophageal reflux disease. *JPGN.* 2006;42:384-391.

Tsou VM, Baker R, Book L, et al. Multicenter, randomized, double-blind study comparing 20 and 40 mg of pantoprazole for symptom relief in adolescents (12 to 16 years of age) with gastroesophageal reflux disease (GERD). *Clin Pediatr.* 2006;45:741-749.

Ward RM, Kearns GL, Tammara B, et al. A multicenter, randomized, open-label, pharmacokinetics and safety study of pantoprazole tablets in children and adolescents aged 6 through 16 years with GERD. *J Clin Pharmacol.* 2011;51(6):876-887.

Ward RM, Tammara B, Sullivan SE, et al. Single-dose, multiple-dose, and population pharmacokinetics of pantoprazole in neonates and preterm infants with a clinical diagnosis of gastroesophageal reflux disease (GERD). *Eur J Clin Pharmacol.* 2010;66:555-561.

Winter H, Kum-Nji P, Mahomedy SH, et al, "Efficacy and Safety of Pantoprazole Delayed-Release Granules for Oral Suspension in a Placebo-Controlled Treatment-Withdrawal Study in Infants 1-11 Months Old With Symptomatic GERD," *J Pediatr Gastroenterol Nutr,* 2010, 50(6):609-18.

◆ **Pantoprazole for Injection (Can)** *see* Pantoprazole *on page 1595*

◆ **Pantoprazole Magnesium** *see* Pantoprazole *on page 1595*

◆ **Pantoprazole Sodium** *see* Pantoprazole *on page 1595*

◆ **Pantoprazole Sodium for Injection (Can)** *see* Pantoprazole *on page 1595*

Papaverine (pa PAV er een)

Medication Safety Issues
Sound-alike/look-alike issues:
Papaverine may be confused with pamidronate
Therapeutic Category Antimigraine Agent; Vasodilator
Generic Availability (U.S.) Yes
Use Relief of peripheral and cerebral ischemia associated with arterial spasm; investigationally for prophylaxis of migraine headache; intracavernosal injection for impotence

Pregnancy Risk Factor C
Pregnancy Considerations Teratogenic effects have not been observed in animal reproduction studies.
Breast-Feeding Considerations It is not known if papaverine is excreted in breast milk. The manufacturer recommends that caution be exercised when administering papaverine to nursing women.
Contraindications Hypersensitivity to papaverine or any component; complete atrioventricular block; Parkinson's disease
Precautions Use with caution in patients with glaucoma; administer I.V. slowly and with caution since arrhythmias and apnea may occur with rapid I.V. use; should **not** be used in neonates due to the increased risk of drug-induced cerebral vasodilation and possibility of an intracranial bleed
Adverse Reactions
Cardiovascular: Arrhythmias (with rapid I.V. use), flushing, mild hypertension, tachycardia
Central nervous system: Headache, malaise, sedation, vertigo
Dermatologic: Rash
Gastrointestinal: Abdominal distress, anorexia, constipation, diarrhea, nausea
Hepatic: Cirrhosis, hepatic hypersensitivity, hepatitis (rare)
Respiratory: Apnea (with rapid I.V. use)
Miscellaneous: Diaphoresis
Drug Interactions
Metabolism/Transport Effects None known.
Avoid Concomitant Use There are no known interactions where it is recommended to avoid concomitant use.
Increased Effect/Toxicity
Papaverine may increase the levels/effects of: DULoxetine; Hypotensive Agents

The levels/effects of Papaverine may be increased by: Barbiturates
Decreased Effect There are no known significant interactions involving a decrease in effect.
Stability Protect from heat or freezing; do not refrigerate injection; solutions should be clear to pale yellow; precipitates with LR
Mechanism of Action Smooth muscle spasmolytic producing a generalized smooth muscle relaxation including: vasodilatation, gastrointestinal sphincter relaxation, bronchiolar muscle relaxation, and potentially a depressed myocardium (with large doses); muscle relaxation may occur due to inhibition or cyclic nucleotide phosphodiesterase, increasing cyclic AMP; muscle relaxation is unrelated to nerve innervation; papaverine increases cerebral blood flow in normal subjects; oxygen uptake is unaltered
Pharmacodynamics Onset of action: Oral: Rapid
Pharmacokinetics (Adult data unless noted)
Protein binding: 90%
Metabolism: Rapid in the liver
Bioavailability: Oral: ~54%
Half-life: 30-120 minutes
Elimination: Primarily as metabolites in urine
Dosing: Neonatal Peripheral arterial catheter patency: Full-term neonates: Add 30 mg preservative-free papaverine to an admixture of 250 mL NS or $^1/_2$NS with heparin 1 unit/mL; infuse via peripheral arterial catheter at ≤1 mL/hour (see Heparin). A double-blind, placebo-controlled trial of 141 neonates (median GA: 27 weeks; median birth weight: 910-952 g) demonstrated prolonged functionality of peripherally inserted arterial catheters (Griffin, 2005). **Note:** Due to the risk of IVH, the use of papaverine in preterm neonates <3 weeks is not recommended (Griffin, 2005); further studies are needed.
Dosing: Usual
Children:
Arterial spasm: I.M., I.V.: 1.5 mg/kg 4 times/day

◀

Peripheral arterial catheter patency: Add 30 mg papaverine to an admixture of 250 mL NS or ½NS with heparin 1 unit/mL (Heulitt, 1993); infuse via peripheral arterial catheter; some centers report infusions at ≤1 mL/hour

Migraine prophylaxis: Children and Adolescents 6-15 years: Oral: Initial: 5 mg/kg/day given once daily; range: 5-10 mg/kg/day divided into 2-3 doses/day

Adults:

Oral: 75-300 mg 3-5 times/day

Oral, sustained release: 150-300 mg every 12 hours

I.M., I.V.: 30-120 mg every 3 hours as needed

Administration

Oral: Administer after or with meals, milk or antacids to decrease nausea; swallow sustained release capsule whole, do not crush or chew

Parenteral: Rapid I.V. administration may result in arrhythmias and fatal apnea; administer slow I.V. over 1-2 minutes

Monitoring Parameters Liver enzymes; intraocular pressure in glaucoma patients

Additional Information Evidence of therapeutic value of systemic use for relief of peripheral and cerebral ischemia related to arterial spasm is lacking

Further studies are needed to determine the benefit of adding papaverine (60 mg/500 mL) to arterial catheter infusions containing NS or ½NS and heparin 1 unit/mL. One investigation showed a lower risk of arterial catheter failure and longer duration of arterial catheter function in patients 7 months to 5.5 years of age who received papaverine in their arterial catheter solutions; these results should be verified by additional studies before the addition of papaverine to arterial catheter solutions can be recommended.

Dosage Forms Excipient information presented when available (limited, particularly for generics); consult specific product labeling.

Solution, Injection, as hydrochloride:

Generic: 30 mg/mL (2 mL, 10 mL)

References

Griffin MP and Siadaty MS, "Papaverine Prolongs Patency of Peripheral Arterial Catheters in Neonates," *J Pediatr*, 2005, 146(1):62-5.

Heulitt MJ, Farrington EA, O'Shea TM, et al, "Double-Blind, Randomized, Controlled Trial of Papaverine-Containing Infusions to Prevent Failure of Arterial Catheters in Pediatric Patients," *Crit Care Med*, 1993, 21(6):825-9.

Sillanpää M and Koponen M, "Papaverine in the Prophylaxis of Migraine and Other Vascular Headache in Children," *Acta Paediatr Scand*, 1978, 67(2):209-12.

♦ **Papaverine Hydrochloride** *see* Papaverine *on page 1599*

Papillomavirus (Types 6, 11, 16, 18) Vaccine (Human, Recombinant)

(pap ih LO ma VYE rus typs six e LEV en SIX teen AYE teen vak SEEN YU man ree KOM be nant)

Medication Safety Issues

Sound-alike/look-alike issues:

Papillomavirus vaccine types 6, 11, 16, 18 (Gardasil) may be confused with Papillomavirus vaccine types 16, 18 (Cervarix)

Related Information

Immunization Administration Recommendations *on page 2368*

Immunization Guidelines *on page 2373*

Brand Names: U.S. Gardasil

Brand Names: Canada Gardasil

Therapeutic Category Vaccine

Generic Availability (U.S.) No

Use

Prevention of cervical, vulvar, vaginal, and anal cancer caused by HPV types 16 and 18; genital warts caused by HPV types 6 and 11; cervical adenocarcinoma *in situ*; and vulvar, vaginal, cervical, or anal intraepithelial neoplasia caused by HPV types 6, 11, 16, 18 (FDA approved in females ages 9 to 26 years)

Prevention of genital warts caused by HPV types 6 and 11; anal cancer caused by HPV types 16 and 18; and anal intraepithelial neoplasia caused by HPV types 6, 11, 16, and 18 (FDA approved in males ages 9 to 26 years)

The Advisory Committee on Immunization Practices (ACIP) recommends routine vaccination for females and males 11 to 12 years of age; catch-up vaccination is recommended for females 13 to 26 years of age and males 13 to 21 years of age. Males 22 to 26 years may also be vaccinated. The ACIP also recommends routine vaccination for men who have sex with men (MSM) through 26 years of age (CDC/ACIP [Markowitz, 2007]; CDC, 59[20], 2010; CDC, 60[50], 2011). Vaccination is also recommended for immunocompromised persons or MSM through 26 years of age who were not previously vaccinated when they were younger.

Pregnancy Risk Factor B

Pregnancy Considerations Teratogenic effects were not observed in animal reproduction studies. In clinical trials, women who were found to be pregnant before the completion of the 3-dose regimen were instructed to defer any remaining dose until pregnancy resolution. Pregnancies detected within 30 days of vaccination had a higher rate of congenital anomalies (pyloric stenosis, congenital megacolon, congenital hydronephrosis, hip dysplasia, club foot) than the placebo group. Pregnancies with onset beyond 30 days of vaccination had a rate of congenital anomalies consistent with the general population. Overall, the types of teratogenic events were the same as those generally observed for this age group. Administration of the vaccine in pregnancy is not recommended; until additional information is available, the vaccine series (or completion of the series) should be delayed until pregnancy is completed (CDC, 2007). Pregnancy testing is not required prior to administration of the vaccine (CDC, 2013a).

A registry has been established for women exposed to the HPV vaccine during pregnancy (1-877-888-4231).

Breast-Feeding Considerations It is not known if this vaccine is excreted into breast milk. Infants had a higher incidence of acute respiratory illness when breast-fed by mothers within 30 days postvaccination. The manufacturer recommends that caution be exercised when administering papilloma virus vaccine to nursing women. Lactating women may receive vaccine (CDC, 2007; CDC, 59[20], 2010).

Contraindications Hypersensitivity to human papillomavirus vaccine, yeast, or any component

Warnings Immediate treatment (including epinephrine 1:1000) for anaphylactic and/or hypersensitivity reactions should be available during vaccine use. There is no evidence that individuals already infected with HPV will be protected; those already infected with one or more HPV types were protected from disease in the remaining HPV types. Not for the treatment of active disease; will not protect against diseases not caused by HPV types 6, 11, 16, and 18. Syncope has been reported with use of injectable vaccines and may be accompanied by transient visual disturbances, weakness, or tonic-clonic movements. Procedures should be in place to avoid injuries from falling and to restore cerebral perfusion if syncope occurs (CDC, 57[17], 2008).

Injection contains polysorbate 80 (Tween 80) which may cause allergic reactions in susceptible individuals.

Precautions The decision to administer or delay vaccination because of current or recent febrile illness depends on the severity of symptoms and the etiology of the disease. Immunization should be delayed during the course of an acute severe febrile illness; may administer to patients with mild acute illness (with or without fever). Use with caution in severely immunocompromised patients (eg, patients receiving chemo/radiation therapy or other immunosuppressive therapy, including high-dose corticosteroids); may have a reduced response to vaccination; inactivated vaccines should be administered ≥2 weeks prior to planned immunosuppression when feasible (IDSA [Rubin, 2013]). In general, household and close contacts of persons with altered immunocompetence may receive all age-appropriate vaccines. Vaccination may not result in effective immunity in all patients. Response depends upon multiple factors (eg, type of vaccine, age of patient) and may be improved by administering the vaccine at the recommended dose, route, and interval (CDC/ACIP [Kroger, 2011]).

Use caution in patients with coagulation, including thrombocytopenia, due to an increased risk for bleeding following I.M. administration; if the patient receives antihemophilia or other similar therapy, I.M. injection can be scheduled shortly after such therapy is administered. Antipyretics have not been shown to prevent febrile seizures; antipyretics may be used to treat fever or discomfort following vaccination (CDC/ACIP [Kroger, 2011]). One study reported that routine prophylactic administration of acetaminophen to prevent fever prior to vaccination decreased the immune response of some vaccines; the clinical significance of this reduction in immune response has not been established (Prymula, 2009).

Use of this vaccine for specific medical and/or other indications (eg, immunocompromising conditions, hepatic or kidney disease, diabetes) is also addressed in the ACIP Recommended Immunization Schedule (CDC/ACIP [Akinsanya-Beysolow, 2014]; CDC/ACIP [Bridges, 2014]).

Adverse Reactions All serious adverse reactions must be reported to the U.S. Department of Health and Human Services (DHHS) Vaccine Adverse Event Reporting System (VAERS) 1-800-822-7967 or online at https://vaers.hhs.gov/esub/index. In Canada, adverse reactions may be reported to local provincial/territorial health agencies or to the Vaccine Safety Section at Public Health Agency of Canada (1-866-844-0018).

Central nervous system: Dizziness, fever, headache, insomnia, malaise
Local: Injection site: Bruising, erythema, hematoma, pain, pruritus, swelling
Gastrointestinal: Diarrhea, nausea, toothache, vomiting
Neuromuscular & skeletal: Arthralgia, myalgia
Respiratory: Cough, nasal congestion, pharyngolaryngeal pain
Rare but important or life-threatening: Acute disseminated encephalomyelitis, alopecia areata, anaphylactic/anaphylactoid reaction, appendicitis, arrhythmia, arthritis, asthma, autoimmune hemolytic anemia and other autoimmune diseases, bronchospasm, cellulitis, cerebrovascular accident, chills, DVT, fatigue, gastroenteritis, Guillain-Barré syndrome, hypersensitivity reaction, hyper-/hypothyroidism, injection site joint movement impairment, ITP, JIA, lymphadenopathy, motor neuron disease, pancreatitis, paralysis, pelvic inflammatory disease, pulmonary embolus, RA, renal failure (acute), seizure, sepsis, syncope (may result in falls with injury or be associated with tonic-clonic movements), transverse myelitis, urticaria, weakness

Drug Interactions
Metabolism/Transport Effects None known.
Avoid Concomitant Use There are no known interactions where it is recommended to avoid concomitant use.
Increased Effect/Toxicity There are no known significant interactions involving an increase in effect.

Decreased Effect
The levels/effects of Papillomavirus (Types 6, 11, 16, 18) Vaccine (Human, Recombinant) may be decreased by: Belimumab; Fingolimod; Immunosuppressants

Stability Store at 2°C to 8°C (36°F to 46°F); do not freeze. Protect from light. May be stored at temperatures ≤25°C (≤77°F) for a total time of ≤72 hours.

Mechanism of Action Contains inactive human papillomavirus (HPV) proteins HPV 6 L1, HPV 11 L1, HPV 16 L1, and HPV 18 L1 which produce neutralizing antibodies to prevent cervical cancer, cervical adenocarcinoma, cervical, vaginal and vulvar neoplasia, and genital warts caused by HPV. The vaccine has not been shown to provide cross-protective efficacy to HPV types not contained in the vaccine. Immunogenicity has been measured by the percentage of persons who became seropositive for antibodies contained in the vaccine; the minimum anti-HPV antibody concentration needed to protect against disease has not been determined. The population benefit to vaccination is influenced by the prevalence of HPV within the geographic area and subject characteristics (eg, lifetime sexual partners).

Pharmacodynamics
Onset of action: Peak seroconversion was observed 1 month following the last dose of vaccine
Duration: Not well defined; at least 5 years

Dosing: Usual
Pediatric:
Primary immunization:
CDC (ACIP) recommended immunization schedule: Children ≥9 years and Adolescents: I.M.: 0.5 mL per dose for a total of 3 doses administered as follows: Initial dose followed by a second dose at 1 to 2 months after initial and third doses at 6 months after the initial. Administer first dose at age 11 to 12 years although series may be initiated as early as 9 years of age. Minimum interval between first and second doses is 4 weeks; the minimum interval between the second and third dose is 12 weeks (16 weeks preferred); the minimum interval between first and third doses is 24 weeks. If the dose is given in an interval shorter than recommended, the dose should be repeated. The HPV vaccine series should be completed with the same product whenever possible (CDC/ACIP [Markowitz, 2007]; CDC/ACIP, 60[50], 2011).
Manufacturer's labeling: Children ≥9 years and Adolescents: I.M.: 0.5 mL per dose for a total of 3 doses; administer the second and third doses at 2 and 6 months after initial dose; immunization with HPV vaccine is usually initiated at 11 to 12 years; optimally, vaccination should be completed prior to onset of sexual activity
Catch-up immunization: CDC (ACIP) recommendations (Akinsanya-Beysolow, 2014): **Note:** Do not restart the series. If doses have been given, begin the below schedule at the applicable dose number. I.M.: 0.5 mL per dose for a total of 3 doses in females ages 13 to 26 years or males 13 through 18 years who were not previously vaccinated, administered as follows:
First dose given on the elected date
Second dose given at least 4 weeks after the first dose
Third dose given at 16 weeks after the second dose (minimum interval: 12 weeks) and at least 24 weeks after the first dose
Adult: **Immunization:**
CDC (ACIP) recommended immunization schedule: I.M.: 0.5 mL per dose for a total of 3 doses administered as follows: Initial dose followed by a second and third dose at 1 to 2 months and 6 months after the first dose. Administer first dose at age 11 to 12 years; begin series in females aged 13 to 26 years or males 13 to 21 years if not previously vaccinated. Males may also be vaccinated through 26 years of age. Minimum interval

between first and second doses is 4 weeks; the minimum interval between the second and third dose is 12 weeks (16 weeks preferred); the minimum interval between first and third doses is 24 weeks. Inadequate doses or doses received following a shorter than recommended dosing interval should be repeated. The HPV vaccine series should be completed with the same product whenever possible (CDC/ACIP [Markowitz, 2007]; CDC, 59[20], 2010; CDC, 60[50] 2011).

Manufacturer's labeling: Adults ≤26 years: I.M.: 0.5 mL per dose for a total of 3 doses; administer the second and third doses at 2 and 6 months after initial dose

Dosage adjustment in renal impairment: There are no dosage adjustments provided in the manufacturer's labeling.

Dosage adjustment in hepatic impairment: There are no dosage adjustments provided in the manufacturer's labeling.

Administration I.M.: Shake suspension well prior to use; do not use suspension if it is discolored or contains particulate matter; do not dilute or mix with other vaccines. Administer I.M. into the deltoid region of the upper arm or in the higher anterolateral area of the thigh; **not for I.V., intradermal, or SubQ administration.** Adolescents and adults should be vaccinated while seated or lying down. U.S. law requires that the date of administration, the vaccine manufacturer, lot number of vaccine, and the administering person's name, title and address be entered into the patient's permanent medical record. Patients who develop syncope associated with tonic-clonic movements usually respond when maintained in a supine or Trendelenburg position.

Monitoring Parameters Observe for syncope for 15 minutes following administration. If seizure-like activity associated with syncope occurs, maintain patient in supine or Trendelenburg position to reestablish adequate cerebral perfusion. Female patients should continue to be screened for cervical cancer per current guidelines after vaccination series is completed.

Additional Information Comparison of HPV vaccines: Cervarix and Gardasil are both vaccines formulated to protect against infection with the human papillomavirus. Both are inactive vaccines which contain proteins HPV16 L1 and HPV 18 L1, the cause of >70% of invasive cervical cancer. The vaccines differ in that Gardasil also contains HPV 6 L1 and HPV 11 L1 proteins which protect against 75% to 90% of genital warts. The vaccines also differ in their preparation and adjuvants used. The viral proteins in Cervarix are prepared using *Trichoplusia ni* (insect cells) which are adsorbed onto an aluminum salt which is also combined with a monophosphoryl lipid. The viral proteins in Gardasil are prepared using *S. cerevisiae* (baker's yeast) which are then adsorbed onto an aluminum salt. Results from a short-term study (measurements obtained 1 month following the third vaccination in the series) have shown that the immune response to HPV 16 and HPV 18 may be greater with Cervarix; although the clinical significance of this difference is not known, local adverse events may also occur more frequently with this preparation. Both vaccines were effective and results from long-term studies are pending (Einstein, 2009).

In order to maximize vaccination rates, the ACIP recommends simultaneous administration (ie, >1 vaccine on the same day at different anatomic sites) of all age-appropriate vaccines (live or inactivated) for which a person is eligible at a single visit, unless contraindications exist. If available, the use of combination vaccines is generally preferred over separate injections, taking into consideration provider assessment, patient preference, and potential adverse events. If separate vaccines being used, evaluate product information regarding same syringe compatibility of vaccines. Separate needles and syringes should be used for each injection. The ACIP prefers each dose of specific vaccine in a series come from the same manufacturer if possible (CDC/ACIP [Kroger, 2011]). HPV vaccine may be administered concomitantly with Recombivax HB or with Menactra and Adacel (Reisinger, 2010).

For additional information, please refer to the following website: http://www.cdc.gov/vaccines/vpd-vac/.

Dosage Forms Excipient information presented when available (limited, particularly for generics); consult specific product labeling.

Injection, suspension [preservative free]:

Gardasil: HPV 6 L1 protein 20 mcg, HPV 11 L1 protein 40 mcg, HPV 16 L1 protein 40 mcg, and HPV 18 L1 protein 20 mcg per 0.5 mL (0.5 mL) [contains aluminum, polysorbate 80; manufactured using *S. cerevisiae* (baker's yeast)]

References

AAP Steering Committee on Quality Improvement and Management, Subcommittee on Febrile Seizures American Academy of Pediatrics, "Febrile Seizures: Clinical Practice Guideline for the Long-Term Management of the Child With Simple Febrile Seizures," *Pediatrics*, 2008, 121(6):1281-6.

Akinsanya-Beysolow I, Advisory Committee on Immunization Practices (ACIP), ACIP Child/Adolescent Immunization Work Group, et al. Advisory committee on immunization practices recommended immunization schedules for persons aged 0 through 18 years - United States, 2014. *MMWR Morb Mortal Wkly Rep*. 2014; 63(5):108-109. Full schedule available at http://www.cdc.gov/vaccines/schedules/downloads/child/0-18yrs-child-combined-schedule.pdf

Block SL, Nolan T, Sattler C, et al, "Comparison of the Immunogenicity and Reactogenicity of a Prophylactic Quadrivalent Human Papillomavirus (Types 6, 11, 16, and 18) L1 Virus-Like Particle Vaccine in Male and Female Adolescents and Young Adult Women," *Pediatrics*, 2006, 118(5):2135-45.

Bridges CB, Coyne-Beasley T, Advisory Committee on Immunization Practices (ACIP), ACIP Adult Immunization Work Group; Centers for Disease Control and Prevention (CDC). Advisory committee on immunization practices recommended immunization schedule for adults aged 19 years or older - United States, 2014. *MMWR Morb Mortal Wkly Rep*. 2014; 63(5):108-109. Available at: http://www.cdc.gov/vaccines/schedules/downloads/adult/adult-combined-schedule.pdf

Centers for Disease Control and Prevention (CDC), "FDA Licensure of Quadrivalent Human Papillomavirus Vaccine (HPV, Gardasil) for Use in Males and Guidance from the Advisory Committee on Immunization Practices (ACIP), 2011," *MMWR Morb Mortal Wkly Rep*, 2010, 59 (20):630-2.

Centers for Disease Control and Prevention (CDC). Recommendations on the use of quadrivalent human papillomavirus vaccine in males - Advisory Committee on Immunization Practices (ACIP), 2011. *MMWR Morb Mortal Wkly Rep*. 2011;60(50):1705-1708.

Centers for Disease Control and Prevention (CDC), "Syncope After Vaccination-United States, January 2005-July 2007," *MMWR Morb Mortal Wkly Rep*, 2008, 2;57(17):457-60.

Einstein MH, Baron M, Levin MJ, et al. Comparison of the immunogenicity and safety of Cervarix and Gardasil human papillomavirus (HPV) cervical cancer vaccines in healthy women aged 18-45 years. *Hum Vaccin*. 2009;5(10):507-519.

Kroger AT, Atkinson WL, Marcuse EK, Pickering LK. General recommendations on immunization - recommendations of the Advisory Committee on Immunization Practices (ACIP). *MMWR Recomm Rep*. 2011;60(RR-2):1-64.

Markowitz LE, Dunne EF, Saraiya M, et al. Quadrivalent human papillomavirus vaccine. Recommendations of the Advisory Committee on Immunization Practices (ACIP). *MMWR Recomm Rep*. 2007;56(RR-2):1-24.

Prymula R, Siegrist CA, Chlibek R, et al, "Effect of Prophylactic Paracetamol Administration at Time of Vaccination on Febrile Reactions and Antibody Responses in Children: Two Open-Label, Randomised Controlled Trials," *Lancet*, 2009, 374(9698):1339-50.

Reisinger KS, Block SL, Collins-Ogle M, et al, "Safety, Tolerability, and Immunogenicity of Gardasil Given Concomitantly With Menactra and Adacel," *Pediatrics*, 2010, 125(6):1142-51.

Rubin LG, Levin MJ, Ljungman P, et al. 2013 IDSA clinical practice guideline for vaccination of the immunocompromised host. *Clin Infect Dis*. 2014;58(3):e44-e100.

Papillomavirus (Types 16, 18) Vaccine (Human, Recombinant)

(pap ih LO ma VYE rus typs SIX teen AYE teen vak SEEN YU man ree KOM be nant)

Medication Safety Issues

Sound-alike/look-alike issues:

Papillomavirus vaccine types 16, 18 (Cervarix®) may be confused with Papillomavirus vaccine types 6, 11, 16, 18 (Gardasil®)

Cervarix® may be confused with Cerebyx®, CeleBREX®

Related Information

Immunization Administration Recommendations *on page 2368*

Immunization Guidelines *on page 2373*

Brand Names: U.S. Cervarix®

Brand Names: Canada Cervarix®

Therapeutic Category Vaccine, Inactivated (Viral)

Generic Availability (U.S.) No

Use

Prevention of cervical cancer and cervical intraepithelial neoplasia with or without cervical adenocarcinoma *in situ* caused by Human Papillomavirus (HPV) types 16 and 18 (FDA approved in girls ≥9 years and women ≤25 years of age)

The Advisory Committee on Immunization Practices (ACIP) recommends routine vaccination for females 11 to 12 years of age; catch-up vaccination is recommended for females 13 to 26 years of age (CDC/ACIP, 59 [20], 2010)

Pregnancy Risk Factor B

Pregnancy Considerations Adverse events were not observed in animal reproduction studies. Vaccination with papilloma virus vaccine is not recommended in pregnant women. In clinical trials, pregnancy testing was conducted prior to each vaccine administration and vaccination was discontinued if the woman was found to be pregnant; women were also instructed to avoid pregnancy for 2 months after receiving the vaccine. Pregnancies detected within 30 days prior or 45 days after vaccination had a higher rate of spontaneous abortions. A registry has been established for women exposed to Cervarix® during pregnancy (888-452-9622).

Administration of the vaccine in pregnancy is not recommended; until additional information is available, the vaccine series (or completion of the series) should be delayed until pregnancy is completed. Pregnancy testing is not required prior to administration of the vaccine (CDC, 2013).

Breast-Feeding Considerations It is not known if this vaccine is excreted into breast milk. The manufacturer recommends that caution be exercised when administering papilloma virus vaccine to nursing women. Lactating women may receive vaccine (CDC, 2010).

Contraindications Hypersensitivity to human papillomavirus vaccine or any component

Warnings Immediate treatment (including epinephrine 1:1000) for anaphylactic reactions should be available during vaccine use. There is no evidence that individuals exposed to or infected with HPV will be protected; those already infected with one or more HPV types were protected from disease in the remaining HPV types. Not for the treatment of active disease; does not protect against diseases caused by nonvaccine HPV types. Syncope has been reported with use of injectable vaccines and may be accompanied by transient visual disturbances, weakness, or tonic-clonic movements. Procedures should be in place to avoid injuries from falling and to restore cerebral perfusion if syncope occurs (CDC, 57[17], 2008).

Precautions The decision to administer or delay vaccination because of current or recent febrile illness depends on the severity of symptoms and the etiology of the disease.

Immunization should be delayed during the course of an acute severe febrile illness; may administer to patients with mild acute illness (with or without fever). Use with caution in severely immunocompromised patients (eg, patients receiving chemo/radiation therapy or other immunosuppressive therapy, including high-dose corticosteroids); may have a reduced response to vaccination; inactivated vaccines should be administered ≥2 weeks prior to planned immunosuppression when feasible (IDSA [Rubin, 2013]). In general, household and close contacts of persons with altered immunocompetence may receive all age-appropriate vaccines. Vaccination may not result in effective immunity in all patients. Response depends upon multiple factors (eg, type of vaccine, age of patient) and may be improved by administering the vaccine at the recommended dose, route, and interval (CDC/ACIP [Kroger, 2011]).

Use with caution in patients with coagulation disorders, including thrombocytopenia, due to an increased risk for bleeding following I.M. administration; if the patient receives antihemophilia or other similar therapy, I.M. injection can be scheduled shortly after such therapy is administered. Antipyretics have not been shown to prevent febrile seizures; antipyretics may be used to treat fever or discomfort following vaccination (CDC/ACIP [Kroger, 2011]). One study reported that routine prophylactic administration of acetaminophen to prevent fever prior to vaccination decreased the immune response of some vaccines; the clinical significance of this reduction in immune response has not been established (Prymula, 2009).

Use of this vaccine for specific medical and/or other indications (eg, immunocompromising conditions, hepatic or kidney disease, diabetes) is also addressed in the ACIP Recommended Immunization Schedule (CDC/ACIP [Akinsanya-Beysolow, 2014]; CDC/ACIP [Bridges, 2014]). Avoid use of prefilled syringes in latex hypersensitive patients; tip cap and plunger contain latex and may cause an allergic reaction to occur. The single dose vial stopper does not contain latex.

Adverse Reactions All serious adverse reactions must be reported to the U.S. Department of Health and Human Services (DHHS) Vaccine Adverse Event Reporting System (VAERS) 1-800-822-7967 or online at https://vaers.hhs.gov/esub/index. In Canada, adverse reactions may be reported to local provincial/territorial health agencies or to the Vaccine Safety Section at Public Health Agency of Canada (1-866-844-0018).

Central nervous system: Fatigue

Dermatologic: Urticaria

Local: Injection site reactions: Pain, pruritus, redness, swelling

Neuromuscular & skeletal: Arthralgia, myalgia

Respiratory: Nasopharyngitis, pharyngitis, pharyngolaryngeal pain, upper respiratory tract infection

Miscellaneous: Chlamydia infection, influenza, vaginal infection

Rare but important or life-threatening: Allergic reactions, anaphylactic/anaphylactoid reactions, angioedema, erythema multiforme, lymphadenopathy, syncope (may be associated with tonic-clonic movements), vasovagal response

Drug Interactions

Metabolism/Transport Effects None known.

Avoid Concomitant Use There are no known interactions where it is recommended to avoid concomitant use.

Increased Effect/Toxicity There are no known significant interactions involving an increase in effect.

Decreased Effect

The levels/effects of Papillomavirus (Types 16, 18) Vaccine (Human, Recombinant) may be decreased by: Belimumab; Fingolimod; Immunosuppressants

◀ **Stability** Store at 2°C to 8°C (36°F to 46°F); do not freeze; discard if frozen. May develop a fine, white deposit with a clear, colorless supernatant during storage (not a sign of deterioration).

Mechanism of Action Contains inactive human papillomavirus (HPV) proteins HPV 16 L1, and HPV 18 L1 which produce neutralizing antibodies to prevent cervical cancer, cervical adenocarcinoma, and cervical neoplasia cause by HPV.

Pharmacodynamics

Onset of action: Peak seroconversion was observed 1 month following the last dose of vaccine

Duration: Not well defined; >5 years

Dosing: Usual

Pediatric:

Primary immunization:

CDC (ACIP) recommendations: Female only: Children ≥9 years and Adolescents: I.M.: 0.5 mL per dose for a total of 3 doses administered as follows: Initial dose followed by a second dose at 1 to 2 months after initial and third dose at 6 months after the initial dose. Administer first dose to females at age 11 to 12 years although series may be initiated as early as 9 years of age. Minimum interval between the first and second dose is 4 weeks; minimum interval between the second and third dose of vaccine is 12 weeks (16 weeks preferred); minimum interval between first and third dose is 24 weeks. If the dose is given in an interval shorter than recommended, the dose should be repeated. The HPV vaccine series should be completed with the same product whenever possible (CDC/ACIP [Markowitz, 2007]; CDC/ACIP, 60 [50], 2011).

Manufacturer's labeling: Females: Children ≥9 years and Adolescents: I.M.: 0.5 mL per dose for a total of 3 doses. Administer the second and third doses at 1 and 6 months after initial dose.

Catch-up immunization: CDC (ACIP) recommendations (Akinsanya-Beysolow, 2014): **Note:** Do not restart the series. If doses have been given, begin the below schedule at the applicable dose number. I.M.: 0.5 mL per dose for a total of 3 doses in females ages 13 to 18 years who were not previously vaccinated, administered as follows:

First dose given on the elected date

Second dose given at least 4 weeks after the first dose

Third dose given at 16 weeks after the second dose (minimum interval: 12 weeks) and at least 24 weeks after the first dose

Adult: **Immunization:**

CDC recommended immunization schedule: I.M.: 0.5 mL per dose for a total of 3 doses. Administer first dose to females at age 11 to 12 years; begin series in females aged 13 to 26 years if not previously vaccinated. Administer the second and third doses at 1 to 2 months and 6 months after the first dose. Minimum interval between first and second doses is 4 weeks; the minimum interval between the second and third dose is 12 weeks (16 weeks preferred); the minimum interval between first and third doses is 24 weeks. Inadequate doses or doses received following a shorter than recommended dosing interval should be repeated. The HPV vaccine series should be completed with the same product whenever possible (CDC/ACIP [Markowitz, 2007]; CDC/ACIP, 60[50], 2011).

Manufacturer's labeling: Females: I.M.: 0.5 mL per dose for a total of 3 doses. Administer the second and third doses at 1 and 6 months after initial dose.

Dosing adjustment in renal impairment: There are no dosage adjustments provided in the manufacturer's labeling.

Dosing adjustment in hepatic impairment: There are no dosage adjustments provided in the manufacturer's labeling.

Administration I.M.: Shake suspension well prior to use; do not use suspension if it is discolored or contains particulate matter; should be a homogenous, turbid, white suspension. Do not dilute or mix with other vaccines. Administer I.M. into the deltoid region of the upper arm; **not for I.V., intradermal, or SubQ administration.** Adolescents and adults should be vaccinated while seated or lying down. U.S. law requires that the date of administration, the vaccine manufacturer, lot number of vaccine, and the administering person's name, title and address be entered into the patient's permanent medical record.

Monitoring Parameters Observe for syncope for 15 minutes following administration. If seizure-like activity associated with syncope occurs, maintain patient in supine or Trendelenburg position to reestablish adequate cerebral perfusion. Patient should continue to be screened for cervical cancer per current guidelines after vaccination series is completed.

Additional Information Comparison of HPV vaccines: Cervarix and Gardasil are both vaccines formulated to protect against infection with the human papillomavirus. Both are inactive vaccines which contain proteins HPV16 L1 and HPV 18 L1, the cause of >70% of invasive cervical cancer. The vaccines differ in that Gardasil also contains HPV 6 L1 and HPV 11 L1 proteins which protect against 75% to 90% of genital warts. The vaccines also differ in their preparation and adjuvants used. The viral proteins in Cervarix are prepared using *Trichoplusia ni* (insect cells) which are adsorbed onto an aluminum salt which is also combined with a monophosphoryl lipid. The viral proteins in Gardasil are prepared using *S. cerevisiae* (baker's yeast) which are then adsorbed onto an aluminum salt. Results from a short-term study (measurements obtained 1 month following the third vaccination in the series) have shown that the immune response to HPV 16 and HPV 18 may be greater with Cervarix; although the clinical significance of these differences is not known, local adverse events may also occur more frequently with this preparation. Both vaccines are effective and results from long-term studies are pending.

In order to maximize vaccination rates, the ACIP recommends simultaneous administration (ie, >1 vaccine on the same day at different anatomic sites) of all age-appropriate vaccines (live or inactivated) for which a person is eligible at a single visit, unless contraindications exist. If available, the use of combination vaccines is generally preferred over separate injections, taking into consideration provider assessment, patient preference, and potential adverse events. If separate vaccines being used, evaluate product information regarding same syringe compatibility of vaccines. Separate needles and syringes should be used for each injection. The ACIP prefers each dose of specific vaccine in a series come from the same manufacturer if possible (CDC/ACIP [Kroger, 2011]).

For additional information, please refer to the following website: http://www.cdc.gov/vaccines/vpd-vac/.

Dosage Forms Excipient information presented when available (limited, particularly for generics); consult specific product labeling. [DSC] = Discontinued product

Injection, suspension [preservative free]:

Cervarix®: HPV 16 L1 protein 20 mcg and HPV 18 L1 protein 20 mcg per 0.5 mL (0.5 mL [DSC]) [contains aluminum; manufactured using *Trichoplusia ni* (insect cells)]

Cervarix®: HPV 16 L1 protein 20 mcg and HPV 18 L1 protein 20 mcg per 0.5 mL (0.5 mL) [contains aluminum, natural rubber/natural latex in prefilled syringe; manufactured using *Trichoplusia ni* (insect cells)]

References

AAP Steering Committee on Quality Improvement and Management, Subcommittee on Febrile Seizures American Academy of Pediatrics, "Febrile Seizures: Clinical Practice Guideline for the Long-Term Management of the Child With Simple Febrile Seizures," *Pediatrics*, 2008, 121(6):1281-6.

Advisory Committee On Immunization Practices, "Vaccines for Children Program, Vaccines to Prevent Human Papillomavirus (HPV) Infection," October 2009. Available at http://www.cdc.gov/vaccines/programs/vfc/downloads/resolutions/1009hpv-508.pdf.

Akinsanya-Beysolow I, Advisory Committee on Immunization Practices (ACIP), ACIP Child/Adolescent Immunization Work Group, et al. Advisory committee on immunization practices recommended immunization schedule for persons aged 0 through 18 years - United States, 2014. *MMWR Morb Mortal Wkly Rep*. 2014; 63(5):108-109. Full schedule available at http://www.cdc.gov/vaccines/schedules/downloads/child/0-18yrs-child-combined-schedule.pdf

Bridges CB, Coyne-Beasley T, Advisory Committee on Immunization Practices (ACIP), ACIP Adult Immunization Work Group; Centers for Disease Control and Prevention (CDC). Advisory committee on immunization practices recommended immunization schedule for adults aged 19 years or older - United States, 2014. *MMWR Morb Mortal Wkly Rep*. 2014; 63(5):108-109. Available at: http://www.cdc.gov/vaccines/schedules/downloads/adult/adult-combined-schedule.pdf

Centers for Disease Control and Prevention (CDC), FDA licensure of bivalent human papillomavirus vaccine (HPV2, Cervarix) for use in females and updated HPV vaccination recommendations from the Advisory Committee on Immunization Practices (ACIP). *MMWR Morb Mortal Wkly Rep*. 2010;59(20):626-629.

Centers for Disease Control and Prevention (CDC). Recommendations on the use of quadrivalent human papillomavirus vaccine in males - Advisory Committee on Immunization Practices (ACIP), 2011. *MMWR Morb Mortal Wkly Rep*. 2011;60(50):1705-1708.

Centers for Disease Control and Prevention (CDC), "Syncope After Vaccination-United States, January 2005-July 2007," *MMWR Morb Mortal Wkly Rep*, 2008, 2;57(17):457-60.

Kroger AT, Atkinson WL, Marcuse EK, Pickering LK. General recommendations on immunization - recommendations of the Advisory Committee on Immunization Practices (ACIP). *MMWR Recomm Rep*. 2011;60(RR-2):1-64.

Markowitz LE, Dunne EF, Saraiya M, et.al. Quadrivalent human papillomavirus vaccine. Recommendations of the Advisory Committee on Immunization Practices (ACIP). *MMWR Recomm Rep*. 2007;56(RR-2):1-24.

Prymula R, Siegrist CA, Chlibek R, et al, "Effect of Prophylactic Paracetamol Administration at Time of Vaccination on Febrile Reactions and Antibody Responses in Children: Two Open-Label, Randomised Controlled Trials," *Lancet*, 2009, 374(9698):1339-50.

Rubin LG, Levin MJ, Ljungman P, et al. 2013 IDSA clinical practice guideline for vaccination of the immunocompromised host. *Clin Infect Dis*. 2014;58(3):e44-e100.

◆ **Papillomavirus Vaccine, Recombinant** *see* Papillomavirus (Types 6, 11, 16, 18) Vaccine (Human, Recombinant) *on page 1600*

◆ **Papillomavirus Vaccine, Recombinant** *see* Papillomavirus (Types 16, 18) Vaccine (Human, Recombinant) *on page 1603*

◆ **Paracetamol** *see* Acetaminophen *on page 47*

◆ **Parafon Forte DSC** *see* Chlorzoxazone *on page 454*

◆ **Paraplatin** *see* CARBOplatin *on page 379*

◆ **Parcaine** *see* Proparacaine *on page 1755*

Paregoric (par e GOR ik)

Medication Safety Issues

Sound-alike/look-alike issues:
Camphorated tincture of opium is an error-prone synonym (mistaken as opium tincture)

Paregoric may be confused with Percogesic®

High alert medication:
The Institute for Safe Medication Practices (ISMP) includes this medication among its list of drug classes which have a heightened risk of causing significant patient harm when used in error.

Administration issues:
Use care when prescribing opium products; paregoric contains the equivalent of morphine 0.4 mg/mL; opium tincture contains the equivalent of morphine 10 mg/mL

Therapeutic Category Analgesic, Narcotic; Antidiarrheal

Generic Availability (U.S.) Yes

Use Treatment of diarrhea or relief of pain; neonatal abstinence syndrome (neonatal opioid withdrawal)

Pregnancy Risk Factor C

Pregnancy Considerations Animal reproduction studies have not been conducted. Paregoric contains morphine; refer to the Morphine (Systemic) monograph for additional information. In addition, this preparation contains large amounts of alcohol (47%).

Breast-Feeding Considerations Paregoric contains morphine, which is excreted into breast milk; refer to the Morphine (Systemic) monograph for additional information. In addition, this preparation contains large amounts of alcohol (47%). The manufacturer recommends that caution be used if administered to a nursing woman.

Contraindications Hypersensitivity to opium or any component; diarrhea caused by poisoning until the toxic material has been removed

Warnings Abrupt discontinuation after prolonged use may result in symptoms of withdrawal. Do **not** confuse this product (paregoric) with opium tincture which is 25 times **more** potent. Each 5 mL of paregoric contains 2 mg morphine equivalent, 0.02 mL anise oil, 20 mg benzoic acid, 20 mg camphor, 0.2 mL glycerin and alcohol; final alcohol content 45%; paregoric also contains papaverine and noscapine; because all of these additives may be harmful to neonates, **a 25-fold dilution of opium tincture** is often preferred for treatment of neonatal abstinence syndrome (opioid withdrawal). Some centers prefer to use morphine oral solution.

Paregoric contains benzoic acid; benzoic acid (benzoate) is a metabolite of benzyl alcohol; large amounts of benzyl alcohol (≥99 mg/kg/day) have been associated with a potentially fatal toxicity ("gasping syndrome") in neonates; the "gasping syndrome" consists of metabolic acidosis, respiratory distress, gasping respirations, CNS dysfunction (including convulsions, intracranial hemorrhage), hypotension and cardiovascular collapse; use paregoric products containing benzoic acid with caution in neonates; *in vitro* and animal studies have shown that benzoate displaces bilirubin from protein binding sites

Precautions Use with caution in patients with respiratory, hepatic or renal dysfunction, severe prostatic hypertrophy, or history of opioid abuse; opium shares the toxic potential of opioid agonists, usual precautions of opioid agonist therapy should be observed; infants <3 months of age are more susceptible to respiratory depression, use with caution and in reduced doses in this age group

Adverse Reactions

Cardiovascular: Hypotension, peripheral vasodilation

Central nervous system: Central nervous system depression, depression, dizziness, drowsiness, drug dependence (physical and psychological), dysphoria, euphoria, headache, increased intracranial pressure, insomnia, malaise, restlessness, sedation

Dermatologic: Pruritus

Gastrointestinal: Anorexia, biliary tract spasm, constipation, nausea, stomach cramps, vomiting

Genitourinary: Decreased urine output, ureteral spasm

Hepatic: Increased liver enzymes

Hypersensitivity: Histamine release

Neuromuscular & skeletal: Weakness

Ophthalmic: Miosis

Respiratory: Respiratory depression

Drug Interactions

Metabolism/Transport Effects None known.

Avoid Concomitant Use

Avoid concomitant use of Paregoric with any of the following: Azelastine (Nasal); Paraldehyde; Thalidomide

Increased Effect/Toxicity

Paregoric may increase the levels/effects of: Alcohol (Ethyl); Alvimopan; Azelastine (Nasal); Buprenorphine; CNS Depressants; Desmopressin; Diuretics; Hydrocodone; Methotrimeprazine; Metyrosine; Mirtazapine; Paraldehyde; Pramipexole; ROPINIRole; Rotigotine; Selective Serotonin Reuptake Inhibitors; Thalidomide; Zolpidem

The levels/effects of Paregoric may be increased by: Amphetamines; Anticholinergic Agents; Antipsychotic Agents (Phenothiazines); Brimonidine (Topical); Cannabis; Doxylamine; Dronabinol; Droperidol; HydrOXYzine; Kava Kava; Magnesium Sulfate; Methotrimeprazine; Nabilone; Perampanel; Rufinamide; Sodium Oxybate; Succinylcholine; Tapentadol; Tetrahydrocannabinol

Decreased Effect

Paregoric may decrease the levels/effects of: Pegvisomant

The levels/effects of Paregoric may be decreased by: Ammonium Chloride; Mixed Agonist / Antagonist Opioids; Naltrexone

Stability Store in light-resistant, tightly closed container; protect from freezing

Mechanism of Action Increases smooth muscle tone in GI tract, decreases motility and peristalsis, diminishes digestive secretions

Pharmacokinetics (Adult data unless noted)

Metabolism: Opium is metabolized in the liver

Elimination: In urine, primarily as morphine glucuronide conjugates and as parent compound (morphine, codeine, papaverine, etc)

Dosing: Neonatal Note: Due to potential adverse effects from the additives in paregoric, other agents are preferred for treatment of neonatal abstinence syndrome.

Oral: Full-term neonates: Neonatal abstinence syndrome (not a preferred agent): Initial: 0.1 mL/kg or 2 drops/kg with feedings every 3-4 hours; increase dosage by 0.1 mL/kg or 2 drops/kg every 3-4 hours until withdrawal symptoms are controlled; it is rare to exceed 0.7 mL/dose. Stabilize withdrawal symptoms for 3-5 days, then gradually decrease the dosage (keeping the same dosing interval) over a 2- to 4-week period.

Dosing: Usual Oral:

Children: 0.25-0.5 mL/kg 1-4 times/day

Adults: 5-10 mL 1-4 times/day

Administration Oral: May administer with food to decrease GI upset; shake well before use

Monitoring Parameters Respiratory rate, blood pressure, heart rate, level of sedation; neonatal abstinence syndrome (opioid withdrawal): Monitor for resolution of withdrawal symptoms (such as irritability, high-pitched cry, stuffy nose, rhinorrhea, vomiting, poor feeding, diarrhea, sneezing, yawning, etc) and signs of over treatment (such as bradycardia, lethargy, hypotonia, irregular respirations, respiratory depression, etc); an abstinence scoring system (eg, Finnegan abstinence scoring system) can be used to more objectively assess neonatal opioid withdrawal symptoms and the need for dosage adjustment

Controlled Substance C-III

Dosage Forms Excipient information presented when available (limited, particularly for generics); consult specific product labeling.

Tincture, Oral:

Generic: 2 mg/5 mL (473 mL)

References

Dow K, Ordean A, Murphy-Oikonen J, et al, "Neonatal Abstinence Syndrome Clinical Practice Guidelines for Ontario," *J Popul Ther Clin Pharmacol*, 2012, 19(3):e488-506.

Hudak ML, Tan RC, Committee On Drugs, et al, "Neonatal Drug Withdrawal," *Pediatrics*, 2012, 129(2):e540-60.

Kraus DM and Pham JT, "Neonatal Therapy," *Applied Therapeutics: The Clinical Use of Drugs*, 9th ed, Koda-Kimble MA, Young LY, Kradjan WA, et al, eds, Baltimore, MD: Lippincott Williams & Wilkins, 2009.

Levy M and Spino M, "Neonatal Withdrawal Syndrome: Associated Drugs and Pharmacologic Management," *Pharmacotherapy*, 1993, 13(3):202-11.

"Neonatal Drug Withdrawal. American Academy of Pediatrics Committee on Drugs," *Pediatrics*, 1998, 101(6):1079-88.

Paricalcitol (pah ri KAL si tole)

Medication Safety Issues

Sound alike/look alike issues:

Paricalcitol may be confused with calcitriol

Zemplar may be confused with zaleplon, Zelapar, zolpidem, ZyPREXA Zydis

Brand Names: U.S. Zemplar

Brand Names: Canada Zemplar

Therapeutic Category Vitamin D Analog; Vitamin, Fat Soluble

Generic Availability (U.S.) May be product dependent

Use

I.V.: Prevention and treatment of secondary hyperparathyroidism associated with stage 5 chronic kidney disease (CKD) (FDA approved in children ≥5 years and adults)

Oral: Prevention and treatment of secondary hyperparathyroidism associated with stages 3 and 4 chronic kidney disease (CKD) and stage 5 CKD patients on hemodialysis or peritoneal dialysis (FDA approved in adults)

Pregnancy Risk Factor C

Pregnancy Considerations Adverse events were observed in some animal reproduction studies.

Breast-Feeding Considerations It is not known if paricalcitol is excreted in breast milk. Due to the potential for serious adverse reactions in the nursing infant, a decision should be made whether to discontinue nursing or to discontinue the drug, taking into account the importance of treatment to the mother.

Contraindications Hypersensitivity to paricalcitol or any component; vitamin D toxicity; hypercalcemia

Warnings Excessive administration may lead to over suppression of PTH, hypercalcemia, hypercalciuria, hyperphosphatemia, and adynamic bone disease. Acute hypercalcemia may increase risk of cardiac arrhythmias and seizures. Chronic hypercalcemia may lead to generalized vascular and other soft-tissue calcification. Risk of hypercalcemia may be increased by concomitant use of calcium-containing supplements and/or medications that increase serum calcium (eg, thiazide diuretics). Phosphate and vitamin D (and its derivatives) should be withheld during therapy to avoid hypercalcemia. Avoid regular administration of aluminum to prevent overload and toxicity. Dialysate concentration of aluminum should be maintained at <10 mcg/L. Not indicated for use in patients with rapidly worsening kidney function or those who are noncompliant with medications or follow-up (K/DOQI Guidelines, 2003).

Precautions Hypercalcemia potentiates digoxin toxicity; use concomitantly with caution

Adverse Reactions

Cardiovascular: Chest pain, diarrhea, edema, hyper-/hypotension, hypervolemia, MI, palpitation, peripheral edema, syncope

Central nervous system: Anxiety, chills, depression, dizziness, fever, headache, insomnia, lightheadedness, pain, vertigo

Dermatologic: Bruising, rash, skin ulcer

Endocrine & metabolic: Dehydration, hypoglycemia

Gastrointestinal: Abdominal pain, constipation, dyspepsia, GI bleeding, vomiting, xerostomia

Genitourinary: Urinary tract infection

Neuromuscular & skeletal: Arthritis, back pain, leg cramps, weakness

Renal: Uremia

Respiratory: Bronchitis, cough, oropharyngeal pain, pneumonia, rhinitis, sinusitis

Miscellaneous: Allergic reaction, flu-like syndrome, peritonitis, sepsis

Rare but important or life-threatening: Agitation, anemia, angioedema (including laryngeal edema), arrhythmia, atrial flutter, bleeding time prolonged, breast cancer, cardiac arrest, cerebrovascular accident, chest discomfort, confusional state, conjunctivitis, delirium, dysphagia, dyspnea, erectile dysfunction, gait disturbance, gastritis, gastroesophageal reflux, glaucoma, hepatic enzyme (abnormal), hirsutism, hypercalciuria, hyper-/hypocalcemia, hyper-/hypoparathyroidism, hyperkalemia, hyperphosphatemia, injection site extravasation, injection site pain, intestinal ischemia, lymphadenopathy, myalgia, myoclonus, nasopharyngitis, night sweats, ocular hyperemia, oral edema, orthopnea, paresthesia, pruritus, pulmonary edema, rectal hemorrhage, skin burning sensation, taste perversion (metallic), upper respiratory tract infection, urticaria, vaginal infection, weight loss, wheezing

Drug Interactions

Metabolism/Transport Effects Substrate of CYP3A4 (minor); **Note:** Assignment of Major/Minor substrate status based on clinically relevant drug interaction potential

Avoid Concomitant Use

Avoid concomitant use of Paricalcitol with any of the following: Aluminum Hydroxide; Multivitamins/Fluoride (with ADE); Multivitamins/Minerals (with ADEK, Folate, Iron); Sucralfate; Sucroferric Oxyhydroxide; Vitamin D Analogs

Increased Effect/Toxicity

Paricalcitol may increase the levels/effects of: Aluminum Hydroxide; Cardiac Glycosides; Digoxin; Sucralfate; Vitamin D Analogs

The levels/effects of Paricalcitol may be increased by: Calcium Salts; CYP3A4 Inhibitors (Strong); Danazol; Multivitamins/Fluoride (with ADE); Multivitamins/Minerals (with ADEK, Folate, Iron); Thiazide Diuretics

Decreased Effect

The levels/effects of Paricalcitol may be decreased by: Bile Acid Sequestrants; Mineral Oil; Orlistat; Sucroferric Oxyhydroxide

Stability Store at 25°C (77°F); excursions permitted between 15°C to 30°C (59°F to 86°F).

Mechanism of Action Decreased renal conversion of vitamin D to its primary active metabolite (1,25-hydroxyvitamin D) in chronic renal failure leads to reduced activation of vitamin D receptor (VDR), which subsequently removes inhibitory suppression of parathyroid hormone (PTH) release; increased serum PTH (secondary hyperparathyroidism) reduces calcium excretion and enhances bone resorption. Paricalcitol is a synthetic vitamin D analog which binds to and activates the VDR in kidney, parathyroid gland, intestine and bone, thus reducing PTH levels and improving calcium and phosphate homeostasis.

Pharmacokinetics (Adult data unless noted)

Distribution: V_d:

Healthy subjects: Oral: 34 L; I.V.: 24 L

Stage 3 and 4 CKD: Oral: 44-46 L

Stage 5 CKD: Oral: 38-49 L; I.V.: 31-35 L

Protein binding: >99%

Metabolism: Hydroxylation and glucuronidation via hepatic and nonhepatic enzymes, including CYP24, CYP3A4, UGT1A4; forms metabolites (at least one active)

Bioavailability: Oral: 72% to 86% in healthy subjects

Time to peak serum concentration: Oral: 3 hours

Half-life: Adults:

Healthy subjects: Oral: 4-6 hours; I.V.: 5-7 hours

Stage 3 and 4 CKD: Oral: 14-20 hours

Stage 5 CKD: Oral: 14-20 hours; I.V.: 14-15 hours

Elimination: Healthy subjects: Feces (Oral: 70%; I.V.: 63%); urine (Oral: 18%, I.V.: 19%); 51% to 59% as metabolites

Dosing: Usual In stage 3-5 CKD maintain Ca x P <55 mg^2/dL^2 (adults and children >12 years) or <65 mg^2/dL^2 (children <12 years), reduce or interrupt dosing if recommended Ca x P is exceeded or hypercalcemia is observed (K/DOQI Clinical Practice Guidelines, 2005).

Secondary hyperparathyroidism associated with chronic renal failure (stage 5 CKD): Children ≥5 years (limited small studies) and Adults: I.V.: 0.04-0.1 mcg/kg no more frequently than every other day; dose may be increased by 2-4 mcg every 2-4 weeks (0.04-0.1 mcg/kg for children); doses as high as 0.24 mcg/kg (16.8 mcg) have been administered safely; children may require higher weight-based doses; 0.2 ± 0.7 mcg/kg/dose (Seeherunvong, 2006); the dose of paricalcitol should be adjusted based on serum intact parathyroid hormone (iPTH) levels, as follows:

Same or increasing iPTH level: Increase paricalcitol dose

iPTH level decreased by <30%: Increase paricalcitol dose

iPTH level decreased by >30% and <60%: Maintain paricalcitol dose

iPTH level decrease by >60%: Decrease paricalcitol dose

iPTH level 1.5-3 times upper limit of normal: Maintain paricalcitol dose

Adults: Oral: Initial dose, in mcg, based on baseline iPTH level divided by 80. Administer 3 times weekly; no more frequently than every other day. **Note:** To reduce the risk of hypercalcemia initiate only after baseline serum calcium has been adjusted to ≤9.5 mg/dL.

Dose titration: Titration dose (mcg) = most recent iPTH level (pg/ml) divided by 80

Note: In situations where monitoring of iPTH, calcium, and phosphorus occurs less frequently than once per week, a more modest initial and dose titration rate may be warranted: Modest titration dose (mcg) = Most recent iPTH level (pg/mL) divided by 100

Dosage adjustment for hypercalcemia or elevated Ca x P: Decrease calculated dose by 2-4 mcg. If further adjustment is required, dose should be reduced or interrupted until these parameters are normalized. If applicable, phosphate binder dosing may also be adjusted or withheld, or switch to a noncalcium-based phosphate binder

Secondary hyperparathyroidism associated with stage 3 and 4 CKD: Adults: Oral: Initial dose based on baseline serum iPTH:

iPTH ≤500 pg/mL: 1 mcg/day or 2 mcg 3 times/week*

iPTH >500 pg/mL: 2 mcg/day or 4 mcg 3 times/week*

*Do not administer 3 times/week regimen more frequently than every other day

Dosage adjustment based on iPTH level relative to baseline, adjust dose at 2-4 week intervals:

iPTH same or increased: Increase paricalcitol dose by 1 mcg/day or 2 mcg 3 times/week

iPTH decreased by <30%: Increase paricalcitol dose by 1 mcg/day or 2 mcg 3 times/week

iPTH decreased by ≥30% and ≤60%: Maintain paricalcitol dose

iPTH decreased by >60%: Decrease paricalcitol dose by 1 mcg/day* or 2 mcg 3 times/week

iPTH <60 pg/mL: Decrease paricalcitol dose by 1 mcg/day* or 2 mcg 3 times/week

◄ *If patient is taking the lowest dose on an every other day regimen, but further dose reduction is needed, decrease dose to 1 mcg 3 times/week. If further dose reduction is required, withhold drug as needed and restart at a lower dose. If applicable, calcium-phosphate binder dosing may also be adjusted or withheld, or switch to noncalcium-based binder.

Dosage adjustment in hepatic impairment: Adjustment not needed for mild-to-moderate impairment. Paricalcitol has not been evaluated in severe hepatic impairment.

Administration

Oral: May be administered with or without food. With the 3 times/week dosing schedule, doses should not be given more frequently than every other day.

Parenteral: Administer undiluted as an I.V. bolus dose at anytime during dialysis. Doses should not be administered more often than every other day.

Monitoring Parameters Signs and symptoms of vitamin D intoxication

Serum calcium and phosphorus (closely monitor levels during dosage titration and after initiation of a strong CYP3A4 inhibitor):

I.V.: Twice weekly during initial phase, then at least monthly once dose established

Oral: At least every 2 weeks for 3 months or following dose adjustment, then monthly for 3 months, then every 3 months

Calcium phosphorus product (Ca x P): Maintain Ca x P <55 mg^2/dL^2 (adults and children >12 years) or <65 mg^2/dL^2 (children <12 years) in stage 3-5 CKD

Serum or plasma intact parathyroid hormone (iPTH): At least every 2 weeks for 3 months or following dose adjustment, then monthly for 3 months, then as per K/DOQI Guidelines below

Per Kidney Disease Outcome Quality Initiative Practice Guidelines - Children (K/DOQI, 2005):

Stage 3 CKD: iPTH every 6 months

Stage 4 CKD: iPTH every 3 months

Stage 5 CKD: iPTH every 3 months

Per Kidney Disease Outcome Quality Initiative Practice Guidelines - Adults (K/DOQI, 2003):

Stage 3 CKD: iPTH every 12 months

Stage 4 CKD: iPTH every 3 months

Stage 5 CKD: iPTH every 3 months

Reference Range Chronic kidney disease (CKD) is defined either as kidney damage or GFR <60 mL/minute/1.73 m^2 for ≥3 months); stages of CKD are described below:

CKD Stage 1: Kidney damage with normal or increased GFR; GFR ≥90 mL/minute/1.73 m^2

CKD Stage 2: Kidney damage with mild decrease in GFR; GFR 60-89 mL/minute/1.73 m^2

CKD Stage 3: Moderate decrease in GFR; GFR 30-59 mL/minute/1.73 m^2

CKD Stage 4: Severe decrease in GFR; GFR 15-29 mL/minute/1.73 m^2

CKD Stage 5: Kidney failure; GFR <15 mL/minute/1.73 m^2 or dialysis

Target range for iPTH:

Stage 2 CKD: Children: 35-70 pg/mL (3.85-7.7 pmol/L) Children and Adults:

Stage 3 CKD: Children and Adults: 35-70 pg/mL (3.85-7.7 pmol/L)

Stage 4 CKD: Children and Adults: 70-110 pg/mL (7.7-12.1 pmol/L)

Stage 5 CKD:

Children: 200-300 pg/mL (22-33 pmol/L)

Adults: 150-300 pg/mL (16.5-33 pmol/L)

Serum phosphorous:

Stages 1-4 CKD: Children: At or above the age-appropriate lower limits and no higher than age-appropriate upper limits

Stage 3 and 4 CKD: Adults: ≥2.7 to <4.6 mg/dL (≥0.87 to <1.49 mmol/L)

Stage 5 CKD:

Children 1-12 years: 4-6 mg/dL (1.29-1.94 mmol/L)

Children >12 years and Adults: 3.5-5.5 mg/dL (1.13-1.78 mmol/L)

Dosage Forms Excipient information presented when available (limited, particularly for generics); consult specific product labeling.

Capsule, Oral:

Zemplar: 1 mcg, 2 mcg, 4 mcg [contains alcohol, usp]

Generic: 1 mcg, 2 mcg, 4 mcg

Solution, Intravenous:

Zemplar: 2 mcg/mL (1 mL); 5 mcg/mL (1 mL, 2 mL) [contains alcohol, usp, propylene glycol]

References

Greenbaum LA, Benador N, Goldstein SL, et al, "Intravenous Paricalcitol for Treatment of Secondary Hyperparathyroidism in Children on Hemodialysis," *Am J Kidney Dis*, 2007, 49(6):814-23.

"K/DOQI Clinical Practice Guidelines for Bone Metabolism and Disease in Children With Chronic Kidney Disease," *Am J Kidney Dis*, 2005, 46 (4 Suppl 1):S1-121.

"K/DOQI Clinical Practice Guidelines for Bone Metabolism and Disease in Chronic Kidney Disease. Guideline 1. Evaluation of Calcium and Phosphorus Metabolism," *Am J Kidney Dis*, 2003, 42(4 Suppl 3):52-7.

"K/DOQI Clinical Practice Guidelines for Bone Metabolism and Disease in Chronic Kidney Disease. Guideline 3. Evaluation of Serum Phosphorus Levels," *Am J Kidney Dis* , 2003, 42(4 Suppl 3):62-3.

"K/DOQI Clinical Practice Guidelines for Chronic Kidney Disease: Evaluation, Classification, and Stratification, Part 4. Definition and Classification of Stages of Chronic Kidney Disease," *Am J Kidney Dis*, 2002, 39(2 Suppl 1):46-75.

Sanchez CP, "Secondary Hyperparathyroidism in Children With Chronic Renal Failure: Pathogenesis and Treatment," *Paediatr Drugs*, 2003, 5 (11): 763-76.

Seeherunvong W, Nwobi, O, Abitbol CL, et al, "Paricalcitol Versus Calcitriol Treatment for Hyperparathyroidism in Pediatric Hemodialysis Patients," *Pediatr Nephrol*, 2006, 21(10):1434-9.

Ziolkowska H, "Minimizing Bone Abnormalities in Children With Renal Failure," *Paediatr Drugs*, 2006, 8(4):205-22.

◆ **Pariet (Can)** see RABEprazole *on page 1797*

◆ **Pariprazole** see RABEprazole *on page 1797*

◆ **Parlodel** see Bromocriptine *on page 304*

◆ **Paroex** see Chlorhexidine Gluconate *on page 441*

Paromomycin (par oh moe MYE sin)

Brand Names: Canada Humatin

Therapeutic Category Amebicide

Generic Availability (U.S.) Yes

Use Treatment of acute and chronic intestinal amebiasis due to susceptible *Entamoeba histolytica* (not effective in the treatment of extraintestinal amebiasis); tapeworm infestations; adjunctive management of hepatic coma; treatment of cryptosporidial diarrhea

Pregnancy Considerations Paromomycin is poorly absorbed when given orally. Information related to the use of paromomycin in pregnancy is limited (Kreutner, 1981). Use may be considered for the treatment of giardiasis throughout pregnancy (Gardner, 2001) or cryptosporidiosis after the first trimester (DHHS, 2013) in pregnant women.

Breast-Feeding Considerations Paromomycin is poorly absorbed when given orally. Available information suggests that paromomycin may be used in nursing women when renal function is normal in both the mother and infant (Davidson, 2009).

Contraindications Hypersensitivity to paromomycin or any component; intestinal obstruction

Warnings May result in overgrowth of nonsusceptible organisms

Precautions Use with caution in patients with impaired GI motility or possible or proven ulcerative bowel lesions; use with caution in patients with impaired renal function

Adverse Reactions
Gastrointestinal: Abdominal cramps, diarrhea, heartburn, nausea, vomiting

Rare but important or life-threatening: Enterocolitis (secondary), eosinophilia, ototoxicity, pruritus, rash, steatorrhea

Drug Interactions
Metabolism/Transport Effects None known.

Avoid Concomitant Use There are no known interactions where it is recommended to avoid concomitant use.

Increased Effect/Toxicity There are no known significant interactions involving an increase in effect.

Decreased Effect There are no known significant interactions involving a decrease in effect.

Mechanism of Action
Acts directly on ameba; has antibacterial activity against normal and pathogenic organisms in the GI tract; interferes with bacterial protein synthesis by binding to 30S ribosomal subunits

Pharmacokinetics (Adult data unless noted)
Absorption: Poor from the GI tract

Elimination: Excreted unchanged in feces; portion of oral dose that may be absorbed is excreted in urine

Dosing: Usual Oral:
Children:

Intestinal amebiasis (*Entamoeba histolytica*): 25-35 mg/kg/day divided every 8 hours for 7 days

Dientamoeba fragilis infection: 25-30 mg/kg/day divided every 8 hours for 7 days

Tapeworm:

T. saginata, T. solium, D. latum: 11 mg/kg/dose every 15 minutes for 4 doses

H. nana: 45 mg/kg/day once daily for 5-7 days

Adults:

Intestinal amebiasis (*Entamoeba histolytica*): 25-35 mg/kg/day divided every 8 hours for 7 days

Dientamoeba fragilis infection: 25-30 mg/kg/day divided every 8 hours for 7 days

Tapeworm:

T. saginata, T. solium, D. latum: 1 g every 15 minutes for 4 doses

H. nana: 45 mg/kg/day once daily for 5-7 days

Hepatic coma: 4 g/day in 2-4 divided doses for 5-6 days

Cryptosporidial diarrhea: 1.5-2 g/day in 3-4 divided doses for 10-14 days

Administration
Oral: Administer with or after meals

Monitoring Parameters
Periodic urinalysis and renal function tests; be alert to ototoxicity

Additional Information
With the treatment of cestodiasis caused by *T. solium*, paromomycin may cause disintegration of worm segments and release of viable eggs resulting in an increased risk for the development of cysticercosis

Dosage Forms
Excipient information presented when available (limited, particularly for generics); consult specific product labeling.

Capsule, Oral:

Generic: 250 mg

References
Danziger LH, Kanyok TP, and Novak RM, "Treatment of Cryptosporidial Diarrhea in an AIDS Patient With Paromomycin," *Ann Pharmacother*, 1993, 27(12):1460-2.

Liu LX and Weller PF, "Antiparasitic Drugs," *N Engl J Med*, 1996, 334 (18):1178-84.

◆ **Paromomycin Sulfate** *see* Paromomycin *on page 1608*

PARoxetine (pa ROKS e teen)

Medication Safety Issues
Sound-alike/look-alike issues:

PARoxetine may be confused with FLUoxetine, PACLitaxel, piroxicam, pyridoxine, vortioxetine

Paxil may be confused with Doxil, PACLitaxel, Plavix, PROzac, Taxol

BEERS Criteria medication:

This drug may be potentially inappropriate for use in geriatric patients (SIADH: Quality of evidence - moderate; Strength of recommendation - strong).

Related Information
Antidepressant Agents *on page 2219*

Oral Medications That Should Not Be Crushed or Altered *on page 2438*

Safe Handling of Hazardous Drugs *on page 2419*

Brand Names: U.S. Brisdelle; Paxil; Paxil CR; Pexeva

Brand Names: Canada Apo-Paroxetine; Auro-Paroxetine; CO Paroxetine; Dom-Paroxetine; JAMP-Paroxetine; Mylan-Paroxetine; Novo-Paroxetine; Paxil; Paxil CR; PHL-Paroxetine; PMS-Paroxetine; Q-Paroxetine; ratio-Paroxetine; Riva-Paroxetine; Sandoz-Paroxetine; Teva-Paroxetine

Therapeutic Category
Antidepressant, Selective Serotonin Reuptake Inhibitor (SSRI)

Generic Availability (U.S.)
May be product dependent

Use
Brisdelle: Treatment of moderate to severe vasomotor symptoms associated with menopause (FDA approved in adults)

Paxil: Treatment of major depressive disorder (MDD), panic disorder (with or without agoraphobia), obsessive-compulsive disorder (OCD), social anxiety disorder (social phobia), generalized anxiety disorder (GAD), and post-traumatic stress disorder (PTSD) (All indications: FDA approved in adults); has also been used for self-injurious behavior

Paxil CR: Treatment of major depressive disorder (MDD), panic disorder (with or without agoraphobia), social anxiety disorder (social phobia), and premenstrual dysphoric disorder (PMDD) (FDA approved in adults)

Pexeva: Treatment of major depressive disorder (MDD), obsessive-compulsive disorder (OCD), panic disorder (with or without agoraphobia), and generalized anxiety disorder (GAD) (FDA approved in adults)

Medication Guide Available
Yes

Pregnancy Risk Factor
D//X (product specific)

Pregnancy Considerations
Studies in pregnant women have demonstrated a risk to the fetus. Paroxetine crosses the placenta. An increased risk of teratogenic effects, including cardiovascular defects, may be associated with maternal use of paroxetine or other SSRIs; however, available information is conflicting. Nonteratogenic effects in the newborn following SSRI/SNRI exposure late in the third trimester include respiratory distress, cyanosis, apnea, seizures, temperature instability, feeding difficulty, vomiting, hypoglycemia, hypo- or hypertonia, hyperreflexia, jitteriness, irritability, constant crying, and tremor. Symptoms may be due to the toxicity of the SSRIs/SNRIs or a discontinuation syndrome and may be consistent with serotonin syndrome associated with SSRI treatment. Persistent pulmonary hypertension of the newborn (PPHN) has also been reported with SSRI exposure. The long-term effects of *in utero* SSRI exposure on infant development and behavior are not known.

Due to pregnancy-induced physiologic changes, some pharmacokinetic parameters of paroxetine may be altered. The maternal CYP2D6 genotype also influences paroxetine plasma concentrations during pregnancy.

The manufacturer suggests discontinuing paroxetine or switching to another antidepressant unless the benefits of therapy justify continuing treatment during pregnancy; consider other treatment options for women who are planning to become pregnant. The ACOG recommends that therapy with SSRIs or SNRIs during pregnancy be individualized; treatment of depression during pregnancy should incorporate the clinical expertise of the mental health clinician, obstetrician, primary healthcare provider, and pediatrician. The ACOG also recommends that therapy with paroxetine be avoided during pregnancy if possible and that fetuses exposed in early pregnancy be assessed with a fetal echocardiography. According to the American Psychiatric Association (APA), the risks of medication treatment should be weighed against other treatment options and untreated depression. The use of paroxetine is not recommended as first line therapy during pregnancy. For women who discontinue antidepressant medications during pregnancy and who may be at high risk for postpartum depression, the medications can be restarted following delivery. Treatment algorithms have been developed by the ACOG and the APA for the management of depression in women prior to conception and during pregnancy. Menopausal vasomotor symptoms do not occur during pregnancy; therefore, the use of paroxetine for the treatment of menopausal vasomotor symptoms is contraindicated in pregnant women.

Breast-Feeding Considerations Paroxetine is excreted in breast milk and concentrations in the hindmilk are higher than in foremilk. Paroxetine has not been detected in the serum of nursing infants. Adverse reactions have been reported in nursing infants exposed to some SSRIs. The manufacturer recommends that caution be exercised when administering paroxetine to nursing women. Maternal use of an SSRI during pregnancy may cause delayed milk secretion. The American Academy of Breastfeeding Medicine suggests that paroxetine may be considered for the treatment of postpartum depression in appropriately selected women who are nursing. Mothers should be monitored for changes in symptoms and infants should be monitored for growth. The long-term effects on development and behavior have not been studied.

Contraindications Hypersensitivity to paroxetine or any component; use of MAO inhibitors intended to treat psychiatric disorder (concurrently or within 14 days of discontinuing either paroxetine or the MAO inhibitor); initiation of paroxetine in a patient receiving linezolid or intravenous methylene blue; concurrent use of thioridazine or pimozide. Additional product-specific contraindications: Brisdelle: Pregnancy

Warnings Hazardous agent; use appropriate precautions for handling and disposal (NIOSH, 2012). Clinical worsening of depression or suicidal ideation and behavior may occur in pediatric and adult patients with major depressive disorder. In clinical trials, antidepressants increased the risk of suicidal thinking and behavior (suicidality) in children, adolescents, and young adults (18-24 years of age) with major depressive disorder and other psychiatric disorders **[U.S. Boxed Warning]**. This risk must be considered before prescribing antidepressants for any clinical use. Short-term studies did **not** show an increased risk of suicidality with antidepressant use in patients >24 years of age and showed a decreased risk in patients ≥65 years.

Patients of all ages who are treated with antidepressants for any indication require appropriate monitoring and close observation for clinical worsening of depression, suicidality, and unusual changes in behavior, especially during the first few months after antidepressant initiation or when the dose is adjusted. Family members and caregivers should be instructed to closely observe the patient (ie, daily) and communicate condition with healthcare provider. All patients should also be monitored for associated behaviors (eg, anxiety, agitation, panic attacks, insomnia, irritability, hostility, aggressiveness, impulsivity, akathisia, hypomania, mania) which may increase the risk for worsening depression or suicidality. Worsening depression or emergence of suicidality (or associated behaviors listed above) that is abrupt in onset, severe, or not part of the presenting symptoms, may require discontinuation or modification of

drug therapy. The FDA recommends that paroxetine **not** be used in pediatric patients for the treatment of depression. Three well-controlled trials in pediatric patients with depression have failed to show therapeutic superiority over placebo; in addition, an increased risk for suicidal behavior was observed in patients receiving paroxetine when compared to other SSRIs (Dopheide, 2006). SSRI-associated behavioral activation (ie, restlessness, hyperkinesis, hyperactivity, agitation) is two- to threefold more prevalent in children compared to adolescents; it is more prevalent in adolescents compared to adults. Somnolence (including sedation and drowsiness) is more common in adults compared to children and adolescents (Safer, 2006).

Avoid abrupt discontinuation; discontinuation symptoms (including agitation, dysphoria, anxiety, confusion, dizziness, hypomania, nightmares, and other symptoms) may occur if therapy is abruptly discontinued or dose reduced; taper dosage gradually in patients receiving >20 mg/day to minimize risks of discontinuation symptoms; if intolerable symptoms occur following a decrease in dosage or upon discontinuation of therapy, consider resuming the previous dose with a more gradual taper. An SSRI discontinuation syndrome similar to that described in adults has been reported in six children (Diler, 2002). To reduce risk of intentional overdose, write prescriptions for the smallest quantity consistent with good patient care.

May worsen psychosis in some patients or precipitate a shift to mania or hypomania in patients with bipolar disorder. Antidepressant monotherapy in patients with bipolar disorder should be avoided. Patients presenting with depressive symptoms should be screened for bipolar disorder. (Using antidepressants alone may induce manic episodes in patients with this condition.) Paroxetine is not FDA approved for the treatment of bipolar disorder.

Potentially fatal serotonin syndrome may occur when SSRIs are used in combination with serotonergic drugs (eg, triptans) or drugs that impair the metabolism of serotonin [eg, MAO inhibitors; including reversible MAO inhibitors (eg, linezolid, methylene blue)]. Monitor patients closely for signs of serotonin syndrome, such as mental status changes (eg, agitation, hallucinations, delirium, coma); autonomic instability (eg, tachycardia, labile blood pressure, diaphoresis); neuromuscular changes (eg, tremor, rigidity, myoclonus); GI symptoms (eg, nausea, vomiting, diarrhea); and/or seizures. Discontinue treatment (and any concomitant serotonergic agent) immediately if signs/symptoms arise. Initiation of paroxetine within 14 days of receiving an MAO inhibitor is contraindicated. If urgent treatment with linezolid or I.V. methylene blue is required in a patient already receiving paroxetine and potential benefits outweigh potential risks, discontinue paroxetine promptly and administer linezolid or I.V. methylene blue. Monitor for serotonin syndrome for 2 weeks or until 24 hours after the last dose of linezolid or I.V. methylene blue, whichever comes first. May resume paroxetine 24 hours after the last dose of linezolid or I.V. methylene blue. Additional potentially significant interactions may exist, requiring dose or frequency adjustment, additional monitoring, and/or selection of alternative therapy. Consult drug interactions database for more detailed information.

An increased risk of birth defects (specifically cardiovascular malformations) has been reported when paroxetine was taken during the first trimester of pregnancy. The majority of heart defects were ventricular and atrial septal defects (VSD and ASD), some of which required surgical correction. Use paroxetine during pregnancy only if the potential benefits to the mother outweigh the possible risks to the fetus. Administration of paroxetine during late third trimester may result in adverse effects or paroxetine withdrawal syndrome in the newborn. Exposure to SSRIs late in pregnancy may also be associated with an increased risk for persistent pulmonary hypertension of the newborn (Chambers, 2006). Postmarketing reports of premature births in pregnant women receiving paroxetine or other SSRIs have been noted.

Inability to remain still due to feelings of agitation or restlessness has been observed with paroxetine and other SSRIs. Usually occurs within the first few weeks of therapy. Has low potential for sedation and anticholinergic effects relative to cyclic antidepressants; however, among the SSRI class these effects are relatively higher.

Brisdelle contains a lower dose than what is required for the treatment of psychiatric conditions. Patients who require paroxetine for the treatment of psychiatric conditions should discontinue Brisdelle and begin treatment with a paroxetine-containing medication which provides an adequate dosage. Paroxetine hydroxide (Paxil and Paxil CR) tablets contain polysorbate 80 (Tween 80) which may cause allergic reactions in susceptible individuals.

Paroxetine oral suspension contains propylene glycol; toxicities have been reported with use of products containing propylene glycol, including hyperosmolality, lactic acidosis, seizures, and respiratory depression; in neonates large amounts of propylene glycol delivered orally, intravenously (eg, >3000 mg/day), or topically have been associated with potentially fatal toxicities which can include metabolic acidosis, seizures, renal failure, and CNS depression; use oral suspension containing propylene glycol with caution (AAP, 1997; Shehab, 2009).

Precautions Use with caution in patients with renal or hepatic impairment; clearance is decreased and plasma concentrations are increased; a lower dosage may be needed. Use with caution in patients with a history of seizures. Use with caution in patients with cardiovascular disease; paroxetine has not been systemically evaluated in patients with a recent history of MI or unstable heart disease. May cause hyponatremia, use with caution in patients with volume depletion or diuretic use. May cause abnormal bleeding (eg, ecchymosis, purpura, upper GI bleeding); use with caution in patients with impaired platelet aggregation and with concurrent use of aspirin, NSAIDs, or other drugs that affect coagulation. A recent report describes five children (age: 8-15 years) who developed epistaxis (n=4) or bruising (n=1) while receiving SSRI therapy (sertraline) (Lake, 2000). Bone fractures have been associated with antidepressant treatment; consider the possibility of a fragility fracture if an antidepressant-treated patient presents with unexplained bone pain, point tenderness, swelling, or bruising. Concurrent use with tamoxifen may decrease the efficacy of tamoxifen; consider an alternative antidepressant with little or no CYP2D6 inhibition when using tamoxifen for the treatment of prevention of breast cancer. SSRI-associated vomiting is two- to threefold more prevalent in children compared to adolescents and is more prevalent in adolescents compared to adults (Safer, 2006). No clinical studies have assessed the combined use of paroxetine and electroconvulsive therapy. May cause or exacerbate sexual dysfunction in both males and females. May cause mydriasis, use with caution in patients at risk of acute narrow-angle glaucoma or with increased intraocular pressure.

Adverse Reactions

Cardiovascular: Chest pain, hypertension, palpitations, tachycardia, vasodilatation

Central nervous system: Abnormal dreams, agitation, amnesia, anxiety, chills, confusion, depersonalization, dizziness, drowsiness, emotional lability, fatigue, headache, insomnia, lack of concentration, myasthenia, myoclonus, nervousness, paresthesia, vertigo, yawning

Dermatologic: Diaphoresis, pruritus, skin rash

Endocrine & metabolic: Decreased libido, dysmenorrhea, orgasm disturbance, weight gain

Gastrointestinal: Abdominal pain, constipation, decreased appetite, diarrhea, dysgeusia, dyspepsia, flatulence, increased appetite, nausea, vomiting, xerostomia

Genitourinary: Ejaculatory disorder, female genital tract disease, impotence, male genital disease, urinary frequency, urinary tract infection

Infection: Infection

Neuromuscular & skeletal: Arthralgia, back pain, myalgia, myopathy, tremor, weakness

Ophthalmic: Blurred vision, visual disturbance

Otic: Tinnitus

Respiratory: Dyspnea, pharyngitis, rhinitis, sinusitis

Rare but important or life-threatening: Abnormal hepatic function tests, acute angle-closure glaucoma, acute renal failure, adrenergic syndrome, agranulocytosis, akathisia, akinesia, anaphylactoid reaction, anaphylaxis, anemia (various), angina pectoris, angioedema, aphasia, aphthous stomatitis, aplastic anemia, asthma, atrial arrhythmia, atrial fibrillation, bilirubinemia, bloody diarrhea, bone marrow aplasia, bradycardia, bronchitis, bulimia nervosa, bundle branch block, cardiac failure, cataract, cellulitis, cerebral ischemia, cerebrovascular accident, change in platelet count, cholelithiasis, colitis, deafness, dehydration, delirium, depression, diabetes mellitus, disorientation, drug dependence, dyskinesia, dysphagia, dystonia, eclampsia, electrolyte disturbance, emphysema, esophageal achalasia, exfoliative dermatitis, extrapyramidal reaction, fecal impaction, fungal skin infection, gastroenteritis, glaucoma, goiter, Guillain-Barre syndrome, hallucination, hematemesis, hematologic abnormality, hematologic disease, hematoma, hemoptysis, hemorrhage, hemorrhagic pancreatitis, hepatic failure, hepatic necrosis, hepatitis, hepatotoxicity, homicidal ideation, hypercholesteremia, hypergammaglobulinemia, hyperglycemia, hyperhidrosis, hypersensitivity reaction, hyperthyroidism, hypoglycemia, hyponatremia, hypotension, hypothyroidism, immune thrombocytopenia, increased blood urea nitrogen, increased creatine phosphokinase, increased lactate dehydrogenase, increased serum alkaline phosphatase, intestinal obstruction, ischemic heart disease, jaundice, ketosis, low cardiac output, lymphadenopathy, meningitis, migraine, mydriasis, myelitis, myocardial infarction, neuroleptic malignant syndrome, neuropathy, osteoarthritis, osteoporosis, pancreatitis, pancytopenia, paralytic ileus, peptic ulcer, peritonitis, phlebitis, pneumonia, prolonged bleeding time, pulmonary edema, pulmonary embolism, pulmonary fibrosis, pulmonary hypertension, restlessness, seizure, sepsis, serotonin syndrome, spermatozoa disorder (activity altered, DNA fragmentation [abnormal] increased), status epilepticus, Stevens-Johnson syndrome, suicidal ideation, suicidal tendencies, syncope, tetany, thrombophlebitis, thrombosis, torsades de pointes, toxic epidermal necrolysis, uncontrolled diabetes mellitus, vasculitis, ventricular arrhythmia, ventricular fibrillation, ventricular tachycardia, withdrawal syndrome (including increased dreaming/nightmares, muscle cramps/spasms/twitching, headache, nervousness/anxiety, fatigue/tiredness, restless feeling in legs, and trouble sleeping/insomnia)

Drug Interactions

Metabolism/Transport Effects Substrate of CYP2D6 (major); **Note:** Assignment of Major/Minor substrate status based on clinically relevant drug interaction potential; **Inhibits** CYP1A2 (weak), CYP2B6 (moderate), CYP2C19 (weak), CYP2C9 (weak), CYP2D6 (strong), CYP3A4 (weak)

Avoid Concomitant Use

Avoid concomitant use of PARoxetine with any of the following: Dosulepin; Iobenguane I 123; Linezolid; MAO Inhibitors; Methylene Blue; Pimozide; Tamoxifen; Thioridazine; Tryptophan; Urokinase

Increased Effect/Toxicity

PARoxetine may increase the levels/effects of: Agents with Antiplatelet Properties; Anticoagulants; Antidepressants (Serotonin Reuptake Inhibitor/Antagonist); Antipsychotics; Apixaban; ARIPiprazole; Asenapine; Aspirin; AtoMOXetine; Beta-Blockers; BusPIRone; CarBAMazepine; CloZAPine; Collagenase (Systemic); CYP2B6 Substrates; CYP2D6 Substrates; Dabigatran Etexilate; Desmopressin; Dextromethorphan; Dosulepin; DOXOrubicin (Conventional); DULoxetine; Fesoterodine; Galantamine; Highest Risk QTc-Prolonging Agents; Hypoglycemic Agents; Ibritumomab; Iloperidone; Lomitapide; Methadone; Methylene Blue; Metoprolol; Mexiletine; Moderate Risk QTc-Prolonging Agents; Nebivolol; NSAID (COX-2 Inhibitor); NSAID (Nonselective); Pimozide; Propafenone; Rivaroxaban; Salicylates; Serotonin Modulators; Tetrabenazine; Thiazide Diuretics; Thioridazine; Thrombolytic Agents; Tositumomab and Iodine I 131 Tositumomab; TraMADol; Tricyclic Antidepressants; Urokinase; Vitamin K Antagonists; Vortioxetine

The levels/effects of PARoxetine may be increased by: Abiraterone Acetate; Alcohol (Ethyl); Analgesics (Opioid); Antiemetics (5HT3 Antagonists); Antipsychotics; ARIPiprazole; Asenapine; BuPROPion; BusPIRone; Cimetidine; CNS Depressants; Cobicistat; CYP2D6 Inhibitors (Moderate); CYP2D6 Inhibitors (Strong); Dasatinib; DULoxetine; Glucosamine; Herbs (Anticoagulant/Antiplatelet Properties); Ibrutinib; Linezolid; Lithium; MAO Inhibitors; Metoclopramide; Metyrosine; Mifepristone; Multivitamins/Fluoride (with ADE); Multivitamins/Minerals (with ADEK, Folate, Iron); Multivitamins/Minerals (with AE, No Iron); Nonsteroidal Anti-Inflammatory Agents; Omega-3 Fatty Acids; Pentosan Polysulfate Sodium; Pentoxifylline; Pravastatin; Prostacyclin Analogues; TraMADol; Tryptophan; Vitamin E

Decreased Effect

PARoxetine may decrease the levels/effects of: Aprepitant; Codeine; Fosaprepitant; Iloperidone; Iobenguane I 123; Ioflupane I 123; Tamoxifen; Thyroid Products

The levels/effects of PARoxetine may be decreased by: Aprepitant; CarBAMazepine; Cyproheptadine; Darunavir; Fosamprenavir; Fosaprepitant; Nonsteroidal Anti-Inflammatory Agents; NSAID (COX-2 Inhibitor); NSAID (Nonselective); Peginterferon Alfa-2b

Food Interactions Peak concentration is increased, but bioavailability is not significantly altered by food. Management: Administer without regard to meals.

Stability Hazardous agent; use appropriate precautions for handling and disposal (NIOSH, 2012).

Immediate release capsule: Brisdelle: Store at 20°C to 25°C (68°F to 77°F); excursions permitted to 15°C to 30°C (59°F to 86°F); protect from light and humidity.

Immediate release tablet:

Hydrochloride salt (Paxil): Store between 15°C to 30°C (59°F to 86°F).

Mesylate salt (Pexeva): Store at 25°C (77°F); excursions permitted to 15°C to 30°C (59°F to 86°F); protect from humidity.

Oral suspension and controlled release tablet: Store at ≤25°C (≤77°F).

Mechanism of Action Paroxetine is a selective serotonin reuptake inhibitor, chemically unrelated to tricyclic, tetracyclic, or other antidepressants; presumably, the inhibition of serotonin reuptake from brain synapse stimulated serotonin activity in the brain

Pharmacodynamics

Onset of action: Antidepressant effects: The onset of action is within a week; however, individual response varies greatly and full response may not be seen until 8-12 weeks after initiation of treatment.

Antiobsessional and antipanic effects: Up to several weeks

Pharmacokinetics (Adult data unless noted)

Absorption: Oral: Well absorbed

Distribution: V_d: Mean: 8.7 L/kg; range: 3-28 L/kg

Protein binding: 93% to 95%

Metabolism: Extensive by cytochrome P450 enzymes via oxidation and methylation followed by glucuronide and sulfate conjugation; nonlinear kinetics may be seen with higher doses and longer duration of therapy due to saturation of P450 2D6 (CYP2D6), an enzyme partially responsible for metabolism. **Note:** Paroxetine pharmacokinetics have not been studied in patients deficient in CYP2D6 (ie, poor metabolizers)

Bioavailability: Immediate release tablet and oral suspension have equal bioavailability

Half-life:

Paxil: 21 hours

Paxil CR: 15-20 hours

Pexeva: 33.2 hours

Time to peak serum concentration:

Immediate release capsule: Brisdelle: Median: 6 hours (range: 3-8 hours)

Immediate release tablet:

Hydrochloride (Paxil): Mean: 5.2 hours

Mesylate (Pexeva): Mean: 8.1 hours

Controlled release tablet: 6-10 hours

Elimination: Urine (64%; 2% as unchanged drug); feces (36% primarily via bile, <1% as unchanged drug)

Dosing: Usual Note: For maintenance therapy, use lowest effective dose and periodically reassess need for continued treatment

Children and Adolescents:

Obsessive-compulsive disorder (OCD): Limited data available: Children and Adolescents 7-17 years: Oral: Initial: 10 mg once daily; titrate every 7-14 days in 10 mg/day increments; maximum daily dose: 60 mg/day. Dosing based on two trials. The first was a 12-week open-label trial of paroxetine in 20 outpatients 8-17 years of age that demonstrated the potential clinical usefulness in pediatric OCD (Rosenberg, 1999). The second trial demonstrated efficacy of paroxetine in a 10-week, randomized, double-blind, placebo-controlled trial conducted in 207 pediatric patients (aged 7-17 years) with OCD; the overall mean dose was 20.3 mg/day for children and 26.8 mg/day for adolescents (Geller, 2004). Further studies are needed.

Social anxiety disorder: Children and Adolescents 8-17 years: Oral: Initial: 10 mg once daily; titrate at intervals of at least 7 days in 10 mg/day increments; maximum daily dose: 50 mg/day. Dosing based on a 16-week multicenter, randomized, double-blind, placebo-controlled trial that reported the efficacy of paroxetine in pediatric patients (aged 8-17 years) with social anxiety disorder; 163 patients were randomized to receive paroxetine; the overall mean dose was 21.7 mg/day for children and 26.1 mg/day for adolescents (Wagner, 2004).

Adults:

Major depressive disorder (MDD): Oral:

Paxil, Pexeva: Initial: 20 mg once daily, preferably in the morning; increase if needed by 10 mg/day increments at intervals of at least 1 week; maximum daily dose: 50 mg/day

Paxil CR: Initial: 25 mg once daily; increase if needed by 12.5 mg/day increments at intervals of at least 1 week; maximum daily dose: 62.5 mg/day

Generalized anxiety disorder (GAD): Paxil, Pexeva: Oral: Initial: 20 mg once daily, preferably in the morning; if dose is increased, adjust in increments of 10 mg/day at 1-week intervals; doses of 20-50 mg/day were used in clinical trials; however, no greater benefit was seen with doses >20 mg.

Obsessive compulsive disorder (OCD): Paxil, Pexeva: Oral: Initial: 20 mg once daily, preferably in the morning;

increase if needed by 10 mg/day increments at intervals of at least 1 week; recommended dose: 40 mg/day; range: 20-60 mg/day; maximum daily dose: 60 mg/**day**

Panic disorder: Oral:

Paxil, Pexeva: Initial: 10 mg once daily, preferably in the morning; increase if needed by 10 mg/day increments at intervals of at least 1 week; recommended dose: 40 mg/day; range: 10-60 mg/day; maximum daily dose: 60 mg/**day**

Paxil CR: Initial: 12.5 mg once daily, preferably in the morning; increase if needed by 12.5 mg/day increments at intervals of at least 1 week; maximum daily dose: 75 mg/**day**

Post-traumatic stress disorder (PTSD): Paxil: Oral: Initial: 20 mg once daily, preferably in the morning; increase if needed by 10 mg/day increments at intervals of at least 1 week; range: 20-50 mg/day. Limited data suggest doses of 40 mg/day were not more efficacious than 20 mg/day.

Premenstrual dysphoric disorder: Paxil CR: Oral: Initial: 12.5 mg once daily in the morning; may be increased to 25 mg/day; dosing changes should occur at intervals of at least 1 week; may be given daily throughout the menstrual cycle **or** limited to the luteal phase

Social anxiety disorder: Oral:

Paxil: Initial: 20 mg once daily, preferably in the morning; recommended dose: 20 mg/day; range: 20-60 mg/day; doses >20 mg may not have additional benefit

Paxil CR: Initial: 12.5 mg once daily, preferably in the morning; may be increased by 12.5 mg/day increments at intervals of at least 1 week; maximum daily dose: 37.5 mg/**day**

Vasomotor symptoms of menopause: Brisdelle: Oral: 7.5 mg once daily at bedtime.

Discontinuation of therapy: Upon discontinuation of antidepressant therapy, gradually taper the dose to minimize the incidence of withdrawal symptoms and allow for the detection of re-emerging symptoms. Evidence supporting ideal taper rates is limited. APA and NICE guidelines suggest tapering therapy over at least several weeks with consideration to the half-life of the antidepressant; antidepressants with a shorter half-life may need to be tapered more conservatively. In addition, for long-term treated patients, WFSBP guidelines recommend tapering over 4-6 months. If intolerable withdrawal symptoms occur following a dose reduction, consider resuming the previously prescribed dose and/or decrease dose at a more gradual rate (APA, 2010; Bauer, 2002; Haddod, 2001; NCCMH, 2010; Schatzberg, 2006; Shelton, 2001; Warner, 2006).

MAO inhibitor recommendations:

Switching to or from an MAO inhibitor intended to treat psychiatric disorders:

Allow 14 days to elapse between discontinuing an MAO inhibitor intended to treat psychiatric disorders and initiation of paroxetine.

Allow 14 days to elapse between discontinuing paroxetine and initiation of an MAO inhibitor intended to treat psychiatric disorders.

Use with other MAO inhibitors (linezolid or I.V. methylene blue):

Do not initiate paroxetine in patients receiving linezolid or I.V. methylene blue; consider other interventions for psychiatric condition.

If urgent treatment with linezolid or I.V. methylene blue is required in a patient already receiving paroxetine and potential benefits outweigh potential risks, discontinue paroxetine promptly and administer linezolid or I.V. methylene blue. Monitor for serotonin syndrome for 2 weeks or until 24 hours after the last dose of linezolid or I.V. methylene blue, whichever

comes first. May resume paroxetine 24 hours after the last dose of linezolid or I.V. methylene blue.

Dosing adjustment in renal impairment: Adults:

Brisdelle: No dosage adjustments necessary

Paxil, Paxil CR, Pexeva:

CrCl >60 mL/minute: No dosage adjustment necessary

CrCl 30-60 mL/minute: Plasma concentration is 2 times that seen in normal function. There are no dosage adjustments provided in manufacturer's labeling.

Severe impairment (CrCl <30 mL/minute): Mean plasma concentration is ~4 times that seen in normal function.

Paxil, Pexeva: Initial: 10 mg/day; increase if needed by 10 mg/day increments at intervals of at least 1 week; maximum dose: 40 mg/day

Paxil CR: Initial: 12.5 mg/day; increase if needed by 12.5 mg/day increments at intervals of at least 1 week; maximum dose: 50 mg/day

Dosing adjustment in hepatic impairment: Adults:

Brisdelle: No dosage adjustments necessary.

Paxil, Paxil CR, Pexeva:

Mild to moderate impairment: There are no dosage adjustments provided in manufacturer's labeling.

Severe impairment:

Paxil, Pexeva: Initial: 10 mg/day; increase if needed by 10 mg/day increments at intervals of at least 1 week; maximum dose: 40 mg/day

Paxil CR: Initial: 12.5 mg/day; increase if needed by 12.5 mg/day increments at intervals of at least 1 week; maximum dose: 50 mg/day

Administration Hazardous agent; use appropriate precautions for handling and disposal (NIOSH, 2012). May be administered without regard to meals; administration with food may decrease GI side effects; shake suspension well before use. Paxil, Paxil CR, and Pexeva should preferentially be administered in the morning; whereas Brisdelle is recommended to be administered at bedtime. Do not chew or crush immediate or controlled release tablet, swallow whole

Monitoring Parameters Blood pressure, heart rate, liver and renal function. Monitor patient periodically for symptom resolution; monitor for worsening depression, suicidality, and associated behaviors (especially at the beginning of therapy or when doses are increased or decreased); signs and symptoms of serotonin syndrome; akathisia

Additional Information Paroxetine is more potent and more selective than other SSRIs (eg, fluoxetine, fluvoxamine, sertraline, and clomipramine) in the inhibition of serotonin reuptake. If used for an extended period of time, long-term usefulness of paroxetine should be periodically re-evaluated for an individual patient. Paxil CR® tablets contain a degradable polymeric matrix (that controls the dissolution rate over ~4-5 hours) and an entering coating (that delays drug release until tablets leave the stomach).

Dosage Forms Excipient information presented when available (limited, particularly for generics); consult specific product labeling.

Capsule, Oral, as mesylate [strength expressed as base]:

Brisdelle: 7.5 mg [contains fd&c red #40, fd&c yellow #6 (sunset yellow)]

Suspension, Oral, as hydrochloride [strength expressed as base]:

Paxil: 10 mg/5 mL (250 mL) [contains fd&c yellow #6 aluminum lake, methylparaben, propylene glycol, propylparaben, saccharin sodium; orange flavor]

Tablet, Oral, as hydrochloride [strength expressed as base]:

Paxil: 10 mg, 20 mg [scored]

Paxil: 30 mg, 40 mg

Generic: 10 mg, 20 mg, 30 mg, 40 mg

Tablet, Oral, as mesylate [strength expressed as base]:

Pexeva: 10 mg

Pexeva: 20 mg [scored]

◄ Pexeva: 30 mg, 40 mg

Tablet Extended Release 24 Hour, Oral, as hydrochloride [strength expressed as base]:

Paxil CR: 12.5 mg [contains fd&c yellow #10 aluminum lake, fd&c yellow #6 aluminum lake]

Paxil CR: 25 mg

Paxil CR: 37.5 mg [contains fd&c blue #2 aluminum lake]

Generic: 12.5 mg, 25 mg, 37.5 mg

References

American Academy of Pediatrics Committee on Drugs. "Inactive" ingredients in pharmaceutical products: update (subject review). *Pediatrics.* 1997;99(2):268-278.

American Psychiatric Association (APA). Treatment recommendations for patients with major depressive disorder. 3rd ed. May 2010. Available at http://www.psychiatryonline.com/pracGuide/pracGuide-Topic_7.aspx

Bauer M, Whybrow PC, Anst J, et al. World Federation of Societies of Biological Psychiatry (WFSBP) guidelines for biological treatment of unipolar depressive disorders, part 2: maintenance treatment of major depressive disorder and treatment of chronic depressive disorders and subthreshold depressions. *World J Biol Psychiatry.* 2002;3 (2):69-86.

Chambers CD, Hernandez-Diaz S, Van Marter LJ, et al, "Selective Serotonin-Reuptake Inhibitors and Risk of Persistent Pulmonary Hypertension of the Newborn," *N Engl J Med*, 2006, 354(6):579-87.

Diler RS and Avci A, "Selective Serotonin Reuptake Inhibitor Discontin-uation Syndrome in Children: Six Case Reports," *Current Therapeutic Reseach*, 2002, 63(3):188-97.

Dopheide JA, "Recognizing and Treating Depression in Children and Adolescents," *Am J Health Syst Pharm*, 2006, 63(3):233-43.

Findling RL, Reed MD, and Blumer JL, "Pharmacological Treatment of Depression in Children and Adolescents," *Paediatr Drugs*, 1999, 1 (3):161-82.

Geller DA, Wagner KD, Emslie G, et al, "Paroxetine Treatment in Children and Adolescents With Obsessive-Compulsive Disorder: A Randomized, Multicenter, Double-Blind, Placebo-Controlled Trial," *J Am Acad Child Adolesc Psychiatry*, 2004, 43(11):1387-96.

Haddad PM. Antidepressant discontinuation syndromes. *Drug Saf.* 2001;24(3):183-197.

Horrigan JP and Barnhill LJ, "Paroxetine-Pimozide Drug Interactions," *J Am Acad Child Adolesc Psychiatry*, 1994, 33(7):1060-1.

Keller MB, Ryan ND, Strober M, et al, "Efficacy of Paroxetine in the Treatment of Adolescent Major Depression: A Randomized, Con-trolled Trial," *J Am Acad Child Adolesc Psychiatry*, 2001, 40 (7):762-72.

Lake MB, Birmaher B, Wassick S, et al, "Bleeding and Selective Serotonin Reuptake Inhibitors in Childhood and Adolescence," *J Child Adolesc Psychopharmacol*, 2000, 10(1):35-8.

Levinson-Castiel R, Merlob P, Linder N, et al, "Neonatal Abstinence Syndrome After *in utero* Exposure to Selective Serotonin Reuptake Inhibitors in Term Infants," *Arch Pediatr Adolesc Med*, 2006, 160 (2):173-6.

Markel H, Lee A, Holmes RD, et al, "LSD Flashback Syndrome Exacerbated by Selective Serotonin Reuptake Inhibitor Antidepres-sants in Adolescents," *J Pediatr*, 1994, 125(5 Pt 1):817-9.

National Collaborating Centre for Mental Health (NCCMH). Depression: the treatment and management of depression in adults (updated edition). National Institute for Health & Clinical Excellence (NICE). 2010.

National Institute for Occupational Safety and Health (NIOSH), "NIOSH List of Antineoplastic and Other Hazardous Drugs in Healthcare Settings 2012." Available at http://www.cdc.gov/niosh/docs/2012-150/pdfs/2012-150.pdf. Accessed January 21, 2013.

Rey-Sanchez F and Guitierrez-Cassares JR, "Paroxetine in Children With Major Depressive Disorder: An Open Trial," *J Am Acad Child Adolesc Psychiatry*, 1997, 36(10):1443-7.

Rosenberg DR, Stewart CM, Fitzgerald KD, et al, "Paroxetine Open-Label Treatment of Pediatric Outpatients With Obsessive-Compulsive Disorder," *J Am Acad Child Adolesc Psychiatry*, 1999, 38(9):1180-5.

Safer DJ and Zito JM, "Treatment Emergent Adverse Effects of Selective Serotonin Reuptake Inhibitors by Age Group: Children vs. Adolescents," *J Child Adolesc Psychopharmacol*, 2006, 16 (1/2):159-69.

Schatzberg AF, Blier P, Delgado PL, Fava M, Haddad PM, Shelton RC. Antidepressant discontinuation syndrome: consensus panel recom-mendations for clinical management and additional research. *J Clin Psychiatry*. 2006;67(Suppl 4):27-30.

Sharp SC and Hellings JA, "Efficacy and Safety of Selective Serotonin Reuptake Inhibitors in the Treatment of Depression in Children and Adolescents: Practitioner Review," *Clin Drug Investig*, 2006, 26 (5):247-55.

Shehab N, Lewis CL, Streetman DD, Donn SM. Exposure to the pharmaceutical excipients benzyl alcohol and propylene glycol among critically ill neonates. *Pediatr Crit Care Med.* 2009;10 (2):256-259.

Shelton, RC. Steps following attainment of remission: discontinuation of antidepressant therapy. *Prim Care Companion J Clin Psychiatry.* 2001;3(4):168-174.

Stiskal JA, Kulin N, Koren G, et al, "Neonatal Paroxetine Withdrawal Syndrome," *Arch Dis Child Fetal Neonatal Ed*, 2001, 84(2):F134-5.

Wagner KD, Berard R, Stein MB, et al, "A Multicenter, Randomized, Double-Blind, Placebo-Controlled Trial of Paroxetine in Children and Adolescents With Social Anxiety Disorder," *Arch Gen Psychiatry*, 2004, 61(11):1153-62.

Wagner KD, "Pharmacotherapy for Major Depression in Children and Adolescents," *Prog Neuropsychopharmacol Biol Psychiatry*, 2005, 29 (5):819-26.

Warner CH, Bobo W, Warner C, Reid S, Rachal J. Antidepressant discontinuation syndrome. *Am Fam Physician.* 2006;74:449-456.

◆ **Paroxetine Hydrochloride** *see* PARoxetine *on page 1609*

◆ **Paroxetine Mesylate** *see* PARoxetine *on page 1609*

◆ **Parvolex® (Can)** *see* Acetylcysteine *on page 60*

◆ **Pat-Rabeprazole (Can)** *see* RABEprazole *on page 1797*

◆ **Pavabid** *see* Papaverine *on page 1599*

◆ **Pavulon [DSC]** *see* Pancuronium *on page 1593*

◆ **Paxil** *see* PARoxetine *on page 1609*

◆ **Paxil CR** *see* PARoxetine *on page 1609*

◆ **PCA (error-prone abbreviation)** *see* Procainamide *on page 1740*

◆ **PCB** *see* Procarbazine *on page 1743*

◆ **PCC (Caution: Confusion-prone synonym)** *see* Factor IX Complex (Human) [(Factors II, IX, X)] *on page 833*

◆ **PCE** *see* Erythromycin (Systemic) *on page 780*

◆ **PCEC** *see* Rabies Vaccine *on page 1801*

◆ **PC-Tar [OTC]** *see* Coal Tar *on page 532*

◆ **PCV13** *see* Pneumococcal Conjugate Vaccine (13-Val-ent) *on page 1688*

◆ **PCZ** *see* Procarbazine *on page 1743*

◆ **PediaCare Childrens Allergy [OTC]** *see* Diphenhydr-AMINE (Systemic) *on page 673*

◆ **PediaCare Childrens Long-Act [OTC]** *see* Dextrome-thorphan *on page 636*

◆ **Pediacel® (Can)** *see* Diphtheria and Tetanus Toxoids, Acellular Pertussis, Poliovirus and *Haemophilus* b Con-jugate Vaccine *on page 684*

◆ **Pediaderm AF Complete** *see* Nystatin (Topical) *on page 1517*

◆ **Pediaderm HC** *see* Hydrocortisone (Topical) *on page 1038*

◆ **Pediaderm TA** *see* Triamcinolone (Topical) *on page 2078*

◆ **Pedia-Lax [OTC]** *see* Docusate *on page 701*

◆ **Pedia-Lax [OTC]** *see* Glycerin *on page 976*

◆ **Pedia-Lax [OTC]** *see* Magnesium Hydroxide *on page 1294*

◆ **Pediapred** *see* PrednisoLONE (Systemic) *on page 1727*

◆ **Pediarix®** *see* Diphtheria, Tetanus Toxoids, Acellular Pertussis, Hepatitis B (Recombinant), and Poliovirus (Inactivated) Vaccine *on page 690*

◆ **Pediatex® TD** *see* Triprolidine and Pseudoephedrine *on page 2090*

◆ **Pediatric Digoxin CSD (Can)** *see* Digoxin *on page 658*

◆ **Pediatrix (Can)** *see* Acetaminophen *on page 47*

◆ **Pediazole® (Can)** *see* Erythromycin and Sulfisoxazole *on page 785*

◆ **Pedi-Boro [OTC]** *see* Aluminum Acetate *on page 110*

◆ **Pedi-Dri** *see* Nystatin (Topical) *on page 1517*

◆ **Pedipirox-4 Nail** *see* Ciclopirox *on page 465*

◆ **Peditrace** *see* Trace Elements *on page 2059*

- **PedvaxHIB** *see Haemophilus* b Conjugate Vaccine *on page 994*
- **PEG** *see Polyethylene Glycol 3350 on page 1696*
- **PEG-L-asparaginase** *see Pegaspargase on page 1615*
- **Peg 3350 (Can)** *see Polyethylene Glycol 3350 on page 1696*
- **Pegalax (Can)** *see Polyethylene Glycol 3350 on page 1696*
- **PEG-ASP** *see Pegaspargase on page 1615*
- **PEG-asparaginase** *see Pegaspargase on page 1615*

Pegaspargase (peg AS par jase)

Medication Safety Issues
Sound-alike/look-alike issues:
Oncaspar may be confused with Elspar
Pegaspargase may be confused with asparaginase (*E. coli*), asparaginase (*Erwinia*), peginesatide
High alert medication:
This medication is in a class the Institute for Safe Medication Practices (ISMP) includes among its list of drug classes that have a heightened risk of causing significant patient harm when used in error.

Related Information
Emetogenic Potential of Antineoplastic Agents in Children *on page 2327*
Safe Handling of Hazardous Drugs *on page 2419*

Brand Names: U.S. Oncaspar

Therapeutic Category Antineoplastic Agent, Enzyme; Antineoplastic Agent, Miscellaneous

Generic Availability (U.S.) No

Use First-line treatment of newly diagnosed acute lymphoblastic leukemia (ALL) as part of a multiple chemotherapeutic drug regimen (FDA approved in ages ≥1 year and adults); induction treatment of acute lymphoblastic leukemia in combination with other chemotherapeutic agents in patients who have developed hypersensitivity to native forms of L-asparaginase derived from *E. coli* and/or *Erwinia chrysanthemia* (FDA approved in ages ≥1 year and adults); has been used for the treatment of lymphoma and acute myelogenous leukemia (AML)

Pregnancy Risk Factor C

Pregnancy Considerations Animal reproduction studies have not been conducted with pegaspargase.

Breast-Feeding Considerations It is not known if pegaspargase is excreted in breast milk. Due to the potential for serious adverse reactions in the nursing infant, the manufacturer recommends a decision be made whether to discontinue nursing or to discontinue the drug, taking into account the importance of treatment to the mother.

Contraindications Hypersensitivity to pegaspargase or any component; history of any of the following with prior L-asparaginase treatment: Pancreatitis, serious hemorrhagic events, serious thrombosis

Warnings Hazardous agent; use appropriate precautions for handling and disposal (NIOSH, 2012); inhalation of vapors and contact with skin, eyes, or mucous membranes must be avoided. Serious allergic reactions may occur; discontinue in patients with serious allergic reaction. Observe patients for at least 1 hour after administration; immediate treatment for hypersensitivity reactions should be available during administration. Pegaspargase is indicated for use in patients who have had hypersensitivity reactions to native L-asparaginase; however, in one study, 32% of patients with a history of allergic reaction to *E. coli* asparaginase products also experienced allergic reaction to pegaspargase. Serious thrombotic events can occur in patients receiving pegaspargase. Pancreatitis can occur in patients receiving pegaspargase (promptly evaluate patients with abdominal pain). Discontinue pegaspargase

if anaphylaxis or serious allergic reaction, thrombosis, or pancreatitis occur.

Glucose intolerance can occur in patients receiving pegaspargase. Coagulopathy with elevated prothrombin time, partial thromboplastin time, and hypofibrinogenemia can occur in patients receiving pegaspargase (monitor coagulation parameters at baseline and periodically during and after treatment). In patients with severe or symptomatic coagulopathy, treat with fresh-frozen plasma. Reversible hepatotoxicity (hyperbilirubinemia and liver enzyme elevation) may occur.

Precautions Use with caution in patients with an underlying coagulopathy or previous hematologic complication from asparaginase; patients receiving anticoagulation therapy, aspirin, or NSAIDs; use with caution in patients with hyperglycemia, diabetes, hepatic dysfunction, or in patients receiving hepatotoxic agents

Adverse Reactions
Cardiovascular: Thrombosis
Central nervous system: Cerebral thrombosis (or hemorrhage of the brain)
Endocrine & metabolic: Hyperglycemia (some patients required insulin therapy)
Gastrointestinal: Pancreatitis (includes 3 deaths)
Hematologic: Blood coagulation disorder (includes increased prothrombin time or partial thromboplastin time or decreased serum fibrogen)
Hepatic: Abnormal hepatic function tests, hyperbilirubinemia, increased serum transaminases (ALT, AST)
Hypersensitivity: Hypersensitivity reaction (includes anaphylaxis, bronchospasm, erythema, hives, hypotension, laryngeal edema, skin rash, swelling, urticaria; relapsed ALL with no prior asparaginase hypersensitivity, relapsed ALL with prior asparaginase hypersensitivity)
Hepatic:
Immunologic: Hypersensitivity to L-asparaginase
Rare but important or life-threatening: Abdominal pain, anemia, arthralgia, bronchospasm, chest pain, coagulation time increased, colitis, confusion, constipation, deep vein thrombosis, disseminated intravascular coagulation, dizziness, dyspnea, emotional lability, endocarditis, facial edema, gastrointestinal pain, headache, hemorrhagic cystitis, hepatic failure, hyperuricemia, hypoglycemia, increased thirst, lip edema, liver steatosis, myalgia, night sweats, ostealgia, pancytopenia, paresthesia, purpura, renal failure, sagittal sinus thrombosis, seizure, septic shock, superficial venous thrombosis

Drug Interactions
Metabolism/Transport Effects None known.
Avoid Concomitant Use
Avoid concomitant use of Pegaspargase with any of the following: BCG; Natalizumab; Pimecrolimus; Tacrolimus (Topical); Tofacitinib; Vaccines (Live)
Increased Effect/Toxicity
Pegaspargase may increase the levels/effects of: Leflunomide; Natalizumab; Tofacitinib; Vaccines (Live)

The levels/effects of Pegaspargase may be increased by: Denosumab; Pimecrolimus; Roflumilast; Tacrolimus (Topical); Trastuzumab
Decreased Effect
Pegaspargase may decrease the levels/effects of: BCG; Coccidioidin Skin Test; Sipuleucel-T; Vaccines (Inactivated); Vaccines (Live)

The levels/effects of Pegaspargase may be decreased by: Echinacea; Pegloticase

Stability Hazardous agent; use appropriate precautions for handling and disposal (NIOSH, 2012). Store intact vials at 2°C to 8°C (36°F to 46°F); do not freeze; do not administer if there is any indication that the drug has been frozen or that vial has been stored at room temperature [15°C to 25°C (59°F to 77°F)] for >48 hours. If not used immediately, solutions for infusion should be refrigerated immediately after preparation and administered within 24 hours of preparation. Avoid excessive agitation, do not shake; do not use if cloudy or discolored or if precipitate is present; use of a 0.2 micron filter may result in some loss of potency.

Mechanism of Action Pegaspargase is a modified version of L-asparaginase, conjugated with polyethylene glycol. In leukemic cells, asparaginase hydrolyzes L-asparagine to ammonia and L-aspartic acid, leading to depletion of asparagine. Leukemia cells, especially lymphoblasts, require exogenous asparagine; normal cells can synthesize asparagine. Asparagine depletion in leukemic cells leads to inhibition of protein synthesis and apoptosis. Asparaginase is cycle-specific for the G_1 phase of the cell cycle.

Pharmacodynamics
Onset of action: Asparagine depletion: I.M.: Within 4 days
Duration: Asparagine depletion:
I.M.: ~21 days
I.V.: 2-4 weeks (in asparaginase-naïve adults)

Pharmacokinetics (Adult data unless noted)
Absorption: Not absorbed from the GI tract; therefore, requires parenteral administration; I.M.: Slow
Distribution:
Apparent V_d: Plasma volume:
I.M.: Children: 1.5 L/m^2
I.V.: Adults (asparaginase-naïve): 2.4 L/m^2
Half-life:
I.M.: Children: 5.8 days; Adults: 5.5-6 days; 3.2 ± 1.8 days in patients who previously had a hypersensitivity reaction to native L-asparaginase
I.V.: Adults (asparaginase-naïve): 7 days
Time to peak serum concentration: I.M.: 3-4 days
Elimination: Clearance is unaffected by age, renal function, or hepatic function; not detected in urine

Dosing: Usual (Refer to individual protocols):Children (>1 year), Adolescents, and Adults: I.M., I.V.: 2500 units/m^2/dose ≥every 14 days (as part of a combination chemotherapy regimen)

Administration Hazardous agent; use appropriate precautions for handling and disposal (NIOSH, 2012).
I.M.: Limit the volume at a single injection site to 2 mL; for I.M. administration, if the volume to be administered is >2 mL, use multiple injection sites
I.V.: Administer dose as an I.V. infusion in 100 mL of D_5W or NS over a period of 1-2 hours through a running I.V. infusion line

Monitoring Parameters Vital signs during administration, CBC with differential, platelet count, urinalysis, serum amylase, liver enzymes, bilirubin, prothrombin time, renal function tests, urine glucose, blood glucose, uric acid, fibrinogen levels. Observe patients for 1 hour after administration for signs of anaphylaxis and serious allergic reactions.

Dosage Forms Excipient information presented when available (limited, particularly for generics); consult specific product labeling.
Solution, Injection [preservative free]:
Oncaspar: 750 units/mL (5 mL)

References
Asselin BL, Whitin JC, Cappola DJ, et al, "Comparative Pharmacokinetic Studies of Three Asparaginase Preparations," *J Clin Oncol*, 1993, 11(9):1780-6.

Avramis VI and Panosyan EH, "Pharmacokinetic/Pharmacodynamic Relationships of Asparaginase Formulations: The Past, the Present and Recommendations for the Future," *Clin Pharmacokinet*, 2005, 44 (4):367-93.

Avramis VI and Spence SA, "Clinical Pharmacology of Asparaginases in the United States: Asparaginase Population Pharmacokinetic and Pharmacodynamic (PK-PD) Models (NONMEM) in Adult and Pediatric ALL Patients," *J Pediatr Hematol Oncol*, 2007, 29(4):239-47.

Avramis VI, Sencer S, Periclou AP, et al, "A Randomized Comparison of Native *Escherichia coli* Asparaginase and Polyethylene Glycol Conjugated Asparaginase for Treatment of Children With Newly Diagnosed Standard-Risk Acute Lymphoblastic Leukemia: A Children's Cancer Group Study," *Blood*, 2002, 99(6):1986-94.

Capizzi RL, "Asparaginase Revisited," *Leuk Lymphoma*, 1993, 10 (Suppl):147-50.

Douer D, Yampolsky H, Cohen LJ, et al, "Pharmacodynamics and Safety of Intravenous Pegaspargase During Remission Induction in Adults Aged 55 Years or Younger With Newly Diagnosed Acute Lymphoblastic Leukemia," *Blood*, 2007, 109(7):2744-50.

Jarrar M, Gaynon PS, Periclou AP, et al, "Asparagine Depletion After Pegylated *E. coli* Asparaginase Treatment and Induction Outcome in Children With Acute Lymphoblastic Leukemia in First Bone Marrow Relapse: A Children's Oncology Group Study (CCG-1941)," *Pediatr Blood Cancer*, 2006, 47(2):141-6.

National Institute for Occupational Safety and Health (NIOSH), "NIOSH List of Antineoplastic and Other Hazardous Drugs in Healthcare Settings 2012." Available at http://www.cdc.gov/niosh/docs/2012-150/pdfs/2012-150.pdf. Accessed January 21, 2013.

◆ **Pegasys** *see* Peginterferon Alfa-2a *on page 1617*

◆ **Pegasys® (Can)** *see* Peginterferon Alfa-2a *on page 1617*

◆ **Pegasys ProClick** *see* Peginterferon Alfa-2a *on page 1617*

Pegfilgrastim (peg fil GRA stim)

Medication Safety Issues
Sound-alike/look-alike issues:
Neulasta may be confused with Neumega, Neupogen, Nuedexta, and Lunesta
Brand Names: U.S. Neulasta
Brand Names: Canada Neulasta
Therapeutic Category Colony Stimulating Factor; Hematopoietic Agent
Generic Availability (U.S.) No
Use Reduction of the duration of neutropenia and the associated risk of infection in patients with nonmyeloid malignancies receiving myelosuppressive chemotherapeutic regimens associated with a significant incidence of febrile neutropenia
Pregnancy Risk Factor C
Pregnancy Considerations Adverse events were observed in some animal reproduction studies.

Women who are exposed to Neulasta during pregnancy are encouraged to enroll in the Amgen Pregnancy Surveillance Program (800-772-6436).

Breast-Feeding Considerations It is not known if pegfilgrastim is excreted in breast milk. The manufacturer recommends that caution be exercised when administering pegfilgrastim to nursing women.

Contraindications Hypersensitivity to filgrastim, pegfilgrastim, or any component; use in the period between 14 days before and 24 hours after administration of cytotoxic chemotherapy

Warnings Splenic rupture, including fatal cases, has been reported following the administration of pegfilgrastim. Patients experiencing left upper abdominal and/or shoulder tip pain should be evaluated for an enlarged spleen or splenic rupture. ARDS has been reported with use; evaluate patients with pulmonary symptoms such as fever, lung infiltrates, or respiratory distress; withhold or discontinue pegfilgrastim if ARDS occurs. Allergic reactions including anaphylaxis, angioedema, skin rash, erythema, and urticaria have occurred primarily with the initial dose and may recur after discontinuation (reaction may be delayed); close follow-up for several days and permanent discontinuation are recommended for severe reactions.

Do not administer 14 days prior to or within 24 hours following the administration of chemotherapy due to the potential sensitivity of rapidly dividing myeloid cells to cytotoxic chemotherapy. Benefit has not been demonstrated with regimens under a 2-week duration. Administration on the same day as chemotherapy is not recommended (NCCN Myeloid Growth Factor Guidelines, v.1, 2009). Safety and efficacy have not been evaluated for use in peripheral blood progenitor cell (PBPC) mobilization or in patients receiving radiation therapy. May precipitate sickle cell crises in patients with sickle cell disease; carefully evaluate potential risks vs benefits when considering use in this patient population. Use has not been evaluated in patients receiving chemotherapy associated with delayed myelosuppression (eg, nitrosoureas, mitomycin C).

Precautions Use with caution in any malignancy with myeloid characteristics due to pegfilgrastim's potential to act as a growth factor; use with caution in patients with gout; psoriasis; monitor patients with preexisting cardiac conditions as cardiac events (MIs, arrhythmias) have been reported in premarketing clinical studies with the parent drug filgrastim. The 6 mg fixed dose should not be used in infants, children, and adolescents weighing <45 kg.

Adverse Reactions
Cardiovascular: Peripheral edema
Central nervous system: Headache
Gastrointestinal: Constipation, vomiting
Neuromuscular & skeletal: Arthralgia, bone pain, myalgia, weakness
Miscellaneous: Antibody formation
Rare but important or life-threatening: Acute respiratory distress syndrome (ARDS), allergic reaction, anaphylaxis, cutaneous vasculitis, erythema, fever, flushing, hyperleukocytosis, hypoxia, injection site reactions (erythema, induration, pain), leukocytosis, rash, sickle cell crisis, splenic rupture, Sweet's syndrome (acute febrile dermatosis), urticaria. Cytopenias resulting from an antibody response to exogenous growth factors have been reported on rare occasions in patients treated with other recombinant growth factors.

Drug Interactions
Metabolism/Transport Effects None known.
Avoid Concomitant Use There are no known interactions where it is recommended to avoid concomitant use.
Increased Effect/Toxicity There are no known significant interactions involving an increase in effect.
Decreased Effect
The levels/effects of Pegfilgrastim may be decreased by: Pegloticase

Stability Store in refrigerator; do not freeze; if inadvertently frozen, allow to thaw in refrigerator; discard if frozen more than one time. Allow to reach room temperature prior to injection. May be kept at room temperature for up to 48 hours. Protect from light.

Mechanism of Action Stimulates the production, maturation, and activation of neutrophils, pegfilgrastim activates neutrophils to increase both their migration and cytotoxicity. Pegfilgrastim has a prolonged duration of effect relative to filgrastim and a reduced renal clearance.

Pharmacokinetics (Adult data unless noted) Half-life: Adults: 15-80 hours; Children (100 mcg/kg dose): ~20-30 hours (range: Up to 68 hours)
Elimination: Primarily through binding to neutrophils

Dosing: Usual SubQ: **Note:** Do not administer in the period between 14 days before and 24 hours after administration of cytotoxic chemotherapy. According to the NCCN guidelines, efficacy has been demonstrated with every 2-week chemotherapy regimens; however, benefit has not been demonstrated with regimens under a 2-week duration (Myeloid Growth Factor Guidelines, v.1, 2009)
Children (limited studies in children): 100 mcg/kg (maximum dose: 6 mg) once per chemotherapy cycle, beginning 24-72 hours after completion of chemotherapy
Adolescents >45 kg and Adults: 6 mg once per chemotherapy cycle, beginning 24-72 hours after completion of chemotherapy

Dosage adjustment in renal impairment: No adjustment necessary

Administration Parenteral: SubQ: Administer undiluted solution; do not shake

Monitoring Parameters Temperature, CBC with differential and platelet count
Evaluate for left upper abdominal pain, shoulder tip pain, or splenomegaly. Monitor for sickle cell crisis (in patients with sickle cell anemia).

Test Interactions May interfere with bone imaging studies; increased hematopoietic activity of the bone marrow may appear as transient positive bone imaging changes

Dosage Forms Excipient information presented when available (limited, particularly for generics); consult specific product labeling.
Solution, Subcutaneous [preservative free]:
Neulasta: 6 mg/0.6 mL (0.6 mL)

References
André N, Kababri ME, Bertrand P, et al, "Safety and Efficacy of Pegfilgrastim in Children With Cancer Receiving Myelosuppressive Chemotherapy," *Anticancer Drugs*, 2007, 18(3):277-81.
André N, Milano E, Rome A, et al, "Safety of Pegfilgrastim in Children," *Ann Pharmacother*, 2008, 42(2):290.
Fox E, Jayaprakash N, Widemann BC, et al, "Randomized Trial and Pharmacokinetic Study of Pegfilgrastim vs. Filgrastim in Children and Young Adults With Newly Diagnosed Sarcoma Treated With Dose Intensive Chemotherapy," *J Clin Oncol*, 2006, 24(18S):9020 [abstract from 2006 ASCO Annual Meeting Proceedings, Part I].
Koontz SE, Mohassel LR, Jaffe N, et al, "Safety and Efficacy of Pegfilgrastim in Pediatric Oncology Patients: The M.D. Anderson Cancer Center Experience," *J Clin Oncol*, 2004, 22(14S):8272.
National Comprehensive Cancer Network (NCCN), "Clinical Practice Guidelines in Oncology™: Myeloid Growth Factors," Version 1, 2009. Available at http://www.nccn.org/professionals/physician_gls/PDF/myeloid_growth.pdf.
Smith TJ, Khatcheressian J, Lyman GH, et al, "2006 Update of Recommendations for the Use of White Blood Cell Growth Factors: An Evidence-Based Clinical Practice Guideline," *J Clin Oncol*, 2006, 24(19):3187-205.
Snyder RL and Stringham DJ, "Pegfilgrastim-Induced Hyperleukocytosis," *Ann of Pharmacother*, 2007, 41(9):1524-30.
te Poele EM, Kamps WA, Tamminga, RY, et al, "Pegfilgrastim in Pediatric Cancer Patients," *J Pediat Hematol Oncol*, 2005, 27 (11):627-9.
Wendelin G, Lackner H, Schwinger W, et al, "Once-Per-Cycle Pegfilgrastim Versus Daily Filgrastim in Pediatric Patients With Ewing Sarcoma," *J Pediatr Hematol Oncol*, 2005, 27(8):449-51.

◆ **PEG-IFN Alfa-2a** *see* Peginterferon Alfa-2a *on page 1617*
◆ **PEG-IFN Alfa-2b** *see* Peginterferon Alfa-2b *on page 1621*

Peginterferon Alfa-2a
(peg in ter FEER on AL fa too aye)

Related Information
Emetogenic Potential of Antineoplastic Agents in Children *on page 2327*
Brand Names: U.S. Pegasys; Pegasys ProClick
Brand Names: Canada Pegasys®
Therapeutic Category Interferon
Generic Availability (U.S.) No
Use
Chronic hepatitis C: Treatment of chronic hepatitis C virus (HCV) infection in patients with compensated liver disease and who have not been previously treated with interferon alfa alone or in combination with ribavirin (monotherapy with peginterferon alfa-2a is not recommended for treatment of chronic hepatitis C infection unless a patient has a contraindication to or significant intolerance of ribavirin) (FDA approved in ages ≥5 years and adults); treatment of chronic hepatitis C virus (HCV) infection in patients with histological evidence of cirrhosis (Child-Pugh class A) and compensated liver disease (FDA approved in adults); treatment of patients ▸

coinfected with HCV and clinically stable HIV disease (CD$_4$ count >100 cells/mm^3) (FDA approved in adults)

Combination with ribavirin is indicated in patients with HCV genotypes other than 1, pediatric patients (5-17 years), or patients with HCV genotype 1 where use of an HCV NS3/4A protease inhibitor is not warranted based on tolerability, contraindications, or other clinical factors.

Combination with ribavirin and an HCV NS3/4A protease inhibitor is indicated in adults with HCV genotype 1.

Chronic hepatitis B: Treatment with hepatitis B e antigen (HBeAg)-positive and HBeAG-negative chronic hepatitis B virus (HBV) infection who have compensated liver disease and evidence of viral replication and liver inflammation (FDA approved in adults)

Medication Guide Available Yes

Pregnancy Risk Factor C / X in combination with ribavirin

Pregnancy Considerations Reproduction studies with pegylated interferon alfa have not been conducted. Animal studies with nonpegylated interferon alfa-2b have demonstrated abortifacient effects. Disruption of the normal menstrual cycle was also observed in animal studies; therefore, the manufacturer recommends that reliable contraception is used in women of childbearing potential. Alfa interferon is endogenous to normal amniotic fluid. *In vitro* administration studies have reported that when administered to the mother, it does not cross the placenta. Case reports of use in pregnant women are limited. The Perinatal HIV Guidelines Working Group does not recommend that peginterferon-alfa be used during pregnancy. Peginterferon monotherapy should only be used in pregnancy when the potential benefit to the mother justifies the possible risk to the fetus. **[U.S. Boxed Warning]: Combination therapy with ribavirin may cause birth defects; avoid pregnancy in females and female partners of male patients;** combination therapy with ribavirin is contraindicated in pregnancy (refer to Ribavirin monograph); a pregnancy registry has been established for women inadvertently exposed to ribavirin while pregnant (800-593-2214).

Breast-Feeding Considerations Breast milk samples obtained from a lactating mother prior to and after administration of interferon alfa-2b showed that interferon alfa is present in breast milk and administration of the medication did not significantly affect endogenous levels. Breast-feeding is not linked to the spread of hepatitis C virus; however, if nipples are cracked or bleeding, breast-feeding is not recommended. Mothers coinfected with HIV are discouraged from breast-feeding to decrease potential transmission of HIV.

Contraindications Hypersensitivity to interferon alfa, polyethylene glycol (PEG), or any component; autoimmune hepatitis; decompensated liver disease in cirrhotic patients (Child-Pugh score >6); in patients with chronic HCV and coinfected with HIV decompensated liver disease (Child-Pugh score ≥6, class B and C); in neonates and infants due to benzyl alcohol excipient. Combination therapy with ribavirin is additionally contraindicated in pregnancy; men whose female partners are pregnant; hypersensitivity (urticaria, angioedema, bronchoconstriction, and anaphylaxis) to ribavirin any component of the tablet; hemoglobinopathies (eg, thalassemia major, sickle-cell anemia); concurrent didanosine use

Warnings May cause or exacerbate life-threatening neuropsychiatric disorders **[U.S. Boxed Warning]**; monitor closely; discontinue treatment with worsening or persistently severe signs/symptoms of neuropsychiatric disorders. In most cases, these effects were reversible following discontinuation, but not all cases. Neuropsychiatric adverse effects include depression, suicidal ideation, suicide attempt, homicidal ideation, drug overdose, and relapse of drug addiction, and may occur in patients with or without a prior history of psychiatric disorder. Avoid use in severe psychiatric disorders; use with extreme caution in patients with a history of depression. May cause CNS effects; patients who experience dizziness, confusion, somnolence, or fatigue should use caution when performing tasks which require mental alertness (eg, operating machinery or driving).

May cause or exacerbate autoimmune disorders **[U.S. Boxed Warning]**; monitor closely; discontinue treatment in patients with worsening or persistently severe signs/symptoms of autoimmune disease. Thyroiditis, thrombotic thrombocytopenic purpura, immune thrombocytopenia (ITP), rheumatoid arthritis, interstitial nephritis, systemic lupus erythematosus, and psoriasis have been reported with interferon therapy; use with caution in patients with autoimmune disorders.

May cause or aggravate infectious disorders; monitor closely; discontinue treatment in patients with worsening or persistently severe signs/symptoms of infectious disorders **[U.S. Boxed Warning]**; serious and severe infections (bacterial, viral, and fungal) have been reported with treatment. Interferon therapy is commonly associated with flu-like symptoms, including fever; however, rule out other causes/infection with persistent or high fever. May cause myelosuppression (including neutropenia, thrombocytopenia, lymphopenia, aplastic anemia). Use caution with baseline neutrophil count <1500/mm^3, platelet count <90,000/mm^3 or hemoglobin <10 g/dL. Discontinue therapy (at least temporarily) if ANC <500/mm^3 or platelet count <25,000/mm^3.

Hepatic decompensation and death have been associated with the use of alpha interferons, including Pegasys®, in cirrhotic chronic hepatitis C patients; patients coinfected with HIV and receiving highly active antiretroviral therapy have shown an increased risk. Monitor hepatic function closely during use; discontinue if decompensation occurs (Child-Pugh score >6) in monoinfected patients and (Child-Pugh score ≥6, class B and C) in patients coinfected with HIV. In hepatitis B patients, flares (transient and potentially severe increases in serum ALT) may occur during or after treatment; more frequent monitoring of LFTs and a dose reduction are recommended. Discontinue if ALT elevation continues despite dose reduction or if increased bilirubin or hepatic decompensation occur.

May cause ocular effects including decreased vision, retinal hemorrhages, retinal detachment (serous), cotton wool spots, and retinal artery or vein obstruction; discontinue if any ocular symptoms occur during use and a complete eye exam should be performed promptly. Prior to use, all patients should have a visual exam and patients with preexisting disorders (eg, diabetic or hypertensive retinopathy) should have periodically during therapy.

Serious cutaneous reactions, including vesiculobullous eruptions, Stevens-Johnson syndrome, and exfoliative dermatitis, have been reported (rarely) with use, with or without ribavirin therapy; discontinue with signs or symptoms of severe skin reactions. Severe acute hypersensitivity reactions have occurred rarely; prompt discontinuation is advised.

Gastrointestinal hemorrhage, ulcerative and hemorrhagic/ischemic colitis have been observed with interferon alfa treatment; may be severe and/or life-threatening; discontinue if symptoms of colitis (eg, abdominal pain, bloody diarrhea, and/or fever) develop. Colitis generally resolves within 1-3 weeks of discontinuation. Use with caution in patients with an increased risk for severe anemia (eg, spherocytosis, history of GI bleeding). May cause pancreatitis; discontinue therapy if known or suspected pancreatitis develops.

May cause or aggravate ischemic disorders and hemorrhagic cerebrovascular events **[U.S. Boxed Warning]**; cerebrovascular events have been reported in patients without risk factors for stroke (including <45 years of age); monitor closely; discontinue treatment in patients with worsening or persistent ischemia.

May cause or aggravate dyspnea, pulmonary infiltrates, pneumonia, bronchiolitis obliterans, interstitial pneumonia, and sarcoidosis, resulting in potentially fatal respiratory failure; may recur upon rechallenge with interferons. Discontinue with unexplained pulmonary infiltrates or evidence of impaired pulmonary function. Use with caution in patients with pulmonary dysfunction or a history of pulmonary disease.

Combination treatment with ribavirin may cause birth defects and/or fetal mortality; hemolytic anemia (which may worsen cardiac disease), genotoxicity, mutagenicity, and may possibly be carcinogenic **[U.S. Boxed Warning]**. Avoid pregnancy in females and female partners of male patients **[U.S. Boxed Warning]**; combination therapy with ribavirin is contraindicated in pregnancy. Pretreatment pregnancy screening (if woman of childbearing age) is recommended.

Due to differences in dosage, patients should not change brands of interferon without the concurrence of their healthcare provider. Solution for injection contains benzyl alcohol and polysorbate 80 (Tween 80®) which may cause allergic reactions in susceptible individuals.

Precautions Use with caution in renal impairment; clearance is decreased; if CrCl <30 mL/minute dosage adjustment recommended and monitor closely for signs/symptoms of interferon toxicity or laboratory abnormalities; if occur, further dosage reductions may be required.

Use with caution in patients with history of cardiovascular disease; hypertension, arrhythmia, chest pain, and MI have been observed with treatment; baseline (pretreatment) hematological and biochemical tests are recommended for all patients and if preexisting cardiac abnormalities, an ECG is also recommended.

Use with caution in thyroid disease; thyroid disorders (hyper- or hypothyroidism) or exacerbations have been reported; discontinue peginterferon alfa-2a if unable to effectively manage with medication. Use with caution in diabetes mellitus; hyper-/hypoglycemia have been reported; may require adjustments in antidiabetic medications; discontinue peginterferon alfa 2a if unable to effectively manage diabetes with medication.

Inhibition of growth velocity in pediatric patients may occur; in clinical trials, growth suppression of ≥15 percentiles on the normal growth curve was reported for weight in 43% of pediatric patients and for height in 25% of patients after 48 weeks of therapy. At the two-year follow up after treatment, most children had returned to their baseline growth curve percentile; monitor growth at baseline and during therapy.

Use caution with concurrent telbivudine therapy; peripheral neuropathy has been reported.

Safety and efficacy have not been established in the following patient types: Failed other alpha interferon therapy; received liver or other organ transplants; been coinfected with HBV and HCV or HIV; coinfection with HCV and HIV and a CD4$^+$ cell count <100 cells/mm^3; or treatment duration >48 weeks.

Adverse Reactions

Central nervous system: Anxiety, concentration impaired, depression, dizziness, fatigue, fever, headache, insomnia, irritability, memory impaired, mood alteration, nervousness, pain

Dermatologic: Alopecia, dermatitis, eczema, pruritus, rash

Endocrine & metabolic: Growth suppression (children) percentile decrease (including weight, height); hyperthyroidism, hypothyroidism

Gastrointestinal: Abdominal pain, anorexia, diarrhea, nausea, vomiting, xerostomia, weight loss

Hematologic: Anemia, platelets decreased <50,000/mm^3, lymphopenia, neutropenia, thrombocytopenia

Hepatic: ALT increases 5-10 x ULN during treatment; ALT increases >10 x ULN during treatment; ALT increases 5-10 x ULN after treatment; ALT increases >10 x ULN after treatment; hepatic decompensation

Local: Injection site reaction

Neuromuscular & skeletal: Arthralgia, back pain, myalgia, rigors, weakness

Ocular: Blurred vision

Respiratory: Cough, dyspnea

Miscellaneous: Bacterial infection, diaphoresis

Rare but important or life-threatening: Aggression, anaphylaxis, angioedema, angina, aplastic anemia, arrhythmia, autoimmune disorders, bronchiolitis obliterans, bronchoconstriction, cerebral hemorrhage, chest pain, cholangitis, colitis, coma, corneal ulcer, cotton wool spots, dehydration, diabetes mellitus, endocarditis, erythema multiforme major, exertional dyspnea, exfoliative dermatitis, fatty liver, gastrointestinal bleeding, hallucination, hearing impairment, hearing loss, hemoglobin decreased, hematocrit decreased, hepatic dysfunction, hepatic graft rejection, hepatitis B flares, hyper-/hypoglycemia, hypersensitivity reactions, hypertension, influenza, interstitial pneumonitis, macular edema, MI, myositis, optic neuritis, papilledema, pancreatitis, peptic ulcer, peripheral neuropathy, pneumonia, psychiatric disorder, psychosis, pulmonary embolism, pulmonary infiltrates, pure red cell aplasia, renal graft rejection, retinal artery/vein thrombosis, retinal detachment, retinal hemorrhage, retinopathy, rheumatoid arthritis, sarcoidosis, seizures, Stevens-Johnson syndrome, substance overdose, suicidal ideation, suicide, supraventricular arrhythmia, systemic lupus erythematosus, thrombotic thrombocytopenic purpura, triglycerides (increased), urticaria, vesiculobullous eruptions, vision decreased/loss

Drug Interactions

Metabolism/Transport Effects Inhibits CYP1A2 (weak)

Avoid Concomitant Use

Avoid concomitant use of Peginterferon Alfa-2a with any of the following: CloZAPine; Dipyrone; Telbivudine

Increased Effect/Toxicity

Peginterferon Alfa-2a may increase the levels/effects of: Aldesleukin; CloZAPine; Methadone; Ribavirin; Telbivudine; Theophylline Derivatives; Zidovudine

The levels/effects of Peginterferon Alfa-2a may be increased by: Dipyrone

Decreased Effect

The levels/effects of Peginterferon Alfa-2a may be decreased by: Pegloticase

Stability Store at 2°C to 8°C (36°F to 46°F); do not freeze or shake; protect from light. The following stability information has also been reported:

Intact vial: May be stored at room temperature for up to 14 days (Cohen, 2007).

Prefilled syringe: May be stored at room temperature for up to 6 days (Cohen, 2007).

Mechanism of Action Alpha interferons are a family of proteins, produced by nucleated cells that have antiviral, antiproliferative, and immune-regulating activity. There are 16 known subtypes of alpha interferons. Interferons interact with cells through high affinity cell surface receptors. Following activation, multiple effects can be detected including induction of gene transcription. Interferons inhibit cellular growth, alter the state of cellular differentiation, interfere with oncogene expression, alter cell surface antigen expression, increase phagocytic activity of macrophages, and augment cytotoxicity of lymphocytes for target cells.

Pharmacokinetics (Adult data unless noted)

Half-life elimination: Terminal: 50-160 hours; increased with renal dysfunction

Time to peak serum concentration: 72-96 hours

Dosing: Usual

Children ≥5 years and Adolescents: **Chronic hepatitis C virus (HCV) infection:** SubQ: 104 mcg/m^2 once weekly; maximum dose: 180 mcg; in combination with ribavirin (Copegus) (Schwartz, 2011); **Note:** Dosing presented is mathematically equivalent to weekly dosing presented in manufacturer's labeling: 180 mcg/1.73 m^2 x Body Surface Area (BSA); adolescents who reach their 18th birthday during treatment should remain on the pediatric regimen

Duration of therapy (based on genotype):

Genotype 1, 4, 5, 6: 48 weeks

Genotype 2, 3: 24 weeks

Adults:

Chronic hepatitis B: SubQ: 180 mcg once weekly for 48 weeks

Chronic hepatitis C virus (HCV) infection (monoinfection or coinfection with HIV): SubQ: 180 mcg once weekly for 48 weeks as monotherapy or in combination with ribavirin (Copegus®)

Duration of therapy: Monoinfection (based on genotype):

Genotypes 1, 4: 48 weeks

Genotypes 2, 3: 24 weeks

Genotypes 5, 6: No dosing recommendations provided; data insufficient

Duration of therapy: Coinfection with HIV: 48 weeks

Note: American Association for the Study of Liver Diseases (AASLD) guidelines recommendation: Adults with chronic HCV infection (Ghany, 2009): Treatment of choice: Ribavirin plus **peginterferon**; clinical condition and ability of patient to tolerate therapy should be evaluated to determine length and/or likely benefit of therapy. Recommended treatment duration (AASLD guidelines): Genotypes 1,4: 48 weeks; Genotypes 2,3: 24 weeks; Coinfection with HIV: 48 weeks

Dosing adjustment for renal impairment:

Children and Adolescents: There are no dosage adjustment provided in manufacturer's labeling; has not been studied.

Adults:

CrCl ≥30 mL/minute: No adjustment required

CrCl <30 mL/minute: Reduce dose to 135 mcg weekly; monitor for interferon toxicity

End-stage renal disease (ESRD) requiring hemodialysis: 135 mcg weekly; monitor for interferon toxicity

Dosing adjustment for hepatic impairment:

Children ≥5 years and Adolescents: *Chronic Hepatitis C:* ALT ≥5 but <10 x ULN: Decrease interferon dose to 78 mcg/m^2 once weekly. Monitor weekly; further modify dose if needed until ALT stabilizes or decreases (Schwartz, 2011). **Note:** Dosing presented is mathematically equivalent to adjusted weekly dose in manufacturer's labeling: 135 mcg/1.73 m^2 x Body Surface Area (BSA)

ALT ≥10 x ULN (persistent): Discontinue interferon

Adults:

Chronic hepatitis C (HCV): ALT progressively rising above baseline: Decrease dose to 135 mcg weekly **and** monitor LFTs more frequently. If ALT continues to rise despite dose reduction or ALT increase is accompanied by increased bilirubin or hepatic decompensation, discontinue therapy immediately. Therapy may resume after ALT flare subsides.

Chronic hepatitis B (HBV):

ALT >5 x ULN: Consider decreasing dose to 135 mcg weekly or temporarily discontinuing (may resume after ALT flare subsides) **and** monitor LFTs more frequently. If ALT continues to rise despite dose reduction or ALT increase is accompanied by increased bilirubin or hepatic decompensation, discontinue therapy immediately.

ALT >10 x ULN: Consider discontinuing

Dosing adjustment for toxicity: Note: Pediatric dosing adjustments shown below correspond to the following doses in manufacturer's labeling: 78 mcg/m^2 = 135 mcg/1.73 m^2; 52 mcg/m^2 = 90 mcg/1.73 m^2; and 26 mcg/m^2 = 45 mcg/1.73 m^2 (Schwartz, 2011).

For moderate to severe adverse reactions:

Children ≥5 years and Adolescents: Decrease to 78 mcg/m^2 once weekly for initial dose reduction; further dose reductions to 52 mcg/m^2 once weekly and then 26 mcg/m^2 once weekly may be necessary in some cases if reaction persists or recurs. Up to three dosing adjustments for toxicity may be made before discontinuation is considered.

Adults: HCV, HBV infection: For moderate to severe adverse reactions: Decrease to 135 mcg/week for initial dose reduction; further dose reductions to 90 mcg/week may be necessary in some cases if reaction persists or recurs

Depression (severity based upon DSM-IV criteria):

Mild depression: Children ≥5 years, Adolescents, and Adults: No dosage adjustment required; evaluate once weekly by visit/phone call. If depression remains stable, continue weekly visits. If depression improves, resume normal visit schedule.

Moderate depression:

Children ≥5 years and Adolescents: Initially decrease interferon dose to 78 mcg/m^2 once weekly and based upon response of adverse effect further dose modifications may be necessary in stepwise approach; next decrease to 52 mcg/m^2 once weekly and then 26 mcg/m^2 once weekly; evaluate once weekly with an office visit at least every other week. If symptoms improve and remain stable for 4 weeks, resume normal visit schedule; may continue reduced dosing or return to normal dose. If depression remains stable, consider psychiatric evaluation and continue reduced dosing. If symptoms worsen, considered further dosage reduction; discontinue therapy if no improvement after three dosage reductions.

Adults: Decrease interferon dose to 135 mcg once weekly (or to 90 mcg once weekly); evaluate once weekly with an office visit at least every other week. If depression remains stable, consider psychiatric evaluation and continue with reduced dosing. If symptoms improve and remain stable for 4 weeks, resume normal visit schedule; continue reduced dosing or return to normal dose.

Severe depression: Children ≥5 years, Adolescents, and Adults: Discontinue interferon permanently. Obtain immediate psychiatric consultation. Discontinue ribavirin.

Based on hematological parameters: **Note:** Management dependent upon weeks of therapy.

Children ≥5 years and Adolescents:

Neutropenia:

ANC 750-999/mm^3:

Week 1-2: Decrease dose to 78 mcg/m^2 once weekly

Weeks 3-48: No modification

ANC 500-749/mm^3:

Week 1-2: Hold dose until ANC >750/mm^3 then resume therapy at 78 mcg/m^2 once weekly. Assess WBC weekly for 3 weeks to verify ANC >750/mm^3.

Weeks 3-48: Decrease dose to 78 mcg/m^2 once weekly

ANC 250-499/mm^3:

Week 1-2: Hold dose until ANC >750/mm^3 then resume dose at 52 mcg/m^2 once weekly

Weeks 3-48: Hold dose until ANC >750/mm^3 then resume dose at 78 mcg/m^2 once weekly

ANC <250/mm^3 or febrile neutropenia: Discontinue treatment.

Thrombocytopenia: Platelet count <50,000/mm^3: Decrease dose to 52 mcg/m^2 once weekly

Adults:

Neutropenia:

ANC <750/mm^3: 135 mcg once weekly

ANC <500/mm^3: Suspend therapy until >1000/mm^3, then restart at 90 mcg once weekly; monitor ANC

Thrombocytopenia:

Platelet count <50,000/mm^3: 90 mcg once weekly

Platelet count <25,000/mm^3: Discontinue therapy

Administration SubQ: Administer in the abdomen or thigh. Rotate injection site. Do not use if solution contains particulate matter or is discolored. Discard unused solution. Administration should be done on the same day and at approximately the same time each week.

Monitoring Parameters

The following were used during clinical trials:

Children ≥5 years and Adolescents: Hematologic and biochemical assessments were made at weeks 1, 3, 5, and 8, and then every 4 weeks thereafter; TSH measured every 12 weeks; growth parameters (height, weight, percentiles on growth curve) (Schwarz, 2011)

Adults: CBC (including hemoglobin, WBC, and platelets) and chemistries (including liver function tests and uric acid) measured at weeks 1, 2, 4, 6, and 8, and then every 4-6 weeks (more frequently if abnormal); TSH measured every 12 weeks

Additionally, the following baseline values were used as entrance criteria in adults:

Platelet count ≥90,000/mm^3 (as low as 75,000/mm^3 in patients with cirrhosis or 70,000/mm^3 in patients with HCV coinfected with HIV)

ANC ≥1500/mm^3

Serum creatinine <1.5 times ULN

TSH and T$_4$ within normal limits or adequately controlled

CD4$^+$ cell count ≥200 cells/mm^3 or CD4$^+$ cell count ≥100 cells/mm^3, but <200 cells/mm^3 and HIV-1 RNA <5000 copies/mL in HCV patients coinfected with HIV

Hemoglobin ≥12 g/dL for women and ≥13 g/dL for men in HCV monoinfected patients

Hemoglobin ≥11 g/dL for women and ≥12 g/dL for men in HCV patients coinfected with HIV

Also in adults, serum HCV RNA levels (pretreatment, 12- and 24 weeks after therapy initiation, 24 weeks after completion of therapy). **Note:** Discontinuation of therapy may be considered after 12 weeks in patients with HCV (genotype 1) who fail to achieve an early virologic response (defined as ≥2-log decrease in HCV RNA compared to pretreatment) or after 24 weeks with detectable HCV RNA (Ghany, 2009).

Prior to treatment, pregnancy screening should occur for women of childbearing age who are receiving treatment or who have male partners who are receiving treatment. In combination therapy with ribavirin, pregnancy tests should continue monthly up to 6 months after discontinuation of therapy. Evaluate for depression and other psychiatric symptoms before and during therapy; baseline eye examination and periodically in patients with baseline disorders; baseline echocardiogram in patients with cardiac disease.

Dosage Forms Excipient information presented when available (limited, particularly for generics); consult specific product labeling.

Kit, Subcutaneous [preservative free]:

Pegasys: 180 mcg/0.5 mL [contains benzyl alcohol]

Solution, Subcutaneous [preservative free]:

Pegasys: 180 mcg/mL (1 mL) [contains benzyl alcohol]

Pegasys: 180 mcg/0.5 mL (0.5 mL) [contains benzyl alcohol, polysorbate 80]

Pegasys ProClick: 135 mcg/0.5 mL (0.5 mL) [contains benzyl alcohol, polysorbate 80]

Pegasys ProClick: 180 mcg/0.5 mL (0.5 mL) [contains benzyl alcohol]

References

ACOG Practice Bulletin No. 86: "Viral Hepatitis in Pregnancy," *Obstet Gynecol*, 2007, 110(4):941-56.

Cohen V, Jellinek SP, Teperikidis L, et al, "Room-Temperature Storage of Medications Labeled for Refrigeration," *Am J Health-Syst Pharm*, 2007, 64(16):1711-5.

Ghany MG, Nelson DR, Strader DB, et al, "An Update on Treatment of Genotype 1 Chronic Hepatitis C Virus Infection: 2011 Practice Guideline by the American Association for the Study of Liver Diseases," *Hepatology*, 2011, 54(4):1433-44.

Ghany MG, Strader DB, Thomas DL, et al, "Diagnosis, Management and Treatment of Hepatitis C: An Update," *Hepatology*, 2009, 49 (4):1335-74.

Lebon P, Girard S, Thepot F, et al, "The Presence of Alpha-Interferon in Human Amniotic Fluid," *J Gen Virol*, 1982, 59(Pt 2):393-6.

Murray KF, Rodrigue JR, González-Peralta RP, et al, "Design of the PEDS-C trial: Pegylated Interferon ± Ribavirin for Children With Chronic Hepatitis C Viral Infection," *Clin Trials*, 2007, 4(6):661-73.

"Perinatal HIV Guidelines Working Group. Public Health Service Task Force Recommendations for Use of Antiretroviral Drugs in Pregnant HIV-Infected Women for Maternal Health and Interventions to Reduce Perinatal HIV Transmission in the United States," April 29, 2009, 1-90. Available at http://aidsinfo.nih.gov/ContentFiles/PerinatalGL.pdf

Schwarz KB, Gonzalez-Peralta RP, Murray KF, et al, "The Combination of Ribavirin and Peginterferon Is Superior to Peginterferon and Placebo for Children and Adolescents With Chronic Hepatitis C," *Gastroenterology*, 2011, 140(2):450-8.

Waysbort A, Giroux M, Mansat V, et al, "Experimental Study of Transplacental Passage of Alpha Interferon by Two Assay Techniques," *Antimicrob Agents Chemother*, 1993, 37(6):1232-7.

Peginterferon Alfa-2b
(peg in ter FEER on AL fa too bee)

Medication Safety Issues

Sound-alike/look-alike issues:

Peginterferon alfa-2b may be confused with interferon alfa-2a, interferon alfa-2b, interferon alfa-n3, peginterferon alfa-2a

PegIntron may be confused with Intron A, Pegasys

International issues:

Peginterferon alfa-2b may be confused with interferon alpha multi-subtype which is available in international markets

Related Information

Emetogenic Potential of Antineoplastic Agents in Children on page 2327

Brand Names: U.S. Peg-Intron; Peg-Intron Redipen; Peg-Intron Redipen Pak 4; Sylatron

Brand Names: Canada PegIntron

Therapeutic Category Antineoplastic Agent, Biologic Response Modulator; Biological Response Modulator; Immunomodulator, Systemic; Interferon

Generic Availability (U.S.) No

Use

PegIntron®: Treatment of chronic hepatitis C (in combination with ribavirin) in patients who have compensated liver disease (FDA approved in ages ≥3 years and adults); treatment of chronic hepatitis C (as monotherapy) in patients with compensated liver disease who have never received alfa interferons (FDA approved in adults); has also be used for treatment of chronic hepatitis C with HIV coinfection and chronic hepatitis B with HIV coinfection

Sylatron™: Adjuvant treatment of melanoma (with microscopic or gross nodal involvement within 84 days of definitive surgical resection, including lymphadenectomy) (FDA approved in ages ≥18 years and adults)

Medication Guide Available Yes

Pregnancy Risk Factor C / X in combination with ribavirin

Pregnancy Considerations Reproduction studies with pegylated interferon alfa have not been conducted. Animal reproduction studies with nonpegylated interferon alfa-2b have demonstrated abortifacient effects. Disruption of the normal menstrual cycle was also observed in animal studies; therefore, the manufacturer recommends that reliable contraception is used in women of childbearing potential. Alfa interferon is endogenous to normal amniotic fluid (Lebon, 1982). *In vitro* administration studies have reported that when administered to the mother, it does not cross the placenta (Waysbort, 1993). Case reports of use in pregnant women are limited. The DHHS Perinatal HIV Guidelines do not recommend that peginterferon alfa be used during pregnancy (DHHS [perinatal], 2012). **[U.S. Boxed Warning]: Combination therapy with ribavirin may cause birth defects and/or fetal mortality; avoid pregnancy in females and female partners of male patients;** combination therapy with ribavirin is contraindicated in pregnancy. Two forms of contraception should be used along with monthly pregnancy tests during combination therapy and for 6 months after therapy has been discontinued.

A pregnancy registry has been established for women inadvertently exposed to ribavirin while pregnant (800-593-2214).

Breast-Feeding Considerations Breast milk samples obtained from a lactating mother prior to and after administration of interferon alfa-2b showed that interferon alfa is present in breast milk and administration of the medication did not significantly affect endogenous levels (Kumar, 2000). Breast-feeding is not linked to the spread of hepatitis C virus (ACOG, 2007); however, if nipples are cracked or bleeding, breast-feeding is not recommended (CDC, 2010). Mothers coinfected with HIV are discouraged from breast-feeding to decrease potential transmission of HIV (DHHS [perinatal], 2012).

Contraindications Hypersensitivity (including urticaria, angioedema, bronchoconstriction, anaphylaxis, Stevens-Johnson syndrome, and toxic epidermal necrolysis) to peginterferon alfa-2b, interferon alfa, other alfa interferons, or any component; autoimmune hepatitis; decompensated liver disease (Child-Pugh score >6; classes B and C). Combination therapy with ribavirin is contraindicated in pregnancy, women who may become pregnant; males with pregnant partners; hemoglobinopathies (eg, thalassemia major, sickle-cell anemia); renal dysfunction (CrCl <50 mL/ minute)

Warnings May cause or aggravate severe depression or other neuropsychiatric adverse events (including suicide and suicidal ideation) in patients with and without a history of psychiatric disorder; may be irreversible; monitor closely with clinical evaluations (periodic); **[U.S. Boxed Warning]**; discontinue treatment permanently with worsening or persistently severe signs/symptoms of neuropsychiatric disorders (eg, depression, encephalopathy, psychosis). Many cases resolve upon discontinuation, although some may persist. Suicidal ideation or attempts may occur more frequently in pediatric patients as compared to adults (2.4% vs 1% respectively). Addiction relapse, aggression, depression, homicidal ideation, and suicidal behavior/ideation have been observed with peginterferon alfa-2b; bipolar disorder, encephalopathy, hallucinations, mania, and psychosis have been observed with other alfa interferons. Onset may be delayed (up to 6 months after discontinuation). Higher doses may be associated with the development of encephalopathy (higher risk in elderly patients). Use with extreme caution in patients with a history of psychiatric disorders, including depression or substance abuse history. New or exacerbated neuropsychiatric or substance abuse disorders are best managed with early intervention. Drug screening and periodic health evaluation (including monitoring of psychiatric symptoms) is recommended if initiating treatment in patients with coexisting psychiatric condition or substance abuse disorders. Monitor all patients for evidence of depression and other psychiatric symptoms; patients being treated for melanoma should be monitored for depression and psychiatric symptoms every 3 weeks during the first 8 weeks of treatment and every 6 months thereafter; discontinue treatment if psychiatric symptoms persist, worsen, or if suicidal behavior develops. All patients should continue to be monitored for 6 months after completion of therapy.

May cause or exacerbate autoimmune disorders; monitor closely; discontinue treatment in patients with worsening or persistently severe signs/symptoms of autoimmune disease **[U.S. Boxed Warning]**. Thyroiditis, thrombotic thrombocytopenic purpura, immune thrombocytopenia (ITP), rheumatoid arthritis, interstitial nephritis, systemic lupus erythematosus, and psoriasis have been reported with therapy; use with caution in patients with autoimmune disorders.

May cause or aggravate infectious disorders; monitor closely; discontinue treatment in patients with worsening or persistently severe signs/symptoms of infectious disorders **[U.S. Boxed Warning]**. Interferon therapy is commonly associated with flu-like symptoms, including fever; rule out other causes/infection with persistent or high fever.

May cause or aggravate ischemic and hemorrhagic cerebrovascular events; monitor closely; discontinue treatment in patients with worsening or persistent ischemia **[U.S. Boxed Warning]**; cerebrovascular events have been reported in patients without risk factors for stroke.

Alpha interferons suppress bone marrow function which may result in severe cytopenias or aplastic anemia (rarely). Use with caution in patients who are chronically immunosuppressed, with low peripheral blood counts or myelosuppression, including concurrent use of myelosuppressive therapy or at increased risk for severe anemia (eg, spherocytosis, history of GI bleeding). Dosage modification may be necessary for hematologic toxicity. Combination therapy with ribavirin may potentiate the neutropenic effects of alfa interferons. When used in combination with ribavirin, an increased incidence of anemia was observed when using ribavirin weight-based dosing, as compared to flat-dose ribavirin.

Patients with chronic hepatitis C (CHC) with cirrhosis receiving alpha interferons may be at risk for hepatic decompensation and death; immediately discontinue therapy if it occurs (Child-Pugh score >6) or evidence of severe hepatic injury. CHC patients coinfected with HIV are at increased risk for hepatic decompensation when receiving highly active antiretroviral therapy (HAART); monitor closely. A transient increase in ALT (2-5 times above baseline) which is not associated with liver dysfunction may occur with peginterferon alfa-2b use (for the treatment of chronic hepatitis C); may continue treatment with monitoring.

Ophthalmologic disorders (including decreased visual acuity, blindness, macular edema, retinal hemorrhages, optic neuritis, papilledema, cotton wool spots, retinal detachment [serous], and retinal artery or vein thrombosis) have occurred with peginterferon alfa-2b and/or with other alfa interferons. Prior to start of therapy, ophthalmic exams are recommended for all patients; patients with diabetic or hypertensive retinopathy should have periodic ophthalmic exams during treatment; a complete eye exam should be done promptly in patients who develop ocular symptoms. Permanently discontinue treatment with new or worsening ophthalmic disorder. May cause or aggravate dyspnea, pulmonary infiltrates, pneumonia, bronchiolitis obliterans, interstitial pneumonitis, pulmonary hypertension, and sarcoidosis which can result in respiratory failure; may recur upon rechallenge with treatment; monitor closely. Use with caution in patients with existing pulmonary disease (eg, chronic obstructive pulmonary disease). Withhold combination therapy with ribavirin for development of pulmonary infiltrate or pulmonary function impairment.

Pancreatitis has been observed with alfa interferon therapy; withhold treatment for suspected pancreatitis; discontinue therapy for known pancreatitis. Hypertriglyceridemia has been reported; monitor; discontinue if persistent and severe (triglycerides >1000 mg/dL), particularly if combined with symptoms of pancreatitis. Ulcerative or hemorrhagic/ischemic colitis has been observed with alfa interferons; discontinue therapy if signs of colitis (abdominal pain, bloody diarrhea, fever) develop; symptoms typically resolve within 1-3 weeks.

Acute hypersensitivity reactions (urticaria, angioedema, bronchoconstriction, anaphylaxis) and cutaneous reactions (Stevens-Johnson syndrome, toxic epidermal necrolysis) have been reported (rarely) with alfa interferons; prompt discontinuation is recommended; transient rashes do not require interruption of therapy.

Combination treatment with ribavirin may cause birth defects and/or fetal mortality (avoid pregnancy in females and female partners of male patients); hemolytic anemia (which may worsen cardiac disease), genotoxicity, mutagenicity, and may possibly be carcinogenic. Combination therapy with ribavirin is contraindicated in pregnancy **[U.S. Boxed Warning]**.

Due to differences in dosage, patients should not change brands of interferon.

Some formulations contain polysorbate 80 (Tween 80®) which may cause allergic reactions in susceptible individuals. In premature neonates, thrombocytopenia, ascites, pulmonary deterioration, and renal and hepatic failure have been reported after receiving parenteral products containing polysorbate 80 (Alade, 1986; *MMWR*, 1984).

Precautions Use with caution in patients with renal impairment (CrCl <50 mL/minute); increases in serum creatinine have been reported in patients with renal impairment. Dosage adjustment may be required; discontinue if serum creatinine >2 mg/dL in children. Do not use combination therapy with ribavirin in adults with CrCl <50 mL/minute; has not been studied in melanoma patients with renal impairment.

Use with caution in patients with a history of cardiovascular disease; hypotension, arrhythmia, bundle branch block, tachycardia, cardiomyopathy, angina pectoris, and MI have been observed with treatment. Patients with preexisting cardiac abnormalities should have baseline ECGs prior to combination treatment with ribavirin; closely monitor patients with a history of MI or arrhythmia. Patients with a history of significant or unstable cardiac disease should not receive combination treatment with ribavirin. Discontinue treatment (permanently) for new-onset ventricular arrhythmia or cardiovascular decompensation. Use with caution in patients with debilitating conditions; interferons are commonly associated with flu-like symptoms.

Use caution in patients with a history of diabetes mellitus (particularly if prone to DKA). Diabetes mellitus (including new-onset type 1 diabetes) and hyperglycemia, have been reported; discontinue peginterferon alfa-2b if diabetes cannot be effectively managed with medication.

Use with caution in patients with thyroid disorders; may cause or aggravate hyper- or hypothyroidism. Discontinue use in patients with thyroid disease who cannot be controlled with medication.

Severe inhibition of growth velocity, <3rd percentile and affecting height and weight, was reported in 70% of pediatric patients during clinical trials on combination therapy; monitor closely; dosage adjustment may be required. After therapy, 20% continued to have severely inhibited growth; however, in majority of patients, growth velocity rates increased such that by 6 months post-treatment, weight gain stabilized to 53rd percentile (similar to predicted based on average baseline weight: 57th percentile) and height gain stabilized to 44th percentile (less than predicted based on average baseline height: 51st percentile).

Dental/periodontal disorders have been reported with combination therapy; dry mouth may affect teeth and mucous membranes; instruct patients to brush teeth twice daily; encourage regular dental exams; rinse mouth after vomiting. A higher incidence in children compared to adults has been reported with fever (80% vs 46%) and vomiting (27% vs 14%).

Combination therapy with ribavirin is preferred over monotherapy for the treatment of chronic hepatitis C (combination therapy provides a better response). Safety and efficacy have not been established in patients who have received organ transplants, or are coinfected with HIV or hepatitis B. Patients with significant bridging fibrosis or cirrhosis, genotype 1 infection, or who have not responded to prior therapy, including previous pegylated interferon treatment are less likely to benefit from combination therapy with peginterferon alfa-2b and ribavirin.

Adverse Reactions

Cardiovascular: Bundle branch block, chest pain, flushing, myocardial infarction, supraventricular arrhythmia, ventricular tachycardia

Central nervous system: Agitation, anxiety, chills, depression (may be severe), dizziness, emotional liability, fatigue, fever, headache, impaired concentration, insomnia, irritability, malaise, nervousness, olfactory nerve disorder, suicidal behavior (ideation/attempt/suicide)

Dermatologic: Alopecia, dry skin, pruritus, rash

Endocrine & metabolic: Hyper-/hypothyroidism, menstrual disorder

Gastrointestinal: Abdominal pain, anorexia, constipation, diarrhea, dyspepsia, nausea, taste perversion, vomiting, weight loss, xerostomia

Hematologic: Anemia (in combination with ribavirin), neutropenia, thrombocytopenia

Hepatic: Alkaline phosphatase increased, ALT/AST increased, GGT increased, hepatomegaly

Local: Injection site inflammation/reaction, injection site pain

Neuromuscular & skeletal: Arthralgia, musculoskeletal pain, myalgia, paresthesia, rigors, weakness

Ocular: Blurred vision, conjunctivitis

Renal: Proteinuria

Respiratory: Cough, dyspnea, pharyngitis, rhinitis, sinusitis

Miscellaneous: Binding antibodies (melanoma patients), diaphoresis, neutralizing antibodies, viral infection

Rare but important or life-threatening: Addiction (drug) relapse, anaphylaxis, angina, angioedema, aphthous stomatitis, aplastic anemia, arrhythmia, autoimmune thrombocytopenia (with or without purpura), bacterial infection, bipolar disorders, blindness, bronchiolitis obliterans, cardiac arrest, cardiomyopathy, cellulitis, colitis, cotton wool spots, cytopenia, diabetes mellitus, diabetic ketoacidosis, drug overdose, emphysema, encephalopathy, erythema multiforme, fungal infection, gastroenteritis, gout, hallucinations, hearing impairment/loss, hemorrhagic colitis, homicidal ideation, hyperglycemia, hyper-/hypotension, hypersensitivity reactions, ▶

hypertriglyceridemia, injection site necrosis, interstitial nephritis, interstitial pneumonitis, ischemic colitis, leukopenia, loss of consciousness, lupus-like syndrome, macular edema, mania, memory loss, migraine, myositis, nerve palsy (facial/oculomotor), optic neuritis, palpitation, pancreatitis, papilledema, pericardial effusion, peripheral neuropathy, phototoxicity, pleural effusion, pneumonia, psoriasis, psychosis, pulmonary hypertension, pulmonary infiltrates, pure red cell aplasia, renal failure, renal insufficiency, retinal artery or vein thrombosis, retinal detachment (serous), retinal hemorrhage, retinal ischemia, retinopathy, rhabdomyolysis, rheumatoid arthritis, sarcoidosis, seizure, sepsis, serum creatinine increased, Stevens-Johnson syndrome, stroke, systemic lupus erythematosus, tachycardia, thrombotic thrombocytopenic purpura, thyroiditis, toxic epidermal necrolysis, transient ischemic attack, ulcerative colitis, vasculitis, vision decrease/loss, Vogt-Koyanagi-Harada syndrome

Drug Interactions

Metabolism/Transport Effects Inhibits CYP1A2 (weak)

Avoid Concomitant Use

Avoid concomitant use of Peginterferon Alfa-2b with any of the following: CloZAPine; Dipyrone; Telbivudine

Increased Effect/Toxicity

Peginterferon Alfa-2b may increase the levels/effects of: Aldesleukin; CloZAPine; Methadone; Ribavirin; Telbivudine; Zidovudine

The levels/effects of Peginterferon Alfa-2b may be increased by: Dipyrone

Decreased Effect

Peginterferon Alfa-2b may decrease the levels/effects of: CYP2C9 Substrates; CYP2D6 Substrates; FLUoxetine

The levels/effects of Peginterferon Alfa-2b may be decreased by: Pegloticase

Stability Store intact vials at 25°C (77°F); excursions permitted to 15°C to 30°C (59°F to 86°F). Store Redipen® at 2°C to 8°C (36°F to 46°F). Do not freeze. Once reconstituted, each product should be used immediately or may be stored for ≤24 hours at 2°C to 8°C (36°F to 46°F); do not freeze. Products do not contain preservatives; do not reuse.

Mechanism of Action Alpha interferons are a family of proteins, produced by nucleated cells, that have antiviral, antiproliferative, and immune-regulating activity. There are 16 known subtypes of alpha interferons. Interferons interact with cells through high affinity cell surface receptors. Following activation, multiple effects can be detected including induction of gene transcription. Inhibits cellular growth, alters the state of cellular differentiation, interferes with oncogene expression, alters cell surface antigen expression, increases phagocytic activity of macrophages, and augments cytotoxicity of lymphocytes for target cells.

Pharmacokinetics (Adult data unless noted) Note: Peginterferon alfa-2b has a prolonged duration of effect relative to interferon alfa-2b and a reduced renal clearance (sevenfold lower). Data in children similar to adult values.

Bioavailability: Increases with chronic dosing

Half-life elimination: Chronic hepatitis C: ~40 hours (range: 22-60 hours)

Time to peak serum concentration: 15-44 hours

Elimination: Urine (30%); clearance reduced in renal impairment by 17% in moderate dysfunction, 44% in severe dysfunction

Dosing: Usual Note: Due to differences in dosage, patients should not change brands of interferon alfa therapy.

Children and Adolescents:

Chronic hepatitis B virus (HBV) infection (HIV-exposed/-positive): Adolescents: PegIntron: SubQ: 1.5 mcg/kg once weekly for 48 weeks (DHHS [adult], 2013)

Chronic hepatitis C virus (HCV) infection:

Non-HIV-exposed/-infected:

Manufacturer's labeling: Children ≥3 years and Adolescents: PegIntron: SubQ: 60 mcg/m^2 once weekly (in combination with ribavirin). Treatment duration: 48 weeks (genotype 1); 24 weeks (genotypes 2 and 3). Consider discontinuation of combination therapy in patients with HCV (genotype 1) at 12 weeks if a 2 log decrease in HCV-RNA has not been achieved or if HCV-RNA is still detectable at 24 weeks.

Note: Adolescents who reach their 18th birthday during treatment should remain on the pediatric regimen.

Alternate dosing: American Association for the Study of Liver Diseases (AASLD) recommendations: Children ≥2 years and Adolescents: PegIntron: SubQ: 60 mcg/m^2 once weekly (in combination with oral ribavirin) for 48 weeks (all genotypes) (Ghany, 2009)

HIV-exposed/-positive (coinfection):

Children ≥3 years: PegIntron: SubQ: 60 mcg/m^2 once weekly (in combination with ribavirin). Treatment duration: 48 weeks, regardless of genotype (DHHS [pediatric], 2013)

Adolescents: PegIntron: SubQ: 1.5 mcg/kg once weekly (in combination with ribavirin). Treatment duration: 48 weeks, regardless of genotype (DHHS [adult], 2013)

Adults:

Melanoma: Sylatron: SubQ: 6 mcg/kg/week for 8 doses, followed by 3 mcg/kg/week for up to 5 years. **Note:** Premedicate with acetaminophen (500-1000 mg orally) 30 minutes prior to the first dose and as needed for subsequent doses thereafter.

Chronic hepatitis C: PegIntron: Sub Q: Administer dose once weekly. **Note:** Discontinue in patients with HCV (genotype 1) after 12 weeks if HCV RNA does not decrease by at least 2 log (compared to pretreatment) or if detectable HCV RNA present at 24 weeks. Discontinuation is also recommended in patients who previously failed therapy (regardless of genotype) if detectable HCV RNA present at 12 or 24 weeks.

Monotherapy: Duration of treatment is 1 year; Initial dose (based on average dose of 1 mcg/kg/week):

≤45 kg: 40 mcg once weekly

46-56 kg: 50 mcg once weekly

57-72 kg: 64 mcg once weekly

73-88 kg: 80 mcg once weekly

89-106 kg: 96 mcg once weekly

107-136 kg: 120 mcg once weekly

137-160 kg: 150 mcg once weekly

Combination therapy with ribavirin: Treatment duration is 48 weeks for genotype 1, 24 weeks for genotypes 2 and 3, or 48 weeks for patients who previously failed therapy (regardless of genotype). Initial dose (based on an average dose of 1.5 mcg/kg/week):

<40 kg: 50 mcg once weekly

40-50 kg: 64 mcg once weekly

51-60 kg: 80 mcg once weekly

61-75 kg: 96 mcg once weekly

76-85 kg: 120 mcg once weekly

86-105 kg: 150 mcg once weekly

>105 kg: 1.5 mcg/kg once weekly

Note: American Association for the Study of Liver Diseases (AASLD) recommendation: Adults with chronic HCV infection: Treatment of choice: Ribavirin plus **peginterferon**; clinical condition and ability of patient to tolerate therapy should be evaluated to determine length and/or likely benefit of therapy. Recommended treatment duration (AASLD guidelines; Ghany, 2009): Genotypes 1,4: 48 weeks; Genotypes 2,3: 24 weeks; Coinfection with HIV: 48 weeks

Dosing adjustment in renal impairment: Chronic hepatitis C:

Children and Adolescents: *Combination therapy with ribavirin:* Serum creatinine >2 mg/dL: Discontinue treatment

Adults:

Monotherapy:

CrCl 30-50 mL/minute: Reduce dose by 25%

CrCl 10-29 mL/minute: Reduce dose by 50%

Hemodialysis: Reduce dose by 50%

Discontinue use if renal function declines during treatment.

Combination therapy with ribavirin: CrCl <50 mL/minute: Combination therapy with ribavirin is not recommended.

Dosing adjustment hepatic impairment:

Decompensated liver disease or autoimmune hepatitis: Use is contraindicated.

Hepatic decompensation or severe hepatic injury during treatment (Child-Pugh class B or C): Discontinue immediately

Dosing adjustment for toxicity:

Chronic hepatitis C: **Dosage adjustment for depression (severity based upon DSM-IV criteria):**

Mild depression: Children, Adolescents, and Adults: No dosage adjustment required; evaluate once weekly by visit/phone call. If depression remains stable, continue weekly visits. If depression improves, resume normal visit schedule. For worsening depression, see "Moderate depression" below.

Moderate depression: Evaluate once weekly with an office visit at least every other week. If depression remains stable, consider psychiatric evaluation and continue with reduced dosing. If symptoms improve and remain stable for 4 weeks, resume normal visit schedule; continue reduced dosing or return to normal dose. For worsening depression or development of severe depression, discontinue therapy permanently and obtain immediate psychiatric consultation. Utilize followup psychiatric therapy as needed.

Children and Adolescents: Decrease to 40 mcg/m^2 once weekly, may further decrease to 20 mcg/m^2 once weekly if needed

Adults:

Monotherapy: Refer to adult weight-based dosage reduction with monotherapy for depression below

Combination therapy: Refer to adult weight-based dosage reduction with combination therapy for depression below

Severe depression: Children, Adolescent, and Adults: Discontinue peginterferon alfa-2b and ribavirin permanently. Obtain immediate psychiatric consultation.

Chronic hepatitis C: **Dosage adjustment in hematologic toxicity:**

Children and Adolescents:

Hemoglobin decrease >2 g/dL in any 4-week period in patients *with stable cardiac disease:* Reduce peginterferon alfa-2b dose by 50%; monitor and evaluate weekly. If after 4 weeks of dose reduction the hemoglobin remains <12 g/dL: Permanently discontinue both peginterferon alfa-2b and ribavirin.

Hemoglobin 8.5 to <10 g/dL in patients *without history of cardiac disease:* No dosage adjustment for peginterferon alfa-2b. Decrease ribavirin dose.

WBC 1000 to <1500/mm^3, neutrophils 500 to <750/mm^3, or platelets 50,000 to <70,000/mm^3: Reduce peginterferon alfa-2b dose to 40 mcg/m^2 once weekly; may further reduce to 20 mcg/m^2 once weekly

Hemoglobin <8.5 g/dL, WBC <1000/mm^3, neutrophils <500/mm^3, or platelets <50,000/mm^3: Permanently discontinue peginterferon alfa-2b and ribavirin

Adults:

Hemoglobin decrease ≥2 g/dL in any 4-week period and stable cardiac disease: Decrease peginterferon alfa-2b dose by 50%; decrease ribavirin dose. If after 4 weeks of dose reduction hemoglobin <12 g/dL: Permanently discontinue both peginterferon alfa-2b and ribavirin.

Hemoglobin 8.5 to <10 g/dL and no history of cardiac disease: No dosage adjustment necessary for peginterferon alfa-2b. Decrease ribavirin dose; may further reduce ribavirin dose if needed

WBC 1000 to <1500/mm^3, neutrophils 500 to <750/mm^3, or platelets <25,000 to <50,000/mm^3:

Peginterferon alfa-2b monotherapy: Refer to adult weight-based dosage reduction with combination therapy for hematologic toxicity below.

Peginterferon alfa-2b combination therapy: Refer to adult weight-based dosage reduction monotherapy for hematologic toxicity below.

Hemoglobin <8.5 g/dL, WBC <1000/mm^3, neutrophils <500/mm^3, or platelets <25,000/mm^3: Permanently discontinue peginterferon alfa-2b and ribavirin.

Chronic hepatitis C: **Adult weight-based dosage reduction for depression or hematologic toxicity:**

Adults:

Peginterferon alfa-2b monotherapy: Reduce to average weekly dose of 0.5 mcg/kg as follows:

≤45 kg: 20 mcg once weekly

46-56 kg: 25 mcg once weekly

57-72 kg: 30 mcg once weekly

73-88 kg: 40 mcg once weekly

89-106 kg: 50 mcg once weekly

107-136 kg: 64 mcg once weekly

≥137 kg: 80 mcg once weekly

Peginterferon alfa-2b combination therapy: Initially reduce to average weekly dose of 1 mcg/kg; may further reduce to average weekly dose 0.5 mcg/kg if needed as follows:

<40 kg: 35 mcg once weekly; may further reduce to 20 mcg once weekly if needed

40-50 kg: 45 mcg once weekly; may further reduce to 25 mcg once weekly if needed

51-60 kg: 50 mcg once weekly; may further reduce to 30 mcg once weekly if needed

61-75 kg: 64 mcg once weekly; may further reduce to 35 mcg once weekly if needed

76-85 kg: 80 mcg once weekly; may further reduce to 45 mcg once weekly if needed

86-104 kg: 96 mcg once weekly; may further reduce to 50 mcg once weekly if needed

105-125 kg: 108 mcg once weekly; may further reduce to 64 mcg once weekly if needed

>125 kg: 135 mcg once weekly; may further reduce to 72 mcg once weekly if needed

Melanoma: Adults:

Discontinue for any of the following: Persistent or worsening severe neuropsychiatric disorders (depression, psychosis, encephalopathy), grade 4 nonhematologic toxicity, new or worsening retinopathy, new-onset ventricular arrhythmia or cardiovascular decompensation, evidence of hepatic injury (severe) or hepatic decompensation, development of hyper- or hypothyroidism or diabetes that cannot be effectively managed with medication, or inability to tolerate a dose of 1 mcg/kg/week

Temporarily withhold for any of the following: ANC <500/mm^3, platelets <50,000/mm^3, ECOG performance status (PS) ≥2, nonhematologic toxicity ≥grade 3

May reinitiate at a reduced dose once ANC ≥500/mm^3, platelets ≥50,000/mm^3, ECOG PS at 0-1, and nonhematologic toxicity completely resolved or improved to grade 1.

Reduced dose schedule, Weeks 1-8:

First dose reduction (if prior dose 6 mcg/kg/week): 3 mcg/kg/week

Second dose reduction (if prior dose 3 mcg/kg/week): 2 mcg/kg/week

Third dose reduction (if prior dose 2 mcg/kg/week): 1 mcg/kg/week

Discontinue permanently if unable to tolerate 1 mcg/kg/week

Reduced dose schedule, Weeks 9-260:

First dose reduction (if prior dose 3 mcg/kg/week): 2 mcg/kg/week

Second dose reduction (if prior dose 2 mcg/kg/week): 1 mcg/kg/week

Discontinue permanently if unable to tolerate 1 mcg/kg/week

Administration PegIntron® Redipen®: Hold cartridge upright and press the two halves together until there is a "click." Gently invert to mix; do not shake; do not reuse (single use).

PegIntron® (vial): Add 0.7 mL of SWI (supplied diluent) to the vial. Gently swirl. Do not re-enter vial after dose removed. Discard unused reconstituted portion; do not reuse.

Sylatron™ (vial): Add 0.7 mL SWI and swirl gently, resulting in the following concentrations:

296 mcg vial: 40 mcg/0.1 mL

444 mcg vial: 60 mcg/0.1 mL

888 mcg vial: 120 mcg/0.1 mL

SubQ: Rotate injection site; thigh, outer surface of upper arm, and abdomen are preferred injection sites; do not inject near navel or waistline; patients who are thin should only use thigh or upper arm. Do not inject into bruised, infected, irritated, red, or scarred skin. The weekly dose may be administered at bedtime to reduce flu-like symptoms. Administration volume depends on the patient's weight and peginterferon concentration used.

Monitoring Parameters CBC with differential and platelets; serum chemistries, liver function tests, renal function, triglycerides. Clinical studies (for combination therapy) tested as follows: CBC (including hemoglobin, WBC, and platelets) and chemistries (including liver function tests and uric acid) measured at weeks 2, 4, 8, and 12, and then every 6 weeks; TSH measured every 12 weeks during treatment. ECG at baseline for patients with preexisting cardiac abnormalities (for combination therapy with ribavirin)

Hepatitis C:

Serum HCV RNA levels (pretreatment, 12 and 24 weeks after therapy initiation, 24 weeks after completion of therapy). **Note:** Discontinuation of therapy may be considered after 12 weeks in patients with HCV (genotype 1) who fail to achieve an early virologic response (EVR) (defined as ≥2-log decrease in HCV RNA compared to pretreatment) or after 24 weeks with detectable HCV RNA. Treat patients with HCV (genotypes 2,3) for 24 weeks (if tolerated) and then evaluate HCV RNA levels (Ghany, 2009).

Evaluate for depression and other psychiatric symptoms before and after initiation of therapy; patients being treated for melanoma should be monitored for depression and psychiatric symptoms every 3 weeks during the first eight weeks of treatment and every 6 months thereafter; baseline ophthalmic eye examination; periodic ophthalmic exam in patients with diabetic or hypertensive retinopathy; baseline ECG in patients with cardiac disease; serum glucose or Hb A1c (for patients with diabetes mellitus). In combination therapy with ribavirin, pregnancy tests (for women of childbearing age who are receiving treatment or who have male partners who are receiving treatment), continue monthly up to 6 months after discontinuation of therapy.

Dosage Forms Excipient information presented when available (limited, particularly for generics); consult specific product labeling.

Kit, Subcutaneous:

Peg-Intron: 50 mcg/0.5 mL, 80 mcg/0.5 mL, 120 mcg/0.5 mL, 150 mcg/0.5 mL

Peg-Intron Redipen: 50 mcg/0.5 mL, 80 mcg/0.5 mL, 120 mcg/0.5 mL, 150 mcg/0.5 mL

Sylatron: 296 mcg, 444 mcg, 888 mcg, 4 x 296 mcg, 4 x 444 mcg [contains polysorbate 80]

Kit, Subcutaneous [preservative free]:

Peg-Intron Redipen Pak 4: 50 mcg/0.5 mL, 80 mcg/0.5 mL, 120 mcg/0.5 mL, 150 mcg/0.5 mL

References

Alade SL, Brown RE, and Paquet A Jr, "Polysorbate 80 and E-Ferol Toxicity," *Pediatrics*, 1986, 77(4):593-7.

American College of Obstetricians and Gynecologists, "ACOG Practice Bulletin No. 86: Viral Hepatitis in Pregnancy," *Obstet Gynecol*, 2007, 110(4):941-56.

Centers for Disease Control and Prevention (CDC). Sexually transmitted diseases treatment guidelines, 2010. *MMWR Recomm Rep.* 2010;59(RR-12):1-110.

Centers for Disease Control and Prevention (CDC), "Unusual Syndrome With Fatalities Among Premature Infants: Association With a New Intravenous Vitamin E Product," *MMWR Morb Mortal Wkly Rep*, 1984, 33(14):198-9.

DHHS. Guidelines for the prevention and treatment of opportunistic infections among HIV-exposed and HIV-infected children: recommendations from the National Institutes of Health, Centers for Disease Control and Prevention, the HIV Medicine Association of the Infectious Diseases Society of America, the Pediatric Infectious Diseases Society, and the American Academy of Pediatrics. November 6, 2013. Available at http://aidsinfo.nih.gov

DHHS Panel on Opportunistic Infections (OI) in HIV-Infected Adults and Adolescents, "Guidelines for Prevention and Treatment of Opportunistic Infections in HIV-Infected Adults and Adolescents: Recommendations from the Centers for Disease Control and Prevention (CDC), the National Institutes of Health (NIH), and the HIV Medicine Association (HIVMA) of the Infectious Diseases Society of America (IDSA)," May 7, 2013. Available at http://aidsinfo.nih.gov/contentfiles/lvguidelines/adult_oi.pdf

DHHS Panel on Treatment of HIV-Infected Pregnant Women and Prevention of Perinatal Transmission. Recommendations for use of antiretroviral drugs in pregnant HIV-1-infected women for maternal health and interventions to reduce perinatal HIV transmission in the United States. July 31, 2012; 1-235. Available at http://aidsinfo.nih.gov/contentfiles/PerinatalGL.pdf

Dienstag JL and McHutchison JG, "American Gastroenterological Association Medical Position Statement on the Management of Hepatitis C," *Gastroenterology*, 2006, 130(1):225-30.

Ghany MG, Strader DB, Thomas DL, et al, "Diagnosis, Management, and Treatment of Hepatitis C: An Update," *Hepatology*, 2009, 49 (4):1335-74.

Kumar AR, Hale TW, and Moke RE, "Transfer of Interferon Alfa Into Human Breast Milk," *J Hum Lact*, 2000, 16:226-8.

Lebon P, Girard S, Thépot F, et al, "The Presence of Alpha-Interferon in Human Amniotic Fluid," *J Gen Virol*, 1982, 59(Pt 2):393-6.

PegIntron prescribing information, Merck & Co. Inc, Whitehouse Station, NJ, 2011.

Waysbort A, Giroux M, Mansat V, et al, "Experimental Study of Transplacental Passage of Alpha Interferon by Two Assay Techniques," *Antimicrob Agents Chemother*, 1993, 37(6):1232-7.

◆ **Peg-Intron** *see* Peginterferon Alfa-2b *on page 1621*

◆ **PegIntron (Can)** *see* Peginterferon Alfa-2b *on page 1621*

◆ **Peg-Intron Redipen** *see* Peginterferon Alfa-2b *on page 1621*

◆ **Peg-Intron Redipen Pak 4** *see* Peginterferon Alfa-2b *on page 1621*

◆ **PEGLA** *see* Pegaspargase *on page 1615*

◆ **PegLyte (Can)** *see* Polyethylene Glycol-Electrolyte Solution *on page 1697*

◆ **Pegylated G-CSF** *see* Pegfilgrastim *on page 1616*

◆ **Pegylated Interferon Alfa-2a** *see* Peginterferon Alfa-2a *on page 1617*

◆ **Pegylated Interferon Alfa-2b** *see* Peginterferon Alfa-2b *on page 1621*

◆ **PEGyLAX** *see* Polyethylene Glycol 3350 *on page 1696*

Penciclovir (pen SYE kloe veer)

Medication Safety Issues
Sound-alike/look-alike issues:
Denavir® may be confused with indinavir
Brand Names: U.S. Denavir
Therapeutic Category Antiviral Agent, Topical
Generic Availability (U.S.) No
Use Topical treatment of recurrent herpes labialis (cold sores, fever blisters) (FDA approved in ages ≥12 years and adults)
Pregnancy Risk Factor B
Pregnancy Considerations Adverse events have not been observed in animal reproduction studies following intravenous administration.
Breast-Feeding Considerations According to the manufacturer, the decision to continue or discontinue breast-feeding during therapy should take into account the risk of exposure to the infant and the benefits of treatment to the mother.
Contraindications Hypersensitivity to penciclovir, famciclovir, or any component
Precautions No data available on safety and efficacy of penciclovir application to mucous membranes; avoid application to mucous membranes or near the eyes. Efficacy has not been established in immunocompromised patients or children <12 years of age.
Adverse Reactions
Central nervous system: Headache
Dermatologic: Mild erythema
Local: Application site reaction
Rare but important or life-threatening: Erythematous rash, local anesthesia, local edema, oropharyngeal edema, pain, paresthesia, parosmia, pruritus, skin discoloration, urticaria
Drug Interactions
Metabolism/Transport Effects None known.
Avoid Concomitant Use There are no known interactions where it is recommended to avoid concomitant use.
Increased Effect/Toxicity There are no known significant interactions involving an increase in effect.
Decreased Effect There are no known significant interactions involving a decrease in effect.
Stability Store at 20°C to 25°C (68°F to 77°F).
Mechanism of Action In cells infected with HSV-1 or HSV-2, viral thymidine kinase phosphorylates penciclovir to a monophosphate form which, in turn, is converted to penciclovir triphosphate by cellular kinases. Penciclovir triphosphate inhibits HSV polymerase competitively with deoxyguanosine triphosphate. Consequently, herpes viral DNA synthesis and, therefore, replication are selectively inhibited
Pharmacodynamics
Resolution of pain: Adults: 3.5 days (Spruance, 1997)
Cutaneous healing: Adults: 4.8 days (Spruance, 1997)
Pharmacokinetics (Adult data unless noted) Absorption: Topical: Negligible
Dosing: Usual Topical: Children ≥12 years, Adolescents, and Adults: Apply every 2 hours during waking hours for 4 days; start at the first sign or symptom of cold sore (eg, tingling, redness, itching, swelling)
Administration Topical: Apply only to herpes labialis on the lips and face. Apply sufficient amount to cover lesions and gently rub into the affected area. Avoid application in or near eyes since it may cause irritation.
Monitoring Parameters Resolution of pain and healing of cold sore lesion
Additional Information Penciclovir is the active metabolite of the prodrug famciclovir.

Dosage Forms Excipient information presented when available (limited, particularly for generics); consult specific product labeling.
Cream, External:
Denavir: 1% (1.5 g, 5 g) [contains cetostearyl alcohol, propylene glycol]
References
Dekker CL and Prober CG, "Pediatric Uses of Valacyclovir, Penciclovir and Famciclovir," *Pediatr Infect Dis J*, 2001, 20(11):1079-81.
Spruance SL, Rea TL, Thoming C, et al, "Penciclovir Cream for the Treatment of Herpes Simplex Labialis. A Randomized, Multicenter, Double-Blind, Placebo-Controlled Trial. Topical Penciclovir Collaborative Study Group," *JAMA*, 1997, 277(17):1374-9.

PenicillAMINE (pen i SIL a meen)

Medication Safety Issues
Sound-alike/look-alike issues:
Penicillamine may be confused with penicillin
International issues:
Depen [U.S.] may be confused with Depin brand name for nifedipine [India]; Depon brand name for acetaminophen [Greece]; Dipen brand name for diltiazem [Greece]
Pemine [Italy] may be confused with Pamine brand name for methscopolamine [U.S., Canada]
Brand Names: U.S. Cuprimine; Depen Titratabs
Brand Names: Canada Cuprimine®
Therapeutic Category Antidote, Copper Toxicity; Antidote, Lead Toxicity; Chelating Agent, Oral
Generic Availability (U.S.) No
Use Treatment of Wilson's disease, cystinuria, adjunct in the treatment of severe rheumatoid arthritis (FDA approved in adults); has also been used for lead poisoning, primary biliary cirrhosis (as adjunctive therapy following initial treatment with calcium EDTA or BAL); has also been used in lead poisoning
Pregnancy Risk Factor D
Pregnancy Considerations Birth defects, including congenital cutix laxa and associated defects, have been reported in infants following penicillamine exposure during pregnancy. Use for the treatment of rheumatoid arthritis during pregnancy is contraindicated. Use for the treatment of cystinuria only if the possible benefits to the mother outweigh the potential risks to the fetus. Continued treatment of Wilson's disease during pregnancy protects the mother against relapse. Discontinuation has detrimental maternal and fetal effects. Daily dosage should be limited to 750 mg. For planned cesarean section, reduce dose to 250 mg/day for the last 6 weeks of pregnancy, and continue at this dosage until wound healing is complete.
Breast-Feeding Considerations It is not known if penicillamine is excreted in breast milk. Use while breast-feeding is contraindicated by the manufacturer.
Contraindications Rheumatoid arthritic patients with renal insufficiency; patients with previous penicillamine-related aplastic anemia or agranulocytosis; concomitant administration with other hematopoietic-depressant drugs (eg, gold, immunosuppressants, antimalarials, phenylbutazone), pregnancy (except for the treatment of Wilson's disease or certain cases of cystinuria), breast-feeding
Warnings Penicillamine has been associated with fatalities due to agranulocytosis, aplastic anemia, thrombocytopenia, Goodpasture's syndrome, and myasthenia gravis; discontinue therapy if WBC <3500/mm³; temporarily discontinue treatment if the platelet count is <100,000/mm³; patients should be warned to promptly report any symptoms suggesting toxicity **[U.S. Boxed Warning]**; due to the potential severity of these effects, patients should be monitored closely. Proteinuria and/or hematuria may develop and are early warning signs of membraneous glomerulopathy which can progress to nephrotic syndrome; these symptoms may disappear with continued ▶

therapy; close observation is warranted; follow 24-hour urine protein excretion rates; excretion >1 g protein in urine per 24 hours or proteinuria which is progressively increasing requires decreasing the dosage or discontinuation in patients treated for rheumatoid arthritis; in Wilson's disease and cystinuria, the risks versus benefits of continuing must be considered.

Drug fever, sometimes accompanied with a skin eruption, necessitates temporary discontinuation of penicillamine in Wilson's disease and cystinuria patients and discontinuation in rheumatoid arthritic patients. Treatment may be resumed with a small dose and gradually increased to the desired dose once the symptoms have subsided. Early rashes (first few months) associated with penicillamine usually disappear within days after discontinuation of therapy and seldom return when treatment is restarted at a lower dose; late rashes (>6 months of treatment) require discontinuation of therapy.

Interruption of continuous therapy for Wilson's disease or cystinuria even for a few days has been associated with sensitivity reactions upon reinstitution of therapy; approximately 33% of patients will experience an allergic reaction. When used for cystinuria, renal stones may develop; an annual x-ray for renal stones is recommended

Precautions Patients on penicillamine for Wilson's disease or cystinuria should receive pyridoxine supplementation 25-50 mg/day; when treating rheumatoid arthritis, daily pyridoxine supplementation is also recommended. A positive ANA for lupus erythematosus may occur possibly progressing to a lupus-like syndrome. Patients who are allergic to penicillin may theoretically have cross-sensitivity to penicillamine. This possibility has been eliminated now that penicillamine is synthetically produced and no longer contains trace amounts of penicillin.

Adverse Reactions
Cardiovascular: Vasculitis

Central nervous system: Anxiety, agitation, fever, Guillain-Barré syndrome, hyperpyrexia, psychiatric disturbances, worsening neurologic symptoms

Dermatologic: Alopecia, cheilosis, dermatomyositis, drug eruptions, exfoliative dermatitis, lichen planus, pemphigus, pruritus, rash (early and late), skin friability increased, toxic epidermal necrolysis, urticaria, wrinkling (excessive), yellow nail syndrome

Endocrine & metabolic: Hypoglycemia, thyroiditis

Gastrointestinal: Anorexia, diarrhea, epigastric pain, gingivostomatitis, glossitis, nausea, oral ulcerations, pancreatitis, peptic ulcer reactivation, taste alteration, vomiting

Hematologic: Agranulocytosis, aplastic anemia, eosinophilia, hemolytic anemia, leukocytosis, leukopenia, monocytosis, red cell aplasia, sideroblastic anemia, thrombocytopenia, thrombotic thrombocytopenia purpura, thrombocytosis

Hepatic: Alkaline phosphatase increased, hepatic failure, intrahepatic cholestasis, toxic hepatitis

Local: Thrombophlebitis, white papules at venipuncture and surgical sites

Neuromuscular & skeletal: Arthralgia, dystonia, myasthenia gravis, muscle weakness, neuropathies, polyarthralgia (migratory, often with objective synovitis), polymyositis

Ocular: Diplopia, extraocular muscle weakness, optic neuritis, ptosis, visual disturbances

Otic: Tinnitus

Renal: Goodpasture's syndrome, hematuria, nephrotic syndrome, proteinuria, renal failure, renal vasculitis

Respiratory: Asthma, interstitial pneumonitis, pulmonary fibrosis, obliterative bronchiolitis

Miscellaneous: Allergic alveolitis, anetoderma, elastosis perforans serpiginosa, lupus-like syndrome, lactic dehydrogenase increased, lymphadenopathy, mammary hyperplasia, positive ANA test

Drug Interactions
Metabolism/Transport Effects None known.

Avoid Concomitant Use There are no known interactions where it is recommended to avoid concomitant use.

Increased Effect/Toxicity
The levels/effects of PenicillAMINE may be increased by: Multivitamins/Minerals (with ADEK, Folate, Iron)

Decreased Effect
PenicillAMINE may decrease the levels/effects of: Digoxin

The levels/effects of PenicillAMINE may be decreased by: Antacids; Iron Salts

Food Interactions Penicillamine serum levels may be decreased if taken with food. Management: Administer on an empty stomach 1 hour before or 2 hours after meals and at least 1 hour apart from other drugs, milk, antacids, and zinc- or iron-containing products. Certain disease states require further diet adjustment.

Mechanism of Action Chelates with lead, copper, mercury and other heavy metals to form stable, soluble complexes that are excreted in urine; depresses circulating IgM rheumatoid factor, depresses T-cell but not B-cell activity; combines with cystine to form a compound which is more soluble, thus cystine calculi are prevented

Pharmacodynamics Onset of action:
Rheumatoid arthritis: 2-3 months
Wilson's disease: 1-3 months

Pharmacokinetics (Adult data unless noted)
Absorption: 40% to 70%
Protein binding: 80%
Metabolism: In the liver
Half-life: 1.7-7 hours
Time to peak serum concentration: Within 1-3 hours
Elimination: Primarily (30% to 60%) in urine as unchanged drug

Dosing: Usual Oral:
Rheumatoid arthritis: **Note:** The optimal duration of therapy has not been determined; in patients experiencing a remission for ≥6 months, the daily dosage may be decreased in a stepwise fashion in 3-month intervals:
Children: Initial: 3 mg/kg/day (≤250 mg/day) for 3 months, then 6 mg/kg/day (≤500 mg/day) in 2 divided doses for 3 months to a maximum of 10 mg/kg/day (≤1-1.5 g/day) in 3-4 divided doses
Adults: 125-250 mg/day, may increase dose by 125-250 mg/day; if therapy still ineffective after 2-3 months of treatment and no signs of adverse effects, increases of 250 mg/day at 2-3 month intervals up to a maximum daily dose of 1.5 g may be done; doses >500 mg/day should be given in divided doses

Wilson's disease: **Note:** Dose that results in an initial 24-hour urinary copper excretion >2 mg/day should be continued for ~3 months; maintenance dose defined by amount resulting in <10 mcg serum free copper/dL.
Children: AASLD guidelines: 20 mg/kg/day in 2-3 divided doses, round off to the nearest 250 mg dose; reduce dose by 25% when clinically stable; administer with a pyridoxine supplement (25-50 mg/day)
Adults: 750-1500 mg/day in divided doses; maximum dose: 2000 mg/day; administer with a pyridoxine supplement (25-50 mg/day)

Note: In pregnant patients, limit daily dose to 1 g; if a cesarean section is planned, limit daily dose to 250 mg during the last 6 weeks before delivery and postoperatively until the wound has healed.

AASLD guidelines recommend to increase tolerability, therapy may be initiated at 250-500 mg/day and then titrated upward by 250 mg every 4-7 days; usual maintenance dose: 750-1000 mg/day in 2 divided doses; maximum: 1000-1500 mg/day in 2-4 divided doses; reduce dose by 25% when clinically stable (Roberts, 2008)

Cystinuria (doses titrated to maintain urinary cystine excretion at <100-200 mg/day in patients without a history of stones and <100 mg/day in patients who have had stone formation and/or pain):
  Children: 30 mg/kg/day in 4 divided doses; maximum dose: 4 g/day
  Adults: Initial: 2 g/day divided every 6 hours (range: 1-4 g/day)
Lead poisoning (treatment duration varies from 4-12 weeks depending upon the pretreatment blood lead level; goal of therapy is to reduce the total body content so that the blood lead level does not rebound to unacceptable levels post-treatment):
  Children: 20-30 mg/kg/day in 3-4 divided doses; initiating treatment at 25% of this dose and gradually increasing to the full dose over 2-3 weeks may minimize adverse reactions; maximum dose: 1.5 g/day; a reduced dosage of 15 mg/kg/day in 2 divided doses has been shown to be effective in the treatment of mild to moderate lead poisoning (blood lead concentration 20-40 mcg/dL) with a reduction in adverse effects (Shannon, 2000)
  Adults: 1-1.5 g/day in 3-4 divided doses; initiating treatment at 25% of this dose and gradually increasing to the full dose over 2-3 weeks may minimize adverse reactions
Primary biliary cirrhosis: Adults: 250 mg/day to start, increase by 250 mg every 2 weeks up to a maintenance dose of 1 g/day, as 250 mg 4 times/day
Dosing adjustment in renal impairment: CrCl <50 mL/minute: Avoid use

Administration Oral: Administer on an empty stomach 1 hour before or 2 hours after meals, milk, or other medications; patients unable to swallow capsules may mix contents of capsule with fruit juice or chilled pureed fruit; patients with cystinuria should drink copious amounts of water

Monitoring Parameters Urinalysis, CBC with differential, hemoglobin, and platelet count are recommended twice weekly for the first month then every 2 weeks for 6 months and monthly thereafter; in addition, monitor the patient's skin, lymph nodes, and body temperature; liver function tests are recommended every 6 months; weekly measurements of urinary and blood concentrations of the intoxicating metal are indicated; quantitative 24-hour urine protein at 1- to 2-week intervals initially (first 2-3 months); annual x-ray for renal stones (when used for cystinuria)

Wilson's disease: Periodic ophthalmic exam; 24-hour urinary copper excretion; copper excretion is highest initially after treatment and may exceed 1000 mcg/day; chronic treatment should produce urinary copper excretion of 200-500 mcg/day on treatment; values <200 mcg/day may be due to either noncompliance or overtreatment which may be differentiated by measuring nonceruloplasmin bound copper (high in noncompliance and low in overtreatment)

Reference Range Wilson's disease: Adequate treatment: "Free" (unbound) serum copper <10 mcg/dL (Free serum copper = Total copper - ceruloplasmin copper); 24-hour urinary copper excretion 200-500 mcg (3-8 micromoles)/day

Additional Information The racemic mixture interferes with pyridoxine action and is no longer used; however, supplemental pyridoxine is still recommended.

Dosage Forms Excipient information presented when available (limited, particularly for generics); consult specific product labeling.
Capsule, Oral:
  Cuprimine: 250 mg [contains fd&c yellow #10 (quinoline yellow)]
Tablet, Oral:
  Depen Titratabs: 250 mg [scored]

Extemporaneous Preparations A 50 mg/mL oral suspension may be made with capsules. Mix the contents of sixty 250 mg capsules with 3 g carboxymethylcellulose, 150 g sucrose, 300 mg citric acid, and parabens (methylparaben 120 mg, propylparaben 12 mg). Add quantity of propylene glycol sufficient to make 100 mL, then add quantity of purified water sufficient to make 300 mL. Cherry flavor may be added. Label "shake well" and "refrigerate". Stable for 30 days refrigerated.
DeCastro FJ, Jaeger RQ, and Rolfe UT, "An Extemporaneously Prepared Penicillamine Suspension Used to Treat Lead Intoxication," *Hosp Pharm*, 1977, 2:446-8.

References
Piomelli S, "Childhood Lead Poisoning," *Pediatr Clin North Am*, 2002, 49(6):1285-304.
Roberts EA, Schilsky ML, and American Association for Study of Liver Diseases (AASLD)," Diagnosis and Treatment of Wilson Disease: An Update," *Hepatology*, 2008, 47(6):2089-111.
Shannon MW and Townsend MK, "Adverse Effects of Reduced-Dose d-Penicillamine in Children With Mild-to-Moderate Lead Poisoning," *Ann Pharmacother*, 2000, 34(1):15-8.
"Treatment Guidelines for Lead Exposure in Children. American Academy of Pediatrics Committee on Drugs," *Pediatrics*, 1995, 96(1 Pt 1):155-60.

Penicillin G Benzathine
(pen i SIL in jee BENZ a theen)

Medication Safety Issues
Sound-alike/look-alike issues:
  Penicillin may be confused with penicillamine
  Bicillin® may be confused with Wycillin®
Administration issues:
  Penicillin G benzathine may only be administered by deep intramuscular injection; intravenous administration of penicillin G benzathine has been associated with cardiopulmonary arrest and death.
Other safety concerns:
  Bicillin® C-R (penicillin G benzathine and penicillin G procaine) may be confused with Bicillin® L-A (penicillin G benzathine). Penicillin G benzathine is the only product currently approved for the treatment of syphilis. Administration of penicillin G benzathine and penicillin G procaine combination instead of Bicillin® L-A may result in inadequate treatment response.

Brand Names: U.S. Bicillin L-A

Brand Names: Canada Bicillin® L-A

Therapeutic Category Antibiotic, Penicillin

Generic Availability (U.S.) No

Use Active against many gram-positive organisms and some spirochetes; treatment of syphilis; used only for the treatment of mild-to-moderate infections (ie, *Streptococcus* pharyngitis) caused by organisms susceptible to low concentrations of penicillin G, or for prophylaxis of infections caused by these organisms, such as rheumatic fever disease and acute glomerulonephritis (FDA approved in all ages)

Pregnancy Risk Factor B

Pregnancy Considerations Adverse events have not been observed in animal reproduction studies. Penicillin crosses the placenta and distributes into amniotic fluid. Maternal use of penicillins has generally not resulted in an increased risk of adverse fetal effects. Penicillin G is the drug of choice for treatment of syphilis during pregnancy.

Breast-Feeding Considerations Penicillins are excreted in breast milk. The manufacturer recommends that caution be exercised when administering penicillin to nursing women. Nondose-related effects could include modification of bowel flora and allergic sensitization.

Contraindications Hypersensitivity to penicillin or any component

Warnings Do not administer I.V.; do not admix with other I.V. solutions; inadvertent I.V. administration has resulted in cardiac arrest and death **[U.S. Boxed Warning]**. Injection ▶

into or near a nerve may result in permanent neurovascular and neurological damage, gangrene requiring amputation of proximal portions of extremities, necrosis, and sloughing at the injection site; effects have most often occurred in infants and small children. Serious hypersensitivity reactions, including anaphylaxis, have been reported; supportive therapy and medication for the management of anaphylactic reactions should be available for immediate use. Superinfection and *C. difficile*-associated diarrhea have been reported with use of penicillin G benzathine.

Precautions Use with caution in patients with impaired renal function, impaired cardiac function, preexisting seizure disorder, history of significant allergies and/or asthma, or hypersensitivity to cephalosporins. Repeated I.M. injections into anterolateral thigh may result in quadriceps femoris fibrosis or atrophy; risk higher in neonates and infants.

Adverse Reactions

Cardiovascular: Cardiac arrest, cerebral vascular accident, cyanosis, gangrene, hypotension, pallor, palpitations, syncope, tachycardia, vasodilation, vasospasm, vasovagal reaction

Central nervous system: Anxiety, coma, confusion, dizziness, euphoria, fatigue, headache, nervousness, pain, seizure, somnolence

In addition, a syndrome of CNS symptoms has been reported which includes: Severe agitation with confusion, hallucinations (auditory and visual), and fear of death (Hoigne's syndrome); other symptoms include cyanosis, dizziness, palpitations, psychosis, seizures, tachycardia, taste disturbance, tinnitus

Gastrointestinal: Bloody stool, intestinal necrosis, nausea, vomiting

Genitourinary: Impotence, priapism

Hepatic: AST increased

Local: Injection site reactions: Abscess, atrophy, bruising, cellulitis, edema, hemorrhage, inflammation, lump, necrosis, pain, skin ulcer

Neuromuscular & skeletal: Arthritis exacerbation, joint disorder, neurovascular damage, numbness, periostitis, rhabdomyolysis, transverse myelitis, tremor, weakness

Ocular: Blindness, blurred vision

Renal: BUN increased, creatinine increased, hematuria, myoglobinuria, neurogenic bladder, proteinuria, renal failure

Miscellaneous: Diaphoresis, hypersensitivity reactions, Jarisch-Herxheimer reaction, lymphadenopathy, mottling, warmth

Drug Interactions

Metabolism/Transport Effects None known.

Avoid Concomitant Use

Avoid concomitant use of Penicillin G Benzathine with any of the following: BCG; Probenecid

Increased Effect/Toxicity

Penicillin G Benzathine may increase the levels/effects of: Methotrexate; Vitamin K Antagonists

The levels/effects of Penicillin G Benzathine may be increased by: Probenecid

Decreased Effect

Penicillin G Benzathine may decrease the levels/effects of: BCG; Mycophenolate; Sodium Picosulfate; Typhoid Vaccine

The levels/effects of Penicillin G Benzathine may be decreased by: Tetracycline Derivatives

Stability Store at 2°C to 8°C (36°F to 46°F); avoid freezing

Mechanism of Action Interferes with bacterial cell wall synthesis during active multiplication, causing cell wall death and resultant bactericidal activity against susceptible bacteria

Pharmacokinetics (Adult data unless noted)

Absorption: I.M.: Slow

Distribution: Minimal concentrations attained in CSF with inflamed or uninflamed meninges; highest levels in the kidneys; lesser amounts in liver, skin, intestine; excreted in breast milk

Protein binding: ~60%

Time to peak serum concentration: Within 12-24 hours; serum levels are usually detectable for 1-4 weeks depending on the dose; larger doses result in more sustained levels rather than higher levels

Elimination: Excreted by renal tubular excretion; penicillin G is detected in urine for up to 12 weeks after a single I.M. injection; renal clearance is delayed in neonates, young infants, and patients with impaired renal function

Dosing: Neonatal Syphilis, congenital: I.M.: 50,000 units/kg as a single dose (*Red Book*, 2012)

Dosing: Usual

Infants, Children, and Adolescents:

Group A streptococcal upper respiratory infection (Gerber, 2009): I.M.:

Rheumatic fever, primary prevention:

≤27 kg: 600,000 units as a single dose

>27 kg: 1.2 million units as a single dose

Rheumatic fever, secondary prevention: **Note:** Duration of secondary rheumatic fever prophylaxis varies: Rheumatic fever with carditis and residual heart disease: 10 years or until 40 years of age (whichever is longer), sometimes lifelong prophylaxis; rheumatic fever with carditis but no residual heart disease: 10 years or until 21 years of age (whichever is longer); rheumatic fever without carditis: 5 years or until 21 years of age (whichever is longer)

≤27 kg: 600,000 units every 3-4 weeks

>27 kg: 1.2 million units every 3-4 weeks

Syphilis: (CDC, 2010; *Red Book*, 2012): I.M.

Primary, Secondary, or Early Latent (<1 year duration): 50,000 units/kg once; maximum dose: 2.4 million units

Late Latent or Latent with unknown duration: 50,000 units/kg once weekly for 3 doses; maximum dose: 2.4 million units

Adults:

Group A streptococcal upper respiratory infection: I.M.: 1.2 million units as a single dose

Rheumatic fever, secondary prevention: I.M.: 600,000 units twice monthly or 1.2 million units every 4 weeks

Syphilis: (CDC, 2010): I.M.:

Primary, Secondary, or Early Latent (<1 year duration): 2.4 million units as a single dose

Late Latent or Latent with unknown duration: 2.4 million units once weekly for 3 doses

Neurosyphilis: Not indicated as single-drug therapy, but may be given once weekly for 3 weeks following I.V. treatment; refer to Penicillin G Parenteral/Aqueous monograph for dosing

Administration Administer undiluted as deep I.M. injection in the upper outer quadrant of the buttock (adolescents and adults) or into the midlateral aspect of the thigh (neonates, infants, and children); do **not** give I.V., intra-arterially or SubQ; **inadvertent I.V. administration has resulted in thrombosis, severe neurovascular damage, cardiac arrest, and death**

Monitoring Parameters CBC, urinalysis, culture, renal function tests, stool frequency

Test Interactions Positive Coombs' [direct], false-positive urinary and/or serum proteins; false-positive or negative urinary glucose using Clinitest®

Additional Information Use a penicillin G benzathine/penicillin G procaine combination (ie, Bicillin® C-R) to achieve early peak levels in acute infections. Do not administer Bicillin® C-R to treat patients infected with syphilis since this may result in inadequate treatment.

Dosage Forms Excipient information presented when available (limited, particularly for generics); consult specific product labeling.

Suspension, Intramuscular:

Bicillin L-A: 600,000 units/mL (1 mL); 1,200,000 units/2 mL (2 mL); 2,400,000 units/4 mL (4 mL) [contains methylparaben, propylparaben]

References

Centers for Disease Control and Prevention, "Sexually Transmitted Diseases Treatment Guidelines - 2006," *MMWR Recomm Rep*, 2006, 55(RR-11):1-100. Available at http://www.cdc.gov/std/treatment/2006/rr5511.pdf. Accessed September 18, 2008.

Gerber MA, Baltimore RS, Eaton CB, et al, "Prevention of Rheumatic Fever and Diagnosis and Treatment of Acute *Streptococcal pharyngitis*: A Scientific Statement from the American Heart Association Rheumatic Fever, Endocarditis, and Kawasaki Disease Committee of the Council on Cardiovascular Disease in the Young, the Interdisciplinary Council on Functional Genomics and Translational Biology, and the Interdisciplinary Council on Quality of Care and Outcomes Research: Endorsed by the American Academy of Pediatrics," *Circulation*, 2009, 119(11):1541-51.

Kaplan EL, Berrios X, Speth J, et al, "Pharmacokinetics of Benzathine Penicillin G: Serum Levels During the 28 Days After Intramuscular Injection of 1,200,000 Units," *J Pediatr*, 1989, 115(1):146-50.

Paryani SG, Vaughn AJ, Crosby M, et al, "Treatment of Asymptomatic Congenital Syphilis: Benzathine Versus Procaine Penicillin G Therapy," *J Pediatr*, 1994, 125(3):471-5.

Shulman ST, Bisno AL, Clegg HW, et al, "Clinical Practice Guideline for the Diagnosis and Management of Group A Streptococcal Pharyngitis: 2012 Update by the Infectious Diseases Society of America," *Clin Infect Dis*, 2012.

Penicillin G (Parenteral/Aqueous)
(pen i SIL in jee, pa REN ter al, AYE kwee us)

Medication Safety Issues
Sound-alike/look-alike issues:
Penicillin may be confused with penicillamine

Brand Names: U.S. Pfizerpen-G

Brand Names: Canada Crystapen®

Therapeutic Category Antibiotic, Penicillin

Generic Availability (U.S.) Yes

Use Treatment of sepsis, meningitis, pericarditis, endocarditis, pneumonia, and other infections due to susceptible gram-positive organisms (except *Staphylococcus aureus*), some gram-negative organisms such as *Neisseria gonorrhoeae*, or *N. meningitidis* and some anaerobes and spirochetes (FDA approved in all ages)

Pregnancy Risk Factor B

Pregnancy Considerations Adverse events have not been observed in animal reproduction studies. Penicillin crosses the placenta and distributes into amniotic fluid. Maternal use of penicillins has generally not resulted in an increased risk of adverse fetal effects. Penicillin G is the drug of choice for treatment of syphilis during pregnancy and penicillin G (parenteral/aqueous) is the drug of choice for the prevention of early-onset Group B Streptococcal (GBS) disease in newborns (consult current guidelines).

Breast-Feeding Considerations Very small amounts of penicillin G transfer into breast milk. Peak milk concentrations occur at approximately 1 hour after an IM dose and are higher if multiple doses are given. The manufacturer recommends that caution be exercised when administering penicillin to nursing women. Nondose-related effects could include modification of bowel flora and allergic sensitization.

Contraindications Hypersensitivity to penicillin or any component

Warnings Serious and occasionally fatal hypersensitivity (anaphylactoid) reactions have been reported in patients on penicillin therapy, especially with a history of beta-lactam hypersensitivity, history of sensitivity to multiple allergens, or previous IgE-mediated reactions (eg, anaphylaxis, angioedema, urticaria); administration to patients with confirmed penicillin allergies should be avoided; in patients with confirmed cephalosporin allergy, consider skin testing to rule out cross-sensitivity to penicillins. Immediate treatment for anaphylactic reaction should be available during administration. In neonates, elimination rate is decreased due to immature hepatic and renal function; dosage adjustment is needed. Prolonged use may result in fungal or bacterial superinfection, including *C. difficile*-associated diarrhea (CDAD) and pseudomembranous colitis; CDAD has been observed >2 months postantibiotic treatment. Large I.V. or intraventricular doses have been associated with neurotoxicity; use caution, especially in patients with concomitant renal and hepatic dysfunction and in patients with preexisting seizure disorders. Avoid intra-arterial administration or injection into or near major peripheral nerves or blood vessels since such injections may cause severe and/or permanent neurovascular damage. Product contains sodium and potassium; high doses of I.V. therapy may alter serum concentrations.

Precautions Use with caution in patients with renal impairment; dosage modification required; further dosage reduction recommended in patients with impaired hepatic and renal function

Adverse Reactions
Cardiovascular: Localized phlebitis, local thrombophlebitis

Central nervous system: Coma (high doses), hyperreflexia (high doses), myoclonus (high doses), seizure (high doses)

Dermatologic: Contact dermatitis, skin rash

Endocrine & metabolic: Electrolyte disturbance (high doses)

Gastrointestinal: Pseudomembranous colitis

Hematologic & oncologic: Neutropenia, positive direct Coombs test (rare, high doses)

Hypersensitivity: Anaphylaxis, hypersensitivity reaction (immediate and delayed), serum sickness

Immunologic: Jarisch-Herxheimer reaction

Local: Injection site reaction

Renal: Acute interstitial nephritis (high doses), renal tubular disease (high doses)

Drug Interactions
Metabolism/Transport Effects None known.

Avoid Concomitant Use
Avoid concomitant use of Penicillin G (Parenteral/Aqueous) with any of the following: BCG; Probenecid

Increased Effect/Toxicity
Penicillin G (Parenteral/Aqueous) may increase the levels/effects of: Methotrexate; Vitamin K Antagonists

The levels/effects of Penicillin G (Parenteral/Aqueous) may be increased by: Probenecid

Decreased Effect
Penicillin G (Parenteral/Aqueous) may decrease the levels/effects of: BCG; Mycophenolate; Sodium Picosulfate; Typhoid Vaccine

The levels/effects of Penicillin G (Parenteral/Aqueous) may be decreased by: Tetracycline Derivatives

Stability
Penicillin G potassium: Store at 20°C to 25°C (68°F to 77°F). Following reconstitution, solution may be stored for up to 7 days under refrigeration. Premixed bags for infusion should be stored in the freezer at or below -20°C (-4°F); frozen bags may be thawed at room temperature or in refrigerator. Once thawed, solution is stable for 14 days if stored in refrigerator or for 24 hours when stored at room temperature. Do not refreeze.

Penicillin G sodium: Store at 20°C to 25°C (68°F to 77°F). Reconstituted solution may be stored for up to 3 days under refrigeration.

Mechanism of Action Interferes with bacterial cell wall synthesis during active multiplication, causing cell wall death and resultant bactericidal activity against susceptible bacteria

Pharmacokinetics (Adult data unless noted)

Distribution: Penetration across the blood-brain barrier is poor with uninflamed meninges

Protein binding: 65%

Metabolism: Hepatic (10% to 30%) to penicilloic acid

Half-life:

Neonates:

<6 days: 3.2-3.4 hours

7-13 days: 1.2-2.2 hours

>14 days: 0.9-1.9 hours

Infants and Children: 0.5-1.2 hours

Adults: 0.5-0.75 hours with normal renal function

Time to peak serum concentration: I.M.: Within 30 minutes

Elimination: Renal (58% to 85% unchanged drug and metabolites); mainly by tubular secretion and bile

Dialysis: Moderately dialyzable (20% to 50%)

Dosing: Neonatal

General dosing, susceptible infection (non-CNS) (*Red Book*, 2012): I.M., I.V.:

Body weight <1 kg:

PNA ≤14 days: 25,000-50,000 units/kg/**dose** every 12 hours

PNA 15-28 days: 25,000-50,000 units/kg/**dose** every 8 hours

Body weight ≥1 kg:

PNA ≤7 days: 25,000-50,000 units/kg/**dose** every 12 hours

PNA 8-28 days: 25,000-50,000 units/kg/**dose** every 8 hours

Meningitis: I.V.:

Group B streptococcus (*Red Book*, 2012):

PNA 0-7 days: 250,000-450,000 units/kg/day in divided doses every 8 hours

PNA 8-28 days: 450,000-500,000 units/kg/day in divided doses every 6 hours

Other susceptible organisms (Tunkel, 2004):

PNA 0-7 days: 50,000 units/kg/day in divided doses every 8-12 hours

PNA 8-28 days: 200,000 units/kg/day in divided doses every 6-8 hours

Syphilis, congenital (CDC, 2010): I.V.:

PNA 0-7 days: 50,000 units/kg/**dose** every 12 hours for 10 days

PNA 8-28 days: 50,000 units/kg/**dose** every 8 hours for 10 days

Dosing: Usual

Infants, Children, and Adolescents:

General dosing, susceptible infection (*Red Book*, 2012): I.M., I.V.:

Mild to moderate infection: 100,000-150,000 units/kg/day in divided doses every 6 hours maximum daily dose: 8 million units/day

Severe infections: 200,000-300,000 units/kg/day in divided doses every 4 hours; maximum daily dose: 24 million units/day

Anthrax, community-acquired: I.V.: 100,000-150,000 units/kg/day in divided doses every 4-6 hours (Stevens, 2005)

Arthritis, gonococcal: I.M., I.V.:

Weight <45 kg: 100,000 units/kg/day divided every 6 hours for 7-10 days

Weight ≥45 kg: 2.5 million units every 6 hours for 7-10 days

Clostridial myonecrosis (gas gangrene): I.V.: 250,000-400,000 units/kg/day in divided doses every 4-6 hours with or without clindamycin (*Red Book*, 2012)

Diphtheria: I.M., I.V.: 150,000-250,000 units/kg/day in divided doses every 6 hours for 7-10 days. AAP suggests a duration of 14 days (*Red Book*, 2012)

Endocarditis, bacterial, treatment (Baddour, 2005): I.V.:

Enterococcal endocarditis (native or prosthetic valve): 300,000 units/kg/day in divided doses every 4-6 hours with gentamicin for 4-6 weeks

Viridans group streptococci and *Streptococcus bovis* (highly penicillin susceptible):

Native valve: 200,000 units/kg/day in divided doses every 4-6 hours for 4 weeks or 2 weeks if given with gentamicin

Prosthetic valve: 300,000 units/kg/day in divided doses every 4-6 hours for 6 weeks with 2-6 weeks of gentamicin

Viridans group streptococci and *Streptococcus bovis* (relatively resistant):

Native valve: 300,000 units/kg/day in divided doses every 4-6 hours for 4 weeks with 2 weeks of gentamicin

Prosthetic valve: 300,000 units/kg/day in divided doses every 4-6 hours for 6 weeks with 2-6 weeks of gentamicin

Lyme disease: I.V.: 200,000-400,000 units/kg/day in divided doses every 4 hours; maximum daily dose: 24 million units/day (Halperin, 2007; Wormser, 2006)

Meningitis: Note: Dosing varies based on organism being treated. I.V.:

Group B streptococcus: Infants: 450,000-500,000 units/kg/day divided every 6 hours (*Red Book*, 2012)

S. pneumonia: 250,000-400,000 units/kg/day divided every 4-6 hours (*Red Book*, 2012)

Other susceptible organisms: 300,000 units/kg/day divided every 4-6 hours; maximum daily dose: 24 million units/day (Tunkel, 2004)

Meningococcal disease: I.V.: 300,000 units/kg/day in divided doses every 4-6 hours; maximum daily dose: 12 million units/day (*Red Book*, 2012)

Pneumonia, community-acquired (CAP): I.V.: Infants and Children >3 months:

Empiric treatment or *S. pneumoniae* (moderate to severe; MICs to penicillin ≤2.0 mcg/mL): 200,000-250,000 units/kg/day divided every 4-6 hours (Bradley, 2011)

Alternate dosing (AAP recommendation): 250,000-400,000 units/kg/day divided every 4-6 hours (*Red Book*, 2012)

Group A *Streptococcus* (moderate to severe): 100,000-250,000 units/kg/day divided every 4-6 hours (Bradley, 2011)

Rat-bite fever/Haverhill fever: I.V.: 150,000-250,000 units/kg/day in divided doses every 4 hours for 4 weeks; maximum daily dose: 20 million units/day (*Red Book*, 2012)

Syphilis: I.V.:

Congenital: Infants ≥1 month: 200,000-300,000 units/kg/day in divided doses every 4-6 hours for 10 days (CDC, 2009)

Neurosyphilis:

Non-HIV-exposed/-positive: 200,000-300,000 units/kg/day in divided doses every 4-6 hours for 10-14 days; maximum dose: 24 million units/day (*Red Book*, 2012)

HIV-exposed/-positive: 200,000-300,000 units/kg/day divided every 6 hours for 10-14 days; maximum dose: 24 million units/day (CDC, 2009)

Tetanus: I.V.: 100,000 units/kg/day in divided doses every 4-6 hours for 10-14 days; maximum daily dose: 12 million units/day (*Red Book*, 2012)

Adults:

***Actinomyces* species:** I.V.: 10-20 million units/day in divided doses every 4-6 hours for 4-6 weeks

Clostridium perfringens: I.V.: 24 million units/day in divided doses every 4-6 hours with clindamycin

Corynebacterium diptheriae: I.V.: 2-3 million units/day in divided doses every 4-6 hours for 10-12 days

Erysipelas: I.V.: 1-2 million units every 4-6 hours

Erysipelothrix: I.V.: 2-4 million units every 4 hours

Fascial space infections: I.V.: 2-4 million units every 4-6 hours with metronidazole

Leptospirosis: I.V.: 1.5 million units every 6 hours for 7 days

Listeria: I.V.: 15-20 million units/day in divided doses every 4-6 hours for 2 weeks (meningitis) or 4 weeks (endocarditis)

Lyme disease (meningitis): I.V.: 20 million units/day in divided doses

Neurosyphilis: I.V.: 18-24 million units/day in divided doses every 4 hours (or by continuous infusion) for 10-14 days (CDC, 2010)

Prosthetic joint infection: I.V.:

Enterococcus spp (penicillin-susceptible), streptococci (beta-hemolytic): 20-24 million units daily continuous infusion every 24 hours or in divided doses every 4 hours for 4-6 weeks (Osmon, 2013); **Note:** For penicillin-susceptible *Enterococcus* spp, consider addition of aminoglycoside.

Propionibacterium acnes: 20 million units daily continuous infusion every 24 hours or in divided doses every 4 hours for 4-6 weeks (Osmon, 2013)

Streptococcus sp.:

Brain abscess: I.V.: 18-24 million units/day in divided doses every 4 hours with metronidazole

Endocarditis or osteomyelitis: I.V.: 3-4 million units every 4 hours for at least 4 weeks

Pregnancy (prophylaxis GBS): I.V.: 5 million units x 1 dose, then 2.5-3 million units every 4 hours until delivery (CDC, 2010)

Skin and soft tissue: I.V.: 3-4 million units every 4 hours for 10 days

Toxic shock: I.V.: 24 million units/day in divided doses with clindamycin

Streptococcal pneumonia: I.V.: 2-3 million units every 4 hours

Whipple's disease: I.V.: 2 million units every 4 hours for 2 weeks, followed by oral trimethoprim/sulfamethoxazole or doxycycline for 1 year

Relapse or CNS involvement: 4 million units every 4 hours for 4 weeks

Dosing adjustment in renal impairment:

Manufacturer's labeling: Infants, Children, Adolescents, and Adults: I.M., I.V.:

Uremic patients with CrCl >10 mL/minute: Administer a normal dose followed by 50% of the normal dose every 4-5 hours

CrCl <10 mL/minute: Administer a normal dose followed by 50% of the normal dose every 8-10 hours

Alternate recommendation: Adults:

GFR >50 mL/minute: No dosage adjustments are necessary (Aronoff, 2007)

GFR 10-50 mL/minute: Administer 75% of the normal dose (Aronoff, 2007)

GFR <10 mL/minute: Administer 20% to 50% of the normal dose (Aronoff, 2007)

Intermittent hemodialysis (IHD) (administer after hemodialysis on dialysis days) (Heintz, 2009): Administer a normal dose followed by either 25% to 50% of normal dose every 4-6 hours **or** 50% to 100% of normal dose every 8-12 hours. *For mild to moderate infections,* administer 0.5-1 million units every 4-6 hours **or** 1-2 million units every 8-12 hours. *For neurosyphilis, endocarditis, or serious infections,* administer up to 2 million units every 4-6 hours; administer after dialysis on dialysis days **or** supplement with 500,000 units after dialysis. **Note:** Dosing dependent on the assumption of 3 times weekly, complete IHD sessions.

Continuous renal replacement therapy (CRRT) (Heintz, 2009; Trotman, 2005): Drug clearance is highly dependent on the method of renal replacement, filter type, and flow rate. Appropriate dosing requires close monitoring of pharmacologic response, signs of adverse reactions due to drug accumulation, as well as drug concentrations in relation to target trough (if appropriate). The following are general recommendations only (based on dialysate flow/ultrafiltration rates of 1-2 L/hour and minimal residual renal function) and should not supersede clinical judgment:

CVVH: Loading dose of 4 million units, followed by 2 million units every 4-6 hours

CVVHD: Loading dose of 4 million units, followed by 2-3 million units every 4-6 hours

CVVHDF: Loading dose of 4 million units, followed by 2-4 million units every 4-6 hours

Dosing adjustment in hepatic impairment: There are no dosage adjustments provided in the manufacturer's labeling.

Administration Parenteral:

I.M.: Administer I.M. by deep injection in the upper outer quadrant of the buttock. Administer injection around-the-clock to promote less variation in peak and trough levels. **Note:** The 20 million unit dosage form may be administered by continuous I.V. infusion only.

I.V.: Usually administered by intermittent infusion. In some centers, large doses may be administered by continuous I.V. infusion. **Note:** The 20 million unit dosage form may be administered by continuous I.V. infusion only. The potassium or sodium content of the dose should be considered when determining the infusion rate.

Intermittent I.V.: May be dissolved in small amounts of SWFI, NS, or D_5W and administered peripherally as a 50,000-100,000 unit/mL solution. In fluid-restricted patients, 146,000 units/mL in SW results in a maximum recommended osmolality for peripheral infusion. Infuse over 15-30 minutes.

Continuous I.V. infusion: Determine the volume of fluid and rate of its administration required by the patient in a 24-hour period. Add the appropriate daily dosage of penicillin to this fluid. For example, if the daily dose is 10 million units and 2 L of fluid/day is required, add 5 million units to 1 L and adjust the rate of flow so the liter will be infused over 12 hours (83 mL/hour). Repeat steps (5 million units/L at 83 mL/hour) for the remaining 12 hours.

Monitoring Parameters Periodic serum electrolytes, renal and hematologic function tests, cardiac and hematologic function tests during prolonged/high-dose therapy; observe for signs and symptoms of anaphylaxis during first dose

Test Interactions False-positive or negative urinary glucose determination using Clinitest®; positive Coombs' [direct]; false-positive urinary and/or serum proteins

Additional Information

Penicillin G potassium: 1.7 mEq of potassium and 0.3 mEq of sodium per 1 million units of penicillin G

Penicillin G sodium: 2 mEq of sodium per 1 million units of penicillin G

Dosage Forms Excipient information presented when available (limited, particularly for generics); consult specific product labeling.

Solution, Intravenous, as potassium:

Generic: 20,000 units/mL (50 mL); 40,000 units/mL (50 mL); 60,000 units/mL (50 mL)

Solution Reconstituted, Injection:

Pfizerpen-G: 5,000,000 units (1 ea)

Solution Reconstituted, Injection, as potassium:

Pfizerpen-G: 5,000,000 units (1 ea); 20,000,000 units (1 ea)

Pfizerpen-G: 5,000,000 units (1 ea); 20,000,000 units (1 ea) [pyrogen free]

Generic: 5,000,000 units (1 ea); 20,000,000 units (1 ea)
Solution Reconstituted, Injection, as potassium [preservative free]:
Generic: 20,000,000 units (1 ea)
Solution Reconstituted, Injection, as sodium:
Generic: 5,000,000 units (1 ea)

References

Aronoff GR, Bennett WM, Berns JS, et al, *Drug Prescribing in Renal Failure: Dosing Guidelines for Adults and Children*, 5th ed, Philadelphia, PA: American College of Physicians, 2007.

Baddour LM, Wilson WR, Bayer AS, et al, "Infective Endocarditis: Diagnosis, Antimicrobial Therapy, and Management of Complications: A Statement for Healthcare Professionals From the Committee on Rheumatic Fever, Endocarditis, and Kawasaki Disease, Council on Cardiovascular Disease in the Young, and the Councils on Clinical Cardiology, Stroke, and Cardiovascular Surgery and Anesthesia, American Heart Association: Endorsed by the Infectious Diseases Society of America," *Circulation*, 2005, 111(23):e394-434.

Bradley JS, Byington CL, Shah SS, et al, "The Management of Community-Acquired Pneumonia in Infants and Children Older Than 3 Months of Age: Clinical Practice Guidelines by the Pediatric Infectious Diseases Society and the Infectious Diseases Society of America", *Clin Infect Dis*, 2011, 53(7):e25-76.

Centers for Disease Control and Prevention, "Guidelines for Prevention and Treatment of Opportunistic Infections in HIV-Infected Adults and Adolescents," *MMWR Recomm Rep*, 2009, 58(RR-4):1-207.

Centers for Disease Control and Prevention, "Guidelines for the Prevention and Treatment of Opportunistic Infections Among HIV-Exposed and HIV-Infected Children," *MMWR Recomm Rep*, 2009, 58(RR-11):1-166.

Centers for Disease Control, "Prevention of Perinatal Group B Streptococcal Disease," *MMWR*, 2010, 59(RR10)1-32.

Centers for Disease Control and Prevention, "Sexually Transmitted Diseases Treatment Guidelines, 2010," *MMWR Recomm Rep*, 2010, 59(RR-12):1-110.

Halperin JJ, Shapiro ED, Logigian E, et al, "Practice Parameter: Treatment of Nervous System Lyme Disease (an Evidence-Based Review)," *Neurology*, 2007, 69(1):91-102.

Heintz BH, Matzke GR, and Dager WE, "Antimicrobial Dosing Concepts and Recommendations for Critically Ill Adult Patients Receiving Continuous Renal Replacement Therapy or Intermittent Hemodialysis," *Pharmacotherapy*, 2009, 29(5):562-77.

Osmon DR, Berbari EF, Berendt AR, et al, "Diagnosis and Management of Prosthetic Joint Infection: Clinical Practice Guidelines by the Infectious Diseases Society of America," *Clin Infect Dis*, 2013, 56 (1):e1-e25.

Red Book: 2012 Report of the Committee on Infectious Diseases, 29th ed, Pickering LK, ed, Elk Grove Village, IL: American Academy of Pediatrics, 2012.

Stevens DL, Bisno AL, Chambers HF, et al, "Practice Guidelines For the Diagnosis and Management of Skin and Soft-Tissue Infections," *Clin Infect Dis*, 2005, 41(10):1373-406.

Trotman RL, Williamson JC, Shoemaker DM, et al, "Antibiotic Dosing in Critically Ill Adult Patients Receiving Continuous Renal Replacement Therapy," *Clin Infect Dis*, 2005, 41(8):1159-66.

Tunkel AR, Hartman BJ, Kaplan SL, et al, "Practice Guidelines For the Management of Bacterial Meningitis," *Clin Infect Dis*, 2004, 39 (9):1267-84.

Wormser GP, Dattwyler RJ, Shapiro ED, et al, "The Clinical Assessment, Treatment, and Prevention of Lyme Disease, Human Granulocytic Anaplasmosis, and Babesiosis: Clinical Practice Guidelines by the Infectious Diseases Society of America," *Clin Infect Dis*, 2006, 43 (9):1089-134.

◆ **Penicillin G Potassium** *see* Penicillin G (Parenteral/Aqueous) *on page 1631*

Penicillin G Procaine (pen i SIL in jee PROE kane)

Medication Safety Issues
Sound-alike/look-alike issues:
Penicillin G procaine may be confused with penicillin V potassium
Wycillin® may be confused with Bicillin®
Brand Names: Canada Pfizerpen-AS®; Wycillin®
Therapeutic Category Antibiotic, Penicillin
Generic Availability (U.S.) Yes
Use Moderately severe infections due to *Treponema pallidum* and other penicillin G-sensitive microorganisms that are susceptible to low but prolonged serum penicillin concentrations

Pregnancy Risk Factor B
Pregnancy Considerations Adverse events have not been observed in animal reproduction studies. Penicillin crosses the placenta and distributes into amniotic fluid. Maternal use of penicillins has generally not resulted in an increased risk of adverse fetal effects.

Breast-Feeding Considerations Penicillins are excreted in breast milk. The manufacturer recommends that caution be used when administering penicillin to nursing women. Nondose-related effects could include modification of bowel flora and allergic sensitization.

Contraindications Hypersensitivity to penicillin, procaine, or any component

Warnings Some formulations contain sulfites which may cause allergic reactions in susceptible individuals

Precautions Use with caution in patients with renal impairment, hypersensitivity to cephalosporins, or history of seizures; modify dosage in patients with severe renal impairment. Avoid repeated I.M. injections into the anterolateral thigh in neonates and infants since quadriceps femoris fibrosis and atrophy may occur.

Adverse Reactions
Cardiovascular: Conduction disturbances, myocardial depression, vasodilation
Central nervous system: CNS stimulation, confusion, drowsiness, myoclonus, seizure
Hematologic: Hemolytic anemia, neutropenia, positive Coombs' reaction
Local: Pain at injection site, sterile abscess at injection site, thrombophlebitis
Renal: Interstitial nephritis
Miscellaneous: Hypersensitivity reactions, Jarisch-Herxheimer reaction, pseudoanaphylactic reactions, serum sickness

Drug Interactions
Metabolism/Transport Effects None known.
Avoid Concomitant Use
Avoid concomitant use of Penicillin G Procaine with any of the following: BCG; Probenecid
Increased Effect/Toxicity
Penicillin G Procaine may increase the levels/effects of: Methotrexate; Vitamin K Antagonists

The levels/effects of Penicillin G Procaine may be increased by: Probenecid
Decreased Effect
Penicillin G Procaine may decrease the levels/effects of: BCG; Mycophenolate; Sodium Picosulfate; Typhoid Vaccine

The levels/effects of Penicillin G Procaine may be decreased by: Tetracycline Derivatives
Stability Store in refrigerator
Mechanism of Action Inhibits bacterial cell wall synthesis by binding to one or more of the penicillin-binding proteins (PBPs); which in turn inhibits the final transpeptidation step of peptidoglycan synthesis in bacterial cell walls, thus inhibiting cell wall biosynthesis. Bacteria eventually lyse due to ongoing activity of cell wall autolytic enzymes (autolysins and murein hydrolases) while cell wall assembly is arrested.

Pharmacokinetics (Adult data unless noted)
Absorption: I.M.: Slow
Distribution: Penetration across the blood-brain barrier is poor, despite inflamed meninges; appears in breast milk
Time to peak serum concentration: Within 1-4 hours and can persist within the therapeutic range for 15-24 hours
Elimination: Renal clearance is delayed in neonates, young infants, and patients with impaired renal function
Dialysis: Moderately dialyzable (20% to 50%)
Dosing: Neonatal Note: Use in this age group should be avoided since sterile abscesses and procaine toxicity occur more frequently with neonates than older patients

Congenital syphilis: I.M.: Patient weight >1200 g: 50,000 units/kg/day once daily for 10 days; if more than 1 day of therapy is missed, the entire course should be restarted

Dosing: Usual

Infants and Children: I.M.: 25,000-50,000 units/kg/day in divided doses every 12-24 hours; not to exceed 4.8 million units/24 hours

Congenital syphilis: I.M.: 50,000 units/kg/day once daily for 10 days; if more than 1 day of therapy is missed, the entire course should be restarted

Adults: I.M.: 0.6-4.8 million units/day in divided doses every 12-24 hours

When used in conjunction with an aminoglycoside for the treatment of endocarditis caused by susceptible *S. viridans*: I.M.: 1.2 million units every 6 hours for 2-4 weeks

Neurosyphilis: I.M.: 2.4 million units once daily for 10 days with probenecid 500 mg every 6 hours

Administration Parenteral: **Do not give I.V., intra-arterially, or SubQ**; procaine suspension for deep I.M. injection only; inadvertent I.V. administration has resulted in neurovascular damage; in infants and children it is preferable to administer I.M. into the midlateral muscles of the thigh; in adults, administer into the gluteus maximus or into the midlateral muscles of the thigh

Monitoring Parameters Periodic renal and hematologic function tests with prolonged therapy

Test Interactions Positive Coombs' [direct], false-positive urinary and/or serum proteins

Dosage Forms Excipient information presented when available (limited, particularly for generics); consult specific product labeling.

Suspension, Intramuscular:

Generic: 600,000 units/mL (1 mL, 2 mL)

References

Paryani SG, Vaughn AJ, Crosby M, et al, "Treatment of Asymptomatic Congenital Syphilis: Benzathine Versus Procaine Penicillin G Therapy," *J Pediatr*, 1994, 125(3):471-5.

◆ **Penicillin G Sodium** *see* Penicillin G (Parenteral/Aqueous) *on page 1631*

Penicillin V Potassium
(pen i SIL in vee poe TASS ee um)

Medication Safety Issues
Sound-alike/look-alike issues:

Penicillin V procaine may be confused with penicillin G potassium

Brand Names: Canada Apo-Pen VK; Novo-Pen-VK; Nu-Pen-VK

Therapeutic Category Antibiotic, Penicillin

Generic Availability (U.S.) Yes

Use Treatment of mild to moderately severe susceptible bacterial infections involving the upper respiratory tract, skin, and soft tissues; prophylaxis of rheumatic fever (all indications: FDA approved in ages ≥12 years and adults); has also been used for prophylaxis of invasive pneumococcal infections in high-risk patients, treatment of community-acquired cutaneous anthrax, and treatment of community-acquired pneumonia caused by group A streptococcus

Pregnancy Considerations Penicillin crosses the placenta and distributes into amniotic fluid. Maternal use of penicillins has generally not resulted in an increased risk of adverse fetal effects. Due to pregnancy-induced physiologic changes, some pharmacokinetic parameters of penicillin V may be altered in the second and third trimester. Higher doses or increased dosing frequency may be required.

Breast-Feeding Considerations Penicillin V is excreted into breast milk (low concentrations) and may be detected in the urine of some breast-feeding infants. Loose stools and rash have been reported in nursing infants.

Contraindications Hypersensitivity to penicillin or any component

Warnings Serious and occasionally severe or fatal hypersensitivity (anaphylactoid) reactions have been reported in patients on penicillin therapy, especially with a history of beta-lactam hypersensitivity, history of sensitivity to multiple allergens, or previous IgE-mediated reactions (eg, anaphylaxis, angioedema, urticaria). Administration to patients with confirmed penicillin allergy is contraindicated; in patients with confirmed cephalosporin allergy, consider skin testing to rule out cross-sensitivity to penicillins. Prolonged use may result in fungal or bacterial superinfection including *C. difficile*-associated diarrhea (CDAD); CDAD has been observed >2 months postantibiotic treatment.

Oral solution contains sodium benzoate; benzoic acid (benzoate) is a metabolite of benzyl alcohol; large amounts of benzyl alcohol (≥99 mg/kg/day) have been associated with a potentially fatal toxicity ("gasping syndrome") in neonates; the "gasping syndrome" consists of metabolic acidosis, respiratory distress, gasping respirations, CNS dysfunction (including convulsions, intracranial hemorrhage), hypotension and cardiovascular collapse; use oral solution containing sodium benzoate with caution in neonates; *in vitro* and animal studies have shown that benzoate displaces bilirubin from protein binding sites

Precautions Use with caution in patients with renal impairment. Use with caution in patients with a history of asthma. Use with caution in patients with a history of seizure disorder; high levels, particularly in the presence of renal impairment; may increase risk of seizures. Extended duration of therapy or use associated with high serum concentrations (eg, in renal insufficiency) may be associated with an increased risk for some adverse reactions (neutropenia, hemolytic anemia, serum sickness). Oral solution may contain aspartame which is metabolized to phenylalanine and must be avoided (or used with caution) in patients with phenylketonuria.

Adverse Reactions

Gastrointestinal: Melanoglossia, mild diarrhea, nausea, oral candidiasis, vomiting

Rare but important or life-threatening: Acute interstitial nephritis, convulsions, exfoliative dermatitis, hemolytic anemia, hypersensitivity reaction, positive Coombs' reaction, serum-sickness like reactions

Drug Interactions

Metabolism/Transport Effects None known.

Avoid Concomitant Use

Avoid concomitant use of Penicillin V Potassium with any of the following: BCG; Probenecid

Increased Effect/Toxicity

Penicillin V Potassium may increase the levels/effects of: Methotrexate; Vitamin K Antagonists

The levels/effects of Penicillin V Potassium may be increased by: Probenecid

Decreased Effect

Penicillin V Potassium may decrease the levels/effects of: BCG; Mycophenolate; Sodium Picosulfate; Typhoid Vaccine

The levels/effects of Penicillin V Potassium may be decreased by: Tetracycline Derivatives

Food Interactions Food decreases drug absorption rate; decreases drug serum concentration. Management: Take on an empty stomach 1 hour before or 2 hours after meals around-the-clock to promote less variation in peak and trough serum levels.

Stability

Powder for oral solution: Store dry powder at 20°C to 25°C (68°F to 77°F). Refrigerate suspension after reconstitution; discard after 14 days.

Tablets: Store at 20°C to 25°C (68°F to 77°F).

Mechanism of Action Inhibits bacterial cell wall synthesis by binding to one or more of the penicillin-binding proteins (PBPs); which in turn inhibits the final transpeptidation step of peptidoglycan synthesis in bacterial cell walls, thus inhibiting cell wall biosynthesis. Bacteria eventually lyse due to ongoing activity of cell wall autolytic enzymes (autolysins and murein hydrolases) while cell wall assembly is arrested.

Pharmacokinetics (Adult data unless noted)

Absorption: Oral: 60% to 73% from the GI tract

Distribution: Widely distributed to kidneys, liver, skin, tonsils, and into synovial, pleural, and pericardial fluids

Protein binding: 80%

Metabolism: 10% to 30%

Half-life: 30 minutes; prolonged in patients with renal impairment

Time to peak serum concentration: Within 30-60 minutes

Elimination: Penicillin V and its metabolites are excreted in urine mainly by tubular secretion

Dosing: Usual

Infants, Children, and Adolescents:

General dosing, susceptible infections: Oral:

Infants and Children <12 years: Mild to moderate infection: 25-50 mg/kg/day in divided doses every 6-8 hours; maximum daily dose: 2000 mg/day (Red Book, 2012)

Children ≥12 years and Adolescents:

Manufacturer's labeling (fixed dosing): 125-500 mg every 6-8 hours

Alternate dosing (weight-based): Mild to moderate infection: 25-50 mg/kg/day in divided doses every 6-8 hours; maximum daily dose: 2000 mg/day (Red Book, 2012)

Anthrax (cutaneous), community-acquired: Oral: Infants, Children, and Adolescents: 25-50 mg/kg/day in divided doses 2 **or** 4 times daily; maximum single dose: 500 mg (Stevens, 2005)

Fusospirochetosis (Vincent infection), mild to moderately severe infections: Oral: Children ≥12 years and Adolescents: 250-500 mg every 6-8 hours

Tonsillopharyngitis; Group A streptococcal infection, treatment and primary prevention of rheumatic fever: Oral:

Acute treatment (Gerber, 2009; Shulman, 2012; WHO, 2004):

Children ≤27 kg: 250 mg 2-3 times daily for 10 days

Children >27 kg and Adolescents: 500 mg 2-3 times daily for 10 days; in adolescents, 250 mg 4 times daily has also been suggested

Chronic carrier treatment (Group A streptococci): 50 mg/kg/day in 4 divided doses for 10 days in combination with oral rifampin; maximum daily dose: 2000 mg/day (Shulman, 2012)

Recurrent rheumatic fever, prophylaxis: Children and Adolescents: 250 mg twice daily (Gerber, 2009)

Pneumococcal infection prophylaxis for anatomic or functional asplenia [eg, sickle cell disease (SCD)] (AAP, 2000; AAP, 2002; Kavanagh, 2011; NHLBI, 2002): Oral: Infants and Children:

Before 2 months of age (or as soon as SCD diagnosed or asplenia occurs) to 3 years of age: 125 mg twice daily

>3 years: 250 mg twice daily; the decision to discontinue penicillin prophylaxis after 5 years of age in children who have not experienced invasive pneumococcal infection and have received recommended pneumococcal immunizations is patient and clinician dependent; **Note:** Some clinicians recommend in

patients <5 years, a lower dose of 125 mg twice daily (Red Book, 2012)

Pneumonia, community-acquired; Group A Streptococcus, mild infection or step-down therapy: Oral: Infants ≥3 months, Children, and Adolescents: 50-75 mg/kg/day in 3-4 divided doses (Bradley, 2011); maximum daily dose: 2000 mg/day

Adults:

Anthrax (cutaneous), community-acquired: Oral: 250-500 mg 4 times daily for 5-9 days (Stevens, 2005)

Fusospirochetosis (Vincent infection): Oral: 250-500 mg 3-4 times daily

Pharyngitis (streptococcal): Oral:

Acute treatment, group A streptococci (IDSA guidelines): 250 mg 4 times daily or 500 mg twice daily for 10 days (Shulman, 2012)

Chronic carrier treatment, group A streptococcal (IDSA guidelines): 500 mg 4 times daily for 10 days in combination with oral rifampin (Shulman, 2012)

Prophylaxis of recurrent rheumatic fever infections: Oral: 250 mg twice daily

Dosing adjustment in renal impairment: Children ≥12 years, Adolescents, and Adults: There are no dosage adjustments provided in manufacturer's labeling. Use with caution; excretion is prolonged in patients with renal impairment.

Dosing adjustment in hepatic impairment: Children ≥12 years, Adolescents, and Adults: There are no dosage adjustments provided in the manufacturer's labeling.

Administration Oral: Administer with water on an empty stomach 1 hour before or 2 hours after meals; may be administered with food to decrease GI upset

Monitoring Parameters With prolonged therapy, monitor renal and hematologic function periodically; observe for change in bowel frequency; monitor for signs of anaphylaxis during first dose

Test Interactions False-positive or negative urinary glucose determination using Clinitest®; positive Coombs' [direct]; false-positive urinary and/or serum proteins

Additional Information 0.7 mEq of potassium/250 mg penicillin V; 250 mg = 400,000 units of penicillin

Dosage Forms Excipient information presented when available (limited, particularly for generics); consult specific product labeling.

Solution Reconstituted, Oral:

Generic: 125 mg/5 mL (100 mL, 200 mL); 250 mg/5 mL (100 mL, 200 mL)

Tablet, Oral:

Generic: 250 mg, 500 mg

References

"American Academy of Pediatrics. Committee on Infectious Diseases. Policy Statement: Recommendations for the Prevention of Pneumococcal Infections, Including the Use of Pneumococcal Conjugate Vaccine (Prevnar™), Pneumococcal Polysaccharide Vaccine, and Antibiotic Prophylaxis," Pediatrics, 2000, 106(2 Pt 1):362-6.

American Academy of Pediatrics. Section on Hematology/Oncology Committee on Genetics. Health supervision for children with sickle cell disease. Pediatrics. 2002;109(3):526-535.

Bradley JS, Byington CL, Shah SS, et al. The management of community-acquired pneumonia in infants and children older than 3 months of age: clinical practice guidelines by the Pediatric Infectious Diseases Society and the Infectious Diseases Society of America. Clin Infect Dis. 2011;53(7):e25-76.

Gerber MA, Baltimore RS, Eaton CB, et al, "Prevention of Rheumatic Fever and Diagnosis and Treatment of Acute Streptococcal pharyngitis: A Scientific Statement from the American Heart Association Rheumatic Fever, Endocarditis, and Kawasaki Disease Committee of the Council on Cardiovascular Disease in the Young, the Interdisciplinary Council on Functional Genomics and Translational Biology, and the Interdisciplinary Council on Quality of Care and Outcomes Research: Endorsed by the American Academy of Pediatrics," Circulation, 2009, 119(11):1541-51.

Kavanagh PL, Sprinz PG, Vinci SR, et al. Management of children with sickle cell disease: a comprehensive review of the literature. Pediatrics. 2011;128(6):e1552-1574.

National Heart Lung and Blood Istitute. The management of sickle cell disease. 4th ed. Bethesda, MD: National Institutes of Health; 2002.

Red Book: 2012 Report of the Committee on Infectious Diseases, 29th ed, Pickering LK, ed, Elk Grove Village, IL: American Academy of Pediatrics, 2012.

Shulman ST, Bisno AL, Clegg HW, et al, "Clinical Practice Guideline for the Diagnosis and Management of Group A Streptococcal Pharyngitis: 2012 Update by the Infectious Diseases Society of America," *Clin Infect Dis*, 2012;55(10):e86-102

Stevens DL, Bisno AL, Chambers HF, et al. Practice guidelines for the diagnosis and management of skin and soft-tissue infections. *Clin Infect Dis*. 2005;41(10):1373-1406.

World Health Organization (WHO). Rheumatic fever and rheumatic heart disease. 2004. Available at http://whqlibdoc.who.int/trs/WHO_TRS_923.pdf

◆ **Penicilloyl-polylysine** *see* Benzylpenicilloyl Polylysine *on page 279*

◆ **Penlac** *see* Ciclopirox *on page 465*

◆ **Pennsaid** *see* Diclofenac (Topical) *on page 649*

◆ **Pentacel®** *see* Diphtheria and Tetanus Toxoids, Acellular Pertussis, Poliovirus and *Haemophilus* b Conjugate Vaccine *on page 684*

◆ **Pentahydrate** *see* Sodium Thiosulfate *on page 1919*

◆ **Pentam** *see* Pentamidine *on page 1637*

Pentamidine (pen TAM i deen)

Related Information
Safe Handling of Hazardous Drugs *on page 2419*
Brand Names: U.S. Nebupent; Pentam
Therapeutic Category Antibiotic, Miscellaneous; Antifungal Agent; Antiprotozoal
Generic Availability (U.S.) No
Use
Aerosol: Prevention of pneumonia caused by *Pneumocystis jirovecii* (formerly *carinii*) (PCP) (FDA approved in ages ≥17 years and adults)

Parenteral: Treatment of pneumonia caused by *Pneumocystis jirovecii* (formerly *carinii*) (PCP) (FDA approved in ages >4 months and adults). **Note:** The CDC recommends pentamidine for patients who cannot tolerate or who fail to respond to sulfamethoxazole and trimethoprim; has also been used in the treatment of African trypanosomiasis, cutaneous leishmaniasis, and amebic meningoencephalitis.

Pregnancy Risk Factor C
Pregnancy Considerations Animal reproduction studies were not conducted by the manufacturer; therefore, pentamidine is classified pregnancy category C. In postmarketing studies, pentamidine was embryocidal but not teratogenic when administered to animals. Pentamidine crosses the human placenta. Administration via the aerosolized route may minimize maternal serum concentrations. Concern regarding occupational exposure of pregnant healthcare workers has been discussed in the literature. Pregnant healthcare workers should avoid aerolized exposure if possible. If avoidance is not possible, they should wear a mask and gloves and ensure proper ventilation. Pentamidine may be used in pregnancy for prophylaxis or treatment of PCP if the patient is unable to take first line medications.

Breast-Feeding Considerations It is not known if pentamidine is excreted in human milk and use of pentamidine during breast-feeding is not recommended by the manufacturer. In the United States where formula is accessible, affordable, safe, and sustainable, complete avoidance of breast-feeding by HIV-infected women is recommended by the AAP and the CDC to decrease potential transmission of HIV.

Contraindications Hypersensitivity to pentamidine isethionate or any component

Warnings Hazardous agent; use appropriate precautions for handling and disposal (NIOSH, 2012). Sudden, severe hypotension (including some fatalities) has been observed, even after a single dose; may occur with either I.V. or I.M. administration, although more common with rapid I.V. administration; monitor blood pressure (during and after infusion); patient should be lying down during administration and emergency equipment should be available. Extravasations which have proceeded to ulceration, tissue necrosis, and/or sloughing at the injection site have been reported; closely monitor I.V. site. Stevens-Johnson syndrome (SJS) has been reported; use with caution in patients with SJS. Nephrotoxicity (eg, increased creatinine, azotemia, renal failure) frequently occurs with parenteral therapy (~30% of patients); concurrent use with other nephrotoxic drugs (eg, aminoglycosides, amphotericin B, cisplatin, foscarnet, vancomycin) may increase risk for nephrotoxicity; use with caution in renal impairment; consider dosage adjustment.

Aerosolized pentamidine may induce bronchospasm or cough, especially in patients with asthma (inhaled bronchodilator therapy prior to pentamidine may control symptoms). Acute pancreatitis has been reported in patients receiving aerosolized pentamidine; use with caution in patients with a history of pancreatic disease or elevated amylase/lipase levels; acute pancreatitis (with fatality) has been reported. Discontinue inhalational pentamidine if signs/symptoms of acute pancreatitis occur. Acute PCP may develop despite aerosolized pentamidine prophylaxis; although rare, extrapulmonary *Pneumocystis jirovecii* disease may occur and has been associated with aerosolized pentamidine; if symptoms of infection occur a thorough evaluation should be conducted. Healthcare personnel who administer aerosolized pentamidine inhalation therapy should be aware of the possibility of secondary exposure to tuberculosis or other infections from patients with undiagnosed pulmonary disease; use appropriate precautions to minimize exposure to healthcare personnel.

Precautions Use with caution in hepatic impairment; has not been studied. Use with caution in patients with diabetes mellitus; hyper-/hypoglycemia and pancreatic islet cell necrosis with hyperinsulinemia has been reported; symptoms may occur months after therapy; monitor blood glucose daily on therapy and periodically thereafter. Use with caution in patients with preexisting cardiovascular disease; hyper-/hypotension, and arrhythmia, including QT prolongation and ventricular tachycardia (eg, torsade de pointes) have been reported; avoid use in patients with diagnosed or suspected congenital long QT syndrome, avoid concurrent use with other drugs known to prolong QT_c interval. Use caution in patients with hypocalcemia.

Use with caution in patients with current evidence and/or prior history of hematologic disorders; anemia, leukopenia, and/or thrombocytopenia have been reported; concurrent use with other bone marrow suppressants may increase the risk for myelotoxicity.

Adverse Reactions
Aerosol:
Central nervous system: Dizziness/lightheadedness, fatigue, fever, headache
Gastrointestinal: Appetite decreased, nausea, oral candida, taste alteration
Hematologic: Anemia
Respiratory: Bronchitis, chest pain, cough, dyspnea, pharyngitis, sinusitis, upper respiratory tract infection, wheezing
Miscellaneous: Herpes infection, infection, influenza, night sweats

Injection:
Cardiovascular: Hypotension
Central nervous system: Confusion/hallucinations
Dermatologic: Rash
Endocrine & metabolic: Hypoglycemia
Gastrointestinal: Nausea/anorexia, taste alteration
Hematologic: Anemia, leukopenia, thrombocytopenia

Hepatic: Liver function tests increased

Local: Local reactions at I.M. injection site (includes sterile abscess, necrosis, pain, induration)

Renal: Azotemia, BUN increased, creatinine increased, renal function impaired

Miscellaneous: Herpes infection, infection, influenza, night sweats

Aerosol or injection: Rare but important or life-threatening: Abdominal pain, allergic reaction, anaphylaxis, anxiety, arthralgia, asthma, blepharitis, blurred vision, bronchitis, bronchospasm, cardiac arrhythmia, central venous line related sepsis, cerebrovascular accident, chest tightness, chills, clotting time prolonged, CMV infection, colitis, confusion, congestion (chest, nasal), conjunctivitis, cough, cryptococcal meningitis, cyanosis, defibrination, depression, dermatitis, desquamation, diabetes mellitus, diabetic ketoacidosis, diarrhea, dizziness, drowsiness, dyspepsia, dyspnea, emotional lability, eosinophilia, erythema, esophagitis, extrapulmonary pneumocystosis, extravasation (tissue ulceration, necrosis, and/or sloughing), facial edema, flank pain, gait unsteady, gagging, gingivitis, headache, hearing loss, hematochezia, hematuria, hemoptysis, hepatic dysfunction, hepatitis, hepatomegaly, histoplasmosis, hyperglycemia, hyperkalemia, hypersalivation, hypertension, hyperventilation, hypesthesia, hypocalcemia, hypomagnesemia, incontinence, insomnia, laryngitis, laryngospasm, leg edema, melena, memory loss, nephritis, nervousness, neuralgia, neuropathy, neutropenia, night sweats, palpitation, pancreatitis, pancytopenia, paranoia, paresthesia, peripheral neuropathy, phlebitis, pleuritis, pneumonitis (eosinophilic or interstitial), pneumothorax, pruritus, rales, renal dysfunction, renal failure, rhinitis, seizure, splenomegaly, Stevens-Johnson syndrome, ST segment abnormal, syncope, syndrome of inappropriate antidiuretic hormone (SIADH), tachycardia, tachypnea, temperature abnormal, torsade de pointes, tremor, vasodilation, vasculitis, ventricular tachycardia, vertigo, vomiting, urticaria, xerostomia

Drug Interactions

Metabolism/Transport Effects Substrate of CYP2C19 (major); **Note:** Assignment of Major/Minor substrate status based on clinically relevant drug interaction potential; **Inhibits** CYP2C19 (weak), CYP2C9 (weak), CYP2D6 (weak), CYP3A4 (weak)

Avoid Concomitant Use

Avoid concomitant use of Pentamidine with any of the following: BCG; Highest Risk QTc-Prolonging Agents; Ivabradine; Mifepristone; Pimozide

Increased Effect/Toxicity

Pentamidine may increase the levels/effects of: ARIPiprazole; Foscarnet; Highest Risk QTc-Prolonging Agents; Lomitapide; Moderate Risk QTc-Prolonging Agents; Pimozide

The levels/effects of Pentamidine may be increased by: CYP2C19 Inhibitors (Moderate); CYP2C19 Inhibitors (Strong); Ivabradine; Luliconazole; Mifepristone; QTc-Prolonging Agents (Indeterminate Risk and Risk Modifying)

Decreased Effect

Pentamidine may decrease the levels/effects of: BCG; Sodium Picosulfate; Typhoid Vaccine

The levels/effects of Pentamidine may be decreased by: CYP2C19 Inducers (Strong); Dabrafenib

Stability Hazardous agent; use appropriate precautions for handling and disposal (NIOSH, 2012). Store intact vials at 20°C to 25°C (68°F to 77°F); protect from light; do not reconstitute with NS because precipitation will occur.

Aerosol: The manufacturer recommends the use of freshly prepared solutions for inhalation; once reconstituted, the solution is stable for up to 48 hours in the vial at room temperature; protect from light. Do **not** mix with other nebulizer solutions.

Injection: After reconstitution with SWI, solution is stable for 48 hours in the vial at room temperature if protected from light. Store at 22°C to 30°C (72°F to 86°F) to avoid crystallization. Solutions for infusion (1-2.5 mg/mL) in D_5W are stable for at least 24 hours at room temperature.

Mechanism of Action Interferes with microbial RNA/DNA, phospholipids and protein synthesis, through inhibition of oxidative phosphorylation and/or incorporation of nucleotides and nucleic acids into RNA and DNA

Pharmacokinetics (Adult data unless noted)

Absorption: I.M.: Well absorbed; Aerosol: Limited systemic absorption

Distribution: Binds to tissues and plasma protein; high concentrations are found in the liver, kidney, adrenals, spleen, lungs and pancreas; poor penetration into CNS; following oral inhalation, high concentrations are found in bronchoalveolar fluid; V_{dss}: I.V.: 821 ± 535 L; I.M.: 2724 ± 1066 L

Half-life: I.V.: 5-8 hours; I.M.: 7-11 hours; half-life may be prolonged in patients with severe renal impairment

Elimination: I.V.: ≤12% in urine as unchanged drug

Dialysis: Not appreciably removed by hemodialysis or peritoneal dialysis

Dosing: Usual

Infants, Children, and Adolescents:

***Pneumocystis jirovecii* (PCP), prophylaxis (primary and secondary):** Limited data available: **Note:** For patients intolerant to sulfamethoxazole and trimethoprim.

HIV-exposed/-positive: Children ≥5 years and Adolescents: Inhalation: 300 mg once monthly via Respirgard® II nebulizer (DHHS [adult and pediatric], 2013)

Oncology patients: Children ≥2 years and Adolescents: I.V.: 4 mg/kg/dose once a month (Kim, 2008; Prasad, 2007)

PCP, treatment (moderate-severe disease): Note: For patients who cannot tolerate or who fail to respond to 5-7 days of sulfamethoxazole and trimethoprim.

Manufacturer's labeling: Infants ≥5 months, Children, and Adolescents: I.M., I.V.: 4 mg/kg/dose once daily for 14-21 days

HIV-exposed/-positive:

Infants and Children: I.V.: 4 mg/kg/dose once daily; if clinical improvement after 7-10 days of therapy, may change to an oral regimen to complete a 21-day course (DHHS [pediatric], 2013)

Adolescents: I.V.: 4 mg/kg/dose once daily for 21 days; some experts recommend a dose reduction to 3 mg/kg/dose for toxicity (DHHS [adult], 2013)

Non-HIV-exposed/-positive: I.V.: 3-4 mg/kg/dose once daily for 21 days (Red Book, 2012)

Trypanosomiasis; treatment (non-CNS disease): I.M.: 4 mg/kg/dose once daily for 7 days (Red Book, 2012)

Cutaneous leishmaniasis; treatment: I.M., I.V.: 2-3 mg/kg/dose once daily or every 2 days for 4-7 doses (Red Book, 2012)

Adults:

***Pneumocystis jirovecii* (PCP), prophylaxis (primary and secondary):** Inhalation: 300 mg/dose every 4 weeks via Respirgard® II nebulizer

PCP, treatment (moderate-severe disease):

Manufacturer's labeling: I.M., I.V.: 4 mg/kg/dose once daily for 14-21 days

CDC recommendation: I.V.: 3-4 mg/kg/dose once daily for 21 days

AIDS*Info* guidelines (HIV-infected/-exposed): I.V.: 4 mg/kg/dose once daily; some experts recommend a dose reduction to 3 mg/kg/dose for toxicity (DHHS [adult], 2013)

Dosing adjustment in renal impairment: The FDA-approved labeling recommends that caution should be used in patients with renal impairment; however, no specific dosage adjustment guidelines are provided. The following guidelines have been used by some clinicians (Aronoff, 2007):

Infants, Children, and Adolescents: I.V.:

GFR >30 mL/minute/1.73 m^2: No adjustment required

GFR 10-30 mL/minute/1.73 m^2: Administer 4 mg/kg/dose every 36 hours

GFR <10 mL/minute/1.73 m^2 and peritoneal dialysis: Administer 4 mg/kg/dose every 48 hours

Hemodialysis: Administer 4 mg/kg/dose every 48 hours, after dialysis on dialysis days

Peritoneal dialysis: 4 mg/kg/dose every 48 hours

Continuous renal replacement therapy: No adjustment required

Adults: I.V.:

CrCl ≥10 mL/minute: No adjustment required

CrCl <10 mL/minute: Administer 4 mg/kg/dose every 24-36 hours

Hemodialysis: Administer 4 mg/kg/dose every 48 hours and 750 mg after each dialysis

Peritoneal dialysis: 4 mg/kg/dose every 48 hours

Continuous renal replacement therapy: No adjustment required

Administration Hazardous agent; use appropriate precautions for handling and disposal (NIOSH, 2012).

Oral inhalation: Reconstitute powder for nebulization with 6 mL SWI. Safe and effective administration via nebulization in children is dependent on patients wearing an appropriately sized pediatric face mask. Deliver via Respirgard® II nebulizer until nebulizer is emptied (30-45 minutes). Use appropriate precautions to minimize exposure to healthcare personnel; refer to individual institutional policy. The manufacturer recommends the use of freshly prepared solutions for inhalation. Do not mix with other nebulizer solutions.

Parenteral:

I.M.: Reconstitute vial with 3 mL SWI to a final concentration of 100 mg/mL; administer deep I.M.

I.V.: Reconstitute with 3-5 mL SWI or D$_5$W; the manufacturer recommends further dilution in D$_5$W; however, stability with further dilution in NS has also been documented. Administer by slow I.V. infusion over a period of at least 60-120 minutes at a final concentration for administration not to exceed 6 mg/mL; rapid I.V. administration can cause severe hypotension. Avoid extravasation; assess catheter position before and during infusion

Vesicant/Extravasation Risk Irritant with vesicant-like properties

Monitoring Parameters Liver function tests, renal function tests (daily), blood glucose (daily), serum potassium and calcium, CBC with differential and platelet count, ECG, blood pressure

Dosage Forms Excipient information presented when available (limited, particularly for generics); consult specific product labeling.

Solution Reconstituted, Inhalation, as isethionate:

Nebupent: 300 mg (1 ea)

Solution Reconstituted, Injection, as isethionate:

Pentam: 300 mg (1 ea)

References

Aronoff GR, Bennett WM, Berns JS, et al, *Drug Prescribing in Renal Failure: Dosing Guidelines for Adults and Children*, 5th ed, Philadelphia, PA: American College of Physicians, 2007, 97, 177.

Centers for Disease Control and Prevention, "Amebic Meningoencephalitis, Primary and Granulomatous." Available at: http://www.dpd.cdc.gov/dpdx/HTML/PDF_Files/MedLetter/AmebicMeningoencephalitis.pdf

Centers for Disease Control and Prevention, "Leishmania." Available at: http://www.dpd.cdc.gov/dpdx/HTML/PDF_Files/MedLetter/Leishmania.pdf

Centers for Disease Control and Prevention, "*Pneumocystis jiroveci* (formerly *carinii*) Pneumonia (PCP)." Available at: http://www.dpd.cdc.gov/dpdx/HTML/PDF_Files/MedLetter/Pneumocystis_jiroveci.pdf

Centers for Disease Control and Prevention, "Trypanosomiasis." Available at: http://www.dpd.cdc.gov/dpdx/HTML/PDF_Files/MedLetter/Trypanosomiasis.pdf.

DHHS. Guidelines for the prevention and treatment of opportunistic infections among HIV-exposed and HIV-infected children: recommendations from the National Institutes of Health, Centers for Disease Control and Prevention, the HIV Medicine Association of the Infectious Diseases Society of America, the Pediatric Infectious Diseases Society, and the American Academy of Pediatrics. November 6, 2013. Available at http://aidsinfo.nih.gov

DHHS Panel on Opportunistic Infections (OI) in HIV-Infected Adults and Adolescents. Guidelines for prevention and treatment of opportunistic infections in HIV-infected adults and adolescents: recommendations from the Centers for Disease Control and Prevention (CDC), the National Institutes of Health (NIH), and the HIV Medicine Association (HIVMA) of the Infectious Diseases Society of America (IDSA). May 7, 2013. Available at http://aidsinfo.nih.gov/contentfiles/lvguidelines/adult_oi.pdf

Kim SY, Dabb AA, Glenn DJ, et al, "Intravenous Pentamidine Is Effective as Second Line Pneumocystis Pneumonia Prophylaxis in Pediatric Oncology Patients," *Pediatr Blood Cancer*, 2008, 50 (4):779-83.

National Institute for Occupational Safety and Health (NIOSH), "NIOSH List of Antineoplastic and Other Hazardous Drugs in Healthcare Settings 2012." Available at http://www.cdc.gov/niosh/docs/2012-150/pdfs/2012-150.pdf. Accessed January 21, 2013.

Prasad P, Nania JJ, and Shankar SM, "Pneumocystis Pneumonia in Children Receiving Chemotherapy," *Pediatr Blood Cancer*, 2008, 50 (4):896-8.

◆ **Pentamidine Isethionate** see Pentamidine on page 1637

◆ **Pentamycetin® (Can)** see Chloramphenicol on page 439

◆ **Pentasa** see Mesalamine on page 1347

◆ **Pentasodium Colistin Methanesulfonate** see Colistimethate on page 541

◆ **Pentavalent Human-Bovine Reassortant Rotavirus Vaccine (PRV)** see Rotavirus Vaccine on page 1855

Pentazocine (pen TAZ oh seen)

Medication Safety Issues

Sound-alike/look-alike issues:

Talwin may be confused with Targin

High alert medication:

The Institute for Safe Medication Practices (ISMP) includes this medication among its list of drug classes which have a heightened risk of causing significant patient harm when used in error.

BEERS Criteria medication:

This drug may be potentially inappropriate for use in geriatric patients (Quality of evidence - low; Strength of recommendation - strong).

Related Information

Opioid Conversion Table on page 2242

Brand Names: U.S. Talwin

Brand Names: Canada Talwin

Therapeutic Category Analgesic, Narcotic; Opioid Partial Agonist; Sedative

Generic Availability (U.S.) No

Use Relief of moderate to severe pain (FDA approved in adults); a sedative prior to surgery (FDA approved in ages ≥1 year and adults); supplement to surgical anesthesia (FDA approved in adults)

Pregnancy Risk Factor C

Pregnancy Considerations Adverse events were not found in animal reproduction studies. Pentazocine is approved for pain relief during labor. When used for pain relief during labor, opioids may temporarily affect the heart rate of the fetus (ACOG, 2002).

If chronic opioid exposure occurs in pregnancy, adverse events in the newborn (including withdrawal) may occur;

monitoring of the neonate is recommended. The minimum effective dose should be used if opioids are needed (Chou, 2009). Neonatal abstinence syndrome following opioid exposure may present with autonomic (eg, fever, temperature instability), gastrointestinal (eg, diarrhea, vomiting, poor feeding/weight gain), or neurologic (eg, high-pitched crying, increased muscle tone, irritability, seizure, tremor) symptoms (Dow, 2012; Hudak, 2012). Neonatal abstinence syndrome has been reported following prolonged use of pentazocine during pregnancy.

Breast-Feeding Considerations It is not known if pentazocine is excreted into breast milk. Parenteral opioids used during labor have the potential to interfere with a newborn's natural reflex to nurse within the first few hours after birth. If pentazocine is administered to a nursing woman, it is recommended to monitor both the mother and baby for psychotomimetic reactions. Nursing infants exposed to large doses of opioids should be monitored for apnea and sedation (Montgomery, 2012).

Contraindications Hypersensitivity to pentazocine or any component

Warnings Pentazocine is a potent opioid analgesic which may cause physical and psychological dependence; abrupt discontinuation after prolonged use may result in withdrawal symptoms or seizures; use with caution in patients with a history of prior opioid dependence or abuse. Pentazocine is also a mild opioid antagonist and may precipitate opioid withdrawal symptoms in patients who have been receiving opioids regularly. Use with extreme caution in patients with head injury, intracranial lesions, or elevated intracranial pressure; exaggerated elevation of ICP may occur. Respiratory depression has been reported (rarely); use with caution in patients with respiratory depression, limited respiratory reserve, severe asthma, other obstructive respiratory conditions, or cyanosis; do not use if appropriate rescue respiratory therapy equipment is unavailable. May cause acute CNS manifestations such as hallucinations, disorientation, and confusion; most cases resolve within a few hours without intervention; monitor closely; use caution if drug is reintroduced after these effects subside; CNS effects may recur.

Severe sclerosis of skin, subcutaneous tissue, and underlying muscle have occurred at injection site; avoid SubQ use unless absolutely necessary; rotate injection site to minimize risk. Injection may contain sodium bisulfite which may cause allergic reactions in susceptible individuals.

Precautions Use with caution in seizure-prone patients, acute MI, patients undergoing biliary tract surgery, and patients with renal, hepatic, or respiratory dysfunction; decrease dosage in patients with decreased hepatic or renal function. Use with caution in ambulatory patients; pentazocine may cause CNS depression and dizziness, which may impair physical or mental abilities; patients must be cautioned against performing tasks which require mental alertness (eg, operating machinery or driving). Use with alcohol or other CNS depressants may increase CNS depressant effects; use with caution.

Adverse Reactions

Cardiovascular: Circulatory depression, facial edema, flushing, hyper-/hypotension, shock, syncope, systemic vascular resistance increased, tachycardia

Central nervous system: Chills, CNS depression, confusion, disorientation, dizziness, drowsiness, euphoria, excitement, hallucinations, headache, insomnia, irritability, lightheadedness, malaise, nightmares, sedation

Dermatologic: Dermatitis, erythema multiforme, pruritus, rash, Stevens-Johnson syndrome, toxic epidermal necrolysis, urticaria

Gastrointestinal: Abdominal distress, anorexia, constipation, diarrhea, nausea, taste alteration, vomiting, xerostomia

Genitourinary: Urinary retention

Hematologic: Agranulocytosis (rare), eosinophilia, WBCs decreased

Local: Injection site reaction (tissue damage and irritation)

Neuromuscular & skeletal: Paresthesia, tremor, weakness

Ocular: Blurred vision, diplopia, miosis, nystagmus

Otic: Tinnitus

Respiratory: Dyspnea, respiratory depression (rare)

Miscellaneous: Anaphylaxis, diaphoresis, physical and psychological dependence

Drug Interactions

Metabolism/Transport Effects None known.

Avoid Concomitant Use

Avoid concomitant use of Pentazocine with any of the following: Azelastine (Nasal); Paraldehyde; Thalidomide

Increased Effect/Toxicity

Pentazocine may increase the levels/effects of: Alcohol (Ethyl); Alvimopan; Azelastine (Nasal); Buprenorphine; CNS Depressants; Desmopressin; Diuretics; Hydrocodone; Methotrimeprazine; Metyrosine; Mirtazapine; Paraldehyde; Pramipexole; ROPINIRole; Rotigotine; Selective Serotonin Reuptake Inhibitors; Thalidomide; Zolpidem

The levels/effects of Pentazocine may be increased by: Amphetamines; Anticholinergic Agents; Antipsychotic Agents (Phenothiazines); Brimonidine (Topical); Cannabis; Doxylamine; Dronabinol; Droperidol; HydrOXYzine; Kava Kava; Magnesium Sulfate; Methotrimeprazine; Nabilone; Perampanel; Rufinamide; Sodium Oxybate; Succinylcholine; Tapentadol; Tetrahydrocannabinol

Decreased Effect

Pentazocine may decrease the levels/effects of: Analgesics (Opioid); Pegvisomant

The levels/effects of Pentazocine may be decreased by: Ammonium Chloride; Naltrexone

Stability Store injection at controlled room temperature at 20°C to 25°C (68°F to 77°F); do not mix injection with barbiturates, precipitation will occur

Mechanism of Action Agonist of kappa opiate receptors and partial agonist of mu opiate receptors in the CNS, causing inhibition of ascending pain pathways, altering the perception of and response to pain; produces analgesia, respiratory depression and sedation similar to opioids

Pharmacodynamics

Onset of action:

I.M., SubQ: Within 15-30 minutes

I.V.: Within 2-3 minutes

Duration: Parenteral: 2-3 hours

Pharmacokinetics (Adult data unless noted)

Distribution: Children 4-8 years (mean ± SD): V_{dss}: 4 ± 1.2 L/kg (Hanunen, 1993)

Protein binding: 60%

Metabolism: In the liver via oxidative and glucuronide conjugation pathways

Half-life: Increased half-life with decreased hepatic function

Neonates: 8-12 hours (estimated; Osifo, 2008)

Children 4-8 years (mean ± SD): 3 ± 1.5 hours (Hanunen, 1993)

Adults: 2-3 hours

Elimination: Small amounts excreted unchanged in urine

Dosing: Neonatal Not recommended for use; safety, efficacy, and dose are not established.

Dosing: Usual

Infants and Children: Limited information available

Preoperative sedation: Manufacturer recommendations:

Infants <1 year: Safety, efficacy, and dose not established

Children 1-16 years: I.M.: 0.5 mg/kg as a single dose
Note: In 300 children (1-14 years) I.M. doses ranging from approximately 0.45-1.5 mg/kg in children <27 kg to 0.65-1.9 mg/kg in children >27 kg were used preoperatively (Rita, 1970)

Postoperative pain: I.M.: Doses of 15 mg for children 5-8 years of age and 30 mg for children 9-14 years of age have been used (n=30) (Waterworth, 1974)

Intraoperative analgesia: I.V.: Titrating doses of 0.5 mg/kg every 30-45 minutes as needed have been given in 50 children 5-9 years of age; total dose required: 1-1.5 mg/kg (Ray, 1994)

Adults:

Analgesia (excluding labor pain):

I.M., SubQ: 30-60 mg every 3-4 hours; do **not** exceed 60 mg/dose; maximum: 360 mg/day

I.V.: 30 mg every 3-4 hours; do **not** exceed 30 mg/dose; maximum: 360 mg/day

Labor pain:

I.M.: 30 mg once

I.V.: 20 mg every 2-3 hours as needed; maximum total dose: 60 mg

Dosing adjustment in renal impairment: Children and Adults:

CrCl 10-50 mL/minute: Administer 75% of normal dose
CrCl <10 mL/minute: Administer 50% of normal dose

Administration SubQ route not advised due to tissue damage; rotate injection site for I.M., SubQ use; avoid intra-arterial injection

Monitoring Parameters Respiratory and cardiovascular status; level of pain relief and sedation; blood pressure

Additional Information Use only in patients who are not tolerant to or physically dependent upon opioids

A retrospective study assessed the use of pentazocine 0.5 mg/kg every 8 hours in neonates undergoing surgery; pentazocine use was associated with life-threatening morbidity and unacceptable high mortality due to persistent respiratory depression; the authors of the study recommend the use of alternative neonatal analgesics (Osifo, 2008).

Controlled Substance C-IV

Dosage Forms Excipient information presented when available (limited, particularly for generics); consult specific product labeling.

Solution, Injection:

Talwin: 30 mg/mL (1 mL)

Talwin: 30 mg/mL (10 mL) [contains methylparaben, sodium bisulfite]

References

ACOG Committee on Practice Bulletins-Obstetrics, "ACOG Practice Bulletin. Clinical Management Guidelines for Obstetrician-Gynecologists Number 36, July 2002. Obstetric Analgesia and Anesthesia," *Obstet Gynecol*, 2002, 100(1):177-91.

Chou R, Fanciullo GJ, Fine PG, et al, "Clinical Guidelines for the Use of Chronic Opioid Therapy in Chronic Noncancer Pain," *J Pain*, 2009, 10 (2):113-30.

Dow K, Ordean A, Murphy-Oikonen J, et al, "Neonatal Abstinence Syndrome Clinical Practice Guidelines for Ontario," *J Popul Ther Clin Pharmacol*, 2012, 19(3):e488-506.

Hanunen K, Olkkola KT, Seppala T, et al, "Pharmacokinetics and Pharmacodynamics of Pentazocine in Children," *Pharmacol Toxicol*, 1993, 73(2):120-3.

Hudak ML, Tan RC, Committee On Drugs, et al, "Neonatal Drug Withdrawal," *Pediatrics*, 2012, 129(2):e540-60.

Montgomery A, Hale TW, and Academy Of Breastfeeding Medicine, "ABM Cinical Protocol #15: Analgesia and Anesthesia for the Breastfeeding Mother, Revised 2012," *Breastfeed Med*, 2012, 7(6):547-53.

Osifo OD and Aghahowa SE, "Hazards of Pentazocine for Neonatal Analgesia: A Single-Centre Experience Over 10 Years," *Ann Trop Paediatr*, 2008, 28(3):205-10.

Ray AD and Gupta M, "Clinical Trial of Pentazocine as Analgesic in Pediatric Cases," *J Indian Med Assoc*, 1994, 92(3):77-9.

Rita L, Seleny FL, and Levin RM, "A Comparison of Pentazocine and Morphine for Pediatric Premedication," *Anesth Analg*, 1970, 49 (3):377-82.

Waterworth TA, "Pentazocine (Fortal) as Postoperative Analgesic in Children," *Arch Dis Child*, 1974, 49(6):488-90.

◆ **Pentazocine Lactate** see Pentazocine on page 1639

PENTobarbital (pen toe BAR bi tal)

Medication Safety Issues

Sound-alike/look-alike issues:

PENTobarbital may be confused with PHENobarbital

Nembutal® may be confused with Myambutol®

BEERS Criteria medication:

This drug may be potentially inappropriate for use in geriatric patients (Quality of evidence - high; Strength of recommendation - strong).

Related Information

Preprocedure Sedatives in Children on page 2402

Brand Names: U.S. Nembutal

Brand Names: Canada Nembutal® Sodium

Therapeutic Category Anticonvulsant, Barbiturate; Barbiturate; General Anesthetic; Hypnotic; Sedative

Generic Availability (U.S.) No

Use Sedation, preanesthetic, short-term treatment of insomnia, and emergency treatment of acute convulsive episodes associated with certain conditions such as status epilepticus, eclampsia, tetanus, cholera, meningitis, and toxic reactions to local anesthetics or strychnine [FDA approved in pediatric patients (age not specified) and adults]; has also been used for procedural sedation (parenteral, oral, and rectal), treatment of increased intracranial pressure, and sedation for the mechanically ventilated ICU patient

Pregnancy Risk Factor D

Pregnancy Considerations Barbiturates can be detected in the placenta, fetal liver and fetal brain. Fetal and maternal blood concentrations may be similar following parenteral administration. An increased incidence of fetal abnormalities may occur following maternal use. When used during the third trimester of pregnancy, withdrawal symptoms may occur in the neonate including seizures and hyperirritability; symptoms may be delayed up to 14 days. Use during labor does not impair uterine activity; however, respiratory depression may occur in the newborn; resuscitation equipment should be available, especially for premature infants.

Breast-Feeding Considerations Small amounts of barbiturates are found in breast milk.

Contraindications Hypersensitivity to barbiturates or any component; manifest or latent porphyria

Warnings Tolerance and/or psychological and physical dependence may occur; abrupt discontinuation after prolonged use may result in withdrawal symptoms, seizures, or status epilepticus; withdraw gradually if used over extended periods of time. Rapid I.V. administration may cause respiratory depression, apnea, laryngospasm, or hypotension (requiring vasopressor support). Pentobarbital may cause CNS depression; effects with alcohol or other sedative drugs may be potentiated. Patients require continuous monitoring and possibly airway management; cardiovascular and respiratory resuscitation equipment should be available with use.

Parenteral solutions are highly alkaline; local tissue irritation and damage (with resultant necrosis) may result from perivascular extravasation; unintentional intra-arterial administration may cause a wide scope of adverse effects ranging from transient pain to gangrene of the limb; discontinue intravenous injection immediately with onset of burning and/or pain and evaluate for arterial injection or perivascular extravasation.

Injection contains 10% alcohol and 40% propylene glycol; toxicities have been reported with use of products containing propylene glycol, including hyperosmolality, lactic ▶

acidosis, seizures, and respiratory depression; in neonates large amounts of propylene glycol delivered orally, intravenously (eg, >3000 mg/day), or topically have been associated with potentially fatal toxicities which can include metabolic acidosis, seizures, renal failure, and CNS depression; use injection containing propylene glycol with caution (AAP, 1997; Shehab, 2009). One case report described an adult patient who developed lactic acidosis possibly secondary to propylene glycol accumulation following a continuous infusion of pentobarbital (Miller, 2008). Consider monitoring for signs of propylene glycol toxicity (eg, lactic acidosis, acute renal failure, osmol gap) in patients who require a continuous infusion of pentobarbital.

Precautions Use with caution in patients with acute or chronic pain; may cause paradoxical responses, including agitation and hyperactivity, particularly in patients with acute pain and in pediatric patients. Use with caution and reduce the dose in patients with hepatic impairment; do not use in patients with hepatic coma. Use with caution in patients who are debilitated and those with hypovolemic shock, or heart failure.

Adverse Reactions

Cardiovascular: Bradycardia, hypotension, syncope

Central nervous system: Abnormal thinking, agitation, anxiety, ataxia, CNS excitation, confusion, depression, dizziness, drowsiness, fever, hallucinations, headache, hyperkinesia, insomnia, nervousness, nightmares, psychiatric disturbances, somnolence

Dermatologic: Angioedema, exfoliative dermatitis, rash

Gastrointestinal: Constipation, nausea, vomiting

Hematologic: Megaloblastic anemia

Hepatic: Hepatotoxicity

Local: Injection site reactions

Respiratory: Apnea (especially with rapid I.V. use), hypoventilation, laryngospasm, respiratory depression

Miscellaneous: Gangrene with inadvertent intra-arterial injection, hypersensitivity reactions

Drug Interactions

Metabolism/Transport Effects Induces CYP2A6 (strong), CYP3A4 (strong)

Avoid Concomitant Use

Avoid concomitant use of PENTobarbital with any of the following: Abiraterone Acetate; Apixaban; Apremilast; Artemether; Axitinib; Azelastine (Nasal); Bedaquiline; Boceprevir; Bortezomib; Bosutinib; Cabozantinib; Ceritinib; CloZAPine; Crizotinib; Dienogest; Dronedarone; Enzalutamide; Everolimus; Ibrutinib; Itraconazole; Ivacaftor; Lapatinib; Lumefantrine; Lurasidone; Macitentan; Mifepristone; NIFEdipine; Nilotinib; Nisoldipine; Paraldehyde; PAZOPanib; Perampanel; PONATinib; Praziquantel; Ranolazine; Regorafenib; Rivaroxaban; Roflumilast; RomiDEPsin; Simeprevir; Somatostatin Acetate; SORAfenib; Tasimelteon; Telaprevir; Thalidomide; Ticagrelor; Tofacitinib; Tolvaptan; Toremifene; Uliprtal; Vandetanib; Vemurafenib; VinCRIStine (Liposomal); Vorapaxar

Increased Effect/Toxicity

PENTobarbital may increase the levels/effects of: Alcohol (Ethyl); Azelastine (Nasal); Buprenorphine; Clarithromycin; CNS Depressants; Hydrocodone; Hypotensive Agents; Meperidine; Methotrimeprazine; Metyrosine; Paraldehyde; Pramipexole; ROPINIRole; Rotigotine; Selective Serotonin Reuptake Inhibitors; Thalidomide; Thiazide Diuretics; Zolpidem

The levels/effects of PENTobarbital may be increased by: Brimonidine (Topical); Cannabis; Carbonic Anhydrase Inhibitors; Chloramphenicol; Clarithromycin; Doxylamine; Dronabinol; Droperidol; HydrOXYzine; Kava Kava; Magnesium Sulfate; Methotrimeprazine; Nabilone; Primidone; Rufinamide; Sodium Oxybate; Somatostatin Acetate; Tapentadol; Tetrahydrocannabinol; Valproic Acid and Derivatives

Decreased Effect

PENTobarbital may decrease the levels/effects of: Abiraterone Acetate; Acetaminophen; Apixaban; Apremilast; ARIPiprazole; Artemether; Axitinib; Bedaquiline; Beta-Blockers; Boceprevir; Bortezomib; Bosutinib; Brentuximab Vedotin; Cabozantinib; Calcium Channel Blockers; Cannabidiol; Cannabis; Ceritinib; Chloramphenicol; Clarithromycin; CloZAPine; Contraceptives (Estrogens); Contraceptives (Progestins); Corticosteroids (Systemic); Crizotinib; CycloSPORINE (Systemic); CYP2A6 Substrates; CYP3A4 Substrates; Dasatinib; Dienogest; DOXOrubicin (Conventional); Doxycycline; Dronabinol; Dronedarone; Enzalutamide; Etoposide; Everolimus; Exemestane; FentaNYL; Gefitinib; Griseofulvin; GuanFACINE; Ibrutinib; Imatinib; Itraconazole; Ivacaftor; Ixabepilone; LamoTRIgine; Lapatinib; Linagliptin; Lumefantrine; Lurasidone; Macitentan; Maraviroc; Mifepristone; NIFEdipine; Nilotinib; Nisoldipine; PAZOPanib; Perampanel; PONATinib; Praziquantel; Propafenone; QUEtiapine; Ranolazine; Regorafenib; Rivaroxaban; Roflumilast; RomiDEPsin; Saxagliptin; Simeprevir; SORAfenib; SUNItinib; Tadalafil; Tasimelteon; Telaprevir; Teniposide; Tetrahydrocannabinol; Ticagrelor; Tofacitinib; Tolvaptan; Toremifene; Tricyclic Antidepressants; Uliprtal; Valproic Acid and Derivatives; Vandetanib; Vemurafenib; Vilazodone; VinCRIStine (Liposomal); Vitamin K Antagonists; Vorapaxar; Vortioxetine; Zuclopenthixol

The levels/effects of PENTobarbital may be decreased by: Ketorolac (Nasal); Ketorolac (Systemic); Mefloquine; Multivitamins/Minerals (with ADEK, Folate, Iron); Orlistat; Pyridoxine; Rifamycin Derivatives

Stability Store at controlled room temperature of 20°C to 25°C (68°F to 77°F); brief excursions of 15°C to 30°C (59°F to 86°F) permitted. Avoid excessive heat; protect from freezing. Aqueous solutions are alkaline and unstable; low pH may cause precipitate; use only clear solution

Mechanism of Action Barbiturate with sedative, hypnotic, and anticonvulsant properties. Barbiturates depress the sensory cortex, decrease motor activity, alter cerebellar function, and produce drowsiness, sedation, and hypnosis. In high doses, barbiturates exhibit anticonvulsant activity; barbiturates produce dose-dependent respiratory depression; reduce brain metabolism and cerebral blood flow in order to decrease intracranial pressure

Pharmacodynamics Note: Values below are for sedation in pediatric and adult patients.

Onset of action (Krauss, 2006):

I.M.: Within 10-15 minutes

I.V.: Almost immediate, within 3-5 minutes

Oral, Rectal: 15-60 minutes

Duration (Krauss, 2006):

I.M.: 1-2 hours

I.V.: 15-45 minutes

Oral, Rectal: 1-4 hours

Pharmacokinetics (Adult data unless noted)

Distribution: V_d:

Children: 0.8 L/kg (Schiable, 1982)

Adults: 1 L/kg (Ehrnebo, 1974)

Protein binding: 45% to 70%

Metabolism: Extensive in the liver via hydroxylation and glucuronidation (Wermeling, 1985)

Half-life, terminal:

Children: 26 ± 16 hours (Schaible, 1982)

Adults (healthy): 22 hours (15-50 hours, dose-dependent) (Ehrnebo, 1974)

Elimination: <1% excreted unchanged in urine

Dosing: Usual Note: Adjust dose based on patient's age, weight, and medical condition.

Infants, Children, and Adolescents: **Note:** Consider the potential for delayed metabolism or elimination in infants <6 months of age (Krauss, 2006).

Hypnotic: Children: I.M.: 2-6 mg/kg; maximum dose: 100 mg/dose
Preoperative sedation: Infants and Children:
I.M.: 2-6 mg/kg; maximum dose: 100 mg/dose
I.V.: 1-3 mg/kg to a maximum of 100 mg to desired effect
Procedural (moderate) sedation:
Infants: Oral: 4 mg/kg, if needed supplemental 2-4 mg/kg every 30 minutes; maximum total dose: 8 mg/kg (Mason, 2004)
Infants and Children:
I.M.: 2-6 mg/kg; maximum dose: 100 mg
I.V.: Initial 1-2 mg/kg; additional doses of 1-2 mg/kg every 3-5 minutes to desired effect; usual effective total dose: 1-6 mg/kg (maximum: 100 mg/dose) (Krauss, 2006; Mason, 2004). **Note:** Patients receiving concurrent barbiturate therapy may require higher total mg/kg doses (up to 9 mg/kg) (Mason, 2004).
Children: Oral, Rectal: (Krauss, 2006):
<4 years: 3-6 mg/kg; maximum dose: 100 mg
≥4 years: 1.5-3 mg/kg; maximum dose: 100 mg
Adolescents: I.V.: 100 mg prior to procedure
Reduction of elevated ICP: I.V.: **Note:** Intubation is required; adjust dose based on hemodynamics, ICP, cerebral perfusion pressure, and EEG.
Low dose: Children and Adolescents: 5 mg/kg every 4-6 hours (Mazzola, 2002)
High-dose pentobarbital coma: Children and Adolescents: Loading dose: 10 mg/kg over 30 minutes, then 5 mg/kg every hour for 3 hours; initial maintenance infusion: 1 mg/kg/**hour**; adjust to maintain burst suppression on EEG; maintenance dose range: 1-2 mg/kg/**hour** (Adelson, 2003; Rangel-Castillo, 2008)
Sedation of mechanically ventilated ICU patient (who failed standard therapy): I.V.: Infants, Children, and Adolescents: Loading dose: 1 mg/kg followed by 1 mg/kg/**hour** infusion. Additional boluses at a dose equal to hourly rate may be given every 2 hours as needed. If ≥4-6 boluses are administered within 24 hours, then increase maintenance rate by 1 mg/kg/**hour**; reported required range: 1-6 mg/kg/**hour** (median: 2 mg/kg/**hour**). Tapering of dose and/or conversion to oral phenobarbital has been reported for therapy ≥5 days (Tobias, 1995; Tobias, 2000; Tobias 2000a). **Note:** Higher rates of adverse effects were observed in a small report that used higher loading and initial maintenance doses (Yanay, 2004).
Status epilepticus refractory to standard therapy: **Note:** Intubation is required; adjust dose based on hemodynamics, seizure activity, and EEG.
I.V.: Infants, Children, and Adolescents: Loading dose: 5 mg/kg; maintenance infusion: Initial: 1 mg/kg/**hour**, may increase up to 3 mg/kg/**hour** (usual range: 1-3 mg/kg/**hour**); maintain burst suppression on EEG for 12-48 hours (no seizure activity), tapering pentobarbital rate by 0.5 mg/kg every 12 hours has been reported (Abend, 2008; Holmes, 1999; Kim, 2001)
High-dose pentobarbital coma: I.V.: Infants and Children: Loading dose: 10-15 mg/kg given slowly over 1-2 hours; monitor blood pressure and respiratory rate. Maintenance infusion: Initial: 1 mg/kg/**hour**; may increase up to 5 mg/kg/**hour** (usual range: 0.5-3 mg/kg/**hour**); maintain burst suppression on EEG (Holmes, 1999). **Note:** Loading doses of 20-35 mg/kg (given over 1-2 hours) have been utilized in pediatric patients for pentobarbital coma, but these higher loading doses often cause hypotension requiring vasopressor therapy.

Adults:
Hypnotic/sedative:
I.M.: 150-200 mg
I.V.: Initial: 100 mg; decrease dose for elderly or debilitated patients. If needed, may administer additional increments after at least 1 minute, up to a total dose of 200-500 mg
Refractory status epilepticus: I.V.: **Note:** Intubation required; adjust dose based on hemodynamics, seizure activity, and EEG (Abou Khaled 2008; Millikan, 2009; Mirski, 2008; Yaffe, 1993). Various regimens available:
Loading dose: 10-15 mg/kg (5-10 mg/kg in patients with preexisting hypotension) administer slowly over 1 hour; initial maintenance infusion: 0.5-1 mg/kg/hour; adjust to maintain burst suppression pattern on EEG; maintenance dose range: 0.5-5 mg/kg/hour (Yaffe, 1993). **Note:** Patients may require infusion rates up to 10 mg/kg/hour (Abou Khaled, 2008; Mirski, 2008).
Loading dose: 5 mg/kg (up to 25-50 mg/minute); repeat 5 mg/kg boluses until seizures stop; maintenance dose: 1 mg/kg/hour (range: 0.5-10 mg/kg/hour) (Abou Khaled, 2008)
When increasing maintenance infusion rate during active seizure activity, some experts suggest administration of an additional 5 mg/kg bolus, given the long half-life of pentobarbital.
Administration
Parenteral:
I.M.: Intramuscular administration should be deep and in a large muscle to avoid tissue irritation. Adults: Do not exceed 5 mL volume at one injection site
I.V.: Do not inject >50 mg/minute; rapid I.V. injection may cause respiratory depression, apnea, laryngospasm, bronchospasm, and hypotension; administer over 10-30 minutes; maximum concentration: 50 mg/mL for slow I.V. push; may dilute in D_5W, $D_{10}W$, NS, LR, Ringer's injection, D_5LR, and dextrose/saline combinations for continuous infusion. Solution highly alkaline (pH=9.5); care should be taken to avoid extravasation; consider administration using large bore vein (not hand or wrist) or via a running I.V. line at port farthest from patient's vein.
Oral: Parenteral solution may be mixed with cherry syrup prior to administration to improve palatability (Chung, 2000; Mason, 2004).
Monitoring Parameters Vital signs, respiratory status (including pulse oximetry for moderate sedation), cardiovascular status, CNS status. Monitor EEG when using pentobarbital to treat status epilepticus or to reduce ICP. Monitor ICP and cerebral perfusion pressure (CPP) (CPP = MAP - ICP) when using pentobarbital coma to reduce ICP. Consider monitoring for signs of propylene glycol toxicity (eg, lactic acidosis, acute renal failure, osmolal gap) in patients who require a continuous infusion of pentobarbital. Periodically monitor renal, hepatic, and hematopoietic function with prolonged therapy.
Reference Range Therapeutic:
Hypnotic: 1-5 mcg/mL (SI: 4-22 micromoles/L)
Coma: 20-50 mcg/mL (SI: 88-221 micromoles/L)
Toxic: >10 mcg/mL (SI: >44 μmol/L)
Additional Information Tolerance to hypnotic effect can occur; taper dose to prevent withdrawal; in pediatric patients, a total cumulative pentobarbital dose ≥25 mg/kg or duration ≥5-7 days have been reported to have a higher probability of withdrawal. To prevent withdrawal in susceptible pediatric patients, the following dosing approach transitioning to PHENobarbital has been described: Discontinue PENTobarbital infusion, administer half of the PHENobarbital I.V. loading dose (see table on the next page) over 1 hour followed 6 hours later by the remaining half of PHENobarbital loading dose I.V. (over 1 hour). Begin maintenance PHENobarbital dose 6 hours after loading dose completed; the maintenance PHENobarbital

dose should be ⅓ of the initial loading dose I.V. given every 12 hours. Once patient is stabilized, may switch to oral therapy and begin tapering 10% to 20% weekly (Tobias, 2000; Tobias, 2000a). **Note:** This conversion method is based on preliminary data and further studies are needed to confirm the efficacy of this regimen.

PENTobarbital Infusion Rate (mg/kg/hour)	PHENobarbital I.V. Loading Dose (mg/kg)
1-2	8
2-3	15
3-4	20

Controlled Substance C-II

Dosage Forms Excipient information presented when available (limited, particularly for generics); consult specific product labeling.
Solution, Injection, as sodium:
Nembutal: 50 mg/mL (20 mL, 50 mL) [latex free; contains alcohol, usp, propylene glycol]

References

Abend NS and Dlugos DJ, "Treatment of Refractory Status Epilepticus: Literature Review and a Proposed Protocol," *Pediatr Neurol*, 2008, 38 (6):377-90.

Abou Khaled KJ and Hirsch LJ, "Updates in the Management of Seizures and Status Epilepticus in Critically Ill Patients," *Neurol Clin*, 2008, 26(2):385-408.

Adelson PD, Bratton SL, Carney NA, et al, "Guidelines for the Acute Medical Management of Severe Traumatic Brain Injury in Infants, Children, and Adolescents. Chapter 13. The Use of Barbiturates in the Control of Intracranial Hypertension in Severe Pediatric Traumatic Brain Injury," *Pediatr Crit Care Med*, 2003, 4(3 Suppl):S49-52.

American Academy of Pediatrics Committee on Drugs. "Inactive" ingredients in pharmaceutical products: update (subject review). *Pediatrics*. 1997;99(2):268-278.

Brain Trauma Foundation, American Association of Neurological Surgeons, Congress of Neurological Surgeons, et al, "Guidelines for the Management of Severe Traumatic Brain Injury. XI. Anesthetics, Analgesics, and Sedatives," *J Neurotrauma*, 2007, 24 Suppl 1:S71-6.

Brain Trauma Foundation, American Association of Neurological Surgeons, and Joint Section on Neurotrauma and Critical Care, "Use of Barbiturates in the Control of Intracranial Hypertension," *J Neurotrauma*, 2000, 17(6-7):527-30.

Chung T, Hoffer FA, Connor L, et al. The use of oral pentobarbital sodium (nembutal) versus chloral hydrate in infants undergoing CT and MR imaging – a pilot study. *Pediatr Radiol*. 2000;30:332-335.

Ehmebo M, "Pharmacokinetics and Distribution Properties of Pentobarbital in Humans Following Oral and Intravenous Administration," *J Pharm Sci*, 1974, 63(7):1114-8.

Fischer JH and Raineri DL, "Pentobarbital Anesthesia for Status Epilepticus," *Clin Pharm*, 1987, 6(8):601-2.

Holmes GL and Riviello JJ, "Midazolam and Pentobarbital for Refractory Status Epilepticus," *Pediatr Neurol*, 1999, 20(4):259-64.

Kim SJ, Lee DY, and Kim JS, "Neurologic Outcomes of Pediatric Epileptic Patients With Pentobarbital Coma," *Pediatr Neurol*, 2001, 25(3):217-20.

Krauss B and Green SM, "Procedural Sedation and Analgesia in Children," *Lancet*, 2006, 367(9512):766-80.

Mason KP, Zurakowski D, Connor L, et al, "Infant Sedation for MR Imaging and CT: Oral Versus Intravenous Pentobarbital," *Radiology*, 2004, 233(3):723-8.

Mazzola CA and Adelson PD, "Critical Care Management of Head Trauma in Children," *Crit Care Med*, 2002, 30(11 Suppl):S393-401.

Miller MA, Forni A, and Yogaratnam D, "Propylene Glycol-Induced Lactic Acidosis in a Patient Receiving Continuous Infusion Pentobarbital," *Ann Pharmacother*, 2008, 42(10):1502-6.

Millikan D, Rice B, and Silbergleit R, "Emergency Treatment of Status Epilepticus: Current Thinking," *Emerg Med Clin North Am*, 2009, 27 (1):101-13, ix.

Pereira JK, Burrows PE, Richards HM, et al, "Comparison of Sedation Regimens for Pediatric Outpatient CT," *Pediatr Radiol*, 1993, 23 (5):341-4.

Rangel-Castilla L, Gopinath S, and Robertson CS, "Management of Intracranial Hypertension," *Neurol Clin*, 2008, 26(2):521-41.

Schaible DH, Cupit GC, Swedlow DB, et al, "High-Dose Pentobarbital Pharmacokinetics in Hypothermic Brain-Injured Children," *J Pediatr*, 1982, 100(4):655-60.

Shehab N, Lewis CL, Streetman DD, Donn SM. Exposure to the pharmaceutical excipients benzyl alcohol and propylene glycol among critically ill neonates. *Pediatr Crit Care Med*. 2009;10 (2):256-259.

Tobias JD, "Pentobarbital for Sedation During Mechanical Ventilation in the Pediatric ICU Patient," *J Intensive Care Med*, 2000, 15:115-20.

Tobias JD, "Tolerance, Withdrawal, and Physical Dependency After Long-Term Sedation and Analgesia of Children in the Pediatric Intensive Care Unit," *Crit Care Med*, 2000a, 28(6):2122-32.

Tobias JD, Deshpande JK, Pietsch JB, et al, "Pentobarbital Sedation for Patients in the Pediatric Intensive Care Unit," *South Med J*, 1995, 88 (3):290-4.

Wermeling D, Record K, Bell R, et al, "Hemodialysis Clearance of Pentobarbital During Continuous Infusion," *Ther Drug Monit*, 1985, 7(4):485-7.

Yaffe K and Lowenstein DH, "Prognostic Factors of Pentobarbital Therapy for Refractory Generalized Status Epilepticus," *Neurology*, 1993, 43(5):895-900.

Yanay O, Brogan TV, and Martin LD, "Continuous Pentobarbital Infusion in Children Is Associated With High Rates of Complications," *J Crit Care*, 2004, 19(3):174-8.

◆ **Pentobarbital Sodium** *see* PENTobarbital *on page 1641*

Pentostatin (pen toe STAT in)

Medication Safety Issues

Sound-alike/look-alike issues:
Pentostatin may be confused with pentamidine, pentosan

High alert medication:
The Institute for Safe Medication Practices (ISMP) includes this medication among its list of drug classes which have a heightened risk of causing significant patient harm when used in error.

International issues:
Nipent [U.S., Canada, and multiple international markets] may be confused with Nipin brand name for nifedipine [Italy, Singapore]

Related Information
Emetogenic Potential of Antineoplastic Agents in Children *on page 2327*
Safe Handling of Hazardous Drugs *on page 2419*

Brand Names: U.S. Nipent

Brand Names: Canada Nipent®

Therapeutic Category Antineoplastic Agent, Antimetabolite; Antineoplastic Agent, Antimetabolite (Purine Analog); Antineoplastic Agent, Antimetabolite (Purine Antagonist)

Generic Availability (U.S.) No

Use Treatment of hairy cell leukemia; other uses include treatment of cutaneous T-cell lymphoma, chronic lymphocytic leukemia (CLL), and acute and chronic graft-versus-host disease (GVHD)

Pregnancy Risk Factor D

Pregnancy Considerations Animal studies have demonstrated teratogenicity, maternal toxicity, and fetal loss. There are no adequate and well-controlled studies in pregnant women. Women of childbearing potential should be advised to avoid becoming pregnant.

Breast-Feeding Considerations Due to the potential for serious adverse reactions in nursing the infant, breast-feeding is not recommended.

Contraindications Hypersensitivity to pentostatin or any component

Warnings Hazardous agent; use appropriate precautions for handling and disposal (NIOSH, 2012). Severe CNS, renal, and liver toxicity have occurred with doses higher than recommended; do not exceed the recommended dose **[U.S. Boxed Warning]**; may cause elevations (reversible) in liver function tests. Severe pulmonary toxicities have occurred with doses higher than recommended; do not exceed the recommended dose. Do not administer concurrently with fludarabine; concomitant use has resulted in serious or fatal pulmonary toxicity **[U.S. Boxed Warning]**. Fatal pulmonary edema and hypotension have also been reported in patients treated with pentostatin in combination with carmustine, etoposide, or high-dose cyclophosphamide as part of a myeloablative regimen for bone marrow transplant. Bone marrow suppression may occur, primarily early in treatment and frequent monitoring of CBC during this time is necessary; if neutropenia persists beyond early cycles, evaluate for disease status. Safety and efficacy have not been established in children.

Precautions Use with caution in patients with renal dysfunction (CrCl <60 mL/minute); the terminal half-life is prolonged; appropriate dosing guidelines in renal insufficiency have not been determined. Severe rashes may occur and worsen with therapy continuation; may require withholding of treatment or discontinuation. Treatment should be temporarily withheld for active infections during therapy. Should be administered under the supervision of an experienced cancer chemotherapy physician **[U.S. Boxed Warning]**.

Adverse Reactions

Cardiovascular: Angina, arrhythmia, AV block, bradycardia, cardiac arrest, chest pain, deep thrombophlebitis, facial edema, heart failure, hypertension, hypotension, pericardial effusion, peripheral edema, sinus arrest, syncope, tachycardia, vasculitis, ventricular extrasystoles

Central nervous system: Abnormal dreams/thinking, amnesia, anxiety, ataxia, chills, CNS toxicity, confusion, depression, dizziness, emotional lability, encephalitis, fatigue, fever, hallucination, headache, hostility, insomnia, meningism, nervousness, neuritis, neurosis, pain, seizure, somnolence, vertigo

Dermatologic: Abscess, acne, alopecia, cellulitis, dry skin, eczema, furunculosis, petechial rash, photosensitivity, pruritus, rash, skin disorder, urticaria

Endocrine & metabolic: Amenorrhea, gout, hypercalcemia, hyponatremia, libido decreased/loss

Gastrointestinal: Abdominal pain, anorexia, constipation, diarrhea, dyspepsia, dysphagia, flatulence, gingivitis, glossitis, ileus, nausea/vomiting, oral moniliasis, stomatitis, taste perversion

Genitourinary: Impotence, urinary tract infection

Hematologic: Acute leukemia, agranulocytosis, anemia, aplastic anemia, hemolytic anemia, hemorrhage, leukopenia, myelosuppression, thrombocytopenia

Hepatic: Transaminases increased

Local: Phlebitis

Neuromuscular & skeletal: Arthralgia, arthritis, dysarthria, hyperkinesia, myalgia, neuralgia, neuropathy, osteomyelitis, paralysis, paresthesia, twitching, weakness

Ocular: Amblyopia, conjunctivitis, eyes nonreactive, lacrimation disorder, photophobia, retinopathy, vision abnormal, watery eyes, xerophthalmia

Otic: Deafness, earache, labyrinthitis, tinnitus

Renal: Creatinine increased, nephropathy, renal failure, renal insufficiency, renal function abnormal, renal stone

Respiratory: Asthma, bronchitis, bronchospasm, cough, dyspnea, laryngeal edema, pharyngitis, pneumonia, pulmonary embolus, rhinitis, sinusitis, upper respiratory infection

Miscellaneous: Allergic reaction, bacterial infection, diaphoresis, flu-like syndrome, herpes simplex, herpes zoster, infection, sepsis, viral infection

Rare but important or life-threatening: Dysuria, fungal infection (skin), hematuria, lethargy, pulmonary edema, pulmonary toxicity (fatal; in combination with fludarabine), uveitis/vision loss

Drug Interactions

Metabolism/Transport Effects None known.

Avoid Concomitant Use

Avoid concomitant use of Pentostatin with any of the following: BCG; CloZAPine; Dipyrone; Fludarabine; Natalizumab; Nelarabine; Pegademase Bovine; Pimecrolimus; Tacrolimus (Topical); Tofacitinib; Vaccines (Live)

Increased Effect/Toxicity

Pentostatin may increase the levels/effects of: CloZAPine; Cyclophosphamide; Fludarabine; Leflunomide; Natalizumab; Tofacitinib; Vaccines (Live)

The levels/effects of Pentostatin may be increased by: Denosumab; Dipyrone; Fludarabine; Pimecrolimus; Roflumilast; Tacrolimus (Topical); Trastuzumab

Decreased Effect

Pentostatin may decrease the levels/effects of: BCG; Coccidioidin Skin Test; Nelarabine; Pegademase Bovine; Sipuleucel-T; Vaccines (Inactivated); Vaccines (Live)

The levels/effects of Pentostatin may be decreased by: Echinacea; Pegademase Bovine

Stability Hazardous agent; use appropriate precautions for handling and disposal (NIOSH, 2012). Store intact vials under refrigeration at 2°C to 8°C (36°F to 46°F); reconstituted vials and further dilutions are stable at room temperature for 8 hours.

Stable in LR, NS; **variable stability (consult detailed reference)** in D_5W

Y-site administration: Compatible: Fludarabine, melphalan, ondansetron, paclitaxel, sargramostim

Mechanism of Action Pentostatin is a purine antimetabolite that inhibits adenosine deaminase, preventing the deamination of adenosine to inosine. Accumulation of deoxyadenosine (dAdo) and deoxyadenosine 5'-triphosphate (dATP) results in a reduction of purine metabolism and DNA synthesis and cell death.

Pharmacokinetics (Adult data unless noted)

Distribution: I.V.: V_d: Adults: 36.1 L (20.1 L/m^2); rapidly to body tissues

Protein binding: ~4%

Half-life elimination: Adults:

Distribution half-life: 11-85 minutes

Terminal half-life: 3-7 hours; renal impairment (CrCl <50 mL/minute): 4-18 hours

Elimination: Urine (~50% to 96%) within 24 hours (30% to 90% as unchanged drug)

Clearance: Adults: 68 mL/minute/m^2 (mean)

Dosing: Usual I.V.: Adults (refer to individual protocols): Hydration with 500-1000 mL fluid prior to infusion and 500 mL after infusion is recommended:

Hairy cell leukemia: 4 mg/m^2 every 2 weeks

CLL: 4 mg/m^2 weekly for 3 weeks, then every 2 weeks

Cutaneous T-cell lymphoma: 3.75-5 mg/m^2 daily for 3 days every 3 weeks

Acute GVHD: 1.5 mg/m^2 daily for 3 days; may repeat after 2 weeks if needed

Chronic GVHD: 4 mg/m^2 every 2 weeks for 12 doses; then 4 mg/m^2 every 3-4 weeks (if still improving)

Dosage adjustment in renal impairment: The FDA-approved labeling does not contain renal dosage adjustment guidelines; use with caution in patients with CrCl <60 mL/minute. Two patients with CrCl 50-60 mL/minute achieved responses when treated with 2 mg/m^2/dose. The following guidelines have been used by some clinicians:

Kintzel, 1995:

CrCl 46-60 mL/minute: Administer 70% of dose

CrCl 31-45 mL/minute: Administer 60% of dose

CrCl <30 mL/minute: Consider use of alternative drug

Lathia, 2002:

CrCl 40-59 mL/minute: Administer 3 mg/m^2/dose

CrCl 20-39 mL/minute: Administer 2 mg/m^2/dose

Administration Hazardous agent; use appropriate precautions for handling and disposal (NIOSH, 2012).

I.V.: Reconstitute with 5 mL SWI to a concentration of 2 mg/mL. The solution may be further diluted in 25-50 mL NS or D_5W for infusion. Administer I.V. as a 20- to 30-minute infusion or as an I.V. bolus over 5 minutes.

Monitoring Parameters CBC with differential, platelet count, liver function, serum uric acid, renal function (creatinine clearance), bone marrow evaluation

Dosage Forms Excipient information presented when available (limited, particularly for generics); consult specific product labeling.

◀ Solution Reconstituted, Intravenous:
Nipent: 10 mg (1 ea)

References

al-Razzak LA, Benedetti AE, Waugh WN, et al, "Chemical Stability of Pentostatin (NSC-218321), a Cytotoxic and Immunosuppressant Agent," *Pharm Res*, 1990, 7(5):452-60.

Bolanos-Meade J, Jacobsohn DA, Margolis J, et al, "Pentostatin in Steroid-Refractory Acute Graft-Versus-Host Disease," *J Clin Oncol*, 2005, 23(12):2661-8.

Brogden RN and Sorkin EM, "Pentostatin. A Review of Its Pharmacodynamic and Pharmacokinetic Properties, and Therapeutic Potential in Lymphoproliferative Disorders," *Drugs*, 1993, 46(4):652-77.

Catovsky D, "Clinical Experience With 2'-Deoxycoformycin," *Hematol Cell Ther*, 1996, 38(Suppl 2):103-7.

Dillman RO, "A New Chemotherapeutic Agent: Deoxycoformycin (Pentostatin)," *Semin Hematol*, 1994, 31(1):16-27.

Dillman RO, Mick R, and McIntyre OR, "Pentostatin in Chronic Lymphocytic Leukemia: A Phase II Trial of Cancer and Leukemia Group B," *J Clin Oncol*, 1989, 7(4):433-8.

Grever MR, Siaw MFE, Jacob WF, et al, "The Biochemical and Clinical Consequences of 2'-Deoxycoformycin in Refractory Lymphoproliferative Malignancy," *Blood*, 1981, 57(3):406-17.

Jacobsohn DA, Chen AR, Zahurak M, et al, "Phase II Study of Pentostatin in Patients With Corticosteroid-Refractory Chronic Graft-Versus-Host Disease," *J Clin Oncol*, 2007, 25(27):4255-61.

Kane BJ, Kuhn JG, and Roush MK, "Pentostatin: An Adenosine Deaminase Inhibitor For the Treatment of Hairy Cell Leukemia," *Ann Pharmacother*, 1992, 26(7-8):939-47.

Kintzel PE and Dorr RT, "Anticancer Drug Renal Toxicity and Elimination: Dosing Guidelines for Altered Renal Function," *Cancer Treat Rev*, 1995, 21(1):33-64.

Kurzrock R, Pilat S, and Duvic M, "Pentostatin Therapy of T-Cell Lymphomas With Cutaneous Manifestations," *J Clin Oncol*, 1999, 17(10):3117-21.

Lathia C, Fleming GF, Meyer M, et al, "Pentostatin Pharmacokinetics and Dosing Recommendations in Patients With Mild Renal Impairment," *Cancer Chemother Pharmacol*, 2002, 50(2):121-6.

Margolis J and Grever MR, "Pentostatin (Nipent): A Review of Potential Toxicity and Its Management," *Semin Oncol*, 2000, 27(2 Suppl 5):9-14.

National Institute for Occupational Safety and Health (NIOSH), "NIOSH List of Antineoplastic and Other Hazardous Drugs in Healthcare Settings 2012." Available at http://www.cdc.gov/niosh/docs/2012-150/pdfs/2012-150.pdf. Accessed January 21, 2013.

Tsimberidou AM, Giles F, Duvic M, et al, "Phase II Study of Pentostatin in Advanced T-Cell Lymphoid Malignancies: Update of an M.D. Anderson Cancer Center Series," *Cancer*, 2004, 100(2):342-9.

Pentoxifylline (pen toks IF i lin)

Medication Safety Issues
Sound-alike/look-alike issues:
Pentoxifylline may be confused with tamoxifen
TRENtal® may be confused with Bentyl®, TEGretol®, Trandate®

Related Information
Oral Medications That Should Not Be Crushed or Altered *on page 2438*

Brand Names: U.S. TRENtal [DSC]
Brand Names: Canada Pentoxifylline SR
Therapeutic Category Blood Viscosity Reducer Agent
Generic Availability (U.S.) Yes
Use Symptomatic management of peripheral vascular disease, mainly intermittent claudication (FDA approved in adults)

Has also been studied for use in AIDS patients with increased tumor necrosis factor, cerebrovascular accidents, cerebrovascular diseases, new onset type I diabetes mellitus, diabetic atherosclerosis, diabetic neuropathy, diabetic nephropathy, gangrene, cutaneous polyarteritis nodosa, hemodialysis shunt thrombosis, cerebral malaria, septic shock, sepsis in premature neonates, sickle cell syndromes, vasculitis, Kawasaki disease, Raynaud's syndrome, cystic fibrosis, bone marrow transplant-related toxicities (ie, graft-versus-host disease, veno-occlusive disease, and interstitial pneumonitis), and persistent pulmonary hypertension of the newborn

Pregnancy Risk Factor C

Pregnancy Considerations Adverse events were observed in animal reproduction studies. Information related to use in pregnant women has not been located. Pentoxifylline may be used to test sperm viability when evaluating nonfertile males (ASRM, 2012). It has also been evaluated for the treatment of infertility due to endometriosis, but use for this purpose is not currently recommended (Lu, 2012).

Breast-Feeding Considerations Pentoxifylline and its metabolites are excreted into breast milk. Five nursing women (~6 weeks postpartum) were given a single dose of pentoxifylline 400 mg and maternal milk and serum samples were measured 2 and 4 hours later. The mean M/P ratio of pentoxifylline was 0.87 at 4 hours; actual milk concentrations ranged from below the limit of detection to 67.4 ng/mL. Three metabolites were also measured in breast milk, with mean M/P ratios ranging from 0.54-1.13 at 4 hours (Witter, 1985). Due to the potential for serious adverse reactions in the nursing infant, the manufacturer recommends a decision be made whether to discontinue nursing or to discontinue the drug, taking into account the importance of treatment to the mother.

Contraindications Hypersensitivity to pentoxifylline, any component, or other xanthine derivatives (eg, caffeine, theophylline, theobromine); recent cerebral or retinal hemorrhage

Warnings Use with caution in patients with renal or hepatic impairment, insulin-treated diabetics, chronic occlusive arterial disease of the limbs, recent surgery, or peptic ulcerations

Adverse Reactions
Gastrointestinal: Nausea, vomiting
Rare but important or life-threatening: Anaphylactic shock, anaphylactoid reaction, anaphylaxis, angioedema, angina, anorexia, aplastic anemia, arrhythmia, aseptic meningitis, blurred vision, chest pain, cholecystitis, conjunctivitis, depression, fibrinogen decreased (serum), hallucinations, hepatitis, hypotension, leukemia, leukopenia, liver enzymes increased, pancytopenia, scotoma, seizure, tachycardia, thrombocytopenia

Drug Interactions
Metabolism/Transport Effects Inhibits CYP1A2 (weak)

Avoid Concomitant Use
Avoid concomitant use of Pentoxifylline with any of the following: Ketorolac (Nasal); Ketorolac (Systemic)

Increased Effect/Toxicity
Pentoxifylline may increase the levels/effects of: Agents with Antiplatelet Properties; Antihypertensives; Heparin; Heparin (Low Molecular Weight); Theophylline Derivatives; Vitamin K Antagonists

The levels/effects of Pentoxifylline may be increased by: Cimetidine; Ciprofloxacin (Systemic); Ketorolac (Nasal); Ketorolac (Systemic)

Decreased Effect There are no known significant interactions involving a decrease in effect.

Food Interactions Food may decrease rate but not extent of absorption. Pentoxifylline peak serum levels may be decreased if taken with food.

Mechanism of Action Reduces blood viscosity via increased leukocyte and erythrocyte deformability and decreased neutrophil adhesion/activation; improves peripheral tissue oxygenation presumably through enhanced blood flow.

Pharmacodynamics Onset of action: 2-4 weeks with multiple doses

Pharmacokinetics (Adult data unless noted)
Absorption: Oral: Well absorbed
Distribution: Pentoxifylline and metabolites distribute into breast milk
Metabolism: Undergoes first-pass in the liver, dose-related (nonlinear) pharmacokinetics; 2 active metabolites (M-I

and M-V); **Note:** Plasma concentrations of M-1 and M-V are 5 and 8 times greater, respectively, than pentoxifylline

Half-life, apparent:

Parent drug: 24-48 minutes

Metabolites: 60-96 minutes

Time to peak serum concentration: Within 2-4 hours

Elimination: Metabolites excreted in urine; 0% eliminated unchanged in the urine: 50% to 80% eliminated as M-V metabolite in the urine; 20% as other metabolites

Dosing: Usual Oral:

Children: Minimal information available; one investigation (Furukawa, 1994) found a lower incidence of coronary artery lesions in 22 children (mean age: 2 years) treated for acute Kawasaki disease with versus without pentoxifylline 20 mg/kg/day (given in 3 divided doses); all patients received aspirin and I.V. gamma globulin therapy; a lower dose (10 mg/kg/day) was not effective; higher doses have been used investigationally for the treatment of cystic fibrosis (Aronoff, 1994)

Adults: 400 mg 3 times/day with meals; decrease to 400 mg twice daily if CNS or GI side effects occur. **Note:** Although clinical benefit may be seen within 2-4 weeks, treatment should be continued for at least 8 weeks.

Dosing adjustment in renal impairment: Use with caution; monitor for enhanced therapeutic and toxic effects; **Note:** Pentoxifylline is not eliminated unchanged in the urine; however, the pharmacologically active metabolite (M-V) is; M-V may accumulate in patients with renal impairment and add to pharmacologic and toxic effects.

Adults: Dosage adjustments not listed by manufacturer; adjust dose based on degree of renal impairment (Aronoff, 2007)

CrCl >50 mL/minute: 400 mg every 8-12 hours

CrCl 10-50 mL/minute: 400 mg every 12-24 hours

CrCl <10 mL/minute: 400 mg every 24 hours; **Note:** Further dosage reduction may be required; Paap (1996) suggests a further reduction to 200 mg once daily but current products (extended or controlled release; unscored) may require adaptation to 400 mg once every other day

Administration Oral: Administer with food or antacids to decrease GI upset. Do not crush, break, or chew extended or controlled release tablet, swallow whole.

Test Interactions False-positive theophylline levels

Dosage Forms Excipient information presented when available (limited, particularly for generics); consult specific product labeling. [DSC] = Discontinued product

Tablet Extended Release, Oral:

TRENtal: 400 mg [DSC] [contains benzyl alcohol]

Generic: 400 mg

Extemporaneous Preparations A 20 mg/mL oral suspension may be made using tablets. Crush ten 400 mg tablets and reduce to a fine powder. Add a small amount of purified water and mix to a uniform paste; mix while adding purified water to **almost** 200 mL; transfer to a calibrated bottle, rinse mortar with vehicle, and add quantity of vehicle sufficient to make 200 mL. Label "shake well" and "refrigerate". Stable 91 days.

Nahata MC, Pai VB, and Hipple TF, *Pediatric Drug Formulations*, 5th ed, Cincinnati, OH: Harvey Whitney Books Co, 2004.

References

Aronoff GR, Bennett WM, Berns JS, et al, *Drug Prescribing in Renal Failure: Dosing Guidelines for Adults and Children*, 5th ed, Philadelphia, PA: American College of Physicians, 2007, 117.

Aronoff SC, Quinn FJ, Carpenter LS, et al, "Effects of Pentoxifylline on Sputum Neutrophil Elastase and Pulmonary Function in Patients With Cystic Fibrosis: Preliminary Observations," *J Pediatr*, 1994, 125(6 Pt 1):992-7.

Berman W Jr, Berman N, Pathak D, et al, "Effects of Pentoxifylline (Trental®) on Blood Flow, Viscosity, and Oxygen Transport in Young Adults With Inoperable Cyanotic Congenital Heart Disease," *Pediatr Cardiol*, 1994, 15(2):66-70.

Furukawa S, Matsubara T, Umezawa Y, et al, "Pentoxifylline and Intravenous Gamma Globulin Combination Therapy for Acute Kawasaki Disease," *Eur J Pediatr*, 1994, 153(9):663-7.

Lauterbach R, "Pentoxifylline Treatment of Persistent Pulmonary Hypertension of Newborn," *Eur J Pediatr*, 1993, 152(5):460. (I.V. use)

Lauterbach R, Pawlik D, Tomaszczyk B, et al, "Pentoxifylline Treatment of Sepsis of Premature Infants; Preliminary Clinical Observations," *Eur J Pediatr*, 1994, 153(9):672-4. (I.V. use)

Lu D, Song H, Li Y, et al, "Pentoxifylline for Endometriosis," *Cochrane Database Syst Rev*, 2012, 1:CD007677.

MacDonald MJ, Shahidi NT, Allen DB, et al, "Pentoxifylline in the Treatment of Children With New-Onset Type I Diabetes Mellitus," *JAMA*, 1994, 271(1):27-8.

Paap CM, Simpson KS, Horton MW, et al, "Multiple-Dose Pharmacokinetics of Pentoxifylline and Its Metabolites During Renal Insufficiency," *Ann Pharmacother*, 1996, 30(7-8):724-9.

Practice Committee of American Society for Reproductive Medicine, "Diagnostic Evaluation of the Infertile Male: A Committee Opinion," *Fertil Steril*, 2012, 98(2):294-301.

Witter FR and Smith RV, "The Excretion of Pentoxifylline and Its Metabolites Into Human Breast Milk," *Am J Obstet Gynecol*, 1985, 151(8):1094-7.

◆ **Pentoxifylline SR (Can)** *see* Pentoxifylline *on page 1646*

◆ **Pentrax Gold [OTC]** *see* Coal Tar *on page 532*

◆ **Pentrax Gold Shampoo [OTC] (Can)** *see* Coal Tar *on page 532*

◆ **Pentrax Tar Shampoo [OTC] (Can)** *see* Coal Tar *on page 532*

◆ **Pen VK** *see* Penicillin V Potassium *on page 1635*

◆ **Pepcid** *see* Famotidine *on page 843*

◆ **Pepcid® (Can)** *see* Famotidine *on page 843*

◆ **Pepcid® AC (Can)** *see* Famotidine *on page 843*

◆ **Pepcid® I.V. (Can)** *see* Famotidine *on page 843*

◆ **Peptic Relief [OTC]** *see* Bismuth *on page 294*

◆ **Pepto-Bismol [OTC]** *see* Bismuth *on page 294*

◆ **Pepto-Bismol To-Go [OTC]** *see* Bismuth *on page 294*

◆ **Percocet** *see* Oxycodone and Acetaminophen *on page 1573*

◆ **Percocet-Demi (Can)** *see* Oxycodone and Acetaminophen *on page 1573*

◆ **Percodan®** *see* Oxycodone and Aspirin *on page 1575*

◆ **Perdiem Overnight Relief [OTC]** *see* Senna *on page 1877*

◆ **Perforomist** *see* Formoterol *on page 929*

◆ **Periactin** *see* Cyproheptadine *on page 569*

◆ **Peri-Colace® [OTC]** *see* Docusate and Senna *on page 702*

◆ **Peridex** *see* Chlorhexidine Gluconate *on page 441*

◆ **Peridex Oral Rinse (Can)** *see* Chlorhexidine Gluconate *on page 441*

◆ **Periogard** *see* Chlorhexidine Gluconate *on page 441*

◆ **PerioMed** *see* Fluoride *on page 894*

◆ **Periostat (Can)** *see* Doxycycline *on page 721*

Permethrin (per METH rin)

Brand Names: U.S. Acticin; Elimite

Brand Names: Canada Kwellada-P [OTC]; Nix [OTC]

Therapeutic Category Antiparasitic Agent, Topical; Pediculocide; Scabicidal Agent

Generic Availability (U.S.) Yes

Use Single application treatment of infestation with *Pediculus humanus capitis* (head louse) and its nits; treatment of *Sarcoptes scabiei* (scabies) (FDA approved in ages ≥2 months and adults)

Pregnancy Risk Factor B

Pregnancy Considerations Adverse effects have not been observed in oral animal reproduction studies. The amount of permethrin available systemically following topical application is ≤2%. The CDC considers the use of permethrin or pyrethrins with piperonyl butoxide the drugs of choice for the treatment of pubic lice during pregnancy (CDC, 2010).

Breast-Feeding Considerations It is not known if permethrin is excreted in breast milk. Because many drugs are excreted in human milk and because of the evidence for tumorigenic potential of permethrin in animal studies, consideration should be given to discontinuing nursing temporarily or withholding the drug while the mother is nursing.

Contraindications Hypersensitivity to pyrethroid, pyrethrin, any component, or to chrysanthemums

Precautions For external use only; do not use near the eyes or on mucous membranes such as inside the nose, mouth, or vagina

Adverse Reactions

Dermatologic: Erythema, pruritus, rash of scalp

Local: Burning, numbness, scalp discomfort, stinging, or tingling; edema

Drug Interactions

Metabolism/Transport Effects None known.

Avoid Concomitant Use There are no known interactions where it is recommended to avoid concomitant use.

Increased Effect/Toxicity There are no known significant interactions involving an increase in effect.

Decreased Effect There are no known significant interactions involving a decrease in effect.

Mechanism of Action Inhibits sodium ion influx through nerve cell membrane channels in parasites resulting in delayed repolarization and thus paralysis and death of the pest

Pharmacokinetics (Adult data unless noted)

Absorption: Topical: Minimal (<2%)

Metabolism: By ester hydrolysis to inactive metabolites

Dosing: Neonatal Topical: Full-term neonates: Scabies: A single application of permethrin 5% cream was shown to be safe and effective in a full-term neonate (PNA: 21 days) when applied from scalp to toes for 6 hours before rinsing with soap and water (Quarterman, 1994).

Dosing: Usual Topical: Infants and Children ≥2 months and Adults:

Head lice: After hair has been washed with shampoo, rinsed with water and towel dried, apply a sufficient volume of creme rinse to saturate the hair and scalp; also apply behind the ears and at the base of the neck; leave on hair for 10 minutes before rinsing off with water; remove remaining nits. May repeat in 1 week if lice or nits still present; in areas of head lice resistance to 1% permethrin, 5% permethrin has been applied to clean, dry hair and left on overnight (8-14 hours) under a shower cap.

Scabies: Apply cream from head to toe; leave on for 8-14 hours before washing off with water; for infants, also apply on the hairline, neck, scalp, temple, and forehead; may reapply in 1 week if live mites appear.

Administration Topical: Avoid contact with eyes during application; shake creme rinse well before using. Apply cream in the evening and leave on overnight to maximize exposure of the mites to the drug.

Additional Information Topical cream formulation contains formaldehyde which is a contact allergen

Dosage Forms Excipient information presented when available (limited, particularly for generics); consult specific product labeling.

Cream, External:

Acticin: 5% (60 g)

Elimite: 5% (60 g) [contains formaldehyde solution]

Generic: 5% (60 g)

Lotion, External:

Generic: 1% (59 mL)

References

Centers for Disease Control and Prevention (CDC), "Sexually Transmitted Diseases Treatment Guidelines, 2010," *MMWR Recomm Rep*, 2010, 59(RR-12):1-110.

Currie BJ and McCarthy JS, "Permethrin and Ivermectin for Scabies," *N Engl J Med*, 2010, 362(8):717-25.

"Drugs for Head Lice," *Med Lett Drugs Ther*, 1997, 39(992):6-7.

Hogan DJ, Schachner L, Tanglertsampan C, "Diagnosis and Treatment of Childhood Scabies and Pediculosis," *Pediatr Clin North Am*, 1991, 38(4):941-57.

Krowchuk DP, Tunnessen WW Jr, and Hurwitz S, "Pediatric Dermatology Update," *Pediatrics*, 1992, 90(2 Pt 1):259-64.

Quarterman MJ and Lesher JL, "Neonatal Scabies Treated With Permethrin 5% Cream," *Pediatr Dermatol*, 1994, 11(3):264-6.

◆ **Pernox® Lemon [OTC]** *see* Sulfur and Salicylic Acid *on page 1956*

◆ **Pernox® Regular [OTC]** *see* Sulfur and Salicylic Acid *on page 1956*

◆ **Peroxide** *see* Hydrogen Peroxide *on page 1040*

Perphenazine (per FEN a zeen)

Medication Safety Issues

Sound-alike/look-alike issues:

Trilafon may be confused with Tri-Levlen®

BEERS Criteria medication:

This drug may be potentially inappropriate for use in geriatric patients (Quality of evidence - moderate; Strength of recommendation - strong).

Brand Names: Canada Apo-Perphenazine®

Therapeutic Category Antiemetic; Antipsychotic Agent, Typical, Phenothiazine; Phenothiazine Derivative

Generic Availability (U.S.) Yes

Use Treatment of schizophrenia (FDA approved in ages ≥12 years and adults); severe nausea and vomiting (FDA approved in adults); other psychotic disorders (eg, schizoaffective disorder), psychotic depression

Pregnancy Considerations Jaundice or hyper/hyporeflexia have been reported in newborn infants following maternal use of phenothiazines. Antipsychotic use during the third trimester of pregnancy has a risk for abnormal muscle movements (extrapyramidal symptoms [EPS]) and withdrawal symptoms in newborns following delivery. Symptoms in the newborn may include agitation, feeding disorder, hypertonia, hypotonia, respiratory distress, somnolence, and tremor; these effects may be self-limiting or require hospitalization.

Breast-Feeding Considerations Based on information from two mother-infant pairs, following maternal use of perphenazine 16-24 mg/day, the estimated exposure to the breast-feeding infant would be 0.1% to 0.2% of the weight-adjusted maternal dose. Adverse events have not been reported in nursing infants (information from four cases). Infants should be monitored for signs of adverse events; routine monitoring of infant serum concentrations is not recommended.

Contraindications Hypersensitivity to perphenazine or any component; cross-sensitivity with other phenothiazines may exist; severe CNS depression; subcortical brain damage; bone marrow suppression; blood dyscrasias; coma

Warnings May cause extrapyramidal symptoms, including pseudoparkinsonism, acute dystonic reactions, akathisia, and tardive dyskinesia (risk of these reactions is moderate-high relative to other neuroleptics, and is dose-dependent; to decrease risk of tardive dyskinesia: Use smallest dose and shortest duration possible; evaluate continued need periodically; risk of dystonia is increased with the use of high potency and higher doses of conventional antipsychotics and in males and younger patients). May be associated with neuroleptic malignant syndrome (NMS); monitor for mental status changes, fever, muscle rigidity, and/or autonomic instability; risk may be increased in patients with Parkinson's disease or Lewy body dementia. Safety for use during pregnancy and lactation has not been established; prolonged jaundice, hyper-reflexia, hyporeflexia, or extrapyramidal signs may occur in newborn infants of mothers who received phenothiazines; clinical benefits should clearly outweigh risks before initiating use during pregnancy. May cause pigmentary retinopathy; discontinue drug if ophthalmoscopic or visual field exam demonstrated retinal changes.

Leukopenia, neutropenia, and agranulocytosis (sometimes fatal) have been reported in clinical trials and postmarketing reports with antipsychotic use; presence of risk factors (eg, preexisting low WBC or history of drug-induced leuko/neutropenia) should prompt periodic blood count assessment. Discontinue therapy at first signs of blood dyscrasias or if absolute neutrophil count <1000/mm^3. Use is contraindicated in patients with existing blood dyscrasias or bone marrow suppression.

An increased risk of death has been reported with the use of antipsychotics in elderly patients with dementia-related psychosis [U.S. Boxed Warning]; most deaths seemed to be cardiovascular (eg, sudden death, heart failure) or infectious (eg, pneumonia) in nature; perphenazine is not approved for this indication.

Precautions Use with caution in patients with hemodynamic instability; may cause hypotension; predisposition to seizures; cardiac, hepatic, renal, or respiratory disease; psychic depression. May cause sedation, which may impair physical or mental abilities; patients must be cautioned about performing tasks which require mental alertness (eg, operating machinery or driving); use with caution in disorders where CNS depression is a feature. Use with caution in Parkinson's disease. Esophageal dysmotility and aspiration have been associated with antipsychotic use; use with caution in patients at risk of pneumonia. Use with caution in breast cancer or other prolactin-dependent tumors; may elevate prolactin levels. May alter temperature regulation; use with caution with strenuous exercise, heat exposure, dehydration, and concomitant medication possessing anticholinergic effects. May mask toxicity of other drugs due to antiemetic effects. May alter cardiac conduction; life-threatening arrhythmias have occurred with therapeutic doses of phenothiazines. May cause orthostatic hypotension; use with caution in patients at risk of this effect or those who would not tolerate transient hypotensive episodes (cerebrovascular disease, cardiovascular disease, or other medications which may predispose). May cause photosensitization; avoid prolonged exposure to sunlight. Perphenazine has not been shown to be effective for the treatment of behavioral complications in patients with mental retardation. Safety and efficacy in children <12 years of age has not been established.

Cholestatic jaundice, liver damage, and hepatitis may occur; obtain appropriate liver tests; discontinue treatment if liver tests are abnormal. Monitor renal function in patients with long-term therapy; discontinue treatment if BUN becomes abnormal. Phenothiazines may cause anticholinergic effects (confusion, agitation, constipation, xerostomia, blurred vision, urinary retention); therefore, they should be used with caution in patients with decreased GI motility, urinary retention, benign prostatic hypertrophy, xerostomia, or visual problems. Conditions which also may be exacerbated by cholinergic blockade include narrow-angle glaucoma (screening is recommended) and worsening of myasthenia gravis. Relative to other neuroleptics, perphenazine has a low potency of cholinergic blockade.

Adverse Reactions

Cardiovascular: Bradycardia, cardiac arrest, ECG changes, hyper-/hypotension, orthostatic hypotension, pallor, peripheral edema, sudden death, tachycardia

Central nervous system: Bizarre dreams, catatonic-like states, cerebral edema, dizziness, drowsiness, extrapyramidal symptoms (pseudoparkinsonism, akathisia, dystonias, tardive dyskinesia), faintness, headache, hyperactivity, hyperpyrexia, impairment of temperature regulation, insomnia, lethargy, neuroleptic malignant syndrome (NMS), nocturnal confusion, paradoxical excitement, paranoid reactions, restlessness, seizure

Dermatologic: Discoloration of skin (blue-gray), photosensitivity

Endocrine & metabolic: Amenorrhea, breast enlargement, hyper-/hypoglycemia, galactorrhea, lactation, libido changes, gynecomastia, menstrual irregularity, parotid swelling (rare), SIADH

Gastrointestinal: Adynamic ileus, anorexia, appetite increased, constipation, diarrhea, fecal impaction, obstipation, nausea, salivation, vomiting, weight gain, xerostomia

Genitourinary: Bladder paralysis, ejaculatory disturbances, incontinence, polyuria, urinary retention

Hematologic: Agranulocytosis, eosinophilia, hemolytic anemia, leukopenia, pancytopenia, thrombocytopenic purpura

Hepatic: Hepatotoxicity, jaundice

Neuromuscular & skeletal: Muscle weakness

Ocular: Blurred vision, cornea and lens changes, epithelial keratopathies, glaucoma, mydriasis, myosis, photophobia, pigmentary retinopathy

Renal: Glycosuria

Respiratory: Nasal congestion

Miscellaneous: Allergic reactions, diaphoresis, systemic lupus erythematosus-like syndrome

Drug Interactions

Metabolism/Transport Effects Substrate of CYP1A2 (minor), CYP2C19 (minor), CYP2C9 (minor), CYP2D6 (major), CYP3A4 (minor); **Note:** Assignment of Major/Minor substrate status based on clinically relevant drug interaction potential; **Inhibits** CYP1A2 (weak), CYP2D6 (weak)

Avoid Concomitant Use

Avoid concomitant use of Perphenazine with any of the following: Aclidinium; Amisulpride; Azelastine (Nasal); Ipratropium (Oral Inhalation); Metoclopramide; Paraldehyde; Potassium Chloride; Sulpiride; Thalidomide; Tiotropium; Umeclidinium

Increased Effect/Toxicity

Perphenazine may increase the levels/effects of: AbobotulinumtoxinA; Alcohol (Ethyl); Amisulpride; Analgesics (Opioid); Anticholinergic Agents; Antidepressants (Serotonin Reuptake Inhibitor/Antagonist); ARIPiprazole; Azelastine (Nasal); Beta-Blockers; Buprenorphine; Cannabinoid-Containing Products; CNS Depressants; Hydrocodone; Methotrimeprazine; Methylphenidate; Metyrosine; Mirabegron; Mirtazapine; OnabotulinumtoxinA; Paraldehyde; Porfimer; Potassium Chloride; RimabotulinumtoxinB; Selective Serotonin Reuptake Inhibitors; Serotonin Modulators; Sulpiride; Thalidomide; Thiazide Diuretics; Thiopental; Tiotropium; Topiramate; Zolpidem

The levels/effects of Perphenazine may be increased by: Abiraterone Acetate; Acetylcholinesterase Inhibitors (Central); Aclidinium; Antidepressants (Serotonin Reuptake Inhibitor/Antagonist); Antimalarial Agents; Beta-Blockers; Brimonidine (Topical); Cannabis; CYP2D6 Inhibitors (Moderate); CYP2D6 Inhibitors (Strong); Darunavir; Doxylamine; Dronabinol; Droperidol; HydrOXYzine; Ipratropium (Oral Inhalation); Kava Kava; Lithium; Magnesium Sulfate; Methotrimeprazine; Methylphenidate; Metoclopramide; Metyrosine; Nabilone; Perampanel; Pramlintide; Rufinamide; Serotonin Modulators; Sodium Oxybate; Tapentadol; Tetrabenazine; Tetrahydrocannabinol; Umeclidinium

Decreased Effect

Perphenazine may decrease the levels/effects of: Acetylcholinesterase Inhibitors (Central); Amphetamines; Anti-Parkinson's Agents (Dopamine Agonist); Quinagolide; Secretin

◄ *The levels/effects of Perphenazine may be decreased by:* Acetylcholinesterase Inhibitors (Central); Antacids; Anti-Parkinson's Agents (Dopamine Agonist); Lithium; Peginterferon Alfa-2b

Stability Store at controlled room temperature at 20°C to 25°C (68°F to 77°F); dispense in tight, light-resistant container

Mechanism of Action Perphenazine is a piperazine phenothiazine antipsychotic which blocks postsynaptic mesolimbic dopaminergic receptors in the brain; exhibits alpha-adrenergic blocking effect and depresses the release of hypothalamic and hypophyseal hormones

Pharmacodynamics

Onset of action: 2-4 weeks for control of psychotic symptoms (hallucinations, disorganized thinking or behavior, delusions)

Adequate trial: 6 weeks at moderate to high dose based on tolerability

Duration: Variable

Pharmacokinetics (Adult data unless noted)

Absorption: Well absorbed

Distribution: Crosses placenta

Metabolism: Extensively hepatic to metabolites via sulfoxidation, hydroxylation, dealkylation, and glucuronidation; **Note:** Metabolism is subject to genetic polymorphism; CYP2D6 poor metabolizers will have higher plasma concentrations of perphenazine compared with normal or extensive metabolizers.

Half-life: Perphenazine: 9-12 hours; 7-hydroxyperphenazine: 9.9-18.8 hours

Time to peak serum concentration: Perphenazine: 1-3 hours; 7-hydroxyperphenazine: 2-4 hours

Elimination: Urine and feces, primarily as metabolites

Dialysis: Not dialyzable (0% to 5%)

Dosing: Usual Oral: **Note:** Dosage should be individualized; use lowest effective dose and shortest effective duration; periodically reassess the need for continued treatment

Children: **Note:** Safety and efficacy have not been established in children <12 years of age; use in this age group is not recommended by manufacturer. Some centers use the following doses:

Schizophrenia/psychoses:

<1 year: Dosage not established

1-6 years: 4-6 mg/day in divided doses

6-12 years: 6 mg/day in divided doses

>12 years: 4-16 mg 2-4 times/day

Postoperative vomiting: Dosage not established; use not recommended. Previous studies used an I.V. dose of 70 mcg/kg (maximum: 5 mg/dose) in children 2-12 years of age to decrease postoperative vomiting; perphenazine was shown to be more effective than placebo (Splinter, 1997), more effective than dexamethasone (Splinter, 1997a), and similar in efficacy to ondansetron (Splinter, 1998). However, I.V. granisetron was shown to be more effective than I.V. perphenazine (Fujii, 1999). Only one study has assessed oral perphenazine; doses of 70 mcg/kg were administered 1 hour prior to surgery to 100 children, 4-10 years of age, to reduce postoperative vomiting; oral granisetron was more effective than oral perphenazine (Fujii, 1999a).

Adults:

Schizophrenia/psychoses: 4-16 mg 2-4 times/day; maximum: 64 mg/day (exceptions occur; indication specific)

Nausea/vomiting: 8-16 mg/day in divided doses; maximum: 24 mg/day

Dosing adjustment in hepatic impairment: Specific guidelines are not available; consider dosage reduction in patients with liver disease

Administration May be administered without regard to meals; do not administer within 2 hours of antacids

Monitoring Parameters Vital signs; periodic eye exam, CBC with differential, liver enzyme tests; renal function in patients with long-term use; fasting blood glucose/Hgb A_{1c}; BMI; therapeutic response (mental status, mood, affect, gait), and adverse reactions at beginning of therapy and periodically with long-term use [eg, excess sedation, extrapyramidal symptoms, tardive dyskinesia, CNS changes, abnormal involuntary movement scale (AIMS)]

Reference Range 2-6 nmol/L

Additional Information Long-term usefulness of perphenazine should be periodically re-evaluated in patients receiving the drug for extended periods; consideration should be given whether to decrease the maintenance dose or discontinue drug therapy

Dosage Forms Excipient information presented when available (limited, particularly for generics); consult specific product labeling.

Tablet, Oral:

Generic: 2 mg, 4 mg, 8 mg, 16 mg

References

Azaz-Livshits TL, Symmer LI, and Fraenkel YM, "Atypical Neuroleptic Malignant Syndrome Presenting as Rhabdomyolysis, Altered Consciousness, and Leukocytosis," *J Pharm Technol*, 1995, 11:173-5.

Fujii Y, Saitoh Y, Tanaka H, et al, "Anti-Emetic Efficacy of Prophylactic Granisetron Compared With Perphenazine for the Prevention of Post-Operative Vomiting in Children," *Eur J Anaesthesiol*, 1999, 16 (5):304-7.

Fujii Y, Saitoh Y, Tanaka H, et al, "Preoperative Oral Antiemetics for Reducing Postoperative Vomiting After Tonsillectomy in Children: Granisetron Versus Perphenazine," *Anesth Analg*, 1999a, 88 (6):1298-301.

Hansen LB and Larsen NE, "Metabolic Interaction Between Perphenazine and Disulfiram," *Lancet*, 1982, 2(8313):1472.

Harper G, Dawes M, Azlin C, et al, "Small Bowel Obstruction in a Child on an Antipsychotic," *J Child Adolesc Psychopharmacol*, 1995, 5:81-4.

Lieberman JA, Stroup TS, McEvoy JP, et al, "Effectiveness of Antipsychotic Drugs in Patients With Chronic Schizophrenia," *N Engl J Med*, 2005, 353(12):1209-23.

Miyamoto S, Duncan GE, Marx CE, et al, "Treatments for Schizophrenia: A Critical Review of Pharmacology and Mechanisms of Action of Antipsychotic Drugs," *Mol Psychiatry*, 2005, 10(1):79-104.

Remington G, "Tardive Dyskinesia: Eliminated, Forgotten, or Overshadowed?" *Curr Opin Psychiatry*, 2007, 20(2):131-7.

Splinter WM and Roberts DJ, "Perphenazine Decreases Vomiting by Children After Tonsillectomy," *Can J Anaesth*, 1997, 44(12):1308-10.

Splinter WM and Roberts DJ, "Prophylaxis for Vomiting by Children After Tonsillectomy: Dexamethasone Versus Perphenazine," *Anesth Analg*, 1997a, 85(3):534-7.

Splinter WM and Rhine EJ, "Prophylaxis for Vomiting by Children After Tonsillectomy: Ondansetron Compared With Perphenazine," *Br J Anaesth*, 1998, 80(2):155-8.

◆ **Persantine** *see* Dipyridamole *on page 693*

◆ **Persantine® (Can)** *see* Dipyridamole *on page 693*

◆ **Pertussis, Acellular (Adsorbed)** *see* Diphtheria and Tetanus Toxoids, Acellular Pertussis, Poliovirus and Haemophilus b Conjugate Vaccine *on page 684*

◆ **Pertzye** *see* Pancrelipase *on page 1591*

◆ **Pethidine Hydrochloride** *see* Meperidine *on page 1337*

◆ **Petrolatum White and Mineral Oil Ophthalmic Ointment** *see* Ocular Lubricant *on page 1521*

◆ **Pexeva** *see* PARoxetine *on page 1609*

◆ **PFA** *see* Foscarnet *on page 936*

◆ **Pfizerpen-AS® (Can)** *see* Penicillin G Procaine *on page 1634*

◆ **Pfizerpen-G** *see* Penicillin G (Parenteral/Aqueous) *on page 1631*

◆ **PGE₁** *see* Alprostadil *on page 103*

◆ **PGI₂** *see* Epoprostenol *on page 770*

◆ **PGX** *see* Epoprostenol *on page 770*

◆ **Pharbechlor [OTC]** *see* Chlorpheniramine *on page 448*

◆ **Pharbedryl [OTC]** *see* DiphenhydrAMINE (Systemic) *on page 673*

- ◆ **Phazyme [OTC]** *see* Simethicone *on page 1891*
- ◆ **Phazyme™ (Can)** *see* Simethicone *on page 1891*
- ◆ **Phenadoz** *see* Promethazine *on page 1748*

Phenazopyridine (fen az oh PEER i deen)

Medication Safety Issues
Sound-alike/look-alike issues:
Phenazopyridine may be confused with phenoxybenzamine
Pyridium® may be confused with Dyrenium®, Perdiem®, pyridoxine, pyrithione
Brand Names: U.S. Azo-Gesic [OTC]; Baridium [OTC]; Pyridium; Urinary Pain Relief [OTC]
Therapeutic Category Analgesic, Urinary; Local Anesthetic, Urinary
Generic Availability (U.S.) Yes
Use Symptomatic relief of urinary burning, itching, frequency and urgency in association with urinary tract infection, or following urologic procedures
Pregnancy Risk Factor B
Pregnancy Considerations Adverse events have not been observed in animal reproduction studies. Phenazopyridine crosses the placenta and can be detected in amniotic fluid (Meyer, 1991).
Breast-Feeding Considerations
It is not known if phenazopyridine is excreted into breast milk.
Contraindications Hypersensitivity to phenazopyridine or any component; liver or kidney disease (do not use in patients with CrCl <50 mL/minute)
Warnings Does not treat infection, acts only as an analgesic; drug should be discontinued if skin or sclera develop a yellow color.
Precautions Use with caution in patients with renal impairment (CrCl 50-80 mL/minute)
Adverse Reactions
Central nervous system: Dizziness, headache
Gastrointestinal: Stomach cramps
Rare but important or life-threatening: Acute renal failure, hemolytic anemia, hepatitis, methemoglobinemia
Drug Interactions
Metabolism/Transport Effects None known.
Avoid Concomitant Use There are no known interactions where it is recommended to avoid concomitant use.
Increased Effect/Toxicity
Phenazopyridine may increase the levels/effects of: Prilocaine; Sodium Nitrite

The levels/effects of Phenazopyridine may be increased by: Nitric Oxide
Decreased Effect There are no known significant interactions involving a decrease in effect.
Mechanism of Action An azo dye which exerts local anesthetic or analgesic action on urinary tract mucosa through an unknown mechanism
Pharmacokinetics (Adult data unless noted)
Metabolism: In the liver and other tissues
Elimination: In urine (where it exerts its action); renal excretion (as unchanged drug) is rapid and accounts for 65% of the drug's elimination
Dosing: Usual Oral:
Children: 12 mg/kg/day in 3 divided doses for 2 days if used concomitantly with an antibacterial agent for UTI
Adults: 95-200 mg 3-4 times/day for 2 days if used concomitantly with an antibacterial agent for UTI
Dosing interval in renal impairment:
CrCl 50-80 mL/minute: Administer every 8-16 hours
CrCl <50 mL/minute: Avoid use
Administration Oral: Administer with food to decrease GI distress

Test Interactions Phenazopyridine may cause delayed reactions with glucose oxidase reagents (Clinistix®, Tes-Tape®); occasional false-positive tests occur with Tes-Tape®; cupric sulfate tests (Clinitest®) are not affected; interference may also occur with urine ketone tests (Acetest®, Ketostix®) and urinary protein tests; tests for urinary steroids and porphyrins may also occur
Dosage Forms Excipient information presented when available (limited, particularly for generics); consult specific product labeling.
Tablet, Oral, as hydrochloride:
Azo-Gesic: 95 mg
Baridium: 97.2 mg
Pyridium: 100 mg, 200 mg
Urinary Pain Relief: 95 mg
Generic: 95 mg, 100 mg, 200 mg
References
Meyer BA, Gonik B, and Creasy RK, "Evaluation of Phenazopyridine Hydrochloride as a Tool in the Diagnosis of Premature Rupture of the Membranes," *Am J Perinatol*, 1991, 8(5):297-9.

- ◆ **Phenazopyridine Hydrochloride** *see* Phenazopyridine *on page 1651*
- ◆ **Phenergan** *see* Promethazine *on page 1748*

PHENobarbital (fee noe BAR bi tal)

Medication Safety Issues
Sound-alike/look-alike issues:
PHENobarbital may be confused with PENTobarbital, Phenergan®, phenytoin
BEERS Criteria medication:
This drug may be potentially inappropriate for use in geriatric patients (Quality of evidence - high; Strength of recommendation - strong).
Brand Names: Canada PMS-Phenobarbital
Therapeutic Category Anticonvulsant, Barbiturate; Barbiturate; Hypnotic; Sedative
Generic Availability (U.S.) Yes
Use
Oral: Management of generalized tonic-clonic and partial seizures [FDA approved in pediatric patients (age not specified) and adults]; sedation (tablets: FDA approved in children and adults; elixir, oral solution: FDA approved in adults); insomnia (hypnotic) (FDA approved in adults)
Parenteral: Treatment of generalized tonic-clonic seizures including status epilepticus and cortical focal seizures (FDA approved in adults); sedation (FDA approved in adults)

Phenobarbital has also been used in neonatal and febrile seizures (treatment and prevention); prevention and treatment of neonatal hyperbilirubinemia; hyperbilirubinemia associated with chronic cholestasis; management of sedative/hypnotic withdrawal; management of neonatal abstinence syndrome
Pregnancy Risk Factor B/D (manufacturer dependent)
Pregnancy Considerations Barbiturates can be detected in the placenta, fetal liver, and fetal brain. Fetal and maternal blood concentrations may be similar following parenteral administration. An increased incidence of fetal abnormalities may occur following maternal use. The use of folic acid throughout pregnancy and vitamin K during the last month of pregnancy is recommended; epilepsy itself, number of medications, genetic factors, or a combination of these probably influence the teratogenicity of anticonvulsant therapy. When used during the third trimester of pregnancy, withdrawal symptoms may occur in the neonate, including seizures and hyperirritability; symptoms of withdrawal may be delayed in the neonate up to 14 days after birth. Use during labor does not impair uterine activity; however, respiratory depression may occur in the

◄ newborn; resuscitation equipment should be available, especially for premature infants.

Breast-Feeding Considerations Phenobarbital is excreted into breast milk. Infantile spasms and other withdrawal symptoms have been reported following the abrupt discontinuation of breast-feeding.

Contraindications Hypersensitivity to phenobarbital, barbiturates, or any component; porphyria (manifest and latent)

Additional dosage form specific contraindications: Oral elixir, solution, and tablets: Marked hepatic impairment; respiratory disease in which dyspnea or obstruction are evident; Tablets: Known previous addiction to sedative/hypnotic medication

Warnings Tolerance and/or psychological and physical dependence may occur; use with caution in patients with a history of drug abuse; potential for drug dependency exists; abrupt discontinuation after prolonged use may result in withdrawal symptoms, seizures, or status epilepticus; withdraw gradually if used over extended periods of time unless safety concerns require a more rapid withdrawal. Rapid I.V. administration may cause respiratory depression, apnea, laryngospasm, or hypotension; use with caution in hemodynamically unstable patients (hypotension or shock). Phenobarbital may cause CNS depression, which may impair physical or mental abilities; patients must be cautioned about performing tasks which require mental alertness (eg, operating machinery or driving). Effects with other sedative drugs or ethanol may be potentiated. When treating status epilepticus, additional respiratory support may be required particularly when maximizing loading dose or if concurrent sedative therapy (Hegenbarth, 2008).

Antiepileptic drugs (AEDs) increase the risk of suicidal behavior and ideation in patients receiving these medications for any indication. Pooled analyses of placebo-controlled trials involving 11 different AEDs (regardless of indication) showed a twofold increased risk of suicidal thoughts or behavior (estimated incidence rate: 0.43% in AED treated patients compared to 0.24% of patients receiving placebo); increased risk was observed as early as 1 week after initiation of AED and continued through duration of trials (most trials ≤24 weeks); risk did not vary significantly with age (age range: 5-100 years). Consider risks and benefits of AEDs before prescribing; use with caution in patients with depression or suicidal tendencies. Monitor all patients receiving an AED for emergence of suicidal thoughts or behavior, thoughts of self-harm, any unusual changes in behavior or mood, or the emergence or worsening of depressive symptoms; notify healthcare provider immediately if symptoms or concerning behavior occur. **Note:** The FDA requires a Medication Guide for all antiepileptic drugs informing patients of this risk.

Parenteral solution contains 10% alcohol and 67.8% propylene glycol; toxicities have been reported with use of products containing propylene glycol, including hyperosmolality, lactic acidosis, seizures, and respiratory depression; in neonates, large amounts of propylene glycol delivered orally, intravenously (eg, >3000 mg/day), or topically have been associated with potentially fatal toxicities which can include metabolic acidosis, seizures, renal failure, and CNS depression; use injectable forms containing propylene glycol with caution (AAP, 1997; Shehab, 2009). Commercially available oral elixir and solution may contain 13.5% to 15% alcohol.

Precautions Use with caution in patients with renal or respiratory diseases; use is contraindicated for marked respiratory disease. Use with caution in patients with acute or chronic pain; paradoxical excitement may occur or important symptoms may be masked. Use with caution in patients with hepatic dysfunction; decreased dosage may be needed; avoid use in patients with premonitory signs of hepatic coma; use is contraindicated in marked hepatic impairment. Use with caution during pregnancy; fetal abnormalities may occur; neonates may experience withdrawal symptoms with chronic maternal use. Use with caution in debilitated patients; paradoxical excitement, depression, or confusion may occur. Use with caution in children requiring chronic therapy; in children treated with phenobarbital for complicated febrile seizures, cognitive deficits have been reported.

Solution for injection is highly alkaline and extravasation may cause local tissue damage leading to necrosis; ensure patient has adequate intravenous access with I.V. use. Intra-arterial administration may cause reactions ranging from transient pain to gangrene and is contraindicated. Subcutaneous administration may cause tissue irritation (eg, redness, tenderness, necrosis) and is not recommended.

Pediatric patients may be at increased risk for vitamin D deficiency; with chronic therapy; phenobarbital may cause catabolism of vitamin D; the daily vitamin D requirement may be increased in these patients (≥400 units/day); vitamin D status should be periodically monitored with laboratory data (Misra, 2008; Wagner, 2008) A retrospective study demonstrated that enzyme-inducing antiepileptic drugs (AEDs) (carbamazepine, phenobarbital, and phenytoin) increased systemic clearance of antileukemic drugs (teniposide and methotrexate) and were associated with a worse event-free survival, CNS relapse, and hematologic relapse (ie, lower efficacy), in B-lineage ALL children receiving chemotherapy; the authors recommend using nonenzyme-inducing AEDs in patients receiving chemotherapy for ALL (Relling, 2000). Barbiturates, including phenobarbital, induce liver enzyme activity; accelerating the metabolism of various drugs; potentially significant interactions may exist, requiring dose or frequency adjustment, additional monitoring, and/or selection of alternative therapy. Consult drug interactions database for more detailed information.

Adverse Reactions

Cardiovascular: Bradycardia, hypotension, syncope

Central nervous system: Agitation, anxiety, ataxia, CNS excitation or depression, confusion, dizziness drowsiness, hallucinations, "hangover" effect, headache, hyperkinesia, impaired judgment, insomnia, lethargy, nervousness, nightmares, somnolence

Dermatologic: Exfoliative dermatitis, rash, Stevens-Johnson syndrome

Gastrointestinal: Constipation, nausea, vomiting

Hematologic: Agranulocytosis, megaloblastic anemia, thrombocytopenia

Local: Pain at injection site, thrombophlebitis with I.V. use

Renal: Oliguria

Respiratory: Apnea (especially with rapid I.V. use), hypoventilation, laryngospasm, respiratory depression

Miscellaneous: Gangrene with inadvertent intra-arterial injection

Drug Interactions

Metabolism/Transport Effects Substrate of CYP2C19 (major), CYP2C9 (minor), CYP2E1 (minor); **Note:** Assignment of Major/Minor substrate status based on clinically relevant drug interaction potential; **Induces** CYP1A2 (strong), CYP2A6 (strong), CYP2B6 (strong), CYP2C8 (strong), CYP2C9 (strong), CYP3A4 (strong), P-glycoprotein

Avoid Concomitant Use

Avoid concomitant use of PHENobarbital with any of the following: Abiraterone Acetate; Apixaban; Apremilast; Artemether; Axitinib; Azelastine (Nasal); Bedaquiline; Boceprevir; Bortezomib; Bosutinib; Cabozantinib; Ceritinib; CloZAPine; Crizotinib; Dabigatran Etexilate; Darunavir; Dienogest; Dolutegravir; Dronedarone; Enzalutamide;

Etravirine; Everolimus; Ibrutinib; Itraconazole; Ivacaftor; Lapatinib; Lumefantrine; Lurasidone; Macitentan; Mifepristone; NIFEdipine; Nilotinib; Nisoldipine; Paraldehyde; PAZOPanib; Perampanel; Pirfenidone; Pomalidomide; PONATinib; Praziquantel; Ranolazine; Regorafenib; Rilpivirine; Rivaroxaban; Roflumilast; RomiDEPsin; Simeprevir; Sofosbuvir; Somatostatin Acetate; SORAfenib; Stiripentol; Tasimelteon; Telaprevir; Thalidomide; Ticagrelor; Tofacitinib; Tolvaptan; Toremifene; Ulipristal; Vandetanib; Vemurafenib; VinCRIStine (Liposomal); Vorapaxar; Voriconazole

Increased Effect/Toxicity

PHENobarbital may increase the levels/effects of: Alcohol (Ethyl); Azelastine (Nasal); Buprenorphine; Clarithromycin; CNS Depressants; Hydrocodone; Hypotensive Agents; Meperidine; Methotrimeprazine; Metyrosine; Paraldehyde; Pramipexole; Prilocaine; QuiNIDine; Rotigotine; Selective Serotonin Reuptake Inhibitors; Sodium Nitrite; Thalidomide; Thiazide Diuretics; Zolpidem

The levels/effects of PHENobarbital may be increased by: Brimonidine (Topical); Cannabis; Carbonic Anhydrase Inhibitors; Chloramphenicol; Clarithromycin; Cosyntropin; CYP2C19 Inhibitors (Moderate); CYP2C19 Inhibitors (Strong); Dexmethylphenidate; Doxylamine; Dronabinol; Droperidol; Felbamate; Fosphenytoin; HydrOXYzine; Kava Kava; Luliconazole; Magnesium Sulfate; Methotrimeprazine; Methylphenidate; Nabilone; Nitric Oxide; OXcarbazepine; Phenytoin; Primidone; QuiNINE; Rufinamide; Sodium Oxybate; Somatostatin Acetate; Tapentadol; Tetrahydrocannabinol; Valproic Acid and Derivatives

Decreased Effect

PHENobarbital may decrease the levels/effects of: Abiraterone Acetate; Acetaminophen; Afatinib; Albendazole; Apixaban; Apremilast; ARIPiprazole; Artemether; Axitinib; Bazedoxifene; Bedaquiline; Bendamustine; Beta-Blockers; Boceprevir; Bortezomib; Bosutinib; Brentuximab Vedotin; Cabozantinib; Calcium Channel Blockers; Canagliflozin; Cannabidiol; Cannabis; Ceritinib; Chloramphenicol; Clarithromycin; CloZAPine; Cobicistat; Contraceptives (Estrogens); Contraceptives (Progestins); Corticosteroids (Systemic); Crizotinib; CycloSPORINE (Systemic); CYP1A2 Substrates; CYP2A6 Substrates; CYP2B6 Substrates; CYP2C8 Substrates; CYP2C9 Substrates; CYP3A4 Substrates; Dabigatran Etexilate; Darunavir; Dasatinib; Deferasirox; Diclofenac (Systemic); Dienogest; Disopyramide; Dolutegravir; DOXOrubicin (Conventional); Doxycycline; Dronabinol; Dronedarone; Elvitegravir; Enzalutamide; Eslicarbazepine; Etoposide; Etravirine; Everolimus; Exemestane; Felbamate; FentaNYL; Fosphenytoin; Gefitinib; Griseofulvin; GuanFACINE; Ibrutinib; Imatinib; Irinotecan; Itraconazole; Ivacaftor; Ixabepilone; Lacosamide; LamoTRIgine; Lapatinib; Linagliptin; Lopinavir; Lumefantrine; Lurasidone; Macitentan; Maraviroc; Methadone; MetroNIDAZOLE (Systemic); Mifepristone; NIFEdipine; Nilotinib; Nisoldipine; OXcarbazepine; PAZOPanib; Perampanel; P-glycoprotein/ABCB1 Substrates; Phenytoin; Pirfenidone; Pomalidomide; PONATinib; Praziquantel; Propafenone; QUEtiapine; QuiNIDine; QuiNINE; Ranolazine; Regorafenib; Rilpivirine; Rivaroxaban; Roflumilast; RomiDEPsin; Rufinamide; Saxagliptin; Simeprevir; Sofosbuvir; SORAfenib; Stiripentol; SUNItinib; Tadalafil; Tasimelteon; Telaprevir; Teniposide; Tetrahydrocannabinol; Ticagrelor; Tipranavir; Tofacitinib; Tolvaptan; Toremifene; Treprostinil; Tricyclic Antidepressants; Ulipristal; Valproic Acid and Derivatives; Vandetanib; Vemurafenib; Vilazodone; VinCRIStine (Liposomal); Vitamin K Antagonists; Vorapaxar; Voriconazole; Vortioxetine; Zonisamide; Zuclopenthixol

The levels/effects of PHENobarbital may be decreased by: Amphetamines; Cholestyramine Resin; CYP2C19 Inducers (Strong); Dabrafenib; Folic Acid; Ketorolac (Nasal); Ketorolac (Systemic); Leucovorin Calcium-Levoleucovorin; Levomefolate; Mefloquine; Methylfolate; Multivitamins/Minerals (with ADEK, Folate, Iron); Orlistat; Pyridoxine; Rifamycin Derivatives; Tipranavir

Food Interactions May cause decrease in vitamin D and calcium.

Stability

Oral elixir, solution, and tablets: Store at 20°C to 25°C (68°F to 77°F); protect from light. Protect tablets from moisture.

Injection: Store at 20°C to 25°C (68°F to 77°F); protect from light. Not stable in aqueous solutions; use only clear solutions; do not add to acidic solutions, precipitation may occur.

Mechanism of Action Long-acting barbiturate with sedative, hypnotic, and anticonvulsant properties. Barbiturates depress the sensory cortex, decrease motor activity, alter cerebellar function, and produce drowsiness, sedation, and hypnosis. In high doses, barbiturates exhibit anticonvulsant activity; barbiturates produce dose-dependent respiratory depression.

Pharmacodynamics Hypnosis:

Onset of action:
Oral: Within 20-60 minutes
I.V.: Within 5 minutes
Maximum effect: I.V.: Within 30 minutes
Duration:
Oral: 6-10 hours
I.V.: 4-10 hours

Pharmacokinetics (Adult data unless noted)

Absorption: Oral: 70% to 90%
Distribution: V_d:
Neonates: 0.8-1 L/kg
Infants: 0.7-0.8 L/kg
Children: 0.6-0.7 L/kg
Protein binding: 35% to 50%, decreased protein binding in neonates
Metabolism: In the liver via hydroxylation and glucuronide conjugation
Half-life:
Neonates: 45-500 hours
Infants: 20-133 hours
Children: 37-73 hours
Adults: 53-140 hours
Time to peak serum concentration: Oral: Within 1-6 hours
Elimination: 20% to 50% excreted unchanged in urine; clearance can be increased with alkalinization of urine or with oral multiple-dose activated charcoal
Dialysis: Moderately dialyzable (20% to 50%)

Dosing: Neonatal

Status epilepticus; neonatal seizures: Limited data available: I.V.: Initial: 15-20 mg/kg as a single dose; may repeat doses of 5-10 mg/kg every 15-20 minutes as needed (maximum total dose: 40 mg/kg) (Cloherty, 2012; Gilman, 1989; Lockman, 1979; Painter, 1978; Painter, 1981). **Note:** Additional respiratory support may be required, especially when maximizing loading dose (Hegenbarth, 2008).

Seizures, maintenance therapy: Oral, I.V.: 3-4 mg/kg/day given once daily; maintenance dose usually starts 12-24 hours after loading dose; assess serum concentrations; increase to 5 mg/kg/day if needed (usually by second week of therapy) (Bourgeois, 1995; Cloherty, 2012; Kleigman, 2011)

Neonatal abstinence syndrome (AAP, 1998; Burgos, 2009; Hudak, 2012): Limited data available:
Loading dose (optional): I.V., Oral: 16 mg/kg
I.V.: Administer as a single dose; follow with maintenance dose 12-24 hours after loading dose
Oral: Administer divided into 2 doses and administered every 4-6 hours; follow with maintenance dose 12-24 hours after loading dose
Maintenance dose: Oral, I.V.: Initial: 5 mg/kg/day divided every 12 hours; adjust dose according to abstinence

scores and serum concentrations; usual required dose: 2-8 mg/kg/day. After patient is stabilized, decrease phenobarbital dose 20% every other day or such that drug concentration decreases by 10% to 20% per day (AAP, 1998; Burgos, 2009; Finnegan, 1979).

Neuroprotectant following anoxic injury (with or without cooling): Limited data available: I.V.: 40 mg/kg once; if introducing therapeutic hypothermia, administer prior to cooling (Hall, 1998; Meyn, 2010).

Dosing: Usual

Pediatric:

Status epilepticus: Infants, Children, and Adolescents: I.V.: Initial: 15-20 mg/kg; maximum dose: 1000 mg; may repeat once after 10-15 minutes if needed; maximum total dose: 40 mg/kg; repeat doses administered sooner than 10-15 minutes may not allow adequate time for peak CNS concentrations to be achieved and may lead to CNS depression (Brophy, 2012; Hegenbarth, 2008). **Note:** Additional respiratory support may be required particularly when maximizing loading dose or if concurrent sedative therapy.

Seizures, maintenance therapy: Note: Maintenance dose usually starts 12 hours after loading dose:

Manufacturer's labeling: Infants, Children, and Adolescents: Oral: 3-6 mg/kg/day

Alternate dosing: Limited data available (Geurinni, 2006; Kliegman, 2011):

Initial: Oral, I.V.:

Infants and Children ≤5 years: 3-5 mg/kg/day in 1-2 divided doses

Children >5 years: 2-3 mg/kg/day in 1-2 divided doses

Adolescents: 1-3 mg/kg/day in 1-2 divided doses (Nelson, 1996)

Usual dosing range: **Note:** Dosage should be individualized based upon clinical response and serum concentration; once daily doses usually administered at bedtime in children and adolescents. Some centers have used:

Infants: 5-6 mg/kg/day in 1-2 divided doses

Children:

1-5 years: 6-8 mg/kg/day in 1-2 divided doses

5-12 years: 4-6 mg/kg/day in 1-2 divided doses

Adolescents: 1-3 mg/kg/day in 1-2 divided doses

Sedation: Note: Newer, shorter-acting agents may be preferable.

Manufacturer's labeling: Children and Adolescents: Oral: 2 mg/kg/**dose** 3 times daily; maximum dose: 40 mg

Alternate dosing: Limited data available: Infants and Children: I.M., Oral: 2-3 mg/kg/day in divided doses every 8-12 hours (Nelson, 1996)

Insomnia (hypnotic): Limited data available; shorter-acting agents may be preferable: Infants and Children: I.M., Oral: 2-3 mg/kg/**dose**; may repeat dose as needed after 12-24 hours (Nelson, 1996); some centers have used: I.M., I.V.: 3-5 mg/kg at bedtime

Hyperbilirubinemia: Limited data available: Infants and Children: Oral: Usual range: 3-8 mg/kg/day in 2-3 divided doses; doses up to 10 mg/kg/day in divided doses have been used in case reports (Cies, 2007; Nelson, 1996); for the treatment of hyperbilirubinemia in Crigler-Najjar Syndrome, a dose of 5 mg/kg/day has been used to reduce serum bilirubin concentrations (Kliegman, 2011); not recommended for management of biliary cirrohisis due to sedation and other adverse effects (Lindor-AASLD, 2009)

Sedative/hypnotic withdrawal; prevention; conversion of PENTobarbital to PHENobarbital (PENTobarbital infusion, a total cumulative PENTobarbital dose ≥25 mg/kg or duration ≥5-7 days): Limited data available: Infants, Children, and Adolescents: The following approach transitioning from PENTobarbital to

PHENobarbital has been described: Discontinue PENTobarbital infusion, administer half of the PHENobarbital I.V. loading dose (see table) over 1 hour followed 6 hours later by the remaining half of PHENobarbital loading dose I.V. (over 1 hour). Begin I.V. maintenance PHENobarbital dose 6 hours after loading dose completed; the maintenance PHENobarbital dose should be 1/3 of the initial loading dose and given every 12 hours. Once patient is stabilized, may switch to oral therapy and begin tapering 10% to 20% weekly (Tobias, 2000; Tobias, 2000a). **Note:** This conversion method is based on preliminary data in mechanically ventilated patients; further studies are needed to confirm the efficacy of this regimen. Closely monitor respiratory status and evaluate patient for withdrawal symptoms.

PENTobarbital Infusion Rate (mg/kg/hour)	PHENobarbital I.V. Loading Dose (mg/kg)
1-2	8
2-3	15
3-4	20

Adult:

Sedation: Oral, I.M.: 30-120 mg/day in 2-3 divided doses

Preoperative sedation: I.M.: 100-200 mg 1-1.5 hours before procedure

Anticonvulsant/status epilepticus:

Loading dose: I.V.: 10-20 mg/kg (maximum rate: ≤60 mg/minute in patients ≥60 kg); may repeat dose in 20-minute intervals as needed; maximum total dose: 30 mg/kg

Maintenance dose: Oral, I.V.: 1-3 mg/kg/day in divided doses or 50-100 mg 2-3 times/day

Dosing adjustment in renal impairment: No specific dosage adjustment provided in manufacturer's labeling; reduced doses are recommended. The following guidelines have been used by some clinicians (Aronoff, 2007):

Infants, Children, and Adolescents: **Note:** Renally adjusted dose recommendations are based on doses of 3-7 mg/kg/day every 12-24 hours

GFR ≥10 mL/minute/1.73 m^2: No adjustment necessary

GFR <10 mL/minute/1.73 m^2: Decrease normal dose by 50% and administer every 24 hours

Intermittent hemodialysis [moderately dialyzable (20% to 50%)]: Supplemental dose may be needed during and after dialysis depending on individual seizure threshold

Peritoneal dialysis (PD): 40% to 50% removed; amount varies depending on number of cycles

Continuous renal replacement therapy (CRRT): Monitor serum concentrations; a case report suggests that clearance and volume of distribution increased with CVVH; more frequent and higher dosing may be necessary in some cases (Pasko, 2004)

Adults:

CrCl ≥10 mL/minute: No dosage adjustment necessary.

CrCl <10 mL/minute: Administer every 12-16 hours.

Hemodialysis [moderately dialyzable (20% to 50%)]: Administer dose before dialysis and 50% of dose after dialysis.

Peritoneal dialysis: Administer 50% of normal dose.

CRRT: Administer normal dose and monitor levels.

Dosing adjustment in hepatic impairment: No specific dosage adjustment provided in manufacturer's labeling; reduced doses are recommended. Phenobarbital exposure is increased with hepatic impairment; use with caution.

Administration

Oral: Administer elixir or solution with water, milk, or juice

Parenteral: Do not inject I.V. faster than 1 mg/kg/minute with a maximum of 30 mg/minute for infants and children and 60 mg/minute for adults ≥60 kg. Neonatal studies that used a loading dose of 40 mg/kg for perinatal asphyxia infused the dose over 60 minutes (Hall, 1998). Do not administer intra-arterially. Avoid extravasation; SubQ administration is not recommended. For I.M. administration, inject deep into muscle; do not exceed 5 mL per injection site (adults) due to potential for tissue irritation.

Monitoring Parameters CNS status, seizure activity, liver enzymes, CBC with differential, renal function, serum concentrations; signs and symptoms of suicidality (eg, anxiety, depression, behavior changes). With I.V. use: Respiratory rate, heart rate, blood pressure, I.V. site (stop injection if patient complains of pain in the limb). For treatment of hyperbilirubinemia: Monitor bilirubin (total and direct)

Reference Range

Therapeutic:

Infants, Children, and Adolescents: 15-40 mcg/mL (SI: 65-172 micromole/L)

Adults: 20-40 mcg/mL (SI: 86-172 micromole/L)

Toxic: >40 mcg/mL (SI: >172 micromole/L)

Toxic concentration: Slowness, ataxia, nystagmus: 35-80 mcg/mL (SI: 150-344 micromole/L)

Coma with reflexes: 65-117 mcg/mL (SI: 279-502 micromole/L)

Coma without reflexes: >100 mcg/mL (SI: >430 micromole/L)

Test Interactions Assay interference of LDH

Controlled Substance C-IV

Dosage Forms Excipient information presented when available (limited, particularly for generics); consult specific product labeling.

Elixir, Oral:

Generic: 20 mg/5 mL (473 mL)

Solution, Oral:

Generic: 20 mg/5 mL (473 mL)

Solution, Injection, as sodium:

Generic: 65 mg/mL (1 mL); 130 mg/mL (1 mL)

Tablet, Oral:

Generic: 15 mg, 16.2 mg, 30 mg, 32.4 mg, 60 mg, 64.8 mg, 97.2 mg, 100 mg

Extemporaneous Preparations An alcohol-free 10 mg/mL phenobarbital oral suspension may be made from tablets and one of two different vehicles (a 1:1 mixture of Ora-Plus® and Ora-Sweet® or a 1:1 mixture of Ora-Plus® and Ora-Sweet® SF). Crush ten phenobarbital 60 mg tablets in a glass mortar and reduce to a fine powder. Mix 30 mL of Ora-Plus® and 30 mL of either Ora-Sweet® or Ora-Sweet® SF; stir vigorously. Add 15 mL of the vehicle to the powder and mix to a uniform paste. Transfer the mixture to a 2 ounce amber plastic prescription bottle. Rinse mortar and pestle with 15 mL of the vehicle; transfer to bottle. Repeat, then add quantity of vehicle sufficient to make 60 mL. Label "shake well." May mix dose with chocolate syrup (1:1 volume) immediately before administration to mask the bitter aftertaste. Stable for 115 days when stored in amber plastic prescription bottles at room temperature.

Cober M and Johnson CE, "Stability of an Extemporaneously Prepared Alcohol-Free Phenobarbital Suspension," *Am J Health Syst Pharm,* 2007, 64(6):644-6.

References

American Academy of Pediatrics Committee on Drugs. "Inactive" ingredients in pharmaceutical products: update (subject review). *Pediatr.* 1997;99(2):268-278.

Aronoff GR, Bennett WM, Berns JS, et al, *Drug Prescribing in Renal Failure: Dosing Guidelines for Adults and Children,* 5th ed. Philadelphia, PA: American College of Physicians; 2007.

Bourgeois BF. Antiepileptic drugs in pediatric practice. *Epilepsia.* 1995;36(Suppl 2):S34-45.

Brophy GM, Bell R, Claassen J, et al, "Guidelines for the Evaluation and Management of Status Epilepticus," *Neurocrit Care,* 2012, 17(1):3-23.

Burgos AE. Burke, Jr BL. Neonatal abstinence syndrome. *Neoreviews.* 2009;10(5):222-229.

Cies JJ and Giamalis JN, "Treatment of Cholestatic Pruritus in Children," *Am J Health Syst Pharm,* 2007, 64(11):1157-62.

Cloherty JP, Eichenwald EC, Stark AR, eds. *Manual of Neonatal Care.* 7th ed. Philadelphia, PA: Lippincott Williams & Wilkins; 2012.

Finnegan LP, Mitros TF, and Hopkins LE, "Management of Neonatal Narcotic Abstinence Utilizing a Phenobarbital Loading Dose Method," *NIDA Res Monogr,* 1979, 27:247-53.

Gilman JT, Gal P, Duchowny MS, et al, "Rapid Sequential Phenobarbital Treatment of Neonatal Seizures," *Pediatrics,* 1989, 83(5):674-8.

Guerrini R, "Epilepsy in Children," *Lancet,* 2006, 367(9509):499-524.

Hall RT, Hall FK, and Daily DK, "High-Dose Phenobarbital Therapy in Term Newborn Infants With Severe Perinatal Asphyxia: A Randomized, Prospective Study With Three-Year Follow-Up," *J Pediatr,* 1998, 132(2):345-8.

Hegenbarth MA and American Academy of Pediatrics Committee on Drugs, "Preparing for Pediatric Emergencies: Drugs to Consider," *Pediatrics,* 2008, 121(2):433-43.

Hudak ML, Tan RC, Committee On Drugs, et al, "Neonatal Drug Withdrawal," *Pediatrics,* 2012, 129(2):e540-60.

Kliegman RM, Stanton BF, St. Gemell JW, et al, eds. *Nelson Textbook of Pediatrics.* 19th ed. Philadelphia, PA: Saunders Elsevier;2011.

Kraus DM, Pham JT. "Neonatal Therapy." *Koda-Kimble & Young's Applied Therapeutics: The Clinical Use of Drugs.* 10th ed. Alldredge BK, Corelli RL, Ernst ME, et al, eds, Baltimore, MD: Wolters Kluwer Health/ Lippincott Williams & Wilkins, 2013.

Lindor KD, Gershwin ME, Poupon R, et al, "Primary Biliary Cirrhosis," *Hepatology,* 2009, 50(1):291-308.

Lockman LA, Kriel R, Zaske D, et al, "Phenobarbital Dosage for Control of Neonatal Seizures," *Neurology,* 1979, 29(11):1445-9.

Meyn DF Jr, Ness J, Ambalavanan N, et al, "Prophylactic Phenobarbital and Whole-Body Cooling for Neonatal Hypoxic-Ischemic Encephalopathy," *J Pediatr,* 2010, 157(2):334-6.

Misra M, Pacaud D, Petryk A, Collett-Solberg PF, Kappy M, Drug and Therapeutics Committee of the Lawson Wilkins Pediatric Endocrine Society. Vitamin D deficiency in children and its management: review of current knowledge and recommendations. *Pediatrics.* 2008;122 (2):398-417.

Nelson WE, Behrman RE, Kliegman RM, et al, eds. *Nelson Textbook of Pediatrics.* 15th ed. Philadelphia, PA: WB Saunders Company; 1996.

"Neonatal Drug Withdrawal. American Academy of Pediatrics Committee on Drugs," *Pediatrics,* 1998, 101(6):1079-88.

Painter MJ, Pippenger C, MacDonald H, et al, "Phenobarbital and Diphenylhydantoin Levels in Neonates With Seizures," *J Pediatr,* 1978, 92(2):315-9.

Painter MJ, Pippenger C, Wasterlain C, et al, "Phenobarbital and Phenytoin in Neonatal Seizures: Metabolism and Tissue Distribution," *Neurology,* 1981, 31(9):1107-12.

Pasko DA, Annich GM. Phenobarbital pharmacokinetics of an infant on ECMO and CVVHD: a case report. Presented to Pediatric CRRT; Orlando FL;2004.

Relling MV, Pui CH, Sandlund JT, et al, "Adverse Effect of Anticonvulsants on Efficacy of Chemotherapy for Acute Lymphoblastic Leukaemia," *Lancet,* 2000, 356(9226):285-90.

Shehab N, Lewis CL, Streetman DD, Donn SM. Exposure to the pharmaceutical excipients benzyl alcohol and propylene glycol among critically ill neonates. *Pediatr Crit Care Med.* 2009;10 (2):256-259.

Tobias JD, "Tolerance, Withdrawal, and Physical Dependency After Long-Term Sedation and Analgesia of Children in the Pediatric Intensive Care Unit," *Crit Care Med,* 2000a, 28(6):2122-32.

Tobias JD, Deshpande JK, Pietsch JB, et al, "Pentobarbital Sedation for Patients in the Pediatric Intensive Care Unit," *South Med J,* 1995, 88 (3):290-4.

Wagner CL, Greer FR, American Academy of Pediatrics Section on Breastfeeding, American Academy of Pediatrics Committee on Nutrition. Prevention of rickets and vitamin D deficiency in infants, children, and adolescents. *Pediatrics.* 2008;122(5):1142-1152.

♦ **Phenobarbital, Hyoscyamine, Atropine, and Scopolamine** *see* Hyoscyamine, Atropine, Scopolamine, and Phenobarbital *on page 1058*

♦ **Phenobarbital Sodium** *see* PHENobarbital *on page 1651*

♦ **Phenobarbitone** *see* PHENobarbital *on page 1651*

♦ **Phenoptin** *see* Sapropterin *on page 1865*

Phenoxybenzamine (fen oks ee BEN za meen)

Medication Safety Issues

Sound-alike/look-alike issues:

Phenoxybenzamine may be confused with phenazopyridine

Related Information

Oral Medications That Should Not Be Crushed or Altered *on page 2438*

Safe Handling of Hazardous Drugs *on page 2419*

Brand Names: U.S. Dibenzyline

Therapeutic Category Alpha-Adrenergic Blocking Agent, Oral; Antihypertensive Agent; Vasodilator

Generic Availability (U.S.) No

Use Symptomatic management of hypertension and sweating in patients with pheochromocytoma

Pregnancy Risk Factor C

Pregnancy Considerations Adequate animal reproduction studies have not been conducted. It is not known whether phenoxybenzamine can cause fetal harm when administered to a pregnant woman or can affect reproduction capacity.

Breast-Feeding Considerations It is not known if phenoxybenzamine is excreted in breast milk. Due to the potential for serious adverse reactions in the nursing infant, a decision should be made whether to discontinue nursing or to discontinue the drug, taking into account the importance of treatment to the mother.

Contraindications Hypersensitivity to phenoxybenzamine or any component; shock

Warnings Hazardous agent; use appropriate precautions for handling and disposal (NIOSH, 2012). Capsule contains benzyl alcohol which may cause allergic reactions in susceptible individuals; large amounts of benzyl alcohol (≥99 mg/kg/day) have been associated with a potentially fatal toxicity ("gasping syndrome") in neonates; avoid use of phenoxybenzamine products containing benzyl alcohol in neonates; *in vitro* and animal studies have shown that benzoate, a metabolite of benzyl alcohol, displaces bilirubin from protein binding sites.

Precautions Use with caution in patients with renal dysfunction, cerebral or coronary arteriosclerosis

Adverse Reactions

Cardiovascular: Orthostatic hypotension, tachycardia

Central nervous system: Drowsiness, fatigue

Gastrointestinal: GI irritation

Genitourinary: Inhibition of ejaculation

Ocular: Miosis

Respiratory: Nasal congestion

Drug Interactions

Metabolism/Transport Effects None known.

Avoid Concomitant Use

Avoid concomitant use of Phenoxybenzamine with any of the following: Alpha1-Blockers

Increased Effect/Toxicity

Phenoxybenzamine may increase the levels/effects of: Alpha1-Blockers; Amifostine; Antihypertensives; Calcium Channel Blockers; Obinutuzumab; RiTUXimab

The levels/effects of Phenoxybenzamine may be increased by: Beta-Blockers; Brimonidine (Topical); Diazoxide; Herbs (Hypotensive Properties); MAO Inhibitors; Pentoxifylline; Phosphodiesterase 5 Inhibitors; Prostacyclin Analogues

Decreased Effect

Phenoxybenzamine may decrease the levels/effects of: Alpha-/Beta-Agonists; Alpha1-Agonists

The levels/effects of Phenoxybenzamine may be decreased by: Herbs (Hypertensive Properties); Methylphenidate; Yohimbine

Stability Hazardous agent; use appropriate precautions for handling and disposal (NIOSH, 2012).

Mechanism of Action Produces long-lasting noncompetitive alpha-adrenergic blockade of postganglionic synapses in exocrine glands and smooth muscle; relaxes urethra and increases opening of the bladder

Pharmacodynamics Oral:

Onset of action: Within 2 hours

Maximum effect: Within 4-6 hours

Duration: Effects can continue for up to 4 days

Pharmacokinetics (Adult data unless noted)

Absorption: Oral: ~20% to 30%

Distribution: Distributes to and may accumulate in adipose tissues

Half-life: Adults: 24 hours

Elimination: Primarily in urine and bile

Dosing: Usual Oral:

Children: Initial: 0.2 mg/kg once daily; maximum dose: 10 mg/dose; increase every 4 days by 0.2 mg/kg/day increments; usual maintenance dose: 0.4-1.2 mg/kg/day every 6-8 hours; maximum doses of up to 2-4 mg/kg/day have been recommended

Adults: Initial: 10 mg twice daily; increase dose every other day to usual dose of 10-40 mg every 8-12 hours; higher doses may be needed

Administration Hazardous agent; use appropriate precautions for handling and disposal (NIOSH, 2012).

Oral: May administer with milk to decrease GI upset

Monitoring Parameters Blood pressure, orthostasis, heart rate

Dosage Forms Excipient information presented when available (limited, particularly for generics); consult specific product labeling.

Capsule, Oral, as hydrochloride:

Dibenzyline: 10 mg [contains benzyl alcohol]

Extemporaneous Preparations Hazardous agent: Use appropriate precautions for handling and disposal.

A 2 mg/mL oral suspension may be made with capsules, propylene glycol 1%, and citric acid 0.15% in distilled water. Prepare the vehicle by dissolving 150 mg citric acid in a minimal amount of distilled water. Add 1 mL propylene glycol and mix well; add quantity of distilled water sufficient to make 100 mL (only a small portion of this vehicle will be used to make the final product). Grind the contents of two phenoxybenzamine 10 mg capsules in a mortar and reduce to a fine powder. Add a small portion of the vehicle and mix to a uniform paste; transfer to a graduated cylinder, rinse mortar with vehicle, and add quantity of prepared vehicle sufficient to make 10 mL. Transfer to an amber glass prescription bottle with tight-fitting cap; label "shake well" and "refrigerate". Stable for 7 days when stored in amber glass prescription bottles and refrigerated.

A stock solution of 10 mg/mL in propylene glycol was stable for 30 days refrigerated. When this stock solution was diluted 1:4 (v/v) with syrup (66.7% sucrose) to 2 mg/mL, the preparation was stable for 1 hour refrigerated. **Note:** Although the stock solution is stable for 30 days, it must be diluted before administration to decrease the amount of propylene glycol delivered to the patient.

Lim LY, Tan LL, Chan EW, et al, "Stability of Phenoxybenzamine Hydrochloride in Various Vehicles," *Am J Health Syst Pharm,* 1997, 54(18):2073-8.

References

National Institute for Occupational Safety and Health (NIOSH), "NIOSH List of Antineoplastic and Other Hazardous Drugs in Healthcare Settings 2012." Available at http://www.cdc.gov/niosh/docs/2012-150/pdfs/2012-150.pdf. Accessed January 21, 2013.

◆ **Phenoxybenzamine Hydrochloride** *see* Phenoxybenzamine *on page 1655*

◆ **Phenoxymethyl Penicillin** *see* Penicillin V Potassium *on page 1635*

Phentolamine (fen TOLE a meen)

Medication Safety Issues

Sound-alike/look-alike issues:

Phentolamine may be confused with phentermine, Ventolin

Regitine may be confused with Reglan

Related Information

Management of Drug Extravasations *on page 2255*

Brand Names: Canada Rogitine®

Therapeutic Category Alpha-Adrenergic Blocking Agent, Parenteral; Antidote, Extravasation; Antihypertensive Agent; Diagnostic Agent, Pheochromocytoma; Vasodilator

Generic Availability (U.S.) Yes

Use Diagnosis of pheochromocytoma; treatment of hypertension associated with pheochromocytoma or other causes of excess sympathomimetic amines; local treatment and prevention of dermal necrosis after extravasation of drugs with alpha-adrenergic effects (dobutamine, dopamine, epinephrine, metaraminol, norepinephrine, phenylephrine)

Pregnancy Risk Factor C

Pregnancy Considerations Adverse events were observed in some oral animal reproduction studies. Diagnosing and treating pheochromocytoma is critical for favorable maternal and fetal outcomes (Schenker, 1971; Schenker, 1982).

Breast-Feeding Considerations It is not known if phentolamine is excreted in breast milk. Due to the potential for serious adverse reaction in the nursing infant, the decision to discontinue phentolamine or discontinue breast-feeding during treatment should take in account the benefits of treatment to the mother.

Contraindications Hypersensitivity to phentolamine or any component; renal impairment; coronary or cerebral arteriosclerosis; MI

Precautions Use with caution in patients with gastritis, peptic ulcer; history of cardiac arrhythmias; MI, cerebrovascular spasm, and cerebrovascular occlusion may occur

Adverse Reactions

Cardiovascular: Bradycardia (OraVerse), cerebrovascular occlusion, hypertension (OraVerse), hypotension, myocardial infarction, tachycardia (OraVerse)

Central nervous system: Cerebrovascular spasm, headache (OraVerse), mouth pain (OraVerse), paresthesia (OraVerse; mild, transient)

Dermatologic: Facial swelling (OraVerse), pruritus (OraVerse)

Gastrointestinal: Diarrhea (OraVerse), nausea, upper abdominal pain (OraVerse), vomiting (OraVerse)

Local: Pain at injection site (OraVerse)

Rare but important or life-threatening: Cardiac arrhythmia, orthostatic hypotension

Drug Interactions

Metabolism/Transport Effects None known.

Avoid Concomitant Use

Avoid concomitant use of Phentolamine with any of the following: Alpha1-Blockers

Increased Effect/Toxicity

Phentolamine may increase the levels/effects of: Alpha1-Blockers; Amifostine; Antihypertensives; Calcium Channel Blockers; Obinutuzumab; RiTUXimab

The levels/effects of Phentolamine may be increased by: Beta-Blockers; Brimonidine (Topical); Diazoxide; Herbs (Hypotensive Properties); MAO Inhibitors; Pentoxifylline; Phosphodiesterase 5 Inhibitors; Prostacyclin Analogues

Decreased Effect

Phentolamine may decrease the levels/effects of: Alpha-/Beta-Agonists; Alpha1-Agonists

The levels/effects of Phentolamine may be decreased by: Herbs (Hypertensive Properties); Methylphenidate; Yohimbine

Stability Reconstituted solution is stable for 48 hours at room temperature and 1 week when refrigerated

Mechanism of Action Competitively blocks alpha-adrenergic receptors (nonselective) to produce brief antagonism of circulating epinephrine and norepinephrine to reduce hypertension caused by alpha effects of these

catecholamines and minimizes tissue injury due to extravasation of these and other sympathomimetic vasoconstrictors (eg, dopamine, phenylephrine); also has a positive inotropic and chronotropic effect on the heart thought to be due to presynaptic alpha-2 receptor blockade which results in release of presynaptic norepinephrine (Hoffman, 1980)

OraVerse™: Causes vasodilation and increased blood flow in injection area via alpha-adrenergic blockade to accelerate reversal of soft tissue anesthesia

Pharmacodynamics

Onset of action:

I.M.: Within 15-20 minutes

I.V.: Immediate

Maximum effect:

I.M.: Within 20 minutes

I.V.: Within 2 minutes

Duration:

I.M.: 30-45 minutes

I.V.: Within 15-30 minutes

Pharmacokinetics (Adult data unless noted)

Metabolism: In the liver

Half-life: Adults: 19 minutes

Elimination: 10% to 13% excreted in urine as unchanged drug

Dosing: Neonatal Treatment of alpha-adrenergic agonist drug extravasation: SubQ: **Note:** Total dose required depends on the size of extravasation; dose may be repeated if required. Infiltrate area of extravasation with a small amount (eg, 1 mL given in 0.1-0.2 mL aliquots) of a 0.25-0.5 mg/mL solution (made by diluting 2.5-5 mg in 10 mL of preservative free NS) within 12 hours of extravasation; in general, do not exceed 2.5 mg total; monitor blood pressure, especially when dose exceeds the recommended I.M./I.V. dose of 0.1 mg/kg

Dosing: Usual

Treatment of alpha-adrenergic agonist drug extravasation: SubQ: **Note:** Total dose required depends on the size of extravasation; dose may be repeated if required: Infants, Children, and Adults: Infiltrate area of extravasation with a small amount (eg, 1 mL given in 0.2 mL aliquots) of a 0.5-1 mg/mL solution (made by diluting 5-10 mg in 10 mL of NS) within 12 hours of extravasation; in general, do not exceed 0.1-0.2 mg/kg or 5 mg total; **Note:** Doses of <5 mg total are usually effective; one **adult** case using a total dose of 50 mg (given over 1 hour in 0.5 ml aliquots of a 1 mg/mL solution) for a large extravasation has been reported (Cooper, 1989).

Diagnosis of pheochromocytoma: I.M., I.V.:

Children: 0.05-0.1 mg/kg/dose, maximum single dose: 5 mg

Adults: 5 mg

Hypertension (prior to surgery for pheochromocytoma): I.M., I.V.:

Children: 0.05-0.1 mg/kg/dose given 1-2 hours before pheochromocytomectomy; repeat as needed to control blood pressure; maximum single dose: 5 mg

Adults: 5 mg given 1-2 hours before pheochromocytomectomy; repeat as needed to control blood pressure

Hypertensive crisis due to MAO inhibitor/sympathomimetic amine interaction: I.M., I.V.: Adults: 5-20 mg

Administration Parenteral: Treatment of extravasation: Infiltrate area of extravasation with multiple small injections of a diluted solution; use 27- or 30-gauge needles and change needle between each skin entry to prevent bacterial contamination and minimize pain; do not inject a volume such that swelling of the extremity or digit with resultant compartment syndrome occurs

Monitoring Parameters Blood pressure, heart rate, orthostasis; treatment of extravasation: site of extravasation, skin color, local perfusion

Additional Information When drugs with alpha-adrenergic effects extravasate, they cause local vasoconstriction ▶

which causes blanching of the skin and a pale, cold, hard appearance; SubQ phentolamine blocks the alpha-adrenergic receptors and reverses the vasoconstriction; the extravasation area should "pink up" and return to normal skin color following SubQ administration of phentolamine. Dobutamine primarily stimulates beta$_1$-adrenergic receptors, but does possess alpha (and beta$_2$) adrenergic effects; the alpha-adrenergic effects (vasoconstriction) may be seen when dobutamine extravasates (since high concentrations of dobutamine would be present locally); although infrequent, cases of dermal necrosis from dobutamine extravasation have been reported; thus, phentolamine may help prevent dermal necrosis following dobutamine extravasations (Hoff, 1979; MacCara, 1983). Injection contains mannitol 25 mg/vial

Dosage Forms Excipient information presented when available (limited, particularly for generics); consult specific product labeling.

Solution, Injection, as mesylate:
Generic: 5 mg/mL (1 mL)
Solution Reconstituted, Injection, as mesylate:
Generic: 5 mg (1 ea)

References

Cooper BE, "High-Dose Phentolamine for Extravasation of Pressors," *Clin Pharm*, 1989, 8(10):689.

Flemmer L and Chan JS, "A Pediatric Protocol for Management of Extravasation Injuries," *Pediatr Nurs*, 1993, 19(4):355-8, 424.

Hoff JV, Peatty PA, and Wade JL, "Dermal Necrosis From Dobutamine," *N Engl J Med*, 1979, 300(22):1280.

MacCara ME, "Extravasation: A Hazard of Intravenous Therapy," *Drug Intell Clin Pharm*, 1983, 17(10):713-7.

Schenker JG and Chowers I, "Pheochromocytoma and Pregnancy. Review of 89 Cases," *Obstet Gynecol Surv*, 1971, 26(11):739-47.

Schenker JG and Granat M, "Phaeochromocytoma and Pregnancy - An Updated Appraisal," *Aust N Z J Obstet Gynaecol*, 1982, 22(1):1-10.

Siwy BK and Sadove AM, "Acute Management of Dopamine Infiltration Injury With Regitine," *Plast Reconstr Surg*, 1987, 80(4):610-2.

Subhani M, Sridhar S, and DeCristofaro JD, "Phentolamine Use in a Neonate for the Prevention of Dermal Necrosis Caused by Dopamine: A Case Report," *J Perinatol*, 2001, 21(5):324-6.

Thigpen JL, "Peripheral Intravenous Extravasation: Nursing Procedure for Initial Treatment," *Neonatal Netw*, 2007, 26(6):379-84.

Zenk KE, "Management of Intravenous Extravasations," *Infusion*, 1981, 5:77-9.

◆ **Phentolamine Mesylate** *see* Phentolamine *on page 1656*

◆ **Phenylalanine Mustard** *see* Melphalan *on page 1328*

◆ **Phenylazo Diamino Pyridine Hydrochloride** *see* Phenazopyridine *on page 1651*

Phenylephrine (Systemic) (fen il EF rin)

Medication Safety Issues

Sound-alike/look-alike issues:
Sudafed PE® may be confused with Sudafed®

High alert medication:
The Institute for Safe Medication Practices (ISMP) includes this medication among its list of drugs which have a heightened risk of causing significant patient harm when used in error.

Related Information

Management of Drug Extravasations *on page 2255*
Serotonin Syndrome *on page 2405*

Brand Names: U.S. Little Colds Decongestant [OTC]; Medi-Phenyl [OTC]; Nasal Decongestant PE Max St [OTC]; Nasal Decongestant [OTC]; Non-Pseudo Sinus Decongestant [OTC]; Sudafed PE Childrens [OTC]; Sudafed PE Maximum Strength [OTC]; Sudogest PE [OTC]

Therapeutic Category Adrenergic Agonist Agent; Alpha-Adrenergic Agonist; Sympathomimetic

Generic Availability (U.S.) May be product dependent

Use

Parenteral: Treatment of hypotension and vascular failure in shock; supraventricular tachycardia; as a vasoconstrictor in regional analgesia (All indications: FDA approved adults); treatment of hypotension during spinal anesthesia (FDA approved in pediatric patients [age not specified] and adults)

Oral: Temporary relief of nasal congestion due to the common cold, hay fever, or other upper respiratory allergies (OTC products: FDA approved in ages ≥4 years and adults; consult specific product formulation for appropriate age group

Pregnancy Risk Factor C

Pregnancy Considerations Animal reproduction studies have not been conducted; therefore, the manufacturer classifies phenylephrine as pregnancy category C. Phenylephrine crosses the placenta at term. Maternal use of phenylephrine during the first trimester of pregnancy is not strongly associated with an increased risk of fetal malformations; maternal dose and duration of therapy were not reported in available publications. Phenylephrine is available over-the-counter (OTC) for the symptomatic relief of nasal congestion. Decongestants are not the preferred agents for the treatment of rhinitis during pregnancy. Oral phenylephrine should be avoided during the first trimester of pregnancy; short-term use (<3 days) of intranasal phenylephrine may be beneficial to some patients although its safety during pregnancy has not been studied. Phenylephrine injection is used at delivery for the prevention and/or treatment of maternal hypotension associated with spinal anesthesia in women undergoing cesarean section. Phenylephrine may be associated with a more favorable fetal acid base status than ephedrine; however, overall fetal outcomes appear to be similar. Nausea or vomiting may be less with phenylephrine than ephedrine but is also dependent upon blood pressure control. Phenylephrine may be preferred in the absence of maternal bradycardia.

Breast-Feeding Considerations It is not known if phenylephrine is excreted into breast milk. The manufacturer recommends that caution be exercised when administering phenylephrine to nursing women.

Contraindications Hypersensitivity to phenylephrine or any component; severe hypertension, ventricular tachycardia

OTC labeling: When used for self-medication, do not use if taking MAO inhibitor or within 2 weeks of discontinuation of MAO inhibitor

Warnings Phenylephrine injection should be administered by adequately trained individuals familiar with its use **[U.S. Boxed Warning]**. Phenylephrine injection is a vesicant; infuse into large veins and ensure proper needle or catheter placement prior to and during infusion; avoid extravasation.

Avoid or use with extreme caution in patients with heart failure or cardiogenic shock; increased systemic vascular resistance may significantly reduce cardiac output. Assure adequate circulatory volume to minimize need for vasoconstrictors. Avoid use in patients with hypertension (contraindicated in severe hypertension); monitor blood pressure closely and adjust infusion rate.

Safety and efficacy for the use of cough and cold products in children <2 years of age is limited. Serious adverse effects including death have been reported. The FDA notes that there are no approved OTC uses for these products in children <2 years of age. Healthcare providers are reminded to ask caregivers about the use of OTC cough and cold products in order to avoid exposure to multiple medications containing the same ingredient. When used for self-medication (OTC), use caution in patients with asthma, bowel obstruction/narrowing, hyperthyroidism, diabetes mellitus, cardiovascular disease, ischemic heart disease, hypertension, increased intraocular pressure, prostatic hyperplasia, or in the elderly. Notify health care provider if symptoms do not improve within 7 days or are accompanied by fever. Discontinue and contact health care provider if nervousness, dizziness, or sleeplessness occur.

Injection may contain sulfites which may cause allergic reactions in susceptible individuals. Some oral formulations contain sodium benzoate; benzoic acid (benzoate) is a metabolite of benzyl alcohol; large amounts of benzyl alcohol (≥99 mg/kg/day) have been associated with a potentially fatal toxicity ("gasping syndrome") in neonates; *in vitro* and animal studies have shown that benzoate displaces bilirubin from protein binding sites; avoid use of benzyl alcohol containing products in neonates.

Precautions Use as pressor therapy for treatment of hypotension and vascular failure is not a substitute for replacement of blood, plasma, and body fluids. Use with caution in patients with hyperthyroidism, bradycardia, partial heart block, myocardial disease, or severe arteriosclerosis. Use parenteral product with extreme caution in patients taking MAO inhibitors; hypertension may result from concurrent use; use in contraindicated with oral products.

Adverse Reactions
Injection:
Cardiovascular: Arrhythmia (rare), decreased cardiac output, hypertension, pallor, precordial pain or discomfort, reflex bradycardia, severe peripheral and visceral vasoconstriction

Central nervous system: Anxiety, dizziness, excitability, giddiness, headache, insomnia, nervousness, restlessness

Endocrine & metabolic: Metabolic acidosis

Gastrointestinal: Gastric irritation, nausea

Local: I.V.: Extravasation which may lead to necrosis and sloughing of surrounding tissue, blanching of skin

Neuromuscular & skeletal: Paresthesia, pilomotor response, tremor, weakness

Renal: Decreased renal perfusion, reduced urine output

Respiratory: Respiratory distress

Miscellaneous: Hypersensitivity reactions (including rash, urticaria, leukopenia, agranulocytosis, thrombocytopenia)

Oral:
Central nervous system: Anxiety, dizziness, excitability, giddiness, headache, insomnia, nervousness, restlessness

Drug Interactions
Metabolism/Transport Effects None known.

Avoid Concomitant Use
Avoid concomitant use of Phenylephrine (Systemic) with any of the following: Ergot Derivatives; Hyaluronidase; Iobenguane I 123; MAO Inhibitors

Increased Effect/Toxicity
Phenylephrine (Systemic) may increase the levels/effects of: Sympathomimetics

The levels/effects of Phenylephrine (Systemic) may be increased by: Acetaminophen; AtoMOXetine; Cannabinoid-Containing Products; Ergot Derivatives; Hyaluronidase; Linezolid; MAO Inhibitors; Tricyclic Antidepressants

Decreased Effect
Phenylephrine (Systemic) may decrease the levels/effects of: Benzylpenicilloyl Polylysine; FentaNYL; Iobenguane I 123; Ioflupane I 123

The levels/effects of Phenylephrine (Systemic) may be decreased by: Alpha1-Blockers

Stability Solution for injection: Store vials at 20°C to 25°C (68°F to 77°F); excursions permitted to 15°C to 30°C (59°F to 86°F); protect from light; do not use if solution turns brown or contains a precipitate.

Oral: Store at 20°C to 25°C (68°F to 77°F); protect oral solution from light.

Mechanism of Action Potent, direct-acting alpha-adrenergic agonist with virtually no beta-adrenergic activity; produces systemic arterial vasoconstriction. Such increases in systemic vascular resistance result in dose dependent increases in systolic and diastolic blood pressure and reductions in heart rate and cardiac output especially in patients with heart failure.

Pharmacodynamics
Onset of action:
Blood pressure increase/vasoconstriction:
I.M., SubQ: Within 10-15 minutes
I.V.: Immediate
Nasal decongestant: Oral: 15-30 minutes (Kollar, 2007)
Duration: Blood pressure increase/vasoconstriction:
I.M.: 1 to 2 hours
I.V.: 15 to 20 minutes
SubQ: 50 minutes
Nasal decongestant: Oral: 2 to 4 hours

Pharmacokinetics (Adult data unless noted)
Absorption: Oral: Rapid and complete (Kanfer, 1993)
Distribution: V_d initial: 26-61 L; V_{dss} 184-543 L (mean 340 L) (Hengstmann, 1982)
Metabolism: Hepatic via oxidative deamination (oral: 24%; I.V.: 50%); undergoes sulfation [oral (mostly within gut wall): 46%; I.V.: 8%] and some glucuronidation; forms inactive metabolites (Kanfer, 1993)
Bioavailability: Oral: ≤38% (Hengstmann, 1982; Kanfer, 1993)
Half-life: Alpha phase: ~5 minutes: terminal phase: 2-3 hours (Hengstmann, 1982; Kanfer, 1993)
Time to peak serum concentration: Oral: 0.75-2 hours (Kanfer, 1993)
Elimination: Urine (mostly as inactive metabolites)

Dosing: Neonatal Hypotension, low cardiac output: Continuous I.V. infusion: Usual initial range: 0.1 to 0.5 mcg/kg/minute; titrate to desired response (Wessel, 2001); in cases of shock or intraoperative hypotension, doses up to 2 mcg/kg/minute have been reported (Kliegman, 2011; Shaddy, 1989) and for management of infundibular spasm (Tet Spell), even higher doses up to 5 mcg/kg/minute may be required (AAP, 1998; Shaddy, 1989)

Dosing: Usual Pediatric: **Note:** Dosing presented in both mg (oral) and mcg (parenteral); use caution when ordering and dispensing.

Nasal congestion: Oral:
Children 4 to 5 years: 2.5 mg every 4 hours; maximum daily dose: 15 mg in 24 hours
Children 6 to 11 years: 5 mg every 4 hours; maximum daily dose: 30 mg in 24 hours
Children ≥12 years and Adolescents: 10 mg every 4 hours; maximum daily dose: 60 mg in 24 hours

Hypotension, low cardiac output: Infants, Children, and Adolescents:
I.M., SubQ: 100 mcg/kg/dose every 1 to 2 hours as needed; maximum dose: 5000 mcg
I.V. bolus: 5 to 20 mcg/kg/dose every 10 to 15 minutes as needed (AAP, 1998; Shaddy, 1989); initial dose should not exceed 500 mcg; maximum dose: 1000 mcg
Continuous I.V. infusion: Usual initial dose: 0.1 to 0.5 mcg/kg/minute; titrate to desired response (Di Gennaro, 2010; Stewart, 2002; Wessel, 2001); in cases of shock or intraoperative hypotension, doses up to 2 mcg/kg/minute have been reported (Di Gennaro, 2010; Kliegman, 2011; Shaddy, 1989; Stewart, 2002) and for management of infundibular spasm (Tet Spell), even higher doses up to 5 mcg/kg/minute may be required (AAP, 1998; Shaddy, 1989)

Hypotension during spinal anesthesia: I.M., SubQ:
Infants, Children, and Adolescents: 44 to 88 mcg/kg/dose; maximum dose: 500 mcg

◄ Adult:

Hypotension/shock:

I.V. bolus: 100 to 500 mcg/dose every 10 to 15 minutes as needed (initial dose should not exceed 500 mcg)

I.V. infusion: 100 to 180 mcg/minute, **or alternatively**, 0.5 mcg/kg/minute; titrate to desired response. Dosing ranges between 0.4 to 9.1 mcg/kg/minute have been reported (Gregory, 1991)

Nasal congestion: Oral: OTC labeling: 10 mg every 4 hours as needed for ≤7 days; maximum total dose: 60 mg in 24 hours

Paroxysmal supraventricular tachycardia: Note: Not recommended for routine use in treatment of supraventricular tachycardias: I.V.: 250 to 500 mcg over 20 to 30 seconds

Usual Infusion Concentrations: Pediatric I.V. infusion: 20 mcg/mL, 40 mcg/mL, or 60 mcg/mL

Administration

Oral: OTC products: Administer without regard to food

Parenteral:

I.V. bolus: Dilute to 1 mg/mL and administer dose over 20 to 30 seconds

Continuous I.V. infusion: Further dilute in appropriate fluid; concentrations are usually 20 to 60 mcg/mL; when administering as a continuous infusion, central line administration is preferred; administration into an umbilical arterial catheter is **not** recommended. I.V. infusions require an infusion pump.

Vesicant; ensure proper needle or catheter placement prior to and during infusion; avoid extravasation. If extravasation occurs, stop infusion immediately and disconnect (leave cannula/needle in place); gently aspirate extravasated solution (do **not** flush the line); remove needle/cannula; elevate extremity. Initiate phentolamine (or alternative antidote). (See Management of Drug Extravasations on page 2255 for more details.) Apply dry warm compresses (Hurst, 2004).

Vesicant/Extravasation Risk Vesicant

Monitoring Parameters Heart rate, blood pressure, central venous pressure, arterial blood gases (hypotension/shock treatment)

Product Availability

Vazculep (10 mg/mL injection): FDA approved July 2014; anticipated availability is currently unknown.

Vazculep is indicated for the treatment of clinically important hypotension resulting primarily from vasodilation in the setting of anesthesia.

Dosage Forms Excipient information presented when available (limited, particularly for generics); consult specific product labeling.

Liquid, Oral, as hydrochloride:

Little Colds Decongestant: 2.5 mg/mL (30 mL) [alcohol free, dye free, saccharin free; contains sodium benzoate; grape flavor]

Solution, Injection, as hydrochloride:

Generic: 10 mg/mL (1 mL, 5 mL, 10 mL)

Solution, Oral, as hydrochloride:

Sudafed PE Childrens: 2.5 mg/5 mL (118 mL) [alcohol free, sugar free; contains edetate disodium, fd&c red #40, sodium benzoate]

Tablet, Oral, as hydrochloride:

Medi-Phenyl: 5 mg

Nasal Decongestant: 10 mg [contains fd&c blue #2 (indigotine), fd&c red #40, fd&c yellow #6 aluminum lake]

Nasal Decongestant PE Max St: 10 mg [pseudoephedrine free; contains fd&c red #40 aluminum lake]

Non-Pseudo Sinus Decongestant: 10 mg [contains fd&c red #40 aluminum lake, fd&c yellow #6 aluminum lake]

Sudafed PE Maximum Strength: 10 mg [contains fd&c red #40 aluminum lake, fd&c yellow #10 aluminum lake, fd&c yellow #6 aluminum lake]

Sudafed PE Maximum Strength: 10 mg [contains fd&c red #40 aluminum lake, fd&c yellow #6 aluminum lake]

Sudafed PE Maximum Strength: 10 mg [pseudoephedrine free; contains fd&c red #40 aluminum lake, fd&c yellow #10 aluminum lake, fd&c yellow #6 aluminum lake]

Sudogest PE: 10 mg [contains fd&c red #40]

References

Brierley J, Carcillo JA, Choong K, et al. Clinical practice parameters for hemodynamic support of pediatric and neonatal septic shock: 2007 update from the American College of Critical Care Medicine. Crit Care Med. 2009;37(2):666-688.

Children's Sudafed PE nasal decongestant (phenylephrine systemic) [prescribing information]. McNeil PPC.

Committee on Drugs, 1996 to 1997, Liaison Representatives, and AAP Section Liaisons. Drugs for pediatric emergencies. Pediatrics. 1998;101(1):E13.

Di Gennaro JL, Mack CD, Malakouti A, Zimmerman JJ, Armstead W, Vavilala MS. Use and effect of vasopressors after pediatric traumatic brain injury. Dev Neurosci. 2010;32(5-6):420-430.

Gregory JS, Bonfiglio MF, Dasta JF, Reilley TE, Townsend MC, Flancbaum L. Experience with phenylephrine as a component of the pharmacologic support of septic shock. Crit Care Med. 1991;19 (11):1395-1400.

Hengstmann JH, Goronzy J. Pharmacokinetics of 3H-phenylephrine in man. Eur J Clin Pharmacol. 1982;21(4):335-341.

Hurst S, McMillan M. Innovative solutions in critical care units: extravasation guidelines. Dimens Crit Care Nurs. 2004;23(3):125-128.

Kanfer I, Dowse R, Vuma V. Pharmacokinetics of oral decongestants. Pharmacotherapy. 1993;13(6 Pt 2):116-128.

Kliegman RM, Stanton BF, St. Gemell JW, et al, eds. Nelson Textbook of Pediatrics. 19th ed. Philadelphia, PA: Saunders Elsevier;2011.

Kollar C, Schneider H, Waksman J, Krusinska E. Meta-analysis of the efficacy of a single dose of phenylephrine 10 mg compared with placebo in adults with acute nasal congestion due to the common cold. Clin Ther. 2007;29(6):1057-1070.

Phenylephrine hydrochloride injection [prescribing information]. Shirley, NY: American regent, Inc; November 2005.

Phenylephrine hydrochloride [prescribing information]. Eatontown, NJ: West-Ward Pharmaceuticals; December 2012.

Phillips MS. Standardizing I.V. infusion concentrations: national survey results. Am J Health Syst Pharm. 2011;68(22):2176-2182.

Shaddy RE, Viney J, Judd VE, McGough EC. Continuous intravenous phenylephrine infusion for treatment of hypoxemic spells in tetralogy of Fallot. J Pediatr. 1989;114(3):468-470.

Stewart JM, Munoz J, Weldon A. Clinical and physiological effects of an acute alpha-1 adrenergic agonist and a beta-1 adrenergic antagonist in chronic orthostatic intolerance. Circulation. 2002;106 (23):2946-2954.

Wessel DL. Managing low cardiac output syndrome after congenital heart surgery. Crit Care Med. 2001;29(10 Suppl):S220-S230.

Phenylephrine (Nasal) (fen il EF rin)

Medication Safety Issues

Sound-alike/look-alike issues:

Neo-Synephrine® (phenylephrine, nasal) may be confused with Neo-Synephrine® (oxymetazoline)

Brand Names: U.S. 4-Way Fast Acting [OTC]; 4-Way Menthol [OTC]; Afrin Childrens [OTC]; Nasal Four [OTC]; Neo-Synephrine [OTC]; Rhinall [OTC]

Brand Names: Canada Neo-Synephrine®

Therapeutic Category Adrenergic Agonist Agent; Alpha-Adrenergic Agonist; Nasal Agent, Vasoconstrictor; Sympathomimetic

Generic Availability (U.S.) Yes

Use Symptomatic relief of nasal and nasopharyngeal mucosal congestion (OTC products: FDA approved in adults; refer to product specific information regarding FDA approval in pediatric patients)

Pregnancy Considerations When administered intravenously, phenylephrine crosses the placenta. Refer to the Phenylephrine (Systemic) monograph for details. Decongestants are not the preferred agents for the treatment of rhinitis during pregnancy. Short-term use (<3 days) of intranasal phenylephrine may be beneficial to some patients, although its safety during pregnancy has not been studied.

Breast-Feeding Considerations It is not known if phenylephrine is excreted into breast milk.

Contraindications Hypersensitivity to phenylephrine or any component

Warnings Safety and efficacy for the use of cough and cold products in children <2 years of age is limited. Serious adverse effects including death have been reported. The FDA notes that there are no approved OTC uses for these products in children <2 years of age. Healthcare providers are reminded to ask caregivers about the use of OTC cough and cold products in order to avoid exposure to multiple medications containing the same ingredient.

Precautions Rebound nasal congestion may occur if abruptly discontinued after prolonged use; do not use beyond 3 days without consulting prescriber. Use with caution in patients with hyperthyroidism, hypertension, cardiovascular disease, including ischemic heart disease, or diabetes.

Adverse Reactions Nasal: Burning, nasal discharge, sneezing, stinging

Drug Interactions

Metabolism/Transport Effects None known.

Avoid Concomitant Use

Avoid concomitant use of Phenylephrine (Nasal) with any of the following: Ergot Derivatives; Iobenguane I 123; MAO Inhibitors

Increased Effect/Toxicity

Phenylephrine (Nasal) may increase the levels/effects of: Sympathomimetics

The levels/effects of Phenylephrine (Nasal) may be increased by: AtoMOXetine; Cannabinoid-Containing Products; Ergot Derivatives; Linezolid; MAO Inhibitors; Tricyclic Antidepressants

Decreased Effect

Phenylephrine (Nasal) may decrease the levels/effects of: FentaNYL; Iobenguane I 123

The levels/effects of Phenylephrine (Nasal) may be decreased by: Alpha1-Blockers

Stability Store at room temperature; protect from light.

Mechanism of Action Potent, direct-acting alpha-adrenergic agonist with virtually no beta-adrenergic activity; produces local vasoconstriction resulting in nasal decongestion.

Pharmacodynamics

Onset of action: Intranasal: ≤2 minutes (Chua, 1989)

Duration of action: Intranasal: 2.5-4 hours (dose dependent) (Chua, 1989)

Dosing: Usual Nasal congestion: Note: Therapy should not exceed 3 days:

Infants and Children <2 years: Limited data available: 0.5% solution: Intranasal: Instill 0.1 mL in each nostril as a single dose (Ralston, 2008; Turner, 1996). In a double-blind, placebo-controlled trial in 20 infants (mean age: 4 months) with bronchiolitis results showed, improved respiratory scores and oxygen saturation; however, statistical significance was not reached (Ralston, 2008). In another randomized, double-blind, placebo-controlled trial, 23 pediatric patients (age range: 6-18 months) with the common cold showed improvement in nasal obstruction which was not considered significant; no effect on middle ear pressures was observed (Turner, 1996).

Children ≥2 years:

2 to <6 years: 0.125% solution: Intranasal: Instill 1 drop in each nostril every 2-4 hours as needed. **Note:** Consult product specific information for further details.

Little Noses® Decongestant: Instill 2-3 drops in each nostril every 4 hours as needed

6-12 years: 0.25% solution: Intranasal: Instill 1-3 sprays in each nostril every 4 hours as needed

Children >12 years and Adolescents: 0.25% to 1% solutions: Intranasal: Instill 1-3 drops or sprays every 4 hours as needed

Adults: 0.25% to 1% solution: Intranasal: Instill 2-3 sprays or 2-3 drops in each nostril every 4 hours as needed

Administration Spray or apply drops into each nostril while gently occluding the other.

Dosage Forms Excipient information presented when available (limited, particularly for generics); consult specific product labeling.

Solution, Nasal, as hydrochloride:

4-Way Fast Acting: 1% (14.8 mL, 29.6 mL) [contains benzalkonium chloride]

4-Way Menthol: 1% (14.8 mL, 29.6 mL) [contains benzalkonium chloride, menthol, polysorbate 80]

Afrin Childrens: 0.25% (15 mL)

Nasal Four: 1% (29.6 mL) [contains benzalkonium chloride]

Neo-Synephrine: 0.25% (15 mL); 0.5% (15 mL); 1% (15 mL)

Rhinall: 0.25% (30 mL, 40 mL)

References

Chua SS, Benrimoj SI, and Triggs EJ, "Pharmacokinetics of Non-Prescription Sympathomimetic Agents," *Biopharm Drug Dispos,* 1989, 10(1):1-14.

Ralston S and Roohi M, "A Randomized, Controlled Trial of Nasal Phenylephrine in Infants Hospitalized for Bronchiolitis," *J Pediatr,* 2008, 153(6):795-8.

Turner RB and Darden PM, "Effect of Topical Adrenergic Decongestants on Middle Ear Pressure in Infants With Common Colds," *Pediatr Infect Dis J,* 1996, 15(7):621-4.

Phenylephrine (Ophthalmic) (fen il EF rin)

Medication Safety Issues

Sound-alike/look-alike issues:

Mydfrin® may be confused with Midrin®

Brand Names: U.S. Altafrin; Mydfrin [DSC]; Neofrin

Brand Names: Canada Dionephrine®; Mydfrin®

Therapeutic Category Adrenergic Agonist Agent; Adrenergic Agonist Agent, Ophthalmic; Alpha-Adrenergic Agonist; Ophthalmic Agent, Mydriatic; Sympathomimetic

Generic Availability (U.S.) Yes

Use As a mydriatic in ophthalmic procedures and treatment of wide-angle glaucoma; OTC use as symptomatic relief of eye irritation

Pregnancy Risk Factor C

Pregnancy Considerations Animal reproduction studies have not been conducted; therefore, the manufacturer classifies phenylephrine ophthalmic as pregnancy category C. When administered intravenously, phenylephrine crosses the placenta (refer to the Phenylephrine (Systemic) monograph for details). The amount of phenylephrine available systemically following ophthalmic application is generally less in comparison to oral or I.V. doses.

Breast-Feeding Considerations It is not known if phenylephrine is excreted into breast milk. The manufacturer recommends that caution be exercised when administering phenylephrine to nursing women.

Contraindications Hypersensitivity to phenylephrine or any component; severe hypertension, ventricular tachycardia; narrow-angle glaucoma

Warnings Do not use if solution turns brown or contains a precipitate. May contain sulfites which may cause allergic reactions in susceptible individuals.

Adverse Reactions Systemic effects are rare at normal dosages.

Cardiovascular: Arrhythmia (rare), hypertension (rare), myocardial infarction (rare), subarachnoid hemorrhage (rare), syncope (rare)

Ocular: Burning, irritation, vision changes, rebound miosis, floaters (transient)

Drug Interactions

Metabolism/Transport Effects None known.

◄ **Avoid Concomitant Use**
Avoid concomitant use of Phenylephrine (Ophthalmic) with any of the following: Ergot Derivatives; Iobenguane I 123; MAO Inhibitors
Increased Effect/Toxicity
Phenylephrine (Ophthalmic) may increase the levels/ effects of: Sympathomimetics

The levels/effects of Phenylephrine (Ophthalmic) may be increased by: AtoMOXetine; Cannabinoid-Containing Products; Ergot Derivatives; Linezolid; MAO Inhibitors; Tricyclic Antidepressants
Decreased Effect
Phenylephrine (Ophthalmic) may decrease the levels/ effects of: Iobenguane I 123

The levels/effects of Phenylephrine (Ophthalmic) may be decreased by: Alpha1-Blockers
Mechanism of Action Potent, direct-acting alpha-adrenergic agonist with virtually no beta-adrenergic activity; produces local vasoconstriction
Pharmacodynamics
Onset of action: Mydriasis: 15-30 minutes
Duration: Mydriasis 2.5% solution: 1-3 hours
Pharmacokinetics (Adult data unless noted)
Absorption: Minimal systemic absorption (Kumar, 1986)
Time to peak serum concentration: ≤20 minutes (Kumar, 1986)
Dosing: Neonatal Ophthalmic procedures: Use combination products containing 1% phenylephrine (see specific monographs for details). In neonates, 2.5% phenylephrine has been shown to cause significant increases in blood pressure compared to 1% preparations (Chew, 2005).
Dosing: Usual
Ophthalmic procedures:
Infants <1 year: Instill 1 drop of 2.5% 15-30 minutes before procedures
Children and Adults: Instill 1 drop of 2.5% or 10% solution, may repeat in 10-60 minutes as needed
Ophthalmic irritation (OTC formulation for relief of eye redness): Adults: Instill 1-2 drops 0.12% solution into affected eye, up to 4 times/day; do not use for >72 hours
Administration Instill drops into conjunctival sac of affected eye(s); avoid contact of bottle tip with skin or eye; finger pressure should be applied to the lacrimal sac during and for 1-2 minutes after instillation to decrease risk of absorption and systemic reactions
Dosage Forms Excipient information presented when available (limited, particularly for generics); consult specific product labeling. [DSC] = Discontinued product
Solution, Ophthalmic, as hydrochloride:
Altafrin: 2.5% (15 mL); 10% (5 mL) [contains benzalkonium chloride]
Mydfrin: 2.5% (3 mL [DSC], 5 mL [DSC]) [contains benzalkonium chloride, edetate disodium]
Neofrin: 2.5% (15 mL) [contains benzalkonium chloride, edetate disodium, sodium bisulfite]
Neofrin: 10% (5 mL) [contains benzalkonium chloride]
Generic: 2.5% (2 mL [DSC], 3 mL, 5 mL, 15 mL); 10% (5 mL)
Solution, Ophthalmic, as hydrochloride [preservative free]:
Generic: 2.5% (1 ea)

References
Chew C, Rahman RA, Shafie SM, et al, "Comparison of Mydriatic Regimens Used in Screening for Retinopathy of Prematurity in Preterm Infants With Dark Irides," *J Pediatr Ophthalmol Strabismus,* 2005, 42(3):166-73.
Kumar V, Schoenwald RD, Barcellos WA, et al, "Aqueous Vs Viscous Phenylephrine. I. Systemic Absorption and Cardiovascular Effects," *Arch Ophthalmol,* 1986, 104(8):1189-91.

Phenylephrine (Topical) (fen il EF rin)

Brand Names: U.S. Anu-Med [OTC]; GRX Hemorrhoidal [OTC]; Hem-Prep [OTC]; Hemorrhoidal [OTC]; Preparation H [OTC]; Rectacaine [OTC]
Therapeutic Category Adrenergic Agonist Agent; Alpha-Adrenergic Agonist; Hemorrhoidal Treatment Agent; Sympathomimetic
Generic Availability (U.S.) Yes
Use Symptomatic relief of hemorrhoidal symptoms
Pregnancy Considerations When administered intravenously, phenylephrine crosses the placenta. Refer to the Phenylephrine (Systemic) monograph for details. There is limited information available supporting the use of topical agents for the treatment of hemorrhoids. Products containing phenylephrine should be used with caution in pregnant women, especially patients with hypertension or diabetes.
Breast-Feeding Considerations It is not known if phenylephrine is excreted into breast milk.
Contraindications Hypersensitivity to phenylephrine or any component; severe hypertension, ventricular tachycardia
Precautions Use with caution in patients with cardiovascular disease, diabetes, hyperthyroidism, ocular hypertension
Adverse Reactions Rare systemic effects may occur.
Drug Interactions
Metabolism/Transport Effects None known.
Avoid Concomitant Use
Avoid concomitant use of Phenylephrine (Topical) with any of the following: Ergot Derivatives; Iobenguane I 123; MAO Inhibitors
Increased Effect/Toxicity
Phenylephrine (Topical) may increase the levels/effects of: Sympathomimetics

The levels/effects of Phenylephrine (Topical) may be increased by: AtoMOXetine; Cannabinoid-Containing Products; Ergot Derivatives; Linezolid; MAO Inhibitors; Tricyclic Antidepressants
Decreased Effect
Phenylephrine (Topical) may decrease the levels/effects of: Iobenguane I 123

The levels/effects of Phenylephrine (Topical) may be decreased by: Alpha1-Blockers
Mechanism of Action Potent, direct-acting alpha-adrenergic agonist with virtually no beta-adrenergic activity; produces local vasoconstriction.
Dosing: Usual Treatment of hemorrhoidal symptoms: Children ≥12 years and Adults: Apply to rectal area or by applicator into rectum up to 4 times/day
Administration Apply to clean and dry rectal area at night, in the morning, or after each bowel movement; when using applicator, remove protective cover from applicator and attach to tube. Lubricate applicator well, then gently insert into rectum. Thoroughly cleanse applicator after each use and replace protective cover.
Dosage Forms Excipient information presented when available (limited, particularly for generics); consult specific product labeling.
Ointment, Rectal, as hydrochloride:
GRX Hemorrhoidal: 0.25% (43 g) [contains benzoic acid, methylparaben, propylparaben]
Hemorrhoidal: 0.25% (57 g) [contains benzoic acid, methylparaben, propylparaben]
Preparation H: 0.25% (28 g, 57 g)
Rectacaine: 0.25% (30 g)
Suppository, Rectal, as hydrochloride:
Anu-Med: 0.25% (12 ea)
Hem-Prep: 0.25% (24 ea)

Hemorrhoidal: 0.25% (12 ea) [contains methylparaben, propylparaben]

Preparation H: 0.25% (12 ea, 24 ea, 48 ea)

Rectacaine: 0.25% (12 ea)

◆ **Phenylephrine and Cyclopentolate** see Cyclopentolate and Phenylephrine on page 560

◆ **Phenylephrine and Promethazine** see Promethazine and Phenylephrine on page 1752

◆ **Phenylephrine Hydrochloride** see Phenylephrine (Nasal) on page 1660

◆ **Phenylephrine Hydrochloride** see Phenylephrine (Ophthalmic) on page 1661

◆ **Phenylephrine Hydrochloride** see Phenylephrine (Systemic) on page 1658

◆ **Phenylephrine Hydrochloride** see Phenylephrine (Topical) on page 1662

◆ **Phenylephrine, Promethazine, and Codeine** see Promethazine, Phenylephrine, and Codeine on page 1752

◆ **Phenylethylmalonylurea** see PHENobarbital on page 1651

◆ **Phenytek** see Phenytoin on page 1663

Phenytoin (FEN i toyn)

Medication Safety Issues
Sound-alike/look-alike issues:
Phenytoin may be confused with phenelzine, phentermine, PHENobarbital

Dilantin may be confused with Dilaudid, diltiazem, Dipentum

High alert medication:
The Institute for Safe Medication Practices (ISMP) includes this medication (I.V. formulation) among its list of drug classes which have a heightened risk of causing significant patient harm when used in error.

International issues:
Dilantin [U.S., Canada, and multiple international markets] may be confused with Dolantine brand name for pethidine [Belgium]

Related Information
Management of Drug Extravasations on page 2255

Brand Names: U.S. Dilantin; Dilantin Infatabs; Phenytek; Phenytoin Infatabs

Brand Names: Canada Dilantin; Novo-Phenytoin; Taro-Phenytoin; Tremytoine Inj

Therapeutic Category Antiarrhythmic Agent, Class I-B; Anticonvulsant, Hydantoin

Generic Availability (U.S.) Yes

Use
Oral: Management of generalized tonic-clonic (grand mal) and complex partial seizures and the prevention of seizures following head trauma/neurosurgery [FDA approved in pediatric (age not specified) and adults]. Has also been used for simple partial seizures; ventricular arrhythmias, including those associated with digitalis intoxication, prolonged QT interval, and surgical repair of congenital heart diseases in children

Parenteral: Management of status epilepticus of the grand mal type and prevention and treatment of seizures occurring during neurosurgery [FDA approved in neonatal and pediatric patients (age not specified) and adults]

Medication Guide Available Yes

Pregnancy Risk Factor D

Pregnancy Considerations Phenytoin crosses the placenta (Harden and Pennell, 2009). An increased risk of congenital malformations and adverse outcomes may occur following in utero phenytoin exposure. Reported malformations include orofacial clefts, cardiac defects, dysmorphic facial features, nail/digit hypoplasia, growth abnormalities including microcephaly, and mental deficiency. Isolated cases of malignancies (including neuroblastoma) and coagulation defects in the neonate (may be life threatening) following delivery have also been reported. Maternal use of phenytoin should be avoided when possible to decrease the risk of cleft palate and poor cognitive outcomes. Polytherapy may also increase the risk of congenital malformations; monotherapy is recommended (Harden and Meador, 2009). The maternal use of folic acid throughout pregnancy is recommended to reduce the risk of major congenital malformations (Harden and Pennell, 2009).

Total plasma concentrations of phenytoin are decreased in the mother during pregnancy; unbound plasma (free) concentrations are also decreased and plasma clearance is increased. Due to pregnancy-induced physiologic changes, women who are pregnant may require dose adjustments of phenytoin in order to maintain clinical response; monitoring during pregnancy should be considered (Harden and Pennell, 2009). For women with epilepsy who are planning a pregnancy in advance, baseline serum concentrations should be measured once or twice prior to pregnancy during a period when seizure control is optimal. Monitoring can then be continued once each trimester during pregnancy and postpartum; more frequent monitoring may be needed in some patients. Monitoring of unbound plasma concentrations is recommended (Patsalos, 2008). In women taking phenytoin who are trying to avoid pregnancy, potentially significant interactions may exist with hormone-containing contraceptives; consult drug interactions database for more detailed information.

Patients exposed to phenytoin during pregnancy are encouraged to enroll themselves into the North American Antiepileptic Drug (NAAED) Pregnancy Registry by calling 1-888-233-2334. Additional information is available at https:\\aedpregnancyregistry.org.

Breast-Feeding Considerations Phenytoin is excreted in breast milk; however, the amount to which the infant is exposed is considered small. The manufacturers of phenytoin do not recommend breast-feeding during therapy.

Contraindications Hypersensitivity to phenytoin, any component, or other hydantoins; concurrent use of delavirdine [due to loss of virologic response and possible resistance to delavirdine or other non-nucleoside reverse transcriptase inhibitors (NNRTIs)]

Injection: Additional contraindications: Sinus bradycardia, sinoatrial block, second and third degree AV block, Adams-Stokes syndrome

Warnings Rapid intravenous administration may cause hypotension **[U.S. Boxed Warning]** and/or cardiac arrhythmias (eg, heart block, ventricular tachycardia, ventricular fibrillation); to reduce these risks, phenytoin must be administered slowly I.V. Intravenous administration should not exceed 50 mg/minute in adult patients. In neonates, the FDA labeled maximum I.V. administration rate is 1-3 mg/kg/minute; **Note:** Most clinicians use a lower maximum rate of infusion in neonates: 0.5-1 mg/kg/minute; in infants and children: 1-3 mg/kg/minute. Adverse cardiac events have been reported at or below the recommended infusion rate; cardiac monitoring is necessary during and after administration of intravenous phenytoin; reduction in rate of administration or discontinuation of infusion may be necessary. For nonemergency use, intravenous phenytoin should be administered more slowly; the use of oral phenytoin should be used whenever possible.

Abrupt withdrawal of phenytoin may precipitate status epilepticus in epileptic patients; do not discontinue abruptly; phenytoin should be withdrawn gradually, unless safety concerns (eg, allergic or hypersensitivity reaction) require a more rapid withdrawal.

Acute hepatotoxicity associated with a hypersensitivity syndrome characterized by fever, skin eruptions, and lymphadenopathy has been reported to occur within the first 2 months of treatment; discontinue if skin rash or lymphadenopathy occurs. Serious skin reactions, including toxic epidermal necrolysis (TEN) and Stevens-Johnson syndrome (SJS), although rarely reported, have resulted in fatalities; phenytoin should be discontinued if there are any signs of rash and patient should be evaluated for signs and symptoms of drug reaction with eosinophilia and systemic symptoms (DRESS). Preliminary data suggests that patients testing positive for the human leukocyte antigen (HLA) allele *HLA-B*1502* have an increased risk of developing SJS and/or TEN. The risk appears to be highest in the early months of therapy initiation. The presence of this genetic variant exists in up to 15% of people of Asian descent in China, Thailand, Malaysia, Indonesia, Taiwan, and the Philippines, and may vary from <1% in Japanese and Koreans, to 2% to 4% of South Asians and Indians; this variant is virtually absent in those of Caucasian, African-American, Hispanic, or European ancestry; consider avoiding phenytoin use in patients *HLA-B*1502* positive if other therapeutic options available. **Note:** Carbamazepine, another antiepileptic with a chemical structure similar to phenytoin, includes in the manufacturer labeling a recommendation to screen patients of Asian descent for the *HLA-B*1502* allele prior to initiating therapy; this is not a current recommendation in the phenytoin manufacturer labeling.

A spectrum of hematologic effects have been reported with use (eg, agranulocytosis, neutropenia, leukopenia, thrombocytopenia, pancytopenia, and anemias); patients with a previous history of adverse hematologic reaction to any drug may be at increased risk. Early detection of hematologic change is important; advise patients of early signs and symptoms including fever, sore throat, mouth ulcers, infections, easy bruising, petechial or purpuric hemorrhage.

Chronic use of phenytoin has been associated with decreased bone mineral density (osteopenia, osteoporosis, and osteomalacia) and bone fractures. Pediatric patients may be at increased risk for vitamin D deficiency; with chronic therapy, phenytoin may cause catabolism of vitamin D; the daily vitamin D requirement may be increased in these patients (≥400 units/day); vitamin D status should be periodically monitored with laboratory data (Misra, 2008; Wagner, 2008).

The "purple glove syndrome" (ie, discoloration with edema and pain of distal limb) may occur following peripheral I.V. administration of phenytoin. This syndrome may or may not be associated with drug extravasation. Symptoms may resolve spontaneously; however, skin necrosis and limb ischemia may occur; interventions such as fasciotomies, skin grafts, and amputation may be required. To decrease the risk of this syndrome, inject phenytoin slowly and directly into a large vein through a large gauge needle or I.V. catheter. Follow the I.V. injection with NS flushes through the same needle or I.V. catheter.

Antiepileptic drugs (AEDs) increase the risk of suicidal behavior and ideation in patients receiving these medications for any indication. Pooled analyses of placebo-controlled trials involving 11 different AEDs (regardless of indication) showed a twofold increased risk of suicidal thoughts or behavior (estimated incidence rate: 0.43% in AED treated patients compared to 0.24% of patients receiving placebo); increased risk was observed as early as 1 week after initiation of AED and continued through duration of trials (most trials ≤24 weeks); risk did not vary significantly by age (age range: 5–100 years). Consider risks and benefits of AEDs before prescribing. Monitor all patients receiving an AED for emergence of suicidal thoughts or behavior, thoughts of self-harm, any unusual changes in behavior or mood, or the emergence or worsening of depressive symptoms; notify healthcare provider immediately if symptoms or concerning behavior occur. **Note:** The FDA requires a Medication Guide for all antiepileptic drugs informing patients of this risk.

Dilantin® 30 mg capsule and oral suspension contain sodium benzoate; benzoic acid (benzoate) is a metabolite of benzyl alcohol; large amounts of benzyl alcohol (≥99 mg/kg/day) have been associated with a potentially fatal toxicity ("gasping syndrome") in neonates; the "gasping syndrome" consists of metabolic acidosis, respiratory distress, gasping respirations, CNS dysfunction (including convulsions, intracranial hemorrhage), hypotension and cardiovascular collapse; use phenytoin products containing sodium benzoate with caution in neonates; *in vitro* and animal studies have shown that benzoate displaces bilirubin from protein binding sites. Injection contains 10% alcohol and 40% propylene glycol; toxicities have been reported with use of products containing propylene glycol, including hyperosmolality, lactic acidosis, seizures, and respiratory depression; in neonates large amounts of propylene glycol delivered orally, intravenously (eg, >3000 mg/day), or topically have been associated with potentially fatal toxicities which can include metabolic acidosis, seizures, renal failure, and CNS depression; use injection containing propylene glycol with caution (AAP, 1997; Shehab, 2009).

Precautions Use with caution in patients with any condition associated with low serum albumin levels, which will increase the free fraction of phenytoin in the serum and, therefore, the pharmacologic response. Use with caution in renal impairment; serum concentrations may be difficult to interpret; consider monitoring free (unbound) concentrations. Use with caution in hepatic impairment; clearance may be substantially reduced in cirrhosis; frequent monitoring of free (unbound) serum concentrations should be considered. Use with caution in patients with underlying cardiac disease; use is contraindicated in bradycardia, sinoatrial block, second and third degree heart block, or Adam-Stokes. Use with caution in patients with porphyria; may cause exacerbations. Should not be used to treat absence seizures; has been shown to increase frequency. May cause sedation, confusional states, or cerebellar dysfunction (loss of motor coordination) at higher total serum concentrations, or at lower total serum concentrations when the free fraction of phenytoin is increased; possible permanent cerebellum damage may occur with chronic toxic serum concentrations; effects with other sedative drugs or ethanol may be potentiated; use with caution in patients who are debilitated.

May cause gingival overgrowth or hyperplasia; reported incidence up to 60%; some data suggest development is associated with higher doses and serum concentrations; folic acid supplementation (0.5 mg/day in pediatric patients ≥6 years) may help to prevent or decrease gingival overgrowth; patients should be counseled regarding the importance of proper dental hygiene (Arya, 2011).

Adverse Reactions I.V. effects: Bradycardia, cardiac arrhythmia, cardiovascular collapse (especially with rapid I.V. use), hypotension, thrombophlebitis, venous irritation and pain

Effects not related to plasma phenytoin concentrations: Carbohydrate intolerance, folic acid deficiency, gingival hypertrophy, hypertrichosis, osteomalacia, peripheral neuropathy, systemic lupus erythematosus, thickening of facial features, vitamin D deficiency

Concentration-related effects: Ataxia, blurred vision, coma, confusion, diplopia, dizziness, drowsiness, fever, folic acid depletion, gum tenderness, hyperglycemia, lethargy, mood changes, nausea, nystagmus, osteomalacia, rash, slurred speech, vomiting

Related to elevated concentrations:
>20 mcg/mL (SI: >79 micromole/L): Far lateral nystagmus
>30 mcg/mL (SI: >119 micromole/L): 45°lateral gaze nystagmus and ataxia
>40 mcg/mL (SI: >158 micromole/L): Decreased mentation
>100 mcg/mL (SI: >396 micromole/L): Death

Cardiovascular: Bradycardia, cardiac arrhythmia, cardiovascular collapse, hypotension

Central nervous system: Dizziness, drowsiness, headache, insomnia, psychiatric changes, slurred speech, vertigo

Dermatologic: Rash

Gastrointestinal: Constipation, enlargement of lips, gingival hyperplasia, hepatic injury, nausea, taste disturbance, vomiting

Genitourinary: Peyronie's disease

Hematologic: Agranulocytosis, granulocytopenia, leukopenia, pancytopenia, thrombocytopenia

Hepatic: Acute hepatic failure, hepatitis, toxic hepatitis

Local: I.V. administration: Inflammation, irritation, necrosis, sloughing, tenderness, thrombophlebitis

Neuromuscular & skeletal: Paresthesia, peripheral neuropathy, tremor

Ocular: Blurred vision, diplopia, nystagmus

Rare but important or life-threatening: Anaphylaxis, blood dyscrasias, coarsening of facial features, drug rash with eosinophilia and systemic symptoms (DRESS), dyskinesias, hepatitis, Hodgkin lymphoma, hypertrichosis, immunoglobulin abnormalities, lymphadenopathy, lymphoma, macrocytosis, megaloblastic anemia, periarteritis nodosa, pseudolymphoma, systemic lupus erythematosus-like syndrome, Stevens-Johnson syndrome, toxic epidermal necrolysis, venous irritation and pain

Drug Interactions
Metabolism/Transport Effects Substrate of CYP2C19 (major), CYP2C9 (major), CYP3A4 (minor); **Note:** Assignment of Major/Minor substrate status based on clinically relevant drug interaction potential; **Induces** CYP2B6 (strong), CYP2C19 (strong), CYP2C8 (strong), CYP2C9 (strong), CYP3A4 (strong), P-glycoprotein

Avoid Concomitant Use
Avoid concomitant use of Phenytoin with any of the following: Abiraterone Acetate; Apixaban; Apremilast; Artemether; Axitinib; Azelastine (Nasal); Bedaquiline; Boceprevir; Bortezomib; Bosutinib; Cabozantinib; Ceritinib; CloZAPine; Crizotinib; Dabigatran Etexilate; Darunavir; Delavirdine; Dienogest; Dolutegravir; Dronedarone; Enzalutamide; Etravirine; Everolimus; Ibrutinib; Itraconazole; Ivacaftor; Lapatinib; Lumefantrine; Lurasidone; Macitentan; Mifepristone; NIFEdipine; Nilotinib; Nisoldipine; Paraldehyde; PAZOPanib; PONATinib; Praziquantel; Ranolazine; Regorafenib; Rilpivirine; Rivaroxaban; Roflumilast; RomiDEPsin; Simeprevir; Sofosbuvir; SORAfenib; Stiripentol; Tasimelteon; Telaprevir; Thalidomide; Ticagrelor; Tofacitinib; Tolvaptan; Toremifene; Ulipristal; Vandetanib; Vemurafenib; VinCRIStine (Liposomal); Vorapaxar

Increased Effect/Toxicity
Phenytoin may increase the levels/effects of: Azelastine (Nasal); Buprenorphine; Clarithromycin; CNS Depressants; Fosamprenavir; Hydrocodone; Lithium; Methotrexate; Methotrimeprazine; Metyrosine; Neuromuscular-Blocking Agents (Nondepolarizing); Paraldehyde; PHENobarbital; Pramipexole; Prilocaine; ROPINIRole; Rotigotine; Selective Serotonin Reuptake Inhibitors; Sodium Nitrite; Thalidomide; Vitamin K Antagonists; Zolpidem

The levels/effects of Phenytoin may be increased by: Alcohol (Ethyl); Allopurinol; Amiodarone; Antifungal Agents (Azole Derivatives, Systemic); Benzodiazepines; Brimonidine (Topical); Calcium Channel Blockers; Cannabis; Capecitabine; CarBAMazepine; Carbonic Anhydrase Inhibitors; CeFAZolin; Chloramphenicol; Cimetidine; Clarithromycin; Cosyntropin; CYP2C19 Inhibitors (Moderate); CYP2C19 Inhibitors (Strong); CYP2C9 Inhibitors (Moderate); CYP2C9 Inhibitors (Strong); Delavirdine; Dexmethylphenidate; Disulfiram; Doxylamine; Dronabinol; Droperidol; Efavirenz; Eslicarbazepine; Ethosuximide; Felbamate; Floxuridine; Fluconazole; Fluorouracil (Systemic); Fluorouracil (Topical); FLUoxetine; FluvoxaMINE; Halothane; HydrOXYzine; Isoniazid; Kava Kava; Luliconazole; Magnesium Sulfate; Methotrimeprazine; Methylphenidate; MetroNIDAZOLE (Systemic); Miconazole (Oral); Nabilone; Nitric Oxide; Omeprazole; OXcarbazepine; Rufinamide; Sertraline; Sodium Oxybate; Tacrolimus (Systemic); Tapentadol; Tegafur; Telaprevir; Tetrahydrocannabinol; Ticlopidine; Topiramate; TraZODone; Trimethoprim; Vitamin K Antagonists

Decreased Effect
Phenytoin may decrease the levels/effects of: Abiraterone Acetate; Acetaminophen; Afatinib; Albendazole; Amiodarone; Antifungal Agents (Azole Derivatives, Systemic); Apixaban; Apremilast; ARIPiprazole; Artemether; Axitinib; Bazedoxifene; Bedaquiline; Boceprevir; Bortezomib; Bosutinib; Brentuximab Vedotin; Busulfan; Cabozantinib; Canagliflozin; Cannabidiol; Cannabis; CarBAMazepine; Caspofungin; Ceritinib; Chloramphenicol; Clarithromycin; CloZAPine; Cobicistat; Contraceptives (Estrogens); Contraceptives (Progestins); Crizotinib; CycloSPORINE (Systemic); CYP2B6 Substrates; CYP2C19 Substrates; CYP2C8 Substrates; CYP2C9 Substrates; CYP3A4 Substrates; Dabigatran Etexilate; Darunavir; Dasatinib; Deferasirox; Delavirdine; Diclofenac (Systemic); Dienogest; Disopyramide; Dolutegravir; DOXOrubicin (Conventional); Doxycycline; Dronabinol; Dronedarone; Efavirenz; Elvitegravir; Enzalutamide; Eslicarbazepine; Ethosuximide; Etoposide; Etoposide Phosphate; Etravirine; Everolimus; Exemestane; Ezogabine; Felbamate; FentaNYL; Flunarizine; Gefitinib; GuanFACINE; HMG-CoA Reductase Inhibitors; Ibrutinib; Imatinib; Irinotecan; Itraconazole; Ivacaftor; Ixabepilone; Lacosamide; LamoTRIgine; Lapatinib; Levodopa; Linagliptin; Loop Diuretics; Lopinavir; Lumefantrine; Lurasidone; Macitentan; Maraviroc; Mebendazole; Meperidine; Methadone; MethylPREDNISolone; MetroNIDAZOLE (Systemic); Metyrapone; Mexiletine; Mifepristone; Nelfinavir; Neuromuscular-Blocking Agents (Nondepolarizing); NIFEdipine; Nilotinib; Nisoldipine; Omeprazole; OXcarbazepine; PAZOPanib; Perampanel; P-glycoprotein/ABCB1 Substrates; PONATinib; Praziquantel; PrednisoLONE (Systemic); PredniSONE; Primidone; QUEtiapine; QuiNIDine; QuiNINE; Ranolazine; Regorafenib; Rilpivirine; Ritonavir; Rivaroxaban; Roflumilast; RomiDEPsin; Rufinamide; Saxagliptin; Sertraline; Simeprevir; Sirolimus; Sofosbuvir; SORAfenib; SUNItinib; Tacrolimus (Systemic); Tadalafil; Tasimelteon; Telaprevir; Temsirolimus; Teniposide; Tetrahydrocannabinol; Theophylline Derivatives; Thyroid Products; Ticagrelor; Tipranavir; Tofacitinib; Tolvaptan; Topiramate; Topotecan; Toremifene; TraZODone; Treprostinil; Trimethoprim; Ulipristal; Valproic Acid and Derivatives; Vandetanib; Vemurafenib; Vilazodone; VinCRIStine; VinCRIStine (Liposomal); Vorapaxar; Vortioxetine; Zonisamide; Zuclopenthixol

The levels/effects of Phenytoin may be decreased by: Alcohol (Ethyl); Amphetamines; Antacids; Bleomycin; CarBAMazepine; Ciprofloxacin (Systemic); Colesevelam; CYP2C19 Inducers (Strong); CYP2C9 Inducers (Strong); Dabrafenib; Diazoxide; Enzalutamide; Folic Acid; Fosamprenavir; Ketorolac (Nasal); Ketorolac (Systemic);

Leucovorin Calcium-Levoleucovorin; Levomefolate; Lopinavir; Mefloquine; Methotrexate; Methylfolate; Multivitamins/Minerals (with ADEK, Folate, Iron); Nelfinavir; Orlistat; Peginterferon Alfa-2b; PHENobarbital; Platinum Derivatives; Pyridoxine; Rifampin; Ritonavir; Stiripentol; Theophylline Derivatives; Tipranavir; Valproic Acid and Derivatives; Vigabatrin; VinCRIStine

Food Interactions

Ethanol:

Acute use: Ethanol inhibits metabolism of phenytoin and may also increase CNS depression. Management: Monitor patients. Caution patients about effects.

Chronic use: Ethanol stimulates metabolism of phenytoin. Management: Monitor patients.

Food: Phenytoin serum concentrations may be altered if taken with food. If taken with enteral nutrition, phenytoin serum concentrations may be decreased. Tube feedings decrease bioavailability. Phenytoin may decrease calcium, folic acid, and vitamin D levels. Supplementing folic acid may lower the seizure threshold. Management: Hold tube feedings 1-2 hours before and 1-2 hours after phenytoin administration. Do not supplement folic acid. Consider vitamin D supplementation. Take preferably on an empty stomach.

Stability

Oral:

Capsule: Store at 20°C to 25°C (68°F to 77°F) in tightly closed container. Protect from light and moisture.

Suspension: Store at 20°C to 25°C (68°F to 77°F); do not freeze. Protect from light.

Tablet, chewable: Store at 20°C to 25°C (68°F to 77°F). Protect from moisture.

Parenteral: Solution for injection: Store intact vial at 20°C to 25°C (68°F to 77°F); excursions permitted to 15°C to 30°C (59°F to 86°F). Parenteral solution may be used as long as there is no precipitate and it is not hazy; slightly yellowed solution may be used; refrigeration may cause precipitate, sometimes the precipitate may be resolved by allowing the solution to reach room temperature again; drug may precipitate with pH ≤11.5; do not mix with other medications.

I.V. intermittent infusion preparations: No consensus exists in the literature regarding phenytoin stability in I.V. solutions; due to a low solubility, phenytoin may precipitate in aqueous solutions; some centers have successfully used dilutions of 1-10 mg/mL in NS or LR; infusions should begin as soon as possible after preparation (eg, within 1 hour); diluted solutions should not be refrigerated; inspect for particulate matter; discard 4 hours after preparation (Gannaway, 1983).

Mechanism of Action Stabilizes neuronal membranes and decreases seizure activity by increasing efflux or decreasing influx of sodium ions across cell membranes in the motor cortex during generation of nerve impulses; prolongs effective refractory period and suppresses ventricular pacemaker automaticity, shortens action potential in the heart

Pharmacokinetics (Adult data unless noted)

Absorption: Oral: Slow, variable; dependent on product formulation; decreased in neonates

Distribution: V_d:

Neonates:

Premature: 1-1.2 L/kg

Full-term: 0.8-0.9 L/kg

Infants: 0.7-0.8 L/kg

Children: 0.7 L/kg

Adults: 0.6-0.7 L/kg

Protein binding: Adults: 90% to 95%; Neonates: Decreased protein binding and increased free fraction of phenytoin (up to 20%); Infants: Decreased protein binding and increased free fraction of phenytoin (up to 15%); also increased free fraction in patients with

hyperbilirubinemia, hypoalbuminemia, renal dysfunction, or uremia

Metabolism: Follows dose-dependent (Michaelis-Menten) pharmacokinetics; "apparent" or calculated half-life is dependent upon serum concentration, therefore, metabolism is best described in terms of K_m and V_{max}; V_{max} is increased in infants >6 months and children compared to adults; major metabolite (via oxidation) HPPA undergoes enterohepatic recycling and elimination in urine as glucuronides

Bioavailability: Formulation dependent

Half-life, elimination (apparent): 7-42 hours; newborns (PNA <7 days): Apparent half-life greatly prolonged (clearance decreased) and then rapidly accelerates to infant levels by 5 weeks of life; **Note:** Elimination is not first-order and follows Michaelis-Menten pharmacokinetics; half-life increases with increasing phenytoin concentrations

Time to peak serum concentration: Oral: Dependent upon formulation

Extended release capsule: Within 4-12 hours

Immediate release preparation: Within 2-3 hours

Elimination: <5% excreted unchanged in urine; increased clearance and decreased serum concentrations with febrile illness; highly variable clearance, dependent upon intrinsic hepatic function and dose administered

Dosing: Neonatal Note: Dosage should be individualized based upon clinical response and serum concentrations. Phenytoin base (eg, oral suspension, chewable tablets) contains ~8% more drug than phenytoin sodium (~92 mg base is equivalent to 100 mg phenytoin sodium). Dosage adjustments and closer serum monitoring may be necessary when switching dosage forms.

Status epilepticus; neonatal seizures:

Manufacturer labeling: I.V.: 15-20 mg/kg in a single or divided dose; then begin maintenance therapy usually 12 hours after dose

Alternate dosing: AAP recommendation: I.V.: 10 mg/kg in a single dose; then begin maintenance therapy usually 12 hours after dose. **Note:** Phenobarbital is the preferred treatment for treatment of neonatal seizures. Fosphenytoin is preferred over phenytoin if available due to lower risk of cardiac adverse effects (Hegenbarth, 2008).

Seizures; maintenance therapy: I.V., Oral: Initial: 5 mg/kg/day in 2 divided doses; usual range: 4-8 mg/kg/day in 2 divided doses; some patients may require dosing every 8 hours

Dosing: Usual Note: Dosage should be individualized based upon clinical response and serum concentrations; maintenance therapy dosage adjustments are typically not made more frequently than every 7 days. Phenytoin base (eg, oral suspension, chewable tablets) contains ~8% more drug than phenytoin sodium (~92 mg base is equivalent to 100 mg phenytoin sodium). Dosage adjustments and closer serum monitoring may be necessary when switching dosage forms.

Infants, Children and Adolescents:

Status epilepticus:

Manufacturer labeling: Loading dose: I.V.: 15-20 mg/kg in a single or divided dose; then begin maintenance therapy usually 12 hours after dose

Alternate dosing: AAP, NCS recommendations: Loading dose: I.V.: 20 mg/kg in a single or divided doses; maximum dose: 1000 mg; then begin maintenance therapy usually 12 hours after dose (Brophy, 2012; Hegenbarth, 2008). An additional load of 5-10 mg/kg if status epilepticus is not resolved has been used; however, some experts recommend trying another agent once a total loading dose of 20 mg/kg has been given (Brophy, 2012).

Seizures:

Loading dose (if not previously on phenytoin): I.V., Oral: 15-20 mg/kg; if currently on phenytoin, reloading dose should be based upon serum concentrations and recent dosing history; an oral loading dose should be divided into 3 doses and administered every 2-4 hours to decrease GI adverse effects and to ensure complete oral absorption

Maintenance therapy: I.V., Oral: Initial: 5 mg/kg/day in divided doses (based upon dosage form, see below); usual range: 4-8 mg/kg/day; maximum daily dose: 300 mg/**day**. Some experts suggest higher maintenance doses (8-10 mg/kg/day) may be necessary in infants and young children (Guerrini, 2006). Dosing should be based upon ideal body weight (IBW).

Usual dosing range (Bauer, 1983; Chiba, 1980; Suzuki, 1994):

6 months to 3 years: 8-10 mg/kg/day

4-6 years: 7.5-9 mg/kg/day

7-9 years: 7-8 mg/kg/day

10-16 years: 6-7 mg/kg/day

Dosing interval (product specific):

Immediate release preparations (including injection, suspension, and chewable tablets): Divide daily dose into 2-3 doses per day

Extended release preparations: In most pediatric patients, usually dosed every 12 hours; however, in adolescent patients with sufficiently long half-life, may be dosed every 24 hours

Seizure prophylaxis, traumatic brain injury: Limited data available; efficacy results variable: I.V.: Initial: 18 mg/kg over 20 minutes; followed by 6 mg/kg/day divided every 8 hours for 48 hours was used in a double-blind, placebo-controlled trial of 102 pediatric patients (n=46 treatment group; median age: 6.4 years) and showed no significance difference in seizure frequency between groups; however, the trial was stopped early due to a very low seizure frequency among both study groups (Young, 2004). In a retrospective trial, reduced seizure frequency with prophylactic phenytoin use was described (Lewis, 1993). **Note:** Current guidelines suggest that prophylactic phenytoin may be considered to reduce the incidence of early post-traumatic seizures in pediatric patients with severe traumatic brain injuries but it does not reduce the risk of long-term seizures or improve neurologic outcome (Kochanek, 2012). Further studies are needed.

Adults: Note: Phenytoin base (eg, oral suspension, chewable tablets) contains ~8% more drug than phenytoin sodium (~92 mg base is equivalent to 100 mg phenytoin sodium). Dosage adjustments and closer serum monitoring may be necessary when switching dosage forms.

Status epilepticus: I.V.: Loading dose: Manufacturer recommends 10-15 mg/kg; however, 15-20 mg/kg at a maximum rate of 50 mg/minute is generally recommended (Kälviäinen, 2007; Lowenstein, 2005); initial maintenance dose: 4-8 mg/kg/day

Anticonvulsant: I.V., Oral: 100 mg every 6-8 hours

Anticonvulsant: Oral: Loading dose: 15-20 mg/kg; consider prior phenytoin serum concentrations and/or recent dosing history if available; administer oral loading dose in 3 divided doses given every 2-4 hours to decrease GI adverse effects and to ensure complete oral absorption; initial maintenance dose: 300 mg/day in 3 divided doses; may also administer in 1-2 divided doses using extended release formulation; adjust dosage based on individual requirements; usual maintenance dose range: 300-600 mg/day

Dosage adjustment in obesity: Loading dose: Use adjusted body weight (ABW) correction based on a pharmacokinetic study of phenytoin loading doses in obese patients (Abernethy, 1985). The larger correction factor (ie, 1.33) is due to a doubling of V_d estimated in these obese patients.

ABW = [(Actual body weight – IBW) x 1.33] + IBW

Maximum loading dose: I.V.: 2000 mg (Erstad, 2004)

Maintenance doses should be based on ideal body weight, conventional daily doses with adjustments based upon therapeutic drug monitoring, and clinical effectiveness (Abernethy, 1985; Erstad, 2002; Erstad, 2004).

Dosing adjustment in renal impairment: Phenytoin serum concentrations may be difficult to interpret in renal failure. Monitoring of free (unbound) concentrations or adjustment to allow interpretation is recommended.

Dosing adjustment in hepatic impairment: Safe in usual doses in mild liver disease; clearance may be substantially reduced in cirrhosis and plasma concentration monitoring with dose adjustment advisable. Free phenytoin concentrations should be monitored closely.

Administration

Oral:

Extended release capsules: May be administered without regard to meals

Suspension: Shake well prior to use; measure and administer dose using a calibrated oral dosing syringe (or other accurate dose-measuring device). Absorption is impaired when phenytoin suspension is given concurrently to patients who are receiving continuous nasogastric feedings. A method to resolve this interaction is to divide the daily dose of phenytoin and withhold the administration of nutritional supplements for 1-2 hours before and after each phenytoin dose.

Parenteral: I.V.: Phenytoin should be administered I.V. directly into a large vein through a large gauge needle or I.V. catheter. I.V. injections should be followed by NS flushes through the same needle or I.V. catheter to avoid local irritation of the vein. I.V. intermittent infusion: Dilute with NS to a concentration of 1-10 mg/mL, use an in-line 0.22 micron filter; avoid extravasation. Avoid I.M. use due to erratic absorption, pain on injection, and precipitation of drug at injection site. pH: 10.0-12.3

Neonates: I.V. infusion rate: Usual maximum rate: 0.5-1 mg/kg/minute; FDA-labeled maximum rate: 1-3 mg/kg/minute; **Note:** Most clinicians use a lower maximum rate of infusion in neonates of 0.5-1 mg/kg/minute

Infants, Children, and Adults: Do not exceed I.V. infusion rate of 1-3 mg/kg/minute; maximum rate: 50 mg/minute

Vesicant/Extravasation Risk Vesicant

Monitoring Parameters CBC with differential, liver function, suicidality (eg, suicidal thoughts, depression, behavioral changes), bone growth or BMD

Serum phenytoin concentrations: If available, free phenytoin concentrations should be obtained in patients with hyperbilirubinemia, renal impairment, uremia, or hypoalbuminemia; in adult patients, if free phenytoin concentrations are unavailable, the adjusted total concentration may be determined based upon equations. Trough serum concentrations are generally recommended for routine monitoring. To ensure therapeutic concentration is attained, peak serum concentrations may be measured 1 hour after the end of an I.V. infusion (particularly after a loading dose).

Additional monitoring with I.V. use: Continuous cardiac monitoring (rate, rhythm, blood pressure) and clinical observation during administration is recommended; blood pressure and pulse should be monitored every 15 minutes for 1 hour after administration with nonemergency use (Meek, 1999); emergency use may require more frequent monitoring and for a longer time after administration; infusion site reactions

◀ ## Reference Range

Timing of serum samples: Because phenytoin is slowly absorbed, peak serum concentrations may occur 4-8 hours after ingestion of an oral dose. The apparent serum half-life varies with the dosage and the drug follows Michaelis-Menten kinetics. In adults, the average apparent half-life is about 24 hours; in pediatric patients, the apparent half-life is age-dependent (longer in neonates). Steady-state concentrations are reached in 5-10 days.

Toxicity is measured clinically, and some patients may require levels outside the suggested therapeutic range.

Therapeutic range:

Total phenytoin:

Neonates: 8-15 mcg/mL

Pediatric patients ≥1 month and Adults: 10-20 mcg/mL

Concentrations of 5-10 mcg/mL may be therapeutic for some patients, but concentrations <5 mcg/mL are not likely to be effective

50% of adult patients show decreased frequency of seizures at concentrations >10 mcg/mL

86% of adult patients show decreased frequency of seizures at concentrations >15 mcg/mL

Add another anticonvulsant if satisfactory therapeutic response is not achieved with a phenytoin concentration of 20 mcg/mL

Free phenytoin: 1-2.5 mcg/mL

Total phenytoin:

Toxic: >30 mcg/mL (SI: >119 micromole/L)

Lethal: >100 mcg/mL (SI: >400 micromole/L)

When to draw serum concentrations: This is dependent on the disease state being treated and the clinical condition of the patient.

Key points:

Slow absorption of extended capsules and prolonged apparent half-life minimize fluctuations between peak and trough concentrations, thus timing of sampling is not crucial.

Trough concentrations are generally recommended for routine monitoring (capsules, oral suspension, chewable tablets, and intermittent I.V. dosing). Daily levels are not necessary and may result in incorrect dosage adjustments. If it is determined essential to monitor free phenytoin concentrations, concomitant monitoring of total phenytoin concentrations is not necessary and expensive.

After a loading dose: If rapid therapeutic serum concentrations are needed, initial concentrations may be drawn after 1 hour (after end of I.V. loading dose) or within 24 hours (after last oral loading dose) to aid in determining maintenance dose or need to reload.

Early assessment of serum concentrations: Draw within 2-3 days of therapy initiation to ensure that the patient's metabolism is not remarkably different from that which would be predicted by average literature-derived pharmacokinetic parameters; early serum concentrations should be used cautiously in design of new dosing regimens.

Second concentration: Draw within 6-7 days with subsequent doses of phenytoin adjusted accordingly.

If plasma concentrations have not changed over a 3- to 5-day period, monitoring interval may be increased to once weekly in the acute clinical setting. In stable patients requiring long-term therapy, generally monitor levels at 3- to 12-month intervals.

Adjustment of serum concentration: See tables.

Note: Although it is ideal to obtain free phenytoin concentrations to assess serum concentrations in patients with hypoalbuminemia or renal failure (CrCl ≤10 mL/minute), it may not always be possible. If free phenytoin concentrations are unavailable, the following equations may be utilized in adult patients.

Adjustment of Serum Concentration in Adults With Low Serum Albumin

Measured Total Phenytoin Concentration (mcg/mL)	Adult Patient's Serum Albumin (g/dL)			
	3.5	3	2.5	2
	Adjusted Total Phenytoin Concentration (mcg/mL)[1]			
5	6	7	8	10
10	13	14	17	20
15	19	21	25	30

[1]Adjusted concentration = measured total concentration divided by [(0.2 x albumin) + 0.1].

Adjustment of Serum Concentration in Adults With Renal Failure (CrCl ≤10 mL/min)

Measured Total Phenytoin Concentration (mcg/mL)	Adult Patient's Serum Albumin (g/dL)				
	4	3.5	3	2.5	2
	Adjusted Total Phenytoin Concentration (mcg/mL)[1]				
5	10	11	13	14	17
10	20	22	25	29	33
15	30	33	38	43	50

[1]Adjusted concentration = measured total concentration divided by [(0.1 x albumin) + 0.1].

Dosage Forms Excipient information presented when available (limited, particularly for generics); consult specific product labeling.

Capsule, Oral, as sodium:

Dilantin: 30 mg [contains fd&c yellow #10 (quinoline yellow)]

Dilantin: 100 mg

Phenytek: 200 mg, 300 mg [contains brilliant blue fcf (fd&c blue #1), fd&c blue #1 aluminum lake, fd&c blue #2 aluminum lake, fd&c red #40 aluminum lake, fd&c yellow #10 aluminum lake]

Generic: 100 mg, 200 mg, 300 mg

Solution, Injection, as sodium:

Generic: 50 mg/mL (2 mL, 5 mL)

Suspension, Oral:

Dilantin: 125 mg/5 mL (237 mL) [orange-vanilla flavor]

Generic: 125 mg/5 mL (4 mL, 237 mL)

Tablet Chewable, Oral:

Dilantin Infatabs: 50 mg [scored]

Phenytoin Infatabs: 50 mg [scored; contains fd&c yellow #10 aluminum lake, fd&c yellow #6 aluminum lake, saccharin sodium]

Generic: 50 mg

References

Abernethy DR and Greenblatt DJ, "Phenytoin Disposition in Obesity. Determination of Loading Dose," *Arch Neurol*, 1985, 42(5):468-71.

American Academy of Pediatrics Committee on Drugs, "'Inactive' Ingredients in Pharmaceutical Products: Update (Subject Review)," *Pediatrics*, 1997, 99(2):268-78.

Arya R, Gulati S, Kabra M, et al, "Folic Acid Supplementation Prevents Phenytoin-Induced Gingival Overgrowth in Children," *Neurology*, 76 (15):1338-43.

Au Yeung SC and Ensom MH, "Phenytoin and Enteral Feedings: Does Evidence Support an Interaction?" *Ann Pharmacother*, 2000, 34 (7-8):896-905.

Bauer LA and Blouin RA, "Phenytoin Michaelis-Menten Pharmacokinetics in Caucasian Pediatric Patients," *Clin Pharmacokinet*, 1983, 8 (6):545-9.

Black J, Hannaman T, and Malone C, "The Relationship of Serum Albumin Level to Phenytoin Toxicity," *J Clin Pharmacol*, 1987, 27 (3):249-50.

Brophy GM, Bell R, Claassen J, et al, "Guidelines for the Evaluation and Management of Status Epilepticus," *Neurocrit Care*, 2012, 17(1):3-23.

Chiba K, Ishizaki T, Miura H, et al, "Michaelis-Menten Pharmacokinetics of Diphenylhydantoin and Application in the Pediatric Age Patient," *J Pediatr*, 1980, 96(3 Pt 1):479-84.

Cook J, Randinitis E, and Wilder BJ, "Effect of Food on the Bioavailability of 100-mg Dilantin® Kapseals," *Neurology*, 2001, 57 (4):698-700.

Erstad BL, "Dosing of Medications in Morbidly Obese Patients in the Intensive Care Unit Setting," *Intensive Care Med*, 2004, 30(1):18-32.

Erstad BL, "Which Weight for Weight-Based Dosage Regimens in Obese Patients?" *Am J Health Syst Pharm*, 2002, 59(21):2105-10.

Guerrini R, "Epilepsy in Children," *Lancet*, 2006, 367(9509):499-524.

Harden CL, Meador KJ, Pennell PB, et al. Practice parameter update: management issues for women with epilepsy-focus on pregnancy (an evidence-based review): teratogenesis and perinatal outcomes: report of the quality standards subcommittee and therapeutics and technology assessment subcommittee of the American Academy of Neurology and American Epilepsy Society. *Neurology*. 2009, 73 (2):133-141.

Harden CL, Pennell PB, Koppel BS, et al. Practice parameter update management issues for women with epilepsy-focus on pregnancy (an evidence-based review): vitamin K, folic acid, blood levels, and breastfeeding: report of the quality standards subcommittee and therapeutics and technology assessment subcommittee of the American Academy of Neurology and American Epilepsy Society. *Neurology*. 2009;73(2):142-149.

Hegenbarth MA and American Academy of Pediatrics Committee on Drugs, "Preparing for Pediatric Emergencies: Drugs to Consider," *Pediatrics*, 2008, 121(2):433-43.

Kälviäinen R, "Status Epilepticus Treatment Guidelines," *Epilepsia*, 2007, 48(Suppl 8):99-102.

Kerrick JM, Wolff DL, and Graves NM, "Predicting Unbound Phenytoin Concentrations in Patients Receiving Valproic Acid: A Comparison of Two Prediction Methods," *Ann Pharmacother*, 1995, 29(5):470-4.

Kochanek PM, Carney N, Adelson PD, et al, "Guidelines for the Acute Medical Management of Severe Traumatic Brain Injury in Infants, Children, and Adolescents-Second Edition," *Pediatr Crit Care Med*, 2012, 13(Suppl 1):S1-82.

Lewis RJ, Yee L, Inkelis SH, et al, "Clinical Predictors of Post-Traumatic Seizures in Children With Head Trauma," *Ann Emerg Med*, 1993, 22 (7):1114-8.

Lowenstein DH, "Treatment Options for Status Epilepticus," *Curr Opin Pharmacol*, 2005, 5(3):334-9.

Mansur LI, Murrow RW, Garrelts JC, et al, "Rebound of Plasma Free Phenytoin Concentration Following Plasmapheresis in a Patient With Thrombotic Thrombocytopenic Purpura," *Ann Pharmacother*, 1995, 29(6):592-5.

Meek PD, Davis SN, Collins DM, et al, "Guidelines for Nonemergency Use of Parenteral Phenytoin Products: Proceedings of an Expert Panel Consensus Process. Panel on Nonemergency Use of Parenteral Phenytoin Products," *Arch Intern Med*, 1999, 159(22):2639-44.

Misra M, Pacaud D, Petryk A, Collett-Solberg PF, Kappy M, Drug and Therapeutics Committee of the Lawson Wilkins Pediatric Endocrine Society. Vitamin D deficiency in children and its management: review of current knowledge and recommendations. *Pediatrics*. 2008;122 (2):398-417.

Patsalos PN, Berry DJ, Bourgeois BF, et al. Antiepileptic drugs-best practice guidelines for therapeutic drug monitoring: a position paper by the Subcommission on Therapeutic Drug Monitoring, ILAE Commission on Therapeutic Strategies. *Epilepsia*. 2008;49(7):1239-1276.

Pfeifle CE, Adler DS, and Gannaway WL, "Phenytoin Sodium Solubility in Three Intravenous Solutions," *Am J Hosp Pharm*, 1981, 38 (3):358-62.

Shearer P and Riviello J, "Generalized Convulsive Status Epilepticus in Adults and Children: Treatment Guidelines and Protocols," *Emerg Med Clin North Am*, 2011, 29(1):51-64.

Suzuki Y, Mimaki T, Cox S, et al, "Phenytoin Age-Dose-Concentration Relationship in Children," *Ther Drug Monit*, 1994, 16(2):145-50.

Wagner CL, Greer FR, American Academy of Pediatrics Section on Breastfeeding, American Academy of Pediatrics Committee on Nutrition. Prevention of rickets and vitamin D deficiency in infants, children, and adolescents. *Pediatrics*. 2008;122(5):1142-1152.

Wilder BJ, Leppik I, Hietpas TJ, et al, "Effect of Food on Absorption of Dilantin® Kapseals and Mylan Extended Phenytoin Sodium Capsules," *Neurology*, 2001, 57(4):582-9.

Young KD, Okada PJ, Sokolove PE, et al, "A Randomized, Double-Blinded, Placebo-Controlled Trial of Phenytoin for the Prevention of Early Posttraumatic Seizures in Children With Moderate to Severe Blunt Head Injury," *Ann Emerg Med*, 2004, 43(4):435-46.

◆ **Phenytoin Infatabs** see Phenytoin on page 1663

◆ **Phenytoin Sodium** see Phenytoin on page 1663

◆ **Phenytoin Sodium, Extended** see Phenytoin on page 1663

◆ **Phenytoin Sodium, Prompt** see Phenytoin on page 1663

◆ **Phisohex [DSC]** see Hexachlorophene on page 1016

◆ **pHisoHex® (Can)** see Hexachlorophene on page 1016

◆ **PHL-Amantadine (Can)** see Amantadine on page 112

◆ **PHL-Amiodarone (Can)** see Amiodarone on page 127

◆ **PHL-Amlodipine (Can)** see AmLODIPine on page 135

◆ **PHL-Amoxicillin (Can)** see Amoxicillin on page 140

◆ **PHL-Azithromycin (Can)** see Azithromycin (Systemic) on page 247

◆ **PHL-Baclofen (Can)** see Baclofen on page 259

◆ **PHL-Bethanechol (Can)** see Bethanechol on page 288

◆ **PHL-Ciprofloxacin (Can)** see Ciprofloxacin (Systemic) on page 471

◆ **PHL-Citalopram (Can)** see Citalopram on page 484

◆ **PHL-Clonazepam (Can)** see ClonazePAM on page 514

◆ **PHL-Clonazepam-R (Can)** see ClonazePAM on page 514

◆ **PHL-Cyclobenzaprine (Can)** see Cyclobenzaprine on page 558

◆ **PHL-Dexamethasone (Can)** see Dexamethasone (Systemic) on page 615

◆ **PHL-Divalproex (Can)** see Valproic Acid and Derivatives on page 2102

◆ **PHL-Docusate Sodium [OTC] (Can)** see Docusate on page 701

◆ **PHL-Doxycycline (Can)** see Doxycycline on page 721

◆ **PHL-Fluconazole (Can)** see Fluconazole on page 877

◆ **PHL-Fluoxetine (Can)** see FLUoxetine on page 901

◆ **PHL-Fluvoxamine (Can)** see FluvoxaMINE on page 922

◆ **PHL-Gabapentin (Can)** see Gabapentin on page 950

◆ **PHL-Levetiracetam (Can)** see LevETIRAcetam on page 1219

◆ **PHL-Lithium Carbonate (Can)** see Lithium on page 1266

◆ **PHL-Lorazepam (Can)** see LORazepam on page 1280

◆ **PHL-Lovastatin (Can)** see Lovastatin on page 1286

◆ **PHL-Meloxicam (Can)** see Meloxicam on page 1325

◆ **PHL-Metformin (Can)** see MetFORMIN on page 1353

◆ **PHL-Methimazole (Can)** see Methimazole on page 1362

◆ **PHL-Methylphenidate (Can)** see Methylphenidate on page 1379

◆ **PHL-Minocycline (Can)** see Minocycline on page 1420

◆ **PHL-Olanzapine (Can)** see OLANZapine on page 1525

◆ **PHL-Olanzapine ODT (Can)** see OLANZapine on page 1525

◆ **PHL-Ondansetron (Can)** see Ondansetron on page 1544

◆ **PHL-Oxybutynin (Can)** see Oxybutynin on page 1568

◆ **PHL-Paroxetine (Can)** see PARoxetine on page 1609

◆ **PHL-Pravastatin (Can)** see Pravastatin on page 1720

◆ **PHL-Quetiapine (Can)** see QUEtiapine on page 1783

◆ **PHL-Ranitidine (Can)** see Ranitidine on page 1805

◆ **PHL-Risperidone (Can)** see RisperiDONE on page 1831

◆ **PHL-Salbutamol (Can)** see Albuterol on page 84

◆ **PHL-Sertraline (Can)** see Sertraline on page 1879

◆ **PHL-Simvastatin (Can)** see Simvastatin on page 1892

◆ **PHL-Sotalol (Can)** see Sotalol on page 1925

◆ **PHL-Sumatriptan (Can)** see SUMAtriptan on page 1958

◆ **PHL-Terazosin (Can)** see Terazosin on page 1981

◆ **PHL-Terbinafine (Can)** see Terbinafine (Systemic) on page 1982

◆ **PHL-Topiramate (Can)** see Topiramate on page 2046

- **PHL-Trazodone (Can)** *see* TraZODone *on page 2065*
- **PHL-Ursodiol C (Can)** *see* Ursodiol *on page 2095*
- **PHL-Valacyclovir (Can)** *see* ValACYclovir *on page 2097*
- **PHL-Valproic Acid (Can)** *see* Valproic Acid and Derivatives *on page 2102*
- **PHL-Valproic Acid E.C. (Can)** *see* Valproic Acid and Derivatives *on page 2102*
- **PHL-Verapamil SR (Can)** *see* Verapamil *on page 2129*
- **Phos-Flur** *see* Fluoride *on page 894*
- **Phos-Flur Rinse [OTC]** *see* Fluoride *on page 894*
- **PhosLo** *see* Calcium Acetate *on page 344*
- **PhosLo® (Can)** *see* Calcium Acetate *on page 344*
- **Phoslyra** *see* Calcium Acetate *on page 344*
- **Phos-NaK** *see* Potassium Phosphate and Sodium Phosphate *on page 1718*
- **Phospha 250™ Neutral** *see* Potassium Phosphate and Sodium Phosphate *on page 1718*
- **Phosphate, Potassium** *see* Potassium Phosphate *on page 1715*
- **Phosphates, Sodium** *see* Sodium Phosphates *on page 1913*
- **Phosphonoformate** *see* Foscarnet *on page 936*
- **Phosphonoformic Acid** *see* Foscarnet *on page 936*
- **p-Hydroxyampicillin** *see* Amoxicillin *on page 140*
- **Phylloquinone** *see* Phytonadione *on page 1671*
- **Physicians EZ Use B-12** *see* Cyanocobalamin *on page 556*
- **Physicians EZ Use Flu** *see* Influenza Virus Vaccine (Inactivated) *on page 1103*

Physostigmine (fye zoe STIG meen)

Medication Safety Issues
Sound-alike/look-alike issues:
Physostigmine may be confused with Prostigmin®, pyridostigmine

Related Information
Safe Handling of Hazardous Drugs *on page 2419*

Therapeutic Category Antidote, Anticholinergic Agent; Cholinergic Agent; Cholinergic Agent, Ophthalmic

Generic Availability (U.S.) Yes

Use Reverse toxic, life-threatening delirium caused by atropine, diphenhydramine, dimenhydrinate, *Atropa belladonna* (deadly nightshade), or jimson weed (*Datura* spp)

Pregnancy Considerations In general, medications used as antidotes should take into consideration the health and prognosis of the mother; antidotes should be administered to pregnant women if there is a clear indication for use and should not be withheld because of fears of teratogenicity (Bailey, 2003).

Breast-Feeding Considerations It is not known if physostigmine is excreted in breast milk. According to the manufacturer, the decision to continue or discontinue breast-feeding during therapy should take into account the risk of exposure to the infant and the benefits of treatment to the mother.

Contraindications Hypersensitivity to physostigmine or any component; GI or GU obstruction, asthma, diabetes mellitus, gangrene, severe cardiovascular disease; patients receiving depolarizing neuromuscular blockers (eg, succinylcholine)

Warnings Hazardous agent; use appropriate precautions for handling and disposal. Because physostigmine has the potential for producing severe adverse effects, (ie, seizures, bradycardia), routine use as an antidote is controversial. Patients must have a normal QRS interval, as measured by ECG, in order to receive; use caution in

poisoning with agents known to prolong intraventricular conduction. Atropine should be readily available to treat severe adverse effects. Injection contains benzyl alcohol and bisulfite which may cause allergic reactions in susceptible individuals; large amounts of benzyl alcohol (≥99 mg/kg/day) have been associated with a potentially fatal toxicity ("gasping syndrome") in neonates; the "gasping syndrome" consists of metabolic acidosis, respiratory distress, gasping respirations, CNS dysfunction (including convulsions, intracranial hemorrhage), hypotension and cardiovascular collapse; *in vitro* and animal studies have shown that benzoate, a metabolite of benzyl alcohol, displaces bilirubin from protein-binding sites; use injection with caution in neonates.

Precautions Use with caution in patients with epilepsy, narrow-angle glaucoma, marked vagotonia, parkinsonism, bradycardia

Adverse Reactions
Cardiovascular: Asystole, bradycardia, palpitation
Central nervous system: Hallucinations, nervousness, restlessness, seizure
Gastrointestinal: Defecation, diarrhea, nausea, salivation, stomach pain, vomiting
Genitourinary: Urinary frequency
Neuromuscular & skeletal: Twitching
Ocular: Lacrimation, miosis
Respiratory: Bronchospasm, dyspnea, pulmonary edema, respiratory distress, respiratory paralysis
Miscellaneous: Diaphoresis, hypersensitivity

Drug Interactions
Metabolism/Transport Effects None known.
Avoid Concomitant Use There are no known interactions where it is recommended to avoid concomitant use.
Increased Effect/Toxicity
Physostigmine may increase the levels/effects of: Beta-Blockers; Cholinergic Agonists; Succinylcholine

The levels/effects of Physostigmine may be increased by: Corticosteroids (Systemic)
Decreased Effect
Physostigmine may decrease the levels/effects of: Neuromuscular-Blocking Agents (Nondepolarizing)

The levels/effects of Physostigmine may be decreased by: Dipyridamole

Mechanism of Action Physostigmine is a carbamate which inhibits the enzyme acetylcholinesterase and prolongs the central and peripheral effects of acetylcholine

Pharmacodynamics Parenteral:
Onset of action: Within 3-8 minutes
Duration: 30 minutes to 1 hour

Pharmacokinetics (Adult data unless noted)
Distribution: Widely distributed throughout the body; crosses into the CNS
Half-life: 1-2 hours
Elimination: Via hydrolysis by cholinesterases

Dosing: Usual
Reversal of toxic anticholinergic effects: **Note:** Administer slowly over 5 minutes to prevent respiratory distress and seizures. Continuous infusions of physostigmine should never be used.
Children: Reserve for life-threatening situations only: I.V.: 0.01-0.03 mg/kg/dose; may repeat after 15-20 minutes to a maximum total dose of 2 mg
Adults: I.M., I.V., SubQ: 0.5-2 mg initially, repeat every 20 minutes until response or adverse effect occurs; repeat 1-4 mg every 30-60 minutes as life-threatening symptoms recur
Preanesthetic reversal: Children and Adults:
I.M., I.V.: Give twice the dose, on a weight basis, of the anticholinergic drug (atropine, scopolamine)

Administration Parenteral: Infuse slowly I.V. without additional dilution over 5 minutes. Too rapid administration can cause bradycardia and hypersalivation leading to respiratory distress and seizures.

Monitoring Parameters Heart rate, respiratory rate, ECG

Test Interactions Increased aminotransferase [ALT/AST] (S), increased amylase (S)

Dosage Forms Excipient information presented when available (limited, particularly for generics); consult specific product labeling.

Solution, Injection, as salicylate:
Generic: 1 mg/mL (2 mL)

References

Bailey B, "Are There Teratogenic Risks Associated With Antidotes Used in the Acute Management of Poisoned Pregnant Women?" *Birth Defects Res A Clin Mol Teratol*, 2003, 67(2):133-40.

◆ **Physostigmine Salicylate** *see* Physostigmine *on page 1670*

◆ **Physostigmine Sulfate** *see* Physostigmine *on page 1670*

◆ **Phytomenadione** *see* Phytonadione *on page 1671*

Phytonadione (fye toe na DYE one)

Medication Safety Issues
Sound-alike/look-alike issues:
Mephyton® may be confused with melphalan, methadone

Brand Names: U.S. Mephyton®

Brand Names: Canada AquaMEPHYTON®; Konakion; Mephyton®

Therapeutic Category Nutritional Supplement; Vitamin, Fat Soluble

Generic Availability (U.S.) Yes

Use

Injection: Prophylaxis and treatment of hemorrhagic disease of the newborn (FDA approved in newborns); prevention and treatment of hypoprothrombinemia caused by vitamin K deficiency, vitamin K antagonist (VKA)-induced (eg, warfarin-induced), other drug-induced vitamin K deficiency, altered activity, or altered metabolism (FDA approved in adults); hypoprothrombinemia caused by malabsorption or inability to synthesize vitamin K (FDA approved in adults)

Oral: Prevention and treatment of hypoprothrombinemia caused by vitamin K deficiency, vitamin K antagonist (VKA)-induced (eg, warfarin-induced), other drug-induced vitamin K deficiency, altered activity, or altered metabolism; hypoprothrombinemia caused by malabsorption or inability to synthesize vitamin K (FDA approved in adults)

Pregnancy Risk Factor C

Pregnancy Considerations Animal reproduction studies have not been conducted. Phytonadione crosses the placenta in limited concentrations (Kazzi, 1990). The dietary requirements of vitamin K are the same in pregnant and nonpregnant women (IOM, 2000). In general, medications used as antidotes should take into consideration the health and prognosis of the mother; antidotes should be administered to pregnant women if there is a clear indication for use and should not be withheld because of fears of teratogenicity (Bailey, 2003).

Breast-Feeding Considerations Small amounts of dietary vitamin K can be detected in breast milk and the dietary requirements of vitamin K are the same in nursing and non-nursing women (IOM, 2000). Information following the use of phytonadione has not been located. The manufacturer recommends caution be used if phytonadione is administered to a nursing woman.

Contraindications Hypersensitivity to phytonadione or any component

Warnings Severe reactions resembling anaphylaxis or hypersensitivity have occurred rarely during or immediately after I.V. administration despite proper dilution and rate of administration) **[U.S. Boxed Warning]** and with I.M. administration; anaphylactoid reactions typically occurred when patients received large I.V. doses administered rapidly with formulations containing polyethoxylated castor oil; proper dosing, dilution, and administration will minimize risk (Ageno, 2012; Riegert-Johnson, 2002); restrict I.V. and I.M. administration for situations where the subcutaneous route is not feasible.

Efficacy (eg, control of bleeding, decrease in INR) is delayed regardless of route of administration; patient management may require other treatments in the interim. In patients receiving a therapeutic vitamin K antagonist (VKA) (eg, warfarin), administer a dose of phytonadione that will quickly lower the INR into a safe range without causing resistance to warfarin. High phytonadione doses may lead to warfarin resistance for at least 1 week. Phytonadione will not counter the effect of heparin.

Ineffective in hereditary hypoprothrombinemia. If initial dose of phytonadione does not reverse coagulopathy in patients with liver disease-induced hypoprothrombinemia, higher doses are unlikely to have any effect. In neonates, severe hemolytic anemia and hyperbilirubinemia have been reported rarely following large doses (10-20 mg) of phytonadione.

Injectable products may contain aluminum; toxic aluminum concentrations may be seen with high doses, prolonged use, or renal dysfunction. Premature neonates are at higher risk due to immature renal function and aluminum intake from other parenteral sources. Parenteral aluminum exposure of >4-5 mcg/kg/day is associated with CNS and bone toxicity and tissue loading may occur at lower doses. Injection products may contain 0.9% benzyl alcohol which may cause allergic reactions in susceptible individuals; large amounts of benzyl alcohol (≥99 mg/kg/day) have been associated with a potentially fatal toxicity ("gasping syndrome") in neonates; the "gasping syndrome" consists of metabolic acidosis, respiratory distress, gasping respirations, CNS dysfunction (including convulsions, intracranial hemorrhage), hypotension and cardiovascular collapse; *in vitro* and animal studies have shown that benzoate, a metabolite of benzyl alcohol, displaces bilirubin from protein-binding sites; injection is safe in neonates when used in appropriate doses. Injection may also contain polysorbate 80 (Tween 80®) which may cause allergic reactions in susceptible individuals. In premature neonates, thrombocytopenia, ascites, pulmonary deterioration, and renal and hepatic failure have been reported after receiving parenteral products containing polysorbate 80 (Alade, 1986; CDC, 1984). Infusion of polysorbate 80-containing solutions through polyvinyl chloride tubing may cause DEHP to leach into the solution; in immature animals, exposure to DEHP may adversely affect the development of the male reproductive tract. Some injectable dosage forms contain polyethoxylated castor oil (Cremophor® EL) which has been associated with anaphylactoid reactions; use these formulations with caution. Injectable products may contain propylene glycol; toxicities have been reported with use of products containing propylene glycol, including hyperosmolality, lactic acidosis, seizures, and respiratory depression; in neonates large amounts of propylene glycol delivered orally, intravenously (eg, >3000 mg/day), or topically have been associated with potentially fatal toxicities which can include metabolic acidosis, seizures, renal failure, and CNS depression; use injectable products containing propylene glycol with caution (AAP, 1997; Shehab, 2009).

Precautions The oral route is the safest method of administration and requires the presence of bile salts for absorption; in obstructive jaundice or with biliary fistulas, concurrent administration of bile salts would be necessary for proper absorption. Manufacturers recommend the SubQ route over other parenteral routes; however, SubQ is less predictable when compared to the oral route and efficacy may be delayed. The American College of Chest Physicians recommends the I.V. route in patients with major bleeding secondary to use of vitamin K antagonists (VKAs) such as warfarin. The I.V. route should be restricted to emergency situations only where oral phytonadione cannot be used.

Adverse Reactions

Cardiovascular: Cyanosis, flushing, hyper-/hypotension

Central nervous system: Dizziness

Dermatologic: Erythematous skin eruptions, pruritus, scleroderma-like lesions

Endocrine & metabolic: Hyperbilirubinemia (newborn; greater than recommended doses)

Gastrointestinal: Abnormal taste

Local: Injection site reactions

Respiratory: Dyspnea

Miscellaneous: Diaphoresis, hypersensitivity reactions, nonimmunologic anaphylaxis (formerly known as anaphylactoid reaction), sweating

Drug Interactions

Metabolism/Transport Effects None known.

Avoid Concomitant Use There are no known interactions where it is recommended to avoid concomitant use.

Increased Effect/Toxicity There are no known significant interactions involving an increase in effect.

Decreased Effect

Phytonadione may decrease the levels/effects of: Vitamin K Antagonists

The levels/effects of Phytonadione may be decreased by: Mineral Oil; Orlistat

Stability

Injection: Store at 15°C to 30°C (59°F to 86°F), protect from light. **Note:** Store Hospira product at 20°C to 25°C (68°F to 77°F).

Oral: Store tablets at 15°C to 30°C (59°F to 86°F); protect from light.

Mechanism of Action Promotes liver synthesis of clotting factors (II, VII, IX, X); however, the exact mechanism as to this stimulation is unknown. Menadiol is a water soluble form of vitamin K; phytonadione has a more rapid and prolonged effect than menadione; menadiol sodium diphosphate (K_4) is half as potent as menadione (K_3).

Pharmacodynamics

Onset of action: Blood coagulation factors increase: Oral: Within 6-12 hours; Parenteral: Within 1-2 hours

Maximum effect: Normalization prothrombin time (INR): Oral: 24-48 hours; Parenteral: 12-14 hours

Pharmacokinetics (Adult data unless noted)

Absorption: Oral: From the intestines in the presence of bile; SubQ: Variable; I.M.: Readily absorbed

Metabolism: Rapidly in the liver

Elimination: In bile and urine as metabolites

Dosing: Neonatal Note: Dosing presented in **mcg** and mg; verify dosing units.

Adequate intake (Vanek, 2012): Oral:
Preterm neonates: 8-10 **mcg**/kg/day
Term neonates: 2 **mcg**/day

Parenteral nutrition, maintenance requirement (Vanek, 2012): I.V.:
Preterm neonate: 10 **mcg**/kg/day
Term neonates: 200 **mcg**/day

Vitamin K deficiency bleeding (formerly known as hemorrhagic disease of the newborn):
Prophylaxis: I.M.: **Note:** Administer within 1 hour of birth AAP recommendations (AAP, 2003; AAP, 2009):
Preterm neonate:
Birth weight <1000 g: 0.3 mg/kg (Costakos, 2003)
Birth weight ≥1000 g: 0.5 mg
Term neonate: 0.5-1 mg

Alternate dosing: GA <32 weeks: 0.2 mg; may repeat dose for prolonged prothrombin time or clinical signs of bleeding (Clarke, 2006)
Treatment: SubQ, I.M.: 1-2 mg/day

Dosing: Usual SubQ route is preferred; I.V. and I.M. routes should be restricted to situations when the SubQ route is not feasible. **Note:** Dosing presented in **mcg** and mg; verify dosing units.

Infants, Children, and Adolescents:
Adequate intake (IOM, 2001; Vanek, 2013):
1-6 months: 2 **mcg**/day
7-12 months: 2.5 **mcg**/day
1-3 years: 30 **mcg**/day
4-8 years: 55 **mcg**/day
9-13 years: 60 **mcg**/day
14-18 years: 75 **mcg**/day

Vitamin K deficiency, prevention, and supplementation (Disease-specific):
Biliary atresia (Shneider, 2012): **Note:** Dose and route are determined by INR value: Infants 1-6 months:
INR >1.2-1.5: 2.5 mg once daily orally
INR >1.5-1.8: Initial: 2-5 mg I.M. once followed by 2.5 mg once daily orally
INR >1.8: Initial: 2-5 mg I.M. once followed by 5 mg once daily orally
Cholestasis: Oral:: 2.4-15 mg/day (Sathe, 2010)
Cystic fibrosis: Oral: 0.3-0.5 mg/day (Borowitz, 2002; Sathe, 2010)
Liver disease: Oral: 2.5-5 mg/day (Nightingale, 2009; Sathe, 2010)

Reversal of Vitamin K antagonists (eg, warfarin):
Weight-based dosing (preferred): *Chest* recommendations: I.V.: 0.03 mg/kg/dose is recommended for excessively prolonged INR (usually INR >8; no evidence of bleeding) due to vitamin K-antagonist (eg, warfarin): if significant bleeding, consider use of fresh frozen plasma, prothrombin complex concentrates, or recombinant factor VIIa (Bolton-Maggs, 2002; Monagle, 2012)
Alternate dosing: Fixed dosing: **Note:** Smaller pediatric patients should receive doses on the low end of dosing range; excessive dosages may cause warfarin-resistance (Bolton-Maggs, 2002; Michelson, 1998)
No bleeding, rapid reversal needed, patient will require further oral anticoagulant therapy: SubQ, I.V.: 0.5-2 mg
No bleeding, rapid reversal needed, patient will not require further oral anticoagulant therapy: SubQ, I.V.: 2-5 mg
Significant bleeding, not life-threatening: SubQ, I.V.: 0.5-2 mg
Significant bleeding, life-threatening: SubQ, I.V.: 5 mg

Parenteral nutrition, maintenance requirement (Vanek, 2012): I.V.: **Note:** Patients receiving warfarin may not require TPN supplementation of phytonadione.
Infants: 10 **mcg**/kg/day
Children and Adolescents: 200 **mcg**/day

Vitamin K deficiency (Hypoprothrombinemia) due to drugs (other than coumarin derivatives) or factors limiting absorption or synthesis of vitamin K:
Infants and Children:
Oral: 2.5-5 mg/24 hours
SubQ, I.M., I.V.: 1-2 mg/dose as a single dose
Adolescents:
Oral: 2.5-25 mg/24 hours
SubQ, I.M., I.V.: 2.5-10 mg
Adults:
Adequate intake (IOM, 2001):
Male: 120 **mcg**/day
Female: 90 **mcg**/day
Pregnant, ≤18 years of age: 75 **mcg**/day

Pregnant, ≥19 years of age: 90 **mcg**/day

Breast-feeding, ≤18 years of age: 75 **mcg**/day

Breast-feeding, ≥19 years of age: 90 **mcg**/day

Vitamin K deficiency due to drugs (other than cou-marin derivatives) or factors limiting absorption or synthesis: Oral, SubQ, I.M., I.V.: Initial: 2.5-25 mg (rarely up to 50 mg)

Vitamin K deficiency (supratherapeutic INR) secondary to VKAs (eg, warfarin):

If INR above therapeutic range to <4.5 (no evidence of bleeding): Lower or hold next VKA dose and monitor frequently; when INR approaches desired range, resume VKA dosing with a lower dose (Patriquin, 2011)

If INR 4.5-10 (no evidence of bleeding): The 2012 *Chest* guidelines recommend against routine phytonadione (ie, vitamin K) administration in this setting (Guyatt, 2012). Previously, the 2008 ACCP guidelines recommended if no risk factors for bleeding exist, to omit next 1 or 2 VKA doses, monitor INR more frequently, and resume with an appropriately adjusted VKA dose when INR in desired range; may consider administering vitamin K orally 1-2.5 mg if other risk factors for bleeding exist (Hirsh, 2008). Others have recommended consideration of vitamin K 1 mg orally or 0.5 mg I.V. (Patriquin, 2011).

If INR >10 (no evidence of bleeding): The 2012 ACCP guidelines recommend administration of oral vitamin K (dose not specified) in this setting (Guyatt, 2012). Previously, the 2008 ACCP guidelines recommended to hold warfarin, administer vitamin K orally 2.5-5 mg, expect INR to be reduced within 24-48 hours, monitor INR more frequently and give additional vitamin K at an appropriate dose if necessary; resume warfarin at an appropriately adjusted dose when INR is in desired range (Hirsh, 2008). Others have recommended consideration of vitamin K 2-2.5 mg orally or 0.5-1 mg I.V. (Patriquin, 2011).

If minor bleeding at any INR elevation: Hold warfarin, may administer vitamin K orally 2.5-5 mg, monitor INR more frequently, may repeat dose after 24 hours if INR correction incomplete; resume warfarin at an appropriately adjusted dose when INR is in desired range (Patriquin, 2011)

If major bleeding at any INR elevation: The 2012 ACCP guidelines recommend administration of four-factor prothrombin complex concentrate (PCC) and I.V. vitamin K 5-10 mg in this setting (Guyatt, 2012); however, in the U.S., the available PCCs (Bebulin®VH and Profilnine® SD) are **three**-factor PCCs and do not contain adequate levels of factor VII. Four-factor PCCs include Beriplex® P/N, Cofact®, Konyne®, or Octaplex® all of which are **not** available in the U.S. Previously, the 2008 ACCP guidelines recommended to hold warfarin, administer vitamin K 10 mg by slow I.V. infusion and supplement with PCC depending on the urgency of the situation; I.V. vitamin K may be repeated every 12 hours (Hirsh, 2008).

Note: Use of high doses of vitamin K (eg, 10-15 mg) may cause warfarin resistance for ≥1 week. During this period of resistance, heparin or low molecular-weight heparin (LMWH) may be given until INR responds (Ansell, 2008).

Preprocedural/surgical INR normalization in patients receiving warfarin (routine use): Oral: 1-2.5 mg once administered on the day before surgery; recheck INR on day of procedure/surgery (Douketis, 2012). Others have recommended the use of vitamin K 1 mg orally for mild INR elevations (ie, INR 3.0-4.5) (Patriquin, 2011).

Administration

Oral: May be administered with or without food. The parenteral formulation may also be used for small oral

doses (eg, 1 mg) or situations in which tablets cannot be swallowed (Crowther, 2000; O'Connor, 1986).

Parenteral: SubQ administration is the preferred method; for I.V. administration, dilute in 5-10 mL I.V. fluid (D_5W or NS) (maximum concentration: 10 mg/mL); infuse over 15-30 minutes; maximum rate of infusion: 1 mg/minute

Monitoring Parameters PT, INR

Dosage Forms Excipient information presented when available (limited, particularly for generics); consult specific product labeling.

Injection, aqueous colloidal: 1 mg/0.5 mL (0.5 mL) [contains benzyl alcohol, polyoxyethylated castor oil]; 10 mg/mL (1 mL) [contains benzyl alcohol, polyoxyethylated castor oil]

Injection, aqueous colloidal [preservative free]: 1 mg/0.5 mL (0.5 mL) [contains polysorbate 80, propylene glycol 10.4 mg/0.5 mL]

Tablet, oral: 100 mcg

Mephyton®: 5 mg [scored]

Extemporaneous Preparations A 1 mg/mL oral suspension may be made with tablets. Crush six 5 mg tablets in a mortar and reduce to a fine powder. Add 5 mL each of water and methylcellulose 1% and mix to a uniform paste. Mix while adding sorbitol in incremental proportions to **almost** 30 mL; transfer to a calibrated bottle, rinse mortar with sorbitol, and add quantity of sorbitol sufficient to make 30 mL. Label "shake well" and "refrigerate". Stable for 3 days.

Nahata MC and Hipple TF, *Pediatric Drug Formulations*, 3rd ed, Cincinnati, OH: Harvey Whitney Books Co, 1997.

Note: The parenteral formulation may also be used for small oral doses (eg, 1 mg) or situations in which tablets cannot be swallowed (Crowther, 2000; O'Connor, 1986).

References

Alade SL, Brown RE, and Paquet A Jr, "Polysorbate 80 and E-Ferol Toxicity," *Pediatrics*, 1986, 77(4):593-7.

American Academy of Pediatrics Committee on Drugs. "Inactive" ingredients in pharmaceutical products: update (subject review). *Pediatrics*. 1997;99(2):268-278.

American Academy of Pediatrics Committee on Fetus and Newborn, "Controversies Concerning Vitamin K and the Newborn. American Academy of Pediatrics Committee on Fetus and Newborn," *Pediatrics*, 2003, 112(1 Pt 1):191-2.

American Academy of Pediatrics Committee on Nutrition, "Micronutrients: Vitamin K," *Pediatric Nutrition Handbook*, 6th ed, Kleinman RE, ed, Elk Grove Village, IL: American Academy of Pediatrics, 2009, 469.

Ansell J, Hirsh J, Hylek E, et al, "Pharmacology and Management of the Vitamin K Antagonists: American College of Chest Physicians Evidence-Based Clinical Practice Guidelines (8th Edition)," *Chest*, 2008, 133(6 Suppl):160-98.

Bailey B, "Are There Teratogenic Risks Associated With Antidotes Used in the Acute Management of Poisoned Pregnant Women?" *Birth Defects Res A Clin Mol Teratol*, 2003, 67(2):133-40.

Bolton-Maggs P and Brook L, "The Use of Vitamin K for Reversal of Over-Warfarinization in Children," *Br J Haematol*, 2008, 118(3):924.

Borowitz D, Baker RD, and Stallings V, "Consensus Report on Nutrition for Pediatric Patients With Cystic Fibrosis," *J Pediatr Gastroenterol Nutr*, 2002, 35(3):246-59.

Centers for Disease Control (CDC), "Unusual Syndrome With Fatalities Among Premature Infants: Association With a New Intravenous Vitamin E Product," *MMWR Morb Mortal Wkly Rep*, 1984, 33 (14):198-9.

Clarke P, Mitchell SJ, Wynn R, et al, "Vitamin K Prophylaxis for Preterm Infants: A Randomized, Controlled Trial of 3 Regimens," *Pediatrics*, 2006, 118(6):e1657-66.

Costakos DT, Greer FR, Love LA, et al, "Vitamin K Prophylaxis for Premature Infants: 1 mg Versus 0.5 mg," *Am J Perinatol*, 2003, 20 (8):485-90.

Crowther MA, Julian J, McCarty D, et al, "Treatment of Warfarin-Associated Coagulopathy With Oral Vitamin K: A Randomised Controlled Trial," *Lancet*, 2000, 356(9241):1551-3.

Department Health & Human Services, Food Drug Administration, "Aluminum in Large and Small Volume Parenterals Used in Total Parenteral Nutrition," *Federal Register*, 2000, 65(17):4103-11.

Douketis JD, Spyropoulos AC, Spencer FA, et al, "Perioperative Management of Antithrombotic Therapy: Antithrombotic Therapy and Prevention of Thrombosis, 9th ed: American College of Chest Physicians Evidence-Based Clinical Practice Guidelines," *Chest*, 2012, 141(2 Suppl):e326-50.

Guyatt GH, Akl EA, Crowther M, et al, "Executive Summary: Antithrombotic Therapy and Prevention of Thrombosis, 9th ed: American College of Chest Physicians Evidence-Based Clinical Practice Guidelines," *Chest*, 2012, 141(2 Suppl):7-47.

Hirsh J, Guyatt G, Albers GW, et al, "Executive Summary: American College of Chest Physicians Evidence-Based Clinical Practice Guidelines (8th Edition), *Chest*, 2008, 133(6 Suppl):71-109.

IOM (Institute of Medicine), *Dietary Reference Intakes for Vitamin A, Vitamin K, Arsenic, Boron, Chromium, Copper, Iodine, Iron, Manganese, Molybdenum, Nickel, Silicon, Vanadium, and Zinc*, Washington, DC: National Academy Press, 2001.

Kazzi NJ, Ilagan NB, Liang KC, et al, "Placental Transfer of Vitamin K1 in Preterm Pregnancy," *Obstet Gynecol*, 1990, 75(3 Pt 1):334-7.

Michelson AD, Bovill E, Monagle P, et al, "Antithrombic Therapy in Children," *Chest*, 1998, 114(5 Suppl):748-69.

Monagle P, Chan AK, Goldenberg NA. et al, "Antithrombotic Therapy in Neonates and Children: Antithrombotic Therapy and Prevention of Thrombosis, 9th ed: American College of Chest Physicians Evidence-Based Clinical Practice Guidelines," *Chest*, 2012, 141(2 Suppl): e737-801.

Nightingale S and Ng VL, "Optimizing Nutritional Management in Children With Chronic Liver Disease," *Pediatr Clin North Am*, 2009, 56(5):1161-83.

O'Connor ME and Addiego JE Jr, "Use of Oral Vitamin K1 to Prevent Hemorrhagic Disease of the Newborn Infant," *J Pediatr*, 1986, 108 (4):616-9.

Patriquin C and Crowther M, "Treatment of Warfarin-Associated Coagulopathy With Vitamin K," *Expert Rev Hematol*, 2011, 4(6):657-65.

Sathe MN and Patel AS, "Update in Pediatrics: Focus on Fat-Soluble Vitamins," *Nutr Clin Pract*, 2010, 25(4):340-6.

Shehab N, Lewis CL, Streetman DD, Donn SM. Exposure to the pharmaceutical excipients benzyl alcohol and propylene glycol among critically ill neonates. *Pediatr Crit Care Med*. 2009;10 (2):256-259.

Shneider BL, Magee JC, Bezerra JA, et al, "Efficacy of Fat-Soluble Vitamin Supplementation in Infants With Biliary Atresia," *Pediatrics*, 2012, 130(3):e607-14.

Vanek VW, Borum P, Buchman A, et al, "A.S.P.E.N. Position Paper: Recommendations for Changes in Commercially Available Parenteral Multivitamin and Multi-trace Element Products," *Nutr Clin Pract*, 2012, 27(4):440-91.

◆ **PIC 200 [OTC]** *see* Polysaccharide-Iron Complex *on page 1701*

Pilocarpine (Systemic) (pye loe KAR peen)

Medication Safety Issues
Sound-alike/look-alike issues:
Salagen® may be confused with selegiline
Brand Names: U.S. Salagen
Brand Names: Canada Salagen®
Therapeutic Category Cholinergic Agent
Generic Availability (U.S.) Yes
Use Symptomatic treatment of xerostomia caused by salivary gland hypofunction resulting from radiotherapy for cancer of the head and neck; and in Sjögren's syndrome
Pregnancy Risk Factor C
Pregnancy Considerations Adverse events were observed in some animal reproduction studies.
Breast-Feeding Considerations It is not known if pilocarpidine systemic is excreted in breast milk. Due to the potential for serious adverse reactions in the nursing infant, a decision should be made whether to discontinue nursing or to discontinue the drug, taking into account the importance of treatment to the mother.
Contraindications Hypersensitivity to pilocarpine or any component; severe hepatic impairment
Warnings Reduce dosage in hepatic impairment
Precautions Use with caution in patients with preexisting CHF, asthma, peptic ulcer, urinary tract obstruction, Parkinson's disease
Adverse Reactions
Cardiovascular: Edema, facial edema, flushing, hypertension, palpitation, tachycardia
Central nervous system: Chills, dizziness, fever, headache, pain, somnolence
Dermatologic: Pruritus, rash

Gastrointestinal: Diarrhea, dyspepsia, constipation, flatulence, glossitis, increased salivation, nausea, stomatitis, taste perversion, vomiting
Genitourinary: Urinary frequency, urinary incontinence, vaginitis
Neuromuscular & skeletal: Myalgias, tremor, weakness
Ocular: Abnormal vision, amblyopia, blurred vision, conjunctivitis lacrimation
Otic: Tinnitus
Respiratory: Dysphagia, epistaxis, increased cough, rhinitis, sinusitis
Miscellaneous: Allergic reaction, diaphoresis, voice alteration
Rare but important or life-threatening: Abnormal dreams, alopecia, angina pectoris, anorexia, anxiety, arrhythmia, body odor, bone disorder, cholelithiasis, colitis, confusion, dry eyes, dry mouth, ECG abnormality, myasthenia, photosensitivity reaction, nervousness, pancreatitis, paresthesia, salivary gland enlargement, sputum increased, taste loss, tongue disorder, urinary impairment, urinary urgency, yawning
Drug Interactions
Metabolism/Transport Effects Inhibits CYP2A6 (weak), CYP2E1 (weak), CYP3A4 (weak)
Avoid Concomitant Use
Avoid concomitant use of Pilocarpine (Systemic) with any of the following: Pimozide
Increased Effect/Toxicity
Pilocarpine (Systemic) may increase the levels/effects of: ARIPiprazole; Dofetilide; Lomitapide; Pimozide

The levels/effects of Pilocarpine (Systemic) may be increased by: Acetylcholinesterase Inhibitors; Beta-Blockers
Decreased Effect There are no known significant interactions involving a decrease in effect.
Food Interactions Fat decreases the rate of absorption, maximum concentration and increases the time it takes to reach maximum concentration. Management: Avoid administering with a high-fat meal.
Pharmacodynamics Increased salivary flow
Onset of action: 20 minutes
Maximum effect: 1 hour
Duration: 3-5 hours
Pharmacokinetics (Adult data unless noted)
Half-life, elimination: 0.76-1.35 hours
Mild to moderate hepatic impairment: 2.1 hours
Elimination: Urine
Dosing: Usual
Xerostomia: Adults: Oral:
Following head and neck cancer: 5 mg 3 times/day, titration up to 10 mg 3 times/day may be considered for patients who have not responded adequately; not to exceed 10 mg/dose
Sjögren's syndrome: 5 mg 4 times/day
Dosage adjustment in hepatic impairment: Adults: Oral: Patients with moderate impairment: 5 mg 2 times/day regardless of indication; avoid use in severe hepatic impairment
Administration May be administered with or without food; avoid administration with high-fat meal
Monitoring Parameters Salivation (xerostomia treatment)
Dosage Forms Excipient information presented when available (limited, particularly for generics); consult specific product labeling.
Tablet, Oral, as hydrochloride:
Salagen: 5 mg
Salagen: 7.5 mg [contains fd&c blue #2 aluminum lake]
Generic: 5 mg, 7.5 mg

Pilocarpine (Ophthalmic) (pye loe KAR peen)

Medication Safety Issues
Sound-alike/look-alike issues:
Isopto® Carpine may be confused with Isopto® Carbachol

Brand Names: U.S. Isopto Carpine; Pilopine HS
Brand Names: Canada Diocarpine; Isopto® Carpine; Pilopine HS®
Therapeutic Category Cholinergic Agent; Cholinergic Agent, Ophthalmic; Ophthalmic Agent, Miotic
Generic Availability (U.S.) May be product dependent
Use Management of chronic simple glaucoma, chronic and acute angle-closure glaucoma; counter effects of cycloplegics
Pregnancy Risk Factor C
Pregnancy Considerations Animal reproduction studies have not been conducted.
Breast-Feeding Considerations It is not known if pilocarpine (ophthalmic) is excreted in breast milk. The manufacturer recommends that caution be exercised when administering pilocarpine (ophthalmic) to nursing women.
Contraindications Hypersensitivity to pilocarpine or any component; when cholinergic effects such as constriction are undesirable (eg, acute inflammatory disease of anterior chamber, acute iritis)
Precautions Use with caution in patients with preexisting retinal disease, corneal abrasion, or those predisposed to retinal tears; may occasionally precipitate angle closure by increased resistance to aqueous flow from the posterior to anterior eye chamber

Adverse Reactions
Cardiovascular: Hypertension, tachycardia
Dermatologic: Diaphoresis
Gastrointestinal: Diarrhea, nausea, salivation, vomiting
Ocular: Burning, ciliary spasm, conjunctival vascular congestion, corneal granularity, lacrimation, lens opacity, myopia, retinal detachment, supraorbital or temporal headache, visual acuity decreased
Respiratory: Bronchial spasm, pulmonary edema

Drug Interactions
Metabolism/Transport Effects Inhibits CYP2A6 (weak), CYP2E1 (weak), CYP3A4 (weak)
Avoid Concomitant Use
Avoid concomitant use of Pilocarpine (Ophthalmic) with any of the following: Pimozide
Increased Effect/Toxicity
Pilocarpine (Ophthalmic) may increase the levels/effects of: ARIPiprazole; Dofetilide; Lomitapide; Pimozide

The levels/effects of Pilocarpine (Ophthalmic) may be increased by: Acetylcholinesterase Inhibitors; Beta-Blockers
Decreased Effect There are no known significant interactions involving a decrease in effect.
Mechanism of Action Directly stimulates cholinergic receptors in the eye causing miosis (by contraction of the iris sphincter), loss of accommodation (by constriction of ciliary muscle), and lowering of intraocular pressure (with decreased resistance to aqueous humor outflow)

Pharmacodynamics
Ophthalmic solution instillation: Miosis:
Onset of action: Within 10-30 minutes
Duration: 4-8 hours
Intraocular pressure reduction:
Onset of action: 1 hour
Duration: 4-12 hours
Dosing: Usual Children and Adults:
Gel: 0.5" (1.3 cm) ribbon applied to lower conjunctival sac once daily at bedtime; adjust dosage as required to control elevated intraocular pressure

Solution: Instill 1-2 drops up to 6 times/day; adjust the concentration and frequency as required to control elevated intraocular pressure
To counteract the mydriatic effects of sympathomimetic agents: Instill 1 drop of a 1% solution in the affected eye
Administration
Gel: Instill gel into affected eye(s); close the eye for 1-2 minutes and instruct patient to roll the eyeball in all directions; avoid contact of bottle tip with eye or skin
Solution: Shake well before use; instill into affected eye(s); apply finger pressure to lacrimal sac during and for 1-2 minutes after instillation to decrease drainage into the nose and throat and minimize possible systemic absorption
Monitoring Parameters Intraocular pressure, funduscopic exam, visual field testing
Dosage Forms Excipient information presented when available (limited, particularly for generics); consult specific product labeling.
Gel, Ophthalmic, as hydrochloride:
Pilopine HS: 4% (4 g) [contains benzalkonium chloride, edetate disodium]
Solution, Ophthalmic, as hydrochloride:
Isopto Carpine: 1% (15 mL); 2% (15 mL); 4% (15 mL)
Generic: 1% (15 mL); 2% (15 mL); 4% (15 mL)

♦ **Pilocarpine Hydrochloride** *see* Pilocarpine (Ophthalmic) *on page 1675*

♦ **Pilocarpine Hydrochloride** *see* Pilocarpine (Systemic) *on page 1674*

♦ **Pilopine HS** *see* Pilocarpine (Ophthalmic) *on page 1675*

♦ **Pilopine HS® (Can)** *see* Pilocarpine (Ophthalmic) *on page 1675*

Pimecrolimus (pim e KROE li mus)

Medication Safety Issues
Sound-alike/look-alike issues:
Pimecrolimus may be confused with tacrolimus
Brand Names: U.S. Elidel
Brand Names: Canada Elidel
Therapeutic Category Immunomodulating Agent, Topical
Generic Availability (U.S.) No
Use Second-line agent for short-term and intermittent treatment of mild to moderate atopic dermatitis in nonimmunocompromised patients unresponsive to, or intolerant of other treatments
Medication Guide Available Yes
Pregnancy Risk Factor C
Pregnancy Considerations Adverse events were not observed in animal reproduction studies following topical application.
Breast-Feeding Considerations It is not known if pimecrolimus is excreted in breast milk. Due to the potential for serious adverse reactions in the nursing infant, the manufacturer recommends a decision be made whether to discontinue nursing or to discontinue the drug, taking into account the importance of treatment to the mother.
Contraindications Hypersensitivity to pimecrolimus or any component; Netherton's syndrome due to potential for increased systemic absorption; application to site with active cutaneous viral infection (treat and clear infection prior to the start of therapy); application on malignant or premalignant skin conditions
Warnings Pimecrolimus therapy may be associated with an increased risk for eczema herpeticum, varicella zoster, or herpes simplex virus infection; consider discontinuing therapy in patients who develop lymphadenopathy or in patients who have skin papillomas which worsen. Cream contains benzyl alcohol which may cause allergic reactions in susceptible individuals; large amounts of benzyl

alcohol (≥99 mg/kg/day) have been associated with a potentially fatal toxicity ("gasping syndrome") in neonates; the "gasping syndrome" consists of metabolic acidosis, respiratory distress, gasping respirations, CNS dysfunction (including convulsions, intracranial hemorrhage), hypotension and cardiovascular collapse.

Precautions Use with caution in immunocompromised patients and in patients who have experienced adverse effects to topical cyclosporine or tacrolimus.

Adverse Reactions

Central nervous system: Fever (more common in children and adolescents), headache (more common in children and adolescents)

Dermatologic: Acne vulgaris, folliculitis (more common in adults), herpes simplex dermatitis, impetigo, molluscum contagiosum (children and adolescents), skin infection, urticaria, warts (children and adolescents)

Gastrointestinal: Abdominal pain, constipation (children and adolescents), diarrhea (more common in children and adolescents), gastroenteritis (more common in children and adolescents), nausea, toothache, vomiting

Genitourinary: Dysmenorrhea

Hypersensitivity: Hypersensitivity

Infection: Bacterial infection, herpes simplex infection, influenza, staphylococcal infection, varicella, viral infection (children and adolescents)

Local: Application site reaction (more common in adults), local burning (more common in adults; tends to resolve/improve as lesions resolve), local irritation (more common in adults), localized erythema, local pruritus

Neuromuscular & skeletal: Arthralgia, back pain

Ocular: Conjunctivitis, eye infection

Otic: Otic infection, otitis media

Respiratory: Asthma, asthma aggravated (children and adolescents), bronchitis (more common in children and adolescents), cough (more common in children and adolescents), dyspnea, epistaxis, flu-like symptoms, nasal congestion, nasopharyngitis (more common in infants, children, and adolescents), pharyngitis (more common in children and adolescents), pneumonia, rhinitis, rhinorrhea (children and adolescents), sinusitis, sore throat, streptococcal pharyngitis (children and adolescents), tonsillitis (more common in children and adolescents), upper respiratory tract infection (more common in children and adolescents), viral upper respiratory tract infection, wheezing (children and adolescents)

Miscellaneous: Laceration (children and adolescents)

Rare but important or life-threatening: Anaphylaxis, angioedema, eczema (herpeticum), lymphadenopathy, malignant neoplasm (basal cell carcinoma, squamous cell carcinoma, malignant melanoma, malignant lymphoma), skin discoloration

Drug Interactions

Metabolism/Transport Effects Substrate of CYP3A4 (minor); **Note:** Assignment of Major/Minor substrate status based on clinically relevant drug interaction potential

Avoid Concomitant Use

Avoid concomitant use of Pimecrolimus with any of the following: Immunosuppressants

Increased Effect/Toxicity

Pimecrolimus may increase the levels/effects of: Immunosuppressants

The levels/effects of Pimecrolimus may be increased by: CYP3A4 Inhibitors (Moderate); CYP3A4 Inhibitors (Strong)

Decreased Effect There are no known significant interactions involving a decrease in effect.

Stability Store at room temperature; do not freeze

Mechanism of Action Penetrates inflamed epidermis to inhibit T cell activation by blocking transcription of proinflammatory cytokine genes such as interleukin-2, interferon gamma (Th1-type), interleukin-4, and interleukin-10 (Th2-type). Pimecrolimus binds to the intracellular protein FKBP-12, inhibiting calcineurin, which blocks cytokine transcription and inhibits T-cell activation. Prevents release of inflammatory cytokines and mediators from mast cells *in vitro* after stimulation by antigen/IgE.

Pharmacodynamics Onset of action: Time to significant improvement: 8 days

Pharmacokinetics (Adult data unless noted)

Absorption: Topical: Low systemic absorption; blood concentration of pimecrolimus was routinely <2 ng/mL with treatment of atopic dermatitis in adult patients (13% to 62% BSA involvement); blood concentration of pimecrolimus was <3 ng/mL in 26 pediatric patients 2-14 years of age with atopic dermatitis (20% to 69% BSA involvement). Detectable blood levels were observed in a higher proportion of children as compared to adults and may be due to the larger surface area to body mass ratio seen in pediatric patients.

Protein binding: 99.5%, primarily to various lipoproteins

Metabolism: In the liver by the cytochrome P450 3A4 system

Half-life: Terminal: 30-40 hours

Time to peak serum concentration: Topical: 2-6 hours

Elimination: 80% in the feces as metabolites

Dosing: Usual Children ≥2 years of age and Adults: Topical: Apply twice daily; use smallest amount of cream needed to control symptoms; continue therapy for as long as symptoms persist; re-evaluate patient at 6 weeks. **Note:** Pimecrolimus is not approved for use in children <2 years of age since the drug's long-term effect on the developing immune system is unknown. Detectable blood levels were observed in a higher proportion of children as compared to adults and may be due to the larger surface area to body mass ratio seen in pediatric patients. Children <2 years of age treated with pimecrolimus had a higher rate of upper respiratory infections than those treated with placebo.

Administration Topical: Avoid contact with eyes, nose, mouth, and cut, scraped, or infected skin areas. Wash hands with soap and water prior to and after cream application. If applying cream after a bath or shower, make sure skin is dry. Apply thin layer of cream by gently rubbing it in over affected skin surfaces which may include head and neck areas. The use of occlusive dressings is not recommended.

Monitoring Parameters Check skin for signs of worsening condition (increase in pruritus, erythema, excoriation, and lichenification)

Dosage Forms Excipient information presented when available (limited, particularly for generics); consult specific product labeling.

Cream, External:

Elidel: 1% (30 g, 60 g, 100 g) [contains benzyl alcohol, cetyl alcohol, propylene glycol]

References

Eichenfield LF, Lucky AW, Boguniewicz M, et al, "Safety and Efficacy of Pimecrolimus (ASM 981) Cream 1% in the Treatment of Mild and Moderate Atopic Dermatitis in Children and Adolescents," *J Am Acad Dermatol*, 2002, 46(4):495-504.

Wahn U, Bos JD, Goodfield M, et al, "Efficacy and Safety of Pimecrolimus Cream in the Long-Term Management of Atopic Dermatitis in Children," *Pediatrics*, 2002, 110(1 Pt 1):e2.

Wellington K and Jarvis B, "Topical Pimecrolimus: A Review of Its Clinical Potential in the Management of Atopic Dermatitis," *Drugs*, 2002, 62(5):817-40.

Pimozide (PI moe zide)

Medication Safety Issues

BEERS Criteria medication:
This drug may be potentially inappropriate for use in geriatric patients (Quality of evidence - moderate; Strength of recommendation - strong).

Brand Names: U.S. Orap

Brand Names: Canada Apo-Pimozide®; Orap®; PMS-Pimozide

Therapeutic Category Antipsychotic Agent, Typical

Generic Availability (U.S.) No

Use Suppression of severe motor and phonic (vocal) tics in patients with Tourette's disorder who have failed to respond satisfactorily to standard treatment and whose daily life function and/or development is severely compromised by the presence of motor and phonic tics (FDA approved in ages ≥2 years and adults)

Note: A trial of standard treatment is currently recommended before a trial of pimozide because of pimozide's potential cardiac toxicity (Scahill, 2006).

Pregnancy Risk Factor C

Pregnancy Considerations Adverse events were observed in some animal reproduction studies. Antipsychotic use during the third trimester of pregnancy has a risk for abnormal muscle movements (extrapyramidal symptoms [EPS]) and withdrawal symptoms in newborns following delivery. Symptoms in the newborn may include agitation, feeding disorder, hypertonia, hypotonia, respiratory distress, somnolence, and tremor; these effects may be self-limiting or require hospitalization. There are no adequate and well-controlled studies in pregnant women. Use only if potential benefit justifies risk to the fetus.

Breast-Feeding Considerations It is not known if pimozide is excreted in breast milk. Due to the potential for serious adverse reactions in the nursing infant, a decision should be made whether to discontinue nursing or to discontinue the drug, taking into account the importance of treatment to the mother.

Contraindications Hypersensitivity to pimozide or any component; simple tics or tics other than Tourette's disorder; patients receiving medications that can cause motor and phonic tics (eg, amphetamines, methylphenidate, pemoline) until these medications can be withdrawn to determine whether or not the drug (rather than Tourette's Disorder) is causing the tics; severe toxic CNS depression; coma; history of cardiac arrhythmias; congenital long QT syndrome; concurrent use with QT$_c$-prolonging agents; hypokalemia or hypomagnesemia; concurrent use of drugs that are inhibitors of cytochrome P450 CYP3A4, including azole antifungals (itraconazole, ketoconazole), macrolide antibiotics [ie, clarithromycin, erythromycin (**Note:** The manufacturer lists azithromycin, dirithromycin, and troleandomycin in its list of contraindicated macrolides; however, azithromycin does not inhibit CYP3A4, but may interact with pimozide on the basis of QT$_c$ prolongation)], citalopram, escitalopram, nefazodone, sertraline, protease inhibitors (eg, atazanavir, indinavir, nelfinavir, ritonavir, saquinavir), and other less potent inhibitors of CYP3A4 (eg, fluvoxamine, zileuton); concurrent use with strong CYP2D6 inhibitors (eg, paroxetine)

Warnings May alter cardiac conduction; sudden unexplained deaths have occurred in patients taking high doses (~1 mg/kg); deaths may be due to prolongation of the QT interval predisposing patients to ventricular arrhythmias; monitor ECG at baseline and periodically during dosage titration; correct any hypokalemia prior to initiation of therapy and maintain normal serum potassium during therapy. Pimozide may cause hypotension; incidence is less than other antipsychotics; use with caution in patients with autonomic instability, hemodynamic instability, hypovolemia, cerebrovascular or cardiovascular disease, or concurrent medications which may predispose to hypotension/bradycardia.

Patients who are genetically poor CYP2D6 metabolizers (~5% to 10% of the population) will display increased pimozide serum concentrations and a prolonged half-life that results in a longer time to achieve steady state (~2 weeks). Concentrations are similar to those seen with concurrent therapy with strong CYP2D6 inhibitors (ie, paroxetine). Dosage adjustments are recommended in these patients.

Pimozide may alter temperature regulation. May cause extrapyramidal symptoms, including pseudoparkinsonism, acute dystonic reactions, akathisia, and tardive dyskinesia; risk of these reactions is high relative to other neuroleptics, and is dose-dependent; to decrease risk of tardive dyskinesia: Use smallest dose and shortest duration possible; evaluate continued need periodically; risk of dystonia is increased with the use of high potency and higher doses of conventional antipsychotics and in males and younger patients. Use may be associated with neuroleptic malignant syndrome (NMS); monitor for mental status changes, fever, muscle rigidity, and/or autonomic instability; may also be associated with increased CPK, myogloburia, and acute renal failure; discontinue use if these symptoms occur; NMS may recur upon rechallenge.

Leukopenia, neutropenia, and agranulocytosis (sometimes fatal) have been reported in clinical trials and postmarketing reports with antipsychotic use; presence of risk factors (eg, preexisting low WBC or history of drug-induced leuko/neutropenia) should prompt periodic blood count assessment. Discontinue therapy at first signs of blood dyscrasias or if absolute neutrophil count <1000/mm^3.

Precautions May cause anticholinergic effects (confusion, agitation, constipation, xerostomia, blurred vision, urinary retention); use with caution in patients with decreased GI motility, urinary retention, BPH, xerostomia, or visual problems. Relative to neuroleptics, pimozide has a moderate potency of cholinergic blockade. Use with caution in patients with narrow-angle glaucoma; condition may be exacerbated by cholinergic blockade; screening is recommended. Use with caution in patients with myasthenia gravis; condition may be exacerbated by cholinergic blockade. Use with caution in patients with renal or hepatic impairment. Use with caution in patients at risk of seizures, including those with a history of seizures, head trauma, brain damage, alcoholism, or concurrent therapy with medications which may lower seizure threshold; antipsychotics may lower seizures threshold. Esophageal dysmotility and aspiration have been associated with antipsychotic use; use with caution in patients at risk of pneumonia (ie, Alzheimer's disease).

May be moderately sedating, use with caution in disorders where CNS depression is a feature; patients must be cautioned about performing tasks which require mental alertness (eg, operating machinery or driving). Pimozide may have a tumorigenic potential; a dose-related increase in pituitary tumors was observed in studies of mice; full significance in humans is unknown; however, this finding should be considered when deciding to use pimozide chronically in a young patient. Limited information about the use of pimozide in children <12 years of age exists. Antipsychotics are associated with increased prolactin levels; clinical significance of hyperprolactinemia in patients with breast cancer or other prolactin-dependent tumors is unknown.

Avoid abrupt discontinuation after prolonged use; abrupt discontinuation in patients receiving maintenance treatment may result in transient dyskinetic signs in some

◀ patients; these dyskinetic movements may not be distinguishable from tardive dyskinesia (except for duration).

Adverse Reactions

Cardiovascular: Abnormal ECG

Central nervous system: Akathisia, akinesia, behavior changes, depression, dreams abnormal, drowsiness, headache, hyperkinesias, insomnia, nervousness, sedation, somnolence

Dermatologic: Rash

Gastrointestinal: Appetite increased, constipation, diarrhea, dysphagia, salivation increased, taste disturbance, thirst, xerostomia

Genitourinary: Impotence

Neuromuscular & skeletal: Handwriting change, muscle tightness, myalgia, rigidity, stooped posture, torticollis, tremor, weakness

Ocular: Accommodation decreased, photophobia, visual disturbance

Rare but important or life-threatening (some reported for other than Tourette's disorder): Anorexia, blurred vision, cataracts, chest pain, diaphoresis, dizziness, excitement; extrapyramidal symptoms (dystonia, pseudoparkinsonism, tardive dyskinesia); GI distress, gingival hyperplasia (case report), hemolytic anemia, hyper-/hypotension, hyponatremia, libido decreased, nausea, neuroleptic malignant syndrome, orthostatic hypotension, nocturia, palpitation, periorbital edema, polyuria, QT$_c$ prolongation, seizure, skin irritation, syncope, tachycardia, ventricular arrhythmia, vomiting, weight gain/loss

Drug Interactions

Metabolism/Transport Effects Substrate of CYP1A2 (major), CYP2D6 (major), CYP3A4 (major); **Note:** Assignment of Major/Minor substrate status based on clinically relevant drug interaction potential; **Inhibits** CYP2C19 (weak), CYP2D6 (weak), CYP2E1 (weak), CYP3A4 (weak)

Avoid Concomitant Use

Avoid concomitant use of Pimozide with any of the following: Aclidinium; Amisulpride; Antifungal Agents (Azole Derivatives, Systemic); Aprepitant; Azelastine (Nasal); Boceprevir; Conivaptan; Crizotinib; CYP2D6 Inhibitors (Strong); CYP3A4 Inhibitors (Moderate); CYP3A4 Inhibitors (Strong); CYP3A4 Inhibitors (Weak); Enzalutamide; FLUoxetine; Fosaprepitant; Fusidic Acid (Systemic); Grapefruit Juice; Highest Risk QTc-Prolonging Agents; Ipratropium (Oral Inhalation); Ivabradine; Macrolide Antibiotics; Metoclopramide; Mifepristone; Moderate Risk QTc-Prolonging Agents; Nefazodone; Paraldehyde; Potassium Chloride; Protease Inhibitors; Selective Serotonin Reuptake Inhibitors; Sulpiride; Telaprevir; Thalidomide; Tiotropium; Umeclidinium; Zileuton

Increased Effect/Toxicity

Pimozide may increase the levels/effects of: AbobotulinumtoxinA; Alcohol (Ethyl); Amisulpride; Analgesics (Opioid); Anticholinergic Agents; Azelastine (Nasal); Buprenorphine; Cannabinoid-Containing Products; CNS Depressants; Highest Risk QTc-Prolonging Agents; Hydrocodone; Methylphenidate; Metyrosine; OnabotulinumtoxinA; Paraldehyde; Potassium Chloride; RimabotulinumtoxinB; Serotonin Modulators; Sulpiride; Thalidomide; Thiazide Diuretics; Tiotropium; Topiramate; Zolpidem

The levels/effects of Pimozide may be increased by: Acetylcholinesterase Inhibitors (Central); Aclidinium; Antifungal Agents (Azole Derivatives, Systemic); Aprepitant; Boceprevir; Brimonidine (Topical); Cannabis; Conivaptan; Crizotinib; CYP1A2 Inhibitors (Moderate); CYP1A2 Inhibitors (Strong); CYP2D6 Inhibitors (Moderate); CYP2D6 Inhibitors (Strong); CYP3A4 Inhibitors (Moderate); CYP3A4 Inhibitors (Strong); CYP3A4 Inhibitors (Weak); Deferasirox; Doxylamine; Dronabinol; FLUoxetine; Fosaprepitant; Fusidic Acid (Systemic);

Grapefruit Juice; HydrOXYzine; Ipratropium (Oral Inhalation); Ivabradine; Kava Kava; Luliconazole; Macrolide Antibiotics; Magnesium Sulfate; Methylphenidate; Metoclopramide; Metyrosine; Mifepristone; Moderate Risk QTc-Prolonging Agents; Nabilone; Nefazodone; Perampanel; Pramlintide; Protease Inhibitors; QTc-Prolonging Agents (Indeterminate Risk and Risk Modifying); Rufinamide; Selective Serotonin Reuptake Inhibitors; Serotonin Modulators; Simeprevir; Sodium Oxybate; Tapentadol; Telaprevir; Tetrahydrocannabinol; Umeclidinium; Zileuton

Decreased Effect

Pimozide may decrease the levels/effects of: Acetylcholinesterase Inhibitors (Central); Amphetamines; Anti-Parkinson's Agents (Dopamine Agonist); Quinagolide; Secretin

The levels/effects of Pimozide may be decreased by: Acetylcholinesterase Inhibitors (Central); Anti-Parkinson's Agents (Dopamine Agonist); Bosentan; Cannabis; CYP1A2 Inducers (Strong); CYP3A4 Inducers (Strong); Dabrafenib; Deferasirox; Enzalutamide; Mitotane; Peginterferon Alfa-2b; Siltuximab; St Johns Wort; Tocilizumab

Food Interactions Pimozide serum concentration may be increased when taken with grapefruit juice due to CYP3A4 inhibition. Management: Avoid concurrent use with grapefruit juice.

Stability Store at 25°C (77°F); excursions permitted to 15°C to 30°C (59°F to 86°F). Dispense in a tight, light-resistant container.

Mechanism of Action Pimozide, a diphenylbutylpiperidine conventional antipsychotic, is a potent centrally-acting dopamine-receptor antagonist resulting in its characteristic neuroleptic effects

Pharmacodynamics Onset of action: Within one week

Maximum effect: 4-6 weeks

Duration: Variable

Pharmacokinetics (Adult data unless noted)

Absorption: Oral: >50%

Protein binding: 99%

Metabolism: Hepatic via N-dealkylation primarily by CYP3A4, but with contributions by CYP1A2 and CYP2D6; significant first-pass effect

Half-life:

Tourette's disorder (Sallee, 1987):

Children 6-13 years (n=4): Mean ± SD: 66 ± 49 hours

Adults 23-39 years (n=7): Mean ± SD: 111 ± 57 hours

Schizophrenia: Adults: Mean: 55 hours

Time to peak serum concentration: 6-8 hours; range: 4-12 hours

Elimination: Urine

Dosing: Usual Note: Slow titration is recommended to improve tolerability; use lowest effective dose. An ECG should be performed baseline and periodically thereafter, especially during dosage adjustment.

Children and Adolescents: **Tourette's disorder:** Oral: Manufacturer's labeling: Children ≥2 years and Adolescents: Initial: 0.05 mg/kg/dose (maximum dose: 1 mg) once daily, preferably at bedtime; may increase dose every third day if needed; maximum daily dose: 0.2 mg/kg/**day** not to exceed 10 mg/**day**; in pediatric trials of children ≥7 years old, reported mean effective dose: 2.4-3.4 mg/day (range: 1-6 mg) (Gilbert, 2004; Sallee, 1997). **Note:** If therapy requires exceeding dose of 0.05 mg/kg/**day**, CYP2D6 geno-/phenotyping should be performed; CYP2D6 poor metabolizers should be dose titrated in ≥14-day increments and should not receive doses in excess of 0.05 mg/kg/**day**.

Adults: **Tourette's disorder:** Oral: Initial: 1-2 mg/day in divided doses, then increase dose as needed every other day; maximum daily dose: 10 mg/**day** or 0.2 mg/kg/**day** (whichever is less). **Note:** If therapy requires exceeding dose of 4 mg/day, CYP2D6 geno-/phenotyping should be performed; CYP2D6 poor metabolizers should be dose titrated in ≥14-day increments and should not receive doses in excess of 4 mg/**day**.

Dosing adjustment in renal impairment: Children ≥2 years, Adolescents, and Adults: There are no dosage adjustments provided in the manufacturer's labeling; use with caution.

Dosing adjustment in hepatic impairment: Children ≥2 years, Adolescents, and Adults: There are no dosage adjustments provided in the manufacturer's labeling; use with caution.

Dosing adjustment for toxicity: Children ≥2 years, Adolescents, and Adults:

ECG changes:

Children: QT_c prolongation >0.47 seconds or >25% above baseline: Decrease dose.

Adults: QT_c prolongation >0.52 seconds or >25% above baseline: Decrease dose.

Neuroleptic malignant syndrome: Discontinue; monitor carefully if therapy is reinitiated.

Tardive dyskinesia signs/symptoms: Consider discontinuing.

Administration May be administered without regard to meals.

Monitoring Parameters ECG should be performed at baseline and periodically thereafter, especially during dosage adjustment; vital signs; serum potassium; magnesium, sodium; renal and hepatic function; height, weight, BMI; mental status, abnormal involuntary movement scale (AIMS), extrapyramidal symptoms (EPS) screening; CBC with differential (patients with a history of low WBC or drug-induced leukopenia or neutropenia)

Test Interactions Increased prolactin (S)

Dosage Forms Excipient information presented when available (limited, particularly for generics); consult specific product labeling.

Tablet, Oral:

Orap: 1 mg, 2 mg [scored]

References

Bruggeman R, van der Linden C, Buitelaar JK, et al, "Risperidone Versus Pimozide in Tourette's Disorder: A Comparative Double-Blind Parallel-Group Study," *J Clin Psychiatry*, 2001, 62(1):50-6.

Bruun RD, "Subtle and Under-Recognized Side Effects of Neuroleptic Treatment in Children With Tourette's Disorder," *Am J Psychiatry*, 1988, 145(5):621-4.

Gilbert DL, Batterson JR, Sethuraman G, et al, "Tic Reduction With Risperidone Versus Pimozide in a Randomized, Double-Blind, Crossover Trial," *J Am Acad Child Adolesc Psychiatry*, 2004, 43(2):206-14.

Jankovic J, "Tourette's Syndrome," *NEJM*, 2001, 345(16):1184-92.

Jimenez-Jimenez FJ and Garcia-Ruiz PJ, "Pharmacological Options for the Treatment of Tourette's Disorder," *Drugs*, 2001, 61(15):2207-20.

Krähenbühl S, Sauter B, Kupferschmidt H, et al, "Case Report: Reversible QT Prolongation With Torsade de Pointes in a Patient With Pimozide Intoxication," *Am J Med Sci*, 1995, 309(6):315-6.

Larkin C, "Epileptogenic Effect of Pimozide," *Am J Psychiatry*, 1983, 140(3):372-3.

Muller-Vahl JT, "The Treatment of Tourette's Syndrome: Current Opinions," *Expert Opin Pharmacother*, 2002, 3(7):899-914.

"Pimozide (Orap) Contraindicated With Clarithromycin (Biaxin™) and Other Macrolide Antibiotics," *FDA Medical Bulletin*, October 1996, 3.

Roessner V, Plessen KJ, Rothenberger A, et al, "European Clinical Guidelines for Tourette Syndrome and Other Tic Disorders. Part II: Pharmacological Treatment," *Eur Child Adolesc Psychiatry*, 2011, 20 (4):173-96.

Sallee FR, Dougherty D, Sethuraman G, et al, "Prolactin Monitoring of Haloperidol and Pimozide Treatment in Children With Tourette's Syndrome," *Biol Psychiatry*, 1996, 40(10):1044-50.

Sallee FR, Nesbitt L, Jackson C, et al, "Relative Efficacy of Haloperidol and Pimozide in Children and Adolescents With Tourette's Disorder," *Am J Psychiatry*, 1997, 154(8):1057-62.

Sallee FR, Pollock BG, Stiller RL, et al, "Pharmacokinetics of Pimozide in Adults and Children With Tourette's Syndrome," *J Clin Pharmacol*, 1987, 27(10):776-81.

Scahill L, Erenberg G, Berlin CM Jr, et al, "Contemporary Assessment and Pharmacotherapy of Tourette Syndrome," *NeuroRx*, 2006, 3 (2):192-206.

◆ **Pin-X [OTC]** see Pyrantel Pamoate on page 1774

◆ **Pink Bismuth** see Bismuth on page 294

◆ **Pink Bismuth [OTC]** see Bismuth on page 294

◆ **Pinnacaine Otic** see Benzocaine on page 273

Piperacillin and Tazobactam

(pi PER a sil in & ta zoe BAK tam)

Medication Safety Issues

Sound-alike/look-alike issues:

Zosyn may be confused with Zofran, Zyvox

International issues:

Tazact [India] may be confused with Tazac brand name for nizatidine [Australia]; Tiazac brand name for diltiazem [U.S., Canada]

Brand Names: U.S. Zosyn

Brand Names: Canada AJ-PIP/TAZ; Piperacillin and Tazobactam for Injection; Tazocin

Therapeutic Category Antibiotic, Beta-lactam and Beta-lactamase Inhibitor Combination; Antibiotic, Penicillin (Antipseudomonal)

Generic Availability (U.S.) Yes: Excludes infusion

Use Treatment of moderate to severe infections caused by susceptible organisms (FDA approved in ages ≥2 months and adults); including sepsis, postpartum endometritis or pelvic inflammatory disease, intra-abdominal infections, uncomplicated or complicated infections involving skin and skin structures, moderate severity community-acquired pneumonia, and moderate to severe nosocomial pneumonia. Tazobactam expands activity of piperacillin to include beta-lactamase producing strains of *S. aureus, H. influenzae, B. fragilis, Klebsiella, E. coli,* and *Acinetobacter.* When piperacillin and tazobactam is used to treat nosocomial pneumonia caused by *P. aeruginosa,* combination therapy with an aminoglycoside is recommended.

Pregnancy Risk Factor B

Pregnancy Considerations Adverse events have not been observed in animal reproduction studies. Piperacillin and tazobactam both cross the placenta and are found in the fetal serum, placenta, amniotic fluid, and fetal urine. When used during pregnancy, the clearance and volume of distribution of piperacillin/tazobactam are increased; half-life and AUC are decreased (Bourget, 1998). Piperacillin/tazobactam is approved for the treatment of postpartum gynecologic infections, including endometritis or pelvic inflammatory disease, caused by susceptible organisms.

Breast-Feeding Considerations Low concentrations of piperacillin are excreted in breast milk; information for tazobactam is not available. The manufacturer recommends that caution be used when administering piperacillin/tazobactam to nursing women. Nondose-related effects could include modification of bowel flora.

Contraindications Hypersensitivity to piperacillin, tazobactam, penicillins, cephalosporins, beta-lactamase inhibitors, or any component

Warnings Serious and occasionally fatal hypersensitivity (anaphylactoid) reactions have been reported in patients on penicillin therapy, especially with a history of beta-lactam hypersensitivity, history of sensitivity to multiple allergens, or previous IgE-mediated reactions (eg, anaphylaxis, angioedema, urticaria); administration to patients with confirmed penicillin or cephalosporin allergies is contraindicated; immediate treatment for anaphylactoid reaction should be available during administration. Prolonged use may result in fungal or bacterial superinfection, including *C. difficile*-associated diarrhea (CDAD) and pseudomembranous colitis; CDAD has been observed >2 months postantibiotic treatment. Abnormal platelet aggregation and prolonged bleeding have been reported in patients with renal failure. Piperacillin therapy has been associated with an increased incidence of fever and rash in cystic fibrosis patients.

Precautions Use with caution in patients with renal impairment or underdeveloped kidneys; due to sodium load and ▶

◀ to the adverse effects of high serum concentrations of penicillins; dosage adjustment recommended. Use with caution in patients with a history of seizure disorder; high levels, particularly in the presence of renal impairment, may increase risk of seizures.

Adverse Reactions

Cardiovascular: Chest pain, edema, hypertension, phlebitis

Central nervous system: Agitation, anxiety, dizziness, headache, insomnia, pain

Dermatologic: Pruritus, skin rash

Gastrointestinal: Abdominal pain, change in stool, constipation, diarrhea, dyspepsia, nausea, oral candidiasis, vomiting

Hepatic: Increased serum AST

Local: Local irritation

Infection: Abscess, candidiasis, infection, sepsis

Respiratory: Dyspnea, pharyngitis, rhinitis

Miscellaneous: Fever

Rare but important or life-threatening: Agranulocytosis, anaphylactoid reaction, anaphylaxis, anemia, aphthous stomatitis, atrial fibrillation, bradycardia, cardiac arrest, cardiac arrhythmia, cardiac failure, change in platelet count, cholestatic jaundice, circulatory arrest, *Clostridium difficile* associated diarrhea, confusion, convulsions, decreased hematocrit, decreased hemoglobin, decreased serum albumin, depression, dysgeusia, dysuria, electrolyte disturbance, eosinophilia, epistaxis, erythema multiforme, gastritis, genital pruritus, hallucination, hematuria, hemolytic anemia, hemorrhage, hepatitis, hiccups, hyperglycemia, hypersensitivity reaction, hypoglycemia, increased blood glucose, increased blood urea nitrogen, increased gamma-glutamyl transferase, increased serum alkaline phosphatase, increased serum ALT, increased serum AST, increased serum bilirubin, increased serum creatinine, increased thirst, inflammation, interstitial nephritis, intestinal obstruction, leukopenia, leukorrhea, melena, mesenteric embolism, myalgia, myocardial infarction, neutropenia, oliguria, pancytopenia, photophobia, positive direct Coombs test, prolonged partial thromboplastin time, prolonged prothrombin time, pulmonary edema, pulmonary embolism, purpura, renal failure, rigors, Stevens-Johnson syndrome, supraventricular tachycardia, syncope, thrombocythemia, thrombocytopenia, thrombophlebitis, toxic epidermal necrolysis, urinary incontinence, urinary retention, vaginitis, ventricular fibrillation, ventricular tachycardia

Drug Interactions

Metabolism/Transport Effects None known.

Avoid Concomitant Use

Avoid concomitant use of Piperacillin and Tazobactam with any of the following: BCG; Probenecid

Increased Effect/Toxicity

Piperacillin and Tazobactam may increase the levels/effects of: Floxacillin; Methotrexate; Vecuronium; Vitamin K Antagonists

The levels/effects of Piperacillin and Tazobactam may be increased by: Probenecid

Decreased Effect

Piperacillin and Tazobactam may decrease the levels/effects of: Aminoglycosides; BCG; Mycophenolate; Sodium Picosulfate; Typhoid Vaccine

The levels/effects of Piperacillin and Tazobactam may be decreased by: Tetracycline Derivatives

Stability Parenteral:

Vials: Store intact vials at 20°C to 25°C (68°F to 77°F). Reconstituted piperacillin/tazobactam solution is stable for 24 hours at room temperature and 48 hours when refrigerated

Premixed solution: Store at -20°C (-4°F); thawed solution is stable for 24 hours at room temperature or 14 days refrigerated; do not refreeze

Mechanism of Action Piperacillin inhibits bacterial cell wall synthesis by binding to one or more of the penicillin-binding proteins (PBPs); which in turn inhibits the final transpeptidation step of peptidoglycan synthesis in bacterial cell walls, thus inhibiting cell wall biosynthesis. Bacteria eventually lyse due to ongoing activity of cell wall autolytic enzymes (autolysins and murein hydrolases) while cell wall assembly is arrested. Piperacillin exhibits time-dependent killing. Tazobactam inhibits many beta-lactamases, including staphylococcal penicillinase and Richmond-Sykes types 2, 3, 4, and 5, including extended spectrum enzymes; it has only limited activity against class 1 beta-lactamases other than class 1C types.

Pharmacokinetics (Adult data unless noted) Both AUC and peak concentrations are dose proportional

Distribution: Widely distributed into tissues and body fluids including lungs, intestinal mucosa, female reproductive tissues, interstitial fluid, gallbladder, and bile; penetration into CSF is poor when meninges are uninflamed

V_d: Children and Adults: 0.243 L/kg

Protein binding:

Piperacillin: ~26% to 33%

Tazobactam: 31% to 32%

Metabolism:

Piperacillin: 6% to 9% to desethyl metabolite (weak activity)

Tazobactam: ~22% to inactive metabolite

Bioavailability: I.M.:

Piperacillin: 71%

Tazobactam: 84%

Half-life (Pediatric data: Reed, 1994):

Piperacillin:

Infants 2-5 months: 1.4 hours

Children 6-23 months: 0.9 hour

Children 2-12 years: 0.7 hour

Adults: 0.7-1.2 hours

Metabolite: 1-1.5 hours

Tazobactam:

Infants 2-5 months: 1.6 hours

Children 6-23 months: 1 hour

Children 2-12 years: 0.8-0.9 hour

Adults: 0.7-0.9 hour

Elimination: Piperacillin and tazobactam are both eliminated by renal tubular secretion and glomerular filtration. Piperacillin, tazobactam, and desethylpiperacillin are also secreted into bile.

Piperacillin: 50% to 70% eliminated unchanged in urine

Tazobactam: Found in urine at 24 hours, with 20% as the inactive metabolite and 80% as unchanged drug

Clearance: Children 9 months to 12 years: 5.64 mL/minute/kg

Dosing: Neonatal Zosyn (piperacillin and tazobactam) is a combination product; each 3.375 g vial contains 3 g piperacillin sodium and 0.375 g tazobactam sodium in an 8:1 ratio. Dosage recommendations are based on the **piperacillin** component.

General dosing, susceptible infection:

Weight-directed dosing (*Red Book*, 2012): I.V.:

Body weight <1 kg:

PNA ≤14 days: 100 mg piperacillin/kg/dose every 12 hours

PNA 15 to 28 days: 100 mg piperacillin/kg/dose every 8 hours

Body weight ≥1 kg:

PNA ≤7 days: 100 mg piperacillin/kg/dose every 12 hours

PNA 8 to 28 days: 100 mg piperacillin/kg/dose every 8 hours

Age-directed dosing: **Note:** Limited data available, positive efficacy results, dosage regimens variable, dosing partially extrapolated from piperacillin data; further studies are needed (Kacet, 1992)

GA <36 weeks:

PNA 0 to 7 days: 75 mg/kg/dose every 12 hours

PNA 8 to 28 days: 75 mg/kg/dose every 8 hours

Meningitis: PNA 0 to 7 days: 200 mg/kg/dose every 12 hours of piperacillin was used in two neonates (GA: 31, 35 weeks) (Placzek, 1983)

GA ≥36 weeks:

PNA 0 to 7 days: 75 mg/kg/dose every 8 hours

PNA 8 to 28 days: 75 mg/kg/dose every 6 hours

Dosing: Usual

Infants, Children, and Adolescents: Zosyn (piperacillin and tazobactam) is a combination product; each 3.375 g vial contains 3 g piperacillin sodium and 0.375 g tazobactam sodium in an 8:1 ratio. Dosage recommendations are based on the **piperacillin** component. **Note:** Some centers divide doses every 6 hours for enhanced pharmacodynamic profile. Unless otherwise specified, dosing presented is based on traditional infusion method (I.V. infusion over 30 minutes).

General dosing, susceptible infection (*Red Book* [AAP], 2012): I.V.: Severe infections:

Infants <2 months: 100 mg piperacillin/kg/dose every 6 hours

Infants 2 to 9 months: 80 mg piperacillin/kg/dose every 8 hours

Infants >9 months, Children, and Adolescents: 100 mg piperacillin/kg/dose every 8 hours; maximum daily dose: 16 g/**day**

Appendicitis and/or peritonitis: I.V.:

Infants 2 to 9 months: 80 mg of piperacillin/kg/dose every 8 hours

Infants >9 months and Children weighing ≤40 kg: 100 mg piperacillin/kg/dose every 8 hours

Children weighing >40 kg and Adolescents: 3000 mg (3.375 g piperacillin/tazobactam product) every 6 hours; maximum daily dose: 16 g/**day**

Cystic fibrosis, pseudomonal lung infection: Note: Multiple dosing approaches have been evaluated; optimal dose may vary based on disease severity, susceptibility patterns (eg, MIC), or patient tolerability:

Standard dosing range: I.V.: 240 to 400 mg piperacillin/kg/day divided every 8 hours (Kleigman, 2011); others have used 350 to 400 mg/kg/day divided every 4 hours in early piperacillin trials (Zobell, 2013)

High-dose: Limited data available: I.V.: 450 mg/kg/day every 4 to 6 hours or 600 mg/kg/day divided every 4 hours has been described from early studies of piperacillin alone; usual maximum daily dose: 18 to 24 g/**day**. **Note:** Piperacillin doses >600 mg/kg/day or an extended duration of therapy (>14 days) have been associated with dose-related adverse effects including serum sickness, immune-mediated hemolytic anemia and bone marrow suppression (Zobell, 2013).

Intra-abdominal infection, complicated: I.V.: 200 to 300 mg piperacillin/kg/day divided every 6 to 8 hours; maximum daily dose: 12 g/**day** (Solomkin, 2010)

Surgical antimicrobial prophylaxis (Bratzler, 2013): I.V.:

Infants 2 to 9 months: 80 mg/kg piperacillin component 30 to 60 minutes prior to procedure; may repeat in 2 hours

Infants >9 months, Children, and Adolescents weighing ≤40 kg: 100 mg/kg piperacillin component 30 to 60 minutes prior to procedure; may repeat in 2 hours

Adolescents weighing >40 kg: 3000 mg (3.375 g piperacillin/tazobactam product) 30 to 60 minutes prior to procedure; may repeat in 2 hours

Extended-infusion method: Limited data available: I.V.: Children and Adolescents: 100 mg piperacillin/kg/dose infused over 4 hours 3 times daily. Dosing based on a prospective, observational study (n=332) in a single

children's hospital comparing the extended interval method to traditional dosing (Nichols, 2012).

Adults: **Note:** Dosing expressed as total dose of combination product (piperacillin/tazobactam); dosing presented is based on traditional infusion method (I.V. infusion over 30 minutes) unless otherwise specified as the extended infusion method (I.V. infusion over 4 hours)

General dosing, susceptible infection: I.V.: 3.375 **g** (3000 mg piperacillin/375 mg tazobactam) every 6 hours

Extended-infusion method: 3.375 to 4.5 **g** I.V. over 4 hours every 8 hours (Kim, 2007; Shea, 2009); an alternative regimen of 4.5 **g** I.V. over 3 hours every 6 hours has also been described (Kim, 2007)

Diverticulitis, intra-abdominal abscess, peritonitis: I.V.: 3.375 **g** every 6 hours; **Note:** Some clinicians use 4.5 **g** every 8 hours for empiric coverage since the% time>MIC is similar between the regimens for most pathogens; however, this regimen is **not** recommended for nosocomial pneumonia or *Pseudomonas* coverage.

Intra-abdominal infection, complicated: I.V.: 3.375 **g** every 6 hours for 4 to 7 days (provided source controlled); **Note:** Increase to 3.375 **g** every 4 hours or 4.5 **g** every 6 hours if *P. aeruginosa* is suspected. Not recommended for mild to moderate, community-acquired intra-abdominal infections due to risk of toxicity and the development of resistant organisms (Solomkin, 2010).

Pneumonia, nosocomial: I.V.: 4.5 **g** every 6 hours for 7 to 14 days (when used empirically, combination with an aminoglycoside or antipseudomonal fluoroquinolone is recommended; consider discontinuation of additional agent if *P. aeruginosa* is not isolated)

Severe infections: I.V.: 3.375 **g** every 6 hours for 7 to 10 days; **Note:** Some clinicians use 4.5 **g** every 8 hours for empiric coverage since the%time>MIC is similar between the regimens for most pathogens; however, this regimen is **not** recommended for nosocomial pneumonia or *Pseudomonas* coverage.

Skin and soft tissue infection: I.V.: 3.375 **g** every 6 to 8 hours for 7 to 14 days. **Notes:** When used for necrotizing infection of skin, fascia, or muscle, combination with clindamycin and ciprofloxacin is recommended (Stevens, 2005); for severe diabetic foot infections, recommended treatment duration is up to 4 weeks depending on severity of infection and response to therapy (Lipsky, 2012).

Dosing adjustment in renal impairment:

Infants, Children, and Adolescents: There are no dosage adjustments provided in the manufacturer's labeling; however, the following have been used by some clinicians (Aronoff, 2007): Dosing based on a usual dose of 200 to 300 piperacillin component mg/kg/day in divided doses every 6 hours.

GFR >50 mL/minute/1.73 m^2: No adjustment required

GFR 30 to 50 mL/minute/1.73 m^2: 35 to 50 mg piperacillin component/kg every 6 hours

GFR <30 mL/minute/1.73 m^2: 35 to 50 mg piperacillin component/kg every 8 hours

Intermittent hemodialysis (IHD): Hemodialysis removes 30% to 40% of a piperacillin/tazobactam dose: 50 to 75 mg piperacillin/kg every 12 hours

Peritoneal dialysis (PD): Peritoneal dialysis removes 21% of tazobactam and 6% of piperacillin: 50 to 75 mg piperacillin/kg every 12 hours

Continuous renal replacement therapy (CRRT): 35 to 50 mg piperacillin/kg every 8 hours

Adults:

Traditional infusion method (ie, I.V. infusion over 30 minutes): Manufacturer's labeling:

Nosocomial pneumonia:

CrCl >40 mL/minute: No adjustment needed

CrCl 20 to 40 mL/minute: 3.375 **g** every 6 hours

◄ CrCl <20 mL/minute: 2.25 **g** every 6 hours
Hemodialysis: 2.25 **g** every 8 hours with an additional dose of 0.75 **g** after each dialysis
CAPD: Adults: 2.25 **g** every 8 hours
All other indications:
CrCl >40 mL/minute: No adjustment needed
CrCl 20 to 40 mL/minute: 2.25 **g** every 6 hours
CrCl <20 mL/minute: 2.25 **g** every 8 hours
Hemodialysis: Hemodialysis removes 30% to 40% of a piperacillin/tazobactam dose: 2.25 **g** every 12 hours with an additional dose of 0.75 **g** after each dialysis
CAPD: Peritoneal dialysis removes 21% of tazobactam and 6% of piperacillin: 2.25 **g** every 12 hours

Dosing adjustment in patients with hepatic cirrhosis: No dosing adjustment required

Administration Parenteral: Intermittent I.V. infusion: May administer over 30 minutes at a maximum concentration of 200 mg/mL (piperacillin component); however, concentrations ≤20 mg/mL are preferred.

Monitoring Parameters Serum electrolytes, bleeding time especially in patients with renal impairment; periodic tests of renal, hepatic, and hematologic function; observe for changes in bowel frequency, CBC with differential; monitor for signs of anaphylaxis during first dose

Test Interactions Positive Coombs' [direct] test; false positive reaction for urine glucose using copper-reduction method (Clinitest®); may result in false positive results with the Platelia® *Aspergillus* enzyme immunoassay (EIA)

Some penicillin derivatives may accelerate the degradation of aminoglycosides *in vitro*, leading to a potential underestimation of aminoglycoside serum concentration. **Note:** Reformulated Zosyn® containing EDTA has been shown to be compatible *in vitro* for Y-site infusion with amikacin and gentamicin diluted in NS or D_5W (applies **only** to specific concentrations and varies by product; consult manufacturer's labeling). Reformulated Zosyn® containing EDTA is **not** compatible with tobramycin.

Additional Information Some penicillins (eg, carbenicillin, ticarcillin, and piperacillin) have been shown to inactivate aminoglycosides *in vitro*. This has been observed to a greater extent with tobramycin and gentamicin, while amikacin has shown greater stability against inactivation. Concurrent use of these agents may pose a risk of reduced antibacterial efficacy *in vivo*, particularly in the setting of profound renal impairment. However, definitive clinical evidence is lacking. If combination penicillin/aminoglycoside therapy is desired in a patient with renal dysfunction, separation of doses (if feasible), and routine monitoring of aminoglycoside levels, CBC, and clinical response should be considered. **Note:** Reformulated Zosyn® containing EDTA has been shown to be compatible *in vitro* for Y-site infusion with amikacin and gentamicin diluted in NS or D_5W (applies only to specific concentrations and varies by product; consult manufacturer's labeling). Reformulated Zosyn® containing EDTA is not compatible with tobramycin.

Dosage Forms Excipient information presented when available (limited, particularly for generics); consult specific product labeling.

Note: 8:1 ratio of piperacillin sodium/tazobactam sodium

Infusion [premixed non-osmotic solution]:
Zosyn®: 2.25 g: Piperacillin 2 g and tazobactam 0.25 g (50 mL) [contains edetate disodium, sodium 128 mg (5.58 mEq)]
Zosyn®: 3.375 g: Piperacillin 3 g and tazobactam 0.375 g (50 mL) [contains edetate disodium, sodium 192 mg (8.38 mEq)]
Zosyn®: 4.5 g: Piperacillin 4 g and tazobactam 0.5 g (100 mL) [contains edetate disodium, sodium 256 mg (11.17 mEq)]

Injection, powder for reconstitution: 2.25 g: Piperacillin 2 g and tazobactam 0.25 g; 3.375 g: Piperacillin 3 g and tazobactam 0.375 g; 4.5 g: Piperacillin 4 g and tazobactam 0.5 g; 40.5 g: Piperacillin 36 g and tazobactam 4.5 g

Zosyn®: 2.25 g: Piperacillin 2 g and tazobactam 0.25 g [contains edetate disodium, sodium 128 mg (5.58 mEq)]
Zosyn®: 3.375 g: Piperacillin 3 g and tazobactam 0.375 g [contains edetate disodium, sodium 192 mg (8.38 mEq)]
Zosyn®: 4.5 g: Piperacillin 4 g and tazobactam 0.5 g [contains edetate disodium, sodium 256 mg (11.17 mEq)]
Zosyn®: 40.5 g: Piperacillin 36 g and tazobactam 4.5 g [contains edetate disodium, sodium 2304 mg (100.4 mEq); bulk pharmacy vial]

References

American Academy of Pediatrics (AAP). In: Pickering LK, Baker CJ, Kimberlin DW, Long SS, eds. *Red Book: 2012 Report of the Committee on Infectious Diseases.* 29th ed. Elk Grove Village, IL: American Academy of Pediatrics; 2012.

Aronoff GR, Bennett WM, Berns JS, et al, *Drug Prescribing in Renal Failure: Dosing Guidelines for Adults and Children,* 5th ed. Philadelphia, PA: American College of Physicians; 2007.

Bourget P, Sertin A, Lesne-Hulin A, et al, "Influence of Pregnancy on the Pharmacokinetic Behaviour and the Transplacental Transfer of the Piperacillin-Tazobactam Combination," *Eur J Obstet Gynecol Reprod Biol,* 1998, 76(1):21-7.

Bratzler DW, Dellinger EP, Olsen KM, et al, "Clinical Practice Guidelines for Antimicrobial Prophylaxis in Surgery," *Am J Health Syst Pharm,* 2013, 70(3):195-283.

Bryson HM and Brogden RN, "Piperacillin/Tazobactam. A Review of its Antibacterial Activity, Pharmacokinetic Properties, and Therapeutic Potential," *Drugs,* 1994, 47(3):506-35.

Flidel-Rimon O, Friedman S, Gradstein S, et al, "Reduction in Multiresistant Nosocomial Infections in Neonates Following Substitution of Ceftazidime With Piperacillin/Tazobactam in Empiric Antibiotic Therapy," *Acta Paediatr,* 2003, 92(10):1205-7.

Flidel-Rimon O, Friedman S, Leibovitz E, et al, "The Use of Piperacillin/Tazobactam (in Association With Amikacin) in Neonatal Sepsis: Efficacy and Safety Data," *Scand J Infect Dis,* 2006, 38(1):36-42.

Kim A, Sutherland CA, Kuti JL, et al, "Optimal Dosing of piperacillin-Tazobactam for the Treatment of *Pseudomonas aeruginosa* Infections: Prolonged or Continuous Infusion?" *Pharmacotherapy,* 2007, 27(11):1490-7.

Kliegman RM, Stanton BF, St. Gemell JW, et al, eds. *Nelson Textbook of Pediatrics.* 19th ed. Philadelphia, PA: Saunders Elsevier;2011.

Lipsky BA, Berendt AR, Cornia PB, et al, "2012 Infectious Diseases Society of America Clinical Practice Guideline for the Diagnosis and Treatment of Diabetic Foot Infections," *Clin Infect Dis,* 2012, 54(12):e132-73.

Nichols KR, Knoderer CA, Cox EG, et al, "System-Wide Implementation of the Use of an Extended-Infusion Piperacillin/Tazobactam Dosing Strategy: Feasibility of Utilization From a Children's Hospital Perspective," *Clin Ther,* 2012, 34(6):1459-65.

Pillay T, Pillay DG, Adhikari M, et al, "Piperacillin/Tazobactam in the Treatment of *Klebsiella pneumoniae* Infections in Neonates," *Am J Perinatol,* 1998, 15(1):47-51.

Reed MD, Goldfarb J, Yamashita T, et al, "Single-Dose Pharmacokinetics of Piperacillin and Tazobactam in Infants and Children," *Antimicrob Agents Chemother,* 1994, 38(12):2817-26.

Rubino CM, Gal P, and Ransom JL, "A Review of the Pharmacokinetic and Pharmacodynamic Characteristics of Beta-Lactam/Beta-Lactamase Inhibitor Combination Antibiotics in Premature Infants," *Pediatr Infect Dis J,* 1998, 17(12):1200-10.

Shea KM, Cheatham SC, Smith DW, et al, "Comparative Pharmacodynamics of Intermittent and Prolonged Infusions of Piperacillin/Tazobactam Using Monte Carlo Simulations and Steady-State Pharmacokinetic Data From Hospitalized Patients," *Ann Pharmacother,* 2009, 43(11):1747-54.

Solomkin JS, Mazuski JE, Bradley JS, et al, "Diagnosis and Management of Complicated Intra-abdominal Infection in Adults and Children: Guidelines by the Surgical Infection Society and the Infectious Diseases Society of America," *Clin Infect Dis,* 2010, 50(2):133-64.

Zobell JT, Waters CD, Young DC, et al, "Optimization of Anti-Pseudomonal Antibiotics for Cystic Fibrosis Pulmonary Exacerbations: II. Cephalosporins and Penicillins," *Pediatr Pulmonol,* 2013, 48(2):107-22.

◆ **Piperacillin and Tazobactam for Injection (Can)** *see* Piperacillin and Tazobactam *on page 1679*

◆ **Piperacillin and Tazobactam Sodium** *see* Piperacillin and Tazobactam *on page 1679*

◆ **Piperacillin Sodium and Tazobactam Sodium** *see* Piperacillin and Tazobactam *on page 1679*

Pirbuterol (peer BYOO ter ole)

Brand Names: U.S. Maxair Autohaler [DSC]
Therapeutic Category Adrenergic Agonist Agent; Antiasthmatic; Beta$_2$-Adrenergic Agonist; Bronchodilator; Sympathomimetic
Generic Availability (U.S.) No
Use Prevention and treatment of bronchospasm in patients with reversible airway obstruction due to asthma or COPD
Pregnancy Risk Factor C
Pregnancy Considerations Adverse events have been observed in some animal reproduction studies. Beta-agonists may interfere with uterine contractility if administered during labor.

Uncontrolled asthma is associated with adverse events on pregnancy (increased risk of perinatal mortality, preeclampsia, preterm birth, low birth weight infants). Other beta$_2$-receptor agonists are preferred for the treatment of asthma during pregnancy (NAEPP, 2005).
Breast-Feeding Considerations It is not known if pirbuterol is excreted into breast milk. The manufacturer recommends that pirbuterol be used in breast-feeding women only if the potential benefit to the mother outweighs the possible risk to the infant. The use of beta$_2$-receptor agonists are not considered a contraindication to breastfeeding (NAEPP, 2005).
Contraindications Hypersensitivity to pirbuterol or or any component
Warnings Paradoxical bronchospasm may occur, especially with the first use of a new cannister
Precautions Use with caution in patients with hyperthyroidism, diabetes mellitus, cardiovascular disorders (including coronary insufficiency or hypertension); excessive or prolonged use can lead to tolerance
Adverse Reactions
Cardiovascular: Palpitations, tachycardia
Central nervous system: Dizziness, headache, nervousness, tremor
Endocrine & metabolic: Decreased serum potassium, increased serum glucose
Gastrointestinal: Nausea
Rare but important or life-threatening: Chest pain, confusion, depression, hypotension, insomnia, numbness of extremities, pruritus, skin rash, sore throat, syncope
Drug Interactions
Metabolism/Transport Effects None known.
Avoid Concomitant Use
Avoid concomitant use of Pirbuterol with any of the following: Beta-Blockers (Nonselective); Iobenguane I 123
Increased Effect/Toxicity
Pirbuterol may increase the levels/effects of: Atosiban; Loop Diuretics; Sympathomimetics; Thiazide Diuretics

The levels/effects of Pirbuterol may be increased by: AtoMOXetine; Cannabinoid-Containing Products; Linezolid; MAO Inhibitors; Tricyclic Antidepressants
Decreased Effect
Pirbuterol may decrease the levels/effects of: Iobenguane I 123

The levels/effects of Pirbuterol may be decreased by: Beta-Blockers (Beta1 Selective); Beta-Blockers (Nonselective); Betahistine
Stability Store at room temperature
Mechanism of Action Pirbuterol is a beta$_2$-adrenergic agonist with a similar structure to albuterol, specifically a pyridine ring has been substituted for the benzene ring in albuterol. The increased beta$_2$ selectivity of pirbuterol

results from the substitution of a tertiary butyl group on the nitrogen of the side chain, which additionally imparts resistance of pirbuterol to degradation by monoamine oxidase and provides a lengthened duration of action in comparison to the less selective beta-agonist agents.
Pharmacodynamics
Onset of action: 5 minutes
Maximum effect: 30-60 minutes
Duration: 5 hours
Pharmacokinetics (Adult data unless noted)
Metabolism: Liver (by sulfate conjugation)
Half-life: 2 hours
Elimination: 51% excreted in the urine as pirbuterol plus its sulfate conjugate
Dosing: Usual Oral inhalation:
Acute asthma exacerbation (NIH guidelines):
Children: 4-8 inhalations every 20 minutes for 3 doses then every 1-4 hours
Children >12 years and Adults: 4-8 inhalations every 20 minutes for up to 4 hours then every 1-4 hours
Maintenance therapy (nonacute) (NIH guidelines): Children and Adults: 2 inhalations 3-4 times/day
Administration Oral inhalation: Shake well before administration; "prime" (test spray) inhaler prior to first use and if it has not been used for 48 hours; use spacer for children <8 years of age (Maxair™ Inhaler only); Maxair™ Autohaler™ is breath activated; after sealing lips around mouthpiece, inhale deeply with steady, moderate force; inhalation triggers the release "puff" of medication; do not stop inhalation when puff occurs, but continue to take a deep, full breath; hold breath for 10 seconds, then exhale slowly
Monitoring Parameters Serum potassium, heart rate, pulmonary function tests, respiratory rate; arterial or capillary blood gases (if patient's condition warrants)
Dosage Forms Considerations
Maxair Autohaler 14 g canisters contain 400 inhalations.
Maxair Autohaler contains chlorofluorocarbons
Dosage Forms Excipient information presented when available (limited, particularly for generics); consult specific product labeling. [DSC] = Discontinued product
Aerosol Breath Activated, Inhalation, as acetate:
Maxair Autohaler: 200 mcg/INH (14 g [DSC])
References
"Guidelines for the Diagnosis and Management of Asthma. NAEPP Expert Panel Report 3," August 2007, www.nhlbi.nih.gov/guidelines/asthma/asthgdln.pdf.
"National Asthma Education and Prevention Program. Expert Panel Report: Guidelines for the Diagnosis and Management of Asthma Update on Selected Topics–2002," *J Allergy Clin Immunol*, 2002, 110 (5 Suppl):S141-219.
National Asthma Education and Prevention Program (NAEPP) Working Group Report on "Managing Asthma During Pregnancy: Recommendations for Pharmacologic Treatment," National Institutes of Health, National Heart, Lung, and Blood Institute, NIH Publication No. 05-5236, March 2005. Available at http://www.nhlbi.nih.gov/health/prof/lung/asthma/astpreg/astpreg_full.pdf

◆ **Pirbuterol Acetate** *see* Pirbuterol *on page 1683*

Piroxicam (peer OKS i kam)

Medication Safety Issues
Sound-alike/look-alike issues:
Feldene may be confused with FLUoxetine
Piroxicam may be confused with PARoxetine
BEERS Criteria medication:
This drug may be potentially inappropriate for use in geriatric patients (Quality of evidence - moderate; Strength of recommendation - strong).
International issues:
Flogene [Brazil] may be confused with Flogen brand name for naproxen [Mexico]; Florone brand name for diflorasone [Germany, Greece]; Flovent brand name for fluticasone [U.S., Canada]

Related Information

Oral Medications That Should Not Be Crushed or Altered
on page 2438

Brand Names: U.S. Feldene

Brand Names: Canada Apo-Piroxicam; Dom-Piroxicam; PMS-Piroxicam

Therapeutic Category Analgesic, Non-narcotic; Anti-inflammatory Agent; Nonsteroidal Anti-inflammatory Drug (NSAID), Oral

Generic Availability (U.S.) Yes

Use Management of rheumatoid arthritis and osteoarthritis (FDA approved in adults); has also been used to treat juvenile idiopathic arthritis

Medication Guide Available Yes

Pregnancy Risk Factor C

Pregnancy Considerations Adverse events were not observed in the initial animal reproduction studies; therefore, the manufacturer classifies piroxicam as pregnancy category C. NSAID exposure during the first trimester is not strongly associated with congenital malformations; however, cardiovascular anomalies and cleft palate have been observed following NSAID exposure in some studies. The use of a NSAID close to conception may be associated with an increased risk of miscarriage. Nonteratogenic effects have been observed following NSAID administration during the third trimester including: Myocardial degenerative changes, prenatal constriction of the ductus arteriosus, fetal tricuspid regurgitation, failure of the ductus arteriosus to close postnatally; renal dysfunction or failure, oligohydramnios; gastrointestinal bleeding or perforation, increased risk of necrotizing enterocolitis; intracranial bleeding (including intraventricular hemorrhage), platelet dysfunction with resultant bleeding; pulmonary hypertension. Because they may cause premature closure of the ductus arteriosus, use of NSAIDs late in pregnancy should be avoided (use after 31 or 32 weeks gestation is not recommended by some clinicians). The chronic use of NSAIDs in women of reproductive age may be associated with infertility that is reversible upon discontinuation of the medication.

Breast-Feeding Considerations Piroxicam is excreted into breast milk. Breast-feeding is not recommended by the manufacturer.

Contraindications Hypersensitivity to piroxicam or any component; history of asthma, urticaria, or allergic-type reaction to aspirin, or other NSAIDs; patients with the "aspirin triad" [asthma, rhinitis (with or without nasal polyps), and aspirin intolerance] (fatal asthmatic and anaphylactoid reactions may occur in these patients); perioperative pain in the setting of coronary artery bypass graft (CABG) surgery; active GI bleeding

Warnings NSAIDs are associated with an increased risk of adverse cardiovascular thrombotic events, including potentially fatal MI and stroke **[U.S. Boxed Warning]**. Risk may be increased with duration of use or preexisting cardiovascular risk factors or disease. Carefully evaluate individual cardiovascular risk profiles prior to prescribing. Use the lowest effective dose for the shortest duration of time, taking into consideration individual patient treatment goals, to reduce risk of cardiovascular events; alternate therapies should be considered for patients at high risk. Use is contraindicated for treatment of perioperative pain in the setting of CABG surgery **[U.S. Boxed Warning]**; an increased incidence of MI and stroke was found in patients receiving COX-2 selective NSAIDs for the treatment of pain within the first 10-14 days after CABG surgery. NSAIDs may cause fluid retention, edema, and new onset or worsening of preexisting hypertension; use with caution in patients with hypertension, CHF, or fluid retention. Use is contraindicated in severe heart failure. Concurrent administration of ibuprofen, and potentially other nonselective NSAIDs, may interfere with aspirin's cardioprotective effect.

NSAIDs may increase the risk of gastrointestinal inflammation, ulceration, bleeding, and perforation **[U.S. Boxed Warning]**. These events, which can be potentially fatal, may occur at any time during therapy, and without warning. Avoid the use of NSAIDs in patients with active GI bleeding or ulcer disease. Use NSAIDs with extreme caution in patients with a history of GI bleeding or ulcers (these patients have a 10-fold increased risk for developing a GI bleed). Use NSAIDs with caution in patients with other risk factors which may increase GI bleeding (eg, concurrent therapy with aspirin, anticoagulants, and/or corticosteroids, longer duration of NSAID use; smoking; use of alcohol; and poor general health). Use the lowest effective dose for the shortest duration of time, taking into consideration individual patient treatment goals; alternate therapies should be considered for patients at high risk.

NSAIDs may compromise existing renal function; dose-dependent decreases in prostaglandin synthesis may result from NSAID use, reducing renal blood flow which may cause renal decompensation. Patients with impaired renal function, dehydration, heart failure, liver dysfunction, those taking diuretics and ACE inhibitors are at greatest risk of renal toxicity; use with caution in these patients; monitor renal function closely. NSAIDs are not recommended for use in patients with advanced renal disease. Long-term use of NSAIDs may cause renal papillary necrosis and other renal injury.

Even in patients without prior exposure anaphylactoid reactions may occur; patients with "aspirin triad" [bronchial asthma, aspirin intolerance, and rhinitis (with or without nasal polyps)] are at increased risk; use is contraindicated in these patients. Do not use in patients who experience bronchospasm, asthma, rhinitis, or urticaria with NSAID or aspirin therapy. NSAIDs may cause serious and potentially fatal dermatologic adverse reactions, including exfoliative dermatitis, Stevens-Johnson syndrome, and toxic epidermal necrolysis; discontinue use at first sign of skin rash or hypersensitivity. A serum sickness-like reaction can rarely occur; watch for arthralgias, pruritus, fever, fatigue, and rash. May cause drowsiness, dizziness, blurred vision, and other neurologic effects which may impair physical or mental abilities; patients must be cautioned about performing tasks which require mental alertness (eg, operating machinery or driving). Discontinue use with blurred or diminished vision and perform ophthalmologic exam. Periodically evaluate vision in all patients receiving long term therapy. Avoid use of NSAIDs in late pregnancy as they may cause premature closure of the ductus arteriosus.

Precautions Use with caution in patients with decreased hepatic function; closely monitor patients with abnormal LFTs; severe hepatic reactions (eg, fulminant hepatitis, liver failure) have occurred with NSAID use, rarely; discontinue if signs or symptoms of liver disease develop, or if systemic manifestations occur. Use with caution in patients with asthma; asthmatic patients may have aspirin-sensitive asthma which may be associated with severe and potentially fatal bronchospasm when aspirin or NSAIDs are administered. Anemia (due to occult or gross blood loss from the GI tract, fluid retention, or other effect on erythropoiesis) may occur; monitor hemoglobin and hematocrit in patients receiving long-term therapy. Use with caution and monitor carefully in patients with coagulation disorders or those receiving anticoagulants, as NSAIDs inhibit platelet aggregation and may prolong bleeding time. Use with caution in patients known or suspected to be poor CYP2C9 metabolizers; hepatic metabolism may be reduced resulting in elevated serum concentrations.

Adverse Reactions

Cardiovascular: Edema

Central nervous system: Dizziness, headache

Dermatologic: Pruritus, skin rash

Gastrointestinal: Abdominal pain, anorexia, constipation, diarrhea, dyspepsia, flatulence, gastrointestinal hemorrhage, gastrointestinal perforation, heartburn, nausea, ulcer, vomiting

Hematologic & oncologic: Anemia, prolonged bleeding time

Hepatic: Increased liver enzymes

Otic: Tinnitus

Renal: Renal function abnormality

Rare but important or life-threatening: Agranulocytosis, anaphylaxis, angioedema, aplastic anemia, aseptic meningitis, blurred vision, bone marrow depression, cardiac arrhythmia, cardiac failure, cystitis, dyspnea, epistaxis, erythema multiforme, exacerbation of angina pectoris, gastritis, glomerulonephritis, hallucination, hearing loss, hemolytic anemia, hepatic failure, hepatitis, hyperkalemia, hypertension, interstitial nephritis, jaundice, leukopenia, myocardial infarction, nephrotic syndrome, pancreatitis, pancytopenia, peripheral neuropathy, polydipsia, polyuria, renal failure, skin photosensitivity, Stevens-Johnson syndrome, tachycardia, thrombocytopenia, toxic amblyopia, toxic epidermal necrolysis

Drug Interactions

Metabolism/Transport Effects Substrate of CYP2C9 (major); **Note:** Assignment of Major/Minor substrate status based on clinically relevant drug interaction potential; **Inhibits** CYP2C9 (weak)

Avoid Concomitant Use

Avoid concomitant use of Piroxicam with any of the following: Floctafenine; Ketorolac (Nasal); Ketorolac (Systemic); NSAID (COX-2 Inhibitor); Omacetaxine; Urokinase

Increased Effect/Toxicity

Piroxicam may increase the levels/effects of: 5-ASA Derivatives; Agents with Antiplatelet Properties; Aliskiren; Aminoglycosides; Anticoagulants; Apixaban; Bisphosphonate Derivatives; Collagenase (Systemic); CycloSPORINE (Systemic); Dabigatran Etexilate; Deferasirox; Desmopressin; Digoxin; Eplerenone; Haloperidol; Ibritumomab; Lithium; Methotrexate; Nonsteroidal Anti-Inflammatory Agents; NSAID (COX-2 Inhibitor); Omacetaxine; PEMEtrexed; Porfimer; Potassium-Sparing Diuretics; PRALAtrexate; Quinolone Antibiotics; Rivaroxaban; Salicylates; Tenofovir; Thrombolytic Agents; Tositumomab and Iodine I 131 Tositumomab; Urokinase; Vancomycin; Vitamin K Antagonists

The levels/effects of Piroxicam may be increased by: ACE Inhibitors; Angiotensin II Receptor Blockers; Antidepressants (Tricyclic, Tertiary Amine); Ceritinib; Corticosteroids (Systemic); CycloSPORINE (Systemic); CYP2C9 Inhibitors (Moderate); CYP2C9 Inhibitors (Strong); Dasatinib; Floctafenine; Glucosamine; Herbs (Anticoagulant/Antiplatelet Properties); Ibrutinib; Ketorolac (Nasal); Ketorolac (Systemic); Mifepristone; Multivitamins/Fluoride (with ADE); Multivitamins/Minerals (with ADEK, Folate, Iron); Multivitamins/Minerals (with AE, No Iron); Nonsteroidal Anti-Inflammatory Agents; Omega-3 Fatty Acids; Pentosan Polysulfate Sodium; Pentoxifylline; Probenecid; Prostacyclin Analogues; Selective Serotonin Reuptake Inhibitors; Serotonin/Norepinephrine Reuptake Inhibitors; Sodium Phosphates; Tipranavir; Treprostinil; Vitamin E

Decreased Effect

Piroxicam may decrease the levels/effects of: ACE Inhibitors; Agents with Antiplatelet Properties; Aliskiren; Angiotensin II Receptor Blockers; Beta-Blockers; Eplerenone; HydrALAZINE; Loop Diuretics; Potassium-Sparing Diuretics; Prostaglandins (Ophthalmic); Salicylates; Selective Serotonin Reuptake Inhibitors; Thiazide Diuretics

The levels/effects of Piroxicam may be decreased by: Bile Acid Sequestrants; CYP2C9 Inducers (Strong); Dabrafenib; Nonsteroidal Anti-Inflammatory Agents; Peginterferon Alfa-2b; Salicylates

Food Interactions Onset of effect may be delayed if piroxicam is taken with food. Management: May administer with food or milk to decrease GI upset.

Mechanism of Action Reversibly inhibits cyclooxygenase-1 and 2 (COX-1 and 2) enzymes, which results in decreased formation of prostaglandin precursors; has antipyretic, analgesic, and anti-inflammatory properties

Other proposed mechanisms not fully elucidated (and possibly contributing to the anti-inflammatory effect to varying degrees), include inhibiting chemotaxis, altering lymphocyte activity, inhibiting neutrophil aggregation/activation, and decreasing proinflammatory cytokine levels.

Pharmacodynamics Analgesia:

Onset of action: Oral: Within 1 hour

Maximum effect: 3-5 hours

Pharmacokinetics (Adult data unless noted)

Absorption: Oral: Well absorbed

Distribution:

V_d:

Children and Adolescents 7-16 years: 0.16 L/kg (range: 0.12-0.25 L/kg) (Mäkelä, 1991)

Adults: 0.14 L/kg

Protein binding: 99%

Metabolism: Hepatic predominantly via CYP2C9; metabolites are inactive

Half-life:

Children and Adolescents 7-16 years: 32.6 hours (range: 22-40 hours) (Mäkelä, 1991)

Adults: 50 hours

Time to peak: 3-5 hours

Elimination: Excreted as metabolites and unchanged drug (~5% to 10%) in the urine; small amount excreted in feces

Dosing: Usual

Children and Adolescents: **Juvenile idiopathic arthritis (JIA):** Oral: 0.2-0.4 mg/kg/**day** once daily; maximum daily dose: 15 mg/day (American Pain Society, 2008); **Note:** 15 mg strength not available in U.S.

Adults: **Osteoarthritis, rheumatoid arthritis:** Oral: 10-20 mg/day in 1-2 divided doses; maximum daily dose: 20 mg/**day**

Dosing adjustment in renal impairment: Adults:

Mild to moderate impairment: There are no dosage adjustments provided in manufacturer's labeling.

Severe impairment: Use is not recommended (has not been studied); if therapy must be initiated, close monitoring is recommended.

Dosing adjustment in hepatic impairment: Adults: There are no specific dosage adjustments provided in manufacturer's labeling; however, a dosage reduction is recommended.

Administration May administer with food or milk to decrease GI upset

Monitoring Parameters Occult blood loss, CBC, BUN, serum creatinine, liver enzymes; periodic ophthalmologic exams with chronic use

Test Interactions Increased bleeding time

Dosage Forms Excipient information presented when available (limited, particularly for generics); consult specific product labeling.

Capsule, Oral:

Feldene: 10 mg, 20 mg

Generic: 10 mg, 20 mg

References

Mäkelä AL, Olkkola KT, and Mattila MJ, "Steady State Pharmacokinetics of Piroxicam in Children With Rheumatic Diseases," *Eur J Clin Pharmacol*, 1991, 41(1):79-81.

"Principles of Analgesic Use in the Treatment of Acute Pain and Cancer Pain," 6th ed, Glenview, IL: American Pain Society, 2008.

- *p*-Isobutylhydratropic Acid *see* Ibuprofen *on page 1059*
- Pitressin Synthetic *see* Vasopressin *on page 2121*
- Pitrex (Can) *see* Tolnaftate *on page 2044*
- Pix Carbonis *see* Coal Tar *on page 532*
- Plantago Seed *see* Psyllium *on page 1773*
- Plantain Seed *see* Psyllium *on page 1773*
- Plaquenil *see* Hydroxychloroquine *on page 1048*
- Plasbumin-5 *see* Albumin *on page 82*
- Plasbumin®-5 (Can) *see* Albumin *on page 82*
- Plasbumin-25 *see* Albumin *on page 82*
- Plasbumin®-25 (Can) *see* Albumin *on page 82*
- Platinol *see* CISplatin *on page 481*
- Platinol-AQ *see* CISplatin *on page 481*
- Plavix *see* Clopidogrel *on page 521*
- Plendil *see* Felodipine *on page 850*
- Pliaglis *see* Lidocaine and Tetracaine *on page 1248*
- PMPA *see* Tenofovir *on page 1977*
- PMS-Adenosine (Can) *see* Adenosine *on page 76*
- PMS-Amantadine (Can) *see* Amantadine *on page 112*
- PMS-Amiodarone (Can) *see* Amiodarone *on page 127*
- PMS-Amitriptyline (Can) *see* Amitriptyline *on page 133*
- PMS-Amlodipine (Can) *see* AmLODIPine *on page 135*
- PMS-Amoxicillin (Can) *see* Amoxicillin *on page 140*
- PMS-Anagrelide (Can) *see* Anagrelide *on page 166*
- PMS-Atenolol (Can) *see* Atenolol *on page 222*
- PMS-Atomoxetine (Can) *see* AtoMOXetine *on page 224*
- PMS-Atorvastatin (Can) *see* AtorvaSTATin *on page 227*
- PMS-Azithromycin (Can) *see* Azithromycin (Systemic) *on page 247*
- PMS-Baclofen (Can) *see* Baclofen *on page 259*
- PMS-Benztropine (Can) *see* Benztropine *on page 276*
- PMS-Bethanechol (Can) *see* Bethanechol *on page 288*
- PMS-Bisacodyl [OTC] (Can) *see* Bisacodyl *on page 293*
- PMS-Bosentan (Can) *see* Bosentan *on page 298*
- PMS-Brimonidine Tartrate (Can) *see* Brimonidine (Ophthalmic) *on page 303*
- PMS-Bromocriptine (Can) *see* Bromocriptine *on page 304*
- PMS-Bupropion SR (Can) *see* BuPROPion *on page 327*
- PMS-Buspirone (Can) *see* BusPIRone *on page 332*
- PMS-Candesartan (Can) *see* Candesartan *on page 363*
- PMS-Captopril (Can) *see* Captopril *on page 368*
- PMS-Carbamazepine (Can) *see* CarBAMazepine *on page 372*
- PMS-Carvedilol (Can) *see* Carvedilol *on page 385*
- PMS-Cefaclor (Can) *see* Cefaclor *on page 391*
- PMS-Cephalexin (Can) *see* Cephalexin *on page 429*
- PMS-Cetirizine (Can) *see* Cetirizine *on page 431*
- PMS-Chloral Hydrate (Can) *see* Chloral Hydrate *on page 436*
- PMS-Cholestyramine (Can) *see* Cholestyramine Resin *on page 457*
- PMS-Ciclopirox (Can) *see* Ciclopirox *on page 465*
- PMS-Cimetidine (Can) *see* Cimetidine *on page 469*
- PMS-Ciprofloxacin (Can) *see* Ciprofloxacin (Systemic) *on page 471*
- PMS-Ciprofloxacin XL (Can) *see* Ciprofloxacin (Systemic) *on page 471*
- PMS-Citalopram (Can) *see* Citalopram *on page 484*
- PMS-Clarithromycin (Can) *see* Clarithromycin *on page 490*
- PMS-Clindamycin (Can) *see* Clindamycin (Systemic) *on page 495*
- PMS-Clobazam (Can) *see* CloBAZam *on page 504*
- PMS-Clobetasol (Can) *see* Clobetasol *on page 506*
- PMS-Clonazepam (Can) *see* ClonazePAM *on page 514*
- PMS-Clonazepam-R (Can) *see* ClonazePAM *on page 514*
- PMS-Clopidogrel (Can) *see* Clopidogrel *on page 521*
- PMS-Codeine (Can) *see* Codeine *on page 534*
- PMS-Colchicine (Can) *see* Colchicine *on page 537*
- PMS-Conjugated Estrogens C.S.D. (Can) *see* Estrogens (Conjugated/Equine, Systemic) *on page 799*
- PMS-Cyclobenzaprine (Can) *see* Cyclobenzaprine *on page 558*
- PMS-Cyclopentolate (Can) *see* Cyclopentolate *on page 560*
- PMS-Cyproheptadine (Can) *see* Cyproheptadine *on page 569*
- PMS-Deferoxamine (Can) *see* Deferoxamine *on page 604*
- PMS-Desipramine (Can) *see* Desipramine *on page 608*
- PMS-Desmopressin (Can) *see* Desmopressin *on page 612*
- PMS-Dexamethasone (Can) *see* Dexamethasone (Systemic) *on page 615*
- PMS-Diazepam (Can) *see* Diazepam *on page 640*
- PMS-Dicitrate (Can) *see* Sodium Citrate and Citric Acid *on page 1906*
- PMS-Diclofenac (Can) *see* Diclofenac (Systemic) *on page 645*
- PMS-Diclofenac K (Can) *see* Diclofenac (Systemic) *on page 645*
- PMS-Diclofenac-SR (Can) *see* Diclofenac (Systemic) *on page 645*
- PMS-Digoxin (Can) *see* Digoxin *on page 658*
- PMS-Diltiazem CD (Can) *see* Diltiazem *on page 667*
- PMS-Dimenhydrinate [OTC] (Can) *see* DimenhyDRINATE *on page 670*
- PMS-Diphenhydramine (Can) *see* DiphenhydrAMINE (Systemic) *on page 673*
- PMS-Dipivefrin (Can) *see* Dipivefrin *on page 692*
- PMS-Divalproex (Can) *see* Valproic Acid and Derivatives *on page 2102*
- PMS-Docusate Calcium [OTC] (Can) *see* Docusate *on page 701*
- PMS-Docusate Sodium [OTC] (Can) *see* Docusate *on page 701*
- PMS-Doxazosin (Can) *see* Doxazosin *on page 712*
- PMS-Doxycycline (Can) *see* Doxycycline *on page 721*
- PMS-Enalapril (Can) *see* Enalapril *on page 744*
- PMS-Erythromycin (Can) *see* Erythromycin (Ophthalmic) *on page 784*
- PMS-Famciclovir (Can) *see* Famciclovir *on page 842*
- PMS-Fentanyl MTX (Can) *see* FentaNYL *on page 853*
- PMS-Fluconazole (Can) *see* Fluconazole *on page 877*

◆ **PMS-Fluorometholone (Can)** *see* Fluorometholone *on page 897*

◆ **PMS-Fluoxetine (Can)** *see* FLUoxetine *on page 901*

◆ **PMS-Fluvoxamine (Can)** *see* FluvoxaMINE *on page 922*

◆ **PMS-Fosinopril (Can)** *see* Fosinopril *on page 938*

◆ **PMS-Furosemide (Can)** *see* Furosemide *on page 948*

◆ **PMS-Gabapentin (Can)** *see* Gabapentin *on page 950*

◆ **PMS-Gentamicin (Can)** *see* Gentamicin (Ophthalmic) *on page 966*

◆ **PMS-Gentamicin (Can)** *see* Gentamicin (Topical) *on page 967*

◆ **PMS-Glyburide (Can)** *see* GlyBURIDE *on page 974*

◆ **PMS-Haloperidol (Can)** *see* Haloperidol *on page 998*

◆ **PMS-Haloperidol LA (Can)** *see* Haloperidol *on page 998*

◆ **PMS-Hydrochlorothiazide (Can)** *see* Hydrochlorothiazide *on page 1023*

◆ **PMS-Hydromorphone (Can)** *see* HYDROmorphone *on page 1041*

◆ **PMS-Hydroxyzine (Can)** *see* HydrOXYzine *on page 1054*

◆ **PMS-Ibuprofen (Can)** *see* Ibuprofen *on page 1059*

◆ **PMS Imipramine (Can)** *see* Imipramine *on page 1080*

◆ **PMS-Ipratropium (Can)** *see* Ipratropium (Oral Inhalation) *on page 1144*

◆ **PMS-Irbesartan (Can)** *see* Irbesartan *on page 1147*

◆ **PMS-Isoniazid (Can)** *see* Isoniazid *on page 1158*

◆ **PMS-Lactulose (Can)** *see* Lactulose *on page 1193*

◆ **PMS-Lamotrigine (Can)** *see* LamoTRIgine *on page 1199*

◆ **PMS-Letrozole (Can)** *see* Letrozole *on page 1211*

◆ **PMS-Levetiracetam (Can)** *see* LevETIRAcetam *on page 1219*

◆ **PMS-Levobunolol (Can)** *see* Levobunolol *on page 1223*

◆ **PMS-Levofloxacin (Can)** *see* Levofloxacin (Systemic) *on page 1228*

◆ **PMS-Lisinopril (Can)** *see* Lisinopril *on page 1262*

◆ **PMS-Lithium Carbonate (Can)** *see* Lithium *on page 1266*

◆ **PMS-Lithium Citrate (Can)** *see* Lithium *on page 1266*

◆ **PMS-Loperamine (Can)** *see* Loperamide *on page 1270*

◆ **PMS-Lorazepam (Can)** *see* LORazepam *on page 1280*

◆ **PMS-Losartan (Can)** *see* Losartan *on page 1283*

◆ **PMS-Lovastatin (Can)** *see* Lovastatin *on page 1286*

◆ **PMS-Medroxyprogesterone (Can)** *see* MedroxyPROGESTERone *on page 1318*

◆ **PMS-Meloxicam (Can)** *see* Meloxicam *on page 1325*

◆ **PMS-Metformin (Can)** *see* MetFORMIN *on page 1353*

◆ **PMS-Methylphenidate (Can)** *see* Methylphenidate *on page 1379*

◆ **PMS-Metoclopramide (Can)** *see* Metoclopramide *on page 1391*

◆ **PMS-Metoprolol-L (Can)** *see* Metoprolol *on page 1396*

◆ **PMS-Metoprolol-B (Can)** *see* Metoprolol *on page 1396*

◆ **PMS-Metronidazole (Can)** *see* MetroNIDAZOLE (Systemic) *on page 1399*

◆ **PMS-Minocycline (Can)** *see* Minocycline *on page 1420*

◆ **PMS-Misoprostol (Can)** *see* Misoprostol *on page 1423*

◆ **PMS-Mometasone (Can)** *see* Mometasone (Topical) *on page 1435*

◆ **PMS-Montelukast (Can)** *see* Montelukast *on page 1438*

◆ **PMS-Montelukast FC (Can)** *see* Montelukast *on page 1438*

◆ **PMS-Morphine Sulfate SR (Can)** *see* Morphine (Systemic) *on page 1440*

◆ **PMS-Nabilone (Can)** *see* Nabilone *on page 1459*

◆ **PMS-Naproxen (Can)** *see* Naproxen *on page 1470*

◆ **PMS-Naproxen EC (Can)** *see* Naproxen *on page 1470*

◆ **PMS-Nifedipine (Can)** *see* NIFEdipine *on page 1497*

◆ **PMS-Nizatidine (Can)** *see* Nizatidine *on page 1508*

◆ **PMS-Nortriptyline (Can)** *see* Nortriptyline *on page 1512*

◆ **PMS-Nystatin (Can)** *see* Nystatin (Oral) *on page 1516*

◆ **PMS-Olanzapine (Can)** *see* OLANZapine *on page 1525*

◆ **PMS-Olanzapine ODT (Can)** *see* OLANZapine *on page 1525*

◆ **PMS-Omeprazole (Can)** *see* Omeprazole *on page 1535*

◆ **PMS-Omeprazole DR (Can)** *see* Omeprazole *on page 1535*

◆ **PMS-Ondansetron (Can)** *see* Ondansetron *on page 1544*

◆ **PMS-Oxybutynin (Can)** *see* Oxybutynin *on page 1568*

◆ **PMS-Oxycodone (Can)** *see* OxyCODONE *on page 1569*

◆ **PMS-Oxycodone-Acetaminophen (Can)** *see* Oxycodone and Acetaminophen *on page 1573*

◆ **PMS-Oxycodone CR (Can)** *see* OxyCODONE *on page 1569*

◆ **PMS-Pamidronate (Can)** *see* Pamidronate *on page 1587*

◆ **PMS-Pantoprazole (Can)** *see* Pantoprazole *on page 1595*

◆ **PMS-Paroxetine (Can)** *see* PARoxetine *on page 1609*

◆ **PMS-Phenobarbital (Can)** *see* PHENobarbital *on page 1651*

◆ **PMS-Pimozide (Can)** *see* Pimozide *on page 1677*

◆ **PMS-Piroxicam (Can)** *see* Piroxicam *on page 1683*

◆ **PMS-Polytrimethoprim (Can)** *see* Trimethoprim and Polymyxin B *on page 2089*

◆ **PMS-Pravastatin (Can)** *see* Pravastatin *on page 1720*

◆ **PMS-Prednisolone Sodium Phosphate Forte (Can)** *see* PrednisoLONE (Ophthalmic) *on page 1730*

◆ **PMS-Prochlorperazine (Can)** *see* Prochlorperazine *on page 1745*

◆ **PMS-Promethazine (Can)** *see* Promethazine *on page 1748*

◆ **PMS-Propofol (Can)** *see* Propofol *on page 1755*

◆ **PMS-Propranolol (Can)** *see* Propranolol *on page 1759*

◆ **PMS-Pseudoephedrine (Can)** *see* Pseudoephedrine *on page 1770*

◆ **PMS-Quetiapine (Can)** *see* QUEtiapine *on page 1783*

◆ **PMS-Quinapril (Can)** *see* Quinapril *on page 1788*

◆ **PMS-Rabeprazole EC (Can)** *see* RABEprazole *on page 1797*

◆ **PMS-Ranitidine (Can)** *see* Ranitidine *on page 1805*

◆ **PMS-Risperidone (Can)** *see* RisperiDONE *on page 1831*

◆ **PMS-Risperidone ODT (Can)** *see* RisperiDONE *on page 1831*

◆ **PMS-Rosuvastatin (Can)** *see* Rosuvastatin *on page 1853*

◆ **PMS-Salbutamol (Can)** *see* Albuterol *on page 84*

◆ **PMS-Sertraline (Can)** *see* Sertraline *on page 1879*

◆ **PMS-Sildenafil (Can)** *see* Sildenafil *on page 1884*

- **PMS-Simvastatin (Can)** *see* Simvastatin *on page 1892*
- **PMS-Sodium Cromoglycate (Can)** *see* Cromolyn (Systemic, Oral Inhalation) *on page 551*
- **PMS-Sodium Polystyrene Sulfonate (Can)** *see* Sodium Polystyrene Sulfonate *on page 1917*
- **PMS-Sotalol (Can)** *see* Sotalol *on page 1925*
- **PMS-Sucralate (Can)** *see* Sucralfate *on page 1940*
- **PMS-Sulfacetamide (Can)** *see* Sulfacetamide (Ophthalmic) *on page 1943*
- **PMS-Sulfasalazine (Can)** *see* SulfaSALAzine *on page 1954*
- **PMS-Sumatriptan (Can)** *see* SUMAtriptan *on page 1958*
- **PMS-Tamoxifen (Can)** *see* Tamoxifen *on page 1968*
- **PMS-Terazosin (Can)** *see* Terazosin *on page 1981*
- **PMS-Terbinafine (Can)** *see* Terbinafine (Systemic) *on page 1982*
- **PMS-Testosterone (Can)** *see* Testosterone *on page 1986*
- **PMS-Theophylline (Can)** *see* Theophylline *on page 2005*
- **PMS-Timolol (Can)** *see* Timolol (Ophthalmic) *on page 2028*
- **PMS-Tobramycin (Can)** *see* Tobramycin (Ophthalmic) *on page 2039*
- **PMS-Topiramate (Can)** *see* Topiramate *on page 2046*
- **PMS-Trazodone (Can)** *see* TraZODone *on page 2065*
- **PMS-Trifluoperazine (Can)** *see* Trifluoperazine *on page 2082*
- **PMS-Trihexyphenidyl (Can)** *see* Trihexyphenidyl *on page 2085*
- **PMS-Ursodiol C (Can)** *see* Ursodiol *on page 2095*
- **PMS-Valacyclovir (Can)** *see* ValACYclovir *on page 2097*
- **PMS-Valproic Acid (Can)** *see* Valproic Acid and Derivatives *on page 2102*
- **PMS-Valproic Acid E.C. (Can)** *see* Valproic Acid and Derivatives *on page 2102*
- **PMS-Valsartan (Can)** *see* Valsartan *on page 2108*
- **PMS-Vancomycin (Can)** *see* Vancomycin *on page 2110*
- **PMS-Venlafaxine XR (Can)** *see* Venlafaxine *on page 2125*
- **PMS-Verapamil SR (Can)** *see* Verapamil *on page 2129*
- **Pneumo 23™ (Can)** *see* Pneumococcal Polysaccharide Vaccine (Polyvalent) *on page 1691*
- **Pneumococcal 13-Valent Conjugate Vaccine** *see* Pneumococcal Conjugate Vaccine (13-Valent) *on page 1688*

Pneumococcal Conjugate Vaccine (13-Valent)
(noo moe KOK al KON ju gate vak SEEN, thur TEEN vay lent)

Medication Safety Issues
Sound-alike/look-alike issues:
Pneumococcal 13-Valent Conjugate Vaccine (Prevnar 13) may be confused with Pneumococcal 7-Valent Conjugate Vaccine (Prevnar) or with Pneumococcal 23-Valent Polysaccharide Vaccine (Pneumovax 23)

Related Information
Immunization Administration Recommendations *on page 2368*
Immunization Guidelines *on page 2373*

Brand Names: U.S. Prevnar 13
Brand Names: Canada Prevnar 13
Therapeutic Category Vaccine, Inactivated (Bacterial)

Generic Availability (U.S.) No
Use
Immunization against *Streptococcus pneumoniae* infection caused by serotypes 1, 3, 4, 5, 6A, 6B, 7F, 9V, 14, 18C, 19A, 19F, and 23F (FDA approved in ages 6 weeks to 17 years and adults ≥50 years). Prevention of otitis media in infants and children caused by *Streptococcus pneumoniae* serotypes 4, 6B, 9V, 14, 18C, 19F, and 23F (FDA approved in ages 6 weeks to 5 years)

The Advisory Committee on Immunization Practices (ACIP) recommends routine vaccination for the following (CDC/ACIP [Nuorti, 2010]):
- All infants and children age 2 to 59 months
- Children 60 to 71 months with underlying medical conditions including:
  - Immunocompetent children with chronic heart disease (particularly cyanotic congenital heart disease and heart failure), chronic lung disease (including asthma if treated with high dose corticosteroids), diabetes, cerebrospinal fluid leaks, or cochlear implants
  - Children with functional or anatomic asplenia, including sickle cell disease or other hemoglobinopathies, congenital or acquired asplenia, or splenic dysfunction
  - Children with immunocompromising conditions, including congenital immunodeficiency (includes B or T cell deficiency, compliment deficiencies and phagocytic disorders; excludes chronic granulomatous disease), HIV infection, chronic renal failure, nephrotic syndrome, leukemia, lymphoma, Hodgkin disease, generalized malignancies, solid organ transplant, or other diseases requiring immunosuppressive drugs (including long-term systemic corticosteroids and radiation therapy)
- Children who received ≥1 dose of 7-valent pneumococcal vaccine (PCV7): **Note:** Routine use is not recommended for healthy children ≥5 years

Children ≥6 years, Adolescents, and Adults with the following immunocompromising conditions (CDC/ACIP, 61[40], 2012; CDC/ACIP, 62[25], 2013):
- Immunocompetent persons with cerebrospinal fluid leaks or cochlear implants
- Persons with functional or anatomic asplenia, including sickle cell disease or other hemoglobinopathies, or congenital or acquired asplenia
- Persons with immunocompromising conditions including congenital or acquired immunodeficiency (includes B or T cell deficiency, compliment deficiencies and phagocytic disorders; excludes chronic granulomatous disease), HIV infection, chronic renal failure, nephrotic syndrome, leukemia, lymphoma, Hodgkin disease, generalized malignancies, solid organ transplant, multiple myeloma, or other diseases requiring immunosuppressive drugs (including long-term systemic corticosteroids and radiation therapy)

Pregnancy Risk Factor B
Pregnancy Considerations Animal reproduction studies have not shown adverse fetal effects. Inactivated vaccines have not been shown to cause increased risks to the fetus (NCIRD/ACIP, 2011).
Breast-Feeding Considerations It is not known if this vaccine is excreted into breast milk. The manufacturer recommends that caution be exercised when administering this vaccine to nursing women. Inactivated vaccines do not affect the safety of breast-feeding for the mother or the infant. Breast-feeding infants should be vaccinated according to the recommended schedules (NCIRD/ACIP, 2011).
Contraindications Hypersensitivity to pneumococcal vaccine or any component, including diphtheria toxoid
Warnings Immediate treatment (including epinephrine 1:1000) for anaphylactic and/or hypersensitivity reactions should be available during vaccine administration. Syncope has been reported with use of injectable vaccines

and may be accompanied by transient visual disturbances, weakness, or tonic-clonic movements. Procedures should be in place to avoid injuries from falling and to restore cerebral perfusion if syncope occurs (CDC, 57[17], 2008). Apnea has occurred following intramuscular vaccine administration in premature neonates; consider clinical status implications. Contains polysorbate 80 (Tween 80®) which may cause allergic reactions in susceptible individuals. In premature neonates, thrombocytopenia, ascites, pulmonary deterioration, and renal and hepatic failure have been reported after receiving parenteral products containing polysorbate 80 (Alade, 1986; CDC, 1984).

Precautions The decision to administer or delay vaccination because of current or recent febrile illness depends on the severity of symptoms and the etiology of the disease. Immunization should be delayed during the course of an acute severe febrile illness; may administer to patients with mild acute illness (with or without fever). Use with caution in severely immunocompromised patients (eg, patients receiving chemo-/radiation therapy or other immunosuppressive therapy including high-dose corticosteroids); may have a reduced response to vaccination; inactivated vaccines should be administered ≥2 weeks prior to planned immunosuppression when feasible (IDSA [Rubin, 2013]). In general, households and close contacts of persons with altered immunocompetence may receive all age-appropriate vaccines. Vaccination may not result in effective immunity in all patients. Response depends upon multiple factors (eg, type of vaccine, age of patient) and may be improved by administering the vaccine at the recommended dose, route, and interval (CDC/ACIP [Kroger, 2011]).

Use of pneumococcal conjugate vaccine does not replace use of the 23-valent pneumococcal polysaccharide vaccine in children ≥24 months of age with asplenia, HIV infection, sickle-cell disease, or other chronic illnesses (CDC/ACIP [Nuorti, 2010]). Use with caution in patients with coagulation disorders, including thrombocytopenia, due to an increased risk for bleeding following I.M. administration; if the patient receives antihemophilia or other similar therapy, I.M. injection can be scheduled shortly after such therapy is administered (CDC/ACIP [Kroger, 2011]).

Febrile seizures have been reported; CDC reports indicate that young children appear to be at increased risk of febrile seizures when given the pneumococcal conjugate vaccine (PCV13) at the same time as the inactivated influenza virus vaccine (TIV); the risk appears to be greatest from ages 12 to 23 months. Because febrile seizures are typically benign and occur in 2% to 5% of all young children, the ACIP does not recommend a delay in administration of either vaccine or altering the vaccine schedule in any manner due to the potential risk of infection. Antipyretics have not been shown to prevent febrile seizures; antipyretics may be used to treat fever or discomfort following vaccination (CDC/ACIP [Kroger, 2011]). One study reported that routine prophylactic administration of acetaminophen to prevent fever due to vaccines has been shown to decrease the immune response of some vaccines; the clinical significance of this reduction in immune response has not been established (Prymula, 2009). Concurrent administration of PCV13 and PPV23 has not been studied and is not recommended (CDC/ACIP [Nuorti, 2010]). Not to be used to treat pneumococcal infections or to provide immunity against diphtheria.

Use of this vaccine for specific medical and/or other indications (eg, immunocompromising conditions, hepatic or kidney disease, diabetes) is also addressed in the ACIP Recommended Immunization Schedule (CDC/ACIP [Akinsanya-Beysolow, 2014]; CDC/ACIP [Bridges, 2014]). Specific recommendations for use of this vaccine in immunocompromised patients with asplenia, cancer, HIV infection, cerebrospinal fluid leaks, cochlear implants, hematopoietic stem cell transplant (prior to or after), sickle cell disease, solid organ transplant (prior to or after), or those receiving immunosuppressive therapy for chronic conditions are available from the IDSA (Rubin, 2014).

Adverse Reactions All serious adverse reactions must be reported to the U.S. Department of Health and Human Services (DHHS) Vaccine Adverse Event Reporting System (VAERS) 1-800-822-7967 or online at https://vaers.hhs.gov/esub/index.

Central nervous system: Chills, drowsiness, fatigue, fever, headache, insomnia, irritability

Dermatologic: Hives, rash

Gastrointestinal: Appetite decreased, diarrhea, vomiting

Local: Erythema, limitation of arm motion, pain, swelling, tenderness

Neuromuscular & skeletal: Arthralgia, myalgia

Rare but important or life-threatening: Abnormal crying, erythema multiforme, febrile seizures, hypersensitivity reaction (bronchospasm, dyspnea, facial edema), seizure, urticaria, urticaria-like rash

Adverse reactions observed with PCV7 which may also be seen with PCV-13: Anaphylactic reaction, angioneurotic edema, apnea, breath holding, edema, hypotonic hyporesponsive episode, injection site reaction (dermatitis, pruritus), lymphadenopathy (localized), shock

Drug Interactions

Metabolism/Transport Effects None known.

Avoid Concomitant Use There are no known interactions where it is recommended to avoid concomitant use.

Increased Effect/Toxicity There are no known significant interactions involving an increase in effect.

Decreased Effect

Pneumococcal Conjugate Vaccine (13-Valent) may decrease the levels/effects of: Influenza Virus Vaccine (Inactivated)

The levels/effects of Pneumococcal Conjugate Vaccine (13-Valent) may be decreased by: Belimumab; Fingolimod; Immunosuppressants; Influenza Virus Vaccine (Inactivated)

Stability Store refrigerated at 2°C to 8°C (36°F to 46°F); do not freeze; discard if frozen.

Mechanism of Action Promotes active immunization against invasive disease caused by *S. pneumoniae* capsular serotypes 1, 3, 4, 5, 6A, 6B, 7F, 9V, 14, 18C, 19A, 19F, and 23F, all which are individually conjugated to CRM197 protein

Dosing: Usual

Pediatric:

Primary immunization; healthy patients: Note: Preterm infants should be vaccinated according to their chronological age from birth.

Infants and Children 6 weeks to 59 months: I.M.: 0.5 mL per dose for a total of 4 doses given as follows: the first dose may be given as young as 6 weeks of age, but is typically given at 8 weeks (2 months of age); the 3 remaining doses are usually given at 4, 6, and 12 to 15 months of age. The recommended dosing interval is 4 to 8 weeks. The minimum interval between doses in infants <1 year of age is 4 weeks. The minimum interval between the third and fourth dose is 8 weeks.

Children and Adolescents 6 to 18 years: I.M.: 0.5 mL as a single dose; at least 8 weeks after any previous doses. **Note:** This dose is not part of the CDC (ACIP) recommended immunization schedule

Catch-up immunization, healthy patients: CDC (ACIP) recommendations (Akinsanya-Beysolow, 2014): **Note:** Do not restart the series. If doses have been given (PCV7 or PCV13), begin the below schedule at the applicable dose number. I.M.: 0.5 mL per dose for a total of 1 to 4 doses administered as follows:

First dose given on the elected date.

Second dose given at least 4 weeks after the first dose (if first dose at age <12 months) **or** at least 8 weeks after the first dose (if first dose at ≥12 months of age). This dose is not needed in healthy patients if the first dose was given at ≥24 months of age.

Third dose given at least 4 weeks after the second dose (if age <12 months) or at least 8 weeks after the first dose (if age ≥12 months). This dose is not needed in healthy patients if the previous dose was given at ≥24 months of age.

Fourth dose given at least 8 weeks after the third dose. This dose is only needed for children 12 to 59 months of age who received 3 doses before age 12 months or for children at high risk who received 3 doses at any age.

High-risk conditions; primary or revaccination:

Children 2 through 5 years [CDC/ACIP [Nuorti, 2010]]:

Pneumococcal vaccine-naïve (no previous PCV13): I.M.: 0.5 mL for a total of 2 doses at least 8 weeks apart

Previously vaccinated with PCV7 and/or PCV13:

Previously received <3 doses of PCV (PCV7 and/or PCV13): I.M.: 0.5 mL dose for a total of 2 doses at least 8 weeks apart and at least 8 weeks after the most recent dose,

Previously received three doses of PCV (PCV7 and/or PCV13): I.M.: 0.5 mL as a single dose ≥8 weeks after most recent dose.

Previously received 4 doses of PCV7 or other age-appropriate complete PCV7 series: I.M.: 0.5 mL as a single dose ≥8 weeks after most recent dose

Children and Adolescents 6 to 18 years (CDC/ACIP 62 [25], 2013):

Pneumococcal vaccine-naïve (no previous PCV13 or PPSV23 vaccine): I.M.: 0.5 mL as a single dose

Previously vaccinated with PPSV23 vaccine: If PCV13 has never been administered, give PCV13 vaccine: I.M.: 0.5 mL as a single dose ≥8 weeks after the last dose of PPSV23 vaccine. The PCV13 vaccine should be administered even if child has previously received PCV7.

Previously completed vaccination series with PCV7 (4 doses) (CDC 59 [RR-11], 2010): I.M.:

CDC (ACIP) recommendations (CDC/ACIP [Nuorti, 2010]):

Children 14 to 59 months: I.M.: 0.5 mL as a single supplemental dose ≥8 weeks after the most recent PCV7 dose

Children 60 to 71 months with an underlying medical condition: I.M.: 0.5 mL as a single supplemental dose ≥8 weeks after the most recent dose of PCV7 or PPSV23

Manufacturer's labeling: Children 15 to 59 months: I.M.: 0.5 mL as a single supplemental dose ≥8 weeks after the most recent PCV7 dose

Adult: **Immunization: Note:** Efficacy of PCV13 administered <5 years after PPSV23 is unknown.

Adults ≥50 years: I.M.: 0.5 mL as a single dose

Adults ≥19 years with specified underlying medical conditions (CDC/ACIP, 61[40], 2012):

Pneumococcal vaccine naïve (no previous PCV13 or PPSV23 vaccine): I.M.: Administer PCV13 0.5 mL as a single dose followed by 1 dose of PPSV23 8 weeks later

Previously vaccinated with PPSV23: I.M.: PCV13 0.5 mL as a single dose ≥1 year after the last dose of PPSV23

Dosing adjustment in renal impairment: There are no dosage adjustments provided in the manufacturer's labeling.

Dosing adjustment in hepatic impairment: There are no dosage adjustments provided in the manufacturer's labeling.

Administration I.M.: Shake vial well before withdrawing the dose; administer I.M. into midlateral aspect of the thigh in infants and small children; administer in the deltoid area to older children and adults; **not for I.V. or SubQ administration.** Adolescents and adults should be vaccinated while seated or lying down. U.S. law requires that the date of administration; the vaccine manufacturer; lot number of vaccine; and the administering person's name, title, and address be entered into the patient's permanent medical record.

Monitoring Parameters Observe for syncope for 15 minutes following administration. If seizure-like activity associated with syncope occurs, maintain patient in supine or Trendelenburg position to reestablish adequate cerebral perfusion.

Additional Information Pneumococcal 13-valent conjugate vaccine (PCV13; Prevnar 13) is the successor to the previously-marketed pneumococcal 7-valent conjugate vaccine (PCV7; Prevnar). Prevnar 13 contains an additional six serotypes of *Streptococcus pneumoniae*, compared to the seven serotypes provided in the original Prevnar formulation.

In order to maximize vaccination rates, the ACIP recommends simultaneous administration (ie, >1 vaccine on the same day at different anatomic sites) of all age-appropriate vaccines (live or inactivated) for which a person is eligible at a single visit, unless contraindications exist. If available, the use of combination vaccines is generally preferred over separate injections, taking into consideration provider assessment, patient preference, and potential adverse events. If separate vaccines being used, evaluate product information regarding same syringe compatibility of vaccines. Separate needles and syringes should be used for each injection. The ACIP prefers each dose of specific vaccine in a series come from the same manufacturer if possible (CDC/ACIP [Kroger, 2011).

For additional information, please refer to the following website: http://www.cdc.gov/vaccines/vpd-vac/.

Dosage Forms Excipient information presented when available (limited, particularly for generics); consult specific product labeling.

Injection, suspension:

Prevnar 13: 2 mcg of each capsular saccharide for serotypes 1, 3, 4, 5, 6A, 7F, 9V, 14, 18C, 19A, 19F, and 23F, and 4 mcg of serotype 6B [bound to diphtheria CRM_{197} protein ~34 mcg] per 0.5 mL (0.5 mL) [contains aluminum, polysorbate 80, and yeast]

References

AAP Steering Committee on Quality Improvement and Management, Subcommittee on Febrile Seizures American Academy of Pediatrics, "Febrile Seizures: Clinical Practice Guideline for the Long-Term Management of the Child With Simple Febrile Seizures," *Pediatrics,* 2008, 121(6):1281-6.

Akinsanya-Beysolow I, Advisory Committee on Immunization Practices (ACIP), ACIP Child/Adolescent Immunization Work Group, et al. Advisory committee on immunization practices recommended immunization schedules for persons aged 0 through 18 years - United States, 2014. *MMWR Morb Mortal Wkly Rep.* 2014; 63(5):108-109. Full schedule available at http://www.cdc.gov/vaccines/schedules/downloads/child/0-18yrs-child-combined-schedule.pdf

Alade SL, Brown RE, and Paquet A Jr, "Polysorbate 80 and E-Ferol Toxicity," *Pediatrics,* 1986, 77(4):593-7.

American Academy of Pediatrics Committee on Infectious Diseases, "Recommendations for the Prevention of *Streptococcus pneumoniae* Infections in Infants and Children: Use of 13-Valent Pneumococcal

Conjugate Vaccine (PCV13) and Pneumococcal Polysaccharide Vaccine (PPSV23)," *Pediatrics*, 2010, 126(1):186-90.

Bridges CB, Coyne-Beasley T, Advisory Committee on Immunization Practices (ACIP), ACIP Adult Immunization Work Group; Centers for Disease Control and Prevention (CDC). Advisory committee on immunization practices recommended immunization schedule for adults aged 19 years or older - United States, 2014. *MMWR Morb Mortal Wkly Rep*. 2014; 63(5):108-109. Available at: http://www.cdc.gov/vaccines/schedules/downloads/adult/adult-combined-schedule.pdf

Centers for Disease Control and Prevention (CDC), "Syncope After Vaccination-United States, January 2005-July 2007," *MMWR Morb Mortal Wkly Rep*, 2008, 2;57(17):457-60.

Centers for Disease Control (CDC), "Unusual Syndrome With Fatalities Among Premature Infants: Association With a New Intravenous Vitamin E Product," *MMWR Morb Mortal Wkly Rep*, 1984, 33 (14):198-9.

Centers for Disease Control and Prevention (CDC), "Use of 13-Valent Pneumococcal Conjugate Vaccine and 23-Valent Pneumococcal Polysaccharide Vaccine Among Children Aged 6-18 Years With Immunocompromising Conditions: Recommendations of the Advisory Committee on Immunization Practices (ACIP)," *MMWR Morb Mortal Wkly Rep*, 2013, 62(25):521-4.

Centers for Disease Control and Prevention (CDC), "Use of 13-Valent Pneumococcal Conjugate Vaccine and 23-Valent Pneumococcal Polysaccharide Vaccine for Adults With Immunocompromising Conditions: Recommendations of the Advisory Committee on Immunization Practices (ACIP)," *MMWR Morb Mortal Wkly Rep*, 2012, 61 (40):816-9.

Kroger AT, Atkinson WL, Marcuse EK, Pickering LK. General recommendations on immunization - recommendations of the Advisory Committee on Immunization Practices (ACIP). *MMWR Recomm Rep*. 2011;60(RR-2):1-64.

Nuorti JP, Whitney CG. Prevention of pneumococcal disease among infants and children - use of 13-valent Ppneumococcal conjugate vaccine and 23-valent pneumococcal polysaccharide vaccine - recommendations of the Advisory Committee on Immunization Practices (ACIP). *MMWR Recomm Rep*. 2010;59(RR-11):1-18.

Prymula R, Siegrist CA, Chlibek R, et al, "Effect of Prophylactic Paracetamol Administration at Time of Vaccination on Febrile Reactions and Antibody Responses in Children: Two Open-Label, Randomised Controlled Trials," *Lancet*, 2009, 374(9698):1339-50.

Reefhuis J, Honein MA, Whitney CG, et al, "Risk of Bacterial Meningitis in Children With Cochlear Implants," *N Engl J Med*, 2003, 349 (5):435-45.

Rubin LG, Levin MJ, Ljungman P, et al. 2013 IDSA clinical practice guideline for vaccination of the immunocompromised host. *Clin Infect Dis*. 2014;58(3):e44-e100.

Pneumococcal Polysaccharide Vaccine (Polyvalent)
(noo moe KOK al pol i SAK a ride vak SEEN, pol i VAY lent)

Medication Safety Issues
Sound-alike/look-alike issues:
Pneumococcal 23-Valent Polysaccharide Vaccine (Pneumovax® 23) may be confused with Pneumococcal 7-Valent Conjugate Vaccine (Prevnar®) or with Pneumococcal 13-Valent Conjugate Vaccine (Prevnar 13®)

Related Information
Immunization Administration Recommendations *on page 2368*

Immunization Guidelines *on page 2373*

Brand Names: U.S. Pneumovax® 23
Brand Names: Canada Pneumo 23™; Pneumovax® 23
Therapeutic Category Vaccine
Generic Availability (U.S.) No
Use To provide immunization against pneumococcal disease caused by serotypes included in the vaccine (FDA approved in ages ≥2 years and adults).

The Advisory Committee on Immunization Practices (ACIP) recommends routine vaccination for patients with the following underlying medical conditions (CDC/ACIP, 59 [34], 2010; CDC/ACIP, 61[40], 2012; CDC/ACIP [Nuorti, 2010]):
- Immunocompromised children ≥2 years, adolescents, and adults ≤64 years with congenital or acquired immunodeficiency (includes B or T cell deficiency, compliment deficiencies and phagocytic disorders; excludes

chronic granulomatous disease), HIV infection, chronic renal failure, nephrotic syndrome, leukemia, lymphoma, Hodgkin disease, generalized malignancies, solid organ transplant, multiple myeloma, or other diseases requiring immunosuppressive drugs (including long-term systemic corticosteroids and radiation therapy)
- Children ≥2 years, adolescents, and adults 19 to 64 years with functional or anatomic asplenia, including sickle cell disease or other hemoglobinopathies, congenital or acquired asplenia, splenic dysfunction, or splenectomy
- Immunocompetent children ≥2 years and adolescents with chronic heart disease (particularly cyanotic congenital heart disease and heart failure), chronic lung disease (including asthma if treated with high dose corticosteroids), diabetes, cerebrospinal fluid leaks, or cochlear implants
- Immunocompetent adults 19 to 64 years with chronic heart disease (including heart failure and cardiomyopathies; excluding hypertension), chronic lung disease (including COPD, emphysema, and asthma), diabetes, cerebrospinal fluid leaks, cochlear implants, alcoholism, chronic liver disease, cirrhosis, and cigarette smokers
- All adults ≥65 years

Pregnancy Risk Factor C
Pregnancy Considerations Animal reproduction studies have not been conducted. Vaccination should be considered in pregnant women at high risk for infection. Inactivated vaccines have not been shown to cause increased risks to the fetus (CDC, 2011)
Breast-Feeding Considerations Inactivated vaccines do not affect the safety of breast-feeding for the mother or the infant. Breast-feeding infants should be vaccinated according to the recommended schedules (CDC, 2011).
Contraindications Hypersensitivity to pneumococcal vaccine or any component
Warnings Immediate treatment (including epinephrine 1:1000) for anaphylactic and/or acute hypersensitivity reactions should be available during vaccine use; intradermal administration may cause severe local reactions. Syncope has been reported with use of injectable vaccines and may be accompanied by transient visual disturbances, weakness, or tonic-clonic movements. Procedures should be in place to avoid injuries from falling and to restore cerebral perfusion if syncope occurs (CDC, 57[17], 2008).
Precautions The decision to administer or delay vaccination because of current or recent febrile illness depends on the severity of symptoms and the etiology of the disease. Immunization should be delayed during the course of an acute severe febrile illness; may administer to patients with mild acute illness (with or without fever). Use with caution in severely immunocompromised patients (eg, patients receiving chemo/radiation therapy or other immunosuppressive therapy, including high-dose corticosteroids); may have a reduced response to vaccination. Patients who will be receiving immunosuppressive therapy (including Hodgkin's disease, cancer chemotherapy, or transplantation) should be vaccinated at least 2 weeks prior to the initiation of immunosuppressive therapy when feasible (IDSA [Rubin, 2014]). Immune responses may be impaired for several months following intensive immunosuppressive therapy (up to 2 years in Hodgkin's disease patients). In general, households and close contacts of persons with altered immunocompetence may receive all age-appropriate vaccines. Vaccination may not result in effective immunity in all patients. Response depends upon multiple factors (eg, type of vaccine, age of patient) and may be improved by administering the vaccine at the recommended dose, route, and interval (CDC/ACIP [Kroger, 2011]).

Use caution in patients with severe cardiovascular or pulmonary disease where a systemic reaction may pose a significant risk. Patients who will undergo splenectomy or cochlear implant should be vaccinated at least 2 weeks prior to surgery, if possible. Patients with HIV should be vaccinated as soon as possible (following confirmation of the diagnosis). Not recommended in children <2 years of age.

Administer with caution to patients with thrombocytopenia or any coagulation disorder that would be compromised by I.M. injection; if the patient receives antihemophilia or other similar therapy, I.M. injection can be scheduled shortly after such therapy is administered. May cause relapse in patients with stable idiopathic thrombocytopenia purpura. Antipyretics have not been shown to prevent febrile seizures; antipyretics may be used to treat fever or discomfort following vaccination (CDC/ACIP [Kroger, 2011]). One study reported that routine prophylactic administration of acetaminophen to prevent fever prior to vaccination decreased the immune response of some vaccines; the clinical significance of this reduction in immune response has not been established (Prymula, 2009).

Use of this vaccine for specific medical and/or other indications (eg, immunocompromising conditions, hepatic or kidney disease, diabetes) is also addressed in the ACIP Recommended Immunization Schedule (CDC/ACIP [Akinsanya-Beysolow, 2014]; CDC/ACIP [Bridges, 2014]). Specific recommendations for use of this vaccine in immunocompromised patients with asplenia, cancer, HIV infection, cerebrospinal fluid leaks, cochlear implants, hematopoietic stem cell transplant (prior to or after), sickle cell disease, solid organ transplant (prior to or after), or those receiving immunosuppressive therapy for chronic conditions as well as contacts of immunocompromised patients are available from the IDSA (Rubin, 2014).

Adverse Reactions All serious adverse reactions must be reported to the U.S. Department of Health and Human Services (DHHS) Vaccine Adverse Event Reporting System (VAERS) 1-800-822-7967 or online at https://vaers.hhs.gov/esub/index. In Canada, adverse reactions may be reported to local provincial/territorial health agencies or to the Vaccine Safety Section at Public Health Agency of Canada (1-866-844-0018).

Central nervous system: Chills, Guillain-Barré syndrome, fever ≤102°F*, fever >102°F, headache, malaise, pain, radiculoneuropathy, seizure (febrile)

Dermatologic: Angioneurotic edema, cellulitis, rash, urticaria

Gastrointestinal: Nausea, vomiting

Hematologic: Hemolytic anemia (in patients with other hematologic disorders), leukocytosis, thrombocytopenia (in patients with stabilized ITP)

Local: Injection site reaction* (erythema, induration, swelling, soreness, warmth); peripheral edema in injected extremity

Neuromuscular & skeletal: Arthralgia, arthritis, limb mobility decreased, myalgia, paresthesia, weakness

Miscellaneous: Anaphylactoid reaction, C-reactive protein increased, lymphadenitis, lymphadenopathy, serum sickness

*Reactions most commonly reported in clinical trials.

Drug Interactions

Metabolism/Transport Effects None known.

Avoid Concomitant Use There are no known interactions where it is recommended to avoid concomitant use.

Increased Effect/Toxicity There are no known significant interactions involving an increase in effect.

Decreased Effect

Pneumococcal Polysaccharide Vaccine (Polyvalent) may decrease the levels/effects of: Zoster Vaccine

The levels/effects of Pneumococcal Polysaccharide Vaccine (Polyvalent) may be decreased by: Belimumab; Fingolimod; Immunosuppressants

Stability Store at 2°C to 8°C (36°F to 46°F).

Mechanism of Action Although there are more than 80 known pneumococcal capsular types, pneumococcal disease is mainly caused by only a few types of pneumococci. Pneumococcal vaccine contains capsular polysaccharides of 23 pneumococcal types of Streptococcal pneumoniae which represent at least 85% to 90% of pneumococcal disease isolates in the United States. The 23 capsular pneumococcal vaccine contains purified capsular polysaccharides of pneumococcal types 1, 2, 3, 4, 5, 6B, 7F, 8, 9N, 9V, 10A, 11A, 12F, 14, 15B, 17F, 18C, 19F, 19A, 20, 22F, 23F, and 33F.

Dosing: Usual

Pediatric:

Primary immunization: Children ≥2 years and Adolescents with specified underlying medical conditions: I.M., SubQ: 0.5 mL as a single dose; immunization with PCV13 should be completed prior to PPSV23 as recommended. The minimum interval between the last dose of PCV13 and PPSV23 is 8 weeks (AAP, 2010; CDC/ACIP [Nuorti, 2010]).

Revaccination: Children with functional or anatomic asplenia or who are immunocompromised: One revaccination dose ≥5 years after the first dose of PPSV23. Revaccination of immunocompetent individuals is generally not recommended (CDC/ACIP [Nuorti, 2010]).

Adult:

Primary immunization:

Adults 19 to 64 years of age with specified underlying medical conditions: Pneumococcal vaccine-naïve (no previous PCV13 or PPSV23 vaccine): I.M., SubQ: 0.5 mL as a single dose. Immunization with PCV13 should be completed prior to PPSV23 as recommended. The minimum interval between the last dose of PCV13 and PPSV23 is 8 weeks (CDC/ACIP, 61[40], 2012).

Adults ≥65 years of age without previous PPSV23 vaccination: I.M., SubQ: 0.5 mL as a single dose (CDC/ACIP, 59[34], 2010).

Revaccination:

Adults 19 to 64 years of age with chronic renal failure or nephrotic syndrome, functional, or anatomic asplenia or who are immunocompromised: One revaccination dose ≥5 years after first dose of PPSV23 (CDC/ACIP, 59[34], 2010) and ≥8 weeks after PCV13 (CDC/ACIP, 61[40], 2012)

Adults ≥65 years: One revaccination dose if ≥5 years after first dose of PPSV23 and if <65 years of age at the time of the initial vaccination (for any indication). Immunocompetent adults who received primary vaccination at ≥65 years do not need to be revaccinated (CDC/ACIP, 59[34], 2010; CDC/ACIP, 61[40], 2012).

Dosing adjustment in renal impairment: There are no dosage adjustments provided in the manufacturer's labeling.

Dosing adjustment in hepatic impairment: There are no dosage adjustments provided in the manufacturer's labeling.

Administration Administer SubQ or I.M. either the anterolateral aspect of the thigh or the deltoid muscle; **not for I.V. or intradermal administration.** Adolescents and adults should be vaccinated while seated or lying down. U.S. law requires that the date of administration; the vaccine manufacturer; lot number of vaccine; and the administering person's name, title, and address be entered into the patient's permanent medical record.

Monitoring Parameters Observe for syncope for 15 minutes following administration. If seizure-like activity associated with syncope occurs, maintain patient in supine or Trendelenburg position to reestablish adequate cerebral perfusion.

Additional Information In order to maximize vaccination rates, the ACIP recommends simultaneous administration (ie, >1 vaccine on the same day at different anatomic sites) of all age-appropriate vaccines (live or inactivated) for which a person is eligible at a single visit, unless contraindications exist. If available, the use of combination vaccines is generally preferred over separate injections, taking into consideration provider assessment, patient preference, and potential adverse events. If separate vaccines being used, evaluate product information regarding same syringe compatibility of vaccines. Separate needles and syringes should be used for each injection. The ACIP prefers each dose of specific vaccine in a series come from the same manufacturer if possible (CDC/ACIP [Kroger, 2011]).

For additional information, please refer to the following website: http://www.cdc.gov/vaccines/vpd-vac/.

Dosage Forms Excipient information presented when available (limited, particularly for generics); consult specific product labeling.

Injection, solution:

Pneumovax® 23: 25 mcg each of 23 capsular polysaccharide isolates/0.5 mL (0.5 mL, 2.5 mL)

References

AAP Steering Committee on Quality Improvement and Management, Subcommittee on Febrile Seizures American Academy of Pediatrics, "Febrile Seizures: Clinical Practice Guideline for the Long-Term Management of the Child With Simple Febrile Seizures," *Pediatrics*, 2008, 121(6):1281-6.

Akinsanya-Beysolow I, Advisory Committee on Immunization Practices (ACIP), ACIP Child/Adolescent Immunization Work Group, et al. Advisory committee on immunization practices recommended immunization schedules for persons aged 0 through 18 years - United States, 2014. *MMWR Morb Mortal Wkly Rep*. 2014; 63(5):108-109. Full schedule available at http://www.cdc.gov/vaccines/schedules/downloads/child/0-18yrs-child-combined-schedule.pdf

American Academy of Pediatrics Committee on Infectious Diseases, "Recommendations for the Prevention of *Streptococcus pneumoniae* Infections in Infants and Children: Use of 13-Valent Pneumococcal Conjugate Vaccine (PCV13) and Pneumococcal Polysaccharide Vaccine (PPSV23)," *Pediatrics*, 2010, 126(1):186-90.

Bridges CB, Coyne-Beasley T, Advisory Committee on Immunization Practices (ACIP), ACIP Adult Immunization Work Group; Centers for Disease Control and Prevention (CDC). Advisory committee on immunization practices recommended immunization schedule for adults aged 19 years or older - United States, 2014. *MMWR Morb Mortal Wkly Rep*. 2014; 63(5):108-109. Available at: http://www.cdc.gov/vaccines/schedules/downloads/adult/adult-combined-schedule.pdf

Centers for Disease Control and Prevention (CDC), "Syncope After Vaccination-United States, January 2005-July 2007," *MMWR Morb Mortal Wkly Rep*, 2008, 2;57(17):457-60.

Centers for Disease Control and Prevention (CDC), "Updated Recommendations for Prevention of Invasive Pneumococcal Disease Among Adults Using the 23-Valent Pneumococcal Polysaccharide Vaccine (PPSV23)," *MMWR Morb Mortal Wkly Rep*, 2010, 59 (34):1102-6.

Centers for Disease Control and Prevention (CDC), "Use of 13-Valent Pneumococcal Conjugate Vaccine and 23-Valent Pneumococcal Polysaccharide Vaccine for Adults With Immunocompromising Conditions: Recommendations of the Advisory Committee on Immunization Practices (ACIP)," *MMWR Morb Mortal Wkly Rep*, 2012, 61 (40):816-9.

Davidson M, Bulkow LR, Grabman J, et al, "Immunogenicity of Pneumococcal Revaccination in Patients With Chronic Disease," *Arch Intern Med*, 1994, 154(19):2209-14.

Kroger AT, Atkinson WL, Marcuse EK, Pickering LK. General recommendations on immunization - recommendations of the Advisory Committee on Immunization Practices (ACIP). *MMWR Recomm Rep*. 2011;60(RR-2):1-64.

Nuorti JP, Whitney CG. Prevention of pneumococcal disease among infants and children - use of 13-valent pneumococcal conjugate vaccine and 23-valent pneumococcal polysaccharide vaccine - recommendations of the Advisory Committee on Immunization Practices (ACIP). *MMWR Recomm Rep*. 2010;59(RR-11):1-18.

Prymula R, Siegrist CA, Chlibek R, et al, "Effect of Prophylactic Paracetamol Administration at Time of Vaccination on Febrile Reactions and Antibody Responses in Children: Two Open-Label, Randomised Controlled Trials," *Lancet*, 2009, 374(9698):1339-50.

Rubin LG, Levin MJ, Ljungman P, et al. 2013 IDSA clinical practice guideline for vaccination of the immunocompromised host. *Clin Infect Dis*. 2014;58(3):e44-e100.

◆ **Pneumovax® 23** *see* Pneumococcal Polysaccharide Vaccine (Polyvalent) *on page 1691*

◆ **PNU-140690E** *see* Tipranavir *on page 2031*

◆ **Podactin [OTC]** *see* Miconazole (Topical) *on page 1410*

◆ **Podactin [OTC]** *see* Tolnaftate *on page 2044*

◆ **Podocon** *see* Podophyllum Resin *on page 1693*

◆ **Podofilm® (Can)** *see* Podophyllum Resin *on page 1693*

◆ **Podophyllin** *see* Podophyllum Resin *on page 1693*

Podophyllum Resin (po DOF fil um REZ in)

Related Information
Medications for Which a Single Dose May Be Fatal When Ingested by a Toddler *on page 2408*
Safe Handling of Hazardous Drugs *on page 2419*
Brand Names: U.S. Podocon
Brand Names: Canada Podofilm®
Therapeutic Category Keratolytic Agent
Generic Availability (U.S.) Yes
Use Topical treatment of benign growths including external genital and perianal warts (condylomata acuminata), papillomas, fibroids
Pregnancy Considerations Reports in pregnant women have shown evidence of fetal abnormalities, fetal death, and stillbirth; use is contraindicated in women who are or may become pregnant
Breast-Feeding Considerations It is not known of podophyllum resin is excreted into breast milk. Use in nursing women is contraindicated by the manufacturer.
Contraindications Not to be used on birthmarks, moles, or warts with hair growth; cervical, urethral, oral warts; not to be used by diabetic patients or patients with poor circulation; pregnant women; do not apply to normal tissue
Warnings Hazardous agent; use appropriate precautions for handling and disposal (NIOSH, 2012). For external use only. Avoid contact with the eyes as it can cause severe corneal damage; 25% solution should not be applied to or near mucous membranes; podophyllum resin has caused teratogenic effects (skin tags, polyneuritis, limb malformations, septal heart defects) and fetal death when used during pregnancy.
Precautions Use of large amounts of drug should be avoided. Do not apply to moles, birthmarks, or unusual warts; do not use if wart or surrounding tissue is inflamed/irritated. To be applied by a physician only.

Adverse Reactions
Central nervous system: Coma, fever, polyneuritis
Gastrointestinal: Paralytic ileus
Hematologic: Leukopenia, thrombocytopenia
Neuromuscular & skeletal: Paresthesia
Miscellaneous: Death

Drug Interactions
Metabolism/Transport Effects None known.
Avoid Concomitant Use There are no known interactions where it is recommended to avoid concomitant use.
Increased Effect/Toxicity There are no known significant interactions involving an increase in effect.
Decreased Effect There are no known significant interactions involving a decrease in effect.
Stability Hazardous agent; use appropriate precautions for handling and disposal (NIOSH, 2012). Protect from light; avoid exposure to excessive heat.
Mechanism of Action Directly affects epithelial cell metabolism by arresting mitosis through binding to a protein subunit of spindle microtubules (tubulin)
Dosing: Usual Children and Adults: Topical: 10% to 25% solution in compound benzoin tincture; use 1 drop at a time

allowing drying between drops until area is covered; total volume should be limited to <0.5 mL to an area <10 cm^2 for genital or perianal warts or <2 cm^2 for vaginal warts per treatment session; therapy may be repeated once weekly for up to 4 applications for the treatment of genital or perianal warts; use 10% solution when applied to or near mucous membranes

Verrucae: 25% solution is applied directly to the wart; remove drug from area of application within 6 hours

Administration Hazardous agent; use appropriate precautions for handling and disposal (NIOSH, 2012).

Topical: Clean and dry affected area prior to application. Use applicator provided with product. When applying for the first time leave on for only 30-40 minutes to determine patient sensitivity. After first use may leave on 1-4 hours depending on severity of lesion; systemic absorption may occur with prolonged contact. Do not treat large areas or many warts at one time. Remove drug with alcohol or soap and water once treatment time has elapsed.

Dosage Forms Excipient information presented when available (limited, particularly for generics); consult specific product labeling.

Solution, External:

Podocon: 25% (15 mL)

References

Goldfarb MT, Gupta AK, Gupta MA, et al, "Office Therapy for Human Papillomavirus Infection in Nongenital Sites," *Dermatol Clin*, 1991, 9 (2):287-96.

National Institute for Occupational Safety and Health (NIOSH), "NIOSH List of Antineoplastic and Other Hazardous Drugs in Healthcare Settings 2012." Available at http://www.cdc.gov/niosh/docs/2012-150/pdfs/2012-150.pdf. Accessed January 21, 2013.

◆ **Polio Vaccine** *see* Poliovirus Vaccine (Inactivated) *on page 1694*

◆ **Poliovirus, Inactivated (IPV)** *see* Diphtheria and Tetanus Toxoids, Acellular Pertussis, and Poliovirus Vaccine *on page 682*

◆ **Poliovirus, Inactivated (IPV)** *see* Diphtheria and Tetanus Toxoids, Acellular Pertussis, Poliovirus and *Haemophilus* b Conjugate Vaccine *on page 684*

Poliovirus Vaccine (Inactivated)
(POE lee oh VYE rus vak SEEN, in ak ti VAY ted)

Medication Safety Issues
Administration issues:
Poliovirus vaccine (inactivated) may be confused with tuberculin products. Medication errors have occurred when poliovirus vaccine (IPV) has been inadvertently administered instead of tuberculin skin tests (PPD). These products are refrigerated and often stored in close proximity to each other.

Related Information
Immunization Administration Recommendations *on page 2368*

Immunization Guidelines *on page 2373*

Brand Names: U.S. IPOL®

Brand Names: Canada Imovax® Polio

Therapeutic Category Vaccine, Inactivated Bacteria

Generic Availability (U.S.) No

Use Provide active immunity to poliovirus (FDA approved in ages ≥6 weeks and adults)

The Advisory Committee on Immunization Practices (ACIP) recommends routine vaccination for the following:
• All infants and children (first dose given at 2 months of age) (CDC, 58[30], 2009)

Routine immunization of adults in the United States is generally not recommended. Adults with previous wild poliovirus disease, who have never been immunized, or those who are incompletely immunized may receive inactivated poliovirus vaccine if they fall into one of the following categories (CDC/ACIP [Prevots, 2000]):
• Travelers to regions or countries where poliomyelitis is endemic or epidemic
• Health care workers in close contact with patients who may be excreting poliovirus
• Laboratory workers handling specimens that may contain poliovirus
• Members of communities or specific population groups with diseases caused by wild poliovirus
• Incompletely vaccinated or unvaccinated adults in a household or with other close contact with children receiving oral poliovirus (may be at increased risk of vaccine associated paralytic poliomyelitis)

Pregnancy Risk Factor C

Pregnancy Considerations Animal reproduction studies have not been conducted. Although adverse effects of IPV have not been documented in pregnant women or their fetuses, vaccination of pregnant women should be avoided on theoretical grounds. Pregnant women at increased risk for infection and requiring immediate protection against polio may be administered the vaccine.

Breast-Feeding Considerations Inactivated virus vaccines do not affect the safety of breast-feeding for the mother or the infant. Breast-feeding infants should be vaccinated according to the recommended schedules (CDC, 2011).

Contraindications Hypersensitivity to any component including neomycin, streptomycin, or polymyxin B

Warnings Immediate treatment (including epinephrine 1:1000) for anaphylactic and/or hypersensitivity reactions should be available during vaccine use. Apnea has occurred following intramuscular vaccine administration in premature infants; consider clinical status implications. Syncope has been reported with use of injectable vaccines and may be accompanied by transient visual disturbances, weakness, or tonic-clonic movements. Procedures should be in place to avoid injuries from falling and to restore cerebral perfusion if syncope occurs (CDC, 57[17], 2008). Products may contain 2-phenoxyethanol, calf serum protein, formaldehyde, neomycin, streptomycin, or polymyxin B.

Precautions The decision to administer or delay vaccination because of current or recent febrile illness depends on the severity of symptoms and the etiology of the disease. Immunization should be delayed during the course of an acute severe febrile illness; may administer to patients with mild acute illness (with or without fever).

Use with caution in severely immunocompromised patients (eg, patients receiving chemo/radiation therapy or other immunosuppressive therapy, including high-dose corticosteroids); may have a reduced response to vaccination;; inactivated vaccines should be administered ≥2 weeks prior to planned immunosuppression when feasible (IDSA [Rubin, 2014]). In general, households and close contacts of persons with altered immunocompetence may receive all age-appropriate vaccines.

Vaccination may not result in effective immunity in all patients. Response depends upon multiple factors (eg, type of vaccine, age of patient) and may be improved by administering the vaccine at the recommended dose, route, and interval (CDC/ACIP [Kroger, 2011]). Patients with prior clinical poliomyelitis or incomplete immunization with oral poliovirus vaccine (OPV) may receive inactivated poliovirus vaccine (IPV). Immune response may be decreased in patients receiving immune globulin. Use of the minimum age and minimum intervals during the first 6 months of life should only be done when the vaccine recipient is at risk for imminent exposure to circulating poliovirus (shorter intervals and earlier start dates may lead to lower seroconversion).

Antipyretics have not been shown to prevent febrile seizures; antipyretics may be used to treat fever or discomfort following vaccination (CDC/ACIP [Kroger, 2011]). One study reported that routine prophylactic administration of acetaminophen to prevent fever prior to vaccination decreased the immune response of some vaccines; the clinical significance of this reduction in immune response has not been established (Prymula, 2009).

Use of this vaccine for specific medical and/or other indications (eg, immunocompromising conditions, hepatic or kidney disease, diabetes) is also addressed in the ACIP Recommended Immunization Schedule (CDC/ACIP [Akinsanya-Beysolow, 2014]; CDC/ACIP [Bridges, 2014]). Specific recommendations for use of this vaccine in immunocompromised patients with asplenia, cancer, HIV infection, cerebrospinal fluid leaks, cochlear implants, hematopoietic stem cell transplant (prior to or after), sickle cell disease, solid organ transplant (prior to or after), or those receiving immunosuppressive therapy for chronic conditions as well as contacts of immunocompromised patients are available from the IDSA (Rubin, 2014).

Adverse Reactions All serious adverse reactions must be reported to the U.S. Department of Health and Human Services (DHHS) Vaccine Adverse Event Reporting System (VAERS) 1-800-822-7967 or online at https://vaers.hhs.gov/esub/index. In Canada, adverse reactions may be reported to local provincial/territorial health agencies or to the Vaccine Safety Section at Public Health Agency of Canada (1-866-844-0018).

Central nervous system: Fever (>39°C), irritability (most common in infants 2 months of age), tiredness
Gastrointestinal: Anorexia
Local: Injection site: Swelling, tenderness
Gastrointestinal: Vomiting
Local: Injection site: Erythema
Miscellaneous: Persistent crying
Rare but important or life-threatening: Allergic reaction, anaphylactic shock, anaphylaxis, febrile seizures, hypersensitivity reactions, lymphadenopathy, seizures; Guillain-Barré syndrome has been temporally related to another inactivated poliovirus vaccine

Drug Interactions
Metabolism/Transport Effects None known.
Avoid Concomitant Use There are no known interactions where it is recommended to avoid concomitant use.
Increased Effect/Toxicity There are no known significant interactions involving an increase in effect.
Decreased Effect
The levels/effects of Poliovirus Vaccine (Inactivated) may be decreased by: Belimumab; Fingolimod; Immunosuppressants

Stability Store at 2°C to 8°C (35°F to 46°F); do not freeze; protect from light.
Dosing: Usual
Pediatric: **Note:** Use of the minimum age and minimum intervals during the first 6 months of life should only be done when the vaccine recipient is at risk for imminent exposure to circulating poliovirus (shorter intervals and earlier start dates may lead to lower seroconversion).
Primary immunization: Infants and Children 6 weeks to 47 months: I.M., SubQ: 0.5 mL per dose for a total of 3 doses administered as follows: 2 months, 4 months, and 6 to 18 months; do not administer more frequently than 4 weeks apart (preferably given more than 8 weeks apart)
Booster immunization: Children 4 to 6 years: I.M., SubQ: 0.5 mL as a single dose; administered at least 6 months from the previous dose

Catch-up immunization: Infants, Children, and Adolescents 4 months to 18 years: **Note:** Do not restart the series if doses have been given (OPV or IPV). Begin the below schedule at the applicable dose number. Exposure to circulating poliovirus (shorter intervals and earlier start dates may lead to lower seroconversion). I.M., SubQ: 0.5 mL per dose for a total of 1 to 4 doses administered as follows:
First dose given on the elected date
Second dose given at least 4 weeks after the first dose
Third dose given at least 4 weeks after the second dose
Fourth dose given at ≥4 years of age and least 6 months after the second dose; fourth dose not needed if the third dose was given at least 6 months after second dose and at ≥4 years of age)
Note: If 4 or more doses were administered before age of 4 years, an additional dose should be given at age 4 to 6 years, at least 6 months after the previous dose.
Adult: **Note:** Not routinely recommended unless at increased risk of exposure.
Immunization:
Poliovirus vaccine-naïve (no previous IPV or OPV vaccine): I.M., SubQ: 0.5 mL per dose for a total of 3 doses given as follows: Two 0.5 mL doses administered at 1- to 2-month intervals, followed by a third dose 6 to 12 months later. If <3 months, but at least 2 months are available before protection is needed, 3 doses may be administered at least 1 month apart. If administration must be completed within 1 to 2 months, give 2 doses at least 1 month apart. If <1 month is available, give 1 dose.
Previously vaccinated with at least at least 1 previous dose of OPV, <3 doses of IPV, or a combination of OPV and IPV equaling <3 doses: Administer at least one 0.5 mL dose of IPV. Additional doses to complete the series may be given if time permits.
Immunization for increased risk of exposure (completely vaccinated): I.M, SubQ: 0.5 mL as a single dose
Dosing adjustment in renal impairment: There are no dosage adjustments provided in the manufacturer's labeling.
Dosing adjustment in hepatic impairment: There are no dosage adjustments provided in the manufacturer's labeling.
Administration Administer I.M. or SubQ into midlateral aspect of the thigh in infants and small children; administer in the deltoid area to older children and adults; **not for I.V. administration.** Adolescents and adults should be vaccinated while seated or lying down. U.S. law requires that the date of administration, the vaccine manufacturer, lot number of vaccine, and the administering person's name, title, and address be entered into the patient's permanent medical record.
Monitoring Parameters Observe for syncope for 15 minutes following administration. If seizure-like activity associated with syncope occurs, maintain patient in supine or Trendelenburg position to reestablish adequate cerebral perfusion.
Test Interactions May temporarily suppress tuberculin skin test sensitivity (4-6 weeks)
Additional Information Oral polio vaccine (OPV) is no longer distributed in the United States; OPV is the vaccine of choice for global eradication in areas with continued or recent circulation of wild-type poliovirus, most developing countries where the higher cost of IPV prohibits its use or where inadequate sanitation necessitates an optimal barrier to wild-type virus circulation (Red Book [AAP], 2012)

In order to maximize vaccination rates, the ACIP recommends simultaneous administration (ie, >1 vaccine on the same day at different anatomic sites) of all age-appropriate vaccines (live or inactivated) for which a person is eligible

◀ at a single visit, unless contraindications exist. If available, the use of combination vaccines is generally preferred over separate injections, taking into consideration provider assessment, patient preference, and potential adverse events. If separate vaccines being used, evaluate product information regarding same syringe compatibility of vaccines. Separate needles and syringes should be used for each injection. The ACIP prefers each dose of specific vaccine in a series come from the same manufacturer if possible (CDC/ACIP [Kroger, 2011]).

For additional information, please refer to the following website: http://www.cdc.gov/vaccines/vpd-vac/.

Dosage Forms Excipient information presented when available (limited, particularly for generics); consult specific product labeling.

Injection, suspension:

IPOL®: Type 1 poliovirus 40 D-antigen units, type 2 poliovirus 8 D-antigen units, and type 3 poliovirus 32 D-antigen units per 0.5 mL (0.5 mL, 5 mL) [contains 2-phenoxyethanol, formaldehyde, calf serum protein, neomycin (may have trace amounts), streptomycin (may have trace amounts), and polymyxin B (may have trace amounts)]

References

AAP Steering Committee on Quality Improvement and Management, Subcommittee on Febrile Seizures American Academy of Pediatrics, "Febrile Seizures: Clinical Practice Guideline for the Long-Term Management of the Child With Simple Febrile Seizures," *Pediatrics*, 2008, 121(6):1281-6.

Akinsanya-Beysolow I, Advisory Committee on Immunization Practices (ACIP), ACIP Child/Adolescent Immunization Work Group, et al. Advisory committee on immunization practices recommended immunization schedule for adults aged 19 years or older - United States, 2014. *MMWR Morb Mortal Wkly Rep*. 2014; 63(5):108-109. Full schedule available at http://www.cdc.gov/vaccines/schedules/downloads/child/0-18yrs-child-combined-schedule.pdf

American Academy of Pediatrics (AAP). In: Pickering LK, Baker CJ, Kimberlin DW, Long SS, eds. *Red Book: 2012 Report of the Committee on Infectious Diseases*. 29th ed. Elk Grove Village, IL: American Academy of Pediatrics; 2012.

Bridges CB, Coyne-Beasley T, Advisory Committee on Immunization Practices (ACIP), et al. Advisory Committee on Immunization Practices recommended immunization schedule for adults aged 19 years or older - United States, 2014. *MMWR Morb Mortal Wkly Rep*. 2014;63 (5):110-112.

Centers for Disease Control and Prevention (CDC), "Syncope After Vaccination-United States, January 2005-July 2007," *MMWR Morb Mortal Wkly Rep*, 2008, 2;57(17):457-60.

Centers for Disease Control and Prevention (CDC). Updated recommendations of the Advisory Committee on Immunization Practices (ACIP) regarding routine poliovirus vaccination. *MMWR Recomm Rep*. 2009;58(30):829-830.

Kroger AT, Atkinson WL, Marcuse EK, Pickering LK. General recommendations on immunization - recommendations of the Advisory Committee on Immunization Practices (ACIP). *MMWR Recomm Rep*. 2011;60(RR-2):1-64.

Prevots DR, Burr RK, and Sutter RW, "Poliomyelitis Prevention in the United States: Updated Recommendations of the Advisory Committee on Immunization Practices (ACIP)," *MMWR Recomm Rep*, 2000, 49(RR-5):1-22.

Prymula R, Siegrist CA, Chlibek R, et al, "Effect of Prophylactic Paracetamol Administration at Time of Vaccination on Febrile Reactions and Antibody Responses in Children: Two Open-Label, Randomised Controlled Trials," *Lancet*, 2009, 374(9698):1339-50.

Rubin LG, Levin MJ, Ljungman P, et al. 2013 IDSA clinical practice guideline for the vaccination of the immunocompromised host. *Clin Infect Dis*. 2014;58(3):e44-e100.

◆ **Polocaine** *see* Mepivacaine *on page 1341*

◆ **Polocaine® (Can)** *see* Mepivacaine *on page 1341*

◆ **Polocaine-MPF** *see* Mepivacaine *on page 1341*

◆ **Polycin™** *see* Bacitracin and Polymyxin B *on page 257*

◆ **Polycitra** *see* Citric Acid, Sodium Citrate, and Potassium Citrate *on page 487*

◆ **Polycitra K** *see* Potassium Citrate and Citric Acid *on page 1710*

◆ **Polyethylene Glycol-L-asparaginase** *see* Pegaspargase *on page 1615*

Polyethylene Glycol 3350
(pol i ETH i leen GLY kol 3350)

Medication Safety Issues
Sound-alike/look-alike issues:
MiraLax may be confused with Mirapex
Polyethylene glycol 3350 may be confused with polyethylene glycol electrolyte solution
International issues:
MiraLax may be confused with Murelax brand name for oxazepam [Australia]
Polyethylene glycol 3350 may be confused with polyethylene glycol 4000 [international markets]

Brand Names: U.S. GaviLAX [OTC]; GlycoLax [OTC]; HealthyLax [OTC]; MiraLax [OTC]; PEGyLAX

Brand Names: Canada Peg 3350; Pegalax; Relaxa

Therapeutic Category Laxative, Osmotic

Generic Availability (U.S.) Yes

Use Treatment of occasional constipation (FDA approved in ages ≥17 years)

Pregnancy Considerations Polyethylene glycol (PEG) has minimal systemic absorption and would be unlikely to cause fetal malformations. However, until additional information is available, use to treat constipation in pregnancy should be avoided unless other preferred methods are inadequate (Mahadevan, 2006). Use as a bowel preparation prior to colonoscopy in pregnant women may be considered (Wexner, 2006).

Contraindications Hypersensitivity to polyethylene glycol or any component; GI obstruction, ileus, gastric retention, bowel perforation, toxic colitis, megacolon

Warnings Evaluate patients with symptoms of bowel obstruction (nausea, vomiting, abdominal pain, or distension) prior to use. 1-3 days may be required to produce bowel movement. Prolonged, frequent, or excessive use may lead to electrolyte imbalance.

Precautions Use with caution in patients with renal dysfunction.

Adverse Reactions
Dermatologic: Urticaria
Gastrointestinal: Abdominal bloating, cramping, diarrhea, flatulence, nausea
Rare but important or life-threatening: Anaphylactic shock (observed with PEG 6000)

Drug Interactions
Metabolism/Transport Effects None known.
Avoid Concomitant Use There are no known interactions where it is recommended to avoid concomitant use.
Increased Effect/Toxicity There are no known significant interactions involving an increase in effect.
Decreased Effect
Polyethylene Glycol 3350 may decrease the levels/effects of: Digoxin

Stability Store at room temperature before reconstitution.

Mechanism of Action An osmotic agent, polyethylene glycol 3350 causes water retention in the stool; increases stool frequency.

Pharmacodynamics Onset of action: Produces bowel movement in 1-3 days

Dosing: Usual
Occasional constipation: Dulcolax Balance®, MiraLax™:
Children >6 months: 0.5-1.5 g/kg daily (initial dose: 0.5 g/kg; titrate to effect); not to exceed 17 g/day
Adults: Oral: 17 g (~1 heaping tablespoon) daily
Fecal impaction: >3 years: 1-1.5 g/kg daily (maximum daily dose: 100 g) for 3 days
Bowel preparation:
Children >2 years: 1.5 g/kg/day (maximum daily dose: 100 g) for 4 days
Adults: Mix 17 g in 8 oz of clear liquid and administer the entire mixture every 10 minutes until 2 liters are

consumed (start within 6 hours after administering 20 mg bisacodyl delayed-release tablets) (Wexner, 2006)

Administration Oral: Dulcolax Balance®, MiraLax™: 17 g (dose may be measured using bottle cap) added to 4-8 ounces of beverage (cold, hot, or room temperature)

Monitoring Parameters Stool frequency

Dosage Forms Excipient information presented when available (limited, particularly for generics); consult specific product labeling.

Packet, Oral:
HealthyLax: (1 ea, 14 ea)
MiraLax: (1 ea, 10 ea, 12 ea, 24 ea)
Generic: (1 ea, 14 ea, 30 ea, 100 ea)

Powder, Oral:
GaviLAX: (238 g, 510 g)
GlycoLax: (119 g, 255 g, 527 g)
MiraLax: (1 ea, 119 g, 238 g, 510 g)
PEGyLAX: (527 g)
Generic: 17 g/dose (119 g, 238 g, 510 g); (119 g, 238 g, 250 g, 255 g, 500 g, 510 g, 527 g, 850 g)

References

Bell EA and Wall GC, "Pediatric Constipation Therapy Using Guidelines and Polyethylene Glycol 3350," *Ann Pharmacother*, 2004, 38 (4):686-93.

Candy D and Belsey J, "Macrogol (Polyethylene Glycol) Laxatives in Children With Functional Constipation and Faecal Impaction: A Systematic Review," *Arch Dis Child*, 2009, 94(2):156-60.

Co-Minh HB, Demoly P, Guillot B, et al, "Anaphylactic Shock After Oral Intake and Contact Urticaria Due to Polyethylene Glycols," *Allergy*, 2007, 62(1):92-3.

Loening-Baucke V, "Prevalence, Symptoms and Outcome of Constipation in Infants and Toddlers," *J Pediatr*, 2005, 146(3):359-63.

Loening-Baucke V, Krishna R, and Pashankar DS, "Polyethylene Glycol 3350 Without Electrolytes for the Treatment of Functional Constipation in Infants and Toddlers," *J Pediatr Gastroenterol Nutr*, 2004, 39 (5):536-9.

Mahadevan U and Kane S, "American Gastroenterological Association Institute Technical Review on the Use of Gastrointestinal Medications in Pregnancy," *Gastroenterology*, 2006, 131(1):283-311.

Michail S, Gendy E, Preud'Homme D, et al, "Polyethylene Glycol for Constipation in Children Younger Than Eighteen Months Old," *J Pediatr Gastroenterol Nutr*, 2004, 39(2):197-9.

North American Society for Pediatric Gastroenterology, Hepatology and Nutrition, "Evaluation and Treatment of Constipation in Children: Summary of Updated Recommendations of the North American Society for Pediatric Gastroenterology, Hepatology and Nutrition," *J Pediatr Gastroenterol Nutr*, 2006, 43(3):405-7.

Nurko S, Youssef NN, Sabri M, et al, "PEG3350 in the Treatment of Childhood Constipation: A Multicenter, Double-Blinded, Placebo-Controlled Trial," *J Pediatr*, 2008, 153(2):254-61, 261.e1.

Pashankar DS, Bishop WP, and Loening-Baucke V, "Long-Term Efficacy of Polyethylene Glycol 3350 for the Treatment of Chronic Constipation in Children With and Without Encopresis," *Clin Pediatr (Phila)*, 2003, 42(9):815-9.

Pashankar DS, Loening-Baucke V, and Bishop WP, "Safety of Polyethylene Glycol 3350 for the Treatment of Chronic Constipation in Children," *Arch Pediatr Adolesc Med*, 2003, 157(7):661-4.

Pashankar DS, Uc A, and Bishop WP, "Polyethylene Glycol 3350 Without Electrolytes: A New Safe, Effective, and Palatable Bowel Preparation for Colonoscopy in Children," *J Pediatr*, 2004, 144 (3):358-62.

Pelham RW, Nix LC, Chavira RE, et al, "Clinical Trial: Single- and Multiple-Dose Pharmacokinetics of Polyethylene Glycol (PEG-3350) in Healthy Young and Elderly Subjects," *Aliment Pharmacol Ther*, 2008, 28(2):256-65.

Safder S, Demintieva Y, Rewalt M, et al, "Stool Consistency and Stool Frequency are Excellent Clinical Markers for Adequate Colon Preparation After Polyethylene Glycol 3350 Cleansing Protocol: A Prospective Clinical Study in Children," *Gastrointest Endosc*, 2008, 68 (6):1131-5.

van den Berg MM, van Rossum CH, de Lorijn F, et al, "Functional Constipation in Infants: A Follow-Up Study," *J Pediatr*, 2005, 147 (5):700-4.

Voskuijl W, de Lorijn F, Verwijs W, et al, "PEG 3350 (Transipeg) Versus Lactulose in the Treatment of Childhood Functional Constipation: A Double Blind, Randomised, Controlled, Multicentre Trial," *Gut*, 2004, 53(11):1590-4.

Wexner SD, Beck DE, Baron TH, et al, "A Consensus Document on Bowel Preparation Before Colonoscopy: Prepared by a Task Force From the American Society of Colon and Rectal Surgeons (ASCRS), the American Society for Gastrointestinal Endoscopy (ASGE), and the Society of American Gastrointestinal and Endoscopic Surgeons (SAGES)," *Surg Endosc*, 2006, 20(7):1161.

Wexner SD, Beck DE, Baron TH, et al, "A Consensus Document on Bowel Preparation Before Colonoscopy: Prepared by a Task Force from The American Society of Colon and Rectal Surgeons (ASCRS), The American Society for Gastrointestinal and Endoscopy (ASGE) and The Society of American Gastrointestinal and Endoscopic Surgeons (SAGES)," *Dis Colon Rectum*, 2006, 49(6):792-809.

Youssef NN, Peters JM, Henderson W, et al, "Dose Response of PEG 3350 for the Treatment of Childhood Fecal Impaction," *J Pediatr*, 2002, 141(3):410-4.

Polyethylene Glycol-Electrolyte Solution
(pol i ETH i leen GLY kol ee LEK troe lite soe LOO shun)

Medication Safety Issues
Sound-alike/look-alike issues:
GoLYTELY may be confused with NuLYTELY
TriLyte may be confused with TriLipix

International issues:
Polyethylene glycol 3350 may be confused with polyethylene glycol 4000 [international markets]

Brand Names: U.S. Colyte; GaviLyte-C; GaviLyte-G; GaviLyte-N; GoLYTELY; MoviPrep; NuLYTELY; TriLyte

Brand Names: Canada Colyte; Klean-Prep; PegLyte

Therapeutic Category Laxative, Bowel Evacuant; Laxative, Osmotic

Generic Availability (U.S.) Yes

Use Bowel cleansing prior to GI procedure (GaviLyte™-N, NuLYTELY®, Trilyte™: FDA approved in ages ≥6 months and adults; MoviPrep®: FDA approved in ages ≥18 and adults; Colyte®, GaviLyte™-C, GaviLyte™-G: FDA approved in adults); has also been used for whole bowel irrigation after toxic ingestions and for treatment of fecal impaction

Medication Guide Available Yes

Pregnancy Risk Factor C

Pregnancy Considerations Animal reproduction studies have not been conducted. Information related to the use of polyethylene glycol-electrolyte solution in pregnancy is limited (Neri, 2004). Colonoscopy in pregnant women is generally reserved for strong indications or life-threatening emergencies; until additional safety data for polyethylene glycol-electrolyte solution is available, other agents may be preferred for this purpose (Siddiqui, 2006; Wexner, 2006).

Breast-Feeding Considerations It is not known if polyethylene glycol-electrolyte solution is excreted into breast milk. Significant changes in the mother's fluid or electrolyte balance would not be expected with most products.

Contraindications Hypersensitivity to polyethylene glycol or any component, GI obstruction, illeus, gastric retention, bowel perforation, toxic colitis, megacolon

Warnings Serious arrhythmias have been reported (rarely) with the use of ionic osmotic laxative products; use with caution in patients who may be at risk of cardiac arrhythmias (eg, patients with a history of prolonged QT, uncontrolled arrhythmias, recent MI, unstable angina, CHF, or cardiomyopathy); consider predose and post-colonoscopy ECGs in these patients. Fluid and electrolyte disturbances can lead to arrhythmias, seizures, and renal impairment; correct electrolyte imbalances prior to use. Advise patients to maintain adequate hydration before, during, and after treatment; if patient becomes dehydrated or experiences significant vomiting after treatment, consider post-colonoscopy lab tests (electrolytes, creatinine, and BUN).

Seizures and/or loss of consciousness have occurred rarely in patients with no prior history of seizures; seizures resolved with the correction of fluid and electrolyte abnormalities. Use caution in patients with a history of seizures or who are at an increased risk of seizures (concomitant administration of medications that lower the seizure threshold, patients withdrawing from alcohol or benzodiazepines) and in patients with known or suspected hyponatremia or low serum osmolality.

Cases of ischemic colitis have been reported; concomitant use of stimulant laxatives may increase the risk and is not recommended. The potential for mucosal aphthous ulcerations as a result of the bowel preparation should be considered, especially when evaluating colonoscopy results in patients with known or suspected inflammatory bowel disease.

Evaluate patients with symptoms of bowel obstruction or perforation (nausea, vomiting, abdominal pain or distension) prior to use; if a patient develops severe bloating, distention, or abdominal pain during administration, slow the rate of administration or temporarily discontinue use until the symptoms subside. No additional ingredients or flavors (other than the flavor packets provided) should be added to the polyethylene glycol-electrolyte solution.

Precautions May interfere with barium coating of intestinal wall using the double contrast technique. Use with caution in patients with ulcerative colitis. Use with caution in patients with renal impairment and/or in patients taking medications that may adversely affect renal function (eg, diuretics, NSAIDs, ACE inhibitors, ARBs). Use with caution and observe closely in patients who are unconscious or semiconscious or patients with impaired gag reflex or those who are otherwise prone to regurgitation or aspiration during administration. Use in patients <2 years of age may result in hypoglycemia, dehydration, and hypokalemia. Use MoviPrep with caution in patients with G6PD deficiency (especially patients with an active infection, history of hemolysis, or taking concomitant medications know to precipitate hemolytic reactions) due to the presence of sodium ascorbate and ascorbic acid in the formulation. MoviPrep also contains phenylalanine which must be avoided (or used with caution) in patients with phenylketonuria.

Adverse Reactions
Central nervous system: Dizziness, headache, malaise, rigors, sleep disorder

Endocrine & metabolic: Increased thirst

Gastrointestinal: Abdominal distention, abdominal pain, anorectal pain, bloating, dyspepsia, hunger, nausea, vomiting

Rare but important or life-threatening: Anaphylaxis, angioedema, aspiration, asystole (older adults >60 years), chest tightness, esophageal perforation (older adults >60 years), hypersensitivity reaction, ischemic colitis, Mallory-Weiss syndrome (older adults >60 years), pulmonary edema (older adults >60 years), rhinorrhea, seizure, shock, tightness in chest and throat, upper gastrointestinal hemorrhage (older adults >60 years), urticaria

Drug Interactions
Metabolism/Transport Effects None known.

Avoid Concomitant Use There are no known interactions where it is recommended to avoid concomitant use.

Increased Effect/Toxicity There are no known significant interactions involving an increase in effect.

Decreased Effect There are no known significant interactions involving a decrease in effect.

Stability
CoLyte®, GaviLyte™-C: Store at 20°C to 25°C (68°F to 77°F); excursions permitted to 15°C to 30°C (59°F to 86°F). Refrigerate reconstituted solution. Use within 48 hours of preparation.

GaviLyte™-G, GoLYTELY®: Store at 15°C to 30°C (59°F to 86°F). Refrigerate reconstituted solution. Use within 48 hours of preparation.

GaviLyte™-N: Store at 25°C (77°F). Refrigerate reconstituted solution. Use within 48 hours of preparation.

MoviPrep®: Store at 20°C to 25°C (68°F to 77°F); excursions permitted to 15°C to 30°C (59°F to 86°F). Refrigerate reconstituted solution. Use within 24 hours of preparation.

NuLYTELY®, TriLyte™: Store at 25°C (77°F); excursions permitted to 15°C to 30°C (59°F to 86°F). Refrigerate reconstituted solution. Use within 48 hours of preparation.

Mechanism of Action Induces catharsis by strong electrolyte and osmotic effects

Pharmacodynamics Onset of action: Bowel cleansing: Within 1-2 hours

Dosing: Usual
Infants ≥6 months, Children, and Adolescents:

Bowel cleansing (to prevent excessive fluid and electrolyte changes, use only products containing supplemental electrolytes for bowel cleansing): Patient should fast at least 2 hours (preferably 3-4 hours) prior to ingestion: Oral, nasogastric: GaviLyte™-N, NuLYTELY®, and TriLyte™: 25 mL/kg/hour until rectal effluent is clear (usually in ~4 hours). One study used 40 mL/kg/hour intermittently by mouth or continuously by nasogastric drip in patients ≥18 months (Sandheimer, 1991). Although not FDA approved for pediatric patients, other preparations have been used in pediatric studies: Colyte®, GoLYTELY® (Sondheimer, 1991; Tuggle, 1987).

Fecal impaction (NASPGHAN, 2006): Nasogastric:
Rapid disimpaction: 25 mL/kg/hour until rectal effluent is clear

Slower disimpaction: 20 mL/kg/hour for 4 hours per day
Maintenance in older children: 5-10 mL/kg/day

Toxic ingestion (AACT, 2004): Nasogastric:
Ages ≥9 months to 6 years: 500 mL/hour until rectal effluent is clear

Ages 6-12 years: 1000 mL/hour until rectal effluent is clear

Adolescents: 1500-2000 mL/hour until rectal effluent is clear

Note: Continue treatment at least until the rectal effluent is clear; treatment duration may be extended based on corroborative evidence of continued presence of poisons in the GI tract as determined by radiographic means or the presence of the poison in the effluent.

Adults: **Bowel cleansing:**
CoLyte, GaviLyte-C, GaviLyte-G, GaviLyte-N, GoLYTELY, NuLYTELY, TriLyte:
Oral: 240 mL (8 oz) every 10 minutes until 4 L are consumed or the rectal effluent is clear; rapid drinking of each portion is preferred to drinking small amounts continuously

Nasogastric: 20-30 mL/minute until 4 L are administered or the rectal effluent is clear

MoviPrep: Oral: Administer 2 L total with an additional 1 L of clear fluid prior to colonoscopy as follows:
Split dose (2-day regimen) (preferred method):
Dose 1: Evening before colonoscopy (10-12 hours before dose 2): 240 mL (8 oz) every 15 minutes until 1 L (entire contents of container) is consumed. Then fill container with 480 mL (16 oz) of clear liquid and consume prior to going to bed.

Dose 2: On the morning of the colonoscopy (beginning at least 3.5 hours prior to procedure): 240 mL (8 oz) every 15 minutes until 1 L (entire contents of container) is consumed. Then fill container with 480 mL (16 oz) of clear liquid and consume at least 2 hours before the procedure.

Evening only dose (1-day regimen) (alternate method):
Dose 1: Evening before colonoscopy (at least 3.5 hours before bedtime): 240 mL (8 oz) every 15 minutes until 1 L (entire contents of container) is consumed

Dose 2: ~90 minutes after starting dose 1: 240 mL (8 oz) every 15 minutes until 1 L (entire contents of container) is consumed. Then fill container with 1 L (32 oz) of clear liquid and consume all of the liquid prior to going to bed.

Dosage adjustment in renal impairment: There are no dosage adjustments provided in manufacturer's labeling (not studied).

Dosage adjustment in hepatic impairment: There are no dosage adjustments provided in manufacturer's labeling (not studied).

Administration Oral: For bowel cleansing, no solid foods for 2-4 hours prior to initiation of therapy; rapid drinking is preferred to drinking small amounts continuously; chilled solution often more palatable, but not recommended for infants; refrigerate reconstituted solution when not in use; do not add ingredients as flavorings before use; discard any unused portion. The solution may be administered via nasogastric tube for bowel cleansing or whole bowel irrigation in patients who are unwilling or unable to drink the solution.

Colyte®, GaviLyte™-C, GaviLyte™-G, GaviLyte™-N, GoLYTELY®, NuLYTELY®, and TriLyte™: If using a flavor packet, add the flavor packet contents to the powder and shake well prior to adding water. Add tap water to "fill-line" for reconstitution and shake well until all ingredients have dissolved.

MoviPrep®: Mix the contents of one pouch A and one pouch B to container. Add 1000 mL of lukewarm water; mix the solution until dissolved. Repeat mixing procedure if second liter is needed.

Monitoring Parameters Electrolytes, BUN, serum glucose, urine osmolality; children <2 years of age should be monitored for hypoglycemia, dehydration, hypokalemia (not studied).

Additional Information Concentrations for reconstituted solutions:

When prepared as recommended by the manufacturer, the solutions will contain:

CoLyte®, GaviLyte™-C: When dissolved in sufficient water to make 4000 mL, the final solution contains PEG-3350 60 g/L, sodium 125 mEq/L, sulfate 80 mEql/L, chloride 35 mEql/L, bicarbonate 20 mEq/L, and potassium 10 mEq/L

GaviLyte™-G, GoLYTELY®: When dissolved in sufficient water to make 4000 mL, the final solution contains PEG-3350 59 g/L, sodium 125 mEq/L, sulfate 40 mEq/L, chloride 35 mEq/L, bicarbonate 20 mEq/L, and potassium 10 mEq/L

GaviLyte™-N, NuLYTELY®, TriLyte®: When dissolved in sufficient water to make 4000 mL, the final solution contains PEG-3350 105 g/L, sodium 65 mEq/L, chloride 53 mEq/L, bicarbonate 17 mEq/L, and potassium 5 mEq/L

Dosage Forms Excipient information presented when available (limited, particularly for generics); consult specific product labeling.

Powder, for solution, oral: PEG 3350 240 g, sodium sulfate 22.72 g, sodium bicarbonate 6.72 g, sodium chloride 5.84 g, and potassium chloride 2.98 g (4000 mL); PEG 3350 236 g, sodium sulfate 22.74 g, sodium bicarbonate 6.74 g, sodium chloride 5.86 g, and potassium chloride 2.97 g (4000 mL); PEG 3350 240 g, sodium bicarbonate 5.72 g, sodium chloride 11.2 g, and potassium chloride 1.48 g (4000 mL)

Colyte: PEG 3350 227.1 g, sodium sulfate 21.5 g, sodium bicarbonate 6.36 g, sodium chloride 5.53 g, and potassium chloride 2.82 g (3785 mL) [supplied with cherry, lemon lime, and orange flavor packs]

Colyte: PEG 3350 240 g, sodium sulfate 22.72 g, sodium bicarbonate 6.72 g, sodium chloride 5.84 g, and potassium chloride 2.98 g (4000 mL) [supplied with cherry, citrus berry, lemon lime, orange, and pineapple flavor packs]

GaviLyte-C: PEG 3350 240 g, sodium sulfate 22.72 g, sodium bicarbonate 6.72 g, sodium chloride 5.84 g, and potassium chloride 2.98 g (4000 mL) [supplied with lemon flavor packet]

GaviLyte-G: PEG 3350 236 g, sodium sulfate 22.74 g, sodium bicarbonate 6.74 g, sodium chloride 5.86 g, and potassium chloride 2.97 g (4000 mL) [supplied with lemon flavor packet]

GaviLyte-N: PEG 3350 420 g, sodium bicarbonate 5.72 g, sodium chloride 11.2 g, and potassium chloride 1.48 g (4000 mL) [supplied with lemon flavor packet]

GoLYTELY: PEG 3350 227.1 g, sodium sulfate 21.5 g, sodium bicarbonate 6.36 g, sodium chloride 5.53 g, and potassium chloride 2.82 g per packet (1s) [regular flavor; makes 1 gallon of solution after mixing]

GoLYTELY: PEG 3350 236 g, sodium sulfate 22.74 g, sodium bicarbonate 6.74 g, sodium chloride 5.86 g, and potassium chloride 2.97 g (4000 mL) [regular and pineapple flavor]

MoviPrep: Pouch A: PEG 3350 100g, sodium sulfate 7.5 g, sodium chloride 2.69 g, potassium chloride 1.02 g; Pouch B: Ascorbic acid 4.7 g, sodium ascorbate 5.9 g (1000 mL) [contains phenylalanine 131 mg/treatment; lemon flavor; packaged with 2 of Pouch A and 2 of Pouch B in carton and a disposable reconstitution container]

NuLYTELY: PEG 3350 420 g, sodium bicarbonate 5.72 g, sodium chloride 11.2 g, and potassium chloride 1.48 g (4000 mL) [supplied with cherry, lemon-lime, orange, and pineapple flavor packs]

TriLyte: PEG 3350 420 g, sodium bicarbonate 5.72 g, sodium chloride 11.2 g, and potassium chloride 1.48 g (4000 mL) [supplied with cherry, citrus berry, lemon lime, orange, and pineapple flavor packs]

References

American Academy of Clinical Toxicology, European Association of Poison Centres and Clinical Toxicologists, "Position Paper: Whole Bowel Irrigation," *J Toxicol Clin Toxicol*, 2004, 42(6):843-54.

Neri I, Blasi I, Castro P, et al, "Polyethylene Glycol Electrolyte Solution (Isocolan) for Constipation During Pregnancy: An Observational Open-Label Study," *J Midwifery Womens Health*, 2004, 49(4):355-8.

North American Society for Pediatric Gastroenterology, Hepatology and Nutrition (NASPGHAN). Evaluation and treatment of constipation in children: recommendations of the North American Society for Pediatric Gastroenterology, Hepatology and Nutrition. *J Pediatr Gastroenterol Nutr.* 2006;43(3):e1-13.

Siddiqui U and Denise Proctor D, "Flexible Sigmoidoscopy and Colonoscopy During Pregnancy," *Gastrointest Endosc Clin N Am*, 2006, 16 (1):59-69.

Sondheimer JM, Sokol RJ, Taylor SF, et al, "Safety, Efficacy and Tolerance of Intestinal Lavage in Pediatric Patients Undergoing Diagnostic Colonoscopy," *J Pediatr*, 1991, 119(1):148-52.

Tuggle DW, Hoelzer DJ, Tunell WP, et al, "The Safety and Cost-Effectiveness of Polyethylene Glycol Electrolyte Solution Bowel: Preparation in Infants and Children," *J Pediatr Surg*, 1987, 22 (6):513-5.

Wexner SD, Beck DE, Baron TH, et al, "A Consensus Document on Bowel Preparation Before Colonoscopy: Prepared by a Task Force from The American Society of Colon and Rectal Surgeons (ASCRS), The American Society for Gastrointestinal and Endoscopy (ASGE) and The Society of American Gastrointestinal and Endoscopic Surgeons (SAGES)," *Dis Colon Rectum*, 2006, 49(6):792-809.

◆ **Polyethylene Glycol Interferon Alfa-2b** *see* Peginterferon Alfa-2b *on page 1621*

◆ **Poly-Iron 150 [OTC]** *see* Polysaccharide-Iron Complex *on page 1701*

Polymyxin B (pol i MIKS in bee)

Medication Safety Issues

High alert medication:

The Institute for Safe Medication Practices (ISMP) includes this medication (intrathecal administration) among its list of drug classes which have a heightened risk of causing significant patient harm when used in error.

Therapeutic Category Antibiotic, Miscellaneous; Antibiotic, Ophthalmic; Antibiotic, Urinary Irrigation

Generic Availability (U.S.) Yes

Use Topically for wound irrigation and bladder irrigation against *Pseudomonas aeruginosa*; used occasionally for gut decontamination. Parenteral use of polymyxin B has mainly been replaced by less toxic antibiotics. Reserved for life-threatening infections caused by organisms resistant to the preferred drugs; used as inhalation therapy for gram-negative respiratory infections resistant to preferred drugs; used intrathecally for meningeal infections due to susceptible organisms which are resistant to less toxic antibiotics

Pregnancy Considerations [U.S. Boxed Warning]: Safety in pregnant women has not been established. Animal reproduction studies are lacking. A teratogenic potential has not been identified for polymyxin b, but very limited data is available (Heinonen, 1977; Kazy, 2005). Based on the relative toxicity compared to other antibiotics, systemic use in pregnancy is not recommended (Knothe, 1985). Due to poor tissue diffusion, topical use would be expected to have only minimal risk to the mother or fetus (Leachman, 2006).

Breast-Feeding Considerations It is not known if polymyxin b is excreted in human milk. If present in breast milk, polymyxin b is not absorbed well from a normal gastrointestinal tract. Nondose-related effects could include modification of the bowel flora.

Contraindications Hypersensitivity to polymyxin or any component

Warnings May cause nephrotoxicity; renal function should be evaluated prior to initiation; patients with renal damage and nitrogen retention should receive reduced dosage **[U.S. Boxed Warning]**; polymyxin B-induced nephrotoxicity may be manifested by albuminuria, cellular casts, and azotemia; discontinue therapy with decreasing urinary output and increasing BUN. May cause neurotoxicity **[U.S. Boxed Warning]**; neurotoxic reactions may be manifested by irritability, weakness, drowsiness, ataxia, perioral paresthesia, numbness of the extremities, and blurring of vision. These reactions are usually associated with high serum levels found in patients with impaired renal function or nephrotoxicity. Avoid concurrent or sequential use of other nephrotoxic and neurotoxic drugs, particularly bacitracin, kanamycin, streptomycin, paromomycin, colistin, tobramycin, neomycin, gentamicin, and amikacin **[U.S. Boxed Warning]**. The drug's neurotoxicity can result in respiratory paralysis from neuromuscular blockade, especially when the drug is given soon after anesthesia or muscle relaxants. Polymyxin B sulfate is toxic when given parenterally; **avoid parenteral use whenever possible**.

Precautions Use with caution in patients with myasthenia gravis, patients receiving neuromuscular blocking agents or anesthetics, and in patients with impaired renal function; modify dosage in patients with renal impairment; **I.M. use is not recommended in infants and children due to severe pain at injection site**. Safety in pregnant women has not been established.

Adverse Reactions

Cardiovascular: Facial flushing

Central nervous system: Neurotoxicity (irritability, drowsiness, ataxia, perioral paresthesia, numbness of the extremities, and blurred vision); dizziness, drug fever, meningeal irritation with intrathecal administration

Dermatologic: Urticarial rash

Endocrine & metabolic: Hypocalcemia, hyponatremia, hypokalemia, hypochloremia

Local: Pain at injection site

Neuromuscular & skeletal: Neuromuscular blockade, weakness

Renal: Nephrotoxicity

Respiratory: Respiratory arrest

Miscellaneous: Anaphylactoid reaction

Drug Interactions

Metabolism/Transport Effects None known.

Avoid Concomitant Use

Avoid concomitant use of Polymyxin B with any of the following: BCG

Increased Effect/Toxicity

Polymyxin B may increase the levels/effects of: Colistimethate; Neuromuscular-Blocking Agents

The levels/effects of Polymyxin B may be increased by: Capreomycin

Decreased Effect

Polymyxin B may decrease the levels/effects of: BCG; Sodium Picosulfate

Stability Protect from light; incompatible with calcium, magnesium, cephalothin, chloramphenicol, heparin, penicillins; inactivated by acidic or alkaline solutions

Mechanism of Action Binds to phospholipids, alters permeability, and damages the bacterial cytoplasmic membrane permitting leakage of intracellular constituents

Pharmacokinetics (Adult data unless noted)

Absorption: Well absorbed from the peritoneum; minimal absorption (<10%) from the GI tract (except in neonates), from mucous membranes or intact skin

Distribution: Widely distributed to body tissues in the liver, kidneys, heart, muscle; does not penetrate into CSF or synovial fluid; does not cross the placenta

Half-life: 4.5-6 hours, increased with reduced renal function

Time to peak serum concentration: I.M.: Within 2 hours

Elimination: Primarily as unchanged drug (>60%) in urine via glomerular filtration

Dialysis: Not removed by hemodialysis

Dosing: Usual Note: Avoid parenteral use when possible

Infants <2 years:

I.M.: 25,000-40,000 units/kg/day divided every 6 hours

I.V.: 15,000-45,000 units/kg/day by continuous I.V. infusion or divided every 12 hours

Intrathecal: 20,000 units once daily for 3-4 days or 25,000 units once every other day; continue 25,000 units once every other day for at least 2 weeks after cultures of the CSF are negative

Children ≥2 years and Adults:

I.M.: 25,000-30,000 units/kg/day divided every 6 hours

I.V.: 15,000-25,000 units/kg/day divided every 12 hours or by continuous infusion; total daily dose should not exceed 2,000,000 units/day

Bladder irrigation: Continuous irrigation of the urinary bladder for up to 10 days using 20 mg (equal to 200,000 units) added to 1 L of NS; usually no more than 1 L of irrigant is used per day unless urine flow rate is high; administration rate is adjusted to patient's urine output

Topical irrigation or topical solution: 0.1% to 0.3% solution used to irrigate infected wounds; should not exceed 2 million units/day in adults

Gut sterilization: Oral: 100,000-200,000 units/kg/day divided every 6-8 hours

Inhalation: 2-2.5 mg/kg/day divided every 6 hours; final concentration for administration should not exceed 10 mg/mL

Intrathecal: 50,000 units once daily for 3-4 days, then reduce to once every other day for at least 2 weeks after cultures of the CSF are negative

Dosing adjustment in renal impairment:

CrCl 5-20 mL/minute: Administer 50% of usual daily dose divided every 12 hours

CrCl <5 mL/minute: Administer 15% of the usual daily dose divided every 12 hours

Administration Parenteral (avoid parenteral use whenever possible):

I.M.: Not recommended for routine use in infants and children because of the severe pain which occurs with I.M. injection; administer I.M. injections deep into the upper outer quadrant of the gluteal muscles at a final concentration of 250,000 units/mL

I.V.: Infuse drug slowly over 60-90 minutes or by continuous infusion at a concentration of 1000-1667 units/mL in D_5W

Intrathecal: Reconstitute vial with 10 mL NS without preservatives to provide a final concentration of 50,000 units/mL

Monitoring Parameters WBC, serum electrolytes, renal function tests, serum drug concentration, urine output

Reference Range Serum concentration >5 mcg/mL are toxic in adults

Additional Information 1 mg = 10,000 units; neuromuscular blockade may be reversed with calcium chloride

Dosage Forms Excipient information presented when available (limited, particularly for generics); consult specific product labeling.

Solution Reconstituted, Injection:
Generic: 500,000 units (1 ea)
Solution Reconstituted, Injection [preservative free]:
Generic: 500,000 units (1 ea)

References

Heinonen OP, Slone D, and Shapiro S, "Birth Defects and Drugs in Pregnancy," Publishing Sciences Group, Inc, Littleton, MA, 1977.

Kazy Z, Puhó E, and Czeizel AE, "Parenteral Polymyxin B Treatment During Pregnancy," *Reprod Toxicol*, 2005, 20(2):181-2

Knothe H and Dette GA, "Antibiotics in Pregnancy: Toxicity and Teratogenicity," *Infection*, 1985, 13(2):49-51.

Leachman SA and Reed BR, "The Use of Dermatologic Drugs in Pregnancy and Lactation," *Dermatol Clin*, 2006, 24(2):167-97.

◆ **Polymyxin B and Bacitracin** see Bacitracin and Polymyxin B on page 257

◆ **Polymyxin B and Neomycin** see Neomycin and Polymyxin B on page 1483

◆ **Polymyxin B and Trimethoprim** see Trimethoprim and Polymyxin B on page 2089

◆ **Polymyxin B, Bacitracin, and Neomycin** see Bacitracin, Neomycin, and Polymyxin B on page 258

◆ **Polymyxin B, Bacitracin, Neomycin, and Hydrocortisone** see Bacitracin, Neomycin, Polymyxin B, and Hydrocortisone on page 258

◆ **Polymyxin B, Neomycin, and Dexamethasone** see Neomycin, Polymyxin B, and Dexamethasone on page 1484

◆ **Polymyxin B, Neomycin, and Hydrocortisone** see Neomycin, Polymyxin B, and Hydrocortisone on page 1485

◆ **Polymyxin B Sulfate** see Polymyxin B on page 1699

◆ **Polymyxin E** see Colistimethate on page 541

Polysaccharide-Iron Complex
(pol i SAK a ride-EYE ern KOM pleks)

Brand Names: U.S. EZFE 200 [OTC]; Ferrex 150 Plus [OTC]; Ferrex 150 [OTC]; FerUS [OTC] [DSC]; iFerex 150 [OTC]; Myferon 150 [OTC]; NovaFerrum 50 [OTC]; NovaFerrum Pediatric Drops [OTC]; Nu-Iron [OTC]; PIC 200 [OTC]; Poly-Iron 150 [OTC]

Therapeutic Category Iron Salt

Generic Availability (U.S.) May be product dependent

Use Prevention and treatment of iron deficiency anemias (OTC: FDA approved in adults); has also been used as supplemental therapy for patients receiving epoetin alfa

Pregnancy Considerations It is recommended that pregnant women meet the dietary requirements of iron with diet and/or supplements in order to prevent adverse events associated with iron deficiency anemia in pregnancy. Treatment of iron deficiency anemia in pregnant women is the same as in nonpregnant women and in most cases, oral iron preparations may be used. Except in severe cases of maternal anemia, the fetus achieves normal iron stores regardless of maternal concentrations.

Breast-Feeding Considerations Iron is normally found in breast milk. Breast milk or iron fortified formulas generally provide enough iron to meet the recommended dietary requirements of infants. The amount of iron in breast milk is generally not influenced by maternal iron status.

Warnings Accidental iron overdose is a leading cause of fatal poisoning in children <6 years of age **[U.S. Boxed Warning]**; in case of accidental overdose, contact poison control center immediately; ingestions of ≥40 mg/kg elemental iron or who have persistent symptoms should seek immediate care; consider all iron sources when evaluating the dose of iron, including combination products, infant formulas, and liquid nutritional supplements; store out of children's reach and in child-resistant containers.

Precautions Routine use for >6 months is not recommended; some patients may require prolonged therapy (eg, continuous bleeding or menorrhagia). Avoid in patients with peptic ulcer, enteritis, or ulcerative colitis. Avoid in patients receiving frequent blood transfusions; patients already prone to chronic iron overload.

Adverse Reactions
Gastrointestinal: Constipation, dark stools, diarrhea, epigastric pain, GI irritation, heartburn, nausea, stomach cramping, vomiting
Genitourinary: Discolored urine
Miscellaneous: Staining of teeth
Rare but important or life-threatening: Contact irritation

Drug Interactions
Metabolism/Transport Effects None known.
Avoid Concomitant Use
Avoid concomitant use of Polysaccharide-Iron Complex with any of the following: Dimercaprol
Increased Effect/Toxicity
The levels/effects of Polysaccharide-Iron Complex may be increased by: Dimercaprol
Decreased Effect
Polysaccharide-Iron Complex may decrease the levels/effects of: Bisphosphonate Derivatives; Cefdinir; Deferiprone; Dolutegravir; Eltrombopag; Levodopa; Levothyroxine; Methyldopa; PenicillAMINE; Phosphate Supplements; Quinolone Antibiotics; Tetracycline Derivatives; Trientine

The levels/effects of Polysaccharide-Iron Complex may be decreased by: Antacids; H2-Antagonists; Pancrelipase; Proton Pump Inhibitors; Trientine

Pharmacodynamics
Onset of action: Hematologic response: Red blood cells form within 3-10 days; similar onset as parenteral iron salts
Maximum effect: Peak reticulocytosis occurs in 5-10 days, and hemoglobin values increase within 2-4 weeks

Pharmacokinetics (Adult data unless noted)
Absorption: Oral: Iron is absorbed in the duodenum and upper jejunum; in persons with normal iron stores 10% of an oral dose is absorbed; this is increased to 20% to 30% in persons with inadequate iron stores; food and achlorhydria will decrease absorption
Protein binding: To transferrin
Elimination: Excreted in the urine, sweat, sloughing of intestinal mucosa, and by menses

Dosing: Usual
Infants, Children, and Adolescents: **Note:** Dosages are expressed in terms of **elemental** iron.
Recommended daily allowance (RDA): Oral:
4-8 years: 10 mg/day
9-13 years: 8 mg/day
14-18 years: Males: 11 mg/day; Females: 15 mg/day;
Iron deficiency: Oral: Children ≥6 years: 50-100 mg/day; may be given in divided doses

Adults:
Recommended daily allowance (RDA): Oral:
19-50 years: Males: 8 mg/day; Females: 18 mg/day; Pregnant females: 27 mg/day; Lactating females: 9 mg/day
≥50 years: 8 mg/day
Iron deficiency: Oral: 150-300 mg/day
Administration Administer with water or juice between meals for maximum absorption; may administer with food if GI upset occurs; do not administer with milk or milk products.
Monitoring Parameters Serum iron, total iron binding capacity, reticulocyte count, hemoglobin, ferritin
Reference Range
Serum iron: 22-184 mcg/dL
Total iron binding capacity:
Infants: 100-400 mcg/dL
Children and Adults: 250-400 mcg/dL
Additional Information 100% elemental iron. When treating iron deficiency anemias, treat for 3-4 months after hemoglobin/hematocrit return to normal in order to replenish total body stores.
Dosage Forms Excipient information presented when available (limited, particularly for generics); consult specific product labeling. [DSC] = Discontinued product
Capsule, Oral:
EZFE 200: 200 mg [non-toxic; contains brilliant blue fcf (fd&c blue #1), fd&c red #40, fd&c yellow #10 (quinoline yellow)]
Ferrex 150: 150 mg [contains fd&c blue #1 aluminum lake, fd&c red #40 aluminum lake, fd&c yellow #5 aluminum lake]
FerUS 150: 150 mg [DSC]
iFerex 150: 150 mg [contains brilliant blue fcf (fd&c blue #1), fd&c red #40, fd&c yellow #10 (quinoline yellow)]
Myferon 150: 150 mg
NovaFerrum 50: 50 mg
Nu-Iron: 150 mg [contains brilliant blue fcf (fd&c blue #1), fd&c red #40]
PIC 200: 200 mg
Poly-Iron 150: 150 mg
Liquid, Oral:
NovaFerrum Pediatric Drops: 15 mg/mL (120 mL) [alcohol free, dye free, gluten free, lactose free, sodium free, sugar free; contains sodium benzoate; raspberry-grape flavor]

References
Carney LN, Nepa A, Cohen SS, et al, "Parenteral and Enteral Nutrition Support: Determining the Best Way to Feed," In: Corkins MR, Balint J, Bobo E, et al, eds, *The A.S.P.E.N Pediatric Nutrition Support Core Curriculum*, Silver Spring: MD: American Society of Parenteral and Enteral Nutrition, 2010, 440-1.
Centers for Disease Control and Prevention (CDC), "Recommendations to Prevent and Control Iron Deficiency in the United States," *MMWR REcomm Rep*, 1998, 47(RR-3):1-36.
Institute of Medicine, National Research Council, "Iron Deficiency Anemia: Recommended Guidelines for the Prevention, Detection, and Management Among U.S. Children and Women of Childbearing Age," Washington, D.C.: The National Academies Press, 1993.
World Health Organization (WHO), "Iron Deficiency Anaemia: Assessment, Prevention, and Control. A Guide for Programme Managers," 2001.

◆ **Polysporin® [OTC]** see Bacitracin and Polymyxin B on page 257
◆ **Polytar [OTC]** see Coal Tar on page 532
◆ **Polytrim®** see Trimethoprim and Polymyxin B on page 2089
◆ **Polytrim™ (Can)** see Trimethoprim and Polymyxin B on page 2089
◆ **Polyvinyl Alcohol** see Artificial Tears on page 205
◆ **Pontocaine (Can)** see Tetracaine (Systemic) on page 1994
◆ **Pontocaine (Can)** see Tetracaine (Topical) on page 1995

Poractant Alfa (por AKT ant AL fa)

Brand Names: U.S. Curosurf
Brand Names: Canada Curosurf®
Therapeutic Category Lung Surfactant
Generic Availability (U.S.) No
Use Treatment of respiratory distress syndrome (RDS) in premature infants
Warnings Rapidly affects oxygenation and lung compliance and should be restricted to a highly supervised use in a clinical setting with immediate availability of clinicians experienced with intubation and ventilatory management of premature infants; if transient episodes of bradycardia and decreased oxygen saturation occur, discontinue the dosing procedure and initiate measures to alleviate the condition; produces rapid improvements in lung oxygenation and compliance that may require immediate reductions in ventilator settings and FiO_2.

Pulmonary hemorrhage is a known complication of premature birth and very low birth weight. It has been reported in both clinical trials and postmarketing reports in infants who have received poractant.
Precautions Correction of acidosis, hypotension, anemia, hypoglycemia, and hypothermia is recommended prior to administration
Adverse Reactions
Cardiovascular: Bradycardia, hypotension
Respiratory: Endotracheal tube blockage, oxygen desaturation
Rare but important or life-threatening: Pulmonary hemorrhage
Drug Interactions
Metabolism/Transport Effects None known.
Avoid Concomitant Use
Avoid concomitant use of Poractant Alfa with any of the following: Ceritinib
Increased Effect/Toxicity
Poractant Alfa may increase the levels/effects of: Bradycardia-Causing Agents; Ceritinib
Decreased Effect There are no known significant interactions involving a decrease in effect.
Stability Store in refrigerator; protect from light; prior to administration, allow to slowly warm to room temperature; artificial warming methods should **not** be used; unused, unopened vials warmed to room temperature may be returned to the refrigerator within 24 hours of warming only once; vials are for single use only
Mechanism of Action Endogenous pulmonary surfactant reduces surface tension at the air-liquid interface of the alveoli during ventilation and stabilizes the alveoli against collapse at resting transpulmonary pressures. A deficiency of pulmonary surfactant in preterm infants results in respiratory distress syndrome characterized by poor lung expansion, inadequate gas exchange, and atelectasis. Poractant alpha compensates for the surfactant deficiency and restores surface activity to the infant's lungs. It reduces mortality and pneumothoraces associated with RDS.
Dosing: Neonatal Endotracheal: Initial: 2.5 mL/kg/dose (200 mg/kg/dose); may repeat 1.25 mL/kg/dose (100 mg/kg/dose) at 12-hour intervals for up to 2 additional doses; maximum total dose: 5 mL/kg
Administration Intratracheal: For intratracheal administration only; suction infant prior to administration; inspect solution to verify complete mixing of the suspension; do not shake; gently turn vial upside-down to obtain uniform suspension; administer intratracheally by instillation through a 5-French end-hole catheter inserted into the infant's endotracheal tube; each dose should be administered as two aliquots, with each aliquot administered into one of the two main bronchi by positioning the infant with

either the right or left side dependent; alternatively, it may be administered through a secondary lumen of a dual lumen endotracheal tube as a single dose administered over 1 minute without interrupting mechanical ventilation

Monitoring Parameters Continuous heart rate and transcutaneous O_2 saturation should be monitored during administration; frequent ABG sampling is necessary to prevent postdosing hyperoxia and hypocarbia

Dosage Forms Excipient information presented when available (limited, particularly for generics); consult specific product labeling.

Suspension, Inhalation [preservative free]:
Curosurf: 80 mg/mL (1.5 mL, 3 mL) [contains sodium chloride]

◆ **Porcine Lung Surfactant** see Poractant Alfa on page 1702

Posaconazole (poe sa KON a zole)

Medication Safety Issues
Sound-alike/look-alike issues:
Noxafil may be confused with minoxidil
Posaconazole may be confused with itraconazole
International issues:
Noxafil [U.S. and multiple international markets] may be confused with Noxidil brand name for minoxidil [Thailand]

Brand Names: U.S. Noxafil
Brand Names: Canada Posanol Suspension
Therapeutic Category Antifungal Agent, Systemic; Antifungal Agent, Triazole
Generic Availability (U.S.) No
Use Prophylaxis of invasive *Aspergillus* and *Candida* infections in high-risk, severely immunocompromised patients [eg, hematopoietic stem cell transplant (HSCT) recipients with graft-versus-host disease or those with hematologic malignancies with prolonged neutropenia secondary to chemotherapy]; treatment of oropharyngeal candidiasis (including patients refractory to itraconazole and/or fluconazole) (All indications: FDA approved in ages ≥13 years and adults); has also been used for treatment of serious invasive fungal infections in patients intolerant of, or refractory to, conventional antifungal therapy
Pregnancy Risk Factor C
Pregnancy Considerations Posaconazole has been shown to be teratogenic in animal studies. There are no adequate and well-controlled studies in pregnant women. Use only if the benefit to the mother justifies potential risk to the fetus.
Breast-Feeding Considerations Excretion in breast milk has not been investigated; use only if the benefit to the mother justifies potential risk to the fetus.
Contraindications Hypersensitivity to posaconazole, any component, or other azole antifungal agent; concurrent therapy with ergot alkaloids, sirolimus, an HMG-CoA reductase inhibitor metabolized by CYP3A4 (eg, atorvastatin, lovastatin, simvastatin), or a CPY3A4 substrate that prolongs the QT interval (eg, cisapride, quinidine, pimozide)
Warnings Hepatic dysfunction has occurred, ranging from reversible mild/moderate increases of ALT, AST, alkaline phosphatase, total bilirubin, and/or clinical hepatitis to severe reactions (cholestasis, hepatic failure including death). Liver function tests and bilirubin should be monitored at the start and during posaconazole therapy. Consider discontinuation of therapy in patients who develop clinical evidence of liver disease that may be secondary to posaconazole.

Concomitant use of posaconazole with some drugs may require cautious use, may not be recommended, or may require dosage adjustments. Posaconazole has been

associated with QT interval prolongation and torsade de pointes (rarely); use caution in patients with an increased risk of arrhythmia (long QT syndrome, concurrent QT_c-prolonging drugs, hypokalemia). Use is contraindicated with medications known to prolong the QT_c interval and are metabolized through the CYP3A4 system. Correct electrolyte abnormalities (eg, potassium, magnesium, and calcium) before initiating therapy. Concurrent use may significantly increase midazolam concentrations and potentiate or prolong sedative or hypnotic effects. Reversal agents should be readily available.

Concurrent use with cyclosporine or tacrolimus may significantly increase the whole blood trough concentrations of cyclosporine or tacrolimus and may result in rare serious adverse events (eg, nephrotoxicity, leukoencephalopathy, and death); dose reductions and close monitoring are recommended with initiation of posaconazole therapy. Concurrent use with sirolimus is contraindicated.

Oral suspension contains sodium benzoate; benzoic acid (benzoate) is a metabolite of benzyl alcohol; large amounts of benzyl alcohol (≥99 mg/kg/day) have been associated with a potentially fatal toxicity ("gasping syndrome") in neonates; use oral suspension containing sodium benzoate with caution in neonates; *in vitro* and animal studies have shown that benzoate displaces bilirubin from protein-binding sites. Oral suspension also contains polysorbate 80 (Tween 80) which may cause allergic reactions in susceptible individuals.

Precautions Use with caution in patients with severe renal impairment (CrCl <20 mL/minute/1.73 m²); monitor for breakthrough fungal infection in patients with severe renal impairment. Patients with severe diarrhea or vomiting should be closely monitored for breakthrough fungal infections. In patients unable to eat or tolerate nutritional supplements, alternative antifungal therapy should be considered or patient should be closely monitored for breakthrough fungal infections.

Adverse Reactions Note: Unless otherwise specified, adverse reactions are identified with oral formulations and reflect data from use in comparator trials with multiple concomitant conditions and medications; some adverse reactions may be due to underlying condition(s). Systemic includes oral and intravenous routes.

Cardiovascular: Edema, hypertension (systemic), hypotension, peripheral edema (systemic), pulmonary embolism, tachycardia, thrombophlebitis (intravenous via peripheral venous catheter), torsades de pointes

Central nervous system: Anxiety, chills (systemic), dizziness, fatigue (systemic), headache (systemic), insomnia, lower extremity edema, pain, paresthesia, rigors

Dermatologic: Diaphoresis, pruritus, skin rash (systemic)

Endocrine & metabolic: Adrenocortical insufficiency, dehydration, hyperglycemia, hypocalcemia, hypokalemia (systemic), hypomagnesemia (systemic), weight loss

Gastrointestinal: Abdominal pain (systemic), anorexia, constipation (systemic), decreased appetite (systemic), diarrhea (systemic), dyspepsia, mucositis, nausea (systemic), oral candidiasis, stomatitis, upper abdominal pain (systemic), vomiting (systemic)

Genitourinary: Vaginal hemorrhage

Hematologic & oncologic: Anemia (systemic), febrile neutropenia, hemolytic-uremic syndrome, neutropenia, petechia (systemic), thrombocytopenia (systemic), thrombotic thrombocytopenic purpura

Hepatic: Hepatic failure, hepatitis, hepatomegaly, hyperbilirubinemia, increased liver enzymes, increased serum alkaline phosphatase, increased serum ALT, increased serum AST, jaundice

Hypersensitivity: Hypersensitivity reaction

Infection: Bacteremia, cytomegalovirus disease, herpes simplex infection

Neuromuscular & skeletal: Arthralgia, back pain, musculoskeletal pain, weakness

Renal: Acute renal failure

Respiratory: Cough (systemic), dyspnea (systemic), epistaxis (systemic), pharyngitis, pneumonia, upper respiratory tract infection

Miscellaneous: Fever (systemic)

Rare but important or life-threatening: Atrial fibrillation, cholestasis, hypersensitivity, prolonged Q-T interval on ECG, reduced ejection fraction, syncope

Drug Interactions

Metabolism/Transport Effects Inhibits CYP3A4 (strong)

Avoid Concomitant Use

Avoid concomitant use of Posaconazole with any of the following: Ado-Trastuzumab Emtansine; Alfuzosin; Apixaban; AtorvaSTATin; Avanafil; Axitinib; Bosutinib; Cabozantinib; Ceritinib; Cisapride; Conivaptan; Crizotinib; Dihydroergotamine; Dofetilide; Dronedarone; Efavirenz; Eletriptan; Eplerenone; Ergoloid Mesylates; Ergonovine; Ergotamine; Everolimus; Halofantrine; Ibrutinib; Ivabradine; Lapatinib; Lomitapide; Lovastatin; Lurasidone; Macitentan; Methadone; Methylergonovine; Nilotinib; Nisoldipine; Pimozide; QuiNIDine; Ranolazine; Red Yeast Rice; Regorafenib; Rivaroxaban; Saccharomyces boulardii; Salmeterol; Silodosin; Simeprevir; Simvastatin; Sirolimus; Tamsulosin; Ticagrelor; Tolvaptan; Toremifene; Ulipristal; Vemurafenib; VinCRIStine (Liposomal); Vorapaxar

Increased Effect/Toxicity

Posaconazole may increase the levels/effects of: Ado-Trastuzumab Emtansine; Alfentanil; Alfuzosin; Almotriptan; Alosetron; Antineoplastic Agents (Vinca Alkaloids); Apixaban; ARIPiprazole; Atazanavir; AtorvaSTATin; Avanafil; Axitinib; Bedaquiline; Benzodiazepines (metabolized by oxidation); Boceprevir; Bortezomib; Bosentan; Bosutinib; Brentuximab Vedotin; Brinzolamide; Budesonide (Nasal); Budesonide (Systemic, Oral Inhalation); BusPIRone; Busulfan; Cabozantinib; Calcium Channel Blockers; Cannabis; Ceritinib; Cilostazol; Cisapride; Colchicine; Conivaptan; Corticosteroids (Orally Inhaled); Corticosteroids (Systemic); Crizotinib; CycloSPORINE (Systemic); CYP3A4 Substrates; Dienogest; Digoxin; Dihydroergotamine; DOCEtaxel; Dofetilide; DOXOrubicin (Conventional); Dronabinol; Dronedarone; Dutasteride; Eletriptan; Enzalutamide; Eplerenone; Ergoloid Mesylates; Ergonovine; Ergotamine; Etravirine; Everolimus; FentaNYL; Fesoterodine; Fluticasone (Nasal); Fluticasone (Oral Inhalation); Fosamprenavir; Fosphenytoin; GlipiZIDE; GuanFACINE; Halofantrine; Highest Risk QTc-Prolonging Agents; Ibrutinib; Iloperidone; Imatinib; Ivabradine; Ivacaftor; Ixabepilone; Lacosamide; Lapatinib; Levomilnacipran; Lomitapide; Losartan; Lovastatin; Lurasidone; Macitentan; Macrolide Antibiotics; Maraviroc; Methadone; Methylergonovine; MethylPREDNISolone; Mifepristone; Moderate Risk QTc-Prolonging Agents; Nilotinib; Nisoldipine; Ospemifene; OxyCODONE; Paricalcitol; PAZOPanib; Phenytoin; Pimecrolimus; Pimozide; PONATinib; Propafenone; QUEtiapine; QuiNIDine; Ranolazine; Red Yeast Rice; Regorafenib; Repaglinide; Rifamycin Derivatives; Rilpivirine; Ritonavir; Rivaroxaban; RomiDEPsin; Ruxolitinib; Salmeterol; Saxagliptin; Sildenafil; Silodosin; Simeprevir; Simvastatin; Sirolimus; Solifenacin; SORAfenib; SUNItinib; Tacrolimus (Systemic); Tacrolimus (Topical); Tadalafil; Tamsulosin; Telaprevir; Temsirolimus; Tetrahydrocannabinol; Ticagrelor; Tofacitinib; Tolterodine; Tolvaptan; Toremifene; Ulipristal; Vardenafil; Vemurafenib; Vilazodone; VinCRIStine (Liposomal); Vitamin K Antagonists; Vorapaxar; Zolpidem; Zuclopenthixol

The levels/effects of Posaconazole may be increased by: Boceprevir; Etravirine; Macrolide Antibiotics; Mifepristone; Telaprevir

Decreased Effect

Posaconazole may decrease the levels/effects of: Amphotericin B; Ifosfamide; Prasugrel; Saccharomyces boulardii; Ticagrelor

The levels/effects of Posaconazole may be decreased by: Didanosine; Efavirenz; Etravirine; Fosamprenavir; Fosphenytoin; H2-Antagonists; Metoclopramide; Phenytoin; Proton Pump Inhibitors; Rifamycin Derivatives; Sucralfate

Food Interactions Bioavailability increased ~3 times when posaconazole is administered with a nonfat meal or an oral liquid nutritional supplement; increased ~4 times when administered with a high-fat meal. Management: Suspension must be administered with or within 20 minutes of a full meal or an oral liquid nutritional supplement, or may be administered with an acidic carbonated beverage (eg, ginger ale). Take tablet with food. Consider alternative antifungal therapy in patients with inadequate oral intake or severe diarrhea/vomiting.

Stability Store at 25°C (77°F); excursions permitted to 15°C to 30°C (59°F to 86°F); do not freeze.

Mechanism of Action Interferes with fungal cytochrome P450 (latosterol-14α-demethylase) activity, decreasing ergosterol synthesis (principal sterol in fungal cell membrane) and inhibiting fungal cell membrane formation.

Pharmacokinetics (Adult data unless noted)

Absorption: Coadministration with food, liquid nutritional supplements, and/or acidic carbonated beverages (eg, ginger ale) increases absorption; fasting states do not provide sufficient absorption to ensure adequate plasma concentrations

Distribution: V_d: 1774 L; extensive extravascular distribution and penetration into body tissues

Protein binding: >98%, predominantly bound to albumin

Metabolism: Not significantly metabolized; ~15% to 17% undergoes non-CYP-mediated metabolism, primarily via hepatic glucuronidation into metabolites

Half-life: 35 hours (range: 20-66 hours)

Time to peak serum concentration: 3-5 hours

Elimination: Feces 71% (66% as unchanged drug); urine 13% (<0.2% as unchanged drug)

Dosing: Usual

Infants, Children, and Adolescents:

Antifungal prophylaxis, HSCT recipients: Limited data available: Oral: Infants ≥8 months and Children <12 years: 4 mg/kg/dose 3 times daily; begin 2-4 days prior to discharge and continue until either day 100 post-HSCT or until CD_3 T cells reach 200/mm³ and CD_4 cells reach 100/mm³ whichever is longer. Dosing based on experience in 60 pediatric patients (median age: 6 years; age range: 0.7-11.5 years); pharmacokinetic analysis showed 12 mg/kg/day (4 mg/kg 3 times daily) produced morning serum trough concentration similar to effective adult values. The other evaluated regimen of 10 mg/kg/day (5 mg/kg twice daily) produced morning trough levels that were approximately 3 times lower than the thrice daily regimen and was subsequently removed from the protocol. Overall, no patients developed invasive mycosis (probable or proven), the median duration of therapy was 127 days (range: 12-188 days), and no severe adverse effects were observed (Döring, 2012).

Aspergillosis, invasive; prophylaxis: Oral: Adolescents ≥13 years: 200 mg 3 times daily; duration of therapy is based on recovery from neutropenia or immunosuppression

Candidiasis: Oral:

Esophageal infection (HIV-exposed/-positive): Treatment: Adolescent: 400 mg twice daily for 14-21 days;

Note: If patient has frequent or severe recurrences may continue for suppressive therapy; consider discontinuing when CD_4 >200/mm^3 (DHHS [adult], 2013)

Invasive infections:

Prophylaxis: Adolescents ≥13 years: 200 mg 3 times daily; duration of therapy is based on recovery from neutropenia or immunosuppression

Treatment (refractory infection): Limited data available: Children ≥8 years and Adolescents: 800 mg/day administered as either 200 mg 4 times daily **or** 400 mg twice daily; this regimen produced similar plasma concentrations in both children (n=12; age range: 8-17 years; weight: 24-76 kg) and adults (Krishna, 2007)

Oropharyngeal infection:

Non-HIV-exposed/-positive: Adolescents ≥13 years:
Treatment: Initial: 100 mg twice daily on day 1; maintenance: 100 mg once daily for 13 days
Treatment (refractory infection): 400 mg twice daily; duration of therapy is based on underlying disease and clinical response

HIV-exposed/-positive: Treatment: Adolescents: Initial: 400 mg twice daily on day 1; then maintenance: 400 mg once daily for 7-14 days (DHHS [adult], 2013)

Adults:

Aspergillosis, invasive: Oral:

Prophylaxis: 200 mg 3 times daily; duration of therapy is based on recovery from neutropenia or immunosuppression; initiate posaconazole in patients with acute myelogenous leukemia (AML) or myelodysplastic syndromes (MDS) several days before the anticipated onset of neutropenia (eg, at the time of chemotherapy initiation) and discontinue once neutropenia is resolved (Cornely, 2007; NCCN, 2009)

Treatment (refractory to or intolerant of conventional therapy): 200 mg 4 times daily initially; after disease stabilization, may decrease frequency to 400 mg twice daily (Walsh, 2007). **Note:** Duration of therapy should be a minimum of 6-12 weeks or throughout period of immunosuppression and until lesions have resolved (Walsh, 2008).

Candidal infections: Oral:

Prophylaxis: 200 mg 3 times daily; duration of therapy is based on recovery from neutropenia or immunosuppression

Treatment:

Oropharyngeal infection: Initial: 100 mg twice daily for 1 day; maintenance: 100 mg once daily for 13 days
Refractory oropharyngeal infection: 400 mg twice daily; duration of therapy is based on underlying disease and clinical response

Dosing adjustment in renal impairment: Adolescents ≥13 years and Adults: No dosage adjustments are recommended; however, patients with CrCl <20 mL/minute/1.73 m^2 should be monitored for breakthrough fungal infections. Not removed by hemodialysis.

Dosage adjustment in hepatic impairment: Adolescents ≥13 years and Adults: No dosage adjustments are recommended.

Administration Oral: Shake suspension before use. Administer during or within 20 minutes following a full meal, liquid nutritional supplement, or an acidic carbonated beverage (eg, ginger ale). In patients able to swallow, administer oral suspension using dosing spoon provided by the manufacturer; spoon should be rinsed clean with water after each use and before storage. For patients who cannot tolerate a full meal or an oral liquid nutritional supplement, alternative antifungal therapy should be considered.

Monitoring Parameters Hepatic function tests and bilirubin prior to initiation and periodically during therapy; serum electrolytes (eg, calcium, potassium and magnesium), serum creatinine, ECG; breakthrough fungal infections

Additional Information Dextrose content (oral suspension): 350 mg/mL

Product Availability Noxafil injection: FDA approved March 2014; availability anticipated in April 2014.

Dosage Forms Excipient information presented when available (limited, particularly for generics); consult specific product labeling.

Solution, Intravenous:

Noxafil: 300 mg/16.7 mL (16.7 mL) [contains edetate disodium]

Suspension, Oral:

Noxafil: 40 mg/mL (105 mL) [contains polysorbate 80, sodium benzoate; cherry flavor]

Tablet Delayed Release, Oral:

Noxafil: 100 mg

References

Cornely OA, Maertens J, Winston DJ, et al, "Posaconazole vs Fluconazole or Itraconazole Prophylaxis in Patients With Neutropenia," *N Engl J Med*, 2007, 356(4):348-59.

Döring M, Müller C, Johann PD, et al, "Analysis of Posaconazole as Oral Antifungal Prophylaxis in Pediatric Patients Under 12 Years of Age Following Allogeneic Stem Cell Transplantation," *BMC Infect Dis*, 2012, 12:263.

DHHS Panel on Opportunistic Infections (OI) in HIV-Infected Adults and Adolescents, "Guidelines for Prevention and Treatment of Opportunistic Infections in HIV-Infected Adults and Adolescents: Recommendations from the Centers for Disease Control and Prevention (CDC), the National Institutes of Health (NIH), and the HIV Medicine Association (HIVMA) of the Infectious Diseases Society of America (IDSA)," May 7, 2013. Available at http://aidsinfo.nih.gov/contentfiles/lvguidelines/adult_oi.pdf

Gubbins PO, Krishna G, Sansone-Parsons A, et al, "Pharmacokinetics and Safety of Oral Posaconazole in Neutropenic Stem Cell Transplant Recipients," *Antimicrob Agents Chemother*, 2006, 50(6):1993-9.

Hope WW, Castagnola E, Groll AH, et al, "ESCMID* Guideline for the Diagnosis and Management of *Candida* Diseases 2012: Prevention and Management of Invasive Infections in Neonates and Children Caused by *Candida spp*," *Clin Microbiol Infect*, 2012, 18(Suppl 7):38-52.

Krishna G, Sansone-Parsons A, Martinho M, et al, "Posaconazole Plasma Concentrations in Juvenile Patients With Invasive Fungal Infection," *Antimicrob Agents Chemother*, 2007, 51(3):812-8.

National Comprehensive Cancer Network® (NCCN), "Clinical Practice Guidelines in Oncology™: Prevention and Treatment of Cancer-Related Infections," Version 2.2009. Available at http://www.nccn.org/professionals/physician_gls/PDF/infections.pdf

Walsh TJ, Anaissie EJ, Denning DW, et al, "Treatment of Aspergillosis: Clinical Practice Guidelines of the Infectious Diseases Society of America," *Clin Infect Dis*, 2008, 46(3):327-60.

Walsh TJ, Raad I, Patterson TF, et al, "Treatment of Invasive Aspergillosis With Posaconazole in Patients Who Are Refractory to or Intolerant of Conventional Therapy: An Externally Controlled Trial," *Clin Infect Dis*, 2007, 44(1):2-12.

◆ **Posanol Suspension (Can)** *see* Posaconazole *on page 1703*

◆ **Posture® [OTC]** *see* Calcium Phosphate (Tribasic) *on page 359*

Potassium Acetate (poe TASS ee um AS e tate)

Medication Safety Issues

Other safety concerns:

Consider special storage requirements for intravenous potassium salts; I.V. potassium salts have been administered IVP in error, leading to fatal outcomes.

Related Information

Management of Drug Extravasations *on page 2255*

Therapeutic Category Electrolyte Supplement, Parenteral

Generic Availability (U.S.) Yes

Use Treatment and prevention of hypokalemia when it is necessary to avoid chloride or acid/base status requires an additional source of bicarbonate

Pregnancy Risk Factor C

Pregnancy Considerations Animal reproduction studies have not been conducted. Potassium requirements are the same in pregnant and nonpregnant women. Adverse events have not been observed following use of potassium supplements in healthy women with normal pregnancies. Use caution in pregnant women with other medical conditions (eg, pre-eclampsia; may be more likely to develop hyperkalemia) (IOM, 2004).

Breast-Feeding Considerations Potassium is excreted into breast milk (IOM, 2004).

Contraindications Hypersensitivity to any component of the potassium supplement; severe renal impairment, untreated Addison's disease, heat cramps, hyperkalemia, severe tissue trauma

Warnings Potassium acetate should be administered only in patients with adequate urine flow; must be diluted before I.V. use and infused slowly

Precautions Use with caution in patients with cardiac disease, patients receiving potassium-sparing drugs; patients should be on a cardiac monitor during intermittent infusions for doses >0.5 mEq/kg/hour or 5 mEq/hour (adults); solution for injection contains aluminum; use caution with impaired renal function and in premature infants

Adverse Reactions

Cardiovascular: Arrhythmias, EEG abnormalities, heart block, hypotension

Central nervous system: Confusion, listlessness

Neuromuscular & skeletal: Paralysis, paresthesia, weakness

Local: Local tissue necrosis with extravasation

Drug Interactions

Metabolism/Transport Effects None known.

Avoid Concomitant Use There are no known interactions where it is recommended to avoid concomitant use.

Increased Effect/Toxicity

Potassium Acetate may increase the levels/effects of: ACE Inhibitors; Angiotensin II Receptor Blockers; Potassium-Sparing Diuretics

The levels/effects of Potassium Acetate may be increased by: Eplerenone; Heparin; Heparin (Low Molecular Weight)

Decreased Effect There are no known significant interactions involving a decrease in effect.

Stability Store at room temperature; do not freeze

Mechanism of Action Potassium is the major cation of intracellular fluid and is essential for the conduction of nerve impulses in heart, brain, and skeletal muscle; contraction of cardiac, skeletal and smooth muscles; maintenance of normal renal function, acid-base balance, carbohydrate metabolism, and gastric secretion

Pharmacokinetics (Adult data unless noted)

Distribution: Enters cells via active transport from extracellular fluid

Elimination: Primarily urine; skin and feces (small amounts); most intestinal potassium reabsorbed

Dosing: Neonatal I.V. doses should be incorporated into the patient's maintenance I.V. fluids; intermittent I.V. potassium administration should be reserved for severe depletion situations; continuous ECG monitoring should be used for intermittent doses >0.5 mEq/kg/**hour**. **Note:** Doses listed as mEq of **potassium**.

Normal daily requirement: I.V.: 2-6 mEq/kg/day

Treatment of hypokalemia: Intermittent I.V. infusion (must be diluted prior to administration): 0.5-1 mEq/kg/dose, infuse at 0.3-0.5 mEq/kg/**hour** (maximum dose/rate: 1 mEq/kg/**hour**); then repeated as needed based on frequently obtained lab values; severe depletion or ongoing losses may require >200% of normal daily limit needs

Dosing: Usual I.V. doses should be incorporated into the patient's maintenance I.V. fluids; intermittent I.V. potassium administration should be reserved for severe depletion

situations; continuous ECG monitoring should be used for intermittent doses >0.5 mEq/kg/**hour**. **Note:** Doses listed as mEq of **potassium**.

Normal daily requirement: I.V.:

Infants: 2-6 mEq/kg/day

Children: 2-3 mEq/kg/day

Adults: 40-80 mEq/day

Treatment of hypokalemia:

Infants and Children:

Intermittent I.V. infusion (must be diluted prior to administration): 0.5-1 mEq/kg/dose (maximum dose: 40 mEq), infuse at 0.3-0.5 mEq/kg/**hour** (maximum dose/rate: 1 mEq/kg/**hour**); then repeated as needed based on frequently obtained lab values; severe depletion or ongoing losses may require >200% of normal daily limit needs

Adults:

Intermittent I.V. infusion: 5-10 mEq/hour (continuous cardiac monitor for rates >5 mEq/hour), not to exceed 40 mEq/hour; usual adult maximum per 24 hours: 400 mEq

Potassium dosage/rate of infusion guidelines:

Serum potassium ≥2.5 mEq/L (and <desired): 10 mEq with additional doses if needed; maximum infusion rate: 10 mEq/hour; maximum 24-hour dose: 200 mEq

Serum potassium <2.5 mEq/L: Up to 40 mEq with additional doses based upon frequent lab monitoring; maximum infusion rate: 40 mEq/hour; maximum 24-hour dose: 400 mEq; deficits at a plasma level of 2 mEq/L may be as high as 400-800 mEq of potassium

Administration Parenteral: Potassium must be diluted prior to parenteral administration; maximum recommended concentration (peripheral line): 80-100 mEq/L; maximum recommended concentration (central line): 150 mEq/L or 15 mEq/100 mL; in severely fluid-restricted patients (with central lines): 200 mEq/L or 20 mEq/100 mL has been used; maximum rate of infusion

Vesicant/Extravasation Risk Vesicant/irritant (at concentrations >0.1 mEq/mL)

Monitoring Parameters Serum potassium, glucose, chloride, pH, urine output (if indicated), cardiac monitor [if intermittent I.V. infusion or potassium I.V. infusion rates >0.5 mEq/kg/hour or 5 mEq/hour (adults)]

Additional Information 1 mEq of acetate is equivalent to the alkalinizing effect of 1 mEq of bicarbonate. Hypokalemia is highly arrhythmogenic, particularly in the setting of ischemia or digitalis toxicity. ECG evidence of hypokalemia includes flattening of the T wave. As the T wave shrinks, U waves may appear. There is no prolongation of the QT interval. Hyperkalemia may present as tall peaked symmetrical T waves. S-T elevation may present in severe hyperkalemia. QRS complex progressively widens with eventual apparent sine waves on the ECG. Hyperkalemia will also induce cardiac slowing and AV conduction abnormalities.

Dosage Forms Excipient information presented when available (limited, particularly for generics); consult specific product labeling.

Solution, Intravenous:

Generic: 2 mEq/mL (20 mL, 50 mL, 100 mL); 4 mEq/mL (50 mL)

References

Hamill RJ, Robinson LM, Wexler HR, et al, "Efficacy and Safety of Potassium Infusion Therapy in Hypokalemic Critically Ill Patients," *Crit Care Med*, 1991, 19(5):694-9.

IOM (Institute of Medicine), *Dietary Reference Intakes for Water, Potassium, Sodium, Chloride, and Sulfate*, Washington, DC: National Academy Press, 2004.

Khilnani P, "Electrolyte Abnormalities in Critically Ill Children," *Crit Care Med*, 1992, 20(2):241-50.

Potassium Bicarbonate

(poe TASS ee um bye KAR bun ate)

Brand Names: U.S. Effer-K; K-Bicarb [OTC]; K-Effervescent

Therapeutic Category Electrolyte Supplement, Oral

Generic Availability (U.S.) May be product dependent

Use Treatment and prevention of hypokalemia when it is necessary to avoid chloride or acid/base status requires bicarbonate

Pregnancy Risk Factor C

Pregnancy Considerations Animal reproduction studies have not been conducted. Potassium requirements are the same in pregnant and nonpregnant women. Adverse events have not been observed following use of potassium supplements in healthy women with normal pregnancies. Use caution in pregnant women with other medical conditions (eg, pre-eclampsia; may be more likely to develop hyperkalemia) (IOM, 2004).

Breast-Feeding Considerations Potassium is excreted into breast milk (IOM, 2004). Breast-feeding is not recommended by the manufacturer.

Contraindications Hypersensitivity to any component of the potassium supplement; severe renal impairment, untreated Addison's disease, heat cramps, hyperkalemia, severe tissue trauma; solid oral dosage forms are contraindicated in patients in whom there is a structural, pathological, and/or pharmacologic cause for delay or arrest in passage through the GI tract

Precautions Use with caution in patients with cardiac and/or renal disease, patients receiving potassium-sparing drugs

Drug Interactions

Metabolism/Transport Effects None known.

Avoid Concomitant Use There are no known interactions where it is recommended to avoid concomitant use.

Increased Effect/Toxicity

Potassium Bicarbonate may increase the levels/effects of: ACE Inhibitors; Angiotensin II Receptor Blockers; Potassium-Sparing Diuretics

The levels/effects of Potassium Bicarbonate may be increased by: Eplerenone; Heparin; Heparin (Low Molecular Weight)

Decreased Effect There are no known significant interactions involving a decrease in effect.

Stability Store at room temperature.

Pharmacokinetics (Adult data unless noted)

Absorption: Well absorbed from upper GI tract

Distribution: Enters cells via active transport from extracellular fluid

Elimination: Primarily urine; skin and feces (small amounts); most intestinal potassium reabsorbed

Dosing: Usual Oral (doses listed as mEq of **potassium**):

Normal daily requirement:

Children: 2-3 mEq/kg/day

Adults: 40-80 mEq/day

Prevention of hypokalemia during diuretic therapy:

Children: 1-2 mEq/kg/day in 1-2 divided doses

Adults: 25-100 mEq/day in 2-4 divided doses

Administration Oral: Dissolve completely in 3-8 oz cold water, juice, or other suitable beverage and drink slowly

Monitoring Parameters Serum potassium, chloride, glucose, pH, urine output (if indicated)

Additional Information Hypokalemia is highly arrhythmogenic, particularly in the setting of ischemia or digitalis toxicity. ECG evidence of hypokalemia includes flattening of the T wave. As the T wave shrinks, U waves may appear. There is no prolongation of the QT interval. Hyperkalemia may present as tall peaked symmetrical T waves. S-T elevation may present in severe hyperkalemia. QRS complex progressively widens with eventual apparent sine waves on the ECG. Hyperkalemia will also induce cardiac slowing and AV conduction abnormalities.

Dosage Forms Excipient information presented when available (limited, particularly for generics); consult specific product labeling.

Capsule, Oral:

K-Bicarb: 99 mg

Tablet Effervescent, Oral:

Effer-K: 25 mEq [lime flavor]

Effer-K: 25 mEq [contains fd&c red #40, fd&c red #40 aluminum lake, saccharin; cherry berry flavor]

Effer-K: 25 mEq [contains fd&c yellow #10 (quinoline yellow), fd&c yellow #10 aluminum lake, saccharin; lemon citrus flavor]

Effer-K: 25 mEq [contains fd&c yellow #6 (sunset yellow), fd&c yellow #6 aluminum lake, saccharin; orange flavor]

Effer-K: 25 mEq [contains saccharin; unflavored flavor]

K-Effervescent: 25 mEq [orange flavor]

References

IOM (Institute of Medicine), *Dietary Reference Intakes for Water, Potassium, Sodium, Chloride, and Sulfate,* Washington, DC: National Academy Press, 2004.

Potassium Bicarbonate and Potassium Chloride

(poe TASS ee um bye KAR bun ate & poe TASS ee um KLOR ide)

Related Information

Oral Medications That Should Not Be Crushed or Altered *on page 2438*

Potassium Bicarbonate *on page 1707*

Potassium Chloride *on page 1708*

Therapeutic Category Electrolyte Supplement, Oral

Generic Availability (U.S.) Yes

Use Treatment or prevention of hypokalemia

Pregnancy Risk Factor C

Pregnancy Considerations Animal reproduction studies have not been conducted with this combination. Refer to individual agents.

Breast-Feeding Considerations Refer to individual agents.

Contraindications Hypersensitivity to any component of the potassium supplement; severe renal impairment, untreated Addison's disease, heat cramps, hyperkalemia, severe tissue trauma

Precautions Use with caution in patients with cardiac and/or renal disease, patients receiving potassium-sparing drugs

Adverse Reactions Gastrointestinal: Abdominal discomfort, diarrhea, nausea, vomiting

Drug Interactions

Metabolism/Transport Effects None known.

Avoid Concomitant Use

Avoid concomitant use of Potassium Bicarbonate and Potassium Chloride with any of the following: Anticholinergic Agents; Glycopyrrolate

Increased Effect/Toxicity

Potassium Bicarbonate and Potassium Chloride may increase the levels/effects of: ACE Inhibitors; Angiotensin II Receptor Blockers; Potassium-Sparing Diuretics

The levels/effects of Potassium Bicarbonate and Potassium Chloride may be increased by: Anticholinergic Agents; Eplerenone; Glycopyrrolate; Heparin; Heparin (Low Molecular Weight)

Decreased Effect There are no known significant interactions involving a decrease in effect.

Stability Store at room temperature.

Dosing: Usual Oral (doses listed as mEq of **potassium**):

Normal daily requirement:

Children: 2-3 mEq/kg/day

Adults: 40-80 mEq/day

Prevention of hypokalemia during diuretic therapy:
Children: 1-2 mEq/kg/day in 1-2 divided doses
Adults: 25-100 mEq/day in 2-4 divided doses

Administration Dissolve tablets in 3-4 ounces cold water or juice; solution should be sipped slowly, over 5-10 minutes; administer with meals

Monitoring Parameters Serum potassium, glucose, chloride, pH, urine output (if indicated)

Additional Information Hypokalemia is highly arrhythmogenic, particularly in the setting of ischemia or digitalis toxicity. ECG evidence of hypokalemia includes flattening of the T wave. As the T wave shrinks, U waves may appear. There is no prolongation of the QT interval. Hyperkalemia may present as tall peaked symmetrical T waves. S-T elevation may present in severe hyperkalemia. QRS complex progressively widens with eventual apparent sine waves on the ECG. Hyperkalemia will also induce cardiac slowing and AV conduction abnormalities.

Dosage Forms Excipient information presented when available (limited, particularly for generics); consult specific product labeling.

Tablet for solution, oral [effervescent]: Potassium chloride 25 mEq [potassium bicarbonate 0.5 g and potassium chloride 1.5 g]

◆ **Potassium Bicarbonate and Potassium Chloride (Effervescent)** see Potassium Bicarbonate and Potassium Chloride on page 1707

Potassium Chloride (poe TASS ee um KLOR ide)

Medication Safety Issues

Sound-alike/look-alike issues:
Kaon-Cl-10 may be confused with kaolin
KCl may be confused with HCl
Klor-Con may be confused with Klaron®
microK may be confused with Macrobid®, Micronase

High alert medication:
The Institute for Safe Medication Practices (ISMP) includes this medication (I.V. formulation) among its list of drugs which have a heightened risk of causing significant patient harm when used in error.

Other safety concerns:
Per JCAHO recommendations, concentrated electrolyte solutions should not be available in patient care areas.
Consider special storage requirements for intravenous potassium salts; I.V. potassium salts have been administered IVP in error, leading to fatal outcomes.

Related Information
Management of Drug Extravasations on page 2255
Oral Medications That Should Not Be Crushed or Altered on page 2438

Brand Names: U.S. K-Tab; K-Vescent; Klor-Con; Klor-Con 10; Klor-Con M10; Klor-Con M15; Klor-Con M20; Micro-K

Brand Names: Canada Apo-K; K-10; K-Dur; Micro-K Extencaps; Roychlor; Slo-Pot; Slow-K

Therapeutic Category Electrolyte Supplement, Oral; Electrolyte Supplement, Parenteral

Generic Availability (U.S.) Yes

Use Treatment or prevention of hypokalemia

Pregnancy Risk Factor C

Pregnancy Considerations Reproduction studies have not been conducted. Potassium requirements are the same in pregnant and nonpregnant women. Adverse events have not been observed following use of potassium supplements in healthy women with normal pregnancies. Use caution in pregnant women with other medical conditions (eg, pre-eclampsia; may be more likely to develop hyperkalemia) (IOM, 2004). Potassium supplementation (that does not cause maternal hyperkalemia) would not be expected to cause adverse fetal events.

Breast-Feeding Considerations Potassium is excreted into breast milk (IOM, 2004). The normal content of potassium in human milk is ~13 mEq/L. Supplementation (that does not cause maternal hyperkalemia) would not be expected to affect normal concentrations.

Contraindications Hypersensitivity to any component of the potassium supplement; severe renal impairment; untreated Addison's disease, heat cramps, hyperkalemia, severe tissue trauma; solid oral dosage forms are contraindicated in patients in whom there is a structural, pathological, and/or pharmacologic cause for delay or arrest in passage through the GI tract; an oral liquid potassium preparation should be used in patients with esophageal compression or delayed gastric emptying time

Warnings Potassium chloride injection should be administered only in patients with adequate urine flow; injection must be diluted before I.V. use and infused slowly

Precautions Use with caution in patients with cardiac disease and/or renal disease, patients receiving potassium-sparing drugs; patients should be on a cardiac monitor during intermittent infusions for doses >0.5 mEq/kg/hour

Adverse Reactions
Dermatologic: Rash
Endocrine & metabolic: Hyperkalemia
Gastrointestinal: Abdominal pain/discomfort, diarrhea, flatulence, GI bleeding (oral), GI obstruction (oral), GI perforation (oral), nausea, vomiting

Drug Interactions
Metabolism/Transport Effects None known.

Avoid Concomitant Use
Avoid concomitant use of Potassium Chloride with any of the following: Anticholinergic Agents; Glycopyrrolate

Increased Effect/Toxicity
Potassium Chloride may increase the levels/effects of: ACE Inhibitors; Angiotensin II Receptor Blockers; Potassium-Sparing Diuretics

The levels/effects of Potassium Chloride may be increased by: Anticholinergic Agents; Eplerenone; Glycopyrrolate; Heparin; Heparin (Low Molecular Weight)

Decreased Effect There are no known significant interactions involving a decrease in effect.

Stability Store at room temperature; do not freeze

Mechanism of Action Potassium is the major cation of intracellular fluid and is essential for the conduction of nerve impulses in heart, brain, and skeletal muscle; contraction of cardiac, skeletal and smooth muscles; maintenance of normal renal function, acid-base balance, carbohydrate metabolism, and gastric secretion

Pharmacokinetics (Adult data unless noted)
Absorption: Well absorbed from upper GI tract; enters cells via active transport from extracellular fluid
Distribution: Enters cells via active transport from extracellular fluid
Elimination: Primarily urine; skin and feces (small amounts); most intestinal potassium reabsorbed

Dosing: Neonatal Note: I.V. doses should be incorporated into the patient's maintenance I.V. fluids; intermittent I.V. potassium administration should be reserved for severe depletion situations; continuous ECG monitoring should be used for intermittent doses >0.5 mEq/kg/**hour**. Doses listed as mEq of **potassium**.

Normal daily requirements: Oral, I.V.: 2-6 mEq/kg/day
Prevention of hypokalemia during diuretic therapy: 1-2 mEq/kg/day in 1-2 divided doses
Treatment of hypokalemia: **Note:** High variability exists in dosing/infusion rate recommendations; therapy should be guided by patient condition and specific institutional guidelines.

Oral: 2-5 mEq/kg/day in divided doses; not to exceed 1-2 mEq/kg as a single dose; if deficits are severe or ongoing losses are great, I.V. route should be considered preferred route of administration

Intermittent I.V. infusion (must be diluted prior to administration): 0.5-1 mEq/kg/dose, infuse at 0.3-0.5 mEq/kg/**hour** (maximum dose/rate: 1 mEq/kg/**hour**); then repeated as needed based on frequently obtained lab values; severe depletion or ongoing losses may require >200% of normal daily limit needs

Dosing: Usual Note: I.V. doses should be incorporated into the patient's maintenance I.V. fluids; intermittent I.V. potassium administration should be reserved for severe depletion situations; continuous ECG monitoring should be used for intermittent doses >0.5 mEq/kg/hour. Doses listed as mEq of **potassium**. When using microencapsulated or wax matrix formulations, use no more than 20 mEq as a single dose.

Normal daily requirements: Oral, I.V.:
Infants: 2-6 mEq/kg/day
Children: 2-3 mEq/kg/day
Adults: 40-80 mEq/day
Prevention of hypokalemia during diuretic therapy: Oral:
Infants and Children: 1-2 mEq/kg/day in 1-2 divided doses
Adults: 20-40 mEq/day in 1-2 divided doses
Treatment of hypokalemia: **Note:** High variability exists in dosing/infusion rate recommendations; therapy should be guided by patient condition and specific institutional guidelines.
Infants and Children:
Oral: 2-5 mEq/kg/day in divided doses; not to exceed 1-2 mEq/kg as a single dose; if deficits are severe or ongoing losses are great, I.V. route should be considered preferred route of administration
Intermittent I.V. infusion (must be diluted prior to administration): 0.5-1 mEq/kg/dose (maximum dose: 40 mEq) to infuse at 0.3-0.5 mEq/kg/hour (maximum dose/rate: 1 mEq/kg/hour); then repeated as needed based on frequently obtained lab values; severe depletion or ongoing losses may require >200% of normal daily limit needs
Adults:
Intermittent I.V. infusion: 5-10 mEq/hour (continuous cardiac monitor recommended for rates >5 mEq/hour), not to exceed 40 mEq/hour; usual adult maximum per 24 hours: 400 mEq
Potassium dosage/rate of infusion guidelines:
Serum potassium ≥2.5 mEq/L (and <desired): 10 mEq with additional doses if needed; maximum infusion rate: 10 mEq/hour; maximum 24-hour dose: 200 mEq
Serum potassium <2.5 mEq/L: Up to 40 mEq, with additional doses based upon frequent lab monitoring; maximum infusion rate: 40 mEq/hour; maximum 24-hour dose: 400 mEq; deficits at a plasma level of 2 mEq/L may be as high as 400-800 mEq of potassium
Oral:
Asymptomatic, mild hypokalemia: Usual dosage range: 40-100 mEq/day divided in 2-5 doses; generally recommended to limit doses to 20-25 mEq/dose to avoid GI discomfort
Mild to moderate hypokalemia: Some clinicians may administer up to 120-240 mEq/day divided in 3-4 doses; limit doses to 40-60 mEq/dose. If deficits are severe or ongoing losses are great, I.V. route should be considered.

Administration
Oral: Sustained release and wax matrix tablets (K-Tab®, Kaon-Cl-10®, Klor-Con®) should be swallowed whole, do not crush or chew; administer with food; powder (Klor-Con®) should be dissolved in 4-5 ounces of water or juice; capsule (microK®) should be swallowed whole, do not chew; may also be opened and contents sprinkled on a spoonful of applesauce or pudding and swallowed immediately without chewing; do not administer liquid formulations full strength, must be diluted in 2-6 parts of water or juice. Klor-Con® M tablet may be broken in half and each half swallowed separately; the whole tablet may be dissolved in approximately 4 ounces of water (allow approximately 2 minutes to dissolve, stir well, and drink immediately).
Parenteral: Potassium must be diluted prior to parenteral administration; maximum recommended concentration (peripheral line): 80 mEq/L; maximum recommended concentration (central line): 150 mEq/L or 15 mEq/100 mL; in severely fluid-restricted patients (with central lines): 200 mEq/L or 20 mEq/100 mL has been used
Infusion rates (including all sources): Pediatric patients: Usual range: 0.3-0.5 mEq/kg/hour; maximum rate: 1 mEq/kg/hour up to 40 mEq/hour; continuous cardiac monitoring recommended for rates >0.5 mEq/kg/hour

Vesicant/Extravasation Risk Vesicant/irritant (at concentrations >0.1 mEq/mL)

Monitoring Parameters Serum potassium, glucose, chloride, pH, urine output (if indicated), cardiac monitor [if intermittent I.V. infusion or potassium I.V. infusion rates >0.5 mEq/kg/hour or >10 mEq/hour (adults)]

Additional Information Hypokalemia is highly arrhythmogenic, particularly in the setting of ischemia or digitalis toxicity. ECG evidence of hypokalemia includes flattening of the T wave. As the T wave shrinks, U waves may appear. There is no prolongation of the QT interval. Hyperkalemia may present as tall peaked symmetrical T waves. S-T elevation may present in severe hyperkalemia. QRS complex progressively widens with eventual apparent sine waves on the ECG. Hyperkalemia will also induce cardiac slowing and AV conduction abnormalities.

Dosage Forms Considerations
750 mg potassium chloride = elemental potassium 390 mg = potassium 10 mEq = potassium 10 mmol

Dosage Forms Excipient information presented when available (limited, particularly for generics); consult specific product labeling. [DSC] = Discontinued product
Capsule Extended Release, Oral:
Micro-K: 8 mEq, 10 mEq
Generic: 8 mEq, 10 mEq
Liquid, Oral:
Generic: 20 mEq/15 mL (10%) (473 mL); 40 mEq/15 mL (20%) (473 mL)
Packet, Oral:
K-Vescent: 20 mEq (100 ea)
Klor-Con: 20 mEq (1 ea, 30 ea, 100 ea); 25 mEq (30 ea, 100 ea) [sugar free; contains fd&c yellow #6 (sunset yellow); fruit flavor]
Generic: 20 mEq (30 ea, 100 ea)
Solution, Intravenous:
Generic: 5 mEq (250 mL); 10 mEq (500 mL, 1000 mL); 20 mEq (1000 mL); 30 mEq (1000 mL); 40 mEq (1000 mL); 0.4 mEq/mL (50 mL); 10 mEq/100 mL (100 mL); 10 mEq/50 mL (50 mL); 20 mEq/100 mL (100 mL); 20 mEq/50 mL (50 mL); 40 mEq/100 mL (100 mL); 2 mEq/mL (5 mL, 10 mL, 15 mL, 20 mL, 30 mL, 250 mL); 20 mEq/L (1000 mL); 40 mEq/L (1000 mL)
Solution, Oral:
Generic: 20 mEq/15 mL (10%) (15 mL, 30 mL, 473 mL [DSC])
Tablet Extended Release, Oral:
K-Tab: 10 mEq [contains fd&c yellow #10 (quinoline yellow)]

K-Tab: 20 mEq

Klor-Con: 8 mEq [contains fd&c blue #1 aluminum lake, fd&c blue #2 aluminum lake]

Klor-Con 10: 10 mEq [contains fd&c yellow #10 aluminum lake, fd&c yellow #6 aluminum lake]

Klor-Con M10: 10 mEq

Klor-Con M15: 15 mEq [scored]

Klor-Con M20: 20 mEq [scored]

Generic: 8 mEq, 10 mEq, 20 mEq

References

Hamill RJ, Robinson LM, Wexler HR, et al, "Efficacy and Safety of Potassium Infusion Therapy in Hypokalemic Critically Ill Patients," *Crit Care Med*, 1991, 19(5):694-9.

IOM (Institute of Medicine), *Dietary Reference Intakes for Water, Potassium, Sodium, Chloride, and Sulfate*, Washington, DC: National Academy Press, 2004.

Khilnani P, "Electrolyte Abnormalities in Critically Ill Children," *Crit Care Med*, 1992, 20(2):241-50.

Potassium Citrate and Citric Acid
(poe TASS ee um SIT rate & SI trik AS id)

Brand Names: U.S. Cytra-K

Therapeutic Category Alkalinizing Agent, Oral

Generic Availability (U.S.) Yes

Use As long-term therapy to alkalinize the urine for control and/or dissolution of uric acid and cystine calculi of the urinary tract [FDA approved in pediatric patients (age not specified) and adults]; treatment of chronic metabolic acidosis secondary to chronic renal insufficiency or syndrome of renal tubular acidosis when use of sodium salt is undesirable [FDA approved in pediatric patients (age not specified) and adults]

Pregnancy Considerations Refer to potassium citrate monograph for information.

Breast-Feeding Considerations Refer to potassium citrate monograph for information.

Contraindications Hypersensitivity to any component; severe renal insufficiency, oliguria, or azotemia; potassium-restricted diet; untreated Addison's disease; adynamia episodica hereditaria (hyperkalemic periodic paralysis); acute dehydration; heat cramps; anuria; severe myocardial damage; hyperkalemia from any cause

Warnings Hyperkalemia and alkalosis may occur with large doses, especially in patients with renal impairment; severe hyperkalemia may lead to muscle weakness/paralysis and cardiac conduction abnormalities (eg, heart block, ventricular arrhythmias, asystole). Monitor serum potassium concentrations closely; concomitant use of potassium-sparing diuretics, potassium supplements, and/or potassium-containing salts, angiotensin-converting enzyme (ACE) inhibitors, or cardiac glycosides should be done cautiously. Use with caution in patients with acid/base alterations; changes in serum potassium concentrations can occur during acid/base correction.

Some oral solutions contain sodium benzoate. Benzoic acid (benzoate) is a metabolite of benzyl alcohol; large amounts of benzyl alcohol (≥99 mg/kg/day) have been associated with a potentially fatal toxicity ("gasping syndrome") in neonates; the "gasping syndrome" consists of metabolic acidosis, respiratory distress, gasping respirations, CNS dysfunction (including convulsions, intracranial hemorrhage), hypotension, and cardiovascular collapse; use oral solution containing sodium benzoate with caution in neonates; *in vitro* and animal studies have shown that benzoate displaces bilirubin from protein binding sites. Some oral solutions contain propylene glycol; toxicities have been reported with use of products containing propylene glycol, including hyperosmolality, lactic acidosis, seizures, and respiratory depression; in neonates large amounts of propylene glycol delivered orally, intravenously (eg, >3000 mg/day), or topically have been associated with potentially fatal toxicities which can include metabolic acidosis, seizures, renal failure, and CNS depression; use oral solutions containing propylene glycol with caution (AAP, 1997; Shehab, 2009).

Precautions Use with caution in patients with renal impairment; monitor serum potassium concentrations closely (contraindicated with severe impairment, oliguria, azotemia). Use with caution in patients with cardiovascular disease (eg, heart failure, cardiac arrhythmias); patients may be more susceptible to life-threatening cardiac effects associated with hyper-/hypokalemia. Use with caution in patients with disorders or conditions likely to contribute to altered serum potassium and hyperkalemia (eg, severe tissue breakdown from trauma or burns). May cause GI upset (eg, nausea, vomiting, diarrhea, abdominal pain, discomfort) and lead to GI ulceration, bleeding, and/or perforation; undiluted solution can cause GI irritation; dilute with water prior to administration. Conversion of citrate to bicarbonate may be impaired in patients with hepatic failure, in shock, or who are severely ill.

Drug Interactions

Metabolism/Transport Effects None known.

Avoid Concomitant Use There are no known interactions where it is recommended to avoid concomitant use.

Increased Effect/Toxicity

Potassium Citrate and Citric Acid may increase the levels/effects of: ACE Inhibitors; Aluminum Hydroxide; Angiotensin II Receptor Blockers; Potassium-Sparing Diuretics

The levels/effects of Potassium Citrate and Citric Acid may be increased by: Eplerenone; Heparin; Heparin (Low Molecular Weight)

Decreased Effect There are no known significant interactions involving a decrease in effect.

Stability Store at controlled room temperature, 20°C to 25°C (68°F to 77°F). Protect from excessive heat and freezing. Keep container tightly closed.

Pharmacokinetics (Adult data unless noted)

Metabolism: ≥95% via hepatic oxidation to bicarbonate; may be impaired in patients with hepatic failure, in shock, or who are severely ill

Elimination: <5% unchanged in the urine

Dosing: Neonatal Oral: **Note:** 1 mL of oral solution contains 2 mEq of bicarbonate and 2 mEq of potassium; 1 packet of crystals contains 30 mEq of bicarbonate and 30 mEq of potassium: 2-3 mEq bicarbonate/kg/**day** (1-1.5 mL/kg/**day**) in 3-4 divided doses

Dosing: Usual Oral: **Note:** 1 mL of oral solution contains 2 mEq of bicarbonate and 2 mEq of potassium; 1 packet of crystals contains 30 mEq of bicarbonate and 30 mEq of potassium.

Manufacturer's recommendation: Pediatric patients: 5-15 mL (10-30 mEq bicarbonate) per dose after meals and at bedtime

Alternative recommendation: Dosing per mEq of bicarbonate:

Infants and Children: 2-3 mEq bicarbonate/kg/**day** (1-1.5 mL/kg/**day**) in 3-4 divided doses

Adults:

Powder: One packet (30 mEq bicarbonate) dissolved in 6 oz water after meals and at bedtime

Solution: 15-30 mL (30-60 mEq bicarbonate) per dose after meals and at bedtime

Note: When using to alkalinize the urine, 10-15 mL doses given 4 times/day typically maintain urinary pH 6.5-7.4; doses 15-20 mL 4 times/day usually maintain urinary pH at 7.0-7.6

Administration Dose should be diluted in water (pediatric patients: 3 oz; adults: 6 oz) to minimize injury due to high concentration of potassium; administer after meals and at bedtime to prevent saline laxative effect; may follow dose with additional water if necessary; dose may be chilled to improve palatability. Shake well before use.

Dosage Forms Excipient information presented when available (limited, particularly for generics); consult specific product labeling. [DSC] = Discontinued product

Powder for solution, oral:

Cytra-K: Potassium citrate monohydrate 3300 mg and citric acid monohydrate 1002 mg per packet (100s) [sugar free; fruit-punch flavor; each packet contains potassium 30 mEq equivalent to bicarbonate 30 mEq]

Solution, oral: Potassium citrate monohydrate 1100 mg and citric acid monohydrate 334 mg per 5 mL (473 mL) [DSC]

Cytra-K: Potassium citrate monohydrate 1100 mg and citric acid monohydrate 334 mg per 5 mL (480 mL) [ethanol free, sugar free; contains propylene glycol; cherry flavor; contains potassium 2 mEq/mL equivalent to bicarbonate 2 mEq /mL]

References

American Academy of Pediatrics Committee on Drugs. "Inactive" ingredients in pharmaceutical products: update (subject review). *Pediatrics.* 1997;99(2):268-278.

Gal P and Reed MD, "Medications," *Nelson Textbook of Pediatrics*, 18th ed, Kliegman RM, Behrman RE, Jenson HB, et al, eds, Philadelphia, PA: Saunders, 2007, 2955-3000.

Shehab N, Lewis CL, Streetman DD, Donn SM. Exposure to the pharmaceutical excipients benzyl alcohol and propylene glycol among critically ill neonates. *Pediatr Crit Care Med.* 2009;10 (2):256-259.

◆ **Potassium Citrate, Citric Acid, and Sodium Citrate** *see* Citric Acid, Sodium Citrate, and Potassium Citrate *on page 487*

Potassium Gluconate
(poe TASS ee um GLOO coe nate)

Brand Names: U.S. K-99 [OTC]

Therapeutic Category Electrolyte Supplement, Oral

Generic Availability (U.S.) Yes

Use Treatment or prevention of hypokalemia

Pregnancy Considerations Potassium requirements are the same in pregnant and non-pregnant women. Adverse events have not been observed following use of potassium supplements in healthy women with normal pregnancies. Use caution in pregnant women with other medical conditions (eg, pre-eclampsia; may be more likely to develop hyperkalemia) (IOM, 2004).

Breast-Feeding Considerations Potassium is excreted into breast milk (IOM, 2004).

Contraindications Hypersensitivity to any component of the potassium supplement; severe renal impairment, untreated Addison's disease, heat cramps, hyperkalemia, severe tissue trauma; solid oral dosage forms are contraindicated in patients in whom there is a structural, pathological, and/or pharmacologic cause for delay or arrest in passage through the GI tract

Precautions Use with caution in patients with cardiac and/ or renal disease, patients receiving potassium-sparing drugs

Drug Interactions

Metabolism/Transport Effects None known.

Avoid Concomitant Use There are no known interactions where it is recommended to avoid concomitant use.

Increased Effect/Toxicity

Potassium Gluconate may increase the levels/effects of: ACE Inhibitors; Angiotensin II Receptor Blockers; Potassium-Sparing Diuretics

The levels/effects of Potassium Gluconate may be increased by: Eplerenone; Heparin; Heparin (Low Molecular Weight)

Decreased Effect There are no known significant interactions involving a decrease in effect.

Stability Store at room temperature.

Mechanism of Action Potassium is the major cation of intracellular fluid and is essential for the conduction of nerve impulses in heart, brain, and skeletal muscle; contraction of cardiac, skeletal and smooth muscles; maintenance of normal renal function, acid-base balance, carbohydrate metabolism, and gastric secretion

Pharmacokinetics (Adult data unless noted)

Absorption: Well absorbed from upper GI tract

Distribution: Enters cells via active transport from extracellular fluid

Elimination: Primarily urine; skin and feces (small amounts); most intestinal potassium reabsorbed

Dosing: Usual Oral: **Note:** Doses listed as mEq of potassium (approximately 4.3 mEq potassium/g potassium gluconate; 1 mEq potassium is equivalent to 39 mg elemental potassium)

Normal daily requirement:

Children: 2-3 mEq/kg/day

Adults: 40-80 mEq/day

Prevention of hypokalemia during diuretic therapy:

Children: 1-2 mEq/kg/day in 1-2 divided doses

Adults: 20-40 mEq/day in 1-2 divided doses

Treatment of hypokalemia:

Children: 2-5 mEq/kg/day in divided doses; not to exceed 1-2 mEq/kg as a single dose; if deficits are severe or ongoing losses are great, I.V. route should be considered preferred route of administration

Adults: 40-100 mEq/day in 2-4 divided doses

Administration Oral: Sustained release and wax matrix tablets should be swallowed whole, do not crush or chew; administer with food

Monitoring Parameters Serum potassium, chloride, glucose, pH, urine output (if indicated)

Test Interactions Decreased ammonia (B)

Additional Information 9.4 g potassium gluconate is approximately equal to 40 mEq potassium (4.3 mEq potassium/g potassium gluconate). Hypokalemia is highly arrhythmogenic, particularly in the setting of ischemia or digitalis toxicity. ECG evidence of hypokalemia includes flattening of the T wave. As the T wave shrinks, U waves may appear. There is no prolongation of the QT interval. Hyperkalemia may present as tall peaked symmetrical T waves. S-T elevation may present in severe hyperkalemia. QRS complex progressively widens with eventual apparent sine waves on the ECG. Hyperkalemia will also induce cardiac slowing and AV conduction abnormalities.

Dosage Forms Considerations

1 g potassium gluconate = elemental potassium 167 mg = potassium 4.3 mEq = potassium 4.3 mmol

Dosage Forms Excipient information presented when available (limited, particularly for generics); consult specific product labeling.

Capsule, Oral [preservative free]:

K-99: 595 mg [dye free, sugar free, yeast free]

Tablet, Oral:

Generic: 2 mEq, 2.5 mEq

Tablet, Oral [strength expressed as base]:

Generic: 80 mg

References

IOM (Institute of Medicine), *Dietary Reference Intakes for Water, Potassium, Sodium, Chloride, and Sulfate*, Washington, DC: National Academy Press, 2004.

Potassium Iodide (poe TASS ee um EYE oh dide)

Medication Safety Issues

Sound-alike/look-alike issues:

Potassium iodide products, including saturated solution of potassium iodide (SSKI®) may be confused with potassium iodide and iodine (Strong Iodide Solution or Lugol's solution)

Other safety concerns:

Dosage volume: Dosing errors have been reported during the prescribing, dispensing, and administration of potassium iodide-containing solutions (eg, Lugol's, SSKI). Errors have occurred when **mL** doses were administered, when only **drops** were indicated for the dose. Carefully review dosage and administration information; appropriate oral dosage is most commonly expressed as drops to provide doses less than 1 mL. Dispensing unit doses is also highly recommended; pharmacists should never dispense quantities that could be lethal if consumed as a single dose. (ISMP, 2011).

Brand Names: U.S. SSKI; ThyroShield [OTC]

Therapeutic Category Antithyroid Agent; Expectorant

Generic Availability (U.S.) No

Use Expectorant for the symptomatic treatment of chronic pulmonary diseases complicated by mucous (SSKI®: FDA approved in adults); block thyroidal uptake of radioactive isotopes of iodine in a radiation emergency or other exposure to radioactive iodine (Iosat™, ThyroSafe™, ThyroShield™: FDA approved in all ages); has also been used to reduce thyroid vascularity prior to thyroidectomy and management of thyrotoxic crisis; lymphocutaneous and cutaneous sporotrichosis

Pregnancy Risk Factor D

Pregnancy Considerations Iodide crosses the placenta (may cause hypothyroidism and goiter in fetus/newborn). Use as an expectorant during pregnancy is contraindicated by the AAP. Use for protection against thyroid cancer secondary to radioactive iodine exposure is considered acceptable based upon risk:benefit, keeping in mind the dose and duration. In general, medications used as antidotes should take into consideration the health and prognosis of the mother; antidotes should be administered to pregnant women if there is a clear indication for use and should not be withheld because of fears of teratogenicity (Bailey, 2003). Pregnant women should take as instructed by public officials and contact their physician. Repeat dosing should be avoided if possible. Refer to Iodine monograph for additional information.

Breast-Feeding Considerations Potassium iodide is excreted in breast milk. May cause skin rash in nursing infant. Nursing mothers should take as instructed by public officials and contact their physician. Refer to Iodine monograph for additional information.

Contraindications Hypersensitivity to iodides or any component; dermatitis herpetiformis, hypocomplementemic vasculitis, nodular thyroid condition with heart disease

Warnings Prolonged use can lead to hypothyroidism.

Precautions Use with caution in patients with cystic fibrosis; may have exaggerated susceptibility to goitrogenic effects; use caution in patients with myotonia congenita, a history of thyroid disease, cardiac disease, renal impairment, Addison's disease, tuberculosis, or acute bronchitis. Treatment with potassium iodide may cause flare-up of acne and/or dermatitis. Use with caution in patients receiving medications that increase serum potassium concentrations. With radiopharmaceutical use, potassium iodide must be administered prior to receiving radiopharmaceuticals that require thyroid protection.

Adverse Reactions

Cardiovascular: Cardiac arrhythmia

Central nervous system: Confusion, fatigue, fever, numbness, tingling sensation

Dermatologic: Skin rash, urticaria

Endocrine & metabolic: Goiter, hyperthyroidism (prolonged use), hypothyroidism (prolonged use), myxedema

Gastrointestinal: Diarrhea, enlargement of salivary glands, gastric distress, gastrointestinal hemorrhage, metallic taste, nausea, stomach pain, vomiting

Hematologic & oncologic: Lymphedema, thyroid adenoma

Hypersensitivity: Hypersensitivity reaction (angioedema, cutaneous and mucosal hemorrhage, serum sickness-like symptoms)

Neuromuscular & skeletal: Weakness

Respiratory: Dyspnea, wheezing

Miscellaneous: Iodine poisoning (with prolonged treatment/high doses)

Drug Interactions

Metabolism/Transport Effects None known.

Avoid Concomitant Use

Avoid concomitant use of Potassium Iodide with any of the following: Sodium Iodide I131

Increased Effect/Toxicity

Potassium Iodide may increase the levels/effects of: ACE Inhibitors; Angiotensin II Receptor Blockers; Cardiac Glycosides; Lithium; Potassium-Sparing Diuretics; Theophylline Derivatives

The levels/effects of Potassium Iodide may be increased by: Eplerenone; Heparin; Heparin (Low Molecular Weight)

Decreased Effect

Potassium Iodide may decrease the levels/effects of: Sodium Iodide I131; Vitamin K Antagonists

Stability Store at 15°C to 30°C (59°F to 86°F); protect from light; keep container tightly closed. SSKI® if exposed to cold temperatures may develop crystallization; warming with shaking will redissolve crystals; if solution becomes brown/yellow in color, it should be discarded.

Mechanism of Action Reduces viscosity of mucus by increasing respiratory tract secretions; inhibits secretion of thyroid hormone, fosters colloid accumulation in thyroid follicles. Following radioactive iodine exposure, potassium iodide blocks the uptake of radioactive iodine by the thyroid, reducing the risk of thyroid cancer.

Pharmacodynamics Antithyroid effects:

Onset of action: 24-48 hours

Maximum effect: 10-15 days after continuous therapy

Duration: May persist up to 6 weeks

Radioactive iodine exposure: Duration: 24 hours

Dosing: Neonatal

Prevention of thyroidal uptake of radioactive isotopes of iodine to reduce risk of thyroid cancer following nuclear accident: Oral: (Iosat™, ThyroSafe™, ThyroShield™): 16.25 mg once daily; **Note:** Continue treatment until the risk of exposure has passed and/or until other measures (evacuation, sheltering, control of the food and milk supply) have been successfully implemented

Thyroid gland protection during radiopharmaceutical use: Oral: ThyroShield™: 16 mg once on the day before radiopharmaceutical use (Olivier, 2003)

Dosing: Usual

Infants, Children, and Adolescents:

Cutaneous sporotrichosis: Limited data available: Children and Adolescents: Oral: SSKI®: Initial: 50 mg (1 drop or 0.05 mL) 3 times daily; increase as tolerated to ≤50 mg/kg/dose (≤1 drop/kg/dose or ≤0.05 mL/kg/dose) 3 times daily; Maximum: 2500 mg/dose (50 drops/dose or 2.5 mL/dose); continued at the maximum tolerated dosage for several weeks after lesions have resolved (Kauffman, 2007; Red Book, 2009)

Expectorant: Children: Oral: SSKI®: 60-250 mg 4 times daily

Prevention of thyroidal uptake of radioactive isotopes of iodine to reduce risk of thyroid cancer following nuclear accident: Oral: Iosat™, ThyroSafe™, ThyroShield™: **Note:** Continue treatment until the risk of exposure has passed and/or until other measures (evacuation, sheltering, control of the food and milk supply) have been successfully implemented.

Infants and Children ≤3 years: 32.5 mg once daily

Children and Adolescents >3-18 years and weight <68 kg (150 lbs): 65 mg once daily

Children and Adolescent 12-18 years and weight ≥68 kg (150 lbs): 130 mg once daily

Thyroid gland protection during radiopharmaceutical use: Limited data available; **Note:** Begin at 1-48 hours prior to exposure; continue potassium iodide after radiopharmaceutical administration until risk of exposure has diminished (treatment duration and time of initiation is dependent on the radiopharmaceutical; consult specific protocol; Oral: Iostat™, ThyroSafe™, ThyroShield™ (Giammarile, 2008; Olivier, 2003):

Infants <5 kg: 16 mg once daily

Infants >5 kg: 32 mg once daily

Children:

1-3 years and 5-15 kg: 32 mg once daily

>3-12 years and 15-50 kg: 65 mg once daily

≥50 kg: 130 mg once daily

Adolescents:

<50 kg: 65 mg once daily

≥50 kg: 130 mg once daily

Thyroidectomy, preoperative preparation: Children and Adolescents: Oral: SSKI®: 150-350 mg (3-7 drops or 0.15-0.35 mL) 3 times daily; administer for 10 days before surgery; if not euthyroid prior to surgery, consider concurrent beta-blockade (eg, propranolol) in the immediate preoperative period to reduce the risk of thyroid storm (Bahn, 2011)

Thyrotoxic crisis/thyroid storm: Note: Administer at least 1 hour after antithyroid drug (eg, methimazole) administration:

Infants: Oral: SSKI®: 100 mg (2 drops or 0.1 mL) 4 times daily

Children and Adolescents: Oral: SSKI®: 250 mg (5 drops or 0.25 mL) 2-4 times daily

Adults:

Expectorant: Oral: SSKI®: 300-600 mg 3-4 times daily

Preparation for thyroidectomy: Oral: 50-100 mg (1-2 drops **or** 0.05-0.1 mL SSKI®) 3 times daily; administer for 10 days before surgery; if not euthyroid prior to surgery, consider concurrent beta-blockade (eg, propranolol) in the immediate preoperative period to reduce the risk of thyroid storm (Bahn, 2011)

Sporotrichosis (cutaneous, lymphocutaneous): Oral: SSKI®: Initial: 5 drops 3 times daily; increase to 40-50 drops 3 times daily as tolerated until 2-4 weeks after lesions have resolved (usual duration: 3-6 months) (Kauffman, 2007)

Thyroid gland protection during radiopharmaceutical use: Oral: Tablet: 130 mg once daily or Solution (SSKI®): 4 drops 3 times daily. **Note:** Begin at 1-48 hours prior to exposure. Continue potassium iodide after radiopharmaceutical administration until risk of exposure has diminished (treatment duration and time of initiation is dependent on the radiopharmaceutical, consult specific protocol).

Thyrotoxic crisis/thyroid storm: Oral: **Note:** Administer at least 1-2 hours after antithyroid drug administration: 250 mg (5 drops **or** 0.25 mL SSKI®) every 6 hours (Bahn, 2011)

To reduce risk of thyroid cancer following nuclear accident (Iosat™, ThyroSafe™, ThyroShield™): Oral: Adults (including pregnant/lactating women): Oral: 130 mg once daily. **Note:** Dosing should continue until risk of exposure has passed or other measures are are implemented.

Administration Oral: Administer after meals with food or milk or dilute with a large quantity of water, fruit juice, milk, or broth

Monitoring Parameters Thyroid function tests; sign/ symptoms of hyperthyroidism; thyroid function should be monitored in pregnant women, neonates, and young infants if repeat doses are required following radioactive iodine exposure

Test Interactions Iodide may alter thyroid function tests.

Additional Information SSKI® 10 drops = potassium iodide 500 mg

Dosage Forms Excipient information presented when available (limited, particularly for generics); consult specific product labeling.

Solution, Oral:

SSKI: 1 g/mL (30 mL, 237 mL)

ThyroShield: 65 mg/mL (30 mL) [contains brilliant blue fcf (fd&c blue #1), fd&c red #40, methylparaben, propylene glycol, propylparaben, saccharin sodium; black raspberry flavor]

Extemporaneous Preparations A 16.25 mg/5 mL oral solution may be made with tablets. Crush one 130 mg tablet and reduce to a fine powder. Add 20 mL of water and mix until powder is dissolved. Add an additional 20 mL of low-fat milk (white or chocolate), orange juice, flat soda, raspberry syrup, or infant formula. Stable for 7 days under refrigeration.

To prepare an 8.125 mg/5 mL oral solution, crush one 65 mg tablet and reduce to a fine powder. Add 20 mL of water and mix until powder is dissolved. Add an additional 20 mL of low-fat milk (white or chocolate), orange juice, flat soda, raspberry syrup, or infant formula. Stable for 7 days under refrigeration.

References

"American Academy of Pediatrics Committee on Environmental Health. Radiation Disasters and Children," *Pediatrics*, 2003, 111(6 Pt 1):1455-66.

Bahn RS (Chair), Burch HB, Cooper DS, et al, "Hyperthyroidism and Other Causes of Thyrotoxicosis: Management Guidelines of the American Thyroid Association and American Association of Clinical Endocrinologists," *Thyroid*, 2011, 21(6):593-646.

Bailey B, "Are There Teratogenic Risks Associated With Antidotes Used in the Acute Management of Poisoned Pregnant Women?" *Birth Defects Res A Clin Mol Teratol*, 2003, 67(2):133-40.

Giammarile F, Chiti A, Lassmann M,et al, "EANM Procedure Guidelines for 131I-meta-iodobenzylguanidine (131I-mIBG) Therapy," *Eur J Nucl Med Mol Imaging*, 2008, 35(5):1039-47.

Kauffman CA, Bustamante B, Chapman SW, et al, "Clinical Practice Guidelines for the Management of Sporotrichosis: 2007 Update by the Infectious Diseases Society of America," *Clin Infect Dis*, 2007, 45 (10):1255-65.

Nayak B and Burman K, "Thyrotoxicosis and Thyroid Storm," *Endocrinol Metab Clin North Am*, 2006, 35(4):663-86.

Olivier P, Colarinha P, Fettich J, et al, "Guidelines for Radioiodinated MIBG Scintigraphy in Children," *Eur J Nucl Med Mol Imaging*, 2003, 30(5):45-50.

"Potassium Iodide as a Thyroid Blocking Agent in a Radiation Emergency: Final Recommendations on Use," Washington DC, Bureau of Radiological Health and Bureau of Drugs, Food and Drug Administration, 1982.

Red Book: 2009 Report of the Committee on Infectious Diseases, "Sporotrichosis," 28th ed, Pickering LK, ed, Elk Grove Village, IL: American Academy of Pediatrics, 2009, 598-9.

U.S. Food and Drug Administration, "FDA's Guidance on Protection of Children and Adults Against Thyroid Cancer in Case of Nuclear Accident," FDA Talk Paper. Available at: http://www.fda.gov/bbs/topics/answers/2001/ans01126.html. Accessed January 11, 2002.

Potassium Iodide and Iodine

(poe TASS ee um EYE oh dide & EYE oh dine)

Medication Safety Issues

Sound-alike/look-alike issues:

Potassium iodide and iodine (Strong Iodide Solution or Lugol's solution) may be confused with potassium iodide products, including saturated solution of potassium iodide (SSKI®)

Other safety concerns:

Dosage volume: Dosing errors have been reported during the prescribing, dispensing, and administration of potassium iodide-containing solutions (eg, Lugol's, SSKI). Errors have occurred when **mL** doses were administered, when only **drops** were indicated for the dose. Carefully review dosage and administration information; appropriate oral dosage is most commonly expressed as drops to provide doses less than 1 mL. Dispensing unit doses is also highly recommended; pharmacists should never dispense quantities that could be lethal if consumed as a single dose. (ISMP, 2011).

Therapeutic Category Antibacterial, Topical; Antithyroid Agent

Generic Availability (U.S.) Yes

Use

Oral solution: Reduce thyroid vascularity prior to thyroidectomy and management of thyrotoxic crisis (FDA approved in adults); has also been used to block thyroidal uptake of radioactive isotopes of iodine in a radiation emergency or after therapeutic/diagnostic use of radioactive iodine

Topical solution: Provide topical antisepsis (FDA approved in adults)

Pregnancy Risk Factor D (potassium iodide)

Pregnancy Considerations Iodide crosses the placenta (may cause hypothyroidism and goiter in fetus/newborn). Use for protection against thyroid cancer secondary to radioactive iodine exposure is considered acceptable based upon risk:benefit, keeping in mind the dose and duration. Repeat dosing should be avoided if possible. Refer to Iodine for additional information.

Breast-Feeding Considerations Skin rash in the nursing infant has been reported with maternal intake of potassium iodide. Refer to Iodine monograph for additional information.

Contraindications Hypersensitivity to iodine or any component; active tuberculosis

Warnings Hypersensitivity reactions to iodine have been reported. Prolonged use can lead to hypothyroidism and iodism (chronic iodide intoxication).

Precautions Use with caution in patients with cystic fibrosis; may have exaggerated susceptibility to goitrogenic effects. Use with caution in patients with myotonia congenital, Addison's disease, acute bronchitis, or a history of thyroid disease and cardiac disease; avoid use in patients with iodine-induced goiter. Use may cause flare-up of acne and/or dermatitis; avoid use in patients with dermatitis herpetiformis or hypocomplementemic vasculitis.

Adverse Reactions

Cardiovascular: Irregular heart beat

Central nervous system: Confusion, tiredness, fever

Dermatologic: Skin rash

Endocrine & metabolic: Goiter, salivary gland swelling/tenderness, thyroid adenoma, swelling of neck/throat, myxedema, lymph node swelling, hyper-/hypothyroidism

Gastrointestinal: Diarrhea, gastrointestinal bleeding, metallic taste, nausea, stomach pain, stomach upset, vomiting

Neuromuscular & skeletal: Numbness, tingling, weakness, joint pain

Miscellaneous: Chronic iodine poisoning (with prolonged treatment/high doses); iodism, hypersensitivity reactions (angioedema, cutaneous and mucosal hemorrhage, serum sickness-like symptoms)

Drug Interactions

Metabolism/Transport Effects None known.

Avoid Concomitant Use

Avoid concomitant use of Potassium Iodide and Iodine with any of the following: Sodium Iodide I131

Increased Effect/Toxicity

Potassium Iodide and Iodine may increase the levels/effects of: ACE Inhibitors; Angiotensin II Receptor Blockers; Cardiac Glycosides; Lithium; Potassium-Sparing Diuretics; Theophylline Derivatives

The levels/effects of Potassium Iodide and Iodine may be increased by: Eplerenone; Heparin; Heparin (Low Molecular Weight)

Decreased Effect

Potassium Iodide and Iodine may decrease the levels/effects of: Sodium Iodide I131; Vitamin K Antagonists

Stability

Oral solution: Store at room temperature; excursions permitted at 15°C to 30°C (59°F to 86°F); protect from light and keep container tightly closed

Topical solution: Store at 15°C to 30°C (59°F to 86°F); protect from light and keep container tightly closed.

Mechanism of Action In hyperthyroidism, iodine temporarily inhibits thyroid hormone synthesis and secretion into the circulation; use also decreases thyroid gland size and vascularity. Serum T_4 and T_3 concentrations can be reduced for several weeks with use but effect will not be maintained.

Following radioactive iodine exposure, potassium iodide blocks uptake of radioiodine by the thyroid, reducing the risk of thyroid cancer.

Pharmacodynamics Antithyroid effects:

Onset of action: 24-48 hours

Maximum effect: 10-15 days after continuous therapy

Duration: May persist up to 6 weeks

Dosing: Neonatal Graves' disease: Oral: Lugol's solution: 1 drop/dose 3 times daily

Dosing: Usual

Children:

Thyroidectomy, preoperative preparation: Oral: Lugol's solution: 3-5 drops (0.1-0.3 mL)/dose 3 times daily; administer for 10 days before surgery

Thyrotoxic crisis: Oral: Lugol's solution: 4-8 drops/dose 3 times daily, begin therapy preferably 2 hours following the initial dose of either propylthiouracil or methimazole

Adults:

Thyroidectomy, preoperative preparation: Oral: Lugol's solution: 5-7 drops (0.25-0.35 mL)/dose 3 times daily; administer for 10 days before surgery; if not euthyroid prior to surgery, consider concurrent beta-blockade (eg, propranolol) in the immediate preoperative period to reduce the risk of thyroid storm (Bahn, 2011)

Thyrotoxic crisis: Oral: Lugol's solution: 4-8 drops/dose every 6-8 hours; begin administration ≥1 hour following the initial dose of either propylthiouracil or methimazole (Nayak, 2006)

Administration

Oral: Dilute with a large quantity of water, fruit juice, or milk or administer after meals with food or milk

Topical: For external use only; apply to area requiring antiseptic

Monitoring Parameters Thyroid function tests; signs/symptoms of hyperthyroidism; thyroid function should be monitored in pregnant women, neonates, and young infants if repeat doses are required following radioactive iodine exposure

Test Interactions Iodide may alter thyroid function tests.

Dosage Forms Excipient information presented when available (limited, particularly for generics); consult specific product labeling.

Solution, oral: Potassium iodide 100 mg/mL and iodine 50 mg/mL (473 mL)

Solution, topical: Potassium iodide 100 mg/mL and iodine 50 mg/mL (8 mL)

References

"American Academy of Pediatrics Committee on Environmental Health. Radiation Disasters and Children," *Pediatrics*, 2003, 111(6 Pt 1):1455-66.

Hassoun A and Oberfield SE, "Renal, Endocrine, and Metabolic Disorders," *Roger's Textbook of Pediatric Intensive Care*, 3rd ed, David G Nichols, ed, Philadelphia, PA: Lippincott, Williams, & Wilkins, 2008;1658.

Kauffman CA, Hajjeh R, and Chapman SW, "Practice Guidelines for the Management of Patients With Sporotrichosis. For the Mycoses Study Group. Infectious Diseases Society of America," *Clin Infect Dis*, 2000, 30(4):684-7.

Nayak B and Burman K, "Thyrotoxicosis and Thyroid Storm," *Endocrinol Metab Clin North Am*, 2006, 35(4):663-86.

"Potassium Iodide as a Thyroid Blocking Agent in a Radiation Emergency: Final Recommendations on Use," Washington DC, Bureau of Radiological Health and Bureau of Drugs, Food and Drug Administration, 1982.

U.S. Food and Drug Administration, "FDA's Guidance on Protection of Children and Adults Against Thyroid Cancer in Case of Nuclear Accident," *FDA Talk Paper*. Available at: http://www.fda.gov/bbs/topics/answers/2001/ans01126.html. Accessed January 11, 2002.

Potassium Phosphate (poe TASS ee um FOS fate)

Medication Safety Issues

High alert medication:

The Institute for Safe Medication Practices (ISMP) includes this medication (I.V. formulation) among its list of drugs which have a heightened risk of causing significant patient harm when used in error.

Other safety concerns:

Per JCAHO recommendations, concentrated electrolyte solutions should not be available in patient care areas.

Consider special storage requirements for intravenous potassium salts; I.V. potassium salts have been administered IVP in error, leading to fatal outcomes.

Safe Prescribing: Because inorganic phosphate exists as monobasic and dibasic anions, with the mixture of valences dependent on pH, ordering by mEq amounts is unreliable and may lead to large dosing errors. In addition, I.V. phosphate is available in the sodium and potassium salt; therefore, the content of these cations must be considered when ordering phosphate. The most reliable method of ordering I.V. phosphate is by millimoles, then specifying the potassium or sodium salt. For example, an order for 15 mmol of phosphate as potassium phosphate in one liter of normal saline.

Brand Names: U.S. Neutra-Phos®-K [OTC] [DSC]

Therapeutic Category Electrolyte Supplement, Parenteral; Phosphate Salt; Potassium Salt

Generic Availability (U.S.) Yes: Injection

Use Treatment and prevention of hypophosphatemia; source of phosphate in large volume I.V. fluids (All indications: FDA approved in all ages)

Pregnancy Risk Factor C

Pregnancy Considerations Reproduction studies have not been conducted. Phosphorus requirements are the same in pregnant and nonpregnant women (IOM, 1997). Although this product is not used for potassium supplementation, adverse events have not been observed following use of potassium supplements in healthy women with normal pregnancies. Use caution in pregnant women with other medical conditions (eg, pre-eclampsia; may be more likely to develop hyperkalemia) (IOM, 2004).

Breast-Feeding Considerations Phosphorus, sodium, and potassium are normal constituents of human milk.

Contraindications Hypersensitivity to phosphate (salts) or any component; hyperphosphatemia, hyperkalemia, hypocalcemia

Warnings Must be diluted before I.V. use and infused slowly. Close monitoring of serum potassium concentrations is needed to avoid hyperkalemia; severe hyperkalemia may lead to muscle weakness/paralysis and cardiac conduction abnormalities (eg, heart block, ventricular arrhythmias, asystole). Use with caution in patients with cardiovascular disease (eg, heart failure, cardiac arrhythmias); these patients may be more susceptible to life-threatening cardiac effects associated with hyper-/hypokalemia; patients must be on a cardiac monitor during intermittent infusions. Use extreme caution when administering potassium phosphate parenterally; evaluate patient's renal function, cardiac and fluid status, and any factors contributing to altered potassium concentrations (eg, acidosis, alkalosis) prior to therapy; parenteral **potassium** salt forms should be administered only in patients with adequate urine flow. Closely monitor potassium and phosphate concentrations and response to therapy. Parenteral potassium may cause pain and phlebitis, requiring a decrease in infusion rate or potassium concentration. Admixture of phosphate and calcium in I.V. fluids can result in calcium phosphate precipitation.

Precautions Use with caution in patients with renal impairment; renal impairment requires close monitoring of serum potassium and phosphorus concentrations to avoid hyperkalemia and/or hyperphosphatemia. Use with caution in patients with acid/base alterations; changes in serum potassium concentrations can occur during acid/base correction, monitor closely. Use with caution in digitalized patients; may be more susceptible to potentially life-threatening cardiac effects with rapid changes in serum potassium concentrations. Use with caution in patients receiving concomitant medications or therapies that increase potassium (eg, ACEI, potassium-sparing diuretics, potassium containing salt substitutes). Injection contains aluminum; toxic aluminum concentrations may be seen with high doses, prolonged use, or renal dysfunction. Premature neonates are at higher risk due to immature renal function and aluminum intake from other parenteral sources. Parenteral aluminum exposure of >4-5 mcg/kg/day is associated with CNS and bone toxicity and tissue loading may occur at lower doses.

Adverse Reactions

Cardiovascular: Arrhythmia, bradycardia, chest pain, ECG changes, edema, heart block, hypotension

Central nervous system: Listlessness, mental confusion, tetany (with large doses of phosphate)

Endocrine & metabolic: Hyperkalemia

Gastrointestinal: Diarrhea, nausea, stomach pain, vomiting

Genitourinary: Urine output decreased

Local: Phlebitis

Neuromuscular & skeletal: Paralysis, paresthesia, weakness

Renal: Acute renal failure

Respiratory: Dyspnea

Drug Interactions

Metabolism/Transport Effects None known.

Avoid Concomitant Use There are no known interactions where it is recommended to avoid concomitant use.

Increased Effect/Toxicity

Potassium Phosphate may increase the levels/effects of: ACE Inhibitors; Angiotensin II Receptor Blockers; Potassium-Sparing Diuretics

The levels/effects of Potassium Phosphate may be increased by: Bisphosphonate Derivatives; Eplerenone; Heparin; Heparin (Low Molecular Weight)

Decreased Effect

The levels/effects of Potassium Phosphate may be decreased by: Antacids; Calcium Salts; Iron Salts; Magnesium Salts; Multivitamins/Minerals (with ADEK, Folate, Iron); Sucralfate

Food Interactions Avoid administering with oxalate (berries, nuts, chocolate, beans, celery, tomato) or phytate-containing foods (bran, whole wheat).

Stability Store intact vials at 20°C to 25°C (68°F to 77°F); excursions permitted between 15°C and 30°C (59°F and 86°F). Calcium phosphate stability in parenteral nutrition solutions is dependent upon the pH of the solution, temperature, and relative concentration of each ion. The pH of the solution is primarily dependent upon the amino acid concentration. The higher the percentage of amino acids, the lower the pH, and the more soluble the calcium and phosphate. Individual commercially available amino acid solutions vary significantly with respect to pH-lowering potential and consequent calcium phosphate compatibility. Check with a pharmacist to determine compatibility.

Mechanism of Action

Phosphorus in the form of organic and inorganic phosphate has a variety of important biochemical functions in the body and is involved in many significant metabolic and enzymatic reactions in almost all organs and tissues. It exerts a modifying influence on the steady state of calcium levels, a buffering effect on acid-base equilibrium and a primary role in the renal excretion of hydrogen ion.

Potassium is the major cation of intracellular fluid and is essential for the conduction of nerve impulses in heart, brain, and skeletal muscle; contraction of cardiac, skeletal and smooth muscles; maintenance of normal renal function, acid-base balance, carbohydrate metabolism, and gastric secretion.

Pharmacokinetics (Adult data unless noted) Elimination: Execreted in the urine with over 80% to 90% of dose reabsorbed by the kidney

Dosing: Neonatal Note: If phosphate repletion is required and a phosphate product is not available at your institution, consider the use of sodium glycerophosphate pentahydrate (Glycophos) as a suitable substitute. Concentration and dosing are different from FDA approved products; use caution when switching between products. Refer to sodium glycerophosphate pentahydrate monograph.

Caution: With orders for I.V. phosphate, there is considerable confusion associated with the use of millimoles (mmol) versus milliequivalents (mEq) to express the phosphate requirement. The most reliable method of ordering I.V. phosphate is by millimoles, then specifying the potassium or sodium salt. Intravenous doses listed as mmol of phosphate. **Note:** Consider the contribution of potassium when determining the appropriate phosphate replacement.

Phosphorus Estimated Average Requirement (EAR):
Oral: 3.2 mmol/day (adequate intake)
Parenteral nutrition, maintenance requirement: I.V.: 1-2 mmol/kg/day (Mirtallo, 2004)

Dosing: Usual Note: If phosphate repletion is required and a phosphate product is not available at your institution, consider the use of sodium glycerophosphate pentahydrate (Glycophos) as a suitable substitute. Concentration and dosing are different from FDA approved products; use caution when switching between products. Refer to sodium glycerophosphate pentahydrate monograph.

Caution: With orders for I.V. phosphate, there is considerable confusion associated with the use of millimoles (mmol) versus milliequivalents (mEq) to express the phosphate requirement. The most reliable method of ordering I.V. phosphate is by millimoles, then specifying the potassium or sodium salt. Intravenous doses listed as mmol of phosphate. **Note:** Consider the contribution of potassium when determining the appropriate phosphate replacement.

Infants, Children, and Adolescents:
Phosphorus - Recommended Daily Allowance (RDA) and Estimated Average Requirement (EAR):
1-6 months:
EAR: 3.2 mmol/day (adequate intake)
7-12 months:
EAR: 8.9 mmol/day (adequate intake)
1-3 years:
RDA: 14.8 mmol/day
EAR: 12.3 mmol/day
4-8 years:
RDA: 16.1 mmol/day
EAR: 13.1 mmol/day

9-18 years:
RDA: 40.3 mmol/day
EAR: 34 mmol/day
19-30 years:
RDA: 22.6 mmol/day
EAR: 18.7 mmol/day

Hypophosphatemia, acute: Hypophosphatemia does not necessarily equate with phosphate depletion. Hypophosphatemia may occur in the presence of low, normal, or high total body phosphate and conversely, phosphate depletion may exist with normal, low, or elevated levels of serum phosphate (Gaasbeek, 2005). It is difficult to provide concrete guidelines for the treatment of severe hypophosphatemia because the extent of total body deficits and response to therapy are difficult to predict. Aggressive doses of phosphate may result in a transient serum elevation followed by redistribution into intracellular compartments or bone tissue. Intermittent I.V. infusion should be reserved for severe depletion situations; requires continuous cardiac monitoring. Guidelines differ based on degree of illness, need/use of TPN, and severity of hypophosphatemia. If hyperkalemia exists, consider phosphate replacement strategy without potassium (eg, sodium phosphates). Various regimens for replacement of phosphate in adults have been studied. The regimens below have only been studied in adult patients, however, many institutions have used them in children safely and successfully. Obese patients and/or severe renal impairment were excluded from phosphate supplement trials. **Note:** 1 mmol phosphate = 31 mg phosphorus; 1 mg phosphorus = 0.032 mmol phosphate

I.V. doses may be incorporated into the patient's maintenance I.V. fluids; intermittent I.V. infusion should be reserved for severe depletion situations. **Note:** Doses listed as mmol of **phosphate**

Children and Adolescents: **Note:** There are no prospective studies of parenteral phosphate replacement in children. The following weight-based guidelines for adult dosing may be cautiously employed in pediatric patients. Guidelines differ based on degree of illness, use of TPN, and severity of hypophosphatemia.

General replacement guidelines (Lentz, 1978): **Note:** The initial dose may be increased by 25% to 50% if the patient is symptomatic secondary to hypophosphatemia and lowered by 25% to 50% if the patient is hypercalcemic.

Low dose: 0.08 mmol/kg over 6 hours; use if losses are recent and uncomplicated

Intermediate dose: 0.16-0.24 mmol/kg over 4-6 hours; use if serum phosphorus level 0.5-1 mg/dL (0.16-0.32 mmol/L)

High dose: 0.36 mmol/kg over 6 hours; use if serum phosphorus <0.5 mg/dL (<0.16 mmol/L)

Patients receiving TPN (Clark, 1995):
Low dose: 0.16 mmol/kg over 4-6 hours; use if serum phosphorus level 2.3-3 mg/dL (0.73- 0.96 mmol/L)

Intermediate dose: 0.32 mmol/kg over 4-6 hours; use if serum phosphorus level 1.6-2.2 mg/dL (0.51-0.72 mmol/L)

High dose: 0.64 mmol/kg over 8-12 hours; use if serum phosphorus <1.5 mg/dL (<0.5 mmol/L)

Critically ill adult trauma patients receiving TPN (Brown, 2006):
Low dose: 0.32 mmol/kg over 4-6 hours; use if serum phosphorus level 2.3-3 mg/dL (0.73-0.96 mmol/L)

Intermediate dose: 0.64 mmol/kg over 4-6 hours; use if serum phosphorus level 1.6-2.2 mg/dL (0.51-0.72 mmol/L)

High dose: 1 mmol/kg over 8-12 hours; use if serum phosphorus <1.5 mg/dL (<0.5 mmol/L)

Alternative method in critically ill patients (Kingston, 1985):

Low dose: 0.25 mmol/kg over 4 hours; use if serum phosphorus level 0.5-1 mg/dL (0.16-0.32 mmol/L)

Moderate dose: 0.5 mmol/kg over 4 hours; use if serum phosphorus level <0.5 mg/dL (<0.16 mmol/L)

Parenteral nutrition, maintenance requirement (Mirtallo, 2004): I.V.:

Infants and Children ≤50 kg: 0.5-2 mmol/kg/day

Children >50 kg and Adolescents: 10-40 mmol/day

Adults: I.V.:

Hypophosphatemia, acute treatment: Repletion of severe hypophosphatemia should be done I.V. because large doses of oral phosphate may cause diarrhea and intestinal absorption may be unreliable. Reserve intermittent I.V. infusion for severe depletion situations; may require continuous cardiac monitoring depending on potassium administration rate. If potassium >4.0 mEq/L consider phosphate replacement strategy without potassium (eg, sodium phosphates). Guidelines differ based on degree of illness, need/use of parenteral nutrition, and severity of hypophosphatemia. Patients with severe renal impairment were excluded from phosphate supplement trials. **Note:** 1 mmol phosphate = 31 mg phosphorus; 1 mg phosphorus = 0.032 mmol phosphate

General replacement guidelines (Lentz, 1978):

Low dose, if serum phosphate losses are recent and uncomplicated: 0.08 mmol/kg over 6 hours

Intermediate dose, if serum phosphorus level 0.5-1 mg/dL (0.16-0.32 mmol/L): 0.16-0.24 mmol/kg over 4-6 hours

Note: The initial dose may be increased by 25% to 50% if the patient is symptomatic secondary to hypophosphatemia and lowered by 25% to 50% if the patient is hypercalcemic.

Critically ill adult patients receiving concurrent enteral/parenteral nutrition (Brown, 2006; Clark, 2006): **Note:** Round doses to the nearest 7.5 mmol for ease of preparation. If administering with phosphate-containing parenteral nutrition, do not exceed 15 mmol/L within parenteral nutrition.

Low dose, serum phosphorus level 2.3-3 mg/dL (0.74-0.96 mmol/L): 0.16-0.32 mmol/kg over 4-6 hours

Intermediate dose, serum phosphorus level 1.6-2.2 mg/dL (0.51-0.71 mmol/L): 0.32-0.64 mmol/kg over 4-6 hours

High dose, serum phosphorus <1.5 mg/dL (<0.5 mmol/L): 0.64-1 mmol/kg over 8-12 hours

Obesity: May use adjusted body weight for patients weighing >130% of ideal body weight (and BMI<40 kg/m^2) by using [IBW + 0.25 (ABW-IBW)].

Parenteral nutrition: I.V.: 10-15 mmol/1000 kcal (Hicks, 2001) **or** 20-40 mmol/24 hours (Mirtallo, 2004)

Administration Parenteral: Intermittent I.V. infusion: Observe the vial for the presence of translucent visible particles. Do not use vial if particles are present. Injection must be diluted in appropriate I.V. solution and volume prior to administration. In general, the dose, concentration of infusion, and rate of administration may be dependent on patient condition and specific institution policy. Must consider administration precautions for phosphate and potassium when prescribing. **Note:** Due to the potential presence of particulates, American Regent, Inc recommends the use of a 5-micron filter when preparing I.V. potassium phosphate-containing solutions (Important Drug Administration Information, American Regent, 2013); a similar recommendation has not been noted by other manufacturers. Maximum concentration: Peripheral line: 0.05 mmol/mL; Central line: 0.12 mmol/mL (maximum concentrations were determined with consideration for maximum potassium concentrations); maximum rate of infusion: 0.06 mmol/kg/hour; do **not** infuse with calcium-containing I.V. fluids. **Note:** Due to the potential presence of translucent visible particles, American Regent, Inc recommends the use of a 0.22-micron in-line filter for I.V. administration (1.2-micron filter if admixture contains lipids) (Important Drug Administration Information, American Regent, 2013); a similar recommendation has not been noted by other manufacturers.

Monitoring Parameters Serum potassium, calcium, and phosphorus concentrations; renal function; in pediatric patients after I.V. phosphate repletion, repeat serum phosphorus concentration should be checked 2 hours later (ASPEN Pediatric Nutrition Support Core Curriculum, 2010; cardiac monitor (if intermittent infusion or potassium infusion rates >0.5 mEq/kg/hour in children or >10 mEq/hour in adults)

Reference Range Note: There is a diurnal variation with the nadir at 1100, plateau at 1600, and peak in the early evening (Gaasbeek, 2005); 1 mmol/L phosphate = 3.1 mg/dL phosphorus

Newborn 0-5 days: 4.8-8.2 mg/dL

1-3 years: 3.8-6.5 mg/dL

4-11 years: 3.7-5.6 mg/dL

12-15 years: 2.9-5.4 mg/dL

16-19 years: 2.7-4.7 mg/dL

Additional Information Cow's milk is a good source of phosphate with 1 mg elemental (0.032 mmol) elemental phosphate per mL.

Dosage Forms Considerations

Potassium 4.4 mEq is equivalent to potassium 170 mg

Phosphorous 3 mmol is equivalent to phosphorus 93 mg

Dosage Forms Excipient information presented when available (limited, particularly for generics); consult specific product labeling.

Injection, solution: Potassium 4.4 mEq and phosphorus 3 mmol per mL (5 mL, 15 mL, 50 mL) [equivalent to potassium 170 mg and elemental phosphorus 93 mg per mL]

References

Brown KA, Dickerson, RN, Morgan, RN, et al, "A New Graduated Dosing Regimen for Phosphorus Replacement in Patients Receiving Nutrition Support," *JPEN*, 2006, 30(3):209-14.

Clark CL, Sacks GS, Dickerson RN, et al, "Treatment of Hypophosphatemia in Patients Receiving Specialized Nutrition Support Using a Graduated Dosing Scheme: Results From a Prospective Clinical Trial," *Crit Care Med*, 1995, 23(9):1504-11.

Department Health and Human Services, Food and Drug Administration, "Aluminum in Large and Small Volume Parenterals Used in Total Parenteral Nutrition," *Federal Register*, 2000, 65(17):4103-11.

Gaasbeek A and Meinders AE, "Hypophosphatemia: An Update on Its Etiology and Treatment," *Am J Med*, 2005, 118(10):1094-101.

IOM (Institute of Medicine), Dietary Reference Intakes for Calcium, Phosphorus, Magnesium, Vitamin D, and Fluoride, National Academy of Sciences, Washington, DC, 1997.

IOM (Institute of Medicine), Dietary Reference Intakes for Water, Potassium, Sodium, Chloride, and Sulfate, Washington, DC: National Academy Press, 2004.

Kingston M and Al-Siba'i MB, "Treatment of Severe Hypophosphatemia," *Crit Care Med*, 1985, 13(1):16-8

Lentz RD, Brown DM, and Kjellstrand CM, "Treatment of Severe Hypophosphatemia," *Ann Intern Med*, 1978, 89(6):941-4.

Lloyd CW and Johnson CE, "Management of Hypophosphatemia," *Clin Pharm*, 1988, 7(2):123-8.

Rosen GH, Boullata JI, O'Rangers EA, et al, "Intravenous Phosphate Repletion Regimen for Critically Ill Patients With Moderate Hypophosphatemia," *Crit Care Med*, 1995, 23(7):1204-10.

Schmidt GL, "Fluids and Electrolytes," In: Corkins MR, Balint J, Bobo E, et al, eds, The A.S.P.E.N Pediatric Nutrition Support Core Curriculum, Silver Spring: MD: American Society of Parenteral and Enteral Nutrition, 2010, 87-102.

Potassium Phosphate and Sodium Phosphate

(poe TASS ee um FOS fate & SOW dee um FOS fate)

Medication Safety Issues

Sound-alike/look-alike issues:
K-Phos® Neutral may be confused with Neutra-Phos-K®

Brand Names: U.S. K-Phos® Neutral; K-Phos® No. 2; Phos-NaK; Phospha 250™ Neutral

Therapeutic Category Electrolyte Supplement, Oral; Phosphate Salt; Potassium Salt; Sodium Salt

Generic Availability (U.S.) Yes

Use Treatment and prevention of hypophosphatemia (FDA approved in ages ≥4 years and adults); urinary acidification (FDA approved in adults)

Pregnancy Risk Factor C

Pregnancy Considerations Animal reproduction studies have not been conducted.

Breast-Feeding Considerations It is not known if the combination product is excreted in breast milk. The manufacturer recommends that caution be exercised when administering potassium phosphate and sodium phosphate to nursing women. Refer to individual agents.

Contraindications Hypersensitivity to phosphate (salts) or any component; hyperphosphatemia, hyperkalemia, hypocalcemia, hypomagnesemia, hypernatremia, severe renal impairment, severe tissue trauma, heat cramps, CHF, patients with phosphate kidney stones

Precautions Use with caution in patients with renal impairment, patients receiving potassium-sparing drugs (potassium salt forms), patients with adrenal insufficiency, cirrhosis

Adverse Reactions

Cardiovascular: Bradycardia, cardiac arrhythmia, chest pain, edema, lower extremity edema, tachycardia

Central nervous system: Confusion, dizziness, fatigue, headache, paresthesia, seizure, tetany (with large doses of phosphate)

Endocrine & metabolic: Alkalosis, hyperkalemia, weight gain

Gastrointestinal: Diarrhea, flatulence, nausea, sore throat, stomach pain, vomiting

Genitourinary: Decreased urine output

Neuromuscular & skeletal: Arthralgia, limb pain, muscle cramps, ostealgia, paralysis, weakness

Renal: Acute renal failure

Respiratory: Dyspnea

Miscellaneous: Increased thirst

Drug Interactions

Metabolism/Transport Effects None known.

Avoid Concomitant Use There are no known interactions where it is recommended to avoid concomitant use.

Increased Effect/Toxicity
Potassium Phosphate and Sodium Phosphate may increase the levels/effects of: ACE Inhibitors; Angiotensin II Receptor Blockers; Potassium-Sparing Diuretics

The levels/effects of Potassium Phosphate and Sodium Phosphate may be increased by: Bisphosphonate Derivatives; Eplerenone; Heparin; Heparin (Low Molecular Weight)

Decreased Effect
The levels/effects of Potassium Phosphate and Sodium Phosphate may be decreased by: Antacids; Calcium Salts; Iron Salts; Magnesium Salts; Multivitamins/Minerals (with ADEK, Folate, Iron); Sucralfate

Stability Store at room temperature.

Pharmacodynamics Onset of action (catharsis): Oral: 3-6 hours

Pharmacokinetics (Adult data unless noted)
Absorption: Oral: 1% to 20%

Elimination: Oral forms excreted in feces

Dosing: Neonatal Note: Consider the contribution of potassium when determining the appropriate phosphate replacement. **Phosphorus Estimated Average Requirement (EAR):** Oral: 3.2 mmol/day (adequate intake)

Dosing: Usual Note: Consider the contribution of sodium and potassium cations when determining appropriate phosphate replacement.

Phosphorus-Recommended Daily Allowance (RDA) and Estimated Average Requirement (EAR):
1-6 months:
  EAR: 3.2 mmol/day (adequate intake)
7-12 months:
  EAR: 8.9 mmol/day (adequate intake)
1-3 years:
  RDA: 14.8 mmol/day
  EAR: 12.3 mmol/day
4-8 years:
  RDA: 16.1 mmol/day
  EAR: 13.1 mmol/day
9-18 years:
  RDA: 40.3 mmol/day
  EAR: 34 mmol/day
19-30 years:
  RDA: 22.6 mmol/day
  EAR: 18.7 mmol/day

Maintenance: Oral:
  Children: 2-3 mmol/kg/day in divided doses
  Adults: 50-150 mmol/day in divided doses

Supplementation:
K-Phos® Neutral, Phospha 250™ Neutral:
  Children >4 years and Adolescents: 1 tablet 4 times/day
  Adults: 1-2 tablets 4 times/day
Phos-NaK:
  Children 4-8 years: 1 packet 2 times/day
  Children ≥9 years, Adolescents, and Adults: 1 packet 4 times/day

Urinary acidification: Oral: **Note:** Packets are **not** an appropriate substitution for this indication due to the higher potassium content.
  Adults: K-Phos® No. 2: 1 tablet 4 times/day; may administer 1 tablet every 2 hours (maximum: 8 tablets/24 hours) when urine is difficult to acidify

Administration Oral: Administer with food to reduce the risk of diarrhea; contents of 1 packet should be diluted in 75 mL water or juice before administration; administer tablets with a full glass of water; maintain adequate fluid intake; dilute oral solution with an equal volume of cool water

Monitoring Parameters Serum potassium, sodium, calcium, phosphorus, renal function, reflexes

Reference Range Note: There is a diurnal variation with the nadir at 1100, plateau at 1600, and peak in the early evening (Gaasbeek, 2005); 1 mmol/L phosphate = 3.1 mg/dL phosphorus
Newborns: 4.2-9 mg/dL phosphorus (1.36-2.91 mmol/L phosphate)
6 weeks to 18 months: 3.8-6.7 mg/dL phosphorus (1.23-2.16 mmol/L phosphate)
18 months to 3 years: 2.9-5.9 mg/dL phosphorus (0.94-1.91 mmol/L phosphate)
3-15 years: 3.6-5.6 mg/dL phosphorus (1.16-1.81 mmol/L phosphate)
>15 years: 2.5-5 mg/dL phosphorus (0.81-1.62 mmol/L phosphate)

Hypophosphatemia:
Moderate: 1-2 mg/dL phosphorus (0.32-0.65 mmol/L phosphate)
Severe: <1 mg/dL phosphorus (<0.32 mmol/L phosphate)

Additional Information Each mmol of phosphate contains 31 mg elemental phosphorus; 1 mmol/L phosphate = 3.1 mg/dL phosphorus; cow's milk is a good source of phosphate with 1 mg elemental (0.032 mmol) phosphate per mL

Dosage Forms Excipient information presented when available (limited, particularly for generics); consult specific product labeling.

Powder for solution, oral:

Phos-NaK: Dibasic potassium phosphate, monobasic potassium phosphate, dibasic sodium phosphate, and monobasic sodium phosphate per packet (100s) [sugar free; equivalent to elemental phosphorus 250 mg (8 mmol), sodium 160 mg (6.9 mEq), and potassium 280 mg (7.1 mEq) per packet; fruit flavor]

Tablet, oral:

K-Phos® Neutral: Monobasic potassium phosphate 155 mg, dibasic sodium phosphate 852 mg, and monobasic sodium phosphate 130 mg [equivalent to elemental phosphorus 250 mg (8 mmol), sodium 298 mg (13 mEq), and potassium 45 mg (1.1 mEq)]

K-Phos® No. 2: Potassium acid phosphate 305 mg and sodium acid phosphate 700 mg [equivalent to elemental phosphorus 250 mg (8 mmol), sodium 134 mg (5.8 mEq), and potassium 88 mg (2.3 mEq)]

Phospha 250™ Neutral: Monobasic potassium phosphate 155 mg, dibasic sodium phosphate 852 mg, and monobasic sodium phosphate 130 mg [equivalent to elemental phosphorus 250 mg (8 mmol), sodium 298 mg (13 mEq), and potassium 45 mg (1.1 mEq)]

References

Gaasbeek A and Meinders AE, "Hypophosphatemia: An Update on Its Etiology and Treatment," *Am J Med*, 2005, 118(10):1094-101.

◆ **PPL** *see* Benzylpenicilloyl Polylysine *on page 279*

◆ **PPSV** *see* Pneumococcal Polysaccharide Vaccine (Polyvalent) *on page 1691*

◆ **PPSV23** *see* Pneumococcal Polysaccharide Vaccine (Polyvalent) *on page 1691*

◆ **PPV23** *see* Pneumococcal Polysaccharide Vaccine (Polyvalent) *on page 1691*

Pralidoxime (pra li DOKS eem)

Medication Safety Issues

Sound-alike/look-alike issues:

Pralidoxime may be confused with pramoxine, pyridoxine

Protopam® may be confused with protamine

Brand Names: U.S. Protopam Chloride

Therapeutic Category Antidote, Anticholinesterase; Antidote, Organophosphate Poisoning

Generic Availability (U.S.) May be product dependent

Use Treatment of muscle weakness and/or respiratory depression secondary to poisoning due to organophosphate anticholinesterase pesticides and chemicals (eg, nerve agents) [FDA approved in pediatric patients (age not specified) and adults]; control of overdose of anticholinesterase medications used to treat myasthenia gravis (ambenonium, neostigmine, pyridostigmine) [FDA approved in pediatric patients (age not specified) and adults]

Pregnancy Risk Factor C

Pregnancy Considerations Animal reproduction studies have not been conducted. A case report did not show evidence of adverse events after pralidoxime administration during the second trimester (Kamha, 2005). In general, medications used as antidotes should take into consideration the health and prognosis of the mother; antidotes should be administered to pregnant women if there is a clear indication for use and should not be withheld because of fears of teratogenicity (Bailey, 2003).

Breast-Feeding Considerations It is not known if pralidoxime is excreted in breast milk. The manufacturer recommends that caution be exercised when administering pralidoxime to nursing women.

Contraindications Hypersensitivity to pralidoxime or any component

Warnings Clinical symptoms that are consistent with suspected organophosphate poisoning should be treated with antidote immediately; administration should not be delayed for confirmatory laboratory tests; treatment should include proper evacuation and decontamination procedures as indicated; medical personnel should protect themselves from inadvertent contamination. Antidote administration is intended only for initial management; definitive and more intensive medical care is required following administration. Individuals should not rely solely on antidote for treatment; the concomitant use of atropine will be necessary and other supportive measures (eg, artificial respiration) may still be required. Pralidoxime is not indicated for the treatment of carbamate poisoning; acetylcholinesterase is weakly, but not permanently, affected by carbamates. Pralidoxime is not indicated for the treatment of poisoning due to phosphorus, inorganic phosphates, or organophosphates without anticholinesterase activity.

Precautions Use with caution in patients with myasthenia gravis; administration may precipitate a myasthenic crisis. Use with caution in patients with renal impairment; dosage modification may be required. Rapid I.V. infusion may be associated with temporary worsening of cholinergic manifestations (eg, tachycardia, laryngospasm, muscle rigidity, cardiac arrest) in adults; in children muscle fasciculations, apnea, and convulsions have also been reported. During the management of anticholinesterase poisoning, the use of medications that may be potentiated by anticholinesterases; avoid use if possible or use extreme caution including theophylline, aminophylline, reserpine, succinylcholine, phenothiazines, respiratory depressants (eg, opioids, barbiturates).

Adverse Reactions

Cardiovascular: Cardiac arrest, hypertension, tachycardia

Central nervous system: Dizziness, drowsiness, headache, paralysis, seizure

Dermatologic: Skin rash

Gastrointestinal: Nausea

Hepatic: Increased serum ALT (transient), increased serum AST (transient)

Local: Pain at injection site (I.M.)

Neuromuscular & skeletal: Fasciculations, increased creatine phosphokinase, laryngospasm, muscle rigidity, weakness

Ophthalmic: Accommodation disturbance, blurred vision, diplopia

Renal: Renal insufficiency

Respiratory: Apnea, hyperventilation

Drug Interactions

Metabolism/Transport Effects None known.

Avoid Concomitant Use There are no known interactions where it is recommended to avoid concomitant use.

Increased Effect/Toxicity There are no known significant interactions involving an increase in effect.

Decreased Effect There are no known significant interactions involving a decrease in effect.

Stability Store at 20°C to 25°C (68°F to 77°F); excursions permitted to 15°C to 30°C (59°F to 86°F).

Mechanism of Action Reactivates cholinesterase that had been inactivated by phosphorylation due to exposure to organophosphate pesticides and cholinesterase-inhibiting nerve agents (eg, terrorism and chemical warfare agents such as sarin) by displacing the enzyme from its receptor sites; removes the phosphoryl group from the active site of the inactivated enzyme

Pharmacokinetics (Adult data unless noted)

Distribution: V_{dss}: 0.6-2.7 L/kg; severely poisoned pediatric patients (n=11; age: 0.8-18 years): ~9 L/kg (range: 1.7-13.8 L/kg) (Schexnayder, 1998); may increase with increasing severity of organophosphate intoxication

Protein binding: None

Metabolism: Hepatic

Half-life: Apparent: 74-77 minutes; pediatric patients (n=11; age: 0.8-18 years): 2.4-5 hours

Time to peak serum concentration: I.M.: 35 minutes

Elimination: Urine (~80% as metabolites and unchanged drug)

Dosing: Usual Note: Use in conjunction with atropine; atropine effects should be established before pralidoxime is administered.

Organophosphate poisoning: Note: I.V. administration is preferable; if I.V. route not feasible, may be given I.M. or SubQ

I.V.:

Infants, Children, and Adolescents ≤16 years: Loading dose: 20-50 mg/kg (maximum: 2000 mg/dose); Maintenance infusion: 10-20 mg/kg/**hour**; alternatively, a repeat bolus of 20-50 mg/kg (maximum: 2000 mg/dose) may be administered after 1 hour if muscle weakness is not relieved and repeated every 10-12 hours thereafter, as needed if muscle weakness persists

Adolescents >16 years and Adults: Loading dose: 1000-2000 mg; Maintenance: Repeat bolus of 1000-2000 mg after 1 hour and repeated every 10-12 hours thereafter, as needed

I.M.:

Infants, Children, and Adolescents <40 kg:

Mild symptoms: 15 mg/kg/dose; repeat as needed for persistent mild symptoms every 15 minutes to a maximum total dose of 45 mg/kg; may administer doses in rapid succession if severe symptoms develop

Severe symptoms: 15 mg/kg/dose; repeat twice in rapid succession to deliver a total dose of 45 mg/kg

Persistent symptoms: May repeat the entire series (45 mg/kg in 3 divided doses) beginning ~1 hour after administration of the last injection

Children and Adolescents ≥40 kg and Adults:

Mild symptoms: 600 mg; repeat as needed for persistent mild symptoms every 15 minutes to a maximum total dose of 1800 mg; may administer doses in rapid succession if severe symptoms develop

Severe symptoms: 600 mg; repeat twice in rapid succession to deliver a total dose of 1800 mg

Persistent symptoms: May repeat the entire series (1800 mg in 3 divided doses) beginning ~1 hour after administration of the last injection

Anticholinesterase poisoning (eg, neostigmine, pyridostigmine): Adults: I.V.: 1000-2000 mg; followed by increments of 250 mg every 5 minutes as needed

Dosage adjustment in renal impairment: Pediatric patients (age not specified) and Adults: Dose should be reduced; no specific recommendations are provided by the manufacturer

Administration Parenteral:

I.M.: May use 300 mg/mL solution autoinjector or dilute 1000 mg vial with 3.3 mL SWI for a final concentration of 300 mg/mL; in children, administer intramuscularly in the anterolateral aspect of the thigh

I.V.: Reconstitute 1000 mg with 20 mL SWI (50 mg/mL); further dilute with NS to a final concentration of 10-20 mg/mL; maximum concentration is 50 mg/mL (in SWI) and should be used when lower concentration is not practical or in cases of fluid overload, pulmonary edema or more rapid administration is needed

Loading dose: Infuse over 15-30 minutes; if maximally concentrated solution (50 mg/mL) must be administered over ≥5 minutes not to exceed 200 mg/minute

Maintenance dose (intermittent infusion): Infuse over 15-30 minutes a rate not to exceed 200 mg/minute

Monitoring Parameters Heart rate, respiratory rate, muscle fasciculations and strength, pulse oximetry, blood pressure and cardiac monitoring with I.V. administration

Additional Information Most effective when given as soon as possible after exposure, typically within 36 hours after termination of exposure to poison.

Dosage Forms Excipient information presented when available (limited, particularly for generics); consult specific product labeling.

Device, Intramuscular, as chloride:

Generic: 600 mg/2 mL (2 mL)

Solution Reconstituted, Intravenous, as chloride:

Protopam Chloride: 1 g (1 ea)

References

Bailey B, "Are There Teratogenic Risks Associated With Antidotes Used in the Acute Management of Poisoned Pregnant Women?" *Birth Defects Res A Clin Mol Teratol*, 2003, 67(2):133-40.

Kamha AA, Al Omary IY, Zalabany HA, et al, "Organophosphate Poisoning in Pregnancy: A Case Report," *Basic Clin Pharmacol Toxicol*, 2005, 96(5):397-8.

◆ **Pralidoxime Chloride** *see* Pralidoxime *on page 1719*

◆ **Pravachol** *see* Pravastatin *on page 1720*

Pravastatin (prav a STAT in)

Medication Safety Issues

Sound-alike/look-alike issues:

Pravachol may be confused with atorvaSTATin, Prevacid, Prinivil, propranolol

Pravastatin may be confused with nystatin, pitavastatin, prasugrel

Brand Names: U.S. Pravachol

Brand Names: Canada Apo-Pravastatin®; CO Pravastatin; Dom-Pravastatin; JAMP-Pravastatin; Mint-Pravastatin; Mylan-Pravastatin; Novo-Pravastatin; Nu-Pravastatin; PHL-Pravastatin; PMS-Pravastatin; Pravachol; RAN-Pravastatin; ratio-Pravastatin; Riva-Pravastatin; Sandoz-Pravastatin; Teva-Pravastatin; ZYM-Pravastatin

Therapeutic Category Antilipemic Agent; HMG-CoA Reductase Inhibitor

Generic Availability (U.S.) Yes

Use Adjunct to dietary therapy in patients with heterozygous familial hypercholesterolemia (HFH) hypercholesterolemia if LDL-C remains ≥190 mg/dL or if ≥160 mg/dL with family history of premature cardiovascular (CVD) or presence of ≥2 cardiovascular risk [FDA approved in children ≥8 years of age and adolescents]. Adjunct to dietary therapy to decrease elevated serum total and low density lipoprotein cholesterol (LDL-C), apolipoprotein B (apo-B), and triglyceride levels, and to increase high density lipoprotein cholesterol (HDL-C) in patients with primary hypercholesterolemia (heterozygous, familial, and nonfamilial) and mixed dyslipidemia (Fredrickson types IIa and IIb) (FDA approved in adults); adjunct to dietary therapy in patients with isolated hypertriglyceridemia (Fredrickson type IV) (FDA approved in adults); treatment of primary dysbetalipoproteinemia (Fredrickson Type III) who do not respond adequately to diet (FDA approved in adults); primary and secondary prevention of cardiovascular disease in high risk patients (FDA approved in adults)

Primary prevention of cardiovascular disease in high-risk patients (FDA approved in adults); risk factors include: Age ≥55 years, smoking, hypertension, low HDL-C, or family history of early coronary heart disease; secondary prevention of cardiovascular disease to reduce the risk of MI, stroke, revascularization procedures, and angina in patients with evidence of coronary heart disease.

Pregnancy Risk Factor X

Pregnancy Considerations Adverse events were observed in some animal reproduction studies. Pravastatin was found to cross the placenta in an *ex vivo* study using term human placentas (Nanovskaya, 2013). There are reports of congenital anomalies following maternal use of HMG-CoA reductase Inhibitors in pregnancy; however, maternal disease, differences in specific agents used, and the low rates of exposure limit the interpretation of the available data (Godfrey, 2012; Lecarpentier, 2012). Cholesterol biosynthesis may be important in fetal development; serum cholesterol and triglycerides increase normally during pregnancy. The discontinuation of lipid lowering medications temporarily during pregnancy is not expected to have significant impact on the long term outcomes of primary hypercholesterolemia treatment.

Use of pravastatin is contraindicated in pregnancy. HMG-CoA reductase inhibitors should be discontinued prior to pregnancy (ADA, 2013). If treatment of dyslipidemias is needed in pregnant women or in women of reproductive age, other agents are preferred (Berglund, 2012; Stone, 2013). The manufacturer recommends administration to women of childbearing potential only when conception is highly unlikely and patients have been informed of potential hazards.

Breast-Feeding Considerations A small amount of pravastatin is excreted into breast milk. Data is available from eight lactating females administered pravastatin 20 mg twice daily for 2.5 days. After the fifth dose, maximum maternal serum concentrations were ~40 ng/mL (pravastatin) and ~26 ng/mL (metabolite) and maximum milk concentrations were ~3.9 ng/mL (pravastatin) and ~2.1 ng/mL (metabolite). Maximum milk concentrations were detected ~3 hours after the dose (Pan, 1988). Due to the potential for serious adverse reactions in a nursing infant, use while breast-feeding is contraindicated by the manufacturer.

Contraindications Hypersensitivity to pravastatin or any component; active liver disease; unexplained persistent elevations of serum transaminases; pregnancy; breast-feeding

Warnings Patients receiving HMG-CoA reductase inhibitors have developed rhabdomyolysis with or without acute renal failure and/or myopathy; patients should be monitored closely; risk is dose related and is increased with concurrent use of other lipid-lowering medications (eg, fibric acid derivatives or niacin at doses >1 g/day). With concurrent use of erythromycin, clarithromycin, or cyclosporine; consider dosage reductions of pravastatin. Ensure patient is on the lowest effective pravastatin dose in all circumstances. Discontinue in any patient in which CPK levels are markedly elevated (>10 times ULN) or if myopathy is suspected/diagnosed; monitoring of CPK may be warranted, but may not prevent severe myopathy. The manufacturer recommends temporary discontinuation for elective major surgery, acute medical or surgical conditions, or in any patient experiencing an acute or serious condition predisposing to renal failure (eg, sepsis, hypotension, trauma, uncontrolled seizures). However, based upon current evidence, HMG-CoA reductase inhibitor therapy should be continued in the perioperative period unless risk outweighs cardioprotective benefit. Use caution in patients with renal impairment, inadequately treated hypothyroidism, and those taking other drugs associated with myopathy (eg, colchicine); these patients are predisposed to myopathy. Patients should be instructed to report unexplained muscle pain, tenderness, weakness, or brown urine.

An autoimmune-mediated myopathy (IMNM) has been reported (rarely) with HMG-CoA reductase inhibitor therapy; presents as proximal muscle weakness with elevated CPK levels, which persists despite discontinuation of HMG-CoA reductase inhibitor therapy; additionally, muscle biopsy may show necrotizing myopathy with limited inflammation; immunosuppressive therapy (eg, corticosteroids, azathioprine) may be used for treatment.

Postmarketing reports of fatal and nonfatal hepatic failure are rare; if serious hepatotoxicity with clinical symptoms and/or hyperbilirubinemia or jaundice occurs during treatment, interrupt therapy. If an alternate etiology is not identified, do not restart pravastatin. Liver enzyme tests should be obtained at baseline and as clinically indicated; routine periodic monitoring of liver enzymes is not necessary. Use with caution in patients with history of heavy alcohol use or a previous history of liver disease

Precautions Increases in Hb A_{1c} and fasting blood glucose have been reported with HMG-CoA reductase inhibitors; however, the benefits of statin therapy far outweigh the risk of dysglycemia. Secondary causes of hyperlipidemia should be ruled out prior to therapy; has not been studied in conditions where the major abnormality is elevation of chylomicrons (hyperlipoproteinemia Types I or V). Use caution in patients with conditions or on medications that reduce steroidogenesis (eg, ketoconazole, spironolactone, cimetidine).

Although rare, reversible cognitive impairment (including confusion, forgetfulness, amnesia, and memory loss) can occur with HMG-CoA reductase inhibitors. These cognitive symptoms have been reported at variable times during therapy (1 day to years after initiation) and are reversible with discontinuation; resolution usually occurs within ~3 weeks. Cases have not been associated with fixed or progressive dementia; nor have they been associated with age, specific HMG-CoA reductase inhibitor, dose, or concomitant medication use.

Adverse Reactions

Cardiovascular: Chest pain

Central nervous system: Dizziness, fatigue, headache

Dermatologic: Rash

Gastrointestinal: Diarrhea, heartburn, nausea, vomiting

Hepatic: Transaminases increased

Neuromuscular & skeletal: Myalgia

Respiratory: Cough

Miscellaneous: Influenza

Rare but important or life-threatening: Allergy, amnesia (reversible), anaphylaxis, angioedema, cholestatic jaundice, cirrhosis, cognitive impairment (reversible), confusion (reversible), cranial nerve dysfunction, dermatomyositis, erythema multiforme, ESR increase, fulminant hepatic necrosis, gynecomastia, hemolytic anemia, hepatitis, hepatoma, lens opacity, libido change, lupus erythematosus-like syndrome, memory disturbance (reversible), memory impairment (reversible), muscle weakness, myopathy, neuropathy, pancreatitis, paresthesia, peripheral nerve palsy, polymyalgia rheumatica, positive ANA, purpura, rhabdomyolysis, Stevens-Johnson syndrome, taste disturbance, tremor, vasculitis, vertigo

Additional class-related events or case reports (not necessarily reported with pravastatin therapy): Angioedema, blood glucose increased, cataracts, depression, diabetes mellitus (new onset), dyspnea, eosinophilia, erectile dysfunction, facial paresis, glycosylated hemoglobin (Hb A_{1c}) increased, hypersensitivity reaction, immune-mediated necrotizing myopathy (IMNM), impaired extraocular muscle movement, impotence, interstitial lung disease, leukopenia, malaise, memory loss, ophthalmoplegia, paresthesia, peripheral neuropathy, photosensitivity, psychic disturbance, skin discoloration, thrombocytopenia, thyroid dysfunction, toxic epidermal necrolysis, transaminases increased, vomiting

Drug Interactions

Metabolism/Transport Effects Substrate of CYP3A4 (minor), P-glycoprotein, SLCO1B1; **Note:** Assignment of

Major/Minor substrate status based on clinically relevant drug interaction potential; **Inhibits** CYP2C9 (weak), CYP2D6 (weak), CYP3A4 (weak)

Avoid Concomitant Use
Avoid concomitant use of Pravastatin with any of the following: Fusidic Acid (Systemic); Gemfibrozil; Pimozide; Red Yeast Rice

Increased Effect/Toxicity
Pravastatin may increase the levels/effects of: ARIPiprazole; CycloSPORINE (Systemic); DAPTOmycin; Dofetilide; Lomitapide; PARoxetine; PAZOPanib; Pimozide; Trabectedin; Vitamin K Antagonists

The levels/effects of Pravastatin may be increased by: Bezafibrate; Boceprevir; Clarithromycin; Colchicine; CycloSPORINE (Systemic); Darunavir; Eltrombopag; Erythromycin (Systemic); Fenofibrate and Derivatives; Fusidic Acid (Systemic); Gemfibrozil; Itraconazole; Niacin; Niacinamide; P-glycoprotein/ABCB1 Inhibitors; Raltegravir; Red Yeast Rice; Simeprevir; Telaprevir; Telithromycin

Decreased Effect
Pravastatin may decrease the levels/effects of: Lanthanum

The levels/effects of Pravastatin may be decreased by: Antacids; Bile Acid Sequestrants; Efavirenz; Fosphenytoin; Nelfinavir; P-glycoprotein/ABCB1 Inducers; Phenytoin; Rifamycin Derivatives; Saquinavir

Stability Store at 25°C (77°F), excursions permitted to 15°C to 30°C (59°F to 86°F); protect from light and moisture; dispense in a tightly closed container.

Mechanism of Action Pravastatin is a competitive inhibitor of 3-hydroxy-3-methylglutaryl coenzyme A (HMG-CoA) reductase, which is the rate-limiting enzyme involved in *de novo* cholesterol synthesis.

Pharmacodynamics
Onset of action: 2 weeks
Maximum effect: After 4 weeks
LDL-reduction: 40 mg/day: 34% (for each doubling of this dose, LDL-C is lowered by ~6%)

Pharmacokinetics (Adult data unless noted)
Absorption: Oral: 34%; Rapidly absorbed
Distribution: V_d: 0.46 L/kg
Protein binding: 50%
Metabolism: Hepatic to multiple metabolites; primary metabolite is 3α-hydroxy-iso-pravastatin (2.5% to 10% activity of parent drug); extensive first-pass metabolism
Bioavailability: Absolute: 17%
Half-life:
Children and Adolescents (4.9-15.6 years): 1.6 hours; range: 0.85-4.2 hours (Hedman, 2003)
Adults: 77 hours (including all metabolites); pravastatin: 2.3 hours; 3α-hydroxy-iso-pravastatin: ~1.5 hours (Gustavson, 2005)
Time to peak serum concentration: 1-1.5 hours
Elimination: ~20% excreted in urine unchanged and 70% in feces

Dosing: Usual Dosage should be individualized according to the baseline LDL-C level, the recommended goal of therapy, and patient response; adjustments should be made at intervals of 4 weeks

Children and Adolescents: Oral: **Hyperlipidemia or heterozygous familial and nonfamilial hypercholesterolemia: Note:** Begin treatment if after adequate trial of diet the following are present: LDL-C ≥190 mg/dL or LDL-C remains ≥160 mg/dL and positive family history of premature cardiovascular disease or meets NCEP classification. (NHLBI 2011). Therapy may be considered for children 8-9 years of age meeting the above criteria or for children with diabetes mellitus and LDL-C ≥130 mg/dL (Daniels, 2008).

Children and Adolescents 8-13 years: 20 mg once daily; doses >20 mg have not been studied
Adolescents 14-18 years: 40 mg once daily; doses >40 mg have not been studied

Adults: **Hyperlipidemias, primary prevention of coronary events, secondary prevention of cardiovascular events:** Oral: Initial: 40 mg once daily; titrate dosage to response (usual range: 10-80 mg) (maximum daily dose: 80 mg/**day**)

Dosing adjustment in renal impairment: Adults: Significant impairment: Initiate dosage at 10 mg once daily

Dosing adjustment in hepatic impairment: There are no dosage adjustments provided in the manufacturer labeling; contraindicated in active liver disease or in patients with unexplained persistent elevations of serum transaminases.

Dosing adjustment for pravastatin with concomitant medications: Adults:
Clarithromycin: Maximum daily dose: 40 mg/**day**
Cyclosporine: Initial: 10 mg pravastatin daily at bedtime; titrate with caution (maximum daily dose: 20 mg/**day**)

Administration Oral: May be taken without regard to meals or time of day. Give at least 1 hour before or 4 hours after bile acid resins.

Monitoring Parameters
Pediatric patients: Baseline: ALT, AST, and creatine phosphokinase levels (CPK); fasting lipid panel (FLP) and repeat ALT and AST should be checked after 4 weeks of therapy; if no myopathy symptoms or laboratory abnormalities, then monitor FLP, ALT, and AST every 3-4 months during the first year and then every 6 months thereafter (NHLBI, 2011).
Adults: Baseline CPK (recheck CPK in any patient with symptoms suggestive of myopathy; discontinue therapy if markedly elevated); baseline liver function tests (LFTs) and repeat when clinically indicated thereafter. Patients with elevated transaminase levels should have a second (confirmatory) test and frequent monitoring until values normalize; discontinue if increase in ALT/AST is persistently >3 times ULN (NCEP, 2002).
Lipid panel (total cholesterol, HDL, LDL, triglycerides):
ATP III recommendations (NCEP, 2002): Baseline; 6-8 weeks after initiation of drug therapy; if dose increased, then at 6-8 weeks until final dose determined. Once treatment goal achieved, follow-up intervals may be reduced to every 4-6 months. Lipid panel should be assessed at least annually, and preferably at each clinic visit.
Manufacturer recommendation: Analyze lipid panel at initiation and 4 weeks after each titration.

Dosage Forms Excipient information presented when available (limited, particularly for generics); consult specific product labeling.
Tablet, Oral, as sodium:
Pravachol: 20 mg, 40 mg, 80 mg
Generic: 10 mg, 20 mg, 40 mg, 80 mg

References
American Diabetes Association, "Standards of Medical Care in Diabetes-2013," *Diabetes Care*, 2013, 36(Suppl 1):S11-66.
Berglund L, Brunzell JD, Goldberg AC, et al, "Evaluation and Treatment of Hypertriglyceridemia: An Endocrine Society Clinical Practice Guideline," *J Clin Endocrinol Metab*, 2012, 97(9):2969-89.
Daniels SR, Greer FR, and Committee on Nutrition, "Lipid Screening and Cardiovascular Health in Childhood," *Pediatrics*, 2008, 122 (1):198-208.
"Executive Summary of The Third Report of The National Cholesterol Education Program (NCEP) Expert Panel on Detection, Evaluation, and Treatment of High Blood Cholesterol in Adults (Adult Treatment Panel III)," *JAMA*, 2001, 285(19):2486-97.
Godfrey LM, Erramouspe J, and Cleveland KW, "Teratogenic Risk of Statins in Pregnancy," *Ann Pharmacother*, 2012, 46(10):1419-24.
Gustavson LE, Schweitzer SM, Koehne-Voss S, et al, "The Effects of Multiple Doses of Fenofibrate on the Pharmacokinetics of Pravastatin and Its 3Alpha-hydroxy Isomeric Metabolite," *J Clin Pharmacol*, 2005, 45(8):947-53.

Hedman M, Neuvonen PJ, Neuvonen M, et al, "Pharmacokinetics and Pharmacodynamics of Pravastatin in Children With Familial Hypercholesterolemia," Clin Pharmacol Ther, 2003, 74(2):178-85.

Lecarpentier E, Morel O, Fournier T, et al, "Statins and Pregnancy: Between Supposed Risks and Theoretical Benefits," Drugs, 2012, 72 (6):773-88.

McCrindle BW, Urbina EM, Dennison BA, et al, "Drug Therapy of High-Risk Lipid Abnormalities in Children and Adolescents: A Scientific Statement from the American Heart Association Atherosclerosis, Hypertension, and Obesity in Youth Committee, Council of Cardiovascular Disease in the Young, With the Council on Cardiovascular Nursing," Circulation, 2007, 115(14):1948-67.

National Heart, Lung, and Blood Institute, "Expert Panel on Integrated Guidelines for Cardiovascular Health and Risk Reduction in Children and Adolescents," Clinical Practice Guidelines, 2011, National Institutes of Health. Available at http://www.nhlbi.nih.gov/guidelines/cvd_ped/peds_guidelines_full.pdf

Pan HY, DeVault AR, Swites BJ, et al, "Pharmacokinetics and Pharmacodynamics of Pravastatin Alone and With Cholestyramine in Hypercholesterolemia," Clin Pharmacol Ther, 1990, 48(2):201-7.

Rodenburg J, Vissers MN, Wiegman A, et al, "Statin Treatment in Children With Familial Hypercholesterolemia: The Younger, the Better," Circulation, 2007, 116(6):664-8.

"Third Report of the National Cholesterol Education Program Expert Panel on Detection, Evaluation, and Treatment of High Blood Cholesterol in Adults (Adult Treatment Panel III)," May 2001, www.nhlbi.nih.gov/guidelines/cholesterol.

Wiegman A, Hutten BA, de Groot E, et al, "Efficacy and Safety of Statin Therapy in Children With Familial Hypercholesterolemia: A Randomized Controlled Trial," JAMA, 2004, 292(3):331-7.

◆ **Pravastatin Sodium** see Pravastatin on page 1720

◆ **Praxis ASA EC 81 Mg Daily Dose (Can)** see Aspirin on page 212

Praziquantel (pray zi KWON tel)

Related Information
Oral Medications That Should Not Be Crushed or Altered on page 2438

Brand Names: U.S. Biltricide

Brand Names: Canada Biltricide

Therapeutic Category Anthelmintic

Generic Availability (U.S.) No

Use Treatment of all stages of schistosomiasis caused by Schistosoma species pathogenic to humans; treatment of clonorchiasis, opisthorchiasis (FDA approved in ages ≥4 years and adults); has also been used in the treatment of cysticercosis and many intestinal tapeworm and trematode infections

Pregnancy Risk Factor B

Pregnancy Considerations Adverse effects have not been observed in animal reproduction studies. Use in pregnant women only if clearly needed.

Breast-Feeding Considerations Appears in breast milk at a concentration of ¼ that of maternal serum. Women should be advised to not breast-feed on the day of treatment and for 72 hours after treatment.

Contraindications Hypersensitivity to praziquantel or any component; ocular cysticercosis; spinal cysticercosis (Red Book, 2009); concurrent use with strong CYP3A4 inducers, particularly rifampin

Warnings Therapeutic concentrations of praziquantel may not be achieved with concurrent administration of strong inducers of cytochrome P450 (eg, rifampin); concurrent use is contraindicated

Precautions Use with caution in patients with moderate to severe hepatic disease (Child-Pugh class B and C) and in patients with heart abnormalities. CSF reaction syndrome in patients being treated for neurocysticercosis has been reported; syndrome includes CSF protein concentrations increased, headache, hyperthermia, intracranial hypertension, and seizures; patients with cerebral cysticercosis should be hospitalized for the duration of treatment. Not recommended for use in patients with a history of epilepsy and/or signs of potential CNS involvement suggestive of cysticercosis.

Adverse Reactions May be more serious in patients with a heavy worm burden.

Central nervous system: Dizziness, headache, malaise

Dermatologic: Urticaria

Gastrointestinal: Abdominal distress, nausea

Miscellaneous: Fever

Rare but important or life-threatening: Abdominal pain, anorexia, atrioventricular block, bloody diarrhea, bradycardia, cardiac arrhythmia, ectopic beats, eosinophilia, hypersensitivity, hypersensitivity reaction, myalgia, paradoxical reaction (in schistosomiasis), polyserositis, pruritus, seizure, serum sickness (in schistosomiasis; Jarisch-Herxheimer-like reaction), ventricular fibrillation,vomiting

Drug Interactions

Metabolism/Transport Effects Substrate of CYP3A4 (major); **Note:** Assignment of Major/Minor substrate status based on clinically relevant drug interaction potential; **Inhibits** CYP2D6 (weak)

Avoid Concomitant Use

Avoid concomitant use of Praziquantel with any of the following: Conivaptan; CYP3A4 Inducers (Strong); Fusidic Acid (Systemic)

Increased Effect/Toxicity

Praziquantel may increase the levels/effects of: ARIPiprazole

The levels/effects of Praziquantel may be increased by: Ceritinib; Cimetidine; Conivaptan; CYP3A4 Inhibitors (Moderate); CYP3A4 Inhibitors (Strong); Dasatinib; Fusidic Acid (Systemic); Ivacaftor; Ketoconazole (Systemic); Luliconazole; Mifepristone; Simeprevir; Stiripentol

Decreased Effect

The levels/effects of Praziquantel may be decreased by: Aminoquinolines (Antimalarial); Bosentan; CYP3A4 Inducers (Strong); Dabrafenib; Deferasirox; Siltuximab; St Johns Wort; Tocilizumab

Stability Store at <30°C (<86°F).

Mechanism of Action Increases the cell permeability to calcium in schistosomes, causing strong contractions and paralysis of worm musculature leading to detachment of suckers from the blood vessel walls and to dislodgment

Pharmacokinetics (Adult data unless noted)

Absorption: Oral: ~80%

Distribution: CSF concentration is 14% to 20% of plasma concentration

Protein binding: ~80%

Metabolism: Extensive first-pass effect; metabolized by the liver to hydroxylated and conjugated metabolites

Half-life: 0.8-1.5 hours

Metabolites: 4.5 hours

Time to peak serum concentration: Within 1-3 hours

Elimination: Praziquantel and metabolites excreted mainly in urine 80% (>99% as metabolites)

Dosing: Usual Oral:

Children and Adolescents:

Flukes:

Clonorchiasis [Clonorchis sinesis (Chinese liver fluke)]; Opisthorchiasis [Opisthorchis viverrini (Southeast Asian liver fluke)]:

Manufacturer's labeling: Children ≥4 years and Adolescents: 25 mg/kg/dose 3 times daily (at 4- to 6-hour intervals) for 1 day

Alternative dosing (Red Book, 2009): 25 mg/kg/dose 3 times daily for 2 days

Fasciolopsis buski, Heterophyes heterophyes, Metagonimus yokogawi (intestinal flukes); Metorchis conjunctus (North American liver fluke): 25 mg/kg/dose 3 times daily for 1 day (Red Book, 2009)

Nanophyetus salmincola: 20 mg/kg/dose 3 times daily for 1 day (Red Book, 2009)

Paragonimus westermani (lung fluke): 25 mg/kg/dose 3 times daily for 2 days (Red Book, 2009)

▶

Schistosomiasis:

Manufacturer's labeling: Children >4 years and Adolescents: 20 mg/kg/dose 3 times daily (at 4- to 6-hour intervals) for 1 day

Alternative dosing (*Red Book*, 2009): **Note:** Praziquantel does not kill developing worms; therapy started within 1-2 months of exposure should be repeated in 1-2 months.

S. mansoni, S. haematobium: 20 mg/kg/dose twice daily for 1 day

S. japonicum, S. mekongi: 20 mg/kg/dose 3 times daily for 1 day

Tapeworms (*Red Book*, 2009):

Cysticercosis [*Taenia solium* (pork tapeworm)]; tissue (larvae) stage: 33.3 mg/kg/dose 3 times daily for 1 day followed by 16.7 mg/kg/dose 3 times daily for 29 days; **Note:** May be used in conjunction with antiseizure medication and/or corticosteroids.

Diphyllobothrium latum (fish), *Taenia saginata* (beef), *Taenia solium* (pork), *Dipylidium caninum* (dog); intestinal (adult) stage: 5-10 mg/kg as a single dose

Hymenolepis nana (dwarf tapeworm): 25 mg/kg as a single dose

Adults:

Schistosomiasis: 20 mg/kg/dose 3 times daily (at 4- to 6-hour intervals) for 1 day

Clonorchiasis/opisthorchiasis: 25 mg/kg/dose 3 times daily (at 4- to 6-hour intervals) for 1 day

Dosage adjustment in renal impairment: No dosage adjustments are recommended

Dosage adjustments in hepatic impairment: Moderate to severe impairment (Child-Pugh classes B and C): Use caution; decreased metabolism may lead to higher and prolonged serum concentrations; there are no dosage adjustments provided in the manufacturer's labeling.

Administration Oral: Administer tablets with water during meals; tablets can be halved or quartered; do not chew tablets due to bitter taste

Dosage Forms Excipient information presented when available (limited, particularly for generics); consult specific product labeling.

Tablet, Oral:

Biltricide: 600 mg [scored]

References

King CH and Mahmoud AA, "Drug Five Years Later: Praziquantel," *Ann Intern Med*, 1989, 110(4):290-6.

Liu LX and Weller PF, "Antiparasitic Drug," *N Engl J Med*, 1996, 334 (18):1178-84.

Red Book: 2009 Report of the Committee on Infectious Diseases, 28th ed, Pickering LK, ed, Elk Grove Village, IL: American Academy of Pediatrics, 2009.

Prazosin (PRAZ oh sin)

Medication Safety Issues

Sound-alike/look-alike issues:

Prazosin may be confused with predniSONE

BEERS Criteria medication:

This drug may be potentially inappropriate for use in geriatric patients (Quality of evidence - moderate; Strength of recommendation - strong).

Brand Names: U.S. Minipress

Brand Names: Canada Apo-Prazo; Minipress; Novo-Prazin; Nu-Prazo; Teva-Prazosin

Therapeutic Category Alpha-Adrenergic Blocking Agent, Oral; Antihypertensive Agent; Vasodilator

Generic Availability (U.S.) Yes

Use Treatment of hypertension alone or in combination with diuretics or beta-blockers (FDA approved in adults); has also been used in the management of the sympathetic stimulatory cardiovascular effects of scorpion envenomation usually due to non-*Centruroides* species stings (typically found outside North America)

Pregnancy Risk Factor C

Pregnancy Considerations Adverse events were observed in some animal reproduction studies. Prazosin crosses the placenta and its pharmacokinetics may be slightly altered during pregnancy (Bourget, 1995; Rubin, 1983). Limited use in pregnant women has not demonstrated any fetal abnormalities or adverse effects (Dommisse, 1983).

Untreated chronic maternal hypertension is associated with adverse events in the fetus, infant, and mother. If treatment for hypertension during pregnancy is needed, other agents are generally preferred (ACOG, 2013).

Breast-Feeding Considerations Small amounts of prazosin are excreted in breast milk. The manufacturer recommends that caution be exercised when administering prazosin to nursing women.

Contraindications Hypersensitivity to prazosin, quinazolines, or any component

Warnings Marked orthostatic hypotension, syncope, and loss of consciousness may occur with first dose, dose increase, or within first few days of therapy; syncope usually occurs 30-90 minutes post-initial dose; occasionally preceded with severe tachycardia (120-160 bpm in adults); anticipate a similar effect if therapy is interrupted for a few days, if dosage is rapidly increased, large initial dose (>1 mg in adults), or if another antihypertensive drug (eg, beta-blockers, diuretics, and particularly vasodilators) or a PDE-5 inhibitor (eg, sildenafil, tadalafil, vardenafil) is introduced. Patients should be cautioned about performing hazardous tasks when starting new therapy or adjusting dosage upward. May cause priapism (rarely).

Precautions Use with caution in patient with cataracts or undergoing corrective cataract surgery; intraoperative floppy iris syndrome (IFIS) has been observed in cataract surgery patients who were on or were previously treated with alpha₁-blockers; there appears to be no benefit in discontinuing alpha₁-blockers prior to surgery. Use with caution in patients with narcolepsy; worsening of symptoms has been reported although causality has not been established.

Adverse Reactions

Cardiovascular: Edema, orthostatic hypotension, palpitation, syncope

Central nervous system: Depression, dizziness, drowsiness, headache, nervousness, vertigo

Dermatologic: Rash

Endocrine & metabolic: Decreased energy

Gastrointestinal: Constipation, diarrhea, nausea, vomiting, xerostomia

Genitourinary: Urinary frequency

Neuromuscular & skeletal: Weakness

Ocular: Blurred vision, reddened sclera

Respiratory: Dyspnea, epistaxis, nasal congestion

Rare but important or life-threatening: Abdominal discomfort, allergic reaction, alopecia, angina, arthralgia, bradycardia, cataplexy, cataracts (both development and disappearance have been reported), diaphoresis, enuresis, eye pain, fever, flushing, gynecomastia, hallucinations, impotence, insomnia, leukopenia, lichen planus, liver function abnormalities, malaise, MI, narcolepsy (worsened), pain, pancreatitis, paresthesia, pigmentary mottling and serous retinopathy, positive ANA titer, priapism, pruritus, systemic lupus erythematosus, tachycardia, tinnitus, urticaria, vasculitis

Reported in association with other alpha₁-blockers: Intraoperative floppy iris syndrome (with cataract surgery)

Drug Interactions

Metabolism/Transport Effects Induces P-glycoprotein

Avoid Concomitant Use

Avoid concomitant use of Prazosin with any of the following: Alpha1-Blockers; Dabigatran Etexilate; Sofosbuvir; VinCRIStine (Liposomal)

Increased Effect/Toxicity

Prazosin may increase the levels/effects of: Alpha1-Blockers; Amifostine; Antihypertensives; Calcium Channel Blockers; DULoxetine; Hypotensive Agents; Obinutuzumab; RiTUXimab

The levels/effects of Prazosin may be increased by: Barbiturates; Beta-Blockers; Brimonidine (Topical); Diazoxide; Herbs (Hypotensive Properties); MAO Inhibitors; Pentoxifylline; Phosphodiesterase 5 Inhibitors; Prostacyclin Analogues

Decreased Effect

Prazosin may decrease the levels/effects of: Afatinib; Alpha-/Beta-Agonists; Alpha1-Agonists; Brentuximab Vedotin; Dabigatran Etexilate; DOXOrubicin (Conventional); Linagliptin; P-glycoprotein/ABCB1 Substrates; Sofosbuvir; VinCRIStine (Liposomal)

The levels/effects of Prazosin may be decreased by: Herbs (Hypertensive Properties); Methylphenidate; Yohimbine

Food Interactions Food has variable effects on absorption. Management: Administer without regard to food.

Mechanism of Action Competitively inhibits postsynaptic alpha-adrenergic receptors which results in vasodilation of veins and arterioles and a decrease in total peripheral resistance and blood pressure

Pharmacodynamics

Onset of action: Antihypertensive: Within 2 hours
Maximum effect: Antihypertensive: 2-4 hours
Duration: 10-24 hours

Pharmacokinetics (Adult data unless noted)

Distribution: V_d: 0.5 L/kg
Protein-binding: 92% to 97%
Metabolism: Extensive in the liver, metabolites may be active
Bioavailability: 43% to 82%
Time to peak serum concentration: ~3 hours
Half-life: 2-3 hours, prolonged with CHF
Elimination: Feces; urine (6% to 10% renally as unchanged drug)

Dosing: Usual

Infants, Children, and Adolescents:

Hypertension: Children and Adolescents: Limited data available: Oral: Initial: 0.05-0.1 mg/kg/**day** in divided doses every 8 hours; may titrate up to 0.5 mg/kg/**day** in divided doses 3 times daily; maximum daily dose: 20 mg/**day** (NHBPEP, 2004; NHLBI, 2011)

Scorpion envenomation: Limited data available:

Weight-directed: Infants ≥4 months, Children, and Adolescents: Oral: 0.03 mg/kg/dose; second dose has been administered at 3 or 6 hours after initial dose; subsequent doses every 6 hours; therapy has been continued for 48 hours or until extremities are warm and dry (Bosnak, 2009; Gupta, 2010)

Fixed dosing: Infants >6 months, Children, and Adolescents: Oral: 0.25 mg every 3 hours until extremities are warm and dry (Bawaskar, 2010)

Adults: **Hypertension:** Oral: Initial: 1 mg/dose 2-3 times/day; usual maintenance dose: 2-20 mg/day in divided doses 2-3 times/day (JNC 7); maximum daily dose: 20 mg

Administration Oral: Administer without regard to meals at the same time each day.

Monitoring Parameters Blood pressure (standing and sitting or supine)

Test Interactions Increased urinary VMA 17%, norepinephrine metabolite 42%; therefore, false positives may occur in screening for pheochromocytoma. If elevated VMA is found, discontinue prazosin and retest after one month.

Dosage Forms Excipient information presented when available (limited, particularly for generics); consult specific product labeling.

Capsule, Oral:
Minipress: 1 mg, 2 mg, 5 mg
Generic: 1 mg, 2 mg, 5 mg

References

American College of Obstetricians and Gynecologists, "ACOG Practice Bulletin No. 125: Chronic Hypertension in Pregnancy," *Obstet Gynecol*, 2012, 119(2 Pt 1):396-407.

Bawaskar HS and Bawaskar PH, "Efficacy and Safety of Scorpion Antivenom Plus Prazosin Compared With Prazosin Alone for Venomous Scorpion *(Mesobuthus tamulus)* Sting: Randomised Open Label Clinical Trial," *BMJ*, 2011, 342:c7136.

Bosnak M, Levent Yilmaz H, Ece A, et al, "Severe Scorpion Envenomation in Children: Management in Pediatric Intensive Care Unit," *Hum Exp Toxicol*, 2009, 28(11):721-8.

Bourget P, Fernandez H, Edouard D, et al, "Disposition of a New Rate-Controlled Formulation of prazosin in the Treatment of Hypertension During Pregnancy: Transplacental Passage of Prazosin," *Eur J Drug Metab Pharmacokinet*, 1995, 20(3):233-41.

Chobanian AV, Bakris GL, Black HR, et al, "The Seventh Report of the Joint National Committee on Prevention, Detection, Evaluation, and Treatment of High Blood Pressure: The JNC 7 report," *JAMA*, 2003, 289(19):2560-72.

Dommisse J, Davey DA, and Roos PJ, "Prazosin and Oxprenolol Therapy in Pregnancy Hypertension," *S Afr Med J*, 1983, 64(7):231-3.

Gupta BD, Parakh M, and Purohit A, "Management of Scorpion Sting: Prazosin or Dobutamine," *J Trop Pediatr*, 2010, 56(2):115-8.

National Heart, Lung, and Blood Institute, "Expert Panel on Integrated Guidelines for Cardiovascular Health and Risk Reduction in Children and Adolescents," Clinical Practice Guidelines, 2011, National Institutes of Health. Available at http://www.nhlbi.nih.gov/guidelines/cvd_ped/peds_guidelines_full.pdf. Accessed: March 16, 2012.

National High Blood Pressure Education Program Working Group on High Blood Pressure in Children and Adolescents, "The Fourth Report on the Diagnosis, Evaluation, and Treatment of High Blood Pressure in Children and Adolescents," *Pediatrics*, 2004, 114(2 Suppl 4th Report):555-76.

Rubin PC, Butters L, Low RA, et al, "Clinical Pharmacological Studies With Prazosin During Pregnancy Complicated by Hypertension," *Br J Clin Pharmacol*, 1983, 16(5):543-7.

Sinaiko AR, "Pharmacologic Management of Childhood Hypertension," *Pediatr Clin North Am*, 1993, 40(1):195-212.

Tuuri RE and Reynolds S, "Scorpion Envenomation and Antivenom Therapy," *Pediatr Emerg Care*, 2011, 27(7):667-72.

◆ **Prazosin Hydrochloride** *see* Prazosin *on page 1724*

◆ **PR Benzoyl Peroxide Wash** *see* Benzoyl Peroxide *on page 275*

◆ **Precedex** *see* Dexmedetomidine *on page 621*

◆ **Precose** *see* Acarbose *on page 46*

◆ **Predator [OTC]** *see* Lidocaine (Topical) *on page 1242*

◆ **Pred Forte** *see* PrednisoLONE (Ophthalmic) *on page 1730*

◆ **Pred-G®** *see* Prednisolone and Gentamicin *on page 1731*

◆ **Pred Mild** *see* PrednisoLONE (Ophthalmic) *on page 1730*

Prednicarbate (pred ni KAR bate)

Medication Safety Issues

Sound-alike/look-alike issues:
Dermatop® may be confused with Dimetapp®

Related Information
Topical Corticosteroids *on page 2224*

Brand Names: U.S. Dermatop

Brand Names: Canada Dermatop®

Therapeutic Category Adrenal Corticosteroid; Anti-inflammatory Agent; Corticosteroid, Topical; Glucocorticoid

Generic Availability (U.S.) Yes

Use

Cream: Relief of the inflammatory and pruritic manifestations of corticosteroid-responsive dermatoses (medium potency topical corticosteroid) (FDA approved in ages ≥1 year and adults) **Note:** In pediatric patients, safety and efficacy ≥3 weeks has not been established)

Ointment: Relief of the inflammatory and pruritic manifestations of corticosteroid-responsive dermatoses (medium-potency topical corticosteroid) (FDA approved in ages ≥10 years and adults)

Pregnancy Risk Factor C

Pregnancy Considerations There are no adequate and well-controlled studies using prednicarbate during pregnancy. However, intrauterine growth retardation has been reported with other topical steroids. Avoid use in large amounts for long periods of time during pregnancy.

Breast-Feeding Considerations Systemic corticosteroids are excreted in human milk. The extent of topical absorption is variable. Use with caution while breast-feeding; do not apply to nipples.

Contraindications Hypersensitivity to prednicarbate or any component

Warnings Hypothalamic-pituitary-adrenal (HPA) suppression may occur; acute adrenal insufficiency (adrenal crisis) may occur with abrupt withdrawal after long-term therapy or with stress; withdrawal and discontinuation of corticosteroids should be done carefully. Adverse systemic effects (eg, hyperglycemia, glycosuria, fluid and electrolyte changes) may occur when topical steroids are used in large areas of the body, denuded areas, for prolonged periods of time, with an occlusive dressing, and/or in infants and small children; infants and small children may be more susceptible to HPA axis suppression or other systemic toxicities due to larger skin surface area to body mass ratio; use with caution in pediatric patients. If HPA suppression occurs, consider withdrawal of prednicarbate, reduction in frequency of application, or substitution with a less potent corticosteroid. Cushing's syndrome and intracranial hypertension have also been reported in pediatric patients. May cause inhibition of bone growth in pediatric patients. Immunosuppression may occur; patients may be more susceptible to infections; avoid exposure to chickenpox and measles. Corticosteroids may activate latent opportunistic infections or exacerbate systemic fungal infections. Prolonged treatment with corticosteroids has been associated with the development of Kaposi's sarcoma (case reports); if noted, discontinuation of therapy should be considered. Allergic contact dermatitis can occur and is usually diagnosed by failure to heal rather than clinical exacerbation; diagnostic patch testing may corroborate observation.

Ointment contains propylene glycol; toxicities have been reported with use of products containing propylene glycol, including hyperosmolality, lactic acidosis, seizures, and respiratory depression; in neonates large amounts of propylene glycol delivered orally, intravenously (eg, >3000 mg/day), or topically have been associated with potentially fatal toxicities which can include metabolic acidosis, seizures, renal failure, and CNS depression; use ointment containing propylene glycol with caution (AAP, 1997; Shehab, 2009).

Precautions Do not use for diaper dermatitis. Avoid use with occlusive dressing or application to denuded skin or to large surface areas. Avoid using higher than recommended doses; suppression of HPA axis function may occur. Reduction in growth velocity may occur when corticosteroids are administered to pediatric patients by any route (monitor growth). Prolonged use may result in fungal or bacterial superinfection. Use may be associated with local sensitization.

Avoid contact with latex-containing products; may damage or reduce effectiveness of latex condoms or diaphragms. If contact occurs, latex product should be disposed. Avoid contact with eyes, face, underarms, or groin area; not for intravaginal use.

Adverse Reactions

Dermatologic: Mild telangiectasia, shininess, skin atrophy, thinness

Rare but important or life-threatening: Acneiform eruptions, allergic contact dermatitis, burning, edema, folliculitis, hypopigmentation, miliaria, paresthesia, perioral dermatitis, pruritus, rash, secondary infection, striae, urticaria

Drug Interactions

Metabolism/Transport Effects None known.

Avoid Concomitant Use

Avoid concomitant use of Prednicarbate with any of the following: Aldesleukin

Increased Effect/Toxicity

Prednicarbate may increase the levels/effects of: Ceritinib; Deferasirox

The levels/effects of Prednicarbate may be increased by: Telaprevir

Decreased Effect

Prednicarbate may decrease the levels/effects of: Aldesleukin; Corticorelin; Hyaluronidase; Telaprevir

Stability

Topical cream: Store at 5°C to 25°C (41°F to 77°F).
Topical ointment: Store at 15°C to 30°C (59°F to 86°F).

Mechanism of Action Topical corticosteroids have anti-inflammatory, antipruritic, vasoconstrictive, and antiproliferative actions

Pharmacokinetics (Adult data unless noted) Absorption: Topical corticosteroids are absorbed percutaneously. The extent is dependent on several factors, including epidermal integrity (intact vs abraded skin), formulation, age of the patient, and the use of occlusive dressings. Percutaneous absorption of topical steroids is increased in neonates (especially preterm neonates), infants, and young children.

Dosing: Usual Topical: **Note:** Therapy should be discontinued once control is achieved; if no improvement is seen within 2 weeks, reassessment of diagnosis may be necessary.

Cream: Children ≥1 year and Adults: Apply a thin film to affected area twice daily

Ointment: Children ≥10 year and Adults: Apply a thin film to affected area twice daily

Administration Apply a thin film to clean, dry skin and rub in gently. For external use only. Do not use on diaper area, face, groin area, underarm, or open wounds. Do not cover with occlusive dressings.

Monitoring Parameters Growth in pediatric patients; assess HPA axis suppression (eg, ACTH stimulation test, morning plasma cortisol test, urinary free cortisol test)

Dosage Forms Excipient information presented when available (limited, particularly for generics); consult specific product labeling.

Cream, External:
Dermatop: 0.1% (60 g)
Generic: 0.1% (15 g, 60 g)
Ointment, External:
Dermatop: 0.1% (60 g)
Generic: 0.1% (15 g, 60 g)

References

American Academy of Pediatrics Committee on Drugs. "Inactive" ingredients in pharmaceutical products: update (subject review). *Pediatrics.* 1997;99(2):268-278.

Goedert JJ, Vitale F, Lauria C, et al, "Risk Factors for Classical Kaposi's Sarcoma," *J Natl Cancer Inst,* 2002, 94(22):1712-8.

Shehab N, Lewis CL, Streetman DD, Donn SM. Exposure to the pharmaceutical excipients benzyl alcohol and propylene glycol among critically ill neonates. *Pediatr Crit Care Med.* 2009;10 (2):256-259.

PrednisoLONE (Systemic) (pred NISS oh lone)

Medication Safety Issues
Sound-alike/look-alike issues:
PrednisoLONE may be confused with predniSONE
Pediapred may be confused with Pediazole
Prelone may be confused with PROzac

Related Information
Corticosteroids Systemic Equivalencies *on page 2222*

Brand Names: U.S. Flo-Pred; Millipred; Millipred DP; Millipred DP 12-Day; Orapred ODT; Orapred [DSC]; Pediapred; Prelone; Veripred 20

Brand Names: Canada Hydeltra T.B.A.; Novo-Prednisolone; Pediapred

Therapeutic Category Adrenal Corticosteroid; Anti-inflammatory Agent; Antiasthmatic; Corticosteroid, Systemic; Glucocorticoid

Generic Availability (U.S.) May be product dependent

Use Treatment of endocrine disorders, rheumatic disorders, collagen diseases, dermatologic diseases, allergic states, respiratory diseases, hematologic disorders, neoplastic diseases, edematous states, and GI diseases

Pregnancy Risk Factor C/D (manufacturer specific)

Pregnancy Considerations Adverse events have been observed with corticosteroids in animal reproduction studies. Prednisolone crosses the placenta; prior to reaching the fetus, prednisolone is converted by placental enzymes to prednisone. As a result, the amount of prednisolone reaching the fetus is ~8-10 times lower than the maternal serum concentration (healthy women at term; similar results observed with preterm pregnancies complicated by HELLP syndrome) (Beitins, 1972; van Runnard Heimel, 2005). Some studies have shown an association between first trimester systemic corticosteroid use and oral clefts (Park-Wyllie, 2000; Pradat, 2003). Systemic corticosteroids may also influence fetal growth (decreased birth weight); however, information is conflicting (Lunghi, 2010). Hypoadrenalism may occur in newborns following maternal use of corticosteroids in pregnancy; monitor.

When systemic corticosteroids are needed in pregnancy, it is generally recommended to use the lowest effective dose for the shortest duration of time, avoiding high doses during the first trimester (Leachman, 2006; Lunghi, 2010; Makol, 2011; Østensen, 2009). Inhaled corticosteroids are preferred for the treatment of asthma during pregnancy. Oral corticosteroids, such as prednisolone, may be used for the treatment of severe persistent asthma if needed; the lowest dose administered on alternate days (if possible) should be used (NAEPP, 2005). Prednisolone may be used to treat women during pregnancy who require therapy for congenital adrenal hyperplasia (Speiser, 2010). Topical agents are preferred for managing atopic dermatitis in pregnancy; for severe symptomatic or recalcitrant atopic dermatitis, a short course of prednisolone may be used during the third trimester (Koutroulis, 2011).

Women exposed to prednisolone during pregnancy for the treatment of an autoimmune disease may contact the OTIS Autoimmune Diseases Study at 877-311-8972.

Breast-Feeding Considerations Prednisolone is excreted into breast milk. In one study (n=6), milk concentrations were 5% to 25% of the maternal serum concentration with peak concentrations occurring ~1 hour after the maternal dose. The milk/plasma ratio was found to be 0.2 with doses ≥30 mg/day and 0.1 with doses <30 mg/day. Following a maternal dose of prednisolone 80 mg/day, it was calculated that a breast-feeding infant would ingest <0.1% of the maternal dose (Ost, 1985). One manufacturer notes that when used systemically, maternal use of corticosteroids have the potential to cause adverse events in a nursing infant (eg, growth suppression, interfere with endogenous corticosteroid production) and therefore caution should be used when administered to nursing women. In order to decrease potential exposure to a nursing infant, one manufacturer recommends administering the dose after nursing, at the time of day with the longest interval between feeds. Other sources recommend waiting 4 hours after the maternal dose before breast-feeding (Bae, 2012; Leachman, 2006; Makol, 2011; Ost, 1985). Other guidelines note that maternal use of systemic corticosteroids is not a contraindication to breast-feeding (NAEPP, 2005).

Contraindications Hypersensitivity to prednisolone or any component; acute superficial herpes simplex keratitis; systemic fungal infections; varicella infections; live or live, attenuated virus vaccines (with immunosuppressive doses of corticosteroids)

Warnings Hypothalamic-pituitary-adrenal (HPA) suppression may occur, particularly in younger children or in patients receiving high doses for prolonged periods; acute adrenal insufficiency (adrenal crisis) may occur with abrupt withdrawal after long-term therapy or with stress; withdrawal and discontinuation of corticosteroids should be tapered slowly and carefully; patients with HPA axis suppression may require doses of systemic glucocorticosteroids prior to, during, and after unusual stress (eg, surgery).

Immunosuppression may occur; patients may be more susceptible to infections; prolonged use of corticosteroids may also increase the incidence of secondary infection, mask acute infection (including fungal infections), prolong or exacerbate viral or fungal infections, activate latent opportunistic infections, or limit response to vaccines. Exposure to chickenpox should be avoided; corticosteroids should not be used to treat ocular herpes simplex; use caution in patients with a history of ocular herpes simplex. Corticosteroids should not be used for cerebral malaria or viral hepatitis. Close observation is required in patients with latent tuberculosis and/or TB reactivity; restrict use in active TB (only in conjunction with antituberculosis treatment).

May cause osteoporosis (at any age) or inhibition of bone growth in pediatric patients. Use with caution in patients with osteoporosis. In a population-based study of children, risk of fracture was shown to be increased with >4 courses of corticosteroids; underlying clinical condition may also impact bone health and osteoporotic effect of corticosteroids (Leonard, 2006).

Corticosteroid use may cause psychiatric disturbances, including depression, euphoria, insomnia, mood swings, and personality changes. preexisting psychiatric conditions may be exacerbated by corticosteroid use. Acute myopathy may occur with high doses, usually in patients with neuromuscular transmission disorders; myopathy may involve ocular and/or respiratory muscles; monitor creatine kinase; recovery may be delayed. Increased IOP may occur, especially with prolonged use; in children, increased IOP has been shown to be dose-dependent and produce a greater IOP in children <6 years than older children (Lam, 2005). Rare cases of anaphylactoid reactions have been reported with corticosteroids.

Orapred® oral solution contains sodium benzoate; benzoic acid (benzoate) is a metabolite of benzyl alcohol; large amounts of benzyl alcohol (≥99 mg/kg/day) have been associated with a potentially fatal toxicity ("gasping syndrome") in neonates; the "gasping syndrome" consists of metabolic acidosis, respiratory distress, gasping respirations, CNS dysfunction (including convulsions, intracranial hemorrhage), hypotension, and cardiovascular collapse; use prednisolone products containing sodium benzoate or benzoic acid with caution in neonates; *in vitro* and animal studies have shown that benzoate displaces bilirubin from protein binding sites. Flo-Pred™ oral suspension contains propylene glycol; toxicities have been reported with use of products containing propylene glycol, including hyperosmolality, lactic acidosis, seizures, and respiratory depression; in neonates large amounts of propylene glycol delivered orally, intravenously (eg, >3000 mg/day), or topically have been associated with potentially fatal toxicities which can include metabolic acidosis, seizures, renal failure, and CNS depression; use oral suspension containing propylene glycol with caution (AAP, 1997; Shehab, 2009).

Precautions Avoid using higher than recommended doses; suppression of HPA function, suppression of linear growth (ie, reduction of growth velocity), reduced bone mineral density, hypercorticism (Cushing's syndrome), hyperglycemia, or glucosuria may occur; titrate to lowest effective dose. Reduction in growth velocity may occur when corticosteroids are administered to pediatric patients by any route (monitor growth). Use with extreme caution in patients with respiratory tuberculosis or untreated systemic infections. Use with caution in patients with hypertension, heart failure, or renal impairment; long-term use has been associated with fluid retention and hypertension. Use with caution in patients with GI diseases (diverticulitis, peptic ulcer, ulcerative colitis) due to risk of GI bleeding and perforation. High-dose corticosteroids should not be used for management of head injury; increased mortality was observed in patients receiving high-dose I.V. methylprednisolone. Use with caution in patients with myasthenia gravis; exacerbation of symptoms has occurred, especially during initial treatment with corticosteroids. Use with caution in patients with hepatic impairment, including cirrhosis; enhanced pharmacologic effect due to decreased metabolism and long-term use has been associated with fluid retention. Use with caution following acute MI; corticosteroids have been associated with myocardial rupture; hypertrophic cardiomyopathy has been reported in premature neonates.

Use with caution in patients with diabetes; corticosteroids may alter glucose regulation, leading to hyperglycemia. Use with caution in patients with cataracts and/or glaucoma; increased intraocular pressure, open-angle glaucoma, and cataracts have occurred with prolonged use; consider routine eye exams in chronic users. Use with caution in patients with a history of seizure disorder; seizures have been reported with adrenal crisis. Use with caution in patients with thyroid dysfunction; changes in thyroid status may necessitate dosage adjustments; metabolic clearance of corticosteroids increases in hyperthyroid patients and decreases in hypothyroid patients. Prolonged treatment with corticosteroids has been associated with the development of Kaposi's sarcoma (case reports); if noted, discontinuation of therapy should be considered. Use with caution in patients with thromboembolic tendencies or thrombophlebitis.

Use with caution in patients with cataracts and/or glaucoma; with prolonged use, corticosteroids may result in ocular hypertension and/or glaucoma, with damage to the optic nerve, defects in visual acuity and fields of vision, and posterior subcapsular cataract formation. Corticosteroids should not be used in active ocular herpes simplex.

Adverse Reactions
Cardiovascular: Cardiomyopathy, CHF, edema, facial edema, hypertension

Central nervous system: Headache, insomnia, malaise, nervousness, pseudotumor cerebri, psychic disorders, seizure, vertigo

Dermatologic: Bruising, facial erythema, hirsutism, petechiae, skin test reaction suppression, thin fragile skin, urticaria

Endocrine & metabolic: Carbohydrate tolerance decreased, Cushing's syndrome, diabetes mellitus, growth suppression, hyperglycemia, hypernatremia, hypokalemia, hypokalemic alkalosis, menstrual irregularities, negative nitrogen balance, pituitary adrenal axis suppression

Gastrointestinal: Abdominal distention, increased appetite, indigestion, nausea, pancreatitis, peptic ulcer, ulcerative esophagitis, weight gain

Hepatic: LFTs increased (usually reversible)

Neuromuscular & skeletal: Arthralgia, aseptic necrosis (humeral/femoral heads), fractures, muscle mass decreased, muscle weakness, osteoporosis, steroid myopathy, tendon rupture, weakness

Ocular: Cataracts, exophthalmus, eyelid edema, glaucoma, intraocular pressure increased, irritation

Respiratory: Epistaxis

Miscellaneous: Diaphoresis increased, impaired wound healing

Rare but important or life-threatening: Venous thrombosis (Johannesdottir, 2013)

Drug Interactions
Metabolism/Transport Effects Substrate of CYP3A4 (minor); **Note:** Assignment of Major/Minor substrate status based on clinically relevant drug interaction potential; **Inhibits** CYP3A4 (weak)

Avoid Concomitant Use
Avoid concomitant use of PrednisoLONE (Systemic) with any of the following: Aldesleukin; BCG; Indium 111 Capromab Pendetide; Mifepristone; Natalizumab; Pimecrolimus; Pimozide; Tacrolimus (Topical); Tofacitinib

Increased Effect/Toxicity
PrednisoLONE (Systemic) may increase the levels/effects of: Acetylcholinesterase Inhibitors; Amphotericin B; Androgens; ARIPiprazole; Ceritinib; CycloSPORINE (Systemic); Deferasirox; Dofetilide; Leflunomide; Lomitapide; Loop Diuretics; Natalizumab; NSAID (COX-2 Inhibitor); NSAID (Nonselective); Pimozide; Thiazide Diuretics; Tofacitinib; Vaccines (Live); Warfarin

The levels/effects of PrednisoLONE (Systemic) may be increased by: Antifungal Agents (Azole Derivatives, Systemic); Aprepitant; Boceprevir; Calcium Channel Blockers (Nondihydropyridine); CycloSPORINE (Systemic); Denosumab; Estrogen Derivatives; Fluconazole; Fosaprepitant; Indacaterol; Macrolide Antibiotics; Mifepristone; Neuromuscular-Blocking Agents (Nondepolarizing); Pimecrolimus; Quinolone Antibiotics; Ritonavir; Roflumilast; Salicylates; Tacrolimus (Topical); Telaprevir; Trastuzumab

Decreased Effect
PrednisoLONE (Systemic) may decrease the levels/effects of: Aldesleukin; Antidiabetic Agents; BCG; Calcitriol; Coccidioidin Skin Test; Corticorelin; CycloSPORINE (Systemic); Hyaluronidase; Indium 111 Capromab Pendetide; Isoniazid; Salicylates; Sipuleucel-T; Telaprevir; Urea Cycle Disorder Agents; Vaccines (Inactivated)

The levels/effects of PrednisoLONE (Systemic) may be decreased by: Aminoglutethimide; Antacids; Barbiturates; Bile Acid Sequestrants; Echinacea; Fosphenytoin; Mifepristone; Mitotane; Phenytoin; Primidone; Rifamycin Derivatives

Stability Dispense oral liquid formulations in tight, light-resistant containers.

Storage:
Flo-Pred™: Store at 20°C to 25°C (68°F to 77°F); do not refrigerate; dispense in original container (to avoid loss of formulation during transfer).

Millipred™: Store at 20°C to 25°C (68°F to 77°F).

Pediapred® oral solution: Store at 4°C to 24°C (39°F to 77°F); may be refrigerated.

Orapred® oral solution: Store in refrigerator at 2°C to 8°C (36°F to 46°F).

Orapred ODT®: Store at controlled room temperature at 20°C to 25°C (68°F to 77°F) in blister pack; protect from moisture.

Mechanism of Action Decreases inflammation by suppression of migration of polymorphonuclear leukocytes and reversal of increased capillary permeability; suppresses the immune system by reducing activity and volume of the lymphatic system

Pharmacokinetics (Adult data unless noted)
Absorption: Well-absorbed
Protein binding: 70% to 90% (concentration dependent)
Metabolism: Primarily in the liver, but also metabolized in most tissues, to inactive compounds
Half-life, serum: 2-4 hours
Elimination: In urine, principally as glucuronide and sulfate-conjugated metabolites

Dosing: Neonatal Bronchopulmonary dysplasia, treatment: **See Dosing: Usual** for dosing in infants

Dosing: Usual Dose depends upon condition being treated and response of patient; dosage for infants and children should be based on disease severity and patient response, rather than by rigid adherence to dosage guidelines by age, weight, or body surface area. Consider alternate day therapy for long-term therapy. Discontinuation of long-term therapy requires gradual withdrawal by tapering the dose.

Infants: Bronchopulmonary dysplasia, treatment: 2 mg/kg/day divided twice daily for 5 days, followed by 1 mg/kg/day once daily for 3 days, followed by 1 mg/kg/dose every other day for 3 doses was used in 131 former premature neonates (postmenstrual age: ≥36 weeks) with BPD; results showed weaning of supplemental oxygen was facilitated in patients with capillary pCO_2 <48.5 mm Hg and pulmonary acuity score <0.5 (Bhandari, 2006)

NIH Asthma Guidelines (NAEPP, 2007): Oral:
Children <12 years:
Asthma exacerbations (emergency care or hospital doses): 1-2 mg/kg/day in 2 divided doses (maximum: 60 mg/day) until peak expiratory flow is 70% of predicted or personal best
Short-course "burst" (acute asthma): 1-2 mg/kg/day in divided doses 1-2 times/day for 3-10 days; maximum dose: 60 mg/day; **Note:** Burst should be continued until symptoms resolve or patient achieves peak expiratory flow 80% of personal best; usually requires 3-10 days of treatment (~5 days on average); longer treatment may be required
Long-term treatment: 0.25-2 mg/kg/day given as a single dose in the morning or every other day as needed for asthma control; maximum dose: 60 mg/day
Children ≥12 years and Adults:
Asthma exacerbations (emergency care or hospital doses): 40-80 mg/day in divided doses 1-2 times/day until peak expiratory flow is 70% of predicted or personal best
Short-course "burst" (acute asthma): 40-60 mg/day in divided doses 1-2 times/day for 3-10 days; **Note:** Burst should be continued until symptoms resolve and peak expiratory flow is at least 80% of personal best; usually requires 3-10 days of treatment (~5 days on average); longer treatment may be required
Long-term treatment: 7.5-60 mg daily given as a single dose in the morning or every other day as needed for asthma control

Children: Oral:
Anti-inflammatory or immunosuppressive dose: 0.1-2 mg/kg/day in divided doses 1-4 times/day
Nephrotic syndrome:
Pediatric Nephrology Panel recommendations (Hogg, 2000):
Initial: 2 mg/kg/day or 60 mg/m²/day given every day in 1-3 divided doses (maximum dose: 80 mg/day) until urine is protein-free or for 4-6 weeks, followed by maintenance dose: 2 mg/kg/dose or 40 mg/m²/dose given every other day in the morning; gradually

taper and discontinue after 4-6 weeks; **Note:** 6-week daily therapy, followed by 6-week alternate day therapy, may induce a higher rate of long remission compared to the standard of 4 weeks of daily therapy, followed by 4 weeks of alternate day therapy; however, a higher incidence of adverse effects may be seen with the longer regimen and the clinical benefit may be variable.
Relapse: Use high-dose daily steroid regimen (listed above) until urine is protein-free for 3 days; follow with maintenance-tapering course of alternate day therapy (maintenance dose listed above) for 4-6 weeks; subsequent therapy is determined by individual's response and number of relapses (Hogg, 2000)
British Pediatric Nephrology Consensus Statement (Report of a Workshop by the British Association for Paediatric Nephrology and Research Unit, 1994):
First 3 episodes: Initial: 2 mg/kg/day or 60 mg/m²/day given every day (maximum dose: 80 mg/day) until urine is protein-free for 3 consecutive days (maximum dose: 28 days), followed by 1-1.5 mg/kg/dose or 40 mg/m²/dose (maximum: 60 mg/dose) given every other day for 4 weeks
Frequent relapses (long-term maintenance dose): 0.5-1 mg/kg/dose given every other day for 3-6 months
Adults: Oral: 5-60 mg/day

Administration Administer after meals or with food or milk to decrease GI upset.
Flo-Pred™: Administer using the provided calibrated syringe (supplied by manufacturer) to accurately measure the dose. Syringe should be washed prior to next use.
Orapred ODT®: Do not cut, split, or break tablets; do not use partial tablets. Remove tablet from blister pack immediately prior to use. May swallow tablet whole or allow to dissolve on tongue.

Monitoring Parameters Blood pressure, weight, electrolytes, serum glucose; IOP (use >6 weeks); bone mineral density (long-term use); children's height and growth

Test Interactions Response to skin tests

Dosage Forms Excipient information presented when available (limited, particularly for generics); consult specific product labeling. [DSC] = Discontinued product
Solution, Oral, as base:
Generic: 15 mg/5 mL (240 mL, 480 mL)
Solution, Oral, as sodium phosphate [strength expressed as base]:
Millipred: 10 mg/5 mL (237 mL) [dye free; contains edetate disodium, methylparaben, saccharin sodium; grape flavor]
Orapred: 15 mg/5 mL (20 mL [DSC], 237 mL [DSC]) [dye free; contains alcohol, usp, sodium benzoate; grape flavor]
Pediapred: 5 mg/5 mL (120 mL) [alcohol free, dye free, sugar free; contains edetate disodium, methylparaben; raspberry flavor]
Veripred 20: 20 mg/5 mL (237 mL) [alcohol free, dye free; contains edetate disodium, methylparaben, saccharin sodium; grape flavor]
Generic: 15 mg/5 mL (237 mL); 25 mg/5 mL (237 mL); 5 mg/5 mL (120 mL)
Suspension, Oral, as acetate [strength expressed as base]:
Flo-Pred: 15 mg/5 mL (30 mL) [contains butylparaben, disodium edta, propylene glycol; cherry flavor]
Syrup, Oral, as base:
Prelone: 15 mg/5 mL (240 mL) [contains alcohol, usp, benzoic acid, brilliant blue fcf (fd&c blue #1), fd&c red #40, propylene glycol, saccharin sodium; cherry flavor]
Generic: 15 mg/5 mL (240 mL, 480 mL)

Tablet, Oral, as base:

Millipred: 5 mg [scored; contains fd&c yellow #10 (quinoline yellow), fd&c yellow #6 (sunset yellow), sodium benzoate]

Millipred DP: 5 mg [scored; contains fd&c yellow #10 (quinoline yellow), fd&c yellow #6 (sunset yellow), sodium benzoate]

Millipred DP 12-Day: 5 mg [scored; contains fd&c yellow #10 (quinoline yellow), fd&c yellow #6 (sunset yellow), sodium benzoate]

Tablet Dispersible, Oral, as sodium phosphate [strength expressed as base]:

Orapred ODT: 10 mg, 15 mg, 30 mg [grape flavor]

References

American Academy of Pediatrics Committee on Drugs. "Inactive" ingredients in pharmaceutical products: update (subject review). *Pediatrics*. 1997;99(2):268-278.

Bae YS, Van Voorhees AS, Hsu S, et al, "Review of Treatment Options For Psoriasis in Pregnant or Lactating Women: From the Medical Board of the National Psoriasis Foundation," *J Am Acad Dermatol*, 2012, 67(3):459-77.

Beitins IZ, Bayard F, Ances IG, et al, "The Transplacental Passage of Prednisone and Prednisolone in Pregnancy Near Term," *J Pediatr*, 1972, 81(5):936-45.

Bhandari A, Schramm CM, Kimble C, et al, "Effect of a Short Course of Prednisolone in Infants With Oxygen-Dependent Bronchopulmonary Dysplasia," *Pediatrics*, 2008, 121(2):e344-9.

Hogg RJ, Portman RJ, Milliner D, et al, "Evaluation and Management of Proteinuria and Nephrotic Syndrome in Children: Recommendations From a Pediatric Nephrology Panel Established at the National Kidney Foundation Conference on Proteinuria, Albuminuria, Risk, Assessment, Detection, and Elimination (PARADE)," *Pediatrics*, 2000, 105(6):1242-9.

"'Inactive' Ingredients in Pharmaceutical Products: Update (Subject Review). American Academy of Pediatrics Committee on Drugs," *Pediatrics*, 1997, 99(2):268-78.

Koutroulis I, Papoutsis J, and Kroumpouzos G, "Atopic Dermatitis in Pregnancy: Current Status and Challenges," *Obstet Gynecol Surv*, 2011, 66(10):654-63.

Lam DS, Fan DS, Ng JS, et al, "Ocular Hypertensive and Anti-Inflammatory Responses to Different Dosages of Topical Dexamethasone in Children: A Randomized Trial," *Clin Experiment Ophthalmol*, 2005, 33 (3):252-8.

Leachman SA and Reed BR, "The Use of Dermatologic Drugs in Pregnancy and Lactation," *Dermatol Clin*, 2006, 24(2):167-97, vi.

Leonard MB, "Glucocorticoid-Induced Osteoporosis in Children: Impact of the Underlying Disease," *Pediatrics*, 2007, 119 Suppl 2:S166-74.

Lunghi L, Pavan B, Biondi C, et al, "Use of Glucocorticoids in Pregnancy," *Curr Pharm Des*, 2010, 16(32):3616-37.

Makol A, Wright K, and Amin S, "Rheumatoid Arthritis and Pregnancy: Safety Considerations in Pharmacological Management," *Drugs*, 2011, 71(15):1973-87.

National Asthma Education and Prevention Program (NAEPP), "Expert Panel Report 3 (EPR-3): Guidelines for the Diagnosis and Management of Asthma," *Clinical Practice Guidelines*, National Institutes of Health, National Heart, Lung, and Blood Institute, NIH Publication No. 08-4051, prepublication 2007. Available at: http://www.nhlbi.nih.gov/guidelines/asthma/asthgdln.htm.

National Asthma Education and Prevention Program (NAEPP) Working Group Report on "Managing Asthma During Pregnancy: Recommendations For Pharmacologic Treatment," National Institutes of Health, National Heart, Lung, and Blood Institute, NIH Publication No. 05-5236, March 2005. Available at http://www.nhlbi.nih.gov/health/prof/lung/asthma/astpreg/astpreg_full.pdf

Østensen M and Forger F, "Management of RA Medications in Pregnant Patients," *Nat Rev Rheumatol*, 2009, 5(7):382-90.

Ost L, Wettrell G, Björkhem I, et al, "Prednisolone Excretion in Human Milk," *J Pediatr*, 1985, 106(6):1008-11.

Park-Wyllie L, Mazzotta P, Pastuszak A, et al, "Birth defects After Maternal Exposure to Corticosteroids: Prospective Cohort Study and Meta-Analysis of Epidemiological Studies," *Teratology*, 2000, 62 (6):385-92.

Pradat P, Robert-Gnansia E, Di Tanna GL, et al, "First Trimester Exposure to Corticosteroids and Oral Clefts," *Birth Defects Res A Clin Mol Teratol*, 2003, 67(12):968-70.

Report of a Workshop by the British Association for Paediatric Nephrology and Research Unit, Royal College of Physicians, "Consensus Statement on Management and Audit Potential for Steroid Responsive Nephrotic Syndrome," *Arch Dis Child*, 1994, 70(2):151-7.

Shehab N, Lewis CL, Streetman DD, Donn SM. Exposure to the pharmaceutical excipients benzyl alcohol and propylene glycol among critically ill neonates. *Pediatr Crit Care Med*. 2009;10 (2):256-259.

Speiser PW, Azziz R, Baskin LS, et al, "Congenital Adrenal Hyperplasia Due to Steroid 21-Hydroxylase Deficiency: An Endocrine Society Clinical Practice Guideline," *J Clin Endocrinol Metab*, 2010, 95 (9):4133-60.

van Runnard Heimel PJ, Schobben AF, Huisjes AJ, et al, "The Transplacental Passage of Prednisolone in Pregnancies Complicated by Early-Onset HELLP Syndrome," *Placenta*, 2005, 26(10):842-5.

PrednisoLONE (Ophthalmic) (pred NISS oh lone)

Medication Safety Issues

Sound-alike/look-alike issues:

PrednisoLONE may be confused with predniSONE

Brand Names: U.S. Omnipred; Pred Forte; Pred Mild

Brand Names: Canada Minims Prednisolone Sodium Phosphate; PMS-Prednisolone Sodium Phosphate Forte; Pred Forte; Pred Mild; Ratio-Prednisolone; Sandoz Prednisolone

Therapeutic Category Anti-inflammatory Agent, Ophthalmic; Corticosteroid, Ophthalmic

Generic Availability (U.S.) Yes

Use Treatment of inflammatory conditions of the palpebral and bulbar conjunctiva, cornea, and anterior segment of the globe; corneal injury from chemical, radiation, thermal burns, or foreign body penetration (All indications: FDA approved in adults)

Pregnancy Risk Factor C

Pregnancy Considerations Ophthalmic prednisolone was shown to be teratogenic in animal studies. When administered systemically, prednisolone crosses the placenta. The amount of prednisolone available systemically following topical application of the ophthalmic drops is unknown; refer to the PrednisoLONE (Systemic) monograph for additional information.

Breast-Feeding Considerations The amount of prednisolone available systemically following topical application of the ophthalmic drops is unknown. Due to the potential for serious adverse reactions in the nursing infant, the manufacturer recommends a decision be made whether to discontinue nursing or to discontinue the drug, taking into account the importance of treatment to the mother. When administered systemically, prednisolone is excreted in breast milk. Refer to the PrednisoLONE, Systemic monograph for additional information.

Contraindications Hypersensitivity to prednisolone or any component; acute superficial herpes simplex keratitis (dendritic keratitis), vaccinia, varicella, and most other viral diseases of the cornea and conjunctiva; mycobacterial or fungal infections of the eye

Additional product-specific indications: Prednisolone sodium phosphate (solution): Use after uncomplicated removal of superficial corneal foreign body

Warnings Immunosuppression may occur; patients may be more susceptible to infections; prolonged use of corticosteroids may also increase the incidence of secondary infection, mask acute infection (including fungal infections), prolong or exacerbate viral or fungal infections, activate latent opportunistic infections, or limit response to vaccines. Exposure to chickenpox should be avoided; corticosteroids should not be used to treat ocular herpes simplex; use caution in patients with a history of ocular herpes simplex. Close observation is required in patients with latent tuberculosis and/or TB reactivity; restrict use in active TB (only in conjunction with antituberculosis treatment). Increased IOP may occur especially with prolonged use; in children, increased IOP has been shown to be dose-dependent and produce a greater IOP in children <6 years than older children (Lam, 2005).

Suspension may contain sodium bisulfite which may cause allergic reactions in susceptible individuals. Prednisolone acetate suspensions contain polysorbate 80 (Tween 80)

which may cause allergic reactions in susceptible individuals.

Precautions Use with caution in patients with cataracts and/or glaucoma; increased intraocular pressure, open-angle glaucoma, and cataracts have occurred with prolonged use, consider routine eye exams in chronic users. Avoid prolonged use of ophthalmic corticosteroids, which may result in ocular hypertension and/or glaucoma, with damage to the optic nerve, defects in visual acuity and fields of vision, and posterior subcapsular cataract formation. Monitor intraocular pressure if ophthalmic solution/suspension used for 10 days or longer. Use following cataract surgery may delay healing or increase the incidence of bleb formation. Various ophthalmic disorders, as well as prolonged use of corticosteroids, may result in corneal and scleral thinning. Continued use in a patient with corneal or sclera, thinning may result in perforation. Withdraw therapy with gradual tapering of dose. Not effective in Sjogren's keratoconjunctivitis or mustard gas keratitis.

Adverse Reactions Ocular: Conjunctival hyperemia, conjunctivitis, corneal ulcers, delayed wound healing, glaucoma, intraocular pressure increased, keratitis, loss of accommodation, optic nerve damage, mydriasis, posterior subcapsular cataract formation, ptosis, secondary ocular infection

Drug Interactions

Metabolism/Transport Effects Substrate of CYP3A4 (minor); **Note:** Assignment of Major/Minor substrate status based on clinically relevant drug interaction potential

Avoid Concomitant Use There are no known interactions where it is recommended to avoid concomitant use.

Increased Effect/Toxicity

PrednisoLONE (Ophthalmic) may increase the levels/effects of: Ceritinib

Decreased Effect There are no known significant interactions involving a decrease in effect.

Stability

Prednisolone acetate (suspension):

Omnipred: Store at 8°C to 24°C (46°F to 75°F); store in an upright position.

Pred Forte: Store at ≤25°C (≤77°F); protect from freezing; store in an upright position.

Prednisolone sodium phosphate (solution): Store at 15°C to 25°C (59°F to 77°F); protect from light; keep tightly closed.

Mechanism of Action Reduces inflammation by inhibiting edema, leukocyte migration, fibrin deposition, capillary proliferation and dilation, collagen deposition and scar formation.

Dosing: Usual

Pediatric: **Ophthalmic inflammation, treatment:** Limited data available: Children and Adolescents: Prednisolone acetate 1% (suspension): Instill 1 to 2 drops into conjunctival sac 3 to 6 times daily. If signs and symptoms fail to improve after 2 days, re-evaluate. Initiate with more frequent dosing, and decrease as clinically indicated. If signs and symptoms fail to improve after 2 days, re-evaluate (Wilson, 2009).

Adult: **Ophthalmic inflammation, treatment:**

Prednisolone acetate 1% (suspension):

Omnipred: Instill 2 drops into conjunctival sac 4 times daily. If signs and symptoms fail to improve after 2 days, re-evaluate.

Pred Forte: Instill 1 to 2 drops into conjunctival sac 2 to 4 times daily. During the initial 24 to 48 hours, the dosing frequency may be increased if necessary. If signs and symptoms fail to improve after 2 days, re-evaluate.

Prednisolone sodium phosphate 1% (solution): Instill 1 to 2 drops into conjunctival sac every hour during the day and every 2 hours at night until favorable response is

obtained, then use 1 drop every 4 hours; later further reduction to 1 drop 3 to 4 times daily may be adequate

Dosing adjustment in renal impairment: There are no dosage adjustments provided in manufacturer's labeling.

Dosing adjustment in hepatic impairment: There are no dosage adjustments provided in manufacturer's labeling.

Administration Not for injection into eye; for topical use only. Shake suspension well before use; instill drops into affected eye(s); avoid contact of container tip with skin or eye; apply finger pressure to lacrimal sac during and for 1-2 minutes after instillation to decrease risk of absorption and systemic effects

Dosage Forms Excipient information presented when available (limited, particularly for generics); consult specific product labeling.

Solution, Ophthalmic, as sodium phosphate:

Generic: 1% (10 mL)

Suspension, Ophthalmic, as acetate:

Omnipred: 1% (5 mL, 10 mL) [contains benzalkonium chloride, edetate disodium, polysorbate 80]

Pred Forte: 1% (1 mL, 5 mL, 10 mL, 15 mL) [contains benzalkonium chloride, edetate disodium, polysorbate 80, sodium bisulfite]

Pred Mild: 0.12% (5 mL, 10 mL)

Generic: 1% (5 mL, 10 mL, 15 mL)

References

Lam DS, Fan DS, Ng JS, Yu CB, Wong CY, Cheung AY. Ocular hypertensive and anti-inflammatory responses to different dosages of topical dexamethasone in children: a randomized trial. *Clin Experiment Ophthalmol.* 2005;33(3):252-258.

Omnipred (prednisolone acetate ophthalmic suspension) [prescribing information]. Fort Worth, TX: Alcon Laboratories; October 2007.

Pred Forte (prednisolone acetate ophthalmic suspension) [prescribing information]. Irvine, CA: Allergan; August 2013.

Prednisolone sodium phosphate ophthalmic solution) [prescribing information]. Tampa, FL: Bausch & Lomb Inc; January 2013.

Wilson ME, Saunders RA, Trivedi RH, eds. *Pediatric Ophthalmology.* Springer; 2009.

◆ **Prednisolone Acetate, Ophthalmic** *see* PrednisoLONE (Ophthalmic) *on page 1730*

Prednisolone and Gentamicin

(pred NIS oh lone & jen ta MYE sin)

Brand Names: U.S. Pred-G®

Therapeutic Category Antibiotic, Ophthalmic; Corticosteroid, Ophthalmic

Generic Availability (U.S.) No

Use Treatment of steroid responsive inflammatory conditions and superficial ocular infections due to strains of microorganisms susceptible to gentamicin such as *Staphylococcus*, *E. coli*, *H. influenzae*, *Klebsiella*, *Neisseria*, *Pseudomonas*, *Proteus*, and *Serratia* species

Pregnancy Risk Factor C

Pregnancy Considerations See individual agents.

Breast-Feeding Considerations See individual agents.

Contraindications Hypersensitivity to prednisolone, gentamicin, or any component; dendritic keratitis, fungal diseases, vaccinia, varicella, most other viral infections, and mycobacterial infection of the eye. Contraindicated after uncomplicated removal of a corneal foreign body.

Warnings Prolonged use may result in glaucoma, damage to the optic nerve, defects in visual acuity, posterior subcapsular cataract formation, and secondary ocular infections

Adverse Reactions

Dermatologic: Delayed wound healing

Local: Discomfort, irritation

Ocular: Glaucoma, intraocular pressure increased, optic nerve damage (infrequent), posterior subcapsular cataract formation, superficial punctate keratitis

Miscellaneous: Secondary infection

Drug Interactions

Metabolism/Transport Effects Refer to individual components.

Avoid Concomitant Use There are no known interactions where it is recommended to avoid concomitant use.

Increased Effect/Toxicity

Prednisolone and Gentamicin may increase the levels/ effects of: Ceritinib

Decreased Effect There are no known significant interactions involving a decrease in effect.

Dosing: Usual Children and Adults: Ophthalmic: Instill 1 drop 2-4 times/day; during the initial 24-48 hours, the dosing frequency may be increased if necessary, up to 1 drop every hour; or small amount (1/2" ribbon) of ointment can be applied into the conjunctival sac 1-3 times/day

Administration Suspension: Shake well before using; instill drop into affected eye; avoid contacting bottle tip with skin or eye; apply finger pressure to lacrimal sac during and for 1-2 minutes after instillation to decrease risk of absorption and systemic effects

Monitoring Parameters With use >10 days, monitor intraocular pressure

Dosage Forms Excipient information presented when available (limited, particularly for generics); consult specific product labeling. [DSC] = Discontinued product

Ointment, ophthalmic:

Pred-G®: Prednisolone acetate 0.6% and gentamicin sulfate 0.3% (3.5 g)

Suspension, ophthalmic:

Pred-G®: Prednisolone acetate 1% and gentamicin sulfate 0.3% (5 mL, 10 mL [DSC]) [contains benzalkonium chloride]

◆ **Prednisolone Sodium Phosphate** *see* PrednisoLONE (Systemic) *on page 1727*

◆ **Prednisolone Sodium Phosphate, Ophthalmic** *see* PrednisoLONE (Ophthalmic) *on page 1730*

PredniSONE (PRED ni sone)

Medication Safety Issues

Sound-alike/look-alike issues:

PredniSONE may be confused with methylPREDNISolone, Pramosone, prazosin, prednisoLONE, PriLOSEC, primidone, promethazine

Related Information

Corticosteroids Systemic Equivalencies *on page 2222*

Brand Names: U.S. PredniSONE Intensol; Rayos

Brand Names: Canada Apo-Prednisone; Novo-Prednisone; Winpred

Therapeutic Category Adrenal Corticosteroid; Anti-inflammatory Agent; Antiasthmatic; Corticosteroid, Systemic; Glucocorticoid

Generic Availability (U.S.) May be product dependent

Use Management of adrenocortical insufficiency; used for its anti-inflammatory or immunosuppressant effects

Pregnancy Risk Factor C

Pregnancy Considerations Adverse events have been observed with corticosteroids in animal reproduction studies. Prednisone and its metabolite, prednisolone, cross the human placenta. In the mother, prednisone is converted to the active metabolite prednisolone by the liver. Prior to reaching the fetus, prednisolone is converted by placental enzymes back to prednisone. As a result, the level of prednisone remaining in the maternal serum and reaching the fetus are similar; however, the amount of prednisolone reaching the fetus is ~8-10 times lower than the maternal serum concentration (healthy women at term) (Beitins, 1972). Some studies have shown an association between first trimester systemic corticosteroid use and oral clefts (Park-Wyllie, 2000; Pradat, 2003). Systemic corticosteroids may also influence fetal growth (decreased birth

weight); however, information is conflicting (Lunghi, 2010). Hypoadrenalism may occur in newborns following maternal use of corticosteroids in pregnancy; monitor.

When systemic corticosteroids are needed in pregnancy, it is generally recommended to use the lowest effective dose for the shortest duration of time, avoiding high doses during the first trimester (Leachman, 2006; Lunghi, 2010; Makol, 2011; Østensen, 2009). Inhaled corticosteroids are preferred for the treatment of asthma during pregnancy. Oral corticosteroids, such as prednisone, may be used for the treatment of severe persistent asthma if needed; the lowest dose administered on alternate days (if possible) should be used (NAEPP, 2005). Prednisone may be used to treat lupus nephritis in pregnant women who have active nephritis or substantial extrarenal disease activity (Hahn, 2012).

Pregnant women exposed to prednisone for antirejection therapy following a transplant may contact the National Transplantation Pregnancy Registry (NTPR) at 215-955-4820. Women exposed to prednisone during pregnancy for the treatment of an autoimmune disease (eg, rheumatoid arthritis) may contact the OTIS Autoimmune Diseases Study at 877-311-8972.

Breast-Feeding Considerations Prednisone and its metabolite, prednisolone, are found in low concentrations in breast milk. Following a maternal dose of 10 mg (n=1), milk concentrations were measured ~2 hours after the maternal dose (prednisone 0.0016 mcg/mL; prednisolone 0.0267 mcg/mL) (Katz, 1975). In a study which included six mother/infant pairs, adverse events were not observed in nursing infants (maternal prednisone dose not provided) (Ito, 1993).

The manufacturer notes that when used systemically, maternal use of corticosteroids have the potential to cause adverse events in a nursing infant (eg, growth suppression, interfere with endogenous corticosteroid production) and therefore, a decision should be made whether to discontinue nursing or to discontinue the drug, taking into account the importance of treatment to the mother. If there is concern about exposure to the infant, some guidelines recommend waiting 4 hours after the maternal dose of an oral systemic corticosteroid before breast-feeding in order to decrease potential exposure to the nursing infant (based on a study using prednisolone) (Bae, 2011; Leachman, 2006; Makol, 2011; Ost, 1985). Other guidelines note that maternal use of prednisone is not a contraindication to breast-feeding (NAEPP, 2005).

Contraindications Hypersensitivity to prednisone or any component; serious infections, except septic shock or tuberculous meningitis; systemic fungal infections; varicella infections; live or live, attenuated virus vaccines (with immunosuppressive doses of corticosteroids)

Warnings Hypothalamic-pituitary-adrenal (HPA) suppression may occur, particularly in younger children or in patients receiving high doses for prolonged periods; acute adrenal insufficiency (adrenal crisis) may occur with abrupt withdrawal after long-term therapy or with stress; withdrawal and discontinuation of corticosteroids should be tapered slowly and carefully; patients with HPA axis suppression may require doses of systemic glucocorticosteroids prior to, during, and after unusual stress (eg, surgery).

Immunosuppression may occur; patients may be more susceptible to infections; prolonged use of corticosteroids may also increase the incidence of secondary infection, mask acute infection (including fungal infections), prolong or exacerbate viral or fungal infections, activate latent opportunistic infections, or limit response to vaccines. Exposure to chickenpox should be avoided; corticosteroids should not be used to treat ocular herpes simplex; use caution in patients with a history of ocular herpes simplex. Corticosteroids should not be used for cerebral malaria or viral hepatitis. Close observation is required in patients with latent tuberculosis and/or TB reactivity; restrict use in active TB (only in conjunction with antituberculosis treatment).

May cause osteoporosis (at any age) or inhibition of bone growth in pediatric patients. Use with caution in patients with osteoporosis. In a population-based study of children, risk of fracture was shown to be increased with >4 courses of corticosteroids; underlying clinical condition may also impact bone health and osteoporotic effect of corticosteroids (Leonard, 2006).

Corticosteroid use may cause psychiatric disturbances, including depression, euphoria, insomnia, mood swings, and personality changes. preexisting psychiatric conditions may be exacerbated by corticosteroid use. Acute myopathy may occur with high doses, usually in patients with neuromuscular transmission disorders; myopathy may involve ocular and/or respiratory muscles; monitor creatine kinase; recovery may be delayed. Increased IOP may occur, especially with prolonged use; in children, increased IOP has been shown to be dose-dependent and produce a greater IOP in children <6 years than older children (Lam, 2005). Rare cases of anaphylactoid reactions have been reported with corticosteroids.

Oral solution contains sodium benzoate; benzoic acid (benzoate) is a metabolite of benzyl alcohol; large amounts of benzyl alcohol (≥99 mg/kg/day) have been associated with a potentially fatal toxicity ("gasping syndrome") in neonates; the "gasping syndrome" consists of metabolic acidosis, respiratory distress, gasping respirations, CNS dysfunction (including convulsions, intracranial hemorrhage), hypotension and cardiovascular collapse; use prednisone products containing sodium benzoate with caution in neonates; in vitro and animal studies have shown that benzoate displaces bilirubin from protein binding sites. Concentrated oral solution (Intensol) contains propylene glycol; toxicities have been reported with use of products containing propylene glycol, including hyperosmolality, lactic acidosis, seizures, and respiratory depression; in neonates large amounts of propylene glycol delivered orally, intravenously (eg, >3000 mg/day), or topically have been associated with potentially fatal toxicities which can include metabolic acidosis, seizures, renal failure, and CNS depression; use oral solutions containing propylene glycol with caution (AAP, 1997; Shehab, 2009).

Precautions Avoid using higher than recommended doses; suppression of HPA function, suppression of linear growth (ie, reduction of growth velocity), reduced bone mineral density, hypercorticism (Cushing's syndrome), hyperglycemia, or glucosuria may occur; titrate to lowest effective dose. Reduction in growth velocity may occur when corticosteroids are administered to pediatric patients by any route (monitor growth). Use with extreme caution in patients with respiratory tuberculosis or untreated systemic infections. Use with caution in patients with hypertension, heart failure, or renal impairment; long-term use has been associated with fluid retention and hypertension. Use with caution in patients with GI diseases (diverticulitis, peptic ulcer, ulcerative colitis) due to risk of GI bleeding and perforation. High-dose corticosteroids should not be used for management of head injury; increased mortality was observed in patients receiving high-dose I.V. methylprednisolone. Use with caution in patients with myasthenia gravis; exacerbation of symptoms has occurred, especially during initial treatment with corticosteroids. Use with caution in patients with hepatic impairment, including cirrhosis; enhanced pharmacologic effect due to decreased metabolism and long-term use has been associated with fluid retention. Use with caution following acute MI; corticosteroids have been associated with myocardial rupture;

hypertrophic cardiomyopathy has been reported in premature neonates.

Use with caution in patients with diabetes; corticosteroids may alter glucose regulation, leading to hyperglycemia. Use with caution in patients with cataracts and/or glaucoma; increased intraocular pressure, open-angle glaucoma, and cataracts have occurred with prolonged use; consider routine eye exams in chronic users. Use with caution in patients with a history of seizure disorder; seizures have been reported with adrenal crisis. Use with caution in patients with thyroid dysfunction; changes in thyroid status may necessitate dosage adjustments; metabolic clearance of corticosteroids increases in hyperthyroid patients and decreases in hypothyroid patients. Prolonged treatment with corticosteroids has been associated with the development of Kaposi's sarcoma (case reports); if noted, discontinuation of therapy should be considered. Use with caution in patients with thromboembolic tendencies or thrombophlebitis.

Adverse Reactions

Cardiovascular: Congestive heart failure (in susceptible patients), hypertension

Central nervous system: Emotional instability, headache, intracranial pressure increased (with papilledema), psychic derangements (including euphoria, insomnia, mood swings, personality changes, severe depression), seizure, vertigo

Dermatologic: Bruising, facial erythema, petechiae, thin fragile skin, urticaria, wound healing impaired

Endocrine & metabolic: Adrenocortical and pituitary unresponsiveness (in times of stress), carbohydrate intolerance, Cushing's syndrome, diabetes mellitus, fluid retention, growth suppression (in children), hypokalemic alkalosis, hypothyroidism enhanced, menstrual irregularities, negative nitrogen balance due to protein catabolism, potassium loss, sodium retention

Gastrointestinal: Abdominal distension, pancreatitis, peptic ulcer (with possible perforation and hemorrhage), ulcerative esophagitis

Hepatic: ALT increased, AST increased, alkaline phosphatase increased

Neuromuscular & skeletal: Aseptic necrosis of femoral and humeral heads, muscle mass loss, muscle weakness, osteoporosis, pathologic fracture of long bones, steroid myopathy, tendon rupture (particularly Achilles tendon), vertebral compression fractures

Ocular: Exophthalmos, glaucoma, intraocular pressure increased, posterior subcapsular cataracts

Miscellaneous: Allergic reactions, anaphylactic reactions, diaphoresis, hypersensitivity reactions, infections, Kaposi's sarcoma

Rare but important or life-threatening: Venous thrombosis (Johannesdottir, 2013)

Drug Interactions

Metabolism/Transport Effects Substrate of CYP3A4 (minor); **Note:** Assignment of Major/Minor substrate status based on clinically relevant drug interaction potential; **Induces** CYP2C19 (weak/moderate), CYP3A4 (weak/moderate)

Avoid Concomitant Use

Avoid concomitant use of PredniSONE with any of the following: Aldesleukin; Axitinib; BCG; Indium 111 Capromab Pendetide; Mifepristone; Natalizumab; Pimecrolimus; Simeprevir; Tacrolimus (Topical); Tofacitinib

Increased Effect/Toxicity

PredniSONE may increase the levels/effects of: Acetylcholinesterase Inhibitors; Amphotericin B; Androgens; Ceritinib; CycloSPORINE (Systemic); Deferasirox; Leflunomide; Loop Diuretics; Natalizumab; NSAID (COX-2 Inhibitor); NSAID (Nonselective); Thiazide Diuretics; Tofacitinib; Vaccines (Live); Warfarin

◄

The levels/effects of PredniSONE may be increased by:
Antifungal Agents (Azole Derivatives, Systemic); Aprepitant; Boceprevir; Calcium Channel Blockers (Nondihydropyridine); CycloSPORINE (Systemic); Denosumab; Estrogen Derivatives; Fluconazole; Fosaprepitant; Indacaterol; Macrolide Antibiotics; Mifepristone; Neuromuscular-Blocking Agents (Nondepolarizing); Pimecrolimus; Quinolone Antibiotics; Ritonavir; Roflumilast; Salicylates; Tacrolimus (Topical); Telaprevir; Trastuzumab

Decreased Effect

PredniSONE may decrease the levels/effects of: Aldesleukin; Antidiabetic Agents; ARIPiprazole; Axitinib; BCG; Calcitriol; Coccidioidin Skin Test; Corticorelin; CycloSPORINE (Systemic); Hyaluronidase; Ibrutinib; Indium 111 Capromab Pendetide; Isoniazid; Salicylates; Saxagliptin; Simeprevir; Sipuleucel-T; Telaprevir; Urea Cycle Disorder Agents; Vaccines (Inactivated)

The levels/effects of PredniSONE may be decreased by: Aminoglutethimide; Antacids; Barbiturates; Bile Acid Sequestrants; Echinacea; Fosphenytoin; Mifepristone; Mitotane; Phenytoin; Primidone; Rifamycin Derivatives; Somatropin; Tesamorelin

Mechanism of Action Decreases inflammation by suppression of migration of polymorphonuclear leukocytes and reversal of increased capillary permeability; suppresses the immune system by reducing activity and volume of the lymphatic system; suppresses adrenal function at high doses. Antitumor effects may be related to inhibition of glucose transport, phosphorylation, or induction of cell death in immature lymphocytes. Antiemetic effects are thought to occur due to blockade of cerebral innervation of the emetic center via inhibition of prostaglandin synthesis.

Pharmacokinetics (Adult data unless noted) Converted rapidly in the liver to prednisolone (active)

Dosing: Usual Dose depends upon condition being treated and response of patient; dosage for infants and children should be based on disease severity and patient response rather than by rigid adherence to dosage guidelines by age, weight, or body surface area. Consider alternate day therapy for long-term therapy. Discontinuation of long-term therapy requires gradual withdrawal by tapering the dose. Oral:

NIH Asthma Guidelines (NAEPP, 2007):
Children <12 years:
Asthma exacerbations (emergency care or hospital doses): 1-2 mg/kg/day in 2 divided doses (maximum: 60 mg/day) until peak expiratory flow is 70% of predicted or personal best
Short-course "burst" (acute asthma): 1-2 mg/kg/day in divided doses 1-2 times/day for 3-10 days; maximum dose: 60 mg/day; **Note:** Burst should be continued until symptoms resolve or patient achieves peak expiratory flow 80% of personal best; usually requires 3-10 days of treatment (~5 days on average); longer treatment may be required
Long-term treatment: 0.25-2 mg/kg/day given as a single dose in the morning or every other day as needed for asthma control; maximum dose: 60 mg/day
Children ≥12 years and Adults:
Asthma exacerbations (emergency care or hospital doses): 40-80 mg/day in divided doses 1-2 times/day until peak expiratory flow is 70% of predicted or personal best
Short-course "burst" (acute asthma): 40-60 mg/day in divided doses 1-2 times/day for 3-10 days; **Note:** Burst should be continued until symptoms resolve and peak expiratory flow is at least 80% of personal best; usually requires 3-10 days of treatment (~5 days on average); longer treatment may be required

Long-term treatment: 7.5-60 mg daily given as a single dose in the morning or every other day as needed for asthma control

Children:
Alternative asthma dosing by age:
Short-course "burst" (acute asthma):
<1 year: 10 mg every 12 hours
1-4 years: 20 mg every 12 hours
5-13 years: 30 mg every 12 hours
>13 years: 40 mg every 12 hours
Long-term treatment:
<1 year: 10 mg every other day
1-4 years: 20 mg every other day
5-13 years: 30 mg every other day
>13 years: 40 mg every other day
Anti-inflammatory or immunosuppressive: 0.05-2 mg/kg/day divided 1-4 times/day
Nephrotic syndrome:
Pediatric Nephrology Panel recommendations (Hogg, 2000):
Initial: 2 mg/kg/day or 60 mg/m^2/day given every day in 1-3 divided doses (maximum dose: 80 mg/day) until urine is protein free for 4-6 weeks; followed by maintenance dose: 2 mg/kg/dose or 40 mg/m^2/dose given every other day in the morning; gradually taper and discontinue after 4-6 weeks; **Note:** 6-week daily therapy followed by 6-week alternate day therapy may induce a higher rate of long remission compared to the standard of 4 weeks of daily therapy followed by 4 weeks of alternate day therapy; however, a higher incidence of adverse effects may be seen with the longer regimen and the clinical benefit may be variable.
Relapse: Use high-dose daily steroid regimen (listed above) until urine is protein free for 3 days; follow with maintenance-tapering course of alternate day therapy (maintenance dose listed above) for 4-6 weeks; subsequent therapy is determined by individual's response and number of relapses (Hogg, 2000)
British Pediatric Nephrology Consensus Statement (Report of a Workshop by the British Association for Paediatric Nephrology and Research Unit, 1994):
First 3 episodes: Initial: 2 mg/kg/day or 60 mg/m^2/day given every day (maximum dose: 80 mg/day) until urine is protein free for 3 consecutive days (maximum dose: 28 days); followed by 1-1.5 mg/kg/dose or 40 mg/m^2/dose (maximum: 60 mg/dose) given every other day for 4 weeks
Frequent relapses (long-term maintenance dose): 0.5-1 mg/kg/dose given every other day for 3-6 months
Children and Adults: Physiologic replacement: 4-5 mg/m^2/day
Adults: 5-60 mg/day in divided doses 1-4 times/day

Administration Oral: Administer after meals or with food or milk to decrease GI upset

Monitoring Parameters Blood pressure, weight, serum electrolytes, glucose; children's height and growth

Test Interactions Decreased response to skin tests

Dosage Forms Excipient information presented when available (limited, particularly for generics); consult specific product labeling.
Concentrate, Oral:
PredniSONE Intensol: 5 mg/mL (30 mL) [contains alcohol, usp; unflavored flavor]
Solution, Oral:
Generic: 5 mg/5 mL (5 mL, 120 mL, 500 mL)
Tablet, Oral:
Generic: 1 mg, 2.5 mg, 5 mg, 10 mg, 20 mg, 50 mg
Tablet Delayed Release, Oral:
Rayos: 1 mg, 2 mg, 5 mg

References

American Academy of Pediatrics Committee on Drugs. "Inactive" ingredients in pharmaceutical products: update (subject review). *Pediatrics*. 1997;99(2):268-278.

Bae YS, Van Voorhees AS, Hsu S, et al, "Review of Treatment Options For Psoriasis in Pregnant or Lactating Women: From the Medical Board of the National Psoriasis Foundation," *J Am Acad Dermatol*, 2012, 67(3):459-77.

Beitins IZ, Bayard F, Ances IG, et al, "The Transplacental Passage of Prednisone and Prednisolone in Pregnancy Near Term," *J Pediatr*, 1972, 81(5):936-45.

Hahn BH, McMahon MA, Wilkinson A, et al, "American College of Rheumatology Guidelines for Screening, Treatment, and Management of Lupus Nephritis," *Arthritis Care Res (Hoboken)*, 2012, 64 (6):797-808.

Hogg RJ, Portman RJ, Milliner D, et al, "Evaluation and Management of Proteinuria and Nephrotic Syndrome in Children: Recommendations From a Pediatric Nephrology Panel Established at the National Kidney Foundation Conference on Proteinuria, Albuminuria, Risk, Assessment, Detection, and Elimination (PARADE)," *Pediatrics*, 2000, 105(6):1242-9.

"'Inactive' Ingredients in Pharmaceutical Products: Update (Subject Review). American Academy of Pediatrics Committee on Drugs," *Pediatrics*, 1997, 99(2):268-78.

Ito S, Blajchman A, Stephenson M, et al, "Prospective Follow-up of Adverse Reactions in Breast-Fed Infants Exposed to Maternal Medication," *Am J Obstet Gynecol*, 1993, 168(5):1393-9.

Katz FH and Duncan BR, "Letter: Entry of Prednisone Into Human Milk," *N Engl J Med*, 1975, 293(22):1154.

Lam DS, Fan DS, Ng JS, et al, "Ocular Hypertensive and Anti-Inflammatory Responses to Different Dosages of Topical Dexamethasone in Children: A Randomized Trial," *Clin Experiment Ophthalmol*, 2005, 33 (3):252-8.

Leachman SA and Reed BR, "The Use of Dermatologic Drugs in Pregnancy and Lactation," *Dermatol Clin*, 2006, 24(2):167-97, vi.

Leonard MB, "Glucocorticoid-Induced Osteoporosis in Children: Impact of the Underlying Disease," *Pediatrics*, 2007, 119 Suppl 2:S166-74.

Lunghi L, Pavan B, Biondi C, et al, "Use of Glucocorticoids in Pregnancy," *Curr Pharm Des*, 2010, 16(32):3616-37.

Makol A, Wright K, and Amin S, "Rheumatoid Arthritis and Pregnancy: Safety Considerations in Pharmacological Management," *Drugs*, 2011, 71(15):1973-87.

Murphy CM, Coonce SL, and Simon PA, "Treatment of Asthma in Children," *Clin Pharm*, 1991, 10(9):685-703.

National Asthma Education and Prevention Program (NAEPP), "Expert Panel Report 3 (EPR-3): Guidelines for the Diagnosis and Management of Asthma," *Clinical Practice Guidelines*, National Institutes of Health, National Heart, Lung, and Blood Institute, NIH Publication No. 08-4051, prepublication 2007; available at http://www.nhlbi.nih.gov/guidelines/asthma/asthgdln.htm.

National Asthma Education and Prevention Program (NAEPP) Working Group Report on "Managing Asthma During Pregnancy: Recommendations for Pharmacologic Treatment," National Institutes of Health, National Heart, Lung, and Blood Institute, NIH Publication No. 05-5236, March 2005. Available at http://www.nhlbi.nih.gov/health/prof/lung/asthma/astpreg/astpreg_full.pdf

Østensen M and Forger F, "Management of RA Medications in Pregnant PATIENTS," *Nat Rev Rheumatol*, 2009, 5(7):382-90.

Ost L, Wettrell G, Bjorkhem I, et al, "Prednisolone Excretion in Human Milk," *J Pediatr*, 1985, 106(6):1008-11.

Park-Wyllie L, Mazzotta P, Pastuszak A, et al, "Birth Defects After Maternal Exposure to Corticosteroids: Prospective Cohort Study and Meta-analysis of Epidemiological Studies," *Teratology*, 2000, 62 (6):385-92.

Pradat P, Robert-Gnansia E, Di Tanna GL, et al, "First Trimester Exposure to Corticosteroids and Oral Clefts," *Birth Defects Res A Clin Mol Teratol*, 2003, 67(12):968-70.

Report of a Workshop by the British Association for Paediatric Nephrology and Research Unit, Royal College of Physicians, "Consensus Statement on Management and Audit Potential for Steroid Responsive Nephrotic Syndrome," *Arch Dis Child*, 1994, 70(2):151-7.

Sagraves R, Kaiser D, and Sharpe GL, "Prednisone and Prednisolone Concentrations in the Milk of a Lactating Mother," *Drug Intell Clin Pharm*, 1981, 15:484.

Shehab N, Lewis CL, Streetman DD, Donn SM. Exposure to the pharmaceutical excipients benzyl alcohol and propylene glycol among critically ill neonates. *Pediatr Crit Care Med*. 2009;10 (2):256-259.

◆ **PredniSONE Intensol** see PredniSONE *on page 1732*

◆ **Pregnyl** see Chorionic Gonadotropin (Human) *on page 460*

◆ **Pregnyl® (Can)** see Chorionic Gonadotropin (Human) *on page 460*

◆ **Prelone** see PrednisoLONE (Systemic) *on page 1727*

◆ **Premarin** see Estrogens (Conjugated/Equine, Systemic) *on page 799*

◆ **Premarin** see Estrogens (Conjugated/Equine, Topical) *on page 801*

◆ **Premarin® (Can)** see Estrogens (Conjugated/Equine, Systemic) *on page 799*

◆ **Premarin® (Can)** see Estrogens (Conjugated/Equine, Topical) *on page 801*

◆ **Premium Activated Charcoal [OTC] (Can)** see Charcoal, Activated *on page 432*

◆ **Preparation H [OTC]** see Phenylephrine (Topical) *on page 1662*

◆ **Preparation H Hydrocortisone [OTC]** see Hydrocortisone (Topical) *on page 1038*

◆ **Pre-Pen®** see Benzylpenicilloyl Polylysine *on page 279*

◆ **Pressyn® (Can)** see Vasopressin *on page 2121*

◆ **Pressyn® AR (Can)** see Vasopressin *on page 2121*

◆ **Pretz [OTC]** see Sodium Chloride *on page 1902*

◆ **Pretz Irrigation [OTC]** see Sodium Chloride *on page 1902*

◆ **Prevacare® [OTC]** see Alcohol (Ethyl) *on page 88*

◆ **Prevacid** see Lansoprazole *on page 1206*

◆ **Prevacid® (Can)** see Lansoprazole *on page 1206*

◆ **Prevacid 24HR [OTC]** see Lansoprazole *on page 1206*

◆ **Prevacid® FasTab (Can)** see Lansoprazole *on page 1206*

◆ **Prevacid SoluTab** see Lansoprazole *on page 1206*

◆ **Prevalite** see Cholestyramine Resin *on page 457*

◆ **Prevex B (Can)** see Betamethasone (Topical) *on page 285*

◆ **Prevex® HC (Can)** see Hydrocortisone (Topical) *on page 1038*

◆ **PreviDent** see Fluoride *on page 894*

◆ **PreviDent 5000 Booster** see Fluoride *on page 894*

◆ **PreviDent 5000 Booster Plus** see Fluoride *on page 894*

◆ **PreviDent 5000 Dry Mouth** see Fluoride *on page 894*

◆ **PreviDent 5000 Plus** see Fluoride *on page 894*

◆ **Prevnar 13** see Pneumococcal Conjugate Vaccine (13-Valent) *on page 1688*

◆ **Prezista** see Darunavir *on page 595*

◆ **Prezista® (Can)** see Darunavir *on page 595*

◆ **Prilocaine and Lidocaine** see Lidocaine and Prilocaine *on page 1246*

◆ **PriLOSEC** see Omeprazole *on page 1535*

◆ **PriLOSEC OTC [OTC]** see Omeprazole *on page 1535*

◆ **Primaclone** see Primidone *on page 1737*

◆ **Primacor (Can)** see Milrinone *on page 1417*

Primaquine (PRIM a kween)

Medication Safety Issues

Sound-alike/look-alike issues:

Primaquine may be confused with primidone

Therapeutic Category Antimalarial Agent

Generic Availability (U.S.) Yes

Use For the radical cure (prevention of relapse) of vivax malaria (*P. vivax*) [FDA approved in adults]; has also been used for prevention relapse of *P. ovale*, prevention of malaria (primarily *P. vivax*), malaria postexposure prophylaxis, and treatment of *Pneumocystis jirovecii* (PCP) pneumonia

Pregnancy Considerations Animal reproduction studies have not been conducted. Primaquine use is not recommended in pregnant women per CDC Guidelines. Consult current CDC guidelines for the treatment of malaria during pregnancy.

Breast-Feeding Considerations It is not known if primaquine is excreted in breast milk. If therapy is needed, the mother and infant should be tested for G6PD deficiency; primaquine before primaquine is given to a woman who is breast-feeding. It may be used in breast-feeding mothers and infants with normal G6PD levelsconcentrations (CDC, 2012).

Contraindications Acutely ill patients who have a tendency to develop granulocytopenia (rheumatoid arthritis, SLE); patients concurrently receiving drugs capable of depressing the bone marrow or receiving other drugs which can cause hemolytic anemia; patients receiving quinacrine

Warnings Hemolytic reactions may occur in patients with G-6-P-D deficiency and in individuals with a history of favism; the CDC recommends screening for G-6-P-D deficiency prior to initiating treatment with primaquine. Anemia, methemoglobinemia, and leukopenia have been associated with primaquine use; promptly discontinue with signs of hemolytic anemia (darkening of urine, marked fall in hemoglobin, or erythrocyte count); do not exceed recommended dosage or duration. Primaquine tablets contain polysorbate 80 (Tween 80) which may cause allergic reactions in susceptible individuals.

Precautions Use with caution in patients with NADH methemoglobin reductase deficiency; methemoglobinemia may occur. Primaquine should only be prescribed by physicians familiar with its use **[U.S. Boxed Warning]**.

Adverse Reactions

Cardiovascular: Arrhythmias (rare)

Central nervous system: Headache

Dermatologic: Pruritus

Gastrointestinal: Abdominal cramps, dyspepsia, nausea, vomiting

Hematologic: Agranulocytosis, anemia, hemolytic anemia (in patients with G6PD deficiency), leukopenia, leukocytosis, methemoglobinemia (in NADH-methemoglobin reductase-deficient individuals)

Ocular: Interference with visual accommodation

Drug Interactions

Metabolism/Transport Effects Substrate of CYP2D6 (major), CYP3A4 (major); **Note:** Assignment of Major/Minor substrate status based on clinically relevant drug interaction potential; **Inhibits** CYP1A2 (strong), CYP2D6 (weak), CYP3A4 (weak); **Induces** CYP1A2 (weak/moderate)

Avoid Concomitant Use

Avoid concomitant use of Primaquine with any of the following: Agomelatine; Artemether; Lumefantrine; Mefloquine; Pimozide; Pirfenidone; Pomalidomide; Tasimelteon

Increased Effect/Toxicity

Primaquine may increase the levels/effects of: Agomelatine; Antipsychotic Agents (Phenothiazines); ARIPiprazole; Bendamustine; Beta-Blockers; Cardiac Glycosides; CloZAPine; CYP1A2 Substrates; Dapsone (Systemic); Dapsone (Topical); Dofetilide; Lomitapide; Lumefantrine; Mefloquine; Pimozide; Pirfenidone; Pomalidomide; Prilocaine; Sodium Nitrite; Tasimelteon

The levels/effects of Primaquine may be increased by: Abiraterone Acetate; Artemether; CYP2D6 Inhibitors (Moderate); CYP2D6 Inhibitors (Strong); Dapsone (Systemic); Darunavir; Mefloquine; Nitric Oxide

Decreased Effect

Primaquine may decrease the levels/effects of: Anthelmintics

The levels/effects of Primaquine may be decreased by: Bosentan; CYP3A4 Inducers (Strong); Dabrafenib; Deferasirox; Mitotane; Peginterferon Alfa-2b; Siltuximab; St Johns Wort; Tocilizumab

Stability Store at 25°C (77°F); excursions permitted to 15°C to 30°C (59°F to 86°F); protect from light.

Mechanism of Action Eliminates the primary tissue exoerythrocytic forms of *P. ovale* and *P. vivax*; disrupts mitochondria and binds to DNA

Pharmacokinetics (Adult data unless noted)

Absorption: Oral: Well absorbed

Metabolism: Hepatic metabolism to carboxyprimaquine, an active metabolite via CYP1A2

Half-life: 7 hours; reported range: 3.7-9.6 hours

Time to peak serum concentration: Within 3 hours

Elimination: Small amount of unchanged drug excreted in urine

Dosing: Usual Oral: **Note:** Dosage expressed as mg of **base** (15 mg base = 26.3 mg primaquine phosphate):

Pediatric:

Malaria: Oral:

Treatment or relapse prevention of *P. vivax* malaria: Infants, Children, and Adolescents: 0.5 mg base/kg once daily for 14 days; maximum single dose: 30 mg base (CDC, 2013)

Treatment of uncomplicated malaria (*P. vivax* and *P. ovale*): Infants, Children, and Adolescents: 0.5 mg base/kg once daily for 14 days with chloroquine or hydroxychloroquine; maximum single dose: 30 mg base (CDC, 2013)

Prevention of malaria (primarily *P. vivax*):

Non-HIV-exposed/-positive: Infants, Children and Adolescents: 0.5 mg base/kg once daily; maximum single dose: 30 mg base; initiate 1 to 2 days prior to travel and continue once daily while in the area with malaria risk, and for 7 days after departure from malaria-endemic area (CDC, 2014)

HIV-exposed/-positive:

Primary prophylaxis: Infants and Children: 0.6 mg base/kg once daily; maximum single dose: 30 mg base; initiate 1 day prior to travel and continue once daily while in the area with malaria risk, and for 3 to 7 days after departure from malaria-endemic area (DHHS [pediatric], 2013)

Secondary prophylaxis and antirelapse therapy: Infants, Children, and Adolescents: 0.5 mg base/kg once daily for 14 days after departure from malaria-endemic area; maximum single dose: 30 mg base (CDC, 2014)

Pneumocystis jirovecii pneumonia (PCP) (HIV-exposed/-positive) treatment: Oral:

Infants and Children: 0.3 mg base/kg once daily for 21 days in combination with clindamycin; maximum single dose: 30 mg base (DHHS [pediatric], 2013)

Adolescents: 30 mg base once daily for 21 days in combination with clindamycin (DHHS [adult], 2013)

Adult:

Malaria: Oral:

Treatment or prevention of relapse of *P. vivax* malaria: 30 mg base once daily for 14 days

Treatment of uncomplicated *P. vivax* and *P. ovale* malaria: 30 mg base once daily for 14 days with chloroquine or hydroxychloroquine; alternative regimen (for mild G-6-P-D deficiency or as an alternative to daily regimen): 45 mg base once weekly for 8 weeks (use only after consultation with an infectious disease/tropical medicine expert) (CDC, 2011)

Chemoprophylaxis: 30 mg base once daily; start 1 to 2 days prior to travel and continue once daily while in the area with malaria risk, and for 7 days after departure from malaria-endemic area (CDC, 2012)

Presumptive antirelapse therapy for *P. vivax* and *P. ovale* malaria: 30 mg base once daily for 14 days after departure from malaria-endemic area (CDC, 2012)

Pneumocystis jirovecii pneumonia (PCP); treatment:
Oral: 30 mg base once daily for 21 days (in combination with clindamycin) (DHHS [adult], 2013)

Administration Oral: Administer with meals to decrease adverse GI effects; drug has a bitter taste

Monitoring Parameters Periodic CBC, visual color check of urine, hemoglobin, glucose; if hemolysis is suspected, monitor CBC, haptoglobin, peripheral smear, urinalysis dipstick for occult blood; G-6-PD deficiency screening (prior to initiating treatment; CDC recommendation)

Dosage Forms Excipient information presented when available (limited, particularly for generics); consult specific product labeling.

Tablet, Oral, as phosphate:
  Generic: 26.3 mg

Extemporaneous Preparations A 6 mg base/5 mL oral suspension may be made using tablets. Crush ten 15 mg base tablets and reduce to a fine powder. In small amounts, add a total of 10 mL Carboxymethylcellulose 1.5% and mix to a uniform paste; mix while adding Simple Syrup, NF to **almost** 125 mL; transfer to a calibrated bottle, rinse mortar with vehicle, and add quantity of vehicle sufficient to make 125 mL. Label "shake well" and "refrigerate". Stable 7 days.

Nahata MC, Pai VB, and Hipple TF, *Pediatric Drug Formulations*, 5th ed, Cincinnati, OH: Harvey Whitney Books Co, 2004.

References

Centers for Disease Control and Prevention (CDC). *CDC Health Information for International Travel*. New York: Oxford University Press; 2014; Chapter 3. Available at http://wwwnc.cdc.gov/travel/page/yellowbook-home-2014

Centers for Disease Control and Prevention (CDC). Guidelines for treatment of malaria in the United States. Treatment Table Update, July 1, 2013. Available at http://www.cdc.gov/malaria/resources/pdf/treatmenttable.pdf

Centers for Disease Control and Prevention (CDC), "Pneumocystis jiroveci (Formerly carinii) Pneumonia (PCP)." Available at http://www.dpd.cdc.gov/DPDx/HTML/PDF_Files/MedLetter/Pneumocystis%20jiroveci.pdf.

Centers for Disease Control and Prevention (CDC). Treatment of malaria (guidelines for clinicians. July 2013b. Available at http://www.cdc.gov/malaria/resources/pdf/clinicalguidance.pdf

DHHS. Guidelines for the prevention and treatment of opportunistic infections among HIV-exposed and HIV-infected children: recommendations from the National Institutes of Health, Centers for Disease Control and Prevention, the HIV Medicine Association of the Infectious Diseases Society of America, the Pediatric Infectious Diseases Society, and the American Academy of Pediatrics. November 6, 2013. Available at http://aidsinfo.nih.gov

DHHS Panel on Opportunistic Infections (OI) in HIV-Infected Adults and Adolescents. Guidelines for prevention and treatment of opportunistic infections in HIV-infected adults and adolescents: recommendations from the Centers for Disease Control and Prevention (CDC), the National Institutes of Health (NIH), and the HIV Medicine Association (HIVMA) of the Infectious Diseases Society of America (IDSA)," May 7, 2013. Available at http://aidsinfo.nih.gov/contentfiles/lvguidelines/adult_oi.pdf

Lynk A and Gold R, "Review of 40 Children With Imported Malaria," *Pediatr Infect Dis J*, 1989, 8(11):745-50.

◆ **Primaquine Phosphate** *see* Primaquine *on page 1735*

◆ **Primaxin I.M. [DSC]** *see* Imipenem and Cilastatin *on page 1077*

◆ **Primaxin® I.V.** *see* Imipenem and Cilastatin *on page 1077*

◆ **Primaxin I.V. Infusion (Can)** *see* Imipenem and Cilastatin *on page 1077*

Primidone (PRI mi done)

Medication Safety Issues
Sound-alike/look-alike issues:
Primidone may be confused with predniSONE, primaquine, pyridoxine

Brand Names: U.S. Mysoline
Brand Names: Canada Apo-Primidone®
Therapeutic Category Anticonvulsant, Barbiturate; Barbiturate
Generic Availability (U.S.) Yes
Use Management of generalized tonic-clonic (grand mal), complex partial and simple partial (focal) seizures
Medication Guide Available Yes
Pregnancy Considerations Primidone and its metabolites (PEMA, phenobarbital, and p-hydroxyphenobarbital) cross the placenta; neonatal serum concentrations at birth are similar to those in the mother. Withdrawal symptoms may occur in the neonate and may be delayed due to the long half-life of primidone and its metabolites. Use may be associated with birth defects and adverse events; the use of folic acid throughout pregnancy and vitamin K during the last month of pregnancy is recommended. Epilepsy itself, number of medications, genetic factors, or a combination of these probably influence the teratogenicity of anticonvulsant therapy.

Patients exposed to primidone during pregnancy are encouraged to enroll themselves into the NAAED Pregnancy Registry by calling 1-888-233-2334. Additional information is available at www.aedpregnancyregistry.org.

Breast-Feeding Considerations Primidone and its metabolites (PEMA, phenobarbital, and p-hydroxyphenobarbital) are found in breast milk (variable concentrations). The manufacturer recommends discontinuing breast-feeding if undue drowsiness and somnolence occur in the newborn.

Contraindications Hypersensitivity to primidone or any component; porphyria

Warnings Antiepileptic drugs (AEDs) increase the risk of suicidal behavior and ideation in patients receiving these medications for any indication. Pooled analyses of placebo-controlled trials involving 11 different AEDs (regardless of indication) showed a twofold increased risk of suicidal thoughts or behavior (estimated incidence rate: 0.43% in AED treated patients compared to 0.24% of patients receiving placebo); increased risk was observed as early as 1 week after initiation of AED and continued through duration of trials (most trials ≤24 weeks); risk did not vary significantly by age (age range: 5–100 years). Consider risks and benefits of AEDs before prescribing. Monitor all patients receiving an AED for emergence of suicidal thoughts or behavior, thoughts of self-harm, any unusual changes in behavior or mood, or the emergence or worsening of depressive symptoms; notify healthcare provider immediately if symptoms or concerning behavior occur. **Note:** The FDA is requiring that a Medication Guide be developed for all antiepileptic drugs informing patients of this risk.

Generic tablet may contain sodium benzoate; benzoic acid (benzoate) is a metabolite of benzyl alcohol; large amounts of benzyl alcohol (≥99 mg/kg/day) have been associated with a potentially fatal toxicity ("gasping syndrome") in neonates; the "gasping syndrome" consists of metabolic acidosis, respiratory distress, gasping respirations, CNS dysfunction (including convulsions, intracranial hemorrhage), hypotension and cardiovascular collapse; avoid use of primidone products containing sodium benzoate in neonates; *in vitro* and animal studies have shown that benzoate displaces bilirubin from protein binding sites

Precautions Use with caution in patients with renal or hepatic impairment. Abrupt discontinuation may precipitate status epilepticus

Adverse Reactions
Central nervous system: Ataxia, drowsiness, emotional disturbances, fatigue, hyperirritability, suicidal ideation, vertigo
Dermatologic: Morbilliform skin eruptions

Gastrointestinal: Anorexia, nausea, vomiting

Genitourinary: Impotence

Hematologic: Agranulocytosis, granulocytopenia, megaloblastic anemia (idiosyncratic), red cell aplasia/hypoplasia

Ocular: Diplopia, nystagmus

Drug Interactions

Metabolism/Transport Effects Induces CYP1A2 (strong), CYP2B6 (strong), CYP2C8 (strong), CYP2C9 (strong), CYP3A4 (strong), P-glycoprotein

Avoid Concomitant Use

Avoid concomitant use of Primidone with any of the following: Abiraterone Acetate; Apixaban; Apremilast; Artemether; Axitinib; Azelastine (Nasal); Bedaquiline; Boceprevir; Bortezomib; Bosutinib; Cabozantinib; Ceritinib; CloZAPine; Crizotinib; Dabigatran Etexilate; Dienogest; Dolutegravir; Dronedarone; Enzalutamide; Etravirine; Everolimus; Ibrutinib; Itraconazole; Ivacaftor; Lapatinib; Lumefantrine; Lurasidone; Macitentan; Mifepristone; NIFEdipine; Nilotinib; Nisoldipine; Paraldehyde; PAZOPanib; Perampanel; Pirfenidone; Pomalidomide; PONATinib; Praziquantel; Ranolazine; Regorafenib; Rilpivirine; Rivaroxaban; Roflumilast; RomiDEPsin; Simeprevir; Sofosbuvir; SORAfenib; Tasimelteon; Telaprevir; Thalidomide; Ticagrelor; Tofacitinib; Tolvaptan; Toremifene; Ulipristal; Vandetanib; Vemurafenib; VinCRIStine (Liposomal); Vorapaxar

Increased Effect/Toxicity

Primidone may increase the levels/effects of: Alcohol (Ethyl); Azelastine (Nasal); Barbiturates; Buprenorphine; Clarithromycin; CNS Depressants; Hydrocodone; Ifosfamide; Methotrimeprazine; Metyrosine; Paraldehyde; Pramipexole; Rotigotine; Selective Serotonin Reuptake Inhibitors; Thalidomide; Valproic Acid and Derivatives; Zolpidem

The levels/effects of Primidone may be increased by: Brimonidine (Topical); Cannabis; Carbonic Anhydrase Inhibitors; Clarithromycin; Cosyntropin; Dexmethylphenidate; Doxylamine; Dronabinol; Droperidol; Felbamate; HydrOXYzine; Kava Kava; Magnesium Sulfate; Methotrimeprazine; Methylphenidate; Nabilone; Sodium Oxybate; Tapentadol; Tetrahydrocannabinol; Valproic Acid and Derivatives

Decreased Effect

Primidone may decrease the levels/effects of: Abiraterone Acetate; Afatinib; Apixaban; Apremilast; ARIPiprazole; Artemether; Axitinib; Bazedoxifene; Bedaquiline; Bendamustine; Boceprevir; Bortezomib; Bosutinib; Brentuximab Vedotin; Cabozantinib; Canagliflozin; Cannabidiol; Cannabis; Ceritinib; Clarithromycin; CloZAPine; Contraceptives (Progestins); Corticosteroids (Systemic); Crizotinib; CYP1A2 Substrates; CYP2B6 Substrates; CYP2C8 Substrates; CYP2C9 Substrates; CYP3A4 Substrates; Dabigatran Etexilate; Dasatinib; Diclofenac (Systemic); Dienogest; Dolutegravir; DOXOrubicin (Conventional); Dronabinol; Dronedarone; Enzalutamide; Eslicarbazepine; Etravirine; Everolimus; Exemestane; Felbamate; FentaNYL; Gefitinib; GuanFACINE; Ibrutinib; Imatinib; Itraconazole; Ivacaftor; Ixabepilone; LamoTRIgine; Lapatinib; Linagliptin; Lumefantrine; Lurasidone; Macitentan; Maraviroc; Methadone; Mifepristone; NIFEdipine; Nilotinib; Nisoldipine; PAZOPanib; Perampanel; P-glycoprotein/ABCB1 Substrates; Pirfenidone; Pomalidomide; PONATinib; Praziquantel; QUEtiapine; QuiNIDine; Ranolazine; Regorafenib; Rilpivirine; Rivaroxaban; Roflumilast; RomiDEPsin; Rufinamide; Saxagliptin; Simeprevir; Sofosbuvir; SORAfenib; SUNItinib; Tadalafil; Tasimelteon; Telaprevir; Tetrahydrocannabinol; Ticagrelor; Tofacitinib; Tolvaptan; Toremifene; Treprostinil; Ulipristal; Vandetanib; Vemurafenib; Vilazodone; VinCRIStine (Liposomal); Vorapaxar; Vortioxetine; Zuclopenthixol

The levels/effects of Primidone may be decreased by: Carbonic Anhydrase Inhibitors; Folic Acid; Fosphenytoin; Ketorolac (Nasal); Ketorolac (Systemic); Leucovorin Calcium-Levoleucovorin; Levomefolate; Mefloquine; Methylfolate; Orlistat; Phenytoin

Food Interactions Protein-deficient diets increase duration of action of primidone.

Mechanism of Action Decreases neuron excitability, raises seizure threshold similar to phenobarbital; primidone has two active metabolites, phenobarbital and phenylethylmalonamide (PEMA); PEMA may enhance the activity of phenobarbital

Pharmacokinetics (Adult data unless noted)

Distribution: V$_d$: Adults: 2-3 L/kg

Protein-binding: 99%

Metabolism: In the liver to phenobarbital (active) and phenylethylmalonamide (PEMA)

Bioavailability: 60% to 80%

Half-life:

Primidone: 10-12 hours

PEMA: 16 hours

Phenobarbital: 52-118 hours (age-dependent)

Time to peak serum concentration: Oral: Within 4 hours

Elimination: Urinary excretion of both active metabolites and unchanged primidone (15% to 25%)

Dosing: Neonatal Oral: Seizure disorder: 12-20 mg/kg/day in 2-4 divided doses; start with lower dosage and titrate upward

Dosing: Usual Oral: Seizure disorder:

Children <8 years: Initial: 50-125 mg/day given at bedtime; increase by 50-125 mg/day increments every 3-7 days; usual dose: 10-25 mg/kg/day in 3-4 divided doses

Children ≥8 years and Adults: Initial: 125-250 mg/day at bedtime; increase by 125-250 mg/day every 3-7 days; usual dose: 750-1500 mg/day in 3-4 divided doses with maximum dosage of 2 g/day

Administration Oral: Administer with food to decrease GI upset

Monitoring Parameters Serum primidone and phenobarbital concentrations; CBC with differential; neurological status, seizure frequency, duration, severity; signs and symptoms of suicidality (eg, anxiety, depression, behavior changes)

Reference Range Monitor both primidone and phenobarbital concentrations.

Primidone:

Therapeutic: 5-12 mcg/mL (SI: 23-55 micromoles/L)

Toxic effects rarely present with levels <10 mcg/mL (SI: 46 micromoles/L) if phenobarbital concentrations are low

Toxic: >15 mcg/mL (SI: >69 micromoles/L)

Phenobarbital:

Therapeutic: 15-40 mcg/mL (SI: 65-172 micromoles/L)

Potentially toxic: >40 mcg/mL (SI: >172 micromoles/L)

Coma: >50 mcg/mL (SI: >215 micromoles/L)

Potentially lethal: >80 mcg/mL (SI: >344 micromoles/L)

Additional Information Mysoline® suspension was discontinued in February 2001

Dosage Forms Excipient information presented when available (limited, particularly for generics); consult specific product labeling.

Tablet, Oral:

Mysoline: 50 mg, 250 mg [scored]

Generic: 50 mg, 250 mg

◆ **Primlev** *see* Oxycodone and Acetaminophen *on page 1573*

◆ **Primsol** *see* Trimethoprim *on page 2087*

◆ **Prinivil** *see* Lisinopril *on page 1262*

◆ **Priorix (Can)** *see* Measles, Mumps, and Rubella Virus Vaccine *on page 1307*

- ◆ **Priorix-Tetra (Can)** *see* Measles, Mumps, Rubella, and Varicella Virus Vaccine *on page 1310*
- ◆ **Privigen** *see* Immune Globulin *on page 1084*
- ◆ **Privine® [OTC]** *see* Naphazoline (Nasal) *on page 1469*
- ◆ **Pro-AAS EC-80 (Can)** *see* Aspirin *on page 212*
- ◆ **ProAir HFA** *see* Albuterol *on page 84*
- ◆ **PRO-Amiodarone (Can)** *see* Amiodarone *on page 127*
- ◆ **Pro-Amox-250 (Can)** *see* Amoxicillin *on page 140*
- ◆ **Pro-Amox-500 (Can)** *see* Amoxicillin *on page 140*
- ◆ **PRO-Azithromycin (Can)** *see* Azithromycin (Systemic) *on page 247*

Probenecid (proe BEN e sid)

Medication Safety Issues
Sound-alike/look-alike issues:
Probenecid may be confused with Procanbid
Brand Names: Canada Benuryl™
Therapeutic Category Adjuvant Therapy, Penicillin Level Prolongation; Antigout Agent; Uric Acid Lowering Agent; Uricosuric Agent
Generic Availability (U.S.) Yes
Use Adjuvant to therapy with penicillins to prolong serum concentrations (FDA approved in ages ≥2 years and adults); treatment of hyperuricemia associated with gout and gouty arthritis (FDA approved in adults); has also been used with cephalosporin therapy to prolong serum concentrations and to prevent nephrotoxicity associated with cidofovir therapy
Pregnancy Considerations Probenecid crosses the placenta. Based on available data, an increased risk of adverse fetal events have not been reported (Gutman, 2012).
Contraindications Hypersensitivity to probenecid or any component; pediatric patients <2 years of age; individuals with blood dyscrasias or uric acid kidney stones; initiation during an acute gout attack; concurrent aspirin therapy (regardless of dose)
Warnings Salicylates may diminish the therapeutic effect of probenecid; this effect may be more pronounced with high, chronic doses; however, the manufacturer recommends the use of an alternative analgesic even in place of small doses of aspirin; probenecid may increase the half-life of acetaminophen and some NSAIDS (eg, ketoprofen, naproxen); consider dosage reductions. Probenecid may increase the serum concentration of methotrexate; avoid concomitant use of probenecid and methotrexate if possible; if concurrent use necessary, consider lower methotrexate doses and monitor for methotrexate toxicity. Therapy with probenecid should not be initiated until an acute gouty attack has subsided; may cause exacerbation of acute gouty attack; if an acute attack occurs during probenecid therapy, usage may continue but other appropriate agents (eg, colchicine) should be used to control the acute attack; the frequency of acute gouty attacks may increase during the first 6-12 months of therapy. Use has been associated with rare, severe hypersensitivity reactions, including anaphylaxis; discontinue therapy if reaction occurs.
Precautions Use with caution in patients with renal impairment; dosage requirements may be increased; monotherapy may not be effective if CrCl <30 mL/minute; concurrent use with penicillin in patients with renal insufficiency is not recommended. Use with caution in patients with peptic ulcer disease. In gouty patients, probenecid may cause hematuria, renal colic, costovertebral pain, and development of uric acid stones; may be prevented by liberal fluid intake and alkalinization of urine. Use caution in patients with G6PD deficiency; may increase risk for hemolytic anemia.

Adverse Reactions
Cardiovascular: Flushing
Central nervous system: Dizziness, fever, headache
Dermatologic: Alopecia, dermatitis, pruritus, rash
Gastrointestinal: Anorexia, dyspepsia, gastroesophageal reflux, nausea, sore gums, vomiting
Genitourinary: Hematuria, polyuria
Hematologic: Anemia, aplastic anemia, hemolytic anemia (in G6PD deficiency), leukopenia
Hepatic: Hepatic necrosis
Neuromuscular & skeletal: Costovertebral pain, gouty arthritis (acute)
Renal: Nephrotic syndrome, renal colic
Miscellaneous: Anaphylaxis, hypersensitivity

Drug Interactions
Metabolism/Transport Effects Inhibits CYP2C19 (weak), UGT1A6
Avoid Concomitant Use
Avoid concomitant use of Probenecid with any of the following: Doripenem; Ketorolac (Nasal); Ketorolac (Systemic); Meropenem; Pegloticase; Penicillins
Increased Effect/Toxicity
Probenecid may increase the levels/effects of: Acetaminophen; Cefotaxime; Cephalosporins; Dapsone (Systemic); Deferiprone; Doripenem; Ertapenem; Ganciclovir-Valganciclovir; Gemifloxacin; Imipenem; Ketoprofen; Ketorolac (Nasal); Ketorolac (Systemic); Loop Diuretics; LORazepam; Meropenem; Methotrexate; Mycophenolate; Nitrofurantoin; Nonsteroidal Anti-Inflammatory Agents; Oseltamivir; Pegloticase; Penicillins; PRALAtrexate; Quinolone Antibiotics; Sodium Benzoate; Sodium Phenylacetate; Sulfonylureas; Theophylline Derivatives; Urea Cycle Disorder Agents; Zidovudine
Decreased Effect
Probenecid may decrease the levels/effects of: Loop Diuretics

The levels/effects of Probenecid may be decreased by: Salicylates
Stability Store at 20°C to 25°C (68°F to 77°F); protect from light.
Mechanism of Action Competitively inhibits the reabsorption of uric acid at the proximal convoluted tubule, thereby promoting its excretion and reducing serum uric acid levels; increases plasma levels of weak organic acids (penicillins, cephalosporins, or other beta-lactam antibiotics) by competitively inhibiting their renal tubular secretion
Pharmacodynamics
Maximum effect:
Penicillin concentrations: After 2 hours
Uric acid renal clearance: 30 minutes
Pharmacokinetics (Adult data unless noted)
Absorption: Rapid and complete from GI tract
Protein binding: 85% to 95%
Metabolism: Hepatic
Half-life: 6-12 hours
Time to peak serum concentration: Within 2-4 hours
Dosing: Usual
Infants, Children, and Adolescents:
Prolongation of penicillin serum levels: Children ≥2 years and Adolescents: **Note:** Dosing per manufacturer; some indication-specific dosing may vary.
Patient weight ≤50 kg: Oral: Initial: 25 mg/kg/dose or 700 mg/m^2/dose as a single dose; maintenance: 40 mg/kg/**day** or 1200 mg /m^2/**day** in 4 divided doses; maximum dose: 500 mg
Patient weight >50 kg: Oral: 500 mg 4 times daily
Gonorrhea, uncomplicated infections of cervix, urethra, and rectum: Adolescents >45 kg: Oral: 1000 mg as a single dose with cefoxitin (CDC, 2010)
Pelvic inflammatory disease: Adolescents >50 kg: Oral: 1000 mg as a single dose with cefoxitin in

combination with doxycycline with/without metronidazole (CDC, 2010)

Neurosyphilis: Adolescents >50 kg: Oral: 500 mg 4 times daily with procaine penicillin for 10-14 days (CDC, 2010)

Prevention of cidofovir nephrotoxicity: Infants, Children, and Adolescents: Limited data available; various regimens have been reported (Anderson, 2008; Bhadri, 2009; Cesaro, 2005; Doan, 2007; Williams, 2009): Oral: Weight-directed dosing: 25-40 mg/kg/dose (maximum dose: 2000 mg) administered 3 hours before cidofovir infusion and 10-20 mg/kg/dose (maximum dose: 1000 mg) at 2-3 hours and 8-9 hours after cidofovir infusion

Body surface area (BSA)-directed dosing: 1000-2000 mg/m^2/dose administered 3 hours prior to cidofovir, followed by 500-1250 mg/m^2/dose 1-2 hours and 8 hours after completion

Adults:

Gonorrhea, uncomplicated infections of cervix, urethra, and rectum: Oral: 1000 mg as a single dose with cefoxitin (CDC, 2010)

Hyperuricemia with gout: Oral: Initial: 250 mg twice daily for 1 week; may increase to 500 mg twice daily; if needed, may increase in 500 mg increments every 4 weeks; maximum daily dose: 2000 mg/**day**. If serum uric acid levels are within normal limits and gout attacks have been absent for 6 months, daily dosage may be reduced by 500 mg increments every 6 months.

Prolongation of penicillin serum levels: Oral: 500 mg 4 times daily; **Note:** Dosing per manufacturer, some indication-specific dosing may vary.

Dosing adjustment in renal impairment: Children ≥2 years, Adolescents, and Adults: CrCl <30 mL/minute: Avoid use

Dosing adjustment in hepatic impairment: There are no dosage adjustments provided in manufacturer's labeling.

Administration Oral: Administer with food or antacids to minimize GI effects

Monitoring Parameters Uric acid, renal function, CBC

Test Interactions False-positive glucosuria with Clinitest®, a falsely high determination of theophylline has occurred and the renal excretion of phenolsulfonphthalein 17-ketosteroids and bromsulfophthalein (BSP) may be inhibited

Dosage Forms Excipient information presented when available (limited, particularly for generics); consult specific product labeling.

Tablet, Oral:

Generic: 500 mg

References

Anderson EJ, Guzman-Cottrill JA, Kletzel M, et al, "High-Risk Adenovirus-Infected Pediatric Allogeneic Hematopoietic Progenitor Cell Transplant Recipients and Preemptive Cidofovir Therapy," *Pediatr Transplant*, 2008, 12(2):219-27.

Bhadri VA, Lee-Horn L, and Shaw PJ, "Safety and Tolerability of Cidofovir in High-Risk Pediatric Patients," *Transpl Infect Dis*, 2009, 11(4):373-9.

Centers for Disease Control and Prevention (CDC), "Sexually Transmitted Diseases Treatment Guidelines, 2010," *MMWR Recomm Rep*, 2010, 59(RR-12):1-110.

Cesaro S, Zhou X, Manzardo C, et al, "Cidofovir for Cytomegalovirus Reactivation in Pediatric Patients After Hematopoietic Stem Cell Transplantation," *J Clin Virol*, 2005, 34(2):129-32.

Doan ML, Mallory GB, Kaplan SL, et al, "Treatment of Adenovirus Pneumonia With Cidofovir in Pediatric Lung Transplant Recipients," *J Heart Lung Transplant*, 2007, 26(9):883-9.

Gutman J, Kachur SP, Slutsker L, et al, "A Clinical Algorithm Identifies Combination of Probenecid-Sulphadoxine-Pyrimethamine for intermittent Preventive Treatment in Pregnancy," *Malar J*, 2012, 11:39.

Ilett KF, Hackett LP, Ingle B, et al, "Transfer of Probenecid and Cephalexin into Breast Milk," *Ann Pharmacother*, 2006, 40(5):986-9.

Williams KM, Agwu AL, Dabb AA, et al, "A Clinical Algorithm Identifies High Risk Pediatric Oncology and Bone Marrow Transplant Patients Likely to Benefit From Treatment of Adenoviral Infection," *J Pediatr Hematol Oncol*, 2009, 31(11):825-31.

Procainamide (pro KANE a mide)

Medication Safety Issues

Sound-alike/look-alike issues:

Procanbid may be confused with probenecid, Procan SR®

Pronestyl may be confused with Ponstel®

High alert medication:

The Institute for Safe Medication Practices (ISMP) includes this medication among its list of drugs which have a heightened risk of causing significant patient harm when used in error.

BEERS Criteria medication:

This drug may be potentially inappropriate for use in geriatric patients (Quality of evidence - high; Strength of recommendation - strong).

Administration issues:

Procainamide hydrochloride is available in 10 mL vials of 100 mg/mL and in 2 mL vials with 500 mg/mL. Note that **BOTH** vials contain 1 gram of drug; confusing the strengths can lead to massive overdoses or underdoses.

Other safety concerns:

PCA is an error-prone abbreviation (mistaken as patient controlled analgesia)

Related Information

Adult ACLS Algorithms *on page 2198*

Medications for Which a Single Dose May Be Fatal When Ingested by a Toddler *on page 2408*

Pediatric ALS (PALS) Algorithms *on page 2195*

Brand Names: Canada Apo-Procainamide®; Procainamide Hydrochloride Injection, USP; Procan SR®

Therapeutic Category Antiarrhythmic Agent, Class I-A

Generic Availability (U.S.) Yes

Use Treatment of life-threatening ventricular arrhythmias (FDA approved in adults); has also been used for treatment of paroxysmal supraventricular tachycardia (PSVT) and symptomatic premature ventricular contractions; and to prevent recurrence of ventricular tachycardia

PALS guidelines: Tachycardia with pulses and poor perfusion (probable SVT [unresponsive to vagal maneuvers and adenosine and/or synchronized cardioversion]; probable VT [unresponsive to synchronized cardioversion or adenosine])

ACLS guidelines: Treatment of the following arrhythmias in patients with preserved left ventricular function: Stable monomorphic VT; pre-excited atrial fibrillation; stable wide complex regular tachycardia (likely VT)

Pregnancy Risk Factor C

Pregnancy Considerations Animal reproduction studies have not been conducted. Procainamide crosses the placenta; procainamide and its active metabolite (N-acetyl procainamide) can be detected in the cord blood and neonatal serum.

Breast-Feeding Considerations Procainamide and its metabolite are found in breast milk and concentrations may be higher than in the maternal serum. In a case report, procainamide was used throughout pregnancy with a dose of 2 g/day prior to delivery. After birth (39 weeks gestation) milk and maternal serum concentrations were obtained over 15 hours of a dosing interval. Mean maternal serum concentrations were procainamide 1.1 mcg/mL and N-acetyl procainamide 1.6 mcg/mL. Mean milk concentrations were procainamide 5.4 mcg/mL and N-acetyl procainamide 3.5 mcg/mL. Due to the potential for adverse events in the nursing infant, breast-feeding is not recommended by the manufacturer.

Contraindications Hypersensitivity to procainamide, procaine, other ester-type local anesthetics, or any component; complete heart block; second degree AV block or various types of hemiblock (without a functional artificial pacemaker); torsade de pointes, SLE

Warnings In the Cardiac Arrhythmia Suppression Trial (CAST), recent (>6 days but <2 years ago) myocardial infarction patients with asymptomatic, nonlife-threatening ventricular arrhythmias did not benefit and may have been harmed by attempts to suppress the arrhythmia with flecainide or encainide **[U.S. Boxed Warning]**. An increased mortality or nonfatal cardiac arrest rate (7.7%) was seen in the active treatment group compared with patients in the placebo group (3%). The applicability of the CAST results to other populations is unknown. Procainamide should be reserved for patients with life-threatening ventricular arrhythmias

Potentially fatal blood dyscrasias (eg, agranulocytosis) have occurred with therapeutic doses **[U.S. Boxed Warning]**; weekly monitoring is recommended during the first 3 months of therapy and periodically thereafter; discontinue procainamide if occurs.

Long-term administration leads to the development of a positive antinuclear antibody (ANA) test in 50% of patients which may lead to a lupus erythematosus-like syndrome (in 20% to 30% of patients) **[U.S. Boxed Warning]**; assess relative benefits and risks if ANA titer becomes positive and consider alternative agent; discontinue procainamide if SLE symptoms develop and change to alternative agent.

Injection solution contains sodium metabisulfite which may cause allergic-type reactions, including anaphylactic symptoms and life-threatening asthmatic episodes in susceptible individuals; more frequently observed in asthmatics.

Precautions Use caution with concurrent use of other antiarrhythmics; may exacerbate or increase the risk of conduction disturbances. Procainamide may increase ventricular response rate in patients with atrial fibrillation or flutter; control AV conduction before initiating. Watch for proarrhythmic effects with procainamide; monitor and adjust dose to prevent QT_c prolongation; avoid use in patients with QT prolongation (ACLS [Neumar, 2010]) and avoid concurrent use with other drugs known to prolong QT_c interval. Reduce dose if first-degree heart block occurs. Correct electrolyte disturbances, especially hypokalemia or hypomagnesemia, prior to use and throughout therapy. Use with caution or avoid (ACLS [Neumar, 2010]) in patients with HF; may precipitate or exacerbate condition due to negative inotropic actions.

Use with caution in patients with renal or hepatic impairment; drug may accumulate; dosage adjustment recommended. Avoid use in myasthenia gravis; may worsen condition. Potentially significant interactions may exist, requiring dose or frequency adjustment, additional monitoring, and/or selection of alternative therapy. Consult drug interactions database for more detailed information.

Adverse Reactions
Cardiovascular: Hypotension
Dermatologic: Rash
Gastrointestinal: Diarrhea, nausea, taste disorder, vomiting
Rare but important or life-threatening: Agranulocytosis, alkaline phosphatase increased, angioedema, anorexia, aplastic anemia, arrhythmia exacerbated, arthralgia, asystole, bone marrow suppression, cerebellar ataxia, confusion, demyelinating polyradiculoneuropathy, disorientation, dizziness, drug fever, fever, first degree heart block, flushing, granulomatous hepatitis, hallucinations, hemolytic anemia, hepatic failure, hyperbilirubinemia, hypoplastic anemia, intrahepatic cholestasis, leukopenia, lightheadedness, maculopapular rash, mania, mental depression, myasthenia gravis worsened, myocardial contractility depressed, myocarditis, myopathy, neuromuscular blockade, neutropenia, pancreatitis, pancytopenia, paradoxical increase in ventricular rate in atrial fibrillation/flutter, peripheral/polyneuropathy, pleural effusion, positive Coombs' test, proarrhythmia, pseudo-

obstruction, psychosis, pulmonary embolism, QT_c-interval prolongation, pruritus, rash, respiratory failure due to myopathy, second-degree heart block, tachycardia, thrombocytopenia, torsade de pointes, transaminases increased, urticaria, vasculitis, ventricular fibrillation, weakness

Drug Interactions
Metabolism/Transport Effects Substrate of CYP2D6 (major); **Note:** Assignment of Major/Minor substrate status based on clinically relevant drug interaction potential

Avoid Concomitant Use
Avoid concomitant use of Procainamide with any of the following: Amiodarone; Fingolimod; Highest Risk QTc-Prolonging Agents; Ivabradine; Mifepristone; Moderate Risk QTc-Prolonging Agents; Propafenone

Increased Effect/Toxicity
Procainamide may increase the levels/effects of: Highest Risk QTc-Prolonging Agents; Neuromuscular-Blocking Agents

The levels/effects of Procainamide may be increased by: Abiraterone Acetate; Amiodarone; Cimetidine; CYP2D6 Inhibitors (Moderate); CYP2D6 Inhibitors (Strong); Darunavir; Fingolimod; Ivabradine; LamoTRIgine; Lurasidone; Mifepristone; Moderate Risk QTc-Prolonging Agents; Propafenone; QTc-Prolonging Agents (Indeterminate Risk and Risk Modifying); Ranitidine; Trimethoprim

Decreased Effect
The levels/effects of Procainamide may be decreased by: Peginterferon Alfa-2b

Food Interactions Acute ethanol administration reduces procainamide serum concentrations. Management: Avoid ethanol.

Stability Store intact vials at 15°C to 30°C (59°F to 86°F). The solution is initially colorless but may turn slightly yellow on standing. Injection of air into the vial causes solution to darken. Discard solutions darker than light amber. Color formation may occur upon refrigeration. When admixed in NS or D_5W to a final concentration of 2 to 4 mg/mL, solution is stable at room temperature for 24 hours and for 7 days under refrigeration.

Mechanism of Action Decreases myocardial excitability and conduction velocity and may depress myocardial contractility, by increasing the electrical stimulation threshold of ventricle, His-Purkinje system and through direct cardiac effects

Pharmacodynamics Onset of action: I.M. 10-30 minutes
Pharmacokinetics (Adult data unless noted)
Distribution: V_d (decreased with CHF or shock):
  Children: 2.2 L/kg
  Adults: 2 L/kg
Protein binding: 15% to 20%
Metabolism: By acetylation in the liver to produce N-acetyl procainamide (NAPA) (active metabolite)
Half-life:
  Procainamide (dependent upon hepatic acetylator phenotype, cardiac function, and renal function):
    Children: 1.7 hours
    Adults with normal renal function: 2.5-4.7 hours
  NAPA (dependent upon renal function):
    Children: 6 hours
    Adults with normal renal function: 6-8 hours
Time to peak serum concentration: I.M.: 15-60 minutes
Elimination: Urinary excretion (25% as NAPA)

Dosing: Neonatal Note: Dose must be individualized and titrated to patient's response; monitor serum concentrations.

Supraventricular tachycardia: Limited data available: I.V.: Loading dose: 7 to 10 mg/kg infused over 60 minutes followed by a continuous I.V. infusion of 20 to 80 **mcg**/kg/minute; a retrospective study of 20 neonates (GA: ≥25 weeks) reported a mean loading dose of 9.6 ± 1.5 mg/kg and a mean continuous infusion rate of 37.56 ± 13.52 **mcg**/kg/minute; **Note:** Procainamide serum concentrations were supratherapeutic in five neonates studied; four of the five were <36 weeks GA and all five had CrCl <30 mL/minute/1.73m^2; these results indicate that doses may need to be decreased in preterm neonates and in those with renal impairment (Moffett, 2006)

Dosing: Usual Note: Dose must be individualized and titrated to patient's response; monitor serum concentrations.

Pediatric: **Antiarrhythmic:** Limited data available:

I.M.: Children and Adolescents: 20 to 30 mg/kg/day divided every 4 to 6 hours; maximum daily dose: 4000 mg/**day** (Nelson, 1996)

I.V., I.O: Infants, Children, and Adolescents:

Loading dose: 10 to 15 mg/kg over 30 to 60 minutes; in adults, maximum dose range: 1000 to 1500 mg (Hegenbarth, 2008; Kliegman, 2011)

Maintenance: Continuous I.V. infusion: 20 to 80 **mcg**/kg/minute; maximum daily dose: 2000 mg/24 hours (Kliegman, 2011)

Stable wide-complex tachycardia of unknown origin (atrial or ventricular) or SVT (PALS [Kleinman, 2010]): Infants, Children, and Adolescents: **Note:** Avoid or use extreme caution when administering procainamide with other drugs that prolong QT interval (eg, amiodarone); consider consulting with cardiology expert

I.V., I.O.: Loading dose: 15 mg/kg infused over 30-60 minutes; monitor ECG and blood pressure; stop the infusion if hypotension occurs or QRS complex widens by >50% of baseline

Adult: **Antiarrhythmic:**

I.M.: 50 mg/kg/day divided every 3 to 6 hours **or** 0.5 to 1 g every 4 to 8 hours (Koch-Weser, 1971)

I.V.: Loading dose: 15 to 18 mg/kg administered as slow infusion over 25 to 30 minutes **or** 100 mg/dose at a rate not to exceed 50 mg/minute repeated every 5 minutes as needed to a total dose of 1000 mg

Hemodynamically stable monomorphic VT or pre-excited atrial fibrillation (ACLS [Neumar, 2010]):

Loading dose: Infuse 20 to 50 mg/minute **or** 100 mg every 5 minutes until arrhythmia controlled, hypotension occurs, QRS complex widens by 50% of its original width, or total of 17 mg/kg is given. Follow with a continuous infusion of 1 to 4 mg/minute. **Note:** Not recommended for use in ongoing ventricular fibrillation (VF) or pulseless ventricular tachycardia (VT) due to prolonged administration time and uncertain efficacy.

Maintenance dose: 1 to 4 mg/minute by continuous I.V. infusion. Maintenance infusions should be reduced by one-third in patients with moderate renal or cardiac impairment and by two-thirds in patients with severe renal or cardiac impairment.

Dosing adjustment in renal impairment:

Infants, Children, and Adolescents: There are no specific recommendations provided in the manufacturer's labeling; dose must be individualized and titrated to patient's response; monitor serum concentrations; some have suggested the following (Aronoff, 2007): **Note:** Renally adjusted dose recommendations are based on a dose of loading dose of 15 mg/kg total.

GFR <10 mL/minute/1.73 m^2:

Loading dose: Reduce dose to 12 mg/kg

Maintenance infusion: Start at lower end of continuous infusion range of 20 to 80 **mcg**/kg/minute

Adults: I.V.:

Loading dose: Reduce dose to 12 mg/kg in severe renal impairment

Maintenance infusion: Reduce dose by one-third in patients with mild renal impairment. Reduce dose by two-thirds in patients with severe renal impairment.

Dialysis: All patients:

Procainamide: Moderately hemodialyzable (20% to 50%): Monitor procainamide/N-acetylprocainamide (NAPA) levels; supplementation may be necessary

NAPA: Not dialyzable (0% to 5%)

Procainamide/NAPA: Not peritoneal dialyzable (0% to 5%)

Procainamide/NAPA: Replace by blood level during continuous arteriovenous or venovenous hemofiltration

Dosing adjustment in hepatic impairment: Reduce dose by 50%.

Administration I.V.: Should dilute prior to I.V. administration to facilitate rate of dosage administration; dilute loading doses to a maximum concentration of 20 to 30 mg/mL (Halpern, 1980; Phelps, 2013) for continuous I.V. infusion, dilute to a usual final concentration of 2 to 4 mg/mL in D$_5$W or NS (Phelps, 2013)

Pediatric: **Note:** Infusion rate should be decreased if QT interval becomes prolonged or patient develops heart block; discontinue the infusion if patient develops hypotension or QRS interval widens to >50% of baseline; severe hypotension can occur with rapid I.V. administration (Hegenbarth, 2008; PALS [Kleinman, 2010])

Neonates: May administer I.V. loading dose over 60 minutes (Moffett, 2006)

Infants and Children: Administer I.V. loading dose over 30 to 60 minutes; not to exceed 50 mg/minute (Hegenberth, 2008; PALS [Kleinman, 2010])

Adolescents: Usual infusion rate: 20 to 50 mg/minute not to exceed 50 mg/minute (Hegenberth, 2008; PALS [Kleinman, 2010]; ACLS [Neumar, 2010])

Adult: Usual rate of infusion: 20 to 50 mg/minute; do not administer faster than 50 mg/minute (ACLS [Neumar, 2010]); severe hypotension can occur with rapid I.V. administration; for continuous I.V. infusion, further dilute to usual final concentration 2 to 8 mg/mL in D$_5$W or NS.

Monitoring Parameters ECG, blood pressure; CBC with differential and platelet counts at weekly intervals for the first 3 months of treatment, periodically thereafter, or if signs of infection, bruising or bleeding occur; antinuclear antibody test (ANA); renal function; serum drug concentrations (procainamide and NAPA) especially in patients with hepatic impairment, renal failure, or those receiving higher maintenance doses (eg, adults: >3 mg/minute) for >24 hours

Reference Range Timing of serum samples: Draw 6 to 12 hours after start of I.V. infusion; half-life is 2.5 to 5 hours in adults

Therapeutic: Optimal ranges must be ascertained for individual patients, with ECG monitoring

Procainamide: 4 to 10 mcg/mL (SI: 15 to 37 micromoles/L)

Sum of procainamide and N-acetyl procainamide: 10 to 30 mcg/mL (SI: <110 micromoles/L)

Toxic (procainamide): >10-12 mcg/mL (SI: >37-44 micromoles/L)

Test Interactions In the presence of propranolol or supra-pharmacologic concentrations of lidocaine or meprobamate, tests which depend on fluorescence to measure procainamide/NAPA concentrations may be affected.

Dosage Forms Excipient information presented when available (limited, particularly for generics); consult specific product labeling.

Solution, Injection, as hydrochloride:

Generic: 100 mg/mL (10 mL); 500 mg/mL (2 mL)

References

Chang PM, Silka MJ, Moromisato DY, et al, "Amiodarone Versus Procainamide for the Acute Treatment of Recurrent Supraventricular Tachycardia in Pediatric Patients," *Circ Arrhythm Electrophysiol*, 2010, 3(2):134-40.

Field JM, Hazinski MF, Sayre MR, et al, "Part 1: Executive Summary: 2010 American Heart Association Guidelines for Cardiopulmonary Resuscitation and Emergency Cardiovascular Care," *Circulation*, 2010, 122(18 Suppl 3):640-56.

Halpern SW, Ellrodt G, Singh BN, Mandel WJ. Efficacy of intravenous procainamide infusion in converting atrial fibrillation to sinus rhythm: relation of left atrial size. *Br Heart J.* 1980;44:589-595.

Hegenbarth MA. American Academy of Pediatrics Committee on Drugs. Preparing for pediatric emergencies: drugs to consider. *Pediatrics.* 2008;121(2):433-443.

Kliegman RM, Stanton BF, St. Gemell JW, et al, eds. *Nelson Textbook of Pediatrics.* 19th ed. Philadelphia, PA: Saunders Elsevier;2011.

Kleinman ME, Chameides L, Schexnayder SM, et al, "Part 14: Pediatric Advanced Life Support: 2010 American Heart Association Guidelines for Cardiopulmonary Resuscitation and Emergency Cardiovascular Care," *Circulation*, 2010, Nov, 122(18 Suppl 3):876-908.

Koch-Weser J and Klein SW, "Procainamide Dosage Schedules, Plasma Concentrations, and Clinical Effects," *JAMA*, 1971, 215 (9):1454-60.

Moffett BS, Cannon BC, Friedman RA, et al, "Therapeutic Levels of Intravenous Procainamide in Neonates: A Retrospective Assessment," *Pharmacotherapy*, 2006, 26(12):1687-93.

Nelson WE, Behrman RE, Kliegman RM, et al, eds. *Nelson Textbook of Pediatrics.* 15th ed. Philadelphia, PA: WB Saunders Company; 1996.

Neumar RW, Otto CW, Link MS, et al, "Part 8: Adult Advanced Cardiovascular Life Support: 2010 American Heart Association Guidelines for Cardiopulmonary Resuscitation and Emergency Cardiovascular Care," *Circulation*, 2010, 122(18 Suppl 3):729-67.

Phelps SJ, Hak EB, Crill CM, eds. *Teddy Bear Book: Pediatric Injectable Drugs.* 10th ed. Bethesda, MD: American Society of Health-System Pharmacists;2013.

Procainamide hydrochloride [prescribing information]. Lake Forest, IL: Hospira, Inc; December 2007.

Singh S, Gelband H, Mehta AV, et al, "Procainamide Elimination Kinetics in Pediatric Patients," *Clin Pharmacol Ther*, 1982, 32 (5):607-11.

◆ **Procainamide Hydrochloride** *see* Procainamide *on page 1740*

◆ **Procainamide Hydrochloride Injection, USP (Can)** *see* Procainamide *on page 1740*

◆ **Procaine Amide Hydrochloride** *see* Procainamide *on page 1740*

◆ **Procaine Benzylpenicillin** *see* Penicillin G Procaine *on page 1634*

◆ **Procaine Penicillin G** *see* Penicillin G Procaine *on page 1634*

◆ **Procanbid** *see* Procainamide *on page 1740*

◆ **Procan SR® (Can)** *see* Procainamide *on page 1740*

Procarbazine (proe KAR ba zeen)

Medication Safety Issues
Sound-alike/look-alike issues:
Procarbazine may be confused with dacarbazine
High alert medication:
This medication is in a class the Institute for Safe Medication Practices (ISMP) includes among its list of drug classes which have a heightened risk of causing significant patient harm when used in error.

Related Information
Emetogenic Potential of Antineoplastic Agents in Children *on page 2327*

Oral Medications That Should Not Be Crushed or Altered *on page 2438*

Safe Handling of Hazardous Drugs *on page 2419*

Brand Names: U.S. Matulane

Brand Names: Canada Matulane; Natulan

Therapeutic Category Antineoplastic Agent, Miscellaneous

Generic Availability (U.S.) No

Use Treatment of Hodgkin lymphoma [FDA approved in pediatrics (age not specified) and adults]

Pregnancy Risk Factor D

Pregnancy Considerations Adverse events were observed in animal reproduction studies. There are case reports of fetal malformations in the offspring of pregnant women exposed to procarbazine as part of a combination chemotherapy regimen. Women of reproductive potential should avoid becoming pregnant during treatment.

Breast-Feeding Considerations It is not known if procarbazine is excreted in breast milk. Due to the potential for serious adverse reactions in the nursing infant, nursing is not recommended during treatment with procarbazine.

Contraindications Hypersensitivity to procarbazine or any component; inadequate bone marrow reserve

Warnings Hazardous agent; use appropriate precautions for handling and disposal (NIOSH, 2012). Hematologic toxicity (leukopenia and thrombocytopenia) may occur 2-8 weeks after treatment initiation; allow ≥1 month interval between radiation therapy or myelosuppressive chemotherapy and initiation of treatment. Withhold treatment for leukopenia (WBC <4000/mm^3) or thrombocytopenia (platelets <100,000/mm^3), hemorrhage, or bleeding tendencies; monitor for infections due to neutropenia. May cause hemolysis and/or presence of Heinz inclusion bodies in erythrocytes.

Procarbazine is associated with a high emetic potential; antiemetics are recommended to prevent nausea and vomiting. May cause diarrhea and stomatitis; withhold treatment for diarrhea or stomatitis. Azoospermia and infertility have been reported with procarbazine when used in combination with other chemotherapy agents. May cause secondary malignancies and is possibly carcinogenic; acute myeloid leukemia and lung cancer have been reported following use. Withhold treatment for hypersensitivity reactions or CNS toxicity (paresthesias, neuropathies, confusion). In pediatric patients, undue toxicity characterized as tremors, coma, and convulsions have been reported rarely; monitor closely with use.

Precautions Use with caution in renal or hepatic impairment; may result in increased toxicity. Avoid ethanol consumption; may cause disulfiram-like reaction. Procarbazine possesses MAO inhibitor activity and has potential for severe drug and food interactions; follow MAOI diet (avoid tyramine-containing foods). May potentiate CNS depression when used with phenothiazine derivatives, barbiturates, opioids, tricyclic antidepressants, or methyldopa. Potentially significant interactions may exist, requiring dose or frequency adjustment, additional monitoring, and/or selection of alternative therapy. Consult drug interactions database for more detailed information. Should be administered under the supervision of an experienced cancer chemotherapy physician **[U.S. Boxed Warning]**.

Adverse Reactions
Cardiovascular: Edema, flushing, hypotension, syncope, tachycardia

Central nervous system: Apprehension, ataxia, chills, coma, confusion, depression, dizziness, drowsiness, falling, fatigue, hallucination, headache, hyporeflexia, insomnia, lethargy, nervousness, neuropathy, nightmares, pain, paresthesia, seizure, slurred speech, unsteadiness

Dermatologic: Alopecia, dermatitis, diaphoresis, hyperpigmentation, pruritus, skin rash, urticaria

Endocrine & metabolic: Gynecomastia (in prepubertal and early pubertal males)

Gastrointestinal: Abdominal pain, anorexia, constipation, diarrhea, dysphagia, hematemesis, melena, nausea and vomiting (increasing the dose in a stepwise fashion over several days may minimize), stomatitis, xerostomia

Genitourinary: Azoospermia (reported with combination chemotherapy), hematuria, nocturia, reduced fertility

Hematologic & oncologic: Anemia, bone marrow depression, eosinophilia, hemolysis (in patients with G6PD deficiency), hemolytic anemia, malignant neoplasm (secondary; nonlymphoid; reported with combination therapy), pancytopenia, petechia, purpura, thrombocytopenia

Hepatic: Hepatic insufficiency, jaundice

Hypersensitivity: Hypersensitivity reaction

Infection: Herpes virus infection, increased susceptibility to infection

Neuromuscular & skeletal: Arthralgia, foot-drop, myalgia, tremor, weakness

Ophthalmic: Accommodation disturbance, diplopia, nystagmus, papilledema, photophobia, retinal hemorrhage

Otic: Hearing loss

Renal: Polyuria

Respiratory: Cough, epistaxis, hemoptysis, hoarseness, pleural effusion, pneumonitis, pulmonary toxicity

Miscellaneous: Fever

Drug Interactions

Metabolism/Transport Effects Inhibits Monoamine Oxidase

Avoid Concomitant Use

Avoid concomitant use of Procarbazine with any of the following: Alpha-/Beta-Agonists (Indirect-Acting); Alpha1-Agonists; Amphetamines; Anilidopiperidine Opioids; Antidepressants (Serotonin Reuptake Inhibitor/Antagonist); Apraclonidine; AtoMOXetine; BCG; Bezafibrate; Buprenorphine; BuPROPion; BusPIRone; CarBAMazepine; CloZAPine; Cyclobenzaprine; Cyproheptadine; Dexmethylphenidate; Dextromethorphan; Diethylpropion; Dipyrone; Hydrocodone; HYDROmorphone; Isometheptene; Levonordefrin; Linezolid; Maprotiline; Meperidine; Methyldopa; Methylene Blue; Methylphenidate; Mirtazapine; Morphine (Liposomal); Morphine (Systemic); Natalizumab; Oxymorphone; Pholcodine; Pimecrolimus; Pizotifen; Selective Serotonin Reuptake Inhibitors; Serotonin 5-HT1D Receptor Agonists; Serotonin/Norepinephrine Reuptake Inhibitors; Tacrolimus (Topical); Tapentadol; Tetrabenazine; Tetrahydrozoline (Nasal); Tofacitinib; Tricyclic Antidepressants; Tryptophan; Vaccines (Live)

Increased Effect/Toxicity

Procarbazine may increase the levels/effects of: Alpha-/Beta-Agonists (Indirect-Acting); Alpha1-Agonists; Amphetamines; Antidepressants (Serotonin Reuptake Inhibitor/Antagonist); Antihypertensives; Antipsychotics; Apraclonidine; AtoMOXetine; Beta2-Agonists; Betahistine; Bezafibrate; Brimonidine (Ophthalmic); Brimonidine (Topical); BuPROPion; Carbocisteine; CloZAPine; Cyproheptadine; Dexmethylphenidate; Dextromethorphan; Diethylpropion; Domperidone; Doxapram; Doxylamine; EPINEPHrine (Nasal); Epinephrine (Racemic); EPINEPHrine (Systemic, Oral Inhalation); Hydrocodone; HYDROmorphone; Hypoglycemic Agents; Isometheptene; Leflunomide; Levonordefrin; Linezolid; Lithium; Meperidine; Methadone; Methyldopa; Methylene Blue; Methylphenidate; Metoclopramide; Mirtazapine; Morphine (Liposomal); Morphine (Systemic); Natalizumab; Norepinephrine; Orthostatic Hypotension Producing Agents; OxyCODONE; Pizotifen; Reserpine; Selective Serotonin Reuptake Inhibitors; Serotonin 5-HT1D Receptor Agonists; Serotonin Modulators; Serotonin/Norepinephrine Reuptake Inhibitors; Tetrahydrozoline (Nasal); Tofacitinib; Tricyclic Antidepressants; Vaccines (Live); Vitamin K Antagonists

The levels/effects of Procarbazine may be increased by: Altretamine; Anilidopiperidine Opioids; Antiemetics (5HT3 Antagonists); Antipsychotics; Buprenorphine; BusPIRone; CarBAMazepine; COMT Inhibitors; Cyclobenzaprine; Denosumab; Dipyrone; Levodopa; MAO Inhibitors; Maprotiline; Oxymorphone; Pholcodine; Pimecrolimus; Roflumilast; Tacrolimus (Topical); Tapentadol; Tetrabenazine; TraMADol; Trastuzumab; Tryptophan

Decreased Effect

Procarbazine may decrease the levels/effects of: BCG; Cardiac Glycosides; Coccidioidin Skin Test; Domperidone; Sipuleucel-T; Vaccines (Inactivated); Vaccines (Live); Vitamin K Antagonists

The levels/effects of Procarbazine may be decreased by: Cyproheptadine; Domperidone; Echinacea

Food Interactions

Ethanol: Ethanol may cause a disulfiram reaction. Management: Avoid ethanol.

Food: Concurrent ingestion of foods rich in tyramine, dopamine, tyrosine, phenylalanine, tryptophan, or caffeine may cause sudden and severe high blood pressure (hypertensive crisis or serotonin syndrome). Management: Avoid tyramine-containing foods (aged or matured cheese; air-dried or cured meats including sausages and salamis; fava or broad bean pods, tap/draft beers, Marmite concentrate, sauerkraut, soy sauce, and other soybean condiments). Food's freshness is also an important concern; improperly stored or spoiled food can create an environment in which tyramine concentrations may increase. Avoid foods containing dopamine, tyrosine, phenylalanine, tryptophan, or caffeine.

Stability Protect from light.

Mechanism of Action Inhibits DNA, RNA, and protein synthesis by inhibiting transmethylation of methionine into transfer RNA; may also damage DNA directly through alkylation.

Pharmacokinetics (Adult data unless noted)

Absorption: Oral: Well absorbed

Distribution: Crosses the blood-brain barrier and distributes into CSF, liver, kidney, intestine, and skin

Metabolism: In the liver; first-pass conversion to cytotoxic metabolites

Half-life: 10 minutes

Time to peak serum concentration: Within 1 hour

Elimination: In urine (<5% as unchanged drug) and 70% as metabolites

Dosing: Usual Note: Refer to individual protocols for specific dosage and interval information. Procarbazine is associated with a high emetic potential; antiemetics are recommended to prevent nausea and vomiting. The manufacturer suggests that an estimated lean body mass be used in obese patients and patients with rapid weight gain due to edema, ascites, or abnormal fluid retention.

Pediatric: **Hodgkin lymphoma:** Oral:

MOPP regimen: **Note:** While procarbazine is approved as part of the MOPP regimen, the MOPP regimen is generally no longer used due to improved toxicity profiles with other combination regimens used in the treatment of Hodgkin lymphoma (Kelly, 2012). Manufacturer's labeling:: Infants, Children, and Adolescents: 50-100 mg/m^2/day once daily for 14 days of a 28-day cycle (Longo, 1986).

BEACOPP regimen: Limited data available: Children and Adolescents: 100 mg/m^2 days 0-6 of a 21-day treatment cycle (in combination with bleomycin, etoposide, doxorubicin, cyclophosphamide, vincristine, and prednisone) for 4 cycles (Kelly, 2011)

Adult: **Hodgkin lymphoma:** Oral:

MOPP regimen: While procarbazine is approved as part of the MOPP regimen, the MOPP regimen is generally no longer used due to improved toxicity profiles with other combination regimens used in the treatment of Hodgkin lymphoma.

BEACOPP, standard or escalated regimen: Limited data available: 100 mg/m^2 days 1-7 every 21 days (in combination with bleomycin, etoposide, doxorubicin, cyclophosphamide, vincristine, and prednisone) for 8 cycles (Diehl, 2003)

Dosing adjustment in renal impairment: All patients: There are no dosage adjustments provided in manufacturer's labeling; use with caution; may result in increased toxicity. However, because predominantly inactive metabolites are excreted via the kidneys, dosage adjustment is not necessary (Kintzel, 1995).

Dosing adjustment in hepatic impairment: All patients: There are no dosage adjustments provided in manufacturer's labeling; use with caution; may result in increased toxicity. The following adjustments have been reported in literature:

Floyd, 2006:
Transaminases 1.6-6 times ULN: Administer 75% of dose
Transaminases >6 times ULN: Use clinical judgment
Serum bilirubin >5 mg/dL or transaminases >3 times ULN: Avoid use
King, 2001: Adults: Serum bilirubin >5 mg/dL or transaminases >180 units/L: Avoid use

Administration Hazardous agent; use appropriate precautions for handling and disposal (NIOSH, 2012).

Oral: Total daily dose may be administered as a single daily dose or in divided doses throughout the day to minimize GI toxicity. Procarbazine is associated with a high emetic potential; antiemetics are recommended to prevent nausea and vomiting.

Monitoring Parameters CBC with differential, platelet and reticulocyte count (at least every 3-4 days); also urinalysis (weekly), liver function test (prior to therapy and weekly), renal function test (prior to therapy and weekly), alkaline phosphatase (weekly). Monitor for infections, CNS toxicity, and gastrointestinal toxicities.

Dosage Forms Excipient information presented when available (limited, particularly for generics); consult specific product labeling.

Capsule, Oral, as hydrochloride:
Matulane: 50 mg

Extemporaneous Preparations Hazardous agent: Use appropriate precautions for handling and disposal.

A 10 mg/mL oral suspension may be prepared using capsules, glycerin, and strawberry syrup. Empty the contents of ten 50 mg capsules into a mortar. Add 2 mL glycerin and mix to a thick uniform paste. Add 10 mL strawberry syrup in incremental proportions; mix until uniform. Transfer the mixture to an amber glass bottle and rinse mortar with small amounts of strawberry syrup; add rinses to the bottle in sufficient quantity to make 50 mL. Label "shake well" and "protect from light". Stable for 7 days at room temperature.

Matulane® data on file, Sigma Tau Pharmaceuticals, Inc.

References

Diehl V, Franklin J, Pfreundschuh M, et al. Standard and increased-dose BEACOPP chemotherapy compared with COPP-ABVD for advanced Hodgkin's disease. *N Engl J Med.* 2003;348 (24):2386-2395.

Floyd J, Mirza I, Sachs B, Perry MC. Hepatotoxicity of chemotherapy. *Semin Oncol.* 2006;33(1):50-67.

Kelly KM, Sposto R, Hutchinson R, et al. BEACOPP chemotherapy is a highly effective regimen in children and adolescents with high-risk Hodgkin lymphoma: a report from the Children's Oncology Group. *Blood.* 2011;117(9):2596-2603.

King PD, Perry MC. Hepatotoxicity of chemotherapy. *Oncologist.* 2001;6(2):162-176.

Kintzel PE, Dorr RT. Anticancer drug renal toxicity and elimination: dosing guidelines for altered renal function. *Cancer Treat Rev.* 1995;21(1):33-64.

Longo DL, Young RC, Wesley M, et al, "Twenty Years of MOPP Therapy for Hodgkin's Disease," *J Clin Oncol,* 1986, 4(9):1295-306.

National Institute for Occupational Safety and Health (NIOSH), "NIOSH List of Antineoplastic and Other Hazardous Drugs in Healthcare Settings 2012." Available at http://www.cdc.gov/niosh/docs/2012-150/pdfs/2012-150.pdf. Accessed January 21, 2013.

Rodriguez LA, Prados M, Silver P, et al, "Re-evaluation of Procarbazine for the Treatment of Recurrent Malignant Central Nervous System Tumors," *Cancer,* 1989, 64(12):2420-3.

◆ **Procarbazine Hydrochloride** *see* Procarbazine *on page 1743*

◆ **Procardia** *see* NIFEdipine *on page 1497*

◆ **Procardia XL** *see* NIFEdipine *on page 1497*

◆ **PRO-Cefadroxil (Can)** *see* Cefadroxil *on page 392*

◆ **PRO-Cefuroxime (Can)** *see* Cefuroxime *on page 422*

◆ **ProCentra** *see* Dextroamphetamine *on page 629*

Prochlorperazine (proe klor PER a zeen)

Medication Safety Issues
Sound-alike/look-alike issues:
Prochlorperazine may be confused with chlorproMAZINE
Compazine may be confused with Copaxone, Coumadin

BEERS Criteria medication:
This drug may be potentially inappropriate for use in geriatric patients (Quality of evidence - varies based on comorbidity; Strength of recommendation - varies based on comorbidity)

Other safety concerns:
CPZ (occasional abbreviation for Compazine) is an error-prone abbreviation (mistaken as chlorpromazine)

Brand Names: U.S. Compazine; Compro

Brand Names: Canada Apo-Prochlorperazine; Nu-Prochlor; PMS-Prochlorperazine; Sandoz-Prochlorperazine

Therapeutic Category Antiemetic; Antipsychotic Agent, Typical, Phenothiazine; Phenothiazine Derivative

Generic Availability (U.S.) Yes

Use
Oral: Management of nonsurgical nausea and vomiting [FDA approved in ages ≥2 years (and at least 9 kg) and adults]; management of surgery-related nausea and vomiting (FDA approved in adults); treatment of acute and chronic psychosis [FDA approved in ages ≥2 years (and at least 9 kg) and adults]; has also been used for treatment of intractable migraine headaches

Parenteral: Management of severe nonsurgical nausea and vomiting [FDA approved in ages ≥2 years (and at least 9 kg) and adults]; treatment of schizophrenia [FDA approved in ages ≥2 years (and at least 9 kg) and adults]

Rectal: Management of severe nausea and vomiting (FDA approved in adults)

Pregnancy Considerations Jaundice or hyper-/hyporeflexia have been reported in newborn infants following maternal use of phenothiazines. Antipsychotic use during the third trimester of pregnancy has a risk for abnormal muscle movements (extrapyramidal symptoms [EPS]) and withdrawal symptoms in newborns following delivery. Symptoms in the newborn may include agitation, feeding disorder, hypertonia, hypotonia, respiratory distress, somnolence, and tremor; these effects may be self-limiting or require hospitalization. Use may interfere with pregnancy tests, causing false positive results. Prochlorperazine has been used for the treatment of nausea and vomiting associated with pregnancy (Levicheck, 2002; Mahadevan, 2006); however, other agents may be preferred (ACOG, 2004).

Breast-Feeding Considerations Other phenothiazines are excreted in human milk; excretion of prochlorperazine is not known.

Contraindications Hypersensitivity to prochlorperazine or any component; cross-sensitivity with other phenothiazines may exist; avoid use in patients with narrow-angle glaucoma; severe liver or cardiac disease, severe toxic CNS depression or coma

Additional contraindications for pediatric patients: Infants and children <2 years or <9 kg (20 pounds); management of postoperative nausea and vomiting (pediatric surgery); pediatric conditions for which dosing not described

◀ **Warnings** High incidence of extrapyramidal reactions especially in children, reserve use in children <5 years of age to those who are unresponsive to other antiemetics; incidence of extrapyramidal reactions is increased with acute illnesses such as chicken pox, measles, CNS infections, gastroenteritis, and dehydration; extrapyramidal reactions may also be confused with CNS signs of Reye's syndrome or other encephalopathies; avoid use in these clinical conditions

Lowers seizure threshold, use cautiously in patients with seizure history; discontinue use at least 48 hours before myelography and do not resume therapy until 24 hours post myelography. Use of antipsychotics in combination with lithium has been associated with an encephalopathy syndrome similar to NMS; monitor patients closely and discontinue treatment if encephalopathic symptomatology develops. Impaired core body temperature regulation may occur; caution with strenuous exercise, heat exposure, dehydration, and concomitant medication possessing anticholinergic effects. May cause sedation; effects may be potentiated when used with other sedative drugs or ethanol; may impair physical or mental abilities; patients must be cautioned about performing tasks which require mental alertness (eg, operating machinery or driving).

Leukopenia, neutropenia, and agranulocytosis (sometimes fatal) have been reported in clinical trials and postmarketing reports with antipsychotic use; presence of risk factors (eg, preexisting low WBC or history of drug-induced leuko/neutropenia) should prompt periodic blood count assessment. Discontinue therapy at first signs of blood dyscrasias or if absolute neutrophil count <1000/mm^3.

An increased risk of death has been reported with the use of antipsychotics in elderly patients with dementia-related psychosis **[U.S. Boxed Warning]**; most deaths seemed to be cardiovascular (eg, sudden death, heart failure) or infectious (eg, pneumonia) in nature; prochlorperazine is not approved for this indication.

Injection contains benzyl alcohol which may cause allergic reactions in susceptible individuals; large amounts of benzyl alcohol (≥99 mg/kg/day) have been associated with a potentially fatal toxicity ("gasping syndrome") in neonates; the "gasping syndrome" consists of metabolic acidosis, respiratory distress, gasping respirations, CNS dysfunction (including convulsions, intracranial hemorrhage), hypotension and cardiovascular collapse; avoid use of injection in neonates.

Precautions Use with caution in hepatic and renal impairment. Use with caution in patients at risk for hypotension or in those who would not tolerate transient hypotensive episodes (cerebrovascular disease, cardiovascular disease, hypovolemia, or concurrent medication use which may predispose to hypotension/bradycardia; hypotension may occur following administration, particularly when parenteral form is used or in high dosages; may also cause orthostatic hypotension.

Use with caution in patients with decreased gastrointestinal motility, paralytic ileus, urinary retention, BPH, xerostomia, or visual problems; may cause anticholinergic effects (constipation, xerostomia, blurred vision, urinary retention). Use with caution in patients with narrow-angle glaucoma or myasthenia gravis; condition may be exacerbated by cholinergic blockade. Use with caution in patients with Parkinson's disease; patients may be more sensitive to adverse effects. Use with caution in patients at risk of pneumonia (ie, Alzheimer's disease); antipsychotic use has been associated with esophageal dysmotility and aspiration. Use associated with increased prolactin levels; clinical significance of hyperprolactinemia in patients with breast cancer or other prolactin-dependent tumors is unknown.

Adverse Reactions Reported with prochlorperazine or other phenothiazines.

Cardiovascular: Cardiac arrest, cerebral edema, hypotension, peripheral edema, Q-wave distortions, sudden death, T-wave distortions

Central nervous system: Agitation, altered cerebrospinal fluid proteins, catatonia, coma, cough reflex suppressed, dizziness, drowsiness, fever (mild [I.M.]), headache, hyperpyrexia, impairment of temperature regulation, insomnia, neuroleptic malignant syndrome (NMS), oculogyric crisis, opisthotonos, restlessness, seizure, somnolence, tremulousness

Dermatologic: Angioedema, contact dermatitis, epithelial keratopathy, erythema, eczema, exfoliative dermatitis, itching, photosensitivity, skin pigmentation, urticaria

Endocrine & metabolic: Amenorrhea, galactorrhea, gynecomastia, glucosuria, hyper-/hypoglycemia, lactation, libido (changes in), menstrual irregularity

Gastrointestinal: Appetite increased, atonic colon, constipation, ileus, nausea, obstipation, vomiting, weight gain, xerostomia

Genitourinary: Ejaculating dysfunction, ejaculatory disturbances, impotence, priapism, urinary retention

Hematologic: Agranulocytosis, aplastic anemia, eosinophilia, hemolytic anemia, leukopenia, pancytopenia, thrombocytopenic purpura

Hepatic: Biliary stasis, cholestatic jaundice, hepatotoxicity

Neuromuscular & skeletal: Dystonias (torticollis, carpopedal spasm, trismus, protrusion of tongue); extrapyramidal symptoms (pseudoparkinsonism, akathisia, dystonias, tardive dyskinesia, hyperreflexia); SLE-like syndrome, tremor

Ocular: Blurred vision, lenticular/corneal deposits, miosis, mydriasis, pigmentary retinopathy

Respiratory: Asthma, laryngeal edema, nasal congestion

Miscellaneous: Allergic reactions, asphyxia, diaphoresis

Drug Interactions

Metabolism/Transport Effects None known.

Avoid Concomitant Use

Avoid concomitant use of Prochlorperazine with any of the following: Aclidinium; Amisulpride; Azelastine (Nasal); Dofetilide; Ipratropium (Oral Inhalation); Metoclopramide; Paraldehyde; Potassium Chloride; Sulpiride; Thalidomide; Tiotropium; Umeclidinium

Increased Effect/Toxicity

Prochlorperazine may increase the levels/effects of: AbobotulinumtoxinA; Alcohol (Ethyl); Amisulpride; Analgesics (Opioid); Anticholinergic Agents; Antidepressants (Serotonin Reuptake Inhibitor/Antagonist); Azelastine (Nasal); Beta-Blockers; Buprenorphine; Cannabinoid-Containing Products; CNS Depressants; Dofetilide; Hydrocodone; Methotrimeprazine; Methylphenidate; Metyrosine; Mirabegron; Mirtazapine; OnabotulinumtoxinA; Paraldehyde; Porfimer; Potassium Chloride; RimabotulinumtoxinB; Selective Serotonin Reuptake Inhibitors; Serotonin Modulators; Sulpiride; Thalidomide; Thiazide Diuretics; Thiopental; Tiotropium; Topiramate; Zolpidem

The levels/effects of Prochlorperazine may be increased by: Acetylcholinesterase Inhibitors (Central); Aclidinium; Antidepressants (Serotonin Reuptake Inhibitor/Antagonist); Antimalarial Agents; Beta-Blockers; Brimonidine (Topical); Cannabis; Deferoxamine; Doxylamine; Dronabinol; Droperidol; HydrOXYzine; Ipratropium (Oral Inhalation); Kava Kava; Lithium; Magnesium Sulfate; Methotrimeprazine; Methylphenidate; Metoclopramide; Metyrosine; Nabilone; Perampanel; Pramlintide; Rufinamide; Serotonin Modulators; Sodium Oxybate; Tapentadol; Tetrabenazine; Tetrahydrocannabinol; Umeclidinium

Decreased Effect

Prochlorperazine may decrease the levels/effects of: Acetylcholinesterase Inhibitors (Central); Amphetamines;

Anti-Parkinson's Agents (Dopamine Agonist); Quinagolide; Secretin

The levels/effects of Prochlorperazine may be decreased by: Acetylcholinesterase Inhibitors (Central); Antacids; Anti-Parkinson's Agents (Dopamine Agonist); Lithium

Stability All dosage forms: Store at controlled room temperature; protect from light. With injection, a clear or slightly yellow solution may be used; incompatible with aminophylline, amphotericin B, ampicillin, calcium salts, cephalothin, foscarnet (Y-site), furosemide, hydrocortisone, hydromorphone, methohexital, midazolam, penicillin G, pentobarbital, phenobarbital, thiopental

Mechanism of Action Prochlorperazine is a piperazine phenothiazine antipsychotic which blocks postsynaptic mesolimbic dopaminergic D_1 and D_2 receptors in the brain, including the chemoreceptor trigger zone; exhibits a strong alpha-adrenergic and anticholinergic blocking effect and depresses the release of hypothalamic and hypophyseal hormones; believed to depress the reticular activating system, thus affecting basal metabolism, body temperature, wakefulness, vasomotor tone and emesis

Pharmacodynamics

Onset of action:
Oral: 30-40 minutes
I.M.: Within 10-20 minutes
Rectal: Within 60 minutes

Duration:
I.M.: 3-4 hours
Rectal, oral immediate release: 3-4 hours

Dosing: Usual

Children and Adolescents: **Note:** Use lowest possible dose in pediatric patients to decrease incidence of extrapyramidal reactions

Antiemetic: Children ≥2 years and weight ≥9 kg and Adolescents:

Oral:
9-13 kg: 2.5 mg every 12-24 hours as needed; maximum daily dose: 7.5 mg/**day**
>13-18 kg: 2.5 mg every 8-12 hours as needed; maximum daily dose: 10 mg/**day**
>18-39 kg: 2.5 mg every 8 hours **or** 5 mg every 12 hours as needed; maximum daily dose: 15 mg/**day**
>39 kg: 5-10 mg every 6-8 hours; usual maximum daily dose: 40 mg/**day**

Parenteral (as edisylate): Administer based upon patient response, typically every 8-12 hours; convert to oral therapy as soon as possible.
Manufacturer's labeling: I.M.: 0.13 mg/kg/dose; maximum single dose: 10 mg
Alternate dosing: I.M., I.V.: 0.1-0.15 mg/kg/dose; maximum single dose: 10 mg

Migraine, intractable: Limited data available: Children ≥8 years and Adolescents: I.V. (as edisylate): 0.1-0.15 mg/kg as a single dose has been studied in 20 children between the ages of 8-17 years combined with I.V. hydration (Kabbouche, 2001)

Psychoses; schizophrenia: Children 2-12 years and ≥9 kg:

Oral: 2.5 mg every 8-12 hours; initial maximum daily dose: 10 mg/day on first day; may increase dosage as needed; maximum daily dose: Children 2-5 years: 20 mg/**day**; Children 6-12 years: 25 mg/**day**
I.M. (as edisylate): 0.13 mg/kg/dose, control usually obtained with single dose; change to oral as soon as possible

Adults:

Antiemetic:

Oral (tablet): 5-10 mg 3-4 times/**day**; usual maximum: 40 mg/day; larger doses may rarely be required
I.M. (as edisylate): 5-10 mg every 3-4 hours; usual maximum: 40 mg/**day**

I.V. (as edisylate): 2.5-10 mg; maximum: 10 mg/dose or 40 mg/**day**; may repeat dose every 3-4 hours as needed
Rectal: 25 mg twice daily

Surgical nausea/vomiting: Note: Should not exceed 40 mg/**day**:

I.M. (as edisylate): 5-10 mg 1-2 hours before induction or to control symptoms during or after surgery; may repeat once if necessary
I.V. (as edisylate): 5-10 mg 15-30 minutes before induction or to control symptoms during or after surgery; may repeat once if necessary

Antipsychotic:

Oral: 5-10 mg 3-4 times/day; titrate dose slowly every 2-3 days; doses up to 150 mg/**day** may be required in some patients for treatment of severe disturbances
I.M. (as edisylate): Initial: 10-20 mg; if necessary repeat initial dose every 1-4 hours to gain control; more than 3-4 doses are rarely needed. If parenteral administration is still required, give 10-20 mg every 4-6 hours; change to oral as soon as possible.

Nonpsychotic anxiety: Oral (tablet): Usual dose: 15-20 mg/**day** in divided doses; do not give doses >20 mg/**day** or for longer than 12 weeks

Administration

Oral: Administer with food or water
Parenteral: I.M. is preferred; avoid I.V. administration; if necessary, may be administered by direct I.V. injection at a maximum rate of 5 mg/minute; do not administer by SubQ route (tissue damage may occur)

Monitoring Parameters CBC with differential and periodic ophthalmic exams (if chronically used)

Test Interactions False-positives for phenylketonuria, pregnancy

Additional Information Previously recommended rectal dosages in pediatric patients were similar to the oral formulation dosages; however, an appropriate dosage form for rectal administration to pediatric patients is no longer available in the U.S.

Dosage Forms Excipient information presented when available (limited, particularly for generics); consult specific product labeling.

Solution, Injection, as edisylate [strength expressed as base]:
Generic: 5 mg/mL (2 mL, 10 mL)

Suppository, Rectal:
Compazine: 25 mg (12 ea)
Compro: 25 mg (12 ea)
Generic: 25 mg (12 ea, 1000 ea)

Tablet, Oral, as maleate [strength expressed as base]:
Compazine: 5 mg, 10 mg
Generic: 5 mg, 10 mg

References

American College of Obstetrics and Gynecology. ACOG practice bulletin: nausea and vomiting of pregnancy. *Obstet Gynecol.* 2004;103 (4):803-814.

Kabbouche MA, Vockell AL, LeCates SL, et al, "Tolerability and Effectiveness of Prochlorperazine for Intractable Migraine in Children," *Pediatrics,* 2001, 107(4):E62, www.pediatrics.org/cgi/content/full/107/4/e62.

Levichek Z, Atanackovic G, Oepkes D, et al. Nausea and vomiting of pregnancy. Evidence-based treatment algorithm. *Can Fam Physician.* 2002;48:267-268, 277.

Mahadevan U, Kane S. American Gastroenterological Association Institute technical review on the use of gastrointestinal medications in pregnancy. *Gastroenterology.* 2006;131(1):283-311.

◆ **Prochlorperazine Edisylate** *see* Prochlorperazine *on page 1745*

◆ **Prochlorperazine Maleate** *see* Prochlorperazine *on page 1745*

◆ **Prochlorperazine Mesylate** *see* Prochlorperazine *on page 1745*

- ◆ **PRO-Ciprofloxacin (Can)** *see* Ciprofloxacin (Systemic) *on page 471*
- ◆ **PRO-Clonazepam (Can)** *see* ClonazePAM *on page 514*
- ◆ **Procrit** *see* Epoetin Alfa *on page 766*
- ◆ **Proctocort** *see* Hydrocortisone (Topical) *on page 1038*
- ◆ **Procto-Pak** *see* Hydrocortisone (Topical) *on page 1038*
- ◆ **Proctosol HC** *see* Hydrocortisone (Topical) *on page 1038*
- ◆ **Proctozone-HC** *see* Hydrocortisone (Topical) *on page 1038*
- ◆ **Procysbi™** *see* Cysteamine (Systemic) *on page 571*
- ◆ **Procysbi** *see* Cysteamine (Systemic) *on page 571*
- ◆ **Procytox (Can)** *see* Cyclophosphamide *on page 561*
- ◆ **PRO-Dexamethasone (Can)** *see* Dexamethasone (Systemic) *on page 615*
- ◆ **PRO-Diclo-Rapide (Can)** *see* Diclofenac (Systemic) *on page 645*
- ◆ **PRO-Enalapril (Can)** *see* Enalapril *on page 744*
- ◆ **Profilnine SD** *see* Factor IX Complex (Human) [(Factors II, IX, X)] *on page 833*
- ◆ **Proflavanol C™ (Can)** *see* Ascorbic Acid *on page 206*
- ◆ **PRO-Fluconazole (Can)** *see* Fluconazole *on page 877*
- ◆ **PRO-Fluoxetine (Can)** *see* FLUoxetine *on page 901*
- ◆ **PRO-Gabapentin (Can)** *see* Gabapentin *on page 950*
- ◆ **PRO-Glyburide (Can)** *see* GlyBURIDE *on page 974*
- ◆ **Proglycem** *see* Diazoxide *on page 643*
- ◆ **Proglycem® (Can)** *see* Diazoxide *on page 643*
- ◆ **Prograf** *see* Tacrolimus (Systemic) *on page 1963*
- ◆ **Proguanil and Atovaquone** *see* Atovaquone and Proguanil *on page 231*
- ◆ **Proguanil Hydrochloride and Atovaquone** *see* Atovaquone and Proguanil *on page 231*
- ◆ **PRO-Hydroxyquine (Can)** *see* Hydroxychloroquine *on page 1048*
- ◆ **Pro-Indo (Can)** *see* Indomethacin *on page 1096*
- ◆ **Prokine** *see* Sargramostim *on page 1870*
- ◆ **Proleukin** *see* Aldesleukin *on page 90*
- ◆ **Proleukin® (Can)** *see* Aldesleukin *on page 90*
- ◆ **PRO-Levetiracetam (Can)** *see* LevETIRAcetam *on page 1219*
- ◆ **PRO-Lisinopril (Can)** *see* Lisinopril *on page 1262*
- ◆ **PRO-Lorazepam (Can)** *see* LORazepam *on page 1280*
- ◆ **PRO-Lovastatin (Can)** *see* Lovastatin *on page 1286*
- ◆ **PRO-Metformin (Can)** *see* MetFORMIN *on page 1353*

Promethazine (proe METH a zeen)

Medication Safety Issues

Sound-alike/look-alike issues:

Promethazine may be confused with chlorproMAZINE, predniSONE

Phenergan® may be confused with PHENobarbital, Phrenilin®, Theragran

High alert medication:

The Institute for Safe Medication Practices (ISMP) includes this medication (I.V. formulation) among its list of drugs which have a heightened risk of causing significant patient harm when used in error.

BEERS Criteria medication:

This drug may be potentially inappropriate for use in geriatric patients (Quality of evidence - high; Strength of recommendation - strong).

Administration issues:

To prevent or minimize tissue damage during I.V. administration, the Institute for Safe Medication Practices (ISMP) has the following recommendations:
- Limit concentration available to the 25 mg/mL product
- Consider limiting initial doses to 6.25-12.5 mg
- Further dilute the 25 mg/mL strength into 10-20 mL NS
- Administer through a large bore vein (not hand or wrist)
- Administer via running I.V. line at port farthest from patient's vein
- Consider administering over 10-15 minutes
- Instruct patients to report immediately signs of pain or burning

International issues:

Sominex: Brand name for promethazine in Great Britain, but also is a brand name for diphenhydrAMINE in the U.S.

Related Information

Management of Drug Extravasations *on page 2255*

Brand Names: U.S. Phenadoz; Phenergan; Promethegan

Brand Names: Canada Bioniche Promethazine; Histantil; Phenergan; PMS-Promethazine

Therapeutic Category Antiemetic; Phenothiazine Derivative; Sedative

Generic Availability (U.S.) Yes

Use Symptomatic treatment of various allergic conditions and motion sickness, sedative, antiemetic; adjunct to postoperative analgesia and anesthesia (FDA approved in ages ≥2 years and adults)

Pregnancy Risk Factor C

Pregnancy Considerations Teratogenic effects were not observed in animal reproduction studies. Promethazine crosses the placenta. Maternal promethazine use has generally not resulted in an increased risk of birth defects. Platelet aggregation may be inhibited in newborns following maternal use of promethazine within 2 weeks of delivery. Promethazine is used for the treatment of nausea and vomiting of pregnancy (refer to current guidelines). Promethazine is also indicated for use during labor for obstetric sedation and may be used alone or as an adjunct to opioid analgesics.

Breast-Feeding Considerations It is not known if promethazine is excreted in breast milk. According to the manufacturer, the decision to continue or discontinue breast-feeding during therapy should take into account the risk of exposure to the infant and the benefits of treatment to the mother. Antihistamines may decrease maternal serum prolactin concentrations when administered prior to the establishment of nursing.

Contraindications Hypersensitivity to promethazine or any component (cross reactivity with other phenothiazines may occur); severe toxic CNS depression or coma; intra-arterial administration; subcutaneous administration; children <2 years; treatment of lower respiratory tract symptoms, including asthma; intra-arterial or subcutaneous administration

Warnings Contraindicated in children <2 years of age due to the potential for severe and potentially fatal respiratory depression **[U.S. Boxed Warning]**. A wide range of weight-based doses have resulted in respiratory depression; excessively high doses have been associated with sudden death in children; use with caution and use the lowest effective dose in children ≥2 years of age and avoid concomitant use with other medications having respiratory depressant effects. Serious tissue injury, including gangrene, has been reported with promethazine injection, regardless of the route of administration **[U.S. Boxed Warning]**. Preferred route of administration is by deep intramuscular (I.M.) injection. Do not give SubQ or intra-arterially due to severe local reactions including necrosis; rapid I.V. administration may produce a transient fall in blood pressure; slow I.V. administration may produce a slightly elevated blood pressure. Injection may contain sodium metabisulfite which may cause allergic reactions in susceptible individuals. Neuroleptic malignant syndrome (NMS) has been reported with promethazine when used alone or in combination with antipsychotic drugs. Children with dehydration are at increased risk for development of dystonic reactions.

Precautions Use with caution in patients with cardiovascular disease, narrow-angle glaucoma, prostatic hypertrophy, GI or GU obstruction, bone marrow depression, impaired liver function, asthma, peptic ulcer, sleep apnea, and hypertensive crisis; avoid in patients with suspected Reye's syndrome or other hepatic diseases; promethazine may lower the seizure threshold; use with caution in patients with seizure disorders or receiving other medications which may also lower the seizure threshold; promethazine has been reported to cause cholestatic jaundice; may cause photosensitivity

Adverse Reactions

Cardiovascular: Bradycardia, hyper-/hypotension, nonspecific QT changes, orthostatic hypotension, tachycardia,

Central nervous system: Agitation akathisia, catatonic states, confusion, delirium, disorientation, dizziness, drowsiness, dystonias, euphoria, excitation, extrapyramidal symptoms, faintness, fatigue, hallucinations, hysteria, insomnia, lassitude, pseudoparkinsonism, tardive dyskinesia, nervousness, neuroleptic malignant syndrome, nightmares, sedation, seizure, somnolence

Dermatologic: Angioneurotic edema, dermatitis, photosensitivity, skin pigmentation (slate gray), urticaria

Endocrine & metabolic: Amenorrhea, breast engorgement, gynecomastia, hyperglycemia, lactation

Gastrointestinal: Constipation, nausea, vomiting, xerostomia

Genitourinary: Ejaculatory disorder, impotence, urinary retention

Hematologic: Agranulocytosis, leukopenia, thrombocytopenia, thrombocytopenic purpura

Hepatic: Jaundice

Local: Abscess, distal vessel spasm, gangrene, injection site reactions (burning, edema, erythema, pain), palsies, paralysis, phlebitis, sensory loss, thrombophlebitis, tissue necrosis, venous thrombosis

Neuromuscular & skeletal: Incoordination, tremor

Ocular: Blurred vision, corneal and lenticular changes, diplopia, epithelial keratopathy, pigmentary retinopathy

Otic: Tinnitus

Respiratory: Apnea, asthma, nasal congestion, respiratory depression

Drug Interactions

Metabolism/Transport Effects Substrate of CYP2B6 (major), CYP2D6 (major); **Note:** Assignment of Major/Minor substrate status based on clinically relevant drug interaction potential; **Inhibits** CYP2D6 (weak)

Avoid Concomitant Use

Avoid concomitant use of Promethazine with any of the following: Aclidinium; Azelastine (Nasal); Ipratropium (Oral Inhalation); Metoclopramide; Paraldehyde; Potassium Chloride; Thalidomide; Tiotropium; Umeclidinium

Increased Effect/Toxicity

Promethazine may increase the levels/effects of: Abobotulinumtoxin A; Alcohol (Ethyl); Analgesics (Opioid); Anticholinergic Agents; Antipsychotics; ARIPiprazole; Azelastine (Nasal); Buprenorphine; Cannabinoid-Containing Products; CNS Depressants; Highest Risk QTc-Prolonging Agents; Hydrocodone; Methotrimeprazine;

Mirabegron; Moderate Risk QTc-Prolonging Agents; Onabotulinumtoxin A; Paraldehyde; Potassium Chloride; Pramipexole; Rimabotulinumtoxin B; ROPINIRole; Rotigotine; Serotonin Modulators; Thalidomide; Thiazide Diuretics; Tiotropium; Topiramate; Zolpidem

The levels/effects of Promethazine may be increased by: Abiraterone Acetate; Aclidinium; Antiemetics (5HT3 Antagonists); Antipsychotics; Brimonidine (Topical); Cannabis; CYP2B6 Inhibitors (Moderate); CYP2B6 Inhibitors (Strong); CYP2D6 Inhibitors (Moderate); CYP2D6 Inhibitors (Strong); Darunavir; Doxylamine; Dronabinol; Droperidol; HydrOXYzine; Ipratropium (Oral Inhalation); Kava Kava; Magnesium Sulfate; MAO Inhibitors; Methotrimeprazine; Metoclopramide; Metyrosine; Mifepristone; Nabilone; Perampanel; Pramlintide; Quazepam; Rufinamide; Sodium Oxybate; Tapentadol; Tetrahydrocannabinol; Umeclidinium

Decreased Effect

Promethazine may decrease the levels/effects of: Acetylcholinesterase Inhibitors (Central); EPINEPHrine (Nasal); Epinephrine (Racemic); EPINEPHrine (Systemic, Oral Inhalation); Secretin

The levels/effects of Promethazine may be decreased by: Acetylcholinesterase Inhibitors (Central); CYP2B6 Inducers (Strong); Dabrafenib; Peginterferon Alfa-2b

Stability

Injection: Prior to dilution, store at 20°C to 25°C (68°F to 77°F). Protect from light. Solutions in NS or D_5W are stable for 24 hours at room temperature.

Oral solution: Store at 15°C to 25°C (59°F to 77°F). Protect from light.

Suppositories: Store refrigerated at 2°C to 8°C (36°F to 46°F).

Tablets: Store at 20°C to 25°C (68°F to 77°F). Protect from light.

Compatible (when comixed in the same syringe) with atropine, chlorpromazine, diphenhydramine, droperidol, fentanyl, glycopyrrolate, hydromorphone, hydroxyzine hydrochloride, meperidine, midazolam, nalbuphine, pentazocine, prochlorperazine, scopolamine; **incompatible** when mixed with aminophylline, cefoperazone (Y-site), ceftriaxone (same syringe), chloramphenicol, dexamethasone (same syringe), dimenhydrinate (same syringe), foscarnet (Y-site), furosemide, heparin, hydrocortisone, methohexital, penicillin G, pentobarbital, phenobarbital, thiopental

Mechanism of Action Phenothiazine derivative; blocks postsynaptic mesolimbic dopaminergic receptors in the brain; exhibits a strong alpha-adrenergic blocking effect and depresses the release of hypothalamic and hypophyseal hormones; competes with histamine for the H_1-receptor; muscarinic-blocking effect may be responsible for antiemetic activity; reduces stimuli to the brainstem reticular system

Pharmacodynamics

Onset of action:
Oral, I.M.: Within 20 minutes
I.V.: 3-5 minutes
Duration: Oral: 4-6 hours

Pharmacokinetics (Adult data unless noted)

Absorption: 88%
Bioavailability: 25% (due to first pass metabolism)
Half-life: 9-16 hours
Metabolism: In the liver
Elimination: Principally as inactive metabolites in the urine and in the feces

Dosing: Usual

Children ≥2 years (use with extreme caution utilizing the lowest most effective dose):

Antihistamine: Oral: 0.1 mg/kg/dose (not to exceed 12.5 mg) every 6 hours during the day and 0.5 mg/kg/dose (not to exceed 25 mg) at bedtime as needed

Antiemetic: Oral, I.M., I.V., rectal: 0.25-1 mg/kg (not to exceed 25 mg) 4-6 times/day as needed

Motion sickness: Oral, rectal: 0.5 mg/kg (not to exceed 25 mg) 30 minutes to 1 hour before departure, then every 12 hours as needed

Preoperative analgesia/hypnotic adjunct: I.M., I.V.: 1.1 mg/kg once in combination with an analgesic or hypnotic (at reduced dosage) and with an atropine-like agent (at appropriate dosage). **Note:** Promethazine dosage should not exceed half of suggested adult dosage.

Sedation: Oral, I.M., I.V., rectal: 0.5-1 mg/kg/dose (not to exceed 25 mg) every 6 hours as needed

Adults:

Antihistamine:

Oral, rectal: 6.25-12.5 mg 3 times/day and 25 mg at bedtime

I.M., I.V.: 25 mg, may repeat in 2 hours when necessary; switch to oral route as soon as feasible

Antiemetic: Oral, I.M., I.V., rectal: 12.5-25 mg every 4 hours as needed

Motion sickness: Oral: 25 mg twice daily with the first dose 30 minutes to 1 hour before departure, then repeat 8-12 hours later as needed

Obstetrics (labor) as adjunct to analgesia: I.M., I.V.: Early labor: 50 mg; established labor: 25-75 mg in combination with analgesic at reduced dosage; may repeat every 4 hours for up to 2 additional doses (maximum: 100 mg/day while in labor)

Pre/postoperative analgesia/hypnotic adjunct: I.M., I.V.: 25-50 mg in combination with analgesic or hypnotic (at reduced dosage)

Sedation: Oral, I.M., I.V., rectal: 25-50 mg/dose; repeat every 4-6 hours if needed

Administration

Oral: Administer with food, water, or milk to decrease GI distress

Parenteral: Deep I.M. administration is preferred; avoid I.V. use; in selected patients, promethazine has been administered I.V. diluted to a maximum concentration of 25 mg/mL and infused at a maximum rate of 25 mg/minute; to minimize phlebitis, consider administering over 10-15 minutes; consider limiting initial dose to 6.25-12.5 mg; further dilute the 25 mg/mL strength into 10-20 mL NS; administer through a large bore vein (not hand or wrist) or via a running I.V. line at port farthest from patient's vein. Not for SubQ administration; promethazine is a chemical irritant which may produce necrosis.

Vesicant/Extravasation Risk Vesicant

Monitoring Parameters Relief of symptoms, mental status; monitor for signs and symptoms of tissue injury (burning or pain at injection site, phlebitis, edema) with I.V. administration

Test Interactions May interfere with urine detection of amphetamine/methamphetamine (false-positive); alters the flare response in intradermal allergen tests; hCG-based pregnancy tests may result in false-negatives or false-positives

Additional Information Although promethazine has been used in combination with meperidine and chlorpromazine as a premedication (lytic cocktail), this combination may have a higher rate of adverse effects compared to alternative sedative/analgesics

Dosage Forms Excipient information presented when available (limited, particularly for generics); consult specific product labeling.

Solution, Injection, as hydrochloride:

Phenergan: 50 mg/mL (1 mL) [contains edetate disodium, phenol, sodium metabisulfite]

Phenergan: 25 mg/mL (1 mL) [pyrogen free; contains edetate disodium, phenol, sodium metabisulfite]

Generic: 25 mg/mL (1 mL); 50 mg/mL (1 mL)

Solution, Oral, as hydrochloride:

Generic: 6.25 mg/5 mL (118 mL, 473 mL)

Suppository, Rectal, as hydrochloride:

Phenadoz: 12.5 mg (12 ea); 25 mg (12 ea)

Promethegan: 12.5 mg (12 ea); 25 mg (12 ea, 1000 ea); 50 mg (12 ea)

Generic: 12.5 mg (1 ea, 12 ea); 25 mg (1 ea, 12 ea)

Syrup, Oral, as hydrochloride:

Generic: 6.25 mg/5 mL (118 mL, 473 mL)

Tablet, Oral, as hydrochloride:

Generic: 12.5 mg, 25 mg, 50 mg

References

Strenkoski-Nix LC, Ermer J, DeCleene S, et al, "Pharmacokinetics of Promethazine Hydrochloride After Administration of Rectal Suppositories and Oral Syrup to Healthy Subjects," *Am J Health Syst Pharm*, 2000, 57(16):1499-505.

Promethazine and Codeine
(proe METH a zeen & KOE deen)

Medication Safety Issues

High alert medication:

The Institute for Safe Medication Practices (ISMP) includes this medication among its list of drug classes which have a heightened risk of causing significant patient harm when used in error.

Therapeutic Category Antitussive; Cough Preparation; Phenothiazine Derivative

Generic Availability (U.S.) Yes

Use Temporary relief of coughs and upper respiratory symptoms associated with allergy or the common cold (FDA approved in ages ≥6 years and adults)

Pregnancy Risk Factor C

Pregnancy Considerations Reproduction studies have not been conducted with this combination. See individual agents.

Breast-Feeding Considerations See individual agents.

Contraindications Hypersensitivity to promethazine or other phenothiazines, codeine, or any component; pediatric patients <6 years of age; lower respiratory tract symptoms, including asthma; coma

Additional contraindication for codeine: Postoperative pain management in pediatric patients who have undergone tonsillectomy and/or adenoidectomy

Warnings Avoid use in children <6 years of age **[U.S. Boxed Warning]**, due to the potential for severe and potentially fatal respiratory depression associated with the combination of promethazine and other respiratory depressants (eg, codeine); fatalities associated with promethazine use alone in children <2 years of age have also been reported. Respiratory depression and death have occurred in children who received codeine following tonsillectomy and/or adenoidectomy and were found to have evidence of being ultrarapid metabolizers of codeine due to a CYP2D6 polymorphism **[U.S. Boxed Warning]**; patients with this phenotype may have extensive conversion of codeine to morphine with resultant increased serum morphine concentrations; this may result in increased opioid-mediated effects and possible life-threatening respiratory depression or signs of overdose (eg, extreme sleepiness, confusion, shallow breathing) at usual therapeutic doses of codeine; codeine use is contraindicated in the postoperative pain management of pediatric patients who have undergone tonsillectomy and/or adenoidectomy. Deaths have also occurred in nursing infants after being exposed to high concentrations of morphine because the mothers were ultrarapid metabolizers of codeine. Ultrarapid metabolizers of codeine [ie, patients with more than two copies of functional alleles (CYP2D6 genotype with gene duplications denoted as *1/*1xN or *1/*2xN)] are at increased risk of opioid toxicity; avoid the use of codeine in these patients; consider alternative analgesics such as morphine or a nonopioid agent (Crews, 2012). The observed occurrence of the CYP2D6 "ultrarapid" phenotype is: North Africans, Ethiopians, and Arabs: 16% to 28%; African-Americans: 3%; Caucasians: 1% to 10%; Hispanics: 0.5% to 1%; and Chinese and Japanese: 0.5% to 1%. Codeine should be prescribed in all patients in the lowest effective dose and for the shortest period of time; patients and caregivers should be informed about risks and signs of morphine overdose. Due to the incidence of serious side effects and fatalities associated with codeine use in children, Health Canada is no longer recommending codeine use in any child <12 years of age.

Use with caution in atopic children. Use the lowest effective dose for the shortest period of time. Dose should not be increased if cough does not respond; re-evaluate within 5 days for possible underlying pathology. Codeine is not recommended for cough control in patients with a productive cough or chronic respiratory disease. Neuroleptic malignant syndrome (NMS) has been reported with promethazine when used alone or in combination with antipsychotic drugs; monitor for mental status changes, fever, muscle rigidity, and/or autonomic instability. May alter temperature regulation or mask toxicity of other drugs due to antiemetic effects. May alter cardiac conduction; life-threatening arrhythmias have occurred with therapeutic doses of phenothiazines.

May cause CNS depression, which may impair physical or mental abilities; patients must be cautioned about performing tasks which require mental alertness (eg, operating machinery or driving). Use with caution in disorders where CNS depression is a feature. Effects may be potentiated when used with other sedative drugs including ethanol. Use with extreme caution in patients with head injury, intracranial lesions, or elevated intracranial pressure; exaggerated elevation of ICP may occur. May cause orthostatic hypotension, use with caution in patients at risk of hypotension or where transient hypotensive episodes would be poorly tolerated (cardiovascular disease, cerebrovascular disease, hypovolemia, or concurrent medication use which may predispose to hypotension/bradycardia). Codeine may obscure diagnosis or clinical course of patients with acute abdominal conditions.

Precautions Use with caution in patients with cardiovascular disease, narrow-angle glaucoma, prostatic hypertrophy, GI or GU obstruction, bone marrow depression, impaired liver function, peptic ulcer, sleep apnea, and hypertensive crisis; avoid in patients with suspected Reye's syndrome; promethazine may lower the seizure threshold; use with caution in patients with seizure disorders or receiving other medications which may also lower the seizure threshold; use with caution in patients with hypersensitivity reactions to morphine, hydrocodone, hydromorphone, levorphanol, oxycodone, oxymorphone. Promethazine has been reported to cause cholestatic jaundice.

Adverse Reactions See individual agents.

Drug Interactions

Metabolism/Transport Effects Refer to individual components.

Avoid Concomitant Use

Avoid concomitant use of Promethazine and Codeine with any of the following: Aclidinium; Azelastine (Nasal); Ipratropium (Oral Inhalation); Metoclopramide; Paraldehyde; Potassium Chloride; Thalidomide; Tiotropium; Umeclidinium

Increased Effect/Toxicity

Promethazine and Codeine may increase the levels/effects of: AbobotulinumtoxinA; Alcohol (Ethyl); Alvimopan; Analgesics (Opioid); Anticholinergic Agents; Antipsychotics; ARIPiprazole; Azelastine (Nasal); Buprenorphine; Cannabinoid-Containing Products; CNS Depressants; Desmopressin; Diuretics; Highest Risk QTc-Prolonging Agents; Hydrocodone; Methotrimeprazine; Mirabegron; Moderate Risk QTc-Prolonging Agents; OnabotulinumtoxinA; Paraldehyde; Potassium Chloride; Pramipexole; RimabotulinumtoxinB; ROPINIRole; Rotigotine; Serotonin Modulators; Thalidomide; Thiazide Diuretics; Tiotropium; Topiramate; Zolpidem

The levels/effects of Promethazine and Codeine may be increased by: Abiraterone Acetate; Aclidinium; Amphetamines; Anticholinergic Agents; Antiemetics (5HT3 Antagonists); Antipsychotic Agents (Phenothiazines); Antipsychotics; Brimonidine (Topical); Cannabis; CYP2B6 Inhibitors (Moderate); CYP2B6 Inhibitors (Strong); Darunavir; Doxylamine; Dronabinol; Droperidol; HydrOXYzine; Ipratropium (Oral Inhalation); Kava Kava; Magnesium Sulfate; MAO Inhibitors; Methotrimeprazine; Metoclopramide; Metyrosine; Mifepristone; Nabilone; Perampanel; Pramlintide; Quazepam; Rufinamide; Sodium Oxybate; Somatostatin Analogs; Succinylcholine; Tapentadol; Tetrahydrocannabinol; Umeclidinium

Decreased Effect

Promethazine and Codeine may decrease the levels/effects of: Acetylcholinesterase Inhibitors (Central); EPINEPHrine (Nasal); Epinephrine (Racemic); EPINEPHrine (Systemic, Oral Inhalation); Pegvisomant; Secretin

The levels/effects of Promethazine and Codeine may be decreased by: Acetylcholinesterase Inhibitors (Central); Ammonium Chloride; CYP2B6 Inducers (Strong); CYP2D6 Inhibitors (Moderate); CYP2D6 Inhibitors (Strong); Dabrafenib; Mixed Agonist / Antagonist Opioids; Naltrexone; Peginterferon Alfa-2b

Stability Store at 20°C to 25°C (68°F to 77°F); protect from light.

Dosing: Usual Note: Dosage expressed as mL based on product formulation: Promethazine 6.25 mg and codeine 10 mg per 5 mL.

Children and Adolescents: **Antitussive (nonproductive cough):** Oral:

Children 6-11 years: 2.5-5 mL every 4-6 hours as needed; maximum total dose: 30 mL/24 hours

Children ≥12 years and Adolescents: 5 mL every 4-6 hours as needed; maximum total dose: 30 mL/24 hours

Adults: **Upper respiratory symptoms:** Oral: 5 mL every 4-6 hours as needed; maximum total dose: 30 mL/24 hours

Dosing adjustment in renal impairment: Children ≥6 years, Adolescents, and Adults: There are no specific dosage adjustments provided in the manufacturer's labeling; use with caution; consider decreasing dose.

Dosing adjustment in hepatic impairment: Children ≥6 years, Adolescents, and Adults: There are no specific dosage adjustments provided in the manufacturer's labeling; use with caution; consider decreasing dose.

Administration Oral: Administer with food or water to decrease GI upset. Administer with accurate measuring device; do not use household teaspoon (overdosage may occur).

Test Interactions

Codeine: Amylase and lipase plasma levels may by unreliable for 24 hours after codeine administration.

Promethazine: Pregnancy tests (hCG-based) may result in false-negatives or false-positives; increased serum glucose may be seen with glucose tolerance tests; may suppress the wheal and flare reactions to skin test antigens

Controlled Substance C-V

Dosage Forms Excipient information presented when available (limited, particularly for generics); consult specific product labeling.

Syrup: Promethazine hydrochloride 6.25 mg and codeine phosphate 10 mg per 5 mL (5 mL, 118 mL, 473 mL)

Promethazine and Phenylephrine
(proe METH a zeen & fen il EF rin)

Related Information
Phenylephrine (Systemic) *on page 1658*
Promethazine *on page 1748*
Brand Names: U.S. Promethazine VC
Therapeutic Category Antihistamine/Decongestant Combination
Generic Availability (U.S.) Yes
Use Temporary relief of upper respiratory symptoms associated with allergy or the common cold
Pregnancy Risk Factor C
Pregnancy Considerations Reproduction studies have not been conducted with this combination. Refer to individual monographs.
Contraindications Hypersensitivity to promethazine, phenylephrine, or any component; cross reactivity with other phenothiazines may occur; asthma, peripheral vascular disease, severe hypertension, cardiovascular disease, liver disease, patients receiving MAO inhibitors; children <2 years
Warnings Avoid use of promethazine in children <2 years of age due to the potential for severe and potentially fatal respiratory depression **[U.S. Boxed Warning]**. A wide range of weight-based doses have resulted in respiratory depression; excessively high doses have been associated with sudden death in children; use with caution and use the lowest effective dose in children >2 years of age and avoid concomitant use with other medications having respiratory depressant effects. Neuroleptic malignant syndrome (NMS) has been reported with promethazine when used alone or in combination with antipsychotic drugs. Children with dehydration are at increased risk for development of dystonic reactions.
Precautions Use with caution in patients with cardiovascular disease, narrow-angle glaucoma, prostatic hypertrophy, GI or GU obstruction, bone marrow depression, impaired liver function, asthma, peptic ulcer, sleep apnea, and hypertensive crisis; avoid in patients with suspected Reye's syndrome; promethazine may lower the seizure threshold; use with caution in patients with seizure disorders or receiving other medications which may also lower the seizure threshold; promethazine has been reported to cause cholestatic jaundice
Adverse Reactions See individual agents.
Drug Interactions
Metabolism/Transport Effects Refer to individual components.
Avoid Concomitant Use
Avoid concomitant use of Promethazine and Phenylephrine with any of the following: Aclidinium; Azelastine (Nasal); Ergot Derivatives; Hyaluronidase; Iobenguane I 123; Ipratropium (Oral Inhalation); MAO Inhibitors; Metoclopramide; Paraldehyde; Potassium Chloride; Thalidomide; Tiotropium; Umeclidinium
Increased Effect/Toxicity
Promethazine and Phenylephrine may increase the levels/effects of: AbobotulinumtoxinA; Alcohol (Ethyl); Analgesics (Opioid); Anticholinergic Agents; Antipsychotics; ARIPiprazole; Azelastine (Nasal); Buprenorphine; Cannabinoid-Containing Products; CNS Depressants; Highest Risk QTc-Prolonging Agents; Hydrocodone; Methotrimeprazine; Mirabegron; Moderate Risk QTc-Prolonging Agents; OnabotulinumtoxinA; Paraldehyde; Potassium Chloride; Pramipexole; RimabotulinumtoxinB; ROPINIRole; Rotigotine; Serotonin Modulators; Sympathomimetics; Thalidomide; Thiazide Diuretics; Tiotropium; Topiramate; Zolpidem

The levels/effects of Promethazine and Phenylephrine may be increased by: Abiraterone Acetate; Acetaminophen; Aclidinium; Antiemetics (5HT3 Antagonists); Antipsychotics; AtoMOXetine; Brimonidine (Topical); Cannabinoid-Containing Products; Cannabis; CYP2B6 Inhibitors (Moderate); CYP2B6 Inhibitors (Strong); CYP2D6 Inhibitors (Moderate); CYP2D6 Inhibitors (Strong); Darunavir; Doxylamine; Dronabinol; Droperidol; Ergot Derivatives; Hyaluronidase; HydrOXYzine; Ipratropium (Oral Inhalation); Kava Kava; Linezolid; Magnesium Sulfate; MAO Inhibitors; Methotrimeprazine; Metoclopramide; Metyrosine; Mifepristone; Nabilone; Perampanel; Pramlintide; Quazepam; Rufinamide; Sodium Oxybate; Tapentadol; Tetrahydrocannabinol; Tricyclic Antidepressants; Umeclidinium

Decreased Effect
Promethazine and Phenylephrine may decrease the levels/effects of: Acetylcholinesterase Inhibitors (Central); Benzylpenicilloyl Polylysine; EPINEPHrine (Nasal); Epinephrine (Racemic); EPINEPHrine (Systemic, Oral Inhalation); FentaNYL; Iobenguane I 123; Ioflupane I 123; Secretin

The levels/effects of Promethazine and Phenylephrine may be decreased by: Acetylcholinesterase Inhibitors (Central); Alpha1-Blockers; CYP2B6 Inducers (Strong); Dabrafenib; Peginterferon Alfa-2b

Dosing: Usual Oral:
Children:
2-6 years: 1.25 mL every 4-6 hours, not to exceed 7.5 mL in 24 hours
6-12 years: 2.5 mL every 4-6 hours, not to exceed 15 mL in 24 hours
Children >12 years and Adults: 5 mL every 4-6 hours, not to exceed 30 mL in 24 hours

Administration Oral: Administer with food, water, or milk to decrease GI distress

Test Interactions May suppress the wheal and flare reactions to skin test antigens; false negative and positive reactions with pregnancy tests relying on immunological reactions between hCG and anti-hCG

Dosage Forms Excipient information presented when available (limited, particularly for generics); consult specific product labeling.
Syrup, oral:
Promethazine VC: Promethazine hydrochloride 6.25 mg and phenylephrine hydrochloride 5 mg per 5 mL (118 mL, 473 mL) [contains ethanol 7%, menthol, propylene glycol, sodium benzoate; apricot-peach flavor]

◆ **Promethazine Hydrochloride** *see* Promethazine *on page 1748*

Promethazine, Phenylephrine, and Codeine (proe METH a zeen, fen il EF rin, & KOE deen)

Brand Names: U.S. Promethazine VC/Codeine
Therapeutic Category Antihistamine/Decongestant Combination; Antitussive; Cough Preparation
Generic Availability (U.S.) Yes
Use Temporary relief of coughs and upper respiratory symptoms including nasal congestion (FDA approved in ages ≥6 years and adults)
Pregnancy Risk Factor C
Pregnancy Considerations Reproduction studies have not been conducted with this combination. See individual agents.

Breast-Feeding Considerations Codeine enters breast milk; excretion of promethazine and phenylephrine is unknown. See individual agents.

Contraindications Hypersensitivity to promethazine or other phenothiazines, codeine, phenylephrine, or any component; children <6 years of age; lower respiratory symptoms, including asthma; coma; peripheral vascular disease; hypertension; concurrent MAO inhibitor

Additional contraindication for codeine: Postoperative pain management in pediatric patients who have undergone tonsillectomy and/or adenoidectomy

Warnings Avoid use in children <6 years of age **[U.S. Boxed Warning]** due to the potential for severe and potentially fatal respiratory depression associated with the combination of promethazine and other respiratory depressants (eg, codeine); fatalities associated with promethazine use alone in children <2 years of age have also been reported. Respiratory depression and death have occurred in children who received codeine following tonsillectomy and/or adenoidectomy and were found to have evidence of being ultrarapid metabolizers of codeine due to a CYP2D6 polymorphism **[U.S. Boxed Warning]**; patients with this phenotype may have extensive conversion of codeine to morphine with resultant increased serum morphine concentrations; this may result in increased opioid-mediated effects and possible life-threatening respiratory depression or signs of overdose (eg, extreme sleepiness, confusion, shallow breathing) at usual therapeutic doses of codeine; codeine use is contraindicated in the postoperative pain management of pediatric patients who have undergone tonsillectomy and/or adenoidectomy. Deaths have also occurred in nursing infants after being exposed to high concentrations of morphine because the mothers were ultrarapid metabolizers of codeine. Ultrarapid metabolizers of codeine [ie, patients with more than two copies of functional alleles (CYP2D6 genotype with gene duplications denoted as *1/*1xN or *1/*2xN)] are at increased risk of opioid toxicity; avoid the use of codeine in these patients; consider alternative analgesics such as morphine or a nonopioid agent (Crews, 2012). The observed occurrence of the CYP2D6 "ultrarapid" phenotype is: North Africans, Ethiopians, and Arabs: 16% to 28%; African-Americans: 3%; Caucasians: 1% to 10%; Hispanics: 0.5% to 1%; and Chinese and Japanese: 0.5% to 1%. Codeine should be prescribed in all patients in the lowest effective dose and for the shortest period of time; patients and caregivers should be informed about risks and signs of morphine overdose. Due to the incidence of serious side effects and fatalities associated with codeine use in children, Health Canada is no longer recommending codeine use in any child <12 years of age.

Use with caution in patients with severe respiratory disease (COPD, sleep apnea); may lead to potentially fatal respiratory depression. Use contraindicated in patients with asthma.

Use the lowest effective dose for the shortest period of time. Dose should not be increased if cough does not respond; re-evaluate within 5 days for possible underlying pathology. Codeine is not recommended for cough control in patients with a productive cough or chronic respiratory disease. Neuroleptic malignant syndrome (NMS) has been reported with promethazine when used alone or in combination with antipsychotic drugs; monitor for mental status changes, fever, muscle rigidity, and/or autonomic instability. May alter temperature regulation or mask toxicity of other drugs due to antiemetic effects. May alter cardiac conduction; life-threatening arrhythmias have occurred with therapeutic doses of phenothiazines.

May cause CNS depression, which may impair physical or mental abilities; patients must be cautioned about performing tasks which require mental alertness (eg, operating machinery or driving). Use with caution in disorders where CNS depression is a feature. Effects may be potentiated when used with other sedative drugs including ethanol. Use with extreme caution in patients with head injury, intracranial lesions, or elevated intracranial pressure; exaggerated elevation of ICP may occur. May cause orthostatic hypotension; use with caution in patients at risk of hypotension or where transient hypotensive episodes would be poorly tolerated (cardiovascular disease, cerebrovascular disease, hypovolemia, or concurrent medication use which may predispose to hypotension/bradycardia). Codeine may obscure diagnosis or clinical course of patients with acute abdominal conditions.

Precautions Use with caution in patients with cardiovascular disease, narrow-angle glaucoma, prostatic hypertrophy, GI or GU obstruction, bone marrow depression, impaired liver function, hyperthyroidism, diabetes mellitus, peptic ulcer, sleep apnea, and hypertensive crisis; avoid in patients with suspected Reye's syndrome; promethazine may lower the seizure threshold; use with caution in patients with seizure disorders or receiving other medications which may also lower the seizure threshold; use with caution in patients with hypersensitivity reactions to morphine, hydrocodone, hydromorphone, levorphanol, oxycodone, oxymorphone. Promethazine has been reported to cause cholestatic jaundice.

Adverse Reactions See individual agents.

Drug Interactions

Metabolism/Transport Effects Refer to individual components.

Avoid Concomitant Use

Avoid concomitant use of Promethazine, Phenylephrine, and Codeine with any of the following: Aclidinium; Azelastine (Nasal); Ergot Derivatives; Hyaluronidase; Iobenguane I 123; Ipratropium (Oral Inhalation); MAO Inhibitors; Metoclopramide; Paraldehyde; Potassium Chloride; Thalidomide; Tiotropium; Umeclidinium

Increased Effect/Toxicity

Promethazine, Phenylephrine, and Codeine may increase the levels/effects of: AbobotulinumtoxinA; Alcohol (Ethyl); Alvimopan; Analgesics (Opioid); Anticholinergic Agents; Antipsychotics; ARIPiprazole; Azelastine (Nasal); Buprenorphine; Cannabinoid-Containing Products; CNS Depressants; Desmopressin; Diuretics; Highest Risk QTc-Prolonging Agents; Hydrocodone; Methotrimeprazine; Mirabegron; Moderate Risk QTc-Prolonging Agents; OnabotulinumtoxinA; Paraldehyde; Potassium Chloride; Pramipexole; RimabotulinumtoxinB; ROPINIRole; Rotigotine; Serotonin Modulators; Sympathomimetics; Thalidomide; Thiazide Diuretics; Tiotropium; Topiramate; Zolpidem

The levels/effects of Promethazine, Phenylephrine, and Codeine may be increased by: Abiraterone Acetate; Acetaminophen; Aclidinium; Amphetamines; Anticholinergic Agents; Antiemetics (5HT3 Antagonists); Antipsychotic Agents (Phenothiazines); Antipsychotics; AtoMOXetine; Brimonidine (Topical); Cannabinoid-Containing Products; Cannabis; CYP2B6 Inhibitors (Moderate); CYP2B6 Inhibitors (Strong); Darunavir; Doxylamine; Dronabinol; Droperidol; Ergot Derivatives; Hyaluronidase; HydrOXYzine; Ipratropium (Oral Inhalation); Kava Kava; Linezolid; Magnesium Sulfate; MAO Inhibitors; Methotrimeprazine; Metoclopramide; Metyrosine; Mifepristone; Nabilone; Perampanel; Pramlintide; Quazepam; Rufinamide; Sodium Oxybate; Somatostatin Analogs; Succinylcholine; Tapentadol; Tetrahydrocannabinol; Tricyclic Antidepressants; Umeclidinium

Decreased Effect

Promethazine, Phenylephrine, and Codeine may decrease the levels/effects of: Acetylcholinesterase Inhibitors (Central); Benzylpenicilloyl Polylysine; EPINEPHrine (Nasal); Epinephrine (Racemic); EPINEPHrine ▶

(Systemic, Oral Inhalation); FentaNYL; Iobenguane I
123; Ioflupane I 123; Pegvisomant; Secretin

*The levels/effects of Promethazine, Phenylephrine, and
Codeine may be decreased by:* Acetylcholinesterase
Inhibitors (Central); Alpha1-Blockers; Ammonium Chloride; CYP2B6 Inducers (Strong); CYP2D6 Inhibitors (Moderate); CYP2D6 Inhibitors (Strong); Dabrafenib; Mixed
Agonist / Antagonist Opioids; Naltrexone; Peginterferon
Alfa-2b

Stability Store at 20°C to 25°C (68°F to 77°F); protect from
light.

Dosing: Usual Note: Dosage expressed as mL based on
product formulation: Promethazine 6.25 mg, phenylephrine 5 mg, and codeine 10 mg per 5 mL

Children and Adolescents: **Antitussive (nonproductive
cough):** Oral:

Children 6-11 years: 2.5-5 mL every 4-6 hours as
needed; maximum total dose: 30 mL/24 hours

Children ≥12 years and Adolescents: 5 mL every 4-6
hours as needed; maximum total dose: 30 mL/24 hours

Adults: **Cough and upper respiratory symptoms:** Oral: 5
mL every 4-6 hours as needed; maximum total dose: 30
mL/24 hours

Dosing adjustment in renal impairment: Children ≥6
years, Adolescents, and Adults: There are no specific
dosage adjustments provided in the manufacturer's labeling; use with caution; consider decreasing dose.

Dosing adjustment in hepatic impairment: Children ≥6
years, Adolescents, and Adults: There are no specific
dosage adjustments provided in the manufacturer's labeling; use with caution; consider decreasing dose.

Administration Oral: Administer with food or water to
decrease GI upset. Administer with an accurate measuring
device; do not use a household teaspoon (overdosage
may occur).

Test Interactions

Codeine: Amylase and lipase plasma levels may by unreliable for 24 hours after codeine administration.

Promethazine: Pregnancy tests (hCG-based) may result in
false-negatives or false-positives; increased serum glucose may be seen with glucose tolerance tests.

Controlled Substance C-V

Dosage Forms Excipient information presented when
available (limited, particularly for generics); consult specific
product labeling.

Syrup, Oral:

Promethazine VC/Codeine: Promethazine hydrochloride
6.25 mg, phenylephrine hydrochloride 5 mg, and
codeine phosphate 10 mg per 5 mL (120 mL, 480 mL)
[contains alcohol, fd&c yellow #6 (sunset yellow),methylparaben,propylene glycol,propylparaben,saccharin
sodium, sodium benzoate]

Generic: Promethazine hydrochloride 6.25 mg, phenylephrine hydrochloride 5 mg, and codeine phosphate
10 mg per 5 mL (120 mL, 480 mL)

◆ **Promethazine VC** *see Promethazine and Phenylephrine
on page 1752*

◆ **Promethazine VC/Codeine** *see Promethazine, Phenylephrine, and Codeine on page 1752*

◆ **Promethegan** *see Promethazine on page 1748*

◆ **Promolaxin [OTC]** *see Docusate on page 701*

◆ **PRO-Naproxen EC (Can)** *see Naproxen on page 1470*

◆ **Pronestyl** *see Procainamide on page 1740*

◆ **Pronutrients Vitamin D3 [OTC]** *see Cholecalciferol
on page 455*

Propantheline (proe PAN the leen)

Medication Safety Issues

BEERS Criteria medication:

This drug may be potentially inappropriate for use in
geriatric patients (Quality of evidence - moderate;
Strength of recommendation - strong).

Therapeutic Category Anticholinergic Agent; Antispasmodic Agent, Gastrointestinal; Antispasmodic Agent, Urinary

Generic Availability (U.S.) Yes

Use Adjunctive treatment of peptic ulcer, irritable bowel
syndrome, pancreatitis, ureteral and urinary bladder
spasm; to reduce duodenal motility during diagnostic
radiologic procedures

Pregnancy Risk Factor C

Pregnancy Considerations Animal reproduction studies
have not been conducted.

Breast-Feeding Considerations It is not known if propantheline is excreted in breast milk. The manufacturer
recommends that caution be exercised when administering propantheline to nursing women.

Contraindications Hypersensitivity to propantheline or
any component; narrow-angle glaucoma; ulcerative colitis;
toxic megacolon; obstructive disease of the GI or urinary
tract

Warnings Infants, patients with Down's syndrome, and
children with spastic paralysis or brain damage may be
hypersensitive to antimuscarinic effects

Precautions Use with caution in febrile patients, patients
with hyperthyroidism, hepatic, cardiac, or renal disease,
hypertension, GI infections, diarrhea, reflux esophagitis

Adverse Reactions

Cardiovascular: Palpitation, tachycardia

Central nervous system: Confusion, dizziness, drowsiness, headache, insomnia, nervousness

Endocrine & metabolic: Suppression of lactation

Gastrointestinal: Bloated feeling, constipation, loss of
taste, nausea, vomiting, xerostomia

Genitourinary: Impotence, urinary hesitancy, urinary
retention

Neuromuscular & skeletal: Weakness

Ocular: Blurred vision, cycloplegia, mydriasis, ocular tension increased

Miscellaneous: Allergic reactions, anaphylaxis, diaphoresis decreased

Drug Interactions

Metabolism/Transport Effects None known.

Avoid Concomitant Use

*Avoid concomitant use of Propantheline with any of the
following:* Aclidinium; Ipratropium (Oral Inhalation);
Potassium Chloride; Tiotropium; Umeclidinium

Increased Effect/Toxicity

Propantheline may increase the levels/effects of: Abobotulinumtoxin A; Analgesics (Opioid); Anticholinergic
Agents; Cannabinoid-Containing Products; Mirabegron;
OnabotulinumtoxinA; Potassium Chloride; RimabotulinumtoxinB; Thiazide Diuretics; Tiotropium; Topiramate

The levels/effects of Propantheline may be increased by:
Aclidinium; Ipratropium (Oral Inhalation); MAO Inhibitors;
Pramlintide; Umeclidinium

Decreased Effect

Propantheline may decrease the levels/effects of: Acetylcholinesterase Inhibitors (Central); Secretin

*The levels/effects of Propantheline may be decreased
by:* Acetylcholinesterase Inhibitors (Central)

Mechanism of Action Competitively blocks the action of
acetylcholine at postganglionic parasympathetic receptor
sites

Pharmacodynamics

Onset of action: Within 30-45 minutes

Duration: 4-6 hours

Pharmacokinetics (Adult data unless noted)

Metabolism: In the liver and GI tract

Elimination: In urine, bile, and other body fluids

Dosing: Usual Oral:

Antisecretory:

Children: 1-2 mg/kg/day in 3-4 divided doses

Adults: 15 mg 3 times/day before meals or food and 30 mg at bedtime; for mild manifestations: 7.5 mg 3 times/day

Antispasmodic:

Children: 2-3 mg/kg/day in divided doses every 4-6 hours and at bedtime

Adults: 15 mg 3 times/day before meals or food and 30 mg at bedtime

Administration Oral: Administer 30 minutes before meals and at bedtime

Dosage Forms Excipient information presented when available (limited, particularly for generics); consult specific product labeling.

Tablet, Oral, as bromide:

Generic: 15 mg

◆ **Propantheline Bromide** see Propantheline
on page 1754

Proparacaine (proe PAR a kane)

Brand Names: U.S. Alcaine; Parcaine

Brand Names: Canada Alcaine®; Diocaine®

Therapeutic Category Local Anesthetic, Ophthalmic

Generic Availability (U.S.) Yes

Use Local anesthesia for tonometry, gonioscopy; suture removal from cornea; removal of corneal foreign body; cataract extraction, glaucoma surgery; short operative procedure involving the cornea and conjunctiva

Pregnancy Risk Factor C

Pregnancy Considerations Animal reproduction studies have not been conducted.

Breast-Feeding Considerations It is not known if proparacaine is excreted in breast milk. The manufacturer recommends that caution be exercised when administering proparacaine to nursing women.

Contraindications Hypersensitivity to proparacaine or any component

Precautions Use with caution in patients with cardiac disease, hyperthyroidism

Adverse Reactions

Dermatologic: Allergic contact dermatitis

Hypersensitivity: Hypersensitivity reaction (corneal; characterized by acute, intense, and diffuse epithelial keratitis; gray, ground glass appearance; exfoliation of skin; corneal filaments; and can include iritis with descemetitis)

Ophthalmic: Burning sensation of eyes, conjunctival hemorrhage, conjunctival hyperemia, corneal erosion, cycloplegia, eye redness, mydriasis, stinging of eyes

Drug Interactions

Metabolism/Transport Effects None known.

Avoid Concomitant Use There are no known interactions where it is recommended to avoid concomitant use.

Increased Effect/Toxicity There are no known significant interactions involving an increase in effect.

Decreased Effect There are no known significant interactions involving a decrease in effect.

Stability Refrigerate and protect from light

Mechanism of Action Prevents initiation and transmission of impulse at the nerve cell membrane by decreasing ion permeability through stabilizing

Pharmacodynamics

Onset of action: Within 20 seconds of instillation

Duration: 15-20 minutes

Dosing: Neonatal Ophthalmic: Instill 2 drops of 0.5% solution 30 seconds prior to procedure; a crossover study in 22 premature neonates (GA: <30 weeks) undergoing examination for retinopathy of prematurity showed decreased pain scores compared to placebo (Marsh, 2005)

Dosing: Usual Children and Adults:

Ophthalmic surgery: Instill 1 drop of 0.5% solution in eye every 5-10 minutes for 5-7 doses

Tonometry, gonioscopy, suture removal: Instill 1-2 drops of 0.5% solution in eye just prior to procedure

Administration Ophthalmic: Instill drops into affected eye(s); avoid contact of bottle tip with skin or eye

Dosage Forms Excipient information presented when available (limited, particularly for generics); consult specific product labeling.

Solution, Ophthalmic, as hydrochloride:

Alcaine: 0.5% (15 mL)

Parcaine: 0.5% (15 mL)

Generic: 0.5% (15 mL)

References

Marsh VA, Young WO, Dunaway KK, et al, "Efficacy of Topical Anesthetics to Reduce Pain in Premature Infants During Eye Examinations for Retinopathy of Prematurity," *Ann Pharmacother*, 2005, 39 (5):829-33.

◆ **Proparacaine Hydrochloride** see Proparacaine
on page 1755

◆ **Propine® (Can)** see Dipivefrin on page 692

Propofol (PROE po fole)

Medication Safety Issues

Sound-alike/look-alike issues:

Diprivan may be confused with Diflucan, Ditropan

Propofol may be confused with fospropofol

High alert medication:

The Institute for Safe Medication Practices (ISMP) includes this medication among its list of drugs which have a heightened risk of causing significant patient harm when used in error.

Administration issues:

Propofol may be confused with bupivacaine liposome injectable suspension (Exparel) in operating rooms and other surgical areas due to their similar white, milky appearance especially when prepared in syringes. Bupivacaine liposome injectable suspension (Exparel) is intended only for administration via infiltration into the surgical site (and **not** for systemic use). Confusion with propofol may lead to accidental intravenous administration of Exparel instead of the intended propofol. Therefore, to avoid potential confusion ISMP recommends that all vials be separated when stocked in common areas and all prepared syringes be labeled.

Brand Names: U.S. Diprivan; Fresenius Propoven

Brand Names: Canada Diprivan; PMS-Propofol; Propofol Injection

Therapeutic Category General Anesthetic

Generic Availability (U.S.) Yes

Use Induction of general anesthesia (FDA approved in ages ≥3 years and adults); maintenance of general anesthesia (FDA approved in ages ≥2 months and adults); initiation and maintenance of monitored anesthesia care sedation (FDA approved in adults); sedation of intubated, mechanically ventilated ICU patients (FDA approved in adults); combined sedation and regional anesthesia (FDA approved in adults)

Note: Consult local regulations and individual institutional policies and procedures.

Pregnancy Risk Factor B

Pregnancy Considerations Propofol crosses the placenta and may be associated with neonatal CNS and respiratory depression. Propofol is not recommended by the manufacturer for obstetrics, including cesarean section deliveries.

Breast-Feeding Considerations Propofol is excreted in breast milk. Breast-feeding is not recommended by the manufacturer. A green discoloration to the breast milk was noted in a woman following administration of propofol during surgery for removal of an ectopic pregnancy. Although other medications were also administered, propofol was detected in the milk and assumed to be the cause; resolution of this effect occurred within 48 hours after surgery (Birkholz, 2009).

Contraindications Hypersensitivity to propofol or any component; hypersensitivity to eggs, egg products, soybeans, or soy products; patients who are not intubated or mechanically ventilated; other contraindications to general anesthesia or sedation apply

Additional product specific contraindications: Fresenius Propoven: Hypersensitivity to peanuts. **Note:** In July 2012, the FDA initiated temporary importation of Fresenius Propoven 1% (propofol) injection into the U.S. market to address a propofol shortage.

Warnings Propofol vials and prefilled syringes have the potential to support the growth of various microorganisms despite product additives intended to suppress microbial growth; to limit the potential for contamination, strictly adhere to recommendations in product labeling for handling and administering propofol.

Propofol-related infusion syndrome (PRIS) is a serious side effect with a high mortality rate (up to 33%) characterized by dysrhythmia (eg, bradycardia or tachycardia), heart failure, hyperkalemia, lipemia, metabolic acidosis, and/or rhabdomyolysis or myoglobinuria with subsequent renal failure. Risk factors include poor oxygen delivery, sepsis, serious cerebral injury, and the administration of high doses of propofol (usually doses >83 mcg/kg/minute or >5 mg/kg/hour for >48 hours), but has also been reported following large dose, short-term infusions during surgical anesthesia. PRIS has also been reported with lower-dose infusions (Chukwuemeka, 2006; Merz, 2006). The onset of the syndrome is rapid, occurring within 4 days of initiation. The mechanism of the syndrome has yet to be determined. Alternate sedation therapy should be considered for patients with escalating doses of vasopressors or inotropes, when cardiac failure occurs during high-dose propofol infusion, when metabolic acidosis is observed, or in whom lengthy and/or high-dose sedation is needed (Barr, 2013; Corbett, 2008). Metabolic acidosis with fatal cardiac failure has occurred in several children (4 weeks to 11 years of age) who received propofol infusions at average rates of infusion of 4.5 to 10 mg/kg/hour for 66 to 115 hours (maximum rates of infusion: 6.2 to 11.5 mg/kg/hour) (Bray, 1995; Parke, 1992; Strickland, 1995). Anecdotal reports of serious adverse events, including death, have been reported in pediatric patients with upper respiratory tract infections receiving propofol for ICU sedation. Not recommended for ICU sedation of pediatric patients; an increased number of deaths was observed in a multicenter clinical trial of pediatric ICU patients who received propofol (9% mortality) versus patients who received other sedative agents (4% mortality); although causality was not established, propofol is not indicated for sedation in PICU patients until further studies can document its safety in this population. Concurrent use of fentanyl and propofol in pediatric patients may result in bradycardia.

Use requires careful patient monitoring, should only be used by experienced personnel who are not actively engaged in the procedure or surgery. If used in a nonintubated and/or nonmechanically ventilated patient, qualified personnel and appropriate equipment for rapid institution of respiratory and/or cardiovascular support must be immediately available. Use to induce moderate (conscious) sedation in patients warrants monitoring equivalent to that seen with deep anesthesia. Consult local regulations and individual institutional policies and procedures. Patients require continuous monitoring and airway management; cardiovascular and respiratory resuscitation equipment should be available. Use with caution in ASA-PS 3 or 4, elderly, or debilitated patients; use a lower induction dose, a slower maintenance rate of administration and avoid rapidly delivered bolus doses to these patients to reduce the incidence of unwanted cardiorespiratory depressive events. Not recommended for use in obstetrics, cesarean deliveries, lactating women, patients with increased ICP, or impaired cerebral circulation.

Avoid abrupt discontinuation prior to weaning or daily wake up assessments. Abrupt discontinuation may result in rapid awakening, anxiety, agitation, and resistance to mechanical ventilation. Abrupt discontinuation in pediatric patients may cause agitation, hyperirritability, tremulousness, and flushing of hands and feet; increased frequency of bradycardia, jitteriness, and agitation have also been observed. Wean the infusion rate so the patient awakens slowly; discontinue opioids and paralytic agents prior to weaning. Long-term infusions can result in some tolerance; taper propofol infusions to prevent withdrawal.

May rarely cause hypersensitivity, anaphylaxis, anaphylactoid reactions, angioedema, bronchospasm, and erythema; medications for the treatment of hypersensitivity reactions should be available for immediate use. Diprivan contains egg lecithin, soybean oil, and disodium edetate; generic products may contain egg lecithin, soybean oil, or sodium metabisulfite; any of which may cause allergic reactions in susceptible individuals. Use is contraindicated in patients who are hypersensitive to eggs, egg products, soybeans, or soy product. Use with caution in patients with history of hypersensitivity/anaphylactic reaction to peanuts; a low risk of cross-reactivity between soy and peanuts may exist; Fresenius Propoven is contraindicated in patients with peanut hypersensitivity. Some formulations that contain edetate disodium can chelate trace metals including zinc; as much as 10 mg of elemental zinc may be lost per day when calcium disodium edetate is used in gram doses to treat heavy metal poisonings; no reports of zinc deficiency or low zinc levels have been reported with Diprivan; mean urinary zinc loss in clinical trials was 1.5 to 2 mg/day in pediatric patients and 2.5 to 3 mg/day in adult patients. Risk of decreased zinc levels may be in patients with prolonged therapy (>5 days) or a predisposition to zinc deficiency (eg, burns, diarrhea, or sepsis). A holiday from propofol infusion should take place after 5 days of therapy to allow for evaluation and necessary replacement of zinc.

Generic products may also contain benzyl alcohol or sodium benzoate; benzoic acid (benzoate) is a metabolite of benzyl alcohol; large amounts of benzyl alcohol (≥99 mg/kg/day) have been associated with a potentially fatal toxicity ("gasping syndrome") in neonates; use propofol products containing benzyl alcohol or sodium benzoate with caution in neonates; *in vitro* and animal studies have shown that benzoate displaces bilirubin from protein binding sites.

Precautions Use with caution in patients with increased intracranial pressure or impaired cerebral circulation; substantial decreases in mean arterial pressure and subsequent decreases in cerebral perfusion pressure may occur; consider continuous infusion or administer as a slow bolus. Use with caution in patients with seizures or history of epilepsy; seizure may occur during recovery phase.

Use with caution in patients who are hemodynamically unstable, hypovolemic, or have abnormally low vascular tone (eg, sepsis); the major cardiovascular effect of propofol is hypotension especially if patient is hypovolemic or if bolus dosing is used. Hypotension may be substantial with a reduction in mean arterial pressure occasionally exceeding 30%.

Use with caution in patients with preexisting hyperlipidemia as evidenced by increased serum triglyceride levels or serum turbidity; propofol is formulated within a 10% fat emulsion, hypertriglyceridemia is an expected side effect. Patients who develop hypertriglyceridemia (eg, >500 mg/dL) are at risk of developing pancreatitis. Serum triglyceride levels should be obtained prior to initiation of therapy and every 3 to 7 days thereafter. Monitoring of serum triglycerides should especially be considered with therapy >48 hours with doses exceeding 50 mcg/kg/minute (Devlin, 2005). An alternative sedative agent should be employed if significant hypertriglyceridemia occurs. Use with caution in patients with preexisting pancreatitis; use of propofol may exacerbate this condition.

I.V. injection may produce transient local pain (especially when administered through a small vein). Perioperative myoclonia may occur. Propofol lacks analgesic properties; pain management requires specific use of analgesic agents, at effective dosages; propofol must be titrated separately from the analgesic agent.

Adverse Reactions

Cardiovascular: Arrhythmia, bradycardia, cardiac output decreased, hyper-/hypotension, tachycardia

Central nervous system: Movement

Dermatologic: Pruritus, rash

Endocrine & metabolic: Hypertriglyceridemia

Local: Injection site burning, stinging, or pain

Respiratory: Apnea, respiratory acidosis during weaning

Rare but important or life-threatening: Agitation, amblyopia, anaphylaxis, anaphylactoid reaction, anticholinergic syndrome, asystole, atrial arrhythmia, bigeminy, cardiac arrest, chills, cough, dizziness, delirium, discoloration (green [urine, hair, or nailbeds]), extremity pain, fever, flushing, hemorrhage, hypersalivation, hypertonia, hypomagnesemia, hypoxia, infusion site reactions (including pain, swelling, blisters and/or tissue necrosis following accidental extravasation); laryngospasm, leukocytosis, lung function decreased, myalgia, myoclonia (rarely including convulsions and opisthotonos), nausea, pancreatitis, paresthesia, phlebitis, postoperative unconsciousness with or without increase in muscle tone, premature atrial contractions, premature ventricular contractions, pulmonary edema, propofol-related infusion syndrome, rhabdomyolysis, somnolence, syncope, thrombosis, urine cloudy, vision abnormality, wheezing

Drug Interactions

Metabolism/Transport Effects Substrate of CYP1A2 (minor), CYP2A6 (minor), CYP2B6 (major), CYP2C19 (minor), CYP2C9 (minor), CYP2D6 (minor), CYP2E1 (minor), CYP3A4 (minor); **Note:** Assignment of Major/Minor substrate status based on clinically relevant drug interaction potential; **Inhibits** CYP1A2 (weak), CYP2C9 (weak), CYP2D6 (weak), CYP2E1 (weak), CYP3A4 (weak)

Avoid Concomitant Use

Avoid concomitant use of Propofol with any of the following: Azelastine (Nasal); Paraldehyde; Pimozide; Thalidomide

Increased Effect/Toxicity

Propofol may increase the levels/effects of: Alcohol (Ethyl); ARIPiprazole; Azelastine (Nasal); Buprenorphine; CNS Depressants; Dofetilide; Hydrocodone; Lomitapide; Methotrimeprazine; Metyrosine; Midazolam; Mirtazapine; Paraldehyde; Pimozide; Pramipexole;

ROPINIRole; Ropivacaine; Rotigotine; Selective Serotonin Reuptake Inhibitors; Thalidomide; Zolpidem

The levels/effects of Propofol may be increased by: Alfentanil; Brimonidine (Topical); Cannabis; CYP2B6 Inhibitors (Moderate); CYP2B6 Inhibitors (Strong); Doxylamine; Dronabinol; Droperidol; HydrOXYzine; Kava Kava; Magnesium Sulfate; Methotrimeprazine; Midazolam; Nabilone; Perampanel; Quazepam; Rifampin; Rufinamide; Sodium Oxybate; Tapentadol; Tetrahydrocannabinol

Decreased Effect

The levels/effects of Propofol may be decreased by: Peginterferon Alfa-2b

Food Interactions Edetate disodium, an ingredient of propofol emulsion, may lead to decreased zinc levels in patients on prolonged therapy (>5 days) or those predisposed to deficiency (burns, diarrhea, and/or major sepsis). Management: Zinc replacement therapy may be needed.

Stability Store at 4°C to 25°C (40°F to 77°F); refrigeration is not recommended; do not freeze. Do not use if contamination is suspected or if there is evidence of separation of phases of emulsion, particulate matter, or discoloration. Discard unused portions at end of surgical procedure or within 12 hours (whichever is less). For ICU use: Discard tubing and unused portions after 12 hours. Unused, undiluted Fresenius Propoven should be discarded within 12 hours after the vial is opened, or within 6 hours if diluted; discard tubing after 12 hours. Solution further diluted in D_5W (concentration <2 mg/mL) is more stable in glass; stability in plastic: 95% potency after 2 hours.

Mechanism of Action Propofol is a short-acting, lipophilic intravenous general anesthetic. The drug is unrelated to any of the currently used barbiturate, opioid, benzodiazepine, arylcyclohexylamine, or imidazole intravenous anesthetic agents. Propofol causes global CNS depression, presumably through agonism of $GABA_A$ receptors and perhaps reduced glutamatergic activity through NMDA receptor blockade.

Pharmacodynamics

Onset of anesthesia: Within 30 seconds after bolus infusion

Duration: ~3-10 minutes depending on the dose, rate and duration of administration; with prolonged use (eg, 10 days ICU sedation), propofol accumulates in tissues and redistributes into plasma when the drug is discontinued, so that the time to awakening (duration of action) is increased; however, if dose is titrated on a daily basis, so that the minimum effective dose is utilized, time to awakening may be within 10-15 minutes even after prolonged use

Pharmacokinetics (Adult data unless noted)

Distribution: Large volume of distribution; highly lipophilic

V_d (apparent): Children 4-12 years: 5-10 L/kg

V_{dss}:

Adults: 170-350 L

Adults (10-day infusion): 60 L/kg

Protein binding: 97% to 99%

Metabolism: Hepatic via glucuronide and sulfate conjugation

Half-life (three-compartment model):

Alpha: 2-8 minutes

Beta (second distribution): ~40 minutes

Terminal: ~200 minutes; range: 300-700 minutes

Terminal (after 10-day infusion): 1-3 days

Elimination: Urine (~88% as metabolites, 40% as glucuronide metabolite); feces (<2%)

Dosing: Usual Consult local regulations and individual institutional policies and procedures. Dosage must be individualized based on total body weight and titrated to the desired clinical effect; wait at least 3-5 minutes between dosage adjustments to clinically assess drug effects; smaller doses are required when used with opioids; the following are general dosing guidelines (see "Abbreviations, Acronyms, and Symbols" section in front section for explanation of ASA-PS classes). **Note:** Increase dose in patients with chronic alcoholism (Fassoulaki, 1993); decrease dose with acutely intoxicated (alcoholic) patients.

Pediatric: **General anesthesia:**

Induction of general anesthesia: Children and Adolescents (healthy) 3 to 16 years, ASA-PS 1 or 2: I.V.: 2.5 to 3.5 mg/kg over 20 to 30 seconds; use a lower dose for ASA-PS 3 or 4

Maintenance of general anesthesia: Infants, Children, and Adolescents (healthy) ≥2 months to ≤16 years, ASA-PS 1 or 2: I.V. infusion: General range: 125 to 300 mcg/kg/minute (7.5 to 18 mg/kg/**hour**); Initial dose immediately following induction: 200 to 300 mcg/kg/minute; then decrease dose after 30 minutes if clinical signs of light anesthesia are absent; usual infusion rate after initial 30 minutes: 125 to 150 mcg/kg/minute (7.5 to 9 mg/kg/hour); infants and children ≤5 years may require higher infusion rates compared to older children.

Adult:

General anesthesia:

Induction of general anesthesia:

Healthy adults, ASA-PS 1 or 2, <55 years: I.V.: 2 to 2.5 mg/kg (~40 mg every 10 seconds until onset of induction)

Debilitated, ASA-PS 3 or 4: I.V.: 1 to 1.5 mg/kg (~20 mg every 10 seconds until onset of induction)

Maintenance of general anesthesia:

Healthy adults, ASA-PS 1 or 2, <55 years:

I.V. infusion: Initial: 100 to 200 mcg/kg/minute (or 6 to 12 mg/kg/**hour**) for 10 to 15 minutes; usual maintenance infusion rate: 50 to 100 mcg/kg/minute (or 3 to 6 mg/kg/**hour**) to optimize recovery time

I.V. intermittent bolus: 25 to 50 mg increments as needed

Debilitated, ASA-PS 3 or 4: I.V. Infusion: 50 to 100 mcg/kg/minute (or 3 to 6 mg/kg/hour)

Monitored anesthesia care sedation:

Healthy adults, ASA-PS 1 or 2, <55 years: Slow I.V. infusion: 100 to 150 mcg/kg/minute (or 6 to 9 mg/kg/**hour**) for 3 to 5 minutes **or** slow injection: 0.5 mg/kg over 3 to 5 minutes followed by I.V. infusion of 25 to 75 mcg/kg/minute (or 1.5 to 4.5 mg/kg/**hour**) **or** incremental bolus doses: 10 mg or 20 mg

Debilitated or ASA-PS 3 or 4 patients: Use 80% of healthy adult dose

ICU sedation in intubated mechanically-ventilated patients: Avoid rapid bolus injection; individualize dose and titrate to response. Continuous I.V. infusion: Initial: 5 mcg/kg/minute (or 0.3 mg/kg/**hour**); increase by 5 to 10 mcg/kg/minute (or 0.3 to 0.6 mg/kg/**hour**) every 5 to 10 minutes until desired sedation level is achieved; usual maintenance: 5 to 50 mcg/kg/minute (or 0.3 to 3 mg/kg/**hour**); reduce dose after adequate sedation established and adjust to response (eg, evaluate frequently to use minimum dose for sedation). Daily interruption with retitration or a light target level of sedation is recommended to minimize prolonged sedative effects (Barr, 2013).

Debilitated or ASA-PS 3 or 4 patients: Use 80% of healthy adult dose; reduce dose after adequate sedation established and adjust to response (eg, evaluate frequently to use minimum dose for sedation). Daily interruption with retitration or a light target level of sedation is recommended to minimize prolonged sedative effects (Barr, 2013).

Dosing adjustment in renal impairment: No dosage adjustment necessary.

Dosing adjustment in hepatic impairment: No dosage adjustment necessary.

Administration Note: Consult local regulations and individual institutional policies and procedures.

Parenteral: I.V.: Strict aseptic technique must be maintained in handling. Prepare drug for single-patient use only. Shake injection well before use. Does not need further diluted prior to administration; however, may further dilute with D₅W at a concentration ≥2 mg/mL; diluted emulsion is more stable in glass (stability in plastic: 95% potency after 2 hours). Administer pediatric induction doses over 20 to 30 seconds. Do not administer via filter with <5-micron pore size. Do not administer through the same I.V. catheter with blood or plasma. To reduce pain associated with injection, use larger veins of forearm or antecubital fossa; lidocaine I.V. (1 mL of a 1% solution) may also be used prior to administration or it may be added to propofol immediately before administration in a quantity not to exceed 20 mg lidocaine per 200 mg propofol.

Monitoring Parameters Cardiac monitor, blood pressure, oxygen saturation (during monitored anesthesia care sedation), arterial blood gas (with prolonged infusions). With prolonged infusions (eg, ICU sedation), monitor for metabolic acidosis, hyperkalemia, rhabdomyolysis or elevated CPK, hepatomegaly, and progression of cardiac and renal failure.

ICU sedation: Adult: Assess and adjust sedation according to scoring system (Richmond Agitation-Sedation Scale [RASS] or Sedation-Agitation Scale [SAS]) (Barr, 2013); assess CNS function daily. Serum triglyceride levels should be obtained prior to initiation of therapy and every 3 to 7 days thereafter, especially if receiving for >48 hours with doses exceeding 50 mcg/kg/minute (Devlin, 2005); use intravenous port opposite propofol infusion or temporarily suspend infusion and flush port prior to blood draw.

Diprivan: Monitor zinc levels in patients predisposed to deficiency (burns, diarrhea, major sepsis) or after 5 days of treatment.

Additional Information Propofol injection contains ~0.1 g of fat/mL (1.1 kcal/mL).

Acute febrile reactions: In June 2007, the FDA alerted clinicians of several reports of chills, fever, and body aches occurring in clusters of patients after administration of propofol for sedation in gastrointestinal suites. These reports were received from several facilities and involved multiple vials and lots. Symptoms appeared 6 to 18 hours following propofol therapy and persisted for ≤3 days. There is no evidence that any patient had sepsis or that the vials were contaminated. The FDA has tested multiple propofol vials and lots used in these patients and presently have found no evidence of bacterial contamination. Regardless, propofol vials and prefilled syringes have the potential to support the growth of various microorganisms despite product additives intended to suppress microbial growth. To limit the potential for contamination, the FDA is reminding healthcare professionals to strictly adhere to recommendations in product labeling for handling and administering propofol. Clinicians should also be vigilant for signs and symptoms of acute febrile reactions and evaluate patients for bacteremia. The FDA is continuing to work with the Centers for Disease Control and Prevention to investigate factors contributing to these occurrences. Additional information is available at http://www.fda.gov/Drugs/DrugSafety/PostmarketDrugSafetyInformationforPatientsandProviders/ucm109357.htm.

Dosage Forms Excipient information presented when available (limited, particularly for generics); consult specific product labeling.

Emulsion, Intravenous:

Diprivan: 10 mg/mL (20 mL, 50 mL, 100 mL) [contains edetate disodium, egg phospholipids (egg lecithin), glycerin, soybean oil]

Generic: 10 mg/mL (20 mL, 50 mL, 100 mL)
Emulsion, Intravenous [preservative free]:
Fresenius Propoven: 10 mg/mL (20 mL, 50 mL, 100 mL)
[contains egg phosphatides, soybean oil]
Generic: 10 mg/mL (20 mL, 50 mL, 100 mL)

References

Barr J, Fraser GL, Puntillo K, et al, "Clinical Practice Guidelines for the Management of Pain, Agitation, and Delirium in Adult Patients in the Intensive Care Unit," *Crit Care Med*, 2013, 41(1):263-306.

Baumeister FAM, Oberhoffer R, Liebhaber GM, et.al. Fatal propofol infusion syndrome in association with ketogenic diet. *Neuropediatrics*. 2004;35: 250-252.

Bennett SN, McNeil MM, Bland LA, et al, "Postoperative Infections Traced to Contamination of an Intravenous Anesthetic, Propofol," *N Engl J Med*, 1995, 333(3):147-54.

Birkholz T, Eckardt G, Renner S, et al. Green breast milk after propofol administration. *Anesthesiology*. 2009;111(5):1168-1169.

Bradley AED, Tober KES, and Brown RE, "Use of Propofol in Patients with Food Allergies," *Anaesthesia*, 2008, 63(4):433-45.

Bray RJ, "Fatal Myocardial Failure Associated With a Propofol Infusion in a Child," *Anaesthesia*, 1995, 50(1):94.

Burow BK, Johnson ME, and Packer DL, "Metabolic Acidosis Associated With Propofol in the Absence of Other Causative Factors," *Anesthesiology*, 2004, 101(1):239-41.

Cawley MJ, Guse TM, Laroia A, et al, "Propofol Withdrawal Syndrome in an Adult Patient With Thermal Injury," *Pharmacotherapy*, 2003, 23 (7):933-9.

Chukwuemeka A, Ko R, and Ralph-Edwards A, "Short-term Low-Dose Propofol Anaesthesia Associated with Severe Metabolic Acidosis," *Anaesth Intensive Care*, 2006, 34(5):651-5.

Corbett SM, Montoya ID, and Moore FA, "Propofol-Related Infusion Syndrome in Intensive Care Patients," *Pharmacotherapy*, 2008, 28 (2):250-58.

Dellinger RP, Levy MM, Rhodes A, et al, "Surviving Sepsis Campaign: International Guidelines for Management of Severe Sepsis and Septic Shock, 2012," *Crit Care Med*, 2013, 41(2):580-637.

Devlin JW, Lau AK, and Tanios MA, "Propofol-Associated Hypertriglyceridemia and Pancreatitis in the Intensive Care Unit: An Analysis of Frequency and Risk Factors," *Pharmacotherapy*, 2005, 25 (10):1348-52.

European Medicines Agency, "Public Statement on the Allergenic Potency of Herbal Medicinal Products Containing Soya or Peanut Protein," London: European Medicines Agency, 2006. Available at http://www.ema.europa.eu/docs/en_GB/document_library/Scientific_-guideline/2010/04/WC500089954.pdf. Accessed April 16, 2013.

Fassoulaki A, Farinotti R, Servin F, et al, "Chronic Alcoholism Increases the Induction Dose of Propofol in Humans," *Anesth Analg*, 1993, 77 (3):553-6.

Fresenius propoven (emulsion for injection or infusion propofol) [prescribing information]. Rapsgatan, Sweden: Fresenious Kabi AB; October 2010.

Gross J, Bailey P, Connis R, et al, "Practice Guidelines for Sedation and Analgesia by Non-Anesthesiologists. An Updated Report by the American Society of Anesthesiologist Task Force on Sedation and Analgesia by Nonanesthesiologists," *Anesthesiology*, 2002, 96 (4):1004-17.

Hofer KN, McCarthy MW, Buck ML, et al, "Possible Anaphylaxis After Propofol in a Child With Food Allergy," *Ann Pharmacother*, 2003; 37 (3): 398–401.

Kress JP and Hall JB, "Sedation in the Mechanically Ventilated Patient," *Crit Care Med*, 2006, 34 (10):2541-46.

Kress JP, Pohlman AS, O'Connor MF, et al, "Daily Interruption of Sedative Infusions in Critically Ill Patients Undergoing Mechanical Ventilation," *N Engl J Med*, 2000, 342(20):1471-7.

Liolios A, Guerit JM, Scholtes JL, et al, "Propofol Infusion Syndrome Associated With Short-term Large-Dose Infusion During Surgical Anesthesia in an Adult," *Anesth Analg*, 2005, 100(6):1804-6.

Merz TM, Regli B, Rothen HU, et al, "Propofol Infusion Syndrome: A Fatal Case at a Low Infusion Rate," *Anesth Analg*, 2006, 103(4):1050.

Parke TJ, Stevens JE, Rice ASC, et al, "Metabolic Acidosis and Fatal Myocardial Failure After Propofol Infusion in Children: Five Case Reports," *BMJ*, 1992, 305(6854):613-6.

Strickland RA and Murray MJ, "Fatal Metabolic Acidosis in a Pediatric Patient Receiving an Infusion of Propofol in the Intensive Care Unit: Is There a Relationship?" *Crit Care Med*, 1995, 23(2):405-9.

◆ **Propofol Injection (Can)** *see* Propofol *on page 1755*

Propranolol (proe PRAN oh lole)

Medication Safety Issues

Sound-alike/look-alike issues:
Propranolol may be confused with prasugrel, Pravachol, Propulsid

Inderal may be confused with Adderall, Enduron, Imdur, Imuran, Inderide, Isordil, Toradol

High alert medication:
The Institute for Safe Medication Practices (ISMP) includes this medication among its list of drugs which have a heightened risk of causing significant patient harm when used in error.

Administration issues:
Significant differences exist between oral and I.V. dosing. Use caution when converting from one route of administration to another.

International issues:
Inderal [Canada and multiple international markets], Inderal LA [U.S.], and Inderal XL [U.S.] may be confused with Indiaral brand name for loperamide [France] or Indamol brand name for indapamide [Italy]

Related Information

Oral Medications That Should Not Be Crushed or Altered *on page 2438*

Serotonin Syndrome *on page 2405*

Brand Names: U.S. Hemangeol; Inderal LA; Inderal XL; InnoPran XL

Brand Names: Canada Apo-Propranolol; Dom-Propranolol; Inderal; Inderal LA; Novo-Pranol; Nu-Propranolol; PMS-Propranolol; Propranolol Hydrochloride Injection, USP; Teva-Propranolol

Therapeutic Category Antianginal Agent; Antiarrhythmic Agent, Class II; Antihypertensive Agent; Antimigraine Agent; Beta-Adrenergic Blocker

Generic Availability (U.S.) Yes

Use

Oral:
Immediate release: Management of hypertension alone or in combination with other agents, angina pectoris, symptomatic treatment of hypertrophic subaortic stenosis, migraine headache prophylaxis, pheochromocytoma, essential tremor, atrial fibrillation, reduction of mortality post-MI (all indications FDA approved in adults); has also been used for tetralogy of Fallot cyanotic spells; short-term adjunctive therapy of thyrotoxicosis

Extended release capsules (InnoPran XL®): Management of hypertension alone or in combination with other agents (FDA approved in adults)

Long acting capsules (Inderal® LA): Management of hypertension alone or in combination with other agents, angina pectoris, symptomatic treatment of hypertrophic subaortic stenosis, migraine headache prophylaxis (all indications: FDA approved in adults)

I.V.: Supraventricular arrhythmias (such as atrial fibrillation and flutter, AV nodal re-entrant tachycardias), ventricular tachycardias (catecholamine-induced arrhythmias, digoxin toxicity) (all indications FDA approved in adults); has also been used for tetralogy of Fallot cyanotic spells; short-term adjunction therapy of thyrotoxicosis

Pregnancy Risk Factor C

Pregnancy Considerations Adverse events have been observed in some animal reproduction studies; therefore, the manufacturer classifies propranolol as pregnancy category C. Propranolol crosses the placenta and is measurable in the newborn serum following maternal use during pregnancy. In a cohort study, an increased risk of cardiovascular defects was observed following maternal use of beta-blockers during pregnancy. Intrauterine growth restriction (IUGR), small placentas, as well as fetal/neonatal bradycardia, hypoglycemia, and/or respiratory depression have been observed following *in utero* exposure to beta-blockers as a class. Adequate facilities for monitoring infants at birth should be available. Untreated chronic maternal hypertension and pre-eclampsia are also associated with adverse events in the fetus, infant, and mother. The peak maternal serum concentrations of propranolol and the active metabolite 4-hydroxypropranolol do not change during pregnancy; peak serum concentrations of naphthoxylactic acid are lower in the third trimester when compared to postpartum. Propranolol is recommended for use in the management of thyrotoxicosis in pregnancy. Propranolol has been evaluated for the treatment of hypertension in pregnancy, but other agents may be more appropriate for use. Propranolol has also been used in the management of hypertrophic obstructive cardiomyopathy in pregnancy and has been studied for use as an adjunctive agent in the management of dysfunctional labor (dystocia).

Breast-Feeding Considerations Propranolol is excreted into breast milk with peak concentrations occurring ~2-3 hours after an oral dose. The inactive metabolites of propranolol have also been detected in breast milk. The manufacturer recommends that caution be exercised when administering propranolol to nursing women. Due to immature hepatic metabolism in newborns, breast-feeding infants should be monitored for adverse events.

Contraindications Hypersensitivity to propranolol or any component; uncompensated CHF, cardiogenic shock, sinus bradycardia, sick sinus syndrome, heart block greater than first-degree (except in patients with a functioning artificial pacemaker), asthma, hyperactive airway disease, chronic obstructive lung disease, Raynaud's syndrome

Warnings May depress myocardial activity and precipitate or worsen CHF; use with caution and monitor closely, especially in patients with compensated heart failure. In patients with angina pectoris, exacerbation of angina and, in some cases, MI occurred following abrupt discontinuance of therapy **[U.S. Boxed Warning]**; reduce dose gradually over at least a few weeks when discontinuing therapy. Beta-blockers should generally be avoided in patients with bronchospastic disease (nonallergic bronchospasm, chronic bronchitis, emphysema), as bronchospasm may occur. Hypoglycemia may occur, particularly in infants and children (whether the patient has diabetes mellitus or not), especially during fasting before surgery; hypoglycemia may also occur after prolonged physical exertion and in patients with renal dysfunction. Propranolol decreases the ability of the heart to respond to reflex adrenergic stimuli and may increase the risks of general anesthesia and surgical procedures. Propranolol may mask clinical signs of hyperthyroidism (exacerbation of symptoms of hyperthyroidism, including thyroid storm, may occur following abrupt discontinuation). Severe bradycardia (requiring pacemaker) may occur in patients with Wolff-Parkinson-White syndrome. In patients with pheochromocytoma, adequate alpha-blockade is required prior to use of any beta-blocker. Hypersensitivity reactions (including anaphylactic and anaphylactoid reactions) and serious cutaneous reactions (including erythema multiforme, exfoliative dermatitis, Stevens-Johnson syndrome, toxic epidermal necrolysis, and urticaria) have been reported with propranolol use. Beta-blocker use has been associated with induction or exacerbation of psoriasis, but cause and effect have not been firmly established.

Precautions Propranolol may block hypoglycemia-induced tachycardia and blood pressure changes, use with caution in patients with diabetes mellitus; acute elevations in blood pressure have been reported after insulin-induced hypoglycemia in patients receiving propranolol. Use with caution in patients with peripheral vascular disease (beta-blockers may aggravate arterial insufficiency). Use with caution in patients with renal or hepatic dysfunction; consider dosage reduction in patients with hepatic insufficiency. Use with caution in patients with underlying skeletal muscle disease; exacerbation of myopathy and myotonia may occur. Avoid I.V. use in patients receiving calcium channel blockers (eg, verapamil) (effects may be potentiated). Patients receiving beta-blockers who have a

history of anaphylactic reactions, may be more reactive to a repeated allergen challenge and may not be responsive to the usual epinephrine doses used to treat an allergic reaction. Use with caution in patients receiving amide anesthetics (eg, lidocaine, bupivicaine, mepivicaine), as anesthetic clearance may be inhibited.

Adverse Reactions

Cardiovascular: Angina pectoris, atrioventricular conduction disturbance, bradycardia, cardiogenic shock, cold extremities, congestive heart failure, hypotension, ineffective myocardial contractions, syncope

Central nervous system: Agitation, amnesia, carpal tunnel syndrome, catatonia, cognitive dysfunction, confusion, dizziness, drowsiness, fatigue, hypersomnia, irritability, lethargy, nightmares, paresthesia, psychosis, sleep disorder, vertigo

Dermatologic: Changes in nails, contact dermatitis, dermal ulcer, eczematous rash, erosive lichen planus, hyperkeratosis, pruritus, skin rash

Endocrine & metabolic: Hyperglycemia, hyperkalemia, hyperlipidemia, hypoglycemia

Gastrointestinal: Abdominal pain, anorexia, constipation, decreased appetite, diarrhea, stomach discomfort

Genitourinary: Oliguria, proteinuria

Hematologic & oncologic: Immune thrombocytopenia, thrombocytopenia

Hepatic: Increased serum alkaline phosphatase, increased serum transaminases

Neuromuscular & skeletal: Arthropathy, oculomucocutaneous syndrome, polyarthritis

Ophthalmic: Conjunctival hyperemia, decreased visual acuity, mydriasis

Renal: Increased blood urea nitrogen, interstitial nephritis (rare)

Respiratory: Bronchiolitis (infants; associated with cough, fever, diarrhea, and vomiting), bronchitis (infants; associated with cough, fever, diarrhea, and vomiting), bronchospasm, dyspnea, pulmonary edema, wheezing

Miscellaneous: Ulcer

Rare but important or life-threatening: Agranulocytosis, alopecia, arterial insufficiency, arterial mesenteric thrombosis, decreased heart rate (infants), decreased serum glucose (infants), depression, emotional lability, epigastric distress, erythema multiforme, fever combined with generalized ache, sore throat, laryngospasm, and respiratory distress), hallucination, hypersensitivity reaction (including anaphylaxis, anaphylactoid reaction), impotence, insomnia, ischemic colitis, lupus-like syndrome, myotonia, myopathy, nonthrombocytopenic purpura, peripheral arterial disease (exacerbation), Peyronie's disease, pharyngitis, psoriasiform eruption, purpura, Raynaud's phenomenon, second degree atrioventricular block (infants; in a patient with an underlying conduction disorder), slightly clouded sensorium, Stevens-Johnson syndrome, systemic lupus erythematosus, temporary amnesia, tingling of extremities (hands), toxic epidermal necrolysis, urticaria, visual disturbance, weakness, xerophthalmia

Drug Interactions

Metabolism/Transport Effects Substrate of CYP1A2 (major), CYP2C19 (minor), CYP2D6 (major), CYP3A4 (minor); **Note:** Assignment of Major/Minor substrate status based on clinically relevant drug interaction potential; **Inhibits** CYP1A2 (weak), CYP2D6 (weak), P-glycoprotein

Avoid Concomitant Use

Avoid concomitant use of Propranolol with any of the following: Beta2-Agonists; Bosutinib; Ceritinib; Floctafenine; Methacholine; PAZOPanib; Silodosin; Topotecan; VinCRIStine (Liposomal)

Increased Effect/Toxicity

Propranolol may increase the levels/effects of: Afatinib; Alpha-/Beta-Agonists (Direct-Acting); Alpha1-Blockers;

Alpha2-Agonists; Amifostine; Antihypertensives; Antipsychotic Agents (Phenothiazines); ARIPiprazole; Bosutinib; Bradycardia-Causing Agents; Brentuximab Vedotin; Bupivacaine; Cardiac Glycosides; Ceritinib; Cholinergic Agonists; Colchicine; Dabigatran Etexilate; DOXOrubicin (Conventional); DULoxetine; Ergot Derivatives; Everolimus; Fingolimod; Grass Pollen Allergen Extract (5 Grass Extract); Hypotensive Agents; Insulin; Lidocaine (Systemic); Lidocaine (Topical); Mepivacaine; Methacholine; Midodrine; Obinutuzumab; PAZOPanib; P-glycoprotein/ABCB1 Substrates; Prucalopride; Rifaximin; RiTUXimab; Rivaroxaban; Rizatriptan; Silodosin; Sulfonylureas; Topotecan; VinCRIStine (Liposomal); ZOLMitriptan

The levels/effects of Propranolol may be increased by: Abiraterone Acetate; Acetylcholinesterase Inhibitors; Alcohol (Ethyl); Alpha2-Agonists; Aminoquinolines (Antimalarial); Amiodarone; Anilidopiperidine Opioids; Antipsychotic Agents (Phenothiazines); Barbiturates; Brimonidine (Topical); Calcium Channel Blockers (Dihydropyridine); Calcium Channel Blockers (Nondihydropyridine); CYP1A2 Inhibitors (Moderate); CYP1A2 Inhibitors (Strong); CYP2D6 Inhibitors (Moderate); CYP2D6 Inhibitors (Strong); Darunavir; Deferasirox; Diazoxide; Dipyridamole; Disopyramide; Dronedarone; Floctafenine; FluvoxaMINE; Herbs (Hypotensive Properties); Lacidipine; MAO Inhibitors; NiCARdipine; Pentoxifylline; Phosphodiesterase 5 Inhibitors; Propafenone; Prostacyclin Analogues; QuiNIDine; Regorafenib; Reserpine; Selective Serotonin Reuptake Inhibitors; Vemurafenib; Zileuton

Decreased Effect

Propranolol may decrease the levels/effects of: Beta2-Agonists; Lacidipine; Theophylline Derivatives

The levels/effects of Propranolol may be decreased by: Alcohol (Ethyl); Barbiturates; Bile Acid Sequestrants; Cannabis; CYP1A2 Inducers (Strong); Cyproterone; Herbs (Hypertensive Properties); Methylphenidate; Nonsteroidal Anti-Inflammatory Agents; Peginterferon Alfa-2b; Rifamycin Derivatives; Yohimbine

Food Interactions

Ethanol: Ethanol may increase or decrease plasma levels of propranolol. Reports are variable and have shown both enhanced as well as inhibited hepatic metabolism (of propranolol). Management: Caution advised with consumption of ethanol and monitor for heart rate and/or blood pressure changes.

Food: Propranolol serum levels may be increased if taken with food. Protein-rich foods may increase bioavailability; a change in diet from high carbohydrate/low protein to low carbohydrate/high protein may result in increased oral clearance. Management: Tablets (immediate release) should be taken on an empty stomach. Capsules (extended release) may be taken with or without food, but be consistent with regard to food.

Stability

Injection: Store at controlled room temperature; protect from freezing or excessive heat; protect from light; injection is compatible in D_5W, NS, D_5NS, $D_5\frac{1}{2}NS$, $\frac{1}{2}NS$, LR; incompatible with bicarbonate

Capsule, tablet: Store at 20°C to 25°C (68°F to 77°F). Protect from freezing or excessive heat. Protect from light and moisture. Dispense in tightly closed, light-resistant container.

Mechanism of Action

Nonselective beta-adrenergic blocker (class II antiarrhythmic); competitively blocks response to beta$_1$- and beta$_2$-adrenergic stimulation which results in decreases in heart rate, myocardial contractility, blood pressure, and myocardial oxygen demand. Nonselective beta-adrenergic blockers (propranolol, nadolol) reduce portal pressure by producing splanchnic vasoconstriction (beta$_2$ effect) thereby reducing portal blood flow.

Pharmacodynamics

Beta blockade: Oral (immediate release):
Onset of action: Within 1-2 hours
Duration: ~6 hours

Pharmacokinetics (Adult data unless noted)

Absorption: Oral: Rapid and complete

Distribution: V_d: 3.9 L/kg; crosses the placenta and blood-brain barrier; small amounts appear in breast milk

Protein-binding: Alpha$_1$-acid glycoprotein and albumin; **Note:** The S-isomer of propranolol preferentially binds to alpha$_1$-acid glycoprotein and the R-isomer preferentially binds to albumin
Newborns: 60% to 68%
Adults: 93%

Metabolism: Extensive first-pass effect, metabolized in the liver to active and inactive compounds; the 3 main metabolic pathways include: Aromatic hydroxylation (primarily 4-hydroxylation), N-dealkylation followed by further side-chain oxidation and direct glucuronidation; the 4 primary metabolites include: Propranolol glucuronide, naphthyloxylactic acid, and sulfate and glucuronic acid conjugates of 4-hydroxy propranolol; **Note:** Aromatic hydroxylation is catalyzed primarily by isoenzyme CYP2D6; side chain oxidation is mainly via CYP1A2, but also CYP2D6; 4-hydroxypropranolol possesses beta-adrenergic receptor blocking activity and is a weak inhibitor of CYP2D6.

Bioavailability: Oral: 26% ± 10%; oral bioavailability may be increased in Down syndrome children; protein-rich foods increase bioavailability of immediate release tablets by ~50%

Half-life, distribution: I.V.: 5-10 minutes

Half-life, elimination (prolonged with hepatic dysfunction):
Neonates and Infants: Possible increased half-life
Children: 3.9-6.4 hours
Adults: 4-6 hours

Time to peak serum concentration:
Immediate release: 1-4 hours
Extended release capsule (InnoPran XL™): 12-14 hours
Sustained release capsule (Inderal® LA): 6 hours

Elimination: Metabolites are excreted primarily in urine (96% to 99%); <1% excreted in urine as unchanged drug
Clearance: Decreased in hepatic dysfunction and in chronic renal failure

Dialysis: Not dialyzable: (0% to 5%)

Dosing: Neonatal

Note: Dosage should be individualized based on patient response.
Oral: Initial: 0.25 mg/kg/dose every 6-8 hours; increase slowly as needed to maximum of 5 mg/kg/day
I.V.: Initial: 0.01 mg/kg slow I.V. push over 10 minutes; may repeat every 6-8 hours as needed; increase slowly to maximum of 0.15 mg/kg/dose every 6-8 hours
Thyrotoxicosis: Oral: 2 mg/kg/day in divided doses every 6-12 hours; occasionally higher doses may be required

Dosing: Usual

Note: Dosage should be individualized based on patient response
Arrhythmias:
Oral:
Children: Initial: 0.5-1 mg/kg/day in divided doses every 6-8 hours; titrate dosage upward every 3-5 days; usual dose: 2-4 mg/kg/day; higher doses may be needed; do not exceed 16 mg/kg/day or 60 mg/kg/day
Adults: 10-30 mg/dose every 6-8 hours
I.V.:
Children: 0.01-0.1 mg/kg slow I.V. over 10 minutes; maximum dose: 1 mg (infants); 3 mg (children)
Adults: 1-3 mg/dose slow IVP; repeat every 2-5 minutes up to a total of 5 mg; titrate initial dose to desired response **or** 0.5-1 mg/dose slow IVP over 1 minute; may repeat, if necessary, up to a total maximum dose of 0.1 mg/kg (Neumar, 2010); **Note:** Once response achieved or maximum dose administered, additional doses should not be given for at least 4 hours.

Hypertension: Oral:

Children: Immediate release formulations: Initial: 0.5-1 mg/kg/day in divided doses every 6-12 hours; increase gradually every 5-7 days; usual dose: 1-5 mg/kg/day; maximum dose: 8 mg/kg/day

Children and Adolescents 1-17 years: Immediate release formulations: Initial: 1-2 mg/kg/day divided in 2-3 doses/ day; titrate dose to effect; maximum dose: 4 mg/kg/day up to 640 mg/day; sustained release formulation may be dosed once daily (National High Blood Pressure Education Program Working Group on High Blood Pressure in Children and Adolescents, 2004)

Adults:

Immediate release formulations: Initial: 40 mg twice daily; increase dosage every 3-7 days; usual dose: 120-240 mg divided in 2-3 doses/day; maximum daily dose: 640 mg; usual dosage range (JNC 7): 40-160 mg/day in 2 divided doses

Extended release formulations:

Inderal® LA: Initial: 80 mg once daily; usual maintenance: 120-160 mg once daily; maximum daily dose: 640 mg; usual dosage range (JNC 7): 60-180 mg/day once daily

InnoPran XL®: Initial: 80 mg once daily at bedtime; if initial response is inadequate, may be increased at 2-3 week intervals to a maximum dose of 120 mg

Migraine headache prophylaxis: Oral:

Children: 0.6-1.5 mg/kg/day divided every 8 hours; maximum dose: 4 mg/kg/day **or**

≤35 kg: 10-20 mg 3 times/day

>35 kg: 20-40 mg 3 times/day

Adults: Initial: 80 mg/day divided every 6-8 hours (or once daily as sustained release capsule); increase by 20-40 mg/dose every 3-4 weeks to a maximum of 160-240 mg/day given in divided doses every 6-8 hours (or once daily as sustained release capsules)

Tetralogy spells:

Oral: Palliation: Infants and Children: Initial: 0.25 mg/kg/ dose every 6 hours (1 mg/kg/day); if ineffective within first week of therapy, may increase by 1 mg/kg/day every 24 hours to maximum of 5 mg/kg/day; if patient becomes refractory may increase slowly to a maximum of 10-15 mg/kg/day but must carefully monitor heart rate, heart size, and cardiac contractility; average dose: 2.3 mg/kg/day; range: 0.8-5 mg/kg/day (Garson, 1981). Some centers use: Initial: 0.5-1 mg/kg/dose every 6 hours; usual: 1-2 mg/kg/dose every 6 hours.

I.V.: Infants and Children: 0.15–0.25 mg/kg/dose infused over 10 minutes; maximum initial dose: 1 mg; may repeat dose once (Hegenbarth, 2008); alternatively, initiate lower doses of 0.015-0.02 mg/kg/dose and titrate to effect, up to 0.1-0.2 mg/kg/dose

Thyrotoxicosis:

Oral: Adolescents and Adults: 10-40 mg/dose every 6 hours

I.V.: Adults: 1-3 mg/dose slow I.V. as a single dose

Administration

Oral: Administer with food; administer extended release capsules consistently either with food or on an empty stomach; do not chew or crush sustained or extended release capsules, swallow whole; mix concentrated oral solution with water, fruit juice, liquid, or semisolid food before administration

Parenteral: I.V. administration should not exceed 1 mg/minute; administer slow I.V. over 10 minutes in children; maximum concentration for injection: 1 mg/mL

Monitoring Parameters ECG, blood pressure, heart rate

Reference Range Therapeutic: 50-100 ng/mL (SI: 190-390 nmol/L) at end of dosing interval

Additional Information Not indicated for hypertensive emergencies. Do not abruptly discontinue therapy, taper dosage gradually over 2 weeks. The pH of solution for injection is adjusted with citric acid.

Product Availability Hemangeol (propranolol oral solution): FDA approved March 2014; availability anticipated in June 2014. Hemangeol is indicated for the treatment of proliferating infantile hemangioma requiring systemic therapy.

Dosage Forms Excipient information presented when available (limited, particularly for generics); consult specific product labeling.

Capsule Extended Release 24 Hour, Oral, as hydrochloride:

Inderal LA: 60 mg, 80 mg, 120 mg, 160 mg [contains brilliant blue fcf (fd&c blue #1)]

Inderal XL: 80 mg, 120 mg

InnoPran XL: 80 mg, 120 mg

Generic: 60 mg, 80 mg, 120 mg, 160 mg

Solution, Intravenous, as hydrochloride:

Generic: 1 mg/mL (1 mL)

Solution, Oral, as hydrochloride:

Hemangeol: 4.28 mg/mL (120 mL) [alcohol free, paraben free, sugar free; contains saccharin sodium]

Generic: 20 mg/5 mL (500 mL); 40 mg/5 mL (500 mL)

Tablet, Oral, as hydrochloride:

Generic: 10 mg, 20 mg, 40 mg, 60 mg, 80 mg

References

Brauchli YB, Jick SS, Curtin F, et al, "Association Between Beta-Blockers, Other Antihypertensive Drugs and Psoriasis: Population-Based Case-Control Study," *Br J Dermatol*, 2008, 158(6):1299-307.

Chobanian AV, Bakris GL, Black HR, et al, "The Seventh Report of the Joint National Committee on Prevention, Detection, Evaluation, and Treatment of High Blood Pressure: The JNC 7 report," *JAMA*, 2003, 289(19):2560-72.

Garson A Jr, Gillette PC, and McNamara DG, "Propranolol: The Preferred Palliation for Tetralogy of Fallot," *Am J Cardiol*, 1981, 47 (5):1098-104.

Gold MH, Holy AK, and Roenigk HH Jr, "Beta-Blocking Drugs and Psoriasis. A Review of Cutaneous Side Effects and Retrospective Analysis of Their Effects on Psoriasis," *J Am Acad Dermatol*, 1988, 19 (5 Pt 1):837-41.

Hegenbarth MA and American Academy of Pediatrics Committee on Drugs, "Preparing for Pediatric Emergencies: Drugs to Consider," *Pediatrics*, 2008, 121(2):433-43.

Lai CW, Ziegler DK, Lansky LL, et al, "Hemiplegic Migraine in Childhood: Diagnostic and Therapeutic Aspects," *J Pediatr*, 1982, 101 (5):696-9.

National High Blood Pressure Education Program Working Group on High Blood Pressure in Children and Adolescents, "The Fourth Report on the Diagnosis, Evaluation, and Treatment of High Blood Pressure in Children and Adolescents," *Pediatrics*, 2004, 114(2 Suppl 4th Report):555-76.

Neumar RW, Otto CW, Link MS, et al, "Part 8: Adult Advanced Cardiovascular Life Support: 2010 American Heart Association Guidelines for Cardiopulmonary Resuscitation and Emergency Cardiovascular Care," *Circulation*, 2010, 122(18 Suppl 3):S729-67.

Pickoff AS, Zies L, Ferrer PL, et al, "High-Dose Propranolol Therapy in the Management of Supraventricular Tachycardia," *J Pediatr*, 1979, 94(1):144-6.

Rasoulpour M and Marinelli KA, "Systemic Hypertension," *Clin Perinatol*, 1992, 19(1):121-37.

Schön MP and Boehncke WH, "Psoriasis," *N Engl J Med*, 2005, 352 (18):1899-912.

Sinaiko AR, "Pharmacologic Management of Childhood Hypertension," *Pediatr Clin North Am*, 1993, 40(1):195-212.

◆ **Propranolol Hydrochloride** *see* Propranolol *on page 1759*

◆ **Propranolol Hydrochloride Injection, USP (Can)** *see* Propranolol *on page 1759*

◆ **Proprinal® Cold and Sinus [OTC]** *see* Pseudoephedrine and Ibuprofen *on page 1772*

◆ **Propulsid®** *see* Cisapride *on page 478*

◆ **2-Propylpentanoic Acid** *see* Valproic Acid and Derivatives *on page 2102*

Propylthiouracil (proe pil thye oh YOOR a sil)

Medication Safety Issues

Sound-alike/look-alike issues:

Propylthiouracil may be confused with Purinethol®

PTU is an error-prone abbreviation (mistaken as mercaptopurine [Purinethol®; 6-MP])

Brand Names: Canada Propyl-Thyracil®

Therapeutic Category Antithyroid Agent

Generic Availability (U.S.) Yes

Use Adjunctive therapy in patients intolerant of methimazole to ameliorate hyperthyroidism symptoms in preparation for surgical treatment or radioactive iodine therapy (FDA approved in adults); treatment of hyperthyroidism in patients intolerant of methimazole and not candidates for surgical/radiotherapy (FDA approved in adults)

Medication Guide Available Yes

Pregnancy Risk Factor D

Pregnancy Considerations Propylthiouracil has been found to readily cross the placenta. Teratogenic effects have not been observed; however, nonteratogenic adverse effects, including fetal and neonatal hypothyroidism, goiter, and hyperthyroidism, have been reported following maternal propylthiouracil use. The transfer of thyroid-stimulating immunoglobulins can stimulate the fetal thyroid *in utero* and transiently after delivery and may increase the risk of fetal or neonatal hyperthyroidism.

Uncontrolled maternal hyperthyroidism may result in adverse neonatal outcomes (eg, prematurity, low birth weight) and adverse maternal outcomes (eg, pre-eclampsia, congestive heart failure, stillbirth, and abortion). To prevent adverse fetal and maternal events, normal maternal thyroid function should be maintained prior to conception and throughout pregnancy. Antithyroid treatment is recommended for the control of hyperthyroidism during pregnancy. Propylthiouracil is considered first-line therapy, especially during the first trimester. Due to an increased risk of liver toxicity, use of methimazole may be preferred during the second and third trimesters. If drug therapy is changed, maternal thyroid function should be monitored after 2 weeks and then every 2-4 weeks. Propylthiouracil, along with other medications, is used for the treatment of thyroid storm in pregnant women; alternative therapy is recommended if oral administration is not possible.

The pharmacokinetics of propylthiouracil are not significantly changed during pregnancy; however, the severity of hyperthyroidism may fluctuate throughout pregnancy. Doses of propylthiouracil may be decreased as pregnancy progresses and discontinued weeks to months prior to delivery.

Breast-Feeding Considerations Propylthiouracil is excreted in human breast milk; however, the infant dose is considered low and unlikely to affect infant thyroid hormones. The American Thyroid Association considers doses <300 mg/day to be safe during breast-feeding (Stagnaro-Green, 2011).

Contraindications Hypersensitivity to propylthiouracil or any component

Warnings May cause significant bone marrow depression; the most severe manifestation is agranulocytosis; aplastic anemia, thrombocytopenia, and leukopenia may also occur. Discontinue in the presence of unexplained fever. Has been associated with a variety of autoimmune reactions, including a lupus-like syndrome, as well as vasculitis; discontinuation may be warranted. Severe liver injury (some fatal) and acute liver failure (some cases requiring transplantation) have been reported **[U.S. Boxed Warning]**. Patients should be counseled to recognize and report symptoms suggestive of hepatic dysfunction (especially in first 6 months of treatment); symptoms suggestive of hepatic dysfunction should prompt immediate discontinuation. Routine liver function test monitoring may not reduce risk due to unpredictable and rapid onset. Has been associated with rare but severe dermatologic reactions; discontinue in the presence of exfoliative dermatitis.

Glomerulonephritis and interstitial nephritis with acute renal failure have been reported.

Precautions May cause hypoprothrombinemia and bleeding; monitor PT/INR. Use with caution in patients receiving other drugs known to cause myelosuppression, particularly agranulocytosis. Use should be limited to patients unable to tolerate methimazole or in whom surgery or radioactive iodine treatment are not appropriate.

Adverse Reactions

Cardiovascular: Periarteritis, vasculitis (ANCA-positive, cutaneous, leukocytoclastic)

Central nervous system: Drowsiness, drug fever, fever, headache, neuritis, vertigo

Dermatologic: Alopecia, erythema nodosum, exfoliative dermatitis, pruritus, skin pigmentation, skin rash, skin ulcers, urticaria

Endocrine & metabolic: Goiter, weight gain

Gastrointestinal: Constipation, loss of taste, nausea, sialoadenopathy, splenomegaly, stomach pain, taste perversion, vomiting

Hematologic: Agranulocytosis, aplastic anemia, bleeding, granulopenia, hypoprothrombinemia, leukopenia, thrombocytopenia

Hepatic: Acute liver failure, cholestatic jaundice, hepatitis

Neuromuscular & skeletal: Arthralgia, myalgia, paresthesia

Renal: Acute renal failure, glomerulonephritis, nephritis

Respiratory: Alveolar hemorrhage, interstitial pneumonitis

Miscellaneous: Lymphadenopathy, SLE-like syndrome

Drug Interactions

Metabolism/Transport Effects None known.

Avoid Concomitant Use

Avoid concomitant use of Propylthiouracil with any of the following: CloZAPine; Dipyrone; Sodium Iodide I131

Increased Effect/Toxicity

Propylthiouracil may increase the levels/effects of: Cardiac Glycosides; CloZAPine; Theophylline Derivatives

The levels/effects of Propylthiouracil may be increased by: Dipyrone

Decreased Effect

Propylthiouracil may decrease the levels/effects of: Sodium Iodide I131; Vitamin K Antagonists

Food Interactions Propylthiouracil serum levels may be altered if taken with food. Management: Administer at the same time in relation to meals each day, either always with meals or always between meals.

Mechanism of Action Inhibits the synthesis of thyroid hormones by blocking the oxidation of iodine in the thyroid gland; blocks synthesis of thyroxine and triiodothyronine

Pharmacodynamics For significant therapeutic effects 24-36 hours are required; remission of hyperthyroidism usually does not occur before 4 months of continued therapy

Pharmacokinetics (Adult data unless noted)

Protein binding: 75% to 80%

Metabolism: Hepatic

Bioavailability: 80% to 95%

Half-life: 1.5-5 hours

End-stage renal disease: 8.5 hours

Time to peak serum concentration: Oral: Within 1 hour; persists for 2-3 hours

Elimination: 35% excreted in urine

Dosing: Neonatal Oral (adjust dosage to maintain T_3, T_4, and TSH in normal range; elevated T_3 may be sole indicator of inadequate treatment. Elevated TSH indicates excessive antithyroid treatment): Initial: 5 mg/kg/day in divided doses every 8 hours; if no response in 36-48 hours, increase dose by 50%; usual range: 5-10 mg/kg/day

Dosing: Usual Oral: Adjust dosage to maintain T_3, T_4, and TSH in normal range; elevated T_3 may be sole indicator of inadequate treatment. Elevated TSH indicates excessive antithyroid treatment.

Children: 5-7 mg/kg/day in divided doses every 8 hours **or**
6-10 years: 50-150 mg/day divided every 8 hours
≥10 years: 150-300 mg/day divided every 8 hours
Maintenance: Determined by patient response or 1/3 to 2/3 of the initial dose in divided doses every 8-12 hours; this begins usually after 2 months on an effective initial dosage

Adults: Initial: 300 mg/day in divided doses every 8 hours. In patients with severe hyperthyroidism, very large goiters, or both, the initial dosage may be increased to 400 mg/day; an occasional patient will require 600-900 mg/day; usual maintenance: 100-150 mg/day in divided doses every 8 hours (Goldberg, 2003; Nayak, 2006)

Dosing adjustment in renal impairment: Adjustment is not necessary

Administration Oral: Administer same time in relation to meals each day, either always with meals or always between meals

Monitoring Parameters CBC with differential, liver function tests, platelets, thyroid function tests (TSH, T_3, T_4), prothrombin time, INR

Reference Range

Thyroid Function Tests

Lab Parameters	Age	Normal Range
T_4 (thyroxine) serum concentration	1-7 days	10.1-20.9 mcg/dL
	8-14 days	9.8-16.6 mcg/dL
	1 month to 1 year	5.5-16.0 mcg/dL
	>1 year	4.0-12.0 mcg/dL
Free thyroxine index (FTI)	1-3 days	9.3-26.6
	1-4 weeks	7.6-20.8
	1-4 months	7.4-17.9
	4-12 months	5.1-14.5
	1-6 years	5.7-13.3
	>6 years	4.8-14.0
T_3 serum concentration	Newborns	100-470 ng/dL
	1-5 years	100-260 ng/dL
	5-10 years	90-240 ng/dL
	10 years to Adult	70-210 ng/dL
T_3 uptake		35%-45%
TSH serum concentration	Cord	3-22 micro international units/mL
	1-3 days	<40 micro international units/mL
	3-7 days	<25 micro international units/mL
	>7 days	0-10 micro international units/mL

Dosage Forms Excipient information presented when available (limited, particularly for generics); consult specific product labeling.

Tablet, Oral:
Generic: 50 mg

Extemporaneous Preparations A 5 mg/mL oral suspension may be made with tablets and a 1:1 mixture of Ora-Plus® and Ora-Sweet®. Crush twenty 50 mg propylthiouracil tablets in a mortar and reduce to a fine powder. Add small portions of vehicle and mix to a uniform paste; mix while adding vehicle in incremental proportions to **almost** 200 mL; transfer to a calibrated bottle, rinse mortar with vehicle, and add quantity of vehicle sufficient to make 200 mL. Label "shake well" and "refrigerate". Stable for 91 days refrigerated (preferred) and 70 days at room temperature.
Nahata MC, Pai VB, and Hipple TF, *Pediatric Drug Formulations*, 5th ed, Cincinnati, OH: Harvey Whitney Books Co, 2004.

References

American College of Obstetricians and Gynecologists, ACOG Practice Bulletin, Clinical Management Guidelines for Obstetrician-Gynecologists, Number 37, August 2002. (Replaces Practice Bulletin Number 32, November 2001), "Thyroid Disease in Pregnancy," *Obstet Gynecol*, 2002, 100(2):387-96.
Clark SM, Saade GR, Snodgrass WR, et al, "Pharmacokinetics and Pharmacotherapy of Thionamides in Pregnancy," *Ther Drug Monit*, 2006, 28(4):477-83.
Cooper DS, "Antithyroid Drugs," *N Engl J Med*, 2005, 352(9):905-17.
Diav-Citrin O and Ornoy A, "Teratogen Update: Antithyroid Drugs – Methimazole, Carbimazole, and Propylthiouracil," *Teratology*, 2002, 65(1):38-44.
Goldberg PA and Inzucchi SE, "Critical Issues in Endocrinology," *Clin Chest Med*, 2003, 24(4):583-606.
Lee A, Moretti ME, Collantes A, et al, "Choice of Breastfeeding and Physicians' Advice: A Cohort Study of Women Receiving Propylthiouracil, *Pediatrics*, 2000, 106(1 Pt 1):27-30.
Lock DR and Sthoeger ZM, "Severe Hepatotoxicity on Beginning Propylthiouracil Therapy," *J Clin Gastroenterol*, 1997, 24(4):267-9.
Mandel SJ and Cooper DS, "The Use of Antithyroid Drugs in Pregnancy and Lactation," *J Clin Endocrinol Metab*, 2001, 86(6):2354-9.
Nayak B and Burman K, "Thyrotoxicosis and Thyroid Storm," *Endocrinol Metab Clin North Am*, 2006, 35(4):663-86.
Raby C, Lagorce JF, Jambut-Absil AC, et al, "The Mechanism of Action of Synthetic Antithyroid Drugs: Iodine Complexation During Oxidation of Iodide," *Endocrinology*, 1990, 126(3):1683-91.
Stagnaro-Green A, Abalovich M, Alexander E, et al, "Guidelines of the American Thyroid Association for the Diagnosis and Management of Thyroid Disease During Pregnancy and Postpartum," *Thyroid*, 2011, 21(10):1081-125.

◆ **Propyl-Thyracil® (Can)** *see* Propylthiouracil *on page 1762*

◆ **2-Propylvaleric Acid** *see* Valproic Acid and Derivatives *on page 2102*

◆ **ProQuad** *see* Measles, Mumps, Rubella, and Varicella Virus Vaccine *on page 1310*

◆ **PRO-Quetiapine (Can)** *see* QUEtiapine *on page 1783*

◆ **PRO-Rabeprazole (Can)** *see* RABEprazole *on page 1797*

◆ **PRO-Risperidone (Can)** *see* RisperiDONE *on page 1831*

◆ **PRO-Sotalol (Can)** *see* Sotalol *on page 1925*

◆ **Prostacyclin** *see* Epoprostenol *on page 770*

◆ **Prostaglandin E₁** *see* Alprostadil *on page 103*

◆ **Prostigmin** *see* Neostigmine *on page 1486*

◆ **Prostin VR** *see* Alprostadil *on page 103*

Protamine (PROE ta meen)

Medication Safety Issues
Sound-alike/look-alike issues:
Protamine may be confused with ProAmatine, Protonix®, Protopam®

Therapeutic Category Antidote, Heparin

Generic Availability (U.S.) Yes

Use Treatment of heparin overdosage; neutralize heparin during surgery or dialysis procedures

Pregnancy Risk Factor C

Pregnancy Considerations Animal reproduction studies have not been conducted. In general, medications used as antidotes should take into consideration the health and prognosis of the mother; antidotes should be administered to pregnant women if there is a clear indication for use and should not be withheld because of fears of teratogenicity (Bailey, 2003). Protamine sulfate may be used during delivery to reduce the risk of bleeding following maternal use of heparin or low molecular weight heparin (LMWH) (Bates, 2012).

Breast-Feeding Considerations It is not known if protamine is excreted in breast milk. The manufacturer recommends that caution be exercised when administering protamine to nursing women.

Contraindications Hypersensitivity to protamine or any component

Warnings Anaphylactic reactions may occur; hypotension and other cardiovascular events (including cardiovascular collapse, noncardiogenic pulmonary edema, pulmonary vasoconstriction, and pulmonary hypertension) may occur **[U.S. Boxed Warning]**; risk factors include rapid administration, high doses or overdose, repeated doses, previous protamine administration (including protamine-containing drugs such as NPH insulin), fish allergy, vasectomy, severe left ventricular dysfunction, and abnormal preoperative pulmonary hemodynamics. Heparin rebound associated with anticoagulation and bleeding has been reported to occur occasionally; symptoms typically occur 8-9 hours after protamine administration, but may occur as long as 18 hours later

Precautions Use with caution in patients allergic to fish, with prior history of vasectomy, and patients receiving protamine-containing insulin or previous protamine therapy.

Adverse Reactions

Cardiovascular: Bradycardia, flushing, hypotension, sudden fall in blood pressure

Central nervous system: Lassitude

Gastrointestinal: Nausea, vomiting

Hematologic: Hemorrhage

Respiratory: Dyspnea, pulmonary hypertension

Miscellaneous: Hypersensitivity reactions

Drug Interactions

Metabolism/Transport Effects None known.

Avoid Concomitant Use There are no known interactions where it is recommended to avoid concomitant use.

Increased Effect/Toxicity There are no known significant interactions involving an increase in effect.

Decreased Effect There are no known significant interactions involving a decrease in effect.

Stability Refrigerate; stable for at least 2 weeks at room temperature

Mechanism of Action Combines with strongly acidic heparin to form a stable complex (salt) neutralizing the anticoagulant activity of both drugs

Pharmacodynamics Onset of action: Heparin neutralization occurs within 5 minutes following I.V. injection

Pharmacokinetics (Adult data unless noted) Elimination: Unknown

Dosing: Neonatal Note: Limited data in neonates. Doses are extrapolated from adult information.

I.V.: Protamine dosage is determined by the most recent dosage of heparin or low molecular weight heparin (LMWH); 1 mg of protamine sulfate neutralizes 90 USP units of heparin (lung), 115 USP units of heparin (intestinal), and 1 mg of enoxaparin; maximum dose: 50 mg

Heparin overdosage: Since blood heparin concentrations decrease rapidly **after** heparin administration, adjust the protamine dosage depending upon the duration of time since heparin administration as follows (see table):

Time Since Last Heparin Dose (min)	Dose of Protamine (mg) to Neutralize 100 units of Heparin
<30	1
30-60	0.5-0.75
60-120	0.375-0.5
>120	0.25-0.375

LMWH overdosage: If most recent LMWH dose has been administered within the last 4 hours, use 1 mg protamine per 1 mg (100 units) LMWH; a second dose of 0.5 mg protamine per 1 mg (100 units) LMWH may be given if APTT remains prolonged 2-4 hours after the first dose; one report described dividing the total protamine dose and administering to a target Anti-Xa level to avoid potential protamine toxicity (Wiernikowski, 2007)

Dosing: Usual I.V.: Infants, Children and Adults: Protamine dosage is determined by the most recent dosage of heparin or low molecular weight heparin (LMWH); 1 mg of protamine neutralizes 90 USP units of heparin (lung), 115 USP units of heparin (intestinal), and 1 mg (100 units) LMWH; maximum dose: 50 mg

Heparin overdosage: Since blood heparin concentrations decrease rapidly **after** heparin administration, adjust the protamine dosage depending upon the duration of time since heparin administration as follows (see table):

Time Since Last Heparin Dose (min)	Dose of Protamine (mg) to Neutralize 100 units of Heparin
<30	1
30-60	0.5-0.75
60-120	0.375-0.5
>120	0.25-0.375

If heparin is administered by deep SubQ injection, use 1-1.5 mg protamine per 100 units heparin; this may be done by administering a portion of the dose (eg, 25-50 mg) slowly I.V. followed by the remaining portion as a continuous infusion over 8-16 hours (the expected absorption time of the SubQ heparin dose)

LMWH overdosage: If most recent LMWH dose has been administered within the last 4 hours, use 1 mg protamine per 1 mg (100 units) LMWH; a second dose of 0.5 mg protamine per 1 mg (100 units) LMWH may be given if APTT remains prolonged 2-4 hours after the first dose

Administration Parenteral: Inject without further dilution over 10 minutes not to exceed 5 mg/minute; maximum of 50 mg in any 10-minute period

Monitoring Parameters Coagulation tests, APTT or ACT, cardiac monitor, and blood pressure monitor required during administration

Dosage Forms Excipient information presented when available (limited, particularly for generics); consult specific product labeling.

Solution, Intravenous, as sulfate:

Generic: 10 mg/mL (5 mL, 25 mL)

Solution, Intravenous, as sulfate [preservative free]:

Generic: 10 mg/mL (5 mL, 25 mL)

References

Bailey B, "Are There Teratogenic Risks Associated With Antidotes Used in the Acute Management of Poisoned Pregnant Women?" *Birth Defects Res A Clin Mol Teratol*, 2003, 67(2):133-40.

Bates SM, Greer IA, Middeldorp S, et al. "VTE, Thrombophilia, Antithrombotic Therapy, and Pregnancy: Antithrombotic Therapy and Prevention of Thrombosis, 9th ed: American College of Chest Physicians Evidence-Based Clinical Practice Guidelines," *Chest*, 2012, 141(2 Suppl):e691-736.

Moganasundram S, Hunt BJ, Sykes K, et al, "The Relationship Among Thromboelastography, Hemostatic Variables, and Bleeding After Cardiopulmonary Bypass Surgery in Children," *Anesth Analg*, 2010, 110 (4):995-1002.

Monagle P, Chalmers E, Chan A, et al, "Antithrombotic Therapy in Neonates and Children: American College of Chest Physicians Evidence-Based Clinical Practice Guidelines (8th Edition)," *Chest*, 2008, 133(6 Suppl):887-968.

Wiernikowski JT, Chan A, and Lo G, "Reversal of Anti-Thrombin Activity Using Protamine Sulfate. Experience in a Neonate With a 10-fold Overdose of Enoxaparin," *Thromb Res*, 2007, 120(2):303-5.

◆ **Protamine Sulfate** *see* Protamine *on page 1764*

◆ **Protease, Lipase, and Amylase** *see* Pancrelipase *on page 1591*

♦ **Protection Plus® [OTC]** *see* Alcohol (Ethyl) *on page 88*

♦ **Protein C** *see* Protein C Concentrate (Human) *on page 1766*

Protein C Concentrate (Human)
(PROE teen cee KON suhn trate HYU man)

Medication Safety Issues
Sound-alike/look-alike issues:
Ceprotin may be confused with aprotinin, Cipro®
Protein C concentrate (human) may be confused with activated protein C (human, recombinant) which refers to drotrecogin alfa

Brand Names: U.S. Ceprotin

Therapeutic Category Anticoagulant; Blood Product Derivative; Enzyme

Generic Availability (U.S.) No

Use Replacement therapy for severe congenital protein C deficiency for the prevention and/or treatment of venous thromboembolism and purpura fulminans (FDA approved in neonatal, pediatric, and adult patients). Has also been used in patients with purpura fulminans secondary to meningococcemia.

Pregnancy Risk Factor C

Pregnancy Considerations Reproductive studies have not been performed. It is unknown if administration during pregnancy will result in fetal harm.

Breast-Feeding Considerations Use in nursing mothers has not been studied.

Contraindications Hypersensitivity to protein C or any component

Warnings Formulation may contain trace amounts of mouse protein and/or heparin from manufacturing process and allergic reactions could occur; discontinue use in the presence of hypersensitivity/allergic reactions. Trace amounts of heparin contained within the formulation may lead to heparin-induced thrombocytopenia (HIT); if HIT suspected, discontinue use and evaluate platelet counts. An increased risk of bleeding may be seen in patients receiving concomitant anticoagulant therapy including thrombolytic agents (tPA), heparin, oral anticoagulants, glycoprotein IIb/IIIa antagonists, platelet aggregation inhibitors, and aspirin.

Precautions Use with caution in sodium-restricted or renally impaired patients; the maximum daily dose of Ceprotin provides >200 mg of sodium. Product of human plasma; may potentially contain infectious agents which could transmit disease. Screening of donors, as well as testing and/or inactivation or removal of certain viruses, reduces this risk. Consideration should be given for patients to receive appropriate vaccinations during therapy (eg, hepatitis A or B vaccine). Use with caution in patients with hepatic or renal impairment; data on the use in these patients is not available.

Adverse Reactions As with all drugs which may affect hemostasis, bleeding may be associated with protein C administration. Hemorrhage may occur at virtually any site. Risk is dependent on multiple variables, including the concurrent use of multiple agents that alter hemostasis and patient susceptibility.
Central nervous system: Lightheadedness
Hematologic: Bleeding
Miscellaneous: Hypersensitivity reactions (itching and rash)
Postmarketing and/or case reports: Fever, hemothorax, hypotension, hyperhidrosis, restlessness

Drug Interactions
Metabolism/Transport Effects None known.
Avoid Concomitant Use
Avoid concomitant use of Protein C Concentrate (Human) with any of the following: Apixaban; Dabigatran

Etexilate; Omacetaxine; Rivaroxaban; Urokinase; Vorapaxar

Increased Effect/Toxicity
Protein C Concentrate (Human) may increase the levels/effects of: Anticoagulants; Collagenase (Systemic); Deferasirox; Ibritumomab; Omacetaxine; Rivaroxaban; Tositumomab and Iodine I 131 Tositumomab

The levels/effects of Protein C Concentrate (Human) may be increased by: Agents with Antiplatelet Properties; Apixaban; Dabigatran Etexilate; Dasatinib; Herbs (Anticoagulant/Antiplatelet Properties); Ibrutinib; Nonsteroidal Anti-Inflammatory Agents; Omega-3 Fatty Acids; Pentosan Polysulfate Sodium; Prostacyclin Analogues; Salicylates; Sugammadex; Thrombolytic Agents; Tibolone; Tipranavir; Urokinase; Vitamin E; Vorapaxar

Decreased Effect
The levels/effects of Protein C Concentrate (Human) may be decreased by: Estrogen Derivatives; Progestins

Stability Store under refrigeration at 2°C to 8°C (36°F to 46°F); do not freeze. Protect from light. After reconstitution administer within 3 hours and discard any unused portion.

Mechanism of Action Converted to activated protein C (APC). APC is a serine protease which inactivates factors Va and VIIIa, limiting thrombotic formation. *In vitro* data also suggest inhibition of plasminogen activator inhibitor-1 (PAF-1) resulting in profibrinolytic activity, inhibition of macrophage production of tumor necrosis factor, blocking of leukocyte adhesion, and limitation of thrombin-induced inflammatory responses.

Pharmacodynamics Onset of action: 30 minutes

Pharmacokinetics (Adult data unless noted) Note: Limited data suggests that infants and very young children may have a faster clearance, lower AUC and maximum serum concentration, larger volume of distribution, and shorter half-life than older subjects.
Distribution: V_d: Median: 0.074L/kg (range: 0.044-0.165 L/kg)
Metabolism: Activated protein C (APC) inactivated by plasma protease inhibitors
Half-life elimination: Median: 9.8 hours (range: 4.9-14.7 hours)
Time to peak, serum concentration: Median: 0.5 hours (range: 0.17-1.33 hours)

Dosing: Neonatal Note: Patient variables (including age, clinical condition, and plasma levels of protein C) will influence dosing and duration of therapy. Individualize dosing based on protein C activity and patient's pharmacokinetic profile.

Severe congenital protein C deficiency: I.V.:

Acute episode/short-term prophylaxis:
Initial dose: 100-120 units/kg/dose (for determination of recovery and half-life); followed by subsequent 3 doses: 60-80 units/kg/dose every 6 hours adjusted to maintain peak protein C activity of 100%
Maintenance dose: 45-60 units/kg/dose every 6 or 12 hours adjusted to maintain recommended maintenance trough protein C activity levels >25%
Long-term prophylaxis: Maintenance dose: 45-60 units/kg/dose every 12 hours (recommended maintenance trough protein C activity levels >25%)
Note: Maintain target peak protein C activity of 100% during acute episodes and short-term prophylaxis. Maintain trough levels of protein C activity >25%. Higher peak levels of protein C may be necessary in prophylactic therapy of patients at increased risk for thrombosis (eg, infection, trauma, surgical intervention).

Purpura fulminans secondary to meningococcemia: Limited data available. I.V.: A retrospective review of 94 pediatric patients (0-18 years including eight newborns) reported a median dose of 100 units/kg/day divided every 4-6 hours was used in the majority of patients (78 of the 94 patients); the other dosing in the remaining patients was an initial bolus with the remainder of daily dose administered as a continuous I.V. infusion (dosing specifics were not provided); median treatment duration of 33 hours (range: 1-645 hours); daily dose range: 28-375 units/kg/day (Veldman, 2010). Further studies needed.

Dosing: Usual Note: Patient variables (including age, clinical condition, and plasma levels of protein C) will influence dosing and duration of therapy. Individualize dosing based on protein C activity and patient's pharmacokinetic profile.

Severe congenital protein C deficiency: I.V.: Infants, Children, Adolescents, and Adults:

Acute episode/short-term prophylaxis:
Initial dose: 100-120 units/kg/dose (for determination of recovery and half-life) followed by subsequent 3 doses: 60-80 units/kg/dose every 6 hours adjusted to maintain peak protein C activity of 100%
Maintenance dose: 45-60 units/kg/dose every 6 or 12 hours adjusted to maintain recommended maintenance trough protein C activity levels >25%
Long-term prophylaxis: Maintenance dose: 45-60 units/kg/dose every 12 hours (recommended maintenance trough protein C activity levels >25%)

Note: Maintain target peak protein C activity of 100% during acute episodes and short-term prophylaxis. Maintain trough levels of protein C activity >25%. Higher peak levels of protein C may be necessary in prophylactic therapy of patients at increased risk for thrombosis (eg, infection, trauma, surgical intervention).

Purpura fulminans secondary to meningococcemia: Limited data available: Infants >1month, Children, and Adolescents: I.V.: 100-150 units/kg/dose every 6 hours for 72 hours then 50-150 units/kg/dose every 12 hours until target symptom/sign resolution or treatment duration reaches 7 days. This protocol was used in a Phase II, double-blind, placebo-controlled, dose-finding study of 40 pediatric patients [median age: 2.3 years (range: 2.4 months-16.1 years)] (de Kleijn, 2003). A retrospective review of 94 pediatric patients (newborn to 18 years) reported a median dose of 100 units/kg/day divided every 4-6 hours or as an initial bolus with the remainder of daily dose administered as a continuous I.V. infusion (dosing specifics were not provided); median treatment duration of 2 days (range: 1-24 days); daily dose range: 28-375 units/kg/day (Veldman, 2010). An open-label, prospective study of 36 patients (3 months to 76 years) reported an initial dose of 100 units/kg followed by a continuous I.V. infusion with an initial rate of 10 units/kg/hour adjusted daily to maintain plasma protein C concentration 80-120 units/mL (White, 2000).

Administration Parenteral: Allow vials and SWI to warm to room temperature prior to reconstitution. Using provided transfer set, reconstitute vial with appropriate volume of SWI for final concentration of ~100 units/mL (ie, 500 units vial with 5 mL and 1000 units vial with 10 mL). Gently swirl vial until powder is completely dissolved. Use provided filter needle to withdraw solution from vial; remove filter needle prior to administration. Administer by I.V. injection:
Neonates, Infants, and Children <10 kg: Rate should not exceed 0.2 mL/kg/minute
Children >10 kg, Adolescents, and Adults: Rate should not exceed 2 mL/minute

Monitoring Parameters Protein C activity (chromogenic assay) prior to and during therapy (if acute thrombotic event, check protein C activity immediately before next injection); signs and symptoms of bleeding; hemoglobin/hematocrit, PT/INR, platelet count

Reference Range Maintain target peak protein C activity of 100% during acute episodes and short-term prophylaxis. Maintain trough levels of protein C activity >25%. Higher peak levels of protein C may be necessary in prophylactic therapy of patients at increased risk for thrombosis (eg, infection, trauma, surgical intervention).

Additional Information Conversion to vitamin K antagonist therapy may cause a transient hypercoagulable state during therapy initiation due to shorter half-life of protein C than other vitamin K-dependent clotting factors. For patients requiring conversion to oral vitamin K antagonists, it is recommended to continue protein C therapy during oral anticoagulant initiation until anticoagulation stabilized. It is also advised to begin with a low dose of oral anticoagulant instead of a loading dose.

Prescribers should register their patients to assist in the collection and assessment of protein C concentration deficiency, treatment, safety, and outcomes of subjects. More information may be found at the following website: http://clinicaltrials.gov/ct2/show/NCT01127529.

Dosage Forms Excipient information presented when available (limited, particularly for generics); consult specific product labeling.
Solution Reconstituted, Intravenous [preservative free]:
Ceprotin: 500 units (1 ea); 1000 units (1 ea) [contains albumin human, heparin, mouse protein (murine) (hamster)]

References
de Kleijn ED, de Groot R, Hack CE, et al, "Activation of Protein C Following Infusion of Protein C Concentrate in Children With Severe Meningococcal Sepsis and Purpura Fulminans: A Randomized, Double-Blinded, Placebo-Controlled, Dose-Finding Study," Crit Care Med, 2003, 31(6):1839-47.

Veldman A, Fischer D, Wong FY, et al, "Human Protein C Concentrate in the Treatment of Purpura Fulminans: A Retrospective Analysis of Safety and Outcome in 94 Pediatric Patients," Crit Care, 2010, 14(4): R156.

White B, Livingstone W, Murphy C, et al, "An Open-Label Study of the Role of Adjuvant Hemostatic Support With Protein C Replacement Therapy in Purpura Fulminans-Associated Meningococcemia," Blood, 2000, 96(12):3719-24.

◆ **Prothrombin Complex Concentrate (Caution: Confusion-prone synonym)** see Factor IX Complex (Human) [(Factors II, IX, X)] on page 833

◆ **Protonix** see Pantoprazole on page 1595

◆ **Protopam Chloride** see Pralidoxime on page 1719

◆ **Protopic** see Tacrolimus (Topical) on page 1967

◆ **Protopic® (Can)** see Tacrolimus (Topical) on page 1967

◆ **PRO-Topiramate (Can)** see Topiramate on page 2046

◆ **Protrin DF (Can)** see Sulfamethoxazole and Trimethoprim on page 1948

Protriptyline (proe TRIP ti leen)

Medication Safety Issues
Sound-alike/look-alike issues:
Vivactil® may be confused with Vyvanse®
BEERS Criteria medication:
This drug may be potentially inappropriate for use in geriatric patients (SIADH: Quality of evidence - moderate; Strength of recommendation - strong).

Related Information
Antidepressant Agents on page 2219

Brand Names: U.S. Vivactil

Therapeutic Category Antidepressant, Tricyclic (Secondary Amine)

Generic Availability (U.S.) Yes

Use Treatment of depression (FDA approved in adults)

Medication Guide Available Yes

Pregnancy Considerations Adverse events have not been observed in animal reproduction studies. Tricyclic antidepressants may be associated with irritability, jitteriness, and convulsions (rare) in the neonate (Yonkers, 2009).

The ACOG recommends that therapy for depression during pregnancy be individualized; treatment should incorporate the clinical expertise of the mental health clinician, obstetrician, primary healthcare provider, and pediatrician (ACOG, 2008). According to the American Psychiatric Association (APA), the risks of medication treatment should be weighed against other treatment options and untreated depression. For women who discontinue antidepressant medications during pregnancy and who may be at high risk for postpartum depression, the medications can be restarted following delivery (APA, 2010). Treatment algorithms have been developed by the ACOG and the APA for the management of depression in women prior to conception and during pregnancy (Yonkers, 2009).

Breast-Feeding Considerations It is not known if protriptyline is excreted in breast milk. According to the manufacturer, the decision to continue or discontinue breast-feeding during therapy should take into account the risk of exposure to the infant and the benefits of treatment to the mother.

Contraindications Hypersensitivity to protriptyline (cross-reactivity to other cyclic antidepressants may occur) or any component; use of MAO inhibitors within 14 days (potentially fatal reactions may occur); concurrent use of cisapride; use in a patient during the acute recovery phase of MI

Warnings Clinical worsening of depression or suicidal ideation and behavior may occur in children and adults with major depressive disorder **[U.S. Boxed Warning]**. In clinical trials, antidepressants increased the risk of suicidal thinking and behavior (suicidality) in children, adolescents, and young adults (18-24 years of age) with major depressive disorder and other psychiatric disorders. This risk must be considered before prescribing antidepressants for any clinical use. Short-term studies did not show an increased risk of suicidality with antidepressant use in patients >24 years of age and showed a decreased risk in patients ≥65 years.

Patients of all ages who are treated with antidepressants for any indication require appropriate monitoring and close observation for clinical worsening of depression, suicidality, and unusual changes in behavior, especially during the first few months after antidepressant initiation or when the dose is adjusted. Family members and caregivers should be instructed to closely observe the patient (ie, daily) and communicate condition with healthcare provider. Patients should also be monitored for associated behaviors (eg, anxiety, agitation, panic attacks, insomnia, irritability, hostility, aggressiveness, impulsivity, akathisia, hypomania, mania) which may increase the risk for worsening depression or suicidality. Worsening depression or emergence of suicidality (or associated behaviors listed above) that is abrupt in onset, severe, or not part of the presenting symptoms, may require discontinuation or modification of drug therapy.

Do not discontinue abruptly in patients receiving high doses chronically (withdrawal symptoms may occur). To reduce risk of intentional overdose, write prescriptions for the smallest quantity consistent with good patient care. Screen individuals for bipolar disorder prior to treatment (using antidepressants alone may induce manic episodes in patients with this condition). May worsen psychosis in some patients. Protriptyline is not FDA approved for the treatment of bipolar depression.

Precautions May cause sedation; more common in adults than adolescents; sedation may result in impaired performance of tasks requiring alertness (eg, operating machinery or driving). Sedative effects may be additive with other CNS depressants and/or ethanol. The degree of sedation is low relative to other antidepressants. May aggravate aggressive behavior; more prevalent in adolescents compared to adults. May increase the risks associated with electroconvulsive therapy; limit such treatment to patients in whom it is essential. Consider discontinuing, when possible, prior to elective surgery. Therapy should not be abruptly discontinued in patients receiving high doses for prolonged periods. May alter glucose regulation; both an increase and decrease in blood glucose has been reported; use with caution in patients with diabetes.

May cause tachycardia and orthostatic hypotension (risk is moderate relative to other antidepressants); use with caution in patients at risk of hypotension or in patients where transient tachycardia or hypotensive episodes would be poorly tolerated (cardiovascular disease or cerebrovascular disease). The degree of anticholinergic blockade produced by this agent is moderate relative to other cyclic antidepressants; however, caution should still be used in patients with urinary retention, benign prostatic hyperplasia, narrow-angle glaucoma, increased IOP, xerostomia, visual problems, constipation, or history of bowel obstruction.

Use with caution in patients with a history of cardiovascular disease (including previous MI, stroke, tachycardia, or conduction abnormalities). The risk of conduction abnormalities with this agent is moderate-high relative to other antidepressants. Use caution in patients with a previous seizure disorder or condition predisposing to seizures such as brain damage, alcoholism, or concurrent therapy with other drugs which lower the seizure threshold. Use with caution in hyperthyroid patients or those receiving thyroid supplementation (cardiac arrhythmias may occur). Use with caution in patients with hepatic or renal dysfunction.

Adverse Reactions

Cardiovascular: Arrhythmias, heart block, hyper-/hypotension, MI, palpitation, stroke, tachycardia

Central nervous system: Agitation, anxiety, ataxia, confusion, delirium, delusions, dizziness, drowsiness, EPS, exacerbation of psychosis, fatigue, hallucinations, headache, hypomania, incoordination, insomnia, nightmares, panic, restlessness, seizure

Dermatologic: Alopecia, itching, petechiae, photosensitivity, rash, urticaria

Endocrine & metabolic: Breast enlargement, galactorrhea, gynecomastia, increased or decreased libido, syndrome of inappropriate ADH secretion (SIADH)

Gastrointestinal: Anorexia, constipation, decreased lower esophageal sphincter tone may cause GE reflux, diarrhea, heartburn, increased appetite, nausea, trouble with gums, unpleasant taste, vomiting, weight gain/loss, xerostomia

Genitourinary: Difficult urination, impotence, testicular edema

Hematologic: Agranulocytosis, eosinophilia, leukopenia, purpura, thrombocytopenia

Hepatic: Cholestatic jaundice, increased liver enzymes

Neuromuscular & skeletal: Fine muscle tremor, numbness, tingling, tremor, weakness

Ocular: Blurred vision, eye pain, increased intraocular pressure

Otic: Tinnitus

Miscellaneous: Allergic reactions, excessive diaphoresis

Drug Interactions

Metabolism/Transport Effects Substrate of CYP2D6 (major); **Note:** Assignment of Major/Minor substrate status based on clinically relevant drug interaction potential

Avoid Concomitant Use

Avoid concomitant use of Protriptyline with any of the following: Aclidinium; Azelastine (Nasal); Cisapride; Iobenguane I 123; Ipratropium (Oral Inhalation); Linezolid; MAO Inhibitors; Methylene Blue; Moxonidine; Paraldehyde; Potassium Chloride; Thalidomide; Tiotropium; Umeclidinium

Increased Effect/Toxicity

Protriptyline may increase the levels/effects of: AbobotulinumtoxinA; Alcohol (Ethyl); Alpha-/Beta-Agonists (Direct-Acting); Alpha1-Agonists; Amphetamines; Analgesics (Opioid); Anticholinergic Agents; Antipsychotics; Azelastine (Nasal); Beta2-Agonists; Buprenorphine; Cannabinoid-Containing Products; Cisapride; Citalopram; CNS Depressants; Desmopressin; Escitalopram; Highest Risk QTc-Prolonging Agents; Hydrocodone; Methotrimeprazine; Methylene Blue; Metyrosine; Mirabegron; Moderate Risk QTc-Prolonging Agents; OnabotulinumtoxinA; Paraldehyde; Potassium Chloride; Pramipexole; QuiNIDine; RimabotulinumtoxinB; ROPINIRole; Rotigotine; Serotonin Modulators; Sodium Phosphates; Sulfonylureas; Thalidomide; Thiazide Diuretics; Tiotropium; Topiramate; TraMADol; Vitamin K Antagonists; Yohimbine; Zolpidem

The levels/effects of Protriptyline may be increased by: Abiraterone Acetate; Aclidinium; Altretamine; Antiemetics (5HT3 Antagonists); Antipsychotics; Brimonidine (Topical); Cannabis; Cimetidine; Cinacalcet; Citalopram; Cobicistat; CYP2D6 Inhibitors (Moderate); CYP2D6 Inhibitors (Strong); Darunavir; Dexmethylphenidate; Doxylamine; Dronabinol; Droperidol; DULoxetine; Escitalopram; FLUoxetine; FluvoxaMINE; HydrOXYzine; Ipratropium (Oral Inhalation); Kava Kava; Linezolid; Lithium; Magnesium Sulfate; MAO Inhibitors; Methotrimeprazine; Methylphenidate; Metoclopramide; Metyrosine; Mifepristone; Nabilone; PARoxetine; Perampanel; Pramlintide; Protease Inhibitors; QuiNIDine; Rufinamide; Sertraline; Sodium Oxybate; Tapentadol; Terbinafine (Systemic); Tetrahydrocannabinol; Thyroid Products; TraMADol; Umeclidinium; Valproic Acid and Derivatives

Decreased Effect

Protriptyline may decrease the levels/effects of: Acetylcholinesterase Inhibitors (Central); Alpha2-Agonists; Alpha2-Agonists (Ophthalmic); Iobenguane I 123; Moxonidine; Secretin

The levels/effects of Protriptyline may be decreased by: Acetylcholinesterase Inhibitors (Central); Barbiturates; CarBAMazepine; Peginterferon Alfa-2b; St Johns Wort

Mechanism of Action Increases the synaptic concentration of serotonin and/or norepinephrine in the central nervous system by inhibition of their reuptake by the presynaptic neuronal membrane

Pharmacodynamics

Onset of action: 1-2 weeks
Maximum effect: 4-12 weeks
Duration: 1-2 days

Pharmacokinetics (Adult data unless noted)

Protein binding: 92%
Metabolism: Extensively hepatic via N-oxidation, hydroxylation, and glucuronidation; first-pass effect (10% to 25%)
Half-life: 54-92 hours (average: 74 hours)
Time to peak serum concentration: 24-30 hours
Elimination: Urine

Dosing: Usual Oral:

Children: **Note:** Safe and effective use in children has not been established; controlled clinical trials have not shown tricyclic antidepressants to be superior to placebo for the treatment of depression in children and adolescents (Dopheide, 2006; Wagner, 2005).

Adolescents: Manufacturer labeling: Initial: 5 mg/dose given 2-3 times/day; may increase in 2 weeks as tolerated; slow titration is recommended in order to facilitate monitoring for adverse effects such as behavioral activation; usual dose: 15-20 mg/day in divided doses

Adults: Initial: 10 mg/dose given twice daily; may increase every week as tolerated to a goal of 30-60 mg/day in 3-4 divided doses

Administration Oral: May administer with food to decrease GI upset; do not administer with grapefruit juice.

Monitoring Parameters Heart rate, blood pressure, mental status, weight. Monitor patient periodically for symptom resolution; monitor for worsening depression, suicidality, and associated behaviors (especially at the beginning of therapy or when doses are increased or decreased).

Reference Range Therapeutic: 70-250 ng/mL (SI: 266-950 nmol/L); Toxic: >500 ng/mL (SI: >1900 nmol/L)

Dosage Forms Excipient information presented when available (limited, particularly for generics); consult specific product labeling.

Tablet, Oral, as hydrochloride:
Vivactil: 5 mg [contains fd&c red #40, fd&c yellow #6 (sunset yellow)]
Vivactil: 10 mg [contains fd&c yellow #10 (quinoline yellow)]
Generic: 5 mg, 10 mg

References

ACOG Committee on Practice Bulletins-Obstetrics. ACOG practice bulletin: clinical management guidelines for obstetrician-gynecologists number 92, April 2008 (replaces practice bulletin number 87, November 2007). Use of psychiatric medications during pregnancy and lactation. *Obstet Gynecol.* 2008;111(4):1001-1020.

American Psychiatric Association (APA). Treatment recommendations for patients with major depressive disorder. 3rd ed, May 2010. Available at http://www.psychiatryonline.com/pracGuide/pracGuideTopic_7.aspx

Dopheide JA, "Recognizing and Treating Depression in Children and Adolescents," *Am J Health Syst Pharm,* 2006, 63(3):233-43.

Larochelle P, Hamet P, and Enjalbert M, "Responses to Tyramine and Norepinephrine After Imipramine and Trazodone," *Clin Pharmacol Ther,* 1979, 26(1):24-30.

Mitchell JR, "Guanethidine and Related Agents. III Antagonism by Drugs Which Inhibit the Norepinephrine Pump in Man," *J Clin Invest,* 1970, 49(8):1596-604.

Pass SE and Simpson RW, "Discontinuation and Reinstitution of Medications During the Perioperative Period," *Am J Health Syst Pharm,* 2004, 61(9):899-912.

Roose SP, Glassman AH, Attia E, et al, "Comparative Efficacy of Selective Serotonin Reuptake Inhibitors and Tricyclics in the Treatment of Melancholia," *Am J Psychiatry,* 1994, 151(12):1735-9.

Rundegren J, van Dijken J, Mörnstad H, et al, "Oral Conditions in Patients Receiving Long-Term Treatment With Cyclic Antidepressant Drugs," *Swed Dent J,* 1985, 9(2):55-64.

Smith IE and Quinnell TG, "Pharmacotherapies for Obstructive Sleep Apnoea: Where Are We Now?" *Drugs,* 2004, 64(13):1385-99.

Svedmyr N, "The Influence of a Tricyclic Antidepressive Agent (Protriptyline) on Some of the Circulatory Effects of Noradrenaline and Adrenalin in Man," *Life Sci,* 1968, 7(1):77-84.

Wagner KD, "Pharmacotherapy for Major Depression in Children and Adolescents," *Prog Neuropsychopharmacol Biol Psychiatry,* 2005, 29 (5):819-26.

Yonkers KA, Wisner KL, Stewart DE, et al. The management of depression during pregnancy: a report from the American Psychiatric Association and the American College of Obstetricians and Gynecologists. *Obstet Gynecol.* 2009;114(3):703-713.

◆ **Protriptyline Hydrochloride** *see* Protriptyline *on page 1767*

◆ **Protylol (Can)** *see* Dicyclomine *on page 652*

◆ **PRO-Valacyclovir (Can)** *see* ValACYclovir *on page 2097*

◆ **Proventil HFA** *see* Albuterol *on page 84*

◆ **Provera** *see* MedroxyPROGESTERone *on page 1318*

◆ **Provera® (Can)** *see* MedroxyPROGESTERone *on page 1318*

◆ **Provera-Pak (Can)** *see* MedroxyPROGESTERone *on page 1318*

◆ **PRO-Verapamil SR (Can)** *see* Verapamil *on page 2129*

◆ **Provigil** see Modafinil on page 1429

◆ **Provil [OTC]** see Ibuprofen on page 1059

◆ **Proxymetacaine** see Proparacaine on page 1755

◆ **PROzac** see FLUoxetine on page 901

◆ **Prozac (Can)** see FLUoxetine on page 901

◆ **PROzac Weekly** see FLUoxetine on page 901

◆ **PRP-OMP (PedvaxHIB)** see Haemophilus b Conjugate Vaccine on page 994

◆ **PRP-T (ActHIB)** see Haemophilus b Conjugate Vaccine on page 994

◆ **PRP-T (Hiberix)** see Haemophilus b Conjugate Vaccine on page 994

◆ **Prudoxin** see Doxepin (Topical) on page 717

◆ **Prymaccone** see Primaquine on page 1735

◆ **P & S [OTC]** see Salicylic Acid on page 1860

◆ **23PS** see Pneumococcal Polysaccharide Vaccine (Polyvalent) on page 1691

Pseudoephedrine (soo doe e FED rin)

Medication Safety Issues
Sound-alike/look-alike issues:
Sudafed® may be confused with sotalol, Sudafed PE®, Sufenta®

Related Information
Oral Medications That Should Not Be Crushed or Altered on page 2438

Brand Names: U.S.
Childrens Silfedrine [OTC]; Decongestant 12Hour Max St [OTC]; ElixSure Congestion [OTC]; Genaphed [OTC]; Nasal Decongestant [OTC]; Nexafed [OTC]; Psudatabs [OTC]; Simply Stuffy [OTC]; Sudafed 12 Hour [OTC]; Sudafed 24 Hour [OTC]; Sudafed Childrens [OTC]; Sudafed [OTC]; Sudanyl [OTC]; SudoGest 12 Hour [OTC]; SudoGest [OTC]; Suphedrine [OTC]; Zephrex-D [OTC]

Brand Names: Canada
Balminil Decongestant; Benylin® D for Infants; Contac® Cold 12 Hour Relief Non Drowsy; Drixoral® ND; Eltor®; PMS-Pseudoephedrine; Pseudofrin; Robidrine®; Sudafed® Decongestant

Therapeutic Category
Adrenergic Agonist Agent; Decongestant; Sympathomimetic

Generic Availability (U.S.)
May be product dependent

Use
Temporary symptomatic relief of nasal congestion due to common cold, upper respiratory allergies, and sinusitis; also promotes nasal or sinus drainage (immediate release formulations: FDA approved in ages >4 years and adults; extended release formulations: FDA approved in ages >12 years and adults)

Pregnancy Considerations
Use of pseudoephedrine during the first trimester may be associated with a possible risk of gastroschisis, small intestinal atresia, and hemifacial microsomia due to pseudoephedrine's vasoconstrictive effects; additional studies are needed to define the magnitude of risk. Single doses of pseudoephedrine were not found to adversely affect the fetus during the third trimester of pregnancy (limited data); however, fetal tachycardia was noted in a case report following maternal use of an extended release product for multiple days. Decongestants are not the preferred agents for the treatment of rhinitis during pregnancy. Oral pseudoephedrine should be avoided during the first trimester.

Breast-Feeding Considerations
Pseudoephedrine is excreted into breast milk in concentrations that are ~4% of the weight adjusted maternal dose. The time to maximum milk concentration is ~1-2 hours after the maternal dose. Irritability has been reported in nursing infants (limited data; dose, duration, relationship to breast-feeding not provided). Milk production may be decreased in some women.

Contraindications
Hypersensitivity to pseudoephedrine or any component; MAO inhibitor therapy, severe hypertension, severe coronary artery disease

Warnings
Safety and efficacy for the use of cough and cold products in children <2 years of age is limited. Serious adverse effects including death have been reported. The FDA notes that there are no approved OTC uses for these products in children <2 years of age. Healthcare providers are reminded to ask caregivers about the use of OTC cough and cold products in order to avoid exposure to multiple medications containing the same ingredient. Some products contain sodium benzoate; benzoic acid (benzoate) is a metabolite of benzyl alcohol; large amounts of benzyl alcohol (≥99 mg/kg/day) have been associated with a potentially fatal toxicity ("gasping syndrome") in neonates; in vitro and animal studies have shown that benzoate displaces bilirubin from protein binding sites; avoid use of sodium benzoate containing products in neonates

Precautions
Use with caution in patients with hyperthyroidism, diabetes mellitus, prostatic hypertrophy, mild-moderate hypertension, arrhythmias, renal impairment, seizure disorders.

When used for self-medication (OTC), notify healthcare provider if symptoms do not improve within 7 days or are accompanied by fever. Discontinue and contact healthcare provider if nervousness, dizziness, or sleeplessness occur.

Adverse Reactions
Cardiovascular: Arrhythmia, cardiovascular collapse with hypotension, hypertension, palpitation, tachycardia

Central nervous system: Chills, confusion, coordination impaired, dizziness, drowsiness, excitability, fatigue, hallucination, headache, insomnia, nervousness, neuritis, restlessness, seizure, transient stimulation, vertigo

Dermatologic: Photosensitivity, rash, urticaria

Gastrointestinal: Anorexia, constipation, diarrhea, dry throat, ischemic colitis, nausea, vomiting, xerostomia

Genitourinary: Difficult urination, dysuria, polyuria, urinary retention

Hematologic: Agranulocytosis, hemolytic anemia, thrombocytopenia

Neuromuscular & skeletal: Tremor, weakness

Ocular: Blurred vision, diplopia

Otic: Tinnitus

Respiratory: Chest/throat tightness, dry nose, dyspnea, nasal congestion, thickening of bronchial secretions, wheezing

Miscellaneous: Anaphylaxis, diaphoresis

Drug Interactions
Metabolism/Transport Effects None known.

Avoid Concomitant Use
Avoid concomitant use of Pseudoephedrine with any of the following: Ergot Derivatives; Iobenguane I 123; MAO Inhibitors

Increased Effect/Toxicity
Pseudoephedrine may increase the levels/effects of: Sympathomimetics

The levels/effects of Pseudoephedrine may be increased by: Alkalinizing Agents; AtoMOXetine; Cannabinoid-Containing Products; Carbonic Anhydrase Inhibitors; Ergot Derivatives; Linezolid; MAO Inhibitors; Serotonin/Norepinephrine Reuptake Inhibitors

Decreased Effect
Pseudoephedrine may decrease the levels/effects of: Benzylpenicilloyl Polylysine; FentaNYL; Iobenguane I 123

The levels/effects of Pseudoephedrine may be decreased by: Alpha1-Blockers; Spironolactone; Urinary Acidifying Agents

Food Interactions Onset of effect may be delayed if pseudoephedrine is taken with food. Management: Administer without regard to food.

Mechanism of Action Directly stimulates alpha-adrenergic receptors of respiratory mucosa causing vasoconstriction; directly stimulates beta-adrenergic receptors causing bronchial relaxation, increased heart rate and contractility

Pharmacodynamics

Onset of action: Decongestant: Oral: 30 minutes (Chua, 1989)

Maximum effect: Decongestant: Oral: ~1-2 hours (Chua, 1989)

Duration: Immediate release tablet: 3-8 hours (Chua, 1989)

Pharmacokinetics (Adult data unless noted)

Absorption: Rapid (Simons, 1996)

Distribution: V_d:

Children: ~2.5 L/kg (Simons, 1996)

Adults: 2.64-3.51 L/kg (Kanfer, 1993)

Metabolism: Undergoes n-demethylation to norpseudoephedrine (active) (Chua, 1989; Kanfer, 1993); hepatic (<1%) (Kanfer, 1993)

Half-life elimination: Varies by urine pH and flow rate; alkaline urine decreases renal elimination of pseudoephedrine (Kanfer, 1993)

Children: ~3 hours (urine pH ~6.5) (Simons, 1996)

Adults: 9-16 hours (pH 8); 3-6 hours (pH 5) (Chua, 1989)

Time to peak serum concentration:

Children: Immediate release tablet: ~2 hours (Simons, 1996)

Adults: Immediate release tablet: 1-3 hours (dose-dependent) (Kanfer, 1993)

Elimination: Urine (43% to 96% as unchanged drug, 1% to 6% as active norpseudoephedrine); dependent on urine pH and flow rate; alkaline urine decreases renal elimination of pseudoephedrine (Kanfer, 1993)

Dosing: Usual Oral:

Infants and Children:

<4 years: 1 mg/kg/dose every 6 hours; maximum single dose: 15 mg (Gentile, 2000)

4-5 years:

Manufacturer's recommendation: 15 mg every 4-6 hours; maximum dose: 60 mg/24 hours

Alternative dosing: 1 mg/kg/dose every 6 hours; maximum dose: 15 mg (Gentile, 2000)

6-12 years: 30 mg every 4-6 hours; maximum dose: 120 mg/24 hours

Adolescents and Adults:

Immediate release: 60 mg every 4-6 hours; maximum dose: 240 mg/day

Extended release: 120 mg every 12 hours or 240 mg once daily

Administration Oral: Administer with water or milk to decrease GI distress; swallow timed release tablets or capsules whole, do not chew or crush; Sudafed® 24 Hour tablet may not completely dissolve and appear in stool

Test Interactions Interferes with urine detection of amphetamine (false-positive)

Additional Information Because ephedrine and pseudoephedrine have been used to synthesize methamphetamine, the DEA has placed them in the category of "Schedule Listed Products"; restrictions are in place to reduce the potential for misuse (diversion) and abuse (eg, storage requirements, additional documentation of sale); the DEA limit for a single transaction to a single individual for drug products containing ephedrine or pseudoephedrine is 3.6 g/24 hours, 9 g/30 days, or if mail-order transaction 7.5 g/30 days.

Dosage Forms Excipient information presented when available (limited, particularly for generics); consult specific product labeling.

Gel, Oral, as hydrochloride:

ElixSure Congestion: 15 mg/5 mL (120 mL) [alcohol free; contains brilliant blue fcf (fd&c blue #1), carbomer 934p, propylene glycol, propylparaben; grape bubblegum flavor]

Liquid, Oral, as hydrochloride:

Childrens Silfedrine: 15 mg/5 mL (118 mL, 237 mL) [grape flavor]

Nasal Decongestant: 30 mg/5 mL (118 mL) [contains fd&c red #40, methylparaben, saccharin sodium, sodium benzoate; raspberry flavor]

Sudafed Childrens: 15 mg/5 mL (118 mL) [alcohol free, sugar free; contains brilliant blue fcf (fd&c blue #1), edetate disodium, fd&c red #40, menthol, polyethylene glycol, saccharin sodium, sodium benzoate; grape flavor]

Syrup, Oral, as hydrochloride:

Nasal Decongestant: 30 mg/5 mL (473 mL) [contains fd&c red #40, methylparaben, saccharin sodium, sodium benzoate; raspberry flavor]

Tablet, Oral, as hydrochloride:

Genaphed: 30 mg

Nasal Decongestant: 30 mg [contains fd&c red #40 aluminum lake, fd&c yellow #6 aluminum lake]

Nasal Decongestant: 30 mg [contains fd&c red #40 aluminum lake, polysorbate 80]

Psudatabs: 30 mg [contains fd&c red #40, fd&c yellow #10 (quinoline yellow), fd&c yellow #6 (sunset yellow)]

Simply Stuffy: 30 mg

Sudafed: 30 mg

Sudafed: 30 mg [contains fd&c red #40 aluminum lake, fd&c yellow #10 aluminum lake, fd&c yellow #6 aluminum lake]

Sudanyl: 30 mg

SudoGest: 30 mg [contains fd&c red #40 aluminum lake, fd&c yellow #10 aluminum lake, fd&c yellow #6 aluminum lake]

SudoGest: 30 mg [contains fd&c red #40 aluminum lake, fd&c yellow #6 aluminum lake]

SudoGest: 60 mg [scored]

Suphedrine: 30 mg

Generic: 30 mg, 60 mg

Tablet Abuse-Deterrent, Oral, as hydrochloride:

Nexafed: 30 mg

Zephrex-D: 30 mg

Tablet Extended Release 12 Hour, Oral, as hydrochloride:

Decongestant 12Hour Max St: 120 mg [contains polysorbate 80]

Sudafed 12 Hour: 120 mg

Sudafed 12 Hour: 120 mg [contains fd&c blue #1 aluminum lake]

SudoGest 12 Hour: 120 mg

Generic: 120 mg

Tablet Extended Release 24 Hour, Oral, as hydrochloride:

Sudafed 24 Hour: 240 mg

References

Chua SS, Benrimoj SI, and Triggs EJ, "Pharmacokinetics of Non-Prescription Sympathomimetic Agents," *Biopharm Drug Dispos*, 1989, 10(1):1-14.

Gentile DA, Friday GA, and Skoner DP, "Management of Allergic Rhinitis: Antihistamines and Decongestants," *Immunol Allergy Clin NA*, 2000, 20(2):355-68.

Kanfer I, Dowse R, and Vuma V, "Pharmacokinetics of Oral Decongestants," *Pharmacotherapy*, 1993, 13(6 Pt 2):116-28.

Simons FE, Gu X, Watson WT, et al, "Pharmacokinetics of the Orally Administered Decongestants Pseudoephedrine and Phenylpropanolamine in Children," *J Pediatr*, 1996, 129(5):729-34.

Werler MM, "Teratogen Update: Pseudoephedrine," *Birth Defects Res A Clin Mol Teratol*, 2006, 76(6):445-52.

◆ **Pseudoephedrine and Brompheniramine** see Brompheniramine and Pseudoephedrine on page 306

Pseudoephedrine and Ibuprofen
(soo doe e FED rin & eye byoo PROE fen)

Brand Names: U.S. Advil® Cold & Sinus [OTC]; Proprinal® Cold and Sinus [OTC]

Brand Names: Canada Advil® Cold & Sinus; Advil® Cold & Sinus Daytime; Children's Advil® Cold; Sudafed® Sinus Advance

Therapeutic Category Decongestant/Analgesic

Generic Availability (U.S.) Yes: Caplet

Use Temporary relief of cold, sinus, and flu symptoms (including nasal congestion, headache, sore throat, minor body aches and pains, and fever)

Pregnancy Considerations Refer to individual agents.

Breast-Feeding Considerations Refer to individual agents.

Contraindications Hypersensitivity to pseudoephedrine, ibuprofen, or any component, aspirin, or other NSAIDs; active GI bleeding, ulcer disease; patients with the "aspirin triad" [asthma, rhinitis (with or without nasal polyps), and aspirin intolerance] (fatal asthmatic and anaphylactoid reactions may occur in these patients); MAO inhibitor therapy, severe hypertension, severe coronary artery disease

Warnings Safety and efficacy for the use of cough and cold products in children <2 years of age is limited. Serious adverse effects including death have been reported (in some cases, high blood concentrations of pseudoephedrine were found). The FDA notes that there are no approved OTC uses for these products in children <2 years of age. Healthcare providers are reminded to ask caregivers about the use of OTC cough and cold products in order to avoid exposure to multiple medications containing the same ingredient.

Some products contain sodium benzoate; benzoic acid (benzoate) is a metabolite of benzyl alcohol; large amounts of benzyl alcohol (≥99 mg/kg/day) have been associated with a potentially fatal toxicity ("gasping syndrome") in neonates; the "gasping syndrome" consists of metabolic acidosis, respiratory distress, gasping respirations, CNS dysfunction (including convulsions, intracranial hemorrhage), hypotension and cardiovascular collapse; avoid use of formulations containing sodium benzoate in neonates; in vitro and animal studies have shown that benzoate displaces bilirubin from protein binding sites

Precautions Use with caution in patients with mild-moderate hypertension, heart disease, arrhythmias, diabetes mellitus, thyroid disease, asthma, glaucoma, prostatic hypertrophy, CHF, decreased renal or hepatic function, dehydration, history of GI disease (bleeding or ulcers), or those receiving anticoagulants.

Adverse Reactions See individual agents.

Drug Interactions

Metabolism/Transport Effects Refer to individual components.

Avoid Concomitant Use

Avoid concomitant use of Pseudoephedrine and Ibuprofen with any of the following: Ergot Derivatives; Floctafenine; Iobenguane I 123; Ketorolac (Nasal); Ketorolac (Systemic); MAO Inhibitors; NSAID (COX-2 Inhibitor); Omacetaxine; Urokinase

Increased Effect/Toxicity

Pseudoephedrine and Ibuprofen may increase the levels/effects of: 5-ASA Derivatives; Agents with Antiplatelet Properties; Aliskiren; Aminoglycosides; Anticoagulants; Apixaban; Bisphosphonate Derivatives; Collagenase (Systemic); CycloSPORINE (Systemic); Dabigatran Etexilate; Deferasirox; Desmopressin; Digoxin; Eplerenone; Haloperidol; Ibritumomab; Lithium; Methotrexate; Nonsteroidal Anti-Inflammatory Agents; NSAID (COX-2 Inhibitor); Omacetaxine; PEMEtrexed; Porfimer;

Potassium-Sparing Diuretics; PRALAtrexate; Quinolone Antibiotics; Rivaroxaban; Salicylates; Sympathomimetics; Tenofovir; Thrombolytic Agents; Tositumomab and Iodine I 131 Tositumomab; Urokinase; Vancomycin; Vitamin K Antagonists

The levels/effects of Pseudoephedrine and Ibuprofen may be increased by: ACE Inhibitors; Alkalinizing Agents; Angiotensin II Receptor Blockers; Antidepressants (Tricyclic, Tertiary Amine); AtoMOXetine; Cannabinoid-Containing Products; Carbonic Anhydrase Inhibitors; Corticosteroids (Systemic); CycloSPORINE (Systemic); Dasatinib; Ergot Derivatives; Floctafenine; Glucosamine; Herbs (Anticoagulant/Antiplatelet Properties); Ibrutinib; Ketorolac (Nasal); Ketorolac (Systemic); Linezolid; MAO Inhibitors; Multivitamins/Fluoride (with ADE); Multivitamins/Minerals (with ADEK, Folate, Iron); Multivitamins/Minerals (with AE, No Iron); Nonsteroidal Anti-Inflammatory Agents; Omega-3 Fatty Acids; Pentosan Polysulfate Sodium; Pentoxifylline; Probenecid; Prostacyclin Analogues; Selective Serotonin Reuptake Inhibitors; Serotonin/Norepinephrine Reuptake Inhibitors; Sodium Phosphates; Tipranavir; Treprostinil; Vitamin E; Voriconazole

Decreased Effect

Pseudoephedrine and Ibuprofen may decrease the levels/effects of: ACE Inhibitors; Agents with Antiplatelet Properties; Aliskiren; Angiotensin II Receptor Blockers; Benzylpenicilloyl Polylysine; Beta-Blockers; Eplerenone; FentaNYL; HydrALAZINE; Imatinib; Iobenguane I 123; Loop Diuretics; Potassium-Sparing Diuretics; Prostaglandins (Ophthalmic); Salicylates; Selective Serotonin Reuptake Inhibitors; Thiazide Diuretics

The levels/effects of Pseudoephedrine and Ibuprofen may be decreased by: Alpha1-Blockers; Bile Acid Sequestrants; Nonsteroidal Anti-Inflammatory Agents; Salicylates; Spironolactone; Urinary Acidifying Agents

Food Interactions See individual agents.

Pharmacodynamics See individual monographs for Pseudoephedrine and Ibuprofen.

Pharmacokinetics (Adult data unless noted) See individual monographs for Pseudoephedrine and Ibuprofen.

Dosing: Usual Oral:

Manufacturer's recommendations:

Advil® Cold & Sinus (capsules): Children >12 years and Adults: 1 capsule (pseudoephedrine 30 mg/ibuprofen 200 mg) every 4-6 hours; if symptoms do not respond; may use 2 capsules/dose; not to exceed 6 capsules/day

Alternative pediatric dosing: May dose according to the pseudoephedrine component:

Children ≥2 years: 4 mg/kg/day in divided doses every 6 hours or as an alternative:

Children 2-5 years: 15 mg every 6 hours; maximum dose: 60 mg/24 hours

Children 6-12 years: 30 mg every 6 hours or extended release product 60 mg every 12 hours; maximum dose: 120 mg/24 hours

Children >12 years and Adults: 30-60 mg every 6 hours; maximum dose: 240 mg/24 hours

Administration Oral: Administer with food

Test Interactions See individual agents.

Dosage Forms Excipient information presented when available (limited, particularly for generics); consult specific product labeling.

Caplet:

Advil® Cold & Sinus, Proprinal® Cold and Sinus: Pseudoephedrine hydrochloride 30 mg and ibuprofen 200 mg

Capsule, liquid filled:

Advil® Cold & Sinus: Pseudoephedrine hydrochloride 30 mg and ibuprofen 200 mg [solubilized ibuprofen as free acid and potassium salt; contains potassium 20 mg/capsule and coconut oil]

◆ **Pseudoephedrine and Loratadine** *see* Loratadine and Pseudoephedrine *on page 1279*

◆ **Pseudoephedrine and Triprolidine** *see* Triprolidine and Pseudoephedrine *on page 2090*

◆ **Pseudoephedrine Hydrochloride** *see* Pseudoephedrine *on page 1770*

◆ **Pseudoephedrine Sulfate** *see* Pseudoephedrine *on page 1770*

◆ **Pseudofrin (Can)** *see* Pseudoephedrine *on page 1770*

◆ **Pseudomonic Acid A** *see* Mupirocin *on page 1452*

◆ **Psoriasin [OTC]** *see* Coal Tar *on page 532*

◆ **Psoriasin [OTC]** *see* Salicylic Acid *on page 1860*

◆ **Psudatabs [OTC]** *see* Pseudoephedrine *on page 1770*

Psyllium (SIL i yum)

Medication Safety Issues
Sound-alike/look-alike issues:
Fiberall® may be confused with Feverall®

Brand Names: U.S. Dietary Fiber Laxative [OTC]; Evac [OTC]; Fiber Therapy [OTC]; Geri-Mucil [OTC]; Konsyl [OTC]; Konsyl-D [OTC]; Metamucil MultiHealth Fiber [OTC]; Natural Fiber Therapy [OTC]; Natural Psyllium Seed [OTC]; Natural Vegetable Fiber [OTC]; Reguloid [OTC]; Sorbulax [OTC]

Brand Names: Canada Metamucil®

Therapeutic Category Laxative, Bulk-Producing

Generic Availability (U.S.) May be product dependent

Use Dietary fiber supplement (OTC: All products: FDA approved in adults; refer to product specific information regarding FDA approval in pediatric patients, most products FDA approved in ages ≥12 years); treatment of occasional constipation (OTC: All products: FDA approved in adults; refer to product specific information regarding FDA approval in pediatric patients, most products FDA approved in ages ≥6 years); has also been used for adjunctive treatment with dietary management for hyperlipidemia (eg, LDL, total cholesterol, or triglycerides) and treatment of chronic constipation; management of irritable bowel syndrome

Pregnancy Considerations Psyllium is not absorbed systemically. When administered with adequate fluids, use is considered safe for the treatment of occasional constipation during pregnancy (Wald, 2003).

Contraindications Hypersensitivity to psyllium or any component; difficulty swallowing

Warnings Hypersensitivity reactions have been reported with ingestion or inhalation of psyllium in susceptible individuals. Products must be taken with at least 8 ounces of fluid in order to prevent choking; if difficulty breathing or swallowing, chest pain, or vomiting occurs after a dose, immediately seek medical attention; do not use in patients with difficulty swallowing. When used for self-medication (OTC), do not use in the presence of abdominal pain, nausea, or vomiting. Healthcare provider should be contacted prior to use if sudden changes of bowel habits have persisted >2 weeks. If rectal bleeding or failure to have a bowel movement occurs or constipation persists beyond 1 week, discontinue use and contact healthcare provider. Not for self-treatment of constipation lasting >1 week.

Precautions Use with caution in patients with esophageal strictures, ulcers, stenosis, or intestinal adhesions; avoid use in patients with or prone to fecal impaction or GI obstruction. To reduce the risk of coronary heart disease, the soluble fiber from psyllium should be used in conjunction with a diet low in saturated fat and cholesterol.

Some products may contain aspartame which is metabolized to phenylalanine and must be avoided (or used with caution) in patients with phenylketonuria. Some products may contain the following (consult detailed product-specific labeling): Calcium, potassium, sodium, or soy lecithin.

Adverse Reactions
Gastrointestinal: Abdominal cramps, constipation, diarrhea, esophageal or bowel obstruction
Respiratory: Bronchospasm
Miscellaneous: Anaphylaxis upon inhalation in susceptible individuals, rhinoconjunctivitis

Drug Interactions
Metabolism/Transport Effects None known.
Avoid Concomitant Use There are no known interactions where it is recommended to avoid concomitant use.
Increased Effect/Toxicity There are no known significant interactions involving an increase in effect.
Decreased Effect There are no known significant interactions involving a decrease in effect.

Stability Store at room temperature; protect from moisture (consult product labeling for specific information).

Mechanism of Action Psyllium is a soluble fiber. It absorbs water in the intestine to form a viscous liquid which promotes peristalsis and reduces transit time.

Pharmacodynamics Onset of action: 12-72 hours

Pharmacokinetics (Adult data unless noted) Absorption: Oral: Generally not absorbed; small amounts of grain extract present in the preparation have been reportedly absorbed following colonic hydrolysis

Dosing: Usual
Children and Adolescents:
Adequate intake for total fiber: Oral: **Note:** The definition of "fiber" varies; however, the soluble fiber in psyllium is only one type of fiber which makes up the daily recommended intake of total fiber; contribution from other food sources should also be considered when assessing intake. Reported requirements variable:
AAP/NHLBI recommendation (NHLBI, 2011): Minimum intake: Children 2-10 years: Daily dietary intake (g/day) = Age (years) + 5 g
IOM recommendation:
Children 1-3 years: 19 g/day
Children 4-8 years: 25 g/day
Children and Adolescents 9-13 years: Male: 31 g/day; Female: 26 g/day
Adolescents: 14-18 years: Male: 38 g/day; Female: 26 g/day
Constipation: Oral: **Note:** General dosing guidelines (Federal Register, 1985); consult specific product labeling.
Children 6-11 years: 1.25-15 g/day in 1-3 divided doses
Children ≥12 years and Adults: 2.5-30 g/day in 1-3 divided doses
Hypercholesterolemia; adjunct treatment with dietary management (NHLBI, 2011): Oral:
Children 2 to <12 years: 6 g/day in 1-3 divided doses
Children ≥12 years and Adolescents: 12 g/day in 1-3 divided doses
Adults:
Adequate intake for total fiber: Oral: **Note:** The definition of "fiber" varies; however, the soluble fiber in psyllium is only one type of fiber which makes up the daily recommended intake of total fiber.
Adults 19-50 years: Male: 38 g/day; Female: 25 g/day
Adults ≥51 years: Male: 30 g/day; Female: 21 g/day
Pregnancy: 28 g/day
Lactation: 29 g/day
Constipation: Oral: Psyllium: 2.5-30 g per day in divided doses

Reduce risk of coronary heart disease: Oral: Soluble fiber ≥7 g (psyllium seed husk ≥10.2 g) per day

Administration Oral: Granules and powder must be mixed in an 8 ounce glass of water or juice; drink an 8 ounce glass of liquid with each dose of wafers or capsules; capsules should be swallowed one at a time. When more than one dose is required, divide throughout the day. Separate dose by at least 2 hours from other drug therapies. Inhalation of psyllium dust may cause sensitivity to psyllium (eg, runny nose, watery eyes, wheezing).

Monitoring Parameters Dependent upon use, may include stool output and frequency; serum lipids, weight

Dosage Forms Considerations Psyllium hydrophilic mucilloid 3.4 g is equivalent to 2 g Soluble fiber

Dosage Forms Excipient information presented when available (limited, particularly for generics); consult specific product labeling. [DSC] = Discontinued product
Capsule, Oral:
  Konsyl: 520 mg [gluten free, sugar free]
  Reguloid: 0.52 g [contains fd&c yellow #6 aluminum lake]
Packet, Oral:
  Konsyl: 28.3% (1 ea) [gluten free, kosher certified; contains fd&c yellow #10 (quinoline yellow), fd&c yellow #6 (sunset yellow)]
  Konsyl: 28.3% (30 ea) [gluten free, kosher certified; contains fd&c yellow #10 (quinoline yellow), fd&c yellow #6 (sunset yellow); orange flavor]
  Konsyl: 60.3% (1 ea, 30 ea) [gluten free, kosher certified, sugar free; contains aspartame, fd&c yellow #6 (sunset yellow); orange flavor]
  Konsyl: 100% (1 ea, 30 ea, 100 ea) [gluten free, kosher certified, sugar free; bland flavor]
Powder, Oral:
  Dietary Fiber Laxative: 28.3% (283 g, 300 g, 425 g, 660 g) [contains fd&c yellow #6 (sunset yellow)]
  Fiber Therapy: 58.6% (283 g) [sugar free; contains aspartame, fd&c yellow #6 (sunset yellow)]
  Geri-Mucil: 68% (368 g)
  Geri-Mucil: 68% (368 g) [contains fd&c yellow #6 aluminum lake]
  Geri-Mucil: 68% (284 g) [sugar free]
  Geri-Mucil: 68% (283 g) [sugar free; contains aspartame, fd&c yellow #6 aluminum lake]
  Konsyl: 28.3% (538 g) [gluten free, kosher certified; contains fd&c yellow #10 (quinoline yellow), fd&c yellow #6 (sunset yellow); orange flavor]
  Konsyl: 30.9% (397 g) [gluten free, kosher certified; contains fd&c yellow #6 (sunset yellow); orange flavor]
  Konsyl: 60.3% (450 g) [gluten free, kosher certified, sugar free; contains aspartame, fd&c yellow #6 (sunset yellow); orange flavor]
  Konsyl: 71.67% (300 g) [gluten free, kosher certified, sugar free; bland flavor]
  Konsyl: 100% (300 g, 450 g) [gluten free, kosher certified, sugar free]
  Konsyl: 100% (300 g, 450 g) [gluten free, kosher certified, sugar free; bland flavor]
  Konsyl: 60.3% (283 g) [sugar free; contains aspartame, fd&c yellow #6 (sunset yellow); orange flavor]
  Konsyl-D: 52.3% (397 g, 500 g [DSC]) [flavor free; sweet flavor]
  Metamucil MultiHealth Fiber: 58.6% (425 g) [gluten free, sugar free; contains aspartame, brilliant blue fcf (fd&c blue #1), fd&c red #40]
  Metamucil MultiHealth Fiber: 63% (660 g) [gluten free, sugar free]
  Natural Fiber Therapy: 30.9% (368 g, 539 g); 48.57% (368 g, 538 g)
  Natural Psyllium Seed: 100% (480 g) [animal products free, gelatin free, gluten free, kosher certified, lactose free, no artificial color(s), no artificial flavor(s), starch free, sugar free, yeast free]
  Natural Vegetable Fiber: 48.57% (368 g)

Reguloid: 48.57% (369 g, 540 g)
Reguloid: 28.3% (369 g, 540 g) [contains fd&c yellow #6 (sunset yellow), fd&c yellow #6 aluminum lake; orange flavor]
Reguloid: 58.6% (284 g, 426 g) [sugar free; natural flavor]
Reguloid: 58.6% (284 g, 426 g) [sugar free; contains aspartame, fd&c yellow #6 (sunset yellow), fd&c yellow #6 aluminum lake]
Sorbulax: 100% (420 g)
Powder, Oral [preservative free]:
  Evac: (480 g) [dye free]

References

Department of Health & Human Services, Food and Drug Administration, *Federal Register*, 1985.
"Dietary Reference Intakes for Energy, Carbohydrate, Fiber, Fat, Fatty Acids, Cholesterol, Protein and Amino Acids," Standing Committee on the Scientific Evaluation of Dietary Reference Intakes, Food and Nutrition Board, Institute of Medicine, National Academy of Sciences, Washington, DC: National Academy Press, 2005. Available at http://www.nap.edu.
James SL, Muir JG, Curtis SL, et al, "Dietary Fibre: A Roughage Guide," *Intern Med J*, 2003, 33(7):291-6.
National Heart, Lung, and Blood Institute, "Expert Panel on Integrated Guidelines for Cardiovascular Health and Risk Reduction in Children and Adolescents," *Clinical Practice Guidelines*, 2011. Available at http://www.nhlbi.nih.gov/guidelines/cvd_ped/peds_guidelines_full.pdf
Singh B, "Psyllium as Therapeutic and Drug Delivery Agent," *Int J Pharm*, 2007, 334(1-2):1-14.
Wald A, "Constipation, Diarrhea, and Symptomatic Hemorrhoids During Pregnancy," *Gastroenterol Clin North Am*, 2003, 32(1):309-22.
Williams CL, Bollella M, and Wynder EL, "A New Recommendation for Dietary Fiber in Childhood," *Pediatrics*, 1995, 96(5 Pt 2):985-8.

◆ **Psyllium Husk** *see* Psyllium *on page* 1773
◆ **Psyllium Hydrophilic Mucilloid** *see* Psyllium *on page* 1773
◆ **Pteroylglutamic Acid** *see* Folic Acid *on page* 925
◆ **PTG** *see* Teniposide *on page* 1976
◆ **PTU (error-prone abbreviation)** *see* Propylthiouracil *on page* 1762
◆ **Pulmicort** *see* Budesonide (Systemic, Oral Inhalation) *on page* 308
◆ **Pulmicort Flexhaler** *see* Budesonide (Systemic, Oral Inhalation) *on page* 308
◆ **Pulmicort Turbuhaler (Can)** *see* Budesonide (Systemic, Oral Inhalation) *on page* 308
◆ **Pulmophylline (Can)** *see* Theophylline *on page* 2005
◆ **PulmoSal** *see* Sodium Chloride *on page* 1902
◆ **Pulmozyme** *see* Dornase Alfa *on page* 709
◆ **Pulmozyme® (Can)** *see* Dornase Alfa *on page* 709
◆ **Purell® [OTC]** *see* Alcohol (Ethyl) *on page* 88
◆ **Purell® 2 in 1 [OTC]** *see* Alcohol (Ethyl) *on page* 88
◆ **Purell® Lasting Care [OTC]** *see* Alcohol (Ethyl) *on page* 88
◆ **Purell® Moisture Therapy [OTC]** *see* Alcohol (Ethyl) *on page* 88
◆ **Purell® with Aloe [OTC]** *see* Alcohol (Ethyl) *on page* 88
◆ **Purified Chick Embryo Cell** *see* Rabies Vaccine *on page* 1801
◆ **Purinethol** *see* Mercaptopurine *on page* 1342
◆ **Purixan** *see* Mercaptopurine *on page* 1342

Pyrantel Pamoate (pi RAN tel PAM oh ate)

Brand Names: U.S. Pamix [OTC]; Pin-X [OTC]; Reeses Pinworm Medicine [OTC]
Brand Names: Canada Combantrin
Therapeutic Category Anthelmintic
Generic Availability (U.S.) May be product dependent

Use Roundworm (*Ascaris lumbricoides*), pinworm (*Enterobius vermicularis*), and hookworm (*Ancylostoma duodenale* and *Necator americanus*) infestations; trichostrongyliasis and moniliformis infections

Pregnancy Considerations Pyrantel pamoate has minimal systemic absorption. Systemic absorption would be required in order for pyrantel pamoate to cross the placenta and reach the fetus.

Contraindications Hypersensitivity to pyrantel pamoate or any component

Warnings Pin-X® contains sodium benzoate; benzoic acid (benzoate) is a metabolite of benzyl alcohol; large amounts of benzyl alcohol (≥99 mg/kg/day) have been associated with a potentially fatal toxicity ("gasping syndrome") in neonates; the "gasping syndrome" consists of metabolic acidosis, respiratory distress, gasping respirations, CNS dysfunction (including convulsions, intracranial hemorrhage), hypotension and cardiovascular collapse; avoid use of pyrantel pamoate products containing sodium benzoate in neonates; *in vitro* and animal studies have shown that benzoate displaces bilirubin from protein binding sites

Precautions Use with caution in patients with liver impairment, anemia, malnutrition. The chewable tablet contains aspartame which is metabolized to phenylalanine and must be avoided or used with caution in patients with phenylketonuria.

Adverse Reactions

Central nervous system: Dizziness, headache

Gastrointestinal: Abdominal cramps, diarrhea, nausea, vomiting

Drug Interactions

Metabolism/Transport Effects Substrate of CYP2D6 (minor); **Note:** Assignment of Major/Minor substrate status based on clinically relevant drug interaction potential

Avoid Concomitant Use There are no known interactions where it is recommended to avoid concomitant use.

Increased Effect/Toxicity There are no known significant interactions involving an increase in effect.

Decreased Effect

The levels/effects of Pyrantel Pamoate may be decreased by: Aminoquinolines (Antimalarial); Peginterferon Alfa-2b

Stability Store at room temperature. Protect from light.

Mechanism of Action Causes the release of acetylcholine and inhibits cholinesterase; acts as a depolarizing neuromuscular blocker, paralyzing the helminths

Pharmacokinetics (Adult data unless noted)

Absorption: Oral: Poor

Metabolism: Undergoes partial hepatic metabolism

Time to peak serum concentration: Within 1-3 hours

Elimination: In feces (50% as unchanged drug) and urine (7% as unchanged drug and metabolites)

Dosing: Usual Children and Adults: Oral:

Roundworm, pinworm, or trichostrongyliasis: 11 mg pyrantel base/kg administered as a single dose; maximum dose: 1 g; dosage should be repeated after 2 weeks for pinworm infection

Hookworm: 11 mg pyrantel base/kg/day once daily for 3 days

Maximum daily dose: 1 g

Moniliformis infection: 11 mg pyrantel base/kg as a single dose; repeat this dose twice at 2-week intervals

Administration Oral: May be mixed with milk or fruit juice. May be administered without regard to meals. Purgation is not required prior to, during, or after use.

Suspension: Shake well before use.

Tablet: Chewable tablet must be chewed thoroughly before swallowing.

Monitoring Parameters Stool for presence of eggs, worms, and occult blood; serum AST and ALT

Dosage Forms Excipient information presented when available (limited, particularly for generics); consult specific product labeling.

Suspension, Oral [strength expressed as base]:

Pamix: 50 mg/mL (30 mL, 60 mL, 240 mL)

Pin-X: 50 mg/mL (30 mL, 60 mL) [sugar free; contains methylparaben, propylene glycol, propylparaben, saccharin sodium, sodium benzoate; caramel flavor]

Reeses Pinworm Medicine: 50 mg/mL (30 mL) [contains saccharin sodium, sodium benzoate]

Tablet, Oral [strength expressed as base]:

Reeses Pinworm Medicine: 62.5 mg [scored]

Tablet Chewable, Oral [strength expressed as base]:

Pin-X: 250 mg [scored; contains aspartame, fd&c yellow #6 aluminum lake; orange flavor]

Pyrazinamide (peer a ZIN a mide)

Brand Names: Canada Tebrazid™

Therapeutic Category Antitubercular Agent

Generic Availability (U.S.) Yes

Use Adjunctive treatment of *Mycobacterium* tuberculosis infection in combination with other antituberculosis agents (FDA approved in children and adults); especially useful in disseminated and meningeal tuberculosis; CDC currently recommends a 3 or 4 multidrug regimen which includes pyrazinamide, rifampin, INH, and at times ethambutol or streptomycin for the treatment of tuberculosis

Pregnancy Risk Factor C

Pregnancy Considerations Teratogenic effects have not been observed in animal reproduction studies. Due to the risk of tuberculosis to the fetus, treatment is recommended when the probability of maternal disease is moderate to high. Although not recommended as the initial treatment regimen, the use of pyrazinamide during pregnancy is recommended by The World Health Organization (Blumberg, 2003).

Breast-Feeding Considerations Low concentrations of pyrazinamide have been detected in breast milk; concentrations are less than maternal plasma concentration (Holdiness, 1984). The amount of drug in breast milk is considered insufficient for the treatment of tuberculosis in breast-fed infants.

Contraindications Hypersensitivity to pyrazinamide or any component; severe hepatic damage

Warnings Dose-related hepatotoxicity ranging from transient ALT/AST elevations to jaundice, hepatitis, and/or liver atrophy (rare) has occurred; the 2-month rifampin-pyrazinamide regimen for the treatment of latent tuberculosis infection (LTBI) has been associated with severe and fatal liver injuries; incidence increased with pyrazinamide doses >30 mg/kg/day. The IDSA and CDC recommend that the 2-month rifampin-pyrazinamide regimen should not generally be used in patients with LTBI.

Precautions Use with caution in patients with renal failure, gout, diabetes mellitus, patients receiving concurrent medications associated with liver injury (particularly with rifampin), or in patients with a history of alcoholism

Adverse Reactions

Central nervous system: Malaise

Gastrointestinal: Anorexia, nausea, vomiting

Neuromuscular & skeletal: Arthralgia, myalgia

Rare but important or life-threatening: Acne, angioedema (rare), anticoagulant effect, dysuria, fever, gout, hepatotoxicity, interstitial nephritis, itching, photosensitivity, porphyria, rash, sideroblastic anemia, thrombocytopenia, urticaria

Drug Interactions

Metabolism/Transport Effects None known.

Avoid Concomitant Use There are no known interactions where it is recommended to avoid concomitant use.

Increased Effect/Toxicity

Pyrazinamide may increase the levels/effects of: Cyclo-SPORINE (Systemic); Rifampin

Decreased Effect There are no known significant interactions involving a decrease in effect.

Stability Store at controlled room temperature of 15°C to 30°C (59°F to 86°F).

Mechanism of Action Converted to pyrazinoic acid in susceptible strains of *Mycobacterium* which lowers the pH of the environment; exact mechanism of action has not been elucidated

Pharmacokinetics (Adult data unless noted)

Absorption: Oral: Well absorbed

Distribution: Widely distributed into body tissues and fluids including the liver, lung, and CSF

Protein binding: 50%

Metabolism: In the liver

Half-life: 9-10 hours, prolonged with reduced renal or hepatic function

Time to peak serum concentration: Within 2 hours

Elimination: In urine (4% as unchanged drug)

Dosing: Usual Oral: Tuberculosis, treatment: **Note:** Used as part of a multidrug regimen. Treatment regimens consist of an initial 2-month phase, followed by a continuation phase of 4 or 7 additional months; frequency of dosing may differ depending on phase of therapy.

Infants, Children <40 kg, and Adolescents ≤14 years and <40 kg:

Non-HIV patients (CDC, 2003):

Daily therapy: 15-30 mg/kg/dose (maximum: 2 g/dose) once daily

Directly observed therapy (DOT): 50 mg/kg/dose (maximum: 2 g/dose) twice weekly

HIV-exposed/infected patients: (CDC, 2009): Daily therapy: 20-40 mg/kg/dose once daily (maximum: 2 g/day) (CDC, 2009)

Adults: Suggested dosing based on lean body weight (Blumberg, 2003):

Daily therapy:

40-55 kg: 1000 mg

56-75 kg: 1500 mg

76-90 kg: 2000 mg (maximum dose regardless of weight)

Twice weekly directly observed therapy (DOT):

40-55 kg: 2000 mg

56-75 kg: 3000 mg

76-90 kg: 4000 mg (maximum dose regardless of weight)

3 times/week DOT:

40-55 kg: 1500 mg

56-75 kg: 2500 mg

76-90 kg: 3000 mg (maximum dose regardless of weight)

Monitoring Parameters Periodic liver function tests, serum uric acid

Test Interactions Reacts with Acetest® and Ketostix® to produce pinkish-brown color

Dosage Forms Excipient information presented when available (limited, particularly for generics); consult specific product labeling.

Tablet, Oral:

Generic: 500 mg

Extemporaneous Preparations A 100 mg/mL oral suspension may be made with tablets. Crush two-hundred pyrazinamide 500 mg tablets and mix with a suspension containing 500 mL methylcellulose 1% and 500 mL simple syrup. Add to this a suspension containing one-hundred forty crushed pyrazinamide tablets in 350 mL methylcellulose 1% and 350 mL simple syrup to make 1.7 L suspension. Label "shake well" and "refrigerate". Stable for 60 days refrigerated (preferred) and 45 days at room temperature.

Nahata MC, Morosco RS, and Peritre SP, "Stability of Pyrazinamide in Two Suspensions," *Am J Health Syst Pharm*, 1995, 52(14):1558-60.

References

Ad Hoc Committee of the Scientific Assembly on Microbiology, Tuberculosis and Pulmonary Infections, "Treatment of Tuberculosis and Tuberculosis Infection in Adults and Children," *Clin Infect Dis*, 1995, 21:9-27.

American Academy of Pediatrics, Committee on Infectious Diseases, "Chemotherapy for Tuberculosis in Infants and Children," *Pediatrics*, 1992, 89(1):161-5.

Blumberg HM, Burman WJ, Chaisson RE, et al, "American Thoracic Society/Centers for Disease Control and Prevention/Infectious Diseases Society of America: Treatment of Tuberculosis," *Am J Respir Crit Care Med*, 2003, 167(4):603-62.

Centers for Disease Control and Prevention (CDC), "Guidelines for the Prevention and Treatment of Opportunistic Infections Among HIV-Exposed and HIV-Infected Children," *MMWR Recomm Rep*, 2009, 58(RR-11):1-166. Available at http://aidsinfo.nih.gov/contentfiles/Pediatric_OI.pdf

Centers for Disease Control and Prevention, "Treatment of Tuberculosis," *MMWR Recomm Rep*, 2003, 52(RR-11):1-77.

Holdiness MR, "Antituberculosis Drugs and Breast-Feeding," *Arch Intern Med*, 1984, 144(9):1888.

Starke JR, "Multidrug Therapy for Tuberculosis in Children," *Pediatr Infect Dis J*, 1990, 9(11):785-93.

Starke JR and Correa AG, "Management of Mycobacterial Infection and Disease in Children," *Pediatr Infect Dis J*, 1995, 14(6):455-70.

"Update: Fatal and Severe Liver Injuries Associated With Rifampin and Pyrazinamide for Latent Tuberculosis Infection, and Revisions in American Thoracic Society/CDC Recommendations - United States, 2001," *MMWR Morb Mortal Wkly Rep*, 2001, 50(34):733-5.

◆ **Pyrazinoic Acid Amide** *see* Pyrazinamide *on page 1775*

◆ **Pyri 500 [OTC]** *see* Pyridoxine *on page 1778*

◆ **2-Pyridine Aldoxime Methochloride** *see* Pralidoxime *on page 1719*

◆ **Pyridium** *see* Phenazopyridine *on page 1651*

Pyridostigmine (peer id oh STIG meen)

Medication Safety Issues

Sound-alike/look-alike issues:

Pyridostigmine may be confused with physostigmine

Regonol® may be confused with Reglan®, Renagel®

Related Information

Oral Medications That Should Not Be Crushed or Altered *on page 2438*

Brand Names: U.S. Mestinon; Regonol

Brand Names: Canada Mestinon®; Mestinon®-SR

Therapeutic Category Antidote; Neuromuscular Blocking Agent; Cholinergic Agent

Generic Availability (U.S.) May be product dependent

Use

Oral: Mestinon®: Treatment of myasthenia gravis (FDA approved in adults); has also been used for treatment of vincristine induced neurotoxicity, congenital myasthenic syndrome, and pretreatment for Soman nerve gas exposure (military use only)

Parenteral: Regonol®: Reversal agent for effects of nondepolarizing neuromuscular blocking agents (FDA approved in adults); has also been used for treatment of myasthenia gravis

Pregnancy Risk Factor B

Pregnancy Considerations Safety has not been established for use during pregnancy. The potential benefit to the mother should outweigh the potential risk to the fetus. When pyridostigmine is needed in myasthenic mothers, giving dose parenterally 1 hour before completion of the second stage of labor may facilitate delivery and protect the neonate during the immediate postnatal state.

Breast-Feeding Considerations Neonates of myasthenia gravis mothers may have difficulty in sucking and swallowing (as well as breathing). Neonatal pyridostigmine may be indicated by symptoms (confirmed by edrophonium test).

Contraindications Hypersensitivity to pyridostigmine, bromides, or any component; GI or GU obstruction

Warnings Overdosage may result in cholinergic crisis; this must be distinguished from myasthenic crisis; discontinue if symptoms of excess cholinergic activity (eg, salivation, sweating, urinary incontinence) occur. Adequate facilities should be available for cardiopulmonary resuscitation when testing and adjusting dose for myasthenia gravis; have atropine and epinephrine ready to treat hypersensitivity reactions. For brief or prolonged periods, anticholinesterase insensitivity can develop. Neonates of myasthenic mothers may have transient difficulties in swallowing, sucking, and breathing; use of pyridostigmine may be of benefit; use edrophonium test to assess neonate with these symptoms.

When used for reversal of muscle relaxants, prior or concurrent doses of atropine or glycopyrrolate should be considered with large doses of pyridostigmine. A peripheral nerve stimulator may be helpful to monitor neuromuscular function and minimize excessive dosing or inadequate reversal.

Some injections contain benzyl alcohol which may cause allergic reactions in susceptible individuals; syrup contains sodium benzoate; large amounts of benzyl alcohol (≥99 mg/kg/day) have been associated with a potentially fatal toxicity ("gasping syndrome") in neonates; the "gasping syndrome" consists of metabolic acidosis, respiratory distress, gasping respirations, CNS dysfunction (including convulsions, intracranial hemorrhage), hypotension and cardiovascular collapse; use injections containing benzyl alcohol with caution in neonates; *in vitro* and animal studies have shown that benzoate, a metabolite of benzyl alcohol, displaces bilirubin from protein binding sites; avoid use of the syrup in neonates

Pretreatment with pyridostigmine alone will not protect against exposure to Soman nerve gas; its efficacy is dependent upon the rapid use of atropine and pralidoxime after exposure. Discontinue use of pyridostigmine after exposure.

Precautions Use with caution in patients with renal impairment; dosage adjustment may be necessary. Use with caution in patients with seizure disorder, asthma or bronchospastic disease, bradycardia or cardiac arrhythmias, hyperthyroidism, or GI disease, including peptic ulcer. Regonol® injection must be administered by trained personnel **[U.S. Boxed Warning]**.

Adverse Reactions

Cardiovascular: Arrhythmias (especially bradycardia), AV block, cardiac arrest, decreased carbon monoxide, flushing, hypotension, nodal rhythm, nonspecific ECG changes, syncope, tachycardia

Central nervous system: Convulsions, dizziness, drowsiness, dysphonia, headache, loss of consciousness

Dermatologic: Skin rash, thrombophlebitis (I.V.), urticaria

Gastrointestinal: Abdominal pain, diarrhea, dysphagia, flatulence, hyperperistalsis, nausea, salivation, stomach cramps, vomiting

Genitourinary: Urinary urgency

Neuromuscular & skeletal: Arthralgia, dysarthria, fasciculations, muscle cramps, myalgia, spasms, weakness

Ocular: Amblyopia, lacrimation, small pupils

Respiratory: Bronchial secretions increased, bronchiolar constriction, bronchospasm, dyspnea, laryngospasm, respiratory arrest, respiratory depression, respiratory muscle paralysis

Miscellaneous: Allergic reactions, anaphylaxis, diaphoresis increased

Drug Interactions

Metabolism/Transport Effects None known.

Avoid Concomitant Use There are no known interactions where it is recommended to avoid concomitant use.

Increased Effect/Toxicity

Pyridostigmine may increase the levels/effects of: Beta-Blockers; Cholinergic Agonists; Succinylcholine

The levels/effects of Pyridostigmine may be increased by: Corticosteroids (Systemic)

Decreased Effect

Pyridostigmine may decrease the levels/effects of: Neuromuscular-Blocking Agents (Nondepolarizing)

The levels/effects of Pyridostigmine may be decreased by: Dipyridamole; Methocarbamol

Stability All dosage forms: Store at 25°C (77°F), excursions permitted to 15°C to 30°C (59°F to 86°F); protect from light. Tablets are extremely moisture sensitive; do not remove desiccant and keep bottle closed tightly. Mottling of the Timespan tablets may occur; however, efficacy is not affected.

Mechanism of Action Inhibits destruction of acetylcholine by acetylcholinesterase which facilitates transmission of impulses across myoneural junction

Pharmacodynamics

Recovery from vincristine neurotoxicity: Onset of action: 1-2 weeks (Akbayram, 2010)

Myasthenia gravis:

Onset of action:

Oral: Within 30 minutes (Maggi, 2011)

I.M.: 15-30 minutes

I.V.: Within 2-5 minutes

Duration:

Oral: 3-4 hours (Maggi, 2011)

I.M., I.V.: 2-3 hours

Pharmacokinetics (Adult data unless noted)

Absorption: Oral: Very poor

Distribution: V_d: 0.53-1.76 L/kg (Aquilonius, 1986)

Protein Binding: None (Aquilonius, 1986)

Metabolism: Hepatic and at tissue site by cholinesterases

Bioavailability: Oral: 10% to 20% (Aquilonius, 1986)

Half-life: 1-2 hours; renal failure: ~6 hours (Aquilonius, 1986)

Time to peak serum concentration: Oral: 1-2 hours (Aquilonius, 1986)

Elimination: Urine (80% to 90% as unchanged drug) (Aquilonius, 1986)

Dosing: Neonatal Myasthenic syndrome; congenital: Limited data available: Oral: 1 mg/kg/dose every 4 hours; maximum daily dose: 7 mg/kg/**day** divided in 5-6 doses (Lorenzoni, 2012)

Dosing: Usual

Infants, Children and Adolescents: **Note:** All pediatric dosing recommendations based on immediate release product formulations.

Myasthenic syndrome, congenital: Limited data available: Oral: 1 mg/kg/dose every 4 hours; maximum daily dose: 7 mg/kg/**day** divided in 5-6 doses (Lorenzoni, 2012)

Myasthenia gravis, autoimmune: Limited data available: **Note:** Dosage should be adjusted such that larger doses administered prior to time of greatest fatigue.

Oral: 1 mg/kg/dose every 4-6 hours; maximum daily dose: 7 mg/kg/**day** divided in 5-6 doses; usual daily dose: 600 mg/**day**; doses as high as 1500 mg/**day** have been used (Andrews, 1998; Maggi, 2011)

I.M., I.V.: 0.05-0.15 mg/kg/dose; maximum dose: 10 mg

Reversal of nondepolarizing neuromuscular blocker: Limited data available: I.M., I.V.: 0.1-0.25 mg/kg/dose. **Note:** Give atropine or glycopyrrolate immediately prior to minimize side effects.

Vincristine-induced neurotoxicity: Limited data available: Children ≥2 years and Adolescents: Oral: 3 mg/kg/day divided in 2 doses, given with pyridoxine for 3 weeks; dosing based on a case series of four children (age: 2-13 years) receiving vincristine for treatment of ALL (Akbayram, 2010) and a 2-year old receiving vincristine for a cervical synovial sarcoma (Muller, 2004)

Adults:

Myasthenia gravis:

Oral:

Immediate release: Highly individualized dosing ranges: 60-1500 mg/day, usually 600 mg/day divided into 5-6 doses, spaced to provide maximum relief

Sustained release formulation: Highly individualized dosing ranges: 180-540 mg once or twice daily (doses separated by at least 6 hours); **Note:** Most clinicians reserve sustained release dosage form for bedtime dose only.

I.M. or slow I.V. push: To supplement oral dosage pre- and postoperatively during labor and postpartum, during myasthenic crisis, or when oral therapy is impractical: ~1/30th of oral dose; observe patient closely for cholinergic reactions

I.V. infusion: To supplement oral dosage pre- and postoperatively, during labor and postpartum, during myasthenic crisis, or when oral therapy is impractical: Initial: 2 mg/hour with gradual titration in increments of 0.5-1 mg/hour, up to a maximum rate of 4 mg/hour

Reversal of nondepolarizing neuromuscular blocker: I.V.: 0.1-0.25 mg/kg/dose; 10-20 mg is usually sufficient (full recovery usually occurs ≤15 minutes, but ≥30 minutes may be required)

Soman nerve gas exposure; pretreatment (military use): Oral: 30 mg every 8 hours beginning several hours before exposure; discontinue at first sign of nerve agent exposure, then begin atropine and pralidoxime

Dosage adjustment in renal impairment: There are no dosage adjustments are provided in the manufacturer's labeling; however, lower doses may be required due to prolonged elimination; dosage titration should be based on drug effects.

Dosage adjustment in hepatic impairment: There are no dosage adjustments are provided in the manufacturer's labeling.

Administration

Oral: Swallow sustained release tablets whole, do not chew or crush

Parenteral: May administer I.M. or as a direct I.V. slowly over 2-4 minutes; patients receiving large parenteral doses should be pretreated with atropine

Monitoring Parameters Muscle strength, heart rate, respiration; vital capacity; observe for cholinergic reactions, particularly when administered I.V.

Dosage Forms Excipient information presented when available (limited, particularly for generics); consult specific product labeling.

Solution, Injection, as bromide:

Regonol: 5 mg/mL (2 mL) [contains benzyl alcohol]

Syrup, Oral, as bromide:

Mestinon: 60 mg/5 mL (473 mL) [contains alcohol, usp, brilliant blue fcf (fd&c blue #1), fd&c red #40, sodium benzoate; raspberry flavor]

Tablet, Oral, as bromide:

Mestinon: 60 mg [scored]

Generic: 60 mg

Tablet Extended Release, Oral, as bromide:

Mestinon: 180 mg [scored]

References

Akbayram S, Akgun C, Doğan M, et al, "Use of Pyridoxine and Pyridostigmine in Children With Vincristine-Induced Neuropathy," *Indian J Pediatr*, 2010, 77(6):681-3.

Andrews PI, "A Treatment Algorithm for Autoimmune Myasthenia Gravis in Childhood," *Ann N Y Acad Sci*, 1998, 841:789-802.

Aquilonius SM and Hartvig P, "Clinical Pharmacokinetics of Cholinesterase Inhibitors," *Clin Pharmacokinet*, 1986, 11(3):236-49.

Lorenzoni PJ, Scola RH, Kay CS, et al, "Congenital Myasthenic Syndrome: A Brief Review," *Pediatr Neurol*, 2012, 46(3):141-8.

Maggi L and Mantegazza R, "Treatment of Myasthenia Gravis: Focus on Pyridostigmine," *Clin Drug Investig*, 2011, 31(10):691-701.

Müller L, Kramm CM, Tenenbaum T, et al, "Treatment of Vincristine-Induced Bilateral Ptosis With Pyridoxine and Pyridostigmine," *Pediatr Blood Cancer*, 2004, 42(3):287-8.

◆ **Pyridostigmine Bromide** see Pyridostigmine on page 1776

Pyridoxine (peer i DOKS een)

Medication Safety Issues

Sound-alike/look-alike issues:

Pyridoxine may be confused with paroxetine, pralidoxime, Pyridium®

International issues:

Doxal [Brazil] may be confused with Doxil brand name for DOXOrubicin [U.S.]

Doxal: Brand name for pyridoxine/thiamine combination [Brazil], but also the brand name for doxepin [Finland]

Brand Names: U.S. Neuro-K-250 T.D. [OTC]; Neuro-K-250 Vitamin B6 [OTC]; Neuro-K-50 [OTC]; Neuro-K-500 [OTC]; Pyri 500 [OTC]

Therapeutic Category Antidote, Cycloserine Toxicity; Antidote, Hydrazine Toxicity; Antidote, Mushroom Toxicity; Drug-induced Neuritis, Treatment Agent; Nutritional Supplement; Vitamin, Water Soluble

Generic Availability (U.S.) May be product dependent

Use Prevention and treatment of vitamin B_6 deficiency; treatment of drug-induced deficiency (eg, isoniazid or oral contraceptives); treatment of inborn errors of metabolism (eg, B_6-dependent seizures or anemia); injection may be used when oral route not feasible (All indications: FDA approved in adults); has also been used for the treatment of pyridoxine-dependent seizures and treatment of acute intoxication of isoniazid, cycloserine, hydrazine, and mushroom (genus *Gyromitra*)

Pregnancy Risk Factor A

Pregnancy Considerations Water soluble vitamins cross the placenta. Maternal pyridoxine plasma concentrations may decrease as pregnancy progresses and requirements may be increased in pregnant women (IOM, 1998). Pyridoxine is used to treat nausea and vomiting of pregnancy (Neibyl, 2010). In general, medications used as antidotes should take into consideration the health and prognosis of the mother; antidotes should be administered to pregnant women if there is a clear indication for use and should not be withheld because of fears of teratogenicity (Bailey, 2003).

Breast-Feeding Considerations Pyridoxine is found in breast milk and concentrations vary by maternal intake. Pyridoxine requirements are increased in nursing women compared to non-nursing women (IOM, 1998). Possible inhibition of lactation at doses >600 mg/day when taken immediately postpartum (Foukas, 1973).

Contraindications Hypersensitivity to pyridoxine or any component

Warnings Severe, permanent peripheral neuropathies have been reported with pyridoxine; neurotoxicity is more common with long-term administration of large doses (>2000 mg/day in adults). Single vitamin deficiency is rare; evaluate for other deficiencies.

Precautions The parenteral product may contain aluminum; toxic aluminum concentrations may be seen with high doses, prolonged use, or renal dysfunction. Premature neonates are at higher risk due to immature renal function and aluminum intake from other parenteral sources. Parenteral aluminum exposure of >4-5 mcg/kg/day is associated with CNS and bone toxicity and tissue loading may occur at lower doses.

Adverse Reactions

Central nervous system: Headache, seizure (following very large I.V. doses), somnolence

Endocrine & metabolic: Acidosis, folic acid decreased

Gastrointestinal: Nausea

Hepatic: AST increased

Neuromuscular & skeletal: Neuropathy, paresthesia

Miscellaneous: Allergic reactions

Drug Interactions

Metabolism/Transport Effects None known.

Avoid Concomitant Use There are no known interactions where it is recommended to avoid concomitant use.

Increased Effect/Toxicity There are no known significant interactions involving an increase in effect.

Decreased Effect

Pyridoxine may decrease the levels/effects of: Altretamine; Barbiturates; Fosphenytoin; Levodopa; Phenytoin

Stability Store at 20°C to 25°C (68°F to 77°F); protect from light.

Mechanism of Action Precursor to pyridoxal, which functions in the metabolism of proteins, carbohydrates, and fats; pyridoxal also aids in the release of liver and muscle-stored glycogen and in the synthesis of GABA (within the central nervous system) and heme

Pharmacokinetics (Adult data unless noted)

Absorption: Readily from the GI tract; primarily in jejunum

Metabolism: Hepatic to pyridoxal phosphate and pyridoxamine phosphate

Half-life, biologic: 15-20 days

Elimination: Urine (as metabolites)

Dosing: Neonatal

Adequate intake (AI): Oral: 0.1 mg/day (0.01 mg/kg/day)

Pyridoxine-dependent seizures: Oral, I.M., I.V.:

Initial: I.V. preferred: 50 to 100 mg (Rajesh, 2003)

Maintenance: Oral preferred: Usual: 50 to 100 mg/day; range: 10 to 200 mg (Rajesh, 2003); an observational study in UK described a usual dose of 30 mg/kg/day (Baxter, 1999)

Dosing: Usual

Pediatric:

Adequate intake (AI): Oral: Infants:

1 to <6 months: 0.1 mg (0.01 mg/kg)

6 to 12 months: 0.3 mg (0.03 mg/kg)

Recommended daily allowance (RDA): Oral:

1 to 3 years: 0.5 mg

4 to 8 years: 0.6 mg

9 to 13 years: 1 mg

14 to 18 years:

Male: 1.3 mg

Female: 1.2 mg

Dietary deficiency; treatment: Oral, I.M., I.V.:

Children: 5 to 25 mg/day for 3 weeks, then 2.5 to 5 mg/day in multivitamin product

Adolescents: 10 to 20 mg/day for 3 weeks, then 2 to 5 mg/day (usual dosage found in multivitamin products)

Pyridoxine-dependent seizures, treatment: Oral, I.M., I.V.: Infants and Children:

Initial: I.V. preferred: 50 to 100 mg (Rajesh, 2003)

Maintenance: Oral preferred: Usual: 50 to 100 mg/day; range: 10 to 200 mg (Rajesh, 2003); an observational study in UK described a usual dose of 30 mg/kg/day (Baxter, 1999)

Drug-induced deficiency/toxicity (cycloserine, isoniazid, penicillamine); chronic use: Oral, I.M., I.V.:

Isoniazid/Cycloserine:

Prevention: **Note:** Recommended for patients at risk: Exclusively breast-fed infants, meat- and milk-deficient diet, nutritional deficiency, pregnant adolescents (*Red Book*, 2012).

Non-HIV-exposed/-positive:

Infants and Children: 1 mg/kg/day; usual range: 10 to 50 mg/day (*Red Book* [AAP], 2012)

Adolescents: 30 mg/day

HIV-exposed/-positive:

Infants and Children: 1 to 2 mg/kg once daily; maximum daily dose: 50 mg/day (DHHS [pediatric], 2013)

Adolescents: 25 mg/day (DHHS [adult], 2013)

Treatment:

Infants and Children: Optimal dose not established, higher doses than prophylaxis are necessary for treatment of neuritis (ataxia), some clinicians have suggested the following: 100 mg/day; higher doses (ie, 200mg/day) may be necessary to alleviate signs/symptoms

Adolescents: Initial: 100 mg/day for 3 weeks followed by 30 mg/day

Penicillamine (in Wilson Disease patients): Limited data available: Children and Adolescents: 25 to 50 mg/day (Roberts, 2008)

Acute isoniazid ingestion:

Treatment of isoniazid-induced seizures and/or coma:

I.V.: Children and Adolescents:

Acute ingestion of known amount: Initial: A total dose of pyridoxine equal to the amount of isoniazid ingested (maximum dose: 70 mg/kg up to 5 g); administer at a rate of 0.5 to 1 g/minute until seizures stop or the maximum initial dose has been administered; may repeat every 5 to 10 minutes as needed to control persistent seizure activity and/or CNS toxicity. If seizures stop prior to the administration of the calculated initial dose, infuse the remaining pyridoxine over 4 to 6 hours (Howland, 2006; Morrow, 2006).

Acute ingestion of unknown amount: Initial: 70 mg/kg (maximum dose: 5 g); administer at a rate of 0.5 to 1 g/minute; may repeat every 5 to 10 minutes as needed to control persistent seizure activity and/or CNS toxicity (Howland, 2006; Morrow, 2006; Santucci, 1999)

Prevention of isoniazid-induced seizures and/or coma:

I.V.: Children: Asymptomatic patients who present within 2 hours of ingesting a potentially toxic amount of isoniazid should receive a prophylactic dose of pyridoxine (Boyer, 2006). Dosing recommendations are the same as for the treatment of symptomatic patients.

Acute intoxication: Children and Adolescents: Mushroom ingestion (genus *Gyromitra*): I.V.: 25 mg/kg/dose; repeat as necessary to a maximum total dose of 15 to 20 g (Lheureaux, 2005)

Adult:

Recommended daily allowance: Oral:

19 to 50 years: 1.3 mg

>50 years:

Female: 1.5 mg

Male: 1.7 mg

Pregnancy: 1.9 mg

Lactation: 2 mg

Dietary deficiency: Oral, I.M., I.V.: Adults: 10 to 20 mg/day for 3 weeks, then 2-5 mg/day (usual dosage found in multivitamin products). Doses up to 600 mg/day may be needed with pyridoxine dependency syndrome.

Drug-induced neuritis (eg, isoniazid): Oral, I.M., I.V.: Prophylaxis: HIV-exposed/-positive: 25 mg/day; 50 mg/day if pregnant (DHHS [adult], 2013)

Treatment of isoniazid-induced seizures and/or coma following acute ingestion: I.V.:

Acute ingestion of known amount: Initial: A total dose of pyridoxine equal to the amount of isoniazid ingested (maximum dose: 5000 mg); administer at a rate of 500 to 1000 mg/minute until seizures stop or the maximum initial dose has been administered; may repeat every 5 to 10 minutes as needed to control persistent seizure activity and/or CNS toxicity. If seizures stop prior to the administration of the calculated initial dose, infuse the remaining pyridoxine over 4 to 6 hours (Howland, 2006; Morrow, 2006).

Acute ingestion of unknown amount: Initial: 5000 mg; administer at a rate of 500 to 1000 mg/minute; may repeat every 5 to 10 minutes as needed to control persistent seizure activity and/or CNS toxicity (Howland, 2006; Morrow, 2006)

Prevention of isoniazid-induced seizures and/or coma following acute ingestion: I.V.: Asymptomatic patients who present within 2 hours of ingesting a potentially toxic amount of isoniazid should receive a prophylactic dose of pyridoxine (Boyer, 2006). Dosing recommendations are the same as for the treatment of symptomatic patients.

Acute intoxication: Mushroom ingestion (genus *Gyromitra*): I.V.: 25 mg/kg/dose; repeat as necessary to a maximum total dose of 15 to 20 g (Lheureaux, 2005)

Administration

Oral: Administer without regard to meals

Parenteral: May be administered I.M. or slow I.V.; seizures have been precipitated following large I.V. doses

Isoniazid toxicity: Initial doses should be administered at a rate of 500-1000 mg/minute. If the parenteral formulation is not available, anecdotal reports suggest that pyridoxine tablets may be crushed and made into a slurry and given at the same dose orally or via nasogastric (NG) tube (Boyer, 2006) or an extemporaneous compounded solution may be used. Oral administration is not recommended for acutely poisoned patients with seizure activity.

Monitoring Parameters When administering large I.V. doses, monitor respiratory rate, heart rate, and blood pressure

For treatment of isoniazid, hydrazine, or gyromitrin-containing mushroom toxicity: Anion gap, arterial blood gases, electrolytes, neurological exam, seizure activity

Reference Range 30-80 ng/mL

Test Interactions False positive urobilinogen spot test using Ehrlich's reagent

Additional Information Toxicology guidelines suggest that at least 8-24 **grams** be stocked for potential overdoses. This is enough to treat 1 patient weighing 100 kg for an initial 8- to 24-hour period. In areas where tuberculosis is common, hospitals should consider stocking 24 **grams**. This is enough to treat 1 patient for 24 hours (Dart, 2009).

Dosage Forms Excipient information presented when available (limited, particularly for generics); consult specific product labeling.

Capsule, Oral, as hydrochloride:
Neuro-K-250 T.D.: 250 mg [corn free, rye free, starch free, sugar free, wheat free]

Solution, Injection, as hydrochloride:
Generic: 100 mg/mL (1 mL)

Tablet, Oral, as hydrochloride:
Neuro-K-50: 50 mg
Neuro-K-500: 500 mg
Neuro-K-250 Vitamin B6: 250 mg
Pyri 500: 500 mg
Generic: 25 mg, 50 mg, 100 mg, 250 mg

Tablet, Oral, as hydrochloride [preservative free]:
Generic: 25 mg, 50 mg, 100 mg

Tablet Extended Release, Oral, as hydrochloride:
Generic: 200 mg

Extemporaneous Preparations A 1 mg/mL oral solution may be made using pyridoxine injection. Withdraw 100 mg (1 mL of a 100 mg/mL injection) from a vial with a needle and syringe; add to 99 mL simple syrup in an amber bottle. Label "refrigerate". Stable for 30 days refrigerated.

Nahata MC, Pai VB, and Hipple TF, *Pediatric Drug Formulations*, 5th ed, Cincinnati, OH: Harvey Whitney Books Co, 2004.

References

Bailey B, "Are There Teratogenic Risks Associated With Antidotes Used in the Acute Management of Poisoned Pregnant Women?" *Birth Defects Res A Clin Mol Teratol*, 2003, 67(2):133-40.

Boyer EW, "Antituberculous Medications," *Goldfrank's Toxicologic Emergencies*, 8th ed, Flomenbaum NE, Goldfrank LR, Hoffman, RS, et al, eds, New York, NY: McGraw-Hill Companies, Inc, 2006, 861-71.

Dart RC, Borron SW, Caravati EM, et al,"Expert Consensus Guidelines for Stocking of Antidotes in Hospitals That Provide Emergency Care," *Ann Emerg Med*, 2009, 54(3):386-94.

Department Health and Human Services, Food Drug Administration, "Aluminum in Large and Small Volume Parenterals Used in Total Parenteral Nutrition," *Federal Register*, 2000, 65(17):4103-11.

DHHS. Guidelines for the prevention and treatment of opportunistic infections among HIV-exposed and HIV-infected children: recommendations from the National Institutes of Health, Centers for Disease Control and Prevention, the HIV Medicine Association of the Infectious Diseases Society of America, the Pediatric Infectious Diseases Society, and the American Academy of Pediatrics. November 6, 2013. Available at http://aidsinfo.nih.gov

DHHS Panel on Opportunistic Infections (OI) in HIV-Infected Adults and Adolescents. Guidelines for prevention and treatment of opportunistic infections in HIV-infected adults and adolescents: recommendations from the Centers for Disease Control and Prevention (CDC), the National Institutes of Health (NIH), and the HIV Medicine Association (HIVMA) of the Infectious Diseases Society of America (IDSA). May 7, 2013. Available at http://aidsinfo.nih.gov/contentfiles/lvguidelines/adult_oi.pdf

Diaz JH, "Syndromic Diagnosis and Management of Confirmed Mushroom Poisonings," *Crit Care Med*, 2005, 33(2):427-36.

Foukas MD, "An Antilactogenic Effect of Pyridoxine," *J Obstet Gynaecol BrCommonw*, 1973, 80(8):718-20.

Howland MA, "Antidotes in Depth: Pyridoxine," *Goldfrank's Toxicologic Emergencies*, 8th ed, Flomenbaum NE, Goldfrank LR, Hoffman RS, et al, eds, New York, NY: McGraw-Hill Companies, Inc, 2006, 872-5.

IOM (Institute of Medicine). Dietary reference intakes for thiamin, riboflavin, niacin, vitamin B₆, folate, vitamin B₁₂, pantothenic acid, biotin, and choline.Washington, DC:The National Academies Press, 1998.

Lheureaux P, Penaol A, and Gri M. Pyridoxine in clinical toxicology: a review. *Eur J of Emerg Med*. 2005;12(2):78-85.

Morrow LE, Wear RE, Schuller D, et al, "Acute Isoniazid Toxicity and the Need for Adequate Pyridoxine Supplies," *Pharmacotherapy*, 2006, 26 (10):1529-32.

Nagappan R and Riddell T, "Pyridoxine Therapy in a Patient With Severe Hydrazine Sulfate Toxicity," *Crit Care Med*, 2000, 28 (6):2116-8.

Niebyl JR, "Clinical Practice. Nausea and Vomiting in Pregnancy," *N Engl J med*, 2010, 363(16):1544-50.

Rajesh R and Girija AS, "Pyridoxine-Dependent Seizures: A Review," *Indian Pediatr*, 2003, 40(7):633-8.

Roberts EA, Schilsky ML, and American Association for Study of Liver Diseases (AASLD). Diagnosis and treatment of Wilson disease: an update. *Hepatology*. 2008;47(6):2089-2111.

Santucci KA, Shah BR, and Linakis JG, "Acute Isoniazid Exposures and Antidote Availability," *Pediatric Emergency Care*, 1999, 15 (2):99-101.

◆ **Pyridoxine Hydrochloride** *see* Pyridoxine *on page 1778*

Pyrimethamine (peer i METH a meen)

Medication Safety Issues

Sound-alike/look-alike issues:

Daraprim® may be confused with Dantrium®, Daranide®

Brand Names: U.S. Daraprim

Brand Names: Canada Daraprim®

Therapeutic Category Antimalarial Agent

Generic Availability (U.S.) No

Use Used in combination with sulfadiazine for treatment of toxoplasmosis [FDA approved in pediatric patients (age not specified) and adults]; chemoprophylaxis and treatment of malaria [FDA approved in pediatric patients (age not specified) and adults]; has also been used in combination with dapsone as primary or secondary prophylaxis for *Pneumocystis jirovecii* in HIV-infected patients. **Note:** Although an FDA labeled indication, the use of pyrimethamine for chemoprophylaxis or treatment of malaria is not routinely recommended due to severe adverse reactions and reports of resistance (CDC, 2013a).

Pregnancy Risk Factor C

Pregnancy Considerations Teratogenic effects have been observed in animal reproduction studies. If administered during pregnancy (ie, for toxoplasmosis), supplementation of folate is strongly recommended. Pregnancy should be avoided during therapy.

Breast-Feeding Considerations Pyrimethamine enters breast milk and may result in significant systemic concentrations in breast-fed infants. The effect of concurrent therapy with sulfonamide or dapsone (frequently used with pyrimethamine as combination treatment) must be considered.

Contraindications Hypersensitivity to pyrimethamine, or any component; megaloblastic anemia secondary to folate deficiency

Warnings Megaloblastic anemia, leukopenia, thrombocytopenia, and pancytopenia have been reported; most commonly with high doses but may also occur in susceptible patients at low doses (eg, G6PD deficiency, folate deficiency); use with caution in patients with possible folate deficiency (eg, malabsorption syndrome, pregnancy, alcoholism); use is contraindicated in patients with known megaloblastic anemia due to folate deficiency; monitor CBC and platelets twice weekly in patients receiving high-dose therapy (eg, toxoplasmosis treatment). When used for more than 3-4 days or with high doses, it may be advisable to administer leucovorin to prevent hematologic complications due to pyrimethamine-induced folic acid deficiency; continue leucovorin during therapy and for 1 week after therapy is discontinued (to account for the long half-life of pyrimethamine) (CDC, 2009; CDC, 2013). Hypersensitivity dermatologic reactions including TEN and SJS have been reported, particularly when coadministered with a sulfonamide; patients should be counseled to discontinue use and notify prescriber at first sign of a rash.

Precautions Use with caution in patients with impaired renal or hepatic function and in patients with a history of seizure disorders.

Adverse Reactions

Cardiovascular: Arrhythmias (large doses)

Dermatologic: Erythema multiforme, rash, Stevens-Johnson syndrome, toxic epidermal necrolysis

Gastrointestinal: Anorexia, atrophic glossitis, vomiting

Hematologic: Leukopenia, megaloblastic anemia, pancytopenia, pulmonary eosinophilia, thrombocytopenia

Genitourinary: Hematuria

Miscellaneous: Anaphylaxis

Drug Interactions

Metabolism/Transport Effects Inhibits CYP2C9 (moderate)

Avoid Concomitant Use

Avoid concomitant use of Pyrimethamine with any of the following: Artemether; Lumefantrine

Increased Effect/Toxicity

Pyrimethamine may increase the levels/effects of: Antipsychotic Agents (Phenothiazines); Bosentan; Cannabis; Carvedilol; CYP2C9 Substrates; Dapsone (Systemic); Dapsone (Topical); Dronabinol; Lumefantrine; Tetrahydrocannabinol

The levels/effects of Pyrimethamine may be increased by: Artemether; Dapsone (Systemic)

Decreased Effect

The levels/effects of Pyrimethamine may be decreased by: Methylfolate

Stability Store at 15°C to 25°C (59°F to 77°F); protect from light.

Mechanism of Action Inhibits parasitic dihydrofolate reductase, resulting in inhibition of vital tetrahydrofolic acid synthesis

Pharmacokinetics (Adult data unless noted)

Absorption: Oral: Well absorbed

Distribution: V_d: Adults: 2.9 L/kg; distributed to the kidneys, lung, liver, and spleen

Protein binding: 80% to 87%

Half-life: 111 hours (range: 54-148 hours)

Time to peak serum concentration: Within 2-6 hours

Elimination: Pyrimethamine and metabolites are excreted in urine

Dosing: Neonatal Congenital toxoplasmosis (independent of HIV status); treatment: Oral: Initial: 2 mg/kg/day once daily for 2 days, then 1 mg/kg/day once daily given with sulfadiazine for the first 6 months; next 6 months: 1 mg/kg/day 3 times/week (eg, MWF) with sulfadiazine; total treatment duration:12 months; oral leucovorin 10 mg 3 times/week should be administered throughout the entire course to prevent hematologic toxicity (CDC, 2009; McAuley, 2008)

Dosing: Usual

Infants and Children:

Toxoplasmosis: Oral:

Treatment:

Congenital toxoplasmosis (independent of HIV status): Infants: Initial: 2 mg/kg/dose once daily for 2 days, then 1 mg/kg/day once daily given with sulfadiazine for the first 6 months; next 6 months: 1 mg/kg/day 3 times/week (eg, MWF) with sulfadiazine; oral leucovorin 10 mg 3 times/week should be administered throughout entire course to prevent hematologic toxicity (total treatment duration: 12 months) (CDC, 2009; McAuley, 2008)

Acquired infection:

HIV-exposed/-positive: 2 mg/kg (maximum dose: 50 mg) once daily for 3 days followed by 1 mg/kg (maximum dose: 25 mg) once daily in combination with sulfadiazine or clindamycin and leucovorin 10-25 mg daily; continue for at least 6 weeks; consider longer duration if clinical or radiologic disease is extensive or incomplete response; follow with chronic suppressive therapy (CDC, 2009)

Non-HIV-exposed/-positive: Children: 2 mg/kg (maximum dose: 50 mg) once daily for 2 days, followed by 1 mg/kg/day (maximum dose: 25 mg) once daily for 3-6 weeks in combination with sulfadiazine or clindamycin; oral leucovorin should be administered to prevent hematologic toxicity. Continue therapy until 1-2 weeks after the resolution of symptoms (*Red Book*, 2012).

Prophylaxis:

First episode of *Toxoplasma gondii*:

HIV-exposed/-positive (CDC, 2009):

In combination with dapsone: 1 mg/kg/day of pyrimethamine once daily (maximum single dose: 25 mg) with dapsone plus oral leucovorin 5 mg every 3 days

In combination with atovaquone: 1 mg/kg or 15 mg/m² of pyrimethamine once daily (maximum single dose: 25 mg) with atovaquone plus oral leucovorin

Hematopoietic cell transplantation recipients: 1 mg/kg/day of pyrimethamine once daily (maximum single dose: 75 mg) with clindamycin and leucovorin. Start after engraftment and administer as long as the patient remains on immunosuppressive therapy (Tomblyn, 2009).

Recurrence of *Toxoplasma gondii*: HIV-exposed/-positive: 1 mg/kg or 15 mg/m^2 once daily (maximum single dose: 25 mg) given with sulfadiazine, clindamycin, or atovaquone, plus oral leucovorin 5 mg every 3 days (CDC, 2009)

Malaria: Note: Current CDC recommendations for malaria prophylaxis or treatment do not include the use of pyrimethamine; resistance to pyrimethamine is prevalent worldwide. (CDC, 2011); however, pyrimethamine is still discussed in the World Health Organization (WHO) treatment guidelines (WHO, 2010; WHO, 2011).

Chemoprophylaxis: Oral: Begin prophylaxis before entering endemic area:
Infants and Children <4 years: 6.25 mg once weekly
Children 4-10 years: 12.5 mg once weekly
Children >10 years: 25 mg once weekly
Treatment [non-*falciparum* malaria; use in conjunction with a sulfonamide (eg, sulfadoxine)]: Oral:
Children 4-10 years: 25 mg daily for 2 days; following clinical cure, administer a once-weekly chemoprophylaxis regimen for ≥10 weeks. **Note:** Pyrimethamine monotherapy is generally not recommended.
Children >10 years: 25 mg daily for 2 days; following clinical cure, administer a once-weekly chemoprophylaxis regimen for ≥10 weeks. **Note:** Pyrimethamine monotherapy is **not** recommended; if circumstances arise where it must be used alone in semi-immune patients, give 50 mg daily for 2 days; then (following clinical cure) administer a once-weekly chemoprophylaxis regimen for ≥10 weeks.

Adolescents:
Isosporiasis (*Isospora belli*), HIV-positive/-exposed (DHHS, 2013): Oral:
Treatment: 50-75 mg once daily in combination with leucovorin calcium
Chronic maintenance: 25 mg once daily in combination with leucovorin calcium
Malaria: Note: Current CDC recommendations for malaria prophylaxis or treatment do not include the use of pyrimethamine; resistance to pyrimethamine is prevalent worldwide (CDC, 2011); however, pyrimethamine is still discussed in the World Health Organization (WHO) treatment guidelines (WHO, 2010; WHO, 2011).

Chemoprophylaxis: Oral: Begin prophylaxis before entering endemic area: 25 mg once weekly
Treatment: Oral: 25 mg daily for 2 days; following clinical cure, administer a once-weekly chemoprophylaxis regimen for ≥10 weeks. **Note:** Pyrimethamine monotherapy is not recommended; if circumstances arise where it must be used alone in semi-immune patients, give 50 mg daily for 2 days; then (following clinical cure) administer a once-weekly chemoprophylaxis regimen for ≥10 weeks.

***Pneumocystis jirovecii* pneumonia (PCP) (HIV-positive/-exposed)** (DHHS, 2013): Primary prophylaxis or chronic maintenance (secondary prophylaxis): Oral:
In combination with dapsone and leucovorin: 50-75 mg pyrimethamine with dapsone and leucovorin 25 mg once weekly
In combination with atovaquone and leucovorin: 25 mg pyrimethamine with atovaquone and leucovorin 10 mg once daily

Toxoplasmosis:
Treatment; encephalitis (HIV-exposed/-positive): Oral: 200 mg once as a single dose, followed by weight-based daily dosing: For weight <60 kg: 50 mg or for weight ≥60 kg: 75 mg once daily, typically used in combination with sulfadiazine and leucovorin; other combination regimens include clindamycin, atovaquone, or azithromycin and leucovorin; continue for at least 6 weeks; consider longer duration if clinical or radiologic disease is extensive or incomplete response (DHHS, 2013)

Prophylaxis:
First episode:
HIV-exposed/-positive: Oral: 50 mg or 75 mg once weekly with dapsone, plus oral leucovorin **or** 25 mg once daily with atovaquone in combination with leucovorin (DHHS, 2013)
Hematopoietic cell transplantation recipients: Oral: 25-75 mg once daily with clindamycin and leucovorin. Start after engraftment and administer as long as the patient remains on immunosuppressive therapy (Tomblyn, 2009)
Recurrence; HIV-exposed/-positive: Oral: 25-50 mg once daily in combination with sulfadiazine plus oral leucovorin **or** 25-50 mg once daily with clindamycin in combination with oral leucovorin **or** 25 mg once daily with atovaquone in combination with leucovorin (DHHS, 2013)

Adults:
Malaria chemoprophylaxis: Oral: **Note:** Current CDC recommendations for malaria prophylaxis do not include the use of pyrimethamine; resistance to pyrimethamine is prevalent worldwide.
Manufacturer's labeling: 25 mg once weekly
Malaria treatment (non-*falciparum* malaria; use in conjunction with a sulfonamide [eg, sulfadoxine]): Oral: **Note:** Current CDC recommendations for malaria treatment do not include the use of pyrimethamine; resistance to pyrimethamine is prevalent worldwide.
Manufacturer's labeling: 25 mg daily for 2 days; following clinical cure, administer a once-weekly chemoprophylaxis regimen for ≥10 weeks. **Note:** Pyrimethamine use alone is **not** recommended; if circumstances arise where it must be used alone in semi-immune patients, give 50 mg daily for 2 days; then (following clinical cure) administer a once-weekly chemoprophylaxis regimen for ≥10 weeks.

Toxoplasmosis: Oral:
Treatment: 50-75 mg/day for 1-3 weeks depending on patient's tolerance and response, then may reduce dose by 50% and continue for 4-5 weeks; use in conjunction with a sulfonamide and leucovorin
Prophylaxis and treatment in HIV-positive/-exposed patients (DHHS, 2013):
Prophylaxis for first episode of *Toxoplasma gondii*: 50 mg or 75 mg once weekly with dapsone, plus oral leucovorin **or** 25 mg once daily with atovaquone in combination with leucovorin
Prophylaxis to prevent recurrence of *Toxoplasma gondii*: 25-50 mg once daily in combination with sulfadiazine plus oral leucovorin **or** 25-50 mg once daily with clindamycin in combination with oral leucovorin **or** 25 mg once daily with atovaquone in combination with leucovorin
Treatment of *Toxoplasma gondii* encephalitis: 200 mg as a single dose, followed by 50 mg (<60 kg patients) or 75 mg (≥60 kg patients) daily, plus sulfadiazine and leucovorin **or** 200 mg as a single dose, followed by 50 mg (<60 kg patients) or 75 mg (≥60 kg patients) daily, with clindamycin, atovaquone, or azithromycin in combination with oral leucovorin calcium; continue treatment for at least 6 weeks; longer if clinical or radiologic disease is extensive or response is incomplete at 6 weeks.

Dosing adjustment in renal impairment: There are no dosage adjustments provided in the manufacturer's labeling.

Dosing adjustment in hepatic impairment: There are no dosage adjustments provided in the manufacturer's labeling.

Administration Oral: Administer with meals to minimize vomiting

Monitoring Parameters CBC, including platelet counts twice weekly with high-dose therapy (eg, when used for toxoplasmosis treatment; frequency not defined for lower doses); liver and renal function

Dosage Forms Excipient information presented when available (limited, particularly for generics); consult specific product labeling.

Tablet, Oral:

Daraprim: 25 mg [scored]

Extemporaneous Preparations A 2 mg/mL oral suspension may be made with tablets and a 1:1 mixture of Simple Syrup, NF and methylcellulose 1%. Crush forty 25 mg tablets in a mortar and reduce to a fine powder. Add small portions of vehicle and mix to a uniform paste; mix while adding vehicle in incremental proportions to **almost** 500 mL; transfer to a calibrated bottle, rinse mortar with vehicle, and add quantity of vehicle sufficient to make 500 mL. Label "shake well" and "refrigerate". Stable for 91 days.
Nahata MC, Pai VB, and Hipple TF, *Pediatric Drug Formulations*, 5th ed, Cincinnati, OH: Harvey Whitney Books Co, 2004.

References
Centers for Disease Control and Prevention (CDC). Guidelines for treatment of malaria in the United States, treatment table update, 2013a. Available at http://www.cdc.gov/malaria/resources/pdf/treatmenttable.pdf
Centers for Disease Control and Prevention (CDC), "Guidelines for the Prevention and Treatment of Opportunistic Infections Among HIV-Exposed and HIV-Infected Children," *MMWR Recomm Rep*, 2009, 58(RR-11):1-166. Available at http://aidsinfo.nih.gov/contentfiles/Pediatric_OI.pdf
DHHS Panel on Opportunistic Infections (OI) in HIV-Infected Adults and Adolescents. Guidelines for prevention and treatment of opportunistic infections in HIV-infected adults and adolescents: recommendations from the Centers for Disease Control and Prevention (CDC), the National Institutes of Health (NIH), and the HIV Medicine Association (HIVMA) of the Infectious Diseases Society of America (IDSA)," May 7, 2013. Available at http://aidsinfo.nih.gov/contentfiles/lvguidelines/adult_oi.pdf
McAuley JB, "Toxoplasmosis in Children," *Pediatr Infect Dis J*, 2008, 27 (2):161-2.
Red Book: 2012 Report of the Committee on Infectious Diseases, "Antibacterial Drugs Dosage Tables," 29th ed, Pickering LK, ed, Elk Grove Village, IL: American Academy of Pediatrics, 2012, 808-16.
Tomblyn M, Chiller T, Einsele H, et al, "Guidelines for Preventing Infectious Complications Among Hematopoietic Cell Transplantation Recipients: A Global Perspective," *Biol Blood Marrow Transplant*, 2009, 15(10):1143-238.
World Health Organization, "Guidelines for the Treatment of Malaria," 2010, World Health Organization, Geneva. Available at http://whqlibdoc.who.int/publications/2010/9789241547925_eng.pdf
World Health Organization, "Guidelines for the Treatment of Malaria, update 2010," World Health Organization, Geneva. Available at http://www.who.int/malaria/publications/atoz/mal_treatchild_revised.pdf

◆ **Pyrimethamine and Sulfadoxine** see Sulfadoxine and Pyrimethamine *on page 1947*

◆ **Q-Amlodipine (Can)** see AmLODIPine *on page 135*

◆ **Q-Citalopram (Can)** see Citalopram *on page 484*

◆ **Q-Cyclobenzaprine (Can)** see Cyclobenzaprine *on page 558*

◆ **Q-Dryl [OTC]** see DiphenhydrAMINE (Systemic) *on page 673*

◆ **Q-Fluoxetine (Can)** see FLUoxetine *on page 901*

◆ **Q-Metformin (Can)** see MetFORMIN *on page 1353*

◆ **Qnasl** see Beclomethasone (Nasal) *on page 267*

◆ **Q-Omeprazole (Can)** see Omeprazole *on page 1535*

◆ **Q-Pantoprazole (Can)** see Pantoprazole *on page 1595*

◆ **Q-Pap [OTC]** see Acetaminophen *on page 47*

◆ **Q-Pap Children's [OTC]** see Acetaminophen *on page 47*

◆ **Q-Pap Extra Strength [OTC]** see Acetaminophen *on page 47*

◆ **Q-Pap Infant's [OTC]** see Acetaminophen *on page 47*

◆ **Q-Paroxetine (Can)** see PARoxetine *on page 1609*

◆ **Q-Sertraline (Can)** see Sertraline *on page 1879*

◆ **Q-Simvastatin (Can)** see Simvastatin *on page 1892*

◆ **Q-Tapp Cold & Allergy [OTC]** see Brompheniramine and Pseudoephedrine *on page 306*

◆ **Q-Terbinafine (Can)** see Terbinafine (Systemic) *on page 1982*

◆ **Q-Topiramate (Can)** see Topiramate *on page 2046*

◆ **Q-Tussin [OTC]** see GuaiFENesin *on page 984*

◆ **Q-Tussin DM [OTC]** see Guaifenesin and Dextromethorphan *on page 987*

◆ **Quadrivalent Human Papillomavirus Vaccine** see Papillomavirus (Types 6, 11, 16, 18) Vaccine (Human, Recombinant) *on page 1600*

◆ **Qualaquin** see QuiNINE *on page 1794*

◆ **Qudexy XR** see Topiramate *on page 2046*

◆ **Quelicin** see Succinylcholine *on page 1938*

◆ **Quelicin® (Can)** see Succinylcholine *on page 1938*

◆ **Quelicin-1000** see Succinylcholine *on page 1938*

◆ **Quenalin [OTC]** see DiphenhydrAMINE (Systemic) *on page 673*

◆ **Questran** see Cholestyramine Resin *on page 457*

◆ **Questran Light** see Cholestyramine Resin *on page 457*

◆ **Questran Light Sugar Free (Can)** see Cholestyramine Resin *on page 457*

QUEtiapine (kwe TYE a peen)

Medication Safety Issues

Sound-alike/look-alike issues:

QUEtiapine may be confused with OLANZapine

SEROquel may be confused with Serzone, SINEquan

BEERS Criteria medication:

This drug may be potentially inappropriate for use in geriatric patients (Quality of evidence - moderate; Strength of recommendation - strong).

Related Information

Oral Medications That Should Not Be Crushed or Altered *on page 2438*

Brand Names: U.S. SEROquel; SEROquel XR

Brand Names: Canada Apo-Quetiapine; Auro-Quetiapine; Ava-Quetiapine; CO Quetiapine; Dom-Quetiapine; JAMP-Quetiapine; Mar-Quetiapine; Mylan-Quetiapine; PHL-Quetiapine; PMS-Quetiapine; PRO-Quetiapine; Quetiapine XR; RAN-Quetiapine; ratio-Quetiapine; Riva-Quetiapine; Sandoz-Quetiapine; Sandoz-Quetiapine XRT; Seroquel; Seroquel XR; Teva-Quetiapine; Teva-Quetiapine XR

Therapeutic Category Antipsychotic Agent, Atypical

Generic Availability (U.S.) May be product dependent

Use

Immediate release (Seroquel®): Acute treatment (adjunct and monotherapy) of manic episodes associated with bipolar I disorder (FDA approved in ages ≥10 years and adults); treatment of schizophrenia (FDA approved in ages ≥13 years and adults); acute treatment of depressive episodes associated with bipolar disorder (FDA approved in adults); adjunct therapy for maintenance in bipolar I disorder (FDA approved in adults); has also been used for autism

Extended release (Seroquel XR®): Acute treatment (adjunct and monotherapy) of manic or mixed episodes associated with bipolar I disorder (FDA approved in ages ≥10 years and adults); treatment of schizophrenia (FDA approved in ages ≥13 years and adults); acute treatment of depressive episodes associated with bipolar disorder (FDA approved in adults); adjunct maintenance therapy of bipolar I disorder (FDA approved in adults); adjunct treatment of major depressive disorder (FDA approved in adults)

◀ **Medication Guide Available** Yes
Pregnancy Risk Factor C
Pregnancy Considerations Adverse events were observed in animal reproduction studies. Quetiapine crosses the placenta and can be detected in cord blood (Newport, 2007). Congenital malformations have not been observed in humans (based on limited data). Antipsychotic use during the third trimester of pregnancy has a risk for abnormal muscle movements (extrapyramidal symptoms [EPS]) and/or withdrawal symptoms in newborns following delivery. Symptoms in the newborn may include agitation, feeding disorder, hypertonia, hypotonia, respiratory distress, somnolence, and tremor; these effects may be self-limiting or require hospitalization. Quetiapine may cause hyperprolactinemia, which may decrease reproductive function in both males and females.

Treatment algorithms have been developed by the ACOG and the APA for the management of depression in women prior to conception and during pregnancy (Yonkers, 2009). The ACOG recommends that therapy during pregnancy be individualized; treatment with psychiatric medications during pregnancy should incorporate the clinical expertise of the mental health clinician, obstetrician, primary healthcare provider, and pediatrician. Safety data related to atypical antipsychotics during pregnancy is limited and routine use is not recommended. However, if a woman is inadvertently exposed to an atypical antipsychotic while pregnant, continuing therapy may be preferable to switching to a typical antipsychotic that the fetus has not yet been exposed to; consider risk:benefit (ACOG, 2008).

Healthcare providers are encouraged to enroll women 18-45 years of age exposed to quetiapine during pregnancy in the Atypical Antipsychotics Pregnancy Registry (1-866-961-2388 or http://www.womensmentalhealth.org/pregnancyregistry).

Breast-Feeding Considerations Quetiapine is excreted into breast milk. Based on information from 8 mother-infant pairs, concentrations of quetiapine in breast milk have been reported from undetectable to 170 mcg/L. The estimated exposure to the breast-feeding infant would be up to 0.1 mg/kg/day (relative infant dose up to 0.43% based on a weight adjusted maternal dose of 400 mg/day). Due to the potential for serious adverse reactions in the nursing infant, the manufacturer recommends a decision be made whether to discontinue nursing or to discontinue the drug, taking into account the importance of treatment to the mother.

Contraindications Hypersensitivity to quetiapine or any component

Warnings Clinical worsening of depression or suicidal ideation and behavior may occur in children and adults with major depressive disorder **[U.S. Boxed Warnings]**. In clinical trials, antidepressants increased the risk of suicidal thinking and behavior (suicidality) in children, adolescents, and young adults (18-24 years of age) with major depressive disorder and other psychiatric disorders. This risk must be considered before prescribing antidepressants for any clinical use. Short-term studies did **not** show an increased risk of suicidality with antidepressant use in patients >24 years of age and showed a decreased risk in patients ≥65 years.

Patients of all ages who are treated with antidepressants for any indication require appropriate monitoring and close observation for clinical worsening of depression, suicidality, and unusual changes in behavior, especially during the first few months after antidepressant initiation or when the dose is adjusted. Family members and caregivers should be instructed to closely observe the patient (ie, daily) and communicate condition with healthcare provider. Patients should also be monitored for associated behaviors (eg, anxiety, agitation, panic attacks, insomnia, irritability, hostility, aggressiveness, impulsivity, akathisia, hypomania, mania) which may increase the risk for worsening depression or suicidality. Worsening depression or emergence of suicidality (or associated behaviors listed above) that is abrupt in onset, severe, or not part of the presenting symptoms, may require discontinuation or modification of drug therapy. To reduce risk of intentional overdose, write prescriptions for the smallest quantity consistent with good patient care. Screen individuals for bipolar disorder prior to treatment of depression (using antidepressants alone may induce manic episodes in patients with this condition). May worsen psychosis in some patients or precipitate a shift to mania or hypomania in patients with bipolar disorder. Quetiapine is FDA approved for the treatment of bipolar depression.

Avoid abrupt discontinuation; discontinuation symptoms (including insomnia, nausea and vomiting, headache, diarrhea, dizziness, irritability, and other symptoms) may occur if therapy is abruptly discontinued or dose reduced; taper the dose to minimize risks of discontinuation symptoms; if intolerable symptoms occur following a decrease in dosage or upon discontinuation of therapy, consider resuming the previous dose with a more gradual taper.

May cause neuroleptic malignant syndrome (symptoms include hyperpyrexia, altered mental status, muscle rigidity, autonomic instability, acute renal failure, rhabdomyolysis, and elevated CPK). May cause extrapyramidal reactions, including pseudoparkinsonism, acute dystonic reactions, akathisia, and tardive dyskinesia (risk of these reactions is low relative to other neuroleptics, and is dose-dependent; to decrease risk of tardive dyskinesia: Use smallest dose and shortest duration possible; evaluate continued need periodically; risk of dystonia is increased with the use of high potency and higher doses of conventional antipsychotics and in males and younger patients).

Hyperglycemia has been reported with atypical antipsychotics, which may be severe and include potentially fatal ketoacidosis or hyperosmolar coma. In pediatric (ages 10-17 years) clinical trials of quetiapine, slight increases in fasting glucose levels were reported (mean change: 3.62 mg/dL), however, no pediatric patients with baseline fasting glucose <126 mg/dL developed treatment-emergent hyperglycemia (≥126 mg/dL). Use with caution and monitor glucose closely in patients with diabetes mellitus (or with risk factors such as family history or obesity); measure fasting blood glucose at the beginning of therapy and periodically during therapy in these patients; monitor for symptoms of hyperglycemia in all patients treated with quetiapine; measure fasting blood glucose in patients who develop symptoms.

Leukopenia, neutropenia, and agranulocytosis (sometimes fatal) have been reported in clinical trials and postmarketing reports with antipsychotic use; presence of risk factors (eg, preexisting low WBC or history of drug-induced leuko/neutropenia) should prompt periodic blood count assessment. Discontinue therapy at first signs of blood dyscrasias or if absolute neutrophil count <1000/mm^3.

In children and adolescents, increases in blood pressure (including hypertensive crisis) have been reported. In pediatric clinical trials (ages: 10-17 years), an increase in SBP (≥20 mm Hg) and DBP (≥10 mm Hg) was observed more frequently than placebo (SBP: 15.2% vs 5.5%; DBP: 40.6% vs 24.5%). Monitor blood pressure at baseline and periodically during therapy with quetiapine.

May alter cardiac conduction; life-threatening arrhythmias have occurred with therapeutic doses of antipsychotics. Quetiapine use has been associated with QT prolongation; postmarketing reports have occurred in patients with concomitant illness, quetiapine overdose, or who were receiving concomitant therapy known to affect QT interval or cause electrolyte imbalance. Avoid use in patients at increased risk of torsade de pointes/sudden death (eg, hypokalemia, hypomagnesemia, history of cardiac arrhythmias, congenital prolongation of QT interval, concomitant medications with QT_c interval-prolonging properties). Use with caution in patients at increased risk of QT prolongation (eg, cardiovascular disease, heart failure, cardiac hypertrophy, elderly, family history of QT prolongation).

May cause dose-related decreases in thyroid hormone levels, including cases requiring thyroid hormone replacement therapy. Reversal of thyroid effects occurred in almost all cases following discontinuation. Use has been noted to cause cataracts in animals; lens changes have been observed in humans during long-term treatment. Lens examination on initiation of therapy and every 6 months is recommended.

An increased risk of death has been reported with the use of antipsychotics in elderly patients with dementia-related psychosis **[U.S. Boxed Warning]**; most deaths seemed to be cardiovascular (eg, sudden death, heart failure) or infectious (eg, pneumonia) in nature. An increased risk of cerebrovascular events (TIAs and CVAs) has also been reported with the use of antipsychotics in these patients. Quetiapine is not approved for the treatment of patients with dementia-related psychosis.

Pediatric psychiatric disorders are frequently serious mental disorders which present with variable symptoms that do not always match adult diagnostic criteria. Conduct a thorough diagnostic evaluation and carefully consider risks of psychotropic medication before initiation in pediatric patients. Medication therapy for pediatric patients with bipolar disorder and schizophrenia is indicated as part of a total treatment program that frequently includes educational, psychological, and social interventions.

Potentially significant interactions may exist, requiring dose or frequency adjustment, additional monitoring, and/or selection of alternative therapy. Consult drug interactions database for more detailed information.

Precautions Use with caution in patients with hepatic disease or impairment; may increase serum transaminases (primarily ALT; transient, reversible). Quetiapine undergoes substantial hepatic metabolism via CYP3A4; may require dose adjustment in patients with hepatic impairment. Use with caution in patients with renal disease; experience is limited. May cause anticholinergic effects (confusion, agitation, constipation, xerostomia, blurred vision, urinary retention); use with caution in patients with decreased GI motility, urinary retention, BPH, xerostomia, or visual problems. Relative to other antipsychotics, quetiapine has a moderate potency of cholinergic blockade. Impaired core body temperature regulation may occur; caution with strenuous exercise, heat exposure, dehydration, and concomitant medication possessing anticholinergic effects. May cause orthostatic hypotension and in some cases syncope; risk increased during dose titration; use with caution in patients at risk of this effect or in those who would not tolerate transient hypotensive episodes (cerebrovascular disease, cardiovascular disease, hypovolemia, or concurrent medication use which may predispose to hypotension/bradycardia).

Increases in cholesterol and triglycerides have been noted; in pediatric trials (ages: 10-17 years), total cholesterol increased to a clinically significant level (≥200 mg/dL) in 10% to 12% of patients, and triglycerides (≥150 mg/dL) in 17% to 22% of patients. Use with caution in patients with preexisting abnormal lipid profile; monitor lipid profile.

Significant weight gain has been observed with antipsychotic therapy; incidence varies with specific drug. Monitor growth (including weight, height, BMI and waist circumference) in pediatric patients receiving quetiapine; compare weight gain to standard growth curves. The SATIETY (Second-Generation Antipsychotic Treatment Indications, Effectiveness and Tolerability in Youth) study showed children and adolescents aged 4-19 years taking second-generation antipsychotics for the first time experienced significant weight gain, increase in BMI from baseline, and an increase in waist circumference with aripiprazole, olanzapine, quetiapine, and risperidone compared to untreated patients. Average weight gain after a median of 10.8 weeks was 8.5 kg with olanzapine, 6.1 kg with quetiapine, 5.3 kg with risperidone, and 4.4 kg with aripiprazole compared to 0.2 kg in untreated group. A significant increase in total cholesterol, triglycerides, and nonhigh density lipoprotein was seen with quetiapine and olanzapine. Biannual monitoring of cardiometabolic indices after the first 3 months of therapy is suggested (Correll, 2009).

Rare cases of priapism have been reported. May be sedating or cause motor or cognitive impairment; particularly during initial dose titration; use with caution in disorders where CNS depression is a feature. Patients must be cautioned about performing tasks which require mental alertness (eg, operating machinery or driving). Use with caution in patients with breast cancer or other prolactin-dependent tumors; quetiapine increases prolactin concentrations; in pediatric clinical trials (ages: 10-17 years), development of clinically significant prolactin levels occurred in 13.4% of male patients and 8.7% of females; high concentrations of prolactin may reduce pituitary gonadotropin secretion; galactorrhea, amenorrhea, gynecomastia, impotence, decreased bone density may occur. Use with caution in children and adolescents; adverse effects due to increased prolactin concentrations have been observed; long-term effects on growth or sexual maturation have not been evaluated. Use with caution in those at risk of aspiration pneumonia; esophageal dysmotility and aspiration have been associated with antipsychotic agents.

Use with caution in patients at risk for seizures, including those with a history of seizures, head trauma, brain damage, alcoholism, or concurrent therapy with medications which may lower seizure threshold; elderly patients may be at increased risk of seizures due to an increased prevalence of predisposing factors.

Adverse Reactions Actual frequency may be dependent upon dose and/or indication.

Cardiovascular: Hypertension (diastolic; children and adolescents), hypertension, hypotension, increased heart rate, orthostatic hypotension (more common in adults), palpitations, peripheral edema, syncope, systolic hypertension (children and adolescents), tachycardia

Central nervous system: Abnormal dreams, abnormality in thinking, aggressive behavior (children and adolescents), agitation, akathisia, anxiety, ataxia, chills, confusion, decreased mental acuity, depression, disorientation, dizziness, drooling, drowsiness, drug-induced Parkinson's disease, dysarthria, dystonia, extrapyramidal reaction, falling, fatigue, headache, hypersomnia, hypertonia, hypoesthesia, insomnia, irritability, lack of concentration, lethargy, migraine, pain, paresthesia, restless leg syndrome, restlessness, tardive dyskinesia, twitching, vertigo

Dermatologic: Acne vulgaris (children and adolescents), diaphoresis, hyperhidrosis, pallor (children and adolescents), skin rash

Endocrine & metabolic: Decreased HDL cholesterol (≤40 mg/dL), decreased libido, hyperglycemia (≥200 mg/dL post glucose challenge or fasting glucose ≥126 mg/dL), hyperprolactinemia, hypothyroidism, increased gamma-glutamyl transferase, increased LDL cholesterol (≥160 mg/dL), increased serum triglycerides (≥200 mg/dL), increased thirst (children and adolescents), total cholesterol increased (≥240 mg/dL), weight gain (dose related)

Gastrointestinal: Abdominal distension, abdominal pain, anorexia, constipation, decreased appetite, dyspepsia (dose related), dysphagia, flatulence, gastroenteritis, gastroesophageal reflux disease, increased appetite, nausea, periodontal abscess (adolescents), toothache, unpleasant taste, vomiting, xerostomia (more common in adults)

Genitourinary: Impotence, lactation (female), pollakiuria, urinary tract infection

Hematologic & oncologic: Hemorrhage, leukopenia, lymphadenopathy, neutropenia

Hepatic: Increased serum transaminases

Hypersensitivity: Seasonal allergy

Neuromuscular & skeletal: Arthralgia, back pain, dyskinesia, limb pain, muscle rigidity, muscle spasm, myalgia, neck pain, neck stiffness, stiffness (children and adolescents), tremor, weakness

Ophthalmic: Amblyopia, blurred vision

Otic: Otalgia

Respiratory: Cough, dry throat, dyspnea, epistaxis (adolescents), flu-like symptoms, nasal congestion, pharyngitis, rhinitis, sinus congestion, sinus headache, sinusitis, upper respiratory tract infection

Miscellaneous: Fever

Rare but important or life-threatening: Abnormal T waves on ECG, acute hepatic failure, acute renal failure, agranulocytosis, amnesia, anemia, angina pectoris, atrial arrhythmia, atrioventricular block, bundle branch block, cardiac failure, cardiomyopathy, cataract, cerebrovascular accident, dehydration, diabetes mellitus, dysuria, eosinophilia, exfoliative dermatitis, galactorrhea, hallucination, hematemesis, hypersensitivity, hypoglycemia, increased ST segment on ECG, intestinal obstruction, involuntary body movements, leukocytosis, myocarditis, neuroleptic malignant syndrome, palpitations, pancreatitis, pneumonia, priapism, prolonged Q-T interval on ECG, rectal hemorrhage, rhabdomyolysis, seizure, SIADH, suicidal ideation, thrombocytopenia, urinary retention, widened QRS complex on ECG

Drug Interactions

Metabolism/Transport Effects Substrate of CYP2D6 (minor), 3A4 (major)

Avoid Concomitant Use

Avoid concomitant use of QUEtiapine with any of the following: Aclidinium; Amisulpride; Azelastine (Nasal); Conivaptan; Fusidic Acid (Systemic); Highest Risk QTc-Prolonging Agents; Ipratropium (Oral Inhalation); Ivabradine; Metoclopramide; Mifepristone; Moderate Risk QTc-Prolonging Agents; Paraldehyde; Potassium Chloride; Sulpiride; Thalidomide; Tiotropium; Umeclidinium

Increased Effect/Toxicity

QUEtiapine may increase the levels/effects of: AbobotulinumtoxinA; Alcohol (Ethyl); Amisulpride; Analgesics (Opioid); Anticholinergic Agents; Azelastine (Nasal); Buprenorphine; Cannabinoid-Containing Products; CNS Depressants; DULoxetine; Highest Risk QTc-Prolonging Agents; Hydrocodone; Hypotensive Agents; Methotrimeprazine; Methylphenidate; Metyrosine; OnabotulinumtoxinA; Paraldehyde; Potassium Chloride; RimabotulinumtoxinB; Selective Serotonin Reuptake Inhibitors; Serotonin Modulators; St Johns Wort; Sulpiride; Thalidomide; Thiazide Diuretics; Tiotropium; Topiramate; Zolpidem

The levels/effects of QUEtiapine may be increased by: Acetylcholinesterase Inhibitors (Central); Aclidinium; Barbiturates; Brimonidine (Topical); Cannabis; Conivaptan; CYP3A4 Inhibitors (Moderate); CYP3A4 Inhibitors (Strong); Doxylamine; Dronabinol; Fusidic Acid (Systemic); HydrOXYzine; Ipratropium (Oral Inhalation); Ivabradine; Ivacaftor; Kava Kava; Luliconazole; Magnesium

Sulfate; Methotrimeprazine; Methylphenidate; Metoclopramide; Metyrosine; Mifepristone; Moderate Risk QTc-Prolonging Agents; Nabilone; Perampanel; Pramlintide; QTc-Prolonging Agents (Indeterminate Risk and Risk Modifying); Rufinamide; Serotonin Modulators; Simeprevir; Sodium Oxybate; Stiripentol; Tapentadol; Tetrahydrocannabinol; Umeclidinium

Decreased Effect

QUEtiapine may decrease the levels/effects of: Acetylcholinesterase Inhibitors (Central); Amphetamines; Anti-Parkinson's Agents (Dopamine Agonist); Quinagolide; Secretin

The levels/effects of QUEtiapine may be decreased by: Acetylcholinesterase Inhibitors (Central); Bosentan; CYP3A4 Inducers (Strong); Dabrafenib; Deferasirox; Mitotane; Peginterferon Alfa-2b; Siltuximab; St Johns Wort; Tocilizumab

Food Interactions In healthy volunteers, administration of quetiapine (immediate release) with food resulted in an increase in the peak serum concentration and AUC by 25% and 15%, respectively, compared to the fasting state. Administration of the extended release formulation with a high-fat meal (~800-1000 calories) resulted in an increase in peak serum concentration by 44% to 52% and AUC by 20% to 22% for the 50 mg and 300 mg tablets; administration with a light meal (≤300 calories) had no significant effect on the C_{max} or AUC. Management: Administer without food or with a light meal (≤300 calories).

Stability Store at 25°C (77°F); excursions permitted to 15°C to 30°C (59°F to 86°F).

Mechanism of Action Quetiapine is a dibenzothiazepine atypical antipsychotic. It has been proposed that this drug's antipsychotic activity is mediated through a combination of dopamine type 2 (D_2) and serotonin type 2 (5-HT_2) antagonism. It is an antagonist at multiple neurotransmitter receptors in the brain: Serotonin 5-HT_{1A} and 5-HT_2, dopamine D_1 and D_2, histamine H_1, and adrenergic alpha$_1$- and alpha$_2$-receptors; but appears to have no appreciable affinity at cholinergic muscarinic and benzodiazepine receptors. Norquetiapine, an active metabolite, differs from its parent molecule by exhibiting high affinity for muscarinic M1 receptors.

Antagonism at receptors other than dopamine and 5-HT_2 with similar receptor affinities may explain some of the other effects of quetiapine. The drug's antagonism of histamine H_1-receptors may explain the somnolence observed. The drug's antagonism of adrenergic alpha$_1$-receptors may explain the orthostatic hypotension observed.

Pharmacokinetics (Adult data unless noted)

Absorption: Rapidly absorbed following oral administration; parent compound AUC and C_{max} were 41% and 39% lower, respectively, in pediatric patients (10-17 years) compared to adults when adjusted for weight, but pharmacokinetics of active metabolite were similar to adult values after adjusting for weight.

Distribution: V_d: 10 ± 4 L/kg

Protein binding, plasma: 83%

Metabolism: Primarily hepatic; via CYP3A4; forms the metabolite N-desalkyl quetiapine (active) and two inactive metabolites [sulfoxide metabolite (major metabolite) and parent acid metabolite]

Bioavailability: 100% (relative to oral solution)

Half-life elimination:

Children and Adolescents (ages 12-17): Quetiapine: 5.3 hours (McConville, 2000)

Adults: Quetiapine: ~6 hours; Extended release: ~7 hours

Time to peak serum concentration:

Children and Adolescents ages 12-17: Immediate release: 0.5-3 hours (McConville, 2000)

Adults: Immediate release: 1.5 hours; Extended release: 6 hours

Elimination: Urine (73% as metabolites, <1% of total dose as unchanged drug); feces (20%)

Dosing: Usual Note: Patients who have interrupted therapy for >1 week should generally be restarted at the initial dosing and retitrated; patients who have interrupted therapy for <1 week can generally be reinitiated on their previous dose.

Children and Adolescents:

Bipolar disorder, mania or mixed episodes: Children and Adolescents ≥10 years: Oral:

Immediate release tablet: Initial: 25 mg twice daily on day 1; increase to 50 mg twice daily on day 2, then 100 mg twice daily on day 3, then 150 mg twice daily on day 4, then continue at the target dose of 200 mg twice daily beginning on day 5. May increase further based on clinical response and tolerability at increments ≤100 mg/day up to 300 mg twice daily; however, no additional benefit was seen with 300 mg twice daily vs 200 mg twice daily. Usual dosage range: 200-300 mg twice daily; maximum daily dose: 600 mg/**day**. Total daily doses may also be divided into 3 doses per day. Continue therapy at lowest dose needed to maintain remission; periodically assess maintenance treatment needs

Extended release: Initial: 50 mg once daily on day 1; increase to 100 mg once daily on day 2, then increase in 100 mg/day increments each day until a target dose of 400 mg once daily is reached on day 5. Usual dosage range: 400-600 mg once daily; maximum daily dose: 600 mg/**day**; continue therapy at lowest dose needed to maintain remission; periodically assess maintenance treatment needs

Switching from immediate release to extended release: May convert patients from immediate release to extended release tablets at the equivalent total daily dose and administer once daily; individual dosage adjustments may be necessary.

Schizophrenia: Adolescents: Oral:

Immediate release tablet: Initial: 25 mg twice daily on day 1; increase to 50 mg twice daily on day 2, 100 mg twice daily on day 3, then 150 mg twice daily on day 4, then continue at a target dose of 200 mg twice daily beginning on day 5. May increase further based on clinical response and tolerability at increments ≤100 mg/day up to 400 mg twice daily; however, no additional benefit was seen with 400 mg twice daily vs 200 mg twice daily. Usual dosage range: 200-400 mg twice daily; maximum daily dose: 800 mg/**day**. Total daily doses may also be divided into 3 doses per day. Periodically assess maintenance treatment needs.

Extended release: Initial: 50 mg once daily on day 1; increase to 100 mg once daily on day 2, then increase in 100 mg/day increments each day until a target dose of 400 mg once daily is reached on day 5. Usual dosage range: 400-800 mg once daily; maximum daily dose: 800 mg/**day**. Periodically assess maintenance treatment needs.

Switching from immediate release to extended release: May convert patients from immediate release to extended release tablets at the equivalent total daily dose and administer once daily; individual dosage adjustments may be necessary.

Adults:

Bipolar disorder: Oral:

Depression:

Immediate release tablet: Initial: 50 mg once daily at bedtime the first day; increase to 100 mg once daily at bedtime on day 2, then increase by 100 mg/day increments each day until a target dose of 300 mg once daily at bedtime is reached by day 4. Further increases up to 600 mg once daily by day 8 have

been evaluated in clinical trials, but no additional antidepressant efficacy was noted. Maximum daily dose: 300 mg/**day**

Extended release tablet: Initial: 50 mg once daily the first day; increase to 100 mg once daily on day 2, then increase by 100 mg/day increments each day until a target dose of 300 mg once daily is reached by day 4. Maximum daily dose: 300 mg/**day**

Switching from immediate release to extended release: May convert patients from immediate release to extended release tablets at the equivalent total daily dose and administer once daily; individual dosage adjustments may be necessary.

Mania:

Immediate release tablet: Initial: 50 mg twice daily on day 1, increase dose in increments of 100 mg/day each day to 200 mg twice daily on day 4; may increase at increments ≤200 mg/day to 400 mg twice daily by day 6. Usual dosage range: 200-400 mg twice daily. Maximum daily dose: 800 mg/**day**

Extended release tablet: Initial: 300 mg once daily on day 1; increase to 600 mg once daily on day 2 and adjust dose to 400-800 mg once daily on day 3, depending on response and tolerance. Maximum daily dose: 800 mg/**day**

Switching from immediate release to extended release: May convert patients from immediate release to extended release tablets at the equivalent total daily dose and administer once daily; individual dosage adjustments may be necessary.

Maintenance therapy:

Immediate release tablet (twice daily dosing) or extended release tablet (once daily dosing): 400-800 mg/day with lithium or divalproex; **Note:** In the maintenance phase, patients generally continue on the same dose on which they were stabilized. Maximum daily dose: 800 mg/**day**. Average time of stabilization was 15 weeks in clinical trials. During maintenance treatment, periodically reassess need for continued therapy and the appropriate dose. Patients who have discontinued therapy for >1 week should generally be retitrated following reinitiation of therapy; patients who have discontinued therapy for <1 week can generally be reinitiated at their previous dose.

Major depressive disorder (adjunct to antidepressants): Oral: Extended release tablet: Initial: 50 mg once daily on days 1 and 2; may be increased to 150 mg once daily on day 3. Usual dosage range: 150-300 mg once daily. Maximum daily dose: 300 mg/**day**

Schizophrenia/psychoses: Oral:

Immediate release tablet: Initial: 25 mg twice daily; followed by increases in the total daily dose on the second and third day in increments of 25-50 mg divided 2-3 doses daily, if tolerated, to a target dose of 300-400 mg/day in 2-3 divided doses by day 4. Make further adjustments of 50-100 mg/day as needed at intervals of at least 2 days. Usual maintenance range: 150-750 mg/day. Maximum daily dose: 750 mg/**day**

Extended release tablet: Initial: 300 mg once daily; increase in increments of up to 300 mg/day (in intervals ≥1 day). Usual maintenance range: 400-800 mg once daily. Maximum daily dose: 800 mg/**day**

Switching from immediate release to extended release: May convert patients from immediate release to extended release tablets at the equivalent total daily dose and administer once daily; individual dosage adjustments may be necessary.

Note: During maintenance treatment, periodically reassess the need for continued therapy and the appropriate dose.

Dosage adjustment for concomitant therapy: Children ≥10 years, Adolescents, and Adults:

Concomitant use with a strong CYP3A4 inhibitor (eg, ketoconazole, itraconazole, indinavir, ritonavir, nefazodone): Immediate release or extended release: Decrease quetiapine to one-sixth of the original dose; when strong CYP3A4 inhibitor is discontinued, increase quetiapine dose by sixfold.

Concomitant use with a strong CYP3A4 inducer (eg, phenytoin, carbamazepine, rifampin, St. John's wort): Immediate release or extended release: Increase quetiapine up to fivefold of the original dose when combined with chronic treatment (>7-14 days) of a strong CYP3A4 inducer; titrate based on clinical response and tolerance; when the strong CYP3A4 inducer is discontinued, decrease quetiapine to the original dose within 7-14 days.

Dosing adjustment in renal impairment: No adjustment required

Dosing adjustment in hepatic impairment: Lower clearance in hepatic impairment (30% lower); higher plasma levels expected; dosage adjustment may be needed.

Adults:

Immediate release tablet: Initial: 25 mg daily; increase dose by 25-50 mg daily increments to effective dose, based on clinical response and tolerability. If initiated with immediate-release formulation, patient may transition to extended-release formulation (at equivalent total daily dose) when effective dose has been reached.

Extended release tablet: Initial: 50 mg once daily; increase dose by 50 mg daily increments to effective dose, based on clinical response and tolerability.

Administration

Oral:

Immediate release tablet: May be administered with or without food.

Extended release tablet: Administer without food or with a light meal (≤300 calories), preferably in the evening. Swallow tablet whole; do not break, crush, or chew.

Nasogastric/enteral tube: Immediate release tablet: Adults: Hold tube feeds for 30 minutes before administration; flush with 25 mL of sterile water. Crush dose, mix in 10 mL water and administer via NG/enteral tube; follow with a 50 mL flush of sterile water. Restart tube feedings after drug administration (Devlin, 2010).

Monitoring Parameters Vital signs, including for children and adolescents; BP at baseline and periodically; CBC with differential; fasting lipid profile and fasting blood glucose/Hb A_{1c} (prior to treatment, at 3 months, then annually); weight, growth, BMI, and waist circumference (especially in children), personal/family history of diabetes, blood pressure, mental status, abnormal involuntary movement scale (AIMS), extrapyramidal symptoms (EPS). In adults, weight should be assessed prior to treatment, at 4 weeks, 8 weeks, 12 weeks, and then at quarterly intervals; consider titrating to a different antipsychotic agent for a weight gain ≥5% of the initial weight. Monitor patient periodically for symptom resolution; monitor for worsening depression, suicidality, and associated behaviors (especially at the beginning of therapy or when doses are increased or decreased). Patients should have eyes checked for cataracts every 6 months while on this medication.

Measure both TSH and free T4, along with clinical assessment, at baseline and follow-up to determine thyroid status; measurement of TSH alone may not be accurate; the exact mechanism of the effect of quetiapine on the thyroid axis is unknown.

Test Interactions May interfere with urine detection of methadone (false-positives); may cause false-positive serum TCA screen

Dosage Forms Excipient information presented when available (limited, particularly for generics); consult specific product labeling.

Tablet, Oral:

SEROquel: 25 mg, 50 mg, 100 mg, 200 mg, 300 mg, 400 mg

Generic: 25 mg, 50 mg, 100 mg, 200 mg, 300 mg, 400 mg

Tablet Extended Release 24 Hour, Oral:

SEROquel XR: 50 mg, 150 mg, 200 mg, 300 mg, 400 mg

References

American College of Obstetricians and Gynecologists, ACOG Practice Bulletin: Clinical Management Guidelines for Obstetricians-Gynecologists No. 92 April 2008 (Replaces Practice Bulletin Number 87, November 2007), "Use of Psychiatric Medications During Pregnancy and Lactation," *Obstet Gynecol*, 2008, 111(4):1001-20.

Correll CU, Manu P, Olshanskiy V, et al, "Cardiometabolic Risk of Second-Generation Antipsychotic Medications During First-Time Use in Children and Adolescents," *JAMA*, 2009, 302(16):1765-73.

DeVane CL and Nemeroff CB, "Clinical Pharmacokinetics of Quetiapine: An Atypical Antipsychotic," *Clin Pharmacokinet*, 2001, 40 (7):509-22.

Devlin JW, Roberts RJ, Fong JJ, et al, "Efficacy and Safety of Quetiapine in Critically Ill Patients With Delirium: A Prospective, Multicenter, Randomized, Double-Blind, Placebo-Controlled Pilot Study," *Crit Care Med*, 2010, 38(2):419-27.

McConville BJ, Arvanitis LA, Thyrum PT, et al, "Pharmacokinetics, Tolerability, and Clinical Effectiveness of Quetiapine Fumarate: An Open-Label Trial in Adolescents With Psychotic Disorders," *J Clin Psychiatry*, 2000, 61(4):252-60.

Newport DJ, Calamaras MR, DeVane CL, et al, "Atypical Antipsychotic Administration During Late Pregnancy: Placental Passage and Obstetrical Outcomes," *Am J Psychiatry*, 2007, 164(8):1214-20.

Yonkers KA, Wisner KL, Stewart DE, et al, "The Management of Depression During Pregnancy: A Report From the American Psychiatric Association and the American College of Obstetricians and Gynecologists," *Obstet Gynecol*, 2009, 114(3):703-13.

◆ **Quetiapine Fumarate** *see* QUEtiapine *on page 1783*

◆ **Quetiapine XR (Can)** *see* QUEtiapine *on page 1783*

◆ **Quillivant XR** *see* Methylphenidate *on page 1379*

◆ **Quinalbarbitone Sodium** *see* Secobarbital *on page 1875*

Quinapril (KWIN a pril)

Medication Safety Issues

Sound-alike/look-alike issues:

Accupril may be confused with Accolate, Accutane, AcipHex, Monopril

International issues:

Accupril [U.S., Canada] may be confused with Acepril which is a brand name for captopril [Great Britain]; enalapril [Hungary, Switzerland]; lisinopril [Malaysia]

Brand Names: U.S. Accupril

Brand Names: Canada Accupril; Apo-Quinapril; PMS-Quinapril

Therapeutic Category Angiotensin-Converting Enzyme (ACE) Inhibitor; Antihypertensive Agent

Generic Availability (U.S.) Yes

Use Treatment of hypertension alone or in combination with thiazide diuretics (FDA approved in adults); management of heart failure as adjunctive therapy in combination with conventional therapy (eg, diuretics, digitalis) (FDA approved in adults)

Pregnancy Risk Factor D

Pregnancy Considerations [U.S. Boxed Warning]: Drugs that act on the renin-angiotensin system can cause injury and death to the developing fetus. Discontinue as soon as possible once pregnancy is detected. Quinapril crosses the placenta; teratogenic effects may occur following maternal use during pregnancy. Drugs that act on the renin-angiotensin system are associated with oligohydramnios. Oligohydramnios, due to decreased fetal renal function, may lead to fetal lung hypoplasia and skeletal malformations. Their use in pregnancy is also associated with anuria, hypotension, renal failure, skull hypoplasia, and death in the fetus/neonate. Chronic maternal hypertension itself is also associated with adverse events in the fetus/infant. ACE inhibitors are not recommended during pregnancy to treat maternal hypertension or heart failure. Use of an ACE inhibitor should also be avoided in any woman of reproductive age. Women who are planning a pregnancy should be considered for other medication options if an ACE inhibitor is currently prescribed or the ACE inhibitor should be discontinued as soon as possible once pregnancy is detected. The exposed fetus should be monitored for fetal growth, amniotic fluid volume, and organ formation. Infants exposed to an ACE inhibitor *in utero* should be monitored for hyperkalemia, hypotension, and oliguria (exchange transfusions or dialysis may be needed). These adverse events are generally associated with maternal use in the second and third trimesters.

Untreated chronic maternal hypertension is also associated with adverse events in the fetus, infant, and mother. The use of ACE inhibitors is not recommended to treat chronic uncomplicated hypertension in pregnant women and should generally be avoided in women of reproductive potential (ACOG, 2013).

Breast-Feeding Considerations Quinapril is excreted in breast milk. The manufacturer recommends that caution be exercised when administering quinapril to nursing women. The Canadian labeling contraindicates use in nursing women.

Contraindications Hypersensitivity to quinapril, any component, or other ACE inhibitors; patients with idiopathic or hereditary angioedema or a history of angioedema with ACE inhibitors

Warnings Angioedema can occur at any time during treatment (especially following first dose). Angioedema may occur in the head, neck, extremities, or intestines; patients with angioedema of the intestines may present with abdominal pain (with or without nausea or vomiting); angioedema of the larynx, glottis, or tongue may cause airway obstruction, especially in patients with a history of airway surgery. Prolonged monitoring may be required, even in patients with swelling of only the tongue (ie, without respiratory distress) because treatment with corticosteroids and antihistamines may not be sufficient; very rare fatalities have occurred with angioedema of the larynx or tongue; appropriate treatment (eg, establishing patent airway and/or SubQ epinephrine) should be readily available for patients with angioedema of larynx, glottis, or tongue, in whom airway obstruction is likely to occur.

Anaphylactic/anaphylactoid reactions can occur with ACE inhibitors. Life-threatening anaphylactoid reactions may be seen during hemodialysis (eg, CVVHD) with high-flux dialysis membranes (eg, AN69), and rarely, during low density lipoprotein apheresis with dextran sulfate cellulose. Rare cases of anaphylactoid reactions have been reported in patients undergoing sensitization treatment with hymenoptera (bee, wasp) venom while receiving ACE inhibitors.

ACE inhibitor therapy has been associated with rare but potentially fatal cases of agranulocytosis, neutropenia, or leukopenia with myeloid hypoplasia; higher risk for development of neutropenia is associated with renal impairment; risk is further increased in patients with both renal impairment and collagen vascular disease (eg, systemic lupus erythematosus); incidence with quinapril is less than other ACE inhibitors. Onset of neutropenia is usually within 3 months of ACEI inhibitor initiation; closely monitor CBC with differential for the first 3 months of therapy and periodically thereafter in these patients; neutrophil count generally returns to baseline within 2 weeks of discontinuation.

ACE inhibitor use has been associated with deterioration of renal function and/or increases in serum creatinine, particularly in patients with low renal blood flow (eg, renal artery stenosis, heart failure) whose glomerular filtration rate (GFR) is dependent on efferent arteriolar vasoconstriction by angiotensin II; deterioration may result in oliguria, acute renal failure, and progressive azotemia. Small increases in serum creatinine may occur following initiation; consider discontinuation only in patients with progressive and/or significant deterioration in renal function.

A rare toxicity associated with ACE inhibitors includes cholestatic jaundice, which may progress to fulminant hepatic necrosis; discontinue if marked elevation of hepatic transaminases or jaundice occurs and initiate appropriate medical treatment.

Drugs that act on the renin-angiotensin system can cause injury and death to the developing fetus. Discontinue as soon as possible once pregnancy is detected **[U.S. Boxed Warning]**.

Concomitant use of an ARB or renin inhibitor (eg, aliskiren) is associated with an increased risk of hypotension, hyperkalemia, and renal dysfunction. Concomitant use with aliskiren should be avoided in patients with GFR <60 mL/minute and is contraindicated in patients with diabetes mellitus (regardless of GFR).

Precautions Use with caution in patients with renal impairment; dosage reduction may be necessary; avoid rapid dosage escalation which may lead to further renal impairment. Use with caution in patients with unstented unilateral/bilateral renal artery stenosis. When unstented bilateral renal artery stenosis is present, use is generally avoided due to the elevated risk of deterioration in renal function unless possible benefits outweigh risks.

Use with caution when initiating therapy and in volume-depleted patients; may cause symptomatic hypotension with or without syncope, usually with the first several doses; correct volume depletion prior to initiation; initiate lower doses in patients with sodium or volume depletion; close monitoring of patient is required especially with initial dosing and dosing increases; blood pressure must be lowered at a rate appropriate for the patient's clinical condition. Although dose reduction may be necessary, hypotension alone is not a reason for discontinuation of future ACE inhibitor use especially in patients with heart failure where a reduction in systolic blood pressure is a desirable observation. Use caution in patients with ischemic heart disease or cerebrovascular disease during therapy initiation; observe closely due to the potential consequences posed by falling blood pressure (eg, MI, stroke); fluid replacement may be required to restore blood pressure; therapy may then be resumed; discontinue therapy in patients whose hypotension recurs. Use with caution in patients with severe aortic stenosis; may reduce coronary perfusion resulting in ischemia. Use with caution in patients with hypertrophic cardiomyopathy (HCM) and outflow tract obstruction since reduction in afterload may worsen symptoms associated with this condition.

May cause hyperkalemia; risk factors include renal dysfunction, diabetes mellitus, concomitant use of potassium-sparing diuretics, potassium supplements, and/or potassium-containing salts; use with caution, if at all, with these agents, and monitor potassium closely. Concurrent use of angiotensin receptor blockers (ARBs) may increase the risk of clinically significant adverse events (eg, renal dysfunction, hyperkalemia).

Use with caution before, during, or immediately after major surgery; cardiopulmonary bypass, intraoperative blood loss or vasodilating anesthesia increases endogenous renin release; use of ACE inhibitors perioperatively will blunt angiotensin II formation and may result in hypotension.

An ACE inhibitor cough is a dry, hacking, nonproductive one that usually occurs within the first few months of treatment and should generally resolve within 1-4 weeks after discontinuation of the ACE inhibitor. In pediatric patients, an isolated dry hacking cough lasting >3 weeks was reported in 7 of 42 pediatric patients (17%) receiving ACE inhibitors (von Vigier, 2000); a review of pediatric randomized-controlled ACE inhibitor trials reported a lower incidence of 3.2% (Baker-Smith, 2010). Other causes of cough should be considered (eg, pulmonary congestion in patients with heart failure) and excluded prior to discontinuation.

Adverse Reactions

Cardiovascular: Chest pain, first-dose hypotension, hypotension

Central nervous system: Dizziness, fatigue, headache

Dermatologic: Rash

Endocrine & metabolic: Hyperkalemia

Gastrointestinal: Diarrhea, nausea, vomiting

Neuromuscular & skeletal: Back pain, myalgia

Renal: BUN/serum creatinine increased, worsening of renal function (in patients with bilateral renal artery stenosis or hypovolemia)

Respiratory: Cough, dyspnea, upper respiratory symptoms,

Rare but important or life-threatening: Acute renal failure, agranulocytosis, alopecia, amblyopia, anaphylactoid reaction, angina, angioedema, arrhythmia, cerebrovascular accident, depression, dermatopolymyositis, eosinophilic pneumonitis, exfoliative dermatitis, gastrointestinal hemorrhage, heart failure, hemolytic anemia, hepatitis, hyperkalemia, hypertensive crisis, impotence, insomnia, MI, orthostatic hypotension, pancreatitis, pemphigus, photosensitivity, shock, stroke, syncope, thrombocytopenia, viral infection, visual hallucinations (Doane, 2013)

A syndrome which may include arthralgia, elevated ESR, eosinophilia and positive ANA, fever, interstitial nephritis, myalgia, rash, and vasculitis has been reported with ACE inhibitors. In addition, hepatic necrosis, neutropenia, pancreatitis, and/or agranulocytosis (particularly in patients with collagen-vascular disease or renal impairment) have been associated with many ACE inhibitors.

Drug Interactions

Metabolism/Transport Effects None known.

Avoid Concomitant Use There are no known interactions where it is recommended to avoid concomitant use.

Increased Effect/Toxicity

Quinapril may increase the levels/effects of: Allopurinol; Amifostine; Antihypertensives; AzaTHIOprine; CycloSPORINE (Systemic); DULoxetine; Ferric Gluconate; Gold Sodium Thiomalate; Grass Pollen Allergen Extract (5 Grass Extract); Hypotensive Agents; Iron Dextran Complex; Lithium; Nonsteroidal Anti-Inflammatory Agents; Obinutuzumab; RiTUXimab; Sodium Phosphates

The levels/effects of Quinapril may be increased by: Alfuzosin; Aliskiren; Angiotensin II Receptor Blockers; Barbiturates; Brimonidine (Topical); Canagliflozin; Diazoxide; DPP-IV Inhibitors; Eplerenone; Everolimus; Heparin; Heparin (Low Molecular Weight); Herbs (Hypotensive Properties); Loop Diuretics; MAO Inhibitors; Pentoxifylline; Phosphodiesterase 5 Inhibitors; Potassium Salts; Potassium-Sparing Diuretics; Prostacyclin Analogues; Sirolimus; Temsirolimus; Thiazide Diuretics; TiZANidine; Tolvaptan; Trimethoprim

Decreased Effect

Quinapril may decrease the levels/effects of: Quinolone Antibiotics; Tetracycline Derivatives

The levels/effects of Quinapril may be decreased by: Antacids; Aprotinin; Herbs (Hypertensive Properties); Icatibant; Lanthanum; Methylphenidate; Nonsteroidal Anti-Inflammatory Agents; Salicylates; Yohimbine

Stability Store at 15°C to 30°C (59°F to 86°F); protect from light.

Mechanism of Action Competitive inhibitor of angiotensin-converting enzyme (ACE); prevents conversion of angiotensin I to angiotensin II, a potent vasoconstrictor; results in lower levels of angiotensin II which causes an increase in plasma renin activity and a reduction in aldosterone secretion; a CNS mechanism may also be involved in hypotensive effect as angiotensin II increases adrenergic outflow from CNS; vasoactive kallikreins may be decreased in conversion to active hormones by ACE inhibitors, thus reducing blood pressure

Pharmacodynamics

Onset of action: Antihypertensive: 1 hour

Maximum effect: Antihypertensive: 2-4 hours postdose

Duration: 24 hours (chronic dosing)

Pharmacokinetics (Adult data unless noted)

Absorption: Quinapril: ≥60%

Distribution:

Infants and Children <6 years: 0.7 L/kg (range: 0.27-1.48 L/kg) (Blumer, 2003)

Adults: 1.5 L/kg (Aronoff, 2007)

Protein binding: Quinapril: 97%; Quinaprilat: 97%

Metabolism: Rapidly hydrolyzed to quinaprilat, the active metabolite (~38% of an oral dose)

Half-life:

Infants and Children <7 years: Quinaprilat: 2.3 hours (Blumer, 2003)

Adults: Quinaprilat: 3 hours; increases as CrCl decreases

Time to peak serum concentration:

Infants and Children <7 years: 1.7 hours (range: 1-4 hours) (Blumer, 2003)

Adults: Quinaprilat: ~2 hours

Elimination: Urine (50% to 60% primarily as quinaprilat)

Dosing: Usual

Children and Adolescents: **Hypertension:** Limited data available: Oral: Initial: 5-10 mg once daily; may titrate every 2 weeks; maximum daily dose: 80 mg/day; for younger patients or those who are small for age, begin at lower end of range. A pharmacokinetic analyses of a 0.2 mg/kg single-dose in 24 pediatric patients <7 years of age, reported similar serum concentrations to those in adults who received a single 10 mg dose (Blumer, 2003; NHLBI, 2011)

Adults:

Heart failure: Oral: Initial: 5 mg once or twice daily, titrated at weekly intervals to 20-40 mg daily in 2 divided doses; target dose (heart failure): 20 mg twice daily (ACC/AHA 2009 Heart Failure Guidelines)

Hypertension: Oral: Initial: 10-20 mg once daily, adjust according to blood pressure response at peak and trough blood levels; initial dose may be reduced to 5 mg in patients receiving diuretic therapy if the diuretic is continued.

Usual dose range (JNC 7): 10-40 mg once daily

Dosing adjustment in renal impairment: Adults: Lower initial doses should be used; after initial dose (if tolerated), administer initial dose twice daily; may be increased at weekly intervals to optimal response:

Heart failure: Oral: Initial:

CrCl >30 mL/minute: Administer 5 mg/day

CrCl 10-30 mL/minute: Administer 2.5 mg/day

CrCl <10 mL/minute: No recommendations; insufficient data available

Hypertension: Oral: Initial:
CrCl >60 mL/minute: Administer 10 mg/day
CrCl 30-60 mL/minute: Administer 5 mg/day
CrCl 10-30 mL/minute: Administer 2.5 mg/day
CrCl <10 mL/minute: No recommendations; insufficient data available

Dosing adjustment in hepatic impairment: Adults: In patients with alcoholic cirrhosis, hydrolysis of quinapril to quinaprilat is impaired; however, the subsequent elimination of quinaprilat is unaltered.

Administration Oral: May be administered without regard to food

Monitoring Parameters Blood pressure, BUN, serum creatinine, renal function, urine dipstick for protein, serum potassium, WBC with differential, especially during first 3 months of therapy for patients with renal impairment and/or collagen vascular disease; monitor for angioedema and anaphylactoid reactions; hypovolemia and postural hypotension when beginning therapy, adjusting dosage, and on a regular basis throughout

Dosage Forms Excipient information presented when available (limited, particularly for generics); consult specific product labeling.
Tablet, Oral:
Accupril: 5 mg [scored; contains magnesium carbonate]
Accupril: 10 mg, 20 mg, 40 mg [contains magnesium carbonate]
Generic: 5 mg, 10 mg, 20 mg, 40 mg

Extemporaneous Preparations A 1 mg/mL quinapril oral suspension may be made with tablets, K-Phos® Neutral (equivalent to 250 mg elemental phosphorus, 13 mEq sodium, and 1.1 mEq potassium per tablet), Bicitra®, and Ora-Sweet SF™. Place ten quinapril 20 mg tablets in an amber plastic prescription bottle (eg, 240 mL). In a separate container, prepare a buffer solution by crushing one K-Phos® Neutral tablet and dissolving it in 100 mL sterile water for irrigation. Add 30 mL of the prepared K-Phos® buffer solution to the quinapril tablets. Shake for at least 2 minutes, then remove cap and allow the concentrate to stand for 15 minutes, then shake the concentrate again for an additional minute. Add 30 mL of Bicitra® and shake for 2 minutes. Add quantity sufficient of Ora-Sweet SF® (~140 mL) to make 200 mL and shake the suspension. Store in amber plastic prescription bottles; label "shake well" and "refrigerate." Stable for 28 days refrigerated (Freed, 2005).

Freed AN, Silbering SB, Kolodsick KJ, et al, "The Development and Stability Assessment of Extemporaneous Pediatric Formulations of Accupril," *Int J Pharm*, 2005, 304(1-2):135-44.

References

Aronoff GR, Bennett WM, Berns JS, et al, *Drug Prescribing in Renal Failure: Dosing Guidelines for Adults and Children*, 5th ed, Philadelphia, PA: American College of Physicians; 2007.

Baker-Smith CM, Benjamin DK Jr, Califf RM, et al, "Cough in Pediatric Patients Receiving Angiotensin-Converting Enzyme Inhibitor Therapy or Angiotensin Receptor Blocker Therapy in Randomized Controlled Trials," *Clin Pharmacol Ther*, 2010, 87(6):668-71.

Blumer JL, Daniels SR, Dreyer WJ, et al, "Pharmacokinetics of Quinapril in Children: Assessment During Substitution for Chronic Angiotensin-Converting Enzyme Inhibitor Treatment," *J Clin Pharmacol*, 2003, 43(2):128-32.

Brown NJ, Ray WA, Snowden M, et al, "Black Americans Have an Increased Rate of Angiotensin Converting Enzyme Inhibitor-Associated Angioedema," *Clin Pharmacol Ther*, 1996, 60(1):8-13.

Chobanian AV, Bakris GL, Black HR, et al, "The Seventh Report of the Joint National Committee on Prevention, Detection, Evaluation, and Treatment of High Blood Pressure: The JNC 7 Report," *JAMA*, 2003, 289(19):2560-71.

Flynn JT, "Management of Hypertension in the Young: Role of Antihypertensive Medications," *J Cardiovasc Pharmacol*, 2011, 58 (2):111-20.

National High Blood Pressure Education Program Working Group on High Blood Pressure in Children and Adolescents, "The Fourth Report on the Diagnosis, Evaluation, and Treatment of High Blood Pressure in Children and Adolescents," *Pediatrics*, 2004, 114(2 Suppl):555-76.

von Vigier RO, Mozzettini S, Truttmann AC, et al, "Cough Is Common in Children Prescribed Converting Enzyme Inhibitors," *Nephron*, 2000, 84(1):98.

◆ **Quinapril Hydrochloride** *see* Quinapril *on page 1788*

◆ **Quinate® (Can)** *see* QuiNIDine *on page 1791*

QuiNIDine (KWIN i deen)

Medication Safety Issues
Sound-alike/look-alike issues:
QuiNIDine may be confused with cloNIDine, quiNINE
High alert medication:
The Institute for Safe Medication Practices (ISMP) includes this medication (I.V. formulation) among its list of drug classes which have a heightened risk of causing significant patient harm when used in error.
BEERS Criteria medication:
This drug may be potentially inappropriate for use in geriatric patients (Quality of evidence - high; Strength of recommendation - strong).

Related Information
Medications for Which a Single Dose May Be Fatal When Ingested by a Toddler *on page 2408*
Oral Medications That Should Not Be Crushed or Altered *on page 2438*

Brand Names: Canada Apo-Quinidine®; BioQuin® Durules™; Novo-Quinidin; Quinate®

Therapeutic Category Antiarrhythmic Agent, Class I-A; Antimalarial Agent

Generic Availability (U.S.) Yes

Use
Quinidine **sulfate**: Treatment of life-threatening *Plasmodium falciparum* malaria [Oral: Immediate release: FDA approved in pediatric patients (age not specified) and adults]; conversion of atrial fibrillation and/or flutter; prophylaxis after cardioversion of atrial fibrillation and/or flutter to maintain normal sinus rhythm; suppression of serious recurrent ventricular arrhythmias (eg, life-threatening ventricular tachycardia) (Oral: Immediate/extended release: FDA approved in adults); has also been used to prevent reoccurrence of paroxysmal supraventricular tachycardia, paroxysmal A-V junctional rhythm, paroxysmal ventricular tachycardia, paroxysmal atrial fibrillation, and atrial or ventricular premature contractions

Quinidine **gluconate**: Treatment of life-threatening *Plasmodium falciparum* malaria [Parenteral: FDA approved in pediatric patients (age not specified) and adults]; conversion of atrial fibrillation and/or flutter; prophylaxis after cardioversion of atrial fibrillation and/or flutter to maintain normal sinus rhythm; suppression of serious recurrent ventricular arrhythmias (eg, life-threatening ventricular tachycardia) (Parenteral, Oral: Extended release: FDA approved in adults); has also been used to prevent reoccurrence of paroxysmal supraventricular tachycardia, paroxysmal A-V junctional rhythm, paroxysmal ventricular tachycardia, paroxysmal atrial fibrillation, and atrial or ventricular premature contractions; **Note:** The use of I.V. quinidine gluconate for these indications has been replaced by more effective/safer antiarrhythmic agents (eg, amiodarone and procainamide).

Pregnancy Risk Factor C

Pregnancy Considerations Animal reproduction studies have not been conducted. Quinidine crosses the placenta and can be detected in the amniotic fluid, cord blood, and neonatal serum. Quinidine is indicated for use in the treatment of severe malaria infection in pregnant women (CDC, 2011; Smereck, 2011) and has also been used to treat arrhythmias in pregnancy when other agents are ineffective (European Society of Cardiology, 2003).

Breast-Feeding Considerations Quinidine can be detected in breast milk at concentrations slightly lower than those in the maternal serum. The manufacturer recommends avoiding use in nursing women.

Contraindications Hypersensitivity to quinidine, any component, or cinchona derivatives; patients who have a ▶

history of thrombocytic purpura during prior therapy with quinidine or quinine; patients with complete A-V block with an A-V junctional or idioventricular pacemaker; patients with intraventricular conduction defects (marked widening of QRS complex); patients who might be adversely affected by anticholinergic agents (eg, myasthenia gravis)

Contraindications from other product labeling: Concurrent use of cisapride, fosamprenavir, ritonavir, or quinolone antibiotics which prolong QT interval

Warnings Antiarrhythmic drugs have not been shown to enhance survival in nonlife-threatening ventricular arrhythmias and may increase mortality; the risk is greatest with structural heart disease. Quinidine may increase mortality in treatment of atrial fibrillation/flutter **[U.S. Boxed Warning]**. Quinidine prolongs the QT$_c$ interval, which may lead to torsade de pointes; risk increased by bradycardia, hypokalemia, hypomagnesemia, or high serum levels of quinidine; avoid use in patients with diagnosed or suspected congenital long QT syndrome; correct electrolyte abnormalities prior to and throughout therapy. May increase ventricular response rate in patients with atrial fibrillation or flutter; control AV conduction before initiating. Use with caution in patients at risk for heart block; can unmask sick sinus syndrome (causes bradycardia). Use with caution in patients with myocardial depression. Quinidine decreases digoxin elimination and may cause digoxin-induced toxicity; a reduction in digoxin dose is required. May cause syncope, most likely due to ventricular tachycardia or fibrillation; syncope may subside spontaneously, but occasionally may be fatal; discontinue quinidine if syncope occurs. Hypersensitivity reactions may occur.

Quinidine is available in gluconate and sulfate salt formulations which are not interchangeable on a mg per mg basis, due to differences in the amount of quinidine base supplied.

Precautions Use with caution in patients with hepatic impairment; reduced dosage recommended; quinidine-induced hepatotoxicity, including granulomatous hepatitis, increased serum AST and alkaline phosphatase concentrations, and jaundice may occur. Use with caution in renal impairment; adjust dose with severe impairment. Use with caution in patients with HF; may precipitate or exacerbate condition. Use with caution in patients with G-6-PD deficiency; hemolysis may occur.

Adverse Reactions

Cardiovascular: Angina, new or worsened arrhythmia (proarrhythmic effect), hypotension, palpitation, QT$_c$ prolongation (modest prolongation is common, however, excessive prolongation is rare and indicates toxicity), syncope

Central nervous system: Fatigue, headache, incoordination, lightheadedness, nervousness, sleep disturbance, syncope, tremor

Dermatologic: Rash

Gastrointestinal: Anorexia, bitter taste, diarrhea, nausea, stomach cramping, upper GI distress, vomiting

Neuromuscular & skeletal: Weakness

Ocular: Blurred vision

Otic: Tinnitus

Respiratory: Wheezing

Rare but important or life-threatening: Abnormal pigmentation, acute psychotic reactions, agranulocytosis, angioedema, arthralgia, bronchospasm, cerebral hypoperfusion (possibly resulting in ataxia, apprehension, and seizure), cholestasis, confusion, CPK increased, delirium, depression, drug-induced lupus-like syndrome, eczematous dermatitis, esophagitis, exacerbated bradycardia (in sick sinus syndrome), exfoliative rash, fever, flushing, granulomatous hepatitis, hallucinations, hearing impaired, heart block, hemolytic anemia, hepatotoxic reaction (rare), lichen planus, livedo reticularis, lymphadenopathy,

melanin pigmentation of the hard palate, myalgia, mydriasis, nephropathy, optic neuritis, pancytopenia, paradoxical increase in ventricular rate during atrial fibrillation/flutter, photosensitivity, pneumonitis, pruritus, psoriaform rash, QT$_c$ prolongation (excessive), respiratory depression, sicca syndrome, tachycardia, thrombocytopenia, thrombocytopenic purpura, torsade de pointes, urticaria, uveitis, vascular collapse, vasculitis, ventricular fibrillation, ventricular tachycardia, vertigo, visual field loss

Note: Cinchonism, a syndrome which may include tinnitus, high-frequency hearing loss, deafness, vertigo, blurred vision, diplopia, photophobia, headache, confusion, and delirium has been associated with quinidine use. Usually associated with chronic toxicity, this syndrome has also been described after brief exposure to a moderate dose in sensitive patients. Vomiting and diarrhea may also occur as isolated reactions to therapeutic quinidine levels.

Drug Interactions

Metabolism/Transport Effects Substrate of CYP2C9 (minor), CYP2E1 (minor), CYP3A4 (major), P-glycoprotein; **Note:** Assignment of Major/Minor substrate status based on clinically relevant drug interaction potential; **Inhibits** CYP2C9 (weak), CYP2D6 (strong), CYP3A4 (weak), P-glycoprotein

Avoid Concomitant Use

Avoid concomitant use of QuiNIDine with any of the following: Amiodarone; Antifungal Agents (Azole Derivatives, Systemic); Bosutinib; Conivaptan; Crizotinib; Enzalutamide; Fingolimod; Fusidic Acid (Systemic); Haloperidol; Highest Risk QTc-Prolonging Agents; Ivabradine; Macrolide Antibiotics; Mefloquine; Mifepristone; Moderate Risk QTc-Prolonging Agents; PAZOPanib; Pimozide; Propafenone; Protease Inhibitors; Silodosin; Tamoxifen; Thioridazine; Topotecan; VinCRIStine (Liposomal)

Increased Effect/Toxicity

QuiNIDine may increase the levels/effects of: Afatinib; ARIPiprazole; AtoMOXetine; Bosutinib; Brentuximab Vedotin; Calcium Channel Blockers (Dihydropyridine); Cardiac Glycosides; Colchicine; CYP2D6 Substrates; Dabigatran Etexilate; Dalfampridine; Dextromethorphan; DOXOrubicin (Conventional); Everolimus; Fesoterodine; Haloperidol; Highest Risk QTc-Prolonging Agents; Lomitapide; Mefloquine; Metoprolol; Nebivolol; Neuromuscular-Blocking Agents; PAZOPanib; P-glycoprotein/ABCB1 Substrates; Pimozide; Propafenone; Propranolol; Prucalopride; Rifaximin; Rivaroxaban; Silodosin; Thioridazine; Topotecan; Tricyclic Antidepressants; Verapamil; VinCRIStine (Liposomal); Vitamin K Antagonists; Vortioxetine

The levels/effects of QuiNIDine may be increased by: Amiodarone; Antacids; Antifungal Agents (Azole Derivatives, Systemic); Boceprevir; Calcium Channel Blockers (Dihydropyridine); Carbonic Anhydrase Inhibitors; Cimetidine; Conivaptan; Crizotinib; CYP3A4 Inhibitors (Moderate); CYP3A4 Inhibitors (Strong); Diltiazem; Fingolimod; Fosphenytoin; Fusidic Acid (Systemic); Haloperidol; Ivabradine; Ivacaftor; Luliconazole; Lurasidone; Macrolide Antibiotics; Mifepristone; Moderate Risk QTc-Prolonging Agents; P-glycoprotein/ABCB1 Inhibitors; PHENobarbital; Protease Inhibitors; QTc-Prolonging Agents (Indeterminate Risk and Risk Modifying); Reserpine; Selective Serotonin Reuptake Inhibitors; Simeprevir; Stiripentol; Telaprevir; Tricyclic Antidepressants; Verapamil

Decreased Effect

QuiNIDine may decrease the levels/effects of: Codeine; Dihydrocodeine; Hydrocodone; Tamoxifen; TraMADol

The levels/effects of QuiNIDine may be decreased by: Bosentan; Calcium Channel Blockers (Dihydropyridine); CYP3A4 Inducers (Strong); Dabrafenib; Deferasirox; Enzalutamide; Etravirine; Fosphenytoin; Kaolin; Mitotane; P-glycoprotein/ABCB1 Inducers; PHENobarbital; Phenytoin; Potassium-Sparing Diuretics; Primidone; Rifamycin Derivatives; Siltuximab; St Johns Wort; Sucralfate; Tocilizumab

Food Interactions Changes in dietary salt intake may alter the rate and extent of quinidine absorption. Quinidine serum levels may be increased if taken with food. Food has a variable effect on absorption of sustained release formulation. The rate of absorption of quinidine may be decreased following the ingestion of grapefruit juice. Excessive intake of fruit juice or vitamin C may decrease urine pH and result in increased clearance of quinidine with decreased serum concentration. Alkaline foods may result in increased quinidine serum concentrations. Management: Avoid changes in dietary salt intake. Grapefruit juice should be avoided. Take around-the-clock to avoid variation in serum levels and with food or milk to avoid GI irritation.

Stability
Oral: Store at 20°C to 25°C (68°F to 77°F); protect from light.
Parenteral: Store at 25°C (77°F); excursions permitted to 15°C to 30°C (59°F to 86°F). Do not use discolored parenteral solution.

Mechanism of Action Class Ia antiarrhythmic agent; depresses phase O of the action potential; decreases myocardial excitability and conduction velocity, and myocardial contractility by decreasing sodium influx during depolarization and potassium efflux in repolarization; also reduces calcium transport across cell membrane

Pharmacokinetics (Adult data unless noted)
Distribution: V_d: Adults: 2-3.5 L/kg, decreased V_d with CHF, malaria; increased V_d with cirrhosis
Protein-binding: Binds mainly to alpha$_1$-acid glycoprotein and to a lesser extent albumin; protein-binding changes may occur in periods of stress due to increased alpha$_1$-acid glycoprotein concentrations (eg, acute myocardial infarction) or in certain disease states due to decreased alpha$_1$-acid glycoprotein concentrations (eg, cirrhosis, hyperthyroidism, malnutrition)
Newborns: 60% to 70%
Adults: 80% to 90%
Metabolism: Extensively hepatic (50% to 90%) to inactive compounds
Bioavailability: Sulfate: ~70% with wide variability between patients (45% to 100%); Gluconate: 70% to 80%
Time to peak serum concentration: Oral: Sulfate: Immediate release: 2 hours; Extended release: 6 hours; Gluconate: Extended release: 3-5 hours
Half-life, plasma (increased half-life with cirrhosis and CHF):
Children: 2.5-6.7 hours
Adults: 6-8 hours
Elimination: Urine (15% to 25% as unchanged drug)
Dialysis: Slightly dialyzable (5% to 20%) by hemodialysis; not removed by peritoneal dialysis

Dosing: Usual Note: Dose expressed in terms of the salt formulation.
Infants, Children, and Adolescents:
Malaria, treatment (severe, life-threatening): I.V.: **Quinidine gluconate:** 10 mg/kg infused over 60-120 minutes, followed by 0.02 mg/kg/minute continuous infusion for ≥24 hours; alternatively, may administer 24 mg/kg loading dose over 4 hours, followed by 12 mg/kg over 4 hours every 8 hours (beginning 8 hours after loading dose). Change to oral quinine once parasite density is <1% and patient can receive oral medication to complete treatment course; total duration of treatment (quinidine/quinine): 3 days in Africa or

South America; 7 days in Southeast Asia; use in combination with doxycycline, tetracycline, or clindamycin; omit quinidine loading dose if patient received >40 mg/kg of quinine in preceding 48 hours or mefloquine within preceding 12 hours (CDC, 2009). **Note:** Close monitoring, including telemetry, is **required**; if severe cardiac adverse effects occur, infusion rate may need to be decreased or drug temporarily discontinued.

Arrhythmias: Children and Adolescents: Limited data available:
Oral: Quinidine **sulfate**; immediate release: Usual: 30 mg/kg/day or 900 mg/m^2/day in 5 daily doses or 6 mg/kg every 4-6 hours; range: 15-60 mg/kg/day in 4-5 divided doses; usual maximum dose: 600 mg; maximum daily dose: 3000-4000 mg/**day**
I.V.: Quinidine **gluconate**: 2-10 mg/kg/dose every 3-6 hours as needed (I.V. route **not** recommended)

Adults:
Malaria: I.V.: Quinidine **gluconate**: 10 mg/kg infused over 60-120 minutes, followed by 0.02 mg/kg/minute continuous infusion for ≥24 hours; alternatively, may administer 24 mg/kg loading dose over 4 hours, followed by 12 mg/kg over 4 hours every 8 hours (beginning 8 hours after loading dose). Change to oral quinine once parasite density is <1% and patient can receive oral medication to complete treatment course; total duration of treatment (quinidine/quinine): 3 days in Africa or South America; 7 days in Southeast Asia; use in combination with doxycycline, tetracycline, or clindamycin; omit quinidine loading dose if patient received >40 mg/kg of quinine in preceding 48 hours or mefloquine within preceding 12 hours (CDC, 2009). **Note:** Close monitoring, including telemetry, is required; if severe cardiac adverse effects occur, infusion rate may need to be decreased or drug temporarily discontinued.

Arrythmias: Oral:
Immediate release formulations: Quinidine **sulfate**: Initial: 200-400 mg/dose every 6 hours; the dose may be increased cautiously to desired effect; maximum daily dose range: 3000-4000 mg/**day**
Extended release formulations:
Quinidine **sulfate**: Initial: 300 mg every 8-12 hours; the dose may be increased cautiously to desired effect
Quinidine **gluconate**: Initial: 324 mg every 8-12 hours; the dose may be increased cautiously to desired effect

Dosing adjustment in renal impairment: The FDA-approved labeling recommends that caution should be used in patients with renal impairment; however, no specific dosage adjustment guidelines are available. The following guidelines have been used by some clinicians (Aronoff, 2007): Oral: Adults:
CrCl ≥10 mL/minute: No adjustment required.
CrCl <10 mL/minute: Administer 75% of normal dose.
Hemodialysis: Administer dose following hemodialysis session.
Peritoneal dialysis: Supplemental dose is not necessary.
CRRT: No dosage adjustment required; monitor serum concentrations.

Dosing adjustment in hepatic impairment: Use caution; hepatic impairment decreases clearance; dosage adjustments are not provided in the manufacturers' labeling although toxicity may occur if the dose is not appropriately adjusted; larger loading dose may be indicated

Administration
Oral: Administer with water on an empty stomach, but may administer with food or milk to decrease GI upset; best to administer in a consistent manner with regards to meals and around-the-clock to promote less variation in peak and trough serum concentrations; swallow extended

release tablets whole, do not chew or crush; some preparations of quinidine **gluconate** extended release tablets may be split in half to facilitate dosage titration; tablets are not scored.

Parenteral: I.V.: Maximum rate of infusion: 10 mg/minute; maximum concentration: 16 mg/mL; I.V. tubing length should be minimized (quinidine may be significantly adsorbed to polyvinyl chloride tubing)

Monitoring Parameters CBC with differential, platelet count, liver and renal function tests. Serum concentrations should be routinely performed during long-term administration. Continuously monitor blood pressure and ECG (for widening QRS complex and lengthening of QT_c interval) and periodically monitor blood glucose for hypoglycemia with I.V. use.

Reference Range Optimal therapeutic level is method dependent

Therapeutic: 2-5 mcg/mL (SI: 6.2-15.4 micromole/L).

Patient-dependent therapeutic response occurs at levels of 3-6 mcg/mL (SI: 9.2-18.5 micromole/L).

Additional Information Quinidine **gluconate**: 267 mg = quinidine **sulfate**: 200 mg

Formation of a concretion of tablets or bezoar in the stomach has been reported following tablet ingestion by a 16-month old infant; diagnostic or therapeutic endoscopy may be required in patients with massive overdose and prolonged elevated serum quinidine concentrations

Dosage Forms Excipient information presented when available (limited, particularly for generics); consult specific product labeling.

Solution, Injection, as gluconate:
Generic: 80 mg/mL (10 mL)
Tablet, Oral, as sulfate:
Generic: 200 mg, 300 mg
Tablet Extended Release, Oral, as gluconate:
Generic: 324 mg
Tablet Extended Release, Oral, as sulfate:
Generic: 300 mg

Extemporaneous Preparations A 10 mg/mL oral liquid preparation may be made with tablets and one of three different vehicles (cherry syrup, a 1:1 mixture of Ora-Sweet® and Ora-Plus®, or a 1:1 mixture of Ora-Sweet® SF and Ora-Plus®). Crush six 200 mg tablets in a mortar and reduce to a fine powder. Add 15 mL of the chosen vehicle and mix to a uniform paste; mix while adding vehicle in incremental proportions to **almost** 120 mL; transfer to a calibrated bottle, rinse mortar with vehicle, and add quantity of vehicle sufficient to make 120 mL. Label "shake well" and "protect from light". Stable for 60 days when stored in amber plastic prescription bottles in the dark at room temperature or refrigerated.

Allen LV and Erickson MA, "Stability of Bethanechol Chloride, Pyrazinamide, Quinidine Sulfate, Rifampin, and Tetracycline in Extemporaneously Compounded Oral Liquids," *Am J Health Syst Pharm*, 1998, 55(17):1804-9.

References

Centers for Disease Control and Prevention, "Guidelines for Treatment of Malaria in the United States, 2009." Available at http://www.cdc.gov/malaria/resources/pdf/treatmenttable.pdf

European Society for Cardiology, Task Force on the Management of Cardiovascular Diseases During Pregnancy of the European Society of Cardiology, "Expert Consensus Document on Management of Cardiovascular Diseases During Pregnancy," *Eur Heart J*, 2003, 24 (8):761-81.

Pickoff AS, Singh S, and Gelband H, *The Medical Management of Cardiac Arrhythmias in Cardiac Arrhythmias in the Neonate, Infant and Child*, Roberts NK and Gelband H, ed, Norwalk, CT: Appleton-Century-Crofts, 1983.

Smereck J, "Malaria in Pregnancy: Update on Emergency Management," *J Emerg Med*, 2011, 40(4):393-6.

Szefler SJ, Pieroni DR, Gingell RL, et al, "Rapid Elimination of Quinidine in Pediatric Patients," *Pediatrics*, 1982, 70(3):370-5.

◆ **Quinidine Gluconate** see QuiNIDine on page 1791

◆ **Quinidine Polygalacturonate** see QuiNIDine on page 1791

◆ **Quinidine Sulfate** see QuiNIDine on page 1791

QuiNINE (KWYE nine)

Medication Safety Issues
Sound-alike/look-alike issues:
QuiNINE may be confused with quiNIDine

Related Information
Medications for Which a Single Dose May Be Fatal When Ingested by a Toddler on page 2408

Brand Names: U.S. Qualaquin

Brand Names: Canada Apo-Quinine®; Novo-Quinine; Quinine-Odan

Therapeutic Category Antimalarial Agent; Skeletal Muscle Relaxant, Miscellaneous

Generic Availability (U.S.) Yes

Use Treatment of chloroquine-resistant, uncomplicated *P. falciparum* malaria infection (inactive against sporozoites, pre-erythrocytic or exoerythrocytic forms of plasmodia) in conjunction with other antimalarial agents [FDA approved in pediatrics (age not specified) and adults]; has also been used for the treatment of uncomplicated chloroquine-resistant *P. vivax* malaria (in conjunction with other antimalarial agents); treatment of *Babesia microti* infection in conjunction with clindamycin

Medication Guide Available Yes

Pregnancy Risk Factor C

Pregnancy Considerations Teratogenic effects have been reported in some animal studies. Quinine crosses the human placenta. Cord plasma to maternal plasma quinine ratios have been reported as 0.18-0.46 and should not be considered therapeutic to the infant. Teratogenic effects, optic nerve hypoplasia, and deafness have been reported in the infant following maternal use of very high doses; however, therapeutic doses used for malaria are generally considered safe. Quinine may also cause significant hypoglycemia when used during pregnancy. Malaria infection in pregnant women may be more severe than in nonpregnant women. Because *P. falciparum* malaria can cause maternal death and fetal loss, pregnant women traveling to malaria-endemic areas must use personal protection against mosquito bites. Quinine may be used for the treatment of malaria in pregnant women; consult current CDC guidelines. Pregnant women should be advised not to travel to areas of *P. falciparum* resistance to chloroquine.

Breast-Feeding Considerations Based on limited data, it is estimated that nursing infants would receive <0.4% of the maternal dose from breast-feeding.

Contraindications Hypersensitivity to quinine or any component or to mefloquine or quinidine (cross sensitivity reported); history of potential hypersensitivity reactions [including black water fever, thrombotic thrombocytopenia purpura (TTP), hemolytic uremic syndrome (HUS), or thrombocytopenia] associated with prior quinine use; prolonged QT interval; myasthenia gravis; optic neuritis, G6PD deficiency

Warnings Quinine is not recommended for the prevention/treatment of nocturnal leg cramps due to the potential for severe and/or life-threatening side effects (eg, cardiac arrhythmias, thrombocytopenia, HUS/TTP, severe hypersensitivity reactions) **[U.S. Boxed Warning]**. These risks, as well as the absence of clinical effectiveness, do not justify its use in the unapproved/unlabeled prevention and/or treatment of leg cramps. Use may cause significant hypoglycemia due to quinine-induced insulin release.

Severe hypersensitivity reactions (eg, Stevens-Johnson syndrome, anaphylactic shock) have occurred; discontinue following any signs of sensitivity. Other events, including acute interstitial nephritis, neutropenia, and granulomatous hepatitis, may also be attributed to hypersensitivity reactions. Immune-mediated thrombocytopenia, including life-threatening cases and hemolytic uremic syndrome/thrombotic thrombocytopenic purpura (HUS/TTP), has occurred with use. Chronic renal failure associated with TTP has also been reported. Thrombocytopenia generally resolves within a week upon discontinuation. Re-exposure may result in increased severity of thrombocytopenia and faster onset.

Precautions Use with caution in patients with clinical conditions or on medications which may prolong the QT interval or cause cardiac arrhythmias (quinine has quinidine-like activity), in patients with myasthenia gravis, and in patients with impaired liver function.

Adverse Reactions

Cardiovascular: Atrial fibrillation, atrioventricular block, bradycardia, cardiac arrest, chest pain, hypotension, irregular rhythm, nodal escape beats, orthostatic hypotension, palpitation, QT prolongation, syncope, tachycardia, torsade de pointes, unifocal premature ventricular contractions, U waves, vasodilation, ventricular fibrillation, ventricular tachycardia

Central nervous system: Aphasia, ataxia, chills, coma, confusion, disorientation, dizziness, dystonic reaction, fever, flushing, headache, mental status altered, restlessness, seizure, suicide, vertigo

Dermatologic: Acral necrosis, allergic contact dermatitis, bullous dermatitis, bruising, cutaneous rash (urticaria, papular, scarlatinal), cutaneous vasculitis, exfoliative dermatitis, erythema multiforme, petechiae, photosensitivity, pruritus, Stevens-Johnson syndrome, toxic epidermal necrolysis

Endocrine & metabolic: Hypoglycemia

Gastrointestinal: Abdominal pain, anorexia, diarrhea, esophagitis, gastric irritation, nausea, vomiting

Hematologic: Agranulocytosis, aplastic anemia, coagulopathy, disseminated intravascular coagulation, hemolytic anemia, hemolytic uremic syndrome, hemorrhage, hypoprothrombinemia, immune thrombocytopenia (ITP), leukopenia, neutropenia, pancytopenia, thrombocytopenia, thrombotic thrombocytopenic purpura

Hepatic: Granulomatous hepatitis, hepatitis, jaundice, liver function test abnormalities

Neuromuscular & skeletal: Myalgia, tremor, weakness

Ocular: Blindness, blurred vision (with or without scotomata), color vision disturbance, diminished visual fields, diplopia, night blindness, optic neuritis, photophobia, pupillary dilation, vision loss (sudden)

Otic: Deafness, hearing impaired, tinnitus

Renal: Acute interstitial nephritis, hemoglobinuria, renal failure, renal impairment

Respiratory: Asthma, dyspnea, pulmonary edema

Miscellaneous: Black water fever, diaphoresis, hypersensitivity reaction, lupus anticoagulant, lupus-like syndrome

Drug Interactions

Metabolism/Transport Effects Substrate of CYP1A2 (minor), CYP2C19 (minor), CYP3A4 (major), P-glycoprotein; **Note:** Assignment of Major/Minor substrate status based on clinically relevant drug interaction potential; **Inhibits** CYP2C8 (moderate), CYP2C9 (moderate), CYP2D6 (moderate), CYP3A4 (weak), P-glycoprotein

Avoid Concomitant Use

Avoid concomitant use of QuiNINE with any of the following: Antacids; Artemether; Bosutinib; Conivaptan; Fusidic Acid (Systemic); Halofantrine; Highest Risk QTc-Prolonging Agents; Ivabradine; Lopinavir; Lumefantrine; Macrolide Antibiotics; Mefloquine; Mifepristone; Moderate Risk QTc-Prolonging Agents; Neuromuscular-Blocking Agents; PAZOPanib; Pimozide; Rifampin; Ritonavir; Silodosin; Thioridazine; Topotecan; VinCRIStine (Liposomal)

Increased Effect/Toxicity

QuiNINE may increase the levels/effects of: Afatinib; Antihypertensives; Antipsychotic Agents (Phenothiazines); Bosentan; Bosutinib; Brentuximab Vedotin; Cannabis; CarBAMazepine; Cardiac Glycosides; Carvedilol; Colchicine; CYP2C8 Substrates; CYP2C9 Substrates; CYP2D6 Substrates; Dabigatran Etexilate; Dapsone (Systemic); Dapsone (Topical); DOXOrubicin (Conventional); Dronabinol; Everolimus; Fesoterodine; Halofantrine; Herbs (Hypotensive Properties); Highest Risk QTc-Prolonging Agents; HMG-CoA Reductase Inhibitors; Hypoglycemic Agents; Lomitapide; Lumefantrine; Mefloquine; Metoprolol; Nebivolol; Neuromuscular-Blocking Agents; PAZOPanib; P-glycoprotein/ABCB1 Substrates; PHENobarbital; Pimozide; Prilocaine; Prucalopride; Rifaximin; Ritonavir; Rivaroxaban; Silodosin; Sodium Nitrite; Tetrahydrocannabinol; Theophylline Derivatives; Thioridazine; Topotecan; VinCRIStine (Liposomal); Vitamin K Antagonists

The levels/effects of QuiNINE may be increased by: Alkalinizing Agents; Artemether; Cimetidine; Conivaptan; CYP3A4 Inhibitors (Moderate); CYP3A4 Inhibitors (Strong); Dapsone (Systemic); Fusidic Acid (Systemic); Herbs (Hypoglycemic Properties); Ivabradine; Ivacaftor; Luliconazole; Macrolide Antibiotics; MAO Inhibitors; Mefloquine; Mifepristone; Moderate Risk QTc-Prolonging Agents; Nitric Oxide; P-glycoprotein/ABCB1 Inhibitors; QTc-Prolonging Agents (Indeterminate Risk and Risk Modifying); Ritonavir; Salicylates; Selective Serotonin Reuptake Inhibitors; Simeprevir; Stiripentol; Tetracycline

Decreased Effect

QuiNINE may decrease the levels/effects of: Codeine; Tamoxifen; TraMADol

The levels/effects of QuiNINE may be decreased by: Antacids; Bosentan; CarBAMazepine; CYP3A4 Inducers (Strong); Dabrafenib; Deferasirox; Fosphenytoin; Loop Diuretics; Lopinavir; Mitotane; P-glycoprotein/ABCB1 Inducers; PHENobarbital; Phenytoin; Rifampin; Ritonavir; Siltuximab; St Johns Wort; Tocilizumab

Stability Store at 20°C to 25°C (68°F to 77°F). Protect from light. Do not refrigerate or freeze.

Mechanism of Action Depresses oxygen uptake and carbohydrate metabolism; intercalates into DNA, disrupting the parasite's replication and transcription; cardiovascular effects similar to quinidine

Pharmacokinetics (Adult data unless noted)

Absorption: Oral: Readily absorbed, mainly from the upper small intestine

Distribution: Widely distributed to body tissues and fluids including small amounts into bile and CSF (2% to 7% of plasma concentration); crosses the placenta; excreted into breast milk

V_d (children): 0.8 L/kg

V_d (adults): 1.9 L/kg

Protein binding: 70% to 90%

Metabolism: Primarily in the liver via hydroxylation pathways

Half-life:

Children: 6-12 hours

Adults: 8-14 hours

Time to peak serum concentration: Within 2-4 hours

Elimination: In bile and saliva with ~20% excreted unchanged in urine; renal excretion is twofold in the presence of acidic urine

Dialysis: Not effectively removed by peritoneal dialysis; removed by hemodialysis

Dosing: Usual Oral: **Note:** Actual duration of quinine treatment for malaria may be dependent upon the geographic region or pathogen. Dosage expressed in terms of the **salt**; 1 capsule Qualaquin® = 324 mg of quinine sulfate = 269 mg of base.

Children:

Treatment of uncomplicated chloroquine-resistant *P. falciparum* malaria: CDC guidelines: 30 mg/kg/day in divided doses every 8 hours for 3-7 days depending on region (maximum dose: 1944 mg/day).Tetracycline, doxycycline, or clindamycin (consider risk versus benefit of using tetracycline or doxycycline in children <8 years of age) should also be given.

Treatment of uncomplicated chloroquine-resistant *P. vivax* malaria: CDC guidelines: 30 mg/kg/day in divided doses every 8 hours for 3-7 days depending on region (maximum dose: 1944 mg/day). Tetracycline or doxycycline (consider risk versus benefit of using tetracycline or doxycycline in children <8 years of age) **plus** primaquine should also be given.

Babesiosis: 30 mg/kg/day, divided every 8 hours for 7-10 days with clindamycin; maximum dose: 648 mg/dose

Adults:

Treatment of uncomplicated chloroquine-resistant *P. falciparum* malaria: CDC guidelines: 648 mg every 8 hours for 3-7 days. Tetracycline, doxycycline, or clindamycin should also be given.

Treatment of uncomplicated chloroquine-resistant *P. vivax* malaria: CDC guidelines: 648 mg every 8 hours for 3-7 days. Tetracycline or doxycycline **plus** primaquine should also be given.

Babesiosis: 648 mg every 8 hours for 7-10 days with clindamycin

Dosing adjustment in renal impairment: Adult:

CrCl 10-50 mL/minute: Administer every 8-12 hours

CrCl <10 mL/minute: Administer every 24 hours

Severe chronic renal failure not on dialysis: Initial dose: 648 mg followed by 324 mg every 12 hours

Administration Oral: Do not crush capsule to avoid bitter taste

Monitoring Parameters CBC with platelet count, liver function tests, blood glucose, ophthalmologic examination

Test Interactions May interfere with urine detection of opioids (false-positive); positive Coombs' [direct]; false elevation of urinary steroids (when assayed by Zimmerman method) and catecholamines; qualitative and quantitative urine dipstick protein assays

Additional Information Parenteral form of quinine (dihydrochloride) is no longer available from the CDC; quinidine gluconate should be used instead; the FDA has banned over-the-counter (OTC) drug products containing quinine sold for treatment and/or prevention of malaria, as well as, products labeled for treatment or prevention of nocturnal leg cramps

Dosage Forms Excipient information presented when available (limited, particularly for generics); consult specific product labeling.

Capsule, Oral, as sulfate:

Qualaquin: 324 mg

Generic: 324 mg

References

Aronoff GR, Berns JS, Brier ME, et al, *Drug Prescribing in Renal Failure: Dosing Guidelines for Adults*, 4th ed. Philadelphia, PA: American College of Physicians; 1999, p 73.

Centers for Disease Control and Prevention (CDC), "Guidelines for Treatment of Malaria in the United States," Treatment Table Update, May 18, 2009. Available at: http://www.cdc.gov/malaria/resources/pdf/treatmenttable.pdf

Centers for Disease Control and Prevention (CDC), "Treatment of Malaria (Guidelines for Clinicians)." Available at: http://www.cdc.gov/malaria/pdf/clinicalguidance.pdf.

"Drugs for Parasitic Infections," *Treatment Guidelines From the Medical Letter*, 2004, 50(Suppl):e1-14.

Schulbe DE, "Quinine Ban Signals Change for Pharmacists, APhA," *Pharmacy Today*, 1995, 1(12):6.

◆ **Quinine-Odan (Can)** *see* QuiNINE *on page 1794*

◆ **Quinine Sulfate** *see* QuiNINE *on page 1794*

Quinupristin and Dalfopristin
(kwi NYOO pris tin & dal FOE pris tin)

Brand Names: U.S. Synercid®

Brand Names: Canada Synercid®

Therapeutic Category Antibiotic, Streptogramin

Generic Availability (U.S.) No

Use Treatment of complicated skin and skin structure infections caused by *Staphylococcus aureus* (methicillin-susceptible) or *Streptococcus pyogenes* (FDA approved in ages ≥12 years and adults); has also been used for salvage therapy for invasive MRSA infections in cases of vancomycin treatment failure

Pregnancy Risk Factor B

Pregnancy Considerations Because adverse effects were not observed in animal reproduction studies, quinupristin/dalfopristin is classified pregnancy category B. There are no adequate and well-controlled studies of quinupristin/dalfopristin in pregnant women.

Breast-Feeding Considerations It is not known if quinupristin/dalfopristin is excreted in human milk. The manufacturer recommends caution if administering quinupristin/dalfopristin to a nursing woman. The increased molecular weight of quinupristin/dalfopristin may minimize excretion into human milk. Nondose-related effects could include modification of bowel flora.

Contraindications Hypersensitivity to quinupristin, dalfopristin, other streptogramins (pristinamycin or virginiamycin), or to any component

Warnings Quinupristin/dalfopristin inhibit cytochrome P450 3A4 metabolism of cyclosporine, midazolam, nifedipine, and terfenadine. A 77% increase in cyclosporine's half-life with a 63% increase in the AUC has been reported; cyclosporine levels should be closely monitored in patients who are receiving quinupristin/dalfopristin therapy concomitantly. Coadministration of quinupristin/dalfopristin with cytochrome P450 3A4 substrates with narrow therapeutic ranges require serum concentration monitoring of these drugs. Concurrent use with astemizole, terfenadine, and cisapride is not recommended. Drugs metabolized by the cytochrome P450 3A4 system that may prolong the QT$_c$ interval should be avoided. Prolonged use may result in fungal or bacterial superinfection, including *C. difficile*-associated diarrhea (CDAD) and pseudomembranous colitis; CDAD has been observed >2 months postantibiotic treatment. Resistance to quinupristin/dalfopristin has been reported in a few cases of *Enterococcus faecium* infections.

Precautions Use with caution in patients with hepatic or renal dysfunction; dosage reduction may be necessary in patients with hepatic cirrhosis. May cause hyperbilirubinemia (primarily conjugated, up to 5 times ULN) in ~25% of patients. May cause pain and phlebitis when infused through a peripheral line; consider increasing the infusion volume, changing infusion sites, or establishing central venous access; administration of hydrocortisone or diphenhydramine does not decrease infusion site reactions. Episodes of severe arthralgia and myalgia have been reported; reduction in dosage frequency may improve symptoms.

Adverse Reactions

Central nervous system: Headache, pain

Dermatologic: Pruritus, rash

Endocrine & metabolic: Hyperglycemia

Gastrointestinal: Diarrhea, nausea, vomiting

Hematologic: Anemia

Hepatic: Hyperbilirubinemia, increased GGT, increased LDH

Local: Inflammation at infusion site, infusion site reaction, local edema, local pain, thrombophlebitis

Neuromuscular & skeletal: Arthralgia, CPK increased, myalgia

Rare but important or life-threatening: Allergic reaction, anaphylactoid reaction, angina, apnea, arrhythmia, cardiac arrest, coagulation disorder, dysautonomia, dyspnea, encephalopathy, gout, hematuria, hemolytic anemia, hepatitis, hyperkalemia, hypotension, maculopapular rash, mesenteric artery occlusion, myasthenia, neuropathy, pancreatitis, pancytopenia, paraplegia, paresthesia, pericarditis, pleural effusion, pseudomembranous colitis, respiratory distress, seizure, shock, stomatitis, syncope, thrombocytopenia, urticaria

Drug Interactions

Metabolism/Transport Effects Refer to individual components.

Avoid Concomitant Use

Avoid concomitant use of Quinupristin and Dalfopristin with any of the following: Pimozide

Increased Effect/Toxicity

Quinupristin and Dalfopristin may increase the levels/effects of: ARIPiprazole; CycloSPORINE (Systemic); Dofetilide; Lomitapide; Pimozide

Decreased Effect There are no known significant interactions involving a decrease in effect.

Stability Store intact vials at 2°C to 8°C (36°F to 46°F); reconstituted drug is stable for 1 hour at room temperature; infusion bag is stable for 5 hours at room temperature and for 54 hours if refrigerated at 2°C to 8°C (36°F to 46°F); **incompatible** with NS and heparin.

Mechanism of Action Quinupristin/dalfopristin inhibits bacterial protein synthesis by binding to different sites on the 50S bacterial ribosomal subunit thereby inhibiting protein synthesis

Pharmacokinetics (Adult data unless noted)

Distribution: V_d: Quinupristin: 0.45 L/kg; Dalfopristin: 0.24 L/kg

Metabolism: Quinupristin is conjugated with glutathione and cysteine to active metabolites; dalfopristin is hydrolyzed to an active metabolite

Half-life:

Quinupristin: 0.85 hour

Dalfopristin: 0.7 hour

Elimination: Feces (75% to 77% as unchanged drug and metabolites); urine (15% to 19%)

Dosing: Usual Dosage is expressed in terms of combined "mg" of quinupristin plus dalfopristin:

Infants, Children, and Adolescents: Limited data in infants and children <12 years:

General dosing, susceptible infection (*Red Book*, 2012): I.V.: Severe infection: 15-22.5 mg/kg/day in divided doses every 8-12 hours

Enterococcus faecium, vancomycin resistant (VREF): Limited data available: I.V.: 7.5 mg/kg/dose every 8 hours; dosing based on an Emergency-Use Program [n=127, mean age: 7.3 years (range: 1.2 months to 17 years)] (Loeffler, 2002) and a case series (n=8, range: 17 months to 18 years) (Gray, 2000)

MRSA, vancomycin failure salvage therapy: I.V.: 7.5 mg/kg/dose every 8 hours (Liu, 2011; Loeffler, 2002)

Skin and skin structure infection; complicated, treatment: I.V.: 7.5 mg/kg/dose every 12 hours for at least 7 days

VP-shunt infection, ventriculitis: Limited data available: Intraventricular/intrathecal **(use a preservative-free preparation):** Usual dose: 1-2 mg/**day**; reported range: 1-5 mg; administered with concurrent I.V. quinupristin/dalfopristin therapy (Nachman, 1995; Tunkel, 2004; Tush, 1998)

Adults:

Bacteremia, MRSA (persistent, vancomycin failure): I.V.: 7.5 mg/kg every 8 hours (Liu, 2011)

Skin and skin structure infection; complicated, treatment: I.V.: 7.5 mg/kg/dose every 12 hours for at least 7 days

Dosing adjustment in renal impairment: No dosage adjustment is required for use in patients with renal impairment or patients undergoing peritoneal dialysis. Not removed by peritoneal dialysis or hemodialysis

Dosing adjustment in hepatic impairment: There are no dosage adjustments provided in the manufacturer labeling; not studied; pharmacokinetic data suggest adjustment may be necessary.

Administration Parenteral: Reconstitute vial by slowly adding 5 mL D_5W or SWI to make a 100 mg/mL solution; gently swirl the vial contents without shaking to minimize foam formation; further dilute the reconstituted solution with D_5W to a final maximum concentration for administration via peripheral line of 2 mg/mL; maximum concentration for administration via a central line is 5 mg/mL; if an injection site reaction occurs, the dose can be further diluted to a final concentration of <1 mg/mL. Administer infusion over 60 minutes; prior to and following administration, the infusion line should be flushed with D_5W to minimize venous irritation; **DO NOT FLUSH** with saline or heparin solutions due to incompatibility.

Monitoring Parameters CBC, liver function test; monitor infusion site closely; number and type of stools/day for diarrhea

Dosage Forms Excipient information presented when available (limited, particularly for generics); consult specific product labeling.

Injection, powder for reconstitution:

Synercid®: 500 mg: Quinupristin 150 mg and dalfopristin 350 mg

References

Garey KW, Tesoro E, Muggia V, et al, "Cerebrospinal Fluid Concentrations of Quinupristin-Dalfopristin in a Patient With Vancomycin-Resistant *Enterococcus faecium* Ventriculitis," *Pharmacotherapy*, 2001, 21(6):748-50.

Gransden WR, King A, Marossy D, et al, "Quinupristin/Dalfopristin in Neonatal *Enterococcus faecium* Meningitis," *Arch Dis Child Fetal Neonatal Ed*, 1998, 78(3):F235-6.

Gray JW, Darbyshire PJ, Beath SV, et al, "Experience With Quinupristin/Dalfopristin in Treating Infections With Vancomycin-Resistant *Enterococcus faecium* in Children," *Pediatr Infect Dis J*, 2000, 19 (3):234-8.

Gupte G, Jyothi S, Graham S, et al, "Synercid Use in Children Is Associated With Arthralgia and Myalgia," *Archives of Disease in Childhood*, 2006, 91(Supp 1):67.

Liu C, Bayer A, Cosgrove SE, et al, "Clinical Practice Guidelines by the Infectious Diseases Society of America for the Treatment of Methicillin-Resistant *Staphylococcus aureus* Infections in Adults and Children: Executive Summary," *Clin Infect Dis*, 2011, 52(3):285-92.

Loeffler AM, Drew RH, Perfect JR, et al, "Safety and Efficacy of Quinupristin/Dalfopristin for Treatment of Invasive Gram-Positive Infections in Pediatric Patients," *Pediatr Infect Dis J*, 2002, 21 (10):950-6.

Nachman SA, Verma R, and Egnor M, "Vancomycin-Resistant *Enterococcus faecium* Shunt Infection in an Infant: An Antibiotic Cure," *Microb Drug Resist*, 1995, 1(1):95-6.

Red Book: 2012 Report of the Committee on Infectious Diseases, 29th ed, Pickering LK, ed, Elk Grove Village, IL: American Academy of Pediatrics, 2012.

◆ **Qutenza™** *see* Capsaicin *on page 367*

◆ **Qvar** *see* Beclomethasone (Oral Inhalation) *on page 265*

◆ **QVAR (Can)** *see* Beclomethasone (Oral Inhalation) *on page 265*

◆ **R-1569** *see* Tocilizumab *on page 2040*

◆ **RabAvert** *see* Rabies Vaccine *on page 1801*

RABEprazole (ra BEP ra zole)

Medication Safety Issues

Sound-alike/look-alike issues:

AcipHex may be confused with Acephen, Accupril, Aricept, pHisoHex

RABEprazole may be confused with ARIPiprazole, donepezil, lansoprazole, omeprazole, raloxifene

Related Information

Oral Medications That Should Not Be Crushed or Altered on page 2438

Brand Names: U.S. Aciphex; AcipHex Sprinkle

Brand Names: Canada Apo-Rabeprazole; Pariet; Pat-Rabeprazole; PMS-Rabeprazole EC; PRO-Rabeprazole; Rabeprazole EC; RAN-Rabeprazole; Riva-Rabeprazole EC; Sandoz-Rabeprazole; Teva-Rabeprazole EC

Therapeutic Category Gastric Acid Secretion Inhibitor; Gastrointestinal Agent, Gastric or Duodenal Ulcer Treatment; Proton Pump Inhibitor

Generic Availability (U.S.) May be product dependent

Use Treatment of symptomatic gastroesophageal reflux disease (GERD) (FDA approved in ages ≥1 year and adults); short-term treatment (4-8 weeks) and maintenance of erosive or ulcerative GERD (FDA approved in adults); short-term treatment (4 weeks) of duodenal ulcers (FDA approved in adults); long-term treatment of pathological hypersecretory conditions (eg, Zollinger-Ellison syndrome) (FDA approved in adults); in combination with clarithromycin and amoxicillin, adjunctive treatment of duodenal ulcers associated with *Helicobacter pylori* (FDA approved in adults)

Medication Guide Available Yes

Pregnancy Risk Factor B

Pregnancy Considerations Adverse events were not observed in animal reproduction studies. Available studies have not shown an increased risk of major birth defects following maternal use of proton pump inhibitors during pregnancy; however, information specific to rabeprazole is limited (Pasternak, 2010); most information available for omeprazole. When treating GERD in pregnancy, PPIs may be used when clinically indicated (Katz, 2013).

Breast-Feeding Considerations It is not known if rabeprazole is excreted into breast milk. The manufacturer recommends that caution be exercised when administering rabeprazole to nursing women.

Contraindications Hypersensitivity to rabeprazole, substituted benzimidazole proton pump inhibitors (eg, lansoprazole, omeprazole), or any component

Warnings Symptomatic response to therapy with rabeprazole does not preclude the presence of gastric malignancy. Use of gastric acid inhibitors including proton pump inhibitors (PPIs) and H$_2$ blockers has been associated with an increased risk for development of acute gastroenteritis and community-acquired pneumonia (Canani, 2006). Use of PPIs may also increase the risk of *Clostridium difficile*-associated diarrhea (CDAD), especially in hospitalized patients; consider CDAD diagnosis in patients with persistent diarrhea that does not improve. Use the lowest dose and shortest duration of PPI therapy appropriate for the condition being treated.

An increased incidence of osteoporosis-related bone fractures of the hip, spine, or wrist may occur with PPI therapy; patients on high-dose (multiple daily doses) or long-term therapy (≥1 year) should be monitored. Use the lowest effective dose for the shortest duration of time, use vitamin D and calcium supplementation, and follow appropriate guidelines to reduce risk of fractures in patients at risk.

Hypomagnesemia has been reported rarely, usually with prolonged PPI use of >3 months (most cases >1 year of therapy), and may be symptomatic or asymptomatic; severe cases may cause tetany, seizures, and cardiac arrhythmias. Consider obtaining serum magnesium concentrations prior to beginning long-term therapy, especially if taking concomitant digoxin, diuretics, or other drugs known to cause hypomagnesemia; and periodically thereafter. Hypomagnesemia may be corrected by magnesium supplementation, although discontinuation of rabeprazole may be necessary; magnesium concentrations typically return to normal within 1 week of stopping.

PPIs may diminish the therapeutic effect of clopidogrel, thought to be due to reduced formation of the active metabolite of clopidogrel. The manufacturer of clopidogrel recommends either avoidance of both omeprazole (even when scheduled 12 hours apart) and esomeprazole or use of a PPI with comparatively less effect on the active metabolite of clopidogrel (eg, pantoprazole). Avoidance of rabeprazole appears prudent due to potent *in vitro* CYP2C19 inhibition (Li, 2004) and lack of sufficient comparative *in vivo* studies with other PPIs. In contrast to these warnings, others have recommended the continued use of PPIs, regardless of the degree of inhibition, in patients with a history of GI bleeding or multiple risk factors for GI bleeding who are also receiving clopidogrel since no evidence has established clinically meaningful differences in outcome; however, a clinically-significant interaction cannot be excluded in those who are poor metabolizers of clopidogrel (Abraham, 2010; Levine, 2011). Concomitant use of PPIs with high dose methotrexate may lead to increased and prolonged serum concentrations of methotrexate and/or its metabolite, possibly causing methotrexate toxicities; temporary discontinuation of PPIs may be considered. Concomitant use of warfarin with PPIs may result in increased INR and prothrombin time; patients must be closely monitored. Potentially significant interactions may exist, requiring dose or frequency adjustment, additional monitoring, and/or selection of alternative therapy. Consult drug interactions database for more detailed information.

Precautions Use with caution in patients with severe hepatic impairment

Adverse Reactions

Cardiovascular: Peripheral edema

Central nervous system: Dizziness, headache, pain

Gastrointestinal: Abdominal pain, constipation, diarrhea, flatulence, nausea, vomiting, xerostomia

Hepatic: Hepatic encephalopathy, hepatitis, increased liver enzymes

Infection: Increased susceptibility to infection

Neuromuscular & skeletal: Arthralgia, myalgia

Respiratory: Pharyngitis

Rare but important or life-threatening:Agranulocytosis, albuminuria, alopecia, amblyopia, anaphylaxis, anemia, angioedema, bone fracture, bullous rash, cholecystitis, cholelithiasis, *Clostridium difficile* associated diarrhea (CDAD), colitis, coma, delirium, disorientation, erythema multiforme, gynecomastia, hematuria, hemolytic anemia, hyperammonemia, hypersensitivity reaction, hypertension, hypokalemia, hypomagnesemia, hyponatremia, increased thyroid stimulating hormone level, interstitial nephritis, jaundice, leukocytosis, leukopenia, melena, migraine, neutropenia, osteoporosis, palpitation, pancreatitis, pancytopenia, pathological fracture due to osteoporosis, pneumonia, rhabdomyolysis, sinus bradycardia, Stevens-Johnson syndrome, thrombocytopenia, toxic epidermal necrolysis

Drug Interactions

Metabolism/Transport Effects Substrate of CYP2C19 (major), CYP3A4 (major); **Note:** Assignment of Major/Minor substrate status based on clinically relevant drug interaction potential; **Inhibits** CYP2C19 (weak), CYP2C8 (moderate), CYP2D6 (weak), CYP3A4 (weak)

Avoid Concomitant Use

Avoid concomitant use of RABEprazole with any of the following: Dasatinib; Delavirdine; Erlotinib; Nelfinavir; PAZOPanib; Pimozide; PONATinib; Rilpivirine; Risedronate

Increased Effect/Toxicity

RABEprazole may increase the levels/effects of: Amphetamine; ARIPiprazole; CYP2C8 Substrates; Dexmethylphenidate; Dextroamphetamine; Dofetilide; Lomitapide; Methotrexate; Methylphenidate; Pimozide;

Raltegravir; Risedronate; Saquinavir; Tacrolimus (Systemic); Voriconazole

The levels/effects of RABEprazole may be increased by: Fluconazole; Ketoconazole (Systemic); Voriconazole

Decreased Effect

RABEprazole may decrease the levels/effects of: Atazanavir; Bisphosphonate Derivatives; Bosutinib; Cefditoren; Clopidogrel; Dabigatran Etexilate; Dabrafenib; Dasatinib; Delavirdine; Erlotinib; Gefitinib; Indinavir; Iron Salts; Itraconazole; Ketoconazole (Systemic); Mesalamine; Multivitamins/Minerals (with ADEK, Folate, Iron); Mycophenolate; Nelfinavir; Nilotinib; PAZOPanib; PONATinib; Posaconazole; Rilpivirine; Riociguat; Risedronate; Vismodegib

The levels/effects of RABEprazole may be decreased by: Bosentan; CYP2C19 Inducers (Strong); CYP3A4 Inducers (Strong); Dabrafenib; Deferasirox; Mitotane; Siltuximab; St Johns Wort; Tipranavir; Tocilizumab

Food Interactions Prolonged treatment (≥2 years) may lead to malabsorption of dietary vitamin B_{12} and subsequent vitamin B_{12} deficiency (Lam, 2013).

Stability Store at 25°C (77°F); excursions permitted to 15°C to 30°C (59°F to 86°F). Protect from moisture.

Mechanism of Action Potent proton pump inhibitor; suppresses gastric acid secretion by inhibiting the parietal cell H+/K+ ATP pump

Pharmacodynamics

Onset of action: 1 hour

Duration: 24 hours

Pharmacokinetics (Adult data unless noted)

Protein binding: 96.3%

Metabolism: Extensive hepatic metabolism via cytochrome isoenzymes CYP3A and CYP2C19 to inactive metabolites; CYP2C19 exhibits a known genetic polymorphism due to its deficiency in some subpopulations (3% to 5% of Caucasians and 17% to 20% of Asians) which results in slower metabolism

Bioavailability: Tablet: 52%

Half-life:

Adolescents: ~0.55-1 hour (James, 2007)

Adults: 1-2 hours

Time to peak serum concentration:

Adolescents: Tablet: 3.3-4.1 hours (James, 2007)

Adults: Capsule: 1-6.5 hours; Tablet: 2-5 hours

Excretion: 90% in urine

Dosing: Usual

Children and Adolescents:

GERD, symptomatic: Oral:

Children 1-11 years:

<15 kg: 5 mg once daily for ≤12 weeks; if inadequate response may increase to 10 mg once daily

≥15 kg: 10 mg once daily for ≤12 weeks

Children ≥12 years and Adolescents: 20 mg once daily for up to 8 weeks

Adults:

GERD, erosive/ulcerative: Oral: Treatment: 20 mg once daily for 4-8 weeks; if inadequate response, may repeat up to an additional 8 weeks; maintenance: 20 mg once daily

GERD, symptomatic: Oral: Treatment: 20 mg once daily for 4 weeks; if inadequate response, may repeat for an additional 4 weeks

Duodenal ulcer: Oral: 20 mg once daily for ≤4 weeks; additional therapy may be required for some patients

Helicobacter pylori **eradication:** Oral: 20 mg twice daily administered for 7 days (in combination with clarithromycin and amoxicillin)

Hypersecretory conditions (eg, Zollinger-Ellison Syndrome): Oral: 60 mg once daily; dose may need to be adjusted as necessary. Doses as high as 100 mg once daily and 60 mg twice daily have been used and

continued as long as necessary (up to 1 year in some patients).

Dosing adjustment in renal impairment: Children ≥1 year, Adolescents, and Adults: No dosage adjustments are recommended

Dosing adjustment in hepatic impairment: Children ≥1 year, Adolescents, and Adults:

Mild to moderate: No dosage adjustments are recommended

Severe impairment: There are no dosage adjustments provided in the manufacturer's labeling (has not been studied). Use with caution; elimination may be decreased.

Administration

Oral: May administer with an antacid.

Capsules: Administer 30 minutes before a meal. Open capsule and sprinkle contents on a small amount of soft food (eg, applesauce, fruit- or vegetable-based baby food, yogurt) or empty contents into a small amount of liquid (eg, infant formula, apple juice, pediatric electrolyte solution); food or liquid should be at or below room temperature. Do not chew or crush granules; administer whole dose within 15 minutes of preparation; do not store for future use.

Tablets: May be administered without regard to food; best if taken 30 minutes before a meal when treating GERD (Lightdale, 2013). Tablets should be swallowed whole, do not chew, crush, or split.

Monitoring Parameters Magnesium levels in patients on long-term treatment or those taking digoxin, diuretics, or other drugs that cause hypomagnesemia; susceptibility testing recommended in patients who fail *H. pylori* eradication regimen.

Dosage Forms Excipient information presented when available (limited, particularly for generics); consult specific product labeling.

Capsule Sprinkle, Oral, as sodium:

AcipHex Sprinkle: 5 mg [contains fd&c blue #2 aluminum lake]

AcipHex Sprinkle: 10 mg [contains fd&c yellow #6 (sunset yellow)]

Tablet Delayed Release, Oral, as sodium:

Aciphex: 20 mg

Generic: 20 mg

References

Abraham NS, Hlatky MA, Antman EM, et al, "ACCF/ACG/AHA 2010 Expert Consensus Document on the Concomitant Use of Proton Pump Inhibitors and Thienopyridines: A Focused Update of the ACCF/ACG/AHA 2008 Expert Consensus Document on Reducing the Gastrointestinal Risks of Antiplatelet Therapy and NSAID Use: A Report of the American College of Cardiology Foundation Task Force on Expert Consensus Documents," *Circulation*, 2010, 122 (24):2619-33.

Canani RB, Cirillo P, Roggero P, et al, "Therapy With Gastric Acidity Inhibitors Increases the Risk of Acute Gastroenteritis and Community-Acquired Pneumonia in Children," *Pediatrics*, 2006, 117(5):e817-20.

Chey WD, Wong BC, and Practice Parameters Committee of the American College of Gastroenterology, "American College of Gastroenterology Guideline on the Management of *Helicobacter pylori* Infection," *Am J Gastroenterol*, 2007, 102(8):1808-25.

Gibbons TE and Gold BD, "The Use of Proton Pump Inhibitors in Children: A Comprehensive Review," *Paediatr Drugs*, 2003, 5 (1):25-40.

James L, Walson P, Lomax K, et al, "Pharmacokinetics and Tolerability of Rabeprazole Sodium in Subjects Aged 12 to 16 Years With Gastroesophageal Reflux Disease: An Open-Label, Single- and Multiple-Dose Study," *Clin Ther*, 2007, 29(9):2082-92.

Katz PO, Gerson LB, and Vela MF, "Guidelines for the Diagnosis and Management of Gastroesophageal Reflux Disease," *Am J Gastroenterol*, 2013, 108(3):308-28.

Levine GN, Bates ER, Blankenship JC, et al, "2011 ACCF/AHA/SCAI Guideline for Percutaneous Coronary Intervention: A Report of the American College of Cardiology Foundation/American Heart Association Task Force on Practice Guidelines and the Society for Cardiovascular Angiography and Interventions," *Circulation*, 2011, 124(23): e574-651.

Li XQ, Andersson TB, Ahlström M, et al, "Comparison of Inhibitory Effects of the Proton Pump-Inhibiting Drugs Omeprazole,

Esomeprazole, Lansoprazole, Pantoprazole, and Rabeprazole on Human Cytochrome P450 Activities," *Drug Metab Dispos*, 2004, 32 (8):821-7.

Lightdale JR, Gremse DA, and the Section on Gastroenterology, Hepatology, and Nutrition, "Gastroesophageal Reflux: Management Guidance for the Pediatrician," *Pediatrics*, 2013, 131(5):e1684-95.

Pasternak B and Hviid A, "Use of Proton-Pump Inhibitors in Early Pregnancy and the Risk of Birth Defects," *N Engl J Med*, 2010, 363 (22):2114-23.

◆ Rabeprazole EC (Can) *see* RABEprazole *on page 1797*

Rabies Immune Globulin (Human)

(RAY beez i MYUN GLOB yoo lin, HYU man)

Related Information
Immunization Administration Recommendations *on page 2368*
Immunization Guidelines *on page 2373*
Brand Names: U.S. HyperRAB S/D; Imogam Rabies-HT
Brand Names: Canada HyperRAB S/D; Imogam Rabies Pasteurized
Therapeutic Category Immune Globulin
Generic Availability (U.S.) No
Use Provide postexposure prophylaxis of persons with suspected rabies exposure who previously have not been vaccinated against rabies; postexposure prophylaxis consists of thorough wound treatment and the administration of rabies vaccine and rabies immune globulin (FDA approved in children and adults)
Pregnancy Risk Factor C
Pregnancy Considerations Animal reproduction studies have not been conducted. Pregnancy is not a contraindication to postexposure prophylaxis. Pre-exposure prophylaxis may be indicated during pregnancy if the risk for exposure to rabies is significant.
Contraindications Hypersensitivity to rabies immune globulin or any component; previously immunized individuals with confirmed adequate rabies antibody titers
Warnings Product of human plasma; may potentially contain infectious agents which could transmit disease. Screening of donors, as well as testing and/or inactivation or removal of certain viruses, reduces this risk. Infections thought to be transmitted by this product should be reported to the manufacturer.
Precautions Use with caution in patients with a history of allergic reactions to human immunoglobulin preparations or with IgA deficiency; hypersensitivity and anaphylactic reactions can occur; immediate treatment [including epinephrine 1 mg/mL (1:1000)] should be available. Use caution in patients with thrombocytopenia or coagulation disorders; I.M. injections may be contraindicated.
Adverse Reactions
Central nervous system: Fever (mild), headache, malaise
Dermatologic: Angioneurotic edema, rash
Local: Injection site: Pain, stiffness, soreness, tenderness
Renal: Nephrotic syndrome
Miscellaneous: Anaphylaxis
Drug Interactions
Metabolism/Transport Effects None known.
Avoid Concomitant Use There are no known interactions where it is recommended to avoid concomitant use.
Increased Effect/Toxicity There are no known significant interactions involving an increase in effect.
Decreased Effect
Rabies Immune Globulin (Human) may decrease the levels/effects of: Vaccines (Live)
Stability Store between 2°C to 8°C (36°F to 46°F); do not freeze. Discard product exposed to freezing.
The following stability information has also been reported for HyperRAB® S/D: May be exposed to room temperature for a cumulative 7 days (Cohen, 2007)

Mechanism of Action Rabies immune globulin is a solution of globulins dried from the plasma or serum of selected adult human donors who have been immunized with rabies vaccine and have developed high titers of rabies antibody. It generally contains 10% to 18% of protein of which not less than 80% is monomeric immunoglobulin G.
Pharmacodynamics
Onset of action: Rabies antibody appears in serum within 24 hours
Peak antibody level: 2-13 days
Pharmacokinetics (Adult data unless noted) Half-life: 24 days
Dosing: Neonatal
Postexposure prophylaxis (ACIP Recommendation): Local wound infiltration: 20 units/kg single dose administered as soon as possible after exposure. If anatomically feasible, the full rabies immune globulin (RIG) dose should be infiltrated around and into the wound(s); any remaining volume should be administered I.M. at a site distant from the vaccine administration site. If rabies vaccine was initiated without rabies immune globulin, rabies immune globulin may be administered through the seventh day after the first vaccine dose. Administration of RIG is not recommended after the seventh day postvaccine since an antibody response to the vaccine is expected during this time period (CDC, 2010).
Dosing: Usual Postexposure prophylaxis: Local wound infiltration: Infants, Children, Adolescents, and Adults: 20 units/kg single dose administered as soon as possible after exposure. If anatomically feasible, the full rabies immune globulin (RIG) dose should be infiltrated around and into the wound(s); any remaining volume should be administered I.M. at a site distant from the vaccine administration site. If rabies vaccine was initiated without rabies immune globulin, rabies immune globulin may be administered through the seventh day after the first vaccine dose. Administration of RIG is not recommended after the seventh day postvaccine since an antibody response to the vaccine is expected during this time period.
Administration Do **not** administer I.V. Do not administer rabies vaccine in the same syringe or at same administration site as RIG.
Wound infiltration: Thoroughly cleanse wound(s) with soap and water; use povidone-iodine solution to irrigate the wound(s); infiltrate with RIG in the area around and into the wound(s); any remaining dose should be administered I.M. If RIG dose volume is insufficient for wound(s) infiltration, dilute RIG two- to threefold in NS to an adequate volume to insure that all wound areas receive infiltrate (*Red Book*, 2012).
I.M.: Inject into the deltoid muscle of the upper arm or lateral thigh muscle at a site distant from rabies vaccine administration. The gluteal area should be avoided to reduce the risk of sciatic nerve damage. Infants and children with small muscle mass may require multiple I.M. sites for dose delivery.
Monitoring Parameters Serum rabies antibody titer (if rabies immune globulin is inadvertently administered after the eighth day from the first rabies vaccine dose).
Dosage Forms Excipient information presented when available (limited, particularly for generics); consult specific product labeling.
Injectable, Intramuscular:
Imogam Rabies-HT: 150 units/mL (2 mL, 10 mL)
Injectable, Intramuscular [preservative free]:
HyperRAB S/D: 150 units/mL (2 mL, 10 mL)
References
Centers for Disease Control and Prevention (CDC), "Recommendations of the Advisory Committee on Immunization Practices (ACIP): General Recommendations on Immunization," *MMWR Recomm Rep*, 2011, 60(2):1-64.

Centers for Disease Control and Prevention (CDC), "Use of a Reduced (4-Dose) Vaccine Schedule for Postexposure Prophylaxis to Prevent Human Rabies," *MMWR Recomm Rep*, 2010, 59(RR-2):1-9. Available at http://www.cdc.gov/mmwr/PDF/rr/rr5902.pdf

Cohen V, Jellinek SP, Teperikidis L, et al, "Room-Temperature Storage of Medications Labeled for Refrigeration," *Am J Health Syst Pharm*, 2007, 64(16):1711-5.

Red Book: 2012 Report of the Committee on Infectious Diseases, 29th ed, Pickering LK, ed, Elk Grove Village, IL: American Academy of Pediatrics, 2012.

Willoughby RE Jr and Hammarin AL, "Prophylaxis Against Rabies in Children Exposed to Bats," *Pediatr Infect Dis Jp*, 2005, 24 (12):1109-10.

Rabies Vaccine (RAY beez vak SEEN)

Related Information
Immunization Administration Recommendations *on page 2368*

Immunization Guidelines *on page 2373*

Brand Names: U.S. Imovax Rabies; RabAvert
Brand Names: Canada Imovax Rabies; RabAvert
Therapeutic Category Vaccine
Generic Availability (U.S.) No

Use
Pre-exposure immunization: To provide protection against rabies virus to persons with unrecognized exposure or to those in areas where postexposure treatment would be delayed (FDA approved in all ages). Vaccinate persons with greater than usual risk due to occupation or avocation, including veterinarians, rangers, animal handlers, certain laboratory workers, and persons living in or visiting countries for longer than 1 month where rabies is a constant threat. **Note:** Routine pre-exposure prophylaxis for the general U.S. population or routine travelers to areas where rabies is not enzootic is not recommended

Postexposure prophylaxis: To provide protection against rabies virus. If a bite from a carrier animal is unprovoked or if the animal is not captured and rabies is present in that species and area, administer rabies immune globulin (RIG) and the vaccine as indicated (FDA approved in all ages)

Pregnancy Risk Factor C

Pregnancy Considerations Animal reproduction studies have not been conducted. Pregnancy is not a contraindication to postexposure prophylaxis. Pre-exposure prophylaxis during pregnancy may also be considered if risk of rabies is great.

Breast-Feeding Considerations Breast-feeding mothers may be vaccinated. Inactivated virus vaccines do not affect the safety of breast-feeding for the mother or the infant. Breast-feeding infants should be vaccinated according to the recommended schedules (CDC, 2011)

Contraindications
Pre-exposure treatment: Hypersensitivity to any component; Imovax® Rabies contains albumin and neomycin; RabAvert® contains albumin, amphotericin B, bovine gelatin, chicken protein, chlortetracycline, and neomycin

Postexposure treatment: Life-threatening allergic reactions to rabies vaccine or any components (carefully consider a patient's risk of rabies before continuing therapy)

Warnings Immediate treatment for anaphylactic/anaphylactoid reaction should be available during administration of this vaccine. Once postexposure prophylaxis has begun, administration should generally not be interrupted or discontinued due to local or mild adverse events. Continuation of vaccination following severe systemic reactions should consider the person's risk of developing rabies. Report serious reactions to VAERS or the manufacturer/distributor. An immune complex reaction characterized by generalized urticaria, arthralgia, arthritis, angioedema, nausea, vomiting, fever, and malaise has been reported 2-21 days following booster doses of rabies vaccine. Immune response may be decreased in immunocompromised patients. Encephalitis, meningitis, and neuroparalytic events (eg, Guillain-Barré syndrome, myelitis, retrobulbar neuritis) and multiple sclerosis have been temporally associated with use; careful consideration of a patient's risk of rabies should be assessed. Pre-exposure immunization does not eliminate the need for prompt prophylaxis following an exposure but does reduce the postexposure treatment regimen. Syncope has been reported with use of injectable vaccines and may be accompanied by transient visual disturbances, weakness, or tonic-clonic movements. Procedures should be in place to avoid injuries from falling and to restore cerebral perfusion if syncope occurs. In general, household and close contacts of persons with altered immune competence may receive all age-appropriate vaccines. Products contain albumin and may carry a remote risk of transmitting Creutzfeldt-Jakob or other viral diseases.

Precautions Administer with caution to patients with thrombocytopenia or any coagulation disorder that would be compromised by I.M. injection. Antipyretics have not been shown to prevent febrile seizures; antipyretics may be used to treat fever or discomfort following vaccination (CDC, 2011). One study reported that routine prophylactic administration of acetaminophen to prevent fever prior to vaccination decreased the immune response of some vaccines; the clinical significance of this reduction in immune response has not been established (Prymula, 2009).

Adverse Reactions All serious adverse reactions must be reported to the U.S. Department of Health and Human Services (DHHS) Vaccine Adverse Event Reporting System (VAERS) 1-800-822-7967 or online at https://vaers.hhs.gov/esub/index. In Canada, adverse reactions may be reported to local provincial/territorial health agencies or to the Vaccine Safety Section at Public Health Agency of Canada (1-866-844-0018).

Cardiovascular: Circulatory reactions, edema, palpitation

Central nervous system: Chills, dizziness, encephalitis, fatigue, fever >38°C (100°F), Guillain-Barré syndrome, headache, malaise, meningitis, multiple sclerosis, myelitis, neuroparalysis, seizures, vertigo

Dermatologic: Pruritus, urticaria, urticaria pigmentosa

Endocrine & metabolic: Hot flashes

Gastrointestinal: Diarrhea, vomiting

Local: Hematoma, limb swelling (extensive)

Neuromuscular & skeletal: Arthralgia, limb pain, monoarthritis, neuropathy, paralysis (transient), paresthesias (transient), weakness

Ocular: Retrobulbar neuritis, visual disturbances

Respiratory: Bronchospasm, dyspnea, wheezing

Miscellaneous: Allergic reactions, anaphylaxis, hypersensitivity reactions, serum sickness, swollen lymph nodes

Drug Interactions
Metabolism/Transport Effects None known.

Avoid Concomitant Use There are no known interactions where it is recommended to avoid concomitant use.

Increased Effect/Toxicity There are no known significant interactions involving an increase in effect.

Decreased Effect
The levels/effects of Rabies Vaccine may be decreased by: Belimumab; Chloroquine; Fingolimod; Immunosuppressants

Stability Store at 2°C to 8°C (36°F to 46°F). Protect from light; do not freeze.

Mechanism of Action Rabies vaccine is an inactivated virus vaccine which promotes immunity by inducing an active immune response. The production of specific antibodies requires about 7-10 days to develop. Rabies immune globulin or antirabies serum, equine (ARS) is given in conjunction with rabies vaccine to provide immune protection until an antibody response can occur.

Pharmacodynamics
Onset of action: I.M.: Rabies antibody: ~7-10 days
Peak effect: ~30-60 days
Duration: ≥1 year

Dosing: Neonatal Postexposure prophylaxis: All post-exposure treatment should begin with immediate cleansing of the wound with soap and water (for ~15 minutes); immunization should begin as soon as possible after exposure.
ACIP Recommendations: I.M.: 1 mL/dose for 4 doses, on days 0, 3, 7, and 14; **Note:** Immunocompromised patients should receive a fifth dose on day 28. Administer rabies immune globulin (RIG) 20 units/kg body weight around and into the wound(s) if anatomically feasible; administer any remaining volume of the RIG dose I.M. at a distant anatomical site (CDC, 2010).

Dosing: Usual Infants, Children, Adolescents, and Adults: I.M.:
Pre-exposure prophylaxis: 1 mL/dose for 3 doses, on days 0, 7, and 28. Frequency of booster doses dependent upon rabies exposure risk and may include using antibody titers drawn every 6 months to 2 years to determine booster dose need. **Note:** Prolonging the interval between doses does not interfere with immunity achieved after the concluding dose of the basic series.
Postexposure prophylaxis: All postexposure treatment should begin with immediate cleansing of the wound with soap and water (for ~15 minutes); immunization should begin as soon as possible after exposure.
Persons not previously immunized (ACIP Recommendation): 1 mL/dose for 4 doses, on days 0, 3, 7, and 14; **Note:** Immunocompromised patients should receive a fifth dose on day 28. Administer rabies immune globulin (RIG) 20 units/kg body weight around and into the wound(s) if anatomically feasible; administer any remaining volume of the RIG dose I.M. at a distant anatomical site (CDC, 2010).
Persons who have previously received vaccine (either previous postexposure prophylaxis or pre-exposure series of vaccination) or have a previously documented rabies antibody titer considered adequate: 1 mL/dose on days 0 and 3; do not administer RIG

Administration I.M.: Reconstitute with provided diluent; **not for I.V. or SubQ administration;** administer injections in the deltoid muscle, not the gluteal; for infants and small children the outer aspect of the thigh may be used. Do not administer in same syringe as RIG. Adolescents and adults should be vaccinated while seated or lying down.

Monitoring Parameters Serum rabies antibody titers are not routinely recommended in postexposure patients unless the patient was immunocompromised; to determine the need for repeat booster treatment, titers may be measured every 6 months to 2 years in persons at high risk for exposure. Observe for syncope for 15 minutes following administration. If seizure-like activity associated with syncope occurs, maintain patient in supine or Trendelenburg position to reestablish adequate cerebral perfusion.

Additional Information In order to maximize vaccination rates, the ACIP recommends simultaneous administration (ie, >1 vaccine on the same day at different anatomic sites) of all age-appropriate vaccines (live or inactivated) for which a person is eligible at a single visit, unless contraindications exist. If available, the use of combination vaccines is generally preferred over separate injections, taking into consideration provider assessment, patient preference, and potential adverse events. If separate vaccines being used, evaluate product information regarding same syringe compatibility of vaccines. Separate needles and syringes should be used for each injection. The ACIP prefers each dose of specific vaccine in a series come from the same manufacturer if possible. (CDC, 2011)

For additional information, please refer to the following website: http://www.cdc.gov/vaccines/vpd-vac/.
Dosage Forms Excipient information presented when available (limited, particularly for generics); consult specific product labeling.
Injectable, Intramuscular [preservative free]:
Imovax Rabies: 2.5 units/mL (1 ea) [contains albumin human, neomycin sulfate]
Suspension Reconstituted, Intramuscular:
RabAvert: (1 ea) [contains albumin human, chicken protein, edetate disodium, gelatin (bovine), neomycin]

References
AAP Steering Committee on Quality Improvement and Management, Subcommittee on Febrile Seizures American Academy of Pediatrics, "Febrile Seizures: Clinical Practice Guideline for the Long-Term Management of the Child With Simple Febrile Seizures," *Pediatrics*, 2008, 121(6):1281-6.
Centers for Disease Control and Prevention (CDC), "Recommendations of the Advisory Committee on Immunization Practices (ACIP): General Recommendations on Immunization," *MMWR Recomm Rep*, 2011, 60(2):1-64.
Centers for Disease Control and Prevention (CDC), "Syncope After Vaccination-United States, January 2005-July 2007," *MMWR Morb Mortal Wkly Rep*, 2008, 2;57(17):457-60.
Centers for Disease Control and Prevention (CDC), "Use of a Reduced (4-Dose) Vaccine Schedule for Postexposure Prophylaxis to Prevent Human Rabies," *MMWR Recomm Rep*, 2010, 59(RR-2):1-9. Available at http://www.cdc.gov/mmwr/PDF/rr/rr5902.pdf
Manning SE, Rupprecht CE, Fishbein D, et al, "Human Rabies Prevention–United States, 2008: Recommendations of the Advisory Committee on Immunization Practices," *MMWR Recomm Rep*, 2008, 57(RR-3):1-28.
National Center for Immunization and Respiratory Diseases, "General Recommendations on Immunization - Recommendations of the Advisory Committee on Immunization Practices (ACIP)," *MMWR Recomm Rep*, 2011, 60(2):1-64.
Prymula R, Siegrist CA, Chlibek R, et al, "Effect of Prophylactic Paracetamol Administration at Time of Vaccination on Febrile Reactions and Antibody Responses in Children: Two Open-Label, Randomised Controlled Trials," *Lancet*, 2009, 374(9698):1339-50.
Rupprecht CE, Briggs D, Brown CM, et al, "Use of a Reduced (4-Dose) Vaccine Schedule for Postexposure Prophylaxis to Prevent Human Rabies: Recommendations of the Advisory Committee on Immunization Practices," *MMWR Recomm Rep*, 2010, 59(RR-2):1-9.

◆ **Racemic Epinephrine** *see* EPINEPHrine (Systemic, Oral Inhalation) *on page 761*

◆ **Racepinephrine** *see* EPINEPHrine (Systemic, Oral Inhalation) *on page 761*

◆ **RAD001** *see* Everolimus *on page 821*

◆ **rAHF** *see* Antihemophilic Factor (Recombinant) *on page 172*

◆ **RAL** *see* Raltegravir *on page 1802*

◆ **R-albuterol** *see* Levalbuterol *on page 1218*

◆ **Ralivia (Can)** *see* TraMADol *on page 2060*

Raltegravir (ral TEG ra vir)

Related Information
Adult and Adolescent HIV *on page 2348*
Pediatric HIV *on page 2338*
Perinatal HIV *on page 2356*
Brand Names: U.S. Isentress
Brand Names: Canada Isentress
Therapeutic Category Antiretroviral, Integrase Inhibitor (Anti-HIV); Antiviral Agent; HIV Agents (Anti-HIV Agents); Integrase Inhibitor
Generic Availability (U.S.) No
Use Treatment of HIV-1 infection in combination with other antiretroviral agents (FDA approved in ages ≥4 weeks weighing ≥3 kg and adults). **Note:** HIV regimens consisting of **three** antiretroviral agents are strongly recommended.
Pregnancy Risk Factor C
Pregnancy Considerations Adverse events were observed in some animal reproduction studies. Raltegravir has high transfer across the human placenta and can be

detected in neonatal serum after delivery. Standard doses appear to be appropriate in pregnant women. The DHHS Perinatal HIV Guidelines consider raltegravir to be an alternative for use in antiretroviral-naïve pregnant patients when drug interactions with protease inhibitors are a concern. Because of its ability to rapidly suppress viral load, some experts have suggested using raltegravir in late pregnancy in women who have high viral loads; however, this use is not routinely recommended at this time. Reversible elevation of liver enzymes occurred in a patient who initiated raltegravir late in pregnancy; monitor liver enzymes if used during pregnancy.

Regardless of CD4 count or HIV RNA copy number, all HIV-infected pregnant women should receive a combination antiretroviral (ARV) drug regimen. A combination of antepartum, intrapartum, and infant ARV prophylaxis is recommended. ARV therapy should be started as soon as possible in women with symptomatic infection. Although earlier initiation may be more effective in reducing the perinatal transmission of HIV, initiation may be delayed until after 12 weeks gestation in women who do not require immediate treatment after careful consideration of maternal conditions (eg nausea and vomiting) and the potential risks of first trimester fetal exposure for specific agents. A scheduled cesarean delivery at 38 weeks gestation is recommended for all women with HIV RNA >1000 copies/mL or unknown concentrations near delivery in order to decrease transmission. If ARV therapy must be interrupted for <24 hours during the peripartum period, stop then restart all medications simultaneously in order to decrease the chance of developing resistance. Long-term follow-up is recommended for all infants exposed to ARV medications. In couples who want to conceive, the HIV-infected partner should attain maximum viral suppression prior to conception.

Health care providers are encouraged to enroll pregnant women exposed to antiretroviral medications in the Antiretroviral Pregnancy Registry (1-800-258-4263 or www.APRegistry.com). Health care providers caring for HIV-infected women and their infants may contact the National Perinatal HIV Hotline (888-448-8765) for clinical consultation (DHHS [perinatal], 2014).

Breast-Feeding Considerations It is not known if raltegravir is excreted into breast milk. Maternal or infant antiretroviral therapy does not completely eliminate the risk of postnatal HIV transmission. In addition, multiclass-resistant virus has been detected in breast-feeding infants despite maternal therapy. Therefore, in the United States, where formula is accessible, affordable, safe, and sustainable, and the risk of infant mortality due to diarrhea and respiratory infections is low, complete avoidance of breast-feeding by HIV-infected women is recommended to decrease potential transmission of HIV (DHHS [perinatal], 2014).

Contraindications Hypersensitivity to raltegravir or any component

Warnings Severe and sometimes fatal cases of Stevens-Johnson syndrome and toxic epidermal necrolysis have been reported with raltegravir. Hypersensitivity reactions including rash with fever, fatigue, malaise, conjunctivitis, or other constitutional symptoms, organ dysfunction, and/or hepatic failure have also been reported. Discontinue immediately if a severe skin reaction or hypersensitivity symptoms develop. Monitor liver transaminases and start supportive therapy.

Precautions Use with caution in patients with risk factors for CK elevations and/or skeletal muscle abnormalities, including those taking other drugs known to cause myopathy or rhabdomyolysis; grade 2 to 4 creatine kinase (CK) increases have been observed; myopathy and rhabdomyolysis have been reported.

Immune reconstitution syndrome (an acute inflammatory response to residual or indolent opportunistic infections) may occur in HIV patients during initial treatment with combination antiretroviral agents; this syndrome may require further patient assessment and therapy. Autoimmune disorders (eg, Graves' disease, Guillain-Barré syndrome, and polymyositis) have been reported in patients experiencing immune reconstitution; time to onset is variable and may occur many months after antiretroviral treatment is initiated.

The chewable tablet and oral suspension are not bioequivalent with the film-coated tablets; do not substitute. Chewable tablets contain aspartame which is metabolized to phenylalanine and must be avoided (or used with caution) in patients with phenylketonuria; each 100 mg tablet contains ~0.1 mg phenylalanine.

Adverse Reactions

Central nervous system: Dizziness, fatigue, headache, insomnia

Endocrine & metabolic: Increased serum glucose

Gastrointestinal: Increased serum amylase, increased serum lipase, nausea

Hematologic: Abnormal absolute neutrophil count, thrombocytopenia

Hepatic: Hyperbilirubinemia, increased serum alkaline phosphatase, increased serum ALT (incidence higher with hepatitis B and/or C coinfection), increased serum AST (incidence higher with hepatitis B and/or C coinfection)

Neuromuscular & skeletal: Increased creatine phosphokinase

Rare but important or life-threatening: Anemia, cerebellar ataxia, depression (particularly in subjects with a preexisting history of psychiatric illness), drug rash with eosinophilia and systemic symptoms (DRESS; Perry, 2013), gastritis, hepatic failure, hepatitis, hypersensitivity, myopathy, nephrolithiasis, psychomotor agitation (children; grade 3), renal failure, rhabdomyolysis, Stevens-Johnson syndrome, suicidal ideation, toxic epidermal necrolysis

Drug Interactions

Metabolism/Transport Effects None known.

Avoid Concomitant Use

Avoid concomitant use of Raltegravir with any of the following: Aluminum Hydroxide; Magnesium Salts

Increased Effect/Toxicity

Raltegravir may increase the levels/effects of: Fibric Acid Derivatives; HMG-CoA Reductase Inhibitors; Zidovudine

The levels/effects of Raltegravir may be increased by: Proton Pump Inhibitors

Decreased Effect

Raltegravir may decrease the levels/effects of: Fosamprenavir

The levels/effects of Raltegravir may be decreased by: Aluminum Hydroxide; Efavirenz; Fosamprenavir; Magnesium Salts; Rifabutin; Rifampin; Tipranavir

Food Interactions Variable absorption depending upon meal type (low- vs high-fat meal) and dosage form. Management: Raltegravir was administered without regard to meals in clinical trials.

Stability Store at 20°C to 25°C (68°F to 77°F); excursions permitted to 15°C to 30°C (59°F to 86°F). Store chewable tablets in original package with bottle tightly closed and desiccant in bottle to protect from moisture. Store oral suspension in the original container; do not open foil packet until ready for use.

Mechanism of Action Incorporation of viral DNA into the host cell's genome is required to produce a self-replicating provirus and propagation of infectious virion particles. The viral cDNA strand produced by reverse transcriptase is subsequently processed and inserted into the human genome by the enzyme HIV-1 integrase (encoded by the pol gene of HIV). Raltegravir inhibits the catalytic activity of integrase, thus preventing integration of the proviral gene into human DNA.

Pharmacokinetics (Adult data unless noted)

Protein binding: ~83%

Metabolism: Primarily hepatic glucuronidation mediated by UGT1A1

Bioavailability: Film-coated tablet: Not established; Chewable tablet: Higher oral bioavailability compared to film-coated tablet; dosage forms are not interchangeable.

Half-life elimination: ~9 hours

Time to peak, serum concentration: Film-coated tablet: ~3 hours

Elimination: Feces (~51% as unchanged drug); urine (~32%; 9% as unchanged drug)

Dosing: Usual Note: Chewable tablets and oral suspension are not bioequivalent with film-coated tablets; dosing is not interchangeable.

Pediatric: **HIV infection, treatment:** Oral: **Note:** Use in combination with other antiretroviral agents.

Oral suspension (20 mg/mL): Infants and Children weighing 3 to <20 kg:

Weight-directed dosing: 6 mg/kg/dose twice daily; maximum dose: 100 mg/dose

Fixed-dosing:

3 to <4 kg: 20 mg (1 mL) twice daily
4 to <6 kg: 30 mg (1.5 mL) twice daily
6 to <8 kg: 40 mg (2 mL) twice daily
8 to <11 kg: 60 mg (3 mL) twice daily
11 to <14 kg: 80 mg (4 mL) twice daily
14 to <20 kg: 100 mg (5 mL) twice daily

Chewable tablets: Children weighing ≥11 kg:

Weight-directed dosing: 6 mg/kg/dose twice daily; maximum dose: 300 mg/dose

Fixed-dosing:

11 to <14 kg: 75 mg (3 x 25 mg tablet) twice daily
14 to <20 kg: 100 mg (1 x 100 mg tablet) twice daily
20 to <28 kg: 150 mg (1.5 x 100 mg tablet) twice daily
28 to <40 kg: 200 mg (2 x 100 mg tablet) twice daily
≥40 kg: 300 mg (3 x 100 mg tablet) twice daily

Film-coated tablets: Children and Adolescents weighing ≥25 kg: 400 mg twice daily

Adult: **HIV infection, treatment:** Oral: **Note:** Use in combination with other antiretroviral agents: Film-coated tablet: 400 mg twice daily

Dosing adjustment for concomitant therapy: Adults: Concomitant rifampin therapy: Raltegravir dose: Film-coated tablet: 800 mg twice daily

Dosing adjustment in renal impairment: Infants, Children, Adolescents, and Adults: No dosage adjustment required

Dosing adjustment in hepatic impairment: Infants, Children, Adolescents, and Adults:

Mild to moderate hepatic impairment: No dosage adjustment required

Severe impairment: No data available

Administration Oral: Take without regard to meals.

Chewable tablets may be chewed or swallowed whole; 100 mg chewable tablet can be broken in half.

Film-coated tablets must be swallowed whole.

Oral suspension: Open foil packet of single dose (100 mg). Measure 5 mL water in provided mixing cup. Pour packet contents into 5 mL water, close lid, and swirl for 30 to 60 seconds; do not turn the mixing cup upside down; resulting concentration: 20 mg/mL. Once mixed, measure recommended suspension dose with an oral syringe. Administer within 30 minutes of mixing with water. Discard any remaining suspension in the trash.

Monitoring Parameters Note: Monitor CD4 percentage (if <5 years of age) or CD4 count (if ≥5 years of age) at least every 3 to 4 months (DHHS [pediatric], 2014).

Prior to initiation of therapy: Genotypic resistance testing, CD4 and viral load (every 3 to 4 months), CBC with differential, LFTs, BUN, creatinine, electrolytes, glucose, urinalysis (every 6 to 12 months), and assessment of readiness for adherence with medication regimen. At initiation and with any change in treatment regimen: CBC with differential, electrolytes, calcium, phosphate, glucose, LFTs, bilirubin, urinalysis (at initiation), BUN, creatinine, albumin, total protein, lipid panel (at initiation), CD4, and viral load. After 1 to 2 weeks of therapy: Signs of medication toxicity and adherence. After 2 to 4 weeks of therapy: CBC with differential, viral load, signs of medication toxicity, and adherence; then every 3 to 4 months: CBC with differential, electrolytes, glucose, LFTs, bilirubin, BUN, creatinine, CD4, viral load, signs of medication toxicity, and adherence. Every 6 to 12 months: Lipid panel and urinalysis. CD4 monitoring frequency may be decreased to every 6 to 12 months in children who are adherent to therapy if the value is well above the threshold for opportunistic infections, viral suppression is sustained, and the clinical status is stable for more than 2 to 3 years (DHHS [pediatric], 2014). Monitor for growth and development, signs of HIV-specific physical conditions, HIV disease progression, opportunistic infections.

Reference Range Trough concentration (Limited data available; range utilized in trials): Median 72 ng/mL (Range: 29 to 118 ng/mL) (DHHS [adult, pediatric], 2014)

Product Availability Isentress (100 mg single use packets for oral suspension): FDA approved December 2013; anticipated availability is the third quarter of 2014.

Dosage Forms Excipient information presented when available (limited, particularly for generics); consult specific product labeling.

Packet, Oral:

Isentress: 100 mg (60 ea) [contains polyethylene glycol; banana flavor]

Tablet, Oral:

Isentress: 400 mg [contains polyethylene glycol]

Tablet Chewable, Oral:

Isentress: 25 mg [contains aspartame, saccharin sodium; orange banana flavor]

Isentress: 100 mg [scored; contains aspartame, saccharin sodium; orange banana flavor]

References

DHHS Panel on Antiretroviral Guidelines for Adults and Adolescents. Guidelines for the use of antiretroviral agents in HIV-1-infected adults and adolescents, Department of Health and Human Services. May 1, 2014. Available at http://www.aidsinfo.nih.gov/ContentFiles/AdultandAdolescentGL.pdf

DHHS Panel on Antiretroviral Therapy and Medical Management of HIV-Infected Children. Guidelines for the use of antiretroviral agents in pediatric HIV infection. February 12, 2014. Available at http://aidsinfo.nih.gov

DHHS Panel on Treatment of HIV-Infected Pregnant Women and Prevention of Perinatal Transmission. Recommendations for the use of antiretroviral drugs in pregnant HIV-1-infected women for maternal health and interventions to reduce perinatal HIV-1 transmission in the United States. March 28, 2014. Available at http://aidsinfo.nih.gov

Grinsztejn B, Nguyen BY, Katlama C, et al. Safety and efficacy of the HIV-1 integrase inhibitor raltegravir (MK-0518) in treatment-experienced patients with multidrug-resistant virus: a phase II randomised controlled trial. *Lancet.* 2007;369(9569):1261-1269.

Kassahun K, McIntosh I, Cui D, et al. Metabolism and disposition in humans of raltegravir (MK-0518), an anti-AIDS drug targeting the human immunodeficiency virus 1 integrase enzyme. *Drug Metab Dispos.* 2007;35(9):1657-1663.

Lennox JL, DeJesus E, Lazzarin A, et al. Safety and efficacy of raltegravir-based versus efavirenz-based combination therapy in treatment-naïve patients with HIV-1 infection: a multicentre, double-blind randomised controlled trial. *Lancet.* 2009;374(9692):796-806.

Nachman S, Acosta E, Zheng N, et al. Interim results from IMPAACT P1066: raltegravir (RAL) oral chewable tablet (CT) formulation in children 2-5 years. 18th Conference on Retroviruses and Opportunistic Infections (CROI). 2011 [Poster abstract 715 from 2011 CROI Conference].

Nair V, Chi G. HIV integrase inhibitors as therapeutic agents in AIDS. *Rev Med Virol.* 2007;17(4):277-295.

◆ **RAN-Amlodipine (Can)** *see* AmLODIPine *on page 135*

◆ **RAN-Atenolol (Can)** *see* Atenolol *on page 222*

◆ **RAN-Atorvastatin (Can)** *see* AtorvaSTATin *on page 227*

◆ **Ran-Candesartan (Can)** *see* Candesartan *on page 363*

◆ **RAN-Carvedilol (Can)** *see* Carvedilol *on page 385*

◆ **RAN™-Cefprozil (Can)** *see* Cefprozil *on page 412*

◆ **RAN-Ciproflox (Can)** *see* Ciprofloxacin (Systemic) *on page 471*

◆ **RAN™-Citalo (Can)** *see* Citalopram *on page 484*

◆ **RAN-Clarithromycin (Can)** *see* Clarithromycin *on page 490*

◆ **RAN-Clopidogrel (Can)** *see* Clopidogrel *on page 521*

◆ **RAN-Enalapril (Can)** *see* Enalapril *on page 744*

◆ **RAN-Fentanyl Matrix Patch (Can)** *see* FentaNYL *on page 853*

◆ **RAN-Fentanyl Transdermal System (Can)** *see* FentaNYL *on page 853*

◆ **RAN-Fosinopril (Can)** *see* Fosinopril *on page 938*

◆ **RAN-Gabapentin (Can)** *see* Gabapentin *on page 950*

◆ **RAN-Imipenem-Cilastatin (Can)** *see* Imipenem and Cilastatin *on page 1077*

◆ **RAN-Irbesartan (Can)** *see* Irbesartan *on page 1147*

Ranitidine (ra NI ti deen)

Medication Safety Issues
Sound-alike/look-alike issues:
Ranitidine may be confused with amantadine, rimantadine

Zantac may be confused with Xanax, Zarontin, Zofran, ZyrTEC

Brand Names: U.S. Acid Reducer Maximum Strength [OTC] [DSC]; Acid Reducer [OTC]; GoodSense Acid Reducer [OTC]; Ranitidine Acid Reducer [OTC]; Zantac; Zantac 150 Maximum Strength [OTC]; Zantac 75 [OTC]

Brand Names: Canada Acid Reducer; Apo-Ranitidine; CO Ranitidine; Dom-Ranitidine; Myl-Ranitidine; Mylan-Ranitidine; Nu-Ranit; PHL-Ranitidine; PMS-Ranitidine; RAN-Ranitidine; Ranitidine Injection, USP; ratio-Ranitidine; Riva-Ranitidine; Sandoz-Ranitidine; ScheinPharm Ranitidine; Teva-Ranitidine; Zantac; Zantac 75; Zantac Maximum Strength Non-Prescription

Therapeutic Category Gastrointestinal Agent, Gastric or Duodenal Ulcer Treatment; Histamine H_2 Antagonist

Generic Availability (U.S.) Yes

Use Short-term treatment of active duodenal ulcers and benign gastric ulcers; long-term prophylaxis of duodenal ulcer and gastric hypersecretory states; gastroesophageal reflux disease (GERD); recurrent postoperative ulcer; treatment and prophylaxis of erosive esophagitis; upper GI bleeding, prevention of acid-aspiration pneumonitis during surgery, and prevention of stress-induced ulcers; over-the-counter (OTC) formulation for use in the relief of heartburn, acid indigestion, and sour stomach

Pregnancy Risk Factor B

Pregnancy Considerations Adverse events were not observed in animal studies; therefore, ranitidine is classified as pregnancy category B. Ranitidine crosses the placenta. An increased risk of congenital malformations or adverse events in the newborn has generally not been observed following maternal use of ranitidine during pregnancy. Histamine H_2 antagonists have been evaluated for the treatment of gastroesophageal reflux disease (GERD) as well as gastric and duodenal ulcers during pregnancy. If needed, ranitidine is the agent of choice. Histamine H_2 antagonists may be used for aspiration prophylaxis prior to cesarean delivery.

Breast-Feeding Considerations Ranitidine is excreted into breast milk. The manufacturer recommends that caution be exercised when administering ranitidine to nursing women. Peak milk concentrations of ranitidine occur ~5.5 hours after the dose (case report).

Contraindications Hypersensitivity to ranitidine or any component or other H_2 antagonists; patients with history of acute porphyria (may precipitate an acute attack)

Warnings Use of gastric acid inhibitors, including proton pump inhibitors and H_2 blockers, has been associated with an increased risk for development of acute gastroenteritis and community-acquired pneumonia (Canani, 2006). A large epidemiological study has suggested an increased risk for developing pneumonia in patients receiving H_2 receptor antagonists; however, a causal relationship with ranitidine has not been demonstrated. Rapid I.V. administration of ranitidine has been associated with bradycardia, particularly in patients predisposed to cardiac rhythm disturbances. A cohort analysis including over 11,000 neonates reported an association of H_2 blocker use and an increased incidence of NEC in VLBW neonates (Guillet, 2006). An approximate sixfold increase in mortality, NEC, and infection (ie, sepsis, pneumonia, UTI) was reported in patients receiving ranitidine in a cohort analysis of 274 VLBW neonates (Terrin, 2011).

Precautions Use with caution in patients with liver and renal impairment; dosage modification required in patients with renal impairment.

Adverse Reactions
Cardiovascular: Asystole, atrioventricular block, bradycardia (with rapid I.V. administration), premature ventricular beats, tachycardia, vasculitis

Central nervous system: Agitation, dizziness, depression, hallucinations, headache, insomnia, malaise, mental confusion, somnolence, vertigo

Dermatologic: Alopecia, erythema multiforme, rash

Endocrine & metabolic: Prolactin levels increased

Gastrointestinal: Abdominal discomfort/pain, constipation, diarrhea, nausea, necrotizing enterocolitis (VLBW neonates; Guillet, 2006), pancreatitis, vomiting

Hematologic: Acquired immune hemolytic anemia, acute porphyritic attack, agranulocytosis, aplastic anemia, granulocytopenia, leukopenia, pancytopenia, thrombocytopenia

Hepatic: Cholestatic hepatitis, hepatic failure, hepatitis, jaundice

Local: Transient pain, burning or itching at the injection site

Neuromuscular & skeletal: Arthralgia, involuntary motor disturbance, myalgia

Ocular: Blurred vision

Renal: Acute interstitial nephritis, serum creatinine increased

Respiratory: Pneumonia (causal relationship not established)

Miscellaneous: Anaphylaxis, angioneurotic edema, hypersensitivity reactions (eg, bronchospasm, fever, eosinophilia)

Drug Interactions
Metabolism/Transport Effects Substrate of CYP1A2 (minor), CYP2C19 (minor), CYP2D6 (minor), P-glycoprotein; **Note:** Assignment of Major/Minor substrate status based on clinically relevant drug interaction potential; Inhibits CYP1A2 (weak), CYP2D6 (weak)

Avoid Concomitant Use
Avoid concomitant use of Ranitidine with any of the following: Dasatinib; Delavirdine; PAZOPanib; PONATinib; Risedronate

Increased Effect/Toxicity
Ranitidine may increase the levels/effects of: ARIPiprazole; Dexmethylphenidate; Methylphenidate; Procainamide; Risedronate; Saquinavir; Sulfonylureas; Varenicline; Warfarin

The levels/effects of Ranitidine may be increased by: P-glycoprotein/ABCB1 Inhibitors

Decreased Effect

Ranitidine may decrease the levels/effects of: Atazanavir; Bosutinib; Cefditoren; Cefpodoxime; Cefuroxime; Dabrafenib; Dasatinib; Delavirdine; Erlotinib; Fosamprenavir; Gefitinib; Indinavir; Iron Salts; Itraconazole; Ketoconazole (Systemic); Mesalamine; Multivitamins/Minerals (with ADEK, Folate, Iron); Nelfinavir; Nilotinib; PAZOPanib; PONATinib; Posaconazole; Prasugrel; Rilpivirine; Vismodegib

The levels/effects of Ranitidine may be decreased by: Peginterferon Alfa-2b; P-glycoprotein/ABCB1 Inducers

Food Interactions Prolonged treatment (≥2 years) may lead to malabsorption of dietary vitamin B_{12} and subsequent vitamin B_{12} deficiency (Lam, 2013).

Stability Protect injection from light; stable for 48 hours at room temperature or 30 days when frozen in D_5W or NS; stable for 24 hours in TPN solutions; stable for 24 hours in 3-in-1 total nutrient admixture

Mechanism of Action Competitive inhibition of histamine at H_2-receptors at the gastric parietal cells, which inhibits gastric acid secretion, gastric volume, and hydrogen ion concentration are reduced. Does not affect pepsin secretion, pentagastrin-stimulated intrinsic factor secretion, or serum gastrin.

Pharmacokinetics (Adult data unless noted)

Distribution: Minimally penetrates the blood-brain barrier; breast milk to plasma ratio: 1.9-6.7

V_d:
Children: 1-1.3 L/kg
Adults: 1.4 L/kg

Protein binding: 15%

Metabolism: In the liver

Bioavailability:
Oral: ~50%
I.M.: 90% to 100%

Half-life:
Neonates (receiving ECMO): 6.6 hours
Infants: 3.5 hours
Children 3.5-16 years: 1.8-2 hours
Adults:
Normal renal and hepatic function: 2-2.5 hours
Decreased renal function (CrCl 25-35 mL/minute): 4.8 hours

Time to peak serum concentration:
Oral: 1-3 hours
I.M.: 15 minutes

Elimination: 30% (oral) or 70% (I.V.) eliminated as unchanged drug in the urine and in feces

Dialysis: Hemodialysis: Slightly dialyzable (5% to 20%)

Dosing: Neonatal Note: Consider judicial use in neonatal population due to an association of H_2 blocker use and an increased incidence of NEC in VLBW neonates (Guillet, 2006) and a reported approximate sixfold increase in mortality, NEC, and infection (ie, sepsis, pneumonia, UTI) in VLBW neonates receiving ranitidine (Terrin, 2011).

Gastroesophageal reflux: Limited data available: Corrected age <44 weeks: Oral: 2 mg/kg/dose every 8 hours (Birch, 2009; Sutphen, 1989, Wheatley, 2012)

GI bleed or stress ulcer; prophylaxis: Limited data available; dosing regimens variable: I.V.:
Intermittent I.V.:
GA <37 weeks: 0.5 mg/kg/dose every 12 hours (Kuusela, 1998); others have used 1.5-3 mg/kg/day divided every 12 hours
GA ≥37 weeks: 1.5-2 mg/kg/day in divided doses every 8 hours (Crill, 1999); others have recommended higher dosing at 1.5 mg/kg/dose every 8 hours (ASHP, 1999; Kuusela, 1998)
Continuous I.V. infusion: **Note:** Reported ranges are similar to the total daily dose with intermittent I.V.

dosing. Loading dose: 1.5 mg/kg/dose, followed by usual range of 0.04-0.08 mg/kg/hour infusion (1-2 mg/kg/**day**); reported range of 0.031-0.125 mg/kg/hour (0.75-3 mg/kg/**day**); in a trial of premature neonates on concurrent dexamethasone, an infusion rate of 0.0625 mg/kg/hour was shown to maintain neonatal gastric pH >4; higher rates of 0.125 mg/kg/hour have been used without additional clinical benefit (Crill, 1999; Kelly, 1993)

ECMO: Term neonates: Loading dose: 2 mg/kg/dose over 10 minutes followed by 0.083 mg/kg/hour infusion (2 mg/kg/**day**), begin infusion 24 hours after loading dose; rate of infusion was increased by 0.042 mg/kg/hour (1 mg/kg/**day**) if gastric pH fell to <4 (Wells, 1998)

Dosing: Usual

Infants, Children, and Adolescents 1 month to 16 years:
Gastric/duodenal ulcer:
Oral:
Treatment: 4-8 mg/kg/day divided twice daily; maximum: 300 mg/day
Maintenance: 2-4 mg/kg/day once daily; maximum: 150 mg/day
I.V.: 2-4 mg/kg/day divided every 6-8 hours; maximum: 200 mg/day
GERD and erosive esophagitis:
Oral: 4-10 mg/kg/day divided twice daily; maximum: GERD: 300 mg/day; erosive esophagitis: 600 mg/day
I.V.: 2-4 mg/kg/day divided every 6-8 hours; maximum: 200 mg/day **or as an alternative**
Continuous infusion: Initial: 1 mg/kg/dose for one dose followed by infusion of 0.08-0.17 mg/kg/hour or 2-4 mg/kg/day

Adolescents ≥16 years and Adults:
Treatment of duodenal or gastric ulcers, GERD, maintenance of erosive esophagitis: Oral: 150 mg/dose twice daily or 300 mg at bedtime
Prophylaxis of recurrent duodenal ulcer: Oral: 150 mg at bedtime
Gastric hypersecretory conditions:
Oral: 150 mg twice daily; maximum: 600 mg/day
I.M., I.V.: 50 mg/dose every 6-8 hours (dose not to exceed 400 mg/day)
Continuous I.V. infusion: Initial 50 mg I.V. followed by 6.25 mg/hour titrated to gastric pH >4.0 for prophylaxis or >7.0 for treatment; **continuous I.V. infusion is preferred in patients with active bleeding**
Erosive esophagitis: Oral: 150 mg 4 times/day
Pathologic hypersecretory conditions (eg, Zollinger-Ellison syndrome):
Continuous I.V. infusion: Initial 50 mg I.V. followed by 1 mg/kg/hour infusion; titrate dosage in 0.5 mg/kg/hour increments to maintain gastric acid output at <10 mEq/hour; doses up to 2.5 mg/kg/hour (220 mg/hour) have been used
Oral: 150 mg twice daily; more frequent administration may be indicated depending upon response; doses up to 6.3 g/day have been used in severe cases
Relief of heartburn, acid indigestion, sour stomach (OTC use): Oral: 75 mg 30-60 minutes before eating; no more than 2 tablets/day

Dosing adjustment in renal impairment:
Children (Aronoff, 2007):
Oral: Based on a usual dose of 2-6 mg/kg/day divided every 8-12 hours
GFR >50 mL/minute/1.73 m^2: No adjustment required
GFR 30-50 mL/minute/1.73 m^2: 2 mg/kg/dose every 12 hours
GFR 10-29 mL/minute/1.73 m^2: 1 mg/kg/dose every 12 hours
GFR <10 mL/minute/1.73 m^2: 1 mg/kg/dose every 24 hours
Hemodialysis: 1 mg/kg/dose every 24 hours

Peritoneal dialysis: 1 mg/kg/dose every 24 hours
Continuous renal replacement therapy: 2 mg/kg/dose every 12 hours
Parenteral (I.V.): Based on a usual dose of 2-4 mg/kg/day divided every 6-24 hours
GFR >50 mL/minute/1.73 m^2: No adjustment required
GFR 30-50 mL/minute/1.73 m^2: 1 mg/kg/dose every 12 hours
GFR 10-29 mL/minute/1.73 m^2: 0.5 mg/kg/dose every 12 hours
GFR <10 mL/minute/1.73 m^2: 0.5 mg/kg/dose every 24 hours
Hemodialysis: 0.5 mg/kg/dose every 24 hours
Peritoneal dialysis: 0.5 mg/kg/dose every 24 hours
Continuous renal replacement therapy: 1 mg/kg/dose every 12 hours
Adults: CrCl <50 mL/minute:
Oral: 150 mg every 24 hours; adjust dose cautiously if needed
I.V.: 50 mg every 18-24 hours; adjust dose cautiously if needed
Hemodialysis: Adjust dose schedule to administer dose at the end of dialysis

Usual Infusion Concentrations: Pediatric Note: Premixed solutions available
I.V. infusion: 0.5 mg/mL
Administration
Oral: Administer with meals and at bedtime
Parenteral: Intermittent I.V. infusion preferred over direct injection to decrease risk of bradycardia; for intermittent infusion, infuse over 15-30 minutes, at a usual concentration of 0.5 mg/mL; for direct I.V. injection, administer over a period of at least 5 minutes, not to exceed 10 mg/minute (4 mL/minute) at a final concentration not to exceed 2.5 mg/mL; For I.M., administer undiluted (25 mg/mL)

Monitoring Parameters AST, ALT, serum creatinine; when used to prevent stress-related GI bleeding, measure the intragastric pH and try to maintain pH >4; gastric acid secretion (<10 mEq/hour)

Reference Range Serum level necessary to inhibit basal acid secretion:
Children: 90% suppression: 40-60 ng/mL
Adults: 50% suppression: 36-94 ng/mL

Test Interactions False-positive urine protein using Multistix®; gastric acid secretion test; skin test allergen extracts. May also interfere with urine detection of amphetamine/methamphetamine (false-positive).

Additional Information Causes fewer CNS adverse reactions and drug interactions compared to cimetidine; safety and efficacy of full-dose therapy extending beyond 8 weeks have not been determined

Dosage Forms Excipient information presented when available (limited, particularly for generics); consult specific product labeling. [DSC] = Discontinued product
Capsule, Oral:
Generic: 150 mg, 300 mg
Solution, Injection:
Zantac: 50 mg/2 mL (2 mL); 150 mg/6 mL (6 mL); 1000 mg/40 mL (40 mL) [contains phenol]
Generic: 50 mg/2 mL (2 mL); 150 mg/6 mL (6 mL); 1000 mg/40 mL (40 mL)
Syrup, Oral:
Zantac: 15 mg/mL (480 mL [DSC]) [contains alcohol, usp, butylparaben, propylparaben, saccharin sodium; peppermint flavor]
Generic: 15 mg/mL (10 mL, 473 mL, 474 mL, 480 mL); 75 mg/5 mL (473 mL, 480 mL); 150 mg/10 mL (10 mL)
Tablet, Oral:
Acid Reducer: 75 mg
Acid Reducer: 75 mg [DSC] [sugar free]
Acid Reducer Maximum Strength: 150 mg [DSC] [sugar free; contains fd&c yellow #6 (sunset yellow)]

GoodSense Acid Reducer: 75 mg [gluten free]
Ranitidine Acid Reducer: 75 mg
Zantac 75: 75 mg
Zantac: 150 mg, 300 mg
Zantac 150 Maximum Strength: 150 mg
Zantac 150 Maximum Strength: 150 mg [sodium free, sugar free; contains brilliant blue fcf (fd&c blue #1); mint flavor]
Generic: 75 mg, 150 mg, 300 mg

References
Aronoff GR, Bennett WM, Berns JS, et al, *Drug Prescribing in Renal Failure: Dosing Guidelines for Adults and Children*, 5th ed. Philadelphia, PA: American College of Physicians, 2007.
Birch JL and Newell SJ, "Gastrooesophageal Reflux Disease in Preterm Infants: Current Management and Diagnostic Dilemmas," *Arch Dis Child Fetal Neonatal Ed*, 2009, 94(5):F379-83.
Blumer JL, Rothstein FC, Kaplan BS, et al, "Pharmacokinetic Determination of Ranitidine Pharmacodynamics in Pediatric Ulcer Disease," *J Pediatr*, 1985, 107(2):301-6.
Canani RB, Cirillo P, Roggero P, et al, "Therapy With Gastric Acidity Inhibitors Increases the Risk of Acute Gastroenteritis and Community-Acquired Pneumonia in Children," *Pediatrics*, 2006, 117(5):e817-20.
Crill CM and Hak EB, "Upper Gastrointestinal Tract Bleeding in Critically III Pediatric Patients," *Pharmacotherapy*, 1999, 19(2):162-80.
Eddleston JM, Booker PD, and Green JR, "Use of Ranitidine in Children Undergoing Cardiopulmonary Bypass," *Crit Care Med*, 1989, 17 (1):26-9.
Fontana M, Massironi E, Rossi A, et al, "Ranitidine Pharmacokinetics in Newborn Infants," *Arch Dis Child*, 1993, 68(5 Spec No):602-3.
Guillet R, Stoll BJ, Cotten CM, et al, "Association of H2-Blocker Therapy and Higher Incidence of Necrotizing Enterocolitis in Very Low Birth Weight Infants," *Pediatrics*, 2006, 117(2):137-42.
Kelly EJ, Chatfield SL, Brownlee KG, et al, "The Effect of Intravenous Ranitidine on the Intragastric pH of Preterm Infants Receiving Dexamethasone," *Arch Dis Child*, 1993, 69(1 Spec No):37-9.
Kuusela AL, "Long-Term Gastric pH Monitoring for Determining Optimal Dose of Ranitidine for Critically III Preterm and Term Neonates," *Arch Dis Child Fetal Neonatal Ed*, 1998, 78(2):F151-3.
Lopez-Herce J, Albajara L, Codoceo R, et al, "Ranitidine Prophylaxis in Acute Gastric Mucosal Damage in Critically III Pediatric Patients," *Crit Care Med*, 1988, 16(6):591-93.
Morris DL, Markham SJ, Beechey A, et al, "Ranitidine-Bolus or Infusion Prophylaxis for Stress Ulcer," *Crit Care Med*, 1988, 16(3):229-32.
Roberts CJ, "Clinical Pharmacokinetics of Ranitidine," *Clin Pharmacokinet*, 1984, 9(3):211-21.
Sutphen JL and Dillard VL, "Effect of Ranitidine on Twenty-Four-Hour Gastric Acidity in Infants," *J Pediatr*, 1989, 114(3):472-4.
Terrin G, Passariello A, De Curtis M, et al, "Ranitidine Is Associated With Infections, Necrotizing Enterocolitis, and Fatal Outcome in Newborns," *Pediatrics*, 2012, 129(1):40-5.
Wells TG, Heuilitt MJ, Taylor BJ, et al, "Pharmacokinetics and Pharmacodynamics of Ranitidine in Neonates Treated With Extracorporeal Membrane Oxygenation," *J Clin Pharmacol*, 1998, 38(5):402-7.
Wheatley E and Kennedy KA, "Cross-Over Trial of Treatment for Bradycardia Attributed to Gastroesophageal Reflux in Preterm Infants," *J Pediatr*, 2009, 155(4):516-21.

◆ **Ranitidine Acid Reducer [OTC]** *see* Ranitidine *on page 1805*

◆ **Ranitidine Hydrochloride** *see* Ranitidine *on page 1805*

◆ **Ranitidine Injection, USP (Can)** *see* Ranitidine *on page 1805*

◆ **RAN-Letrozole (Can)** *see* Letrozole *on page 1211*

◆ **RAN-Levetiracetam (Can)** *see* LevETIRAcetam *on page 1219*

◆ **RAN-Lisinopril (Can)** *see* Lisinopril *on page 1262*

◆ **RAN-Losartan (Can)** *see* Losartan *on page 1283*

◆ **RAN™-Metformin (Can)** *see* MetFORMIN *on page 1353*

◆ **RAN-Montelukast (Can)** *see* Montelukast *on page 1438*

◆ **RAN™-Nabilone (Can)** *see* Nabilone *on page 1459*

◆ **RAN-Omeprazole (Can)** *see* Omeprazole *on page 1535*

◆ **RAN™-Ondansetron (Can)** *see* Ondansetron *on page 1544*

◆ **RAN-Pantoprazole (Can)** *see* Pantoprazole *on page 1595*

◆ **RAN-Pravastatin (Can)** *see* Pravastatin *on page 1720*

◆ **RAN-Quetiapine (Can)** *see* QUEtiapine *on page 1783*

◆ **RAN-Rabeprazole (Can)** *see* RABEprazole *on page 1797*

◆ **RAN-Ranitidine (Can)** *see* Ranitidine *on page 1805*

◆ **RAN-Risperidone (Can)** *see* RisperiDONE *on page 1831*

◆ **RAN-Rosuvastatin (Can)** *see* Rosuvastatin *on page 1853*

◆ **Ran-Sertraline (Can)** *see* Sertraline *on page 1879*

◆ **RAN-Simvastatin (Can)** *see* Simvastatin *on page 1892*

◆ **RAN-Topiramate (Can)** *see* Topiramate *on page 2046*

◆ **Ran-Valsartan (Can)** *see* Valsartan *on page 2108*

◆ **Ran-Venlafaxine XR (Can)** *see* Venlafaxine *on page 2125*

◆ **Rapamune** *see* Sirolimus *on page 1895*

◆ **Rapamune® (Can)** *see* Sirolimus *on page 1895*

◆ **Rapamycin** *see* Sirolimus *on page 1895*

◆ **RapiMed Children's [OTC]** *see* Acetaminophen *on page 47*

◆ **RapiMed Junior [OTC]** *see* Acetaminophen *on page 47*

Rasburicase (ras BYOOR i kayse)

Brand Names: U.S. Elitek

Brand Names: Canada Fasturtec®

Therapeutic Category Enzyme; Uric Acid Lowering Agent

Generic Availability (U.S.) No

Use Initial management of plasma uric acid levels in patients with leukemia, lymphoma, and solid tumor malignancies who are receiving anticancer therapy expected to result in tumor lysis and subsequent elevation of plasma uric acid (FDA approved in ages ≥1 month and adults)

Pregnancy Risk Factor C

Pregnancy Considerations Adverse effects were observed in animal reproduction studies. There are no adequate and well-controlled studies in pregnant women. Use during pregnancy only if the benefit to the mother outweighs the potential risk to the fetus.

Breast-Feeding Considerations Due to the potential for serious adverse reactions in the nursing infant, the decision to discontinue breast-feeding or to discontinue rasburicase should take into account the benefits of treatment to the mother.

Contraindications History of anaphylaxis or severe hypersensitivity to rasburicase or any component; history of hemolytic reaction or methemoglobinemia associated with rasburicase; glucose-6-phosphatase dehydrogenase (G6PD) deficiency

Warnings Severe hypersensitivity reactions (including anaphylaxis) have been reported; immediately and permanently discontinue in patients developing serious hypersensitivity reaction **[U.S. Boxed Warning]**. Reactions may occur at any time during treatment (including the initial dose); signs and symptoms may include bronchospasm, chest pain/tightness, dyspnea, hypotension, hypoxia, shock, or urticaria. The safety and efficacy of more than one course of administration has not been established.

Patients at higher risk for G6PD deficiency (eg, African, Mediterranean, or Southeast Asian descent) should be screened prior to therapy **[U.S. Boxed Warning]**. Severe hemolytic reactions occurred within 2-4 days of rasburicase initiation. Due to the risk for hemolysis (<1%), rasburicase is contraindicated in patients with G6PD deficiency. Discontinue immediately and permanently in any patient developing hemolysis. Methemoglobinemia has been reported (<1%). Discontinue immediately and permanently in any patient developing methemoglobinemia **[U.S. Boxed Warning]**. Initiate appropriate treatment (eg, transfusion, methylene blue) if methemoglobinemia occurs.

Precautions Patients at risk for tumor lysis syndrome should receive appropriate I.V. hydration as part of uric acid management; however, alkalinization (with sodium bicarbonate) concurrently with rasburicase is not recommended (Coiffier, 2008). Enzymatic degradation of uric acid in blood samples will occur if left at room temperature **[U.S. Boxed Warning]; may interfere with serum uric acid measurements;** specific guidelines for the collection of plasma uric acid samples must be followed including collection in prechilled tubes with heparin anticoagulant, immediate ice water bath immersion and assay within 4 hours. Rasburicase is immunogenic and can elicit an antibody response; efficacy may be reduced with subsequent courses of therapy; the safety and efficacy of more than one course of administration has not been established.

Data suggest that children <2 years of age may experience a higher frequency of adverse effects than adults, particularly vomiting (75% vs 55%), diarrhea (63% vs 20%), fever (50% vs 38%), and rash (38% vs 10%).

Adverse Reactions

Cardiovascular: Fluid overload, ischemic coronary disease, peripheral edema, supraventricular arrhythmia

Central nervous system: Anxiety, fever, headache,

Dermatologic: Rash

Endocrine & metabolic: Hyper-/hypophosphatemia

Gastrointestinal: Abdominal/gastrointestinal infection, abdominal pain, constipation, diarrhea, mucositis, nausea, vomiting

Hematologic: Neutropenia, neutropenia with fever

Hepatic: ALT increased, hyperbilirubinemia

Respiratory: Pharyngolaryngeal pain, pulmonary hemorrhage, respiratory distress/failure

Miscellaneous: Antibody formation, hypersensitivity, sepsis

Rare but important or life-threatening: Acute renal failure, anaphylaxis, arrhythmia, cardiac arrest, cardiac failure, cellulitis, cerebrovascular disorder, chest pain, cyanosis, dehydration, hemolysis, hemorrhage, hot flashes, ileus, infection, intestinal obstruction, liver enzymes increased, methemoglobinemia, MI, pancytopenia, paresthesia, pneumonia, pulmonary edema, pulmonary hypertension, retinal hemorrhage, rigors, seizure, thrombosis, thrombophlebitis

Drug Interactions

Metabolism/Transport Effects None known.

Avoid Concomitant Use There are no known interactions where it is recommended to avoid concomitant use.

Increased Effect/Toxicity There are no known significant interactions involving an increase in effect.

Decreased Effect There are no known significant interactions involving a decrease in effect.

Stability Prior to reconstitution, store intact vial with diluent at 2°C to 8°C (36°F to 46°F); do not freeze. Protect from light. Reconstituted and final solution may be stored up to 24 hours at 2°C to 8°C (36°F to 46°F). Discard unused product.

Mechanism of Action Rasburicase is a recombinant urate-oxidase enzyme, which converts uric acid to allantoin (an inactive and soluble metabolite of uric acid); it does not inhibit the formation of uric acid.

Pharmacodynamics Onset: Uric acid levels decrease within 4 hours of initial administration

Pharmacokinetics (Adult data unless noted)

Distribution: V_d: Children: 110-127 mL/kg

Half-life: Children: 18 hours

Dosing: Usual

Infants, Children, and Adolescents: **Hyperuricemia associated with malignancy:** I.V.:

Multiple-dosing:

Manufacturer's labeling (Elitek): 0.2 mg/kg/dose once daily for up to 5 days. **Note:** Limited data suggest that a single prechemotherapy dose (versus multiple-day administration) may be sufficiently efficacious. Monitoring electrolytes, hydration status, and uric acid concentrations are necessary to identify the need for additional doses. Other clinical manifestations of tumor lysis syndrome (eg, hyperphosphatemia, hypocalcemia, and hyperkalemia) may occur.

Alternate dosing (Coiffier, 2008): Limited data available: 0.05-0.2 mg/kg once daily for 1-7 days (average of 2-3 days) with the duration of treatment dependent on plasma uric acid levels and clinical judgment (patients with significant tumor burden may require an increase to twice daily); the following dose levels are recommended based on risk of tumor lysis syndrome (TLS):

High risk and baseline uric acid level >7.5 mg/dL: 0.2 mg/kg once daily (duration is based on plasma uric acid levels)

Intermediate risk and baseline uric acid level <7.5 mg/dL: 0.15 mg/kg once daily (duration is based on plasma uric acid levels); may consider managing initially with a single dose

Low risk and baseline uric acid level <7.5 mg/dL: 0.1 mg/kg once daily (duration is based on clinical judgment); a dose of 0.05 mg/kg was used (with good results) in one trial

Single-dose: Limited data available: 0.15 mg/kg; additional doses may be needed based on serum uric acid levels (Liu, 2005)

Adults: **Hyperuricemia associated with malignancy:** I.V.:

Manufacturer's labeling: 0.2 mg/kg once daily for up to 5 days (manufacturer recommended dose) **or**

Alternate dosing (Coiffier, 2008): 0.05-0.2 mg/kg once daily for 1-7 days (average: 2-3 days) with the duration of treatment dependent on plasma uric acid levels and clinical judgment (patients with significant tumor burden may require an increase to twice daily); the following dose levels are recommended based on risk of tumor lysis syndrome (TLS):

High risk: 0.2 mg/kg once daily (duration is based on plasma uric acid levels)

Intermediate risk: 0.15 mg/kg once daily (duration is based on plasma uric acid levels)

Low risk: 0.1 mg/kg once daily (duration is based on clinical judgment); a dose of 0.05 mg/kg was used effectively in one trial

Dosing adjustment in renal impairment: There is no dosage adjustment provided in manufacturer's labeling.

Dosing adjustment in hepatic impairment: There is no dosage adjustment provided in manufacturer's labeling.

Administration I.V.: Dilute each 1.5 mg vial with 1 mL or 7.5 mg vial with 5 mL of provided diluent; gently swirl, do not shake; further dilute desired dose in NS to a final volume of 50 mL; infuse over 30 minutes, do not bolus; do not filter or mix with other medications. The optimal timing of rasburicase administration (with respect to chemotherapy administration) is not specified in the manufacturer's labeling. In some studies, chemotherapy was administered 4-24 hours after the first rasburicase dose (Cortes, 2010; Kikuchi, 2009; Vadhan-Raj, 2012); however, rasburicase generally may be administered irrespective of chemotherapy timing.

Monitoring Parameters Plasma uric acid levels (4 hours after rasburicase administration, then every 6-8 hours until TLS resolution), CBC, G6PD deficiency screening (in patients at high risk for deficiency); monitor for hypersensitivity

Test Interactions Specific handling procedures must be followed to prevent the degradation of uric acid in plasma samples. Blood must be collected in prechilled tubes containing heparin anticoagulant. Samples must then be **immediately** immersed in an ice water bath. Prepare samples by centrifugation in a precooled centrifuge (4°C). Samples must be kept in ice water bath and analyzed within 4 hours of collection.

Dosage Forms Excipient information presented when available (limited, particularly for generics); consult specific product labeling.

Solution Reconstituted, Intravenous:

Elitek: 1.5 mg (1 ea); 7.5 mg (1 ea)

References

Coiffier B, Altman A, Pui CH, et al, "Guidelines for the Management of Pediatric and Adult Tumor Lysis Syndrome: An Evidence-Based Review," *J Clin Oncol*, 2008, 26(16):2767-78.

Coiffier B, Mounier N, Bologna S, et al, "Efficacy and Safety of Rasburicase (Recombinant Urate Oxidase) for the Prevention and Treatment of Hyperuricemia During Induction Chemotherapy of Aggressive Non-Hodgkin's Lymphoma: Results of the GRAAL1 (Groupe d'Etude des Lymphomes de l'Adulte Trial on Rasburicase Activity in Adult Lymphoma) Study," *J Clin Oncol*, 2003, 21(23):4402-6.

Cortes J, Moore JO, Maziarz RT, et al, "Control of Plasma Uric Acid in Adults at Risk for Tumor Lysis Syndrome: Efficacy and Safety of Rasburicase Alone and Rasburicase Followed by Allopurinol Compared With Allopurinol Alone – Results of a Multicenter Phase III Study," *J Clin Oncol*, 2010, 28(27):4207-13.

Goldman SC, Holcenberg JS, Finklestein JZ, et al, "A Randomized Comparison Between Rasburicase and Allopurinol in Children With Lymphoma or Leukemia at High Risk for Tumor Lysis," *Blood*, 2001, 97(10):2998-3003.

Jeha S, Kantarjian H, Irwin D, et al, "Efficacy and Safety of Rasburicase, a Recombinant Urate Oxidase (Elitek), in the Management of Malignancy-Associated Hyperuricemia in Pediatric and Adult Patients: Final Results of a Multicenter Compassionate Use Trial," *Leukemia*, 2005, 19(1):34-8.

Kikuchi A, Kigasawa H, Tsurusawa M, et al, "A Study of Rasburicase for the Management of Hyperuricemia in Pediatric Patients With Newly Diagnosed Hematologic Malignancies at High Risk for Tumor Lysis Syndrome," *Int J Hematol*, 2009, 90(4):492-500.

Liu CY, Sims-McCallum RP, and Schiffer CA, "A Single Dose of Rasburicase Is Sufficient for the Treatment of Hyperuricemia in Patients Receiving Chemotherapy," *Leuk Res*, 2005, 29(4):463-5.

Pui CH, Mahmoud HH, Wiley JM, et al, "Recombinant Urate Oxidase for the Prophylaxis or Treatment of Hyperuricemia in Patients With Leukemia or Lymphoma," *J Clin Oncol*, 2001, 19(3):697-704.

Vadhan-Raj S, Fayad LE, Fanale MA, et al, "A Randomized Trial of a Single-Dose Rasburicase Versus Five-Daily Doses in Patients at Risk for Tumor Lysis Syndrome," *Ann Oncol*, 2012, 23(6):1640-5.

◆ **rATG** *see* Antithymocyte Globulin (Rabbit) *on page 184*

◆ **ratio-Aclavulanate (Can)** *see* Amoxicillin and Clavulanate *on page 144*

◆ **ratio-Acyclovir (Can)** *see* Acyclovir (Systemic) *on page 63*

◆ **ratio-Amiodarone (Can)** *see* Amiodarone *on page 127*

◆ **ratio-Amlodipine (Can)** *see* AmLODIPine *on page 135*

◆ **ratio-Atenolol (Can)** *see* Atenolol *on page 222*

◆ **ratio-Atorvastatin (Can)** *see* AtorvaSTATin *on page 227*

◆ **ratio-Azithromycin (Can)** *see* Azithromycin (Systemic) *on page 247*

◆ **ratio-Baclofen (Can)** *see* Baclofen *on page 259*

◆ **ratio-Bisacodyl [OTC] (Can)** *see* Bisacodyl *on page 293*

◆ **ratio-Brimonidine (Can)** *see* Brimonidine (Ophthalmic) *on page 303*

◆ **ratio-Bupropion SR (Can)** *see* BuPROPion *on page 327*

◆ **ratio-Carvedilol (Can)** *see* Carvedilol *on page 385*

◆ **ratio-Cefuroxime (Can)** *see* Cefuroxime *on page 422*

◆ **ratio-Ciprofloxacin (Can)** *see* Ciprofloxacin (Systemic) *on page 471*

◆ **ratio-Citalopram (Can)** *see* Citalopram *on page 484*

◆ **ratio-Clarithromycin (Can)** *see* Clarithromycin *on page 490*

◆ **ratio-Clobetasol (Can)** *see* Clobetasol *on page 506*

◆ **ratio-Clonazepam (Can)** *see* ClonazePAM *on page 514*

◆ **ratio-Codeine (Can)** *see* Codeine *on page 534*

◆ **ratio-Cyclobenzaprine (Can)** *see* Cyclobenzaprine *on page 558*

◆ **ratio-Dexamethasone (Can)** *see* Dexamethasone (Systemic) *on page 615*

◆ **ratio-Diltiazem CD (Can)** *see* Diltiazem *on page 667*

◆ **ratio-Docusate Sodium [OTC] (Can)** *see* Docusate *on page 701*

◆ **ratio-Ectosone (Can)** *see* Betamethasone (Topical) *on page 285*

◆ **ratio-Emtec-30 (Can)** *see* Acetaminophen and Codeine *on page 53*

◆ **ratio-Enalapril (Can)** *see* Enalapril *on page 744*

◆ **ratio-Fentanyl (Can)** *see* FentaNYL *on page 853*

◆ **ratio-Fluoxetine (Can)** *see* FLUoxetine *on page 901*

◆ **ratio-Fluticasone (Can)** *see* Fluticasone (Nasal) *on page 913*

◆ **ratio-Fluvoxamine (Can)** *see* FluvoxaMINE *on page 922*

◆ **ratio-Gabapentin (Can)** *see* Gabapentin *on page 950*

◆ **ratio-Gentamicin (Can)** *see* Gentamicin (Topical) *on page 967*

◆ **ratio-Glyburide (Can)** *see* GlyBURIDE *on page 974*

◆ **ratio-Indomethacin (Can)** *see* Indomethacin *on page 1096*

◆ **ratio-Ipra-Sal (Can)** *see* Albuterol *on page 84*

◆ **ratio-Ipratropium UDV (Can)** *see* Ipratropium (Oral Inhalation) *on page 1144*

◆ **ratio-Irbesartan (Can)** *see* Irbesartan *on page 1147*

◆ **ratio-Ketorolac (Can)** *see* Ketorolac (Ophthalmic) *on page 1184*

◆ **ratio-Lamotrigine (Can)** *see* LamoTRIgine *on page 1199*

◆ **ratio-Lenoltec (Can)** *see* Acetaminophen and Codeine *on page 53*

◆ **Ratio-Levobunolol (Can)** *see* Levobunolol *on page 1223*

◆ **ratio-Lisinopril P (Can)** *see* Lisinopril *on page 1262*

◆ **ratio-Lisinopril Z (Can)** *see* Lisinopril *on page 1262*

◆ **ratio-Meloxicam (Can)** *see* Meloxicam *on page 1325*

◆ **ratio-Metformin (Can)** *see* MetFORMIN *on page 1353*

◆ **ratio-Methotrexate Sodium (Can)** *see* Methotrexate *on page 1367*

◆ **ratio-Methylphenidate (Can)** *see* Methylphenidate *on page 1379*

◆ **ratio-Minocycline (Can)** *see* Minocycline *on page 1420*

◆ **ratio-Mometasone (Can)** *see* Mometasone (Topical) *on page 1435*

◆ **ratio-Morphine (Can)** *see* Morphine (Systemic) *on page 1440*

◆ **ratio-Morphine SR (Can)** *see* Morphine (Systemic) *on page 1440*

◆ **ratio-Omeprazole (Can)** *see* Omeprazole *on page 1535*

◆ **ratio-Ondansetron (Can)** *see* Ondansetron *on page 1544*

◆ **ratio-Orciprenaline® (Can)** *see* Metaproterenol *on page 1352*

◆ **Ratio-Oxycocet (Can)** *see* Oxycodone and Acetaminophen *on page 1573*

◆ **ratio-Pantoprazole (Can)** *see* Pantoprazole *on page 1595*

◆ **ratio-Paroxetine (Can)** *see* PARoxetine *on page 1609*

◆ **ratio-Pravastatin (Can)** *see* Pravastatin *on page 1720*

◆ **Ratio-Prednisolone (Can)** *see* PrednisoLONE (Ophthalmic) *on page 1730*

◆ **ratio-Quetiapine (Can)** *see* QUEtiapine *on page 1783*

◆ **ratio-Ranitidine (Can)** *see* Ranitidine *on page 1805*

◆ **ratio-Risperidone (Can)** *see* RisperiDONE *on page 1831*

◆ **ratio-Salbutamol (Can)** *see* Albuterol *on page 84*

◆ **ratio-Sertraline (Can)** *see* Sertraline *on page 1879*

◆ **ratio-Sildenafil R (Can)** *see* Sildenafil *on page 1884*

◆ **ratio-Simvastatin (Can)** *see* Simvastatin *on page 1892*

◆ **ratio-Sotalol (Can)** *see* Sotalol *on page 1925*

◆ **ratio-Terazosin (Can)** *see* Terazosin *on page 1981*

◆ **ratio-Theo-Bronc (Can)** *see* Theophylline *on page 2005*

◆ **Ratio-Topilene (Can)** *see* Betamethasone (Topical) *on page 285*

◆ **Ratio-Topisone (Can)** *see* Betamethasone (Topical) *on page 285*

◆ **ratio-Trazodone (Can)** *see* TraZODone *on page 2065*

◆ **ratio-Valproic (Can)** *see* Valproic Acid and Derivatives *on page 2102*

◆ **Rayos** *see* PredniSONE *on page 1732*

◆ **6R-BH4** *see* Sapropterin *on page 1865*

◆ **Reactine [OTC] (Can)** *see* Cetirizine *on page 431*

◆ **Rebetol** *see* Ribavirin *on page 1818*

◆ **Recombinant α-L-Iduronidase (Glycosaminoglycan α-L-Iduronohydrolase)** *see* Laronidase *on page 1210*

◆ **Recombinant Granulocyte-Macrophage Colony Stimulating Factor** *see* Sargramostim *on page 1870*

◆ **Recombinant Human Deoxyribonuclease** *see* Dornase Alfa *on page 709*

◆ **Recombinant Human Insulin-Like Growth Factor-1** *see* Mecasermin *on page 1313*

◆ **Recombinant Human Interleukin-2** *see* Aldesleukin *on page 90*

◆ **Recombinant Human Interleukin-11** *see* Oprelvekin *on page 1549*

◆ **Recombinant Influenza Vaccine, Trivalent** *see* Influenza Virus Vaccine (Recombinant) *on page 1112*

◆ **Recombinant Interleukin-11** *see* Oprelvekin *on page 1549*

◆ **Recombinant N-Acetylgalactosamine 4-Sulfatase** *see* Galsulfase *on page 953*

◆ **Recombinant Urate Oxidase** *see* Rasburicase *on page 1808*

◆ **Recombinate** *see* Antihemophilic Factor (Recombinant) *on page 172*

◆ **Recombivax HB** *see* Hepatitis B Vaccine (Recombinant) *on page 1009*

◆ **Recort Plus [OTC]** *see* Hydrocortisone (Topical) *on page 1038*

◆ **Recothrom®** *see* Thrombin (Topical) *on page 2017*

◆ **Rectacaine [OTC]** *see* Phenylephrine (Topical) *on page 1662*

◆ **Rectacort-HC** *see* Hydrocortisone (Topical) *on page 1038*

◆ **RectiCare [OTC]** *see* Lidocaine (Topical) *on page 1242*

◆ **Rectiv** *see* Nitroglycerin *on page 1504*

◆ **Rederm [OTC]** *see* Hydrocortisone (Topical) *on page 1038*

◆ **Reeses Pinworm Medicine [OTC]** *see* Pyrantel Pamoate *on page 1774*

◆ **Refenesen [OTC]** *see* GuaiFENesin *on page 984*

◆ **Refenesen 400 [OTC]** *see* GuaiFENesin *on page 984*

◆ **Refenesen DM [OTC]** *see* Guaifenesin and Dextromethorphan *on page 987*

◆ **Refissa** *see* Tretinoin (Topical) *on page 2071*

◆ **Refresh® Lacri-Lube® [OTC]** *see* Ocular Lubricant *on page 1521*

◆ **Regitine [DSC]** *see* Phentolamine *on page 1656*

◆ **Reglan** *see* Metoclopramide *on page 1391*

◆ **Regonol** *see* Pyridostigmine *on page 1776*

◆ **Regular Insulin** *see* Insulin Regular *on page 1134*

◆ **Reguloid [OTC]** *see* Psyllium *on page 1773*

◆ **Rejuva-A (Can)** *see* Tretinoin (Topical) *on page 2071*

◆ **Relaxa (Can)** *see* Polyethylene Glycol 3350 *on page 1696*

◆ **Relenza® (Can)** *see* Zanamivir *on page 2166*

◆ **Relenza Diskhaler** *see* Zanamivir *on page 2166*

◆ **Remedy Antifungal [OTC]** *see* Miconazole (Topical) *on page 1410*

◆ **Remicade** *see* InFLIXimab *on page 1099*

◆ **Remicade® (Can)** *see* InFLIXimab *on page 1099*

Remifentanil (rem i FEN ta nil)

Medication Safety Issues
Sound-alike/look-alike issues:
Remifentanil may be confused with alfentanil
High alert medication:
The Institute for Safe Medication Practices (ISMP) includes this medication among its list of drug classes which have a heightened risk of causing significant patient harm when used in error.

Brand Names: U.S. Ultiva

Brand Names: Canada Ultiva®

Therapeutic Category Analgesic, Narcotic; General Anesthetic

Generic Availability (U.S.) No

Use Analgesic for use during the induction of general anesthesia (FDA approved in adults); maintenance of general anesthesia (FDA approved in ages 0-2 months, 1-12 years, and adults); continued analgesia into the immediate postoperative period (FDA approved in adults); as the analgesic component of monitored anesthesia (FDA approved in adults); has also been used as adjunct for analgesia during endotracheal intubation, for total intravenous anesthesia (TIVA), and for continuous analgesia/sedation in critically ill mechanically ventilated patients.

Pregnancy Risk Factor C

Pregnancy Considerations Adverse events were not observed in animal reproduction studies. Remifentanil has been shown to cross the placenta; fetal and maternal concentrations may be similar.

Breast-Feeding Considerations It is not known if remifentanil is excreted into breast milk. The manufacturer recommends that caution be used if administered to a nursing woman. Remifentanil has a limited duration of action; use may be appropriate for breast-feeding women undergoing short procedures (Montgomery, 2012).

Contraindications Hypersensitivity to remifentanil, fentanyl or fentanyl analogs, or any component; **not for intrathecal or epidural administration,** due to the presence of glycine in the formulation

Warnings Remifentanil is not recommended as the sole agent in general anesthesia, because the loss of consciousness cannot be assured and due to the high incidence of apnea, hypotension, tachycardia, and muscle rigidity; it should be administered by individuals specifically trained in the use of anesthetic agents and should not be used in diagnostic or therapeutic procedures outside the monitored anesthesia setting; resuscitative and intubation equipment should be readily available; monitor vital signs and oxygenation continuously during administration. May cause hypotension; use with caution in patients with hypovolemia, cardiovascular disease (including acute MI), or drugs which may exaggerate hypotensive effects (including phenothiazines or general anesthetics).

May cause chest wall or skeletal muscle rigidity leading to impaired ventilation or respiratory distress/arrest; has been reported with rapid I.V. infusion (eg, single doses of >1 mcg/kg administered over 30-60 seconds or infusion rates >0.1 mcg/kg/minute), single doses <1 mcg/kg when used concurrently with continuous infusion of remifentanil, and inadequate clearing of I.V. tubing following remifentanil administration when another fluid is administered through the same line (ensure line clear upon completion of administration). If muscle rigidity occurs, slow infusion rate, administration of a neuromuscular blocking agent may be necessary. Use of a skeletal muscle relaxant, propofol, or thiopental prior to or during remifentanil infusion may also reduce muscle rigidity. Limit use of single doses of >1 mcg/kg administered over 30-60 seconds or infusion rates >0.1 mcg/kg/minute to maintenance of general anesthesia.

Interruption of an infusion will result in offset of effects within 5-10 minutes; the discontinuation of remifentanil infusion should be preceded by the establishment of adequate postoperative analgesia orders, especially for patients in whom postoperative pain is anticipated

Precautions Use with caution in the morbidly obese due to differences in cardiovascular and respiratory physiology. Use with caution when administering to patients with bradycardia. In patients <55 years of age, intraoperative awareness has been reported when used with propofol rates of ≤75 mcg/kg/minute. Use with caution in patients with a history of drug abuse or acute alcoholism; potential for drug dependency exists; tolerance, psychological and physical dependence may occur with prolonged use.

Adverse Reactions
Cardiovascular: Bradycardia (dose dependent), flushing, hypertension (dose dependent), hypotension, tachycardia (dose dependent)

Central nervous system: Agitation, chills, dizziness, fever, headache, postoperative pain

Dermatologic: Pruritus

Gastrointestinal: Nausea, vomiting

Local: Pain at injection site

Neuromuscular & skeletal: Muscle rigidity

Respiratory: Apnea, hypoxia, respiratory depression

Miscellaneous: Diaphoresis, shivering, warm sensation

Rare but important or life-threatening: Abdominal discomfort, amnesia, anaphylaxis, anxiety, arrhythmias, awareness under anesthesia without pain, bronchitis, bronchospasm, chest pain, confusion, constipation, cough, CPK increased, diarrhea, disorientation, dysphagia, dysphoria, dyspnea, dysuria, ECG changes, electrolyte disorders, erythema, gastroesophageal reflux, hallucinations, heart block, heartburn, hiccups, hyperglycemia, ileus, incontinence, involuntary movement, laryngospasm, leukocytosis, liver dysfunction, lymphopenia, nasal congestion, nightmares, nystagmus, oliguria, paresthesia, pharyngitis, pleural effusion, prolonged emergence from anesthesia, pulmonary edema, rales, rapid awakening from anesthesia, rash, rhinorrhea, rhonchi, seizure, sleep disturbance, stridor, syncope, temperature regulation impaired, thrombocytopenia, tremors, twitching, urine retention, urticaria, xerostomia

Drug Interactions
Metabolism/Transport Effects None known.

Avoid Concomitant Use
Avoid concomitant use of Remifentanil with any of the following: Azelastine (Nasal); MAO Inhibitors; Paraldehyde; Thalidomide

Increased Effect/Toxicity
Remifentanil may increase the levels/effects of: Alcohol (Ethyl); Alvimopan; Azelastine (Nasal); Beta-Blockers; Buprenorphine; Calcium Channel Blockers

◄ (Nondihydropyridine); CNS Depressants; Desmopressin; Diuretics; Hydrocodone; MAO Inhibitors; Methotrimeprazine; Metyrosine; Mirtazapine; Paraldehyde; Pramipexole; ROPINIRole; Rotigotine; Selective Serotonin Reuptake Inhibitors; Thalidomide; Zolpidem

The levels/effects of Remifentanil may be increased by: Amphetamines; Anticholinergic Agents; Antipsychotic Agents (Phenothiazines); Brimonidine (Topical); Cannabis; Doxylamine; Dronabinol; Droperidol; HydrOXYzine; Kava Kava; Magnesium Sulfate; Methotrimeprazine; Nabilone; Perampanel; Rufinamide; Sodium Oxybate; Succinylcholine; Tapentadol; Tetrahydrocannabinol

Decreased Effect

Remifentanil may decrease the levels/effects of: Pegvisomant

The levels/effects of Remifentanil may be decreased by: Ammonium Chloride; Mixed Agonist / Antagonist Opioids; Naltrexone

Stability Prior to reconstitution, store at 2°C to 25°C (36°F to 77°F). Stable for 24 hours at room temperature after reconstitution and further dilution to concentrations of 20-250 mcg/mL in D_5LR, D_5NS, D_5W, 1/2NS, NS, (4 hours if diluted with LR).

Y-site administration: Compatible: Acyclovir, alfentanil, amikacin, aminophylline, ampicillin, ampicillin/sulbactam, aztreonam, bretylium, bumetanide, buprenorphine, butorphanol, calcium gluconate, cefazolin, cefotaxime, cefotetan, cefoxitin, ceftazidime, ceftizoxime, ceftriaxone, cefuroxime, cimetidine, ciprofloxacin, cisatracurium, clindamycin, dexamethasone sodium phosphate, digoxin, diphenhydramine, dobutamine, dopamine, doxycycline, droperidol, enalaprilat, epinephrine, esmolol, famotidine, fentanyl, fluconazole, furosemide, ganciclovir gatifloxacin, gentamicin, haloperidol, heparin, hydrocortisone sodium succinate, hydromorphone, hydroxyzine, imipenem/cilastatin, inamrinone, isoproterenol, ketorolac, lidocaine, linezolid, lorazepam, magnesium sulfate, mannitol, meperidine, methylprednisolone sodium succinate, metoclopramide, metronidazole, midazolam, minocycline, morphine, nalbuphine, netilmicin, nitroglycerin, norepinephrine, ofloxacin, ondansetron, phenylephrine, piperacillin, piperacillin/tazobactam, potassium chloride, procainamide, prochlorperazine, propofol, promethazine, ranitidine, sodium bicarbonate, sufentanil, theophylline, thiopental, ticarcillin, ticarcillin/clavulanate potassium, tobramycin, trimethoprim/sulfamethoxazole, vancomycin, zidovudine.

Mechanism of Action Binds with stereospecific mu-opioid receptors at many sites within the CNS, increases pain threshold, alters pain reception, inhibits ascending pain pathways

Pharmacodynamics

Analgesia:

Onset of action: 1-3 minutes

Maximum effect: 3-5 minutes

Duration: 3-10 minutes (Scott, 2005)

Pharmacokinetics (Adult data unless noted) Note: In pediatric patients (neonates through adolescents), pharmacokinetic data showed variable age-related changes with distribution (ie, highest V_d associated with lowest age) and clearance (ie, fastest clearance in the youngest patients); however, no age-related changes with half-life (Ross, 2001).

Distribution:

Pediatric patients (Ross, 2001): V_{dss}:

Neonates ≤2 months: 453 ± 145 mL/kg

Infants and Children >2 months to <2 years: 308 ± 89 mL/kg

Children 2-6 years: 240 mL/kg ± 131 mL/kg

Children 7-12 years: 249 mL/kg ± 91 mL/kg

Adolescents 13 to <16 years: 223 ± 31 mL/kg

Adolescents 16-18 years: 243 ± 109 mL/kg

Adults: V_d: Initial: 100 mL/kg; V_{dss}: 350 mL/kg

Protein binding: ~70% (primarily alpha$_1$ acid glycoprotein)

Metabolism: Rapid via blood and tissue esterases; not metabolized by plasma cholinesterase (pseudocholinesterase) and is not appreciably metabolized by the liver

Half-life (dose dependent):

Pediatric patients (Ross, 2001): Effective:

Neonates ≤2 months: 5.4 minutes (range: 3-8 minutes)

Infants and Children >2 months to <2 years: 3.4 minutes (range: 2-6 minutes)

Children 2-6 years: 3.6 minutes (range: 1-6 minutes)

Children 7-12 years: 5.3 minutes (range: 3-7 minutes)

Adolescents: 13 to <16 years: 3.7 minutes (range: 2-5 minutes)

Adolescents 16-18 years: 5.7 minutes (range: 5-6 minutes)

Adults: Terminal: 10-20 minutes; effective: 3-10 minutes

Time to peak serum concentration: Intranasal: Children ≤7 years: ~3.5 minutes (Verghese, 2008)

Elimination: Clearance:

Pediatric patients (Ross, 2001):

Neonates ≤2 months of age: 90.5 ± 36.8 mL/minute/kg

Infants and Children >2 months to <2 years: 92.1 ± 25.8 mL/minute/kg

Children 2-6 years: 76.0 ± 22.4 mL/minute/kg

Children 7-12 years: 59.7 ± 22.5 mL/minute/kg

Adolescents 13 to <16 years: 57.2 ± 21.2 mL/minute/kg

Adolescents 16-18 years: 46.5 ± 2.1 mL/minute/kg

Adults: ~40 mL/minute/kg

Dosing: Neonatal

Anesthesia, maintenance of anesthesia with nitrous oxide (70%): Continuous I.V. infusion: 0.4 mcg/kg/minute (range: 0.4-1 mcg/kg/minute); supplemental bolus dose of 1 mcg/kg may be administered; smaller bolus dose may be required with potent inhalation agents, potent neuraxial anesthesia, significant comorbidities, significant fluid shifts, or without atropine pretreatment. Clearance in neonates is highly variable; dose should be carefully titrated.

Analgesia/sedation in mechanically ventilated patients: Limited data available, dosage not established: Continuous I.V. infusion:

Preterm infants: Initial: 0.075 mcg/kg/minute, titrate to effect; dosing based on a trial in 48 preterm infants requiring mechanical ventilation (GA: Mean: 28.5 weeks, range: 25-33 weeks; PNA: 1-17 days); in a large majority of the patients (73%), dose escalation from the initial dose was required within the first 6 hours of therapy; mean effective dose: 0.11 ±0.05 mcg/kg/minute, maximum reported dose: 0.94 mcg/kg/minute. No cardiovascular or respiratory adverse effects were observed (Giannantonio, 2009).

Term infants: Initial: 0.15 mcg/kg/minute, titrate to effect; dosing based on a randomized, double-blind, comparative study of neonates and young infants (n=23; GA: ≥36 weeks; PNA: <60 days) requiring mechanical ventilation who were given a combination of either midazolam/remifentanil (n=11) or midazolam/fentanyl (n=12); mean remifentanil effective dose: 0.23 mcg/kg/minute; maximum reported dose: 0.5 mcg/kg/minute; efficacy data and adverse effect profile were similar to fentanyl (Welzing, 2012)

Endotracheal intubation, nonemergent: Limited data available: I.V.: 1-3 mcg/kg/dose; may repeat dose in 2-3 minutes if needed (Choong, 2010; Kumar, 2010; Silva, 2008)

Dosing: Usual

Infants, Children, and Adolescents: **Note:** Continuous I.V. infusion: Dose should be based on ideal body weight (IBW) in obese patients (>30% over IBW).

Analgesia (postoperative); mechanically ventilated patient: Limited data available: Children and

Adolescents 3-16 years: Continuous I.V. infusion: 0.1 mcg/kg/minute with or without adjunctive medication, titrate to effect; dosing based on a randomized, double-blind comparative trial of remifentanil versus fentanyl in 22 postoperative orthopedic spinal surgery patients requiring mechanical ventilation (remifentanil group, n=11; age: Mean:13 years, range: 3-16 years); similar efficacy and adverse effect profile were reported with both treatment groups (Akinci, 2005)

Analgesia/sedation in mechanically ventilated patients: Limited data available: Infants ≤2 months: Continuous I.V. infusion: Initial: 0.15 mcg/kg/minute, titrate to effect; dosing based on a randomized, double-blind, comparative study of neonates and young infants (n=23; GA: ≥36 weeks; PNA: <60 days) requiring mechanical ventilation who were given a combination of either midazolam/remifentanil (n=11) or midazolam/fentanyl (n=12); mean remifentanil effective dose: 0.23 mcg/kg/minute; maximum reported dose: 0.5 mcg/kg/minute; efficacy data and adverse effect profile were similar to fentanyl (Welzing, 2012)

Anesthesia, maintenance of anesthesia: Continuous I.V. infusion:

Infants 1-2 months: Maintenance of anesthesia with nitrous oxide (70%): 0.4 mcg/kg/minute (range: 0.4-1 mcg/kg/minute); supplemental bolus dose of 1 mcg/kg may be administered, smaller bolus dose may be required with potent inhalation agents, potent neuraxial anesthesia, significant comorbidities, significant fluid shifts, or without atropine pretreatment

Infants ≥3 months, Children, and Adolescents: Limited data available: Maintenance of anesthesia with halothane, sevoflurane, or isoflurane: 0.25 mcg/kg/minute (range: 0.05-1.3 mcg/kg/minute); supplemental bolus dose of 1 mcg/kg may be administered every 2-5 minutes. Consider increasing concomitant anesthetics with infusion rate >1 mcg/kg/minute. Infusion rate can be titrated upward in increments up to 50% or titrated downward in decrements of 25% to 50%. May titrate every 2-5 minutes.

Anesthesia, total intravenous (TIVA); with or without propofol induction: Limited data available: I.V.: Loading dose (may omit if propofol induction used): 0.5 mcg/kg/minute for 3 minutes (total dose: 1.5 mcg/kg) or 1 mcg/kg over 1 minute; followed by an initial maintenance dose: 0.05-1 mcg/kg/minute; titrate in 0.05 mcg/kg/minute increments every 3 minutes to effect; usual effective range: 0.2-0.5 mcg/kg/minute; has been used in combination with propofol (bolus and/or infusion) (Malherbe, 2010a; Malherbe, 2010b; Mani, 2010; Shen, 2012)

Endotracheal intubation for elective procedures: Limited data available:

I.V.: Usual range: 1-3 mcg/kg/dose, doses as high as 4 mcg/kg have been used. Dosing based on multiple trials in patients undergoing elective procedures requiring intubation who were not receiving neuromuscular blockers and remifentanil administered in combination with other induction agents such as propofol, ketamine, or sevoflurane. (Begec, 2009; Blair, 2004; Hume-Smith, 2010; Klemola, 2000; Morgan, 2007; Park, 2009)

Intranasal (using parenteral 100 mcg/mL formulation): Children ≤7 years: 4 mcg/kg/dose; administer half of the total dose in each nostril; wait 2-3 minutes before attempting intubation. Dosing based on a double-blind, randomized, controlled trial (n=188), remifentanil was administered after sevoflurane induction and overall, was found more effective than saline placebo at both endpoints of 2 minutes and 3 minutes postdose. Results also showed that within the remifentanil treatment groups, good or excellent intubation conditions were reported more often at 3 minutes postdose than at 2 minutes (91.7% vs 68.2%) (Verghese, 2008).

Procedural sedation: Limited data available, dosage not established: I.V.: 0.5 mcg/kg with propofol has been used to induce analgesia and adjunct sedation prior to esophagogastroduodenoscopy (n=22; age range: 2-12 years) and short hemato-oncologic invasive procedures (n=30, age range: 2-18 years) (Hirsh, 2010; Ince, 2013). A higher dose of 3 mcg/kg was used in already sedated (sevoflurane) infants and young children who required apnea for CT or MRI imaging (n=12, age range: 6-16 months) (Joshi, 2009). In a dose-finding trial, continuous I.V. infusion of remifentanil at 0.2 mcg/kg/minute has been shown more effective than a lower 0.1 mcg/kg/minute in 60 children 2-12 years undergoing diagnostic cardiac catheterization; pretreatment with oral midazolam and local groin anesthetic also utilized (Kaynar, 2011).

Adults:

Induction of anesthesia: 0.5-1 mcg/kg/minute; if endotracheal intubation is to occur in <8 minutes, an initial dose of 1 mcg/kg may be given over 30-60 seconds; in coronary bypass surgery: 1 mcg/kg/minute

Maintenance of anesthesia: Note: Supplemental bolus dose of 1 mcg/kg may be administered every 2-5 minutes. Consider increasing concomitant anesthetics with infusion rate >1 mcg/kg/minute. Infusion rate can be titrated upward in increments of 25% to 100% or downward in decrements of 25% to 50%. May titrate every 2-5 minutes.

With nitrous oxide (66%): 0.4 mcg/kg/minute (range: 0.1-2 mcg/kg/minute)

With isoflurane: 0.25 mcg/kg/minute (range: 0.05-2 mcg/kg/minute)

With propofol: 0.25 mcg/kg/minute (range: 0.05-2 mcg/kg/minute)

Coronary bypass surgery: 1 mcg/kg/minute (range: 0.125-4 mcg/kg/minute); supplemental dose: 0.5-1 mcg/kg

Continuation as an analgesic in immediate postoperative period: 0.1 mcg/kg/minute (range: 0.025-0.2 mcg/kg/minute). Infusion rate may be adjusted every 5 minutes in increments of 0.025 mcg/kg/minute. Bolus doses are not recommended. Infusion rates >0.2 mcg/kg/minute are associated with respiratory depression.

Coronary bypass surgery, continuation as an analgesic into the ICU: 1 mcg/kg/minute (range: 0.05-1 mcg/kg/minute)

Analgesic component of monitored anesthesia care: Note: Supplemental oxygen is recommended:

Single I.V. dose given 90 seconds prior to local anesthetic:

Remifentanil alone: 1 mcg/kg over 30-60 seconds

With midazolam: 0.5 mcg/kg over 30-60 seconds

Continuous infusion beginning 5 minutes prior to local anesthetic:

Remifentanil alone: 0.1 mcg/kg/minute

With midazolam: 0.05 mcg/kg/minute

Continuous infusion given after local anesthetic:

Remifentanil alone: 0.05 mcg/kg/minute (range: 0.025-0.2 mcg/kg/minute)

With midazolam: 0.025 mcg/kg/minute (range: 0.025-0.2 mcg/kg/minute)

Note: Following local or anesthetic block, infusion rate should be decreased to 0.05 mcg/kg/minute; rate adjustments of 0.025 mcg/kg/minute may be done at 5-minute intervals

Dosing adjustment in renal impairment: Removed by hemodialysis (30%). There are no dosage adjustments provided in the manufacturer's labeling; however, remifentanil pharmacokinetics are unchanged in patients with end stage renal disease.

Dosing adjustment in hepatic impairment: There are no dosage adjustments provided in the manufacturer's labeling; however, remifentanil pharmacokinetics are unchanged in patients with severe hepatic impairment.

Administration I.V.: Prepare solution by adding 1 mL of diluent per 1 mg of remifentanil. Shake well. Further dilute to a final concentration of 20, 25, 50, or 250 mcg/mL in compatible I.V. solution. An infusion device should be used to administer continuous infusions. During the maintenance of general anesthesia, I.V. boluses ≤1 mcg/kg may be administered over 30-60 seconds; for doses >1 mcg/kg, administer over >60 seconds (to reduce the potential to develop skeletal muscle and chest wall rigidity). Injections should be given into I.V. tubing close to the venous cannula; tubing should be cleared after treatment to prevent residual effects when other fluids are administered through the same I.V. line.

Monitoring Parameters Respiratory and cardiovascular status, blood pressure, heart rate

Controlled Substance C-II

Dosage Forms Excipient information presented when available (limited, particularly for generics); consult specific product labeling.

Solution Reconstituted, Intravenous [preservative free]:
Ultiva: 1 mg (1 ea); 2 mg (1 ea); 5 mg (1 ea)

References

Abu-Kishk I, Hod-Feins R, Anekstein Y, et al. Remifentanil use in pediatric scoliosis surgery – an effective alternative to morphine (a retrospective study). Yonsei Med J. 2012;53(5): 1014-1021.

Akinci SB, Kanbak M, Guler A, et al. Remifentanil versus fentanyl for short-term analgesia-based sedation in mechanically ventilated postoperative children. Pediatric Anesthesia. 2005;15:870-878.

Barr J, Fraser GL, Puntillo K, et al. Clinical practice guidelines for the management of pain, agitation, and delirium in adult patients in the intensive care unit. Crit Care Med. 2013;41(1):263-306.

Begec Z, Demirbilek S, Ozturk E, et al. Remifentanil and propofol for tracheal intubation without muscle relaxant in children: the effects of ketamine. Eur J Anaesthesiol. 2009;26:213-217.

Blair JM, Hill DA, Wilson CM, et al. Assessment of tracheal intubation in children after induction with propofol and different doses of remifentanil. Anesthesia. 2004;59:27-33.

Choong L, AlFaleh K, Doucette J, et al. Remifentanil for endotracheal intubation in neonates: a randomized controlled trial. Arch Dis Child Fetal Neonatal Ed. 2010;95,F80-84.

Fotopoulou G, Theocharis S, Vasileiou I, et al. Management of the airway without the use of neuromuscular blocking agents: the use of remifentanil. Fundamental and Clinical Pharmacology. 2012;72-85.

Giannantonio C, Sammartino M, Valente E, et al. Remifentanil analgosedation in preterm newborns during mechanical ventilation. Acta Paediatrica. 2009;98(7):1111-1115.

Hirsh I, Lerner A, Schnaider I, et al. Remifentanil versus fentanyl for esophagogastroduodenoscopy in children. JPGN. 2010;51:618-621.

Hume-Smith H, McCormack J, Montgomery C, et al. The effect of age on the dose of remifentanil for tracheal intubation in infants and children. Pediatric Anesthesia. 2010;20:19-27.

Ince IE, Iyilikci L, Yilmaz S, et al.. Sedation for short hemato-oncologic invasive procedures in children: comparison of propofol-remifentanil and propofol-fentanyl. J Pediatr Hematol Oncol. 2013;35:112-117.

Joshi G and Tobias J. Remifentanil to facilitate high-resolution computed tomography imagine of the chest or magnetic resonance imaging in infants. Southern Medical Journal. 2009;102 (11):1121-1124.

Kaynar A, Kelsaka E, Karakaya D, et al. Effects of different doses of remifentanil infusion on hemodynamics and recovery in children undergoing pediatric diagnostic cardiac catheterization. Journal of Cardiothoracic and Vascular Anesthesia. 2011;25(4):660-664.

Klemola U, Hiller A. Tracheal intubation after induction of anesthesia in children with propofol – remifentanil or propofol-rocuronium. Can J Anesth. 2000;47(9):854-859.

Kumar P, Denson SE, Mancuso TJ, et al. Premedication for non-emergency endotracheal intubation in the neonate. Pediatrics. 2010;125(3):608-615.

Malherbe S, Ansermino JM. Total intravenous anesthesia and spontaneous ventilation for foreign body removal in children: how much drug? Anesth Analg. 2010a;111(6):1566.

Malherbe S, Whyte S, Singh P, et al. Total intravenous anesthesia and spontaneous respiration for airway endoscopy in children – a prospective evaluation. Pediatric Anesthesia. 2010b;20:434-438.

Mani V, Morton N. Overview of total intravenous anesthesia in children. Pediatric Anesthesia. 2010;20:211-222.

Montgomery A, Hale TW, Academy Of Breastfeeding Medicine. ABM cinical protocol #15: analgesia and anesthesia for the breastfeeding mother, revised 2012. Breastfeed Med. 2012;7(6):547-553.

Morgan JM, Barker I, Peacock JE, et al. A comparison of intubating conditions in children following induction of anaesthesia with propofol and suxamethonium or propofol and remifentanil. Anesthesia. 2007;62:135-139.

Park KS, Park SY, Kim JW, et al. Effect of remifentanil on tracheal intubation conditions and haemodynamics in children anaesthetized with sevoflurane and nitrous oxide. Anaesth Intensive Care. 2009;37:577-583.

Ross AK, Davis PJ, Dear GD GL, et al. Pharmacokinetics of remifentanil in anesthetized pediatric patients undergoing elective surgery or diagnostic procedures. Anesth Analg. 2001;93:1393-1401.

Scott LJ, Perry CM. Remifentanil: a review of its use during the induction and maintenance of general anaesthesia. Drugs. 2005;65 (13):1793-1823.

Shen X, Hu C, Ye M, et al. Profol-remifentanil intravenous anesthesia and spontaneous ventilation for airway foreign body removal in children with preoperative respiratory impairment. Pediatric Anesthesia. 2012;22:1166-1170.

Silva YPE, Gomez RS, Marcatto JDO, et al.. Early awakening and extubation with remifentanil in ventilated premature neonates. Pediatric Anesthesia. 2008;18:176-183.

Verghese ST, Hannallah RS, Brennan M, et al. The effect of intranasal administration of remifentanil on intubating conditions and airway response after sevoflurane induction of anesthesia in children. Anesth Analf. 2008;107:1176-1181.

Welzing L, Oberthuer A, Junghaenel S, et al. Remifentanil/midazolam versus fentanyl/midazolam for analgesia and sedation of mechanically ventilated neonates and young infants: a randomized controlled trial. Intensive Care Med. 2012;38:1017-1024.

◆ **Renagel** see Sevelamer on page 1882

◆ **Renedil (Can)** see Felodipine on page 850

◆ **Renova** see Tretinoin (Topical) on page 2071

◆ **Renova Pump** see Tretinoin (Topical) on page 2071

◆ **Renvela** see Sevelamer on page 1882

◆ **Resectisol** see Mannitol on page 1301

◆ **Restasis** see CycloSPORINE (Ophthalmic) on page 569

◆ **Restasis® (Can)** see CycloSPORINE (Ophthalmic) on page 569

◆ **Retin-A** see Tretinoin (Topical) on page 2071

◆ **Retin-A Micro** see Tretinoin (Topical) on page 2071

◆ **Retin-A Micro Pump** see Tretinoin (Topical) on page 2071

◆ **Retinoic Acid** see Tretinoin (Topical) on page 2071

◆ **Retinova (Can)** see Tretinoin (Topical) on page 2071

◆ **Retisert** see Fluocinolone (Ophthalmic) on page 891

◆ **Retisert® (Can)** see Fluocinolone (Ophthalmic) on page 891

◆ **Retrovir** see Zidovudine on page 2168

◆ **Retrovir® (Can)** see Zidovudine on page 2168

◆ **Retrovir® (AZT™) (Can)** see Zidovudine on page 2168

◆ **Revatio** see Sildenafil on page 1884

◆ **Revitalose C-1000® (Can)** see Ascorbic Acid on page 206

◆ **Revonto** see Dantrolene on page 583

◆ **Reyataz** see Atazanavir on page 218

◆ **rFVIIa** see Factor VIIa (Recombinant) on page 831

◆ **R-Gene 10** see Arginine on page 195

◆ **rhASB** see Galsulfase on page 953

◆ **rhDNase** see Dornase Alfa on page 709

◆ **Rheumatrex** see Methotrexate on page 1367

◆ **rhGAA** see Alglucosidase Alfa on page 95

◆ **r-h α-GAL** see Agalsidase Beta on page 79

◆ **RhIG** see Rh$_o$(D) Immune Globulin on page 1815

◆ **rhIGF-1 (Mecasermin [Increlex®])** see Mecasermin on page 1313

◆ **rhIL-11** see Oprelvekin on page 1549

◆ **Rhinalar® (Can)** *see* Flunisolide (Nasal) *on page 890*

◆ **Rhinall [OTC]** *see* Phenylephrine (Nasal) *on page 1660*

◆ **Rhinaris [OTC]** *see* Sodium Chloride *on page 1902*

◆ **Rhinaris-CS Anti-Allergic Nasal Mist (Can)** *see* Cromolyn (Nasal) *on page 553*

◆ **Rhinocort Aqua** *see* Budesonide (Nasal) *on page 313*

◆ **Rhinocort® Aqua® (Can)** *see* Budesonide (Nasal) *on page 313*

◆ **Rhinocort® Turbuhaler® (Can)** *see* Budesonide (Nasal) *on page 313*

◆ **Rho(D) Immune Globulin (Human)** *see* Rhₒ(D) Immune Globulin *on page 1815*

Rhₒ(D) Immune Globulin
(ar aych oh (dee) i MYUN GLOB yoo lin)

Brand Names: U.S. HyperRHO S/D; MICRhoGAM Ultra-Filtered Plus; RhoGAM Ultra-Filtered Plus; Rhophylac; WinRho SDF

Brand Names: Canada WinRho® SDF

Therapeutic Category Immune Globulin

Generic Availability (U.S.) No

Use

Suppression of Rh isoimmunization: Use in the following situations when an Rhₒ(D)-negative individual is exposed to Rhₒ(D)-positive blood: During delivery of an Rhₒ(D)-positive infant; abortion; amniocentesis; chorionic villus sampling; ruptured tubal pregnancy; abdominal trauma; transplacental hemorrhage. Used when the mother is Rhₒ(D) negative, the father of the child is either Rhₒ(D) positive or Rhₒ(D) unknown, the baby is either Rhₒ(D) positive or Rhₒ(D) unknown (FDA approved in pregnant women)

Transfusion: Suppression of Rh isoimmunization in Rhₒ(D)-negative individuals transfused with Rhₒ(D) antigen-positive RBCs or blood components containing Rhₒ(D) antigen-positive RBCs (FDA approved in adults)

Treatment of immune thrombocytopenia (ITP): Used intravenously in the following nonsplenectomized Rhₒ(D) positive individuals: Acute ITP (WinRho SDF: FDA approved in children), chronic ITP (Rhophylac: FDA approved in adults; WinRho SDF: FDA approved in children and adults), ITP secondary to HIV infection (WinRho SDF: FDA approved in ages <16 years and adults)

Pregnancy Risk Factor C

Pregnancy Considerations Animal studies have not been conducted. Available evidence suggests that Rhₒ(D) immune globulin administration during pregnancy does not harm the fetus or affect future pregnancies.

Breast-Feeding Considerations Adverse events in the nursing infant have not been observed when administered to women for the suppression of Rh isoimmunization.

Contraindications Hypersensitivity to immune globulin or any component

Additional product-specific contraindications:

MICRhoGAM UF Plus, RhoGAM UF Plus: Rh-positive patients

Rhophylac: IgA deficiency with antibodies against IgA and history of hypersensitivity

WinRho SDF: Autoimmune hemolytic anemia; preexisting hemolysis or high risk for hemolysis; IgA deficiency with antibodies against IgA and history of hypersensitivity; suppression of isoimmunization in infants

Warnings WinRho SDF and Rhophylac are the only products approved for treatment of ITP; administer I.V. only when treating ITP. Severe, sometimes fatal, cases of intravascular hemolysis (IVH) have been reported in patients treated for ITP **[U.S. Boxed Warning]**; rare but serious signs and symptoms (eg, back pain, shaking chills, fever, and discolored urine) have occurred within 4 hours of administration; IVH has been reported in postmarketing experience in patients treated for ITP and may result in clinically compromising anemia and multiorgan system failure including acute respiratory distress syndrome. Acute renal insufficiency and disseminated intravascular coagulation (DIC) have also been reported. Patients with ITP should be advised of the signs and symptoms of IVH and instructed to report them immediately. Reduce WinRho SDF dosage in ITP patients with serum Hgb concentration <10 g/dL to minimize the risk of increasing the severity of anemia; consider alternative treatment with hemoglobin <8 g/dL; monitor for signs and/or symptoms of intravascular hemolysis, clinically compromising anemia, and renal insufficiency.

Product of human plasma; may potentially contain infectious agents which could transmit disease. Screening of donors, as well as testing and/or inactivation or removal of certain viruses, reduces the risk. Infections thought to be transmitted by this product should be reported to the manufacturer. Not intended for use as immunoglobulin replacement therapy for immune deficiency syndromes. When used to suppress Rh isoimmunization, the drug is administered to the mother **not** the infant.

Noncardiogenic pulmonary edema has been reported with intravenous immune globulin use. Transfusion-related acute lung injury (TRALI) is characterized by severe respiratory distress, pulmonary edema, hypoxemia, and fever in the presence of normal left ventricular function and usually occurs within 1-6 hours after the infusion. Thrombotic events have been reported with administration of intravenous immune globulins (IVIG); use with caution in patients with a history of atherosclerosis or cardiovascular and/or thrombotic risk factors or patients with known/suspected hyperviscosity. Consider a baseline assessment of blood viscosity in patients at risk for hyperviscosity. Administer at the minimum practical infusion rate.

MICRhoGAM UF Plus, RhoGAM UF Plus, and WinRho SDF contain polysorbate 80 (Tween 80) which may cause allergic reactions in susceptible individuals. In premature neonates, thrombocytopenia, ascites, pulmonary deterioration, and renal and hepatic failure have been reported after receiving parenteral products containing polysorbate 80 (Alade, 1986; CDC, 1984). Infusion of polysorbate 80-containing solutions through polyvinyl chloride tubing may cause DEHP to leach into the solution; in immature animals, exposure to DEHP may adversely affect the development of the male reproductive tract.

Precautions Anaphylactic hypersensitivity reactions can occur; use with caution in IgA deficiency; may increase risk of hypersensitivity especially in patients with anti-IgA antibodies present. Use with caution in patients with thrombocytopenia or bleeding disorders; bleeding/hematoma may occur from I.M. administration. For treatment of ITP, use should be considered only in those patients who are Rh-positive and nonsplenectomized (Neunert, 2011; Provan, 2010); alternative treatment should be used in ITP patients with hemoglobin concentrations <8 g/dL. WinRho SDF contains maltose; may cause false-positive glucose concentrations.

Adverse Reactions

Cardiovascular: Hyper-/hypotension, pallor, vasodilation

Central nervous system: Chills, dizziness, fever, headache, malaise, somnolence

Dermatologic: Pruritus, rash

Gastrointestinal: Abdominal pain, diarrhea, nausea, vomiting

Hematologic: Haptoglobin decreased, hemoglobin decreased (patients with ITP), intravascular hemolysis (patients with ITP)

Hepatic: Bilirubin increased, LDH increased

Local: Injection site reaction: Discomfort, induration, mild pain, redness, swelling

Neuromuscular & skeletal: Arthralgia, back pain, hyperkinesia, myalgia, weakness

Renal: Acute renal insufficiency

Miscellaneous: Anaphylaxis, diaphoresis, infusion-related reactions, positive anti-C antibody test (transient), shivering

Postmarketing and/or case reports: Anemia (clinically-compromising), anuria, ARDS, cardiac arrest, cardiac failure, chest pain, chromaturia, DIC, edema, erythema, fatigue, hematuria, hemoglobinemia, hemoglobinuria (transient in patients with ITP), hyperhidrosis, hypersensitivity, injection site irritation, jaundice, myocardial infarction, muscle spasm, nausea, pain in extremities, renal failure, renal impairment, tachycardia, transfusion-related acute lung injury

Drug Interactions

Metabolism/Transport Effects None known.

Avoid Concomitant Use There are no known interactions where it is recommended to avoid concomitant use.

Increased Effect/Toxicity There are no known significant interactions involving an increase in effect.

Decreased Effect

Rho(D) Immune Globulin may decrease the levels/effects of: Vaccines (Live)

Stability Store at 2°C to 8°C (35°F to 46°F), do not freeze. RhoGAM UF Plus, MICRhoGAM UF Plus: May be stored at 25°C (77°F) for up to 10 days [data on file (Ortho Clinical Diagnostics, 2011)]; however, the manufacturer recommends storage under refrigeration. Room temperature stability information should only be utilized in situations where the drug has been inadvertently exposed to prolonged room temperature.

HyperRHO S/D: May be stored at 25°C (77°F) for ~2 weeks [data on file (Talecris Biotherapeutics, 2011)]; however, the manufacturer recommends storage under refrigeration. Room temperature stability information should only be utilized in situations where the drug has been inadvertently exposed to prolonged room temperature.

Rhophylac: Protect from light.

Mechanism of Action

Rh suppression: Prevents isoimmunization by suppressing the immune response and antibody formation by $Rh_o(D)$ negative individuals to $Rh_o(D)$ positive red blood cells.

ITP: Not completely characterized; $Rh_o(D)$ immune globulin is thought to form anti-D-coated red blood cell complexes which bind to macrophage Fc receptors within the spleen; blocking or saturating the spleens ability to clear antibody-coated cells, including platelets. In this manner, platelets are spared from destruction.

Pharmacodynamics

Onset of action:
Rh isoimmunization: I.V.: 8 hours
ITP: I.V.: 1-2 days
Maximum effect: ITP: 7-14 days
Duration:
ITP (single dose): I.V.: 30 days
Passive anti-$Rh_o(D)$ antibodies (after 120 mcg dose): I.V.: 6 weeks

Pharmacokinetics (Adult data unless noted)

Distribution: Appears in breast milk, however, not absorbed by the nursing infant
Half-life, elimination:
I.M.: 18-30 days
I.V.: 16-24 days
Time to peak serum concentration:
I.M.: 5-10 days
I.V.: 2 hours

Dosing: Usual

Infants, Children, and Adolescents: **ITP:**
Manufacturer's labeling: WinRho SDF: I.V.: Children and Adolescents <16 years:
Initial:
Hemoglobin <10 g/dL: 25-40 mcg/kg as single dose or divided into 2 doses given on separate days
Hemoglobin ≥10 g/dL: 50 mcg/kg as single dose or divided into 2 doses given on separate days
Maintenance: **Note:** Usage dependent upon clinical response, platelet count, hemoglobin, red blood cell counts, and reticulocyte levels; platelet counts >50,000/mm³ rarely require treatment
Response to initial dose: 25-60 mcg/kg as single dose
Nonresponse to initial therapy:
Hemoglobin <8 g/dL: Alternative therapy should be used
Hemoglobin 8-10 g/dL: 25-40 mcg/kg as single dose
Hemoglobin >10 g/dL: 50-60 mcg/kg as single dose
Alternate dosing: I.V.: **Note:** Recommended as first-line in Rh-positive, nonsplenectomized pediatric patients (Neunert, 2011; Provan, 2010)
First-line; initial treatment or chronic: 50-75 mcg/kg (Provan, 2010)
Serious or life-threatening bleeding: 75 mcg/kg in combination with platelet infusion(s) and corticosteroids (Provan, 2010)

Adults:
ITP:
Rhophylac: I.V.: 50 mcg/kg
WinRho SDF: I.V.:
Initial: 50 mcg/kg as a single injection, or can be given as a divided dose on separate days. If hemoglobin is <10 g/dL: Dose should be reduced to 25-40 mcg/kg
Subsequent dosing: 25-60 mcg/kg can be used if required to increase platelet count
Maintenance dosing if patient **did respond** to initial dosing: 25-60 mcg/kg based on platelet count and hemoglobin concentration
Maintenance dosing if patient **did not respond** to initial dosing:
Hemoglobin <8 g/dL: Alternative treatment should be used
Hemoglobin 8-10 g/dL: Redose between 25-40 mcg/kg
Hemoglobin >10 g/dL: Redose between 50-60 mcg/kg

$Rh_o(D)$ suppression: **Note:** One "full dose" (300 mcg) provides enough antibody to prevent Rh sensitization if the volume of RBC entering the circulation is ≤15 mL. When >15 mL is suspected, a fetal red cell count should be performed to determine the appropriate dose.
Pregnancy:
Antepartum prophylaxis: In general, single dose is given at 28 weeks. If given early in pregnancy, administer every 12 weeks to ensure adequate levels of passively acquired anti-Rh.
HyperRHO S/D Full Dose, RhoGAM: I.M.: 300 mcg
Rhophylac, WinRho SDF: I.M., I.V.: 300 mcg
Postpartum: In general, dose is administered as soon as possible after delivery, preferably within 72 hours. Can be given up to 28 days following delivery
HyperRHO S/D Full Dose, RhoGAM: I.M.: 300 mcg
Rhophylac: I.M., I.V.: 300 mcg
WinRho SDF: I.M., I.V.: 120 mcg
Threatened abortion, any time during pregnancy (with continuation of pregnancy):
HyperRHO S/D Full Dose, RhoGAM: I.M.: 300 mcg; administer as soon as possible
Rhophylac, WinRho SDF: I.M., I.V.: 300 mcg; administer as soon as possible
Abortion, miscarriage, termination of ectopic pregnancy:
RhoGAM: I.M.: ≥13 weeks gestation: 300 mcg

HyperRHO S/D Mini Dose, MICRhoGAM: I.M.: <13 weeks gestation: 50 mcg

Rhophylac: I.M., I.V.: 300 mcg

WinRho SDF: I.M., I.V.: After 34 weeks gestation: 120 mcg; administer immediately or within 72 hours

Amniocentesis, chorionic villus sampling:

HyperRHO S/D Full Dose, RhoGAM: I.M.: At 15-18 weeks gestation or during the 3rd trimester: 300 mcg. If dose is given between 13-18 weeks, repeat at 26-28 weeks and within 72 hours of delivery.

Rhophylac: I.M., I.V.: 300 mcg

WinRho SDF: I.M., I.V.:

Before 34 weeks gestation: 300 mcg; administer immediately, repeat dose every 12 weeks during pregnancy

After 34 weeks gestation: 120 mcg, administered immediately or within 72 hours

Excessive fetomaternal hemorrhage (>15 mL): Rhophylac: I.M., I.V.: 300 mcg within 72 hours plus 20 mcg/mL fetal RBCs in excess of 15 mL if excess transplacental bleeding is quantified or 300 mcg/dose if bleeding cannot be quantified

Abdominal trauma, manipulation:

HyperRHO S/D Full Dose, RhoGAM: I.M.: 2nd or 3rd trimester: 300 mcg. If dose is given between 13-18 weeks, repeat at 26-28 weeks and within 72 hours of delivery.

Rhophylac: I.M., I.V.: 300 mcg within 72 hours

WinRho SDF: I.M., I.V.: After 34 weeks gestation: 120 mcg; administer immediately or within 72 hours

Transfusion:

HyperRHO S/D Full Dose, RhoGAM: I.M.: Multiply the volume of Rh positive whole blood administered by the hematocrit of the donor unit to equal the volume of RBCs transfused. The volume of RBCs is then divided by 15 mL, providing the number of 300 mcg doses (vials/syringes) to administer. If the dose calculated results in a fraction, round up to the next higher whole 300 mcg dose (vial/syringe).

WinRho SDF: Administer within 72 hours after exposure of incompatible blood transfusions or massive fetal hemorrhage.

I.V.: Calculate dose as follows; administer 600 mcg every 8 hours until the total dose is administered:

Exposure to Rh$_O$(D) positive whole blood: 9 mcg/mL blood

Exposure to Rh$_O$(D) positive red blood cells: 18 mcg/mL cells

I.M.: Calculate dose as follows; administer 1200 mcg every 12 hours until the total dose is administered:

Exposure to Rh$_O$(D) positive whole blood: 12 mcg/mL blood

Exposure to Rh$_O$(D) positive red blood cells: 24 mcg/mL cells

Rhophylac: I.M., I.V.: 20 mcg per 2 mL transfused blood or 1 mL erythrocyte concentrate

Administration Parenteral: WinRho SDF and Rhophylac are the only immune globulin products available that can be administered both I.M. and I.V.; however, **for the treatment of ITP, it must be administered I.V.**

I.M.: Administer into the deltoid muscle of upper arm or the anterolateral aspect of the upper thigh; the gluteal region is not recommended for routine administration due to the potential risk of sciatic nerve injury; if gluteal area is used, administer only in the upper, outer quadrant. The total volume can be given in divided doses at different sites at one time or may be divided and given at intervals provided the total dosage is given within 72 hours of the fetomaternal hemorrhage or transfusion.

I.V.:

WinRho SDF: Infuse over 3-5 minutes; if further dilution is desired, use NS as diluent

Rhophylac: ITP: Infuse at 2 mL per 15-60 seconds

Monitoring Parameters Signs and symptoms of intravascular hemolysis (IVH), anemia, renal insufficiency, back pain, shaking, chills, discolored urine, or hematuria; observe patient for side effects for 8 hours following administration

Patients with suspected IVH: CBC, haptoglobin, plasma hemoglobin, urine dipstick, BUN, serum creatinine, liver function tests, DIC-specific tests [D-dimer, fibrin degradation products (FDP) or fibrin split products (FSP)] for differential diagnosis. In patients at increased risk of developing acute renal failure, periodically monitor renal function and urine output. Clinical response may be determined by monitoring platelets, red blood cell (RBC) counts, hemoglobin, and reticulocyte levels.

ITP: Check blood type, CBC, reticulocyte count, DAT before initiating treatment with WinRho SDF; check urine dipstick before initiating treatment with WinRho SDF or Rhophylac and repeat urine dipstick at 2 and 4 hours after administration and prior to end of the 8-hour monitoring period.

Test Interactions Some infants born to women given Rh$_O$(D) antepartum have a weakly positive Coombs' test at birth. Fetal-maternal hemorrhage may cause false blood-typing result in the mother; when there is any doubt to the patients' Rh type, Rh$_O$(D) immune globulin should be administered. WinRho® SDF liquid contains maltose; may result in falsely elevated blood glucose levels with dehydrogenase pyrroloquinolinequinone or glucose-dye-oxidoreductase testing methods. WinRho® SDF contains trace amounts of anti-A, B, C and E; may alter Coombs' tests following administration.

Additional Information 1 mcg = 5 units

Treatment of ITP in Rh-positive patients with an intact spleen appears to be about as effective as IVIG.

HyperRho S/D and RhoGAM, which are prepared using cold ethanol fraction and ultrafiltration, must be administered intramuscularly because trace amounts of IgA and other plasma proteins in the product could cause anaphylaxis if they were given intravenously. Rhophylac and WinRho SDF are prepared by ion-exchange chromatography isolation and are purer, allowing them to be given intramuscularly or intravenously.

Dosage Forms Excipient information presented when available (limited, particularly for generics); consult specific product labeling. [DSC] = Discontinued product

Injectable, Intramuscular:

HyperRHO S/D: 50 mcg (1 ea [DSC])

Injectable, Intramuscular [preservative free]:

HyperRHO S/D: 50 mcg (1 ea); 300 mcg (1 ea) [latex free]

MICRhoGAM Ultra-Filtered Plus: 50 mcg (1 ea) [latex free, thimerosal free; contains polysorbate 80]

RhoGAM Ultra-Filtered Plus: 300 mcg (1 ea) [latex free, thimerosal free; contains polysorbate 80]

Solution, Injection:

WinRho SDF: 2500 units/2.2 mL (2.2 mL); 5000 units/4.4 mL (4.4 mL); 1500 units/1.3 mL (1.3 mL); 15,000 units/13 mL (13 mL)

Solution, Injection [preservative free]:

Rhophylac: 1500 units/2 mL (2 mL)

WinRho SDF: 2500 units/2.2 mL (2.2 mL); 5000 units/4.4 mL (4.4 mL); 1500 units/1.3 mL (1.3 mL); 15,000 units/13 mL (13 mL) [contains polysorbate 80]

References

Alade SL, Brown RE, and Paquet A Jr, "Polysorbate 80 and E-Ferol Toxicity," *Pediatrics*, 1986, 77(4):593-7.

Centers for Disease Control (CDC), "Unusual Syndrome With Fatalities Among Premature Infants: Association With a New Intravenous Vitamin E Product," *MMWR Morb Mortal Wkly Rep*, 1984, 33 (14):198-9.

Gaines AR, "Acute Onset Hemoglobinemia and/or Hemoglobinuria and Sequelae Following Rh(o)(D) Immune Globulin Intravenous

Administration in Immune Thrombocytopenic Purpura Patients," *Blood*, 2000, 95(8):2523-9.

Neunert C, Lim W, Crowther M, et al. The American Society of Hematology 2011 evidence-based practice guideline for immune thrombocytopenia. *Blood*. 2011;117(16):4190-4207.

Provan D, Stasi R, Newland A, et al. International consensus report on the investigation and management of primary immune thrombocytopenia. *Blood*. 2010;115:168-186.

Shahgholi E, Vosough P, Sotoudeh K, et al, "Intravenous Immune Globulin Versus Intravenous Anti-D Immune Globulin for the Treatment of Acute Immune Thrombocytopenic Purpura," *Indian J Pediatr*, 2008, 75(12):1231-5.

◆ **RhoGAM Ultra-Filtered Plus** see Rhₒ(D) Immune Globulin on page 1815

◆ **RhoIGIV** see Rhₒ(D) Immune Globulin on page 1815

◆ **RhoIVIM** see Rhₒ(D) Immune Globulin on page 1815

◆ **Rho®-Loperamine (Can)** see Loperamide on page 1270

◆ **Rho-Nitro Pump Spray (Can)** see Nitroglycerin on page 1504

◆ **Rhophylac** see Rhₒ(D) Immune Globulin on page 1815

◆ **Rhoxal-loperamide (Can)** see Loperamide on page 1270

◆ **Rhoxal-sotalol (Can)** see Sotalol on page 1925

◆ **rHuEPO** see Epoetin Alfa on page 766

◆ **rhuGM-CSF** see Sargramostim on page 1870

◆ **rhuMAb-E25** see Omalizumab on page 1533

◆ **rhuMAb-VEGF** see Bevacizumab on page 288

◆ **Riax** see Benzoyl Peroxide on page 275

◆ **Ribasphere** see Ribavirin on page 1818

◆ **Ribasphere RibaPak** see Ribavirin on page 1818

Ribavirin (rye ba VYE rin)

Medication Safety Issues

Sound-alike/look-alike issues:
Ribavirin may be confused with riboflavin, rifampin, Robaxin

Related Information
Safe Handling of Hazardous Drugs on page 2419

Brand Names: U.S. Copegus; Moderiba; Rebetol; Ribasphere; Ribasphere RibaPak; Virazole

Brand Names: Canada Virazole

Therapeutic Category Antiviral Agent, Inhalation Therapy

Generic Availability (U.S.) Yes: Capsule, tablet

Use
Inhalation: Treatment of hospitalized patients with severe RSV infections (FDA approved in infants and young children); specially indicated for treatment of severe lower respiratory tract RSV infections in patients with an underlying compromising condition (prematurity, BPD and other chronic lung conditions, congenital heart disease, immunodeficiency, immunosuppression), and recent transplant recipients; has also been used in other viral infections including influenza A and B and adenovirus

Oral: Used in combination with pegylated or nonpegylated interferon alfa-2b, recombinant injection for the treatment of chronic hepatitis C in patients with compensated liver disease who were previously untreated with alpha interferon (Rebetol®: FDA approved in ages ≥3 years and adults; all other products: FDA approved in adults); or used in combination with pegylated or nonpegylated interferon alfa-2b, recombinant injection for the treatment of chronic hepatitis C in patients with compensated liver disease who have relapsed after alpha interferon therapy (FDA approved in adults)

Medication Guide Available Yes

Pregnancy Risk Factor X

Pregnancy Considerations [U.S. Boxed Warning]: Significant teratogenic effects have been observed in all animal studies at ~0.01 times the maximum recommended daily human dose. Use is contraindicated in pregnancy. Negative pregnancy test is required before initiation and monthly thereafter. Avoid pregnancy in female patients and female partners of male patients during therapy by using two effective forms of contraception; continue contraceptive measures for at least 6 months after completion of therapy. If patient or female partner becomes pregnant during treatment, she should be counseled about potential risks of exposure. If pregnancy occurs during use or within 6 months after treatment, report to the ribavirin pregnancy registry (800-593-2214).

Breast-Feeding Considerations It is not known if ribavirin is excreted in breast milk. Due to the potential for serious adverse reactions in the nursing infant, a decision should be made whether to discontinue nursing or to discontinue the drug, taking into account the importance of treatment to the mother.

Contraindications Hypersensitivity to ribavirin or any component; pregnancy

Additional contraindications for oral formulation: Men whose female partners are pregnant; patients with hemoglobinopathies (ie, thalassemia major, sickle cell anemia); autoimmune hepatitis; as monotherapy for treatment of chronic hepatitis C; pancreatitis; patients with significant or unstable cardiac disease; CrCl <50 mL/minute; coadministration with didanosine (cases of fatal hepatic failure, peripheral neuropathy, pancreatitis, and hyperlactatemia/lactic acidosis have been reported)

Additional contraindications for ribavirin tablet used in combination with peginterferon alfa-2a: Hepatic impairment (Child-Pugh score >6; class B or C) in cirrhotic chronic hepatitis C monoinfected patients before or during treatment; hepatic impairment (Child-Pugh score ≥6) in cirrhotic chronic hepatitis C patients coinfected with HIV before or during treatment

Warnings Hazardous agent; use appropriate precautions for handling and disposal (NIOSH, 2012). Ribavirin is potentially mutagenic, tumor-promoting, and gonadotoxic; ribavirin may cause birth defects and/or death of the exposed fetus **[U.S. Boxed Warning]**. Avoid pregnancy in female patients and female partners of male patients for 6 months after therapy. Pregnant healthcare workers should not be administering aerosolized ribavirin due to risk of exposure. A primary adverse effect of oral ribavirin is hemolytic anemia which may worsen cardiac disease and lead to myocardial infarction **[U.S. Boxed Warning]**. The anemia usually occurs within 1-2 weeks of therapy initiation. Closely monitor hemoglobin or hematocrit pretreatment and during the first 4 weeks of therapy. Patients with underlying cardiac disease should have an ECG performed prior to initiation of oral ribavirin therapy. With combination therapy, neuropsychiatric effects (some life-threatening or fatal) including depression, suicidal/homicidal ideation, suicidal attempts, suicides, addiction relapse, and aggression in association with interferon alfa therapy in patients with and without previous psychiatric symptoms have been reported. Suicidal ideation or attempts may occur more frequently in pediatric patients as compared to adults (2.4% vs 1%, respectively). Also observed are psychoses, hallucinations, bipolar disorders, and mania. Use with extreme caution in patients with a history of psychiatric disorders, including depression. Patients should be monitored for signs and symptoms; if they occur, continued monitoring throughout therapy and for 6 months post-treatment recommended. If symptoms persist, worsen, or if suicidal behavior or aggression towards others develops, peginterferon should be discontinued and the patient should be followed with psychiatric care given when appropriate. In severe cases, discontinue immediately and complete a psychiatric intervention. Severe acute hypersensitivity reactions have been reported (rarely); reactions include urticaria, angioedema, bronchoconstriction, and anaphylaxis; discontinue use if hypersensitivity occurs. Serious skin reactions have been reported (including Stevens-Johnson syndrome and erythema multiforme major) rarely; discontinue use if patient develops signs or symptoms of severe skin reactions. Serious ophthalmologic disorders have occurred with combination therapy; may require discontinuation of combination therapy in patients who experience new or worsening ophthalmologic disorders. Severe inhibition of growth velocity, <3rd percentile, and affecting height and weight was reported in 70% of pediatric patients during clinical trials on combination therapy; monitor closely, dosage adjustment may be required. After therapy, 20% continued to have severely inhibited growth; however, in majority of patients, growth velocity rates increased such that by 6 months post-treatment, weight gain stabilized to 53rd percentile (similar to predicted based on average baseline weight: 57th percentile) and height gain stabilized to 44th percentile (less than predicted based on average baseline height: 51st percentile). Dental and periodontal disorders have been reported with combination therapy.

Ribavirin oral solution contains sodium benzoate; benzoic acid (benzoate) is a metabolite of benzyl alcohol; large amounts of benzyl alcohol (≥99 mg/kg/day) have been associated with a potentially fatal toxicity ("gasping syndrome") in neonates; the "gasping syndrome" consists of metabolic acidosis, respiratory distress, gasping respirations, CNS dysfunction (including convulsions, intracranial hemorrhage), hypotension and cardiovascular collapse; avoid use of ribavirin products containing sodium benzoate in neonates; *in vitro* and animal studies have shown that benzoate displaces bilirubin from protein binding sites.

Inhalation: Use with caution in patients requiring assisted ventilation because precipitation of the drug in the respiratory equipment may interfere with safe and effective patient ventilation **[U.S. Boxed Warning]**. Sudden respiratory deterioration has been observed during the initiation of aerosolized ribavirin in infants **[U.S. Boxed Warning]**; carefully monitor infants and carefully monitor patients with COPD and asthma for deterioration of respiratory function

Precautions Oral: Use with caution in patients with preexisting cardiac disease, patients with evidence of pulmonary infiltrates or pulmonary function impairment (closely monitor), or patients with sarcoidosis (may exacerbate sarcoidosis).

Adverse Reactions

Inhalation:
Cardiovascular: Cardiac arrest, digitalis toxicity, hypotension
Central nervous system: Fatigue, headache, insomnia
Gastrointestinal: Nausea, anorexia
Hematologic: Anemia
Ocular: Conjunctivitis
Respiratory: Apnea, mild bronchospasm, worsening of respiratory function

Oral (all adverse reactions are documented while receiving combination therapy with alfa interferons; as reported in adults unless noted; most common pediatric adverse reactions were similar to adults):
Cardiovascular: Chest pain, flushing
Central nervous system: Agitation, anxiety, depression, dizziness, emotional lability, fatigue (children and adults), fever, headache, insomnia (children and adults), impaired concentration, irritability, malaise, memory impairment, mood alteration, nervousness, pain, suicidal ideation

Dermatologic: Alopecia (children and adults), dermatitis, dry skin, eczema, pruritus (children and adults), rash
Endocrine & metabolic: Growth suppression (pediatric), hyperuricemia, hypothyroidism, menstrual disorder
Gastrointestinal: Abdominal pain, anorexia, constipation, diarrhea, dyspepsia, nausea (children and adults), RUQ pain, taste perversion, vomiting, weight loss, xerostomia
Hematologic: Anemia, hemoglobin decreased, hemolytic anemia, leukopenia, lymphopenia, neutropenia, thrombocytopenia
Hepatic: Bilirubin increased, hepatic decompensation, hepatomegaly, transaminases increased
Local: Inflammation at injection site, injection site reaction
Neuromuscular & skeletal: Arthralgia, back pain, decreased linear skeletal growth (including lagging weight gain), musculoskeletal pain (children and adults), myalgia (children and adults), rigors, weakness
Ocular: Blurred vision, conjunctivitis
Respiratory: Cough, dyspnea (including exertional), pharyngitis, rhinitis, sinusitis, upper respiratory tract infection (children)
Miscellaneous: Bacterial infection, diaphoresis, flu-like syndrome (children and adults), fungal infection, viral infection

Rare but important or life-threatening: Aggression, angina, aplastic anemia, arrhythmia; autoimmune disorders (systemic lupus erythematosus, rheumatoid arthritis, sarcoidosis); bone marrow suppression, cerebral hemorrhage, cholangitis, colitis, coma, corneal ulcer, dehydration, diabetes mellitus, drug abuse relapse/overdose, exfoliative dermatitis, fatty liver, hearing impairment/loss, gastrointestinal bleeding, gout, hallucination, hepatic dysfunction, hyper-/hypothyroidism, hypersensitivity (including anaphylaxis, angioedema, bronchoconstriction, and urticaria), macular edema, myositis, optic neuritis, papilledema, pancreatitis, peptic ulcer, peripheral neuropathy, pneumonitis, psychosis, psychotic disorder, pulmonary dysfunction, pulmonary embolism, pulmonary infiltrates, pure red cell aplasia, retinal artery/vein thrombosis, retinal detachment, retinal hemorrhage, retinopathy, sarcoidosis exacerbation; skin reactions (erythema multiforme, exfoliative dermatitis, urticaria, vesiculobullous eruptions); Stevens-Johnson syndrome, suicide, thrombotic thrombocytopenic purpura, thyroid function test abnormalities; transplant rejection (kidney, liver); vision loss

Note: Incidence of headache, fever, suicidal ideation, and vomiting are higher in children.

Drug Interactions

Metabolism/Transport Effects None known.

Avoid Concomitant Use
Avoid concomitant use of Ribavirin with any of the following: Didanosine

Increased Effect/Toxicity
Ribavirin may increase the levels/effects of: AzaTHIOprine; Didanosine; Reverse Transcriptase Inhibitors (Nucleoside)

The levels/effects of Ribavirin may be increased by: Interferons (Alfa); Zidovudine

Decreased Effect
Ribavirin may decrease the levels/effects of: Influenza Virus Vaccine (Live/Attenuated)

Food Interactions Oral: High-fat meal increases the AUC and C_{max}. Management: Capsule (in combination with peginterferon alfa-2b) and tablet should be administered with food. Other dosage forms and combinations should be taken consistently in regards to food.

Stability Hazardous agent; use appropriate precautions for handling and disposal (NIOSH, 2012).

Inhalation: Store vials in a dry place at 15°C to 30°C (59°F to 86°F). Reconstituted solution is stable for 24 hours at

◀ room temperature; do not mix with other aerosolized medications

Oral: Store at controlled room temperature of 25°C (77°F); excursions permitted to 15°C to 30°C (59°F to 86°F). Solution may also be refrigerated at 2°C to 8°C (36°F to 46°F).

Mechanism of Action Inhibits replication of RNA and DNA viruses; inhibits influenza virus RNA polymerase activity and inhibits the initiation and elongation of RNA fragments resulting in inhibition of viral protein synthesis

Pharmacokinetics (Adult data unless noted)

Absorption: Inhalation: Systemically absorbed from the respiratory tract following nasal and oral inhalation; absorption is dependent upon respiratory factors and method of drug delivery; maximal absorption occurs with the use of the aerosol generator via an endotracheal tube

Distribution: Highest concentrations are found in the respiratory tract and erythrocytes; with chronic oral administration, ribavirin distributes slowly into CSF

Metabolism: Occurs intracellularly and may be necessary for drug action; metabolized by the liver to deribosylated ribavirin (active metabolite)

Bioavailability: Oral: 64%

Half-life:

Respiratory tract secretions: ~2 hours

Plasma:

Children: Inhalation: 6.5-11 hours

Adults: Oral: 24-36 hours after a single dose; half-life is much longer in the erythrocyte (16-40 days), which can be used as a marker for intracellular metabolism; terminal half-life after multiple doses is 151 hours

Time to peak serum concentration: Aerosol inhalation: At the end of the inhalation period

Oral capsule: 3 hours

Tablet: 2 hours

Elimination: Hepatic metabolism is the major route of elimination with 40% of the drug cleared renally as unchanged drug and metabolites

Dosing: Usual

Infants, Children, and Adults: Aerosol inhalation:

Use with Viratek® small particle aerosol generator (SPAG-2) at a concentration of 20 mg/mL (6 g reconstituted with 300 mL of sterile water without preservatives); 6 g ribavirin vial has also been diluted with 300 mL of sterile NS solution rather than sterile water to achieve a near isotonic solution.

Note: Dose actually delivered to the patient will depend on patient's minute ventilation

Continuous aerosolization: 12-18 hours/day for 3 days, or up to 7 days in length

Intermittent aerosolization (high-dose, short-duration aerosol): 2 g over 2 hours 3 times/day at a concentration of 60 mg/mL (6 g reconstituted with 100 mL of sterile water without preservatives) in **nonmechanically ventilated** patients for 3-7 days has been used to permit easier accessibility for patient care and limit environmental exposure of healthcare worker. Due to apparent increased potential for crystallization of the high-dose 60 mg/mL solution around areas of turbulent flow such as bends in tubing or connector pieces, use of high-dose therapy in individuals with an endotracheal tube in place is **not** recommended (Englund, 1994).

Children ≥3 years and Adolescents: Chronic hepatitis C (in combination with interferon alfa-2b):

Oral capsule or solution: 15 mg/kg/day in 2 divided doses (morning and evening). Treatment duration: 48 weeks (genotype 1); 24 weeks (genotypes 2 and 3). Consider discontinuation of combination therapy in patients with HCV (genotype 1) at 12 weeks if a 2 log decrease in HCV-RNA has not been achieved or if HCV-RNA is still detectable at 24 weeks.

Manufacturer's recommendations (for capsule administration):

<47 kg: Use solution

47-59 kg: 400 mg twice daily

60-73 kg: 400 mg in the morning; 600 mg in the evening

>73 kg: 600 mg twice daily

Alternate dosing: (*Red Book*, 2009):

25-36 kg: 200 mg twice daily

37-49 kg: 200 mg in morning; 400 mg in evening

50-61 kg: 400 mg twice daily

>61-75 kg: 400 mg in the morning; 600 mg in the evening

>75 kg: 600 mg twice daily

Adults:

Oral capsule (Rebetol®, Ribasphere®):

Chronic hepatitis C (in combination with interferon alfa-2b):

≤75 kg: 400 mg in morning and 600 mg in evening

>75 kg: 600 mg twice daily

Chronic hepatitis C (in combination with peginterferon alfa-2b): 400 mg twice daily

Oral tablet (Copegus®):

Chronic hepatitis C, genotype 1,4 (in combination with peginterferon alfa-2a):

<75 kg: 500 mg twice daily for 48 weeks

≥75 kg: 600 mg twice daily for 48 weeks

Chronic hepatitis C, genotype 2,3 (in combination with peginterferon alfa-2a): 400 mg twice daily for 24 weeks

Chronic hepatitis C in HIV coinfected patient (in combination with peginterferon alfa-2a): 400 mg twice daily for 48 weeks, regardless of genotype

Dosage adjustment in renal impairment: CrCl <50 mL/minute: Oral route is contraindicated

Children: Serum creatinine >2 mg/dL: Discontinue treatment

Dosage adjustment in hematologic toxicity: Oral:

Children:

Patient **without** cardiac history:

Hemoglobin <10 g/dL: Decrease ribavirin dose to 12 mg/kg/day; may further reduce to 8 mg/kg/day

Hemoglobin <8.5 g/dL: Permanently discontinue ribavirin

Patient **with** cardiac history:

Hemoglobin decrease ≥2 g/dL in any 4-week period in patients: Decrease ribavirin dose to 12 mg/kg/day; may further reduce to 8 mg/kg/day; monitor and evaluate weekly

Hemoglobin <12 g/dL after 4 weeks of reduced dose: Permanently discontinue ribavirin

Adults:

Patient **without** cardiac history:

Hemoglobin <10 g/dL: Decrease dose to 600 mg/day

Hemoglobin <8.5 g/dL: Permanently discontinue treatment

Patient **with** cardiac history:

Hemoglobin has decreased ≥2 g/dL during any 4-week period of treatment: Decrease dose to 600 mg/day

Hemoglobin <12 g/dL after 4 weeks of reduced dose: Permanently discontinue treatment

Administration Hazardous agent; use appropriate precautions for handling and disposal (NIOSH, 2012).

Inhalation: Ribavirin should be administered in well-ventilated rooms (at least 6 air changes/hour)

Mechanically ventilated patients: Ribavirin can potentially be deposited in the ventilator delivery system depending on temperature, humidity, and electrostatic forces; this deposition can lead to malfunction or obstruction of the expiratory valve, resulting in inadvertently high positive end-expiratory pressures. The use of one-way valves in the inspiratory lines, a breathing circuit filter in the expiratory line, and frequent monitoring and filter replacement have been effective in preventing these problems.

Oral: Administer concurrently with interferon alfa injection (pegylated or nonpegylated). Capsule should not be opened, crushed, chewed, or broken. Use oral solution in children ≤5 years of age, those ≤25 kg, or those who cannot swallow capsules.

Capsule or solution in combination with interferon alfa-2b: May be administered with or without food

Capsule in combination with peginterferon alfa-2b: Administer with food

Tablet: Administer with food

Monitoring Parameters

Inhalation: Respiratory function, hemoglobin, reticulocyte count, CBC, I & O

Oral: Hemoglobin, hematocrit, CBC with differential, platelet count, liver function tests, TSH, dental and ophthalmologic exam; close attention to growth during therapy and post-treatment

Serum HCV RNA levels (pretreatment, 12- and 24 weeks after therapy initiation, 24 weeks after completion of therapy). **Note:** Discontinuation of therapy may be considered after 12 weeks in patients with HCV (genotype 1) who fail to achieve an early virologic response (EVR) (defined as ≥2-log decrease in HCV RNA compared to pretreatment) or after 24 weeks with detectable HCV RNA. Treat patients with HCV (genotypes 2,3) for 24 weeks (if tolerated) and then evaluate HCV RNA levels (Ghany, 2009).

Prior to treatment, pregnancy screening should occur for women of childbearing age who are receiving treatment or who have male partners who are receiving treatment. In combination therapy with ribavirin, pregnancy tests should continue monthly up to 6 months after discontinuation of therapy. Evaluate for depression and other psychiatric symptoms before and during therapy; baseline eye examination and periodically in patients with baseline disorders; baseline echocardiogram in patients with cardiac disease.

Additional Information RSV season is usually October to May; varies based on regional climate. Viral shedding period for RSV is usually 3-8 days.

Dosage Forms Excipient information presented when available (limited, particularly for generics); consult specific product labeling.

Capsule, oral: 200 mg
  Rebetol: 200 mg
  Ribasphere: 200 mg

Powder for solution, for nebulization:
  Virazole: 6 g [reconstituted product contains ribavirin 20 mg/mL]

Solution, oral:
  Rebetol: 40 mg/mL (100 mL) [contains propylene glycol, sodium benzoate; bubblegum flavor]

Tablet, oral: 200 mg
  Copegus: 200 mg
  Ribasphere: 200 mg, 400 mg, 600 mg

Tablet, oral [dose-pack]:
  Ribasphere RibaPak 600: 200 mg AM dose, 400 mg PM dose (14s, 56s)
  Ribasphere RibaPak 800: 400 mg AM dose, 400 mg PM dose (14s, 56s)
  Ribasphere RibaPak 1000: 600 mg AM dose, 400 mg PM dose (14s, 56s)
  Ribasphere RibaPak 1200: 600 mg AM dose, 600 mg PM dose (14s, 56s)

References

American Academy of Pediatrics Committee on Infectious Diseases, "Reassessment of the Indications for Ribavirin Therapy in Respiratory Syncytial Virus Infections," *Pediatrics*, 1996, 97(1):137-40.

Centers for Disease Control and Prevention (CDC), "Guidelines for the Prevention and Treatment of Opportunistic Infections Among HIV-Exposed and HIV-Infected Children," *MMWR Recomm Rep*, 2009, 58(RR-11):1-166. Available at http://aidsinfo.nih.gov/contentfiles/Pediatric_OI.pdf

Englund JA, Piedra PA, Ahn Y-M, et al, "High-Dose, Short-Duration Ribavirin Aerosol Therapy Compared With Standard Ribavirin Therapy in Children With Suspected Respiratory Syncytial Virus Infection," *J Pediatr*, 1994, 125:635-41.

Janai HK, Marks MI, Zaleska M, et al, "Ribavirin: Adverse Drug Reactions 1986 to 1988," *Pediatr Infect Dis J*, 1990, 9(3):209-11.

Meert KL, Sarnaik AP, Gelmini MJ, et al, "Aerosolized Ribavirin in Mechanically Ventilated Children With Respiratory Syncytial Virus Lower Respiratory Tract Disease: A Prospective, Double-Blind, Randomized Trial," *Crit Care Med*, 1994, 22(4):566-72.

National Institute for Occupational Safety and Health (NIOSH), "NIOSH List of Antineoplastic and Other Hazardous Drugs in Healthcare Settings 2012." Available at http://www.cdc.gov/niosh/docs/2012-150/pdfs/2012-150.pdf. Accessed January 21, 2013.

"NIH Consensus Statement on Management of Hepatitis C: 2002," *NIH Consens State Sci Statements*, 2002, 19(3):1-46.

Red Book: 2009 Report of the Committee on Infectious Diseases, "Antiviral Drug," 28th ed, Pickering LK, ed, Elk Grove Village, IL: American Academy of Pediatrics, 2009, 777-82.

Smith DW, Frankel LR, Mathers LH, et al, "A Controlled Trial of Aerosolized Ribavirin in Infants Receiving Mechanical Ventilation for Severe Respiratory Syncytial Virus Infection," *N Engl J Med*, 1991, 325(1):24-9.

Wirth S, Lang T, Gehring S, et al, "Recombinant Alfa-Interferon Plus Ribavirin Therapy in Children and Adolescents With Chronic Hepatitis C," *Hepatology*, 2002, 36(5):1280-4.

Riboflavin (RYE boe flay vin)

Medication Safety Issues

Sound-alike/look-alike issues:
Riboflavin may be confused with ribavirin

Brand Names: U.S. B-2-400 [OTC]

Therapeutic Category Nutritional Supplement; Vitamin, Water Soluble

Generic Availability (U.S.) Yes

Use Prevention of riboflavin deficiency and treatment of ariboflavinosis; microcytic anemia associated with glutathione reductase deficiency

Pregnancy Considerations Water-soluble vitamins cross the placenta. Riboflavin requirements may be increased in pregnant women compared to nonpregnant women (IOM, 1998).

Breast-Feeding Considerations Riboflavin is found in breast milk. Concentrations may be influenced by supplements or maternal deficiency. Riboflavin requirements may be increased in nursing women compared to non-nursing women (IOM, 1998).

Contraindications Hypersensitivity to riboflavin or any component

Adverse Reactions Genitourinary: Discoloration of urine (yellow-orange)

Drug Interactions

Metabolism/Transport Effects None known.

Avoid Concomitant Use There are no known interactions where it is recommended to avoid concomitant use.

Increased Effect/Toxicity There are no known significant interactions involving an increase in effect.

Decreased Effect There are no known significant interactions involving a decrease in effect.

Stability Protect from light

Mechanism of Action Component of flavoprotein enzymes that work together, which are necessary for normal tissue respiration; also needed for activation of pyridoxine and conversion of tryptophan to niacin

Pharmacokinetics (Adult data unless noted)

Absorption: Readily via GI tract; GI absorption is decreased in patients with hepatitis, cirrhosis, or biliary obstruction

Metabolism: Metabolic fate unknown

Half-life, biologic: 66-84 minutes

Elimination: 9% eliminated unchanged in urine

Dosing: Neonatal Oral: Adequate intake: 0.3 mg/day (0.04 mg/kg/day)

Dosing: Usual Oral:

Riboflavin deficiency:

Children: 3-10 mg/day in divided doses

Adults: 5-30 mg/day in divided doses

Adequate intake: Infants:

1 to <6 months: 0.3 mg (0.04 mg/kg)

6-12 months: 0.4 mg (0.04 mg/kg)

Recommended daily allowance (RDA): Children and Adults:

1-3 years: 0.5 mg

4-8 years: 0.6 mg

9-13 years: 0.9 mg

14-18 years:

Male: 1.3 mg

Female: 1 mg

19-70 years:

Male: 1.3 mg

Female: 1.1 mg

Microcytic anemia associated with glutathione reductase deficiency: Adults: 10 mg daily for 10 days

Administration Oral: Administer with food

Monitoring Parameters CBC and reticulocyte counts (if anemic when treating deficiency)

Test Interactions Large doses may interfere with urinalysis based on spectrometry; may cause false elevations in fluorometric determinations of catecholamines and urobilinogen

Dosage Forms Excipient information presented when available (limited, particularly for generics); consult specific product labeling.

Capsule, Oral:

B-2-400: 400 mg

Generic: 50 mg

Tablet, Oral:

Generic: 25 mg, 50 mg, 100 mg

Tablet, Oral [preservative free]:

Generic: 100 mg

References

IOM (Institute of Medicine), "Dietary Reference Intakes for Thiamin, Riboflavin, Niacin, Vitamin B$_6$, Folate, Vitamin B$_{12}$, Pantothenic Acid, Biotin, and Choline," Washington, DC: The National Academies Press, 1998.

◆ **Ridaura** see Auranofin on page 239

◆ **Ridaura® (Can)** see Auranofin on page 239

Rifabutin (rif a BYOO tin)

Medication Safety Issues

Sound-alike/look-alike issues:

Rifabutin may be confused with rifampin

Brand Names: U.S. Mycobutin

Brand Names: Canada Mycobutin®

Therapeutic Category Antibiotic, Miscellaneous; Antitubercular Agent

Generic Availability (U.S.) Yes

Use Prevention of disseminated *Mycobacterium avium* complex (MAC) in patients with advanced HIV infection (FDA approved in adults); has also been utilized in multiple drug regimens for treatment of MAC; alternative to rifampin as prophylaxis for latent tuberculosis infection (LTBI) or part of multidrug regimen for treatment active tuberculosis infection; alternative as agent for prophylaxis of *Mycobacterium avium* complex in children >6 years; add-on therapy for severe *Mycobacterium avium* complex add-on infection

Pregnancy Risk Factor B

Pregnancy Considerations Adverse events were seen in some animal reproduction studies.

Breast-Feeding Considerations In the United States, where formula is accessible, affordable, safe, and sustainable, and the risk of infant mortality due to diarrhea and respiratory infections is low, complete avoidance of breast-feeding by HIV-infected women is recommended to decrease potential transmission of HIV (DHHS [perinatal], 2011).

Contraindications Hypersensitivity to rifabutin, any component, or other rifamycin

Warnings Rifabutin as a single agent must not be administered to patients with active tuberculosis since its use may lead to the development of tuberculosis that is resistant to both rifabutin and rifampin; rifabutin should be discontinued in patients with AST >3x ULN (symptomatic) or ≥5x ULN (regardless of symptoms) or if significant bilirubin and/or alkaline phosphatase elevations occur. Tiny, asymptomatic peripheral and central corneal deposits have been observed during routine ophthalmologic exams in HIV-positive patients receiving rifabutin. *C. difficile*-associated diarrhea has been reported with use of rifabutin.

Precautions Use with caution in patients with liver or renal impairment; modify dose in patients with CrCl <30 mL/minute. Rifabutin is a CYP3A3/4 isoenzyme inducer which may reduce the plasma concentrations of itraconazole, clarithromycin, and saquinavir. CYP3A3/4 isoenzyme inhibitors such as fluconazole and clarithromycin may elevate levels of rifabutin increasing the risk of adverse reactions. Monitor patients, and in some cases, reduce the rifabutin dose when coadministered with fluconazole or clarithromycin. Rifabutin decreases plasma concentrations of delavirdine; delavirdine increases plasma concentrations of rifabutin (coadministration of rifabutin and delavirdine is not recommended). May be associated with neutropenia and/or thrombocytopenia (rarely); consider hematologic monitoring and discontinue permanently if signs of thrombocytopenia (eg, petechial rash) occur.

Adverse Reactions

Central nervous system: Headache, fever

Dermatologic: Rash

Gastrointestinal: Abdominal pain, dyspepsia, eructation, flatulence, nausea, taste perversion, vomiting

Genitourinary: Discoloration of urine

Hematologic: Leukopenia, neutropenia, thrombocytopenia

Hepatic: ALT increased, AST increased

Neuromuscular & skeletal: Myalgia

Rare but important or life-threatening: Aphasia, arthralgia, chest pain, confusion, dyspnea, flu-like syndrome, hepatitis, hemolysis, myositis, parasthesia, seizures, skin discoloration, T-wave abnormalities, uveitis

Drug Interactions

Metabolism/Transport Effects Substrate of CYP1A2 (minor), CYP3A4 (major); **Note:** Assignment of Major/Minor substrate status based on clinically relevant drug interaction potential; **Induces** CYP3A4 (strong)

Avoid Concomitant Use

Avoid concomitant use of Rifabutin with any of the following: Abiraterone Acetate; Apixaban; Apremilast; Artemether; Atovaquone; Axitinib; BCG; Bedaquiline; Boceprevir; Bortezomib; Bosutinib; Cabozantinib; Ceritinib; CloZAPine; Cobicistat; Crizotinib; Dienogest; Dronedarone; Elvitegravir; Enzalutamide; Everolimus; Ibrutinib; Itraconazole; Ivacaftor; Lapatinib; Lumefantrine; Lurasidone; Macitentan; Mifepristone; Mycophenolate; NIFEdipine; Nilotinib; Nisoldipine; PAZOPanib; Perampanel; PONATinib; Praziquantel; Ranolazine; Regorafenib; Rivaroxaban; Roflumilast; RomiDEPsin; Simeprevir; Sofosbuvir; SORAfenib; Tasimelteon; Telaprevir; Ticagrelor; Tofacitinib; Tolvaptan; Toremifene; Ulipristal; Vandetanib; Vemurafenib; VinCRIStine (Liposomal); Vorapaxar; Voriconazole

Increased Effect/Toxicity

Rifabutin may increase the levels/effects of: Clarithromycin; Clopidogrel; Darunavir; Fosamprenavir; Ifosfamide; Isoniazid; Lopinavir; Pitavastatin

The levels/effects of Rifabutin may be increased by: Antifungal Agents (Azole Derivatives, Systemic); Atazanavir; Boceprevir; Clarithromycin; Darunavir; Delavirdine;

Fosamprenavir; Indinavir; Lopinavir; Macrolide Antibiotics; Nelfinavir; Nevirapine; Ritonavir; Saquinavir; Telaprevir; Tipranavir; Voriconazole

Decreased Effect

Rifabutin may decrease the levels/effects of: Abiraterone Acetate; Alfentanil; Angiotensin II Receptor Blockers; Antiemetics (5HT3 Antagonists); Antifungal Agents (Azole Derivatives, Systemic); Apixaban; Apremilast; ARIPiprazole; Artemether; Atovaquone; Axitinib; Barbiturates; BCG; Bedaquiline; Benzodiazepines (metabolized by oxidation); Boceprevir; Bortezomib; Bosutinib; Brentuximab Vedotin; BusPIRone; Cabozantinib; Calcium Channel Blockers; Cannabidiol; Cannabis; Ceritinib; Clarithromycin; CloZAPine; Cobicistat; Contraceptives (Estrogens); Contraceptives (Progestins); Corticosteroids (Systemic); Crizotinib; CycloSPORINE (Systemic); CYP3A4 Substrates; Dapsone (Systemic); Dasatinib; Delavirdine; Dienogest; DOXOrubicin (Conventional); Dronabinol; Dronedarone; Efavirenz; Elvitegravir; Enzalutamide; Etravirine; Everolimus; Exemestane; FentaNYL; Gefitinib; GuanFACINE; HMG-CoA Reductase Inhibitors; Ibrutinib; Imatinib; Indinavir; Itraconazole; Ivacaftor; Ixabepilone; Lapatinib; Linagliptin; Lumefantrine; Lurasidone; Macitentan; Maraviroc; Mifepristone; Morphine (Systemic); Mycophenolate; Nelfinavir; Nevirapine; NIFEdipine; Nilotinib; Nisoldipine; PAZOPanib; Perampanel; PONATinib; Praziquantel; Propafenone; QUEtiapine; QuiNIDine; Raltegravir; Ramelteon; Ranolazine; Regorafenib; Rilpivirine; Rivaroxaban; Roflumilast; RomiDEPsin; Saxagliptin; Simeprevir; Sodium Picosulfate; Sofosbuvir; SORAfenib; SUNItinib; Tacrolimus (Systemic); Tadalafil; Tamoxifen; Tasimelteon; Telaprevir; Temsirolimus; Tetrahydrocannabinol; Ticagrelor; Tofacitinib; Tolvaptan; Toremifene; Typhoid Vaccine; Ulipristal; Vandetanib; Vemurafenib; Vilazodone; VinCRIStine (Liposomal); Vitamin K Antagonists; Vorapaxar; Voriconazole; Vortioxetine; Zaleplon; Zolpidem; Zuclopenthixol

The levels/effects of Rifabutin may be decreased by: Bosentan; CYP3A4 Inducers (Strong); Dabrafenib; Deferasirox; Efavirenz; Mitotane; Nevirapine; Siltuximab; St Johns Wort; Tocilizumab

Food Interactions High-fat meal may decrease the rate but not the extent of absorption. Management: May administer with meals.

Stability Capsules should be stored in a well-closed container at 25°C (77°F) with excursions permitted to 15°C to 30°C (59°F to 86 °F)

Mechanism of Action Inhibits DNA-dependent RNA polymerase at the beta subunit which prevents chain initiation

Pharmacokinetics (Adult data unless noted)

Absorption: Oral: Readily absorbed

Distribution: To body tissues including the lungs, liver, spleen, eyes, and kidneys

V_d: Adults: 9.3 ± 1.5 L/kg

Protein binding: 85%

Metabolism: Hepatically to 5 metabolites; predominantly 25-O-desacetyl-rifabutin (antimicrobial activity equivalent to parent drug; serum AUC 10% of parent drug) and 31-hydroxy-rifabutin (serum AUC 7% of parent drug)

Bioavailability: 20% in HIV patients

Half-life, terminal: 45 hours (range: 16-69 hours)

Time to peak serum concentration: 2-4 hours

Elimination: Renal and biliary clearance of unchanged drug is 10%; 30% excreted in feces; 53% excreted in urine

Dosing: Usual Oral:

Infants and Children:

Mycobacterium avium complex (MAC) (CDC, 2009):

Treatment, add-on therapy for severe infection: 10-20 mg/kg once daily (maximum: 300 mg)

Prophylaxis for first episode (HIV-positive/exposed patients ≥6 years): 300 mg once daily

Prophylaxis for recurrence (HIV positive-/exposed patients): 5 mg/kg (maximum dose: 300 mg) once daily as an optional add-on to primary therapy of clarithromycin and ethambutol

Tuberculosis, treatment (alternative to rifampin): 10-20 mg/kg (maximum dose: 300 mg) once daily or intermittently 2-3 times weekly

Adolescents and Adults (CDC, 2009a):

Disseminated MAC in advanced HIV infection:

Prophylaxis: 300 mg once daily or 150 mg twice daily to reduce gastrointestinal upset

Treatment: 300 mg once daily as an optional add-on to primary therapy of clarithromycin and ethambutol

Tuberculosis (alternative to rifampin):

Prophylaxis of LTBI: 300 mg once daily for 4 months

Treatment of active TB: 300 mg once daily or intermittently 2-3 times weekly as part of multidrug regimen

Dosage adjustment for concurrent efavirenz (no concomitant protease inhibitor): Adolescents and Adults: Increase rifabutin dose to 450-600 mg daily or 600 mg 3 times/week

Dosage adjustment for concurrent nelfinavir, amprenavir, indinavir: Adolescents and Adults: Reduce rifabutin dose to 150 mg/day; no change in dose if administered twice weekly

Dosage adjustment in renal impairment: CrCl <30 mL/minute: Reduce dose by 50%

Administration Oral: May administer with or without food or mix with applesauce if patient unable to swallow capsule; administer with food to decrease GI upset

Monitoring Parameters Periodic liver function tests, CBC with differential, platelet count, hemoglobin, hematocrit, ophthalmologic exam, number and type of stools/day for diarrhea

Dosage Forms Excipient information presented when available (limited, particularly for generics); consult specific product labeling.

Capsule, Oral:

Mycobutin: 150 mg

Generic: 150 mg

Extemporaneous Preparations A 20 mg/mL rifabutin oral suspension may be made with capsules and a 1:1 mixture of Ora-Sweet® and Ora-Plus®. Empty the the powder from eight 150 mg rifabutin capsules into a glass mortar; add 20 mL of vehicle and mix to a uniform paste. Mix while adding vehicle in incremental proportions to almost 60 mL; transfer to a calibrated bottle, rinse mortar with vehicle, and add quantity of vehicle sufficient to make 60 mL. Label "shake well". Stable for 12 weeks at 4°C, 25°C, 30°C, and 40°C.

Haslam JL, Egodage KL, Chen Y, et al, "Stability of Rifabutin in Two Extemporaneously Compounded Oral Liquids," *Am J Health Syst Pharm*, 1999, 56(4):333-6.

References

Adult Prevention and Treatment of Opportunistic Infections Guidelines Working Group, "Guidelines for Prevention and Treatment of Opportunistic Infections in HIV-Infected Adults and Adolescents. March 24, 2009," *MMWR*, 2009; 58 (early release): 1-198. Available at: http://www.cdc.gov/mmwr/preview/mmwrhtml/rr58e324a1.htm. Accessed May 21, 2009.

Centers for Disease Control and Prevention (CDC), "Guidelines for the Prevention and Treatment of Opportunistic Infections Among HIV-Exposed and HIV-Infected Children," *MMWR Recomm Rep*, 2009, 58(RR-11):1-166. Available at http://aidsinfo.nih.gov/contentfiles/Pediatric_OI.pdf

DHHS Panel on Treatment of HIV-Infected Pregnant Women and Prevention of Perinatal Transmission, "Recommendations for Use of Antiretroviral Drugs in Pregnant HIV-1-Infected Women for Maternal Health and Interventions to Reduce Perinatal HIV Transmission in the United States," September 14, 2011, 1-207.

Krause PJ, Hight DW, Schwartz AN, et al, "Successful Management of *Mycobacterium intracellulare* Pneumonia in a Child," *Pediatr Infect Dis*, 1986, 5(2):269-71.

Levin RH and Bolinger AM, "Treatment of Nontuberculous Mycobacterial Infections in Pediatric Patients," *Clin Pharm*, 1988, 7(7):545-51.

Starke JR and Correa AG, "Management of Mycobacterial Infection and Disease in Children," *Pediatr Infect Dis J*, 1995, 14(6):455-70.

Working Group on Guidelines for the Prevention and Treatment of Opportunistic Infections Among HIV-Exposed and HIV-Infected Children, "Guidelines for Prevention and Treatment of Opportunistic Infections in HIV-Exposed and HIV-Infected Children [DRAFT]," June 20, 2008," 2008, 1-250. Available at: http://aidsinfo.nih.gov/content-files/Pediatric_OI.pdf. Accessed May 21, 2009.

♦ **Rifadin** see Rifampin on page 1824

♦ **Rifadin® (Can)** see Rifampin on page 1824

♦ **Rifampicin** see Rifampin on page 1824

Rifampin (rif AM pin)

Medication Safety Issues
Sound-alike/look-alike issues:
Rifadin® may be confused with Rifater®, Ritalin®
Rifampin may be confused with ribavirin, rifabutin, Rifamate®, rifapentine, rifaximin
Brand Names: U.S. Rifadin
Brand Names: Canada Rifadin®; Rofact™
Therapeutic Category Antibiotic, Miscellaneous; Antitubercular Agent
Generic Availability (U.S.) Yes
Use Management of active tuberculosis in combination with other agents [FDA approved in pediatric patients (age not specified) and adults]; elimination of meningococci from asymptomatic carriers [FDA approved in pediatric patients (age not specified) and adults]; has also been used for prophylaxis in contacts of patients with *Haemophilus influenzae* type B infection; used in combination with other anti-infectives in the treatment of staphylococcal infections
Pregnancy Risk Factor C
Pregnancy Considerations Teratogenic effects have been reported in animal studies. Rifampin crosses the human placenta. Due to the risk of tuberculosis to the fetus, treatment is recommended when the probability of maternal disease is moderate to high. Postnatal hemorrhages have been reported in the infant and mother with isoniazid administration during the last few weeks of pregnancy.
Breast-Feeding Considerations The manufacturer does not recommend breast-feeding due to tumorigenicity observed in animal studies; however, the CDC does not consider rifampin a contraindication to breast-feeding.
Contraindications Hypersensitivity to rifampin, rifamycins, or any component; concurrent use with amprenavir, saquinavir/ritonavir (possibly other protease inhibitors)
Warnings Two month rifampin-pyrazinamide regimen for the treatment of latent tuberculosis infection (LTBI) has been associated with severe and fatal liver injuries. The IDSA and CDC now recommend that this regimen should not generally be used in patients with LTBI.
Precautions Use with caution in patients with liver impairment, patients receiving concurrent medications associated with liver injury (particularly with pyrazinamide), or in patients with a history of alcoholism; modification of dosage should be considered in patients with severe liver impairment
Adverse Reactions
Cardiovascular: Edema, flushing
Central nervous system: Ataxia, behavioral changes, concentration impaired, confusion, dizziness, drowsiness, fatigue, fever, headache, numbness, psychosis
Dermatologic: Pemphigoid reaction, pruritus, rash, urticaria
Endocrine & metabolic: Adrenal insufficiency, menstrual disorders
Gastrointestinal: Anorexia, cramps, diarrhea, epigastric distress, flatulence, heartburn, nausea, pseudomembranous colitis, pancreatitis, vomiting
Hematologic: Agranulocytosis (rare), DIC, eosinophilia, hemoglobin decreased, hemolysis, hemolytic anemia, leukopenia, thrombocytopenia (especially with high-dose therapy)
Hepatic: Hepatitis (rare), jaundice, LFTs increased
Neuromuscular & skeletal: Myalgia, osteomalacia, weakness
Ocular: Exudative conjunctivitis, visual changes
Renal: Acute renal failure, BUN increased, hemoglobinuria, hematuria, interstitial nephritis, uric acid increased
Miscellaneous: Flu-like syndrome
Drug Interactions
Metabolism/Transport Effects Substrate of P-glycoprotein, SLCO1B1; **Induces** CYP1A2 (strong), CYP2A6 (strong), CYP2B6 (strong), CYP2C19 (strong), CYP2C8 (strong), CYP2C9 (strong), CYP3A4 (strong), P-glycoprotein
Avoid Concomitant Use
Avoid concomitant use of Rifampin with any of the following: Abiraterone Acetate; Apixaban; Apremilast; Artemether; Atazanavir; Atovaquone; Axitinib; BCG; Bedaquiline; Boceprevir; Bortezomib; Bosutinib; Cabozantinib; Ceritinib; CloZAPine; Cobicistat; Crizotinib; Dabigatran Etexilate; Darunavir; Dienogest; Dronedarone; Elvitegravir; Enzalutamide; Esomeprazole; Etravirine; Everolimus; Fosamprenavir; Ibrutinib; Indinavir; Itraconazole; Ivacaftor; Lapatinib; Lopinavir; Lumefantrine; Lurasidone; Macitentan; Mifepristone; Mycophenolate; Nelfinavir; NIFEdipine; Nilotinib; Nisoldipine; Omeprazole; PAZOPanib; Perampanel; Pirfenidone; Pomalidomide; PONATinib; Praziquantel; QuiNINE; Ranolazine; Regorafenib; Rilpivirine; Ritonavir; Rivaroxaban; Roflumilast; RomiDEPsin; Saquinavir; Simeprevir; Sofosbuvir; SORAfenib; Tasimelteon; Telaprevir; Ticagrelor; Tipranavir; Tofacitinib; Tolvaptan; Toremifene; Ulipristal; Vandetanib; Vemurafenib; VinCRIStine (Liposomal); Vorapaxar; Voriconazole
Increased Effect/Toxicity
Rifampin may increase the levels/effects of: Bosentan; Clarithromycin; Clopidogrel; Fexofenadine; Isoniazid; Leflunomide; Lopinavir; Pitavastatin; Propofol; RomiDEPsin; Saquinavir

The levels/effects of Rifampin may be increased by: Antifungal Agents (Azole Derivatives, Systemic); Clarithromycin; Delavirdine; Eltrombopag; Macrolide Antibiotics; P-glycoprotein/ABCB1 Inhibitors; Pyrazinamide; Voriconazole
Decreased Effect
Rifampin may decrease the levels/effects of: Abiraterone Acetate; Afatinib; Alfentanil; Amiodarone; Angiotensin II Receptor Blockers; Antidiabetic Agents (Thiazolidinedione); Antiemetics (5HT3 Antagonists); Antifungal Agents (Azole Derivatives, Systemic); Apixaban; Apremilast; Aprepitant; ARIPiprazole; Artemether; Atazanavir; Atovaquone; Axitinib; Barbiturates; Bazedoxifene; BCG; Bedaquiline; Bendamustine; Benzodiazepines (metabolized by oxidation); Beta-Blockers; Boceprevir; Bortezomib; Bosentan; Bosutinib; Brentuximab Vedotin; BusPIRone; Cabozantinib; Calcium Channel Blockers; Canagliflozin; Cannabidiol; Cannabis; Caspofungin; Ceritinib; Chloramphenicol; Citalopram; Clarithromycin; CloZAPine; Cobicistat; Contraceptives (Estrogens); Contraceptives (Progestins); Corticosteroids (Systemic); Crizotinib; CycloSPORINE (Systemic); CYP1A2 Substrates; CYP2A6 Substrates; CYP2B6 Substrates; CYP2C19 Substrates; CYP2C8 Substrates; CYP2C9 Substrates; CYP3A4 Substrates; Dabigatran Etexilate; Dapsone (Systemic); Darunavir; Dasatinib; Deferasirox; Delavirdine; Diclofenac (Systemic); Dienogest; Disopyramide; Dolutegravir; DOXOrubicin (Conventional); Doxycycline; Dronabinol; Dronedarone; Efavirenz; Elvitegravir; Enzalutamide; Erlotinib; Esomeprazole; Etravirine; Everolimus; Exemestane; FentaNYL; Fexofenadine; Fosamprenavir; Fosaprepitant; Fosphenytoin;

Gefitinib; GuanFACINE; HMG-CoA Reductase Inhibitors; Ibrutinib; Imatinib; Indinavir; Itraconazole; Ivacaftor; Ixabepilone; LamoTRIgine; Lapatinib; Linagliptin; Lopinavir; Lumefantrine; Lurasidone; Macitentan; Maraviroc; Methadone; Mifepristone; Mirabegron; Morphine (Systemic); Mycophenolate; Nelfinavir; Nevirapine; NIFEdipine; Nilotinib; Nisoldipine; Omeprazole; OxyCODONE; PAZOPanib; Perampanel; P-glycoprotein/ABCB1 Substrates; Phenytoin; Pirfenidone; Pomalidomide; PONATinib; Prasugrel; Praziquantel; Propafenone; QUEtiapine; QuiNIDine; QuiNINE; Raltegravir; Ramelteon; Ranolazine; Regorafenib; Repaglinide; Rilpivirine; Ritonavir; Rivaroxaban; Roflumilast; Saquinavir; Saxagliptin; Simeprevir; Sirolimus; Sodium Picosulfate; Sofosbuvir; SORAfenib; Sulfonylureas; SUNItinib; Tacrolimus (Systemic); Tadalafil; Tamoxifen; Tasimelteon; Telaprevir; Temsirolimus; Terbinafine (Systemic); Tetrahydrocannabinol; Thyroid Products; Ticagrelor; Tipranavir; Tofacitinib; Tolvaptan; Toremifene; Treprostinil; Typhoid Vaccine; Ulipristal; Valproic Acid and Derivatives; Vandetanib; Vemurafenib; Vilazodone; VinCRIStine (Liposomal); Vorapaxar; Voriconazole; Vortioxetine; Zaleplon; Zidovudine; Zolpidem; Zuclopenthixol

The levels/effects of Rifampin may be decreased by: P-glycoprotein/ABCB1 Inducers

Food Interactions Food decreases the extent of absorption; rifampin concentrations may be decreased if taken with food. Management: Administer on an empty stomach with a glass of water (ie, 1 hour prior to, or 2 hours after meals or antacids).

Stability
Oral: Store capsules at 25°C (77°F); excursions permitted to 15°C to 30°C (59°F to 86°F); avoid excessive heat [>40°C (104°F)]; store in a dry place.
Parenteral: Store intact vials at 25°C (77°F); excursions permitted to 15°C to 30°C (59°F to 86°F); avoid excessive heat [>40°C (104°F)]; protect from light. Reconstituted I.V. solution is stable for 24 hours at room temperature; upon further dilution, it is stable for 4 hours in D_5W and up to 24 hours in NS at room temperature; however, 11% to 13% rifampin decomposition has been reported to occur in 24 hours for solutions diluted in NS. Administer rifampin I.V. solution within 4 hours after preparation to avoid potential for precipitation and decomposition beyond this period.

Mechanism of Action Inhibits bacterial RNA synthesis by binding to the beta subunit of DNA-dependent RNA polymerase, blocking RNA transcription

Pharmacokinetics (Adult data unless noted)
Absorption: Oral: Well absorbed
Distribution: Highly lipophilic; crosses the blood-brain barrier and is widely distributed into body tissues and fluids such as the liver, lungs, gallbladder, bile, tears, and breast milk; distributes into CSF when meninges are inflamed
Protein binding: 80%
Metabolism: Undergoes enterohepatic recycling; metabolized in the liver to a deacetylated metabolite (active)
Half-life: 3-4 hours, prolonged with hepatic impairment
Time to peak serum concentration: Oral: Within 2-4 hours
Elimination: Principally in feces (60% to 65%) and urine (~30%)
Dialysis: Plasma rifampin concentrations are not significantly affected by hemodialysis or peritoneal dialysis

Dosing: Neonatal I.V., Oral:
H. influenzae prophylaxis: 10 mg/kg/day once daily for 4 days
Meningococcal prophylaxis: 10 mg/kg/day in divided doses every 12 hours for 2 days
Staphylococcus aureus, synergy for infections: 5-20 mg/kg/day in divided doses every 12 hours with other antibiotics

Dosing: Usual Oral, I.V.:
Tuberculosis:
Active infection, treatment: **Note:** A four-drug regimen (isoniazid, rifampin, pyrazinamide, and ethambutol) is preferred for the initial, empiric treatment of TB. The regimen should be altered based on drug susceptibility results as appropriate. In HIV-exposed/positive patients, rifabutin may be used an alternative to rifampin. American Thoracic Society and CDC currently recommend twice weekly therapy as part of a short-course regimen, which follows 1-2 months of daily treatment of uncomplicated pulmonary tuberculosis in the compliant patient.
Daily therapy:
Infants and Children: 10-20 mg/kg/day (maximum dose: 600 mg)
Adults: 10 mg/kg/day administered once daily (maximum dose: 600 mg)
Directly observed therapy (DOT):
Infants and Children: 10-20 mg/kg (maximum dose: 600 mg) administered 2 times/week if HIV negative **or** administered 3 times weekly if HIV-exposed/positive.
Adults: 10 mg/kg (maximum dose: 600 mg) administered 2 or 3 times/week
Latent tuberculosis infection (LTBI) treatment (as an alternative to isoniazid): **Note:** Combination with pyrazinamide should not generally be offered (*MMWR*, Aug 8, 2003). In HIV-exposed/positive patients, isoniazid is preferred due to potential for drug interactions of rifampin with antiretroviral therapy.
Infants and Children: 10-20 mg/kg/day once daily for 4 months (maximum dose: 600 mg/day)
Adults: 10 mg/kg/dose once daily for 4 months (maximum dose: 600 mg/day)
Primary prophylaxis of isoniazid-resistant tuberculosis in HIV-exposed/positive patients: Infants and Children: 10-20 mg/kg/dose once daily for 4-6 months (maximum dose: 600 mg/day)

Endocarditis, prosthetic valve due to MRSA (Baddour, 2005; Lui, 2011):
Infants and Children: 15-20 mg/kg/day divided every 8 hours
Adults: 300 mg every 8 hours for at least 6 weeks (combine with vancomycin for the entire duration of therapy and gentamicin for the first 2 weeks)

H. influenzae **prophylaxis:**
Infants and Children: 20 mg/kg/day once daily for 4 days, not to exceed 600 mg/dose
Adults: 600 mg once daily for 4 days

Meningococcal prophylaxis:
Infants and Children: 20 mg/kg/day in divided doses every 12 hours for 2 days, not to exceed 600 mg/dose
Adults: 600 mg every 12 hours for 2 days

Staphylococcus aureus, nasal carriers:
Children: 15 mg/kg/day divided every 12 hours for 5-10 days; **Note: Must use in combination with at least one other systemic antistaphylococcal antibiotic.** Not recommended as first-line drug for decolonization; evidence is weak for use in patients with recurrent infections (Liu, 2011).
Adults: 600 mg/day for 5-10 days; **Note: Must use in combination with at least one other systemic antistaphylococcal antibiotic.** Not recommended as first-line drug for decolonization; evidence is weak for use in patients with recurrent infections (Liu, 2011).

Staphylococcus aureus, synergy for infections: Adults: 600 mg once daily or 300-450 mg every 12 hours with other antibiotics. **Note:** Must be used in combination with another antistaphylococcal antibiotic to avoid rapid development of resistance (Liu, 2011).

Administration

Oral: Administer on an empty stomach with a glass of water (ie, 1 hour prior to or 2 hours after meals or antacids) to increase total absorption (food may delay and reduce the amount of rifampin absorbed). The compounded oral suspension must be shaken well before using. May mix contents of capsule with applesauce or jelly

Parenteral: Do not administer I.M. or SubQ. Reconstitute vial with 10 mL SWI; further dilute in an appropriate volume of a compatible solution at a final concentration not to exceed 6 mg/mL; administer I.V. preparation once daily by slow I.V. infusion over 30 minutes to 3 hours

Monitoring Parameters Periodic monitoring of liver function (AST, ALT); bilirubin, CBC, platelet count

Test Interactions May interfere with urine detection of opioids (false-positive); positive Coombs' reaction [direct], rifampin inhibits standard assay's ability to measure serum folate and B$_{12}$; transient increase in LFTs and decreased biliary excretion of contrast media

Dosage Forms Excipient information presented when available (limited, particularly for generics); consult specific product labeling.

Capsule, Oral:
  Rifadin: 150 mg, 300 mg
  Generic: 150 mg, 300 mg
Solution Reconstituted, Intravenous:
  Rifadin: 600 mg (1 ea)
  Generic: 600 mg (1 ea)

Extemporaneous Preparations A rifampin 1% w/v suspension (10 mg/mL) may be made with capsules and one of four syrups (Syrup NF, simple syrup, Syrpalta® syrup, or raspberry syrup). Empty the contents of four 300 mg capsules or eight 150 mg capsules onto a piece of weighing paper. If necessary, crush contents to produce a fine powder. Transfer powder to a 4-ounce amber glass or plastic prescription bottle. Rinse paper and spatula with 20 mL of chosen syrup and add the rinse to bottle; shake vigorously. Add 100 mL syrup to the bottle and shake vigorously. Label "shake well". Stable for 4 weeks at room temperature or refrigerated.

A 25 mg/mL oral suspension may be made with capsules and cherry syrup concentrate diluted 1:4 with simple syrup, NF. Empty the contents of ten 300 mg capsules into a mortar and reduce to a fine powder. Add 20 mL of the vehicle and mix to a uniform paste; mix while adding the vehicle in incremental proportions to **almost** 120 mL; transfer to a calibrated bottle, rinse mortar with vehicle, and add quantity of vehicle sufficient to make 120 mL. Label "shake well" and "refrigerate". Stable for 28 days refrigerated (preferred) or at room temperature.

Nahata MC, Pai VB, and Hipple TF, *Pediatric Drug Formulations*, 5th ed, Cincinnati, OH: Harvey Whitney Books Co, 2004.

References

American Academy of Pediatrics Committee on Infectious Diseases, "Chemotherapy for Tuberculosis in Infants and Children," *Pediatrics*, 1992, 89(1):161-5.

Baddour LM, Wilson WR, Bayer AS, et al, "Infective Endocarditis: Diagnosis, Antimicrobial Therapy, and Management of Complications: A Statement for Healthcare Professionals From the Committee on Rheumatic Fever, Endocarditis, and Kawasaki Disease, Council on Cardiovascular Disease in the Young, and the Councils on Clinical Cardiology, Stroke, and Cardiovascular Surgery and Anesthesia, American Heart Association: Endorsed by the Infectious Diseases Society of America," *Circulation*, 2005, 111(23):394-434.

Centers for Disease Control and Prevention (CDC), "Guidelines for the Prevention and Treatment of Opportunistic Infections Among HIV-Exposed and HIV-Infected Children," *MMWR Recomm Rep*, 2009, 58(RR-11):1-166. Available at http://aidsinfo.nih.gov/contentfiles/Pediatric_OI.pdf

Centers for Disease Control and Prevention, "Treatment of Tuberculosis. American Thoracic Society, CDC, and Infectious Diseases Society of America 2003," *MMWR Recomm Rep*, 2003, 52 (RR11):3-5.

Liu C, Bayer A, Cosgrove SE, et al, "Clinical Practice Guidelines by the Infectious Diseases Society of America for the Treatment of Methicillin-Resistant *Staphylococcus aureus* Infections in Adults and Children: Executive Summary," *Clin Infect Dis*, 2011, 52(3):285-92.

Shulman ST, Bisno AL, Clegg HW, et al, "Clinical Practice Guideline for the Diagnosis and Management of Group A Streptococcal Pharyngitis: 2012 Update by the Infectious Diseases Society of America," *Clin Infect Dis*, 2012.

Starke JR, "Modern Approach to the Diagnosis and Treatment of Tuberculosis in Children," *Pediatr Clin North Am*, 1988, 35(3):441-64.

Starke JR, "Multidrug Therapy for Tuberculosis in Children," *Pediatr Infect Dis J*, 1990, 9(11):785-93.

Tan TQ, Mason EO Jr, Ou CN, et al, "Use of Intravenous Rifampin in Neonates With Persistent Staphylococcal Bacteremia," *Antimicrob Agents Chemother*, 1993, 37(11):2401-6.

Rifaximin (rif AX i min)

Medication Safety Issues
Sound-alike/look-alike issues:
  Rifaximin may be confused with rifampin
Brand Names: U.S. Xifaxan
Therapeutic Category Antibiotic, Miscellaneous
Generic Availability (U.S.) No
Use Treatment of travelers' diarrhea caused by noninvasive strains of *E. coli* (FDA approved in ages ≥12 years and adults); reduction in the risk of overt hepatic encephalopathy (HE) recurrence (FDA approved in ages ≥18 years and adults); has also been used in inflammatory bowel disease and irritable bowel syndrome
Pregnancy Risk Factor C
Pregnancy Considerations Adverse events have been observed in some animal reproduction studies. Due to the limited oral absorption of rifaximin in patients with normal hepatic function, exposure to the fetus is expected to be low.
Breast-Feeding Considerations It is not known if rifaximin is excreted in human milk. Due to the potential for serious adverse reactions in the nursing infant, the manufacturer recommends a decision be made whether to discontinue nursing or to discontinue the drug, taking into account the importance of treatment to the mother. Because of the limited oral absorption of rifaximin in patients with normal hepatic function, exposure to the nursing infant is expected to be low.
Contraindications Hypersensitivity to rifaximin, other rifamycin antibiotics, or any component
Warnings Hypersensitivity reactions have been reported; including exfoliative dermatitis, angioneurotic edema, and anaphylaxis. Prolonged use may result in fungal or bacterial superinfection, including *C. difficile*-associated diarrhea (CDAD) and pseudomembranous colitis; CDAD has been observed >2 months postantibiotic treatment. Efficacy has not been established for the treatment of diarrhea due to pathogens other than *E. coli*, including *C. jejuni*, *Shigella*, and *Salmonella*; consider alternative therapy if symptoms persist or worsen after 24-48 hours of treatment; avoid use in diarrhea with fever or blood in the stool. Rifaximin tablets contain propylene glycol; toxicities have been reported with use of propylene glycol containing medications, including hyperosmolality, lactic acidosis, seizures, and respiratory depression; in neonates large amounts of propylene glycol delivered orally, intravenously (eg, >3000 mg/day), or topically have been associated with potentially fatal toxicities which can include metabolic acidosis, seizures, renal failure, and CNS depression; use tablets containing propylene glycol with caution (AAP, 1997; Shehab, 2009).
Precautions Use with caution in patients with severe hepatic impairment (Child-Pugh class C); efficacy for prevention of hepatic encephalopathy has not been established in patients with a Model for End-Stage Liver Disease (MELD) score >25. Rifaximin should not be used for treatment of systemic infections; <1% is absorbed orally.

Adverse Reactions

Cardiovascular: Chest pain, edema, hypotension, peripheral edema

Central nervous system: Attention disturbance, amnesia, confusion, depression, dizziness, fatigue, fever, headache, hypoesthesia, pain, tremor, vertigo

Dermatological: Cellulitis, pruritus, rash

Endocrine and metabolism: Hyper-/hypoglycemia, hyperkalemia, hyponatremia

Hepatic: Ascites

Gastrointestinal: Abdominal pain, abdominal tenderness, anorexia, dehydration, esophageal varices, nausea, weight gain, xerostomia

Hematologic: Anemia

Neuromuscular & skeletal: Arthralgia, muscle spasms, myalgia

Respiratory: Dyspnea, epistaxis, nasopharyngitis, pneumonia, rhinitis, upper respiratory tract infection

Miscellaneous: Influenza-like illness

All indications: Rare but important or life-threatening: Abnormal dreams, allergic dermatitis, anaphylaxis, angioneurotic edema, AST increased, choluria, CDAD, dry lips, dysuria, ear pain, exfoliative dermatitis, flushing, gingival disorder, hematuria, hot flashes, hypersensitivity reactions, lymphocytosis, migraine, monocytosis, motion sickness, nasal irritation, nasopharyngitis, neck pain, neutropenia, pharyngitis, pharyngolaryngeal pain, polyuria, proteinuria, sunburn, syncope, taste loss, tinnitus, urticaria, weakness, weight loss

Drug Interactions

Metabolism/Transport Effects Induces CYP3A4 (minor)

Avoid Concomitant Use

Avoid concomitant use of Rifaximin with any of the following: BCG

Increased Effect/Toxicity

The levels/effects of Rifaximin may be increased by: CycloSPORINE (Systemic); P-glycoprotein/ABCB1 Inhibitors

Decreased Effect

Rifaximin may decrease the levels/effects of: BCG; Sodium Picosulfate

Stability Store at 20°C to 25°C (68°F to 77°F); excursions permitted to 15°C to 30°C (59°F to 86°F).

Mechanism of Action Rifaximin inhibits bacterial RNA synthesis by binding to bacterial DNA-dependent RNA polymerase.

Pharmacokinetics (Adult data unless noted)

Absorption: Low and variable; increased with worsening hepatic impairment (patients with Child-Pugh class C have greater exposure than Child-Pugh class A patients)

Protein binding: Healthy subjects: ~68%; Hepatic impairment: 62%

Half-life elimination: Mean range: 2-5 hours

Time to peak serum concentration: 1 hour

Elimination: Feces (~97% as unchanged drug); urine (<1%)

Dosing: Usual

Pediatric:

Diarrhea, travelers': Oral: **Note:** Efficacy has not been established for the treatment of diarrhea due to pathogens other than E. coli, including C. jejuni, Shigella, and Salmonella; avoid use in diarrhea with fever or blood in the stool; consider alternative therapy if symptoms persist or worsen after 24-48 hours of treatment

Children 3-11 years: Limited data available: 100 mg 4 times daily for up to 5 days has been used in 38 children (age range: 3-8 years) to treat infectious diarrhea (Beseghi, 1998; Frisari, 1997)

Children ≥12 years and Adolescents: 200 mg 3 times daily for 3 days

Hepatic encephalopathy: Oral: Adolescents ≥18 years: Reduction of overt hepatic encephalopathy recurrence: 550 mg 2 times daily

Inflammatory bowel disease (IBD) (Crohn's disease, ulcerative colitis): Limited data available: Oral: Children ≥8 years and Adolescents: 10-30 mg/kg/day in divided doses; maximum daily dose: 1200 mg/**day**. Dosing based on a retrospective experience of 23 pediatric patients (age range: 8-21 years) with IBD flare (Crohn's disease, n=12; ulcerative colitis: n=11); patients received rifaximin 400-1200 mg/day (10-30 mg/kg/day); improvements in diarrhea and abdominal pain were reported within the first 4 weeks of therapy for the majority of patients (~74%), and within a week in some cases; higher total daily doses (1200 mg/day vs 400 mg/day) were associated with better symptom control (Muniyappa, 2009).

Small intestinal bacterial overgrowth (SIBO) [eg, irritable bowel syndrome (IBS), chronic abdominal pain]: Limited data available; efficacy results variable: Oral: Children ≥3 years and Adolescents: 200 mg 3 times daily, dosing based on prospective study of 50 pediatric patients with IBS (age range: 3-15 years); results showed 7 days of therapy resulted in improved symptoms and a reduction in bacterial overgrowth based on lactulose breath test (LBT) results (Scarpellini, 2013); however, a double-blind placebo-controlled trial in pediatric patients (n=75 including 49 who received rifaximin, age range: 8-18 years) with chronic abdominal pain showed very low efficacy in normalizing LBT (20% response rate) and treating SIBO compared to placebo at a higher dose of 550 mg 3 times daily for 7 days (Collins, 2011). Further studies are needed.

Adults:

Hepatic encephalopathy: Oral: Reduction of overt hepatic encephalopathy recurrence: 550 mg 2 times daily

Travelers' diarrhea: Oral: 200 mg 3 times daily for 3 days

Dosing adjustment for renal impairment: There are no dosage adjustments provided in the manufacturer's labeling (has not been studied).

Dosing adjustment for hepatic impairment: No dosage adjustment necessary. Use with caution in patients with severe impairment (Child-Pugh class C) as systemic absorption does occur and pharmacokinetic parameters are highly variable.

Administration Oral: May be administered with or without food.

Monitoring Parameters Temperature, blood in stool, change in symptoms; monitor changes in mental status in hepatic encephalopathy

Dosage Forms Excipient information presented when available (limited, particularly for generics); consult specific product labeling.

Tablet, Oral:

Xifaxan: 200 mg, 550 mg [contains edetate disodium]

Extemporaneous Preparations A 20 mg/mL oral suspension may be made using tablets. Crush six 200 mg tablets and reduce to a fine powder. Add 30 mL of a 1:1 mixture of Ora-Sweet® and Ora-Plus® or a 1:1 mixture of Ora-Sweet® SF and Ora-Plus®; mix well while adding the vehicle in geometric proportions to **almost** 60 mL; transfer to a calibrated bottle, rinse mortar with vehicle, and add quantity of vehicle sufficient to make 60 mL. Label "shake well". Stable 60 days at room temperature.

Cober MP, Johnson CE, Lee J, et al, "Stability of Extemporaneously Prepared Rifaximin Oral Suspensions," Am J Health Syst Pharm, 2010, 67(4):287-89.

References

American Academy of Pediatrics Committee on Drugs. "Inactive" ingredients in pharmaceutical products: update (subject review). *Pediatrics*. 1997;99(2):268-278.

Beseghi U, De'Angelis GL. Comparison of two non-absorbable antibiotics for treatment of bacterial enteritis in children. *Eur Rev Med Pharmacol Sci*. 1998;2(3-4):131-136.

Collins BS, Lin HC. Double-blind, placebo-controlled antibiotic treatment study of small intestinal bacterial overgrowth in children with chronic abdominal pain. *J Pediatr Gastroenterol Nutr*. 2011;52:382-386.

Frisari L, Viggiano V, Pelagalli M. An open, controlled study of two nonabsorbable antibiotics for the oral treatment of paediatric infectious diarrhea. *Current Medical Research and Opinion*. 1997;14(1):39-45.

Muniyappa P, Gulati R, Mohr F, Hupertz V. Use and safety of rifaximin in children with inflammatory bowel disease. *Journal of Pediatric Gastroenterology and Nutrition*. 2009;49:400-404.

Scarpellini E, Giorgio V, Gabrielli M, et al. Rifaximin treatment for small intestinal bacterial overgrowth in children with irritable bowel syndrome: a preliminary study. *European Review for Medical and Pharmacological Sciences*. 2013;17:1314-1320.

Shehab N, Lewis CL, Streetman DD, Donn SM. Exposure to the pharmaceutical excipients benzyl alcohol and propylene glycol among critically ill neonates. *Pediatr Crit Care Med*. 2009;10(2):256-259.

◆ **RIG** *see* Rabies Immune Globulin (Human) *on page 1800*

Rilonacept (ri LON a sept)

Brand Names: U.S. Arcalyst

Therapeutic Category Interleukin-1 Receptor Antagonist

Generic Availability (U.S.) No

Use Treatment of cryopyrin-associated periodic syndromes (CAPS), including familial cold autoinflammatory syndrome (FCAS) and Muckle-Wells syndrome (MWS) (FDA approved in ages ≥12 years and adults)

Pregnancy Risk Factor C

Pregnancy Considerations Adverse events have been observed in animal reproduction studies.

Breast-Feeding Considerations It is not known if rilonacept is excreted in breast milk. The manufacturer recommends that caution be exercised when administering rilonacept to nursing women.

Contraindications Hypersensitivity to rilonacept or any component

Warnings May decrease immune response to infection due to interleukin-1 (IL-1) blockade; serious infections have been reported during rilonacept therapy. Exercise caution when considering use in patients with a history of new or recurrent infections, conditions that predispose them to infections, latent infections [eg, tuberculosis (TB)] or opportunistic infections. Patients who develop a new infection while undergoing treatment should be monitored closely; discontinue therapy if serious infection develops. Risk of serious infection increased with concurrent tumor necrosis factor (TNF)-blocker (eg, etanercept) use; manufacturer recommends avoiding concurrent therapy with TNF blockers and other IL-1 blocking agents (eg, canakinumab, anakinra). Avoid use in patients with active TB; patients should be evaluated for latent tuberculosis infection with a tuberculin skin test prior to starting therapy. Latent TB infections should be treated prior to initiating rilonacept therapy; monitor for signs/symptoms of active TB during therapy. May cause hypersensitivity reactions (rare); discontinue use if occurs.

Precautions Use may affect defenses against malignancies; impact on the development and course of malignancies is not fully defined. Patients should be brought up-to-date with all immunizations, including pneumococcal and influenza, before initiating therapy; live vaccines should not be given concurrently. No data are available concerning the effects of therapy on vaccine effectiveness or secondary transmission of live vaccines in patients receiving therapy. May increase serum lipids (eg, total cholesterol, HDL, LDL, triglycerides); monitor lipid profile periodically

(eg, after 2-3 months of therapy); in some cases, initiation of lipid-lowering therapy may be necessary. Local injection site reactions frequently reported; majority mild-moderate; typically lasting 1-2 days; characterized by erythema, bruising, dermatitis, inflammation, pain, pruritus, swelling, urticaria, vesicles, warmth, and hemorrhage. Antibody-formation to rilonacept has been reported (incidence: 35%); clinical impact is not fully defined; however, no correlation with clinical effectiveness or safety was noted during trials.

Adverse Reactions

Central nervous system: Hypoesthesia

Immunologic: Antibody development

Infection: Increased susceptibility to infection

Local: Injection site reaction (majority mild-moderate; typically lasting 1-2 days; characterized by bleeding, bruising, erythema, induration, inflammation, itching, pain, swelling, urticaria; other local reactions include dermatitis, vesicles)

Respiratory: Cough, sinusitis, upper respiratory tract infection

Rare but important or life-threatening: Bacterial meningitis (*Streptococcus pneumoniae*), bronchitis, colitis, gastrointestinal hemorrhage, hypercholesterolemia, hypersensitivity reaction, increased HDL cholesterol, increased LDL cholesterol, increased serum triglycerides, mycobacterium infection (*Mycobacterium intracellulare*), neutropenia (transient)

Drug Interactions

Metabolism/Transport Effects None known.

Avoid Concomitant Use

Avoid concomitant use of Rilonacept with any of the following: Anti-TNF Agents; BCG; Canakinumab; Natalizumab; Pimecrolimus; Tacrolimus (Topical); Tofacitinib; Vaccines (Live)

Increased Effect/Toxicity

Rilonacept may increase the levels/effects of: Canakinumab; Leflunomide; Natalizumab; Tofacitinib; Vaccines (Live)

The levels/effects of Rilonacept may be increased by: Anti-TNF Agents; Denosumab; Pimecrolimus; Roflumilast; Tacrolimus (Topical); Trastuzumab

Decreased Effect

Rilonacept may decrease the levels/effects of: BCG; Coccidioidin Skin Test; Sipuleucel-T; Vaccines (Inactivated); Vaccines (Live)

The levels/effects of Rilonacept may be decreased by: Echinacea

Stability Store intact vial at 2°C to 8°C (36°F to 46°F); do not freeze; protect from light. After reconstitution, protect from light and store at room temperature; use within 3 hours of reconstitution. Reconstituted solution is described as viscous, clear, and colorless to pale yellow.

Mechanism of Action Cryopyrin-associated periodic syndromes (CAPS) refers to rare genetic syndromes caused by mutations in the nucleotide-binding domain, leucine rich family (NLR), pyrin domain containing 3 (NLRP-3) gene or the cold-induced autoinflammatory syndrome-1 (*CIAS1*) gene. Cryopyrin, a protein encoded by this gene, regulates interleukin-1 beta (IL-1β) activation. Deficiency of cryopyrin results in excessive inflammation. Rilonacept reduces inflammation by binding to IL-1β (some binding of IL-1α and IL-1 receptor antagonist) and preventing interaction with cell surface receptors.

Pharmacodynamics Onset of action: Steady-state concentrations reached in ~6 weeks

Dosing: Usual SubQ: Cryopyrin-associated periodic syndromes (CAPS):

Children and Adolescents 12-17 years:

Initial: Loading dose 4.4 mg/kg; maximum dose: 320 mg/dose; **Note:** Loading dose may be divided into 1 or 2 separate injections (maximum injection volume: 2 mL/injection) and given on the same day at different sites

Maintenance dose: Begin 1 week after loading dose: 2.2 mg/kg/dose once weekly; maximum dose: 160 mg/dose; **Note:** Do not administer more frequently than once weekly.

Adolescents ≥18 years and Adults:

Initial: Loading dose: 320 mg administered as 2 separate injections (160 mg each) on the same day at different sites

Maintenance: Begin 1 week after loading dose: 160 mg once weekly; **Note:** Do not administer more frequently than once weekly.

Administration SubQ: Reconstitute with 2.3 mL of preservative-free SWI; shake vial for 1 minute then let sit for 1 minute; resulting solution is 80 mg/mL. Administer subcutaneously, if total dose exceeds 2 mL, dose should be divided into 2 injections at different sites; rotate injection sites (thigh, abdomen, upper arm); avoid sites that are bruised, red, tender, or hard.

Monitoring Parameters CBC with differential, C-reactive protein (CRP), serum amyloid A; signs or symptoms of infection; latent TB screening (prior to initiating therapy), lipid profile (2-3 months after initiating therapy and periodically thereafter)

Dosage Forms Excipient information presented when available (limited, particularly for generics); consult specific product labeling.

Solution Reconstituted, Subcutaneous [preservative free]:
Arcalyst: 220 mg (1 ea) [contains polyethylene glycol]

RimabotulinumtoxinB

(rime uh BOT yoo lin num TOKS in bee)

Medication Safety Issues

Other safety concerns:

Botulinum products are not interchangeable; potency differences may exist between the products.

Brand Names: U.S. Myobloc

Therapeutic Category Muscle Contracture, Treatment

Generic Availability (U.S.) No

Use Treatment of cervical dystonia (FDA approved in adults)

Medication Guide Available Yes

Pregnancy Risk Factor C (manufacturer)

Pregnancy Considerations Reproduction studies have not been conducted. Based on limited case reports using onabotulinumtoxinA, adverse fetal effects have not been observed with inadvertent administration during pregnancy. It is currently recommended to ensure adequate contraception in women of childbearing years.

Breast-Feeding Considerations It is not known if rimabotulinumtoxinB is excreted in breast milk. The manufacturer recommends that caution be exercised when administering rimabotulinumtoxinB to nursing women.

Contraindications Hypersensitivity to botulinum toxin or any component of the formulation

Warnings Use of rimabotulinumtoxinB should be reserved for healthcare providers familiar and experienced in the assessment and management of patients with cervical dystonia

The U.S. Food and Drug Administration (FDA) and Health Canada have issued respective early communications to healthcare professionals alerting them of serious adverse events (including fatalities) in association with the use of onabotulinumtoxinA (Botox®, Botox® Cosmetic) and rimabotulinumtoxinB (Myobloc®). Events reported are suggestive of botulism, indicating systemic spread of the botulinum toxin beyond the site of injection. Reactions were observed in both adult and pediatric patients treated for a variety of conditions with varying doses. However, the most serious outcomes, including respiratory failure and death, were associated with the use in children for cerebral palsy limb spasticity. The FDA has evaluated postmarketing cases and now reports that systemic and potentially fatal toxicity may result from local injection of the botulinum toxins in the treatment of other underlying conditions such as cerebral palsy associated with limb spasticity. Monitor patients closely for signs/symptoms of systemic toxic effects (possibly occurring 1 day to several weeks after treatment) and instruct patients to seek immediate medical attention with worsening symptoms or dysphagia, dyspnea, muscle weakness, or difficulty speaking.

Precautions Use with caution in patients with peripheral motor neuropathic diseases (eg, amyotrophic lateral sclerosis or motor neuropathy) or neuromuscular junction disorders (eg, myasthenia gravis or Lambert-Eaton syndrome) as these patients may be at increased risk for development of significant systemic side effects including severe dysphagia and respiratory compromise; use cautiously if there is inflammation present at the proposed injection site or when excessive weakness or atrophy is present in the target muscles

Adverse Reactions

Cardiovascular: Chest pain, edema, peripheral edema, vasodilation

Central nervous system: Anxiety, chills, confusion, dizziness, fever, headache, hyperesthesia, malaise, migraine, pain, somnolence, tremor, vertigo

Dermatologic: Bruising, pruritus

Endocrine & metabolic: Hypercholesterolemia

Gastrointestinal: Dyspepsia, dysphagia, glossitis, nausea, stomatitis, taste perversion, vomiting, xerostomia

Genitourinary: Cystitis, urinary tract infection, vaginal moniliasis

Hematologic: Serum neutralizing activity

Local: Injection site pain

Neuromuscular & skeletal: Arthralgia, arthritis, back pain, hernia, myasthenia, neck pain, torticollis, weakness

Ocular: Amblyopia, vision abnormal

Otic: Otitis media, tinnitus

Respiratory: Cough, dyspnea, pneumonia, rhinitis

Miscellaneous: Abscess, allergic reaction, antibody formation, cyst, flu-like syndrome, infection, neoplasm, viral infection

Rare but important or life-threatening: Constipation

Drug Interactions

Metabolism/Transport Effects None known.

Avoid Concomitant Use There are no known interactions where it is recommended to avoid concomitant use.

Increased Effect/Toxicity

The levels/effects of RimabotulinumtoxinB may be increased by: AbobotulinumtoxinA; Aminoglycosides; Anticholinergic Agents; Neuromuscular-Blocking Agents; OnabotulinumtoxinA

Decreased Effect There are no known significant interactions involving a decrease in effect.

Stability Store solution in refrigerator at 2°C to 8°C (36°F to 46°F); stable for 4 hours at room temperature after dilution with NS

Mechanism of Action RimabotulinumtoxinB (previously known as botulinum toxin type B) is a neurotoxin produced by *Clostridium botulinum*, spore-forming anaerobic bacillus. It cleaves synaptic Vesicle Association Membrane Protein (VAMP; synaptobrevin) which is a component of the protein complex responsible for docking and fusion of the synaptic vesicle to the presynaptic membrane. By blocking neurotransmitter release, rimabotulinumtoxinB paralyzes the muscle.

Pharmacodynamics Duration of paralysis: 12-16 weeks

Dosing: Usual I.M.: Adults: 2500-5000 units divided among affected muscles; patients without a prior history of tolerating botulinum toxin injections should receive a lower initial dose; subsequent doses should be individualized related to the patient's response; doses up to 10,000 units have been used

Administration Parenteral: For I.M. administration only by individuals understanding the relevant neuromuscular anatomy and any alterations to the anatomy due to prior surgical procedures and standard electromyographic techniques; solution may be diluted with NS prior to administration

Monitoring Parameters Monitor patients closely for signs/symptoms of systemic toxic effects (possibly occurring 1 day to several weeks after treatment)

Toronto Western Spasmodic Torticollis Rating Scale (TWSTRS) which evaluates severity, disability, and pain

Dosage Forms Excipient information presented when available (limited, particularly for generics); consult specific product labeling.

Solution, Intramuscular [preservative free]:
Myobloc: 2500 units/0.5 mL (0.5 mL); 5000 units/mL (1 mL); 10,000 units/2 mL (2 mL) [contains albumin human]

References

"Botulinum Toxin," *NIH Consens Statement*, 1990, 12-14, 8(8):1-20.

Figgitt DP and Noble S, "Botulinum Toxin B: A Review of Its Therapeutic Potential in the Management of Cervical Dystonia," *Drugs*, 2002, 62 (4):705-22.

Rimantadine (ri MAN ta deen)

Medication Safety Issues
Sound-alike/look-alike issues:
Rimantadine may be confused with amantadine, ranitidine, Rimactane
Flumadine® may be confused with fludarabine, flunisolide, flutamide

Brand Names: U.S. Flumadine

Brand Names: Canada Flumadine®

Therapeutic Category Antiviral Agent, Oral

Generic Availability (U.S.) Yes

Use Treatment of influenza A viral infection (FDA approved in ages ≥17 years and adults); prophylaxis of influenza A virus (FDA approved in ages ≥1 year and adults); please refer to current ACIP guidelines for recommendations during current flu season)

Pregnancy Risk Factor C

Pregnancy Considerations Animal data suggest embryotoxicity, maternal toxicity, and offspring mortality at doses 7-11 times the recommended human dose. There are no adequate and well-controlled studies in pregnant women.

Influenza infection may be more severe in pregnant women. Untreated influenza infection is associated with an increased risk of adverse events to the fetus and an increased risk of complications or death to the mother. Oseltamivir and zanamivir are currently recommended for the treatment or prophylaxis influenza in pregnant women and women up to 2 weeks postpartum. Appropriate antiviral agents are currently recommended as an adjunct to vaccination and should not be used as a substitute for vaccination in pregnant women (consult current CDC guidelines).

Healthcare providers are encouraged to refer women exposed to influenza vaccine, or who have taken an antiviral medication during pregnancy to the Vaccines and Medications in Pregnancy Surveillance System (VAMPSS) by contacting The Organization of Teratology Information Specialists (OTIS) at (877) 311-8972.

Breast-Feeding Considerations Do not use in nursing mothers due to potential adverse effect in infants. The CDC recommends that women infected with the influenza virus follow general precautions (eg, frequent hand washing) to decrease viral transmission to the child. Mothers with influenza-like illnesses at delivery should consider avoiding close contact with the infant until they have received 48 hours of antiviral medication, fever has resolved, and cough and secretions can be controlled. These measures may help decrease (but not eliminate) the risk of transmitting influenza to the newborn during breast-feeding. During this time, breast milk can be expressed and bottle-fed to the infant by another person who is not infected. Protective measures, such as wearing a face mask, changing into a clean gown or clothing, and strict hand hygiene should be continued by the mother for ≥7 days after the onset of symptoms or until symptom-free for 24 hours. Infant care should be performed by a non-infected person when possible (consult current CDC guidelines).

Contraindications Hypersensitivity to rimantadine, amantadine, or any component

Warnings Resistance of influenza A virus to rimantadine may develop spontaneously or rapidly during treatment; cross-resistance between amantadine and rimantadine occurs. Due to increased resistance, the CDC has recommended that rimantadine and amantadine no longer be used as monotherapy for the treatment or prophylaxis of influenza A in the United States until susceptibility has been re-established. Consult current CDC guidelines for additional information.

Precautions Use with caution in patients with liver disease, renal impairment, epilepsy, uncontrolled psychosis, severe psychoneurosis, and in patients receiving CNS stimulant drugs. May increase seizure activity in patients with preexisting seizure disorders; discontinue use if seizure occurs. Modify dosage in patients with severe renal impairment, severe hepatic dysfunction, or active seizure disorder; use in patients <1 year of age has not been adequately assessed

Adverse Reactions
Central nervous system: Concentration impaired, dizziness, headache, insomnia
Gastrointestinal: Abdominal pain, anorexia, nausea, vomiting, xerostomia
Neuromuscular & skeletal: Weakness
Rare but important or life-threatening: Agitation, ataxia, bronchospasm, cardiac failure, confusion, convulsions, depression, diarrhea, dyspnea, euphoria, gait abnormality, hallucinations, heart block, hyperkinesias, hypertension, lactation, palpitation, parosmia, pedal edema, rash, syncope, tachycardia, taste alteration, tremor

Drug Interactions

Metabolism/Transport Effects None known.

Avoid Concomitant Use There are no known interactions where it is recommended to avoid concomitant use.

Increased Effect/Toxicity
The levels/effects of Rimantadine may be increased by: MAO Inhibitors

Decreased Effect
Rimantadine may decrease the levels/effects of: Influenza Virus Vaccine (Live/Attenuated)

Food Interactions Food does not affect rate or extent of absorption.

Stability Store at 25°C (77°F); excursions permitted to 15°C to 30°C (59°F to 86°F).

Mechanism of Action Exerts its inhibitory effect on three antigenic subtypes of influenza A virus (H1N1, H2N2, H3N2) early in the viral replicative cycle, possibly inhibiting the uncoating process; it has no activity against influenza B virus and is two- to eightfold more active than amantadine

Pharmacokinetics (Adult data unless noted)

Absorption: Oral: Well absorbed

Distribution: 17-25 L/kg

Protein binding: ~40%

Metabolism: Extensively in the liver via hydroxylation and glucuronidation

Half-life:

Children 4-8 years: 13-38 hours

Adults: 25.4 hours

Time to peak serum concentration: 6 hours

Elimination: <25% excreted unchanged in the urine

Dialysis: Hemodialysis: Negligible effect

Dosing: Usual Oral:

Prophylaxis: Note: Monotherapy is not recommended. In order to control outbreaks in institutions, if influenza A virus subtyping is unavailable and oseltamivir-resistant viruses are circulating, rimantadine may be used in combination with oseltamivir if zanamivir cannot be used. Therapy should continue for ≥2 weeks and until ~10 days after illness onset in the last patient (CDC, 2011; Harper, 2009)

Children 1-9 years: 5 mg/kg/day in 1-2 divided doses; maximum dose: 150 mg/day

Children ≥10 years who weigh <40 kg: 5 mg/kg/day in 2 divided doses

Children ≥10 years who weigh ≥40 kg and Adults: 100 mg twice daily

Treatment: Note: Dosages for treatment and prophylaxis are the same; duration of treatment: 5-7 days; optimal duration not established; discontinue as soon as clinically warranted to reduce the emergence of antiviral drug resistant viruses.

Dosage adjustment in renal impairment: Adults:

CrCl ≥30 mL/minute: Dose adjustment not required

CrCl <30 mL/minute: 100 mg/day

Dosage adjustment in hepatic impairment: Adults: Severe dysfunction: 100 mg/day

Administration Oral: May administer with food

Additional Information Not active against influenza B; treatment or prophylaxis in immunosuppressed patients has not been fully evaluated; duration of fever and other symptoms can be reduced if rimantadine therapy is started within the first 48 hours of influenza A illness

During an outbreak of influenza, administer rimantadine prophylaxis for 2-3 weeks after influenza vaccination until vaccine antibody titers are sufficient to provide protection

Dosage Forms Excipient information presented when available (limited, particularly for generics); consult specific product labeling.

Tablet, Oral, as hydrochloride:

Flumadine: 100 mg [contains fd&c yellow #6 (sunset yellow), fd&c yellow #6 aluminum lake]

Generic: 100 mg

Extemporaneous Preparations Rimantadine 10 mg/mL Suspension:

To prepare suspension, 10 mL of Ora-Sweet® will be required for every 100 mg tablet of rimantadine. (Do not prepare more than a 14-day supply).

- Calculate the total dose needed (daily dose x number of days = mg of rimantadine needed) and round the final mg of rimantadine needed up to the next 100 mg (eg, 750 mg would be 800 mg, or eight 100 mg tablets).
- Calculate the total volume of Ora-Sweet® by taking the rounded mg of rimantadine and dividing by 10 mg/mL (eg, 800 mg divided by 10 mg/mL = 80 mL).
- Grind required number of tablets in mortar and triturate to a fine powder. Slowly add 1/3 of the total volume of Ora-Sweet® to the mortar and triturate until a uniform suspension is achieved.
- Transfer to an amber glass or PET plastic bottle. Slowly add another 1/3 of the total volume of Ora-Sweet® to the mortar, rinsing the mortar, then transferring the contents

into the bottle. Repeat using the final 1/3 of Ora-Sweet®. Add additional vehicle to bottle, if needed, to achieve the total calculated volume.

- Shake well to ensure homogeneous suspension. Some inert ingredients in the tablet may be insoluble.
- Label: Shake gently prior to each use.
- Suspension is stable for 14 days when stored at room temperature (25°C/77°F).

References

Bradley JS, Byington CL, Shah SS, et al, "The Management of Community-Acquired Pneumonia in Infants and Children Older Than 3 Months of Age: Clinical Practice Guidelines by the Pediatric Infectious Diseases Society and the Infectious Diseases Society of America", Clin Infect Dis, 2011, 53(7):e25-76.

Centers for Disease Control, "Antiviral Agents for the Treatment and Chemoprophylaxis of Influenza. Recommendations of the Advisory Committee on Immunization Practices (ACIP)," MMWR Recomm Rep, 2011, 60(1):1-24.

Harper SA, Bradley JS, Englund JA, et al, "Seasonal Influenza in Adults and Children - Diagnosis, Treatment, Chemoprophylaxis, and Institutional Outbreak Management: Clinical Practice Guidelines of the Infectious Diseases Society of America," Clin Infect Dis, 2009, 48 (8):1003-32.

Red Book: 2009 Report of the Committee on Infectious Diseases, "Influenza," 28th ed, Pickering LK, ed, Elk Grove Village, IL: American Academy of Pediatrics, 2009.

◆ **Rimantadine Hydrochloride** see Rimantadine on page 1830

◆ **Riomet** see MetFORMIN on page 1353

◆ **RisaQuad™ [OTC]** see Lactobacillus on page 1191

◆ **RisaQuad®-2 [OTC]** see Lactobacillus on page 1191

◆ **RisperDAL** see RisperiDONE on page 1831

◆ **Risperdal (Can)** see RisperiDONE on page 1831

◆ **Risperdal M-Tab** see RisperiDONE on page 1831

◆ **RisperDAL M-TAB** see RisperiDONE on page 1831

◆ **RisperDAL Consta** see RisperiDONE on page 1831

◆ **Risperdal Consta (Can)** see RisperiDONE on page 1831

RisperiDONE (ris PER i done)

Medication Safety Issues

Sound-alike/look-alike issues:

RisperiDONE may be confused with reserpine, rOPINIRole

RisperDAL may be confused with lisinopril, reserpine, Restoril

BEERS Criteria medication:

This drug may be potentially inappropriate for use in geriatric patients (Quality of evidence - moderate; Strength of recommendation - strong).

Related Information

Oral Medications That Should Not Be Crushed or Altered on page 2438

Safe Handling of Hazardous Drugs on page 2419

Brand Names: U.S. RisperDAL; RisperDAL Consta; RisperDAL M-TAB; RisperiDONE M-TAB

Brand Names: Canada Apo-Risperidone; Ava-Risperidone; CO Risperidone; Dom-Risperidone; JAMP-Risperidone; Mar-Risperidone; Mint-Risperidon; Mylan-Risperidone; PHL-Risperidone; PMS-Risperidone; PMS-Risperidone ODT; PRO-Risperidone; RAN-Risperidone; ratio-Risperidone; Risperdal; Risperdal Consta; Risperdal M-Tab; Riva-Risperidone; Sandoz-Risperidone; Teva-Risperidone

Therapeutic Category Antipsychotic Agent, Atypical; Antipsychotic Agent, Benzisoxazole

Generic Availability (U.S.) May be product dependent

Use

Oral: Management of schizophrenia (FDA approved in ages ≥13 years and adults); treatment of acute mania or mixed episodes associated with bipolar I disorder (FDA approved as monotherapy in ages ≥10 years and adults; FDA approved in combination with lithium or valproate in adults); treatment of irritability (including aggression, temper tantrums, self-injurious behavior, and quickly changing moods) associated with autistic disorder in children and adolescents (FDA approved in ages 5-16 years); has also been used for treatment of Tourette syndrome (tics), disruptive behavior disorders, and delirium and irritability in the management of pervasive development disorders.

I.M.: Management of schizophrenia (FDA approved in adults); maintenance treatment of bipolar I disorder as monotherapy or in combination with lithium or valproate (FDA approved in adults)

Pregnancy Risk Factor C

Pregnancy Considerations Adverse events were observed in animal reproduction studies. In human studies, risperidone and its metabolite cross the placenta (Newport, 2007). An increased risk of teratogenic effects has not been observed following maternal use of risperidone (limited data) (Coppola, 2007). Agenesis of the corpus callosum has been noted in one case report of an infant exposed *in utero*; relationship to risperidone exposure is not known. Antipsychotic use during the third trimester of pregnancy has a risk for extrapyramidal symptoms (EPS) and/or withdrawal symptoms in newborns following delivery. Symptoms in the newborn may include agitation, feeding disorder, hypertonia, hypotonia, respiratory distress, somnolence, and tremor. These effects may be self-limiting and allow recovery within hours or days with no specific treatment, or they may be severe requiring prolonged hospitalization. When using Risperdal® Consta®, patients should notify healthcare provider if they become or intend to become pregnant during therapy or within 12 weeks of last injection. Risperidone may cause hyperprolactinemia, which may decrease reproductive function in both males and females.

The ACOG recommends that therapy during pregnancy be individualized; treatment with psychiatric medications during pregnancy should incorporate the clinical expertise of the mental health clinician, obstetrician, primary healthcare provider, and pediatrician. Safety data related to atypical antipsychotics during pregnancy is limited and routine use is not recommended. However, if a woman is inadvertently exposed to an atypical antipsychotic while pregnant, continuing therapy may be preferable to switching to a typical antipsychotic that the fetus has not yet been exposed to; consider risk:benefit (ACOG, 2008).

Healthcare providers are encouraged to enroll women 18-45 years of age exposed to risperidone during pregnancy in the Atypical Antipsychotics Pregnancy Registry (1-866-961-2388 or http://www.womensmentalhealth.org/pregnancyregistry).

Breast-Feeding Considerations Risperidone and its metabolite are excreted in breast milk. Due to the potential for serious adverse reactions in the nursing infant, the manufacturer recommends a decision be made whether to discontinue nursing or to discontinue the drug, taking into account the importance of treatment to the mother. It is also recommended that women using Risperdal Consta not breast-feed during therapy or for 12 weeks after the last injection.

Contraindications Hypersensitivity to risperidone or any component

Warnings Hazardous agent; use appropriate precautions for handling and disposal (NIOSH, 2012). May cause neuroleptic malignant syndrome (symptoms include hyperpyrexia, altered mental status, muscle rigidity, autonomic instability, acute renal failure, rhabdomyolysis, and elevated CPK). May cause extrapyramidal reactions, including pseudoparkinsonism, acute dystonic reactions, akathisia, and tardive dyskinesia (risk of these reactions is low relative to other neuroleptics, and is dose-dependent; to decrease risk of tardive dyskinesia: Use smallest dose and shortest duration possible; evaluate continued need periodically; risk of dystonia is increased with the use of high potency and higher doses of conventional antipsychotics and in males and younger patients; occurring in up to 18% of children). May cause hyperglycemia, which may be severe and include potentially fatal ketoacidosis or hyperosmolar coma; use with caution and monitor glucose closely in patients with diabetes mellitus (or with risk factors such as family history or obesity); measure fasting blood glucose at the beginning of therapy and periodically during therapy in these patients; monitor for symptoms of hyperglycemia in all patients treated with risperidone; measure fasting blood glucose in patients who develop symptoms. May alter cardiac conduction (low risk relative to other neuroleptics); QT prolongation and life-threatening arrhythmias have occurred with therapeutic doses of neuroleptics; use with caution in patients with conduction abnormalities.

Leukopenia, neutropenia, and agranulocytosis (sometimes fatal) have been reported in clinical trials and postmarketing reports with antipsychotic use; presence of risk factors (eg, preexisting low WBC or history of drug-induced leuko/neutropenia) should prompt periodic blood count assessment. Discontinue therapy at first signs of blood dyscrasias or if absolute neutrophil count <1000/mm^3.

Intraoperative floppy iris syndrome (IFIS) has been reported in adult patients (case reports) receiving risperidone and undergoing cataract surgery (Ford, 2011). Prior to cataract surgery, evaluate for prior or current risperidone use. The benefits or risks of interrupting risperidone prior to surgery have not been established; clinicians are advised to proceed with surgery cautiously.

An increased risk of death has been reported with the use of antipsychotics in elderly patients with dementia-related psychosis **[U.S. Boxed Warning]**; most deaths seemed to be cardiovascular (eg, sudden death, heart failure) or infectious (eg, pneumonia) in nature; a higher risk of mortality was seen with the use of furosemide plus risperidone (compared to risperidone alone or compared with placebo plus furosemide). An increased incidence of cerebrovascular adverse events (eg, transient ischemic attack, stroke), including fatalities, has been reported with the use of risperidone in elderly patients with dementia-related psychosis. Risperidone is not approved for the treatment of patients with dementia-related psychosis

Oral solution contains benzoic acid; benzoic acid (benzoate) is a metabolite of benzyl alcohol; large amounts of benzyl alcohol (≥99 mg/kg/day) have been associated with a potentially fatal toxicity ("gasping") in neonates; avoid use of risperidone products containing benzoic acid in neonates; *in vitro* and animal studies have shown that benzoate displaces bilirubin from protein binding sites. Vehicle used in injectable product (polylactide-co-glycolide microspheres) has rarely been associated with retinal artery occlusion in patients with abnormal arteriovenous anastomosis (eg, patent foramen ovale).

Precautions Use with caution and decrease the dose in patients with renal or hepatic impairment. Use with caution in patients with breast cancer or other prolactin-dependent tumors; risperidone elevates prolactin levels to a greater degree than other antipsychotic agents; high levels of prolactin may reduce pituitary gonadotropin secretion; galactorrhea, amenorrhea, gynecomastia, impotence, decreased bone density may occur. Use with caution in children and adolescents; adverse effects due to elevated prolactin levels have been observed; long-term effects on growth or sexual maturation have not been evaluated.

Risperidone may cause a higher than normal weight gain in children and adolescents; monitor growth (including weight, height, BMI, and waist circumference) in pediatric patients receiving risperidone; compare weight gain to standard growth curves. Risperidone may cause increases in metabolic indices (eg, serum cholesterol, triglycerides).
Note: A prospective, nonrandomized cohort study followed 338 antipsychotic naïve pediatric patients (age 4-19 years) for a median 10.8 weeks (range 10.5-11.2 weeks) and reported the following significant mean increases in weight in kg (and% change from baseline): Olanzapine: 8.5 kg (15.2%), quetiapine: 6.1 kg (10.4%), risperidone: 5.3 kg (10.4%), and aripiprazole: 4.4 kg (8.1%) compared to the control cohort: 0.2 kg (0.65%). Increases in metabolic indices (eg, serum cholesterol, triglycerides, glucose) were also reported; a significant increase in serum triglycerides of 9.7 mg/mL was observed for patients receiving risperidone. Biannual monitoring of cardiometabolic indices after the first 3 months of therapy is suggested (Correll, 2009).

Use with caution in patients with seizure disorders or patients with conditions that lower seizure threshold; seizures have been rarely reported. Use with caution in patients with concomitant illnesses that may affect hepatic metabolism or hemodynamic responses (eg, unstable cardiac disease, recent MI), Parkinson's disease, or dementia with Lewy Bodies; an increased sensitivity to antipsychotic medications and adverse effects have been reported. Use with caution in suicidal patients. Use with caution in those at risk of aspiration pneumonia; esophageal dysmotility and aspiration have been associated with antipsychotic agents. May cause orthostatic hypotension with resultant dizziness, tachycardia, or syncope (especially during initial dose titration); use with caution in patients with cardiovascular disease (heart failure, past MI, or myocardia ischemia), cerebrovascular disease, dehydration, hypovolemia, or other conditions which may predispose patients to hypotension; may cause hypotension when used with antihypertensive agents. May cause somnolence (dose-related), priapism (rarely), thrombotic thrombocytopenic purpura (case report), alteration of temperature regulation (use with caution in patients exposed to temperature extremes); may mask diseases or toxicity of other drugs due to antiemetic effects. Rare cases of hepatotoxicity have been reported (Kumra, 1997; McDougle, 2000).

Children may experience a higher frequency of certain adverse effects than adults, particularly fatigue (18% to 42% vs ≤3%), somnolence (12% to 67% vs ≤14%), fever (20% vs 2%), constipation (21% vs 9%), increased salivation (22% vs 3%), abdominal pain (18% vs 4%), and dry mouth (13% vs 4%).

Orally disintegrating tablets contain aspartame which is metabolized to phenylalanine and must be avoided or used with caution in patients with phenylketonuria.

Adverse Reactions

Cardiovascular: Bradycardia, bundle branch block, buttock pain, chest pain, ECG changes, facial edema, first degree atrioventricular block, hypertension, hypotension, orthostatic hypotension, palpitations, paresthesia, peripheral edema, prolonged Q-T interval on ECG, syncope, tachycardia (more common in adults)

Central nervous system: Abnormal gait, agitation, akathisia, anxiety, ataxia, decreased attention span, depression, disturbed sleep, dizziness, drooling (more common in children), drowsiness (more common in adults), dystonia, falling, fatigue (more common in children), headache, hypoesthesia, insomnia, lethargy, malaise, nervousness, orthostatic dizziness, pain, parkinsonian-like syndrome (more common in children), sedation (more common in children), seizure, tardive dyskinesia, vertigo

Dermatologic: Acne vulgaris, eczema, pruritus, skin sclerosis, skin rash, xeroderma

Endocrine & metabolic: Amenorrhea, decreased libido, galactorrhea, gynecomastia, hyperglycemia, hyperprolactinemia, increased gamma-glutamyl transferase, increased thirst (more common in children), oligomenorrhea, weight gain (more common in children), weight loss

Gastrointestinal: Abdominal pain (more common in children), anorexia, constipation, decreased appetite, diarrhea, dyspepsia, gastritis, gastroenteritis, increased appetite (more common in children), nausea, sialorrhea, toothache, vomiting (more common in children), xerostomia

Genitourinary: Cystitis, ejaculatory disorder, erectile dysfunction, glycosuria, irregular menses, mastalgia, menstruation, sexual disorder, urinary incontinence (more common in children), urinary tract infection

Hematologic & oncologic: Anemia, neutropenia

Hepatic: Increased serum ALT, increased serum AST

Hypersensitivity: Hypersensitivity

Infection: Infection, influenza, localized infection, subcutaneous abscess, viral infection

Local: Induration at injection site, injection site reaction, pain at injection site, swelling at injection site

Neuromuscular & skeletal: Abnormal posture, akinesia, arthralgia, back pain, dyskinesia (more common in adults), hypokinesia, increased creatine phosphokinase, limb pain, musculoskeletal chest pain, myalgia, neck pain, tremor (more common in adults), weakness

Ophthalmic: Blurred vision, conjunctivitis, reduced visual acuity

Otic: Otalgia, otic infection

Respiratory: bronchitis, cough (more common in children), dyspnea, epistaxis, flu-like symptoms, nasal congestion, nasopharyngitis (more common in children), pharyngitis, pharyngolaryngeal pain, pneumonia, respiratory tract infection, rhinitis, rhinorrhea (more common in children), sinus congestion, sinusitis

Miscellaneous: Fever (more common in children)

Rare but important or life-threatening: Abnormal erythrocytes, abscess at injection site, acariasis, agranulocytosis, alopecia, anaphylaxis, angioedema, apnea, aspiration, atrial fibrillation, atrial premature contractions, cardiorespiratory arrest, cerebral ischemia, cerebrovascular accident, cholestatic hepatitis, cholinergic syndrome, coma, cyst, delirium, depression of ST segment on ECG, dermal ulcer, diabetes mellitus, diabetic coma, diabetic ketoacidosis, disruption of body temperature regulation, diverticulitis, esophageal motility disorder, eye infection, fecal incontinence, fecaloma, glaucoma, granulocytopenia, hematoma, hemorrhage, hepatic failure, hepatic injury, hyperkeratosis, hyperthermia, hypertonia, hypertriglyceridemia, hyperuricemia, hypoglycemia, hypokalemia, hyponatremia, hypothermia, impaired consciousness, increased serum cholesterol, intestinal obstruction, intraoperative floppy iris syndrome, leukocytosis, leukopenia, leukorrhea, lower respiratory tract infection, lymphadenopathy, mania, migraine, myocardial infarction, myocarditis, neuroleptic malignant syndrome, nystagmus, ocular hyperemia, pancreatitis, Pelger-Huët anomaly, phlebitis, pituitary neoplasm, precocious puberty, priapism, pulmonary embolism, renal insufficiency, retinal artery occlusion, retrograde ejaculation, rhabdomyolysis, SIADH, sleep apnea, swelling of eye, synostosis, thrombocytopenia, thrombophlebitis, thrombotic thrombocytopenic purpura, tissue necrosis, tongue paralysis, torticollis, transient ischemic attacks, unresponsive to stimuli, urinary retention, ventricular premature contractions, ventricular tachycardia, water intoxication, withdrawal syndrome

Drug Interactions

Metabolism/Transport Effects Substrate of CYP2D6 (major), CYP3A4 (minor), P-glycoprotein; **Note:** Assignment of Major/Minor substrate status based on clinically relevant drug interaction potential; **Inhibits** CYP2D6 (weak), CYP3A4 (weak)

Avoid Concomitant Use

Avoid concomitant use of RisperiDONE with any of the following: Aclidinium; Amisulpride; Azelastine (Nasal); Ipratropium (Oral Inhalation); Metoclopramide; Paraldehyde; Pimozide; Potassium Chloride; Sulpiride; Thalidomide; Tiotropium; Umeclidinium

Increased Effect/Toxicity

RisperiDONE may increase the levels/effects of: AbobotulinumtoxinA; Alcohol (Ethyl); Amisulpride; Analgesics (Opioid); Anticholinergic Agents; ARIPiprazole; Azelastine (Nasal); Buprenorphine; Cannabinoid-Containing Products; CNS Depressants; Highest Risk QTc-Prolonging Agents; Hydrocodone; Lomitapide; Methotrimeprazine; Methylphenidate; Metyrosine; Mirabegron; Mirtazapine; Moderate Risk QTc-Prolonging Agents; OnabotulinumtoxinA; Paliperidone; Paraldehyde; Pimozide; Potassium Chloride; RimabotulinumtoxinB; Selective Serotonin Reuptake Inhibitors; Serotonin Modulators; Sulpiride; Thalidomide; Thiazide Diuretics; Tiotropium; Topiramate; Zolpidem

The levels/effects of RisperiDONE may be increased by: Abiraterone Acetate; Acetylcholinesterase Inhibitors (Central); Aclidinium; Brimonidine (Topical); Cannabis; CYP2D6 Inhibitors (Moderate); CYP2D6 Inhibitors (Strong); Darunavir; Doxylamine; Dronabinol; Droperidol; HydrOXYzine; Ipratropium (Oral Inhalation); Kava Kava; Lithium; Loop Diuretics; Magnesium Sulfate; Methotrimeprazine; Methylphenidate; Metoclopramide; Metyrosine; Mifepristone; Nabilone; Perampanel; P-glycoprotein/ABCB1 Inhibitors; Pramlintide; Rufinamide; Selective Serotonin Reuptake Inhibitors; Serotonin Modulators; Sodium Oxybate; Tapentadol; Tetrahydrocannabinol; Umeclidinium; Valproic Acid and Derivatives; Verapamil

Decreased Effect

RisperiDONE may decrease the levels/effects of: Acetylcholinesterase Inhibitors (Central); Amphetamines; Anti-Parkinson's Agents (Dopamine Agonist); Quinagolide; Secretin

The levels/effects of RisperiDONE may be decreased by: Acetylcholinesterase Inhibitors (Central); CarBAMazepine; Lithium; Peginterferon Alfa-2b; P-glycoprotein/ABCB1 Inducers

Food Interactions Oral solution is not compatible with beverages containing tannin or pectinate (cola or tea). Management: Administer oral solution with water, coffee, orange juice, or low-fat milk.

Stability Hazardous agent; use appropriate precautions for handling and disposal (NIOSH, 2012).
Oral solution, tablet: Store at controlled room temperature 15°C to 25°C (59°F to 77°F); protect from light; protect tablets from moisture; protect oral solution from freezing; do not store orally-disintegrating tablets once removed from blister unit.
Injection: Store undiluted vials and diluent at 2°C to 8°C (36°F to 46°F); protect from light; may store at room temperature ≤77°F (25°C) for ≤7 days prior to reconstitution; reconstituted suspension must be used within 6 hours.

Mechanism of Action Risperidone is a benzisoxazole atypical antipsychotic with mixed serotonin-dopamine antagonist activity that binds to 5-HT_2-receptors in the CNS and in the periphery with a very high affinity; binds to dopamine-D_2 receptors with less affinity. The binding affinity to the dopamine-D_2 receptor is 20 times lower than the 5-HT_2 affinity. The addition of serotonin antagonism to dopamine antagonism (classic neuroleptic mechanism) is thought to improve negative symptoms of psychoses and reduce the incidence of extrapyramidal side effects. Alpha$_1$, alpha$_2$ adrenergic, and histaminergic receptors are also antagonized with high affinity. Risperidone has low to moderate affinity for 5-HT_{1C}, 5-HT_{1D}, and 5-HT_{1A} receptors, weak affinity for D_1 and no affinity for muscarinics or beta$_1$ and beta$_2$ receptors

Pharmacokinetics (Adult data unless noted) Note: Following oral administration, the pharmacokinetics of risperidone and 9-hydroxyrisperidone in children were found to be similar to values in adults (after adjusting for differences in body weight).

Absorption:
Oral: Well absorbed
I.M.: Initial: <1% of dose released from microspheres; main release starts at ≥3 weeks; release is maintained from 4-6 weeks; release ends by 7 weeks

Distribution: Distributes into breast milk; breast milk to plasma ratio (n=1): Risperidone: 0.42; 9-hydroxyrisperidone: 0.24 (Hill, 2000)
V_d: Risperidone: 1-2 L/kg

Protein binding: Risperidone: 90%, plasma protein binding increases with increasing concentrations of alpha$_1$-acid glycoprotein; 9-hydroxyrisperidone: 77%; **Note:** Risperidone free fraction may be increased by ~35% in patients with hepatic impairment due to decreased concentrations of albumin and alpha$_1$-acid glycoprotein

Metabolism: Extensive in the liver via cytochrome P450 CYP2D6 to 9-hydroxyrisperidone (major active metabolite); also undergoes N-dealkylation (minor pathway); **Note:** 9-hydroxyrisperidone is the predominant circulating form and is approximately equal to risperidone in receptor binding activity; clinical effects are from combined concentrations of risperidone and 9-hydroxyrisperidone; clinically important differences between CYP2D6 poor and extensive metabolizers are not expected (pharmacokinetics of the sum of risperidone and 9-hydroxyrisperidone were similar in poor and extensive metabolizers)

Bioavailability:
Oral: 70%; tablet (relative to solution): 94%; **Note:** Orally-disintegrating tablets and oral solution are bioequivalent to tablets.
IM: Deltoid I.M. injection is bioequivalent to gluteal I.M. injection

Half-life (apparent):
Oral:
Risperidone: Extensive metabolizers: 3 hours; poor metabolizers: 20 hours
9-hydroxyrisperidone: Extensive metabolizers: 21 hours; poor metabolizers: 30 hours
Sum of risperidone and 9-hydroxyrisperidone: Overall mean: 20 hours
I.M.: 3-6 days (due to extended release of drug from microspheres and subsequent absorption)

Time to peak serum concentration: Oral: Solution or tablet:
Risperidone: 1 hour
9-hydroxyrisperidone: Extensive metabolizers: 3 hours; poor metabolizers: 17 hours

Elimination: Excreted as risperidone and metabolites in urine (70%) and feces (14%)
Clearance: Moderate to severe renal impairment (sum of risperidone and 9-hydroxyrisperidone): Decreased by 60%

Dosing: Usual
Children and Adolescents:
Autism, associated irritability, including aggression, temper, tantrums, self-injurious behavior, and quickly changing moods:
Children ≥5 years and Adolescents: **Note:** Individualize dose according to patient response and tolerability:
15-20 kg: Oral: Initial: 0.25 mg/day; after ≥4 days, may increase dose to 0.5 mg/day; maintain this dose for ≥14 days. In patients not achieving sufficient clinical response, may increase dose in increments of 0.25 mg/day at ≥2-week intervals. Doses ranging from 0.5-3 mg/day have been evaluated; however, therapeutic effect reached plateau at 1 mg/day in clinical trials. Following clinical response, consider gradually decreasing dose to lowest effective dose. May be administered once daily or in divided doses twice daily.
≥20 kg: Oral: Initial: 0.5 mg/day; after ≥4 days, may increase dose to 1 mg/day; maintain this dose for ≥14 days. In patients not achieving sufficient clinical response, may increase dose in increments of 0.5 mg/day at ≥2-week intervals. Doses ranging from 0.5-3 mg/day have been evaluated; however, therapeutic effect reached plateau at 2.5 mg/day (3 mg/day in pediatric patients >45 kg) in clinical trials. Following clinical response, consider gradually decreasing to lowest effective dose. May be administered once daily or in divided doses twice daily.
Bipolar mania: Children and Adolescents 10-17 years: Oral: Initial: 0.5 mg once daily; dose may be adjusted if needed, in increments of 0.5-1 mg/day at intervals ≥24 hours, as tolerated, to a dose of 2.5 mg/day. Doses ranging from 0.5-6 mg/day have been evaluated; however, doses >2.5 mg/day do not confer additional benefit and are associated with increased adverse events; doses >6 mg/day have not been studied. **Note:** May administer 1/2 the daily dose twice daily in patients who experience persistent somnolence.
Delirium: Limited data available; further studies are needed:
Children <5 years: Oral: Initial: 0.1-0.2 mg once daily at bedtime; dosing based on retrospective review of 10 pediatric patients (ages: 4 months to 16 years) which included three patients <5 years of age (Schieveld, 2007)
Children ≥5 years and Adolescents: Oral: Initial: 0.2-0.5 mg once daily at bedtime; may titrate to lowest effective dose every 1-2 days; usual range: 0.2-2.5 mg/day in divided doses 2-4 times daily; maximum daily dose dependent upon patient weight: <20 kg: 1 mg/day; 20-45 kg: 2.5 mg/day, >45 kg: 3 mg/day (Karnik, 2007; Schieveld, 2007; Silver, 2010)
Disruptive behavior disorders (eg, conduct disorder, oppositional defiant disorder): Limited data available: Children ≥4 years and Adolescents: Oral: Initial: 0.01 mg/kg/dose once daily for 2 days, then 0.02 mg/kg/dose once daily, may further increase on weekly basis as tolerated to 0.06 mg/kg/dose once daily; usual maximum daily dose: 2 mg/**day**; improvement in target symptoms typically within 1-4 weeks (Aman, 2002; Findling, 2004; Kutcher, 2004; Pandina, 2006). **Note:** May administer 1/2 the daily dose twice daily if breakthrough symptoms occur in the afternoon or evening.
Pervasive developmental disorders (PDD) (eg, disruptive behavior, aggression, irritability): Limited data available: Children ≥5 years and Adolescents: Oral: Initial: 0.01 mg/kg/dose once daily for 2 days, then 0.02 mg/kg/dose once daily; may further increase on weekly basis by ≤0.02 mg/kg/day increments as tolerated to 0.06 mg/kg/dose once daily; reported mean dose: 0.05 mg/kg/day (1.48 mg/day); other trials have

reported similar optimal doses: 0.75-1.8 mg/day; improvement in target symptoms typically within 2-4 weeks (Fisman, 1996; McDougle, 1997; Shea, 2004). **Note:** May administer 1/2 the daily dose twice daily if breakthrough symptoms occur in the afternoon or evening.
Schizophrenia: Adolescents 13-17 years: Oral: Initial: 0.5 mg once daily; dose may be adjusted if needed, in increments of 0.5-1 mg/day at intervals ≥24 hours, as tolerated, to a dose of 3 mg/day. Doses ranging from 1-6 mg/day have been evaluated; however, doses >3 mg/day do not confer additional benefit and are associated with increased adverse events. **Note:** May administer 1/2 the daily dose twice daily in patients who experience persistent somnolence.
Tourette syndrome, tics: Limited data available: Children ≥7 years and Adolescents: Oral: Initial: 0.25-0.5 mg once daily at night; may gradually titrate every 4-5 days in 0.25-0.5 mg increments to usual reported therapeutic range: 0.25-6 mg/day divided in twice daily doses (Dion, 2002; Roessner, 2011; Scahill, 2003; Singer, 2010)
Adults: **Note:** When reinitiating treatment after discontinuation, the initial titration schedule should be followed.
Bipolar mania: Oral: Initial: 2-3 mg/dose once daily; adjust dose as needed, by 1 mg/day increments at intervals ≥24 hours; dosing range: 1-6 mg/day; no dosing recommendation available for treatment >3 weeks duration
Bipolar I, maintenance: I.M. (RisperDAL® Consta®): 25 mg every 2 weeks; if unresponsive, some may benefit from larger doses (37.5-50 mg); maximum dose: 50 mg every 2 weeks. Dosage adjustments should not be made more frequently than every 4 weeks. A lower initial dose of 12.5 mg may be appropriate in some patients (eg, demonstrated poor tolerability to other psychotropic medications).
Note: Oral risperidone (or other antipsychotic) should be administered with the initial injection of RisperDAL® Consta® and continued for 3 weeks (then discontinued) to maintain adequate therapeutic plasma concentrations prior to main release phase of risperidone from injection site. When switching from depot administration to a short-acting formulation, administer short-acting agent in place of the next regularly scheduled depot injection.
Schizophrenia:
Oral: Initial: 2 mg/day in 1-2 divided doses; may be increased by 1-2 mg/day at intervals ≥24 hours to a recommended dosage range of 4-8 mg/day; may be given as a single daily dose once maintenance dose is achieved; daily dosages >6 mg do not appear to confer any additional benefit and the incidence of extrapyramidal symptoms is higher than with lower doses. Further dose adjustments should be made in increments/decrements of 1-2 mg/day on a weekly basis. Dose range studied in clinical trials: 4-16 mg/day. Maintenance: Recommended dosage range: 2-8 mg/day
I.M.: (RisperDAL® Consta®): Initial: 25 mg every 2 weeks; if unresponsive, some may benefit from larger doses (37.5-50 mg); maximum dose: 50 mg every 2 weeks. Dosage adjustments should not be made more frequently than every 4 weeks. A lower initial dose of 12.5 mg may be appropriate in some patients (eg, demonstrated poor tolerability to psychotropic medications).
Note: Oral risperidone (or other antipsychotic) should be administered with the initial injection of RisperDAL® Consta® and continued for 3 weeks (then discontinued) to maintain adequate therapeutic plasma concentrations prior to main release phase of risperidone from injection site. When switching

from depot administration to a short-acting formulation, administer short-acting agent in place of the next regularly scheduled depot injection.

Dosing adjustment in renal impairment:

Children and Adolescents: There are no dosage adjustments provided in manufacturer's labeling.

Adults:

Oral: CrCl <30 mL/minute: Initial: 0.5 mg twice daily; increase (as tolerated) in increments of ≤0.5 mg twice daily; increases to dosages >1.5 mg twice daily should be made at intervals of ≥1 week; slower titration may be required in some patients. Clearance of the active moiety (sum of parent drug and active metabolite) is decreased by 60% in patients with moderate-to-severe renal disease (CrCl <60 mL/minute) compared to healthy subjects.

I.M.: Initiate with **oral** dosing (0.5 mg twice daily for 1 week, then 2 mg/day for 1 week); if tolerated, begin 25 mg **I.M.** every 2 weeks; continue oral dosing for 3 weeks after the first I.M. injection. An initial I.M. dose of 12.5 mg may also be considered.

Dosing adjustment in hepatic impairment:

Children and Adolescents: There are no dosage adjustments provided in manufacturer's labeling.

Adults:

Oral: Child-Pugh Class C: Initial: 0.5 mg twice daily; increase (as tolerated) in increments of ≤0.5 mg twice daily; increases to dosages >1.5 mg twice daily should be made at intervals of ≥1 week; slower titration may be required in some patients. The mean free fraction of risperidone in plasma was increased by 35% in patients with hepatic impairment compared to healthy subjects.

I.M.: Initiate with **oral** dosing (0.5 mg twice daily for 1 week, then 2 mg/day for 1 week); if tolerated, begin 25 mg **I.M.** every 2 weeks; continue oral dosing for 3 weeks after the first I.M. injection. An initial I.M. dose of 12.5 mg may also be considered.

Administration Hazardous agent; use appropriate precautions for handling and disposal (NIOSH, 2012).

Oral: May be administered without regard to meals.

Oral solution: May administer directly from the manufacturer provided calibrated pipette or may mix with water, coffee, orange juice, or low-fat milk; do not mix with cola or tea; **Note:** Manufacturer provided calibrated pipette is calibrated in milligrams and milliliters; minimum calibrated volume: 0.25 mL; maximum calibrated volume: 3 mL

Orally-disintegrating tablets: Do not remove tablet from blister pack until ready to administer; do not push tablet through foil (tablet may become damaged); peel back foil to expose tablet; use dry hands to remove tablet and place immediately on tongue; tablet will dissolve within seconds and may be swallowed with or without liquid; do not split or chew tablet

I.M.: Before reconstitution, bring injection and diluent to room temperature; reconstitute with provided diluent only; shake vial vigorously for a minimum of 10 seconds to properly mix; suspension should appear thick, milky, and uniform; use immediately (or within 6 hours of reconstitution); if suspension settles prior to use, shake vigorously to resuspend. Administer deep I.M. into either the deltoid muscle or the upper-outer quadrant of the gluteal area; avoid inadvertent injection into blood vessel; **do not administer I.V.;** alternate injection site between the two arms or buttocks; do not combine two different dosage strengths into one single administration; administer with needle provided (1-inch needle for deltoid administration or 2-inch needle for gluteal administration); do not substitute any components of the dose pack.

Monitoring Parameters Blood pressure (including orthostatic) and heart rate, particularly during dosage titration;

mental status, abnormal involuntary movement scale (AIMS), and extrapyramidal symptoms; growth, BMI, waist circumference, and weight (in adults, weight should be assessed prior to treatment and at 4 weeks, 8 weeks, 12 weeks, and then at quarterly intervals; consider titrating to a different antipsychotic agent for a weight gain ≥5% of the initial weight); CBC with differential; liver enzymes in children (especially obese children or those who are rapidly gaining weight while receiving therapy); lipid profile; fasting blood glucose/Hgb A_{1c} (prior to treatment, at 3 months, then annually); prolactin serum concentrations

Additional Information Long-term usefulness of risperidone should be periodically re-evaluated in patients receiving the drug for extended periods of time. Risperdal® Consta® is a long-acting injection comprised of an extended release microsphere formulation; prior to injection, the microspheres are suspended in the provided diluent; the small polymeric microspheres degrade slowly, releasing the medication at a controlled rate.

Dosage Forms Excipient information presented when available (limited, particularly for generics); consult specific product labeling.

Solution, Oral:

RisperDAL: 1 mg/mL (30 mL) [contains benzoic acid]

Generic: 1 mg/mL (30 mL)

Suspension Reconstituted, Intramuscular:

RisperDAL Consta: 12.5 mg (1 ea); 25 mg (1 ea); 37.5 mg (1 ea); 50 mg (1 ea)

Tablet, Oral:

RisperDAL: 0.25 mg, 0.5 mg, 1 mg

RisperDAL: 2 mg [contains fd&c yellow #6 aluminum lake]

RisperDAL: 3 mg [contains fd&c yellow #10 (quinoline yellow)]

RisperDAL: 4 mg [contains fd&c blue #2 aluminum lake, fd&c yellow #10 (quinoline yellow)]

Generic: 0.25 mg, 0.5 mg, 1 mg, 2 mg, 3 mg, 4 mg

Tablet Dispersible, Oral:

RisperDAL M-TAB: 0.5 mg, 1 mg, 2 mg, 3 mg, 4 mg [contains aspartame, peppermint oil (mentha piperita oil)]

RisperiDONE M-TAB: 0.5 mg, 1 mg, 2 mg, 3 mg, 4 mg [contains aspartame]

Generic: 0.25 mg, 0.5 mg, 1 mg, 2 mg, 3 mg, 4 mg

References

Aman MG, De Smedt G, Derivan A, et al, "Double-Blind, Placebo-Controlled Study of Risperidone for the Treatment of Disruptive Behaviors in Children With Subaverage Intelligence," *Am J Psychiatry*, 2002, 159(8):1337-46.

American College of Obstetricians and Gynecologists, ACOG Practice Bulletin: Clinical Management Guidelines for Obstetricians-Gynecologists No. 92 April 2008 (Replaces Practice Bulletin Number 87, November 2007), "Use of Psychiatric Medications During Pregnancy and Lactation," *Obstet Gynecol*, 2008, 111(4):1001-20.

American Diabetes Association, American Psychiatric Association, American Association of Clinical Endocrinologists, and North American Association for the Study of Obesity, "Consensus Development Conference on Antipsychotic Drugs and Obesity and Diabetes," *Diabetes Care*, 2004, 27(2):596-601.

Bruggeman R, van der Linden C, Buitelaar JK, et al, "Risperidone Versus Pimozide in Tourette's Disorder: A Comparative Double-Blind Parallel-Group Study," *J Clin Psychiatry*, 2001, 62(1):50-6.

Coppola D, Russo LJ, Kwarta RF Jr, et al, "Evaluating the Postmarketing Experience of Risperidone Use During Pregnancy: Pregnancy and Neonatal Outcomes," *Drug Saf*, 2007, 30(3):247-64.

Correll CU, Manu P, Olshanskiy V, et al, "Cardiometabolic Risk of Second-Generation Antipsychotic Medications During First-Time Use in Children and Adolescents," *JAMA*, 2009, 302(16):1765-73.

Dion Y, Annable L, Sandor P, et al, "Risperidone in the Treatment of Tourette Syndrome: A Double-Blind, Placebo-Controlled Trial," *J Clin Psychopharmacol*, 2002, 22(1):31-9.

Donfrancesco R, Calderoni D, and Vitiello B, "Open-Label Amantadine in Children With Attention-Deficit/Hyperactivity Disorder," *J Child Adolesc Psychopharmacol*, 2007, 17(5):657-64.

Findling RL, Aman MG, Eerdekens M, et al, "Long-Term, Open-Label Study of Risperidone in Children With Severe Disruptive Behaviors and Below-Average IQ," *Am J Psychiatry*, 2004, 161(4):677-84.

Fisman S and Steele M, "Use of Risperidone in Pervasive Developmental Disorders: A Case Series," *J Child Adolesc Psychopharmacol*, 1996, 6(3):177-90.

Ford RL, Sallam A, Towler HM. Intraoperative floppy iris syndrome associated with risperidone intake. *Eur J Ophthalmol*. 2011;21 (2):210-211.

Fu-I L, Boarati MA, Stravogiannis A, et al, "Use of Risperidone Long-Acting Injection to Support Treatment Adherence and Mood Stabilization in Pediatric Bipolar Patients: A Case Series," *J Clin Psychiatry*, 2009, 70(4):604-6.

Hill RC, McIvor RJ, Wojnar-Horton RE, et al, "Risperidone Distribution and Excretion Into Human Milk: Case Report and Estimated Infant Exposure During Breast-Feeding," *J Clin Psychopharmacol*, 2000, 20 (2):285-6.

Ipser J and Stein DJ, "Systematic Review of Pharmacotherapy of Disruptive Behavior Disorders in Children and Adolescents," *Psychopharmacology (Berl)*, 2007, 191(1):127-40.

Karnik NS, Joshi SV, Paterno C, et al, "Subtypes of Pediatric Delirium: A Treatment Algorithm," *Psychosomatics*, 2007, 48(3):253-7.

Kumra S, Herion D, Jacobsen LK, et al, "Case Study: Risperidone-Induced Hepatotoxicity in Pediatric Patients," *J Am Acad Child Adolesc Psychiatry*, 1997, 36(5):701-5.

Kutcher S, Aman M, Brooks SJ, et al, "International Consensus Statement on Attention-Deficit/Hyperactivity Disorder (ADHD) and Disruptive Behaviour Disorders (DBDs): Clinical Implications and Treatment Practice Suggestions," *Eur Neuropsychopharmacol*, 2004, 14 (1):11-28.

Lombroso PJ, Scahill L, King RA, et al, "Risperidone Treatment of Children and Adolescents With Chronic Tic Disorders: A Preliminary Report," *J Am Acad Child Adolesc Psychiatry*, 1995, 34(9):1147-52.

McDougle CJ, Holmes JP, Bronson MR, et al, "Risperidone Treatment of Children and Adolescents With Pervasive Developmental Disorders: A Prospective Open-Label Study," *J Am Acad Child Adolesc Psychiatry*, 1997, 36(5):685-93.

National Institute for Occupational Safety and Health (NIOSH), "NIOSH List of Antineoplastic and Other Hazardous Drugs in Healthcare Settings 2012." Available at http://www.cdc.gov/niosh/docs/2012-150/pdfs/2012-150.pdf. Accessed January 21, 2013.

Newport DJ, Calamaras MR, DeVane CL, et al, "Atypical Antipsychotic Administration During Late Pregnancy: Placental Passage and Obstetrical Outcomes," *Am J Psychiatry*, 2007, 164(8):1214-20.

Pandina GJ, Aman MG, and Findling RL, "Risperidone in the Management of Disruptive Behavior Disorders," *J Child Adolesc Psychopharmacol*, 2006, 16(4):379-92.

Roessner V, Plessen KJ, Rothenberger A, et al, "European Clinical Guidelines for Tourette Syndrome and Other Tic Disorders. Part II: Pharmacological Treatment," *Eur Child Adolesc Psychiatry*, 2011, 20 (4):173-96.

Sandor P and Stephens RJ, "Risperidone Treatment of Aggressive Behavior in Children With Tourette Syndrome," *J Clin Psychopharmacol*, 2000, 20(6):710-2.

Scahill L, Leckman JF, Schultz RT, et al, "A Placebo-Controlled Trial of Risperidone in Tourette Syndrome," *Neurology*, 2003, 60(7):1130-5.

Schieveld JN, Leroy PL, van Os J, et al, "Pediatric Delirium in Critical Illness: Phenomenology, Clinical Correlates and Treatment Response in 40 Cases in the Pediatric Intensive Care Unit," *Intensive Care Med*, 2007, 33(6):1033-40.

Shea S, Turgay A, Carroll A, et al, "Risperidone in the Treatment of Disruptive Behavioral Symptoms in Children With Autistic and Other Pervasive Developmental Disorders," *Pediatrics*, 2004, 114(5): e634-41.

Silver GH, Kearney JA, Kutko MC, et al, "Infant Delirium in Pediatric Critical Care Settings," *Am J Psychiatry*, 2010, 167(10):1172-7.

Singer HS, "Treatment of Tics and Tourette Syndrome," *Curr Treat Options Neurol*, 2010, 12(6):539-61.

Smith HA, Fuchs DC, Pandharipande PP, et al, "Delirium: An Emerging Frontier in the Management of Critically Ill Children," *Crit Care Clin*, 2009, 25(3):593-614.

◆ **RisperiDONE M-TAB** *see* RisperiDONE *on page 1831*

◆ **Ritalin** *see* Methylphenidate *on page 1379*

◆ **Ritalin LA** *see* Methylphenidate *on page 1379*

◆ **Ritalin SR** *see* Methylphenidate *on page 1379*

Ritonavir (ri TOE na veer)

Medication Safety Issues
Sound-alike/look-alike issues:
Ritonavir may be confused with Retrovir®
Norvir® may be confused with Norvasc®

Related Information
Adult and Adolescent HIV *on page 2348*
Oral Medications That Should Not Be Crushed or Altered *on page 2438*
Pediatric HIV *on page 2338*
Perinatal HIV *on page 2356*
Brand Names: U.S. Norvir
Brand Names: Canada Norvir®; Norvir® SEC
Therapeutic Category Antiretroviral Agent; HIV Agents (Anti-HIV Agents); Protease Inhibitor
Generic Availability (U.S.) No
Use Treatment of HIV infection in combination with other antiretroviral agents (FDA approved in ages >1 month and adults); has also been used as a pharmacokinetic "booster" for other protease inhibitors. **Note:** HIV regimens consisting of **three** antiretroviral agents are strongly recommended.

Pregnancy Risk Factor B
Pregnancy Considerations Adverse events were observed in animal reproduction studies only with doses which were also maternally toxic. Ritonavir has a low level of transfer across the human placenta; no increased risk of overall birth defects has been observed following first trimester exposure according to data collected by the antiretroviral pregnancy registry. Early studies have shown lower plasma levels during pregnancy compared to postpartum, however dosage adjustment is not needed when used as a low-dose booster in pregnant women. The DHHS Perinatal HIV Guidelines consider ritonavir to be a preferred protease inhibitor (PI) for use during pregnancy when used as a booster for other PIs (not recommended as a single protease inhibitor in ART naïve pregnant women). The oral solution contains alcohol and therefore may not be the best formulation for use in pregnancy. A small increased risk of preterm birth has been associated with maternal use of protease inhibitor-based combination antiretroviral (ARV) therapy during pregnancy; however, the benefits of use generally outweigh this risk and PIs should not be withheld if otherwise recommended. Hyperglycemia, new onset of diabetes mellitus, or diabetic ketoacidosis have been reported with protease inhibitors; it is not clear if pregnancy increases this risk.

Regardless of CD4 count or HIV RNA copy number, all HIV-infected pregnant women should receive a combination antiretroviral ARV drug regimen. A combination of antepartum, intrapartum, and infant ARV prophylaxis is recommended. ARV therapy should be started as soon as possible in women with symptomatic infection. Although earlier initiation may be more effective in reducing the perinatal transmission of HIV, initiation may be delayed until after 12 weeks gestation in women who do not require immediate treatment after careful consideration of maternal conditions (eg, nausea and vomiting) and the potential risks of first trimester fetal exposure for specific agents. A scheduled cesarean delivery at 38 weeks gestation is recommended for all women with HIV RNA >1000 copies/mL or unknown concentrations near delivery in order to decrease transmission. If ARV therapy must be interrupted for <24 hours during the peripartum period, stop then restart all medications simultaneously in order to decrease the chance of developing resistance. Long-term follow-up is recommended for all infants exposed to ARV medications. In couples who want to conceive, the HIV-infected partner should attain maximum viral suppression prior to conception.

Health care providers are encouraged to enroll pregnant women exposed to antiretroviral medications in the Antiretroviral Pregnancy Registry (1-800-258-4263 or www.APRegistry.com). Health care providers caring for HIV-infected women and their infants may contact the National

Perinatal HIV Hotline (888-448-8765) for clinical consultation (DHHS [perinatal], 2014).

Breast-Feeding Considerations It is not known if ritonavir is excreted into breast milk; serum concentrations in nursing infants were undetectable at 12 weeks of age. Maternal or infant antiretroviral therapy does not completely eliminate the risk of postnatal HIV transmission. In addition, multiclass-resistant virus has been detected in breast-feeding infants despite maternal therapy. Therefore, in the United States, where formula is accessible, affordable, safe, and sustainable, and the risk of infant mortality due to diarrhea and respiratory infections is low, complete avoidance of breast-feeding by HIV-infected women is recommended to decrease potential transmission of HIV (DHHS [perinatal], 2014).

Warnings Ritonavir is a potent CYP3A enzyme inhibitor that interacts with numerous drugs **[U.S. Boxed Warnings]**. Due to potential serious and/or life-threatening drug interactions, some drugs are contraindicated. Concomitant use with fluticasone, salmeterol, high-dose ketoconazole, high-dose itraconazole, or high-dose or long-term use of meperidine is **not** recommended. Alteration of dose or serum concentration monitoring may be required with other medications. Use of ritonavir with other antiretroviral agents (eg, certain protease inhibitors) may require dosage adjustment of both agents (see individual monographs for specific dosage recommendations).

Potentially fatal pancreatitis may occur; advanced HIV disease and elevated serum triglycerides may place patient at increased risk; monitor serum lipase and amylase, and for symptoms of nausea, vomiting, and/or abdominal pain. Temporary or permanent discontinuation may be clinically indicated; discontinue ritonavir in patients with pancreatitis. Hepatic reactions, including elevated liver enzymes, hepatitis, and jaundice may occur; coinfection with hepatitis B or C may increase risk; use with caution in patients with underlying hepatic disease, hepatitis B or C, cirrhosis, or those with high baseline transaminases; consider increased monitoring of transaminases in these patients; hepatic dysfunction with fatalities have also been reported. Significant elevations of serum triglycerides and cholesterol may occur; monitor and manage appropriately.

New onset diabetes mellitus, exacerbation of diabetes, and hyperglycemia have been reported in HIV-infected patients receiving protease inhibitors. Protease inhibitors have been associated with a variety of hypersensitivity reactions (some severe), including rash, anaphylaxis (rare), angioedema, bronchospasm, erythema multiforme, toxic epidermal necrolysis, and/or Stevens-Johnson syndrome (rare). It is generally recommended to discontinue treatment if severe rash or moderate symptoms accompanied by other systemic symptoms occur.

Ritonavir oral solution contains 43% ethanol (v/v) and 26.6% propylene glycol (w/v); accidental ingestion could result in alcohol-related toxicity. Ethanol competitively inhibits propylene glycol metabolism, which may lead to propylene glycol toxicity in neonates due to impaired elimination. Preterm neonates may be at increased risk of adverse events from propylene glycol toxicity, including cardiotoxicity (complete AV block, bradycardia, cardiomyopathy), lactic acidosis, CNS depression, respiratory complications, acute renal failure, and death. Do not use oral solution in neonates with a PMA <44 weeks, unless benefit outweighs risk and neonate is closely monitored for increases in serum osmolality, serum creatinine, and other signs of propylene glycol toxicity (eg, CNS depression, seizures, cardiac arrhythmias, hemolysis); in neonates particularly, symptoms should be distinguished from sepsis. Toxicities have been reported with the use of products containing propylene glycol in all ages, including hyperosmolality, lactic acidosis, seizures, and respiratory depression. Due to concentration of ethanol in oral solution, an overdose in a child may cause potentially lethal alcohol toxicity. Treatment for overdose should be supportive and include general poisoning management; activated charcoal may help remove unabsorbed medication; dialysis unlikely to be of benefit; however, dialysis can remove alcohol and propylene glycol. In pediatric patients <6 months of age, the total amounts of ethanol and propylene glycol delivered from all medications should be considered to avoid toxicity.

Precautions Use with caution in patients with hepatic insufficiency, elevated liver enzymes, or hepatitis. Ritonavir may prolong the PR interval; cases of second- or third-degree AV block have been reported; use with caution in patients with cardiomyopathy, ischemic heart disease, preexisting conduction abnormalities, or structural heart disease [these patients may be at increased risk of conduction abnormalities (eg, second- or third-degree AV block)]; use with caution with drugs that prolong the PR interval. Spontaneous bleeding episodes have been reported in patients with hemophilia type A and B receiving protease inhibitors; additional factor VIII may be needed.

Fat redistribution and accumulation [ie, central obesity, peripheral wasting, facial wasting, breast enlargement, dorsocervical fat enlargement (buffalo hump), and cushingoid appearance] have been observed in patients receiving antiretroviral agents (causal relationship not established).

Immune reconstitution syndrome (an acute inflammatory response to residual or indolent opportunistic infections) may occur in HIV patients during treatment with combination antiretroviral agents, including ritonavir; this syndrome may require further patient assessment and therapy. Autoimmune disorders (eg, Grave's disease, Guillain-Barré syndrome, and polymyositis) have been reported in patients experiencing immune reconstitution; time to onset is variable and may occur many months after antiretroviral treatment is initiated.

Norvir® tablets are **not** bioequivalent to Norvir® capsules. Gastrointestinal side effects (eg, nausea, vomiting, abdominal pain, diarrhea) or paresthesias may be more common when patients are switching from the capsule to the tablet formulation due to a higher peak concentration (26% increase) observed with the tablet formulation compared to the capsule. These side effects may decrease as therapy is continued.

Adverse Reactions

Cardiovascular: Edema (including peripheral edema), flushing, hypertension, syncope, vasodilatation

Central nervous system: Anxiety, confusion, depression, disturbance in attention, dizziness, drowsiness, fatigue, headache, insomnia, malaise, paresthesia, peripheral neuropathy

Dermatologic: Acne vulgaris, diaphoresis, pruritus, skin rash

Endocrine & metabolic: Hypercholesterolemia, increased serum triglycerides, increased uric acid, lipodystrophy (acquired)

Gastrointestinal: Abdominal pain, anorexia, diarrhea, dysgeusia, dyspepsia, flatulence, gastrointestinal hemorrhage, increased serum amylase (pediatric), nausea, throat irritation (local), vomiting

Hematologic & oncologic: Anemia (pediatric), neutropenia (pediatric), thrombocytopenia (pediatric)

Hepatic: Hepatitis, increased gamma-glutamyl transferase, increased serum ALT, increased serum AST

Hypersensitivity: Hypersensitivity reaction

Neuromuscular & skeletal: Increased creatine phosphokinase, musculoskeletal pain (arthralgia and back pain), myalgia, weakness

Ophthalmic: Blurred vision
Renal: Polyuria
Respiratory: Cough, oropharyngeal pain, pharyngitis
Miscellaneous: Fever
Rare but important or life-threatening: Adrenal suppression, adrenocortical cortex insufficiency, anaphylaxis, amnesia, angioedema, aphasia, asthma, atrioventricular block (first, second, or third degree), cachexia, cerebral ischemia, chest pain, cholestatic jaundice, coma, Cushing's syndrome, dementia, depersonalization, diabetes mellitus, diabetic ketoacidosis, esophageal ulcer, gastroenteritis, gastroesophageal reflux disease, gout, hallucination, hematologic disease (myeloproliferative), hemorrhage (in patients with hemophilia A or B), hepatic coma, hepatitis, hepatomegaly, hepatosplenomegaly, hyperglycemia, hypotension, hypothermia, hypoventilation, immune reconstitution syndrome, intestinal obstruction, leukemia (acute myeloblastic), leukopenia, lymphadenopathy, lymphocytosis, malignant melanoma, manic behavior, myocardial infarction, neuropathy, orthostatic hypotension, palpitations, pancreatitis, paralysis, pneumonia, prolongation P-R interval on ECG, prolonged Q-T interval on ECG, pseudomembranous colitis, rectal hemorrhage, redistribution of body fat, renal failure, renal insufficiency, right bundle branch block, seizure, Stevens-Johnson syndrome, subdural hematoma, syncope, tachycardia, torsades de pointes, toxic epidermal necrolysis, ulcerative colitis, vasospasm, venous thrombosis (cerebral)

Drug Interactions

Metabolism/Transport Effects Substrate of CYP1A2 (minor), CYP2B6 (minor), CYP2D6 (minor), CYP3A4 (major), P-glycoprotein; **Note:** Assignment of Major/Minor substrate status based on clinically relevant drug interaction potential; **Inhibits** CYP2C19 (weak), CYP2C8 (strong), CYP2C9 (weak), CYP2D6 (strong), CYP2E1 (weak), CYP3A4 (strong), P-glycoprotein; **Induces** CYP1A2 (weak/moderate), CYP2C9 (weak/moderate), CYP3A4 (weak/moderate)

Avoid Concomitant Use

Avoid concomitant use of Ritonavir with any of the following: Ado-Trastuzumab Emtansine; Alfuzosin; Amiodarone; Apixaban; Atovaquone; Avanafil; Axitinib; Bosutinib; Cabozantinib; Ceritinib; Cisapride; Conivaptan; Crizotinib; Disulfiram; Dronedarone; Enzalutamide; Eplerenone; Ergot Derivatives; Etravirine; Everolimus; Flecainide; Fluticasone (Nasal); Fusidic Acid (Systemic); Halofantrine; Ibrutinib; Ivabradine; Lapatinib; Lomitapide; Lovastatin; Lurasidone; Macitentan; Midazolam; Nilotinib; Nisoldipine; PAZOPanib; Pimozide; Propafenone; QuiNIDine; QuiNINE; Ranolazine; Red Yeast Rice; Regorafenib; Rifampin; Rivaroxaban; Salmeterol; Silodosin; Simeprevir; Simvastatin; St Johns Wort; Tamoxifen; Tamsulosin; Thioridazine; Ticagrelor; Tipranavir; Tolvaptan; Topotecan; Toremifene; Triazolam; Ulipristal; Vemurafenib; VinCRIStine (Liposomal); Vorapaxar; Voriconazole

Increased Effect/Toxicity

Ritonavir may increase the levels/effects of: Ado-Trastuzumab Emtansine; Afatinib; Alfuzosin; Almotriptan; Alosetron; ALPRAZolam; Amiodarone; Apixaban; ARIPiprazole; AtoMOXetine; AtorvaSTATin; Avanafil; Axitinib; Bedaquiline; Bortezomib; Bosentan; Bosutinib; Brentuximab Vedotin; Brinzolamide; Budesonide (Nasal); Budesonide (Systemic, Oral Inhalation); Cabozantinib; Calcium Channel Blockers (Dihydropyridine); Calcium Channel Blockers (Nondihydropyridine); Cannabis; CarBAMazepine; Ceritinib; Cisapride; Clarithromycin; Clorazepate; Colchicine; Conivaptan; Corticosteroids (Orally Inhaled); Crizotinib; Cyclophosphamide; CycloSPORINE (Systemic); CYP2C8 Substrates; CYP2D6 Substrates; CYP3A4 Substrates; Dabigatran Etexilate; Diazepam; Dienogest; Digoxin; DOXOrubicin (Conventional); Dronabinol; Dronedarone; Dutasteride; Efavirenz; Enfuvirtide;

Enzalutamide; Eplerenone; Ergot Derivatives; Estazolam; Everolimus; FentaNYL; Fesoterodine; Flecainide; Flurazepam; Fluticasone (Nasal); Fluticasone (Oral Inhalation); Fusidic Acid (Systemic); GuanFACINE; Halofantrine; Highest Risk QTc-Prolonging Agents; Ibrutinib; Iloperidone; Imatinib; Itraconazole; Ivabradine; Ivacaftor; Ixabepilone; Ketoconazole (Systemic); Lacosamide; Lapatinib; Levomilnacipran; Linagliptin; Lomitapide; Lovastatin; Lurasidone; Macitentan; Maraviroc; Meperidine; MethylPREDNISolone; Metoprolol; Midazolam; Mifepristone; Moderate Risk QTc-Prolonging Agents; Nebivolol; Nefazodone; Nilotinib; Nisoldipine; Ospemifene; OxyCODONE; Paricalcitol; PAZOPanib; P-glycoprotein/ABCB1 Substrates; Pimecrolimus; Pimozide; Pioglitazone; PONATinib; PrednisoLONE (Systemic); PredniSONE; Propafenone; Protease Inhibitors; Prucalopride; QUEtiapine; QuiNIDine; QuiNINE; Ranolazine; Red Yeast Rice; Regorafenib; Rifabutin; Rifaximin; Rilpivirine; Riociguat; Rivaroxaban; RomiDEPsin; Rosuvastatin; Ruxolitinib; Salmeterol; Saxagliptin; Sildenafil; Silodosin; Simeprevir; Simvastatin; SORAfenib; Tacrolimus (Systemic); Tacrolimus (Topical); Tadalafil; Tamsulosin; Telaprevir; Temsirolimus; Tetrabenazine; Tetrahydrocannabinol; Thioridazine; Ticagrelor; Tofacitinib; Tolterodine; Tolvaptan; Topotecan; Toremifene; TraZODone; Treprostinil; Triamcinolone (Systemic); Triazolam; Ulipristal; Vardenafil; Vemurafenib; Vilazodone; VinBLAStine; VinCRIStine; VinCRIStine (Liposomal); Vorapaxar; Vortioxetine; Zuclopenthixol

The levels/effects of Ritonavir may be increased by: ARIPiprazole; Clarithromycin; CycloSPORINE (Systemic); Delavirdine; Disulfiram; Efavirenz; Enfuvirtide; Fusidic Acid (Systemic); MetroNIDAZOLE (Topical); Mifepristone; P-glycoprotein/ABCB1 Inhibitors; Posaconazole; QuiNINE; Simeprevir

Decreased Effect

Ritonavir may decrease the levels/effects of: Abacavir; Atovaquone; Axitinib; Boceprevir; BuPROPion; Canagliflozin; Clarithromycin; Codeine; Contraceptives (Estrogens); Deferasirox; Delavirdine; Etravirine; Fosphenytoin; Ifosfamide; Iloperidone; LamoTRIgine; Meperidine; Methadone; Phenytoin; Prasugrel; Proguanil; QuiNINE; Simeprevir; Tamoxifen; Telaprevir; Ticagrelor; Valproic Acid and Derivatives; Voriconazole; Warfarin; Zidovudine

The levels/effects of Ritonavir may be decreased by: Antacids; Boceprevir; CarBAMazepine; CYP3A4 Inducers (Strong); Dabrafenib; Fosphenytoin; Garlic; Mitotane; Peginterferon Alfa-2b; P-glycoprotein/ABCB1 Inducers; Phenytoin; Rifampin; Siltuximab; St Johns Wort; Tipranavir; Tocilizumab

Food Interactions Food enhances absorption. Management: Manufacturer recommends taking with food. Maintain adequate hydration, unless instructed to restrict fluid intake.

Stability

Oral capsules: Store at 2°C to 8°C (36°F to 46°F) until dispensed; dispense and store in original container. Refrigeration after dispensing is recommended but not required; stable for 30 days at <77°F (25°C); protect from light; avoid exposure to excessive heat; keep bottle tightly closed.
Oral tablets: Store at <30°C (<86°F); excursions permitted to 50°C (122°F) for up to 7 days. Dispense in original container or USP equivalent tight container (60 mL or less). Exposure to high humidity outside the original or USP equivalent tight container for >2 weeks is **not** recommended.
Oral solution: Store at 20°C to 25°C (68°F to 77°F); dispense and store in original container; do not refrigerate; avoid exposure to excessive heat; keep bottle tightly

closed; use by product expiration date (limited shelf life of 6 months).

Mechanism of Action Binds to the site of HIV-1 protease activity and inhibits cleavage of viral Gag-Pol polyprotein precursors into individual functional proteins required for infectious HIV. This results in the formation of immature, noninfectious viral particles.

Pharmacokinetics (Adult data unless noted)

Absorption: Well absorbed

Distribution: High concentrations in serum and lymph nodes; V_d (apparent): 0.41 ± 0.25 L/kg

Protein binding: 98% to 99%

Metabolism: In the liver by cytochrome P450 isoenzyme CYP3A and (to a lesser extent) CYP2D6; five metabolites have been identified; the major metabolite (M-2), an isopropylthiazole oxidation metabolite, is active at a level similar to ritonavir, but is found in low concentrations in the plasma

Bioavailability: Absolute bioavailability unknown; tablets are **not** bioequivalent to capsules; mean peak concentration of tablet was found to be 26% higher than capsule in a single dose study, in patients fed a moderate-fat meal

Half-life:

Children: 2 to 4 hours

Adults: 3 to 5 hours

Time to peak serum concentration: Oral solution: Fasting: 2 hours; nonfasting: 4 hours

Elimination: Renal clearance is negligible; 3.5% of dose is excreted as unchanged drug in the urine; 34% excreted as unchanged drug in the feces

Clearance: Pediatric patients: 1.5 to 1.7 times faster than adults

Dosing: Neonatal PMA <44 weeks: Do not use due to potential toxicity from excipients; no data about appropriate dose or safety exists (DHHS [pediatric], 2014)

Dosing: Usual

Pediatric: **HIV infection, treatment: Note:** Use in combination with other antiretroviral agents: Oral:

Ritonavir as sole protease inhibitor: **Note:** Not recommended as the sole protease inhibitor in any regimen (DHHS [pediatric], 2014)

Infants >1 month (PMA ≥44 weeks) and Children:

Initial: 250 mg/m²/dose every 12 hours; titrate upward at 2- to 3-day intervals by 50 mg/m²/dose twice daily increments to 350 to 400 mg/m²/dose twice daily; maximum dose: 600 mg/dose twice daily; **Note:** Patients who do not tolerate 400 mg/m² twice daily (due to adverse effects) may be treated with the highest tolerated dose; however, an alternative antiretroviral agent should be considered.

Serum concentrations comparable to those seen in adults receiving standard doses were obtained in children >2 years of age who received 350 to 400 mg/m² twice daily. In younger patients (1 month to 2 years of age) who received 350 or 450 mg/m²/dose twice daily, ritonavir AUCs were 16% lower and trough concentrations were 60% lower than those observed in adults receiving standard doses; higher ritonavir AUCs were not observed with the 450 mg/m²/dose twice daily compared to the 350 mg/m²/dose twice daily dosing.

Adolescents: **Note:** Ritonavir as sole protease inhibitor is no longer commonly used in clinical practice and is not recommended in any initial antiretroviral regimen (DHHS [adults], 2014): 600 mg twice daily; may use a dose titration schedule to reduce adverse events (nausea/vomiting) by initiating therapy at 300 mg twice daily; increase dose at 2- to 3-day intervals by 100 mg twice daily increments up to a maximum dose of 600 mg twice daily

Ritonavir as pharmacokinetic enhancer ("booster doses" of ritonavir): **Note:** Ritonavir is used at lower doses to increase the serum concentrations of other protease inhibitors; the recommended dose of ritonavir varies when used with different protease inhibitors; see monographs for individual protease inhibitors for recommended doses; appropriate pediatric "booster doses" of ritonavir have not been established for use with every protease inhibitor or for all pediatric age groups.

Adult: **HIV infection, treatment: Note:** Use in combination with other antiretroviral agents: Oral:

Ritonavir as sole protease inhibitor: **Note:** Ritonavir as sole protease inhibitor is no longer commonly used in clinical practice and is not recommended in any initial antiretroviral regimen (DHHS [adults], 2014): 600 mg twice daily; may use a dose titration schedule to reduce adverse events (nausea/vomiting) by initiating therapy at 300 mg twice daily; increase dose at 2- to 3-day intervals by 100 mg twice daily increments up to a maximum dose of 600 mg twice daily

Ritonavir as pharmacokinetic enhancer ("booster doses" of ritonavir): **Note:** Ritonavir is used at lower doses to increase the serum concentrations of other protease inhibitors; the recommended dose of ritonavir varies when used with different protease inhibitors; see monographs for individual protease inhibitors for recommended doses

Usual dose: 100 to 400 mg/day, as 100 to 200 mg once or twice daily; range: 100 to 800 mg/day; dose depends on the protease inhibitor. In patients without evidence of PI resistance, once daily booster-dosing of 100 mg ritonavir may be preferred to 200 mg/day due to less gastrointestinal and metabolic adverse events.

Dosing adjustment in renal impairment: No adjustment recommended; renal clearance is negligible (DHHS [adult], 2014)

Dosing adjustment in hepatic impairment:

Mild to moderate hepatic impairment: No adjustment recommended; lower ritonavir serum concentrations have been reported in patients with moderate hepatic impairment (use with caution; monitor closely for adequate response)

Severe hepatic impairment: Use not recommended; pharmacokinetics of ritonavir has not been studied in these patients

Administration Administer with meals to improve tolerability. Swallow tablets whole; do not chew, break, or crush. Consider reserving liquid formulation for use in patients receiving tube feeding due to its bad taste. Shake liquid well before use. May mix liquid formulation with milk, chocolate milk, vanilla or chocolate pudding or ice cream, or a liquid nutritional supplement. Other techniques used to increase tolerance in children include dulling the taste buds by chewing ice, giving popsicles or spoonfuls of partially frozen orange or grape juice concentrates before administration of ritonavir; coating the mouth with peanut butter to eat before the dose; administration of strong-tasting foods such as maple syrup, cheese, or strong-flavored chewing gum immediately after a dose. Oral solution is highly concentrated; use a calibrated oral dosing syringe to measure and administer. Separate administration of ritonavir and didanosine by 2 hours (DHHS [pediatric], 2014).

Monitoring Parameters Note: Monitor CD4 percentage (if <5 years of age) or CD4 count (if ≥5 years of age) at least every 3 to 4 months (DHHS [pediatric], 2014).

Prior to initiation of therapy: Genotypic resistance testing, CD4 and viral load (every 3 to 4 months), CBC with differential, LFTs, BUN, creatinine, electrolytes, glucose, and urinalysis (every 6 to 12 months), and assessment of readiness for adherence with medication regimen. At initiation and with any change in treatment regimen: CBC with differential, electrolytes, calcium, phosphate, glucose,

LFTs, bilirubin, urinalysis (at initiation), BUN, creatinine, albumin, total protein, lipid panel (at initiation), CD4, and viral load. After 1 to 2 weeks of therapy: Signs of medication toxicity and adherence. After 2 to 4 weeks of therapy: CBC with differential, viral load, signs of medication toxicity, and adherence; then every 3 to 4 months: CBC with differential, electrolytes, glucose, LFTs, bilirubin, BUN, creatinine, CD4, viral load, signs of medication toxicity, and adherence. Every 6 to 12 months: Lipid panel and urinalysis. CD4 monitoring frequency may be decreased to every 6 to 12 months in children who are adherent to therapy if the value is well above the threshold for opportunistic infections, viral suppression is sustained, and the clinical status is stable for more than 2 to 3 years (DHHS [pediatric], 2014). Monitor for growth and development, signs of HIV-specific physical conditions, HIV disease progression, opportunistic infections, hepatitis, or pancreatitis.

Dosage Forms Excipient information presented when available (limited, particularly for generics); consult specific product labeling.

Capsule, Oral:
Norvir: 100 mg [contains alcohol, usp]

Solution, Oral:
Norvir: 80 mg/mL (240 mL) [contains alcohol, usp, fd&c yellow #6 (sunset yellow), propylene glycol, saccharin sodium; peppermint-caramel flavor]

Tablet, Oral:
Norvir: 100 mg

References

Danner SA, Carr A, Leonard JM, et al. A short-term study of the safety, pharmacokinetics, and efficacy of ritonavir, an inhibitor of HIV-1 protease. European-Australian Collaborative Ritonavir Study Group. *N Engl J Med*. 1995;333(23):1528-1533.

DeSilva KE, Le Flore DB, Marston BJ, Rimland D. Serotonin syndrome in HIV-infected individuals receiving antiretroviral therapy and fluoxetine. *AIDS*. 2001;15(10)1281-1285.

DHHS Panel on Antiretroviral Guidelines for Adults and Adolescents. Guidelines for the use of antiretroviral agents in HIV-1-infected adults and adolescents, Department of Health and Human Services. May 1, 2014. Available at http://www.aidsinfo.nih.gov/ContentFiles/AdultandAdolescentGL.pdf

DHHS Panel on Antiretroviral Therapy and Medical Management of HIV-Infected Children. Guidelines for the use of antiretroviral agents in pediatric HIV infection. February 12, 2014. Available at http://aidsinfo.nih.gov

DHHS Panel on Treatment of HIV-Infected Pregnant Women and Prevention of Perinatal Transmission. Recommendations for the use of antiretroviral drugs in pregnant HIV-1-infected women for maternal health and interventions to reduce perinatal HIV-1 transmission in the United States. March 28, 2014. Available at http://aidsinfo.nih.gov

Gatti G, Pontali E, Boni S, De Pascalis CR, Bassetti M, Bassetti D. The relationship between ritonavir plasma trough concentration and virological and immunological response in HIV-infected children. *HIV Med*. 2002;3(2):125-128.

Nachman SA, Lindsey JC, Pelton S, et al. Growth in human immunodeficiency virus-infected children receiving ritonavir-containing antiretroviral therapy. *Arch Pediatr Adolesc Med*. 2002;156(5):497-503.

Nachman SA, Stanley K, Yogev R, et al. Nucleoside analogs plus ritonavir in stable antiretroviral therapy-experienced HIV-infected children: a randomized controlled trial. Pediatric AIDS Clinical Trials Group 338 Study Team. *JAMA*. 2000;283(4):492-498.

◆ **Ritonavir and Lopinavir** see Lopinavir and Ritonavir on page 1272

◆ **Rituxan** see RiTUXimab on page 1841

RiTUXimab (ri TUK si mab)

Medication Safety Issues

Sound-alike/look-alike issues:
Rituxan may be confused with Remicade
RiTUXimab may be confused with brentuximab, bevacizumab, inFLIXimab, ramucirumab, ruxolitinib

High alert medication:
The medication is in a class the Institute for Safe Medication Practices (ISMP) includes among its list of drug classes which have a heightened risk of causing significant patient harm when used in error.

Administration issues:
The rituximab dose for rheumatoid arthritis is a flat dose (1000 mg) and is not based on body surface area (BSA).

Related Information

Emetogenic Potential of Antineoplastic Agents in Children on page 2327

Brand Names: U.S. Rituxan

Brand Names: Canada Rituxan

Therapeutic Category Antineoplastic Agent, Anti-CD20; Antineoplastic Agent, Monoclonal Antibody; Antirheumatic Miscellaneous; Immunosuppressant Agent; Monoclonal Antibody

Generic Availability (U.S.) No

Use Treatment of CD20-positive, B-cell non-Hodgkin's lymphoma (NHL) [including relapsed or refractory, low-grade or follicular B-cell NHL (as a single agent); follicular B-cell NHL, previously untreated (in combination with first-line chemotherapy, and as single-agent maintenance therapy if response to first-line rituximab with chemotherapy); nonprogressing, low-grade B-cell NHL (as a single agent after first-line CVP treatment), diffuse large B-cell NHL, previously untreated (in combination with CHOP chemotherapy or other anthracycline-based regimen)]; treatment of CD20-positive chronic lymphocytic leukemia (CLL) (in combination with cyclophosphamide and fludarabine); treatment of moderately- to severely-active rheumatoid arthritis (in combination with methotrexate) in patients with inadequate response to one or more TNF antagonists; treatment of granulomatosis with polyangiitis (GPA; Wegener's Granulomatosis) and microscopic polyangiitis (MPA) in combination with glucocorticoids (FDA approved in adults); has also been used for the treatment of systemic autoimmune disorders (other than rheumatoid arthritis; ie, autoimmune hemolytic anemia in children); refractory systemic lupus erythematosus; steroid-refractory chronic graft-versus-host disease (GVHD); refractory nephrotic syndrome, chronic immune thrombocytopenia (ITP); post-transplant lymphoproliferative disorder (PTLD)

Medication Guide Available Yes

Pregnancy Risk Factor C

Pregnancy Considerations Animal reproduction studies have demonstrated adverse effects including decreased (reversible) B-cells and immunosuppression. Rituximab crosses the placenta and can be detected in the newborn. In one infant born at 41 weeks gestation, in utero exposure occurred from week 16-37; rituximab concentrations were higher in the neonate at birth (32,095 ng/mL) than the mother (9750 ng/mL) and still measurable at 18 weeks of age (700 ng/mL infant; 500 ng/mL mother) (Friedrichs, 2006).

B-cell lymphocytopenia lasting <6 months may occur in exposed infants. Limited information is available following maternal use of rituximab for the treatment of lymphomas and hematologic disorders (Ton, 2011). Retrospective case reports of inadvertent pregnancy during rituximab treatment collected by the manufacturer (often combined with concomitant teratogenic therapies) describe premature births and infant hematologic abnormalities and infections; no specific pattern of birth defects has been observed (limited data) (Chakravarty, 2010). Use is not recommended to treat non-life-threatening maternal conditions (eg, rheumatoid arthritis) during pregnancy (Makol, 2011; Østensen, 2008) and other agents are preferred for treating lupus nephritis in pregnant women (Hahn, 2012).

Effective contraception should be used during and for 12 months following treatment. Healthcare providers are encouraged to enroll women with rheumatoid arthritis exposed to rituximab during pregnancy in the ▶

MotherToBabyAutoImmune Diseases Study by contacting the Organization of Teratology Information Specialists (OTIS) (877-311-8972).

Breast-Feeding Considerations It is not known if rituximab is excreted in human milk. However, human IgG is excreted in breast milk, and therefore, rituximab may also be excreted in milk. Although rituximab would not be expected to enter the circulation of a nursing infant in significant amounts, the decision to discontinue rituximab or discontinue breast-feeding should take into account the benefits of treatment to the mother.

Contraindications Hypersensitivity to rituximab or any component

Warnings Progressive multifocal leukoencephalopathy (PML) due to JC virus has been reported with rituximab use (may be fatal) **[U.S. Boxed Warning]**. Cases were reported in patients with hematologic malignancies or autoimmune diseases receiving rituximab either with combination chemotherapy or with hematopoietic stem cell transplant. Cases were also reported in patients receiving rituximab for autoimmune disease and may have received concurrent or prior immunosuppressant therapy. Onset may be delayed, although most cases were diagnosed within 12 months of the last rituximab dose. Symptoms may include confusion/disorientation, motor weakness/hemiparesis, altered vision/speech, and poor motor coordination; may progress over weeks to months. Evaluate any neurological change promptly; discontinue rituximab in patients who develop PML; consider reduction/discontinuation of concurrent chemotherapy or immunosuppressants.

Severe (sometimes fatal) infusion reactions which may include hypotension, angioedema, hypoxia, bronchospasm, pulmonary infiltrates, acute respiratory distress syndrome, MI, ventricular fibrillation, cardiogenic shock, urticaria, and anaphylaxis have occurred within 24 hours of rituximab administration; monitor closely during infusion **[U.S. Boxed Warning]**. Most of these reactions occurred during the first infusion with time to onset of 30-120 minutes. Fatal infusion reactions were more frequently associated with female gender, pulmonary infiltrates, CLL, or mantle cell lymphoma. Close monitoring required during first and subsequent infusions, especially in patients with preexisting cardiac and pulmonary conditions, patients with prior cardiopulmonary adverse events, and those with high numbers of circulating malignant cells (≥25,000/mm^3). Prior to infusion, premedicate patients with acetaminophen and an antihistamine (and methylprednisolone for patients with RA). Medications for the treatment of hypersensitivity reactions (eg, bronchodilators, epinephrine, antihistamines, corticosteroids) should be available for immediate use. In the event of a severe reaction, interrupt the rituximab infusion and institute supportive care measures (eg, I.V. fluids, vasopressors, oxygen, bronchodilators, diphenhydramine, and acetaminophen). When symptoms completely resolve, may resume rituximab at a 50% reduction from the previous infusion rate. Discontinue rituximab with grades 3 or 4 infusion reactions or in the event of serious or life-threatening cardiac arrhythmias. Mild to moderate infusion-related reactions (eg, chills, fever, rigors) occur frequently in 80% of patients after first infusion, decreasing to 40% in subsequent infusions and are typically managed through slowing or interrupting the infusion; infusion may be resumed at a 50% infusion rate reduction upon resolution of symptoms. Due to the potential for hypotension, consider withholding antihypertensives 12 hours prior to treatment. Rheumatoid arthritis patients are at increased risk for cardiovascular events; monitor closely during and after each infusion.

Tumor lysis syndrome leading to acute renal failure requiring dialysis may occur 12-24 hours following the first dose when used as a single agent to treat NHL **[U.S. Boxed**

Warning]. Hyperkalemia, hypocalcemia, hyperuricemia, and/or hyperphosphatemia may occur. Prophylaxis for tumor lysis syndrome (allopurinol and hydration) should be considered for patients at risk (patients with high tumor burden or with high numbers of circulating malignant cells). Monitor for signs of renal failure; discontinue rituximab with increasing serum creatinine or oliguria. Correct electrolyte abnormalities; monitor hydration status. May cause fatal renal toxicity in patients with hematologic malignancies. Patients who received combination therapy with cisplatin and rituximab for NHL experienced renal toxicity during clinical trials; this combination is not an approved treatment regimen. Severe and sometimes fatal mucocutaneous reactions (lichenoid dermatitis, paraneoplastic pemphigus, Stevens-Johnson syndrome, toxic epidermal necrolysis, and vesiculobullous dermatitis) have been reported **[U.S. Boxed Warning]**; onset has been variable but has occurred as early as the first day of exposure. Patients experiencing severe mucocutaneous skin reactions should not receive further infusions and should seek prompt medical evaluation. Abdominal pain, bowel obstruction, and perforation have been reported (rarely fatal) with an average onset of symptoms of ~6 days; complaints of abdominal pain should be evaluated, especially if early in the treatment course.

Reactivation of hepatitis B (with fulminant hepatitis, hepatic failure, and death) has been reported in association with use; consider screening high-risk patients prior to therapy initiation. Do not use if severe active infection is present. Serious and potentially fatal bacterial, fungal, and either new or reactivated viral infections may occur during treatment and up to 1 year after completing rituximab. Infections have been observed in patients with prolonged hypogammaglobulinemia, defined as hypogammaglobulinemia >11 months after rituximab exposure; monitor immunoglobulin levels as necessary. Associated new or reactivated viral infections have included cytomegalovirus, herpes simplex virus, parvovirus B19, varicella zoster virus, West Nile virus, and hepatitis B and C. Discontinue rituximab (and concomitant chemotherapy) in patients who develop viral hepatitis and initiate antiviral therapy. Discontinue rituximab in patients who develop other serious infections and initiate appropriate anti-infective treatment.

Injection contains polysorbate 80 (Tween 80®) which may cause allergic reactions in susceptible individuals. In premature neonates, thrombocytopenia, ascites, pulmonary deterioration, and renal and hepatic failure have been reported after receiving parenteral products containing polysorbate 80 (Alade, 1986; CDC, 1984). Infusion of polysorbate 80-containing solutions through polyvinyl chloride tubing may cause DEHP to leach into the solution; in immature animals, exposure to DEHP may adversely affect the development of the male reproductive tract.

Precautions Use with caution in patients with preexisting cardiac or pulmonary conditions, renal impairment, and patients at risk for developing tumor lysis syndrome. Patients should be brought up to date with all recommended immunizations before initiating therapy. Live vaccines should not be given concurrently; there are no data available concerning secondary transmission of live vaccines in patients receiving therapy; evaluate risks of therapy delay versus benefit (of inactivated vaccines) for NHL patients. Safety and efficacy of rituximab in combination with biologic agents or disease-modifying antirheumatic drugs (DMARD) other than methotrexate or for retreatment of RA have not been established. Rituximab is not recommended for use in RA patients who have not had prior inadequate response to TNF antagonists. The safety of concomitant immunosuppressants other than corticosteroids has not been evaluated in patients with WG and MPA after rituximab-induced B-cell depletion. There are only limited data on subsequent courses of rituximab for

WG or MPA; safety and efficacy of retreatment has not been established.

Adverse Reactions Note: Patients treated with rituximab for rheumatoid arthritis (RA) may experience fewer adverse reactions.

Cardiovascular: Flushing, hyper-/hypotension, peripheral edema

Central nervous system: Anxiety, chills, dizziness, fatigue, fever, headache, insomnia, migraine, pain

Dermatologic: Angioedema, pruritus, rash, urticaria

Endocrine & metabolic: Hyperglycemia

Gastrointestinal: Abdominal pain, diarrhea, dyspepsia, nausea, vomiting, weight gain

Hematologic: Anemia, cytopenia, lymphopenia, leukopenia, neutropenia, neutropenic fever, thrombocytopenia

Hepatic: ALT increased

Neuromuscular & skeletal: Arthralgia, back pain, muscle spasm, myalgia, neuropathy, paresthesia, weakness

Respiratory: Bronchospasm, cough, dyspnea, epistaxis, rhinitis, sinusitis, throat irritation, upper respiratory tract infection

Miscellaneous: Infusion-related reactions (may include angioedema, bronchospasm, chills, dizziness, fever, headache, hyper-/hypotension, myalgia, nausea, pruritus, rash, rigors, urticaria, and vomiting); infection (including bacterial, viral, fungal); night sweats; human antichimeric antibody (HACA) positive

Rare but important or life-threatening: Acute renal failure, anaphylactoid reaction/anaphylaxis, angina, aplastic anemia, ARDS, arrhythmia, bowel obstruction/perforation, bronchiolitis obliterans, cardiac failure, cardiogenic shock, encephalomyelitis, fatal infusion-related reactions, fulminant hepatitis, gastrointestinal perforation, hemolytic anemia, hepatic failure, hepatitis, hepatitis B reactivation, hyperviscosity syndrome (in Waldenström's macroglobulinemia), hypogammaglobulinemia (prolonged), hypoxia, interstitial pneumonitis, laryngeal edema, lichenoid dermatitis, lupus-like syndrome, marrow hypoplasia, MI, mucositis, mucocutaneous reaction, neutropenia (late-onset occurring >40 days after last dose), optic neuritis, pancytopenia (prolonged), paraneoplastic pemphigus (uncommon), pleuritis, pneumonia, pneumonitis, polyarticular arthritis, polymyositis, posterior reversible encephalopathy syndrome (PRES), progressive multifocal leukoencephalopathy (PML), pure red cell aplasia, renal toxicity, reversible posterior leukoencephalopathy syndrome (RPLS), serum sickness, Stevens-Johnson syndrome, supraventricular arrhythmia, systemic vasculitis, toxic epidermal necrolysis, tuberculosis reactivation, tumor lysis syndrome, uveitis, vasculitis with rash, ventricular fibrillation, ventricular tachycardia, vesiculobullous dermatitis, viral reactivation (includes JC virus, cytomegalovirus, herpes simplex virus, parvovirus B19, varicella zoster virus, West Nile virus, and hepatitis C), wheezing

Drug Interactions

Metabolism/Transport Effects None known.

Avoid Concomitant Use

Avoid concomitant use of RiTUXimab with any of the following: Abatacept; BCG; Belimumab; Certolizumab Pegol; CloZAPine; Dipyrone; Natalizumab; Pimecrolimus; Tacrolimus (Topical); Tofacitinib; Vaccines (Live)

Increased Effect/Toxicity

RiTUXimab may increase the levels/effects of: Abatacept; Belimumab; Certolizumab Pegol; CloZAPine; Leflunomide; Natalizumab; Tofacitinib; Vaccines (Live)

The levels/effects of RiTUXimab may be increased by: Abciximab; Antihypertensives; Denosumab; Dipyrone; Pimecrolimus; Roflumilast; Tacrolimus (Topical); Trastuzumab

Decreased Effect

RiTUXimab may decrease the levels/effects of: BCG; Coccidioidin Skin Test; Sipuleucel-T; Vaccines (Inactivated); Vaccines (Live)

The levels/effects of RiTUXimab may be decreased by: Echinacea

Stability Store intact vials at 2°C to 8°C (36°F to 46°F); do not freeze or shake; protect vials from direct sunlight; dilution of rituximab to a final concentration of 1-4 mg/mL in NS or D_5W is stable for 24 hours if refrigerated or stored at room temperature

Mechanism of Action Rituximab is a monoclonal antibody directed against the CD20 antigen on B-lymphocytes. CD20 regulates cell cycle initiation; and, possibly, functions as a calcium channel. Rituximab binds to the antigen on the cell surface, activating complement-dependent B-cell cytotoxicity; and to human Fc receptors, mediating cell killing through an antibody-dependent cellular toxicity. B-cells are believed to play a role in the development and progression of rheumatoid arthritis. Signs and symptoms of RA are reduced by targeting B-cells and the progression of structural damage is delayed.

Pharmacodynamics Duration: B-cell recovery begins ~6 months following completion of treatment; medium B-cell levels return to normal by 12 months

Pharmacokinetics (Adult data unless noted)

Distribution: Binds to lymphoid cells in the thymus, spleen, and B lymphocytes in peripheral blood and lymph nodes

Half-life: Adults:

NHL: Median terminal half-life: 22 days (range: 6-52 days)

CLL: Median terminal half-life: 32 days (range: 14-62 days)

Rheumatoid arthritis: 18 days (range: 5-78 days)

Dosing: Usual Refer to individual protocols. Pretreatment with acetaminophen and an antihistamine is recommended for all indications. For oncology uses, a uricostatic agent (eg, allopurinol) and aggressive hydration is recommended for patients at risk for tumor lysis syndrome (high tumor burden or lymphocytes >25,000/mm^3). In patients with CLL, *pneumocystis jiroveci* pneumonia (PCP) and antiherpetic viral prophylaxis is recommended during treatment (and for up to 12 months following treatment). In patients with WG and MPA, PCP prophylaxis is recommended during and for 6 months after rituximab treatment.

Infants, Children, and Adolescents:

Autoimmune hemolytic anemia: Infants ≥4 months, Children, and Adolescents: I.V. infusion: 375 mg/m^2 once weekly for 2-4 doses (Zecca, 2003)

Chronic ITP: Children and Adolescents: I.V. infusion: 375 mg/m^2 once weekly for 4 doses (Parodi, 2009; Wang, 2005)

Post-transplant lymphoproliferative disorder: Infants ≥11 months, Children, and Adolescents: I.V. infusion: 375 mg/m^2 once weekly for 3-4 doses (Milpied, 2000; Serinet, 2002)

Refractory SLE: Children ≥8 years and Adolescents: I.V. infusion: 375 mg/m^2 once weekly for 2-4 doses; or 750 mg/m^2 on days 1 and 15 (maximum dose: 1000 mg) (Marks, 2005)

Refractory severe nephrotic syndrome: Infants ≥11 months, Children, and Adolescents: I.V. infusion: 375 mg/m^2 once weekly for 1-4 doses has been used in small case series, case reports, and retrospective analyses, including reports of successful remission induction of severe or refractory nephrotic syndromes that are poorly responsive to standard therapies (Della Strologo, 2009; Fujinaga, 2010; Gugonis, 2008; Kaito, 2010; Prytula, 2010)

Adults:

CLL: I.V. infusion: 375 mg/m^2 on the day prior to fludarabine/cyclophosphamide in cycle 1, then 500 mg/m^2 on day 1 (every 28 days) of cycles 2-6

Granulomatosis with polyangiitis (GPA; Wegener's granulomatosis) and Microscopic polyangiitis (MPA): I.V. infusion: 375 mg/m^2 once weekly for 4 doses (in combination with methylprednisolone I.V. for 1-3 days followed by daily prednisone)

NHL (relapsed/refractory, low-grade or follicular CD20-positive, B-cell): I.V. infusion: 375 mg/m^2 once weekly for 4 or 8 doses

Retreatment following disease progression: I.V. infusion: 375 mg/m^2 once weekly for 4 doses

NHL (diffuse large B-cell): I.V. infusion: 375 mg/m^2 given on day 1 of each chemotherapy cycle for up to 8 doses

NHL (follicular, CD20-positive, B-cell, previously untreated): I.V. infusion: 375 mg/m^2 given on day 1 of each chemotherapy cycle for up to 8 doses

Maintenance therapy (as a single agent, in patients with partial or complete response to rituximab plus chemotherapy; begin 8 weeks after completion of combination chemotherapy): I.V. infusion: 375 mg/m^2 every 8 weeks for 12 doses

NHL (nonprogressing, low-grade, CD20-positive, B-cell, after first-line CVP): I.V. infusion: 375 mg/m^2 once weekly for 4 doses every 6 months for up to 4 cycles (initiate after 6-8 cycles of chemotherapy are completed)

NHL: Combination therapy with ibritumomab: I.V. infusion: 250 mg/m^2 I.V. day 1; repeat in 7-9 days with ibritumomab

Rheumatoid arthritis: I.V. infusion: 1000 mg on days 1 and 15 in combination with methotrexate; subsequent courses may be administered every 24 weeks (based on clinical evaluation), if necessary may be repeated no sooner than every 16 weeks. **Note:** Premedication with methylprednisolone 100 mg I.V. (or equivalent) is recommended 30 minutes prior to each dose.

Administration DO NOT ADMINISTER UNDILUTED OR as an I.V. push or rapid injection: I.V. infusion:

Initial infusion: Start at a rate of 50 mg/hour at a final concentration for administration of 1-4 mg/mL in NS or D$_5$W. If no hypersensitivity or infusion-related reactions occur, increase infusion rate in 50 mg/hour increments every 30 minutes to a maximum infusion rate of 400 mg/hour as tolerated.

Subsequent infusions:

Standard infusion: If patient tolerated initial infusion, start at 100 mg/hour and increased by 100 mg/hour increments at 30 minute intervals to a maximum infusion rate of 400 mg/hour. If hypersensitivity or infusion-related reactions occur, slow or interrupt the infusion. If symptoms completely resolve, resume infusion at 50% of the previous rate.

Accelerated infusion rate (90 minutes): For adult patients with previously untreated follicular NHL and diffuse large B-cell NHL who are receiving a corticosteroid as part of their combination chemotherapy regimen, have a circulating lymphocyte count <5000/mm^3, or have no significant cardiovascular disease. After tolerance has been established (no grade 3 or 4 infusion-related event) at the recommended infusion rate in cycle 1, a rapid infusion rate may be used beginning with cycle 2. The daily corticosteroid, acetaminophen, and diphenhydramine are administered prior to treatment, then the rituximab dose is administered over 90 minutes, with 20% of the dose administered over the first 30 minutes and the remaining 80% is given over 60 minutes (Sehn, 2007). If the 90-minute infusion in cycle 2 is tolerated, the same rate may be used for the remainder of the treatment regimen (through cycles 6 or 8).

Monitoring Parameters Vital signs, CBC with differential and platelet counts (obtain at weekly to monthly intervals and more frequently in patients with cytopenias, or at 2-4 month intervals in rheumatoid arthritis patients, WG and MPA), serum electrolytes, uric acid, renal function tests, liver function tests, fluid balance; monitor for infusion reactions, cardiac monitoring for patients with preexisting cardiac condition; peripheral CD20$^+$ cells; human antimurine antibody and human antichimeric antibody titers (high levels may increase the risk of allergic reactions); screening for hepatitis B, signs or symptoms of PML, signs or symptoms of bowel obstruction/perforation

Dosage Forms Excipient information presented when available (limited, particularly for generics); consult specific product labeling.

Concentrate, Intravenous [preservative free]:

Rituxan: 10 mg/mL (10 mL, 50 mL) [contains polysorbate 80]

References

Alade SL, Brown RE, and Paquet A Jr, "Polysorbate 80 and E-Ferol Toxicity," *Pediatrics*, 1986, 77(4):593-7.

Centers for Disease Control (CDC), "Unusual Syndrome With Fatalities Among Premature Infants: Association With a New Intravenous Vitamin E Product," *MMWR Morb Mortal Wkly Rep*, 1984, 33 (14):198-9.

Chakravarty EF, Murray ER, Kelman A, et al, "Pregnancy Outcomes After Maternal Exposure to Rituximab," *Blood*, 2011, 117(5):1499-506.

Dello Strologo L, Guzzo I, Laurenzi C, et al, "Use of Rituximab in Focal Glomerulosclerosis Relapses After Renal Transplantation," *Transplantation*, 2009, 88(3):417-20.

Edwards JC, Szczepanski L, Szechinski J, et al, "Efficacy of B-Cell-Targeted Therapy With Rituximab in Patients With Rheumatoid Arthritis," *N Engl J Med*, 2004, 350(25):2572-81.

Friedrichs B, Tiemann M, Salwender H, et al. The effects of rituximab treatment during pregnancy on a neonate. *Haematologica*. 2006;91 (10):1426-1427.

Fujinaga S, Hirano D, Nishizaki N, et al, "Single Infusion of Rituximab for Persistent Steroid-Dependent Minimal-Change Nephrotic Syndrome After Long-Term Cyclosporine," *Pediatr Nephrol*, 2010, 25 (3):539-44.

Guigonis V, Dallocchio A, Baudouin V, et al, "Rituximab Treatment for Severe Steroid- or Cyclosporine-Dependent Nephrotic Syndrome: A Multicentric Series of 22 Cases," *Pediatr Nephrol*, 2008, 23 (8):1269-79.

Hahn BH, McMahon MA, Wilkinson A, et al, "American College of Rheumatology Guidelines for Screening, Treatment, and Management of Lupus Nephritis," *Arthritis Care Res (Hoboken)*, 2012, 64 (6):797-808.

Kaito H, Kamei K, Kikuchi E, et al, "Successful Treatment of Collapsing Focal Segmental Glomerulosclerosis With a Combination of Rituximab, Steroids and Ciclosporin," *Pediatr Nephrol*, 2010, 25(5):957-9.

Makol A, Wright K, Amin S. Rheumatoid arthritis and pregnancy: safety considerations in pharmacological management. *Drugs*. 2011;71 (15):1973-1987.

Marks SD, Patey S, Brogan PA, et al, "B Lymphocyte Depletion Therapy in Children With Refractory Systemic Lupus Erythematosus," *Arthritis Rheum*, 2005, 52(10):3168-74.

Milpied N, Vasseur B, Parquet N, et al, "Humanized Anti-CD20 Monoclonal Antibody (Rituximab) in Post Transplant B-lymphoproliferative Disorder: A Retrospective Analysis on 32 Patients," *Ann Oncol*, 2000, 11 Suppl 1:113-6.

Østensen M, Lockshin M, Doria A, et al. Update on safety during pregnancy of biological agents and some immunosuppressive antirheumatic drugs. *Rheumatology (Oxford)*. 2008;47 Suppl 3:28-31.

Parodi E, Rivetti E, Amendola G, et al, "Long-Term Follow-Up Analysis After Rituximab Therapy in Children With Refractory Symptomatic ITP: Identification of Factors Predictive of a Sustained Response," *Br J Haematol*, 2009, 144(4):552-8.

Provan D, Stasi R, Newland AC, et al, "International Consensus Report on the Investigation and Management of Primary Immune Thrombocytopenia," *Blood*, 2010, 115(2):168-86.

Prytuła A, Iijima K, Kamei K, et al, "Rituximab in Refractory Nephrotic Syndrome," *Pediatr Nephrol*, 2010, 25(3):461-8.

Serinet MO, Jacquenin E, Habes D, et al, "Anti-CD20 Monoclonal Antibody (Rituximab) Treatment for Epstein-Barr Virus-Associated, B-Cell Lymphoproliferative Disease in Pediatric Liver Transplant Recipients," *J Ped Gastroenterology & Nutrition*, 2002, 34(4):389-93.

Ton E, Tekstra J, Hellmann PM, et al. Safety of rituximab therapy during twins' pregnancy. *Rheumatology (Oxford)*. 2011;50(4):806-808.

Wang J, Wiley JM, Luddy R, et al, "Chronic Immune Thrombocytopenic Purpura in Children: Assessment of Rituximab Treatment," *J Pediatr*, 2005, 146(2):217-21.

Zecca M, Nobili B, Ramenghi U, et al, "Rituximab for the Treatment of Refractory Autoimmune Hemolytic Anemia in Children," *Blood*, 2003, 101(10):3857-61.

◆ **RIV** see Influenza Virus Vaccine (Recombinant) on page 1112

◆ **RIV₃** see Influenza Virus Vaccine (Recombinant) on page 1112

◆ **Riva-Amiodarone (Can)** see Amiodarone on page 127

◆ **Riva-Amlodipine (Can)** see AmLODIPine on page 135

◆ **Riva-Atenolol (Can)** see Atenolol on page 222

◆ **RIVA-Atomoxetine (Can)** see AtoMOXetine on page 224

◆ **Riva-Azithromycin (Can)** see Azithromycin (Systemic) on page 247

◆ **Riva-Baclofen (Can)** see Baclofen on page 259

◆ **Riva-Buspirone (Can)** see BusPIRone on page 332

◆ **Riva-Ciprofloxacin (Can)** see Ciprofloxacin (Systemic) on page 471

◆ **Riva-Citalopram (Can)** see Citalopram on page 484

◆ **Riva-Clarithromycin (Can)** see Clarithromycin on page 490

◆ **Riva-Clindamycin (Can)** see Clindamycin (Systemic) on page 495

◆ **Riva-Clonazepam (Can)** see ClonazePAM on page 514

◆ **Rivacocet (Can)** see Oxycodone and Acetaminophen on page 1573

◆ **Riva-Cycloprine (Can)** see Cyclobenzaprine on page 558

◆ **Riva-Dicyclomine (Can)** see Dicyclomine on page 652

◆ **Riva-Enalapril (Can)** see Enalapril on page 744

◆ **Riva-Fluconazole (Can)** see Fluconazole on page 877

◆ **Riva-Fluoxetine (Can)** see FLUoxetine on page 901

◆ **Riva-Fluvox (Can)** see FluvoxaMINE on page 922

◆ **Riva-Fosinopril (Can)** see Fosinopril on page 938

◆ **Riva-Gabapentin (Can)** see Gabapentin on page 950

◆ **Riva-Glyburide (Can)** see GlyBURIDE on page 974

◆ **Riva-Hydroxyzine (Can)** see HydrOXYzine on page 1054

◆ **Riva-Lisinopril (Can)** see Lisinopril on page 1262

◆ **Riva-Loperamide (Can)** see Loperamide on page 1270

◆ **Riva-Lovastatin (Can)** see Lovastatin on page 1286

◆ **Riva-Metformin (Can)** see MetFORMIN on page 1353

◆ **Riva-Metoprolol-L (Can)** see Metoprolol on page 1396

◆ **Riva-Minocycline (Can)** see Minocycline on page 1420

◆ **Rivanase AQ (Can)** see Beclomethasone (Nasal) on page 267

◆ **Riva-Olanzapine (Can)** see OLANZapine on page 1525

◆ **Riva-Olanzapine ODT (Can)** see OLANZapine on page 1525

◆ **Riva-Omeprazole DR (Can)** see Omeprazole on page 1535

◆ **Riva-Oxybutynin (Can)** see Oxybutynin on page 1568

◆ **Riva-Pantoprazole (Can)** see Pantoprazole on page 1595

◆ **Riva-Paroxetine (Can)** see PARoxetine on page 1609

◆ **Riva-Pravastatin (Can)** see Pravastatin on page 1720

◆ **Riva-Quetiapine (Can)** see QUEtiapine on page 1783

◆ **Riva-Rabeprazole EC (Can)** see RABEprazole on page 1797

◆ **Riva-Ranitidine (Can)** see Ranitidine on page 1805

◆ **Riva-Risperidone (Can)** see RisperiDONE on page 1831

◆ **Riva-Rosuvastatin (Can)** see Rosuvastatin on page 1853

◆ **Riva-Sertraline (Can)** see Sertraline on page 1879

◆ **Riva-Simvastatin (Can)** see Simvastatin on page 1892

◆ **Rivasol (Can)** see Zinc Sulfate on page 2176

◆ **Rivasone (Can)** see Betamethasone (Topical) on page 285

◆ **Riva-Sotalol (Can)** see Sotalol on page 1925

◆ **Riva-Terbinafine (Can)** see Terbinafine (Systemic) on page 1982

◆ **Riva-Valacyclovir (Can)** see ValACYclovir on page 2097

◆ **Riva-Venlafaxine XR (Can)** see Venlafaxine on page 2125

◆ **Riva-Verapamil SR (Can)** see Verapamil on page 2129

◆ **Rivotril (Can)** see ClonazePAM on page 514

◆ **Rixubis** see Factor IX (Recombinant) on page 838

Rizatriptan (rye za TRIP tan)

Brand Names: U.S. Maxalt; Maxalt-MLT

Brand Names: Canada Apo-Rizatriptan®; CO Rizatriptan; CO Rizatriptan ODT; JAMP-Rizatriptan; Mar-Rizatriptan; Maxalt RPD™; Maxalt™; Mylan-Rizatriptan ODT; Sandoz-Rizatriptan ODT

Therapeutic Category Antimigraine Agent; Serotonin 5-HT₁D Receptor Agonist

Generic Availability (U.S.) Yes

Use Acute treatment of migraine with or without aura (FDA approved in ages ≥6 years and adults)

Pregnancy Risk Factor C

Pregnancy Considerations Adverse events were observed in animal reproduction studies. Information related to rizatriptan use in pregnancy is limited (Källén, 2011; Nezvalová-Henriksen, 2010; Nezvalová-Henriksen, 2012).

A pregnancy registry has been established to monitor outcomes of women exposed to rizatriptan during pregnancy (800-986-8999). Preliminary data from the pregnancy registry (prospectively collected from 65 live births 1998-2004) does not show an increased risk of congenital malformations (Fiore, 2005). Until additional information is available, other agents are preferred for the initial treatment of migraine in pregnancy (Da Silva, 2012; MacGregor, 2012; Williams, 2012).

Breast-Feeding Considerations It is not known if rizatriptan is excreted in breast milk. The manufacturer recommends that caution be exercised when administering rizatriptan to nursing women.

Contraindications Hypersensitivity to rizatriptan or any component; known or suspected ischemic heart disease (eg, angina pectoris, MI, silent MI); other significant underlying cardiovascular diseases; coronary artery vasospasm, including Prinzmetal's angina; uncontrolled hypertension; history of stroke or transient ischemic attack; peripheral vascular disease; ischemic bowel disease; management of hemiplegic or basilar migraine; concomitant use (within last 24 hours) of ergotamine derivatives and/or ergotamine-containing medications (eg, methysergide, dihydroergotamine) or other 5-HT₁ agonist (eg, triptans); concomitant use (within 2 weeks) of MAO inhibitors

Warnings Serious coronary events, including coronary artery vasospasm, transient ischemia, acute MI, life-threatening arrhythmias (eg, ventricular tachycardia/fibrillation), and death have been reported with 5-HT₁ agonist administration; avoid use in patients with risk factors for coronary artery disease, unless cardiovascular disease can be ruled ▶

out; consider administering first dose under close supervision to patients at high risk for coronary disease. Patients who experience sensations of chest pain/pressure/tightness or symptoms suggestive of angina following dosing should be evaluated for coronary artery disease or Prinzmetal's angina before receiving additional doses. If dosing resumed and symptoms recur, ECG monitoring is recommended. Periodically evaluate cardiovascular system in patients with risk factors for coronary artery disease. Cerebrovascular events (eg, cerebral hemorrhage, subarachnoid hemorrhage, stroke) have been reported with 5-HT$_1$ agonist (triptan) administration. Vasospasm-related events (eg, peripheral vascular ischemia, Raynaud's syndrome, and colonic ischemia with abdominal pain and bloody diarrhea) have been reported with 5-HT$_1$ agonists; transient and permanent blindness and significant partial vision loss have been very rarely reported; further evaluation is recommended in patients with signs and symptoms suggestive of reduced peripheral arterial blood flow following 5-HT$_1$ agonist (eg, triptan) use. Medication overuse headache may occur with overuse of acute migraine medications; a significant increase in frequency of migraine attacks or migraine-like daily headaches may occur; withdrawal of overused medication and treatment of withdrawal symptoms may be required. Potentially fatal serotonin syndrome may occur when triptans are used in combination with SSRIs (eg, fluoxetine, sertraline) or SNRIs (eg, venlafaxine); monitor carefully if the two drugs are used concomitantly. Maxalt-MLT® tablets contain phenylalanine which should be used with caution in patients with phenylketonuria.

Precautions Use with caution in patients with controlled hypertension; temporary increases in peripheral vascular resistance and blood pressure may occur; significant elevation in blood pressure, including hypertensive crisis, has also been reported on rare occasions in patients with and without a history of hypertension. Use with caution in patients with impaired hepatic function or receiving dialysis. Other potentially serious neurological conditions should be ruled out prior to acute migraine therapy; if a patient does not respond to the first dose of rizatriptan, the diagnosis of migraine should be reconsidered. Rizatriptan could potentially bind to melanin-containing tissues (eg, eye) due to chemical properties leading to toxicity with extended use; animal data did not show ophthalmologic toxicities. Some adverse effects may be dose-related including: Fatigue, somnolence, chest pain, and weakness; fatigue more common in adults than pediatric patients (≤30% vs ~1%).

Adverse Reactions

Cardiovascular: Chest pain, flushing, palpitation

Central nervous system: Dizziness, euphoria, fatigue (dose related; more common in adults), headache, hypoesthesia, pain, somnolence

Dermatologic: Skin flushing

Gastrointestinal: Abdominal discomfort, diarrhea, nausea, vomiting, xerostomia

Neuromuscular & skeletal: Neck, throat, and jaw pain/tightness/pressure; paresthesia; tremor; weakness

Respiratory: Dyspnea

Miscellaneous: Feeling of heaviness

Rare but important or life-threatening: Anaphylaxis/anaphylactoid reactions, angina, angioedema, blurred vision, bradycardia, confusion, edema, hallucination (children), hearing impairment, hypertensive crisis, memory impairment, MI, myocardial ischemia, pruritus, seizure, syncope, tachycardia, tinnitus, tongue edema, toxic epidermal necrolysis, vasospasm, vertigo, wheezing

Drug Interactions

Metabolism/Transport Effects None known.

Avoid Concomitant Use

Avoid concomitant use of Rizatriptan with any of the following: Ergot Derivatives; MAO Inhibitors

Increased Effect/Toxicity

Rizatriptan may increase the levels/effects of: Antipsychotics; Droxidopa; Ergot Derivatives; Metoclopramide; Serotonin Modulators

The levels/effects of Rizatriptan may be increased by: Antiemetics (5HT3 Antagonists); Antipsychotics; Ergot Derivatives; MAO Inhibitors; Propranolol

Decreased Effect There are no known significant interactions involving a decrease in effect.

Food Interactions Food delays absorption. Management: Administer without regard to meals.

Stability Store at 15°C to 30°C (59°F to 86°F). MLT tablets should remain in blister pack until administration.

Mechanism of Action Selective agonist for serotonin (5-HT$_{1B}$ and 5-HT$_{1D}$ receptors) in cranial arteries; causes vasoconstriction and reduces sterile inflammation associated with antidromic neuronal transmission correlating with relief of migraine

Pharmacokinetics (Adult data unless noted)

Absorption: Complete

Distribution: V_d: 110-140 L

Protein binding: 14%

Metabolism: Via monoamine oxidase-A to a major inactive and a minor (14%) active metabolite; first-pass effect

Bioavailability: ~45%; AUC in females reported to be 30% higher than males

Half-life: 2-3 hours

Time to peak serum concentration: Maxalt®: 1-1.5 hours; Maxalt-MLT®: 1.6-2.5 hours

Elimination: Urine (82%, ~14% as unchanged drug); feces (12%)

Dialysis: Reported AUC 44% higher in dialysis patients compared to normal renal function; effects of hemodialysis or peritoneal dialysis are unknown

Dosing: Usual Oral: **Migraine, acute treatment:**

Children and Adolescents ≥6 years: **Note:** Safety and efficacy of multiple rizatriptan doses in a 24-hour period has not been established for pediatric patients.

<40 kg: 5 mg as a single dose

≥40 kg: 10 mg as a single dose

Adults: 5-10 mg, repeat after 2 hours if significant relief is not attained; maximum: 30 mg in a 24-hour period; **Note:** In patients with risk factors for coronary artery disease, following adequate evaluation to establish the absence of coronary artery disease, the initial dose should be administered in a setting where response may be evaluated (physician's office or similarly staffed setting). ECG monitoring may be considered.

Dosage adjustment with concomitant propranolol:

Children and Adolescents 6-17 years:

<40 kg: Do not use rizatriptan

≥40 kg: 5 mg as a single dose; maximum: 5 mg in a 24-hour period

Adults: 5 mg; may repeat after 2 hours; maximum daily dose: 15 mg in a 24-hour period

Administration Oral: Orally disintegrating tablets (Maxalt-MLT®): Do not remove the blister from the pouch until ready to use; blister pouch should be opened by peeling back (not pushing through foil) and with dry hands; place tablet on the tongue to dissolve; do not crush, break, or chew; additional liquids are not necessary.

Monitoring Parameters Headache severity

Additional Information Safety of treating >4 migraines per month is not established; rizatriptan is not indicated for migraine prophylaxis; safety and efficacy for cluster headaches has not been established.

Dosage Forms Excipient information presented when available (limited, particularly for generics); consult specific product labeling.

Tablet, Oral:

Maxalt: 5 mg, 10 mg

Generic: 5 mg, 10 mg

Tablet Dispersible, Oral:
Maxalt-MLT: 5 mg, 10 mg [contains aspartame; peppermint flavor]
Generic: 5 mg, 10 mg

References

Ahonen K, Hämäläinen ML, Eerola M. et al, "A Randomized Trial of Rizatriptan in Migraine Attacks in Children," *Neurology*, 2006, 67 (7):1135-40.

Da Silva AN and Tepper SJ, "Acute Treatment of Migraines," *CNS Drugs*, 2012, 26(10):823-39.

Fiore M, Shields KE, Santanello N, et al, "Exposure to Rizatriptan During Pregnancy: Post-Marketing Experience Up to 30 June 2004," *Cephalalgia*, 2005, 25(9):685-8.

Källén B, Nilsson E, and Otterblad Olausson P, "Delivery Outcome After Maternal Use of Drugs for Migraine: A Register Study in Sweden," *Drug Saf*, 2011, 34(8):691-703.

Lewis D, Ashwal S, Hershey A, et al, "Practice Parameter: Pharmacological Treatment of Migraine Headache in Children and Adolescents: Report of the American Academy of Neurology Quality Standards Subcommittee and the Practice Committee of the Child Neurology Society," *Neurology*, 2004, 63(12):2215-24.

Visser WH, Winner P, Strohmaier K, et al, "Rizatriptan 5 mg for the Acute Treatment of Migraine in Adolescents: Results From a Double-Blind, Single-Attack Study and Two Open-Label, Multiple-Attack Studies," *Headache*, 2004, 44(9):891-9.

MacGregor EA, "Headache in Pregnancy," *Neurol Clin*, 2012, 30 (3):835-66.

Nezvalová-Henriksen K, Spigset O, and Nordeng HM, "Errata in 'Triptan Exposure During Pregnancy and the Risk of Major Congenital Malformations and Adverse Pregnancy Outcomes: Results From the Norwegian Mother and Child Sohort Study,'" *Headache*, 2012, 52 (8):1319-20.

Nezvalová-Henriksen K, Spigset O, and Nordeng H, "Triptan Exposure During Pregnancy and the Risk of Major Congenital Malformations and Adverse Pregnancy Outcomes: Results From the Norwegian Mother and Child Cohort Study," *Headache*, 2010, 50(4):563-75.

Williams SH and Kehr HA, "An Update in the Treatment of Neurologic Disorders During Pregnancy-Focus on Migraines and Seizures," *J Pharm Pract*, 2012, 25(3):341-51.

Winner P, Lewis D, Visser WH, et al, "Rizatriptan 5 mg for the Acute Treatment of Migraine in Adolescents: A Randomized, Double-Blind, Placebo-Controlled Study," *Headache*, 2002, 42(1):49-55.

- **rLFN-α2** *see* Interferon Alfa-2b *on page 1138*
- **Ro 5488** *see* Tretinoin (Systemic) *on page 2068*
- **RoActemra** *see* Tocilizumab *on page 2040*
- **Robafen [OTC]** *see* GuaiFENesin *on page 984*
- **Robafen AC** *see* Guaifenesin and Codeine *on page 985*
- **Robafen Cough [OTC]** *see* Dextromethorphan *on page 636*
- **Robafen DM [OTC]** *see* Guaifenesin and Dextromethorphan *on page 987*
- **Robaxin** *see* Methocarbamol *on page 1364*
- **Robaxin® (Can)** *see* Methocarbamol *on page 1364*
- **Robaxin-750** *see* Methocarbamol *on page 1364*
- **Robidrine® (Can)** *see* Pseudoephedrine *on page 1770*
- **Robinul** *see* Glycopyrrolate *on page 977*
- **Robinul-Forte** *see* Glycopyrrolate *on page 977*
- **Robitussin® (Can)** *see* GuaiFENesin *on page 984*
- **Robitussin AC** *see* Guaifenesin and Codeine *on page 985*
- **Robitussin Chest Congestion [OTC]** *see* GuaiFENesin *on page 984*
- **Robitussin Childrens Cough LA [OTC]** *see* Dextromethorphan *on page 636*
- **Robitussin CoughGels [OTC]** *see* Dextromethorphan *on page 636*
- **Robitussin Lingering CoughGels [OTC]** *see* Dextromethorphan *on page 636*
- **Robitussin Lingering LA Cough [OTC]** *see* Dextromethorphan *on page 636*
- **Robitussin Maximum Strength [OTC]** *see* Dextromethorphan *on page 636*

- **Robitussin Mucus+Chest Congest [OTC]** *see* GuaiFENesin *on page 984*
- **Robitussin Peak Cold Cough + Chest Congestion DM [OTC]** *see* Guaifenesin and Dextromethorphan *on page 987*
- **Robitussin Peak Cold Maximum Strength Cough + Chest Congestion DM [OTC]** *see* Guaifenesin and Dextromethorphan *on page 987*
- **Robitussin Peak Cold Sugar-Free Cough + Chest Congestion DM [OTC]** *see* Guaifenesin and Dextromethorphan *on page 987*
- **Rocaltrol** *see* Calcitriol *on page 342*
- **Rocephin** *see* CefTRIAXone *on page 417*

Rocuronium (roe kyoor OH nee um)

Medication Safety Issues

Sound-alike/look-alike issues:
Zemuron® may be confused with Remeron®

High alert medication:
The Institute for Safe Medication Practices (ISMP) includes this medication among its list of drugs which have a heightened risk of causing significant patient harm when used in error.

Other safety concerns:
United States Pharmacopeia (USP) 2006: The Interdisciplinary Safe Medication Use Expert Committee of the USP has recommended the following:
- Hospitals, clinics, and other practice sites should institute special safeguards in the storage, labeling, and use of these agents and should include these safeguards in staff orientation and competency training.
- Healthcare professionals should be on high alert (especially vigilant) whenever a neuromuscular-blocking agent (NMBA) is stocked, ordered, prepared, or administered.

Brand Names: U.S. Zemuron

Brand Names: Canada Rocuronium Bromide Injection; Zemuron®

Therapeutic Category Neuromuscular Blocker Agent, Nondepolarizing; Skeletal Muscle Relaxant, Paralytic

Generic Availability (U.S.) Yes

Use Adjunct to general anesthesia, to facilitate endotracheal intubation, and provide skeletal muscle relaxation during surgery or mechanical ventilation (FDA approved in all ages); to facilitate rapid sequence intubation (FDA approved in adults)

Pregnancy Risk Factor C

Pregnancy Considerations Teratogenic effects were not observed in animal reproduction studies. Rocuronium crosses the placenta; umbilical venous plasma levels are ~18% of the maternal concentration following a maternal dose of 0.6 mg/kg (Abouleish, 1994). The manufacturer does not recommend use for rapid sequence induction during cesarean section.

Breast-Feeding Considerations Information related to rocuronium use and breast-feeding has not been located. If present in breast milk, oral absorption by a nursing infant would be expected to be minimal (Lee, 1993).

Contraindications Hypersensitivity to rocuronium, other neuromuscular blocking agents, or any component

Warnings Ventilation must be supported during neuromuscular blockade; rocuronium should only be used by individuals who are experienced in the maintenance of an adequate airway and respiratory support. Rocuronium does not alter consciousness; use in conjunction with adequate sedation or anesthesia. Severe allergic reactions have been reported with neuromuscular-blocking agents including rocuronium; cross-sensitivity with other neuromuscular-blocking agents may occur; use extreme caution in patients with previous anaphylactic reactions. Some patients may experience prolonged recovery of neuromuscular function after administration (especially after prolonged use); patients should be adequately recovered prior to extubation.

Precautions Use with caution in patients with hepatic impairment; consider dosage reduction for severe hepatic disease. Many clinical conditions may potentiate or antagonize neuromuscular blockade, see table. Increased sensitivity in patients with myasthenia gravis, Eaton-Lambert syndrome; resistance to neuromuscular blockade in burn patients (>30% of body) for period of 5-70 days postinjury; resistance to neuromuscular blockade in patients with muscle trauma, denervation, immobilization, infection.

Clinical Conditions Affecting Neuromuscular Blockade

Potentiation	Antagonism
Acidosis	Alkalosis
Acute intermittent porphyria	Demyelinating lesions
Electrolyte abnormalities	Diabetes mellitus
Hypermagnesemia	Hypercalcemia
Severe hypocalcemia	Peripheral neuropathies
Severe hypokalemia	
Severe hyponatremia	
Hepatic failure	
Neuromuscular diseases	
Renal failure	

Adverse Reactions

Cardiovascular: Hypertension, hypotension (transient)

Rare but important or life-threatening: Abnormal ECG, anaphylactoid reaction, anaphylaxis, arrhythmia, bronchospasm, injection site edema, hiccups, pruritus, nausea, pulmonary vascular resistance (increased), rash, rhonchi, shock, tachycardia, vomiting, wheezing

Drug Interactions

Metabolism/Transport Effects None known.

Avoid Concomitant Use

Avoid concomitant use of Rocuronium with any of the following: QuiNINE

Increased Effect/Toxicity

Rocuronium may increase the levels/effects of: Cardiac Glycosides; Corticosteroids (Systemic); OnabotulinumtoxinA; RimabotulinumtoxinB

The levels/effects of Rocuronium may be increased by: AbobotulinumtoxinA; Aminoglycosides; Calcium Channel Blockers; Capreomycin; Clindamycin (Topical); Colistimethate; CycloSPORINE (Systemic); Fosphenytoin-Phenytoin; Inhalational Anesthetics; Ketorolac (Nasal); Ketorolac (Systemic); Lincosamide Antibiotics; Lithium; Loop Diuretics; Magnesium Salts; Polymyxin B; Procainamide; QuiNIDine; QuiNINE; Spironolactone; Tetracycline Derivatives; Vancomycin

Decreased Effect

The levels/effects of Rocuronium may be decreased by: Acetylcholinesterase Inhibitors; Fosphenytoin-Phenytoin; Loop Diuretics

Stability Store intact vials at 2°C to 8°C (36°F to 46°F); do not freeze; intact vials are stable 60 days at room temperature; open vials are stable for 30 days at room temperature. Dilutions up to 5 mg/mL in NS, D_5W, D_5NS, and LR are stable for up to 24 hours at room temperature; do not mix with alkaline solutions

Mechanism of Action Blocks acetylcholine from binding to receptors on motor endplate inhibiting depolarization

Pharmacodynamics

Maximum effect:
Infants ≥3 months and Children: 30 seconds to 1 minute
Adults: 1-3.7 minutes

Duration:
Infants: 3-12 months: 40 minutes
Children: 1-12 years: 26-30 minutes

Adults: 20-94 minutes (dose-related) (most prolonged in elderly ≥65 years of age)

Pharmacokinetics (Adult data unless noted)

Distribution: V_d:
Children: 0.21-0.3 L/kg
Adults: 0.22-0.26 L/kg
  Hepatic dysfunction: 0.53 L/kg
  Renal dysfunction: 0.34 L/kg

Protein binding: ~30%

Half-life:
Alpha elimination: 1-2 minutes
Beta elimination:
  Infants 3-12 months: 1.3 ± 0.5 hours
  Children 1 to <3 years: 1.1 ± 0.7 hours
  Children 3 to <8 years: 0.8 ± 0.3 hours
  Adults: 1.4-2.4 hours
  Hepatic dysfunction: 4.3 hours
  Renal dysfunction: 2.4 hours

Elimination: Primarily biliary excretion (70%); up to 30% of dose excreted unchanged in urine

Clearance: Pediatric patients:
  Infants 3 to <12 months: 0.35 L/kg/hour
  Children 1 to <3 years: 0.32 L/kg/hour
  Children 3 to <8 years: 0.44 L/kg/hour

Dosing: Neonatal Note: Dose to effect; doses will vary due to interpatient variability. Dosing also dependent on anesthetic technique and age of patient. In general, the onset of effect is shortened and duration is prolonged as the dose increases. The time to maximum nerve block is longest in neonates.

Tracheal intubation, surgical:
Initial: I.V.: 0.45-0.6 mg/kg
Maintenance for continued surgical relaxation:
  I.V.: 0.075-0.15 mg/kg; dosing interval as determined by monitoring
  Continuous I.V. infusion: 7-10 mcg/kg/minute

Dosing: Usual Note: Dose to effect; doses will vary due to interpatient variability. Dosing also dependent on anesthetic technique and age of patient. The manufacturer recommends dosing based on actual body weight in all obese patients; however, may use ideal body weight (IBW) for morbidly obese (BMI >40 kg/m²) adult patients (Leykin, 2004); onset time may be slightly delayed using IBW. In general, the onset of effect is shortened and duration is prolonged as the dose increases. The time to maximum nerve block is shortest in infants 1-3 months; the duration of relaxation is shortest in children 2-11 years and longest in infants.

Rapid sequence intubation: Children, Adolescents, and Adults: I.V.: 0.6-1.2 mg/kg; (Cheng, 2002; Fuchs-Buder, 1996; Mazurek, 1998; Naguib, 1997)

Tracheal intubation, surgical: Infants, Children, Adolescents, and Adults: **Note:** Inhaled anesthetic agents prolong the duration of action of rocuronium; use lower end of the dosing range; dosing interval guided by monitoring with a peripheral nerve stimulator.
Initial:
  I.V.: 0.45-0.6 mg/kg
  I.M. (Kaplan, 1999):
    Infants ≥3 months: 1 mg/kg administered as a single dose
    Children 1-6 years: 1.8 mg/kg administered as a single dose
Maintenance for continued surgical relaxation:
  I.V.:
    Infants, Children, and Adolescents: 0.075-0.15 mg/kg; repeat as needed
    Adults: 0.1-0.2 mg/kg; repeat as needed
  Continuous I.V. infusion:
    Infants, Children, and Adolescents: 7-12 mcg/kg/minute; use the lower end of dosing range for infants and upper end for children >2 to ≤11 years of age
    Adults: 4-16 mcg/kg/minute

Administration Parenteral: May be administered undiluted by rapid I.V. injection; for continuous I.V. infusion, dilute with NS, D$_5$W, or LR to a final concentration of 0.5-1 mg/mL

Monitoring Parameters Peripheral nerve stimulator measuring twitch response, heart rate, blood pressure, assisted ventilation status

Dosage Forms Excipient information presented when available (limited, particularly for generics); consult specific product labeling.

Solution, Intravenous, as bromide:
Zemuron: 50 mg/5 mL (5 mL); 100 mg/10 mL (10 mL)
Generic: 50 mg/5 mL (5 mL); 100 mg/10 mL (10 mL)
Solution, Intravenous, as bromide [preservative free]:
Generic: 50 mg/5 mL (5 mL); 100 mg/10 mL (10 mL)

References

Abouleish E, Abboud T, Lechevalier T, et al, "Rocuronium (Org 9426) for Caesarean Section," Br J Anaesth, 1994, 73(3):336-41.

Cheng CA, Aun CST, and Gin T, "Comparison of Rocuronium and Suxamethonium for Rapid Tracheal Intubation in Children," Paediatr Anaesth, 2002, 12(2):140-5.

Fuchs-Buder T and Tassonyi E, "Intubating Conditions and Time Course of Rocuronium-Induced Neuromuscular Block in Children," Br J Anaesth, 1996, 77(3):335-8.

Kaplan RF, Uejima T, Lobel G, et al, "Intramuscular Rocuronium in Infants and Children: A Multicenter Study to Evaluate Tracheal Intubating Conditions, Onset, and Duration of Action," Anesthesiology, 1999, 91(3):633-8.

Lee JJ and Rubin AP, "Breast Feeding and Anaesthesia," Anaesthesia, 1993, 48(7):616-25.

Leykin Y, Pellis T, Lucca M, et al, "The Pharmacodynamic Effects of Rocuronium When Dosed According to Real Body Weight or Ideal Body Weight in Morbidly Obese Patients," Anesth Analg, 2004, 99 (4):1086-9.

Martin LD, Bratton SL, and O'Rourke PP, "Clinical Uses and Controversies of Neuromuscular Blocking Agents in Infants and Children," Crit Care Med, 1999, 27(7):1358-68.

Mazurek AJ, Rae B, Hann S, et al, "Rocuronium Versus Succinylcholine: Are They Equally Effective During Rapid-Sequence Induction of Anesthesia?" Anesth Analg, 1998, 87:1259-62.

Naguib M, Samarkandi AH, Ammar A, et al, "Comparison of Suxamethonium and Different Combinations of Rocuronium and Mivacurium for Rapid Tracheal Intubation in Children," Br J Anaesth, 1997, 79 (4):450-5.

Reynolds LM, Lau M, Brown R, et al, "Bioavailability of Intramuscular Rocuronium in Infants and Children," Anesthesiology, 1997, 87 (5):1096-105.

Willets LS, "Rocuronium for Tracheal Intubation," Ped Pharmacotherapy, 2000, 6(10):1-6.

◆ **Rocuronium Bromide** see Rocuronium on page 1847

◆ **Rocuronium Bromide Injection (Can)** see Rocuronium on page 1847

◆ **Rofact™ (Can)** see Rifampin on page 1824

◆ **Rogitine® (Can)** see Phentolamine on page 1656

◆ **Rolene (Can)** see Betamethasone (Topical) on page 285

◆ **Romazicon (Can)** see Flumazenil on page 888

◆ **Romycin** see Erythromycin (Ophthalmic) on page 784

Ropivacaine (roe PIV a kane)

Medication Safety Issues
Sound-alike/look-alike issues:
Ropivacaine may be confused with bupivacaine, rOPI-NIRole

High alert medication:
The Institute for Safe Medication Practices (ISMP) includes this medication (epidural administration) among its list of drug classes which have a heightened risk of causing significant patient harm when used in error.

Brand Names: U.S. Naropin

Brand Names: Canada Naropin®; Ropivacaine Hydrochloride Injection, USP

Therapeutic Category Local Anesthetic, Injectable

Generic Availability (U.S.) No

Use Production of local or regional anesthesia for surgery, obstetrical procedures, and for acute pain management: peripheral nerve block, local infiltration, sympathetic block, caudal or epidural block

Pregnancy Risk Factor B

Pregnancy Considerations Teratogenic events were not observed in animal studies. When used for epidural block during labor and delivery, systemically absorbed ropivacaine may cross the placenta, resulting in varying degrees of fetal or neonatal effects (eg, CNS or cardiovascular depression). Fetal or neonatal adverse events include fetal bradycardia (12%), neonatal jaundice (8%), low Apgar scores (3%), fetal distress (2%), neonatal respiratory disorder (3%). Maternal hypotension may also result from systemic absorption. In cases of hypotension, position pregnant woman in left lateral decubitus position to prevent aortocaval compression by the gravid uterus. Epidural anesthesia may prolong the second stage of labor.

Breast-Feeding Considerations It is not known if ropivacaine is excreted into breast milk; however, exposure to a nursing infant is expected to be low. The manufacturer recommends that caution be exercised when administering ropivacaine to nursing women.

Contraindications Hypersensitivity to ropivacaine hydrochloride, any anesthetic of the amide type (eg, bupivacaine, lidocaine, mepivacaine), or any component; not recommended for I.V. regional anesthesia (Bier block)

Warnings Convulsions and cardiac arrhythmias, due to systemic toxicity leading to cardiac arrest have been reported, presumably following unintentional I.V. injection; should be administered in small incremental doses; not for use in emergency situations when rapid onset of surgical anesthesia is necessary; not for use for the production of obstetrical paracervical block anesthesia, retrobulbar block, or spinal anesthesia (subarachnoid block); unlike other local anesthetics, administration with epinephrine does not affect onset, duration of action, or the systemic absorption of ropivacaine. Supraclavicular brachial plexus blocks may be associated with a higher frequency of serious adverse effects; major peripheral nerve blocks, often close to large blood vessels pose an increased risk of intravenous systemic absorption due to the proximity and large volume of dosage. Chondrolysis has been reported following continuous intra-articular infusion; intra-articular administration of local anesthetics is not an FDA-approved route of administration.

Precautions Use with caution in patients with liver disease, impaired cardiovascular function, particularly CHF, hypotension, hypovolemia, heart block, and neurological or psychiatric disorders. Patients treated with class III antiarrhythmics may be at increased risk for additive cardiac effects and should be monitored closely (consider ECG monitoring). For epidural use, it is recommended that a test dose of either a local anesthetic with rapid onset alone or in combination with epinephrine be administered prior to ropivacaine to detect unintentional intravascular or intrathecal injection which would result in systemic toxicity (CNS or cardiovascular)

Adverse Reactions

Cardiovascular: Bradycardia, chest pain, hypo- or hypertension, tachycardia

Central nervous system: Anxiety, chills, dizziness, headache, lightheadedness

Dermatologic: Pruritus

Endocrine & metabolic: Hypokalemia

Gastrointestinal: Nausea, vomiting

Hematologic: Anemia

Neuromuscular & skeletal: Back pain, circumoral paresthesia, hypoesthesia, rigors, paresthesia

Renal: Oliguria

Respiratory: Dyspnea

Miscellaneous: Shivering

Rare but important or life-threatening: Angioedema, apnea (usually associated with epidural block in head/neck region), bronchospasm, cardiac arrest, cardiovascular collapse, chondrolysis (continuous intra-articular administration), dyskinesia, hallucinations, hyperthermia, myocardial depression, MI, rash, seizure, syncope, tinnitus, ventricular arrhythmia

Drug Interactions

Metabolism/Transport Effects Substrate of CYP1A2 (major), CYP2B6 (minor), CYP2D6 (minor), CYP3A4 (minor); **Note:** Assignment of Major/Minor substrate status based on clinically relevant drug interaction potential

Avoid Concomitant Use There are no known interactions where it is recommended to avoid concomitant use.

Increased Effect/Toxicity

The levels/effects of Ropivacaine may be increased by: Abiraterone Acetate; Ciprofloxacin (Systemic); CYP1A2 Inhibitors (Moderate); CYP1A2 Inhibitors (Strong); Deferasirox; FluvoxaMINE; Hyaluronidase; Propofol; Vemurafenib

Decreased Effect

Ropivacaine may decrease the levels/effects of: Technetium Tc 99m Tilmanocept

The levels/effects of Ropivacaine may be decreased by: Peginterferon Alfa-2b

Stability Store at controlled room temperature; preservative-free, discard promptly after use; do not mix with alkaline solutions as precipitation will occur

Mechanism of Action Blocks both the initiation and conduction of nerve impulses by decreasing the neuronal membrane's permeability to sodium ions, which results in inhibition of depolarization with resultant blockade of conduction

Pharmacodynamics

Onset of anesthetic action (dependent on dose and route of administration):

Epidural block (100-200 mg): T10 sensory block: 10 minutes (range: 5-13 minutes)

Epidural block, Cesarean section (up to 150 mg): T6 sensory block: 11-26 minutes

Duration (dependent upon dose and route of administration):

Epidural block (100-200 mg): 4 hours (range: 3-5 hours)

Epidural block, Cesarean section (up to 150 mg):

Sensory block: 1.7-3.2 hours

Motor block: 1.4-2.9 hours

Pharmacokinetics (Adult data unless noted)

Absorption: Well absorbed systemically in a biphasic manner following epidural administration; addition of epinephrine has no affect on the absorption of ropivacaine

Distribution: Distributes into breast milk

V_d (after intravascular infusion):

Children: 2.1-4.2 L/kg

Adults: 41 ± 7 L

Protein binding: 94%

Metabolism: In the liver via cytochrome P450 isoenzyme, predominantly CYP1A2 and CYP3A4 (10 metabolites with 2 active)

Bioavailability: 87% to 98% (epidural)

Half-life:

Epidural: Terminal phase:

Children: 4.9 hours (range: 3-6.7 hours)

Adults: 4.2 ± 1 hour

I.V.: Adults: 1.9 ± 0.5 hours

Time to peak serum concentration (dose and route dependent):

Caudal (children): 0.33-2.05 hours

Cesarean section: 14-65 minutes

Epidural (adults): 17-97 minutes

Elimination: 1% to 2% excreted unchanged in urine

Dosing: Usual Dose varies with procedure, depth of anesthesia, vascularity of tissues, duration of anesthesia, and condition of patient

Caudal block: Children (limited data): 2 mg/kg

Epidural block (other than caudal block): Children: 1.7 mg/kg

Lumbar epidural surgery: Adults: 75-150 mg (15-30 mL 0.5%); maximum: 200 mg (40 mL 0.5%)

Lumbar epidural Cesarean section: Adults: 100-150 mg (20-30 mL 0.5% **or** 15-20 mL 0.75%)

Thoracic epidural surgery: Adults: 25-75 mg (5-15 mL 0.5%)

Epidural continuous infusion:

Children 4 months to 7 years (limited data) (Hansen, 2000): 1 mg/kg loading dose followed by 0.4 mg/kg/hour continuous **epidural** infusion

Adults: 10-14 mg loading dose (5-7 mL 0.2%) followed by 12-28 mg/hour (6-14 mL/hour 0.2%) continuous **epidural** infusion

Major nerve block (eg, brachial plexus block): Adults: 75-300 mg (10-40 mL 0.75%)

Minor nerve block and infiltration: Adults: 5-200 mg (1-40 mL 0.5%)

Administration Parenteral: Administer in small incremental doses; when using continuous intermittent catheter techniques, use frequent aspirations before and during the injection to avoid intravascular injection

Monitoring Parameters After epidural or subarachnoid administration: Blood pressure, heart rate, respiration, signs of CNS toxicity (lightheadedness, dizziness, tinnitus, restlessness, tremors, twitching, drowsiness, circumoral paresthesia)

Dosage Forms Excipient information presented when available (limited, particularly for generics); consult specific product labeling.

Solution, Injection, as hydrochloride [preservative free]:

Naropin: 2 mg/mL (10 mL, 20 mL, 100 mL, 200 mL); 5 mg/mL (20 mL, 30 mL, 100 mL, 200 mL); 7.5 mg/mL (20 mL); 10 mg/mL (10 mL, 20 mL)

References

Hansen TG, Ilett KF, Lim SI, et al, "Pharmacokinetics and Clinical Efficacy of Long-Term Epidural Ropivacaine Infusion in Children," *Br J Anaesth*, 2000, 85(3):347-53.

Hansen TG, Ilett KF, Reid C, et al, "Caudal Ropivacaine in Infants: Population Pharmacokinetics and Plasma Concentrations," *Anesthesiology*, 2001, 94(4):579-84.

Lonnqvist PA, Westrin P, Larsson BA, et al, "Ropivacaine Pharmacokinetics After Caudal Block in 1-8 Year Old Children," *Br J Anaesth*, 2000, 85(4):506-11.

Wulf H, Peters C, and Behnke H, "The Pharmacokinetics of Caudal Ropivacaine 0.2% in Children. A Study of Infants Aged Less Than 1 Year and Toddlers Aged 1-5 Years Undergoing Inguinal Hernia Repair," *Anaesthesia*, 2000, 55(8):757-60.

◆ **Ropivacaine Hydrochloride** see Ropivacaine on page 1849

◆ **Ropivacaine Hydrochloride Injection, USP (Can)** see Ropivacaine on page 1849

◆ **Rosadan** see MetroNIDAZOLE (Topical) on page 1404

◆ **Rosasol (Can)** see MetroNIDAZOLE (Topical) on page 1404

Rosiglitazone (roh si GLI ta zone)

Medication Safety Issues

Sound-alike/look-alike issues:

Avandia may be confused with Avalide, Coumadin, Prandin

High alert medication:

The Institute for Safe Medication Practices (ISMP) includes this medication among its list of drug classes

which have a heightened risk of causing significant patient harm when used in error.

International issues:
Avandia [U.S., Canada, and multiple international markets] may be confused with Avanza brand name for mirtazapine [Australia]

Brand Names: U.S. Avandia

Brand Names: Canada Avandia

Therapeutic Category Antidiabetic Agent, Oral; Antidiabetic Agent, Thiazolidinedione

Generic Availability (U.S.) No

Use Adjunct treatment of type 2 diabetes mellitus (non-insulin-dependent, NIDDM) to improve glycemic control in patients who do not achieve control with diet and exercise alone or diet and exercise in combination with diabetic medication and for whom pioglitazone therapy is not an option (FDA approved in adults)

Prescribing and Access Restrictions Health Canada requires written informed consent for new and current patients receiving rosiglitazone.

Medication Guide Available Yes

Pregnancy Risk Factor C

Pregnancy Considerations Adverse effects were observed in initial animal reproduction studies. Rosiglitazone has been found to cross the placenta during the first trimester of pregnancy. Inadvertent use early in pregnancy has not been shown to increase the rate of adverse fetal effects, although in the majority of cases, the medication was stopped as soon as pregnancy was detected (Chan, 2005; Kalyoncu, 2005; Yaris, 2004). For women with diabetes, maternal hyperglycemia itself can be associated with adverse effects in the fetus, neonate, and mother. To prevent adverse events, prior to conception and throughout pregnancy the maternal HbA$_{1c}$ should be kept close to normal but without causing significant hypoglycemia. Maternal hyperglycemia can be associated with adverse effects in the mother. The use of thiazolidinediones in pregnant women is not recommended; insulin is the drug of choice for the control of diabetes mellitus during pregnancy (ACOG, 2005; ADA, 2013; Kitzmiller, 2008; Metzger, 2007).

Thiazolidinediones may cause ovulation in anovulatory premenopausal women, increasing the risk of pregnancy; adequate contraception in premenopausal women is recommended. Insulin-sensitizing agents, including rosiglitazone, have been evaluated for the treatment of polycystic ovary syndrome (POS) (ASRM, 2008). However, due to long-term safety concerns associated with their use, thiazolidinediones should be avoided in women of reproductive age (Fauser, 2012).

Breast-Feeding Considerations It is not known if rosiglitazone is excreted in breast milk. Although breast-feeding is encouraged for all women, including those with diabetes, the safety of rosiglitazone during breast-feeding has not yet been established (Metzger, 2007). According to the manufacturer, the decision to continue or discontinue breast-feeding during therapy should take into account the risk of exposure to the infant and the benefits of treatment to the mother.

Contraindications Hypersensitivity to rosiglitazone or any component; initiation of therapy in patients with NYHA Class III/IV heart failure

Warnings Thiazolidinediones, including rosiglitazone, may cause or exacerbate congestive heart failure (CHF) **[U.S. Boxed Warning]**; patients should be closely monitored for signs and symptoms of CHF (eg, rapid weight gain, dyspnea, edema), particularly after initiation or dose increases; discontinue use if any deterioration of cardiac function occurs. Rosiglitazone is not recommended for use in patients with symptomatic heart failure **[U.S. Boxed Warning]**; initiation of therapy is contraindicated in patients with NYHA class III or IV heart failure.

Rosiglitazone use may also be associated with an increased risk of MI **[U.S. Boxed Warning]** and cardiovascular death; use with caution in patients at risk for cardiovascular events and monitor closely. Discontinue if any deterioration in cardiac status occurs. Avoid concurrent use of rosiglitazone with insulin due to an increased risk of edema, congestive heart failure, and myocardial ischemic events. Concomitant use with nitrates is not recommended; an increased risk of MI has been observed in nitrate users vs non-nitrate users in clinical trials.

Because of cardiovascular risks, rosiglitazone-containing medications are only available through the Avandia-Rosiglitazone Medicines Access Program™ **[U.S. Boxed Warning]**; patients and prescribers must be registered with and meet conditions of the program.

A dose-related weight gain has been observed with use; mechanism unknown but likely associated with fluid retention and fat accumulation; a more rapid onset of weight gain may be suggestive of excessive edema and heart failure.

Idiosyncratic hepatotoxicity has been reported with thiazolidinedione agents including rosiglitazone (rare); avoid use in patients who previously experienced jaundice during troglitazone therapy; discontinue use in patients who develop jaundice during therapy. Use with caution in patients with elevated transaminases (AST or ALT); do not initiate in patients with active liver disease or ALT >2.5 times the upper limit of normal (ULN) at baseline; evaluate patients with ALT ≤2.5 times ULN at baseline or during therapy for cause of enzyme elevation; during therapy, if ALT >3 times ULN, re-evaluate levels promptly and discontinue if elevation persists or if jaundice occurs at any time during use.

An increased incidence of bone fractures in females treated with rosiglitazone was observed during analysis of long-term trial; majority of fractures occurred in the upper arm, hand, and foot (differing from the hip or spine fractures usually associated with postmenopausal osteoporosis). Consider risk of fracture prior to initiation and during use. May decrease hemoglobin, hematocrit, and/or WBC count (slight); effects may be related to increased plasma volume and/or dose-related; use with caution in patients with anemia.

Should not be used in Type 1 diabetes mellitus or diabetic ketoacidosis as the mechanism of action of rosiglitazone requires the presence of insulin.

Precautions Use with caution in premenopausal, anovulatory women; use may induce ovulation increasing the risk of pregnancy; adequate contraception in premenopausal women is recommended. Use with caution in patients with preexisting macular edema or diabetic retinopathy; postmarketing events of new-onset or worsening diabetic macular edema with decreased visual acuity have been reported; most patients had peripheral edema at the time of diagnosis; regular ophthalmic exams are recommended.

Adverse Reactions Note: As reported in monotherapy studies. Rare cases of hepatocellular injury have been reported in men in their 60s within 2 to 3 weeks after initiation of rosiglitazone therapy. LFTs in these patients revealed severe hepatocellular injury which responded with rapid improvement of liver function and resolution of symptoms upon discontinuation of rosiglitazone. Patients were also receiving other potentially hepatotoxic medications (Al-Salman, 2000; Freid, 2000).

Cardiovascular: Cardiac failure (incidence likely higher in patients with preexisting cardiac failure), edema, hypertension, ischemic heart disease (incidence likely higher in patients with preexisting CAD)

Central nervous system: Headache

Endocrine & metabolic: hypoglycemia, increased HDL cholesterol, increased LDL cholesterol, increased serum cholesterol (total), weight gain

Gastrointestinal: Diarrhea

Hematologic & oncologic: Anemia

Neuromuscular & skeletal: Arthralgia, back pain, bone fracture (incidence greater in females; usually upper arm, hand, or foot)

Respiratory: Nasopharyngitis, upper respiratory tract infection

Miscellaneous: Trauma

Rare but important or life-threatening: Anaphylaxis, angina pectoris, angioedema, cardiac arrest, coronary artery disease, coronary thrombosis, decreased HDL cholesterol, decreased hematocrit, decreased hemoglobin, decreased visual acuity, decreased white blood cell count, dyspnea, hepatic failure, hepatitis, increased serum bilirubin, increased serum transaminases, jaundice (reversible), macular edema, myocardial infarction, pleural effusion, pulmonary edema, Stevens-Johnson syndrome, thrombocytopenia, weight gain (rapid, excessive; usually due to fluid accumulation)

Drug Interactions

Metabolism/Transport Effects Substrate of CYP2C8 (major), CYP2C9 (minor); **Note:** Assignment of Major/Minor substrate status based on clinically relevant drug interaction potential; **Inhibits** CYP2C19 (weak), CYP2C8 (moderate), CYP2C9 (weak)

Avoid Concomitant Use There are no known interactions where it is recommended to avoid concomitant use.

Increased Effect/Toxicity

Rosiglitazone may increase the levels/effects of: CYP2C8 Substrates; Hypoglycemic Agents

The levels/effects of Rosiglitazone may be increased by: Androgens; CYP2C8 Inhibitors (Moderate); CYP2C8 Inhibitors (Strong); Deferasirox; Gemfibrozil; Herbs (Hypoglycemic Properties); Insulin; MAO Inhibitors; Mifepristone; Pegvisomant; Pregabalin; Salicylates; Selective Serotonin Reuptake Inhibitors; Trimethoprim; Vasodilators (Organic Nitrates)

Decreased Effect

The levels/effects of Rosiglitazone may be decreased by: Cholestyramine Resin; Corticosteroids (Orally Inhaled); Corticosteroids (Systemic); CYP2C8 Inducers (Strong); Dabrafenib; Danazol; Loop Diuretics; Luteinizing Hormone-Releasing Hormone Analogs; Rifampin; Somatropin; Thiazide Diuretics

Stability Store at 25°C (77°F); excursions permitted 15°C to 30°C (59°F to 86°F); protect from light.

Mechanism of Action Thiazolidinedione antidiabetic agent that lowers blood glucose by improving target cell response to insulin, without increasing pancreatic insulin secretion. It has a mechanism of action that is dependent on the presence of insulin for activity. Rosiglitazone is an agonist for peroxisome proliferator-activated receptor-gamma (PPARgamma). Activation of nuclear PPAR-gamma receptors influences the production of a number of gene products involved in glucose and lipid metabolism. PPARgamma is abundant in the cells within the renal collecting tubules; fluid retention results from stimulation by thiazolidinediones which increases sodium reabsorption.

Pharmacodynamics Maximum effect: Up to 12 weeks

Pharmacokinetics (Adult data unless noted)

Distribution: V_{dss} (apparent): 17.6 L

Protein binding: 99.8%; primarily albumin

Metabolism: Hepatic (99%), metabolism by cytochrome P450 isoenzyme CYP2C8, minor metabolism via CYP2C9

Bioavailability: 99%

Half-life: 3-4 hours

Time to peak serum concentration: 1 hour, delayed with food

Elimination: Urine (64%) and feces (23%) as metabolites

Dosing: Usual Type 2 diabetes:

Children ≥10 years and Adolescents: Limited data available: Oral: Initial: 2 mg twice daily; then increase to 4 mg twice daily after 8 weeks; in combination with metformin; dosing presented was used 233 pediatric patients as part of a larger multicenter comparative trial of treatments (n=699) and results showed rosiglitazone and metformin more effective than other treatment arms (ie, metformin alone or metformin and lifestyle changes) at maintaining glycemic control (Copeland, 2011; The TODAY Study Group, 2007; The TODAY Study Group, 2012).

Adults: **Note:** All patients should be initiated at the lowest recommended dose:

Monotherapy: Oral: Initial: 4 mg as a single daily dose or in divided doses twice daily; if response is inadequate after 8-12 weeks of treatment the dosage may be increased to 8 mg daily as a single daily dose or in divided doses twice daily

Combination therapy (with sulfonylureas, metformin, or sulfonylurea plus metformin): Oral: Initial: 4 mg daily as a single daily dose or in divided doses twice daily. If response is inadequate after 8-12 weeks of treatment, the dosage may be increased to 8 mg daily as a single daily dose or in divided doses twice daily. Reduce dose of sulfonylurea if hypoglycemia occurs. It is unlikely that the dose of metformin will need to be reduced due to hypoglycemia.

Dosage adjustment in renal impairment: No dosage adjustment is required

Dosage adjustment in hepatic impairment: Clearance is significantly lower in hepatic impairment. Therapy should not be initiated if the patient exhibits active liver disease or increased transaminases (>2.5 times the upper limit of normal) at baseline

Administration Oral: May be taken without regard to meals

Monitoring Parameters Signs and symptoms of hypoglycemia, fluid retention, or heart failure, fasting blood glucose, hemoglobin A_{1c}; liver enzymes: Baseline, every 2 months for the first 12 months of therapy, and periodically thereafter; patients with an elevation in ALT >3 times the upper limit of normal should be rechecked as soon as possible; if the ALT levels remain >3 times the upper limit of normal, therapy with rosiglitazone should be discontinued; ophthalmic exams

Reference Range Indicators of optimal glycemic control in children and adolescents (IDF/ISPAD, 2011; Rewers, 2009): **Note:** Targets must be adjusted based on individual needs/circumstances (eg, patients who experience severe hypoglycemia, patients with hypoglycemic unawareness): Blood glucose:

Fasting/Preprandial: 90-145 mg/dL

Postprandial: 90-180 mg/dL

Bedtime: 120-180 mg/dL

Hb A_{1c}: <7.5%

Dosage Forms Excipient information presented when available (limited, particularly for generics); consult specific product labeling.

Tablet, Oral:

Avandia: 2 mg, 4 mg, 8 mg

References

Al-Salman J, Arjomand H, Kemp DG, et al, "Hepatocellular Injury in a Patient Receiving Rosiglitazone. A Case Report," *Ann Intern Med*, 2000, 132(2):121-4.

American College of Obstetricians and Gynecologists, "ACOG Practice Bulletin. Clinical Management Guidelines for Obstetrician-Gynecologists. Number 60, March 2005. Pregestational Diabetes Mellitus," *Obstet Gynecol*, 2005, 105(3):675-85.

American Diabetes Association, "Standards of Medical Care in Diabetes – 2013," *Diabetes Care*, 2013, 36(Suppl 1):S11-66.

Chan LY, Yeung JH, and Lau TK, "Placental Transfer of Rosiglitazone in the First Trimester of Human Pregnancy," *Fertil Steril*, 2005, 83 (4):955-8.

Copeland KC, Zeitler P, Geffner M, et al, "Characteristics of Adolescents and Youth With Recent-Onset Type 2 Diabetes: The TODAY Cohort at Baseline," *J Clin Endocrinol Metab*, 2011, 96(1):159-67.

DeFronzo RA, "Pharmacologic Therapy for Type 2 Diabetes Mellitus," *Ann Intern Med*, 1999, 131(4):281-303.

Fauser BC, Tarlatzis BC, Rebar RW, et al, "Consensus on Women's Health Aspects of Polycystic Ovary Syndrome (PCOS): The Amsterdam ESHRE/ASRM-Sponsored 3rd PCOS Consensus Workshop Group," *Fertil Steril*, 2012, 97(1):28-38.

Forman LM, Simmons DA, and Diamond RH, "Hepatic Failure in a Patient Taking Rosiglitazone," *Ann Intern Med*, 2000, 132(2):118-21.

Freid J, Everitt D, and Boscia J, "Rosiglitazone and Hepatic Failure," *Ann Intern Med*, 2000, 132(2):164-6.

IDF/ISPAD, "Global Guideline for Diabetes in Childhood and Adolescence," 2011. Available at http://www.ispad.org/FileCenter.html?CategoryID=30

Kahn SE, Haffner SM, Heise MA, et al, "Glycemic Durability of Rosiglitazone, Metformin, or Glyburide Monotherapy," *N Engl J Med*, 2006, 355(23):2427-43.

Kalyoncu NI, Yaris F, Ulku C, et al, "A Case of Rosiglitazone Exposure in the Second Trimester of Pregnancy," *Reprod Toxicol*, 2005, 19 (4):563-4.

Kitzmiller JL, Block JM, Brown FM, et al, "Managing Preexisting Diabetes for Pregnancy: Summary of Evidence and Consensus Recommendations for Care," *Diabetes Care*, 2008, 31(5):1060-79.

Metzger BE, Buchanan TA, Coustan DR, et al, "Summary and Recommendations of the Fifth International Workshop-Conference on Gestational Diabetes Mellitus," *Diabetes Care*, 2007, 30(Suppl 2):S251-60.

Practice Committee of American Society for Reproductive Medicine, "Use of Insulin-Sensitizing Agents in the Treatment of Polycystic Ovary Syndrome," *Fertil Steril*, 2008, 90(5 Suppl):S69-73.

Rewers M, Pihoker C, Donaghue K, "Assessment and Monitoring of Glycemic Control in Children and Adolescents With Diabetes," *Pediatr Diabetes*, 2009, (10 Suppl)12:71-87.

TODAY Study Group, Zeitler P, Epstein L, et al, "Treatment Options for Type 2 Diabetes in Adolescents and Youth: A Study of the Comparative Efficacy of Metformin Alone or in Combination With Rosiglitazone or Lifestyle Intervention in Adolescents With Type 2 Diabetes," *Pediatr Diabetes*, 2007, 8(2):74-87.

TODAY Study Group, Zeitler P, Hirst K, et al, "A Clinical Trial to Maintain Glycemic Control in Youth With Type 2 Diabetes," *N Engl J Med*, 2012, 366(24):2247-56.

Yaris F, Yaris E, Kadioglu M, et al, "Normal Pregnancy Outcome Following Inadvertent Exposure to Rosiglitazone, Gliclazide, and Atorvastatin in a Diabetic and Hypertensive Woman," *Reprod Toxicol*, 2004, 18(4):619-21.

◆ **Rosone (Can)** *see* Betamethasone (Topical) on page 285

Rosuvastatin (roe soo va STAT in)

Medication Safety Issues
Sound-alike/look-alike issues:
Rosuvastatin may be confused with atorvaSTATin, nystatin, pitavastatin

Brand Names: U.S. Crestor

Brand Names: Canada Apo-Rosuvastatin; CO Rosuvastatin; Crestor; Dom-Rosuvastatin; Jamp-Rosuvastatin; Med-Rosuvastatin; Mint-Rosuvastatin; Mylan-Rosuvastatin; PMS-Rosuvastatin; RAN-Rosuvastatin; Riva-Rosuvastatin; Sandoz-Rosuvastatin; Teva-Rosuvastatin

Therapeutic Category Antilipemic Agent, HMG-CoA Reductase Inhibitor

Generic Availability (U.S.) No

Use Adjunct to dietary therapy to reduce elevated total-C, LDL-C, and apo-B levels in patients with heterozygous familial hypercholesterolemia (HeFH) [FDA approved in ages 10-17 years (girls ≥1 year postmenarche)]. Adjunct to dietary therapy for hyperlipidemias to reduce elevations in total cholesterol (TC), LDL-C, apo-B, nonHDL-C, and triglycerides (TG) in patients with primary hypercholesterolemia (elevations of 1 or more components are present in Fredrickson type IIa, IIb, and IV hyperlipidemias) (FDA approved in adults); treatment of hypertriglyceridemia (FDA approved in adults); treatment of primary dysbetalipoproteinemia (Fredrickson type III hyperlipidemia) (FDA approved in adults); treatment of homozygous familial hypercholesterolemia (FH) (FDA approved in adults); to slow progression of atherosclerosis as an adjunct to diet to lower TC and LDL-C (FDA approved in adults)

Pregnancy Risk Factor X

Pregnancy Considerations Adverse events were observed in some animal reproduction studies. There are reports of congenital anomalies following maternal use of HMG-CoA reductase inhibitors in pregnancy; however, maternal disease, differences in specific agents used, and the low rates of exposure limit the interpretation of the available data (Godfrey, 2012; Lecarpentier, 2012). Cholesterol biosynthesis may be important in fetal development; serum cholesterol and triglycerides increase normally during pregnancy. The discontinuation of lipid lowering medications temporarily during pregnancy is not expected to have significant impact on the long term outcomes of primary hypercholesterolemia treatment.

Use of rosuvastatin is contraindicated in pregnancy. HMG-CoA reductase inhibitors should be discontinued prior to pregnancy (ADA, 2013). If treatment of dyslipidemias is needed in pregnant women or in women of reproductive age, other agents are preferred (Berglund, 2012; Stone, 2013). The manufacturer recommends administration to women of childbearing potential only when conception is highly unlikely and patients have been informed of potential hazards.

Breast-Feeding Considerations It is not known if rosuvastatin is excreted into breast milk. Due to the potential for serious adverse reactions in a nursing infant, use while breast-feeding is contraindicated by the manufacturer.

Contraindications Hypersensitivity to rosuvastatin or any component; active liver disease; unexplained persistent elevations of hepatic serum transaminases (>3 times ULN); pregnancy; breast-feeding

Warnings Patients receiving HMG-CoA reductase inhibitors have developed rhabdomyolysis with or without acute renal failure and/or myopathy; patients should be monitored closely; risk is dose-related and is increased with concurrent use of other lipid-lowering medications (eg, fibric acid derivatives or niacin at doses >1 g/day) or large quantities of grapefruit juice (>1 quart/day). With concurrent use of cyclosporine, lopinavir/ritonavir, or atazanavir/ritonavir; dosage reductions of rosuvastatin recommended. Ensure patient is on the lowest effective rosuvastatin dose in all circumstances. Discontinue in any patient in which CPK levels are markedly elevated (>10 times ULN) or if myopathy is suspected/diagnosed; monitoring of CPK may be warranted, but may not prevent severe myopathy. The manufacturer recommends temporary discontinuation for elective major surgery, acute medical or surgical conditions, or in any patient experiencing an acute or serious condition predisposing to renal failure (eg, sepsis, hypotension, trauma, uncontrolled seizures). However, based upon current evidence, HMG-CoA reductase inhibitor therapy should be continued in the perioperative period unless risk outweighs cardioprotective benefit. Use caution in patients with renal impairment, inadequately treated hypothyroidism, and those taking other drugs associated with myopathy (eg, colchicine); these patients are predisposed to myopathy. Patients should be instructed to report unexplained muscle pain, tenderness, weakness, or brown urine.

An autoimmune-mediated myopathy (IMNM), has been reported (rarely) with HMG-CoA reductase inhibitor therapy; presents as proximal muscle weakness with elevated CPK levels, which persists despite discontinuation of HMG-CoA reductase inhibitor therapy; additionally, muscle biopsy may show necrotizing myopathy with limited inflammation; immunosuppressive therapy (eg, corticosteroids, azathioprine) may be used for treatment. Hematuria (microscopic) and proteinuria have been observed; more ▶

commonly reported in patients receiving rosuvastatin 40 mg daily. Typically, transient and not associated with a decrease in renal function. Consider dosage reduction if unexplained hematuria and proteinuria persists.

Postmarketing reports of fatal and nonfatal hepatic failure are rare; if serious hepatotoxicity with clinical symptoms and/or hyperbilirubinemia or jaundice occurs during treatment, interrupt therapy. If an alternate etiology is not identified, do not restart rosuvastatin. Liver enzyme tests should be obtained at baseline and as clinically indicated; routine periodic monitoring of liver enzymes is not necessary. Use with caution in patients with history of heavy alcohol use or a previous history of liver disease.

Precautions Rosuvastatin significantly increases INR in patients on warfarin. INR should be monitored before starting rosuvastatin and frequently during therapy. Transient proteinuria and hematuria have been reported; consider dose reduction if finding persists. Use caution in patients with conditions or on medications that reduce steroidogenesis (eg, ketoconazole, spironolactone, cimetidine). Increases in Hb A_{1c} and fasting blood glucose have been reported with HMG-CoA reductase inhibitors; however, the benefits of statin therapy far outweigh the risk of dysglycemia. Secondary causes of hyperlipidemia should be ruled out prior to therapy; has not been studied in conditions where the major abnormality is elevation of chylomicrons (hyperlipoproteinemia Types I or V). Use caution in patients with severe renal impairment not receiving dialysis; dosage adjustment required.

Although rare, reversible cognitive impairment (including confusion, forgetfulness, amnesia, and memory loss) can occur with HMG-CoA reductase inhibitors. These cognitive symptoms have been reported at variable times during therapy (1 day to years after initiation) and are reversible with discontinuation; resolution usually occurs within ~3 weeks. Cases have not been associated with fixed or progressive dementia; nor have they been associated with age, specific HMG-CoA reductase inhibitor, dose, or concomitant medication use.

Adverse Reactions

Central nervous system: Dizziness, headache

Endocrine & metabolic: Diabetes mellitus

Gastrointestinal: Abdominal pain, constipation, nausea

Hepatic: Increased serum ALT (>3 times ULN)

Neuromuscular & skeletal: Arthralgia, increased creatine phosphokinase, myalgia, weakness

Rare but important or life-threatening: Abnormal thyroid function test, amnesia (reversible), cataract, cognitive dysfunction (reversible), confusion (reversible), depression, elevated glycosylated hemoglobin (Hb A_{1c}), gynecomastia, hematuria (microscopic), hepatic failure, hepatitis, hyperglycemia, hypersensitivity reaction (including angioedema, pruritus, rash, urticaria), immune-mediated necrotizing myopathy, increased gamma-glutamyl transferase, increased serum alkaline phosphatase, increased serum AST, increased serum bilirubin, increased serum glucose, insomnia, jaundice, memory impairment (reversible), myoglobinuria, myositis, myopathy, nightmares, pancreatitis, proteinuria (dose related), renal failure, rhabdomyolysis, thrombocytopenia

Drug Interactions

Metabolism/Transport Effects Substrate of CYP2C9 (minor), CYP3A4 (minor), SLCO1B1; **Note:** Assignment of Major/Minor substrate status based on clinically relevant drug interaction potential

Avoid Concomitant Use

Avoid concomitant use of Rosuvastatin with any of the following: Fusidic Acid (Systemic); Gemfibrozil; Red Yeast Rice

Increased Effect/Toxicity

Rosuvastatin may increase the levels/effects of: DAPTOmycin; PAZOPanib; Trabectedin; Vitamin K Antagonists

The levels/effects of Rosuvastatin may be increased by: Amiodarone; Bezafibrate; Boceprevir; Colchicine; CycloSPORINE (Systemic); Dronedarone; Eltrombopag; Fenofibrate and Derivatives; Fusidic Acid (Systemic); Gemfibrozil; Itraconazole; Niacin; Niacinamide; Protease Inhibitors; Raltegravir; Red Yeast Rice; Simeprevir; Telaprevir

Decreased Effect

Rosuvastatin may decrease the levels/effects of: Lanthanum

The levels/effects of Rosuvastatin may be decreased by: Antacids; Eslicarbazepine

Stability Store between 20°C and 25°C (68°F to 77°F). Protect from moisture.

Mechanism of Action Inhibitor of 3-hydroxy-3-methylglutaryl coenzyme A (HMG-CoA) reductase, the rate-limiting enzyme in cholesterol synthesis (reduces the production of mevalonic acid from HMG-CoA); this then results in a compensatory increase in the expression of LDL receptors on hepatocyte membranes and a stimulation of LDL catabolism

Pharmacodynamics

Onset of action: Within 1 week

Maximum effect: 4 weeks

Pharmacokinetics (Adult data unless noted) Note: In pediatric patients (10-17 years of age), maximum serum concentration and AUC have been shown to be similar to adult values.

Distribution: V_d: 134 L

Protein binding: 88%, mostly to albumin

Metabolism: Hepatic (10%), via CYP2C9; N-desmethyl rosuvastatin, one-sixth to one-half the HMG-CoA reductase activity of the parent compound

Bioavailability: ~20% (high first-pass extraction by liver); increased in Asian patients (twofold increase in median exposure)

Half-life elimination: ~19 hours

Time to peak serum concentration: 3-5 hours

Elimination: Feces (90%), primarily as unchanged drug

Dosing: Usual Doses should be individualized according to the baseline LDL-cholesterol levels, the recommended goal of therapy, and patient response; adjustments should be made at intervals of 4 weeks or more.

Children and Adolescents: **Note:** A lower, conservative dosing regimen may be necessary in patient populations predisposed to myopathy, including patients of Asian descent or concurrently receiving other lipid-lowering agents (eg, gemfibrozil, niacin, fibric acid derivatives), amiodarone, atazanavir/ritonavir, cyclosporine, lopinavir/ritonavir, or indinavir (see conservative, maximum adult doses below).

Heterozygous familial hypercholesterolemia: Children and Adolescents 10-17 years: Oral: 5-20 mg once daily; may titrate dose at 4-week intervals; maximum daily dose: 20 mg/**day**

Homozygous familial hypercholesterolemia: Limited data available: Children and Adolescents (≥8 years and ≥32 kg): Oral: Initial dose: 20 mg once daily; titrate at 6-week intervals to 40 mg once daily. Although higher doses have been used (ie, 80 mg/day), additional benefit has not been reported. Dosing based on an open-label, forced-titration study of 44 patients (n=8 pediatric patients ≥8 years) which reported 72% of patients responded to rosuvastatin treatment (Marias, 2008).

Adults:

Hyperlipidemia, mixed dyslipidemia, hypertriglyceridemia, primary dysbetalipoproteinemia, slowing progression of atherosclerosis: Oral:

Initial dose:

General dosing: 10 mg once daily; 20 mg once daily may be used in patients with severe hyperlipidemia (LDL >190 mg/dL) and aggressive lipid targets

Conservative dosing: Patients requiring less aggressive treatment or predisposed to myopathy (including patients of Asian descent): 5 mg once daily

Titration: After 2 weeks, may be increased by 5-10 mg once daily; dosing range: 5-40 mg/day; maximum daily dose: 40 mg/**day**

Note: The 40 mg dose should be reserved for patients who have not achieved goal cholesterol levels on a dose of 20 mg/day, including patients switched from another HMG-CoA reductase inhibitor.

Homozygous familial hypercholesterolemia (FH): Initial: 20 mg once daily; maximum dose: 40 mg/day

Dosing adjustment with concomitant medications: Adults:

Atazanavir/ritonavir or lopinavir/ritonavir: Initiate rosuvastatin at 5 mg once daily; rosuvastatin dose should not exceed 10 mg/day

Cyclosporine: Rosuvastatin dose should not exceed 5 mg/day

Gemfibrozil: Avoid concurrent use; if unable to avoid concurrent use, initiate rosuvastatin at 5 mg once daily; rosuvastatin dose should not exceed 10 mg/day

Dosing adjustment in renal impairment: Adults:

Mild to moderate impairment: No dosage adjustment required.

CrCl <30 mL/minute/1.73 m^2 and not receiving hemodialysis: Initial: 5 mg once daily; do not exceed 10 mg once daily

Dosing adjustments in hepatic impairment: There are no dosage adjustments provided in the manufacturer labeling; systemic exposure may be increased in patients with liver disease; use is contraindicated in patients with active liver disease or unexplained transaminase elevations.

Administration May be taken with or without food; may be taken at any time of the day.

Monitoring Parameters

Pediatric patients: Baseline: ALT, AST, and creatine phosphokinase levels (CPK); fasting lipid panel (FLP) and repeat ALT and AST should be checked after 4 weeks of therapy; if no myopathy symptoms or laboratory abnormalities, then monitor FLP, ALT, and AST every 3-4 months during the first year and then every 6 months thereafter (NHLBI, 2011).

Adults: Baseline CPK (recheck CPK in any patient with symptoms suggestive of myopathy; discontinue therapy if markedly elevated); baseline liver function tests (LFTs) and repeat when clinically indicated thereafter. Patients with elevated transaminase levels should have a second (confirmatory) test and frequent monitoring until values normalize; discontinue if increase in ALT/AST is persistently >3 times ULN (NCEP, 2002).

Lipid panel (total cholesterol, HDL, LDL, triglycerides):

ATP III recommendations (NCEP, 2002): Baseline; 6-8 weeks after initiation of drug therapy; if dose increased, then at 6-8 weeks until final dose determined. Once treatment goal achieved, follow-up intervals may be reduced to every 4-6 months. Lipid panel should be assessed at least annually, and preferably at each clinic visit.

Manufacturer's recommendation: Analyze lipid panel at initiation and every 2-4 weeks during therapy.

Dosage Forms Excipient information presented when available (limited, particularly for generics); consult specific product labeling.

Tablet, Oral:

Crestor: 5 mg, 10 mg, 20 mg, 40 mg

References

American Diabetes Association, "Standards of Medical Care in Diabetes-2013," *Diabetes Care*, 2013, 36(Suppl 1):S11-66.

Berglund L, Brunzell JD, Goldberg AC, et al, "Evaluation and Treatment of Hypertriglyceridemia: An Endocrine Society Clinical Practice Guideline," *J Clin Endocrinol Metab*, 2012, 97(9):2969-89.

Daniels SR, Greer FR, and Committee on Nutrition, "Lipid Screening and Cardiovascular Health in Childhood," *Pediatrics*, 2008, 122 (1):198-208.

"Executive Summary of the Third Report of the National Cholesterol Education Program (NCEP) Expert Panel on Detection, Evaluation, and Treatment of High Blood Cholesterol in Adults (Adult Treatment Panel III)," *JAMA*, 2001, 285(19):2486-97.

Godfrey LM, Erramouspe J, and Cleveland KW, "Teratogenic Risk of Statins in Pregnancy," *Ann Pharmacother*, 2012, 46(10):1419-24.

Lecarpentier E, Morel O, Fournier T, et al, "Statins and Pregnancy: Between Supposed Risks and Theoretical Benefits," *Drugs*, 2012, 72 (6):773-88.

Marais AD, Raal FJ, Stein EA, et al, "A Dose-Titration and Comparative Study of Rosuvastatin and Atorvastatin in Patients With Homozygous Familial Hypercholesterolaemia," *Atherosclerosis*, 2008, 197 (1):400-6.

McCrindle BW, Urbina EM, Dennison BA, et al, "Drug Therapy of High-Risk Lipid Abnormalities in Children and Adolescents: A Scientific Statement From the American Heart Association Atherosclerosis, Hypertension, and Obesity in Youth Committee, Council of Cardiovascular Disease in the Young, With the Council on Cardiovascular Nursing," *Circulation*, 2007, 115(14):1948-67.

National Heart, Lung, and Blood Institute, "Expert Panel on Integrated Guidelines for Cardiovascular Health and Risk Reduction in Children and Adolescents," Clinical Practice Guidelines, 2011, National Institutes of Health. Available at http://www.nhlbi.nih.gov/guidelines/cvd_ped/peds_guidelines_full.pdf

◆ **Rosuvastatin Calcium** see Rosuvastatin *on page 1853*

◆ **Rotarix** see Rotavirus Vaccine *on page 1855*

◆ **RotaTeq** see Rotavirus Vaccine *on page 1855*

Rotavirus Vaccine (ROE ta vye rus vak SEEN)

Medication Safety Issues

Administration issues:

Rotavirus vaccines (Rotarix and RotaTeq) are only available for **ORAL** administration. Occasionally, the live oral rotavirus vaccines have been administered as an injection, thereby making the vaccine ineffective (ISMP, 2014). Avoid the administration of oral rotavirus vaccines as an injection. An oral dose should still be given if the dose was inadvertently administered as an injection (JAMA, 2014).

Related Information

Immunization Administration Recommendations *on page 2368*

Immunization Guidelines *on page 2373*

Brand Names: U.S. Rotarix; RotaTeq

Brand Names: Canada Rotarix; RotaTeq

Therapeutic Category Vaccine, Live Virus

Generic Availability (U.S.) No

Use Routine immunization to prevent rotavirus gastroenteritis caused by serotypes G1, G2, G3, and G4 (RotaTeq) or serotypes G1, G3, G4, and G9 (Rotarix) (Rotarix: FDA approved in ages 6 to24 weeks; RotaTeq: FDA approved in ages 6 to 32 weeks)

The Advisory Committee on Immunization Practices (ACIP) recommends routine vaccination of all infants (CDC/ACIP [Cortese, 2009]).

Pregnancy Risk Factor C

Pregnancy Considerations Reproduction studies have not been conducted. Not indicated for use in women of reproductive age. Infants living in households with pregnant women may be vaccinated (CDC, 2009).

Breast-Feeding Considerations Infants receiving vaccine may be breast fed (CDC, 2009).

Contraindications Hypersensitivity to rotavirus vaccine or any component; infants with severe combined immunodeficiency disease (SCID); infants with history of intussusception. Additional product specific contraindication: Rotarix: History of uncorrected congenital GI malformations (including Meckel's diverticulum) that may be a predisposition to intussusception.

Warnings Rotavirus vaccine should not be administered to infants with acute, moderate to severe gastroenteritis until the condition improves. The decision to administer or delay vaccination because of current or recent febrile illness depends on the severity of symptoms and the etiology of the disease. Patients with mild low-grade fever (<38.1°C), mild gastroenteritis, or mild upper respiratory infection may receive vaccine. Information is not available for use of rotavirus vaccine in postexposure prophylaxis. Live virus vaccines may be transmitted to nonvaccinated contacts; use with caution in the presence of immunocompromised family members. Viral shedding occurs within the first weeks of administration; peak viral shedding generally occurs ~7 days after the first dose. The ACIP recommends vaccination of infants living in households with persons who are immunocompromised (CDC/ACIP [Cortese, 2009]).

An increased risk of intussusception was observed with a previously licensed rotavirus vaccine. Cases have been noted in postmarketing reports and a temporal association has been observed in postmarketing observational studies with current vaccines. Cases were noted within 21 to 31 days of the first dose, with a clustering of cases within the first 7 days following administration. RotaTeq and Rotarix are contraindicated in patients with a history of intussusception. Use with caution in infants with a history of gastrointestinal disorders (eg, active acute gastrointestinal disorders, chronic diarrhea, failure to thrive, history of congenital abdominal disorders, abdominal surgery); vaccine may be used with controlled gastroesophageal reflux disease. Rotarix is contraindicated in patients with a history of uncorrected congenital malformation of the GI tract.

Immediate treatment (including epinephrine 1:1000) for anaphylactoid and/or hypersensitivity reactions should be available during vaccine use.

Administration errors have been reported. This vaccine is for oral administration only; doses inadvertently administered by injection are not considered valid and an oral replacement dose should be given according to the appropriate age and schedule. Eye splashes to the provider, parent, or infant have been reported; to minimize risk of coughing, sneezing, and spitting, administer gently inside the cheek (CDC [Hibbs, 2014]).

Precautions Use with caution in immunocompromised infants (including blood dyscrasias, leukemia, lymphoma, malignant neoplasms affecting bone marrow or lymphatic system), infants on immunosuppressants (including high-dose corticosteroids; may be administered with topical corticosteroids or inhaled steroids), or infants with primary and acquired immunodeficiencies (including HIV/AIDS, cellular immune deficiencies, hypogammaglobulinemic and dysgammaglobulinemic states); safety and efficacy have not been established. The ACIP recommendations support vaccination of HIV-exposed or infected infants, since the diagnosis of infection may not be made prior to the first dose of the vaccine and also because strains of rotavirus vaccine are considerably attenuated (CDC/ACIP [Cortese, 2009]). Vaccination may not result in effective immunity in all patients. Response to vaccine depends upon multiple factors (eg, type of vaccine, age of patient) and may be improved by administering the vaccine at the recommended dose, route, and interval. Vaccines may not be effective if administered during periods of altered immune competence (CDC/ACIP [Kroger, 2011]).

Antipyretics have not been shown to prevent febrile seizures. Antipyretics may be used to treat fever or discomfort following vaccination (CDC/ACIP [Kroger, 2011]). One study reported that routine prophylactic administration of acetaminophen to prevent fever due to vaccines has been shown to decrease the immune response of some vaccines; the clinical significance of this reduction in immune response has not been established (Prymula, 2009). Some packaging may contain natural latex/natural rubber; the oral applicator of Rotarix contains latex. The RotaTeq dosing tube is latex-free.

Adverse Reactions All serious adverse reactions must be reported to the U.S. Department of Health and Human Services (DHHS) Vaccine Adverse Event Reporting System (VAERS) 1-800-822-7967 or online at https://vaers.hhs.gov/esub/index.

Central nervous system: Fever >38.1°C, fussiness, irritability

Gastrointestinal: Diarrhea, flatulence, vomiting

Otic: Otitis media

Respiratory: Bronchospasm, nasopharyngitis

Rare but important or life-threatening: Anaphylaxis, angioedema, gastroenteritis with severe diarrhea and prolonged vaccine viral shedding in infants with SCID, hematochezia, immune thrombocytopenia (ITP), intussusception, Kawasaki disease, seizure, transmission of vaccine virus from recipient to nonvaccinated contacts, urticaria

Drug Interactions

Metabolism/Transport Effects None known.

Avoid Concomitant Use

Avoid concomitant use of Rotavirus Vaccine with any of the following: Belimumab; Fingolimod; Immunosuppressants

Increased Effect/Toxicity

The levels/effects of Rotavirus Vaccine may be increased by: Belimumab; Corticosteroids (Systemic); Dimethyl Fumarate; Fingolimod; Hydroxychloroquine; Immunosuppressants; Leflunomide; Mercaptopurine; Methotrexate

Decreased Effect

Rotavirus Vaccine may decrease the levels/effects of: Tuberculin Tests

The levels/effects of Rotavirus Vaccine may be decreased by: Dimethyl Fumarate; Fingolimod; Immune Globulins; Immunosuppressants

Stability

Rotarix: Prior to reconstitution, store powder at 2°C to 8°C (36°F to 46°F); diluent may be stored at 20°C to 25°C (68°F to 77°F). Protect from light; discard if frozen. Following reconstitution, may be refrigerated or stored at room temperature for up to 24 hours. Discard if frozen.

RotaTeq: Store and transport at 2°C to 8°C (36°F to 46°F). Administer as soon as possible once removed from refrigerator. Protect from light.

Mechanism of Action A live vaccine; replicates in the small intestine and promotes active immunity to rotavirus gastroenteritis. Rotarix is specifically indicated for prevention of rotavirus gastroenteritis caused by serotypes G1, G3, G4, and G9 and RotaTeq is specifically indicated for prevention of rotavirus gastroenteritis caused by serotypes G1, G2, G3, and G4. However, vaccines may provide immunity to other serotypes.

Pharmacodynamics Note: There is no established relationship between antibody response and protection against gastroenteritis.

Seroconversion:

Rotarix: Antirotavirus IgA antibodies were noted 1 to 2 months following completion of the 2-dose series in 77% to 87% of infants.

RotaTeq: A threefold increase in antirotavirus IgA was noted following completion of the 3-dose regimen in 93% to 100% of infants.

Duration: Following administration of rotavirus vaccine, efficacy of protecting against any grade of rotavirus gastroenteritis through two seasons was 70% to 79%.

Dosing: Usual

Pediatric: **Note:** In the event a dose is regurgitated, spit out, or infant vomits, AAP does not recommend readministration of the dose; subsequent doses should be administered on routine schedule (AAP, 2009).

Note: The ACIP recommendations for vaccination recommend completing the vaccine series with the same product whenever possible. If continuing with same product will cause vaccination to be deferred, or if product used previously is unknown, vaccination should be completed with the product available. If RotaTeq was used in any previous doses, or if the specific product used was unknown, a total of 3 doses should be given.

Primary immunization:

Rotarix: Infants 6 to 24 weeks of age: Oral: 1 mL per dose for a total of 2 doses given as follows: 2 and 4 months of age. Initial dose should be administered from 6 weeks through 14 weeks 6 days of age; the first and second dose should be separated by ≥4 weeks. The 2-dose series should be completed by 24 weeks of age; maximum age for last dose: 8 months 0 days of age

RotaTeq: Infants 6 to 32 weeks of age: Oral: 2 mL per dose for a total of 3 doses given as follows: 2, 4, and 6 months of age. Initial dose should be administered from 6 weeks through 12 weeks; subsequent doses administered at 4- to 10-week intervals. Routine administration of the first dose at >12 weeks of age is not recommended (insufficient data). Administer all doses by 32 weeks of age. Infants who have had rotavirus gastroenteritis before getting the full course of vaccine should still initiate or complete the 3-dose schedule; initial infection provides only partial immunity.

Catch-up immunization: CDC (ACIP) Recommendations: **Note:** Do not restart the series. If doses have been given, begin the below schedule at the applicable dose number. The series should not be started in infants ≥15 weeks. The final dose in the series should be administered by 8 months 0 days of age. For infants inadvertently administered rotavirus vaccine at ≥15 weeks of age, the vaccine series may be completed according to schedule and prior to 8 months and 0 days of age. If RotaTeq was used in any previous doses, or if the specific product used was unknown, a total of 3 doses should be given. Oral:

First dose given at <15 weeks of age

Second dose given at least 4 weeks after the first dose

Third dose given at least 4 weeks after the second dose (not needed if first 2 doses were Rotarix)

Dosing adjustment in renal impairment: There are no dosage adjustments provided in the manufacturer's labeling.

Dosing adjustment in hepatic impairment: There are no dosage adjustments provided in the manufacturer's labeling.

Administration Oral use only; **not for injection.** To avoid potential eye splashes caused by coughing, sneezing, and spitting, administer gently inside the cheek (CDC [Hibbs, 2014]).

Rotarix: Connect transfer adapter onto vial and push downwards until transfer adapter is in place. Shake oral applicator containing liquid diluent (suspension will be a turbid liquid). Connect oral applicator to transfer adapter and transfer entire contents of oral applicator into the lyophilized vaccine. With transfer adapter in place, shake vigorously. Withdraw entire mixture back into oral applicator. Infant should be in reclining position. Using oral applicator, administer contents into infant's inner cheek. If most of dose is spit out or regurgitated, may administer a replacement dose at the same visit. Dispose of applicator and vaccine vial in biologic waste container.

RotaTeq: Clear fluid from the dispensing tip by holding dosing tube vertically and tapping cap; puncture dispensing tip by screwing cap clockwise; remove cap by turning counterclockwise; gently squeeze liquid dose into infant's mouth toward the inner cheek until dosing tube is empty. If an incomplete dose is given (eg, infant spits or regurgitates dose), do not administer replacement dose. The infant can continue to receive any remaining doses of the series at the designated time interval. Do not mix or dilute vaccine with any other vaccine or solution.

Test Interactions Tuberculin tests: Rotavirus vaccine may diminish the diagnostic effect of tuberculin tests.

Additional Information Diphtheria and tetanus antigens in DTaP, HIB, IPV, hepatitis B vaccine, and pneumococcal conjugate vaccine may be given concurrently with rotavirus vaccine.

In the United States, rotavirus outbreaks occur from late fall to early spring. In the Southwest, the peak rotavirus season is November through December; the peak epidemic travels across the United States from west to east terminating in April through May in the Northeast.

In order to maximize vaccination rates, the ACIP recommends simultaneous administration (ie, >1 vaccine on the same day at different anatomic sites) of all age-appropriate vaccines (live or inactivated) for which a person is eligible at a single visit, unless contraindications exist. If available, the use of combination vaccines is generally preferred over separate injections, taking into consideration provider assessment, patient preference, and potential adverse events. The ACIP prefers each dose of specific vaccine in a series come from the same manufacturer if possible (CDC/ACIP [Kroger, 2011]).

For additional information, please refer to the following website: http://www.cdc.gov/vaccines/vpd-vac/.

Dosage Forms Excipient information presented when available (limited, particularly for generics); consult specific product labeling.

Powder, for suspension, oral [preservative free; human derived]:

Rotarix: G1P[8] ≥10^6 CCID$_{50}$ per 1 mL [contains sorbitol, sucrose; supplied with diluent which may contain natural rubber/natural latex in packaging]

Solution, oral [preservative free; bovine and human derived]:

RotaTeq: G1 ≥2.2 x 10^6 infectious units, G2 ≥2.8 x 10^6 infectious units, G3 ≥2.2 x 10^6 infectious units, G4 ≥2 x 10^6 infectious units, and P1A [8] ≥2.3 x 10^6 infectious units per 2 mL (2 mL)

References

AAP Steering Committee on Quality Improvement and Management, Subcommittee on Febrile Seizures American Academy of Pediatrics, "Febrile Seizures: Clinical Practice Guideline for the Long-Term Management of the Child With Simple Febrile Seizures," *Pediatrics*, 2008, 121(6):1281-6.

Akinsanya-Beysolow I, Advisory Committee on Immunization Practices (ACIP), ACIP Child/Adolescent Immunization Work Group, et al. Advisory committee on immunization practices recommended immunization schedule for adults aged 19 years or older - United States, 2014. *MMWR Morb Mortal Wkly Rep*. 2014; 63(5):108-109. Full schedule available at http://www.cdc.gov/vaccines/schedules/downloads/child/0-18yrs-child-combined-schedule.pdf

American Academy of Pediatrics, Committee on Infectious Diseases. Prevention of rotavirus disease: updated guidelines for use of rotavirus vaccine. *Pediatrics*. 2009;123(5):1412-1420.

Cortese MM, Parashar UD. Prevention of rotavirus gastroenteritis among infants and children: recommendations of the Advisory Committee on Immunization Practices (ACIP). *MMWR Recomm Rep*. 2009;58(RR-2):1-25.

Centers for Disease Control and Prevention (CDC), "Syncope After Vaccination-United States, January 2005-July 2007," *MMWR Morb Mortal Wkly Rep*, 2008, 2;57(17):457-60.

Hibbs BF, Miller ER, Shimabukuro T, Centers for Disease Control and Prevention (CDC). Notes from the field: rotavirus vaccine administration errors--United States, 2006-2013. *MMWR Morb Mortal Wkly Rep*. 2014;63(4):81.

Kroger AT, Atkinson WL, Marcuse EK, Pickering LK. General recommendations on immunization - recommendations of the Advisory Committee on Immunization Practices (ACIP). *MMWR Recomm Rep*. 2011;60(RR-2):1-64.

Prymula R, Siegrist CA, Chlibek R, et al, "Effect of Prophylactic Para-cetamol Administration at Time of Vaccination on Febrile Reactions and Antibody Responses in Children: Two Open-Label, Randomised Controlled Trials," *Lancet*, 2009, 374(9698):1339-50.

Vesikari T, Matson DO, Dennehy P, et al, "Safety and Efficacy of a Pentavalent Human-Bovine (WC3) Reassortant Rotavirus Vaccine," *N Engl J Med*, 2006, 354(1):23-33.

◆ **Rotavirus Vaccine, Pentavalent** *see* Rotavirus Vaccine *on page 1855*

◆ **Rowasa** *see* Mesalamine *on page 1347*

◆ **Roxanol** *see* Morphine (Systemic) *on page 1440*

◆ **Roxicet** *see* Oxycodone and Acetaminophen *on page 1573*

◆ **Roxicodone** *see* OxyCODONE *on page 1569*

◆ **Roychlor (Can)** *see* Potassium Chloride *on page 1708*

◆ **RP-6976** *see* DOCEtaxel *on page 697*

◆ **RP-59500** *see* Quinupristin and Dalfopristin *on page 1796*

◆ **RS-25259** *see* Palonosetron *on page 1586*

◆ **RS-25259-197** *see* Palonosetron *on page 1586*

◆ **RTCA** *see* Ribavirin *on page 1818*

◆ **Rubella, Measles and Mumps Vaccines** *see* Measles, Mumps, and Rubella Virus Vaccine *on page 1307*

◆ **Rubella, Varicella, Measles, and Mumps Vaccine** *see* Measles, Mumps, Rubella, and Varicella Virus Vaccine *on page 1310*

◆ **Rubidomycin Hydrochloride** *see* DAUNOrubicin (Conventional) *on page 599*

◆ **RUF 331** *see* Rufinamide *on page 1858*

Rufinamide (roo FIN a mide)

Brand Names: U.S. Banzel
Brand Names: Canada Banzel™
Therapeutic Category Anticonvulsant, Triazole Derivative
Generic Availability (U.S.) No
Use Adjunctive therapy of seizures associated with Lennox-Gastaut syndrome (FDA approved in ages ≥4 years and adults)
Medication Guide Available Yes
Pregnancy Risk Factor C
Pregnancy Considerations Adverse effects were seen in animal studies. There are no adequate and well-controlled studies in pregnant women; use during pregnancy only if clearly needed. Hormonal contraceptives may be less effective with concurrent rufinamide use; additional forms of nonhormonal contraceptives should be used.

Patients exposed to rufinamide during pregnancy are encouraged to enroll themselves into the AED Pregnancy Registry by calling 1-888-233-2334. Additional information is available at www.aedpregnancyregistry.org.

Breast-Feeding Considerations Excretion into breast milk is unknown, but may be expected. Breast-feeding is not recommended by the manufacturer due to the potential for adverse effects in the nursing infant.

Contraindications Hypersensitivity to rufinamide or any component; patients with familial short QT syndrome

Warnings Antiepileptic drugs (AEDs) increase the risk of suicidal behavior and ideation in patients receiving these medications for any indication. Pooled analyses of placebo-controlled trials involving 11 different AEDs (regardless of indication) showed a twofold increased risk of suicidal thoughts or behavior (estimated incidence rate: 0.43% in AED treated patients compared to 0.24% of patients receiving placebo); increased risk was observed as early as 1 week after initiation of AED and continued through duration of trials (most trials ≤24 weeks); risk did

not vary significantly by age (age range: 5-100 years). Consider risks and benefits of AEDs before prescribing. Monitor all patients receiving an AED for emergence of suicidal thoughts or behavior, thoughts of self-harm, any unusual changes in behavior or mood, or the emergence or worsening of depressive symptoms; notify healthcare provider immediately if symptoms or concerning behavior occur. **Note:** The FDA requires a Medication Guide for all antiepileptic drugs informing patients of this risk.

Central nervous system adverse events including somnolence, fatigue, coordination abnormalities, dizziness, gait disturbances, and ataxia may occur; effects with other sedative drugs or ethanol may be potentiated; patients should be cautioned about performing tasks which require mental alertness (eg, operating machinery or driving). Avoid abrupt discontinuation of therapy; withdraw gradually (~25% dose reduction every 2 days) to lessen chance for increased seizure frequency; if abrupt discontinuation is medically necessary, close medical supervision is recommended.

Potentially serious, sometimes fatal, multiorgan hypersensitivity reactions (including severe hepatitis) have been reported with some antiepileptic drugs, including rufinamide; cases reported with rufinamide occurred in children <12 years and presented within the first 4 weeks of therapy. Monitor for rash, fever, and signs and symptoms of possible disparate manifestations associated with lymphatic, hepatic, renal, and/or hematologic organ systems. Patients who develop rash should be closely monitored for other signs and symptoms of reaction; if hypersensitivity reaction(s) is suspected; discontinue therapy.

Shortening of the QT interval has been reported; in a placebo-controlled QT interval study, ECG findings showed 46% to 65% of rufinamide-treated patients experienced a possible dose-dependent QT shortening of >20 msec at the time of maximum serum concentrations compared to 5% to 10% of placebo patients; however, QT interval reductions did not fall below 300 msec and no signs of ventricular arrhythmias or sudden death reported. Do not use in patients with familial short QT syndrome and use with caution in patients receiving concurrent medications that shorten the QT interval.

Precautions Use with caution in patients with mild to moderate hepatic impairment; use is not recommended in patients with severe hepatic impairment. May cause leukopenia. Concomitant use with valproic acid may increase rufinamide serum concentrations; rufinamide dosage adjustment recommended. Children may experience some adverse effects not reported in adults, including aggression, attention disturbance, hyperactivity, pruritus, rash, nasopharyngitis, and seizures.

Suspension contains propylene glycol; in neonates large amounts of propylene glycol delivered orally, intravenously (eg, >3000 mg/day), or topically have been associated with potentially fatal toxicities which can include metabolic acidosis, seizures, renal failure, and CNS depression; use rufinamide suspension containing propylene glycol with caution in neonates.

Adverse Reactions
Cardiovascular: QT shortening (dose related)
Central nervous system: Aggression, anxiety, ataxia, attention disturbance, dizziness, fatigue, headache, hyperactivity, seizure, somnolence, status epilepticus, vertigo
Dermatologic: Pruritus, rash
Gastrointestinal: Abdominal pain, appetite decreased/increased, constipation, dyspepsia, nausea, vomiting
Hematologic: Anemia, leukopenia
Neuromuscular & skeletal: Back pain, gait disturbance, tremor
Ocular: Blurred vision, diplopia, nystagmus
Otic: Otitis media

Renal: Pollakiuria

Respiratory: Bronchitis, nasopharyngitis, sinusitis

Miscellaneous: Influenza

Rare but important or life-threatening: Atrioventricular block (first degree), bundle branch block (right), dysuria, enuresis, hematuria; hypersensitivity (multiorgan; includes eosinophilia, facial edema, fever, hepatitis [severe], LFTs increased, rash, stupor, urticaria); incontinence, iron-deficiency anemia, lymphadenopathy, nephrolithiasis, neutropenia, nocturia, polyuria, thrombocytopenia, urinary incontinence

Drug Interactions

Metabolism/Transport Effects Inhibits CYP2E1 (weak); **Induces** CYP3A4 (weak/moderate)

Avoid Concomitant Use

Avoid concomitant use of Rufinamide with any of the following: Axitinib; Simeprevir

Increased Effect/Toxicity

Rufinamide may increase the levels/effects of: CNS Depressants; Fosphenytoin; PHENobarbital; Phenytoin

The levels/effects of Rufinamide may be increased by: Alcohol (Ethyl); Valproic Acid and Derivatives

Decreased Effect

Rufinamide may decrease the levels/effects of: ARIPiprazole; Axitinib; CarBAMazepine; Ethinyl Estradiol; Ibrutinib; Norethindrone; Saxagliptin; Simeprevir

The levels/effects of Rufinamide may be decreased by: CarBAMazepine; Fosphenytoin; PHENobarbital; Phenytoin; Primidone

Food Interactions Food increases the absorption of rufinamide. Management: Take with food.

Stability Store at 25°C (77°F); excursions permitted to 15°C to 30°C (59°F to 86°F); protect tablets from moisture. Oral suspension: Discard within 90 days after opening; cap of bottle fits over the adapter.

Mechanism of Action A triazole-derivative antiepileptic whose exact mechanism is unknown. *In vitro*, it prolongs the inactive state of the sodium channels, thereby limiting repetitive firing of sodium-dependent action potentials mediating anticonvulsant effects.

Pharmacokinetics (Adult data unless noted) Note: Pharmacokinetic data in pediatric patients (4-17 years) has been shown to be similar to adult data.

Absorption: Slow; extensive ≥85%

Distribution: Apparent V_d: ~50 L (dose-dependent, dose: 3200 mg/day)

Protein binding: 34%, primarily to albumin

Metabolism: Extensively via carboxylesterase-mediated hydrolysis of the carboxylamide group to CGP 47292 (inactive metabolite); weak inhibitor of CYP2E1 and weak inducer of CYP3A4

Bioavailability: Extent decreased with increased dose; oral tablets and oral suspension are bioequivalent

Half-life: ~6-10 hours

Time to peak serum concentration: 4-6 hours

Elimination: Urine [85%, ~66% as CGP 47292 (inactive metabolite), <2% as unchanged drug]

Dialysis: Decreased AUC by 30% and maximum serum concentration by 16%; consider dosage adjustment

Dosing: Usual Oral: Lennox-Gastaut syndrome:

Children ≥4 years: Initial: 10 mg/kg/day in 2 equally divided doses; increase dose by ~10 mg/kg increments every other day to a target dose of 45 mg/kg/day in 2 equally divided doses (maximum dose: 3200 mg/day); effectiveness of doses lower than the target dose is unknown.

Adults: Initial: 400-800 mg/day in 2 equally divided doses; increase dose by 400-800 mg/day every other day to a maximum dose of 3200 mg/day in 2 equally divided doses; effectiveness of doses lower than 3200 mg/day is unknown.

Dosage adjustment for concomitant medications: Valproate: Initial rufinamide dose should be <10 mg/kg/day (children) or 400 mg/day (adults)

Dosage adjustment in renal impairment:

CrCl <30 mL/minute: No dosage adjustment needed

Hemodialysis: No specific guidelines available; consider dosage adjustment for loss of drug

Dosage adjustment in hepatic impairment:

Mild to moderate impairment: Use with caution

Severe impairment: Use in severe impairment has not been studied and is not recommended

Administration Administer with food.

Tablets: May be swallowed whole, split in half, or crushed.

Oral suspension: Shake well; use provided adapter and calibrated oral syringe to measure dose.

Monitoring Parameters Seizure frequency, duration, and severity; CBC; signs and symptoms of suicidality (eg, anxiety, depression, behavior changes); consider ECG (with concurrent medications that can shorten QT interval)

Dosage Forms Excipient information presented when available (limited, particularly for generics); consult specific product labeling.

Suspension, Oral:

Banzel: 40 mg/mL (460 mL) [contains methylparaben, propylene glycol, propylparaben; orange flavor]

Tablet, Oral:

Banzel: 200 mg, 400 mg [scored]

Extemporaneous Preparations A 40 mg/mL oral suspension may be made using tablets. Crush twelve 400 mg tablets (or twenty-four 200 mg tablets) and reduce to a fine powder. Add 60 mL of Ora-Plus® in incremental proportions until a smooth suspension is obtained; then mix well while adding 60 mL of Ora-Sweet® or Ora-Sweet® SF; transfer to a calibrated bottle. Label "shake well". Stable 90 days at room temperature.

Hutchinson DJ, Liou Y, Best R, et al, "Stability of Extemporaneously Prepared Rufinamide Oral Suspensions," *Ann Pharmacother*, 2010, 44(3):462-5.

References

American Academy of Pediatrics Committee on Drugs, "'Inactive' Ingredients in Pharmaceutical Products: Update (Subject Review)," *Pediatr*, 1997, 99(2):268-78.

Glauser T, Kluger G, Sachdeo R, et al, "Rufinamide for Generalized Seizures Associated With Lennox-Gastaut Syndrome," *Neurology*, 2008, 70(21):1950-8.

◆ **RV1 (Rotarix)** *see* Rotavirus Vaccine *on page 1855*

◆ **RV5 (RotaTeq)** *see* Rotavirus Vaccine *on page 1855*

◆ **Rylosol (Can)** *see* Sotalol *on page 1925*

◆ **Rythmodan® (Can)** *see* Disopyramide *on page 694*

◆ **Rythmodan®-LA (Can)** *see* Disopyramide *on page 694*

◆ **S2 [OTC]** *see* EPINEPHrine (Systemic, Oral Inhalation) *on page 761*

◆ **Sabril** *see* Vigabatrin *on page 2134*

Sacrosidase (sak ROE si dase)

Brand Names: U.S. Sucraid

Brand Names: Canada Sucraid®

Therapeutic Category Sucrase Deficiency, Treatment Agent

Generic Availability (U.S.) No

Use Replacement therapy in congenital sucrase-isomaltase deficiency (CSID) [FDA approved in pediatric patients (age not specified) and adults]

Prescribing and Access Restrictions Sucraid® is not available in retail pharmacies or via mail-order pharmacies. To obtain the product, please refer to http://www.sucraid.net/how-to-order-sucraid or call 1-866-740-2743.

Pregnancy Risk Factor C

Pregnancy Considerations Animal reproduction studies have not been conducted. Use is not expected to cause fetal harm when used during pregnancy; administer to a pregnant woman only when indicated.

Breast-Feeding Considerations Sacrosidase is broken down in the stomach and intestines and the component amino acids and peptides are then absorbed as nutrients.

Contraindications Hypersensitivity to sacrosidase or any component, yeast, yeast products, glycerin (glycerol), or papain

Warnings Hypersensitivity reactions to sacrosidase, including bronchospasm, have been reported; administer initial doses in a setting where acute hypersensitivity reactions may be treated within a few minutes; skin testing may be performed prior to administration to potentially identify patients at risk for hypersensitivity reactions. Product may contain papain; severe hypersensitivity reactions, including anaphylaxis, have been observed with papain exposure. Tachycardia and hypotension, in association with some papain-induced hypersensitivity reactions, have also been observed. In addition, inconclusive data suggests a possible cross-sensitivity may exist between patients with natural rubber latex hypersensitivity and papaya, the source of papain. Use is contraindicated in patients with a known papain hypersensitivity. Oral solution contains 50% glycerol.

Precautions Use with caution in diabetes mellitus; sacrosidase enables absorption of the by-products of sucrose hydrolysis (glucose and fructose); monitor serum glucose; diet and/or insulin dosage may need to be adjusted.

Adverse Reactions

Central nervous system: Headache, insomnia, nervousness

Endocrine & metabolic: Dehydration

Gastrointestinal: Abdominal pain, constipation, diarrhea, nausea, vomiting

Rare but important or life-threatening: Hypersensitivity reactions, wheezing

Drug Interactions

Metabolism/Transport Effects None known.

Avoid Concomitant Use There are no known interactions where it is recommended to avoid concomitant use.

Increased Effect/Toxicity There are no known significant interactions involving an increase in effect.

Decreased Effect There are no known significant interactions involving a decrease in effect.

Food Interactions May be inactivated or denatured if administered with fruit juice or warm or hot food/liquids. Isomaltase deficiency is not addressed by supplementation of sacrosidase. Management: Administer with 2-4 oz of water, milk, or formula. Because isomaltase deficiency is not addressed by supplementation of sacrosidase, adherence to a low-starch diet may be required.

Stability Store at 2°C to 8°C (36°F to 46°F); protect from light; discard 4 weeks after opening

Mechanism of Action Sacrosidase is a naturally-occurring gastrointestinal enzyme derived from baker's yeast (*Saccharomyces cerevisiae*) which breaks down the disaccharide sucrose to its monosaccharide components. Hydrolysis is necessary to allow absorption of these nutrients.

Pharmacokinetics (Adult data unless noted) Metabolism: Sacrosidase is metabolized in the GI tract to individual amino acids which are systemically absorbed

Dosing: Usual Congenital sucrose-isomaltase deficiency (CSID) or sucrase deficiency; oral replacement (CSID): Oral:

Infants and Children ≤15 kg: 8500 units (1 mL) per meal or snack

Children >15 kg, Adolescents, and Adults: 17,000 units (2 mL) per meal or snack

Administration Oral: Dilute in 2-4 ounces of water, milk, or formula; approximately ¹/₂ of the dose may be taken before, and the remainder of the dose at the completion of, each meal or snack; do not administer with fruit juices, warm or hot food or liquids

Monitoring Parameters Breath hydrogen test, oral sucrose tolerance test, urinary disaccharides, intestinal disaccharidases (measured from small bowel biopsy)

CSID symptomatology: Diarrhea, abdominal pain, gas, and bloating

Additional Information 1 mL = 22 drops from sacrosidase container tip

Dosage Forms Excipient information presented when available (limited, particularly for generics); consult specific product labeling.

Solution, Oral:

Sucraid: 8500 units/mL (118 mL) [contains papain]

References

Treem WR, McAdams L, Stanford L, et al, "Sacrosidase Therapy for Congenital Sucrose-Isomaltase Deficiency," *J Pediatr Gastroenterol Nutr*, 1999, 28(2):137-42.

◆ **Safe Tussin DM [OTC]** *see* Guaifenesin and Dextromethorphan *on page 987*

◆ **Safe Wash [OTC]** *see* Sodium Chloride *on page 1902*

◆ **Saizen** *see* Somatropin *on page 1920*

◆ **Saizen Click.Easy** *see* Somatropin *on page 1920*

◆ **SalAc [OTC]** *see* Salicylic Acid *on page 1860*

◆ **Salactic Film [OTC]** *see* Salicylic Acid *on page 1860*

◆ **Salacyn** *see* Salicylic Acid *on page 1860*

◆ **Salagen** *see* Pilocarpine (Systemic) *on page 1674*

◆ **Salagen® (Can)** *see* Pilocarpine (Systemic) *on page 1674*

◆ **Salazopyrin (Can)** *see* SulfaSALAzine *on page 1954*

◆ **Salazopyrin En-Tabs (Can)** *see* SulfaSALAzine *on page 1954*

◆ **Salbutamol** *see* Albuterol *on page 84*

◆ **Salbutamol HFA (Can)** *see* Albuterol *on page 84*

◆ **Salbutamol Sulphate** *see* Albuterol *on page 84*

◆ **Salex** *see* Salicylic Acid *on page 1860*

◆ **Salicylazosulfapyridine** *see* SulfaSALAzine *on page 1954*

Salicylic Acid (sal i SIL ik AS id)

Medication Safety Issues

Sound-alike/look-alike issues:

Occlusal™-HP may be confused with Ocuflox®

Other safety concerns:

Transdermal patch may contain conducting metal (eg, aluminum); remove patch prior to MRI.

Brand Names: U.S. Bensal HP; Betasal [OTC]; Calicylic [OTC]; Clear Away 1-Step Wart Remover [OTC]; Corn Remover One Step [OTC]; Corn Remover Ultra Thin [OTC]; DHS Sal [OTC]; Exuviance Blemish Treatment [OTC]; Gordofilm; Hydrisalic [OTC]; Ionil [OTC]; Keralyt; Keralyt Scalp; Keralyt [OTC]; Mediplast [OTC]; Neutrogena Oil-Free Acne Wash [OTC]; One Step Callus Remover [OTC]; P & S [OTC]; Psoriasin [OTC]; Sal-Plant [OTC]; SalAc [OTC]; Salactic Film [OTC]; Salacyn; Salex; Salicylic Acid Wart Remover; Salkera; Salvax; Scalpicin 2 in 1 [OTC]; Scholls Callus Removers [OTC] [DSC]; Scholls Corn Removers Extra [OTC] [DSC]; Scholls Corn Removers Small [OTC] [DSC]; Scholls Corn Removers [OTC] [DSC]; Sebasorb [OTC]; Stri-Dex Maximum Strength [OTC]; Stri-Dex Sensitive Skin [OTC]; Stridex Essential [OTC]; Tinamed Corn/Callus Remover [OTC]; Tinamed Wart Remover [OTC]; Trans-Ver-Sal AdultPatch [OTC]; Trans-Ver-Sal PediaPatch [OTC]; Trans-Ver-Sal PlantarPatch [OTC]; UltraSal-ER; Virasal

Brand Names: Canada Duofilm®; Duoforte® 27; Occlusal™-HP; Sebcur®; Soluver®; Soluver® Plus; Trans-Plantar®; Trans-Ver-Sal®

Therapeutic Category Keratolytic Agent

Generic Availability (U.S.) May be product dependent

Use Topically for its keratolytic effect in controlling seborrheic dermatitis or psoriasis of body and scalp, dandruff, and other scaling dermatoses; removing excessive keratin in hyperkeratotic skin disorders (eg, verrucae, ichthyoses, keratosis palmaris and plantaris, keratosis pilaris, and pityriasis rubra pilaris); removing warts, corns, calluses; used in the treatment of acne

Pregnancy Risk Factor C

Pregnancy Considerations Adverse events have been observed in animal reproduction studies when administered orally. Salicylates cross the placenta (Østensen, 1998). Systemic absorption of topically applied salicylic acid varies depending on duration and vehicle (9% to 25%) (Akhavan, 2003).

Breast-Feeding Considerations Oral salicylates are found in breast milk (Bar-Oz, 2003). Systemic absorption of topically applied salicylic acid varies depending on duration and vehicle (9% to 25%) (Akhavan, 2003). Breast-feeding is not recommended by the manufacturer.

Contraindications Hypersensitivity to salicylic acid or any component; children <2 years of age

Warnings Should not be used systemically due to severe irritating effect on GI mucosa; prolonged use over large areas, especially in children, may result in salicylate toxicity; do not apply on irritated, reddened, or infected skin; do not use on moles, birthmarks, warts with hair growing from them, or genital warts; topical liquid may contain tartrazine which may cause allergic reactions in susceptible individuals

Precautions For external use only; avoid contact with eyes, face, lips, and other mucous membranes

Adverse Reactions

Central nervous system: Dizziness, headache, mental confusion

Local: Burning and irritation at site of exposure on normal tissue, peeling, scaling

Otic: Tinnitus

Respiratory: Hyperventilation

Drug Interactions

Metabolism/Transport Effects None known.

Avoid Concomitant Use There are no known interactions where it is recommended to avoid concomitant use.

Increased Effect/Toxicity There are no known significant interactions involving an increase in effect.

Decreased Effect There are no known significant interactions involving a decrease in effect.

Mechanism of Action Produces desquamation of hyperkeratotic epithelium via dissolution of the intercellular cement which causes the cornified tissue to swell, soften, macerate, and desquamate. Salicylic acid is keratolytic at concentrations of 3% to 6%; it becomes destructive to tissue at concentrations >6%. Concentrations of 6% to 60% are used to remove corns and warts and in the treatment of psoriasis and other hyperkeratotic disorders.

Pharmacokinetics (Adult data unless noted)

Absorption: Topical: Readily absorbed

Time to peak serum concentration: Within 5 hours when applied with an occlusive dressing

Elimination: Salicyluric acid (52%), salicylate glucuronides (42%), and salicylic acid (6%) are the major metabolites identified in urine after percutaneous absorption

Dosing: Usual Children ≥2 years and Adults: Topical:

Foam: Apply to the affected area twice daily. Rub into skin until completely absorbed.

Lotion, cream, gel: Apply a thin layer to the affected area once or twice daily

Shampoo: Initial: Use daily or every other day; app hair and massage vigorously into the scalp; rins thoroughly after shampooing; 1-2 treatments/week usually maintain control

Solution: Apply a thin layer directly to wart using brush applicator once daily as directed for 1 week or until the wart is removed

Administration Topical: For external use only. Not for ophthalmic, oral, anal, or intravaginal use. When applying in concentrations >10%, protect surrounding normal tissue with petrolatum

Monitoring Parameters Signs and symptoms of salicylate toxicity: Nausea, vomiting, dizziness, tinnitus, loss of hearing, lethargy, diarrhea, psychic disturbances

Dosage Forms Excipient information presented when available (limited, particularly for generics); consult specific product labeling. [DSC] = Discontinued product

Cream, External:

Calicylic: 10% (60 g)

Salacyn: 6% (400 g) [contains cetyl alcohol, disodium edta, methylparaben, propylparaben, trolamine (triethanolamine)]

Generic: 6% (400 g, 454 g)

Foam, External:

SalAc: 2% (100 g) [contains alcohol, usp]

Salkera: 6% (60 g) [contains cetostearyl alcohol, edetate disodium dihydrate, methylparaben, propylene glycol, propylparaben]

Salvax: 6% (70 g, 200 g) [contains ethylparaben, methylparaben, polysorbate 80, propylene glycol, propylparaben, trolamine (triethanolamine)]

Generic: 6% (70 g, 200 g)

Gel, External:

Exuviance Blemish Treatment: 2% (15 g) [contains denatured alcohol, peanut oil, propylene glycol]

Hydrisalic: 17% (14 g) [contains fd&c red #40, isopropyl alcohol]

Keralyt: 3% (28.4 g) [contains alcohol, usp]

Keralyt: 6% (40 g, 100 g) [contains hydroxypropyl cellulose, propylene glycol, sd alcohol 40]

Sal-Plant: 17% (14 g)

Generic: 6% (40 g)

Kit, External:

Keralyt Scalp: 6% [contains edetate sodium (tetrasodium), propylene glycol, sd alcohol 40]

Salex: 6% [contains cetyl alcohol, disodium edta, methylparaben, propylparaben, trolamine (triethanolamine)]

Generic: 6%

Liquid, External:

Ionil: (360 mL)

Neutrogena Oil-Free Acne Wash: 2% (124 mL) [contains benzalkonium chloride, disodium edta, fd&c red #40, propylene glycol]

Psoriasin: 3% (177 mL) [dye free, fragrance free]

Salicylic Acid Wart Remover: 27.5% (10 mL) [contains isopropyl alcohol]

Scalpicin 2 in 1: 3% (44 mL) [fragrance free; contains menthol, propylene glycol]

Tinamed Corn/Callus Remover: 17% (14.8 mL)

Tinamed Wart Remover: 17% (14.8 mL) [contains alcohol, usp]

Virasal: 27.5% (10 mL) [contains isopropyl alcohol, isopropyl-metacresol (isopropyl-m-cresol]

Generic: 26% (10 mL); 27.5% (10 mL)

Lotion, External:

Salacyn: 6% (414 mL) [contains cetyl alcohol, disodium edta, methylparaben, propylparaben, trolamine (triethanolamine)]

Sebasorb: Attapulgite 10% and salicylic acid 2% (42 g)

Generic: 6% (400 g, 414 mL, 473 mL)

Ointment, External:

Bensal HP: 3% (4 g, 15 g, 30 g)

Pad, External:
Clear Away 1-Step Wart Remover: 40% (14 ea)
Corn Remover One Step: 40% (6 ea)
Corn Remover Ultra Thin: 40% (9 ea)
Mediplast: 40% (1 ea, 25 ea)
One Step Callus Remover: 40% (4 ea)
Scholls Callus Removers: 40% (4 ea [DSC], 6 ea [DSC])
Scholls Corn Removers: 40% (9 ea [DSC])
Scholls Corn Removers Extra: 40% (9 ea [DSC])
Scholls Corn Removers Small: 40% (9 ea [DSC])
Stri-Dex Maximum Strength: 2% (55 ea, 90 ea) [alcohol free]
Stri-Dex Sensitive Skin: 0.5% (55 ea, 90 ea) [alcohol free]
Stridex Essential: 1% (55 ea) [alcohol free; contains menthol, tetrasodium etidronate]
Patch, External:
Trans-Ver-Sal AdultPatch: 15% (12 ea, 40 ea)
Trans-Ver-Sal PediaPatch: 15% (15 ea, 40 ea)
Trans-Ver-Sal PlantarPatch: 15% (10 ea)
Shampoo, External:
Betasal: 3% (480 mL)
DHS Sal: 3% (120 mL)
DHS Sal: 3% (120 mL) [contains disodium edta]
Ionil: 2% (120 mL)
P & S: 2% (236 mL) [contains edetate sodium (tetrasodium), methylparaben, propylparaben, trolamine (triethanolamine)]
Salex: 6% (177 mL) [contains methylparaben, propylparaben, trolamine (triethanolamine)]
Generic: 6% (177 mL)
Solution, External:
Gordofilm: 16.7% (15 mL)
Salactic Film: 17% (15 mL)
UltraSal-ER: 28.5% (10 mL) [contains isopropyl alcohol, phenol, polysorbate 80]

References
Akhavan A and Bershad S, "Topical Acne Drugs: Review of Clinical Properties, Systemic Exposure, and Safety," *Am J Clin Dermatol*, 2003, 4(7):473-92.
Bar-Oz B, Bulkowstein M, Benyamini L, et al, "Use of Antibiotic and Analgesic Drugs During Lactation," *Drug Saf*, 2003, 26(13):925-35.
Østensen M, "Nonsteroidal Anti-inflammatory Drugs During Pregnancy," *Scand J Rheumatol Suppl*, 1998, 107:128-32.

◆ **Salicylic Acid and Sulfur** *see* Sulfur and Salicylic Acid *on page 1956*

◆ **Salicylic Acid Wart Remover** *see* Salicylic Acid *on page 1860*

◆ **Saline** *see* Sodium Chloride *on page 1902*

◆ **Saline Flush ZR** *see* Sodium Chloride *on page 1902*

◆ **Saline Mist Spray [OTC]** *see* Sodium Chloride *on page 1902*

◆ **Saljet [OTC]** *see* Sodium Chloride *on page 1902*

◆ **Saljet Rinse [OTC]** *see* Sodium Chloride *on page 1902*

◆ **Salkera** *see* Salicylic Acid *on page 1860*

◆ **Salk Vaccine** *see* Poliovirus Vaccine (Inactivated) *on page 1694*

Salmeterol (sal ME te role)

Medication Safety Issues
Sound-alike/look-alike issues:
Salmeterol may be confused with Salbutamol, Solu-Medrol
Serevent may be confused with Atrovent, Combivent, sertraline, Sinemet, Spiriva, Zoloft
Brand Names: U.S. Serevent Diskus
Brand Names: Canada Serevent Diskhaler Disk; Serevent Diskus
Therapeutic Category Adrenergic Agonist Agent; Antiasthmatic; Beta₂-Adrenergic Agonist; Bronchodilator
Generic Availability (U.S.) No

Use Concomitant therapy with inhaled corticosteroids for maintenance treatment of asthma and prevention of bronchospasm in patients with reversible obstructive airway disease, including patients with nocturnal symptoms (FDA approved in ages ≥4 years and adults); prevention of exercise-induced bronchospasm as concomitant therapy in patients with persistent asthma and as monotherapy in those without persistent asthma (FDA approved in ages ≥4 years and adults); maintenance treatment of bronchospasm associated with COPD (FDA approved in adults); **NOT** indicated for the relief of acute bronchospasm
Medication Guide Available Yes
Pregnancy Risk Factor C
Pregnancy Considerations Adverse events were observed in some animal reproduction studies. Beta-agonists have the potential to affect uterine contractility if administered during labor.

Uncontrolled asthma is associated with adverse events on pregnancy (increased risk of perinatal mortality, preeclampsia, preterm birth, low birth weight infants). Although data related to its use in pregnancy is limited, salmeterol may be used when a long-acting beta agonist is needed to treat moderate persistent or severe persistent asthma in pregnant women (NAEPP, 2005).
Breast-Feeding Considerations It is not known if salmeterol is excreted into breast milk. The manufacturer recommends that caution be exercised when administering salmeterol to nursing women. The use of beta₂-receptor agonists are not considered a contraindication to breast-feeding (NAEPP, 2005).
Contraindications Hypersensitivity to salmeterol, adrenergic amines, or any component; severe hypersensitivity to milk proteins; monotherapy in the treatment of asthma (ie, use without a concomitant long-term asthma control medication, such as an inhaled corticosteroid); treatment of status asthmaticus or other acute episodes of asthma or COPD
Warnings Long-acting beta₂-adrenergic agents (LABAs), including salmeterol, increase the risk of asthma-related deaths **[U.S. Boxed Warning]**. Salmeterol should only be prescribed in patients not adequately controlled on long-term asthma-controller medications (ie, inhaled corticosteroid) or whose disease severity requires initiation of two maintenance therapies. Monotherapy with a LABA is contraindicated in the treatment of asthma. In a large clinical trial, LABA (salmeterol) use was associated with an increase in asthma-related deaths compared to placebo (when added to usual asthma therapy); risk is considered a class effect among all LABAs. Data are not available to determine if the addition of an inhaled corticosteroid lessens this increased risk of death associated with LABA use or if LABA use also increases the risk of death in patients with COPD. Assess patients at regular intervals once asthma control is maintained on combination therapy to determine if step-down therapy is appropriate (without loss of asthma control), and the patient can be maintained on an inhaled corticosteroid only. LABAs are not appropriate in patients whose asthma is adequately controlled on low- or medium-dose inhaled corticosteroids. LABAs may increase the risk of asthma-related hospitalization in pediatric and adolescent patients **[U.S. Boxed Warning]**; when addition of a LABA is clinically indicated in patients <18 years of age, a combination product containing a LABA and an inhaled corticosteroid is preferred to ensure compliance.

Salmeterol should not be used to relieve acute asthmatic or COPD symptoms, rapidly deteriorating, or potentially life-threatening episodes of asthma or COPD; acute episodes should be treated with short-acting beta₂-agonist. Routine use of inhaled, short-acting beta₂-agonists should be discontinued prior to initiation of salmeterol. Corticosteroids should not be stopped or reduced when salmeterol is initiated. Salmeterol should not be used more frequently than recommended (twice daily), at higher doses or with any additional long-acting beta₂-adrenergic agonist; adverse cardiovascular effects (possibly fatal) have been reported with excessive beta₂-adrenergic over-stimulation. Not recommended for use with strong CYP3A4 inhibitors (eg, ketoconazole, ritonavir, atazanavir, clarithromycin, indinavir, itraconazole, nefazodone, nelfinavir, saquinavir, telithromycin) due to potential for an increased risk of cardiovascular events. Paroxysmal bronchospasm (which can be fatal) has been reported with salmeterol and other beta₂-agonist inhaled agents; if this occurs, discontinue treatment; most commonly occurs with first use of a new canister or vial. Symptoms of laryngeal spasm, irritation, or swelling, such as stridor and choking, have been reported; if occurs, discontinue treatment. Because LABAs may disguise poorly-controlled persistent asthma, frequent or chronic use of LABAs for exercise-induced bronchospasm is discouraged by the NAEPP Asthma Guidelines (NAEPP, 2007).

Precautions Use with caution in patients with cardiovascular disorders (especially coronary insufficiency, arrhythmias, hypertension, heart failure), although uncommon at recommended doses, beta-agonists may cause elevation in BP and HR and result in CNS stimulation and excitation. Caution should also be used in patients with thyrotoxicosis, seizure disorders, or conditions that are unusually sensitive to sympathomimetic amines. Transient hypokalemia from intracellular shunting may occur and produce adverse cardiovascular effects. Use with caution in patients with diabetes mellitus (DM); beta₂-agonists can increase serum glucose aggravating preexisting DM and ketoacidosis. Use caution in patients with hepatic impairment. Immediate hypersensitivity reactions (urticaria, angioedema, rash, bronchospasm) have been reported. Powder for oral inhalation contains lactose; very rare anaphylactic reactions have been reported in patients with severe milk protein allergy.

Adverse Reactions

Cardiovascular: Edema, hypertension, pallor

Central nervous system: Anxiety, dizziness, fever, headache, migraine, sleep disturbance

Dermatologic: Contact dermatitis, eczema, photodermatitis, rash, urticaria

Endocrine & metabolic: Hyperglycemia

Gastrointestinal: Dental pain, dyspepsia, gastrointestinal infection, nausea, oropharyngeal candidiasis, throat irritation, xerostomia

Hepatic: Liver enzymes increased

Neuromuscular & skeletal: Arthralgia, articular rheumatism, joint pain, muscular cramps/spasm/stiffness, pain, paresthesia, rigidity

Ocular: Keratitis/conjunctivitis

Respiratory: Asthma, cough, influenza, nasal congestion, pharyngitis, rhinitis, sinusitis, tracheitis/bronchitis, viral respiratory tract infection

Rare but important or life-threatening: Abdominal pain, agitation, aggression, anaphylactic reaction (some in patients with severe milk allergy [Diskus®]), angioedema, aphonia, arrhythmia, atrial fibrillation, cataracts, chest congestion, chest tightness, choking, contusions, Cushing syndrome, Cushingoid features, depression, dysmenorrhea, dyspnea, earache, ecchymoses, edema (facial, oropharyngeal), eosinophilic conditions, glaucoma, growth velocity reduction in children/adolescents, hypercorticism, hypersensitivity reaction (immediate and delayed), hypokalemia, hypothyroidism, intraocular pressure increased, laryngeal spasm/irritation, irregular menstruation, myositis, oropharyngeal irritation, osteoporosis, pallor, paradoxical bronchospasm, paradoxical tracheitis, paranasal sinus pain, PID, QTc prolongation, restlessness, stridor, supraventricular tachycardia, syncope, tremor, vaginal candidiasis, vaginitis, vulvovaginitis, rare

cases of vasculitis (Churg-Strauss syndrome), ventricular tachycardia, weight gain

Drug Interactions

Metabolism/Transport Effects Substrate of CYP3A4 (major); **Note:** Assignment of Major/Minor substrate status based on clinically relevant drug interaction potential

Avoid Concomitant Use

Avoid concomitant use of Salmeterol with any of the following: Beta-Blockers (Nonselective); Cobicistat; Conivaptan; CYP3A4 Inhibitors (Strong); Fusidic Acid (Systemic); Iobenguane I 123; Long-Acting Beta2-Agonists; Telaprevir; Tipranavir

Increased Effect/Toxicity

Salmeterol may increase the levels/effects of: Atosiban; Highest Risk QTc-Prolonging Agents; Long-Acting Beta2-Agonists; Loop Diuretics; Moderate Risk QTc-Prolonging Agents; Sympathomimetics; Thiazide Diuretics

The levels/effects of Salmeterol may be increased by: AtoMOXetine; Cannabinoid-Containing Products; Ceritinib; Cobicistat; Conivaptan; CYP3A4 Inhibitors (Moderate); CYP3A4 Inhibitors (Strong); Dasatinib; Fusidic Acid (Systemic); Ivacaftor; Linezolid; Luliconazole; MAO Inhibitors; Mifepristone; Simeprevir; Telaprevir; Tipranavir; Tricyclic Antidepressants

Decreased Effect

Salmeterol may decrease the levels/effects of: Iobenguane I 123

The levels/effects of Salmeterol may be decreased by: Beta-Blockers (Beta1 Selective); Beta-Blockers (Nonselective); Betahistine

Stability Store at controlled room temperature 20°C to 25°C (68°F to 77°F) in a dry place away from direct heat or sunlight; stable for 6 weeks after removal from protective foil pouch.

Mechanism of Action Relaxes bronchial smooth muscle by selective action on beta₂-receptors with little effect on heart rate; salmeterol acts locally in the lung.

Pharmacodynamics

Onset of action: Asthma: 30-48 minutes; COPD: 2 hours

Peak effect: Asthma: 3 hours; COPD: 2-5 hours

Duration: Up to 12 hours

Pharmacokinetics (Adult data unless noted)

Protein binding: 96%

Metabolism: Extensive hydroxylation via CYP3A4

Half-life: 5.5 hours

Elimination: 60% in feces and 25% in urine over a 7-day period

Dosing: Usual Children ≥4 years and Adults:

Asthma, maintenance treatment; prevention: Inhalation, oral: 50 mcg (1 actuation/puff) twice daily, 12 hours apart; **Note:** For long-term asthma control, long-acting beta₂-agonists should be used in combination with inhaled corticosteroids and **not** as monotherapy.

Exercise-induced bronchospasm, prevention: Inhalation: 50 mcg (1 inhalation/puff) 30 minutes prior to exercise; additional doses should not be used for 12 hours; patients who are using salmeterol twice daily should **not** use an additional salmeterol dose prior to exercise; if twice daily use is not effective during exercise, consider other appropriate therapy; **Note:** Because long-acting beta₂-agonists (LABAs) may disguise poorly-controlled persistent asthma, frequent or chronic use of LABAs for exercise-induced bronchospasm is discouraged by the NAEPP Asthma Guidelines (NAEPP, 2007).

COPD, maintenance treatment: Adults: 50 mcg (1 inhalation/puff) twice daily (~12 hours apart); maximum: 1 inhalation twice daily

Administration Inhalation: Not for use with a spacer

Monitoring Parameters Pulmonary function tests, vital signs, CNS stimulation, serum glucose, serum potassium

Additional Information When salmeterol is initiated in patients previously receiving a short-acting beta agonist, instruct the patient to discontinue the regular use of the short-acting beta agonist and to utilize the shorter-acting agent for symptomatic or acute episodes only.

Dosage Forms Excipient information presented when available (limited, particularly for generics); consult specific product labeling.

Aerosol Powder Breath Activated, Inhalation:
Serevent Diskus: 50 mcg/dose (28 ea, 60 ea) [contains lactose]

References

Meyer JM, Wenzel CL, and Kradjan WA, "Salmeterol: A Novel, Long-Acting Beta$_2$-Agonist," *Ann Pharmacother*, 1993, 27(12):1478-87.

National Asthma Education and Prevention Program (NAEPP), "Expert Panel Report 3 (EPR-3): Guidelines for the Diagnosis and Management of Asthma," Clinical Practice Guidelines, National Institutes of Health, National Heart, Lung, and Blood Institute, NIH Publication No. 08-4051, prepublication 2007. Available at http://www.nhlbi.nih.gov/guidelines/asthma/asthgdln.htm

National Asthma Education and Prevention Program (NAEPP) Working Group Report on "Managing Asthma During Pregnancy: Recommendations for Pharmacologic Treatment," National Institutes of Health, National Heart, Lung, and Blood Institute, NIH Publication No. 05-5236, March 2005. Available at http://www.nhlbi.nih.gov/health/prof/lung/asthma/astpreg/astpreg_full.pdf

◆ **Salmeterol and Fluticasone** *see* Fluticasone and Salmeterol *on page 916*

◆ **Salmeterol Xinafoate** *see* Salmeterol *on page 1862*

◆ **Salofalk (Can)** *see* Mesalamine *on page 1347*

◆ **Salonpas® Gel-Patch Hot [OTC]** *see* Capsaicin *on page 367*

◆ **Salonpas® Hot [OTC] [DSC]** *see* Capsaicin *on page 367*

◆ **Sal-Plant [OTC]** *see* Salicylic Acid *on page 1860*

◆ **Salt** *see* Sodium Chloride *on page 1902*

◆ **Salt Poor Albumin** *see* Albumin *on page 82*

◆ **Salvax** *see* Salicylic Acid *on page 1860*

◆ **Sancuso** *see* Granisetron *on page 980*

◆ **SandIMMUNE** *see* CycloSPORINE (Systemic) *on page 564*

◆ **Sandimmune I.V. (Can)** *see* CycloSPORINE (Systemic) *on page 564*

◆ **SandoSTATIN** *see* Octreotide *on page 1518*

◆ **Sandostatin® (Can)** *see* Octreotide *on page 1518*

◆ **Sandostatin LAR** *see* Octreotide *on page 1518*

◆ **SandoSTATIN LAR Depot** *see* Octreotide *on page 1518*

◆ **Sandoz-Almotriptan (Can)** *see* Almotriptan *on page 99*

◆ **Sandoz-Amiodarone (Can)** *see* Amiodarone *on page 127*

◆ **Sandoz Amlodipine (Can)** *see* AmLODIPine *on page 135*

◆ **Sandoz-Anagrelide (Can)** *see* Anagrelide *on page 166*

◆ **Sandoz-Atenolol (Can)** *see* Atenolol *on page 222*

◆ **Sandoz-Atomoxetine (Can)** *see* AtoMOXetine *on page 224*

◆ **Sandoz-Atorvastatin (Can)** *see* AtorvaSTATin *on page 227*

◆ **Sandoz-Azithromycin (Can)** *see* Azithromycin (Systemic) *on page 247*

◆ **Sandoz-Bosentan (Can)** *see* Bosentan *on page 298*

◆ **Sandoz-Brimonidine (Can)** *see* Brimonidine (Ophthalmic) *on page 303*

◆ **Sandoz-Bupropion SR (Can)** *see* BuPROPion *on page 327*

◆ **Sandoz-Candesartan (Can)** *see* Candesartan *on page 363*

◆ **Sandoz-Carbamazepine (Can)** *see* CarBAMazepine *on page 372*

◆ **Sandoz-Cefprozil (Can)** *see* Cefprozil *on page 412*

◆ **Sandoz-Ciprofloxacin (Can)** *see* Ciprofloxacin (Systemic) *on page 471*

◆ **Sandoz-Citalopram (Can)** *see* Citalopram *on page 484*

◆ **Sandoz-Clarithromycin (Can)** *see* Clarithromycin *on page 490*

◆ **Sandoz-Clonazepam (Can)** *see* ClonazePAM *on page 514*

◆ **Sandoz-Clopidogrel (Can)** *see* Clopidogrel *on page 521*

◆ **Sandoz-Cyclosporine (Can)** *see* CycloSPORINE (Systemic) *on page 564*

◆ **Sandoz-Diclofenac (Can)** *see* Diclofenac (Systemic) *on page 645*

◆ **Sandoz-Diclofenac Rapide (Can)** *see* Diclofenac (Systemic) *on page 645*

◆ **Sandoz-Diclofenac SR (Can)** *see* Diclofenac (Systemic) *on page 645*

◆ **Sandoz-Diltiazem CD (Can)** *see* Diltiazem *on page 667*

◆ **Sandoz-Diltiazem T (Can)** *see* Diltiazem *on page 667*

◆ **Sandoz-Dimenhydrinate [OTC] (Can)** *see* DimenhyDRINATE *on page 670*

◆ **Sandoz-Dorzolamide (Can)** *see* Dorzolamide *on page 710*

◆ **Sandoz-Enalapril (Can)** *see* Enalapril *on page 744*

◆ **Sandoz-Estradiol Derm 50 (Can)** *see* Estradiol (Systemic) *on page 796*

◆ **Sandoz-Estradiol Derm 75 (Can)** *see* Estradiol (Systemic) *on page 796*

◆ **Sandoz-Estradiol Derm 100 (Can)** *see* Estradiol (Systemic) *on page 796*

◆ **Sandoz-Famciclovir (Can)** *see* Famciclovir *on page 842*

◆ **Sandoz-Felodipine (Can)** *see* Felodipine *on page 850*

◆ **Sandoz Fentanyl Patch (Can)** *see* FentaNYL *on page 853*

◆ **Sandoz-Fluoxetine (Can)** *see* FLUoxetine *on page 901*

◆ **Sandoz-Fluvoxamine (Can)** *see* FluvoxaMINE *on page 922*

◆ **Sandoz-Glyburide (Can)** *see* GlyBURIDE *on page 974*

◆ **Sandoz-Indomethacin (Can)** *see* Indomethacin *on page 1096*

◆ **Sandoz-Irbesartan (Can)** *see* Irbesartan *on page 1147*

◆ **Sandoz-Letrozole (Can)** *see* Letrozole *on page 1211*

◆ **Sandoz-Levobunolol (Can)** *see* Levobunolol *on page 1223*

◆ **Sandoz-Levofloxacin (Can)** *see* Levofloxacin (Systemic) *on page 1228*

◆ **Sandoz-Lisinopril (Can)** *see* Lisinopril *on page 1262*

◆ **Sandoz-Loperamide (Can)** *see* Loperamide *on page 1270*

◆ **Sandoz Losartan (Can)** *see* Losartan *on page 1283*

◆ **Sandoz-Lovastatin (Can)** *see* Lovastatin *on page 1286*

◆ **Sandoz-Metformin FC (Can)** *see* MetFORMIN *on page 1353*

◆ **Sandoz-Methylphenidate SR (Can)** *see* Methylphenidate *on page 1379*

◆ **Sandoz-Metoprolol SR (Can)** *see* Metoprolol *on page 1396*

◆ **Sandoz-Metoprolol (Type L) (Can)** *see* Metoprolol *on page 1396*

◆ **Sandoz-Minocycline (Can)** *see* Minocycline *on page 1420*

- **Sandoz-Montelukast (Can)** *see* Montelukast *on page 1438*
- **Sandoz-Montelukast Granules (Can)** *see* Montelukast *on page 1438*
- **Sandoz-Morphine SR (Can)** *see* Morphine (Systemic) *on page 1440*
- **Sandoz-Mycophenolate (Can)** *see* Mycophenolate *on page 1453*
- **Sandoz-Mycophenolate Mofetil (Can)** *see* Mycophenolate *on page 1453*
- **Sandoz-Olanzapine (Can)** *see* OLANZapine *on page 1525*
- **Sandoz-Olanzapine ODT (Can)** *see* OLANZapine *on page 1525*
- **Sandoz-Omeprazole (Can)** *see* Omeprazole *on page 1535*
- **Sandoz-Ondansetron (Can)** *see* Ondansetron *on page 1544*
- **Sandoz-Oxycodone/Acetaminophen (Can)** *see* Oxycodone and Acetaminophen *on page 1573*
- **Sandoz-Pantoprazole (Can)** *see* Pantoprazole *on page 1595*
- **Sandoz-Paroxetine (Can)** *see* PARoxetine *on page 1609*
- **Sandoz-Pravastatin (Can)** *see* Pravastatin *on page 1720*
- **Sandoz Prednisolone (Can)** *see* PrednisoLONE (Ophthalmic) *on page 1730*
- **Sandoz-Prochlorperazine (Can)** *see* Prochlorperazine *on page 1745*
- **Sandoz-Quetiapine (Can)** *see* QUEtiapine *on page 1783*
- **Sandoz-Quetiapine XRT (Can)** *see* QUEtiapine *on page 1783*
- **Sandoz-Rabeprazole (Can)** *see* RABEprazole *on page 1797*
- **Sandoz-Ranitidine (Can)** *see* Ranitidine *on page 1805*
- **Sandoz-Risperidone (Can)** *see* RisperiDONE *on page 1831*
- **Sandoz-Rizatriptan ODT (Can)** *see* Rizatriptan *on page 1845*
- **Sandoz-Rosuvastatin (Can)** *see* Rosuvastatin *on page 1853*
- **Sandoz-Salbutamol (Can)** *see* Albuterol *on page 84*
- **Sandoz-Sertraline (Can)** *see* Sertraline *on page 1879*
- **Sandoz-Simvastatin (Can)** *see* Simvastatin *on page 1892*
- **Sandoz-Sotalol (Can)** *see* Sotalol *on page 1925*
- **Sandoz-Sumatriptan (Can)** *see* SUMAtriptan *on page 1958*
- **Sandoz-Tacrolimus (Can)** *see* Tacrolimus (Systemic) *on page 1963*
- **Sandoz-Terbinafine (Can)** *see* Terbinafine (Systemic) *on page 1982*
- **Sandoz-Timolol (Can)** *see* Timolol (Ophthalmic) *on page 2028*
- **Sandoz-Tobramycin (Can)** *see* Tobramycin (Ophthalmic) *on page 2039*
- **Sandoz-Topiramate (Can)** *see* Topiramate *on page 2046*
- **Sandoz-Trifluridine (Can)** *see* Trifluridine *on page 2084*
- **Sandoz-Valproic (Can)** *see* Valproic Acid and Derivatives *on page 2102*
- **Sandoz-Valsartan (Can)** *see* Valsartan *on page 2108*

- **Sandoz-Venlafaxine XR (Can)** *see* Venlafaxine *on page 2125*
- **Sani-Supp Adult [OTC]** *see* Glycerin *on page 976*
- **Sani-Supp Pediatric [OTC]** *see* Glycerin *on page 976*

Sapropterin (sap roe TER in)

Medication Safety Issues
Sound-alike/look-alike issues:
  Sapropterin may be confused with cyproterone
Brand Names: U.S. Kuvan
Generic Availability (U.S.) No
Use Adjunct to dietary restriction for the treatment of tetrahydrobiopterin (BH4) responsive phenylketonuria (PKU) to reduce blood phenylalanine (Phe) concentrations (FDA approved in ages ≥4 years and adults)
Pregnancy Risk Factor C
Pregnancy Considerations Adverse events have been observed in some animal reproduction studies. High levels of maternal phenylalanine are associated with congenital heart disease, developmental delay, facial dysmorphism, learning difficulties, and microcephaly. Phenylalanine (PHE) concentrations should be normalized prior to conception. Fetal development is optimal when PHE concentrations <360 micromol/L are achieved prior to conception (Vockley, 2014). Dietary control with proper supplementation is recommended during pregnancy. Maternal PHE requirements may change throughout pregnancy; frequent testing and dietary modifications may be necessary (Vockley, 2014). Some clinicians recommend that dietary control be achieved for at least 4 weeks prior to conception; however, studies suggest that as long as control is achieved by 10 weeks of pregnancy, teratogenic effects of untreated maternal phenylketonuria can be decreased (Koch, 2003; Maillot, 2007). In addition to standard fetal monitoring, fetal echocardiography is recommended at 18-22 weeks gestation (Vockley, 2014). Pregnant women exposed to sapropterin are encouraged to enroll in the Kuvan pregnancy registry (866-906-6100).
Breast-Feeding Considerations It is not known if sapropterin is excreted in breast milk. The manufacturer recommends that caution be exercised when administering sapropterin to nursing women. Infants unaffected by phenylalanine hydroxylase (PHA) deficiency are able to metabolize the slightly higher PHE concentrations from breast milk of mothers with PHA deficiency (Vockley, 2014).
Contraindications Hypersensitivity to sapropterin or any component
Warnings Phenylalanine (Phe) serum concentrations should be monitored and maintained within the patient's target range during sapropterin treatment; elevated Phe serum concentrations may cause severe neurological damage (including mental retardation, microcephaly, delayed speech, seizures, and behavioral abnormalities) and low Phe serum concentrations are associated with catabolism and protein breakdown; dietary management of Phe intake is required to ensure nutritional balance and adequate phenylalanine control. Response rate to sapropterin during clinical trials was variable (~20% to 56%); assessment of response is established through therapeutic trial only and cannot be predetermined by lab testing; if Phe serum concentrations do not decrease after treatment at a dose of 20 mg/kg/day for 1 month, the patient should be considered a nonresponder and sapropterin discontinued.

Severe allergic reactions were not observed in clinical trials; however, patients with mild to moderate allergy (eg, rash) should be evaluated for risk vs benefit prior to continuing therapy.

Precautions Sapropterin should be used in conjunction with a phenylalanine-restricted diet as prescribed by clinician experienced in management of PKU patients. Use with caution in patients with hepatic or renal impairment; monitor carefully; use has not been studied in these patients; hepatic damage has been associated with impaired phenylalanine metabolism. Use with caution in patients taking concurrent medications that affect nitric oxide-mediated vasorelaxation, including phosphodiesterase 5 (PDE-5) inhibitors (eg, sildenafil, tadalafil, vardenafil); additive effects may potentially lead to decreased blood pressure; combination has not been evaluated in humans. Use with caution with concomitant folic acid antagonists (eg, methotrexate) and derivatives therapy; folic acid antagonists may decrease tetrahydrobiopterin (BH4) levels via dihydropteridine reductase enzyme inhibition. Use with caution in patients with neurological disorders or receiving levodopa; seizure, overstimulation, and irritability were reported in postmarketing safety data.

Adverse Reactions

Central nervous system: Headache

Respiratory: Rhinorrhea

Gastrointestinal: Diarrhea, vomiting

Respiratory: Cough, nasal congestion, pharyngolaryngeal pain

Rare but important or life-threatening: Anaphylaxis, gastritis, gastrointestinal hemorrhage, hemorrhage (postprocedural), hyperactivity, increased gamma-glutamyl transferase, myocardial infarction, peripheral edema, seizure (including seizure exacerbation), upper respiratory tract infection

Drug Interactions

Metabolism/Transport Effects None known.

Avoid Concomitant Use There are no known interactions where it is recommended to avoid concomitant use.

Increased Effect/Toxicity

Sapropterin may increase the levels/effects of: Levodopa; Phosphodiesterase 5 Inhibitors

Decreased Effect

The levels/effects of Sapropterin may be decreased by: Methotrexate; PRALAtrexate

Stability Store at 20°C to 25°C (68°F to 77°F); excursions permitted to 15°C to 30°C (59°F to 86°F); protect from moisture; may change to light yellow color over time, normal occurrence and safe to use.

Mechanism of Action Sapropterin is a synthetic form of the cofactor BH4 (tetrahydrobiopterin) for the enzyme phenylalanine hydroxylase (PAH). PAH hydroxylates phenylalanine to form tyrosine. BH4 activates residual PAH enzyme, improving normal phenylalanine metabolism and decreasing phenylalanine levels in sapropterin responders. Approximately 25% to 50% of patients with PAH deficiency are responsive to sapropterin (Vockley, 2014).

Pharmacodynamics

Onset of action: Within 24 hours of initial dose, decreases in serum Phe concentrations

Maximum effect: 1-2 months

Duration: 24 hours

Pharmacokinetics (Adult data unless noted)

Absorption: Enhanced with food; high-fat/high-calorie

Half-life: 6.7 hours (range: ~4-17 hours)

Dosing: Usual Phenylketonuria (PKU), adjunct treatment:

Infants ≥7 months and Children <4 years: Limited data available: Oral: Initial: 10-20 mg/kg/dose once daily; some clinicians report beginning with a lower dose and adjusting upward to effect while others began at high end of range and once response established decreased dosage to lowest effective dose; dosing based on a multicenter, case series (n=6). Reported dosing tended to round to the nearest 100 mg increment so dosages up to 24 mg/kg/day were used; clinicians also reported

positive response to therapy through dietary increases of phenylalanine consumption as opposed to significant decreases in serum Phe concentrations (Burton, 2011)

Children ≥4 years, Adolescents: Oral:

Initial: 10 mg/kg/dose once daily; may increase to 20 mg/kg/dose once daily if serum Phe concentration has not decreased after 1 month. Serum Phe concentrations should be evaluated after the initial week of therapy or with any dosage adjustment and periodically to assess response to therapy. If positive response to therapy occurs, begin maintenance dosing and monitoring. If serum Phe concentration has not decreased from baseline after 1 month at 20 mg/kg/dose once daily, discontinue therapy (nonresponder).

Maintenance: 5-20 mg/kg/dose once daily

Adults: Oral: Initial: 10 mg/kg/dose once daily; adjust after 1 month based on blood phenylalanine levels (if phenylalanine levels do not decrease from baseline, increase dose to 20 mg/kg once daily); discontinue if phenylalanine levels do not decrease after 1 month of treatment at 20 mg/kg/day (nonresponder). Maintenance range: 5-20 mg/kg once daily

Administration Administer with food, preferably at the same time each day. Dissolve tablets in 120-240 mL (4-8 oz) water or apple juice; may crush or stir to aid in dissolution; dissolution may take several minutes and may not be complete (eg, small piece floating on surface of liquid); this is expected. Dose should be consumed within 15 minutes of dissolution; may rinse remaining tablet residue (with more water or apple juice) and drink. For use in infants and young children, sapropterin has shown similar stability when mixed with phenylalanine-free formula, applesauce, and pudding (Burton, 2011a).

Monitoring Parameters Phenylalanine serum concentrations (baseline, after 1 week of treatment, periodically for first month, regularly thereafter); children may require more frequent monitoring

Dosage Forms Excipient information presented when available (limited, particularly for generics); consult specific product labeling.

Packet, Oral, as dihydrochloride:

Kuvan: 100 mg (1 ea, 30 ea)

Tablet Soluble, Oral, as dihydrochloride:

Kuvan: 100 mg

References

Burton BK, Adams DJ, Grange DK, et al, "Letters to the Editor: Reply: Tetrahydrobiopterin and Phenylketonuria," J Pediatr, 2011a, 158:864-5.

Burton BK, Adams DJ, Grange DK, et al, "Tetrahydrobiopterin Therapy for Phenylketonuria in Infants and Young Children," J Pediatr, 2011, 158(3):410-5.

Burton BK, Grange DK, Milanowski A, et al, "The Response of Patients With Phenylketonuria and Elevated Serum Phenylalanine to Treatment With Oral Sapropterin Dihydrochloride (6R-Tetrahydrobiopterin): A Phase II, Multicentre, Open-Label, Screening Study," J Inherit Metab Dis, 2007, 30(5):700-7.

Koch R, Hanley W, Levy H, et al, "The Maternal Phenylketonuria International Study: 1984-2002," Pediatrics, 2003, 112(6 Pt 2):1523-9.

Levy H, Burton B, Cederbaum S, et al, "Recommendations for Evaluation of Responsiveness to Tetrahydrobiopterin (BH4) in Phenylketonuria and Its Use in Treatment," Mol Genet Metab, 2007, 92 (4):287-291.

Levy HL, Milanowski A, Chakrapani A, et al, "Efficacy of Sapropterin Dihydrochloride (Tetrahydrobiopterin, 6R-BH4) for Reduction of Phenylalanine Concentration in Patients With Phenylketonuria: A Phase III Randomised Placebo-Controlled Study," Lancet, 2007, 370 (9586):504-10.

Maillot F, Cook P, Lilburn M, et al, "A Practical Approach to Maternal Phenylketonuria Management," J Inherit Metab Dis, 2007, 30 (2):198-201.

◆ **Sapropterin Dihydrochloride** see Sapropterin on page 1865

Saquinavir (sa KWIN a veer)

Medication Safety Issues
Sound-alike/look-alike issues:
Saquinavir may be confused with SINEquan®

Related Information
Adult and Adolescent HIV *on page 2348*
Pediatric HIV *on page 2338*
Perinatal HIV *on page 2356*

Brand Names: U.S. Invirase
Brand Names: Canada Invirase®
Therapeutic Category Antiretroviral Agent; HIV Agents (Anti-HIV Agents); Protease Inhibitor
Generic Availability (U.S.) No
Use Treatment of HIV infection in combination with other antiretroviral agents (FDA approved in ages ≥16 years and adults); **Note:** HIV regimens consisting of three antiretroviral agents are strongly recommended; due to its low bioavailability, Invirase must only be used in combination regimens that include ritonavir "booster doses" so that adequate plasma saquinavir concentrations are attained
Medication Guide Available Yes
Pregnancy Risk Factor B
Pregnancy Considerations Adverse events were not observed in animal reproduction studies. Saquinavir has a low level of transfer across the human placenta. Based on available data, saquinavir administered twice daily with ritonavir 100 mg twice daily provide adequate levels in pregnant women. The DHHS Perinatal HIV Guidelines consider saquinavir and ritonavir to be an alternative combination for use in antiretroviral-naïve pregnant women; use without ritonavir is **not** recommended. A small increased risk of preterm birth has been associated with maternal use of protease inhibitor-based combination antiretroviral (ARV) therapy during pregnancy; however, the benefits of use generally outweigh this risk and protease inhibitors (PIs) should not be withheld if otherwise recommended. Hyperglycemia, new onset of diabetes mellitus, or diabetic ketoacidosis have been reported with PIs; it is not clear if pregnancy increases this risk.

Regardless of CD4 count or HIV RNA copy number, all HIV-infected pregnant women should receive a combination antiretroviral ARV drug regimen. A combination of antepartum, intrapartum, and infant ARV prophylaxis is recommended.ARV therapy should be started as soon as possible in women with symptomatic infection. Although earlier initiation may be more effective in reducing the perinatal transmission of HIV, initiation may be delayed until after 12 weeks gestation in women who do not require immediate treatment after careful consideration of maternal conditions (eg, nausea and vomiting) and the potential risks of first trimester fetal exposure for specific agents. A scheduled cesarean delivery at 38 weeks gestation is recommended for all women with HIV RNA >1000 copies/mL or unknown concentrations near delivery in order to decrease transmission. If ARV therapy must be interrupted for <24 hours during the peripartum period, stop then restart all medications simultaneously in order to decrease the chance of developing resistance. Long-term follow-up is recommended for all infants exposed to ARV medications. In couples who want to conceive, the HIV-infected partner should attain maximum viral suppression prior to conception.

Health care providers are encouraged to enroll pregnant women exposed to antiretroviral medications in the Antiretroviral Pregnancy Registry (1-800-258-4263 or www.APRegistry.com). Health care providers caring for HIV-infected women and their infants may contact the National Perinatal HIV Hotline (888-448-8765) for clinical consultation (DHHS [perinatal], 2014).

Breast-Feeding Considerations It is not known if saquinavir is excreted into breast milk. Maternal or infant antiretroviral therapy does not completely eliminate the risk of postnatal HIV transmission. In addition, multiclass-resistant virus has been detected in breast-feeding infants despite maternal therapy. Therefore, in the United States, where formula is accessible, affordable, safe, and sustainable, and the risk of infant mortality due to diarrhea and respiratory infections is low, complete avoidance of breast-feeding by HIV-infected women is recommended to decrease potential transmission of HIV (DHHS [perinatal], 2014).

Contraindications Hypersensitivity (eg, anaphylaxis, Stevens-Johnson syndrome) to saquinavir, saquinavir mesylate, or any component; congenital or acquired QT prolongation, refractory hypokalemia or hypomagnesemia; concomitant use of other medications that both increase saquinavir plasma concentrations and prolong the QT interval; complete AV block (without implanted ventricular pacemaker) or patients at high risk of complete AV block; severe hepatic impairment; concurrent therapy with alfuzosin, amiodarone, bepridil, cisapride, dihydroergotamine, dofetilide, ergonovine, ergotamine, flecainide, lidocaine (systemic), lovastatin, methylergonovine, midazolam (oral), pimozide, propafenone, quinidine, rifampin, sildenafil [when used for pulmonary artery hypertension (Revatio®)], simvastatin, trazodone, or triazolam

Warnings Saquinavir must be used in combination with ritonavir. Continued administration of saquinavir after loss of viral suppression may increase the likelihood of cross-resistance to other protease inhibitors.

Saquinavir is a potent CYP3A4 isoenzyme inhibitor that interacts with numerous drugs. Due to potential serious and/or life-threatening drug interactions, some drugs are contraindicated. Concurrent use with St John's wort or garlic capsules is **not** recommended. Alteration of dose or serum concentration monitoring may be required with other medications.

Saquinavir/ritonavir causes dose-dependent PR interval prolongation, potentially leading to heart block; second or third degree AV block has been reported (rare); risk may be increased in patients with structural heart disease, preexisting conduction abnormalities, cardiomyopathy, and ischemic heart disease; ECG monitoring is recommended.

Saquinavir/ritonavir may cause dose-dependent QT interval prolongation, potentially leading to torsade de pointes; avoid use in patients with long QT syndrome (saquinavir is contraindicated in patients with congenital or acquired QT prolongation); patients who may be at increased risk are those with congestive heart failure, bradyarrhythmias, hepatic impairment, and electrolyte abnormalities (particularly potassium, magnesium). Correct electrolyte abnormalities (hypokalemia and hypomagnesemia) and monitor electrolytes periodically during therapy. Perform baseline ECG in all patients prior to initiating therapy; do not initiate saquinavir/ritonavir in patients with a baseline QT interval >450 msec. If baseline QT interval <450 msec, may initiate therapy but a subsequent ECG is recommended after ~3 to 4 days of therapy. If subsequent QT interval is >480 msec or is prolonged over baseline by >20 msec, therapy should be discontinued.

Spontaneous bleeding episodes have been reported in patients with hemophilia receiving an HIV protease inhibitor. New onset diabetes mellitus, exacerbation of diabetes and hyperglycemia have been reported in HIV-infected patients receiving protease inhibitors. Significant elevations of serum triglycerides and cholesterol may occur (monitor and manage appropriately).

May cause photosensitivity reactions (eg, exposure to sunlight may cause severe sunburn, skin rash, redness, or itching); advise patient to avoid exposure to sunlight and artificial light sources (eg, sunlamps, tanning bed/booth) and to wear protective clothing, wide-brimmed hats, sunglasses, and lip sunscreen (SPF ≥15). Sunscreen should be used (broad-spectrum sunscreen or physical sunscreen [preferred] or sunblock with SPF ≥15) (DHHS [pediatric], 2014).

Precautions Use with caution in patients with mild to moderate hepatic disease including hepatitis B or C, cirrhosis, or chronic alcoholism; increased liver enzymes, or worsening liver disease may occur. Use is contraindicated in patients with severe hepatic impairment.

Fat redistribution and accumulation [ie, central obesity, peripheral wasting, facial wasting, breast enlargement, dorsocervical fat enlargement (buffalo hump), and cushingoid appearance] have been observed in patients receiving antiretroviral agents (causal relationship not established).

Immune reconstitution syndrome (an acute inflammatory response to residual or indolent opportunistic infections) may occur in HIV patients during initial treatment with combination antiretroviral agents, including saquinavir; this syndrome may require further patient assessment and therapy. Autoimmune disorders (eg, Graves' disease, Guillain-Barré syndrome, and polymyositis) have been reported in patients experiencing immune reconstitution; time to onset is variable and may occur many months after antiretroviral treatment is initiated.

Adverse Reactions
Incidence data shown for saquinavir soft gel capsule formulation (no longer available) in combination with ritonavir.
Cardiovascular: Chest pain
Central nervous system: Anxiety, depression, fatigue, fever, headache, insomnia, pain
Dermatologic: Dry lips/skin, eczema, pruritus, rash, verruca
Endocrine & metabolic: Hyper-/hypoglycemia, hyperkalemia, libido disorder, lipodystrophy, serum amylase increased
Gastrointestinal: Abdominal discomfort, abdominal pain, appetite decreased, buccal mucosa ulceration, constipation, diarrhea, dyspepsia, flatulence, nausea, taste alteration, vomiting
Hepatic: AST increased, ALT increased, bilirubin increased
Neuromuscular & skeletal: Back pain, CPK increased, paresthesia, weakness
Renal: Creatinine kinase increased
Respiratory: Bronchitis, pneumonia, sinusitis
Miscellaneous: Influenza

Incidence not currently defined (limited to significant reactions; reported for hard or soft gel capsule with/without ritonavir)
Cardiovascular: Cyanosis, heart valve disorder (including murmur), hyper-/hypotension, peripheral vasoconstriction, prolonged QT interval, prolonged PR interval, syncope, thrombophlebitis
Central nervous system: Agitation, amnesia, ataxia, confusion, hallucination, hyper-/hyporeflexia, myelopolyradiculoneuritis, neuropathies, poliomyelitis, progressive multifocal encephalopathy, psychosis, seizures, somnolence, speech disorder, suicide attempt
Dermatologic: Alopecia, bullous eruption, dermatitis, erythema, maculopapular rash, photosensitivity, Stevens-Johnson syndrome, skin ulceration, urticaria
Endocrine & metabolic: Dehydration, diabetes, electrolyte changes, TSH increased

Gastrointestinal: Ascites, colic, dysphagia, esophagitis, bloody stools, gastritis, intestinal obstruction, hemorrhage (rectal), pancreatitis, stomatitis
Genitourinary: impotence, prostate enlarged, hematuria, UTI
Hematologic: Acute myeloblastic leukemia, anemia (including hemolytic), leukopenia, neutropenia, pancytopenia, splenomegaly, thrombocytopenia
Hepatic: Alkaline phosphatase increased, GGT increased, hepatitis, hepatomegaly, hepatosplenomegaly, jaundice, liver disease exacerbation
Neuromuscular & skeletal: Arthritis, LDH increased
Ocular: Blepharitis, visual disturbance
Otic: Otitis, hearing decreased, tinnitus
Renal: Nephrolithiasis, renal calculus
Respiratory: Dyspnea, hemoptysis, pharyngitis, upper respiratory tract infection
Miscellaneous: Immune reconstitution syndrome, infections (bacterial, fungal, viral)
Postmarketing and/or case reports: AV block (second or third degree), torsade de pointes

Drug Interactions
Metabolism/Transport Effects Substrate of CYP2D6 (minor), CYP3A4 (major), P-glycoprotein; **Note:** Assignment of Major/Minor substrate status based on clinically relevant drug interaction potential; **Inhibits** CYP2C19 (weak), CYP2C9 (weak), CYP2D6 (weak), CYP3A4 (strong), P-glycoprotein

Avoid Concomitant Use
Avoid concomitant use of Saquinavir with any of the following: Ado-Trastuzumab Emtansine; Alfuzosin; Amiodarone; Apixaban; Avanafil; Axitinib; Bepridil [Off Market]; Bosutinib; Cabozantinib; Ceritinib; Cisapride; Conivaptan; Crizotinib; Darunavir; Dofetilide; Dronedarone; Eplerenone; Ergot Derivatives; Everolimus; Flecainide; Fusidic Acid (Systemic); Halofantrine; Highest Risk QTc-Prolonging Agents; Ibrutinib; Ivabradine; Lapatinib; Lidocaine (Systemic); Lomitapide; Lovastatin; Lurasidone; Macitentan; Midazolam; Mifepristone; Nilotinib; Nisoldipine; PAZOPanib; Pimozide; Propafenone; QuiNIDine; Ranolazine; Red Yeast Rice; Regorafenib; Rifampin; Rivaroxaban; Salmeterol; Silodosin; Simeprevir; Simvastatin; St Johns Wort; Tamsulosin; Ticagrelor; Tipranavir; Tolvaptan; Topotecan; Toremifene; TraZODone; Triazolam; Ulipristal; Vemurafenib; VinCRIStine (Liposomal); Vorapaxar

Increased Effect/Toxicity
Saquinavir may increase the levels/effects of: Ado-Trastuzumab Emtansine; Afatinib; Alfuzosin; Almotriptan; Alosetron; ALPRAZolam; Amiodarone; Apixaban; ARIPiprazole; AtorvaSTATin; Avanafil; Axitinib; Bedaquiline; Bepridil [Off Market]; Bortezomib; Bosentan; Bosutinib; Brentuximab Vedotin; Brinzolamide; Budesonide (Nasal); Budesonide (Systemic, Oral Inhalation); Cabozantinib; Calcium Channel Blockers (Dihydropyridine); Calcium Channel Blockers (Nondihydropyridine); Cannabis; CarBAMazepine; Ceritinib; Cisapride; Clarithromycin; Clorazepate; Colchicine; Conivaptan; Corticosteroids (Orally Inhaled); Crizotinib; Cyclophosphamide; CycloSPORINE (Systemic); CYP3A4 Substrates; Dabigatran Etexilate; Diazepam; Digoxin; Dofetilide; DOXOrubicin (Conventional); Dronabinol; Dronedarone; Dutasteride; Efavirenz; Enfuvirtide; Eplerenone; Ergot Derivatives; Everolimus; FentaNYL; Fesoterodine; Flecainide; Flurazepam; Fluticasone (Nasal); Fluticasone (Oral Inhalation); Fusidic Acid (Systemic); GuanFACINE; Halofantrine; Highest Risk QTc-Prolonging Agents; Ibrutinib; Imatinib; Itraconazole; Ivabradine; Ivacaftor; Ixabepilone; Ketoconazole (Systemic); Lacosamide; Lapatinib; Levomilnacipran; Lidocaine (Systemic); Lomitapide; Lovastatin; Lurasidone; Macitentan; Maraviroc; Meperidine; MethylPREDNISolone; Midazolam; Moderate Risk QTc-Prolonging Agents; Nefazodone; Nilotinib; Nisoldipine;

Ospemifene; OxyCODONE; Paricalcitol; PAZOPanib; P-glycoprotein/ABCB1 Substrates; Pimecrolimus; Pimozide; PONATinib; Propafenone; Protease Inhibitors; Prucalopride; QuiNIDine; Ranolazine; Red Yeast Rice; Regorafenib; Repaglinide; Rifabutin; Rifaximin; Rilpivirine; Riociguat; Rivaroxaban; Rosuvastatin; Ruxolitinib; Salmeterol; Saxagliptin; Sildenafil; Silodosin; Simeprevir; Simvastatin; Tacrolimus (Systemic); Tacrolimus (Topical); Tadalafil; Tamsulosin; Temsirolimus; Tetrahydrocannabinol; Ticagrelor; Tofacitinib; Tolterodine; Tolvaptan; Topotecan; Toremifene; TraZODone; Triazolam; Tricyclic Antidepressants; Ulipristal; Vardenafil; Vemurafenib; Vilazodone; VinCRIStine (Liposomal); Vorapaxar; Warfarin

The levels/effects of Saquinavir may be increased by: Bepridil [Off Market]; Clarithromycin; CycloSPORINE (Systemic); Delavirdine; Enfuvirtide; Etravirine; Fusidic Acid (Systemic); H2-Antagonists; Itraconazole; Ivabradine; Ketoconazole (Systemic); Methadone; Mifepristone; P-glycoprotein/ABCB1 Inhibitors; Proton Pump Inhibitors; QTc-Prolonging Agents (Indeterminate Risk and Risk Modifying); Rifampin; Simeprevir

Decreased Effect

Saquinavir may decrease the levels/effects of: Abacavir; Boceprevir; Clarithromycin; Contraceptives (Estrogens); Contraceptives (Progestins); Darunavir; Delavirdine; Etravirine; Ifosfamide; Meperidine; Methadone; Prasugrel; Pravastatin; Ticagrelor; Valproic Acid and Derivatives; Zidovudine

The levels/effects of Saquinavir may be decreased by: Antacids; Boceprevir; Bosentan; CarBAMazepine; CYP3A4 Inducers (Strong); Dabrafenib; Deferasirox; Efavirenz; Garlic; Mitotane; Nevirapine; Peginterferon Alfa-2b; P-glycoprotein/ABCB1 Inducers; Rifampin; Siltuximab; St Johns Wort; Tipranavir; Tocilizumab

Food Interactions A high-fat meal maximizes bioavailability. Saquinavir levels may increase if taken with grapefruit juice. Management: Administer within 2 hours of a full meal. Monitor closely with concurrent grapefruit juice use.

Stability Invirase® capsules and tablets: Store at 25°C (77°F); excursions permitted to 15°C to 30°C (59°F to 86°F); store in tightly closed bottles

Mechanism of Action Binds to the site of HIV-1 protease activity and inhibits cleavage of viral Gag-Pol polyprotein precursors into individual functional proteins required for infectious HIV. This results in the formation of immature, noninfectious viral particles.

Pharmacokinetics (Adult data unless noted)

Distribution: CSF concentration is negligible when compared to concentrations from matched plasma samples; partitions into tissues

V_d: 700 L

Protein binding: 98%

Metabolism: Extensive first-pass effect; hepatic metabolism by cytochrome P450 3A system to inactive mono- and dihydroxylated metabolites

Bioavailability:

Invirase capsules: 4% (increased in the presence of food); bioavailability of Invirase® capsules and tablets are similar when administered with low dose ritonavir (ie, booster doses of ritonavir)

Half-life, serum: 1 to 2 hours

Elimination: 81% to 88% of dose eliminated in feces; 1% to 3% excreted in urine within 5 days

Clearance: Children: Significantly higher than adults

Dosing: Neonatal Not approved for use; appropriate dose is unknown.

Dosing: Usual

Pediatric: **HIV Infection, treatment:** Oral: Use in combination with other antiretroviral agents. **Note:** ECG should be done prior to starting therapy; do not initiate therapy if pretreatment QT interval >450 msec or if there is a diagnosis of long QT syndrome. Saquinavir must only be used in regimens that include ritonavir "booster doses" so that adequate saquinavir serum concentrations are attained; do not use without ritonavir booster doses.

Infants and Children <2 years: Not approved for use; appropriate dose is unknown.

Children ≥2 years and Adolescents <16 years: Limited data available (DHHS [pediatric], 2014): Oral:

Treatment-experienced, ritonavir-boosted regimen: Children ≥2 years and Adolescents <16 years:

5 kg to <15 kg: Saquinavir 50 mg/kg/dose **plus** ritonavir 3 mg/kg/dose twice daily; maximum single saquinavir dose: 1000 mg

15 kg to <40 kg: Saquinavir 50 mg/kg/dose **plus** ritonavir 2.5 mg/kg/dose twice daily;; maximum single saquinavir dose: 1000 mg

≥40 kg: Saquinavir 1000 mg **plus** ritonavir 100 mg twice daily

Salvage therapy, lopinavir/ritonavir-boosted regimen: Children ≥7 years and Adolescents <16 years: Saquinavir 750 mg/m²/dose or 50 mg/kg/dose **plus** lopinavir/ritonavir twice daily; maximum single saquinavir dose: 1600 mg

Adolescents ≥16 years: Oral:

Ritonavir-boosted regimen: Saquinavir 1000 mg (five 200 mg capsules or two 500 mg tablets) **plus** ritonavir 100 mg twice daily

Lopinavir/ritonavir-boosted regimen: Saquinavir 1000 mg **plus** lopinavir 400 mg/ritonavir 100 mg twice daily; no additional ritonavir is necessary

Adult: **HIV Infection, treatment:** Oral: Use in combination with other antiretroviral agents. **Note:** ECG should be done prior to starting therapy; do not initiate therapy if pretreatment QT interval >450 msec or if there is a diagnosis of long QT syndrome. Saquinavir must only be used in regimens that include ritonavir "booster doses" so that adequate saquinavir serum concentrations are attained; do not use without ritonavir booster doses.

Ritonavir-boosted regimen: Saquinavir 1000 mg (five 200 mg capsules or two 500 mg tablets) **plus** ritonavir 100 mg twice daily

Lopinavir/ritonavir-boosted regimen: Saquinavir 1000 mg **plus** lopinavir 400 mg/ritonavir 100 mg twice daily; no additional ritonavir is necessary

Dosing adjustment in renal impairment:

Mild to moderate renal impairment: No initial dosage adjustment needed

Severe renal impairment or end-stage renal disease: Studies have not been conducted; use with caution; serum concentrations may be elevated

Dosing adjustment in hepatic impairment: Mild or moderate hepatic impairment: No dosage adjustment needed; use with caution; **Note:** Worsening of liver disease may occur in patients with underlying hepatitis B or C, cirrhosis, chronic alcoholism, or other underlying liver abnormalities. Use is contraindicated in severe hepatic impairment.

Administration Oral: Administer saquinavir (along with ritonavir) within 2 hours after a full meal to increase absorption; administer at same time as ritonavir-containing products. For patients unable to swallow a capsule, open the capsule and place the contents into an empty container. Add 15 mL of either sugar syrup or sorbitol syrup **or** 3 teaspoons of jam, stir for 30 to 60 seconds, and immediately administer full amount; mixture should be at room temperature before administration.

Monitoring Parameters Note: Monitor CD4 percentage (if <5 years of age) or CD4 count (if ≥5 years of age) at least every 3 to 4 months (DHHS [pediatric], 2014).

ECG (baseline and after 3 to 4 days of therapy); Prior to initiation of therapy: Genotypic resistance testing, CD4 and viral load (every 3 to 4 months), CBC with differential, LFTs, BUN, creatinine, lipid panel, electrolytes, glucose, and urinalysis (every 6 to 12 months), and assessment of readiness for adherence with medication regimen. At initiation and with any change in treatment regimen: CBC with differential, electrolytes, calcium, phosphate, glucose, LFTs, bilirubin, urinalysis (at initiation), BUN, creatinine, albumin, total protein, lipid panel (at initiation), CD4, and viral load. After 1 to 2 weeks of therapy: Signs of medication toxicity and adherence. After 2 to 4 weeks of therapy: CBC with differential, viral load, signs of medication toxicity, and adherence; then every 3 to 4 months: CBC with differential, electrolytes, glucose, LFTs, bilirubin, BUN, creatinine, CD4, viral load, signs of medication toxicity, and adherence. Every 6 to 12 months: Lipid panel and urinalysis. CD4 monitoring frequency may be decreased to every 6 to 12 months in children who are adherent to therapy if the value is well above the threshold for opportunistic infections, viral suppression is sustained, and the clinical status is stable for more than 2 to 3 years (DHHS [pediatric], 2014). Monitor for growth and development, signs of HIV-specific physical conditions, HIV disease progression, opportunistic infections or arrhythmias.

Reference Range Plasma trough concentration: 100 to 250 ng/mL (DHHS [adult/pediatric], 2014)

Additional Information Fortovase (saquinavir soft gel capsules) has been discontinued in the U.S. because ritonavir-boosted Invirase tablet-containing regimens result in fewer GI side effects and a lower pill burden compared to ritonavir-boosted Fortovase regimens.

Dosage Forms Excipient information presented when available (limited, particularly for generics); consult specific product labeling.

Capsule, Oral:
Invirase: 200 mg
Tablet, Oral:
Invirase: 500 mg

References

DHHS Panel on Antiretroviral Guidelines for Adults and Adolescents. Guidelines for the use of antiretroviral agents in HIV-1-infected adults and adolescents, Department of Health and Human Services. May 1, 2014. Available at http://www.aidsinfo.nih.gov/ContentFiles/AdultandAdolescentGL.pdf

DHHS Panel on Antiretroviral Therapy and Medical Management of HIV-Infected Children. Guidelines for the use of antiretroviral agents in pediatric HIV infection. February 12, 2014. Available at http://aidsinfo.nih.gov

DHHS Panel on Treatment of HIV-Infected Pregnant Women and Prevention of Perinatal Transmission. Recommendations for the use of antiretroviral drugs in pregnant HIV-1-infected women for maternal health and interventions to reduce perinatal HIV-1 transmission in the United States. March 28, 2014. Available at http://aidsinfo.nih.gov

Singh M, Arora R, Jawad E. HIV protease inhibitors induced prolongation of the QT interval: electrophysiology and clinical implications. *Am J Ther.* 2009.

◆ **Saquinavir Mesylate** *see* Saquinavir *on page 1867*

◆ **Sarafem** *see* FLUoxetine *on page 901*

Sargramostim (sar GRAM oh stim)

Medication Safety Issues
Sound-alike/look-alike issues:
Leukine may be confused with Leukeran, leucovorin
Brand Names: U.S. Leukine
Brand Names: Canada Leukine
Therapeutic Category Colony-Stimulating Factor; Hematopoietic Agent
Generic Availability (U.S.) No
Use Accelerates myeloid recovery in patients undergoing autologous or allogeneic BMT, mobilizes hematopoietic progenitor cells into peripheral blood for collection by leukapheresis, and accelerates myeloid recovery following autologous peripheral stem cell transplantation and prolong survival in patients with graft failure or engraftment delay after BMT (FDA approved in adults); shortens time to neutrophil recovery and reduces the incidence of severe and life-threatening infections and infections resulting in death following induction chemotherapy in older adults with acute myelogenous leukemia (AML) (FDA approved in adults ≥55 years of age). Has also been used to increase neutrophil counts in patients with malignancies receiving myelosuppressive chemotherapy (beginning >24 hour after chemotherapy) and for management of neonatal neutropenia.

Pregnancy Risk Factor C

Pregnancy Considerations Animal reproduction studies have not been conducted.

Breast-Feeding Considerations It is not known if sargramostim is excreted in breast milk. Breast-feeding is not recommended by the manufacturer.

Contraindications Hypersensitivity to GM-CSF, yeast-derived products, or any component; excessive leukemic myeloid blasts in bone marrow or peripheral blood (≥10%); concurrent or the 24 hours preceding or following chemotherapy or radiation therapy

Warnings Anaphylaxis or other serious allergic reactions have been reported; discontinue immediately and initiate appropriate therapy if a serious allergic or anaphylactic reaction occurs. A "first-dose effect", characterized by respiratory distress, hypoxia, flushing, hypotension, syncope, and/or tachycardia, may occur (rarely) with the first dose of a cycle and resolve with appropriate symptomatic treatment; does not usually occur with subsequent doses within that cycle.

Edema, capillary leak syndrome, pleural and/or pericardial effusion have been reported with use; fluid retention has been shown to be reversible with dosage reduction or discontinuation of sargramostim with or without concomitant use of diuretics. Use with caution in patients with preexisting fluid retention, pulmonary infiltrates, or congestive heart failure; may exacerbate fluid retention. Reversible transient supraventricular arrhythmias have been reported, especially in patients with a history of arrhythmias; use with caution in patients with preexisting cardiac disease. May cause sequestration of granulocytes in the pulmonary circulation; dyspnea may occur. If dyspnea occurs, decrease infusion rate by 50%; discontinue drug if persists despite reduction in administration rate; use with caution in patients with hypoxia or preexisting pulmonary disease.

Injection solution may contain benzyl alcohol which may cause allergic reactions in susceptible individuals; large amounts of benzyl alcohol (≥99 mg/kg/day) have been associated with a potentially fatal toxicity ("gasping syndrome") in neonates; the "gasping syndrome" consists of metabolic acidosis, respiratory distress, gasping respirations, CNS dysfunction (including convulsions, intracranial hemorrhage), hypotension and cardiovascular collapse; use sargramostim injection products containing benzyl alcohol with caution in neonates; *in vitro* and animal studies have shown that benzoate, a metabolite of benzyl alcohol, displaces bilirubin from protein binding sites

Precautions Use with caution in patients with autoimmune or chronic inflammatory disease, hypertension, cardiovascular disease, or pulmonary disease. Use with caution in patients with hepatic impairment; reversible hyperbilirubinemia and elevated transaminases have been reported. Use with caution in patients with renal impairment; reversible elevations in serum creatinine have been reported. Monitor hepatic and renal function prior to therapy and at least every other week in patients with history of renal or hepatic impairment.

May cause rapid increase in peripheral blood counts: If ANC is >20,000/mm^3 or platelets >500,000/mm^3, decrease dose by 50% or discontinue drug (based on patient's clinical condition); counts will fall to normal within 3-7 days after discontinuing drug; monitor CBC with differential twice weekly during therapy.

Sargramostim may act as a growth factor for any tumor type, particularly myeloid malignancies; use with caution in any malignancy with myeloid characteristics; discontinue use if disease progression occurs during treatment. Limited response to sargramostim may be seen in patients who have received bone marrow purged by chemical agents which do not preserve an adequate number of responsive hematopoietic progenitors (eg, <1.2 x 10^4/kg progenitors). In patients receiving autologous bone marrow transplant, response to sargramostim may be limited if extensive radiotherapy to the abdomen or chest or multiple myelotoxic agents were administered prior to transplant. Simultaneous administration or administration 24 hours preceding/following cytotoxic chemotherapy or radiotherapy is contraindicated due to the sensitivity of rapidly dividing hematopoietic progenitor cells.

Adverse Reactions

Cardiovascular: Chest pain, edema, hypertension, pericardial effusion, peripheral edema, tachycardia, thrombosis

Central nervous system: Anxiety, chills, headache, insomnia, malaise

Dermatologic: Pruritus, skin rash

Endocrine & metabolic: Hypercholesterolemia, hyperglycemia, hypomagnesemia, weight loss

Gastrointestinal: Abdominal pain, anorexia, diarrhea, dysphagia, gastric ulcer, gastrointestinal hemorrhage, hematemesis, nausea, vomiting

Hepatic: Hyperbilirubinemia

Immunologic: Antibody development

Neuromuscular & skeletal: Arthralgia, myalgia, ostealgia, weakness

Ophthalmic: Retinal hemorrhage

Renal: Increased blood urea nitrogen, increased serum creatinine

Respiratory: Dyspnea, epistaxis, pharyngitis, pleural effusion

Miscellaneous: Fever

Rare but important or life-threatening: Anaphylaxis, capillary leak syndrome, cardiac arrhythmia, eosinophilia, hypoxia, leukocytosis, liver function impairment (transient), pericarditis, prolonged prothrombin time, respiratory distress, rigors, sore throat, supraventricular cardiac arrhythmia, syncope, thrombocythemia, thrombophlebitis

Drug Interactions

Metabolism/Transport Effects None known.

Avoid Concomitant Use There are no known interactions where it is recommended to avoid concomitant use.

Increased Effect/Toxicity

Sargramostim may increase the levels/effects of: Bleomycin

The levels/effects of Sargramostim may be increased by: Cyclophosphamide

Decreased Effect There are no known significant interactions involving a decrease in effect.

Stability

Powder for injection: Store intact vial at 2°C to 8°C (36°F to 46°F); do not freeze; do not shake. Preparations made with SWI should be administered as soon as possible and discarded within 6 hours of reconstitution. Solutions reconstituted with bacteriostatic water may be stored for up to 20 days at 2°C to 8°C (36°F to 46°F).

Solution for injection: Store at 2°C to 8°C (36°F to 46°F); do not freeze; do not shake. May be stored for up to 20 days at 2°C to 8°C (36°F to 46°F) once the vial has been entered. Discard remaining solution after 20 days.

Mechanism of Action Stimulates proliferation, differentiation and functional activity of neutrophils, eosinophils, monocytes, and macrophages.

Pharmacodynamics

Onset of action: Increase in WBC in 7-14 days

Duration: WBC will return to baseline within 1 week after discontinuing drug

Pharmacokinetics (Adult data unless noted)

Half-life:

Pediatric patients 6 months to 15 years: I.V.: Median: 1.6 hours; range: 0.9-2.5 hours; SubQ: Median: 2.3 hours (0.3-3.8 hours) (Stute, 1995)

Adults: I.V.: 60 minutes: SubQ: 2.7 hours

Time to peak serum concentration: SubQ: 1-3 hours

Dosing: Neonatal Neutropenia: Limited data available; efficacy result variable: SubQ: 10 mcg/kg/dose once daily for 5 days. The PROGRAMS trial (single-blind, multicenter) evaluated use in 280 premature neonates (GA: ≤31 weeks; weight: ≤10th percentile body weight) and showed a correction of neutropenia but no reduction in sepsis or improved survival (Carr, 2009); an extension study also reported no difference in developmental, neurological, or general health outcomes in former premature neonates who received sargramostim compared to placebo (Marlow, 2013)

Dosing: Usual

Infants, Children, and Adolescents: **Neutrophil recovery following bone marrow transplant:** Limited data available: I.V.: 250 mcg/m^2/day (infused over 2-4 hours or SubQ) once daily for 21 days to begin 2-4 hours after the marrow infusion on day 0 of BMT or not less than 24 hours after chemotherapy (Trigg, 2000; Nemunaitis, 1991)

Adults: **Note:** May round the dose to the nearest vial size (Ozer, 2000).

Acute myeloid leukemia (AML), neutrophil recovery following chemotherapy: Adults ≥55 years: I.V.: 250 mcg/m^2/day (infused over 4 hours) starting approximately on day 11 or 4 days following the completion of induction chemotherapy (if day 10 bone marrow is hypoplastic with <5% blasts), continue until ANC >1500/mm^3 for 3 consecutive days or a maximum of 42 days.

If a second cycle of chemotherapy is necessary, administer ~4 days after the completion of chemotherapy if the bone marrow is hypoplastic with <5% blasts.

Discontinue sargramostim immediately if leukemic regrowth occurs.

Bone marrow transplant (BMT), failure or engraftment delay: I.V.: 250 mcg/m^2/day (infused over 2 hours) for 14 days; if engraftment has not occurred after 7 days off sargramostim, may repeat. If engraftment still has not occurred after 7 days off sargramostim, a third course of 500 mcg/m^2/day for 14 days may be attempted. If there is still no improvement, it is unlikely that further dose escalation will be of benefit. If blast cells appear or disease progression occurs, discontinue treatment.

Myeloid reconstitution after allogeneic or autologous bone marrow transplant: I.V.: 250 mcg/m^2/day (infused over 2 hours), begin 2-4 hours after the marrow infusion and ≥24 hours after chemotherapy or radiotherapy, when the post marrow infusion ANC is <500/mm^3, and continue until ANC >1500/mm^3 for 3 consecutive days. If blast cells appear or progression of the underlying disease occurs, discontinue treatment.

Peripheral stem cell transplant, mobilization of peripheral blood progenitor cells (PBPC): I.V., SubQ: 250 mcg/m^2/day I.V. (infused over 24 hours) or SubQ once daily; continue the same dose throughout PBPC collection.

Postperipheral blood progenitor cell transplantation: I.V., SubQ: 250 mcg/m^2/day I.V. (infused over 24 hours)

or SubQ once daily beginning immediately following infusion of progenitor cells; continue until ANC is >1500/mm^3 for 3 consecutive days.

Dosing adjustment for adverse effects (hematologic) or "first dose" effect: Infants, Children, Adolescents, and Adults: If WBC >50,000/mm^3, ANC is >20,000/mm^3, or platelets >500,000/mm^3, or severe adverse reaction occurs: Decrease dose by 50% or discontinue drug (based on protocol or patient's clinical condition).

Administration Parenteral:

I.V.: Administer as 2-hour or 4-hour I.V. infusion or by continuous I.V. infusion. Do not shake solution to avoid foaming. Dilute in NS; if the final concentration of GM-CSF in NS is <10 mcg/mL, then add 1 mg albumin per mL of I.V. fluid. Albumin acts as a carrier molecule to prevent drug adsorption to the I.V. tubing. Albumin should be added to NS prior to addition of GM-CSF. An in-line membrane filter should **not** be used for intravenous administration.

SubQ: Reconstituted 250 mcg/mL or 500 mcg/mL solution may be administered without further dilution; rotate injection sites; avoiding naval/waistline

Monitoring Parameters CBC with differential (at least twice weekly during therapy), platelets; renal/liver function tests (at least every 2 weeks); vital signs, weight; hydration status; pulmonary function

Test Interactions May interfere with bone imaging studies; increased hematopoietic activity of the bone marrow may appear as transient positive bone imaging changes

Additional Information Produced by recombinant DNA technology using a yeast-derived expression system

Dosage Forms Excipient information presented when available (limited, particularly for generics); consult specific product labeling. [DSC] = Discontinued product

Solution, Injection:
Leukine: 500 mcg/mL (1 mL [DSC]) [contains benzyl alcohol]

Solution Reconstituted, Intravenous:
Leukine: 250 mcg (1 ea [DSC])

Solution Reconstituted, Intravenous [preservative free]:
Leukine: 250 mcg (1 ea)

References

Carr R, Brocklehurst P, Doré CJ, et al, "Granulocyte-Macrophage Colony Stimulating Factor Administered as Prophylaxis for Reduction of Sepsis in Extremely Preterm, Small for Gestational Age Neonates (the PROGRAMS Trial): A Single-Blind, Multicentre, Randomised Controlled Trial," *Lancet*, 2009, 373(9659):226-33.

Carr R, Modi N, Dore CJ, et al, "A Randomized, Controlled Trial of Prophylactic Granulocyte-Macrophage Colony-Stimulating Factor in Human Newborns Less Than 32 Weeks Gestation," *Pediatrics*, 1999, 103(4 Pt 1):796-802.

Lieschke GJ and Burgess AW, "Granulocyte Colony-Stimulating Factor and Granulocyte-Macrophage Colony-Stimulating Factor," (1) *N Engl J Med*, 1992, 327(1):28-35.

Lieschke GJ and Burgess AW, "Granulocyte Colony-Stimulating Factor and Granulocyte-Macrophage Colony-Stimulating Factor," (2) *N Engl J Med*, 1992, 327(2):99-106.

Marlow N, Morris T, Brocklehurst P, et al. A randomised trial of granulocyte-macrophage colong-stimulating factor for neonatal sepsis: outcomes at 2 years. *Arch Dis Child Fetal Neonatal Ed.* 2013;98:46-53.

Nemunaitis J, Rabinowe SN, Singer JW, et.al. Recombinant granulocyte-macrophage coloney-stimulating factor after autologous bone marrow transplantation for lymphoid cancer. *NEJM.* 1991;324:1773-1778.

Ozer H, Armitage JO, Bennett CL, et al. 2000 update of recommendations for the use of hematopoietic colony-stimulating factors: evidence-based, clinical practice guidelines. American Society of Clinical Oncology Growth Factors Expert Panel. *J Clin Oncol.* 2000;18(20):3558-3585.

Stute N, Furman WL, Schell M, et al, "Pharmacokinetics of Recombinant Human Granulocyte - Macrophage Colony - Stimulating Factor in Children After Intravenous and Subcutaneous Administration," *J Pharm Sci*, 1995, 84(7):824-8.

Trigg ME, Peters C, Zimmerman MB. Administration of recombinant human granulocyte-macrophage colony-stimulating factor to children undergoing allogeneic marrow transplantation; a prospective,

randomized, double-masked, placebo-controlled trial. *Pediatr Transplantation.* 2000; 4:123-131.

Trissel LA, Bready BB, Kwan JW, et al, "Visual Compatibility of Sargramostim With Selected Antineoplastic Agents, Anti-infectives, or Other Drugs During Simulated Y-Site Injection," *Am J Hosp Pharm*, 1992, 49(2):402-6.

◆ **Sarna® HC (Can)** *see* Hydrocortisone (Topical) *on page 1038*

◆ **Sarnol-HC [OTC]** *see* Hydrocortisone (Topical) *on page 1038*

◆ **Saturated Potassium Iodide Solution** *see* Potassium Iodide *on page 1711*

◆ **Saturated Solution of Potassium Iodide** *see* Potassium Iodide *on page 1711*

◆ **SC 33428** *see* IDArubicin *on page 1067*

◆ **Scalacort** *see* Hydrocortisone (Topical) *on page 1038*

◆ **Scalacort DK** *see* Hydrocortisone (Topical) *on page 1038*

◆ **Scalpicin 2 in 1 [OTC]** *see* Salicylic Acid *on page 1860*

◆ **Scalpicin Maximum Strength [OTC]** *see* Hydrocortisone (Topical) *on page 1038*

◆ **SCH 52365** *see* Temozolomide *on page 1972*

◆ **SCH 56592** *see* Posaconazole *on page 1703*

◆ **ScheinPharm Ranitidine (Can)** *see* Ranitidine *on page 1805*

◆ **Scholls Callus Removers [OTC] [DSC]** *see* Salicylic Acid *on page 1860*

◆ **Scholls Corn Removers [OTC] [DSC]** *see* Salicylic Acid *on page 1860*

◆ **Scholls Corn Removers Extra [OTC] [DSC]** *see* Salicylic Acid *on page 1860*

◆ **Scholls Corn Removers Small [OTC] [DSC]** *see* Salicylic Acid *on page 1860*

◆ **SCIG** *see* Immune Globulin *on page 1084*

◆ **S-Citalopram** *see* Escitalopram *on page 788*

Scopolamine (Systemic) (skoe POL a meen)

Medication Safety Issues

BEERS Criteria medication:
This drug may be potentially inappropriate for use in geriatric patients (Quality of evidence - moderate; Strength of recommendation - strong).

Other safety concerns:
Transdermal patch may contain conducting metal (eg, aluminum); remove patch prior to MRI.

Brand Names: U.S. Transderm-Scop

Brand Names: Canada Buscopan®; Scopolamine Hydrobromide Injection; Transderm-V®

Therapeutic Category Anticholinergic Agent; Anticholinergic Agent, Transdermal

Generic Availability (U.S.) May be product dependent

Use Preoperative medication to produce amnesia and decrease salivary and respiratory secretions; prevention of motion sickness (oral and transdermal formulations) and prevention of postoperative nausea and vomiting (transdermal formulation); inhibits excessive motility and hypertonus of the GI tract in such conditions as the irritable colon syndrome, mild dysentery, diverticulitis, and pylorospasm (oral formulation)

Pregnancy Risk Factor C

Pregnancy Considerations Adverse events were observed in some animal reproduction studies. Scopolamine crosses the placenta; may cause respiratory depression and/or neonatal hemorrhage when used during pregnancy. Transdermal scopolamine has been used as an adjunct to epidural anesthesia for cesarean delivery without adverse CNS effects on the newborn. Parenteral administration does not increase the duration of labor or affect uterine contractions. Except when used prior to cesarean section, use during pregnancy only if the benefit to the mother outweighs the potential risk to the fetus.

Breast-Feeding Considerations Scopolamine is excreted into breast milk. The manufacturer recommends caution be used if scopolamine is administered to a nursing woman.

Contraindications Hypersensitivity to scopolamine or any component; patients hypersensitive to belladonna or barbiturates may be hypersensitive to scopolamine; GI or GU obstruction, thyrotoxicosis, tachycardia secondary to cardiac insufficiency, paralytic ileus, myasthenia gravis

Warnings Drug withdrawal symptoms such as nausea, vomiting, headache, dizziness, and equilibrium disturbance have been reported following removal of transdermal system, primarily in patients using the system for more than 3 days; discontinue if patient reports unusual visual disturbances or pain within the eye. Patients with idiosyncratic reactions to anticholinergics, including scopolamine, may experience disorientation, delirium, and/or marked somnolence; may be accompanied by dilated pupils, rapid pulse, and xerostomia. Safety and efficacy have not been established for use of transdermal and oral scopolamine in children.

Transdermal patch may contain conducting metal (eg, aluminum); remove patch prior to MRI. Scopolamine (hyoscine) hydrobromide should not be interchanged with scopolamine butylbromide formulations; dosages are not equivalent.

Precautions Use with caution with hepatic or renal dysfunction since adverse CNS effects occur more often in these patients; use with caution in infants and children since they may be more susceptible to adverse effects of scopolamine; use with caution in patients with cardiac disease, seizures, or psychoses

Adverse Reactions

Cardiovascular: Bradycardia, flushing, orthostatic hypotension, tachycardia

Central nervous system: Acute toxic psychosis (rare), agitation (rare), ataxia, confusion, delusion (rare), disorientation, dizziness, drowsiness, fatigue, hallucination (rare), headache, irritability, loss of memory, paranoid behavior (rare), restlessness, sedation

Dermatologic: Drug eruptions, dry skin, dyshidrosis, erythema, pruritus, rash, urticaria

Endocrine & metabolic: Thirst

Gastrointestinal: Constipation, diarrhea, dry throat, dysphagia, nausea, vomiting, xerostomia

Genitourinary: Dysuria, urinary retention

Neuromuscular & skeletal: Tremor, weakness

Ocular: Accommodation impaired, blurred vision, conjunctival infection, cycloplegia, dryness, glaucoma (narrowangle), increased intraocular pain, itching, photophobia, pupil dilation, retinal pigmentation

Respiratory: Dry nose, dyspnea

Miscellaneous: Anaphylaxis (rare), anaphylactic shock (rare), angioedema, diaphoresis decreased, heat intolerance, hypersensitivity reactions

Drug Interactions

Metabolism/Transport Effects None known.

Avoid Concomitant Use

Avoid concomitant use of Scopolamine (Systemic) with any of the following: Aclidinium; Azelastine (Nasal); Ipratropium (Oral Inhalation); Paraldehyde; Potassium Chloride; Thalidomide; Tiotropium; Umeclidinium

Increased Effect/Toxicity

Scopolamine (Systemic) may increase the levels/effects of: AbobotulinumtoxinA; Alcohol (Ethyl); Analgesics (Opioid); Anticholinergic Agents; Azelastine (Nasal); Buprenorphine; Cannabinoid-Containing Products; CNS Depressants; Hydrocodone; Methotrimeprazine;

Metyrosine; Mirabegron; Mirtazapine; OnabotulinumtoxinA; Paraldehyde; Potassium Chloride; Pramipexole; RimabotulinumtoxinB; ROPINIRole; Rotigotine; Selective Serotonin Reuptake Inhibitors; Thalidomide; Thiazide Diuretics; Tiotropium; Topiramate; Zolpidem

The levels/effects of Scopolamine (Systemic) may be increased by: Aclidinium; Brimonidine (Topical); Cannabis; Doxylamine; Dronabinol; Droperidol; HydrOXYzine; Ipratropium (Oral Inhalation); Kava Kava; Magnesium Sulfate; Methotrimeprazine; Nabilone; Perampanel; Pramlintide; Rufinamide; Sodium Oxybate; Tapentadol; Tetrahydrocannabinol; Umeclidinium

Decreased Effect

Scopolamine (Systemic) may decrease the levels/effects of: Acetylcholinesterase Inhibitors (Central); Secretin

The levels/effects of Scopolamine (Systemic) may be decreased by: Acetylcholinesterase Inhibitors (Central)

Stability

Injection and tablet: Store at room temperature 15°C to 30°C (58°F to 86°F)

Transdermal system: Store at 20°C to 25°C (68°F to 77°F) Physically compatible when mixed in the same syringe with atropine, butorphanol, chlorpromazine, dimenhydrinate, diphenhydramine, droperidol, fentanyl, glycopyrrolate, hydromorphone, hydroxyzine, meperidine, metoclopramide, morphine, pentazocine, pentobarbital, perphenazine, prochlorperazine, promazine, promethazine, or thiopental

Mechanism of Action Blocks the action of acetylcholine at parasympathetic sites in smooth muscle, secretory glands and the CNS; increases cardiac output, dries secretions, antagonizes histamine and serotonin

Pharmacodynamics

Onset of action:

Oral, I.M.: 30 minutes to 1 hour

I.V.: 10 minutes

Transdermal: 4 hours

Duration:

Oral, I.M.: 4-6 hours

I.V.: 2 hours

Transdermal: 72 hours

Pharmacokinetics (Adult data unless noted)

Absorption: Well absorbed by all routes of administration

Metabolism: In the liver

Half-life: 9.5 hours

Excretion: <5% excreted unchanged in the urine

Dosing: Usual

Preoperatively and antiemetic:

I.M., I.V., SubQ:

Children: 6 mcg/kg/dose (maximum dose: 0.3 mg/ dose); may be repeated every 6-8 hours

Adults: 0.3-0.65 mg; may be repeated 3-4 times/day

Transdermal: Adults: Apply 1 disc behind the ear the evening before surgery; if prior to cesarean section, apply 1 hour prior to minimize exposure to infant

Motion sickness:

Oral: Children >12 years and Adults: 1-2 tablets 1 hour prior to exposure; may repeat after 8 hours of continued exposure

Transdermal: Children >12 years and Adults: Apply 1 disc behind the ear at least 4 hours prior to exposure every 3 days as needed

Administration

Oral: May be administered without regard to food

Parenteral: I.V.: Dilute with an equal volume of SWI and administer by direct I.V. injection over 2-3 minutes

Transdermal: Transdermal patch is programmed to deliver 1 mg over 3 days. Once applied, do not remove the patch for 3 full days. Apply patch to hairless area behind one ear; wash hands before and after application; if becomes ▶

dislodged, replace with fresh patch. Do not use any patch that has been damaged, cut, or manipulated in any way.

Test Interactions Interferes with gastric secretion test

Dosage Forms Excipient information presented when available (limited, particularly for generics); consult specific product labeling.

Patch 72 Hour, Transdermal:
Transderm-Scop: 1.5 mg (1 ea, 4 ea, 10 ea, 24 ea)

Solution, Injection, as hydrobromide:
Generic: 0.4 mg/mL (1 mL)

Scopolamine (Ophthalmic) (skoe POL a meen)

Brand Names: U.S. Isopto Hyoscine

Therapeutic Category Anticholinergic Agent, Ophthalmic; Ophthalmic Agent, Mydriatic

Generic Availability (U.S.) No

Use To produce cycloplegia and mydriasis; treatment of iridocyclitis

Pregnancy Considerations When administered intravenously or transdermally, scopolamine crosses the placenta; refer to Scopolamine (Systemic) monograph for details. Scopolamine is rapidly absorbed systemically after ocular application (Lahdes, 1990).

Contraindications Hypersensitivity to scopolamine or any component; patients hypersensitive to belladonna or barbiturates may be hypersensitive to scopolamine; narrow-angle glaucoma

Warnings Discontinue if patient reports unusual visual disturbances or pain within the eye.

Adverse Reactions Note: Systemic adverse effects have been reported following ophthalmic administration.

Central nervous system: Drowsiness, somnolence, visual hallucination

Dermatologic: Eczematoid dermatitis

Gastrointestinal: Xerostomia

Ocular: Blurred vision, edema, exudate, follicular conjunctivitis, increased intraocular pressure, local irritation, photophobia, vascular congestion

Drug Interactions

Metabolism/Transport Effects None known.

Avoid Concomitant Use

Avoid concomitant use of Scopolamine (Ophthalmic) with any of the following: Aclidinium; Azelastine (Nasal); Ipratropium (Oral Inhalation); Paraldehyde; Potassium Chloride; Thalidomide; Tiotropium; Umeclidinium

Increased Effect/Toxicity

Scopolamine (Ophthalmic) may increase the levels/effects of: AbobotulinumtoxinA; Alcohol (Ethyl); Analgesics (Opioid); Anticholinergic Agents; Azelastine (Nasal); Buprenorphine; Cannabinoid-Containing Products; CNS Depressants; Hydrocodone; Methotrimeprazine; Metyrosine; Mirabegron; Mirtazapine; OnabotulinumtoxinA; Paraldehyde; Potassium Chloride; Pramipexole; RimabotulinumtoxinB; ROPINIRole; Rotigotine; Selective Serotonin Reuptake Inhibitors; Thalidomide; Thiazide Diuretics; Tiotropium; Topiramate; Zolpidem

The levels/effects of Scopolamine (Ophthalmic) may be increased by: Aclidinium; Brimonidine (Topical); Cannabis; Doxylamine; Dronabinol; Droperidol; HydrOXYzine; Ipratropium (Oral Inhalation); Kava Kava; Magnesium Sulfate; Methotrimeprazine; Nabilone; Perampanel; Pramlintide; Rufinamide; Sodium Oxybate; Tapentadol; Tetrahydrocannabinol; Umeclidinium

Decreased Effect

Scopolamine (Ophthalmic) may decrease the levels/effects of: Acetylcholinesterase Inhibitors (Central); Secretin

The levels/effects of Scopolamine (Ophthalmic) may be decreased by: Acetylcholinesterase Inhibitors (Central)

Stability Store at 8°C to 27°C (46°F to 80°F); protect from light

Mechanism of Action Blocks the action of acetylcholine at parasympathetic sites in sphincter muscle of the iris and the accommodative muscle of the ciliary body; prevents accommodation; dilates pupils

Dosing: Usual

Refraction:
Children: Instill 1 drop of 0.25% to eye(s) twice daily for 2 days before procedure
Adults: Instill 1-2 drops of 0.25% to eye(s) 1 hour before procedure

Iridocyclitis:
Children: Instill 1 drop of 0.25% to eye(s) up to 3 times/day
Adults: Instill 1-2 drops of 0.25% to eye(s) up to 3 times/day

Administration Instill drops to conjunctival sac of affected eye(s); avoid contact of bottle tip with skin or eye; finger pressure should be applied to lacrimal sac during and for 1-2 minutes after instillation to decrease risk of absorption and systemic reactions. Remove contact lenses prior to administration; wait 15 minutes before reinserting if using products containing benzalkonium chloride. Wash hands following administration.

Dosage Forms Excipient information presented when available (limited, particularly for generics); consult specific product labeling.

Solution, Ophthalmic, as hydrobromide:
Isopto Hyoscine: 0.25% (5 mL)

References

Lahdes K, Huupponen R, Kaila T, et al. "Systemic Absorption of Ocular Scopolamine in Patients," *J Ocul Pharmacol*, 1990 6(1):61-6.

◆ **Scopolamine Base** *see* Scopolamine (Systemic) *on page 1872*

◆ **Scopolamine Butylbromide** *see* Scopolamine (Systemic) *on page 1872*

◆ **Scopolamine Hydrobromide** *see* Scopolamine (Ophthalmic) *on page 1874*

◆ **Scopolamine Hydrobromide** *see* Scopolamine (Systemic) *on page 1872*

◆ **Scopolamine Hydrobromide Injection (Can)** *see* Scopolamine (Systemic) *on page 1872*

◆ **Scopolamine, Hyoscyamine, Atropine, and Phenobarbital** *see* Hyoscyamine, Atropine, Scopolamine, and Phenobarbital *on page 1058*

◆ **Scorpion Antivenin** *see* Centruroides Immune F(ab')₂ (Equine) *on page 428*

◆ **Scorpion Antivenom** *see* Centruroides Immune F(ab')₂ (Equine) *on page 428*

◆ **Scot-Tussin Allergy Relief [OTC]** *see* DiphenhydrAMINE (Systemic) *on page 673*

◆ **Scot-Tussin Diabetes CF [OTC]** *see* Dextromethorphan *on page 636*

◆ **Scot-Tussin Expectorant [OTC]** *see* GuaiFENesin *on page 984*

◆ **Scot-Tussin Senior [OTC]** *see* Guaifenesin and Dextromethorphan *on page 987*

◆ **Scytera [OTC]** *see* Coal Tar *on page 532*

◆ **SD/01** *see* Pegfilgrastim *on page 1616*

◆ **Sea-Clens Wound Cleanser [OTC]** *see* Sodium Chloride *on page 1902*

◆ **Sea Soft Nasal Mist [OTC]** *see* Sodium Chloride *on page 1902*

◆ **Sebasorb [OTC]** *see* Salicylic Acid *on page 1860*

◆ **Sebcur® (Can)** *see* Salicylic Acid *on page 1860*

◆ **Sebex [OTC]** *see* Sulfur and Salicylic Acid *on page 1956*

- **SE BPO Wash** *see* Benzoyl Peroxide *on page 275*
- **Seb-Prev [DSC]** *see* Sulfacetamide (Topical) *on page 1944*
- **Seb-Prev Wash** *see* Sulfacetamide (Topical) *on page 1944*
- **Sebulex® [OTC]** *see* Sulfur and Salicylic Acid *on page 1956*

Secobarbital (see koe BAR bi tal)

Medication Safety Issues
Sound-alike/look-alike issues:
Seconal® may be confused with Sectral®
BEERS Criteria medication:
This drug may be potentially inappropriate for use in geriatric patients (Quality of evidence - high; Strength of recommendation - strong).

Brand Names: U.S. Seconal
Therapeutic Category Barbiturate; Hypnotic; Sedative
Generic Availability (U.S.) No
Use Short-term treatment of insomnia; preanesthetic agent
Pregnancy Risk Factor D
Pregnancy Considerations Barbiturates can be detected in the placenta, fetal liver, and fetal brain. Fetal and maternal blood concentrations may be similar following parenteral administration. An increased incidence of fetal abnormalities may occur following maternal use. When used during the third trimester of pregnancy, withdrawal symptoms may occur in the neonate including seizures and hyperirritability; symptoms may be delayed up to 14 days. Use during labor does not impair uterine activity; however, respiratory depression may occur in the newborn; resuscitation equipment should be available, especially for premature infants.
Breast-Feeding Considerations Small amounts of barbiturates are found in breast milk.
Contraindications Hypersensitivity to secobarbital or any component; preexisting CNS depression, severe uncontrolled pain, porphyria, severe respiratory disease with dyspnea or obstruction
Warnings Hypersensitivity reactions including anaphylaxis and angioedema may occur. Hazardous sleep-related activities, such as sleep-driving (driving while not fully awake without any recollection of driving), preparing and eating food, and making phone calls while asleep have also been reported. Effects with other sedative drugs or ethanol may be potentiated.
Precautions Use with caution in patients with hypovolemic shock, CHF, hepatic impairment, respiratory dysfunction or depression, previous addiction to the sedative/hypnotic group, chronic or acute pain, renal dysfunction; tolerance or psychological and physical dependence may occur with prolonged use; abrupt discontinuation after prolonged use may result in withdrawal symptoms

Adverse Reactions
Central nervous system: Somnolence
Rare but important or life-threatening: Abnormal thinking, agitation, angioedema, anxiety, apnea, ataxia, bradycardia, CNS depression, complex sleep-related behavior (sleep-driving, cooking or eating food, making phone calls), confusion, constipation, dizziness, exfoliative dermatitis, fever, hallucinations, headache, hyperkinesis, hypotension, hypoventilation, insomnia, liver injury, megaloblastic anemia, nausea, nervousness, nightmares, pain at injection site, rash, syncope, unusual excitement, vomiting

Drug Interactions
Metabolism/Transport Effects Induces CYP2A6 (strong), CYP2C8 (strong), CYP2C9 (strong)

Avoid Concomitant Use
Avoid concomitant use of Secobarbital with any of the following: Azelastine (Nasal); Enzalutamide; Paraldehyde; Somatostatin Acetate; Thalidomide
Increased Effect/Toxicity
Secobarbital may increase the levels/effects of: Alcohol (Ethyl); Azelastine (Nasal); Buprenorphine; CNS Depressants; Hydrocodone; Hypotensive Agents; Meperidine; Methotrimeprazine; Metyrosine; Mirtazapine; Paraldehyde; Pramipexole; ROPINIRole; Rotigotine; Selective Serotonin Reuptake Inhibitors; Thalidomide; Thiazide Diuretics; Zolpidem

The levels/effects of Secobarbital may be increased by: Brimonidine (Topical); Cannabis; Chloramphenicol; Doxylamine; Dronabinol; Droperidol; Felbamate; HydrOXYzine; Kava Kava; Magnesium Sulfate; Methotrimeprazine; Nabilone; Perampanel; Primidone; Rufinamide; Sodium Oxybate; Somatostatin Acetate; Tapentadol; Tetrahydrocannabinol; Valproic Acid and Derivatives

Decreased Effect
Secobarbital may decrease the levels/effects of: Acetaminophen; Beta-Blockers; Calcium Channel Blockers; Chloramphenicol; Contraceptives (Estrogens); Contraceptives (Progestins); Corticosteroids (Systemic); CycloSPORINE (Systemic); CYP2A6 Substrates; CYP2C8 Substrates; CYP2C9 Substrates; Diclofenac (Systemic); Doxycycline; Enzalutamide; Etoposide; Etoposide Phosphate; Felbamate; Griseofulvin; LamoTRIgine; Propafenone; Teniposide; Theophylline Derivatives; Treprostinil; Tricyclic Antidepressants; Valproic Acid and Derivatives; Vitamin K Antagonists

The levels/effects of Secobarbital may be decreased by: Multivitamins/Minerals (with ADEK, Folate, Iron); Pyridoxine; Rifamycin Derivatives
Mechanism of Action Depresses CNS activity by binding to barbiturate site at GABA-receptor complex enhancing GABA activity, depressing reticular activity system; higher doses may be gabamimetic
Pharmacodynamics
Onset of action: Hypnosis: Oral: 15-30 minutes
Duration: Hypnosis: Oral: 3-4 hours with 100 mg dose
Pharmacokinetics (Adult data unless noted)
Absorption: Oral: Well absorbed (90%)
Distribution: V_d: Adults: 1.5 L/kg; crosses the placenta; appears in breast milk
Protein binding: 45% to 60%
Metabolism: In the liver by the microsomal enzyme system
Half-life:
Children: 2-13 years: 2.7-13.5 hours
Adults: 15-40 hours; mean 28 hours
Time to peak serum concentration: Oral: Within 2-4 hours
Elimination: Renally as inactive metabolites and small amounts as unchanged drug
Dialysis: Hemodialysis: Slightly dialyzable (5% to 20%)
Dosing: Usual Oral:
Children:
Preoperative sedation: 2-6 mg/kg (maximum dose: 100 mg/dose) 1-2 hours before procedure
Sedation: 6 mg/kg/day divided every 8 hours
Adults:
Hypnotic: Usual: 100 mg/dose at bedtime; range 100-200 mg/dose
Preoperative sedation: 100-300 mg 1-2 hours before procedure
Monitoring Parameters Blood pressure, heart rate, respiratory rate, pulse oximetry, CNS status
Additional Information Effectiveness for insomnia decreases greatly after 2 weeks of use; alkalinization of urine does not significantly increase excretion; withdraw

slowly over 5-6 days after prolonged use to avoid sleep disturbances and rapid eye movement (REM) rebound

In March 2007, the FDA requested that all manufacturers of sedative-hypnotic drug products, including Seconal® (secobarbital), revise the labeling to include a greater emphasis on the risks of adverse events. The events include severe hypersensitivity reactions including anaphylaxis and/or angioedema, as well as hazardous sleep-related activities (eg, sleep-driving - driving while not fully awake after consumption of sedative-hypnotic drug, with no recollection of the event). Other activities may include preparing and ingesting food, and the use of the telephone, while asleep. These events may occur at any time during therapy including with the first dose administered.

Manufacturers must provide written notification to healthcare providers regarding the new warnings. In addition, manufacturers are to develop "Patient Medication Guides" designed to educate consumers about the potential risks and to advise them of precautionary measures that can be taken. This advice will contain recommendations on correct utilization of the medication as well as the avoidance of the consumption of ethanol and/or other CNS-depressant agents. The FDA is also recommending manufacturers conduct studies evaluating the frequencies of sleep-driving (and other sleep-related behaviors) with the individual products.

Patients should be instructed not to discontinue these medications without first speaking with their healthcare provider. Patients should also be informed of the potential for an allergic reaction, the signs and symptoms of anaphylaxis, and the appropriate emergency self-treatment of an anaphylactic reaction.

Additional information on the sedative-hypnotic products and sleep disorders is available at http://www.fda.gov/NewsEvents/Newsroom/PressAnnouncements/2007/ucm108868.htm

Controlled Substance C-II

Dosage Forms Excipient information presented when available (limited, particularly for generics); consult specific product labeling.

Capsule, Oral, as sodium:
  Seconal: 100 mg [contains fd&c yellow #10 (quinoline yellow)]

References

Levine HL, Cohen ME, Duffner PK, et al, "Rectal Absorption and Disposition of Secobarbital in Epileptic Children," *Pediatr Pharmacol (New York)*, 1982, 2(1):33-8.

Nahata MC, Starling S, and Edwards RC, "Prolonged Sedation Associated With Secobarbital in Newborn Infants Receiving Ventilatory Support," *Am J Perinatol*, 1991, 8(1):35-6.

Wolfert RR and Cox RM, "Room Temperature Stability of Drug Products Labeled for Refrigerated Storage," *Am J Hosp Pharm*, 1975, 32 (6):585-7.

◆ **Secobarbital Sodium** *see* Secobarbital *on page 1875*

◆ **Seconal** *see* Secobarbital *on page 1875*

◆ **SecreFlo** *see* Secretin *on page 1876*

Secretin (SEE kr tin)

Brand Names: U.S. ChiRhoStim; SecreFlo

Therapeutic Category Diagnostic Agent, Gastrinoma (Zollinger-Ellison Syndrome); Diagnostic Agent, Pancreatic Exocrine Insufficiency

Generic Availability (U.S.) No

Use Diagnosis of gastrinoma (Zollinger-Ellison syndrome) and diagnosis of pancreatic exocrine dysfunction (chronic pancreatitis); facilitation of endoscopic retrograde cholangiopancreatography (ERCP) visualization

Pregnancy Risk Factor C

Pregnancy Considerations Reproduction studies have not been conducted.

Breast-Feeding Considerations It is not known if secretin is excreted in breast milk. The manufacturer recommends that caution be exercised when administering secretin to nursing women.

Contraindications Hypersensitivity to secretin or any component; do not give to patients with acute pancreatitis until attack has subsided

Precautions Administer an I.V. test dose of 0.2 mcg (0.1 mL) particularly in patients with a history of hypersensitivity, allergy or asthma; use with caution in patients who are highly nervous or have an excessive gag reflex; patients receiving anticholinergics, patients who have had a vagotomy, or patients with inflammatory bowel disease may have a reduced response to secretin; patients with alcoholic or other liver diseases may have an increased response to secretin

Adverse Reactions

Cardiovascular: Flushing

Gastrointestinal: Abdominal discomfort/pain, nausea, vomiting

Miscellaneous: Bleeding (sphincterectomy)

Rare but important or life-threatening: Abdominal cramps, anxiety, bloating, bradycardia (mild), diaphoresis, diarrhea, dyspepsia, faintness, fatigue, fever, headache, heart rate increased, hypotension, leukocytoplastic vasculitis, lightheadedness, numbness/tingling in the extremities, oral secretions increased, oxygen saturation decreased, pallor, pancreatitis (mild), rash (abdominal), respiratory distress (transient), sedation, seizure, warm sensation (abdomen/face)

Drug Interactions

Metabolism/Transport Effects None known.

Avoid Concomitant Use There are no known interactions where it is recommended to avoid concomitant use.

Increased Effect/Toxicity There are no known significant interactions involving an increase in effect.

Decreased Effect

The levels/effects of Secretin may be decreased by: Anticholinergic Agents

Stability Store in freezer (-20°C); SecreFlo™ should be used immediately after reconstitution; human secretin is also stable for 1 year refrigerated and 6 months at room temperature

Mechanism of Action Human and porcine secretin are both synthetically derived products and are equally potent on an osmolar basis. Secretin is a hormone which is normally secreted by duodenal mucosa and upper jejunal mucosa. It increases the volume and bicarbonate content of pancreatic juice; stimulates the flow of hepatic bile with a high bicarbonate concentration; stimulates gastrin release in patients with Zollinger-Ellison syndrome.

Pharmacodynamics

Maximum output of pancreatic secretions: Within 30 minutes

Duration: At least 2 hours

Pharmacokinetics (Adult data unless noted)

Distribution: V_d: Porcine formulation: 2 L (approximately); human formulation: 2.7 L

Protein binding: 40%

Inactivated by proteolytic enzymes if administered orally

Metabolism: Metabolic fate is thought to be hydrolysis to smaller peptides

Half-life: Porcine formulation: 27 minutes; human formulation: 45 minutes

Elimination: Clearance: Porcine formulation: 487 ± 136 mL/minute; human formulation: 580.9 ± 51.3 mL/minute

Dosing: Usual Children and Adults: I.V.:

Diagnostic agent for pancreatic function: 0.2 mcg/kg as single dose

Diagnostic agent for gastrinoma (Zollinger-Ellison): 0.4 mcg/kg as single dose

Facilitation of ERCP visualization: 0.2 mcg/kg as a single dose

Administration Parenteral: Reconstitute with 8 mL of NS resulting in a 2 mcg/mL solution; shake vigorously to ensure dissolution; use immediately by direct I.V. injection slowly over 1 minute

Monitoring Parameters Peak bicarbonate concentration of duodenal fluid aspirate (chronic pancreatitis); serum gastrin (gastrinoma)

Reference Range

Peak gastric bicarbonate concentration:
Normal: 94-134 mEq/L
Chronic pancreatitis: <80 mEq/L
Severe pancreatitis: <50 mEq/L
Serum gastrin:
Normal: ≤110 pg/mL
Gastrinoma: >110 pg/mL

Additional Information SecreFlo™ is available currently as an orphan drug by contacting the manufacturer Repligen; a double-blind crossover study of secretin 0.2 clinical units/kg versus placebo in 56 autistic children revealed no significant differences between the 2 groups (1 clinical unit is equivalent to 0.2 mcg) (Owley, 2001)

Dosage Forms Excipient information presented when available (limited, particularly for generics); consult specific product labeling.

Solution Reconstituted, Intravenous:
ChiRhoStim: 16 mcg (1 ea)
SecreFlo: 16 mcg (1 ea)

References

Owley T, McMahon W, Cook EH, et al, "Multisite, Double-Blind, Placebo-Controlled Trial of Porcine Secretin in Autism," *J Am Acad Child Adolesc Psychiatry*, 2001, 40(11):1293-9.

♦ **Secretin, Human** see Secretin *on page 1876*

♦ **Secretin, Porcine** see Secretin *on page 1876*

♦ **Secura Antifungal [OTC]** see Miconazole (Topical) *on page 1410*

♦ **Secura Antifungal Extra Thick [OTC]** see Miconazole (Topical) *on page 1410*

♦ **Seebri Breezhaler (Can)** see Glycopyrrolate *on page 977*

♦ **Selax [OTC] (Can)** see Docusate *on page 701*

♦ **Selenium** see Trace Elements *on page 2059*

Selenium Sulfide (se LEE nee um SUL fide)

Brand Names: U.S. Anti-Dandruff [OTC]; Dandrex [OTC]; Selsun [DSC]; Tersi

Brand Names: Canada Versel®

Therapeutic Category Antiseborrheic Agent, Topical; Shampoos

Generic Availability (U.S.) May be product dependent

Use To treat itching and flaking of the scalp associated with dandruff; to control scalp seborrheic dermatitis; treatment of tinea versicolor

Pregnancy Risk Factor C

Pregnancy Considerations Animal reproduction studies have not been conducted.

Breast-Feeding Considerations It is not known if selenium sulfide is found in breast milk following topical application. The manufacturer recommends that caution be used if administered to nursing women.

Contraindications Hypersensitivity to selenium or any component

Warnings Hazardous agent; use appropriate precautions for handling and disposal. Safety in infants has not been established; avoid use in children <2 years of age

Precautions Do not use on damaged skin to avoid any systemic toxicity

Adverse Reactions

Central nervous system: Lethargy

Dermatologic: Alopecia, hair discoloration, unusual dryness or oiliness of scalp

Gastrointestinal: Abdominal pain, garlic breath, vomiting following long-term use on damaged skin

Local: Burning, itching, irritation, stinging (transient)

Neuromuscular & skeletal: Tremor

Miscellaneous: Diaphoresis

Drug Interactions

Metabolism/Transport Effects None known.

Avoid Concomitant Use There are no known interactions where it is recommended to avoid concomitant use.

Increased Effect/Toxicity There are no known significant interactions involving an increase in effect.

Decreased Effect There are no known significant interactions involving a decrease in effect.

Mechanism of Action May block the enzymes involved in growth of epithelial tissue

Pharmacokinetics (Adult data unless noted) Absorption: Not absorbed topically through intact skin, but can be absorbed topically through damaged skin

Dosing: Usual Children ≥2 years and Adults: Topical:

Dandruff, seborrhea: Massage 5-10 mL into wet scalp, leave on scalp 2-3 minutes, rinse thoroughly and repeat application; alternatively, 5-10 mL of shampoo is applied and allowed to remain on scalp for 5-10 minutes before being rinsed off thoroughly without a repeat application; shampoo twice weekly for 2 weeks initially, then use once every 1-4 weeks as indicated depending upon control

Tinea versicolor: Apply the 2.5% lotion in a thin layer covering the body surface from the face to the knees; leave on skin for 10 minutes, then rinse thoroughly; apply every day for 7 days; then follow with monthly applications for 3 months to prevent recurrences

Administration Topical: For external use only; avoid contact with eyes or acutely inflamed skin

Dosage Forms Excipient information presented when available (limited, particularly for generics); consult specific product labeling. [DSC] = Discontinued product

Foam, External:
Tersi: 2.25% (70 g) [contains trolamine (triethanolamine)]
Lotion, External:
Selsun: 2.5% (120 mL [DSC])
Generic: 2.5% (118 mL, 120 mL)
Shampoo, External:
Anti-Dandruff: 1% (207 mL) [contains brilliant blue fcf (fd&c blue #1), menthol]
Dandrex: 1% (240 mL)

References

Lester RS, "Topical Formulary for the Pediatrician," *Pediatr Clin North Am*, 1983, 30(4):749-65.

♦ **Selsun [DSC]** see Selenium Sulfide *on page 1877*

♦ **Selzentry** see Maraviroc *on page 1304*

♦ **Senexon [OTC]** see Senna *on page 1877*

♦ **Senexon®-S [OTC]** see Docusate and Senna *on page 702*

Senna (SEN na)

Medication Safety Issues

Sound-alike/look-alike issues:

Perdiem may be confused with Pyridium

Senexon may be confused with Cenestin

Senokot may be confused with Depakote

Brand Names: U.S. Ex-Lax Maximum Strength [OTC]; Ex-Lax [OTC]; Geri-kot [OTC]; GoodSense Senna Laxative [OTC]; Natural Senna Laxative [OTC]; Perdiem Overnight Relief [OTC]; Senexon [OTC]; Senna Lax [OTC];

Senna Laxative [OTC]; Senna Maximum Strength [OTC]; Senna Smooth [OTC]; Senna-Gen [OTC] [DSC]; Senna-GRX [OTC]; Senna-Lax [OTC]; Senna-Tabs [OTC]; Senna-Time [OTC]; SennaCon [OTC]; Senno [OTC]; Senokot To Go [OTC]; Senokot XTRA [OTC]; Senokot [OTC]

Therapeutic Category Laxative, Stimulant

Generic Availability (U.S.) May be product dependent

Use Short-term treatment of constipation; evacuate the colon for bowel or rectal examinations

Pregnancy Considerations An increased risk of congenital abnormalities was not observed following maternal use of senna during pregnancy (Acs, 2009). Short-term use of senna is generally considered safe during pregnancy (Mahadevan, 2006).

Breast-Feeding Considerations Maternal use of senna is considered compatible with breast-feeding (Mahadevan, 2006).

Contraindications Hypersensitivity to senna or any component; nausea and vomiting; undiagnosed abdominal pain, appendicitis, intestinal obstruction or perforation

Warnings Concentrated liquid contains sodium benzoate which may cause allergic reactions in susceptible individuals; use products containing sodium benzoate with caution in neonates; *in vitro* and animal studies have shown that benzoate displaces bilirubin from protein binding sites

Precautions Avoid prolonged use (>1 week); chronic use may lead to dependency, fluid and electrolyte imbalance, vitamin and mineral deficiencies

Adverse Reactions Gastrointestinal: Abdominal cramps, diarrhea, nausea, vomiting

Drug Interactions

Metabolism/Transport Effects None known.

Avoid Concomitant Use There are no known interactions where it is recommended to avoid concomitant use.

Increased Effect/Toxicity There are no known significant interactions involving an increase in effect.

Decreased Effect There are no known significant interactions involving a decrease in effect.

Pharmacodynamics Onset of action:

Oral: Within 6-24 hours

Rectal: Evacuation occurs in 30 minutes to 2 hours

Pharmacokinetics (Adult data unless noted)

Metabolism: In the liver

Elimination: In the feces (via bile) and in urine

Dosing: Usual Oral:

Constipation:

Infants 1 month to 2 years: Syrup: 1.25-2.5 mL (2.2-4.4 mg sennosides) at bedtime, not to exceed 5 mL (8.8 mg sennosides)/day

Children:

Syrup:

2 to <6 years: 2.5-3.75 mL (4.4-6.6 mg sennosides) at bedtime, not to exceed 3.75 mL (6.6 mg sennosides) twice daily

6-12 years: 5-7.5 mL (8.8-13.2 mg sennosides) at bedtime, not to exceed 7.5 mL (13.2 mg sennosides) twice daily

Tablet:

2 to <6 years: 1/2 tablet (4.3 mg sennosides) at bedtime, not to exceed 1 tablet (8.6 mg sennosides) twice daily

6-12 years: 1 tablet (8.6 mg sennosides) at bedtime, not to exceed 2 tablets (17.2 mg sennosides) twice daily

Children ≥12 years and Adults:

Syrup: 10-15 mL (17.6-26.4 mg sennosides) at bedtime, not to exceed 15 mL (26.4 mg sennosides) twice daily

Tablet: 2 tablets (17.2 mg sennosides) at bedtime, not to exceed 4 tablets (34.4 mg sennosides) twice daily

Bowel evacuation: Children ≥12 years and Adults: 130 mg sennosides (X-Prep® 75 mL) between 2:00 PM to 4:00 PM on the day prior to procedure

Administration Oral: Administer with water; syrup can be taken with juice or milk or mixed with ice cream to mask taste.

Monitoring Parameters I & O, frequency of bowel movements, serum electrolytes if severe diarrhea occurs

Dosage Forms Excipient information presented when available (limited, particularly for generics); consult specific product labeling. [DSC] = Discontinued product

Leaves, Oral:

Generic: (454 g)

Syrup, Oral:

Senna-GRX: 8.8 mg/5 mL (236 mL) [contains parabens]

Generic: 8.8 mg/5 mL (236 mL, 237 mL); 176 mg/5 mL (15 mL, 237 mL)

Tablet, Oral:

Ex-Lax: 15 mg [sodium free]

Ex-Lax Maximum Strength: 25 mg [sodium free]

Geri-kot: 8.6 mg

GoodSense Senna Laxative: 8.6 mg

Perdiem Overnight Relief: 15 mg

Senexon: 8.6 mg

Senna Lax: 8.6 mg

Senna Laxative: 8.6 mg

Senna Maximum Strength: 25 mg

Senna Smooth: 15 mg [contains sodium benzoate]

Senna-Gen: 8.6 mg [DSC]

Senna-Lax: 8.6 mg

Senna-Tabs: 8.6 mg

Senna-Time: 8.6 mg

SennaCon: 8.6 mg

Senno: 8.6 mg

Senokot: 8.6 mg

Senokot To Go: 8.6 mg

Senokot XTRA: 17.2 mg

Generic: 8.6 mg, 15 mg

Tablet Chewable, Oral:

Ex-Lax: 15 mg

Ex-Lax: 15 mg [chocolate flavor]

References

Acs N, Bánhidy F, Puhó EH, et al, "Senna Treatment in Pregnant Women and Congenital Abnormalities in Their Offspring - A Population-Based Case-Control Study," *Reprod Toxicol*, 2009, 28(1):100-4.

Mahadevan U and Kane S, "American Gastroenterological Association Institute Medical Position Statement on the Use of Gastrointestinal Medications in Pregnancy," *Gastroenterology*, 2006, 131(1):278-82.

Perkin JM, "Constipation in Childhood: A Controlled Comparison Between Lactulose and Standardized Senna," *Curr Med Res Opin*, 1977, 4(8):540-3.

◆ **Senna and Docusate** *see* Docusate and Senna *on page 702*

◆ **SennaCon [OTC]** *see* Senna *on page 1877*

◆ **Senna-Gen [OTC] [DSC]** *see* Senna *on page 1877*

◆ **Senna-GRX [OTC]** *see* Senna *on page 1877*

◆ **Senna Lax [OTC]** *see* Senna *on page 1877*

◆ **Senna Laxative [OTC]** *see* Senna *on page 1877*

◆ **SennaLax-S [OTC]** *see* Docusate and Senna *on page 702*

◆ **Senna Maximum Strength [OTC]** *see* Senna *on page 1877*

◆ **Senna Plus [OTC]** *see* Docusate and Senna *on page 702*

◆ **Senna-S** *see* Docusate and Senna *on page 702*

◆ **Senna Smooth [OTC]** *see* Senna *on page 1877*

◆ **Senna-Tabs [OTC]** *see* Senna *on page 1877*

◆ **Senna-Time [OTC]** *see* Senna *on page 1877*

◆ **Senno [OTC]** *see* Senna *on page 1877*

◆ **Sennosides** *see* Senna *on page 1877*

◆ **Senokot [OTC]** see Senna on page 1877

◆ **Senokot-S® [OTC]** see Docusate and Senna on page 702

◆ **Senokot To Go [OTC]** see Senna on page 1877

◆ **Senokot XTRA [OTC]** see Senna on page 1877

◆ **SenoSol™-SS [OTC]** see Docusate and Senna on page 702

◆ **Sensorcaine** see Bupivacaine on page 318

◆ **Sensorcaine® (Can)** see Bupivacaine on page 318

◆ **Sensorcaine-MPF** see Bupivacaine on page 318

◆ **Sensorcaine-MPF Spinal** see Bupivacaine on page 318

◆ **Septa-Amlodipine (Can)** see AmLODIPine on page 135

◆ **Septa-Atenolol (Can)** see Atenolol on page 222

◆ **Septa-Ciprofloxacin (Can)** see Ciprofloxacin (Systemic) on page 471

◆ **Septa-Citalopram (Can)** see Citalopram on page 484

◆ **Septa-Metformin (Can)** see MetFORMIN on page 1353

◆ **Septra** see Sulfamethoxazole and Trimethoprim on page 1948

◆ **Septra DS** see Sulfamethoxazole and Trimethoprim on page 1948

◆ **Septra Injection (Can)** see Sulfamethoxazole and Trimethoprim on page 1948

◆ **Serevent Diskhaler Disk (Can)** see Salmeterol on page 1862

◆ **Serevent Diskus** see Salmeterol on page 1862

◆ **Seromycin [DSC]** see CycloSERINE on page 563

◆ **SEROquel** see QUEtiapine on page 1783

◆ **Seroquel (Can)** see QUEtiapine on page 1783

◆ **SEROquel XR** see QUEtiapine on page 1783

◆ **Seroquel XR (Can)** see QUEtiapine on page 1783

◆ **Serostim** see Somatropin on page 1920

Sertraline (SER tra leen)

Medication Safety Issues
Sound-alike/look-alike issues:
Sertraline may be confused with cetirizine, selegiline, Serevent, Soriatane

Zoloft may be confused with Zocor

BEERS Criteria medication:
This drug may be potentially inappropriate for use in geriatric patients (Quality of evidence - moderate; Strength of recommendation - strong).

Related Information
Antidepressant Agents on page 2219

Brand Names: U.S. Zoloft

Brand Names: Canada Apo-Sertraline; Auro-Sertraline; CO Sertraline; Dom-Sertraline; GD-Sertraline; JAMP-Sertraline; MINT-Sertraline; Mylan-Sertraline; PHL-Sertraline; PMS-Sertraline; Q-Sertraline; Ran-Sertraline; ratio-Sertraline; Riva-Sertraline; Sandoz-Sertraline; Teva-Sertraline; Zoloft

Therapeutic Category Antidepressant, Selective Serotonin Reuptake Inhibitor (SSRI)

Generic Availability (U.S.) Yes

Use Treatment of obsessive-compulsive disorder (FDA approved in ages ≥6 years and adults); treatment of major depressive disorder, panic disorder (with or without agoraphobia), post-traumatic stress disorder, premenstrual dysphoric disorder, and social anxiety disorder (social phobia) (FDA approved in adults)

Medication Guide Available Yes

Pregnancy Risk Factor C

Pregnancy Considerations Adverse events have been observed in animal reproduction studies. Sertraline crosses the human placenta. An increased risk of teratogenic effects, including cardiovascular defects, may be associated with maternal use of sertraline or other SSRIs; however, available information is conflicting. Nonteratogenic effects in the newborn following SSRI/SNRI exposure late in the third trimester include respiratory distress, cyanosis, apnea, seizures, temperature instability, feeding difficulty, vomiting, hypoglycemia, hypo- or hypertonia, hyper-reflexia, jitteriness, irritability, constant crying, and tremor. Symptoms may be due to the toxicity of the SSRIs/SNRIs or a discontinuation syndrome and may be consistent with serotonin syndrome associated with SSRI treatment. Persistent pulmonary hypertension of the newborn (PPHN) has also been reported with SSRI exposure. The long-term effects of in utero SSRI exposure on infant development and behavior are not known.

Due to pregnancy-induced physiologic changes, women who are pregnant may require adjusted doses of sertraline to achieve euthymia. The ACOG recommends that therapy with SSRIs or SNRIs during pregnancy be individualized; treatment of depression during pregnancy should incorporate the clinical expertise of the mental health clinician, obstetrician, primary healthcare provider, and pediatrician. According to the American Psychiatric Association (APA), the risks of medication treatment should be weighed against other treatment options and untreated depression. For women who discontinue antidepressant medications during pregnancy and who may be at high risk for postpartum depression, the medications can be restarted following delivery. Treatment algorithms have been developed by the ACOG and the APA for the management of depression in women prior to conception and during pregnancy.

Breast-Feeding Considerations Sertraline and desmethylsertraline are excreted in breast milk. Adverse events have been reported in nursing infants exposed to some SSRIs. The American Academy of Breastfeeding Medicine suggests that sertraline may be considered for the treatment of postpartum depression in appropriately selected women who are nursing. Infants exposed to sertraline while breast-feeding generally receive a low relative dose and serum concentrations are not detectable in most infants. Sertraline concentrations in the hindmilk are higher than in foremilk. If the benefits of the mother receiving the sertraline and breast-feeding outweigh the risks, the mother may consider pumping and discarding breast milk with the feeding 7-9 hours after the daily dose to decrease sertraline exposure to the infant. The long-term effects on development and behavior have not been studied. The manufacturer recommends that caution be exercised when administering sertraline to nursing women. Maternal use of an SSRI during pregnancy may cause delayed milk secretion.

Contraindications Hypersensitivity to sertraline or any component; use of MAO inhibitors within 14 days (potentially fatal reactions may occur); concurrent use of pimozide; oral concentrate is contraindicated in patients receiving disulfiram (contains 12% alcohol)

Warnings Clinical worsening of depression or suicidal ideation and behavior may occur in children and adults with major depressive disorder **[U.S. Boxed Warnings]**. In clinical trials, antidepressants increased the risk of suicidal thinking and behavior (suicidality) in children, adolescents, and young adults (18-24 years of age) with major depressive disorder and other psychiatric disorders. This risk must be considered before prescribing antidepressants for any clinical use. Short-term studies did **not** show an increased risk of suicidality with antidepressant use in patients >24 years of age and showed a decreased risk in patients ≥65 years.

Patients of all ages who are treated with antidepressants for any indication require appropriate monitoring and close observation for clinical worsening of depression, suicidality, and unusual changes in behavior, especially during the first few months after antidepressant initiation or when the dose is adjusted. Family members and caregivers should be instructed to closely observe the patient (ie, daily) and communicate condition with healthcare provider. Patients should also be monitored for associated behaviors (eg, anxiety, agitation, panic attacks, insomnia, irritability, hostility, aggressiveness, impulsivity, akathisia, hypomania, mania) which may increase the risk for worsening depression or suicidality. Worsening depression or emergence of suicidality (or associated behaviors listed above) that is abrupt in onset, severe, or not part of the presenting symptoms, may require discontinuation or modification of drug therapy. SSRI-associated behavioral activation (ie, restlessness, hyperkinesis, hyperactivity, agitation) is two- to threefold more prevalent in children compared to adolescents; it is more prevalent in adolescents compared to adults. Somnolence (including sedation and drowsiness) is more common in adults compared to children and adolescents (Safer, 2006).

Avoid abrupt discontinuation; discontinuation symptoms (including agitation, dysphoria, anxiety, confusion, dizziness, hypomania, nightmares, and other symptoms) may occur if therapy is abruptly discontinued or dose reduced; taper the dose to minimize risks of discontinuation symptoms; if intolerable symptoms occur following a decrease in dosage or upon discontinuation of therapy, consider resuming the previous dose with a more gradual taper.

To reduce risk of intentional overdose, write prescriptions for the smallest quantity consistent with good patient care. Screen individuals for bipolar disorder prior to treatment (using antidepressants alone may induce manic episodes in patients with this condition). Potentially fatal serotonin syndrome may occur when SSRIs are used in combination with serotonergic drugs (eg, triptans) or drugs that impair the metabolism of serotonin (eg, MAO inhibitors).

Dropper for oral concentrate contains natural rubber latex which may cause allergic reactions in susceptible individuals; avoid use in patients with allergy to latex. Some tablets contain polysorbate 80 (Tween 80) which may cause allergic reactions in susceptible individuals.

Precautions Use with caution in patients with seizure disorders, concomitant illnesses that may effect hepatic metabolism or hemodynamic responses (eg, unstable cardiac disease, recent MI), and in suicidal patients; use with caution and decrease dose in patients with hepatic dysfunction; may result in hyponatremia, SIADH, significant weight loss (monitor weight and growth in pediatric patients), decrease in serum uric acid (mild uricosuric effect, use with caution in patient at risk of uric acid nephropathy), activation of mania/hypomania, or abnormal bleeding; SSRIs may increase risk of bleeding (eg, upper GI bleeding) especially in patients receiving nonselective NSAIDs, aspirin, or other drugs that affect coagulation. Use with caution during late third trimester of pregnancy [newborns may experience adverse effects or withdrawal symptoms (consider risk and benefits); exposure to SSRIs late in pregnancy may also be associated with an increased risk for persistent pulmonary hypertension of the newborn (Chambers, 2006)]. SSRI-associated vomiting is two- to threefold more prevalent in children compared to adolescents; it is more prevalent in adolescents compared to adults (Safer, 2006). Children may experience some adverse effects not reported in adults, including aggressive reaction, epistaxis, hyperkinesia, purpura, sinusitis, urinary incontinence.

Adverse Reactions

Cardiovascular: Chest pain, palpitations

Central nervous system: Agitation, aggressive behavior (children ≥2%), anxiety, dizziness, drowsiness, fatigue, headache, hypertonia, hypoesthesia, insomnia, malaise, nervousness, pain, paresthesia, yawning

Dermatologic: Diaphoresis, skin rash

Endocrine & metabolic: Decreased libido, weight gain

Gastrointestinal: Abdominal pain, anorexia, constipation, diarrhea, dyspepsia, flatulence, increased appetite, nausea, vomiting, xerostomia

Genitourinary: Ejaculatory disorder, impotence, urinary incontinence (children ≥2%)

Hematologic & oncologic: Purpura (children)

Neuromuscular & skeletal: Back pain (≥1%), hyperkinesia (children ≥2%), myalgia(≥1%), tremor, weakness

Ophthalmic: Visual disturbance

Otic: Tinnitus

Respiratory: Epistaxis (children ≥2%), rhinitis, sinusitis (children ≥2%)

Miscellaneous: Fever (children ≥2%)

Rare but important or life-threatening: Acute renal failure, agranulocytosis, altered platelet function, anaphylactoid reaction, aplastic anemia, apnea, ataxia, atrial arrhythmia, atrioventricular block, bradycardia, cerebrovascular spasm, choreoathetosis, colitis, coma, cystitis, depression, diverticulitis, dystonia, edema, esophagitis, extrapyramidal reaction, hematuria, hemoptysis, hepatic failure, hepatitis, hepatomegaly, hypertension, hypoglycemia, hyponatremia, increased INR, increased serum bilirubin, increased serum transaminases, leukopenia, myocardial infarction, neuroleptic malignant syndrome, oculogyric crisis, orthostatic hypotension, pancreatitis, peptic ulcer bleed, peripheral ischemia, proctitis, prolonged Q-T interval on ECG, pulmonary hypertension, pyelonephritis, rectal hemorrhage, serotonin syndrome, SIADH, Stevens-Johnson syndrome, suicidal ideation, thrombocytopenia, torsades de pointes, ventricular tachycardia, withdrawal syndrome

Drug Interactions

Metabolism/Transport Effects Substrate of CYP2B6 (minor), CYP2C19 (minor), CYP2C9 (minor), CYP2D6 (minor), CYP3A4 (minor); **Note:** Assignment of Major/Minor substrate status based on clinically relevant drug interaction potential; **Inhibits** CYP1A2 (weak), CYP2B6 (moderate), CYP2C19 (moderate), CYP2C8 (weak), CYP2C9 (weak), CYP2D6 (moderate), CYP3A4 (weak)

Avoid Concomitant Use

Avoid concomitant use of Sertraline with any of the following: Disulfiram; Dosulepin; Iobenguane I 123; Linezolid; MAO Inhibitors; Methylene Blue; Pimozide; Thioridazine; Tryptophan; Urokinase

Increased Effect/Toxicity

Sertraline may increase the levels/effects of: Agents with Antiplatelet Properties; Anticoagulants; Antidepressants (Serotonin Reuptake Inhibitor/Antagonist); Antipsychotics; Apixaban; ARIPiprazole; Aspirin; Beta-Blockers; BusPIRone; CarBAMazepine; Citalopram; CloZAPine; Collagenase (Systemic); CYP2B6 Substrates; CYP2C19 Substrates; CYP2D6 Substrates; Dabigatran Etexilate; Desmopressin; Dextromethorphan; Dosulepin; DOXOrubicin (Conventional); Fesoterodine; Fosphenytoin; Galantamine; Highest Risk QTc-Prolonging Agents; Hypoglycemic Agents; Ibritumomab; Lomitapide; Methadone; Methylene Blue; Metoprolol; Moderate Risk QTc-Prolonging Agents; Nebivolol; NSAID (COX-2 Inhibitor); NSAID (Nonselective); Phenytoin; Pimozide; Propafenone; RisperIDONE; Rivaroxaban; Salicylates; Serotonin Modulators; Thiazide Diuretics; Thioridazine; Thrombolytic Agents; Tositumomab and Iodine I 131 Tositumomab; TraMADol; Tricyclic Antidepressants; Urokinase; Vitamin K Antagonists

The levels/effects of Sertraline may be increased by: Alcohol (Ethyl); Analgesics (Opioid); Antiemetics (5HT3 Antagonists); Antipsychotics; BusPIRone; Cimetidine; CNS Depressants; Cobicistat; Dasatinib; Disulfiram; Glucosamine; Grapefruit Juice; Herbs (Anticoagulant/Antiplatelet Properties); Ibrutinib; Linezolid; Lithium; Macrolide Antibiotics; MAO Inhibitors; Metoclopramide; Metyrosine; Mifepristone; Multivitamins/Fluoride (with ADE); Multivitamins/Minerals (with ADEK, Folate, Iron); Multivitamins/Minerals (with AE, No Iron); Nonsteroidal Anti-Inflammatory Agents; Omega-3 Fatty Acids; Pentosan Polysulfate Sodium; Pentoxifylline; Prostacyclin Analogues; Tipranavir; TraMADol; Tryptophan; Vitamin E

Decreased Effect

Sertraline may decrease the levels/effects of: Clopidogrel; Codeine; Iobenguane I 123; Ioflupane I 123; Tamoxifen; Thyroid Products

The levels/effects of Sertraline may be decreased by: CarBAMazepine; Cyproheptadine; Darunavir; Efavirenz; Fosphenytoin; Nonsteroidal Anti-Inflammatory Agents; NSAID (COX-2 Inhibitor); NSAID (Nonselective); Peginterferon Alfa-2b; Phenytoin

Food Interactions Sertraline average peak serum levels may be increased if taken with food. Management: Administer consistently with or without food.

Stability Store at room temperature

Mechanism of Action Antidepressant with selective inhibitory effects on presynaptic serotonin (5-HT) reuptake and only very weak effects on norepinephrine and dopamine neuronal uptake. *In vitro* studies demonstrate no significant affinity for adrenergic, cholinergic, GABA, dopaminergic, histaminergic, serotonergic, or benzodiazepine receptors.

Pharmacodynamics Maximum effect may take several weeks

Pharmacokinetics (Adult data unless noted)

Protein binding: 98%

Metabolism: Significant first pass effect; undergoes N-demethylation to N-desmethylsertraline (significantly less active than sertraline); both parent and metabolite undergo oxidative deamination, followed by reduction, hydroxylation and conjugation with glucuronide (**Note:** Children 6-17 years may metabolize sertraline slightly better than adults, as pediatric AUCs and peak concentrations were 22% lower than adults when adjusted for weight; however, lower doses are recommended for younger pediatric patients to avoid excessive drug levels)

Bioavailability: Tablets approximately equal to oral solution

Half-life: Parent: Mean: 26 hours; metabolite (N-desmethylsertraline): 62-104 hours

Children: 6-12 years: Mean: 26.2 hours

Children: 13-17 years: Mean: 27.8 hours

Adults: 18-45 years: Mean: 27.2 hours

Elimination: 40% to 45% of dose eliminated in urine (none as unchanged drug); 40% to 45% eliminated in feces (12% to 14% as unchanged drug)

Clearance: May be decreased in patients with hepatic impairment

Dialysis: Not likely to remove significant amount of drug due to large V_d

Dosing: Usual Oral:

Children 6-12 years:

Depression: **Note:** Not FDA approved: Initial: 12.5-25 mg once daily; titrate dose upwards if clinically needed; may increase by 25-50 mg/day increments at intervals of at least 1 week; mean final dose in 21 children (8-18 years of age) was 100 ± 53 mg or 1.6 mg/kg/day (n=11); range: 25-200 mg/day; maximum dose: 200 mg/day (Dopheide, 2006; Tierney, 1995); avoid excessive dosing

Obsessive-compulsive disorder: Initial: 25 mg once daily; titrate dose upwards if clinically needed; increase by 25-50 mg/day increments at intervals of at least 1 week; range: 25-200 mg/day; maximum dose: 200 mg/day; avoid excessive dosing

Adolescents 13-17 years:

Depression: Initial 25-50 mg once daily; titrate dose upwards if clinically needed; may increase by 50 mg/day increments at intervals of at least 1 week; mean final dose in 13 adolescents was 110 ± 50 mg or about 2 mg/kg/day (McConville, 1996); in another study using a slower titration, the mean dose at week 6 was 93 mg (n=41) and at week 10 was 127 mg (n=34) (Ambrosini, 1999); range: 25-200 mg/day; maximum dose: 200 mg/day (Dopheide, 2006).

Obsessive-compulsive disorder: Initial: 50 mg once daily; titrate dose upwards if clinically needed; increase by 50 mg/day increments at intervals of at least 1 week; range: 25-200 mg/day; maximum dose: 200 mg/day

Adults:

Depression and obsessive-compulsive disorder: Initial: 50 mg once daily; titrate dose upwards if clinically needed; increase by 50 mg/day increments at intervals of at least 1 week; range: 50-200 mg/day; maximum dose: 200 mg/day

Panic disorder, post-traumatic stress disorder, and social anxiety disorder: Initial: 25 mg once daily; increase dose after 1 week to 50 mg once daily; titrate dose further if clinically needed; increase by 50 mg/day increments at intervals of at least 1 week; range: 50-200 mg/day; maximum dose: 200 mg/day

Premenstrual dysphoric disorder: Initial: 50 mg/day given daily throughout the menstrual cycle **or** only during the luteal phase of the menstrual cycle (depending on assessment of physician); may increase if needed by 50 mg increments per menstrual cycle; maximum dose when using daily dosing throughout the menstrual cycle: 150 mg/day; maximum dose when dosing only during the luteal phase of the menstrual cycle: 100 mg/day. **Note:** If using a 100 mg/day dose with luteal phase dosing, use a 50 mg/day titration step for 3 days at the beginning of each luteal phase dosing period.

Dosing adjustment in renal impairment: None needed

Dosing adjustment in hepatic impairment: Use with caution and in reduced doses

Administration Oral: May be administered without regard to food; do not administer with grapefruit juice; administer once daily dosage in morning or evening. Must dilute oral concentrate before use; measure dose with dropper provided and mix with 4 ounces of water, orange juice, lemonade, ginger ale, or lemon/lime soda; do not mix with other liquids; take dose immediately after mixing, do not mix ahead of time; sometimes a slight haze may be seen after mixing (this is normal)

Monitoring Parameters Weight and growth in children if long-term therapy; uric acid, CBC, liver function, serum sodium, urine output. Monitor patient periodically for symptom resolution; monitor for worsening depression, suicidality, and associated behaviors (especially at the beginning of therapy or when doses are increased or decreased)

Test Interactions May interfere with urine detection of benzodiazepines (false-positive)

Additional Information Two larger studies of children and adolescents with depression and obsessive-compulsive disorder utilized a forced upward dosage titration of sertraline to 200 mg/day; these studies conclude that the adult dosage titration regimen can be used in children ≥6 years and adolescents (Alderman, 1998; March, 1998); however, other studies in adults (Fabre, 1995) demonstrate that lower sertraline doses (50 mg/day) are as effective as higher doses with fewer adverse effects and discontinuations of therapy. Further studies are needed in pediatric patients to identify optimal doses; clinically, doses should be individually titrated based on patient response and adverse effects.

A recent report (Lake, 2000) describes 5 children (age 8-15 years) who developed epistaxis (n=4) or bruising (n=1) while receiving sertraline therapy. Another recent report describes the SSRI discontinuation syndrome in 6 children; the syndrome was similar to that reported in adults (Diler, 2002). Due to limited long-term studies, the clinical usefulness of sertraline should be periodically re-evaluated in patients receiving the drug for extended intervals; effects of long term use of sertraline on pediatric growth, development, and maturation have not been directly assessed.

Neonates born to women receiving SSRIs late during the third trimester may experience respiratory distress, apnea, cyanosis, temperature instability, vomiting, feeding difficulty, hypoglycemia, constant crying, irritability, hypotonia, hypertonia, hyper-reflexia, tremor, jitteriness, and seizures; these symptoms may be due to a direct toxic effect, withdrawal syndrome, or (in some cases) serotonin syndrome. Withdrawal symptoms occur in 30% of neonates exposed to SSRIs *in utero*; monitor newborns for at least 48 hours after birth; long-term effects of *in utero* exposure to SSRIs are unknown (Levinson-Castiel, 2006).

Dosage Forms Excipient information presented when available (limited, particularly for generics); consult specific product labeling.

Concentrate, Oral:

Zoloft: 20 mg/mL (60 mL) [contains alcohol, usp, menthol]

Generic: 20 mg/mL (60 mL)

Tablet, Oral:

Zoloft: 25 mg [scored; contains fd&c blue #1 aluminum lake, fd&c red #40 aluminum lake, fd&c yellow #10 aluminum lake, polysorbate 80]

Zoloft: 50 mg [scored; contains fd&c blue #2 aluminum lake]

Zoloft: 100 mg [scored; contains polysorbate 80]

Generic: 25 mg, 50 mg, 100 mg

References

Alderman J, Wolkow R, Chung M, et al, "Sertraline Treatment of Children and Adolescents With Obsessive-Compulsive Disorder or Depression: Pharmacokinetics, Tolerability, and Efficacy," *J Am Acad Child Adolesc Psychiatry*, 1998, 37(4):386-94.

Ambrosini PJ, Wagner KD, Biederman J, et al, "Multicenter Open-Label Sertraline Study in Adolescent Outpatients With Major Depression," *J Am Acad Child Adolesc Psychiatry*, 1999, 38(5):566-72.

Chambers CD, Hernandez-Diaz S, Van Marter LJ, et al, "Selective Serotonin-Reuptake Inhibitors and Risk of Persistent Pulmonary Hypertension of the Newborn," *N Engl J Med*, 2006, 354(6):579-87.

Diler R and Avci A, "Selective Serotonin Reuptake Inhibitor Discontinuation Syndrome in Children: Six Case Reports," *Current Therapeutic Research*, 2002, 63(3):188-97.

Dopheide JA, "Recognizing and Treating Depression in Children and Adolescents," *Am J Health Syst Pharm*, 2006, 63(3):233-43.

Fabre LF, Abuzzahab FS, Amin M, et al, "Sertraline Safety and Efficacy in Major Depression: A Double-Blind Fixed-Dose Comparison With Placebo," *Biol Psychiatry*, 1995, 38(9):592-602.

Findling RL, Reed MD, and Blumer JL, "Pharmacological Treatment of Depression in Children and Adolescents," *Paediatr Drugs*, 1999, 1 (3):161-82.

Lake MB, Birmaher B, Wassick S, et al, "Bleeding and Selective Serotonin Reuptake Inhibitors in Childhood and Adolescence," *J Child Adolesc Psychopharmacol*, 2000, 10(1):35-8.

Levinson-Castiel R, Merlob P, Linder N, et al, "Neonatal Abstinence Syndrome After *in utero* Exposure to Selective Serotonin Reuptake Inhibitors in Term Infants," *Arch Pediatr Adolesc Med*, 2006, 160 (2):173-6.

March JS, Biederman J, Wolkow R, et al, "Sertraline in Children and Adolescents With Obsessive-Compulsive Disorder: A Multicenter Randomized Controlled Trial," *JAMA*, 1998, 280(20):1752-6.

McConville BJ, Minnery KL, Sorter MT, et al, "An Open Study of the Effects of Sertraline on Adolescent Major Depression," *J Child Adolesc Psychopharmacol*, 1996, 6(1):41-51.

Safer DJ and Zito JM, "Treatment Emergent Adverse Effects of Selective Serotonin Reuptake Inhibitors by Age Group: Children vs. Adolescents," *J Child Adolesc Psychopharmacol*, 2006, 16 (1/2):159-69.

Sharp SC and Hellings JA, "Efficacy and Safety of Selective Serotonin Reuptake Inhibitors in the Treatment of Depression in Children and Adolescents: Practitioner Review," *Clin Drug Investig*, 2006, 26 (5):247-55.

Thomsen PH, "Obsessive-Compulsive Disorder: Pharmacological Treatment," *Eur Child Adolesc Psychiatry*, 2000, 9 (Suppl 1):I76-84.

Tierney E, Joshi PT, Llinas JF, et al, "Sertraline for Major Depression in Children and Adolescents: Preliminary Clinical Experience," *J Child Adolesc Psychopharmacol*, 1995; 5(1):13-27.

Wagner KD, "Pharmacotherapy for Major Depression in Children and Adolescents," *Prog Neuropsychopharmacol Biol Psychiatry*, 2005, 29 (5):819-26.

◆ **Sertraline Hydrochloride** *see* Sertraline *on page 1879*

◆ **Serzone** *see* Nefazodone *on page 1474*

Sevelamer (se VEL a mer)

Medication Safety Issues

Sound-alike/look-alike issues:

Renagel® may be confused with Reglan®, Regonol®, Renvela®

Renvela® may be confused with Reglan®, Regonol®, Renagel®

Sevelamer may be confused with Savella®

International issues:

Renagel [U.S., Canada, and multiple international markets] may be confused with Remegel brand name for aluminium hydroxide and magnesium carbonate [Netherlands] and for calcium carbonate [Hungary, Great Britain and Ireland] and with Remegel Wind Relief brand name for calcium carbonate and simethicone [Great Britain]

Related Information

Oral Medications That Should Not Be Crushed or Altered *on page 2438*

Brand Names: U.S. Renagel; Renvela

Brand Names: Canada Renagel; Renvela

Therapeutic Category Phosphate Binder

Generic Availability (U.S.) May be product dependent

Use Reduction of serum phosphorus in patients with chronic kidney disease on hemodialysis (FDA approved in adults)

Pregnancy Risk Factor C

Pregnancy Considerations Adverse events were observed in animal reproduction studies. Sevelamer is not absorbed systemically; however, it may cause a reduction in the absorption of some vitamins.

Breast-Feeding Considerations Sevelamer is not absorbed systemically; however, it may cause a reduction in the absorption of some vitamins.

Contraindications Hypersensitivity to sevelamer or any component; bowel obstruction

Warnings In preclinical animal studies, sevelamer (at doses of 6-100 times the recommended human dose) reduced the levels of vitamin D, E, K, and folic acid; no evidence of decreased vitamin levels has been shown in human trials; however, most patients were receiving vitamin supplements.

Precautions Use tablet dosage form with caution in patients with gastrointestinal disorders including dysphagia, swallowing disorders, severe gastrointestinal motility disorders (including constipation), or major gastrointestinal surgery; broken or crushed tablets will rapidly expand in water/saliva and may be a choking hazard; consider use of powder for suspension in these patients. Bowel obstruction and perforation have also been reported with sevelamer use.

Sevelamer may bind to some drugs in the gastrointestinal tract and decrease their absorption; when changes in absorption of oral medications may have significant clinical consequences (such as antiarrhythmic and antiseizure medications), these medications should be taken at least 1 hour before or 3 hours after a dose of sevelamer.

In a trial conducted in pediatric patients (n=18; age range: 10 months to 18 years), an increase in metabolic acidosis was noted in the sevelamer HCl group (incidence: 34.4%) (Pieper, 2006); in another pediatric trial (n=17, age range: 2-18 years), no untoward effects were reported (Mahdavi, 2003). Patients should be closely monitored.

Adverse Reactions

Endocrine & metabolic: Hypercalcemia, metabolic acidosis (more common in children)

Gastrointestinal: Abdominal pain, constipation, diarrhea, dyspepsia, flatulence, nausea, peritonitis (peritoneal dialysis), vomiting

Rare but important or life-threatening: Fecal impaction, intestinal obstruction (rare), intestinal perforation (rare)

Drug Interactions

Metabolism/Transport Effects None known.

Avoid Concomitant Use There are no known interactions where it is recommended to avoid concomitant use.

Increased Effect/Toxicity There are no known significant interactions involving an increase in effect.

Decreased Effect

Sevelamer may decrease the levels/effects of: Calcitriol; Levothyroxine; Mycophenolate; Quinolone Antibiotics

Food Interactions May cause reductions in vitamin D, E, K, or folic acid absorption. Management: Must be administered with meals. Consider vitamin supplementation.

Stability Store at 25°C (77°F); excursions permitted to 15°C to 30°C (59°F to 86°F); protect from moisture.

Mechanism of Action Sevelamer (a polymeric compound) binds phosphate within the intestinal lumen, limiting absorption and decreasing serum phosphate concentrations without altering calcium, aluminum, or bicarbonate concentrations.

Pharmacodynamics Onset of Action: Reduction in serum phosphorus: 1-2 weeks (Burke, 1997; Chertow, 1997)

Pharmacokinetics (Adult data unless noted)

Absorption: Not systemically absorbed

Elimination: Feces 100%

Dosing: Usual Note: Phosphate binding capacity: Sevelamer HCl 400 mg binds 32 mg of phosphate; 800 mg binds 64 mg of phosphate.

Infants, Children, and Adolescents:

Hyperphosphatemia: Limited data available: Oral:

Infants ≥10 months and Children <2 years: Sevelamer HCl (Renagel): Mean final dose: 140 ± 86 mg/kg/day (5.38 ± 3.24 **g**/day) was reported in a small trial (n=18, age range: 10 months to 18 years) to achieve the targeted serum phosphorus level. Initial dosing was based upon prior phosphate binder dose and serum phosphorus concentrations (Pieper, 2006). In a case report of a 19-month old, an initial dose of 100 mg/kg/day divided every 8 hours with titration up to 130 mg/kg/day was reported to effectively lower serum phosphorus levels (Storms, 2006).

Children ≥2 years and Adolescents: Sevelamer HCl (Renagel): Initial dose: 400 or 800 mg three times daily administered with meals; titrate at monthly intervals in 1200 mg/day increments (ie, 400 mg at each meal) to target phosphorus level; final mean range: 140-163 mg/kg/day (5.38-6.7 **g**/day); dosing based on experience in 46 patients; prior or final comparative calcium salt phosphate-binder dose: 4 ± 3 **g**/day (Gulati, 2010; Mahdavi, 2003; Pieper, 2006). Sevelamer carbonate (Renvela) has also been used in pediatric patients with similar efficacy as sevelamer hydrochloride (Renagel) (Gonzalez, 2010).

Hyperphosphatemia, pretreatment of oral and enteral nutrition: Limited data available: Oral: 800 mg (tablets or powder) added to up to 400 mL of breast milk or 100 mL of infant formula, tube feeding, and cow's milk; after sitting for 10 minutes, decant liquid from the precipitate at the bottom; reported experience has shown a decrease in phosphate of >85% in breast milk, 42% in cow's milk, 48% in tube feeding, and 68% in infant formula (KDOQI, 2009; Raaijmakers, 2013)

Adults: **Control of serum phosphorus:** Oral:

Patients not taking a phosphate binder: 800-1600 mg 3 times daily with meals; the initial dose may be based on the serum phosphorus:

Serum phosphorus >5.5 mg/dL and <7.5 mg/dL: 800 mg 3 times daily

Serum phosphorus ≥7.5 mg/dL and <9 mg/dL: 1200-1600 mg 3 times daily

Serum phosphorus ≥9 mg/dL: 1600 mg 3 times daily

Maintenance dose adjustment based on serum phosphorous concentration [goal range: 3.5-5.5 mg/dL; maximum dose studied was equivalent to 13 **g**/day (sevelamer hydrochloride) or 14 **g**/day (sevelamer carbonate)]:

Serum phosphorus >5.5 mg/dL: Increase by 400-800 mg per meal at 2-week intervals

Serum phosphorus 3.5-5.5 mg/dL: Maintain current dose

Serum phosphorus <3.5 mg/dL: Decrease by 400-800 mg per meal

Dosage adjustment when switching between phosphate-binder products: 667 mg of calcium acetate is equivalent to ~800 mg sevelamer (carbonate or hydrochloride); conversion based on dose per meal:

Calcium acetate 667 mg: Convert to 800 mg Renagel/Renvela

Calcium acetate 1334 mg: Convert to 1600 mg as Renagel/Renvela (800 mg tablets x 2) **or** 1200 mg as Renagel (400 mg tablets x 3)

Calcium acetate 2001 mg: Convert to 2400 mg as Renagel/Renvela (800 mg tablets x 3) **or** 2000 mg as Renagel (400 mg tablets x 5)

Administration

Oral: Administer with meals, at least 1 hour before or 3 hours after other medications.

Tablets: Swallow tablets whole; do not break, chew, or crush; contents will expand with water.

Packets for oral suspension: Mix powder with water prior to administration. The 0.8 g packet should be mixed with 30 mL of water and the 2.4 g packet should be mixed with 60 mL of water (multiple packets may be mixed together using the appropriate amount of water). Stir vigorously to suspend mixture just prior to drinking; powder does not dissolve. Drink within 30 minutes of preparing or resuspend just prior to drinking.

Monitoring Parameters

Serum chemistries, including bicarbonate and chloride

Serum calcium and phosphorus: Frequency of measurement may be dependent upon the presence and magnitude of abnormalities, the rate of progression of CKD, and the use of treatments for CKD-mineral and bone disorders. In children initial assessment should occur at CKD stage 2 (KDIGO, 2009):

CKD stage 3: Every 6-12 months

CKD stage 4: Every 3-6 months

CKD stage 5 and 5D: Every 1-3 months

Periodic 24-hour urinary calcium and phosphorus; magnesium; alkaline phosphatase every 12 months or more frequently in the presence of elevated PTH; creatinine, BUN, albumin; intact parathyroid hormone (iPTH) every 3-12 months depending on CKD severity

Reference Range

Corrected total serum calcium: Children, Adolescents, and Adults: CKD stages 2-5D: Maintain normal ranges; preferably on the lower end for stage 5 (KDIGO, 2009; KDOQI, 2005)

Phosphorus (KDIGO, 2009):

CKD stages 3-5: Maintain normal ranges

CKD stage 5D: Lower elevated phosphorus levels toward the normal range

Additional Information Chronic kidney disease (CKD) (KDIGO, 2013; KDOQI, 2002): Children ≥2 years, Adolescents, and Adults: GFR <60 mL/minute/1.73 m^2 or kidney damage for >3 months; stages of CKD are described below:

CKD Stage 1: Kidney damage with normal or increased GFR; GFR >90 mL/minute/1.73 m^2

CKD Stage 2: Kidney damage with mild decrease in GFR; GFR 60-89 mL/minute/1.73 m^2

CKD Stage 3: Moderate decrease in GFR; GFR 30-59 mL/minute/1.73 m^2

CKD Stage 4: Severe decrease in GFR; GFR 15-29 mL/minute/1.73 m^2

CKD Stage 5: Kidney failure; GFR <15 mL/minute/1.73 m^2 or dialysis

Dosage Forms

Excipient information presented when available (limited, particularly for generics); consult specific product labeling.

Packet, Oral, as carbonate:

Renvela: 0.8 g (1 ea, 90 ea); 2.4 g (1 ea, 90 ea) [citrus flavor]

Tablet, Oral, as carbonate:

Renvela: 800 mg

Generic: 800 mg

Tablet, Oral, as hydrochloride:

Renagel: 400 mg, 800 mg

References

Burke SK, Slatopolsky EA, Goldberg DI. RenaGel, a novel calcium- and aluminium-free phosphate binder, inhibits phosphate absorption in normal volunteers. *Nephrol Dial Transplant.* 1997;12(8):1640-1644.

Chertow GM, Burke SK, Lazarus JM, et al. Poly[allylamine hydrochloride] (RenaGel): a noncalcemic phosphate binder for the treatment of hyperphosphatemia in chronic renal failure. *Am J Kidney Dis.* 1997;29(1):66-71.

Kidney Disease: Improving Global Outcomes (KDIGO) CKD-MBD Work Group. KDIGO clinical practice guideline for the diagnosis, evaluation, prevention, and treatment of chronic kidney disease-mineral and bone disorder (CKD-MBD). *Kidney Int Suppl.* 2009;76(S113):1-130.

Kidney Disease: Improving Global Outcomes (KDIGO) CKD Work Group. KDIGO 2012 clinical practice guideline for the evaluation and management of chronic kidney disease. *Kidney Inter.* 2013;3:1-150.

Mahdavi H, Kuizon BD, Gales B, et al, "Sevelamer Hydrochloride: An Effective Phosphate Binder in Dialyzed Children," *Pediatr Nephrol,* 2003, 18(12):1260-4.

National Kidney Foundation. K/DOQI clinical practice guidelines for chronic kidney disease: evaluation, classification and stratification. *Am J Kidney Dis.* 2002;39:S1-S266.

National Kidney Foundation. K/DOQI clinical practice guidelines for bone metabolism and disease in children with chronic kidney disease. *Am J Kidney Dis.* 2005;46:S1-S122.

National Kidney Foundation. KDOQI clinical practice guideline for nutrition in children with CKD: 2008 update. *Am J Kidney Dis.* 2009;53:S1-S124.

Pieper AK, Haffner D, Hoppe B, et al, "A Randomized Crossover Trial Comparing Sevelamer With Calcium Acetate in Children With CKD," *Am J Kidney Dis,* 2006, 47(4):625-35.

Raaijmakers R, Houkes LM, Schröder CH, et al. Pre-treatment of dairy and breast milk with sevelamer hydrochloride and sevelamer carbonate to reduce phosphate. *Perit Dial Int.* 2013;33(5):565-572.

Storms LE, Chicella MF, Dice JE. Sevelamer therapy for pediatric end-stage renal disease. *Pharmacotherapy.* 2006;26(3):410-413.

◆ **Sevelamer Carbonate** see Sevelamer on page 1882

◆ **Sevelamer Hydrochloride** see Sevelamer on page 1882

◆ **SfRowasa** see Mesalamine on page 1347

◆ **S/GSK1349572** see Dolutegravir on page 705

◆ **Shohl's Solution (Modified)** see Sodium Citrate and Citric Acid on page 1906

◆ **Sig-Enalapril (Can)** see Enalapril on page 744

◆ **Silace [OTC]** see Docusate on page 701

◆ **Siladryl Allergy [OTC]** see DiphenhydrAMINE (Systemic) on page 673

◆ **Silapap Children's [OTC]** see Acetaminophen on page 47

◆ **Silapap Infant's [OTC]** see Acetaminophen on page 47

Sildenafil (sil DEN a fil)

Medication Safety Issues

Sound-alike/look-alike issues:

Revatio may be confused with ReVia, Revonto

Sildenafil may be confused with silodosin, tadalafil, vardenafil

Viagra may be confused with Allegra, Vaniqa

Brand Names: U.S. Revatio; Viagra

Brand Names: Canada Apo-Sildenafil; CO Sildenafil; GD-Sildenafil; PMS-Sildenafil; ratio-Sildenafil R; Revatio; Teva-Sildenafil; Viagra

Therapeutic Category Phosphodiesterase Type-5 (PDE5) Inhibitor

Generic Availability (U.S.) May be product dependent

Use Treatment of WHO Group I pulmonary arterial hypertension (PAH) (Revatio®: FDA approved in adults); treatment of erectile dysfunction (Viagra®: FDA approved in male adults). Has also been used for treatment of persistent pulmonary hypertension of the newborn (PPHN) refractory to treatment with inhaled nitric oxide; facilitation of weaning from nitric oxide (ie, to attenuate rebound effects after discontinuing inhaled nitric oxide); secondary pulmonary hypertension following cardiac surgery; **Note:** The FDA recommends against the use of sildenafil (Revatio®) for treatment of pulmonary arterial hypertension (PAH) in pediatric patients (1-17 years of age) due to a dose-dependent increased mortality risk observed in a long-term (median follow-up: 4 years; range: 0.3-7 years) study.

Pregnancy Risk Factor B

Pregnancy Considerations Adverse events were not observed in animal reproduction studies. Information related to the use of sildenafil for the treatment of pulmonary arterial hypertension (PAH) in pregnant women is limited (Hsu, 2011). Current guidelines recommend that women with PAH use effective contraception and avoid pregnancy (Badesch, 2007; McLaughlin, 2009). Less than 0.001% appears in the semen.

Breast-Feeding Considerations It is not known if sildenafil is excreted in breast milk. The manufacturer recommends that caution be exercised when administering sildenafil to nursing women.

Contraindications Hypersensitivity to sildenafil or any component; concurrent use of organic nitrates (eg, nitroglycerin, isosorbide dinitrate) in any form (potentiates the hypotensive effects)

Warnings The Food and Drug Administration (FDA) recommends that sildenafil (Revatio®) not be used to treat pulmonary arterial hypertension (PAH) in pediatric patients (1-17 years of age) due to a dose-dependent increased mortality risk observed in a long-term study (median follow-up: 4 years; range: 0.3-7 years). The Sildenafil in Treatment-Naive Children, Aged 1–17 Years, With Pulmonary Arterial Hypertension (STARTS-1, 2) study, a randomized, double-blind, international, multicenter, placebo-controlled, parallel-group trial, included 234 pediatric patients (1-17 years, weight ≥8 kg) with PAH (mild-to-moderate symptoms), and evaluated 3 doses (low, medium, and high) of sildenafil on efficacy and safety (eg, long-term mortality). High doses were in the range of 0.88-2.5 mg/kg/dose (rounded to the nearest 20, 40, or 80 mg fixed dose) administered three times daily and were based upon a desired steady state concentration of 373 ng/mL with the expected inhibition of 90% of phosphodiesterase type 5 activity *in vitro*. An increased risk of death was observed after 2 years of therapy and appeared to be dose-dependent with the highest risk in the high-dose group after ≥3 years of treatment (20% vs 9% and 14% in the low- and medium-dose groups, respectively); most deaths (74%) occurred in patients with idiopathic and hereditary PAH. The most frequent causes of death in the trial were pulmonary hypertension and heart failure and were determined to be part of disease progression by the authors; pulmonary hypertension and heart failure are also the most common causes of death in patients with PAH (Barst, 2012). The FDA is requesting additional long-term studies in adult patients.

Decreases in blood pressure may occur due to vasodilator effects; the cardiovascular status of the patient should be considered prior to initiating treatment; certain patients may be adversely affected by vasodilator effects (eg, patients with resting hypotension, fluid depletion, severe left ventricular outflow obstruction, or autonomic dysfunction). Sildenafil is not recommended for use in patients with pulmonary veno-occlusive disease; consider diagnosis of pulmonary veno-occlusive disease in patients who develop pulmonary edema when receiving sildenafil. Vaso-occlusive crisis requiring hospitalization may occur in patients with PAH secondary to sickle cell disease who are treated with sildenafil; the effectiveness of sildenafil in this patient population has not been established. In the presence of increased left atrial pressure unresponsive to afterload reduction, the use of sildenafil may result in pulmonary capillary hypertension. Sildenafil may cause transient dose-related impairment of blue/green color discrimination.

A sudden decrease or loss of hearing has been reported rarely, in patients receiving sildenafil for the treatment of pulmonary arterial hypertension and for erectile dysfunction. Hearing changes may be accompanied by vestibular symptoms (eg, tinnitus, vertigo, dizziness). It is not known if PDE5 inhibitors cause this condition or if other related factors are responsible. Patients receiving sildenafil for the treatment of pulmonary arterial hypertension who experience sudden hearing changes should **not** stop taking the medication, but should contact their healthcare provider immediately. Patients receiving sildenafil for erectile dysfunction who experience a sudden hearing change should discontinue the drug and notify a healthcare provider immediately. Ritonavir or other potent CYP3A inhibitors can increase sildenafil serum concentrations; concurrent use not recommended.

The oral suspension contains sodium benzoate; benzoic acid (benzoate) is a metabolite of benzyl alcohol; large amounts of benzyl alcohol (≥99 mg/kg/day) have been associated with a potentially fatal toxicity ("gasping syndrome") in neonates; the "gasping syndrome" consists of metabolic acidosis, respiratory distress, gasping respirations, CNS dysfunction (including convulsions, intracranial hemorrhage), hypotension and cardiovascular collapse; use the oral suspension containing sodium benzoate with caution in neonates; *in vitro* and animal studies have shown that benzoate displaces bilirubin from protein binding sites.

Additional warnings for patients treated for erectile dysfunction: Rare cases of sudden vision loss attributed to nonarteritic ischemic optic neuropathy (NAION) have been reported with the use of phosphodiesterase type-5 (PDE5) inhibitors when used for the treatment of male erectile dysfunction; NAION is a condition where blood flow is blocked to the optic nerve. NAION is more common in individuals with heart disease, diabetes, hypertension, certain eye problems, smokers, or those >50 years of age. Vision loss in one eye has been reported in some men after taking PDE5 inhibitors. It is not known if PDE5 inhibitors cause this condition or if other related factors are responsible. Patients taking a PDE5 inhibitor and who experience vision loss should stop taking the drug and notify a healthcare provider immediately.

A degree of cardiac risk is associated with sexual activity in patients with preexisting cardiovascular disease; sildenafil should not generally be used to treat erectile dysfunction in men with underlying cardiovascular disease which would deem sexual activity inadvisable. Prolonged or painful erections may occur; patients should seek immediate medical assistance if erection lasts >4 hours; permanent damage to the penis may occur without immediate treatment. The safety and efficacy of sildenafil with other treatments for erectile dysfunction have not been established; concurrent use is not recommended.

One possible case of retinopathy of prematurity reported after treatment with I.V. sildenafil (Marsh, 2004; Pierce, 2005)

Precautions Use with caution in patients with resting hypotension or hypertension; cardiovascular disease, including cardiac failure, unstable angina, or a recent history (within the last 6 months) of MI, stroke, or life-threatening arrhythmia; patients with retinitis pigmentosa (subpopulation of these patients have a retinal phosphodiesterase disorder); patients receiving concurrent bosentan (efficacy has not been evaluated; bosentan decreases sildenafil serum concentrations); patients receiving alpha-blockers or other antihypertensive agents (additive hypotensive effects; symptomatic hypotension may occur). Combination therapy of sildenafil products or use with other PDE-5 inhibitors has not been evaluated and should be avoided. Use with caution in patients with hepatic or renal impairment; dosage adjustment may be needed.

Use with caution in patients with anatomical deformation of the penis (angulation, cavernosal fibrosis, Peyronie's disease); conditions which may predispose patients to priapism (sickle cell anemia, multiple myeloma, leukemia). Epistaxis may occur and at a higher incidence in patients with pulmonary arterial hypertension due to connective tissue disorders or in patients receiving concurrent oral vitamin K antagonists. Use with caution in patients with bleeding disorders or with active peptic ulcer disease; safety of sildenafil is not known in these patients; may cause platelet dysfunction; *in vitro* study with human platelets indicates that sildenafil potentiates the antiaggregatory effect of nitric oxide.

Adverse Reactions Based upon normal doses for either indication or route. (Adverse effects such as flushing, diarrhea, myalgia, and visual disturbances may be increased with adult doses >100 mg/24 hours.)

Cardiovascular: Flushing

Central nervous system: Dizziness, headache, insomnia, paresthesia

Dermatologic: Erythema, skin rash

Gastrointestinal: Diarrhea, dyspepsia, gastritis, nausea

Genitourinary: Urinary tract infection

Hepatic: Increased liver enzymes

Neuromuscular & skeletal: Back pain, myalgia

Ophthalmic: Visual disturbance (including vision color changes, blurred vision, and photophobia)

Respiratory: Epistaxis, exacerbation of dyspnea, nasal congestion, rhinitis, sinusitis

Miscellaneous: Fever

Rare but important or life-threatening: Abnormal hepatic function tests, absent reflexes, amnesia (transient global), anemia, anorgasmia, anterior chamber eye hemorrhage, anterior ischemic optic neuropathy, arthritis, auditory impairment, breast hypertrophy, burning sensation of eyes, cardiac failure, cataract, cerebrovascular hemorrhage, colitis, cystitis, depression, diaphoresis, diplopia, dry eye syndrome, dysphagia, ECG abnormality, ejaculatory disorder, exfoliative dermatitis, falling, gastroenteritis, genital edema, gingivitis, glossitis, gout, herpes simplex infection, hyperglycemia, hypernatremia, hypersensitivity reaction, hypertension, hypertonia, hypoglycemia, increased bronchial secretions, increased intraocular pressure, ischemic heart disease, laryngitis, leukopenia, malignant melanoma (Li, 2014), migraine, myasthenia, mydriasis, myocardial infarction, neuralgia, neuropathy, orthostatic hypotension, otalgia, peripheral edema, pharyngitis, photophobia, priapism, prolonged erection, pulmonary hemorrhage, rectal hemorrhage, retinal edema, retinal hemorrhage, retinal vascular disease, rupture of tendon, seizure, severe sickle cell crisis (vaso-occlusive crisis in patients with pulmonary hypertension associated with sickle cell disease), skin photosensitivity, stomatitis, syncope, synovitis, tachycardia, transient ischemic attacks, unstable diabetes, urinary incontinence, ventricular arrhythmia, vitreous detachment, vitreous traction

Drug Interactions

Metabolism/Transport Effects Substrate of CYP1A2 (minor), CYP2C19 (minor), CYP2C9 (minor), CYP2D6 (minor), CYP2E1 (minor), CYP3A4 (major); **Note:** Assignment of Major/Minor substrate status based on clinically relevant drug interaction potential; **Inhibits** CYP2C9 (weak), CYP3A4 (weak)

Avoid Concomitant Use

Avoid concomitant use of Sildenafil with any of the following: Alprostadil; Amyl Nitrite; Boceprevir; Cobicistat; Conivaptan; Fusidic Acid (Systemic); Phosphodiesterase 5 Inhibitors; Pimozide; Riociguat; Telaprevir; Vasodilators (Organic Nitrates)

Increased Effect/Toxicity

Sildenafil may increase the levels/effects of: Alpha1-Blockers; Alprostadil; Amyl Nitrite; Antihypertensives; ARIPiprazole; Bosentan; Dofetilide; HMG-CoA Reductase Inhibitors; Lomitapide; Phosphodiesterase 5 Inhibitors; Pimozide; Riociguat; Vasodilators (Organic Nitrates)

The levels/effects of Sildenafil may be increased by: Alcohol (Ethyl); Boceprevir; Ceritinib; Cobicistat; Conivaptan; CYP3A4 Inhibitors (Moderate); CYP3A4 Inhibitors (Strong); Dasatinib; Erythromycin (Systemic); Fluconazole; Fusidic Acid (Systemic); Itraconazole; Ivacaftor; Ketoconazole (Systemic); Lorcaserin; Luliconazole; Mifepristone; Posaconazole; Protease Inhibitors; Sapropterin; Simeprevir; Stiripentol; Telaprevir; Voriconazole

Decreased Effect

The levels/effects of Sildenafil may be decreased by: Bosentan; CYP3A4 Inducers (Strong); Dabrafenib; Deferasirox; Etravirine; Mitotane; Peginterferon Alfa-2b; Siltuximab; St Johns Wort; Tocilizumab

Food Interactions Grapefruit juice may increase serum levels/toxicity of sildenafil. Management: Avoid grapefruit juice.

Stability

Revatio®:

Oral:

Tablets: Store at 20°C to 25°C (68°F to 77°F); excursions permitted to 15°C to 30°C (59°F to 86°F).

Powder for oral suspension: Store dry powder at <30°C (<86°F); protect from moisture. Following reconstitution, may store at <30°C (<86°F) or at 2°C to 8°C (36°F to 46°F). Discard unused portion after 30 days. Do not freeze.

Parenteral: Store at 20°C to 25°C (68°F to77°F); excursions permitted to 15°C to 30°C (59°F to 86°F).

Parenteral solution further diluted to 0.067-0.667 mg/mL in D_5W has been reported to be stable for 1 week when stored in polypropylene syringes at room temperature 20°C to 25°C (68°F to 77°F) (Al Hadithy, 2011).

Viagra®: Tablets: Store at 25°C (77°F); excursions permitted to 15°C to 30°C (59°F to 86°F).

Mechanism of Action

Erectile dysfunction: Does not directly cause penile erections, but affects the response to sexual stimulation. The physiologic mechanism of erection of the penis involves release of nitric oxide (NO) in the corpus cavernosum during sexual stimulation. NO then activates the enzyme guanylate cyclase, which results in increased levels of cyclic guanosine monophosphate (cGMP), producing smooth muscle relaxation and inflow of blood to the corpus cavernosum. Sildenafil enhances the effect of NO by inhibiting phosphodiesterase type 5 (PDE-5), which is responsible for degradation of cGMP in the corpus cavernosum; when sexual stimulation causes local release of NO, inhibition of PDE-5 by sildenafil causes increased levels of cGMP in the corpus cavernosum, resulting in smooth muscle relaxation and inflow of blood to the corpus cavernosum; at recommended doses, it has no effect in the absence of sexual stimulation.

Pulmonary arterial hypertension (PAH): Inhibits phosphodiesterase type 5 (PDE-5) in smooth muscle of pulmonary vasculature where PDE-5 is responsible for the degradation of cyclic guanosine monophosphate (cGMP). Increased cGMP concentration results in pulmonary vasculature relaxation; vasodilation in the pulmonary bed and the systemic circulation (to a lesser degree) may occur.

Pharmacodynamics

Maximum effect: Decrease blood pressure: Oral: 1-2 hours

Duration of Action: Decrease blood pressure: <8 hours

Pharmacokinetics (Adult data unless noted)

Absorption: Oral: Rapid; slower with a high-fat meal; tablet and suspension are bioequivalent

Distribution: Distributes into tissues

V_d total: Neonates: 22.4 L (or 456 L/70 kg) (Mukherjee, 2009)

V_{dss}: Adults: 105 L

Protein binding:

Neonates: Sildenafil: 93.9% ± 2.5%; N-desmethyl metabolite: 92% ± 3% (Mukherjee, 2009)

Adults: Sildenafil and N-desmethyl metabolite: ~96%

Metabolism: Via the liver via cytochrome P450 isoenzyme CYP3A4 (major route) and CYP2C9 (minor route). Major metabolite (UK-103320 or desmethylsildenafil) is formed via N-desmethylation pathway and has 50% of the activity as sildenafil.

Bioavailability: Oral: Mean: 41%; range: 25% to 63%; may be higher in patients with PAH compared to healthy volunteers; **Note:** A 10 mg dose of the injection is predicted to have an effect equal to a 20 mg oral dose taking into consideration the parent drug and active metabolite

Half-life (terminal):

Sildenafil:

Neonates: PNA 1 day: 55.9 hours (Mukherjee, 2009)

Neonates: PNA 7 days: 47.7 hours (Mukherjee, 2009)

Adults: 4 hours

Active N-desmethyl metabolite:

Neonates: 11.9 hours (Mukherjee, 2009)

Adults: 4 hours

Time to peak serum concentration: Oral: Fasting: 30-120 minutes (median 60 minutes); delayed by 60 minutes with a high-fat meal

Elimination: Excreted as metabolites; 80% of dose excreted in feces, 13% in urine

Clearance: Decreased in patients with hepatic cirrhosis or severe renal impairment; clearance may be lower in patients with PAH compared to normal volunteers. Sildenafil clearance in newborns is significantly decreased compared to adults, but approaches adult (allometrically scaled) values by the first week of life (Mukherjee, 2009). Clearance of N-desmethyl active metabolite is decreased in patients with severe renal impairment.

Dialysis: Not likely to be beneficial due to high protein binding

Dosing: Neonatal Note: In pediatric patients (1-17 years of age) with PAH, an increased mortality risk was associated with long-term use (>2 years) at dosage levels of 0.88-2.5 mg/kg/dose administered three times daily (Barst, 2012); the FDA recommends against the use of sildenafil (Revatio®) for treatment of PAH in children and adolescents; the mortality risk of long-term use in neonates is unknown.

Pulmonary hypertension: Note: Limited data available; dose not established; a wide range of doses and interpatient variability has been reported; careful dose titration is necessary; most literature consists of case reports or small studies; further studies are needed.

Oral: Full-term neonates: Usual range: 0.5-3 mg/kg/dose every 6-12 hours; the largest study was a double-blind, randomized, placebo-controlled trial and used an initial dose of 3 mg/kg/dose every 6 hours in 31 patients (Vargas-Origel, 2010); earlier studies used 0.3-2 mg/kg/dose every 6-24 hours; optimal duration not established (Ahsman, 2009; Baquero, 2006; Noori, 2007)

I.V.: GA >34 weeks and PNA <72 hours: PPHN: 0.4 mg/kg loading dose administered over 3 hours followed by continuous infusion of 1.6 mg/kg/**day** for up to 7 days was used in four patients in an open-label, dose-escalation trial of 36 neonates with an oxygenation index (OI) ≥15 on two occasions at least 30 minutes apart; 29 patients were also receiving iNO (Steinhorn, 2009); **Note:** The dose listed here is the dose recommended by the authors for use in future clinical trials.

Pulmonary hypertension, facilitation of inhaled nitric oxide (iNO) wean (in patients who previously failed iNO wean): Note: Limited information exists; dose not established; a wide range of doses and interpatient variability has been reported; careful dose titration is necessary; most literature consists of case reports or small studies; further studies are needed.

Oral: Full-term neonates:

Single dose: ~0.3 mg/kg/dose given once 70-90 minutes prior to iNO discontinuation was used in three patients (3 days, 6 weeks, and 4 months of age) (Atz, 1999)

Multiple dose: Initial: 0.3 mg/kg/dose (range: 0.22-0.47 mg/kg/dose) every 6 hours (average duration: 28 days) was used in seven patients (median age: 12 months; range: 3 days to 21 months); optimal duration of treatment not established (Lee, 2008).

Dosing: Usual

Infants, Children, and Adolescents: **Note:** In pediatric patients (1-17 years of age) with PAH, an increased mortality risk was associated with long-term use (>2 years) at dosage levels of 0.88-2.5 mg/kg/dose administered three times daily (Barst, 2012); the FDA recommends against the use of sildenafil (Revatio®) for treatment of PAH in children and adolescents; the mortality risk of long-term use in infants is unknown.

Pulmonary hypertension: Limited data available; dose and duration of therapy not established; interpatient variability has been reported; further studies are needed; Oral:

Infants: Initial: 0.25 mg/kg/dose every 6 hours **or** 0.5 mg/kg/dose every 8 hours; titrate as needed;

maximum reported dose range: 1-2 mg/kg/dose every 6-8 hours (Humpl, 2011; Mourani, 2009).

An open-label, prospective trial of 25 pediatric patients <5 years of age (median age: 6 months; age range: 10 days to 4.9 years) reported statistically significant improvement in echocardiography outcome measures; in 15 patients, sildenafil abolished rebound pulmonary hypertension following NO withdrawal; the initial dose of 0.25 mg/kg/dose four times daily was titrated as tolerated to a target of 1 mg/kg/dose four times daily; the reported median dose was 0.7 mg/kg/dose four times daily (range: 0.5-2.25 mg/kg/dose); reported duration of therapy was 9 days to 4.3 years (n=25); 11 patients were discontinued on sildenafil therapy due to clinical resolution; nine deaths were reported [severe lung hypoplasia (n=3); veno-occlusive disease post-chemotherapy (n=1); severe BPD (n=1); cause of death unrelated to pulmonary vascular disease (n=4)] (Humpl, 2011).

A retrospective trial of 25 pediatric patients <2 years of age (which included at least 16 infants) evaluated long-term safety and efficacy in patients with chronic lung disease (72% with BPD); at therapy initiation, the subject ages ranged from 14 days to 96 weeks (median: ~6 months); the initial dose of 0.5 mg/kg/dose every 8 hours was titrated as tolerated; the majority of patients were treated with 8 mg/kg/**day** (2 mg/kg/dose four times daily); echocardiogram showed clinical improvement in 88% of patients; reported duration of therapy was 28-950 days (median: 241 days); five deaths were reported during therapy (day 25-241 of therapy; median: 135 days); causes of death included sepsis, meningitis, and refractory respiratory disease (Mourani, 2009).

Children and Adolescents <18 years of age: **Note:** Dosage should not be increased; higher doses and long-term use are associated with an increased mortality risk (Barst, 2012).

8-20 kg: 10 mg three times daily

>20 kg to 45 kg: 20 mg three times daily

>45 kg: 40 mg three times daily

Dosing based on the STARTS-1and 2 trial, a randomized, double-blind, placebo-controlled study in 235 pediatric patients (1-17 years of age) which evaluated short-term and long-term safety and efficacy of 3 dose levels (low, medium, and high-dose); results suggested that the medium dose level (shown above) is efficacious at improving exercise capacity, functional class and hemodynamic status in the short-term (16 weeks duration); the low dosage level was not shown to be efficacious. The long-term safety and efficacy data showed a dose-dependent increased risk of mortality which was highest among the high-dose group. It was estimated that the dosing presented will produce serum concentration of 140 ng/mL and would be expected to inhibit 77% of phosphodiesterase type 5 activity *in vitro* (Barst, 2012).

Pulmonary hypertension, congenital heart surgery (postoperative): Limited data available; dosing regimens variable:

Oral (or nasogastric tube): Initial: 0.5 mg/kg/dose upon admission to ICU; increase in 0.5 mg/kg/dose increments every 4-6 hours up to a maximum dose of 2 mg/kg/dose as tolerated; upon discontinuation of mechanical ventilation, sildenafil therapy can be tapered over 5-7 days; dosing based on a retrospective report of 100 pediatric patients (including neonates through >10 years of age) which showed reduction in pulmonary arterial pressures and/or prevention of severe pulmonary hypertension (Nemoto, 2010). A lower dose of 0.35 mg/kg/dose every 4 hours for 1 week postoperatively was used in a retrospective, case-controlled trial of 38 pediatric patients (age range: 5-33 months) (Palma, 2011). In another retrospective report (n=45, median age: 32.6 months; range: 6 days to 17 years), a mean dose of 0.9 ± 0.3 mg/kg/dose four times daily was reported (Uhm, 2010). Further studies are needed. **Note:** Use of preoperative sildenafil therapy for the prevention of pulmonary hypertension following congenital heart surgery has produced variable efficacy results (Palma, 2011); a double-blind, placebo-controlled trial showed a negative impact on oxygenation and ventricular function (Vassalos, 2011).

I.V.: Infants >60 days and Children: Loading dose: Range: 0.04-0.35 mg/kg administered over 5 minutes, followed by a maintenance infusion: Reported range: 0.015-0.4 mg/kg/**hour** continued for 24-72 hours was used for pulmonary hypertension occurring within 48 hours of the end of cardiac surgery in a multicenter, randomized, double-blind, placebo-controlled dose-finding trial (n=17; median age: 5 months; age range: 3 months to 14 years; neonates and infants <60 days were excluded from the trial); dosages were either low, medium, or high dose (n=4 each treatment group; n=5 placebo) designed to attain serum concentrations of 40, 120, and 360 ng/mL, respectively; patients receiving sildenafil at all dosages were found to have lower pulmonary artery pressure and when compared to placebo, shorter duration of mechanical ventilation (median: 3 days vs 8 days), shorter ICU stay (median: 6 days vs 15 days), and shorter hospitalization (median: 12 days vs 21 days); study closed early due to slow patient accrual leading to underpowered results; no conclusions about dosage were able to be determined (Fraisse, 2011). Further studies are needed.

Pulmonary hypertension, facilitation of inhaled nitric oxide (iNO) wean (in patients who have not previously failed iNO wean): Limited data available: Oral: Single dose: 0.4 mg/kg/dose (range: 0.3-0.5 mg/kg/dose) given once 60 minutes prior to iNO discontinuation; dosing based on a randomized, double-blind, placebo-controlled trial in 29 infants and young children (median age: 5.6 months; age range: 1-15 months; n=15 treatment arm) (Namachivayam, 2006). Further studies are needed.

Adults:

Erectile dysfunction (Viagra®): Oral: Usual: 50 mg taken as needed, ~1 hour before sexual activity (dose may be taken 30 minutes to 4 hours before sexual activity). Based on effectiveness and tolerance, may increase dose to a maximum of 100 mg or decrease to 25 mg. Maximum recommended dosing frequency: Once daily

Pulmonary arterial hypertension (Revatio®):

Oral: 20 mg 3 times daily taken at least 4-6 hours apart; no evidence for additional efficacy was observed with higher doses; treatment with higher doses is not recommended

I.V.: 10 mg 3 times daily

Dosage adjustment in hepatic impairment: Adults:

Revatio®:

Mild-to-moderate hepatic impairment (Child Pugh class A and B): No dosage adjustment needed

Severe hepatic impairment (Child Pugh class C): Has not been studied

Viagra®:

Mild-to-moderate hepatic impairment (Child Pugh class A and B): Initial: 25 mg should be considered

Severe hepatic impairment (Child Pugh class C): Has not been studied

Dosage adjustment in renal impairment: Adults:

Revatio®: No dosage adjustments needed

Viagra®: Severe renal impairment (creatinine clearance <30 mL/minute): Initial: 25 mg should be considered

Dosage considerations for patients taking alpha blockers: Adults: Viagra®: Initial: 25 mg

Dosage adjustment for concomitant use of potent CYP34A inhibitors: Adults:

Revatio®:

Erythromycin: No dosage adjustment needed

Itraconazole, ketoconazole: Use is not recommended

Protease inhibitors: Contraindicated

Viagra®:

Erythromycin, itraconazole, ketoconazole: Initial: 25 mg should be considered

Protease inhibitors: Maximum sildenafil dose: 25 mg every 48 hours

Administration

Oral:

Revatio®: Administer doses at least 4-6 hours apart; may be administered without regard to meals; shake oral suspension well prior to use

Viagra®: Administer dose ~1 hour before sexual activity (may be administered 30 minutes to 4 hours before sexual activity).

I.V.: Revatio®:

Neonates: In clinical trials, loading dose was administered over 3 hours, followed by a continuous I.V. infusion (Steinhorn, 2009)

Infant, Children, and Adolescents: In clinical trials, loading dose was administered as a bolus over 5 minutes, followed by a continuous I.V. infusion (Fraisse, 2011)

Adults: Administer as an I.V. bolus

Monitoring Parameters Heart rate, blood pressure, oxygen saturation, PaO_2

Additional Information Sildenafil is ~10 times more selective for PDE-5 as compared to PDE-6. PDE-6 is found in the retina and is involved in phototransduction. At higher plasma levels, inhibition of PDE-6 may occur and may account for the abnormalities in color vision noted in some patients.

Product Availability Revatio oral suspension is not currently available in the U.S. Launch date for U.S. availability is unknown.

Dosage Forms Excipient information presented when available (limited, particularly for generics); consult specific product labeling.

Solution, Intravenous:

Revatio: 10 mg/12.5 mL (12.5 mL)

Tablet, Oral:

Revatio: 20 mg

Viagra: 25 mg, 50 mg, 100 mg [contains fd&c blue #2 aluminum lake]

Generic: 20 mg

Extemporaneous Preparations A 2.5 mg/mL sildenafil citrate oral suspension may be made with tablets and either a 1:1 mixture of methylcellulose 1% and simple syrup NF or a 1:1 mixture of Ora-Sweet and Ora-Plus. Crush thirty sildenafil 25 mg tablets (Viagra) in a mortar and reduce to a fine powder. Add small portions of chosen vehicle and mix to a uniform paste; mix while adding vehicle in incremental proportions to **almost** 300 mL; transfer to a graduated cylinder, rinse mortar with vehicle, and add quantity of vehicle sufficient to make 300 mL. Store in amber plastic bottles and label "shake well". Stable for 90 days at room temperature or refrigerated.

Nahata MC, Morosco RS, and Brady MT, "Extemporaneous Sildenafil Citrate Oral Suspensions for the Treatment of Pulmonary Hypertension in Children," *Am J Health-Syst Pharm*, 2006, 63(3):254-7.

References

Al Hadithy AF, de Goede AL, Eckhardt M, et al, "Stability of Sildenafil (Revatio®) Dilutions in Dextrose 5%," *Intensive Care Med*, 2011, 37 (11):1899.

Ahsman MJ, Witjes BC, Wildschut ED, et al, "Sildenafil Exposure in Neonates With Pulmonary Hypertension After Administration Via a Nasogastric Tube," *Arch Dis Child Fetal Neonatal Ed*, 2010, 95(2): F109-14.

Apitz C, Reyes JT, Holtby H, et al, "Pharmacokinetic and Hemodynamic Responses to Oral Sildenafil During Invasive Testing in Children With Pulmonary Hypertension," *J Am Coll Cardiol*, 2010, 55(14):1456-62.

Atz AM and Wessel DL, "Sildenafil Ameliorates Effects of Inhaled Nitric Oxide Withdrawal," *Anesthesiology*, 1999, 91(1):307-10.

Badesch DB, Abman SH, Simonneau G, et al, "Medical Therapy for Pulmonary Arterial Hypertension: Updated ACCP Evidence-Based Clinical Practice Guidelines," *Chest*, 2007, 131(6):1917-28.

Baquero H, Soliz A, Neira F, et al, "Oral Sildenafil in Infants With Persistent Pulmonary Hypertension of the Newborn: A Pilot Randomized Blinded Study," *Pediatrics*, 2006, 117(4):1077-83.

Barst RJ, Ivy DD, Gaitan G, et al, "A Randomized, Double-Blind, Placebo-Controlled, Dose-Ranging Study of Oral Sildenafil Citrate in Treatment-Naive Children With Pulmonary Arterial Hypertension," *Circulation*, 2012, 125(2):324-34.

Carroll WD and Dhillon R, "Sildenafil as a Treatment for Pulmonary Hypertension," *Arch Dis Child*, 2003, 88(9):827-8.

Erickson S, Reyes J, Bohn D, et al, "Sildenafil (Viagra) in Childhood and Neonatal Pulmonary Hypertension," *J Am Coll Cardiol*, 2002, 39 (Suppl):S402.

Fraisse A and Wessel DL, "Acute Pulmonary Hypertension in Infants and Children: cGMP-Related Drugs," *Pediatr Crit Care Med*, 2010, 11 (2 Suppl):S37-40.

Haworth SG and Hislop AA, "Treatment and Survival in Children With Pulmonary Arterial Hypertension: The UK Pulmonary Hypertension Service for Children 2001-2006," *Heart*, 2009, 95(4):312-7.

Humpl T, Reyes JT, Erickson S, et al, "Sildenafil Therapy for Neonatal and Childhood Pulmonary Hypertensive Vascular Disease," *Cardiol Young*, 2011, 21(2):187-93.

Humpl T, Reyes JT, Holtby H, et al, "Beneficial Effect of Oral Sildenafil Therapy on Childhood Pulmonary Arterial Hypertension: Twelve-Month Clinical Trial of a Single-Drug, Open-Label, Pilot Study," *Circulation*, 2005, 111(24):3274-80.

Hsu CH, Gomberg-Maitland M, Glassner C, et al, "The Management of Pregnancy and Pregnancy-Related Medical Conditions in Pulmonary Arterial Hypertension Patients," *Int J Clin Pract Suppl*, 2011, 172:6-14.

Karatza AA, Bush A, and Magee AG, "Safety and Efficacy of Sildenafil Therapy in Children With Pulmonary Hypertension," *Int J Cardiol*, 2005, 100(2):267-73.

Karatza AA, Narang I, Rosenthal M, et al, "Treatment of Primary Pulmonary Hypertension With Oral Sildenafil," *Respiration*, 2004, 71 (2):192-4.

König K and Henschke P, "Successful Weaning of Nitric Oxide Facilitated by a Single Dose of Sildenafil in a Baby With Persistent Pulmonary Hypertension of the Newborn," *Pediatr Pulmonol*, 2009, 44(8):837.

Kothari SS and Duggal B, "Chronic Oral Sildenafil Therapy in Severe Pulmonary Artery Hypertension," *Indian Heart J*, 2002, 54(4):404-9.

Krishnan U, Krishnan S, and Gewitz M, "Treatment of Pulmonary Hypertension in Children With Chronic Lung Disease With Newer Oral Therapies," *Pediatr Cardiol*, 2008, 29(6):1082-6.

Lammers AE, Haworth SG, and Pierce CM, "Intravenous Sildenafil as an Effective Treatment of Pulmonary Hypertensive Crises During Acute Intestinal Malabsorption," *Cardiol Young*, 2006, 16(1):84-6.

Lee JE, Hillier SC, and Knoderer CA, "Use of Sildenafil to Facilitate Weaning From Inhaled Nitric Oxide in Children With Pulmonary Hypertension Following Surgery for Congenital Heart Disease," *J Intensive Care Med*, 2008, 23(5):329-34.

Marsh CS, Marden B, and Newsom R, "Severe Retinopathy of Prematurity (ROP) in a Premature Baby Treated With Sildenafil Acetate (Viagra) for Pulmonary Hypertension," *Br J Ophthalmol*, 2004, 88 (2):306-7.

McLaughlin VV, Archer SL, Badesch DB, et al, "ACCF/AHA 2009 Expert Consensus Document on Pulmonary Hypertension. A Report of the American College of Cardiology Foundation Task Force on Expert Consensus Documents and the American Heart Association Developed in Collaboration With the American College of Chest Physicians; American Thoracic Society, Inc.; and the Pulmonary Hypertension Association," *J Am Coll Cardiol*, 2009, 53(17):1573-619.

Mourani PM, Sontag MK, Ivy DD, et al, "Effects of Long-Term Sildenafil Treatment for Pulmonary Hypertension in Infants With Chronic Lung Disease," *J Pediatr*, 2009, 154(3):379-84.

Mukherjee A, Dombi T, Wittke B, et al, "Population Pharmacokinetics of Sildenafil in Term Neonates: Evidence of Rapid Maturation of Metabolic Clearance in the Early Postnatal Period," *Clin Pharmacol Ther*, 2009, 85(1):56-63.

Nagdyman N, Fleck T, Bitterling B, et al, "Influence of Intravenous Sildenafil on Cerebral Oxygenation Measured by Near-Infrared Spectroscopy in Infants After Cardiac Surgery," *Pediatr Res*, 2006, 59(3):462-5.

Namachivayam P, Theilen U, Butt WW, et al, "Sildenafil Prevents Rebound Pulmonary Hypertension After Withdrawal of Nitric Oxide in Children," *Am J Respir Crit Care Med*, 2006, 174(9):1042-7.

Nemoto S, Sasaki T, Ozawa H, et al, "Oral Sildenafil for Persistent Pulmonary Hypertension Early After Congenital Cardiac Surgery in Children," *Eur J Cardiothorac Surg*, 2010, 38(1):71-7.

Noori S, Friedlich P, Wong P, et al, "Cardiovascular Effects of Sildenafil in Neonates and Infants With Congenital Diaphragmatic Hernia and Pulmonary Hypertension," *Neonatology*, 2007, 91(2):92-100.

Palma G, Giordano R, Russolillo V, et al, "Sildenafil Therapy for Pulmonary Hypertension Before and After Pediatric Congenital Heart Surgery," *Tex Heart Inst J*, 2011, 38(3):238-42.

Pierce CM, Petros AJ, and Fielder AR, "No Evidence for Severe Retinopathy of Prematurity Following Sildenafil," *Br J Ophthalmol*, 2005, 89(2):250.

Raja SG, Danton MD, MacArthur KJ, et al, "Effects of Escalating Doses of Sildenafil on Hemodynamics and Gas Exchange in Children With Pulmonary Hypertension and Congenital Cardiac Defects," *J Cardiothorac Vasc Anesth*, 2007, 21(2):203-7.

Raposo-Sonnenfeld I, Otero-González I, Blanco-Aparicio M, et al, "Treatment With Sildenafil, Bosentan, or Both in Children and Young People With Idiopathic Pulmonary Arterial Hypertension and Eisenmenger's Syndrome," *Rev Esp Cardiol*, 2007, 60(4):366-72.

Samada K, Shiraishi H, Aoyagi J, et al, "Cerebral Hemorrhage Associated With Sildenafil (Revatio) in an Infant," *Pediatr Cardiol*, 2009, 30 (7):998-9.

Singh TP, Rohit M, Grover A, et al, "A Randomized, Placebo-Controlled, Double-Blind, Crossover Study to Evaluate the Efficacy of Oral Sildenafil Therapy in Severe Pulmonary Artery Hypertension," *Am Heart J*, 2006, 151(4):851.e1-5.

Spillers J, "PPHN: Is Sildenafil the New Nitric? A Review of the Literature," *Adv Neonatal Care*, 2010, 10(2):69-74.

Steinhorn RH, Kinsella JP, Pierce C, et al, "Intravenous Sildenafil in the Treatment of Neonates With Persistent Pulmonary Hypertension," *J Pediatr*, 2009, 155(6):841-847.

Uhm JY, Jhang WK, Park JJ, et al, "Postoperative Use of Oral Sildenafil in Pediatric Patients With Congenital Heart Disease," *Pediatr Cardiol*, 2010, 31(4):515-20.

Vargas-Origel A, Gómez-Rodríguez G, Aldana-Valenzuela C, et al, "The Use of Sildenafil in Persistent Pulmonary Hypertension of the Newborn," *Am J Perinatol*, 2010, 27(3):225-30.

Vassalos A, Peng E, Young D, et al, "Pre-Operative Sildenafil and Pulmonary Endothelial-Related Complications Following Cardiopulmonary Bypass: A Randomised Trial in Children Undergoing Cardiac Surgery," *Anaesthesia*, 2011, 66(6):472-80.

◆ **Sildenafil Citrate** *see* Sildenafil *on page 1884*

◆ **Silenor** *see* Doxepin (Systemic) *on page 715*

◆ **Silexin [OTC]** *see* Guaifenesin and Dextromethorphan *on page 987*

◆ **Silkis (Can)** *see* Calcitriol *on page 342*

◆ **Silphen Cough [OTC]** *see* DiphenhydrAMINE (Systemic) *on page 673*

◆ **Silphen DM Cough [OTC]** *see* Dextromethorphan *on page 636*

◆ **Siltussin DAS [OTC]** *see* GuaiFENesin *on page 984*

◆ **Siltussin DM [OTC]** *see* Guaifenesin and Dextromethorphan *on page 987*

◆ **Siltussin DM DAS [OTC]** *see* Guaifenesin and Dextromethorphan *on page 987*

◆ **Siltussin SA [OTC]** *see* GuaiFENesin *on page 984*

◆ **Silvadene** *see* Silver Sulfadiazine *on page 1890*

◆ **Silver Bullet Suppository [OTC] (Can)** *see* Bisacodyl *on page 293*

Silver Nitrate (SIL ver NYE trate)

Therapeutic Category Ophthalmic Agent, Miscellaneous; Topical Skin Product

Generic Availability (U.S.) Yes

Use Astringent; cauterization of wounds; germicidal; removal of granulation tissue, corns, and warts

Contraindications Hypersensitivity to silver nitrate or any component; not for use on broken skin or cuts

Warnings Do not use applicator sticks on the eyes. Prolonged use may result in skin discoloration. Silver nitrate is a caustic agent and inappropriate use may cause chemical burns. Skin contact time with applicator sticks should be extremely short when used in neonates or on thin delicate skin contact.

Adverse Reactions
Dermatologic: Burning and skin irritation, staining of the skin
Hematologic: Methemoglobinemia

Drug Interactions
Metabolism/Transport Effects None known.
Avoid Concomitant Use
Avoid concomitant use of Silver Nitrate with any of the following: BCG
Increased Effect/Toxicity There are no known significant interactions involving an increase in effect.
Decreased Effect
Silver Nitrate may decrease the levels/effects of: BCG; Sodium Picosulfate

Stability Store applicator sticks in a dry place since moisture causes the oxidized film to dissolve; protect from light

Mechanism of Action Free silver ions precipitate bacterial proteins by combining with chloride in tissue forming silver chloride; coagulates cellular protein to form an eschar; silver ions or salts or colloidal silver preparations can inhibit the growth of both gram-positive and gram-negative bacteria. This germicidal action is attributed to the precipitation of bacterial proteins by liberated silver ions. Silver nitrate coagulates cellular protein to form an eschar, and this mode of action is the postulated mechanism for control of benign hematuria, rhinitis, and recurrent pneumothorax.

Pharmacokinetics (Adult data unless noted) Absorption: Not readily absorbed from mucous membranes

Dosing: Usual Children and Adults:
Sticks: Apply to mucous membranes and other moist skin surfaces only on area to be treated
Topical solution: Apply a cotton applicator dipped in solution on the affected area 2-3 times/week for 2-3 weeks

Dosage Forms Excipient information presented when available (limited, particularly for generics); consult specific product labeling.
Applicator sticks, topical: Silver nitrate 75% and potassium nitrate 25%
Solution, topical: 0.5% (960 mL); 10% (30 mL); 25% (30 mL); 50% (30 mL)

References
Cushing AH and Smith S, "Methemoglobinemia With Silver Nitrate Therapy of a Burn: Report of a Case," *J Pediatr*, 1969, 74(4):613-5.

Silver Sulfadiazine (SIL ver sul fa DYE a zeen)

Brand Names: U.S. Silvadene; SSD; Thermazene
Brand Names: Canada Flamazine®
Therapeutic Category Antibiotic, Topical
Generic Availability (U.S.) Yes
Use Adjunct in the prevention and treatment of infection in second and third degree burns
Pregnancy Risk Factor B
Pregnancy Considerations Adverse events were not observed in animal reproduction studies. Because of the theoretical increased risk for hyperbilirubinemia and kernicterus, sulfadiazine is contraindicated for use near term, on premature infants, or on newborn infants during the first 2 months of life (refer to Sulfadiazine monograph).
Breast-Feeding Considerations It is not known if sulfadiazine is found in breast milk following topical application; however, sulfonamide serum concentrations may reach therapeutic levels following application to extensive areas. Oral sulfadiazine is contraindicated in nursing mothers since sulfonamides cross into the milk and may cause

kernicterus in the newborn (refer to Sulfadiazine monograph).

Contraindications Hypersensitivity to silver sulfadiazine or any component; premature infants or neonates <2 months of age since sulfas may displace bilirubin from protein binding sites and cause kernicterus

Precautions Use with caution in patients with G-6-PD deficiency and renal impairment; sulfadiazine may accumulate in patients with impaired hepatic or renal function

Adverse Reactions
Dermatologic: Discoloration of skin, erythema multiforme, itching, photosensitivity, rash
Hematologic: Agranulocytosis, aplastic anemia, hemolytic anemia, leukopenia
Hepatic: Hepatitis
Renal: Interstitial nephritis
Miscellaneous: Allergic reactions may be related to sulfa component

Drug Interactions
Metabolism/Transport Effects None known.
Avoid Concomitant Use
Avoid concomitant use of Silver Sulfadiazine with any of the following: BCG
Increased Effect/Toxicity There are no known significant interactions involving an increase in effect.
Decreased Effect
Silver Sulfadiazine may decrease the levels/effects of: BCG; Sodium Picosulfate

Stability Discard if cream is darkened (reacts with heavy metals resulting in release of silver)

Mechanism of Action Acts upon the bacterial cell wall and cell membrane. Bactericidal for many gram-negative and gram-positive bacteria and is effective against yeast. Active against *Pseudomonas aeruginosa*, *Pseudomonas maltophilia*, *Enterobacter* species, *Klebsiella* species, *Serratia* species, *Escherichia coli*, *Proteus mirabilis*, *Morganella morganii*, *Providencia rettgeri*, *Proteus vulgaris*, *Providencia* species, *Citrobacter* species, *Acinetobacter calcoaceticus*, *Staphylococcus aureus*, *Staphylococcus epidermidis*, *Enterococcus* species, *Candida albicans*, *Corynebacterium diphtheriae*, and *Clostridium perfringens*

Pharmacokinetics (Adult data unless noted)
Absorption: Significant percutaneous absorption of sulfadiazine can occur especially when applied to extensive burns
Half-life: 10 hours and is prolonged in patients with renal insufficiency
Time to peak serum concentration: Within 3-11 days of continuous topical therapy
Elimination: ~50% excreted unchanged in urine

Dosing: Usual Children and Adults: Topical: Apply once or twice daily with a sterile gloved hand; apply to a thickness of 1/16"; burned area should be covered with cream at all times

Administration Topical: Apply to cleansed, debrided burned areas

Monitoring Parameters Serum electrolytes, UA, renal function test, CBC in patients with extensive burns on long-term treatment

Additional Information Contains methylparaben

Dosage Forms Excipient information presented when available (limited, particularly for generics); consult specific product labeling.
Cream, External:
Silvadene: 1% (20 g, 50 g, 85 g, 400 g, 1000 g) [contains methylparaben, propylene glycol]
SSD: 1% (25 g, 50 g, 85 g, 400 g) [contains cetyl alcohol, methylparaben, propylene glycol]
Thermazene: 1% (20 g, 50 g, 85 g, 400 g, 1000 g) [contains methylparaben, propylene glycol]
Generic: 1% (20 g, 25 g, 50 g, 85 g, 400 g)

References

Kulick MI, Wong R, Okarma TB, et al, "Prospective Study of Side Effects Associated With the Use of Silver Sulfadiazine in Severely Burned Patients," *Ann Plast Surg*, 1985, 14(5):407-18.

Lockhart SP, Rushworth A, Azmy AA, et al, "Topical Silver Sulfadiazine: Side Effects and Urinary Excretion," *Burns Incl Therm Inj*, 1983, 10 (1):9-12.

Simethicone (sye METH i kone)

Medication Safety Issues
Sound-alike/look-alike issues:
Simethicone may be confused with cimetidine

Mylanta® may be confused with Mynatal®

Mylicon® may be confused with Modicon®, Myleran®

Brand Names: U.S. Equalizer Gas Relief [OTC]; Gas Free Extra Strength [OTC]; Gas Relief Extra Strength [OTC]; Gas Relief Ultra Strength [OTC]; Gas Relief [OTC]; Gas-X Childrens [OTC]; Gas-X Extra Strength [OTC]; Gas-X Infant Drops [OTC]; Gas-X Ultra Strength [OTC]; Gas-X [OTC]; GasAid [OTC]; Infants Gas Relief [OTC]; Infants Simethicone [OTC]; Mi-Acid Gas Relief [OTC]; Mytab Gas Maximum Strength [OTC]; Mytab Gas [OTC]; Phazyme [OTC]

Brand Names: Canada Ovol®; Phazyme™

Therapeutic Category Antiflatulent

Generic Availability (U.S.) May be product dependent

Use Relieve flatulence, functional gastric bloating, and postoperative gas pains

Pregnancy Considerations Simethicone is not absorbed systemically following oral administration. Systemic absorption would be required in order for simethicone to cross the placenta and reach the fetus.

Breast-Feeding Considerations Due to lack of systemic absorption, simethicone is not expected to be excreted in breast milk.

Contraindications Hypersensitivity to simethicone or any component

Warnings Mylicon® Infant drops contain sodium benzoate; benzoic acid (benzoate) is a metabolite of benzyl alcohol; large amounts of benzyl alcohol (≥99 mg/kg/day) have been associated with a potentially fatal toxicity ("gasping syndrome") in neonates; *in vitro* and animal studies have shown that benzoate displaces bilirubin from protein binding sites; avoid use of Mylicon® Infant drops in neonates.

Precautions Phazyme® Quick Dissolve contains phenylalanine; avoid use or use with caution in phenylketonurics

Adverse Reactions Gastrointestinal: Loose stools

Drug Interactions
Metabolism/Transport Effects None known.
Avoid Concomitant Use There are no known interactions where it is recommended to avoid concomitant use.

Increased Effect/Toxicity There are no known significant interactions involving an increase in effect.

Decreased Effect There are no known significant interactions involving a decrease in effect.

Food Interactions Avoid carbonated beverages and gas-forming foods.

Mechanism of Action Decreases the surface tension of gas bubbles thereby disperses and prevents gas pockets in the GI system

Pharmacokinetics (Adult data unless noted) Elimination: In feces

Dosing: Usual Oral:

Infants and Children <2 years: 20 mg 4 times/day

Children 2-12 years: 40 mg 4 times/day

Children >12 years and Adults: 40-250 mg after meals and at bedtime as needed, not to exceed 500 mg/day

Administration Oral: Administer after meals or at bedtime; chew tablets thoroughly before swallowing; mix with water, infant formula or other liquid; place strips (Gas-X® Children's Tongue Twisters™ or Gas-X® Thin Strips™) directly on the tongue

Dosage Forms Excipient information presented when available (limited, particularly for generics); consult specific product labeling.

Capsule, Oral:

Gas Free Extra Strength: 125 mg [contains brilliant blue fcf (fd&c blue #1), fd&c red #40, fd&c yellow #10 (quinoline yellow)]

Gas Relief Extra Strength: 125 mg [contains brilliant blue fcf (fd&c blue #1), fd&c red #40, fd&c yellow #10 (quinoline yellow)]

Gas Relief Ultra Strength: 180 mg [contains fd&c red #40, fd&c yellow #6 (sunset yellow)]

Gas Relief Ultra Strength: 180 mg [contains fd&c yellow #6 (sunset yellow)]

Gas-X Extra Strength: 125 mg [contains brilliant blue fcf (fd&c blue #1), fd&c red #40, fd&c yellow #10 (quinoline yellow)]

Gas-X Ultra Strength: 180 mg [contains fd&c yellow #6 (sunset yellow)]

GasAid: 125 mg

Phazyme: 180 mg

Generic: 180 mg

Liquid, Oral:

Gas-X Infant Drops: 20 mg/0.3 mL (30 mL) [alcohol free, no artificial color(s), no artificial flavor(s), saccharin free; contains polyethylene glycol, sodium benzoate]

Strip, Oral:

Gas-X Childrens: 40 mg (16 ea) [contains alcohol, usp, fd&c red #40; sweet cinnamon flavor]

Gas-X Extra Strength: 62.5 mg (18 ea, 30 ea) [contains alcohol, usp, brilliant blue fcf (fd&c blue #1); peppermint flavor]

Gas-X Extra Strength: 62.5 mg (18 ea) [contains alcohol, usp, fd&c red #40]

Suspension, Oral:

Equalizer Gas Relief: 40 mg/0.6 mL (30 mL) [vanilla flavor]

Gas Relief: 20 mg/0.3 mL (30 mL) [dye free; contains sodium benzoate; fruit flavor]

Infants Gas Relief: 20 mg/0.3 mL (30 mL) [contains sodium benzoate]

Infants Simethicone: 20 mg/0.3 mL (30 mL) [alcohol free, no artificial color(s), no artificial flavor(s), saccharin free; contains polyethylene glycol, sodium benzoate]

Generic: 40 mg/0.6 mL (30 mL)

Tablet Chewable, Oral:

Gas-X: 80 mg [scored; cherry creme flavor]

Gas-X: 80 mg [scored; peppermint creme flavor]

Gas-X Extra Strength: 125 mg

Gas-X Extra Strength: 125 mg [scored; peppermint creme flavor]

Gas-X Extra Strength: 125 mg [contains fd&c yellow #10 aluminum lake; peppermint creme flavor]

Gas-X Extra Strength: 125 mg [contains soy protein; cherry cream flavor]

Mi-Acid Gas Relief: 80 mg

Mytab Gas: 80 mg [peppermint flavor]

Mytab Gas Maximum Strength: 125 mg [scored; peppermint flavor]

Phazyme: 125 mg [cool mint flavor]

Phazyme: 125 mg [contains aspartame; cool mint flavor]

Generic: 80 mg, 125 mg

◆ **Simply Allergy [OTC]** *see* DiphenhydrAMINE (Systemic) *on page 673*

◆ **Simply Cough [OTC]** *see* Dextromethorphan *on page 636*

◆ **Simply Sleep [OTC]** *see* DiphenhydrAMINE (Systemic) *on page 673*

◆ **Simply Sleep® (Can)** *see* DiphenhydrAMINE (Systemic) *on page 673*

◆ **Simply Stuffy [OTC]** *see* Pseudoephedrine *on page 1770*

◆ **Simulect** *see* Basiliximab *on page 263*

◆ **Simulect® (Can)** *see* Basiliximab *on page 263*

Simvastatin (sim va STAT in)

Medication Safety Issues
Sound-alike/look-alike issues:
Simvastatin may be confused with atorvaSTATin, nystatin, pitavastatin

Zocor may be confused with Cozaar, Lipitor, Zoloft, ZyrTEC

International issues:
Cardin [Poland] may be confused with Cardem brand name for celiprolol [Spain]; Cardene brand name for nicardipine [U.S., Great Britain, Netherlands]

Brand Names: U.S. Zocor

Brand Names: Canada Apo-Simvastatin; Auro-Simvastatin; Ava-Simvastatin; CO Simvastatin; Dom-Simvastatin; JAMP-Simvastatin; Mar-Simvastatin; Mint-Simvastatin; Mylan-Simvastatin; Nu-Simvastatin; PHL-Simvastatin; PMS-Simvastatin; Q-Simvastatin; RAN-Simvastatin; ratio-Simvastatin; Riva-Simvastatin; Sandoz-Simvastatin; Simvastatin-Odan; Taro-Simvastatin; Teva-Simvastatin; Zocor; ZYM-Simvastatin

Therapeutic Category Antilipemic Agent; HMG-CoA Reductase Inhibitor

Generic Availability (U.S.) Yes

Use Adjunct to dietary therapy to decrease elevated serum total (total-C) and low density lipoprotein cholesterol (LDL-C), and apolipoprotein B (apo-B) in patients with heterozygous familial hypercholesterolemia if LDL-C remains ≥190 mg/dL, if ≥160 mg/dL with family history of premature cardiovascular disease (CVD) or presence of ≥2 cardiovascular risk factors (FDA approved in boys and postmenarcheal girls 10-17 years); adjunct to dietary therapy to decrease elevated serum total-C, LDL-C, apo-B, and triglyceride (TG) levels and to increase high-density lipoprotein cholesterol (HDL-C) in patients with primary hypercholesterolemia (heterozygous, familial, and nonfamilial) and mixed dyslipidemia (Fredrickson types IIa and IIb) (FDA approved in adults); reduce elevated TG in patients with hypertriglyceridemia (Fredrickson type IV) (FDA approved in adults); reduce elevated TG and VLDL-C in patients with primary dysbetalipoproteinemia (Fredrickson Type III) (FDA approved in adults); reduce elevated total-C and LDL-C in patients with homozygous familial hypercholesterolemia (FDA approved in adults)

Secondary prevention of cardiovascular events in hypercholesterolemic patients with established coronary heart disease (CHD) or at high risk for CHD: To reduce cardiovascular morbidity (myocardial infarction, coronary/noncoronary revascularization procedures) and mortality; to reduce the risk of stroke (FDA approved in adults)

Pregnancy Risk Factor X

Pregnancy Considerations Adverse events were not observed in animal reproduction studies. There are reports of congenital anomalies following maternal use of HMG-CoA reductase inhibitors in pregnancy; however, maternal disease, differences in specific agents used, and the low rates of exposure limit the interpretation of the available data (Godfrey, 2012; Lecarpentier, 2012). Cholesterol biosynthesis may be important in fetal development; serum cholesterol and triglycerides increase normally during pregnancy. The discontinuation of lipid lowering medications temporarily during pregnancy is not expected to have significant impact on the long term outcomes of primary hypercholesterolemia treatment.

Use of simvastatin is contraindicated in pregnancy. HMG-CoA reductase inhibitors should be discontinued prior to pregnancy (ADA, 2013). If treatment of dyslipidemias is needed in pregnant women or in women of reproductive age, other agents are preferred (Berglund, 2012; Stone, 2013). The manufacturer recommends administration to women of childbearing potential only when conception is highly unlikely and patients have been informed of potential hazards.

Breast-Feeding Considerations It is not known if simvastatin is excreted into breast milk. Due to the potential for serious adverse reactions in a nursing infant, breast-feeding is contraindicated by the manufacturer.

Contraindications Hypersensitivity to simvastatin or any component; active liver disease; unexplained persistent elevations of serum transaminases; pregnancy; breast-feeding; concomitant use of strong CYP3A4 inhibitors (eg, boceprevir, clarithromycin, erythromycin, HIV protease inhibitors, itraconazole, ketoconazole, nefazodone, posaconazole, telaprevir, telithromycin, voriconazole), cyclosporine, danazol, and gemfibrozil

Warnings Patients receiving HMG-CoA reductase inhibitors have developed rhabdomyolysis with or without acute renal failure and/or myopathy; patients should be monitored closely; risk is dose-related and greater in patients receiving simvastatin 80 mg than those receiving other HMG-CoA reductase inhibitors at similar efficacy dose. High dose (80 mg) is limited to patients who have been taking this dose for >12 consecutive months without evidence of myopathy and are not currently taking or beginning to take a simvastatin dose-limiting or contraindicated interacting medication. Risk is also increased with concurrent use of other lipid-lowering medications (eg, fibric acid derivatives or niacin at doses >1 g/day) or during concurrent use with potent CYP3A4 inhibitor (some are contraindicated) or large quantities of grapefruit juice (>1 quart/day). With concurrent use of verapamil, diltiazem, dronedarone, amiodarone, amlodipine, lomitapide and ranolazine; dosage reductions of simvastatin recommended. Concomitant use of high-dose simvastatin (80 mg) with niacin ≥1 g/day may increase risk of myopathy in Chinese patients. Ensure patient is on the lowest effective simvastatin dose in all circumstances. Discontinue in any patient in which CPK levels are markedly elevated (>10 times ULN) or if myopathy is suspected/diagnosed; monitoring of CPK may be warranted, but may not prevent severe myopathy. The manufacturer recommends temporary discontinuation for elective major surgery, acute medical or surgical conditions, or in any patient experiencing an acute or serious condition predisposing to renal failure (eg, sepsis, hypotension, trauma, uncontrolled seizures). However, based upon current evidence, HMG-CoA reductase inhibitor therapy should be continued in the perioperative period unless risk outweighs cardioprotective benefit. Use caution in patients with renal impairment, inadequately treated hypothyroidism, and those taking other drugs associated with myopathy (eg, colchicine); these patients are predisposed to myopathy. Patients should be instructed to report unexplained muscle pain, tenderness, weakness, or brown urine.

An autoimmune-mediated myopathy (IMNM) has been reported (rarely) with HMG-CoA reductase inhibitor therapy; presents as proximal muscle weakness with elevated CPK levels, which persists despite discontinuation of HMG-CoA reductase inhibitor therapy; additionally, muscle biopsy may show necrotizing myopathy with limited inflammation; immunosuppressive therapy (eg, corticosteroids, azathioprine) may be used for treatment.

Postmarketing reports of fatal and nonfatal hepatic failure are rare; if serious hepatotoxicity with clinical symptoms and/or hyperbilirubinemia or jaundice occurs during treatment, interrupt therapy. If an alternate etiology is not identified, do not restart atorvastatin. Liver enzyme tests should be obtained at baseline and as clinically indicated; routine periodic monitoring of liver enzymes is not necessary. Use with caution in patients with history of heavy alcohol use or a previous history of liver disease.

Precautions Increases in Hb A_{1c} and fasting blood glucose have been reported with HMG-CoA reductase inhibitors; however, the benefits of statin therapy far outweigh the risk of dysglycemia. Secondary causes of hyperlipidemia should be ruled out prior to therapy; has not been studied when the primary lipid abnormality is chylomicron elevation (Fredrickson types I and V).

Although rare, reversible cognitive impairment (including confusion, forgetfulness, amnesia, and memory loss) can occur with HMG-CoA reductase inhibitors. These cognitive symptoms have been reported at variable times during therapy (1 day to years after initiation) and are reversible with discontinuation; resolution usually occurs within ~3 weeks. Cases have not been associated with fixed or progressive dementia; nor have they been associated with age, specific HMG-CoA reductase inhibitor, dose or concomitant medication use.

Adverse Reactions
Cardiovascular: Atrial fibrillation, edema
Central nervous system: Headache, vertigo
Dermatologic: Eczema
Gastrointestinal: Abdominal pain, constipation, gastritis, nausea
Hepatic: Transaminases increased (>3 x ULN)
Neuromuscular & skeletal: CPK increased (>3 x normal), myalgia
Respiratory: Bronchitis, upper respiratory infections
Rare but important or life-threatening: Alkaline phosphatase increased, alopecia, amnesia (reversible), anaphylaxis, anemia, angioedema, arthralgia, arthritis, blood glucose increased, chills, cognitive impairment (reversible), confusion (reversible), depression, dermatomyositis, diabetes mellitus (new onset), diarrhea, dizziness, dryness of skin/mucous membranes, dyspepsia, dyspnea, eosinophilia, erythema multiforme, ESR increased, fever, flatulence, flushing, glycosylated hemoglobin (Hb A_{1c}) increased, GGT increased, hemolytic anemia, hepatic failure, hepatitis, hypersensitivity reaction, jaundice, leukopenia, malaise, memory disturbance (reversible), memory impairment (reversible), muscle cramps, nail changes, nodules, pancreatitis, paresthesia, peripheral neuropathy, photosensitivity, polymyalgia rheumatica, positive ANA, pruritus, purpura, rash, rhabdomyolysis, skin discoloration, Stevens-Johnson syndrome, systemic lupus erythematosus-like syndrome, thrombocytopenia, toxic epidermal necrolysis, urticaria, vasculitis, vomiting, weakness

Additional class-related events or case reports (not necessarily reported with simvastatin therapy): Alteration in taste, anorexia, anxiety, bilirubin increased, cataracts, cholestatic jaundice, cirrhosis, decreased libido, depression, erectile dysfunction/impotence, facial paresis, fatty liver, fulminant hepatic necrosis, gynecomastia, hepatoma, hyperbilirubinemia, immune-mediated necrotizing myopathy (IMNM), impaired extraocular muscle movement, increased CPK (>10 x normal), interstitial lung disease, ophthalmoplegia, peripheral nerve palsy, psychic disturbance, renal failure (secondary to rhabdomyolysis), thyroid dysfunction, tremor, vertigo

Drug Interactions
Metabolism/Transport Effects Substrate of CYP3A4 (major), SLCO1B1; **Note:** Assignment of Major/Minor substrate status based on clinically relevant drug interaction potential; **Inhibits** CYP2C8 (weak), CYP2C9 (weak), CYP2D6 (weak)

Avoid Concomitant Use
Avoid concomitant use of Simvastatin with any of the following: Boceprevir; Clarithromycin; Conivaptan; CycloSPORINE (Systemic); CYP3A4 Inhibitors (Strong); Erythromycin (Systemic); Fusidic Acid (Systemic); Gemfibrozil; Mifepristone; Protease Inhibitors; Red Yeast Rice; Telaprevir; Telithromycin

Increased Effect/Toxicity
Simvastatin may increase the levels/effects of: ARIPiprazole; DAPTOmycin; Diltiazem; PAZOPanib; Trabectedin; Vitamin K Antagonists

The levels/effects of Simvastatin may be increased by: Amiodarone; AmLODIPine; Azithromycin (Systemic); Bezafibrate; Boceprevir; Ceritinib; Clarithromycin; Colchicine; Conivaptan; CycloSPORINE (Systemic); CYP3A4 Inhibitors (Moderate); CYP3A4 Inhibitors (Strong); Cyproterone; Danazol; Dasatinib; Diltiazem; Dronedarone; Eltrombopag; Erythromycin (Systemic); Fenofibrate and Derivatives; Fluconazole; Fusidic Acid (Systemic); Gemfibrozil; Grapefruit Juice; Green Tea; Imatinib; Ivacaftor; Lomitapide; Luliconazole; Mifepristone; Niacin; Niacinamide; Protease Inhibitors; QuiNINE; Raltegravir; Ranolazine; Red Yeast Rice; Sildenafil; Simeprevir; Telaprevir; Telithromycin; Ticagrelor; Verapamil

Decreased Effect
Simvastatin may decrease the levels/effects of: Lanthanum

The levels/effects of Simvastatin may be decreased by: Antacids; Bosentan; CYP3A4 Inducers (Strong); Dabrafenib; Deferasirox; Efavirenz; Eslicarbazepine; Etravirine; Fosphenytoin; Mitotane; Phenytoin; Rifamycin Derivatives; Siltuximab; St Johns Wort; Tocilizumab

Food Interactions Simvastatin serum concentration may be increased when taken with grapefruit juice. Management: Avoid concurrent intake of large quantities of grapefruit juice (>1 quart/day).

Stability Store at 5°C to 30°C (41°F to 86°F).

Mechanism of Action Simvastatin is a methylated derivative of lovastatin that acts by competitively inhibiting 3-hydroxy-3-methylglutaryl-coenzyme A (HMG-CoA) reductase, the enzyme that catalyzes the rate-limiting step in cholesterol biosynthesis

Pharmacodynamics
Onset of action: >3 days
Maximum effect: After 2 weeks
LDL-C reduction: 20-40 mg/day: 35% to 41% (for each doubling of this dose, LDL-C is lowered ~6%)
Average HDL-C increase: 5% to 15%
Average triglyceride reduction: 7% to 30%

Pharmacokinetics (Adult data unless noted)
Absorption: Oral: Although 85% is absorbed following administration, <5% reaches the general circulation due to an extensive first-pass effect
Protein binding: ~95%
Metabolism: Hepatic via CYP3A4; extensive first-pass effect
Time to peak serum concentration: 1.3-2.4 hours
Elimination: 13% excreted in urine and 60% in feces

Dosing: Usual
Children and Adolescents: **Note:** A lower, conservative dosing regimen may be necessary in patient populations predisposed to myopathy including patients of Chinese descent or those concurrently receiving other lipid-lowering agents (eg, niacin, fibric acid derivatives), amiodarone, amlodipine, diltiazem, dronedarone, ranolazine, verapamil (see the following conservative, maximum adult doses)

Heterozygous familial hypercholesterolemia: Children and Adolescents 10-17 years: Oral: Initial: 10 mg once daily in the evening; may increase dose in intervals of 4 weeks or more to a maximum daily dose: 40 mg/**day**

Hyperlipidemia: Limited data available: Children and Adolescents: Oral:

Children <10 years: Initial: 5 mg once daily in the evening increasing to 10 mg once daily after 4 weeks and to 20 mg once daily after another 4 weeks as tolerated; dosing based on initial compassionate use study (Ducobu, 1992)

Children ≥10 years and Adolescents: Initial: 10 mg once daily in the evening increasing to 20 mg once daily after 6 weeks and to 40 mg once daily after another 6 weeks as tolerated

Adults: **Note:** Doses should be individualized according to the baseline LDL-cholesterol levels, the recommended goal of therapy, and the patient's response; adjustments should be made at intervals of 4 weeks or more; doses may need adjusted based on concomitant medications

Note: Dosing limitation: **Simvastatin 80 mg is limited to patients that have been taking this dose for >12 consecutive months without evidence of myopathy and are not currently taking or beginning to take a simvastatin dose-limiting or contraindicated interacting medication.** If patient is unable to achieve LDL-C goal using the 40 mg dose of simvastatin, increasing to 80 mg dose is not recommended. Instead, switch patient to an alternative LDL-C-lowering treatment providing greater LDL-C reduction.

Homozygous familial hypercholesterolemia: Oral: 40 mg once daily in the evening

Prevention of cardiovascular events, hyperlipidemias: Oral: 10-20 mg once daily in the evening (range: 5-40 mg/day)

Patients requiring only moderate reduction of LDL-cholesterol: May be started at 5-10 mg once daily in the evening; adjust to achieve recommended LDL-C goal

Patients requiring reduction of >40% in low-density lipoprotein (LDL) cholesterol: May be started at 40 mg once daily in the evening; adjust to achieve recommended LDL-C goal

Patients with CHD or at high risk for cardiovascular events (patients with diabetes, PVD, history of stroke, or other cerebrovascular disease): Dosing should be started at 40 mg once daily in the evening; simvastatin should be started simultaneously with diet therapy

Dosing adjustment in patients receiving concomitant diltiazem, dronedarone, or verapamil: Adults: Dose should not exceed 10 mg/day

Dosing adjustment in patients receiving concomitant amiodarone, amlodipine, or ranolazine: Adults: Dose should not exceed 20 mg/day

Dosing adjustment in patients receiving concomitant lomitapide: Adults: Simvastatin dose should not exceed 20 mg/day (or 40 mg daily for those who previously tolerated simvastatin 80 mg daily for ≥1 year without evidence of muscle toxicity)

Dosing adjustment in Chinese patients on niacin doses ≥1 g/day: Adults: Use caution with simvastatin doses exceeding 20 mg/day; because of an increased risk of myopathy, do not increase simvastatin dose to 80 mg.

Dosing adjustment in renal impairment: Adults: Manufacturer's recommendations:

Mild to moderate renal impairment: No dosage adjustment necessary; simvastatin does not undergo significant renal excretion

Severe renal impairment: CrCl <30 mL/minute; Initial: 5 mg/day with close monitoring

Alternative recommendation: No dosage adjustment necessary for any degree of renal impairment (Aronoff, 2007)

Dosing adjustments in hepatic impairment: Contraindicated in patients with active liver disease, including unexplained persistent elevations in hepatic transaminases.

Administration Oral: May be taken without regard to meals. Administration with the evening meal or at bedtime has been associated with somewhat greater LDL-C reduction

Monitoring Parameters

Pediatric patients: Baseline: ALT, AST, and creatine phosphokinase levels (CPK); fasting lipid panel (FLP) and repeat ALT and AST should be checked after 4 weeks of therapy; if no myopathy symptoms or laboratory abnormalities, then monitor FLP, ALT, and AST every 3-4 months during the first year and then every 6 months thereafter (NHLBI, 2011)

Adults: Baseline CPK (recheck CPK in any patient with symptoms suggestive of myopathy; discontinue therapy if markedly elevated); baseline liver function tests (LFTs) and repeat when clinically indicated thereafter. Patients with elevated transaminase levels should have a second (confirmatory) test and frequent monitoring until values normalize; discontinue if increase in ALT/AST is persistently >3 times ULN (NCEP, 2002).

Lipid panel (total cholesterol, HDL, LDL, triglycerides):

ATP III recommendations (NCEP, 2002): Baseline; 6-8 weeks after initiation of drug therapy; if dose increased, then at 6-8 weeks until final dose determined. Once treatment goal achieved, follow-up intervals may be reduced to every 4-6 months. Lipid panel should be assessed at least annually, and preferably at each clinic visit.

Manufacturer recommendation: Analyze lipid panel at initiation, after 4 weeks of therapy and periodically thereafter

Dosage Forms Excipient information presented when available (limited, particularly for generics); consult specific product labeling.

Tablet, Oral:

Zocor: 5 mg, 10 mg, 20 mg, 40 mg, 80 mg

Generic: 5 mg, 10 mg, 20 mg, 40 mg, 80 mg

References

American Diabetes Association, "Standards of Medical Care in Diabetes-2013," *Diabetes Care*, 2013, 36(Suppl 1):S11-66.

Berglund L, Brunzell JD, Goldberg AC, et al, "Evaluation and Treatment of Hypertriglyceridemia: An Endocrine Society Clinical Practice Guideline," *J Clin Endocrinol Metab*, 2012, 97(9):2969-89.

Daniels SR, Greer FR, and Committee on Nutrition, "Lipid Screening and Cardiovascular Health in Childhood," *Pediatrics*, 2008, 122 (1):198-208.

DeJongh S, et al, "Efficacy, Safety, and Tolerability of Simvastatin in Children With Familial Hypercholesterolemia," *Clin Drug Invest*, 2002, 22(8): 533-40.

Ducobu J, Brasseur D, Chaudron JM, et al, "Simvastatin Use in Children," *Lancet*, 1992, 339(8807):1488.

"Executive Summary of The Third Report of The National Cholesterol Education Program (NCEP) Expert Panel on Detection, Evaluation, and Treatment of High Blood Cholesterol in Adults (Adult Treatment Panel III)," *JAMA*, 2001, 285(19):2486-97.

Godfrey LM, Erramouspe J, and Cleveland KW, "Teratogenic Risk of Statins in Pregnancy," *Ann Pharmacother*, 2012, 46(10):1419-24.

Lecarpentier E, Morel O, Fournier T, et al, "Statins and Pregnancy: Between Supposed Risks and Theoretical Benefits," *Drugs*, 2012, 72 (6):773-88.

McCrindle BW, Urbina EM, Dennison BA, et al, "Drug Therapy of High-Risk Lipid Abnormalities in Children and Adolescents: A Scientific Statement from the American Heart Association Atherosclerosis, Hypertension, and Obesity in Youth Committee, Council of Cardiovascular Disease in the Young, With the Council on Cardiovascular Nursing," *Circulation*, 2007, 115(14):1948-67.

National Heart, Lung, and Blood Institute, "Expert Panel on Integrated Guidelines for Cardiovascular Health and Risk Reduction in Children and Adolescents," Clinical Practice Guidelines, 2011, National Institutes of Health. Available at http://www.nhlbi.nih.gov/guidelines/cvd_ped/peds_guidelines_full.pdf

"Third Report of the National Cholesterol Education Program Expert Panel on Detection, Evaluation, and Treatment of High Blood Cholesterol in Adults (Adult Treatment Panel III)," May 2001, www.nhlbi.nih.gov/guidelines/cholesterol.

- **Simvastatin and Ezetimibe** *see* Ezetimibe and Simvastatin *on page 829*
- **Simvastatin-Odan (Can)** *see* Simvastatin *on page 1892*
- **Sinequan (Can)** *see* Doxepin (Systemic) *on page 715*
- **Singulair** *see* Montelukast *on page 1438*
- **Sinus Nasal Spray [OTC]** *see* Oxymetazoline (Nasal) *on page 1577*

Sirolimus (sir OH li mus)

Medication Safety Issues
Sound-alike/look-alike issues:
Rapamune® may be confused with Rapaflo®
Sirolimus may be confused with everolimus, pimecrolimus, tacrolimus, temsirolimus

Related Information
Oral Medications That Should Not Be Crushed or Altered *on page 2438*
Safe Handling of Hazardous Drugs *on page 2419*

Brand Names: U.S. Rapamune
Brand Names: Canada Rapamune®
Therapeutic Category Immunosuppressant Agent; mTOR Kinase Inhibitor
Generic Availability (U.S.) May be product dependent
Use Prophylaxis of organ rejection in renal transplant patients at low-moderate immunologic risk in combination with corticosteroids and cyclosporine (cyclosporine may be withdrawn after 2-4 months in conjunction with an increase in sirolimus dosage) (FDA approved in ages ≥13 years and adults); prophylaxis of organ rejection in renal transplant patients at high immunologic risk in combination with cyclosporine and corticosteroids for the first year (FDA approved in ages ≥18 years and adults); has also been used for primary immunosuppression in heart and intestinal transplantation (given in conjunction with a calcineurin inhibitor, as a substitute for a calcineurin inhibitor to reduce side effects, or to eliminate steroid use); rescue agent for acute and chronic organ rejection (rescue due to calcineurin toxicity or to treat resistant acute or chronic rejection despite calcineurin inhibitor therapy); prevention of acute graft-versus-host disease (GVHD) in allogeneic stem cell transplantation; treatment of refractory acute or chronic GVHD; treatment of vascular anomalies
Medication Guide Available Yes
Pregnancy Risk Factor C
Pregnancy Considerations Adverse events have been observed in animal reproduction studies. Effective contraception must be initiated before therapy with sirolimus and continued for 12 weeks after discontinuation.

The National Transplantation Pregnancy Registry (NTPR, Temple University) is a registry for pregnant women taking immunosuppressants following any solid organ transplant. The NTPR encourages reporting of all immunosuppressant exposures during pregnancy in transplant recipients at 877-955-6877.
Breast-Feeding Considerations It is not known if sirolimus is excreted in breast milk. Due to the potential for adverse reactions in the breast-fed infant, including possible immunosuppression, breast-feeding is not recommended.
Contraindications Hypersensitivity to sirolimus or any component
Warnings Hazardous agent; use appropriate precautions for handling and disposal (NIOSH, 2012). Immunosuppression with sirolimus may result in increased susceptibility to infection **[U.S. Boxed Warning]**. Immune suppression may increase the risk of opportunistic infections (including activation of latent viral infections including BK virus-associated nephropathy), fatal infections, and sepsis. Prophylactic treatment for *Pneumocystis jirovecii*

pneumonia (PCP) should be administered for 1 year post-transplant; prophylaxis for cytomegalovirus (CMV) should be taken for 3 months post-transplant in patients at risk for CMV. Progressive multifocal leukoencephalopathy (PML), an opportunistic CNS infection caused by reactivation of the JC virus, has been reported in patients receiving immunosuppressive therapy, including sirolimus. Clinical findings of PML include apathy, ataxia, cognitive deficiency, confusion, and hemiparesis; promptly evaluate any patient presenting with neurological changes; consider decreasing the degree of immunosuppression with consideration to the risk of organ rejection in transplant patients.

Immunosuppressive agents, including sirolimus, may be associated with the development of lymphoma or other malignancies **[U.S. Boxed Warning]**. Immunosuppressant therapy is associated with an increased risk of skin cancer; limit sun and ultraviolet light exposure; use appropriate sun protection.

Hypersensitivity reactions including anaphylactic/anaphylactoid reactions, exfoliative dermatitis, and hypersensitivity vasculitis have been reported following administration of sirolimus. Angioedema has been reported; concurrent use with other drugs known to cause angioedema (eg, ACE inhibitors) may increase risk.

Sirolimus is not recommended for use in lung transplant patients **[U.S. Boxed Warning]**. Bronchial anastomotic dehiscence cases have been reported in lung transplant patients when sirolimus was used as part of an immunosuppressive regimen; most of these reactions were fatal.

Sirolimus is not recommended for use in liver transplant patients **[U.S. Boxed Warning]**; studies indicate an association with an increased risk of hepatic artery thrombosis (HAT), graft failure, and increased mortality (with evidence of infection) in these patients when sirolimus is used in combination with cyclosporine and/or tacrolimus. Most cases of HAT occurred within 30 days of transplant.

Increased urinary protein excretion has been observed when converting renal transplant patients from calcineurin inhibitors to sirolimus during maintenance therapy. A higher severity of proteinuria prior to sirolimus conversion correlates with a higher degree of proteinuria after conversion. In some patients, proteinuria may reach nephrotic levels; new onset nephrotic syndrome has been reported. Increased risk of BK viral-associated nephropathy which may impair renal function and cause graft loss; consider decreasing immunosuppressive burden if evidence of deteriorating renal function.

Use has been associated with an increased risk of fluid accumulation, impaired wound healing, and lymphocele. Peripheral edema, lymphedema, and pleural and pericardial effusions (including significant effusions and tamponade) were reported; use with caution in patients in whom fluid accumulation may be poorly tolerated, such as in cardiovascular disease (heart failure or hypertension) and pulmonary disease. Cases of interstitial lung disease [eg, pneumonitis, bronchiolitis obliterans organizing pneumonia (BOOP), pulmonary fibrosis] have been observed (some fatal); risk may be increased with higher trough concentrations.

Concurrent use with strong inhibitors of CYP3A4 and/or p-glycoprotein (ie, erythromycin, ketoconazole, voriconazole, itraconazole, telithromycin, or clarithromycin) or strong inducers of CYP3A4 and/or p-glycoprotein (rifampin or rifabutin) is not recommended. Concurrent use with a calcineurin inhibitor (cyclosporine, tacrolimus) may increase the risk of calcineurin inhibitor-induced hemolytic uremic syndrome/thrombotic thrombocytopenic purpura/thrombotic microangiopathy (HUS/TTP/TMA). The risk for thrombotic microangiopathy after allogeneic hematopoietic cell transplantation is increased when trough levels are above 10 ng/mL (Shayani, 2013) Potentially significant interactions may exist, requiring dose or frequency adjustment, additional monitoring, and/or selection of alternative therapy. Consult drug interactions database for more detailed information.

Oral solution contains 1.5% to 2.5% ethanol. Oral solution contains propylene glycol; toxicities have been reported with use of products containing propylene glycol, including hyperosmolality, lactic acidosis, seizures, and respiratory depression; in neonates large amounts of propylene glycol delivered orally, intravenously (eg, >3000 mg/day), or topically have been associated with potentially fatal toxicities which can include metabolic acidosis, seizures, renal failure, and CNS depression; use oral solutions containing propylene glycol with caution (AAP, 1997; Shehab, 2009).

Precautions Use with caution in patients with hepatic impairment; a reduction in the maintenance dose is recommended. Use with caution in patients with hyperlipidemia; may increase serum cholesterol and triglycerides.

Use with caution in renal impairment, or when used concurrently with medications which alter renal function; sirolimus may decrease GFR and increase serum creatinine. In renal transplant patients, *de novo* use without cyclosporine has been associated with higher rates of acute rejection. Sirolimus should be used in combination with cyclosporine initially. Sirolimus may delay recovery of renal function in patients with delayed allograft function. Monitor renal function closely when combined with cyclosporine; consider dosage adjustment or discontinue in patients with increasing serum creatinine. Separate dosing; sirolimus should be administered 4 hours after oral cyclosporine doses.

Use caution in the perioperative period due to increased chance of surgical complications from wound dehiscence and impaired wound and tissue healing; patients with a body mass index >30 kg/m² are at increased risk for abnormal wound healing.

Adequate laboratory and supportive medical resources must be readily available. Sirolimus concentrations are dependent on the assay method (eg, chromatographic and immunoassay) used; assay methods are not interchangeable. Variations in methods to determine sirolimus whole blood concentrations, as well as interlaboratory variations, may result in improper dosage adjustments, which may lead to subtherapeutic or toxic concentrations. Determine the assay method used to assure consistency (or accommodations if changes occur) and for monitoring purposes, be aware of alterations to assay method or reference range. The manufacturer recommends high performance liquid chromatography (HPLC) as the reference standard to determine sirolimus trough concentrations.

Animal studies have indicated that sirolimus may inhibit skeletal and muscle growth. There has been at least one human case report of growth failure in a child. Further studies needed (Hymes, 2011). Should only be used by physicians experienced in immunosuppressive therapy and management of transplant patients **[U.S. Boxed Warning]**.

Adverse Reactions

Cardiovascular: Atrial fibrillation, CHF, DVT, edema, facial edema, hyper-/hypotension, hypervolemia, orthostatic hypotension, palpitation, peripheral edema, peripheral vascular disorder, syncope, tachycardia, thrombosis, vasodilation

Central nervous system: Anxiety, chills, confusion, depression, dizziness, emotional lability, headache, hypoesthesia, insomnia, malaise, neuropathy, pain, somnolence

Dermatologic: Acne, cellulitis, dermal ulcer, dermatitis (fungal), ecchymosis, hirsutism, pruritus, rash, skin carcinoma (includes basal cell carcinoma, squamous cell carcinoma, melanoma), skin hypertrophy, wound healing abnormal

Endocrine & metabolic: Acidosis, Cushing's syndrome, dehydration, diabetes mellitus, glycosuria, hypercalcemia, hypercholesterolemia, hyperglycemia, hyperphosphatemia, hypertriglyceridemia, hypocalcemia, hypoglycemia, hypomagnesemia, hyponatremia

Gastrointestinal: Abdomen enlarged, abdominal pain, anorexia, constipation, diarrhea, dysphagia, eructation, esophagitis, flatulence, gastritis, gastroenteritis, gingival hyperplasia, gingivitis, ileus, mouth ulceration, nausea, oral moniliasis, stomatitis, weight loss

Genitourinary: Amenorrhea, hypermenorrhea, impotence, menstrual disease, ovarian cyst, pelvic pain, scrotal edema, testis disorder, urinary tract infection

Hematologic: Anemia, hemolytic-uremic syndrome, hemorrhage, leukopenia, leukocytosis, polycythemia, thrombocytopenia, TTP

Hepatic: Abnormal liver function tests, alkaline phosphatase increased, ascites, LDH increased

Local: Thrombophlebitis

Neuromuscular & skeletal: Arthralgia, arthrosis, bone necrosis, CPK increased, hyper-/hypotonia, leg cramps, myalgia, osteoporosis, paresthesia, tetany

Renal: Albuminuria, bladder pain, BUN increased, dysuria, hematuria, hydronephrosis, kidney pain, nephropathy (toxic), nocturia, oliguria, pyelonephritis, pyuria, serum creatinine increased, tubular necrosis, urinary frequency, urinary incontinence, urinary retention

Respiratory: Asthma, atelectasis, bronchitis, cough, epistaxis, hypoxia, lung edema, pleural effusion, pneumonia, pulmonary embolism, rhinitis, sinusitis

Ocular: Abnormal vision, cataract, conjunctivitis

Otic: Ear pain, otitis media, tinnitus

Miscellaneous: Abscess, diaphoresis, flu-like syndrome, hernia, herpesvirus infection, infection (including opportunistic), lymphadenopathy, lymphocele, lymphoproliferative disease/lymphoma, peritonitis, sepsis

Rare but important or life-threatening: ALT increased, alveolar proteinosis, anaphylactoid reaction, anaphylaxis, anastomotic disruption, angioedema, ascites, AST increased, azoospermia, *Clostridium difficile* colitis, cytomegalovirus, Epstein-Barr virus, exfoliative dermatitis, fascial dehiscence, focal segmental glomerulosclerosis, hepatic necrosis, hepatotoxicity, hypersensitivity reaction, hypersensitivity vasculitis, hypophosphatemia, incisional hernia; interstitial lung disease (dose-related; includes pneumonitis, pulmonary fibrosis, and bronchiolitis obliterans organizing pneumonia [BOOP] with no identified infectious etiology); joint disorders, lymphedema, myocardial infarction, mycobacterial infection, nephropathy (BK virus-associated), nephrotic syndrome, neutropenia, pancreatitis, pancytopenia, pericardial effusion, *Pneumocystis* pneumonia, progressive multifocal leukoencephalopathy (PML), proteinuria, pulmonary hemorrhage, reversible posterior leukoencephalopathy syndrome (RPLS), tamponade, tuberculosis, wound dehiscence

Note: Hepatic artery thrombosis [HAT] and graft failure have been reported in liver transplant patients (not an approved use); bronchial anastomotic dehiscence has been reported in lung transplant patients (not an approved use).

Drug Interactions

Metabolism/Transport Effects Substrate of CYP3A4 (major), P-glycoprotein; **Note:** Assignment of Major/Minor substrate status based on clinically relevant drug interaction potential; **Inhibits** CYP3A4 (weak)

Avoid Concomitant Use

Avoid concomitant use of Sirolimus with any of the following: BCG; CloZAPine; Conivaptan; Crizotinib; Dipyrone; Enzalutamide; Fusidic Acid (Systemic);

Mifepristone; Natalizumab; Pimecrolimus; Pimozide; Posaconazole; Tacrolimus (Systemic); Tacrolimus (Topical); Tofacitinib; Vaccines (Live); Voriconazole

Increased Effect/Toxicity

Sirolimus may increase the levels/effects of: ACE Inhibitors; ARIPiprazole; CloZAPine; CycloSPORINE (Systemic); Dofetilide; Leflunomide; Lomitapide; Natalizumab; Pimozide; Tacrolimus (Systemic); Tacrolimus (Topical); Tofacitinib; Vaccines (Live)

The levels/effects of Sirolimus may be increased by: Boceprevir; Ceritinib; Clotrimazole (Topical); Conivaptan; Crizotinib; CycloSPORINE (Systemic); CYP3A4 Inhibitors (Moderate); CYP3A4 Inhibitors (Strong); Dasatinib; Denosumab; Dipyrone; Fluconazole; Fusidic Acid (Systemic); Itraconazole; Ivacaftor; Ketoconazole (Systemic); Luliconazole; Macrolide Antibiotics; Mifepristone; Nelfinavir; P-glycoprotein/ABCB1 Inhibitors; Pimecrolimus; Posaconazole; Roflumilast; Stiripentol; Tacrolimus (Systemic); Tacrolimus (Topical); Telaprevir; Trastuzumab; Voriconazole

Decreased Effect

Sirolimus may decrease the levels/effects of: BCG; Coccidioidin Skin Test; Sipuleucel-T; Tacrolimus (Systemic); Vaccines (Inactivated); Vaccines (Live)

The levels/effects of Sirolimus may be decreased by: Bosentan; CYP3A4 Inducers (Strong); Dabrafenib; Deferasirox; Echinacea; Efavirenz; Enzalutamide; Fosphenytoin; Mitotane; P-glycoprotein/ABCB1 Inducers; Phenytoin; Rifampin; Siltuximab; St Johns Wort; Tocilizumab

Food Interactions Grapefruit juice may decrease clearance of sirolimus. Ingestion with high-fat meals decreases peak concentrations but increases AUC by 23% to 35%. Management: Avoid grapefruit juice. Take consistently (either with or without food) to minimize variability.

Stability Hazardous agent; use appropriate precautions for handling and disposal (NIOSH, 2012).

Oral solution: Store at 2°C to 8°C (36°F to 46°F); protect from light. A slight haze may develop in refrigerated solutions, but the quality of the product is not affected. After opening, solution should be used in 1 month. If necessary, may be stored at temperatures up to 25°C (77°F) for ≤15 days after opening. Product may be stored in amber syringe for a maximum of 24 hours (at room temperature or refrigerated). Discard syringe after single use. Solution should be used immediately following dilution.

Tablet: Store at 20°C to 25°C (68°F to 77°F); protect from light.

Mechanism of Action Sirolimus inhibits T-lymphocyte activation and proliferation in response to antigenic and cytokine stimulation and inhibits antibody production. Its mechanism differs from other immunosuppressants. Sirolimus binds to FKBP-12, an intracellular protein, to form an immunosuppressive complex which inhibits the regulatory kinase, mTOR (mammalian target of rapamycin). This inhibition suppresses cytokine mediated T-cell proliferation, halting progression from the G1 to the S phase of the cell cycle. It inhibits acute rejection of allografts and prolongs graft survival.

Pharmacokinetics (Adult data unless noted)

Absorption: Rapid

Distribution: V_{dss}: 12 ± 8 L/kg

Protein binding: ~92%; primarily to albumin

Metabolism: Extensive; in intestinal wall via P-glycoprotein and hepatic via CYP3A4; to 7 major metabolites

Bioavailability: Oral solution: 14%; tablet: 27% (relative to the oral solution); oral solution and tablets are not bioequivalent however, clinical equivalence shown at 2 mg dose

Half-life:

Children: 13.7 ± 6.2 hours

Adults: 62 ± 16 hours; extended in hepatic impairment (Child-Pugh class A or B) to 113 hours

Time to peak serum concentration: Oral solution: 1-3 hours; tablet: 1-6 hours

Elimination: Primarily eliminated via feces (91%) and urine (2.2%)

Dosing: Usual Note: Sirolimus tablets and oral solution are not bioequivalent due to differences in absorption; however, clinical equivalence has been demonstrated at the 2 mg dose

Pediatric: Note: Dosage should be individualized and based on monitoring of serum trough concentrations; target range is variable and may depend upon transplantation type, length of time since transplant, renal function, infection, rejection history, drug combinations used, and side effects of individual agents.

Heart transplantation: Limited data available: Children and Adolescents: Oral: **Note:** Not used first-line; most data describes an alternative immunosuppression in combination with either cyclosporine or tacrolimus in patients for renal-sparing effects, following retransplantation (treatment of rejection) or to prevent or promote regression of transplant coronary artery disease (Denfield, 2010)

BSA/weight-directed dosing:

Loading dose: 3 mg/m^2 on day 1 (Balfour, 2006; Denfield, 2010)

Maintenance dose: Evaluate serum trough concentrations and adjust dose to overall target range: 4-12 ng/mL (ISHLT, Costanzo 2010). Some trials report using lower target ranges of 4-10 ng/mL (Chinnock, 2011; Lobach, 2005; Matthews, 2010). In children, a specific maintenance dose has not been reported in the majority of trials. In 16 pediatric patients (age range: 2-18 years), the mean reported dose to reach target serum concentration of 5-10 ng/mL was 7 mg/m^2 (or 0.25 mg/kg) (Lobach, 2005). One trial used an initial median dose of 1 mg once daily (range: 0.3-2 mg once daily) and adjusted to achieve target concentration of 4-8 ng/mL (final dosage range 0.3-4 mg once daily) (Matthews, 2010). In adolescents <40 kg, an initial maintenance dose of 1 mg/m^2/day in 1-2 divided doses has been suggested (Denfield, 2010).

Alternative fixed dosing: Adolescents with weight ≥40 kg: Loading dose: 6 mg on day 1; then maintenance: 2 mg once daily; evaluate serum trough concentrations and adjust dose to overall target range: 4-12 ng/mL (Denfield, 2010; ISHLT Costanzo, 2010); some suggest higher initial targets when sirolimus therapy initiated and then decrease to 4-8 ng/mL (Balfour, 2005; Chinnock, 2011; Lobach, 2005).

Renal transplantation, prophylaxis of organ rejection (low to moderate immunologic risk): Oral:

Conversion from tacrolimus in patients with stable graft function: Children and Adolescents: Limited data available: Initial maintenance dose: 3 mg/m^2/day divided every 12 hours; adjust dose to achieve target sirolimus serum trough concentration (Hymes, 2008; Hymes, 2011). In one trial, a loading dose of 5 mg/m^2 on day 1 was used, followed by maintenance doses of 3 mg/m^2/day divided every 12 hours (Hymes, 2008).

Manufacturer's recommendations: Adolescents:

Weight <40 kg: Loading dose: 3 mg/m^2 on day 1; initial maintenance dose: 1 mg/m^2/day divided every 12 hours or once daily; adjust dose to achieve target sirolimus trough blood concentration

Weight ≥40 kg: Loading dose: 6 mg on day 1; maintenance: 2 mg once daily; adjust dose to achieve target sirolimus trough blood concentration.

Dosage adjustment: Sirolimus dosages should be adjusted to maintain trough concentrations within desired range based on risk and concomitant therapy; maximum daily dose: 40 mg/**day**. Dosage should be adjusted at intervals of 7-14 days to account for the long half-life of sirolimus; in children receiving twice-daily dosing, serum concentrations should be checked earlier due to pharmacokinetic differences. In general, dose proportionality may be assumed. New sirolimus dose **equals** current dose **multiplied by** (target concentration/current concentration). **Note:** If large dose increase is required, consider loading dose calculated as:

Loading dose **equals** (new maintenance dose **minus** current maintenance dose) **multiplied by** 3

Maximum daily dose: 40 mg/day; if required dose is >40 mg (due to loading dose), divide over 2 days. Serum concentrations should not be used as the sole basis for dosage adjustment (monitor clinical signs/symptoms, tissue biopsy, and laboratory parameters).

Maintenance therapy after withdrawal of cyclosporine: Following 2-4 months of combined therapy, withdrawal of cyclosporine may be considered in low to moderate risk patients. Cyclosporine should be discontinued over 4-8 weeks, and a necessary increase in the dosage of sirolimus (up to fourfold) should be anticipated due to removal of metabolic inhibition by cyclosporine and to maintain adequate immunosuppressive effects.

Vascular anomalies/tumors (eg, Kaposiform hemangioendothelioma); refractory: Very limited data available: Infants ≥7 months, Children, and Adolescents ≤14 years: Oral: Oral solution: Initial: 0.8 mg/m^2 twice daily (approximately every 12 hours); titrate to a serum trough concentration of 10-15 ng/mL; dosing based on a pilot case series (n=6), the mean response time was 25 days (range: 8-65 days) (Hammill, 2011). Further studies are needed.

Adults: **Renal transplantation, prophylaxis of organ rejection:** Oral:

Low- to moderate-immunologic risk patients: Dosing by body weight:
<40 kg: Loading dose: 3 mg/m^2 on day 1, followed by maintenance dosing of 1 mg/m^2 once daily
≥40 kg: Loading dose: 6 mg on day 1; maintenance: 2 mg once daily

High-immunologic risk patients: Oral: Loading dose: Up to 15 mg on day 1; maintenance: 5 mg/day; obtain trough concentration between days 5-7 and adjust accordingly. Continue concurrent cyclosporine/sirolimus therapy for 1 year following transplantation. Further adjustment of the regimen must be based on clinical status.

Dosage adjustment: Sirolimus dosages should be adjusted to maintain trough concentrations within desired range based on risk and concomitant therapy. Maximum daily dose: 40 mg. Dosage should be adjusted at intervals of 7-14 days to account for the long half-life of sirolimus. In general, dose proportionality may be assumed. New sirolimus dose **equals** current dose **multiplied by** (target concentration/current concentration). **Note:** If large dose increase is required, consider loading dose calculated as:

Loading dose **equals** (new maintenance dose **minus** current maintenance dose) **multiplied by** 3

Maximum daily dose: 40 mg/**day**; if required dose is >40 mg (due to loading dose), divide over 2 days. Serum concentrations should not be used as the sole basis for dosage adjustment (monitor clinical signs/symptoms, tissue biopsy, and laboratory parameters).

Maintenance therapy after withdrawal of cyclosporine: Cyclosporine withdrawal is not recommended in high-immunological risk patients. Following 2-4 months of combined therapy, withdrawal of cyclosporine may be considered in low-to-moderate risk patients. Cyclosporine should be discontinued over 4-8 weeks, and a necessary increase in the dosage of sirolimus (up to fourfold) should be anticipated due to removal of metabolic inhibition by cyclosporine and to maintain adequate immunosuppressive effects. Dose-adjusted trough target concentrations are typically 16-24 ng/mL for the first year post-transplant and 12-20 ng/mL thereafter (measured by chromatographic methodology).

Dosing adjustment in renal impairment: No dosage adjustment necessary (in loading or maintenance dose); however, adjustment of regimen (including discontinuation of therapy) should be considered when used concurrently with cyclosporine and elevated or increasing serum creatinine is noted.

Dosing adjustment in hepatic impairment:
Loading dose: No dosage adjustment required
Maintenance dose:
Mild to moderate hepatic impairment (Child-Pugh classes A and B): Reduce maintenance dose by ~33%
Severe hepatic impairment (Child-Pugh class C): Reduce maintenance dose by ~50%

Administration Hazardous agent; use appropriate precautions for handling and disposal (NIOSH, 2012). May be taken with or without food, but take medication consistently with respect to meals to minimize absorption variability. Initial dose should be administered as soon as possible after transplant. Sirolimus should be taken 4 hours after oral cyclosporine (Neoral or Gengraf).

Oral solution: Use amber oral syringe to withdraw solution from the bottle. Empty dose from syringe into a glass or plastic cup and mix with at least 2 ounces of water or orange juice. No other liquids should be used for dilution. Patient should stir vigorously and drink the diluted sirolimus solution immediately. Then refill cup with an additional 4 ounces of water or orange juice; stir contents vigorously and have patient drink solution at once.

Oral tablets: Do not crush, split, or chew.

Monitoring Parameters Monitor LFTs and CBC during treatment. Monitor sirolimus levels in all patients (especially in pediatric patients, patients ≥13 years of age weighing <40 kg, patients with hepatic impairment, or on concurrent potent inhibitors or inducers of CYP3A4 or P-gp, and/or if cyclosporine dosing is markedly reduced or discontinued), and when changing dosage forms of sirolimus. Also monitor serum cholesterol and triglycerides, blood pressure, serum creatinine, and urinary protein. Serum drug concentrations should be determined 3-4 days after loading doses and 7-14 days after dosage adjustments; however, these concentrations should not be used as the sole basis for dosage adjustment, especially during withdrawal of cyclosporine (monitor clinical signs/symptoms, tissue biopsy, and laboratory parameters). **Note:** Concentrations and ranges are dependent on and will vary with assay methodology (chromatographic or immunoassay); assay methods are not interchangeable.

Reference Range Note: Sirolimus concentrations are dependent on the assay method (eg, chromatographic and immunoassay) used; assay methods are not interchangeable. Determine the assay method used to assure consistency (or accommodations if changes occur) and for monitoring purposes, be aware of alterations to assay method or reference range.

Children and Adolescents: **Note:** See institution specific guidelines:
Target serum trough concentration for heart transplantation: 4-12 (ISHLT, Costanzo 2010)

Target serum trough concentration for renal transplantation (based on HPLC methods):

Low to moderate immunologic risk (after cyclosporine withdrawal):

First year after transplant:16-24 ng/mL

After 1 year: 12-20 ng/mL

High immunologic risk (with cyclosporine): 10-15 ng/mL

Target serum trough concentration for vascular anomalies: 10-15 ng/mL (Hammill, 2011)

Adults: **Note:** Trough concentrations vary based on clinical context and use of additional immunosuppressants. The following represents typical adult ranges.

When combined with tacrolimus and mycophenolate mofetil (MMF) without steroids: 6-8 ng/mL

As a substitute for tacrolimus (starting 4-8 weeks post-transplant), in combination with MMF and steroids: 8-12 ng/mL

Following conversion from tacrolimus to sirolimus >6 months post-transplant due to chronic allograft nephropathy: 4-6 ng/mL

Dosage Forms Excipient information presented when available (limited, particularly for generics); consult specific product labeling.

Solution, Oral:

Rapamune: 1 mg/mL (60 mL) [contains alcohol, usp]

Tablet, Oral:

Rapamune: 0.5 mg, 1 mg, 2 mg

Generic: 0.5 mg

References

American Academy of Pediatrics Committee on Drugs. "Inactive" ingredients in pharmaceutical products: update (subject review). *Pediatrics.* 1997;99(2):268-278.

Balfour IC, Srun SW, Wood EG, et al, "Early Renal Benefit of Rapamycin Combined With Reduced Calcineurin Inhibitor Dose in Pediatric Heart Transplantation Patients," *J Heart Lung Transplant*, 2006, 25 (5):518-22.

Chinnock TJ, Shankel T, Deming D, et.al. Calcineurin inhibitor minimization using sirolimus leads to improved renal function in pediatric heart transplant recipients. *Pediatric Transplantation.* 2011;15:746-749.

Costanzo MR. The international society of heart and lung transplantation guidelines for the care of heart transplant recipients. *J Heart Lung Transplant.* 2010;29:914-956.

Denfield SW. Strategies to prevent cellular rejection in pediatric heart transplant recipients. *Pediatric Drugs.* 2010;12(6):391-403.

Ettenger RB and Grimm EM, "Safety and Efficacy of TOR Inhibitors in Pediatric Renal Transplant Recipients," *Am J Kidney Dis*, 2001, 38(4 Suppl 2):S22-8.

Gupta P, Kaufman S, and Fishbein TM, "Sirolimus for Solid Organ Transplantation in Children," *Pediatr Transplant*, 2005, 9(3):269-76.

Hammill AM, Wentzel M, Gupta A, et.al. Sirolimus for the treatment of complicated vascular anomalies in children. *Pediatr Blood Cancer.* 2011;57:1018-1024.

Hymes LC, Warshaw BL. Five-year experience using sirolimus-based calcineurun inhibitor-free immunosuppression in pediatric renal transplantation. *Pediatric Transplantation.* 2011;15:437-441.

Hymes LC, Warshaw BL.Sirolimus in pediatric patients: results in the first 6 months post-renal transplant. *Pediatric Transplantation.* 2005;9:520-522.

Hymes LC, Warshaw BL, Amaral SG, et.al. Tacrolimus withdrawal and conversion to sirolimus at three months post-pediatric renal transplantation. *Pediatr Transplantation.* 2008;12:773-777.

Lobach NE, Pollock-Barziv SM, West LJ, et al, "Sirolimus Immunosuppression in Pediatric Heart Transplant Recipients: A Single-Center Experience," *J Heart Lung Transplant*, 2005, 24(2):184-9.

Matthews KL, Gossett J, Vande Kappelle P, et.al. Indications, tolerance and complications of a sirolimus and calineurin inhibitor immunosuppression regimen: intermediate experience in pediatric heart transplantation recipients. *Pediatric Transplantation.* 2010;14:402-408.

National Institute for Occupational Safety and Health (NIOSH), "NIOSH List of Antineoplastic and Other Hazardous Drugs in Healthcare Settings 2012." Available at http://www.cdc.gov/niosh/docs/2012-150/pdfs/2012-150.pdf. Accessed January 21, 2013.

Sarwal M and Pascual J, "Immunosuppression Minimization in Pediatric Transplantation," *Am J Transplant*, 2007, 7(10):2227-35.

Schubert M, Venkataramanan R, Holt DW, et al, "Pharmacokinetics of Sirolimus and Tacrolimus in Pediatric Transplant Patients," *Am J Transplant*, 2004, 4(5):767-73.

Shayani S, Palmer J, Stiller T, et.al. Thombotic microangiopathy associated with sirolimus level after allogeneic hematopoietic cell

transplantation with tacrolimus/sirolimus-based graft-versus-host disease prophylaxis. *Biol Blood Marrow Transplant.* 2013;19:298-304.

Shehab N, Lewis CL, Streetman DD, Donn SM. Exposure to the pharmaceutical excipients benzyl alcohol and propylene glycol among critically ill neonates. *Pediatr Crit Care Med.* 2009;10 (2):256-259.

◆ **Sirop Docusate De Sodium [OTC] (Can)** *see* Docusate *on page 701*

◆ **Sitavig** *see* Acyclovir (Topical) *on page 68*

◆ **SKF 104864** *see* Topotecan *on page 2053*

◆ **SKF 104864-A** *see* Topotecan *on page 2053*

◆ **Sklice** *see* Ivermectin (Topical) *on page 1172*

◆ **Sleep Tabs [OTC]** *see* DiphenhydrAMINE (Systemic) *on page 673*

◆ **Slo-Niacin [OTC]** *see* Niacin *on page 1491*

◆ **Slo-Pot (Can)** *see* Potassium Chloride *on page 1708*

◆ **Slow Fe [OTC]** *see* Ferrous Sulfate *on page 868*

◆ **Slow Iron [OTC]** *see* Ferrous Sulfate *on page 868*

◆ **Slow-K (Can)** *see* Potassium Chloride *on page 1708*

◆ **Slow-Mag [OTC]** *see* Magnesium Chloride *on page 1291*

◆ **Slow Magnesium/Calcium [OTC]** *see* Magnesium Chloride *on page 1291*

◆ **Slow Release Iron [OTC] [DSC]** *see* Ferrous Sulfate *on page 868*

◆ **SMX-TMP** *see* Sulfamethoxazole and Trimethoprim *on page 1948*

◆ **SMZ-TMP** *see* Sulfamethoxazole and Trimethoprim *on page 1948*

◆ **Snake Antivenin, FAB (Ovine)** *see* Crotalidae Polyvalent Immune Fab (Ovine) *on page 553*

◆ **Snake Antivenom, FAB (Ovine)** *see* Crotalidae Polyvalent Immune Fab (Ovine) *on page 553*

◆ **Sochlor [OTC]** *see* Sodium Chloride *on page 1902*

◆ **Sodium 2-Mercaptoethane Sulfonate** *see* Mesna *on page 1350*

◆ **Sodium *L*-Triiodothyronine** *see* Liothyronine *on page 1256*

Sodium Acetate (SOW dee um AS e tate)

Therapeutic Category Alkalinizing Agent, Parenteral; Electrolyte Supplement, Parenteral; Sodium Salt

Generic Availability (U.S.) Yes

Use Sodium salt replacement; correction of acidosis through conversion of acetate to bicarbonate

Pregnancy Risk Factor C

Pregnancy Considerations Animal reproduction studies have not been conducted. Sodium requirements do not change during pregnancy (IOM, 2004).

Breast-Feeding Considerations Sodium is found in breast milk. Sodium requirements do not change during lactation (IOM, 2004).

Contraindications Hypersensitivity to sodium acetate or any component; alkalosis, hypocalcemia, edema, cirrhosis, excessive chloride losses, hypernatremia

Warnings Avoid extravasation

Precautions Use with caution in patients with hepatic failure, CHF or other sodium-retaining conditions

Adverse Reactions

Cardiovascular: Hypervolemia, thrombosis

Dermatologic: Chemical cellulitis at injection site (extravasation)

Endocrine & metabolic: dilution of serum electrolytes, hypernatremia, hypocalcemia, hypokalemia, metabolic alkalosis, overhydration

Gastrointestinal: Flatulence, gastric distension

Local: Phlebitis

Respiratory: Pulmonary edema
Miscellaneous: Congestive conditions

Drug Interactions

Metabolism/Transport Effects None known.

Avoid Concomitant Use There are no known interactions where it is recommended to avoid concomitant use.

Increased Effect/Toxicity There are no known significant interactions involving an increase in effect.

Decreased Effect There are no known significant interactions involving a decrease in effect.

Stability Store at room temperature of 20°C to 25°C (68°F to 77°F); **incompatible** with acids, acidic salts, catecholamines, atropine

Dosing: Neonatal Sodium acetate is metabolized to bicarbonate on an equimolar basis outside the liver; administer in large volume I.V. fluids as a sodium source. Dosage is dependent upon the clinical condition, fluid, electrolytes and acid-base balance of the patient.

Maintenance sodium requirements: I.V.: 3-4 mEq/kg/day; maximum dose: 100-150 mEq/day

Dosing: Usual Sodium acetate is metabolized to bicarbonate on an equimolar basis outside the liver; administer in large volume I.V. fluids as a sodium source. Dosage is dependent upon the clinical condition, fluid, electrolytes, and acid-base balance of the patient.

Maintenance sodium requirements: I.V.:
Infants and Children: 3-4 mEq/kg/day; maximum dose: 100-150 mEq/day
Adults: 154 mEq/day
Metabolic acidosis: If sodium acetate is desired over sodium bicarbonate, the amount of acetate may be dosed utilizing the equation found in the sodium bicarbonate monograph as each mEq acetate is converted to a mEq of HCO_3; see Sodium Bicarbonate monograph

Administration Parenteral: Must be diluted prior to I.V. administration; dose and rate of administration are dependent on patient condition. Consult individual institutional policies and procedures; in general, central-line administration is preferred for hypertonic solutions (>0.9%) if available and/or if infusion is to be continued; peripheral administration may be necessary for initiation of treatment in critical patients; use of peripheral administration should be limited (Luu, 2011). Some suggest central line administration is not needed until infusing solutions >2.8% sodium acetate in sterile water (2.8% sodium acetate in sterile water has osmolarity approximately equivalent to 2% sodium chloride) (Mortimer, 2006; Suarez, 2004). If diluted in D_5W or other solution, the osmolarity may be higher requiring central line administration at a lower sodium acetate concentration.

Monitoring Parameters Serum electrolytes including calcium, arterial blood gases (if indicated)

Additional Information Sodium and acetate content of 1 g: 7.3 mEq

Dosage Forms Excipient information presented when available (limited, particularly for generics); consult specific product labeling.

Solution, Intravenous, as anhydrous:
Generic: 2 mEq/mL (20 mL, 50 mL, 100 mL); 4 mEq/mL (50 mL, 100 mL)

References

IOM (Institute of Medicine), *Dietary Reference Intakes for Water, Potassium, Sodium, Chloride, and Sulfate*, Washington, DC: National Academy Press, 2004.

Luu JL, Wendtland CL, Gross MF, et al. Three-percent saline administration during pediatric critical care transport. *Pediatr Emerg Care.* 2011;27(12):1113-1117.

Mortimer DS, Jancik J. Administering hypertonic saline to patients with severe traumatic brain injury. *J Neurosci Nurs.* 2006;38(3):142-146.

Suarez, JI. Hypertonic saline for cerebral edema and elevated intracranial pressure.*Cleve Clin J Med.* 2004;71(Suppl 1):S9-S13.

◆ **Sodium Acid Carbonate** *see* Sodium Bicarbonate
on page 1901

◆ **Sodium Aurothiomalate** *see* Gold Sodium Thiomalate *on page 979*

Sodium Benzoate (SOW dee um BENZ oh ate)

Therapeutic Category Ammonium Detoxicant; Hyperammonemia Agent; Urea Cycle Disorder (UCD) Treatment Agent

Use Adjunctive therapy for the prevention and treatment of hyperammonemia due to suspected or proven urea cycle disorders

Precautions Use with caution in patients with Reye's syndrome, propionic or methylmalonic acidemia. *In vitro* and animal studies have shown that benzoate, a metabolite of benzyl alcohol, displaces bilirubin from protein binding sites; use cautiously in neonates, particularly those with hyperbilirubinemia.

Drug Interactions

Metabolism/Transport Effects None known.

Avoid Concomitant Use There are no known interactions where it is recommended to avoid concomitant use.

Increased Effect/Toxicity
The levels/effects of Sodium Benzoate may be increased by: Probenecid

Decreased Effect There are no known significant interactions involving a decrease in effect.

Mechanism of Action Assists in lowering serum ammonia levels by activation of a nonurea cycle pathway (the benzoate-hippurate pathway); ammonia in the presence of benzoate will conjugate with glycine to form hippurate which is excreted by the kidney

Pharmacokinetics (Adult data unless noted)
Half-life: 0.75-7.4 hours
Elimination: Clearance is largely attributable to metabolism with urinary excretion of hippurate, the major metabolite

Dosing: Neonatal Oral: Investigational use (not an FDA-approved drug): Initial loading dose: 0.25 g/kg/dose followed by 0.25 g/kg/day divided every 6-8 hours (Enns, 2007). **Note:** If I.V. administration is necessary, see the Sodium Phenylacetate and Sodium Benzoate monograph for information about a commercially available parenteral product.

Dosing: Usual Oral: Investigational use (not an FDA-approved drug): **Note:** If I.V. administration is necessary, see the Sodium Phenylacetate and Sodium Benzoate monograph for information about a commercially available parenteral product.

Infants and Children: Initial loading dose: 0.25 g/kg/dose followed by 0.25 g/kg/day divided every 6-8 hours (Enns, 2007).
Adolescents and Adults: Initial 5.5 g/m² followed by 5.5 g/ m²/day divided every 6-8 hours

Administration Not available commercially; Oral: Must be compounded using chemical powder

Monitoring Parameters Plasma ammonia and amino acids

Additional Information Used to treat urea cycle enzyme deficiency in combination with arginine; a maximum of 1 mole nitrogen is removed for every 1 mole of benzoate administered

Dosage Forms Powder: 454 g

References

Batshaw ML, "Hyperammonemia," *Curr Probl Pediatr*, 1984, 14 (11):1-69.

Batshaw ML and Brusilow SW, "Treatment of Hyperammonemic Coma Caused by Inborn Errors of Urea Synthesis," *J Pediatr*, 1980, 97 (6):893-900.

Batshaw ML, MacArthur RB, and Tuchman M, "Alternative Pathway Therapy for Urea Cycle Disorders: Twenty Years Later," *J Pediatr*, 2001, 138(1 Suppl):S46-54.

Enns GM, Berry SA, Berry GT, et al, "Survival After Treatment With Phenylacetate and Benzoate for Urea-Cycle Disorders," *N Engl J Med*, 2007, 356(22):2282-92.

Green TP, Marchessault RP, and Freese DK, "Disposition of Sodium Benzoate in Newborn Infants With Hyperammonemia," *J Pediatr*, 1983, 102(5):785-90.

Maestri NE, Hauser ER, Bartholomew D, et al, "Prospective Treatment of Urea Cycle Disorders," *J Pediatr*, 1991, 119(6):923-8.

Summar M, "Current Strategies for the Management of Neonatal Urea Cycle Disorders," *J Pediatr*, 2001, 138(1 Suppl):S30-9.

◆ **Sodium Benzoate and Caffeine** *see* Caffeine *on page 338*

◆ **Sodium Benzoate and Sodium Phenylacetate** *see* Sodium Phenylacetate and Sodium Benzoate *on page 1911*

Sodium Bicarbonate (SOW dee um bye KAR bun ate)

Related Information
Management of Drug Extravasations *on page 2255*

Brand Names: U.S. Neut

Therapeutic Category Alkalinizing Agent, Oral; Alkalinizing Agent, Parenteral; Antacid; Electrolyte Supplement, Oral; Electrolyte Supplement, Parenteral; Sodium Salt

Generic Availability (U.S.) Yes

Use Management of metabolic acidosis; antacid; alkalinization of urine; stabilization of acid base status in cardiac arrest and treatment of life-threatening hyperkalemia

Pregnancy Risk Factor C

Pregnancy Considerations Animal reproduction studies have not been conducted. The use of sodium bicarbonate in pregnant women for the management of cardiac arrest and metabolic acidosis is the same as in nonpregnant women (Campbell, 2009; Vanden Hoek, 2010). Antacids containing sodium bicarbonate should not be used during pregnancy due to their potential to cause metabolic alkalosis and fluid overload (Mahadevan, 2007).

Breast-Feeding Considerations Sodium is found in breast milk (IOM, 2004).

Contraindications Hypersensitivity to sodium bicarbonate or any component; alkalosis, hypocalcemia, hypernatremia; unknown abdominal pain, inadequate ventilation during cardiopulmonary resuscitation; excessive chloride losses

Warnings Avoid extravasation, tissue necrosis can occur due to the hypertonicity of $NaHCO_3$; use of I.V. $NaHCO_3$ should be reserved for documented metabolic acidosis and for life-threatening hyperkalemia; routine use in cardiac arrest is not recommended; patient should be adequately ventilated before administering in cardiac arrest; administration of excessive amounts of sodium bicarbonate may result in metabolic alkalosis which decreases the delivery of oxygen to tissues; monitor use closely

Precautions Use with caution in patients with CHF or other sodium-retaining conditions and renal insufficiency. Rapid administration of hyperosmotic solution in neonates, infants, and children <2 years of age has led to hypernatremia, decreased CSF pressure, and intracranial hemorrhage.

Adverse Reactions
Cardiovascular: Cerebral hemorrhage, CHF (aggravated), edema

Central nervous system: Tetany

Gastrointestinal: Belching, flatulence (with oral), gastric distension

Endocrine & metabolic: Hypernatremia, hyperosmolality, hypocalcemia, hypokalemia, increased affinity of hemoglobin for oxygen-reduced pH in myocardial tissue necrosis when extravasated, intracranial acidosis, metabolic alkalosis, milk-alkali syndrome (especially with renal dysfunction)

Respiratory: Pulmonary edema

Drug Interactions
Metabolism/Transport Effects None known.

Avoid Concomitant Use
Avoid concomitant use of *Sodium Bicarbonate* with any of the following: PONATinib

Increased Effect/Toxicity
Sodium Bicarbonate may increase the levels/effects of: Alpha-/Beta-Agonists (Indirect-Acting); Amphetamines; Calcium Polystyrene Sulfonate; Dexmethylphenidate; Flecainide; Memantine; Methylphenidate; QuiNIDine; QuiNINE

The levels/effects of *Sodium Bicarbonate* may be increased by: AcetaZOLAMIDE

Decreased Effect
Sodium Bicarbonate may decrease the levels/effects of: ACE Inhibitors; Anticonvulsants (Hydantoin); Antipsychotic Agents (Phenothiazines); Atazanavir; Bisacodyl; Bosutinib; Cefditoren; Cefpodoxime; Cefuroxime; Chloroquine; Corticosteroids (Oral); Dabigatran Etexilate; Dabrafenib; Dasatinib; Delavirdine; Elvitegravir; Erlotinib; Flecainide; Gabapentin; HMG-CoA Reductase Inhibitors; Hyoscyamine; Iron Salts; Isoniazid; Itraconazole; Ketoconazole (Systemic); Lithium; Mesalamine; Methenamine; Multivitamins/Minerals (with ADEK, Folate, Iron); Nilotinib; PAZOPanib; PenicillAMINE; Phosphate Supplements; PONATinib; Potassium Acid Phosphate; Protease Inhibitors; Rilpivirine; Riociguat; Sulpiride; Tetracycline Derivatives; Trientine; Vismodegib

Stability Do not mix $NaHCO_3$ with calcium salts, catecholamines, atropine

Mechanism of Action
Dissociates to provide bicarbonate ion which neutralizes hydrogen ion concentration and raises blood and urinary pH

Neutralizing additive (dental use): Increases pH of lidocaine and epinephrine solution to improve tolerability and increase tissue uptake

Pharmacodynamics
Onset of action:
Oral, as antacid: 15 minutes
I.V.: Rapid

Duration:
Oral: 1-3 hours
I.V.: 8-10 minutes

Pharmacokinetics (Adult data unless noted)
Absorption: Oral: Well absorbed

Elimination: Reabsorbed by kidney and <1% is excreted in urine

Dosing: Neonatal Note: Rapid administration at a high concentration may be associated with fluctuation in cerebral blood flow and possibly ICH; carefully consider clinical need before administering (Aschner, 2008).

Metabolic acidosis: Dosage should be based on the following formula if blood gases and pH measurements are available: HCO_3^- (mEq) = 0.3 x weight (kg) x base deficit (mEq/L) or HCO_3^- (mEq) = 0.5 x weight (kg) x [24 - serum HCO_3^- (mEq/L)]; usual dosage: 1-2 mEq/kg/dose (Berg, 2010)

Note: In 55 asphyxiated neonates, a fixed dose of 1.8 mEq/kg/dose over 3-5 minutes administered within first 5 minutes of life did not show clinical benefit (eg, survival, acid-base status, neurodevelopmental outcomes) compared to control group; further studies needed (Lokesh, 2004; Murki, 2004).

Dosing: Usual
Cardiac arrest: Patient should be adequately ventilated before administering $NaHCO_3$
Infants: 1 mEq/kg slow IVP initially; may repeat with 0.5 mEq/kg in 10 minutes one time, or as indicated by the patient's acid-base status
Children and Adults: 1 mEq/kg IVP initially; may repeat with 0.5 mEq/kg in 10 minutes one time, or as indicated by the patient's acid-base status

Metabolic acidosis: Dosage should be based on the following formula if blood gases and pH measurements are available:

Infants and Children: HCO_3^-(mEq) = 0.3 x weight (kg) x base deficit (mEq/L) **or** HCO_3^-(mEq) = 0.5 x weight (kg) x [24 - serum HCO_3^-(mEq/L)]

Adults: HCO_3^-(mEq) = 0.2 x weight (kg) x base deficit (mEq/L) **or** HCO_3^-(mEq) = 0.5 x weight (kg) x [24 - serum HCO_3^-(mEq/L)]

If acid-base status is not available: Dose for older Children and Adults: 2-5 mEq/kg I.V. infusion over 4-8 hours; subsequent doses should be based on patient's acid-base status

Prevention of hyperuricemia secondary to tumor lysis syndrome (urinary alkalinization) (refer to individual protocols):

Infants and Children:

I.V.: 120-200 mEq/m²/day diluted in maintenance I.V. fluids of 3000 mL/m²/day; titrate to maintain urine pH between 6-7

Oral: 12 g/m²/day divided into 4 doses; titrate to maintain urine pH between 6-7

Chronic renal failure: Oral: Initiate when plasma HCO_3^- <15 mEq/L:

Children: 1-3 mEq/kg/day in divided doses

Adults: 20-36 mEq/day in divided doses

Renal tubular acidosis: Oral:

Distal:

Children: 2-3 mEq/kg/day in divided doses

Adults: 0.5-2 mEq/kg/day given in 4-5 divided doses

Proximal: Children and Adults: Initial: 5-10 mEq/kg/day in divided doses; maintenance: Increase as required to maintain serum bicarbonate in the normal range

Urine alkalinization: Oral:

Children: 1-10 mEq (84-840 mg)/kg/day in divided doses; dose should be titrated to desired urinary pH

Adults: 48 mEq (4 g) initially, then 12-24 mEq (1-2 g) every 4 hours; dose should be titrated to desired urinary pH; doses up to 16 g/day have been used

Antacid: Oral: Adults: 325 mg to 2 grams 1-4 times/day

Administration

Oral: Administer 1-3 hours after meals

Parenteral: For direct I.V. administration: In neonates and infants, use the 0.5 mEq/mL solution or dilute the 1 mEq/mL solution 1:1 with **SWI**; in children and adults, the 1 mEq/mL solution may be used; administer slowly (maximum rate in neonates and infants: 10 mEq/minute); for infusion, dilute to a maximum concentration of 0.5 mEq/mL in dextrose solution and infuse over 2 hours (maximum rate of administration: 1 mEq/kg/hour)

Vesicant/Extravasation Risk Vesicant (at concentrations ≥8.4%)

Monitoring Parameters Serum electrolytes including calcium, urinary pH, arterial blood gases (if indicated)

Additional Information 1 mEq $NaHCO_3$ is equivalent to 84 mg; each g of $NaHCO_3$ provides 12 mEq each of sodium and bicarbonate ions; the osmolarity of 0.5 mEq/mL is 1000 mOsm/L and 1 mEq/mL is 2000 mOsm/L

Dosage Forms Considerations

Sodium bicarbonate solution 4.2% [42 mg/mL] provides 0.5 mEq/mL each of sodium and bicarbonate

Sodium bicarbonate solution 7.5% [75 mg/mL] provides 0.9 mEq/mL each of sodium and bicarbonate

Sodium bicarbonate solution 8.4% [84 mg/mL] provides 1 mEq/mL each of sodium and bicarbonate

Dosage Forms Excipient information presented when available (limited, particularly for generics); consult specific product labeling.

Powder, Oral:

Generic: (1 g, 120 g, 454 g, 500 g, 1000 g, 2500 g, 12000 g, 25000 g, 45000 g)

Solution, Intravenous:

Neut: 4% (5 mL)

Generic: 4.2% (5 mL, 10 mL); 7.5% (50 mL); 8.4% (10 mL, 50 mL)

Tablet, Oral:

Generic: 325 mg, 650 mg

References

Aschner JL and Poland RL, "Sodium Bicarbonate: Basically Useless Therapy," *Pediatrics*, 2008, 122(4):831-5.

Berg CS, Barnette AR, Myers BJ, et al, "Sodium Bicarbonate Administration and Outcome in Preterm Infants," *J Pediatr*, 2010, 157 (4):684-7.

Campbell TA and Sanson TG, "Cardiac Arrest and Pregnancy," *J Emerg Trauma Shock*, 2009, 2(1):34-42.

IOM (Institute of Medicine), *Dietary Reference Intakes for Water, Potassium, Sodium, Chloride, and Sulfate*, Washington, DC: National Academy Press, 2004.

Lokesh L, Kumar P, Murki S, et al, "A Randomized Controlled Trial of Sodium Bicarbonate in Neonatal Resuscitation-Effect on Immediate Outcome," *Resuscitation*, 2004, 60(2):219-23.

Mahadevan U, "Gastrointestinal Medications in Pregnancy," *Best Pract Res Clin Gastroenterol*, 2007, 21(5):849-77.

Murki S, Kumar P, Lingappa L, et al, "Effect of a Single Dose of Sodium Bicarbonate Given During Neonatal Resuscitation at Birth on the Acid-Base Status on First Day of Life," *J Perinatol*, 2004, 24 (11):696-9.

Vanden Hoek TL, Morrison LJ, Shuster M, et al, "Part 12: Cardiac Arrest in Special Situations: 2010 American Heart Association Guidelines for Cardiopulmonary Resuscitation and Emergency Cardiovascular Care," *Circulation*, 2010, 122(18 Suppl 3):829-61.

◆ **Sodium Bicarbonate and Omeprazole** *see* Omeprazole and Sodium Bicarbonate *on page 1538*

Sodium Chloride (SOW dee um KLOR ide)

Medication Safety Issues

High alert medication:

The Institute for Safe Medication Practices (ISMP) includes this medication (I.V. formulation >0.9% concentration) among its list of drugs which have a heightened risk of causing significant patient harm when used in error.

Other safety concerns:

Per The Joint Commission (TJC) recommendations, concentrated electrolyte solutions (eg, NaCl >0.9%) should not be available in patient care areas.

Inappropriate use of low sodium or sodium-free intravenous fluids (eg, D_5W, hypotonic saline) in pediatric patients can lead to significant morbidity and mortality due to hyponatremia (ISMP, 2009).

Related Information

Management of Drug Extravasations *on page 2255*

Pediatric Parenteral Nutrition *on page 2312*

Brand Names: U.S. 4-Way Saline [OTC]; Afrin Saline Nasal Mist [OTC]; Altachlore [OTC]; Altamist Spray [OTC]; Ayr Nasal Mist Allergy/Sinus [OTC]; Ayr Saline Nasal Drops [OTC]; Ayr Saline Nasal Gel [OTC]; Ayr Saline Nasal No-Drip [OTC]; AYR Saline Nasal Rinse [OTC]; Ayr Saline Nasal [OTC]; Ayr [OTC]; Baby Ayr Saline [OTC]; Broncho Saline [OTC]; Deep Sea Nasal Spray [OTC]; Entsol Nasal Wash [OTC]; Entsol Nasal [OTC]; Entsol [OTC]; Humist [OTC]; HyperSal; Muro 128 [OTC]; Na-Zone [OTC]; Nasal Moist [OTC]; Nebusal; Ocean Complete Sinus Rinse [OTC]; Ocean for Kids [OTC]; Ocean Nasal Spray [OTC]; Ocean Ultra Saline Mist [OTC]; Pretz Irrigation [OTC]; Pretz [OTC]; PulmoSal; Rhinaris [OTC]; Safe Wash [OTC]; Saline Flush ZR; Saline Mist Spray [OTC]; Saljet Rinse [OTC]; Saljet [OTC]; Sea Soft Nasal Mist [OTC]; Sea-Clens Wound Cleanser [OTC]; Sochlor [OTC]; Sodium Chloride Thermoject Sys; Swab-Flush Saline Flush; Wound Wash Saline [OTC]

Therapeutic Category Electrolyte Supplement, Oral; Electrolyte Supplement, Parenteral; Lubricant, Ocular; Sodium Salt

Generic Availability (U.S.) May be product dependent

Use Restoration of sodium ion in hyponatremia [FDA approved in pediatric patients (age not specified) and adults], restores moisture to nasal membranes [FDA approved in pediatric patients (age not specified) and adults], source of electrolytes and water for expansion of the extracellular fluid compartment [FDA approved in pediatric patients (age not specified) and adults], diluent and delivery system of compatible drug additives [FDA approved in pediatric patients (age not specified) and adults]; has also been used for reduction of intracranial pressure (ICP), improvement of mucociliary clearance and airway hydration in CF and acute viral bronchiolitis, reduction of corneal edema, and prevention of muscle cramps and heat prostration

Pregnancy Risk Factor C

Pregnancy Considerations Animal reproduction studies have not been conducted. Sodium requirements do not change during pregnancy (IOM, 2004). Nasal saline rinses may be used for the treatment of pregnancy rhinitis (Wallace, 2008)

Breast-Feeding Considerations Sodium is found in breast milk. Sodium requirements do not change during lactation (IOM, 2004).

Contraindications Hypersensitivity to sodium chloride or any component; hypertonic uterus, hypernatremia (except when used for increased intracranial pressure), fluid retention

Warnings With systemic therapy, sodium toxicity is almost exclusively related to how fast a sodium deficit is corrected; both rate and magnitude of correction are extremely important; in neonates, maximum serum correction rate should generally not exceed 10 mEq/L/day; in infants, children, adolescents, and adults, do not exceed a maximum serum correction rate of 12 mEq/L/day. Administration of low sodium or sodium free I.V. solutions may result in significant hyponatremia or water intoxication in pediatric patients; monitor serum sodium concentration.

Bacteriostatic products may contain benzyl alcohol which may cause allergic reactions in susceptible individuals; large amounts of benzyl alcohol (≥99 mg/kg/day) have been associated with a potentially fatal toxicity ("gasping syndrome") in neonates; the "gasping syndrome" consists of metabolic acidosis, respiratory distress, gasping respirations, CNS dysfunction (including convulsions, intracranial hemorrhage), hypotension and cardiovascular collapse; avoid using products containing benzyl alcohol in neonates and bacteriostatic NS should not be used for diluting or reconstituting drugs for administration in a neonate; *in vitro* and animal studies have shown that benzoate, a metabolite of benzyl alcohol, displaces bilirubin from protein binding sites

Precautions Use with caution in patients with heart failure, renal insufficiency, cirrhosis, hypertension, and edema

Adverse Reactions

Cardiovascular: Congestive heart failure, transient hypotension (especially with adult administration of 23.4% NaCl)

Central nervous system: Central pontine myelinolysis (due to rapid correction of hyponatremia)

Endocrine & metabolic: Dilution of serum electrolytes, extravasation, hypernatremia, hypervolemia, hypokalemia, overhydration

Gastrointestinal: Nausea, vomiting (oral use)

Local: Thrombosis, phlebitis, extravasation

Respiratory: Bronchospasm (inhalation with hypertonic solutions), pulmonary edema

Drug Interactions

Metabolism/Transport Effects None known.

Avoid Concomitant Use

Avoid concomitant use of Sodium Chloride with any of the following: Tolvaptan

Increased Effect/Toxicity

Sodium Chloride may increase the levels/effects of: Tolvaptan

Decreased Effect

Sodium Chloride may decrease the levels/effects of: Lithium

Stability Store injection at room temperature; do not freeze; protect from heat. Use only clear solutions.

Mechanism of Action Principal extracellular cation; functions in fluid and electrolyte balance, osmotic pressure control, and water distribution

Pharmacokinetics (Adult data unless noted)

Absorption: Oral, I.V.: Rapid

Distribution: Widely distributed

Elimination: Mainly in urine but also in sweat, tears, and saliva

Dosing: Neonatal Dosage depends upon clinical condition, fluid, electrolyte, and acid-base balance of patient.

Normal daily requirement:

Premature neonates: Oral, I.V.: 2-5 mEq/kg/day (Mirtallo, 2004); infants born at ≤32 weeks gestation may require higher dosage (up to 8 mEq/kg/day) for the first 2 weeks of life (Al-Dahhan, 2002)

Term neonates: Oral, I.V.: 2-5 mEq/kg/day (Mirtallo, 2004)

Hyponatremia: I.V.: **0.9% isotonic solution:**

Dose (mEq sodium) = [desired serum sodium (mEq/L) − actual serum sodium (mEq/L)] x 0.6 x wt (kg)

Note: For acute correction, use 125 mEq/L as the "desired serum sodium"; acutely correct serum sodium by 5 mEq/L/dose increments (eg, from a serum concentration of 120 mEq/L to 125 mEq/L) using a serum correction rate of <0.4-0.5 mEq/L/hour; goal serum correction rate: ≤8-10 mEq/L/day. Hypertonic saline should be used with caution and only for severe cases of hyponatremia with a serum sodium <120 mEq/L and patient experiencing symptoms (Marcialis, 2011).

Nasal dryness/congestion: Intranasal: 0.9% intranasal solution: 2-6 drops per nostril as needed

Ocular dryness:

Ophthalmic, ointment: Apply once daily or more often as needed

Ophthalmic solution: Instill 1-2 drops into affected eye(s) every 3-4 hours

Volume expansion, resuscitation: AHA, AAP: Neonatal resuscitation recommendation: I.V.: **0.9% isotonic solution:** 10 mL/kg; may repeat (Kattwinkel, 2010); in a retrospective analysis of neonates requiring CPR at birth, 21 ± 14 mL/kg was the effective dose (n=13, GA: ≥34 weeks) (Wyckoff, 2005)

Dosing: Usual Dosage depends upon clinical condition, fluid, electrolyte, and acid-base balance of patient; systemic hypertonic solutions (>0.9%) should only be used for the initial treatment of acute serious symptomatic hyponatremia or increased intracranial pressure.

Pediatric:

Normal daily requirements:

Infants and Children ≤50 kg: Oral, I.V: 2-5 mEq/kg/day (Mirtallo, 2004)

Children >50 kg and Adolescents: Oral, I.V: 1-2 mEq/kg/day (Mirtallo, 2004)

Bronchiolitis, viral (inpatient): Infants and Children 1-24 months: Inhalation: **3% solution:** 4 mL inhaled every 2 hours for 3 doses followed by every 4 hours for 5 doses and continued every 6 hours until discharge (Kuzik, 2007); pretreatment with a bronchodilator may be necessary to prevent potential bronchospasm

Bronchodilator diluent: Infants, Children, and Adolescents: Inhalation: 1-3 sprays (1-3 mL) to dilute bronchodilator solution in nebulizer before administration

Cystic fibrosis: Children ≥6 years and Adolescents: Inhalation: **7% solution:** 4 mL inhaled twice daily. **Note:** Clinically, some CF centers use 3% or 3.5% inhaled solutions if patients cannot tolerate 7%; pretreatment with a bronchodilator is recommended to prevent potential bronchospasm

Dehydration: Infants, Children, and Adolescents: I.V.: **0.9% isotonic solution:** Initial: 20 mL/kg/dose; maximum dose: 1000 mL followed by remaining replacement using sodium chloride concentration appropriate for age over 24 hours for dehydration (Meyers, 2009)

Hyponatremia: Infants, Children, and Adolescents: I.V.:
Note: Use **0.9% isotonic solution or 3% hypertonic solution** depending on clinical severity and etiology.

Dose (mEq sodium) = [desired serum sodium (mEq/L) - actual serum sodium (mEq/L)] x 0.6 x wt (kg)

Note: For acute correction, use 125 mEq/L as the "desired serum sodium"; acutely correct serum sodium by 5 mEq/L/dose increments (eg, from a serum concentration of 120 mEq/L to 125 mEq/L) using a serum correction rate of ≤2 mEq/L/hour for the first few hours followed by a serum correction rate of ≤0.5 mEq/L/hour; goal serum correction rate: ≤12 mEq/L/day; more gradual correction in increments of 10 mEq/L/day is indicated in the asymptomatic patient

Hypovolemic shock: Infants, Children, and Adolescents: I.V.: **0.9% isotonic solution:** 20 mL/kg/dose; may repeat up to ≥60 mL/kg until capillary perfusion improves or signs of fluid overload occur (Ceneviva, 1998; Parker, 2004)

Increased intracranial pressure (ICP): Infants, Children, and Adolescents: I.V.: **3% hypertonic solution:**
Bolus: Limited data available; optimal dose not established; further studies are needed

Traumatic brain injury guidelines: 6.5-10 mL/kg/dose (Fisher, 1992; Kochanek, 2012)

Alternate dosing: 5 mL/kg/dose administered early in presentation (during critical care transport) was reported in a retrospective trial of 101 pediatric patients (age range: 2 months to 17 years) with suspected increased ICP (Luu, 2011); some centers use 2-5 mL/kg/dose; boluses are typically infused over 30 minutes but are occasionally administered more rapidly depending on the clinical scenario (Abd-Allah, 2012)

Continuous I.V. infusion: 0.1-1 mL/kg/hour titrated to maintain ICP <20 mm Hg (Kochanek, 2012); monitor serum sodium concentration closely; some centers utilize titration protocols with rate adjustments varying with serum sodium concentration; maintain serum osmolarity <360 mOsmol/L

Nasal dryness/congestion:
Infants: Intranasal: **0.9% intranasal solution:** 2-6 drops per nostril as needed

Children and Adolescents: Intranasal: Use as often as needed

Ocular dryness: Infants, Children, and Adolescents:
Ophthalmic, ointment: Apply once daily or more often as needed

Ophthalmic, solution: Instill 1-2 drops into affected eye(s) every 3-4 hours

Adult:
Bronchodilator diluent: Inhalation: 1-3 sprays (1-3 mL) to dilute bronchodilator solution in nebulizer before administration

Chloride maintenance electrolyte requirement in parenteral nutrition: I.V.: As needed to maintain acid-base balance with parenteral nutrition; use equal amounts of chloride and acetate to maintain balance and adjust ratio based on individual patient needs (Mirtallo, 2004).

GU irrigant: Irrigation: 1-3 L/day by intermittent irrigation

Hyponatremia: I.V.: To correct acute (<24 hours) or chronic (>48 hours), severe (<120 mEq/L) hyponatremia: In general, a serum sodium concentration increase of 4-6 mEq/L within a 24-hour period is sufficient to improve most symptoms of hyponatremia. In chronic severe hyponatremia, overcorrection risks iatrogenic osmotic demyelination syndrome. For patients with severe symptoms or other need for urgent correction, one approach is to increase serum sodium concentration by 4-6 mEq/L within the first 6 hours and postpone any further correction until the next day at a correction rate of 4-6 mEq/L per day. Choice of sodium correction fluid concentration is dependent upon the severity of the hyponatremia with more concentrated solutions (eg, 3% NaCl) for more severe cases; monitor serum sodium closely during administration (Sterns, 2013).

Irrigation: Spray affected area

Nasal congestion: Intranasal: 2-3 sprays in each nostril as needed

Ophthalmic:
Ointment: Apply once daily or more often
Solution: Instill 1-2 drops into affected eye(s) every 3-4 hours

Replacement: I.V.: Determined by laboratory determinations mEq

Sodium maintenance electrolyte requirement in parenteral nutrition: I.V.: 1-2 mEq/kg/24 hours; customize amounts based on individual patient needs (Mirtallo, 2004).

Administration

Inhalation: Nebulization; studies administering hypertonic saline utilized varying types of nebulizers, including jet and ultrasonic

Nasal: Spray into 1 nostril while gently occluding other

Ophthalmic: Apply to affected eye(s); avoid contact of bottle tip with eye or skin

Oral: Administer with full glass of water

Parenteral: Central-line administration is preferred for hypertonic saline (>0.9%) if available and/or if infusion is to be continued; peripheral administration may be necessary for initiation of treatment in critical patients; use of peripheral administration should be limited; intraosseous administration may be used if unable to obtain intravenous access (Luu, 2011)

Rate of administration:
Bolus:
0.9% isotonic solution:
Hypotension, shock:
Neonates: Published data not available; consider slower administration to avoid IVH (Kattwinkel, 2010)
Infants, Children, and Adolescents: Administer boluses over 5 minutes (Brierley, 2009)
Dehydration: Bolus: Administer over 20-60 minutes
3% hypertonic solution: In pediatric patients, typically infused over 30 minutes (Abd-Allah, 2012); some trials have described administering at a rate of 10 mEq/kg/hour when treating acute, life-threatening ICP elevation (Kamat, 2003)
Continuous I.V. infusion: Maximum rate: 1 mEq/kg/hour

Vesicant/Extravasation Risk Vesicant (at concentrations >1%)

Monitoring Parameters Serum sodium, chloride, I & O, weight; ICP, serum osmolarity (when used to treat increased ICP), capillary perfusion, MAP, CVP (fluid resuscitation)

Reference Range Serum/plasma sodium concentration:
Premature neonates: 132-140 mEq/L
Full-term neonates: 133-142 mEq/L
Infants ≥2 months to Adults: 135-145 mEq/L

Additional Information

I.V. solutions: NS (0.9%) = 154 mEq/L; 3% NaCl = 513 mEq/L; 5% NaCl = 856 mEq/L
Tablet 1 g = 17.1 mEq
3% NaCl: Osmolarity: 1027 mOsm/L

Dosage Forms Considerations 1 g sodium chloride = elemental sodium 393.3 mg = 17.1 mEq sodium = sodium 17.1 mmol

Dosage Forms Excipient information presented when available (limited, particularly for generics); consult specific product labeling.

Aerosol Solution, Inhalation:
  Broncho Saline: 0.9% (90 mL, 240 mL)
Aerosol Solution, Nasal [preservative free]:
  Ocean Complete Sinus Rinse: (177 mL) [drug free]
Gel, Nasal:
  Ayr Saline Nasal: (14.1 g) [contains aloe barbadensis, brilliant blue fcf (fd&c blue #1), methylparaben, propylparaben, soybean oil]
  Ayr Saline Nasal No-Drip: (22 mL) [contains aloe barbadensis, benzalkonium chloride, benzyl alcohol, soybean oil]
  Entsol Nasal: (20 g)
  Rhinaris: 0.2% (28.4 g) [contains benzalkonium chloride, propylene glycol]
Liquid, External:
  Sea-Clens Wound Cleanser: (355 mL)
Nebulization Solution, Inhalation:
  Generic: 0.9% (3 mL)
Nebulization Solution, Inhalation [preservative free]:
  HyperSal: 3.5% (4 mL) [latex free]
  HyperSal: 7% (4 mL)
  Nebusal: 3% (4 mL); 6% (4 mL)
  PulmoSal: 7% (4 mL)
  Generic: 0.9% (3 mL, 5 mL, 15 mL); 3% (4 mL, 15 mL); 7% (4 mL); 10% (4 mL, 15 mL)
Ointment, Ophthalmic:
  Altachlore: 5% (3.5 g)
  Muro 128: 5% (3.5 g)
  Generic: 5% (3.5 g)
Packet, Nasal [preservative free]:
  AYR Saline Nasal Rinse: 1.57 g (50 ea, 100 ea) [iodine free]
Solution, External:
  Saljet: 0.9% (30 mL)
  Wound Wash Saline: 0.9% (210 mL)
Solution, External [preservative free]:
  Safe Wash: 0.9% (210 mL) [drug free, latex free]
  Saljet Rinse: 0.9% (30 mL)
Solution, Injection:
  Sodium Chloride Thermoject Sys: 0.9% (10 mL)
  Generic: 0.9% (2 mL, 2.5 mL, 3 mL, 5 mL, 10 mL, 20 mL, 30 mL, 100 mL); 23.4% (20 mL, 40 mL)
Solution, Injection [preservative free]:
  Generic: 0.9% (1 mL, 2 mL, 2.5 mL, 3 mL, 5 mL, 10 mL, 20 mL, 30 mL, 50 mL)
Solution, Intravenous:
  SwabFlush Saline Flush: 0.9% (10 mL)
  Generic: 0.45% (25 mL, 50 mL, 100 mL, 250 mL, 500 mL, 1000 mL); 0.9% (2.5 mL, 3 mL, 10 mL, 25 mL, 50 mL, 100 mL, 150 mL, 250 mL, 500 mL, 1000 mL); 3% (500 mL); 5% (500 mL); 14.6% (30 mL, 100 mL, 200 mL, 250 mL)
Solution, Intravenous [preservative free]:
  Saline Flush ZR: 0.9% (2.5 mL, 5 mL, 10 mL) [latex free]
  Generic: 0.9% (1 mL, 2 mL, 2.5 mL, 3 mL, 5 mL, 10 mL, 50 mL, 100 mL, 500 mL, 1000 mL)
Solution, Irrigation:
  Generic: 0.9% (250 mL, 500 mL, 1000 mL, 1500 mL, 2000 mL, 3000 mL, 4000 mL, 5000 mL)
Solution, Nasal:
  4-Way Saline: (29.6 mL)
  Afrin Saline Nasal Mist: 0.65% (30 mL, 45 mL)
  Altamist Spray: 0.65% (45 mL, 60 mL)
  Ayr: 0.65% (50 mL)
  Ayr Nasal Mist Allergy/Sinus: 2.65% (50 mL) [contains benzalkonium chloride]
  Ayr Saline Nasal Drops: 0.65% (50 mL)
  Baby Ayr Saline: 0.65% (30 mL)
  Deep Sea Nasal Spray: 0.65% (44 mL) [contains benzalkonium chloride]

Entsol: (30 mL)
Humist: 0.65% (45 mL)
Na-Zone: 0.65% (59 mL)
Nasal Moist: 0.65% (15 mL, 45 mL)
Ocean for Kids: 0.65% (37.5 mL) [alcohol free, drug free; contains benzalkonium chloride]
Ocean Nasal Spray: 0.65% (45 mL, 104 mL, 480 mL) [contains benzalkonium chloride]
Pretz: (50 mL, 946 mL)
Pretz Irrigation: (237 mL)
Rhinaris: 0.2% (30 mL) [contains benzalkonium chloride, propylene glycol]
Saline Mist Spray: 0.65% (45 mL) [contains benzalkonium chloride]
Sea Soft Nasal Mist: 0.65% (45 mL)
Generic: 0.65% (44 mL, 45 mL)
Solution, Nasal [preservative free]:
  Entsol Nasal: 3% (100 mL) [drug free]
  Entsol Nasal Wash: (237 mL)
  Ocean Ultra Saline Mist: (90 mL) [drug free]
Solution, Ophthalmic:
  Altachlore: 5% (15 mL, 30 mL)
  Muro 128: 2% (15 mL); 5% (15 mL, 30 mL)
  Sochlor: 5% (15 mL)
  Generic: 5% (15 mL)
Swab, Nasal:
  Ayr Saline Nasal Gel: (20 ea) [contains methylparaben, propylparaben, soybean oil, trolamine (triethanolamine)]
Tablet, Oral:
  Generic: 1 g

References

Abd-Allah, S. Personal communication. February 2012.

Al-Dahhan J, Jannoun L, and Haycock GB, "Effect of Salt Supplementation of Newborn Premature Infants on Neurodevelopmental Outcome at 10-13 Years of Age," Arch Dis Child Fetal Neonatal Ed, 2002, 86(2):F120-3.

Brierley J, Carcillo JA, Choong K, et al, "Clinical Practice Parameters for Hemodynamic Support of Pediatric and Neonatal Septic Shock: 2007 Update From the American College of Critical Care Medicine," Crit Care Med, 2009, 37(2):666-88.

Ceneviva G, Paschall JA, Maffei F, et al, "Hemodynamic Support in Fluid-Refractory Pediatric Septic Shock," Pediatrics, 1998, 102(2):e19.

Dellon EP, Donaldson SH, Johnson R, et al, "Safety and Tolerability of Inhaled Hypertonic Saline in Young Children With Cystic Fibrosis," Pediatr Pulmonol, 2008, 43(11):1100-6.

Elkins MR, Robinson M, Rose BR, et al, "A Controlled Trial of Long-Term Inhaled Hypertonic Saline in Patients With Cystic Fibrosis," N Engl J Med, 2006, 354(3):229-40.

Fisher B, Thomas D, and Peterson B, "Hypertonic Saline Lowers Raised Intracranial Pressure in Children After Head Trauma," J Neurosurg Anesthesiol, 1992, 4(1):4-10.

Institute for Safe Medication Practice, "Plain D_5W or Hypotonic Saline Solutions Post-Op Could Result in Acute Hyponatremia and Death in Healthy Children," ISMP Medication Safety Alert, August 13, 2009. Available online at http://www.ismp.org/Newsletters/acutecare/articles/20090813.asp.

IOM (Institute of Medicine), Dietary Reference Intakes for Water, Potassium, Sodium, Chloride, and Sulfate, Washington, DC: National Academy Press, 2004.

Kamat P, Vats A, Gross M, et al. Use of hypertonic saline for the treatment of altered mental status associated with diabetic ketoacidosis. Pediatr Crit Care Med. 2003;4(2):239-242.

Kattwinkel J, Perlman JM, Aziz K, et al, "Part 15: Neonatal Resuscitation: 2010 American Heart Association Guidelines for Cardiopulmonary Resuscitation and Emergency Cardiovascular Care," Circulation, 2010, 122(18 Suppl 3):909-19.

Khanna S, Davis D, Peterson B, et al, "Use of Hypertonic Saline in the Treatment of Severe Refractory Posttraumatic Intracranial Hypertension in Pediatric Traumatic Brain Injury," Crit Care Med, 2000, 28(4):1144-51.

Kochanek PM, Carney N, Adelson PD, et al, "Guidelines for the Acute Medical Management of Severe Traumatic Brain Injury in Infants, Children, and Adolescents - Second Edition," Pediatr Crit Care Med, 2012, 139(Suppl 10):1-82.

Kuzik BA, Al-Qadhi SA, Kent S, et al, "Nebulized Hypertonic Saline in the Treatment of Viral Bronchiolitis in Infants," J Pediatr, 2007, 151(3):266-70, 270.e1.

Luu JL, Wendtland CL, Gross MF, et al, "Three-Percent Saline Administration During Pediatric Critical Care Transport," *Pediatr Emerg Care*, 2011, 27(12):1113-7.

Marcialis MA, Dessi A, Pintus MC, et al, "Neonatal Hyponatremia: Differential Diagnosis and Treatment," *J Matern Fetal Neonatal Med*, 2011, 24(Suppl 1):75-9.

Meyers R, "Pediatric Fluid and Electrolyte Therapy," *J Pediatr Pharmacol Ther*, 2009, 14:204–11

Mirtallo J, Canada T, Johnson D, et al, "Safe Practices for Parenteral Nutrition," *JPEN J Parenter Enteral Nutr*, 2004, 28(6):39-70.

Parker MM, Hazelzet JA, and Carcillo JA, "Pediatric Considerations," *Crit Care Med*, 2004, 32(11 Suppl):S591-4.

Subbarao P, Balkovec S, Solomon M, et al, "Pilot Study of Safety and Tolerability of Inhaled Hypertonic Saline in Infants With Cystic Fibrosis," *Pediatr Pulmonol*, 2007, 42(5):471-6.

Wallace DV, Dykewicz MS, Bernstein DI, et al, "The Diagnosis and Management of Rhinitis: An Updated Practice Parameter," *J Allergy Clin Immunol*, 2008, 122(2 Suppl):1-84.

Wyckoff MH, Perlman JM, and Laptook AR, "Use of Volume Expansion During Delivery Room Resuscitation in Near-Term and Term Infants," *Pediatrics*, 2005, 115(4):950-5.

◆ **Sodium Chloride Thermoject Sys** *see* Sodium Chloride on page 1902

Sodium Citrate and Citric Acid
(SOW dee um SIT rate & SI trik AS id)

Medication Safety Issues
Sound-alike/look-alike issues:
Bicitra may be confused with Polycitra
Brand Names: U.S. Cytra-2; Oracit®; Shohl's Solution (Modified)
Brand Names: Canada PMS-Dicitrate
Therapeutic Category Alkalinizing Agent, Oral
Generic Availability (U.S.) Yes
Use As long-term therapy to alkalinize the urine for control and/or dissolution of uric acid and cystine calculi of the urinary tract (FDA approved in children and adults); treatment of chronic metabolic acidosis secondary to chronic renal insufficiency or syndrome of renal tubular acidosis when use of potassium salt is contraindicated or undesirable (FDA approved in children and adults); buffer and neutralize gastric hydrochloric acid (FDA approved in adults).
Pregnancy Risk Factor Not established
Pregnancy Considerations Use caution with toxemia of pregnancy.
Contraindications Hypersensitivity to sodium citrate, citric acid, or any component; severe renal insufficiency, oliguria, or azotemia; untreated Addison's disease, adynamia episodica hereditaria (hyperkalemic periodic paralysis), acute dehydration, heat cramp, anuria, severe myocardial damage, hyperkalemia, sodium-restricted diet
Warnings Some oral solutions contain sodium benzoate; benzoic acid (benzoate) is a metabolite of benzyl alcohol; large amounts of benzyl alcohol (≥99 mg/kg/day) have been associated with a potentially fatal toxicity ("gasping syndrome") in neonates; the "gasping syndrome" consists of metabolic acidosis, respiratory distress, gasping respirations, CNS dysfunction (including convulsions, intracranial hemorrhage), hypotension, and cardiovascular collapse; use oral solution containing sodium benzoate with caution in neonates; *in vitro* and animal studies have shown that benzoate displaces bilirubin from protein binding sites. Some oral solutions contain propylene glycol; toxicities have been reported with use of products containing propylene glycol, including hyperosmolality, lactic acidosis, seizures, and respiratory depression; in neonates large amounts of propylene glycol delivered orally, intravenously (eg, >3000 mg/day), or topically have been associated with potentially fatal toxicities which can include metabolic acidosis, seizures, renal failure, and CNS depression; use oral solutions containing propylene glycol with caution (AAP, 1997; Shehab, 2009).

Precautions Use caution in patients with impaired renal function to prevent hypernatremia or alkalosis in the presence of hypocalcemia. Use caution in patients with cardiac disease, sodium- or fluid-retaining conditions (eg, cardiac failure, hypertension, peripheral/pulmonary edema, toxemia of pregnancy); conversion of citrate to bicarbonate may be impaired in patients with hepatic failure, in shock, or who are severely ill. Avoid concurrent use of aluminum-based antacids; dilute with water prior to administration to prevent saline laxative effect.
Adverse Reactions Generally well tolerated with normal renal function.
Central nervous system: Tetany
Endocrine & metabolic: Metabolic alkalosis
Gastrointestinal: Diarrhea, nausea, vomiting
Drug Interactions
Metabolism/Transport Effects None known.
Avoid Concomitant Use There are no known interactions where it is recommended to avoid concomitant use.
Increased Effect/Toxicity
Sodium Citrate and Citric Acid may increase the levels/ effects of: Aluminum Hydroxide
Decreased Effect There are no known significant interactions involving a decrease in effect.
Stability Store at controlled room temperature of 15°C to 30°C (59°F to 86°F); do not freeze. Protect from excessive heat.
Pharmacokinetics (Adult data unless noted)
Metabolism: ≥95% via hepatic oxidation to bicarbonate; may be impaired in patients with hepatic failure, shock, or severe illness
Elimination: Urine (<5% as sodium citrate)
Dosing: Neonatal Oral: **Note:** 1 mL of oral solution contains 1 mEq of bicarbonate:
Systemic alkalinization: 2-3 mEq bicarbonate/kg/day (2-3 mL/kg/day) in 3-4 divided doses
Dosing: Usual Oral: **Note:** 1 mL of oral solution contains 1 mEq of bicarbonate:
Systemic alkalinization:
Manufacturer's recommendation: Children ≥2 years: 5-15 mL (5-15 mEq bicarbonate) per dose after meals and at bedtime
Alternative recommendation: Dosing per mEq of bicarbonate: Infants and Children: 2–3 mEq bicarbonate/kg/ **day** (2-3 mL/kg/**day**) in 3-4 divided doses
Adults: 10-30 mL (10-30 mEq bicarbonate) per dose after meals and at bedtime
Administration Dilute with 30-90 mL of water and administer after meals to avoid saline laxative effect; chilling solution prior to dosing helps to enhance palatability. Shake well before use.
Monitoring Parameters Periodic serum (sodium, potassium, calcium, bicarbonate)
Dosage Forms Considerations
Each mL provides 1 mEq sodium, and is equivalent to 1 mEq bicarbonate
Dosage Forms Excipient information presented when available (limited, particularly for generics); consult specific product labeling.
Solution, oral:
Generic: Sodium citrate 500 mg and citric acid 334 mg per 5 mL (480 mL)
Cytra-2: Sodium citrate 500 mg and citric acid 334 mg per 5 mL (480 mL) [alcohol free, dye free, sugar free; contains propylene glycol and sodium benzoate; grape flavor]
Oracit®: Sodium citrate 490 mg and citric acid 640 mg per 5 mL (15 mL, 30 mL, 500 mL, 3840 mL)
Shohl's Solution (Modified): Sodium citrate 500 mg and citric acid 300 mg per 5 mL (480 mL) [contains alcohol]

References

American Academy of Pediatrics Committee on Drugs. "Inactive" ingredients in pharmaceutical products: update (subject review). *Pediatrics.* 1997;99(2):268-278.

Shehab N, Lewis CL, Streetman DD, Donn SM. Exposure to the pharmaceutical excipients benzyl alcohol and propylene glycol among critically ill neonates. *Pediatr Crit Care Med.* 2009;10 (2):256-259.

◆ **Sodium Citrate, Citric Acid, and Potassium Citrate** *see* Citric Acid, Sodium Citrate, and Potassium Citrate *on page 487*

◆ **Sodium Cromoglicate** *see* Cromolyn (Nasal) *on page 553*

◆ **Sodium Cromoglicate** *see* Cromolyn (Ophthalmic) *on page 553*

◆ **Sodium Cromoglicate** *see* Cromolyn (Systemic, Oral Inhalation) *on page 551*

◆ **Sodium Diuril** *see* Chlorothiazide *on page 446*

◆ **Sodium Edecrin** *see* Ethacrynic Acid *on page 806*

◆ **Sodium Etidronate** *see* Etidronate *on page 810*

◆ **Sodium Ferric Gluconate** *see* Ferric Gluconate *on page 864*

◆ **Sodium Ferric Gluconate Complex** *see* Ferric Gluconate *on page 864*

◆ **Sodium Fluoride** *see* Fluoride *on page 894*

Sodium Glycerophosphate Pentahydrate
(SOE dee um glis er oh FOS fate pen ta HYE drate)

Related Information
Potassium Phosphate *on page 1715*
Sodium Phosphates *on page 1913*

Therapeutic Category Electrolyte Supplement, Parenteral

Use Supplement in parenteral nutrition to meet the requirements of phosphate; has also been used for general phosphate repletion during sodium phosphate and potassium phosphate shortages

Pregnancy Considerations Animal reproduction studies have not been conducted. Phosphorus requirements are similar in pregnant and nonpregnant women (IOM, 1997).

Breast-Feeding Considerations Phosphorus is a normal constituent of human milk (IOM, 1997).

Contraindications Hypersensitivity to sodium glycerophosphate or any component; dehydration; hypernatremia, hyperphosphatemia; severe renal insufficiency; shock

Warnings Unlike phosphate products available in the U.S., sodium glycerophosphate pentahydrate is an organic phosphate product and varies from other phosphate products in terms of concentration, dosing, and preservative content; use caution when switching between products. Parenteral sodium phosphate formulations may cause electrolyte disturbances (hyponatremia, hypokalemia, hypocalcemia, hypomagnesemia) and low serum osmolarity which has been associated with generalized tonicclonic seizures and/or loss of consciousness in patients with no prior history of seizures; seizures were associated with electrolyte abnormalities; neurologic abnormalities resolved after correction of fluid and electrolyte abnormalities. Use with caution in patients with a history of seizures, those at higher risk of seizures, or on medication that lowers seizure threshold.

Precautions Use with caution in patients with preexisting electrolyte imbalances or risk of electrolyte disturbance (eg, hypocalcemia, hyperphosphatemia, hypernatremia). Use is contraindicated in patients who are dehydrated. Use with caution in patients with renal impairment. Monitor closely for hyperphosphatemia, particularly when GFR is ≤20% of mean adult normal values (IOM, 1997). Use is contraindicated in patients with severe renal impairment.

Adverse Reactions None reported by manufacturer. Adverse drug reactions listed have been reported in one small clinical trial (n=27) (Topp, 2011a).
Central nervous system: Headache
Endocrine & metabolic: Hypocalcemia
Gastrointestinal: Nausea, xerostomia

Drug Interactions
Metabolism/Transport Effects None known.
Avoid Concomitant Use There are no known interactions where it is recommended to avoid concomitant use.
Increased Effect/Toxicity
The levels/effects of Sodium Glycerophosphate Pentahydrate may be increased by: Bisphosphonate Derivatives
Decreased Effect There are no known significant interactions involving a decrease in effect.

Stability Store intact vials at ≤25°C (77°F); do not freeze.

Mechanism of Action Phosphorous participates in bone deposition, calcium metabolism, utilization of B complex vitamins, and as a buffer in acid-base equilibrium.

Pharmacokinetics (Adult data unless noted)
Metabolism: Hydrolyzed to inorganic phosphate
Half-life elimination: Inorganic phosphate: 2.06 hours (Topp, 2011a)
Time to peak serum concentration: 4 hours (Topp, 2011a)
Elimination: Inorganic phosphate: Urine

Note: One study involving 27 healthy adult volunteers compared pharmacokinetic data from infusions of 80 mmol sodium phosphate and 80 mmol sodium glycerophosphate pentahydrate delivered over a 4-hour period in a randomized, double-blind, crossover study. Bioequivalence was demonstrated between the two drugs in terms of serum AUC (0-24 hours) and C_{max} levels of inorganic phosphate; however, the corrected excretion of inorganic phosphate in a 24-hour urine collection failed to demonstrate bioequivalence between sodium phosphate and sodium glycerophosphate pentahydrate. It is suggested that a small amount of unhydrolyzed sodium glycerophosphate in the urine, undetectable by the assay, is responsible for this discrepancy (Topp, 2011a).

Inorganic phosphate is released from the glycerophosphate molecule by hydrolysis. The maximum amount of glycerophosphate that can be hydrolyzed per day is dependent on serum alkaline phosphatase activity; use caution in patients with reduced alkaline phosphatase activity.

Dosing: Neonatal Note: When converting from inorganic phosphate products (ie, sodium phosphate and potassium phosphate), maintain the same mmol amount of phosphate. Doses are listed as mmol of phosphate. Sodium glycerophosphate pentahydrate 306.1 mg = sodium glycerophosphate 216 mg = phosphate 1 **mmol**. Sodium glycerophosphate pentahydrate will provide 2 mEq of sodium for every 1 mmol of phosphate delivered.

Caution: With orders for I.V. phosphate, there is considerable confusion associated with the use of millimoles (mmol) versus milliequivalents (mEq) to express the phosphate requirement. The most reliable method of ordering I.V. phosphate is by millimoles.

Parenteral nutrition, maintenance requirement: I.V.:
Manufacturer's labeling: 1-1.5 mmol/kg/day admixed within parenteral nutrition solution. Dosage should be individualized.
ASPEN recommendations (Mirtallo, 2004): 1-2 mmol/ kg/day

Dosing: Usual Note: When converting from inorganic phosphate products (ie, sodium phosphate and potassium phosphate), maintain the same mmol amount of phosphate. Doses are listed as mmol of phosphate. Sodium glycerophosphate pentahydrate 306.1 mg = sodium glycerophosphate 216 mg = phosphate 1 **mmol**. Sodium glycerophosphate pentahydrate will provide 2 mEq of sodium for every 1 mmol of phosphate delivered.

Caution: With orders for I.V. phosphate, there is considerable confusion associated with the use of millimoles (mmol) versus milliequivalents (mEq) to express the phosphate requirement. The most reliable method of ordering I.V. phosphate is by millimoles.

Infants, Children, and Adolescents:
Parenteral nutrition, maintenance requirement: I.V.:
Manufacturer's labeling: Infants: 1-1.5 mmol/kg/day admixed within parenteral nutrition solution. Dosage should be individualized.
ASPEN recommendations (Mirtallo, 2004):
Infants and Children ≤50 kg: 0.5-2 mmol/kg/day
Children >50 kg and Adolescents: 10-40 mmol/day
Hypophosphatemia, acute: Hypophosphatemia does not necessarily equate with phosphate depletion. Hypophosphatemia may occur in the presence of low, normal, or high total body phosphate and conversely, phosphate depletion may exist with normal, low, or elevated levels of serum phosphate (Gaasbeek, 2005). It is difficult to provide concrete guidelines for the treatment of severe hypophosphatemia because the extent of total body deficits and response to therapy are difficult to predict. Aggressive doses of phosphate may result in a transient serum elevation followed by redistribution into intracellular compartments or bone tissue. Intermittent I.V. infusion should be reserved for severe depletion situations; requires continuous cardiac monitoring. Guidelines differ based on degree of illness, need/use of TPN, and severity of hypophosphatemia. If hyperkalemia exists, consider phosphate replacement strategy without potassium (eg, sodium phosphates). Various regimens for replacement of phosphate in adults have been studied. The regimens below have only been studied in adult patients, however, many institutions have used them in children safely and successfully. Obese patients and/or severe renal impairment were excluded from phosphate supplement trials. **Note:** 1 mmol phosphate = 31 mg phosphorus; 1 mg phosphorus = 0.032 mmol phosphate.
I.V. doses may be incorporated into the patient's maintenance I.V. fluids; intermittent I.V. infusion should be reserved for severe depletion situations. **Note:** Doses listed as mmol of phosphate.
Infants, Children, and Adolescents: **Note:** There are no prospective studies of parenteral phosphate replacement in children. The following weight-based guidelines for adult dosing may be cautiously employed in pediatric patients. Guidelines differ based on degree of illness, use of TPN, and severity of hypophosphatemia.
General replacement guidelines (Lentz, 1978): **Note:** The initial dose may be increased by 25% to 50% if the patient is symptomatic secondary to hypophosphatemia and lowered by 25% to 50% if the patient is hypercalcemic.
Low dose: 0.08 mmol/kg over 6 hours; use if losses are recent and uncomplicated
Intermediate dose: 0.16-0.24 mmol/kg over 4-6 hours; use if serum phosphorus level 0.5-1 mg/dL (0.16-0.32 mmol/L)
High dose: 0.36 mmol/kg over 6 hours; use if serum phosphorus <0.5 mg/dL (<0.16 mmol/L)
Patients receiving TPN (Clark, 1995):
Low dose: 0.16 mmol/kg over 4-6 hours; use if serum phosphorus level 2.3-3 mg/dL (0.73-0.96 mmol/L)
Intermediate dose: 0.32 mmol/kg over 4-6 hours; use if serum phosphorus level 1.6-2.2 mg/dL (0.51-0.72 mmol/L)

High dose: 0.64 mmol/kg over 8-12 hours; use if serum phosphorus <1.5 mg/dL (<0.5 mmol/L)
Critically ill adult trauma patients receiving TPN (Brown, 2006):
Low dose: 0.32 mmol/kg over 4-6 hours; use if serum phosphorus level 2.3-3 mg/dL (0.73-0.96 mmol/L)
Intermediate dose: 0.64 mmol/kg over 4-6 hours; use if serum phosphorus level 1.6-2.2 mg/dL (0.51-0.72 mmol/L)
High dose: 1 mmol/kg over 8-12 hours; use if serum phosphorus <1.5 mg/dL (<0.5 mmol/L)
Alternative method in critically ill patients (Kingston, 1985):
Low dose: 0.25 mmol/kg over 4 hours; use if serum phosphorus level 0.5-1 mg/dL (0.16-0.32 mmol/L)
Moderate dose: 0.5 mmol/kg over 4 hours; use if serum phosphorus level <0.5 mg/dL (<0.16 mmol/L)
Adults:
Phosphate replacement, parenteral nutrition: Manufacturer's labeling: I.V.: 10-20 mmol/day admixed within parenteral nutrition solution. Dosage should be individualized.
Phosphate repletion, general (unlabeled use):
Hypophosphatemia, acute treatment: I.V.: It is difficult to provide concrete guidelines for the treatment of severe hypophosphatemia because the extent of total body deficits and response to therapy are difficult to predict. Aggressive doses of phosphate may result in a transient serum elevation followed by redistribution into intracellular compartments or bone tissue. It is recommended that repletion of severe hypophosphatemia be done I.V. because large doses of oral phosphate may cause diarrhea and intestinal absorption may be unreliable. Intermittent I.V. infusion should be reserved for severe depletion situations; requires continuous cardiac monitoring. Guidelines differ based on degree of illness, need/use of TPN, and severity of hypophosphatemia. Obese patients and/or severe renal impairment were excluded from phosphate supplement trials. **Note:** 1 mmol phosphate = 31 mg phosphorus; 1 mg phosphorus = 0.032 mmol phosphate.
Critically ill adult patients receiving concurrent enteral/parenteral nutrition (Brown, 2006; Clark, 1995): **Note:** Round doses to the nearest 7.5 mmol for ease of preparation. If administering with phosphate-containing parenteral nutrition, do not exceed 15 mmol/L within parenteral nutrition. May use adjusted body weight for patients weighing >130% of ideal body weight (and BMI <40 kg/m^2) by using [IBW + 0.25 (ABW-IBW)]:
Low dose, serum phosphorus level 2.3-3 mg/dL (0.74-0.96 mmol/L): 0.16-0.32 mmol/kg over 4-6 hours
Intermediate dose, serum phosphorus level 1.6-2.2 mg/dL (0.51-0.71 mmol/L): 0.32-0.64 mmol/kg over 4-6 hours
High dose, serum phosphorus <1.5 mg/dL (<0.5 mmol/L): 0.64-1 mmol/kg over 8-12 hours
Parenteral nutrition: I.V.: 10-15 mmol/1000 kcal (Hicks, 2001) **or** 20-40 mmol/24 hours (Mirtallo, 2004)
Dosing adjustment in renal impairment: There are no dosing adjustments provided in the manufacturer's labeling (has not been studied); use with caution since phosphate excretion is primarily renal.
Dosing adjustments in hepatic impairment: There are no dosing adjustments provided in the manufacturer's labeling (has not been studied); however, phosphate excretion is primarily renal.
Administration Must be diluted prior to parenteral administration. In general, the dose, concentration of infusion,

and rate of administration may be dependent on patient condition and specific institution policy. Per the manufacturer, infusion time should not be <8 hours and not >24 hours.

Monitoring Parameters Serum sodium, calcium, and phosphorus concentrations; renal function; in pediatric patients after I.V. phosphate repletion, repeat serum phosphorus concentration should be checked 2 hours later (ASPEN Pediatric Nutrition Support Core Curriculum, 2010)

Reference Range Note: There is a diurnal variation with the nadir at 1100, plateau at 1600, and peak in the early evening (Gaasbeek, 2005); 1 mmol/L phosphate = 3.1 mg/dL phosphorus
Newborn 0-5 days: 4.8-8.2 mg/dL
1-3 years: 3.8-6.5 mg/dL
4-11 years: 3.7-5.6 mg/dL
12-15 years: 2.9-5.4 mg/dL
16-19 years: 2.7-4.7 mg/dL

Additional Information Cow's milk is a good source of phosphate with 1 mg elemental (0.032 mmol) elemental phosphate per mL.

References

Brown KA, Dickerson RN, Morgan LM, et al, "A New Graduated Dosing Regimen for Phosphorus Replacement in Patients Receiving Nutrition Support," *JPEN J Parenter Enteral Nutr*, 2006, 30(3):209-14.
Clark CL, Sacks GS, Dickerson RN, et al, "Treatment of Hypophosphatemia in Patients Receiving Specialized Nutrition Support Using a Graduated Dosing Scheme: Results from a Prospective Clinical Trial," *Crit Care Med*, 1995, 23(9):1504-11.
Gaasbeek A and Meinders AE, "Hypophosphatemia: An Update on Its Etiology and Treatment," *Am J Med*, 2005, 118(10):1094-101.
Hicks W and Hardy G, "Phosphate Supplementation for Hypophosphataemia and Parenteral Nutrition," *Curr Opin Clin Nutr Metab Care*, 2001, 4(3):227-33.
IOM (Institute of Medicine), *Dietary Reference Intakes for Calcium, Phosphorus, Magnesium, Vitamin D, and Fluoride*, National Academy of Sciences, Washington, DC, 1997.
Kingston M and Al-Siba'i MB, "Treatment of Severe Hypophosphatemia," *Crit Care Med*, 1985, 13(1):16-8.
Lentz RD, Brown DM, and Kjellstrand CM, "Treatment of Severe Hypophosphatemia," *Ann Intern Med*, 1978, 89(6):941-4.
Mirtallo J, Canada T, Johnson D, et al, "Safe Practices for Parenteral Nutrition," *JPEN J Parenter Enteral Nutr*, 2004, 28(6):S39-70.
Schmidt GL, "Fluids and Electrolytes," *The A.S.P.E.N. Pediatric Nutrition Support Core Curriculum*, Corkins MR, Balint J, Bobo E, et al, eds, Silver Springs, MD: American Society of Parenteral and Enteral Nutrition, 2010, 87-102.
Topp H, Hochfeld O, Bark S, et al, "Glycerophosphate Does Not Interact With Components of Parenteral Nutrition," *Pharmacology*, 2011, 88 (1-2):114-20.
Topp H, Hochfeld O, Bark S, et al, "Glycerophosphate Is Interchangeable With Inorganic Phosphate in Terms of Safety and Serum Pharmacokinetics," *Pharmacology*, 2011a, 88(3-4):193-200.

◆ **Sodium Hydrogen Carbonate** *see* Sodium Bicarbonate *on page 1901*

◆ **Sodium Hyposulfate** *see* Sodium Thiosulfate *on page 1919*

◆ **Sodium Nafcillin** *see* Nafcillin *on page 1462*

Sodium Nitrite and Sodium Thiosulfate
(SOW dee um NYE trite & SOW dee um thye oh SUL fate)

Brand Names: U.S. Nithiodote
Therapeutic Category Antidote
Use Treatment of acute, life-threatening cyanide poisoning (FDA approved in all ages)
Pregnancy Risk Factor C
Pregnancy Considerations Teratogenic effects have been observed following maternal exposure to high concentrations of sodium nitrite in drinking water. Teratogenic effects were not observed in animal reproduction studies of sodium nitrite or sodium thiosulfate. Embryotoxic and nonteratogenic effects were observed in animal reproduction studies of sodium nitrite. Methemoglobin reductase is lower in the fetus compared to adults and may result in adverse effects due to nitrite-induced prenatal hypoxia. There are no adequate and well-controlled studies of Nithiodote in pregnant women. In general, medications used as antidotes should take into consideration the health and prognosis of the mother; antidotes should be administered to pregnant women if there is a clear indication for use and should not be withheld because of fears of teratogenicity (Bailey, 2003).

Breast-Feeding Considerations It is not known if sodium nitrite or sodium thiosulfate is excreted in breast milk. The manufacturer recommends that caution be exercised when administering sodium nitrite and sodium thiosulfate to nursing women.

Contraindications Hypersensitivity to sodium nitrite, sodium thiosulfate or any component

Warnings Sodium nitrite may cause methemoglobin formation and severe hypotension resulting in diminished oxygen-carrying capacity and even death **[U.S. Boxed Warning]**; serious adverse effects may occur at doses less than twice the recommended therapeutic dose. Monitor for adequate perfusion and oxygenation; ensure patient is euvolemic. Use with caution in patients with preexisting diminished oxygen or cardiovascular reserve [eg, smoke inhalation victims, anemia (dosage reduction in proportion to oxygen carrying capacity is recommended), substantial blood loss, and cardiac or respiratory compromise], in patients at greater risk for developing methemoglobinemia (eg, neonates and infants <6 months or congenital methemoglobin reductase deficiency), and in patients who may be susceptible to injury from vasodilation; the use of hydroxocobalamin is recommended in these patients.

Due to the risk for serious adverse effects, use with caution in patients where the diagnosis of cyanide poisoning is uncertain; however, if clinical suspicion of cyanide poisoning is high, treatment should not be delayed. Treatment of cyanide poisoning should include decontamination and supportive therapy. Collection of pretreatment blood cyanide concentrations does not preclude administration and should not delay administration in the emergency management of highly suspected or confirmed cyanide toxicity. Pretreatment levels may be useful as postinfusion levels may be inaccurate. Monitor patients for return of symptoms for 24-48 hours; repeat treatment should be administered if symptoms return. Consider consultation with a poison control center at 1-800-222-1222.

Fire victims may present with both cyanide and carbon monoxide poisoning. Carbon monoxide poisoning leads to carboxyhemoglobinemia which decreases the oxygen-carrying capacity; use of sodium nitrite which induces methemoglobinemia may worsen oxygen-carrying capacity. In this scenario, sodium thiosulfate may be used alone to promote the clearance of cyanide. Due to the slow onset of action of sodium thiosulfate, may consider using hydroxocobalamin alone or in combination with sodium thiosulfate (Howland, 2011). The presence of sulfite hypersensitivity should not preclude the use of this medication.

Precautions Use with caution in patients with G6PD deficiency; increased risk for hemolytic crisis following sodium nitrite administration; monitor for an acute drop in hematocrit. Use caution with concurrent use of antihypertensives, diuretics, phosphodiesterase-5 enzyme (PDE5) inhibitors, and medications known to cause methemoglobinemia.

Adverse Reactions
Sodium nitrite:
Cardiovascular: Arrhythmias, cyanosis, flushing, hypotension, palpitations, syncope, tachycardia
Central nervous system: Anxiety, coma, confusion, dizziness, fatigue, headache, lightheadedness, seizure
Dermatologic: Urticaria

Endocrine & metabolic: Acidosis

Gastrointestinal: Abdominal pain, nausea, vomiting

Hematologic: Methemoglobinemia

Local: Injection site tingling

Neuromuscular & skeletal: Numbness, paresthesia, weakness

Ocular: Blurred vision

Respiratory: Dyspnea, tachypnea

Miscellaneous: Diaphoresis

Sodium thiosulfate:

Cardiovascular: Hypotension

Central nervous system: Disorientation, headache

Gastrointestinal: Nausea, salty taste, vomiting

Hematologic: Bleeding time prolonged

Miscellaneous: Warmth

Drug Interactions

Metabolism/Transport Effects None known.

Avoid Concomitant Use There are no known interactions where it is recommended to avoid concomitant use.

Increased Effect/Toxicity

Sodium Nitrite and Sodium Thiosulfate may increase the levels/effects of: Prilocaine

The levels/effects of Sodium Nitrite and Sodium Thiosulfate may be increased by: Methemoglobinemia Associated Agents; Nitric Oxide

Decreased Effect There are no known significant interactions involving a decrease in effect.

Stability Store at 20°C to 25°C (68°F to 77°F); excursions permitted to 15°C to 30°C (59°F to 86°F); do not freeze. Protect from direct light.

Mechanism of Action

Sodium nitrite: Promotes the formation of methemoglobin which competes with cytochrome oxidase for the cyanide ion. Cyanide combines with methemoglobin to form cyanomethemoglobin, thereby freeing the cytochrome oxidase and allowing aerobic metabolism to continue.

Sodium thiosulfate: Serves as a sulfur donor in rhodanese-catalyzed formation of thiocyanate (much less toxic than cyanide).

Pharmacodynamics

Sodium nitrite:

Onset: Peak effect: Methemoglobinemia: 30-60 minutes

Duration: Methemoglobinemia: ~55 minutes

Pharmacokinetics (Adult data unless noted)

Sodium nitrite:

Metabolism: To ammonia and other metabolites

Excretion: Urine (~40% as unchanged drug)

Sodium thiosulfate:

Half-life elimination:

Thiosulfate: ~3 hours (Howland, 2011)

Thiocyanate: ~3 hours; renal impairment: ≤9 days

Elimination: Urine (~20% to 50% as unchanged drug)

Dosing: Neonatal Cyanide poisoning: Refer to Infant, Children, and Adolescent dosing.

Dosing: Usual Cyanide poisoning: Note: Administer sodium nitrite first, followed immediately by the administration of sodium thiosulfate. Monitor the patient for 24-48 hours following doses.

Step 1:

Sodium nitrite:

Manufacturer's labeling:

Infants, Children, and Adolescents: I.V.: Initial: 3% solution: 0.2 mL/kg; maximum dose: 10 mL (300 mg); if repeat dosing is necessary due to symptom return, use 50% of the original dose; **Note:** Presented dose equates to 6 mg/kg of sodium nitrite or 6-8 mL/m² of the 3% solution.

Adults: I.V.: Initial: 3% solution: 10 mL (300 mg); if repeat dosing is necessary due to symptom return, use 50% of the original dose

Alternate dosing: Hemoglobin-dependent dosing: Infants, Children, Adolescents, and Adults: I.V.: For patients who are unable to tolerate significant methemoglobinemia (eg, patients with comorbidities that compromise oxygen delivery, such as heart disease, lung disease, etc), dosing may be based on hemoglobin levels (when rapid bedside testing is available) to prevent fatal methemoglobinemia; see table (Berlin, 1970):

Dosing Based on Hgb Level	
Hemoglobin Level (g/dL)	Dose of 3% Sodium Nitrite Solution (Maximum dose: 10 mL)
7	0.19 mL/kg
8	0.22 mL/kg
9	0.25 mL/kg
10	0.27 mL/kg
11	0.3 mL/kg
12	0.33 mL/kg
13	0.36 mL/kg
14	0.39 mL/kg

Step 2:

Sodium thiosulfate: Note: Dosing information provided based upon contents of Nithiodote™ kit. Sodium thiosulfate is also available as an individual product; see Sodium Thiosulfate monograph for additional information.

Infants, Children, and Adolescents: I.V.: Initial: 25% solution: 1 mL/kg; maximum dose: 50 mL (12.5 **g**); if repeat dosing necessary due to symptom return, use 50% of the original dose. **Note:** Presented dose equates to 250 mg/kg of sodium thiosulfate or 30-40 mL/m² of the 25% solution.

Adults: I.V.: Initial: 25% solution: 50 mL (12.5 **g**); if repeat dosing is necessary due symptom return, use 50% of the original dose

Dosage adjustment in renal impairment: No dosage adjustment provided in the manufacturer's labeling; however, renal elimination of sodium nitrite and sodium thiosulfate is significant and risk of adverse effects may be increased in patients with renal impairment.

Dosage adjustment in hepatic impairment: No dosage adjustment provided in the manufacturer's labeling (has not been studied).

Administration Administer both components undiluted via slow I.V. injection as soon as possible after diagnosis of acute, life-threatening cyanide poisoning. Administer sodium nitrite first at a rate of 2.5-5 mL/minute, followed immediately by the administration of sodium thiosulfate over 10-20 minutes. Decrease rate of infusion in the event of significant hypotension, nausea, or vomiting.

Monitoring Parameters Monitor for at least 24-48 hours after administration; blood pressure and heart rate during and after infusion; hemoglobin/hematocrit; co-oximetry; serum lactate levels; venous-arterial PO2 gradient; serum methemoglobin and oxyhemoglobin. Pretreatment cyanide levels may be useful diagnostically.

Reference Range Symptoms associated with blood cyanide levels:

Flushing and tachycardia: 0.5-1 mcg/mL

Obtundation: 1-2.5 mcg/mL

Coma and respiratory depression: >2.5 mcg/mL

Death: >3 mcg/mL

Dosage Forms Excipient information presented when available (limited, particularly for generics); consult specific product labeling.

Injection, solution [combination package]:
Nithiodote: Sodium nitrite 300 mg/10 mL (10 mL) and sodium thiosulfate 12.5 g/50 mL (50 mL)

References

Agency for Toxic Substances and Disease Registry (ATSDR), "Medical Management Guidelines for Hydrogen Cyanide (HCN)." Available at http://www.atsdr.cdc.gov/MHMI/mmg8.pdf

Bailey B, "Are There Teratogenic Risks Associated With Antidotes Used in the Acute Management of Poisoned Pregnant Women?" *Birth Defects Res A Clin Mol Teratol*, 2003, 67(2):133-40.

Berlin CM, "The Treatment of Cyanide Poisoning in Children," *Pediatrics*, 1970, 46(5):793-6.

Geller RJ, Barthold C, Saiers JA, et al, "Pediatric Cyanide Poisoning: Causes, Manifestations, Management, and Unmet Needs," *Pediatrics*, 2006, 118(5):2146-58.

Gracia R and Shepherd G, "Cyanide Poisoning and Its Treatment," *Pharmacotherapy*, 2004, 24(10):1358-65.

Hall AH, Dart R, and Bogdan G, "Sodium Thiosulfate or Hydroxocobalamin For The Empiric Treatment of Cyanide Poisoning?" *Ann Emerg Med*, 2007, 49(6):806-13.

Howland MA, "Antidotes in Depth: Sodium and Amyl Nitrite," *Goldfrank's Toxicologic Emergencies*, 9th ed, Nelson LS, Hoffman RS, Lewin NA, et al, eds, New York, NY: McGraw-Hill Companies, Inc, 2011, 1519-22.

Howland MA, "Antidotes in Depth: Sodium Thiosulfate," *Goldfrank's Toxicologic Emergencies*, 9th ed, Nelson LS, Hoffman RS, Lewin NA, et al, eds, New York, NY: McGraw-Hill Companies, Inc, 2011.

◆ **Sodium Nitroferricyanide** *see* Nitroprusside *on page 1507*

◆ **Sodium Nitroprusside** *see* Nitroprusside *on page 1507*

Sodium Phenylacetate and Sodium Benzoate

(SOW dee um fen il AS e tate & SOW dee um BENZ oh ate)

Brand Names: U.S. Ammonul®

Therapeutic Category Ammonium Detoxicant; Hyperammonemia Agent; Urea Cycle Disorder (UCD) Treatment Agent

Generic Availability (U.S.) No

Use Adjunct to treatment of acute hyperammonemia and encephalopathy in patients with urea cycle disorders involving partial or complete deficiencies of carbamylphosphate synthetase (CPS), ornithine transcarbamoylase (OTC), argininosuccinate lyase (ASL), or argininosuccinate synthetase (ASS); for use with hemodialysis in acute neonatal hyperammonemic coma, moderate-to-severe hyperammonemic encephalopathy and hyperammonemia which fails to respond to initial therapy

Pregnancy Risk Factor C

Pregnancy Considerations In animal studies, phenylacetate was shown to cause neurological toxicity. Reproduction studies have not been conducted with this combination.

Contraindications Hypersensitivity to sodium phenylacetate, sodium benzoate, or any component of the formulation

Warnings Severity of hyperammonemia may require hemodialysis, as well as nutritional management and medical support; due to enhanced potassium excretion, monitor potassium level closely; potential tissue extravasant which may result in skin necrosis, administer only through central I.V. line. Repeat loading doses are not indicated due to prolonged plasma levels noted in pharmacokinetic studies.

Precautions Due to high sodium content use with caution in patients with congestive heart failure, renal or hepatic dysfunction, or sodium retention associated with edema; maintain caloric intake at 80 cal/kg/day

Adverse Reactions Nonspecific adverse reactions include: Nervous system disorders; metabolism and nutrition disorders; respiratory, thoracic, and mediastinal disorders; general disorders and injection site reactions; gastrointestinal disorders; blood and lymphatic system disorders; cardiac disorders; skin and subcutaneous tissue disorders; vascular disorders; psychiatric disorders; injury, poisoning, and procedural complications; renal and urinary disorders

More blood and lymphatic system, and vascular disorders were reported for patients ≤30 days of age; more gastrointestinal disorders were reported for patients >30 days.

Cardiovascular: Hypotension

Central nervous system: Agitation, brain edema, coma, mental impairment, pyrexia, seizures

Endocrine & metabolic: Acidosis, hyperammonemia, hyperglycemia, hypocalcemia, hypokalemia, metabolic acidosis

Gastrointestinal: Diarrhea, nausea, vomiting

Genitourinary: Urinary tract infection

Hematologic: Anemia, disseminated intravascular coagulation (DIC)

Local: Injection site reaction

Respiratory: Respiratory distress

Miscellaneous: Infection

Rare but important or life-threatening: Abdominal distention, acute psychosis, acute respiratory distress syndrome, aggression, alkalosis, alopecia, anuria, areflexia, ataxia, atrial rupture, blindness, blood carbon dioxide changes, blood glucose changes, blood pH increased, bradycardia, brain death, brain hemorrhage, brain herniation, brain infarction, cardiac arrest/failure, cardiac output decreased, cardiogenic shock, cardiomyopathy, cardiopulmonary arrest/failure, cerebral atrophy, chest pain, cholestasis, clonus, coagulopathy, confusion, consciousness depressed, dehydration, dyspnea, edema, encephalopathy, fluid overload/retention, flushing, gastrointestinal hemorrhage, hallucinations, hemangioma, hemorrhage, hepatic artery stenosis, hepatic failure, hepatotoxicity, hypercapnia, hyperkalemia, hypernatremia, hypertension, hyperventilation, injection site reaction (blistering, extravasation, hemorrhage), intracranial pressure increased, jaundice, Kussmaul respiration, maculopapular rash, multiorgan failure, nerve paralysis, pancytopenia, pCO_2 changes, pericardial effusion, phlebothrombosis, pneumonia aspiration, pneumothorax, pruritus, pulmonary edema, pulmonary hemorrhage, rash, renal failure, respiratory alkalosis/acidosis, respiratory arrest/failure, respiratory rate increased, sepsis, septic shock, subdural hematoma, tetany, thrombocytopenia, thrombosis, tremor, urinary retention, urticaria, weakness

Drug Interactions

Metabolism/Transport Effects None known.

Avoid Concomitant Use There are no known interactions where it is recommended to avoid concomitant use.

Increased Effect/Toxicity
The levels/effects of Sodium Phenylacetate and Sodium Benzoate may be increased by: Probenecid

Decreased Effect There are no known significant interactions involving a decrease in effect.

Stability Prior to dilution, store at room temperature of 25°C (77°F). Following dilution in $D_{10}W$, solution for infusion may be stored at room temperature for up to 24 hours. Stable when mixed with arginine HCl 10% injection

Mechanism of Action Sodium phenylacetate and sodium benzoate provide alternate pathways for the removal of ammonia through the formation of their metabolites. One mole of sodium phenylacetate removes two moles of nitrogen; one mole of sodium benzoate removes one mole of nitrogen.

Pharmacokinetics (Adult data unless noted)

Metabolism: Hepatic and renal; sodium phenylacetate conjugates with glutamine, forming the active metabolite, phenylacetylglutamine (PAG); sodium benzoate combines with glycine to form the active metabolite hippuric acid (HIP)

◀ Excretion: Urine

Dosing: Neonatal I.V.: Administer as a loading dose over 90-120 minutes, followed by an equivalent dose as a maintenance infusion over 24 hours. Arginine HCl is administered concomitantly. Dosage based on weight and specific enzyme deficiency; therapy should continue until ammonia levels are in normal range. Do not repeat loading dose.

CPS and OTC deficiency: Ammonul® 2.5 mL/kg and arginine 10% 2 mL/kg (provides sodium phenylacetate 250 mg/kg, sodium benzoate 250 mg/kg and arginine hydrochloride 200 mg/kg)

ASS and ASL deficiency: Ammonul® 2.5 mL/kg and arginine 10% 6 mL/kg (provides sodium phenylacetate 250 mg/kg, sodium benzoate 250 mg/kg and arginine hydrochloride 600 mg/kg)

Note: Pending a specific diagnosis, the bolus and maintenance dose of arginine should be 6 mL/kg. If ASS or ASL are excluded as diagnostic possibilities, reduce dose of arginine to 2 mL/kg/day.

Dosing: Usual I.V.: Administer as a loading dose over 90-120 minutes, followed by an equivalent dose as a maintenance infusion over 24 hours. Arginine HCl is administered concomitantly. Dosage based on weight and specific enzyme deficiency; therapy should continue until ammonia levels are in normal range. Do not repeat loading dose.

Infants and Children ≤20 kg:
CPS and OTC deficiency: Ammonul® 2.5 mL/kg and arginine 10% 2 mL/kg (provides sodium phenylacetate 250 mg/kg, sodium benzoate 250 mg/kg and arginine hydrochloride 200 mg/kg)

ASS and ASL deficiency: Ammonul® 2.5 mL/kg and arginine 10% 6 mL/kg (provides sodium phenylacetate 250 mg/kg, sodium benzoate 250 mg/kg and arginine hydrochloride 600 mg/kg)

Note: Pending a specific diagnosis in infants, the bolus and maintenance dose of arginine should be 6 mL/kg. If ASS or ASL are excluded as diagnostic possibilities, reduce dose of arginine to 2 mL/kg/day.

Children >20 kg:
CPS and OTC deficiency: Ammonul® 55 mL/m^2 and arginine 10% 2 mL/kg (provides sodium phenylacetate 5.5 g/m^2, sodium benzoate 5.5 g/m^2 and arginine hydrochloride 200 mg/kg)

ASS and ASL deficiency: Ammonul® 55 mL/m^2 and arginine 10% 6 mL/kg (provides sodium phenylacetate 5.5 g/m^2, sodium benzoate 5.5 g/m^2, and arginine hydrochloride 600 mg/kg)

Dosage adjustment in renal impairment: Use with caution; monitor closely

Dialysis: Ammonia clearance is ~10 times greater with hemodialysis than by peritoneal dialysis or hemofiltration. Exchange transfusion is ineffective.

Dosage adjustment in hepatic impairment: Use with caution

Administration I.V.: Must be administered via central line; administration via peripheral line may cause burns. Dilute in D$_{10}$W at ≥25 mL/kg prior to administration. May mix with arginine HCl. In case of extravasation, discontinue infusion and resume at new injection site.

Monitoring Parameters Neurologic status, plasma ammonia, plasma glutamine, clinical response, serum electrolytes (potassium or bicarbonate supplementation may be required), acid-base balance, infusion site

Reference Range Long-term target levels (may not be appropriate for every patient):

Plasma ammonia: <40 μmol/L

Plasma glutamine: <1000 μmol/L

Normal plasma levels of alanine, glycine, lysine, arginine (except in arginase deficiency); normal urinary orotate excretion; normal plasma protein concentration

Additional Information Ucephan® (sodium phenylacetate and sodium benzoate), was previously available as an oral liquid for chronic treatment of urea cycle disorders. Although no longer commercially available, this combination may be compounded for patients not responsive to or tolerant of other treatments.

Dosage Forms Excipient information presented when available (limited, particularly for generics); consult specific product labeling.

Injection, solution [concentrate]:
Ammonul®: Sodium phenylacetate 100 mg and sodium benzoate 100 mg per 1 mL (50 mL)

References

Batshaw ML, MacArthur RB, and Tuchman M, "Alternative Pathway Therapy for Urea Cycle Disorders: Twenty Years Later," *J Pediatr*, 2001, 138(1 Suppl):46-54.

Berry GT and Steiner RD, "Long-Term Management of Patients With Urea Cycle Disorders," *J Pediatr*, 2001, 138(1 Suppl):56-60.

Brusilow SW, Danney M, Waber LJ, et al, "Treatment of Episodic Hyperammonemia in Children With Inborn Errors of Urea Synthesis," *N Engl J Med*, 1984, 310(25):1630-4.

"Consensus Statement From a Conference for the Management of Patients With Urea Cycle Disorders. Urea Cycle Disorders Conference Group," *J Pediatr*, 2001, 138(1 Suppl):1-5.

Gutteridge C and Kuhn RJ, "Compatibility of 10% Sodium Benzoate Plus 10% Sodium Phenylacetate With Various Flavored Vehicles," *Am J Hosp Pharm*, 1994, 51(19):2508, 2510.

Sodium Phenylbutyrate
(SOW dee um fen il BYOO ti rate)

Brand Names: U.S. Buphenyl

Therapeutic Category Ammonium Detoxicant; Hyperammonemia Agent; Urea Cycle Disorder (UCD) Treatment Agent

Generic Availability (U.S.) May be product dependent

Use Adjunctive therapy in the chronic management of patients with urea cycle disorder involving deficiencies of carbamoylphosphate synthetase, ornithine transcarbamylase, or argininosuccinic acid synthetase; provides an alternative pathway for waste nitrogen excretion

Pregnancy Risk Factor C

Pregnancy Considerations Animal reproduction studies have not been conducted.

Breast-Feeding Considerations It is not known if sodium phenylbutyrate is excreted in breast milk. The manufacturer recommends that caution be exercised when administering sodium phenylbutyrate to nursing women.

Contraindications Hypersensitivity to phenylbutyrate, or any component; patients with severe hypertension, heart failure or renal dysfunction; **phenylbutyrate is not indicated in the treatment of acute hyperammonemia**

Precautions Use cautiously in patients with renal or hepatic dysfunction and in patients who must maintain a low sodium diet as each gram of drug contains 125 mg sodium

Adverse Reactions

Cardiovascular: Syncope

Central nervous system: Depression, headache

Dermatologic: Rash

Endocrine & metabolic: Acidosis, alkalosis, amenorrhea/menstrual dysfunction, hyperbilirubinemia, hyperchloremia, hyper-/hypophosphatemia, hypernatremia, hyperuricemia, hypokalemia, total protein decreased

Gastrointestinal: Abdominal pain, abnormal taste, anorexia, gastritis, nausea, vomiting

Hematologic: Anemia, leukocytosis, leukopenia, thrombocytopenia, thrombocytosis

Hepatic: Alkaline phosphatase increased, transaminases increased

Renal: Renal tubular acidosis

Miscellaneous: Offensive body odor

Rare but important or life-threatening: Aplastic anemia, arrhythmia, bruising, constipation, edema, fatigue, lightheadedness, memory impairment, neuropathy (exacerbation), pancreatitis, peptic ulcer disease, rectal bleeding, somnolence

Drug Interactions

Metabolism/Transport Effects Inhibits CYP1A2 (weak), CYP2C19 (weak), CYP2C8 (weak), CYP2C9 (weak), CYP2D6 (weak), CYP3A4 (weak)

Avoid Concomitant Use

Avoid concomitant use of Sodium Phenylbutyrate with any of the following: Pimozide

Increased Effect/Toxicity

Sodium Phenylbutyrate may increase the levels/effects of: ARIPiprazole; Dofetilide; Lomitapide; Pimozide

The levels/effects of Sodium Phenylbutyrate may be increased by: Probenecid

Decreased Effect

The levels/effects of Sodium Phenylbutyrate may be decreased by: Corticosteroids (Systemic); Haloperidol; Valproic Acid and Derivatives

Stability Store at room temperature (59°F to 86°F); after opening, containers should be kept tightly closed

Mechanism of Action Sodium phenylbutyrate is a pro-drug which is rapidly converted to phenylacetate, followed by conjugation with glutamine to form phenylacetylglutamine; phenylacetylglutamine serves as a substitute for urea as it is clears nitrogenous waste from the body when excreted in the urine.

Pharmacokinetics (Adult data unless noted)

Distribution: V_d: 0.2 L/kg

Metabolism: conjugation to phenylacetylglutamine (active form); undergoes nonlinear Michaelis-Menten elimination kinetics

Half-life: 0.8 hours (parent compound); 1.2 hours (phenyl-acetate)

Time to peak serum concentration:

Powder: 1 hour

Tablet: 1.35 hours

Elimination: 80% of metabolite excreted in urine in 24 hours

Dosing: Neonatal Oral: 300-600 mg/kg/day divided 4-6 times daily dependent upon deficiency type (Berry, 2001)

Arginase deficiency: 300-600 mg/kg/day divided 4 times daily

Argininosuccinic acid lyase (ASL), argininosuccinic synthetase (ASS), carbamyl phosphate synthetase I (CPS), or ornithine transcarbamylase (OTC) deficiency: 450-600 mg/kg/day divided 4 times daily

Dosing: Usual Oral:

Infants and Children <20 kg: 300-600 mg/kg/day divided 4-6 times daily dependent upon on deficiency type; maximum daily dose: 20 g/day (Berry, 2001)

Arginase deficiency: 300-600 mg/kg/day divided 4 times daily

Argininosuccinic acid lyase (ASL), argininosuccinic synthetase (ASS), carbamyl phosphate synthetase I (CPS), or ornithine transcarbamylase (OTC) deficiency: 450-600 mg/kg/day divided 4 times daily

Children >20 kg and Adults: 9.9-13 g/m^2/day, divided 4-6 times daily; maximum daily dose: 20 g/day (Berry, 2001)

Administration Oral: Administer with meals or feedings; mix powder with food or drink; avoid mixing with acidic beverages (eg, most fruit juices or colas)

Monitoring Parameters Plasma ammonia and glutamine concentrations, serum electrolytes, proteins, hepatic and renal function tests, physical signs/symptoms of hyper-ammonemia (ie, lethargy, ataxia, confusion, vomiting, seizures, and memory impairment)

Additional Information Teaspoon and tablespoon measuring devices are provided with the powder; each 1 g powder contains 0.94 g sodium phenylbutyrate = 125 mg sodium; each tablet contains 0.5 g sodium phenylbutyrate = 62 mg sodium

Dosage Forms Considerations Powder products: 1 level teaspoon provides 3 g sodium phenylbutyrate, 1 level tablespoon provides 8.6 g sodium phenylbutyrate. Measurers provided with the product.

Dosage Forms Excipient information presented when available (limited, particularly for generics); consult specific product labeling.

Powder, Oral:

Buphenyl: (250 g) [contains sodium 125 mg/g]

Generic: (250 g)

Tablet, Oral:

Buphenyl: 500 mg [contains sodium 62 mg/tablet]

Extemporaneous Preparations A 200 mg/mL oral suspension may be prepared with sodium phenylbutyrate powder, USP; Ora-Plus®; and either Ora-Sweet® or Ora-Sweet® SF. Place 12 g of sodium phenylbutyrate in a glass mortar and reduce to a fine powder. Separately, mix 30 mL Ora-Plus® and 30 mL of either Ora-Sweet® or Ora-Sweet® SF for a total volume of 60 mL. Add 30 mL of the vehicle mixture to the powder and mix to a uniform smooth suspension. Transfer the mixture into a 2 oz amber prescription bottle; rinse mortar with vehicle, and add quantity of vehicle sufficient to make 60 mL. Label "shake well". Stable for 90 days at room temperature. **Note:** Authors recommend administering a masking agent such as chocolate syrup or peanut butter, before and after medication administration, to mask the bitter taste.

Caruthers RL and Johnson CE, "Stability of Extemporaneously Prepared Sodium Phenylbutyrate Oral Suspensions," *Am J Health Syst Pharm*, 2007, 64(14):1513-5.

References

Batshaw ML, MacArthur RB, and Tuchman M, "Alternative Pathway Therapy for Urea Cycle Disorders: Twenty Years Later," *J Pediatr*, 2001, 138(1 Suppl):S46-S55.

Berry GT and Steiner RD, "Long-Term Management of Patients With Urea Cycle Disorders," *J Pediatr*, 2001, 138(1 Suppl):S56-60.

Brusilow SW, "Phenylacetylglutamine May Replace Urea as a Vehicle for Waste Nitrogen Excretion," *Pediatr Res*, 1991, 29(2):147-50.

Maestri NE, Brusilow SW, Clissold DB, et al, "Long-Term Treatment of Girls With Ornithine Transcarbamylase Deficiency," *N Engl J Med*, 1996, 335(12):855-9.

◆ **Sodium Phosphate and Potassium Phosphate** *see* Potassium Phosphate and Sodium Phosphate *on page 1718*

Sodium Phosphates (SOW dee um FOS fates)

Medication Safety Issues

Administration issues:

Enemas and oral solution are available in pediatric and adult sizes; prescribe by "volume" not by "bottle."

Because inorganic phosphate exists as monobasic and dibasic anions, with the mixture of valences dependent on pH, ordering by mEq amounts is unreliable and may lead to large dosing errors. In addition, I.V. phosphate is available in the sodium and potassium salt; therefore, the content of these cations must be considered when ordering phosphate. The most reliable method of ordering I.V. phosphate is by millimoles, then specifying the potassium or sodium salt.

Brand Names: U.S. Fleet Enema Extra [OTC]; Fleet Enema [OTC]; Fleet Pedia-Lax Enema [OTC]; LaCrosse Complete [OTC]; OsmoPrep

Brand Names: Canada Fleet Enema

Therapeutic Category Electrolyte Supplement, Oral; Electrolyte Supplement, Parenteral; Laxative, Saline; Sodium Salt

Generic Availability (U.S.) Yes: Enema, injection, oral solution

Use

Injection: Treatment and prevention of hypophosphatemia; source of phosphate in large-volume I.V. fluids (FDA approved in all ages)

Oral:

Solution: Treatment of occasional constipation (OTC product: FDA approved in ages ≥5 years and adults)

Tablets (OsmoPrep): Bowel cleansing for colonoscopy (FDA approved in adults)

Rectal: Treatment of occasional constipation (OTC product: Fleet Pedia-Lax Enema: FDA approved in ages 2-11 years; Fleet Enema, Fleet Enema Extra: FDA approved in ages ≥12 years and adults. Refer to product-specific information to determine FDA approved ages for additional products).

Medication Guide Available Yes

Pregnancy Risk Factor C

Pregnancy Considerations Reproduction studies have not been conducted with these products. Use with caution in pregnant women.

Breast-Feeding Considerations Phosphorus, sodium, and potassium are normal constituents of human milk.

Contraindications Hypersensitivity to sodium phosphate salts or any component

Additional product-specific contraindications:

Injection: Hyperphosphatemia, hypocalcemia, hypernatremia, severe renal impairment (CrCl <30 mL/minute), severe tissue trauma, heat cramps

Oral solution: Dehydration, heart failure, renal impairment, electrolyte abnormalities; use for bowel cleansing

Oral tablets: Acute phosphate nephropathy (biopsy proven), bowel obstruction, bowel perforation, gastric bypass or stapling surgery, toxic colitis, toxic megacolon

Enema: Dehydration, GI obstruction (known or suspected), heart failure, imperforate anus, inflammatory bowel disease (active), megacolon (congenital or acquired), paralytic ileus, perforation, renal impairment (clinically significant)

Warnings Acute phosphate nephropathy has been reported (rarely) with use of oral sodium phosphate products as a colon cleanser prior to colonoscopy. Some cases have resulted in permanent renal impairment (some requiring dialysis) **[U.S. Boxed Warning]**. Risk factors for acute phosphate nephropathy may include increased age (>55 years of age), preexisting renal dysfunction, bowel obstruction, active colitis, dehydration, and the use of medicines that affect renal perfusion or function (eg, ACE inhibitors, ARBs, diuretics, and possibly NSAIDs), although some cases have been reported in patients without apparent risk factors; avoid use if possible in patients with risk factors. Other preventive measures may include not exceeding the maximum recommended dose and avoiding the concurrent use of other laxatives containing sodium phosphate; encourage patients to adequately hydrate before, during, and after use; obtain baseline and postprocedure labs in patients at risk; consider hospitalization and intravenous hydration during bowel cleansing for patients unable to hydrate themselves (eg, frail patients). Use is contraindicated in patients with acute phosphate nephropathy (biopsy proven). Use with caution in patients with renal impairment; patients may be at risk for sodium retention and edema. Close monitoring required to avoid hyperphosphatemia. Administration of oral sodium phosphate products as a bowel preparation in adults has been associated with metabolic acidosis, tetany, and death; fatalities have been observed in patients with renal insufficiency, bowel perforation, and in patients who misused or overdosed sodium phosphate products.

Serious cardiac arrhythmias including QT prolongation have been associated (rarely) with use of oral sodium phosphate products used as bowel prep prior to colonoscopy; use caution in patients with or at risk for arrhythmias (eg, cardiomyopathy, prolonged QT interval, history of uncontrolled arrhythmias, recent MI) or with concurrent use of other QT-prolonging medications; pre-/postdose ECGs should be considered in high-risk patients.

Sodium phosphate products may cause electrolyte disturbances (hyponatremia, hypokalemia, hypocalcemia, hypomagnesemia) and low serum osmolarity which has been associated with generalized tonic-clonic seizures and/or loss of consciousness in patients with no prior history of seizures; seizures were associated with electrolyte abnormalities; neurologic abnormalities resolved after correction of fluid and electrolyte abnormalities. Use with caution in patients with a history of seizures, those at higher risk of seizures, or on medication that lowers seizure threshold.

Oral solution contains sodium benzoate; benzoic acid (benzoate) is a metabolite of benzyl alcohol; large amounts of benzyl alcohol (≥99 mg/kg/day) have been associated with a potentially fatal toxicity ("gasping syndrome") in neonates; the "gasping syndrome" consists of metabolic acidosis, respiratory distress, gasping respirations, CNS dysfunction (including convulsions, intracranial hemorrhage), hypotension and cardiovascular collapse; use oral solution containing sodium benzoate with caution in neonates; *in vitro* and animal studies have shown that benzoate displaces bilirubin from protein binding sites.

Precautions Use with caution in patients with preexisting electrolyte imbalances, dehydration, or risk of electrolyte disturbance (hypocalcemia, hyperphosphatemia, hypernatremia); correct dehydration and electrolyte disturbances prior to use for bowel preparations. Use with caution in patients with chronic inflammatory bowel disease or severe active ulcerative colitis; may induce colonic aphthous ulceration and ischemic colitis (some requiring hospitalization). Colitis has been associated with acute phosphate nephropathy. Use oral sodium phosphate tablets with caution in patients with impaired gag reflex and those prone to regurgitation or aspiration.

Enemas/oral solutions are available in pediatric and adult sizes; prescribe by "volume" not by "bottle." Some products contain phenylalanine; use with caution in patients with phenylketonuria. The parenteral product contains aluminum; toxic aluminum concentrations may be seen with high doses, prolonged use, or renal dysfunction. Premature neonates are at higher risk due to immature renal function and aluminum intake from other parenteral sources. Parenteral aluminum exposure of >4-5 mcg/kg/day is associated with CNS and bone toxicity and tissue loading may occur at lower doses.

Adverse Reactions

Central nervous system: Dizziness, headache

Gastrointestinal: Abdominal pain, bloating, mucosal bleeding, nausea, superficial mucosal ulcerations, vomiting

Endocrine & metabolic: Hypernatremia, hyperphosphatemia, hypocalcemia (on colonoscopy day), hypokalemia (on colonoscopy day), hypophosphatemia (2-3 days postcolonoscopy)

Postmarketing and/or case reports: Acute phosphate nephropathy, anaphylaxis, bronchospasm, calcium nephrolithiasis, cardiac arrhythmia, dehydration, dysphagia, dyspnea, facial edema, increased blood urea nitrogen, increased serum creatinine, ischemic colitis, lip edema, paresthesia, pharyngeal edema, pruritus, rectal bleeding, renal failure, renal insufficiency, renal tubular necrosis, seizure, skin rash, tightness in throat, tongue edema, urticaria

Drug Interactions

Metabolism/Transport Effects None known.

Avoid Concomitant Use There are no known interactions where it is recommended to avoid concomitant use.

Increased Effect/Toxicity

Sodium Phosphates may increase the levels/effects of: Nonsteroidal Anti-Inflammatory Agents

The levels/effects of Sodium Phosphates may be increased by: ACE Inhibitors; Angiotensin II Receptor

Blockers; Bisphosphonate Derivatives; Diuretics; Tricyclic Antidepressants

Decreased Effect

The levels/effects of Sodium Phosphates may be decreased by: Antacids; Calcium Salts; Iron Salts; Magnesium Salts; Multivitamins/Minerals (with ADEK, Folate, Iron); Sucralfate

Stability

Enema: Store at room temperature.

Oral:

Solution: Store at room temperature; do not freeze.

Tablet: Store at 25°C (77°F); excursions permitted between 15°C and 30°C (59°F and 86°F).

Solution for injection: Store intact vials at 20°C to 25°C (68°F to 77°F); excursions permitted between 15°C and 30°C (59°F and 86°F). Phosphate salts may precipitate when mixed with calcium salts. Calcium-phosphate stability in parenteral nutrition solutions is dependent upon the pH of the solution, temperature, and relative concentration of each ion. The pH of the solution is primarily dependent upon the amino acid concentration. The higher the percentage of amino acids, the lower the pH, and the more soluble the calcium and phosphate. Individual commercially available amino acid solutions vary significantly with respect to pH-lowering potential and consequent calcium phosphate compatibility. Check with a pharmacist to determine compatibility.

Mechanism of Action As a laxative, exerts osmotic effect in the small intestine by drawing water into the lumen of the gut, producing distention and promoting peristalsis and evacuation of the bowel; phosphorous participates in bone deposition, calcium metabolism, utilization of B complex vitamins, and as a buffer in acid-base equilibrium

Pharmacodynamics Onset of action (catharsis):

Oral: 3-6 hours

Rectal: 2-5 minutes

Pharmacokinetics (Adult data unless noted)

Absorption: Oral: 1% to 20%

Elimination: Oral forms excreted in feces; I.V. forms are excreted in the urine with over 80% to 90% of dose reabsorbed by the kidney

Dosing: Neonatal Note: If phosphate repletion is required and a phosphate product is not available at your institution, consider the use of sodium glycerophosphate pentahydrate (Glycophos) as a suitable substitute. Concentration and dosing are different from FDA approved products; use caution when switching between products. Refer to sodium glycerophosphate pentahydrate monograph.

Caution: With orders for I.V. phosphate, there is considerable confusion associated with the use of millimoles (mmol) versus milliequivalents (mEq) to express the phosphate requirement. The most reliable method of ordering I.V. phosphate is by millimoles, then specifying the potassium or sodium salt. Intravenous doses listed as mmol of phosphate. **Note:** Consider the contribution of sodium when determining the appropriate phosphate replacement.

Phosphorus Estimated Average Requirement (EAR): Dietary Intake Reference (DIR) (1997 National Academy of Science Recommendations) (**Note:** DIR is under review as of March 2009): Oral: 3.2 mmol/day (adequate intake)

Parenteral nutrition, maintenance requirement (Mirtallo, 2004): I.V.: 1-2 mmol/kg/day

Dosing: Usual Note: If phosphate repletion is required and a phosphate product is not available at your institution, consider the use of sodium glycerophosphate pentahydrate (Glycophos) as a suitable substitute. Concentration and dosing are different from FDA approved products; use caution when switching between products. Refer to sodium glycerophosphate pentahydrate monograph.

Caution: With orders for I.V. phosphate, there is considerable confusion associated with the use of millimoles (mmol) versus milliequivalents (mEq) to express the phosphate requirement. The most reliable method of ordering I.V. phosphate is by millimoles, then specifying the potassium or sodium salt. Intravenous doses listed as mmol of phosphate. **Note:** Consider the contribution of sodium when determining the appropriate phosphate replacement.

Infants, Children, and Adolescents: Phosphorus: Oral: See table.

Phosphorus – Recommended Daily Allowance (RDA) and Estimated Average Requirement (EAR)

Age	RDA (mmol/day)	EAR (mmol/day)
1-6 mo	–	3.2[A]
7-12 mo	–	8.9[A]
1-3 y	14.8	12.3
4-8 y	16.1	13.1
9-18 y	40.3	34
19-30 y	22.6	18.7

[A]Adequate intake (AI)

Hypophosphatemia, acute: Hypophosphatemia does not necessarily equate with phosphate depletion. Hypophosphatemia may occur in the presence of low, normal, or high total body phosphate and conversely, phosphate depletion may exist with normal, low, or elevated levels of serum phosphate (Gaasbeek, 2005). It is difficult to provide concrete guidelines for the treatment of severe hypophosphatemia because the extent of total body deficits and response to therapy are difficult to predict. Aggressive doses of phosphate may result in a transient serum elevation followed by redistribution into intracellular compartments or bone tissue. Intermittent I.V. infusion should be reserved for severe depletion situations; requires continuous cardiac monitoring. Guidelines differ based on degree of illness, need/use of TPN, and severity of hypophosphatemia. If hypokalemia exists, consider phosphate replacement strategy with potassium (eg, potassium phosphates). Various regimens for replacement of phosphate in adults have been studied. The regimens below have only been studied in adult patients; however, many institutions have used them in children safely and successfully. Obese patients and/or severe renal impairment were excluded from phosphate supplement trials. **Note:** 1 mmol phosphate = 31 mg phosphorus; 1 mg phosphorus = 0.032 mmol phosphate.

I.V. doses may be incorporated into the patient's maintenance I.V. fluids; intermittent I.V. infusion should be reserved for severe depletion situations. **Note:** Doses listed as mmol of **phosphate**.

Children and Adolescents: **Note:** There are no prospective studies of parenteral phosphate replacement in children. The following weight-based guidelines for adult dosing may be cautiously employed in pediatric patients. Guidelines differ based on degree of illness, use of TPN, and severity of hypophosphatemia.

General replacement guidelines (Lentz, 1978): **Note:** The initial dose may be increased by 25% to 50% if the patient is symptomatic secondary to hypophosphatemia and lowered by 25% to 50% if the patient is hypercalcemic.

Low dose: 0.08 mmol/kg over 6 hours; use if losses are recent and uncomplicated

Intermediate dose: 0.16-0.24 mmol/kg over 4-6 hours; use if serum phosphorus level 0.5-1 mg/dL (0.16-0.32 mmol/L)

High dose: 0.36 mmol/kg over 6 hours; use if serum phosphorus <0.5 mg/dL (<0.16 mmol/L)

Patients receiving TPN (Clark, 1995):
Low dose: 0.16 mmol/kg over 4-6 hours; use if serum phosphorus level 2.3-3 mg/dL (0.73- 0.96 mmol/L)
Intermediate dose: 0.32 mmol/kg over 4-6 hours; use if serum phosphorus level 1.6-2.2 mg/dL (0.51-0.72 mmol/L)
High dose: 0.64 mmol/kg over 8-12 hours; use if serum phosphorus <1.5 mg/dL (<0.5 mmol/L)

Critically ill adult trauma patients receiving TPN (Brown, 2006):
Low dose: 0.32 mmol/kg over 4-6 hours; use if serum phosphorus level 2.3-3 mg/dL (0.73-0.96 mmol/L)
Intermediate dose: 0.64 mmol/kg over 4-6 hours; use if serum phosphorus level 1.6-2.2 mg/dL (0.51-0.72 mmol/L)
High dose: 1 mmol/kg over 8-12 hours; use if serum phosphorus <1.5 mg/dL (<0.5 mmol/L)

Alternative method in critically ill patients (Kingston, 1985):
Low dose: 0.25 mmol/kg over 4 hours; use if serum phosphorus level 0.5-1 mg/dL (0.16-0.32 mmol/L)
Moderate dose: 0.5 mmol/kg over 4 hours; use if serum phosphorus level <0.5 mg/dL (<0.16 mmol/L)

Maintenance: Oral: 2-3 mmol/kg/day in divided doses (including dietary intake)

Parenteral nutrition, maintenance requirement (Mirtallo, 2004): I.V.:
Infants and Children ≤50 kg: 0.5-2 mmol/kg/day
Children >50 kg and Adolescents: 10-40 mmol/day

Constipation:
Oral, solution (Monobasic sodium phosphate monohydrate 2.4 g and dibasic sodium phosphate heptahydrate 0.9 g per 5 mL): **Note:** Must be diluted in a full glass of water:
Children 5-9 years: 7.5 mL as a single dose
Children 10-11 years: 15 mL as a single dose
Children ≥12 years and Adolescents: 15 mL as a single dose; maximum single daily dose: 45 mL/**day**
Rectal: Fleet Enema:
Children 2-4 years: Administer **one half** contents of one 2.25 ounce pediatric enema
Children 5-11 years: Administer the contents of one 2.25 ounce pediatric enema
Children ≥12 years and Adolescents: Administer the contents of one 4.5 ounce enema as a single dose

Adults:
Hypophosphatemia, acute treatment: I.V.: It is difficult to provide concrete guidelines for the treatment of severe hypophosphatemia because the extent of total body deficits and response to therapy are difficult to predict. Aggressive doses of phosphate may result in a transient serum elevation followed by redistribution into intracellular compartments or bone tissue. It is recommended that repletion of severe hypophosphatemia be done I.V. because large doses of oral phosphate may cause diarrhea and intestinal absorption may be unreliable. Intermittent I.V. infusion should be reserved for severe depletion situations; requires continuous cardiac monitoring. Guidelines differ based on degree of illness, need/use of TPN, and severity of hypophosphatemia. If hypokalemia exists (some clinicians recommend threshold of <4 mmol/L), consider phosphate replacement strategy with potassium (eg, potassium phosphates). Obese patients and/or severe renal

impairment patients were excluded from phosphate supplement trials. **Note:** 1 mmol phosphate = 31 mg phosphorus; 1 mg phosphorus = 0.032 mmol phosphate.

General replacement guidelines (Lentz, 1978):
Low dose, serum phosphorus losses are recent and uncomplicated: 0.08 mmol/kg over 6 hours
Intermediate dose, serum phosphorus level 0.5-1 mg/dL (0.16-0.32 mmol/L): 0.16-0.24 mmol/kg over 6 hours
Note: The initial dose may be increased by 25% to 50% if the patient is symptomatic secondary to hypophosphatemia and lowered by 25% to 50% if the patient is hypercalcemic.

Critically ill adult patients receiving concurrent enteral/parenteral nutrition (Brown, 2006; Clark, 1995): **Note:** Round doses to the nearest 7.5 mmol for ease of preparation. If administering with phosphate-containing parenteral nutrition, do not exceed 15 mmol/L within parenteral nutrition. May use adjusted body weight for patients weighing >130% of ideal body weight (and BMI <40 kg/m^2) by using [IBW + 0.25 (ABW-IBW)]:
Low dose, serum phosphorus level 2.3-3 mg/dL (0.74-0.96 mmol/L): 0.16-0.32 mmol/kg over 4-6 hours
Intermediate dose, serum phosphorus level 1.6-2.2 mg/dL (0.51-0.71 mmol/L): 0.32-0.64 mmol/kg over 4-6 hours
High dose, serum phosphorus <1.5 mg/dL (<0.5 mmol/L): 0.64-1 mmol/kg over 8-12 hours
Parenteral nutrition: I.V.: 10-15 mmol/1000 kcal (Hicks, 2001) **or** 20-40 mmol/24 hours (Mirtallo, 2004)
Laxative (Fleet): Rectal: Contents of one 4.5 oz enema as a single dose
Laxative: Oral solution: 15 mL as a single dose; maximum single daily dose: 45 mL
Bowel cleansing prior to colonoscopy: Oral tablets: **Note:** Do not use additional agents, especially other sodium phosphate products.
OsmoPrep: A total of 32 tablets and 2 quarts of clear liquids (8 ounces of clear liquids with each dose) divided as follows:
Evening before colonoscopy: 4 tablets every 15 minutes for 5 doses (total of 20 tablets)
3-5 hours prior to colonoscopy: 4 tablets every 15 minutes for 3 doses (total of 12 tablets)

Administration
Oral: Administer with food to reduce the risk of diarrhea (unless using for bowel preparation); maintain adequate fluid intake; dilute oral solution in 8 ounces of cool water, follow with an additional 8 ounces of water. Products used as preparation for colonoscopy (OsmoPrep) should be administered with at least 8 ounces water for each dose.

Parenteral: Intermittent I.V. infusion; do not administer I.V. push. Observe the vial for the presence of crystals. Do not use vial if crystals are present. Dilute in a compatible I.V. fluid. **Note:** Due to the potential for solution crystallization, American Regent, Inc recommends the use of a 5-micron filter when preparing I.V. sodium phosphate containing solutions (Important Drug Administration Safety Information, American Regent, 2013); a similar recommendation has not been noted by other manufacturers. Maximum concentration: Peripheral line: 0.05 mmol/mL; Central line: 0.12 mmol/mL (maximum concentrations were determined with consideration for maximum sodium concentration); maximum rate of infusion: 0.06 mmol/kg/hour; do **not** infuse with calcium-containing I.V. fluids. **Note:** Due to the potential for solution crystallization, American Regent, Inc recommends the use of a 0.22-micron in-line filter for I.V. administration (1.2-micron filter if admixture contains lipids) (Important Drug Safety

Information, American Regent, 2013); a similar recommendation has not been noted by other manufacturers.

Rectal: Gently insert enema tip into rectum with a slight side-to-side movement and tip pointing toward the navel; have patient bear down. Administer with patient lying on left side and knees bent or with patient kneeling and head and chest leaning forward until left side of face is resting comfortably. **Note:** Preparation for **one half** bottle administration: Unscrew cap and remove 30 mL of liquid; replace cap and administer as usual.

Monitoring Parameters

I.V.: Serum sodium, calcium, and phosphorus concentrations; renal function; in pediatric patients after I.V. phosphate repletion, repeat serum phosphorus concentration should be checked 2 hours later (ASPEN Pediatric Nutrition Support Core Curriculum, 2010)

Oral: Bowel cleansing: Baseline and postprocedure labs (electrolytes, calcium, phosphorus, BUN, creatinine) in patients at risk for acute renal nephropathy, seizure, or who have a history of electrolyte abnormality; ECG in patients with risks for prolonged QT or arrhythmias. Ensure euvolemia before initiating bowel preparation.

Rectal: Stool output

Reference Range Note: There is a diurnal variation with the nadir at 1100, plateau at 1600, and peak in the early evening (Gaasbeek, 2005); 1 mmol/L phosphate = 3.1 mg/dL phosphorus

Newborn 0-5 days: 4.8-8.2 mg/dL

1-3 years: 3.8-6.5 mg/dL

4-11 years: 3.7-5.6 mg/dL

12-15 years: 2.9-5.4 mg/dL

16-19 years: 2.7-4.7 mg/dL

Additional Information Cow's milk is a good source of phosphate with 1 mg elemental (0.032 mmol) elemental phosphate per mL

Fleet Pedia-Lax Enema: 2.25 oz bottle administers 59 mL

Fleet Enema: 4.5 oz bottle administers 118 mL

Dosage Forms Considerations

Sodium 4 mEq is equivalent to sodium 92 mg

Phosphorous 3 mmol is equivalent to phosphorus 93 mg

Dosage Forms Excipient information presented when available (limited, particularly for generics); consult specific product labeling.

Injection, solution [concentrate; preservative free]: Phosphorus 3 mmol and sodium 4 mEq per 1 mL (5 mL, 15 mL, 50 mL) [equivalent to phosphorus 93 mg and sodium 92 mg per 1 mL; source of electrolytes: monobasic and dibasic sodium phosphate]

Solution, oral: Monobasic sodium phosphate monohydrate 2.4 g and dibasic sodium phosphate heptahydrate 0.9 g per 5 mL (45 mL) [sugar free; contains sodium 556 mg/5 mL, sodium benzoate; ginger-lemon flavor]

Solution, rectal [enema]: Monobasic sodium phosphate monohydrate 19 g and dibasic sodium phosphate heptahydrate 7 g per 118 mL delivered dose (133 mL)

Fleet Enema: Monobasic sodium phosphate monohydrate 19 g and dibasic sodium phosphate heptahydrate 7 g per 118 mL delivered dose (133 mL) [contains sodium 4.4 g/118 mL]

Fleet Enema Extra: Monobasic sodium phosphate monohydrate 19 g and dibasic sodium phosphate heptahydrate 7 g per 197 mL delivered dose (230 mL) [contains sodium 4.4 g/197 mL]

Fleet Pedia-Lax™ Enema: Monobasic sodium phosphate monohydrate 9.5 g and dibasic sodium phosphate heptahydrate 3.5 g per 59 mL delivered dose (66 mL) [contains sodium 2.2 g/59 mL]

LaCrosse Complete: Monobasic sodium phosphate monohydrate 19 g and dibasic sodium phosphate heptahydrate 7 g per 118 mL delivered dose (133 mL) [contains sodium 4.4 g/118 mL]

Tablet, oral [scored]:

OsmoPrep: Monobasic sodium phosphate monohydrate 1.102 g and dibasic sodium phosphate anhydrous 0.398 g [sodium phosphate 1.5 g per tablet; gluten free]

References

Brown KA, Dickerson RN, Morgan LM, et al, "A New Graduated Dosing Regimen for Phosphorus Replacement in Patients Receiving Nutrition Support," JPEN, 2006, 30(3):209-14.

Clark CL, Sacks GS, Dickerson RN, et al, "Treatment of Hypophosphatemia in Patients Receiving Specialized Nutrition Support Using a Graduated Dosing Scheme: Results From a Prospective Clinical Trial," Crit Care Med, 1995, 23(9):1504-11.

Department Health and Human Services, Food and Drug Administration, "Aluminum in Large and Small Volume Parenterals Used in Total Parenteral Nutrition," Federal Register, 2000, 65(17):4103-11.

"Dietary Reference Intakes for Calcium, Phosphorus, Magnesium, Vitamin D, and Fluoride. Standing Committee on the Scientific Evaluation of Dietary Reference Intakes, Food and Nutrition Board, Institute of Medicine," National Academy of Sciences, Washington, DC: National Academy Press, 1997.

Gaasbeek A and Meinders AE, "Hypophosphatemia: An Update on Its Etiology and Treatment", Am J Med, 2005, 118(10):1094-101.

Kingston M and Al-Siba'i MB, "Treatment of Severe Hypophosphatemia," Crit Care Med, 1985, 13(1):16-8

Lentz RD, Brown BM, and Kjellstrand CM, "Treatment of Severe Hypophosphatemia," Ann Intern Med, 1978, 89(6):941-4.

Lloyd CW and Johnson CE, "Management of Hypophosphatemia," Clin Pharm, 1988, 7(2):123-8.

Rosen GH, Boullata JI, O'Rangers EA, et al, "Intravenous Phosphate Repletion Regimen for Critically Ill Patients With Moderate Hypophosphatemia," Crit Care Med, 1995, 23(7):1204-10.

Schmidt GL, "Fluids and Electrolytes," In: Corkins MR, Balint J, Bobo E, et al, eds, The A.S.P.E.N Pediatric Nutrition Support Core Curriculum, Silver Spring: MD: American Society of Parenteral and Enteral Nutrition, 2010, 87-102.

Sodium Polystyrene Sulfonate

(SOW dee um pol ee STYE reen SUL fon ate)

Medication Safety Issues

Sound-alike/look-alike issues:

Kayexalate® may be confused with Kaopectate®

Sodium polystyrene sulfonate may be confused with calcium polystyrene sulfonate

Administration issues:

Always prescribe either one-time doses or as a specific number of doses (eg, 15 g q6h x 2 doses). Scheduled doses with no dosage limit could be given for days leading to dangerous hypokalemia.

International issues:

Kionex [U.S.] may be confused with Kinex brand name for biperiden [Mexico]

Brand Names: U.S. Kalexate; Kayexalate; Kionex; SPS

Brand Names: Canada Kayexalate®; PMS-Sodium Polystyrene Sulfonate

Therapeutic Category Antidote, Hyperkalemia

Generic Availability (U.S.) Yes

Use Treatment of hyperkalemia (FDA approved in adults)

Pregnancy Risk Factor C

Pregnancy Considerations Animal reproduction studies have not been conducted. There are no adequate and well-controlled studies in pregnant women. Use during pregnancy only if benefits outweigh the risks.

Breast-Feeding Considerations It is not known if sodium polystyrene sulfonate is excreted in breast milk. The manufacturer recommends that caution be exercised when administering sodium polystyrene sulfonate to nursing women.

Contraindications Hypersensitivity to sodium polystyrene sulfonate or any component; hypokalemia; obstructive bowel disease; neonates with reduced gut motility (postoperatively or drug-induced); oral administration in neonates.

Additional contraindications: Sodium polystyrene sulfonate suspension (**with** sorbitol): Rectal administration in ▶

neonates (particularly in premature infants); any postoperative patient until normal bowel function resumes

Warnings Treatment with this drug alone may be insufficient to rapidly correct severe hyperkalemia; other more rapidly effective appropriate measures should be used; enema will reduce the serum potassium faster than oral administration, but the oral route will result in a greater reduction over several hours; severe hypokalemia may occur; daily evaluation of serum potassium is recommended at minimum; ECG monitoring may be appropriate in select patients; systemic alkalosis has been reported when administered in conjunction with nonabsorbable cation-donating antacids and laxatives such as magnesium hydroxide. Intestinal obstructions due to concretions of aluminum hydroxide have been reported when administered with sodium polystyrene sulfonate; colonic necrosis and other serious gastrointestinal events (eg, bleeding, ischemic colitis, perforation) have been reported, especially when administered with sorbitol; increased risk may be associated with a history of intestinal disease or surgery, hypovolemia, prematurity, and renal insufficiency or failure; use with sorbitol is not recommended.

Precautions Use with caution in patients with severe HF, hypertension, or edema; sodium load may exacerbate condition. In addition to serum potassium lowering effects, cation-exchange resins may also affect other cation concentrations possibly resulting in decreased serum magnesium and calcium. Commercially available liquid product contains propylene glycol; in neonates, large amounts of propylene glycol (eg, >3000 mg/day I.V.) have been associated with potentially fatal toxicities which can include metabolic acidosis, seizures, renal failure, and CNS depression; use (dosage form) containing propylene glycol with caution in neonates. Use caution in premature or low birth-weight infants due to risk of digestive hemorrhage and colonic necrosis. Use with caution in children when administering rectally; excessive dosage or inadequate dilution may result in fecal impaction.

Adverse Reactions

Endocrine & metabolic: Hypernatremia, hypocalcemia, hypokalemia, hypomagnesemia, sodium retention

Gastrointestinal: Anorexia, constipation, diarrhea, fecal impaction, intestinal necrosis (rare), intestinal obstruction (due to concretions in association with aluminum hydroxide), nausea, vomiting

Rare but important or life-threatening: Acute bronchitis (rare; associated with inhalation of particles), concretions, gastrointestinal bleeding, gastrointestinal ulceration, intestinal perforation, ischemic colitis

Drug Interactions

Metabolism/Transport Effects None known.

Avoid Concomitant Use

Avoid concomitant use of Sodium Polystyrene Sulfonate with any of the following: Laxatives (Magnesium Containing); Meloxicam; Sorbitol

Increased Effect/Toxicity

Sodium Polystyrene Sulfonate may increase the levels/effects of: Aluminum Hydroxide; Digoxin

The levels/effects of Sodium Polystyrene Sulfonate may be increased by: Antacids; Laxatives (Magnesium Containing); Meloxicam; Sorbitol

Decreased Effect

Sodium Polystyrene Sulfonate may decrease the levels/effects of: Lithium; Thyroid Products

Food Interactions Some liquids may contain potassium: Management: Do not mix in orange juice or in any fruit juice known to contain potassium.

Stability Store at 25°C (77°F); excursions permitted to 15°C to 30°C (59°F to 86°F); suspensions made from powder should be freshly prepared and used within 24 hours of preparation

Mechanism of Action Removes potassium by exchanging sodium ions for potassium ions in the intestine (especially the large intestine) before the resin is passed from the body; exchange capacity is 1 mEq/g *in vivo*, and *in vitro* capacity is 3.1 mEq/g, therefore, a wide range of exchange capacity exists such that close monitoring of serum electrolytes is necessary

Pharmacodynamics Onset of action: Within 2-24 hours

Pharmacokinetics (Adult data unless noted) Elimination: Remains in the GI tract to be completely excreted in the feces (primarily as potassium polystyrene sulfonate)

Dosing: Neonatal Hyperkalemia (not preferred): Rectal: 1 g/kg/dose every 2-6 hours (Malone, 1991; Yaseen 2008); may employ lower doses by using the practical exchange ratio of 1 mEq K$^+$/g of resin as the basis for calculation. **Note:** Due to complications of hypernatremia and NEC, use in neonates should be reserved for refractory cases.

Dosing: Usual Hyperkalemia:

Infants and Children:

Oral: 1 g/kg/dose every 6 hours

Rectal: 1 g/kg/dose every 2-6 hours; in small children and infants, employ lower doses by using the practical exchange ratio of 1 mEq K$^+$/g of resin as the basis for calculation.

Adults:

Oral: 15 g 1-4 times/day

Rectal: 30-50 g every 6 hours

Administration

Oral or NG: Shake commercially available suspension well before use. **Do not mix in orange juice.** Chilling the oral mixture will increase palatability.

Powder for suspension: For each 1 g of the powdered resin, add 3-4 mL of water or syrup (amount of fluid usually ranges from 20-100 mL).

Enema: Route is less effective than oral administration. Administer cleansing enema first. Each dose of the powder for suspension should be suspended in 100 mL of aqueous vehicle and administered as a warm emulsion (body temperature). The commercially available suspension should also be warmed to body temperature. During administration, the solution should be agitated gently. Retain enema in colon for at least 30-60 minutes and for several hours, if possible. Once retention time is complete, irrigate colon with a nonsodium-containing solution to remove resin

Monitoring Parameters Serum sodium, potassium, calcium, magnesium, ECG (if applicable)

Additional Information 1 g of resin binds ~1 mEq of potassium; 4.1 mEq sodium per g of powder; 1 level teaspoon contains 3.5 g polystyrene sulfonate

Dosage Forms Excipient information presented when available (limited, particularly for generics); consult specific product labeling.

Powder, Oral:

Kalexate: (454 g) [sorbitol free; contains sodium 100 mg (4.1 mEq)/g]

Kayexalate: (453.6 g) [contains sodium 100 mg (4.1 mEq)/g]

Kionex: (454 g) [contains sodium 100 mg (4.1 mEq)/g]

Generic: (453.6 g, 454 g)

Suspension, Oral:

Kionex: 15 g/60 mL (60 mL, 473 mL) [contains alcohol, usp, methylparaben, propylene glycol, propylparaben, saccharin sodium, sodium 1500 mg (65 mEq)/60 mL, sorbitol; raspberry flavor]

SPS: 15 g/60 mL (60 mL, 120 mL, 473 mL) [contains alcohol, usp, methylparaben, propylene glycol, propylparaben, saccharin sodium, sodium 1500 mg (65 mEq)/60 mL, sorbitol; cherry flavor]

Generic: 15 g/60 mL (60 mL, 480 mL, 500 mL)

Suspension, Rectal:

Generic: 30 g/120 mL (120 mL); 50 g/200 mL (200 mL)

References

American Academy of Pediatrics Committee on Drugs, " 'Inactive' Ingredients in Pharmaceutical Products: Update (Subject Review)," *Pediatrics*, 1997, 99(2):268-78.

Malone TA, "Glucose and Insulin Versus Cation-Exchange Resin for the Treatment of Hyperkalemia in Very Low Birth Weight Infants," *J Pediatr*, 1991, 118(1):121-3.

Vemgal P and Ohlsson A, "Interventions for Non-Oliguric Hyperkalaemia in Preterm Neonates," *Cochrane Database Syst Rev*, 2007, (1): CD005257.

Yaseen H, Khalaf M, Dana A, et al, "Salbutamol Versus Cation-Exchange Resin (Kayexalate) for the Treatment of Nonoliguric Hyperkalemia in Preterm Infants," *Am J Perinatol*, 2008, 25(3):193-7.

◆ **Sodium Sulamyd (Can)** *see* Sulfacetamide (Ophthalmic) *on page 1943*

◆ **Sodium Sulfacetamide** *see* Sulfacetamide (Ophthalmic) *on page 1943*

◆ **Sodium Sulfacetamide** *see* Sulfacetamide (Topical) *on page 1944*

Sodium Thiosulfate (SOW dee um thye oh SUL fate)

Related Information
Management of Drug Extravasations *on page 2255*

Therapeutic Category Antidote, Cyanide; Antidote, Extravasation

Generic Availability (U.S.) Yes

Use Treatment of cyanide poisoning [FDA approved in pediatric patients (age not specified) and adults]; has also been used for used in the management of mechlorethamine extravasation

Pregnancy Risk Factor C

Pregnancy Considerations Teratogenic effects were not observed in animal reproduction studies of sodium thiosulfate. In general, medications used as antidotes should take into consideration the health and prognosis of the mother; antidotes should be administered to pregnant women if there is a clear indication for use and should not be withheld because of fears of teratogenicity (Bailey, 2003).

Breast-Feeding Considerations It is not known if sodium thiosulfate is excreted in breast milk. Because sodium thiosulfate may be used as an antidote in life-threatening situations, breast-feeding is not a contraindication to use. It is not known when breast-feeding may safely be restarted following administration; the manufacturer recommends caution be used following administration to nursing women.

Contraindications Hypersensitivity to sodium thiosulfate or any component

Precautions The presence of sulfite hypersensitivity should not preclude the use of this medication. Due to the risk for serious adverse effects, use with caution in patients where the diagnosis of cyanide poisoning is uncertain. However, if clinical suspicion of cyanide poisoning is high, treatment should not be delayed. Treatment of cyanide poisoning should include decontamination and supportive therapy. Collection of pretreatment blood cyanide concentrations does not preclude administration and should not delay administration in the emergency management of highly suspected or confirmed cyanide toxicity. Pretreatment levels may be useful as postinfusion levels may be inaccurate. Monitor patients for return of symptoms for 24-48 hours; repeat treatment should be administered if symptoms return. Consider consultation with a poison control center at 1-800-222-1222.

Fire victims may present with both cyanide and carbon monoxide poisoning. In this scenario, sodium thiosulfate may be used alone to promote the clearance of cyanide. Due to the slow onset of action of sodium thiosulfate, may consider using hydroxocobalamin alone or in combination with sodium thiosulfate (Howland, 2011).

Adverse Reactions
Cardiovascular: Hypotension
Central nervous system: Disorientation, headache
Gastrointestinal: Nausea, salty taste, vomiting
Hematologic: Bleeding time prolonged
Miscellaneous: Warmth

Drug Interactions
Metabolism/Transport Effects None known.
Avoid Concomitant Use There are no known interactions where it is recommended to avoid concomitant use.
Increased Effect/Toxicity There are no known significant interactions involving an increase in effect.
Decreased Effect There are no known significant interactions involving a decrease in effect.
Stability Store intact vials at 20°C to 25°C (68°F to 77°F); excursions permitted to 15°C to 30°C (59°F to 86°F)

Compounded SubQ solution: Store the 1/6 M (~4%) solution at 15°C to 30°C (59°F to 86°F) (Polovich, 2009)

Mechanism of Action
Cyanide toxicity: Serves as a sulfur donor in rhodanese-catalyzed formation of thiocyanate (much less toxic than cyanide)
Extravasation management: Neutralizes the reactive species of mechlorethamine; reduces the formation of hydroxyl radicals which cause tissue injury

Pharmacokinetics (Adult data unless noted)
Half-life, elimination:
Thiosulfate: ~3 hours (Howland, 2011)
Thiocyanate: ~3 hours; renal impairment: ≤9 days
Elimination: Urine (~20% to 50% as unchanged drug)

Dosing: Usual Note: Sodium thiosulfate is available as a 10% and 25% concentration and as part of various antidote kits or as a single product. Some dosing is concentration-dependent; verify product strength prior to dose calculation.

Cyanide poisoning: Note: Usually given in conjunction with sodium nitrite. Administer sodium nitrite first, followed immediately by the administration of sodium thiosulfate. Monitor the patient for 24-48 hours following doses.

Infants, Children, and Adolescents:
Manufacturer's labeling: I.V.: Initial: 7 g/m^2; maximum dose: 12.5 g; if repeat dosing is necessary due to symptom return, use 50% of original dose.
Alternate dosing (volume-based): I.V.: Initial: 25% solution: 1 mL/kg; maximum dose: 50 mL (12.5 g); if repeat dosing is necessary due to symptom return, use 50% of original dose. **Note:** Presented dose equates to 250 mg/kg of sodium thiosulfate or 28-40 mL/m^2 of the 25% solution. Dosing is from Nithiodote™ manufacturer's labeling.
Adults: I.V.: Initial: 12.5 g (50 mL of a 25% solution); if repeat dosing is necessary due symptom return, use 50% of the original dose

Mechlorethamine extravasation: Children, Adolescents, and Adults: SubQ: 1/6 M (~4%) solution: Inject 2 mL for each mg of mechlorethamine suspected to have extravasated (Polovich, 2009)

Dosage adjustment in renal impairment: No dosage adjustment provided in the manufacturer's labeling; however, renal elimination of sodium thiosulfate is significant and risk of adverse effects may be increased in patients with renal impairment.

Dosage adjustment in hepatic impairment: No dosage adjustment provided in the manufacturer's labeling (has not been studied).

Administration
Cyanide poisoning: I.V.: Inject slowly, over at least 10-20 minutes using a 0.22 micron in-line filter; rapid administration may cause hypotension

Mechlorethamine extravasation: SubQ: Inject into the extravasation site using ≤25-gauge needle; change needle with each injection (Polovich, 2009)

Preparation of compounded SubQ solution: Final concentration: 1/6 M (~4%) solution:

If using 10% sodium thiosulfate, add 4 mL to 6 mL SWI

If using 25% sodium thiosulfate, add 1.6 mL to 8.4 mL SWI

Monitoring Parameters

Cyanide poisoning: Monitor for at least 24-48 hours after administration; blood pressure and heart rate during and after infusion; hemoglobin/hematocrit; co-oximetry; serum lactate levels; venous-arterial PO_2 gradient; serum methemoglobin and oxyhemoglobin. Pretreatment cyanide levels may be useful diagnostically.

Mechlorethamine extravasation: Monitor extravasation site for pain, blister formation, skin sloughing, arm/hand swelling/stiffness; monitor for fever, chills, or worsening pain

Dosage Forms
Excipient information presented when available (limited, particularly for generics); consult specific product labeling.

Injection, solution [preservative free]: 100 mg/mL (10 mL); 250 mg/mL (50 mL)

Injection, solution: 250 mg/mL (50 mL)

References

Bailey B, "Are There Teratogenic Risks Associated With Antidotes Used in the Acute Management of Poisoned Pregnant Women?" *Birth Defects Res A Clin Mol Teratol*, 2003, 67(2):133-40.

Geller RJ, Barthold C, Saiers JA, et al, "Pediatric Cyanide Poisoning: Causes, Manifestations, Management, and Unmet Needs," *Pediatrics*, 2006, 118(5):2146-58.

Gracia R and Shepherd G, "Cyanide Poisoning and Its Treatment," *Pharmacotherapy*, 2004, 24(10):1358-65.

Hall AH, Dart R, and Bogdan G, "Sodium Thiosulfate or Hydroxocobalamin for the Empiric Treatment of Cyanide Poisoning?" *Ann Emerg Med*, 2007, 49(6):806-13.

Howland MA, "Antidotes in Depth: Sodium and Amyl Nitrite," *Goldfrank's Toxicologic Emergencies*, 9th ed, Nelson LS, Hoffman RS, Lewin NA, et al, eds, New York, NY: McGraw-Hill Companies, Inc, 2011, 1519-22.

Howland MA, "Antidotes in Depth: Sodium Thiosulfate," *Goldfrank's Toxicologic Emergencies*, 9th ed, Nelson LS, Hoffman RS, Lewin NA, et al, eds, New York, NY: McGraw-Hill Companies, Inc, 2011.

Mokhlesi B, Leikin JB, Murray P, et al, "Adult Toxicology in Critical Care: Part II: Specific Poisonings," *Chest*, 2003, 123(3):897-922.

Polovich M, Whitford JN and Olsen M, *Chemotherapy and Biotherapy Guidelines and Reccomendations for Practice*, 3rd ed, Pittsburgh, PA: Oncology Nursing Society, 2009.

♦ **Sodium Thiosulfate and Sodium Nitrite** see Sodium Nitrite and Sodium Thiosulfate *on page 1909*

♦ **Sodium Thiosulphate** see Sodium Thiosulfate *on page 1919*

♦ **Sof-Lax [OTC]** see Docusate *on page 701*

♦ **Soflax [OTC] (Can)** see Docusate *on page 701*

♦ **Soflax C [OTC] (Can)** see Docusate *on page 701*

♦ **Soflax EX [OTC] (Can)** see Bisacodyl *on page 293*

♦ **Soflax Pediatric Drops [OTC] (Can)** see Docusate *on page 701*

♦ **Solaraze** see Diclofenac (Topical) *on page 649*

♦ **Solodyn** see Minocycline *on page 1420*

♦ **Soltamox** see Tamoxifen *on page 1968*

♦ **Solu-CORTEF** see Hydrocortisone (Systemic) *on page 1034*

♦ **Solu-Cortef® (Can)** see Hydrocortisone (Systemic) *on page 1034*

♦ **Solugel® (Can)** see Benzoyl Peroxide *on page 275*

♦ **Solumedrol** see MethylPREDNISolone *on page 1386*

♦ **Solu-MEDROL** see MethylPREDNISolone *on page 1386*

♦ **Solu-Medrol (Can)** see MethylPREDNISolone *on page 1386*

♦ **Soluver® (Can)** see Salicylic Acid *on page 1860*

♦ **Soluver® Plus (Can)** see Salicylic Acid *on page 1860*

Somatropin (soe ma TROE pin)

Medication Safety Issues

Sound-alike/look-alike issues:

Humatrope may be confused with homatropine

Somatrem may be confused with somatropin

Somatropin may be confused with homatropine, sumatriptan

BEERS Criteria medication:

This drug may be potentially inappropriate for use in geriatric patients (Quality of evidence - high; Strength of recommendation - strong).

Brand Names: U.S. Genotropin; Genotropin MiniQuick; Humatrope; Norditropin FlexPro; Norditropin NordiFlex Pen; Nutropin AQ NuSpin 10; Nutropin AQ NuSpin 20; Nutropin AQ NuSpin 5; Nutropin AQ Pen; Nutropin [DSC]; Omnitrope; Saizen; Saizen Click.Easy; Serostim; Tev-Tropin; Zorbtive

Brand Names: Canada Humatrope; Norditropin Simplexx; Nutropin; Nutropin AQ; Nutropin AQ NuSpin; Nutropin AQ Pen; Omnitrope; Saizen; Serostim

Therapeutic Category Growth Hormone

Generic Availability (U.S.) No

Use

Children:

Treatment of growth failure due to inadequate endogenous growth hormone secretion (Genotropin®, Humatrope®, Norditropin®, Nutropin®, Nutropin AQ®, Omnitrope®, Saizen®, Tev-Tropin®: FDA approved in children)

Treatment of short stature associated with Turner syndrome (Genotropin®, Humatrope®, Norditropin®, Nutropin®, Nutropin AQ®, Omnitrope®: FDA approved in children)

Treatment of Prader-Willi syndrome (Genotropin®, Omnitrope®: FDA approved in ages >2 years)

Treatment of growth failure associated with chronic renal insufficiency (CRI) up until the time of renal transplantation (Nutropin®, Nutropin AQ®: FDA approved in children)

Treatment of growth failure in children born small for gestational age (SGA) who fail to manifest catch-up growth by 2-4 years of age (Genotropin®, Humatrope®, Norditropin® Omnitrope®: FDA approved in children)

Treatment of idiopathic short stature (nongrowth hormone-deficient short stature) defined by height standard deviation score (SDS) ≤2.25 and growth rate not likely to attain normal adult height (Genotropin®, Humatrope®, Nutropin®, Nutropin AQ®, Omnitrope®: FDA approved in children)

Treatment of short stature or growth failure associated with short stature homeobox gene (SHOX) deficiency (Humatrope®: FDA approved in children)

Treatment of short stature associated with Noonan syndrome (Norditropin®: FDA approved in children)

Adults: All indications: FDA approved in adults

HIV patients with wasting or cachexia with concomitant antiviral therapy (Serostim®)

Replacement of endogenous growth hormone in patients with adult growth hormone deficiency who meet both of the following criteria (Genotropin®, Humatrope®, Norditropin®, Nutropin®, Nutropin AQ®, Omnitrope®, Saizen®):

Biochemical diagnosis of adult growth hormone deficiency by means of a subnormal response to a standard growth hormone stimulation test (peak growth hormone ≤5 mcg/L). Confirmatory testing may not be required in patients with congenital/genetic growth hormone deficiency or multiple pituitary hormone deficiencies due to organic diseases.

and

Adult-onset: Patients who have adult growth hormone deficiency whether alone or with multiple hormone deficiencies (hypopituitarism) as a result of pituitary disease, hypothalamic disease, surgery, radiation therapy, or trauma

or

Childhood-onset: Patients who were growth hormone-deficient during childhood, confirmed as an adult before replacement therapy is initiated
Treatment of short-bowel syndrome (Zorbtive®)

Pregnancy Risk Factor B/C (depending upon manufacturer)

Pregnancy Considerations Teratogenic effects were not observed in animal studies. Reproduction studies have not been conducted with all agents. During normal pregnancy, maternal production of endogenous growth hormone decreases as placental growth hormone production increases. Data with somatropin use during pregnancy is limited.

Breast-Feeding Considerations It is not known if somatropin is excreted in breast milk. The manufacturer recommends that caution be exercised when administering somatropin to nursing women.

Contraindications Hypersensitivity to human growth hormone or any component; patients with Prader-Willi syndrome who are severely obese or have severe respiratory impairment; do not use for growth promotion in pediatric patients with closed epiphyses; patients with acute critical illness due to complications following open heart or abdominal surgery, multiple accidental trauma, or acute respiratory failure; patients with active neoplasia, patients with proliferative or preproliferative diabetic retinopathy

Warnings Fatalities in pediatric patients with Prader-Willi syndrome following the use of growth hormone have been reported; these fatalities occurred in patients with one or more risk factors, including severe obesity, sleep apnea, respiratory impairment, or unidentified respiratory infection. In addition, male patients may be at increased risk. Treatment interruption is recommended in patients who show signs of upper airway obstruction, including the onset of or increased snoring. In addition, evaluation of and/or monitoring for sleep apnea and respiratory infections are recommended. 35% of childhood-onset adult GH-deficient subjects treated with growth hormone 0.025 mg/kg/day for 2 years had supraphysiologic levels of insulin-like growth factor-1 (IGF-1) detected during research studies; the risks of this elevation are unknown at this time; the manufacturer recommends reduction in dosage if IGF-1 levels are excessive.

Diluents for Nutropin®, Saizen®, and Zorbtive™ contain benzyl alcohol which may cause allergic reactions in susceptible individuals; large amounts of benzyl alcohol (≥99 mg/kg/day) have been associated with a potentially fatal toxicity ("gasping syndrome") in neonates; the "gasping syndrome" consists of metabolic acidosis, respiratory distress, gasping respirations, CNS dysfunction (including convulsions, intracranial hemorrhage), hypotension and cardiovascular collapse; *in vitro* and animal studies have shown that benzoate, a metabolite of benzyl alcohol, displaces bilirubin from protein-binding sites; avoid use of benzyl alcohol containing diluents in neonates.

Intracranial hypertension with papilledema, visual changes, headache, nausea, and/or vomiting has been reported; this has occurred during the first 8 weeks of therapy; all reported cases were reversible upon discontinuation of therapy; baseline and regular fundoscopic exams are recommended for assistance in recognizing this potential adverse effect.

Pancreatitis (rare) has been reported; incidence in children (especially girls) with Turner syndrome may be greater than adults.

Precautions Use with caution in patients with diabetes or family history of diabetes; use with caution in patients with evidence of active malignancy, progression of any underlying intracranial lesion, or actively growing intracranial tumor; monitor these patients closely for progression or recurrence of the underlying disease process; insulin dosage may require adjustment when growth hormone therapy is instituted; patients with hypopituitarism may develop hypothyroidism during growth hormone therapy; children may develop slipped capital epiphyses during therapy; progression of scoliosis may occur in patients with a history of scoliosis. SubQ administration can cause local lipoatrophy or lipodystrophy and may enhance the development of neutralizing antibodies.

Adverse Reactions

Growth hormone deficiency: Adverse reactions reported with growth hormone deficiency vary greatly by age. Generally, percentages are less in pediatric patients than adults, and many of the reactions reported in adults are dose related. Percentages reported also vary by product. Below is a listing by age group; events reported more commonly overall are noted with an asterisk (*).

Children: Antibodies development, arthralgia, benign intracranial hypertension, edema, eosinophilia, glycosuria, Hb A_{1c} increased, headache, hematoma, hematuria, hyperglycemia (mild), hypertriglyceridemia, hypoglycemia, hypothyroidism, injection site reaction, intracranial tumor, leg pain, lipoatrophy, leukemia, meningioma, muscle pain, papilledema, pseudotumor cerebri, psoriasis exacerbation, rash, scoliosis progression, seizure, slipped capital femoral epiphysis, weakness

Adults: Acne, ALT increased, AST increased, arthralgia*, back pain, bronchitis, carpal tunnel syndrome, chest pain, cough, depression, diabetes mellitus (type 2), diaphoresis, dizziness, edema*, fatigue, flu-like syndrome*, gastritis, glucose intolerance, glucosuria, headache*, hyperglycemia (mild), hypertension, hypoesthesia, hypothyroidism, infection, insomnia, insulin resistance, joint disorder, leg edema, muscle pain, myalgia*, nausea, pain in extremities, paresthesia*, peripheral edema*, pharyngitis, retinopathy, rhinitis, skeletal pain*, stiffness in extremities, surgical procedure, upper respiratory tract infection, weakness

Additional/postmarketing reactions observed with growth hormone deficiency: Gynecomastia, increased growth of preexisting nevi, pancreatitis

HARS: Serostim®: Arthralgia, blood glucose increased, edema (peripheral), headache, hypoesthesia, myalgia, pain (extremity), paresthesia

Idiopathic short stature: Humatrope®: Arthralgia, arthrosis, gynecomastia, hip pain, hyperlipidemia, hypertension, myalgia, otitis media, scoliosis. Additional adverse reactions listed as reported using other products from ISS NCGS Cohort: Aggressiveness, benign intracranial hypertension, diabetes, edema, hair loss, headache, injection site reaction

Prader-Willi syndrome: Genotropin®: Aggressiveness, arthralgia, edema, hair loss, headache, benign intracranial hypertension, myalgia; fatalities associated with use in this population have been reported

Turner syndrome: Humatrope®: Ear disorders, otitis media, joint pain, respiratory illness, surgical procedures, urinary tract infection

HIV patients with wasting or cachexia: Serostim®: Edema, gynecomastia, headache, hypoesthesial; musculoskeletal disorders (arthralgia, arthrosis, myalgia); nausea, paresthesia, peripheral edema,

Short-bowel syndrome: Zorbtive®: Abdominal pain, arthralgia, chest pain, dehydration, diaphoresis, dizziness, facial edema, flatulence, generalized edema, ▶

hearing symptoms, infection, injection site pain, injection site reaction, malaise, moniliasis, myalgia, nausea, pain, peripheral edema, rash, rhinitis, vomiting

SHOX deficiency: Humatrope®: Arthralgia, excessive cutaneous nevi, gynecomastia, scoliosis

Small for gestational age: Genotropin®, Humatrope®: Mild, transient hyperglycemia; benign intracranial hypertension (rare); central precocious puberty; jaw prominence (rare); aggravation of preexisting scoliosis (rare); injection site reactions; progression of pigmented nevi; carpal tunnel syndrome (rare) diabetes mellitus (rare); otitis media; headache; slipped capital femoral epiphysis

Drug Interactions

Metabolism/Transport Effects None known.

Avoid Concomitant Use There are no known interactions where it is recommended to avoid concomitant use.

Increased Effect/Toxicity There are no known significant interactions involving an increase in effect.

Decreased Effect

Somatropin may decrease the levels/effects of: Antidiabetic Agents; Cortisone; PredniSONE

The levels/effects of Somatropin may be decreased by: Estrogen Derivatives

Stability

Genotropin®: Store at 2°C to 8°C (36°F to 46°F); do not freeze. Protect from light. Following reconstitution, may store under refrigeration and use within 28 days.

Genotropin® Miniquick®: Store in refrigerator prior to dispensing, but may be stored ≤25°C (77°F) for up to 3 months after dispensing. Once reconstituted, solution must be refrigerated and used within 24 hours. Discard unused portion.

Humatrope®:

Vial: Store intact vial at 2°C to 8°C (36°F to 46°F); do not freeze. If reconstitute with provided diluent or bacteriostatic water for injection, use within 14 days; if reconstituted with SWI, use within 24 hours and discard unused portion.

Cartridge: Store intact cartridge at 2°C to 8°C (36°F to 46°F); do not freeze. Following reconstitution with provided diluent, stable for 28 days under refrigeration.

Norditropin®: Store at 2°C to 8°C (36°F to 46°F); do not freeze. Avoid direct light.

Cartridge: If refrigerated, use within 4 weeks once inserted into pen. Orange cartridges (5 mg/1.5 mL) may also be stored up to 3 weeks at ≤25°C (77°F).

Prefilled pen: If refrigerated, use within 4 weeks after initial injection. Orange and blue prefilled pens may also be stored up to 3 weeks at ≤25°C (77°F).

Nutropin®: Store intact vial at 2°C to 8°C (36°F to 46°F); do not freeze. If reconstituted with provided diluent use within 14 days; if reconstitute with SWI, use immediately and discard unused portion.

Nutropin® AQ formulations: Store intact vial at 2°C to 8°C (36°F to 46°F); do not freeze. Use within 28 days following initial use.

Omnitrope®:

Powder for injection: Store intact vial under refrigeration at 2°C to 8°C (36°F to 46°F); do not freeze. Protect from light. Following reconstitution with provided diluent, may be stored under refrigeration for up to 3 weeks. Store vial in carton to protect from light.

Solution: Store intact vial refrigeration at 2°C to 8°C (36°F to 46°F). Once the cartridge is loaded into the pen delivery system, store under refrigeration for up to 21 days after first use.

Saizen®: Store intact vial at 15°C to 30°C (59°F to 86°F). Following reconstitution with bacteriostatic water for injection, reconstituted solution should be refrigerated and used within 14 days. When reconstituted with SWI, use immediately and discard unused portion. The Saizen® easy click cartridge, when reconstituted with the

provided bacteriostatic water, should be stored under refrigeration and used within 21 days.

Serostim®: Store intact vial at 15°C to 30°C (59°F to 86°F); after reconstitution with SWI, use immediately and discard unused portion.

Tev-Tropin®: Store intact vial at 2°C to 8°C (36°F to 46°F). Following reconstitution with bacteriostatic NS, solution is stable for 14 days under refrigeration. Some cloudiness may occur; do not use if cloudiness persists after warming to room temperature.

Zorbtive®: Store intact vials and diluent at room temperature of 15°C to 30°C (59°F to 86°F). Store reconstituted vial under refrigeration at 2°C to 8°C (36°F to 46°F) for up to 14 days; do not freeze.

Mechanism of Action Somatropin is a purified polypeptide hormones of recombinant DNA origin; somatropin contains the identical sequence of amino acids found in human growth hormone; human growth hormone assists growth of linear bone, skeletal muscle, and organs by stimulating chondrocyte proliferation and differentiation, lipolysis, protein synthesis, and hepatic glucose output; stimulates erythropoietin which increases red blood cell mass; exerts both insulin-like and diabetogenic effects; enhances the transmucosal transport of water, electrolytes, and nutrients across the gut

Pharmacokinetics (Adult data unless noted)

Absorption: I.M., SubQ: Well absorbed

Distribution: V_d:

Somatrem: 50 mL/kg

Somatropin: 70 mL/kg

Metabolism: ~90% of dose metabolized in the liver and kidney cells

Bioavailability:

SubQ:

Somatrem: 81% ± 20%

Somatropin: 75%

I.M.: Somatropin: 63%

Half-life:

SubQ:

Somatrem: 2.3 ± 0.42 hours

Somatropin: 3.8 hours

I.M.: Somatropin: 4.9 hours

Elimination: 0.1% of dose excreted in urine unchanged

Dosing: Usual

Children:

AIDS-related wasting or cachexia: Serostim®: Children ≥6 years and Adolescents: Limited data available: SubQ: 0.04-0.07 mg/kg/day for 4 weeks; dosing based on two small trials of pediatric patients (n=11; age: 6-17 years)

Chronic renal insufficiency: Nutropin®, Nutropin® AQ: SubQ: 0.35 mg/kg **weekly** divided into daily injections; continue until the time of renal transplantation

Dosage recommendations in patients treated for CRI who require dialysis:

Hemodialysis: Administer dose at night prior to bedtime or at least 3-4 hours after hemodialysis to prevent hematoma formation from heparin

CCPD: Administer dose in the morning following dialysis

CAPD: Administer dose in the evening at the time of overnight exchange

Growth hormone inadequacy: Note: Therapy should be discontinued when patient has reached satisfactory adult height, when epiphyses have fused, or when the patient ceases to respond. Growth of 5 cm/year or more is expected; if growth rate does not exceed 2.5 cm in a 6-month period, double the dose for the next 6 months; if there is still no satisfactory response, discontinue therapy.

Genotropin®, Omnitrope®: SubQ: 0.16-0.24 mg/kg **weekly** divided into daily doses (6-7 doses)

Humatrope®: SubQ: 0.18-0.3 mg/kg **weekly** divided into equal doses 6-7 days/week

Norditropin®: SubQ: 0.024-0.034 mg/kg/dose 6-7 times per week

Nutropin®, Nutropin® AQ: SubQ: 0.3 mg/kg **weekly** divided into daily doses; in pubertal patients, dosage may be increased to 0.7 mg/kg **weekly** divided into daily doses

Saizen®: I.M., SubQ: 0.18 mg/kg **weekly** divided into equal daily doses **or** as 0.06 mg/kg/dose administered 3 days per week **or** as 0.03 mg/kg/dose administered 6 days per week

Tev-Tropin™: SubQ: 0.3 mg/kg divided 3 times per week

Idiopathic short stature:

Genotropin®, Omnitrope®: SubQ: 0.47 mg/kg **weekly** divided into equal doses 6-7 days/week

Humatrope®: SubQ: 0.37 mg/kg **weekly** divided into daily doses (6-7 days)

Nutropin®, Nutropin® AQ: SubQ: Up to 0.3 mg/kg **weekly** divided into daily doses

Noonan syndrome: Norditropin®: SubQ: Up to 0.066 mg/kg/day

Prader-Willi syndrome: Genotropin®, Omnitrope®: SubQ: 0.24 mg/kg **weekly** divided daily into 6-7 doses per week

SGA at birth who fail to catch-up by 2-4 years of age:

Genotropin®, Omnitrope: 0.48 mg/kg **weekly** divided daily into 6-7 doses per week

Humatrope®: SubQ: 0.47 mg/kg **weekly**divided into equal doses 6-7 days/week

Norditropin®: SubQ: Up to 0.469 mg/kg **weekly** divided into equal doses 7 days/week

Alternate dosing (small for gestational age): In older/ early pubertal children or children with very short stature, consider initiating therapy at higher doses (0.469 mg/kg weekly divided into equal doses 7 days/week); then consider reducing the dose (0.231 mg/kg weekly) if substantial catch-up growth observed. In younger children (<4 years) with less severe short stature, consider initiating therapy with lower doses (0.231 mg/kg weekly) and then titrating the dose upwards as needed.

SHOX deficiency: Humatrope®: SubQ: 0.35 mg/kg **weekly** divided into equal doses 6-7 days per week

Turner syndrome:

Genotropin®; Omnitrope®: SubQ: 0.33 mg/kg **weekly** divided into 6-7 doses/week

Humatrope®: SubQ: 0.375 mg/kg **weekly** divided into equal doses 6-7 days/week

Nutropin®, Nutropin® AQ: SubQ: Up to 0.375 mg/kg **weekly** divided into equal doses 3-7 times/week

Adults:

AIDS-related wasting or cachexia: Serostim®: SubQ: Administered once daily at bedtime:

<35 kg: 0.1 mg/kg

35-44 kg: 4 mg

45-55 kg: 5 mg

>55 kg: 6 mg

Growth hormone deficiency: Note: To minimize adverse events in older or overweight patients, reduced dosages may be necessary. During therapy, dosage should be decreased if required by the occurrence of side effects or excessive IGF-1 levels.

Weight-based dosing:

Norditropin®: SubQ: Initial dose ≤0.028 mg/kg **weekly** divided into equal doses 7 days/week; after 6 weeks of therapy, may increase dose to 0.112 mg/kg weekly divided into equal doses 7 days/week

Nutropin®, Nutropin® AQ: SubQ: ≤0.006 mg/kg/day; dose may be increased according to individual requirements, up to a maximum of 0.025 mg/kg/ day in patients <35 years of age, or up to a maximum of 0.0125 mg/kg/day in patients ≥35 years of age

Humatrope®: SubQ: ≤0.006 mg/kg/day; dose may be increased according to individual requirements, up to a maximum of 0.0125 mg/kg/day

Genotropin®, Omnitrope®: SubQ: ≤0.04 mg/kg **weekly** divided into 6-7 doses; dose may be increased at 4- to 8-week intervals according to individual requirements, to a maximum of 0.08 mg/kg/week

Saizen®: SubQ: ≤0.005 mg/kg/day; dose may be increased to not more than 0.01 mg/kg/day after 4 weeks, based on individual requirements

Nonweight-based dosing: SubQ: Initial: 0.2 mg/day (range: 0.15-0.3 mg/day); may increase every 1-2 months by 0.1-0.2 mg/day based on response and/ or serum IGF-I levels

Dosage adjustment with estrogen supplementation (growth hormone deficiency): Larger doses of somatropin may be needed for women taking oral estrogen replacement products; dosing not affected by topical products

Short-bowel syndrome: Zorbtive®: SubQ: 0.1 mg/kg daily not to exceed 8 mg/day; treatment >4 weeks has not been studied adequately. Excessive fluid retention or arthralgias may be treated symptomatically or by a 50% dosage reduction; stop therapy for up to 5 days prior to lowering dosage if symptoms are severe; if symptoms do not resolve after 5 days or recur with the lowered dosage, discontinue treatment.

Dosage adjustment in renal impairment: Reports indicate patients with chronic renal failure tend to have decreased clearance; specific dosing suggestions not available

Dosage adjustment in hepatic impairment: Clearance may be reduced in patients with severe hepatic dysfunction; specific dosing suggestions not available

Administration Parenteral: Administer SubQ (preferred route) or I.M.; not for I.V. injection; do not shake vial; rotate injection site; administer into the thigh, buttock, or abdomen; limit SubQ injection volume to 1 mL per site

Genotropin® cartridges: Reconstitute with provided diluent resulting in the following concentrations: 1.5 mg cartridge = 1.3 mg/mL, 5.8 mg cartridge = 5 mg/mL, and 13.8 mg cartridge = 12 mg/mL

Nutropin®: Reconstitute each 5 mg vial with 1.5-5 mL diluent

Norditropin® Cartridges: Must be used with the NordiPen® injection pen (each cartridge has a color-coded injection pen which is graduated to deliver the appropriate dose); do not interchange

Omnitrope®: Reconstitute with provided diluent; swirl gently; do not shake

Saizen®: Reconstitute 5 mg vial with 1-3 mL provided diluent and 8.8 mg vial with 2-3 mL provided diluent (diluent contains benzyl alcohol); swirl vial with gentle rotary motion; do not shake

Tev-Tropin®: Reconstitute with 1-5 mL NS (bacteriostatic NS is provided; NS without preservative may be used in neonates); swirl gently; do not shake. Cloudiness may occur when stored in the refrigerator after reconstitution. Allow solution to warm to room temperature. If cloudiness persists, do not use.

Zorbtive®: Reconstitute each 4 mg, 5 mg, or 6 mg vial with 0.5 mL or 1 mL preservative free SWI; reconstitute 8.8 mg vial with 1 mL or 2 mL diluent (contains benzyl alcohol)

Note: When treating chronic renal insufficiency patients, growth hormone should be administered as follows: in hemodialysis patients, administer injection at night just prior to sleeping and at least 3-4 hours after dialysis; in chronic cycling peritoneal dialysis patients, administer injection in the morning after dialysis; in chronic ambulatory peritoneal dialysis patients administer injection in the evening at the time of the overnight exchange.

Monitoring Parameters Growth curve, periodic thyroid function tests, bone age (annually), periodical urine testing for glucose, somatomedin C levels; fundoscopic exams; progression of scoliosis and clinical evidence of slipped capital femoral epiphysis such as a limp or hip or knee pain

Dosage Forms Excipient information presented when available (limited, particularly for generics); consult specific product labeling. [DSC] = Discontinued product

Solution, Subcutaneous:
Norditropin FlexPro: 5 mg/1.5 mL (1.5 mL); 10 mg/1.5 mL (1.5 mL); 15 mg/1.5 mL (1.5 mL) [contains phenol]
Norditropin NordiFlex Pen: 30 mg/3 mL (3 mL) [contains phenol]
Nutropin AQ NuSpin 5: 5 mg/2 mL (2 mL) [contains phenol]
Nutropin AQ NuSpin 10: 10 mg/2 mL (2 mL) [contains phenol]
Nutropin AQ NuSpin 20: 20 mg/2 mL (2 mL) [contains phenol]
Nutropin AQ Pen: 10 mg/2 mL (2 mL)
Nutropin AQ Pen: 20 mg/2 mL (2 mL) [contains phenol]
Omnitrope: 5 mg/1.5 mL (1.5 mL) [contains benzyl alcohol]
Omnitrope: 10 mg/1.5 mL (1.5 mL) [contains phenol]
Solution Reconstituted, Injection:
Humatrope: 5 mg (1 ea)
Humatrope: 6 mg (1 ea); 12 mg (1 ea); 24 mg (1 ea) [contains glycerin, metacresol]
Saizen: 5 mg (1 ea); 8.8 mg (1 ea)
Saizen Click.Easy: 8.8 mg (1 ea)
Solution Reconstituted, Subcutaneous:
Genotropin: 5 mg (1 ea); 12 mg (1 ea) [contains metacresol]
Nutropin: 10 mg (1 ea [DSC]) [contains benzyl alcohol]
Omnitrope: 5.8 mg (1 ea)
Serostim: 4 mg (1 ea); 5 mg (1 ea); 6 mg (1 ea)
Tev-Tropin: 5 mg (1 ea)
Zorbtive: 8.8 mg (1 ea) [contains benzyl alcohol]
Solution Reconstituted, Subcutaneous [preservative free]:
Genotropin MiniQuick: 0.2 mg (1 ea); 0.4 mg (1 ea); 0.6 mg (1 ea); 0.8 mg (1 ea); 1 mg (1 ea); 1.2 mg (1 ea); 1.4 mg (1 ea); 1.6 mg (1 ea); 1.8 mg (1 ea); 2 mg (1 ea)

References

Cohen P, Rogol AD, Deal CL, et al, "Consensus Statement on the Diagnosis and Treatment of Children With Idiopathic Short Stature: A Summary of the Growth Hormone Research Society, the Lawson Wilkins Pediatric Endocrine Society, and the European Society for Paediatric Endocrinology Workshop," *J Clin Endocrinol Metab*, 2008, 93(11):4210-7.

Gharib H, Cook DM, Saenger PH, et al, "American Association of Clinical Endocrinologists Medical Guidelines for Clinical Practice for Growth Hormone Use in Adults and Children - 2003 Update," *Endocr Pract*, 2003, 9(1):64-76.

Howrie DL, "Growth Hormone for the Treatment of Growth Failure in Children," *Clin Pharm*, 1987, 6(4):283-91.

Molitch ME, Clemmons DR, Malozowski S, et al, "Evaluation and Treatment of Adult Growth Hormone Deficiency: An Endocrine Society Clinical Practice Guideline," *J Clin Endocrinol Metab*, 2006, 91 (5):1621-34.

◆ **Sominex [OTC]** *see* DiphenhydrAMINE (Systemic) *on page 673*

◆ **Sominex® (Can)** *see* DiphenhydrAMINE (Systemic) *on page 673*

◆ **Sominex Maximum Strength [OTC]** *see* DiphenhydrAMINE (Systemic) *on page 673*

◆ **Som Pam (Can)** *see* Flurazepam *on page 907*

◆ **Soothe® [OTC]** *see* Artificial Tears *on page 205*

◆ **Soothe & Cool INZO Antifungal [OTC]** *see* Miconazole (Topical) *on page 1410*

◆ **Soothe® Hydration [OTC]** *see* Artificial Tears *on page 205*

Sorbitol (SOR bi tole)

Therapeutic Category Laxative, Hyperosmolar; Laxative, Osmotic

Generic Availability (U.S.) Yes

Use
Solution:
Oral: Hyperosmotic laxative; sweetening agent (OTC product: FDA approved in ages ≥12 years and adults); has also been used as a humectant; facilitates the passage of charcoal-toxin complex through the intestinal tract
Rectal: Hyperosmotic laxative (OTC product: FDA approved in ages ≥12 years and adults); has also been used as a humectant; facilitates the passage of charcoal-toxin complex through the intestinal tract
Irrigation solution: Genitourinary irrigant in transurethral prostatic resection or other transurethral resection or other transurethral surgical procedures; irrigant for indwelling catheter to maintain patency (FDA approved in adults)

Pregnancy Risk Factor C

Pregnancy Considerations Animal reproduction studies have not been conducted.

Breast-Feeding Considerations The manufacturer recommends that caution be exercised when administering sorbitol to nursing women.

Contraindications Hypersensitivity to sorbitol or any component
Solution: Abdominal pain, nausea, vomiting
Management of ingestions (poisonous): Absent bowel sounds, recent abdominal/rectal trauma, recent bowel surgery, intestinal obstruction, intestinal perforation; volume depletion, hypotension or significant electrolyte imbalance (AACT/EAPCCT, 2004)
Irrigation solution: Anuria

Warnings Large doses may cause fluid shifts and electrolyte imbalances. For the management of acute ingestions, administration of sorbitol with charcoal is not routinely recommended and if used, therapy should be limited (eg, single dose) to prevent excessive fluid and electrolyte losses; excessive amounts of activated charcoal with sorbitol may cause hypernatremic dehydration in pediatric patients. Current toxicologic data does not support the use of charcoal/sorbitol combination to reduce the bioavailability of ingested drugs nor improve the outcome of poisoned patients (AACT/EAPCCT, 2004).

Precautions Use with caution in infants; other causes of constipation should be evaluated prior to initiating therapy. Use with caution in patients with renal impairment, severe cardiopulmonary disease, dehydration, electrolyte imbalance, and in patients unable to metabolize sorbitol.

Adverse Reactions
Cardiovascular: Edema
Endocrine & metabolic: Fluid and electrolyte losses, hyperglycemia, lactic acidosis
Gastrointestinal: Abdominal discomfort, diarrhea, dry mouth, nausea, vomiting, xerostomia

Drug Interactions
Metabolism/Transport Effects None known.
Avoid Concomitant Use
Avoid concomitant use of Sorbitol with any of the following: Calcium Polystyrene Sulfonate; Sodium Polystyrene Sulfonate
Increased Effect/Toxicity
Sorbitol may increase the levels/effects of: Calcium Polystyrene Sulfonate; Sodium Polystyrene Sulfonate

Decreased Effect There are no known significant interactions involving a decrease in effect.

Stability
Solution: Store at 15°C to 30°C (59°F to 86°F); do not freeze; below 15°C (59°F) cloudiness and thickening may occur; warming will restore clarity and fluidity without affecting product quality
Irrigation solution: Store at 25°C; brief exposure to 40°C does not adversely affect the product. Avoid excessive heat.

Mechanism of Action A polyalcoholic sugar with osmotic cathartic actions

Pharmacokinetics (Adult data unless noted)
Absorption: Oral, rectal: Poor
Metabolism: Mainly in the liver to fructose

Dosing: Usual
Infants, Children, and Adolescents:
Constipation, chronic: Oral: 70% solution: 1-3 mL/kg/day in divided doses, usually twice daily (NASPGHAN, 2006)
Hyperosmotic laxative, intermittent use: Note: Usually as single dose, at infrequent intervals:
Children 2-11 years:
Oral: 70% solution: 2 mL/kg
Rectal enema: 25% to 30% solution: 30-60 mL once daily as needed
Children ≥12 years and Adolescents:
Oral: 70% solution: 30-150 mL
Rectal enema: 25% to 30% solution: 120 mL once daily as needed
Toxic ingestion, adjunct with charcoal: Children ≥1 year and Adolescents: Oral: 35% solution: 4.3 mL/kg; **Note:** Current guidelines recommend limiting use to a single dose administered with the initial charcoal dose of 1 g/kg (AACT/EAPCCT, 2004).
Adults:
Hyperosmotic laxative (as single dose, at infrequent intervals):
Oral: 70% solution: 30-150 mL
Rectal enema: 25% to 30% solution: 120 mL
Transurethral surgical procedures: Irrigation: Topical: 3% to 3.3% as transurethral surgical procedure irrigation

Monitoring Parameters Fluid status, serum electrolytes (changes may be delayed due to slow absorption)

Dosage Forms Excipient information presented when available (limited, particularly for generics); consult specific product labeling.
Solution, Irrigation:
Generic: 3% (3000 mL); 3.3% (2000 mL, 4000 mL)
Solution, Oral:
Generic: 70% (30 mL, 473 mL, 474 mL, 480 mL, 3840 mL)

References
American Academy of Clinical Toxicology and European Association of Poisons Centres and Clinical Toxicologists, "Position Paper: Cathartics," *J Toxicol Clin Toxicol*, 2004, 42(3):243–53.
American Academy of Clinical Toxicology and European Association of Poison Centres and Clinical Toxicologists,"Position Statement and Practice Guidelines on the Use of Multi-dose Activated Charcoal in the Treatment of Acute Poisoning," *J Toxicol Clin Toxicol*, 1999, 37 (6):731–51.
Charney EB and Bodurtha JN, "Intractable Diarrhea Associated With the Use of Sorbitol," *J Pediatr*, 1981, 98:157-8.
James LP, Nichols MH, and King WD, "A Comparison of Cathartics in Pediatric Ingestions," *Pediatrics*, 1995, 96(2 Pt 1):235-8.
Kumar A, Weatherly MR, and Beaman DC, "Sweeteners, Flavorings, and Dyes in Antibiotic Preparations," *Pediatrics*, 1991, 87(3):352-60.
North American Society for Pediatric Gastroenterology, Hepatology and Nutrition, "Evaluation and Treatment of Constipation in Infants and Children: Recommendations of the North American Society for Pediatric Gastroenterology, Hepatology and Nutrition," *J Pediatr Gastroenterol Nutr*, 2006, 43(3):1-13.

◆ **Sorbulax [OTC]** *see* Psyllium *on page 1773*
◆ **Sore Throat Relief [OTC]** *see* Benzocaine *on page 273*

◆ **Sorine** *see* Sotalol *on page 1925*

Sotalol (SOE ta lole)

Medication Safety Issues
Sound-alike/look-alike issues:
Sotalol may be confused with Stadol, Sudafed
Betapace may be confused with Betapace AF
BEERS Criteria medication:
This drug may be potentially inappropriate for use in geriatric patients (Quality of evidence - high; Strength of recommendation - strong).

Related Information
Adult ACLS Algorithms *on page 2198*
Brand Names: U.S. Betapace; Betapace AF; Sorine
Brand Names: Canada Apo-Sotalol; CO Sotalol; Dom-Sotalol; Med-Sotalol; Mylan-Sotalol; Novo-Sotalol; Nu-Sotalol; PHL-Sotalol; PMS-Sotalol; PRO-Sotalol; ratio-Sotalol; Rhoxal-sotalol; Riva-Sotalol; Rylosol; Sandoz-Sotalol; ZYM-Sotalol
Therapeutic Category Antiarrhythmic Agent, Class II; Antiarrhythmic Agent, Class III; Beta-Adrenergic Blocker
Generic Availability (U.S.) Yes
Use
Betapace®, Sorine®, generic: Treatment of life-threatening ventricular arrhythmias (eg, sustained ventricular tachycardia) (Betapace®: FDA approved in ages ≥3 days and adults; Sorine®, generic: FDA approved in adults)
Betapace AF®: Maintenance of normal sinus rhythm in patients who have highly symptomatic atrial fibrillation and atrial flutter, but who are currently in normal sinus rhythm [not usually for use in patients with paroxysmal atrial fibrillation/flutter that is easily reversed (eg, by Valsalva maneuver)] (FDA approved in ages ≥3 days and adults)
Note: Do not substitute Betapace AF® for other products (and vice versa); significant differences in FDA approved labeling exist [eg, dosage and administration, safety information and patient package insert (Betapace AF® labeling contains a patient package insert specific for atrial fibrillation/flutter)]
Injection: Substitution for oral sotalol in those who are unable to take sotalol orally (FDA approved in ages ≥3 years and adults); used in adult ACLS algorithm for hemodynamically stable monomorphic ventricular tachycardia

Pregnancy Risk Factor B
Pregnancy Considerations Adverse events were not observed in the initial animal reproduction studies; therefore, the manufacturer classifies sotalol as pregnancy category B. Sotalol crosses the placenta and is found in amniotic fluid. In a cohort study, an increased risk of cardiovascular defects was observed following maternal use of beta-blockers during pregnancy. Intrauterine growth restriction (IUGR), small placentas, as well as fetal/neonatal bradycardia, hypoglycemia, and/or respiratory depression have been observed following in utero exposure to beta-blockers as a class. Adequate facilities for monitoring infants at birth should be available. Untreated chronic maternal hypertension and pre-eclampsia are also associated with adverse events in the fetus, infant, and mother; however, sotalol is currently not recommended for the initial treatment of hypertension in pregnancy. Because sotalol crosses the placenta in concentrations similar to the maternal serum, it has been used for the treatment of fetal atrial flutter or fetal supraventricular tachycardia without hydrops. The clearance of sotalol is increased during the third trimester of pregnancy, but other pharmacokinetic parameters do not significantly differ from nonpregnant values.

Breast-Feeding Considerations Sotalol is excreted into breast milk in concentrations higher than those found in the maternal serum. Although adverse events in nursing infants have not been observed in case reports, close monitoring for bradycardia, hypotension, respiratory distress, and hypoglycemia is advised. According to the manufacturer, the decision to continue or discontinue breast-feeding during therapy should take into account the risk of exposure to the infant and the benefits of treatment to the mother.

Contraindications Hypersensitivity to sotalol or any component; sinus bradycardia; second or third degree AV heart block (except in patients with a functioning artificial pacemaker); congenital or acquired long QT syndromes; uncontrolled heart failure; cardiogenic shock; asthma

Additional contraindications: Betapace AF® and the injectable formulation: Baseline QT$_c$ interval >450 msec; bronchospastic conditions; CrCl <40 mL/minute; serum potassium <4 mEq/L; sick sinus syndrome (except in patients with a functioning artificial pacemaker)

Warnings Initiation, reinitiation, and dosage increases of sotalol must occur in a facility that can provide continuous ECG monitoring, recognition and treatment of life-threatening arrhythmias, and CPR **[U.S. Boxed Warning]**. Patients must be monitored with continuous ECG for a minimum of 3 days (on their maintenance dose). Use with caution and adjust the dose in patients with renal impairment; creatinine clearance must be calculated prior to dosing.

May cause serious and life-threatening proarrhythmias [may cause or worsen ventricular arrhythmias (eg, sustained ventricular tachycardia, torsade de pointes, ventricular fibrillation)] **[U.S. Boxed Warning]**; risk factors for torsade de pointes include: Higher sotalol doses, presence of sustained VT, female gender, excessive prolongation of the QT$_c$ interval, history of heart failure or cardiomegaly, decreased renal function, hypokalemia, hypomagnesemia, and bradycardia; monitor ECG for proarrhythmic effects; adjust dose to prevent QT$_c$ prolongation; correct electrolyte imbalances (especially hypokalemia and hypomagnesemia) before initiating sotalol. Do not initiate I.V. therapy if baseline QT$_c$ interval is >450 msec; if QT$_c$ exceeds 500 msec during therapy, reduce the dose, prolong the infusion duration, or discontinue use **[U.S. Boxed Warning]**.

Bradycardia, heart block, or hypotension may occur. Use oral formulation only with extreme caution in patients with sick sinus syndrome; do not use I.V. product in patients with sick sinus syndrome unless functioning artificial pacemaker is present. May cause or worsen heart failure (use with caution in patients with compensated heart failure); use with caution and titrate dose carefully within the first 2 weeks post-MI (experience is limited); use with caution in patients with peripheral vascular disease (may aggravate arterial insufficiency). Concomitant use with other drugs that prolong the QT interval (eg, Class I and Class III antiarrhythmics, phenothiazines, tricyclic antidepressants, and certain oral macrolide and quinolone antibiotics) or prolong refractoriness (eg, disopyramide, quinidine, procainamide, and amiodarone) is not recommended; Class I or Class III antiarrhythmic agents should be withheld for at least three half-lives prior to starting sotalol.

Exacerbation of angina, arrhythmias, and in some cases MI may occur following abrupt discontinuation of beta-blockers; avoid abrupt discontinuation, wean slowly, monitor for signs and symptoms of ischemia. Beta-blockers should generally be avoided in patients with bronchospastic disease; if administered, use the lowest possible dose and monitor patients carefully. Patients receiving beta-blockers, who have a history of anaphylactic reactions, may be more reactive to a repeated allergen challenge and may not be responsive to the usual epinephrine doses used to treat an allergic reaction. Beta-blockers may block hypoglycemia-induced tachycardia and blood pressure

changes; use with caution in patients with diabetes mellitus. May mask signs of thyrotoxicosis. Use caution with anesthetic agents that decrease myocardial function.

Precautions Use with caution in patients receiving calcium channel blockers.

Adverse Reactions

Cardiovascular: Angina pectoris, bradycardia (dose related), cardiac failure, cardiovascular signs and symptoms, cerebrovascular accident, chest pain, ECG abnormality, edema, hypertension, hypotension, palpitations, peripheral vascular disease, presyncope, proarrhythmia, prolonged Q-T interval on ECG (dose related), syncope, torsades de pointes (dose related), vasodilation, worsened ventricular tachycardia

Central nervous system: Anxiety, confusion, depression, dizziness, fatigue (dose related), headache, impaired consciousness, insomnia, mood changes, sensation of cold, sleep disorder

Dermatologic: Diaphoresis, hyperhidrosis, skin rash

Endocrine & metabolic: Sexual disorder, weight changes

Gastrointestinal: Abdominal distention, abdominal pain, change in appetite, colonic disease, decreased appetite, diarrhea, dyspepsia, flatulence, nausea and vomiting, stomach pain

Genitourinary: Genitourinary complaint, impotence

Hematologic & oncologic: Hemorrhage

Infection: Infection, influenza

Local: Local pain

Neuromuscular & skeletal: Back pain, limb pain, musculoskeletal chest pain, musculoskeletal pain, weakness

Ophthalmic: Visual disturbance

Respiratory: Asthma, dyspnea (dose related), pulmonary disease, tracheobronchitis, upper respiratory complaint

Miscellaneous: AICD discharge, fever, laboratory test abnormality

Rare but important or life-threatening: Alopecia, bronchiolitis obliterans organizing pneumonia, crusted skin (red), eosinophilia, hypersensitivity angiitis, increased liver enzymes, increased serum transaminases, leukopenia, paralysis, phlebitis, pruritus, pulmonary edema, Raynaud's phenomenon, retroperitoneal fibrosis, serum transaminases increased, skin necrosis (after extravasation), skin photosensitivity, thrombocytopenia

Drug Interactions

Metabolism/Transport Effects None known.

Avoid Concomitant Use

Avoid concomitant use of Sotalol with any of the following: Beta2-Agonists; Ceritinib; Fingolimod; Floctafenine; Highest Risk QTc-Prolonging Agents; Ivabradine; Methacholine; Mifepristone; Moderate Risk QTc-Prolonging Agents; Propafenone

Increased Effect/Toxicity

Sotalol may increase the levels/effects of: Alpha-/Beta-Agonists (Direct-Acting); Alpha1-Blockers; Alpha2-Agonists; Amifostine; Antihypertensives; Antipsychotic Agents (Phenothiazines); Bradycardia-Causing Agents; Bupivacaine; Cardiac Glycosides; Ceritinib; Cholinergic Agonists; DULoxetine; Ergot Derivatives; Grass Pollen Allergen Extract (5 Grass Extract); Highest Risk QTc-Prolonging Agents; Hypotensive Agents; Insulin; Lidocaine (Systemic); Lidocaine (Topical); Mepivacaine; Methacholine; Midodrine; Obinutuzumab; RiTUXimab; Sulfonylureas

The levels/effects of Sotalol may be increased by: Acetylcholinesterase Inhibitors; Alpha2-Agonists; Aminoquinolines (Antimalarial); Anilidopiperidine Opioids; Antipsychotic Agents (Phenothiazines); Barbiturates; Brimonidine (Topical); Calcium Channel Blockers (Dihydropyridine); Calcium Channel Blockers (Nondihydropyridine); Diazoxide; Dipyridamole; Fingolimod; Floctafenine; Herbs (Hypotensive Properties); Ivabradine; Lidocaine (Topical); MAO Inhibitors; Mifepristone;

Moderate Risk QTc-Prolonging Agents; Pentoxifylline; Phosphodiesterase 5 Inhibitors; Propafenone; Prostacyclin Analogues; QTc-Prolonging Agents (Indeterminate Risk and Risk Modifying); Regorafenib; Reserpine

Decreased Effect

Sotalol may decrease the levels/effects of: Beta2-Agonists; Theophylline Derivatives

The levels/effects of Sotalol may be decreased by: Barbiturates; Herbs (Hypertensive Properties); Methylphenidate; Nonsteroidal Anti-Inflammatory Agents; Rifamycin Derivatives; Yohimbine

Food Interactions Sotalol peak serum concentrations may be decreased if taken with food. Management: Administer without regard to meals.

Stability

Tablets and injection: Store at controlled room temperature 25°C (77°F); excursions permitted to 15°C to 30°C (59°F to 86°F)

Tablets: Dispense in tight, light-resistant container

Injection: Protect from light; do not freeze. Stable in D_5W, NS, or lactated ringers.

Mechanism of Action

Beta-blocker which contains both beta-adrenoreceptor-blocking (Vaughan Williams Class II) and cardiac action potential duration prolongation (Vaughan Williams Class III) properties

Class II effects: Increased sinus cycle length, slowed heart rate, decreased AV nodal conduction, and increased AV nodal refractoriness Sotalol has both beta$_1$- and beta$_2$-receptor blocking activity. The beta-blocking effect of sotalol is a noncardioselective (half maximal at about 80 mg/day and maximal at doses of 320-640 mg/day). Significant beta-blockade occurs at oral doses as low as 25 mg/day.

Class III effects: Prolongation of the atrial and ventricular monophasic action potentials, and effective refractory prolongation of atrial muscle, ventricular muscle, and atrioventricular accessory pathways in both the antegrade and retrograde directions. Sotalol is a racemic mixture of *d*- and *l*-sotalol; both isomers have similar Class III antiarrhythmic effects while the *l*-isomer is responsible for virtually all of the beta-blocking activity. The Class III effects are seen only at oral doses ≥160 mg/day

Pharmacodynamics Onset of action: Oral: Rapid: 1-2 hours; when administered I.V. for ongoing VT over 5 minutes, onset of action is ~5-10 minutes (Ho, 1994)

Pharmacokinetics (Adult data unless noted)

Distribution: Poor penetration across blood-brain barrier; distributes into breast milk; breast milk to plasma ratio: 2.2-8.8 (mean: 5.4) (O'Hare, 1980)

Protein binding: Sotalol is not protein bound

Metabolism: Sotalol is not metabolized

Bioavailability: Oral: 90% to 100%

Half-life (mean):

Neonates ≤1 month: 8.4 hours

Infants and children >1 month to 24 months: 7.4 hours

Children >2 years to <7 years: 9.1 hours

Children 7-12 years: 9.2 hours

Adults: 12 hours

Adults with renal failure (anuric): Up to 69 hours

Time to peak serum concentration: Oral:

Children 4 days to 12 years: Mean: 2-3 hours

Adults: 2.5-4 hours

Elimination: Primarily as unchanged drug via the kidney

Clearance (apparent):

Neonates ≤1 month: 11 mL/minute

Infants and children >1 month to 24 months: 32 mL/minute

Children >2 years to <7 years: 63 mL/minute

Children 7-12 years: 95 mL/minute

Dialysis: Partially removed by hemodialysis; partial rebound in serum concentrations may occur following dialysis

Dosing: Neonatal Oral: **Note:** Baseline QT_c interval and CrCl must be determined prior to initiation. Dosage must be adjusted to individual response and tolerance; doses should be initiated or increased in a hospital facility that can provide continuous ECG monitoring, recognition and treatment of life-threatening arrhythmias, and CPR.

Note: Manufacturer's dosing recommendations are based on doses per m^2 (that are equivalent to the doses recommended in adults) and on pediatric pharmacokinetic and pharmacodynamic studies (Saul, 2001; Saul, 2001a). BSA, rather than body weight, better predicted apparent clearance of sotalol; however, for a given dose per m^2, a larger drug exposure (larger AUC) and greater pharmacologic effects were observed in smaller subjects (ie, those with BSA <0.33 m^2 versus those with BSA ≥0.33 m^2). For infants and children ≤2 years of age, the manufacturer recommends a dosage reduction based on an age factor determined from a graph (see below).

Manufacturer's recommendations: **Note:** Use with extreme caution if QT_c is >500 msec while receiving sotalol; reduce the dose or discontinue drug if QT_c >550 msec.

The manufacturer recommended pediatric dosage of 30 mg/m²/dose given 3 times/day must be **REDUCED** by an age-related factor that is obtained from the graph (see graph). First, obtain the patient's age in months; use the graph to determine where the patient's age (on the logarithmic scale) intersects the age factor curve; read the age factor from the Y-axis; then multiply the age factor by the pediatric dose listed below (ie, the dose for children >2 years); this will result in the proper reduction in dose for age. For example, the age factor for a neonate (PNA: 14 days) is 0.5, so the initial dosage would be (0.5 x 30 mg/m²/dose) = 15 mg/m²/dose given 3 times daily. Similar calculations should be made for dosage titrations; increase dosage gradually, if needed; allow adequate time between dosage increments to achieve new steady-state and to monitor clinical response, heart rate and QT_c intervals; half-life is prolonged with decreasing age (<2 years), so time to reach new steady-state will increase; for example, the time to reach steady-state in a neonate may be ≥1 week.

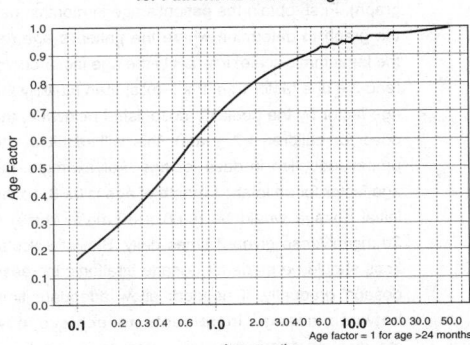

**Sotalol Age Factor Nomogram
for Patients ≤2 Years of Age**

Adapted from U.S. Food and Drug Administration.
http://www.fda.gov/cder/foi/label/2001/2115s3lbl.PDF

Alternative dosing:

Initial: 2 mg/kg/day divided every 8 hours; if needed, increase dosage gradually by 1-2 mg/kg/day increments; allow at least 3 days between dosage increments to achieve new steady-state and to monitor clinical response, heart rate, and QT_c intervals (Läer, 2005)

Proposed required dose: 4 mg/kg/day divided every 8 hours; **Note:** It is not necessary to increase to required dosage if desired clinical effect has been achieved at a lower dosage

Dosing: Usual

Oral: **Note:** Baseline QT_c interval and CrCl must be determined prior to initiation. Dosage must be adjusted to individual response and tolerance; doses should be initiated or increased in a hospital facility that can provide continuous ECG monitoring, recognition and treatment of life-threatening arrhythmias, and CPR:

Infants and Children: Manufacturer's dosing recommendations are based on doses per m² (that are equivalent to the doses recommended in adults) and on pediatric pharmacokinetic and pharmacodynamic studies (Saul, 2001; Saul, 2001a). BSA, rather than body weight, better predicted apparent clearance of sotalol; however, for a given dose per m², a larger drug exposure (larger AUC) and greater pharmacologic effects were observed in smaller subjects (ie, those with BSA <0.33 m² versus those with BSA ≥0.33 m²). For infants and children ≤2 years of age, the manufacturer recommends a dosage reduction based on an age factor determined from a graph (see below).

Manufacturer's recommendations: **Note:** Use with extreme caution if QT_c is >500 msec while receiving sotalol; reduce the dose or discontinue drug if QT_c >550 msec.

Infants and Children ≤2 years: The manufacturer recommended pediatric dosage of 30 mg/m²/dose 3 times/day must be **REDUCED** using an age-related factor that is obtained from the graph (see graph). First, obtain the patient's age in months; use the graph to determine where the patient's age (on the logarithmic scale) intersects the age factor curve; read the age factor from the Y-axis; then multiply the age factor by the pediatric dose listed below (ie, the dose for children >2 years); this will result in the proper reduction in dose for age. For example, the age factor for an infant 1 month of age is 0.68, so the initial dosage would be (0.68 x 30 mg/m²/dose) = 20 mg/m²/dose given 3 times daily. Similar calculations should be made for dosage titrations; increase dosage gradually, if needed; allow adequate time between dosage increments to achieve new steady-state and to monitor clinical response, heart rate and QT_c intervals; half-life is prolonged with decreasing age (<2 years), so time to reach new steady-state will increase.

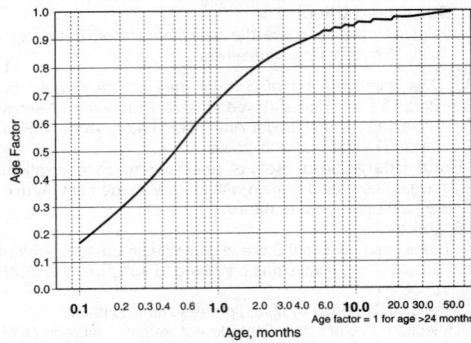

Sotalol Age Factor Nomogram for Patients ≤2 Years of Age

Adapted from U.S. Food and Drug Administration.
http://www.fda.gov/cder/foi/label/2001/2115s3lbl.PDF

Children >2 years: Initial: 30 mg/m²/dose given 3 times daily; increase dosage gradually if needed; allow at least 36 hours between dosage increments to achieve new steady-state and to monitor clinical response, heart rate, and QT_c intervals; may increase gradually to a maximum of 60 mg/m²/dose given 3 times daily

Alternative pediatric dosing:

Initial: 2 mg/kg/day divided every 8 hours; if needed, increase dosage gradually by 1-2 mg/kg/day increments; allow 3 days between dosage increments to achieve new steady-state and to monitor clinical response, heart rate, and QT_c intervals; maximum: 10 mg/kg/day (if no limiting side effects occur) (Beaufort-Krol, 1997; Colloridi, 1992; Läer, 2005; Maragnes, 1992; Pfammatter, 1995; Pfammatter, 1997; Tipple, 1991); do not exceed adult doses

Proposed required doses: **Note:** It is not necessary to increase to required dosage if desired clinical effect has been achieved at a lower dosage.

Infants and Children 1 month to 6 years: 6 mg/kg/day divided every 8 hours

Children >6 years: 4 mg/kg/day divided every 8 hours

Adults:

Ventricular arrhythmias (Betapace®, Sorine®, generic) (**Note:** Use with extreme caution if QT_c is >500 msec while receiving sotalol; reduce the dose or discontinue drug if QT_c >550 msec): Initial: 80 mg twice daily; increase dosage gradually if needed; allow 3 days between dosage increments to achieve new steady-state and to determine maximum effects on QT interval; may increase gradually to 240-320 mg/day in 2 divided doses; usual effective dose: 160-320 mg/day given in 2-3 divided doses; **Note:** Doses as high as 480-640 mg/day may be required in some patients with life-threatening refractory ventricular arrhythmias; however, potential benefit must outweigh increased risk of adverse effects (eg, proarrhythmias).

Atrial fibrillation or atrial flutter (Betapace AF®): [**Note:** If baseline QT interval is >450 msec, do not initiate therapy. During initiation and dose titration, if the QT interval is ≥500 msec, reduce the dose or discontinue the drug. During maintenance therapy, monitor the QT interval regularly; if the QT interval is ≥520 msec, reduce the dose or discontinue the drug]: Initial: 80 mg twice daily; increase dosage gradually after 3 days, if needed [ie, if frequency of relapses of atrial fibrillation/flutter is not reduced and the dose is toler-ated without excessive QT prolongation (ie, if QT interval is <520 msec)]; allow 3 days between dosage increments to achieve new steady-state and to deter-mine maximum effects on QT interval; reduce the dose or discontinue the drug if the QT interval is ≥500 msec; dose may be increased to 120 mg twice daily (usual effective dose); the dosage may be further increased to 160 mg twice daily if response is inad-equate and the dose is tolerated without excessive QT prolongation; maximum dose: 160 mg twice daily.

I.V.: Adults: Note: Baseline QT_c interval and CrCl must be determined prior to initiation. The effects of the initial I.V. dose must be monitored and the dose titrated either upward or downward, if needed, based on clinical effect, QT_c interval, or adverse reactions. Doses should be initiated or increased in a hospital facility that can provide continuous ECG monitoring, recognition, and treatment of life-threatening arrhythmias, and CPR:

Conversion from oral sotalol to I.V. sotalol:
80 mg oral equivalent to 75 mg I.V.
120 mg oral equivalent to 112.5 mg I.V.
160 mg oral equivalent to 150 mg I.V.

Ventricular arrhythmias:
Substitution for oral sotalol: Initial dose: 75 mg infused over 5 hours twice daily
Dose adjustment: If the frequency of relapse does not reduce and excessive QT_c prolongation does not occur, may increase to 112.5 mg twice daily. For ventricular arrhythmias, may increase dose every 3 days in increments of 75 mg/day.
Dose range: Usual therapeutic dose: 75-150 mg twice daily; maximum dose: 300 mg twice daily

Hemodynamically stable monomorphic VT, ongoing: 1.5 mg/kg over 5 minutes (ACLS, 2010); Note: One clinical trial employed standard dose of 100 mg (Ho, 1994).

Atrial fibrillation or atrial flutter:
Substitution for oral sotalol: Initial dose: 75 mg infused over 5 hours twice daily
Dose adjustment: If the frequency of relapse does not reduce and excessive QT_c prolongation does not occur, may increase to 112.5 mg twice daily. For ventricular arrhythmias, may increase dose every 3 days in increments of 75 mg/day.
Dose range: Usual therapeutic dose: 112.5 mg twice daily; maximum dose: 150 mg twice daily

Dosing adjustment in renal impairment:
Children: Dosing in children with renal impairment has not been investigated; use lower doses or increased dosing intervals; closely monitor clinical response, heart rate and QT_c interval; allow adequate time between dosage increments to achieve new steady-state, since half-life will be prolonged with renal impairment

Adults: Administer the initial dose (ie, 80 mg) and sub-sequent doses at the following intervals:
Ventricular arrhythmias (Betapace®, Sorine®, generic):
CrCl >60 mL/minute: Administer every 12 hours
CrCl 30-60 mL/minute: Administer every 24 hours
CrCl 10-29 mL/minute: Administer every 36-48 hours
CrCl <10 mL/minute: Individualize dose
Atrial fibrillation/flutter (Betapace AF®):
CrCl >60 mL/minute: Administer every 12 hours
CrCl 40-60 mL/minute: Administer every 24 hours
CrCl <40 mL/minute: Use is contraindicated (per product labeling)
Note: The manufacturer of the injectable formulation recommends adjustment similar to that used for Beta-pace AF®; however, the injectable formulation may be used for either indication.
Note: Due to the prolonged half-life in patients with renal dysfunction, allow at least 5-6 doses (at the above

recommended interval) between dosage increments to achieve a new steady-state and to monitor QT intervals
Dosing adjustment in hepatic impairment: Not needed

Administration
Oral: May be administered without regard to meals, but should be administered at the same time each day
I.V.:
Substitution for oral: Dilute in NS, D_5W, or LR to final concentration of 0.75-1.5 mg/mL and infuse over 5 hours
Hemodynamically stable monomorphic VT: Administer I.V. push over 5 minutes; use with caution due to increased risk of adverse events (eg, bradycardia, hypotension, torsades de pointes) (ACLS, 2010)

Monitoring Parameters Continuous ECG for a minimum of 3 days with initiation of therapy or dosage increase, QT interval, heart rate, renal function, serum potassium, and magnesium
Betapace AF®: In addition, during initiation and dosage titration, monitor the QT interval 2-4 hours after each dose.
Injectable formulation: Monitor QT interval after completion of each infusion.

Test Interactions May falsely increase urinary metanephr-ine values when fluorimetric or photometric methods are used; does not interact with HPLC assay with solid phase extraction for determination of urinary catecholamines

Additional Information Betapace AF®: Do not discharge patients from the hospital within 12 hours of electrical or pharmacological conversion from atrial fibrillation/flutter to normal sinus rhythm.

Dosage Forms Excipient information presented when available (limited, particularly for generics); consult specific product labeling.
Tablet, Oral, as hydrochloride:
Betapace: 80 mg, 120 mg, 160 mg [scored]
Betapace AF: 80 mg, 120 mg, 160 mg [scored]
Sorine: 80 mg, 120 mg, 160 mg, 240 mg [scored]
Generic: 80 mg, 120 mg, 160 mg, 240 mg

Extemporaneous Preparations A 5 mg/mL sotalol syrup may be made with Betapace, Sorine, or Betapace AF tablets and Simple Syrup containing sodium benzoate 0.1% (Syrup, NF). Place 120 mL Syrup, NF in a 6-ounce amber plastic (polyethylene terephthalate) prescription bottle; add five Betapace, Sorine, or Betapace AF 120 mg tablets and shake the bottle to wet the tablets. Allow tablets to hydrate for at least 2 hours, then shake intermittently over ≥2 hours until the tablets are completely disintegrated; a dispersion of fine particles (water-insoluble inactive ingredients) in syrup should be obtained. Note: To simplify the disintegration process, tablets can hydrate overnight; tablets may also be crushed, carefully trans-ferred into the bottle and shaken well until a dispersion of fine particles in syrup is obtained. Label "shake well". Stable for 3 months at 15°C to 30°C (59°F to 86°F) and ambient humidity.

Betapace prescribing information, Bayer HealthCare Pharmaceuticals Inc, Wayne, NJ, 2011.
Betapace AF prescribing information, Bayer HealthCare Pharmaceut-icals Inc, Wayne, NJ, 2011.
Sorine prescribing information, Upsher-Smith, Minneapolis, MN, 2012.

References
Beaufort-Krol GC and Bink-Boelkens MT, "Effectiveness of Sotalol for Atrial Flutter in Children After Surgery for Congenital Heart Disease," Am J Cardiol, 1997, 79(1):92-4.
Colloridi V, Perri C, Ventriglia F, et al, "Oral Sotalol in Pediatric Atrial Ectopic Tachycardia," Am Heart J, 1992, 123(1):254-6.
Field JM, Hazinski MF, Sayre MR, et al, "Part 1: Executive Summary: 2010 American Heart Association Guidelines for Cardiopulmonary Resuscitation and Emergency Cardiovascular Care," Circulation, 2010, 122(18 Suppl 3):S640-56.
Ho DS, Zecchin RP, Richards DA, et al, "Double-Blind Trial of Ligno-caine Versus Sotalol for Acute Termination of Spontaneous Sustained Ventricular Tachycardia," Lancet, 1994, 344(8914):18-23.
Läer S, Elshoff JP, Meibohm B, et al, "Development of a Safe and Effective Pediatric Dosing Regimen for Sotalol Based on Population

Pharmacokinetics and Pharmacodynamics in Children With Supraventricular Tachycardia," *J Am Coll Cardiol*, 2005, 46(7):1322-30.

Maragnes P, Tipple M, and Fournier A, "Effectiveness of Oral Sotalol for Treatment of Pediatric Arrhythmias," *Am J Cardiol*, 1992, 69(8):751-4.

Neumar RW, Otto CW, Link MS, et al, "Part 8: Adult Advanced Cardiovascular Life Support: 2010 American Heart Association Guidelines for Cardiopulmonary Resuscitation and Emergency Cardiovascular Care," *Circulation*, 2010, 122(18 Suppl 3):S729-67.

O'Hare MF, Murnaghan GA, Russell CJ, et al, "Sotalol as a Hypotensive Agent in Pregnancy," *Br J Obstet Gynaecol*, 1980, 87(9):814-20.

Pfammatter JP and Paul T, "New Antiarrhythmic Drug in Pediatric Use: Sotalol," *Pediatr Cardiol*, 1997, 18(1):28-34.

Pfammatter JP, Paul T, Lehmann C, et al, "Efficacy and Proarrhythmia of Oral Sotalol in Pediatric Patients," *J Am Coll Cardiol*, 1995, 26 (4):1002-7.

Saul JP, Ross B, Schaffer MS, et al, "Pharmacokinetics and Pharmacodynamics of Sotalol in a Pediatric Population With Supraventricular and Ventricular Tachyarrhythmia," *Clin Pharmacol Ther*, 2001, 69 (3):145-57.

Saul JP, Schaffer MS, Karpawich PP, et al, "Single-Dose Pharmacokinetics of Sotalol in a Pediatric Population With Supraventricular and/or Ventricular Tachyarrhythmia," *J Clin Pharmacol*, 2001, 41(1):35-43.

Tanel RE, Walsh EP, Lulu JA, et al, "Sotalol for Refractory Arrhythmias in Pediatric and Young Adult Patients: Initial Efficacy and Long-Term Outcome," *Am Heart J*, 1995, 130(4):791-7.

Tipple M and Sandor G, "Efficacy and Safety of Oral Sotalol in Early Infancy," *Pacing Clin Electrophysiol*, 1991, 14(1 Pt 2):2062-5.

◆ **Sotalol Hydrochloride** *see* Sotalol *on page 1925*

◆ **SPA** *see* Albumin *on page 82*

◆ **SPD417** *see* CarBAMazepine *on page 372*

◆ **Spectracef** *see* Cefditoren *on page 397*

Spinosad (SPIN oh sad)

Brand Names: U.S. Natroba

Therapeutic Category Antiparasitic Agent, Topical; Pediculocide

Generic Availability (U.S.) Yes

Use Topical treatment of head lice (*Pediculosis capitis*) infestation (FDA approved in ages ≥4 years and adults)

Pregnancy Risk Factor B

Pregnancy Considerations Teratogenic effects were not observed in animal reproduction studies. Human studies did not assess the absorption of benzyl alcohol, an ingredient in the product.

Breast-Feeding Considerations Spinosad used topically is not systemically absorbed and will not be present in human milk. The suspension formulation does include benzyl alcohol, which may be systemically absorbed and may be excreted in human milk. Lactating women may choose to pump and discard breast milk for five benzyl alcohol half-lives (8 hours) after use to avoid ingestion of benzyl alcohol by an infant.

Contraindications Hypersensitivity to spinosad or any component

Warnings Topical lotion contains benzyl alcohol which may cause allergic reactions in susceptible individuals; large amounts of benzyl alcohol (≥99 mg/kg/day) have been associated with a potentially fatal toxicity ("gasping syndrome") in neonates; the "gasping syndrome" consists of metabolic acidosis, respiratory distress, gasping respirations, CNS dysfunction (including convulsions, intracranial hemorrhage), hypotension, and cardiovascular collapse; avoid use in neonates; *in vitro* and animal studies have shown that benzoate, a metabolite of benzyl alcohol, displaces bilirubin from protein binding sites.

Precautions For topical use on scalp and scalp hair only; not for oral, ophthalmic, or intravaginal use. Avoid contact with eyes; if contact occurs, rinse thoroughly with water. Wash hands after application. Avoid use in infants <6 months of age due to higher potential for increased absorption due to an immature skin barrier and high skin surface area to body mass ratio.

Adverse Reactions

Dermatologic: Application site erythema, application site irritation, skin irritation

Ocular: Erythema, hyperemia, irritation

Rare: Alopecia, application site reactions (dryness, exfoliation), dry skin

Drug Interactions

Metabolism/Transport Effects None known.

Avoid Concomitant Use There are no known interactions where it is recommended to avoid concomitant use.

Increased Effect/Toxicity There are no known significant interactions involving an increase in effect.

Decreased Effect There are no known significant interactions involving a decrease in effect.

Stability Store at 25°C (77°F); excursions permitted between 15°C to 30°C (59°F to 86°F).

Mechanism of Action Insect paralysis and death is caused by central nervous system excitation and involuntary muscle contractions. Spinosad is thought to be both pediculocidal and ovicidal (Stough, 2009).

Pharmacokinetics (Adult data unless noted) Absorption: Not absorbed topically [not detectable in a plasma sampling study of pediatric patients (4-15 years of age); absorption of the benzyl alcohol was not analyzed in the study].

Dosing: Usual Head lice: Infants ≥6 months, Children, Adolescents and Adults: Topical: Apply sufficient amount to cover dry scalp and completely cover dry hair (maximum dose: 120 mL); if live lice are seen after 7 days after first treatment, repeat with second application (Stough, 2009)

Administration For external use only. Shake bottle well. Apply to dry scalp and rub gently until the scalp is thoroughly moistened, then apply to dry hair, completely covering scalp and hair. Leave on for 10 minutes (start timing treatment after the scalp and hair have been completely covered). The hair should then be rinsed thoroughly with warm water. Shampoo may be used immediately after the product is completely rinsed off. If live lice are seen 7 days after the first treatment, repeat with second application. Avoid contact with the eyes; wash hands after use. Nit combing is not required, although a fine-tooth comb may be used to remove treated lice and nits from hair and scalp.

Dosage Forms Excipient information presented when available (limited, particularly for generics); consult specific product labeling.

Suspension, External:

Natroba: 0.9% (120 mL) [contains benzyl alcohol, cetearyl alcohol, fd&c yellow #6 (sunset yellow), isopropyl alcohol, propylene glycol]

Generic: 0.9% (120 mL)

References

Frankowski BL, Bocchini JA Jr, and Council on School Health and Committee on Infectious Diseases, "Head Lice," *Pediatrics*, 2010, 126 (2):392-403.

Stough D, Shellabarger S, Quiring J, et al, "Efficacy and Safety of Spinosad and Permethrin Creme Rinses for Pediculosis Capitis (Head Lice)," *Pediatrics*, 2009, 124(3):389-95.

Spironolactone (speer on oh LAK tone)

Medication Safety Issues

Sound-alike/look-alike issues:

Aldactone may be confused with Aldactazide

BEERS Criteria medication:

This drug may be potentially inappropriate for use in geriatric patients (Quality of evidence - moderate; Strength of recommendation - strong).

International issues:

Aldactone: Brand name for spironolactone [U.S., Canada, multiple international markets], but also the brand name for potassium canrenoate [Austria, Czech Republic, Germany, Hungary, Poland]

Brand Names: U.S. Aldactone

Brand Names: Canada Aldactone; Teva-Spironolactone

Therapeutic Category Antihypertensive Agent; Diuretic, Potassium Sparing

Generic Availability (U.S.) Yes

Use Management of edema associated with CHF, cirrhosis of the liver accompanied by edema or ascites, and nephrotic syndrome; treatment of primary hypertension, primary hyperaldosteronism, hypokalemia, and hirsutism; treatment of severe heart failure (NYHA class III-IV) to increase survival and reduce hospitalizations when used in addition to standard therapy

Pregnancy Risk Factor C

Pregnancy Considerations Adverse events were observed in some animal reproduction studies. The antiandrogen effects of spironolactone have been shown to cause feminization of the male fetus in animal studies. Spironolactone crosses the placenta (Regitz-Zagrosek, 2011).

The treatment of heart failure is generally the same in pregnant and nonpregnant women; however, spironolactone should be avoided in the first trimester due to its antiandrogenic effects (Regitz-Zagrosek, 2011). The use of mineralocorticoid receptor antagonists is not recommended to treat chronic uncomplicated hypertension in pregnant women and should generally be avoided in women of reproductive potential. When treatment for hypertension in pregnancy is needed, other agents are preferred (ACOG, 2013). Use of diuretics to treat edema during normal pregnancies is not appropriate; use may be considered when edema is due to pathologic causes (as in the nonpregnant patient); monitor.

Breast-Feeding Considerations The active metabolite of spironolactone (canrenone) has been found in breast milk. Information is available from a case report following maternal use of spironolactone 25 mg twice daily throughout pregnancy, then 4 times daily after delivery. Milk and maternal serum samples were obtained 17 days after birth. Two hours after the maternal dose, canrenone concentrations were ~144 ng/mL (serum) and ~104 ng/mL (milk). When measured 14.5 hours after the dose, canrenone concentrations were ~92 ng/mL (serum) and ~47 ng/mL (milk). The authors calculated the estimated maximum amount of canrenone to the nursing infant to be ~0.2% of the maternal dose (Phelps, 1977). Effects to humans are not known; however, this metabolite was found to be carcinogenic in rats. Diuretics have the potential to decrease milk volume and suppress lactation. According to the manufacturer, the decision to continue or discontinue breast-feeding during therapy should take into account the risk of exposure to the infant and the benefits of treatment to the mother; if use of spironolactone is essential, an alternative method of feeding should be used.

Contraindications Hypersensitivity to spironolactone or any component; renal failure, anuria, hyperkalemia

Warnings Spironolactone has been shown to be tumorigenic in toxicity studies using 25-250 times the usual human dose in rats **[U.S. Boxed Warning]**.

Precautions Concomitant administration of potassium-sparing diuretics (eg, amiloride and triamterene) and ACE inhibitors or NSAIDs has been associated with severe hyperkalemia; may cause transient elevation of BUN, possibly due to a concentration effect; sustained elevations should be evaluated; monitor potassium levels closely; in CHF, potassium levels and renal function should be checked in 3 days and 1 week after beginning therapy, then every 2-4 weeks for 3-12 months, then every 3-6 months. Discontinue or interrupt therapy for serum potassium >5 mEq/L or for serum creatinine >4 mg/dL in patients with heart failure. Use with caution in patients with dehydration, hyponatremia, impaired renal clearance (CrCl <50 mL/minute) or hepatic dysfunction

Adverse Reactions

Cardiovascular: Vasculitis

Central nervous system: Ataxia, confusion, drowsiness, headache, lethargy

Dermatologic: Erythematous maculopapular rash, Stevens-Johnson syndrome, toxic epidermal necrolysis, urticaria

Endocrine & metabolic: Amenorrhea, gynecomastia, hyperkalemia

Gastrointestinal: Abdominal cramps, diarrhea, gastritis, gastrointestinal hemorrhage, gastrointestinal ulcer, nausea, vomiting

Genitourinary: Impotence, irregular menses, postmenopausal bleeding

Hematologic & oncologic: Agranulocytosis, malignant neoplasm of breast

Hepatic: Hepatotoxicity

Hypersensitivity: Anaphylaxis

Immunologic: DRESS syndrome

Renal: Increased blood urea nitrogen, renal failure, renal insufficiency

Miscellaneous: Fever

Drug Interactions

Metabolism/Transport Effects None known.

Avoid Concomitant Use

Avoid concomitant use of Spironolactone with any of the following: AMILoride; CycloSPORINE (Systemic); Tacrolimus (Systemic); Triamterene

Increased Effect/Toxicity

Spironolactone may increase the levels/effects of: ACE Inhibitors; Amifostine; Ammonium Chloride; Antihypertensives; Cardiac Glycosides; CycloSPORINE (Systemic); Digoxin; DULoxetine; Hypotensive Agents; Neuromuscular-Blocking Agents (Nondepolarizing); Obinutuzumab; RiTUXimab; Sodium Phosphates; Tacrolimus (Systemic)

The levels/effects of Spironolactone may be increased by: Alfuzosin; AMILoride; Analgesics (Opioid); Angiotensin II Receptor Blockers; AtorvaSTATin; Barbiturates; Brimonidine (Topical); Canagliflozin; Cholestyramine Resin; Diazoxide; Drospirenone; Eplerenone; Heparin; Heparin (Low Molecular Weight); Herbs (Hypotensive Properties); MAO Inhibitors; Nitrofurantoin; Nonsteroidal Anti-Inflammatory Agents; Pentoxifylline; Phosphodiesterase 5 Inhibitors; Potassium Salts; Prostacyclin Analogues; Tolvaptan; Triamterene; Trimethoprim

Decreased Effect

Spironolactone may decrease the levels/effects of: Abiraterone Acetate; Alpha-/Beta-Agonists; Cardiac Glycosides; Mitotane; QuiNIDine

The levels/effects of Spironolactone may be decreased by: Herbs (Hypertensive Properties); Methylphenidate; Nonsteroidal Anti-Inflammatory Agents; Yohimbine

Food Interactions Food increases absorption. Management: Administer with food to increase absorption and decrease GI upset.

Mechanism of Action Competes with aldosterone for receptor sites in the distal renal tubules, increasing sodium chloride and water excretion while conserving potassium and hydrogen ions; may block the effect of aldosterone on arteriolar smooth muscle as well

Pharmacokinetics (Adult data unless noted)

Distribution: V_d: Breast milk to plasma ratio: 0.51-0.72

Protein binding: 91% to 98%

Metabolism: In the liver to multiple metabolites, including canrenone (active)

Half-life:

Spironolactone: 78-84 minutes

Canrenone: 13-24 hours

Time to peak serum concentration: Within 1-3 hours (primarily as the active metabolite)

Elimination: Urinary and biliary

Dosing: Neonatal Oral: Diuretic: 1-3 mg/kg/day divided every 12-24 hours

Dosing: Usual Oral:

Children:

Diuretic, hypertension: 1-3.3 mg/kg/day or 60 mg/m^2/day in divided doses every 6-12 hours; not to exceed 100 mg/day

Diagnosis of primary aldosteronism: 100-400 mg/m^2/day in 1-2 divided doses

Adults:

Edema, hypokalemia: 25-200 mg/day in 1-2 divided doses

Hypertension (JNC 7): 25-50 mg/day divided once or twice daily

Heart failure, severe (NYHA class III-IV; with ACE inhibitor and a loop diuretic ± digoxin): 12.5-25 mg/day; maximum daily dose: 50 mg. If 25 mg once daily not tolerated, reduction to 25 mg every other day was the lowest maintenance dose possible.

Diagnosis of primary aldosteronism: 100-400 mg/day in 1-2 divided doses

Acne in women: 25-200 mg once daily

Hirsutism in women: 50-200 mg/day in 1-2 divided doses

CHF: Patients with severe heart failure already using an ACE inhibitor and a loop diuretic ± digoxin: 12.5-25 mg/day, increase or reduce depending on individual response and evidence of hyperkalemia; maximum daily dose: 50 mg

Dosing interval in renal impairment:

CrCl 10-50 mL/minute: Administer every 12-24 hours

CrCl <10 mL/minute: Avoid use

Administration Oral: Administer with food

Monitoring Parameters Serum potassium, sodium, and renal function

Test Interactions May interfere with the radioimmunoassay for digoxin.

Dosage Forms Excipient information presented when available (limited, particularly for generics); consult specific product labeling.

Tablet, Oral:

Aldactone: 25 mg

Aldactone: 50 mg, 100 mg [scored]

Generic: 25 mg, 50 mg, 100 mg

Extemporaneous Preparations A 1 mg/mL oral suspension may be made with tablets. Crush ten 25 mg tablets in a mortar and reduce to a fine powder. Add a small amount of purified water and soak for 5 minutes; add 50 mL 1.5% carboxymethylcellulose, 100 mL syrup NF, and mix to a uniform paste; mix while adding purified water in incremental proportions to **almost** 250 mL; transfer to a calibrated bottle, rinse mortar with purified water, and add quantity of purified water sufficient to make 250 mL. Label "shake well". Stable for 3 months at room temperature or refrigerated (Nahata, 1993).

A 2.5 mg/mL oral suspension may be made with tablets. Crush twelve 25 mg tablets in a mortar and reduce to a fine powder. Add small portions of distilled water or glycerin and mix to a uniform paste; mix while adding cherry syrup to **almost** 120 mL; transfer to a calibrated bottle, rinse mortar with cherry syrup, and add quantity of cherry syrup sufficient to make 120 mL. Label "shake well" and "refrigerate". This method may also be used with twenty-four 25 mg tablets for a 5 mg/mL oral suspension. Both concentrations are stable for 28 days refrigerated (Mathur, 1989).

A 25 mg/mL oral suspension may be made with tablets and either a 1:1 mixture of Ora-Sweet and Ora-Plus or a 1:1 mixture of Ora-Sweet SF and Ora-Plus. Crush one-hundred-twenty 25 mg tablets in a mortar and reduce to a fine powder. Add small portions of chosen vehicle and mix to a uniform paste; mix while adding vehicle in incremental

proportions to **almost** 120 mL; transfer to a calibrated bottle, rinse mortar with vehicle, and add quantity of vehicle sufficient to make 120 mL. Store in amber bottles; label "shake well" and "refrigerate". Stable for 60 days refrigerated (Allen, 1996).

Allen LV Jr and Erickson MA 3rd, "Stability of Ketoconazole, Metolazone, Metronidazole, Procainamide Hydrochloride, and Spironolactone in Extemporaneously Compounded Oral Liquids," *Am J Health Syst Pharm*, 1996, 53(17):2073-8.

Mathur LK and Wickman A, "Stability of Extemporaneously Compounded Spironolactone Suspensions," *Am J Hosp Pharm*, 1989, 46(10):2040-2.

Nahata MC, Morosco RS, and Hipple TF, "Stability of Spironolactone in an Extemporaneously Prepared Suspension at Two Temperatures," *Ann Pharmacother*, 1993, 27(10):1198-9.

References

Chobanian AV, Bakris GL, Black HR, et al, "The Seventh Report of the Joint National Committee on Prevention, Detection, Evaluation, and Treatment of High Blood Pressure: The JNC 7 Report," *JAMA*, 2003, 289(19):2560-72.

Hunt SA, Abraham WT, Chin MH, et al, "ACC/AHA 2005 Guideline Update for the Diagnosis and Management of Chronic Heart Failure in the Adult-Summary Article: A Report of the American College of Cardiology/American Heart Association Task Force on Practice Guidelines (Writing Committee to Update the 2001 Guidelines for the Evaluation and Management of Heart Failure)," *J Am Coll Cardiol*, 2005, 46(6):1116-43.

Juurlink DN, Mamdani MM, Lee DS, et al, "Rates of Hyperkalemia After Publication of the Randomized Aldactone Evaluation Study," *N Engl J Med*, 2004, 351(6):543-51.

National High Blood Pressure Education Program Working Group on High Blood Pressure in Children and Adolescents, "The Fourth Report on the Diagnosis, Evaluation, and Treatment of High Blood Pressure in Children and Adolescents," *Pediatrics*, 2004, 114(2 Suppl):555-76.

Phelps DL, Karim A. Spironolactone: relationship between concentrations of dethioacetylated metabolite in human serum and milk. *J Pharm Sci*. 1977;66(8):1203.

Pitt B, Zannad F, Remme WJ, et al, "The Effect of Spironolactone on Morbidity and Mortality in Patients With Severe Heart Failure. Randomized Aldactone Evaluation Study Investigators," *N Engl J Med*, 1999, 341(10):709-17.

Regitz-Zagrosek V, Blomstrom Lundqvist C, et al. ESC Guidelines on the management of cardiovascular diseases during pregnancy: the Task Force on the Management of Cardiovascular Diseases during Pregnancy of the European Society of Cardiology (ESC). *Eur Heart J.* 2011;32(24):3147-3197.

van der Vorst MM, Kist JE, van der Heijden AJ, et al, "Diuretics in Pediatrics: Current Knowledge and Future Prospects," *Paediatr Drugs*, 2006, 8(4):245-64.

◆ **Spironolactone and Hydrochlorothiazide** *see* Hydrochlorothiazide and Spironolactone *on page 1025*

◆ **SPM 927** *see* Lacosamide *on page 1189*

◆ **Sporanox** *see* Itraconazole *on page 1166*

◆ **Sporanox Pulsepak** *see* Itraconazole *on page 1166*

◆ **SPS** *see* Sodium Polystyrene Sulfonate *on page 1917*

◆ **SQV** *see* Saquinavir *on page 1867*

◆ **SS734** *see* Besifloxacin *on page 281*

◆ **SSD** *see* Silver Sulfadiazine *on page 1890*

◆ **SSKI** *see* Potassium Iodide *on page 1711*

◆ **Stagesic™ [DSC]** *see* Hydrocodone and Acetaminophen *on page 1027*

◆ **StanGard Perio** *see* Fluoride *on page 894*

◆ **Stannous Fluoride** *see* Fluoride *on page 894*

◆ **Statex (Can)** *see* Morphine (Systemic) *on page 1440*

Stavudine (STAV yoo deen)

Medication Safety Issues

Sound-alike/look-alike issues:

Zerit® may be confused with Zestril®, Ziac®, ZyrTEC®

Related Information

Adult and Adolescent HIV *on page 2348*

Pediatric HIV *on page 2338*

Perinatal HIV *on page 2356*

Brand Names: U.S. Zerit

Brand Names: Canada Zerit®

Therapeutic Category Antiretroviral Agent; HIV Agents (Anti-HIV Agents); Nucleoside Reverse Transcriptase Inhibitor (NRTI)

Generic Availability (U.S.) Yes

Use Treatment of HIV infection in combination with other antiretroviral agents (FDA approved in all ages). **Note:** HIV regimens consisting of **three** antiretroviral agents are strongly recommended.

Medication Guide Available Yes

Pregnancy Risk Factor C

Pregnancy Considerations Adverse events were observed in some animal reproduction studies. Stavudine has a high level of transfer across the human placenta. No increased risk of overall birth defects has been observed following first trimester exposure according to data collected by the antiretroviral pregnancy registry. Pharmacokinetics of stavudine are not significantly altered during pregnancy; dose adjustments are not needed. Cases of lactic acidosis/hepatic steatosis syndrome related to mitochondrial toxicity have been reported in pregnant women with prolonged use of nucleoside analogues. It is not known if pregnancy itself potentiates this known side effect; however, women may be at increased risk of lactic acidosis and liver damage. In addition, these adverse events are similar to other rare but life-threatening syndromes which occur during pregnancy (eg, HELLP syndrome). Combination treatment with didanosine may also contribute to the risk of lactic acidosis and is not recommended. Hepatic enzymes and electrolytes should be monitored in women receiving nucleoside analogues and clinicians should watch for early signs of the syndrome. In addition, mitochondrial dysfunction may develop in infants following *in utero* exposure. The DHHS Perinatal HIV Guidelines recommend stavudine to be used only in special circumstances during pregnancy; do not use with didanosine or zidovudine; not recommended for initial therapy in antiretroviral-naïve pregnant women due to toxicity (DHHS [perinatal], 2014).

Regardless of CD4 count or HIV RNA copy number, all HIV-infected pregnant women should receive a combination antiretroviral (ARV) drug regimen. A combination of antepartum, intrapartum, and infant ARV prophylaxis is recommended. ARV therapy should be started as soon as possible in women with symptomatic infection. Although earlier initiation may be more effective in reducing the perinatal transmission of HIV, initiation may be delayed until after 12 weeks gestation in women who do not require immediate treatment after careful consideration of maternal conditions (eg, nausea and vomiting) and the potential risks of first trimester fetal exposure for specific agents. A scheduled cesarean delivery at 38 weeks gestation is recommended for all women with HIV RNA >1000 copies/mL or unknown concentrations near delivery in order to decrease transmission. If ARV therapy must be interrupted for <24 hours during the peripartum period, stop then restart all medications simultaneously in order to decrease the chance of developing resistance. Long-term follow-up is recommended for all infants exposed to ARV medications. In couples who want to conceive, the HIV-infected partner should attain maximum viral suppression prior to conception.

Health care providers are encouraged to enroll pregnant women exposed to antiretroviral medications in the Antiretroviral Pregnancy Registry (1-800-258-4263 or www.APRegistry.com). Health care providers caring for HIV-infected women and their infants may contact the National Perinatal HIV Hotline (888-448-8765) for clinical consultation (DHHS [perinatal], 2014).

Breast-Feeding Considerations Stavudine is excreted into breast milk; concentrations in nursing infants are negligible. Maternal or infant antiretroviral therapy does not completely eliminate the risk of postnatal HIV transmission. In addition, multiclass-resistant virus has been detected in breast-feeding infants despite maternal therapy. Therefore, in the United States, where formula is accessible, affordable, safe, and sustainable, and the risk of infant mortality due to diarrhea and respiratory infections is low, complete avoidance of breast-feeding by HIV-infected women is recommended to decrease potential transmission of HIV (DHHS [perinatal], 2014).

Contraindications Hypersensitivity to stavudine or any component

Warnings The major clinical toxicity of stavudine is peripheral neuropathy which has occurred in 8% to 21% of patients in controlled trials; it can be dose-limiting and occurs more frequently in patients with a history of neuropathy, advanced HIV, and in patients receiving other drugs known to cause neuropathy (eg, didanosine). Lactic acidosis and severe hepatomegaly with steatosis, including fatal cases, have been reported with the use of NRTIs **[U.S. Boxed Warning]**; it may be more common with antiretroviral regimens containing stavudine. Risk may be increased in obesity, prolonged nucleoside exposure, prior liver disease, or in female patients. Increased risk of hepatotoxicity also occurs with combined use of stavudine with didanosine and hydroxyurea (avoid this combination). Fatal lactic acidosis has occurred in pregnant women who received stavudine plus didanosine with other antiretroviral agents; use stavudine plus didanosine with caution during pregnancy (and in other patients) and only if benefit clearly outweighs risks. Severe motor weakness (resembling Guillain-Barré syndrome) has been reported, usually in association with lactic acidosis. Manufacturer recommends prompt suspension of all antiretroviral therapy in suspected cases of symptomatic hyperlactatemia, lactic acidosis (with or without neuromuscular weakness), or pronounced hepatotoxicity; signs and symptoms of symptomatic hyperlactemia or lactic acidosis syndrome may include generalized fatigue, GI symptoms (nausea, vomiting, abdominal pain, unexplained weight loss), respiratory symptoms (tachypnea, dyspnea), or neurologic symptoms (motor weakness, Guillain-Barré-type syndrome).

Fatal and nonfatal pancreatitis has occurred during combination antiretroviral therapy which included stavudine and didanosine **[U.S. Boxed Warning]**; avoid the use of stavudine with didanosine; discontinue these drugs (and any other drugs that are toxic to the pancreas) if pancreatitis is suspected; use extreme caution and closely monitor patient if stavudine is restarted in patients with confirmed pancreatitis; the new medication regimen should **not** contain didanosine. **Note:** The incidence of stavudine-associated toxicities may be increased when stavudine is used in combination with other medications that have similar toxicities. An increased risk of pancreatitis and hepatotoxicity (either of which may be fatal) and severe peripheral neuropathy may occur when patients are treated with stavudine in combination with didanosine (with or without hydroxyurea). The combined use of stavudine and hydroxyurea (with or without didanosine) should be avoided. According to AIDS*info* guidelines, the combined use of stavudine and didanosine is **not** recommended for use in adults and adolescents (DHHS [adult], 2014) and is not recommended as part of an initial antiretroviral regimen in pediatric patients; however, it may be considered for use in pediatric salvage regimens if the potential benefit clearly outweighs the risks (DHHS [pediatric], 2014).

Safety and efficacy have not been established in patients with significant liver disease; patients with liver impairment, including chronic active hepatitis, may be at increased risk for liver function abnormalities, including hepatic adverse events that may be severe and potentially fatal; monitor patients carefully; if liver function worsens, consider interruption or discontinuation of therapy. Concomitant use of combination antiretroviral therapy with interferon alfa (with or without ribavirin) has resulted in hepatic decompensation (with some fatalities) in patients coinfected with HIV and HCV; monitor patients closely, especially for hepatic decompensation, neutropenia, and anemia; consider discontinuation of stavudine if needed; consider dose reduction or discontinuation of interferon alfa, ribavirin, or both if clinical toxicities, including hepatic decompensation, worsen. Use of stavudine with zidovudine is **not** recommended due to antagonistic effects.

Precautions Use with caution in patients with a history of peripheral neuropathy, or hepatic or renal impairment; dosage adjustment required in patients with impaired renal function. Fat redistribution and accumulation [ie, central obesity, peripheral wasting, facial wasting, breast enlargement, dorsocervical fat enlargement (buffalo hump), and cushingoid appearance] have been observed in patients receiving antiretroviral agents (causal relationship not established).

Immune reconstitution syndrome (an acute inflammatory response to residual or indolent opportunistic infections) may occur in HIV patients during initial treatment with combination antiretroviral agents; this syndrome may require further patient assessment and therapy. Autoimmune disorders (eg, Grave's disease, Guillain-Barré syndrome, polymyositis) have been reported in patients experiencing immune reconstitution; time to onset is variable and may occur many months after antiretroviral treatment is initiated.

Oral solution contains sucrose (50 mg/mL); diabetic patients should be counseled.

Adverse Reactions Adverse reactions reported below represent experience with combination therapy with other nucleoside analogues and protease inhibitors.
Central nervous system: Headache
Dermatologic: Rash
Gastrointestinal: Diarrhea, nausea, vomiting
Hepatic: ALT increased, AST increased, GGT increased, hyperbilirubinemia
Neuromuscular & skeletal: Peripheral neuropathy
Miscellaneous: Amylase increased, lipase increased
Rare but important or life-threatening: Abdominal pain, allergic reaction, anemia, anorexia, chills, diabetes mellitus, fever, hepatic failure, hepatitis, hepatomegaly (with steatosis; some fatal), hyperglycemia, hyperlactatemia (symptomatic), hyperlipidemia, immune reconstitution syndrome, insomnia, insulin resistance, lactic acidosis (some fatal), leukopenia, macrocytosis, myalgia, neuromuscular weakness (severe-resembling Guillain-Barré), neutropenia, pancreatitis (some fatal), redistribution/accumulation/atrophy of body fat, thrombocytopenia

Drug Interactions
Metabolism/Transport Effects None known.
Avoid Concomitant Use
Avoid concomitant use of Stavudine with any of the following: Hydroxyurea; Zidovudine
Increased Effect/Toxicity
Stavudine may increase the levels/effects of: Didanosine; Hydroxyurea

The levels/effects of Stavudine may be increased by: Hydroxyurea; Ribavirin
Decreased Effect
The levels/effects of Stavudine may be decreased by: DOXOrubicin (Conventional); DOXOrubicin (Liposomal); Zidovudine
Stability
Capsules: Store at 25°C (77°F); excursions permitted to 15°C to 30°C (59°F to 86°F). Dispense in a tightly closed container.

Oral solution: Store intact bottle of powder at 25°C (77°F); excursions permitted to 15°C to 30°C (59°F to 86°F); protect from moisture. Dispense reconstituted solution in original container; store at 2°C to 8°C (36°F to 46°F); solution is stable for 30 days; discard any unused portion after that time.

Mechanism of Action Stavudine is a thymidine analog which interferes with HIV viral DNA dependent DNA polymerase resulting in inhibition of HIV viral replication; nucleoside reverse transcriptase inhibitor

Pharmacokinetics (Adult data unless noted)
Absorption: Rapid
Distribution: Penetrates into the CSF achieving 16% to 97% (mean: 59%) of concomitant plasma concentrations; distributes into extravascular spaces and equally between RBCs and plasma
V_d:
Children: 0.73 ± 0.32 L/kg
Adults: 46 ± 21 L
Protein binding: Negligible
Metabolism: Converted intracellularly to active triphosphate form; metabolism of stavudine plays minimal role in its clearance; minor metabolites include oxidized stavudine and its glucuronide conjugate, glucuronide conjugate of stavudine, N-acetylcysteine conjugate of the ribose after glycosidic cleavage
Bioavailability: Capsule and solution are bioequivalent
Children: 77%
Adults: 86%
Half-life, elimination:
Newborns (at birth): 5.3 ± 2 hours
Neonates 14 to 28 days old: 1.6 ± 0.3 hours
Pediatric patients 5 weeks to 15 years: 0.9 ± 0.3 hours
Adults: 1.6 ± 0.2 hours
Note: Half-life is prolonged with renal dysfunction
Half-life, intracellular: Adults: 3.5 to 7 hours
Time to peak serum concentration: Within 1 hour
Elimination: Urine: 95% of dose (74% as unchanged drug); feces: 3% (62% as unchanged drug); undergoes glomerular filtration and active tubular secretion
Dialysis: 31 ± 5% of the dose is removed by hemodialysis; hemodialysis clearance (n=12) (mean ± SD): 120 ± 18 mL/minute

Dosing: Neonatal HIV infection, treatment: Use in combination with other antiretroviral agents.
PNA 0 to 13 days: Oral: 0.5 mg/kg/dose every 12 hours
PNA ≥14 days: Oral: 1 mg/kg/dose every 12 hours

Dosing: Usual
Pediatric: **HIV infection, treatment:** Use in combination with other antiretroviral agents.
Infants and Children <30 kg: Oral: 1 mg/kg/dose every 12 hours; maximum dose: 30 mg/dose
Children and Adolescents weighing 30 to 59 kg: Oral: 30 mg every 12 hours
Adolescents weighing ≥60 kg: Oral:
AIDS*Info* and WHO recommendations: 30 mg every 12 hours (DHHS [pediatric], 2014)
Manufacturer's labeling: 40 mg every 12 hours
Adult: **HIV infection, treatment:** Use in combination with other antiretroviral agents.
30 to 59 kg: Oral: 30 mg every 12 hours
≥60 kg: Oral: 40 mg every 12 hours
Note: The World Health Organization recommends 30 mg every 12 hours in all adult patients regardless of body weight (DHHS, [adult], 2014).

Dosing adjustment in renal impairment:

Infants, Children, and Adolescents: Insufficient data exists to recommend a specific dosage adjustment; however, a decrease in the dose should be considered in pediatric patients with renal impairment. The following guidelines have been used by some clinicians (Aronoff, 2007):

Weight <30 kg:
GFR >50 mL/minute/1.73 m²: No adjustment required
GFR 30-50 mL/minute/1.73 m²: 0.5 mg/kg/dose every 12 hours
GFR <30 mL/minute/1.73 m²: 0.25 mg/kg/dose every 24 hours
Hemodialysis or peritoneal dialysis: 0.25 mg/kg/dose every 24 hours
Continuous renal replacement therapy (CRRT): 0.5 mg/kg/dose every 12 hours

Weight 30-59 kg:
GFR >50 mL/minute/1.73 m²: No adjustment required
GFR 30-50 mL/minute/1.73 m²: 15 mg every 12 hours
GFR <30 mL/minute/1.73 m²: 7.5 mg every 24 hours
Hemodialysis or peritoneal dialysis: 7.5 mg every 24 hours
Continuous renal replacement therapy (CRRT): 15 mg every 12 hours

Adults:
Weight <60 kg:
CrCl ≥50 mL/minute: No dosage adjustment required
CrCl 26-50 mL/minute: 15 mg every 12 hours
CrCl 10-25 mL/minute: 15 mg every 24 hours
Hemodialysis: 15 mg every 24 hours

Weight ≥60 kg:
CrCl ≥50 mL/minute: No dosage adjustment required
CrCl 26-50 mL/minute: 20 mg every 12 hours
CrCl 10-25 mL/minute: 20 mg every 24 hours
Hemodialysis: 20 mg every 24 hours

Dosing adjustment in hepatic impairment: There are no dosage adjustments provided in the manufacturer labeling.

Administration

Oral: Administer with or without food

Oral capsule: May be opened and dispersed in a small amount of water; administer immediately (DHHS [pediatric] 2014).

Oral solution: Reconstitute with purified water to a final concentration of 1 mg/mL; shake well during reconstitution to ensure complete powder dissolution; shake well before using

Monitoring Parameters Note: Monitor CD4 percentage (if <5 years of age) or CD4 count (if ≥5 years of age) at least every 3-4 months (DHHS [pediatric], 2014).

Prior to initiation of therapy: Genotypic resistance testing, CD4 and viral load (every 3 to 4 months), CBC with differential, LFTs, BUN, creatinine, electrolytes, glucose, urinalysis (every 6 to 12 months), and assessment of readiness for adherence with medication regimen. At initiation and with any change in treatment regimen: CBC with differential, electrolytes, calcium, phosphate, glucose, LFTs, bilirubin, urinalysis (at initiation), BUN, creatinine, albumin, total protein, lipid panel (at initiation), CD4, and viral load. After 1 to 2 weeks of therapy: Signs of medication toxicity and adherence. After 2 to 4 weeks of therapy: CBC with differential, viral load, signs of medication toxicity, and adherence; then every 3 to 4 months: CBC with differential, electrolytes, glucose, LFTs, bilirubin, BUN, creatinine, CD4, viral load, signs of medication toxicity, and adherence. Lipid panel and urinalysis every 6 to 12 months. CD4 monitoring frequency may be decreased to every 6 to 12 months in children who are adherent to therapy if the value is well above the threshold for opportunistic infections, viral suppression is sustained, and the clinical status is stable for more than 2 to 3 years

(DHHS [pediatric], 2014). Monitor for growth and development, signs of HIV-specific physical conditions, HIV disease progression, opportunistic infections peripheral neuropathy, pancreatitis, hepatotoxicity, or lactic acidosis.

Dosage Forms Excipient information presented when available (limited, particularly for generics); consult specific product labeling.

Capsule, Oral:
Zerit: 15 mg, 20 mg, 30 mg, 40 mg
Generic: 15 mg, 20 mg, 30 mg, 40 mg
Solution Reconstituted, Oral:
Zerit: 1 mg/mL (200 mL) [dye free; fruit flavor]
Generic: 1 mg/mL (200 mL)

References

Aronoff GR, Bennett WM, Berns JS, et al, *Drug Prescribing in Renal Failure: Dosing Guidelines for Adults and Children*, 5th ed, Philadelphia, PA: American College of Physicians, 2007.

DHHS Panel on Antiretroviral Guidelines for Adults and Adolescents, "Guidelines for the Use of Antiretroviral Agents in HIV-Infected Adults and Adolescents," May 1, 2014. Available at http://www.aidsinfo.nih.gov

DHHS Panel on Antiretroviral Therapy and Medical Management of HIV-Infected Children, "Guidelines for the Use of Antiretroviral Agents in Pediatric HIV Infection," February 12, 2014. Available at http://aidsinfo.nih.gov

DHHS Panel on Treatment of HIV-Infected Pregnant Women and Prevention of Perinatal Transmission, "Recommendations for the Use of Antiretroviral Drugs in Pregnant HIV-1-Infected Women for Maternal Health and Interventions to Reduce Perinatal HIV-1 Transmission in the United States," March 28, 2014. Available at http://aidsinfo.nih.gov

◆ **Stavzor** *see* Valproic Acid and Derivatives *on page* 2102

◆ **Stelazine** *see* Trifluoperazine *on page* 2082

◆ **Sterile Vancomycin Hydrochloride, USP (Can)** *see* Vancomycin *on page* 2110

◆ **STI-571** *see* Imatinib *on page* 1072

◆ **Stieprox (Can)** *see* Ciclopirox *on page* 465

◆ **Stieva-A (Can)** *see* Tretinoin (Topical) *on page* 2071

◆ **Stimate** *see* Desmopressin *on page* 612

◆ **Stimulant Laxative [OTC]** *see* Bisacodyl *on page* 293

◆ **St Joseph Adult Aspirin [OTC]** *see* Aspirin *on page* 212

◆ **Stomach Relief [OTC]** *see* Bismuth *on page* 294

◆ **Stomach Relief Max St [OTC]** *see* Bismuth *on page* 294

◆ **Stomach Relief Plus [OTC]** *see* Bismuth *on page* 294

◆ **Stool Softener [OTC]** *see* Docusate *on page* 701

◆ **Stool Softener Laxative DC [OTC]** *see* Docusate *on page* 701

◆ **Stop** *see* Fluoride *on page* 894

◆ **Strattera** *see* AtoMOXetine *on page* 224

Streptomycin (strep toe MYE sin)

Medication Safety Issues

Sound-alike/look-alike issues:
Streptomycin may be confused with streptozocin

Brand Names: Canada Streptomycin for Injection

Therapeutic Category Antibiotic, Aminoglycoside; Antitubercular Agent

Generic Availability (U.S.) Yes

Use Combination therapy of active tuberculosis; used in combination with other agents for treatment of streptococcal or enterococcal endocarditis, mycobacterial infections, plague, tularemia, and brucellosis

Pregnancy Risk Factor D

Pregnancy Considerations Streptomycin crosses the placenta. Many case reports of hearing impairment in children exposed *in utero* have been published. Impairment has ranged from mild hearing loss to bilateral deafness. Because of several reports of total irreversible bilateral congenital deafness in children whose mothers received streptomycin during pregnancy, the manufacturer classifies streptomycin as pregnancy risk factor D.

Breast-Feeding Considerations Streptomycin is excreted into breast milk; however, it is not well absorbed when taken orally. This limited oral absorption may minimize exposure to the nursing infant. Nondose-related effects could include modification of bowel flora. Breast-feeding is not recommended by the manufacturer.

Contraindications Hypersensitivity to streptomycin or any component

Warnings Aminoglycosides are associated with significant nephrotoxicity; risk of nephrotoxicity is increased in patients with impaired renal function, high dose therapy, or prolonged therapy. Risk of nephrotoxicity increases when used concurrently with other potentially nephrotoxic drugs **[U.S. Boxed Warning]**; renal damage is usually reversible. May cause severe neurotoxic reactions; risk of neurotoxic reactions increased in patients with impaired renal function **[U.S. Boxed Warning]**; neurotoxicity is manifested as disturbances in vestibular and cochlear function, optic nerve dysfunction, peripheral neuritis, arachnoiditis, and encephalopathy. Headache, nausea, vomiting, and disequilibrium may be indications of vestibular injury. Loss of high frequency hearing is indicative of cochlear toxicity. Risk of ototoxicity increases with use of potent diuretics. May cause neuromuscular blockade and respiratory paralysis **[U.S. Boxed Warning]**; especially when given soon after anesthesia or muscle relaxants. Aminoglycosides can cause fetal harm when administered to a pregnant woman aminoglycosides have been associated with several reports of total irreversible bilateral congenital deafness in pediatric patients exposed *in utero*.

Precautions Use with caution in patients with preexisting vertigo, tinnitus, hearing loss, or neuromuscular disorders. Use with caution in patients with renal impairment; modify dosage in patients with renal impairment; monitor renal function carefully during therapy **[U.S. Boxed Warning]**. Parenteral form should be used only where appropriate audiometric and laboratory testing facilities are available **[U.S. Boxed Warning]**.

Adverse Reactions

Cardiovascular: Hypotension

Central nervous system: Drug fever, headache, neurotoxicity, paresthesia of face

Dermatologic: Angioedema, exfoliative dermatitis, skin rash, urticaria

Gastrointestinal: Nausea, vomiting

Hematologic: Eosinophilia, hemolytic anemia, leukopenia, pancytopenia, thrombocytopenia

Neuromuscular & skeletal: Arthralgia, tremor, weakness

Ocular: Amblyopia

Otic: Ototoxicity (auditory), ototoxicity (vestibular)

Renal: Azotemia, nephrotoxicity

Respiratory: Difficulty in breathing

Miscellaneous: Anaphylaxis

Rare but important or life-threatening: Drug reaction with eosinophilia and systemic symptoms (DRESS), toxic epidermal necrolysis

Drug Interactions

Metabolism/Transport Effects None known.

Avoid Concomitant Use

Avoid concomitant use of Streptomycin with any of the following: BCG; Mannitol

Increased Effect/Toxicity

Streptomycin may increase the levels/effects of: Abobotulinumtoxin A; Bisphosphonate Derivatives; CARBOplatin; Colistimethate; CycloSPORINE (Systemic); Neuromuscular-Blocking Agents; OnabotulinumtoxinA; RimabotulinumtoxinB; Tenofovir

The levels/effects of Streptomycin may be increased by: Amphotericin B; Capreomycin; Cephalosporins (2nd Generation); Cephalosporins (3rd Generation);

Cephalosporins (4th Generation); CISplatin; Loop Diuretics; Mannitol; Nonsteroidal Anti-Inflammatory Agents; Tenofovir; Vancomycin

Decreased Effect

Streptomycin may decrease the levels/effects of: BCG; Sodium Picosulfate; Typhoid Vaccine

The levels/effects of Streptomycin may be decreased by: Penicillins

Stability Streptomycin injection should be stored in the refrigerator

Mechanism of Action Inhibits bacterial protein synthesis by binding directly to the 30S ribosomal subunits causing faulty peptide sequence to form in the protein chain

Pharmacokinetics (Adult data unless noted)

Distribution: Distributes into most body tissues and fluids except the brain; small amounts enter the CSF only with inflamed meninges; crosses the placenta; small amounts appear in breast milk

Protein binding: 34%

Half-life (prolonged with renal impairment):

Newborns: 4-10 hours

Adults: 2-4.7 hours

Time to peak serum concentration: I.M.: Within 1-2 hours

Elimination: 30% to 90% of dose excreted as unchanged drug in urine, with small amount (1%) excreted in bile, saliva, sweat, and tears

Dosing: Neonatal I.M., I.V. (Reserve I.V. for patient who cannot tolerate I.M. injections): 10-20 mg/kg/day once daily

Congenital tuberculosis: 20-40 mg/kg/day (*Red Book*, 2009)

Dosing: Usual I.M., I.V. (Reserve I.V. for patient who cannot tolerate I.M. injections):

Infants: 20-30 mg/kg/day in divided doses every 12 hours

Children:

Tuberculosis: 20-40 mg/kg/day once daily, not to exceed 1 g/day; **or** 20-40 mg/kg/dose twice weekly under direct observation, not to exceed 1.5 g/dose; usually discontinued after 2-3 months of therapy or as soon as isoniazid and rifampin susceptibility is established

Other infections: 20-40 mg/kg/day in combination with other antibiotics divided every 6-12 hours

Plague: 30 mg/kg/day divided every 8-12 hours

Adults:

Tuberculosis: 15 mg/kg/day once daily, not to exceed 1 g/day; **or** 25-30 mg/kg/dose twice weekly under direct observation, not to exceed 1.5 g/dose

Enterococcal endocarditis: 1 g every 12 hours for 2 weeks, then 500 mg every 12 hours for 4 weeks in combination with penicillin

Streptococcal endocarditis: 1 g every 12 hours for 1 week, then 500 mg every 12 hours for 1 week

Tularemia: 1-2 g/day in divided doses for 7-10 days or until patient is afebrile for 5-7 days

Plague: 2 g/day in divided doses until the patient is afebrile for at least 3 days

Dosing adjustment in renal impairment:

CrCl 50-80 mL/minute: Administer 7.5 mg/kg/dose every 24 hours

CrCl 10-50 mL/minute: Administer 7.5 mg/kg/dose every 24-72 hours

CrCl <10 mL/minute: Administer 7.5 mg/kg/dose every 72-96 hours

Administration Parenteral:

I.M.: Inject deep I.M. into a large muscle mass; administer at a concentration not to exceed 500 mg/mL; rotate injection sites

I.V.: I.V. infusion through a peripheral or central line; 12-15 mg/kg/dose is diluted in 100 mL of NS; infuse over 30-60 minutes

Monitoring Parameters Hearing (audiogram), BUN, creatinine; serum concentration of the drug should be monitored in patients with renal impairment; eighth cranial nerve damage is usually preceded by high-pitched tinnitus, roaring noises, sense of fullness in ears, or impaired hearing and may persist for weeks after drug is discontinued

Reference Range Therapeutic serum concentrations: Peak: 15-40 mcg/mL; trough: <5 mcg/mL

Additional Information For use by patients with active tuberculosis that is resistant to isoniazid and rifampin or patients with active tuberculosis in areas where resistance is common and whose drug susceptibility is not yet known. Pfizer will distribute streptomycin directly to physicians and health clinics at no charge. Call Pfizer at 1-800-254-4445.

Dosage Forms Excipient information presented when available (limited, particularly for generics); consult specific product labeling.

Solution Reconstituted, Intramuscular:
Generic: 1 g (1 ea)

References

Ad Hoc Committee of the Scientific Assembly on Microbiology, Tuberculosis, and Pulmonary Infections, "Treatment of Tuberculosis and Tuberculosis Infection in Adults and Children," *Clin Infect Dis*, 1995, 21:9-27.

American Academy of Pediatrics Committee on Infectious Diseases, "Chemotherapy for Tuberculosis in Infants and Children," *Pediatrics* 1992, 89(1):161-5.

Arguedas AG and Wehrle PP, "New Concepts for Antimicrobial Use in Central Nervous System Infections," *Semin Pediatr Infect Dis*, 1991, 2 (1):36-42.

Centers for Disease Control and Prevention (CDC), "Guidelines for the Prevention and Treatment of Opportunistic Infections Among HIV-Exposed and HIV-Infected Children," *MMWR Recomm Rep*, 2009, 58(RR-11):1-166. Available at http://aidsinfo.nih.gov/contentfiles/Pediatric_OI.pdf

Lorin MI, Hsu KH, and Jacob SC, "Treatment of Tuberculosis in Children," *Pediatr Clin North Am*, 1983, 30(2):333-48.

Red Book: 2009 Report of the Committee on Infectious Diseases, 28th ed, Pickering LK, ed, Elk Grove Village, IL: American Academy of Pediatrics, 2009.

◆ **Streptomycin for Injection (Can)** see Streptomycin *on page 1935*

◆ **Streptomycin Sulfate** see Streptomycin *on page 1935*

◆ **Striant** see Testosterone *on page 1986*

◆ **Stridex Essential [OTC]** see Salicylic Acid *on page 1860*

◆ **Stri-Dex Maximum Strength [OTC]** see Salicylic Acid *on page 1860*

◆ **Stri-Dex Sensitive Skin [OTC]** see Salicylic Acid *on page 1860*

◆ **Stromectol** see Ivermectin (Systemic) *on page 1170*

◆ **Strong Iodine Solution** see Potassium Iodide and Iodine *on page 1713*

◆ **Sublinox (Can)** see Zolpidem *on page 2182*

◆ **Suboxone** see Buprenorphine and Naloxone *on page 324*

◆ **Subsys** see FentaNYL *on page 853*

Succimer (SUKS si mer)

Brand Names: U.S. Chemet
Brand Names: Canada Chemet
Therapeutic Category Antidote, Lead Toxicity; Chelating Agent, Oral
Generic Availability (U.S.) No
Use Treatment of lead poisoning in children with blood levels >45 mcg/dL; not indicated for prophylaxis of lead poisoning in a lead-containing environment
Pregnancy Risk Factor C
Pregnancy Considerations Adverse events were observed in animal reproduction studies.

Lead poisoning: Lead is known to cross the placenta in amounts related to maternal plasma levels. Prenatal lead

exposure may be associated with adverse events such as spontaneous abortion, preterm delivery, decreased birth weight, and impaired neurodevelopment. Some adverse outcomes may occur with maternal blood lead levels <10 mcg/dL. In addition, pregnant women exposed to lead may have an increased risk of gestational hypertension. Consider chelation therapy in pregnant women with confirmed blood lead levels ≥45 mcg/dL (pregnant women with blood lead levels ≥70 mcg/dL should be considered for chelation regardless of trimester); consultation with experts in lead poisoning and high-risk pregnancy is recommended. Encephalopathic pregnant women should be chelated regardless of trimester (CDC, 2010).

Breast-Feeding Considerations It is not known if succimer is excreted in breast milk. When used for the treatment of lead poisoning, the amount of lead in breast milk may range from 0.6% to 3% of the maternal serum concentration. Women with confirmed blood lead levels ≥40 mcg/dL should not initiate breast-feeding; pumping and discarding breast milk is recommended until blood lead levels are <40 mcg/dL, at which point breast-feeding may resume (CDC, 2010). Calcium supplementation may reduce the amount of lead in breast milk.

Contraindications Hypersensitivity to succimer or any component

Warnings Elevated blood lead levels and associated symptoms may return rapidly after discontinuation due to redistribution of lead from bone stores to soft tissues and blood; monitor blood lead levels for "rebound" after therapy; mild to moderate neutropenia has been reported; monitor CBC with differential prior to and during therapy; discontinue treatment if ANC <1200/microliter

Precautions Use with caution in patients with renal or hepatic impairment; adequate hydration should be maintained during therapy

Adverse Reactions

Cardiovascular: Arrhythmia (adults)

Central nervous system: Chills, dizziness, drowsiness, fatigue, fever, headache, sleepiness

Dermatologic: Rash (including papular rash, herpetic rash and mucocutaneous eruptions); pruritus

Endocrine & metabolic: Cholesterol increased

Gastrointestinal: Abdominal cramps, appetite decreased, diarrhea, hemorrhoid symptoms, metallic taste, loose stools, mucosal irritation, nausea, sore throat, vomiting

Genitourinary: Proteinuria (adults), urine output decreased (adults), voiding difficulty (adults)

Hematologic & oncologic: Eosinophilia, increased platelet count

Hepatic: Alkaline phosphatase increased, ALT increased, AST increased

Infection: Common cold

Neuromuscular & skeletal: Back pain, flank pain, knee pain (adults), leg pain (adults), neuropathy, paresthesia, rib pain

Ocular: Cloudy film in eye, watery eyes

Otic: Otitis media, plugged ears

Respiratory: Cough, nasal congestion, rhinorrhea

Miscellaneous: Flu-like syndrome, moniliasis

Rare but important or life-threatening: Allergic reactions (especially with retreatment), neutropenia (causal relationship not established)

Drug Interactions

Metabolism/Transport Effects None known.

Avoid Concomitant Use There are no known interactions where it is recommended to avoid concomitant use.

Increased Effect/Toxicity There are no known significant interactions involving an increase in effect.

Decreased Effect There are no known significant interactions involving a decrease in effect.

Mechanism of Action Succimer is an analog of dimercaprol. It forms water soluble chelates with heavy metals ▶

◄ which are subsequently excreted renally. Succimer binds heavy metals; however, the chemical form of these chelates is not known.

Pharmacokinetics (Adult data unless noted)

Absorption: Oral: Rapid, variable

Metabolism: Extensive to mixed succimer-cysteine disulfides

Half-life, elimination: 2 days

Time to peak serum concentration: ~1-2 hours

Elimination: ~25% in urine with peak urinary excretion occurring between 2-4 hours after dosing; of the total amount of succimer eliminated in urine, 90% is eliminated as mixed succimer-cysteine disulfide conjugates; 10% is excreted unchanged; fecal excretion of succimer probably represents unabsorbed drug

Dialysis: Succimer is dialyzable but lead chelates are not

Dosing: Usual Children and Adults: Oral: 10 mg/kg/dose (or 350 mg/m^2/dose) every 8 hours for 5 days followed by 10 mg/kg/dose (or 350 mg/m^2/dose) every 12 hours for 14 days

Succimer Dosing

Weight		Dosage[1] (mg)
18-35 lbs	8-15 kg	100
36-55 lbs	16-23 kg	200
56-75 lbs	24-34 kg	300
76-100 lbs	35-44 kg	400
>100 lbs	>45 kg	500

[1]To be administered every 8 hours.

Note: Concomitant iron therapy has been reported in a small number of children without the formation of a toxic complex with iron (as seen with dimercaprol); courses of therapy may be repeated if indicated by weekly monitoring of blood lead levels; lead levels should be stabilized to <15 mcg/dL; 2 weeks between courses is recommended unless more timely treatment is indicated by lead levels; patients who have received calcium disodium EDTA with or without BAL may be treated with succimer after at least 4 weeks have passed since treatment

Dosing adjustment in renal/hepatic impairment: Administer with caution and monitor closely

Administration Oral: Ensure adequate patient hydration; for patients who cannot swallow the capsule, sprinkle the medicated beads on a small amount of soft food or administer with a fruit juice to mask the odor

Monitoring Parameters Blood lead levels; liver enzymes and CBC with differential (prior to therapy and weekly during therapy)

Test Interactions False-positive ketones (U) using nitroprusside methods, falsely decreased serum CPK; falsely decreased uric acid measurement

Dosage Forms Excipient information presented when available (limited, particularly for generics); consult specific product labeling.

Capsule, Oral:

Chemet: 100 mg

References

American Academy of Pediatrics Committee on Environmental Health, "Lead Exposure in Children: Prevention, Detection, and Management," *Pediatrics*, 2005, 116(4):1036-46.

Binns HJ, Campbell C, Brown MJ, et al, "Interpreting and Managing Blood Lead Levels of Less Than 10 micrograms/dL in Children and Reducing Childhood Exposure to Lead: Recommendations of the Centers for Disease Control and Prevention Advisory Committee on Childhood Lead Poisoning Prevention," *Pediatrics*, 2007, 120(5): e1285-98.

Centers for Disease Control and Prevention (CDC), *Guidelines for the Identification and Management of Lead Exposure in Pregnant and Lactating Women*, Atlanta: CDC; 2010.

Gracia RC and Snodgrass WR, "Lead Toxicity and Chelation Therapy," *Am J Health Syst Pharm*, 2007, 64(1):45-53.

Mann KV and Travers JD, "Succimer, An Oral Lead Chelator," *Clin Pharm*, 1991, 10(12):914-22.

Succinylcholine (suks in il KOE leen)

Medication Safety Issues

High alert medication:

The Institute for Safe Medication Practices (ISMP) includes this medication among its list of drugs which have a heightened risk of causing significant patient harm when used in error.

Other safety concerns:

United States Pharmacopeia (USP) 2006: The Interdisciplinary Safe Medication Use Expert Committee of the USP has recommended the following:

- Hospitals, clinics, and other practice sites should institute special safeguards in the storage, labeling, and use of these agents and should include these safeguards in staff orientation and competency training.

- Healthcare professionals should be on high alert (especially vigilant) whenever a neuromuscular-blocking agent (NMBA) is stocked, ordered, prepared, or administered.

International issues:

Quelicin [U.S., Brazil, Canada, Indonesia] may be confused with Keflin brand name for cefalotin [Argentina, Brazil, Mexico, Netherlands, Norway]

Related Information

Serotonin Syndrome *on page 2405*

Brand Names: U.S. Anectine; Quelicin; Quelicin-1000

Brand Names: Canada Quelicin®

Therapeutic Category Neuromuscular Blocker Agent, Depolarizing; Skeletal Muscle Relaxant, Paralytic

Generic Availability (U.S.) No

Use Adjunct to anesthesia, to facilitate endotracheal intubation, and to provide skeletal muscle relaxation during surgery or mechanical ventilation (FDA approved in all ages)

Pregnancy Risk Factor C

Pregnancy Considerations Reproduction studies have not been conducted. Small amounts cross the placenta. Sensitivity to succinylcholine may be increased due to a ~24% decrease in plasma cholinesterase activity during pregnancy and several days postpartum.

Breast-Feeding Considerations It is not known if succinylcholine is excreted in breast milk. The manufacturer recommends that caution be exercised when administering succinylcholine to nursing women.

Contraindications Hypersensitivity to succinylcholine chloride, or any component; personal or familial history of malignant hyperthermia; skeletal muscle myopathies; acute phase injury following major burns, multiple trauma, extensive denervation of skeletal muscle, or upper motor neuron injury

Warnings Ventilation must be supported during neuromuscular blockade; succinylcholine should only be administered by individuals who are experienced in the maintenance of an adequate airway and respiratory support. Succinylcholine does not alter consciousness; use in conjunction with adequate sedation or anesthesia. Severe allergic reactions have been reported with neuromuscular blocking agents including succinylcholine; cross-sensitivity with other neuromuscular-blocking agents may occur; use extreme caution in patients with previous anaphylactic reactions. Malignant hyperthermia may be triggered by succinylcholine use; risk increases with the concomitant administration of volatile anesthetics; monitor closely for signs/symptoms. Use with caution in children and adolescents; rare reports of acute rhabdomyolysis with hyperkalemia followed by ventricular dysrhythmias, cardiac arrest, and death have been reported in children with undiagnosed skeletal muscle myopathy, most frequently Duchenne's muscular dystrophy **[U.S. Boxed Warning]**. This syndrome presents as peaked T-waves and sudden cardiac arrest within minutes after the administration of succinylcholine. Bradycardia and rarely asystole have been reported; higher incidence in children, particularly those receiving doses >1.5 mg/kg, and following repeat dosing in both children and adults. Also, if sudden cardiac arrest occurs immediately after administration of succinylcholine, consider hyperkalemia as potential etiology and manage accordingly. Since it is difficult to predict which patients may develop this reaction, it is recommended that the use of succinylcholine be limited to emergency intubation or instances where immediate securing of the airway is necessary (eg, laryngospasm, difficult airway, full stomach, or for intramuscular use when a suitable vein is inaccessible). Avoid use in patients with serum potassium >5.5 mEq/L. Metabolized by plasma cholinesterase; use with caution (if at all) in patients suspected of being homozygous for the atypical plasma cholinesterase gene. Plasma cholinesterase activity may also be reduced by burns, decompensated heart disease, infections, malignant tumors, myxedema, pregnancy, severe hepatic or renal dysfunction, ulcer, and certain medications and chemicals. May increase IOP; use caution with narrow-angle glaucoma or penetrating eye injuries; do not use when increase in intraocular pressure is undesirable unless benefit outweighs the risk.

Precautions Use with extreme caution in patients recovering from severe trauma, extensive or severe burns, extensive denervation of skeletal muscle because of disease or injury to the CNS, or with degenerative or dystrophic neuromuscular disease due to increased risk for development of hyperkalemia; risk for hyperkalemia in these patients increases over time and usually peaks at 7-10 days after the injury; risk is dependent upon the extent and location of the injury.

Use with caution in patients with fractures or muscle spasms as initial muscle fasciculations from succinylcholine may cause additional trauma. Tachyphylaxis occurs with repeated administration. Neuromuscular blockade may be prolonged in patients with severe hypokalemia, severe hypocalcemia, severe hyponatremia, hypermagnesemia, neuromuscular diseases, acidosis, acute intermittent porphyria, Eaton-Lambert syndrome, myasthenia gravis, renal failure, and hepatic failure.

Adverse Reactions
Cardiovascular: Arrhythmias, bradycardia (higher with second dose, more frequent in children), cardiac arrest, hyper-/hypotension, tachycardia
Dermatologic: Rash
Endocrine & metabolic: Hyperkalemia
Gastrointestinal: Salivation (excessive)
Neuromuscular & skeletal: Jaw rigidity, muscle fasciculation, postoperative muscle pain, rhabdomyolysis (with possible myoglobinuric acute renal failure)
Ocular: Intraocular pressure increased
Renal: Acute renal failure (secondary to rhabdomyolysis)
Respiratory: Apnea, respiratory depression (prolonged)
Miscellaneous: Anaphylaxis, malignant hyperthermia
Rare but important or life-threatening: Acute quadriplegic myopathy syndrome (prolonged use), myositis ossificans (prolonged use)

Drug Interactions
Metabolism/Transport Effects None known.
Avoid Concomitant Use
Avoid concomitant use of Succinylcholine with any of the following: QuiNINE
Increased Effect/Toxicity
Succinylcholine may increase the levels/effects of: Analgesics (Opioid); Cardiac Glycosides; OnabotulinumtoxinA; RimabotulinumtoxinB

The levels/effects of Succinylcholine may be increased by: AbobotulinumtoxinA; Acetylcholinesterase Inhibitors; Aminoglycosides; Bambuterol; Capreomycin; Clindamycin (Topical); Colistimethate; Cyclophosphamide; Cyclo-SPORINE (Systemic); Echothiophate Iodide; Lincosamide Antibiotics; Lithium; Loop Diuretics; Magnesium Salts; Phenelzine; Polymyxin B; Procainamide; QuiNIDine; QuiNINE; Tetracycline Derivatives; Vancomycin
Decreased Effect
The levels/effects of Succinylcholine may be decreased by: Loop Diuretics
Stability Store at 2°C to 8°C (36°F to 46°F) and may be stored at room temperature for 14 days; injection is incompatible with alkaline solutions
Mechanism of Action Acts similar to acetylcholine, produces depolarization of the motor endplate at the myoneural junction which causes sustained flaccid skeletal muscle paralysis produced by state of accommodation that develops in adjacent excitable muscle membranes
Pharmacodynamics
I.M.:
  Onset of action: 2-3 minutes
  Duration: 10-30 minutes
I.V.:
  Onset of action: Within 30-60 seconds
  Duration: ~4-6 minutes
Pharmacokinetics (Adult data unless noted)
Metabolism: Succinylcholine is rapidly hydrolyzed by plasma pseudocholinesterase to inactive metabolites
Elimination: 10% excreted unchanged in urine
Dosing: Neonatal Note: Because of the risk of malignant hyperthermia, use of continuous I.V. infusion is **not** recommended.
Endotracheal intubation, nonemergent (Kumar, 2010):
  I.M.: 2 mg/kg/dose if no I.V. access
  I.V.: 1-2 mg/kg/dose
Dosing: Usual
Paralysis/skeletal muscle relaxation: Infants, Children, and Adolescents: **Note:** Because of the risk of malignant hyperthermia, use of continuous I.V. infusion is **not** recommended in infants and children.
  I.M.: 3-4 mg/kg; maximum dose: 150 mg
  I.V.:
    Infants: Initial: 2 mg/kg; maintenance: 0.3-0.6 mg/kg every 5-10 minutes as needed
    Children and Adolescents: Initial: 1 mg/kg; maintenance: 0.3-0.6 mg/kg every 5-10 minutes as needed
  Adults:
    I.M.: Up to 3-4 mg/kg; total dose should not exceed 150 mg
    I.V.: Intubation: 0.6 mg/kg (range: 0.3-1.1 mg/kg; rapid sequence intubation: 1-1.5 mg/kg
  Note: Pretreatment with atropine may reduce occurrence of bradycardia. Initial dose of succinylcholine must be increased when nondepolarizing agent pretreatment used because of the antagonism between succinylcholine and nondepolarizing neuromuscular-blocking agents.
Dosing adjustment in renal impairment: Use carefully and/or consider dose reduction; prolonged neuromuscular blockade may occur if reduced plasma cholinesterase activity coexists.
Dosing adjustment in hepatic impairment: Use carefully and/or consider dose reduction; prolonged neuromuscular blockade may occur if reduced plasma cholinesterase activity coexists.
Administration Parenteral:
  I.M.: Injection should be made deeply. Use only when I.V. access is not available.
  I.V.: May be administered by rapid I.V. injection without further dilution; for continuous infusion: Further dilute to 1-2 mg/mL in NS or D_5W

◄ **Monitoring Parameters** Heart rate, blood pressure, serum potassium, assisted ventilator status, peripheral nerve stimulator measuring twitch response

Dosage Forms Excipient information presented when available (limited, particularly for generics); consult specific product labeling.

Solution, Injection, as chloride:
Anectine: 20 mg/mL (10 mL) [contains methylparaben]
Quelicin: 20 mg/mL (10 mL) [contains methylparaben, propylparaben]
Quelicin-1000: 100 mg/mL (10 mL)

References
Kumar P, Denson SE, Mancuso TJ, et al, "Premedication for Non-emergency Endotracheal Intubation in the Neonate," *Pediatrics,* 2010, 125(3):608-15.

♦ **Succinylcholine Chloride** see Succinylcholine on page 1938

♦ **Sucraid** see Sacrosidase on page 1859

♦ **Sucraid® (Can)** see Sacrosidase on page 1859

Sucralfate (soo KRAL fate)

Medication Safety Issues
Sound-alike/look-alike issues:
Sucralfate may be confused with salsalate
Carafate® may be confused with Cafergot®
Administration issues:
For oral administration only. Fatal pulmonary or cerebral embolism has been reported following inadvertent I.V. administration of sucralfate.

Brand Names: U.S. Carafate
Brand Names: Canada Apo-Sucralfate; Dom-Sucralfate; Novo-Sucralate; Nu-Sucralate; PMS-Sucralate; Sucralfate-1; Sulcrate®; Sulcrate® Suspension Plus; Teva-Sucralfate
Therapeutic Category Gastrointestinal Agent, Gastric or Duodenal Ulcer Treatment
Generic Availability (U.S.) May be product dependent
Use Short-term management of duodenal ulcers; gastric ulcers; suspension may be used topically for treatment of stomatitis due to cancer chemotherapy or other causes of esophageal, gastric, and rectal erosions; treatment of NSAID mucosal damage; prevention of stress ulcers
Pregnancy Risk Factor B
Pregnancy Considerations Adverse events were not observed in animal reproduction studies. Sucralfate is only minimally absorbed following oral administration. Based on available data, use of sucralfate does not appear to increase the risk of adverse fetal events when used during the first trimester (Mahadevan, 2006).
Breast-Feeding Considerations It is not known if sucralfate is excreted in breast milk. Sucralfate is only minimally absorbed following oral administration. The manufacturer recommends that caution be exercised when administering sucralfate to nursing women.
Contraindications Hypersensitivity to sucralfate or any component
Warnings Because of the potential for sucralfate to alter the absorption of some drugs, separate administration times (administer other medications 2 hours before or after sucralfate) should be considered when alterations in bioavailability are believed to be critical
Precautions Use with caution in renal failure due to accumulation of aluminum
Adverse Reactions
Gastrointestinal: Constipation
Rare but important or life-threatening: Anaphylaxis, bezoar formation; hypersensitivity (urticaria, angioedema, facial swelling, laryngospasm, respiratory difficulty, rhinitis)
Drug Interactions
Metabolism/Transport Effects None known.

Avoid Concomitant Use
Avoid concomitant use of Sucralfate with any of the following: Multivitamins/Minerals (with ADEK, Folate, Iron); Vitamin D Analogs
Increased Effect/Toxicity
The levels/effects of Sucralfate may be increased by: Multivitamins/Fluoride (with ADE); Multivitamins/Minerals (with ADEK, Folate, Iron); Vitamin D Analogs
Decreased Effect
Sucralfate may decrease the levels/effects of: Antifungal Agents (Azole Derivatives, Systemic); Digoxin; Dolutegravir; Eltrombopag; Furosemide; Levothyroxine; Multivitamins/Fluoride (with ADE); Phosphate Supplements; QuiNIDine; Quinolone Antibiotics; Sulpiride; Tetracycline Derivatives; Vitamin K Antagonists
Mechanism of Action Forms a complex by binding with positively charged proteins in exudates, forming a viscous paste-like, adhesive substance. This selectively forms a protective coating that acts locally to protect the gastric lining against peptic acid, pepsin, and bile salts.
Pharmacodynamics GI protection effect:
Acid neutralizing capacity: 14-17 mEq/1 g dose of sucralfate
Onset of action: 1-2 hours
Duration: Up to 6 hours
Pharmacokinetics (Adult data unless noted)
Absorption: Oral: <5%
Metabolism: Not metabolized
Elimination: 90% excreted in stool; small amounts that are absorbed are excreted in the urine as unchanged compounds
Dosing: Usual Oral:
Children: Dose not established; doses of 40-80 mg/kg/day divided every 6 hours have been used
Stomatitis: 5-10 mL (1 g/10 mL); swish and spit or swish and swallow 4 times/day
Adults:
Stress ulcer prophylaxis: 1 g 4 times/day
Stress ulcer treatment: 1 g every 4 hours
Duodenal ulcer:
Treatment: 1 g 4 times/day for 4-8 weeks, or alternatively 2 g twice daily; treatment is recommended for 4-8 weeks in adults
Maintenance: Prophylaxis: 1 g twice daily
Stomatitis: 1 g/10 mL suspension, swish and spit or swish and swallow 4 times/day
Proctitis: Rectal enema: 2 g/20 mL once or twice daily
Dosage comment in renal impairment: Aluminum salt is minimally absorbed (<5%), however, may accumulate in renal failure
Administration
Oral: Administer on an empty stomach 1 hour before meals and at bedtime; tablet may be broken or dissolved in water before ingestion; do not administer antacids within 30 minutes of administration; shake suspension well before use
Rectal: May administer oral suspension as rectal enema; shake suspension well before use
Additional Information There is approximately 14-16 mEq acid neutralizing capacity per 1 g sucralfate
Dosage Forms Excipient information presented when available (limited, particularly for generics); consult specific product labeling.
Suspension, Oral:
Carafate: 1 g/10 mL (420 mL) [contains fd&c red #40, methylparaben; cherry flavor]
Tablet, Oral:
Carafate: 1 g [scored; contains fd&c blue #1 aluminum lake]
Generic: 1 g
Extemporaneous Preparations Note: Commercial oral suspension is available (100 mg/mL)

A 100 mg/mL oral suspension may be made with tablets. Crush eight 1 g tablets in a mortar and reduce to a fine powder. Add ~20 mL of Sterile Water for Injection and mix to a uniform paste; add an additional 20 mL of Sterile Water for Injection and mix thoroughly making a smooth slurry. Add 40 mL of 70% Sorbitol solution. In a separate container, dissolve two flavor packets (Vari-Flavors; Ross Laboratories) with 10 mL of water, add to mortar, and mix well. Transfer to a calibrated bottle, rinse mortar with Sterile Water for Injection, and add quantity of vehicle sufficient to make 120 mL. Label "shake well" and "refrigerate". Stable for 14 days.

Nahata MC, Pai VB, and Hipple TF, *Pediatric Drug Formulations*, 5th ed, Cincinnati, OH: Harvey Whitney Books Co, 2004.

References

Mahadevan U, Kane S. American Gastroenterological Association Institute technical review on the use of gastrointestinal medications in pregnancy. *Gastroenterology*. 2006;131(1):283-311.

Melko GP, Turco TF, Phelan TF, et al, "Treatment of Radiation-Induced Proctitis With Sucralfate Enemas," *Ann Pharmacother*, 1999, 33 (12):1274-6.

◆ **Sucralfate-1 (Can)** *see* Sucralfate *on page 1940*

◆ **Sucrets® Children's [OTC]** *see* Dyclonine *on page 727*

◆ **Sucrets® Maximum Strength [OTC]** *see* Dyclonine *on page 727*

◆ **Sucrets® Regular Strength [OTC]** *see* Dyclonine *on page 727*

Sucrose (SOO krose)

Brand Names: U.S. Sweet-Ease® [OTC]; TootSweet™ [OTC]

Therapeutic Category Analgesic, Nonopioid

Generic Availability (U.S.) No

Use Provide short-term analgesia in neonates during minor procedures (eg, heel stick, eye exam for retinopathy of prematurity, circumcision, immunization, venipuncture, ET intubation and suctioning, NG tube insertion, I.M. or subcutaneous injection); provide short-term analgesia in infants during immunization administration

Contraindications Hypersensitivity to sucrose, corn, corn products, or any component

Warnings Patients should have a functioning gastrointestinal tract; avoid use in patients with gastrointestinal tract abnormalities (eg, esophageal atresia or tracheal esophageal fistula); while necrotizing enterocolitis (NEC) has not been reported with sucrose administration, risk:benefit assessment should be considered in patients at high risk for NEC. Avoid use in patients at risk for aspiration; sucrose should not be used for patients requiring ongoing analgesia. Oxygen desaturation or brief apnea in premature neonates (spontaneous resolution) has been reported. Concentration of some products has been shown to increase (up to 40%) when stored over a 6-month period.

Precautions Efficacy in unstable or extremely low birthweight, premature neonates has not been established.

Adverse Reactions

Cardiovascular: Bradycardia (self-limiting)

Respiratory: Oxygen desaturation or brief apnea in premature neonates (spontaneous resolution)

Stability Store at 4°C to 32°C (40°F to 90°F); for some products, concentration may increase (up to 40%) when stored over a 6-month period. Unused portion should be discarded.

Mechanism of Action Exact mechanism is not known; it has been proposed that sucrose induces endogenous opioid release.

Pharmacodynamics

Maximum effect: 2 minutes
Duration: 3-5 minutes

Dosing: Neonatal Oral: 0.1-0.2 mL of 24% solution placed on the tongue or buccal surface 2 minutes prior to procedure; various regimens reported, effective range: 0.05-0.5 mL (maximum dose: 2 mL). For doses >0.1 mL, some studies have administered in aliquots with first dose 2 minutes prior to procedure and remainder of dose given intermittently (typically 3 times) during or after procedure (Johnston, 1999; Stevens, 2010).

Dosing: Usual Oral: Infants prior to immunization: 2 mL of 24% solution administered 1-2 minutes prior to vaccine administration has been used; others have shown 10 mL of 25% effective in infants receiving their 2-month vaccinations (Reis, 2003). For older infants, higher concentration of solution for analgesic effect: 2 mL of 50% or 75% solution has been shown effective (Harrison, 2010; Shah, 2009)

Administration For single oral use only. May be administered directly into baby's mouth or via a pacifier dipped into solution. Do not reuse or sterilize; dispose product after use.

Monitoring Parameters Heart rate, respiratory rate, pain relief

Dosage Forms Excipient information presented when available (limited, particularly for generics); consult specific product labeling.

Solution, oral:
Sweet-Ease® Preserved: 24% (15 mL)
TootSweet™: 24% (0.5 mL, 1 mL, 2 mL, 12 mL)
Solution, oral [preservative free]:
Sweet-Ease Natural®: 24% (15 mL)

References

Blass EM and Hoffmeyer LB, "Sucrose as an Analgesic for Newborn Infants," *Pediatrics*, 1991, 87(2):215-8.

Harrison D, Stevens B, Bueno M, et al, "Efficacy of Sweet Solutions for Analgesia in Infants Between 1 and 12 Months of Age: A Systematic Review," *Arch Dis Child*, 2010, 95(6):406-13.

Johnston CC, Stremler R, Horton L, et al, "Effect of Repeated Doses of Sucrose During Heel Stick Procedure in Preterm Neonates," *Biol Neonate*, 1999, 75(3):160-6.

Reis EC, Roth EK, Syphan JL, et al, "Effective Pain Reduction for Multiple Immunization Injections in Young Infants," *Arch Pediatr Adolesc Med*, 2003, 157(11):1115-20.

Shah V, Taddio A, Rieder MJ, et al, "Effectiveness and Tolerability of Pharmacologic and Combined Interventions for Reducing Injection Pain During Routine Childhood Immunizations: Systematic Review and Meta-Analyses," *Clin Ther*, 2009, 31(Suppl 2):S104-51.

Stevens B, Yamada J, and Ohlsson A, "Sucrose for Analgesia in Newborn Infants Undergoing Painful Procedures," *Cochrane Database Syst Rev*, 2010, (1):CD001069.

◆ **Sudafed** *see* Pseudoephedrine *on page 1770*

◆ **Sudafed [OTC]** *see* Pseudoephedrine *on page 1770*

◆ **Sudafed 12 Hour [OTC]** *see* Pseudoephedrine *on page 1770*

◆ **Sudafed 24 Hour [OTC]** *see* Pseudoephedrine *on page 1770*

◆ **Sudafed Childrens [OTC]** *see* Pseudoephedrine *on page 1770*

◆ **Sudafed® Decongestant (Can)** *see* Pseudoephedrine *on page 1770*

◆ **Sudafed PE Childrens [OTC]** *see* Phenylephrine (Systemic) *on page 1658*

◆ **Sudafed PE Maximum Strength [OTC]** *see* Phenylephrine (Systemic) *on page 1658*

◆ **Sudafed® Sinus Advance (Can)** *see* Pseudoephedrine and Ibuprofen *on page 1772*

◆ **Sudanyl [OTC]** *see* Pseudoephedrine *on page 1770*

◆ **SudoGest [OTC]** *see* Pseudoephedrine *on page 1770*

◆ **SudoGest 12 Hour [OTC]** *see* Pseudoephedrine *on page 1770*

◆ **Sudogest PE [OTC]** *see* Phenylephrine (Systemic) *on page 1658*

◆ **Sufenta** see SUFentanil on page 1942

SUFentanil (soo FEN ta nil)

Medication Safety Issues

Sound-alike/look-alike issues:
SUFentanil may be confused with alfentanil, fentaNYL
Sufenta® may be confused with Alfenta, Sudafed, Survanta

High alert medication:
The Institute for Safe Medication Practices (ISMP) includes this medication among its list of drugs which have a heightened risk of causing significant patient harm when used in error.

Brand Names: U.S. Sufenta

Brand Names: Canada Sufenta; Sufentanil Citrate Injection, USP

Therapeutic Category Analgesic, Narcotic; General Anesthetic

Generic Availability (U.S.) Yes

Use Analgesia; analgesia adjunct; anesthetic agent

Pregnancy Risk Factor C

Pregnancy Considerations Adverse event were observed in some animal reproduction studies. Administration of epidural sufentanil with bupivacaine with or without epinephrine is indicated in labor and delivery. Intravenous use or larger epidural doses are not recommended in pregnant women. When used for pain relief during labor, opioids may temporarily affect the heart rate of the fetus (ACOG, 2002).

Breast-Feeding Considerations It is not known if sufentanil is excreted in breast milk. The manufacturer recommends that caution be exercised when administering sufentanil to nursing women. Parenteral opioids used during labor have the potential to interfere with a newborns natural reflex to nurse within the first few hours after birth. When needed, a short-acting opioid such as sufentanil is preferred for women who will be nursing. Nursing infants exposed to large doses of opioids should be monitored for apnea and sedation (Montgomery, 2012).

Contraindications Hypersensitivity to sufentanil or any component; increased intracranial pressure; severe respiratory depression

Warnings May cause severe respiratory depression; rapid I.V. infusion may result in skeletal muscle and chest wall rigidity, impaired ventilation, respiratory distress, apnea, bronchoconstriction, laryngospasm, arrest; inject slowly over 3-5 minutes; nondepolarizing skeletal muscle relaxant may be required; abrupt discontinuation after prolonged use may result in withdrawal symptoms

Precautions Use with caution in patients with head injuries, hepatic impairment, pulmonary disease, or with use of MAO inhibitors within past 14 days; sufentanil shares the toxic potential of opioid agonists, precautions of opioid agonist therapy should be observed

Adverse Reactions
Cardiovascular: Bradycardia, cardiac arrhythmia, hyper-/hypotension

Central nervous system: CNS depression, confusion, somnolence

Dermatologic: Pruritus

Gastrointestinal: Nausea, vomiting

Ocular: Blurred vision

Neuromuscular & Skeletal: Chest wall rigidity

Rare but important or life-threatening: Anaphylaxis, apnea, arrhythmia, biliary spasm, bronchospasm, cardiac arrest, chills, circulatory depression; cold, clammy skin; dizziness, dysesthesia, erythema, itching, laryngospasm, mental depression, paradoxical CNS excitation or delirium, physical and psychological dependence with prolonged use, respiratory depression (dose related), seizure, skeletal muscle rigidity, skin rash, tachycardia, urinary retention, urinary tract spasm, urticaria

Drug Interactions
Metabolism/Transport Effects Substrate of CYP3A4 (major); **Note:** Assignment of Major/Minor substrate status based on clinically relevant drug interaction potential

Avoid Concomitant Use
Avoid concomitant use of SUFentanil with any of the following: Azelastine (Nasal); Ceritinib; Conivaptan; Fusidic Acid (Systemic); MAO Inhibitors; Paraldehyde; Thalidomide

Increased Effect/Toxicity
SUFentanil may increase the levels/effects of: Alcohol (Ethyl); Alvimopan; Azelastine (Nasal); Beta-Blockers; Bradycardia-Causing Agents; Buprenorphine; Calcium Channel Blockers (Nondihydropyridine); Ceritinib; CNS Depressants; Desmopressin; Diuretics; Hydrocodone; MAO Inhibitors; Methotrimeprazine; Metyrosine; Mirtazapine; Paraldehyde; Pramipexole; ROPINIRole; Rotigotine; Selective Serotonin Reuptake Inhibitors; Thalidomide; Zolpidem

The levels/effects of SUFentanil may be increased by: Amphetamines; Anticholinergic Agents; Antipsychotic Agents (Phenothiazines); Brimonidine (Topical); Cannabis; Conivaptan; CYP3A4 Inhibitors (Moderate); CYP3A4 Inhibitors (Strong); Dasatinib; Doxylamine; Dronabinol; Droperidol; Fusidic Acid (Systemic); HydrOXYzine; Ivacaftor; Kava Kava; Luliconazole; Magnesium Sulfate; Methotrimeprazine; Mifepristone; Nabilone; Perampanel; Rufinamide; Simeprevir; Sodium Oxybate; Stiripentol; Succinylcholine; Tapentadol; Tetrahydrocannabinol

Decreased Effect
SUFentanil may decrease the levels/effects of: Pegvisomant

The levels/effects of SUFentanil may be decreased by: Ammonium Chloride; Mixed Agonist / Antagonist Opioids; Naltrexone

Mechanism of Action Binds to opioid receptors throughout the CNS. Once receptor binding occurs, effects are exerted by opening K+ channels and inhibiting Ca++ channels. These mechanisms increase pain threshold, alter pain perception, inhibit ascending pain pathways; short-acting opioid; dose-related inhibition of catecholamine release (up to 30 mcg/kg) controls sympathetic response to surgical stress.

Pharmacodynamics
Onset of action: 1-3 minutes

Duration: Dose dependent; anesthesia adjunct doses: 5 minutes

Pharmacokinetics (Adult data unless noted)
Distribution: V_{dss}:
Children 2-8 years: 2.9 ± 0.6 L/kg
Adults: 1.7 ± 0.2 L/kg

Protein binding (alpha$_1$-acid glycoprotein):
Neonates: 79%
Adults:
Male: 93%
Postpartum women: 91%

Metabolism: Primarily by the liver via demethylation and dealkylation

Half-life, elimination:
Neonates: 382-1162 minutes
Children 2-8 years: 97 ± 42 minutes
Adolescents 10-15 years: 76 ± 33 minutes
Adults: 164 ± 22 minutes

Elimination: ~2% excreted unchanged in the urine; 80% of dose excreted in urine (mostly as metabolites) within 24 hours

Clearance:
Children 2-8 years: 30.5 ± 8.8 mL/minute/kg
Adolescents: 12.8 ± 12 mL/minute/kg

Adults: 12.7 ± 0.8 mL/minute/kg

Dosing: Neonatal Doses should be titrated to appropriate effects; wide range of doses, dependent upon desired degree of analgesia or anesthesia.

General anesthesia, adjunct (deep intraoperative anesthesia for neonatal cardiac surgery): Full-term neonates: I.V.: 5-10 mcg/kg/dose as needed; followed by a continuous I.V. infusion (for postoperative anesthesia): 2 mcg/kg/**hour** for 24 hours (Anand, 1992)

Analgesia/sedation in mechanically ventilated patients: Preterm neonates: I.V.: Loading dose: 0.5 mcg/kg/dose administered over 10 minutes, followed by 0.2 mcg/kg/**hour** continuous infusion was used in 15 mechanically ventilated premature neonates (mean GA: 29.1 weeks (26-34 weeks) and produced "burst-suppression-like" EEG patterns (Tich, 2010)

Dosing: Usual Doses should be titrated to appropriate effects; wide range of doses, dependent upon desired degree of analgesia or anesthesia; use lean body weight to dose patients who are >20% above ideal body weight.

Children <12 years: Anesthesia: I.V.: Initial: 10-25 mcg/kg; maintenance: Up to 25-50 mcg as needed

Adults: I.V.:

Adjunct to general anesthesia:

Low dose: Initial: 0.5-1 mcg/kg; maintenance: 10-25 mcg as needed

Moderate dose: Initial: 2-8 mcg/kg; maintenance: 10-50 mcg as needed

Anesthesia: Initial: 8-30 mcg/kg; maintenance: 10-50 mcg as needed

Administration Parenteral: I.V.: Slow I.V. injection or by infusion

Monitoring Parameters Respiratory rate, blood pressure, heart rate, oxygen saturation, neurological status (for degree of analgesia/anesthesia)

Controlled Substance C-II

Dosage Forms Excipient information presented when available (limited, particularly for generics); consult specific product labeling.

Solution, Intravenous [preservative free]:

Sufenta: 50 mcg/mL (1 mL); 100 mcg/2 mL (2 mL); 250 mcg/5 mL (5 mL)

Generic: 50 mcg/mL (1 mL); 100 mcg/2 mL (2 mL); 250 mcg/5 mL (5 mL)

References

ACOG Committee on Practice Bulletins-Obstetrics, "ACOG Practice Bulletin. Clinical Management Guidelines for Obstetrician-Gynecologists Number 36, July 2002. Obstetric Analgesia and Anesthesia," *Obstet Gynecol*, 2002, 100(1):177-91.

Anand KJ and Hickey PR, "Halothane-Morphine Compared With High-Dose Sufentanil for Anesthesia and Postoperative Analgesia in Neonatal Cardiac Surgery," *N Engl J Med*, 1992, 326(1):1-9.

Guay J, Gaudreault P, Tang A, et al, "Pharmacokinetics of Sufentanil in Normal Children," *Can J Anaesth*, 1992, 39(1):14-20.

Montgomery A, Hale TW, and Academy Of Breastfeeding Medicine, "ABM Cinical Protocol #15: Analgesia and Anesthesia for the Breastfeeding Mother, Revised 2012," *Breastfeed Med*, 2012, 7(6):547-53.

Nguyen The Tich S, Vecchierini MF, Debillon T, et al, "Effects of Sufentanil on Electroencephalogram in Very and Extremely Preterm Neonates," *Pediatrics*, 2003, 111(1):123-8.

Seguin JH, Erenberg A, and Leff RD, "Safety and Efficacy of Sufentanil Therapy in the Ventilated Infant," *Neonatal Netw*, 1994, 13(4):37-40.

◆ **Sufentanil Citrate** see SUFentanil on page 1942

◆ **Sufentanil Citrate Injection, USP (Can)** see SUFentanil on page 1942

◆ **Sulamyd** see Sulfacetamide (Ophthalmic) on page 1943

◆ **Sulamyd** see Sulfacetamide (Topical) on page 1944

◆ **Sulbactam and Ampicillin** see Ampicillin and Sulbactam on page 162

◆ **Sulcrate® (Can)** see Sucralfate on page 1940

◆ **Sulcrate® Suspension Plus (Can)** see Sucralfate on page 1940

Sulfacetamide (Ophthalmic) (sul fa SEE ta mide)

Medication Safety Issues

Sound-alike/look-alike issues:

Bleph®-10 may be confused with Blephamide®

Brand Names: U.S. Bleph-10

Brand Names: Canada AK Sulf Liq; Bleph 10 DPS; Diosulf™; PMS-Sulfacetamide; Sodium Sulamyd

Therapeutic Category Antibiotic, Ophthalmic; Antibiotic, Sulfonamide Derivative

Generic Availability (U.S.) Yes

Use Ophthalmic: Treatment of conjunctivitis and other superficial ocular infections due to susceptible organisms (Ointment; solution: FDA approved in ages ≥2 months and adults); adjunctive treatment with systemic sulfonamides for therapy of trachoma (Solution: FDA approved in ages ≥2 months and adults)

Pregnancy Risk Factor C

Pregnancy Considerations Animal reproduction studies have not been conducted. Use of systemic sulfonamides during pregnancy may cause kernicterus in the newborn. Use during pregnancy only if clearly needed.

Breast-Feeding Considerations The amount of systemic absorption following ophthalmic administration is not known. Use of systemic sulfonamides while breast-feeding may cause kernicterus in the newborn; the amount of systemic absorption following ophthalmic administration is not known.

Contraindications Hypersensitivity to sulfacetamide, any component, or sulfonamides

Warnings Severe reactions to sulfonamides have been reported, regardless of route of administration; reactions may include Stevens-Johnson syndrome, toxic epidermal necrolysis, fulminant hepatic necrosis, or blood dyscrasias. Hypersensitivity reactions may occur when a sulfonamide is readministered, irrespective of the route of administration. At the first sign of hypersensitivity, skin rash, or other reactions, inform physician and discontinue use. Chemical similarities are present among sulfonamides, sulfonylureas, carbonic anhydrase inhibitors, thiazides, and loop diuretics (except ethacrynic acid). Use in patients with sulfonamide allergy is specifically contraindicated in product labeling; however, a risk of cross-reaction exists in patients with allergy to any of these compounds; avoid use when previous reaction has been severe.

Antibacterial activity may be decreased in the presence of purulent exudates containing para-aminobenzoic acid (PABA); nonsusceptible organisms, such as fungi, may proliferate with prolonged or repeated use of sulfonamide preparations. Incompatible with silver preparations; do not administer concurrently.

Precautions For topical ophthalmic use only; do not inject subconjunctivally or introduce directly into the anterior chamber of the eye. Use with caution in patients with severe dry eye or G-6-PD deficiency; hemolysis may occur in patients with G-6-PD deficiency.

Adverse Reactions

Cardiovascular: Edema

Ocular (following ophthalmic application): Burning, conjunctivitis, conjunctival hyperemia, corneal ulcers, irritation, stinging

Miscellaneous: Allergic reactions, systemic lupus erythematosus

Drug Interactions

Metabolism/Transport Effects None known.

Avoid Concomitant Use There are no known interactions where it is recommended to avoid concomitant use.

Increased Effect/Toxicity There are no known significant interactions involving an increase in effect.

Decreased Effect There are no known significant interactions involving a decrease in effect.

◄ **Stability**
Solution: Store at 8°C to 25°C (46°F to 77°F); protect from light. Discolored or cloudy solutions should not be used.
Ointment: Store at 20°C to 25°C (68°F to 77°F).

Mechanism of Action Interferes with bacterial growth by inhibiting bacterial folic acid synthesis through competitive antagonism of PABA

Pharmacodynamics Onset of action: Improvement of conjunctivitis is usually seen within 3-6 days

Dosing: Usual Infants ≥2 months, Children, Adolescents, and Adults:

Conjunctivitis: Ophthalmic:
Ointment: Instill ½" ribbon into the lower conjunctival sac of affected eye(s) every 3-4 hours and at bedtime; increase dosing interval as condition responds. Ointment may be used as an adjunct to the solution; usual duration of treatment: 7-10 days
Solution: Instill 1-2 drops into the lower conjunctival sac of affected eye(s) every 2-3 hours initially; increase dosing interval as condition responds; usual duration of treatment: 7-10 days
Trachoma: Ophthalmic: Solution: Instill 2 drops into the conjunctival sac of affected eye(s) every 2 hours; must be used in conjunction with systemic therapy

Administration For topical application to the eye only; not for injection. Avoid contact of tube or bottle tip with skin or eye. Apply finger pressure to lacrimal sac during and for 1-2 minutes after instillation to decrease risk of absorption and systemic effects.

Monitoring Parameters Response to therapy

Dosage Forms Excipient information presented when available (limited, particularly for generics); consult specific product labeling.
Ointment, Ophthalmic, as sodium:
Generic: 10% (3.5 g)
Solution, Ophthalmic, as sodium:
Bleph-10: 10% (5 mL)
Generic: 10% (15 mL)

References
Lohr JA, Austin RD, Grossman M, et al, "Comparison of Three Topical Antimicrobials for Acute Bacterial Conjunctivitis," *Pediatr Infect Dis J*, 1988, 7(9):626-9.

Sulfacetamide (Topical) (sul fa SEE ta mide)

Medication Safety Issues
Sound-alike/look-alike issues:
Klaron may be confused with Klor-Con

Brand Names: U.S. Klaron; Ovace Plus; Ovace Plus Wash; Ovace Wash; Seb-Prev Wash; Seb-Prev [DSC]

Brand Names: Canada Sulfacet-R

Therapeutic Category Acne Products; Antibiotic, Sulfonamide Derivative; Topical Skin Product

Generic Availability (U.S.) May be product dependent

Use Treatment of seborrheic dermatitis, seborrhea sicca, acne vulgaris, and secondary cutaneous bacterial infections due to organisms susceptible to sulfonamides (FDA approved in ages ≥12 years and adults; refer to product specific information for FDA approved indications)

Pregnancy Risk Factor C

Pregnancy Considerations Animal reproduction studies have not been conducted. The amount of sulfacetamide available systemically following topical administration is unknown. Use of systemic sulfonamides during pregnancy may cause kernicterus in the newborn.

Breast-Feeding Considerations Small amounts of sulfonamides administered orally are excreted in breast milk; it is not known if sulfacetamide administered topically is excreted in breast milk. Use of systemic sulfonamides while breast-feeding may cause kernicterus in the newborn.

Contraindications Hypersensitivity to sulfacetamide, any component, or sulfonamides; infants <2 months of age

Warnings Fatalities associated with sulfonamides, although rare, have occurred due to severe reactions, including Stevens-Johnson syndrome, toxic epidermal necrolysis, systemic lupus erythematosus, hepatic necrosis, agranulocytosis, aplastic anemia, and other blood dyscrasias; discontinue use at first sign of rash or other adverse reaction. Hypersensitivity reactions may occur when a sulfonamide is readministered, irrespective of the route of administration. Antibacterial activity may be decreased in the presence of purulent exudates containing para-aminobenzoic acid (PABA); nonsusceptible organisms, such as fungi, may proliferate with prolonged or repeated use of sulfonamide preparations; hemolysis may occur in patients with G-6-PD deficiency. Some products contain sulfites which may cause allergic reactions in susceptible individuals.

Precautions For external use only; avoid contact with eyes and mucous membranes. May cause reddening and/or scaling of the skin; use caution when applying to denuded or abraded skin. If irritation occurs, discontinue use. Use with caution in patients with G-6-PD deficiency.

Adverse Reactions
Dermatologic: Burning sensation of skin, erythema, pruritus, Stevens-Johnson syndrome, stinging of the skin, toxic epidermal necrolysis
Hematologic & oncologic: Agranulocytosis, aplastic anemia, hematologic abnormality
Hepatic: Fulminant hepatic necrosis
Hypersensitivity: Hypersensitivity reaction
Local: Local irritation, localized edema
Neuromuscular & skeletal: Systemic lupus erythematosus

Drug Interactions
Metabolism/Transport Effects None known.
Avoid Concomitant Use
Avoid concomitant use of Sulfacetamide (Topical) with any of the following: BCG
Increased Effect/Toxicity There are no known significant interactions involving an increase in effect.
Decreased Effect
Sulfacetamide (Topical) may decrease the levels/effects of: BCG; Sodium Picosulfate

Stability
Klaron®: Store at 20°C to 25°C (68°F to 77°F); do not freeze.
Ovace® Plus Shampoo; Ovace® Plus Wash; Ovace® Wash: Store at 25°C (77°F); excursions permitted to 15°C to 30°C (59°F to 86°F); protect from freezing or excessive heat.
Topical sulfacetamide preparations are incompatible with silver preparations.

Mechanism of Action Interferes with bacterial growth by inhibiting bacterial folic acid synthesis through competitive antagonism of PABA

Pharmacokinetics (Adult data unless noted) Absorption: Poor through intact skin

Dosing: Usual Children ≥12 years and Adults:
Acne: Topical: Klaron® Lotion: Apply thin film to affected area twice daily
Seborrheic dermatitis, including seborrhea sicca: Topical:
Ovace® Plus Wash; Ovace® Wash: Wash affected area twice daily; repeat application for 8-10 days. Dosing interval may be increased as eruption subsides. Applications once or twice weekly, or every other week may be used for prevention. If treatment needs to be reinitiated, start therapy as a twice daily regimen.
Ovace® Plus Shampoo: Wash hair at least twice weekly
Secondary cutaneous bacterial infections: Topical:
Ovace® Plus Wash; Ovace® Wash: Wash affected area once daily for 8-10 days

Administration For external use only; avoid contact with eyes and mucous membranes.

Lotion: Shake lotion well before using; apply a thin film to affected area.

Shampoo: Apply to wet hair and massage vigorously into scalp; thoroughly rinse hair.

Wash: Apply to wet hair or skin and massage into a full lather; rinse thoroughly and pat dry; repeat after 10-20 seconds (for seborrheic dermatitis). If skin dryness occurs, rinse off early or use less frequently. Regular shampooing after use on hair is not necessary; however, hair should be shampooed at least once weekly.

Monitoring Parameters Response to therapy

Dosage Forms Excipient information presented when available (limited, particularly for generics); consult specific product labeling. [DSC] = Discontinued product

Cream, External, as sodium:
Ovace Plus: 10% (57 g) [contains benzyl alcohol, butylparaben, cetyl alcohol, disodium edta, ethylparaben, methylparaben, propylparaben]

Gel, External, as sodium:
Ovace Plus Wash: 10% (355 mL) [contains cetearyl alcohol, edetate disodium dihydrate, methylparaben]
Generic: 10% (355 mL)

Liquid, External, as sodium:
Ovace Plus Wash: 10% (180 mL, 473 mL) [contains cetearyl alcohol, edetate disodium, methylparaben]
Ovace Wash: 10% (180 mL, 355 mL, 480 mL) [contains edetate disodium, methylparaben]
Seb-Prev Wash: 10% (340 mL) [contains edetate disodium, methylparaben]
Generic: 10% (177 mL, 354.8 mL, 355 mL, 480 mL)

Lotion, External, as sodium:
Klaron: 10% (118 mL)
Klaron: 10% (118 mL) [contains disodium edta, methylparaben, propylene glycol, sodium metabisulfite]
Ovace Plus: 9.8% (57 g) [contains benzyl alcohol, cetyl alcohol, disodium edta]
Seb-Prev: 10% (118 mL [DSC]) [contains methylparaben, sodium metabisulfite]
Generic: 10% (118 mL)

Shampoo, External, as sodium:
Ovace Plus: 10% (237 mL) [contains cetearyl alcohol, methylparaben, propylparaben]
Generic: 10% (237 mL)

Suspension, External, as sodium:
Generic: 10% (118 mL)

♦ **Sulfacetamide Sodium** see Sulfacetamide (Ophthalmic) on page 1943

♦ **Sulfacetamide Sodium** see Sulfacetamide (Topical) on page 1944

♦ **Sulfacet-R (Can)** see Sulfacetamide (Topical) on page 1944

SulfADIAZINE (sul fa DYE a zeen)

Medication Safety Issues
Sound-alike/look-alike issues:
SulfADIAZINE may be confused with sulfaSALAzine, sulfiSOXAZOLE

Therapeutic Category Antibiotic, Sulfonamide Derivative

Generic Availability (U.S.) Yes

Use Adjunctive treatment in toxoplasmosis with pyrimethamine [FDA approved in ages ≥2 months and adults (may be used in ages <2 months for treatment of congenital toxoplasmosis)]

Treatment of chancroid, trachoma, inclusion conjunctivitis, urinary tract infections, and nocardiosis (not first line), treatment and prophylaxis of meningococcal meningitis, treatment of *H. influenza* meningitis, prophylaxis of rheumatic fever prophylaxis in penicillin-allergic patient,

treatment of uncomplicated attack of malaria due to chloroquine-resistant *Plasmodium falciparum* (FDA approved in ages ≥2 months and adults)

Pregnancy Risk Factor C

Pregnancy Considerations Adverse events have been observed in animal reproduction studies. Sulfadiazine crosses the placenta (Speert, 1943). Available studies and case reports have failed to show an increased risk for congenital malformations after sulfadiazine use (Heinonen, 1977); however, studies with sulfonamides as a class have shown mixed results (ACOG, 2011).

Sulfadiazine is recommended for use in pregnant women to prevent *T. gondii* infection of the fetus, for the maternal treatment of *Toxoplasmic gondii* encephalitis, and as an alternative agent for the secondary prevention of rheumatic fever (CDC, 2009; DHHS, 2013; Gerber, 2009). Sulfonamides may be used to treat other infections in pregnant women when clinically appropriate for confirmed infections caused by susceptible organisms; use during the first trimester should be limited to situations where no alternative therapies are available (ACOG, 2011). Because safer options are available for the treatment of urinary tract infections in pregnant women, use of sulfonamide-containing products >32 weeks gestation should be avoided (Lee, 2008). Due to the theoretical increased risk for hyperbilirubinemia and kernicterus, sulfadiazine is contraindicated by the manufacturer for use near term. Neonatal healthcare providers should be informed if maternal sulfonamide therapy is used near the time of delivery (DHHS, 2013).

Breast-Feeding Considerations Sulfadiazine distributes into human milk. Sulfonamides should not be used while nursing an infant with G6PD deficiency or hyperbilirubinemia (Della-Giustina, 2003). Per the manufacturer, sulfadiazine is contraindicated in nursing mothers since sulfonamides cross into the milk and may cause kernicterus in the newborn. Nondose-related effects could include modification of bowel flora.

Contraindications Hypersensitivity to any sulfa drug or any component; porphyria; infants <2 months of age due to competition with bilirubin for protein-binding sites (unless indicated for the treatment of congenital toxoplasmosis); pregnant women during third trimester and during the breast-feeding period

Warnings Fatalities associated with sulfonamides, although rare, have occurred due to severe reactions, including Stevens-Johnson syndrome, toxic epidermal necrolysis, hepatic necrosis, agranulocytosis, aplastic anemia, and other blood dyscrasias; discontinue use at first sign of rash or any sign of adverse reaction, including sore throat, fever, arthralgia, pallor, purpura, jaundice, cough, shortness of breath, and pulmonary infiltrates. Chemical similarities are present among sulfonamides, sulfonylureas, carbonic anhydrase inhibitors, thiazides, and loop diuretics (except ethacrynic acid); potential for crossreaction exists in patients with allergy to any of these compounds; avoid use when previous reaction has been severe. In an established infection, sulfonamides do not eradicate streptococcus nor prevent sequelae, such as rheumatic fever, and should not be used for the treatment of group A beta-hemolytic streptococcal infection. Prolonged use may result in fungal or bacterial superinfection, including *C. difficile*-associated diarrhea (CDAD) and pseudomembranous colitis; CDAD has been observed >2 months postantibiotic treatment.

Sulfa antibiotics have been shown to displace bilirubin from protein binding sites which may potentially lead to hyperbilirubinemia and kernicterus in neonates and young infants; do not use in neonates; avoid use in infants <2 months unless other options are not available. Tablets or oral suspension extemporaneously compounded with tablets may contain sodium benzoate; benzoic acid (benzoate) is a metabolite of benzyl alcohol; large amounts of benzyl alcohol (≥99 mg/kg/day) have been associated with a potentially fatal toxicity ("gasping syndrome") in neonates; the "gasping syndrome" consists of metabolic acidosis, respiratory distress, gasping respirations, CNS dysfunction (including convulsions, intracranial hemorrhage), hypotension and cardiovascular collapse; use tablets containing sodium benzoate with caution in neonates; *in vitro* and animal studies have shown that benzoate displaces bilirubin from protein binding sites.

Precautions Use with caution in patients with impaired hepatic function or impaired renal function or urinary obstruction; dosage modification may be required in patients with renal impairment; maintain adequate hydration to prevent crystalluria. Use with caution in patients with G6PD deficiency; dose-related hemolysis may occur. Use with caution in patients with allergies or asthma.

Adverse Reactions

Cardiovascular: Allergic myocarditis, periarteritis nodosa

Central nervous system: Ataxia, chills, convulsions, depression, fever, hallucinations, headache, insomnia, vertigo

Dermatologic: Epidermal necrolysis, erythema multiforme, exfoliative dermatitis, photosensitivity, pruritus, purpura, rash, skin eruptions, Stevens-Johnson syndrome, urticaria

Endocrine & metabolic: Hypoglycemia, thyroid function disturbance

Gastrointestinal: Abdominal pain, anorexia, diarrhea, nausea, pancreatitis, stomatitis, vomiting

Genitourinary: Crystalluria, stone formation, toxic nephrosis with oliguria and anuria

Hematologic: Agranulocytopenia, aplastic anemia, hemolytic anemia, hypoprothrombinemia, leukopenia, methemoglobinemia, thrombocytopenia

Hepatic: Hepatitis

Neuromuscular & skeletal: Arthralgia, peripheral neuritis

Ocular: Conjunctival/scleral injection, periorbital edema

Otic: Tinnitus

Renal: Diuresis

Miscellaneous: Anaphylactoid reactions, lupus erythematosus, serum sickness-like reactions

Drug Interactions

Metabolism/Transport Effects Substrate of CYP2C9 (major), CYP2E1 (minor), CYP3A4 (minor); **Note:** Assignment of Major/Minor substrate status based on clinically relevant drug interaction potential; **Inhibits** CYP2C9 (strong)

Avoid Concomitant Use

Avoid concomitant use of SulfADIAZINE with any of the following: BCG; Methenamine; Potassium P-Aminobenzoate; Procaine

Increased Effect/Toxicity

SulfADIAZINE may increase the levels/effects of: Bosentan; Carvedilol; CycloSPORINE (Systemic); CYP2C9 Substrates; Diclofenac (Systemic); Dronabinol; Lacosamide; Methotrexate; Ospemifene; Porfimer; Prilocaine; Sodium Nitrite; Sulfonylureas; Tetrahydrocannabinol; Vitamin K Antagonists

The levels/effects of SulfADIAZINE may be increased by: Cannabis; Ceritinib; CYP2C9 Inhibitors (Moderate); CYP2C9 Inhibitors (Strong); Methenamine; Mifepristone; Nitric Oxide

Decreased Effect

SulfADIAZINE may decrease the levels/effects of: BCG; CycloSPORINE (Systemic); Sodium Picosulfate; Typhoid Vaccine

The levels/effects of SulfADIAZINE may be decreased by: CYP2C9 Inducers (Strong); Dabrafenib; Peginterferon Alfa-2b; Potassium P-Aminobenzoate; Procaine

Food Interactions Vitamin C or acidifying agents (cranberry juice) may cause crystalluria. Management: Avoid large quantities of vitamin C or acidifying agents (cranberry juice).

Stability Store at 20°C to 25°C (68°F to 77°F); protect from light

Mechanism of Action Interferes with bacterial growth by inhibiting bacterial folic acid synthesis through competitive antagonism of PABA

Pharmacokinetics (Adult data unless noted)

Absorption: Oral: Well absorbed

Distribution: Excreted in breast milk; diffuses into CSF with higher concentrations reached when meninges are inflamed; distributed into most body tissues

Protein binding: 38% to 48%

Metabolism: Metabolized by N-acetylation

Half-life: 10 hours

Time to peak serum concentration: Within 4 hours

Elimination: In urine as metabolites (15% to 40%) and as unchanged drug (43% to 60%)

Dosing: Neonatal Congenital toxoplasmosis: Oral:
100 mg/kg/day divided every 12 hours for 12 months in conjunction with pyrimethamine and supplemental leucovorin (CDC, 2009)

Dosing: Usual

Infants <2 months: **Congenital toxoplasmosis:** Oral: 100 mg/kg/day divided every 12 hours for 12 months in conjunction with pyrimethamine and supplemental leucovorin (CDC, 2009)

Infants ≥2 months, Children, and Adolescents:

General dosing, susceptible infection: Oral:

Manufacturer's labeling: Initial: 75 mg/kg/dose or 2000 mg/m^2/dose once followed by maintenance: 150 mg/kg/day or 4000 mg/m^2/day divided every 4-6 hours; maximum daily dose: 6 g/day

Alternate dosing: 120-150 mg/kg/day in divided doses 4-6 times daily; maximum daily dose: 6 g/**day** (*Red Book*, 2012)

Toxoplasmosis (CDC, 2009; *Red Book*, 2012): Oral:

Congenital: Infants: 100 mg/kg/day divided every 12 hours for 12 months in conjunction with pyrimethamine

Acquired: Acute induction therapy: Infants ≥2 months, Children, and Adolescents: 100-200 mg/kg/day divided every 4-6 hours in conjunction with pyrimethamine and supplemental leucovorin; maximum daily dose: 6 g/**day**. Continue acute induction therapy for at least 6 weeks, then follow with chronic suppressive therapy.

Secondary prophylaxis (HIV-exposed/-positive): Infants ≥2 months and Children: 85-120 mg/kg/day divided every 6-12 hours; in combination with pyrimethamine and leucovorin; maximum daily dose: 4000 mg/**day**

Encephalitis; Toxoplasma gondii; treatment (HIV-exposed/-positive) (CDC, 2013): Adolescents: Oral:

Acute therapy: At least 6 weeks of therapy recommended; use in conjunction with pyrimethamine and supplemental leucovorin combination therapy or with atovaquone

Patient weight <60 kg: 1000 mg every 6 hours

Patient weight ≥60 kg: 1500 mg every 6 hours

Chronic maintenance therapy: 2000-4000 mg/day in divided doses 2-4 times daily in conjunction with pyrimethamine and leucovorin or with atovaquone; begin after completion of acute therapy

Rheumatic fever; secondary prophylaxis: Oral:

Manufacturer's labeling:

≤30 kg: 500 mg once daily

≥30 kg: 1000 mg/day

Alternate dosing (Gerber, 2009; *Red Book*, 2012):

Patient weight ≤27 kg: 500 mg once daily

Patient weight >27 kg: 1000 mg once daily

Adults:

General dosing: Oral: Initial 2000-4000 mg once, followed by 2000-4000 mg/day in divided doses 3-6 times daily

***Toxoplasma gondii* encephalitis (HIV-exposed/-positive patients)** (CDC, 2013a): Oral:

Acute therapy: At least 6 weeks of therapy necessary; use in conjunction with pyrimethamine and leucovorin combination therapy or with atovaquone

Patient weight <60 kg: 1000 mg every 6 hours

Patient weight ≥60 kg: 1500 mg every 6 hours

Chronic maintenance therapy: 2000-4000 mg/day in divided doses 2-4 times daily in conjunction with pyrimethamine and leucovorin or with atovaquone; begin after completion of acute therapy

Rheumatic fever prophylaxis: Oral:

<30 kg: 500 mg/day

≥30 kg: 1000 mg/day

Dosing adjustment in renal impairment: There are no dosage adjustments in the manufacturer's labeling.

Dosing adjustment in hepatic impairment: There are no dosage adjustments in the manufacturer's labeling.

Administration Oral: Administer with at least 8 ounces of water and around-the-clock to promote less variation in peak and trough serum levels. In adults, oral sodium bicarbonate may be used to alkalinize the urine of patients unable to maintain adequate fluid intake (in order to prevent crystalluria, azotemia, oliguria) (Lerner, 1996)

Monitoring Parameters CBC, renal function tests, urinalysis; signs of serious blood disorders (sore throat, fever, pallor, purpura, jaundice); CD4+ count in HIV-exposed/-positive patients treated for toxoplasmosis; sulfonamide blood concentrations may be monitored for severe infections (target: 12-15 mg/100 mL); observe for change in bowel frequency

Additional Information Sulfadiazine plus pyrimethamine confers protection against *Pneumocystis jirovecii* so additional PCP prophylaxis not required (CDC, 2009).

Dosage Forms Excipient information presented when available (limited, particularly for generics); consult specific product labeling.

Tablet, Oral:

Generic: 500 mg

Extemporaneous Preparations A 200 mg/mL oral suspension may be made with sulfadiazine powder and sterile water. Place 50 g sulfadiazine powder in a glass mortar. Add small portions of sterile water and mix to a uniform paste; mix while incrementally adding sterile water to **almost** 250 mL; transfer to a calibrated bottle, rinse mortar with sterile water, and add sufficient quantity of sterile water to make 250 mL. Label "shake well" and "refrigerate". Stable for 3 days refrigerated. **Note:** Suspension may also be prepared by crushing one-hundred 500 mg tablets; however, it is stable for only 2 days.

Pathmanathan U, Halgrain D, Chiadmi F, et al, "Stability of Sulfadiazine Oral Liquids Prepared From Tablets and Powder," *J Pharm Pharm Sci*, 2004, 7(1):84-7.

References

American College of Obstetricians and Gynecologists (ACOG) Committee on Obstetric Practice, "ACOG Committee Opinion No. 494: Sulfonamides, Nitrofurantoin, and Risk of Birth Defects," *Obstet Gynecol*, 2011, 117(6):1484-5.

Centers for Disease Control and Prevention (CDC), "Guidelines for the Prevention and Treatment of Opportunistic Infections Among HIV-Exposed and HIV-Infected Children: Recommendations from CDC, the National Institutes of Health, the HIV Medicine Association of the Infectious Diseases Society of America, the Pediatric Infectious Diseases Society, and the American Academy of Pediatrics," *MMWR Recomm Rep*, 2009, 58(RR-11):1-166. Available at http://aidsinfo.nih.gov/contentfiles/Pediatric_OI.pdf

Centers for Disease Control and Prevention (CDC). Guidelines for prevention and treatment of opportunistic infections in HIV-infected adults and adolescents: recommendations from CDC, the National Institutes of Health, and the HIV Medicine Association of the Infectious Diseases Society of America. *MMWR Recomm Rep*. 2009a;58(RR-4):1-207.

Della-Giustina K and Chow G, "Medications in Pregnancy and Lactation," *Emerg Med Clin North Am*, 2003, 21(3):585-613.

DHHS Panel on Opportunistic Infections (OI) in HIV-Infected Adults and Adolescents, "Guidelines for Prevention and Treatment of Opportunistic Infections in HIV-Infected Adults and Adolescents: Recommendations From the Centers for Disease Control and Prevention (CDC), the National Institutes of Health (NIH), and the HIV Medicine Association (HIVMA) of the Infectious Diseases Society of America (IDSA)," May 7, 2013. Available at http://aidsinfo.nih.gov/contentfiles/lvguidelines/adult_oi.pdf

Frenkel JK, "Toxoplasmosis," *Pediatr Clin North Am*, 1985, 32(4):917-32.

Gerber MA, Baltimore RS, Eaton CB, et al, "Prevention of Rheumatic Fever and Diagnosis and Treatment of Acute *Streptococcal pharyngitis*: A Scientific Statement From the American Heart Association Rheumatic Fever, Endocarditis, and Kawasaki Disease Committee of the Council on Cardiovascular Disease in the Young, the Interdisciplinary Council on Functional Genomics and Translational Biology, and the Interdisciplinary Council on Quality of Care and Outcomes Research: Endorsed by the American Academy of Pediatrics," Circulation, 2009, 119(11):1541-51.

Heinonen OP, Slone D, and Shapiro S, *Birth Defects and Drugs in Pregnancy*, Littleton, MA: Publishing Sciences Group, Inc, 1977.

Lee M, Bozzo P, Einarson A, et al, "Urinary Tract Infections in Pregnancy," *Can Fam Physician*, 2008, 54(6):853-4.

Lerner PI. Nocardiosis. *Clin Infect Dis*. 1996;22(6):891-903.

Red Book: 2012 Report of the Committee on Infectious Diseases, "Antibacterial Drugs Dosage Tables," 29th ed, Pickering LK, ed, Elk Grove Village, IL: American Academy of Pediatrics, 2012, 808-16.

Schmidt DR, Hogh B, Andersen O, et al, "Treatment of Infants With Congenital Toxoplasmosis: Tolerability and Plasma Concentrations of Sulfadiazine and Pyrimethamine," *Eur J Pediatr*, 2006, 165(1):19-25.

Speert H, "Placental Transmission of Sulfathiazole and Sulfadiazine and its Significance for Fetal Chemotherapy," *Am J Obstet Gynecol*, 1943, 45:200-7.

Sulfadoxine and Pyrimethamine

(sul fa DOKS een & peer i METH a meen)

Brand Names: U.S. Fansidar® [DSC]

Therapeutic Category Antimalarial Agent

Generic Availability (U.S.) No

Use Treatment of *Plasmodium falciparum* malaria in patients in whom chloroquine resistance is suspected; malaria prophylaxis for travelers to areas where chloroquine-resistant malaria is endemic

Pregnancy Risk Factor C

Pregnancy Considerations Adverse events have been observed in animal reproduction studies. Pyrimethamine and sulfadoxine both cross the placenta. Prophylactic use near term is contraindicated by the manufacturer.

Breast-Feeding Considerations Pyrimethamine and sulfadoxine both enter breast milk. Prophylactic use in lactating women is contraindicated by the manufacturer.

Contraindications Hypersensitivity to any sulfa drug, pyrimethamine, or any component; megaloblastic anemia due to folate deficiency; children <2 months of age (due to competition with bilirubin for protein binding sites); pregnant women at term; breast-feeding; repeated prophylactic use in patients with renal or hepatic failure or with blood dyscrasias

Warnings Fatalities associated with sulfonamides, although rare, have occurred due to severe reactions including Stevens-Johnson syndrome, toxic epidermal necrolysis, hepatic necrosis, agranulocytosis, aplastic anemia and other blood dyscrasias **[U.S. Boxed Warning]**; discontinue use at first sign of rash or any sign of adverse reaction; hemolysis may occur in patients with G-6-PD deficiency

Precautions Use with caution in patients with renal or hepatic impairment, patients with possible folate deficiency, patients with bronchial asthma, and patients with seizure disorders. Avoid excess sun exposure.

Adverse Reactions

Cardiovascular: Myocarditis (allergic), pericarditis (allergic), periorbital edema

Central nervous system: Ataxia, hallucinations, headache, polyneuritis, seizure

Dermatologic: Erythema multiforme, photosensitivity, rash, Stevens-Johnson syndrome, toxic epidermal necrolysis

Endocrine & metabolic: Thyroid function dysfunction

Gastrointestinal: Anorexia, atrophic glossitis, gastritis, pancreatitis, vomiting

Genitourinary: Crystalluria

Hematologic: Megaloblastic anemia, leukopenia, pancytopenia, thrombocytopenia

Hepatic: Hepatic necrosis, hepatitis

Neuromuscular & skeletal: Tremors

Renal: increased BUN, increased serum creatinine, interstitial nephritis, renal failure

Respiratory: Alveolitis (resembling eosinophilic or allergic) respiratory failure

Miscellaneous: Anaphylactoid reaction, drug fever, hypersensitivity, lupus-like syndrome, periarteritis nodosum

Drug Interactions

Metabolism/Transport Effects Refer to individual components.

Avoid Concomitant Use

Avoid concomitant use of Sulfadoxine and Pyrimethamine with any of the following: Artemether; BCG; Lumefantrine; Methenamine; Potassium P-Aminobenzoate; Procaine

Increased Effect/Toxicity

Sulfadoxine and Pyrimethamine may increase the levels/effects of: Antipsychotic Agents (Phenothiazines); Bosentan; Cannabis; Carvedilol; CycloSPORINE (Systemic); CYP2C9 Substrates; Dapsone (Systemic); Dapsone (Topical); Dronabinol; Lumefantrine; Methotrexate; Porfimer; Sulfonylureas; Tetrahydrocannabinol; Vitamin K Antagonists

The levels/effects of Sulfadoxine and Pyrimethamine may be increased by: Artemether; Dapsone (Systemic); Methenamine

Decreased Effect

Sulfadoxine and Pyrimethamine may decrease the levels/effects of: BCG; CycloSPORINE (Systemic); Sodium Picosulfate; Typhoid Vaccine

The levels/effects of Sulfadoxine and Pyrimethamine may be decreased by: Methylfolate; Potassium P-Aminobenzoate; Procaine

Stability Protect from light

Mechanism of Action Sulfadoxine interferes with bacterial folic acid synthesis and growth via competitive inhibition of para-aminiobenzoic acid; pyrimethamine inhibits microbial dihydrofolate reductase, resulting in inhibition of tetrahydrofolic acid synthesis

Pharmacokinetics (Adult data unless noted)

Absorption: Oral: Well absorbed

Distribution: Excreted in breast milk; pyrimethamine is distributed to kidneys, lungs, liver, and spleen; sulfadoxine is widely distributed in the body

Protein binding:
Pyrimethamine: 80% to 87%
Sulfadoxine: 90% to 95%

Half-life:
Pyrimethamine: 111 hours
Sulfadoxine: 169 hours

Time to peak serum concentration: Within 2-8 hours

Elimination: In urine as parent compounds and several unidentified metabolites

Dosing: Usual Children ≥2 months and Adults: Oral:

Treatment of acute attack of malaria: A single dose of the following number of Fansidar® tablets is used in sequence with quinine on last day of quinine therapy:

2-11 months: 1/4 tablet
1-3 years: 1/2 tablet
4-8 years: 1 tablet
9-14 years: 2 tablets
>14 years: 3 tablets

Adults: 3 tablets on last day of quinine therapy

Malaria prophylaxis (for areas where chloroquine-resistant *P. falciparum* exists):

Short-term travel (≤3 weeks): Travelers should carry pyrimethamine-sulfadoxine for use as presumptive self-treatment if a febrile illness develops while taking chloroquine for prophylaxis. Take single dose in the event of febrile illness when medical attention is not immediately available:

2-11 months: 1/4 tablet
1-3 years: 1/2 tablet
4-8 years: 1 tablet
9-14 years: 2 tablets
>14 years and Adults: 3 tablets

Administration Oral: Administer with meals

Monitoring Parameters Liver function tests, CBC including platelet counts, renal function tests and urinalysis should be performed periodically

Additional Information Leucovorin calcium should be administered to reverse signs and symptoms of folic acid deficiency

Dosage Forms Excipient information presented when available (limited, particularly for generics); consult specific product labeling. [DSC] = Discontinued product

Tablet:
Fansidar®: Sulfadoxine 500 mg and pyrimethamine 25 mg [DSC]

References

Lynk A and Gold R, "Review of 40 Children With Imported Malaria," *Pediatr Infect Dis J*, 1989, 8(11):745-50.

Randall G and Seidel JS, "Malaria," *Pediatr Clin North Am*, 1985, 32 (4):893-916.

Sulfamethoxazole and Trimethoprim
(sul fa meth OKS a zole & trye METH oh prim)

Medication Safety Issues

Sound-alike/look-alike issues:

Bactrim may be confused with bacitracin, Bactine, Bactroban

Co-trimoxazole may be confused with clotrimazole

Septra may be confused with Ceptaz, Sectral

Septra DS may be confused with Semprex-D

Brand Names: U.S. Bactrim; Bactrim DS; Septra DS; Sulfatrim

Brand Names: Canada Apo-Sulfatrim; Apo-Sulfatrim DS; Apo-Sulfatrim Pediatric; Protrin DF; Septra Injection; Teva-Trimel; Teva-Trimel DS; Trisulfa; Trisulfa DS; Trisulfa S

Therapeutic Category Antibiotic, Sulfonamide Derivative

Generic Availability (U.S.) Yes

Use

Oral: Treatment of urinary tract infections caused by susceptible *E. coli*, *Klebsiella* and *Enterobacter* sp., *M. morganii*, *P. mirabilis* and *P. vulgaris* (FDA approved in ages ≥2 months and adults); single course treatment of acute otitis media due to *H. influenzae*, *S. pneumoniae*, and *M. catarrhalis* (FDA approved in ages ≥2 months and adults); prophylaxis and treatment of *Pneumocystis jirovecii* pneumonitis (PCP) [FDA approved in pediatric patients (age not specified) and adults]; treatment of enteritis caused by *Shigella flexneri* or *Shigella sonnei* (FDA approved in ages ≥2 months and adults); acute exacerbations of chronic bronchitis due to susceptible strains of *H. influenzae* or *S. pneumoniae* (FDA approved in adults); traveler's diarrhea due to enterotoxigenic *E. coli* (FDA approved in adults). Has also been used for treatment of typhoid fever, *Nocardia asteroids*, MRSA, and *Stenotrophomonas maltophilia* infections

Parenteral: Treatment of *Pneumocystis jirovecii* pneumonitis (PCP), *Shigella*, and severe urinary tract infections due to *E. coli*, *Klebsiella*, and *Enterobacter* spp, *M. morganii*, *P. mirabilis*, and *P. vulgaris* (FDA approved in children and adults); has also been used in treatment of severe or complicated infections caused by susceptible bacteria when oral therapy is not feasible, including typhoid fever and *Nocardia asteroides* infection

Pregnancy Risk Factor D

Pregnancy Considerations Adverse events have been observed in animal reproduction studies. Trimethoprim-sulfamethoxazole (TMP-SMX) crosses the placenta and distributes to amniotic fluid (Ylikorkala, 1973). An increased risk of congenital malformations (neural tube defects, cardiovascular malformations, urinary tract defects, oral clefts, club foot) following maternal use of TMP-SMX during pregnancy has been observed in some studies. Folic acid supplementation may decrease this risk (Crider, 2009; Czeizel, 2001; Hernandez-Diaz, 2000; Hernandez-Diaz, 2001; Matok, 2009). Due to theoretical concerns that sulfonamides pass the placenta and may cause kernicterus in the newborn, neonatal healthcare providers should be informed if maternal sulfonamide therapy is used near the time of delivery (DHHS, 2013).

The pharmacokinetics of TMP-SMX are similar to non-pregnant values in early pregnancy (Ylikorkala, 1973). TMP-SMX is recommended for the prophylaxis or treatment of *Pneumocystis jirovecii* pneumonia (PCP), prophylaxis of *Toxoplasmic gondii* encephalitis (TE), and for the acute and chronic treatment of Q fever in pregnancy (CDC, 2013; DHHS, 2013). Sulfonamides may also be used to treat other infections in pregnant women when clinically appropriate; use during the first trimester should be limited to situations where no alternative therapies are available (ACOG, 2011). Because safer options are available for the treatment of urinary tract infections in pregnant women, use of TMP-containing products in the first trimester and sulfonamide-containing products >32 weeks gestation should be avoided (Lee, 2008).

Breast-Feeding Considerations Small amounts of TMP and SMX are transferred into breast milk. The manufacturer recommends that caution be used if administered to nursing women, especially if breast-feeding ill, jaundiced, premature, or stressed infants due to the potential risk of bilirubin displacement and kernicterus. Sulfonamides should not be used while nursing an infant with G6PD deficiency or hyperbilirubinemia (Della-Giustina, 2003). Maternal indications for TMP-SMX must also be considered prior to nursing. Nondose-related effects could include modification of bowel flora.

Contraindications Hypersensitivity to sulfonamides, trimethoprim, or any component; history of drug-induced immune thrombocytopenia with use of sulfonamides or trimethoprim; megaloblastic anemia due to folate deficiency; marked hepatic damage or severe renal disease (if patient not monitored); infants <2 months of age (manufacturer's information), infants <4 weeks of age (CDC, 2009; Pediatric HIV Opportunistic Infections Guidelines)

Warnings Fatalities associated with sulfonamides, although rare, have occurred due to severe reactions, including Stevens-Johnson syndrome, toxic epidermal necrolysis, hepatic necrosis, agranulocytosis, aplastic anemia, thrombocytopenia, and other blood dyscrasias; discontinue use at first sign of rash or any sign of adverse reaction, including sore throat, fever, arthralgia, pallor, purpura, jaundice, cough, shortness of breath, and pulmonary infiltrates. Chemical similarities are present among sulfonamides, sulfonylureas, carbonic anhydrase inhibitors, thiazides, and loop diuretics (except ethacrynic acid); potential for cross-reaction exists in patients with allergy to any of these compounds; avoid use when previous reaction has been severe. In an established infection, sulfonamides do not eradicate streptococcus nor prevent sequelae, such as rheumatic fever, and should not be used for the treatment of group A beta-hemolytic streptococcal infection. When used for uncomplicated urinary tract infections, this combination should not be used if a single agent is effective. Prolonged use may result in fungal or bacterial superinfection, including *C. difficile*-associated diarrhea (CDAD) and pseudomembranous colitis; CDAD has been observed >2 months postantibiotic treatment. Sulfa antibiotics have been shown to displace bilirubin from protein binding sites which may potentially lead to hyperbilirubinemia and kernicterus in neonates and young infants; do not use in neonates; avoid use in infants <2 months unless other options are not available (eg, *Pneumocystis*). Concomitant use with leucovorin for the acute treatment of *Pneumocystis jirovecii* pneumonia in patients with HIV infection has been associated with increased rates of treatment failure and morbidity.

Trimethoprim may cause folate deficiencies with subsequent bone marrow suppression and blood dyscrasias; monitor patients for fever, sore throat, purpura, or pallor; obtain CBC if any of these symptoms occur; risk may be increased with high dose or prolonged use; discontinue trimethoprim if bone marrow depression occurs; leucovorin calcium may be needed to restore normal hematopoiesis. Immune mediated thrombocytopenia may occur with sulfamethoxazole/trimethoprim therapy; severe cases which may be life-threatening or fatal have been reported; thrombocytopenia usually resolves within 1 week following discontinuation of therapy.

Use during pregnancy may be associated with embryofetal toxicity. Oral suspension and tablets may contain sodium metabisulfite which may cause allergic reactions in susceptible individuals. Injection and oral suspension contain propylene glycol; toxicities have been reported with use of products containing propylene glycol, including hyperosmolality, lactic acidosis, seizures, and respiratory depression; in neonates large amounts of propylene glycol delivered orally, intravenously (eg, >3000 mg/day), or topically have been associated with potentially fatal toxicities which can include metabolic acidosis, seizures, renal failure, and CNS depression; use injections and oral suspensions containing propylene glycol with caution (AAP, 1997; Shehab, 2009). Injection and oral suspension contain benzyl alcohol which may cause allergic reactions in susceptible individuals; large amounts of benzyl alcohol (≥99 mg/kg/day) have been associated with a potentially fatal toxicity ("gasping syndrome") in neonates; the "gasping syndrome" consists of metabolic acidosis, respiratory distress, gasping respirations, CNS dysfunction (including convulsions, intracranial hemorrhage), hypotension and cardiovascular collapse; use products containing benzyl alcohol with caution in neonates; *in vitro* and animal studies have shown that benzoate, a metabolite of benzyl alcohol, displaces bilirubin from protein binding sites.

Precautions Use with caution in patients with renal impairment; dosage adjustment recommended and maintain adequate hydration to prevent crystalluria. Use with caution in patients with porphyria. Use with caution in patients with G-6-PD deficiency; dose-related hemolysis may occur. Use with caution in patients with potential folate deficiency (eg, the elderly, chronic alcoholics, anticonvulsant therapy, malabsorption syndrome, and malnourished), in patients with allergies, asthma, or thyroid dysfunction. Severe and symptomatic hyponatremia may occur, particularly in patients treated for *Pneumocystis jirovecii* pneumonia (PCP). May cause hyperkalemia (associated with high doses of trimethoprim), use with caution in patients receiving potassium-sparing diuretics, potassium supplements, and/or potassium-containing salts. May cause hypoglycemia, particularly in malnourished or patients with renal or hepatic impairment. Incidence of adverse effects appears to be increased in patients with AIDS. Slow acetylators may be more prone to adverse reactions.

◀ **Adverse Reactions**

Cardiovascular: Allergic myocarditis, periarteritis nodosa (rare)

Central nervous system: Apathy, aseptic meningitis, ataxia, chills, depression, fatigue, hallucination, headache, insomnia, nervousness, peripheral neuritis, seizure, vertigo

Dermatologic: Erythema multiforme (rare), exfoliative dermatitis (rare), pruritus, skin photosensitivity, skin rash, Stevens-Johnson syndrome (rare), toxic epidermal necrolysis (rare), urticaria

Endocrine & metabolic: Hyperkalemia (generally at high dosages), hypoglycemia (rare), hyponatremia

Gastrointestinal: Abdominal pain, anorexia, diarrhea, glottis edema, kernicterus (in neonates), nausea, pancreatitis, pseudomembranous colitis, stomatitis, vomiting

Genitourinary: Crystalluria, diuresis (rare), nephrotoxicity (in association with cyclosporine), toxic nephrosis (with anuria and oliguria)

Hematologic & oncologic: Agranulocytosis, anaphylactoid purpura (IgA vasculitis; rare), aplastic anemia, eosinophilia, hemolysis (with G6PD deficiency), hemolytic anemia, hypoprothrombinemia, leukopenia, megaloblastic anemia, methemoglobinemia, neutropenia, thrombocytopenia

Hepatic: Cholestatic jaundice, hepatotoxicity (including hepatitis, cholestasis, and hepatic necrosis), hyperbilirubinemia, increased transaminases

Hypersensitivity: Anaphylaxis, angioedema, hypersensitivity reaction, serum sickness

Neuromuscular & skeletal: Arthralgia, myalgia, rhabdomyolysis (mainly in AIDS patients), systemic lupus erythematosus (rare), weakness

Ophthalmic: Conjunctival injection, injected sclera

Otic: Tinnitus

Renal: Increased blood urea nitrogen, increased serum creatinine, interstitial nephritis, renal failure

Respiratory: Cough, dyspnea, pulmonary infiltrates

Miscellaneous: Fever

Rare but important or life-threatening: Idiopathic thrombocytopenic purpura, prolonged Q-T interval on ECG, thrombotic thrombocytopenic purpura

Drug Interactions

Metabolism/Transport Effects Refer to individual components.

Avoid Concomitant Use

Avoid concomitant use of Sulfamethoxazole and Trimethoprim with any of the following: BCG; Dofetilide; Leucovorin Calcium-Levoleucovorin; Methenamine; Potassium P-Aminobenzoate; Procaine

Increased Effect/Toxicity

Sulfamethoxazole and Trimethoprim may increase the levels/effects of: ACE Inhibitors; Amantadine; Angiotensin II Receptor Blockers; Antidiabetic Agents (Thiazolidinedione); AzaTHIOprine; Bosentan; Cannabis; Carvedilol; CycloSPORINE (Systemic); CYP2C8 Substrates; CYP2C9 Substrates; Dapsone (Systemic); Dapsone (Topical); Digoxin; Dofetilide; Dronabinol; Eplerenone; Fosphenytoin; Highest Risk QTc-Prolonging Agents; LamiVUDine; Memantine; Mercaptopurine; MetFORMIN; Methotrexate; Moderate Risk QTc-Prolonging Agents; Phenytoin; Porfimer; PRALAtrexate; Prilocaine; Procainamide; Repaglinide; Sodium Nitrite; Spironolactone; Sulfonylureas; Tetrahydrocannabinol; Varenicline; Vitamin K Antagonists

The levels/effects of Sulfamethoxazole and Trimethoprim may be increased by: Amantadine; Ceritinib; CYP2C9 Inhibitors (Moderate); CYP2C9 Inhibitors (Strong); Dapsone (Systemic); Memantine; Methenamine; Mifepristone; Nitric Oxide

Decreased Effect

Sulfamethoxazole and Trimethoprim may decrease the levels/effects of: BCG; CycloSPORINE (Systemic); Sodium Picosulfate; Typhoid Vaccine

The levels/effects of Sulfamethoxazole and Trimethoprim may be decreased by: Bosentan; CYP2C9 Inducers (Strong); CYP3A4 Inducers (Strong); Dabrafenib; Deferasirox; Fosphenytoin; Leucovorin Calcium-Levoleucovorin; Mitotane; Peginterferon Alfa-2b; Phenytoin; Potassium P-Aminobenzoate; Procaine; Siltuximab; St Johns Wort; Tocilizumab

Stability

Injection: Store intact vials at 20°C to 25°C (68°F to 77°F); do not refrigerate. Protect from light. Less soluble in alkaline pH. Solution must be diluted prior to administration; do not mix with other drugs or solutions. Following dilution, store at room temperature; do not refrigerate. Manufacturer recommended dilutions and stability of parenteral admixture at room temperature (25°C):

5 mL/125 mL D_5W (1:25 dilution); stable for 6 hours

5 mL/100 mL D_5W (1:20 dilution); stable for 4 hours

5 mL/75 mL D_5W (1:15 dilution); stable for 2 hours

5 mL/50 mL D_5W (1:10 highly concentrated admixture) may precipitate in 1-2 hours

Studies have also confirmed limited stability in NS; detailed references should be consulted.

Oral: Suspension, tablet:

Bactrim™: Store at 20°C to 25°C (68°F to 77°F). Protect from light.

Septra®: Store at 15°C to 25°C (59°F to 77°F). Protect from light.

Mechanism of Action Sulfamethoxazole interferes with bacterial folic acid synthesis and growth via inhibition of dihydrofolic acid formation from para-aminobenzoic acid; trimethoprim inhibits dihydrofolic acid reduction to tetrahydrofolate resulting in sequential inhibition of enzymes of the folic acid pathway

Pharmacokinetics (Adult data unless noted)

Absorption: Oral: Almost completely (90% to 100%)

Distribution: Joint fluid, sputum, middle ear fluid, bile, and CSF

V_d: TMP:

Newborns: ~2.7 L/kg (range: 1.3-4.1 hours) (Springer, 1982)

Infants: 1.5 L/kg (Hoppu, 1989)

Children 1-10 years: 0.86-1 L/kg (Hoppu, 1987)

Adults: ~1.3 L/kg (Hoppu, 1987)

Protein binding:

TMP: ~44%

SMX: 68%

Metabolism: Hepatic, both to multiple metabolites; SMX to hydroxy (via CYP2C9) and acetyl derivatives, and also conjugated with glucuronide; TMP to oxide and hydroxy derivatives; the free forms of both SMX and TMP are therapeutically active

Half-life:

TMP: Prolonged in renal failure

Newborns: ~19 hours; range: 11-27 hours (Springer, 1982)

Infants 2 months to 1 year: ~4.6 hours; range: 3-6 hours (Hoppu, 1989)

Children 1-10 years: 3.7-5.5 hours (Hoppu, 1987)

Children and Adolescents >10 years: 8.19 hours

Adults: 6-11 hours

SMX: 9-12 hours, prolonged in renal failure

Time to peak serum concentration: Oral: Within 1-4 hours

Elimination: Both excreted in urine as metabolites and unchanged drug

Dosing: Usual Note: Dosage recommendations are based on the trimethoprim (TMP) component:

Infants 4 weeks to <2 months (HIV-exposed/-positive):

Pneumocystis **prophylaxis:** Oral: 150 mg TMP/m²/day or 5 mg TMP/kg/day for 3-7 days of every week; total daily dose may be given in divided doses every 12 hours for 3 consecutive or alternating days, in divided doses every 12 hours every day or as a single daily dose for 3 consecutive days (CDC, 2009; *Red Book*, 2012)

Infants ≥2 months, Children, and Adolescents:

General dosing, susceptible infection: Oral, I.V.: 8-12 mg TMP/kg/day in divided doses every 12 hours; maximum single dose: 160 mg TMP (*Red Book*, 2012)

Acute otitis media: Oral: 6-10 mg TMP/kg/day in divided doses every 12 hours for 10 days. **Note:** Due to resistance of *S. pneumoniae*, should not be used in patients that fail first-line amoxicillin therapy (Lieberthal, 2013).

Blastomycosis; South African (Paracoccidioiodomycosis): I.V.: 8-10 mg TMP/kg/day in divided doses 3 times daily for 3-6 weeks; after clinical improvement, may transition to oral therapy: 10 mg TMP/kg/day in divided doses 2 times daily for 2 years or longer (*Red Book*, 2012)

Cyclosporiasis: Limited data available: Oral: 10 mg TMP/kg/day in divided doses twice daily for 7-10 days; maximum single dose: 160 mg TMP (*Red Book*, 2012)

Meningitis: I.V.: 10-20 mg TMP/kg/day divided every 6-12 hours for 7-21 days; duration dependent on the pathogen and clinical course (Tunkel, 2004)

MRSA, community-acquired mild to moderate skin/soft tissue infection: Oral: 8-12 mg TMP/kg/day in divided doses every 12 hours (Liu, 2011); alternatively, use of 20 mg TMP/kg/day in divided doses every 6 hours has been reported (Norrby-Teglund, 2008). If using empirically, consider addition of group A streptococcal coverage.

Pneumocystis jirovecii **pneumonia (PCP) (HIV-exposed/-positive):**

Infants ≥2 months and Children (CDC, 2009):

Treatment: Oral, I.V.: 15-20 mg TMP/kg/day in divided doses every 6-8 hours for 21 days (CDC, 2009)

Prophylaxis: Oral: 150 mg TMP/m²/day or 5 mg TMP/kg/day for 3-7 days of every week; total daily dose may be given in divided doses every 12 hours for 3 consecutive or alternating days, in divided doses every 12 hours every day or as a single daily dose for 3 consecutive days; maximum daily dose: TMP 320 mg/**day** (CDC, 2009)

Adolescents (DHHS, 2013):

Treatment:

Mild to moderate: Oral: 15-20 mg TMP/kg/day in 3 divided doses for 21 days **or** alternatively, 320 mg TMP 3 times daily for 21 days

Moderate to severe: Initial: I.V.: 15-20 mg TMP/kg/day in 3-4 divided doses for 21 days; may switch to oral after clinical improvement

Prophylaxis: Oral: 80-160 mg TMP daily **or** alternatively, 160 mg TMP 3 times weekly

Q-Fever (*Coxiella burnetii*); mild infection (doxycycline therapeutic failure): Children <8 years: Oral: 8 mg TMP/kg/day in divided doses twice daily for 14 days; maximum daily dose 320 mg TMP/**day** (CDC, 2013)

Shigellosis: Note: Due to reported widespread resistance empiric therapy with sulfamethoxazole and trimethoprim is not recommended (CDC-NARMS, 2010; WHO, 2005)

Oral:

Manufacturer's labeling: 8 mg TMP/kg/day in divided doses every 12 hours for 5 days; maximum single dose: 160 mg TMP

Alternate dosing: IDSA recommendations for infectious diarrhea: 10 mg TMP/kg/day in divided doses every 12 hours for 3 days (for immunocompetent patients) or 7-10 days (for immunocompromised patients); maximum single dose: 160 mg TMP (Guerrant, 2001)

I.V.: 8-10 mg TMP/kg/day in divided doses every 6, 8, or 12 hours for up to 5 days

Toxoplasmosis (HIV-exposed/infected):

Prophylaxis, primary:

Infants ≥2 months and Children: Oral: 150 mg TMP/m²/day for 3-7 days of every week; total daily dose may be given in divided doses every 12 hours for 3 consecutive or alternating days, in divided doses every 12 hours every day or as a single daily dose for 3 consecutive days (CDC, 2009)

Adolescents: Oral: 160 mg TMP daily (preferred) **or** 160 mg TMP 3 times weekly **or** 80 mg TMP daily (DHHS, 2013)

Treatment, encephalitis: Adolescents: Oral, I.V.: 10 mg/kg/day TMP in two divided doses for at least 6 weeks; longer duration may be required in some patients followed by chronic maintenance therapy (DHHS, 2013)

Chronic maintenance therapy; postencephalitis treatment: Adolescents: Oral: 160 mg TMP twice daily (DHHS, 2013)

Urinary tract infection:

Treatment:

Oral:

Infants and Children 2-24 months: 6-12 mg TMP/kg/day in divided doses every 12 hours for 7-14 days (AAP, 2011)

Children >24 months and Adolescents: 8 mg TMP/kg/day in divided doses every 12 hours for 3 days; longer duration may be required in some patients; maximum single dose: 160 mg TMP

I.V.: 8-10 mg TMP/kg/day in divided doses every 6, 8, or 12 hours for up to 14 days with serious infections

Prophylaxis: Oral: 2 mg TMP/kg/dose once daily (Mattoo, 2007; *Red Book*, 2012)

Adults:

General dosing, susceptible infection:

Oral: 1-2 double strength tablets (sulfamethoxazole 800 mg; trimethoprim 160 mg) every 12-24 hours

I.V.: 8-20 mg TMP/kg/day divided every 6-12 hours

Chronic bronchitis, acute exacerbation: Oral: One double strength tablet every 12 hours for 10-14 days

Dialysis-related infections:

Exit-site and tunnel infections: Oral: One single-strength tablet daily (Li, 2010)

Peritonitis:

Oral: One double-strength tablet twice daily (Li, 2010)

Intraperitoneal: Loading dose: TMP 320 mg/L; Maintenance: TMP 80 mg/L (Aronoff, 2007; Warady, 2000)

Meningitis, bacterial: I.V.: 10-20 mg TMP/kg/day in divided doses every 6-12 hours

Nocardia: Oral, I.V.:

Cutaneous infections: 5-10 mg TMP/kg/day in 2-4 divided doses

Severe infections (pulmonary/cerebral): 15 mg TMP/kg/day in 2-4 divided doses for 3-4 weeks, then 10 mg TMP/kg/day in 2-4 divided doses. Treatment duration is controversial; an average of 7 months has been reported.

Note: Therapy for severe infection may be initiated I.V. and converted to oral therapy (frequently converted to approximate dosages of oral solid dosage forms: 2 DS tablets every 8-12 hours). Although not widely available, sulfonamide levels should be considered in patients with questionable absorption, at risk for ▶

dose-related toxicity or those with poor therapeutic response.

***Pneumocystis jirovecii* pneumonia (PCP) prophylaxis and treatment in HIV-positive patients** (DHHS, 2013):

Prophylaxis: Oral: 80-160 mg TMP daily or alternatively, 160 mg TMP 3 times weekly

Treatment:

Mild to moderate: Oral: 15-20 mg TMP/kg/day in 3 divided doses for 21 days **or** alternatively, 320 mg TMP 3 times daily for 21 days

Moderate to severe: Oral, I.V.: 15-20 mg TMP/kg/day in 3-4 divided doses for 21 days

Sepsis: I.V.: 20 mg TMP/kg/day divided every 6 hours

Shigellosis: Note: Due to reported widespread resistance, empiric therapy with sulfamethoxazole and trimethoprim is not recommended (CDC-NARMS, 2010; WHO, 2005).

Oral: One double strength tablet every 12 hours for 5 days

I.V.: 8-10 mg TMP/kg/day in divided doses every 6, 8, or 12 hours for up to 5 days

Skin/soft tissue infection due to community-acquired MRSA: Oral: 1-2 double strength tablets every 12 hours (Liu, 2011; Stevens, 2005); **Note:** If beta-hemolytic *Streptococcus* spp are also suspected, a beta-lactam antibiotic should be added to the regimen (Liu, 2011)

***Toxoplasma gondii* encephalitis** (DHHS, 2013):

Primary prophylaxis: Oral: 160 mg TMP daily (preferred) **or** 160 mg TMP 3 times weekly **or** 80 mg TMP daily

Treatment (alternative to sulfadiazine, pyrimethamine, and leucovorin calcium): Oral, I.V.: 5 mg/kg TMP twice daily

Travelers' diarrhea: Oral: One double strength tablet every 12 hours for 5 days

Urinary tract infection:

Oral: One double strength tablet every 12 hours

Duration of therapy: Uncomplicated: 3-5 days; Complicated: 7-10 days

Pyelonephritis: 14 days

Prostatitis: Acute: 2 weeks; Chronic: 2-3 months

I.V.: 8-10 mg TMP/kg/day in divided doses every 6, 8, or 12 hours for up to 14 days with severe infections

Dosing adjustment in renal impairment:

Manufacturer's labeling: Infants ≥2 months, Children, Adolescents, and Adults: Oral, I.V.:

CrCl >30 mL/minute: No adjustment required

CrCl 15-30 mL/minute: Administer 50% of recommended dose

CrCl <15 mL/minute: Use is not recommended

Alternate recommendations:

CrCl 15-30 mL/minute:

Treatment: Children, Adolescents, and Adults: Oral, I.V.: Administer full daily dose (divided every 12 hours) for 24-48 hours, then decrease daily dose by 50% and administer every 24 hours; **Note:** For serious infections, including *Pneumocystis jirovecii* pneumonia (PCP), full daily dose is given in divided doses every 6-8 hours for 2 days, followed by reduction to 50% daily dose divided every 12 hours (Nahata, 1995).

PCP prophylaxis: Adolescents and Adults: Oral: One-half single-strength tablet (40 mg trimethoprim) daily **or** one single-strength tablet (80 mg trimethoprim) daily **or** 3 times weekly (Masur, 2002).

CrCl <15 mL/minute:

Treatment: Children, Adolescents, and Adults: Oral, I.V.: Administer 50% of the daily dose every 48 hours (Nahata, 1995); **Note:** In pediatric patients with GFR <10 mL/minute/1.73 m^2, use is not recommended by some clinicians; if use is required, administer 5-10 mg trimethoprim/kg every 24 hours (Aronoff, 2007).

PCP prophylaxis: Adolescents and Adults: Oral: One-half single-strength tablet (40 mg trimethoprim) daily **or** one single-strength tablet (80 mg trimethoprim) 3 times weekly (Masur, 2002). While the guidelines do acknowledge the alternative of giving one single-strength tablet daily, this may be inadvisable in the uremic/ESRD patient.

Hemodialysis:

Treatment:

Infants, Children, and Adolescents: Not recommended, but if required, administer 5-10 mg TMP/kg every 24 hours (Aronoff, 2007)

Adults: 2.5-10 mg/kg trimethoprim every 24 hours **or** 5-20 mg/kg trimethoprim 3 times weekly after IHD. **Note:** Dosing is highly dependent upon indication for use (eg, treatment of cystitis versus treatment of PCP pneumonia (Heinz, 2009).

PCP prophylaxis: Adolescents and Adults: Oral: One single-strength tablet (80 mg trimethoprim) after each dialysis session (Masur, 2002)

Note: Dosing dependent on the assumption of 3 times/week, complete IHD sessions.

Peritoneal dialysis (PD): Not significantly removed by CAPD; supplemental dosing is not required (Aronoff, 2007):

Treatment: Children, Adolescents, and Adults: Oral, I.V.: Administer 50% of daily dose every 48 hours (Nahata, 1995); **Note:** In pediatric PD patients, use is not recommended by some clinicians, if use is required, administer 5-10 mg trimethoprim/kg every 24 hours (Aronoff, 2007).

PCP prophylaxis: Adolescents and Adults: Oral: One-half single-strength tablet (40 mg trimethoprim) daily **or** 1 single-strength tablet (80 mg trimethoprim) 3 times weekly (Masur, 2002). While the guidelines do acknowledge the alternative of giving 1 single-strength tablet daily, this may be inadvisable in the uremic/ESRD patient.

CRRT:

Infants, Children, and Adolescents: 5 mg TMP/kg/dose every 8 hours (Aronoff, 2007)

Adults (Heintz, 2009; Trotman, 2005): Drug clearance is highly dependent on the method of renal replacement, filter type, and flow rate. Appropriate dosing requires close monitoring of pharmacologic response, signs of adverse reactions due to drug accumulation, as well as drug concentrations in relation to target trough (if appropriate). The following are general recommendations only (based on dialysate flow/ultrafiltration rates of 1-2 L/hour and minimal residual renal function) and should not supersede clinical judgment:

CVVH/CVVHD/CVVHDF: 2.5-7.5 mg/kg of TMP every 12 hours. **Note:** Dosing regimen dependent on clinical indication. Critically-ill patients with *P. jirovecii* pneumonia receiving CVVHDF may require up to 10 mg/kg every 12 hours (Heintz, 2009).

Dosing adjustment in hepatic impairment: There are no dosage adjustments provided in the manufacturer's labeling.

Administration

Oral: May administer with water on an empty stomach; shake suspension well before use

Parenteral: **Do not administer I.M.**

I.V. infusion: Further dilute prior to administration [ie, diluted 1:25 (5 mL drug to 125 mL diluent, ie, D$_5$W); in patients who require fluid restriction, a 1:15 dilution (5 mL drug to 75 mL diluent, ie, D$_5$W) or a 1:10 dilution (5 mL drug to 50 mL diluent, ie, D$_5$W)]. Inspect solution for evidence of cloudiness or precipitation prior to administration; infuse over 60-90 minutes; pH: 10

Monitoring Parameters CBC, renal function test, liver function test, urinalysis; observe for change in bowel frequency

Test Interactions Increased creatinine (Jaffé alkaline picrate reaction); increased serum methotrexate by dihydrofolate reductase method

Additional Information Leucovorin calcium should be given if bone marrow suppression occurs. Guidelines for prophylaxis of *Pneumocystis jirovecii* pneumonia: Initiate PCP prophylaxis in the following patients (CDC, 2009):

- All infants born to HIV-infected mothers should be given prophylaxis with TMP-SMZ beginning at 4-6 weeks of age and continue until HIV infection has been reasonably excluded
- All HIV-infected infants <12 months, regardless of CD4+ count or percentage, should continue prophylaxis through the first year of life and reassess based on defined thresholds
- Children 1-5 years of age with CD4+ count <500/mm^3 or CD4+ percentage <15%
- Children ≥6 years of age with CD4+ count <200 or CD4+ percentage <15%
- Adolescents and Adults with CD4+ count <200 or oropharyngeal candidiasis

Dosage Forms Excipient information presented when available (limited, particularly for generics); consult specific product labeling. **Note:** The 5:1 ratio (SMX:TMP) remains constant in all dosage forms.

Injection, solution: Sulfamethoxazole 80 mg and trimethoprim 16 mg per mL (5 mL, 10 mL, 30 mL)

Suspension, oral: Sulfamethoxazole 200 mg and trimethoprim 40 mg per 5 mL (20 mL, 480 mL)

Sulfatrim: Sulfamethoxazole 200 mg and trimethoprim 40 mg per 5 mL (480 mL) [contains alcohol <0.5%, propylene glycol; cherry flavor]

Tablet, oral: Sulfamethoxazole 400 mg and trimethoprim 80 mg

Bactrim: Sulfamethoxazole 400 mg and trimethoprim 80 mg

Tablet, double-strength, oral: Sulfamethoxazole 800 mg and trimethoprim 160 mg

Bactrim DS: Sulfamethoxazole 800 mg and trimethoprim 160 mg

Septra DS: Sulfamethoxazole 800 mg and trimethoprim 160 mg

References

American Academy of Pediatrics Committee on Drugs. "Inactive" ingredients in pharmaceutical products: update (subject review). *Pediatrics.* 1997;99(2):268-278.

American Academy of Pediatrics Subcommittee on Urinary Tract Infection, "Urinary Tract Infection: Clinical Practice Guideline for the Diagnosis and Management of the Initial UTI in Febrile Infants and Children 2 to 24 Months," *Pediatrics,* 2011, 128(3):595-610.

American College of Obstetricians and Gynecologists (ACOG) Committee on Obstetric Practice, "ACOG Committee Opinion No. 494: Sulfonamides, Nitrofurantoin, and Risk of Birth Defects," *Obstet Gynecol,* 2011, 117(5):1484-5.

Aronoff GR, Bennett WM, Berns JS, et al, *Drug Prescribing in Renal Failure: Dosing Guidelines for Adults and Children,* 5th ed. Philadelphia, PA: American College of Physicians, 2007, 154.

Ashkenazi S, Amir J, Waisman Y, et al, "A Randomized, Double-Blind Study Comparing Cefixime and Trimethoprim-Sulfamethoxazole in the Treatment of Childhood Shigellosis," *J Pediatr,* 1993, 123 (5):817-21.

Centers for Disease Control and Prevention (CDC), "Diagnosis and Management of Q Fever - United States, 2013: Recommendations From CDC and the Q Fever Working Group," *MMWR Recomm Rep,* 2013, 62(RR-03):1-30.

Centers for Disease Control and Prevention (CDC), "Guidelines for the Prevention and Treatment of Opportunistic Infections Among HIV-Exposed and HIV-Infected Children," *MMWR Recomm Rep,* 2009, 58(RR-11):1-166. Available at http://aidsinfo.nih.gov/contentfiles/Pediatric_OI.pdf

Centers for Disease Control and Prevention (CDC), "National Antimicrobial Resistance Monitoring System for Enteric Bacteria (NARMS): Human Isolates Final Report, 2010," Atlanta, Georgia: U.S. Department of Health and Human Services, CDC, 2012.

Crider KS, Cleves MA, Reefhuis J, et al, "Antibacterial Medication Use During Pregnancy and Risk of Birth Defects: National Birth Defects Prevention Study," *Arch Pediatr Adolesc Med,* 2009, 163(11):978-85.

Czeizel AE, Rockenbauer M, Sørensen HT, et al, "The Teratogenic Risk of Trimethoprim-Sulfonamides: A Population Based Case-Control Study," *Reprod Toxicol,* 2001, 15(6):637-46.

Della-Giustina K and Chow G, "Medications in Pregnancy and Lactation," *Emerg Med Clin North Am,* 2003, 21(3):585-613.

DHHS Panel on Opportunistic Infections (OI) in HIV-Infected Adults and Adolescents, "Guidelines for Prevention and Treatment of Opportunistic Infections in HIV-Infected Adults and Adolescents: Recommendations from the Centers for Disease Control and Prevention (CDC), the National Institutes of Health (NIH), and the HIV Medicine Association (HIVMA) of the Infectious Diseases Society of America (IDSA)," May 7, 2013. Available at http://aidsinfo.nih.gov/contentfiles/lvguidelines/adult_oi.pdf

Guerrant RL, Van Gilder T, Steiner TS, et al, "Practice Guidelines for the Management of Infectious Diarrhea," *Clin Infect Dis,* 2001, 32 (3):331-51.

Heintz BH, Matzke GR, Dager WE, "Antimicrobial Dosing Concepts and Recommendations for Critically Ill Adult Patients Receiving Continuous Renal Replacement Therapy or Intermittent Hemodialysis," *Pharmacotherapy,* 2009, 29(5):562-77.

Hernández-Díaz S and Mitchell AA, Author reply, *NEJM,* 2001, 344(12): 934-5.

Hernández-Díaz S, Werler MM, Walker AM, et al, "Folic Acid Antagonists During Pregnancy and the Risk of Birth Defects," *N Engl J Med,* 2000, 343(22):1608-14.

Hoppu K, "Age Differences in Trimethoprim Pharmacokinetics: Need for Revised Dosing in Children?" *Clin Pharmacol Ther,* 1987, 41 (3):336-43.

Hoppu K, "Changes in Trimethoprim Pharmacokinetics After the Newborn Period," *Arch Dis Child,* 1989, 64(3):343-5.

Jarosinki PF, Kennedy PE, and Gallelli JF, "Stability of Concentrated Trimethoprim-Sulfamethoxazole Admixtures," *AJHP,* 1989, 46 (4):732-7.

Lee M, Bozzo P, Einarson A, et al, "Urinary Tract Infections in Pregnancy," *Can Fam Physician,* 2008, 54(6):853-4.

Li PK, Szeto CC, Piraino B, et al, "Peritoneal Dialysis-Related Infections Recommendations: 2010 Update," *Perit Dial Int,* 2010, 30(4):393-423

Lieberthal AS, Carroll AE, Chonmaitree T, et al, "The Diagnosis and Management of Acute Otitis Media," *Pediatrics,* 2013, 131(3): e964-99.

Liu C, Bayer A, Cosgrow SE, et al, "Clinical Practice Guidelines by the Infectious Diseases Society of America for the Treatment of Methicillin-Resistant *Staphylococcus aureus* Infections in Adults and Children," *Clin Infect Dis,* 2011,52:1-38.

Matok I, Gorodischer R, Koren G, et al, "Exposure to Folic Acid Antagonists During the First Trimester of Pregnancy and the Risk of Major Malformations," *Br J Clin Pharmacol,* 2009, 68(6):956-62.

Mattoo TK, "Medical Management of Vesicoureteral Reflux - Quiz Within the Article. Don't Overlook Placebos," *Pediatr Nephrol,* 2007, 22(8):1113-20.

Nahata MC, "Dosing Regimens of Trimethoprim/Sulfamethoxazole (TPM/SMX) in Patients With Renal Dysfunction.," *Ann Pharmacother,* 1995, 29(12):1300.

Paap CM and Nahata MC, "Trimethoprim/Sulfamethoxazole Dosing During Renal Dysfunction," *Annals Pharmacother,* 1995, 29:1300.

Red Book: 2012 Report of the Committee on Infectious Diseases, 29th ed, Pickering LK, ed, Elk Grove Village, IL: American Academy of Pediatrics, 2012.

Shehab N, Lewis CL, Streetman DD, Donn SM. Exposure to the pharmaceutical excipients benzyl alcohol and propylene glycol among critically ill neonates. *Pediatr Crit Care Med.* 2009;10 (2):256-259.

Springer C, Eyal F, and Michel J, "Pharmacology of Trimethoprim-Sulfamethoxazole in Newborn Infants," *J Pediatr,* 1982, 100 (4):647-50.

Stevens DL, Bisno AL, Chambers HF, et al, "Practice Guidelines for the Diagnosis and Management of Skin and Soft-Tissue Infections," *Clin Infect Dis,* 2005, 41(10):1373-406.

Tunkel AR, Hartman BJ, Kaplan SL, et al, "Practice Guidelines for the Management of Bacterial Meningitis," *Clin Infect Dis,* 2004, 39 (9):1267-84.

Warady BA, Schaefer F, Holloway M, et al, "Consensus Guidelines for the Treatment of Peritonitis in Pediatric Patients Receiving Peritoneal Dialysis," *Perit Dial Int,* 2000, 20(6):610-24.

World Health Organization (WHO), "Guidelines for the Control of Shigellosis, Including Epidemics Due to *Shigella dysenteriae* Type 1," 2005. Available at http://whqlibdoc.who.int/publications/2005/9241592330.pdf

Ylikorkala O, Sjöstedt E, Järvinen PA, et al, "Trimethoprim-Sulfonamide Combination Administered Orally and Intravaginally in the First Trimester of Pregnancy: Its Absorption Into Serum and Transfer to Amniotic Fluid," *Acta Obstet Gynecol Scand,* 1973, 52(3):229-34.

◆ **Sulfamylon** *see* Mafenide *on page 1290*

SulfaSALAzine (sul fa SAL a zeen)

Medication Safety Issues
Sound-alike/look-alike issues:
SulfaSALAzine may be confused with salsalate, sulfA-DIAZINE, sulfiSOXAZOLE
Azulfidine may be confused with Augmentin, azaTHIO-prine

Related Information
Oral Medications That Should Not Be Crushed or Altered *on page 2438*

Brand Names: U.S. Azulfidine; Azulfidine EN-tabs; Sulfazine; Sulfazine EC

Brand Names: Canada Apo-Sulfasalazine; PMS-Sulfasalazine; Salazopyrin; Salazopyrin En-Tabs

Therapeutic Category 5-Aminosalicylic Acid Derivative; Anti-inflammatory Agent

Generic Availability (U.S.) Yes

Use Oral:
Tablet: Treatment of mild to moderate ulcerative colitis, adjunct therapy for severe ulcerative colitis and prolongation of remission of ulcerative colitis episodes (FDA approved in ages ≥6 years and adults)

Enteric coated tablet: Management of ulcerative colitis (FDA approved in ages ≥6 years and adults); treatment of juvenile idiopathic arthritis (JIA) in patients with an inadequate response to NSAIDs or salicylates (FDA approved in ages 6-16 years), and treatment of rheumatoid arthritis in an inadequate response to, or intolerance of, an adequate trial of full doses of one or more NSAIDs (FDA approved in adults); has also been used for induction therapy for Crohn's disease. **Note:** Although it is an FDA-labeled indication, the use of sulfasalazine for treatment of JIA is not recommended (per manufacturer; Ringold, 2013).

Pregnancy Risk Factor B

Pregnancy Considerations Adverse events have not been observed in animal reproduction studies. Sulfasalazine and sulfapyridine cross the placenta; a potential for kernicterus in the newborn exists. Agranulocytosis was noted in an infant following maternal use of sulfasalazine during pregnancy. Additionally, cases of neural tube defects have been reported (causation undetermined); sulfasalazine is known to inhibit the absorption and metabolism of folic acid and may diminish the effects of folic acid supplementation. Based on available data, an increase in fetal malformations has not been observed following maternal use of sulfasalazine for the treatment of inflammatory bowel disease or ulcerative colitis. When treatment for inflammatory bowel disease is needed during pregnancy, sulfasalazine may be used, although supplementation with folic acid is recommended (Habal, 2012; Mahadevan, 2009; Mottet, 2007).

Breast-Feeding Considerations Sulfasalazine is excreted in breast milk; sulfapyridine concentrations are ~30% to 60% of the maternal serum. Bloody stools or diarrhea have been reported in nursing infants. Although sulfapyridine has poor bilirubin-displacing ability, exposure may cause kernicterus in the newborn. The manufacturer recommends that caution be used in women who are breast-feeding. Other sources consider use of sulfasalazine to be safe while breast-feeding; monitoring of the infant is recommended (Habal, 2012; Mahadevan, 2009; Mottet, 2007).

Contraindications Hypersensitivity to sulfasalazine, sulfa drugs, salicylates, or any component; porphyria, GI or GU obstruction

Warnings Deaths from irreversible neuromuscular and central nervous system changes have been reported. Fatalities associated with severe reactions including agranulocytosis, aplastic anemia, and other blood dyscrasias have occurred; discontinue use at first sign of rash or signs of serious adverse reactions. Use with extreme caution in patients with blood dyscrasias. May decrease folic acid absorption leading to folate deficiency; consider providing folate supplementation.

Severe skin reactions (some fatal), including Stevens-Johnson syndrome, exfoliative dermatitis, and toxic epidermal necrolysis have occurred with sulfonamides; mostly commonly occurring during the first month of therapy; discontinue use at first sign of rash. Deaths from fibrosing alveolitis have been reported.

Fatalities associated with hepatic damage have occurred; discontinue use at first sign of jaundice or hepatotoxicity; use with extreme caution in patients with impaired hepatic function.

In males, oligospermia (rare) and infertility have been reported; usually reverses upon discontinuation.

Chemical similarities are present among sulfonamides, sulfonylureas, carbonic anhydrase inhibitors, thiazides, and loop diuretics (except ethacrynic acid). Use in patients with sulfonamide allergy is specifically contraindicated in product labeling; however, a risk of cross-reaction exists in patients with allergy to any of these compounds; avoid use when previous reaction has been severe. Severe reactions, including drug rash with eosinophilia and systemic symptoms (DRESS) syndrome have been reported. Fever or lymphadenopathy may be present prior to rash development. Discontinue treatment for severe reactions. Pediatric patients treated with sulfasalazine for JIA have a high incidence of adverse events, including a serum-sickness-like reaction which presents with fever, nausea, vomiting, headache, rash, and altered LFT's; discontinue treatment if these occur; use of sulfasalazine for treatment of JIA is not recommended (per manufacturer; Ringold, 2013).

Precautions Use with caution in patients with renal impairment; maintain adequate hydration to prevent crystalluria and stone formation. Use with caution in patients with G-6-PD deficiency; hemolytic anemia may occur. Use with caution in patients with severe allergies or asthma. Patients classified as slow acetylators may be at increased risk for adverse reactions due to a prolonged half-life of sulfapyrazine (metabolite of sulfasalazine). Nausea, vomiting, and abdominal discomfort commonly occur; titration of dose and/or using the enteric coated formulation may decrease GI adverse effects. If enteric coated tablets are noted to pass without disintegrating, discontinue use of that dosage form.

Adverse Reactions
Central nervous system: Dizziness, headache
Dermatologic: Pruritus, skin rash, urticaria
Gastrointestinal: Abdominal pain, anorexia, dyspepsia, gastric distress, nausea, stomatitis, vomiting
Genitourinary: Oligospermia (reversible)
Hematologic & oncologic: Heinz body anemia, hemolytic anemia, leukopenia, thrombocytopenia
Hepatic: Abnormal hepatic function tests
Respiratory: Cyanosis
Miscellaneous: Fever
Rare but important or life-threatening (includes reactions reported with mesalamine or other sulfonamides): Agranulocytosis, alopecia, anaphylaxis, angioedema, aplastic anemia, arthralgia, cauda equina syndrome, cholestatic hepatitis, cholestatic jaundice, conjunctival injection, crystalluria, depression, diarrhea, DRESS syndrome, drowsiness, eosinophilia, exfoliative dermatitis, folate deficiency, fulminant hepatitis, Guillain-Barré syndrome, hallucination, hearing loss, hematologic abnormality, hematologic disease (pseudomononucleosis), hematuria, hemolytic-uremic syndrome, hepatic cirrhosis, hepatic failure, hepatic necrosis, hepatitis, hypoglycemia, hypoprothrombinemia, injected sclera, insomnia, interstitial nephritis, interstitial pulmonary disease, jaundice,

Kawasaki syndrome (single case report), lupus-like syndrome, megaloblastic anemia, meningitis, methemoglobinemia, myelitis, myelodysplastic syndrome, myocarditis (allergic), nephritis, nephrolithiasis, nephrotic syndrome, neutropenia (congenital), neutropenic enterocolitis, oropharyngeal pain, pancreatitis, parapsoriasis varioliformis acuta, periarteritis nodosa, pericarditis, periorbital edema, peripheral neuropathy, pleurisy, pneumonia, pneumonitis, proteinuria, pulmonary alveolitis, purpura, renal disease (acute), rhabdomyolysis, seizure, sepsis, serum sickness-like reaction (children with JRA have frequent and severe reaction), skin discoloration, skin photosensitivity, Stevens-Johnson syndrome, thyroid function impairment, toxic epidermal necrolysis, toxic nephrosis, urine discoloration, vasculitis

Drug Interactions

Metabolism/Transport Effects None known.

Avoid Concomitant Use There are no known interactions where it is recommended to avoid concomitant use.

Increased Effect/Toxicity

SulfaSALAzine may increase the levels/effects of: Heparin; Heparin (Low Molecular Weight); Methotrexate; Prilocaine; Sodium Nitrite; Thiopurine Analogs; Varicella Virus-Containing Vaccines

The levels/effects of SulfaSALAzine may be increased by: Nitric Oxide; Nonsteroidal Anti-Inflammatory Agents

Decreased Effect

SulfaSALAzine may decrease the levels/effects of: Cardiac Glycosides; Folic Acid; Methylfolate

Mechanism of Action 5-aminosalicylic acid (5-ASA) is the active component of sulfasalazine; the specific mechanism of action of 5-ASA is unknown; however, it is thought that it modulates local chemical mediators of the inflammatory response, especially leukotrienes, and is also postulated to be a free radical scavenger or an inhibitor of tumor necrosis factor (TNF); action appears topical rather than systemic

Pharmacodynamics Onset of action:

JIA: Minimum trial of 3 months is necessary

Ulcerative colitis: >3-4 weeks

Pharmacokinetics (Adult data unless noted)

Absorption: Oral: 10% to 15% as unchanged drug from the small intestine; upon administration, the drug is split into sulfapyridine and 5-aminosalicylic acid (5-ASA) in the colon

Bioavailability: Sulfasalazine: <15%; sulfapyridine: ~60%; 5-aminosalicylic acid: ~10% to 30%

Distribution: Breast milk to plasma ratio: 0.09-0.17

Metabolism: Both components are metabolized in the liver; slow acetylators have higher plasma sulfapyridine concentrations

Half-life:

Sulfasalazine:

Single dose: 5.7 hours

Multiple doses: 7.6 hours

Sulfapyridine:

Single dose: 8.4 hours

Multiple doses: 10.4 hours

Time to peak serum concentration:

Serum sulfasalazine: Within 1.5-6 hours

Serum sulfapyridine (active metabolite): Within 6-24 hours

Elimination: Primarily in urine (as unchanged drug, components, and acetylated metabolites); small amounts appear in feces

Dosing: Usual

Children and Adolescents:

Inflammatory bowel disease (eg, ulcerative colitis; Crohn's disease): Oral:

Weight-based dosing:

Manufacturer's labeling: Ulcerative colitis: Children ≥6 years and Adolescents:

Induction: 40-60 mg/kg/day in 3-6 divided doses; maximum daily dose: 4000 mg/**day**

Maintenance: 30 mg/kg/day in 4 divided doses; maximum daily dose: 2000 mg/**day**

Alternate dosing:

Induction: Crohn disease, ulcerative colitis: 40-70 mg/kg/day in 4-6 divided doses; in some cases, higher induction doses up to 100 mg/kg/day may be required; maximum daily dose: 4000 mg/**day** (Rufo, 2012; Sandu, 2010; Turner, 2012)

Maintenance: Ulcerative colitis: 30-70 mg/kg/day in 2-6 divided doses; maximum daily dose: 4000 mg/**day** (Sandu, 2010; Turner, 2012)

Fixed dosing [Salazopyrin prescribing information (Canada), 2013]: Children ≥25 kg and Adolescents: **Note:** Consider dose reduction or use of enteric coated tablet in patients experiencing adverse gastrointestinal effects with uncoated tablet.

Acute attacks:

25 to <35 kg: 500 mg 3 times daily

35-50 kg: 1000 mg 2-3 times daily

Maintenance of remission:

25 to <35 kg: 500 mg 2 times daily

35-50 kg: 500 mg 2-3 times daily

Desensitization regimen: Children ≥6 years and Adolescents: For patients who may be sensitive to treatment, it is suggested to start with a total dose of 50-250 mg daily and double it every 4-7 days until the desired dose is achieved. Discontinue if symptoms of sensitivity occur. Do not attempt in patients with a history of agranulocytosis or those who have had a previous anaphylactoid reaction on sulfasalazine therapy.

Juvenile idiopathic arthritis: Children and Adolescents 6-16 years: Oral: Enteric coated tablet: 30-50 mg/kg/day in 2 divided doses; maximum daily dose: 2000 mg/**day** (Beukelman, 2011); **Note:** Although it is an FDA-labeled indication, the use of sulfasalazine for treatment of JIA is not recommended (per manufacturer; Ringold, 2013).

Adults:

Rheumatoid arthritis: Oral: Enteric coated tablet: Initial: 0.5-1 g daily; increase weekly to maintenance dose of 2 g daily in 2 divided doses; maximum: 3 g daily (if response to 2 g daily is inadequate after 12 weeks of treatment)

Ulcerative colitis: Oral:

Initial: 3-4 g daily in evenly divided doses at ≤8-hour intervals; may initiate therapy with 1-2 g daily to reduce GI intolerance. **Note:** American College of Gastroenterology guideline recommendations: Titrate to 4-6 g daily in 4 divided doses (Kornbluth, 2010)

Maintenance dose: 2 g daily in evenly divided doses at ≤8-hour intervals; if GI intolerance occurs reduce dosage by 50% and gradually increase to target dose after several days. If GI intolerance persists, stop drug for 5-7 days and reintroduce at a lower daily dose.

Desensitization regimen: For patients who may be sensitive to treatment, it is suggested to start with a total dose of 50-250 mg daily and double it every 4-7 days until the desired dose is achieved. Discontinue if symptoms of sensitivity occur. Do not attempt in patients with a history of agranulocytosis or those who have had a previous anaphylactoid reaction on sulfasalazine therapy.

Dosing adjustment in renal impairment: There are no dosage adjustments provided in manufacturer's labeling; use with extreme caution.

Dosing adjustment in hepatic impairment: There are no dosage adjustments provided in manufacturer's labeling; use with extreme caution.

Administration Tablets should be administered in evenly divided doses, preferably after meals. Do not crush enteric coated tablets.

Monitoring Parameters CBC, liver function tests (prior to therapy, then every other week for first 3 months of therapy, followed by every month for the second 3 months, then once every 3 months thereafter), urinalysis, renal function tests, liver function tests, stool frequency, hematocrit, reticulocyte count

Test Interactions Reports of possible interference with measurements, by liquid chromatography, of urinary normetanephrine causing a false-positive test result have been observed in patients exposed to sulfasalazine or its metabolite, mesalamine/mesalazine.

Dosage Forms Excipient information presented when available (limited, particularly for generics); consult specific product labeling.

Tablet, Oral:
Azulfidine: 500 mg [scored]
Sulfazine: 500 mg [scored]
Generic: 500 mg
Tablet Delayed Release, Oral:
Azulfidine EN-tabs: 500 mg
Sulfazine EC: 500 mg
Generic: 500 mg

Extemporaneous Preparations A 100 mg/mL oral suspension may be made with tablets. Place twenty 500 mg tablets in a mortar and add a small amount of a 1:1 mixture of Ora-Sweet® and Ora-Plus® to cover the tablets. Let soak for 20-30 minutes. Crush the tablets and mix to a uniform paste; mix while adding the vehicle in equal proportions to **almost** 100 mL; transfer to a calibrated bottle, rinse mortar with vehicle, and add sufficient quantity of vehicle to make 100 mL. Label "shake well". Stable 91 days under refrigeration or at room temperature.
Lingertat-Walsh K, Walker SE, Law S, et al, "Stability of Sulfasalazine Oral Suspension," *Can J Hosp Pharm*, 2006, 59(4):194-200.

References

Beukelman T, Patkar NM, Saag KG, et al. 2011 American College of Rheumatology recommendations for the treatment of juvenile idiopathic arthritis: initiation and safety monitoring of therapeutic agents for the treatment of arthritis and systemic features. *Arthritis Care Res*. 2011;63(4):465-482.

Habal FM, Huang VW. Review article: A decision-making algorithm for the management of pregnancy in the inflammatory bowel disease patient. *Aliment Pharmacol Ther*. 2012;35(5):501-15.

Kornbluth, Sachar DB. Ulcerative colitis practice guidelines in adults: American College of Gastroenterology, Practice Parameters Committee. *Am J Gastroenterol*. 2010;105(3):501-523.

Mahadevan U. Pregnancy and inflammatory bowel disease. *Gastroenterol Clin North Am*. 2009;38(4):629-49.

Mottet C, Juillerat P, Pittet V, et al. Pregnancy and breastfeeding in patients with Crohn's disease. *Digestion*. 2007;76(2):149-60.

Ringold S, Weiss PF, Beukelman T, et al. 2013 update of the 2011 American College of Rheumatology recommendations for the treatment of juvenile idiopathic arthritis: recommendations for the medical therapy of children with systemic juvenile idiopathic arthritis and tuberculosis screening among children receiving biologic medications. *Arthritis Rheum*. 2013;65(10):2499-2512.

Rufo PA, Denson LA, Sylvester FA, et al. Health supervision in the management of children and adolescents with IBD: NASPGHAN recommendations. *J Pediatr Gastroenterol Nutr*. 2012;55(1):93-108.

Sandhu BK, Fell JME, Beattie RM, et al. Guidelines for the management of inflammatory bowel disease in children in the United Kingdom. *JPGN*. 2010;50:1-13.

Turner D, Levine A, Escher J, et al. Management of pediatric ulcerative colitis: joint ECCO and ESPGHAN evidence-based consensus guidelines. *J Pediatr Gastroenterol Nutrit*. 2012;55(3):340-361.

◆ **Sulfatrim** *see* Sulfamethoxazole and Trimethoprim *on page 1948*

◆ **Sulfatrim** *see* Sulfamethoxazole and Trimethoprim *on page 1948*

◆ **Sulfazine** *see* SulfaSALAzine *on page 1954*

◆ **Sulfazine EC** *see* SulfaSALAzine *on page 1954*

◆ **Sulfisoxazole and Erythromycin** *see* Erythromycin and Sulfisoxazole *on page 785*

Sulfur and Salicylic Acid
(SUL fyoor & sal i SIL ik AS id)

Brand Names: U.S. ala seb [OTC]; Pernox® Lemon [OTC]; Pernox® Regular [OTC]; Sebex [OTC]; Sebulex® [OTC]

Therapeutic Category Antiseborrheic Agent, Topical

Generic Availability (U.S.) Yes

Use Therapeutic shampoo for dandruff and seborrheal dermatitis; acne skin cleanser

Pregnancy Considerations Refer to salicylic acid monograph.

Breast-Feeding Considerations Refer to salicylic acid monograph.

Contraindications Hypersensitivity to sulfur, salicylic acid, or any component

Warnings For external use only; avoid contact with eyes; discontinue use if skin irritation develops

Precautions Infants are more sensitive to sulfur than adults; do not use in children <2 years of age. Topical preparations containing 2% to 5% sulfur generally are well tolerated; concentration >15% is very irritating to the skin; higher concentrations (eg, 10% or higher) may cause systemic toxicity.

Adverse Reactions Local: Topical preparations containing 2% to 5% sulfur generally are well tolerated, local irritation may occur, concentration >15% is very irritating to the skin, higher concentration (eg, 10% or higher) may cause systemic toxicity (eg, headache, vomiting, muscle cramps, dizziness, collapse)

Stability Preparations containing sulfur may react with metals including silver and copper, resulting in discoloration of the metal

Mechanism of Action Salicylic acid works synergistically with sulfur in its keratolytic action to break down keratin and promote skin peeling

Pharmacokinetics (Adult data unless noted) Absorption: 1% of topically applied sulfur is absorbed; sulfur is reduced to hydrogen sulfide

Dosing: Usual General guidelines; consult specific product labeling. Children ≥2 years and Adults: Topical:
Shampoo: Initial: Massage onto wet scalp; leave lather on scalp for 5 minutes, rinse, repeat application, then rinse thoroughly; use daily or every other day; 1-2 treatments/week will usually maintain control
Soap: Use daily or every other day

Administration Topical: Avoid contact with the eyes; for external use only

Dosage Forms Excipient information presented when available (limited, particularly for generics); consult specific product labeling.
Cleanser, topical [scrub]:
Pernox® Lemon: Sulfur 2% and salicylic acid 1.5% (56 g, 113 g)
Pernox® Regular: Sulfur 2% and salicylic acid 1.5% (113 g)
Shampoo, topical:
ala seb: Sulfur 2% and salicylic acid 2% (118 mL, 355 mL) [contains soya lecithin]
Sebex: Sulfur 2% and salicylic acid 2% (118 mL)
Sebulex®: Sulfur 2% and salicylic acid 2% (200 g)

Sulindac (SUL in dak)

Medication Safety Issues
Sound-alike/look-alike issues:
Clinoril may be confused with Cleocin, Clozaril
BEERS Criteria medication:
This drug may be potentially inappropriate for use in geriatric patients (Quality of evidence - moderate; Strength of recommendation - strong).

Brand Names: Canada Apo-Sulin; Teva-Sulindac

Therapeutic Category Analgesic, Non-narcotic; Anti-inflammatory Agent; Nonsteroidal Anti-inflammatory Drug (NSAID), Oral

Generic Availability (U.S.) Yes

Use Management of inflammatory diseases including osteoarthritis, rheumatoid arthritis, acute gouty arthritis, ankylosing spondylitis, and acute painful shoulder (acute subacromial bursitis/supraspinatus tendonitis) (FDA approved in adults)

Medication Guide Available Yes

Pregnancy Risk Factor C

Pregnancy Considerations Adverse events were not observed in the initial animal reproduction studies; therefore, the manufacturer classifies sulindac as pregnancy category C. Sulindac and the sulfide metabolite have been found to cross the placenta. NSAID exposure during the first trimester is not strongly associated with congenital malformations; however, cardiovascular anomalies and cleft palate have been observed following NSAID exposure in some studies. The use of an NSAID in the first trimester may be associated with an increased risk of miscarriage. Nonteratogenic effects have been observed following NSAID administration during the third trimester including myocardial degenerative changes, prenatal constriction of the ductus arteriosus, failure of the ductus arteriosus to close postnatally, and fetal tricuspid regurgitation; renal dysfunction or failure, oligohydramnios; gastrointestinal bleeding or perforation, increased risk of necrotizing enterocolitis; intracranial bleeding, platelet dysfunction with resultant bleeding; or pulmonary hypertension. Because they may cause premature closure of the ductus arteriosus, use of NSAIDs late in pregnancy should be avoided (use after 31-32 weeks gestation is not recommended by some clinicians). Sulindac has been used in the management of preterm labor. The chronic use of NSAIDs in women of reproductive age may be associated with infertility that is reversible upon discontinuation of the medication. A registry is available for pregnant women exposed to autoimmune medications including sulindac. For additional information contact the Organization of Teratology Information Specialists, OTIS Autoimmune Diseases Study, at (877) 311-8972.

Breast-Feeding Considerations It is not known if sulindac is excreted into breast milk. Breast-feeding is not recommended by the manufacturer.

Contraindications Hypersensitivity to sulindac or any component; history of asthma, urticaria, or allergic-type reaction to aspirin, or other NSAIDs; patients with the "aspirin triad" [asthma, rhinitis (with or without nasal polyps), and aspirin intolerance] (fatal asthmatic and anaphylactoid reactions may occur in these patients); perioperative pain in the setting of coronary artery bypass graft (CABG)

Warnings NSAIDs are associated with an increased risk of adverse cardiovascular thrombotic events, including potentially fatal MI and stroke **[U.S. Boxed Warning]**; risk may be increased with duration of use or preexisting cardiovascular risk factors or disease; carefully evaluate cardiovascular risk profile prior to prescribing; use the lowest effective dose for the shortest duration of time, taking into consideration individual patient treatment goals; alternate therapies should be considered for patients at high risk. Use is contraindicated for treatment of perioperative pain in the setting of CABG surgery **[U.S. Boxed Warning]**; an increased incidence of MI and stroke was found in patients receiving COX-2 selective NSAIDs for the treatment of pain within the first 10-14 days after CABG surgery. NSAIDs may cause fluid retention, edema, and new onset or worsening of preexisting hypertension; use with caution in patients with hypertension, CHF, or fluid retention. Concurrent administration of ibuprofen, and potentially other nonselective NSAIDs, may interfere with aspirin's cardioprotective effect.

NSAIDs may increase the risk of GI inflammation, ulceration, bleeding, and perforation **[U.S. Boxed Warning]**. These events, which can be potentially fatal, may occur at any time during therapy and without warning. Avoid the use of NSAIDs in patients with active GI bleeding or ulcer disease. Use NSAIDs with extreme caution in patients with a history of GI bleeding or ulcers (these patients have a 10-fold increased risk for developing a GI bleed). Use NSAIDs with caution in patients with other risk factors which may increase GI bleeding (eg, concurrent therapy with aspirin, anticoagulants, and/or corticosteroids, longer duration of NSAID use, smoking, use of alcohol, and poor general health). Use the lowest effective dose for the shortest duration of time, taking into consideration individual patient treatment goals; alternate therapies should be considered for patients at high risk.

NSAIDs may compromise existing renal function. Renal toxicity may occur in patients with impaired renal function, dehydration, heart failure, liver dysfunction, or those taking diuretics and ACE inhibitors; use with caution in these patients; monitor renal function closely. NSAIDs are not recommended for use in patients with advanced renal disease. Long-term use of NSAIDs may cause renal papillary necrosis and other renal injury. Use caution in patients with renal lithiasis; sulindac metabolites have been reported as components of renal stones; use hydration in patients with a history of renal stones. Use with caution in patients with decreased hepatic function. Closely monitor patients with any abnormal LFT. Severe hepatic reactions (eg, fulminant hepatitis, liver failure) have occurred with NSAID use, rarely; discontinue if signs or symptoms of liver disease develop or if systemic manifestations occur. May require dosage adjustment in hepatic dysfunction; sulfide and sulfone metabolites may accumulate. Pancreatitis has been reported; discontinue with suspected pancreatitis. May increase the risk of aseptic meningitis, especially in patients with systemic lupus erythematosus (SLE) and mixed connective tissue disorders.

Fatal asthmatic and anaphylactoid reactions may occur in patients with the "aspirin triad" who receive NSAIDs. NSAIDs may cause serious dermatologic adverse reactions including exfoliative dermatitis, Stevens-Johnson syndrome, and toxic epidermal necrolysis. Avoid use of NSAIDs in late pregnancy as they may cause premature closure of the ductus arteriosus.

Precautions Use with caution in patients with peptic ulcer disease, GI bleeding, bleeding abnormalities, impaired renal or hepatic function, CHF, hypertension, and patients receiving anticoagulants

Adverse Reactions
Cardiovascular: Edema
Central nervous system: Dizziness, headache, nervousness
Dermatologic: Pruritus, rash
Gastrointestinal: Abdominal cramps, anorexia, constipation, diarrhea, flatulence, GI pain, heartburn, nausea, vomiting
Otic: Tinnitus
Rare but important or life-threatening: Agranulocytosis, ageusia, alopecia, anaphylaxis, angioneurotic edema,

aplastic anemia, arrhythmia, aseptic meningitis, bitter taste, blurred vision, bone marrow depression, bronchial spasm, bruising, CHF, cholestasis, colitis, conjunctivitis, crystalluria, depression, dry mucous membranes, dyspnea, dysuria, epistaxis, erythema multiforme, exfoliative dermatitis, fever, gastritis, GI bleeding, GI perforation, glossitis, gynecomastia, hearing decreased, hematuria, hemolytic anemia, hepatitis, hepatic failure, hyperglycemia, hyperkalemia, hypersensitivity reaction, hypersensitivity syndrome (includes chills, diaphoresis, fever, flushing), hypersensitivity vasculitis, hypertension, insomnia, intestinal stricture, interstitial nephritis, jaundice, leukopenia, liver function abnormal, metallic taste, necrotizing fascitis, nephrotic syndrome, neuritis, neutropenia, palpitation, pancreatitis, paresthesia, peptic ulcer, photosensitivity, proteinuria, psychosis, purpura, renal calculi, renal failure, renal impairment, retinal disturbances, seizure, somnolence, Stevens-Johnson syndrome, stomatitis, syncope, thrombocytopenia, toxic epidermal necrolysis, urine discoloration, urticaria, vaginal bleeding, vertigo, visual disturbance, weakness

Drug Interactions

Metabolism/Transport Effects None known.

Avoid Concomitant Use

Avoid concomitant use of Sulindac with any of the following: Floctafenine; Ketorolac (Nasal); Ketorolac (Systemic); NSAID (COX-2 Inhibitor); Omacetaxine; Urokinase

Increased Effect/Toxicity

Sulindac may increase the levels/effects of: 5-ASA Derivatives; Agents with Antiplatelet Properties; Aliskiren; Aminoglycosides; Anticoagulants; Apixaban; Bisphosphonate Derivatives; Collagenase (Systemic); CycloSPORINE (Systemic); Dabigatran Etexilate; Deferasirox; Desmopressin; Digoxin; Eplerenone; Haloperidol; Ibritumomab; Methotrexate; Nonsteroidal Anti-Inflammatory Agents; NSAID (COX-2 Inhibitor); Omacetaxine; PEMEtrexed; Porfimer; Potassium-Sparing Diuretics; PRALAtrexate; Quinolone Antibiotics; Rivaroxaban; Salicylates; Tenofovir; Thrombolytic Agents; Tositumomab and Iodine I 131 Tositumomab; Urokinase; Vancomycin; Vitamin K Antagonists

The levels/effects of Sulindac may be increased by: ACE Inhibitors; Angiotensin II Receptor Blockers; Antidepressants (Tricyclic, Tertiary Amine); Corticosteroids (Systemic); CycloSPORINE (Systemic); Dasatinib; Dimethyl Sulfoxide; Floctafenine; Glucosamine; Herbs (Anticoagulant/Antiplatelet Properties); Ibrutinib; Ketorolac (Nasal); Ketorolac (Systemic); Multivitamins/Fluoride (with ADE); Multivitamins/Minerals (with ADEK, Folate, Iron); Multivitamins/Minerals (with AE, No Iron); Nonsteroidal Anti-Inflammatory Agents; Omega-3 Fatty Acids; Pentosan Polysulfate Sodium; Pentoxifylline; Probenecid; Prostacyclin Analogues; Selective Serotonin Reuptake Inhibitors; Serotonin/Norepinephrine Reuptake Inhibitors; Sodium Phosphates; Tipranavir; Treprostinil; Vitamin E

Decreased Effect

Sulindac may decrease the levels/effects of: ACE Inhibitors; Agents with Antiplatelet Properties; Aliskiren; Angiotensin II Receptor Blockers; Beta-Blockers; Eplerenone; HydrALAZINE; Loop Diuretics; Potassium-Sparing Diuretics; Prostaglandins (Ophthalmic); Salicylates; Selective Serotonin Reuptake Inhibitors; Thiazide Diuretics

The levels/effects of Sulindac may be decreased by: Bile Acid Sequestrants; Nonsteroidal Anti-Inflammatory Agents; Salicylates

Stability Store at room temperature of 15°C to 30°C (59°F to 86°F) in tightly closed container.

Mechanism of Action Reversibly inhibits cyclooxygenase-1 and 2 (COX-1 and 2) enzymes, which results in decreased formation of prostaglandin precursors; has antipyretic, analgesic, and anti-inflammatory properties

Other proposed mechanisms not fully elucidated (and possibly contributing to the anti-inflammatory effect to varying degrees), include inhibiting chemotaxis, altering lymphocyte activity, inhibiting neutrophil aggregation/activation, and decreasing proinflammatory cytokine levels.

Pharmacokinetics (Adult data unless noted)

Absorption: 90%

Distribution: Crosses blood-brain barrier (brain concentrations <4% of plasma concentrations)

Protein binding: Sulindac: 93%, sulfone metabolite: 95%, sulfide metabolite: 98%; primarily to albumin

Metabolism: Hepatic; prodrug metabolized to sulfide metabolite (active) for therapeutic effects and to sulfone metabolites (inactive); parent and inactive sulfone metabolite undergo extensive enterohepatic recirculation; metabolites undergo glucuronide conjugation

Half-life elimination: Sulindac: ~8 hours; sulfide metabolite: ~16 hours

Time to peak serum concentration: Sulindac: 3-4 hours; sulfide and sulfone metabolites: 5-6 hours

Elimination: Urine (~50%, primarily as inactive metabolites, <1% as active metabolite); feces (~25%, primarily as metabolites); **Note:** Metabolites appear principally as glucuronide conjugates in urine and bile.

Dosing: Usual Oral:

Children: Limited information exists; some centers use the following: 2-4 mg/kg/day in 2 divided doses; maximum: 6 mg/kg/day; do not exceed 400 mg/day (Giannini, 1995; Skeith, 1991)

Adults: 150-200 mg twice daily; not to exceed 400 mg/day

Dosing adjustment in renal impairment: Not recommended with advanced renal impairment; if required, decrease dose and monitor closely.

Dosing adjustment in hepatic impairment: Dose reduction is necessary; discontinue if abnormal liver function tests occur.

Administration Oral: Administer with food or milk to decrease GI upset

Monitoring Parameters Liver enzymes, BUN, serum creatinine, CBC with differential, platelet count; periodic ophthalmologic exams with chronic use

Test Interactions Increased chloride (S), increased sodium (S), increased bleeding time

Dosage Forms Excipient information presented when available (limited, particularly for generics); consult specific product labeling.

Tablet, Oral:

Generic: 150 mg, 200 mg

References

Giannini EH and Cawkwell GD, "Drug Treatment in Children With Juvenile Rheumatoid Arthritis. Past, Present, and Future," *Pediatr Clin North Am*, 1995, 42(5):1099-125.

Skeith KJ and Jamali F, "Clinical Pharmacokinetics of Drugs Used in Juvenile Arthritis," *Clin Pharmacokinet*, 1991, 21(2):129-49.

SUMAtriptan (soo ma TRIP tan)

Medication Safety Issues

Sound-alike/look-alike issues:

SUMAtriptan may be confused with saxagliptin, sitaGLIPtin, somatropin, ZOLMitriptan

Brand Names: U.S. Alsuma; Imitrex; Imitrex STATdose Refill; Imitrex STATdose System; Sumavel DosePro

Brand Names: Canada Apo-Sumatriptan; Ava-Sumatriptan; CO Sumatriptan; Dom-Sumatriptan; Imitrex; Imitrex DF; Imitrex Injection; Imitrex Nasal Spray; Mylan-Sumatriptan; PHL-Sumatriptan; PMS-Sumatriptan; Sandoz-Sumatriptan; Sumatriptan DF; Taro-Sumatriptan; Teva-Sumatriptan; Teva-Sumatriptan DF

Therapeutic Category Antimigraine Agent

Generic Availability (U.S.) May be product dependent

Use

Injection, intranasal, and tablets: Acute treatment of migraine with or without aura (FDA approved in adults)

Injection: Acute treatment of cluster headaches (FDA approved in adults)

Pregnancy Risk Factor C

Pregnancy Considerations Adverse events were observed in animal reproduction studies. In a study using full term healthy human placentas, limited amounts of sumatriptan were found to cross the placenta (Schenker, 1995).

An overall increased risk of major congenital malformations has not been observed following first trimester exposure to sumatriptan in several studies. Pregnancy outcome information for sumatriptan is available from a pregnancy registry sponsored by GlaxoSmithKline. As of October 2008, data was available for 558 infants/fetuses exposed to sumatriptan, and seven exposed to both sumatriptan and naratriptan. The risk of major birth defects following sumatriptan exposure was 4.6% (95% CI: 2.9-7.2) (Cunnington, 2009). The pregnancy registry was closed in January, 2012 and additional information may be obtained from the manufacturer (800-336-2176). An analysis of data collected between 1995-2008 using the Swedish Medical Birth Register reported pregnancy outcomes following 5-HT$_{1B/1D}$ agonist exposure. An increased risk of major congenital malformations was not observed following sumatriptan exposure (2229 exposed during the first trimester) (Källén, 2011). An increased risk of major congenital malformations was not observed in the prospective Norwegian Mother and Child Cohort Study. The study included women with 5-HT$_{1B/1D}$ agonist exposure between 1999-2006 (n=455); of these, 217 were exposed to sumatriptan (Nezvalová-Henriksen, 2010; Nezvalová-Henriksen, 2012).

If treatment for cluster headaches is needed during pregnancy, sumatriptan may be used (Jürgens, 2009). Other agents are preferred for the initial treatment of migraine in pregnancy (Da Silva, 2012; MacGregor, 2012; Williams, 2012); however, sumatriptan may be considered if first-line agents fail (MacGregor, 2012).

Breast-Feeding Considerations The excretion of sumatriptan into breast milk was studied in five lactating women, 10-28 weeks postpartum (mean: 22.2 weeks). Sumatriptan 6 mg SubQ was administered and maternal milk and blood samples were collected over 8 hours after the dose. Sumatriptan was detected in breast milk. Maximum concentrations in the maternal blood (mean: 80.2 mcg/L; 0.25 hours after the dose) and milk (mean: 87.2 mcg/L; 2.5 hours after the dose) were similar. However, the amount of sumatriptan an infant would be exposed to following breast-feeding is considered to be small (although the mean milk-to-plasma ratio is ~4.9, weight-adjusted doses estimates suggest breast-fed infants receive 3.5% of a maternal dose). Expressing and discarding the milk for 8-12 hours after a single dose is suggested to reduce the amount present even further (Wojnar-Horton, 1996). Breast-feeding is not recommended by some manufacturers; however, according to other sources if treatment is needed, breast-feeding does not need to be discontinued (Jürgens, 2009; MacGregor, 2012).

Contraindications Hypersensitivity to sumatriptan or any component; I.V. administration (coronary vasospasm may occur); patients with ischemic heart disease or signs or symptoms of ischemic heart disease (eg, angina pectoris, Prinzmetal angina, MI, silent MI); other significant underlying cardiovascular diseases); cerebrovascular syndromes (eg, stroke, TIA); peripheral vascular diseases (eg, ischemic bowel disease), severe hepatic impairment (oral and nasal sumatriptan, and injectable Imitrex® only); uncontrolled hypertension; concomitant use (within last 24 hours) of ergotamine, ergotamine derivatives (eg, dihydroergotamine, methysergide), other 5-HT$_1$ agonists (triptans), or MAO inhibitors; use of MAO inhibitors within past 2 weeks (oral and nasal sumatriptan formulations only); management of hemiplegic or basilar migraine

Warnings Life-threatening or fatal hypersensitivity reactions may occur. Rarely, serious coronary events, including coronary artery vasospasm, transient ischemia, acute MI, life-threatening arrhythmias, cardiac arrest, and death, may occur; avoid use in patients with risk factors for coronary artery disease, unless cardiovascular disease can be ruled out; consider administering first dose under close supervision to patients at high risk for coronary disease; ECG should be performed if angina-like symptoms occur; periodically evaluate cardiovascular system in patients with risk factors for coronary artery disease. Cerebrovascular events (eg, cerebral hemorrhage, subarachnoid hemorrhage, stroke) have been reported with 5-HT$_1$ agonist (triptan) administration. Vasospasm-related events (eg, peripheral vascular ischemia, colonic ischemia) have been reported with 5-HT$_1$ agonists. Transient and permanent blindness and significant partial vision loss have been very rarely reported. Potentially fatal serotonin syndrome may occur when triptans are used in combination with SSRIs (eg, fluoxetine, sertraline) or SNRIs (eg, venlafaxine); monitor carefully if the two drugs are used concomitantly.

Precautions Use with caution in patients with controlled hypertension; temporary increases in peripheral vascular resistance and blood pressure may occur; significant elevation in blood pressure, including hypertensive crisis, has also been reported on rare occasions in patients with and without a history of hypertension; use is contraindicated in patients with uncontrolled hypertension. Use oral formulations of sumatriptan with caution and in reduced doses in patients with impaired hepatic function; presystemic clearance of orally administered sumatriptan is reduced in hepatic impairment, leading to increased plasma concentrations. Nonoral routes of administration (nasal, subcutaneous formulations) do not undergo similar hepatic first-pass metabolism and are not expected to result in significantly altered pharmacokinetics in patients with hepatic impairment. Use of the oral, nasal, or Imitrex® injectable dosage form is contraindicated in severe hepatic impairment.

Use with caution in patients with a history of seizure disorder or conditions associated with a decrease in the seizure threshold. Although generally not recommended, if concomitant use of an MAO inhibitor with injectable sumatriptan is deemed necessary, careful monitoring and appropriate dosage adjustments are required (**Note:** Use of MAO inhibitors within past 2 weeks is contraindicated with oral and nasal sumatriptan). Other potentially serious neurological conditions should be ruled out prior to acute migraine therapy. Sumatriptan (given at 5 times the maximum oral single dose) has caused corneal opacities in dogs; other animal studies suggest it may bind to the melanin of the eye; human studies are not available

Serious adverse effects, such as MI, stroke, visual loss, and death have been reported in pediatric patients after sumatriptan use by the oral, intranasal, and/or SubQ route; frequency of such adverse effects cannot currently be determined, thus the use of sumatriptan in patients <18 years of age is not recommended.

Adverse Reactions

Injection:

Cardiovascular: Chest discomfort, flushing

Central nervous system: Anxiety, burning sensation, cold sensation, dizziness, drowsiness, feeling of heaviness, feeling of tightness, feeling strange, headache, localized warm feeling, malaise, paresthesia, pressure sensation, tight feeling in head

Dermatologic: Diaphoresis

Gastrointestinal: Abdominal distress, dysphagia, nausea and vomiting, sore throat

Local: Injection site reaction (includes bleeding, bruising, swelling, and erythema)

Neuromuscular & skeletal: Jaw pain, muscle cramps, myalgia, neck pain, numbness, weakness

Ophthalmic: Visual disturbance

Respiratory: Bronchospasm, nasal signs and symptoms

Nasal spray:

Central nervous system: Dizziness

Gastrointestinal: Nausea, sore throat, unpleasant taste, vomiting

Respiratory: Nasal signs and symptoms

Tablet:

Cardiovascular: Chest pain, hot and cold flashes, palpitations, syncope

Central nervous system: Burning sensation, dizziness, drowsiness, headache, hyperacusis, malaise, migraine, numbness, pain (nonspecified), paresthesia, sensation of pressure (neck/throat/jaw or nonspecified), sleepiness, vertigo

Gastrointestinal: Diarrhea, nausea, reduced salivation, vomiting

Genitourinary: Hematuria

Hematologic & oncologic: Hemolytic anemia, hemorrhage (ear or nose/throat)

Hypersensitivity: Hypersensitivity reaction

Neuromuscular & skeletal: Myalgia

Otic: Hearing loss, tinnitus

Respiratory: Allergic rhinitis, dyspnea, rhinitis, sinusitis, upper respiratory tract inflammation

Transdermal system:

Central nervous system: Feeling abnormal (paresthesia, warm/cold sensation), localized warm feeling, sensation of pressure (chest/neck/throat/jaw)

Dermatologic: Allergic contact dermatitis, skin discoloration (application site), skin vesicle (application site)

Hematologic & oncologic: Bruise (application site)

Local: Localized irritation, localized pain, localized pruritus

Rare but important or life-threatening: Skin erosion (application site)

Route unspecified: Rare but important or life-threatening: Abdominal aortic aneurysm, abnormal hepatic function tests, accommodation disturbance, acute renal failure, anaphylactoid reaction, anaphylaxis, anemia, angioedema, atrial fibrillation, cardiac arrhythmia, cardiomyopathy, cerebral ischemia, cerebrovascular accident, colonic ischemia, coronary artery vasospasm, cyanosis, deafness, dystonic reaction, ECG changes, fluid retention, hallucination, heart block, hemorrhage (nose/throat), hematuria, hemolytic anemia, hypersensitivity reaction, hypertensive crisis, hypertension, hypotension, increased intracranial pressure, increased serum transaminases, increased thyroid stimulating hormone level, intestinal obstruction, ischemic colitis, muscle rigidity, myocardial infarction, myocardial ischemia (transient), optic neuropathy (ischemic), pancytopenia, phlebitis, Prinzmetal angina, psychomotor disturbance, pulmonary embolism, Raynaud's phenomenon, retinal blood vessel · occlusion (artery), retinal thrombosis, seizure, serotonin syndrome, shock, skin photosensitivity, subarachnoid hemorrhage, syncope, giant-cell arteritis, thrombocytopenia, thrombophlebitis, thrombosis, vasculitis, ventricular fibrillation, ventricular tachycardia, vision loss

Drug Interactions

Metabolism/Transport Effects None known.

Avoid Concomitant Use

Avoid concomitant use of SUMAtriptan with any of the following: Ergot Derivatives; MAO Inhibitors

Increased Effect/Toxicity

SUMAtriptan may increase the levels/effects of: Antipsychotics; Droxidopa; Ergot Derivatives; Metoclopramide; Serotonin Modulators

The levels/effects of SUMAtriptan may be increased by: Antiemetics (5HT3 Antagonists); Antipsychotics; Ergot Derivatives; MAO Inhibitors

Decreased Effect There are no known significant interactions involving a decrease in effect.

Stability

Alsuma™: Store at 25°C (77°F); excursions permitted between 15°C and 30°C (59°F to 86°F); do not refrigerate; protect from light. Store each autoinjector in its storage and disposal case; remove from case only prior to use.

Injection (Imitrex®), nasal spray, tablets: Store at 2°C to 30°C (36°F to 86°F); protect from light

Sumavel® DosePro®: Store at 20°C to 25°C (68°F to 77°F); excursions permitted between 15°C and 30°C (59°F to 86°F); do not freeze

Mechanism of Action Selective agonist for serotonin (5-HT$_{1B}$ and 5-HT$_{1D}$ receptors) in cranial arteries; causes vasoconstriction and reduces neurogenic inflammation associated with antidromic neuronal transmission correlating with relief of migraine

Pharmacodynamics Migraine pain relief:

Onset of action:

Oral: 1-1.5 hours

Nasal: ~15-30 minutes

SubQ: 10 minutes to 2 hours

Maximum effect: Oral: 2-4 hours

Pharmacokinetics (Adult data unless noted)

Distribution: Distributes to breast milk following SubQ administration

V_d (central): 50 L

V_d (apparent): 2.4 L/kg

Protein binding: 14% to 21%

Metabolism: In the liver to an indole acetic acid metabolite (inactive) which then undergoes ester glucuronide conjugation; may be metabolized by monoamine oxidase (MAO); extensive first-pass metabolism following oral administration

Bioavailability:

Oral: ~15%; may be significantly increased with liver disease

Intranasal: 17% (compared to SubQ)

SubQ: 97%; **Note:** Sumavel® DosePro® is bioequivalent to sumatriptan SubQ injection via needle when administered into the thigh or abdomen

Half-life:

Distribution: 15 minutes

Terminal: 2 hours; range: 1-4 hours

Time to peak serum concentration:

Oral: Healthy adults: 2 hours; during migraine attacks: 2.5 hours

SubQ: Range: 5-20 minutes; mean: 12 minutes

Elimination: 60% of an oral dose is renally excreted (primarily as metabolites), 40% is eliminated via the feces, and only 3% as unchanged drug; 42% of an intranasal dose is excreted as the indole acetic acid metabolite with 3% excreted in the urine unchanged; 22% of a SubQ dose is excreted in urine unchanged and 38% as the indole acetic acid metabolite

Dosing: Usual Note: Use in children and adolescents <18 years of age not recommended by manufacturer. Results of clinical studies are mixed with regards to efficacy, particularly with oral and injectable sumatriptan; a 2004 practice parameter concluded that sumatriptan nasal spray was effective for the acute treatment of migraines in adolescent patients (Lewis, 2004); additional studies are needed.

Intranasal:

Children 5-12 years: 5 mg, 10 mg, or 20 mg administered in one nostril **as a single dose**, given as soon as possible after the onset of migraine; dose should be selected on an individual basis; optimal dose not established. A double-blind, placebo controlled study of 129 patients (8-17 years; mean 12.4 years) used a weight-based dosing regimen: Body weight: 20-39 kg: 10 mg/dose; body weight ≥40 kg: 20 mg/dose; however, relatively few children <12 years old were included in the study (Ahonen, 2004). A small, randomized, double-blind, placebo-controlled study of 14 children (6-9 years; median: 8.2 years) used intranasal doses of 20 mg/dose (Ueberall, 1999). A small, retrospective review of 10 children (5-12 years; mean: 9.9 years), used intranasal doses of 5 mg (n=2) or 20 mg (n=8) (Hershey, 2001).

Adolescents ≥12 years: 5 mg, 10 mg, or 20 mg administered in one nostril **as a single dose** given as soon as possible after the onset of migraine; dose should be selected on an individual basis (Lewis, 2004; Rothner, 2000; Winner, 2000; Winner, 2006)

Adults: Initial single dose: 5 mg, 10 mg, or 20 mg administered in one nostril, given as soon as possible after the onset of migraine; dose should be selected on an individual basis; 10 mg dose may be administered as 5 mg in each nostril; may repeat after 2 hours; maximum: 40 mg/day

SubQ:

Children and Adolescents 6-18 years: 3-6 mg single dose. An open-labeled prospective trial of 17 children 6-16 years with juvenile migraine used SubQ doses of 6 mg in 15 children (30-70 kg), and 3 mg/dose in two children (22 kg and 30 kg) (MacDonald, 1994). Another open-labeled prospective trial in 50 consecutive children (ages 6-18 years) with severe migraine used SubQ doses of 0.06 mg/kg/dose. Relief was reported as good/excellent in 84% of the patients; 16% reported fair to poor relief; additional studies are needed (Linder, 1996).

Adults: Initial: 4-6 mg; may repeat if needed ≥1 hour after initial dose; maximum: 12 mg/day

Oral:

Adolescents: Efficacy of oral sumatriptan was **not** established in five controlled trials in adolescent patients; frequency of adverse events was dose-related and age-dependent (ie, younger patients reported more adverse events)

Adults: Initial single dose: 25 mg given as soon as possible after the onset of a migraine; range: 25-100 mg/dose; dose should be selected on an individual basis; maximum single dose: 100 mg; may repeat after 2 hours; maximum: 200 mg/day

Dosing adjustment in hepatic impairment: Adults:

Mild to moderate hepatic impairment:

Oral: Bioavailability of oral sumatriptan is increased with liver disease. If treatment is needed, do not exceed single doses of 50 mg.

Intranasal: Has not been studied in patients with hepatic impairment; however, because the intranasally administered drug does not undergo first-pass metabolism, serum concentrations would not be expected to be altered.

SubQ: Has been studied and pharmacokinetics were not altered in patients with hepatic impairment compared to healthy patients.

Severe hepatic impairment: Oral, nasal, and SubQ (limited to Imitrex® injection, per prescribing information) formulations are contraindicated with severe hepatic impairment.

Dosing adjustment in renal impairment: No dosage adjustments are recommended.

Administration

Intranasal: Each nasal spray unit is preloaded with 1 dose; **do not** test the spray unit before use; remove unit from plastic pack when ready to use; while sitting down, gently blow nose to clear nasal passages; keep head upright and close one nostril gently with index finger; hold container with other hand, with thumb supporting bottom and index and middle fingers on either side of nozzle; insert nozzle into nostril about 1/2 inch; close mouth; take a breath through nose while releasing spray into nostril by pressing firmly on blue plunger; remove nozzle from nostril; keep head level for 10-20 seconds and gently breathe in through nose and out through mouth; **do not breathe deeply**

Oral: Administer with water or other fluids; swallow tablet whole; do not split tablet

Parenteral: SubQ use only; do **not** administer I.M.; do **not** administer I.V. (may cause coronary vasospasm). Needle penetrates 1/4 inch of skin; use in areas of the body with adequate skin and subcutaneous thickness.

Alsuma™ is a prefilled single use autoinjector device; product information suggests SubQ administration into lateral thigh or upper arm (adults). Discard after use.

Needleless administration (Sumavel® DosePro®): Do **not** administer I.M.; do **not** administer I.V. (may cause coronary vasospasm). Administer SubQ to the abdomen (>2 inches from the navel) or thigh; do not administer to other areas of the body (eg, arm). Sumavel® DosePro® device is for single use only; discard after use; do not use if the tip of the device is tilted or broken; **Note:** A loud burst of air will be heard and a sensation in the skin will be felt at the time a dose is delivered with this device.

Additional Information The safety of treating an average of >4 headaches in a 30-day period has not been established. Sumatriptan is **not** indicated for migraine prophylaxis.

Sumavel® DosePro® is a single-use, prefilled, disposable, needle-free SubQ delivery system; it uses pressure from a compressed nitrogen gas source to deliver medication via a small, precise hole in the glass medication chamber; medication is propelled through the skin and delivered SubQ without a needle.

Product Availability Zecuity (transdermal system): FDA approved January 2013; anticipated availability is currently unknown. Refer to prescribing information for additional information.

Dosage Forms Excipient information presented when available (limited, particularly for generics); consult specific product labeling.

Solution, Nasal:

Imitrex: 5 mg/actuation (1 ea); 20 mg/actuation (1 ea)

Generic: 5 mg/actuation (1 ea); 20 mg/actuation (1 ea)

Solution, Subcutaneous, as succinate [strength expressed as base]:

Alsuma: 6 mg/0.5 mL (0.5 mL)

Imitrex: 6 mg/0.5 mL (0.5 mL)

Imitrex STATdose Refill: 4 mg/0.5 mL (0.5 mL)

Imitrex STATdose System: 4 mg/0.5 mL (0.5 mL)

Generic: 4 mg/0.5 mL (0.5 mL); 6 mg/0.5 mL (0.5 mL)

Solution, Subcutaneous, as succinate [strength expressed as base, preservative free]:

Generic: 6 mg/0.5 mL (0.5 mL)

Solution Auto-injector, Subcutaneous, as succinate [strength expressed as base]:

Imitrex STATdose System: 6 mg/0.5 mL (0.5 mL)

Generic: 6 mg/0.5 mL (0.5 mL)

Solution Cartridge, Subcutaneous, as succinate [strength expressed as base]:

Imitrex STATdose Refill: 6 mg/0.5 mL (0.5 mL)

Solution Jet-injector, Subcutaneous, as succinate [strength expressed as base]:

Sumavel DosePro: 6 mg/0.5 mL (0.5 mL)

Solution Prefilled Syringe, Subcutaneous, as succinate [strength expressed as base, preservative free]:

Generic: 6 mg/0.5 mL (0.5 mL)

Tablet, Oral, as succinate [strength expressed as base]:

Imitrex: 25 mg, 50 mg, 100 mg

Generic: 25 mg, 50 mg, 100 mg

Extemporaneous Preparations A 5 mg/mL oral liquid preparation made from tablets and one of three different vehicles (Ora-Sweet®, Ora-Sweet® SF, or Syrpalta® syrups). **Note:** Ora-Plus® Suspending Vehicle is used with Ora-Sweet® or Ora-Sweet® SF to facilitate dispersion of the tablets (Ora-Plus® is not necessary if Syrpalta® is the vehicle). Crush nine 100 mg tablets in a mortar and reduce to a fine powder. Add 40 mL of Ora-Plus® in 5 mL increments and mix thoroughly between each addition; rinse mortar and pestle 5 times with 10 mL of Ora-Plus®, pouring into bottle each time, and add quantity of appropriate syrup (Ora-Sweet® or Ora-Sweet® SF) sufficient to make 180 mL. Store in amber glass bottles in the dark; label "shake well", "refrigerate", and "protect from light". Stable for 21 days refrigerated.

Fish DN, Beall HD, Goodwin JD, et al, "Stability of Sumatriptan Succinate in Extemporaneously Prepared Oral Liquids," *Am J Health Syst Pharm*, 1997, 54(14):1619-22.

References

Ahonen K, Hämäläinen ML, Rantala H, et al, "Nasal Sumatriptan Is Effective in Treatment of Migraine Attacks in Children: A Randomized Trial," *Neurology*, 2004, 62(6):883-7.

Cunnington M, Ephross S, and Churchill P, "The Safety of Sumatriptan and Naratriptan in Pregnancy: What Have We Learned?" *Headache*, 2009, 49(10):1414-22.

Da Silva AN and Tepper SJ, "Acute Treatment of Migraines," *CNS Drugs*, 2012, 26(10):823-39.

Gunner KB, Smith HD, and Ferguson LE, "Practice Guideline for Diagnosis and Management of Migraine Headaches in Children and Adolescents: Part Two," *J Pediatr Health Care*, 2008, 22(1):52-9.

Hershey AD, Powers SW, LeCates S, et al, "Effectiveness of Nasal Sumatriptan in 5- to 12-Year-Old Children," *Headache*, 2001, 41 (7):693-7.

Jürgens TP, Schaefer C, and May A, "Treatment of cluster headache in pregnancy and lactation," Cephalalgia. 2009 Apr;29(4):391-400.

Källén B, Nilsson E, and Otterblad Olausson P, "Delivery Outcome After Maternal Use of Drugs for Migraine: A Register Study in Sweden," *Drug Saf*, 2011, 34(8):691-703.

Lewis D, Ashwal S, Hershey A, et al, "Practice Parameter: Pharmacological Treatment of Migraine Headache in Children and Adolescents: Report of the American Academy of Neurology Quality Standards Subcommittee and the Practice Committee of the Child Neurology Society," *Neurology*, 2004, 63(12):2215-24.

Linder SL, "Subcutaneous Sumatriptan in the Clinical Setting: The First 50 Consecutive Patients With Acute Migraine in a Pediatric Neurology Office Practice," *Headache*, 1996, 36(7):419-22.

MacDonald JT, "Treatment of Juvenile Migraine With Subcutaneous Sumatriptan," *Headache*, 1994, 34(10):581-2.

MacGregor EA, "Headache in Pregnancy," *Neurol Clin*, 2012, 30 (3):835-66.

Nezvalová-Henriksen K, Spigset O, and Nordeng HM, "Errata in 'Triptan Exposure During Pregnancy and the Risk of Major Congenital Malformations and Adverse Pregnancy Outcomes: Results From the Norwegian Mother and Child Sohort Study,'" *Headache*, 2012, 52 (8):1319-20.

Nezvalová-Henriksen K, Spigset O, and Nordeng H, "Triptan Exposure During Pregnancy and the Risk of Major Congenital Malformations and Adverse Pregnancy Outcomes: Results From the Norwegian Mother and Child Cohort Study," *Headache*, 2010, 50(4):563-75.

Rothner AD, Winner P, Nett R, et al, "One-Year Tolerability and Efficacy of Sumatriptan Nasal Spray in Adolescents With Migraine: Results of a Multicenter, Open-Label Study," *Clin Ther*, 2000, 22(12):1533-46.

Schenker S, Yang Y, Perez A, et al, "Sumatriptan (Imitrex) Transport by the Human Placenta," *Proc Soc Exp Biol Med*, 1995, 210(3):213-20.

Scott AK, "Sumatriptan Clinical Pharmacokinetics," *Clin Pharmacokinet*, 1994, 27(5):337-44.

Silver S, Gano D, and Gerretsen P, "Acute Treatment of Paediatric Migraine: A Meta-analysis of Efficacy," *J Paediatr Child Health*, 2008, 44(1-2):3-9.

Ueberall MA and Wenzel D, "Intranasal Sumatriptan for the Acute Treatment of Migraine in Children," *Neurology*, 1999, 52(7):1507-10.

Williams SH and Kehr HA, "An Update in the Treatment of Neurologic Disorders During Pregnancy-Focus on Migraines and Seizures," *J Pharm Pract*, 2012, 25(3):341-51.

Winner P, Rothner AD, Saper J, et al, "A Randomized, Double-Blind, Placebo-Controlled Study of Sumatriptan Nasal Spray in the Treatment of Acute Migraine in Adolescents," *Pediatrics*, 2000, 106 (5):989-97.

Winner P, Rothner AD, Wooten JD, et al, "Sumatriptan Nasal Spray in Adolescent Migraineurs: A Randomized, Double-Blind, Placebo-Controlled, Acute Study," *Headache*, 2006, 46(2):212-22.

Wojnar-Horton RE, Hackett LP, Yapp P, et al, "Distribution and Excretion of Sumatriptan in Human Milk," *Br J Clin Pharmacol*, 1996, 41 (3):217-21.

◆ **Sumatriptan DF (Can)** *see* SUMAtriptan *on page 1958*

◆ **Sumatriptan Succinate** *see* SUMAtriptan *on page 1958*

◆ **Sumavel DosePro** *see* SUMAtriptan *on page 1958*

◆ **Superdophilus® [OTC]** *see* Lactobacillus *on page 1191*

◆ **Super Strength Motrin IB Liquid Gel Capsules (Can)** *see* Ibuprofen *on page 1059*

◆ **Supeudol (Can)** *see* OxyCODONE *on page 1569*

◆ **Suphedrine [OTC]** *see* Pseudoephedrine *on page 1770*

◆ **Supprelin LA** *see* Histrelin *on page 1016*

◆ **Suprax** *see* Cefixime *on page 401*

◆ **Suprax® (Can)** *see* Cefixime *on page 401*

◆ **Surfaxin** *see* Lucinactant *on page 1289*

◆ **Sur-Q-Lax [OTC]** *see* Docusate *on page 701*

◆ **Survanta** *see* Beractant *on page 280*

◆ **Survanta® (Can)** *see* Beractant *on page 280*

◆ **Sustiva** *see* Efavirenz *on page 731*

◆ **Suxamethonium Chloride** *see* Succinylcholine *on page 1938*

◆ **SwabFlush Saline Flush** *see* Sodium Chloride *on page 1902*

◆ **Sweet-Ease® [OTC]** *see* Sucrose *on page 1941*

◆ **Sylatron** *see* Peginterferon Alfa-2b *on page 1621*

◆ **Symax Duotab** *see* Hyoscyamine *on page 1056*

◆ **Symax FasTabs** *see* Hyoscyamine *on page 1056*

◆ **Symax-SL** *see* Hyoscyamine *on page 1056*

◆ **Symax-SR** *see* Hyoscyamine *on page 1056*

◆ **Symbicort** *see* Budesonide and Formoterol *on page 314*

◆ **Symmetrel** *see* Amantadine *on page 112*

◆ **Synacthen** *see* Cosyntropin *on page 549*

◆ **Synacthen Depot (Can)** *see* Cosyntropin *on page 549*

◆ **Synagis** *see* Palivizumab *on page 1584*

◆ **Synalar** *see* Fluocinolone (Topical) *on page 892*

◆ **Synalar® (Can)** *see* Fluocinolone (Topical) *on page 892*

◆ **Synalar (Cream)** *see* Fluocinolone (Topical) *on page 892*

◆ **Synalar (Ointment)** *see* Fluocinolone (Topical) *on page 892*

◆ **Synalar TS** *see* Fluocinolone (Topical) *on page 892*

◆ **Synera** *see* Lidocaine and Tetracaine *on page 1248*

◆ **Synercid®** *see* Quinupristin and Dalfopristin *on page 1796*

◆ **Synthroid** *see* Levothyroxine *on page 1234*

◆ **Systane® [OTC]** *see* Artificial Tears *on page 205*

◆ **Systane® Ultra [OTC]** *see* Artificial Tears *on page 205*

◆ **T₃ Sodium (error-prone abbreviation)** *see* Liothyronine *on page 1256*

◆ **T₃/T₄ Liotrix** *see* Liotrix *on page 1258*

◆ **T₄** *see* Levothyroxine *on page 1234*

◆ **T-20** *see* Enfuvirtide *on page 750*

◆ **Tabloid** *see* Thioguanine *on page 2010*

Tacrolimus (Systemic) (ta KROE li mus)

Medication Safety Issues
Sound-alike/look-alike issues:
Prograf may be confused with Gengraf, PROzac

Tacrolimus may be confused with everolimus, pimecrolimus, sirolimus, temsirolimus

Other safety concerns:
The immediate release (Hecoria, Prograf) and extended release (Astagraf XL, Advagraf [Canadian product]) oral formulations are not interchangeable and are not substitutable.

Related Information
Safe Handling of Hazardous Drugs *on page 2419*

Brand Names: U.S. Astagraf XL; Hecoria; Prograf

Brand Names: Canada Advagraf; Prograf; Sandoz-Tacrolimus

Therapeutic Category Immunosuppressant Agent

Generic Availability (U.S.) May be product dependent

Use Prevention of organ rejection in solid organ transplantation patients (FDA approved in children and adults) or prevention and treatment of graft-versus-host disease (GVHD) in allogeneic stem cell transplantation patients

Medication Guide Available Yes

Pregnancy Risk Factor C

Pregnancy Considerations Adverse events were observed in animal reproduction studies. Tacrolimus crosses the human placenta and is measurable in the cord blood, amniotic fluid, and newborn serum. Tacrolimus concentrations in the placenta may be higher than the maternal serum (Jain, 1997). Infants with lower birth weights have been found to have higher tacrolimus concentrations (Bramham, 2013). Transient neonatal hyperkalemia and renal dysfunction have been reported.

Tacrolimus pharmacokinetics are altered during pregnancy. Whole blood concentrations decrease as pregnancy progresses; however, unbound concentrations increase. Measuring unbound concentrations may be preferred, especially in women with anemia or hypoalbuminemia. If unbound concentration measurement is not available, interpretation of whole blood concentrations should account for RBC count and serum albumin concentration (Hebert, 2013; Zheng, 2012).

In general, women who have had a kidney transplant should be instructed that fertility will be restored following the transplant but that pregnancy should be avoided for ~2 years. Tacrolimus may be used as an immunosuppressant during pregnancy. The risk of infection, hypertension, and pre-eclampsia may be increased in pregnant women who have had a kidney transplant (EPBG, 2002).

The National Transplantation Pregnancy Registry (NTPR) is a registry which follows pregnancies which occur in maternal transplant recipients or those fathered by male transplant recipients. The NTPR encourages reporting of pregnancies following solid organ transplant by contacting them at 877-955-6877.

Breast-Feeding Considerations Tacrolimus is excreted into breast milk; concentrations are variable and lower than that of the maternal serum. The low bioavailability of tacrolimus following oral absorption may also decrease the amount of exposure to a nursing infant (Bramham, 2013; French, 2003; Gardiner, 2006). In one study, tacrolimus serum concentrations in the infants did not differ between those who were bottle fed or breast-fed (all infants were exposed to tacrolimus throughout pregnancy) (Bramham, 2013). Available information suggests that tacrolimus exposure to the nursing infant is ≤0.5% of the weight-adjusted maternal dose (Bramham, 2013; French, 2003; Gardiner, 2006). The manufacturer recommends that nursing be discontinued, taking into consideration the importance of the drug to the mother.

Contraindications Hypersensitivity to tacrolimus, polyoxyl 60 hydrogenated castor oil, or any component

Warnings Hazardous agent; use appropriate precautions for handling and disposal (NIOSH, 2012). Immunosuppression with tacrolimus may result in increased susceptibility to infection and the possible development of lymphoma **[U.S. Boxed Warning]**. Increased risk of other malignancies, including skin malignancies; risk is related to intensity and duration of immunosuppression. Lymphoproliferative disorder related to EBV infection has been reported in immunosuppressed organ transplant patients; risk highest in young children; use combination immunosuppressant therapy with caution. Insulin-dependent posttransplant diabetes mellitus has been reported with use; risk increases in African-American and Hispanic kidney transplant patients. Neurotoxicity and nephrotoxicity have been reported especially when used in high doses. To avoid excess nephrotoxicity, do not administer simultaneously with cyclosporine; 24 hours should elapse before one is given after the other. Monitor serum potassium levels during therapy; hyperkalemia and hypokalemia have been reported. May cause hypertension; antihypertensive therapy may be required. Myocardial hypertrophy has been reported; ECG evaluation should be considered in any patient who develops renal failure or clinical manifestations of ventricular dysfunction. Closely monitor tacrolimus levels to assist in dose adjustment, monitor compliance, prevent organ rejection, and reduce drug-related toxicity.

Each mL of injection contains polyoxyl 60 hydrogenated castor oil (HCO-60) (200 mg) and dehydrated alcohol USP 80% v/v. Anaphylaxis has been reported with the injection; use should be reserved for those patients not able to take oral medication. Adequate airway, supportive measures, and agents for treating anaphylaxis should be available when tacrolimus is administered I.V.

Precautions Use with caution and modify dosage in patients with hepatic or renal impairment. Systemic therapy should be administered under the supervision of a physician experienced in immunosuppressive therapy in a facility appropriate for monitoring and managing therapy **[U.S. Boxed Warning]**.

Adverse Reactions As reported for kidney, liver, and heart transplantation:

Cardiovascular: Angina pectoris, atrial fibrillation, atrial flutter, bradycardia, cardiac arrest, cardiac arrhythmia, cardiac failure, cardiorespiratory arrest, cerebral infarction, cerebral ischemia, chest pain, decreased heart rate, deep vein thrombophlebitis, deep vein thrombosis, ECG abnormality (QRS or ST segment or T wave), edema, flushing, hemorrhagic stroke, hypertension, hypertrophic cardiomyopathy, hypotension, ischemic heart disease, myocardial infarction, orthostatic hypotension, pericardial effusion (heart transplant), peripheral edema, peripheral vascular disease, phlebitis, syncope, tachycardia, thrombosis, vasodilatation, ventricular premature contractions

Central nervous system: Abnormal dreams, abnormality in thinking, agitation, amnesia, anxiety, aphasia, ataxia, brain disease, carpal tunnel syndrome, chills, confusion, convulsions, depression, dizziness, drowsiness, emotional lability, excessive crying, falling, fatigue, flaccid paralysis, hallucinations, headache, hypertonia, hypoesthesia, insomnia, mental status changes, mood elevation, myasthenia, myoclonus, nervousness, neurotoxicity, nightmares, pain, paresis, paresthesia, peripheral neuropathy, psychosis, seizure, vertigo, voice disorder, writing difficulty

Dermatologic: Acne vulgaris, alopecia, bruise, cellulitis, condyloma acuminatum, dermal ulcer, dermatological reaction, dermatitis (including fungal), diaphoresis, exfoliative dermatitis, hypotrichosis, pruritus, skin discoloration, skin photosensitivity, skin rash

Endocrine & metabolic: Acidosis, albuminuria, alkalosis, anasarca, Cushing's syndrome, decreased serum bicarbonate, decreased serum iron, dehydration, diabetes mellitus (post-transplant), gout, hirsutism, hypercalcemia, hypercholesterolemia, hyperglycemia, hyperkalemia, hyperlipidemia, hypertriglyceridemia, hyperuricemia, hypervolemia, hypocalcemia, hypoglycemia, hypokalemia, hypomagnesemia, hyponatremia, hypophosphatemia, increased gamma-glutamyl transferase, increased lactate dehydrogenase, weight changes

Gastrointestinal: Abdominal pain, anorexia, aphthous stomatitis, cholangitis, colitis, constipation, delayed gastric emptying, diarrhea, duodenitis, dyspepsia, dysphagia, enlargement of abdomen, esophagitis (including ulcerative), flatulence, gastric ulcer, gastritis, gastroenteritis, gastroesophageal reflux disease, gastrointestinal hemorrhage, gastrointestinal perforation, hernia, hiccups, increased appetite, intestinal obstruction, nausea, oral candidiasis, pancreatic disease (pseudocyst), pancreatitis (including hemorrhagic and necrotizing), peritonitis, rectal disease, stomach cramps, stomatitis, vomiting

Genitourinary: Anuria, bladder spasm, cystitis, dysuria, hematuria, nocturia, oliguria, proteinuria, toxic nephrosis, urinary frequency, urinary incontinence, urinary retention, urinary tract infection, urinary urgency, vaginitis

Hematologic & oncologic: Anemia, blood coagulation disorder, decreased prothrombin time, hemolytic anemia, hemorrhage, hypochromic anemia, hypoproteinemia, increased hematocrit, increased INR, Kaposi's sarcoma, leukocytosis, leukopenia, malignant neoplasm of bladder, malignant neoplasm of thyroid (papillary), neutropenia, pancytopenia, polycythemia, skin neoplasm, thrombocytopenia

Hepatic: Abnormal hepatic function tests, ascites, cholestatic jaundice, hepatic injury, hepatitis (including acute, chronic, and granulomatous), hyperbilirubinemia, increased liver enzymes, increased serum alkaline phosphatase, jaundice

Hypersensitivity: Hypersensitivity reaction

Infection: Abscess, bacterial infection, cytomegalovirus disease, Epstein Barr virus infection, herpes simplex infection, infection, polyoma virus infection, sepsis, serious infection, tinea versicolor

Local: Localized phlebitis, postoperative wound complication

Neuromuscular & skeletal: Arthralgia, arthropathy, back pain, leg cramps, muscle spasm, muscle weakness of the extremities, myalgia, neuropathy (including compression), osteopenia, osteoporosis, tremor, weakness

Ophthalmic: Amblyopia, blurred vision, conjunctivitis, visual disturbance

Otic: Hearing loss, otalgia, otitis externa, otitis media, tinnitus

Renal: Acute renal failure, hydronephrosis, increased blood urea nitrogen, increased serum creatinine, renal disease (BK nephropathy), renal function abnormality, renal tubular necrosis

Respiratory: Allergic rhinitis, asthma, atelectasis, bronchitis, cough, dyspnea, emphysema, flu-like symptoms, pharyngitis, pleural effusion, pneumonia, pneumothorax, pulmonary disease, pulmonary edema, pulmonary infiltrates, respiratory depression, respiratory failure, respiratory tract infection, rhinitis, sinusitis

Miscellaneous: Fever, graft complications, postoperative pain, wound healing impairment

Rare but important or life-threatening: Adult respiratory distress syndrome, agranulocytosis, anaphylactoid reaction, anaphylaxis, angioedema, basal cell carcinoma, biliary tract disease (stenosis), blindness, cerebrovascular accident, coma, deafness, decreased serum fibrinogen, delirium, disseminated intravascular coagulation, dysarthria, graft versus host disease (acute and chronic), hemiparesis, hemolytic-uremic syndrome, hemorrhagic cystitis, hepatic cirrhosis, hepatic failure, hepatic necrosis, hepatic veno-occlusive disease, hepatosplenic T-cell lymphomas, hepatotoxicity, hyperpigmentation, interstitial pulmonary disease, leukemia, leukoencephalopathy, liver steatosis, lymphoproliferative disorder (post-transplant or related to EBV), malignant melanoma, multiorgan failure, mutism, optic atrophy, osteomyelitis, photophobia, polyarthritis, progressive multifocal leukoencephalopathy (PML), prolonged partial thromboplastin time, prolonged Q-T interval on ECG, pulmonary hypertension, pure red cell aplasia, quadriplegia, reversible posterior leukoencephalopathy syndrome, rhabdomyolysis, septicemia, squamous cell carcinoma, status epilepticus, Stevens-Johnson syndrome, supraventricular extrasystole, supraventricular tachycardia, thrombocytopenic purpura, thrombotic thrombocytopenic purpura, torsades de pointes, toxic epidermal necrolysis, venous thrombosis, ventricular fibrillation

Note: Calcineurin inhibitor-induced hemolytic uremic syndrome/thrombotic thrombocytopenic purpura/thrombotic microangiopathy (HUS/TTP/TMA) have been reported (with concurrent sirolimus).

Drug Interactions

Metabolism/Transport Effects Substrate of CYP3A4 (major), P-glycoprotein; **Note:** Assignment of Major/Minor substrate status based on clinically relevant drug interaction potential; **Inhibits** CYP3A4 (weak), P-glycoprotein

Avoid Concomitant Use

Avoid concomitant use of Tacrolimus (Systemic) with any of the following: BCG; Bosutinib; CloZAPine; Conivaptan; Crizotinib; CycloSPORINE (Systemic); Dipyrone; Enzalutamide; Eplerenone; Fusidic Acid (Systemic); Grapefruit Juice; Mifepristone; Natalizumab; PAZOPanib; Pimecrolimus; Pimozide; Potassium-Sparing Diuretics; Silodosin; Sirolimus; Tacrolimus (Topical); Temsirolimus; Tofacitinib; Topotecan; Vaccines (Live); VinCRIStine (Liposomal)

Increased Effect/Toxicity

Tacrolimus (Systemic) may increase the levels/effects of: Afatinib; ARIPiprazole; Bosutinib; Brentuximab Vedotin; CloZAPine; Colchicine; CycloSPORINE (Systemic); Dabigatran Etexilate; DOXOrubicin (Conventional); Everolimus; Fenofibrate and Derivatives; Fosphenytoin; Highest Risk QTc-Prolonging Agents; Leflunomide; Lomitapide; Moderate Risk QTc-Prolonging Agents; Natalizumab; PAZOPanib; P-glycoprotein/ABCB1 Substrates; Phenytoin; Pimozide; Prucalopride; Rifaximin; Rivaroxaban; Silodosin; Sirolimus; Temsirolimus; Tofacitinib; Topotecan; Vaccines (Live); VinCRIStine (Liposomal)

The levels/effects of Tacrolimus (Systemic) may be increased by: Alcohol (Ethyl); Antidepressants (Serotonin Reuptake Inhibitor/Antagonist); Boceprevir; Calcium Channel Blockers (Dihydropyridine); Calcium Channel Blockers (Nondihydropyridine); Ceritinib; Chloramphenicol; Clotrimazole (Oral); Clotrimazole (Topical); Conivaptan; Crizotinib; CycloSPORINE (Systemic); CYP3A4 Inhibitors (Moderate); CYP3A4 Inhibitors (Strong); Danazol; Dasatinib; Denosumab; Dipyrone; Eplerenone; Ertapenem; Fluconazole; Fusidic Acid (Systemic); Grapefruit Juice; Itraconazole; Ivacaftor; Ketoconazole (Systemic); Levofloxacin (Systemic); Luliconazole; Macrolide Antibiotics; MetroNIDAZOLE (Systemic); Mifepristone; P-glycoprotein/ABCB1 Inhibitors; Pimecrolimus; Posaconazole; Potassium-Sparing Diuretics; Protease Inhibitors; Proton Pump Inhibitors; Ranolazine; Roflumilast; Sirolimus; Stiripentol; Tacrolimus (Topical); Telaprevir; Temsirolimus; Trastuzumab; Voriconazole

Decreased Effect

Tacrolimus (Systemic) may decrease the levels/effects of: BCG; Coccidioidin Skin Test; Sipuleucel-T; Vaccines (Inactivated); Vaccines (Live)

The levels/effects of Tacrolimus (Systemic) may be decreased by: Bosentan; Caspofungin; Cinacalcet; CYP3A4 Inducers (Strong); Dabrafenib; Deferasirox; Echinacea; Efavirenz; Enzalutamide; Fosphenytoin; Mitotane; P-glycoprotein/ABCB1 Inducers; Phenytoin; Rifamycin Derivatives; Siltuximab; Sirolimus; St Johns Wort; Temsirolimus; Tocilizumab

Food Interactions

Ethanol: Alcohol may increase the rate of release of extended-release tacrolimus and adversely affect tacrolimus safety and/or efficacy. Management: Avoid alcohol.

Food: Food decreases rate and extent of absorption. High-fat meals have most pronounced effect (37% and 25% decrease in AUC, respectively, and 77% and 25% decrease in C_{max}, respectively, for immediately release and extended release formulations). Grapefruit juice, a CYP3A4 inhibitor, may increase serum level and/or toxicity of tacrolimus. Management: Administer with or without food (immediate release), but be consistent. Administer extended release on an empty stomach. Avoid concurrent use of grapefruit juice.

Stability Hazardous agent; use appropriate precautions for handling and disposal (NIOSH, 2012). Stable for 24 hours when mixed in D_5W or NS in glass or polyolefin containers; 24-hour stability in plastic syringes stored at 24°C; no need to protect from light; do not store in polyvinyl chloride containers since the polyoxyl 60 hydrogenated castor oil injectable vehicle may leach phthalates from polyvinyl chloride containers; polyvinyl-containing administration sets adsorb drug and may lead to a lower dose being delivered to the patient; tacrolimus is unstable in alkaline media; do not mix with acyclovir or ganciclovir.

Mechanism of Action Suppresses cellular immunity (inhibits T-lymphocyte activation), by binding to an intracellular protein, FKBP-12 and complexes with calcineurin dependent proteins to inhibit calcineurin phosphatase activity

Pharmacokinetics (Adult data unless noted)

Absorption: Erratic and incomplete oral absorption (5% to 67%); food within 15 minutes of administration decreases absorption (27%)

Distribution: Distributes to erythrocytes, breast milk, lung, kidneys, pancreas, liver, placenta, heart, and spleen:
Children: 2.6 L/kg (mean)
Adults: 0.85-1.41 L/kg (mean) in liver and renal transplant patients

Protein binding: 99% to alpha-acid glycoprotein (some binding to albumin)

Metabolism: Hepatic metabolism through the cytochrome P450 system (CYP3A) to eight possible metabolites (major metabolite: 31-demethyl tacrolimus has same activity as tacrolimus *in vitro*)

Bioavailability: Oral:
Children: 7% to 55%
Adults: 7% to 32%

Half-life:
Children: 7.7-15.3 hours
Adults: 23-46 hours (in healthy volunteers)

Time to peak serum concentration: Oral: 0.5-6 hours

Elimination: Primarily in bile; <1% excreted unchanged in urine

Clearance: 7-103 mL/minute/kg (average: 30 mL/minute/kg); clearance higher in children

Dosing: Usual

Children: **Note:** Younger children generally require higher maintenance doses on a mg/kg basis than older children, adolescents, or adults (Kim, 2005; Montini, 2006)

Oral:
Liver transplant: Initial: 0.15-0.2 mg/kg/day divided every 12 hours
Heart transplant: Initial: 0.1-0.3 mg/kg/day divided every 12 hours (Pollock-Barziv, 2005; Swenson, 1995)
Kidney transplant: Initial: 0.2-0.3 mg/kg/day divided every 12 hours (Filler, 2005; Kim, 2005; Montini, 2006)
Prevention of graft-vs-host disease (unlabeled use): Convert from I.V. to oral dose (1:4 ratio): Multiply total daily I.V. dose times 4 and administer in 2 divided oral doses per day, every 12 hours (Yanik, 2000)

I.V.:
Liver transplant: 0.03-0.05 mg/kg/day as a continuous infusion
Heart transplant: 0.01-0.03 mg/kg/day as a continuous infusion (Groetzner, 2005)
Kidney transplant: 0.06 mg/kg/day as a continuous infusion (Trompeter, 2002)
Prevention of graft-vs-host disease (unlabeled use): Initial: 0.03 mg/kg/day (based on lean body weight) as continuous infusion. Treatment should begin at least 24 hours prior to stem cell infusion and continued only until oral medication can be tolerated (Yanik, 2000).

Adults:
Oral: 0.075-0.2 mg/kg/day divided every 12 hours
Liver transplant: Initial: 0.1-0.15 mg/kg/day divided every 12 hours
Heart transplant: Initial: 0.075 mg/kg/day divided every 12 hours
Kidney transplant: Initial: 0.2 mg/kg/day in combination with azathioprine or 0.1 mg/kg/day in combination with mycophenolate mofetil. Administer in 2 divided doses every 12 hours.
Prevention of graft-vs-host disease (unlabeled use): Convert from I.V. to oral dose (1:4 ratio): Multiply total daily I.V. dose times 4 and administer in 2 divided oral doses per day, every 12 hours (Uberti, 1999)

I.V. continuous infusion: 0.01-0.05 mg/kg/day
Liver or kidney transplant: Initial: 0.03-0.05 mg/kg/day
Heart transplant: Initial: 0.01 mg/kg/day
Graft-vs-host disease (unlabeled use):
Prevention: 0.03 mg/kg/day (based on lean body weight) as continuous infusion. Treatment should begin at least 24 hours prior to stem cell infusion and continued only until oral medication can be tolerated (Przepiorka, 1999).
Treatment: Initial: 0.03 mg/kg/day (based on lean body weight) as continuous infusion (Furlong, 2000; Przepiorka, 1999)

Dosing adjustment in renal or hepatic impairment: Patients with renal or hepatic impairment should receive the lowest dose in the recommended dosage range; further reductions in dose below these ranges may be required

Hemodialysis: Not removed by hemodialysis

Administration

Oral: Administer on an empty stomach; use oral syringe or glass container (not plastic or foam cup) when administering this medication; do not administer with grapefruit juice; do not administer within 2 hours before or after antacids

Parenteral: May administer by I.V. continuous infusion; I.V. concentrate for injection must be diluted to 0.004-0.02 mg/mL in NS or D_5W prior to administration; polyvinyl chloride-free administration tubing should be used to minimize the potential for significant drug absorption onto the tubing; begin no sooner than 6 hours post-transplant; continue only until oral medication can be tolerated

Hazardous agent; use appropriate precautions for handling and disposal (NIOSH, 2012).

Monitoring Parameters Liver enzymes, BUN, serum creatinine, glucose, potassium, magnesium, phosphorus, blood tacrolimus concentrations; CBC with differential; blood pressure, neurologic status, ECG

Reference Range Limited data correlating serum concentration to therapeutic efficacy/toxicity:

Trough (whole blood ELISA): 5-20 ng/mL

Trough (HPLC): 0.5-1.5 ng/mL

Heart transplant: Typical whole blood trough concentrations:

Months 1-3: 10-20 ng/mL

Months ≥4: 6-18 ng/mL

Kidney transplant: Whole blood trough concentrations:

In combination with azathioprine:

Months 1-3: 7-20 ng/mL

Months 4-12: 5-15 ng/mL

In combination with mycophenolate mofetil/IL-2 receptor antagonist (eg, daclizumab): Months 1-12: 4-11 ng/mL

Liver transplant: Whole blood trough concentrations:

Months 1-12: 5-20 ng/mL

Prevention of graft-vs-host disease: 10-20 ng/mL (Uberti, 1999); although some institutions use a lower limit of 5 ng/mL and an upper limit of 15 ng/mL (Przepiorka, 1999; Yanik, 2000)

Additional Information Tacrolimus should be initiated no sooner than 6 hours after transplant; convert I.V. tacrolimus to oral form as soon as possible or within 2-3 days (the oral formulation should be started 8-12 hours after stopping the I.V. infusion); when switching a patient from cyclosporine to tacrolimus, allow at least 24 hours after discontinuing cyclosporine before initiating tacrolimus therapy to minimize the risk of nephrotoxicity

Additional dosing considerations:

Switch from I.V. to oral therapy: Approximately threefold increase in dose compared to I.V.

Pediatric patients: Approximately two times higher dose compared to adults

Dosage Forms Excipient information presented when available (limited, particularly for generics); consult specific product labeling.

Capsule, Oral:

Hecoria: 0.5 mg, 1 mg, 5 mg

Prograf: 0.5 mg, 1 mg, 5 mg

Generic: 0.5 mg, 1 mg, 5 mg

Capsule Extended Release 24 Hour, Oral:

Astagraf XL: 0.5 mg, 1 mg, 5 mg

Solution, Intravenous:

Prograf: 5 mg/mL (1 mL) [contains alcohol, usp, cremophor el]

Extemporaneous Preparations Hazardous agent: Use appropriate precautions for handling and disposal.

A 0.5 mg/mL tacrolimus oral suspension may be made with immediate release capsules and a 1:1 mixture of Ora-Plus® and Simple Syrup, N.F. Mix the contents of six 5 mg tacrolimus capsules with quantity of vehicle sufficient to make 60 mL. Store in glass or plastic amber prescription bottles; label "shake well". Stable for 56 days at room temperature (Esquivel, 1996; Foster, 1996).

A 1 mg/mL tacrolimus oral suspension may be made with immediate release capsules, sterile water, Ora-Plus®, and Ora-Sweet®. Pour the contents of six 5 mg capsules into a plastic amber prescription bottle. Add ~5 mL of sterile water and agitate bottle until drug disperses into a slurry. Add equal parts Ora-Plus® and Ora-Sweet® in sufficient quantity to make 30 mL. Store in plastic amber prescription bottles; label "shake well". Stable for 4 months at room temperature (Elefante, 2006).

Elefante A, Muindi J, West K, et al, "Long-Term Stability of a Patient-Convenient 1 mg/mL Suspension of Tacrolimus for Accurate Maintenance of Stable Therapeutic Levels," Bone Marrow Transplant, 2006, 37(8):781-4.

Esquivel C, So S, McDiarmid S, Andrews W, and Colombani PM, "Suggested Guidelines for the Use of Tacrolimus in Pediatric Liver Transplant Patients," Transplantation, 1996, 61(5):847-8.

Foster JA, Jacobson PA, Johnson CE, et al, "Stability of Tacrolimus in an Extemporaneously Compounded Oral Liquid (Abstract of Meeting Presentation)," American Society of Health-System Pharmacists Annual Meeting, 1996, 53:P-52(E).

References

Asante-Korang A, Boyle GJ, Webber SA, et al, "Experience of FK506 Immune Suppression in Pediatric Heart Transplantation: A Study of Long-Term Adverse Effects," J Heart Lung Transplant, 1996, 15 (4):415-22.

Bramham K, Chusney G, Lee J, et al, "Breastfeeding and Tacrolimus: Serial Monitoring in Breast-Fed and Bottle-Fed Infants," Clin J Am Soc Nephrol, 2013, Apr;8(4):563-7.

EBPG Expert Group on Renal Transplantation, "European Best Practice Guidelines For Renal Transplantation. Section IV: Long-Term Management of the Transplant Recipient, IV.10. Pregnancy in Renal Transplant Recipients," Nephrol Dial Transplant, 2002, 17 Suppl 4:50-5.

Filler G, Webb NJ, Milford DV, et al, "Four-Year Data After Pediatric Renal Transplantation: A Randomized Trial of Tacrolimus Vs Cyclosporin Microemulsion," Pediatr Transplant, 2005, 9(4):498-503.

French AE, Soldin SJ, Soldin OP, et al, "Milk Transfer and Neonatal Safety of Tacrolimus," Ann Pharmacother, 2003, 37(6):815-8.

Furlong T, Storb R, Anasetti C, et al, "Clinical Outcome After Conversion to FK 506 (Tacrolimus) Therapy for Acute Graft-Versus-Host Disease Resistant to Cyclosporine or for Cyclosporine-Associated Toxicities," Bone Marrow Transplant, 2000, 26(9):985-91.

Gardiner SJ and Begg EJ, "Breastfeeding During Tacrolimus Therapy," Obstet Gynecol, 2006, 107(2 Pt 2):453-5.

Groetzner J, Reichart B, Roemer U, et al, "Cardiac Transplantation in Pediatric Patients: Fifteen-Year Experience of a Single Center," Ann Thorac Surg, 2005, 79(1):53-60.

Hebert MF, Zheng S, Hays K, et al, "Interpreting Tacrolimus Concentrations During Pregnancy and Postpartum," Transplantation, 2013, 95(7):908-15.

Jain A, Venkataramanan R, Fung JJ, et al, "Pregnancy After Liver Transplantation Under Tacrolimus," Transplantation, 1997, 64 (4):559-65.

Kim JS, Aviles DH, Silverstein DM, et al, "Effect of Age, Ethnicity, and Glucocorticoid Use on Tacrolimus Pharmacokinetics in Pediatric Renal Transplant Patients," Pediatr Transplant, 2005, 9(2):162-9.

McDiarmid SV, Colonna JO, Shaked A, et al, "Differences in Oral FK506 Dose Requirements Between Adults and Pediatric Liver Transplant Patients," Transplantation, 1993, 55(6):1328-32.

Menegaux F, Keeffe EB, Andrews BT, et al, "Neurological Complications of Liver Transplantation in Adult Versus Pediatric Patients," Transplantation, 1994, 58(4):447-50.

Montini G, Ujka F, Varagnolo C, et al, "The Pharmacokinetics and Immunosuppressive Response of Tacrolimus in Paediatric Renal Transplant Recipients," Pediatr Nephrol, 2006, 21(5):719-24.

National Institute for Occupational Safety and Health (NIOSH), "NIOSH List of Antineoplastic and Other Hazardous Drugs in Healthcare Settings 2012." Available at http://www.cdc.gov/niosh/docs/2012-150/pdfs/2012-150.pdf. Accessed January 21, 2013.

Pollock-Barziv SM, Dipchand AI, McCrindle BW, et al, "Randomized Clinical Trial of Tacrolimus- Vs Cyclosporine-Based Immunosuppression in Pediatric Heart Transplantation: Preliminary Results at 15-Month Follow-Up," J Heart Lung Transplant, 2005, 24(2):190-4.

Przepiorka D, Devine S, Fay J, et al, "Practical Considerations in the Use of Tacrolimus for Allogeneic Marrow Transplantation," Bone Marrow Transplant, 1999, 24(10):1053-6.

Swenson JM, Fricker FJ, and Armitage JM, "Immunosuppression Switch in Pediatric Heart Transplant Recipients: Cyclosporine to FK 506," J Am Coll Cardiol, 1995, 25(5):1183-8.

Taormina D, Abdallah HY, Venkataramanan R, et al, "Stability and Sorption of FK 506 in 5% Dextrose Injection and 0.9% Sodium Chloride Injection in Glass, Polyvinyl Chloride, and Polyolefin Containers," Am J Hosp Pharm, 1992, 49(1):119-22.

Trompeter R, Filler G, Webb NJ, et al, "Randomized Trial of Tacrolimus Versus Cyclosporin Microemulsion in Renal Transplantation," Pediatr Nephrol, 2002, 17(3):141-9.

Uberti JP, Cronin S, and Ratanatharathorn V, "Optimum Use of Tacrolimus in the Prophylaxis of Graft Versus Host Disease," BioDrugs, 1999, 11(5):343-58.

Yanik G, Levine JE, Ratanatharathorn V, et al, "Tacrolimus (FK506) and Methotrexate as Prophylaxis for Acute Graft-Versus-Host Disease in Pediatric Allogeneic Stem Cell Transplantation," Bone Marrow Transplant, 2000, 26(2):161-7.

Zheng S, Easterling TR, Umans JG, et al, "Pharmacokinetics of Tacrolimus During Pregnancy," Ther Drug Monit, 2012, 34(6):660-70.

Tacrolimus (Topical) (ta KROE li mus)

Medication Safety Issues
Sound-alike/look-alike issues:
Tacrolimus may be confused with everolimus, pimecrolimus, sirolimus, temsirolimus

Related Information
Safe Handling of Hazardous Drugs *on page 2419*

Brand Names: U.S. Protopic

Brand Names: Canada Protopic®

Generic Availability (U.S.) No

Use Second-line agent for short-term and intermittent treatment of moderate to severe atopic dermatitis in nonimmunocompromised patients not responsive to conventional therapy or when conventional therapy is not appropriate (0.03% ointment: FDA approved in ages ≥2 years and adults; 0.1% ointment: FDA approved in ages ≥16 years and adults)

Medication Guide Available Yes

Pregnancy Risk Factor C

Pregnancy Considerations Adverse events were observed in animal reproduction studies. Tacrolimus crosses the human placenta and is measurable in the cord blood, amniotic fluid, and newborn serum following systemic use. Refer to the Tacrolimus, Systemic monograph for additional information.

Breast-Feeding Considerations Tacrolimus is excreted into breast milk following systemic administration. Refer to the Tacrolimus, Systemic monograph for additional information.

Contraindications Hypersensitivity to tacrolimus or any component

Warnings Hazardous agent; use appropriate precautions for handling and disposal (NIOSH, 2012). Topical calcineurin inhibitors have been associated with rare cases of malignancy (including skin and lymphoma); therefore, limit to short-term and intermittent treatment using the minimum amount necessary for the control of symptoms and only on involved areas **[U.S. Boxed Warning]**. Avoid use on malignant or premalignant skin conditions (eg, cutaneous T-cell lymphoma). Should not be used in immunocompromised patients. Do not apply to areas of active bacterial or viral infection; infections at the treatment site should be cleared prior to therapy. Patients with atopic dermatitis are predisposed to skin infections and tacrolimus therapy has been associated with risk of developing eczema herpeticum, varicella zoster, and herpes simplex. May be associated with development of lymphadenopathy; possible infectious causes should be investigated. Discontinue use in patients with unknown cause of lymphadenopathy or acute infectious mononucleosis. If symptoms of atopic dermatitis not improved within 6 weeks, re-evaluate to confirm diagnosis. Not recommended for use in patients with skin disease which may increase systemic absorption (eg, Netherton's syndrome or cutaneous GVHD). Safety of intermittent use for >1 year has not been established. The use of Protopic® in children <2 years of age is not recommended [U.S. Boxed Warning]; only 0.03% ointment is indicated for children 2-15 years. Acute renal failure has been reported (rarely) with topical tacrolimus therapy.

Precautions Minimize exposure to sunlight while on topical therapy

Adverse Reactions
Cardiovascular: Peripheral edema

Central nervous system: Fever, headache, hyperesthesia, pain

Dermatologic: Acne, alopecia, contact dermatitis, cyst, dry skin, eczema herpeticum, erythema, flushing (localized; following ethanol consumption), folliculitis, fungal dermatitis, pruritus, pustular rash, skin burning (tends to improve as lesions resolve), skin tingling, sunburn, urticaria, vesiculobullous rash

Endocrine & metabolic: Dysmenorrhea

Gastrointestinal: Abdominal pain, diarrhea, dyspepsia, gastroenteritis, nausea, vomiting

Neuromuscular & skeletal: Arthralgia, back pain, myalgia, paresthesia

Ocular: Conjunctivitis

Otic: Otitis media

Respiratory: Bronchitis, cough increased, pneumonia, rhinitis, sinusitis

Miscellaneous: Allergic reaction, flu-like syndrome, lymphadenopathy, varicella/herpes zoster

Rare but important or life-threatening: Acute renal failure, anaphylaxis, anaphylactoid reaction, anemia, basal cell carcinoma, chest pain, hypercholesterolemia, malignant melanoma, osteomyelitis, photosensitivity reaction, seizure, septicemia, skin discoloration, squamous cell carcinoma

Drug Interactions
Metabolism/Transport Effects Substrate of CYP3A4 (minor), P-glycoprotein; **Note:** Assignment of Major/Minor substrate status based on clinically relevant drug interaction potential

Avoid Concomitant Use
Avoid concomitant use of Tacrolimus (Topical) with any of the following: CycloSPORINE (Systemic); Immunosuppressants; Sirolimus; Temsirolimus

Increased Effect/Toxicity
Tacrolimus (Topical) may increase the levels/effects of: Alcohol (Ethyl); CycloSPORINE (Systemic); Immunosuppressants; Sirolimus; Temsirolimus

The levels/effects of Tacrolimus (Topical) may be increased by: Antidepressants (Serotonin Reuptake Inhibitor/Antagonist); Antifungal Agents (Azole Derivatives, Systemic); Calcium Channel Blockers (Nondihydropyridine); CycloSPORINE (Systemic); Danazol; Fluconazole; Grapefruit Juice; Macrolide Antibiotics; Protease Inhibitors; Sirolimus; Temsirolimus

Decreased Effect There are no known significant interactions involving a decrease in effect.

Stability Hazardous agent; use appropriate precautions for handling and disposal (NIOSH, 2012). Store at room temperature of 25°C (77°F); excursions permitted to 15°C to 30°C (59°F to 86°F).

Mechanism of Action Suppresses cellular immunity (inhibits T-lymphocyte activation), by binding to an intracellular protein, FKBP-12 and complexes with calcineurin dependent proteins to inhibit calcineurin phosphatase activity

Pharmacokinetics (Adult data unless noted)
Absorption: Minimally absorbed
Bioavailability: <0.5%

Dosing: Usual Moderate to severe atopic dermatitis:
Note: Discontinue use when symptoms have cleared. If no improvement occurs within 6 weeks, patients should be re-examined to confirm diagnosis.

Children and Adolescents ≥2-15 years: Apply a thin layer of 0.03% ointment to affected area twice daily; rub in gently and completely

Adolescents ≥16 years and Adults: Apply a thin layer of 0.03% or 0.1% ointment to affected area twice daily; rub in gently and completely

Administration For external use only; do not cover with occlusive dressings; apply thin layer and rub ointment in gently and completely onto clean, dry skin. Do not bathe, shower, or swim right after ointment application. Moisturizers can be applied after ointment application.

Hazardous agent; use appropriate precautions for handling and disposal (NIOSH, 2012).

Dosage Forms Excipient information presented when available (limited, particularly for generics); consult specific product labeling.

Ointment, External:

Protopic: 0.03% (30 g, 60 g, 100 g); 0.1% (30 g, 60 g, 100 g)

References

National Institute for Occupational Safety and Health (NIOSH), "NIOSH List of Antineoplastic and Other Hazardous Drugs in Healthcare Settings 2012." Available at http://www.cdc.gov/niosh/docs/2012-150/pdfs/2012-150.pdf. Accessed January 21, 2013.

Schachner LA, Lamerson C, Sheehan MP, et al, "Tacrolimus Ointment 0.03% Is Safe and Effective for the Treatment of Mild to Moderate Atopic Dermatitis in Pediatric Patients: Results From a Randomized, Double-Blind, Vehicle-Controlled Study," *Pediatrics*, 2005, 116(3): e334-42.

◆ **Tactuo™ (Can)** *see* Adapalene and Benzoyl Peroxide *on page 74*

◆ **Tagamet HB [OTC]** *see* Cimetidine *on page 469*

◆ **Talwin** *see* Pentazocine *on page 1639*

◆ **Tambocor [DSC]** *see* Flecainide *on page 874*

◆ **Tambocor™ (Can)** *see* Flecainide *on page 874*

◆ **Tamiflu** *see* Oseltamivir *on page 1551*

Tamoxifen (ta MOKS i fen)

Medication Safety Issues

Sound-alike/look-alike issues:

Tamoxifen may be confused with pentoxifylline, Tambocor™, tamsulosin, temazepam

Related Information

Oral Medications That Should Not Be Crushed or Altered *on page 2438*

Safe Handling of Hazardous Drugs *on page 2419*

Brand Names: U.S. Soltamox

Brand Names: Canada Apo-Tamox®; Mylan-Tamoxifen; Nolvadex®-D; PMS-Tamoxifen; Teva-Tamoxifen

Therapeutic Category Antineoplastic Agent, Estrogen Receptor Antagonist

Generic Availability (U.S.) May be product dependent

Use Treatment of metastatic (female and male) breast cancer; adjuvant treatment of breast cancer after primary treatment with surgery and radiation; reduce risk of invasive breast cancer in women with ductal carcinoma *in situ* (DCIS) after surgery and radiation; reduce the incidence of breast cancer in women at high risk (all indications: FDA approved in adults); has also been used in treatment of McCune-Albright Syndrome (MAS) in girls associated with precocious puberty

Medication Guide Available Yes

Pregnancy Risk Factor D

Pregnancy Considerations Animal reproduction studies have demonstrated fetal adverse effects and fetal loss. There have been reports of vaginal bleeding, birth defects and fetal loss in pregnant women. Tamoxifen use during pregnancy may have a potential long term risk to the fetus of a DES-like syndrome. For sexually-active women of childbearing age, initiate during menstruation (negative β-hCG immediately prior to initiation in women with irregular cycles). Tamoxifen may induce ovulation. Barrier or non-hormonal contraceptives are recommended. Pregnancy should be avoided during treatment and for 2 months after treatment has been discontinued.

Breast-Feeding Considerations It is not known if tamoxifen is excreted in breast milk, however, it has been shown to inhibit lactation. Due to the potential for adverse reactions, women taking tamoxifen should not breast-feed.

Contraindications Hypersensitivity to tamoxifen or any component; concurrent warfarin therapy or history of deep vein thrombosis or pulmonary embolism (when tamoxifen is used for cancer risk reduction in women at high risk for breast cancer and in women with DCIS)

Warnings Hazardous agent; use appropriate precautions for handling and disposal (NIOSH, 2012). Tamoxifen use for breast cancer risk reduction in women at high risk for breast cancer and in women with DCIS is associated with an increased incidence of uterine or endometrial cancers **[U. S. Boxed Warning]**; endometrial hyperplasia, polyps, endometriosis, uterine fibroids, and ovarian cysts have occurred; amenorrhea and menstrual irregularities have been reported with tamoxifen use; monitor and promptly evaluate any report of abnormal vaginal bleeding. In a year-long clinical trial of girls (2-10 years) with McCune-Albright syndrome (MAS) associated with precocious puberty, mean uterine volumes were increased after 6 months of therapy, and by study completion had doubled in volume; a causal relationship has not been determined; long-term effects of tamoxifen in this population have not been established; pelvic ultrasound monitoring is recommended (Eugester, 2003).

Serious and life-threatening thromboembolic events, including stroke and pulmonary emboli have occurred at an incidence greater than placebo during use for breast cancer risk reduction in women at high risk for breast cancer and in women with DCIS **[U.S. Boxed Warning]**; these events are rare, but require consideration in risk: benefit evaluation. In patients already diagnosed with breast cancer, the benefits of tamoxifen use are greater than the risks. An increased incidence of thromboembolic events has been associated with use; risk is increased with concomitant chemotherapy; use with caution in individuals with a history of thromboembolic events.

Tamoxifen use may be associated with changes in bone mineral density (BMD) and the effects may be dependent upon menstrual status; in postmenopausal women, tamoxifen use is associated with a protective effect on bone mineral density (BMD), preventing loss of BMD which lasts over the 5-year treatment period. In premenopausal women, a decline (from baseline) in BMD mineral density has been observed in women who continued to menstruate; this may be associated with an increased risk of fractures.

Liver abnormalities such as cholestasis, fatty liver, hepatitis, and hepatic necrosis have occurred; hepatocellular carcinomas have been reported in some studies; relationship to treatment is unclear. Thrombocytopenia and/or leukopenia may occur; neutropenia and pancytopenia have been reported rarely; hemorrhagic episodes have occurred in patients with significant thrombocytopenia. Decreased visual acuity, retinal vein thrombosis, retinopathy, corneal changes, color perception changes, and increased incidence of cataracts along with the need for cataract surgery have been reported.

Precautions Use with caution in patients with hyperlipidemia; infrequent postmarketing cases of hyperlipidemias have been reported. Use with caution in patient with metastatic breast cancer; local disease flare and increased bone and tumor pain may occur; may be associated with (good) tumor response; onset is shortly after therapy initiation and usually resolves rapidly. In patients with bone metastasis, hypercalcemia has occurred, usually within a few weeks of therapy initiation; monitor and institute appropriate hypercalcemia management; discontinue if severe.

Use with caution with concomitant drug therapy affecting CYP and Pgp metabolic pathways; tamoxifen is associated with a high potential for drug interactions; decreased efficacy and an increased risk of breast cancer recurrence has been reported with concurrent moderate or strong

CYP2D6 inhibitors (Aubert, 2009; Dezentje, 2009). Concomitant use with select SSRIs may result in decreased tamoxifen efficacy. Strong CYP2D6 inhibitors (eg, fluoxetine, paroxetine) and moderate CYP2D6 inhibitors (eg, sertraline) are reported to interfere with transformation to the active metabolite endoxifen. Weak CYP2D6 inhibitors (eg, venlafaxine, citalopram) have minimal effect on the conversion to endoxifen (Jin, 2005; NCCN Breast Cancer Risk Reduction Guidelines v.2.2010); escitalopram is also a weak CYP2D6 inhibitor. In a retrospective analysis of breast cancer patients taking tamoxifen and SSRIs, concomitant use of paroxetine and tamoxifen was associated with an increased risk of death due to breast cancer (Kelly, 2010). Lower plasma concentrations of endoxifen (active metabolite) have been observed in patients associated with reduced CYP2D6 activity (Jin, 2005) and may be associated with reduced efficacy.

Adverse Reactions

Cardiovascular: Angina, cardiovascular ischemia, chest pain, deep venous thrombus, edema, flushing, hypertension, MI, peripheral edema, vasodilation, venous thrombotic events

Central nervous system: Anxiety, depression, dizziness, fatigue, headache, insomnia, mood changes, pain

Dermatologic: Alopecia, rash, skin changes

Endocrine & metabolic: Altered menses, amenorrhea, breast neoplasm, breast pain, fluid retention, hot flashes, hypercholesterolemia, menstrual disorder, oligomenorrhea

Gastrointestinal: Abdominal cramps, abdominal pain, anorexia, constipation, diarrhea, dyspepsia, nausea, throat irritation (oral solution), vomiting, weight gain/loss

Genitourinary: Leukorrhea, ovarian cyst, urinary tract infection, vaginal bleeding, vaginal discharge, vaginal hemorrhage, vaginitis, vulvovaginitis

Hematologic: Anemia, thrombocytopenia

Hepatic: AST increased, serum bilirubin increased

Neuromuscular & skeletal: Arthralgia, arthritis, arthrosis, back pain, bone pain, fracture, joint disorder, musculoskeletal pain, myalgia, osteoporosis, paresthesia, weakness

Ocular: Cataract

Renal: Serum creatinine increased

Respiratory: Bronchitis, cough, dyspnea, pharyngitis, sinusitis

Miscellaneous: Allergic reaction, cyst, diaphoresis, flu-like syndrome, infection/sepsis, lymphedema, neoplasm

Rare but important or life-threatening: Angioedema, bullous pemphigoid, cholestasis, corneal changes, endometrial cancer, endometrial hyperplasia, endometrial polyps, endometriosis, erythema multiforme, fatty liver, hepatic necrosis, hepatitis, hypercalcemia, hyperlipidemia, hypersensitivity reactions, hypertriglyceridemia, impotence (males), interstitial pneumonitis, loss of libido (males), pancreatitis, phlebitis, pruritus vulvae, pulmonary embolism, retinal vein thrombosis, retinopathy, second primary tumors, Stevens-Johnson syndrome, stroke,; tumor pain and local disease flare (including increase in lesion size and erythema) during treatment of metastatic breast cancer (generally resolves with continuation); uterine fibroids, vaginal dryness, visual color perception changes

Drug Interactions

Metabolism/Transport Effects Substrate of CYP2A6 (minor), CYP2B6 (minor), CYP2C9 (major), CYP2D6 (major), CYP2E1 (minor), CYP3A4 (major); **Note:** Assignment of Major/Minor substrate status based on clinically relevant drug interaction potential; **Inhibits** CYP2B6 (weak), CYP2C8 (moderate), CYP2C9 (weak), CYP3A4 (weak), P-glycoprotein

Avoid Concomitant Use

Avoid concomitant use of Tamoxifen with any of the following: Bosutinib; Conivaptan; CYP2D6 Inhibitors (Strong); Fusidic Acid (Systemic); Ospemifene; PAZOPanib; Pimozide; Silodosin; Topotecan; VinCRIStine (Liposomal); Vitamin K Antagonists

Increased Effect/Toxicity

Tamoxifen may increase the levels/effects of: Afatinib; ARIPiprazole; Bosutinib; Brentuximab Vedotin; Colchicine; CYP2C8 Substrates; Dabigatran Etexilate; DOXOrubicin (Conventional); Everolimus; Highest Risk QTc-Prolonging Agents; Lomitapide; Mipomersen; Moderate Risk QTc-Prolonging Agents; Ospemifene; PAZOPanib; P-glycoprotein/ABCB1 Substrates; Pimozide; Prucalopride; Rifaximin; Rivaroxaban; Silodosin; Topotecan; VinCRIStine (Liposomal); Vitamin K Antagonists

The levels/effects of Tamoxifen may be increased by: Abiraterone Acetate; Ceritinib; Conivaptan; CYP2C9 Inhibitors (Moderate); CYP2C9 Inhibitors (Strong); CYP3A4 Inhibitors (Moderate); CYP3A4 Inhibitors (Strong); Dasatinib; Fusidic Acid (Systemic); Ivacaftor; Luliconazole; Mifepristone; Simeprevir

Decreased Effect

Tamoxifen may decrease the levels/effects of: Anastrozole; Letrozole; Ospemifene

The levels/effects of Tamoxifen may be decreased by: Aminoglutethimide; Bexarotene (Systemic); Bosentan; CYP2C9 Inducers (Strong); CYP2D6 Inducers (Moderate); CYP2D6 Inhibitors (Strong); CYP3A4 Inducers (Strong); Dabrafenib; Deferasirox; Mitotane; Peginterferon Alfa-2b; Rifamycin Derivatives; Siltuximab; St Johns Wort; Tocilizumab

Food Interactions Grapefruit juice may decrease the metabolism of tamoxifen. Management: Avoid grapefruit juice.

Stability Hazardous agent; use appropriate precautions for handling and disposal (NIOSH, 2012).

Oral solution: Store at ≤25°C (77°F); do not freeze or refrigerate. Protect from light. Discard opened bottle after 3 months.

Tablets: Store at 20°C to 25°C (68°F to 77°F); avoid excessive heat >40°C (>104°F). Protect from light.

Mechanism of Action Competitively binds to estrogen receptors on tumors and other tissue targets, producing a nuclear complex that decreases DNA synthesis and inhibits estrogen effects; nonsteroidal agent with potent antiestrogenic properties which compete with estrogen for binding sites in breast and other tissues; cells accumulate in the G_0 and G_1 phases; therefore, tamoxifen is cytostatic rather than cytocidal.

Pharmacokinetics (Adult data unless noted)

Absorption: Well absorbed

Distribution: High concentrations found in uterus, endometrial, and breast tissue

Protein binding: 99%

Metabolism: Hepatic; via CYP2D6 to 4-hydroxytamoxifen and via CYP3A4/5 to N-desmethyl-tamoxifen. Each is then further metabolized into endoxifen (4-hydroxytamoxifen via CYP3A4 and N-desmethyl-tamoxifen via CYP2D6); both 4-hydroxy-tamoxifen and endoxifen are 30- to 100-fold more potent than tamoxifen.

Half-life elimination: Tamoxifen: ~5-7 days; N-desmethyl tamoxifen: ~14 days

Time to peak, serum concentrations:
Children 2-10 years (female): ~8 hours
Adults: ~5 hours

Elimination: Feces (26% to 51%); urine (9% to 13%)
Clearance: Higher (~2.3 fold) in female pediatric patients (2-10 years) compared to adult breast cancer patients; within pediatric population, clearance faster in children 2-6 years compared to older children

Dosing: Usual

Children 2-10 years: **McCune-Albright syndrome; precocious puberty:** Limited data available: Oral: 20 mg once daily; dosing based on a trial of 25 girls ≤10 years of age (range: 2.9-10.9 years) who received treatment for 1 year; frequency of vaginal bleeding episodes were decreased; growth velocity was significantly decreased prior to pretreatment rates as was skeletal maturation; ovarian and uterine volumes were increased; further studies are needed (Eugester, 2003)

Adults: **Note:** For the treatment of breast cancer, patients receiving both tamoxifen and chemotherapy should receive treatment sequentially, with tamoxifen following completion of chemotherapy.

Breast cancer treatment:
Adjuvant therapy (females): 20 mg once daily for 5 years

Metastatic (males and females): 20-40 mg/day (doses >20 mg should be given in 2 divided doses). **Note:** Although the FDA-approved labeling recommends dosing up to 40 mg/day, clinical benefit has not been demonstrated with doses above 20 mg/day (Bratherton, 1984).

Premenopausal women: Duration of treatment is 5 years (NCCN Breast Cancer guidelines v.1.2011)

Postmenopausal women: Duration of tamoxifen treatment is 2-3 years followed by an aromatase inhibitor (AI) to complete 5 years; if contraindications or intolerant to AI, may take tamoxifen for the full 5 years **or** extended therapy: 4.5-6 years of tamoxifen followed by 5 years of an AI (NCCN Breast Cancer guidelines v.1.2011)

DCIS (females), to reduce the risk for invasive breast cancer: 20 mg once daily for 5 years

Breast cancer risk reduction (pre- and postmenopausal high-risk females): 20 mg once daily for 5 years

Dosing adjustment in renal impairment: There are no dosage adjustments provided in the manufacturer's labeling (not studied).

Dosing adjustment in hepatic impairment: There are no dosage adjustments provided in the manufacturer's labeling; the effect of hepatic dysfunction on tamoxifen pharmacokinetics has not been determined.

Administration Hazardous agent; use appropriate precautions for handling and disposal (NIOSH, 2012). Administer tablets or oral solution with or without food; use supplied dosing cup for oral solution.

Monitoring Parameters CBC with platelets, serum calcium, LFTs; triglycerides and cholesterol (in patients with preexisting hyperlipidemias); INR and PT (in patients on vitamin K antagonists); abnormal vaginal bleeding; breast and gynecologic exams (baseline and routine), mammogram (baseline and routine); signs/symptoms of DVT (leg swelling, tenderness) or PE (shortness of breath); ophthalmic exam (if vision problem or cataracts); bone mineral density (premenopausal women)

McCune-Albright syndrome: In the pediatric clinical trial (study duration: 12 months), the following were monitored: Serum estradiol, estrone, DHEAS, LH, FSH, and IGF-1 (baseline, and at 6 and 12 months of therapy); liver function test (baseline and at 3, 6, and 12 months of therapy); CBC and INR at baseline; assessments of puberty status and growth at baseline and periodically during therapy (6 and 12 months); Height, weight, Tanner stage, bone age (radiographs), vaginal bleeding data, and pelvic ultrasounds (Eugester, 2003)

Test Interactions T_4 elevations (which may be explained by increases in thyroid-binding globulin) have been reported; not accompanied by clinical hyperthyroidism

Dosage Forms Excipient information presented when available (limited, particularly for generics); consult specific product labeling.

Solution, Oral:
Soltamox: 10 mg/5 mL (150 mL) [sugar free; contains alcohol, usp, propylene glycol; licorice-aniseed flavor]

Tablet, Oral:
Generic: 10 mg, 20 mg

Extemporaneous Preparations Hazardous agent: Use appropriate precautions for handling and disposal.

A 0.5 mg/mL oral suspension may be prepared with tablets. Place two 10 mg tablets into 40 mL purified water and let stand ~2-5 minutes. Stir until tablets are completely disintegrated (dispersion time for each 10 mg tablet is ~2-5 minutes). Administer immediately after preparation. To ensure the full dose is administered, rinse glass several times with water and administer residue.

Lam MS, "Extemporaneous Compounding of Oral Liquid Dosage Formulations and Alternative Drug Delivery Methods for Anticancer Drugs," *Pharmacotherapy*, 2011, 31(2):164-92.

References

Aubert RE, Stanek EJ, Yao J, et al, "Risk of Breast Cancer Recurrence in Women Initiating Tamoxifen With CYP2D6 Inhibitors," *J Clin Oncol*, 2009, 27(18S):CRA508 [abstract CRA508 from 2009 ASCO Annual Meeting].

Bratherton DG, Brown CH, Buchanan R, et al, "A Comparison of Two Doses of Tamoxifen (Nolvadex) in Postmenopausal Women With Advanced Breast Cancer: 10 mg bd Versus 20 mg bd," *Br J Cancer*, 1984, 50(2):199-205.

Dezentje V, Van Blijderveen NJ, Gelderblom H, et al, "Concomitant CYP2D6 Inhibitor Use and Tamoxifen Adherence in Early-Stage Breast Cancer: A Pharmacoepidemiologic Study," *J Clin Oncol*, 2009, 27(18S):CRA509 [abstract CRA509 from 2009 ASCO Annual Meeting].

Early Breast Cancer Trialists' Collaborative Group (EBCTCG), "Effects of Chemotherapy and Hormonal Therapy for Early Breast Cancer on Recurrence and 15-Year Survival: An Overview of the Randomised Trials," *Lancet*, 2005, 365(9472):1687-717.

Eastell R, Adams JE, Coleman RE, et al, "Effect of Anastrozole on Bone Mineral Density: 5-Year Results From the Anastrozole, Tamoxifen, Alone or in Combination Trial 18233230," *J Clin Oncol*, 2008, 26 (7):1051-7.

Eugster EA, Rubin SD, Reiter EO, et al, "Tamoxifen Treatment for Precocious Puberty in McCune-Albright Syndrome: A Multicenter Trial," *J Pediatr*, 2003, 143(1):60-6.

Goetz MP, Kamal A, and Ames MM, "Tamoxifen Pharmacogenomics: The Role of CYP2D6 as a Predictor of Drug Response," *Clin Pharmacol Ther*, 2008, 83(1):160-6.

Jin Y, Desta Z, Stearns V, et al, "CYP2D6 Genotype, Antidepressant Use, and Tamoxifen Metabolism During Adjuvant Breast Cancer Treatment," *J Natl Cancer Inst*, 2005, 97(1):30-9.

Kelly CM, Juurlink DN, Gomes T, et al, "Selective Serotonin Reuptake Inhibitors and Breast Cancer Mortality in Women Receiving Tamoxifen: A Population Based Cohort Study," *BMJ*, 2010, 340:c693.

National Comprehensive Cancer Network® (NCCN), "Clinical Practice Guidelines in Oncology™: Breast Cancer," Version 1.2011. Available at http://www.nccn.org/professionals/physician_gls/PDF/breast.pdf

National Comprehensive Cancer Network® (NCCN), "Clinical Practice Guidelines in Oncology™: Breast Cancer Risk Reduction, Version 2.2010." Available at http://www.nccn.org/professionals/physician_gls/PDF/breast_risk.pdf

National Comprehensive Cancer Network® (NCCN), "Clinical Practice Guidelines in Oncology™: Ovarian Cancer," Version 2.2011. Available at http://www.nccn.org/professionals/physician_gls/PDF/ovarian.pdf

National Comprehensive Cancer Network® (NCCN), "Clinical Practice Guidelines in Oncology™: Uterine Neoplasms," Version 1.2011. Available at http://www.nccn.org/professionals/physician_gls/PDF/uterine.pdf

National Institute for Occupational Safety and Health (NIOSH), "NIOSH List of Antineoplastic and Other Hazardous Drugs in Healthcare Settings 2012." Available at http://www.cdc.gov/niosh/docs/2012-150/pdfs/2012-150.pdf. Accessed January 21, 2013.

Sideras K, Ingle JN, Ames MM, et al, "Coprescription of Tamoxifen and Medications That Inhibit CYP2D6," *J Clin Oncol*, 2010, 28 (16):2768-76.

Vehmanen L, Elomaa I, Blomqvist C, et al, "Tamoxifen Treatment After Adjuvant Chemotherapy Has Opposite Effects on Bone Mineral Density in Premenopausal Patients Depending on Menstrual Status," *J Clin Oncol*, 2006, 24(4):675-80.

Visvanathan K, Chlebowski RT, Hurley P, et al, "American Society of Clinical Oncology Clinical Practice Guideline Update on the Use of Pharmacologic Interventions Including Tamoxifen, Raloxifene, and Aromatase Inhibition for Breast Cancer Risk Reduction," *J Clin Oncol*, 2009, 27(19):3235-58.

◆ **Tamoxifen Citras** *see* Tamoxifen *on page 1968*
◆ **Tamoxifen Citrate** *see* Tamoxifen *on page 1968*

◆ **Tanta-Orciprenaline® (Can)** *see* Metaproterenol *on page 1352*

◆ **TAP-144** *see* Leuprolide *on page 1215*

◆ **Tapazole** *see* Methimazole *on page 1362*

◆ **Tapazole® (Can)** *see* Methimazole *on page 1362*

◆ **Targel® [OTC] (Can)** *see* Coal Tar *on page 532*

◆ **Taro-Carbamazepine Chewable (Can)** *see* CarBAMazepine *on page 372*

◆ **Taro-Ciclopirox (Can)** *see* Ciclopirox *on page 465*

◆ **Taro-Ciprofloxacin (Can)** *see* Ciprofloxacin (Systemic) *on page 471*

◆ **Taro-Clindamycin (Can)** *see* Clindamycin (Topical) *on page 500*

◆ **Taro-Clobetasol (Can)** *see* Clobetasol *on page 506*

◆ **Taro-Docusate [OTC] (Can)** *see* Docusate *on page 701*

◆ **Taro-Enalapril (Can)** *see* Enalapril *on page 744*

◆ **Taro-Fluconazole (Can)** *see* Fluconazole *on page 877*

◆ **Taro-Mometasone (Can)** *see* Mometasone (Topical) *on page 1435*

◆ **Taro-Phenytoin (Can)** *see* Phenytoin *on page 1663*

◆ **Taro-Simvastatin (Can)** *see* Simvastatin *on page 1892*

◆ **Taro-Sone (Can)** *see* Betamethasone (Topical) *on page 285*

◆ **Taro-Sumatriptan (Can)** *see* SUMAtriptan *on page 1958*

◆ **Taro-Warfarin (Can)** *see* Warfarin *on page 2156*

◆ **Tavist Allergy [OTC]** *see* Clemastine *on page 494*

◆ **Tavist ND** *see* Loratadine *on page 1278*

◆ **Taxol** *see* PACLitaxel *on page 1579*

◆ **Taxotere** *see* DOCEtaxel *on page 697*

Tazarotene (taz AR oh teen)

Brand Names: U.S. Avage; Fabior; Tazorac
Brand Names: Canada Tazorac
Therapeutic Category Acne Products; Keratolytic Agent
Generic Availability (U.S.) No
Use
  Cream: Treatment of acne vulgaris [Tazorac (0.1%): FDA approved in ages ≥12 years and adults]; treatment of plaque psoriasis [Tazorac (0.05% and 0.1%): FDA approved in ages ≥18 years and adults]; mitigation (palliation) of facial skin wrinkling, facial mottled hyper-/hypopigmentation, and benign facial lentigines as adjunct to comprehensive skin care and sunlight avoidance [Avage (0.1%): FDA approved in ages ≥17 years and adults]
  Gel: Treatment of mild to moderate facial acne vulgaris [Tazorac (0.1%): FDA approved in ages ≥12 years and adults]; treatment of stable plaque psoriasis of up to 20% body surface area involvement [Tazorac (0.05% and 0.1%): FDA approved in ages ≥12 years and adults]
Pregnancy Risk Factor X
Pregnancy Considerations Adverse events were observed in animal reproduction studies. Use in pregnancy is contraindicated. A negative pregnancy test should be obtained within 2 weeks prior to treatment; treatment should begin during a normal menstrual period.
Breast-Feeding Considerations It is not known if tazarotene is excreted in breast milk; recommendations for use differ by manufacturers' labeling. Systemic absorption depends on formulation and size of surface area.
Contraindications Hypersensitivity to tazarotene, other retinoids, vitamin A derivatives (eg, isotretinoin, tretinoin), or any component; pregnancy; use in women of childbearing potential who are unable to comply with birth control requirements

Warnings Women of childbearing potential must use adequate birth control measures; a negative pregnancy test within 2 weeks prior to beginning treatment is recommended; begin treatment during a normal menstrual period. Tazarotene may cause photosensitivity; exposure to sunlight (including sunlamps) should be avoided unless deemed medically necessary, and in such cases, exposure should be minimized (including use of sunscreens/protective clothing). Risk may be increased by concurrent therapy with known photosensitizers (thiazides, tetracyclines, fluoroquinolones, phenothiazines, sulfonamides).
Precautions For external use only; avoid contact with eyes and mouth; also avoid contact with the eyelids when used for acne or psoriasis. Not for use on eczematous, broken, or sunburned skin; may cause severe irritation. Treatment with tazarotene may increase skin sensitivity to weather extremes of wind or cold; concomitant topical medications (eg, medicated or abrasive soaps, cleansers, or cosmetics with a strong drying effect) should be used with caution due to increased skin irritation. Should not be used to treat lentigo maligna. Avoid application over extensive areas; specifically, safety and efficacy of gel applied over >20% of BSA have not been established.
Adverse Reactions
  Cardiovascular: Peripheral edema
  Dermatologic: Burning sensation of skin, cheilitis, contact dermatitis, dermatitis, desquamation, eczema, erythema, exacerbation of psoriasis, pruritus, skin discoloration, skin fissure, skin irritation, skin pain, skin photosensitivity, skin rash, stinging of the skin, xeroderma
  Endocrine & metabolic: Hypertriglyceridemia
  Local: Application site pain, local hemorrhage
  Ophthalmic: Ocular irritation (including edema, irritation, and inflammation of the eye or eyelid)
  Rare but important or life-threatening: Impetigo, skin blister
Drug Interactions
  Metabolism/Transport Effects None known.
  Avoid Concomitant Use There are no known interactions where it is recommended to avoid concomitant use.
  Increased Effect/Toxicity There are no known significant interactions involving an increase in effect.
  Decreased Effect There are no known significant interactions involving a decrease in effect.
Stability
  Cream: Store at 25°C (77°F); excursions permitted to -5°C to 30°C (23°F to 86°F).
  Gel: Store at 25°C (77°F); excursions permitted to 15°C to 30°C (59°F to 86°F).
Mechanism of Action Synthetic, acetylenic retinoid which modulates differentiation and proliferation of epithelial tissue and exerts some degree of anti-inflammatory and immunological activity
Pharmacodynamics
  Onset of action: Psoriasis: 1 week
  Duration: Psoriasis: Up to 12 weeks after discontinuation when initially treated for 2-3 months (duration may be less if initial treatment was shorter)
Pharmacokinetics (Adult data unless noted)
  Absorption: Minimal following cutaneous application (≤6% of dose)
  Protein binding: Metabolite: >99%
  Metabolism: Prodrug, rapidly metabolized via esterases to an active metabolite (tazarotenic acid) following topical application and systemic absorption; tazarotenic acid undergoes further hepatic metabolism
  Half-life: Metabolite: 18 hours
  Elimination: Urine and feces as metabolites
Dosing: Usual
  Children and Adolescents:
    Acne vulgaris: Children ≥12 years and Adolescents: Topical: Tazorac (0.1% cream or gel): Apply as a thin ▶

film (2 mg/cm^2) to affected areas once daily in the evening for up to 12 weeks

Psoriasis: Topical:

Cream: Adolescents ≥18 years: Tazorac (0.05%): Initial: Apply a thin film (2 mg/cm^2) to affected area once daily in the evening; may increase strength to 0.1% if tolerated and necessary

Gel: Children ≥12 years and Adolescents: Tazorac (0.05%): Initial: Apply a thin film (2 mg/cm^2) to affected area once daily in the evening for up to 12 months; may increase strength to 0.1% if tolerated and necessary; apply to no more than 20% of the body surface area

Palliation of fine facial wrinkles, facial mottled hyper-/ hypopigmentation, benign facial lentigines: Adolescents ≥17 years: Topical: Avage: Apply a pea-sized amount once daily at bedtime; lightly cover entire face including eyelids if desired

Adults:

Acne vulgaris: Topical: Tazorac (0.1% cream or gel): Apply as a thin film (2 mg/cm^2) to affected areas once daily in the evening for up to 12 weeks

Psoriasis: Topical:

Cream: Tazorac (0.05%): Initial: Apply a thin film (2 mg/cm^2) to affected area once daily in the evening; may increase strength to 0.1% if tolerated and necessary

Gel: Tazorac (0.05%): Initial: Apply a thin film (2 mg/cm^2) to affected area once daily in the evening for up to 12 months; may increase strength to 0.1% if tolerated and necessary; apply to no more than 20% of the body surface area

Palliation of fine facial wrinkles, facial mottled hyper-/ hypopigmentation, benign facial lentigines: Topical: Avage: Apply a pea-sized amount once daily at bedtime; lightly cover entire face including eyelids if desired

Dosing adjustment in renal impairment: There are no dosage adjustments provided in the manufacturer's labeling; however, dosage adjustment unlikely necessary due to low systemic absorption.

Dosing adjustment in hepatic impairment: There are no dosage adjustments provided in the manufacturer's labeling; however, dosage adjustment unlikely necessary due to low systemic absorption.

Administration For external use only; avoid contact with eyes and mouth; also avoid contact with the eyelids when used for acne or psoriasis. Do not apply to eczematous or sunburned skin.

Acne: Apply in evening after gently cleansing and drying face; apply enough to cover entire affected area.

Palliation of fine facial wrinkles, facial mottled hyper-/ hypopigmentation, benign facial lentigines: Apply to clean, dry face at bedtime; lightly cover entire face including eyelids if desired. Emollients or moisturizers may be applied before or after; if applied before tazarotene, ensure cream or lotion has absorbed into the skin and has dried completely.

Psoriasis: Apply in evening. If a bath or shower is taken prior to application, dry the skin before applying. If emollients are used, apply them at least 1 hour prior to application. Unaffected skin may be more susceptible to irritation; avoid application to these areas.

Monitoring Parameters Disease severity in plaque psoriasis (reduction in erythema, scaling, induration); pregnancy test prior to treatment of females of childbearing age

Dosage Forms Excipient information presented when available (limited, particularly for generics); consult specific product labeling.

Cream, External:

Avage: 0.1% (30 g) [contains benzyl alcohol]

Tazorac: 0.05% (30 g, 60 g); 0.1% (30 g, 60 g) [contains benzyl alcohol]

Foam, External:

Fabior: 0.1% (50 g, 100 g)

Gel, External:

Tazorac: 0.05% (30 g, 100 g); 0.1% (30 g, 100 g) [contains benzyl alcohol]

◆ **Tazicef** see CefTAZidime on page 413

◆ **Tazobactam and Piperacillin** see Piperacillin and Tazobactam on page 1679

◆ **Tazocin (Can)** see Piperacillin and Tazobactam on page 1679

◆ **Tazorac** see Tazarotene on page 1971

◆ **Taztia XT** see Diltiazem on page 667

◆ **Tbo-Filgrastim** see Filgrastim on page 872

◆ **3TC** see LamiVUDine on page 1194

◆ **3TC, Abacavir, and Zidovudine** see Abacavir, Lamivudine, and Zidovudine on page 41

◆ **T-Cell Growth Factor** see Aldesleukin on page 90

◆ **TCGF** see Aldesleukin on page 90

◆ **TCN** see Tetracycline on page 1996

◆ **Td** see Diphtheria and Tetanus Toxoids on page 679

◆ **Td Adsorbed (Can)** see Diphtheria and Tetanus Toxoids on page 679

◆ **Tdap** see Diphtheria and Tetanus Toxoids, and Acellular Pertussis Vaccine on page 686

◆ **TDF** see Tenofovir on page 1977

◆ **Teardrops® (Can)** see Artificial Tears on page 205

◆ **Tears Again® [OTC]** see Artificial Tears on page 205

◆ **Tears Naturale® II [OTC]** see Artificial Tears on page 205

◆ **Tears Naturale® Forte [OTC]** see Artificial Tears on page 205

◆ **Tears Naturale® Free [OTC]** see Artificial Tears on page 205

◆ **Tears Renewed® [OTC]** see Ocular Lubricant on page 1521

◆ **Tebrazid™ (Can)** see Pyrazinamide on page 1775

◆ **Tecnu First Aid [OTC]** see Lidocaine (Topical) on page 1242

◆ **Tecta (Can)** see Pantoprazole on page 1595

◆ **Tegaderm CHG Dressing [OTC]** see Chlorhexidine Gluconate on page 441

◆ **TEGretol** see CarBAMazepine on page 372

◆ **Tegretol (Can)** see CarBAMazepine on page 372

◆ **TEGretol-XR** see CarBAMazepine on page 372

◆ **Telzir® (Can)** see Fosamprenavir on page 931

◆ **Temodal (Can)** see Temozolomide on page 1972

◆ **Temodar** see Temozolomide on page 1972

◆ **Temovate** see Clobetasol on page 506

◆ **Temovate E** see Clobetasol on page 506

Temozolomide (te moe ZOE loe mide)

Medication Safety Issues

Sound-alike/look-alike issues:

Temodar may be confused with Tambocor

Temozolomide may be confused with temsirolimus

High alert medication:

This medication is in a class the Institute for Safe Medication Practices (ISMP) includes among its list of drug classes which have a heightened risk of causing significant patient harm when used in error.

Related Information

Emetogenic Potential of Antineoplastic Agents in Children *on page 2327*

Oral Medications That Should Not Be Crushed or Altered *on page 2438*

Safe Handling of Hazardous Drugs *on page 2419*

Brand Names: U.S. Temodar

Brand Names: Canada Ahi-Temozolomide Capsules; Co-Temozolomide; Temodal

Therapeutic Category Antineoplastic Agent, Alkylating Agent

Generic Availability (U.S.) May be product dependent

Use Treatment of refractory anaplastic astrocytoma with progression after initial therapy with a nitrosourea and procarbazine (FDA approved in adults); treatment of newly-diagnosed glioblastoma multiforme (initially in combination with radiotherapy, then as maintenance treatment) (FDA approved in adults)

Active against recurrent glioblastoma multiforme, low-grade astrocytoma, low-grade oligodendroglioma, metastatic CNS lesions, refractory primary CNS lymphoma, anaplastic oligodendroglioma, primitive neuroectodermal tumors (PNET), including medulloblastoma, pediatric neuroblastoma, advanced or metastatic melanoma, cutaneous T-cell lymphomas [mycosis fungoides (MF) and Sezary Syndrome (SS)], carcinoid tumors, advanced neuroendocrine tumors (carcinoid or islet cell), Ewing's sarcoma (recurrent or progressive), soft tissue sarcomas (extremity/retroperitoneal/intra-abdominal or hemangiopericytoma/solitary fibrous tumor)

Pregnancy Risk Factor D

Pregnancy Considerations Adverse events were observed in animal reproduction studies. May cause fetal harm when administered to pregnant women. Male and female patients should avoid pregnancy while receiving temozolomide.

Breast-Feeding Considerations It is not known if temozolomide is excreted in breast milk. Due to the potential for serious adverse reactions in the nursing infant, a decision should be made to discontinue nursing or to discontinue temozolomide, taking into account the importance of treatment to the mother.

Contraindications Hypersensitivity to temozolomide, dacarbazine, or any component

Warnings Hazardous agent; use appropriate precautions for handling and disposal (NIOSH, 2012). Thrombocytopenia and neutropenia are dose-limiting toxicities which occur late in the treatment cycle and usually resolve within 14 days; prior to therapy initiation patients must have an absolute neutrophil count (ANC) ≥1.5 x 10^9/L and a platelet count ≥100 x 10^9/L; obtain a CBC on day 22 and weekly until the ANC >1.5 x 10^9/L and platelet count >100 x 10^9/L. Prolonged pancytopenia resulting in aplastic anemia has been reported; concurrent use of temozolomide with medications associated with aplastic anemia (eg, carbamazepine, sulfamethoxazole and trimethoprim, phenytoin) may obscure assessment for development of aplastic anemia. *Pneumocystis jirovecii* pneumonia (PCP) may occur; risk is increased in those patients receiving steroids or longer dosing regimens; PCP prophylaxis is required in patients receiving radiotherapy in combination with the 42-day temozolomide regimen. Rare cases of myelodysplastic syndrome and secondary malignancies, including myeloid leukemia, have been reported. May cause fetal harm; pregnancy should be avoided during therapy. Injection contains polysorbate 80 (Tween 80®) which may cause allergic reactions in susceptible individuals. In premature neonates, thrombocytopenia, ascites, pulmonary deterioration, and renal and hepatic failure have been reported after receiving parenteral products containing polysorbate 80 (Alade, 1986; CDC, 1984). Infusion of polysorbate 80-containing solutions through polyvinyl chloride tubing may cause DEHP to leach into the solution; in immature animals, exposure to DEHP may adversely affect the development of the male reproductive tract.

Precautions Use with caution in patients with severe renal or hepatic impairment.

Adverse Reactions Note: With CNS malignancies, it may be difficult to distinguish between CNS adverse events caused by temozolomide versus the effects of progressive disease.

Cardiovascular: Peripheral edema

Central nervous system: Amnesia, anxiety, ataxia, confusion, coordination abnormality, depression, dizziness, fatigue, fever, headache, hemiparesis, insomnia, memory impairment, paresis, seizure, somnolence

Dermatologic: Alopecia, dry skin, erythema, pruritus, radiation injury (maintenance phase after radiotherapy), rash

Endocrine & metabolic: Breast pain, hypercorticism

Gastrointestinal: Abdominal pain, anorexia, constipation, diarrhea, dysphagia, nausea, stomatitis, taste perversion, vomiting, weight gain

Genitourinary: Incontinence, urinary tract infection, urinary frequency

Hematologic: Anemia, leukopenia, lymphopenia, neutropenia, thrombocytopenia

Neuromuscular & skeletal: Abnormal gait, arthralgia, back pain, myalgia, paresthesia, weakness

Ocular: Blurred vision, diplopia, vision abnormality (visual deficit/vision changes)

Respiratory: Cough, dyspnea, pharyngitis, sinusitis, upper respiratory tract infection

Miscellaneous: Allergic reaction, viral infection

Rare but important or life-threatening: Alkaline phosphatase increased, alveolitis, anaphylaxis, aplastic anemia, cholestasis, emotional lability, erythema multiforme, febrile neutropenia, flu-like syndrome, hallucination, hematoma, hemorrhage, hepatitis, hepatotoxicity, herpes simplex, herpes zoster, hyperbilirubinemia, hyperglycemia, hypokalemia, injection site reactions (erythema, irritation, pain, pruritus, swelling, warmth), interstitial pneumonia/pneumonitis, myelodysplastic syndrome, opportunistic infection (eg, PCP), oral candidiasis, pancytopenia (may be prolonged), peripheral neuropathy, petechiae, pneumonitis, pulmonary fibrosis, secondary malignancies (including myeloid leukemia), Stevens-Johnson syndrome, toxic epidermal necrolysis, transaminases increased

Drug Interactions

Metabolism/Transport Effects None known.

Avoid Concomitant Use

Avoid concomitant use of Temozolomide with any of the following: BCG; CloZAPine; Dipyrone; Natalizumab; Pimecrolimus; Tacrolimus (Topical); Tofacitinib; Vaccines (Live)

Increased Effect/Toxicity

Temozolomide may increase the levels/effects of: CloZAPine; Leflunomide; Natalizumab; Tofacitinib; Vaccines (Live)

The levels/effects of Temozolomide may be increased by: Denosumab; Dipyrone; Pimecrolimus; Roflumilast; Tacrolimus (Topical); Trastuzumab; Valproic Acid and Derivatives

Decreased Effect

Temozolomide may decrease the levels/effects of: BCG; Coccidioidin Skin Test; Sipuleucel-T; Vaccines (Inactivated); Vaccines (Live)

The levels/effects of Temozolomide may be decreased by: Echinacea

Food Interactions Food reduces rate and extent of absorption. Management: Administer consistently either with food or without food (was administered in studies under fasting and nonfasting conditions).

Stability Hazardous agent; use appropriate precautions for handling and disposal (NIOSH, 2012).

Capsules: Store at 25°C (77°F); excursions permitted to 15°C to 30°C (59°F to 86°F).

Injection: Refrigerate intact vials for injection at 2°C to 8°C (36°F to 46°F). Reconstituted vials may be stored for up to 14 hours at room temperature (25°C or 77°F). Infusion must be completed within 14 hours of reconstitution.

Mechanism of Action Temozolomide is a prodrug which is rapidly and nonenzymatically converted to the active alkylating metabolite MTIC [(methyl-triazene-1-yl)-imidazole-4-carboxamide]; this conversion is spontaneous, nonenzymatic, and occurs under physiologic conditions in all tissues to which it distributes. The cytotoxic effects of MTIC are manifested through alkylation (methylation) of DNA at the O^6, N^7 guanine positions which lead to DNA double strand breaks and apoptosis. Non-cell cycle specific.

Pharmacokinetics (Adult data unless noted)

Absorption: Oral: Rapidly and completely absorbed

Distribution: Extensive tissue distribution; crosses the blood brain barrier; V_d: 0.4 L/kg

Protein binding: 14%

Bioavailability: Oral: 100% (on a mg-per-mg basis, I.V. temozolomide, infused over 90 minutes, is bioequivalent to an oral dose)

Metabolism: At a neutral or alkaline pH, hydrolyzes to active MTIC (3-methyl-(triazen-1-yl) imidazole-4-carboxamide) and temozolomide acid metabolite; MTIC is further metabolized to 5-amino-imidazole-4-carboxamide (AIC) and methylhydrazine (active alkylating agent); CYP isoenzymes play only a minor role in metabolism (of temozolomide and MTIC)

Half-life:

Children: 1.7 hours

Adults: 1.6-1.8 hours

Time to peak serum concentration: Oral: 1 hour; 2.3 hours after high fat meal

Elimination: <1% excreted in feces; 5% to 7% of unchanged temozolomide excreted renally

Clearance: 5.5 L/hour/m²; women have a ~5% lower clearance than men (adjusted for body surface area); children 3-17 years have similar temozolomide clearance as adults

Dosing: Usual Oral, I.V. (refer to individual protocols):

Infants, Children, and Adolescents: Limited data available; further studies are needed:

Neuroblastoma, relapsed or refractory: Infants, Children, and Adolescents: Oral: 100 mg/m²/dose once daily for 5 days, repeat cycle every 21 days for up to 6 cycles; use in combination with irinotecan; administer 1 hour prior to irinotecan (Bagatell, 2011). **Note:** Temozolomide doses were rounded to the nearest capsule size.

Ewing's sarcoma, recurrent or progressive: Children ≥2 years and Adolescents: Oral: 100 mg/m²/dose once daily for 5 days, repeat cycle every 21 days (in combination with irinotecan; administer 1 hour prior to irinotecan) (Casey, 2009); dosing based on a retrospective review

Solid tumors, relapsed or refractory [including but not limited to brain tumor (astrocytomas, gliomas, medulloblastoma), neuroblastoma, and sarcomas]: Infants, Children, and Adolescents: Oral:

Manufacturer's labeling: Children ≥3 years and Adolescents: 160-200 mg/m²/dose once daily for 5 days every 28 days

Alternative dosing: 200-215 mg/m²/dose days 1-5 every 21-28 days; dose was decreased to 180 mg/m²/dose for patients who received prior craniospinal irradiation or relapsed after bone marrow transplant (De Sio, 2006; Nicholson, 2007)

Adults:

Anaplastic astrocytoma, refractory: Initial dose: 150 mg/m²/dose once daily for 5 days; repeat every 28 days. Subsequent doses of 100-200 mg/m²/dose once daily for 5 days per treatment cycle; based upon hematologic tolerance

Dosage modification for toxicity:

ANC <1000/mm³ or platelets <50,000/mm³ on day 22 or day 29 (day 1 of next cycle): Postpone therapy until ANC >1500/mm³ and platelets >100,000/mm³; reduce dose by 50 mg/m²/dose for subsequent cycle

ANC 1000-1500/mm³ or platelets 50,000-100,000/mm³ on day 22 or day 29 (day 1 of next cycle): Postpone therapy until ANC >1500/mm³ and platelets >100,000/mm³; maintain initial dose

ANC ≥1500/mm³ and platelets ≥100,000/mm³ on day 22 or day 29 (day 1 of next cycle): Increase dose to or maintain dose at 200 mg/m²/dose for 5 days for subsequent cycle

Glioblastoma multiforme (newly diagnosed, high-grade glioma):

Concomitant phase: 75 mg/m²/dose once daily for 42 days with focal radiotherapy (60 Gy administered in 30 fractions). **Note:** PCP prophylaxis is required during concomitant phase and should continue in patients who develop lymphocytopenia until lymphocyte recovery to ≤grade 1. Obtain weekly CBC.

Continue at 75 mg/m²/dose once daily throughout the 42-day concomitant phase (up to 49 days) as long as ANC ≥1500/mm³, platelet count ≥100,000/mm³, and nonhematologic toxicity ≤grade 1 (excludes alopecia, nausea/vomiting)

Dosage modification for toxicity:

ANC ≥500/mm³ but <1500/mm³ or platelet count ≥10,000/mm³ but <100,000/mm³ or grade 2 nonhematologic toxicity (excludes alopecia, nausea/vomiting): Interrupt therapy

ANC <500/mm³ or platelet count <10,000/mm³ or grade 3/4 nonhematologic toxicity (excludes alopecia, nausea/vomiting): Discontinue therapy

Maintenance phase (consists of 6 treatment cycles): Begin 4 weeks after concomitant phase completion **Note:** Each subsequent cycle is 28 days (consisting of 5 days of drug treatment followed by 23 days without treatment). Draw CBC within 48 hours of day 22; hold next cycle and do weekly CBC until ANC >1500/mm³ and platelet count >100,000/mm³; dosing modification should be based on lowest blood counts and worst nonhematologic toxicity during the previous cycle.

Cycle 1: 150 mg/m²/dose once daily for 5 days; repeat every 28 days

Cycles 2-6: May increase to 200 mg/m²/dose once daily for 5 days every 28 days [if ANC ≥1500/mm³, platelets ≥100,000/mm³, and nonhematologic toxicities for cycle 1 are ≤grade 2 (excludes alopecia, nausea/vomiting)]; **Note:** If dose was not escalated at the onset of cycle 2, do not increase for cycles 3-6

Dosage modification (during maintenance phase) for toxicity:

ANC <1000/mm³, platelet count <50,000/mm³, or grade 3 nonhematologic toxicity (excludes alopecia, nausea/vomiting) during previous cycle: Decrease dose by 1 dose level (50 mg/m²/dose for 5 days), unless dose has already been lowered to 100 mg/m²/dose, then discontinue therapy.

If dose reduction <100 mg/m²/dose is required or grade 4 nonhematologic toxicity (excludes alopecia, nausea/vomiting), or if the same grade 3 nonhematologic toxicity occurs after dose reduction: Discontinue therapy.

Dosage adjustment in renal impairment: Adults: Oral: CrCl ≥36 mL/minute/m²: No effect on temozolomide clearance was demonstrated

Severe renal impairment (CrCl <36 mL/minute/m²): Use with caution; no dosage adjustments provided in manufacturers labeling

Dialysis patients: Use has not been studied

Dosage adjustment in hepatic impairment: Adults: Severe hepatic impairment: Use with caution; no dosage adjustments provided in manufacturer's labeling

Administration Hazardous agent; use appropriate precautions for handling and disposal (NIOSH, 2012). Standard antiemetics may be administered if needed.

Oral: Swallow capsule intact with a glass of water; do not chew; if patient is unable to swallow capsule, open capsule and dissolve in apple juice or applesauce taking precautions to avoid exposure to the cytotoxic agent; administer on an empty stomach or at bedtime to reduce the incidence of nausea and vomiting; absorption is affected by food; may administer with food as long as food intake and administration are performed at the same time each day to ensure consistent bioavailability. Do not repeat if vomiting occurs after dose is administered; wait until the next scheduled dose.

Parenteral: I.V.: Bring to room temperature prior to reconstitution. Reconstitute each 100 mg vial with 41 mL sterile water for injection to a final concentration of 2.5 mg/mL. Swirl gently; do not shake. Place dose without further dilution into an empty sterile polyvinyl chloride infusion bag. Infuse over 90 minutes. Infusion must be completed within 14 hours of reconstitution. Flush line before and after administration; may be administered through the same I.V. line as NS. Do not administer other medications through the same I.V. line.

Monitoring Parameters CBC with ANC (absolute neutrophil count) and platelet count; monitor for CNS effects, gastrointestinal disturbance, myelosuppression, opportunistic infection, vision disturbance, and cough on a regular basis; dosage adjustments may be necessary for toxicity.

Additional Information To minimize the risk of a wrong dose error, each strength of temozolomide must be packaged and dispensed in a separate vial or in its original glass bottle. Label each container with the appropriate number of capsules to be taken each day.

Increased MGMT (O-6-methylguanine-DNA methyltransferase) activity/levels within tumor tissue is associated with temozolomide resistance. Glioblastoma patients with decreased levels (due to methylated MGMT promoter) may be more likely to benefit from the combination of radiation therapy and temozolomide (Hegi, 2008; Stupp, 2009). Determination of MGMT status may be predictive for response to alkylating agents.

Dosage Forms Excipient information presented when available (limited, particularly for generics); consult specific product labeling.

Capsule, Oral:

Temodar: 5 mg [contains fd&c blue #2 (indigotine)]

Temodar: 20 mg, 100 mg

Temodar: 140 mg [contains fd&c blue #2 (indigotine)]

Temodar: 180 mg, 250 mg

Generic: 5 mg, 20 mg, 100 mg, 140 mg, 180 mg, 250 mg

Solution Reconstituted, Intravenous:

Temodar: 100 mg (1 ea) [pyrogen free; contains polysorbate 80]

Extemporaneous Preparations Hazardous agent: Use appropriate precautions for handling and disposal.

A 10 mg/mL temozolomide oral suspension may be compounded in a vertical flow hood. Mix the contents of ten 100 mg capsules and 500 mg of povidone K-30 powder in a glass mortar; add 25 mg anhydrous citric acid dissolved in 1.5 mL purified water and mix to a uniform paste; mix

while adding 50 mL Ora-Plus® in incremental proportions. Transfer to an amber plastic bottle, rinse mortar 4 times with small portions of either Ora-Sweet® or Ora-Sweet® SF, and add quantity of Ora-Sweet® or Ora-Sweet® SF sufficient to make 100 mL. Store in plastic amber prescription bottles; label "shake well" and "refrigerate"; include the beyond-use date. Stable for 7 days at room temperature or 60 days refrigerated (preferred).

Trissel LA, Yanping Z, and Koontz SE, "Temozolomide Stability in Extemporaneously Compounded Oral Suspension," *Int J Pharm Compound*, 2006, 10(5):396-9.

References

Alade SL, Brown RE, and Paquet A Jr, "Polysorbate 80 and E-Ferol Toxicity," *Pediatrics*, 1986, 77(4):593-7.

Bagatell R, London WB, Wagner LM, "Phase II Study of Irinotecan and Temozolomide in Children With Relapsed or Refractory Neuroblastoma: A Children's Oncology Group Study," *J Clin Oncol*, 2011, 29 (2):208-13.

Bagatell R, Wagner LM, Cohn SL, et al, "Irinotecan Plus Temozolomide in Children With Recurrent or Refractory Neuroblastoma: A Phase II Children's Oncology Group Study," *J Clin Oncol*, 2009, 27(15S) (abstract).

Casey DA, Wexler LH, Merchant MS, et al, "Irinotecan and Temozolomide for Ewing Sarcoma: The Memorial Sloan-Kettering Experience," *Pediatr Blood Cancer*, 2009, 53(6):1029-34.

Centers for Disease Control (CDC), "Unusual Syndrome With Fatalities Among Premature Infants: Association With a New Intravenous Vitamin E Product," *MMWR Morb Mortal Wkly Rep*, 1984, 33 (14):198-9.

De Sio L, Milano GM, Castellano A, et al, "Temozolomide in Resistant or Relapsed Pediatric Solid Tumors," *Pediatr Blood Cancer*, 2006, 47 (1):30-6.

Esteller M, Garcia-Foncillas J, Andion E, et al, "Inactivation of the DNA-Repair Gene MGMT and the Clinical Response of Gliomas to Alkylating Agents," *N Engl J Med*, 2000, 343(19):1350-4.

Hegi ME, Diserens AC, Gorlia T, et al, "MGMT Gene Silencing and Benefit From Temozolomide in Glioblastoma," *N Engl J Med*, 2005, 352(10):997-1003.

Hegi ME, Liu L, Herman JG, et al, "Correlation of O6-Methylguanine Methyltransferase (MGMT) Promoter Methylation With Clinical Outcomes in Glioblastoma and Clinical Strategies to Modulate MGMT Activity," *J Clin Oncol*, 2008, 26(25):4189-99.

Horton TM, Thompson PA, Berg SL, et al, "Phase I Pharmacokinetic and Pharmacodynamic Study of Temozolomide in Pediatric Patients With Refractory or Recurrent Leukemia: A Children's Oncology Group Study," *J Clin Oncol*, 2007, 25(31):4922-8.

Loh KC, Willert J, Meltzer H, et al, "Temozolomide and Radiation for Aggressive Pediatric Central Nervous System Malignancies," *J Pediatr Hematol Oncol*, 2005, 27(5):254-8.

Marchesi F, Turriziani M, Tortorelli G, et al, "Triazene Compounds: Mechanism of Action and Related DNA Repair Systems," *Pharmacol Res*, 2007, 56(4):275-87.

National Comprehensive Cancer Network® (NCCN), "Clinical Practice Guidelines in Oncology™: Central Nervous System Cancers," Version 2.2011. Available at http://www.nccn.org/professionals/physician_gls/PDF/cns.pdf

National Comprehensive Cancer Network® (NCCN), "Clinical Practice Guidelines in Oncology™: Non-Hodgkin's Lymphomas," Version 3.2011. Available at http://www.nccn.org/professionals/physician_gls/PDF/nhl.pdf

National Institute for Occupational Safety and Health (NIOSH), "NIOSH List of Antineoplastic and Other Hazardous Drugs in Healthcare Settings 2012." Available at http://www.cdc.gov/niosh/docs/2012-150/pdfs/2012-150.pdf. Accessed January 21, 2013.

Nicholson HS, Kretschmar CS, Krailo M, et al, "Phase 2 Study of Temozolomide in Children and Adolescents With Recurrent Central Nervous System Tumors: A Report From the Children's Oncology Group," *Cancer*, 2007, 110(7):1542-50.

Nicholson HS, Krailo M, Ames MM, et al, "Phase I Study of Temozolomide in Children and Adolescents With Recurrent Solid Tumors: A Report From the Children's Cancer Group," *J Clin Oncol*, 1998, 16 (9):3037-43.

Stupp R, Hegi ME, Mason WP, et al, "Effects of Radiotherapy With Concomitant and Adjuvant Temozolomide Versus Radiotherapy Alone on Survival in Glioblastoma in a Randomised Phase III Study: 5-Year Analysis of the EORTC-NCIC Trial," *Lancet Oncol*, 2009, 10 (5):459-66.

Villano JL, Seery TE, and Bressler LR, "Temozolomide in Malignant Gliomas: Current Use and Future Targets," *Cancer Chemother Pharmacol*, 2009, 64(4):647-55.

◆ **Tempra (Can)** see Acetaminophen on page 47

◆ **Tenex** see GuanFACINE on page 989

Teniposide (ten i POE side)

Medication Safety Issues
Sound-alike/look-alike issues:
Teniposide may be confused with etoposide
High alert medication:
This medication is in a class the Institute for Safe Medication Practices (ISMP) includes among its list of drug classes which have a heightened risk of causing significant patient harm when used in error.

Related Information
Emetogenic Potential of Antineoplastic Agents in Children on page 2327
Management of Drug Extravasations on page 2255
Safe Handling of Hazardous Drugs on page 2419

Brand Names: Canada Vumon®

Therapeutic Category Antineoplastic Agent, Podophyllotoxin Derivative; Antineoplastic Agent, Topoisomerase II Inhibitor

Generic Availability (U.S.) Yes

Use Treatment of childhood acute lymphoblastic leukemia (ALL) refractory to induction with other therapy (FDA approved in pediatric patients ages ≥6 months)

Pregnancy Risk Factor D

Pregnancy Considerations Adverse effects were observed in animal reproduction studies. May cause fetal harm if administered during pregnancy. Women of childbearing potential should avoid becoming pregnant during teniposide treatment.

Breast-Feeding Considerations It is not known if teniposide is excreted in breast milk. Due to the potential for serious adverse reactions in the nursing infant, the decision to discontinue teniposide or to discontinue breastfeeding should take into account the benefits of treatment to the mother.

Contraindications Hypersensitivity to teniposide, polyoxyethylated castor oil (Cremophor® EL), or any component

Warnings Hazardous agent; use appropriate precautions for handling and disposal (NIOSH, 2012). Severe, dose-related myelosuppression with resulting infection or bleeding may occur **[U.S. Boxed Warning]**; monitor for infection and bleeding. Patients with Down syndrome and leukemia may be more sensitive to the myelosuppressive effects; reduced initial doses are recommended.

Hypersensitivity reactions, including anaphylaxis-like reactions, have been reported **[U.S. Boxed Warning]**; hypersensitivity reactions may include bronchospasm, dyspnea, hypertension, hypotension, tachycardia, flushing, chills, fever, or urticaria. Monitor closely during infusion; observe continuously for first 60 minutes, frequently thereafter. Stop infusion for signs of anaphylaxis; immediate treatment for anaphylactic reaction should be available during administration; may require treatment with epinephrine, corticosteroids, antihistamines, pressors, or volume expanders. Patients experiencing prior hypersensitivity are at risk for recurrence; retreat only if the potential benefit outweighs the risk of hypersensitivity; premedication (with corticosteroids and antihistamines) is recommended for retreatment.

Hypotension may occur with rapid infusion; infuse slowly over at least 30-60 minutes; discontinue for clinically significant hypotension. If infusion is restarted after being withheld for hypotension, reinitiate at a slower infusion rate. Acute CNS depression, hypotension, and metabolic acidosis have been reported; these events occurred in patients who received high-dose teniposide (investigational protocol) and were premedicated with antiemetics, which along with the alcohol content of teniposide, may have contributed to the depression. Neurotoxicity and severe neuropathy have been reported when teniposide is used in combination with vincristine.

Teniposide injection contains benzyl alcohol which may cause allergic reactions in susceptible individuals; large amounts of benzyl alcohol (≥99 mg/kg/day) have been associated with a potentially fatal toxicity ("gasping syndrome") in neonates; use teniposide injection with caution in neonates. The injection contains polyoxyl 35 castor oil (Cremophor® EL) which may be associated with hypotension and hypersensitivity reactions. Teniposide formulation contains ~43% alcohol and may contribute to adverse effects such as CNS depression, somnolence, lethargy, hypotension, and metabolic acidosis.

Teniposide may cause local tissue necrosis or thrombophlebitis if extravasation occurs. Teniposide is a potential carcinogen; may cause fetal harm when administered to pregnant women; may induce a secondary leukemia.

Precautions Use with caution in patients with renal or hepatic impairment; may require dosage reduction in patients with significant impairment. Use with caution in patients with hypoalbuminemia; teniposide is highly bound to albumin plasma protein. Should be administered under the supervision of an experienced cancer chemotherapy physician **[U.S. Boxed Warning]**.

Adverse Reactions
Cardiovascular: Hypotension (associated with rapid [<30 minutes] infusions)

Central nervous system: Fever

Dermatologic: Alopecia (usually reversible), rash

Gastrointestinal: Diarrhea, mucositis, nausea/vomiting (mild to moderate)

Hematologic: Anemia, leukopenia, myelosuppression, neutropenia, thrombocytopenia

Hematologic: Bleeding

Miscellaneous: Hypersensitivity reactions (includes bronchospasm, chills, dyspnea, fever, flushing, hyper-/hypotension, tachycardia, or urticaria); infection

Rare but important or life-threatening: Arrhythmia, CNS depression, confusion, headache, hepatic dysfunction, intractable hypotension, metabolic abnormality, metabolic acidosis, neuropathy (severe), neurotoxicity, renal dysfunction, thrombophlebitis, tissue necrosis (upon extravasation), weakness

Drug Interactions
Metabolism/Transport Effects Substrate of CYP3A4 (major), P-glycoprotein; **Note:** Assignment of Major/Minor substrate status based on clinically relevant drug interaction potential; **Inhibits** CYP2C9 (weak), CYP3A4 (weak)

Avoid Concomitant Use
Avoid concomitant use of Teniposide with any of the following: BCG; CloZAPine; Conivaptan; Dipyrone; Fusidic Acid (Systemic); Natalizumab; Pimecrolimus; Pimozide; Tacrolimus (Topical); Tofacitinib; Vaccines (Live)

Increased Effect/Toxicity
Teniposide may increase the levels/effects of: ARIPiprazole; CloZAPine; Dofetilide; Leflunomide; Lomitapide; Natalizumab; Pimozide; Tofacitinib; Vaccines (Live); VinCRIStine; VinCRIStine (Liposomal)

The levels/effects of Teniposide may be increased by: Ceritinib; Conivaptan; CYP3A4 Inhibitors (Moderate); CYP3A4 Inhibitors (Strong); Dasatinib; Denosumab; Dipyrone; Fusidic Acid (Systemic); Ivacaftor; Luliconazole; Mifepristone; P-glycoprotein/ABCB1 Inhibitors; Pimecrolimus; Roflumilast; Simeprevir; Stiripentol; Tacrolimus (Topical); Trastuzumab

Decreased Effect

Teniposide may decrease the levels/effects of: BCG; Coccidioidin Skin Test; Sipuleucel-T; Vaccines (Inactivated); Vaccines (Live)

The levels/effects of Teniposide may be decreased by: Barbiturates; Bosentan; CYP3A4 Inducers (Strong); Dabrafenib; Deferasirox; Echinacea; Fosphenytoin; Mitotane; P-glycoprotein/ABCB1 Inducers; Phenytoin; Siltuximab; St Johns Wort; Tocilizumab

Stability Hazardous agent; use appropriate precautions for handling and disposal (NIOSH, 2012). Store ampuls at 2°C to 8°C (36°F to 46°F). Protect from light. Solutions diluted in D_5W or NS for infusion to a concentration of 0.1-0.4 mg/mL are stable at room temperature for up to 24 hours after preparation; solutions diluted to 1 mg/mL should be used within 4 hours of preparation. Refrigeration of diluted solutions is not recommended. Because precipitation may occur at any concentration, the manufacturer recommends administrating as soon as possible after preparation. In order to prevent extraction of the plasticizer DEHP, **solutions should be prepared in non-DEHP-containing containers, such as glass or polyolefin containers.** The use of polyvinyl chloride containers is not recommended.

Mechanism of Action Teniposide does not inhibit microtubular assembly; it has been shown to delay transit of cells through the S phase and arrest cells in late S or early G_2 phase, preventing cells from entering mitosis. Teniposide is a topoisomerase II inhibitor, and appears to cause DNA strand breaks by inhibition of strand-passing and DNA ligase action.

Pharmacokinetics (Adult data unless noted)

Distribution: Mainly into liver, kidneys, small intestine, and adrenals; limited distribution into CSF <1%

Children: V_d: 3-11 L/m²

Adults: V_d: 8-44 L/m²

Protein binding: >99%; primarily albumin

Metabolism: Hepatic, extensive

Half-life: Children: 5 hours

Elimination: Urine (44%, 4% to 12% as unchanged drug); feces (≤10%)

Clearance: Renal: 10% of total body clearance

Dosing: Usual Note: Patients with Down syndrome may be more sensitive to the myelosuppressive effects; administer the first course at half the usual dose and adjust dose in subsequent cycles upward based on degree of toxicities (myelosuppression and mucositis) in the previous course(s).

Infants ≥6 months, Children, and Adolescents: **Acute lymphoblastic leukemia (ALL; combination therapy):**

Manufacturer's labeling: Regimens may vary: I.V.: 165 mg/m² twice weekly for 8-9 doses or 250 mg/m² weekly for 4-8 weeks

Alternate dosing: I.V.: 165 mg/m²/dose days 1 and 2 of weeks 3, 13, and 23 (Lauer, 2001)

Dosing adjustment in renal or hepatic impairment: No specific recommendation (insufficient data). Dose adjustments may be necessary in patient with significant renal or hepatic impairment.

Administration Hazardous agent; use appropriate precautions for handling and disposal (NIOSH, 2012).

Parenteral: I.V. infusion: Further dilute with either D_5W or NS to a final concentration of 0.1, 0.2, 0.4, or 1 mg/mL. Precipitation may occur at any concentration; inspect closely for particulates and administer as soon as possible after preparation. Administer slowly by I.V. infusion over at least 30-60 minutes to minimize the risk of hypotensive reactions; do not administer by rapid I.V. Administer through non-DEHP-containing administration sets; flush infusion line with D_5W or NS before and after infusion; incompatible with heparin. Observe patient continuously for at least the first 60 minutes of infusion,

observe frequently thereafter. Stop infusion and treat accordingly for signs of anaphylaxis or clinically significant hypotension; if infusion is restarted after being withheld for hypotension, reinitiate at a slower infusion rate.

Vesicant/Extravasation Risk Irritant

Monitoring Parameters CBC, platelet count, renal and hepatic function tests; blood pressure; monitor for hypersensitivity reaction (observe continuously for first 60 minutes of infusion, frequently thereafter)

Dosage Forms Excipient information presented when available (limited, particularly for generics); consult specific product labeling.

Solution, Intravenous:

Generic: 10 mg/mL (5 mL)

References

Clark PI and Slevin ML, "The Clinical Pharmacology of Etoposide and Teniposide," *Clin Pharmacokinet*, 1987, 12(4):223-52.

Lauer SJ, Shuster JJ, Mahoney DH Jr, et al, "A Comparison of Early Intensive Methotrexate/Mercaptopurine With Early Intensive Alternating Combination Chemotherapy for High-Risk B-Precursor Acute Lymphoblastic Leukemia: A Pediatric Oncology Group Phase III Randomized Trial," *Leukemia*, 2001, 15(7):1038-45.

National Institute for Occupational Safety and Health (NIOSH), "NIOSH List of Antineoplastic and Other Hazardous Drugs in Healthcare Settings 2012." Available at http://www.cdc.gov/niosh/docs/ 2012-150/pdfs/2012-150.pdf. Accessed January 21, 2013.

Sinkule JA, Stewart CF, Crom WR, et al, "Teniposide (VM26) Disposition in Children With Leukemia," *Cancer Res*, 1984, 44(3):1235-7.

◆ **Tenivac** *see* Diphtheria and Tetanus Toxoids *on page* 679

Tenofovir (ten OF oh vir)

Related Information

Adult and Adolescent HIV *on page* 2348

Pediatric HIV *on page* 2338

Perinatal HIV *on page* 2356

Brand Names: U.S. Viread

Brand Names: Canada Viread

Therapeutic Category Antiretroviral Agent; HIV Agents (Anti-HIV Agents); Nucleotide Reverse Transcriptase Inhibitor (NRTI)

Generic Availability (U.S.) No

Use Treatment of HIV-1 infection in combination with other antiretroviral agents (FDA approved in ages ≥2 years and adults); **Note:** HIV regimens consisting of three antiretroviral agents are strongly recommended; treatment of chronic hepatitis B virus (HBV) (FDA approved in ages ≥12 years and adults)

Pregnancy Risk Factor B

Pregnancy Considerations Adverse events were observed in some animal reproduction studies. Tenofovir has a high level of transfer across the human placenta. Intrauterine growth has not been affected in human studies, but one study found lower length and head circumference. Clinical studies in children have shown bone demineralization with chronic use. No increased risk of overall birth defects has been observed following first trimester exposure according to data collected by the antiretroviral pregnancy registry. Limited data indicate decreased maternal bioavailability during the third trimester; dose adjustments are not needed. Cases of lactic acidosis/hepatic steatosis syndrome related to mitochondrial toxicity have been reported in pregnant women with prolonged use of nucleoside analogues. It is not known if pregnancy itself potentiates this known side effect; however, women may be at increased risk of lactic acidosis and liver damage. In addition, these adverse events are similar to other rare but life-threatening syndromes which occur during pregnancy (eg, HELLP syndrome). Hepatic enzymes and electrolytes should be monitored in women receiving nucleoside analogues and clinicians should watch for early signs of the syndrome. In addition, mitochondrial dysfunction may develop in infants following *in utero* exposure. Renal function should also be monitored. The DHHS Perinatal HIV Guidelines consider tenofovir in combination with either emtricitabine or lamivudine to be a preferred NRTI backbone for use in antiretroviral-naïve pregnant women. The DHHS Perinatal HIV Guidelines consider emtricitabine plus tenofovir, or lamivudine plus tenofovir as recommended dual NRTI/NtRTI backbones for HIV/HBV coinfected pregnant women. Hepatitis B flare may occur if tenofovir is discontinued postpartum.

Regardless of CD4 count or HIV RNA copy number, all HIV-infected pregnant women should receive a combination antiretroviral (ARV) drug regimen. A combination of antepartum, intrapartum, and infant ARV prophylaxis is recommended. ARV therapy should be started as soon as possible in women with symptomatic infection.. Although earlier initiation may be more effective in reducing the perinatal transmission of HIV, also consider maternal conditions (eg, nausea and vomiting) and the potential risks of first trimester fetal exposure for specific agents. A scheduled cesarean delivery at 38 weeks gestation is recommended for all women with HIV RNA >1000 copies/mL or unknown concentrations near delivery in order to decrease transmission. If ARV therapy must be interrupted for <24 hours during the peripartum period, stop then restart all medications simultaneously in order to decrease the chance of developing resistance. Long-term follow-up is recommended for all infants exposed to ARV medications. In couples who want to conceive, the HIV-infected partner should attain maximum viral suppression prior to conception.

Health care providers are encouraged to enroll pregnant women exposed to antiretroviral medications in the Antiretroviral Pregnancy Registry (1-800-258-4263 or www.-APRegistry.com). Health care providers caring for HIV-infected women and their infants may contact the National Perinatal HIV Hotline (888-448-8765) for clinical consultation (DHHS [perinatal], 2014).

Breast-Feeding Considerations Tenofovir is excreted in breast milk. Maternal or infant antiretroviral therapy does not completely eliminate the risk of postnatal HIV transmission. In addition, multiclass-resistant virus has been detected in breast-feeding infants despite maternal therapy. Therefore, in the United States, where formula is accessible, affordable, safe, and sustainable, and the risk of infant mortality due to diarrhea and respiratory infections is low, complete avoidance of breast-feeding by HIV-infected women is recommended to decrease potential transmission of HIV (DHHS [perinatal], 2014).

Contraindications Hypersensitivity to tenofovir or any component

Warnings Cases of lactic acidosis, severe hepatomegaly with steatosis and death have been reported in patients receiving tenofovir and other nucleoside analogues **[U.S. Boxed Warning]**; most of these cases have been in women; prolonged nucleoside use, obesity, and prior liver disease may be risk factors; use with extreme caution in patients with other risk factors for liver disease; discontinue therapy in patients who develop laboratory or clinical evidence of lactic acidosis or pronounced hepatotoxicity.

May cause renal toxicity including acute renal failure and/or Fanconi syndrome (renal tubular injury with severe hypophosphatemia); risk may be increased in patients with preexisting renal disease, underlying systemic disease, or those taking nephrotoxic medications; adults with a low body weight and those taking medications that increase tenofovir serum concentration may also be at increased risk for tenofovir-associated nephrotoxicity; cases of nephrotoxicity have been reported in adolescents receiving tenofovir-containing regimens. Avoid use with concurrent or recent nephrotoxic therapy. Evaluate and monitor renal function, including calculation of creatinine clearance, at baseline and during therapy in all patients receiving tenofovir (regardless of age); monitor serum phosphorus. Dosage adjustment is required in patients with CrCl <50 mL/minute. Use with caution in patients with low body weight or concurrent medications which increase tenofovir levels.

Severe acute exacerbations of HBV have occurred after tenofovir discontinuation in patients infected with HBV **[U.S. Boxed Warning]**; follow hepatic function of HBV-infected patients closely (clinically and with laboratory tests) for at least several months after discontinuing tenofovir therapy; initiate antihepatitis B therapy if needed. Testing for HBV and HIV is recommended prior to the initiation of tenofovir therapy (treatment of HBV in patients with unrecognized/untreated HIV may lead to HIV resistance; treatment of HIV in patients with unrecognized/untreated HBV may lead to rapid HBV resistance). In patients who are coinfected with HIV and HBV, tenofovir should only be used as part of an appropriate combination antiretroviral regimen.

Do not use Viread (tenofovir) with other tenofovir-containing combination formulations (ie, Atripla, Complera, Stribild, Truvada). Do not use tenofovir or tenofovir-containing products with adefovir for the treatment of chronic HBV.

Precautions Use with caution in patients with hepatic impairment; no dosage adjustment is required; limited studies indicate the pharmacokinetics of tenofovir are not significantly altered in hepatic dysfunction. Limited data exists supporting the treatment of chronic hepatitis B in patients with decompensated liver disease exists; observe for increased adverse reactions, including renal dysfunction.

Do not use concurrently with didanosine for the treatment of HIV infection; didanosine toxicity (including pancreatitis and lactic acidosis) is increased and virologic failures have been reported (DHHS [adult, pediatric], 2014).

Fat redistribution and accumulation [ie, central obesity, peripheral wasting, facial wasting, breast enlargement, dorsocervical fat enlargement (buffalo hump), and cushingoid appearance] have been observed in patients receiving antiretroviral agents; causal relationship not established.

Immune reconstitution syndrome (an acute inflammatory response to residual or indolent opportunistic infections) may occur in HIV patients during initial treatment with combination antiretroviral agents including tenofovir; this syndrome may require further patient assessment and therapy. Autoimmune disorders (eg, Graves' disease, polymyositis, and Guillain-Barré syndrome) have been reported in patients experiencing immune reconstitution; time to onset is variable and may occur after many months of therapy.

Osteomalacia and reduced bone mineral density (BMD) may occur; long-term effects in humans are not known. Postmarketing cases of osteomalacia which may increase risk of bone fractures have also been reported in association with proximal renal tubulopathy. Recent studies suggest that tenofovir-related bone loss may be greater in children who are less mature (eg, Tanner stage 1 to 2) than in those who are more physically mature (Tanner ≥3). A significant decrease in lumbar spine BMD (>6%) was reported in 5 of 15 pediatric patients who received a tenofovir-containing regimen for 48 weeks. No orthopedic fractures occurred, but two patients required discontinuation of tenofovir. All five patients with a decrease in BMD were virologic responders and prepubertal (Tanner Stage 1). This study found a moderately strong correlation between decreases in bone mineral density z scores at week 48 and age at baseline. No correlation between decreases in bone mineral density z scores and tenofovir dose or pharmacokinetics was observed; BMD loss may limit the usefulness of tenofovir in prepubertal children [DHHS (pediatric), 2014; Giacomet, 2005; Hazra, 2005; Purdy, 2008]. Monitor BMD for potential bone toxicities during therapy; supplementation with calcium and vitamin D may be beneficial but has not been studied.

The use of antiretroviral regimens that only contain triple nucleoside reverse transcriptase inhibitors (NRTIs) are generally less effective than regimens containing 2 NRTIs and either an NNRTI or protease inhibitor; use triple NRTI-containing regimens with great caution; early virological failure and high rates of resistance may occur; closely monitor for virologic failure and consider treatment modification.

Adverse Reactions Includes data from both treatment-naive and treatment-experienced HIV patients and in chronic hepatitis B.

Cardiovascular: Chest pain

Central nervous system: Anxiety, depression, dizziness, fatigue, headache, insomnia, pain, peripheral neuropathy

Dermatologic: Diaphoresis, pruritus, skin rash (includes maculopapular, pustular, or vesiculobullous rash; pruritus; or urticaria)

Endocrine & metabolic: Glycosuria, hypercholesterolemia, hyperglycemia, increased serum triglycerides, lipodystrophy, weight loss

Gastrointestinal: Abdominal pain, anorexia, diarrhea, dyspepsia, flatulence, increased serum amylase, nausea, vomiting

Genitourinary: Hematuria

Hematologic & oncologic: Neutropenia

Hepatic: Increased serum alkaline phosphatase, increased serum ALT, increased serum AST, increased serum transaminases

Neuromuscular & skeletal: Arthralgia, back pain, decreased bone mineral density, increased creatine phosphokinase, myalgia, weakness

Renal: Increased serum creatinine, renal failure

Respiratory: Nasopharyngitis, pneumonia, sinusitis, upper respiratory tract infection

Miscellaneous: Fever

Rare but important or life-threatening: Angioedema, exacerbation of hepatitis B (following discontinuation), Fanconi's syndrome, hepatitis, hypersensitivity reaction, hypokalemia, hypophosphatemia, immune reconstitution syndrome, increased gamma-glutamyl transferase, interstitial nephritis, lactic acidosis, myopathy, nephrogenic diabetes insipidus, nephrotoxicity, osteomalacia, pancreatitis, polyuria, proteinuria, proximal tubular nephropathy, renal insufficiency, renal tubular necrosis, rhabdomyolysis, severe hepatomegaly with steatosis

Drug Interactions

Metabolism/Transport Effects Inhibits CYP1A2 (weak); **Induces** P-glycoprotein

Avoid Concomitant Use

Avoid concomitant use of Tenofovir with any of the following: Adefovir; Dabigatran Etexilate; Didanosine; VinCRIStine (Liposomal)

Increased Effect/Toxicity

Tenofovir may increase the levels/effects of: Adefovir; Aminoglycosides; Darunavir; Didanosine; Ganciclovir-Valganciclovir

The levels/effects of Tenofovir may be increased by: Acyclovir-Valacyclovir; Adefovir; Aminoglycosides; Atazanavir; Cidofovir; Darunavir; Diclofenac (Systemic); Ganciclovir-Valganciclovir; Lopinavir; Nonsteroidal Anti-Inflammatory Agents; Simeprevir; Telaprevir

Decreased Effect

Tenofovir may decrease the levels/effects of: Afatinib; Atazanavir; Brentuximab Vedotin; Dabigatran Etexilate; Didanosine; DOXOrubicin (Conventional); Linagliptin;

P-glycoprotein/ABCB1 Substrates; Simeprevir; Tipranavir; VinCRIStine (Liposomal)

The levels/effects of Tenofovir may be decreased by: Adefovir; Tipranavir

Food Interactions Fatty meals may increase the bioavailability of tenofovir. Management: May administer with or without food.

Stability Store at 25°C (77°F); excursions permitted to 15°C to 30°C (59°F to 86°F). Dispense in original container only. Keep container tightly closed.

Mechanism of Action Tenofovir disoproxil fumarate (TDF), a nucleotide reverse transcriptase inhibitor, is an analog of adenosine 5'-monophosphate; it interferes with the HIV viral RNA dependent DNA polymerase resulting in inhibition of viral replication. TDF is first converted intracellularly by hydrolysis to tenofovir and subsequently phosphorylated to the active tenofovir diphosphate. Tenofovir inhibits replication of HBV by inhibiting HBV polymerase.

Pharmacokinetics (Adult data unless noted)

Distribution: V_d: 1.2 to 1.3 L/kg

Protein binding: Minimal (7.2% to serum proteins)

Metabolism: Not metabolized by CYP isoenzymes; tenofovir disoproxil fumarate (a prodrug) undergoes diester hydrolysis to tenofovir; tenofovir undergoes phosphorylation to the active tenofovir diphosphate

Bioavailability: Oral:

Tablets: 25% (fasting); high-fat meals will increase AUC by 40%

Powder: Peak serum concentrations are 26% lower compared to tablet, but the mean AUCs are similar

Half-life: Serum: 17 hours; intracellular: 10 to 50 hours

Time to peak serum concentration: Fasting: 1 hour

Elimination: Excreted via glomerular filtration and active tubular secretion; after I.V. administration: 70% to 80% is excreted in the urine as unchanged drug within 72 hours; after multiple oral doses (administered with food): 32% ± 10% is excreted in the urine within 24 hours

Clearance: Total body clearance is decreased in patients with renal impairment

Dosing: Usual

Pediatric:

HIV infection, treatment: Use in combination with other antiretroviral agents: **Note:** Some experts recommend avoiding tenofovir (especially for initial therapy) in prepubertal patients and those in early puberty (Tanner stages 1 and 2), due to concerns about the potential increased risk of bone mineral density loss. Other experts recommend measuring bone mineral density prior to initiation of therapy and 6 months later in these patients [DHHS (pediatric), 2014]:

Infants and Children <2 years: Not approved for use; dose is unknown

Children 2 to <12 years; weighing <35 kg: Oral: 8 mg/kg/dose once daily; maximum daily dose: 300 mg/**day**

Dosage form specific:

Oral powder: **Note:** One level scoop = 40 mg tenofovir disoproxil fumarate

10 to <12 kg: 80 mg (2 scoops) once daily

12 to <14 kg: 100 mg (2.5 scoops) once daily

14 to <17 kg: 120 mg (3 scoops) once daily

17 to <19 kg: 140 mg (3.5 scoops) once daily

19 to <22 kg: 160 mg (4 scoops) once daily

22 to <24 kg: 180 mg (4.5 scoops) once daily

24 to <27 kg: 200 mg (5 scoops) once daily

27 to <29 kg: 220 mg (5.5 scoops) once daily

29 to <32 kg: 240 mg (6 scoops) once daily

32 to <34 kg: 260 mg (6.5 scoops) once daily

34 to <35 kg: 280 mg (7 scoops) once daily

≥35 kg: 300 mg (7.5 scoops) once daily

Oral tablets:
17 to <22 kg: 150 mg once daily
22 to <28 kg: 200 mg once daily
28 to <35 kg: 250 mg once daily
≥35 kg: 300 mg once daily

Children ≥12 years and Adolescents; weight ≥35 kg: Oral: 300 mg once daily

Hepatitis B infection, chronic: Children and Adolescents ≥12 years weighing ≥35 kg: Oral: 300 mg once daily; **Note:** Optimal duration of therapy is unknown.

Adult:

HIV infection, treatment: Oral: 300 mg once daily; **Note:** Use in combination with other antiretroviral agents

Hepatitis B infection, chronic: Oral: 300 mg once daily; **Note:** Tenofovir is recommended for first-line treatment of HBV (Lok, 2009). Concurrent use with adefovir and/or tenofovir combination products should be avoided.

Treatment duration (AASLD practice guidelines; Lok, 2009): **Note:** Patients not achieving <2 log decrease in serum HBV DNA after at least 6 months of therapy should either receive additional treatment or be switched to an alternative therapy.

Hepatitis Be antigen (HBeAg) positive chronic hepatitis: Treat ≥1 year until HBeAg seroconversion and undetectable serum HBV DNA; continue therapy for ≥6 months after HBeAg seroconversion

HBeAg negative chronic hepatitis: Treat >1 year until hepatitis B surface antigen (HB$_s$Ag) clearance

Decompensated liver disease: Lifelong treatment is recommended

Dosing adjustment in renal impairment:

Children and Adolescents: There are no dosage adjustments provided in manufacturer's labeling; has not been studied. Dosage should be decreased in patients with CrCl <50 mL/minute (DHHS [pediatric], 2014)

Adult: Oral: **Note:** Use of powder formulation has not been evaluated in renal impairment. Closely monitor clinical response and renal function in these patients; clinical effectiveness and safety of these guidelines have not been evaluated.

CrCl ≥50 mL/minute: No adjustment necessary
CrCl 30 to 49 mL/minute: 300 mg every 48 hours
CrCl 10 to 29 mL/minute: 300 mg every 72 to 96 hours
CrCl <10 mL/minute without dialysis: There are no dosage adjustments provided in manufacturer's labeling; has not been studied.

Hemodialysis: 4 hours of hemodialysis removed ~10% of a single 300 mg dose; 300 mg every 7 days or after a total of ~12 hours of dialysis (eg, once weekly with 3 hemodialysis sessions of ~4 hours in length); administer dose after completion of dialysis

Dosing adjustment in hepatic impairment: No dosage adjustment required; in adults, limited number of patients have been studied (especially HBV patients with decompensated liver disease); observe for increased adverse reactions, including renal dysfunction.

Administration Oral:

Powder: Must administer with food. Measure dose only using the supplied dosing scoop. Mix powder well with 2-4 ounces of soft food (applesauce, baby food, yogurt) and swallow immediately (avoids bitter taste); ensure that entire mixture is ingested. Do **not** mix in liquid (powder may float on top of the liquid even after stirring).

Tablets: May be administered without regard to meals

Monitoring Parameters

Hepatitis B, treatment: Test patients for HIV prior to starting therapy; CBC with differential, hemoglobin, MCV, reticulocyte count, liver enzymes, bilirubin, renal and hepatic function tests, and HBV RNA plasma levels. Monitor for potential bone and renal abnormalities. Calculate creatinine clearance in all patients prior to starting tenofovir therapy and as clinically needed; monitor for

alterations in calculated creatinine clearance and serum phosphorus in patients at risk or with a history of renal dysfunction and patients receiving concurrent nephrotoxic agents. Monitor weight and growth in children. Consider bone mineral density assessment for all patients with a history of pathologic bone fractures or other risk factors for osteoporosis or bone loss. Monitor hepatic function closely (clinically and with laboratory tests) for at least several months after discontinuing tenofovir therapy.

HIV treatment: Note: Monitor CD4 percentage (if <5 years of age) or CD4 count (if ≥5 years of age) at least every 3 to 4 months (DHHS [pediatric], 2014). Screen for hepatitis B before starting tenofovir. Also prior to initiation of therapy: Genotypic resistance testing, CD4 and viral load (every 3 to 4 months), CBC with differential, LFTs, BUN, creatinine, urine dipstick for protein and glucose, electrolytes, and glucose, urinalysis (every 6 to 12 months), and assessment of readiness for adherence with medication regimen. At initiation and with any change in treatment regimen: CBC with differential, electrolytes, calcium, phosphate, glucose, LFTs, bilirubin, urinalysis (at initiation), BUN, creatinine, albumin, total protein, lipid panel (at initiation), CD4, and viral load. After 1 to 2 weeks of therapy: Signs of medication toxicity and adherence. After 2 to 4 weeks of therapy: CBC with differential, viral load, and signs of medication toxicity, and adherence; then every 3 to 4 months: CBC with differential, electrolytes, glucose, LFTs, bilirubin, BUN, creatinine, CD4, viral load, signs of medication toxicity, and adherence. Every 6 to 12 months: Lipid panel and urinalysis. CD4 monitoring frequency may be decreased to every 6 to 12 months in children who are adherent to therapy if the value is well above the threshold for opportunistic infections, viral suppression is sustained, and the clinical status is stable for more than 2 to 3 years (DHHS [pediatric], 2014). Monitor for growth and development, signs of HIV-specific physical conditions, HIV disease progression, opportunistic infections, bone loss, or lactic acidosis. Consider bone mineral density assessment for all patients with a history of pathologic bone fractures or other risk factors for osteoporosis or bone loss. Some experts recommend obtaining a DXA scan prior to therapy and 6 months into therapy, especially for patients in pre- and early puberty (Tanner stages 1 and 2) (DHHS [pediatric], 2014).

Additional Information Long term studies demonstrating a decrease of clinical progression of HIV in patients receiving tenofovir are needed. Consider tenofovir in patients with HIV strains that would be susceptible as assessed by treatment history or laboratory tests. Mutation of reverse transcriptase at the 65 codon (K65R mutation) confers *in vitro* resistance to tenofovir; the K65R mutation is selected in some patients after treatment with didanosine, zalcitabine, or abacavir; thus, cross-resistance may occur. Multiple nucleoside mutations with a T69S double insertion showed decreased *in vitro* susceptibility to tenofovir; patients with HIV strains that had ≥3 zidovudine-associated mutations that included M41L or L210W showed decreased responses to tenofovir (but these responses were still better than placebo); patients with mutations at K65R, or L74V without zidovudine-associated mutations seemed to have a decreased response to tenofovir

A high rate of early virologic failure in therapy-naïve adult HIV patients has been observed with the once-daily three-drug combination therapy of didanosine enteric-coated beadlets (Videx EC), lamivudine, and tenofovir and the once-daily three-drug combination therapy of abacavir, lamivudine, and tenofovir. These combinations should not be used as a new treatment regimen for naïve or pretreated patients. Any patient currently receiving either of these regimens should be closely monitored for virologic failure and considered for treatment modification. Early virologic failure was also observed in therapy-naïve adult HIV patients treated with tenofovir, didanosine enteric-coated beadlets (Videx EC) and either efavirenz or nevirapine; rapid emergence of resistant mutations has also been reported with this combination; the combination of tenofovir, didanosine, and any non-nucleoside reverse transcriptase inhibitor is **not** recommended as initial antiretroviral therapy. Current guidelines warn **not** to use tenofovir concurrently with didanosine for the treatment of HIV infection; risk of didanosine toxicity (including pancreatitis and lactic acidosis) is increased and virologic failures have been reported (DHHS [adult], 2014).

Dosage Forms Excipient information presented when available (limited, particularly for generics); consult specific product labeling.

Powder, Oral, as disoproxil fumarate:
Viread: 40 mg/g (60 g)

Tablet, Oral, as disoproxil fumarate:
Viread: 150 mg, 200 mg, 250 mg
Viread: 300 mg [contains fd&c blue #2 aluminum lake]

References

DHHS Panel on Antiretroviral Guidelines for Adults and Adolescents. Guidelines for the use of antiretroviral agents in HIV-1-infected adults and adolescents, Department of Health and Human Services. May 1, 2014. Available at http://www.aidsinfo.nih.gov/ContentFiles/AdultandAdolescentGL.pdf

DHHS Panel on Antiretroviral Therapy and Medical Management of HIV-Infected Children. Guidelines for the use of antiretroviral agents in pediatric HIV infection. February 12, 2014. Available at http://aidsinfo.nih.gov

DHHS Panel on Treatment of HIV-Infected Pregnant Women and Prevention of Perinatal Transmission. Recommendations for the use of antiretroviral drugs in pregnant HIV-1-infected women for maternal health and interventions to reduce perinatal HIV-1 transmission in the United States. March 28, 2014. Available at http://aidsinfo.nih.gov

Giacomet V, Mora S, Martelli L, Merlo M, Sciannamblo M, Viganò A. A 12-month treatment with tenofovir does not impair bone mineral accrual in HIV-infected children. *J Acquir Immune Defic Syndr.* 2005;40(4):448-450.

Hazra R, Balis FM, Tullio AN, et al, "Single-Dose and Steady-State Pharmacokinetics of Tenofovir Disoproxil Fumarate in Human Immunodeficiency Virus-Infected Children," *Antimicrob Agents Chemother,* 2004, 48(1):124-9.

Hazra R, Gafni RI, Maldarelli F, et al. Tenofovir disoproxil fumarate and an optimized background regimen of antiretroviral agents as salvage therapy for pediatric HIV infection. *Pediatrics.* 2005;116(6):e846-e854.

Lok AS, McMahon BJ. Chronic hepatitis B: update 2009. *Hepatology.* 2009. Available at http://www.aasld.org/practiceguidelines/Documents/Bookmarked%20Practice%20Guidelines/Chronic_Hep_B_Update_2009%208_24_2009.pdf

Lyseng-Williamson KA, Reynolds NA, Plosker GL. Tenofovir disoproxil fumarate: a review of its use in the management of HIV infection. *Drugs.* 2005;65(3):413-432.

Purdy JB, Gafni RI, Reynolds JC, Zeichner S, Hazra R. Decreased bone mineral density with off-label use of tenofovir in children and adolescents infected with human immunodeficiency virus. *J Pediatr.* 2008;152(4):582-584.

◆ **Tenofovir and Emtricitabine** *see* Emtricitabine and Tenofovir *on page 741*

◆ **Tenofovir Disoproxil Fumarate** *see* Tenofovir *on page 1977*

◆ **Tenofovir Disoproxil Fumarate, Efavirenz, and Emtricitabine** *see* Efavirenz, Emtricitabine, and Tenofovir *on page 735*

◆ **Tenormin** *see* Atenolol *on page 222*

◆ **Tensilon® (Can)** *see* Edrophonium *on page 730*

◆ **Tera-Gel Tar [OTC]** *see* Coal Tar *on page 532*

Terazosin (ter AY zoe sin)

Medication Safety Issues

BEERS Criteria medication:
This drug may be potentially inappropriate for use in geriatric patients (Quality of evidence - moderate; Strength of recommendation - strong).

Brand Names: Canada Apo-Terazosin®; Dom-Terazosin; Hytrin®; Nu-Terazosin; PHL-Terazosin; PMS-Terazosin; ratio-Terazosin; Teva-Terazosin

Therapeutic Category Alpha-Adrenergic Blocking Agent, Oral; Antihypertensive Agent; Vasodilator

Generic Availability (U.S.) Yes

Use Treatment of benign prostate hyperplasia (BPH) (FDA approved in adults); treatment of hypertension alone or in combination with other agents, such as diuretics or beta-blockers (FDA approved in adults)

Pregnancy Risk Factor C

Pregnancy Considerations Teratogenic effects have not been observed in animal studies. Decreased fetal weight and increased risk of fetal mortality were noted in some animal reproduction studies. There are no adequate and well-controlled studies in pregnant women. Use only if benefit outweighs risk.

Untreated chronic maternal hypertension is associated with adverse events in the fetus, infant, and mother. If treatment for hypertension during pregnancy is needed, other agents are generally preferred (ACOG, 2013).

Breast-Feeding Considerations It is not known if terazosin is excreted in breast milk. The manufacturer recommends that caution be exercised when administering terazosin to nursing women.

Contraindications Hypersensitivity to terazosin, quinazolines (prazosin, doxazosin), or any component

Warnings Marked orthostatic hypotension, syncope, and loss of consciousness may occur with first dose or first few days of therapy; syncope usually occurs 30-90 minutes after initial dose; occasionally preceded with severe supraventricular tachycardia (120-160 bpm in adults); anticipate a similar effect if therapy is interrupted for a few days, if dosage is rapidly increased, if large initial dose ($\geq$2 mg in adults), or if another antihypertensive drug (eg, beta-blockers, diuretics, and particularly vasodilators) or a PDE-5 inhibitor (eg, sildenafil, tadalafil, vardenafil) is introduced. Patients should be cautioned about performing hazardous tasks when starting new therapy, after an interruption of therapy, or when adjusting dosage upward. May cause priapism (rarely).

Precautions Use with caution in patient with cataracts or undergoing corrective cataract surgery; intraoperative floppy iris syndrome (IFIS) has been observed in cataract surgery patients receiving or who were previously treated with alpha$_1$-blockers; there appears to be no benefit in discontinuing alpha$_1$-blockers prior to surgery.

Adverse Reactions

Cardiovascular: Orthostatic hypotension, palpitation, peripheral edema, syncope, tachycardia

Central nervous system: Dizziness, somnolence, vertigo

Gastrointestinal: Nausea, weight gain

Genitourinary: Impotence, libido decreased

Neuromuscular & skeletal: Back pain, extremity pain, muscle weakness, paresthesia

Ocular: Blurred vision

Respiratory: Dyspnea, nasal congestion, sinusitis

Rare but important or life-threatening: Abdominal pain, abnormal vision, allergic reactions, anaphylaxis, anxiety, arrhythmia, arthralgia, arthritis, atrial fibrillation, bronchitis, chest pain, conjunctivitis, constipation, cough, diaphoresis, diarrhea, dyspepsia, epistaxis, facial edema, fever, flatulence, flu-like syndrome, gout, insomnia, intraoperative floppy iris syndrome (IFIS), joint disorder, myalgia, neck pain, pharyngitis, polyuria, priapism, pruritus, rash, rhinitis, shoulder pain, thrombocytopenia, tinnitus, urinary incontinence, urinary tract infection, vasodilation, vomiting, xerostomia

Drug Interactions

Metabolism/Transport Effects None known.

Avoid Concomitant Use
Avoid concomitant use of Terazosin with any of the following: Alpha1-Blockers

Increased Effect/Toxicity
Terazosin may increase the levels/effects of: Alpha1-Blockers; Amifostine; Antihypertensives; Calcium Channel Blockers; DULoxetine; Hypotensive Agents; Obinutuzumab; RiTUXimab

The levels/effects of Terazosin may be increased by: Barbiturates; Beta-Blockers; Brimonidine (Topical); Diazoxide; Herbs (Hypotensive Properties); MAO Inhibitors; Pentoxifylline; Phosphodiesterase 5 Inhibitors; Prostacyclin Analogues

Decreased Effect
Terazosin may decrease the levels/effects of: Alpha-/Beta-Agonists; Alpha1-Agonists

The levels/effects of Terazosin may be decreased by: Herbs (Hypertensive Properties); Methylphenidate; Yohimbine

Stability Store at 20°C to 25°C (68°F to 77°F); protect from light and moisture.

Mechanism of Action Alpha$_1$-specific blocking agent with minimal alpha$_2$ effects; this allows peripheral postsynaptic blockade, with the resultant decrease in arterial tone, while preserving the negative feedback loop which is mediated by the peripheral presynaptic alpha$_2$-receptors; terazosin relaxes the smooth muscle of the bladder neck, thus reducing bladder outlet obstruction

Pharmacodynamics
Onset of action: Antihypertensive effect: 15 minutes
Maximum effect: Antihypertensive effect: 2-3 hours
Duration: Antihypertensive effect: 24 hours

Pharmacokinetics (Adult data unless noted)
Absorption: Rapid, complete
Protein binding: 90% to 94%
Metabolism: Hepatic; minimal first pass
Half-life: ~12 hours
Time to peak serum concentration: ~1 hour
Elimination: Feces (~60%, ~20% as unchanged drug); urine (~40%, ~10% as unchanged drug)
Dialysis: ~10% removed during hemodialysis

Dosing: Usual Note: If drug is discontinued for greater than several days, consider beginning with initial dose and retitrate as needed.

Children and Adolescents: **Hypertension:** Oral: Initial: 1 mg once daily typically administered at bedtime; slowly increase dose to achieve desired blood pressure as tolerated; maximum daily dose: 20 mg/**day** (NHBPEP, 2004; NHLBI, 2011)

Adults:

Benign prostatic hyperplasia: Oral: Initial: 1 mg at bedtime; thereafter, titrate upwards, if needed, over several weeks, balancing therapeutic benefit with terazosin-induced postural hypotension; most patients require 10 mg day; if no response after 4-6 weeks of 10 mg/day, may increase to 20 mg/day

Hypertension: Oral: Initial: 1 mg at bedtime; slowly increase dose to achieve desired blood pressure, up to 20 mg/day; usual dose range (JNC 7): 1-20 mg once daily. **Note:** Dosage may be given on a twice-daily regimen if response is diminished at 24 hours.

Administration Oral: Administer without regard to meals at the same time each day.

Monitoring Parameters Standing and sitting/supine blood pressure, especially 2-3 hours after the initial dose, then prior to doses (to ensure adequate control throughout the dosing interval); urinary symptoms if used for BPH treatment

Dosage Forms Excipient information presented when available (limited, particularly for generics); consult specific product labeling.

Capsule, Oral:
Generic: 1 mg, 2 mg, 5 mg, 10 mg

References
Chobanian AV, Bakris GL, Black HR, et al, "The Seventh Report of the Joint National Committee on Prevention, Detection, Evaluation, and Treatment of High Blood Pressure: The JNC 7 Report," *JAMA*, 2003, 289(19):2560-71.

National Heart, Lung, and Blood Institute, "Expert Panel on Integrated Guidelines for Cardiovascular Health and Risk Reduction in Children and Adolescents," Clinical Practice Guidelines, 2011, National Institutes of Health. Available at http://www.nhlbi.nih.gov/guidelines/cvd_ped/peds_guidelines_full.pdf

National High Blood Pressure Education Program Working Group on High Blood Pressure in Children and Adolescents, "The Fourth Report on the Diagnosis, Evaluation, and Treatment of High Blood Pressure in Children and Adolescents," *Pediatrics*, 2004, 114(2 Suppl 4th Report):555-76.

Terbinafine (Systemic) (TER bin a feen)

Medication Safety Issues
Sound-alike/look-alike issues:
Terbinafine may be confused with terbutaline
LamISIL may be confused with LaMICtal, Lomotil

Brand Names: U.S. LamISIL; Terbinex

Brand Names: Canada Apo-Terbinafine; Auro-Terbinafine; CO Terbinafine; Dom-Terbinafine; GD-Terbinafine; JAMP-Terbinafine; Lamisil; Mylan-Terbinafine; PHL-Terbinafine; PMS-Terbinafine; Q-Terbinafine; Riva-Terbinafine; Sandoz-Terbinafine; Teva-Terbinafine

Generic Availability (U.S.) May be product dependent

Use Oral:
Granules: Treatment of tinea capitis (FDA approved in ages ≥4 years and adults)
Tablet: Treatment of onychomycosis of the toenail or fingernail due to susceptible dermatophytes (FDA approved in adults)

Pregnancy Risk Factor B

Pregnancy Considerations Adverse events were not observed in animal reproduction studies. Avoid use in pregnancy since treatment of onychomycosis is postponable.

Breast-Feeding Considerations Terbinafine is excreted in breast milk; the milk/plasma ratio is 7:1. Breast-feeding is not recommended by the manufacturer.

Contraindications Hypersensitivity to terbinafine or any component

Warnings Although rare, Stevens-Johnson syndrome and toxic epidermal necrolysis have been reported; discontinue therapy if progressive skin rash occurs. Transient decreases in absolute lymphocyte counts were observed in clinical trials; severe neutropenia (reversible upon discontinuation) has also been reported. Monitor CBC in patients with preexisting immunosuppression if therapy is to continue >6 weeks. Discontinue therapy if ANC ≤1000/mm^3. Rare cases of hepatic failure (including fatal cases) have been reported; not recommended for use in patients with active or chronic liver disease including hepatic cirrhosis. Discontinue if symptoms or signs of hepatobiliary dysfunction or cholestatic hepatitis develop and assess hepatic function immediately. Not recommended for use in patients with renal impairment (CrCl ≤50 mL/minute); clearance is reduced by approximately 50%.

Taste disturbance (including loss of taste) may occur and and severe cases resulting in weight loss or depression have been reported; resolution may be delayed (eg, several weeks to >1 year) following discontinuation of therapy or in some cases, disturbance may be permanent. Discontinue therapy in patients with symptoms of taste disturbance. Smell disturbance (including loss of smell) has been reported; resolution may be delayed (eg, >1 year) following discontinuation of therapy or in some cases, disturbance may be permanent. Discontinue therapy in patients with symptoms of smell disturbance. Although rare, changes in the ocular lens and retina have been reported; discontinuation of therapy may be required.

Some tablet formulations may contain lactose and should be avoided in patients with galactose intolerance, Lapp lactase deficiency, or glucose-galactose malabsorption syndromes.

Precautions Use with caution in patients sensitive to allylamine antifungals (eg, naftifine, butenafine); cross-sensitivity to terbinafine may exist. Use with caution in patients with lupus; precipitation or exacerbation of cutaneous or systemic lupus erythematosus has been observed; discontinue if signs and/or symptoms develop. Depression has been reported with use; instruct patients to report depressive symptoms/mood changes. Due to potential toxicity, confirmation of diagnostic testing of nail or skin specimens prior to treatment of onychomycosis or dermatomycosis is recommended.

Adverse Reactions Adverse events listed for tablets unless otherwise specified. Granules were studied in patients 4-12 years of age.

Central nervous system: Headache

Dermatologic: Pruritus, skin rash, urticaria

Gastrointestinal: Abdominal pain, diarrhea, dysgeusia, dyspepsia, flatulence, nausea, sore throat (granules), toothache (granules), vomiting

Hepatic: Liver enzyme disorder

Infection: Influenza (granules)

Ophthalmic: Visual disturbance

Respiratory: Cough (granules), nasal congestion (granules), nasopharyngitis (granules), rhinorrhea (granules), upper respiratory tract infection (children, granules)

Miscellaneous: Fever (granules)

Rare but important or life-threatening: Acute generalized exanthematous pustulosis, acute pancreatitis, agranulocytosis, alopecia, altered sense of smell, anaphylaxis, angioedema, depression, DRESS syndrome, exacerbation of psoriasis, exacerbation of systemic lupus erythematosus, hepatic disease, hepatic failure, hypersensitivity reaction, pancytopenia, rhabdomyolysis, severe neutropenia, Stevens-Johnson syndrome, thrombocytopenia, toxic epidermal necrolysis, vasculitis, visual field loss

Drug Interactions

Metabolism/Transport Effects Substrate of CYP1A2 (minor), CYP2C19 (minor), CYP2C9 (minor), CYP3A4 (minor); **Note:** Assignment of Major/Minor substrate status based on clinically relevant drug interaction potential; **Inhibits** CYP2D6 (strong); **Induces** CYP3A4 (weak/moderate)

Avoid Concomitant Use

Avoid concomitant use of Terbinafine (Systemic) with any of the following: Axitinib; Pimozide; Saccharomyces boulardii; Simeprevir; Tamoxifen; Thioridazine

Increased Effect/Toxicity

Terbinafine (Systemic) may increase the levels/effects of: ARIPiprazole; AtoMOXetine; CYP2D6 Substrates; DOXOrubicin (Conventional); Fesoterodine; Iloperidone; Metoprolol; Nebivolol; Pimozide; Propafenone; Tetrabenazine; Thioridazine; Tricyclic Antidepressants; Vortioxetine

Decreased Effect

Terbinafine (Systemic) may decrease the levels/effects of: ARIPiprazole; Axitinib; Codeine; Ibrutinib; Iloperidone; Saccharomyces boulardii; Saxagliptin; Simeprevir; Tamoxifen; TraMADol

The levels/effects of Terbinafine (Systemic) may be decreased by: Rifampin

Stability

Granules: Store at controlled room temperature of 15°C to 30°C (59°F to 86°F).

Tablet: Store below 25°C (77°F); protect from light

Mechanism of Action Synthetic allylamine derivative which inhibits squalene epoxidase, a key enzyme in sterol biosynthesis in fungi. This results in a deficiency in ergosterol within the fungal cell wall and results in fungal cell death.

Pharmacokinetics (Adult data unless noted)

Absorption: Children and Adults: >70%

Distribution: Distributed to sebum and skin predominantly

Protein binding: Plasma: >99%

Metabolism: Hepatic predominantly via CYP1A2, 3A4, 2C8, 2C9, and 2C19 to inactive metabolites

Bioavailability:

Children: 36% to 64%

Adults: 40%

Half-life, terminal: 200-400 hours; very slow release of drug from skin and adipose tissues occurs; effective half-life: Children: 27-31 hours; Adults: ~36 hours

Time to peak serum concentration: Children and Adults: 1-2 hours

Elimination: Children and Adults: 70% in urine

Clearance: Children (14-68 kg): 15.6-26.7 L/hour

Dosing: Usual

Children and Adolescents:

Tinea capitis: Children ≥4 years and Adolescents: Oral: Granules:

<25 kg: 125 mg once daily for 6 weeks

25-35 kg: 187.5 mg once daily for 6 weeks

>35 kg: 250 mg once daily for 6 weeks

Onychomycosis (Gupta, 1997): Limited data available: Children and Adolescents: Oral: Tablets:

10-20 kg: 62.5 mg once daily for 6 weeks (fingernails) or 12 weeks (toenails)

20-40 kg: 125 mg once daily for 6 weeks (fingernails) or 12 weeks (toenails)

>40 kg: 250 mg once daily for 6 weeks (fingernails) or 12 weeks (toenails)

Adults: **Onychomycosis:** Oral: Tablet: Fingernail: 250 mg once daily for 6 weeks; Toenail: 250 mg once daily for 12 weeks

Dosing adjustment in renal impairment: No dosage adjustment provided in manufacturer's U.S. labeling; however, clearance is decreased 50% in patients with CrCl ≤50 mL/minute.

Dosing adjustment in hepatic impairment: Hepatic cirrhosis: Use is not recommended in chronic or active hepatic disease.

Administration Tablets may be administered without regard to meals. Granules should be taken with food; sprinkle on a spoonful of nonacidic food (eg, pudding, mashed potatoes); do not use applesauce or fruit-based foods; swallow granules whole without chewing

Monitoring Parameters AST/ALT prior to initiation, repeat if used >6 weeks; CBC

Additional Information Patients should not be considered therapeutic failures until they have been symptom-free for 2-4 weeks following a course of treatment; GI complaints usually subside with continued administration

Dosage Forms Considerations

Terbinex Kit contains terbinafine 250 mg tablets and hydroxypropyl-chitosan 1% nail lacquer

Dosage Forms Excipient information presented when available (limited, particularly for generics); consult specific product labeling.

Kit, Combination:

Terbinex: 250 mg & 1%

Packet, Oral:

LamISIL: 125 mg (1 ea, 14 ea); 187.5 mg (1 ea, 14 ea) [contains polyethylene glycol]

Tablet, Oral:

LamISIL: 250 mg

Generic: 250 mg

Extemporaneous Preparations A 25 mg/mL oral suspension may be made using tablets. Crush twenty 250 mg tablets and reduce to a fine powder. Add small amount of a 1:1 mixture of Ora-Sweet® and Ora-Plus® and mix to a uniform paste; mix while adding the vehicle in geometric proportions to **almost** 200 mL; transfer to a calibrated bottle, rinse mortar with vehicle, and add quantity of vehicle sufficient to make 200 mL. Label "shake well" and "refrigerate". Stable 42 days.

Nahata MC, Pai VB, and Hipple TF, *Pediatric Drug Formulations*, 5th ed, Cincinnati, OH: Harvey Whitney Books Co, 2004.

References

Abdel-Rahman SM and Nahata MC, "Oral Terbinafine: A New Antifungal Agent," *Ann Pharmacother*, 1997, 31(4):445-56.

Abdel-Rahman SM, Herron J, Fallon-Friedlander S, et al, "Pharmacokinetics of Terbinafine in Young Children Treated for Tinea Capitis," *Pediatr Infect Dis J*, 2005, 24(10):886-91.

Amichai B and Grunwald MH, "Adverse Drug Reactions of the New Oral Antifungal Agents - Terbinafine, Fluconazole, and Itraconazole," *Int J Dermatol*, 1998, 37(6):410-5.

Angello JT, Voytovich RM, and Jan SA, "A Cost/Efficacy Analysis of Oral Antifungals Indicated for the Treatment of Onychomycosis: Griseofulvin, Itraconazole, and Terbinafine," *Am J Manag Care*, 1997, 3(3):443-50.

De Backer M, De Vroey C, Lesaffre E, et al, "Twelve Weeks of Continuous Oral Therapy for Toenail Onychomycosis Caused by Dermatophytes: A Double-Blind Comparative Trial of Terbinafine 250 mg/day Versus Itraconazole 200 mg/day," *J Am Acad Dermatol*, 1998, 38(5 Pt 3):S57-63.

Dwyer CM, White MI, and Sinclair TS, "Cholestatic Jaundice Due to Terbinafine," *Br J Dermatol*, 1997, 136(6):976-7.

Friedlander SF, Aly R, Krafchik B, et al, "Terbinafine in the Treatment of Trichophyton Tinea Capitis: A Randomized, Double-Blind, Parallel-Group, Duration-Finding Study," *Pediatrics*, 2002, 109(4):602-7.

Gupta AK and Shear NH, "Terbinafine: An Update," *J Am Acad Dermatol*, 1997, 37:979-88.

Gupta AK, Sibbald RG, Knowles SR, et al, "Terbinafine Therapy May Be Associated With the Development of Psoriasis De Novo or Its Exacerbation: Four Case Reports and a Review of Drug Induced Psoriasis," *J Am Acad Dermatol*, 1997, 36(5 Part 2):858-62.

Gupta AK, Sibbald RG, Lynde CW, et al, "Onychomycosis in Children: Prevalence and Treatment Strategies," *J Am Acad Dermatol*, 1997, 36(3 Pt 1):395-402.

Jones TC, "Overview of the Use of Terbinafine in Children," *Br J Dermatol*, 1995, 132(5):683-9.

Trepanier EF and Amsden GW, "Current Issues in Onychomycosis," *Ann Pharmacother*, 1998, 32(2):204-14.

Vickers AE, Sinclair JR, Zollinger M, et al, "Multiple Cytochrome P-450s Involved in the Metabolism of Terbinafine Suggest a Limited Potential for Drug-Drug Interactions," *Drug Metab Dispos*, 1999, 27(9):1029-38.

Terbinafine (Topical) (TER bin a feen)

Medication Safety Issues
Sound-alike/look-alike issues:
Terbinafine may be confused with terbutaline

Brand Names: U.S. LamISIL Advanced [OTC]; LamISIL AT Jock Itch [OTC]; LamISIL AT Spray [OTC]; LamISIL AT [OTC]; LamISIL Spray

Brand Names: Canada Lamisil

Therapeutic Category Antifungal Agent, Topical

Generic Availability (U.S.) May be product dependent

Use Antifungal for the treatment of tinea pedis (athlete's foot), tinea cruris (jock itch), and tinea corporis (ringworm) (OTC/prescription formulations); tinea versicolor (prescription formulations)

Pregnancy Considerations Adverse events were not observed in animal reproduction studies with systemic terbinafine. Systemic absorption is limited following topical application.

Breast-Feeding Considerations Following oral administration, terbinafine is excreted into breast milk. (Refer to the Terbinafine, Systemic monograph for additional information). Systemic absorption is limited following topical application. Nursing mothers should not apply topical formulations to the breast.

Contraindications Hypersensitivity to terbinafine or any component

Warnings Topical formulations (gel, cream, or solution) are not for ophthalmic, oral, or intravaginal use.

Adverse Reactions
Dermatologic: Burning, contact dermatitis, dryness, exfoliation, irritation, pruritus, rash
Local: Irritation, stinging

Drug Interactions
Metabolism/Transport Effects None known.
Avoid Concomitant Use There are no known interactions where it is recommended to avoid concomitant use.
Increased Effect/Toxicity There are no known significant interactions involving an increase in effect.
Decreased Effect There are no known significant interactions involving a decrease in effect.

Stability
Cream: Store at 5°C to 30°C (41°F to 86°F).
Solution: Store at 5°C to 25°C (41°F to 77°F); do not refrigerate.

Mechanism of Action Synthetic allylamine derivative which inhibits squalene epoxidase, a key enzyme in sterol biosynthesis in fungi. This results in a deficiency in ergosterol within the fungal cell wall and results in fungal cell death.

Pharmacokinetics (Adult data unless noted)
Absorption: Children and Adults: Limited (<5%)
Distribution: Distributed to sebum and skin predominantly
Half-life: 14-35 hours

Dosing: Usual
Cream, gel, solution: Children ≥12 years and Adults:
Athlete's foot (tinea pedis): OTC/prescription formulations: Apply to affected area twice daily for at least 1 week, not to exceed 4 weeks
Ringworm (tinea corporis) and jock itch (tinea cruris): OTC formulations: Apply cream to affected area once or twice daily for at least 1 week, not to exceed 4 weeks; apply gel or solution once daily for 7 days
Cream, solution: Adults: Tinea versicolor: Prescription formulation: Apply to affected area twice daily for 1 week

Administration Apply to clean, dry affected area in sufficient quantity to cover; avoid contact with eyes, nose, mouth, or other mucous membranes. Do not use occlusive dressings.

Dosage Forms Excipient information presented when available (limited, particularly for generics); consult specific product labeling.
Cream, External, as hydrochloride:
LamISIL AT: 1% (12 g, 24 g, 30 g, 36 g, 42 g) [contains benzyl alcohol, cetyl alcohol]
LamISIL AT Jock Itch: 1% (12 g) [contains benzyl alcohol, cetyl alcohol]
Generic: 1% (12 g, 15 g, 24 g, 30 g)
Gel, External:
LamISIL Advanced: 1% (12 g) [contains alcohol, usp]
Solution, External, as hydrochloride:
LamISIL AT Spray: 1% (30 mL, 125 mL) [contains alcohol, usp, propylene glycol]
LamISIL Spray: 1% (30 mL) [contains alcohol, usp]

◆ **Terbinafine Hydrochloride** *see* Terbinafine (Systemic) *on page 1982*

◆ **Terbinafine Hydrochloride** *see* Terbinafine (Topical) *on page 1984*

◆ **Terbinex** *see* Terbinafine (Systemic) *on page 1982*

Terbutaline (ter BYOO ta leen)

Medication Safety Issues
Sound-alike/look-alike issues:
Brethine may be confused with Methergine®
Terbutaline may be confused with terbinafine, TOLBUTamide

Terbutaline and methylergonovine parenteral dosage forms look similar. Due to their contrasting indications, use care when administering these agents.

Related Information
Management of Drug Extravasations *on page 2255*
Brand Names: Canada Bricanyl® Turbuhaler®
Therapeutic Category Adrenergic Agonist Agent; Anti-asthmatic; Beta$_2$-Adrenergic Agonist; Bronchodilator; Sympathomimetic; Tocolytic Agent
Generic Availability (U.S.) Yes
Use Bronchodilator for relief of reversible bronchospasm in patients with asthma, bronchitis, and emphysema
Pregnancy Risk Factor C
Pregnancy Considerations Adverse events have been observed in animal reproduction studies. Terbutaline crosses the placenta; umbilical cord concentrations are ~11% to 48% of maternal blood levels.

Uncontrolled asthma is associated with adverse events on pregnancy (increased risk of perinatal mortality, pre-eclampsia, preterm birth, low birth weight infants). Terbutaline is not recommended for the treatment of asthma during pregnancy; inhaled beta$_2$-receptor agonists are preferred (NAEPP, 2005).

[U.S. Boxed Warning]: Terbutaline is not FDA approved for and should not be used for prolonged tocolysis (>48-72 hours). Use for maintenance tocolysis should not be done in the outpatient setting. Adverse events observed in pregnant women include arrhythmias, increased heart rate, hyperglycemia (transient), hypokalemia, myocardial ischemia, and pulmonary edema. Heart rate may be increased in the fetus and hypoglycemia may occur in the neonate. Terbutaline has been used in the management of preterm labor. Tocolytics may be used for the short-term (48 hour) prolongation of pregnancy to allow for the administration of antenatal steroids and should not be used prior to fetal viability or when the risks of use to the fetus or mother are greater than the risk of preterm birth (ACOG, 2012).

Breast-Feeding Considerations Terbutaline is excreted in breast milk; concentrations are similar to or higher than those in the maternal plasma. Based on information from four cases, exposure to the breast-fed infant would be <1% of the weight-adjusted maternal dose. Adverse events were not observed in nursing infants (Boréus, 1982; Lönnerholm, 1982). The manufacturer recommends that terbutaline be used in breast-feeding women only if the potential benefit to the mother outweighs the possible risk to the infant. The use of beta$_2$-receptor agonists are not considered a contraindication to breast-feeding (NAEPP, 2005).

Contraindications Hypersensitivity to terbutaline, other sympathomimetic amines, or any component; cardiac arrhythmias associated with tachycardia; tachycardia caused by digitalis intoxication
Injection: Additional contraindications: Prolonged (>72 hours) prevention or management of preterm labor
Oral: Additional contraindications: Prevention or treatment of preterm labor
Warnings Terbutaline is not FDA approved for and should not be used for prolonged tocolysis (>48-72 hours) **[U.S. Boxed Warning]**; use for maintenance tocolysis should not be done in the outpatient setting. Adverse events observed in pregnant women include arrhythmias, increased heart rate, hyperglycemia (transient), hypokalemia, myocardial ischemia, and pulmonary edema. Heart rate may be increased in the fetus and hypoglycemia may occur in the neonate. Oral terbutaline is contraindicated for acute or chronic use in the management of preterm labor. Paradoxical bronchoconstriction may occur with excessive use; if it occurs, discontinue terbutaline immediately

Precautions Use with caution in patients with diabetes mellitus, hypertension, hyperthyroidism, history of seizures, or cardiac disease; excessive or prolonged use may lead to tolerance. Children may experience a higher frequency of some adverse effects than adults, including: Congestion, cough, fever, nasopharyngitis, pharyngeal pain, rhinorrhea, toothache, and vomiting.
Adverse Reactions
Cardiovascular: Hypertension, pounding heartbeat, tachycardia
Central nervous system: Nervousness, restlessness
Endocrine & metabolic: Decreased serum potassium, increased serum glucose
Gastrointestinal: Bad taste in mouth, dry mouth, nausea, vomiting
Neuromuscular & skeletal: Dizziness, drowsiness, headache, insomnia, lightheadedness, muscle cramps, trembling, weakness
Miscellaneous: Diaphoresis
Rare but important or life-threatening: Arrhythmia, cardiac arrest (preterm labor), chest pain, hyperglycemia (preterm labor), hypokalemia (preterm labor), hypotension (preterm labor), paradoxical bronchospasm, myocardial infarction (preterm labor), myocardial ischemia (preterm labor), pulmonary edema (preterm labor)
Drug Interactions
Metabolism/Transport Effects None known.
Avoid Concomitant Use
Avoid concomitant use of Terbutaline with any of the following: Beta-Blockers (Nonselective); Iobenguane I 123
Increased Effect/Toxicity
Terbutaline may increase the levels/effects of: Atosiban; Loop Diuretics; Sympathomimetics; Thiazide Diuretics

The levels/effects of Terbutaline may be increased by: AtoMOXetine; Cannabinoid-Containing Products; Linezolid; MAO Inhibitors; Tricyclic Antidepressants
Decreased Effect
Terbutaline may decrease the levels/effects of: Iobenguane I 123

The levels/effects of Terbutaline may be decreased by: Beta-Blockers (Beta1 Selective); Beta-Blockers (Nonselective); Betahistine
Mechanism of Action Relaxes bronchial and uterine smooth muscle by action on beta$_2$-receptors with less effect on heart rate
Pharmacodynamics
Onset of action:
Oral: 30 minutes
Oral inhalation: 5-30 minutes
SubQ: 6-15 minutes
Duration:
Oral: 4-8 hours
Oral inhalation: 3-6 hours
SubQ: 1.5-4 hours
Pharmacokinetics (Adult data unless noted)
Absorption: 33% to 50%
Distribution: Breast milk to plasma ratio: <2.9
Metabolism: Possible first-pass metabolism after oral use
Half-life: 5.7 hours (range: 2.9-14 hours)
Time to peak serum concentration: SubQ: 0.5 hours
Elimination: Primarily (60%) unchanged in urine after parenteral use
Dosing: Usual
Children <12 years:
Oral: Initial: 0.05 mg/kg/dose every 8 hours, increase gradually, up to 0.15 mg/kg/dose; maximum daily dose: 5 mg
SubQ: 0.005-0.01 mg/kg/dose to a maximum of 0.4 mg/dose every 15-20 minutes for 3 doses; may repeat every 2-6 hours as needed

Note: Continuous I.V. infusion has been used successfully in children with asthma; a 2-10 mcg/kg loading dose followed by an 0.08-0.4 mcg/kg/minute continuous infusion; depending upon the clinical response, the dosage may require titration in increments of 0.1-0.2 mcg/kg/minute every 30 minutes; doses as high as 10 mcg/kg/minute have been used.

Children ≥12 years and Adults:
Oral: 2.5-5 mg/dose every 6-8 hours; maximum daily dose:
12-15 years: 7.5 mg
>15 years: 15 mg
SubQ: 0.25 mg/dose repeated in 20 minutes for 3 doses; a total dose of 0.75 mg should not be exceeded
Nebulization: Children and Adults: 0.01-0.03 mL/kg (1 mg = 1 mL using injection); minimum dose: 0.1 mL; maximum dose: 2.5 mL every 4-6 hours

Administration
Oral: May administer without regard to food
Parenteral: May administer undiluted, direct I.V. over 5-10 minutes; for continuous infusion, dilute to a maximum concentration of 1 mg/mL in D_5W or NS
Inhalation: Nebulization: Dilute dose with 1-2 mL NS

Monitoring Parameters Heart rate, blood pressure, respiratory rate, serum potassium, arterial or capillary blood gases (if applicable)

Dosage Forms Excipient information presented when available (limited, particularly for generics); consult specific product labeling.
Solution, Injection, as sulfate:
Generic: 1 mg/mL (1 mL)
Tablet, Oral, as sulfate:
Generic: 2.5 mg, 5 mg

Extemporaneous Preparations A 1 mg/mL oral suspension may be made with tablets. Crush twenty-four 5 mg tablets in a mortar and reduce to a fine powder. Add 5 mL purified water USP and mix to a uniform paste; mix while adding simple syrup, NF in incremental proportions to **almost** 120 mL; transfer to a calibrated bottle, rinse mortar with vehicle, and add quantity of simple syrup, NF sufficient to make 120 mL. Label "shake well" and "refrigerate". Stable for 30 days.
Nahata MC, Pai VB, and Hipple TF, *Pediatric Drug Formulations*, 5th ed, Cincinnati, OH: Harvey Whitney Books Co, 2004.

References
ACOG Practice Bulletin No. 127: "Management of Preterm Labor,"*Obstet Gynecol*, 2012, 119(6):1308.
Bohn D, Kalloghlian A, Jenkins J, et al, "Intravenous Salbutamol in the Treatment of Status Asthmaticus in Children," *Crit Care Med*, 1984, 12(10):892-6.
Boréus LO and de Château PU, "Terbutaline in Breast Milk," *Br J Clin Pharmacol*, 1982, 13(5):731-2.
Canny GJ and Levison H, "Aerosols - Therapeutic Use and Delivery in Childhood Asthma," *Ann Allergy*, 1988, 60(1):11-9.
Expert Panel Report 2, "Guidelines for the Diagnosis and Management of Asthma," *Clinical Practice Guidelines*, National Institutes of Health, National Heart, Lung, and Blood Institute, NIH Publication No. 94-4051, April, 1997.
Fuglsang G, Pedersen S, and Borgstrom L, "Dose-Response Relationships of I.V. Administered Terbutaline in Children With Asthma," *J Pediatr*, 1989, 114(2):315-20.
Goldenhersh M and Rachelefsky GS, "Childhood Asthma: Management," *Pediatr Rev*, 1989, 10(9):259-67.
"Guidelines for the Diagnosis and Management of Asthma. NAEPP Expert Panel Report 3," August 2007, www.nhlbi.nih.gov/guidelines/asthma/asthgdln.pdf.
Hearne AE and Nagey DA, "Therapeutic Agents in Preterm Labor: Tocolytic Agents," *Clin Obstet Gynecol*, 2000, 43(4):787-801.
Lönnerholm G and Lindström B, "Terbutaline Excretion Into Breast Milk," *Br J Clin Pharmacol*, 1982, 13(5):729-30.
National Asthma Education and Prevention Program (NAEPP), "Expert Panel Report 3 (EPR-3): Guidelines for the Diagnosis and Management of Asthma," *Clinical Practice Guidelines*, National Institutes of Health, National Heart, Lung, and Blood Institute, NIH Publication No. 08-4051, prepublication 2007; available at http://www.nhlbi.nih.gov/guidelines/asthma/asthgdln.htm.
National Asthma Education and Prevention Program (NAEPP) Working Group Report on "Managing Asthma During Pregnancy:

Recommendations for Pharmacologic Treatment," National Institutes of Health, National Heart, Lung, and Blood Institute, NIH Publication No. 05-5236, March 2005. Available at http://www.nhlbi.nih.gov/health/prof/lung/asthma/astpreg/astpreg_full.pdf
Rachelefsky GS and Siegel SC, "Asthma in Infants and Children - Treatment of Childhood Asthma: Part II," *J Allergy Clin Immunol*, 1985, 76(3):409-25.
Tipton WR and Nelson HS, "Frequent Parenteral Terbutaline in the Treatment of Status Asthmaticus in Children," *Ann Allergy*, 1987, 58 (4):252-6.

◆ **Terbutaline Sulfate** *see* Terbutaline *on page 1984*

◆ **Terfluzine (Can)** *see* Trifluoperazine *on page 2082*

◆ **Tersa Tar Shp [OTC] (Can)** *see* Coal Tar *on page 532*

◆ **Tersi** *see* Selenium Sulfide *on page 1877*

◆ **TESPA** *see* Thiotepa *on page 2014*

◆ **Testim** *see* Testosterone *on page 1986*

◆ **Testopel** *see* Testosterone *on page 1986*

Testosterone (tes TOS ter one)

Medication Safety Issues
Sound-alike/look-alike issues:
Testosterone may be confused with testolactone
Testoderm may be confused with Estraderm
AndroGel 1% may be confused with AndroGel 1.62%
Bio-T-Gel may be confused with T-Gel

BEERS Criteria medication:
This drug may be potentially inappropriate for use in geriatric patients (Quality of evidence - moderate; Strength of recommendation - weak).

Other safety concerns:
Transdermal patch may contain conducting metal (eg, aluminum); remove patch prior to MRI.

Related Information
Safe Handling of Hazardous Drugs *on page 2419*

Brand Names: U.S. Androderm; AndroGel; AndroGel Pump; Aveed; Axiron; Depo-Testosterone; First-Testosterone; First-Testosterone MC; Fortesta; Striant; Testim; Testopel; Vogelxo; Vogelxo Pump

Brand Names: Canada Andriol; Androderm; AndroGel; Andropository; Delatestryl; Depotest 100; Everone 200; PMS-Testosterone; Testim

Therapeutic Category Androgen

Generic Availability (U.S.) May be product dependent

Use
Parenteral:
Cypionate injection: Testosterone hormone replacement therapy in males for conditions associated with a deficiency or absence of endogenous testosterone; primary hypogonadism (congenital or acquired) and hypogonadotropic hypogonadism (congenital or acquired) (All indications: FDA approved in ages ≥12 years and adults)
Enanthate injection:
Male patients: Testosterone hormone replacement therapy in males for conditions associated with a deficiency or absence of endogenous testosterone; primary hypogonadism (congenital or acquired) and hypogonadotropic hypogonadism (congenital or acquired); delayed puberty (All indications: FDA approved in adolescents and adults)
Female patients: Inoperable metastatic breast cancer (FDA approved in adults)
Pellet (subcutaneous implant): Testosterone hormone replacement therapy in males for conditions associated with a deficiency or absence of endogenous testosterone; primary hypogonadism (congenital or acquired) and hypogonadotropic hypogonadism (congenital or acquired) (All indications: FDA approved in adolescents and adults)
Buccal system, topical gel, topical solution, transdermal system: Testosterone hormone replacement therapy in

males for conditions associated with a deficiency or absence of endogenous testosterone; primary hypogonadism (congenital or acquired) and hypogonadotropic hypogonadism(congenital or acquired) (All indications: FDA approved in ages ≥18 years and adults)

Medication Guide Available Yes

Pregnancy Risk Factor X

Pregnancy Considerations Testosterone may cause adverse effects, including masculinization of the female fetus, if used during pregnancy. Females who are or may become pregnant should also avoid skin-to-skin contact to areas where testosterone has been applied topically on another person.

Breast-Feeding Considerations High levels of endogenous maternal testosterone, such as those caused by certain ovarian cysts, suppress milk production. Maternal serum testosterone levels generally fall following pregnancy and return to normal once breast-feeding is stopped. The amount of testosterone present in breast milk or the effect to the nursing infant following maternal supplementation is not known. Some products are contraindicated while breast-feeding. Females who are nursing should avoid skin-to-skin contact to areas where testosterone has been applied topically on another person.

Contraindications Hypersensitivity to testosterone or any component (see manufacturer labeling for specific information); males with known or suspected carcinoma of the breast or prostate; specific products are contraindicated in women (see manufacturer labeling)

Depo®-Testosterone: Serious renal, hepatic, or cardiac disease

Warnings Hazardous agent; use appropriate precautions for handling and disposal (NIOSH, 2012). May accelerate bone maturation without producing compensating gain in linear growth; in prepubertal children perform radiographic examination of the hand and wrist every 6 months to determine the rate of bone maturation and to assess the effect of treatment on the epiphyseal centers. Virilization in children has been reported following contact with unwashed or unclothed application sites of men using the topical testosterone **[U.S. Boxed Warning]**; symptoms include advanced bone age, aggressive behavior, enlargement of clitoris requiring surgery, enlargement of penis, erections increased, libido increased, pubic hair development. Patients should strictly adhere to instructions for use in order to prevent secondary exposure. Virilization of female sexual partners has also been reported with male use of the topical testosterone. Symptoms of virilization generally regress following removal of exposure; however, some children did not fully return to age appropriate normal. Signs of inappropriate virilization in women or children following secondary exposure to topical testosterone should be brought to the attention of a healthcare provider. In the event that unwashed or unclothed skin comes in direct contact with testosterone gel, wash with soap and water. In females being treated for metastatic breast cancer, virilization may occur; monitor for signs of virilization; discontinue if mild virilization is present to prevent irreversible symptoms. High initial doses may cause priapism in adolescent males.

Urethral obstruction may develop in patients with BPH; discontinue therapy if occurs; may increase risk of prostatic cancer. If restarted a lower dose should be used. Withhold therapy pending urological evaluation in patients with palpable prostate nodule or induration, PSA >4 ng/mL, or PSA >3 ng/mL in men at high risk of prostate cancer (Bhasin, 2010). Prolonged use of high doses of androgens has been associated with serious hepatic effects (peliosis hepatis, hepatic neoplasms, cholestatic hepatitis, jaundice). Prolonged use of intramuscular testosterone enanthate has been associated with multiple hepatic adenomas. May cause reversible increases in hematocrit

(polycythemia) due to increases of red blood cell mass which may increase risk of thromboembolic events; monitor hematocrit at baseline, 3-6 months after initiation and then annually; discontinue therapy if hematocrit exceeds 54%; may require reinitiation at a lower dose (Bhasin, 2010).

Some dosage forms (see manufacturer's labeling) contain benzyl alcohol which may cause allergic reactions in susceptible individuals; large amounts of benzyl alcohol (≥99 mg/kg/day) have been associated with a potentially fatal toxicity ("gasping syndrome") in neonates; in vitro and animal studies have shown that benzoate, a metabolite of benzyl alcohol, displaces bilirubin from protein binding sites. Some testosterone products may be chemically synthesized from soy which may cause allergic reactions in susceptible individuals. May contain other excipients (eg, sesame oil cottonseed oil) which may cause allergic reactions in susceptible individuals (see manufacturer's labeling). Some products may contain ethanol (see manufacturer's labeling); patients should be instructed on appropriate storage and application precautions to avoid heat and flame. Fortesta™ is not interchangeable with other topical testosterone products. AndroGel® 1% and AndroGel® 1.62% are not interchangeable. Axiron® is not interchangeable with other topical testosterone products; safety and efficacy of Axiron® use in male patients with BMI >35 kg/m² has not been established. Transdermal patch may contain conducting metal (eg, aluminum) which may cause a burn to the skin during an MRI scan; remove patch prior to MRI; reapply patch after scan is completed.

Precautions Use with caution in patients with conditions influenced by edema (eg, cardiovascular disease, migraine, seizure disorder, renal or hepatic impairment) or medications that enhance edema formation (eg, corticosteroids); testosterone may cause fluid retention. Use with caution in obesity or chronic lung disease; may potentiate sleep apnea. Use with caution in diabetes; testosterone may alter insulin sensitivity and glycemic control; additionally, the anabolic activity of testosterone activity may enhance hypoglycemia. Use caution with history of MI or coronary artery disease; may alter lipid profile. Use with caution in cancer or immobile patients; may cause hypercalcemia associated with hypercalciuria; monitor serum calcium concentrations. May cause gynecomastia in male patients. Long-term effects on gum safety when using the buccal formulation are not available; instruct patients to regularly inspect gum region where buccal formulation has been applied.

Adverse Reactions

Cardiovascular: Decreased blood pressure, deep vein thrombosis, edema, hypertension, increased blood pressure, vasodilatation

Central nervous system: Abnormal dreams, aggressive behavior, altered sense of smell, amnesia, anxiety, chills, depression, dizziness, emotional lability, excitement, fatigue, headache, hostility, insomnia, irritability, malaise, mood swings, nervousness, outbursts of anger, paresthesia, seizure, sleep apnea, suicidal ideation, taste disorder

Dermatologic: Acne vulgaris, alopecia, contact dermatitis, diaphoresis, erythema, folliculitis, hair discoloration, hyperhidrosis, pruritus, seborrhea, skin rash, xeroderma

Endocrine & metabolic: Change in libido, decreased gonadotropin, fluid retention, gynecomastia, hirsutism (increase in pubic hair growth), hot flash, hypercalcemia, hyperchloremia, hypercholesterolemia, hyperglycemia, hyperkalemia, hyperlipidemia, hypernatremia, hypoglycemia, hypokalemia, increased plasma estradiol concentration, inorganic phosphate retention, menstrual disease (including amenorrhea), weight gain

Gastrointestinal: Diarrhea, gastroesophageal reflux disease, gastrointestinal hemorrhage, gastrointestinal irritation, increased appetite, nausea, vomiting

Following buccal administration (most common): Dysgeusia, gingival pain, gingival swelling, mouth irritation (including gums), unpleasant taste

Genitourinary: Benign prostatic hypertrophy, difficulty in micturition, ejaculatory disorder, hematuria, impotence, irritable bladder, mastalgia, oligospermia, priapism, prostate induration, prostate specific antigen increase, prostatitis, spontaneous erections, testicular atrophy, urinary tract infection, virilization

Hepatic: Abnormal hepatic function tests, cholestatic hepatitis, cholestatic jaundice, hepatic insufficiency, hepatic necrosis, hepatocellular neoplasms, increased serum bilirubin, peliosis hepatis

Hematologic & oncologic: Anemia, clotting factors suppression, hemorrhage, increased hematocrit, increased hemoglobin, leukopenia, malignant neoplasm of prostate, polycythemia, prostate carcinoma

Hypersensitivity: Anaphylactoid reaction, hypersensitivity reaction (including pulmomary oil microembolism)

Local: Application site reaction (gel, solution), erythema at injection site, inflammation at injection site, pain at injection site

Transdermal system: Application site burning, application site erythema, application site induration, application site pruritus, application site vesicles (including burn-like blisters under system), local allergic contact dermatitis, local skin exfoliation

Neuromuscular & skeletal: Abnormal bone growth (accelerated), arthralgia, back pain, hemarthrosis, hyperkinesia, weakness

Ophthalmic: Increased lacrimation

Renal: Increased serum creatinine, polyuria

Respiratory: Bronchitis (≥3%), nasopharyngitis (≥3%), sinusitis (≥3%), upper respiratory tract infection (≥3%), dyspnea

Rare but important or life-threatening: Injection, gel: Abnormal erythropoiesis, abscess at injection site, anaphylactic shock, anaphylaxis, androgenetic alopecia, angina pectoris, asthma, cardiac arrest, cardiac failure, cerebral infarction, cerebrovascular accident, cerebrovascular insufficiency, chest pain, chronic obstructive pulmonary disease, circulatory shock, cognitive dysfunction, confusion, coronary occlusion, diabetes mellitus, epididymitis, hearing loss (sudden), hematoma at injection site, hyperparathyroidism, hypersensitivity angiitis, hypertriglyceridemia, impaired glucose tolerance, increased intraocular pressure, Korsakoff's psychosis (nonalcoholic), migraine, myocardial infarction, nephrolithiasis, osteoporosis, personality disorder, prolonged partial thromboplastin time, prolonged prothrombin time, prostatic intraepithelial neoplasia, pulmonary embolism pure red cell aplasia, renal colic, respiratory distress, reversible ischemic neurological deficit, spermatocele, systemic lupus erythematosus, tachycardia, thrombocytopenia, thromboembolism, thrombosis, transient ischemic attacks, urinary incontinence, urolithiasis, venous insufficiency, vesicobullous rash, virilization (of children, following secondary exposure to topical gel [advanced bone age, aggressive behavior, enlargement of clitoris requiring surgery, enlargement of penis, increased erections, increased libido, pubic hair development]), vitreous detachment

Drug Interactions

Metabolism/Transport Effects Substrate of CYP2B6 (minor), CYP2C19 (minor), CYP2C9 (minor), CYP3A4 (minor); **Note:** Assignment of Major/Minor substrate status based on clinically relevant drug interaction potential

Avoid Concomitant Use

Avoid concomitant use of Testosterone with any of the following: Dehydroepiandrosterone

Increased Effect/Toxicity

Testosterone may increase the levels/effects of: Antidiabetic Agents; CycloSPORINE (Systemic); Vitamin K Antagonists

The levels/effects of Testosterone may be increased by: Corticosteroids (Systemic); Dehydroepiandrosterone

Decreased Effect There are no known significant interactions involving a decrease in effect.

Stability Hazardous agent; use appropriate precautions for handling and disposal (NIOSH, 2012).

Androderm®: Store at room temperature. Do not store outside of pouch; excessive heat may cause system to burst.

AndroGel® 1%, AndroGel® 1.62%, Axiron®, Delatestryl®, Striant®, Testim®: Store at room temperature.

Depo® Testosterone: Store at room temperature; protect from light.

Fortesta™: Store at room temperature; do not freeze.

Testopel®: Store in a cool, dry location.

Mechanism of Action Principal endogenous androgen responsible for promoting the growth and development of the male sex organs and maintaining secondary sex characteristics in androgen-deficient males

Pharmacodynamics Duration (route and ester dependent): Cypionate and enanthate esters (I.M. administration) have the longest duration: ≤2-4 weeks; pellets: 3-4 months; gel: 24-48 hours

Pharmacokinetics (Adult data unless noted)

Absorption: Transdermal gel: ~10%

Protein binding: 98%, bound to sex hormone-binding globulin (40%) and albumin

Metabolism: Hepatic; forms metabolites including estradiol and dihydrotestosterone (DHT); both are active

Half-life: Variable: 10-100 minutes; Cypionate: I.M.: 8 days

Elimination: Urine (90%), feces (6%)

Dosing: Usual

Infants, Children ≥12 years, and Adolescents <18 years: **Note:** Dosage and duration of therapy depend upon age, sex, diagnosis, patient's response to therapy, and appearance of adverse effects; in general total doses >400 mg/month are not required due to the prolonged action of the drug.

Delayed puberty: Children ≥12 years and Adolescents: Typically not recommended for use before 14 years of age (Palmert, 2012)

I.M.:

Manufacturer labeling: Enanthate: 50-200 mg every 2-4 weeks; usual duration 4-6 months; various regimens evaluated, some begin with high initial doses and taper down as puberty progresses, and others begin low and titrate upward to effect and then taper

Alternate dosing: Initial: Enanthate or cypionate: 50 mg/dose every 4 weeks for 3-6 months; may increase dose in 25-50 mg increments for another 3-6 months to effect; maximum dose: 100 mg; typical duration of therapy: 12 months; if no response or inadequate response after 1 year of treatment, diagnosis should be reconsidered and additional testing performed (Palmert, 2012)

Subcutaneous implant: Pellet: Usual range: 150-450 mg every 3-6 months; usual duration: 4-6 months; dosing typically on the lower end of range; various regimens have been used

Male hypogonadism: Children ≥12 years and Adolescents:

I.M.: Enanthate or cypionate:

Initiation of pubertal growth: 25-75 mg every 3-4 weeks, gradually titrate dose every 6-9 months to 100-150 mg; typical duration of initiation therapy 3-4 years (Han, 2010; Wales, 2011)

Maintenance therapy: 200-250 mg every 3-4 weeks; once expected adult height and adequate virilization achieved, may convert to other testosterone replacement dosage form (eg, patch, gel, etc) (Han, 2010; Wales, 2011)

Subcutaneous implant: Pellet:

Manufacturer's labeling: Usual range: 150-450 mg every 3-6 months; various regimens have been used

Alternate dosing: 8-10 mg/kg/dose every 6 months (Zacharin, 1997)

Multiple pituitary hormone deficiency (with microphallus): Limited data available: Infants: I.M.: Enanthate or cypionate: 25 mg every 4 weeks for 1-3 months

Adolescents ≥18 years and Adults:

Inoperable metastatic breast cancer (females): I.M.: Enanthate: 200-400 mg every 2-4 weeks

Hypogonadism or hypogonadotropic hypogonadism (males):

I.M.: Enanthate or cypionate: 50-400 mg every 2-4 weeks (FDA-approved dosing range); 75-100 mg/week or 150-200 mg every 2 weeks (Bhasin, 2010)

Subcutaneous implant: Pellet: 150-450 mg every 3-6 months

Topical:

Buccal: 30 mg twice daily (every 12 hours) applied to the gum region above the incisor tooth

Gel: Apply to clean, dry, intact skin. **Do not apply testosterone gel to the genitals.**

AndroGel® 1%: 50 mg applied once daily in the morning to the shoulder and upper arms or abdomen. Dosage may be increased to a maximum of 100 mg.

Dose adjustment based on testosterone levels:

Less than normal range: Increase dose from 50 mg to 75 mg or from 75 mg to 100 mg once daily

Greater than normal range: Decrease dose. Discontinue if consistently above normal at 50 mg daily

AndroGel® 1.62%: 40.5 mg applied once daily in the morning to the shoulder and upper arms. Dosage may be increased to a maximum of 81 mg

Dose adjustment based on testosterone levels:

>750 ng/dL: Decrease dose by 20.25 mg/day

350-750 ng/dL: Maintain current dose

<350 ng/dL: Increase dose by 20.25 mg/day

Fortesta™: 40 mg once daily in the morning. Apply to the thighs. Dosing range: 10-70 mg/day

Dose adjustment based on serum testosterone levels:

≥2500 ng/dL: Decrease dose by 20 mg/day

1250 to <2500 ng/dL: Decrease dose by 10 mg/day

500 and <1250 ng/dL: Maintain current dose

<500 ng/dL: Increase dose by 10 mg/day

Testim®: 5 g (containing 50 mg of testosterone) applied once daily (preferably in the morning) to the shoulder and upper arms. Dosage may be increased to a maximum of 10 g (containing 100 mg of testosterone) daily

Dose adjustment based on testosterone levels:

Less than normal range: Increase dose from 5 g (50 mg testosterone) to 10 g (100 mg testosterone) once daily

Greater than normal range: Decrease dose. Discontinue if consistently above normal at 5 g (50 mg testosterone) daily

Solution (Axiron®): 60 mg once daily; dosage range: 30-120 mg/day. Apply to the axilla at the same time each morning; do not apply to other parts of the body. Apply to clean, dry, intact skin. **Do not apply testosterone solution to the genitals.**

Dose adjustment based on serum testosterone levels:

>1050 ng/dL: Decrease 60 mg/day dose to 30 mg/day; if levels >1050 ng/dL persist after dose reduction discontinue therapy

<300 ng/dL: Increase 60 mg/day dose to 90 mg/day, or increase 90 mg/day dose to 120 mg/day

Transdermal system (Androderm®): **Note:** Initial dose is either 4 mg/day or 5 mg/day and dose adjustment varies as follows:

Initial: 4 mg/day (as one 4 mg/day patch; do **not** use two 2 mg/day patches)

Dose adjustment based on testosterone levels:

>930 ng/dL: Decrease dose to 2 mg/day

400-930 ng/dL: Continue 4 mg/day

<400 ng/dL: Increase dose to 6 mg/day (as one 4 mg/day and one 2 mg/day patch)

Initial: 5 mg/day (as one 5 mg/day or two 2.5 mg/day patches)

Dose adjustment based on testosterone levels:

>1030 ng/dL: Decrease dose to 2.5 mg/day

300-1030 ng/dL: Continue 5 mg/day

<300 ng/dL: Increase dose to 7.5 mg/day (as one 5 mg/day and one 2.5 mg/day patch)

Dosing conversion: If needed, patients may be switched from the 2.5 mg/day, 5 mg/day, and 7.5 mg/day patches as follows. Patch change should occur at their next scheduled dosing. Measure early morning testosterone concentrations ~2 weeks after switching therapy:

From 2.5 mg/day patch to 2 mg/day patch

From 5 mg/day patch to 4 mg/day patch

From 7.5 mg/day patch to 6 mg/day patch (one 2 mg/day and one 4 mg/day patch)

Delayed puberty (males):

I.M.: Enanthate: 50-200 mg every 2-4 weeks for a limited duration

Pellet (for subcutaneous implantation): 150-450 mg every 3-6 months

Dosing adjustment in renal impairment: No dosage adjustment provided in manufacturer's labeling (has not been studied). Use with caution; may enhance edema formation.

Dosing adjustment in hepatic impairment: No dosage adjustment provided in manufacturer's labeling (has not been studied). Use with caution; may enhance edema formation.

Administration Hazardous agent; use appropriate precautions for handling and disposal (NIOSH, 2012).

Oral, buccal: Striant™: One mucoadhesive for buccal application (buccal system) should be applied to a comfortable area above the incisor tooth. Apply flat side of system on fingertip. Gently push the curved side against upper gum. Rotate to alternate sides of mouth with each application. Hold buccal system firmly in place for 30 seconds to ensure adhesion. The buccal system should adhere to gum for 12 hours. If the buccal system falls out, replace with a new system. If the system falls out within 4 hours of next dose, the new buccal system should remain in place until the time of the following scheduled dose. System will soften and mold to shape of gum as it absorbs moisture from mouth. Do not chew or swallow the buccal system; check to ensure buccal system is in place following toothbrushing, use of mouthwash, and consumption of food or beverages. The buccal system will not dissolve; gently remove by sliding downwards from gum; avoid scratching gum.

Parenteral: I.M. (cypionate, enanthate): Warming injection to room temperature and shaking vial will help redissolve crystals that have formed after storage. Administer by deep I.M. injection into the gluteal muscle.

Topical:

Transdermal patch: Androderm®: Apply patch to clean, dry area of skin on the back, abdomen, upper arms, or thigh. Do not apply to bony areas or parts of the body that are subject to prolonged pressure while sleeping or sitting. **Do not apply to the scrotum.** Avoid showering, washing the site, or swimming for 3 hours after application. Following patch removal, mild skin irritation may be treated with OTC hydrocortisone cream. A small amount of triamcinolone acetonide 0.1% cream may be applied under the system to decrease irritation; do not use ointment. Patch should be applied nightly. Rotate administration sites, allowing 7 days between applying to the same site.

Topical gel and solution: Apply to clean, dry, intact skin. Application sites should be allowed to dry for a few minutes prior to dressing. Hands should be washed with soap and water after application. **Do not apply testosterone gel or solution to the genitals.** Alcohol-based gels and solutions are flammable; avoid fire or smoking until dry. Testosterone may be transferred to another person following skin-to-skin contact with the application site. Strict adherence to application instructions is needed in order to decrease secondary exposure. Thoroughly wash hands after application and cover application site with clothing (ie, shirt) once gel or solution has dried, or clean application site thoroughly with soap and water prior to contact in order to minimize transfer. In addition to skin-to-skin contact, secondary exposure has also been reported following exposure to secondary items (eg, towel, shirt, sheets). If secondary exposure occurs, the other person should thoroughly wash the skin with soap and water as soon as possible.

AndroGel® 1%, AndroGel® 1.62%, Testim®: Apply (preferably in the morning) to clean, dry, intact skin of the shoulder and upper arms. AndroGel® 1% may also be applied to the abdomen; do not apply Andro-Gel® 1.62% or Testim® to the abdomen. Area of application should be limited to what will be covered by a short-sleeve t-shirt. Apply at the same time each day. Upon opening the packet(s), the entire contents should be squeezed into the palm of the hand and immediately applied to the application site(s). Alternatively, a portion may be squeezed onto palm of hand and applied, repeating the process until entire packet has been applied. Application site should not be washed for ≥2 hours following application of Andro-Gel® 1.62% or Testim®, or >5 hours for Andro-Gel® 1%.

AndroGel® 1% multidose pump: Prime pump 3 times (and discard this portion of product) prior to initial use. Each actuation delivers 12.5 mg of testosterone (4 actuations = 50 mg; 6 actuations = 75 mg; 8 actuations = 100 mg); each actuation may be applied individually or all at the same time. Application site should not be washed for >5 hours following application.

AndroGel® 1.62% multidose pump: Prime pump 3 times (and discard this portion of product) prior to initial use. Each actuation delivers 20.25 mg of gel (2 actuations = 40.5 mg; 3 actuations = 60.75 mg; 4 actuations = 81 mg); each actuation may be applied individually or all at the same time.

Axiron®: Apply using the applicator to the axilla at the same time each morning. Do not apply to other parts of the body (eg, abdomen, genitals, shoulders, upper arms). Avoid washing the site or swimming for 2 hours after application. Prior to first use, prime the applicator pump by depressing it 3 times (discard this portion of the product). After priming, position the nozzle over the applicator cup and depress pump fully one time; ensure liquid enters cup. Each pump actuation delivers testosterone 30 mg. No more than 30 mg (one pump) should be added to the cup at one time. The total dose should be divided between axilla (eg, 30 mg/day: Apply to one axilla only; 60 mg/day: Apply 30 mg to each axilla; 90 mg/day: Apply 30 mg to each axilla, allow to dry, then apply an additional 30 mg to one axilla; etc). To apply dose, keep applicator upright and wipe into the axilla; if solution runs or drips, use cup to wipe. Do not rub into skin with fingers or hand. If more than one 30 mg dose is needed, repeat process. Apply roll-on or stick antiperspirants or deodorants prior to testosterone. Once application site is dry, cover with clothing. After use, rinse applicator under running water and pat dry with a tissue. The application site and dose of this product are not interchangeable with other topical testosterone products.

Fortesta™: Apply to skin of front and inner thighs. Do not apply to other parts of the body. Use one finger to rub gel evenly onto skin of each thigh. Avoid showering, washing the site, or swimming for 2 hours after application. Prior to first dose, prime the pump by holding canister upright and fully depressing the pump 8 times (discard this portion of the product). Each pump actuation delivers testosterone 10 mg. The total dose should be divided between thighs (eg, 10 mg/day: Apply 10 mg to one thigh only; 20 mg/day: Apply 10 mg to each thigh; 30 mg/day: Apply 20 mg to one thigh and 10 mg to the other thigh; etc). Once application site is dry, cover with clothing. The application site and dose of this product are not interchangeable with other topical testosterone products.

Monitoring Parameters Periodic liver function tests, cholesterol, hemoglobin and hematocrit (prior to therapy, at 3-6 months, then annually); radiologic examination of wrist and hand every 6 months (when using in prepubertal children). Withhold initial treatment with hematocrit >50%, hyperviscosity, untreated obstructive sleep apnea, or uncontrolled severe heart failure. Monitor urine and serum calcium and signs of virilization in women treated for breast cancer. Serum glucose (may be decreased by testosterone, monitor patients with diabetes). Evaluate males for response to treatment and adverse events 3-6 months after initiation and then annually.

Bone mineral density: Monitor after 1-2 years of therapy in hypogonadal men with osteoporosis or low trauma fracture (Bhasin, 2010)

Adults:

PSA: In men >40 years of age with baseline PSA >0.6 ng/mL, PSA and prostate exam (prior to therapy, at 3-6 months, then as based on current guidelines). Withhold treatment pending urological evaluation in patients with palpable prostate nodule or induration or PSA >4 ng/mL or if PSA >3 ng/mL in men at high risk of prostate cancer (Bhasin, 2010).

Do not treat with severe untreated BPH with IPSS symptom score >19.

Serum testosterone: After initial dose titration (if applicable), monitor 3-6 months after initiating treatment, then annually

Injection: Measure midway between injections. Adjust dose or frequency if testosterone concentration is <400 ng/dL or >700 ng/dL (Bhasin, 2010)

AndroGel® 1%, Testim®: Morning serum testosterone levels ~14 days after start of therapy or dose adjustments

AndroGel® 1.62%: Morning serum testosterone levels after 14 and 28 days of starting therapy or dose adjustments and periodically thereafter

Androderm®: Morning serum testosterone levels (following application the previous evening) ~14 days after start of therapy or dose adjustments

Axiron®: Serum testosterone levels can be measured 2-8 hours after application and after 14 days of starting therapy or dose adjustments

Fortesta™: Serum testosterone levels can be measured 2 hours after application and after 14 and 35 days of starting therapy or dose adjustments

Striant®: Application area of gums; total serum testosterone 4-12 weeks after initiating treatment, prior to morning dose

Testopel®: Measure at the end of the dosing interval (Bhasin, 2010)

Reference Range Total testosterone, males:

12-13 years: <800 ng/dL
14 years: <1200 ng/dL
15-16 years: 100-1200 ng/dL
17-18 years: 300-1200 ng/dL
19-40 years: 300-950 ng/dL
>40 years: 240-950 ng/dL

Free testosterone, males: 9-30 ng/dL

Test Interactions Testosterone may decrease thyroxine-binding globulin, resulting in decreased total T_4; free thyroid hormone levels are not changed.

Product Availability Natesto (testosterone nasal gel): FDA approved May 2014; anticipated availability is currently unknown.

Controlled Substance C-III

Dosage Forms Excipient information presented when available (limited, particularly for generics); consult specific product labeling.

Cream, Transdermal:
First-Testosterone MC: 2% (60 g) [contains benzyl alcohol, sesame oil]

Gel, Transdermal:
AndroGel: 25 mg/2.5 g (2.5 g); 50 mg/5 g (5 g); 40.5 mg/2.5 g (1.62%) (2.5 g); 20.25 mg/1.25 g (1.62%) (1.25 g) [contains alcohol, usp]
AndroGel Pump: 12.5 mg/actuation (1%) (75 g); 20.25 mg/actuation (1.62%) (75 g) [contains alcohol, usp]
Fortesta: 10 mg/actuation (2%) (60 g) [odorless; contains propylene glycol, trolamine (triethanolamine)]
Testim: 50 mg/5 g (5 g) [contains alcohol, usp, propylene glycol, tromethamine]
Vogelxo: 50 mg/5 g (5 g) [contains alcohol, usp, tromethamine]
Vogelxo Pump: 12.5 mg/actuation (1%) (75 g) [contains alcohol, usp, tromethamine]
Generic: 50 mg/5 g (5 g); 12.5 mg/actuation (1%) (75 g)

Miscellaneous, Buccal:
Striant: 30 mg (60 ea)

Oil, Intramuscular, as cypionate:
Depo-Testosterone: 100 mg/mL (10 mL); 200 mg/mL (1 mL, 10 mL) [contains benzyl alcohol, benzyl benzoate]
Generic: 100 mg/mL (10 mL); 200 mg/mL (1 mL, 10 mL)

Oil, Intramuscular, as enanthate:
Generic: 200 mg/mL (5 mL)

Ointment, Transdermal:
First-Testosterone: 2% (60 g) [contains benzyl alcohol, butylated hydroxytoluene (bht), petrolatum, sesame oil]

Patch 24 Hour, Transdermal:
Androderm: 2 mg/24 hr (1 ea, 60 ea); 4 mg/24 hr (1 ea, 30 ea)

Pellet, Implant:
Testopel: 75 mg (10 ea, 100 ea)

Solution, Transdermal:
Axiron: 30 mg/actuation (90 mL)

Solution, Intramuscular, as undecanoate:
Aveed: 750 mg/3 mL (3 mL) [contains benzyl benzoate, castor oil (ricine oil)]

References

Bhasin S, Cunningham GR, Hayes FJ, et al, "Testosterone Therapy in Men With Androgen Deficiency Syndromes: An Endocrine Society Clinical Practice Guideline," *J Clin Endocrinol Metab*, 2010, 95 (6):2536-59.

Han TS and Bouloux PM, "What Is the Optimal Therapy for Young Males With Hypogonadotropic Hypogonadism?" *Clin Endocrinol (Oxf)*, 2010, 72(6):731-7.

National Institute for Occupational Safety and Health (NIOSH), "NIOSH List of Antineoplastic and Other Hazardous Drugs in Healthcare Settings 2012." Available at http://www.cdc.gov/niosh/docs/2012-150/pdfs/2012-150.pdf. Accessed January 21, 2013.

Palmert MR and Dunkel L, "Clinical Practice. Delayed Puberty," *N Engl J Med*, 2012, 366(5):443-53.

Wales JK, "Disordered Pubertal Development," *Arch Dis Child Educ Pract Ed*, 2012, 97(1):9-16.

Zacharin MR and Warne GL, "Treatment of Hypogonadal Adolescent Boys With Long Acting Subcutaneous Testosterone Pellets," *Arch Dis Child*, 1997, 76(6):495-9.

◆ **Testosterone Cypionate** *see* Testosterone *on page 1986*

◆ **Testosterone Enanthate** *see* Testosterone *on page 1986*

◆ **Testosterone Undecanoate** *see* Testosterone *on page 1986*

◆ **Tetanus and Diphtheria Toxoid** *see* Diphtheria and Tetanus Toxoids *on page 679*

Tetanus Immune Globulin (Human)
(TET a nus i MYUN GLOB yoo lin HYU man)

Related Information

Immunization Administration Recommendations *on page 2368*

Immunization Guidelines *on page 2373*

Brand Names: U.S. HyperTET S/D

Brand Names: Canada HyperTET™ S/D

Therapeutic Category Immune Globulin

Generic Availability (U.S.) No

Use Prophylaxis for tetanus following injury in patients whose immunization for tetanus is incomplete or uncertain [FDA approved in pediatric patients (age not specified) and adults]

The Advisory Committee on Immunization Practices (ACIP) recommends passive immunization with tetanus immune globulin (TIG) for the following:

• Persons with a wound that is not clean or minor and in whom contraindications to a tetanus toxoid-containing vaccine exist and they have not completed a primary series of tetanus toxoid immunization.

• Persons who are wounded in bombings or similar mass casualty events who have penetrating injuries or non-intact skin exposure and who cannot confirm receipt of a tetanus booster within the previous 5 years. In case of shortage, use should be reserved for persons ≥60 years of age.

Pregnancy Risk Factor C

Pregnancy Considerations Animal reproduction studies have not been conducted. Tetanus immune globulin and a tetanus toxoid containing vaccine are recommended by the ACIP as part of the standard wound management to prevent tetanus in pregnant women.

Contraindications Hypersensitivity to tetanus immune globulin, thimerosal, or any component

Warnings As a product of human plasma, this product may potentially transmit infectious agents such as viruses; screening of donors, as well as testing and/or inactivation of certain viruses has reduced this risk. Infections thought to be transmitted by this product should be reported to the manufacturer. Although extremely rare, severe hypersensitivity reactions including anaphylaxis may occur; epinephrine and other anaphylactic treatment agents should be readily available. Not for I.V. administration; serious systemic reactions including hypotension have occurred with inadvertent I.V. administration.

Precautions Administer with caution to patients with thrombocytopenia or any coagulation disorder that would be compromised by I.M. injection; administer with caution in patients with IgA deficiency or a prior history of systemic allergic reactions following the administration of human immunoglobulin preparations. Skin testing should not be performed as local irritation can occur and be misinterpreted as a positive reaction.

Adverse Reactions

Central nervous system: Temperature increased

Dermatologic: Angioneurotic edema (rare)

Local: Injection site: Pain, soreness, tenderness

Renal: Nephritic syndrome (rare)

Miscellaneous: Anaphylactic shock (rare)

Drug Interactions

Metabolism/Transport Effects None known.

Avoid Concomitant Use There are no known interactions where it is recommended to avoid concomitant use.

Increased Effect/Toxicity There are no known significant interactions involving an increase in effect.

Decreased Effect

Tetanus Immune Globulin (Human) may decrease the levels/effects of: Vaccines (Live)

Stability Store at 2°C to 8°C (26°F to 46°F). Do not use if frozen. The following stability information has also been reported for HyperTET™ S/D: May be exposed to room temperature for a cumulative 7 days (Cohen, 2007).

Mechanism of Action Passive immunity toward tetanus

Pharmacodynamics Duration: A single dose may provide protection for up to 14 weeks

Pharmacokinetics (Adult data unless noted)

Absorption: Well absorbed

Time to peak serum concentration: 2 days

Dosing: Neonatal

Prophylaxis of tetanus: I.M.: 4 units/kg as a single dose; some experts recommend administering 250 units regardless of weight or age

Treatment of tetanus: I.M.: 500 units

Dosing: Usual

Prophylaxis of tetanus:

Infants and Children <7 years: I.M.: 4 units/kg as a single dose; some experts recommend administering 250 units regardless of weight or age

Children ≥7 years and Adults: I.M.: 250 units as a single dose; may be increased to 500 units if there has been a delay in initiating prophylaxis or when the wound is considered very tetanus prone

Note: Additional doses of TIG can be given at 4-week intervals in situations where the risk of tetanus infection persists.

Treatment of tetanus: Children and Adults: I.M.: 500-6000 units. Infiltration of part of the dose around the wound is recommended. Tetanus prophylaxis in patients with wounds should consider if the wound is clean or contaminated, the immunization status of the patient, proper use of tetanus toxoid and/or tetanus immune globulin (TIG), wound cleaning, and (if required) surgical debridement and the proper use of antibiotics. Patients with an uncertain or incomplete tetanus immunization status should have additional follow-up to ensure a series is completed. Patients with a history of Arthus reaction following a previous dose of a tetanus toxoid-containing vaccine should not receive a tetanus toxoid-containing vaccine until >10 years after the most recent dose even if they have a wound that is neither clean nor minor. See table.

Tetanus Prophylaxis Wound Management

History of Tetanus Immunization (Doses)	Clean, Minor Wounds		All Other Wounds[1]	
	Tetanus toxoid[2]	TIG	Tetanus toxoid[2]	TIG
Uncertain or <3 doses	Yes	No	Yes	Yes
3 or more doses	No[3]	No	No[4]	No

[1]Such as, but not limited to, wounds contaminated with dirt, feces, soil, and saliva; puncture wounds; wounds from crushing, tears, burns, and frostbite.

[2]Tetanus toxoid in this chart refers to a tetanus toxoid containing vaccine. For children <7 years old DTaP (DT, if pertussis vaccine contraindicated) is preferred to tetanus toxoid alone. For children ≥7 years of age and Adults, Td preferred to tetanus toxoid alone; Tdap may be preferred if the patient has not previously been vaccinated with Tdap.

[3]Yes, if ≥10 years since last dose.

[4]Yes, if ≥5 years since last dose.

Abbreviations: **DT** = Diphtheria and Tetanus Toxoids (formulation for age ≤6 years); **DTaP** = Diphtheria and Tetanus Toxoids, and Acellular Pertussis (formulation for age ≤6 years; Daptacel®, Infanrix®); **Td** = Diphtheria and Tetanus Toxoids (formulation for age ≥7 years; Decavac®, Tenivac™); **TT** = Tetanus toxoid (adsorbed [formulation for age ≥7 years]); **Tdap** = Diphtheria and Tetanus Toxoids, and Acellular Pertussis (Adacel® or Boostrix® [formulations for age ≥7 years]); TIG = Tetanus Immune Globulin

Adapted from the Yellow Book 2010, Chapter 2, *Routine Vaccine-Preventable Diseases, Tetanus*; Available at www.cdc.gov/yellowbook; and *MMWR*, 2006, 55:RR-17.

Administration I.M.: Administer into lateral aspect of mid-thigh or deltoid muscle of upper arm; **not for I.V. administration**. Avoid gluteal region due to risk of injury to sciatic nerve; if gluteal region is used, administer only in the upper outer quadrant. When administered for treatment of tetanus, may be infiltrated locally around the wound site. Do not administer tetanus toxoid and TIG in same syringe (toxoid will be neutralized); tetanus toxoid may be administered at the same time at a separate site.

Dosage Forms Excipient information presented when available (limited, particularly for generics); consult specific product labeling.

Injectable, Intramuscular:

HyperTET S/D: 250 units/mL (1 ea)

References

Centers for Disease Control, "Diphtheria, Tetanus, and Pertussis: Recommendations for Vaccine Use and Other Preventive Measures," *MMWR Recomm Rep*, 1991, 40(RR-10):1-28.

Centers for Disease Control, "Prevention of Pertussis, Tetanus, and Diphtheria Among Pregnant and Postpartum Women and Their Infants, Recommendations of the Advisory Committee on Immunization Practices (ACIP)," *MMWR Recomm Rep*, 2008, 57(early release):1-47. Available at http://www.cdc.gov/mmwr/preview/mmwrhtml/rr57e0514a1.htm?s_cid=rr57e0514a1_e

Centers for Disease Control, "Recommendations for Postexposure Interventions to Prevent Infection With Hepatitis B Virus, Hepatitis C Virus, or Human Immunodeficiency Virus, and Tetanus in Persons Wounded During Bombings and Other Mass-Casualty Events-United States, 2008: Recommendations of the Centers for Disease Control and Prevention (CDC)," *MMWR Recomm Rep*, 2008, 57(RR-6):1-21.

Cohen V, Jellinek SP, Teperikidis L, et al, "Room-Temperature Storage of Medications Labeled for Refrigeration," *Am J Health-Syst Pharm*, 2007, 64(16):1711-15.

National Center for Immunization and Respiratory Diseases, "General Recommendations on Immunization - Recommendations of the Advisory Committee on Immunization Practices (ACIP)," *MMWR Recomm Rep*, 2011, 60(2):1-64.

Red Book: 2009 Report of the Committee on Infectious Diseases, 28th ed, Pickering LK, ed, Elk Grove Village, IL: American Academy of Pediatrics, 2009.

◆ **Tetanus Toxoid** *see* Diphtheria and Tetanus Toxoids, Acellular Pertussis, Poliovirus and *Haemophilus* b Conjugate Vaccine *on page 684*

Tetanus Toxoid (Adsorbed)
(TET a nus TOKS oyd, ad SORBED)

Medication Safety Issues
Sound-alike/look-alike issues:
Tetanus toxoid products may be confused with influenza virus vaccine and tuberculin products. Medication errors have occurred when tetanus toxoid products have been inadvertently administered instead of tuberculin skin tests (PPD) and influenza virus vaccine. These products are refrigerated and often stored in close proximity to each other.

Related Information
Immunization Administration Recommendations *on page 2368*

Immunization Guidelines *on page 2373*

Therapeutic Category Vaccine

Generic Availability (U.S.) Yes

Use Indicated as booster dose in the active immunization against tetanus when combined antigen preparations are not indicated (FDA approved in ages ≥7 years and adults). **Note:** Tetanus and diphtheria toxoids for adult use (Td) is the preferred immunizing agent for most adults and for children after their seventh birthday. Young children should receive trivalent DTaP (diphtheria and tetanus toxoids, and acellular pertussis vaccine) as part of their childhood immunization program, unless pertussis is contraindicated, then DT is warranted.

Pregnancy Risk Factor C

Pregnancy Considerations Animal studies have not been conducted. Inactivated bacterial vaccines have not been shown to cause increased risks to the fetus (CDC, 2011). The ACIP recommends vaccination in previously unvaccinated women or in women with an incomplete vaccination series, whose child may be born in unhygienic conditions. Tetanus immune globulin and a tetanus toxoid-containing vaccine are recommended by the ACIP as part of the standard wound management to prevent tetanus in pregnant women. Vaccination using Td is preferred.

Breast-Feeding Considerations Inactivated vaccines do not affect the safety of breast-feeding for the mother or the infant. Breast-feeding infants should be vaccinated according to the recommended schedules (CDC, 2011).

Contraindications Hypersensitivity to tetanus toxoid or any component

Warnings Immediate treatment (including epinephrine 1:1000) for anaphylactic and/or hypersensitivity reactions should be available during vaccine use. Patients with a history of severe local reaction (Arthus-type) following a previous dose should not be given further routine or emergency doses of tetanus toxoid more frequently than every 10 years, even if using for wound management with wounds that are not clean or minor; these patients generally have high serum antitoxin levels. Guillain-Barré syndrome occurring within 6 weeks of tetanus toxoid vaccination has been reported. Syncope has been reported with use of injectable vaccines and may may be accompanied by transient visual disturbances, weakness, or tonic-clonic movements. Procedures should be in place to avoid injuries from falling and to restore cerebral perfusion if syncope occurs (CDC, 57[17], 2008).

Precautions The decision to administer or delay vaccination because of current or recent febrile illness depends on the severity of symptoms and the etiology of the disease. Immunization should be delayed during the course of an acute severe febrile illness; may administer to patients with mild acute illness (with or without fever). Use with caution in severely immunocompromised patients (eg, patients receiving chemo/radiation therapy or other immunosuppressive therapy, including high-dose corticosteroids); may have a reduced response to vaccination; may be used in patients with HIV infection; inactivated vaccines

should be administered ≥2 weeks prior to planned immunosuppression when feasible (IDSA [Rubin, 2014]). In general, household and close contacts of persons with altered immunocompetence may receive all age-appropriate vaccines. Vaccination may not result in effective immunity in all patients. Response depends upon multiple factors (eg, type of vaccine, age of patient) and may be improved by administering the vaccine at the recommended dose, route, and interval (CDC/ACIP [Kroger, 2011]).

Use with caution in patients with coagulation disorders, including thrombocytopenia, due to an increased risk for bleeding following I.M. administration; if the patient receives antihemophilia or other similar therapy, I.M. injection can be scheduled shortly after such therapy is administered. Antipyretics have not been shown to prevent febrile seizures; antipyretics may be used to treat fever or discomfort following vaccination (CDC/ACIP [Kroger, 2011]). One study reported that routine prophylactic administration of acetaminophen to prevent fever prior to vaccination decreased the immune response of some vaccines; the clinical significance of this reduction in immune response has not been established (Prymula, 2009). Products may contain thimerosal; vial stopper may contain natural latex rubber.

Adverse Reactions All serious adverse reactions must be reported to the U.S. Department of Health and Human Services (DHHS) Vaccine Adverse Event Reporting System (VAERS) 1-800-822-7967 or online at https://vaers.hhs.gov/esub/index.
Cardiovascular: Hypotension

Central nervous system: Brachial neuritis, fever, malaise, pain

Gastrointestinal: Nausea

Local: Edema, induration (with or without tenderness), rash, redness, urticaria, warmth

Neuromuscular: Arthralgia, Guillain-Barré syndrome

Miscellaneous: Anaphylactic reaction, Arthus-type hypersensitivity reaction

Drug Interactions
Metabolism/Transport Effects None known.

Avoid Concomitant Use There are no known interactions where it is recommended to avoid concomitant use.

Increased Effect/Toxicity There are no known significant interactions involving an increase in effect.

Decreased Effect
The levels/effects of Tetanus Toxoid (Adsorbed) may be decreased by: Belimumab; Fingolimod; Immunosuppressants; Meningococcal Polysaccharide (Groups A / C / Y and W-135) Tetanus Toxoid Conjugate Vaccine

Stability Store at 2°C to 8°C (35°F to 46°F). Do not freeze.

Mechanism of Action Tetanus toxoid preparations contain the toxin produced by virulent tetanus bacilli (detoxified growth products of *Clostridium tetani*). The toxin has been modified by treatment with formaldehyde so that it has lost toxicity but still retains ability to act as antigen and produce active immunity; the aluminum salt, a mineral adjuvant, delays the rate of absorption and prolongs and enhances its properties; duration ~10 years.

Pharmacodynamics Duration: Primary immunization: ~10 years

Dosing: Usual
Children ≥7 years, Adolescents, and Adults:
Primary immunization: Not indicated for this use; combined antigen vaccines are recommended. **Note:** In most patients, Td is the recommended product for primary immunization, booster doses, and tetanus immunization in wound management (refer to diphtheria and tetanus toxoid monograph):

Booster doses: I.M: 0.5 mL every 10 years

Tetanus prophylaxis in wound management: Tetanus prophylaxis in patients with wounds should consider if

◀ the wound is clean or contaminated, the immunization status of the patient, proper use of tetanus toxoid and/or tetanus immune globulin (TIG), wound cleaning, and (if required) surgical debridement and the proper use of antibiotics. Patients with an uncertain or incomplete tetanus immunization status should have additional follow-up to ensure a series is completed. Patients with a history of Arthus reaction following a previous dose of a tetanus toxoid-containing vaccine should not receive a tetanus toxoid-containing vaccine until >10 years after the most recent dose even if they have a wound that is neither clean nor minor. See table.

Tetanus Prophylaxis Wound Management

History of Tetanus Immunization (Doses)	Clean, Minor Wounds		All Other Wounds[1]	
	Tetanus toxoid[2]	TIG	Tetanus toxoid[2]	TIG
Uncertain or <3 doses	Yes	No	Yes	Yes
3 or more doses	No[3]	No	No[4]	No

[1]Such as, but not limited to, wounds contaminated with dirt, feces, soil, and saliva; puncture wounds; wounds from crushing, tears, burns, and frostbite.

[2]Tetanus toxoid in this chart refers to a tetanus toxoid containing vaccine. For children <7 years old DTaP (DT, if pertussis vaccine contraindicated) is preferred to tetanus toxoid alone. For children ≥7 years of age and Adults, Td preferred to tetanus toxoid alone; Tdap may be preferred if the patient has not previously been vaccinated with Tdap.

[3]Yes, if ≥10 years since last dose.

[4]Yes, if ≥5 years since last dose.

Abbreviations: **DT** = Diphtheria and Tetanus Toxoids (formulation for age ≤6 years); **DTaP** = Diphtheria and Tetanus Toxoids, and Acellular Pertussis (formulation for age ≤6 years; Daptacel®, Infanrix®); **Td** = Diphtheria and Tetanus Toxoids (formulation for age ≥7 years; Decavac®, Tenivac™); **TT** = Tetanus toxoid (adsorbed [formulation for age ≥7 years]); **Tdap** = Diphtheria and Tetanus Toxoids, and Acellular Pertussis (Adacel® or Boostrix® [formulations for age ≥7 years]); **TIG** = Tetanus Immune Globulin

Adapted from the Yellow Book 2010, Chapter 2, *Routine Vaccine-Preventable Diseases, Tetanus*; Available at www.cdc. gov/yellowbook; and *MMWR*, 2006, 55:RR-17.

Administration I.M.: Shake well prior to use. Administer into lateral aspect of midthigh or deltoid muscle of upper arm; may be administered SubQ if intramuscular route cannot be used; **not for I.V. administration**. Adolescents and adults should be vaccinated while seated or lying down. U.S. law requires that the date of administration, the vaccine manufacturer, lot number of vaccine, and the administering person's name, title, and address be entered into the patient's permanent medical record.

Monitoring Parameters Observe for syncope for 15 minutes following administration. If seizure-like activity associated with syncope occurs, maintain patient in supine or Trendelenburg position to reestablish adequate cerebral perfusion.

Additional Information In order to maximize vaccination rates, the ACIP recommends simultaneous administration (ie, >1 vaccine on the same day at different anatomic sites) of all age-appropriate vaccines (live or inactivated) for which a person is eligible at a single visit, unless contraindications exist. If available, the use of combination vaccines is generally preferred over separate injections, taking into consideration provider assessment, patient preference, and potential adverse events. If separate vaccines being used, evaluate product information regarding same syringe compatibility of vaccines. Separate needles and syringes should be used for each injection. The ACIP prefers each dose of specific vaccine in a series come from the same manufacturer if possible (CDC, 2011).

For additional information, please refer to the following website: http://www.cdc.gov/vaccines/vpd-vac/.

Dosage Forms Excipient information presented when available (limited, particularly for generics); consult specific product labeling.
Solution, Intramuscular:
Generic: 5 units (0.5 mL)

References

AAP Steering Committee on Quality Improvement and Management, Subcommittee on Febrile Seizures American Academy of Pediatrics, "Febrile Seizures: Clinical Practice Guideline for the Long-Term Management of the Child With Simple Febrile Seizures," *Pediatrics*, 2008, 121(6):1281-6.

Centers for Disease Control and Prevention (CDC). Advisory committee on immunization practices recommended immunization schedules for persons aged 0 through 18 years - United States, 2014. *MMWR Morb Mortal Wkly Rep*. 2014;63(5):108-109. Full schedule available at http://www.cdc.gov/vaccines/schedules/downloads/child/0-18yrs-child-combined-schedule.pdf

Centers for Disease Control and Prevention (CDC), "Prevention of Pertussis, Tetanus, and Diphtheria Among Pregnant and Postpartum Women and Their Infants. Recommendations of the Advisory Committee on Immunization Practices (ACIP)," *MMWR Recomm Rep*, 2008, 57(RR-4):1-51; published erratum appears in *MMWR Morb Mortal Wkly Rep*, 2008, 57(26):723.

Centers for Disease Control and Prevention (CDC), "Recommendations of the Advisory Committee on Immunization Practices (ACIP): General Recommendations on Immunization," *MMWR Recomm Rep*, 2011, 60(2):1-64.

Centers for Disease Control and Prevention (CDC), "Syncope After Vaccination-United States, January 2005-July 2007," *MMWR Morb Mortal Wkly Rep*, 2008, 2;57(17):457-60.

Kroger AT, Sumaya CV, Pickering LK, et al. General recommendations on immunization - recommendations of the Advisory Committee on Immunization Practices (ACIP). *MMWR Recomm Rep*. 2011; 60(RR-2):1-64.

Prymula R, Siegrist CA, Chlibek R, et al, "Effect of Prophylactic Paracetamol Administration at Time of Vaccination on Febrile Reactions and Antibody Responses in Children: Two Open-Label, Randomised Controlled Trials," *Lancet*, 2009, 374(9698):1339-50.

Rubin LG, Levin MJ, Ljungman P, et al. 2013 IDSA clinical practice guideline for vaccination of the immunocompromised host. *Clin Infect Dis*. 2014;58(3):e44-e100.

◆ **Tetanus Toxoid, Reduced Diphtheria Toxoid, and Acellular Pertussis, Adsorbed** *see* Diphtheria and Tetanus Toxoids, and Acellular Pertussis Vaccine *on page 686*

◆ **Tetcaine** *see* Tetracaine (Ophthalmic) *on page 1995*

Tetracaine (Systemic) (TET ra kane)

Brand Names: Canada Pontocaine
Therapeutic Category Local Anesthetic, Injectable
Generic Availability (U.S.) Yes
Use Spinal anesthesia
Pregnancy Risk Factor C
Pregnancy Considerations Animal reproduction studies have not been conducted.
Breast-Feeding Considerations It is not known if tetracaine (systemic) is excreted in breast milk. The manufacturer recommends that caution be exercised when administering tetracaine (systemic) to nursing women.
Contraindications Hypersensitivity to tetracaine or any component; CNS disease, meningitis; myasthenia gravis, impaired cardiac conduction
Precautions Use with caution in patients with cardiac disease and hyperthyroidism
Adverse Reactions Note: Adverse effects listed are those characteristics of local anesthetics. Systemic adverse effects are generally associated with excessive doses or rapid absorption.
Cardiovascular: Cardiac arrest, hypotension
Central nervous system: Chills, convulsions, dizziness, drowsiness, nervousness, unconsciousness
Dermatologic: Urticaria
Gastrointestinal: Nausea, vomiting
Hematologic: Methemoglobinemia
Neuromuscular & skeletal: Tremors
Ocular: Blurred vision, pupil constriction
Otic: Tinnitus

Respiratory: Respiratory arrest
Miscellaneous: Allergic reaction, anaphylaxis

Drug Interactions

Metabolism/Transport Effects None known.

Avoid Concomitant Use There are no known interactions where it is recommended to avoid concomitant use.

Increased Effect/Toxicity
The levels/effects of Tetracaine (Systemic) may be increased by: Hyaluronidase

Decreased Effect
Tetracaine (Systemic) may decrease the levels/effects of: Technetium Tc 99m Tilmanocept

Mechanism of Action Ester local anesthetic blocks both the initiation and conduction of nerve impulses by decreasing the neuronal membrane's permeability to sodium ions, which results in inhibition of depolarization with resultant blockade of conduction

Pharmacodynamics Duration: 1.5-3 hours

Pharmacokinetics (Adult data unless noted)
Metabolism: By the liver
Elimination: Metabolites are renally excreted

Dosing: Usual
Children: Safety and efficacy have not been established
Adults:
Injection: Dosage varies with the anesthetic procedure, the degree of anesthesia required, and the individual patient response; it is administered by subarachnoid injection for spinal anesthesia. High, medium, low, or saddle blocks use 0.2% or 0.3% solution. Prolonged effect (2-3 hours): Use 1% solution (a 1% solution should be diluted with an equal volume of CSF before administration)
Perineal anesthesia: 5 mg
Perineal and lower extremities: 10 mg
Anesthesia extending up to the costal margin: 15-20 mg
Low spinal anesthesia (saddle block): 2-5 mg

Administration Subarachnoid administration by experienced individuals only

Dosage Forms Excipient information presented when available (limited, particularly for generics); consult specific product labeling.
Solution, Injection, as hydrochloride [preservative free]:
Generic: 1% (2 mL)

Tetracaine (Ophthalmic) (TET ra kane)

Brand Names: U.S. Altacaine; Tetcaine; TetraVisc; Tetra-Visc Forte

Therapeutic Category Local Anesthetic, Ophthalmic

Generic Availability (U.S.) Yes

Use Local anesthesia for various ophthalmic procedures of short duration (eg, tonometry, gonioscopy), minor ophthalmic surgical procedures (eg, removal of corneal foreign bodies, suture removal), and for various diagnostic purposes (eg, conjunctival scrapings) (FDA approved in adults)

Pregnancy Risk Factor C

Pregnancy Considerations Animal reproduction studies have not been conducted.

Breast-Feeding Considerations It is not known if tetracaine (ophthalmic) is excreted in breast milk. The manufacturer recommends that caution be exercised when administering tetracaine (ophthalmic) to nursing women.

Contraindications Hypersensitivity to tetracaine or any component

Warnings Hypersensitivity reactions may occur; immediate type allergic corneal reactions, characterized by epithelial keratitis/filament formation, necrotic epithelium sloughing, stromal edema, descemetitis, and iritis, have been reported rarely. May delay wound healing. Prolonged use is not recommended. The anesthetized eye should be protected from irritation, foreign bodies, and rubbing to prevent inadvertent damage.

Precautions Some formulations may contain benzalkonium chloride which may be adsorbed by soft contact lenses; remove contacts prior to administration and wait 15 minutes before reinserting.

Adverse Reactions Ocular: Allergic corneal reaction (rare), burning (transient), chemosis, conjunctival redness (transient), lacrimation, photophobia, stinging (transient)

Drug Interactions

Metabolism/Transport Effects None known.

Avoid Concomitant Use There are no known interactions where it is recommended to avoid concomitant use.

Increased Effect/Toxicity There are no known significant interactions involving an increase in effect.

Decreased Effect There are no known significant interactions involving a decrease in effect.

Stability Store at 15°C to 30°C (59°F to 86°F); protect from light; keep container closed tightly

Mechanism of Action Ester local anesthetic blocks both the initiation and conduction of nerve impulses by decreasing the neuronal membrane's permeability to sodium, potassium, and other ions, which results in inhibition of depolarization with resultant blockade of conduction

Pharmacodynamics
Onset of action: Anesthetic effects: Within 30 seconds
Duration: 1.5-3 hours

Pharmacokinetics (Adult data unless noted)
Metabolism: Hepatic; detoxified by plasma esterases to aminobenzoic acid
Elimination: Urine

Dosing: Usual Adults:
Short-term (nonsurgical procedures) anesthesia: Instill 1-2 drops just prior to evaluation
Minor surgical procedures: Instill 1-2 drops every 5-10 minutes for up to 3 doses
Prolonged surgical procedures (such as cataract extraction): Instill 1-2 drops every 5-10 minutes for up to 5 doses

Administration Apply drops to conjunctiva of affected eye(s); avoid contact of bottle tip with skin or eye; finger pressure should be applied to lacrimal sac during and for 1-2 minutes after instillation to decrease risk of absorption and systemic reactions

Dosage Forms Excipient information presented when available (limited, particularly for generics); consult specific product labeling.
Solution, Ophthalmic, as hydrochloride:
Altacaine: 0.5% (1 ea, 15 mL, 30 mL)
Tetcaine: 0.5% (15 mL) [contains chlorobutanol (chlorobutol), edetate disodium]
TetraVisc: 0.5% (1 ea, 5 mL) [contains benzalkonium chloride]
TetraVisc Forte: 0.5% (1 ea, 5 mL) [contains benzalkonium chloride, edetate disodium]
Generic: 0.5% (1 mL, 2 mL, 15 mL)

Tetracaine (Topical) (TET ra kane)

Brand Names: Canada Ametop; Pontocaine

Therapeutic Category Analgesic, Topical; Local Anesthetic, Topical

Generic Availability (U.S.) Yes

Use Local anesthesia for mucous membranes

Pregnancy Risk Factor C

Pregnancy Considerations Animal reproduction studies have not been conducted.

Contraindications Hypersensitivity to tetracaine or any component

Warnings Use prior to cosmetic procedures can result in high systemic levels and lead to toxic effects (eg, arrhythmias, seizures, coma, respiratory depression, and death), particularly when applied in large amounts to cover large areas and/or left on for long periods of time or used with materials, wraps, or dressings to cover the skin after anesthetic application. These practices may increase the degree of systemic absorption and should be avoided. The FDA is recommending consumers consult their healthcare provider for instructions on safe use prior to applying topical anesthetics for medical or cosmetic purposes. Use of products with the lowest amount of anesthetic with the least amount of application possible to relieve pain is also recommended.

Precautions Use with caution in patients with cardiac disease and hyperthyroidism

Adverse Reactions Note: Adverse effects listed are those characteristics of local anesthetics. Systemic adverse effects are generally associated with excessive doses or rapid absorption.

Cardiovascular: Cardiac arrest, hypotension

Central nervous system: Chills, convulsions, dizziness, drowsiness, nervousness, unconsciousness

Dermatologic: Urticaria

Gastrointestinal: Nausea, vomiting

Hematologic: Methemoglobinemia

Neuromuscular & skeletal: Tremors

Ocular: Blurred vision, pupil constriction

Otic: Tinnitus

Respiratory: Respiratory arrest

Miscellaneous: Allergic reaction, anaphylaxis

Drug Interactions

Metabolism/Transport Effects None known.

Avoid Concomitant Use There are no known interactions where it is recommended to avoid concomitant use.

Increased Effect/Toxicity There are no known significant interactions involving an increase in effect.

Decreased Effect There are no known significant interactions involving a decrease in effect.

Mechanism of Action Ester local anesthetic blocks both the initiation and conduction of nerve impulses by decreasing the neuronal membrane's permeability to sodium ions, which results in inhibition of depolarization with resultant blockade of conduction

Pharmacodynamics

Onset of action: Within 3 minutes when applied to mucous membranes

Duration: 1.5-3 hours

Pharmacokinetics (Adult data unless noted)

Metabolism: By the liver

Elimination: Metabolites are renally excreted

Dosing: Usual

Children: Safety and efficacy have not been established

Adults: Apply 2% solution as needed; do not exceed 20 mg (1 mL) per application

- ◆ **Tetracaine and Lidocaine** see Lidocaine and Tetracaine on page 1248

- ◆ **Tetracaine Hydrochloride** see Tetracaine (Ophthalmic) on page 1995

- ◆ **Tetracaine Hydrochloride** see Tetracaine (Systemic) on page 1994

- ◆ **Tetracaine Hydrochloride** see Tetracaine (Topical) on page 1995

- ◆ **Tetracosactide** see Cosyntropin on page 549

Tetracycline (tet ra SYE kleen)

Medication Safety Issues

Sound-alike/look-alike issues:

Tetracycline may be confused with tetradecyl sulfate

Achromycin may be confused with actinomycin, Adriamycin

Related Information

H. pylori Treatment in Pediatric Patients on page 2311

Oral Medications That Should Not Be Crushed or Altered on page 2438

Safe Handling of Hazardous Drugs on page 2419

Brand Names: Canada Apo-Tetra; Nu-Tetra

Therapeutic Category Acne Products; Antibiotic, Ophthalmic; Antibiotic, Tetracycline Derivative; Antibiotic, Topical

Generic Availability (U.S.) Yes

Use

Children, Adolescents and Adults: Treatment of Rocky Mountain spotted fever caused by susceptible *Rickettsia* or brucellosis

Adolescents and Adults: Presumptive treatment of chlamydial infection in patients with gonorrhea

Children >8 years, Adolescents and Adults: Treatment of moderate to severe inflammatory acne vulgaris, Lyme disease, mycoplasmal disease or *Legionella*

Pregnancy Risk Factor D

Pregnancy Considerations Tetracyclines cross the placenta and accumulate in developing teeth and long tubular bones. Tetracyclines may discolor fetal teeth following maternal use during pregnancy; the specific teeth involved and the portion of the tooth affected depends on the timing and duration of exposure relative to tooth calcification. The pharmacokinetics of tetracycline are not altered in pregnant patients with normal renal function. Hepatic toxicity during pregnancy, potentially associated with tetracycline use, has been widely reported in the literature. As a class, tetracyclines are generally considered second-line antibiotics in pregnant women and their use should be avoided (Mylonas, 2011; Whalley, 1966; Whalley, 1970).

Breast-Feeding Considerations Tetracycline is excreted into breast milk (Matsuda, 1984). According to the manufacturer, the decision to continue or discontinue breast-feeding during therapy should take into account the risk of exposure to the infant and the benefits of treatment to the mother. Tetracycline binds to calcium. The calcium in the maternal milk will decrease the amount of tetracycline absorbed by the breast-feeding infant (Mitrano, 2009). Nondose-related effects could include modification of bowel flora.

Contraindications Hypersensitivity to tetracycline or any component

Warnings Hazardous agent; use appropriate precautions for handling and disposal (NIOSH, 2012). Use of tetracyclines during tooth development may cause permanent discoloration of the teeth (yellow-gray to brown) and enamel hypoplasia; adult-onset tooth discoloration following long-term administration of tetracyclines has also been reported. Do not administer to children <8 years of age due to permanent discoloration of teeth and retardation of skeletal development and bone growth (risk being greatest for children <4 years and in those receiving high doses). Tetracyclines have been associated with increases in BUN secondary to antianabolic effects. Pseudotumor cerebri has been reported rarely in infants and adolescents; use with isotretinoin has been associated with cases of pseudotumor cerebri; avoid concomitant treatment with isotretinoin. Photosensitivity reaction may occur; avoid prolonged exposure to sunlight or tanning equipment; discontinue if skin erythema occurs. Prolonged use may result in superinfection, including *C. difficile*-associated diarrhea and pseudomembraneous colitis. Tetratcycline can cause fetal harm if used during pregnancy; avoid use during pregnancy. Hepatotoxicity has been reported rarely; risk may be increased in patients with preexisting hepatic or renal impairment.

Precautions Use with caution in patients with renal and liver impairment; dosage modification required in patients with renal impairment; outdated drug may cause nephropathy

Adverse Reactions

Cardiovascular: Pericarditis

Central nervous system: Bulging fontanels in infants, increased intracranial pressure, paresthesia, pseudotumor cerebri

Dermatologic: Exfoliative dermatitis, photosensitivity, pigmentation of nails, pruritus

Gastrointestinal: Abdominal cramps, anorexia, antibiotic-associated pseudomembranous colitis, diarrhea, discoloration of teeth and enamel hypoplasia (young children), esophagitis, nausea, pancreatitis, staphylococcal enterocolitis, vomiting

Hematologic: Thrombophlebitis

Hepatic: Hepatotoxicity

Renal: Acute renal failure, azotemia, renal damage

Miscellaneous: Anaphylaxis, candidal superinfection, hypersensitivity reactions, superinfection

Drug Interactions

Metabolism/Transport Effects Substrate of CYP3A4 (major); **Note:** Assignment of Major/Minor substrate status based on clinically relevant drug interaction potential; **Inhibits** CYP3A4 (moderate)

Avoid Concomitant Use

Avoid concomitant use of Tetracycline with any of the following: BCG; Bosutinib; Ibrutinib; Ivabradine; Lomitapide; Pimozide; Retinoic Acid Derivatives; Simeprevir; Strontium Ranelate; Tolvaptan; Ulipristal

Increased Effect/Toxicity

Tetracycline may increase the levels/effects of: ARIPiprazole; Avanafil; Bosentan; Bosutinib; Budesonide (Systemic, Oral Inhalation); Cannabis; Colchicine; CYP3A4 Substrates; Dofetilide; DOXOrubicin (Conventional); Dronabinol; Eplerenone; Everolimus; FentaNYL; Halofantrine; Ibrutinib; Imatinib; Ivabradine; Ivacaftor; Lomitapide; Lurasidone; Mipomersen; Neuromuscular-Blocking Agents; OxyCODONE; Pimecrolimus; Pimozide; Porfimer; Propafenone; QuiNINE; Ranolazine; Retinoic Acid Derivatives; Rivaroxaban; Salmeterol; Saxagliptin; Simeprevir; Tetrahydrocannabinol; Tolvaptan; Ulipristal; Vilazodone; Vitamin K Antagonists; Zuclopenthixol

Decreased Effect

Tetracycline may decrease the levels/effects of: Atovaquone; BCG; Ifosfamide; Penicillins; Sodium Picosulfate; Typhoid Vaccine

The levels/effects of Tetracycline may be decreased by: Antacids; Bile Acid Sequestrants; Bismuth; Bismuth Subsalicylate; Bosentan; Calcium Salts; CYP3A4 Inducers (Strong); Dabrafenib; Deferasirox; Iron Salts; Lanthanum; Magnesium Salts; Mitotane; Multivitamins/Minerals (with ADEK, Folate, Iron); Multivitamins/Minerals (with AE, No Iron); Quinapril; Siltuximab; St Johns Wort; Strontium Ranelate; Sucralfate; Sucroferric Oxyhydroxide; Tocilizumab; Zinc Salts

Food Interactions Serum concentrations may be decreased if taken with dairy products. Management: Take on an empty stomach 1 hour before or 2 hours after meals to increase total absorption. Administer around-the-clock to promote less variation in peak and trough serum levels.

Stability Hazardous agent; use appropriate precautions for handling and disposal (NIOSH, 2012). Store at 20°C to 25°C (68°F to 77°F); protect from light. Use of outdated tetracyclines has caused a Fanconi-like syndrome.

Mechanism of Action Inhibits bacterial protein synthesis by binding with the 30S and possibly the 50S ribosomal subunit(s) of susceptible bacteria; may also cause alterations in the cytoplasmic membrane

Pharmacokinetics (Adult data unless noted)

Distribution: Widely distributed to most body fluids and tissues including ascitic, synovial and pleural fluids; bronchial secretions; appears in breast milk; poor penetration into CSF

Absorption:

Oral: 75%

I.M.: Poor, with less than 60% of dose absorbed

Protein binding: 30% to 60%

Half-life: 6-12 hours with normal renal function and is prolonged with renal impairment

Time to peak serum concentration: Within 2-4 hours

Elimination: Primary route is the kidney, with 60% of a dose excreted as unchanged drug in urine, small amounts appear in bile

Dialysis: Slightly dialyzable (5% to 20%)

Dosing: Usual Oral:

Children >8 years: 25-50 mg/kg/day in divided doses every 6 hours; not to exceed 3 g/day

Adolescents and Adults: 250-500 mg/dose every 6-12 hours

Dosing adjustment in renal impairment:

CrCl 50-80 mL/minute: Administer every 8-12 hours

CrCl 10-50 mL/minute: Administer every 12-24 hours

CrCl <10 mL/minute: Administer every 24 hours

Administration Hazardous agent; use appropriate precautions for handling and disposal (NIOSH, 2012).

Oral: Administer 1 hour before or 2 hours after meals with adequate amounts of fluid; avoid taking antacids, calcium, iron, dairy products, or milk formulas within 3 hours of tetracyclines

Topical: Small amount of ointment should be applied to cleansed affected area.

Monitoring Parameters Renal, hepatic, and hematologic function tests; observe for changes in bowel frequency

Dosage Forms Excipient information presented when available (limited, particularly for generics); consult specific product labeling.

Capsule, Oral, as hydrochloride:

Generic: 250 mg, 500 mg

Extemporaneous Preparations Hazardous agent: Use appropriate precautions for handling and disposal.

A 25 mg/mL oral suspension may be made using capsules. Empty the contents of six 500 mg capsules into mortar. Add a small amount (~20 mL) of a 1:1 mixture of Ora-Sweet® and Ora-Plus® and mix to a uniform paste; mix while adding the vehicle in geometric proportions to **almost** 120 mL; transfer to a calibrated bottle, rinse mortar with vehicle, and add quantity of vehicle sufficient to make 120 mL. Label "shake well" and "refrigerate". Stable 28 days refrigerated.

Nahata MC, Pai VB, and Hipple TF, *Pediatric Drug Formulations*, 5th ed, Cincinnati, OH: Harvey Whitney Books Co, 2004.

References

American Academy of Pediatrics. Committee on Drugs. "Requiem for Tetracyclines," *Pediatrics*, 1975, 55(1):142-3.

Matsuda S, "Transfer of Antibiotics Into Maternal Milk," *Biol Res Pregnancy Perinatol*, 1984, 5(2):57-60.

Mitrano JA, Spooner LM, and Belliveau P, "Excretion of Antimicrobials Used to Treat Methicillin-Resistant *Staphylococcus aureus* Infections During Lactation: Safety in Breastfeeding Infants," *Pharmacotherapy*, 2009, 29(9):1103-9.

Mylonas I, "Antibiotic Chemotherapy During Pregnancy and Lactation Period: Aspects for Consideration," *Arch Gynecol Obstet*, 2011, 283 (1):7-18.

National Institute for Occupational Safety and Health (NIOSH), "NIOSH List of Antineoplastic and Other Hazardous Drugs in Healthcare Settings 2012." Available at http://www.cdc.gov/niosh/docs/2012-150/pdfs/2012-150.pdf. Accessed January 21, 2013.

Whalley PJ, Adams RH, and Combes B, "Tetracycline Toxicity in Pregnancy. Liver and Pancreatic Dysfunction," *JAMA*, 1964, 189:357-62.

Whalley PJ, Martin FG, Adams RH, et al, "Disposition of Tetracycline By Pregnant Women With Acute Pyelonephritis," *Obstet Gynecol*, 1970, 36(6):821-6.

◆ **Tetracycline Hydrochloride** see Tetracycline *on page 1996*

◆ **Tetra-Formula Nighttime Sleep [OTC]** *see* Diphenhydr-AMINE (Systemic) *on page 673*

◆ **Tetrahydrocannabinol** *see* Dronabinol *on page 725*

◆ **Tetraiodothyronine and Triiodothyronine** *see* Thyroid, Desiccated *on page 2018*

Tetrastarch (TET ra starch)

Brand Names: U.S. Voluven

Brand Names: Canada Volulyte; Voluven

Therapeutic Category Plasma Volume Expander, Colloid

Generic Availability (U.S.) No

Use Treatment and prophylaxis of hypovolemia (FDA approved in all ages); **Note:** This is not a substitute for blood or plasma; does not have oxygen-carrying capacity.

Pregnancy Risk Factor C

Pregnancy Considerations Adverse events have been observed in animal reproduction studies.

Breast-Feeding Considerations It is not known if tetrastarch is excreted in breast milk. The manufacturer recommends that caution be exercised when administering tetrastarch to nursing women.

Contraindications Hypersensitivity to hydroxyethyl starch or any component; fluid overload (eg, pulmonary edema and CHF), intracranial bleeding, renal failure with oliguria or anuria (not related to hypovolemia), dialysis, or severe hypernatremia or hyperchloremia

Warnings Anaphylactoid reactions (eg, mild influenza-like symptoms, bradycardia, tachycardia, bronchospasm, noncardiac pulmonary edema) to hydroxyethyl starch (HES) solutions have been reported; if signs of hypersensitivity occur, discontinue use immediately and administer appropriate therapy. Administration of large volume may cause a reduction in hematocrit, coagulation factors, and other plasma proteins due to hemodilution; coagulation may be impaired (eg, prolonged PT, PTT, and clotting times) and a transient prolongation of bleeding time may be observed. Avoid use in patients undergoing open heart surgery in association with cardiopulmonary bypass. HES solutions have been associated with excess bleeding in these patients. If used in other patient populations, discontinue use of HES at the first sign of coagulopathy. Administration may cause fluid overload; use with caution in patients at risk from overexpansion of blood volume, including the very young or aged patients and those at risk for developing CHF or pulmonary edema; use is contraindicated in heart failure or any preexisting condition where volume overload is a potential concern. Monitor fluid status and rate of infusion periodically with use; in cases of severe dehydration, crystalloid should be administered first.

Avoid use in critically ill adult patients, including those with sepsis and those admitted to the ICU. HES solutions have been associated with an increased risk of mortality in the critically ill (Brunkhorst, 2008; Perel, 2011; Perner, 2012; Zarychanski, 2009) **[U.S. Boxed Warning (per the FDA; labeling updates pending)]**. The Society of Critical Care Medicine (SCCM) also recommends against the use of HES solutions for fluid resuscitation of severe sepsis and septic shock; crystalloids (eg, sodium chloride) are recommended instead (Dellinger, 2013). HES solutions have also been associated with renal injury requiring renal replacement therapy in critically ill patients (Reinhart, 2012) **[U.S. Boxed Warning (per the FDA; labeling updates pending)]**. If used in patients who are not critically ill, avoid use in patients with preexisting renal dysfunction and discontinue use at the first sign of renal injury. Since the need for renal replacement therapy has been reported up to 90 days after HES administration, continue to monitor renal function in all patients for at least 90 days. HES use has also been associated with acute kidney injury in pediatric patients (Reinhart, 2012).

Precautions Use with caution in patients with severe liver disease or bleeding disorders; may result in further reduction of coagulation factors, increasing the risk of bleeding. Use with caution in patients with renal impairment; fluid status including urine output should be monitored closely; use is contraindicated with oliguria or anuria unrelated to hypovolemia or patients receiving hemodialysis. May temporarily increase serum amylase concentrations.

Adverse Reactions

Dermatologic: Pruritus (dose dependent; may be delayed), skin rash

Gastrointestinal: Increased serum amylase

Hematologic & oncologic: Anemia, coagulation time increased, decreased clotting factors, decreased hematocrit, prolonged prothrombin time, wound hemorrhage

Rare but important or life-threatening: Acute renal failure, anaphylactoid reaction, anaphylaxis, bradycardia, bronchospasm, circulatory shock, flu-like symptoms, hypersensitivity reaction, hypotension, non-cardiogenic pulmonary edema, shock, tachycardia

Drug Interactions

Metabolism/Transport Effects None known.

Avoid Concomitant Use There are no known interactions where it is recommended to avoid concomitant use.

Increased Effect/Toxicity There are no known significant interactions involving an increase in effect.

Decreased Effect There are no known significant interactions involving a decrease in effect.

Stability Store at 15°C to 25°C (59°F to 77°F); do not freeze; use only if solution is clear and free from particles.

Mechanism of Action Produces plasma volume expansion by virtue of its highly colloidal starch structure

Pharmacodynamics

Duration of action: ≥6 hours

Pharmacokinetics (Adult data unless noted)

Distribution: 5.9 L

Metabolism: Molecules >50,000 daltons are metabolized by plasma α-amylase

Half-life: 12 hours

Elimination: Urine [smaller hydroxyethyl starch (<50,000 daltons) unchanged, metabolites]

Clearance: 31.4 mL/minute

Dosing: Neonatal Note: With severe dehydration, administer crystalloid first. Dose and rate of infusion dependent on amount of blood lost, on maintenance or restoration of hemodynamics, and on amount of hemodilution. Titrate to individual colloid needs, hemodynamics, and hydration status. Do not use in critically ill patients, those undergoing open heart surgery with cardiopulmonary bypass, or those with preexisting renal dysfunction.

Volume expansion: I.V. infusion: Usual range: 7-25 mL/kg/dose; maximum daily dose: 50 mL/kg/**day**; in clinical trials of intraoperative use, a dose of 10 mL/kg/dose has been reported (Osthaus, 2008; Witt, 2008)

Dosing: Usual Note: With severe dehydration, administer crystalloid first. Dose and rate of infusion dependent on amount of blood lost, on maintenance or restoration of hemodynamics, and on amount of hemodilution. Titrate to individual colloid needs, hemodynamics, and hydration status. Do not use in critically ill patients, those undergoing open heart surgery with cardiopulmonary bypass, or those with preexisting renal dysfunction.

Infants, Children, and Adolescents: **Volume expansion:**

Infants and Children <2 years: I.V. infusion: Usual range: 7-25 mL/kg/dose; mean reported dose: 16 ± 9 mL/kg/dose; maximum daily dose: 50 mL/kg/**day**; in clinical trials of intraoperative use, a dose of 10 mL/kg/dose has been reported (Chong Sung, 2006; Osthaus, 2008; Witt, 2008).

Children 2-12 years: I.V. infusion: Usual range: 25-47 mL/kg/dose; mean reported dose: 36 ± 11 mL/kg/dose; maximum daily dose: 50 mL/kg/**day**; in clinical trials of intraoperative use, a dose of 10 mL/kg/dose has been reported (Chong Sung, 2006; Osthaus, 2008; Witt, 2008).

Adolescents >12 years: I.V. Infusion: Administer up to 50 mL/kg/**day** (or up to 3500 mL daily in a 70 kg patient); may administer repetitively over several days.

Adults: **Volume expansion:** I.V. infusion: Administer up to 50 mL/kg/**day** (or up to 3500 mL daily in a 70 kg patient); may administer repetitively over several days.

Dosing adjustment in renal impairment: Avoid use in patients with preexisting renal dysfunction; discontinue use at the first sign of renal injury.

Dosing adjustment in hepatic impairment: No dosage adjustments provided in manufacturer's labeling; use with caution in severe impairment.

Administration Administer I.V. only; may be administered via infusion pump or pressure infusion; if administered by pressure infusion, air should be withdrawn or expelled from bag prior to infusion to prevent air embolism. Infuse the first 10-20 mL slowly to observe for anaphylaxis; have epinephrine and resuscitative equipment available. Change I.V. tubing at least once every 24 hours.

Monitoring Parameters Blood pressure, heart rate, capillary refill time, CVP, RAP, MAP; if pulmonary artery catheter in place, monitor cardiac index, PCWP, SVR, and PVR; hemoglobin, coagulation parameters, renal function (continue to monitor for at least 90 days after administration), urine output, acid-base balance

Test Interactions

Serum amylase levels may be temporarily elevated following administration; could interfere with the diagnosis of pancreatitis.

Administration of large volumes may result in decreased coagulation factors, plasma proteins, and /or hematocrit due to dilutional effect.

Additional Information Voluven®: 6% hetastarch (130/0.4) in 0.9% sodium chloride

Molecular weight: ~130,000
Sodium: 154 mEq/L
Chloride: 154 mEq/L
Osmolarity: 308 mOsm/L

Dosage Forms Excipient information presented when available (limited, particularly for generics); consult specific product labeling.

Solution, Intravenous:
Voluven: 6% (500 mL) [dehp free, latex free, pvc free]

References

Brunkhorst FM, Engel C, Bloos F, et al, "Intensive Insulin Therapy and Pentastarch Resuscitation in Severe Sepsis," *N Engl J Med*, 2008, 358(2):125-39.

Chong Sung K, Kum Suk P, Mi Ja Y, et al, "Effects of Intravascular Volume Therapy Using Hydroxyethyl Starch (130/0.4) on Post-Operative Bleeding and Transfusion Requirements in Children Undergoing Cardiac Surgery: A Randomized Clinical Trial," *Acta Anaesthesiol Scand*, 2006, 50(1):108-11.

Dellinger RP, Levy MM, Rhodes A, et al, "Surviving Sepsis Campaign: International Guidelines For Management of Severe Sepsis and Septic Shock: 2012," *Crit Care Med*, 2013, 41(2):580-637.

Hanart C, Khalife M, De Villé A, et al, "Perioperative Volume Replacement in Children Undergoing Cardiac Surgery: Albumin Versus Hydroxyethyl Starch 130/0.4," *Crit Care Med*, 2009, 37(2):696-701.

Lochbuhler H, Galli C, and Hagemann H, "Hydroxyethyl Starch HES 130/0.4 in Paediatric Surgery: Results on an Explorative, Controlled, Multicenter Safety Study," *Crit Care*, 2003, 7(2 Suppl): 107.

Osthaus WA, Witt L, Johanning K, et al, "Equal Effects of Gelatin and Hydroxyethyl Starch (6% HES 130/0.42) on Modified Thrombelastography in Children," *Acta Anaesthesiol Scand*, 2009, 53(3):305-10.

Perel P and Roberts I, "Colloids versus Crystalloids for Fluid Resuscitation in Critically Ill Patients," *Cochrane Database Syst Rev*, 2012, 6: CD000567.

Perner A, Haase N, Guttormsen AB, et al, "Hydroxyethyl Starch 130/0.4 versus Ringer's Acetate in Severe Sepsis," *N Engl J Med*, 2012, 367 (2):124-34; published erratum appears in *N Engl J Med*, 2012, 367 (5):481.

Reinhart K, Perner A, Sprung CL, et al, "Consensus Statement of the ESICM Task Force on Colloid Volume Therapy in Critically Ill Patients," *Intensive Care Med*, 2012, 38(3):368-83.

Sümpelmann R, Kretz FJ, Gäbler R, et al, "Hydroxyethyl Starch 130/0.42/6:1 for Perioperative Plasma Volume Replacement in Children: Preliminary Results of a European Prospective Multicenter Observational Postauthorization Safety Study (PASS)," *Paediatr Anaesth*, 2008, 18(10):929-33.

Witt L, Osthaus WA, Jüttner B, et al, "Alteration of Anion Gap and Strong Ion Difference Caused by Hydroxyethyl Starch 6% (130/0.42) and Gelatin 4% in Children," *Paediatr Anaesth*, 2008, 18(10):934-9.

Zarychanski R, Turgeon AF, Fergusson DA, et al, "Renal Outcomes and Mortality Following Hydroxyethyl Starch Resuscitation of Critically Ill Patients: Systematic Review and Meta-Analysis of Randomized Trials" ATTENTION: The analysis and conclusions of this article are being revised by the authors. This is due to the journal Anesthesia and Analgesia's retraction of a paper by Dr. Joachim Boldt, an author in seven of the studies analyzed in this review. As such, the editors of Open Medicine recommend interpreting this review with extreme caution until Zarychanski et al. publish a new analysis and interpretation in Open Medicine. For more information, see Anesthesia and Analgesia's press release. Open Med, 2009, 3(4):e196-209.

◆ **TetraVisc** *see* Tetracaine (Ophthalmic) *on page 1995*
◆ **TetraVisc Forte** *see* Tetracaine (Ophthalmic) *on page 1995*
◆ **Teva-Acyclovir (Can)** *see* Acyclovir (Systemic) *on page 63*
◆ **Teva-Alprazolam (Can)** *see* ALPRAZolam *on page 100*
◆ **Teva-Amiodarone (Can)** *see* Amiodarone *on page 127*
◆ **Teva-Amlodipine (Can)** *see* AmLODIPine *on page 135*
◆ **Teva-Atenolol (Can)** *see* Atenolol *on page 222*
◆ **Teva-Atomoxetine (Can)** *see* AtoMOXetine *on page 224*
◆ **Teva-Azathioprine (Can)** *see* AzaTHIOprine *on page 241*
◆ **Teva-Candesartan (Can)** *see* Candesartan *on page 363*
◆ **Teva-Carbamazepine (Can)** *see* CarBAMazepine *on page 372*
◆ **Teva-Cefadroxil (Can)** *see* Cefadroxil *on page 392*
◆ **Teva-Chlorpromazine (Can)** *see* ChlorproMAZINE *on page 450*
◆ **Teva-Citalopram (Can)** *see* Citalopram *on page 484*
◆ **Teva-Clarithromycin (Can)** *see* Clarithromycin *on page 490*
◆ **Teva-Clindamycin (Can)** *see* Clindamycin (Systemic) *on page 495*
◆ **Teva-Clonazepam (Can)** *see* ClonazePAM *on page 514*
◆ **Teva-Clopidogrel (Can)** *see* Clopidogrel *on page 521*
◆ **Teva-Diclofenac (Can)** *see* Diclofenac (Systemic) *on page 645*
◆ **Teva-Diclofenac EC (Can)** *see* Diclofenac (Systemic) *on page 645*
◆ **Teva-Diclofenac K (Can)** *see* Diclofenac (Systemic) *on page 645*
◆ **Teva-Diclofenac SR (Can)** *see* Diclofenac (Systemic) *on page 645*
◆ **Teva-Diltiazem (Can)** *see* Diltiazem *on page 667*
◆ **Teva-Diltiazem CD (Can)** *see* Diltiazem *on page 667*
◆ **Teva-Diltiazem HCL ER Capsules (Can)** *see* Diltiazem *on page 667*
◆ **Teva-Docusate Sodium [OTC] (Can)** *see* Docusate *on page 701*
◆ **Teva-Doxazosin (Can)** *see* Doxazosin *on page 712*
◆ **Teva-Doxycycline (Can)** *see* Doxycycline *on page 721*
◆ **Teva-Efavirenz (Can)** *see* Efavirenz *on page 731*
◆ **Teva-Enalapril (Can)** *see* Enalapril *on page 744*
◆ **Teva-Fentanyl (Can)** *see* FentaNYL *on page 853*
◆ **Teva-Fluoxetine (Can)** *see* FLUoxetine *on page 901*
◆ **Teva-Fluvastatin (Can)** *see* Fluvastatin *on page 920*
◆ **Teva-Fosinopril (Can)** *see* Fosinopril *on page 938*

- **Teva-Furosemide (Can)** *see* Furosemide *on page 948*
- **Teva-Gabapentin (Can)** *see* Gabapentin *on page 950*
- **Teva-Glyburide (Can)** *see* GlyBURIDE *on page 974*
- **Tevagrastim** *see* Filgrastim *on page 872*
- **Teva-Hydrochlorothiazide (Can)** *see* Hydrochlorothiazide *on page 1023*
- **Teva-Hydromorphone (Can)** *see* HYDROmorphone *on page 1041*
- **Teva-Imatinib (Can)** *see* Imatinib *on page 1072*
- **Teva-Ipratropium Sterinebs (Can)** *see* Ipratropium (Oral Inhalation) *on page 1144*
- **Teva-Irbesartan (Can)** *see* Irbesartan *on page 1147*
- **Teva-Ketoconazole (Can)** *see* Ketoconazole (Systemic) *on page 1177*
- **Teva-Lamivudine/Zidovudine (Can)** *see* Lamivudine and Zidovudine *on page 1198*
- **Teva-Lamotrigine (Can)** *see* LamoTRIgine *on page 1199*
- **Teva-Lansoprazole (Can)** *see* Lansoprazole *on page 1206*
- **Teva-Letrozole (Can)** *see* Letrozole *on page 1211*
- **Teva-Lisinopril (Type P) (Can)** *see* Lisinopril *on page 1262*
- **Teva-Lisinopril (Type Z) (Can)** *see* Lisinopril *on page 1262*
- **Teva-Lorazepam (Can)** *see* LORazepam *on page 1280*
- **Teva-Losartan (Can)** *see* Losartan *on page 1283*
- **Teva-Lovastatin (Can)** *see* Lovastatin *on page 1286*
- **Teva-Medroxyprogesterone (Can)** *see* MedroxyPROGESTERone *on page 1318*
- **Teva-Meloxicam (Can)** *see* Meloxicam *on page 1325*
- **Teva-Metformin (Can)** *see* MetFORMIN *on page 1353*
- **Teva-Methylphenidate ER-C (Can)** *see* Methylphenidate *on page 1379*
- **Teva-Metoprolol (Can)** *see* Metoprolol *on page 1396*
- **Teva-Montelukast (Can)** *see* Montelukast *on page 1438*
- **Teva-Morphine SR (Can)** *see* Morphine (Systemic) *on page 1440*
- **Teva-Nabilone (Can)** *see* Nabilone *on page 1459*
- **Teva-Nadolol (Can)** *see* Nadolol *on page 1460*
- **Teva-Naproxen (Can)** *see* Naproxen *on page 1470*
- **Teva-Naproxen EC (Can)** *see* Naproxen *on page 1470*
- **Teva-Naproxen Sodium (Can)** *see* Naproxen *on page 1470*
- **Teva-Naproxen Sodium DS (Can)** *see* Naproxen *on page 1470*
- **Teva-Naproxen SR (Can)** *see* Naproxen *on page 1470*
- **Teva-Nevirapine (Can)** *see* Nevirapine *on page 1487*
- **Teva-Nitrofurantoin (Can)** *see* Nitrofurantoin *on page 1502*
- **Teva-Nortriptyline (Can)** *see* Nortriptyline *on page 1512*
- **Teva-Olanzapine (Can)** *see* OLANZapine *on page 1525*
- **Teva-Olanzapine OD (Can)** *see* OLANZapine *on page 1525*
- **Teva-Omeprazole (Can)** *see* Omeprazole *on page 1535*
- **Teva-Ondansetron (Can)** *see* Ondansetron *on page 1544*
- **Teva-Pantoprazole (Can)** *see* Pantoprazole *on page 1595*
- **Teva-Paroxetine (Can)** *see* PARoxetine *on page 1609*
- **Teva-Pravastatin (Can)** *see* Pravastatin *on page 1720*

- **Teva-Prazosin (Can)** *see* Prazosin *on page 1724*
- **Teva-Propranolol (Can)** *see* Propranolol *on page 1759*
- **Teva-Quetiapine (Can)** *see* QUEtiapine *on page 1783*
- **Teva-Quetiapine XR (Can)** *see* QUEtiapine *on page 1783*
- **Teva-Rabeprazole EC (Can)** *see* RABEprazole *on page 1797*
- **Teva-Ranitidine (Can)** *see* Ranitidine *on page 1805*
- **Teva-Risperidone (Can)** *see* RisperiDONE *on page 1831*
- **Teva-Rosuvastatin (Can)** *see* Rosuvastatin *on page 1853*
- **Teva-Salbutamol (Can)** *see* Albuterol *on page 84*
- **Teva-Salbutamol Sterinebs P.F. (Can)** *see* Albuterol *on page 84*
- **Teva-Sertraline (Can)** *see* Sertraline *on page 1879*
- **Teva-Sildenafil (Can)** *see* Sildenafil *on page 1884*
- **Teva-Simvastatin (Can)** *see* Simvastatin *on page 1892*
- **Teva-Spironolactone (Can)** *see* Spironolactone *on page 1930*
- **Teva-Spironolactone/HCTZ (Can)** *see* Hydrochlorothiazide and Spironolactone *on page 1025*
- **Teva-Sucralfate (Can)** *see* Sucralfate *on page 1940*
- **Teva-Sulindac (Can)** *see* Sulindac *on page 1957*
- **Teva-Sumatriptan (Can)** *see* SUMAtriptan *on page 1958*
- **Teva-Sumatriptan DF (Can)** *see* SUMAtriptan *on page 1958*
- **Teva-Tamoxifen (Can)** *see* Tamoxifen *on page 1968*
- **Teva-Terazosin (Can)** *see* Terazosin *on page 1981*
- **Teva-Terbinafine (Can)** *see* Terbinafine (Systemic) *on page 1982*
- **Teva-Theophylline SR (Can)** *see* Theophylline *on page 2005*
- **Teva-Timolol (Can)** *see* Timolol (Systemic) *on page 2026*
- **TEVA-Topiramate (Can)** *see* Topiramate *on page 2046*
- **Teva-Trazodone (Can)** *see* TraZODone *on page 2065*
- **Teva-Trimel (Can)** *see* Sulfamethoxazole and Trimethoprim *on page 1948*
- **Teva-Trimel DS (Can)** *see* Sulfamethoxazole and Trimethoprim *on page 1948*
- **Teva-Valsartan (Can)** *see* Valsartan *on page 2108*
- **Teva-Venlafaxine XR (Can)** *see* Venlafaxine *on page 2125*
- **Tev-Tropin** *see* Somatropin *on page 1920*
- **Texacort** *see* Hydrocortisone (Topical) *on page 1038*
- **TG** *see* Thioguanine *on page 2010*
- **T/Gel Therapeutic Shampoo Extra Strength [OTC] (Can)** *see* Coal Tar *on page 532*
- **6-TG (error-prone abbreviation)** *see* Thioguanine *on page 2010*

Thalidomide (tha LI doe mide)

Medication Safety Issues
Sound-alike/look-alike issues:
Thalidomide may be confused with flutamide, lenalidomide, pomalidomide
Thalomid may be confused with Revlimid, thiamine
High alert medication:
This medication is in a class the Institute for Safe Medication Practices (ISMP) includes among its list of

drug classes that have a heightened risk of causing significant patient harm when used in error.

International issues:

Thalomid [U.S., Canada] may be confused with Thilomide brand name for Iodoxamide [Greece, Turkey]

Related Information

Emetogenic Potential of Antineoplastic Agents in Children *on page 2327*

Oral Medications That Should Not Be Crushed or Altered *on page 2438*

Safe Handling of Hazardous Drugs *on page 2419*

Brand Names: U.S. Thalomid

Brand Names: Canada Thalomid

Therapeutic Category Angiogenesis Inhibitor; Immunosuppressant Agent; Tumor Necrosis Factor (TNF) Blocking Agent

Generic Availability (U.S.) No

Use Treatment of multiple myeloma in combination with dexamethasone (FDA approved in ages ≥12 years and adults); treatment and maintenance of cutaneous manifestations of erythema nodosum leprosum (ENL) (FDA approved in ≥12 years and adults). Has also been used in children when other therapies have failed for treatment of Crohn's disease/ulcerative colitis; refractory chronic graft-versus-host disease (cGVHD); AIDS-related aphthous stomatitis; systemic-onset juvenile idiopathic arthritis (SOJIA); various malignancies

Prescribing and Access Restrictions U.S.: As a requirement of the REMS program, access to this medication is restricted. Thalidomide is approved for marketing only under a special distribution program, the Thalomid REMS (https://www.celgeneriskmanagement.com or 1-888-423-5436), which has been approved by the FDA. Prescribers, patients, and pharmacies must be certified with the program to prescribe or dispense thalidomide. No more than a 4-week supply should be dispensed. Blister packs should be dispensed intact (do not repackage capsules). Prescriptions must be filled within 7 days (for females of reproductive potential) or within 30 days (for all other patients) after authorization number obtained. Subsequent prescriptions may be filled only if fewer than 7 days of therapy remain on the previous prescription. A new prescription is required for further dispensing (a telephone prescription may not be accepted.) Pregnancy testing is required for females of childbearing potential.

Canada: Access to thalidomide is restricted through a controlled distribution program called RevAid. Only physicians and pharmacists enrolled in this program are authorized to prescribe or dispense thalidomide. Patients must be enrolled in the program by their physicians. Further information is available at www.RevAid.ca or by calling 1-888-738-2431.

Medication Guide Available Yes

Pregnancy Risk Factor X

Pregnancy Considerations [U.S. Boxed Warning]: Thalidomide may cause severe birth defects or embryo-fetal death if taken during pregnancy. Thalidomide cannot be used in women who are pregnant or may become pregnant during therapy as even a single dose may cause severe birth defects. In order to decrease the risk of fetal exposure, thalidomide is available only through a special restricted distribution program (Thalomid REMS). Reproduction studies in animals and data from pregnant women have shown evidence of fetal abnormalities; use is contraindicated in women who are or may become pregnant. Anomalies observed in humans include amelia, phocomelia, bone defects, ear and eye abnormalities, facial palsy, congenital heart defects, urinary and genital tract malformations; mortality in ~40% of infants at or shortly after birth has also been reported.

Women of reproductive potential must avoid pregnancy 4 weeks prior to therapy, during therapy, during therapy interruptions, and for ≥4 weeks after therapy is discontinued. Two forms of effective contraception or total abstinence from heterosexual intercourse must be used by females who are not infertile or who have not had a hysterectomy. A negative pregnancy test (sensitivity of at least 50 mIU/mL) 10-14 days prior to therapy, within 24 hours prior to beginning therapy, weekly during the first 4 weeks, and every 4 weeks (every 2 weeks for women with irregular menstrual cycles) thereafter is required for women of childbearing potential. Thalidomide must be immediately discontinued for a missed period, abnormal pregnancy test or abnormal menstrual bleeding; refer patient to a reproductive toxicity specialist if pregnancy occurs during treatment.

Females of reproductive potential (including health care workers and caregivers) must also avoid contact with thalidomide capsules.

Thalidomide is also present in the semen of males. Males (even those vasectomized) must use a latex or synthetic condom during any sexual contact with women of childbearing potential and for up to 28 days following discontinuation of therapy. Males taking thalidomide must not donate sperm.

The parent or legal guardian for patients between 12-18 years of age must agree to ensure compliance with the required guidelines.

If pregnancy occurs during treatment, thalidomide must be immediately discontinued and the patient referred to a reproductive toxicity specialist. Any suspected fetal exposure to thalidomide must be reported to the FDA via the MedWatch program (1-800-FDA-1088) and to Celgene Corporation (1-888-423-5436). In Canada, thalidomide is available only through a restricted-distribution program called RevAid (1-888-738-2431).

Breast-Feeding Considerations It is not known if thalidomide is excreted in breast milk. Due to the potential for serious adverse reactions in the infant, a decision should be made to discontinue nursing or discontinue treatment with thalidomide, taking into account the importance of treatment to the mother. Use in breast-feeding women is contraindicated in the Canadian labeling.

Contraindications Hypersensitivity to thalidomide or any component; pregnancy; women of childbearing potential, unless alternative therapies are inappropriate and adequate precautions are taken to avoid pregnancy; patients unable to comply with S.T.E.P.S.® program (including males)

Warnings Hazardous agent; use appropriate precautions for handling and disposal (NIOSH, 2012). Thalidomide is a known teratogen, even following a single dose **[U.S. Boxed Warning]:** embryotoxic with limb defects noted from the 27th to 40th gestational day of exposure; all cases of phocomelia occur from the 27th to 42nd gestational day; fetal cardiac, gastrointestinal, bone, external ear, eye, and genitourinary tract abnormalities have also been described. Mortality at or shortly after birth has also been reported. Two reliable forms of contraception or abstinence must be used for at least 4 weeks before initiating therapy, during therapy, and for 4 weeks following discontinuation of thalidomide for women of childbearing potential. A negative pregnancy test (sensitivity of at least 50 mIU/mL) within 24 hours prior to beginning therapy, weekly during the first 4 weeks, and every 4 weeks (every 2 weeks for women with irregular menstrual cycles) thereafter is required. Males (even those vasectomized) must use a latex condom during any sexual contact with women of childbearing age. Risk to the fetus from semen of male patients is unknown. Thalidomide must be immediately discontinued and the patient referred to a reproductive

▶

toxicity specialist if pregnancy occurs during treatment. Any suspected fetal exposure to thalidomide must be reported to the FDA via the MedWatch program (800) FDA-1088 and to Celgene Corporation (888) 423-5436.

Use in multiple myeloma patients results in an increased risk of thrombotic events such as deep vein thrombosis and pulmonary embolism **[U.S. Boxed Warning]**. Risk significantly increases when used in combination with standard chemotherapeutic agents, including dexamethasone. Monitor for signs and symptoms of thromboembolism; some patients at risk may benefit from prophylactic anticoagulation or aspirin therapy.

Frequently causes drowsiness and somnolence. Patients must be cautioned about performing tasks which require mental alertness (eg, operating machinery or driving). May cause peripheral neuropathy which may be irreversible; usually associated with chronic use, but has been seen following short-term therapy; no correlation with cumulative dose identified in adults. In children, significant correlations with cumulative dose (>20 g) and duration of therapy (>10 months) have been reported (Priolo, 2008). Patients should be monitored for signs and symptoms of peripheral neuropathy; consider immediate discontinuation (if clinically appropriate) in patients who develop neuropathy.

May cause dizziness and orthostatic hypotension. May cause neutropenia; discontinue therapy if absolute neutrophil count decreases to <750/mm³. Increase HIV viral load has been reported in clinical trials; clinical significance is unknown.

Thalidomide should only be prescribed under the restricted S.T.E.P.S.® program **[U.S. Boxed Warning]**. Thalidomide should only be prescribed to patients (male and female) who can understand and comply with the conditions of the S.T.E.P.S.® program. Distribution is restricted; if the patient is 12-18 years of age, a parent or legal guardian must be able to understand and ensure compliance with the S.T.E.P.S.® program; physicians, pharmacists, and patients must be registered with the S.T.E.P.S.® program.

Precautions Hypersensitivity reactions, Stevens-Johnson syndrome (SJS), and toxic epidermal necrolysis (TEN) have been reported; withhold therapy and evaluate skin rashes; permanently discontinue if rash is exfoliative, purpuric, bullous, or if SJS or TEN is suspected. May cause bradycardia; in some cases, medical intervention may be required; use with caution in patients with cardiovascular disease. May cause seizures; use with caution in patients with a history of seizures, concurrent therapy with drugs which alter seizure threshold, or conditions which predispose to seizures.

Adverse Reactions

Cardiovascular: Edema, facial edema, hypotension, peripheral edema, thrombosis/embolism

Central nervous system: Agitation/anxiety, confusion, dizziness, fatigue, fever, headache, insomnia, malaise, motor neuropathy, nervousness, pain, sensory neuropathy, somnolence, vertigo

Dermatologic: Acne, dermatitis (fungal), desquamation, dry skin, maculopapular rash, nail disorder, pruritus, rash

Endocrine & metabolic: Hyperlipemia, hypocalcemia

Gastrointestinal: Anorexia, constipation, diarrhea, flatulence, nausea, oral moniliasis, tooth pain, weight gain/loss, xerostomia

Genitourinary: Impotence

Hematologic: Anemia, leukopenia, lymphadenopathy, neutropenia

Hepatic: AST increased, bilirubin increased, LFTs abnormal

Neuromuscular & skeletal: Arthralgia, back pain, muscle weakness, myalgia, neck pain/rigidity, neuropathy, paresthesia, tremor, weakness

Renal: Albuminuria, hematuria

Respiratory: Dyspnea, pharyngitis, rhinitis, sinusitis

Miscellaneous: Diaphoresis, infection

Rare but important or life-threatening: Acute renal failure, alkaline phosphatase increased, ALT increased, amenorrhea, angioedema, aphthous stomatitis, arrhythmia, atrial fibrillation, bile duct obstruction, bradycardia, BUN increased, carpal tunnel, cerebral vascular accident, CML, creatinine clearance decreased, creatinine increased, deafness, depression, diplopia, dysesthesia, ECG abnormalities, enuresis, eosinophilia, epistaxis, erythema multiforme, erythema nodosum, erythroleukemia, exfoliative dermatitis, febrile neutropenia, foot drop, galactorrhea, granulocytopenia, gynecomastia, hearing loss, hepatomegaly, Hodgkin's disease, hypercalcemia, hyper-/hypokalemia, hypersensitivity, hypertension, hyper-/hypothyroidism, hypersensitivity, hyperuricemia, hypomagnesemia, hyponatremia, hypoproteinemia, intestinal obstruction, intestinal perforation, interstitial pneumonitis, LDH increased, lethargy, leukocytosis, loss of consciousness, lymphedema, lymphopenia, mental status changes, metrorrhagia, MI, myxedema, nystagmus, oliguria, orthostatic hypotension, pancytopenia, paresthesia, petechiae, peripheral neuritis, photosensitivity, pleural effusion, prothrombin time changes, psychosis, pulmonary embolus, pulmonary hypertension, purpura, Raynaud's syndrome, renal failure, secondary malignancy (AML, MDS, solid tumors), seizure, sepsis, septic shock, sexual dysfunction, sick sinus syndrome, status epilepticus, Stevens-Johnson syndrome, stomach ulcer, stupor, suicide attempt, syncope, tachycardia, thrombocytopenia, toxic epidermal necrolysis, transient ischemic attack, tumor lysis syndrome, urticaria

Drug Interactions

Metabolism/Transport Effects None known.

Avoid Concomitant Use

Avoid concomitant use of Thalidomide with any of the following: Abatacept; Anakinra; Azelastine (Nasal); BCG; Canakinumab; Certolizumab Pegol; CloZAPine; CNS Depressants; Dipyrone; Natalizumab; Paraldehyde; Pimecrolimus; Rilonacept; Tacrolimus (Topical); Tocilizumab; Tofacitinib; Vaccines (Live); Vedolizumab

Increased Effect/Toxicity

Thalidomide may increase the levels/effects of: Abatacept; Alcohol (Ethyl); Anakinra; Azelastine (Nasal); Bisphosphonate Derivatives; Canakinumab; Certolizumab Pegol; CloZAPine; Leflunomide; Metyrosine; Natalizumab; Pamidronate; Paraldehyde; Pramipexole; Rilonacept; ROPINIRole; Rotigotine; Selective Serotonin Reuptake Inhibitors; Tofacitinib; Vaccines (Live); Vedolizumab; Zoledronic Acid

The levels/effects of Thalidomide may be increased by: Brimonidine (Topical); Cannabis; CNS Depressants; Contraceptives (Estrogens); Contraceptives (Progestins); Denosumab; Dexamethasone (Systemic); Dipyrone; Dronabinol; Kava Kava; Magnesium Sulfate; Nabilone; Pimecrolimus; Roflumilast; Rufinamide; Tacrolimus (Topical); Tetrahydrocannabinol; Tocilizumab; Trastuzumab

Decreased Effect

Thalidomide may decrease the levels/effects of: BCG; Coccidioidin Skin Test; Sipuleucel-T; Vaccines (Inactivated); Vaccines (Live)

The levels/effects of Thalidomide may be decreased by: Echinacea

Stability Hazardous agent; use appropriate precautions for handling and disposal (NIOSH, 2012). Store at 25°C (77°F); excursions permitted to 15°C to 30°C (50°F to 86°F). Protect from light. Keep in original package.

Mechanism of Action Immunomodulatory and antiangiogenic characteristics; immunologic effects may vary based on conditions; may suppress excessive tumor necrosis factor-alpha production in patients with ENL, yet may increase plasma tumor necrosis factor-alpha levels in

HIV-positive patients. In multiple myeloma, thalidomide is associated with an increase in natural killer cells and increased levels of interleukin-2 and interferon gamma. Other proposed mechanisms of action include suppression of angiogenesis, prevention of free-radical-mediated DNA damage, increased cell mediated cytotoxic effects, and altered expression of cellular adhesion molecules.

Pharmacokinetics (Adult data unless noted)

Distribution: V_d: 70-120 L

Protein binding: 55% to 66%

Metabolism: Nonenzymatic hydrolysis in plasma; forms multiple metabolites

Half-life elimination: 5-7 hours

Time to peak, plasma: 3-6 hours

Excretion: Urine (<1% as unchanged drug)

Dosing: Usual

Children and Adolescents:

AIDS-related aphthous stomatitis: Limited data available: Adolescents ≥13 years: Oral: 200 mg once daily at bedtime for 4 weeks or sooner if resolution. May be increased to 200 mg twice daily if no improvement after 4 weeks. Dosing based on double-blind, placebo-controlled trial by AIDS Clinical Trials Group (n=57, age: ≥13 years) which showed 55% healing in treatment group vs 7% in placebo (Jacobson, 1997).

Chronic graft-versus-host disease (refractory), treatment: Limited data available: Children ≥2 years and Adolescents: Oral: Initial: 3-6 mg/kg/**day** (maximum initial daily dose: 100 mg/**day**) at bedtime or in 2-4 divided doses before meals; may be adjusted at ≥2 week intervals based on patient response up to 12 mg/kg/**day** in 3-4 divided doses (maximum daily dose: 800 mg/**day**) (Browne, 2000; Rovelli, 1998; Wolff, 2010); one trial using initial doses of 3 mg/kg/dose every 6 hours (dose adjusted to attain goal thalidomide concentration of ≥5 mcg/mL 2 hours postdose) (Vogelsang, 1992)

Crohn's disease/ulcerative colitis (refractory), treatment: Limited data available: Children ≥1 year and Adolescents: Oral: 0.5-3 mg/kg/**day** (maximum daily dose: 300 mg/**day**), usually dosed once daily in the evening; titrate to lowest effective dose after remission is achieved (Facchini, 2001; Lazzerini, 2007; Martelossi, 2004; Zheng, 2011)

Cutaneous erythema nodosum leprosum (ENL): Children ≥12 years and Adolescents: Oral:

Initial: 100-300 mg once daily at bedtime; may increase to 400 mg/day in severe cases or in patients who had previously required a high dose for treatment; for patients <50 kg, initiate at lower end of dosage range.

Maintenance: Continue initial dose until active reaction subsides then taper in 50 mg decrements every 2-4 weeks. Doses may be divided and taken 1 hour after meals. Patients who flare during tapering or with a history of requiring prolonged maintenance should be maintained on the minimum dosage necessary to control the reaction. Efforts to taper should be repeated every 3-6 months, in increments of 50 mg every 2-4 weeks.

Systemic-onset juvenile idiopathic arthritis: Limited data available: Children ≥3 years and Adolescents: Oral: Initial 2 mg/kg/**day**, if necessary may increase at 2-week intervals to 3-5 mg/kg/**day**. Data based on a multicenter, open-labeled prospective study (n=13, age: 3-23 years); within 4 weeks, 11 of 13 patients showed improvement in JRA scores, significant decreases in ESR, and significant increase in hemoglobin (Lehman, 2004).

Adults:

Chronic graft-versus-host disease (refractory), treatment: Oral: Initial: 100 mg at bedtime, with dose escalation up to 400 mg/day in 3-4 divided doses (Wolff, 2010) **or** Initial: 50-100 mg 3 times daily; maximum

dose: 600-1200 mg/day (Kulkarni, 2003) **or** 200 mg 4 times daily (dose adjusted to goal thalidomide concentration of ≥5 mcg/mL 2 hours postdose) (Vogelsang, 1992) **or** 100-300 mg 4 times daily (Parker, 1995)

Crohn's disease, refractory: Oral: 50-100 mg/day at bedtime (Vasiliauskas, 1999) **or** 200-300 mg/day at bedtime (Ehrenpreis, 1999)

Cutaneous erythema nodosum leprosum (ENL): Oral: Initial: 100-300 mg once daily

Adjustments to initial dose:

Patients weighing <50 kg: Initiate at lower end of the dosing range

Severe cutaneous reaction or patients previously requiring high dose may be initiated at 400 mg/day; doses may be divided, but taken 1 hour after meals

Duration and tapering/maintenance:

Maintenance: Dosing should continue until active reaction subsides (usually at least 2 weeks), then tapered in 50 mg decrements every 2-4 weeks

Patients who flare during tapering or with a history of requiring prolonged maintenance should be maintained on the minimum dosage necessary to control the reaction. Efforts to taper should be repeated every 3-6 months, in decrements of 50 mg every 2-4 weeks.

Multiple myeloma: Note: Details concerning dosing for multiple myeloma with combination regimens should also be consulted.

200 mg once daily at bedtime (in combination with dexamethasone 40 mg daily on days 1-4, 9-12, and 17-20 of a 28-day treatment cycle)

In combination with melphalan and prednisone: 200-400 mg once daily (Facon, 2007) **or** 100 mg once daily (Palumbo, 2008)

Dosage adjustment for renal impairment: No adjustment is required for patients with renal impairment and on dialysis (per manufacturer). In a study of six adult patients with end-stage renal disease on dialysis, although clearance was increased by dialysis, a supplemental dose was not needed (Eriksson, 2003).

Multiple myeloma: An evaluation of 29 newly diagnosed adult myeloma patients with renal failure (serum creatinine ≥2 mg/dL) treated with thalidomide and dexamethasone (some also received cyclophosphamide) found that toxicities and efficacy were similar to patients with normal renal function (Seol, 2010). A study evaluating induction therapy with thalidomide and dexamethasone in 31 newly diagnosed adult myeloma patients with renal failure (CrCl <50 mL/minute), including 16 patients with severe renal impairment (CrCl <30 mL/minute) and seven patients on chronic hemodialysis found that toxicities were similar to patients without renal impairment and that thalidomide and dexamethasone could be administered safely (Tosi, 2009).

Dosage adjustment for hepatic impairment: Thalidomide does not appear to undergo significant hepatic metabolism; the pharmacokinetics of thalidomide have not been studied in patients with liver dysfunction.

Dosage adjustment for toxicity:

ANC ≤750/mm^3: Withhold treatment if clinically appropriate

Multiple myeloma: Constipation, oversedation, peripheral neuropathy: Temporarily withhold or continue with a reduced dose

Administration Hazardous agent; use appropriate precautions for handling and disposal (NIOSH, 2012). Administer with water, preferably at bedtime, once daily on an empty stomach, at least 1 hour after the evening meal. Doses >400 mg/day may be given in 2-3 divided doses. Avoid extensive handling of capsules; capsules should remain in blister pack until ingestion. If exposed to the powder content from broken capsules or body fluids from patients receiving thalidomide, the exposed area should be washed with soap and water. For missed doses, if <12 hours have passed, patient may receive dose; if >12 hours have passed, wait until next dose is due.

Monitoring Parameters Monitor for signs and symptoms of thromboembolism (shortness of breath, chest pain, arm/leg swelling). CBC with differential, platelets. Pregnancy testing (sensitivity of at least 50 mIU/mL) is required within 24 hours prior to initiation of therapy, weekly during the first 4 weeks, then every 4 weeks in women with regular menstrual cycles or every 2 weeks in women with irregular menstrual cycles. Signs of neuropathy monthly for the first 3 months, then periodically during treatment; consider monitoring of sensory nerve application potential amplitudes (at baseline and every 6 months) to detect asymptomatic neuropathy. In HIV-seropositive patients: Viral load after 1 and 3 months, then every 3 months.

Reference Range One study suggests that therapeutic plasma thalidomide concentrations in graft-vs-host reactions are 5-8 mcg/mL 2 hours postdose (Vogelsang, 1992).

Additional Information Thalidomide-associated birth defects have only been reported as a result of direct oral ingestion of drug; data is not available regarding cutaneous absorption or inhalation exposures and whether these exposures may result in birth defects.

Dosage Forms Excipient information presented when available (limited, particularly for generics); consult specific product labeling.

Capsule, Oral:

Thalomid: 50 mg, 100 mg

Thalomid: 150 mg, 200 mg [contains fd&c blue #2 (indigotine)]

Extemporaneous Preparations Hazardous agent: Use appropriate precautions for handling and disposal.

A 20 mg/mL oral suspension may be prepared with capsules and a 1:1 mixture of Ora-Sweet and Ora-Plus. Empty the contents of twelve 100 mg capsules into a glass mortar. Add small portions of the vehicle and mix to a uniform paste; mix while adding the vehicle in incremental proportions to almost 60 mL; transfer to an amber calibrated bottle, rinse mortar with vehicle, and add quantity of vehicle sufficient to make 60 mL. Label "shake well," "protect from light," and "refrigerate". Stable for 35 days refrigerated.

Kraft S, Johnson CE, and Tyler RP, "Stability of an Extemporaneously Prepared Thalidomide Suspension," *Am J Health Syst Pharm*, 2011, 69(1):56-8.

References

Bessmertny O and Pham T, "Thalidomide Use in Pediatric Patients," *Ann Pharmacother*, 2002, 36(3):521-5.

Britton WJ and Lockwood DN, "Leprosy," *Lancet*, 2004, 363 (9416):1209-19.

Browne PV, Weisdorf DJ, DeFor T, et al, "Response to Thalidomide Therapy in Refractory Chronic Graft-Versus-Host Disease," *Bone Marrow Transplant*, 2000, 26(8):865-9.

Ehrenpreis ED, Kane SV, Cohen LB, et al, "Thalidomide Therapy for Patients With Refractory Crohn's Disease: An Open-Label Trial," *Gastroenterology*, 1999, 117(6):1271-7.

Eriksson T, Höglund P, Turesson I, et al, "Pharmacokinetics of Thalidomide in Patients With Impaired Renal Function and While On and Off Dialysis," *J Pharm Pharmacol*, 2003, 55(12):1701-6.

Facchini S, Candusso M, Martelossi S, et al, "Efficacy of Long-Term Treatment With Thalidomide in Children and Young Adults With Crohn Disease: Preliminary Results," *J Pediatr Gastroenterol Nutr*, 2001, 32 (2):178-81.

Facon T, Mary JY, Hulin C, et al, "Melphalan and Prednisone Plus Thalidomide Versus Melphalan and Prednisone Alone or Reduced-Intensity Autologous Stem Cell Transplantation in Elderly Patients With Multiple Myeloma (IFM 99-06): A Randomised Trial," *Lancet*, 2007, 370(9594):1209-18.

Jacobson JM, Greenspan JS, Spritzler J, et al, "Thalidomide for the Treatment of Oral Aphthous Ulcers in Patients With Human Immunodeficiency Virus Infection. National Institute of Allergy and Infectious Diseases AIDS Clinical Trials Group," *N Engl J Med*, 1997, 336 (21):1487-93.

Kulkarni S, Powles R, Sirohi B, et al, "Thalidomide After Allogeneic Haematopoietic Stem Cell Transplantation: Activity in Chronic But Not

in Acute Graft-Versus-Host Disease," *Bone Marrow Transplant*, 2003, 32(2):165-70.

Lazzerini M, Martelossi S, Marchetti F, et al, "Efficacy and Safety of Thalidomide in Children and Young Adults With Intractable Inflammatory Bowel Disease: Long-Term Results," *Aliment Pharmacol Ther*, 2007, 25(4):419-27.

Lehman TJ, Schechter SJ, Sundel RP, et al, "Thalidomide for Severe Systemic Onset Juvenile Rheumatoid Arthritis: A Multicenter Study," *J Pediatr*, 2004, 145(6):856-7.

Martelossi S, Marchetti F, Lenhard A, et al, "Treatment With Thalidomide in Children and Adolescents With Inflammatory Bowel Disease," *J Pediatr Gastroenterol Nutr*, 2004, 39(1):S282-3.

Matthews SJ and McCoy C, "Thalidomide: A Review of Approved and Investigational Uses," *Clin Ther*, 2003, 25(2):342-95.

Mehta P, Kedar A, Graham-Pole J, et al, "Thalidomide in Children Undergoing Bone Marrow Transplantation: Series at a Single Institution and Review of the Literature," *Pediatrics*, 1999, 103(4):e44.

National Institute for Occupational Safety and Health (NIOSH), "NIOSH List of Antineoplastic and Other Hazardous Drugs in Healthcare Settings 2012." Available at http://www.cdc.gov/niosh/docs/2012-150/pdfs/2012-150.pdf. Accessed January 21, 2013.

Okafor MC, "Thalidomide for Erythema Nodosum Leprosum and Other Applications," *Pharmacotherapy*, 2003, 23(4):481-93.

Palumbo A, Rajkumar SV, Dimopoulos MA, et al, "Prevention of Thalidomide- and Lenalidomide-Associated Thrombosis in Myeloma," *Leukemia*, 2008, 22(2):414-23.

Parker PM, Chao N, Nademanee A, et al, "Thalidomide as Salvage Therapy for Chronic Graft-Versus-Host Disease," *Blood*, 1995, 86 (9):3604-9.

Priolo T, Lamba LD, Giribaldi G, et al, "Childhood Thalidomide Neuropathy: A Clinical and Neurophysiologic Study," *Pediatr Neurol*, 2008, 38(3):196-9.

Rovelli A, Arrigo C, Nesi F, et al, "The Role of Thalidomide in the Treatment of Refractory Chronic Graft-Versus-Host Disease Following Bone Marrow Transplantation in Children," *Bone Marrow Transplant*, 1998, 21(6):577-81.

Seol Y, Chung J, Kwon B, et al, "Treatment for Patients With Multiple Myeloma Complicated by Renal Failure by Thalidomide-Based Regimens," *J Clin Oncol*, 2010, 28(Suppl):e13093 [Abstract e13093 From 2010 ASCO Annual Meeting].

Teo SK, Colburn WA, Tracewell WG, et al, "Clinical Pharmacokinetics of Thalidomide," *Clin Pharmacokinet*, 2004, 43(5):311-27.

Thompson JL and Hansen LA, "Thalidomide Dosing in Patients With Relapsed or Refractory Multiple Myeloma," *Ann Pharmacother*, 2003, 37(4):571-6.

Tosi P, Zamagni E, Tacchetti P, et al, "Thalidomide-Dexamethasone as Induction Therapy Prior to Autologous Stem-Cell Transplantation in Patients With Newly Diagnosed Multiple Myeloma and Renal Failure," *Blood*, 2009, 114(22):4934 [Abstract 4934 From 2009 ASH Annual Meeting].

Vasiliauskas EA, Kam LY, Abreu-Martin MT, et al, "An Open-Label Pilot Study of Low-Dose Thalidomide in Chronically Active, Steroid-Dependent Crohn's Disease," *Gastroenterology*, 1999, 117 (6):1278-87.

Vogelsang GB, Farmer ER, Hess AD, et al, "Thalidomide for the Treatment of Chronic Graft-Versus-Host Disease," *N Engl J Med*, 1992, 326(16):1055-8.

Wolff D, Schleuning M, von Harsdorf S, et al, "Consensus Conference on Clinical Practice in Chronic GVHD: Second-Line Treatment of Chronic Graft-Versus-Host Disease," *Biol Blood Marrow Transplant*, 2011, 17(1):1-17.

Zheng CF, Xu JH, Huang Y, et al, "Treatment of Pediatric Refractory Crohn's Disease With Thalidomide," *World J Gastroenterol*, 2011, 17 (10):1286-91.

◆ **Thalomid** *see* Thalidomide *on page 2000*

◆ **Tham** *see* Tromethamine *on page 2091*

◆ **THC** *see* Dronabinol *on page 725*

◆ **The Magic Bullett [OTC] (Can)** *see* Bisacodyl *on page 293*

◆ **Theo-24** *see* Theophylline *on page 2005*

◆ **Theochron** *see* Theophylline *on page 2005*

◆ **Theo ER (Can)** *see* Theophylline *on page 2005*

◆ **Theolair (Can)** *see* Theophylline *on page 2005*

Theophylline (thee OFF i lin)

Related Information

Medications for Which a Single Dose May Be Fatal When Ingested by a Toddler *on page 2408*

Oral Medications That Should Not Be Crushed or Altered *on page 2438*

Brand Names: U.S. Elixophyllin; Theo-24; Theochron

Brand Names: Canada Apo-Theo LA®; Novo-Theophyl SR; PMS-Theophylline; Pulmophylline; ratio-Theo-Bronc; Teva-Theophylline SR; Theo ER; Theolair; Uniphyl

Therapeutic Category Antiasthmatic; Bronchodilator; Respiratory Stimulant; Theophylline Derivative

Generic Availability (U.S.) May be product dependent

Use

Oral: Treatment of symptoms and reversible airway obstruction due to chronic asthma, chronic bronchitis, COPD, or other chronic lung diseases [Immediate release oral solution: FDA approved in all ages; Extended release 12 hour tablets: FDA approved in ages ≥6 years and adults; Extended release 24 hour capsules (Theo-24®) and tablets: FDA approved in ages ≥12 years and adults); has also been used for treatment of idiopathic apnea of prematurity and to increase diaphragmatic contractility

Note: The Global Initiative for Asthma Guidelines (2009) and the National Asthma Education and Prevention Program Guidelines (2007) do not recommend oral theophylline as a long-term control medication for asthma in children ≤5 years of age; use has been shown to be effective as an add-on (but not preferred) agent in older children, adolescents, and adults with severe asthma treated with inhaled or oral glucocorticoids. The guidelines do not recommend theophylline for the treatment of exacerbations of asthma.

Parenteral: Adjunctive treatment of acute exacerbations of asthma and other chronic lung diseases (eg, chronic bronchitis, emphysema) (FDA approved in all ages)

Pregnancy Risk Factor C

Pregnancy Considerations Teratogenic effects were observed in animal reproduction studies. Theophylline crosses the placenta; adverse effects may be seen in the newborn. Use is generally safe when used at the recommended doses (serum concentrations 5-12 mcg/mL) however maternal adverse events may be increased and efficacy may be decreased in pregnant women. Theophylline metabolism may change during pregnancy; the half-life is similar to that observed in otherwise healthy, non-smoking adults with asthma during the first and second trimesters (~8.7 hours), but may increase to 13 hours (range: 8-18 hours) during the third trimester. The volume of distribution is also increased during the third trimester. Monitor serum levels. The recommendations for the use of theophylline in pregnant women with asthma are similar to those used in nonpregnant adults (National Heart, Lung, and Blood Institute Guidelines, 2004).

Breast-Feeding Considerations The concentration of theophylline in breast milk is similar to the maternal serum concentration. Irritability may be observed in the nursing infant. Serious adverse events in the infant are unlikely unless toxic serum levels are present in the mother.

Contraindications Hypersensitivity to theophylline or any component

Warnings Due to wide interpatient variability, theophylline serum concentration measurements must be used to optimize therapy and prevent serious toxicity. If a patient develops signs and symptoms of theophylline toxicity (eg, persistent, repetitive vomiting), a serum theophylline concentration should be measured and subsequent doses held. Theophylline clearance may be decreased in neonates, infants <3 months of age with decreased renal function, infants <1 year, elderly patients >60 years of age, in patients following cessation of smoking, in patients with certain disease states (ie, acute pulmonary edema, congestive heart failure, cor pulmonale, fever, hepatic disease, hypothyroidism, acute hepatitis, cirrhosis, sepsis with multiorgan failure, and shock), and when metabolic inhibitors (eg, cimetidine, erythromycin, tacrine) are administered or metabolic inducers (eg, carbamazepine, rifampin) are discontinued. Due to potential saturation of theophylline clearance at serum concentrations within or in some patients less than the therapeutic range, dosage adjustments should be made in small increments (maximum: 25% dose increase). Additional increases in dose due to an exacerbation of symptoms should not be made unless the steady state serum theophylline concentration is <10 mcg/mL.

Some oral solutions may contain propylene glycol; toxicities have been reported with use of products containing propylene glycol, including hyperosmolality, lactic acidosis, seizures, and respiratory depression; in neonates large amounts of propylene glycol delivered orally, intravenously (eg, >3000 mg/day), or topically have been associated with potentially fatal toxicities which can include metabolic acidosis, seizures, renal failure, and CNS depression; use oral solutions containing propylene glycol with caution (AAP, 1997; Shehab, 2009).

Precautions Prior to initiation of therapy or dosage increase, various drug interactions and disease states that may alter theophylline clearance should be considered. Theophylline may exacerbate certain medical conditions [eg, peptic ulcer disease, hyperthyroidism, seizure disorders, hypertension, and cardiac arrhythmias (excluding bradyarrhythmias)]; use with extreme caution in patients with these underlying conditions.

Adverse Reactions Adverse events observed at therapeutic serum levels:

Cardiovascular: Flutter, tachycardia

Central nervous system: Headache, hyperactivity (children), insomnia, restlessness, seizures, status epilepticus (nonconvulsive)

Endocrine & metabolic: Hypercalcemia (with concomitant hyperthyroid disease)

Gastrointestinal: Nausea, reflux or ulcer aggravation, vomiting

Genitourinary: Difficulty urinating (elderly males with prostatism)

Neuromuscular & skeletal: Tremor

Renal: Diuresis (transient)

Drug Interactions

Metabolism/Transport Effects Substrate of CYP1A2 (major), CYP2C9 (minor), CYP2D6 (minor), CYP2E1 (major), CYP3A4 (major); **Note:** Assignment of Major/Minor substrate status based on clinically relevant drug interaction potential; **Inhibits** CYP1A2 (weak)

Avoid Concomitant Use

Avoid concomitant use of Theophylline with any of the following: Conivaptan; Deferasirox; Fusidic Acid (Systemic); Iobenguane I 123; Riociguat; Stiripentol

Increased Effect/Toxicity

Theophylline may increase the levels/effects of: Formoterol; Indacaterol; Pancuronium; Riociguat; Sympathomimetics

The levels/effects of Theophylline may be increased by: Abiraterone Acetate; Alcohol (Ethyl); Allopurinol; Antithyroid Agents; AtoMOXetine; Cannabinoid-Containing Products; Ceritinib; Cimetidine; Conivaptan; CYP1A2 Inhibitors (Moderate); CYP1A2 Inhibitors (Strong); CYP3A4 Inhibitors (Moderate); CYP3A4 Inhibitors (Strong); Dasatinib; Deferasirox; Disulfiram; Estrogen Derivatives; Febuxostat; FluvoxaMINE; Fusidic Acid (Systemic); Interferons; Isoniazid; Ivacaftor; Linezolid; Luliconazole; Macrolide Antibiotics; Methotrexate; Metreleptin; Mexiletine; Mifepristone; Pentoxifylline; Propafenone; QuiNINE; Quinolone Antibiotics; Simeprevir; Stiripentol; Thiabendazole; Ticlopidine; Vemurafenib; Zafirlukast; Zileuton

Decreased Effect

Theophylline may decrease the levels/effects of: Adenosine; Benzodiazepines; CarBAMazepine; Fosphenytoin; Iobenguane I 123; Lithium; Pancuronium; Phenytoin; Regadenoson; Zafirlukast

The levels/effects of Theophylline may be decreased by: Adalimumab; Aminoglutethimide; Barbiturates; Beta-Blockers (Beta1 Selective); Beta-Blockers (Nonselective); Bosentan; Cannabis; CarBAMazepine; CYP1A2 Inducers (Strong); CYP3A4 Inducers (Strong); Cyproterone; Dabrafenib; Fosphenytoin; Isoproterenol; Metreleptin; Mitotane; Peginterferon Alfa-2b; Phenytoin; Protease Inhibitors; Siltuximab; St Johns Wort; Thyroid Products; Tocilizumab

Food Interactions

Ethanol: Ethanol may decrease theophylline clearance. Management: Avoid or limit ethanol.

Food: Food does not appreciably affect the absorption of liquid, fast-release products, and most sustained release products; however, food may induce a sudden release (dose-dumping) of once-daily sustained release products resulting in an increase in serum drug levels and potential toxicity. Changes in diet may affect the elimination of theophylline; charbroiled foods may increase elimination, reducing half-life by 50%. Management: Should be taken with water 1 hour before or 2 hours after meals. Avoid extremes of dietary protein and carbohydrate intake.

Stability Oral solution, tablet, premixed infusion: Store at 25°C (77°F).

Mechanism of Action Causes bronchodilatation, diuresis, CNS and cardiac stimulation, and gastric acid secretion by blocking phosphodiesterase which increases tissue concentrations of cyclic adenine monophosphate (cAMP) which in turn promotes catecholamine stimulation of lipolysis, glycogenolysis, and gluconeogenesis and induces release of epinephrine from adrenal medulla cells

Pharmacokinetics (Adult data unless noted)

Absorption: Oral: Rapid and complete with up to 100% absorption depending upon the formulation used

Distribution: V_d: 0.45 L/kg (range: 0.3-0.7 L/kg) based on ideal body weight; crosses into the CSF; poorly distributes into body fat

Protein binding: 40%; primarily to albumin; decreased protein binding in neonates (due to a greater percentage of fetal albumin), hepatic cirrhosis, uncorrected acidemia, third trimester of pregnancy, and geriatric patients

Metabolism: Hepatic via demethylation (CYP 1A2) and hydroxylation (CYP 2E1 and 3A4); theophylline is metabolized to active metabolites, caffeine and 3-methylxanthine; in neonates this theophylline-derived caffeine accumulates due to decreased hepatic metabolism and significant concentrations of caffeine may occur; a substantial decrease in serum caffeine concentrations occurs after 40 weeks postmenstrual age

Half-life: See table.

Theophylline Mean Clearance and Half-Life With Respect to Age and Altered Physiological States[A]

Patient Group	Clearance (mL/kg/minute)	Half-life (hours)
Premature infants		
postnatal age 3-15 days	0.29	30
postnatal age 25-57 days	0.64	20
Term infants		
postnatal age 1-2 days	Not reported[B]	25
postnatal age 3-30 weeks[C]	Not reported[B]	11
Children and Adolescents		
1-4 years	1.7	3.4
4-12 years	1.6	Not reported[B]
13-15 years	0.9	Not reported[B]
16-17 years	1.4	3.7 (range: 1.5-5.9)
≥18 years (nonsmoking asthmatic)	0.65	8.2
Adults		
≤60 years (nonsmoking asthmatic)	0.65	8.2
>60 years (nonsmoking, healthy)	0.41	9.8
Acute pulmonary edema	0.33	19
Cystic fibrosis (14-28 years)	1.25	6
Liver disease		
acute hepatitis	0.35	19.2
cholestasis	0.65	14.4
cirrhosis	0.31	32
Sepsis with multiorgan failure	0.46	18.8
Hypothyroid	0.38	11.6
Hyperthyroid	0.8	4.5

[A]From Hendeles L, 1995.

[B]Either not reported or not reported in a comparable format.

[C]Maturation of clearance in premature infants and term infants is most closely related to postmenstrual age (PMA); adult clearance values are reached at approximately 55 weeks PMA and higher pediatric values at approximately 60 weeks PMA (Kraus, 1993).

Elimination: Urine; neonates excrete approximately 50% of the dose unchanged in urine; Infants >3 months, children, adolescents, and adults excrete 10% in urine as unchanged drug

Dosing: Neonatal

Note: Dose should be calculated using ideal body weight and individualized by serum concentrations. Due to the longer half-life compared to older patients, the time to achieve steady-state serum concentrations is prolonged in neonates (see theophylline half-life table); serum theophylline concentrations should be drawn after 48-72 hours of therapy (usually 72 hours in neonates); repeat values should be obtained 3 days after each change in dosage or weekly if on a stabilized dosage. If renal function decreased, consider dose reduction and additional monitoring.

Apnea of prematurity: Oral: Immediate release oral solution:

Loading dose: 5-6 mg/kg/dose (Bhatta-Metta, 2003)

Maintenance: 2-6 mg/kg/**day** divided every 8-12 hours (Bhatta-Mehta, 2003; Henderson-Smart, 2011; Skouroliakou, 2009)

Bronchospasm, neonatal lung disease: Oral:

Loading dose: 4.6 mg/kg/dose

Maintenance:

Premature neonates PNA <24 days: 1 mg/kg/dose every 12 hours

Premature neonates PNA ≥24 days: 1.5 mg/kg/dose every 12 hours

Full-term neonates: Total daily dose may be calculated using equation below; divide into 3 equal doses and administer at 8-hour intervals

Total daily dose (mg/**day**) = [(0.2 x age in weeks) +5] x (weight in kg)

Conversion from aminophylline (I.V.) to theophylline therapy: In premature neonates, the same dose may be used; evaluate serum concentrations at 48 hours or sooner if symptoms indicate.

Dosing adjustment in renal impairment: Dose reduction and frequent monitoring of serum theophylline concentrations are required in neonates with decreased renal function; 50% of dose is excreted unchanged in the urine of neonates.

Dosing: Usual Doses should be individualized based on steady-state serum concentrations; theophylline pharmacokinetics have age-dependent factors which may alter required doses particularly in pediatric patients. For obese patients, ideal body weight should be used for dosage calculation.

Infants, Children, and Adolescents:

Acute symptoms: Manufacturer's labeling: **Note:** Not recommended for the treatment of asthma exacerbations (NAEPP, 2007).

Loading dose: **Note:** Doses presented intended to achieve a serum level of approximately 10 mcg/mL; loading doses should be given intravenously (preferred) or with a rapidly absorbed oral product (not an extended release product). On the average, for every 1 mg/kg theophylline given, blood concentrations will rise 2 mcg/mL.

Patients **not** currently receiving methylxanthines:

I.V.: 4.6 mg/kg/dose

Oral: Immediate release product: 5 mg/kg

Patients currently receiving methylxanthines: A loading dose is not recommended without first obtaining a serum theophylline concentration in patients who have received aminophylline or theophylline within the past 24 hours. The loading dose should be calculated as follows:

Dose = (C desired − C measured) (V_d)

C desired = desired serum theophylline concentration

C measured = measured serum theophylline concentration

Maintenance dose: Continuous I.V. infusion: **Note:** Dosing presented is to achieve a target concentration of 10 mcg/mL. Lower initial doses may be required in patients with reduced theophylline clearance. Dosage should be adjusted according to serum concentration measurements during the first 12- to 24-hour period.

Infants 4-6 weeks: 1.5 mg/kg/dose every 12 hours

Infants 6-52 weeks: Dose (mg/kg/**hour**) = (0.008 X age in weeks) + 0.21

Children 1 to <9 years: 0.8 mg/kg/**hour**

Children 9 to <12 years: 0.7 mg/kg/**hour**

Adolescents 12 to <16 years (otherwise healthy, nonsmokers): 0.5 mg/kg/**hour**; maximum daily dose: 900 mg/**day** unless serum concentrations indicate need for larger dose

Adolescents 12 to <16 years (cigarette or marijuana smokers): 0.7 mg/kg/**hour**

Adolescents 16-18 years (otherwise healthy, nonsmokers): 0.4 mg/kg/**hour**; maximum dose: 900 mg/**day** unless serum concentrations indicate need for larger dose

Cardiac decompensation, cor pulmonale, hepatic dysfunction, sepsis with multiorgan failure, shock: Initial: 0.2 mg/kg/**hour**; maximum dose: 400 mg/**day** unless serum concentrations indicate need for larger dose

Chronic conditions: Note: Increase dose only if tolerated. Consider lowering dose or using a slower titration if caffeine-like adverse events occur. Smaller doses given more frequently may be used in patients with a more rapid metabolism to prevent breakthrough symptoms which could occur due to low trough concentration prior to the next dose.

Immediate release formulation: Oral: **Note:** If at risk for impaired clearance or not feasible to monitor serum theophylline concentrations: Do not exceed 16 mg/kg/**day**; maximum daily dose: 400 mg/**day**

Manufacturer's labeling: Frequency based upon age.

Infants: Total daily dose (mg/day) = [(0.2 x age in weeks) + 5] x (weight in kg); frequency is based on age

Dosing interval:

≤26 weeks: Divide in 3 equal doses and administer every 8 hours

>26 weeks: Divide in 4 equal doses and administer every 6 hours

Children and Adolescents 1-15 years and ≤45 kg: Initial:

Days 1-3: 12-14 mg/kg/**day** in divided doses every 4-6 hours; maximum daily dose: 300 mg/**day**

Days 4-6: 16 mg/kg/**day** in divided doses every 4-6 hours; maximum daily dose: 400 mg/**day**

Maintenance: 20 mg/kg/**day** in divided doses every 4-6 hours; maximum daily dose: 600 mg/**day**

Children and Adolescents >45 kg or Adolescents ≥16 years:

Initial:

Days 1-3: 300 mg/**day** in divided doses every 6-8 hours

Days 4-6: 400 mg/**day** in divided doses every 6-8 hours

Maintenance: 600 mg/**day** in divided doses every 6-8 hour

Alternate dosing; age-directed: Some centers have used the following based on age-dependent pharmacokinetics of theophylline:

Children 1 to <9 years: 20-24 mg/kg/**day**; maximum daily dose: 600 mg/**day**

Children 9-12 years: 16 mg/kg/**day**; maximum daily dose: 600 mg/**day**

Children and Adolescents >12-16 years (nonsmokers): 13 mg/kg/**day**; maximum daily dose: 600 mg/**day**

Children >12 years and Adolescents (smokers): 16 mg/kg/**day**; maximum daily dose: 600 mg/**day**

Adolescents >16 years (nonsmokers): 10 mg/kg/**day**; maximum daily dose: 600 mg/**day**

Extended release formulations: Oral: **Note:** If at risk for impaired clearance or not feasible to monitor serum theophylline concentrations: Do not exceed 16 mg/kg/**day**; maximum daily dose: 400 mg/**day**

Children ≥6 years and Adolescents <16 years, weighing ≤45 kg:

Initial:

Days 1-3: 12-14 mg/kg/**day**; maximum daily dose: 300 mg/**day**

Days 4-6: 16 mg/kg/**day**; maximum daily dose: 400 mg/**day**

Maintenance: 20 mg/kg/**day**; maximum daily dose: 600 mg/**day**

Dosing interval (product specific):

12-hour extended release tablets: Children ≥6 years and Adolescents: Divide in 2 equal doses and administer every 12 hours

24-hour extended release tablets: Children ≥12 years and Adolescents: Administer every 24 hours

Children ≥6 years and Adolescents, weighing >45 kg or Adolescents ≥16 years:

12-hour extended release tablets: Children ≥6 years and Adolescents, weighing >45 kg or Adolescents ≥16 years:

Initial:

Days 1-3: 300 mg/**day** in divided doses every 12 hours

Days 4-6: 400 mg/**day** in divided doses every 12 hours

Maintenance: 600 mg/**day** in divided doses every 12 hours

24-hour extended release tablets: Children ≥12 years and Adolescents, weighing >45 kg or Adolescents ≥16 years:

Initial:

Days 1-3: 300-400 mg once daily

Days 4-6: 400-600 mg once daily

Maintenance: Titrate according to serum concentrations

Alternate dosing: Age-directed: Some centers have used the following based on age-dependent pharmacokinetics of theophylline:

Children 6 to <9 years: 20-24 mg/kg/**day**; maximum daily dose: 600 mg/**day**

Children 9-12 years: 16 mg/kg/**day**; maximum daily dose: 600 mg/**day**

Children and Adolescents >12-16 years (nonsmokers): 13 mg/kg/**day**; maximum daily dose: 600 mg/**day**

Children >12 years and Adolescents (smokers): 16 mg/kg/**day**; maximum daily dose: 600 mg/**day**

Adolescents >16 years (nonsmokers): 10 mg/kg/**day**; maximum daily dose: 600 mg/**day**

Adults:

Acute symptoms: Manufacturer's labeling: **Note:** Not recommended for the treatment of asthma exacerbations (NAEPP, 2007).

Loading dose: **Note:** Doses presented intended to achieve a serum concentration of approximately 10 mcg/mL; loading doses should be given intravenously (preferred) or with a rapidly absorbed oral product (not an extended release product). On the average, for every 1 mg/kg theophylline given, blood concentrations will rise 2 mcg/mL.

Patients **not** currently receiving aminophylline or theophylline:

I.V.: 4.6 mg/kg/dose

Oral: Immediate release product: 5 mg/kg/dose

Patients currently receiving aminophylline or theophylline: A loading dose is not recommended without first obtaining a serum theophylline concentration in patients who have received aminophylline or theophylline within the past 24 hours. The loading dose should be calculated as follows:

Dose = (C desired – C measured) (V$_d$)

C desired = desired serum theophylline concentration

C measured = measured serum theophylline concentration

Maintenance dose: Continuous I.V. infusion: **Note:** Dosing presented is to achieve a target concentration of 10 mcg/mL. Lower initial doses may be required in patients with reduced theophylline clearance. Dosage should be adjusted according to serum concentration measurements during the first 12- to 24-hour period.

Adults ≤60 years (otherwise healthy, nonsmokers): 0.4 mg/kg/**hour**; maximum daily dose: 900 mg/**day** unless serum concentrations indicate need for larger dose

Adults >60 years: 0.3 mg/kg/**hour**; maximum daily dose: 400 mg/**day** unless serum levels indicate need for larger dose

Chronic conditions: Oral: **Note:** Increase dose only if tolerated. Consider lowering dose or using a slower titration if caffeine-like adverse events occur. Smaller doses given more frequently may be used in patients with a more rapid metabolism to prevent breakthrough symptoms which could occur due to low trough concentration prior to the next dose.

Immediate release oral solution: Initial dose: 300 mg/**day** administered in divided doses every 6-8 hours; maintenance: 400-600 mg/day (maximum daily dose: 600 mg/**day**)

Extended release formulations: Initial dose: 300-400 mg once daily; maintenance: 400-600 mg once daily (maximum daily dose: 600 mg/**day**)

Dosage adjustment based on serum theophylline concentrations: Infants, Children, Adolescents, and Adults: **Note:** Recheck serum theophylline concentrations after 3 days when using oral dosing, or after 12 hours (children) or 24 hours (adults) when dosing intravenously. Patients maintained with oral therapy should be reassessed at 6- to 12-month intervals, when clinically indicated or if concomitant medication is added which may affect theophylline serum concentration.

<9.9 mcg/mL: If tolerated, but symptoms remain, increase dose by ~25%. Recheck serum theophylline concentrations.

10-14.9 mcg/mL: Maintain dosage if tolerated. Recheck serum concentrations at 24-hour intervals (for acute I.V. dosing) or at 6- to 12-month intervals (for oral dosing).

15-19.9 mcg/mL: Consider 10% dose reduction to improve safety margin even if dose is tolerated.

20-24.9 mcg/mL: Decrease dose by ~25%. Recheck serum concentrations.

25-30 mcg/mL: Skip next dose (oral) or stop infusion for 12 hours (children) or 24 hours (adults) and decrease subsequent doses by at least 25%. Recheck serum concentrations.

>30 mcg/mL: Stop dosing and treat overdose; if resumed, decrease subsequent doses by at least 50%. Recheck serum concentrations.

Dosing adjustment in renal impairment: Oral, I.V.:

Infants 1-3 months: Consider dose reduction and frequent monitoring of serum theophylline concentrations

Infants >3 months, Children, Adolescents, and Adults: No adjustment necessary

Dosing adjustment in hepatic impairment:

Oral: Infants, Children, Adolescents, and Adults: Dose reduction and frequent monitoring of serum theophylline concentration are required in patients with decreased hepatic function (eg, cirrhosis, acute hepatitis, cholestasis)

I.V.: Manufacturer's labeling: Infants, Children, Adolescents, and Adults: Initial: 0.2 mg/kg/**hour**; maximum daily dose: 400 mg/**day** unless serum concentrations indicate need for larger dose

Administration

Oral: Administer on an empty stomach, 1 hour before or 2 hours after a meal. Sustained release preparations should be administered with a full glass of water, whole or cut by half only; do not crush; sustained release capsule forms may be opened and sprinkled on soft foods; do not chew or crush beads

Parenteral: Premix I.V. infusion bags available, administer loading dose over 30 minutes; rate for continuous I.V. infusion dependent upon dosage

Monitoring Parameters Respiratory rate, heart rate, serum theophylline concentration, pulmonary function tests, arterial or capillary blood gases (if applicable); number and severity of apnea spells (apnea of prematurity)

Reference Range

Therapeutic concentrations:

Asthma: 5-15 mcg/mL

Apnea of prematurity: 6-12 mcg/mL; goal concentration is reduced due to decreased protein binding and higher free fraction

Toxic concentration: >20 mcg/mL

Guidelines for Drawing Theophylline Serum Samples

Dosage Form	When to Obtain Sample[A]
I.V. bolus	30 minutes after end of 30-minute infusion
I.V. continuous infusion	12-24 hours after initiation of infusion
Oral immediate release formulations	Peak: 1 hour postdose after at least 1 day of therapy Trough: Just before a dose after at least 1 day of therapy

[A]The time to achieve steady-state serum concentrations is prolonged in patients with longer half-lives (eg, infants and adults with cardiac or liver failure (see theophylline half-life table). In these patients, serum theophylline concentrations should be drawn after 48-72 hours of therapy; serum concentrations may need to be done prior to steady-state to assess the patient's current progress or evaluate potential toxicity.

Test Interactions Plasma glucose, uric acid, free fatty acids, total cholesterol, HDL, HDL/LDL ratio, and urinary free cortisol excretion may be increased by theophylline. Theophylline may decrease triiodothyronine.

Additional Information Due to improved theophylline clearance during the first year of life, serum concentration determinations and dosage adjustments may be needed to optimize therapy

Dosage Forms Excipient information presented when available (limited, particularly for generics); consult specific product labeling.

Capsule Extended Release 24 Hour, Oral:

Theo-24: 100 mg, 200 mg, 300 mg, 400 mg

Elixir, Oral:

Elixophyllin: 80 mg/15 mL (473 mL) [contains fd&c red #40, saccharin sodium; mixed fruit flavor]

Solution, Intravenous:

Generic: 400 mg (250 mL, 500 mL); 800 mg (500 mL)

Solution, Oral:

Generic: 80 mg/15 mL (473 mL)

Tablet Extended Release 12 Hour, Oral:

Theochron: 100 mg, 200 mg, 300 mg [scored]

Generic: 100 mg, 200 mg, 300 mg, 450 mg

Tablet Extended Release 24 Hour, Oral:

Generic: 400 mg, 600 mg

Extemporaneous Preparations Note: An alcohol-containing commercial oral solution is available (80 mg/15mL).

A 5 mg/mL oral suspension may be made with tablets. Crush one 300 mg extended release tablet in a mortar and reduce to a fine powder. Add small portions of a 1:1 mixture of Ora-Sweet® and Ora-Plus® and mix to a uniform paste; mix while adding the vehicle in equal proportions to **almost** 60 mL; transfer to a calibrated bottle, rinse mortar with vehicle, and add sufficient quantity of vehicle to make 60 mL. Label "shake well". Stable for 90 days at room temperature.

Johnson CE, VanDeKoppel S, and Myers E, "Stability of Anhydrous Theophylline in Extemporaneously Prepared Alcohol-Free Oral Suspensions," Am J Health-Syst Pharm, 2005, 62(23):2518-20.

References

American Academy of Pediatrics Committee on Drugs. "Inactive" ingredients in pharmaceutical products: update (subject review). Pediatrics. 1997;99(2):268-278.

Bhatt-Mehta V and Schumacher RE, "Treatment of Apnea of Prematurity," Paediatr Drugs, 2003, 5(3):195-210.

Hendeles L, Jenkins J, and Temple R, "Revised FDA Labeling Guideline for Theophylline Oral Dosage Forms," Pharmacotherapy, 1995, 15(4):409-427.

Henderson-Smart DJ and De Paoli AG, "Methylxanthine Treatment for Apnoea in Preterm Infants," Cochrane Database Syst Rev, 2010, 12: CD000140.

Kearney TE, Manoguerra AS, Curtis GP, et al, "Theophylline Toxicity and the Beta-Adrenergic System," Ann Intern Med, 1985, 102 (6):766-9.

Kraus DM, Fischer JH, Reitz SJ, et al, "Alterations in Theophylline Metabolism During the First Year of Life," Clin Pharmacol Ther, 1993, 54(4):351-9.

National Asthma Education and Prevention Program (NAEPP), "Expert Panel Report 3 (EPR-3): Guidelines for the Diagnosis and Management of Asthma," Clinical Practice Guidelines, National Institutes of Health, National Heart, Lung, and Blood Institute, NIH Publication No. 08-4051, prepublication 2007; available at http://www.nhlbi.nih.gov/guidelines/asthma/asthgdln.htm.

National Heart, Lung, and Blood Institute; National Asthma Education and Prevention Program Asthma and Pregnancy Working Group, "NAEPP Expert Panel Report. Managing Asthma During Pregnancy: Recommendations for Pharmacologic Treatment - 2004 Update," J Allergy Clin Immunol, 2005, 115(1):34-46.

Shehab N, Lewis CL, Streetman DD, Donn SM. Exposure to the pharmaceutical excipients benzyl alcohol and propylene glycol among critically ill neonates. Pediatr Crit Care Med. 2009;10 (2):256-259.

Skouroliakou M, Bacopoulou F, and Markantonis SL, "Caffeine Versus Theophylline for Apnea of Prematurity: A Randomised Controlled Trial," J Paediatr Child Health, 2009, 45(10):587-92.

Upton RA, "Pharmacokinetic Interactions Between Theophylline and Other Medication (Part I)," Clin Pharmacokinet, 1991, 20(1):66-80.

◆ **Theophylline Anhydrous** see Theophylline on page 2005

◆ **Theophylline Ethylenediamine** see Aminophylline on page 124

◆ **TheraCort [OTC]** see Hydrocortisone (Topical) on page 1038

◆ **Thera-Ear [OTC]** see Carbamide Peroxide on page 377

◆ **Therapeutic [OTC]** see Coal Tar on page 532

◆ **Theraplex T [OTC]** see Coal Tar on page 532

◆ **Thermazene** see Silver Sulfadiazine on page 1890

◆ **Thiamazole** see Methimazole on page 1362

◆ **Thiamin** see Thiamine on page 2009

Thiamine (THYE a min)

Medication Safety Issues

Sound-alike/look-alike issues:

Thiamine may be confused with Tenormin, Thalomid, Thorazine

International issues:

Doxal [Brazil] may be confused with Doxil brand name for doxorubicin [U.S.]

Doxal: Brand name for pyridoxine/thiamine [Brazil], but also the brand name for doxepin [Finland]

Brand Names: Canada Betaxin

Therapeutic Category Nutritional Supplement; Vitamin, Water Soluble

Generic Availability (U.S.) Yes

Use Treatment of thiamine deficiency including beriberi, Wernicke's encephalopathy syndrome, and peripheral neuritis associated with pellagra; alcoholic patients with altered sensorium; various genetic metabolic disorders

Pregnancy Risk Factor A

Pregnancy Considerations Water soluble vitamins cross the placenta. Thiamine requirements may be increased during pregnancy (IOM, 1998). Severe nausea and vomiting (hyperemesis gravidarum) may lead to thiamine deficiency manifested as Wernicke's encephalopathy (Chiossi, 2006).

Breast-Feeding Considerations Thiamine is found in breast milk and concentrations are similar in well-nourished mothers who use supplements and those that do not. Thiamine requirements may be increased in nursing women compared to non-nursing women (IOM, 1998).

Contraindications Hypersensitivity to thiamine or any component

Warnings Large doses should be given in divided doses for better oral absorption

Precautions Use parenteral route cautiously

Adverse Reactions Adverse reactions reported with injection.

Cardiovascular: Cyanosis

Central nervous system: Restlessness

Dermatologic: Angioneurotic edema, pruritus, urticaria

Gastrointestinal: Hemorrhage into GI tract, nausea, tightness of the throat

Local: Induration and/or tenderness at the injection site (following I.M. administration)

Neuromuscular & skeletal: Weakness

Respiratory: Pulmonary edema

Miscellaneous: Anaphylactic/hypersensitivity reactions (following I.V. administration), diaphoresis, warmth

Drug Interactions

Metabolism/Transport Effects None known.

Avoid Concomitant Use There are no known interactions where it is recommended to avoid concomitant use.

Increased Effect/Toxicity There are no known significant interactions involving an increase in effect.

Decreased Effect There are no known significant interactions involving a decrease in effect.

Food Interactions

Ethanol: May decrease thiamine absorption. Management: Higher doses may be needed in patients with history of ethanol abuse.

Food: High carbohydrate diets may increase thiamine requirement.

Stability Unstable with alkaline or neutral solutions

Mechanism of Action An essential coenzyme in carbohydrate metabolism by combining with adenosine triphosphate to form thiamine pyrophosphate

Pharmacokinetics (Adult data unless noted)

Absorption:

Oral: Poor

I.M.: Rapid and complete

Metabolism: In the liver

Elimination: Renally as unchanged drug only after body storage sites become saturated

Dosing: Neonatal Adequate intake: Oral: 0.2 mg (0.03 mg/kg)

Dosing: Usual

Adequate intake: Oral: Infants:

1 to <6 months: 0.2 mg (0.03 mg/kg)

6-12 months: 0.3 mg (0.03 mg/kg)

Recommended daily allowance (RDA): Oral:

1-3 years: 0.5 mg

4-8 years: 0.6 mg

9-13 years: 0.9 mg

14-18 years:

Male: 1.2 mg

Female: 1 mg

≥19 years:

Male: 1.2 mg

Female: 1.1 mg

Dietary supplement (depends on caloric or carbohydrate content of the diet):

Oral:

Infants: 0.3-0.5 mg/day

Children: 0.5-1 mg/day

Adults: 1-2 mg/day

Note: The above doses can be found in multivitamin preparations

Thiamine deficiency (beriberi):

Children: 10-25 mg/dose I.M. or I.V. daily (if critically ill), or 10-50 mg/dose orally every day for 2 weeks, then 5-10 mg/dose orally daily for 1 month

Adults: 5-30 mg/dose I.M. or I.V. 3 times/day (if critically ill); then orally 5-30 mg/day in single or divided doses 3 times/day for 1 month

Wernicke's encephalopathy: Adults: Initial: 100 mg I.V., then 50-100 mg/day I.M. or I.V. until consuming a regular, balanced diet

Metabolic disorders: Oral: Adults: 10-20 mg/day (dosages up to 4 g/day in divided doses have been used)

Administration

Oral: May administer with or without food

Parenteral: Administer by slow I.V. injection or I.M.

Reference Range Normal values: 1.6-4 mg/dL

Test Interactions False-positive for uric acid using the phosphotungstate method and for urobilinogen using the Ehrlich's reagent; large doses may interfere with the spectrophotometric determination of serum theophylline concentration

Additional Information Dietary sources include legumes, pork, beef, whole grains, yeast, fresh vegetables; a deficiency state can occur in as little as 3 weeks following total dietary absence

Dosage Forms Excipient information presented when available (limited, particularly for generics); consult specific product labeling.

Capsule, Oral, as hydrochloride:

Generic: 50 mg

Solution, Injection, as hydrochloride:

Generic: 100 mg/mL (2 mL)

Tablet, Oral, as hydrochloride:

Generic: 50 mg, 100 mg, 250 mg

Tablet, Oral, as hydrochloride [preservative free]:

Generic: 100 mg

Extemporaneous Preparations A 100 mg/mL oral suspension may be made with commercially available thiamine powder. Add 10 g of powder to a mortar. Add small portions of a 1:1 mixture of Ora-Sweet® and Ora-Plus® and mix to a uniform paste; mix while adding the vehicle in equal proportions to **almost** 100 mL; transfer to a calibrated bottle, rinse mortar with vehicle, and add sufficient quantity of vehicle to make 100 mL. Label "shake well". Stable 91 days under refrigeration or at room temperature.

Ensom MH and Decarie D, "Stability of Thiamine in Extemporaneously Compounded Suspensions," *Can J Hosp Pharm*, 2005, 58(1):26-30.

References

Chiossi G, Neri I, Cavazzuti M, et al, "Hyperemesis Gravidarum Complicated by Wernicke Encephalopathy: Background, Case Report, and Review of the Literature," *Obstet Gynecol Surv*, 2006, 61(4):255-68.

IOM (Institute of Medicine), *Dietary Reference Intakes for Thiamin, Riboflavin, Niacin, Vitamin B₆, Folate, Vitamin B₁₂, Pantothenic Acid, Biotin and Choline*, Washington, DC: National Academy Press, 1998.

◆ **Thiamine Hydrochloride** see Thiamine on page 2009

◆ **Thiaminium Chloride Hydrochloride** see Thiamine on page 2009

Thioguanine (thye oh GWAH neen)

Medication Safety Issues

Sound-alike/look-alike issues:

Thioguanine may be confused with thiotepa

High alert medication:

This medication is in a class the Institute for Safe Medication Practices (ISMP) includes among its list of

drug classes which have a heightened risk of causing significant patient harm when used in error.

Other safety concerns:

6-thioguanine and 6-TG are error-prone abbreviations (associated with sixfold overdoses of thioguanine)

International issues:

Lanvis [Canada and multiple international markets] may be confused with Lantus brand name for insulin glargine [U.S., Canada, and multiple international markets]

Related Information

Emetogenic Potential of Antineoplastic Agents in Children on page 2327

Oral Medications That Should Not Be Crushed or Altered on page 2438

Safe Handling of Hazardous Drugs on page 2419

Brand Names: U.S. Tabloid

Brand Names: Canada Lanvis®

Therapeutic Category Antineoplastic Agent, Antimetabolite; Antineoplastic Agent, Antimetabolite (Purine Analog)

Generic Availability (U.S.) No

Use Remission induction and remission consolidation treatment of acute nonlymphocytic leukemia (ANLL, AML) [FDA approved in pediatrics (age not specified) and adults]; has also been used for treatment of acute lymphoblastic leukemia (ALL)

Pregnancy Risk Factor D

Pregnancy Considerations Animal studies have demonstrated adverse effects. There are no adequate and well-controlled studies in pregnant women. May cause fetal harm if administered during pregnancy. Women of child-bearing potential should avoid becoming pregnant during treatment.

Breast-Feeding Considerations Due to the potential for serious adverse reactions in the nursing infant, the manufacturer recommends to discontinue breast-feeding during therapy.

Contraindications Hypersensitivity to thioguanine or any component; history of previous therapy resistance with thioguanine and in patients resistant to mercaptopurine (usual to find cross-resistance between thioguanine and mercaptopurine)

Warnings Hazardous agent; use appropriate precautions for handling and disposal (NIOSH, 2012). Not recommended for maintenance therapy or long-term continuous treatment; thioguanine is potentially carcinogenic and teratogenic. Liver toxicity associated with vascular endothelial damage has been reported in patients receiving long-term thioguanine maintenance therapy; liver toxicity is particularly prevalent in children (up to 25%) receiving maintenance therapy for acute lymphoblastic leukemia and in males; liver toxicity usually presents as hepatic sinusoidal obstruction syndrome [SOS; formerly called veno-occlusive disease (VOD)] or portal hypertension; monitor liver function carefully for liver toxicity and discontinue in patients with evidence of hepatic SOS (eg, hyperbilirubinemia, hepatomegaly [tender], and weight gain due to ascites and fluid retention) or portal hypertension (eg, splenomegaly, thrombocytopenia, esophageal varices). Hepatotoxicity with or without transaminase elevations may occur. Pathologic findings of hepatotoxicity include hepatoportal sclerosis, nodular regenerative hyperplasia, peliosis hepatitis, and periportal fibrosis. Avoid ethanol; may increase the risk for hepatotoxicity. Myelosuppression (anemia, leukopenia, and/or thrombocytopenia) is a common dose-related toxicity (may be delayed); monitor for infection (due to leukopenia) or bleeding (due to thrombocytopenia); withhold treatment for abnormally significant drop in blood counts. Patients with genetic enzyme deficiency of thiopurine methyltransferase (TPMT) or who are receiving drugs which inhibit this enzyme (eg, mesalazine, olsalazine, sulfasalazine) may be highly sensitive to myelosuppressive effects and may require substantial dose reductions.

Precautions Thioguanine is potentially carcinogenic and teratogenic. Hyperuricemia occurs commonly with treatment; institute adequate hydration, urine alkalinization, and prophylactic allopurinol. Cross resistance with mercaptopurine generally occurs. Avoid vaccination with live vaccines during treatment.

Adverse Reactions

Endocrine & metabolic: Fluid retention, hyperuricemia (common)

Gastrointestinal: Anorexia, intestinal necrosis, intestinal perforation, nausea, splenomegaly, stomatitis, vomiting, weight gain

Hematologic: Anemia (may be delayed), bleeding, granulocytopenia, leukopenia (common; may be delayed), marrow hypoplasia, pancytopenia, thrombocytopenia (common; may be delayed)

Hepatic: Ascites, esophageal varices, hepatic necrosis (centrilobular), hepatic sinusoidal obstruction syndrome (SOS; veno-occlusive disease), hepatitis, hepatomegaly [tender], hepatoportal sclerosis, hepatotoxicity, hyperbilirubinemia, jaundice, LFTs increased, nodular regenerative hyperplasia, peliosis hepatitis, periportal fibrosis, portal hypertension

Miscellaneous: Infection

Drug Interactions

Metabolism/Transport Effects None known.

Avoid Concomitant Use

Avoid concomitant use of Thioguanine with any of the following: BCG; CloZAPine; Dipyrone; Natalizumab; Pimecrolimus; Tacrolimus (Topical); Tofacitinib; Vaccines (Live)

Increased Effect/Toxicity

Thioguanine may increase the levels/effects of: CloZAPine; Leflunomide; Natalizumab; Tofacitinib; Vaccines (Live)

The levels/effects of Thioguanine may be increased by: 5-ASA Derivatives; Denosumab; Dipyrone; Pimecrolimus; Roflumilast; Tacrolimus (Topical); Trastuzumab

Decreased Effect

Thioguanine may decrease the levels/effects of: BCG; Coccidioidin Skin Test; Sipuleucel-T; Vaccines (Inactivated); Vaccines (Live)

The levels/effects of Thioguanine may be decreased by: Echinacea

Stability Hazardous agent; use appropriate precautions for handling and disposal (NIOSH, 2012). Store at 15°C to 25°C (59°F to 77°F) in a dry location.

Mechanism of Action Purine analog that is incorporated into DNA and RNA resulting in the blockage of synthesis and metabolism of purine nucleotides

Pharmacokinetics (Adult data unless noted)

Absorption: Oral: 30% (range: 14% to 46%), variable and incomplete

Distribution: Does not reach therapeutic concentrations in the CSF

Metabolism: Rapid and extensive hepatic metabolism by thiopurine methyltransferase (TPMT) to 2-amino-6-methylthioguanine (MTG; active) and inactive compounds

Half-life, terminal: 5-9 hours

Time to peak serum concentration: 8 hours

Elimination: Metabolites excreted in urine

Dosing: Usual Oral (refer to individual protocols): **Acute lymphoblastic leukemia (ALL); delayed intensification treatment phase (combination therapy):** Children ≥1 year: 60 mg/m²/dose once daily for 14 days (Lange, 2002; Nachman, 1998)

Dosage adjustment in renal impairment: Children: No adjustment required (Aronoff, 2007).

Dosage adjustment in hepatic impairment: Deterioration in transaminases, alkaline phosphatase or bilirubin, toxic hepatitis, biliary stasis, clinical jaundice, evidence of hepatic sinusoidal obstruction syndrome (veno-occlusive disease), or evidence of portal hypertension: Discontinue treatment.

Administration Hazardous agent; use appropriate precautions for handling and disposal (NIOSH, 2012).

Oral: Total daily dose can be given at one time.

Monitoring Parameters CBC with differential and platelet count, liver function tests (serum transaminases, alkaline phosphatase, bilirubin), hemoglobin, hematocrit, serum uric acid; testing for thiopurine methyltransferase (TPMT) deficiency is available; clinical signs of portal hypertension or hepatic sinusoidal obstruction syndrome (SOS; veno-occlusive disease)

Additional Information Myelosuppressive effects:

WBC: Moderate

Platelets: Moderate

Onset (days): 7-10

Nadir (days): 14

Recovery (days): 21

Note: Myelosuppressive effects may be delayed; continuation of treatment should be evaluated at first sign of decreased hematologic parameter.

Dosage Forms Excipient information presented when available (limited, particularly for generics); consult specific product labeling.

Tablet, Oral:

Tabloid: 40 mg

Extemporaneous Preparations Hazardous agent: Use appropriate precautions for handling and disposal.

A 20 mg/mL oral suspension may be made with tablets, methylcellulose 1%, and simple syrup NF. Crush fifteen 40 mg tablets in a mortar and reduce to a fine powder. Add 10 mL methylcellulose 1% in incremental proportions and mix to a uniform paste. Transfer to a graduated cylinder, rinse mortar with simple syrup, and add quantity of simple syrup sufficient to make 30 mL. Label "shake well" and "refrigerate". Stable for 84 days refrigerated (preferred) or at room temperature.

Dressman JB and Poust RI, "Stability of Allopurinol and Five Antineoplastics in Suspension," *Am J Hosp Pharm*, 1983, 40(4):616-8.

Nahata MC, Pai VB, and Hipple TF, *Pediatric Drug Formulations*, 5th ed, Cincinnati, OH: Harvey Whitney Books Co, 2004.

References

Aronoff GR, Bennett WM, Berns JS, et al, *Drug Prescribing in Renal Failure: Dosing Guidelines for Adults and Children*, 5th ed. Philadelphia, PA: American College of Physicians, 2007, 173.

Broxson EH, Dole M, Wong R, et al, "Portal Hypertension Develops in a Subset of Children With Standard Risk Acute Lymphoblastic Leukemia Treated With Oral 6-Thioguanine During Maintenance Therapy," *Pediatr Blood Cancer*, 2005, 44(3):226-31.

Culbert SJ, Shuster JJ, Land VJ, et al, "Remission Induction and Continuation Therapy in Children With Their First Relapse of Acute Lymphoid Leukemia: A Pediatric Oncology Group Study," *Cancer*, 1991, 67(1):37-42.

Lange BJ, Bostrom BC, Cherlow JM, et al, "Double-Delayed Intensification Improves Event-Free Survival for Children With Intermediate-Risk Acute Lymphoblastic Leukemia: A Report From the Children's Cancer Group," *Blood*, 2002, 99(3):825-33.

Nachman JB, Sather HN, Sensel MG, et al, "Augmented Post-Induction Therapy for Children With High-Risk Acute Lymphoblastic Leukemia and a Slow Response to Initial Therapy," *N Engl J Med*, 1998, 338 (23):1663-71.

National Institute for Occupational Safety and Health (NIOSH), "NIOSH List of Antineoplastic and Other Hazardous Drugs in Healthcare Settings 2012." Available at http://www.cdc.gov/niosh/docs/2012-150/pdfs/2012-150.pdf. Accessed January 21, 2013.

Steuber CP, Civin C, Krischer J, et al, "A Comparison of Induction and Maintenance Therapy for Acute Nonlymphocytic Leukemia in Childhood: Results of a Pediatric Oncology Group Study," *J Clin Oncol*, 1991, 9(2):247-58.

Stork LC, Matloub Y, Broxson E, et al, "Oral 6-Mercaptopurine Versus Oral 6-Thioguanine and Veno-occlusive Disease in Children With Standard-Risk Acute Lymphoblastic Leukemia: Report of the Children's Oncology Group CCG-1952 Clinical Trial," *Blood*, 2010, 115 (14):2740-8.

Vora A, Mitchell CD, Lennard L, et al, "Toxicity and Efficacy of 6-Thioguanine Versus 6-Mercaptopurine in Childhood Lymphoblastic Leukaemia: A Randomised Trial," *Lancet*, 2006, 368(9544):1339-48.

◆ **6-Thioguanine (error-prone abbreviation)** *see* Thioguanine *on page* 2010

◆ **Thiophosphoramide** *see* Thiotepa *on page* 2014

◆ **Thioplex** *see* Thiotepa *on page* 2014

Thioridazine (thye oh RID a zeen)

Medication Safety Issues

Sound-alike/look-alike issues:

Thioridazine may be confused with thiothixene, Thorazine

Mellaril may be confused with Elavil, Mebaral®

BEERS Criteria medication:

This drug may be potentially inappropriate for use in geriatric patients (Quality of evidence - moderate; Strength of recommendation - strong).

Related Information

Medications for Which a Single Dose May Be Fatal When Ingested by a Toddler *on page* 2408

Therapeutic Category Antipsychotic Agent, Typical, Phenothiazine; Phenothiazine Derivative

Generic Availability (U.S.) Yes

Use Due to prolongation of the QT_c interval, thioridazine is currently indicated only for the treatment of refractory schizophrenic patients [FDA approved in pediatric patients (age not specified) and adults]; in the past, the drug had been used for management of psychotic disorders; depressive neurosis; dementia in elderly; severe behavioral problems in children

Pregnancy Considerations Jaundice or hyper-/hyporeflexia have been reported in newborn infants following maternal use of phenothiazines. Antipsychotic use during the third trimester of pregnancy has a risk for abnormal muscle movements (extrapyramidal symptoms [EPS]) and withdrawal symptoms in newborns following delivery. Symptoms in the newborn may include agitation, feeding disorder, hypertonia, hypotonia, respiratory distress, somnolence, and tremor; these effects may be self-limiting or require hospitalization.

Breast-Feeding Considerations Other phenothiazines are excreted in human milk; excretion of thioridazine is not known.

Contraindications Hypersensitivity to thioridazine or any component; cross-sensitivity to other phenothiazines may exist; concurrent therapy with propranolol, pindolol, fluvoxamine, fluoxetine, paroxetine, drugs that inhibit cytochrome P450 isoenzyme CYP2D6, drugs that prolong the QT_c interval, and patients with reduced levels of CYP2D6, a history of cardiac arrhythmias, congenital long QT syndrome, or a QT_c interval >450 msec (adults); severe CNS depression; avoid use in patients with narrow-angle glaucoma, blood dyscrasias, severe liver or cardiac disease

Warnings Dose-related prolongation of the QT_c interval may occur and may be associated with torsade de pointes arrhythmias and sudden death **[U.S. Boxed Warning]**; reserve use for schizophrenic patients who do not respond to adequate treatment with other antipsychotic agents. May cause extrapyramidal symptoms, including pseudoparkinsonism, acute dystonic reactions, akathisia, and tardive dyskinesia (risk of these reactions is low relative to other neuroleptics, and is dose-dependent; to decrease risk of tardive dyskinesia: Use smallest dose and shortest duration possible; evaluate continued need periodically; risk of dystonia is increased with the use of high potency and higher doses of conventional antipsychotics and in males and younger patients). May cause neuroleptic malignant syndrome; monitor for mental status changes, fever, muscle rigidity, and/or autonomic instability (risk may be increased in patients with Parkinson's disease or Lewy body dementia).

Leukopenia, neutropenia, and agranulocytosis (sometimes fatal) have been reported in clinical trials and postmarketing reports with antipsychotic use; presence of risk factors (eg, preexisting low WBC or history of drug-induced leuko/neutropenia) should prompt periodic blood count assessment. Discontinue therapy at first signs of blood dyscrasias or if absolute neutrophil count <1000/mm³.

An increased risk of death has been reported with the use of antipsychotics in elderly patients with dementia-related psychosis **[U.S. Boxed Warning]**; most deaths seemed to be cardiovascular (eg, sudden death, heart failure) or infectious (eg, pneumonia) in nature; thioridazine is not approved for this indication.

Precautions Use with caution in patients with severe cardiovascular disorder or seizures

Adverse Reactions
Cardiovascular: ECG changes, hypotension, orthostatic hypotension, peripheral edema

Central nervous system: Dizziness, drowsiness, EPS (akathisia, dystonias, pseudoparkinsonism, tardive dyskinesia), impairment of temperature regulation, lowering of seizure threshold, neuroleptic malignant syndrome (NMS)

Dermatologic: Discoloration of skin (blue-gray), increased sensitivity to sun, rash

Endocrine & metabolic: Amenorrhea, breast pain, libido (changes in), changes in menstrual cycle, galactorrhea

Gastrointestinal: constipation, diarrhea, nausea, stomach pain, vomiting, weight gain, xerostomia

Genitourinary: Difficulty in urination, ejaculatory disturbances, priapism, urinary retention

Hematologic: Agranulocytosis, leukopenia

Hepatic: Cholestatic jaundice, hepatotoxicity

Neuromuscular & skeletal: Seizure, tremor

Ocular: Blurred vision, cornea and lens changes, pigmentary retinopathy

Respiratory: Nasal congestion

Drug Interactions
Metabolism/Transport Effects Substrate of CYP2C19 (minor), CYP2D6 (major); **Note:** Assignment of Major/Minor substrate status based on clinically relevant drug interaction potential; **Inhibits** CYP1A2 (weak), CYP2C9 (weak), CYP2D6 (strong), CYP2E1 (weak)

Avoid Concomitant Use

Avoid concomitant use of Thioridazine with any of the following: Aclidinium; Amisulpride; Azelastine (Nasal); CYP2D6 Inhibitors; FLUoxetine; FluvoxaMINE; Highest Risk QTc-Prolonging Agents; Ipratropium (Oral Inhalation); Ivabradine; Metoclopramide; Mifepristone; Moclobemide; Moderate Risk QTc-Prolonging Agents; Paraldehyde; Pimozide; Potassium Chloride; Sulpiride; Tamoxifen; Thalidomide; Tiotropium; Umeclidinium

Increased Effect/Toxicity

Thioridazine may increase the levels/effects of: Abobotulinumtoxin A; Alcohol (Ethyl); Amisulpride; Analgesics (Opioid); Anticholinergic Agents; ARIPiprazole; AtoMOXetine; Azelastine (Nasal); Beta-Blockers; Buprenorphine; Cannabinoid-Containing Products; Chlorpheniramine; CNS Depressants; CYP2D6 Substrates; DOXOrubicin (Conventional); Fesoterodine; Highest Risk QTc-Prolonging Agents; Hydrocodone; Methylphenidate; Metoprolol; Metyrosine; Nebivolol; OnabotulinumtoxinA; Paraldehyde; Pimozide; Porfimer; Potassium Chloride; RimabotulinumtoxinB; Selective Serotonin Reuptake Inhibitors; Serotonin Modulators; Sulpiride; Thalidomide; Thiazide Diuretics; Thiopental; Tiotropium; Topiramate; Vortioxetine; Zolpidem

The levels/effects of Thioridazine may be increased by: Acetylcholinesterase Inhibitors (Central); Aclidinium; Antimalarial Agents; Beta-Blockers; Brimonidine (Topical); Cannabis; Chlorpheniramine; CYP2D6 Inhibitors; Darunavir; Doxylamine; Dronabinol; FLUoxetine; FluvoxaMINE; HydrOXYzine; Ipratropium (Oral Inhalation); Ivabradine; Kava Kava; Magnesium Sulfate; Methylphenidate; Metoclopramide; Metyrosine; Mifepristone; Moclobemide; Moderate Risk QTc-Prolonging Agents; Nabilone; Perampanel; Pramlintide; QTc-Prolonging Agents (Indeterminate Risk and Risk Modifying); Rufinamide; Serotonin Modulators; Sodium Oxybate; Tapentadol; Tetrahydrocannabinol; Umeclidinium

Decreased Effect

Thioridazine may decrease the levels/effects of: Acetylcholinesterase Inhibitors (Central); Amphetamines; Anti-Parkinson's Agents (Dopamine Agonist); Codeine; Quinagolide; Secretin; Tamoxifen; TraMADol

The levels/effects of Thioridazine may be decreased by: Acetylcholinesterase Inhibitors (Central); Antacids; Anti-Parkinson's Agents (Dopamine Agonist); Peginterferon Alfa-2b

Mechanism of Action Thioridazine is a piperidine phenothiazine which blocks postsynaptic mesolimbic dopaminergic receptors in the brain; exhibits a strong alpha-adrenergic blocking effect and depresses the release of hypothalamic and hypophyseal hormones

Pharmacokinetics (Adult data unless noted)
Protein binding: 99%
Metabolism: In the liver to active and inactive metabolites
Bioavailability: 25% to 33%
Half-life: Adults: 9-30 hours
Dialysis: Not dialyzable: (0% to 5%)

Dosing: Usual Oral:
Children >2 years: Initial: 0.5 mg/kg/day in 2-3 divided doses; range: 0.5-3 mg/kg/day; usual: 1 mg/kg/day in 2-3 divided doses; maximum dose: 3 mg/kg/day

Behavior problems: Initial: 10 mg 2-3 times/day, increase gradually

Severe psychoses: Initial: 25 mg 2-3 times/day, increase gradually

Children >12 years and Adults:
Schizophrenia/psychoses: Initial: 25-100 mg 3 times/day with gradual increments as needed and tolerated; maximum daily dose: 800 mg/day in 2-4 divided doses; maintenance: 10-200 mg/dose 2-4 times/day

Depressive disorders, dementia: Initial: 25 mg 3 times/day; maintenance dose: 20-200 mg/day

Administration Oral: Administer with water, food, or milk to decrease GI upset; dilute the oral concentrate with water or juice before administration; do not administer liquid thioridazine simultaneously with carbamazepine suspension; do not mix liquid thioridazine with enteric formulas

Monitoring Parameters Baseline and periodic ECG and serum potassium; periodic eye exam, CBC with differential, blood pressure, liver enzyme tests

Test Interactions False-positives for phenylketonuria, urinary amylase, uroporphyrins, urobilinogen; may interfere with urine detection of methadone and phencyclidine (false-positives)

Additional Information In cases of overdoses, cardiovascular monitoring and continuous ECG monitoring should be performed; avoid drugs (such as quinidine, disopyramide, and procainamide) that may further prolong the QT interval

Note: All Mellaril® (brand name) products have been discontinued; Mellaril® suspension was discontinued October, 2000; oral concentrate 100 mg/mL was discontinued March 2001; tablets and 30 mg/mL oral concentrate were discontinued in January 2002.

◀ **Dosage Forms** Excipient information presented when available (limited, particularly for generics); consult specific product labeling.

Tablet, Oral, as hydrochloride:

Generic: 10 mg, 25 mg, 50 mg, 100 mg

References

Aman MG, Marks RE, Turbott SH, et al, "Clinical Effects of Methylphenidate and Thioridazine in Intellectually Subaverage Children," *J Am Acad Child Adolesc Psychiatry*, 1991, 30(2):246-56.

◆ **Thioridazine Hydrochloride** *see* Thioridazine *on page 2012*

◆ **Thiosulfuric Acid Disodium Salt** *see* Sodium Thiosulfate *on page 1919*

Thiotepa (thye oh TEP a)

Medication Safety Issues

Sound-alike/look-alike issues:

Thiotepa may be confused with thioguanine

High alert medication:

This medication is in a class the Institute for Safe Medication Practices (ISMP) includes among its list of drug classes which have a heightened risk of causing significant patient harm when used in error.

Administration issues:

Intrathecal medication safety: The American Society of Clinical Oncology (ASCO)/Oncology Nursing Society (ONS) chemotherapy administration safety standards (Jacobson, 2009) encourage the following safety measures for intrathecal chemotherapy:

- Intrathecal medication should not be prepared during the preparation of any other agents
- After preparation, keep in an isolated location or container clearly marked with a label identifying as "intrathecal" use only
- Delivery to the patient should only be with other medications intended for administration into the central nervous system

Related Information

Emetogenic Potential of Antineoplastic Agents in Children *on page 2327*

Management of Drug Extravasations *on page 2255*

Safe Handling of Hazardous Drugs *on page 2419*

Therapeutic Category Antineoplastic Agent, Alkylating Agent

Generic Availability (U.S.) May be product dependent

Use Treatment of superficial tumors of the bladder; palliative treatment of adenocarcinoma of breast or ovary; control of pleural, pericardial, or peritoneal effusions caused by metastatic tumors (FDA approved in adults); has also been used for intrathecal treatment of leptomeningeal metastases (in adults) and as part of a conditioning regimen prior to autologous or allogeneic hematopoietic stem cell transplantation

Pregnancy Risk Factor D

Pregnancy Considerations Animal reproduction studies have demonstrated teratogenicity and fetal loss. There are no adequate and well-controlled studies in pregnant women. May cause harm if administered during pregnancy. Effective contraception is recommended for men and women of childbearing potential.

Breast-Feeding Considerations Due to the potential for serious adverse reactions in the nursing infant, breast-feeding is not recommended.

Contraindications Hypersensitivity to thiotepa or any component; **Note:** May be contraindicated in certain circumstances of hepatic, renal, and/or bone marrow failure; evaluate on an individual basis as lower dose treatment may still be appropriate if the potential benefit outweighs the risks.

Warnings Hazardous agent; use appropriate precautions for handling and disposal (NIOSH, 2012). Myelosuppression is common; monitor for infection or bleeding. Death due to sepsis and hemorrhage as a result of thiotepa administration has been reported. Thiotepa is potentially mutagenic, carcinogenic, teratogenic, and may cause fertility impairment. May be contraindicated with hepatic, renal, and/or bone marrow impairment/damage; use should be limited to cases in which benefit outweighs risk.

Precautions Reduce dosage in patients with hepatic, renal, or bone marrow dysfunction.

Adverse Reactions

Central nervous system: Chills, dizziness, fatigue, fever, headache

Dermatologic: Alopecia, contact dermatitis, depigmentation (with topical treatment), dermatitis, rash, urticaria

Endocrine & metabolic: Amenorrhea, spermatogenesis inhibition

Gastrointestinal: Abdominal pain, anorexia, nausea, vomiting

Genitourinary: Dysuria, urinary retention

Hematologic: Anemia, bleeding, leukopenia, thrombocytopenia

Local: Injection site pain

Neuromuscular & skeletal: Weakness

Ocular: Blurred vision, conjunctivitis

Renal: Hematuria

Respiratory: Asthma, epistaxis, laryngeal edema, wheezing

Miscellaneous: Allergic reaction, anaphylactic shock, infection

Rare but important or life-threatening: Acute myeloid leukemia (AML), chemical cystitis (bladder instillation), hemorrhagic cystitis (bladder instillation), myelodysplastic syndrome

Drug Interactions

Metabolism/Transport Effects Inhibits CYP2B6 (strong)

Avoid Concomitant Use

Avoid concomitant use of Thiotepa with any of the following: BCG; CloZAPine; Dipyrone; Natalizumab; Pimecrolimus; Tacrolimus (Topical); Tofacitinib; Vaccines (Live)

Increased Effect/Toxicity

Thiotepa may increase the levels/effects of: CloZAPine; CYP2B6 Substrates; Leflunomide; Natalizumab; Tofacitinib; Vaccines (Live)

The levels/effects of Thiotepa may be increased by: Denosumab; Dipyrone; Pimecrolimus; Roflumilast; Tacrolimus (Topical); Trastuzumab

Decreased Effect

Thiotepa may decrease the levels/effects of: BCG; Coccidioidin Skin Test; Sipuleucel-T; Vaccines (Inactivated); Vaccines (Live)

The levels/effects of Thiotepa may be decreased by: Echinacea

Stability Hazardous agent; use appropriate precautions for handling and disposal (NIOSH, 2012). Store intact vials under refrigeration (2°C to 8°C). Protect from light. Reconstituted solutions (10 mg/mL) are stable for up to 28 days under refrigeration (4°C to 8°C) or 7 days at room temperature (25°C), although the manufacturer recommends use within 8 hours when reconstituted solutions are stored under refrigeration. Solutions further diluted (for I.V. use) in NS to 1 mg/mL in NS are stable for 24 hours and to 3 mg/mL are stable for 48 hours at room temperature, although the manufacturer recommends immediate use.

Mechanism of Action Alkylating agent that reacts with DNA phosphate groups to produce cross-linking of DNA strands leading to inhibition of DNA, RNA, and protein synthesis; mechanism of action has not been explored as thoroughly as the other alkylating agents, it is presumed that the aziridine rings open and react as nitrogen mustard; reactivity is enhanced at a lower pH

Pharmacokinetics (Adult data unless noted)

Absorption: Variable absorption through serous membranes and from I.M. injection sites; bladder mucosa: 10% to 100% and is increased with mucosal inflammation or tumor infiltration

Distribution: V_{dss}: 0.7-1.6 L/kg; distributes into CSF

Protein binding: 8% to 13%

Metabolism: In the liver via oxidative desulfuration (cytochrome P450 microsomal enzyme system) primarily to TEPA (active metabolite)

Half-life, terminal:

Thiotepa: 109 minutes (51.6-212 minutes) with dose-dependent clearance

TEPA: 10-21 hours

Elimination: Very little thiotepa or active metabolite are excreted unchanged in urine (1.5% of thiotepa dose)

Dosing: Usual Refer to individual protocols

Infants, Children, and Adolescents: I.V.:

HSCT for CNS malignancy (combination chemotherapy): 300 mg/m²/dose daily for 3 days (Dunkel, 2010; Finlay, 2008; Gilheeney, 2010; Grodman, 2009)

HSCT for neuroblastoma/solid tumors (combination chemotherapy): Children and Adolescents: 300 mg/m²/dose daily for 3 days (Kletzel, 1998; Kushner, 2001; Kushner, 2006)

Adults:

I.V.: Ovarian, breast cancer: 0.3-0.4 mg/kg/dose every 1-4 weeks

Intracavitary: Effusions: 0.6-0.8 mg/kg/dose

Intrathecal: Leptomeningeal metastases: 10 mg twice a week for 4 weeks, then weekly for 4 weeks, then monthly for 4 doses (NCCN CNS cancer guidelines v.1.2010)

Intravesical: Bladder cancer: 60 mg in 30-60 mL NS retained for 2 hours once weekly for 4 weeks

Dosing adjustment in renal impairment: Use with extreme caution; reduced dose may be warranted. Use may be contraindicated with existing renal impairment and should be limited to cases where benefit outweighs risk.

Dosing adjustment in hepatic impairment: Use with extreme caution; reduced dose may be warranted. Use may be contraindicated with existing hepatic impairment and should be limited to cases where benefit outweighs risk.

Dosage adjustment for hematologic toxicity: I.V.:

WBC ≤3000/mm³: Discontinue treatment

Platelets ≤150,000/mm³: Discontinue treatment

Note: Use may be contraindicated with preexisting marrow damage and should be limited to cases where benefit outweighs risk.

Administration Hazardous agent; use appropriate precautions for handling and disposal (NIOSH, 2012).

Bladder instillation: Prepare with 60 mg diluted in 30-60 mL NS and instill by catheter and retain for 2 hours; patients should reposition every 15-30 minutes

Intrapleural or pericardial: Dose is further diluted to a volume of 10-20 mL in NS or D_5W

Intrathecal: Reconstitute each 15 mg vial with 1.5 mL preservative-free SWI then further dilute to a final concentration of 1-5 mg/mL with preservative-free NS. Intrathecal dilutions are preservative-free and should be used as soon as possible after preparation. After preparation, store intrathecal medications (until use) in an isolated location or container clearly marked with a label identifying as "intrathecal" use only.

I.V.: Use appropriate precautions for handling and disposal. Reconstitute each 15 mg vial with 1.5 mL SWI to a concentration of 10 mg/mL. Solutions for I.V. use should be further diluted in NS prior to infusion. Filter

through a 0.22 micron filter (polysulfone membrane [eg, Sterile Aerodisc®] or triton-free cellulose mixed ester [eg, Millex®-GS]) prior to administration; do not use solutions which precipitate or remain opaque after filtering. Low doses (adult) may be administered as a rapid injection over 5 minutes. High doses (pediatric) have longer infusion times (eg, over 2- to 4-hour infusion); refer to specific protocols.

Vesicant/Extravasation Risk May be an irritant

Monitoring Parameters CBC with differential and platelet count, uric acid, urinalysis, renal and hepatic function tests

Additional Information Myelosuppressive effects:

WBC: Moderate

Platelets: Severe

Onset (days): 7-10

Nadir (days): 14-20

Recovery (days): 28

References

Dunkel IJ, Gardner SL, Garvin JH Jr, et al, "High-Dose Carboplatin, Thiotepa, and Etoposide With Autologous Stem Cell Rescue for Patients With Previously Irradiated Recurrent Medulloblastoma," Neuro Oncol, 2010, 12(3):297-303.

Finlay JL, Dhall G, Boyett JM, et al, "Myeloablative Chemotherapy With Autologous Bone Marrow Rescue in Children and Adolescents With Recurrent Malignant Astrocytoma: Outcome Compared With Conventional Chemotherapy: A Report From the Children's Oncology Group," Pediatr Blood Cancer, 2008, 51(6):806-11.

Gilheeney SW, Khakoo Y, Souweidane M, et al, "Thiotepa/Topotecan/ Carboplatin With Autologous Stem Cell Rescue in Recurrent/Refractory/Poor Prognosis Pediatric Malignancies of the Central Nervous System," Pediatr Blood Cancer, 2010, 54(4):591-5.

Grodman H, Wolfe L, and Kretschmar C, "Outcome of Patients With Recurrent Medulloblastoma or Central Nervous System Germinoma Treated With Low Dose Continuous Intravenous Etoposide Along With Dose-Intensive Chemotherapy Followed by Autologous Hematopoietic Stem Cell Rescue," Pediatr Blood Cancer, 2009, 53(1):33-6.

Grossman SA, Finkelstein DM, Ruckdeschel JC, et al, "Randomized Prospective Comparison of Intraventricular Methotrexate and Thiotepa in Patients With Previously Untreated Neoplastic Meningitis. Eastern Cooperative Oncology Group," J Clin Oncol, 1993, 11 (3):561-9.

Jacobson JO, Polovich M, McNiff KK, et al, "American Society of Clinical Oncology/Oncology Nursing Society Chemotherapy Administration Safety Standards," J Clin Oncol, 2009, 27(32):5469-75.

Heideman R, Cole D, Balis F, et al, "Phase I and Pharmacokinetic Evaluation of Thiotepa in the Cerebrospinal Fluid and Plasma of Pediatric Patients: Evidence for Dose-Dependent Plasma Clearance of Thiotepa," Cancer Res, 1989, 49(3):736-41.

Kletzel M, Abella EM, Sandler ES, et al, "Thiotepa and Cyclophosphamide With Stem Cell Rescue for Consolidation Therapy for Children With High-Risk Neuroblastoma: A Phase I/II Study of the Pediatric Blood and Marrow Transplant Consortium," J Pediatr Hematol Oncol, 1998, 20(1):49-54.

Kushner BH, Cheung NK, Kramer K, et al, "Topotecan Combined With Myeloablative Doses of Thiotepa and Carboplatin for Neuroblastoma, Brain Tumors, and Other Poor-Risk Solid Tumors in Children and Young Adults," Bone Marrow Transplant, 2001, 28(6):551-6.

Kushner BH, Kramer K, Modak S, et al, "Topotecan, Thiotepa, and Carboplatin for Neuroblastoma: Failure to Prevent Relapse in the Central Nervous System," Bone Marrow Transplant, 2006, 37 (3):271-6.

National Comprehensive Cancer Network® (NCCN), "Clinical Practice Guidelines in Oncology™: Central Nervous System Cancers," Version 2.2009. Available at: http://www.nccn.org/professionals/physician_gls/PDF/cns.pdf.

National Institute for Occupational Safety and Health (NIOSH), "NIOSH List of Antineoplastic and Other Hazardous Drugs in Healthcare Settings 2012." Available at http://www.cdc.gov/niosh/docs/2012-150/pdfs/2012-150.pdf. Accessed January 21, 2013.

Soussain C, Hoang-Xuan K, Taillandier L, et al, "Intensive Chemotherapy Followed by Hematopoietic Stem-Cell Rescue for Refractory and Recurrent Primary CNS and Intraocular Lymphoma: Société Française de Greffe de Moëlle Osseuse-Thérapie Cellulaire," J Clin Oncol, 2008, 26(15):2512-8.

Thiothixene (thye oh THIKS een)

Medication Safety Issues

Sound-alike/look-alike issues:

Thiothixene may be confused with FLUoxetine, thioridazine

Navane may be confused with Norvasc, Nubain

BEERS Criteria medication:
This drug may be potentially inappropriate for use in geriatric patients (Quality of evidence - moderate; Strength of recommendation - strong).

Brand Names: Canada Navane

Therapeutic Category Antipsychotic Agent, Typical, Phenothiazine; Phenothiazine Derivative

Generic Availability (U.S.) Yes

Use Management of schizophrenia (FDA approved in ages ≥12 years and adults); also used for management of psychotic disorders

Pregnancy Considerations Adverse events were observed in some animal reproduction studies. Antipsychotic use during the third trimester of pregnancy has a risk for abnormal muscle movements (extrapyramidal symptoms [EPS]) and withdrawal symptoms in newborns following delivery. Symptoms in the newborn may include agitation, feeding disorder, hypertonia, hypotonia, respiratory distress, somnolence, and tremor; these effects may be self-limiting or require hospitalization. The ACOG recommends that therapy during pregnancy be individualized; treatment with psychiatric medications during pregnancy should incorporate the clinical expertise of the mental health clinician, obstetrician, primary healthcare provider, and pediatrician. When treating schizophrenia during pregnancy, atypical antipsychotics may be better tolerated by the mother however more information related to fetal effects may be available for agents considered typical (or first generation) antipsychotics (ACOG, 2008). Information related to the use of thiothixene in pregnancy is limited and other agents may be preferred.

Breast-Feeding Considerations It is not known if thiothixene is excreted into breast milk; other agents are preferred for use in nursing women (Klinger, 2013).

Contraindications Hypersensitivity to thiothixene or any component; cross-sensitivity with other phenothiazines may exist; patients with CNS depression, comatose states, circulatory collapse, or blood dyscrasias; avoid use in patients with narrow-angle glaucoma, bone marrow suppression, severe liver or cardiac disease

Warnings May alter cardiac conduction; life-threatening arrhythmias have occurred with therapeutic doses of neuroleptics. May mask toxicity of other drugs or conditions (eg, intestinal obstruction, Reye's syndrome, brain tumor) due to antiemetic effects. Elevates prolactin levels; use with caution in patients with breast cancer or other prolactin-dependent tumors.

May cause extrapyramidal symptoms (EPS), including pseudoparkinsonism, acute dystonic reactions, akathisia, and tardive dyskinesia (risk of these reactions is high relative to other neuroleptics, and is dose-dependent; to decrease risk of tardive dyskinesia: Use smallest dose and shortest duration possible; evaluate continued need periodically; risk of dystonia is increased with the use of high potency and higher doses of conventional antipsychotics and in males and younger patients). Use may be associated with neuroleptic malignant syndrome (NMS); monitor for mental status changes, fever, muscle rigidity, and/or autonomic instability; risk may be increased in patients with Parkinson's disease or Lewy body dementia.

May cause pigmentary retinopathy, and lenticular and corneal deposits, particularly with prolonged therapy. May be sedating, use with caution in disorders in which CNS depression is a feature; patients must be cautioned about performing tasks which require mental alertness (eg, operating machinery or driving). Impaired core body temperature regulation may occur; caution with strenuous exercise, heat exposure, dehydration, and concomitant medication possessing anticholinergic effects. Thiothixene has not been evaluated for the treatment of behavioral complications in patients with mental retardation. Safety and efficacy have not been established in children <12 years of age.

Leukopenia, neutropenia, and agranulocytosis (sometimes fatal) have been reported in clinical trials and postmarketing reports with antipsychotic use; presence of risk factors (eg, preexisting low WBC or history of drug-induced leuko/neutropenia) should prompt periodic blood count assessment. Discontinue therapy at first signs of blood dyscrasias or if absolute neutrophil count <1000/mm³. Use is contraindicated in patients with blood dyscrasia.

An increased risk of death has been reported with the use of antipsychotics in elderly patients with dementia-related psychosis **[U.S. Boxed Warning]**; most deaths seemed to be cardiovascular (eg, sudden death, heart failure) or infectious (eg, pneumonia) in nature; thiothixene is not approved for this indication.

Precautions Use with caution in patients with cardiovascular disease or seizures

Adverse Reactions

Cardiovascular: Cardiac arrest, ECG changes, hypotension, peripheral edema, syncope, tachycardia

Central nervous system: Abnormal cerebrospinal fluid, agitation, cerebral edema, dizziness, drowsiness, extrapyramidal reaction (akathisia, dystonias, pseudoparkinsonism, tardive dyskinesia), fatigue, hyperreflexia (infants), hypertonia (neonates), hypotonia (neonates), insomnia, Neuroleptic Malignant Syndrome, restlessness, seizure

Dermatologic: Contact dermatitis, diaphoresis, exfoliative dermatitis, pruritus, skin discoloration (blue-gray), skin photosensitivity, skin rash, urticaria

Endocrine & metabolic: Amenorrhea, change in libido, galactorrhea, glycosuria, gynecomastia, hyperglycemia, hyperprolactinemia, hypoglycemia, menstrual disease, polydipsia, weight gain

Gastrointestinal: Anorexia, constipation, diarrhea, increased appetite, nausea, paralytic ileus, sialorrhea, stomach pain, vomiting, xerostomia

Genitourinary: Breast hypertrophy, difficulty in micturition, ejaculatory disorder, impotence, lactation, mastalgia

Hematologic & oncologic: Leukocytosis, leukopenia

Hepatic: Increased serum alkaline phosphatase, increased serum transaminase

Hypersensitivity: Anaphylaxis (rare)

Neuromuscular & skeletal: Lupus-like syndrome, tremor, weakness

Ophthalmic: Blurred vision, miosis, mydriasis, retinitis pigmentosa

Respiratory: Asphyxia, nasal congestion, respiratory distress (neonates)

Miscellaneous: Fever, paradoxical reaction (excerbation of psychotic symptoms)

Drug Interactions

Metabolism/Transport Effects Substrate of CYP1A2 (major); **Note:** Assignment of Major/Minor substrate status based on clinically relevant drug interaction potential; **Inhibits** CYP2D6 (weak)

Avoid Concomitant Use

Avoid concomitant use of Thiothixene with any of the following: Aclidinium; Amisulpride; Azelastine (Nasal); Ipratropium (Oral Inhalation); Metoclopramide; Paraldehyde; Potassium Chloride; Sulpiride; Thalidomide; Tiotropium; Umeclidinium

Increased Effect/Toxicity

Thiothixene may increase the levels/effects of: AbobotulinumtoxinA; Alcohol (Ethyl); Amisulpride; Analgesics (Opioid); Anticholinergic Agents; ARIPiprazole; Azelastine (Nasal); Buprenorphine; Cannabinoid-Containing Products; CNS Depressants; Highest Risk QTc-Prolonging Agents; Hydrocodone; Methotrimeprazine; Methylphenidate; Metyrosine; Mirabegron; Mirtazapine; Moderate Risk QTc-Prolonging Agents;

OnabotulinumtoxinA; Paraldehyde; Potassium Chloride; RimabotulinumtoxinB; Selective Serotonin Reuptake Inhibitors; Serotonin Modulators; Sulpiride; Thalidomide; Thiazide Diuretics; Tiotropium; Topiramate; Zolpidem

The levels/effects of Thiothixene may be increased by: Abiraterone Acetate; Acetylcholinesterase Inhibitors (Central); Aclidinium; Brimonidine (Topical); Cannabis; CYP1A2 Inhibitors (Moderate); CYP1A2 Inhibitors (Strong); Deferasirox; Doxylamine; Dronabinol; Droperidol; HydrOXYzine; Ipratropium (Oral Inhalation); Kava Kava; Lithium; Magnesium Sulfate; Methotrimeprazine; Methylphenidate; Metoclopramide; Metyrosine; Mifepristone; Nabilone; Perampanel; Pramlintide; Rufinamide; Serotonin Modulators; Sodium Oxybate; Tapentadol; Tetrahydrocannabinol; Umeclidinium; Vemurafenib

Decreased Effect

Thiothixene may decrease the levels/effects of: Acetylcholinesterase Inhibitors (Central); Amphetamines; Anti-Parkinson's Agents (Dopamine Agonist); Quinagolide; Secretin

The levels/effects of Thiothixene may be decreased by: Acetylcholinesterase Inhibitors (Central); Anti-Parkinson's Agents (Dopamine Agonist); Cannabis; CYP1A2 Inducers (Strong); Cyproterone; Lithium

Mechanism of Action Thiothixene is a thioxanthene antipsychotic which elicits antipsychotic activity by postsynaptic blockade of CNS dopamine receptors resulting in inhibition of dopamine-mediated effects; also has alpha-adrenergic blocking activity

Dosing: Usual Oral:
Children <12 years: Dose not well established (use not recommended); 0.25 mg/kg/day in divided doses
Children ≥12 years and Adults: Initial: 2 mg 3 times/day, up to 20-30 mg/day; maximum dose: 60 mg/day

Administration Oral: Administer with food or water

Monitoring Parameters Periodic eye exam, CBC with differential, blood pressure, liver enzyme tests

Test Interactions May cause false-positive pregnancy test

Dosage Forms Excipient information presented when available (limited, particularly for generics); consult specific product labeling.
Capsule, Oral:
Generic: 1 mg, 2 mg, 5 mg, 10 mg

References
Wiener JM, "Psychopharmacology in Childhood Disorders," *Psychiatr Clin North Am*, 1984, 7(4):831-43.

◆ **Thorazine** *see* ChlorproMAZINE *on page 450*
◆ **Three-Factor PCC** *see* Factor IX Complex (Human) [(Factors II, IX, X)] *on page 833*
◆ **Thrombi-Gel®** *see* Thrombin (Topical) *on page 2017*
◆ **Thrombin-JMI®** *see* Thrombin (Topical) *on page 2017*
◆ **Thrombin-JMI® Epistaxis Kit** *see* Thrombin (Topical) *on page 2017*
◆ **Thrombin-JMI® Pump Spray Kit** *see* Thrombin (Topical) *on page 2017*
◆ **Thrombin-JMI® Syringe Spray Kit** *see* Thrombin (Topical) *on page 2017*

Thrombin (Topical) (THROM bin, TOP i kal)

Medication Safety Issues
Administration issues:
For topical use only. Do not administer intravenously or intra-arterially.

To reduce the risk of intravascular administration, the Institute for Safe Medication Practices (ISMP) has the following recommendations:
- Prepare, label, and dispense topical thrombin from the pharmacy department (including doses used in the operating room).
- Do not leave vial or syringe at bedside.
- Add auxiliary label to all labels and syringes stating "For topical use only - do not inject".
- When appropriate, use solutions which can be applied with an absorbable gelatin sponge or use a dry form on oozing surfaces.
- When appropriate, use spray kits to help differentiate between parenteral products.

Brand Names: U.S. Evithrom®; Recothrom®; Thrombi-Gel®; Thrombi-Pad®; Thrombin-JMI®; Thrombin-JMI® Epistaxis Kit; Thrombin-JMI® Pump Spray Kit; Thrombin-JMI® Syringe Spray Kit

Therapeutic Category Hemostatic Agent

Generic Availability (U.S.) No

Use Hemostasis whenever minor bleeding from capillaries and small venules is accessible
Thrombi-Gel®; Thrombi-Pad®: Temporary control as trauma dressing for moderate-to-severe bleeding wounds; control of surface bleeding from vascular access sites and percutaneous catheter/ tubes

Pregnancy Risk Factor C

Pregnancy Considerations Animal reproduction studies have not been conducted. Reproduction studies conducted with the solvent/detergent used in processing the human-derived product (Evithrom®) showed adverse events in animals. Only residual levels of the solvent/detergent would be expected to remain in the finished product.

Breast-Feeding Considerations Breast-feeding is not recommended by the manufacturer.

Contraindications Hypersensitivity to thrombin or any component; not to be injected directly into circulatory system; Evithrom® is contraindicated for the treatment of massive or brisk arterial bleeding and in patients with a known anaphylactic or severe systemic reaction to blood products; Recothrom® is contraindicated for the treatment of severe or brisk arterial bleeding and in patients with hypersensitivity to hamster or snake proteins; Thrombin-JMI® and Thrombi-Pad® are contraindicated in patients with hypersensitivity to material of bovine origin; Thrombi-Gel® should not be used in closure of skin incisions due to possible interference with healing of skin edges

Warnings For topical use only - do not inject; injection may result in extensive intravascular clotting and death. Use of bovine-source topical thrombin has been associated with abnormalities in hemostasis ranging from asymptomatic alterations in PT and PTT to severe bleeding or thrombosis which have rarely been fatal **[U.S. Boxed Warning]**. These hemostatic effects may be related to formation of antibodies against bovine thrombin and/or factor V which in some cases may cross react with human factor V resulting in factor V deficiency; patients with antibodies to bovine thrombin should not receive topical thrombin again. Thrombi-Gel®, Thrombi-Pad® should not be used in the presence of infection; use caution in areas of contamination. Thrombi-Pad® is nonabsorbable and should not be left in the body.

Adverse Reactions
Cardiovascular: Thromboembolism
Dermatologic: Pruritus
Gastrointestinal: Nausea, vomiting
Hematologic and oncologic: Increased INR, increased neutrophils, lymphocytopenia, prolonged partial thromboplastin time, prolonged prothrombin time
Hypersensitivity: Hypersensitivity reaction
Immunologic: Antibody development

Local: Postoperative wound complication

Drug Interactions

Metabolism/Transport Effects None known.

Avoid Concomitant Use There are no known interactions where it is recommended to avoid concomitant use.

Increased Effect/Toxicity There are no known significant interactions involving an increase in effect.

Decreased Effect There are no known significant interactions involving a decrease in effect.

Stability

Evithrom®: Store frozen vials at -18°C for up to 2 years; unopened vials may be stored at 2°C to 8°C for up to 30 days; stable at room temperature for 24 hours; do not refreeze after thawing; do not refrigerate once at room temperature.

Recothrom®: Store at room temperature; reconstituted solutions may be stored refrigerated for 24 hours.

Thrombi-Gel®: Store at 2°C to 25°C (36°F to 77°F). After wetting with SWI or 0.9% sodium chloride, use within 3 hours.

Thrombi-Pad®: Store at 2°C to 25°C (36°F to 77°F). If pad is wetted with 0.9% sodium chloride, use within 1 hour.

Thrombin-JMI®: Store vials at room temperature; reconstituted vials may be stored in refrigerator for 24 hours or at room temperature for 8 hours.

Mechanism of Action Activates platelets and catalyzes the conversion of fibrinogen to fibrin to promote hemostasis.

Dosing: Usual Topical: Hemostasis:

Powder or solution formulations: Apply 1000-2000 units/mL solution directly or via absorbable gelatin sponge to the site of bleeding or oozing surface; Thrombin-JMI® may also be applied in dry powder form directly to the site. For general use in plastic surgery, dental extractions, skin grafting, etc, solutions containing approximately 100 units/mL are frequently used.

Thrombi-Gel®10, 40, 100: Adults: Wet product with up to 3 mL, 10 mL, or 20 mL, respectively, of 0.9% sodium chloride or SWI; apply directly over source of the bleeding with manual pressure

Thrombi-Pad®: Adults: Apply pad directly over source of bleeding. May apply dry or wetted with up to 10 mL of 0.9% sodium chloride. If desired, product may be left in place for up to 24 hours; do not leave in the body

Administration Not for injection

Topical: Powder or solution formulations: May be applied directly as a powder (Thrombin-JMI®) or as reconstituted solution; the most effective hemostasis results when the thrombin mixes freely with blood as it appears; use NS to reconstitute powder to 1000-2000 units/mL concentration; (Evithrom® must be thawed prior to use and requires no further dilution). The recipient surface should be sponged (not wiped) free of blood before application; do not sponge **treated** surfaces to assure that clot remains securely in place. Refer to manufacturer's information for more specific application information.

Pad or sponge formulations: May cut or roll Thrombi-Gel® to desired shape prior to wetting; once wetted and prior to applying, knead thoroughly to saturate the pad remove trapped air bubbles. Thrombi-Pad® may be applied dry or wet.

Additional Information One unit is amount required to clot 1 mL of standardized fibrinogen solution in 15 seconds

Dosage Forms Excipient information presented when available (limited, particularly for generics); consult specific product labeling.

Pad, topical [preservative free; bovine derived]:
Thrombi-Pad® 3x3: ≥200 units (10s)

Powder for reconstitution, topical [bovine derived]:
Thrombin-JMI®: 5000 units, 20,000 units [supplied with diluent]

Thrombin-JMI® Epistaxis kit: 5000 units [supplied with diluent]

Thrombin-JMI® Pump Spray Kit: 20,000 units [supplied with diluents]

Thrombin-JMI® Syringe Spray Kit: 5000 units; 20,000 units [supplied with diluent]

Powder for reconstitution, topical [preservative free; recombinant]:
Recothrom®: 5000 units; 20,000 units [production involves products derived from hamster and snake sources; supplied with diluent]

Solution, topical [human derived]:
Evithrom®: 800-1200 units/mL (2 mL, 5 mL, 20 mL)

Sponge, topical [preservative free; bovine derived]:
Thrombi-Gel® 10: ≥1000 units (10s)
Thrombi-Gel® 40: ≥1000 units (5s)
Thrombi-Gel® 100: ≥2000 units (5s)

◆ **Thrombi-Pad®** see Thrombin (Topical) on page 2017

◆ **Thymocyte Stimulating Factor** see Aldesleukin on page 90

◆ **Thymoglobulin** see Antithymocyte Globulin (Rabbit) on page 184

Thyroid, Desiccated (THYE roid DES i kay tid)

Medication Safety Issues

BEERS Criteria medication:

This drug may be potentially inappropriate for use in geriatric patients (Quality of evidence - low; Strength of recommendation - strong).

Brand Names: U.S. Armour Thyroid; Nature-Throid; NP Thyroid; Westhroid; Westhroid-P [DSC]; WP Thyroid

Therapeutic Category Thyroid Product

Generic Availability (U.S.) Yes

Use Replacement or supplemental therapy in hypothyroidism of any etiology (FDA approved in all ages); pituitary TSH suppressant for the treatment or prevention of various types of euthyroid goiter, thyroid nodules, thyroiditis, multinodular goiter, and thyroid cancer (FDA approved in adults); **Note:** Not indicated for treatment of transient hypothyroidism associated with subacute thyroiditis.

Pregnancy Risk Factor A

Pregnancy Considerations Endogenous thyroid hormones minimally cross the placenta; the fetal thyroid becomes active around the end of the first trimester. Liothyronine has not been found to increase the risk of teratogenic or adverse effects following maternal use during pregnancy.

Uncontrolled maternal hypothyroidism may result in adverse neonatal and maternal outcomes. To prevent adverse events, normal maternal thyroid function should be maintained prior to conception and throughout pregnancy. Levothyroxine is considered the treatment of choice for the control of hypothyroidism during pregnancy.

Breast-Feeding Considerations Endogenous thyroid hormones are minimally found in breast milk and are not associated with adverse events.

Contraindications Hypersensitivity to pork or any component; untreated thyrotoxicosis; uncorrected adrenal insufficiency

Warnings Not for use in the treatment of obesity or for weight loss **[U.S. Boxed Warning]**; in euthyroid patients, doses within the range of daily hormonal requirements are ineffective for weight reduction; larger doses may produce serious or even life-threatening toxic effects particularly when used with some anorectic drugs (sympathomimetic amines). Overtreatment may result in craniosynostosis in infants and premature closure of epiphyses in children; monitor use closely. Should not be used for treatment of infertility without unrelated hypothyroidism.

Precautions Use with extreme caution in patients with adrenal insufficiency; symptoms may be exaggerated or aggravated. Use with caution and reduce dosage in patients with angina pectoris or other cardiovascular disease; chronic hypothyroidism predisposes patients to coronary artery disease. Use with caution in patients with diabetes mellitus and insipidus; symptoms may be exaggerated or aggravated. May cause transient alopecia in children during the first few months of therapy. In neonates and infants, cardiac overload, arrhythmias, and aspiration from avid suckling may occur during initiation of therapy (eg, first 2 weeks); monitor closely.

Adverse Reactions Note: Adverse reactions often indicative of excess thyroid replacement and/or hyperthyroidism.

Rare but important or life-threatening: Alopecia, cardiac arrhythmia, chest pain, dyspnea, excessive bone loss with overtreatment (excess thyroid replacement), hand tremor, myalgia, palpitation, tachycardia, tremor

Drug Interactions

Metabolism/Transport Effects None known.

Avoid Concomitant Use

Avoid concomitant use of Thyroid, Desiccated with any of the following: Sodium Iodide I131

Increased Effect/Toxicity

Thyroid, Desiccated may increase the levels/effects of: Tricyclic Antidepressants; Vitamin K Antagonists

The levels/effects of Thyroid, Desiccated may be increased by: Piracetam

Decreased Effect

Thyroid, Desiccated may decrease the levels/effects of: Sodium Iodide I131; Theophylline Derivatives

The levels/effects of Thyroid, Desiccated may be decreased by: Bile Acid Sequestrants; Calcium Polystyrene Sulfonate; Calcium Salts; CarBAMazepine; Estrogen Derivatives; Fosphenytoin; Lanthanum; Phenytoin; Rifampin; Selective Serotonin Reuptake Inhibitors; Sodium Polystyrene Sulfonate

Stability Store at 15°C to 30°C (59°F to 86°F).

Mechanism of Action The primary active compound is T_3 (triiodothyronine), which may be converted from T_4 (thyroxine) and then circulates throughout the body to influence growth and maturation of various tissues; exact mechanism of action is unknown; however, it is believed the thyroid hormone exerts its many metabolic effects through control of DNA transcription and protein synthesis; involved in normal metabolism, growth, and development; promotes gluconeogenesis, increases utilization and mobilization of glycogen stores and stimulates protein synthesis, increases basal metabolic rate

Pharmacodynamics Onset of action: Liothyronine (T_3): ~3 hours

Pharmacokinetics (Adult data unless noted)

Absorption: T_4: 40% to 80%; T_3: 95%; desiccated thyroid contains T_4, T_3, and iodine (primarily bound)

Protein binding: T_4: >99% bound to plasma proteins including thyroxine-binding globulin, thyroxine-binding prealbumin, and albumin

Metabolism: Hepatic to triiodothyronine (active); ~80% T_4 deiodinated in kidney and periphery; glucuronidation/conjugation also occurs; undergoes enterohepatic recirculation

Half-life elimination, serum:

T_4: Euthyroid: 6-7 days; Hyperthyroid: 3-4 days; Hypothyroid: 9-10 days

T_3: 2.5 days

Time to peak serum concentration: T_4: 2-4 hours; T_3: 2-3 days

Elimination: Urine (major route of elimination); partially feces

Dosing: Neonatal Note: Doses presented as mg/kg/dose or mg/dose; closely review dosing units; adjust dose based upon clinical response and laboratory parameters

Congenital hypothyroidism: Oral: 4.8-6 mg/kg/dose or 15-30 mg/dose once daily. **Note:** AAP recommends levothyroxine as the preferred treatment for hypothyroidism in neonates (AAP, 2006). Neonates should have therapy initiated at full doses.

Dosing: Usual

Infants, Children, and Adolescents: **Note:** Doses presented as mg/kg/dose or mg/dose; closely review dosing units; adjust dose based upon clinical response and laboratory parameters.

Congenital Hypothyroidism: Note: Infants should have therapy initiated at full doses; Oral:

Infants 1–6 months: 4.8-6 mg/kg/dose or 15-30 mg/dose once daily

Infants >6-12 months: 3.6-4.8 mg/kg/dose or 30-45 mg/dose once daily

Children 1-5 years: 3-3.6 mg/kg/dose or 45-60 mg/dose once daily

Children 6-12 years: 2.4-3 mg/kg/dose or 60-90 mg/dose once daily

Adolescents: Typical doses >1.2-1.8 mg/kg/dose or 90 mg/dose once daily

Adults: **Note:** The American Association of Clinical Endocrinologists does not recommend the use of desiccated thyroid for thyroid replacement therapy for hypothyroidism (Baskin, 2002).

Hypothyroidism: Oral: Initial: 15-30 mg; increase with 15 mg increments every 2-3 weeks; use 15 mg in patients with cardiovascular disease or long-standing myxedema. Maintenance dose: Usually 60-120 mg/day; monitor TSH and clinical symptoms.

Administration Oral: Administer on an empty stomach in the morning before breakfast.

Monitoring Parameters T_4, TSH, heart rate, blood pressure, clinical signs of hypo- and hyperthyroidism; growth, bone development (children); TSH is the most reliable guide for evaluating adequacy of thyroid replacement dosage. TSH may be elevated during the first few months of thyroid replacement despite patients being clinically euthyroid. In cases where T_4 remains low and TSH is within normal limits, an evaluation of "free" (unbound) T_4 is needed to evaluate further increase in dosage.

In congenital hypothyroidism, adequacy of replacement should be determined using both TSH and total- or free-T_4. During the first 3 years of life, total- or free-T_4 should be maintained in the upper 1/2 of the normal range; this should result in normalization of the TSH. In some patients, TSH may not normalize due to a resetting of the pituitary-thyroid feedback as a result of *in utero* hypothyroidism. Monitor closely for cardiac overload, arrhythmias and aspiration from avid suckling.

Pediatric patients: Monitor closely for under/overtreatment. Undertreatment may decrease intellectual development and linear growth, and lead to poor school performance due to impaired concentration and slowed mentation. Overtreatment may adversely affect brain maturation, accelerate bone age (leading to premature closure of the epiphyses and reduced adult height); craniosynostosis has been reported in infants. Perform routine clinical examinations at regular intervals (to assess mental and physical growth and development). Suggested frequency for monitoring thyroid function tests: Every 1-2 months during the first year of life, every 2-3 months between ages 1-3 years, and every 3-12 months thereafter until growth is completed; repeat tests 2 weeks after any change in dosage.

Reference Range

Thyroid Function Tests

Lab Parameters	Age	Normal Range
T_4 (thyroxine) serum concentration	1-7 days	10.1-20.9 mcg/dL
	8-14 days	9.8-16.6 mcg/dL
	1 month to 1 year	5.5-16.0 mcg/dL
	>1 year	4.0-12.0 mcg/dL
Free thyroxine index (FTI)	1-3 days	9.3-26.6
	1-4 weeks	7.6-20.8
	1-4 months	7.4-17.9
	4-12 months	5.1-14.5
	1-6 years	5.7-13.3
	>6 years	4.8-14.0
T_3 serum concentration	Newborns	100-470 ng/dL
	1-5 years	100-260 ng/dL
	5-10 years	90-240 ng/dL
	10 years to Adult	70-210 ng/dL
T_3 uptake		35%-45%
TSH serum concentration	Cord	3-22 micro international units/mL
	1-3 days	<40 micro international units/mL
	3-7 days	<25 micro international units/mL
	>7 days	0-10 micro international units/mL

Additional Information Equivalent doses: The following statement on relative potency of thyroid products is included in a joint statement by American Thyroid Association (ATA), American Association of Clinical Endocrinologists (AACE) and The Endocrine Society (TES): For purposes of conversion, levothyroxine sodium (T_4) 100 mcg is usually considered equivalent to desiccated thyroid 60 mg, thyroglobulin 60 mg, or liothyronine sodium (T_3) 25 mcg. However, these are rough guidelines only and do not obviate the careful re-evaluation of a patient when switching thyroid hormone preparations, including a change from one brand of levothyroxine to another. Joint position statement is available at http://www.thyroid.org/professionals/advocacy/04_12_08_thyroxine.html.

Dosage Forms Excipient information presented when available (limited, particularly for generics); consult specific product labeling. [DSC] = Discontinued product
Tablet, Oral:
Armour Thyroid: 15 mg, 30 mg, 60 mg, 90 mg, 120 mg
Armour Thyroid: 180 mg [scored]
Armour Thyroid: 240 mg
Armour Thyroid: 300 mg [scored]
Nature-Throid: 16.25 mg, 32.5 mg
Nature-Throid: 48.75 mg, 65 mg, 81.25 mg, 97.5 mg, 113.75 mg, 130 mg, 146.25 mg, 162.5 mg, 195 mg, 260 mg, 325 mg [scored]
NP Thyroid: 30 mg, 60 mg, 90 mg
Westhroid: 16.25 mg, 32.5 mg
Westhroid: 48.75 mg, 65 mg [scored]
Westhroid: 81.25 mg
Westhroid: 97.5 mg, 113.75 mg, 130 mg, 146.25 mg, 162.5 mg, 195 mg, 260 mg, 325 mg [scored]
Westhroid-P: 16.25 mg [DSC], 32.5 mg [DSC]
Westhroid-P: 48.75 mg [DSC], 65 mg [DSC], 97.5 mg [DSC], 130 mg [DSC] [scored]
WP Thyroid: 16.25 mg, 32.5 mg
WP Thyroid: 48.75 mg, 65 mg [scored]
WP Thyroid: 81.25 mg
WP Thyroid: 97.5 mg, 113.75 mg, 130 mg [scored]

References
American Academy of Pediatrics, Rose SR, Section on Endocrinology and Committee on Genetics, American Thyroid Association, et al, "Update of Newborn Screening and Therapy for Congenital Hypothyroidism," *Pediatrics*, 2006, 117(6):2290-303.
Baskin HJ, Cobin RH, Duick DS, et al, "American Association of Clinical Endocrinologists Medical Guidelines for Clinical Practice for the Evaluation and Treatment of Hyperthyroidism and Hypothyroidism," *Endocr Pract*, 2002, 8(6):457-69.
Bhasin S, Wallace W, Lawrence JB, et al, "Sudden Death Associated With Thyroid Hormone Abuse," *Am J Med*, 1981, 71(5):887-90.

◆ **Thyroid Extract** see Thyroid, Desiccated on page 2018
◆ **Thyroid USP** see Thyroid, Desiccated on page 2018
◆ **Thyrolar®** see Liotrix on page 1258
◆ **ThyroShield [OTC]** see Potassium Iodide on page 1711

TiaGABine (tye AG a been)

Medication Safety Issues
Sound-alike/look-alike issues:
TiaGABine may be confused with tiZANidine
Brand Names: U.S. Gabitril
Therapeutic Category Anticonvulsant, Miscellaneous
Generic Availability (U.S.) Yes
Use Adjunctive therapy in the treatment of partial seizures (FDA approved in ages ≥12 years and adults)
Medication Guide Available Yes
Pregnancy Risk Factor C
Pregnancy Considerations Adverse events were observed in animal reproduction studies. Patients exposed to tiagabine during pregnancy are encouraged to enroll themselves into the AED Pregnancy Registry by calling 1-888-233-2334. Additional information is available at www.aedpregnancyregistry.org.
Breast-Feeding Considerations Levels of excretion of tiagabine and/or its metabolites in human milk have not been determined and effects on the nursing infant are unknown. According to the manufacturer, the decision to continue or discontinue breast-feeding during therapy should take into account the risk of exposure to the infant and the benefits of treatment to the mother.
Contraindications Hypersensitivity to tiagabine or any component
Warnings Current tiagabine dosing recommendations are based on studies in which most patients also received enzyme-inducing AEDs. Use of recommended tiagabine doses in patients **not** receiving enzyme-inducing AEDs may result in serum concentrations more than twice that of patients receiving enzyme-inducing AEDs. Use with caution and decrease the dose in patients who are **not** receiving enzyme-inducing AEDs; a slower titration of the drug may also be required in these patients.

New-onset seizures and status epilepticus have been reported with tiagabine use (for unlabeled indications) in patients without epilepsy. Higher doses may be a risk factor, but seizures have occurred in patients taking doses as low as 4 mg/day. Seizures have also occurred shortly after a dosage increase. In most cases, patients were also receiving concomitant medications that are thought to lower the seizure threshold (eg, antidepressants, antipsychotics, stimulants, opioids). Discontinue tiagabine and evaluate patients for an underlying seizure disorder in nonepileptic patients who develop seizures while receiving tiagabine.

When used to treat epilepsy, do not abruptly discontinue therapy; withdraw gradually to lessen chance for increased seizure frequency (unless a more rapid withdrawal is required due to safety concerns). Cognitive and neuropsychiatric adverse effects may occur. Exacerbation of

EEG abnormalities associated with CNS adverse events (cognitive and neuropsychiatric) may occur in patients with an EEG history of spike and wave discharges and may require dosage adjustment. Nonconvulsant status epilepticus has also been reported and may respond to dosage reduction or discontinuation. Seizures and status epilepticus may also occur with tiagabine overdose.

Antiepileptic drugs (AEDs) increase the risk of suicidal behavior and ideation in patients receiving these medications for any indication. Pooled analyses of placebo-controlled trials involving 11 different AEDs (regardless of indication) showed a twofold increased risk of suicidal thoughts or behavior (estimated incidence rate: 0.43% in AED treated patients compared to 0.24% of patients receiving placebo); increased risk was observed as early as 1 week after initiation of AED and continued through duration of trials (most trials ≤24 weeks); risk did not vary significantly by age (age range: 5–100 years). Consider risks and benefits of AEDs before prescribing. Monitor all patients receiving an AED for emergence of suicidal thoughts or behavior, thoughts of self-harm, any unusual changes in behavior or mood, or the emergence or worsening of depressive symptoms; notify healthcare provider immediately if symptoms or concerning behavior occur. **Note:** The FDA is requiring that a Medication Guide be developed for all antiepileptic drugs informing patients of this risk.

Precautions Use with caution in patients with hepatic impairment. Possible long-term ophthalmologic effects exist (more studies are needed). Use with caution with alcohol or other CNS depressants. Safety and effectiveness have not been established in children <12 years of age or for any indication other than as adjunctive therapy for partial seizures.

Adverse Reactions

Cardiovascular: Chest pain, edema, hypertension, palpitation, peripheral edema, syncope, tachycardia, vasodilation

Central nervous system: Agitation, ataxia, chills, concentration decreased, confusion, confusion, depersonalization, depression, difficulty with memory, dizziness, euphoria, hallucination, hostility, insomnia, malaise, migraine, nervousness, paranoid reaction, personality disorder, somnolence, speech disorder

Dermatologic: Alopecia, bruising, dry skin, pruritus, rash

Gastrointestinal: Abdominal pain, diarrhea, gingivitis, increased appetite, mouth ulceration, nausea, stomatitis, vomiting, weight gain/loss

Neuromuscular & skeletal: Abnormal gait, arthralgia, dysarthria, hyper-/hypokinesia, hyper-/hypotonia, myasthenia, myalgia, myoclonus, neck pain, paresthesia, reflexes decreased, stupor, tremor, twitching, vertigo, weakness

Ocular: Abnormal vision, amblyopia, nystagmus

Otic: Ear pain, hearing impairment, otitis media, tinnitus

Respiratory: Bronchitis, cough, dyspnea, epistaxis, pneumonia

Miscellaneous: Allergic reaction, cyst, diaphoresis, flu-like syndrome, lymphadenopathy

Rare but important or life-threatening: Abortion, abscess, anemia, angina, apnea, asthma, blepharitis, blindness, cellulitis, cerebral ischemia, cholelithiasis, CNS neoplasm, coma, deafness, dehydration, dysphagia, dystonia, electrocardiogram abnormal, encephalopathy, hemorrhage, erythrocytes abnormal, fecal incontinence, herpes simplex/zoster, glossitis, goiter, hematuria, hemoptysis, hepatomegaly, hypercholesteremia, hyper-/hypoglycemia, hyperlipemia, hypokalemia, hyponatremia, hypotension, hypothyroidism, impotence, kidney failure, leukopenia, liver function tests abnormal, MI, neoplasm, peripheral vascular disorder, paralysis, photophobia, psychosis, petechia, photosensitivity, seizure

(when used for unlabeled uses), sepsis, spasm, suicide attempt, thrombocytopenia, thrombophlebitis, urinary retention, urinary urgency, urticaria, visual field defect

Drug Interactions

Metabolism/Transport Effects Substrate of CYP3A4 (major); **Note:** Assignment of Major/Minor substrate status based on clinically relevant drug interaction potential

Avoid Concomitant Use

Avoid concomitant use of TiaGABine with any of the following: Azelastine (Nasal); Conivaptan; Fusidic Acid (Systemic); Paraldehyde; Thalidomide

Increased Effect/Toxicity

TiaGABine may increase the levels/effects of: Alcohol (Ethyl); Azelastine (Nasal); Buprenorphine; CNS Depressants; Hydrocodone; Methotrimeprazine; Metyrosine; Mirtazapine; Paraldehyde; Pramipexole; ROPINIRole; Rotigotine; Selective Serotonin Reuptake Inhibitors; Thalidomide; Zolpidem

The levels/effects of TiaGABine may be increased by: Brimonidine (Topical); Cannabis; Ceritinib; Conivaptan; CYP3A4 Inhibitors (Moderate); CYP3A4 Inhibitors (Strong); Dasatinib; Doxylamine; Droperidol; Fusidic Acid (Systemic); HydrOXYzine; Ivacaftor; Kava Kava; Luliconazole; Magnesium Sulfate; Methotrimeprazine; Mifepristone; Nabilone; Perampanel; Rufinamide; Simeprevir; Sodium Oxybate; Stiripentol; Tapentadol; Tetrahydrocannabinol

Decreased Effect

The levels/effects of TiaGABine may be decreased by: Bosentan; CYP3A4 Inducers (Strong); Dabrafenib; Deferasirox; Ketorolac (Nasal); Ketorolac (Systemic); Mefloquine; Mitotane; Orlistat; Siltuximab; St Johns Wort; Tocilizumab

Food Interactions Food reduces the rate but not the extent of absorption. Management: Administer with food.

Stability Protect from moisture and light; store at room temperature

Mechanism of Action The exact mechanism by which tiagabine exerts antiseizure activity is not definitively known; however, *in vitro* experiments demonstrate that it enhances the activity of gamma aminobutyric acid (GABA), the major neuroinhibitory transmitter in the nervous system; it is thought that binding to the GABA uptake carrier inhibits the uptake of GABA into presynaptic neurons, allowing an increased amount of GABA to be available to postsynaptic neurons; based on *in vitro* studies, tiagabine does not inhibit the uptake of dopamine, norepinephrine, serotonin, glutamate, or choline

Pharmacokinetics (Adult data unless noted)

Absorption: Rapid and nearly complete (>95%)

Distribution: Mean V_d:

Children 3-10 years: 2.4 L/kg

Adults: 1.3-1.6 L/kg

Note: V_d values are more similar between children and adults when expressed as L/m^2 (Gustavson, 1997)

Protein binding: 96%, mainly to albumin and alpha$_1$-acid glycoprotein

Metabolism: Extensive in the liver via oxidation and glucuronidation; undergoes enterohepatic recirculation

Bioavailability: Oral: 90%

Diurnal effect: Trough concentrations and AUC are lower in the evening versus morning

Half-life:

Children 3-10 years: Mean: 5.7 hours (range: 2-10 hours)

Children 3-10 years receiving enzyme-inducing AEDs: Mean: 3.2 hours (range: 2-7.8 hours)

Adults (normal volunteers): 7-9 hours

Adult patients receiving enzyme-inducing AEDs: 2-5 hours

Time to peak serum concentration: Fasting state: ~45 minutes

Elimination: ~2% excreted unchanged in urine; 25% excreted in urine and 63% excreted in feces as metabolites

Clearance:
Children 3-10 years: 4.2 ± 1.6 mL/minute/kg
Children 3-10 years receiving enzyme-inducing AEDs: 8.6 ± 3.3 mL/minute/kg
Adults (normal volunteers): 109 mL/minute
Adult patients: 1.9 ± 0.5 mL/minute/kg
Adult patients receiving enzyme-inducing AEDs: 6.3 ± 3.5 mL/minute/kg
Note: Clearance values are more similar between children and adults when expressed as mL/minute/m^2 (Gustavson, 1997)
Hepatic impairment: Clearance of unbound drug is decreased by 60%

Dosing: Usual Oral: **Note:** Doses were determined in patients receiving enzyme-inducing AEDs; use of these doses in patients **not** receiving enzyme-inducing AEDs may result in serum concentrations more than twice those of patients receiving enzyme-inducing AEDS; **lower doses are required in patients not receiving enzyme-inducing agents;** a slower titration may also be necessary in these patients. Consider tiagabine dosage adjustment if enzyme-inducing agent is added, discontinued, or dose is changed. Do **not** use loading doses of tiagabine in any patient; do **not** use a rapid dosage escalation or increase the dose in large increments.

Children <12 years: Only limited preliminary information is available; dosing guidelines are not established (Adkins, 1998; Pellock, 1999)

Children 12-18 years: Initial: 4 mg once daily for 1 week, then 8 mg/day given in 2 divided doses for 1 week, then increase weekly by 4-8 mg/day; administer in 2-4 divided doses per day; titrate dose to response; maximum dose: 32 mg/day (doses >32 mg/day have been used in select adolescent patients for short periods of time)

Adults: Initial: 4 mg once daily for 1 week, then increase weekly by 4-8 mg/day; administer in 2-4 divided doses per day; titrate dose to response; usual maintenance: 32-56 mg/day in 2-4 divided doses; maximum dose: 56 mg/day. **Note:** Twice daily dosing may not be well tolerated and dosing 3 times/day is the currently favored dosing frequency (Kalviainen, 1998).

Dosing adjustment in renal impairment: None needed

Dosing adjustment in hepatic impairment: Reduced doses and longer dosing intervals may be required

Administration Oral: Administer with food (to avoid rapid increase in plasma concentrations and adverse CNS effects)

Monitoring Parameters Seizure frequency, duration, and severity; signs and symptoms of suicidality (eg, anxiety, depression, behavior changes)

Reference Range Not established

Additional Information Population pharmacokinetic analysis suggests that tiagabine may be administered at similar doses without adjustment for age, gender, or body weight in epilepsy patients ≥11 years of age (Samara, 1998)

Dosage Forms Excipient information presented when available (limited, particularly for generics); consult specific product labeling.
Tablet, Oral, as hydrochloride:
Gabitril: 2 mg [contains fd&c yellow #6 (sunset yellow)]
Gabitril: 4 mg [contains fd&c yellow #10 (quinoline yellow)]
Gabitril: 12 mg [contains brilliant blue fcf (fd&c blue #1), fd&c yellow #10 (quinoline yellow)]
Gabitril: 16 mg [contains fd&c blue #2 (indigotine)]
Generic: 2 mg, 4 mg

Extemporaneous Preparations A 1 mg/mL tiagabine hydrochloride oral suspension may be made with tablets and a 1:1 mixture of Ora-Sweet® and Ora-Plus®. Crush ten 12 mg tablets in a mortar and reduce to a fine powder.

Add small portions of the vehicle and mix to a uniform paste; mix while adding the vehicle in incremental proportions to **almost** 120 mL; transfer to a graduated cylinder; rinse mortar with vehicle, and add quantity of vehicle sufficient to make 120 mL. Label "shake well" and "refrigerate". Store in amber plastic prescription bottles; stable for 70 days at room temperature or 91 days refrigerated (preferred).

A 1 mg/mL oral suspension may be made with tablets and a 6:1 mixture of simple syrup, NF and methylcellulose 1%. Crush ten 12 mg tablets in a mortar and reduce to a fine powder. Add 17 mL of methylcellulose 1% gel and mix to a uniform paste; mix while adding simple syrup, NF in incremental proportions to **almost** 120 mL; transfer to a graduated cylinder, rinse mortar with syrup, and add quantity of syrup sufficient to make 120 mL. Label "shake well" and "refrigerate". Store in amber plastic prescription bottles; stable for 42 days at room temperature or 91 days refrigerated (preferred).

Nahata MC, Pai VB, and Hipple TF, *Pediatric Drug Formulations*, 5th ed, Cincinnati, OH: Harvey Whitney Books Co, 2004.

References

Adkins JC and Noble S, "Tiagabine. A Review of Its Pharmacodynamic and Pharmacokinetic Properties and Therapeutic Potential in the Management of Epilepsy," *Drugs*, 1998, 55(3):437-60.

Gustavson LE, Boellner SW, Granneman GR, et al, "A Single-Dose Study to Define Tiagabine Pharmacokinetics in Pediatric Patients With Complex Partial Seizures," *Neurology*, 1997, 48(4):1032-7.

Kalviainen R, Brodie MJ, Duncan J, et al, "A Double-Blind, Placebo-Controlled Trial of Tiagabine Given Three-Times Daily as Add-On Therapy for Refractory Partial Seizures. Northern European Tiagabine Study Group," *Epilepsy Res*, 1998, 30(1):31-40.

Leach JP and Brodie MJ, "Tiagabine," *Lancet*, 1998, 351(9097):203-7.

Pellock JM, "Managing Pediatric Epilepsy Syndromes With New Antiepileptic Drugs," *Pediatrics*, 1999, 104(5 Pt 1):1106-16.

Samara EE, Gustavson LE, El-Shourbagy T, et al, "Population Analysis of the Pharmacokinetics of Tiagabine in Patients With Epilepsy," *Epilepsy*, 1998, 39(8):868-73.

◆ **Tiagabine Hydrochloride** see TiaGABine on page 2020
◆ **Tiamol® (Can)** see Fluocinonide on page 894
◆ **Tiazac** see Diltiazem on page 667
◆ **Tiazac XC (Can)** see Diltiazem on page 667

Ticarcillin and Clavulanate Potassium
(tye kar SIL in & klav yoo LAN ate poe TASS ee um)

Brand Names: U.S. Timentin
Brand Names: Canada Timentin
Therapeutic Category Antibiotic, Beta-lactam and Beta-lactamase Combination; Antibiotic, Penicillin (Antipseudomonal)
Generic Availability (U.S.) No
Use Treatment of infections caused by susceptible organisms involving the lower respiratory tract, urinary tract, skin and skin structures, bone and joint, gynecologic, intra-abdominal infections, and septicemia (FDA approved in ages ≥3 months and adults). Clavulanate expands activity of ticarcillin to include beta-lactamase producing strains of *S. aureus, H. influenzae, Moraxella catarrhalis, B. fragilis, Klebsiella, Prevotella, P. aeruginosa, Stenotrophomonas maltophilia, E. coli,* and *Proteus* species
Pregnancy Risk Factor B
Pregnancy Considerations Adverse events were not observed in animal reproduction studies. Ticarcillin and clavulanate cross the placenta (Maberry, 1992). Maternal use of penicillins has generally not resulted in an increased risk of adverse fetal effects (Crider, 2009; Santos, 2011). Ticarcillin/clavulanate is approved for the treatment of postpartum gynecologic infections, including endometritis, caused by susceptible organisms.
Breast-Feeding Considerations Small amounts of ticarcillin are found in breast milk (Matsuda, 1984; von Kobyletzki, 1983); however, it is not orally absorbed (Brogden,

1980). The manufacturer recommends that caution be exercised when administering ticarcillin/clavulanate to nursing women.

Contraindications Hypersensitivity to ticarcillin, clavulanate, any of the penicillins, cephalosporins, or any component

Warnings Serious and occasionally fatal hypersensitivity (anaphylactoid) reactions have been reported in patients receiving ticarcillin/clavulanate therapy, especially with a history of beta-lactam hypersensitivity, history of sensitivity to multiple allergens, or previous IgE-mediated reactions (eg, anaphylaxis, angioedema, urticaria); administration to patients with confirmed penicillin or cephalosporin allergies should be avoided; immediate treatment for anaphylactic reaction should be available during administration. Seizures, abnormal platelet aggregation, and prolonged bleeding have been reported in patients with renal impairment receiving high doses. Prolonged use may result in fungal or bacterial superinfection, including *C. difficile*-associated diarrhea (CDAD) and pseudomembranous colitis; CDAD has been observed >2 months postantibiotic treatment.

Precautions Use with caution and modify dosage in patients with renal impairment; use with caution in patients with heart failure due to high sodium content of the formulation and in patients with preexisting seizure disorder. Use an alternative agent in patients with meningeal seeding from a distant infection site, in whom meningitis is suspected or documented, or in patients who require prophylaxis against central nervous system infection.

Adverse Reactions

Central nervous system: Confusion, drowsiness, fever, headache, Jarisch-Herxheimer reaction, seizure

Dermatologic: Erythema multiforme, pruritus, rash, Stevens-Johnson syndrome, toxic epidermal necrolysis, urticaria

Endocrine & metabolic: Electrolyte imbalance

Gastrointestinal: *Clostridium difficile* colitis, diarrhea, nausea, vomiting

Hematologic: Bleeding, eosinophilia, hemolytic anemia, leukopenia, neutropenia, positive Coombs' reaction, prothrombin time prolonged, thrombocytopenia

Hepatic: Hepatotoxicity, jaundice

Local: Injection site reaction (pain, burning, induration); thrombophlebitis

Neuromuscular & skeletal: Myoclonus

Renal: BUN increased, interstitial nephritis (acute), serum creatinine increased

Miscellaneous: Anaphylaxis, hypersensitivity reactions

Drug Interactions

Metabolism/Transport Effects None known.

Avoid Concomitant Use

Avoid concomitant use of Ticarcillin and Clavulanate Potassium with any of the following: BCG; Probenecid

Increased Effect/Toxicity

Ticarcillin and Clavulanate Potassium may increase the levels/effects of: Methotrexate; Vitamin K Antagonists

The levels/effects of Ticarcillin and Clavulanate Potassium may be increased by: Probenecid

Decreased Effect

Ticarcillin and Clavulanate Potassium may decrease the levels/effects of: Aminoglycosides; BCG; Mycophenolate; Sodium Picosulfate; Typhoid Vaccine

The levels/effects of Ticarcillin and Clavulanate Potassium may be decreased by: Tetracycline Derivatives

Stability Parenteral:

Injection, powder for reconstitution: Store intact vials at or below 24°C (75°F). Reconstituted 200 mg/mL solution is stable for 6 hours at room temperature and 72 hours when refrigerated; when further diluted in D_5W or NS to 10-100 mg/mL is stable for 24 hours at room temperature. Solution diluted in D_5W is stable 3 days if refrigerated; solution diluted in NS is stable 7 days if refrigerated; darkening of drug indicates loss of potency of clavulanate potassium.

Premixed solution: Store at or below -20°C (-4°F); thawed solution is stable for 24 hours at 22°C (77°F) or 7 days at 4°C (39°F); do not refreeze.

Mechanism of Action Inhibits bacterial cell wall synthesis by binding to one or more of the penicillin-binding proteins (PBPs), which in turn inhibits the final transpeptidation step of peptidoglycan synthesis in bacterial cell walls, thus inhibiting cell wall biosynthesis. Bacteria eventually lyse due to ongoing activity of cell wall autolytic enzymes (autolysins and murein hydrolases) while cell wall assembly is arrested.

Pharmacokinetics (Adult data unless noted)

Distribution: Ticarcillin is distributed into tissue, interstitial fluid, pleural fluid, and bile; low concentrations of ticarcillin distribute into the CSF but increase when meninges are inflamed

V_{dss} ticarcillin: 0.22 L/kg

V_{dss} clavulanic acid: 0.4 L/kg

Protein binding:

Ticarcillin: 45%

Clavulanic acid: 25%

Metabolism: Clavulanic acid is metabolized hepatically

Half-life: In patients with normal renal function

Neonates:

Clavulanic acid: 1.9 hours

Ticarcillin: 4.4 hours

Children (1 month to 9.3 years):

Clavulanic acid: 54 minutes

Ticarcillin: 66 minutes

Adults:

Clavulanic acid: 66-90 minutes

Ticarcillin: 66-72 minutes; 13 hours (in patients with renal failure)

Clavulanic acid does not affect the clearance of ticarcillin

Elimination:

Children: 71% of the ticarcillin and 50% of the clavulanic acid dose are excreted unchanged in the urine over 4 hours

Adults: Ticarcillin: Urine (60% to 70% as unchanged drug); Clavulanic acid: Urine (35% to 45% as unchanged drug)

Dialysis: Removed by hemodialysis

Dosing: Neonatal I.V.: **Note:** Timentin® (ticarcillin/clavulanate) is a combination product; each 3.1 g contains 3 g ticarcillin disodium and 0.1 g clavulanic acid. Dosage recommendations are based on **ticarcillin** component:

General dosing, susceptible infection (*Red Book*, 2012): I.V.:

Body weight <1 kg:

PNA ≤14 days: 75 mg ticarcillin/kg/dose every 12 hours

PNA 15-28 days: 75 mg ticarcillin/kg/dose every 8 hours

Body weight ≥1 kg:

PNA ≤7 days: 75 mg ticarcillin/kg/dose every 12 hours

PNA 8-28 days: 75 mg ticarcillin/kg/dose every 8 hours

Dosing: Usual

Infants, Children, and Adolescents: **Note:** Timentin® (ticarcillin/clavulanate) is a combination product; each 3.1 g contains 3 g ticarcillin disodium and 0.1 g clavulanic acid. Dosage recommendations are based on **ticarcillin** component:

General dosing, susceptible infection: I.V.:

Mild to moderate infections: 200 mg ticarcillin/kg/day in divided doses every 6 hours; maximum daily dose: 12 g ticarcillin/**day**

Severe infections:

Manufacturer's labeling: 300 mg ticarcillin/kg/day in divided doses every 4 hours

AAP recommendations: 200-300 mg ticarcillin/kg/day in divided doses every 4-6 hours

Maximum daily dose: 18 **g** ticarcillin/**day**

Cystic fibrosis: I.V.: 400 mg ticarcillin/kg/day in divided doses every 6 hours; higher doses have been used: 400-750 mg ticarcillin/kg/day in divided doses every 6 hours (Zobell, 2013)

Adults:

Systemic infections: I.V.: 3.1 **g** (ticarcillin 3000 mg plus clavulanic acid 100 mg) every 4-6 hours (maximum: 24 g of ticarcillin/day)

Amnionitis, cholangitis, diverticulitis, endometritis, epididymo-orchitis, mastoiditis, orbital cellulitis, peritonitis, pneumonia (aspiration): I.V.: 3.1 **g** (ticarcillin 3000 mg plus clavulanic acid 100 mg) every 6 hours

Intra-abdominal infection, complicated, community-acquired, mild to moderate: I.V.: 3.1 **g** (ticarcillin 3000 mg plus clavulanic acid 100 mg) every 6 hours for 4-7 days (provided source controlled)

Liver abscess, parafascial space infections, septic thrombophlebitis: I.V.: 3.1 **g** (ticarcillin 3000 mg plus clavulanic acid 100 mg) every 4 hours

***Pseudomonas* infections:** I.V.: 3.1 **g** (ticarcillin 3000 mg plus clavulanic acid 100 mg) every 4 hours

Urinary tract infections: I.V.: 3.1 **g** (ticarcillin 3000 mg plus clavulanic acid 100 mg) every 6-8 hours

Dosing adjustment in renal impairment: Note: Dosage recommendations are based on **ticarcillin** component:

Infants, Children, and Adolescents: There are no dosage adjustments provided in the manufacturer's labeling; however, the following have been used by some clinicians (Aronoff, 2007): Dosing based on a usual dose of 200-300 ticarcillin mg/kg/day in divided doses every 6 hours.

GFR >30 mL/minute/1.73 m^2: No adjustment required.

GFR 10-29 mL/minute/1.73 m^2: 50-75 mg ticarcillin/kg every 8 hours

GFR <10 mL/minute/1.73 m^2 (without concomitant hepatic failure): 50-75 mg ticarcillin/kg every 12 hours

GFR <10 mL/minute/1.73 m^2 (with concomitant hepatic failure): 50-75 mg ticarcillin/kg every 24 hours

Intermittent hemodialysis (without concomitant hepatic failure): 50-75 mg ticarcillin/kg every 12 hours

Intermittent hemodialysis (with concomitant hepatic failure): 50-75 mg ticarcillin/kg every 24 hours

Peritoneal dialysis (without concomitant hepatic failure): 50-75 mg ticarcillin/kg every 12 hours

Peritoneal dialysis (with concomitant hepatic failure): 50-75 mg ticarcillin/kg every 24 hours

Continuous renal replacement therapy (CRRT): 50-75 mg ticarcillin/kg every 8 hours

Adults:

CrCl >60 mL/minute: No dosage adjustment required.

CrCl 30-60 mL/minute: 2000 mg ticarcillin component every 4 hours or 3.1 **g** (3000 mg ticarcillin component) every 8 hours

CrCl 10-30 mL/minute: 2000 mg ticarcillin component every 8 hours or 3.1 **g** (3000 mg ticarcillin component) every 12 hours

CrCl <10 mL/minute without concomitant hepatic dysfunction: 2000 mg ticarcillin component every 12 hours

CrCl <10 mL/minute with concomitant hepatic dysfunction: 2000 mg ticarcillin component every 24 hours

Intermittent hemodialysis (IHD) (administer after hemodialysis on dialysis days): Dialyzable (20% to 50%): 2000 mg of ticarcillin component every 12 hours; supplemented with 3.1 **g** (3000 mg ticarcillin component) after each dialysis session. Alternatively, administer 2000 mg of ticarcillin component every 8 hours without a supplemental dose for deep-seated infections (Heintz, 2009). **Note:** Dosing dependent on the assumption of 3 times/week, complete IHD sessions.

Peritoneal dialysis (PD): 3.1 **g** (3000 mg ticarcillin component) every 12 hours

Continuous renal replacement therapy (CRRT) (Heintz, 2009; Trotman, 2005): Drug clearance is highly dependent on the method of renal replacement, filter type, and flow rate. Appropriate dosing requires close monitoring of pharmacologic response, signs of adverse reactions due to drug accumulation, as well as drug concentrations in relation to target trough (if appropriate). The following are general recommendations only (based on dialysate flow/ultrafiltration rates of 1-2 L/hour and minimal residual renal function) and should not supersede clinical judgment:

CVVH: Loading dose of 3.1 **g** (3000 mg ticarcillin component) followed by 2000 mg ticarcillin component every 6-8 hours

CVVHD: Loading dose of 3.1 **g** (3000 mg ticarcillin component) followed by 3.1 **g** (3000 mg ticarcillin component) every 6-8 hours

CVVHDF: Loading dose of 3.1 **g** (3000 mg ticarcillin component) followed by 3.1 **g** (3000 mg ticarcillin component) every 6 hours

Note: Do not administer in intervals exceeding every 8 hours. Clavulanate component is hepatically eliminated; extending the dosing interval beyond 8 hours may result in loss of beta-lactamase inhibition.

CVVH: Dose as for CrCl 10-50 mL/minute

Hemodialysis: 2 g every 12 hours; supplement with 3 g after each dialysis

Peritoneal Dialysis: 3 g every 12 hours

Dosing in hepatic impairment: Adults: With concomitant renal dysfunction (CrCl <10 mL/minute) 2000 mg ticarcillin component every 24 hours

Administration Parenteral: Administer by I.V. intermittent infusion over 30 minutes; final concentration for administration should not exceed 100 mg/mL of ticarcillin; however, concentrations ≤50 mg/mL are preferred. Some penicillins (eg, carbenicillin, ticarcillin, and piperacillin) have been shown to inactivate aminoglycosides *in vitro*. This has been observed to a greater extent with tobramycin and gentamicin, while amikacin has shown greater stability against inactivation. Concurrent use of these agents may pose a risk of reduced antibacterial efficacy *in vivo*, particularly in the setting of profound renal impairment. However, definitive clinical evidence is lacking. If combination penicillin/aminoglycoside therapy is desired in a patient with renal dysfunction, separation of doses (if feasible), and routine monitoring of aminoglycoside levels, CBC, and clinical response should be considered.

Monitoring Parameters Serum electrolytes, periodic renal, hepatic and hematologic function tests; observe I.V. injection site for signs of extravasation; observe for signs and symptoms of anaphylaxis during first dose

Test Interactions Positive Coombs' test, false-positive urinary proteins

Some penicillin derivatives may accelerate the degradation of aminoglycosides *in vitro*, leading to a potential underestimation of aminoglycoside serum concentration.

Dosage Forms Excipient information presented when available (limited, particularly for generics); consult specific product labeling.

Infusion [premixed, frozen]: Ticarcillin 3 g and clavulanic acid 0.1 g (100 mL) [contains sodium 4.51 mEq and potassium 0.15 mEq per g]

Injection, powder for reconstitution: Ticarcillin 3 g and clavulanic acid 0.1 g (3.1 g, 31 g) [contains sodium 4.51 mEq and potassium 0.15 mEq per g]

References

Aronoff GR, Bennett WM, Berns JS, et al, *Drug Prescribing in Renal Failure: Dosing Guidelines for Adults and Children*, 5th ed, Philadelphia, PA: American College of Physicians, 2007.

Begue P, Quiniou F, Quinet B, "Efficacy and Pharmacokinetics of Timentin® in Paediatric Infections," *J Antimicrob Chemother*, 1986, 17(Suppl C):81-91.

Fricke G, Doerck M, Hafner D, et al, "The Pharmacokinetics of Ticarcillin/Clavulanate Acid in Neonates," *J Antimicrob Chemother*, 1989, 24(Suppl B):111-20.

Heintz BH, Matzke GR, and Dager WE, "Antimicrobial Dosing Concepts and Recommendations for Critically Ill Adult Patients Receiving Continuous Renal Replacement Therapy or Intermittent Hemodialysis," *Pharmacotherapy*, 2009, 29(5):562-77.

Red Book: 2012 Report of the Committee on Infectious Diseases, 29th ed, Pickering LK, ed, Elk Grove Village, IL: American Academy of Pediatrics, 2012.

Reed MD, Yamashita TS, and Blumer JL, "Pharmacokinetic-Based Ticarcillin/Clavulanic Acid Dose Recommendations for Infants and Children," *J Clin Pharmacol*, 1995, 35(7):658-65.

Trotman RL, Williamson JC, Shoemaker DM, et al, "Antibiotic Dosing in Critically Ill Adult Patients Receiving Continuous Renal Replacement Therapy," *Clin Infect Dis*, 2005, 41(8):1159-66.

Zobell JT, Waters CD, Young DC, et al, "Optimization of Anti-pseudomonal Antibiotics for Cystic Fibrosis Pulmonary Exacerbations: II. Cephalosporins and Penicillins," *Pediatr Pulmonol*, 2013, 48 (2):107-22.

◆ **Ticarcillin and Clavulanic Acid** see Ticarcillin and Clavulanate Potassium *on page 2022*

◆ **TIG** see Tetanus Immune Globulin (Human) *on page 1991*

◆ **Tigan** see Trimethobenzamide *on page 2086*

Tigecycline (tye ge SYE kleen)

Brand Names: U.S. Tygacil
Brand Names: Canada Tygacil
Therapeutic Category Antibiotic, Glycylcycline
Generic Availability (U.S.) No

Use Treatment of complicated skin and skin structure infections, complicated intra-abdominal infections (eg, appendicitis, cholecystitis, peritonitis, liver abscess), and community-acquired bacterial pneumonia caused by susceptible organisms (FDA approved in ages ≥18 years and adults). **Note:** Not indicated for the treatment of diabetic foot infections nor hospital-acquired pneumonia (HAP), including ventilator-associated pneumonia (VAP). Subgroup of patients with ventilator-associated pneumonia who received tigecycline demonstrated inferior efficacy, including lower cure rates and increased mortality than the comparator group.

Pregnancy Risk Factor D

Pregnancy Considerations Because adverse effects were observed in animals and because of the potential for permanent tooth discoloration, tigecycline is classified pregnancy category D. Tigecycline frequently causes nausea and vomiting and, therefore, may not be ideal for use in a patient with pregnancy-related nausea.

Breast-Feeding Considerations It is not known if tigecycline is found in breast milk. The manufacturer recommends caution if giving tigecycline to a nursing woman. Nondose-related effects could include modification of bowel flora.

Contraindications Hypersensitivity to tigecycline or any component

Warnings All-cause mortality was higher in adult patients treated with tigecycline (4%) compared to those treated with comparator antibiotics (3%) in phase 3 and 4 clinical trials **[U.S. Boxed Warning]**; cause has not been established. In general, deaths were the result of worsening infection, complications of infection, or underlying comorbidity. Not indicated for the treatment of hospital-acquired pneumonia (HAP), including healthcare-associated pneumonia (HCAP) and ventilator-associated pneumonia (VAP). Tigecycline demonstrated inferior efficacy (versus a comparator antibiotic), including lower cure rates and increased mortality in the subgroup of patients with VAP (particularly those with VAP and concurrent bacteremia at baseline).

Life-threatening anaphylaxis/anaphylactoid reactions have been reported; use with caution in patients with prior tetracycline hypersensitivity and/or severe adverse reactions associated with tetracycline use. May cause fetal harm if used during pregnancy; patients should be advised of potential risks associated with use. Due to structural similarity with tetracyclines, permanent discoloration of teeth (brown-yellow-gray) may occur if used during tooth development (fetal stage through children up to 8 years of age). Cases of significant hepatic dysfunction and hepatic failure have been reported with tigecycline use; use with caution in patients with hepatic impairment; monitor patients for abnormal liver function tests; may need to modify dose with severe hepatic impairment. Use may be associated with photosensitivity, pseudotumor cerebri, pancreatitis (including fatalities), and antianabolic effects (including increased BUN, azotemia, acidosis, and hyperphosphatemia). Prolonged use may result in fungal or bacterial superinfection, including *C. difficile*-associated diarrhea (CDAD) or pseudomembranous colitis; CDAD has been observed >2 months postantibiotic treatment.

Precautions Use caution in patients with intestinal perforation (septic shock occurred more frequently than in patients treated with imipenem/cilastatin).

Adverse Reactions
Cardiovascular: Localized phlebitis
Central nervous system: Dizziness, headache
Dermatologic: Skin rash
Endocrine & metabolic: Hyponatremia, increased amylase
Gastrointestinal: Abdominal pain, diarrhea, dyspepsia, nausea, vomiting
Hematologic & oncologic: Anemia, hypoproteinemia
Hepatic: Hyperbilirubinemia, increased serum ALT, increased serum AST, increased serum alkaline phosphatase
Infection: Abscess, infection
Neuromuscular & skeletal: Weakness
Renal: Increased blood urea nitrogen
Respiratory: Pneumonia
Miscellaneous: Abnormal healing
Rare but important or life-threatening: Acute pancreatitis, allergic skin reaction, anaphylactoid reaction, anaphylaxis, anorexia, *Clostridium difficile* associated diarrhea, dysgeusia, eosinophilia, hepatic insufficiency, hepatic failure, hypocalcemia, hypoglycemia, increased INR, increased serum creatinine, increased serum transaminases, increased INR, increased serum creatinine, increased serum transaminases, prolonged partial thromboplastin time, prolonged prothrombin time, pruritus, septic shock, Stevens-Johnson syndrome, swelling at injection site, thrombocytopenia, thrombophlebitis, vaginal moniliasis, vaginitis

Drug Interactions
Metabolism/Transport Effects None known.
Avoid Concomitant Use There are no known interactions where it is recommended to avoid concomitant use.
Increased Effect/Toxicity
Tigecycline may increase the levels/effects of: Warfarin
Decreased Effect There are no known significant interactions involving a decrease in effect.

Stability Store intact vial at 20°C to 25°C (68°F to 77°F); excursions permitted to 15°C to 30°C (59°F to 86°F). Reconstituted solution may be stored at room temperature for up to 6 hours in the vial or up to 24 hours if further diluted in a compatible I.V. solution. Alternatively, may be stored refrigerated for up to 48 hours following immediate transfer of the reconstituted solution into NS or D_5W.

◀ Reconstituted solution is yellow-orange; discard if not yellow-orange.

Mechanism of Action A glycylcycline antibiotic that binds to the 30S ribosomal subunit of susceptible bacteria, thereby, inhibiting protein synthesis. Generally considered bacteriostatic; however, bactericidal activity has been demonstrated against isolates of *S. pneumoniae* and *L. pneumophila*. Tigecycline is a derivative of minocycline (9-t-butylglycylamido minocycline), and while not classified as a tetracycline, it may share some class-associated adverse effects. Tigecycline has demonstrated activity against a variety of gram-positive and -negative bacterial pathogens including methicillin-resistant staphylococci.

Pharmacokinetics (Adult data unless noted)
Distribution: Extensive tissue distribution; distributes into gallbladder, lung, and colon
V_d:
Children (8-11 years): 2.84 L/kg (range: 0.397-11.2 L/kg) (Purdy, 2012)
Adults: 7-9 L/kg
Protein binding: 71% to 89%
Metabolism: Hepatic (not extensively), via glucuronidation, N-acetylation, and epimerization to several metabolites, each <10% of the dose. Clearance is reduced by 55% and half-life increased by 43% in moderate hepatic impairment.
Half-life elimination: Single dose: 27 hours; Multiple doses: 42 hours
Elimination: 22% excreted in urine as unchanged drug; 59% in feces, primarily as unchanged drug

Dosing: Usual Note: Duration of therapy dependent on severity/site of infection and clinical status and response to therapy.
Children ≥8 years and Adolescents: Limited data available:
Note: Use should be reserved for situations when no effective alternative therapy is available; should not be used in pediatric patients <8 years due to adverse effects on tooth development.
General dosing, susceptible infection: I.V.: Dosing based on data from pharmacokinetic trials.
Children 8-11 years: 1.2 mg/kg/dose every 12 hours; maximum single dose: 50 mg
Children ≥12 years and Adolescents: 50 mg every 12 hours
Adults:
Intra-abdominal infection, complicated: I.V.: 100 mg as a single dose, then 50 mg every 12 hours for 5-14 days. **Note:** 2010 IDSA guidelines recommend a treatment duration of 4-7 days (provided source controlled) for community-acquired, mild to moderate infection (Solomkin, 2010).
Skin and skin structure infection, complicated: I.V.: 100 mg as a single dose, then 50 mg every 12 hours for 5-14 days
Pneumonia, community-acquired: I.V.: 100 mg as a single dose, then 50 mg every 12 hours for 7-14 days
Dosing adjustment in renal impairment: Not dialyzable; no dosage adjustment necessary.
Dosing adjustment in hepatic impairment:
Mild to moderate impairment (Child-Pugh class A or B): No dosage adjustment needed.
Severe impairment (Child-Pugh class C): Adults: 100 mg as a single dose, then 25 mg every 12 hours
Administration Reconstitute by adding 5.3 mL NS, D_5W, or LR to each 50 mg vial; swirl gently to dissolve; resulting solution is 10 mg/mL and should be yellow-orange in color; discard if it is not. Further dilute to a concentration not to exceed 1 mg/mL and infuse over 30-60 minutes.
Monitoring Parameters Periodic hepatic function tests; resolution of infection; observe patient for diarrhea
Dosage Forms Excipient information presented when available (limited, particularly for generics); consult specific product labeling.

Solution Reconstituted, Intravenous:
Tygacil: 50 mg (1 ea)

References
Purdy J, Jouve S, Yan JL, et al. Pharmacokinetics and safety profile of tigecycline in children aged 8 to 11 years with selected serious infections: a multicenter, open-label, ascending-dose study. *Clinical Therapeutics*. 2012;34(2): 496-507.
Solomkin JS, Mazuski JE, Bradley JS, et al. Diagnosis and management of complicated intra-abdominal infections in adults and children: guidelines by the Surgical Infection Society and the Infectious Diseases Society of America. *Clin Infect Dis*. 2010;50(2):133-164.

◆ **Tim-AK (Can)** *see* Timolol (Ophthalmic) *on page 2028*
◆ **Timentin** *see* Ticarcillin and Clavulanate Potassium *on page 2022*

Timolol (Systemic) (TIM oh lol)

Medication Safety Issues
Sound-alike/look-alike issues:
Timolol may be confused with atenolol, Tylenol®
Brand Names: Canada Apo-Timol®; Nu-Timolol; Teva-Timolol
Therapeutic Category Antihypertensive Agent; Antimigraine Agent; Beta-Adrenergic Blocker
Generic Availability (U.S.) Yes
Use Treatment of hypertension, alone or in combination with other agents (FDA approved in adults); reduction of cardiovascular mortality and risk of reinfarction in stable post-MI patients (FDA approved in adults); prevention of migraine headaches (FDA approved in adults); treatment of angina
Pregnancy Risk Factor C
Pregnancy Considerations Adverse events were not observed in the initial animal reproduction studies; therefore, the manufacturer classifies timolol as pregnancy category C. Timolol crosses the placenta and decreased fetal heart rate has been observed following maternal use of oral and ophthalmic timolol during pregnancy. In a cohort study, an increased risk of cardiovascular defects was observed following maternal use of beta-blockers during pregnancy. Intrauterine growth restriction (IUGR), small placentas, as well as fetal/neonatal bradycardia, hypoglycemia, and/or respiratory depression have been observed following *in utero* exposure to beta-blockers as a class. Adequate facilities for monitoring infants at birth should be available. Untreated chronic maternal hypertension and pre-eclampsia are also associated with adverse events in the fetus, infant, and mother; however, timolol is currently not recommended for the initial treatment of hypertension in pregnancy. If timolol is required for the treatment of glaucoma during pregnancy, the minimum effective dose should be used in combination with punctual occlusion to decrease exposure to the fetus.
Breast-Feeding Considerations Timolol is excreted into breast milk. According to the manufacturer, the decision to continue or discontinue breast-feeding during therapy should take into account the risk of exposure to the infant and the benefits of treatment to the mother. Due to the potential for adverse events, nursing infants (especially those with cardiorespiratory problems) should be monitored.
Contraindications Hypersensitivity to timolol or any component; uncompensated CHF, cardiogenic shock, bradycardia or heart block, bronchial asthma, severe chronic obstructive pulmonary disease or history of asthma, CHF or bradycardia
Warnings Exacerbation of angina, arrhythmias, and in some cases MI may occur following abrupt discontinuation of beta-blockers **[U.S. Boxed Warning]**; avoid abrupt discontinuation, wean slowly, monitor for signs and symptoms of ischemia. Timolol decreases the ability of the heart to respond to reflex adrenergic stimuli and may increase

the risk of general anesthesia and surgical procedures; beta-blockers should generally be avoided in patients with bronchospastic disease; if administered, use the lowest possible dose and monitor patients carefully. Patients receiving beta-blockers, who have a history of anaphylactic reactions, may be more reactive to a repeated allergen challenge and may not be responsive to the usual epinephrine doses used to treat an allergic reaction. Beta-blockers may block hypoglycemia-induced tachycardia and blood pressure changes; use with caution in patients with diabetes mellitus. May mask signs of thyrotoxicosis (exacerbation of symptoms of hyperthyroidism, including thyroid storm, may occur following abrupt discontinuation). Use caution with anesthetic agents that decrease myocardial function. Beta-blocker use has been associated with induction or exacerbation of psoriasis, but cause and effect have not been firmly established.

Precautions Similar to other beta-blockers; use with caution in patients with decreased renal or hepatic function (dosage adjustment required); use with caution in patients with diabetes mellitus, may block hypoglycemia-induced tachycardia and blood pressure changes. Use with caution in patients with myasthenia gravis or myasthenic symptoms; may potentiate muscle weakness.

Adverse Reactions

Cardiovascular: Angina pectoris, arrhythmia, bradycardia, cardiac failure, cardiac arrest, cerebral vascular accident, cerebral ischemia, edema, hypotension, heart block, palpitation, Raynaud's phenomenon

Central nervous system: Anxiety, confusion, depression, dizziness, disorientation, fatigue, hallucinations, insomnia, memory loss, nervousness, nightmares, somnolence

Dermatologic: Alopecia, angioedema, pseudopemphigoid, psoriasiform rash, psoriasis exacerbation, rash, urticaria

Endocrine & metabolic: Hypoglycemia masked, libido decreased

Gastrointestinal: Anorexia, diarrhea, dyspepsia, nausea, xerostomia

Genitourinary: Impotence, retoperitoneal fibrosis

Hematologic: Claudication

Neuromuscular & skeletal: Myasthenia gravis exacerbation, paresthesia

Ocular: Blepharitis, conjunctivitis, cystoid macular edema, decreased corneal sensitivity, diplopia, dry eyes, foreign body sensation, keratitis, ocular discharge, ocular pain, ptosis, refractive changes, tearing, visual disturbances

Otic: Tinnitus

Respiratory: Bronchospasm, cough, dyspnea, nasal congestion, pulmonary edema, respiratory failure

Miscellaneous: Allergic reactions, cold hands/feet, Peyronie's disease, systemic lupus erythematosus

Drug Interactions

Metabolism/Transport Effects Substrate of CYP2D6 (major); **Note:** Assignment of Major/Minor substrate status based on clinically relevant drug interaction potential; **Inhibits** CYP2D6 (weak)

Avoid Concomitant Use

Avoid concomitant use of Timolol (Systemic) with any of the following: Beta2-Agonists; Ceritinib; Floctafenine; Methacholine

Increased Effect/Toxicity

Timolol (Systemic) may increase the levels/effects of: Alpha-/Beta-Agonists (Direct-Acting); Alpha1-Blockers; Alpha2-Agonists; Amifostine; Antihypertensives; Antipsychotic Agents (Phenothiazines); ARIPiprazole; Bradycardia-Causing Agents; Bupivacaine; Cardiac Glycosides; Ceritinib; Cholinergic Agonists; DULoxetine; Ergot Derivatives; Fingolimod; Grass Pollen Allergen Extract (5 Grass Extract); Hypotensive Agents; Insulin; Lidocaine (Systemic); Lidocaine (Topical); Mepivacaine; Methacholine; Midodrine; Obinutuzumab; RiTUXimab; Sulfonylureas

The levels/effects of Timolol (Systemic) may be increased by: Abiraterone Acetate; Acetylcholinesterase Inhibitors; Alpha2-Agonists; Aminoquinolines (Antimalarial); Amiodarone; Anilidopiperidine Opioids; Antipsychotic Agents (Phenothiazines); Barbiturates; Brimonidine (Topical); Calcium Channel Blockers (Dihydropyridine); Calcium Channel Blockers (Nondihydropyridine); CYP2D6 Inhibitors (Moderate); CYP2D6 Inhibitors (Strong); Darunavir; Diazoxide; Dipyridamole; Disopyramide; Dronedarone; Floctafenine; Herbs (Hypotensive Properties); MAO Inhibitors; Pentoxifylline; Phosphodiesterase 5 Inhibitors; Propafenone; Prostacyclin Analogues; Regorafenib; Reserpine; Selective Serotonin Reuptake Inhibitors

Decreased Effect

Timolol (Systemic) may decrease the levels/effects of: Beta2-Agonists; Theophylline Derivatives

The levels/effects of Timolol (Systemic) may be decreased by: Barbiturates; Herbs (Hypertensive Properties); Methylphenidate; Nonsteroidal Anti-Inflammatory Agents; Peginterferon Alfa-2b; Rifamycin Derivatives; Yohimbine

Mechanism of Action Blocks both beta$_1$- and beta$_2$-adrenergic receptors; reduces blood pressure by blocking adrenergic receptors and decreasing sympathetic outflow, produces a negative chronotropic and inotropic activity through an unknown mechanism

Pharmacodynamics Hypotensive effects:

Onset of action: Within 15-45 minutes

Maximum effect: 30-150 minutes

Duration: 4 hours

Pharmacokinetics (Adult data unless noted)

Distribution: Distributes into human breast milk

Protein binding: <10%

Metabolism: Extensively in the liver, extensive first-pass effect

Bioavailability: ~60%

Half-life: Adults: 2-4 hours; prolonged with reduced renal function

Elimination: Urinary excretion (15% to 20% as unchanged drug)

Dialysis: Not readily dialyzable

Dosing: Usual Oral:

Children: No information regarding pediatric dose is currently available in literature

Adults:

Hypertension: Initial: 10 mg twice daily, increase gradually every 7 days, usual dosage: 20-40 mg/day in 2 divided doses; maximum dose: 60 mg/day; usual dosage range (JNC 7): 20-40 mg/day in 2 divided doses

Prevention of MI: 10 mg twice daily initiated within 1-4 weeks after infarction

Migraine headache: Initial: 10 mg twice daily, increase to maximum of 30 mg/day

Administration May be administered without regard to food

Monitoring Parameters Heart rate, blood pressure; liver enzymes, BUN, serum creatinine with long-term oral use

Dosage Forms Excipient information presented when available (limited, particularly for generics); consult specific product labeling.

Tablet, Oral, as maleate:

Generic: 5 mg, 10 mg, 20 mg

References

Brauchli YB, Jick SS, Curtin F, et al, "Association Between Beta-Blockers, Other Antihypertensive Drugs and Psoriasis: Population-Based Case-Control Study," *Br J Dermatol*, 2008, 158(6):1299-307.

Chobanian AV, Bakris GL, Black HR, et al, "The Seventh Report of the Joint National Committee on Prevention, Detection, Evaluation, and Treatment of High Blood Pressure: The JNC 7 report," *JAMA*, 2003, 289(19):2560-72.

Gold MH, Holy AK, and Roenigk HH Jr, "Beta-Blocking Drugs and Psoriasis. A Review of Cutaneous Side Effects and Retrospective

Analysis of Their Effects on Psoriasis," *J Am Acad Dermatol*, 1988, 19 (5 Pt 1):837-41.

Schön MP and Boehncke WH, "Psoriasis," *N Engl J Med*, 2005, 352 (18):1899-912.

Timolol (Ophthalmic) (TIM oh lol)

Medication Safety Issues
Sound-alike/look-alike issues:
Timolol may be confused with atenolol, Tylenol®

Timoptic® may be confused with Betoptic S®, Talacen, Viroptic®

Other safety concerns:
Bottle cap color change: Timoptic®: Both the 0.25% and 0.5% strengths are now packaged in bottles with yellow caps; previously, the color of the cap on the product corresponded to different strengths.

International issues:
Betimol [U.S.] may be confused with Betanol brand name for metipranolol [Monaco]

Brand Names: U.S. Betimol; Istalol; Timoptic; Timoptic Ocudose; Timoptic-XE

Brand Names: Canada Apo-Timop®; Dom-Timolol; Mylan-Timolol; Novo-Timol; PMS-Timolol; Sandoz-Timolol; Tim-AK; Timolol Maleate-EX; Timoptic-XE®; Timoptic®

Therapeutic Category Beta-Adrenergic Blocker; Beta-Adrenergic Blocker, Ophthalmic

Generic Availability (U.S.) Yes

Use Treatment of elevated intraocular pressure in patients with open-angle glaucoma or ocular hypertension (FDA approved in adults)

Pregnancy Risk Factor C

Pregnancy Considerations Adverse events were not observed in animal reproduction studies; therefore, the manufacturer classifies timolol ophthalmic as pregnancy category C. Timolol crosses the placenta. Decreased fetal heart rate has been observed following maternal use of oral and ophthalmic timolol during pregnancy. In a cohort study, an increased risk of cardiovascular defects was observed following maternal use of beta-blockers during pregnancy. Intrauterine growth restriction (IUGR), small placentas, as well as fetal/neonatal bradycardia, hypoglycemia, and/or respiratory depression have been observed following *in utero* exposure to beta-blockers as a class. Adequate facilities for monitoring infants at birth should be available. Untreated chronic maternal hypertension and pre-eclampsia are also associated with adverse events in the fetus, infant, and mother. If timolol is required for the treatment of glaucoma during pregnancy, the minimum effective dose should be used in combination with punctual occlusion to decrease exposure to the fetus. Also refer to the Timolol (Systemic) monograph for additional information.

Breast-Feeding Considerations Timolol is excreted into breast milk following ophthalmic administration. According to the manufacturer, the decision to continue or discontinue breast-feeding during therapy should take into account the risk of exposure to the infant and the benefits of treatment to the mother. Due to the potential for adverse events, nursing infants (especially those with cardiorespiratory problems) should be monitored. Also refer to the Timolol (Systemic) monograph for additional information.

Contraindications Hypersensitivity to timolol or any component; uncompensated CHF, cardiogenic shock, bradycardia or heart block, bronchial asthma, severe chronic obstructive pulmonary disease or history of asthma, CHF or bradycardia

Warnings Severe CNS, cardiovascular and respiratory adverse effects have been seen following ophthalmic use; same adverse reactions seen with systemic therapy may occur with ocular therapy. Some products do contain benzalkonium chloride which may be absorbed by soft contact lenses; remove lens prior to administration and wait 15 minutes before reinserting.

Precautions Use with a miotic in angle-closure or narrow-angle glaucoma; multi-use ocular products have been associated with bacterial keratitis; avoid touching tip of applicator to eye or other surfaces.

Adverse Reactions
Cardiovascular: Angina pectoris, arrhythmia, bradycardia, cardiac arrest, cardiac failure, cerebral ischemia, cerebral vascular accident, edema, heart block, hypertension, hypotension, palpitation, Raynaud's phenomenon

Central nervous system: Anxiety, confusion, depression, disorientation, dizziness, hallucinations, headache, insomnia, memory loss, nervousness, nightmares, somnolence

Dermatologic: Alopecia, angioedema, pseudopemphigoid, psoriasiform rash, psoriasis exacerbation, rash, urticaria

Endocrine & metabolic: Hypoglycemia masked, libido decreased

Gastrointestinal: Anorexia, diarrhea, dyspepsia, nausea, xerostomia

Genitourinary: Impotence, retoperitoneal fibrosis

Hematologic: Claudication

Neuromuscular & skeletal: Myasthenia gravis exacerbation, paresthesia

Ocular: Blepharitis, blurred vision, burning, cataract, choroidal detachment (following filtration surgery), conjunctival injection, conjunctivitis, corneal sensitivity decreased, cystoid macular edema, diplopia, dry eyes, foreign body sensation, hyperemia, itching, keratitis, ocular discharge, ocular pain, ptosis, stinging, tearing, visual acuity decreased refractive changes, visual disturbances

Otic: Tinnitus

Respiratory: Bronchospasm, cough, dyspnea, nasal congestion, pulmonary edema, respiratory failure

Miscellaneous: Allergic reactions, cold hands/feet, Peyronie's disease, systemic lupus erythematosus

Drug Interactions
Metabolism/Transport Effects Substrate of CYP2D6 (major); **Note:** Assignment of Major/Minor substrate status based on clinically relevant drug interaction potential; **Inhibits** CYP2D6 (weak)

Avoid Concomitant Use
Avoid concomitant use of Timolol (Ophthalmic) with any of the following: Beta2-Agonists; Ceritinib; Floctafenine; Methacholine

Increased Effect/Toxicity
Timolol (Ophthalmic) may increase the levels/effects of: Alpha-/Beta-Agonists (Direct-Acting); Alpha1-Blockers; Alpha2-Agonists; Amifostine; Antihypertensives; Antipsychotic Agents (Phenothiazines); ARIPiprazole; Bradycardia-Causing Agents; Bupivacaine; Cardiac Glycosides; Ceritinib; Cholinergic Agonists; DULoxetine; Ergot Derivatives; Fingolimod; Grass Pollen Allergen Extract (5 Grass Extract); Hypotensive Agents; Insulin; Lidocaine (Systemic); Lidocaine (Topical); Mepivacaine; Methacholine; Midodrine; Obinutuzumab; RiTUXimab; Sulfonylureas

The levels/effects of Timolol (Ophthalmic) may be increased by: Abiraterone Acetate; Acetylcholinesterase Inhibitors; Alpha2-Agonists; Aminoquinolines (Antimalarial); Amiodarone; Anilidopiperidine Opioids; Antipsychotic Agents (Phenothiazines); Barbiturates; Brimonidine (Topical); Calcium Channel Blockers (Dihydropyridine); Calcium Channel Blockers (Nondihydropyridine); CYP2D6 Inhibitors (Moderate); CYP2D6 Inhibitors (Strong); Darunavir; Diazoxide; Dipyridamole; Disopyramide; Dronedarone; Floctafenine; Herbs (Hypotensive Properties); MAO Inhibitors; Pentoxifylline; Phosphodiesterase 5 Inhibitors; Propafenone; Prostacyclin Analogues;

Regorafenib; Reserpine; Selective Serotonin Reuptake Inhibitors

Decreased Effect

Timolol (Ophthalmic) may decrease the levels/effects of: Beta2-Agonists; Theophylline Derivatives

The levels/effects of Timolol (Ophthalmic) may be decreased by: Barbiturates; Herbs (Hypertensive Properties); Methylphenidate; Nonsteroidal Anti-Inflammatory Agents; Rifamycin Derivatives; Yohimbine

Stability Drops: Store at room temperature of 15°C to 25°C (59°F to 77°F); do not freeze. Protect from light.

Timolol GFS: Store at 2°C to 25°C (36°F to 77°F). Protect from light.

Timoptic® OcuDose®: Store in protective foil wrap; use within 1 month after opening foil package

Mechanism of Action Blocks both beta$_1$- and beta$_2$-adrenergic receptors, reduces intraocular pressure by reducing aqueous humor production or possibly outflow; reduces blood pressure by blocking adrenergic receptors and decreasing sympathetic outflow, produces a negative chronotropic and inotropic activity through an unknown mechanism

Pharmacodynamics Intraocular pressure reduction:
Onset of action: Within 30 minutes
Maximum effect: 1-2 hours
Duration: 24 hours

Pharmacokinetics (Adult data unless noted)
Absorption: Timolol is measurable in the serum following ophthalmic use.
Distribution: Distributes into human breast milk

Dosing: Usual
Gel (Timoptic-XE®): Adults: 0.25% or 0.5% gel, instill 1 drop once daily; do not exceed 1 drop once daily of 0.5% gel
Solution (Timoptic®): Children and Adults: Initial: 0.25% solution, instill 1 drop twice daily; increase to 0.5% solution if response not adequate; decrease to 1 drop/day if controlled; do not exceed 1 drop twice daily of 0.5% solution
Solution (Istalol™): Adults: Initial: 0.5% solution: Instill 1 drop once daily in the morning

Administration Apply gentle pressure to lacrimal sac during and immediately following instillation (1 minute) or instruct patient to gently close eyelid after administration, to decrease systemic absorption of ophthalmic drops; avoid contact of bottle tip with skin or eye. Remove contact lenses prior to administration (ophthalmic solution contains benzalkonium chloride which may adsorb to soft contact lenses); lenses may be inserted 15 minutes after administration. Gel: Invert container, shake once before use; administer other topical ophthalmic medications at least 10 minutes before Timoptic-XE®

Monitoring Parameters Monitor IOP

Additional Information Use lowest effective dose in pediatric patients. Children had higher plasma concentrations vs adults; some achieved therapeutic levels; this may result in increased adverse systemic effects. The concurrent use of 2 ophthalmic beta blockers is not recommended.

Dosage Forms Excipient information presented when available (limited, particularly for generics); consult specific product labeling.
Gel Forming Solution, Ophthalmic, as maleate [strength expressed as base]:
Timoptic-XE: 0.25% (5 mL); 0.5% (5 mL)
Generic: 0.25% (5 mL); 0.5% (5 mL)
Solution, Ophthalmic, as hemihydrate [strength expressed as base]:
Betimol: 0.25% (5 mL); 0.5% (5 mL, 10 mL, 15 mL) [contains benzalkonium chloride]

Solution, Ophthalmic, as maleate [strength expressed as base]:
Istalol: 0.5% (2.5 mL, 5 mL) [contains benzalkonium chloride]
Timoptic: 0.25% (5 mL); 0.5% (5 mL, 10 mL) [contains benzalkonium chloride]
Generic: 0.25% (5 mL, 10 mL, 15 mL); 0.5% (5 mL, 10 mL, 15 mL)
Solution, Ophthalmic, as maleate [strength expressed as base, preservative free]:
Timoptic Ocudose: 0.25% (60 ea); 0.5% (60 ea)

References
Hoskins HD, Hetherington J Jr, Magee SD, et al, "Clinical Experience With Timolol in Childhood Glaucoma," *Arch Ophthalmol*, 1985, 103 (8):1163-5.

◆ **Timolol Hemihydrate** *see* Timolol (Ophthalmic) *on page 2028*

◆ **Timolol Maleate** *see* Timolol (Ophthalmic) *on page 2028*

◆ **Timolol Maleate** *see* Timolol (Systemic) *on page 2026*

◆ **Timolol Maleate-EX (Can)** *see* Timolol (Ophthalmic) *on page 2028*

◆ **Timoptic** *see* Timolol (Ophthalmic) *on page 2028*

◆ **Timoptic® (Can)** *see* Timolol (Ophthalmic) *on page 2028*

◆ **Timoptic Ocudose** *see* Timolol (Ophthalmic) *on page 2028*

◆ **Timoptic-XE** *see* Timolol (Ophthalmic) *on page 2028*

◆ **Timoptic-XE® (Can)** *see* Timolol (Ophthalmic) *on page 2028*

◆ **Tinactin [OTC]** *see* Tolnaftate *on page 2044*

◆ **Tinactin Deodorant [OTC]** *see* Tolnaftate *on page 2044*

◆ **Tinactin Jock Itch [OTC]** *see* Tolnaftate *on page 2044*

◆ **Tinamed Corn/Callus Remover [OTC]** *see* Salicylic Acid *on page 1860*

◆ **Tinamed Wart Remover [OTC]** *see* Salicylic Acid *on page 1860*

◆ **Tinaspore [OTC]** *see* Tolnaftate *on page 2044*

◆ **Tincture of Opium** *see* Opium Tincture *on page 1548*

◆ **Tindamax** *see* Tinidazole *on page 2029*

Tinidazole (tye NI da zole)

Brand Names: U.S. Tindamax

Therapeutic Category Amebicide; Antibiotic, Miscellaneous; Antiprotozoal, Nitroimidazole

Generic Availability (U.S.) Yes

Use Treatment of giardiasis caused by *G. duodenalis* (*G. lamblia*) (FDA approved in ages >3 years and adults); treatment of intestinal amebiasis and amebic liver abscess caused by *E. histolytica* (FDA approved in ages >3 years and adults); treatment of trichomoniasis caused by *T. vaginalis* (FDA approved in adults); treatment of bacterial vaginosis caused by *Bacteroides* spp, *Gardnerella vaginalis*, and *Prevotella* spp (FDA approved in nonpregnant adult females)

Pregnancy Risk Factor C

Pregnancy Considerations Adverse events have been observed in some animal reproduction studies. Carcinogenicity studies have not been completed with tinidazole; however, metronidazole has a similar chemical structure and has caused carcinogenic effects in rats and mice. Tinidazole crosses the human placenta and enters the fetal circulation. Use of tinidazole is contraindicated during the first trimester of pregnancy.

Breast-Feeding Considerations Tinidazole is excreted into breast milk in concentrations similar to those in the maternal serum and can be detected for up to 72 hours after administration. Tinidazole is contraindicated in nursing mothers unless breast-feeding is interrupted during therapy and for 3 days after the last dose.

Contraindications Hypersensitivity to tinidazole, nitroimidazole derivatives (including metronidazole), or any component; first trimester of pregnancy; breast-feeding (requires temporary interruption of breast-feeding)

Warnings Carcinogenicity has been observed with chronic use of another nitroimidazole derivative (metronidazole) in animal studies **[U.S. Boxed Warning]**; per the manufacturer, use should be reserved for approved indications only. Seizures and peripheral neuropathy have been reported with tinidazole and other nitroimidazole derivatives; monitor and promptly discontinue therapy if signs/symptoms occur; use with caution in patients with CNS diseases. Prolonged use may result in fungal or bacterial superinfection, including *C. difficile*-associated diarrhea (CDAD), pseudomembranous colitis, and/or vaginal candidiasis. CDAD has been observed >2 months postantibiotic treatment.

Precautions Use with caution in patients with current or a history of blood dyscrasias or hepatic impairment. When used for amebiasis, tinidazole is not indicated for the treatment of asymptomatic cyst passage. Disulfiram-like reactions to ethanol may occur; avoid alcoholic beverages during therapy and for 72 hours after therapy.

Adverse Reactions

Cardiovascular: Flushing, palpitation

Central nervous system: Ataxia, coma (rare), confusion (rare), depression (rare), dizziness, drowsiness, fatigue/malaise, fever, giddiness, headache, insomnia, seizure, vertigo

Dermatologic: Angioedema, pruritus, rash, urticaria

Endocrine & metabolic: Menorrhagia

Gastrointestinal: Abdominal pain, anorexia, appetite decreased, constipation, diarrhea, dyspepsia/cramps/epigastric discomfort, flatulence, furry tongue (rare), metallic/bitter taste, nausea, oral candidiasis, salivation, stomatitis, thirst, tongue discoloration, vomiting, xerostomia

Genitourinary: *Candida* vaginitis, painful urination, pelvic pain, urine abnormality/darkened, vaginal discharge increased, vaginal odor, vulvovaginal discomfort

Hematologic: Leukopenia (transient), neutropenia (transient), thrombocytopenia (reversible; rare)

Hepatic: Transaminases increased

Neuromuscular & skeletal: Arthralgia, arthritis, myalgia, peripheral neuropathy (transient, includes numbness and paresthesia), weakness

Renal: Urinary tract infection

Respiratory: Bronchospasm (rare), dyspnea (rare), pharyngitis (rare), upper respiratory tract infection

Miscellaneous: Burning sensation, *Candida* overgrowth, diaphoresis

Rare but important or life-threatening: Acute hypersensitivity reaction (severe), erythema multiforme, Stevens-Johnson syndrome

Drug Interactions

Metabolism/Transport Effects Substrate of CYP3A4 (minor)

Avoid Concomitant Use

Avoid concomitant use of Tinidazole with any of the following: Alcohol (Ethyl); Disulfiram

Increased Effect/Toxicity Specific interaction studies have not been conducted. Refer to Metronidazole monograph.

Decreased Effect Specific interaction studies have not been conducted. Refer to Metronidazole monograph.

Food Interactions

Ethanol: Concurrent ethanol use may cause a disulfiram-like reaction characterized by flushing, headache, nausea, vomiting, sweating or tachycardia. Management: The manufacturer recommends to avoid all ethanol or any ethanol-containing drugs during and for at least 3 days after completion of treatment.

Food: Peak antibiotic serum concentration lowered and delayed, but total drug absorbed not affected. Management: Administer with food.

Stability Store at 20°C to 25°C (68°F to 77°F); excursions permitted to 15°C to 30°C (59°F to 86°F); protect from light.

Mechanism of Action After diffusing into the organism, it is proposed that tinidazole causes cytotoxicity by damaging DNA and preventing further DNA synthesis.

Pharmacokinetics (Adult data unless noted)

Absorption: Rapid and complete

Distribution: V_d: 50 L; distributes to most body tissues and fluids; crosses the blood-brain barrier

Protein binding: 12%

Metabolism: Hepatic via CYP3A4 (primarily); undergoes oxidation, hydroxylation and conjugation

Half-life elimination: 12-14 hours

Time to peak serum concentration: ~1.6 hours (fasting, delayed ~2 hours when given with food)

Excretion: Urine (20% to 25%); feces (12%)

Dosing: Usual

Pediatric:

Amebiasis, intestinal: Children >3 years and Adolescents: Oral: 50 mg/kg/day for 3 days; maximum daily dose: 2000 mg/**day**; for patients with severe and extraintestinal disease, administer for 5 days (*Red Book* [AAP], 2012)

Amebiasis, liver abscess: Children >3 years and Adolescents: Oral: 50 mg/kg/day for 3 to 5 days; maximum daily dose: 2000 mg/**day**

Bacterial vaginosis: Adolescents: Oral: 2000 mg once daily for 2 days **or** 1000 mg once daily for 5 days (CDC, 2010)

Giardiasis: Children >3 years and Adolescents: Oral: 50 mg/kg as a single dose; maximum dose: 2000 mg

Helicobacter pylori **infection:** Limited data available: Children >3 years and Adolescents: Oral: 20 mg/kg/day in 1 to 2 divided doses for 5 to 7 days in combination with other agents; some studies have used a longer duration of 2 to 6 weeks; maximum daily dose: 1000 mg/**day** (Francavilla, 2005; Moshkowitz, 1998; Nijevitch, 2000; Oderda, 1992)

Nongonococcal urethritis, recurrent/persistent: Adolescents: Oral: 2000 mg as a single dose in combination with azithromycin (CDC, 2010)

Trichomoniasis:

Children >3 years: Oral: 50 mg/kg as a single dose; maximum dose: 2000 mg (*Red Book* [AAP], 2012)

Adolescents: Oral: 2000 mg as a single dose; sexual partners should be treated at the same time; if treatment failure, can consider extended regimen of 2000 mg once daily for 5 days (CDC, 2010; *Red Book* [AAP], 2012)

Adult:

Amebiasis, intestinal: Oral: 2000 mg/day for 3 days

Amebiasis, liver abscess: Oral: 2000 mg/day for 3 to 5 days

Bacterial vaginosis: Oral: 2000 mg/day for 2 days **or** 1000 mg/day for 5 days

Giardiasis: Oral: 2000 mg as a single dose

Trichomoniasis: Oral: 2000 mg as a single dose; sexual partners should be treated at the same time

Dosing adjustment in renal impairment: Children >3 years, Adolescents, and Adults: No dosage adjustment necessary

Hemodialysis: Approximately 43% removed during a 6-hour session; an additional dose equal to 1/2 the usual dose should be administered at the end of hemodialysis if tinidazole is administered prior to hemodialysis on dialysis days

Dosing adjustment in hepatic impairment: There are no dosage adjustments provided in the manufacturer's labeling (has not been studied); use with caution.

Administration Oral: Administer with food to minimize gastrointestinal adverse effects.

Test Interactions May interfere with AST, ALT, triglycerides, glucose, and LDH testing

Dosage Forms Excipient information presented when available (limited, particularly for generics); consult specific product labeling.

Tablet, Oral:

Tindamax: 250 mg, 500 mg [scored; contains fd&c red #40 aluminum lake, fd&c yellow #6 aluminum lake]

Generic: 250 mg, 500 mg

Extemporaneous Preparations A 67 mg/mL suspension may be made with tablets and cherry syrup. Crush four 500 mg tablets in a mortar and reduce to a fine powder. Add 10 mL cherry syrup and mix to a uniform paste; mix while adding cherry syrup in incremental proportions to **almost** 30 mL; transfer to a calibrated bottle, rinse mortar with vehicle, and add quantity of vehicle sufficient to make 30 mL. Label "shake well". Stable for 7 days.

Tindamax® prescribing information, Mission Pharmacal Company, San Antonio, TX, 2007. Available at http://www.accessdata.fda.gov/drug-satfda_docs/label/2007/021618s003lbl.pdf

References

American Academy of Pediatrics (AAP). In: Pickering LK, Baker CJ, Kimberlin DW, Long SS, eds. *Red Book: 2012 Report of the Committee on Infectious Diseases.* 29th ed. Elk Grove Village, IL: American Academy of Pediatrics; 2012.

Centers for Disease Control and Prevention (CDC), "Sexually Transmitted Diseases Treatment Guidelines, 2010," *MMWR Recomm Rep,* 2010, 59(RR-12):1-110.

Francavilla R, Lionetti E, Castellaneta SP, et al. Improved efficacy of 10-day sequential treatment for *Helicobacter pylori* eradication in children: a randomized trial. *Gastroenterology.* 2005;129:1414-1419.

Lamp KC, Freeman CD, Klutman NE, "Pharmacokinetics and pharmacodynamics of the nitroimidazole antimicrobials," *Clin Pharmacokinet,* 1999, 36(5):353-73.

Moshkowitz M, Reif S, Brill S, Ringel Y, Arber N, Halpern Z, Bujanover Y. One-week triple therapy with omeprazole, clarithromycin, and nitroimidazole for *Helicobacter pylori* infection in children and adolescents. *Pediatrics.* 1998;102(1):e14.

Nijevitch AA, Farztdinov KM, Sataev VU, et al. *Helicobacter pylori* infection in childhood: results of management with ranitidine bismuth citrate plus amoxicillin and tinidazole. *Journal of Gastroenterology and Hepatology.* 2000;15:1243-1250.

Odera G, Vaira D, Ainley C, et al. Eighteen month follow up of *Helicobacter pylori* positive children treated with amoxicillin and tinidazole. *Gut.* 1992;33:1328-1330.

◆ **Tioguanine** *see* Thioguanine *on page 2010*

◆ **Tiotixene** *see* Thiothixene *on page 2015*

Tipranavir (tip RA na veer)

Related Information

Adult and Adolescent HIV *on page 2348*

Oral Medications That Should Not Be Crushed or Altered *on page 2438*

Pediatric HIV *on page 2338*

Perinatal HIV *on page 2356*

Brand Names: U.S. Aptivus

Brand Names: Canada Aptivus®

Therapeutic Category Antiviral Agent; HIV Agents (Anti-HIV Agents); Protease Inhibitor

Generic Availability (U.S.) No

Use Treatment of HIV-1 infections in combination with ritonavir and other antiretroviral agents in patients who are highly treatment-experienced or multiprotease inhibitor-resistant (FDA approved in ages ≥2 years and adults).

Note: HIV regimens consisting of **three** antiretroviral agents are strongly recommended.

Pregnancy Risk Factor C

Pregnancy Considerations Adverse events were observed in some animal reproduction studies. Tipranavir crosses the human placenta. The DHHS Perinatal HIV Guidelines note there are insufficient data to recommend use during pregnancy; however, if used, tipranavir must be given with low-dose ritonavir boosting. A small increased risk of preterm birth has been associated with maternal use of protease inhibitor-based combination antiretroviral (ARV) therapy during pregnancy; however, the benefits of use generally outweigh this risk and protease inhibitors (PIs) should not be withheld if otherwise recommended. Hyperglycemia, new onset of diabetes mellitus, or diabetic ketoacidosis have been reported with PIs; it is not clear if pregnancy increases this risk.

Regardless of CD4 count or HIV RNA copy number, all HIV-infected pregnant women should receive a combination ARV drug regimen. A combination of antepartum, intrapartum, and infant ARV prophylaxis is recommended. ARV therapy should be started as soon as possible in women with symptomatic infection. Although earlier initiation may be more effective in reducing the perinatal transmission of HIV, initiation may be delayed until after 12 weeks gestation in women who do not require immediate treatment after careful consideration of maternal conditions (eg, nausea and vomiting) and the potential risks of first trimester fetal exposure for specific agents. A scheduled cesarean delivery at 38 weeks gestation is recommended for all women with HIV RNA >1000 copies/mL or unknown concentrations near delivery in order to decrease transmission. If ARV therapy must be interrupted for <24 hours during the peripartum period, stop then restart all medications simultaneously in order to decrease the chance of developing resistance. Long-term follow-up is recommended for all infants exposed to ARV medications. In couples who want to conceive, the HIV-infected partner should attain maximum viral suppression prior to conception.

Health care providers are encouraged to enroll pregnant women exposed to antiretroviral medications in the Antiretroviral Pregnancy Registry (1-800-258-4263 or www.APRegistry.com). Health care providers caring for HIV-infected women and their infants may contact the National Perinatal HIV Hotline (888-448-8765) for clinical consultation (DHHS [perinatal], 2014).

Women receiving estrogen (as hormonal contraception or replacement therapy) may have an increased incidence of rash.

Breast-Feeding Considerations It is not known if tipranavir is excreted into breast milk. Maternal or infant antiretroviral therapy does not completely eliminate the risk of postnatal HIV transmission. In addition, multiclass-resistant virus has been detected in breast-feeding infants despite maternal therapy. Therefore, in the United States, where formula is accessible, affordable, safe, and sustainable, and the risk of infant mortality due to diarrhea and respiratory infections is low, complete avoidance of breast-feeding by HIV-infected women is recommended to decrease potential transmission of HIV (DHHS [perinatal], 2014).

Contraindications Hypersensitivity to tipranavir or any component; moderate to severe hepatic impairment (Child-Pugh class B or C); concurrent therapy of tipranavir/ritonavir with alfuzosin, amiodarone, bepridil, cisapride, ergot derivatives (eg, dihydroergotamine, ergonovine, ergotamine, methylergonovine), flecainide, lovastatin, midazolam (oral), pimozide, propafenone, quinidine, rifampin, sildenafil [for pulmonary arterial hypertension (eg, Revatio)], simvastatin, St John's wort, and triazolam

Warnings Do not use without ritonavir; use without ritonavir will result in low plasma levels, altering both therapeutic effect and drug interactions. Tipranavir plus ritonavir may ▶

cause hepatitis (including fatalities) and/or exacerbate preexisting hepatic dysfunction **[U.S. Boxed Warning]**; causal relationship not established; most cases reported in patients with advanced HIV-1 disease and receiving multiple concomitant medications; patients with chronic hepatitis B or C coinfection or elevated liver enzymes (transaminases) are at additional increased risk (approximately twofold). Monitor patients closely; discontinue use if signs or symptoms of toxicity occur or if asymptomatic AST/ALT elevations >10 times upper limit of normal or AST/ALT elevations >5 to 10 times upper limit of normal concurrently with total bilirubin >2.5 times the upper limit of normal occur. Use is contraindicated in patients with moderate to severe hepatic impairment (Child-Pugh class B or C); use with caution in patients with mild hepatic impairment (Child-Pugh class A); serum tipranavir concentrations may be increased.

Use of tipranavir plus ritonavir has been associated with rare reports of fatal and nonfatal intracranial hemorrhage **[U.S. Boxed Warning]**; causal relationship not established. Events often occurred in patients with medical conditions (eg, CNS lesions, head trauma, recent neurosurgery, coagulopathy, hypertension, alcohol abuse) or concurrent therapy which may have influenced these events.

Tipranavir plus ritonavir is an inhibitor of cytochrome P450 isoenzyme CYP3A. Administration with drugs that are primarily metabolized by CYP3A may result in increased serum concentrations of the other drug and lead to an increase or prolongation of adverse effects. Due to potential serious and/or life-threatening drug interactions, some drugs are contraindicated or not recommended for concurrent use; other drug interactions require dosage or regimen adjustment or monitoring of serum concentrations.

Skin rash may occur with tipranavir plus ritonavir use, including urticarial rash, maculopapular rash, or photosensitivity; may be accompanied by joint pain or stiffness, throat tightness, or generalized pruritus; reported incidence (all grades): Pediatric patients: 21%, adults: 8% to 10%; median onset: 53 days; treatment may be continued if rash is mild to moderate (rash may resolve; median duration: 22 days); discontinue therapy in cases of severe rash. Use with caution in patients with sulfonamide allergy; tipranavir contains sulfonamide moiety; cross-sensitivity may occur.

May impair platelet aggregation, resulting in bleeding; use with caution in patients who may be at risk for increased bleeding (trauma, surgery or other medical conditions); use with caution in patients with hemophilia A or B; increased bleeding during protease inhibitor therapy has been reported. Changes in glucose tolerance, hyperglycemia, exacerbation of diabetes, DKA, and new-onset diabetes mellitus have been reported in patients receiving protease inhibitors. Increases in total cholesterol and triglycerides have been reported; screening should be done prior to therapy and periodically throughout treatment. May cause hypercholesterolemia less frequently than with other protease inhibitors.

Tipranavir oral solution contains vitamin E (116 units/mL), which is significantly higher than the RDA; avoid taking additional vitamin E (other than a daily multivitamin). The recommended pediatric dose of tipranavir (14 mg/kg body weight) results in a vitamin E dose of 16 units/kg body weight per day, significantly higher than the reference daily intake for vitamin E (10 units) and close to the upper limit of tolerability for children.

Precautions Fat redistribution and accumulation [ie, central obesity, peripheral wasting, facial wasting, breast enlargement, dorsocervical fat enlargement (buffalo hump), and cushingoid appearance] have been observed in patients receiving antiretroviral agents (causal relationship not established).

Immune reconstitution syndrome (an acute inflammatory response to residual or indolent opportunistic infections) may occur in HIV patients during initial treatment with combination antiretroviral agents; this syndrome may require further patient assessment and therapy. Autoimmune disorders (eg, Graves' disease, Guillain-Barré syndrome, and polymyositis) have been reported in patients experiencing immune reconstitution; time to onset is variable and may occur many months after antiretroviral treatment is initiated.

Adverse Reactions

Central nervous system: Fatigue, fever, headache

Dermatologic: Rash

Endocrine & metabolic: Dehydration, hypercholesterolemia, hypertriglyceridemia

Gastrointestinal: Abdominal pain, amylase increased, diarrhea, nausea, vomiting, weight loss

Hepatic: ALT increased, AST increased, GGT increased, transaminases increased

Hematologic: Anemia, bleeding, neutropenia, WBC decreased

Neuromuscular & skeletal: CPK increased, myalgia

Respiratory: Cough, dyspnea, epistaxis

Rare but important or life-threatening: Abdominal distension, anorexia, appetite decreased, diabetes mellitus, dizziness, dyspepsia, exanthem, facial wasting, flatulence, flu-like syndrome, gastroesophageal reflux, hepatic failure, hepatic steatosis, hepatitis, hyperbilirubinemia, hyperglycemia, hypersensitivity, immune reconstitution syndrome, insomnia, intracranial hemorrhage, lipase increased, lipoatrophy, lipodystrophy (acquired), lipohypertrophy, malaise, mitochondrial toxicity, muscle cramp, neuropathy (peripheral), pancreatitis, pruritus, renal insufficiency, sleep disorder, somnolence, thrombocytopenia

Drug Interactions

Metabolism/Transport Effects Substrate of CYP3A4 (major); **Note:** Assignment of Major/Minor substrate status based on clinically relevant drug interaction potential; **Inhibits** CYP2D6 (strong); **Induces** P-glycoprotein

Avoid Concomitant Use

Avoid concomitant use of Tipranavir with any of the following: Alfuzosin; Amiodarone; AtorvaSTATin; Bepridil [Off Market]; Cisapride; Dabigatran Etexilate; Ergot Derivatives; Etravirine; Flecainide; Lovastatin; Midazolam; Pimozide; Propafenone; Protease Inhibitors; QuiNIDine; Rifampin; Salmeterol; Simeprevir; Simvastatin; Sofosbuvir; St Johns Wort; Tamoxifen; Thioridazine; Triazolam; VinCRIStine (Liposomal)

Increased Effect/Toxicity

Tipranavir may increase the levels/effects of: Agents with Antiplatelet Properties; Alfuzosin; ALPRAZolam; Amiodarone; Anticoagulants; ARIPiprazole; AtoMOXetine; AtorvaSTATin; Bepridil [Off Market]; Bosentan; Calcium Channel Blockers (Dihydropyridine); Calcium Channel Blockers (Nondihydropyridine); CarBAMazepine; Cisapride; Clarithromycin; Colchicine; Contraceptives (Progestins); Cyclophosphamide; CycloSPORINE (Systemic); CYP2D6 Substrates; Digoxin; DOXOrubicin (Conventional); Enfuvirtide; Ergot Derivatives; Fesoterodine; Flecainide; Iloperidone; Itraconazole; Ketoconazole (Systemic); Lovastatin; Meperidine; Metoprolol; Midazolam; Nebivolol; Nefazodone; Pimozide; Propafenone; QuiNIDine; Rifabutin; Riociguat; Rosuvastatin; Salmeterol; Sildenafil; Simeprevir; Simvastatin; Tacrolimus (Systemic); Tacrolimus (Topical); Temsirolimus; Tetrabenazine; Thioridazine; TraZODone; Triazolam; Tricyclic Antidepressants; Vardenafil; Vitamin E; Vortioxetine

The levels/effects of Tipranavir may be increased by: Clarithromycin; CycloSPORINE (Systemic); Delavirdine; Disulfiram; Enfuvirtide; Estrogen Derivatives; Fluconazole; MetroNIDAZOLE (Systemic); MetroNIDAZOLE (Topical); Simeprevir

Decreased Effect

Tipranavir may decrease the levels/effects of: Abacavir; Afatinib; Boceprevir; Brentuximab Vedotin; Clarithromycin; Codeine; Dabigatran Etexilate; Delavirdine; Didanosine; Dolutegravir; DOXOrubicin (Conventional); Estrogen Derivatives; Etravirine; Fosphenytoin; Iloperidone; Linagliptin; Meperidine; Methadone; P-glycoprotein/ABCB1 Substrates; PHENobarbital; Phenytoin; Protease Inhibitors; Proton Pump Inhibitors; Raltegravir; Sofosbuvir; Tamoxifen; Tenofovir; Theophylline Derivatives; TraMADol; Valproic Acid and Derivatives; VinCRIStine (Liposomal); Zidovudine

The levels/effects of Tipranavir may be decreased by: Antacids; Boceprevir; Bosentan; CarBAMazepine; CYP3A4 Inducers (Strong); Dabrafenib; Deferasirox; Fosphenytoin; Garlic; Mitotane; PHENobarbital; Phenytoin; Rifampin; Siltuximab; St Johns Wort; Tenofovir; Tocilizumab

Stability

Oral capsule: Store intact bottle at 2°C to 8°C (36°F to 46°F). After bottle is opened, may be stored at 25°C (77°F); excursions permitted to 15°C to 30°C (59°F to 86°F) for up to 60 days.

Oral solution: Store at 25°C (77°F); excursions permitted to 15°C to 30°C (59°F to 86°F). After bottle is open, use within 60 days. Do not refrigerate or freeze oral solution.

Mechanism of Action

Binds to the site of HIV-1 protease activity and inhibits cleavage of viral Gag-Pol polyprotein precursors into individual functional proteins required for infectious HIV. This results in the formation of immature, noninfectious viral particles.

Pharmacokinetics (Adult data unless noted)

Absorption: Incomplete (percentage not established)

Distribution: V_d:

Children:

2 to <6 years: 4 L

6 to <12 years: 4.7 L

Children and Adolescents 12 to 18 years: 5.3 L

Adults: 7.7 to 10.2 L

Protein binding: >99% (albumin, alpha$_1$-acid glycoprotein)

Metabolism: Hepatic, via CYP3A4 (minimal when coadministered with ritonavir)

Bioavailability: Not established

Half-life:

Children:

2 to <6 years of age: ~8 hours

6 to <12 years of age: ~7 hours

Children and Adolescents 12 to 18 years: ~5 hours

Adults: Males: 6 hours; Females: 5.5 hours

Time to peak serum concentration:

Children and Adolescents 2 to 18 years: 2.5 to 2.7 hours

Adults: ~3 hours

Elimination: Feces (82%); urine (4%); primarily as unchanged drug (when coadministered with ritonavir)

Dosing: Usual

Pediatric: **HIV infection, treatment:** Oral: **Note:** Use in combination with other antiretroviral agents. Not recommended for treatment-naïve patients. Coadministration with ritonavir is required.

Infants and Children <2 years: Not recommended for use

Children ≥2 years and Adolescents:

Weight-directed dosing: Tipranavir 14 mg/kg (maximum: 500 mg) twice daily **plus** ritonavir 6 mg/kg (maximum: 200 mg) twice daily

If intolerance or toxicity develops and virus is not resistant to multiple protease inhibitors: May decrease dose to: Tipranavir 12 mg/kg **plus** ritonavir 5 mg/kg twice daily; do not exceed adult doses

BSA-directed dosing: Tipranavir 375 mg/m^2 (maximum: 500 mg) twice daily **plus** ritonavir 150 mg/m^2 (maximum: 200 mg) twice daily

If intolerance or toxicity develops and virus is not resistant to multiple protease inhibitors: May decrease dose to: Tipranavir 290 mg/m^2 **plus** ritonavir 115 mg/m^2 twice daily; do not exceed adult doses

Adult: **HIV infection, treatment:** Oral: Use in combination with other antiretroviral agents. Not recommended for treatment naïve patients. **Note:** Coadministration with ritonavir is required. Tipranavir 500 mg **plus** ritonavir 200 mg twice daily

Dosing adjustment in renal impairment: No adjustment required (DHHS [adult, pediatric], 2014)

Dosing adjustment in hepatic impairment:

Mild impairment (Child-Pugh class A): No adjustment required; use with caution

Moderate to severe impairment (Child-Pugh class B or C): Use is contraindicated

Administration

Coadministration with ritonavir is required. In pediatric patients, may administer tipranavir **plus** ritonavir **capsules** or **solution** together with food (DHHS [pediatric], 2014) and in adults without regard to meals (DHHS [adult], 2014). Administer tipranavir **plus** ritonavir **tablets** at the same time with food.

Monitoring Parameters

Note: Monitor CD4 percentage (if <5 years of age) or CD4 count (if ≥5 years of age) at least every 3 to 4 months (DHHS [pediatric], 2014).

Prior to initiation of therapy: Genotypic resistance testing, CD4 and viral load (every 3 to 4 months), CBC with differential, LFTs, BUN, creatinine, lipid panel, electrolytes, glucose, urinalysis (every 6 to 12 months), and assessment of readiness for adherence with medication regimen. At initiation and with any change in treatment regimen: CBC with differential, electrolytes, calcium, phosphate, glucose, LFTs, bilirubin, urinalysis (at initiation), BUN, creatinine, albumin, total protein, lipid panel (at initiation), CD4, and viral load. After 1 to 2 weeks of therapy: Signs of medication toxicity and adherence. After 2 to 4 weeks of therapy: CBC with differential, viral load, and signs of medication toxicity, and adherence; then every 3 to 4 months: CBC with differential, electrolytes, glucose, LFTs, bilirubin, BUN, creatinine, CD4, viral load, signs of medication toxicity, and adherence. Every 6 to 12 months: Lipid panel and urinalysis. CD4 monitoring frequency may be decreased to every 6 to 12 months in children who are adherent to therapy if the value is well above the threshold for opportunistic infections, viral suppression is sustained, and the clinical status is stable for more than 2 to 3 years (DHHS [pediatric], 2014). Monitor for growth and development, signs of HIV-specific physical conditions, HIV disease progression, opportunistic infections, hepatitis, or pancreatitis.

Reference Range

Plasma trough concentration ≥20,500 ng/mL (based on data from treatment-experienced patient with resistant HIV-1 strains) (DHHS [adult, pediatric], 2014)

Dosage Forms

Excipient information presented when available (limited, particularly for generics); consult specific product labeling.

Capsule, Oral:

Aptivus: 250 mg

Solution, Oral:

Aptivus: 100 mg/mL (95 mL) [contains polyethylene glycol, propylene glycol, tocophersolan; buttermint-butter toffee flavor]

References

DHHS Panel on Antiretroviral Guidelines for Adults and Adolescents. Guidelines for the Use of Antiretroviral Agents in HIV-1-Infected Adults and Adolescents, Department of Health and Human Services. Updated May 1, 2014. Available at http://www.aidsinfo.nih.gov/ContentFiles/AdultandAdolescentGL.pdf.

DHHS Panel on Antiretroviral Therapy and Medical Management of HIV-Infected Children. Guidelines for the use of antiretroviral agents in pediatric HIV infection. February 12, 2014. Available at http://aidsinfo.nih.gov

DHHS Panel on Treatment of HIV-Infected Pregnant Women and Prevention of Perinatal Transmission. Recommendations for the use of antiretroviral drugs in pregnant HIV-1-infected women for maternal health and interventions to reduce perinatal HIV-1 transmission in the United States. March 28, 2014. Available at http://aidsinfo.nih.gov

Graff J, von Hentig N, Kuczka, K, et al. Significant effects of tipranavir on platelet aggregation and thromboxane B_2 formation *in vitro* and *in vivo*. J Antimicrob Chemother. 2008;61(2):394-399.

◆ **Tirosint** *see* Levothyroxine *on page 1234*

◆ **Titralac [OTC]** *see* Calcium Carbonate *on page 346*

◆ **Tivicay** *see* Dolutegravir *on page 705*

◆ **TIV (Trivalent Inactivated Influenza Vaccine)** *see* Influenza Virus Vaccine (Inactivated) *on page 1103*

◆ **TMC-114** *see* Darunavir *on page 595*

◆ **TMC125** *see* Etravirine *on page 819*

◆ **TMP** *see* Trimethoprim *on page 2087*

◆ **TMP-SMX** *see* Sulfamethoxazole and Trimethoprim *on page 1948*

◆ **TMP-SMZ** *see* Sulfamethoxazole and Trimethoprim *on page 1948*

◆ **TMZ** *see* Temozolomide *on page 1972*

◆ **TNG** *see* Nitroglycerin *on page 1504*

◆ **Tobi** *see* Tobramycin (Systemic, Oral Inhalation) *on page 2034*

◆ **TOBI (Can)** *see* Tobramycin (Systemic, Oral Inhalation) *on page 2034*

◆ **Tobi Podhaler** *see* Tobramycin (Systemic, Oral Inhalation) *on page 2034*

◆ **TOBI Podhaler (Can)** *see* Tobramycin (Systemic, Oral Inhalation) *on page 2034*

Tobramycin (Systemic, Oral Inhalation)
(toe bra MYE sin)

Medication Safety Issues
Sound-alike/look-alike issues:
Tobramycin may be confused with Trobicin, vancomycin

International issues:
Nebcin [Multiple international markets] may be confused with Naprosyn brand name for naproxen [U.S., Canada, and multiple international markets]; Nubain brand name for nalbuphine [Multiple international markets]

High alert medication:
The Institute for Safe Medication Practices (ISMP) includes this medication (intrathecal administration) among its list of drug classes which have a heightened risk of causing significant patient harm when used in error.

Brand Names: U.S. Bethkis; Tobi; Tobi Podhaler

Brand Names: Canada Apo-Tobramycin; JAMP-Tobramycin; TOBI; TOBI Podhaler; Tobramycin Injection, USP

Therapeutic Category Antibiotic, Aminoglycoside

Generic Availability (U.S.) May be product dependent

Use
Parenteral: Treatment of documented or suspected infections caused by susceptible gram-negative bacilli, including *Pseudomonas aeruginosa*; nonpseudomonal enteric bacillus infection which is more susceptible to tobramycin than gentamicin based on microbiology testing; susceptible organisms in lower respiratory tract infections (FDA approved in adults), serious central nervous system infection caused by susceptible organisms (FDA approved in adults), septicemia (FDA approved in all ages); intra-abdominal, skin, bone, soft tissue, and urinary tract infections (FDA approved in adults); has also been used for empiric therapy in cystic fibrosis and immunocompromised patients

Inhalation: Management of cystic fibrosis patients with *P. aeruginosa* (FDA approved in ages ≥6 years and adults)

Pregnancy Risk Factor D

Pregnancy Considerations [U.S. Boxed Warning]: Aminoglycosides may cause fetal harm if administered to a pregnant woman. There are several reports of total irreversible bilateral congenital deafness in children whose mothers received another aminoglycoside (streptomycin) during pregnancy; therefore, tobramycin is classified as pregnancy category D. Tobramycin crosses the placenta and produces detectable serum levels in the fetus. Although serious side effects to the fetus have not been reported following maternal use of tobramycin, a potential for harm exists.

Due to pregnancy-induced physiologic changes, some pharmacokinetic parameters of tobramycin may be altered. Pregnant women have an average-to-larger volume of distribution which may result in lower serum peak levels than for the same dose in nonpregnant women. Serum half-life is also shorter.

Breast-Feeding Considerations Tobramycin is excreted into breast milk and breast-feeding is not recommended by the manufacturer; however, tobramycin is not well absorbed when taken orally. This limited oral absorption may minimize exposure to the nursing infant. Nondose-related effects could include modification of bowel flora.

Contraindications Hypersensitivity to tobramycin, any component or other aminoglycosides

Warnings Aminoglycosides are associated with significant nephrotoxicity **[U.S. Boxed Warning]**. Neurotoxicity, manifested as vestibular and permanent bilateral auditory ototoxicity, can occur **[U.S. Boxed Warning]**; tinnitus or vertigo are indications of vestibular injury and impending bilateral irreversible deafness; early ototoxicity usually affects high-pitched sound. Risk of nephrotoxicity and ototoxicity is increased in patients with impaired renal function, dehydration, high-dose therapy, or prolonged therapy. Peak and trough serum concentrations of aminoglycosides should be monitored periodically during therapy to assure adequate levels and to avoid potentially toxic levels **[U.S. Boxed Warning]**. Ototoxicity is associated with high serum concentrations persisting for prolonged periods; nephrotoxicity is associated with high serum trough concentrations. Risk of nephrotoxicity increases when used concurrently with other potentially nephrotoxic drugs **[U.S. Boxed Warning]**; renal damage is usually reversible. Risk of ototoxicity increases with use of potent diuretics **[U.S. Boxed Warning]**. Prolonged use may result in fungal or bacterial superinfection, including *C. difficile*-associated diarrhea (CDAD) and pseudomembranous colitis; CDAD has been observed >2 months postantibiotic treatment. Aminoglycosides can cause fetal harm when administered to a pregnant woman **[U.S. Boxed Warning]**; aminoglycosides have been associated with several reports of total irreversible bilateral congenital deafness in pediatric patients exposed *in utero*. Use with caution in premature infants and neonates **[U.S. Boxed Warning]**; immature renal function may increase risk of accumulation and related toxicity. Some formulations contain sulfites which may cause allergic reactions in susceptible individuals. Not intended for long-term therapy due to toxic hazards associated with extended administration.

Inhalation: Transient tinnitus and hearing loss have been reported in tobramycin inhalation-treated patients; bronchospasm can occur with inhalation of tobramycin. Bronchospasm may occur with tobramycin inhalation;

bronchospasm or wheezing should be treated appropriately if either arise. Safety and efficacy have not been demonstrated in patients with FEV_1 <40% or >80% predicted (Bethkis, TOBI) or FEV_1 <25% or >80% predicted (TOBI Podhaler), in patients colonized with *Burkholderia cepacia*, or in patients <6 years of age.

Precautions Use with caution in patients with preexisting renal impairment; modify dosage in patients with renal impairment; monitor renal and eighth nerve function in patients with known or suspected renal impairment **[U.S. Boxed Warning]**. Use with caution in patients with auditory or vestibular impairment. Use with caution in patients with myasthenia gravis, hypocalcemia, and in conditions which depress neuromuscular transmission; may cause neuromuscular blockade and respiratory paralysis; risk increased with concomitant use of anesthesia or muscle relaxants. Use with caution in pediatric patients on extracorporeal membrane oxygenation (ECMO); pharmacokinetics of aminoglycosides may be altered; dosage adjustment and close monitoring necessary.

Cross-allergenicity with other aminoglycosides has been observed. Avoid intramuscular administration in paralyzed patients due to poor circulation in the atrophic muscles which may result in slower absorption and lower peak serum concentrations; use intravenous route.

With use of Tobi podhaler (oral capsule powder for inhalation), taste disturbance (dysgeusia) was reported more frequently in pediatric patients ≥6 years (7.4%) than adults (2.7%).

Adverse Reactions

Injection: Frequency not defined:

Central nervous system: Confusion, disorientation, dizziness, headache, lethargy, vertigo

Dermatologic: Exfoliative dermatitis, pruritus, skin rash, urticaria

Endocrine & metabolic: Decreased serum calcium, decreased serum magnesium, decreased serum potassium and/or decreased serum sodium, increased lactate dehydrogenase

Gastrointestinal: Diarrhea, nausea, vomiting

Genitourinary: Casts in urine, oliguria, proteinuria

Hematologic & oncologic: Anemia, eosinophilia, granulocytopenia, leukocytosis, leukopenia, thrombocytopenia

Hepatic: Increased serum ALT, increased serum AST, increased serum bilirubin

Local: Pain at injection site

Miscellaneous: Fever

Otic: Auditory ototoxicity, hearing loss, tinnitus, vestibular ototoxicity

Renal: Increased blood urea nitrogen, increased serum creatinine

Inhalation

Cardiovascular: Chest discomfort

Central nervous system: Headache, malaise, voice disorder

Dermatologic: Skin rash

Endocrine: Increased serum glucose

Gastrointestinal: Diarrhea, dysgeusia, nausea, vomiting, xerostomia

Hematologic & oncologic: Eosinophilia, increased erythrocyte sedimentation rate, increased serum immunoglobulins

Miscellaneous: Fever

Neuromuscular & skeletal: Musculoskeletal chest pain, myalgia

Otic: Deafness (including unilateral deafness, reported as mild to moderate hearing loss or increased hearing loss), hypoacusis, tinnitus

Respiratory: Bronchitis, bronchospasm, cough, discoloration of sputum, dyspnea, epistaxis, hemoptysis, laryngitis, nasal congestion, oropharyngeal pain, pharyngolaryngeal pain, productive cough, pulmonary disease (includes pulmonary or cystic fibrosis exacerbations), rales, reduced forced expiratory volume, respiratory depression, rhinitis, throat irritation, tonsillitis, upper respiratory tract infection, wheezing

Rare but important or life-threatening: Abnormal breath sounds, decreased exercise tolerance, decrease in forced vital capacity, hypersensitivity reaction, increased bronchial secretions, lower respiratory tract infection, obstructive pulmonary disease, oral candidiasis, pneumonitis, pruritus, pulmonary congestion, urticaria

Drug Interactions

Metabolism/Transport Effects None known.

Avoid Concomitant Use

Avoid concomitant use of Tobramycin (Systemic, Oral Inhalation) with any of the following: BCG; Mannitol

Increased Effect/Toxicity

Tobramycin (Systemic, Oral Inhalation) may increase the levels/effects of: AbobotulinumtoxinA; Bisphosphonate Derivatives; CARBOplatin; Colistimethate; CycloSPORINE (Systemic); Neuromuscular-Blocking Agents; OnabotulinumtoxinA; RimabotulinumtoxinB; Tenofovir

The levels/effects of Tobramycin (Systemic, Oral Inhalation) may be increased by: Amphotericin B; Capreomycin; Cephalosporins (2nd Generation); Cephalosporins (3rd Generation); Cephalosporins (4th Generation); CISplatin; Loop Diuretics; Mannitol; Nonsteroidal Anti-Inflammatory Agents; Tenofovir; Vancomycin

Decreased Effect

Tobramycin (Systemic, Oral Inhalation) may decrease the levels/effects of: BCG; Sodium Picosulfate; Typhoid Vaccine

The levels/effects of Tobramycin (Systemic, Oral Inhalation) may be decreased by: Penicillins

Stability

Injection:

Powder for injection: Store intact vials at 20°C to 25°C (68°F to 77°F). After reconstitution, solutions remain stable for 24 hours at room temperature and 96 hours when refrigerated.

Solution for injection: Store intact vials at 15°C to 30°C (59°F to 86°F).

Premixed solution (manufacturer premixed): Store at 20°C to 25°C (68°F to 77°F); protect from freezing.

Inhalation:

Powder for inhalation (TOBI podhaler): Store in original packaging at 25°C (77°F), excursions permitted to 15°C to 30°C (59°F to 86°F); protect from moisture.

Solution for inhalation (Bethkis, TOBI): Store at 2°C to 8°C (36°F to 46°F). May be stored in foil pouch at room temperature of 25°C (77°F) for up to 28 days. Avoid intense light. Do not use if cloudy or contains particles; a darkened yellow solution does not indicate loss of potency; incompatible with dornase alfa (may precipitate).

Mechanism of Action Interferes with bacterial protein synthesis by binding to 30S and 50S ribosomal subunits, resulting in a defective bacterial cell membrane

Pharmacodynamics Displays concentration-dependent killing; bacteriocidal

Pharmacokinetics (Adult data unless noted)

Absorption:

Oral: Poor

I.M.: Rapid and complete

Inhalation: Low systemic bioavailability; accumulation can occur in patients with a low glomerular filtration rate

Peak serum concentration following inhalation:

Solution for inhalation: ~1 mcg/mL following a 300 mg dose

Powder for inhalation: ~1 mcg/mL (range: 0.49-1.55 mcg/mL) following a 112 mg dose

Distribution: Distributes primarily in the extracellular fluid volume; poor penetration into the CSF; drug accumulates in the renal cortex; small amounts distribute into bile, sputum, saliva, and tears

V_d: Higher in neonates than older pediatric and adult patients; also increased in patients with edema, ascites, fluid overload; decreased in patients with dehydration

Systemic:
Neonates: 0.45 ± 0.1 L/kg
Infants: 0.4 ± 0.1 L/kg
Children: 0.35 ± 0.15 L/kg
Adolescents: 0.3 ± 0.1 L/kg
Adults: 0.2-0.3 L/kg

Inhalation: Tobramycin remains concentrated primarily in the airways

Protein binding: <30%

Half-life:
I.V.:
Neonates:
≤1200 g: 11 hours
>1200 g: 2-9 hours
Infants: 4 ± 1 hour
Children: 2 ± 1 hour
Adolescents: 1.5 ± 1 hour
Adults with normal renal function: 2-3 hours, directly dependent upon glomerular filtration rate; impaired renal function: 5-70 hours

Inhalation:
Bethkis: 4.4 hours
TOBI/TOBI podhaler: CF patients: 3 hours

Time to peak serum concentration:
I.M.: Within 30-90 minutes
I.V.: 30 minutes after a 30-minute infusion; **Note:** Distribution may be prolonged after larger doses. One study reported a 1.7-hour distribution period after a 60-minute, high-dose aminoglycoside infusion (Demczar, 1997).
Inhalation (TOBI podhaler): 60 minutes

Elimination: With normal renal function, 93% of dose excreted in urine within 24 hours

Dosing: Neonatal Note: Dosage should be based on actual weight unless the patient has hydrops fetalis. Dosage should be individualized based upon serum concentration monitoring.

General dosing; susceptible infection: Limited data available: I.V.: Dosing strategies may vary by institution as a wide variety of dosing regimens have been studied. Consider single-dose administration with serum concentration monitoring in patients with urine output <1 mL/kg/hour or serum creatinine >1.3 mg/dL rather than scheduled dosing. Consider prolongation of dosing interval when coadministered with ibuprofen or indomethacin or in neonates with history of the following: Birth depression, birth hypoxia/asphyxia, or cyanotic congenital heart disease. Some dosing based on gentamicin studies.

Age-directed dosing (de Hoog, 2002; DiCenzo, 2003; Hagen, 2009; Hansen, 2003; Ohler, 2000; Serane, 2009):
GA <32 weeks: 4-5 mg/kg/dose every 48 hours
GA 32-36 weeks: 4-5 mg/kg/dose every 36 hours
GA ≥37 weeks: 4-5 mg/kg/dose every 24 hours
Note: In some trials, a fixed interval of every 24 hours was used with dosages ranging from 2.5-4 mg/kg/dose based on GA (ie, lower doses were used for younger GA).

Weight-directed dosing (Red Book, 2012): I.M., I.V.:
Body weight <1 kg:
PNA ≤14 days: 5 mg/kg/dose every 48 hours
PNA 15-28 days: 4-5 mg/kg/dose every 24-48 hours
Body weight 1-2 kg:
PNA ≤7 days: 5 mg/kg/dose every 48 hours
PNA 8-28 days: 4-5 mg/kg/dose every 24-48 hours

Body weight >2 kg:
PNA ≤7 days: 4 mg/kg/dose every 24 hours
PNA 8-28 days: 4 mg/kg/dose every 12-24 hours

Dosing: Usual Note: Dosage should be based on an estimate of ideal body weight. Some dosing is based on gentamicin studies. In morbidly obese children, adolescents, and adults, dosage requirement may best be estimated using a dosing weight of IBW + 0.4 (TBW - IBW). Dosage should be individualized based upon serum concentration monitoring.

Infants, Children, and Adolescents:
General dosing, susceptible infection:
Conventional dosing: I.M., I.V.: 2.5 mg/kg/dose every 8 hours; some pediatric patients may require larger doses (ie, patients undergoing continuous hemofiltration, patients with major burns, febrile granulocytopenic patients); modify dose based on individual patient requirements as determined by renal function, serum drug concentrations, and patient-specific clinical parameters
Manufacturer's labeling: I.M., I.V.: 2-2.5 mg/kg/dose every 8 hours
Extended-interval dosing: I.V.:
Weight-directed: 4.5-7.5 mg/kg/dose every 24 hours (Contopoulos-Ioannidis, 2004; *Red Book*, 2012)
Age-directed: Based on data from 114 patients, the following has been suggested (McDade, 2010):
3 months to <2 years: 9.5 mg/kg/dose every 24 hours
2 to <8 years: 8.5 mg/kg/dose every 24 hours
≥8 years: 7 mg/kg/dose every 24 hours

Cystic fibrosis, pulmonary infection:
Conventional dosing: I.M., I.V.: 3.3 mg/kg/dose every 8 hours
Extended-interval dosing: I.V.: Initial: 10-12 mg/kg/dose every 24 hours (Flume, 2009; Smyth, 2005; Van Meter, 2009); **Note:** The CF Foundation recommends extended-interval dosing as preferred over conventional dosing.

Intra-abdominal infection, complicated: I.V.: 3-7.5 mg/kg/**day** divided every 8-24 hours (Solomkin, 2010)

CNS infection:
Meningitis (Tunkel, 2004):
Infants and Children: I.V.: 7.5 mg/kg/**day** divided every 8 hours
Adolescents: I.V.: 5 mg/kg/**day** divided every 8 hours
VP-shunt infection, ventriculitis: Limited data available: Intraventricular/intrathecal (**use a preservative-free preparation**): 5-20 mg/**day**

Peritonitis (CAPD) (Warady, 2012): Intraperitoneal: Continuous: Loading dose: 8 mg per liter of dialysate; maintenance dose: 4 mg per liter

Pulmonary infection: Inhalation:
Cystic fibrosis patients: Children ≥6 years and Adolescents:
Bethkis, TOBI: 300 mg every 12 hours; administer in repeated cycles of 28 days on drug, followed by 28 days off drug
TOBI Podhaler: 112 mg (4 x 28 mg capsules) every 12 hours; administer in repeated cycles of 28 days on drug followed by 28 days off drug
Noncystic fibrosis patients: Limited data available:
Note: Used by some centers; no published data are available): Children and Adolescents: 40-80 mg/dose 2-3 times daily

Urinary tract infection:
Traditional dosing: Infants and Children 2-24 months: I.V.: 5 mg/kg/**day** divided every 8 hours (AAP, 2011)

Extended-interval dosing: Limited data available: I.V.: Based on data from 179 patients, the following age-directed dosing has been suggested (Carapetis, 2001):
1 month to <5 years: 7.5 mg/kg/dose every 24 hours
5-10 years: 6 mg/kg/dose every 24 hours
>10 years: 4.5 mg/kg/dose every 24 hours
Adults: In underweight and nonobese patients, use of total body weight (TBW) instead of ideal body weight for determining the initial mg/kg/dose is widely accepted (Nicolau, 1995). Ideal body weight (IBW) also may be used to determine doses for patients who are neither underweight nor obese (Gilbert, 2009).

General dosing, susceptible infection:
Conventional: I.M., I.V.: 1-2.5 mg/kg/dose every 8-12 hours; to ensure adequate peak concentrations early in therapy, higher initial dosage may be considered in selected patients when extracellular water is increased (edema, septic shock, postsurgical, or trauma)
Once daily: I.V.: 4-7 mg/kg/dose once daily; some clinicians recommend this approach for all patients with normal renal function; this dose is at least as efficacious with similar, if not less, toxicity than conventional dosing

Cystic fibrosis: Inhalation:
Bethkis, TOBI: 300 mg every 12 hours (do not administer doses <6 hours apart); administer in repeated cycles of 28 days on drug followed by 28 days off drug
TOBI podhaler: 112 mg (4 x 28 mg capsules) every 12 hours (do not administer doses <6 hours apart); administer in repeated cycles of 28 days on drug followed by 28 days off drug

Dosage adjustment in renal impairment:
Inhalation: Children ≥6 years, Adolescents, and Adults: There are no dosage adjustments provided in manufacturer's labeling (has not been studied).
Parenteral:
Infants, Children, and Adolescents: I.M., I.V.:
The following adjustments have been recommended (Aronoff, 2007): **Note:** Renally adjusted dose recommendations are based on doses of 2.5 mg/kg/dose every 8 hours.
GFR >50 mL/minute/1.73 m^2: No adjustment required
GFR 30-50 mL/minute/1.73 m^2: Administer every 12-18 hours
GFR 10-29 mL/minute/1.73 m^2: Administer every 18-24 hours
GFR <10 mL/minute/1.73 m^2: Administer every 48-72 hours
Intermittent hemodialysis: Dialyzable (25% to 70%): 2 mg/kg/dose; redose as indicated by serum concentrations
Peritoneal dialysis (PD): 2 mg/kg/dose; redose as indicated by serum concentrations
Continuous renal replacement therapy (CRRT): 2-2.5 mg/kg/dose every 12-24 hours, monitor serum concentrations
Adults:
Conventional dosing: I.M., I.V.:
CrCl ≥60 mL/minute: Administer every 8 hours
CrCl 40-60 mL/minute: Administer every 12 hours
CrCl 20-40 mL/minute: Administer every 24 hours
CrCl 10-20 mL/minute: Administer every 48 hours
CrCl <10 mL/minute: Administer every 72 hours
High-dose therapy: I.V.: Interval may be extended (eg, every 48 hours) in patients with moderate renal impairment (CrCl 30-59 mL/minute) and/or adjusted based on serum concentration determinations.

Intermittent hemodialysis (IHD) (administer after hemodialysis on dialysis days) (Heintz, 2009): Dialyzable (25% to 75%; variable; dependent on filter, duration, and type of IHD); **Note:** Dosing dependent on the assumption of 3 times/week, complete IHD sessions: I.V.:
Loading dose of 2-3 mg/kg loading dose followed by:
Mild UTI or synergy: 1 mg/kg every 48-72 hours; consider redosing for pre-HD or post-HD serum concentrations <1 mcg/mL
Moderate to severe UTI: 1-1.5 mg/kg every 48-72 hours; consider redosing for pre-HD serum concentrations <1.5-2 mcg/mL or post-HD serum concentrations <1 mcg/mL
Systemic gram negative rod infection: 1.5-2 mg/kg every 48-72 hours; consider redosing for pre-HD concentrations <3-5 mcg/mL or post-HD serum concentrations <2 mcg/mL
Peritoneal dialysis (PD):
Administration via PD fluid:
Gram-positive infection (eg, synergy): 3-4 mg/L (3-4 mcg/mL) of PD fluid
Gram-negative infection: 4-8 mg/L (4-8 mcg/mL) of PD fluid
Administration via I.V., I.M. route during PD: Dose as for CrCl <10 mL/minute and follow serum concentrations
Continuous renal replacement therapy (CRRT) (Heintz, 2009; Trotman, 2005): Drug clearance is highly dependent on the method of renal replacement, filter type, and flow rate. Appropriate dosing requires close monitoring of pharmacologic response, signs of adverse reactions due to drug accumulation, as well as drug concentrations in relation to target trough (if appropriate). The following are general recommendations only (based on dialysate flow/ultrafiltration rates of 1-2 L/hour and minimal residual renal function) and should not supersede clinical judgment:
CVVH/CVVHD/CVVHDF: I.V.: Loading dose of 2-3 mg/kg followed by:
Mild UTI or synergy: I.V.: 1 mg/kg every 24-36 hours (redose when serum concentration <1 mcg/mL)
Moderate to severe UTI: I.V.: 1-1.5 mg/kg every 24-36 hours (redose when serum concentration <1.5-2 mcg/mL)
Systemic gram-negative infection: I.V.: 1.5-2.5 mg/kg every 24-48 hours (redose when serum concentration <3-5 mcg/mL)

Dosage adjustment in hepatic impairment:
Inhalation: Children ≥6 years, Adolescents, and Adults: No dosage adjustment necessary
Parenteral: Adults: I.M., I.V.: No dosage adjustment necessary

Administration
Inhalation: Doses should be administered as close to a 12-hour schedule as possible; do not administer less than 6 hours apart
Bethkis, Tobi: Use a PARI LC Plus reusable nebulizer and a PARI Vios air compressor (Bethkis) or a DeVilbiss Pulmo-Aide air compressor (Tobi) for administration; patient should be sitting or standing upright and breathing normally through the mouthpiece of the nebulizer. Nebulizer treatment period is usually over 15 minutes. If patient receiving multiple inhalation products, administer Bethkis or TOBI last.
TOBI Podhaler: Capsules should be administered by oral inhalation via Podhaler device following manufacturer recommendations for use and handling. Capsules should not be swallowed. Patients requiring bronchodilator therapy should administer the bronchodilator 15-90 minutes prior to TOBI Podhaler. The sequence of chest physiotherapy and additional inhaled therapies is at the ▶

discretion of the healthcare provider; however, TOBI Podhaler should always be administered last. Use the new podhaler device provided with each weekly pack.

Parenteral:

I.M.: Administer undiluted by deep I.M. route if possible. Slower absorption and lower peak concentrations, probably due to poor circulation in the atrophic muscle, may occur following I.M. injection in paralyzed patients, suggest I.V. route.

I.V.: Administer by slow intermittent infusion over 30-60 minutes (administer higher doses over 60 minutes) or by direct injection over 15 minutes; final I.V. concentration for administration should not exceed 10 mg/mL; administer beta-lactam antibiotics, such as penicillins and cephalosporins, at least 1 hour before or after tobramycin; simultaneous administration may result in reduced antibacterial efficacy

Monitoring Parameters Urinalysis, urine output, BUN, serum creatinine, peak and trough serum tobramycin concentrations; **Note:** Do not use fingerstick for obtaining blood sample in patients concurrently receiving inhaled tobramycin as it may result in falsely elevated drug concentrations); be alert to ototoxicity, audiograms

With conventional dosing, typically obtain serum concentration after the third dose; exceptions for earlier monitoring may include neonates, patients with rapidly changing renal function, or patients receiving extended-interval dosing. Not all pediatric patients who receive aminoglycosides require monitoring of serum aminoglycoside concentrations. Indications for use of aminoglycoside serum concentration monitoring include:

Treatment course >5 days

Patients with decreased or changing renal function

Patients with a poor therapeutic response

Neonates and Infants <3 months of age

Atypical body constituency (obesity, expanded extracellular fluid volume)

Clinical need for higher doses or shorter intervals (cystic fibrosis, burns, endocarditis, meningitis, relatively resistant organism)

Patients on hemodialysis or chronic ambulatory peritoneal dialysis

Signs of nephrotoxicity or ototoxicity

Concomitant use of other nephrotoxic agents

Patients on high-dose aerosolized tobramycin: The utility of monitoring serum concentrations in patients with renal impairment should be per clinician's discretion; serum concentrations achieved following inhalation are significantly less than those achieved following parenteral therapy in patients with normal renal function. Obtaining peak tobramycin concentration 1 hour following inhalation to identify patients who are significant absorbers, in patients with decreased glomerular filtration rate, in patients on concomitant parenteral therapy, and in infants have been recommended by some clinicians (Abdulhamid, 2008).

Reference Range

Traditional dosing: Timing of serum samples: Draw peak 30 minutes after 30-minute infusion has been completed or 1 hour following I.M. injection or beginning of infusion; draw trough immediately before next dose

Therapeutic concentrations:

Peak:

Serious infections: 6-8 mcg/mL (12-17 micromole/L)

Life-threatening infections: 8-10 mcg/mL (17-21 micromole/L)

Urinary tract infections: 4-6 mcg/mL

Synergy against gram-positive organisms: 3-5 mcg/mL

Trough:

Serious infections: 0.5-1 mcg/mL

Life-threatening infections: 1-2 mcg/mL

The American Thoracic Society (ATS) recommends trough levels of <1 mcg/mL for adult patients with hospital-acquired pneumonia.

Timing of serum samples: Draw peak 30 minutes after completion of 30-minute infusion or at 1 hour following initiation of infusion or I.M. injection; draw trough within 30 minutes prior to next dose; aminoglycoside levels measured from blood taken from Silastic® central catheters can sometimes give falsely elevated readings

Extended-interval: **Note:** Pediatric therapeutic monitoring protocols have not been standardized; peak values are 2-3 times greater with extended-interval dosing regimens compared to traditional dosing

Noncystic fibrosis patients: Consider monitoring tobramycin serum concentration 18-20 hours after the start of the infusion to ensure the drug-free interval does not exceed typical postantibiotic effect (PAE) duration

Cystic fibrosis patients: Clinically two methods are utilized. Peak: 25-35 mcg/mL (some centers use 20-30 mcg/mL); 18- to 20-hour value: Detectable but <1 mcg/mL; trough: Nondetectable

Method A: Obtain two serum concentrations at least 1 half-life apart after distribution is complete (eg, obtain a serum concentration 2 hours and 10 hours after the start of the infusion), calculate elimination rate and extrapolate a C_{max} and C_{min}

Method B: Obtain a peak serum concentration 60 minutes after a 60-minute infusion and a serum concentration 18-20 hours after the start of the infusion to ensure the drug-free interval does not exceed typical postantibiotic effect (PAE) duration (4-6 hours)

Test Interactions Some penicillin derivatives may accelerate the degradation of aminoglycosides *in vitro*, leading to a potential underestimation of aminoglycoside serum concentration.

Additional Information Some penicillins (eg, carbenicillin, ticarcillin, and piperacillin) have been shown to inactivate aminoglycosides *in vitro*. This has been observed to a greater extent with tobramycin and gentamicin, while amikacin has shown greater stability against inactivation. Concurrent use of these agents may pose a risk of reduced antibacterial efficacy *in vivo*, particularly in the setting of profound renal impairment; however, definitive clinical evidence is lacking. If combination penicillin/aminoglycoside therapy is desired in a patient with renal dysfunction, separation of doses (if feasible), and routine monitoring of aminoglycoside levels, CBC, and clinical response should be considered.

Dosage Forms Excipient information presented when available (limited, particularly for generics); consult specific product labeling.

Capsule, Inhalation:

Tobi Podhaler: 28 mg

Nebulization Solution, Inhalation [preservative free]:

Bethkis: 300 mg/4 mL (4 mL)

Tobi: 300 mg/5 mL (5 mL) [contains sodium chloride, sodium hydroxide, sulfuric acid]

Generic: 300 mg/5 mL (5 mL)

Solution, Injection:

Generic: 10 mg/mL (2 mL); 80 mg/2 mL (2 mL); 1.2 g/30 mL (30 mL); 2 g/50 mL (50 mL)

Solution, Intravenous:

Generic: 80 mg (100 mL)

Solution Reconstituted, Injection:

Generic: 1.2 g (1 ea)

Solution Reconstituted, Injection [preservative free]:

Generic: 1.2 g (1 ea)

References

Abdulhamid I, Wise TL, Andrews S, et al, "Elevated Serum Tobramycin Concentrations After Treatment With Tobramycin Inhalation in a Preterm Infant," *Pharmacotherapy*, 2008, 28(7):939-44.

American Academy of Pediatrics, Subcommittee on Urinary Tract Infection, Steering Committee on Quality Improvement and Management, Roberts KB. Urinary tract infection: clinical practice guideline for the diagnosis and management of the initial UTI in febrile infants and children 2 to 24 months. *Pediatrics.* 2011;128(3):595-610.

Aronoff GR, Bennett WM, Berns JS, et al, *Drug Prescribing in Renal Failure: Dosing Guidelines for Adults and Children*, 5th ed, Philadelphia, PA: American College of Physicians, 2007.

Bartel K, Habash T, Lugauer S, et al, "Optimal Tobramycin Dosage in Patients With Cystic Fibrosis – Evidence for Predictability Based on Previous Drug Monitoring," *Infection*, 1999, 27(4-5):268-71.

Carapetis JR, Jaquiery AL, Buttery JP, et al, "Randomized, Controlled Trial Comparing Once Daily and Three Times Daily Gentamicin in Children With Urinary Tract Infections," *Pediatr Infect Dis J*, 2001, 20 (3):240-6.

Contopoulos-Ioannidis DG, Giotis ND, Baliatsa DV, et al, "Extended-Interval Aminoglycoside Administration for Children: A Meta-Analysis," *Pediatrics*, 2004, 114(1):e111-8.

de Hoog M, Mouton JW, Schoemaker RC, et al, "Extended-Interval Dosing of Tobramycin in Neonates: Implications for Therapeutic Drug Monitoring," *Clin Pharmacol Ther*, 2002, 71(5):349-58.

Demczar DJ, Nafziger AN, and Bertino JS Jr, "Pharmacokinetics of Gentamicin at Traditional Versus High Doses: Implications for Once-Daily Aminoglycoside Dosing," *Antimicrob Agents Chemother*, 1997, 41(5):1115-9.

DiCenzo R, Forrest A, Slish JC, et al, "A Gentamicin Pharmacokinetic Population Model and Once-Daily Dosing Algorithm for Neonates," *Pharmacotherapy*, 2003, 23(5):585-91.

Flume PA, Mogayzel PJ Jr, Robinson KA, et al, "Cystic Fibrosis Pulmonary Guidelines: Treatment of Pulmonary Exacerbations," *Am J Respir Crit Care Med*, 2009, 180(9):802-8.

Mandell GL, Bennett JE, Dolin R, eds, *Aminoglycosides. Mandell, Douglas, and Bennett's Principles and Practice of Infectious Diseases*. 7th ed. Chapter 26. Philadelphia, PA: Churchill Linvingstone Elsevier; 2009.

Gilbert DN, "Once-Daily Aminoglycoside Therapy," *Antimicrob Agents Chemother*, 1991, 35(3):399-405.

Green TP, Mirkin BL, Peterson PK, et al, "Tobramycin Serum Level Monitoring in Young Patients With Normal Renal Function," *Clin Pharmacokinet*, 1984, 9(5):457-68.

Hagen I and Øymar K, "Pharmacological Differences Between Once Daily and Twice Daily Gentamicin Dosage in Newborns With Suspected Sepsis," *Pharm World Sci*, 2009, 31(1):18-23.

Hansen A, Forbes P, Arnold A, et al, "Once-Daily Gentamicin Dosing for the Preterm and Term Newborn: Proposal for a Simple Regimen That Achieves Target Levels," *J Perinatol*, 2003, 23(8):635-9.

Heintz BH, Matzke GR, and Dager WE, "Antimicrobial Dosing Concepts and Recommendations for Critically Ill Adult Patients Receiving Continuous Renal Replacement Therapy or Intermittent Hemodialysis," *Pharmacotherapy*, 2009, 29(5):562-77.

Knoderer CA, Everett JA, and Buss WF, "Clinical Issues Surrounding Once-Daily Aminoglycoside Dosing in Children," *Pharmacotherapy*, 2003, 23(1):44-56.

Kraus DM, Pai MP, and Rodvold KA, "Efficacy and Tolerability of Extended-Interval Aminoglycoside Administration in Pediatric Patients," *Paediatr Drugs*, 2002, 4(7):469-84.

Massie J and Cranswick N, "Pharmacokinetic Profile of Once Daily Intravenous Tobramycin in Children With Cystic Fibrosis," *J Paediatr Child Health*, 2006, 42(10):601-5.

McDade EJ, Wagner JL, Moffett BS, et al, "Once-Daily Gentamicin Dosing in Pediatric Patients Without Cystic Fibrosis," *Pharmacotherapy*, 2010, 30(3):248-53.

Mouton JW, Jacobs N, Tiddens H, et al, "Pharmacodynamics of Tobramycin in Patients With Cystic Fibrosis," *Diagn Microbiol Infect Dis*, 2005, 52(2):123-7.

Nahata MC, Powell DA, Durrell DE, et al, "Effect of Gestational Age and Birth Weight on Tobramycin Kinetics in Newborn Infants," *J Antimicrob Chemother*, 1984, 14(1):59-65.

Nicolau DP, Freeman OD, Belliveau PP, et al. Experience with a once-daily aminoglycoside program administered to 2184 adult patients. *Antimicrob Agents Chemother*. 1995;39(3):650-655.

Ohler KH, Menke JA, and Fuller L, "Use of Higher Dose Extended Interval Aminoglycosides in a Neonatal Intensive Care Unit," *Am J Perinatol*, 2000, 17(6):285-90.

Ramsey BW, Pepe MS, Quan JM, et al, "Intermittent Administration of Inhaled Tobramycin in Patients With Cystic Fibrosis. Cystic Fibrosis Inhaled Tobramycin Study Group," *N Engl J Med*, 1999, 340(1):23-30.

Red Book: 2012 Report of the Committee on Infectious Diseases, 29th ed, Pickering LK, ed, Elk Grove Village, IL: American Academy of Pediatrics, 2012, 808-16.

Redmann S, Wainwright C, Stacey S, et al, "Misleading High Tobramycin Plasma Concentrations Can Be Caused by Skin Contamination of Fingerprick Blood Following Inhalation of Nebulized Tobramycin (TOBI): A Short Report," *Ther Drug Monit*, 2005, 27(2):205-7.

Serane TV, Zengeya S, Penford G, et al, "Once Daily Dose Gentamicin in Neonates - Is Our Dosing Correct?" *Acta Paediatr*, 2009, 98 (7):1100-5.

Shaw PK, Braun TL, Liebergen A, et al, "Aerosolized Tobramycin Pharmacokinetics in Cystic Fibrosis Patients," *J Pediatr Pharm Pract*, 1997, 2(1):23-6.

Smyth A, Tan KH, Hyman-Taylor P, et al, "Once Versus Three-Times Daily Regimens of Tobramycin Treatment for Pulmonary Exacerbations of Cystic Fibrosis – The TOPIC Study: A Randomised Controlled Trial," *Lancet*, 2005, 365(9459):573-8.

Solomkin JS, Mazuski JE, Bradley JS, et al, "Diagnosis and Management of Complicated Intra-Abdominal Infections in Adults and Children: Guidelines by the Surgical Infection Society and the Infectious Diseases Society of America," *Clin Infect Dis*, 2010, 50(2):133-64.

Trotman RL, Williamson JC, Shoemaker DM, et al, "Antibiotic Dosing in Critically Ill Adult Patients Receiving Continuous Renal Replacement Therapy," *Clin Infect Dis*, 2005, 41(8):1159-66.

Van Meter DJ, Corriveau M, Ahern JW, et al, "A Survey of Once-Daily Dosage Tobramycin Therapy in Patients With Cystic Fibrosis," *Pediatr Pulmonol*, 2009, 44(4):325-9.

Warady BA, Bakkaloglu S, Newland J, et al, "Consensus Guidelines for the Prevention and Treatment of Catheter-Related Infections and Peritonitis in Pediatric Patients Receiving Peritoneal Dialysis: 2012 Update," *Perit Dial Int*, 2012, (32 Suppl 2):S32-86.

Tobramycin (Ophthalmic) (toe bra MYE sin)

Medication Safety Issues

Sound-alike/look-alike issues:

Tobramycin may be confused with Trobicin®, vancomycin

Tobrex® may be confused with TobraDex®

Brand Names: U.S. Tobrex

Brand Names: Canada PMS-Tobramycin; Sandoz-Tobramycin; Tobrex®

Therapeutic Category Antibiotic, Aminoglycoside; Antibiotic, Ophthalmic

Generic Availability (U.S.) May be product dependent

Use Used topically to treat superficial ophthalmic infections caused by susceptible bacteria

Pregnancy Risk Factor B

Pregnancy Considerations Adverse events were not observed following systemic administration of tobramycin in animal reproduction studies; therefore, tobramycin ophthalmic is classified as pregnancy category B. When administered I.M. or I.V., tobramycin crosses the placenta. Refer to the Tobramycin (Systemic) monograph for details. The amount of tobramycin available systemically following topical application of the ophthalmic drops is undetectable (<0.2 mcg/mL). Systemic absorption would be required in order for tobramycin ophthalmic to cross the placenta and reach the fetus.

Breast-Feeding Considerations Due to undetectable (<0.2 mcg/mL) systemic absorption of tobramycin ophthalmic drops, excretion of tobramycin into breast milk would not be expected; however, because of the potential for adverse events in a nursing infant, breast-feeding is not recommended by the manufacturer. When administered I.M. or I.V., tobramycin is detected in breast milk. Refer to the Tobramycin (Systemic) monograph for details.

Contraindications Hypersensitivity to tobramycin or any component

Adverse Reactions Rare but important or life-threatening: Conjunctival erythema, lid itching, lid swelling

Drug Interactions

Metabolism/Transport Effects None known.

Avoid Concomitant Use There are no known interactions where it is recommended to avoid concomitant use.

Increased Effect/Toxicity There are no known significant interactions involving an increase in effect.

Decreased Effect There are no known significant interactions involving a decrease in effect.

Mechanism of Action Interferes with bacterial protein synthesis by binding to 30S and 50S ribosomal subunits resulting in a defective bacterial cell membrane

Dosing: Usual

Children ≥2 months and Adults:

Ointment: Apply 0.5" ribbon into the affected eye 2-3 times/day; for severe infections, apply ointment every 3-4 hours

Solution:

Mild to moderate infections: Instill 1-2 drops every 4 hours

Severe infections: Instill 2 drops every 30-60 minutes initially, then reduce to less frequent intervals

Administration Avoid contact of tube or bottle tip with skin or eye; apply finger pressure to lacrimal sac during and for 1-2 minutes after instillation of drops to decrease risk of absorption and systemic effects.

Dosage Forms Excipient information presented when available (limited, particularly for generics); consult specific product labeling.

Ointment, Ophthalmic:

Tobrex: 0.3% (3.5 g)

Solution, Ophthalmic:

Tobrex: 0.3% (5 mL)

Generic: 0.3% (5 mL)

◆ **Tobramycin Injection, USP (Can)** see Tobramycin (Systemic, Oral Inhalation) on page 2034

◆ **Tobramycin Sulfate** see Tobramycin (Ophthalmic) on page 2039

◆ **Tobramycin Sulfate** see Tobramycin (Systemic, Oral Inhalation) on page 2034

◆ **Tobrex** see Tobramycin (Ophthalmic) on page 2039

◆ **Tobrex® (Can)** see Tobramycin (Ophthalmic) on page 2039

Tocilizumab (toe si LIZ oo mab)

Brand Names: U.S. Actemra

Brand Names: Canada Actemra

Therapeutic Category Antirheumatic, Disease Modifying; Interleukin-6 Receptor Antagonist; Monoclonal Antibody

Generic Availability (U.S.) No

Use Treatment of active systemic juvenile idiopathic arthritis (SJIA) (FDA approved in ages ≥2 years); treatment of active polyarticular juvenile idiopathic arthritis (PJIA) (FDA approved in ages ≥2 years); treatment of moderately- to severely-active rheumatoid arthritis in patients who have had an inadequate response to one or more disease-modifying antirheumatic drugs (DMARDs) (FDA approved in adults)

Medication Guide Available Yes

Pregnancy Risk Factor C

Pregnancy Considerations Adverse events have been observed in some animal reproduction studies. Monoclonal antibodies cross the placenta, with the largest amount transferred during the third trimester. A pregnancy registry has been established to monitor outcomes of women exposed to tocilizumab during pregnancy (877-311-8972).

Breast-Feeding Considerations It is not known if tocilizumab is excreted in human milk. Because many immunoglobulins are excreted in human milk and the potential for serious adverse reactions exists, a decision should be made whether to discontinue nursing or to discontinue the drug, taking into account the importance of the drug to the mother.

Contraindications Hypersensitivity to tocilizumab or any component

Warnings

Serious and potentially fatal infections have been reported with use **[U.S. Boxed Warning]**; reported infections include tuberculosis (TB), bacterial, viral, and protozoal infections, invasive fungal infections, and infections due to other opportunistic pathogens (eg, mycobacterial infection, pneumocystis); patients should be monitored closely for signs and symptoms of infection during and after treatment. Tocilizumab therapy should be interrupted if a patient develops a serious infection, opportunistic infection, or sepsis during treatment until the infection is controlled **[U.S. Boxed Warning]**. Patients frequently present with disseminated disease rather than localized disease and concomitant immunosuppressive therapy (eg, methotrexate or corticosteroids) is often present. The most common serious infections occurring have included pneumonia, UTI, cellulitis, herpes zoster, gastroenteritis, diverticulitis, sepsis, and bacterial arthritis. Do not initiate therapy in patients who have an active or localized infection. Consider the risks and benefits of therapy in patients with the following: A chronic or recurrent infection, exposure to tuberculosis, a history of an opportunistic infection, lived in or traveled to areas where tuberculosis or mycoses are endemic, or predisposing underlying conditions. Concomitant use with other biological DMARDs (eg, TNF blockers, IL-1 receptor blockers, anti-CD20 monoclonal antibodies, selective costimulation modulators) should be avoided due to the increased risk of infection.

Tuberculosis, both reactivation and new infection, has been reported in patients receiving tocilizumab. Perform test for latent TB before use **[U.S. Boxed Warning]**; if positive (induration >5 mm, regardless if previously vaccinated with BCG), initiate treatment for latent TB prior to starting tocilizumab; consider antituberculosis treatment for patients with history of latent or active TB in which complete course of therapy cannot be confirmed or those with risk factors for TB despite testing negative for latent TB. Monitor all patients for active TB during treatment, even if initial latent TB test is negative **[U.S. Boxed Warning]**, particularly those with close contact to a person with active TB or recent travel to an endemic area.

Neutropenia and thrombocytopenia may occur with tocilizumab therapy; dosage adjustment, interruption of therapy, or discontinuation may be required. Therapy should not be initiated in patients with an ANC <2000/mm^3; treatment should be discontinued in patients who develop an ANC <500/mm^3. Therapy should not be initiated in patients with a platelet count <100,000/mm^3; treatment should be discontinued in patients who develop a platelet count <50,000/mm^3.

Tocilizumab may cause liver enzyme abnormalities; therapy should not be initiated in patients with ALT or AST >1.5 times the upper limit of normal (ULN). Tocilizumab is not recommended in patients with active hepatic disease or hepatic impairment. If AST or ALT rise significantly during therapy, dosage and/or therapy adjustment may be necessary; treatment should be discontinued in patients who develop elevated ALT or AST >5 x ULN. Patients receiving concomitant hepatotoxic drugs (eg, methotrexate) are at an increased risk of developing elevated transaminases; elevations are typically reversible and do not result in clinically evident hepatic injury.

Potentially significant interactions may exist, requiring dose or frequency adjustment, additional monitoring, and/or selection of alternative therapy. Consult drug interactions database for more detailed information. Use of tocilizumab may affect defenses against malignancies; impact on the development and course of malignancies is not fully defined; however, malignancies were observed in clinical trials. May cause hypersensitivity, anaphylaxis, or anaphylactoid reactions; permanently discontinue treatment in patients who develop a hypersensitivity reaction to tocilizumab; medications for the treatment of hypersensitivity reactions should be available for immediate use. Patients should seek medical attention if symptoms of hypersensitivity reaction occur with subcutaneous use. Stop immediately and permanently discontinue treatment in patients who develop a hypersensitivity reaction. In clinical studies, reactions requiring treatment discontinuation included generalized erythema, rash, and urticaria.

Injection contains polysorbate 80 (Tween 80®) which may cause allergic reactions in susceptible individuals. Infusion of polysorbate 80-containing solutions through polyvinyl chloride tubing may cause DEHP to leach into the solution; in immature animals, exposure to DEHP may adversely affect the development of the male reproductive tract.

Precautions Use with caution in patients with preexisting or recent onset central or peripheral nervous system demyelinating disorders; rare cases of new-onset or exacerbation of demyelinating disorders (eg, multiple sclerosis, Guillain-Barré syndrome) have been reported; consider discontinuing use in patients who develop peripheral or central nervous system demyelinating disorders during treatment. Therapy is associated with increases in total cholesterol, triglycerides, LDL, and/or HDL; monitor ~4-8 weeks after initiation, then approximately every 6 months; hyperlipidemia should be managed according to current guidelines. Use with caution in patients with a history of herpes zoster; exacerbations have been reported. Use with caution in patients at increased risk for gastrointestinal perforation; perforation has been reported, typically secondary to diverticulitis; monitor for new-onset abdominal symptoms; promptly evaluate if new symptoms occur. Patients should be brought up to date with all immunizations before initiating therapy; live vaccines should not be given concurrently; there is no data available concerning secondary transmission of infection from live vaccines in patients receiving therapy.

Adverse Reactions As reported for monotherapy, except where noted. Combination therapy refers to use in rheumatoid arthritis with nonbiological DMARDs or use in SJIA or PJIA in trials where most patients (~70% to 80%) were taking methotrexate at baseline.
Cardiovascular: Hypertension, peripheral edema
Central nervous system: Dizziness, headache
Dermatologic: Dermatological reaction (combination therapy; includes pruritus, urticaria), skin rash
Endocrine & metabolic: Hypothyroidism, increased LDL cholesterol (>1.5-2 x ULN; combination therapy; children and adolescents), increased serum cholesterol (>240 mg/dL; >1.5-2 x ULN; combination therapy; children and adolescents)
Gastrointestinal: Abdominal pain, diarrhea (children and adolescents), gastric ulcer, gastritis, oral mucosa ulcer, stomatitis, weight gain
Hematologic & oncologic: Leukopenia, neutropenia (combination therapy), thrombocytopenia (combination therapy)
Hepatic: Increased serum ALT, increased serum AST, increased serum bilirubin
Immunologic: Antibody development
Infection: Herpes simplex infection
Local: Injection site reaction (SubQ: Including erythema, pruritus, pain, and hematoma)
Ophthalmic: Conjunctivitis
Renal: Nephrolithiasis
Respiratory: Bronchitis, cough, dyspnea, nasopharyngitis, upper respiratory tract infection
Miscellaneous: Infusion-related reaction (combination therapy)
Rare but important or life-threatening: Anaphylaxis, anaphylactoid reaction, angioedema, aspergillosis, candidiasis, cellulitis, chronic inflammatory demyelinating polyneuropathy, cryptococcosis, diverticulitis, gastroenteritis, gastrointestinal perforation, herpes zoster, hypersensitivity, hypersensitivity pneumonitis, hypertriglyceridemia, hypotension, increased HDL cholesterol, malignant neoplasm (including breast and colon cancer), multiple sclerosis, otitis media, pneumonia, pneumocystosis, reactivation of latent Epstein-Barr virus, septic arthritis, sepsis, tuberculosis, urinary tract infection, varicella

Drug Interactions
Metabolism/Transport Effects None known.
Avoid Concomitant Use
Avoid concomitant use of Tocilizumab with any of the following: Abatacept; Anti-TNF Agents; BCG; Belimumab; Natalizumab; Pimecrolimus; Tacrolimus (Topical); Tofacitinib; Vaccines (Live)
Increased Effect/Toxicity
Tocilizumab may increase the levels/effects of: Abatacept; Anti-TNF Agents; Belimumab; Leflunomide; Natalizumab; Tofacitinib; Vaccines (Live)

The levels/effects of Tocilizumab may be increased by: Abciximab; Denosumab; Pimecrolimus; Roflumilast; Tacrolimus (Topical); Trastuzumab
Decreased Effect
Tocilizumab may decrease the levels/effects of: BCG; Coccidioidin Skin Test; CYP3A4 Substrates; Sipuleucel-T; Vaccines (Inactivated); Vaccines (Live)

The levels/effects of Tocilizumab may be decreased by: Echinacea
Stability Store intact vials at 2°C to 8°C (36°F to 46°F); do not freeze. Protect from light. Diluted solutions may be stored under refrigeration or at room temperature for up to 24 hours and are compatible with polypropylene, polyethylene (PE), polyvinyl chloride (PVC), and glass infusion containers. To mix the solution, gently invert the bag to avoid foaming; diluted solution should reach room temperature prior to administration.
Mechanism of Action Antagonist of the interleukin-6 (IL-6) receptor. Endogenous IL-6 is induced by inflammatory stimuli and mediates a variety of immunological responses. Inhibition of IL-6 receptors by tocilizumab leads to a reduction in cytokine and acute phase reactant production.
Pharmacokinetics (Adult data unless noted)
Distribution: V_{dss}: Children: 2.54 L (SJIA), 4.08 L (PJIA); Adults: 6.4 L
Bioavailability: SubQ: 80%
Half-life elimination:
I.V.: Terminal, single dose: 6.3 days (concentration-dependent); may be increased at steady state up to: Children: 16 days (PJIA), 23 days (SJIA); Adults: 13 days
SubQ: Concentration dependent: Adults: Up to 5 days (every other week dosing) or 13 days (every week dosing)
Dosing: Usual Note: Do not initiate if ANC is <2000/mm³, platelets are <100,000/mm³ or if ALT or AST are >1.5 times ULN.
Pediatric: **Note:** Dose adjustment should not be made based solely on a single-visit body weight measurement due to fluctuations in body weight. May be used as monotherapy or in combination with methotrexate.
Polyarticular juvenile idiopathic arthritis (PJIA): Children ≥2 years and Adolescents:
<30 kg: I.V.: 10 mg/kg every 4 weeks
≥30 kg: I.V.: 8 mg/kg every 4 weeks; maximum single dose: 800 mg
Systemic juvenile idiopathic arthritis (SJIA): Children ≥2 years and Adolescents:
<30 kg: I.V.: 12 mg/kg/dose every 2 weeks
≥30 kg: I.V.: 8 mg/kg/dose every 2 weeks; maximum single dose: 800 mg
Adult: **Rheumatoid arthritis: Note:** Methotrexate or other *nonbiologic* disease-modifying antirheumatic drugs (DMARDs) may be continued for the treatment of rheumatoid arthritis. Tocilizumab should not be used in combination with *biologic* DMARDs.
I.V.: Initial: 4 mg/kg/dose every 4 weeks; may be increased to 8 mg/kg/dose based on clinical response; maximum single dose: 800 mg

SubQ:
<100 kg: 162 mg every other week; increase to every week based on clinical response
≥100 kg: 162 mg every week
Transitioning from I.V. therapy to SubQ therapy: Administer the first SubQ dose instead of the next scheduled I.V. dose.

Dosing adjustment in renal impairment: Children ≥2 years, Adolescents, and Adults:
Mild renal impairment: No dosage adjustment required.
Moderate to severe renal impairment: There are no dosage adjustments provided in the manufacturer labeling (not studied).

Dosing adjustment in hepatic impairment: Children ≥2 years, Adolescents, and Adults: There are no dosage adjustments provided in the manufacturer's labeling (not studied); not recommended for use in patients with active hepatic disease or hepatic impairment.

Dosing adjustment for toxicity:
Children ≥2 years and Adolescents: Polyarticular and systemic juvenile idiopathic arthritis (SJIA): Dose reductions have not been studied; however, dose interruptions are recommended for liver enzyme abnormalities, low neutrophil counts, and low platelets similar to recommendations provided for adult rheumatoid arthritis patients (see below). In addition, consider interrupting or discontinuing concomitant methotrexate and/or other medications and hold tocilizumab dosing until the clinical situation has been assessed.

Adults: Rheumatoid arthritis (RA):
Liver enzyme abnormalities:
>1 to 3 x ULN: For persistent increases in this range, reduce I.V. tocilizumab dose to 4 mg/kg or SubQ therapy to every other week or interrupt therapy until ALT/AST have normalized; adjust concomitant DMARDs as appropriate
>3 to 5 x ULN (confirm with repeat testing): Interrupt tocilizumab therapy until ALT/AST <3 x ULN, then resume tocilizumab I.V. dose at 4 mg/kg or resume SubQ therapy at every other week. For persistent increases in this range, discontinue therapy
>5 x ULN: Discontinue therapy
Low absolute neutrophil counts (ANC):
ANC >1000 cells/mm³: Maintain dose
ANC 500-1000 cells/mm³: Interrupt therapy; when ANC >1000 cells/mm³, resume tocilizumab I.V. dose at 4 mg/kg or resume SubQ therapy at every other week dosing; may increase I.V. dose to 8 mg/kg or SubQ therapy to every week as clinically appropriate
ANC <500 cells/mm³: Discontinue therapy
Low platelet counts:
Platelets 50,000-100,000 cells/mm³: Interrupt therapy; when platelet count is >100,000 cells/mm³, resume tocilizumab I.V. dose at 4 mg/kg or resume SubQ therapy at every other week dosing; may increase I.V. dose to 8 mg/kg or SubQ therapy to every week as clinically appropriate
Platelets <50,000 cells/mm³: Discontinue therapy

Administration
Intravenous: Do not use prefilled subcutaneous syringes to prepare I.V. infusions. Further dilute dose in NS: Children <30 kg: Use 50 mL infusion bag or bottle; or Children ≥30 kg, Adolescents, and Adults: Use 100 mL infusion bag or bottle. Allow diluted solution to reach room temperature prior to administration; infuse over 60 minutes using a dedicated I.V. line. Do not administer I.V. push or I.V. bolus. Do not use if opaque particles or discoloration are visible.
Subcutaneous: Adults: Administer the full amount in the prefilled syringe. Allow to reach room temperature prior to use. Do not use if particulate matter or discoloration is visible; solution should be clear and colorless to pale yellow. Rotate injection sites; avoid injecting into moles,

scars, or tender, bruised, red, or hard skin. Prefilled syringe is available for use by patients (self-administration).

Monitoring Parameters Latent TB screening prior to therapy initiation; neutrophils, platelets, ALT/AST (prior to therapy, 4-8 weeks after start of therapy, and every 3 months thereafter [RA]); neutrophils, platelets, ALT/AST (prior to therapy, at second infusion, and every 2-4 weeks [SJIA] or 4-8 weeks [PJIA] thereafter); additional liver function tests (eg, bilirubin) as clinically indicated; lipid panel (prior to, at 4-8 weeks following initiation, and every ~6 months during therapy); signs and symptoms of infection (prior to, during, and after therapy); signs and symptoms of CNS demyelinating disorder.

The following lab schedule has been used in patients with SJIA: 1-2 weeks, and 1, 2, 6, and 9 months: CBC with differential, C-reactive protein, erythrocyte sedimentation rate, ferritin, and LDH (Dewitt, 2012).

Dosage Forms Excipient information presented when available (limited, particularly for generics); consult specific product labeling.
Solution, Intravenous [preservative free]:
Actemra: 80 mg/4 mL (4 mL); 200 mg/10 mL (10 mL); 400 mg/20 mL (20 mL) [contains polysorbate 80]
Solution Prefilled Syringe, Subcutaneous [preservative free]:
Actemra: 162 mg/0.9 mL (0.9 mL) [contains polysorbate 80]

References
DeWitt EM, Kimura Y, Beukelman T, et al, "Consensus Treatment Plans for New-Onset Systemic Juvenile Idiopathic Arthritis," *Arthritis Care Res (Hoboken)*, 2012, 64(7):1001-10.
Imagawa T, Yokota S, Mori M, et al. Safety and efficacy of tocilizumab, an anti-IL-6-receptor monoclonal antibody, in patients with polyarticular-course juvenile idiopathic arthritis. *Mod Rheumatol.* 2012;22(1):109-115.

◆ **Tofranil** *see* Imipramine *on page 1080*

◆ **Tofranil-PM** *see* Imipramine *on page 1080*

◆ **Tolectin** *see* Tolmetin *on page 2042*

Tolmetin (TOLE met in)

Medication Safety Issues
Sound-alike/look-alike issues:
Tolmetin may be confused wit tolcapone
BEERS Criteria medication:
This drug may be potentially inappropriate for use in geriatric patients (Quality of evidence - moderate; Strength of recommendation - strong).

Therapeutic Category Analgesic, Non-narcotic; Nonsteroidal Anti-inflammatory Drug (NSAID), Oral

Generic Availability (U.S.) Yes

Use Treatment of inflammatory and rheumatoid disorders, including juvenile idiopathic arthritis

Medication Guide Available Yes

Pregnancy Risk Factor C

Pregnancy Considerations Adverse events were not observed in the initial animal reproduction studies; therefore, the manufacturer classifies tolmetin as pregnancy category C. NSAID exposure during the first trimester is not strongly associated with congenital malformations; however, cardiovascular anomalies and cleft palate have been observed following NSAID exposure in some studies. The use of an NSAID close to conception may be associated with an increased risk of miscarriage. Nonteratogenic effects have been observed following NSAID administration during the third trimester including myocardial degenerative changes, prenatal constriction of the ductus arteriosus, fetal tricuspid regurgitation, failure of the ductus arteriosus to close postnatally; renal dysfunction or failure, oligohydramnios; gastrointestinal bleeding or perforation, increased risk of necrotizing enterocolitis; intracranial bleeding (including intraventricular hemorrhage), platelet dysfunction with resultant bleeding; pulmonary hypertension. Because they may cause premature closure of the ductus arteriosus, use of NSAIDs late in pregnancy should be avoided (use after 31 or 32 weeks gestation is not recommended by some clinicians). The chronic use of NSAIDs in women of reproductive age may be associated with infertility that is reversible upon discontinuation of the medication.

Breast-Feeding Considerations Tolmetin is found in breast milk and breast-feeding is not recommended by the manufacturer.

Contraindications Hypersensitivity to tolmetin or any component; history of asthma, urticaria, or allergic-type reaction to aspirin, or other NSAIDs; patients with the "aspirin triad" [asthma, rhinitis (with or without nasal polyps), and aspirin intolerance] (fatal asthmatic and anaphylactoid reactions may occur in these patients); perioperative pain in the setting of coronary artery bypass graft (CABG)

Warnings NSAIDs are associated with an increased risk of adverse cardiovascular thrombotic events, including potentially fatal MI and stroke **[U.S. Boxed Warning]**; risk may be increased with duration of use or preexisting cardiovascular risk factors or disease; carefully evaluate cardiovascular risk profile prior to prescribing; use the lowest effective dose for the shortest duration of time, taking into consideration individual patient treatment goals; alternate therapies should be considered for patients at high risk. Use is contraindicated for treatment of perioperative pain in the setting of CABG surgery **[U.S. Boxed Warning]**; an increased incidence of MI and stroke was found in patients receiving COX-2 selective NSAIDs for the treatment of pain within the first 10-14 days after CABG surgery. NSAIDs may cause fluid retention, edema, and new onset or worsening of preexisting hypertension; use with caution in patients with hypertension, CHF, or fluid retention. Concurrent administration of ibuprofen and potentially other nonselective NSAIDs may interfere with aspirin's cardioprotective effect.

NSAIDs may increase the risk of gastrointestinal inflammation, ulceration, bleeding, and perforation **[U.S. Boxed Warning]**. These events, which can be potentially fatal, may occur at any time during therapy and without warning. Avoid the use of NSAIDs in patients with active GI bleeding or ulcer disease. Use NSAIDs with extreme caution in patients with a history of GI bleeding or ulcers (these patients have a 10-fold increased risk for developing a GI bleed). Use NSAIDs with caution in patients with other risk factors which may increase GI bleeding (eg, concurrent therapy with aspirin, anticoagulants, and/or corticosteroids, longer duration of NSAID use, smoking, use of alcohol, and poor general health). Use the lowest effective dose for the shortest duration of time, taking into consideration individual patient treatment goals; alternate therapies should be considered for patients at high risk

NSAIDs may compromise existing renal function. Renal toxicity may occur in patients with impaired renal function, dehydration, heart failure, liver dysfunction, those taking diuretics and ACE inhibitors; use with caution in these patients; monitor renal function closely. NSAIDs are not recommended for use in patients with advanced renal disease. Long-term use of NSAIDs may cause renal papillary necrosis and other renal injury. Rare cases of severe hepatic reactions (eg, fulminant hepatitis, liver failure) have occurred with NSAID use; closely monitor patients with any abnormal LFT; discontinue if signs or symptoms of liver disease develop or if systemic manifestations occur

Fatal asthmatic and anaphylactoid reactions may occur in patients with the "aspirin triad" who receive NSAIDs. NSAIDs may cause serious dermatologic adverse reactions including exfoliative dermatitis, Stevens-Johnson syndrome, and toxic epidermal necrolysis. Avoid use of NSAIDs in late pregnancy as they may cause premature closure of the ductus arteriosus.

Precautions Use with caution in patients with upper GI disease, impaired renal function, CHF, hypertension, and patients receiving anticoagulants; although rare, anaphylactoid reactions occur more commonly with tolmetin than other NSAIDs

Adverse Reactions

Cardiovascular: Chest pain, hypertension, edema

Central nervous system: Depression, dizziness, drowsiness, headache

Dermatologic: Skin irritation

Endocrine & metabolic: Weight gain/loss

Gastrointestinal: Abdominal pain, constipation, diarrhea, flatulence, gastritis, heartburn, nausea, peptic ulcer, vomiting

Genitourinary: Urinary tract infection

Hematologic: Hemoglobin/hematocrit decreases (transient)

Neuromuscular & skeletal: Weakness

Ocular: Visual disturbances

Otic: Tinnitus

Renal: BUN increased

Rare but important or life-threatening: Agranulocytosis, anaphylactoid reactions, CHF, dysuria, epistaxis, erythema multiforme, exfoliative dermatitis, fever, fluid retention, GI bleeding, GI perforation, glossitis, granulocytopenia, hematuria, hemolytic anemia, hepatic failure, hepatic necrosis, hepatitis, hepatitis (fulminant), interstitial nephritis, jaundice, liver function tests (abnormal), lymphadenopathy, macular changes, nephrotic syndrome, optic neuropathy, proteinuria, purpura, renal failure, retinal changes, serum sickness, stomatitis, Stevens-Johnson syndrome, thrombocytopenia, toxic epidermal necrolysis, urticaria

Drug Interactions

Metabolism/Transport Effects None known.

Avoid Concomitant Use

Avoid concomitant use of Tolmetin with any of the following: Floctafenine; Ketorolac (Nasal); Ketorolac (Systemic); NSAID (COX-2 Inhibitor); Omacetaxine; Urokinase

Increased Effect/Toxicity

Tolmetin may increase the levels/effects of: 5-ASA Derivatives; Agents with Antiplatelet Properties; Aliskiren; Aminoglycosides; Anticoagulants; Apixaban; Bisphosphonate Derivatives; Collagenase (Systemic); CycloSPORINE (Systemic); Dabigatran Etexilate; Deferasirox; Desmopressin; Digoxin; Eplerenone; Haloperidol; Ibritumomab; Lithium; Methotrexate; Nonsteroidal Anti-Inflammatory Agents; NSAID (COX-2 Inhibitor); Omacetaxine; PEMEtrexed; Porfimer; Potassium-Sparing Diuretics; PRALAtrexate; Quinolone Antibiotics; Rivaroxaban; Salicylates; Tenofovir; Thrombolytic Agents; Tositumomab and Iodine I 131 Tositumomab; Urokinase; Vancomycin; Vitamin K Antagonists

The levels/effects of Tolmetin may be increased by: ACE Inhibitors; Angiotensin II Receptor Blockers; Antidepressants (Tricyclic, Tertiary Amine); Corticosteroids (Systemic); CycloSPORINE (Systemic); Dasatinib; Floctafenine; Glucosamine; Herbs (Anticoagulant/Antiplatelet Properties); Ibrutinib; Ketorolac (Nasal); Ketorolac (Systemic); Multivitamins/Fluoride (with ADE); Multivitamins/Minerals (with ADEK, Folate, Iron); Multivitamins/Minerals (with AE, No Iron); Omega-3 Fatty Acids; Pentosan Polysulfate Sodium; Pentoxifylline; Probenecid; Prostacyclin Analogues; Selective Serotonin

Reuptake Inhibitors; Serotonin/Norepinephrine Reuptake Inhibitors; Sodium Phosphates; Tipranavir; Treprostinil; Vitamin E

Decreased Effect

Tolmetin may decrease the levels/effects of: ACE Inhibitors; Agents with Antiplatelet Properties; Aliskiren; Angiotensin II Receptor Blockers; Beta-Blockers; Eplerenone; HydrALAZINE; Loop Diuretics; Potassium-Sparing Diuretics; Prostaglandins (Ophthalmic); Salicylates; Selective Serotonin Reuptake Inhibitors; Thiazide Diuretics

The levels/effects of Tolmetin may be decreased by: Bile Acid Sequestrants; Salicylates

Food Interactions Tolmetin peak serum concentrations may be decreased if taken with food or milk. Management: May be administered with antacids to decrease GI upset.

Mechanism of Action Reversibly inhibits cyclooxygenase-1 and 2 (COX-1 and 2) enzymes, which results in decreased formation of prostaglandin precursors; has antipyretic, analgesic, and anti-inflammatory properties.

Other proposed mechanisms not fully elucidated (and possibly contributing to the anti-inflammatory effect to varying degrees) include inhibiting chemotaxis, altering lymphocyte activity, inhibiting neutrophil aggregation/activation, and decreasing proinflammatory cytokine levels.

Pharmacokinetics (Adult data unless noted)

Absorption: Oral: Well absorbed

Protein binding: 99%

Metabolism: In the liver via oxidation and conjugation

Half-life, elimination: 5 hours

Time to peak serum concentration: Within 30-60 minutes

Elimination: Excreted in the urine as metabolites or conjugates

Dosing: Usual Oral:

Children ≥2 years:

Anti-inflammatory: Initial: 20 mg/kg/day in 3-4 divided doses, then 15-30 mg/kg/day in 3-4 divided doses; maximum dose: 30 mg/kg/day in 4 divided doses; do not exceed 1800 mg/day

Analgesic: 5-7 mg/kg/dose every 6-8 hours

Adults: 400 mg 3 times/day; usual dose: 600 mg to 1.8 g/day; maximum dose: 2 g/day

Administration Oral: May administer with food, milk, or antacids to decrease GI adverse effects

Monitoring Parameters CBC with differential, liver enzymes, occult blood loss, BUN, serum creatinine; periodic ophthalmologic exams

Test Interactions Increased protein, bleeding time; may interfere with urine detection of cannabinoids (false-positive)

Dosage Forms Excipient information presented when available (limited, particularly for generics); consult specific product labeling.

Capsule, Oral:

Generic: 400 mg

Tablet, Oral:

Generic: 200 mg, 600 mg

References

Berde C, Ablin A, Glazer J, et al, "American Academy of Pediatrics Report of the Subcommittee on Disease-Related Pain in Childhood Cancer," *Pediatrics*, 1990, 86(5 Pt 2):818-25.

Giannini EH and Cawkwell GD, "Drug Treatment in Children With Juvenile Rheumatoid Arthritis. Past, Present, and Future," *Pediatr Clin North Am*, 1995, 42(5):1099-125.

Hollingworth P, "The Use of Non-Steroidal Anti-inflammatory Drugs in Paediatric Rheumatic Diseases," *Br J Rheumatol*, 1993, 32(1):73-7.

Rose CD and Doughty RA, "Pharmacological Management of Juvenile Rheumatoid Arthritis," *Drugs*, 1992, 43(6):849-63.

◆ **Tolmetin Sodium** *see* Tolmetin *on page 2042*

Tolnaftate (tole NAF tate)

Medication Safety Issues

Sound-alike/look-alike issues:

Tinactin® may be confused with Talacen

Brand Names: U.S. Anti-Fungal [OTC]; Antifungal [OTC]; Athletes Foot Spray [OTC]; Dr Gs Clear Nail [OTC]; FungiGuard [OTC]; Fungoid-D [OTC]; Jock Itch Spray [OTC]; LamISIL AF Defense [OTC]; Medi-First Anti-Fungal [OTC]; Mycocide Clinical NS [OTC]; Podactin [OTC]; Tinactin Deodorant [OTC]; Tinactin Jock Itch [OTC]; Tinactin [OTC]; Tinaspore [OTC]; Tolnaftate Antifungal [OTC]

Brand Names: Canada Pitrex

Therapeutic Category Antifungal Agent, Topical

Generic Availability (U.S.) Yes

Use Treatment of tinea pedis, tinea cruris, tinea corporis, tinea manuum caused by *Trichophyton rubrum*, *T. mentagrophytes*, *T. tonsurans*, *M. canis*, *M. audouinii*, and *E. floccosum*; also effective in the treatment of tinea versicolor infections due to *Malassezia furfur*

Contraindications Hypersensitivity to tolnaftate or any component; nail and scalp infections

Adverse Reactions

Dermatologic: Contact dermatitis, pruritus

Local: Irritation, stinging

Drug Interactions

Metabolism/Transport Effects None known.

Avoid Concomitant Use There are no known interactions where it is recommended to avoid concomitant use.

Increased Effect/Toxicity There are no known significant interactions involving an increase in effect.

Decreased Effect There are no known significant interactions involving a decrease in effect.

Mechanism of Action Distorts the hyphae and stunts mycelial growth in susceptible fungi

Pharmacodynamics Onset of action: Response may be seen 24-72 hours after initiation of therapy

Dosing: Usual Children and Adults: Topical: Spray aerosol or apply 1-3 drops of solution or a small amount of cream or powder and rub into the affected areas 2-3 times/day for 2-4 weeks

Administration Topical: Wash and dry affected area before drug application; avoid contact with eyes

Monitoring Parameters Resolution of skin infection

Additional Information Usually not effective alone for the treatment of infections involving hair follicles or nails

Dosage Forms Excipient information presented when available (limited, particularly for generics); consult specific product labeling.

Aerosol, External:

Athletes Foot Spray: 1% (150 g) [contains sd alcohol 40]

Aerosol Powder, External:

Jock Itch Spray: 1% (130 g) [contains sd alcohol 40b]

LamISIL AF Defense: 1% (133 g)

Tinactin: 1% (133 g)

Tinactin Deodorant: 1% (133 g)

Cream, External:

Antifungal: 1% (15 g) [odorless]

Fungi-Guard: 1% (15 g)

Fungoid-D: 1% (113 g) [contains cetyl alcohol, methylparaben, propylene glycol, propylparaben, trolamine (triethanolamine)]

Medi-First Anti-Fungal: 1% (1 ea)

Tinactin: 1% (15 g, 30 g)

Tinactin Jock Itch: 1% (15 g)

Tolnaftate Antifungal: 1% (114 g) [contains cetyl alcohol, methylparaben, polysorbate 80, propylene glycol, propylparaben]

Generic: 1% (15 g, 20 g, 28.3 g, 30 g)

Powder, External:

Anti-Fungal: 1% (45 g)

LamISIL AF Defense: 1% (113 g)
Podactin: 1% (45 g)
Tinactin: 1% (108 g)
Generic: 1% (45 g)
Solution, External:
Dr Gs Clear Nail: 1% (18 mL) [contains propylene glycol]
Mycocide Clinical NS: 1% (30 mL) [contains propylene glycol]
Tinaspore: 1% (10 mL)
Generic: 1% (10 mL)

◆ **Tolnaftate Antifungal [OTC]** *see* Tolnaftate *on page 2044*

◆ **Toloxin (Can)** *see* Digoxin *on page 658*

Tolterodine (tole TER oh deen)

Medication Safety Issues
Sound-alike/look-alike issues:
Tolterodine may be confused with fesoterodine, tolcapone

Detrol® may be confused with Ditropan
BEERS Criteria medication:
This drug may be potentially inappropriate for use in geriatric patients (Quality of evidence - varies based on comorbidity; Strength of recommendation - varies based on comorbidity)

Related Information
Oral Medications That Should Not Be Crushed or Altered *on page 2438*

Brand Names: U.S. Detrol; Detrol LA
Brand Names: Canada Detrol®; Detrol® LA; Unidet®
Therapeutic Category Anticholinergic Agent
Generic Availability (U.S.) Yes
Use Treatment of patients with an overactive bladder with symptoms of urinary frequency, urgency, or urge incontinence

Pregnancy Risk Factor C
Pregnancy Considerations Teratogenic effects were observed in some animal reproduction studies.
Breast-Feeding Considerations It is not known if tolterodine is excreted in breast milk. Due to the potential for serious adverse reactions in the nursing infant, a decision should be made whether to discontinue nursing or to discontinue the drug, taking into account the importance of treatment to the mother.
Contraindications Hypersensitivity to tolterodine or fesoterodine (both are metabolized to 5-hydroxymethyl tolterodine) or any component; urinary retention; gastric retention; uncontrolled narrow-angle glaucoma
Warnings May cause drowsiness and/or blurred vision, which may impair physical or mental abilities; patients must be cautioned about performing tasks which require mental alertness (eg, operating machinery or driving). Cases of angioedema have been reported with oral tolterodine; some cases have occurred after a single dose. Discontinue immediately if develops. Has been associated with QT$_c$ prolongation at high (supratherapeutic) doses. The manufacturer recommends caution in patients with congenital prolonged QT or in patients receiving concurrent therapy with QT$_c$-prolonging drugs (class IA or III antiarrhythmics). However, the extent of QT$_c$ prolongation even at supratherapeutic dosages was <15 msec. Individuals who are poor metabolizers via CYP2D6 or in the presence of inhibitors of CYP2D6 and CYP3A4 may be more likely to exhibit prolongation.

Dosage adjustment is recommended in patients receiving CYP3A4 inhibitors; a lower dose of tolterodine is recommended. Also see QT prolongation in "Concerns related to adverse effects" above.

Precautions Use with caution in patients with bladder flow obstruction; may increase the risk of urinary retention. Use with caution in patients with gastrointestinal obstructive disorders (ie, pyloric stenosis); may increase the risk of gastric retention. Use with caution in patients with myasthenia gravis. Use with caution in patients with controlled (treated) narrow-angle glaucoma, hepatic impairment (dosage adjustment is required), and renal impairment (dosage adjustment is required).

Adverse Reactions
Cardiovascular: Chest pain
Central nervous system: Anxiety, dizziness, fatigue, headache, somnolence
Dermatologic: Dry skin
Gastrointestinal: Dry mouth
Gastrointestinal: Abdominal pain, constipation, diarrhea, dyspepsia, weight gain
Genitourinary: Dysuria
Neuromuscular & skeletal: Arthralgia
Ocular: Abnormal vision, dry eyes
Respiratory: Bronchitis, sinusitis
Miscellaneous: Flu-like syndrome, infection
Rare but important or life-threatening: Anaphylaxis, angioedema, confusion, dementia aggravated, disorientation, hallucinations, memory impairment, palpitation, peripheral edema, QT$_c$ prolongation, tachycardia

Drug Interactions
Metabolism/Transport Effects Substrate of CYP2C19 (minor), CYP2C9 (minor), CYP2D6 (major), CYP3A4 (major); **Note:** Assignment of Major/Minor substrate status based on clinically relevant drug interaction potential

Avoid Concomitant Use
Avoid concomitant use of Tolterodine with any of the following: Aclidinium; Conivaptan; Fusidic Acid (Systemic); Ipratropium (Oral Inhalation); Potassium Chloride; Tiotropium; Umeclidinium

Increased Effect/Toxicity
Tolterodine may increase the levels/effects of: AbobotulinumtoxinA; Analgesics (Opioid); Anticholinergic Agents; Cannabinoid-Containing Products; Highest Risk QTc-Prolonging Agents; Mirabegron; Moderate Risk QTc-Prolonging Agents; OnabotulinumtoxinA; Potassium Chloride; RimabotulinumtoxinB; Thiazide Diuretics; Tiotropium; Topiramate; Warfarin

The levels/effects of Tolterodine may be increased by: Abiraterone Acetate; Aclidinium; Antifungal Agents (Azole Derivatives, Systemic); Ceritinib; Conivaptan; CYP2D6 Inhibitors (Moderate); CYP2D6 Inhibitors (Strong); CYP3A4 Inhibitors (Moderate); CYP3A4 Inhibitors (Strong); Dasatinib; Fluconazole; Fusidic Acid (Systemic); Ipratropium (Oral Inhalation); Ivacaftor; Luliconazole; Mifepristone; Pramlintide; Simeprevir; Stiripentol; Umeclidinium; VinBLAStine

Decreased Effect
Tolterodine may decrease the levels/effects of: Acetylcholinesterase Inhibitors (Central); Secretin

The levels/effects of Tolterodine may be decreased by: Acetylcholinesterase Inhibitors (Central); Bosentan; CYP3A4 Inducers (Strong); Dabrafenib; Deferasirox; Mitotane; Peginterferon Alfa-2b; Siltuximab; St Johns Wort; Tocilizumab

Food Interactions Food increases bioavailability (~53% increase) of tolterodine tablets (dose adjustment not necessary); does not affect the pharmacokinetics of tolterodine extended release capsules. As a CYP3A4 inhibitor, grapefruit juice may increase the serum level and/or toxicity of tolterodine, but unlikely secondary to high oral bioavailability. Management: Monitor patients closely with concurrent grapefruit juice use.

Stability Store at 15°C to 30°C (59°F to 86°F); protect from light.

Mechanism of Action Tolterodine is a competitive antagonist of muscarinic receptors. In animal models, tolterodine demonstrates selectivity for urinary bladder receptors over salivary receptors. Urinary bladder contraction is mediated by muscarinic receptors. Tolterodine increases residual urine volume and decreases detrusor muscle pressure.

Pharmacokinetics (Adult data unless noted)
Absorption: Immediate release tablet: Rapid; ≥77%
Distribution: I.V.: V_d: Adults: 113 ± 27 L
Protein binding: >96% (primarily bound to alpha$_1$-acid glycoprotein)
Metabolism: Extensively hepatic, primarily via CYP2D6 (some metabolites share activity) and CYP3A4 usually (minor pathway). In patients with a genetic deficiency of CYP2D6, metabolism via CYP3A4 predominates. Forms three active metabolites.
Half-life elimination:
Immediate release tablet: Extensive metabolizers: ~2 hours; poor metabolizers: ~10 hours
Extended release capsule: Extensive metabolizers: ~7 hours; poor metabolizers: ~18 hours
Time to peak serum concentration:
Immediate release tablet: 1-2 hours
Extended release capsule: 2-6 hours
Excretion: Urine (77%); feces (17%); excreted primarily as metabolites (<1% unchanged drug) of which the active 5-hydroxymethyl metabolite accounts for 5% to 14% (<1% in poor metabolizers)

Dosing: Usual Oral: Adults: Treatment of overactive bladder:
Immediate release tablet: 2 mg twice daily; the dose may be lowered to 1 mg twice daily based on individual response and tolerability
Dosing adjustment in patients concurrently taking strong CYP3A4 inhibitors (eg, ketoconazole, clarithromycin, ritonavir): 1 mg twice daily
Extended release capsule: 4 mg once daily; dose may be lowered to 2 mg once daily based on individual response and tolerability
Dosing adjustment in patients concurrently taking strong CYP3A4 inhibitors (eg, ketoconazole, clarithromycin, ritonavir): 2 mg once daily

Dosing adjustment in renal impairment:
Immediate release tablet: Significantly reduced renal function (studies conducted in patients with CrCl 10-30 mL/minute): 1 mg twice daily; use with caution
Extended release capsule:
CrCl 10-30 mL/minute: 2 mg once daily
CrCl <10 mL/minute: Use is not recommended; has not been studied

Dosing adjustment in hepatic impairment:
Immediate release tablet: Significantly reduced hepatic function: 1 mg twice daily; use with caution
Extended release capsule:
Mild to moderate impairment (Child-Pugh class A or B): 2 mg once daily
Severe impairment (Child-Pugh class C): Use is not recommended; has not been studied

Administration Oral: Administer without regard to food; do not break, crush, or chew extended release capsules.

Dosage Forms Excipient information presented when available (limited, particularly for generics); consult specific product labeling.
Capsule Extended Release 24 Hour, Oral, as tartrate:
Detrol LA: 2 mg, 4 mg
Generic: 2 mg, 4 mg
Tablet, Oral, as tartrate:
Detrol: 1 mg, 2 mg
Generic: 1 mg, 2 mg

◆ **Tolterodine Tartrate** see Tolterodine on page 2045

◆ **Tomoxetine** see AtoMOXetine on page 224
◆ **TootSweet™ [OTC]** see Sucrose on page 1941
◆ **Topactin (Can)** see Fluocinonide on page 894
◆ **Topamax** see Topiramate on page 2046
◆ **Topamax Sprinkle** see Topiramate on page 2046
◆ **Topex Topical Anesthetic** see Benzocaine on page 273
◆ **Topicaine [OTC]** see Lidocaine (Topical) on page 1242
◆ **Topicaine 5 [OTC]** see Lidocaine (Topical) on page 1242
◆ **Topiragen** see Topiramate on page 2046

Topiramate (toe PYRE a mate)

Medication Safety Issues
Sound-alike/look-alike issues:
Topamax may be confused with Sporanox, TEGretol, TEGretol-XR, Toprol-XL

Administration issues
Bioequivalence has not been demonstrated between Trokendi XR and Qudexy XR.
Qudexy XR capsules may be opened to sprinkle the entire contents on a small amount (~1 teaspoon) of soft food. Do not open and sprinkle Trokendi XR capsules on food, chew, or crush; doing so may disrupt the triphasic release properties.
Avoid alcohol use with Trokendi XR within 6 hours prior to and 6 hours after administration; concurrent use may result in dose dumping.

Related Information
Oral Medications That Should Not Be Crushed or Altered on page 2438

Brand Names: U.S. Qudexy XR; Topamax; Topamax Sprinkle; Topiragen; Trokendi XR

Brand Names: Canada Apo-Topiramate; AURO-Topiramate; AVA-Topiramate; CO Topiramate; Dom-Topiramate; GD-Topiramate; Mint-Topiramate; Mylan-Topiramate; PHL-Topiramate; PMS-Topiramate; PRO-Topiramate; Q-Topiramate; RAN-Topiramate; Sandoz-Topiramate; TEVA-Topiramate; Topamax; ZYM-Topiramate

Therapeutic Category Anticonvulsant, Miscellaneous

Generic Availability (U.S.) May be product dependent

Use Oral:
Immediate release: Topamax: Initial monotherapy of primary generalized tonic-clonic seizures or partial onset seizures (FDA approved in ages ≥2 years and adults); adjunctive treatment of primary generalized tonic-clonic seizures or partial onset seizures (FDA approved in ages ≥2 years and adults); adjunctive treatment of seizures associated with Lennox-Gastaut syndrome (FDA approved in ages ≥2 years); prophylaxis of migraine headache (FDA approved in ages ≥12 years and adults); has also been used for infantile spasms
Extended release: Trokendi XR: Initial monotherapy of primary generalized tonic-clonic seizures or partial onset seizures (FDA approved in ages ≥10 years and adults); adjunctive treatment of primary generalized tonic-clonic seizures or partial onset seizures (FDA approved in ages ≥6 years and adults); adjunctive treatment of seizures associated with Lennox-Gastaut syndrome (FDA approved in ages ≥6 years)

Medication Guide Available Yes

Pregnancy Risk Factor D

Pregnancy Considerations Adverse events have been observed in animal reproduction studies. Based on limited data (n=5), topiramate was found to cross the placenta and could be detected in neonatal serum (Ohman, 2002). Topiramate may cause fetal harm if administered to a pregnant woman. An increased risk of oral clefts (cleft lip and/or palate) has been observed following first trimester exposure. Data from the North American Antiepileptic Drug (NAAED) Pregnancy Registry reported that the prevalence of oral clefts was 1.2% for infants exposed to topiramate during the first trimester of pregnancy, versus 0.39% to 0.46% for infants exposed to other antiepileptic drugs and 0.12% with no exposure. Although not evaluated during pregnancy, metabolic acidosis may be induced by topiramate. In general, metabolic acidosis during pregnancy may result in adverse effects and fetal death. Pregnant women and their newborns should be monitored for metabolic acidosis. Maternal serum concentrations may decrease during the second and third trimesters of pregnancy therefore therapeutic drug monitoring should be considered in pregnant women who require therapy (Ohman, 2009; Westin, 2009).

Use for migraine prophylaxis is contraindicated per the Canadian labeling in pregnant women or women of childbearing potential who are not using effective contraception.

Patients exposed to topiramate during pregnancy are encouraged to enroll themselves into the AED Pregnancy Registry by calling 1-888-233-2334. Additional information is available at www.aedpregnancyregistry.org.

Breast-Feeding Considerations Topiramate is excreted into breast milk. Based on information from five nursing infants, infant plasma concentrations of topiramate have been reported as 10% to 20% of the maternal plasma concentration. The manufacturer recommends that caution be used if administered to a nursing woman.

Contraindications Hypersensitivity to topiramate or any component

Additional product-specific contraindications: Trokendi XR: Recent alcohol use (ie, within 6 hours prior to and 6 hours after administration); patients with metabolic acidosis who are taking concomitant metformin

Warnings Hyperchloremic metabolic acidosis may occur in patients receiving topiramate; decreases in serum bicarbonate are relatively common (up to 67% of epilepsy patients and 77% of migraine patients); usually a mild to moderate decrease in serum bicarbonate concentrations (average decrease of 4 mEq/L at dose of 400 mg/day in adults and 6 mg/kg/day in children) and are due to inhibition of carbonic anhydrase and increased renal bicarbonate loss. Bicarbonate loss may be severe (serum bicarbonate <10 mEq/L) in rare cases. In pediatric clinical trials for adjunctive treatment of seizures, persistent decreases in serum bicarbonate occurred in 67% of patients receiving topiramate (versus 10% of those receiving placebo). Markedly low serum bicarbonate values were reported in 11% of pediatric patients receiving topiramate (versus 0% of those receiving placebo). In pediatric monotherapy trials, persistent decreases in serum bicarbonate occurred in 9% of patients receiving 50 mg/day and 25% of patients receiving 400 mg/day. Markedly low serum bicarbonate values were reported in 1% to 6% of pediatric patients receiving topiramate monotherapy. The risk of topiramate-induced metabolic acidosis may be increased in patients with predisposing conditions (eg, diarrhea, status epilepticus, hepatic impairment, renal dysfunction, severe respiratory disorders, ketogenic diet, surgery) or concurrent treatment with other drugs that may cause acidosis. Metabolic acidosis may be more common and more severe in infants and children <2 years of age with up to 45% of patients receiving 25 mg/kg/day developing metabolic acidosis in clinical trials. Monitor for potential complications of chronic acidosis including nephrolithiasis, nephrocalcinosis, osteomalacia/osteoporosis, and reduction in growth rates (including weight). Reductions in Z scores (from baseline) for length, weight, and head circumference were observed in infants and toddlers who received long-term topiramate (for up to 1 year) for intractable partial epilepsy; reductions in Z scores for length and weight correlated to the severity of metabolic acidosis.

Serum bicarbonate should be monitored at baseline and periodically during topiramate therapy. Patients should also be monitored for symptoms of metabolic acidosis (eg, hyperventilation, fatigue, anorexia, stupor, cardiac arrhythmias). Dose reduction or discontinuation (by tapering the dose) should be considered in patients with persistent or severe metabolic acidosis. If treatment is continued, alkali supplementation should be considered.

An ocular syndrome (characterized by secondary acute angle closure glaucoma and acute myopia) has been reported in adult and pediatric patients. Symptoms generally occur within 1 month of treatment initiation and include an acute decrease in visual acuity and/or ocular pain. Ophthalmologic findings may include increased IOP, anterior chamber shallowing, ocular hyperemia, mydriasis, and supracilliary effusion with anterior displacement of lens and iris. Patients experiencing blurred vision and/or eye pain should contact their physician immediately. Primary treatment of this syndrome is discontinuation of topiramate as soon as possible, based on physician judgment. If left untreated, this syndrome may cause serious damage to the eye, including permanent vision loss. Visual field defects have been reported independent of increased intraocular pressure; generally reversible upon discontinuation; consider discontinuation if visual problems occur at any time during treatment.

Rare, but significant, reports of oligohydrosis (decreased sweating) and hyperthermia have occurred in patients receiving topiramate. Most cases occurred in children, and were associated with vigorous exercise and/or high environmental temperatures. Due to the potential for serious sequelae, the use of preventative strategies (hydration before and during exercise or exposure to warm temperatures) is recommended. Monitor patients, especially pediatric patients, for decreased sweating and hyperthermia, especially in warm or hot weather. Use topiramate with caution in patients receiving drugs that predispose to heat-related disorders (eg, anticholinergic agents, carbonic anhydrase inhibitors).

Do not abruptly discontinue therapy in patients with or without a history of epilepsy or seizures; withdraw gradually to lessen the chance for seizures or increased seizure frequency; in pediatric epilepsy clinical trials, doses were gradually withdrawn over 2-8 weeks; in adult trials, daily doses were decreased in weekly intervals by 50-100 mg in epilepsy patients and by 25-50 mg in adult patients with migraines; monitor patients carefully if rapid withdrawal of topiramate is medically required.

CNS adverse effects are common. Cognitive dysfunction (confusion, psychomotor slowing, difficulty with concentration/attention, difficulty with memory, speech or language problems), psychiatric disturbances (depression or mood disorders), and sedation (somnolence or fatigue) may occur with use; incidence may be related to rapid titration and higher doses; patients must be cautioned about performing tasks which require mental alertness (eg, operating machinery or driving). Paresthesia (usually tingling of extremities) may occur; avoid use with alcohol, CNS depressants, or carbonic anhydrase inhibitors. May also cause dizziness and ataxia. The most common adverse effects of topiramate observed in children include the following: Anorexia, cognitive problems, dizziness, fatigue, fever, flushing, headache, mood problems, paresthesia, somnolence, and weight loss; neuropsychiatric and cognitive adverse effects were reported with a lower incidence in children than adults.

Hyperammonemia with or without encephalopathy has been reported with topiramate monotherapy or when topiramate was used concurrently with valproic acid; use with caution in patients with inborn errors of metabolism or ▶

decreased hepatic mitochondrial activity; these patients may be at increased risk. Pediatric patients <24 months of age may be at increased risk for topiramate-associated hyperammonemia, especially when used concurrently with valproic acid. Monitor all patients for lethargy, vomiting, or unexplained changes in mental status. Hypothermia [core body temperature <35°C (95°F)] has been reported with concomitant use of topiramate and valproic acid; symptoms may include lethargy, confusion, coma, or alteration in other major organ system (eg, cardiovascular or respiratory); may occur with or without associated hyperammonemia, and may develop after topiramate initiation or dosage increase; discontinuation of topiramate or valproic acid may be necessary.

Nephrolithiasis (kidney stones) has been reported with use due to carbonic anhydrase activity of topiramate which reduces urinary citrate excretion and increases urinary pH thereby promoting stone formation. Risk is higher in children; reported incidence in adults: 1.5%; in pediatric patients <24 months with long-term use (up to 1 year): 7% (kidney or bladder stones); one retrospective study evaluating long-term use (1 year) in children with epilepsy (n=96; mean age: 6.9 ± 3.8 years) reported an incidence of 5.2% (Mahmoud, 2011); risk may be increased with ketogenic diet or concomitant drugs that produce metabolic acidosis; avoid use while on topiramate therapy; maintain adequate hydration during therapy; monitor for signs or symptoms of kidney or bladder or kidney stone development.

Antiepileptic drugs (AEDs) increase the risk of suicidal behavior and ideation in patients receiving these medications for any indication. Pooled analyses of placebo-controlled trials involving 11 different AEDs (regardless of indication) showed a twofold increased risk of suicidal thoughts or behavior (estimated incidence rate: 0.43% in AED treated patients compared to 0.24% of patients receiving placebo); increased risk was observed as early as 1 week after initiation of AED and continued through duration of trials (most trials ≤24 weeks); risk did not vary significantly by age (age range: 5–100 years). Consider risks and benefits of AEDs before prescribing. Monitor all patients receiving an AED for emergence of suicidal thoughts or behavior, thoughts of self-harm, any unusual changes in behavior or mood, or the emergence or worsening of depressive symptoms; notify health care provider immediately if symptoms or concerning behavior occur. **Note:** The FDA requires a Medication Guide for all antiepileptic drugs informing patients of this risk.

Precautions Use with caution and decrease the dose in patients with renal dysfunction. Use caution with hepatic impairment; clearance may be reduced; dosage adjustment may be required. Potentially significant interactions may exist, requiring dose or frequency adjustment, additional monitoring, and/or selection of alternative therapy. Consult drug interactions database for more detailed information.

Adverse Reactions Adverse events are reported for adult and pediatric patients for various indications and regimens. **Note:** A wide range of dosages were studied. Incidence of adverse events was frequently lower in the pediatric population studied.

Cardiovascular: Angina pectoris, atrioventricular block, bradycardia (adjunctive therapy for epilepsy in children 2 to 16 years, chest pain, deep vein thrombosis, edema, facial edema, flushing, hypertension, hypotension, orthostatic hypotension, phlebitis, pulmonary embolism, syncope, vasodilatation

Central nervous system: Abnormal electroencephalogram, abnormal gait, aggressive behavior, agitation, altered sense of smell, anxiety, apathy, aphasia, apraxia, ataxia, behavioral problems (adjunctive therapy for epilepsy in children 2 to 16 years), brain disease, cognitive dysfunction, confusion, delirium, delusions, depersonalization, depression, dizziness, drowsiness, dysarthria, dystonia, emotional lability, euphoria, exacerbation of depression, exacerbation of migraine headache, fatigue, hallucination, headache, hyperesthesia, hypertonia, hypoesthesia, hyporeflexia (adjunctive therapy for epilepsy in children 2 to 16 years), insomnia, irritability, lack of concentration, language problems, memory impairment, mood disorder, nervousness, neuropathy, pain, paranoia, paresthesia, psychomotor retardation, psychosis, psychoneurosis (adjunctive therapy for epilepsy in children 2 to 16 years), rigors, sensory disturbance, speech disturbance, stupor, tonic-clonic seizures (adjunctive therapy for epilepsy in children 2 to 16 years), vertigo, voice disorder, weight loss

Dermatologic: Abnormal hair texture, acne vulgaris, alopecia, body odor, dermatitis (adjunctive therapy for epilepsy in children 2 to 16 years), dermatological disease, diaphoresis, eczema (adjunctive therapy for epilepsy in children 2 to 16 years), erythematous rash, hypertrichosis (adjunctive therapy for epilepsy in children 2 to 16 years), pallor (adjunctive therapy for epilepsy in children 2 to 16 years), pruritus, seborrhea (adjunctive therapy for epilepsy in children 2 to 16 years), skin discoloration (adjunctive therapy for epilepsy in children 2 to 16 years), skin photosensitivity, skin rash, urticaria

Endocrine & metabolic: Albuminuria, amenorrhea, decreased libido, decreased serum bicarbonate, decreased serum phosphate, dehydration, diabetes mellitus, hot flash, hyperammonemia with/without encephalopathy with/without valproate (migraine therapy in adolescents 12 to 17 years), hyperglycemia, hyperlipidemia, hypermenorrhea, hyperthyroidism (migraine therapy in adolescents 12 to 17 years), hypocalcemia, hypoglycemia (adjunctive therapy for epilepsy in children 2 to 16 years), increased gamma-glutamyl transferase, increased thirst, intermenstrual bleeding, menstrual disease, weight gain (adjunctive therapy for epilepsy in children 2 to 16 years)

Gastrointestinal: Abdominal pain, ageusia, anorexia, constipation, decreased appetite, diarrhea, dysgeusia, dyspepsia, dysphagia (adjunctive therapy for epilepsy in children 2 to 16 years), enlargement of abdomen, esophagitis, fecal incontinence (adjunctive therapy for epilepsy in children 2 to 16 years), flatulence (adjunctive therapy for epilepsy in children 2 to 16 years), gastritis, gastroenteritis, gastroesophageal reflux disease, gastrointestinal disease, gingival hemorrhage, gingival hyperplasia (adjunctive therapy for epilepsy in children 2 to 16 years), gingivitis, glossitis (adjunctive therapy for epilepsy in children 2 to 16 years), hemorrhoids, increased appetite (adjunctive therapy for epilepsy in children 2 to 16 years), melena, nausea, sialorrhea (adjunctive therapy for epilepsy in children 2 to 16 years), stomatitis, vomiting, xerostomia

Genitourinary: Cystitis, dysuria, ejaculatory disorder, genital candidiasis, hematuria, impotence, leukorrhea (adjunctive therapy for epilepsy in children 2 to 16 years), mastalgia, nipple discharge, nocturia (adjunctive therapy for epilepsy in children 2 to 16 years), oliguria, premature ejaculation, prostatic disease, urinary frequency, urinary incontinence, urinary retention, urinary tract infection, urine abnormality, vaginal hemorrhage

Hematologic & oncologic: anemia, eosinophilia, granulocytopenia, hematoma (adjunctive therapy for epilepsy in children 2 to 16 years), leukopenia, lymphadenopathy, lymphocytopenia, neoplasm, prolonged prothrombin time (adjunctive therapy for epilepsy in children 2 to 16 years), purpura (adjunctive therapy for epilepsy in children 2 to 16 years), thrombocythemia, thrombocytopenia (adjunctive therapy for epilepsy in children 2 to 16 years)

Hepatic: Increased serum alkaline phosphatase, increased serum ALT, increased serum AST

Hypersensitivity: Hypersensitivity reaction

Infection: Candidiasis, infection, viral infection

Neuromuscular & skeletal: Arthralgia, arthropathy, back pain, dyskinesia, hyperkinesia (adjunctive therapy for epilepsy in children 2 to 16 years), leg cramps, leg pain, muscle spasm, myalgia, skeletal pain, tremor, weakness

Ophthalmic: Abnormal lacrimation (adjunctive therapy for epilepsy in children 2 to 16 years), accommodation disturbance, blepharoptosis, blurred vision, conjunctivitis, diplopia, eye disease, eye pain, myopia (adjunctive therapy for epilepsy in children 2 to 16 years), nystagmus, photophobia, scotoma, strabismus, visual disturbance, visual field defect, xerophthalmia

Otic: Hearing loss, otitis media, tinnitus

Renal: Increased serum creatinine, nephrolithiasis, polyuria, renal pain

Respiratory: Asthma, bronchitis, cough, dyspnea, epistaxis, flu-like symptoms, laryngitis (migraine therapy in adolescents 12 to 17 years), pharyngeal edema (migraine therapy in adolescents 12 to 17 years), pharyngitis, pneumonia, respiratory tract disease (adjunctive therapy for epilepsy in children 2 to 16 years), rhinitis, sinusitis, upper respiratory tract infection

Miscellaneous: Fever, trauma

Rare but important or life-threatening: Acute myopia with secondary angle-closure glaucoma, bone marrow depression (epilepsy), cerebellar syndrome (epilepsy), decreased serum phosphate (migraine therapy in adolescents 12 to 17 years), erythema multiforme, hepatic failure (including fatalities), hyperthermia, hypohidrosis, hypothermia (with valproate, with or without hyperammonemia), hypokalemia (adjunctive therapy in adults with partial-onset seizures), lymphocytosis (epilepsy), maculopathy, metabolic acidosis (hyperchloremia, nonanion gap), pancreatitis, pancytopenia (epilepsy), pemphigus, renal tubular acidosis, Stevens-Johnson syndrome, suicidal ideation, tongue edema (epilepsy), upper motor neuron lesion (epilepsy), vasospasm (epilepsy)

Drug Interactions

Metabolism/Transport Effects Inhibits CYP2C19 (weak); **Induces** CYP3A4 (weak/moderate)

Avoid Concomitant Use

Avoid concomitant use of Topiramate with any of the following: Alcohol (Ethyl); Axitinib; Azelastine (Nasal); Carbonic Anhydrase Inhibitors; Paraldehyde; Simeprevir; Thalidomide

Increased Effect/Toxicity

Topiramate may increase the levels/effects of: Alpha-/Beta-Agonists (Indirect-Acting); Amitriptyline; Amphetamines; Anticonvulsants (Barbiturate); Anticonvulsants (Hydantoin); Azelastine (Nasal); Buprenorphine; Carbonic Anhydrase Inhibitors; CNS Depressants; Flecainide; Fosphenytoin; Hydrocodone; Lithium; Memantine; MetFORMIN; Methotrimeprazine; Metyrosine; Mirtazapine; Paraldehyde; Phenytoin; Pramipexole; Primidone; QuiNIDine; ROPINIRole; Rotigotine; Selective Serotonin Reuptake Inhibitors; Thalidomide; Valproic Acid and Derivatives; Zolpidem

The levels/effects of Topiramate may be increased by: Alcohol (Ethyl); Anticholinergic Agents; Brimonidine (Topical); Cannabis; Doxylamine; Dronabinol; Droperidol; HydrOXYzine; Kava Kava; Loop Diuretics; Magnesium Sulfate; Methotrimeprazine; Nabilone; Perampanel; Rufinamide; Salicylates; Sodium Oxybate; Tapentadol; Tetrahydrocannabinol; Thiazide Diuretics

Decreased Effect

Topiramate may decrease the levels/effects of: ARIPiprazole; Axitinib; Contraceptives (Estrogens); Contraceptives (Progestins); Ibrutinib; Methenamine; Primidone; Saxagliptin; Simeprevir

The levels/effects of Topiramate may be decreased by: CarBAMazepine; Fosphenytoin; Ketorolac (Nasal); Ketorolac (Systemic); Mefloquine; Orlistat; Phenytoin

Food Interactions Ketogenic diet may increase the possibility of acidosis and/or kidney stones. Management: Monitor for symptoms of acidosis or kidney stones.

Stability

Immediate release: Topamax:

Tablets: Store at 15°C to 30°C (59°F to 86°F); protect from moisture.

Sprinkle capsules: Store at ≤25°C (77°F); protect from moisture.

Extended release: Trokendi XR: Store at 25°C (77°F), excursions permitted 15°C to 30°C (59°F to 86°F); protect from moisture and light.

Mechanism of Action Anticonvulsant activity may be due to a combination of potential mechanisms: Blocks neuronal voltage-dependent sodium channels, enhances GABA(A) activity, antagonizes AMPA/kainate glutamate receptors, and weakly inhibits carbonic anhydrase.

Pharmacokinetics (Adult data unless noted) Note: Immediate release preparations are bioequivalent (sprinkle capsule and tablet); extended release capsules (Trokendi XR) administered once daily is bioequivalent to twice daily administration of immediate release formulations.

Absorption: Rapid; Immediate release formulation: Unaffected by food; Extended release capsule: A single Trokendi XR dose with a high-fat meal increased the C_{max} by 37%, shortened the T_{max} to approximately 8 hours; this effect is significantly reduced following repeat administrations.

Distribution:

V_d: 0.6 to 0.8 L/kg

Protein binding: 15% to 41%; percent protein bound decreases as blood concentrations increase

Metabolism: Minor amounts metabolized hepatically via hydroxylation, hydrolysis, and glucuronidation; percentage of dose metabolized in liver and clearance are increased in patients receiving enzyme inducers (eg, carbamazepine, phenytoin)

Bioavailability: Immediate release: Tablet: 80% (relative to a prepared solution)

Half-life:

Immediate release:

Not receiving concomitant enzyme inducers or valproic acid:

Neonates (full-term) with hypothermia: ~43 hours (Fillipi, 2009)

Infants and Children 9 months to <4 years: 10.4 hours (range: 8.5 to 15.3 hours) (Mikaeloff, 2004)

Children 4 to 7 years: Mean range: 7.7 to 8 hours (Rosenfeld, 1999)

Children 8 to 11 years: Mean range: 11.3 to 11.7 hours (Rosenfeld, 1999)

Children and Adolescents 12 to 17 years: Mean range: 12.3 to 12.8 hours (Rosenfeld, 1999)

Receiving concomitant enzyme inducers (eg, carbamazepine, phenytoin, phenobarbital):

Neonates (full-term) with hypothermia: 26.5 hours (Fillipi, 2009)

Infants and Children 9 months to <4 years: 6.5 hours (range: 3.75 to 10.2 hours) (Mikaeloff, 2004)

Children and Adolescents 4 to 17 years: 7.5 hours (Rosenfeld, 1999)

Receiving valproic acid: Infants and Children 9 months to 4 years: 9.2 hours (range: 7.23 to 12 hours) (Mikaeloff, 2004)

Adults: 19 to 23 hours (mean: 21 hours)

Adults with renal impairment: 59 ± 11 hours

Extended release: Trokendi XR: ~31 hours

Time to peak serum concentration:

Immediate release:

Neonates (full-term) with hypothermia: 3.8 hours (Fillipi, 2009)

Infants and Children 9 months to <4 years: 3.7 hours (range: 1.5 to 10.2 hours) (Michealoff, 2004)

Children 4 to 17 years: Mean range: 1 to 2.8 hours (Rosenfeld, 1999)

Adults: 2 hours; range: 1.4 to 4.3 hours

Extended release: Trokendi XR: ~24 hours

Elimination: Urine (~70% as unchanged drug); may undergo renal tubular reabsorption

Clearance:

Not receiving concomitant enzyme inducers or valproic acid:

Neonates (full-term) with hypothermia: 13.4 mL/kg/hour (Fillipi, 2009)

Infants and Children 9 months to <4 years: 46.5 mL/kg/hour (range: 30.5 to 70.9 mL/kg/hour) (Mikaeloff, 2004)

Children 4 to 17 years: 27.6 mL/kg/hour (Rosenfeld, 1999)

Receiving concomitant enzyme inducers:

Neonates (full-term) with hypothermia: 17.9 mL/kg/hour (Fillipi, 2009)

Infants and Children 9 months to <4 years: 85.4 mL/kg/hour (range: 46.2 to 135 mL/kg/hour) (Mikaeloff, 2004)

Children and Adolescents 4 to 17 years: 60.6 mL/kg/hour (Rosenfeld, 1999)

Receiving valproic acid: Infants and Children 9 months to <4 years: 49.6 mL/kg/hour (range: 26.6 to 60.2 mL/kg/h) (Mikaeloff, 2004)

Adults: 20 to 30 mL/minute

Dosing: Neonatal

Neonatal seizures; refractory: Full-term: Limited data available; efficacy results variable: Oral: Immediate release: 10 mg/kg/day was used in five neonates and 3 mg/kg/day was used in one neonate who were refractory to phenobarbital. In four of the five patients who received the higher dose, an absence or reduction in seizure frequency was observed; the neonate who received low dose (3 mg/kg) had no apparent change in seizures; no adverse effects noted required discontinuation of therapy. Further studies are needed (Glass, 2011).

Neuroprotectant following anoxic injury (with cooling): Full-term: Limited data available; efficacy results variable: Oral: Immediate release: 5 mg/kg/dose on day 1 followed by 3 mg/kg/dose once daily on day 2 and 3 was used in 11 neonates in study of safety; no adverse effects were noted (Filippi, 2010). In an earlier pharmacokinetic pilot study of 13 neonates, the same investigators used 5 mg/kg/dose once daily for 3 days; results showed targeted serum concentrations (5-20 ng/mL) were achieved in 11 of 13 patients with some accumulation in patients treated with deep hypothermia (Filippi, 2009). Further studies are needed.

Dosing: Usual

Pediatric: **Note:** Do not abruptly discontinue therapy; taper dosage gradually to prevent rebound effects.

Infantile spasms: Oral: Limited data available; dosing regimens variable. Consider twice-daily therapy once dose titration begins:

Newly diagnosed infantile spasm: Weight-directed dosing: Infants and Children 3 to 24 months: Immediate release: Initial: 1 to 3 mg/kg/day given as 1 or 2 daily doses; titrate every 3 to 7 days in 1 to 3 mg/kg/day increments as tolerated until seizures controlled; reported mean dose range: 9.1 to 14 mg/kg/day; reported range: 4 to 27 mg/kg/day. Dosing based on two small studies; first was an open-label trial of 15 pediatric patients (mean age: 8 months; age range: 4 to 14 months) with newly diagnosed infantile spasms which used an initial dose of 3 mg/kg/day given in 2 divided doses; doses were increased by 3 mg/kg/day every 3 days until seizures or toxicity developed; mean dose required: 14 mg/kg/day (9 to 27 mg/kg/day); median rate of spasm reduction was 41% within the first 2 months of therapy with 20% of patients becoming spasm free (three of 15 patients) and 33% achieving a 50% reduction in spasm frequency (five of 15 patients) (Hosain, 2006). In another trial of 20 pediatric patients (median age: 6.5 months; range: 3 to 24 months) with newly diagnosed infantile spasms, an initial dose of 1 mg/kg/day was used; dose was increased by 1 mg/kg/day at weekly intervals until seizures were controlled up to a maximum daily dose: 12 mg/kg/day; reported mean stabilizing dose: 9.1 mg/kg/day (4 to 12 mg/kg/day); results showed 30% of patients became spasm free (six of 20 patients) and 70% achieved at least a 50% reduction in spasm frequency (Kwon, 2006)

Refractory: Fixed dosing: Infants ≥3 months to Children ≤4 years; weight ≥7 kg: Immediate release: Initial: 25 mg/day once daily; titrate in 25 mg/day increments every 2 to 3 days as tolerated until seizures controlled up to a maximum daily dose: 24 mg/kg/day; dosing is from an open-label trial of 11 pediatric patients (mean age: 24 months) which reported a mean stabilizing dose of 15 mg/kg/day (8.3 to 23.7 mg/kg/day); results showed statistically significant decrease in spasm frequency with 45% of patients becoming spasm free (Glauser, 1998). In an extension phase of this study in eight of the initial subjects, the mean dose was 29 mg/kg/day (maximum daily dose: 50 mg/kg/day); 50% of the remaining patients (four of eight) were seizure free and all patients except one maintained a ≥50% reduction in spasm frequency (Glauser, 2000).

Anticonvulsant, adjunctive therapy: Oral:

Children and Adolescents 2 to 16 years:

Partial onset seizures or Lennox-Gastaut syndrome:

Immediate release: Children and Adolescents 2 to 16 years: Initial: 1 to 3 mg/kg/day (maximum dose: 25 mg/dose) given nightly for 1 week; increase at 1- to 2-week intervals by 1 to 3 mg/kg/day given in 2 divided doses; titrate dose to response; usual maintenance: 5 to 9 mg/kg/day given in 2 divided doses

Extended release: Trokendi XR: Children and Adolescents 6 to 16 years, able to swallow capsule whole: Initial: 25 mg once daily (approximately 1 to 3 mg/kg/day) given nightly for 1 week; increase at 1- to 2-week intervals in increments of 1 to 3 mg/kg/day rounded to appropriate capsule size given once daily; titrate dose to response; usual maintenance: 5 to 9 mg/kg/dose once daily

Primary generalized tonic-clonic seizures:

Immediate release: Children and Adolescents 2 to 16 years: Initial: 1 to 3 mg/kg/day (maximum dose: 25 mg/dose) given nightly for 1 week; increase over 8 weeks in 1 to 3 mg/kg/day increments given in 2 divided doses to a target dose of 6 mg/kg/day given in 2 divided doses

Extended release: Trokendi XR: Children and Adolescents 6 to 16 years, able to swallow capsule whole: Initial: 25 mg once daily (approximately 1 to 3 mg/kg/day) given nightly for 1 week; increase over 8 weeks in 1 to 3 mg/kg/day increments (rounded to appropriate capsule size) to a target dose of 6 mg/kg/day given once daily

Adolescents ≥17 years:

Partial onset seizures or Lennox-Gastaut syndrome:

Immediate release: Initial: 25 to 50 mg/day given daily for 1 week; increase at weekly intervals by 25 to 50 mg/day; give in 2 divided doses; titrate dose to response; usual maintenance dose: 100 to 200 mg twice daily; maximum daily dose: 1600 mg/day; **Note:** Doses above 400 mg/day have not been shown to increase efficacy in dose-response studies in adults.

Extended release: Trokendi XR: Initial: 25 to 50 mg once daily for 1 week; increase at weekly intervals by 25 to 50 mg/day once daily; titrate dose to response; longer intervals between dosage adjustment may be used; usual maintenance dose: 200 to 400 mg once daily; maximum daily dose: 1600 mg/**day**; higher doses have not been studied

Primary generalized tonic-clonic seizures:

Immediate release: Initial: 25 to 50 mg/day given once daily for 1 week; increase over 8 weeks in 25 to 50 mg/day increments given in 2 divided doses; titrate dose to response; usual maintenance dose: 200 mg twice daily; use slower initial titration rate (>2 week intervals); maximum daily dose: 1600 mg/**day**; **Note:** Doses above 400 mg/day have not been shown to increase efficacy in dose-response studies in adults.

Extended release: Trokendi XR: Initial: 25 mg to 50 mg once daily for 1 week; increase at weekly intervals by 25 to 50 mg/day increments given once daily; titrate dose to response; usual maintenance dose: 400 mg once daily; maximum daily dose: 1600 mg/**day**; higher doses have not been studied

Anticonvulsant, monotherapy: Partial onset seizures or primary generalized tonic-clonic seizures: Oral:

Immediate release:

Children 2 to <10 years: Initial: 25 mg once daily (in evening); may increase if tolerated to 25 mg twice daily in week 2; thereafter, may increase by 25 to 50 mg/day at weekly intervals over 5 to 7 weeks up to the lower end of the target daily maintenance dosing range (ie, to the minimum recommended maintenance dose); if additional seizure control is needed and therapy is tolerated, may further increase by 25 to 50 mg/day at weekly intervals up to the upper end of the target daily maintenance dosing range (ie, to the maximum recommended maintenance dose):

Target daily maintenance dosing range:

≤11 kg: 150-250 mg/day in 2 divided doses

12 to 22 kg: 200-300 mg/day in 2 divided doses

23 to 31 kg: 200-350 mg/day in 2 divided doses

32 to 38 kg: 250-350 mg/day in 2 divided doses

>38 kg: 250-400 mg/day in 2 divided doses

Children ≥10 years and Adolescents: Initial: 25 mg twice daily; increase at weekly intervals by 50 mg/day up to a dose of 100 mg twice daily (week 4 dose); thereafter, may further increase at weekly intervals by 100 mg/day up to the recommended maximum dose of 200 mg twice daily

Extended release: Trokendi XR: Children ≥10 years and Adolescents: Initial: 50 mg once daily for 1 week; increase at weekly intervals by 50 mg/day increments up to a dose of 200 mg/day (week 4 dose); thereafter, may increase at weekly intervals by 100 mg/day up to the recommended dose of 400 mg once daily

Migraine prophylaxis: Oral:

Children 6 to <12 years; weight: ≥20 kg: Limited data available: Immediate release: Initial: 15 mg/day for 1 week; then increase to 15 mg twice daily for 1 week; then increase to 25 mg twice daily for 7 days; continue

to gradually titrate to effect up to target dose of 2 to 3 mg/kg/day divided twice daily; maximum daily dose: 200 mg/day; dosing based on a double-randomized, placebo-controlled trial of 90 pediatric patients <12 years (treatment arm: n= 59; mean age: 11.3 years as part of a larger trial with a total of 108 pediatric patients receiving topiramate compared to 49 receiving placebo) which showed a mean reduction in migraine days/month with topiramate and significantly more topiramate patients experienced ≥75% reduction in mean monthly migraine days compared to placebo (32% vs 14%) for overall study population; mean maintenance dose: 2 mg/kg/day; treatment duration of maintenance dose: 12 weeks (Winner, 2005)

Children ≥12 years and Adolescents: Initial: 25 mg/day given at night for 1 week; increase at weekly intervals in 25 mg/day increments as tolerated and indicated to recommended dose of 50 mg twice daily; in a double-blind, placebo-controlled, dose-finding trial of 103 pediatric patients ≥12 years (mean age: 14.2 years), the daily dose of 100 mg/day was shown to significantly decrease frequency of migraine attacks compared to a lower dose of 50 mg/day (Lewis, 2009)

Adult: **Note:** Do not abruptly discontinue therapy; taper dosage gradually to prevent rebound effects. In clinical trials, adult doses were withdrawn by decreasing in weekly intervals of 50-100 mg/day gradually over 2 to 8 weeks for seizure treatment, and by decreasing in weekly intervals by 25-50 mg/day for migraine prophylaxis.

Epilepsy, monotherapy: Partial onset seizure and primary generalized tonic-clonic seizure: Oral:

Immediate release: Initial: 25 mg twice daily; may increase weekly by 50 mg daily up to 100 mg twice daily (week 4 dose); thereafter, may further increase weekly by 100 mg daily up to the recommended dose of 200 mg twice daily

Extended release: Initial: 50 mg daily for 1 week; may increase weekly by 50 mg daily up to 200 mg once daily (week 4 dose); thereafter, may further increase weekly by 100 mg daily up to the recommended dose of 400 mg once daily.

Epilepsy, adjunctive therapy: Partial onset seizure, primary generalized tonic-clonic seizure, Lennox-Gastaut syndrome: Oral: **Note:** Doses >1600 mg have not been studied.

Immediate release: Initial: 25 mg once or twice daily for 1 week; may increase weekly by 25 to 50 mg daily until response; usual maintenance dose: 100 to 200 mg twice daily (partial-onset seizures) or 200 mg twice daily (primary generalized tonic-clonic seizures). Doses >400 mg have not shown additional benefit for treatment of partial-onset seizures.

Extended release: Initial: 25 to 50 mg once daily for 1 week; may increase weekly by 25 to 50 mg daily until response; usual maintenance dose: 200 to 400 mg once daily (partial-onset seizures, Lennox-Gastaut syndrome) or 400 mg once daily (primary generalized tonic-clonic seizures). Doses >400 mg daily have not shown additional benefit for treatment of partial-onset seizure

Migraine prophylaxis: Oral: Immediate release: Initial: 25 mg once daily (in evening); may increase weekly by 25 mg daily up to the recommended dose of 100 mg daily given in 2 divided doses. Increased intervals between dose adjustments may be considered. Doses >100 mg daily have shown no additional benefit.

Dosing adjustment in renal impairment: Oral:

Infants, Children, and Adolescents: There are no dosage adjustments provided in the manufacturer's labeling; however, the following guidelines have been used by some clinicians (Aronoff, 2007):

GFR >50 mL/minute/1.73 m^2: No dosage adjustment necessary

GFR 10 to 50 mL/minute/1.73 m^2: Administer 50% of dose

GFR <10 mL/minute/1.73 m^2: Administer 25% of dose

Hemodialysis/peritoneal dialysis (PD): Administer 25% of dose; supplemental dose after hemodialysis needed

Continuous renal replacement therapy (CRRT): Administer 50% of dose

Adults: Manufacturer's labeling: CrCl <70 mL/minute/1.73 m^2: Administer 50% of the usual dose; titrate more slowly due to prolonged half-life; significantly hemodialyzed; cleared by hemodialysis at a rate that is 4 to 6 times greater than a normal individual; supplemental doses may be required

Dosing adjustment in hepatic impairment: Children, Adolescents, and Adults: There are no dosage adjustments provided in the manufacturer's labeling; however, clearance may be reduced. Carefully adjust dose as plasma concentrations may be increased if normal dosing is used.

Administration May be administered without regard to food.

Immediate release:

Tablets: Broken tablets have a bitter taste; tablets may be crushed, mixed with water, and administered immediately.

Sprinkle capsules: Swallow sprinkle capsules whole or open and sprinkle contents on small amount of soft food (eg, 1 teaspoonful of applesauce, oatmeal, ice cream, pudding, custard, or yogurt); swallow sprinkle/food mixture immediately; do not chew; do not store for later use; drink fluids after dose to make sure mixture is completely swallowed.

Extended release: Trokendi XR: Swallow capsules whole; do not sprinkle capsules on food, chew, or crush. Avoid alcohol use with within 6 hours prior to and 6 hours after administration.

Monitoring Parameters Frequency, duration, and severity of seizure episodes or migraine headaches; renal function; monitor serum electrolytes including baseline and periodic serum bicarbonate, symptoms of metabolic acidosis, complications of chronic acidosis (eg, nephrolithiasis, rickets, and reduced growth rates); monitor body temperature and for decreased sweating, especially in warm or hot weather; monitor serum ammonia concentration in patients with unexplained lethargy, vomiting, or mental status changes; intraocular pressure, symptoms of secondary angle closure glaucoma; signs and symptoms of suicidality (eg, anxiety, depression, behavior changes)

Reference Range Not applicable; plasma topiramate concentrations have not been shown to correlate with clinical efficacy

Dosage Forms Excipient information presented when available (limited, particularly for generics); consult specific product labeling.

Capsule ER 24 Hour Sprinkle, Oral:

Qudexy XR: 25 mg (30 ea, 500 ea); 50 mg (30 ea, 500 ea); 100 mg (30 ea, 500 ea); 150 mg (30 ea, 500 ea); 200 mg (30 ea, 500 ea)

Capsule Extended Release 24 Hour, Oral:

Trokendi XR: 25 mg [contains brilliant blue fcf (fd&c blue #1), sodium benzoate]

Trokendi XR: 50 mg, 100 mg, 200 mg [contains brilliant blue fcf (fd&c blue #1), fd&c yellow #6 (sunset yellow), sodium benzoate]

Capsule Sprinkle, Oral:

Topamax Sprinkle: 15 mg, 25 mg

Generic: 15 mg, 25 mg

Tablet, Oral:

Topamax: 25 mg, 50 mg, 100 mg, 200 mg

Topiragen: 25 mg, 50 mg, 100 mg, 200 mg

Generic: 25 mg, 50 mg, 100 mg, 200 mg

Extemporaneous Preparations Hazardous agent; use appropriate precautions for handling and disposal (meets NIOSH, 2012 criteria).

A 6 mg/mL topiramate oral suspension may be made with tablets and one of two different vehicles (a 1:1 mixture of Ora-Sweet and Ora-Plus, or a mixture of Simple Syrup, NF and methylcellulose 1% with parabens. Crush six 100 mg tablets in a mortar and reduce to a fine powder. Add a small amount of methylcellulose gel and mix to a uniform paste (**Note:** Use a small amount of methylcellulose gel when using the 1:1 Ora-Sweet and Ora-Plus mixture as the vehicle; use 10 mL methylcellulose 1% with parabens when using Simple Syrup, NF as the vehicle); mix while adding the chosen vehicle in incremental proportions to almost 100 mL; transfer to a graduated cylinder; rinse mortar with vehicle, and add quantity of vehicle sufficient to make 100 mL. Store in plastic prescription bottles; label "shake well" and "refrigerate". Stable for 90 days refrigerated (preferred) or at room temperature.

Nahata MC, Pai VB, and Hipple TF, *Pediatric Drug Formulations*, 5th ed, Cincinnati, OH: Harvey Whitney Books Co, 2004.

References

Brandes JL, Saper JR, Diamond M, et al, "Topiramate for Migraine Prevention: A Randomized Controlled Trial," *JAMA*, 2004, 291 (8):965-73.

Brophy GM, Bell R, Claassen J, et al, "Guidelines For the Evaluation and Management of Status Epilepticus," *Neurocrit Care*, 2012, 17 (1):3-23.

Doose DR, Walker SA, Gisclon LG, et al, "Single-Dose Pharmacokinetics and Effect of Food on the Bioavailability of Topiramate, a Novel Antiepileptic Drug," *J Clin Pharmacol*, 1996, 36(10):884-91.

Filippi L, la Marca G, Fiorini P, et al, "Topiramate Concentrations in Neonates Treated With Prolonged Whole Body Hypothermia for Hypoxic Ischemic Encephalopathy," *Epilepsia*, 2009, 50(11):2355-61.

Filippi L, Poggi C, la Marca G, et al, "Oral Topiramate in Neonates With Hypoxic Ischemic Encephalopathy Treated With Hypothermia: A Safety Study," *J Pediatr*, 2010, 157(3):361-6.

Glass HC, Poulin C, and Shevell MI, "Topiramate For the Treatment of Neonatal Seizures," *Pediatr Neurol*, 2011, 44(6):439-42.

Glauser TA, "Preliminary Observations on Topiramate in Pediatric Epilepsies," *Epilepsia*, 1997, 38(Suppl 1):S37-41.

Glauser TA, "Topiramate Use in Pediatric Patients," *Can J Neurol Sci*, 1998, 25(3):S8-12.

Glauser T, Ben-Menachem E, Bourgeois B, et al, "ILAE Treatment Guidelines: Evidence-Based Analysis of Antiepileptic Drug Efficacy and Effectiveness as Initial Monotherapy For Epileptic Seizures and Syndromes," *Epilepsia*, 2006, 47(7):1094-120.

Glauser TA, Clark PO, and McGee K, "Long-Term Response to Topiramate in Patients With West Syndrome," *Epilepsia*, 2000, 41 Suppl 1:S91-4.

Glauser TA, Clark PO, and Strawsburg R, "A Pilot Study of Topiramate in the Treatment of Infantile Spasms," *Epilepsia*, 1998, 39(12):1324-8.

Go CY, Mackay MT, Weiss SK, et al, "Evidence-Based Guideline Update: Medical Treatment of Infantile Spasms. Report of the Guideline Development Subcommittee of the American Academy of Neurology and the Practice Committee of the Child Neurology Society," *Neurology*, 2012, 78(24):1974-80.

Hershey AD, Powers SW, Vockell AL, et al, "Effectiveness of Topiramate in the Prevention of Childhood Headaches," *Headache*, 2002, 42(8):810-8.

Hosain SA, Merchant S, Solomon GE, Chutorian A. Topiramate for the treatment of infantile spasms. J Child Neurol. 2006;21(1):17-19.

Kwon YS, Jun YH, Hong YJ, et al, "Topiramate Monotherapy in Infantile Spasm," *Yonsei Med J*, 2006, 47(4):498-504.

Lewis D, Winner P, Saper J, et al, "Randomized, Double-Blind, Placebo-Controlled Study to Evaluate the Efficacy and Safety of Topiramate For Migraine Prevention in Pediatric Subjects 12 to 17 Years of Age," *Pediatrics*, 2009, 123(3):924-34.

Mahmoud AA, Rizk T, El-Bakri NK, et al, "Incidence of Kidney Stones With Topiramate Treatment in Pediatric Patients," *Epilepsia*, 2011, 52 (10):1890-3.

Mikaeloff Y, Rey E, Soufflet C, et al, "Topiramate Pharmacokinetics in Children With Epilepsy Aged From 6 Months to 4 Years," *Epilepsia*, 2004, 45(11):1448-52.

Ohman I, Sabers A, de Flon P, et al, "Pharmacokinetics of Topiramate During Pregnancy," *Epilepsy Res*, 2009, 87(2-3):124-9.

Ohman I, Vitols S, Luef G, et al, "Topiramate Kinetics During Delivery, Lactation, and in the Neonate: Preliminary Observations," *Epilepsia*, 2002, 43(10):1157-60.

Patsalos PN, Berry DJ, Bourgeois BF, et al, "Antiepileptic Drugs – Best Practice Guidelines For Therapeutic Drug Monitoring: A Position Paper by the Subcommission on Therapeutic Drug Monitoring, ILAE

Commission on Therapeutic Strategies," *Epilepsia*, 2008, 49 (7):1239-76.

Pellock JM, "Managing Pediatric Epilepsy Syndromes With New Antiepileptic Drugs," *Pediatrics*, 1999, 104(5 Pt 1):1106-16.

Rosenfeld WE, Doose DR, Walker SA, et al, "A Study of Topiramate Pharmacokinetics and Tolerability in Children With Epilepsy," *Pediatr Neurol*, 1999, 20(5):339-44.

Sachdeo RC, "Topiramate. Clinical Profile in Epilepsy," *Clin Pharmacokinet*, 1998, 34(5):335-46.

Silverstein FS and Ferriero DM, "Off-Label Use of Antiepileptic Drugs For the Treatment of Neonatal Seizures," *Pediatr Neurol*, 2008, 39 (2):77-9.

Topamax (topiramate) [prescribing information]. Titusville, NJ: Janssen Pharmaceutical, Inc; April 2014.

Trokendi XR (topiramate) [prescribing information]. Rockville, MD: Supernus Pharmaceuticals, Inc; August 2013.

Westin AA, Nakken KO, Johannessen SI, et al, "Serum Concentration/ dose Ratio of Topiramate During Pregnancy," *Epilepsia*, 2009, 50 (3):480-5.

Winner P, Pearlman EM, Linder SL, et al, "Topiramate For Migraine Prevention in Children: A Randomized, Double-Blind, Placebo-Controlled Trial," *Headache*, 2005, 45(10):1304-12.

◆ **Toposar** *see* Etoposide *on page 815*

Topotecan (toe poe TEE kan)

Medication Safety Issues
Sound-alike/look-alike issues:
Hycamtin may be confused with Mycamine

Topotecan may be confused with irinotecan

High alert medication:
This medication is in a class the Institute for Safe Medication Practices (ISMP) includes among its list of drug classes which have a heightened risk of causing significant patient harm when used in error.

Other safety concerns:
Topotecan overdoses have been reported; potential causes include omission of the leading zero and missing the decimal point when prescribing, preparing, and administering. Recommended intravenous doses should generally not exceed 4 mg; verify dose prior to administration.

Related Information
Emetogenic Potential of Antineoplastic Agents in Children *on page 2327*

Management of Drug Extravasations *on page 2255*

Oral Medications That Should Not Be Crushed or Altered *on page 2438*

Safe Handling of Hazardous Drugs *on page 2419*

Brand Names: U.S. Hycamtin

Brand Names: Canada Hycamtin; Topotecan For Injection; Topotecan Hydrochloride For Injection

Therapeutic Category Antineoplastic Agent, Camptothecin; Antineoplastic Agent, Topoisomerase Inhibitor

Generic Availability (U.S.) May be product dependent

Use Treatment of metastatic ovarian cancer; relapsed or refractory small cell lung cancer; recurrent or resistant (stage IVB) cervical cancer (in combination with cisplatin) (All indications: FDA approved in adults); has also been used in pediatric solid tumors including Ewing's sarcoma, osteosarcoma, rhabdomyosarcoma, and neuroblastoma and acute leukemias (ALL, AML)

Pregnancy Risk Factor D

Pregnancy Considerations Adverse effects were observed in animal reproduction studies. May cause fetal harm in pregnant women. Women of childbearing potential should use effective contraception to prevent pregnancy during treatment.

Breast-Feeding Considerations It is not known if topotecan is excreted in breast milk. Due to the potential for serious adverse reactions in the nursing infant, the manufacturer recommends to discontinue breast-feeding in women who are receiving topotecan.

Contraindications Hypersensitivity to topotecan or any component; severe bone marrow depression

Warnings Hazardous agent; use appropriate precautions for handling and disposal (NIOSH, 2012). The dose-limiting toxicity is bone marrow suppression, primarily neutropenia, which may be severe and lead to infection or fatalities. Monitor bone counts frequently. Do **NOT** administer to patients with baseline neutrophils <1500 cells/mm^3 **[U.S. Boxed Warning]**. Neutropenia is not cumulative over time. In an adult clinical study comparing I.V. to oral topotecan, G-CSF support was administered in a higher percentage of patients receiving oral topotecan (Eckardt, 2007). May also cause thrombocytopenia and anemia. Do **NOT** administer to patients with a platelet count <100,000/mm^3.

Topotecan-induced neutropenia may lead to neutropenic colitis, including fatalities; consider diagnosis in patients presenting with neutropenia, fever, and abdominal pain. Diarrhea has been reported with oral topotecan; may be severe (requiring hospitalization); educate patients on early recognition and proper management, including diet changes, increase in fluid intake, antidiarrheals, and antibiotics. The incidence of diarrhea may be higher in the elderly.

Interstitial lung disease (ILD) (with fatalities) has been reported; monitor for pulmonary signs/symptoms (eg, dyspnea, fever, cough, hypoxia) and discontinue use in patients with confirmed ILD diagnosis. Risk factors for ILD include a history of ILD, pulmonary fibrosis, lung cancer, thoracic radiation, and the use of colony-stimulating factors or medications with pulmonary toxicity.

May cause fetal harm when administered to pregnant women.

Precautions Use caution in patients with renal impairment; may require dosage adjustment. May cause fatigue which may impair physical or mental abilities; patients must be cautioned about performing tasks which require mental alertness (eg, operating machinery or driving). Potentially significant drug interactions may exist, requiring dose or frequency adjustment, additional monitoring, and/or selection of alternative therapy. Consult drug interactions database for more detailed information. Topotecan exposure is increased when oral topotecan is used concurrently with P-glycoprotein inhibitors (eg, cyclosporine A, ketoconazole, ritonavir, saquinavir); avoid concurrent use.

Adverse Reactions
Central nervous system: Fatigue, fever, headache, pain

Dermatologic: Alopecia (reversible), rash

Gastrointestinal: Abdominal pain, anorexia, constipation, diarrhea, nausea, obstruction, stomatitis, vomiting

Hematologic: Anemia, leukopenia, neutropenia (nadir 8-11 days; recovery <21 days), neutropenic fever/sepsis, thrombocytopenia

Hepatic: BUN increased, liver enzymes increased (transient)

Neuromuscular & skeletal: Paresthesia, weakness

Respiratory: Cough, dyspnea, pneumonia

Miscellaneous: Infection, sepsis

Rare but important or life-threatening: Allergic reactions, anaphylactoid reactions, angioedema, bleeding (severe, associated with thrombocytopenia), dermatitis (severe), extravasation (inadvertent), interstitial lung disease (ILD), neutropenic colitis, pancytopenia, pruritus (severe)

Drug Interactions
Metabolism/Transport Effects None known.

Avoid Concomitant Use
Avoid concomitant use of Topotecan with any of the following: BCG; CloZAPine; Dipyrone; Natalizumab; P-glycoprotein/ABCB1 Inhibitors; Pimecrolimus; Tacrolimus (Topical); Tofacitinib; Vaccines (Live)

Increased Effect/Toxicity
Topotecan may increase the levels/effects of: CloZAPine; Leflunomide; Natalizumab; Tofacitinib; Vaccines (Live)

▶

The levels/effects of Topotecan may be increased by:
BCRP/ABCG2 Inhibitors; Denosumab; Dipyrone; Filgrastim; P-glycoprotein/ABCB1 Inhibitors; Pimecrolimus; Platinum Derivatives; Roflumilast; Tacrolimus (Topical); Trastuzumab

Decreased Effect

Topotecan may decrease the levels/effects of: BCG; Coccidioidin Skin Test; Sipuleucel-T; Vaccines (Inactivated); Vaccines (Live)

The levels/effects of Topotecan may be decreased by: Echinacea; Fosphenytoin-Phenytoin

Stability Hazardous agent; use appropriate precautions for handling and disposal (NIOSH, 2012).

Oral capsules: Store at 2°C to 8°C (36°F to 46°F); protect from light; store in the original outer cartons.

Parenteral:

Lyophilized powder for injection: Store intact vials at 20°C and 25°C (68°F and 77°F); protect from light. Reconstituted solution is stable for up to 28 days at 20°C to 25°C (68°F to 77°F), although the manufacturer recommends use immediately after reconstitution. When further diluted in 50-100 mL D_5W or NS; solution is stable for 24 hours at room temperature (manufacturer recommendation) or up to 7 days under refrigeration (Craig, 1997). Reconstituted solution for injection at 1 mg/mL with bacteriostatic SWI for oral administration is stable for 14 days at 4°C in plastic syringes (Daw, 2004).

Solution for injection: Store intact vials at 2°C to 8°C (36°F to 45°F); protect from light. Single-use vials should be discarded after initial vial entry; solutions for infusion are stable for 24 hours at room temperature after diluted.

Mechanism of Action Binds to topoisomerase I and stabilizes the cleavable complex so that religation of the cleaved DNA strand cannot occur. This results in the accumulation of cleavable complexes and single-strand DNA breaks. Topotecan acts in S phase of the cell cycle.

Pharmacokinetics (Adult data unless noted) Note: Pharmacokinetic data in pediatric patients and young adults (0.4-22 years) demonstrated a high level of interpatient variability (43% to 57% dependent upon parameter evaluated) as well as intrapatient variability (20% to 22% dependent upon parameter evaluated) (Schaiquevich, 2007)

Absorption: Oral: Rapid

Distribution:

Pediatric patients and young adults (0.4-22 years): Mean range: 32.2-32.7 L/m^2 (Schaiquevich, 2007)

Adults: 25-75 L/m^2 (Hartmann, 2006)

Protein binding: 35%

Metabolism: Undergoes pH dependent hydrolysis of its active lactone moiety to yield a relatively inactive openring hydroxy acid form in plasma; metabolized in the liver to N-demethylated topotecan

Bioavailability: Oral: Capsule: Adults: ~40%; data from pediatric patients (1-18 years) showed that, while highly variable, the reported median oral bioavailability with oral administration of the reconstituted parenteral solution is similar to adults (Daw, 2004; Zamboni, 1999)

Half-life:

Pediatric patients (0-18 years): Lactone moiety: 2.58 hours ± 0.15 (range: 0.2-7.1 hours) (Santana, 2005)

Adults:

I.V.: 2-3 hours; renal impairment: ~5 hours

Oral: 3-6 hours

Time to peak serum concentration: Oral:

Pediatric patients (1-18 years): Parenteral formulation (reconstituted lyophilized formulation): 0.75-2 hours (Zamboni, 1999)

Adults: Capsules: 1-2 hours; delayed with high-fat meal (3-4 hours)

Elimination:

I.V.: Urine (51%; 3% as N-desmethyl topotecan); feces (18%; 2% as N-desmethyl topotecan)

Oral: Urine (20%; 2% as N-desmethyl topotecan); feces (33%; <2% as N-desmethyl topotecan)

Clearance:

Pediatric patients (0.4-18 years): GFR most significant determinant of clearance; a linear model with GFR has been observed; BSA is also a significant determinant of clearance and AUC more so than patient weight; infants <6 months have decreased clearance (Schaiquevich, 2007). However, pharmacokinetic data from six pediatric patients with severe renal impairment (n=5: Unilateral nephrectomy; n=1: Anephric on hemodialysis) suggests that other mechanisms than GFR may assist with renal clearance; in these patients, overall systemic clearance was shown to be similar to matched controls (age, BSA, and Scr) despite decreased GFR (Iacono, 2003; Iacono, 2004)

Adults: Topotecan plasma clearance is 24% higher in males than in female patients

Dosing: Usual Note: In adults, baseline neutrophil count should be ≥1500/mm^3 and platelets should be ≥100,000/mm^3 prior to treatment; for retreatment, neutrophil count should be >1000/mm^3; platelets >100,000/mm^3 and hemoglobin ≥9 g/dL; consult individual pediatric protocols for details regarding baseline neutrophil and platelet counts and hemoglobin.

Infants, Children, and Adolescents: **Note:** Dosing and frequency may vary by protocol and/or treatment phase; refer to specific protocol. In pediatric patients, dosing may be based on either BSA (mg/m^2) or weight (mg/kg); use extra precaution to verify dosing parameters during calculations.

Acute lymphoblastic leukemia; recurrent (first relapse): Limited data available: I.V.: Children and Adolescents: Induction therapy: 2.4 mg/m^2/dose once daily for 7-9 days (Furman, 2002; Hijiya, 2008)

Acute myeloid leukemia; recurrent, refractory: Limited data available: I.V.: Children and Adolescents: Initial: 4 mg/m^2/dose once on day 1; subsequent daily doses (days 2-5) determined by pharmacokinetic analysis (target AUC: 140 ± 20 ng/mL/hour) and administered once daily (in combination with cladribine); the median reported topotecan dose was 4 mg/m^2/day (range: 1.7-6 mg/m^2/day) (Inaba, 2010)

CNS malignancies, including gliomas: Limited data available; dosing regimens variable: Oral (using reconstituted lyophilized parenteral formulation):

Fixed dosing: 0.8 mg/m^2/dose once daily for 21 days of a 28-day cycle was used in 25 pediatric patients (median age: 9.2 years; range 0.8-23 years) with recurrent brain tumors, including gliomas, medulloblastoma, and ependymoma; the reported median number of cycles: 1.9 [range: 0.5-15 cycles (months)] (Minturn, 2011); further studies are needed

Dose escalation: Children ≥3 years and Adolescents: Initial: 0.4 mg/m^2/dose once daily was used in a trial of 32 pediatric patients (median age: 9.5 years, range: 3-18 years) with recurrent or progression of high-grade glioma; dosage was increased based upon patient tolerance and individual dose-limiting toxicity; doses were increased in 0.2 mg/m^2 increments at weekly intervals for the first 2 weeks of therapy and then increased in 0.1 mg/m^2 increments at weekly intervals up to the maximum dose of 2 mg/m^2/day; once the patient's maximum tolerated dose was reached, the daily dose was decreased until toxicity became acceptable; reported final median maximum tolerated dose: 0.9 mg/m^2/day (range: 0.6-2 mg/m^2/day); median duration of therapy: 3 months (range: 21 days to 1 year) (Wagner, 2004); further studies are needed

Neuroblastoma: Limited data available:

Induction: I.V.:

Patient weight ≤12 kg: 0.04 mg/**kg**/dose once daily for 5 days (in combination with cyclophosphamide); repeat cycle every 21 days for 6 cycles (Park, 2011)

Patient weight >12 kg: Initial: 1.2 mg/m²/dose once daily for 5 days (in combination with cyclophosphamide); repeat cycle every 21 days for 6 cycles (Park, 2011)

Note: Pharmacokinetic analysis was used to guide topotecan therapy during the first 2 cycles using a target AUC: 50-70 ng/mL/hour; median dose for cycle 1 was 1.2 mg/m²/day (range: 0.75-2.1 mg/m²/day) and for cycle 2, the median dose was 1.3 mg/m²/day (range: 1.2-2.9 mg/m²/day) (Park, 2011)

Recurrent, refractory, or untreated metastatic disease: Children and Adolescents:

I.V.:

Combination therapy: 0.75 mg/m²/dose once daily for 5 days (in combination with cyclophosphamide); repeat cycle every 21 days (Ashraf, 2013; Kretschmar, 2004; London, 2010; Saylors, 2001; Zage, 2008)

Monotherapy: 2 mg/m²/day for 5 days (London, 2010)

Oral (using reconstituted lyophilized parenteral formulation): Children ≥2 years and Adolescents: 0.8 mg/m²/dose once daily for 14 days (in combination with oral cyclophosphamide); repeat cycle every 21-28 days (Bowers, 2004). In a Phase I dose escalation trial of 20 pediatric patients (median age: 10.6 years) with refractory solid tumors including neuroblastoma, a daily dose of 1.8 mg/m² once daily for 5 days, followed by 2 days rest, then another 5 days of therapy (one cycle: 10 doses over 12 days); repeat cycle every 28 days was shown to stabilize disease in some patients (Daw, 2004); further studies are needed.

Hematopoietic stem-cell transplant; conditioning: Limited data available: I.V.: Children and Adolescents: 2 mg/m²/dose on days -8 through -4 prior to stem cell transfusion (total dose: 10 mg/m²), in combination with carboplatin and thiotepa, was used in 21 patients (median age: 4.1 years; range: 1-29 years) with refractory solid tumors (neuroblastoma: n=11) (Kushner, 2001). In a Phase I/II trial of 51 patients (median age: 5.1 years; range: 1.5-21 years), an initial dose of: 3 mg/m²/dose on day -11 was used with subsequent doses (days -10 through -2; 10 days total of topotecan therapy) determined by pharmacokinetic analysis (target AUC: 100 ± 20 ng/mL/hour) and administered once daily (in combination with cyclophosphamide on days -6 through -2); the median reported topotecan dose was 3.1 mg/m²/day (range: 1.1-4.6 mg/m²/day) (Kaskow, 2012); further studies are needed

Pediatric solid tumors; recurrent or refractory or untreated metastatic including rhabdosarcoma, Ewing sarcoma: Limited data available:

I.V.:

Combination therapy: 0.75 mg/m²/dose once daily for 5 days every 21 days in combination with cyclophosphamide (Bernstien, 2006; Hunhold, 2006; Saylors, 2001; Waterhouse, 2004) or with cyclophosphamide and vincristine (VTC regimen) (Pappo, 2001); this dosing has also been administered in combination with temozolomide in 28-day cycles (TOTEM regimen) (Rubie, 2010)

Single-agent therapy (window therapy): 2-2.4 mg/m²/dose once daily for 5 days every 21 days (Pappo, 2001)

Oral [using reconstituted lyophilized parenteral formulation or oral capsules (for patients able to swallow)]: Children ≥3 years and Adolescents: 1.8 mg/m² once daily for 5 days, followed by 2 days rest, then another 5 days of therapy (one cycle: 10 doses over 12 days); repeat cycle every 28 days; when using oral capsules, doses were rounded to the nearest 0.25 mg; dosing based on a Phase I trial dose escalation trial of 20 pediatric patients (median age: 10.6 years) with refractory solid tumors (Daw, 2004); further studies are needed

Adults:

Cervical cancer, recurrent or resistant: I.V.: 0.75 mg/m²/day for 3 days [followed by cisplatin on day 1 only (with hydration)] every 21 days

Ovarian cancer, metastatic: I.V.: 1.5 mg/m²/day for 5 consecutive days every 21 days, minimum of 4 cycles recommended in the absence of tumor progression **or** (weekly administration) 4 mg/m² on days 1, 8, and 15 every 28 days until disease progression or unacceptable toxicity or a maximum of 12 months (Sehouli, 2011)

Small cell lung cancer, relapsed or refractory:

I.V.: 1.5 mg/m²/day for 5 consecutive days every 21 days, minimum of 4 cycles recommended in the absence of tumor progression

Oral: 2.3 mg/m²/day for 5 consecutive days every 21 days (round dose to the nearest 0.25 mg); if patient vomits after dose is administered, do not give a replacement dose

Dosing adjustment in renal impairment:

Infants, Children, and Adolescents: Consult protocol for specific recommendations. Some centers have considered the following adjustments: I.V.:

Baseline: Initial dosing:

CrCl >40 mL/minute/1.73 m²: No adjustment necessary

CrCl 20-40 mL/minute/1.73 m²: Administer 50% of dose

CrCl <20 mL/minute/1.73 m²: Hold doses until renal function recovers (CrCl >20 mL/minute/1.73 m²)

During therapy:

CrCl >60 mL/minute/1.73 m²: No adjustment necessary

CrCl 40-60 mL/minute/1.73 m²: Administer 50% of dose

CrCl 20 to <40 mL/minute/1.73 m²: Administer 25% to 50% of dose

CrCl <20 mL/minute/1.73 m²: Hold doses until renal function recovers (CrCl >20 mL/minute/1.73 m²)

Hemodialysis: Very limited data available; some data suggest that clearance of the lactone metabolite is similar to pediatric patients with normal renal function; a case report describes topotecan use in an anephric 6-year old diagnosed with Wilms tumor; the patient received 0.75 mg/m²/dose once daily for 5 days every 21 days with hemodialysis on day 2 and 4; on dialysis days, topotecan was administered ~2 hours before the start of the dialysis session; dosage reductions required for toxicity (myelosuppression) after cycle 4 (Aronoff, 2007; Iacono, 2004)

Continuous renal replacement therapy (CRRT): Administer 50% of dose or reduce dose by 0.75 mg/m²/dose, if appropriate (Aronoff, 2007)

Adults:

Manufacturer's recommendations:

I.V.:

CrCl ≥40 mL/minute: No dosage adjustment necessary.

CrCl 20-39 mL/minute: Reduce dose to 0.75 mg/m²/dose

CrCl <20 mL/minute: There are no dosage adjustments provided in manufacturer's U.S. labeling ▶

(insufficient data available for dosing recommendation).

Note: For topotecan in combination with cisplatin for cervical cancer, do not initiate treatment in patients with serum creatinine >1.5 mg/dL; consider discontinuing treatment in patients with serum creatinine >1.5 mg/dL in subsequent cycles.

Oral:
CrCl ≥50 mL/minute: No dosage adjustment necessary
CrCl 30-49 mL/minute: Reduce dose to 1.8 mg/m^2/day
CrCl <30 mL/minute: There are no dosage adjustments provided in manufacturer's U.S. labeling (insufficient data available for dosing recommendation).

Alternate recommendations:
Aronoff, 2007: I.V.:
CrCl >50 mL/minute: Administer 75% of dose
CrCl 10-50 mL/minute: Administer 50% of dose
CrCl <10 mL/minute: Administer 25% of dose
Hemodialysis: Avoid use
Continuous ambulatory peritoneal dialysis (CAPD): Avoid use
Continuous renal replacement therapy (CRRT): 0.75 mg/m^2

Kintzel, 1995: I.V.:
CrCl 46-60 mL/minute: Administer 80% of dose
CrCl 31-45 mL/minute: Administer 75% of dose
CrCl ≤30 mL/minute: Administer 70% of dose

Dosing adjustment in hepatic impairment: Adults:
I.V.: Bilirubin 1.7-15 mg/dL: No adjustment necessary; the half-life is increased slightly; usual doses are generally tolerated
Oral: Bilirubin >1.5 mg/dL: No adjustment necessary

Dosing adjustment for toxicity: Adults:
Cervical cancer: I.V.: Severe febrile neutropenia (<1000/mm^3 with temperature of 38°C) or platelet count <25,000/mm^3: Reduce topotecan to 0.6 mg/m^2/day for subsequent cycles [may consider GCSF support (beginning on day 4) prior to instituting dose reduction for neutropenic fever]. **Note:** Cisplatin may also require dose adjustment.
For neutropenic fever despite G-SCF use, reduce dose to 0.45 mg/m^2/day for subsequent cycles.

Ovarian cancer: I.V.: Dosage adjustment for hematological effects: Severe neutropenia (<500/mm^3) or platelet count <25,000/mm^3: Reduce dose to 1.25 mg/m^2/day for subsequent cycles [may consider G-CSF support (beginning on day 6) prior to instituting dose reduction for neutropenia]

Small cell lung cancer:
I.V.: Dosage adjustment for hematological effects: Severe neutropenia (<500/mm^3) or platelet count <25,000/mm^3: Reduce dose to 1.25 mg/m^2/day for subsequent cycles [may consider G-CSF support (beginning on day 6) prior to instituting dose reduction for severe neutropenia]
Oral: Severe neutropenia (neutrophils <500/mm^3 associated with fever or infection or lasting ≥7 days) or prolonged neutropenia (neutrophils ≥500/mm^3 to ≤1000/mm^3 lasting beyond day 21) or platelets <25,000/mm^3 or grades 3 or 4 diarrhea: Reduce dose by 0.4 mg/m^2/day for subsequent cycles (may consider same dosage reduction for grade 2 diarrhea if clinically indicated)

Administration Hazardous agent; use appropriate precautions for handling and disposal (NIOSH, 2012).
Parenteral: I.V.: Reconstitute lyophilized powder with 4 mL SWI. Further dilute reconstituted solution or solution for injection in 50-250 mL in D$_5$W or NS and administer by intermittent infusion over 30 minutes.

Oral:
Capsules: May administer with or without food. Swallow capsule whole; do not crush, chew, or divide capsule.
Parenteral formulation; lyophilized powder for oral use: Reconstitute with 4 mL SWI to a final concentration of 1 mg/mL; mix dose in 30 mL of an acidic medium (eg, apple, grape, or orange juice); **Note:** The reconstituted injectable solution is tasteless; the acidic medium serves as the vehicle only, not to mask the taste (Bowers, 2004; Daw, 2004; Minturn, 2001; Wagner, 2004)

Vesicant/Extravasation Risk Irritant

Monitoring Parameters CBC with differential and platelet count; renal function tests; bilirubin; monitor for signs and symptoms of interstitial lung disease; diarrhea symptoms/hydration status

Dosage Forms Excipient information presented when available (limited, particularly for generics); consult specific product labeling.
Capsule, Oral:
Hycamtin: 0.25 mg, 1 mg
Solution, Intravenous:
Generic: 4 mg/4 mL (4 mL)
Solution Reconstituted, Intravenous:
Hycamtin: 4 mg (1 ea)
Generic: 4 mg (1 ea)
Solution Reconstituted, Intravenous [preservative free]:
Generic: 4 mg (1 ea)

References

Ashraf K, Shaikh F, Gibson P, et al. Treatment with topotecan plus cyclophosphamide in children with first relapse of neuroblastoma. *Pediatr Blood Cancer.* 2013;60(10):1636-1641.

Bernstein ML, Devidas M, Lafreniere D, et al. Intensive therapy with growth factor support for patients with Ewing tumor metastatic at diagnosis: Pediatric Oncology Group/Children's Cancer Group Phase II Study 9457–a report from the Children's Oncology Group. *J Clin Oncol.* 2006;24(1):152-159.

Bowers DC, Aquino VM, Leavey PJ, et al. Phase I study of oral cyclophosphamide and oral topotecan for children with recurrent or refractory solid tumors. *Pediatr Blood Cancer.* 2004;42(1):93-98.

Craig SB, Bhatt UH, and Patel K. Stability and compatibility of topotecan hydrochloride for injection with common infusion solutions and containers. *J Pharm Biomed Anal.* 1997;16(2):199-205.

Daw NC, Santana VM, Iacono LC, et al. Phase I and pharmacokinetic study of topotecan administered orally once daily for 5 days for 2 consecutive weeks to pediatric patients with refractory solid tumors. *J Clin Oncol.* 2004;22(5):829-837.

Eckardt JR, von Pawel J, Pujol JL, et al. Phase III study of oral compared with intravenous topotecan as second-line therapy in small-cell lung cancer. *J Clin Oncol.* 2007;25(15):2086-2092.

Furman WL, Stewart CF, Kirstein M, et al, "Protracted Intermittent Schedule of Topotecan in Children With Refractory Acute Leukemia: A Pediatric Oncology Group Study," *J of Clin Oncology,* 2002, 20(6):1617-1624.

Hartmann JT and Lipp HP. Camptothecin and podophyllotoxin derivatives: inhibitors of topoisomerase I and II - mechanisms of action, pharmacokinetics and toxicity profile. *Drug Saf.* 2006;29(3):209-230.

Hijiya N, Stewart CF, Zhou Y, et al. Phase II study of topotecan in combination with dexamethasone, asparaginase, and vincristine in pediatric patients with acute lymphoblastic leukemia in first relapse. *Cancer.* 2008;112(9):1983-1991.

Hunold A, Weddeling N, Paulussen M, et al. Topotecan and cyclophosphamide in patients with refractory or relapsed Ewing tumors. *Pediatr Blood Cancer.* 2006;47(6):795-800.

Iacono LC, Adams D, Homans AC, et al. Topotecan disposition in an anephric child. *J Pediatr Hematol Oncol.* 2004;26(9):596-600.

Iacono LC, Dome JS, Panetta JC, et al. Topotecan pharmacokinetics in children with Wilms tumor and unilateral nephrectomy. *Pharmacotherapy.* 2003;23:410.

Inaba H, Stewart CF, Crews KR, et al. Combination of cladribine plus topotecan for recurrent or refractory pediatric acute myeloid leukemia. *Cancer.* 2010;116(1):98-105.

Kasow KA, Stewart CF, Barfield RC, et al. A phase I/II study of CY and topotecan in patients with high-risk malignancies undergoing autologous hematopoietic cell transplantation: the St Jude long-term follow-up. *Bone Marrow Transplant.* 2012;47(11):1448-1454.

Kintzel PE and Dorr RT. Anticancer drug renal toxicity and elimination: dosing guidelines for altered renal function. *Cancer Treat Rev.* 1995;21(1):33-64.

Kretschmar CS, Kletzel M, Murray K, et al. Response to paclitaxel, topotecan, and topotecan-cyclophosphamide in children with untreated disseminated neuroblastoma treated in an upfront phase II investigational window: a pediatric oncology group study. *J Clin Oncol.* 2004;22(20):4119-4126.

Kushner BH, Cheung NK, Kramer K, et al. Topotecan combined with myeloablative doses of thiotepa and carboplatin for neuroblastoma, brain tumors, and other poor-risk solid tumors in children and young adults. *Bone Marrow Transplant.* 2001;28(6):551-556.

London WB, Frantz CN, Campbell LA, et al. Phase II randomized comparison of topotecan plus cyclophosphamide versus topotecan alone in children with recurrent or refractory neuroblastoma: a Children's Oncology Group study. *J Clin Oncol.* 2010;28(24):3808-3815.

Minturn JE, Janss AJ, Fisher PG, et al, A phase II study of metronomic oral topotecan for recurrent childhood brain tumors. *Pediatr Blood Cancer.* 2011;56(1):39-44.

National Institute for Occupational Safety and Health (NIOSH), "NIOSH List of Antineoplastic and Other Hazardous Drugs in Healthcare Settings 2012." Available at http://www.cdc.gov/niosh/docs/2012-150/pdfs/2012-150.pdf. Accessed January 21, 2013.

Pappo AS, Lyden E, Breneman J, et al. Up-front window trial of topotecan in previously untreated children and adolescents with metastatic rhabdomyosarcoma: an intergroup rhabdomyosarcoma study. *J Clin Oncol.* 2001;19(1):213-219.

Park JR, Scott JR, Stewart CF, et al. Pilot induction regimen incorporating pharmacokinetically guided topotecan for treatment of newly diagnosed high-risk neuroblastoma: a Children's Oncology Group study. *J Clin Oncol.* 2011;29(33):4351-4357.

Rubie H, Geoerger B, Frappaz D, et al. Phase I study of topotecan in combination with temozolomide (TOTEM) in relapsed or refractory paediatric solid tumours. *Eur J Cancer.* 2010;46(15):2763-2770.

Santana VM, Furman WL, Billups CA, et al. Improved response in high-risk neuroblastoma with protracted topotecan administration using a pharmacokinetically guided dosing approach. *J Clin Oncol.* 2005;23(18):4039-4047.

Santana VM, Zamboni WC, Kirstein MN, et al, "A Pilot Study of Protracted Topotecan Dosing Using a Pharmacokinetically Guided Dosing Approach in Children With Solid Tumors," *Clin Cancer Res,* 2003, 9(2):633-640.

Saylors RL 3rd, Stine KC, Sullivan J, et al, "Cyclophosphamide Plus Topotecan in Children With Recurrent or Refractory Solid Tumors: A Pediatric Oncology Group Phase II Study," *J Clin Oncol,* 2001, 19 (15):3463-3469.

Schaiquevich P, Panetta JC, Iacono LC, et al. Population pharmacokinetic analysis of topotecan in pediatric cancer patients. *Clin Cancer Res.* 2007;13(22 Pt 1):6703-6711.

Sehouli J, Stengel D, Harter P, et al. Topotecan Weekly Versus Conventional 5-Day Schedule in Patients With Platinum-Resistant Ovarian Cancer: a randomized multicenter phase II trial of the North-Eastern German Society of Gynecological Oncology Ovarian Cancer Study Group. *J Clin Oncol.* 2011;29(2):242-248.

Wagner S, Erdlenbruch B, Längler A, et al. Oral topotecan in children with recurrent or progressive high-grade glioma: a Phase I/II study by the German Society for Pediatric Oncology and Hematology. *Cancer.* 2004;100(8):1750-1757.

Walterhouse DO, Lyden ER, Breitfeld PP, et al, "Efficacy of Topotecan and Cyclophosphamide Given in a Phase II Window Trial in Children With Newly Diagnosed Metastatic Rhabdomyosarcoma: A Children's Oncology Group Study," *J Clin Oncol,* 2004, 22(8):1398-1403.

Wells RJ, Reid JM, Ames MM, et al, "Phase I Trial of Cisplatin and Topotecan in Children With Recurrent Solid Tumors: Children's Cancer Group Study 0942," *J Pediatr Hematol Oncol,* 2002, 24(2):89-93.

Zage PE, Kletzel M, Murray K, et al. Outcomes of the POG 9340/9341/9342 trials for children with high-risk neuroblastoma: a report from the Children's Oncology Group. *Pediatr Blood Cancer.* 2008;51 (6):747-753.

Zamboni WC, Bowman LC, Tan M, et al. Interpatient variability in bioavailability of the intravenous formulation of topotecan given orally to children with recurrent solid tumors. *Cancer Chemother Pharmacol.* 1999;43(6):454-460.

◆ **Topotecan For Injection (Can)** see Topotecan on page 2053

◆ **Topotecan Hydrochloride** see Topotecan on page 2053

◆ **Topotecan Hydrochloride For Injection (Can)** see Topotecan on page 2053

◆ **Toprol XL** see Metoprolol on page 1396

◆ **Topsyn® (Can)** see Fluocinonide on page 894

◆ **Toradol** see Ketorolac (Systemic) on page 1180

◆ **Toradol® (Can)** see Ketorolac (Systemic) on page 1180

◆ **Toradol® IM (Can)** see Ketorolac (Systemic) on page 1180

Torsemide (TORE se mide)

Medication Safety Issues
Sound-alike/look-alike issues:
Torsemide may be confused with furosemide
Demadex may be confused with Denorex

Brand Names: U.S. Demadex

Therapeutic Category Antihypertensive Agent; Diuretic, Loop

Generic Availability (U.S.) Yes

Use Management of edema associated with CHF and hepatic or renal disease (including chronic renal failure); used alone or in combination with antihypertensives in treatment of hypertension (FDA approved in adults)

Pregnancy Risk Factor B

Pregnancy Considerations A decrease in fetal weight, an increase in fetal resorption, and delayed fetal ossification has occurred in animal studies.

Breast-Feeding Considerations It is not known if torsemide is excreted in breast milk. The manufacturer recommends that caution be exercised when administering torsemide to nursing women.

Contraindications Hypersensitivity to torsemide, any component, or other sulfonylureas; anuria

Warnings Loop diuretics are potent diuretics, excess amounts can lead to profound diuresis with fluid and electrolyte loss; close medical supervision and dose evaluation is required. Potassium supplementation and/or use of potassium-sparing diuretics may be necessary to prevent hypokalemia. Monitor fluid status and renal function in an attempt to prevent oliguria, azotemia, and reversible increases in BUN and creatinine; close medical supervision of aggressive diuresis required. Coadministration of antihypertensives may increase the risk of hypotension.

Ototoxicity has been demonstrated following oral administration of torsemide and following rapid I.V. administration of other loop diuretics. Other possible risk factors may include use in renal impairment, excessive doses, and concurrent use of other ototoxins (eg, aminoglycosides).

Precautions Use with caution in patients with cirrhosis; avoid sudden changes in fluid and electrolyte balance and acid/base status which may lead to hepatic encephalopathy. Administration with an aldosterone antagonist or potassium-sparing diuretic may provide additional diuretic efficacy and maintain normokalemia. Chemical similarities are present among sulfonamides, sulfonylureas, carbonic anhydrase inhibitors, thiazides, and loop diuretics (except ethacrynic acid). Use in patients with sulfonylurea allergy is specifically contraindicated in product labeling; a risk of cross-reaction exists in patients with allergy to any of these compounds; avoid use when previous reaction has been severe. Discontinue if signs of hypersensitivity are noted.

Adverse Reactions
Cardiovascular: Chest pain, ECG abnormality
Central nervous system: Nervousness
Gastrointestinal: Constipation, diarrhea, dyspepsia, nausea, sore throat
Genitourinary: Excessive urination
Neuromuscular & skeletal: Arthralgia, myalgia, weakness
Respiratory: Cough, rhinitis
Rare but important or life-threatening: Angioedema, arthritis, atrial fibrillation, esophageal hemorrhage, GI hemorrhage, hyperglycemia, hyperuricemia, hypokalemia, hyponatremia, hypotension, hypovolemia, impotence, leukopenia, pancreatitis, rash, rectal bleeding, shunt thrombosis, Stevens-Johnson syndrome, syncope, thirst, thrombocytopenia, toxic epidermal necrolysis, ventricular tachycardia, vomiting

Drug Interactions

Metabolism/Transport Effects Substrate of CYP2C8 (minor), CYP2C9 (major), SLCO1B1; **Note:** Assignment of Major/Minor substrate status based on clinically relevant drug interaction potential; **Inhibits** CYP2C19 (weak)

Avoid Concomitant Use There are no known interactions where it is recommended to avoid concomitant use.

Increased Effect/Toxicity

Torsemide may increase the levels/effects of: ACE Inhibitors; Allopurinol; Amifostine; Aminoglycosides; Antihypertensives; Cardiac Glycosides; CISplatin; Dofetilide; DULoxetine; Hypotensive Agents; Ivabradine; Lithium; Methotrexate; Neuromuscular-Blocking Agents; Obinutuzumab; RisperiDONE; RiTUXimab; Salicylates; Sodium Phosphates; Topiramate; Warfarin

The levels/effects of Torsemide may be increased by: Alfuzosin; Analgesics (Opioid); Barbiturates; Beta2-Agonists; Brimonidine (Topical); Canagliflozin; Ceritinib; Corticosteroids (Orally Inhaled); Corticosteroids (Systemic); CycloSPORINE (Systemic); CYP2C9 Inhibitors (Moderate); CYP2C9 Inhibitors (Strong); Diazoxide; Eltrombopag; Herbs (Hypotensive Properties); Licorice; MAO Inhibitors; Methotrexate; Mifepristone; Pentoxifylline; Phosphodiesterase 5 Inhibitors; Probenecid; Prostacyclin Analogues

Decreased Effect

Torsemide may decrease the levels/effects of: Hypoglycemic Agents; Lithium; Neuromuscular-Blocking Agents

The levels/effects of Torsemide may be decreased by: Bile Acid Sequestrants; CYP2C9 Inducers (Strong); Dabrafenib; Herbs (Hypertensive Properties); Methotrexate; Methylphenidate; Nonsteroidal Anti-Inflammatory Agents; Peginterferon Alfa-2b; Probenecid; Salicylates; Yohimbine

Stability

I.V.: Store at 15°C to 30°C (59°F to 86°F). For continuous infusion, a 10 mg/mL dilution in D_5W, NS, or 0.45% sodium chloride is stable for 24 hours at room temperature.

Tablets: Store at 15°C to 30°C (59°F to 86°F).

Mechanism of Action Inhibits reabsorption of sodium and chloride in the ascending loop of Henle and distal renal tubule, interfering with the chloride-binding cotransport system, thus causing increased excretion of water, sodium, chloride, magnesium, and calcium; does not alter GFR, renal plasma flow, or acid-base balance

Pharmacodynamics

Onset of action:
Oral: 60 minutes
I.V.: 10 minutes
Maximum effect:
Oral: 60-120 minutes
I.V.: Within 60 minutes
Duration: Oral, I.V.: 6-8 hours

Pharmacokinetics (Adult data unless noted)

Absorption: Oral: Rapid
Distribution: V_d: 12-15 L; cirrhosis: approximately doubled
Protein binding: Plasma: ≥99%
Metabolism: Hepatic by cytochrome P450, 80%

Bioavailability: ~80%
Half-life: 3.5 hours; 7-8 hours in cirrhosis (dose modification appears unnecessary)
Time to peak serum concentration: Oral: 1 hour; delayed ~30 minutes when administered with food
Elimination: 20% eliminated unchanged in urine

Dosing: Usual Adults (**Note:** I.V. and oral dosing are equivalent):
Edema:
Chronic renal failure: Oral, I.V.: Initial: 20 mg once daily; may increase gradually by doubling dose until the desired diuretic response is obtained (maximum recommended daily dose: 200 mg)
Heart failure:
Oral: Initial: 10-20 mg once daily; may increase gradually by doubling dose until the desired diuretic response is obtained. **Note:** ACC/AHA 2009 guidelines for heart failure maximum daily dose: 200 mg (Hunt, 2009)
I.V.: Initial: 10-20 mg; may repeat every 2 hours with double the dose as needed. **Note:** ACC/AHA 2009 guidelines for heart failure recommend maximum single dose:100-200 mg (Hunt, 2009)
Hepatic cirrhosis: Oral: Initial: 5-10 mg once daily; may increase gradually by doubling dose until the desired diuretic response is obtained (maximum recommended single dose: 40 mg). **Note:** Administer with an aldosterone antagonist or a potassium-sparing diuretic.
Hypertension: Oral: Initial: 5 mg once daily; may increase to 10 mg once daily after 4-6 weeks if adequate antihypertensive response is not apparent; if still not effective, an additional antihypertensive agent may be added. Usual dosage range (JNC 7): 2.5-10 mg once daily. **Note:** Thiazide-type diuretics are preferred in the treatment of hypertension (Chobanian, 2003)

Administration

I.V.: Administer over ≥2 minutes; reserve I.V. administration for situations which require rapid onset of action
Oral: Administer without regard to meals; patients may be switched from the I.V. form to the oral (and vice-versa) with no change in dose

Monitoring Parameters Renal function, serum electrolytes, fluid balance, blood pressure, body weight

Additional Information 10-20 mg torsemide is approximately equivalent to:
Furosemide 40 mg
Bumetanide 1 mg

Dosage Forms Excipient information presented when available (limited, particularly for generics); consult specific product labeling.
Solution, Intravenous:
Generic: 20 mg/2 mL (2 mL); 50 mg/5 mL (5 mL)
Tablet, Oral:
Demadex: 5 mg, 10 mg, 20 mg, 100 mg [scored]
Generic: 5 mg, 10 mg, 20 mg, 100 mg

References

Bard RL, Bleske BE, and Nicklas JM, "Food: An Unrecognized Source of Loop Diuretic Resistance," *Pharmacotherapy*, 2004, 24(5):630-7.
Chobanian AV, Bakris GL, Black HR, et al, "The Seventh Report of the Joint National Committee on Prevention, Detection, Evaluation, and Treatment of High Blood Pressure: The JNC 7 Report," *JAMA*, 2003, 289(19):2560-72.

◆ **Total Allergy [OTC]** *see* DiphenhydrAMINE (Systemic) *on page 673*

◆ **Total Allergy Medicine [OTC]** *see* DiphenhydrAMINE (Systemic) *on page 673*

◆ **Totect** *see* Dexrazoxane *on page 626*

◆ **tPA** *see* Alteplase *on page 104*

◆ **TPV** *see* Tipranavir *on page 2031*

◆ **tRA** *see* Tretinoin (Systemic) *on page 2068*

Trace Elements (trase EL e ments)

Related Information

Pediatric Parenteral Nutrition *on page 2312*

Brand Names: U.S. Multitrace-4; Multitrace-4 Concentrate; Multitrace-4 Neonatal; Multitrace-4 Pediatric; Multitrace-5; Multitrace-5 Concentrate; Trace Elements 4 Pediatric

Therapeutic Category Mineral, Parenteral; Trace Element, Multiple, Neonatal; Trace Element, Parenteral

Generic Availability (U.S.) Yes

Use Prevent and correct trace metal deficiencies (FDA approved in all ages)

Pregnancy Risk Factor C

Pregnancy Considerations Refer to individual elements for requirements in pregnancy.

Breast-Feeding Considerations Refer to individual elements for requirements while breast-feeding.

Contraindications Hypersensitivity to a specific trace metal or component of the trace metal solution; do not give undiluted, direct injection due to potential for phlebitis and tissue irritation

Warnings Metals may accumulate in conditions of renal failure or biliary obstruction; consider reduction in dosage or deletion of copper and manganese in patients with biliary obstruction; avoid copper use in patients with Wilson's disease; administration of copper in the absence of zinc or zinc in the absence of copper may cause decreases in their respective plasma levels; multiple trace metal solutions present a risk of overdosage when the need for one trace element is appreciably higher than for others in the formulation; utilization of individual trace metal solutions may be needed. Consider reduction in dosage or deletion of selenium and chromium in patients with renal dysfunction.

Some products contain benzyl alcohol which may cause allergic reactions in susceptible individuals; large amounts of benzyl alcohol (≥99 mg/kg/day) have been associated with a potentially fatal toxicity ("gasping syndrome") in neonates; the "gasping syndrome" consists of metabolic acidosis, respiratory distress, gasping respirations, CNS dysfunction (including convulsions, intracranial hemorrhage), hypotension and cardiovascular collapse; *in vitro* and animal studies have shown that benzoate, a metabolite of benzyl alcohol, displaces bilirubin from protein-binding sites; use benzyl alcohol-containing products with caution in neonates.

Precautions The parenteral product contains aluminum; toxic aluminum concentrations may be seen with high doses, prolonged use, or renal dysfunction. Premature neonates are at higher risk due to immature renal function and aluminum intake from other parenteral sources. Parenteral aluminum exposure of >4-5 mcg/kg/day is associated with CNS and bone toxicity and tissue loading may occur at lower doses.

Food Interactions Decreased absorption of oral zinc when administered with bran products, protein, and phytates.

Pharmacokinetics (Adult data unless noted)

Chromium: 10% to 20% oral absorption; excretion primarily via kidneys and bile

Copper: 30% oral absorption; 80% elimination via bile; intestinal wall 16% and urine 4%

Manganese: 10% oral absorption; excretion primarily via bile; ancillary routes via pancreatic secretions or reabsorption into the intestinal lumen occur during periods of biliary obstruction

Selenium: Very poor oral absorption; 75% excretion via kidneys, remainder via feces, lung, and skin

Zinc: 20% to 30% oral absorption; 90% excretion in stools, remainder via urine and perspiration

Dosing: Neonatal

ASPEN Guidelines: Trace Mineral Daily Requirements[1] (Mirtallo, 2004)

	Preterm Neonates (<3 kg)	Term Neonates (3-10 kg)
Chromium[2]	0.05-0.2 mcg/kg	0.2 mcg/kg
Copper[3]	20 mcg/kg	20 mcg/kg
Manganese[4]	1 mcg/kg	1 mcg/kg
Selenium[2,5]	1.5-2 mcg/kg	2 mcg/kg
Zinc	400 mcg/kg	50-250 mcg/kg

[1]Recommended intakes of trace elements **cannot** be achieved through the use of a commercially available combination trace element product. Only through the use of individualized trace element products can recommended intakes be achieved.

[2]Reduce dose in patients with renal dysfunction.

[3]Reduce dose by 50% in patients with impaired biliary excretion or cholestatic liver disease.

[4]Omit in patients with impaired biliary excretion or cholestatic liver disease.

[5]Indicated for use in long-term parenteral nutrition patients.

Term neonates (3-10 kg): 20 mcg/kg

Dosing: Usual

Infants, Children, and Adolescents:

ASPEN Guidelines: Trace Mineral Daily Requirements[1] (Mirtallo, 2004)

	Infants 3-10 kg	Infants, Children, and Adolescents 10-40 kg	Adolescents >40 kg
Chromium[2]	0.2 mcg/kg	0.14-0.2 mcg/kg	5-15 mcg
Copper[3]	20 mcg/kg	5-20 mcg/kg	200-500 mcg
Manganese[4]	1 mcg/kg	1 mcg/kg	40-100 mcg
Selenium[2,5]	2 mcg/kg	1-2 mcg/kg	40-60 mcg
Zinc	50-250 mcg/kg	50-125 mcg/kg	2-5 **mg**

[1]Recommended intakes of trace elements **cannot** be achieved through the use of a commercially available combination trace element product. Only through the use of individualized trace element products can recommended intakes be achieved.

[2]Reduce dose in patients with renal dysfunction.

[3]Reduce dose by 50% in patients with impaired biliary excretion or cholestatic liver disease.

[4]Omit in patients with impaired biliary excretion or cholestatic liver disease.

[5]Indicated for use in long-term parenteral nutrition patients.

Adults: **Recommended daily parenteral dosage: Manufacturer labeling:**

Chromium: 10-15 mcg; use caution in renal dysfunction

Copper: 0.5-1.5 **mg**; decrease dose or omit in patients with severe liver dysfunction and/or biliary tract obstruction

Manganese: 150-800 mcg; decrease dose or omit in patients with severe liver dysfunction and/or biliary tract obstruction

Selenium: 20-40 mcg; decrease dose or omit in patients with renal dysfunction and/or gastrointestinal malfunction

Zinc: 2.5-4 **mg**

◀ **Administration** Parenteral: Must be diluted prior to use and infused as component of parenteral nutrition or parenteral solutions

Reference Range

Chromium: 0.18-0.47 ng/mL (SI: 35-90 nmol/L); some laboratories report much higher

Copper: ~0.7-1.5 mcg/mL (SI: 11-24 micromoles/L); levels are higher in pregnant women and children; Note: May not be a meaningful measurement of body stores.

Manganese: 18-30 mcg/dL (SI: 2.3-3.8 micromoles/L)

Selenium: 95-165 ng/mL (SI: 120-209 nmol/L)

Zinc: 70-120 mcg/dL (SI: 10-18.4 micromoles/L)

Additional Information The following describe the symptomatology associated with excess trace elements:

Chromium: Nausea, vomiting, GI ulcers, renal and hepatic dysfunction, convulsions, coma

Copper: Prostration, behavioral changes, diarrhea, progressive marasmus, hypotonia, photophobia, hepatic dysfunction, peripheral edema

Manganese: Irritability, speech disturbances, abnormal gait, headache, anorexia, apathy, impotence, cholestatic jaundice, movement disorders

Selenium: Alopecia, weak nails, dermatitis, dental defects, GI disorders, nervousness, mental depression, metallic taste, garlic odor of breath and sweat

Zinc: Profuse diaphoresis, consciousness decreased, blurred vision, tachycardia, hypothermia

Dosage Forms Excipient information presented when available (limited, particularly for generics); consult specific product labeling.

Injection, solution [combination products]:

Multitrace-4: Chromium 4 mcg, copper 0.4 mg, manganese 0.1 mg, and zinc 1 mg per 1 mL (10 mL) [contains aluminum, benzyl alcohol]

Multitrace-4 Concentrate: Chromium 10 mcg, copper 1 mg, manganese 0.5 mg, and zinc 5 mg per 1 mL (1 mL) [contains aluminum]; chromium 10 mcg, copper 1 mg, manganese 0.5 mg, and zinc 5 mg per 1 mL (10 mL) [contains benzyl alcohol]

Multitrace-4 Neonatal: Chromium 0.85 mcg, copper 0.1 mg, manganese 0.025 mg, and zinc 1.5 mg per 1 mL (2 mL) [contains aluminum]

Multitrace-5: Chromium 4 mcg, copper 0.4 mg, manganese 0.1 mg, selenium 20 mcg, and zinc 1 mg per 1 mL (10 mL) [contains aluminum, benzyl alcohol]

Multitrace-5 Concentrate: Chromium 10 mcg, copper 1 mg, manganese 0.5 mg, selenium 60 mcg, and zinc 5 mg per 1 mL (1 mL) [contains aluminum]; chromium 10 mcg, copper 1 mg, manganese 0.5 mg, selenium 60 mcg, and zinc 5 mg per 1 mL (10 mL) [contains benzyl alcohol]

Trace Elements 4 Pediatric: Chromium 1 mcg, copper 0.1 mg, manganese 0.03 mg, and zinc 0.5 mg per 1 mL (10 mL) [contains aluminum, benzyl alcohol]

Injection, solution [combination products, preservative free]:

Multitrace-4 Pediatric: Chromium 1 mcg, copper 0.1 mg, manganese 0.025 mg, and zinc 1 mg per 1 mL (3 mL) [contains aluminum]

References

Carney LN, Nepa A, Cohen SS, et al, "Parenteral and Enteral Nutrition Support: Determining the Best Way to Feed," In: Corkins MR, Balint J, Bobo E, et al, eds, The A.S.P.E.N Pediatric Nutrition Support Core Curriculum, Silver Spring, MD: American Society of Parenteral and Enteral Nutrition, 2010, 440-1.

Dahlstrom KA, Ament ME, Medhin MG, et al, "Serum Trace Elements in Children Receiving Long-Term Parenteral Nutrition," J Pediatr, 1986, 109(4):625-30.

Department Health and Human Services, Food Drug Administration, "Aluminum in Large and Small Volume Parenterals Used in Total Parenteral Nutrition," Federal Register, 2000, 65(17):4103-11.

Fell JM, Reynolds AP, Meadows N, et al, "Manganese Toxicity in Children Receiving Long-Term Parenteral Nutrition," Lancet, 1996, 347(9010):1218-21.

Greene HL, Hambridge KM, Schanler R, et al, "Guidelines for the Use of Vitamins, Trace Elements, Calcium, Magnesium and Phosphorus in Infants and Children Receiving Total Parenteral Nutrition: Report of the Subcommittee on Pediatric Nutrient Requirements From the Committee on Clinical Practice Issues of The American Society for Clinical Nutrition," Am J Clin Nutr, 1988, 48(5):1324-42.

Litov RE and Combs GF Jr, "Selenium in Pediatric Nutrition," Pediatrics, 1991, 87(3):339-51.

Mirtallo J, Canada T, Johnson D, et al, "Safe Practices for Parenteral Nutrition," JPEN J Parenter Enteral Nutr, 2004, 28(6):S39-70.

◆ **Trace Elements 4 Pediatric** see Trace Elements on page 2059

◆ **Trace Metals** see Trace Elements on page 2059

◆ **Trace Minerals** see Trace Elements on page 2059

◆ **Tracleer** see Bosentan on page 298

◆ **Tracleer® (Can)** see Bosentan on page 298

TraMADol (TRA ma dole)

Medication Safety Issues

Sound-alike/look-alike issues:

TraMADol may be confused with tapentadol, Toradol Trandate, traZODone, Voltaren

Ultram may be confused with Ultane, Ultracet, Voltaren

International issues:

Theradol [Netherlands] may be confused with Foradil brand name for formoterol [U.S., Canada, and multiple international markets], Terazol brand name for terconazole [U.S. and Canada], and Toradol brand name for ketorolac [Canada and multiple international markets]

Trexol [Mexico] may be confused with Trexall brand name for methotrexate [U.S.]; Truxal brand name for chlorprothixene [multiple international markets]

Related Information

Oral Medications That Should Not Be Crushed or Altered on page 2438

Brand Names: U.S. Active-Tramadol; ConZip; EnovaRX-Tramadol; Ultram; Ultram ER

Brand Names: Canada Durela; Ralivia; Tridural; Ultram; Zytram XL

Therapeutic Category Analgesic, Opioid

Generic Availability (U.S.) Yes

Use

Immediate release formulations: Relief of moderate to moderately-severe pain (Ultram: FDA approved in ages ≥17 years and adults; Rybix™ ODT: FDA approved in ages ≥16 years and adults), including postoperative, cancer, neuropathic, low back pain, and pain associated with orthopedic disorders)

Extended release formulations: For patients requiring around-the-clock management of moderate to moderately-severe pain for an extended period of time (Ultram ER: FDA approved in ages ≥18 years and adults)

Pregnancy Risk Factor C

Pregnancy Considerations Adverse events were observed in animal reproduction studies. Tramadol has been shown to cross the human placenta when administered during labor. Postmarketing reports following tramadol use during pregnancy include neonatal seizures, withdrawal syndrome, fetal death, and stillbirth. Tramadol is not recommended for use during labor and delivery. Some Canadian products are contraindicated for use in pregnant women.

If chronic opioid exposure occurs in pregnancy, adverse events in the newborn (including withdrawal) may occur; monitoring of the neonate is recommended (Chou, 2009). Neonatal abstinence syndrome following opioid exposure may present with autonomic (eg, fever, temperature instability), gastrointestinal (eg, diarrhea, vomiting, poor feeding/weight gain), or neurologic (eg, high-pitched crying, increased muscle tone, irritability, seizure, tremor) symptoms (Dow, 2012; Hudak, 2012).

Breast-Feeding Considerations Tramadol is excreted into breast milk. Sixteen hours following a single 100 mg I.V. dose, the amount of tramadol found in breast milk was 0.1% of the maternal dose. Use is not recommended by the manufacturer for postdelivery analgesia in nursing mothers. Some Canadian products are contraindicated for use in nursing women. Nursing infants exposed to large doses of opioids should be monitored for apnea and sedation (Montgomery, 2012).

Contraindications Hypersensitivity to tramadol, opioids, or any component; opioid-dependent patients; acute intoxication with alcohol, hypnotics, centrally-acting analgesics, opioids, or psychotropic drugs

Tramadol extended release tablets: Patients with severe renal impairment (CrCl <30 mL/minute) or severe hepatic impairment (Child-Pugh Class C) since the extended release dosage form does not permit dosing flexibility required in this patient population; patients with severe/ acute bronchial asthma, hypercapnia, or significant respiratory depression in the absence of an appropriately monitored setting and resuscitation equipment

Warnings Tramadol should only be used with **EXTREME** caution in patients receiving MAO inhibitors due to increased risk of seizures and serotonin syndrome. Serotonin syndrome (eg, agitation, hallucinations, coma, tachycardia, labile blood pressure, hyperthermia, hyper-reflexia, incoordination, nausea, vomiting, diarrhea) may occur with concomitant use of tramadol and SSRIs, tricyclic antidepressants, MAOIs, triptans, linezolid, SNRIs, or drugs which impair tramadol metabolism (CYP2D6 and CYP3A4 inhibitors). An increased risk of seizures has been reported; the risk of seizures increases with doses above the recommended range or if naloxone administration is used to treat tramadol overdose; use with caution in patients with a history or an increased risk of seizures (eg, head trauma, increased intracranial pressure, metabolic disorders, CNS infection, malignancy, drug withdrawal).

Use associated with increased risk of suicide in patients already prone to addiction and/or taking tranquilizers or antidepressant drugs. Avoid use in patients who are suicidal or addiction prone. Tramadol interacts with alcohol and drugs of abuse and is subject to overdose, misuse, abuse, and diversion. Tolerance or drug dependence may result from extended use (withdrawal symptoms have been reported); abrupt discontinuation should be avoided. Tapering of dose at the time of discontinuation reduces the risk of withdrawal symptoms.

Not recommended for use during pregnancy or in nursing mothers; neonatal seizures, neonatal withdrawal syndrome, and fetal death have been reported.

Precautions Use with caution and reduce dosage when administered to patients receiving other CNS depressants (may cause CNS depression and/or respiratory depression when combined with other CNS depressants). Use with caution and reduce dosage in patients with liver disease, renal impairment, myxedema, hypothyroidism, or hypoadrenalism. Orally disintegrating tablet (Rybix ODT) contains aspartame which is metabolized to phenylalanine and must be used with caution in patients with phenylketonuria. Use may complicate clinical assessment of patients with acute abdominal conditions.

Adverse Reactions

Cardiovascular: Chest pain, flushing, hypertension, peripheral edema, orthostatic hypotension, vasodilation

Central nervous system: Agitation, anxiety, apathy, chills, confusion, coordination impaired, depersonalization, depression, dizziness, euphoria, fatigue, fever, headache, hypoesthesia, insomnia, lethargy, malaise, nervousness, pain, pyrexia, restlessness, somnolence, vertigo

Dermatologic: Dermatitis, pruritus, rash

Endocrine & metabolic: Hot flashes, hyperglycemia, menopausal symptoms

Gastrointestinal: Abdominal pain, anorexia, appetite decreased, constipation, diarrhea, dyspepsia, flatulence, nausea, vomiting, weight loss, xerostomia

Genitourinary: Pelvic pain, prostatic disorder, urinary frequency, urinary retention, urinary tract infection, urine abnormalities

Neuromuscular & skeletal: Arthralgia, back pain, creatine phosphokinase increased, hypertonia, myalgia, neck pain, paresthesia, rigors, tremor, weakness

Ocular: Blurred vision, miosis

Respiratory: Bronchitis, congestion (nasal/sinus), cough, dyspnea, nasopharyngitis, pharyngitis, rhinitis, rhinorrhea, sinusitis, sneezing, sore throat, upper respiratory infection

Miscellaneous: Diaphoresis, flu-like syndrome, shivering, withdrawal syndrome

Rare but important or life-threatening: Abnormal gait, allergic reaction, amnesia, anaphylactoid reactions, anaphylaxis, anemia, angioedema, appendicitis, ALT increased/decreased, AST increased/decreased, bradycardia, bronchospasm, BUN increased, cataracts, cellulitis, cholecystitis, cholelithiasis, clamminess, cognitive dysfunction, concentration difficulty, creatinine increased, deafness, disorientation, diverticulitis, dreams abnormal, dysphagia, dysuria, ear infection, ECG abnormalities, edema, fecal impaction, gastroenteritis, gastrointestinal bleeding, GGT increased, gout, hallucination, hematuria, hemoglobin decreased, hepatitis, hypotension, hypersensitivity, irritability, joint stiffness, libido decreased, liver enzymes increased, liver failure, menstrual disorder, MI, migraine, muscle cramps, muscle spasms, muscle twitching, myocardial ischemia, night sweats, palpitation, pancreatitis, peripheral edema, peripheral ischemia, pneumonia, proteinuria, pulmonary edema, pulmonary embolism, sedation, seizure, serotonin syndrome, sleep disorder, speech disorder, Stevens-Johnson syndrome, stomatitis, suicidal tendency, syncope, taste perversion, tachycardia, thrombocytopenia, tinnitus, toxic epidermal necrolysis, urticaria, vesicles, visual disturbance

A withdrawal syndrome may include anxiety, diarrhea, hallucinations (rare), nausea, pain, piloerection, rigors, sweating, and tremor. Uncommon discontinuation symptoms may include severe anxiety, panic attacks, or paresthesia.

Drug Interactions

Metabolism/Transport Effects Substrate of CYP2B6 (minor), CYP2D6 (major), CYP3A4 (major); **Note:** Assignment of Major/Minor substrate status based on clinically relevant drug interaction potential

Avoid Concomitant Use

Avoid concomitant use of TraMADol with any of the following: Azelastine (Nasal); CarBAMazepine; Conivaptan; Fusidic Acid (Systemic); Paraldehyde; Thalidomide

Increased Effect/Toxicity

TraMADol may increase the levels/effects of: Alcohol (Ethyl); Alvimopan; Antipsychotics; Azelastine (Nasal); Buprenorphine; CarBAMazepine; CNS Depressants; Desmopressin; Diuretics; Hydrocodone; MAO Inhibitors; Methotrimeprazine; Metoclopramide; Metyrosine; Paraldehyde; Pramipexole; ROPINIRole; Rotigotine; Selective Serotonin Reuptake Inhibitors; Serotonin Modulators; Thalidomide; Tricyclic Antidepressants; Vitamin K Antagonists; Zolpidem

The levels/effects of TraMADol may be increased by: Amphetamines; Anticholinergic Agents; Antipsychotic Agents (Phenothiazines); Antipsychotics; Brimonidine (Topical); Cannabis; Ceritinib; Conivaptan; ►

Cyclobenzaprine; CYP3A4 Inhibitors (Moderate); CYP3A4 Inhibitors (Strong); Dasatinib; Doxylamine; Dronabinol; Droperidol; Fusidic Acid (Systemic); HydrOXYzine; Ivacaftor; Kava Kava; Luliconazole; Magnesium Sulfate; Methotrimeprazine; Mifepristone; Nabilone; Perampanel; Rufinamide; Selective Serotonin Reuptake Inhibitors; Simeprevir; Sodium Oxybate; Stiripentol; Succinylcholine; Tapentadol; Tetrahydrocannabinol; Tricyclic Antidepressants

Decreased Effect

TraMADol may decrease the levels/effects of: CarBAMazepine; Pegvisomant

The levels/effects of TraMADol may be decreased by: Ammonium Chloride; Antiemetics (5HT3 Antagonists); Bosentan; CarBAMazepine; CYP2D6 Inhibitors (Moderate); CYP2D6 Inhibitors (Strong); CYP3A4 Inducers (Strong); Dabrafenib; Deferasirox; Mitotane; Mixed Agonist / Antagonist Opioids; Naltrexone; Siltuximab; St Johns Wort; Tocilizumab

Food Interactions

Immediate release tablet: Rate and extent of absorption were not significantly affected by food. Management: Administer without regard to meals.

Extended release:

ConZip™: Rate and extent of absorption were unaffected by food. Management: Administer without regard to meals.

Ultram® ER: High-fat meal reduced C_{max} and AUC, and increased T_{max} by 3 hours. Management: Administer with or without food, but keep consistent.

Orally disintegrating tablet: Food delays the time to peak serum concentration by 30 minutes; extent of absorption was not significantly affected. Management: Administer without regard to meals.

Stability Store at 25°C (77°F); excursions permitted to 15°C to 30°C (59°F to 86°F); protect from light; dispense in a tight container.

Mechanism of Action Tramadol and its active metabolite (M1) binds to μ-opiate receptors in the CNS causing inhibition of ascending pain pathways, altering the perception of and response to pain; also inhibits the reuptake of norepinephrine and serotonin, which are neurotransmitters involved in the descending inhibitory pain pathway responsible for pain relief (Grond, 2004)

Pharmacodynamics Immediate release formulations:

Onset of action: ~1 hour

Maximum effect: 2-4 hours

Duration: 3-6 hours

Pharmacokinetics (Adult data unless noted)

Absorption: Immediate release formulation: Rapid and complete; extended release formulation: Delayed

Distribution: V_d: 2.5-3 L/kg

Protein binding: 20%

Metabolism: Primarily hepatic via demethylation, glucuronidation, and sulfation; N-demethylation via CYP3A4; active O-desmethyltramadol metabolite formed by CYP2D6

Bioavailability: Immediate release: 75%; extended release: Ultram ER: 85% to 90% as compared to the immediate-release dosage form

Half-life:

Tramadol: ~6-8 hours

Active metabolite: 7-9 hours (prolonged in hepatic or renal impairment)

Time to peak serum concentration: Immediate release formulations: 2 hours; extended release (formulation specific): Ultram ER: ~12 hours; orally disintegrating tablet: Food delays the time to peak serum concentration by 30 minutes

Elimination: Excreted in urine as unchanged drug (30%) and metabolites (60%)

Dialysis: <7% removed in a 4-hour hemodialysis period

Dosing: Usual Moderate to severe pain: Oral:

Children and Adolescents 4-16 years: Immediate release tablet or liquid: 1-2 mg/kg/dose every 4-6 hours; maximum single dose: 100 mg; maximum total daily dose is the lesser of: 8 mg/kg/day **or** 400 mg/day (Finkel, 2002; Payne, 2002; Rose, 2003)

Adolescents ≥16 years and Adults:

Immediate release formulations:

Tablet: 50-100 mg every 4-6 hours; maximum total daily dose: 400 mg/day. For patients not requiring rapid onset of effect, tolerability to adverse effects may be improved by initiating therapy at 25 mg/day and titrating dose by 25 mg every 3 days until 25 mg 4 times/day is reached. Dose may then be increased by 50 mg every 3 days as tolerated to reach 50 mg 4 times/day.

Orally-disintegrating tablet (Rybix ODT): 50-100 mg every 4-6 hours; maximum total daily dose: 400 mg/day. For patients not requiring rapid onset of effect, tolerability to adverse effects may be improved by initiating therapy at 50 mg/day and titrating dose by 50 mg every 3 days until 50 mg 4 times/day is reached; maximum total daily dose: 400 mg/day

Extended release formulations: Ultram ER: Adults ≥18 years: 100 mg once daily; titrate by 100 mg increments every 5 days if needed for pain relief; maximum: 300 mg/day

Dosing adjustment in hepatic impairment:

Immediate release formulations: Adults: Cirrhosis: Recommended dose: 50 mg every 12 hours

Extended release formulations: Ultram ER: Do not use in patients with severe (Child-Pugh Class C) hepatic impairment

Dosing adjustment in renal impairment:

Immediate release formulations: Adults: CrCl <30 mL/minute: Administer 50-100 mg dose every 12 hours (maximum: 200 mg/day)

Extended release formulations: Do not use in patients with CrCl <30 mL/minute

Administration Oral:

Immediate release tablet: May administer with or without food, but it is recommended that it be administered in a consistent manner.

Extended release tablet: Swallow whole with a sufficient amount of liquid. Do not crush, cut, dissolve, or chew extended release tablet; tablet should be taken once daily at approximately the same time each day.

Orally disintegrating tablet: Remove from foil blister by peeling back (do not push tablet through the foil). Place tablet on tongue and allow to dissolve (may take ~1 minute); water is not needed but may be administered with water. Do not chew, break, or split tablet.

Monitoring Parameters Pain relief, respiratory rate, blood pressure, and pulse; signs of tolerance, oversedation, withdrawal, abuse or suicidal ideation; renal and hepatic function

Test Interactions May interfere with urine detection of phencyclidine (false-positive).

Dosage Forms Considerations

EnovaRX-Tramadol and Active-Tramadol are compounding kits. Refer to manufacturer's package insert for compounding instructions.

ConZip extended release capsules are formulated as a biphasic product, providing immediate and extended release components:

100 mg: 25 mg (immediate release) and 75 mg (extended release)

200 mg: 50 mg (immediate release) and 150 mg (extended release)

300 mg: 50 mg (immediate release) and 250 mg (extended release)

Dosage Forms Excipient information presented when available (limited, particularly for generics); consult specific product labeling.

Capsule Extended Release 24 Hour, Oral, as hydrochloride:

ConZip: 100 mg, 200 mg, 300 mg [contains fd&c blue #2 aluminum lake, fd&c yellow #10 aluminum lake]

Generic: 150 mg

Cream, External:

Active-Tramadol: 8% (120 g) [contains chlorocresol (chloro-m-cresol)]

Cream, External, as hydrochloride:

EnovaRX-Tramadol: 5% (60 g, 120 g) [contains cetyl alcohol]

Tablet, Oral, as hydrochloride:

Ultram: 50 mg [scored]

Generic: 50 mg

Tablet Extended Release 24 Hour, Oral, as hydrochloride:

Ultram ER: 100 mg, 200 mg, 300 mg

Generic: 100 mg, 200 mg, 300 mg

Extemporaneous Preparations A 5 mg/mL oral suspension may be made with tablets and either Ora-Sweet® SF or a mixture of 30 mL Ora-Plus® and 30 mL strawberry syrup. Crush six 50 mg tramadol tablets in a mortar and reduce to a fine powder. Add small portions of the chosen vehicle and mix to a uniform paste; mix while adding vehicle in incremental proportions to almost 60 mL; transfer to a calibrated bottle, rinse mortar with vehicle, and add quantity of vehicle sufficient to make 60 mL. Label "shake well before use". Stable for 90 days refrigerated or at room temperature.

Wagner DS, Johnson CE, Cichon-Hensley BK, et al, "Stability of Oral Liquid Preparations of Tramadol in Strawberry Syrup and a Sugar-Free Vehicle," *Am J Health Syst Pharm*, 2003, 60(12):1268-70.

References

Chou R, Fanciullo GJ, Fine PG, et al, "Clinical Guidelines for the Use of Chronic Opioid Therapy in Chronic Noncancer Pain," *J Pain*, 2009, 10 (2):113-30.

Dow K, Ordean A, Murphy-Oikonen J, et al, "Neonatal Abstinence Syndrome Clinical Practice Guidelines for Ontario," *J Popul Ther Clin Pharmacol*, 2012, 19(3):e488-506.

Finkel KJ, Rose JB, Schmitz ML, et al, "An Evaluation of the Efficacy and Tolerability of Oral Tramadol Hydrochloride Tablets for the Treatment of Postsurgical Pain in Children," *Anesth Analg*, 2002, 94 (6):1469-73.

Grond S, Sablotzki A. Clinical pharmacology of tramadol. *Clin Pharmacokinet*. 2004;43(13):879-923.

Hudak ML, Tan RC, Committee On Drugs, et al, "Neonatal Drug Withdrawal," *Pediatrics*, 2012, 129(2):e540-60.

Montgomery A, Hale TW, and Academy Of Breastfeeding Medicine, "ABM Cinical Protocol #15: Analgesia and Anesthesia for the Breastfeeding Mother, Revised 2012," *Breastfeed Med*, 2012, 7(6):547-53.

Payne KA, Roelofse JA, and Shipton EA, "Pharmacokinetics of Oral Tramadol Drops for Postoperative Pain Relief in Children Aged 4 to 7 Years – A Pilot Study," *Anesth Prog*, 2002, 49(4):109-12.

Rose JB, Finkel JC, Arquedas-Mohs A, et al, "Oral Tramadol for the Treatment of Pain of 7-30 Days' Duration in Children," *Anesth Analg*, 2003, 96(1):78-81.

◆ **Tramadol Hydrochloride** *see* TraMADol *on page 2060*

◆ **Trandate** *see* Labetalol *on page 1186*

Tranexamic Acid (tran eks AM ik AS id)

Medication Safety Issues

Sound-alike/look-alike issues:

Cyklokapron may be confused with cycloSPORINE

Brand Names: U.S. Cyklokapron; Lysteda

Brand Names: Canada Cyklokapron; Tranexamic Acid Injection BP

Therapeutic Category Antifibrinolytic Agent; Antihemophilic Agent; Hemostatic Agent

Generic Availability (U.S.) Yes

Use Injection: Short-term use (2-8 days) in hemophilia patients to reduce or prevent hemorrhage and reduce need for blood factor replacement therapy during and following tooth extraction [FDA approved in pediatric patients (age not specified) and adults]; primary menorrhagia; prevention of GI hemorrhage and hemorrhage following ocular trauma; recurrent epistaxis; hereditary angioneurotic edema; prophylactic use to decrease perioperative blood loss and the need for transfusion in patients undergoing congenital heart disease or scoliosis-related surgery

Tablet: Treatment of cyclic heavy menstrual bleeding (FDA approved in postmenarcheal women >18 years)

Pregnancy Risk Factor B

Pregnancy Considerations Adverse events were not observed in animal reproduction studies. Tranexamic acid crosses the placenta and concentrations within cord blood are similar to maternal concentrations. Tranexamic acid has been evaluated for the treatment of postpartum hemorrhage (Ducloy-Bouthors, 2011; Gungorduk, 2011). Lysteda is not indicated for use in pregnant women.

Breast-Feeding Considerations Small amounts of tranexamic acid are excreted in breast milk. The manufacturer recommends that caution be used if administered to a nursing woman.

Contraindications Hypersensitivity to tranexamic acid or any component; subarachnoid hemorrhage; acquired defective color vision, active intravascular clotting process; active thromboembolic disease (eg, cerebral thrombosis, DVT, or PE); history of thrombosis or thromboembolism, including retinal vein or retinal artery occlusion; intrinsic risk of thrombosis or thromboembolism (eg, hypercoagulopathy, thrombogenic cardiac rhythm disease, thrombogenic valvular disease)

Warnings Do not administer concomitantly with factor IX complex concentrates or anti-inhibitor coagulant concentrates due to increased risk of thrombosis. Concomitant use with combination hormonal contraception may further increase risk of thromboembolism; patients taking hormonal contraceptives were excluded from clinical trials. Visual defects (eg, color vision change, visual loss), and retinal venous and arterial occlusions have been reported; discontinue treatment if changes in vision occur; prompt ophthalmic examination should be performed by an ophthalmologist. Avoid use in patients with acquired defective color vision since this would prohibit monitoring one endpoint as a measure of ophthalmic toxicity. Ligneous conjunctivitis has been reported with the tablet, but usually resolves upon discontinuation of therapy. Severe hypersensitivity reactions have been reported rarely. Seizures have been reported with use; most often with intraoperative use (eg, open chamber cardiac surgery) and in older patients (Murkin, 2010). The mechanism by which tranexamic acid use results in seizures may be secondary to neuronal gamma aminobutyric acid (GABA) inhibition.

Precautions Dosage modification required in patients with renal impairment; use with caution in patients with cardiovascular, renal, cerebrovascular disease, or transurethral prostatectomy. Use with caution in patients with upper urinary tract bleeding; ureteral obstruction due to clot formation has been reported. Use with extreme caution in patients with DIC requiring antifibrinolytic therapy; patients should be under strict supervision of a physician experienced in treating this disorder. Use with caution with concurrent tretinoin use; may exacerbate procoagulant effects.

Adverse Reactions

Injection:

Cardiovascular: Hypotension (with rapid I.V. injection)

Central nervous system: Giddiness

Dermatologic: Allergic dermatitis

Endocrine & metabolic: Unusual menstrual discomfort

Gastrointestinal: Diarrhea, nausea, vomiting

Ocular: Blurred vision

Oral:
Central nervous system: Fatigue, headache
Gastrointestinal: Abdominal pain
Hematologic: Anemia
Neuromuscular & skeletal: Arthralgia, back pain, muscle cramps/spasms, muscle pain
Respiratory: Nasal/sinus symptoms

All formulations: Rare but important or life-threatening: Allergic skin reaction, anaphylactic shock, anaphylactoid reactions, cerebral thrombosis, deep vein thrombosis (DVT), diarrhea, dizziness, nausea, pulmonary embolism, renal cortical necrosis, retinal artery/vein obstruction, seizure, ureteral obstruction, visual disturbances (including impaired color vision and loss), vomiting

Drug Interactions
Metabolism/Transport Effects None known.
Avoid Concomitant Use
Avoid concomitant use of Tranexamic Acid with any of the following: Anti-inhibitor Coagulant Complex (Human); Contraceptives (Estrogens); Contraceptives (Progestins)
Increased Effect/Toxicity
Tranexamic Acid may increase the levels/effects of: Anti-inhibitor Coagulant Complex (Human); Fibrinogen Concentrate (Human)

The levels/effects of Tranexamic Acid may be increased by: Contraceptives (Estrogens); Contraceptives (Progestins); Fibrinogen Concentrate (Human); Tretinoin (Systemic)
Decreased Effect There are no known significant interactions involving a decrease in effect.
Stability Store at 25°C (77°F); excursions permitted to 15°C to 30°C (59°F to 86°F). Prepare on same day as infusion. Incompatible with solutions containing penicillin; compatible with dextrose, saline, and heparin, as well as with electrolyte, amino acid, or dextran solutions
Mechanism of Action Forms a reversible complex that displaces plasminogen from fibrin resulting in inhibition of fibrinolysis; it also inhibits the proteolytic activity of plasmin

With reduction in plasmin activity, tranexamic acid also reduces activation of complement and consumption of C1 esterase inhibitor (C1-INH), thereby decreasing inflammation associated with hereditary angioedema.
Pharmacokinetics (Adult data unless noted)
Distribution: Breast milk levels are 1% of serum; CSF levels are 10% of plasma
V_d: Adults: 9-27 L
Protein binding: 3%
Bioavailability: I.M.: 100%; oral: ~45%
Half-life: 2 hours
Time to peak serum concentration:
I.M.: 1 hour
I.V.: 5 minutes
Oral: ~3 hours
Elimination: Elimination characteristics differ by route of administration: after I.V. administration 95% excreted as unchanged drug in urine vs 39% after oral administration
Dosing: Neonatal I.V.: **Note:** Limited data available: Surgery for congenital diaphragmatic hernia during ECMO (bleeding reduction): 4 mg/kg as a single dose 30 minutes before repair, followed by a continuous infusion of 1 mg/kg/ **hour** for 24 hours, was reported to reduce blood loss and hemorrhagic complications in neonates (van der Staak, 1997)
Dosing: Usual Children: I.V.:
Tooth extraction in patients with hemophilia (in combination with replacement therapy): 10 mg/kg immediately before surgery, then 10 mg/kg/dose 3-4 times/day; may be used for 2-8 days
Surgery for congenital heart disease (to reduce perioperative blood loss and need for transfusions): Infants and Children 2 months to 15 years: Limited data available;

dose not established: Reported dosing regimens variable; ideal dose-response not established: Loading dose: 10 mg/kg, priming dose: 10 mg/kg and 10 mg/kg after protamine (Chauhan, 2004; Chauhan, 2004; Eaton, 2008); also reported: Loading dose: 100 mg/kg, followed by 10 mg/kg/hour infusion (continued until ICU transport) and 100 mg/kg priming dose when by-pass initiated (Reid, 1997)
Surgery for scoliosis (to reduce perioperative blood loss and need for transfusions): Children and Adolescents 8-18 years: Limited data available; dose not established: Reported dosing regimens variable; ideal dose-response not established: Loading dose: 100 mg/kg, followed by infusion: 10 mg/kg/hour until skin closure (Sethna, 2005; Shapiro 2007). Other regimens reported with positive results: Loading dose: 20 mg/kg, followed by 10 mg/kg/hour infusion (Grant, 2009) or loading dose: 10 mg/kg and 1 mg/kg/hour infusion (Grant, 2009; Neilipovitz, 2001)
Adults:
I.V.: Tooth extraction in patients with hemophilia (in combination with replacement therapy): 10 mg/kg immediately before surgery, then 10 mg/kg/dose 3-4 times/day; may be used for 2-8 days
Oral: Menorrhagia: 1300 mg 3 times daily (3900 mg/day) for up to 5 days during monthly menstruation

Dosing adjustment in renal impairment: Adults: See table.

Serum Creatinine (mg/dL)	I.V. Dose
1.36-2.83	10 mg/kg twice daily
>2.83-5.66	10 mg/kg once daily
>5.66	10 mg/kg every 48 h or 5 mg/kg every 24 h

Oral: Adult:
Serum creatinine >1.4-2.8 mg/dL: 1300 mg twice daily (2600 mg/day) for up to 5 days
Serum creatinine 2.9-5.7 mg/dL: 1300 mg once daily for up to 5 days
Serum creatinine >5.7 mg/dL: 650 mg once daily for up to 5 days
Administration Oral: Administer without regard to meals. Should be swallowed whole; do not break, chew, or crush.

Parenteral: May be administered by direct I.V. injection at a maximum rate of 100 mg/minute (1 mL/minute); in pediatric scoliosis studies, loading dose infused over 15 minutes
Monitoring Parameters Ophthalmologic exams (baseline and at regular intervals) of chronic therapy
Reference Range 5-10 mcg/mL is required to decrease fibrinolysis
Dosage Forms Excipient information presented when available (limited, particularly for generics); consult specific product labeling.
Solution, Intravenous:
Cyklokapron: 100 mg/mL (10 mL)
Generic: 100 mg/mL (10 mL)
Solution, Intravenous [preservative free]:
Generic: 100 mg/mL (10 mL)
Tablet, Oral:
Lysteda: 650 mg
Generic: 650 mg
Extemporaneous Preparations A 5% (50 mg/mL) oral solution may be prepared by diluting 5 mL of 10% (100 mg/mL) tranexamic acid injection with 5 mL sterile water. Label "refrigerate". Stable for 5 days refrigerated.

A 25 mg/mL oral suspension may be prepared with tablets. Place one 500 mg tablet (strength not available in U.S.) into 20 mL water and let stand ~2-5 minutes. Begin stirring and continue until the tablet is completely disintegrated, forming a fine particulate suspension (dispersion time for each 500 mg tablet is ~2-5 minutes). Administer immediately after preparation.

Lam MS, "Extemporaneous Compounding of Oral Liquid Dosage Formulations and Alternative Drug Delivery Methods for Anticancer Drugs," *Pharmacotherapy*, 2011, 31(2):164-92.

References

Chauhan S, Bisoi A, Kumar N, et al, "Dose Comparison of Tranexamic Acid in Pediatric Cardiac Surgery," *Asian Cardiovasc Thorac Ann*, 2004, 12(2):121-4.

Chauhan S, Das SN, Bisoi A, et al, "Comparison of Epsilon Aminocaproic Acid and Tranexamic Acid in Pediatric Cardiac Surgery," *J Cardiothorac Vasc Anesth*, 2004, 18(2):141-3.

Ducloy-Bouthors A, Jude B, Duhamel A, et al, "High-Dose Tranexamic Acid Reduces Blood Loss in Postpartum Heamorrhage," *Crit Care*, 2011, 15(2):R117.

Eaton MP, "Antifibrinolytic Therapy in Surgery for Congenital Heart Disease," *Anesth Analg*, 2008, 106(4):1087-100.

Grant JA, Howard J, Luntley J, et al, "Perioperative Blood Transfusion Requirements in Pediatric Scoliosis Surgery: The Efficacy of Tranexamic Acid," *J Pediatr Orthop*, 2009, 29(3):300-4.

Gungorduk K, Yildirim G, Asıcıoğlu O, et al, "Efficacy of Intravenous Tranexamic Acid In Reducing Blood Loss After Elective Cesarean Section: A Prospective, Randomized, Double-Blind, Placebo-Controlled Study," *Am J Perinatol*, 2011, 28(3):233-40.

Levin E, Wu J, Devine DV, et al, "Hemostatic Parameters and Platelet Activation Marker Expression in Cyanotic and Acyanotic Pediatric Patients Undergoing Cardiac Surgery in the Presence of Tranexamic Acid," *Thromb Haemost*, 2000, 83(1):54-9.

Murkin JM, Falter F, Granton J, et al, "High-Dose Tranexamic Acid Is Associated With Nonischemic Clinical Seizures in Cardiac Surgical Patients," *Anesth Analg*, 2010, 110(2):350-3.

Neilipovitz DT, Murto K, Hall L, et al, "A Randomized Trial of Tranexamic Acid to Reduce Blood Transfusion for Scoliosis Surgery," *Anesth Analg*, 2001, 93(1):82-7.

Reid RW, Zimmerman AA, Laussen PC, et al, "The Efficacy of Tranexamic Acid Versus Placebo in Decreasing Blood Loss in Pediatric Patients Undergoing Repeat Cardiac Surgery," *Anesth Analg*, 1997, 84(5):990-6.

Sethna NF, Zurakowski D, Brustowicz RM, et al, "Tranexamic Acid Reduces Intraoperative Blood Loss in Pediatric Patients Undergoing Scoliosis Surgery," *Anesthesiology*, 2005, 102(4):727-32.

Shapiro F, Zurakowski D, and Sethna NF, "Tranexamic Acid Diminishes Intraoperative Blood Loss and Transfusion in Spinal Fusions for Duchenne Muscular Dystrophy Scoliosis," *Spine (Phila Pa 1976)*, 2007, 32(20):2278-83.

van der Staak FH, de Haan AF, Geven WB, et al, "Surgical Repair of Congenital Diaphragmatic Hernia During Extracorporeal Membrane Oxygenation: Hemorrhagic Complications and the Effect of Tranexamic Acid," *J Pediatr Surg*, 1997, 32(4):594-9.

Zonis Z, Seear M, Reichert C, et al, "The Effect of Preoperative Tranexamic Acid on Blood Loss After Cardiac Operations in Children," *J Thorac Cardiovasc Surg*, 1996, 111(5):982-7.

◆ **Tranexamic Acid Injection BP (Can)** *see* Tranexamic Acid *on page 2063*

◆ **Transderm-V® (Can)** *see* Scopolamine (Systemic) *on page 1872*

◆ **Transderm-Nitro (Can)** *see* Nitroglycerin *on page 1504*

◆ **Transderm-Scop** *see* Scopolamine (Systemic) *on page 1872*

◆ **Trans-Plantar® (Can)** *see* Salicylic Acid *on page 1860*

◆ ***trans*-Retinoic Acid** *see* Tretinoin (Systemic) *on page 2068*

◆ ***trans*-Retinoic Acid** *see* Tretinoin (Topical) *on page 2071*

◆ **Trans-Ver-Sal® (Can)** *see* Salicylic Acid *on page 1860*

◆ **Trans-Ver-Sal AdultPatch [OTC]** *see* Salicylic Acid *on page 1860*

◆ **Trans-Ver-Sal PediaPatch [OTC]** *see* Salicylic Acid *on page 1860*

◆ **Trans-Ver-Sal PlantarPatch [OTC]** *see* Salicylic Acid *on page 1860*

◆ ***trans* Vitamin A Acid** *see* Tretinoin (Systemic) *on page 2068*

◆ **Tranxene-T** *see* Clorazepate *on page 524*

◆ **Tranxene T-Tab** *see* Clorazepate *on page 524*

◆ **Travel Sickness [OTC]** *see* Meclizine *on page 1317*

◆ **Travel Tabs [OTC] (Can)** *see* DimenhyDRINATE *on page 670*

TraZODone (TRAZ oh done)

Medication Safety Issues

Sound-alike/look-alike issues:

Desyrel may be confused with deferoxamine, Demerol, Delsym, Zestril

TraZODone may be confused with traMADol, ziprasidone

International issues:

Desyrel [Canada, Turkey] may be confused with Deseril brand name for methysergide [Australia, Belgium, Great Britain, Netherlands]

Related Information

Antidepressant Agents *on page 2219*

Oral Medications That Should Not Be Crushed or Altered *on page 2438*

Brand Names: U.S. Oleptro

Brand Names: Canada Apo-Trazodone; Apo-Trazodone D; Dom-Trazodone; Mylan-Trazodone; Novo-Trazodone; Nu-Trazodone; Nu-Trazodone D; Oleptro; PHL-Trazodone; PMS-Trazodone; ratio-Trazodone; Teva-Trazodone; Trazorel; ZYM-Trazodone

Therapeutic Category Antidepressant, Serotonin Reuptake Inhibitor/Antagonist

Generic Availability (U.S.) May be product dependent

Use Treatment of depression, including major depressive disorder (FDA approved in adults); has also been used for treatment of insomnia and prevention of migraines

Medication Guide Available Yes

Pregnancy Risk Factor C

Pregnancy Considerations Adverse effects were observed in some animal reproduction studies. When trazodone is taken during pregnancy, an increased risk of major malformations has not been observed in the limited number of pregnancies studied (Einarson, 2003; Einarson, 2009). The long-term effects of *in utero* trazodone exposure on infant development and behavior are not known.

The ACOG recommends that therapy with antidepressants during pregnancy be individualized; treatment of depression during pregnancy should incorporate the clinical expertise of the mental health clinician, obstetrician, primary healthcare provider, and pediatrician. According to the American Psychiatric Association (APA), the risks of medication treatment should be weighed against other treatment options and untreated depression. Consideration should be given to using agents with safety data in pregnancy. For women who discontinue antidepressant medications during pregnancy and who may be at high risk for postpartum depression, the medications can be restarted following delivery. Treatment algorithms have been developed by the ACOG and the APA for the management of depression in women prior to conception and during pregnancy (ACOG, 2008; APA, 2010; Yonkers, 2009).

Breast-Feeding Considerations Trazodone is excreted into breast milk; breast milk concentrations peak ~2 hours following administration. It is not known if the trazodone metabolite is found in breast milk (Verbeeck, 1986). The long-term effects on neurobehavior have not been studied. The manufacturer recommends that caution be exercised when administering trazodone to nursing women.

Contraindications Hypersensitivity to trazodone or any component

Warnings Trazodone is not approved for use in pediatric patients. Clinical worsening of depression or suicidal ideation and behavior may occur in children and adults with major depressive disorder **[U.S. Boxed Warning]**. In clinical trials, antidepressants increased the risk of suicidal thinking and behavior (suicidality) in children, adolescents, and young adults (18-24 years of age) with major depressive disorder and other psychiatric disorders. This risk must be considered before prescribing antidepressants for any clinical use. Short-term studies did **not** show an increased risk of suicidality with antidepressant use in patients >24 years of age and showed a decreased risk in patients ≥65 years.

Patients of all ages who are treated with antidepressants for any indication require appropriate monitoring and close observation for clinical worsening of depression, suicidality, and unusual changes in behavior, especially during the first few months after antidepressant initiation or when the dose is adjusted. Family members and caregivers should be instructed to closely observe the patient (ie, daily) and communicate condition with healthcare provider. Patients should also be monitored for associated behaviors (eg, anxiety, agitation, panic attacks, insomnia, irritability, hostility, aggressiveness, impulsivity, akathisia, hypomania, mania) which may increase the risk for worsening depression or suicidality. Worsening depression or emergence of suicidality (or associated behaviors listed above) that is abrupt in onset, severe, or not part of the presenting symptoms, may require discontinuation or modification of drug therapy.

To reduce risk of intentional overdose, write prescriptions for the smallest quantity consistent with good patient care. Screen individuals for bipolar disorder prior to treatment (using antidepressants alone may induce manic episodes in patients with this condition).

Serotonin syndrome (SS) and neuroleptic malignant syndrome (NMS)-like reactions may occur with trazodone when used alone, or particularly if used with other serotonergic agents (eg, SSRIs, SNRIs, or triptans), drugs that impair serotonin metabolism [eg, MAO inhibitors (use within 14 days)], or antidopaminergic agents (eg, antipsychotics). Identification and differentiation of SS (eg, tremor, myoclonus, agitation) and more severe NMS-like reactions (eg, hyperthermia, muscle rigidity, autonomic instability, mental status changes) can be complex; monitor patients closely for either syndrome. Discontinue treatment (and any concomitant serotonergic and/or antidopaminergic agents) immediately if signs/symptoms arise. If concurrent use is clinically warranted, carefully observe patient during treatment initiation and dose increases; concurrent use of serotonin precursors (eg, tryptophan) should be avoided.

Although the risk of conduction abnormalities is low with trazodone relative to other antidepressants, QT prolongation (with or without torsade de pointes) and ventricular tachycardia have been observed; use with caution in patients with preexisting cardiac disease or arrhythmias. Other arrhythmias reported include isolated PVCs, ventricular couplets, and tachycardia with syncope. Concurrent use of CYP3A4 inhibitors or drugs that prolong the QT interval may increase the risk of QT prolongation and/or proarrhythmia. Trazodone is not recommended for use during post-MI initial recovery phase. May cause rare (1:6000), prolonged, painful priapism (>6 hours in duration); instruct patient to seek medical assistance for erection lasting >4 hours; use with caution in patients who have conditions which may predispose them to priapism (eg, sickle cell anemia, multiple myeloma, leukemia).

Precautions Use with caution in patients with hepatic or renal impairment. Hypotension and syncope may occur; risk is high relative to other antidepressants; use with caution in patients at risk for these effects or in those who would not tolerate transient hypotensive episodes (eg, cerebrovascular disease, cardiovascular disease, hypovolemia, or concurrent medication use which may predispose to hypotension/bradycardia). May cause sedation (incidence: 20% to 50%), which may impair physical or mental abilities; the degree of sedation is very high with trazodone relative to other antidepressants; patients must be cautioned about performing tasks which require mental alertness (eg, operating machinery or driving). Some antidepressant agents (eg, SSRIs) have been associated with the development of SIADH; hyponatremia has been reported (including severe cases with serum sodium <110 mmol/L), predominately in the elderly; volume depletion and/or concurrent use of diuretics likely increases risk. Relative to tricyclic antidepressants, trazodone is associated with fewer anticholinergic adverse effects.

Drugs that interfere with serotonin reuptake (eg, SSRIs) have been associated with bleeding ranging from relatively minor bruising and epistaxis to life-threatening hemorrhage; similar to these agents, trazodone may also impair platelet aggregation resulting in increased risk of bleeding events, particularly if used concomitantly with aspirin, NSAIDs, warfarin or other anticoagulants. Discontinue use prior to elective surgery (unknown interactions with general anesthetics may exist).

Trazodone therapy should not be abruptly discontinued in patients receiving high doses for prolonged periods; gradually reduce dosage prior to complete discontinuation to avoid withdrawal symptoms (eg, anxiety, agitation, sleep disturbance). Trazodone may increase the risks associated with electroconvulsive therapy (ECT); consider discontinuing, when possible, prior to ECT treatment.

Adverse Reactions

Cardiovascular: Edema, hyper-/hypotension, syncope

Central nervous system: Agitation, concentration decreased, confusion, disorientation, dizziness, fatigue, headache, incoordination, memory impairment, migraine, sedation

Endocrine & metabolic: Libido decreased

Gastrointestinal: Abnormal taste, abdominal pain, constipation, diarrhea, flatulence, nausea, vomiting, weight gain/loss, xerostomia

Genitourinary: Ejaculation disorder, urinary urgency

Neuromuscular & skeletal: Back pain, myalgia, paresthesia, tremor

Ocular: Blurred vision, visual disturbance

Respiratory: Dyspnea, nasal congestion

Miscellaneous: Night sweats

Rare but important and life-threatening: Abnormal dreams, abnormal orgasm, acne, akathisia, allergic reactions, alopecia, amylase increased, anemia, anxiety, aphasia, apnea, appetite increased, arrhythmia, ataxia, atrial fibrillation, bladder pain, bradycardia, breast enlargement/engorgement, cardiac arrest, cardiospasm, cerebrovascular accident, chest pain, CHF, chills, cholestasis, clitorism, conduction block, diplopia, early menses, erectile dysfunction, extrapyramidal symptoms, eye pain, flushing, gait disturbance, hallucination, hearing loss (partial), hematuria, hemolytic anemia, hepatitis, hirsutism, hyperbilirubinemia, hyperhidrosis, hypersalivation, hypersensitivity, hypoesthesia, hypomania, impaired speech, impotence, insomnia, jaundice, lactation, leukocytosis, leukonychia, libido increased, liver enzyme alteration, methemoglobinemia, MI, muscle twitching, orthostatic hypotension, palpitation, paranoia, photophobia, photosensitivity reaction, priapism, pruritus, psoriasis, psychosis, QT prolongation, rash, reflux esophagitis, retrograde ejaculation, salivation increased, seizure, SIADH, speech impairment, stupor, tachycardia, tardive dyskinesia, tinnitus, torsade de pointes, urinary frequency increased, urinary retention, urinary incontinence, urticaria, vasodilation, ventricular ectopy, ventricular tachycardia, vertigo, dry eyes, weakness

Drug Interactions

Metabolism/Transport Effects Substrate of CYP2D6 (minor), CYP3A4 (major); **Note:** Assignment of Major/Minor substrate status based on clinically relevant drug interaction potential; **Inhibits** CYP3A4 (weak); **Induces** P-glycoprotein

Avoid Concomitant Use

Avoid concomitant use of TraZODone with any of the following: Conivaptan; Fusidic Acid (Systemic); Highest Risk QTc-Prolonging Agents; Ivabradine; Linezolid; Lopinavir; MAO Inhibitors; Methylene Blue; Mifepristone; Pimozide; Saquinavir

Increased Effect/Toxicity

TraZODone may increase the levels/effects of: Antipsychotic Agents (Phenothiazines); Antipsychotics; ARIPiprazole; Fosphenytoin; Highest Risk QTc-Prolonging Agents; Lomitapide; Methylene Blue; Metoclopramide; Moderate Risk QTc-Prolonging Agents; Phenytoin; Pimozide; Serotonin Modulators

The levels/effects of TraZODone may be increased by: Alcohol (Ethyl); Antiemetics (5HT3 Antagonists); Antipsychotic Agents (Phenothiazines); Antipsychotics; Atazanavir; Boceprevir; BusPIRone; Cobicistat; Conivaptan; CYP3A4 Inhibitors (Moderate); CYP3A4 Inhibitors (Strong); Darunavir; Dasatinib; Fosamprenavir; Fusidic Acid (Systemic); Indinavir; Ivabradine; Ivacaftor; Linezolid; Lopinavir; Luliconazole; MAO Inhibitors; Mifepristone; Nelfinavir; QTc-Prolonging Agents (Indeterminate Risk and Risk Modifying); Ritonavir; Saquinavir; Selective Serotonin Reuptake Inhibitors; Simeprevir; Stiripentol; Telaprevir; Tipranavir; Venlafaxine

Decreased Effect

TraZODone may decrease the levels/effects of: Warfarin

The levels/effects of TraZODone may be decreased by: Bosentan; CYP3A4 Inducers (Strong); Dabrafenib; Deferasirox; Fosphenytoin; Mitotane; Peginterferon Alfa-2b; Phenytoin; Siltuximab; St Johns Wort; Tocilizumab

Food Interactions Time to peak serum levels may be increased if immediate release trazodone is taken with food. Management: Administer immediate release after meals to decrease lightheadedness and postural hypotension. Administer extended release on an empty stomach.

Stability

Immediate release tablets: Store at 20°C to 25°C (68°F to 77°F); dispense in tight, light-resistant container

Extended release tablets: Store at room temperature 15°C to 30°C (59°F to 86°F); dispense in tight, light-resistant container

Mechanism of Action Inhibits reuptake of serotonin, causes adrenoreceptor subsensitivity, and induces significant changes in 5-HT presynaptic receptor adrenoreceptors. Trazodone also significantly blocks histamine (H_1) and alpha$_1$-adrenergic receptors.

Pharmacodynamics Onset of action: Antidepressant effect:

Immediate release: 1-4 weeks

Extended release: ~6 weeks

Pharmacokinetics (Adult data unless noted)

Absorption: Well absorbed

Protein binding: 85% to 95%

Metabolism: Hepatic via hydroxylation and oxidation; metabolized extensively by CYP3A4 to active metabolite, m-chlorophenylpiperazine (mCPP)

Half-life, elimination: 5-9 hours, prolonged in obese patients

Time to peak serum concentration:

Immediate release: Fasting: 1 hour; food: 2 hours

Extended release: 9 hours; not significantly affected by food

Elimination: Primarily in urine (74%, <1% excreted unchanged) with ~21% excreted in feces

Dosing: Usual

Children and Adolescents: Oral: Immediate release formulation:

Depression: Limited data available; efficacy results variable (Dopheide, 2006); **Note:** Not recommended for first- or second-line treatment of depression (AACAP, 2007):

Weight-based dosing: Children and Adolescents 6-18 years: Initial: 1.5-2 mg/kg/**day** in divided doses; increase gradually every 3-4 days as needed; maximum dose: 6 mg/kg/**day** in 3 divided doses

Fixed-dose: Adolescents: Initial: 25-50 mg/**day**; increase to 100-150 mg/**day** in divided doses

Insomnia; sleep disturbances (in children with comorbid psychiatric disorders): Limited trial or case report data available; however, frequently used clinically in children with comorbid psychiatric disorders (eg, mood disorder, anxiety disorder, developmental delay with ADHD) (Owens, 2010):

Children 18 months to 5 years: Limited data available; dosing based on a subset of pediatric trial including young children (n=16; range: 20 months to 5 years) with opsoclonus-myoclonus syndrome and used fixed doses (see below); however, the median overall dose (n=19) reported was 2.6 mg/kg/**day** (range: 1.2-6.9 mg/kg/**day**) (Pranzatelli, 2005); further studies are needed

Children 18 months to <3 years: Initial: 25 mg/dose at bedtime; may increase dose at 2-week intervals in 25 mg increments; maximum dose: 100 mg/dose

Children 3-5 years: Initial 50 mg/dose at bedtime; may increase dose at 2-week intervals in 25 mg increments; maximum dose: 150 mg/dose

Children >5 years and Adolescents: Initial: 0.75-1 mg/kg/dose or 25-50 mg at bedtime; reported range: 0.5-2 mg/kg/**day** (do not to exceed adult dosing: 200 mg/day); reported trials conducted in pediatric patients with comorbid psychiatric disorders (eg, ADHD, autism, developmental delay), or sleep bruxism (Hollway, 2011; Kratochvil, 2005); when used for palliative care, multiple daily dosing may be necessary; 25-50 mg/dose increase gradually to twice or three times daily as needed (do not exceed adult dosing)

Migraine, prophylaxis: Children and Adolescents ≥7 years: Limited data available: 1 mg/kg/**day** in 3 divided doses; maximum dose: 150 mg/dose; efficacy results variable, further studies are needed (Battistella, 1993; Damen, 2005; Lewis, 2004)

Adults: **Depression: Note:** Therapeutic effects may take up to 6 weeks. Therapy is normally maintained for 6-12 months after optimum response is reached to prevent recurrence of depression.

Immediate release: Initial: 150 mg/day in 3 divided doses (may increase by 50 mg/day every 3-7 days); maximum dose: 600 mg/day

Extended release: Initial: 150 mg once daily at bedtime (may increase by 75 mg/day every 3 days); maximum dose: 375 mg/day; once adequate response obtained, gradually reduce with adjustment based on therapeutic response

Dosing adjustment in renal impairment: Has not been studied; use with caution.

Dosing adjustment in hepatic impairment: Has not been studied; use with caution.

Administration Oral:

Immediate release: Administer after meals or a snack to decrease lightheadedness, sedation, and postural hypotension

Extended release: Take on an empty stomach; swallow whole or as a half tablet without food. Tablet may be broken along the score line, but do not crush or chew.

Monitoring Parameters Blood pressure, mental status, liver enzymes. Monitor patient periodically for symptom resolution; monitor for worsening depression, suicidality, and associated behaviors (especially at the beginning of therapy or when doses are increased or decreased).

Reference Range Note: Plasma levels do not always correlate with clinical effectiveness.
Therapeutic: 0.5-2.5 mcg/mL (SI: 1-6 micromoles/L)
Potentially toxic: >2.5 mcg/mL (SI: >6 micromoles/L)
Toxic: >4 mcg/mL (SI: >10 micromoles/L)

Test Interactions May interfere with urine detection of amphetamine/methamphetamine (false-positive).

Dosage Forms Excipient information presented when available (limited, particularly for generics); consult specific product labeling.
Tablet, Oral, as hydrochloride:
Generic: 50 mg, 100 mg, 150 mg, 300 mg
Tablet Extended Release 24 Hour, Oral, as hydrochloride:
Oleptro: 150 mg, 300 mg [scored]

References

AACAP Work Group on Quality Issues, "Practice Parameter for the Assessment and Treatment of Children and Adolescents With Depressive Disorders," *J Am Acad Child Adolesc Psychiatry,* 2007, 46(11):1503-26.

ACOG Committee on Practice Bulletins–Obstetrics, "ACOG Practice Bulletin: Clinical Management Guidelines for Obstetrician-Gynecologists Number 92, April 2008 (Replaces Practice Bulletin Number 87, November 2007). Use of Psychiatric Medications During Pregnancy and Lactation," *Obstet Gynecol,* 2008, 111(4):1001-20.

American Psychiatric Association, "Treatment Recommendations for Patients With Major Depressive Disorder," 3rd ed, May 2010. Available at http://www.psychiatryonline.com/pracGuide/pracGuideTopic_7.aspx

Dopheide JA, "Recognizing and treating Depression in Children and Adolescents," *Am J Health Syst Pharm,* 2006, 63(3):233-43.

Einarson A, Choi J, Einarson TR, et al, "Incidence of Major Malformations in Infants Following Antidepressant Exposure in Pregnancy: Results of a large Prospective Cohort Study," *Can J Psychiatry,* 2009, 54(4):242-6.

Hollway JA and Aman MG, "Pharmacological Treatment of Sleep Disturbance in Developmental Disabilities: A Review of the Literature," *Res Dev Disabil,* 2011, 32(3):939-62.

Klier CM, Mossaheb N, Saria A, et al, "Pharmacokinetics and Elimination of Quetiapine, Venlafaxine, and Trazodone During Pregnancy and Postpartum," *J Clin Psychopharmacol,* 2007, 27(6):720-2.

Kratochvil CJ, Lake M, Pliszka SR, et al, "Pharmacological Management of Treatment-Induced Insomnia in ADHD," *J Am Acad Child Adolesc Psychiatry,* 2005, 44(5):499-501.

Lewis D, Ashwal S, Hershey A, et al, "Practice Parameter: Pharmacological Treatment of Migraine Headache in Children and Adolescents: Report of the American Academy of Neurology Quality Standards Subcommittee and the Practice Committee of the Child Neurology Society," *Neurology,* 2004, 63(12):2215-24.

Owens JA, Rosen CL, Mindell JA, et al, "Use of Pharmacotherapy for Insomnia in Child Psychiatry Practice: A National Survey," *Sleep Med,* 2010, 11(7):692-700.

Pranzatelli MR, Tate ED, Dukart WS, et al, "Sleep Disturbance and Rage Attacks in Opsoclonus-Myoclonus Syndrome: Response to Trazodone," *J Pediatr,* 2005, 147(3):372-8.

US Preventive Services Task Force, "Screening and Treatment for major Depressive Disorder in Children and Adolescents: US Preventive Services Task Force Recommendation Statement," *Pediatrics,* 2009, 123(4):1223-8.

Verbeeck RK, Ross SG, and McKenna EA, "Excretion of Trazodone in Breast Milk," *Br J Clin Pharmacol,* 1986, 22(3):367-70.

Yonkers KA, Wisner KL, Stewart DE, et al, "The Management of Depression During Pregnancy: A Report From the American Psychiatric Association and the American College of Obstetricians and Gynecologists," *Obstet Gynecol,* 2009, 114(3):703-13.

Zubieta JK and Alessi NE, "Acute and Chronic Administration of Trazodone in the Treatment of Disruptive Behavior Disorders in Children," *J Clin Psychopharmacol,* 1992, 12(5):346-51.

◆ **Trazodone Hydrochloride** *see* TraZODone *on page 2065*

◆ **Trazorel (Can)** *see* TraZODone *on page 2065*

◆ **Trecator** *see* Ethionamide *on page 808*

◆ **Trecator® (Can)** *see* Ethionamide *on page 808*

◆ **Tremytoine Inj (Can)** *see* Phenytoin *on page 1663*

◆ **TRENtal [DSC]** *see* Pentoxifylline *on page 1646*

◆ **Tretin-X** *see* Tretinoin (Topical) *on page 2071*

Tretinoin (Systemic) (TRET i noyn)

Medication Safety Issues
Sound-alike/look-alike issues:
Tretinoin may be confused with ISOtretinoin
Other safety concerns:
Tretinoin (which is also called all-*trans* retinoic acid, or ATRA) may be confused with isotretinoin; while both products may have uses in cancer treatment, they are **not** interchangeable.

Related Information
Emetogenic Potential of Antineoplastic Agents in Children *on page 2327*
Oral Medications That Should Not Be Crushed or Altered *on page 2438*
Safe Handling of Hazardous Drugs *on page 2419*

Brand Names: Canada Vesanoid®

Therapeutic Category Antineoplastic Agent, Miscellaneous; Antineoplastic Agent, Retinoic Acid Derivatives; Retinoic Acid Derivative

Generic Availability (U.S.) Yes

Use Induction of remission in patients with acute promyelocytic leukemia (APL), French American British (FAB) classification M3 (including the M3 variant) characterized by t(15;17) translocation and/or PML/RARα gene presence (FDA approved in adults); has also been used in post consolidation and maintenance therapy in APL and combination therapy (with arsenic trioxide) for remission induction in APL

Pregnancy Risk Factor D

Pregnancy Considerations Adverse events were observed in animal reproduction studies. **[U.S. Boxed Warning]: High risk of teratogenicity; if treatment with tretinoin is required in women of childbearing potential, two reliable forms of contraception should be used simultaneously during and for 1 month after treatment, unless abstinence is the chosen method. Within 1 week prior to starting therapy, serum or urine pregnancy test (sensitivity at least 50 mIU/mL) should be collected. If possible, delay therapy until results are available. Repeat pregnancy testing and contraception counseling monthly throughout the period of treatment.** Contraception must be used even when there is a history of infertility or menopause, unless a hysterectomy has been preformed. Tretinoin was detected in the serum of a neonate at birth following maternal use of standard doses during pregnancy (Takitani, 2005). Use in humans for the treatment of acute promyelocytic leukemia (APL) is limited and exposure occurred after the first trimester in most cases (Valappil, 2007). However, major fetal abnormalities and spontaneous abortions have been reported with other retinoids; some of these abnormalities were fatal. If the clinical condition of a patient presenting with APL during pregnancy warrants immediate treatment, tretinoin use should be avoided in the first trimester; treatment with tretinoin may be considered in the second and third trimester with careful fetal monitoring, including cardiac monitoring (Sanz, 2009).

Breast-Feeding Considerations It is not known if tretinoin is excreted in breast milk. Due to the potential for serious adverse reactions in the nursing infant, breastfeeding should be discontinued prior to treatment initiation.

Contraindications Hypersensitivity to tretinoin, other retinoids, parabens, or any component

Warnings Hazardous agent; use appropriate precautions for handling and disposal (NIOSH, 2012). About 25% of patients with APL treated with tretinoin have experienced APL differentiation syndrome (DS); formerly called retinoic acid-APL [RA-APL] syndrome, which is characterized by fever, dyspnea, acute respiratory distress, weight gain, radiographic pulmonary infiltrates, and pleural or pericardial effusions, edema, and hepatic, renal, and/or multiorgan failure **[U.S. Boxed Warning]**. DS usually occurs during the first month of treatment with some cases reported following the first dose. DS has been observed with or without concomitant leukocytosis and has occasionally been accompanied by impaired myocardial contractility and episodic hypotension. Endotracheal intubation and mechanical ventilation have been required in some cases due to progressive hypoxemia and several patients have expired with multiorgan failure. About one half of DS cases are severe, which is associated with increased mortality. Management has not been defined, although high-dose steroids given at the first suspicion appear to reduce morbidity and mortality. Regardless of the leukocyte count, at the first signs suggestive of DS, immediately initiate steroid therapy with dexamethasone (10 mg I.V. every 12 hours for 3-5 days); taper off over 2 weeks. Most patients do not require termination of tretinoin therapy during treatment of DS.

During treatment, ~40% of patients will develop rapidly evolving leukocytosis **[U.S. Boxed Warning]**. A high WBC at diagnosis increases the risk for further leukocytosis and may be associated with a higher risk of life-threatening complications. If signs and symptoms of the APL-DS syndrome are present together with leukocytosis, initiate treatment with high-dose steroids immediately. Consider adding full-dose chemotherapy (including an anthracycline if not contraindicated) to the tretinoin therapy on day 1 or 2 for patients presenting with a WBC count of >5 x 10^9/L; or start immediately if WBC is <5 x 10^9/L at presentation or reaches ≥6 x 10^9/L by day 5 or ≥10 x 10^9/L by day 10 or ≥15 x 10^9/L by day 28.

Retinoids have been associated with pseudotumor cerebri (benign intracranial hypertension), especially in children. Concurrent use of other drugs associated with this effect (eg, tetracyclines) may increase risk. Early signs and symptoms include papilledema, headache, nausea, vomiting, visual disturbances, intracranial noises, or pulsate tinnitus.

There is a high risk of teratogenicity **[U.S. Boxed Warning]**. Increased risk of spontaneous abortion and major fetal abnormalities have been reported with use of other retinoids. If treatment with tretinoin is required in women of childbearing potential, two reliable forms of contraception should be used during and for 1 month after treatment. Microdosed progesterone preparations (eg, "minipill") may be inadequate during tretinoin treatment. Pregnancy testing and contraception counseling should be repeated monthly throughout the period of treatment. If possible, initiation of treatment with tretinoin should be delayed until negative pregnancy test result is confirmed.

Tretinoin treatment for APL should be initiated early; discontinue and consider alternate therapy if pending cytogenetic analysis does not confirm APL by t(15;17) translocation or the presence of the PML/RARα fusion protein (caused by translocation of the promyelocytic [PML] gene on chromosome 15 and retinoic acid receptor [RAR] alpha gene on chromosome 17).

Hypercholesterolemia and hypertriglyceridemia have been reported in up to 60% of patients, which was reversible upon completion of treatment. Elevated liver function test results occur in 50% to 60% of patients during treatment. Carefully monitor liver function test results during treatment and give consideration to a temporary withdrawal of tretinoin if test results reach >5 times the upper limit of normal. Most liver function test abnormalities will resolve without interruption of treatment or after therapy completion.

Precautions Tretinoin (which is also known as all-*trans* retinoic acid, or ATRA) and isotretinoin may be confused;

while both products may be used in cancer treatment, they are **not** interchangeable; verify product prior to dispensing and administration to prevent medication errors. The risk for thrombosis (arterial and venous) is increased during the first month of treatment. Use with caution with antifibrinolytic agents (eg, tranexamic acid, aminocaproic acid, aprotinin); thrombotic complications have been reported (rarely) with concomitant use. May cause headache, malaise, and/or dizziness; caution patients about performing tasks which require mental alertness (eg, operating machinery or driving). Avoid additional vitamin A supplementation; may lead to vitamin A toxicity. Tretinoin should only be administered under the supervision of a physician who is experienced in the management of patients with acute leukemia, including assessment of possible benefit outweighing risks of known adverse effects **[U.S. Boxed Warning]** since patients with APL are at high risk and can have severe adverse reactions to tretinoin.

Adverse Reactions Most patients will experience drug-related toxicity, especially headache, fever, weakness and fatigue. These are seldom permanent or irreversible and do not typically require therapy interruption.

Cardiovascular: Arrhythmias, cardiac arrest, cardiac failure, cardiomyopathy, chest discomfort, cerebral hemorrhage, edema, facial edema, flushing, heart enlarged, heart murmur, hyper-/hypotension, ischemia, MI, myocarditis, pallor, pericarditis, peripheral edema, secondary cardiomyopathy, stroke

Central nervous system: Agitation, anxiety, aphasia, cerebellar edema, CNS depression, coma, confusion, dementia, depression, dizziness, encephalopathy, facial paralysis, fever, forgetfulness, hallucination, headache, hypotaxia, hypothermia, insomnia, Intracranial hypertension, light reflex absent, malaise, pain, seizure, slow speech, somnolence, spinal cord disorder, unconsciousness

Dermatologic: Alopecia, cellulitis, pruritus, rash, skin changes, skin/mucous membrane dryness

Endocrine & metabolic: Acidosis, fluid imbalance, hypercholesterolemia and/or hypertriglyceridemia

Gastrointestinal: Abdominal distention, abdominal pain, anorexia, constipation, diarrhea, dyspepsia, GI hemorrhage, hepatitis, hepatosplenomegaly, liver function tests increased, mucositis, nausea/vomiting, ulcer, weight gain/loss

Genitourinary: Dysuria, micturition frequency, prostate enlarged

Hematologic: Disseminated intravascular coagulation, hemorrhage, leukocytosis

Hepatic: Ascites, hepatitis, liver function tests increased

Local: Phlebitis

Neuromuscular & skeletal: Abnormal gait, asterixis, bone inflammation, bone pain, dysarthria, flank pain, hemiplegia hyporeflexia leg weakness, myalgia, paresthesia, tremor

Ocular: Agnosia, ocular disorder, visual acuity change, visual disturbance, visual field deficit

Otic: Earache/ear fullness, hearing loss

Renal: Acute renal failure, renal insufficiency, renal tubular necrosis

Respiratory: Bronchial asthma, dyspnea, expiratory wheezing, larynx edema, lower respiratory tract disorders, pleural effusion, pneumonia, pulmonary hypertension, pulmonary infiltration, rales, respiratory insufficiency, upper respiratory tract disorders

Miscellaneous: Diaphoresis, infection, lymph disorder, shivering, retinoic acid-acute promyelocytic leukemia syndrome/differentiation syndrome

Rare but important or life-threatening: Arterial thrombosis, basophilia, erythema nodosum, genital ulceration, hypercalcemia, hyperhistaminemia, irreversible hearing loss, myositis, organomegaly, pancreatitis, pseudotumor

◄ cerebri, renal infarct, Sweet's syndrome, thrombocytosis, vasculitis (skin), venous thrombosis

Drug Interactions

Metabolism/Transport Effects Substrate of CYP2A6 (minor), CYP2B6 (minor), CYP2C8 (major), CYP2C9 (minor); **Note:** Assignment of Major/Minor substrate status based on clinically relevant drug interaction potential; **Inhibits** CYP2C9 (weak); **Induces** CYP2E1 (weak/moderate)

Avoid Concomitant Use

Avoid concomitant use of Tretinoin (Systemic) with any of the following: BCG; Multivitamins/Fluoride (with ADE); Multivitamins/Minerals (with ADEK, Folate, Iron); Multivitamins/Minerals (with AE, No Iron); Natalizumab; Pimecrolimus; Tacrolimus (Topical); Tetracycline Derivatives; Tofacitinib; Vaccines (Live); Vitamin A

Increased Effect/Toxicity

Tretinoin (Systemic) may increase the levels/effects of: Antifibrinolytic Agents; Leflunomide; Natalizumab; Porfimer; Tofacitinib; Vaccines (Live); Vitamin A

The levels/effects of Tretinoin (Systemic) may be increased by: CYP2C8 Inhibitors (Moderate); CYP2C8 Inhibitors (Strong); Deferasirox; Denosumab; Mifepristone; Multivitamins/Fluoride (with ADE); Multivitamins/Minerals (with ADEK, Folate, Iron); Multivitamins/Minerals (with AE, No Iron); Pimecrolimus; Roflumilast; Tacrolimus (Topical); Tetracycline Derivatives; Trastuzumab

Decreased Effect

Tretinoin (Systemic) may decrease the levels/effects of: BCG; Coccidioidin Skin Test; Contraceptives (Estrogens); Contraceptives (Progestins); Sipuleucel-T; Vaccines (Inactivated); Vaccines (Live)

The levels/effects of Tretinoin (Systemic) may be decreased by: CYP2C8 Inducers (Strong); Dabrafenib; Echinacea

Food Interactions Absorption of retinoids has been shown to be enhanced when taken with food. Management: Administer with a meal.

Stability Hazardous agent; use appropriate precautions for handling and disposal (NIOSH, 2012). Store at 20°C to 25°C (68°F to 77°F); protect from light.

Mechanism of Action Tretinoin appears to bind one or more nuclear receptors and decreases proliferation and induces differentiation of APL cells; initially produces maturation of primitive promyelocytes and repopulates the marrow and peripheral blood with normal hematopoietic cells to achieve complete remission

Pharmacokinetics (Adult data unless noted) Note:

Reported pediatric values similar to adult (Smith, 1992; Takitani, 2004)

Absorption: Well-absorbed

Protein binding: >95%, predominantly to albumin

Metabolism: Hepatic via CYP; primary metabolite: 4-oxo-all-*trans*-retinoic acid; displays autometabolism

Half-life: 0.5-2 hours

Time to peak serum concentration: 1-2 hours

Elimination: Urine (63%); feces (30%)

Dosing: Usual Refer to individual protocols: **Note:** Induction treatment of APL with tretinoin should be initiated early; discontinue if pending cytogenetic analysis does not confirm t(15;17) translocation or the presence of the PML/RARα fusion protein.

Acute promyelocytic leukemia (APL): Oral:

Children and Adolescents: Limited data available (de Botton, 2004; Gregory, 2009; Mann, 2001; Ortega, 2005; Sanz, 2009; Testi, 2005):

Remission induction: 45 mg/m^2/day in two equally divided doses until documentation of complete remission (CR); discontinue after CR or after 90 days of treatment, whichever occurs first

Remission induction (in combination with an anthracycline): 25 mg/m^2/day in two equally divided doses until complete remission or 90 days

Consolidation therapy, intermediate- and high-risk patients: 25 mg/m^2/day in two equally divided doses for 15 days each month for 3 months

Maintenance therapy, intermediate- and high-risk patients: 25 mg/m^2/day in two equally divided doses for 15 days every 3 months for 2 years

Adults:

Remission induction: 45 mg/m^2/day in two equally divided doses until documentation of complete remission (CR); discontinue 30 days after CR or after 90 days of treatment, whichever occurs first

Remission induction (in combination with an anthracycline +/- cytarabine): 45 mg/m^2/day in two equally divided doses until complete remission or 90 days (Powell, 2010) or until complete hematologic remission (Adès, 2008; Sanz, 2008; Sanz, 2010)

Remission induction (in combination with arsenic trioxide): 45 mg/m^2/day in two equally divided doses until <5% blasts in marrow and no abnormal promyelocytes or up to 85 days (Estey, 2006; Ravandi, 2009)

Consolidation therapy: 45 mg/m^2/day in two equally divided doses for 15 days each month for 3 months (in combination with chemotherapy) (Lo-Coco, 2010; Sanz, 2010) **or** 45 mg/m^2/day for 14 days every 4 weeks for 7 cycles (in combination with arsenic trioxide) (Ravandi, 2009)

Maintenance therapy, intermediate- and high-risk patients: 45 mg/m^2/day in two equally divided doses for 15 days every 3 months for 2 years (Sanz, 2004)

Dosing adjustment in renal impairment: There are no dosage adjustments provided in the manufacturer's labeling.

Dosing adjustment in hepatic impairment: Adults:

Hepatic impairment prior to treatment: There are no dosage adjustments provided in the manufacturer's labeling.

Hepatotoxicity during treatment: Liver enzymes may normalize with dosage reduction or with continued treatment; discontinue if normalization does not readily occur or if hepatitis is suspected.

Administration Hazardous agent; use appropriate precautions for handling and disposal (NIOSH, 2012). Administer with a meal; do not crush capsules.

It is not recommended to use the capsule contents to extemporaneously prepare tretinoin suspension; however, there are limited case reports of use in patients who are unable to swallow the capsules whole. In a patient with a nasogastric (NG) tube, tretinoin capsules were cut open, with partial aspiration of the contents into a glass syringe, the residual capsule contents were mixed with soy bean oil and aspirated into the same syringe and administered (Shaw, 1995). Tretinoin capsules have also been mixed with sterile water (~20 mL) and heated in a water bath (37°C) to melt the capsules and create an oily suspension for NG tube administration (Bargetzi, 1996). Tretinoin has also been administered sublingually by squeezing the capsule contents beneath the tongue (Kueh, 1999). Low plasma levels have been reported when contents of tretinoin capsules were administered directly through a feeding tube, although patient-specific impaired absorption may have been a contributing factor (Takitani, 2004).

Monitoring Parameters Bone marrow cytology to confirm t(15;17) translocation or the presence of the PML/RARα fusion protein (do not withhold treatment initiation for results); monitor CBC with differential, coagulation profile, liver function test results, and triglyceride and cholesterol levels frequently; monitor closely for signs of APL differentiation syndrome (eg, monitor volume status, pulmonary status, temperature, respiration)

Additional Information For management of APL differentiation syndrome, initiate at first signs of DS: Dexamethasone 10 mg I.V. every 12 hours for 3-5 days; consider interrupting tretinoin until resolution of hypoxia

Dosage Forms Excipient information presented when available (limited, particularly for generics); consult specific product labeling.

Capsule, Oral:

Generic: 10 mg

Extemporaneous Preparations Hazardous agent: Use appropriate precautions for handling and disposal.

Although the manufacturer does not recommend the use of the capsule contents to extemporaneously prepare a suspension of tretinoin (due to reports of low plasma levels) (Vesanoid® data on file), there are limited case reports of use in patients who are unable to swallow the capsules whole. In a patient with a nasogastric (NG) tube, tretinoin capsules were cut open, with partial aspiration of the contents aspirated into a glass syringe. The residual capsule contents were mixed with soybean oil, aspirated into the syringe, and administered (Shaw, 1995). Tretinoin capsules have also been mixed with sterile water (~20 mL) and heated in a water bath to melt the capsules and create an oily suspension for NG tube administration (Bargetzi, 1996). Tretinoin has also been administered sublingually by squeezing the capsule contents beneath the tongue (Kueh, 1999).

Bargetzi MJ, Tichelli A, Gratwohl A, et al, "Oral All-Transretinoic Acid Administration in Intubated Patients With Acute Promyelocytic Leukemia," *Schweiz Med Wochenschr*, 1996, 126(45):1944-5.

Kueh YK, Liew PP, Ho PC, et al, "Sublingual Administration of All-*Trans*-Retinoic Acid to a Comatose Patient With Acute Promyelocytic Leukemia," *Ann Pharmacother*, 1999, 33(4):503-5.

Shaw PJ, Atkins MC, Nath CE, et al, "ATRA Administration in the Critically III Patient," *Leukemia*, 1995, 9(7):1288.

Vesanoid® data on file, Roche Pharmaceuticals

References

Adès L, Sanz MA, Chevret S, et al, "Treatment of Newly Diagnosed Acute Promyelocytic Leukemia (APL): A Comparison of French-Belgian-Swiss and PETHEMA Results," *Blood*, 2008, 111(3):1078-84.

Bargetzi MJ, Tichelli A, Gratwohl A, et al, "Oral All-transretinoic Acid Administration in Intubated Patients With Acute Promyelocytic Leukemia," *Schweiz Med Wochenschr*, 1996, 126(45):1944-5.

de Botton S, Coiteux V, Chevret S, et al, "Outcome of Childhood Acute Promyelocytic Leukemia With All-*Trans*-Retinoic Acid and Chemotherapy," *J Clin Oncol*, 2004, 22(8):1404-12.

Estey E, Garcia-Manero G, Ferrajoli A, et al, "Use of All-*Trans* Retinoic Acid Plus Arsenic Trioxide as an Alternative to Chemotherapy in Untreated Acute Promyelocytic Leukemia," *Blood*, 2006, 107 (9):3469-73.

Gregory J, Kim H, Alonzo T, et al, "Treatment of Children With Acute Promyelocytic Leukemia: Results of the First North American Intergroup Trial INT0129," *Pediatr Blood Cancer*, 2009, 53(6):1005-10.

Kueh YK, Liew PP, Ho PC, et al, "Sublingual Administration of All-*Trans*-retinoic Acid to a Comatose Patient With Acute Promyelocytic Leukemia," *Ann Pharmacother*, 1999, 33(4):503-5.

Lo-Coco F, Avvisati G, Vignetti M, et al, "Front-Line Treatment of Acute Promyelocytic Leukemia With AIDA Induction Followed by Risk-Adapted Consolidation for Adults Younger Than 61 Years: Results of the AIDA-2000 Trial of the GIMEMA Group," *Blood*, 2010, 116 (17):3171-9.

Mann G, Reinhardt D, Ritter J, et al, "Treatment With All-trans Retinoic Acid in Acute Promyelocytic Leukemia Reduces Early Deaths in Children," *Ann Hematol*, 2001, 80(7):417-22.

National Comprehensive Cancer Network® (NCCN), "Practice Guidelines in Oncology™: Acute Myeloid Leukemia," Version 1, 2010. Available at http://www.nccn.org/professionals/physician_gls/PDF/aml.pdf.

National Institute for Occupational Safety and Health (NIOSH), "NIOSH List of Antineoplastic and Other Hazardous Drugs in Healthcare Settings 2012." Available at http://www.cdc.gov/niosh/docs/2012-150/pdfs/2012-150.pdf. Accessed January 21, 2013.

Ortega JJ, Madero L, Martín G, et al, "Treatment With All-*trans* Retinoic Acid and Anthracycline Monochemotherapy for Children With Acute Promyelocytic Leukemia: A Multicenter Study by the PETHEMA Group," *J Clin Oncol*, 2005, 23(30):7632-40.

Powell BL, Moser B, Stock W, et al, "Arsenic Trioxide Improves Event-Free and Over-All Survival for Adults With Acute Promyelocytic Leukemia: North American Leukemia Intergroup Study C9710," *Blood*, 2010, 116(19):3751-7.

Ravandi F, Estey E, Jones D, et al, "Effective Treatment of Acute Promyelocytic Leukemia With All-*Trans*-Retinoic Acid, Arsenic Trioxide, and Gemtuzumab Ozogamicin," *J Clin Oncol*, 2009, 27 (4):504-10.

Sanz MA, Grimwade D, Tallman MS, et al, "Management of Acute Promyelocytic Leukemia: Recommendations From an Expert Panel on Behalf of the European LeukemiaNet," *Blood*, 2009, 113 (9):1875-91.

Sanz MA, Martín G, González M, et al, "Risk-Adapted Treatment of Acute Promyelocytic Leukemia With All-*trans*-retinoic Acid and Anthracycline Monochemotherapy: A Multicenter Study by the PETHEMA Group," *Blood*, 2004, 103(4):1237-43.

Sanz MA, Montesinos P, Rayón C, et al, "Risk-Adapted Treatment of Acute Promyelocytic Leukemia Based on All-*trans* Retinoic Acid and Anthracycline With Addition of Cytarabine in Consolidation Therapy for High-Risk Patients: Further Improvements in Treatment Outcome," *Blood*, 2010, 115(25):5137-46.

Sanz MA, Montesinos P, Vellenga E, et al, "Risk-Adapted Treatment of Acute Promyelocytic Leukemia With All-*trans* Retinoic Acid and Anthracycline Monochemotherapy: Long-Term Outcome of the LPA 99 Multicenter Study by the PETHEMA Group," *Blood*, 2008, 112 (8):3130-4.

Shaw PJ, Atkins MC, Nath CE, et al, "ATRA Administration in the Critically III Patient," *Leukemia*, 1995, 9(7):1288.

Takitani K, Hino N, Terada Y, et al. Plasma all-trans retinoic acid level in neonates of mothers with acute promyelocytic leukemia. *Acta Haematol*. 2005;114(3):167-169.

Takitani K, Koh M, Inoue A, et al, "Pharmacokinetics of All-*Trans* Retinoic Acid in Adults and Children With Acute Promyelocytic Leukemia," *Am J Hematol*, 2006, 81(9):720-1.

Takitani K, Nakao Y, Kosaka Y, et al, "Low Plasma Level of All-*trans* Retinoic Acid After Feeding Tube Administration for Acute Promyelocytic Leukemia," *Am J Hematol*, 2004, 76(1):97-8.

Testi AM, Biondi A, Lo Coco F, et al, "GIMEMA-AIEOPAIDA Protocol for the Treatment of Newly Diagnosed Acute Promyelocytic Leukemia (APL) in Children," *Blood*, 2005, 106(2):447-53.

Valappil S, Kurkar M, Howell R. Outcome of pregnancy in women treated with all-trans retinoic acid; a case report and review of literature. *Hematology*. 2007;12(5):415-418.

Vesanoid® data on file, Roche Pharmaceuticals.

Tretinoin (Topical) (TRET i noyn)

Medication Safety Issues

Sound-alike/look-alike issues:

Tretinoin may be confused with ISOtretinoin, Tenormin, triamcinolone, trientine

International issues:

Renova [U.S., Canada] may be confused with Remov brand name for nimesulide [Italy]

Related Information

Safe Handling of Hazardous Drugs *on page 2419*

Brand Names: U.S. Atralin; Avita; Refissa; Renova; Renova Pump; Retin-A; Retin-A Micro; Retin-A Micro Pump; Tretin-X

Brand Names: Canada Rejuva-A; Renova; Retin-A; Retin-A Micro; Retinova; Stieva-A; Vitamin A Acid

Therapeutic Category Acne Products; Retinoic Acid Derivative; Vitamin, Topical

Generic Availability (U.S.) May be product dependent

Use Treatment of acne vulgaris, photodamaged skin, and some skin cancers

Pregnancy Risk Factor C

Pregnancy Considerations Adverse events were observed in animal reproduction studies following topical application of tretinoin. Teratogenic effects were also observed in pregnant women following topical use; however, a causal association has not been established. When treatment for acne is needed during pregnancy, other agents are preferred (Kong, 2013). These products should not be used for palliation of fine wrinkles, mottled hyperpigmentation, and tactile roughness of facial skin in women who are pregnant, attempting to conceive, or at high risk for pregnancy.

Breast-Feeding Considerations It is not known if tretinoin (topical) is excreted into breast milk. The manufacturer recommends that caution be exercised when administering tretinoin (topical) to nursing women.

Contraindications Hypersensitivity to tretinoin or any component; sunburn

Warnings Hazardous agent; use appropriate precautions for handling and disposal (NIOSH, 2012). Avoid contact with abraded skin, mucous membranes, eyes, mouth, angles of the nose; avoid excessive exposure to sunlight or sunlamps.

Precautions Use with caution in patients with eczema

Adverse Reactions
Dermatologic: Burning sensation of the skin, dermatitis, erythema, skin irritation
Local: Skin edema

Drug Interactions
Metabolism/Transport Effects None known.
Avoid Concomitant Use
Avoid concomitant use of Tretinoin (Topical) with any of the following: Multivitamins/Fluoride (with ADE); Multivitamins/Minerals (with ADEK, Folate, Iron); Multivitamins/Minerals (with AE, No Iron)
Increased Effect/Toxicity
Tretinoin (Topical) may increase the levels/effects of: Porfimer

The levels/effects of Tretinoin (Topical) may be increased by: Multivitamins/Fluoride (with ADE); Multivitamins/Minerals (with ADEK, Folate, Iron); Multivitamins/Minerals (with AE, No Iron)
Decreased Effect
Tretinoin (Topical) may decrease the levels/effects of: Contraceptives (Progestins)
Food Interactions Vitamin A toxicity may rarely occur. Management: Avoid excessive intake of vitamin A (cod liver oil, halibut fish oil).

Stability Hazardous agent; use appropriate precautions for handling and disposal (NIOSH, 2012).

Mechanism of Action Tretinoin is a derivative of vitamin A. When used topically, it modifies epithelial growth and differentiation. In patients with acne, it decreases the cohesiveness of follicular epithelial cells and decreases micromedo formation. Additionally, tretinoin stimulates mitotic activity and increased turnover of follicular epithelial cells causing extrusion of the comedones.

Pharmacodynamics
Onset of action: 2-3 weeks
Maximum effect: May require 6 weeks or longer
Pharmacokinetics (Adult data unless noted)
Absorption: Topical: Minimum absorption
Metabolism: In the liver
Elimination: In bile and urine

Dosing: Usual Children >12 years and Adults: Topical: Begin therapy with a weaker formulation of tretinoin (0.025% cream or 0.01% gel) and increase the concentration as tolerated; apply once daily before retiring or on alternate days; if stinging or irritation develop, decrease frequency of application

Administration Topical: Apply to dry skin (wait at least 15-30 minutes to apply after cleansing); avoid contact with eyes, mucous membranes, mouth, or open wounds

Hazardous agent; use appropriate precautions for handling and disposal (NIOSH, 2012).

Additional Information Liquid preparation generally is more irritating

Product Availability Retin-A Micro Gel 0.08%: FDA approved January 2014; anticipated availability is currently unknown.

Dosage Forms Excipient information presented when available (limited, particularly for generics); consult specific product labeling.
Cream, External:
Avita: 0.025% (20 g, 45 g)
Refissa: 0.05% (20 g, 40 g) [contains edetate disodium, methylparaben, propylparaben]

Renova: 0.02% (40 g, 60 g) [contains benzyl alcohol, cetyl alcohol, edetate disodium, methylparaben, propylparaben]
Renova Pump: 0.02% (44 g) [contains benzyl alcohol, cetyl alcohol, edetate disodium, methylparaben, propylparaben]
Retin-A: 0.025% (20 g, 45 g); 0.05% (20 g, 45 g); 0.1% (20 g, 45 g)
Tretin-X: 0.0375% (35 g); 0.075% (35 g)
Generic: 0.025% (20 g, 45 g); 0.05% (20 g, 40 g, 45 g, 60 g); 0.1% (20 g, 45 g)
Gel, External:
Atralin: 0.05% (45 g) [contains benzyl alcohol, butylparaben, ethylparaben, fish collagen hydrolyzates, isobutylparaben, methylparaben, propylparaben, trolamine (triethanolamine)]
Avita: 0.025% (20 g, 45 g)
Retin-A: 0.01% (15 g, 45 g); 0.025% (15 g, 45 g) [contains alcohol, usp]
Retin-A Micro: 0.04% (20 g, 45 g); 0.1% (20 g, 45 g) [contains benzyl alcohol, disodium edta, propylene glycol, trolamine (triethanolamine)]
Retin-A Micro Pump: 0.04% (50 g); 0.08% (50 g); 0.1% (50 g) [contains benzyl alcohol, disodium edta, propylene glycol, trolamine (triethanolamine)]
Generic: 0.01% (15 g, 45 g); 0.025% (15 g, 45 g); 0.04% (20 g, 45 g, 50 g); 0.1% (20 g, 45 g, 50 g)
Kit, External:
Tretin-X: 0.025%, 0.05%, 0.1% [contains benzyl alcohol, cetearyl alcohol, disodium edta, fd&c red #40, methylparaben, propylparaben, tartrazine (fd&c yellow #5), trolamine (triethanolamine)]

References
National Institute for Occupational Safety and Health (NIOSH), "NIOSH List of Antineoplastic and Other Hazardous Drugs in Healthcare Settings 2012." Available at http://www.cdc.gov/niosh/docs/2012-150/pdfs/2012-150.pdf. Accessed January 21, 2013.
Winston MH, Shalita AR, "Acne Vulgaris, Pathogenesis and Treatment," *Pediatr Clin North Am*, 1991, 38(4):889-903.

◆ **Tretinoin and Clindamycin** see Clindamycin and Tretinoin on page 503

◆ **Tretinoinum** see Tretinoin (Systemic) on page 2068

◆ **Trexall** see Methotrexate on page 1367

◆ **Triaderm (Can)** see Triamcinolone (Topical) on page 2078

Triamcinolone (Systemic) (trye am SIN oh lone)

Medication Safety Issues
Sound-alike/look-alike issues:
Kenalog® may be confused with Ketalar®
Other safety concerns:
TAC (occasional abbreviation for triamcinolone) is an error-prone abbreviation (mistaken as tetracaine-adrenaline-cocaine)

Related Information
Corticosteroids Systemic Equivalencies on page 2222
Brand Names: U.S. Aristospan Intra-Articular; Aristospan Intralesional; Kenalog
Brand Names: Canada Aristospan®
Therapeutic Category Adrenal Corticosteroid; Antiinflammatory Agent; Antiasthmatic; Corticosteroid, Systemic; Glucocorticoid
Generic Availability (U.S.) No
Use
Intra-articular (Aristospan 20 mg/mL, Kenalog-10 and -40): Adjunct therapy for acute gouty arthritis, acute/subacute bursitis, acute tenosynovitis, epicondylitis, rheumatoid arthritis, synovitis, or osteoarthritis [FDA approved in pediatric patients (age not specified) and adults]; has also been used intrabursally and into tendon sheaths

Intralesional (Aristospan 5 mg/mL, Kenalog-10): Alopecia areata; discoid lupus erythematosus; infiltrated, inflammatory lesions associated with granuloma annulare, lichen planus, neurodermatitis, and psoriatic plaques; keloids; necrobiosis lipoidica diabeticorum; possibly helpful in cystic tumors of an aponeurosis or tendon (ganglia) [FDA approved in pediatric patients (age not specified) and adults]; has also been used for infantile hemangioma

Intramuscular: Kenalog-40: Anti-inflammatory or immunosuppressant agent in the treatment of a variety of diseases, including those of allergic, hematologic, dermatologic, neoplastic, rheumatic, endocrine, gastrointestinal, ophthalmic, renal, or respiratory origin [FDA approved in pediatric patients (age not specified) and adults]

Pregnancy Risk Factor C

Pregnancy Considerations Adverse events have been observed with corticosteroids in animal reproduction studies. Some studies have shown an association between first trimester systemic corticosteroid use and oral clefts (Park-Wyllie, 2000; Pradat, 2003). Systemic corticosteroids may also influence fetal growth (decreased birth weight); however, information is conflicting (Lunghi, 2010). Hypoadrenalism may occur in newborns following maternal use of corticosteroids in pregnancy; monitor.

Breast-Feeding Considerations Corticosteroids are excreted in human milk; information specific to triamcinolone has not been located. The manufacturer notes that when used systemically, maternal use of corticosteroids have the potential to cause adverse events in a nursing infant (eg, growth suppression, interfere with endogenous corticosteroid production); therefore, caution should be used if administered to a nursing woman. A case report notes a decrease in milk production following a high-dose triamcinolone injection in a nursing mother with a previously abundant milk supply (McGuire, 2012).

Contraindications Hypersensitivity to triamcinolone or any component

Additional dose- or route-specific contraindications:

Immunosuppressive doses: Immunization with live or live-attenuated vaccines

I.M. (Kenalog 40): Immune thrombocytopenia (ITP)

Warnings Hypothalamic-pituitary-adrenal (HPA) suppression may occur, particularly in younger children or in patients receiving high doses for prolonged periods; acute adrenal insufficiency (adrenal crisis) may occur with abrupt withdrawal after long-term therapy or with stress; withdrawal and discontinuation of corticosteroids should be tapered slowly and carefully; patients with HPA axis suppression may require doses of systemic glucocorticosteroids prior to, during, and after unusual stress (eg, surgery). **Note:** Adrenal suppression with failure to thrive has been reported in infants and young children receiving intralesional corticosteroid injections for the treatment of infantile hemangioma; failure to gain weight may persist until HPA axis recovers; time to recovery of adrenal function may be prolonged (mean: 19.5 weeks; range 4 to 65 weeks) (DeBoer, 2008; Morkane, 2011).

Immunosuppression may occur; patients may be more susceptible to infections; prolonged use of corticosteroids may also increase the incidence of secondary infection, mask acute infection (including fungal infections), prolong or exacerbate viral or fungal infections, activate latent opportunistic infections, or limit response to vaccines. Exposure to chickenpox should be avoided; corticosteroids should not be used to treat ocular herpes simplex; use caution in patients with a history of ocular herpes simplex. Corticosteroids should not be used for cerebral malaria or viral hepatitis. Close observation is required in patients with latent tuberculosis and/or TB reactivity; restrict use in active TB (only in conjunction with antituberculosis treatment). Use with extreme caution in patients

with threadworm infection; may cause serious hyperinfection.

May cause osteoporosis (at any age) or inhibition of bone growth in pediatric patients. Use with caution in patients with osteoporosis. In a population-based study of children, risk of fracture was shown to be increased with >4 courses of corticosteroids; underlying clinical condition may also impact bone health and osteoporotic effect of corticosteroids (Leonard, 2006).

Corticosteroid use may cause psychiatric disturbances, including depression, euphoria, insomnia, mood swings, and personality changes. preexisting psychiatric conditions may be exacerbated by corticosteroid use. Acute myopathy may occur with high doses, usually in patients with neuromuscular transmission disorders; myopathy may involve ocular and/or respiratory muscles; monitor creatine kinase; recovery may be delayed.

Rare cases of anaphylactoid reactions have been reported with corticosteroids.

Route of administration is product-specific; administer products only via recommended route. Do **not** administer any triamcinolone product via the epidural or intrathecal route; serious adverse events, including fatalities, have been reported following epidural or intrathecal administration of corticosteroids. Tissue atrophy at the site of I.M. injection has been reported; avoid intramuscular injections into the deltoid area. Cutaneous atrophy was reported in 2.5% of pediatric patients when given intra-articularly (Bloom, 2011). Prevention of periarticular subcutaneous atrophy via injecting small amounts of saline into the joint and applying pressure following the injection has been recommended (Hashkas, 2005).

Injection may contain benzyl alcohol which may cause allergic reactions in susceptible individuals; large amounts of benzyl alcohol (≥99 mg/kg/day) have been associated with a potentially fatal toxicity ("gasping syndrome") in neonates; *in vitro* and animal studies have shown that benzoate displaces bilirubin from protein binding sites; the injection is not indicated for use in neonates. Injection also contains polysorbate 80 (Tween 80) which may cause allergic reactions in susceptible individuals. In premature neonates, thrombocytopenia, ascites, pulmonary deterioration, and renal and hepatic failure have been reported after receiving parenteral products containing polysorbate 80 (Alade, 1986; CDC, 1984).

Precautions Avoid using higher than recommended doses; suppression of HPA axis function, suppression of linear growth (ie, reduction of growth velocity), reduced bone mineral density, hypercorticism (Cushing's syndrome), hyperglycemia, or glucosuria may occur; titrate to lowest effective dose. Reduction in growth velocity may occur when corticosteroids are administered to pediatric patients by any route (monitor growth). Use with extreme caution in patients with respiratory tuberculosis or untreated systemic infections. Use with caution in patients with hypertension, HF, or renal impairment; long-term use has been associated with fluid retention and hypertension. Use with caution in patients with GI diseases (diverticulitis, peptic ulcer, ulcerative colitis) due to risk of GI bleeding and perforation. High-dose corticosteroids should not be used for management of head injury; increased mortality was observed in patients receiving high-dose I.V. methylprednisolone. Use with caution in patients with myasthenia gravis; exacerbation of symptoms has occurred especially during initial treatment with corticosteroids. Use with caution in patients with hepatic impairment, including cirrhosis; enhanced pharmacologic effect due to decreased metabolism and long-term use has been associated with fluid retention. Use with caution following acute MI; corticosteroids have been associated with myocardial rupture.

Use with caution in patients with diabetes; corticosteroids may alter glucose regulation leading to hyperglycemia. Use with caution in patients with cataracts and/or glaucoma; increased IOP, open-angle glaucoma, and cataracts have occurred with prolonged use, consider routine eye exams in chronic users. Use with caution in patients with a history of seizure disorder; seizures have been reported with adrenal crisis. Use with caution in patients with thyroid dysfunction; changes in thyroid status may necessitate dosage adjustments; metabolic clearance of corticosteroids increases in hyperthyroid patients and decreases in hypothyroid ones. Prolonged treatment with corticosteroids has been associated with the development of Kaposi's sarcoma (case reports); if noted, discontinuation of therapy should be considered. Use with caution in patients with thromboembolic tendencies or thrombophlebitis. Avoid injection into an infected site. Response to killed or inactivated vaccines cannot be predicted in patients receiving immunosuppressive doses of corticosteroids.

Adverse Reactions

Cardiovascular: Arrhythmia, bradycardia, cardiac arrest, cardiac enlargement, CHF, circulatory collapse, edema, hypertension, hypertrophic cardiomyopathy (premature infants), myocardial rupture (following recent MI), syncope, tachycardia, thromboembolism, vasculitis

Central nervous system: Arachnoiditis (I.T.), depression, emotional instability, euphoria, headache, insomnia, intracranial pressure increased, malaise, meningitis (I.T.), mood changes, neuritis, neuropathy, personality change, pseudotumor cerebri (with discontinuation), seizure, spinal cord infarction, stroke, vertigo

Dermatologic: Abscess (sterile), acne, allergic dermatitis, angioedema, atrophy (cutaneous/subcutaneous), bruising, dry skin, erythema, hair thinning, hirsutism, hyper-/hypopigmentation, hypertrichosis, impaired wound healing, lupus erythematosus-like lesions, petechiae, purpura, rash, skin test suppression, striae, thin skin

Endocrine & metabolic: Carbohydrate intolerance, Cushingoid state, diabetes mellitus, fluid retention, glucose intolerance, growth suppression (children), hypokalemia, hypokalemic alkalosis, menstrual irregularities, negative nitrogen balance, sodium retention, sperm motility altered

Gastrointestinal: Abdominal distention, appetite increased, GI hemorrhage, GI perforation, nausea, pancreatitis, peptic ulcer, ulcerative esophagitis, weight gain

Hepatic: Hepatomegaly, liver function tests increased

Local: Thrombophlebitis

Neuromuscular & skeletal: Aseptic necrosis of femoral and humeral heads, calcinosis, Charcot-like arthropathy, fractures, joint tissue damage, muscle mass loss, myopathy, osteoporosis, parasthesia, paraplegia, quadriplegia, tendon rupture, vertebral compression fractures, weakness

Ocular: Cataracts, cortical blindness, exophthalmos, glaucoma, ocular pressure increased, papilledema

Renal: Glycosuria

Respiratory: Pulmonary edema

Miscellaneous: Abnormal fat deposits, anaphylactoid reaction, anaphylaxis, diaphoresis, hiccups, infection, moon face

Drug Interactions

Metabolism/Transport Effects Substrate of CYP3A4 (minor); **Note:** Assignment of Major/Minor substrate status based on clinically relevant drug interaction potential

Avoid Concomitant Use

Avoid concomitant use of Triamcinolone (Systemic) with any of the following: Aldesleukin; BCG; Indium 111 Capromab Pendetide; Mifepristone; Natalizumab; Pimecrolimus; Tacrolimus (Topical); Tofacitinib

Increased Effect/Toxicity

Triamcinolone (Systemic) may increase the levels/effects of: Acetylcholinesterase Inhibitors; Amphotericin B; Androgens; Ceritinib; Deferasirox; Leflunomide; Loop Diuretics; Natalizumab; NSAID (COX-2 Inhibitor); NSAID (Nonselective); Thiazide Diuretics; Tofacitinib; Vaccines (Live); Warfarin

The levels/effects of Triamcinolone (Systemic) may be increased by: Antifungal Agents (Azole Derivatives, Systemic); Aprepitant; Calcium Channel Blockers (Nondihydropyridine); Denosumab; Estrogen Derivatives; Fluconazole; Fosaprepitant; Indacaterol; Macrolide Antibiotics; Mifepristone; Neuromuscular-Blocking Agents (Nondepolarizing); Pimecrolimus; Quinolone Antibiotics; Ritonavir; Roflumilast; Salicylates; Tacrolimus (Topical); Telaprevir; Trastuzumab

Decreased Effect

Triamcinolone (Systemic) may decrease the levels/effects of: Aldesleukin; Antidiabetic Agents; BCG; Calcitriol; Coccidioidin Skin Test; Corticorelin; Hyaluronidase; Indium 111 Capromab Pendetide; Isoniazid; Salicylates; Sipuleucel-T; Telaprevir; Urea Cycle Disorder Agents; Vaccines (Inactivated)

The levels/effects of Triamcinolone (Systemic) may be decreased by: Aminoglutethimide; Barbiturates; Echinacea; Mifepristone; Mitotane; Primidone; Rifamycin Derivatives

Stability

Acetonide (Kenalog): Store at 20°C to 25°C (68°F to 77°F); avoid freezing; protect from light; do not autoclave vials.

Hexacetonide (Aristospan): Store at 20°C to 25°C (68°F to 77°F); avoid freezing; protect from light; do not autoclave. Avoid diluents containing parabens, phenol, or other preservatives; may cause flocculation. Diluted suspension stable up to 1 week.

Mechanism of Action Decreases inflammation by suppression of migration of polymorphonuclear leukocytes and reversal of increased capillary permeability; suppresses the immune system by reducing activity and volume of the lymphatic system; suppresses adrenal function at high doses

Pharmacokinetics (Adult data unless noted)

Distribution: V_d: 99.5 ± 27.5 L

Protein binding: ~68%

Metabolism: Hepatic to 3 identified metabolites (significantly less active than parent drug)

Half-life: Elimination: 88 minutes; Biologic: 18-36 hours

Time to peak serum concentration: I.M.: Within 8-10 hours

Elimination: 40% of dose is excreted in urine; 60% in feces

Dosing: Usual Adjust dose depending upon condition being treated and response of patient. The lowest possible dose should be used to control the condition; when dose reduction is possible, the dose should be reduced gradually.

Pediatric:

General dosing, treatment of inflammatory and allergic conditions: Children and Adolescents:

Manufacturer's labeling: Acetonide (Kenolog-40): I.M.: Initial: 0.11 to 1.6 mg/kg/day (or 3.2 to 48 mg/m²/day) in 3 to 4 divided doses

Alternate dosing: Limited data available: Acetonide: Children 6 to 12 years: I.M.: 0.03 to 0.2 mg/kg/dose every 1 to 7 days (Kliegman, 2011)

Juvenile idiopathic arthritis (JIA), other rheumatic conditions:

Manufacturer's labeling: Children and Adolescents:

Acetonide (Kenalog-10 or -40): Intra-articular, intra-bursal, tendon sheaths: Initial: Smaller joints: 2.5 to 5 mg, larger joints: 5 to 15 mg; maximum dose/treatment (several joints at one time): 20 to 80 mg

Hexacetonide (Aristospan 20 mg/mL): Intra-articular: Average dose: 2 to 20 mg; smaller joints: 2 to 6 mg;

larger joints: 10 to 20 mg. Frequency of injection into a single joint is every 3 to 4 weeks as necessary; to avoid possible joint destruction use as infrequently as possible

Alternate dosing: Limited data available: Children and Adolescents: Hexacetonide: Intra-articular: Large joints (typically knees, ankles): 1 to 1.5 mg/kg/dose; maximum dose: 40 mg; doses greater than 1.5 mg/kg have not been associated with additional clinical benefit; similar dosing for the acetonide salt can be used; however, data shows that the response is greater and lasts longer with hexacetonide (Bloom, 2011; Hashkes, 2005; Zulian, 2003; Zulian 2004)

Infantile hemangioma, severe: Limited data available: Infants and Children ≤49 months: Intralesional: Dosage dependent upon size of lesion: Commonly reported: 1 to 2 mg/kg/dose of the acetonide suspension (either 10 mg/mL or 40 mg/mL) administered in divided doses along the lesion perimeter ~monthly (4 to 5 weeks most frequently reported interval); a maximum dose up to 30 mg/dose has been used; others have reported: 1 to 30 mg of the 10 mg/mL acetonide injection divided into multiple injections along the lesion; has also been used in combination with betamethasone intralesional injections (Chen, 2000; Maguiness, 2012; Pandey, 2009; Praseyono, 2011). From the largest reported experience (n=1514, age range: 1 to 49 months), triamcinolone (1 to 2 mg/kg once every month) alone or in combination with oral corticosteroid (if no response after 6 injections of monotherapy) showed lesion size decrease of 50% or more in 90.3% of infants (age <1 year) and 80% in those >1 year (Pandey, 2009). Another trial (n=155, age range at first injection: 2 to 12 months) which used 1 to 30 mg of a 10 mg/mL concentration administered approximately once monthly (mean interval: 5 weeks) for 3 to 6 months showed lesion size decreased by at least 50% in 85% of the patients (Chen, 2000)

Dermatoses (steroid-responsive, including contact/ atopic dermatitis):

Acetonide (Kenalog-10): Intradermal: Adolescents: Up to 1 mg per injection site and may be repeated 1 or more times weekly; multiple sites may be injected if they are 1 cm or more apart, not to exceed 30 mg

Hexacetonide (Aristospan 5 mg/mL): Intralesional, sublesional: Adolescents: Up to 0.5 mg/square inch of affected skin; initial range: 2 to 48 mg; frequency of dose is determined by clinical response

Adult:

Dermatoses (steroid-responsive, including contact/ atopic dermatitis):

Acetonide (Kenalog-10): Intradermal: Initial: 1 mg

Hexacetonide (Aristospan 5 mg/mL): Intralesional, sublesional: Up to 0.5 mg/square inch of affected skin; range: 2 to 48 mg/day

Hay fever/pollen asthma: Kenalog-40: I.M.: 40 to 100 mg as a single injection/season

Multiple sclerosis (acute exacerbation): Kenalog-40: I.M.: 160 mg daily for 1 week, followed by 64 mg every other day for 1 month

Rheumatic or arthritic disorders:

Intra-articular (or similar injection as designated):

Acetonide (Kenalog-10 or -40): Intra-articular, intrabursal, tendon sheaths: Initial: Smaller joints: 2.5 to 5 mg, larger joints: 5 to 15 mg; may require up to 10 mg for small joints and up to 40 mg for large joints; maximum dose/treatment (several joints at one time): 20 to 80 mg

Hexacetonide (Aristospan 20 mg/mL): Intra-articular: Average dose: 2 to 20 mg; smaller joints: 2 to 6 mg; larger joints: 10 to 20 mg. Frequency of injection into a single joint is every 3 to 4 weeks as necessary; to

avoid possible joint destruction use as infrequently as possible

I.M.: Acetonide (Kenalog-40): Initial: 60 mg; range: 2.5 to 100 mg/day

Dosing adjustment in renal impairment: There are no dosage adjustments provided in the manufacturer's labeling.

Dosing adjustment in hepatic impairment: There are no dosage adjustments provided in the manufacturer's labeling.

Administration Shake well before use to ensure suspension is uniform. Inspect visually to ensure no clumping; administer immediately after withdrawal so settling does not occur in the syringe. Do **not** administer any product I.V. or via the epidural or intrathecal route. When preparing suspension for intralesional administration, may dilute with D_5NS, $D_{10}NS$, NS, or SWI to a 1:1, 1:2, or 1:4 concentration. Solutions for intra-articular use may be diluted with lidocaine 1% or 2%.

Acetonide:

Kenalog-10 injection: For intra-articular or intralesional administration only. When administered intralesionally, inject directly into the lesion (ie, intradermally or subcutaneously). Tuberculin syringes with a 23- to 25-gauge needle are preferable for intralesional injections. For infantile hemangioma, 27- and 30-gauge needles have been used (Chen, 2000; Prasetyono, 2011).

Kenalog-40 injection: For intra-articular, soft tissue or I.M. administration. When administered I.M., inject deep into the gluteal muscle using a minimum needle length of 1 1/2 inches for adults. Obese patients may require a longer needle. Alternate sites for subsequent injections. Avoid I.M. injections into deltoid area.

Hexacetonide:

Aristospan (5 mg/mL): For intralesional or sublesional administration only; use a ≥23-gauge needle

Aristospan (20 mg/mL): For intra-articular and soft tissue administration only; use a ≥23-gauge needle

Monitoring Parameters Intraocular pressure (if therapy >6 weeks); weight, height, and linear growth of pediatric patients (with chronic use); assess HPA suppression. Monitor blood pressure, serum glucose, potassium, calcium, hemoglobin, occult blood loss, and clinical presence of adverse effects.

Dosage Forms Excipient information presented when available (limited, particularly for generics); consult specific product labeling.

Suspension, Injection, as acetonide:

Kenalog: 10 mg/mL (5 mL); 40 mg/mL (1 mL, 5 mL, 10 mL) [contains benzyl alcohol, polysorbate 80]

Suspension, Injection, as hexacetonide:

Aristospan Intra-Articular: 20 mg/mL (1 mL, 5 mL) [contains benzyl alcohol]

Aristospan Intralesional: 5 mg/mL (5 mL) [contains benzyl alcohol]

References

Alade SL, Brown RE, and Paquet A Jr, "Polysorbate 80 and E-Ferol Toxicity," *Pediatrics*, 1986, 77(4):593-7.

Bloom SL, Alario AJ, Miller LC. Intra-articular corticosteroid therapy for juvenile idiopathic arthritis: report of an experiential cohort and literature review. *Rheumatol Int.* 2011;31:749-756.

Centers for Disease Control (CDC), "Unusual Syndrome With Fatalities Among Premature Infants: Association With a New Intravenous Vitamin E Product," *MMWR Morb Mortal Wkly Rep*, 1984, 33 (14):198-9.

Chen MT, Yeong EK, Horng SY. Intralesional corticosteroid therapy in proliferating head and neck hemangiomas: a review of 155 cases. *J Pediatr Surg.* 2000;35(3):420-423.

DeBoer MD, Boston BA. Failure-to-thrive in an infant following injection of capillary hemangioma with triamcinolone acetonide. *Clin Pediatr.* 2008;47(3):296-299.

Hashkes PJ, Laxer RM. Medical treatment of juvenile idiopathic arthritis. *JAMA.* 2005;294(13):1671-1684.

Kliegman RM, Stanton BF, St. Gemell JW, et al, eds. *Nelson Textbook of Pediatrics.* 19th ed. Philadelphia, PA: Saunders Elsevier;2011.

Leonard MB, "Glucocorticoid-Induced Osteoporosis in Children: Impact of the Underlying Disease," *Pediatrics*, 2007, 119 (Suppl 2):S166-74.

Lunghi L, Pavan B, Biondi C, et al, "Use of Glucocorticoids in Pregnancy," *Curr Pharm Des*, 2010, 16(32):3616-12.

Maguiness SM, Frieden IJ. Management of difficult infantile haemangiomas. *Arch Dis Child*. 2012;97(3):266-271.

McGuire E, "Sudden Loss of Milk Supply Following High-Dose Triamcinolone (Kenacort) Injection," *Breastfeed Rev*, 2012, 20(1):32-4.

Morkane C, Gregory JW, Watts P, Warner JT. Adrenal suppression following intralesional corticosteroids for periocular haemangiomas. *Arch Dis Child*. 2011;96:587-589.

Pandey A, Gangopadhyay AN, Gopal SC, et al. Twenty years' experience of steroids in infantile hemangioma - a developing country's perspective. *J Pediatr Surg*. 2009;44(4):688-694.

Park-Wyllie L, Mazzotta P, Pastuszak A, et al, "Birth Defects After Maternal Exposure to Corticosteroids: Prospective Cohort Study and Meta-Analysis of Epidemiological Studies," *Teratology*, 2000, 62 (6):385-92.

Pradat P, Robert-Gnansia E, Di Tanna GL, et al, "First Trimester Exposure to Corticosteroids and Oral Clefts," *Birth Defects Res A Clin Mol Teratol*, 2003, 67(12):968-70.

Prasetyono TOH, Djoenaedi I. Efficacy of intralesional steroid injection in head and neck hemangioma. *Ann Plast Surg*. 2011;66:98-106.

Zulian F, Martini G, Gobber D, Agosto C, Gigante C, Zacchello F. Comparison of intra-articular triamcinolone hexacetonide and triamcinolone acetonide in oligoarticular juvenile idiopathic arthritis. *Rheumatology*. 2003;42:1254-1259.

Zulian F, Martini G, Gobber D, Plebani M, Zacchello F, Manners P. Triamcinolone acetonide and hexacetonide intra-articular treatment of symmetrical joints in juvenile idiopathic arthritis: a double-blind trial. *Rheumatology*. 2004;43:1288-1291.

Triamcinolone (Nasal) (trye am SIN oh lone)

Medication Safety Issues
Sound-alike/look-alike issues:
Nasacort may be confused with NasalCrom
Other safety concerns:
TAC (occasional abbreviation for triamcinolone) is an error-prone abbreviation (mistaken as tetracaine-adrenaline-cocaine)

Brand Names: U.S. Nasacort Allergy 24HR [OTC]; Nasacort AQ

Brand Names: Canada Nasacort AQ; Trinasal

Therapeutic Category Anti-inflammatory Agent; Corticosteroid, Intranasal; Glucocorticoid

Generic Availability (U.S.) May be product dependent

Use Management of nasal symptoms associated with seasonal and perennial allergic rhinitis (FDA approved in ages ≥2 years and adults)

Intranasal corticosteroids have also been used as an adjunct to antibiotics in empiric treatment of acute bacterial rhinosinusitis primarily in patients with history of allergic rhinitis (Chow, 2012) and in pediatric patients with mild obstructive sleep apnea syndrome who cannot undergo adenotonsillectomy or who still have symptoms after surgery (Marcus, 2012).

Pregnancy Risk Factor C

Pregnancy Considerations Adverse events were observed in some animal reproduction studies. Intranasal corticosteroids are recommended for the treatment of rhinitis during pregnancy; the lowest effective dose should be used (NAEPP, 2005; Wallace, 2008).

Breast-Feeding Considerations Corticosteroids are excreted in human milk; information specific to triamcinolone has not been located. The use of inhaled corticosteroids is not considered a contraindication to breast-feeding (NAEPP, 2005). The manufacturer recommends that caution be used if administered to a nursing woman.

Contraindications Hypersensitivity to triamcinolone or any component

Warnings HPA suppression or hypercorticism (Cushing's syndrome) may occur with use of higher than recommended doses or at typical doses in susceptible patients. Acute adrenal insufficiency may occur with abrupt withdrawal after long-term use, with stress, or when converting from systemic to topical corticosteroid therapy; withdrawal or discontinuation of corticosteroids should be done carefully; patients with HPA axis suppression may require doses of systemic glucocorticoids prior to, during, and after unusual stress (eg, surgery). Immunosuppression may occur; patients may be more susceptible to infections; avoid exposure to chickenpox and measles. Epistaxis may occur.

Precautions Avoid using higher than recommended dosages; suppression of HPA function, suppression of linear growth (ie, reduction of growth velocity), reduced bone mineral density, or hypercorticism (Cushing's syndrome) may occur; titrate to lowest effective dose. Reduction in growth velocity may occur when corticosteroids are administered to pediatric patients, even at recommended doses via intranasal route (monitor growth). Use triamcinolone with extreme caution in patients with respiratory tuberculosis; untreated bacterial, fungal, systemic viral or parasitic infections; or ocular herpes simplex. Localized *Candida* infections of the nose and pharynx have been reported rarely; interruption of therapy may be necessary while antifungal therapy is employed. Corticosteroids impair wound healing; avoid use in patients with recent nasal ulcers, nasal surgery, or nasal trauma; allow healing to occur before use. Glaucoma, increased intraocular pressure, and cataracts have been reported following the intranasal application of corticosteroids; monitor patients who have change in vision and in patients with a history of increased ocular pressure, glaucoma, or cataracts. Use of nasal triamcinolone in place of systemic corticosteroids may unmask allergies (eg, eczema, rhinitis) that were previously controlled by the systemic corticosteroids. Rare cases of immediate hypersensitivity reactions or nasal septum perforation may occur with intranasal corticosteroids

Adverse Reactions
Cardiovascular: Facial edema

Central nervous system: Headache, pain

Dermatologic: Photosensitivity, rash

Endocrine & metabolic: Dysmenorrhea

Gastrointestinal: Abdominal pain, diarrhea, dyspepsia, nausea, oral moniliasis, taste perversion, toothache, vomiting, weight gain, xerostomia

Genitourinary: Cystitis, urinary tract infection, vaginal moniliasis

Local: Nasal burning (transient), nasal stinging (transient)

Neuromuscular & skeletal: Back pain, bursitis, myalgia, tenosynovitis

Ocular: Conjunctivitis

Otic: Otitis media

Respiratory: Asthma, bronchitis, chest congestion, cough, epistaxis, pharyngitis, sinusitis

Miscellaneous: Allergic reaction, flu-like syndrome, infection, voice alteration

Rare but important or life-threatening: Anaphylaxis, blood cortisol decreased, bone mineral density loss (rare; prolonged use), cataracts, dizziness, dry throat, dyspnea, fatigue, glaucoma, growth suppression, hoarseness, hypersensitivity, insomnia, intraocular pressure increased, nasal septum perforation, oral candidiasis, osteoporosis (rare; prolonged use), pruritus, sneezing, throat irritation, urticaria (rare), wheezing, wound healing impaired

Drug Interactions
Metabolism/Transport Effects Substrate of CYP3A4 (minor); **Note:** Assignment of Major/Minor substrate status based on clinically relevant drug interaction potential

Avoid Concomitant Use There are no known interactions where it is recommended to avoid concomitant use.

Increased Effect/Toxicity
Triamcinolone (Nasal) may increase the levels/effects of: Ceritinib

Decreased Effect There are no known significant interactions involving a decrease in effect.

Stability Store at controlled room temperature of 20°C to 25°C (68°F to 77°F); do not freeze.

Mechanism of Action Suppresses the immune system by reducing activity and volume of the lymphatic system

Pharmacokinetics (Adult data unless noted)
Absorption: Systemic absorption may occur following intranasal administration.

Half-life:
Terminal (intranasal): 3.1 hours

Elimination: 40% of dose is excreted in urine; 60% in feces

Dosing: Usual
Children and Adolescents: **Seasonal or perennial rhinitis:** Intranasal: Nasacort® AQ: Discontinue treatment if adequate control of symptoms has not occurred after 3 weeks of use.

Children 2-5 years: 110 mcg once daily delivered as 55 mcg (1 spray) **per nostril** once daily

Children 6-11 years: Initial: 110 mcg once daily delivered as 55 mcg (1 spray) **per nostril** once daily; may increase to 220 mcg once daily delivered as 110 mcg (2 sprays) **per nostril** once daily if response not adequate; once symptoms are controlled, reduce to 110 mcg once daily delivered as 55 mcg (1 spray) **per nostril** once daily

Children ≥12 years and Adolescents: Initial: 220 mcg once daily delivered as 110 mcg (2 sprays) **per nostril** once daily; once symptoms are controlled, reduce dose to 110 mcg once daily delivered as 55 mcg (1 spray) **per nostril** once daily.

Adults: **Seasonal or perennial rhinitis:** Intranasal: Nasacort® AQ: Initial: 220 mcg once daily delivered as 110 mcg (2 sprays) **per nostril** once daily; once symptoms are controlled, reduce dose to 110 mcg once daily delivered as 55 mcg (1 spray) **per nostril** once daily

Administration Shake container well before each use. Before first use, prime by pressing pump 5 times or until a fine spray appears. Repeat priming with 1 spray if ≥14 days between use. Blow nose to clear nostrils. Insert applicator into nostril, keeping bottle upright, and close off the other nostril. Breathe in through nose. While inhaling, press pump to release spray. Avoid blowing nose for 15 minutes after use. Do not spray into eyes or mouth. Discard after labeled number of doses has been used, even if bottle is not completely empty.

Monitoring Parameters Mucous membranes for signs of fungal infection, growth (pediatric patients), signs/symptoms of HPA axis suppression/adrenal insufficiency; ocular changes

Additional Information When used short term as adjunctive therapy in acute bacterial rhinosinusitis (ABRS), intranasal steroids show modest symptomatic improvement and few adverse effects; improvement is primarily due to increased sinus drainage. Use should be considered optional in ABRS; however, intranasal corticosteroids should be routinely prescribed to ABRS patients who have a history of or concurrent allergic rhinitis (Chow, 2012).

Dosage Forms Considerations
Nasacort AQ 16.5 g bottles contain 120 sprays.

Dosage Forms Excipient information presented when available (limited, particularly for generics); consult specific product labeling.

Aerosol, Nasal, as acetonide:
Nasacort Allergy 24HR: 55 mcg/actuation (10.8 mL, 16.9 mL) [contains benzalkonium chloride, edetate disodium, polysorbate 80]

Aerosol Solution, Nasal, as acetonide:
Nasacort AQ: 55 mcg/actuation (16.5 g)

Inhaler, Nasal, as acetonide:
Generic: 55 mcg/actuation (16.5 g)

References
Chow AW, Benninger MS, Brook I, et al, "IDSA Clinical Practice Guideline For Acute Bacterial Rhinosinusitis in Children and Adults," *Clin Infect Dis*, 2012, 54(8):e72-e112.

Marcus CL, Brooks LJ, Draper KA, et al, "Diagnosis and Management of Childhood Obstructive Sleep Apnea Syndrome," *Pediatrics*, 2012, 130(3):576-84.

NAEPP Working Group Report on "Managing Asthma During Pregnancy: Recommendations for Pharmacologic Treatment," National Institutes of Health, National Heart, Lung, and Blood Institute, NIH Publication No. 05-5236, March 2005. Available at http://www.nhlbi.nih.gov/health/prof/lung/asthma/astpreg/astpreg_full.pdf

Wallace DV, Dykewicz MS, Bernstein DI, et al, "The Diagnosis and Management of Rhinitis: An Updated Practice Parameter," *J Allergy Clin Immunol*, 2008, 122(2 Suppl):S1-84.

Triamcinolone (Ophthalmic)
(trye am SIN oh lone)

Medication Safety Issues
Other safety concerns:
TAC (occasional abbreviation for triamcinolone) is an error-prone abbreviation (mistaken as tetracaine-adrenaline-cocaine)

Brand Names: U.S. Triesence

Therapeutic Category Anti-inflammatory Agent, Ophthalmic; Corticosteroid, Ophthalmic

Generic Availability (U.S.) No

Use Intravitreal: Treatment of sympathetic ophthalmia, temporal arteritis, uveitis, ocular inflammatory conditions unresponsive to topical corticosteroids; visualization during vitrectomy

Pregnancy Risk Factor D

Pregnancy Considerations Triamcinolone was shown to be teratogenic in animal reproduction studies. Some studies have shown an association between first trimester corticosteroid use and oral clefts; adverse events in the fetus/neonate have been noted in case reports following large doses of systemic corticosteroids during pregnancy. The amount of triamcinolone absorbed systemically following ophthalmic administration is not known.

Breast-Feeding Considerations Corticosteroids are excreted in human milk; information specific to triamcinolone has not been located. The amount of triamcinolone absorbed systemically following ophthalmic administration is not known.

Contraindications Hypersensitivity to triamcinolone or any component; systemic fungal infections; cerebral malaria; serious infections (except septic shock or tuberculous meningitis); idiopathic thrombocytopenia purpura

Warnings Immunosuppression may occur; patients may be more susceptible to infections. Intravitreal injection has been associated with endophthalmitis and visual disturbances. Blindness has been reported following injection into nasal turbinates and intralesional injections into the head. Safety of intraturbinal, subconjunctival, subtenons, or retrobulbar injection has not been demonstrated. Injection contains polysorbate 80 (Tween 80®) which may cause allergic reactions in susceptible individuals.

Precautions Use with caution in patients with cataracts and/or glaucoma; increased intraocular pressure, openangle glaucoma, and cataracts have occurred with prolonged use. Corticosteroids should not be used in active ocular herpes simplex.

Adverse Reactions
Blurred vision, cataract progression, conjunctival hemorrhage, discomfort (transient), endophthalmitis, glaucoma, hypopyon, inflammation, intraocular pressure increase, optic disc vascular disorder, retinal detachment, vitreous floaters, visual acuity decreased

Rare but important or life-threatening: Exophthalmos

Drug Interactions
Metabolism/Transport Effects None known.

◀ **Avoid Concomitant Use** There are no known interactions where it is recommended to avoid concomitant use.

Increased Effect/Toxicity

Triamcinolone (Ophthalmic) may increase the levels/effects of: Ceritinib

Decreased Effect There are no known significant interactions involving a decrease in effect.

Stability Store at 4°C to 25°C (39°F to 77°F)

Mechanism of Action Suppresses the immune system by reducing activity and volume of the lymphatic system

Pharmacokinetics (Adult data unless noted) Half-life elimination: Biologic: 18-36 hours

Dosing: Usual Ophthalmic injection: Intravitreal: Children and Adults:

Ocular disease: Initial: 4 mg as a single dose; additional doses may be given as needed over the course of treatment

Visualization during vitrectomy: 1-4 mg

Administration Not for I.V. use. Shake vial well prior to use. Administer under controlled aseptic conditions (eg, sterile gloves, sterile drape, sterile eyelid speculum). Adequate anesthesia and a broad-spectrum bactericidal agent should be administered prior to injection. Inject immediately after withdrawing from vial. If administration is required in the second eye, a new vial should be used. Do not use if agglomerated (clumpy or granular appearance).

Monitoring Parameters Following injection, monitor for increased intraocular pressure and endophthalmitis; check for perfusion of optic nerve head immediately after injection, tonometry within 30 minutes, biomicroscopy between 2-7 days after injection.

Dosage Forms Excipient information presented when available (limited, particularly for generics); consult specific product labeling.

Suspension, Intraocular, as acetonide:

Triesence: 40 mg/mL (1 mL) [contains polysorbate 80]

Triamcinolone (Topical) (trye am SIN oh lone)

Medication Safety Issues

Sound-alike/look-alike issues:

Kenalog® may be confused with Ketalar®

Other safety concerns:

TAC (occasional abbreviation for triamcinolone) is an error-prone abbreviation (mistaken as tetracaine-adrenaline-cocaine)

Related Information

Topical Corticosteroids *on page 2224*

Brand Names: U.S. Dermasorb TA; Kenalog; Oralone; Pediaderm TA; Trianex; Triderm

Brand Names: Canada Kenalog®; Oracort; Triaderm

Therapeutic Category Anti-inflammatory Agent, Topical; Corticosteroid, Topical; Glucocorticoid

Generic Availability (U.S.) May be product dependent

Use

Cream, lotion, ointment, and spray: Relief of inflammation and pruritus associated with corticosteroid-responsive dermatoses [FDA approved in pediatric patients (age not specified) and adults]

Dental paste: Adjunctive treatment and temporary relief of symptoms related to oral inflammatory lesions and ulcerative lesions due to trauma (FDA approved in adults)

Pregnancy Risk Factor C

Pregnancy Considerations Corticosteroids were found to be teratogenic following topical application in animal reproduction studies. In general, the use of topical corticosteroids during pregnancy is not considered to have significant risk, however, intrauterine growth retardation in the infant has been reported (rare). The use of large amounts or for prolonged periods of time should be avoided.

Breast-Feeding Considerations Corticosteroids are excreted in human milk; information specific to triamcinolone has not been located. The amount of triamcinolone absorbed systemically following topical administration is variable. Hypertension in the nursing infant has been reported following corticosteroid ointment applied to the nipples. Use with caution.

Contraindications Hypersensitivity to triamcinolone or any component

Dental paste also contraindicated with fungal, viral, or bacterial infections of mouth or throat

Warnings Hypothalamic-pituitary-adrenal (HPA) suppression may occur; acute adrenal insufficiency (adrenal crisis) may occur with abrupt withdrawal after long-term therapy or with stress; withdrawal and discontinuation of corticosteroids should be done carefully. Adverse systemic effects (eg, hyperglycemia, glycosuria, fluid and electrolyte changes) may occur when topical steroids are used in large areas of the body, denuded areas, for prolonged periods of time, with an occlusive dressing, and/or in infants and small children; infants and small children may be more susceptible to HPA axis suppression or other systemic toxicities due to larger skin surface area to body mass ratio; use with caution in pediatric patients. If HPA suppression occurs, consider withdrawal of triamcinolone, reduction in frequency of application, or substitution with a less potent corticosteroid. Cushing's syndrome and intracranial hypertension have also been reported in pediatric patients. May cause inhibition of bone growth in pediatric patients. Immunosuppression may occur; patients may be more susceptible to infections; avoid exposure to chickenpox and measles. Corticosteroids may activate latent opportunistic infections or exacerbate systemic fungal infections. Allergic contact dermatitis can occur and is usually diagnosed by failure to heal rather than clinical exacerbation; diagnostic patch testing may corroborate observation.

Dental paste: When used as a topical agent in the oral cavity, if significant regeneration or repair of oral tissues has not occurred in seven days, re-evaluation of the etiology of the oral lesion is advised.

Some creams and lotions may contain polysorbate 80 which may cause allergic reactions in susceptible individuals; consult product-specific information for more detail. Some creams and lotions may contain propylene glycol; toxicities have been reported with use of products containing propylene glycol, including hyperosmolality, lactic acidosis, seizures, and respiratory depression; in neonates large amounts of propylene glycol delivered orally, intravenously (eg, >3000 mg/day), or topically have been associated with potentially fatal toxicities which can include metabolic acidosis, seizures, renal failure, and CNS depression; use creams and lotions containing propylene glycol with caution (AAP, 1997; Shehab, 2009).

Precautions Use caution with occlusive dressings or wraps (including diapers); may increase systemic absorption. Avoid application to denuded skin or to large surface areas; may increase systemic absorption. Prolonged use may result in fungal or bacterial superinfection. Use may be associated with local sensitization.

Topical spray: Product is flammable; avoid open flame. Product for topical use only; avoid spraying into eyes or mouth.

Adverse Reactions

Dermatologic: Acneiform eruptions, allergic contact dermatitis, dryness, folliculitis, hypertrichosis, hypopigmentation, miliaria, perioral dermatitis, pruritus, skin atrophy, skin infection (secondary), skin maceration, striae

Endocrine: HPA axis suppression; metabolic effects (hyperglycemia, hypokalemia)

Local: Burning, irritation

Drug Interactions
Metabolism/Transport Effects None known.
Avoid Concomitant Use
Avoid concomitant use of Triamcinolone (Topical) with any of the following: Aldesleukin
Increased Effect/Toxicity
Triamcinolone (Topical) may increase the levels/effects of: Ceritinib; Deferasirox

The levels/effects of Triamcinolone (Topical) may be increased by: Telaprevir
Decreased Effect
Triamcinolone (Topical) may decrease the levels/effects of: Aldesleukin; Corticorelin; Hyaluronidase; Telaprevir
Stability
Cream: Store at room temperature (see product-specific labeling for detail); avoid freezing.
Dental paste: Store at 20°C to 25°C (68°F to 77°F).
Lotion: Store at room temperature; avoid freezing.
Ointment: Store at 15°C to 30°C (59°F to 86°F).
Spray: Store at room temperature; avoid excessive heat. Do not puncture or incinerate aerosol can.
Mechanism of Action Decreases inflammation by suppression of migration of polymorphonuclear leukocytes and reversal of increased capillary permeability; suppresses the immune system by reducing activity and volume of the lymphatic system
Pharmacokinetics (Adult data unless noted)
Absorption: Topical corticosteroids are absorbed percutaneously. The extent is dependent on several factors, including epidermal integrity (intact vs abraded skin), formulation, and the use of occlusive dressings.
Metabolism: Hepatic
Half-life: Biologic: 18-36 hours
Elimination: 40% of dose is excreted in urine; 60% in feces
Dosing: Usual
Infants, Children, and Adolescents: **Dermatoses (steroid-responsive, including contact/atopic dermatitis):** Topical: **Note:** Frequency based upon severity of condition:
Cream, Ointment:
0.025% or 0.05%: Apply thin film to affected areas 2-4 times daily
0.1% or 0.5%: Apply thin film to affected areas 2-3 times daily
Lotion:
0.025%: Apply 2-4 times daily
0.1%: Apply 2-3 times daily
Spray: Apply to affected area up to 3-4 times daily
Adult:
Dermatoses (steroid-responsive, including contact/atopic dermatitis): Topical:
Cream, Ointment:
0.025% or 0.05%: Apply thin film to affected areas 2-4 times/daily
0.1% or 0.5%: Apply thin film to affected areas 2-3 times daily
Spray: Apply to affected area 3-4 times daily
Oral inflammatory lesions/ulcers: Oral topical (dental paste): Press a small dab (about 1/4 inch) to the lesion 1-3 times daily until a thin film develops; a larger quantity may be required for coverage of some lesions. For optimal results, use only enough to coat the lesion with a thin film; do not rub in.
Administration
Topical: Apply sparingly to affected area and gently rub in until disappears; do not occlude area, unless directed; do not use on open skin; avoid contact with eyes
Dental: Apply small dab until thin, smooth film develops; do not rub in; spreading the paste may result in a granular, gritty sensation and crumbling; apply at bedtime to allow contact of the medication with the lesion overnight; if more frequent application is necessary, apply after meals.

Monitoring Parameters Growth in pediatric patients; assess HPA axis suppression (eg, ACTH stimulation test, morning plasma cortisol test, urinary free cortisol test)
Dosage Forms Excipient information presented when available (limited, particularly for generics); consult specific product labeling.
Aerosol Solution, External, as acetonide:
Kenalog: (63 g, 100 g)
Cream, External, as acetonide:
Triderm: 0.1% (28.4 g, 85.2 g) [contains propylene glycol]
Generic: 0.025% (15 g, 80 g, 454 g); 0.1% (15 g, 30 g, 80 g, 453.6 g, 454 g); 0.5% (15 g)
Kit, External, as acetonide:
Dermasorb TA: 0.1% [contains cetyl alcohol, milk protein, propylene glycol]
Pediaderm TA: 0.1% [contains cetyl alcohol, methylparaben, polysorbate 80, propylene glycol, propylparaben]
Lotion, External, as acetonide:
Generic: 0.025% (60 mL); 0.1% (60 mL)
Ointment, External, as acetonide:
Trianex: 0.05% (17 g, 85 g)
Generic: 0.025% (15 g, 80 g, 454 g); 0.1% (15 g, 80 g, 453.6 g, 454 g); 0.5% (15 g)
Paste, Mouth/Throat, as acetonide:
Oralone: 0.1% (5 g)
Generic: 0.1% (5 g)
References
American Academy of Pediatrics Committee on Drugs. "Inactive" ingredients in pharmaceutical products: update (subject review). *Pediatrics.* 1997;99(2):268-278.
Lewis-Jones S, Mugglestone MA, Guideline Development Group. Management of atopic eczema in children aged up to 12 years: summary of NICE guidance. *BMJ.* 2007;335(7632):1263-1264.
Shehab N, Lewis CL, Streetman DD, Donn SM. Exposure to the pharmaceutical excipients benzyl alcohol and propylene glycol among critically ill neonates. *Pediatr Crit Care Med.* 2009;10(2):256-259.

◆ **Triamcinolone Acetonide** see Triamcinolone (Nasal) on page 2076

◆ **Triamcinolone acetonide** see Triamcinolone (Ophthalmic) on page 2077

◆ **Triamcinolone Acetonide, Parenteral** see Triamcinolone (Systemic) on page 2072

◆ **Triamcinolone Hexacetonide** see Triamcinolone (Systemic) on page 2072

◆ **Triaminic Allerchews [OTC]** see Loratadine on page 1278

◆ **Triaminic Children's Fever Reducer Pain Reliever [OTC]** see Acetaminophen on page 47

◆ **Triaminic Cough/Runny Nose [OTC]** see DiphenhydrAMINE (Systemic) on page 673

◆ **Triaminic Long Acting Cough [OTC]** see Dextromethorphan on page 636

Triamterene (trye AM ter een)

Medication Safety Issues
Sound-alike/look-alike issues:
Triamterene may be confused with trimipramine
Dyrenium may be confused with Pyridium
Brand Names: U.S. Dyrenium
Therapeutic Category Antihypertensive Agent; Diuretic, Potassium Sparing
Generic Availability (U.S.) No
Use Used alone or in combination with other diuretics to treat edema and hypertension; decreases potassium excretion caused by kaliuretic diuretics
Pregnancy Risk Factor C
Pregnancy Considerations Adverse events have not been observed in animal reproduction studies.

Triamterene crosses the placenta and is found in cord blood. Use of triamterene to treat edema during normal pregnancies is not appropriate; use may be considered when edema is due to pathologic causes (as in the non-pregnant patient); monitor.

Breast-Feeding Considerations It is not known if triamterene is excreted in breast milk. Breast-feeding is not recommended by the manufacturer.

Contraindications Hypersensitivity to triamterene or any component; severe renal or hepatic impairment, hyperkalemia; patients receiving other potassium-sparing diuretics

Warnings Hyperkalemia (serum potassium ≥5.5 mEq/L) can occur; patients at risk include those with renal impairment, diabetes, the elderly, and the severely ill **[U.S. Boxed Warning]**. Serum potassium levels must be monitored at frequent intervals especially when dosages are changed or with any illness that may cause renal dysfunction. Hypersensitivity reactions have been reported; monitor for possible occurrence of blood dyscrasias, liver damage, or other idiosyncratic reactions.

Precautions Use with caution in patients with impaired hepatic or renal function, history of renal calculi, diabetes mellitus; patients receiving other potassium-sparing diuretics or potassium supplements may cause uric acid elevations; use with caution in patients with gouty arthritis

Adverse Reactions

Central nervous system: Dizziness, fatigue, headache

Dermatologic: Skin photosensitivity, skin rash

Endocrine & metabolic: Hyperkalemia, hypokalemia, increased uric acid, metabolic acidosis

Gastrointestinal: Diarrhea, nausea, vomiting, xerostomia

Genitourinary: Azotemia

Hematologic & oncologic: Hematologic abnormality, megaloblastic anemia, thrombocytopenia

Hepatic: Jaundice, liver enzyme disorder

Hypersensitivity: Anaphylaxis

Neuromuscular & skeletal: Weakness

Renal: Acute interstitial nephritis (rare), acute renal failure (rare), increased blood urea nitrogen, increased serum creatinine, nephrolithiasis

Drug Interactions

Metabolism/Transport Effects None known.

Avoid Concomitant Use

Avoid concomitant use of Triamterene with any of the following: CycloSPORINE (Systemic); Spironolactone; Tacrolimus (Systemic)

Increased Effect/Toxicity

Triamterene may increase the levels/effects of: ACE Inhibitors; Amifostine; Ammonium Chloride; Antihypertensives; Cardiac Glycosides; CycloSPORINE (Systemic); Dofetilide; DULoxetine; Hypotensive Agents; Obinutuzumab; RiTUXimab; Sodium Phosphates; Spironolactone; Tacrolimus (Systemic)

The levels/effects of Triamterene may be increased by: Alfuzosin; Analgesics (Opioid); Angiotensin II Receptor Blockers; Barbiturates; Brimonidine (Topical); Canagliflozin; Diazoxide; Drospirenone; Eplerenone; Heparin; Heparin (Low Molecular Weight); Herbs (Hypotensive Properties); Indomethacin; MAO Inhibitors; Nonsteroidal Anti-Inflammatory Agents; Pentoxifylline; Phosphodiesterase 5 Inhibitors; Potassium Salts; Prostacyclin Analogues; Tolvaptan

Decreased Effect

Triamterene may decrease the levels/effects of: Cardiac Glycosides; QuiNIDine

The levels/effects of Triamterene may be decreased by: Herbs (Hypertensive Properties); Methylphenidate; Nonsteroidal Anti-Inflammatory Agents; Yohimbine

Mechanism of Action Blocks epithelial sodium channels in the late distal convoluted tubule (DCT) and collecting duct which inhibits sodium reabsorption from the lumen. This effectively reduces intracellular sodium, decreasing the function of Na+/K+ ATPase, leading to potassium retention and decreased calcium, magnesium, and hydrogen excretion. As sodium uptake capacity in the DCT/collecting duct is limited, the natriuretic, diuretic, and antihypertensive effects are generally considered weak.

Pharmacodynamics

Onset of action: Diuresis occurs within 2-4 hours

Duration: 7-9 hours

Note: Maximum therapeutic effect may not occur until after several days of therapy

Pharmacokinetics (Adult data unless noted)

Absorption: Oral: Unreliably absorbed

Metabolism: Hepatic conjugation

Half-life: 100-150 minutes

Elimination: 21% excreted unchanged in urine

Dosing: Usual Oral:

Children: 1-2 mg/kg/day in 1-2 divided doses; maximum dose: 3-4 mg/kg/day and not to exceed 300 mg/day

Adults: 100-300 mg/day in 1-2 divided doses; usual dosage range (JNC 7): 50-100 mg/day

Dosage adjustment in renal impairment: CrCl <10 mL/minute: Avoid use

Dosage adjustment in hepatic impairment: Dose reduction is recommended in patients with cirrhosis

Administration Oral: Administer with food to avoid GI upset

Monitoring Parameters Electrolytes (sodium, potassium, magnesium, HCO$_3$, chloride), CBC, BUN, creatinine, platelets

Test Interactions Interferes with fluorometric assay of quinidine

Additional Information Abrupt discontinuation of therapy may result in rebound kaliuresis; taper off gradually

Dosage Forms Excipient information presented when available (limited, particularly for generics); consult specific product labeling.

Capsule, Oral:

Dyrenium: 50 mg, 100 mg

References

American College of Obstetricians and Gynecologists. ACOG Practice Bulletin No. 125: Chronic hypertension in pregnancy. *Obstet Gynecol.* 2012;119(2, pt 1):396-407.

Chobanian AV, Bakris GL, Black HR, et al, "The Seventh Report of the Joint National Committee on Prevention, Detection, Evaluation, and Treatment of High Blood Pressure: The JNC 7 Report.", *JAMA*, 2003, 289(19):2560-72.

National High Blood Pressure Education Program Working Group on High Blood Pressure in Children and Adolescents, "The Fourth Report on the Diagnosis, Evaluation, and Treatment of High Blood Pressure in Children and Adolescents," *Pediatrics*, 2004, 114(2 Suppl):555-76.

van der Vorst MM, Kist JE, van der Heijden AJ, et al, "Diuretics in Pediatrics: Current Knowledge and Future Prospects," *Paediatr Drugs*, 2006, 8(4):245-64.

◆ **Trianex** *see* Triamcinolone (Topical) *on page* 2078

◆ **Triatec-8 (Can)** *see* Acetaminophen and Codeine *on page* 53

◆ **Triatec-8 Strong (Can)** *see* Acetaminophen and Codeine *on page* 53

◆ **Triatec-30 (Can)** *see* Acetaminophen and Codeine *on page* 53

Triazolam (trye AY zoe lam)

Medication Safety Issues

Sound-alike/look-alike issues:

Triazolam may be confused with alPRAZolam

Halcion® may be confused with halcinonide, Haldol®

BEERS Criteria medication:

This drug may be potentially inappropriate for use in geriatric patients (Quality of evidence - high; Strength of recommendation - strong).

Brand Names: U.S. Halcion

Brand Names: Canada Apo-Triazo®; Gen-Triazolam; Halcion®; Mylan-Triazolam

Therapeutic Category Benzodiazepine; Hypnotic; Sedative

Generic Availability (U.S.) Yes

Use Short-term (generally 7-10 days) treatment of insomnia (FDA approved in ages ≥18 years and adults)

Medication Guide Available Yes

Pregnancy Risk Factor X

Pregnancy Considerations A case report describes placental transfer of triazolam following a maternal overdose. Teratogenic effects have been observed with some benzodiazepines; however, additional studies are needed. The incidence of premature birth and low birth weights may be increased following maternal use of benzodiazepines; hypoglycemia and respiratory problems in the neonate may occur following exposure late in pregnancy. Neonatal withdrawal symptoms may occur within days to weeks after birth and "floppy infant syndrome" (which also includes withdrawal symptoms) have been reported with some benzodiazepines (Bergman, 1992; Iqbal, 2002; Sakai, 1996; Wikner, 2007). Use of triazolam is contraindicated in pregnant women.

Breast-Feeding Considerations Although information specific to triazolam has not been located, all benzodiazepines are expected to be excreted into breast milk. Drowsiness, lethargy, or weight loss in nursing infants have been observed in case reports following maternal use of some benzodiazepines (Iqbal, 2002). Breast-feeding is not recommended by the manufacturer.

Contraindications Hypersensitivity to triazolam or any component; cross-sensitivity with other benzodiazepines may occur; pregnancy; concomitant use with ketoconazole, itraconazole, and nefazodone

Warnings Evaluate patient carefully for medical or psychiatric causes of insomnia prior to initiation of drug treatment; failure of triazolam to treat insomnia (after 7-10 days of therapy), a worsening of insomnia, or the emergence of behavioral changes or thinking abnormalities, may indicate a medical or psychiatric illness requiring evaluation; these effects also have been reported with triazolam use. Due to possible adverse effects, use lowest effective dose. Prescription should be written for a maximum of 7-10 days and should not be prescribed in quantities exceeding a 1-month supply. Abrupt discontinuation after prolonged use may result in withdrawal symptoms or rebound insomnia. Use caution when reducing dose or withdrawing therapy; decrease slowly and monitor for withdrawal symptoms. Flumazenil may cause withdrawal in patients receiving long-term benzodiazepine therapy. An increase in daytime anxiety may occur after as few as 10 days of continuous use, which may be related to withdrawal reaction in some patients.

Triazolam is a substrate of cytochrome P450 isoenzyme CYP3A4; avoid use in patients taking strong CYP3A4 inhibitors; use is contraindicated with certain potent CYP3A4 inhibitors (ketoconazole, itraconazole, nefazodone). Use with caution in patients taking moderate CYP3A4 inducers and major CYP3A4 substrates (see Drug Interactions); consider alternative agents that avoid or lessen the potential for CYP-mediated interactions.

Postmarketing studies have indicated that the use of hypnotic/sedative agents for sleep has been associated with hypersensitivity reactions, including anaphylaxis, as well as angioedema. Hazardous sleep-related activities, such as sleep-driving (driving while not fully awake without any recollection of driving), preparing and eating food, and making phone calls while asleep have also been reported. May cause CNS depression, which may impair physical or mental abilities; patients must be cautioned about performing tasks which require mental alertness (eg, operating machinery or driving); use with caution in patients receiving other CNS depressants or psychoactive medication; effects with other sedative drugs or ethanol may be potentiated. Benzodiazepines have been associated with anterograde amnesia, particularly benzodiazepines with short half-lives such as triazolam. Paradoxical reactions, including hyperactive or aggressive behavior, have been reported with benzodiazepines, particularly in adolescent/pediatric or psychiatric patients. Evaluate any new or unusual changes in behavior.

Precautions Use with caution in patients with hepatic impairment; undergoes extensive hepatic metabolism. Use with caution in patients with renal impairment. Use with caution in patients with a history of drug abuse or acute alcoholism; potential for drug dependency exists; tolerance and psychological and physical dependence may occur with prolonged use. Use with caution in patients with depression, particularly if suicidal risk may be present. Use with caution in patients with an impaired gag reflex. Use with caution in patients with respiratory compromise, COPD, or sleep apnea. Use with caution in debilitated patients; potential for oversedation, impaired coordination, and dizziness with use. Use with extreme caution in patients who are at risk of falls; benzodiazepines have been associated with falls and traumatic injury. Does not have analgesic, antidepressant, or antipsychotic properties.

Adverse Reactions

Central nervous system: Ataxia, dizziness, drowsiness, headache, lightheadedness, nervousness

Gastrointestinal: Nausea, vomiting

Rare but important or life-threatening: Anaphylaxis, angioedema, anterograde amnesia; complex sleep-related behavior (sleep-driving, cooking or eating food, making phone calls); confusion, cramps, depression, dermatitis, dreaming/nightmares, dysesthesia, euphoria, fatigue, hepatic failure (fulminant), memory impairment, pain, paresthesia, tachycardia, violent acts, visual disturbance, weakness, xerostomia

In addition, the following have been reported in association with triazolam and other benzodiazepines: Burning tongue/glossitis/stomatitis, chest pain, dysarthria, jaundice, libido changes, menstrual irregularities; paradoxical reactions (eg, aggressiveness, agitational state, delusions, falling, hallucination, mania, sleep disturbances, syncope); pruritus, sedation, slurred speech, urinary incontinence, urinary retention

Drug Interactions

Metabolism/Transport Effects Substrate of CYP3A4 (major); **Note:** Assignment of Major/Minor substrate status based on clinically relevant drug interaction potential; **Inhibits** CYP2C8 (weak), CYP2C9 (weak)

Avoid Concomitant Use

Avoid concomitant use of Triazolam with any of the following: Azelastine (Nasal); Boceprevir; Cobicistat; Conivaptan; Fusidic Acid (Systemic); Itraconazole; Ketoconazole (Systemic); Methadone; OLANZapine; Paraldehyde; Protease Inhibitors; Sodium Oxybate; Telaprevir; Thalidomide

Increased Effect/Toxicity

Triazolam may increase the levels/effects of: Alcohol (Ethyl); Azelastine (Nasal); Buprenorphine; CloZAPine; CNS Depressants; Hydrocodone; Methadone; Methotrimeprazine; Metyrosine; Mirtazapine; Paraldehyde; Pramipexole; ROPINIRole; Rotigotine; Selective Serotonin Reuptake Inhibitors; Sodium Oxybate; Thalidomide; Zolpidem

The levels/effects of Triazolam may be increased by: Antifungal Agents (Azole Derivatives, Systemic); Aprepitant; Boceprevir; Brimonidine (Topical); Calcium Channel Blockers (Nondihydropyridine); Cannabis; Ceritinib;

Cimetidine; Cobicistat; Conivaptan; Contraceptives (Estrogens); Contraceptives (Progestins); CYP3A4 Inhibitors (Moderate); CYP3A4 Inhibitors (Strong); Dasatinib; Doxylamine; Dronabinol; Droperidol; Fosaprepitant; Fusidic Acid (Systemic); Grapefruit Juice; HydrOXYzine; Isoniazid; Itraconazole; Ivacaftor; Kava Kava; Ketoconazole (Systemic); Luliconazole; Macrolide Antibiotics; Magnesium Sulfate; Methotrimeprazine; Mifepristone; Nabilone; OLANZapine; Perampanel; Protease Inhibitors; Proton Pump Inhibitors; Rufinamide; Selective Serotonin Reuptake Inhibitors; Simeprevir; Stiripentol; Tapentadol; Telaprevir; Tetrahydrocannabinol

Decreased Effect
The levels/effects of Triazolam may be decreased by: Bosentan; CarBAMazepine; CYP3A4 Inducers (Strong); Dabrafenib; Deferasirox; Dexamethasone (Systemic); Mitotane; Rifamycin Derivatives; Siltuximab; St Johns Wort; Theophylline Derivatives; Tocilizumab; Yohimbine

Food Interactions Food may decrease the rate of absorption. Benzodiazepine serum concentrations may be increased by grapefruit juice. Management: Limit or avoid grapefruit juice.

Stability Store at 25°C (77°F); excursions permitted between 15°C to 30°C (59°F to 86°F).

Mechanism of Action Binds to stereospecific benzodiazepine receptors on the postsynaptic GABA neuron at several sites within the central nervous system, including the limbic system, reticular formation. Enhancement of the inhibitory effect of GABA on neuronal excitability results by increased neuronal membrane permeability to chloride ions. This shift in chloride ions results in hyperpolarization (a less excitable state) and stabilization.

Pharmacodynamics Hypnotic effects:
Onset of action: Within 15-30 minutes
Duration: 6-7 hours

Pharmacokinetics (Adult data unless noted)
Distribution: V_d: 0.8-1.8 L/kg
Protein binding: 89%
Metabolism: Extensive in the liver; primary metabolites are conjugated glucuronides
Half-life: 1.5-5.5 hours
Time to peak serum concentration: Within 2 hours
Elimination: In urine as unchanged drug (minor amounts) and metabolites

Dosing: Usual
Children and Adolescents <18 years: **Dental preprocedural sedation:** Limited data available; dosage not established: Oral: 0.02 mg/kg administered as an elixir has been used in children (n=20) for sedation prior to dental procedures (Meyer, 1990); further studies are needed; do not exceed adult doses.
Adolescents ≥18 years and Adults: **Insomnia:** Oral: 0.125-0.25 mg at bedtime; the lower dose of 0.125 mg at bedtime may be sufficient in some patients, such as those with low body weight; maximum daily dose: 0.5 mg/**day**

Administration Oral: Administer dose in bed, since onset of hypnotic effect is rapid; tablet may be crushed or swallowed whole

Monitoring Parameters Daytime alertness; respiratory rate; behavior profile

Controlled Substance C-IV

Dosage Forms Excipient information presented when available (limited, particularly for generics); consult specific product labeling.
Tablet, Oral:
Halcion: 0.25 mg [scored]
Generic: 0.125 mg, 0.25 mg

References
Bergman U, Rosa FW, Baum C, et al, "Effects of Exposure to Benzodiazepine During Fetal Life," *Lancet*, 1992, 340(8821):694-6.

Iqbal MM, Sobhan T, Ryals T, et al, "Effects of Commonly Used Benzodiazepines on the Fetus, the Neonate, and the Nursing Infant," *Psychiatr Serv*, 2002, 53(1):39-49.

Meyer ML, Mourino AP, and Farrington FH, "Comparison of Triazolam to a Chloral Hydrate/Hydroxyzine Combination in the Sedation of Pediatric Dental Patients," *Pediatr Dent*, 1990, 12(5):283-7.

Sakai T, Matsuda H, and Watanabe N, "Triazolam (Halcion) Intoxication in a Neonate-A First Report," *Eur J Pediatr*, 1996, 155(12):1065-6.

Wikner BN, Stiller CO, Bergman U, et al, "Use of Benzodiazepines and Benzodiazepine Receptor Agonists During Pregnancy: Neonatal Outcome and Congenital Malformations," *Pharmacoepidemiol Drug Saf*, 2007, 16(11):1203-10.

◆ **Tribavirin** *see* Ribavirin *on page 1818*

◆ **Tri-Buffered Aspirin [OTC]** *see* Aspirin *on page 212*

◆ **Tricalcium Phosphate** *see* Calcium Phosphate (Tribasic) *on page 359*

◆ **Trichloroacetaldehyde Monohydrate** *see* Chloral Hydrate *on page 436*

◆ **Tricitrates** *see* Citric Acid, Sodium Citrate, and Potassium Citrate *on page 487*

◆ **Tricosal** *see* Choline Magnesium Trisalicylate *on page 459*

◆ **Triderm** *see* Triamcinolone (Topical) *on page 2078*

◆ **Tridil** *see* Nitroglycerin *on page 1504*

◆ **Tridural (Can)** *see* TraMADol *on page 2060*

◆ **Triesence** *see* Triamcinolone (Ophthalmic) *on page 2077*

◆ **Triethylenethiophosphoramide** *see* Thiotepa *on page 2014*

Trifluoperazine (trye floo oh PER a zeen)

Medication Safety Issues
Sound-alike/look-alike issues:
Trifluoperazine may be confused with trihexyphenidyl
Stelazine may be confused with selegiline

BEERS Criteria medication:
This drug may be potentially inappropriate for use in geriatric patients (Quality of evidence - moderate; Strength of recommendation - strong).

Brand Names: Canada Apo-Trifluoperazine®; Novo-Trifluzine; PMS-Trifluoperazine; Terfluzine

Therapeutic Category Antipsychotic Agent, Typical, Phenothiazine; Phenothiazine Derivative

Generic Availability (U.S.) Yes

Use Treatment of schizophrenia (FDA approved in ages ≥6 years and adults); short-term treatment of generalized nonpsychotic anxiety (not a drug of choice) (FDA approved in adults); also used for management of psychotic disorders

Pregnancy Considerations Adverse events were not observed in animal reproduction studies, except when using doses that were also maternally toxic. Jaundice or hyper-/hyporeflexia have been reported in newborn infants following maternal use of phenothiazines. Antipsychotic use during the third trimester of pregnancy has a risk for abnormal muscle movements (extrapyramidal symptoms [EPS]) and withdrawal symptoms in newborns following delivery. Symptoms in the newborn may include agitation, feeding disorder, hypertonia, hypotonia, respiratory distress, somnolence, and tremor; these effects may be self-limiting or require hospitalization.

Breast-Feeding Considerations Trifluoperazine is excreted into breast milk and was measurable in the serum of three nursing infants (adverse events were not reported). Milk concentrations may be higher than those found in the maternal serum. Infants should be monitored for signs of adverse events.

Contraindications Hypersensitivity to trifluoperazine or any component; cross-sensitivity with other phenothiazines may exist; severe CNS depression; bone marrow suppression; blood dyscrasias; severe hepatic disease; coma

Warnings May cause extrapyramidal symptoms, including pseudoparkinsonism, acute dystonic reactions, akathisia, and tardive dyskinesia (risk of these reactions is high relative to other typical antipsychotics, and is dose-dependent; to decrease risk of tardive dyskinesia: Use smallest dose and shortest duration possible; evaluate continued need periodically; risk of dystonia is increased with the use of high potency and higher doses of conventional antipsychotics and in males and younger patients). May be associated with neuroleptic malignant syndrome (NMS); monitor for mental status changes, fever, muscle rigidity, and/or autonomic instability (risk may be increased in patients with Parkinson's disease or Lewy body dementia). Safety for use during pregnancy has not been established; prolonged jaundice, hyper-reflexia, hyporeflexia, or extrapyramidal signs may occur in newborn infants of mothers who received phenothiazines; clinical benefits should clearly outweigh risks before initiating use during pregnancy. May cause pigmentary retinopathy (discontinue drug if ophthalmoscopic or visual field exam demonstrates retinal changes).

Leukopenia, neutropenia, and agranulocytosis (sometimes fatal) have been reported in clinical trials and postmarketing reports with antipsychotic use; presence of risk factors (eg, preexisting low WBC or history of drug-induced leuko/neutropenia) should prompt periodic blood count assessment. Thrombocytopenia, anemia, agranulocytosis, and pancytopenia have been reported with trifluoperazine use. Discontinue therapy at first signs of blood dyscrasias or if absolute neutrophil count <1000/mm³. Use is contraindicated in patients with existing blood dyscrasias or bone marrow suppression.

An increased risk of death has been reported with the use of antipsychotics in elderly patients with dementia-related psychosis **[U.S. Boxed Warning]**; most deaths seemed to be cardiovascular (eg, sudden death, heart failure) or infectious (eg, pneumonia) in nature; trifluoperazine is not approved for this indication.

Precautions Use with caution in patients with hemodynamic instability; predisposition to seizures; subcortical brain damage; hepatic impairment; severe cardiac, renal, or respiratory disease. May cause sedation, which may impair physical or mental abilities; patients must be cautioned about performing tasks which require mental alertness (eg, operating machinery or driving); use with caution in disorders where CNS depression is a feature. Use with caution in Parkinson's disease. Esophageal dysmotility and aspiration have been associated with antipsychotic use; use with caution in patients at risk of pneumonia. Use with caution in breast cancer or other prolactin-dependent tumors (may elevate prolactin levels). May alter temperature regulation (use with caution with strenuous exercise, heat exposure, dehydration, and concomitant medication possessing anticholinergic effects). May mask toxicity of other drugs due to antiemetic effects. May alter cardiac conduction; life-threatening arrhythmias have occurred with therapeutic doses of phenothiazines. May cause orthostatic hypotension; use with caution in patients at risk of this effect or those who would not tolerate transient hypotensive episodes (cerebrovascular disease, cardiovascular disease, or other medications which may predispose). Trifluoperazine has not been shown to be effective for the treatment of behavioral complications in patients with mental retardation. Safety and efficacy in children <6 years of age have not been established.

Cholestatic jaundice, liver damage, and hepatitis may occur; obtain appropriate liver tests if patient develops fever with grippe-like symptoms; discontinue treatment if liver tests are abnormal. Phenothiazines may cause anticholinergic effects (confusion, agitation, constipation, xerostomia, blurred vision, urinary retention); therefore, they should be used with caution in patients with decreased GI motility, urinary retention, benign prostatic hypertrophy, xerostomia, or visual problems. Conditions which also may be exacerbated by cholinergic blockade include narrow-angle glaucoma (screening is recommended) and worsening of myasthenia gravis. Relative to other antipsychotics, trifluoperazine has a low potency of cholinergic blockade.

Adverse Reactions

Cardiovascular: Cardiac arrest, hypotension, orthostatic hypotension

Central nervous system: Dizziness; extrapyramidal symptoms (akathisia, dystonias, pseudoparkinsonism, tardive dyskinesia); headache, impairment of temperature regulation, lowering of seizure threshold, neuroleptic malignant syndrome (NMS)

Dermatologic: Discoloration of skin (blue-gray), increased sensitivity to sun, photosensitivity, rash

Endocrine & metabolic: Breast pain, galactorrhea, gynecomastia, hyperglycemia, hypoglycemia, lactation, libido (changes in), menstrual cycle (changes in)

Gastrointestinal: Constipation, nausea, stomach pain, vomiting, weight gain, xerostomia

Genitourinary: Difficulty in urination, ejaculatory disturbances, priapism, urinary retention

Hematologic: Agranulocytosis, aplastic anemia, eosinophilia, hemolytic anemia, leukopenia, pancytopenia, thrombocytopenic purpura

Hepatic: Cholestatic jaundice, hepatotoxicity

Neuromuscular & skeletal: Tremor

Ocular: Cornea and lens changes, pigmentary retinopathy

Respiratory: Nasal congestion

Drug Interactions

Metabolism/Transport Effects Substrate of CYP1A2 (major); **Note:** Assignment of Major/Minor substrate status based on clinically relevant drug interaction potential

Avoid Concomitant Use

Avoid concomitant use of Trifluoperazine with any of the following: Aclidinium; Amisulpride; Azelastine (Nasal); Ipratropium (Oral Inhalation); Metoclopramide; Paraldehyde; Potassium Chloride; Sulpiride; Thalidomide; Tiotropium; Umeclidinium

Increased Effect/Toxicity

Trifluoperazine may increase the levels/effects of: AbobotulinumtoxinA; Alcohol (Ethyl); Amisulpride; Analgesics (Opioid); Anticholinergic Agents; Antidepressants (Serotonin Reuptake Inhibitor/Antagonist); Azelastine (Nasal); Beta-Blockers; Buprenorphine; Cannabinoid-Containing Products; CNS Depressants; Hydrocodone; Methotrimeprazine; Methylphenidate; Metyrosine; Mirabegron; Mirtazapine; OnabotulinumtoxinA; Paraldehyde; Porfimer; Potassium Chloride; RimabotulinumtoxinB; Selective Serotonin Reuptake Inhibitors; Serotonin Modulators; Sulpiride; Thalidomide; Thiazide Diuretics; Thiopental; Tiotropium; Topiramate; Zolpidem

The levels/effects of Trifluoperazine may be increased by: Abiraterone Acetate; Acetylcholinesterase Inhibitors (Central); Aclidinium; Antidepressants (Serotonin Reuptake Inhibitor/Antagonist); Antimalarial Agents; Beta-Blockers; Brimonidine (Topical); Cannabis; CYP1A2 Inhibitors (Moderate); CYP1A2 Inhibitors (Strong); Deferasirox; Doxylamine; Dronabinol; Droperidol; HydrOXYzine; Ipratropium (Oral Inhalation); Kava Kava; Lithium; Magnesium Sulfate; Methotrimeprazine; Methylphenidate; Metoclopramide; Metyrosine; Nabilone; Perampanel; Pramlintide; Rufinamide; Serotonin Modulators; Sodium Oxybate; Tapentadol; Tetrabenazine; Tetrahydrocannabinol; Umeclidinium; Vemurafenib

Decreased Effect

Trifluoperazine may decrease the levels/effects of: Acetylcholinesterase Inhibitors (Central); Amphetamines; Anti-Parkinson's Agents (Dopamine Agonist); Quinagolide; Secretin

The levels/effects of Trifluoperazine may be decreased by: Acetylcholinesterase Inhibitors (Central); Antacids; Anti-Parkinson's Agents (Dopamine Agonist); Cannabis; CYP1A2 Inducers (Strong); Cyproterone; Lithium

Stability Store at controlled room temperature at 20°C to 25°C (68°F to 77°F); dispense in tight, light-resistant container

Mechanism of Action Trifluoperazine is a piperazine phenothiazine antipsychotic which blocks postsynaptic mesolimbic dopaminergic receptors in the brain; exhibits alpha-adrenergic blocking effect and depresses the release of hypothalamic and hypophyseal hormones

Pharmacodynamics

Onset of action: For control of agitation, aggression, hostility: 2-4 weeks; for control of psychotic symptoms (hallucinations, disorganized thinking or behavior, delusions): Within 1 week

Adequate trial: 6 weeks at moderate to high dose based on tolerability

Duration: Variable

Pharmacokinetics (Adult data unless noted)

Metabolism: Extensively hepatic

Half-life: >24 hours with chronic use

Dialysis: Not dialyzable (0% to 5%)

Dosing: Usual Oral:

Schizophrenia/psychoses (**Note:** Dosage should be individualized; use lowest effective dose and shortest effective duration; periodically reassess the need for continued treatment):

Children <6 years: Dosage not established

Children 6-12 years: Hospitalized or well-supervised patients: Initial: 1 mg 1-2 times/day; gradually increase dose until symptoms are controlled or adverse effects have become troublesome; maintenance: 1-15 mg/day in 1-2 divided doses (maximum: 15 mg/day)

Children >12 years:

Inpatient: Initial: 2-5 mg twice daily; gradually increase dose; usual maintenance: 15-20 mg/day in 2 divided doses (maximum: 40 mg/day)

Outpatient: Initial: 1-3 mg twice daily (maximum: 6 mg/day)

Adults:

Inpatient: Initial: 2-5 mg twice daily; gradually increase dose; usual maintenance: 15-20 mg/day in 2 divided doses (maximum dose: 40 mg/day)

Outpatient: Initial: 1-3 mg twice daily (maximum: 40 mg/day; exceptions occur-indication specific)

Nonpsychotic anxiety: Adults: 1-2 mg twice daily; maximum: 6 mg/day; therapy for anxiety should not exceed 12 weeks; do not exceed 6 mg/day for longer than 12 weeks when treating anxiety; agitation, jitteriness, or insomnia may be confused with original neurotic or psychotic symptoms

Administration May be taken with food to decrease GI upset; do not take within 2 hours of any antacids

Monitoring Parameters Vital signs; periodic eye exam, CBC with differential; liver enzyme tests; fasting blood glucose/Hgb A$_{1c}$; BMI; therapeutic response (mental status, mood, affect, gait), and adverse reactions at beginning of therapy and periodically with long-term use [eg, excess sedation, extrapyramidal symptoms, tardive dyskinesia, CNS changes, abnormal involuntary movement scale (AIMS)]

Test Interactions False-positive for phenylketonuria

Additional Information Long-term usefulness of trifluoperazine should be periodically re-evaluated in patients receiving the drug for extended periods; consideration

should be given whether to decrease the maintenance dose or discontinue drug therapy

Dosage Forms Excipient information presented when available (limited, particularly for generics); consult specific product labeling.

Tablet, Oral:

Generic: 1 mg, 2 mg, 5 mg, 10 mg

References

Miyamoto S, Duncan GE, Marx CE, et al, "Treatments for Schizophrenia: A Critical Review of Pharmacology and Mechanisms of Action of Antipsychotic Drugs," *Mol Psychiatry*, 2005, 10(1):79-104.

Remington G, "Tardive Dyskinesia: Eliminated, Forgotten, or Overshadowed?" *Curr Opin Psychiatry*, 2007, 20(2):131-7.

◆ **Trifluoperazine Hydrochloride** *see* Trifluoperazine *on page 2082*

◆ **Trifluorothymidine** *see* Trifluridine *on page 2084*

Trifluridine (trye FLURE i deen)

Medication Safety Issues

Sound-alike/look-alike issues:

Viroptic® may be confused with Timoptic®

Related Information

Safe Handling of Hazardous Drugs *on page 2419*

Brand Names: U.S. Viroptic

Brand Names: Canada Sandoz-Trifluridine; Viroptic®

Therapeutic Category Antiviral Agent, Ophthalmic

Generic Availability (U.S.) Yes

Use Treatment of primary keratoconjunctivitis and recurrent epithelial keratitis caused by herpes simplex virus types I and II

Pregnancy Risk Factor C

Pregnancy Considerations Adverse effects were not observed during animal reproduction studies of the ophthalmic solution.

Breast-Feeding Considerations The amount of trifluridine available systemically following topical application of the ophthalmic drops is negligible.

Contraindications Hypersensitivity to trifluridine or any component

Warnings Hazardous agent; use appropriate precautions for handling and disposal (NIOSH, 2012).

Adverse Reactions Ocular: Burning or stinging (5%), palpebral edema (3%), epithelial keratopathy, hyperemia, hypersensitivity reactions, irritation, keratitis sicca, ocular pressure increased, stromal edema, superficial punctate keratopathy

Drug Interactions

Metabolism/Transport Effects None known.

Avoid Concomitant Use There are no known interactions where it is recommended to avoid concomitant use.

Increased Effect/Toxicity There are no known significant interactions involving an increase in effect.

Decreased Effect There are no known significant interactions involving a decrease in effect.

Stability Hazardous agent; use appropriate precautions for handling and disposal (NIOSH, 2012). Store in refrigerator; storage at room temperature may result in a solution with altered pH which could result in ocular discomfort upon administration and/or decreased potency.

Mechanism of Action Interferes with viral replication by inhibiting thymidylate synthetase and incorporating into viral DNA in place of thymidine.

Pharmacodynamics Onset of action: Response to treatment occurs within 2-7 days; epithelial healing is complete in 1-2 weeks

Pharmacokinetics (Adult data unless noted) Absorption: Ophthalmic: Systemic absorption is negligible, while corneal penetration is adequate

Dosing: Usual Children and Adults: Ophthalmic: Instill 1 drop into affected eye every 2 hours while awake, to a maximum of 9 drops/day, until re-epithelialization of corneal ulcer occurs; then use 1 drop every 4 hours for another 7 days; do **not** exceed 21 days of treatment

Administration Hazardous agent; use appropriate precautions for handling and disposal (NIOSH, 2012).

Ophthalmic: Avoid contact of bottle tip with skin or eye; instill drops onto the cornea of the affected eye(s); apply finger pressure to lacrimal sac during and for 1-2 minutes after instillation to decrease risk of absorption and systemic effects

Monitoring Parameters Ophthalmologic exam (test for corneal staining with fluorescein or rose Bengal)

Additional Information Found to be effective in 138 of 150 patients unresponsive or intolerant to idoxuridine or vidarabine

Dosage Forms Excipient information presented when available (limited, particularly for generics); consult specific product labeling.

Solution, Ophthalmic:
Viroptic: 1% (7.5 mL) [contains thimerosal]
Generic: 1% (7.5 mL)

References
National Institute for Occupational Safety and Health (NIOSH), "NIOSH List of Antineoplastic and Other Hazardous Drugs in Healthcare Settings 2012." Available at http://www.cdc.gov/niosh/docs/2012-150/pdfs/2012-150.pdf. Accessed January 21, 2013.

◆ **Triglycerides, Medium Chain** *see* Medium Chain Triglycerides *on page 1318*

◆ **Trihexyphen (Can)** *see* Trihexyphenidyl *on page 2085*

Trihexyphenidyl (trye heks ee FEN i dil)

Medication Safety Issues
Sound-alike/look-alike issues:
Trihexyphenidyl may be confused with trifluoperazine
BEERS Criteria medication:
This drug may be potentially inappropriate for use in geriatric patients (Quality of evidence - moderate; Strength of recommendation - strong).

Brand Names: Canada PMS-Trihexyphenidyl; Trihexyphen; Trihexyphenidyl

Therapeutic Category Anti-Parkinson's Agent; Anticholinergic Agent; Antidote, Drug-induced Dystonic Reactions

Generic Availability (U.S.) Yes

Use Adjunctive treatment of Parkinson's disease and treatment of drug-induced extrapyramidal symptoms (EPS) (FDA approved in adults); has also been used for treatment of dystonia in cerebral palsy

Pregnancy Risk Factor C

Pregnancy Considerations Animal reproduction studies have not been conducted. One case report did not show evidence of adverse events after trihexyphenidyl administration during pregnancy (Robottom, 2011).

Breast-Feeding Considerations Anticholinergic agents may suppress lactation.

Contraindications Hypersensitivity to trihexyphenidyl or any component

Precautions Use with caution in patients with hyperthyroidism, renal or hepatic dysfunction, cardiovascular disease (including hypertension), glaucoma, prostatic hyperplasia, obstructive disease of the GI tract, and/or urinary stricture or retention. Does not relieve symptoms of tardive dyskinesia; may exacerbate mental symptoms when used to treat extrapyramidal symptoms. May cause anhidrosis and hyperthermia, which may be severe; use with caution in hot weather or during exercise, especially when administered concomitantly with other anticholinergic drugs to chronically-ill patients, alcoholics, patients with CNS disease, or persons doing manual labor in a hot environment. Trihexyphenidyl may impair physical or mental abilities; until effects on an individual patient are known, patients should be warned to use caution when performing tasks which require mental alertness (eg, operating machinery or driving). When given in large doses or to susceptible patients, may cause weakness and inability to move particular muscle groups.

Adverse Reactions
Cardiovascular: Tachycardia
Central nervous system: Agitation, confusion, delusions, dizziness, drowsiness, euphoria, hallucination, headache, nervousness, paranoia, psychiatric disturbance
Dermatologic: Skin rash
Gastrointestinal: Constipation, intestinal obstruction, nausea, parotitis, toxic megacolon, vomiting, xerostomia
Genitourinary: Urinary retention
Neuromuscular & skeletal: Weakness
Ophthalmic: Blurred vision, glaucoma, increased intraocular pressure, mydriasis

Drug Interactions
Metabolism/Transport Effects None known.

Avoid Concomitant Use
Avoid concomitant use of Trihexyphenidyl with any of the following: Aclidinium; Ipratropium (Oral Inhalation); Potassium Chloride; Tiotropium; Umeclidinium

Increased Effect/Toxicity
Trihexyphenidyl may increase the levels/effects of: Abobotulinumtoxin A; Analgesics (Opioid); Anticholinergic Agents; Cannabinoid-Containing Products; Mirabegron; OnabotulinumtoxinA; Potassium Chloride; RimabotulinumtoxinB; Thiazide Diuretics; Tiotropium; Topiramate

The levels/effects of Trihexyphenidyl may be increased by: Aclidinium; Ipratropium (Oral Inhalation); Pramlintide; Umeclidinium

Decreased Effect
Trihexyphenidyl may decrease the levels/effects of: Acetylcholinesterase Inhibitors (Central); Secretin

The levels/effects of Trihexyphenidyl may be decreased by: Acetylcholinesterase Inhibitors (Central)

Stability Store at 20°C to 25°C (68°F to 77°F).

Mechanism of Action Exerts a direct inhibitory effect on the parasympathetic nervous system. It also has a relaxing effect on smooth musculature; exerted both directly on the muscle itself and indirectly through parasympathetic nervous system (inhibitory effect)

Pharmacokinetics (Adult data unless noted)
Metabolism: Hydroxylation of the alicyclic groups
Time to peak serum concentration: 1.3 hours
Half-life: 33 hours
Elimination: Urine and bile

Dosing: Usual Oral:
Children 2-17 years: Dystonia in cerebral palsy: Initial: 0.1-0.2 mg/kg/day in three divided doses for 1 week; increase by 0.05-0.3 mg/kg/day in three divided doses for the second week; thereafter, titrate up weekly by 0.05-0.5 mg/kg/day in three divided doses as clinically tolerated; dosage is based on a prospective trial of 23 patients (Sanger, 2007); maximum dose: 0.75 mg/kg/day; however, a double-blind, prospective crossover study of 16 patients evaluating the effects of higher dosage resulted in improved clinical outcomes with doses ranging between 0.05-2.6 mg/kg/day in three divided doses although adverse reactions were common per author report (n=8 doses ≥2 mg/kg/day; Rice, 2009)
Adults:
Parkinson's disease: Initial: 1 mg/day; increase by 2 mg increments at intervals of 3-5 days; usual dose: 6-10 mg/day in 3-4 divided doses; doses of 12-15 mg/day may be required
Drug-induced extrapyramidal symptoms: Initial: 1 mg/day; increase as necessary to usual range: 5-15 mg/day in 3-4 divided doses
Use in combination with levodopa: Usual range: 3-6 mg/day in divided doses

Administration Oral: May be taken before or after meals; tolerated best if given in 3 daily doses and with food. High doses (>10 mg/day) may be divided into 4 doses, at meal times and at bedtime.

Monitoring Parameters Intraocular pressure monitoring and gonioscopic evaluations (baseline and at regular intervals)

Dosage Forms Excipient information presented when available (limited, particularly for generics); consult specific product labeling.

Elixir, Oral, as hydrochloride:
Generic: 0.4 mg/mL (473 mL)
Tablet, Oral, as hydrochloride:
Generic: 2 mg, 5 mg

References
Brocks DR, "Anticholinergic Drugs Used in Parkinson's Disease: An Overlooked Class of Drugs From a Pharmacokinetic Perspective," *J Pharm Pharm Sci*, 1999, 2(2):39-46.

He H, McKay G, Wirshing B, et al, "Development and Application of a Specific and Sensitive Radioimmunoassay for Trihexyphenidyl to a Pharmacokinetic Study in Humans," *J Pharm Sci*, 1995, 84(5):561-7.

Rice J and Waugh MC, "Pilot Study on Trihexyphenidyl in the Treatment of Dystonia in Children With Cerebral Palsy," *Child Neurol*, 2009, 24 (2):176-82.

Robottom BJ and Reich SG, "Exposure to High Dosage Trihexyphenidyl During Pregnancy for Treatment of Generalized Dystonia: Case Report and Literature Review," *Neurologist*, 2011, 17(6):340-1.

Sanger TD, Bastian A, Brunstrom J, et al, "Prospective Open-Label Clinical Trial of Trihexyphenidyl in Children With Secondary Dystonia Due to Cerebral Palsy," *J Child Neurol*, 2007, 22(5):530-7.

♦ **Trihexyphenidyl Hydrochloride** *see* Trihexyphenidyl *on page 2085*

♦ **Trilafon** *see* Perphenazine *on page 1648*

♦ **Trileptal** *see* OXcarbazepine *on page 1564*

♦ **Trileptal® (Can)** *see* OXcarbazepine *on page 1564*

♦ **Trilisate** *see* Choline Magnesium Trisalicylate *on page 459*

♦ **TriLyte** *see* Polyethylene Glycol-Electrolyte Solution *on page 1697*

Trimethobenzamide (trye meth oh BEN za mide)

Medication Safety Issues
Sound-alike/look-alike issues:
Tigan may be confused with Tiazac, Ticlid
Trimethobenzamide may be confused with metoclopramide, trimethoprim

BEERS Criteria medication:
This drug may be potentially inappropriate for use in geriatric patients (Quality of evidence - moderate; Strength of recommendation - strong).

Brand Names: U.S. Tigan

Brand Names: Canada Tigan

Therapeutic Category Antiemetic

Generic Availability (U.S.) Yes

Use Treatment of postoperative nausea and vomiting; treatment of nausea and vomiting associated with gastroenteritis

Pregnancy Considerations Teratogenic effects were not observed in animal reproduction studies. Trimethobenzamide has been used to treat nausea and vomiting of pregnancy (ACOG, 2004).

Breast-Feeding Considerations It is not known if trimethobenzamide is excreted in breast milk.

Contraindications Hypersensitivity to trimethobenzamide or any component; injection is contraindicated in children

Warnings Use cautiously in infants and children; antiemetics are not recommended for uncomplicated vomiting in children; limit antiemetic use to prolonged vomiting of known etiology; may mask emesis due to Reye's syndrome, may mimic CNS effects of Reye's syndrome in patients with emesis of other etiologies, and may cause extrapyramidal symptoms (EPS) which may be confused with CNS symptoms of primary disease responsible for emesis. May produce drowsiness and concomitant use with alcohol may result in an adverse interaction.

Precautions Risk of adverse effects (eg, EPS, seizure) may be increased in patients with acute febrile illness, dehydration, electrolyte imbalance, encephalitides, or gastroenteritis; use with caution. Allergic-type skin reactions have been reported with use; discontinue with signs of sensitization. Trimethobenzamide clearance is predominantly renal; consider dosage reductions in patients with renal impairment.

Adverse Reactions
Cardiovascular: Hypotension (I.V. administration)
Central nervous system: Coma, depression, disorientation, dizziness, drowsiness, EPS, headache, Parkinson-like symptoms, seizure
Dermatologic: Allergic-type skin reactions
Gastrointestinal: Diarrhea
Hematologic: Blood dyscrasias
Hepatic: Jaundice
Local: Injection site burning, pain, redness, stinging, or swelling
Neuromuscular & skeletal: Muscle cramps, opisthotonos
Ocular: Blurred vision
Miscellaneous: Hypersensitivity reactions

Drug Interactions
Metabolism/Transport Effects None known.
Avoid Concomitant Use
Avoid concomitant use of Trimethobenzamide with any of the following: Aclidinium; Ipratropium (Oral Inhalation); Potassium Chloride; Tiotropium; Umeclidinium

Increased Effect/Toxicity
Trimethobenzamide may increase the levels/effects of: AbobotulinumtoxinA; Analgesics (Opioid); Anticholinergic Agents; Cannabinoid-Containing Products; Mirabegron; OnabotulinumtoxinA; Potassium Chloride; Rimabotulinumtoxin B; Thiazide Diuretics; Tiotropium; Topiramate

The levels/effects of Trimethobenzamide may be increased by: Aclidinium; Alcohol (Ethyl); Ipratropium (Oral Inhalation); Pramlintide; Umeclidinium

Decreased Effect
Trimethobenzamide may decrease the levels/effects of: Acetylcholinesterase Inhibitors (Central); Secretin

The levels/effects of Trimethobenzamide may be decreased by: Acetylcholinesterase Inhibitors (Central)

Stability Store at room temperature.

Mechanism of Action Acts centrally to inhibit the medullary chemoreceptor trigger zone by blocking emetic impulses to the vomiting center

Pharmacodynamics
Onset of action:
Oral: 10-40 minutes
I.M.: 15-35 minutes
Duration:
Oral: 3-4 hours
I.M.: 2-3 hours

Pharmacokinetics (Adult data unless noted)
Metabolism: Via oxidation, forms metabolite trimethobenzamide N-oxide
Bioavailability: Oral dose is 100% of I.M. dose
Half-life: Adults: 7-9 hours
Time to peak serum concentration:
Oral: 45 minutes
I.M.: 30 minutes
Elimination: 30% to 50% excreted unchanged in urine in 24 hours

Dosing: Usual

Children:

Oral: 15-20 mg/kg/day (400-500 mg/m²/day) divided into 3-4 doses; **or as an alternative**

<13.6 kg: 100 mg 3-4 times/day

13.6-40 kg: 100-200 mg 3-4 times/day

>40 kg: 300 mg 3-4 times/day

I.M.: Not recommended

Adults:

Oral: 300 mg 3-4 times/day

I.M.: 200 mg 3-4 times/day

Postoperative nausea and vomiting (PONV): I.M.: 200 mg, followed 1 hour later by a second 200 mg dose

Dosage adjustment in renal impairment: CrCl ≤70 mL/ minute: Consider dosage reduction or increasing dosing interval (specific adjustment guidelines are not provided in the manufacturer's labeling)

Administration

Oral: May administer without regard to food

Parenteral: I.M. use only by deep injection into upper outer quadrant of gluteal region; **not** for I.V. use

Additional Information Note: Less effective than phenothiazines but may be associated with fewer side effects

Dosage Forms Excipient information presented when available (limited, particularly for generics); consult specific product labeling. [DSC] = Discontinued product

Capsule, Oral, as hydrochloride:

Tigan: 300 mg

Generic: 300 mg

Solution, Intramuscular, as hydrochloride:

Tigan: 100 mg/mL (2 mL)

Tigan: 100 mg/mL (20 mL) [contains phenol]

Generic: 100 mg/mL (2 mL [DSC], 20 mL [DSC])

References

Leung AK and Robson WL, "Acute Gastroenteritis in Children: Role of Anti-Emetic Medication for Gastroenteritis-Related Vomiting," *Paediatr Drugs*, 2007, 9(3):175-84.

◆ **Trimethobenzamide HCl** *see* Trimethobenzamide *on page 2086*

◆ **Trimethobenzamide Hydrochloride** *see* Trimethobenzamide *on page 2086*

Trimethoprim (trye METH oh prim)

Brand Names: U.S. Primsol

Brand Names: Canada Apo-Trimethoprim®

Therapeutic Category Antibiotic, Miscellaneous

Generic Availability (U.S.) May be product dependent

Use Treatment of otitis media caused by susceptible *Streptococcus pneumoniae* and *Haemophilus influenzae* (oral solution: FDA approved in pediatric patients ≥6 months); treatment of urinary tract infections caused by susceptible *Escherichia coli, Proteus mirabilis, Klebsiella pneumoniae, Enterobacter* spp, and coagulase-negative *Staphylococcus* (including *S. saprophyticus*) (FDA approved in adults). Has also been used in combination with other agents for treatment of *Pneumocystis jirovecii* pneumonia (PCP)

Pregnancy Risk Factor C

Pregnancy Considerations Adverse effects have been observed in animal reproduction studies. Trimethoprim crosses the placenta and can be detected in the fetal serum and amniotic fluid (Reid, 1975). Adverse events may be associated with trimethoprim use during pregnancy (Andersen, 2012; Andersen, 2013; Mølgaard-Nielsen, 2012). Untreated urinary tract infections may cause adverse pregnancy outcomes (Nicolle, 2005); because safer options are available for the treatment of UTIs in pregnant women, use of TMP containing products in the first trimester should be avoided (Lee, 2008). Studies evaluating the effects of trimethoprim administration in pregnancy have also been conducted with sulfamethoxazole/trimethoprim (see the Sulfamethoxazole and Trimethoprim monograph for details).

Breast-Feeding Considerations Trimethoprim is excreted in breast milk. The manufacturer recommends caution while using trimethoprim in a breast-feeding woman because trimethoprim may interfere with folic acid metabolism. Nondose-related effects could include modification of bowel flora. Also see the Sulfamethoxazole and Trimethoprim monograph for additional information.

Contraindications Hypersensitivity to trimethoprim or any component; megaloblastic anemia due to folate deficiency

Warnings May cause folate deficiencies with subsequent bone marrow suppression and blood dyscrasias; monitor patients for fever, sore throat, purpura, or pallor; obtain CBC if any of these symptoms occur; risk may be increased with high dose or prolonged use; discontinue trimethoprim if bone marrow depression occurs; leucovorin calcium may be needed to restore normal hematopoiesis.

Prolonged use may result in fungal or bacterial superinfection, including *C. difficile*-associated diarrhea (CDAD) and pseudomembranous colitis; CDAD has been observed >2 months postantibiotic treatment.

Oral solution contains sodium benzoate. Benzoic acid (benzoate) is a metabolite of benzyl alcohol; large amounts of benzyl alcohol (≥99 mg/kg/day) have been associated with a potentially fatal toxicity ("gasping syndrome") in neonates; *in vitro* and animal studies have shown that benzoate displaces bilirubin from protein binding sites. Oral solution contains propylene glycol; toxicities have been reported with use of products containing propylene glycol, including hyperosmolality, lactic acidosis, seizures, and respiratory depression; in neonates large amounts of propylene glycol delivered orally, intravenously (eg, >3000 mg/day), or topically have been associated with potentially fatal toxicities which can include metabolic acidosis, seizures, renal failure, and CNS depression; use oral solution containing propylene glycol with caution (AAP, 1997; Shehab, 2009). Avoid use of trimethoprim products containing sodium benzoate and propylene glycol in neonates.

Precautions Use with caution in patients with impaired renal or hepatic function; decrease dose in patients with renal dysfunction. Use with caution in patients with potential folate deficiency (malnourished, chronic anticonvulsant therapy, or elderly). Due to resistance, should not be used for treatment of acute otitis media caused by *Moraxella catarrhalis*. Trimethoprim is not indicated for prolonged administration or prophylaxis of otitis media in any age.

Adverse Reactions

Central nervous system: Aseptic meningitis (rare), fever

Dermatologic: Erythema multiforme (rare), exfoliative dermatitis (rare), maculopapular rash, phototoxic skin eruptions, pruritus (common), Stevens-Johnson syndrome (rare), toxic epidermal necrolysis (rare)

Endocrine & metabolic: Hyperkalemia, hyponatremia

Gastrointestinal: Epigastric distress, glossitis, nausea, vomiting

Hematologic: Leukopenia, megaloblastic anemia, methemoglobinemia, neutropenia, thrombocytopenia

Hepatic: Cholestatic jaundice (rare), liver enzymes increased

Renal: Increased BUN and creatinine

Miscellaneous: Anaphylaxis, hypersensitivity reactions

Drug Interactions

Metabolism/Transport Effects Substrate of CYP2C9 (major), CYP3A4 (major); **Note:** Assignment of Major/ Minor substrate status based on clinically relevant drug interaction potential; **Inhibits** CYP2C8 (moderate), CYP2C9 (moderate)

Avoid Concomitant Use

Avoid concomitant use of Trimethoprim with any of the following: BCG; Dofetilide; Leucovorin Calcium-Levoleucovorin

Increased Effect/Toxicity

Trimethoprim may increase the levels/effects of: ACE Inhibitors; Amantadine; Angiotensin II Receptor Blockers; Antidiabetic Agents (Thiazolidinedione); AzaTHIOprine; Bosentan; Cannabis; Carvedilol; CYP2C8 Substrates; CYP2C9 Substrates; Dapsone (Systemic); Dapsone (Topical); Digoxin; Dofetilide; Dronabinol; Eplerenone; Fosphenytoin; Highest Risk QTc-Prolonging Agents; LamiVUDine; Memantine; Mercaptopurine; MetFORMIN; Methotrexate; Moderate Risk QTc-Prolonging Agents; Phenytoin; PRALAtrexate; Procainamide; Repaglinide; Spironolactone; Tetrahydrocannabinol; Varenicline

The levels/effects of Trimethoprim may be increased by: Amantadine; Ceritinib; CYP2C9 Inhibitors (Moderate); CYP2C9 Inhibitors (Strong); Dapsone (Systemic); Memantine; Mifepristone

Decreased Effect

Trimethoprim may decrease the levels/effects of: BCG; Sodium Picosulfate; Typhoid Vaccine

The levels/effects of Trimethoprim may be decreased by: Bosentan; CYP2C9 Inducers (Strong); CYP3A4 Inducers (Strong); Dabrafenib; Deferasirox; Fosphenytoin; Leucovorin Calcium-Levoleucovorin; Mitotane; Peginterferon Alfa-2b; Phenytoin; Siltuximab; St Johns Wort; Tocilizumab

Stability Oral:

Solution: Store at 15°C to 25°C (59°F to 77°F); protect from light.

Tablets: Store at 20°C to 25°C (68°F to 77°F); protect from light.

Mechanism of Action Inhibits folic acid reduction to tetrahydrofolate, and thereby inhibits microbial growth

Pharmacokinetics (Adult data unless noted)

Absorption: Oral: Readily and extensively absorbed

Distribution: Penetrates into middle ear fluid with a mean peak middle ear fluid concentration in children 1-12 years of 2 mcg/mL after a single 4 mg/kg dose

V_d:

Newborns: 2.7 L/kg (range: 1.3-4.1 hours) (Springer, 1982)

Infants: 1.5 L/kg (Hoppu, 1989)

Children (Hoppu, 1987):

1-3 years: 0.86 L/kg

8-10 years: 1 L/kg

Adults: ~1.3 L/kg (Hoppu, 1987)

Protein binding: ~44%

Metabolism: Partially hepatic (10% to 20%) via demethylation, oxidation, and hydroxylation

Bioavailability: Similar for tablets and solution

Half-life: Prolonged with renal impairment

Newborns: 19 hours; range: 11-27 hours (Springer, 1982)

Infants 2 months to 1 year: 4.6 hours; range: 3-6 hours (Hoppu, 1989)

Children (Hoppu, 1987):

1-3 years: 3.7 hours

8-10 years: 5.4 hours

Adults, normal renal function: 8-10 hours

Time to peak serum concentration: 1-4 hours

Elimination: Significantly excreted in urine (50% to 60%); 80% as unchanged drug via glomerular filtration and tubular secretion

Dialysis: Moderately dialyzable (20% to 50%)

Dosing: Usual

Infants, Children, and Adolescents:

Otitis media, acute: Infants ≥6 months, Children, and Adolescents: Oral: 10 mg/kg/day in divided doses every 12 hours for 10 days; maximum daily dose: 400 mg/day

Urinary tract infection (uncomplicated), treatment: Infants ≥2 months, Children, and Adolescents: Oral: 4-6 mg/kg/day in divided doses every 12 hours; **Note:** Preferred therapy is sulfamethoxazole and trimethoprim combined product (AAP, 2011).

***Pneumocystis jirovecii* pneumonia (PCP), treatment:** Children and Adolescents: Oral: 15 mg/kg/day in 3 divided doses for 21 days; in combination with dapsone; data in children is limited; preferred therapy is sulfamethoxazole and trimethoprim combined product (DHHS [adult and pediatric], 2013)

Adults:

Urinary tract infection (uncomplicated), treatment: Oral: 100 mg every 12 hours or 200 mg every 24 hours for 10 days; alternative duration of 3 days has been recommended (Gupta, 2011)

***Pneumocystis jirovecii* pneumonia (PCP); treatment:** Oral: 15 mg/kg/day in 3 divided doses for 21 days in combination with dapsone (DHHS [adult], 2013)

Dosing adjustment in renal impairment: Manufacturer's recommendation: Children and Adults:

CrCl 15-30 mL/minute: Administer 50% of recommended dose.

CrCl <15 mL/minute: Use is not recommended.

Dosing adjustment in hepatic impairment: No dosage adjustments are provided in the manufacturer labeling.

Administration Oral: Administer on an empty stomach; may administer with milk or food if GI upset occurs

Monitoring Parameters CBC with differential, platelet count, liver enzyme tests, bilirubin, serum potassium, serum creatinine and BUN

Reference Range Therapeutic:

Peak: 5-15 mg/L

Trough: 2-8 mg/L

Test Interactions May falsely increase creatinine determination measured by the Jaffé alkaline picrate assay; may interfere with determination of serum methotrexate when measured by methods that use a bacterial dihydrofolate reductase as the binding protein (eg, the competitive binding protein technique); does **not** interfere with RIA for methotrexate

Dosage Forms Excipient information presented when available (limited, particularly for generics); consult specific product labeling.

Solution, Oral [strength expressed as base]:

Primsol: 50 mg/5 mL (473 mL) [alcohol free, dye free]

Tablet, Oral:

Generic: 100 mg

Extemporaneous Preparations Note: Commercial oral solution is available (10 mg/mL [dye free, ethanol free; contains propylene glycol, sodium benzoate; bubblegum flavor])

A 10 mg/mL oral suspension may be made with tablets. Crush ten 100 mg tablets in a mortar and reduce to a fine powder. Add 20 mL of a 1:1 mixture of Simple Syrup, NF, and Methylcellulose 1% and mix to a uniform paste; mix while adding the vehicle in incremental proportions to **almost** 100 mL; transfer to a calibrated bottle, rinse mortar with vehicle, and add quantity of vehicle sufficient to make 100 mL. Label "shake well" and "refrigerate". Stable for 91 days.

Nahata MC, Pai VB, and Hipple TF, *Pediatric Drug Formulations*, 5th ed, Cincinnati, OH: Harvey Whitney Books Co, 2004.

References

American Academy of Pediatrics Committee on Drugs. "Inactive" ingredients in pharmaceutical products: update (subject review). *Pediatrics*. 1997;99(2):268-278.

American Academy of Pediatrics, "Urinary Tract Infection: Clinical Practice Guideline for the Diagnosis and Management of the Initial UTI in Febrile Infants and Children 2 to 24 Months," *Pediatrics*, 2011, 128(3):595-610.

Andersen JT, Petersen M, Jimenez-Solem E, et al, "Trimethoprim Use in Early Pregnancy and the Risk of Miscarriage: A Register-Based Nationwide Cohort Study," *Epidemiol Infect*, 2013, 141(8):1749-55.

Andersen JT, Petersen M, Jimenez-Solem E, et al, "Trimethoprim Use Prior to Pregnancy and the Risk of Congenital Malformation: A Register-Based Nationwide Cohort Study," *Obstet Gynecol Int*, 2013, 2013:364526.

DHHS. Guidelines for the prevention and treatment of opportunistic infections among HIV-exposed and HIV-infected children: recommendations from the National Institutes of Health, Centers for Disease Control and Prevention, the HIV Medicine Association of the Infectious Diseases Society of America, the Pediatric Infectious Diseases Society, and the American Academy of Pediatrics. November 6, 2013. Available at http://aidsinfo.nih.gov

DHHS Panel on Opportunistic Infections (OI) in HIV-Infected Adults and Adolescents. Guidelines for prevention and treatment of opportunistic infections in HIV-infected adults and adolescents: recommendations from the Centers for Disease Control and Prevention (CDC), the National Institutes of Health (NIH), and the HIV Medicine Association (HIVMA) of the Infectious Diseases Society of America (IDSA). May 7, 2013. Available at http://aidsinfo.nih.gov/contentfiles/lvguidelines/adult_oi.pdf

Gupta K, Hooton TM, Naber KG, et al, "International Clinical Practice Guidelines for the Treatment of Acute Uncomplicated Cystitis and Pyelonephritis in Women: A 2010 Update by the Infectious Diseases Society of America and the European Society for Microbiology and Infectious Diseases," *Clin Infect Dis*, 2011, 52(5):e103-20.

Hoppu K, "Age Differences in Trimethoprim Pharmacokinetics: Need for Revised Dosing in Children?" *Clin Pharmacol Ther*, 1987, 41 (3):336-43.

Hoppu K, "Changes in Trimethoprim Pharmacokinetics After the Newborn Period," *Arch Dis Child*, 1989, 64(3):343-5.

Lee M, Bozzo P, Einarson A, et al, "Urinary Tract Infections in Pregnancy," *Can Fam Physician*, 2008, 54(6):853-4.

Mølgaard-Nielsen D and Hviid A, "Maternal Use of Antibiotics and the Risk of Orofacial Clefts: A Nationwide Cohort Study," *Pharmacoepidemiol Drug Saf*, 2012, 21(3):246-53.

Nicolle LE, Bradley S, Colgan R, et al, "Infectious Diseases Society of America Guidelines for the Diagnosis and Treatment of Asymptomatic Bacteriuria in Adults," *Clin Infect Dis*, 2005, 40(5):643-54.

Reid DW, Caille G, and Kaufmann NR, "Maternal and Transplacental Kinetics of Trimethoprim and Sulfamethoxazole, Separately and in Combination," *Can Med Assoc J*, 1975, 112(13 Spec No):67-72.

Shehab N, Lewis CL, Streetman DD, Donn SM. Exposure to the pharmaceutical excipients benzyl alcohol and propylene glycol among critically ill neonates. *Pediatr Crit Care Med*. 2009;10 (2):256-259.

Springer C, Eyal F, and Michel J, "Pharmacology of Trimethoprim-Sulfamethoxazole in Newborn Infants," *J Pediatr*, 1982, 100 (4):647-50.

Trimethoprim and Polymyxin B
(trye METH oh prim & pol i MIKS in bee)

Brand Names: U.S. Polytrim®
Brand Names: Canada PMS-Polytrimethoprim; Polytrim™
Therapeutic Category Antibiotic, Ophthalmic
Generic Availability (U.S.) Yes
Use Treatment of surface ocular conjunctivitis and blepharoconjunctivitis caused by susceptible *S. aureus*, *S. epidermidis*, *S. pneumoniae*, *S. viridans*, *H. influenzae*, and *P. aeruginosa* (FDA approved in ages ≥2 months and adults)
Pregnancy Risk Factor C
Pregnancy Considerations Adverse events have been observed with trimethoprim in animal reproduction studies; animal reproduction studies have not been conducted with polymyxin B. See individual agents. If ophthalmic agents are needed during pregnancy, the minimum effective dose should be used in combination with punctual occlusion to decrease potential exposure to the fetus (Samples, 1988).
Breast-Feeding Considerations It is not known if trimethoprim or polymyxin B can be detected in breast milk following ophthalmic administration. The manufacturer recommends that caution be exercised when administering trimethoprim/polymyxin B to nursing women. See individual agents.
Contraindications Hypersensitivity to trimethoprim, polymyxin B, or any component
Warnings Not indicated for prophylaxis or treatment of ophthalmia neonatorum. **Not for injection into the eye.**
Precautions Prolonged use may result in overgrowth of nonsusceptible organisms

Adverse Reactions Ocular: Burning, itching, edema, rash, redness increased, stinging, tearing
Drug Interactions
Metabolism/Transport Effects Refer to individual components.
Avoid Concomitant Use
Avoid concomitant use of Trimethoprim and Polymyxin B with any of the following: BCG; Dofetilide; Leucovorin Calcium-Levoleucovorin
Increased Effect/Toxicity
Trimethoprim and Polymyxin B may increase the levels/effects of: ACE Inhibitors; Amantadine; Angiotensin II Receptor Blockers; Antidiabetic Agents (Thiazolidinedione); AzaTHIOprine; Bosentan; Cannabis; Carvedilol; Colistimethate; CYP2C8 Substrates; CYP2C9 Substrates; Dapsone (Systemic); Dapsone (Topical); Digoxin; Dofetilide; Dronabinol; Eplerenone; Fosphenytoin; Highest Risk QTc-Prolonging Agents; LamiVUDine; Memantine; Mercaptopurine; MetFORMIN; Methotrexate; Moderate Risk QTc-Prolonging Agents; Neuromuscular-Blocking Agents; Phenytoin; PRALAtrexate; Procainamide; Repaglinide; Spironolactone; Tetrahydrocannabinol; Varenicline

The levels/effects of Trimethoprim and Polymyxin B may be increased by: Amantadine; Capreomycin; Ceritinib; CYP2C9 Inhibitors (Moderate); CYP2C9 Inhibitors (Strong); Dapsone (Systemic); Memantine; Mifepristone
Decreased Effect
Trimethoprim and Polymyxin B may decrease the levels/effects of: BCG; Sodium Picosulfate; Typhoid Vaccine

The levels/effects of Trimethoprim and Polymyxin B may be decreased by: Bosentan; CYP2C9 Inducers (Strong); CYP3A4 Inducers (Strong); Dabrafenib; Deferasirox; Fosphenytoin; Leucovorin Calcium-Levoleucovorin; Mitotane; Peginterferon Alfa-2b; Phenytoin; Siltuximab; St Johns Wort; Tocilizumab
Stability Store at 15°C to 25°C (59°F to 77°F); protect from light
Dosing: Usual Infants ≥2 months, Children, Adolescents, and Adults: Ophthalmic: Instill 1 drop in eye(s) every 3 hours (maximum: 6 doses/day) for 7-10 days (manufacturer's recommendation for mild to moderate infection)
Administration For topical use in eye only; avoid contamination of the applicator tip. Apply finger pressure to lacrimal sac during and for 1-2 minutes after instillation to decrease risk of absorption and systemic effects.
Additional Information Polytrim®: pH 4-6.2; osmolality: 270-310 mOsm/kg
Dosage Forms Excipient information presented when available (limited, particularly for generics); consult specific product labeling.
Solution, ophthalmic: Trimethoprim 1 mg and polymyxin B sulfate 10,000 units per 1 mL (10 mL)
Polytrim®: Trimethoprim 1 mg and polymyxin B sulfate 10,000 units per 1 mL (10 mL) [contains benzalkonium chloride]
References
Samples JR and Meyer SM, "Use of Ophthalmic Medications in Pregnant and Nursing Women," *Am J Ophthalmol*, 1988, 106 (5):616-23.

◆ **Trimethoprim and Sulfamethoxazole** *see* Sulfamethoxazole and Trimethoprim *on page 1948*

◆ **Trinasal (Can)** *see* Triamcinolone (Nasal) *on page 2076*

◆ **Trinipatch (Can)** *see* Nitroglycerin *on page 1504*

◆ **Triostat** *see* Liothyronine *on page 1256*

◆ **Tripedia** *see* Diphtheria and Tetanus Toxoids, and Acellular Pertussis Vaccine *on page 686*

◆ **Triple Antibiotic** *see* Bacitracin, Neomycin, and Polymyxin B *on page 258*

◆ **Triple Paste AF [OTC]** *see* Miconazole (Topical) on page 1410

Triprolidine and Pseudoephedrine
(trye PROE li deen & soo doe e FED rin)

Medication Safety Issues
BEERS Criteria medication:
This drug may be potentially inappropriate for use in geriatric patients (Quality of evidence - moderate; Strength of recommendation - strong).

Brand Names: U.S. Aprodine [OTC]; Pediatex® TD
Brand Names: Canada Actifed®
Therapeutic Category Antihistamine/Decongestant Combination; Sympathomimetic
Generic Availability (U.S.) Yes
Use Temporary relief of nasal congestion, running nose, sneezing, itching of nose or throat and itchy, watery eyes due to common cold, hay fever or other upper respiratory allergies (FDA approved in ages ≥6 years and adults)
Pregnancy Considerations Maternal antihistamine use has generally not resulted in an increased risk of birth defects; however, information related to triprolidine is limited. Refer to the Pseudoephedrine monograph for information related to decongestants.
Breast-Feeding Considerations Triprolidine is excreted into breast milk. Based on data from three cases, the estimated exposure to the nursing infant is <1% of the weight-adjusted maternal dose. Antihistamines may decrease maternal serum prolactin concentrations when administered prior to the establishment of nursing. Pseudoephedrine is also excreted into breast milk. Refer to the Pseudoephedrine monograph for information related to decongestants.
Contraindications Hypersensitivity to triprolidine, pseudoephedrine, or any component; severe hypertension or coronary artery disease; MAO inhibitor therapy, GI or GU obstruction, narrow-angle glaucoma
Warnings Safety and efficacy for the use of cough and cold products in children <2 years of age is limited. Serious adverse effects including death have been reported. The FDA notes that there are no approved OTC uses for these products in children <2 years of age. Healthcare providers are reminded to ask caregivers about the use of OTC cough and cold products in order to avoid exposure to multiple medications containing the same ingredient.
Precautions Use with caution in patients with mild to moderate high blood pressure, heart disease, diabetes mellitus, asthma, thyroid disease, or prostatic hypertrophy

Adverse Reactions
Cardiovascular: Tachycardia
Central nervous system: Dizziness, drowsiness, fatigue, headache, insomnia, nervousness, transient stimulation
Gastrointestinal: Abdominal pain, appetite increase, diarrhea, nausea, weight gain, xerostomia
Genitourinary: Dysuria
Neuromuscular & skeletal: Arthralgia, weakness
Respiratory: Pharyngitis, thickening of bronchial secretions
Miscellaneous: Diaphoresis

Drug Interactions
Metabolism/Transport Effects Refer to individual components.

Avoid Concomitant Use
Avoid concomitant use of Triprolidine and Pseudoephedrine with any of the following: Aclidinium; Azelastine (Nasal); Ergot Derivatives; Iobenguane I 123; Ipratropium (Oral Inhalation); MAO Inhibitors; Paraldehyde; Potassium Chloride; Thalidomide; Tiotropium; Umeclidinium

Increased Effect/Toxicity
Triprolidine and Pseudoephedrine may increase the levels/effects of: AbobotulinumtoxinA; Alcohol (Ethyl); Analgesics (Opioid); Anticholinergic Agents; ARIPiprazole;

Azelastine (Nasal); Buprenorphine; Cannabinoid-Containing Products; CNS Depressants; Hydrocodone; Methotrimeprazine; Metyrosine; Mirabegron; Mirtazapine; OnabotulinumtoxinA; Paraldehyde; Potassium Chloride; Pramipexole; RimabotulinumtoxinB; ROPINIRole; Rotigotine; Selective Serotonin Reuptake Inhibitors; Sympathomimetics; Thalidomide; Thiazide Diuretics; Tiotropium; Topiramate; Zolpidem

The levels/effects of Triprolidine and Pseudoephedrine may be increased by: Aclidinium; Alkalinizing Agents; AtoMOXetine; Brimonidine (Topical); Cannabinoid-Containing Products; Cannabis; Carbonic Anhydrase Inhibitors; Doxylamine; Dronabinol; Droperidol; Ergot Derivatives; HydrOXYzine; Ipratropium (Oral Inhalation); Kava Kava; Linezolid; Magnesium Sulfate; MAO Inhibitors; Methotrimeprazine; Nabilone; Perampanel; Pramlintide; Rufinamide; Serotonin/Norepinephrine Reuptake Inhibitors; Sodium Oxybate; Tapentadol; Tetrahydrocannabinol; Umeclidinium

Decreased Effect
Triprolidine and Pseudoephedrine may decrease the levels/effects of: Acetylcholinesterase Inhibitors (Central); Benzylpenicilloyl Polylysine; Betahistine; FentaNYL; Hyaluronidase; Iobenguane I 123; Secretin

The levels/effects of Triprolidine and Pseudoephedrine may be decreased by: Acetylcholinesterase Inhibitors (Central); Alpha1-Blockers; Amphetamines; Spironolactone; Urinary Acidifying Agents

Mechanism of Action Refer to Pseudoephedrine (Systemic) monograph.
Triprolidine is a member of the propylamine (alkylamine) chemical class of H_1-antagonist antihistamines. As such, it is considered to be relatively less sedating than traditional antihistamines of the ethanolamine, phenothiazine, and ethylenediamine classes of antihistamines. Triprolidine has a shorter half-life and duration of action than most of the other alkylamine antihistamines. Like all H_1-antagonist antihistamines, the mechanism of action of triprolidine is believed to involve competitive blockade of H_1-receptor sites resulting in the inability of histamine to combine with its receptor sites and exert its usual effects on target cells. Antihistamines do not interrupt any effects of histamine which have already occurred. Therefore, these agents are used more successfully in the prevention rather than the treatment of histamine-induced reactions.

Dosing: Usual Oral:
≥2 years: May dose according to **pseudoephedrine** component: 4 mg/kg/day in divided doses 3-4 times/day not to exceed a maximum of 60 mg pseudoephedrine per dose
Liquid:
Children 6-12 years: Pediatex® TD: 1.33 mL every 6 hours (maximum: 4 doses/24 hours)
Children ≥12 years and Adults: Pediatex® TD: 2.67 mL every 6 hours (maximum: 4 doses/24 hours)
Syrup (Aprodine):
Children 6-12 years: 5 mL every 4-6 hours; do not exceed 4 doses in 24 hours
Children >12 years and Adults: 10 mL every 4-6 hours; do not exceed 4 doses in 24 hours
Tablet (Aprodine):
Children 6-12 years: 1/2 tablet every 4-6 hours; do not exceed 4 doses in 24 hours
Children >12 years and Adults: One tablet every 4-6 hours; do not exceed 4 doses in 24 hours
Administration Oral: Administer with food or milk to decrease GI irritation
Test Interactions
Pseudoephedrine: Interferes with urine detection of amphetamine (false-positive).

Triprolidine: May suppress the wheal and flare reactions to skin test antigens.

Dosage Forms Excipient information presented when available (limited, particularly for generics); consult specific product labeling. [DSC] = Discontinued product

Liquid, oral:

Pediatex® TD: Triprolidine hydrochloride 0.938 mg and pseudoephedrine hydrochloride 10 mg per 1 mL (30 mL) [cotton candy flavor]

Syrup, oral: Triprolidine hydrochloride 1.25 mg and pseudoephedrine hydrochloride 30 mg per 5 mL (120 mL) [DSC]

Aprodine: Triprolidine hydrochloride 1.25 mg and pseudoephedrine hydrochloride 30 mg per 5 mL (120 mL)

Tablet, oral:

Aprodine: Triprolidine hydrochloride 2.5 mg and pseudoephedrine hydrochloride 60 mg

◆ **Tris Buffer** *see* Tromethamine *on page 2091*

◆ **Trisenox** *see* Arsenic Trioxide *on page 201*

◆ **Tris(hydroxymethyl)aminomethane** *see* Tromethamine *on page 2091*

◆ **Trisulfa (Can)** *see* Sulfamethoxazole and Trimethoprim *on page 1948*

◆ **Trisulfa DS (Can)** *see* Sulfamethoxazole and Trimethoprim *on page 1948*

◆ **Trisulfa S (Can)** *see* Sulfamethoxazole and Trimethoprim *on page 1948*

◆ **Trivagizole-3® (Can)** *see* Clotrimazole (Topical) *on page 527*

◆ **Trivalent Recombinant Hemagglutinin (rHA) Vaccine** *see* Influenza Virus Vaccine (Recombinant) *on page 1112*

◆ **Trixaicin [OTC]** *see* Capsaicin *on page 367*

◆ **Trixaicin HP [OTC]** *see* Capsaicin *on page 367*

◆ **Trizivir®** *see* Abacavir, Lamivudine, and Zidovudine *on page 41*

◆ **Trocaine Throat [OTC]** *see* Benzocaine *on page 273*

◆ **Trocal Cough Suppressant [OTC]** *see* Dextromethorphan *on page 636*

◆ **Trokendi XR** *see* Topiramate *on page 2046*

Tromethamine (troe METH a meen)

Medication Safety Issues
Sound-alike/look-alike issues:
Tromethamine may be confused with TrophAmine®

Related Information
Management of Drug Extravasations *on page 2255*

Brand Names: U.S. Tham

Therapeutic Category Alkalinizing Agent, Parenteral

Generic Availability (U.S.) No

Use Correction of metabolic acidosis associated with cardiac bypass surgery or cardiac arrest; to correct excess acidity of stored blood that is preserved with acid citrate dextrose (ACD); to prime the pump-oxygenator during cardiac bypass surgery; indicated in severe metabolic acidosis in patients in whom sodium or carbon dioxide elimination is restricted [eg, infants needing alkalinization after receiving maximum sodium bicarbonate (8-10 mEq/kg/24 hours)]

Pregnancy Risk Factor C

Pregnancy Considerations Animal studies have not been conducted. There are no adequate and well-controlled studies in pregnant women. Use only if potential benefit outweighs possible risk to the fetus.

Breast-Feeding Considerations It is not known if tromethamine is excreted in breast milk. The manufacturer recommends that caution be exercised when administering tromethamine to nursing women.

Contraindications Hypersensitivity to tromethamine or any component; uremia or anuria; chronic respiratory acidosis (neonates); salicylate intoxication (neonates)

Warnings Avoid infusion via low-lying umbilical venous catheters (particularly with concentrations ≥1.2 M) due to associated risk of hepatocellular necrosis; severe local tissue necrosis and sloughing may occur if solution extravasates; administer via central line or large vein slowly. Due to tromethamine's greater osmotic effects, use of sodium bicarbonate for the treatment of acidotic neonates and infants with RDS may be preferred; may cause prolonged hypoglycemia in neonates or with rapid I.V. infusion and overdosage. Monitor pH carefully as large doses may increase blood pH greater than normal which may result in depressed respiration.

Precautions Reduce dose and monitor pH and serum potassium carefully in renal impairment.

Adverse Reactions
Cardiovascular: Hypervolemia, venospasm
Endocrine & metabolic: Hyperkalemia, hypoglycemia (usually doses >500 mg/kg administered over <1 hour)
Hepatic: Hepatic necrosis (resulted during delivery via umbilical venous catheter)
Local: Necrosis with extravasation, phlebitis, tissue irritation
Respiratory: Apnea, pulmonary edema, respiratory depression

Drug Interactions
Metabolism/Transport Effects None known.
Avoid Concomitant Use There are no known interactions where it is recommended to avoid concomitant use.
Increased Effect/Toxicity
Tromethamine may increase the levels/effects of: Alpha-/Beta-Agonists (Indirect-Acting); Amphetamines; Flecainide; QuiNINE
Decreased Effect There are no known significant interactions involving a decrease in effect.

Stability Store at room temperature; protect from freezing

Mechanism of Action Acts as a proton acceptor, which combines with hydrogen ions, liberating bicarbonate buffer, to correct acidosis. It buffers both metabolic and respiratory acids, limiting carbon dioxide generation. Also an osmotic diuretic.

Pharmacokinetics (Adult data unless noted) 30% of dose is not ionized; rapidly eliminated by kidneys

Dosing: Neonatal I.V.: Dose depends on severity and progression of acidosis: Manufacturer's recommendation: 1 mL/kg for each pH unit below 7.4; additional doses to be determined by changes in PaO_2, pH, and pCO_2

Dosing: Usual I.V.: Dose depends on severity and progression of acidosis: Infants, Children, and Adults:
Empiric dosage based upon base deficit: Tromethamine mL of 0.3 M solution = body weight (kg) x base deficit (mEq/L) x 1.1*; maximum: 500 mg/kg/dose = 13.9 mL/kg/dose using 0.3 M solution
*Factor of 1.1 accounts for an approximate reduction of 10% in buffering capacity due to the presence of sufficient acetic acid to lower the pH of the 0.3 M solution to approximately 8.6
Metabolic acidosis with cardiac arrest: Tromethamine mL of 0.3 M solution: 3.5-6 mL/kg/dose (126-216 mg/kg/dose); maximum: 500 mg/kg/dose = 13.9 mL/kg/dose
Metabolic acidosis with cardiac arrest: Direct instillation to ventricle: Adults: Tromethamine 0.3 M solution: 2-6 g (62-185 mL); do not inject into cardiac muscle
Excess acidity of acid citrate dextrose priming blood: Tromethamine mL of 0.3 M solution: 15-77 mL added to each 500 mL of ACD blood used for priming the pump-oxygenator
Acidosis during cardiac bypass surgery: Tromethamine mL of 0.3 M solution: 9 mL/kg (324 mg/kg/dose); maximum: 1000 mL (36 g) as single dose dose in severe cases and

not to exceed 500 mg/kg over a period of 1 hour (eg, for 70 kg patient, not to exceed 35 g/hour)

Administration Parenteral: Maximum concentration: 0.3 molar; infuse slowly over at least 1 hour or 3-16 mL/kg/hour up to 33-40 mL/kg/day; administer into a central venous line and avoid administration into low-lying umbilical venous lines

Vesicant/Extravasation Risk Vesicant

Monitoring Parameters Serum electrolytes, arterial blood gases, serum pH, blood sugar, ECG monitoring, renal function tests

Additional Information 1 mM = 120 mg = 3.3 mL = 1 mEq of THAM®

Dosage Forms Excipient information presented when available (limited, particularly for generics); consult specific product labeling.

Solution, Intravenous:

Tham: 30 mEq/100 mL (500 mL)

Tropicamide (troe PIK a mide)

Brand Names: U.S. Mydral; Mydriacyl

Brand Names: Canada Diotrope®; Mydriacyl®

Therapeutic Category Ophthalmic Agent, Mydriatic

Generic Availability (U.S.) Yes

Use Short-acting mydriatic used in diagnostic procedures; as well as preoperatively and postoperatively; treatment of some cases of acute iritis, iridocyclitis, and keratitis

Pregnancy Risk Factor C

Pregnancy Considerations Animal reproduction studies have not been conducted. If ophthalmic agents are needed during pregnancy, the minimum effective dose should be used in combination with punctual occlusion to decrease potential exposure to the fetus (Samples, 1988).

Breast-Feeding Considerations It is not known if tropicamide is excreted in breast milk. The manufacturer recommends that caution be used if administered to nursing women.

Contraindications Hypersensitivity to tropicamide or any component; glaucoma, adhesions between the iris and the lens

Warnings Tropicamide may cause an increase in intraocular pressure

Precautions Use with caution in infants and children since tropicamide may cause potentially dangerous CNS disturbances and psychotic reactions

Adverse Reactions

Cardiovascular: Edema, tachycardia, vascular congestion

Central nervous system: Headache, parasympathetic stimulations, somnolence

Dermatologic: Eczematoid dermatitis

Gastrointestinal: Dryness of mouth

Local: Transient stinging

Ocular: Blurred vision, follicular conjunctivitis, increased intraocular pressure, photophobia with or without corneal staining

Drug Interactions

Metabolism/Transport Effects None known.

Avoid Concomitant Use There are no known interactions where it is recommended to avoid concomitant use.

Increased Effect/Toxicity There are no known significant interactions involving an increase in effect.

Decreased Effect There are no known significant interactions involving a decrease in effect.

Stability Store at room temperature; do not refrigerate

Mechanism of Action Prevents the sphincter muscle of the iris and the muscle of the ciliary body from responding to cholinergic stimulation

Pharmacodynamics

Maximum mydriatic effect: ~20-40 minutes

Duration: ~6-7 hours

Maximum cycloplegic effect:

Peak: 20-35 minutes

Duration: <6 hours

Dosing: Neonatal Ophthalmic: Mydriasis: Instill 1 drop (0.5%) 15-20 minutes prior to procedure (1% concentration may be required in patients with heavily pigmented irides); **Note:** In premature neonates, use of 1% solution, while effective, has been associated with significant increases in mean blood pressure when used simultaneously with phenylephrine eye drops (Chew, 2005).

Dosing: Usual Children and Adults: Ophthalmic:

Cycloplegia: Instill 1-2 drops (1%); may repeat in 5 minutes. The exam must be performed within 30 minutes after the repeat dose; if the patient is not examined within 20-30 minutes, instill an additional drop. Concentrations <1% are inadequate for producing satisfactory cycloplegia.

Mydriasis: Instill 1-2 drops (0.5%) 15-20 minutes before exam; may repeat every 30 minutes as needed

Administration Ophthalmic: To minimize systemic absorption, apply finger pressure on the lacrimal sac for 1-2 minutes following instillation of the ophthalmic solution; avoid contact of bottle tip with skin or eye

Dosage Forms Excipient information presented when available (limited, particularly for generics); consult specific product labeling.

Solution, Ophthalmic:

Mydral: 0.5% (15 mL); 1% (15 mL)

Mydriacyl: 1% (3 mL, 15 mL)

Generic: 0.5% (15 mL); 1% (2 mL, 3 mL, 15 mL)

References

Caputo AR and Schnitzer RE, "Systemic Response to Mydriatic Eyedrops in Neonates: Mydriatics in Neonates," *J Pediatr Ophthalmol Strabismus*, 1978, 15(2):109-22.

Chew C, Rahman RA, Shafie SM, et al, "Comparison of Mydriatic Regimens Used in Screening for Retinopathy of Prematurity in Preterm Infants With Dark Irides," *J Pediatr Ophthalmol Strabismus*, 2005, 42(3):166-73.

Samples JR and Meyer SM, "Use of Ophthalmic Medications in Pregnant and Nursing Women," *Am J Ophthalmol*, 1988, 106 (5):616-23.

◆ **Trusopt** *see* Dorzolamide *on page 710*

◆ **Trusopt® (Can)** *see* Dorzolamide *on page 710*

◆ **Truvada** *see* Emtricitabine and Tenofovir *on page 741*

◆ **TSPA** *see* Thiotepa *on page 2014*

◆ **TT** *see* Tetanus Toxoid (Adsorbed) *on page 1993*

◆ **Tums [OTC]** *see* Calcium Carbonate *on page 346*

◆ **Tums Chews Extra Strength (Can)** *see* Calcium Carbonate *on page 346*

◆ **Tums E-X 750 [OTC]** *see* Calcium Carbonate *on page 346*

◆ **Tums Extra Strength (Can)** *see* Calcium Carbonate *on page 346*

◆ **Tums Freshers [OTC]** *see* Calcium Carbonate *on page 346*

◆ **Tums Kids [OTC]** *see* Calcium Carbonate *on page 346*

◆ **Tums Lasting Effects [OTC]** *see* Calcium Carbonate *on page 346*

◆ **Tums Regular Strength (Can)** *see* Calcium Carbonate *on page 346*

◆ **Tums Smoothies [OTC]** *see* Calcium Carbonate *on page 346*

◆ **Tums Smoothies (Can)** *see* Calcium Carbonate *on page 346*

◆ **Tums Ultra 1000 [OTC]** *see* Calcium Carbonate *on page 346*

◆ **Tums Ultra Strength (Can)** *see* Calcium Carbonate *on page 346*

◆ **TussiCaps** *see* Hydrocodone and Chlorpheniramine *on page 1030*

◆ **Tussigon®** *see* Hydrocodone and Homatropine *on page 1032*

◆ **Tussin [OTC]** *see* GuaiFENesin *on page 984*

◆ **Tussionex** *see* Hydrocodone and Chlorpheniramine *on page 1030*

◆ **Tussionex Pennkinetic** *see* Hydrocodone and Chlorpheniramine *on page 1030*

◆ **Twinject (Can)** *see* EPINEPHrine (Systemic, Oral Inhalation) *on page 761*

◆ **Ty21a Vaccine** *see* Typhoid Vaccine *on page 2093*

◆ **Tygacil** *see* Tigecycline *on page 2025*

◆ **Tylenol [OTC]** *see* Acetaminophen *on page 47*

◆ **Tylenol (Can)** *see* Acetaminophen *on page 47*

◆ **Tylenol #2** *see* Acetaminophen and Codeine *on page 53*

◆ **Tylenol #3** *see* Acetaminophen and Codeine *on page 53*

◆ **Tylenol 8 Hour [OTC]** *see* Acetaminophen *on page 47*

◆ **Tylenol Arthritis Pain Extended Relief [OTC]** *see* Acetaminophen *on page 47*

◆ **Tylenol Children's [OTC]** *see* Acetaminophen *on page 47*

◆ **Tylenol Children's Meltaways [OTC]** *see* Acetaminophen *on page 47*

◆ **Tylenol Codeine** *see* Acetaminophen and Codeine *on page 53*

◆ **Tylenol Elixir with Codeine (Can)** *see* Acetaminophen and Codeine *on page 53*

◆ **Tylenol Extra Strength [OTC]** *see* Acetaminophen *on page 47*

◆ **Tylenol Jr. Meltaways [OTC]** *see* Acetaminophen *on page 47*

◆ **Tylenol No. 1 (Can)** *see* Acetaminophen and Codeine *on page 53*

◆ **Tylenol No. 1 Forte (Can)** *see* Acetaminophen and Codeine *on page 53*

◆ **Tylenol No. 2 with Codeine (Can)** *see* Acetaminophen and Codeine *on page 53*

◆ **Tylenol No. 3 with Codeine (Can)** *see* Acetaminophen and Codeine *on page 53*

◆ **Tylenol No. 4 with Codeine (Can)** *see* Acetaminophen and Codeine *on page 53*

◆ **Tylenol® with Codeine No. 3** *see* Acetaminophen and Codeine *on page 53*

◆ **Tylenol® with Codeine No. 4** *see* Acetaminophen and Codeine *on page 53*

◆ **Tylox** *see* Oxycodone and Acetaminophen *on page 1573*

◆ **Typherix (Can)** *see* Typhoid Vaccine *on page 2093*

◆ **Typhim Vi** *see* Typhoid Vaccine *on page 2093*

Typhoid Vaccine (TYE foid vak SEEN)

Related Information
Immunization Administration Recommendations *on page 2368*

Immunization Guidelines *on page 2373*

Brand Names: U.S. Typhim Vi; Vivotif

Brand Names: Canada Typherix; Typhim Vi; Vivotif

Therapeutic Category Vaccine

Generic Availability (U.S.) No

Use Immunization to prevent disease from exposure to *Salmonella typhi*; use is not routinely recommended in the U.S. but is reserved for selected individuals who are either traveling to an area in which there is a recognized risk of exposure to *S. typhi*, who have intimate exposure (eg, household contact) to a *S. typhi* carrier, or who work frequently with *S. typhi* in laboratory settings

Parenteral: Typhim Vi®: Approved for use in children ≥2 years and adults

Oral: Live attenuated Ty21a vaccine (Vivotif®): Approved for use in children ≥6 years and adults

Pregnancy Risk Factor C

Pregnancy Considerations Animal reproduction studies have not been conducted. The manufacturer of the Typhim Vi injection suggests delaying vaccination until the second or third trimester if possible. Untreated typhoid fever may lead to miscarriage or vertical intrauterine transmission causing neonatal typhoid (rare).

Breast-Feeding Considerations It is not known if typhoid vaccine is excreted in breast milk.

Contraindications Hypersensitivity to the vaccine or any component; individuals with blood dyscrasias, leukemia, lymphomas, or other malignant neoplasms affecting the bone marrow or lymphatic systems; concurrent immunosuppressive therapy; primary and acquired immunodeficiency states; family history of congenital or hereditary immunodeficiency; current febrile illness or active febrile infection, oral formulation only: Acute GI illness, persistent diarrhea or vomiting, concurrent systemic antibiotics

Warnings Not all recipients of typhoid vaccine will be fully protected against typhoid fever; demonstrated efficacy ranges from 50% to 80%. Travelers should take all necessary precautions to avoid contact or ingestion of potentially contaminated food or water sources. Unless a complete immunization schedule with oral live attenuated Ty21a vaccine (Vivotif®) is followed, an optimum immune response may not be achieved. Syncope has been reported with use of injectable vaccines and may be accompanied by transient visual disturbances, weakness, or tonic-clonic movements. Procedures should be in place to avoid injuries from falling and to restore cerebral perfusion if syncope occurs.

Precautions Vivotif® should not be administered to immunocompromised persons, including those known to be infected with HIV. Parenteral inactivated vaccine may be an alternative for these individuals. Use with caution to parenteral inactivated vaccine (Typhim Vi®) in severely immunocompromised patients (eg, patients receiving chemo/radiation therapy or other immunosuppressive therapy, including high-dose corticosteroids); may have a reduced response to vaccination and vaccination may not result in effective immunity in all patients. Response depends upon multiple factors (eg, type of vaccine, age of patient) and may be improved by administering the vaccine at the recommended dose, route, and interval (CDC, 2011). In general, household and close contacts of persons with altered immunocompetence may receive all age-appropriate vaccines.

Administer Typhim Vi® with caution to patients with thrombocytopenia or any coagulation disorder that would be compromised by I.M. injection. Antipyretics have not been shown to prevent febrile seizures; antipyretics may be used to treat fever or discomfort following vaccination (CDC, 2011). One study reported that routine prophylactic administration of acetaminophen to prevent fever prior to vaccination decreased the immune response of some vaccines; the clinical significance of this reduction in immune response has not been established (Prymula, 2009).

◀ **Adverse Reactions** In the U.S., all serious adverse reactions must be reported to the Department of Health and Human Services (DHHS) Vaccine Adverse Event Reporting System (VAERS) 1-800-822-7967 or online at https://vaers.hhs.gov/esub/index. In Canada, adverse reactions may be reported to local provincial/territorial health agencies or to the Vaccine Safety Section at Public Health Agency of Canada (1-866-844-0018).

Injection:
Central nervous system: Generalized ache, headache, malaise
Dermatologic: Pruritus
Gastrointestinal: Nausea, vomiting
Local: Erythema at injection site, induration at injection site, pain at injection site, swelling at injection site, tenderness at injection site
Neuromuscular & skeletal: Muscle tenderness, myalgia
Miscellaneous: Fever greater than 100 to 101 degrees, fever (undefined)
Rare but important or life-threatening: Anaphylaxis, angioedema, asthma, diarrhea, flu-like symptoms, Guillain-Barré syndrome, hypersensitivity reaction, intestinal perforation (jejunum), loss of consciousness, lymphadenopathy, neck pain, serum sickness, skin rash, syncope (with and without convulsions)

Oral:
Central nervous system: Headache
Dermatologic: Skin rash
Gastrointestinal: Abdominal pain, diarrhea, nausea, vomiting
Miscellaneous: Fever
Rare but important or life-threatening: Anaphylaxis, demyelinating disease, myalgia, pain, rheumatoid arthritis, sepsis

Drug Interactions

Metabolism/Transport Effects None known.

Avoid Concomitant Use
Avoid concomitant use of Typhoid Vaccine with any of the following: Belimumab; Fingolimod; Immunosuppressants

Increased Effect/Toxicity
The levels/effects of Typhoid Vaccine may be increased by: Belimumab; Corticosteroids (Systemic); Dimethyl Fumarate; Fingolimod; Hydroxychloroquine; Immunosuppressants; Leflunomide; Mercaptopurine; Methotrexate

Decreased Effect
Typhoid Vaccine may decrease the levels/effects of: Tuberculin Tests

The levels/effects of Typhoid Vaccine may be decreased by: Antibiotics; Dimethyl Fumarate; Fingolimod; Immune Globulins; Immunosuppressants

Stability Refrigerate at 2°C to 8°C (35°F to 46°F); do not freeze

Mechanism of Action Virulent strains of Salmonella typhi cause disease by penetrating the intestinal mucosa and entering the systemic circulation via the lymphatic vasculature. One possible mechanism of conferring immunity may be the provocation of a local immune response in the intestinal tract induced by oral ingesting of a live strain with subsequent aborted infection. The ability of S. typhi to produce clinical disease (and to elicit an immune response) is dependent on the bacteria having a complete lipopolysaccharide. The live attenuate Ty21a strain lacks the enzyme UDP-4-galactose epimerase so that lipopolysaccharide is only synthesized under conditions that induce bacterial autolysis. Thus, the strain remains avirulent despite the production of sufficient lipopolysaccharide to evoke a protective immune response. Despite low levels of lipopolysaccharide synthesis, cells lyse before gaining a virulent phenotype due to the intracellular accumulation of metabolic intermediates.

Efficacy: Although no randomized trials comparing the U.S. licensed typhoid vaccine have been conducted, several field trials have demonstrated the efficacy of each vaccine.
Injection: Vaccine induces 4-fold rise in antibody concentration in 88% to 96% of healthy American adults. Vaccine reduced disease incidence 49% to 87% in a trial among adults and children in Nepal. In a study of South African children, blood culture-confirmed cases were reduced 61%, 52%, and 50% in the first, second, and third years, respectively, after a single dose.
Oral: Vaccine reduced disease incidence by 67% to 95% in children older than 6 years.

Pharmacokinetics (Adult data unless noted)
Onset of action: Immunity to Salmonella typhi: Oral: ~1 week; I.M.: ~2 weeks
Duration: Immunity: Oral: ~5 years; Parenteral: ~3 years

Dosing: Usual Immunization:
Oral (Vivotif®): Children ≥6 years and Adults:
Primary immunization: One capsule on alternate days (day 1, 3, 5, and 7) for a total of 4 doses; all doses should be completed at least 1 week prior to potential exposure
Reimmunization: Repeat full course of primary immunization every 5 years
I.M. (Typhim Vi®): Children ≥2 years and Adults:
Primary immunization: 0.5 mL given at least 2 weeks prior to expected exposure
Reimmunization: 0.5 mL; optimal schedule has not been established; a single dose every 2 years is currently recommended for repeated or continued exposure
Note: There is no data concerning using one vaccine (oral vs. I.M.) as a booster after primary immunization with the other vaccine.

Administration
Parenteral: Administer by I.M. injection into the anterolateral aspect of the thigh or arm; **not for I.V. or SubQ administration**. Adolescents and adults should be vaccinated while seated or lying down.
Oral: Oral capsule should be taken 1 hour before a meal with cold or lukewarm drink on alternate days (days 1, 3, 5, and 7); swallow capsule whole, do not chew
U.S. law requires that the date of administration, the vaccine manufacturer, lot number of vaccine, and the administering person's name, title, and address be entered into the patient's permanent medical record.

Monitoring Parameters Observe for syncope for 15 minutes following administration. If seizure-like activity associated with syncope occurs, maintain patient in supine or Trendelenburg position to reestablish adequate cerebral perfusion.

Additional Information In order to maximize vaccination rates, the ACIP recommends simultaneous administration (ie, >1 vaccine on the same day at different anatomic sites) of all age-appropriate vaccines (live or inactivated) for which a person is eligible at a single visit, unless contraindications exist. If available, the use of combination vaccines is generally preferred over separate injections, taking into consideration provider assessment, patient preference, and potential adverse events. If separate vaccines being used, evaluate product information regarding same syringe compatibility of vaccines. Separate needles and syringes should be used for each injection. The ACIP prefers each dose of specific vaccine in a series come from the same manufacturer if possible (CDC, 2011).

For additional information, please refer to the following website: http://www.cdc.gov/vaccines/vpd-vac/.

Dosage Forms Excipient information presented when available (limited, particularly for generics); consult specific product labeling.

Capsule, enteric coated [live]:
Vivotif: Viable *S. typhi* Ty21a 2-6.8 x 10⁹ colony-forming units and nonviable *S. typhi* Ty21a 5-50 x 10⁹ bacterial cells [contains lactose 100-180 mg/capsule and sucrose 26-130 mg/capsule]

Injection, solution [inactivated]:
Typhim Vi: Purified Vi capsular polysaccharide 25 mcg/ 0.5 mL (0.5 mL, 10 mL) [derived from *S. typhi* Ty2 strain]

References
AAP Steering Committee on Quality Improvement and Management, Subcommittee on Febrile Seizures American Academy of Pediatrics, "Febrile Seizures: Clinical Practice Guideline for the Long-Term Management of the Child With Simple Febrile Seizures," *Pediatrics*, 2008, 121(6):1281-6.

Centers for Disease Control and Prevention (CDC), "Syncope After Vaccination-United States, January 2005-July 2007," *MMWR Morb Mortal Wkly Rep*, 2008, 2;57(17):457-60.

Centers for Disease Control and Prevention (CDC), "Typhoid Immunization. Recommendations of the advisory Committee on Immunization Practices (ACIP)," *MMWR Morb Mortal Wkly Rep*, 1994, 43(RR-14):1-7.

National Center for Immunization and Respiratory Diseases, "General Recommendations on Immunization - Recommendations of the Advisory Committee on Immunization Practices (ACIP)," *MMWR Recomm Rep*, 2011, 60(2):1-64.

Prymula R, Siegrist CA, Chlibek R, et al, "Effect of Prophylactic Paracetamol Administration at Time of Vaccination on Febrile Reactions and Antibody Responses in Children: Two Open-Label, Randomised Controlled Trials," *Lancet*, 2009, 374(9698):1339-50.

Red Book: 2006 Report of the Committee on Infectious Diseases, 27th ed, Pickering LK, ed, Elk Grove Village, IL: American Academy of Pediatrics, 2006.

◆ **Typhoid Vaccine Live Oral Ty21a** *see* Typhoid Vaccine *on page* 2093

◆ **506U78** *see* Nelarabine *on page* 1477

◆ **UCB-P071** *see* Cetirizine *on page* 431

◆ **Uceris** *see* Budesonide (Systemic, Oral Inhalation) *on page* 308

◆ **Uceris** *see* Budesonide (Systemic, Oral Inhalation) *on page* 308

◆ **UK-427,857** *see* Maraviroc *on page* 1304

◆ **UK92480** *see* Sildenafil *on page* 1884

◆ **UK109496** *see* Voriconazole *on page* 2150

◆ **Ulcidine (Can)** *see* Famotidine *on page* 843

◆ **Ulesfia** *see* Benzyl Alcohol *on page* 278

◆ **Ultiva** *see* Remifentanil *on page* 1811

◆ **Ultiva® (Can)** *see* Remifentanil *on page* 1811

◆ **Ultram** *see* TraMADol *on page* 2060

◆ **Ultram ER** *see* TraMADol *on page* 2060

◆ **UltraSal-ER** *see* Salicylic Acid *on page* 1860

◆ **Ultrase (Can)** *see* Pancrelipase *on page* 1591

◆ **Ultrase MT (Can)** *see* Pancrelipase *on page* 1591

◆ **Ultravate** *see* Halobetasol *on page* 997

◆ **Ultravate® (Can)** *see* Halobetasol *on page* 997

◆ **Ultresa** *see* Pancrelipase *on page* 1591

◆ **Unasyn®** *see* Ampicillin and Sulbactam *on page* 162

Undecylenic Acid and Derivatives
(un de sil EN ik AS id & dah RIV ah tivs)

Brand Names: U.S. Fungi-Nail® [OTC]
Therapeutic Category Antifungal Agent, Topical
Generic Availability (U.S.) No
Use Treatment of athlete's foot (tinea pedis), ringworm (except nails and scalp), prickly heat, jock itch (tinea cruris), diaper rash, and other minor skin irritations due to superficial dermatophytes
Contraindications Hypersensitivity to undecylenic acid and derivatives or any component; fungal infections of the scalp or nails

Warnings Do not apply to blistered, raw, or oozing areas of skin or over deep wounds or puncture wounds
Drug Interactions
Metabolism/Transport Effects None known.
Avoid Concomitant Use There are no known interactions where it is recommended to avoid concomitant use.
Increased Effect/Toxicity There are no known significant interactions involving an increase in effect.
Decreased Effect There are no known significant interactions involving a decrease in effect.
Pharmacodynamics Onset of action: Improvement in erythema and pruritus may be seen within 1 week after initiation of therapy
Dosing: Usual Children and Adults: Topical: Apply as needed twice daily for 2-4 weeks
Administration Topical: Clean and dry the affected area before topical application; if the solution is sprayed or applied onto the affected area, allow area to air dry; ointment or cream should be applied at night, the powder may be applied during the day or used alone when a drying effect is needed
Monitoring Parameters Resolution of skin infection
Dosage Forms Excipient information presented when available (limited, particularly for generics); consult specific product labeling.
Solution, topical:
Fungi-Nail®: Undecylenic acid 25% (29.57 mL)

◆ **Unidet® (Can)** *see* Tolterodine *on page* 2045

◆ **Uniphyl (Can)** *see* Theophylline *on page* 2005

◆ **Unithroid** *see* Levothyroxine *on page* 1234

◆ **Unithroid Direct** *see* Levothyroxine *on page* 1234

◆ **UniVert** *see* Meclizine *on page* 1317

◆ **Urasal® (Can)** *see* Methenamine *on page* 1361

◆ **Urate Oxidase** *see* Rasburicase *on page* 1808

◆ **Urea Peroxide** *see* Carbamide Peroxide *on page* 377

◆ **Urecholine** *see* Bethanechol *on page* 288

◆ **Urex** *see* Methenamine *on page* 1361

◆ **Urinary Pain Relief [OTC]** *see* Phenazopyridine *on page* 1651

◆ **Uro-Mag [OTC]** *see* Magnesium Oxide *on page* 1296

◆ **Uromax (Can)** *see* Oxybutynin *on page* 1568

◆ **Uromitexan (Can)** *see* Mesna *on page* 1350

◆ **Urozide (Can)** *see* Hydrochlorothiazide *on page* 1023

◆ **Urso (Can)** *see* Ursodiol *on page* 2095

◆ **Urso 250** *see* Ursodiol *on page* 2095

◆ **Ursodeoxycholic Acid** *see* Ursodiol *on page* 2095

Ursodiol (ur soe DYE ol)

Medication Safety Issues
Sound-alike/look-alike issues:
Ursodiol may be confused with ulipristal
Brand Names: U.S. Actigall; Urso 250; Urso Forte
Brand Names: Canada Dom-Ursodiol C; PHL-Ursodiol C; PMS-Ursodiol C; Urso; Urso DS
Therapeutic Category Gallstone Dissolution Agent
Generic Availability (U.S.) Yes
Use Gallbladder stone dissolution (FDA approved in adults); prevention of gallstone formation (obese patients experiencing rapid weight loss) (FDA approved in adults); primary biliary cirrhosis (Urso®) (FDA approved in adults). Other uses include facilitate bile excretion in infants with biliary atresia; treatment of cholestasis secondary to PN; improve the hepatic metabolism of essential fatty acids in patients with cystic fibrosis

◄ **Pregnancy Risk Factor** B

Pregnancy Considerations Adverse events have not been observed in animal reproduction studies. Ursodiol (ursodeoxycholic acid) is the treatment of choice for intrahepatic cholestasis of pregnancy (Kremer, 2011).

Breast-Feeding Considerations It is not known if ursodiol is excreted in breast milk. The manufacturer recommends that caution be exercised when administering ursodiol to nursing women.

Contraindications Hypersensitivity to ursodiol, bile acids, or any component; not to be used with calcified cholesterol stones, radiopaque stones, or bile pigment stones; patients with compelling reasons for cholecystectomy (eg, unremitting acute cholecystitis, cholangitis, biliary obstruction)

Warnings Gallbladder stone dissolution may take several months of therapy; complete dissolution may not occur and recurrence of stones within 5 years has been observed in 50% of patients; use with caution in patients with a reduced metabolic capacity to detoxify via sulfation as lithocholic acid (a naturally occurring bile acid) is a known hepatotoxic metabolite that is cleared via sulfation

Precautions Use with caution in patients with a nonvisualizing gallbladder and those with chronic liver disease

Adverse Reactions

Central nervous system: Dizziness, headache

Dermatologic: Alopecia, rash

Endocrine & metabolic: Hyperglycemia

Gastrointestinal: Constipation, diarrhea, dyspepsia, nausea, peptic ulcer, vomiting

Genitourinary: Urinary tract infection

Hematologic & oncologic: Leukopenia, thrombocytopenia

Hepatic: Cholecystitis

Hypersensitivity: Hypersensitivity reaction

Infection: Viral infection

Neuromuscular & skeletal: Arthritis, back pain, musculoskeletal pain, myalgia

Renal: Increased serum creatinine

Respiratory: Bronchitis, cough, flu-like symptoms, pharyngitis, upper respiratory tract infection

Rare but important or life-threatening: Abdominal distress, abdominal pain, abnormal hepatic function tests, angioedema, anorexia, biliary colic, esophagitis, facial edema, fever, hepatobiliary disease, increased gamma-glutamyl transferase, increased liver enzymes, increased serum alkaline phosphatase, increased serum ALT, increased serum AST, increased serum bilirubin, jaundice, laryngeal edema, malaise, metallic taste, myalgia, peripheral edema, pruritus, transaminases increased, urticaria, weakness

Drug Interactions

Metabolism/Transport Effects None known.

Avoid Concomitant Use There are no known interactions where it is recommended to avoid concomitant use.

Increased Effect/Toxicity There are no known significant interactions involving an increase in effect.

Decreased Effect

Ursodiol may decrease the levels/effects of: Nitrendipine

The levels/effects of Ursodiol may be decreased by: Aluminum Hydroxide; Bile Acid Sequestrants; Estrogen Derivatives; Fibric Acid Derivatives

Stability Store at 20°C to 25°C (68°F to 77°F). Half-tablets (scored URSO Forte 500 mg tablets broken in half) maintain acceptable quality for up to 28 days when stored in the current packaging (bottles) at 20°C to 25°C (68°F to 77°F). Due to the bitter taste, the halved segments should be stored separately from the whole tablets.

Mechanism of Action Decreases the cholesterol content of bile and bile stones by reducing the secretion of cholesterol from the liver and the fractional reabsorption of cholesterol by the intestines. Mechanism of action in primary biliary cirrhosis is not clearly defined.

Pharmacokinetics (Adult data unless noted)

Absorption: 90%

Protein binding: 70%

Metabolism: Undergoes extensive enterohepatic recycling; following hepatic conjugation and biliary secretion, the drug is hydrolyzed to active ursodiol, where it is recycled or transformed to lithocholic acid by colonic microbial flora; during chronic administration, ursodiol becomes a major biliary and plasma bile acid constituting 30% to 50% of biliary and plasma bile acids

Elimination: In feces via bile

Dosing: Neonatal Oral:

Parenteral nutrition-induced cholestasis, treatment: 30 mg/kg/day in 3 divided doses (Chen, 2004); some centers divide in 2 daily doses

Parenteral nutrition-induced cholestasis, prevention: 5 mg/kg/day in 4 divided doses beginning on day of life 3 with initiation of parenteral nutrition; increase dose to 10 mg/kg/day in 4 divided doses with initiation of enteral feeding; increase dose to 20 mg/kg/day in 4 divided doses when full enteral feedings reached. Dosing based on a double-blind, placebo-controlled study of 30 premature neonates (birth weight ≤900 g; GA: <34 weeks) which showed earlier achievement of full feeds and slight decrease of fecal fat excretion in the treatment group (Arslanoglu, 2008)

Dosing: Usual Oral:

Biliary atresia: Infants: 10-15 mg/kg/day once daily

Improvement in the hepatic metabolism of essential fatty acids in cystic fibrosis: Children: 30 mg/kg/day in 2 divided doses

TPN-induced cholestasis, treatment: Infants and Children: 30 mg/kg/day in 3 divided doses (Spagnuolo, 1996)

Gallstone dissolution: Adults: 8-10 mg/kg/day in 2-3 divided doses; maintenance therapy: 250 mg/day at bedtime for 6 months to 1 year; use beyond 24 months is not established

Gallstone prevention: Adults: 300 mg twice daily

Primary biliary cirrhosis: Adults: 13-15 mg/kg/day in 4 divided doses

Administration Oral: Administer with food or, if a single dosage, at bedtime

Monitoring Parameters ALT, AST, sonogram, oral cholecystogram before therapy and every 6 months during therapy; obtain ultrasound images of gallbladder at 6-month intervals for the first year of therapy

Additional Information 30% to 50% of patients have stone recurrence after dissolution

Dosage Forms Excipient information presented when available (limited, particularly for generics); consult specific product labeling.

Capsule, Oral:

Actigall: 300 mg

Generic: 300 mg

Tablet, Oral:

Urso 250: 250 mg

Urso Forte: 500 mg [scored]

Generic: 250 mg, 500 mg

Extemporaneous Preparations A 20 mg/mL ursodiol oral suspension may be made with capsules and either a 1:1 mixture of Ora-Sweet and Ora-Plus or a 1:1 mixture of methylcellulose 1% and syrup NF. Empty the contents of seventeen 300 mg capsules into a mortar. Add small portions of the chosen vehicle and mix to a uniform paste; mix while adding the vehicle in incremental proportions to almost 255 mL; transfer to a calibrated bottle, rinse mortar with vehicle, and add quantity of vehicle sufficient to make 255 mL. Label "shake well" and "refrigerate". Stable for 91 days refrigerated (Nahata, 1999).

A 25 mg/mL ursodiol oral suspension may be made with capsules. Empty the contents of ten 300 mg capsules into a mortar; add 10 mL Glycerin, USP and mix until smooth.

Mix while adding 60 mL Ora-Plus; transfer mixture to a light-resistant bottle, rinse mortar with a small amount of Orange Syrup, NF, and add quantity of syrup sufficient to make 120 mL. Label "shake well". Stable for 60 days at room temperature or refrigerated (Mallett, 1997).

A 50 mg/mL ursodiol oral suspension may be made with tablets and 60 mL of either a 1:1 mixture of Ora-Plus and strawberry syrup or a 1:1 mixture of Ora-Plus and Ora-Sweet SF. Crush twelve 250 mg tablets in a mortar and reduce to a fine powder. Add small portions of the chosen vehicle and mix to a uniform paste; mix while adding the vehicle in incremental proportions to **almost** 60 mL; transfer to a calibrated bottle, rinse mortar with vehicle, and add quantity of vehicle sufficient to make 60 mL. Label "shake well" and "refrigerate". Stable for 90 days refrigerated (Johnson, 2002).

A 60 mg/mL ursodiol oral suspension may be made with capsules. Empty the contents of twelve 300 mg capsules into a mortar. Add small portions of glycerin and mix to a uniform paste; mix while adding simple syrup in incremental proportions to **almost** 60 mL; transfer to a calibrated bottle, rinse mortar with vehicle, and add quantity of vehicle sufficient to make 60 mL. Label "shake well" and "refrigerate". Stable for 35 days refrigerated (Johnson, 1995).

Johnson CE and Nesbitt J, "Stability of Ursodiol in an Extemporaneously Compounded Oral Liquid," *Am J Health Syst Pharm*, 1995, 52 (16):1798-1800.

Johnson CE and Streetman DD, "Stability of Oral Suspensions of Ursodiol Made From Tablets," *Am J Health Syst Pharm*, 2002, 59 (4):361-3.

Mallett MS, Hagan RL, and Peters DA, "Stability of Ursodiol 25 mg/mL in an Extemporaneously Prepared Oral Liquid," *Am J Health Syst Pharm*, 1997, 54(12):1401-4.

Nahata MC, Morosco RS, and Hipple TF, "Stability of Ursodiol in Two Extemporaneously Prepared Oral Suspensions," *J Appl Ther Res*, 1999, 2:221-4.

References

Arslanoglu S, Moro GE, Tauschel HD, et al, "Ursodeoxycholic Acid Treatment in Preterm Infants: A Pilot Study for the Prevention of Cholestasis Associated With Total Parenteral Nutrition," *J Pediatr Gastroenterol Nutr*, 2008, 46(2):228-31.

Chen CY, Tsao PN, Chen HL, et al, "Ursodeoxycholic Acid (UDCA) Therapy in Very-Low-Birth-Weight Infants With Parenteral Nutrition-Associated Cholestasis," *J Pediatr*, 2004, 145(3):317-21.

Colombo C, Setchell KD, Podda M, et al, "Effect of Ursodeoxycholic Acid Therapy for Liver Disease Associated With Cystic Fibrosis," *J Pediatr*, 1990, 117(3):482-9.

Kremer AE, Oude Elferink RP, and Beuers U, "Pathophysiology and Current Management of Pruritus in Liver Disease," *Clin Res Hepatol Gastroenterol*, 2011, 35(2):89-97.

Lepage G, Paradis K, Lacaille F, et al, "Ursodeoxycholic Acid Improves the Hepatic Metabolism of Essential Fatty Acids and Retinol in Children With Cystic Fibrosis," *J Pediatr*, 1997, 130(1)52-8.

Spagnuolo MI, Iorio R, Vegnente A, et al, "Ursodeoxycholic Acid for Treatment of Cholestasis in Children on Long-Term Total Parenteral Nutrition - A Pilot Study," *Gastroenterology*, 1996, 111(3):716-9.

Ullrich D, Rating D, Schroter W, et al, "Treatment With Ursodeoxycholic Acid Renders Children With Biliary Atresia Suitable for Liver Transplantation," *Lancet*, 1987, 2(8571):1324.

◆ **Urso DS (Can)** *see* Ursodiol *on page 2095*

◆ **Urso Forte** *see* Ursodiol *on page 2095*

◆ **Utradol (Can)** *see* Etodolac *on page 812*

◆ **Vacuant Mini-Enema [OTC] [DSC]** *see* Docusate *on page 701*

◆ **Vagistat-3 [OTC]** *see* Miconazole (Topical) *on page 1410*

ValACYclovir (val ay SYE kloe veer)

Medication Safety Issues

Sound-alike/look-alike issues:

Valtrex® may be confused with Keflex®, Valcyte®, Zovirax®

ValACYclovir may be confused with acyclovir, valGANciclovir, vancomycin

Brand Names: U.S. Valtrex

Brand Names: Canada Apo-Valacyclovir®; CO Valacyclovir; DOM-Valacyclovir; Mylan-Valacyclovir; PHL-Valacyclovir; PMS-Valacyclovir; PRO-Valacyclovir; Riva-Valacyclovir; Valtrex®

Therapeutic Category Antiviral Agent, Oral

Generic Availability (U.S.) Yes

Use Treatment of herpes labialis (cold sores) (FDA approved in ages ≥12 years and adults); treatment of chickenpox in immunocompetent patients (FDA approved in ages 2 to <18 years); treatment of herpes zoster (shingles) in immunocompetent patients (FDA approved in adults); treatment of initial and recurrent episodes of genital herpes (FDA approved in adults); suppression of recurrent genital herpes and reduction of heterosexual transmission of genital herpes in immunocompetent patients (FDA approved in adults); has also been used for suppression of genital herpes in HIV-infected individuals; suppression and prevention of vertical transmission of recurrent genital herpes during labor and delivery; for prevention and treatment of herpes infections in both immunocompromised and immunocompetent patients

Pregnancy Risk Factor B

Pregnancy Considerations Adverse events were not observed in animal reproduction studies. Valacyclovir is metabolized to acyclovir. In a pharmacokinetic study, maternal acyclovir serum concentrations were higher in pregnant women receiving valacyclovir than those given acyclovir for the suppression of recurrent herpes simplex virus (HSV) infection late in pregnancy. Amniotic fluid concentrations were also higher; however, there was no evidence that fetal exposure differed between the groups (Kimberlin, 1998). Data from an acyclovir pregnancy registry has shown no increased rate of birth defects than that of the general population; however, the registry is small and the manufacturer notes that use during pregnancy is only warranted if the potential benefit to the mother justifies the risk of the fetus. Because more data is available for acyclovir, that agent is preferred for the treatment of genital herpes in pregnant women (ACOG, 2000; CDC, 2010); however, valacyclovir may be considered for use due to its simplified dosing schedule (DHHS, 2013). Pregnant women who have a history of genital herpes recurrence, suppressive therapy is recommended starting at 36 weeks gestation (ACOG, 2000; DHHS, 2013).

Breast-Feeding Considerations Valacyclovir is metabolized to acyclovir; acyclovir (but not unchanged valacyclovir) can be detected in breast milk. Peak concentrations in breast milk range from 0.5-2.3 times the corresponding maternal acyclovir serum concentration. This is expected to provide a nursing infant with a dose of acyclovir equivalent to ~0.6 mg/kg/day following ingestion of valacyclovir 500 mg twice daily by the mother. The manufacturer recommends that caution be used if administered to a nursing woman. Other sources note that women with HSV infection taking valacyclovir may breast-feed as long as there are not lesions on the breast, body lesions are covered, and strict hand hygiene is practiced (ACOG, 2000; Jaiyeoba, 2012). Women with HSV who also have HIV infection should not breast-feed; complete avoidance of breast-feeding by HIV-infected women is recommended to decrease potential transmission of HIV (DHHS [perinatal], 2012).

Contraindications Hypersensitivity to valacyclovir, acyclovir, or any component

Warnings Thrombotic thrombocytopenic purpura/hemolytic uremic syndrome (TTP/HUS) has occurred in immunocompromised patients (bone marrow or renal transplant or advanced HIV disease) receiving 8 g/day.

Precautions CNS adverse events (eg, agitation, hallucinations, confusion, delirium, seizures, and encephalopathy) have been reported in children with and without renal dysfunction receiving doses exceeding those recommended for current renal function. Use with caution in patients with renal impairment, patients receiving concomitant nephrotoxic drugs, or inadequately hydrated patients; modify dose in patients with renal impairment.

Adverse Reactions

Central nervous system: Depression, dizziness, fatigue, fever, headache

Dermatologic: Rash

Endocrine: Dehydration, dysmenorrhea

Gastrointestinal: Abdominal pain, diarrhea, nausea, vomiting

Hematologic: Mild leukopenia, thrombocytopenia

Hepatic: Alkaline phosphatase increased, ALT increased, AST increased

Neuromuscular & skeletal: Arthralgia

Respiratory: Nasopharyngitis, rhinorrhea

Miscellaneous: Herpes simplex

Rare but important or life-threatening: Acute hypersensitivity reactions (angioedema, anaphylaxis, dyspnea, pruritus, rash, urticaria); aggression, agitation, alopecia, anemia, aplastic anemia, ataxia, creatinine increased, coma, confusion, consciousness decreased, delirium, dysarthria, encephalopathy, erythema multiforme, facial edema, hallucinations (auditory and visual), hemolytic uremic syndrome (HUS), hepatitis, hypertension, leukocytoclastic vasculitis, mania, photosensitivity reaction, psychosis, renal failure, renal pain, seizure, tachycardia, thrombotic thrombocytopenic purpura (TTP), tremor, urinary precipitation, visual disturbances

Drug Interactions

Metabolism/Transport Effects None known.

Avoid Concomitant Use

Avoid concomitant use of ValACYclovir with any of the following: Zoster Vaccine

Increased Effect/Toxicity

ValACYclovir may increase the levels/effects of: Mycophenolate; Tenofovir; Zidovudine

The levels/effects of ValACYclovir may be increased by: Mycophenolate

Decreased Effect

ValACYclovir may decrease the levels/effects of: Zoster Vaccine

Stability Store at 15°C to 25°C (59°F to 77°F).

Mechanism of Action Valacyclovir is rapidly and nearly completely converted to acyclovir by intestinal and hepatic metabolism. Acyclovir is converted to acyclovir monophosphate by virus-specific thymidine kinase then further converted to acyclovir triphosphate by other cellular enzymes. Acyclovir triphosphate inhibits DNA synthesis and viral replication by competing with deoxyguanosine triphosphate for viral DNA polymerase and being incorporated into viral DNA.

Pharmacokinetics (Adult data unless noted)

Absorption: Rapid

Distribution: Acyclovir is widely distributed throughout the body including brain, kidney, lungs, liver, spleen, muscle, uterus, vagina, and CSF; CSF acyclovir concentration is 50% of serum concentration; crosses the placenta; excreted into breast milk

Protein binding: 13.5% to 17.9%

Metabolism: Valacyclovir is converted to acyclovir and L-valine by first-pass intestinal and/or hepatic metabolism; acyclovir is metabolized to a small extent by aldehyde oxidase, alcohol, and aldehyde dehydrogenase to inactive metabolites

Bioavailability: ~42% to 64%, decreased bioavailability with higher doses in children

Half-life:

Normal renal function:

Acyclovir:

Children: 1.3-2.5 hours, slower clearance with increased age

Adults: 2-3.5 hours

Valacyclovir: Adults: ~30 minutes

End-stage renal disease: Acyclovir: 14-20 hours

Time to peak serum concentration:

Children: 1.4-2.6 hours

Adults: 1.5 hours

Elimination: 88% as acyclovir in the urine. **Note:** Following oral radiolabeled valacyclovir administration, 46% of the label is eliminated in feces and 47% is eliminated in urine.

Dialysis: 33% removed during 4-hour hemodialysis session; administer dose postdialysis

Dosing: Usual Oral:

Infants, Children, and Adolescents:

Chickenpox, treatment (immunocompetent patients): 2 years to <18 years: 20 mg/kg/dose 3 times daily for 5 days (maximum: 1000 mg/dose), initiate within 24 hours of rash onset

Herpes labialis (cold sores), treatment: ≥12 years: 2000 mg every 12 hours for 1 day (2 doses), initiate at earliest symptom onset

HSV or VZV, prophylaxis (immunocompromised patients with normal renal function): Children and Adolescents: Limited data available: 15-30 mg/kg/dose given 3 times daily have been reported in pharmacokinetic studies (maximum: 2000 mg/dose)

HSV, treatment (immunocompetent patients): 3 months to 11 years: 20 mg/kg/dose twice daily (maximum: 1000 mg/dose) (Kimberlin, 2010)

Adults:

CMV prophylaxis in allogeneic HSCT recipients: 2000 mg 4 times daily

Herpes labialis (cold sores): 2000 mg every 12 hours for 1 day, initiate at earliest symptom onset

Herpes zoster (shingles): 1000 mg 3 times daily for 7 days

HSV, VZV in cancer patients:

Prophylaxis: 500 mg 2-3 times daily

Treatment: 1000 mg 3 times daily

Genital herpes:

Initial episode: 1000 mg twice daily for 10 days

Recurrent episode: 500 mg twice daily for 3 days

Reduction of transmission: 500 mg once daily (source partner)

Suppressive therapy:

Immunocompetent patients: 1000 mg once daily (500 mg once daily in patients with <9 recurrences/year)

HIV-infected patients (CD4 ≥100 cells/mm^3): 500 mg twice daily

Suppressive therapy during pregnancy: 500 mg twice daily from 36 weeks estimated gestational age until delivery

Dosing interval in renal impairment:

Herpes labialis: Adolescents and Adults:

CrCl 30-49 mL/minute: 1000 mg every 12 hours for 2 doses

CrCl 10-29 mL/minute: 500 mg every 12 hours for 2 doses

CrCl <10 mL/minute: 500 mg as a single dose

Herpes zoster: Adults:

CrCl 30-49 mL/minute: 1000 mg every 12 hours

CrCl 10-29 mL/minute: 1000 mg every 24 hours

CrCl <10 mL/minute: 500 mg every 24 hours

Genital herpes: Adolescents and Adults:

Initial episode:

CrCl 10-29 mL/minute: 1000 mg every 24 hours

CrCl <10 mL/minute: 500 mg every 24 hours

Recurrent episode: CrCl ≤29 mL/minute: 500 mg every 24 hours

Suppressive therapy: CrCl ≤29 mL/minute:
For usual dose of 1000 mg every 24 hours, decrease dose to 500 mg every 24 hours
For usual dose of 500 mg every 24 hours, decrease dose to 500 mg every 48 hours
HIV-infected patients: 500 mg every 24 hours

Administration Oral: May administer with or without food

Monitoring Parameters Urinalysis, BUN, serum creatinine, liver enzymes, CBC

Additional Information
Nadal (2002) suggests the following dosage equivalency: 30 mg/kg/dose 3 times/day valacyclovir corresponds to I.V. acyclovir 250 mg/m^2 or 10 mg/kg/dose 3 times/day 20 mg/kg/dose 3 times/day valacyclovir corresponds to oral acyclovir 20 mg/kg 4-5 times/day

Eksborg, et al (2002) suggests the following dosage equivalency: 500 mg valacyclovir equivalent to 349 mg of I.V. acyclovir

Dosage Forms Excipient information presented when available (limited, particularly for generics); consult specific product labeling.
Tablet, Oral:
Valtrex: 500 mg [contains fd&c blue #2 aluminum lake]
Valtrex: 1 g [scored; contains fd&c blue #2 aluminum lake]
Generic: 500 mg, 1 g

Extemporaneous Preparations A 50 mg/mL oral suspension may be made with caplets and either Ora-Sweet® or Ora-Sweet SF®. Crush eighteen 500 mg caplets in a mortar and reduce to a fine powder. Add 5 mL portions of chosen vehicle (40 mL total) and mix to a uniform paste; transfer to a 180 mL calibrated amber glass bottle, rinse mortar with 10 mL of vehicle 5 times, and add quantity of vehicle sufficient to make 180 mL. Label "shake well" and "refrigerate". Stable for 21 days refrigerated.
Fish DN, Vidaurri VA, and Deeter RG, "Stability of Valacyclovir Hydrochloride in Extemporaneously Prepared Oral Liquids," *Am J Health Syst Pharm*, 1999, 56(19):1957-60.

References
ACOG Committee on Practice Bulletins, "ACOG Practice Bulletin. Clinical Management Guidelines for Obstetrician-Gynecologists. No. 82 June 2007. Management of Herpes in Pregnancy," *Obstet Gynecol*, 2007, 109(6):1489-98.
"ACOG Practice Bulletin. Management of Herpes in Pregnancy. Number 8 October 1999. Clinical Management Guidelines For Obstetrician-Gynecologists," *Int J Gynaecol Obstet*, 2000, 68(2):165-73.
Balfour HH Jr, Hokanson KM, Schacherer RM, et al, "A Virologic Pilot Study of Valacyclovir in Infectious Mononucleosis," *J Clin Virol*, 2007, 39(1):16-21.
Bomgaars L, Thompson P, Berg S, et al, "Valacyclovir and Acyclovir Pharmacokinetics in Immunocompromised Children," *Pediatr Blood Cancer*, 2008, 51(4):504-8.
Centers for Disease Control and Prevention (CDC), "Guidelines for the Prevention and Treatment of Opportunistic Infections Among HIV-Exposed and HIV-Infected Children," *MMWR Recomm Rep*, 2009, 58(RR-11):1-166. Available at http://aidsinfo.nih.gov/contentfiles/Pediatric_OI.pdf
Centers for Disease Control and Prevention (CDC), "Sexually Transmitted Diseases Treatment Guidelines, 2010," *MMWR Recomm Rep*, 2010, 59(RR-12):1-110.
DHHS Panel on Opportunistic Infections (OI) in HIV-Infected Adults and Adolescents, "Guidelines for Prevention and Treatment of Opportunistic Infections in HIV-Infected Adults and Adolescents: Recommendations from the Centers for Disease Control and Prevention (CDC), the National Institutes of Health (NIH), and the HIV Medicine Association (HIVMA) of the Infectious Diseases Society of America (IDSA)," May 7, 2013. Available at http://aidsinfo.nih.gov/contentfiles/lvguidelines/adult_oi.pdf
DHHS Panel on Treatment of HIV-Infected Pregnant Women and Prevention of Perinatal Transmission, "Recommendations For Use of Antiretroviral Drugs in Pregnant HIV-1-Infected Women For Maternal Health and Interventions to Reduce Perinatal HIV Transmission in the United States," July 31, 2012. Available at http://aidsinfo.nih.gov/contentfiles/lvguidelines/perinatalgl.pdf
Eksborg S, Pal N, Kalin M, et al, "Pharmacokinetics of Acyclovir in Immunocompromised Children With Leukopenia and Mucositis After

Chemotherapy: Can Intravenous Acyclovir Be Substituted by Oral Valacyclovir?" *Med Pediatr Oncol*, 2002, 38(4):240-6.
Fish DN, Vidaurri VA, and Deeter RG, "Stability of Valacyclovir Hydrochloride in Extemporaneously Prepared Oral Liquids," *Am J Health Syst Pharm*, 1999, 56(19):1957-60.
Jaiyeoba O, Amaya MI, Soper DE, et al, "Preventing Neonatal Transmission of Herpes Simplex Virus," *Clin Obstet Gynecol*, 2012, 55(2):510-20.
Kimberlin DW, Jacobs RF, Weller S, et al, "Pharmacokinetics and Safety of Extemporaneously Compounded Valacyclovir Oral Suspension in Pediatric Patients From 1 Month Through 11 years of Age," *Clin Infect Dis*, 2010, 50(2):221-8.
Kimberlin DF, Weller S, Whitley RJ, et al, "Pharmacokinetics of Oral Valacyclovir and Acyclovir in Late Pregnancy," *Am J Obstet Gynecol*, 1998, 179(4):846-51.
Nadal D, Leverger G, Sokal EM, et al, "An Investigation of the Steady-State Pharmacokinetics of Oral Valacyclovir in Immunocompromised Children," *J Infect Dis*, 2002, 186(Suppl 1):S123-30.
Simon MW, Fish DN, and Deeter RG, "Pharmacokinetics and Safety of Valaciclovir in Children With Epstein-Barr Virus Illness," *Drugs R D*, 2002, 3(6):365-73.

◆ **Valacyclovir Hydrochloride** *see* ValACYclovir *on page 2097*

◆ **Valcyte** *see* ValGANciclovir *on page 2099*

◆ **23-Valent Pneumococcal Polysaccharide Vaccine** *see* Pneumococcal Polysaccharide Vaccine (Polyvalent) *on page 1691*

ValGANciclovir (val gan SYE kloh veer)

Medication Safety Issues
Sound-alike/look-alike issues:
Valcyte® may be confused with Valium®, Valtrex®
ValGANciclovir may be confused with valACYclovir, ganciclovir

Related Information
Oral Medications That Should Not Be Crushed or Altered *on page 2438*
Safe Handling of Hazardous Drugs *on page 2419*

Brand Names: U.S. Valcyte
Brand Names: Canada Apo-Valganciclovir; Valcyte
Therapeutic Category Antiviral Agent
Generic Availability (U.S.) No

Use Prevention of CMV disease in high-risk patients undergoing heart or kidney transplantation (FDA approved in ages 4 months to 16 years and adults); treatment of cytomegalovirus (CMV) retinitis in patients with acquired immunodeficiency syndrome (AIDS) (FDA approved in adults); prevention of CMV disease in high-risk patients (donor CMV positive/recipient CMV negative) undergoing kidney/pancreas transplantation (FDA approved in adults); has also been used for prevention of CMV disease in high-risk pediatric patients undergoing BMT or hematopoietic stem cell transplant, solid organ transplants other than those indicated above, and congenital CMV disease (Acosta, 2007; Galli, 2007; Lombardi, 2009)

Pregnancy Risk Factor C

Pregnancy Considerations Valganciclovir is converted to ganciclovir and shares its reproductive toxicity. **[U.S. Boxed Warning]: Ganciclovir may be teratogenic and cause aspermatogenesis.** Based on animal data, temporary or permanent impairment of fertility may occur in males and females. Ganciclovir is also teratogenic in animals. Females should use effective contraception during treatment and for 30 days after; males should use barrier contraception during treatment and for 90 days after.

Breast-Feeding Considerations HIV-infected mothers are discouraged from breast-feeding to decrease the potential transmission of HIV.

Contraindications Hypersensitivity to valganciclovir, ganciclovir, or any component

Warnings Hazardous agent; use appropriate precautions for handling and disposal (NIOSH, 2012). May cause dose- or therapy-limiting granulocytopenia, anemia, and/or thrombocytopenia **[U.S. Boxed Warning]**; do not use if ANC <500 cells/mm^3, platelets <25,000/mm^3, or hemoglobin <8 g/dL. Valganciclovir is converted to ganciclovir and shares its reproductive toxicity. Animal studies have demonstrated carcinogenic and teratogenic effects, inhibition of spermatogenesis, and impairment of fertility with ganciclovir **[U.S. Boxed Warning]**. Due to its teratogenic potential, contraceptive precautions need to be followed during and for at least 30 days after therapy for women and 90 days after therapy for men. Studies in liver transplant patients reported a higher incidence of tissue-invasive CMV with valganciclovir relative to oral ganciclovir.

Precautions The bioavailability of ganciclovir from valganciclovir tablets is significantly higher than with ganciclovir capsules; valganciclovir tablets cannot be substituted for ganciclovir capsules on a one-to-one basis. In pediatric patients, the preferred dosage form is oral solution; however, if calculated dose is within 10% of the lowest tablet strength (450 mg), then valganciclovir tablets may be used for doses. Use with caution in patients with preexisting bone marrow suppression, cytopenias, or in those patients receiving myelosuppressive drugs or irradiation; adjust dose or interrupt valganciclovir therapy in patients with neutropenia and/or thrombocytopenia. Use with caution and modify dosage in patients with impaired renal function or in patients receiving concomitant nephrotoxic drugs; maintain adequate hydration.

Oral solution contains sodium benzoate; benzoic acid (benzoate) is a metabolite of benzyl alcohol; large amounts of benzyl alcohol (≥99 mg/kg/day) have been associated with a potentially fatal toxicity ("gasping syndrome") in neonates; the "gasping syndrome" consists of metabolic acidosis, respiratory distress, gasping respirations, CNS dysfunction (including convulsions, intracranial hemorrhage), hypotension, and cardiovascular collapse; use oral solution containing sodium benzoate with caution in neonates; *in vitro* and animal studies have shown that benzoate displaces bilirubin from protein binding sites.

Adverse Reactions Valganciclovir is expected to share similar idiosyncratic or low incidence toxicities associated with ganciclovir.

Cardiovascular: Edema, hyper-/hypotension, peripheral edema

Central nervous system: Agitation, confusion, depression, dizziness, fatigue, fever, hallucination, headache, insomnia, pain, paresthesia, peripheral neuropathy, psychosis, seizure

Dermatologic: Acne, dermatitis, pruritus

Endocrine & metabolic: Dehydration, hyperglycemia, hyper-/hypokalemia, hypocalcemia, hypomagnesemia, hypophosphatemia

Gastrointestinal: Abdominal distention/pain, appetite (decreased), constipation, diarrhea, dyspepsia, nausea, vomiting

Genitourinary: Urinary tract infection

Hematologic: Anemia, aplastic anemia, bleeding (potentially life-threatening due to thrombocytopenia), bone marrow depression, neutropenia, pancytopenia,

Hepatic: Ascites, hepatic insufficiency

Immunologic: Graft rejection, organ transplant rejection

Local: Catheter infection

Neuromuscular & skeletal: Arthralgia, back pain, limb pain, muscle cramps, tremor, weakness

Ocular: Retinal detachment

Renal: Creatinine clearance (decreased), dysuria, renal impairment, serum creatinine increased

Respiratory: Cough, dyspnea, nasopharyngitis, pharyngitis, pleural effusion, rhinorrhea, upper respiratory tract infection

Miscellaneous: Allergic reaction, local and systemic infection (including sepsis)

Rare but important or life-threatening: Bone marrow aplasia, postoperative complication, postoperative pain, postoperative wound complication (infection, increased drainage, dehiscence)

Drug Interactions

Metabolism/Transport Effects None known.

Avoid Concomitant Use

Avoid concomitant use of ValGANciclovir with any of the following: Imipenem

Increased Effect/Toxicity

ValGANciclovir may increase the levels/effects of: Imipenem; Mycophenolate; Reverse Transcriptase Inhibitors (Nucleoside); Tenofovir

The levels/effects of ValGANciclovir may be increased by: Mycophenolate; Probenecid; Tenofovir

Decreased Effect There are no known significant interactions involving a decrease in effect.

Food Interactions Coadministration with a high-fat meal increased AUC by 30%. Management: Valganciclovir should be taken with meals.

Stability Hazardous agent; use appropriate precautions for handling and disposal (NIOSH, 2012).

Oral solution: Store dry powder at 25°C (77°F); excursions permitted to 15°C to 30°C (59°F to 86°F). Prior to dispensing, prepare the oral solution by adding 91 mL of purified water to the bottle; shake well. Store oral solution under refrigeration at 2°C to 8°C (36°F to 46°F); do not freeze. Discard any unused medication after 49 days. A reconstituted 100 mL bottle will only provide 88 mL of solution for administration.

Tablets: Store at 25°C (77°F); excursions permitted to 15°C to 30°C (59°F to 86°F).

Mechanism of Action Valganciclovir is rapidly converted to ganciclovir in the body. The bioavailability of ganciclovir from valganciclovir is increased 10-fold compared to oral ganciclovir. A dose of 900 mg achieved systemic exposure of ganciclovir comparable to that achieved with the recommended doses of intravenous ganciclovir of 5 mg/kg. Ganciclovir is phosphorylated to a substrate which competitively inhibits the binding of deoxyguanosine triphosphate to DNA polymerase resulting in inhibition of viral DNA synthesis.

Pharmacokinetics (Adult data unless noted)

Absorption: Well absorbed; high-fat meal increases AUC by 30%

Distribution: V_{dss}: Ganciclovir: 0.7 L/kg; distributes to most body fluids, tissues, and organs including CSF, ocular tissue, and brain

Protein binding: Ganciclovir: 1% to 2%

Metabolism: Prodrug converted to ganciclovir by intestinal mucosal cells and hepatocytes

Bioavailability: 60% (with food)

Half-life: Ganciclovir:

In either healthy or HIV-positive/CMV-positive patients: 4.08 hours; prolonged with renal impairment (up to 68 hours with severe renal impairment): 4.08 hours

In heart, kidney, kidney-pancreas, or liver transplant patients: 6.48 hours

Time to peak serum concentration: Ganciclovir: 1-3 hours

Elimination: Majority (80% to 90%) excreted as ganciclovir in the urine

Dialysis: 50% removed by a 4-hour hemodialysis

Dosing: Neonatal Oral: **Note:** Valganciclovir tablets and ganciclovir capsules cannot be substituted on a mg-per-mg basis since they are **NOT BIOEQUIVALENT.**

PNA >7 days: 16 mg/kg/dose every 12 hours; a pharmacokinetic study of 24 neonates demonstrated that 16 mg/kg/dose twice daily produced similar serum concentrations to ganciclovir 6 mg/kg intravenously twice daily (Acosta, 2007; Kimberlin, 2008)

Dosing: Usual Oral: **Note:** Valganciclovir tablets and ganciclovir capsules cannot be substituted on a mg-per-mg basis since they are **NOT BIOEQUIVALENT.**

Infants 1-3 months of age: 16 mg/kg/dose every 12 hours; a pharmacokinetic study of 24 neonates demonstrated that 16 mg/kg/dose twice daily produced similar serum concentrations to ganciclovir 6 mg/kg intravenously twice daily; treatment course extended into the infant period and can be considered for this population (Acosta, 2007; Kimberlin, 2008)

Infants, Children, and Adolescents 4 months to 16 years: Manufacturer's recommendations:

Prevention of CMV disease following kidney or heart transplantation:

Once daily dose (mg) = 7 x body surface area x creatinine clearance*

Begin therapy within 10 days of transplantation; continue therapy until 100 days post-transplantation. Doses should be rounded to the nearest 25 mg increment; maximum dose: 900 mg/day

* $CrCl \ (mL/minute/1.73 \ m^2) = [k \ x \ height \ (cm)] \div serum \ creatinine \ (mg/dL)$

Note: If the calculated CrCl is >150 mL/minute/1.73 m^2, then a maximum value of 150 mL/minute/1.73 m^2 should be used to calculate the dose.

Note: Calculated using a *modified* Schwartz formula where k =

• 0.45 in patients <2 years
• 0.55 in boys age 2 to <13 years
• 0.55 in girls age 2-16 years
• 0.7 in boys age 13-16 years

Alternate dosing: Limited information available: 15-18 mg/kg/day once daily for the first 100 days post liver transplant in patients considered low-risk for CMV disease reported by one center for the prevention of CMV disease following transplantation (Clark, 2004)

Adolescents >16 years and Adults:

CMV retinitis:

Induction: 900 mg twice daily for 21 days

Maintenance: Following induction treatment or for patients with inactive CMV retinitis who require maintenance therapy: 900 mg once daily

Prevention of CMV disease following transplantation: 900 mg once daily beginning within 10 days of transplantation; continue therapy until 100 days (heart or kidney-pancreas transplant) or 200 days (kidney transplant) post-transplantation

Dosage adjustment in renal impairment:

Infants, Children, and Adolescents 4 months to 16 years: No additional dosage adjustments required; use of equation adjusts for renal function

Adolescents >16 years and Adults (tablet formulation):

Induction dose:

CrCl 40-59 mL/minute: 450 mg twice daily
CrCl 25-39 mL/minute: 450 mg once daily
CrCl 10-24 mL/minute: 450 mg every 2 days

Maintenance dose:

CrCl 40-59 mL/minute: 450 mg once daily
CrCl 25-39 mL/minute: 450 mg every 2 days
CrCl 10-24 mL/minute: 450 mg twice weekly

Note: Valganciclovir is not recommended in patients receiving hemodialysis. For patients on hemodialysis (CrCl <10 mL/minute), it is recommended that ganciclovir be used instead of valganciclovir with dose adjusted as specified for ganciclovir.

Dosage adjustment in hepatic impairment: Use has not been studied.

Administration Hazardous agent; use appropriate precautions for handling and disposal (NIOSH, 2012).

Oral: Administer with meals.

Monitoring Parameters Retinal exam at least every 4-6 weeks; CBC with differential, platelet count, serum creatinine

Dosage Forms Excipient information presented when available (limited, particularly for generics); consult specific product labeling.

Solution Reconstituted, Oral:

Valcyte: 50 mg/mL (88 mL) [contains saccharin sodium, sodium benzoate; tutti-frutti flavor]

Tablet, Oral:

Valcyte: 450 mg

Extemporaneous Preparations Hazardous agent: Use appropriate precautions for handling and disposal.

Note: Commercial preparation is available (50 mg/mL)

A 60 mg/mL oral suspension may be with tablets and a 1:1 mixture of Ora-Sweet® and Ora-Plus®. Crush sixteen 450 mg tablets and reduce to a fine powder. Add 1 mL portions of chosen vehicle (10 mL total) and mix to a uniform paste; mix while adding the vehicle in incremental proportions to **almost** 120 mL; transfer to a calibrated amber glass bottle, rinse mortar with vehicle, and add quantity of vehicle sufficient to make 120 mL. Label "shake well" and "refrigerate". Stable for 35 days refrigerated.

Henkin CC, Griener JC, and Ten Eick AP, "Stability of Valganciclovir in Extemporaneously Compounded Liquid Formulations," *Am J Health Syst Pharm*, 2003, 60(7):687-90.

References

Acosta EP, Brundage RC, King JR, et al, "Ganciclovir Population Pharmacokinetics in Neonates Following Intravenous Administration of Ganciclovir and Oral Administration of a Liquid Valganciclovir Formulation," *Clin Pharmacol Ther*, 2007, 81(6):867-72.

Burri M, Wiltshire H, Kahlert C, et al, "Oral Valganciclovir in Children: Single Dose Pharmacokinetics in a Six-Year-Old Girl," *Pediatr Infect Dis J*, 2004, 23(3):263-6.

Centers for Disease Control and Prevention (CDC), "Guidelines for the Prevention and Treatment of Opportunistic Infections Among HIV-Exposed and HIV-Infected Children," *MMWR Recomm Rep*, 2009, 58(RR-11):1-166. Available at http://aidsinfo.nih.gov/contentfiles/Pediatric_OI.pdf

Clark BS, Chang IF, Karpen SJ, et al, "Valganciclovir for the Prophylaxis of Cytomegalovirus Disease in Pediatric Liver Transplant Recipients," *Transplantation*, 2004, 77(9):1480.

Galli L, Novelli A, Chiappini E, et al, "Valganciclovir for Congenital CMV Infection: A Pilot Study on Plasma Concentration in Newborns and Infants," *Pediatr Infect Dis J*, 2007, 26(5):451-3.

Kimberlin DW, Acosta EP, Sánchez PJ, et al, "Pharmacokinetic and Pharmacodynamic Assessment of Oral Valganciclovir in the Treatment of Symptomatic Congenital Cytomegalovirus Disease," *J Infect Dis*, 2008, 197(6):836-45.

Lombardi G, Garofoli F, Villani P, et al, "Oral Valganciclovir Treatment in Newborns With Symptomatic Congenital Cytomegalovirus Infection," *Eur J Clin Microbiol Infect Dis*, 2009, 28(12):1465-70.

National Institute for Occupational Safety and Health (NIOSH), "NIOSH List of Antineoplastic and Other Hazardous Drugs in Healthcare Settings 2012." Available at http://www.cdc.gov/niosh/docs/2012-150/pdfs/2012-150.pdf. Accessed January 21, 2013.

Peyriere H, Jeziorsky E, Jalabert A, et al, "Neurotoxicity Related to Valganciclovir in a Child With Impaired Renal Function: Usefulness of Therapeutic Drug Monitoring," *Ann Pharmacother*, 2006, 40(1):143-6.

◆ **Valganciclovir Hydrochloride** see ValGANciclovir on page 2099

◆ **Valisone Scalp Lotion (Can)** see Betamethasone (Topical) on page 285

◆ **Valium** see Diazepam on page 640

◆ **Valium® (Can)** see Diazepam on page 640

◆ **Valorin [OTC]** see Acetaminophen on page 47

◆ **Valorin Extra [OTC]** see Acetaminophen on page 47

◆ **Valproate Semisodium** see Valproic Acid and Derivatives on page 2102

◆ **Valproate Sodium** see Valproic Acid and Derivatives on page 2102

◆ **Valproic Acid** see Valproic Acid and Derivatives on page 2102

◆ **Valproic Acid Derivative** see Valproic Acid and Derivatives on page 2102

Valproic Acid and Derivatives
(val PROE ik AS id & dah RIV ah tives)

Medication Safety Issues
Sound-alike/look-alike issues:
Depakene may be confused with Depakote
Depakote may be confused with Depakene, Depakote ER, Senokot
Depakote ER may be confused with divalproex enteric coated
Valproate sodium may be confused with vecuronium

Related Information
Oral Medications That Should Not Be Crushed or Altered *on page 2438*
Safe Handling of Hazardous Drugs *on page 2419*
Brand Names: U.S. Depacon; Depakene; Depakote; Depakote ER; Depakote Sprinkles; Stavzor
Brand Names: Canada Apo-Divalproex; Apo-Valproic; Depakene; Dom-Divalproex; Dom-Valproic Acid; Dom-Valproic Acid E.C.; Epival; Mylan-Divalproex; Mylan-Valproic; Novo-Divalproex; PHL-Divalproex; PHL-Valproic Acid; PHL-Valproic Acid E.C.; PMS-Divalproex; PMS-Valproic Acid; PMS-Valproic Acid E.C.; ratio-Valproic; Sandoz-Valproic

Therapeutic Category Anticonvulsant, Miscellaneous; Infantile Spasms, Treatment
Generic Availability (U.S.) May be product dependent
Use
Oral:
Immediate release capsules and syrup (Depakene®): Monotherapy and adjunctive therapy in the treatment of patients with complex partial seizures (FDA approved in ages ≥10 years and adults), monotherapy and adjunctive therapy of simple and complex absence seizures [FDA approved in pediatric patients (age not specified) and adults], and adjunctive therapy in patients with multiple seizure types that include absence seizures [FDA approved in pediatric patients (age not specified) and adults]; has also been used to treat mixed seizure types, myoclonic and generalized tonic-clonic (grand mal) seizures; may be effective in infantile spasms; oral syrup has also been used rectally for treatment of seizure disorders when oral route is not available
Delayed release capsules (Stavzor™): Monotherapy and adjunctive therapy in the treatment of patients with complex partial seizures (FDA approved in ages ≥10 years and adults); monotherapy and adjunctive therapy of simple and complex absence seizures and adjunctive therapy in patients with multiple seizure types that include absence seizures [FDA approved pediatric patients (age not specified) and adults]; prophylaxis of migraine headaches (FDA approved in ages ≥12 years and adults); treatment of manic episodes of bipolar disorders (FDA approved in adults)
Delayed release tablets (Depakote®): Monotherapy and adjunctive therapy in the treatment of patients with complex partial seizures, monotherapy and adjunctive therapy of simple and complex absence seizures and adjunctive therapy in patients with multiple seizure types that include absence seizures [FDA approved in pediatric patients (age not specified) and adults]; prophylaxis of migraine headaches (FDA approved in ages ≥16 years and adults); treatment of manic episodes of bipolar disorders (FDA approved in adults)
Extended release tablets (Depakote ER®): Monotherapy and adjunctive therapy in the treatment of patients with complex partial seizures; monotherapy and adjunctive therapy of simple and complex absence seizures and adjunctive therapy in patients with multiple seizure types that include absence seizures (all epilepsy types listed: FDA approved in ages ≥10 years and adults);

prophylaxis of migraine headaches (FDA approved in ages ≥12 years and adults); treatment of manic episodes of bipolar disorders (FDA approved in adults)
Sprinkle capsules (Depakote®): Monotherapy and adjunctive therapy in the treatment of patients with complex partial seizures (FDA approved in ages ≥10 years and adults); monotherapy and adjunctive therapy of simple and complex absence seizures and adjunctive therapy in patients with multiple seizure types that include absence seizures [FDA approved in pediatric patients (age not specified) and adults]; has also been used to treat mixed seizure types, myoclonic and generalized tonic-clonic (grand mal) seizures; may be effective in infantile spasms
Parenteral: Injection (Depacon®): Monotherapy and adjunctive therapy in the treatment of patients with complex partial seizures (FDA approved in ages ≥10 years and adults); monotherapy and adjunctive therapy of simple and complex absence seizures, and adjunctive therapy in patients with multiple seizure types that include absence seizures [FDA approved in pediatric patients (age not specified) and adults]; has also been used to treat mixed seizure types, myoclonic and generalized tonic-clonic (grand mal) seizures; may be effective in infantile spasms. **Note:** Parenteral formulation is indicated for patients in whom oral administration of valproic acid or derivatives is temporarily not feasible; has also been used in patients with absence status epilepticus.

Medication Guide Available Yes
Pregnancy Risk Factor X (migraine prophylaxis)/D (all other indications)
Pregnancy Considerations [U.S. Boxed Warning]: May cause teratogenic effects such as neural tube defects (eg, spina bifida) and decreased IQ scores following *in utero* exposure. Teratogenic effects have been reported in animals and humans. Valproic acid crosses the placenta (Harden, 2009b). Neural tube, cardiac, facial (characteristic pattern of dysmorphic facial features), skeletal, multiple other defects reported. Information from the North American Antiepileptic Drug Pregnancy Registry notes a fourfold increase in congenital malformations with exposure to valproic acid monotherapy during the 1st trimester of pregnancy when compared to monotherapy with other antiepileptic drugs (AED). The risk of spinal bifida is ~1% to 2% (general population risk estimated to be 0.06% to 0.07%). The effect of folic acid supplementation to decrease this risk is unknown, however, folic acid supplementation is recommended for all women contemplating pregnancy.

Nonteratogenic adverse effects have also been reported. Afibrinogenemia leading to fatal hemorrhage and hepatotoxicity have been noted in case reports of infants following *in utero* exposure to valproic acid. Developmental delay, decreased IQ scores, autism and/or autism spectrum disorder have also been reported.

Use is contraindicated in pregnant women for the prevention of migraine. Current guidelines recommend complete avoidance of valproic acid and derivatives for the treatment of epilepsy in pregnant women whenever possible (Harden, 2009a). **Use is not recommended in women of childbearing potential for any condition unless alternative therapies are not appropriate,** especially when used for conditions not associated with permanent injury or risk of death. Effective contraception should be used during treatment. When pregnancy is being planned, consider tapering off of therapy prior to conception if appropriate and supplementing with folic acid.

A pregnancy registry is available for women who have been exposed to valproic acid. Patients may enroll themselves in the North American Antiepileptic Drug (NAAED)

Pregnancy Registry by calling (888) 233-2334. Additional information is available at www.aedpregnancyregistry.org.

Breast-Feeding Considerations Valproate is excreted into breast milk. Breast milk concentrations of valproic acid have been reported as 1% to 10% of maternal concentration. The weight-adjusted dose to the infant has been calculated to be ~4% (Hagg, 2000). The manufacturer recommends that caution be used if administered to nursing women.

Contraindications Hypersensitivity to valproic acid, any derivative, or any component; hepatic disease or significant hepatic dysfunction; urea cycle disorders (UCD); pregnancy when used for the prevention of migraine; known mitochondrial disorders caused by mutations in mitochondrial DNA polymerase gamma (POLG; eg, Alpers-Huttenlocher Syndrome); children <2 years suspected of having a POLG-related disorder

Warnings Hazardous agent; use appropriate precautions for handling and disposal (NIOSH, 2012).

Hepatic failure resulting in death may occur, usually in the initial 6 months of therapy **[U.S. Boxed Warning]**; neonates, infants, and children <2 years of age are at considerably increased risk, especially those on anticonvulsant polytherapy, with congenital metabolic disorders, with severe seizure disorders and mental retardation, or with organic brain disease; monitor patients closely for appearance of malaise, loss of seizure control, weakness, facial edema, anorexia, jaundice, and vomiting; monitor liver enzymes prior to therapy and at frequent intervals, especially during the first 6 months; discontinue valproic acid and derivatives if hepatotoxicity occurs; hepatic dysfunction may progress despite discontinuing treatment. Although carnitine is clearly indicated for the management of valproic acid overdose and hepatotoxicity (and strongly recommended for select patients at high risk of valproic acid-associated hepatotoxicity), the role of routine prophylactic carnitine supplementation is unclear (Freeman, 1994; Raskind, 2000). A case of a fatal hepatotoxic reaction has been reported in a child receiving valproic acid despite carnitine supplementation (Murphy, 1993). A valproic acid-associated Reye's-like syndrome has also been reported (Hilmas, 2000). Risk for hepatic failure and resultant deaths is also increased in patients with hereditary neurometabolic syndromes caused by DNA mutations of the mitochondrial DNA Polymerase gamma (POLG) gene (eg, Alpers-Huttenlocher Syndrome) **[U.S. Boxed Warning]**. Use is contraindicated in patients with known mitochondrial disorders caused by POLG mutations and children <2 years of age suspected of having a POLG-related disorder. A POLG-related disorder may be present in patients with a family history or suggestive symptoms of a POLG-related disorder [unexplained encephalopathy, refractory epilepsy (focal, myoclonic), status epilepticus at presentation, developmental delays, psychomotor regression, axonal sensorimotor neuropathy, myopathy cerebellar ataxia, opthalmoplegia, or complicated migraine with occipital aura.]. Valproic acid use in children ≥2 years of age suspected of having a POLG-related disorder should only be considered after other anticonvulsants have failed and with close monitoring for the development of acute liver injury. POLG mutation testing should be performed in accordance with current clinical practice.

Cases of life-threatening pancreatitis (including fatalities) have been reported in children and adults **[U.S. Boxed Warning]**; pancreatitis may be hemorrhagic and rapidly progress to death; onset has occurred shortly after starting therapy and after several years of treatment; monitor patients closely for nausea, vomiting, anorexia, and abdominal pain and evaluate promptly; discontinue valproic acid and derivatives if pancreatitis occurs.

Dose-related thrombocytopenia, inhibition of platelet aggregation, and bleeding may occur; risk of thrombocytopenia increases significantly with serum valproic acid concentrations ≥110 mcg/mL in females or ≥135 mcg/mL in males; in some cases, platelet counts may normalize with continued treatment; however, reduce dose or discontinue drug if patient develops evidence of hemorrhage, bruising, or a disorder of hemostasis/coagulation. Evaluate platelet counts prior to initiating therapy and periodically thereafter.

Reversible and irreversible cerebral and cerebellar atrophy have been reported; motor and cognitive function should be routinely monitored to assess for signs and symptoms of brain atrophy. Parenteral valproate is not recommended for the prophylaxis of post-traumatic seizures in patients with acute head trauma; study results for this use suggested increased mortality with parenteral valproate compared to parenteral phenytoin.

Hyperammonemic encephalopathy, which may be fatal, has been reported following initiation of valproic acid and derivatives in patients with known or suspected urea cycle disorders (UCD), particularly ornithine transcarbamylase deficiency. Valproic acid and derivatives are contraindicated in patients with UCD. Before valproic acid or a derivative is started, evaluation for UCD should be considered in patients with 1) a history of unexplained coma or encephalopathy, encephalopathy associated with a protein load, unexplained mental retardation, pregnancy or postpartum encephalopathy, or history of increased plasma ammonia or glutamine; 2) cyclical vomiting and lethargy, episodic extreme irritability, ataxia, low BUN, or protein avoidance; 3) family history of UCD or family history of unexplained infant deaths (especially males); or 4) other signs and symptoms of UCD.

Hyperammonemia may occur, even in the absence of liver enzyme abnormalities; asymptomatic elevations of ammonia require continued monitoring; discontinuation of valproate should be considered if elevations persist. Ammonia concentrations should be measured in patients who develop symptoms of hyperammonemic encephalopathy: Unexplained lethargy, vomiting, changes in mental status, or in patients who present with hypothermia; discontinue therapy if ammonia concentrations are increased, treat hyperammonemia promptly, and evaluate for possible urea cycle disorder (UCD).

Concurrent use of valproic acid or a derivative with topiramate may result in hyperammonemia with or without encephalopathy; use with caution in patients with inborn errors of metabolism or decreased hepatic mitochondrial activity; these patients may be at increased risk. Hyperammonemia should also be considered when patients present with hypothermia. Hypothermia [unintentional drop in core body temperature to <35°C (95°F) has been reported with valproic acid and derivatives; hypothermia may or may not be associated with hyperammonemia; may also occur with concomitant topiramate therapy following topiramate initiation or dosage increase.

Congenital malformations such as neural tube defects (eg, spina bifida), craniofacial defects, cardiovascular malformations, anomalies of other body systems, and decreased IQ scores following *in utero* exposure may occur **[U.S. Boxed Warning]**. Use in women of childbearing potential requires that benefits of use in the mother be weighed against the potential risk to the fetus, especially when used for conditions not associated with permanent injury or risk of death (eg, migraine). Maternal use of valproic acid or a derivative during pregnancy may result in clotting abnormalities or hepatic failure in the newborn.

Multiorgan hypersensitivity reactions have been rarely reported in adults and pediatric patients in association with ▶

initiation of valproic acid and derivatives; at least one death has been reported; patient may present with fever and rash in association with symptoms of organ system dysfunction [eg, lymphadenopathy, hepatitis, abnormalities in liver function tests, hematologic abnormalities (eosinophilia, neutropenia, thrombocytopenia), pruritus, oliguria, nephritis, arthralgia, asthenia]; valproic acid and derivatives should be discontinued in patients suspected of having multiorgan hypersensitivity reactions.

Antiepileptic drugs (AEDs) increase the risk of suicidal behavior and ideation in patients receiving these medications for any indication. Pooled analyses of placebo-controlled trials involving 11 different AEDs (regardless of indication) showed a twofold increased risk of suicidal thoughts or behavior (estimated incidence rate: 0.43% in AED-treated patients compared to 0.24% of patients receiving placebo); increased risk was observed as early as 1 week after initiation of AED and continued through duration of trials (most trials ≤24 weeks); risk did not vary significantly by age (age range: 5-100 years). Consider risks and benefits of AEDs before prescribing. Monitor all patients receiving an AED for emergence of suicidal thoughts or behavior, thoughts of self-harm, any unusual changes in behavior or mood, or the emergence or worsening of depressive symptoms; notify healthcare provider immediately if symptoms or concerning behavior occur. **Note:** The FDA requires a Medication Guide for all anti-epileptic drugs, informing patients of this risk.

Precautions Valproic acid and derivatives may stimulate the replication of HIV and CMV *in vitro*; clinical effects are unknown. CNS depression may occur with use of valproic acid or a derivative. Patients must be cautioned about performing tasks which require mental alertness (operating machinery or driving). Effects with other sedative drugs or ethanol may be potentiated. Anticonvulsants should not be discontinued abruptly because of the possibility of increasing seizure frequency; valproic acid and derivatives should be withdrawn gradually to minimize the potential of increased seizure frequency, unless safety concerns require a more rapid withdrawal. Patients treated for bipolar disorder should be monitored closely for clinical worsening or suicidality; prescriptions should be written for the smallest quantity consistent with good patient care.

Medication residue in stool has been reported (rarely) with oral Depakote® (divalproex sodium) formulations; some reports have occurred in patients with shortened GI transit times (eg, diarrhea) or anatomic GI disorders (eg, ileostomy, colostomy). In patients reporting medication residue in stool, it is recommended to monitor valproate level and clinical condition.

Adverse Reactions

Cardiovascular: Arrhythmia, chest pain, edema, facial edema, hyper-/hypotension, orthostatic hypotension, palpitation, peripheral edema, tachycardia, vasodilatation

Central nervous system: Abnormal dreams, abnormal thinking, agitation, amnesia, anxiety, ataxia, chills, confusion, coordination abnormal, depression catatonia, dizziness, dyskinesia, emotional lability, euphoria, fever, hallucination, headache, hypoesthesia, insomnia, malaise, nervousness, pain, personality disorder, somnolence, speech disorder, tardive dyskinesia, vertigo

Dermatologic: Alopecia, bruising, discoid lupus erythematosus, dry skin, furunculosis, petechia, pruritus, rash, seborrhea

Endocrine & metabolic: Amenorrhea, dysmenorrhea, hypoproteinemia, metrorrhagia

Gastrointestinal: Abdominal pain, anorexia, appetite increased, constipation, diarrhea, dyspepsia, dysphagia, eructation, fecal incontinence, flatulence, gastroenteritis, glossitis, gum hemorrhage, hematemesis, incontinence, mouth ulceration, nausea, pancreatitis, periodontal abscess, stomatitis, taste perversion, vomiting, weight gain/loss, xerostomia

Genitourinary: Cystitis, dysuria, urinary frequency, urinary incontinence, vaginal hemorrhage, vaginitis

Hematologic: Thrombocytopenia (dose related)

Hepatic: ALT increased, AST increased

Local: Injection site inflammation, injection site pain, injection site reaction

Neuromuscular & skeletal: Abnormal gait, arthralgia, arthrosis, back pain, dysarthria, hypertonia, hypokinesia, leg cramps. myalgia, myasthenia, neck pain, neck rigidity, paresthesia, reflex increased, tremor, twitching, weakness

Ocular: Abnormal vision, amblyopia, blurred vision, conjunctivitis, diplopia, dry eyes, eye pain, nystagmus

Otic: Deafness, ear pain, otitis media, tinnitus

Respiratory: Bronchitis, cough, dyspnea, epistaxis, pharyngitis, pneumonia, rhinitis, sinusitis

Miscellaneous: Diaphoresis, flu-like syndrome, hiccups, infection

Rare but important or life-threatening: Aggression, agranulocytosis, allergic reaction, anaphylaxis, anemia, aplastic anemia, asterixis, behavioral deterioration, bilirubin increased, bleeding time altered, bone marrow suppression, bone pain, bradycardia, breast enlargement, cutaneous vasculitis, carnitine decreased, cerebral atrophy (reversible), coma (rare), dementia, encephalopathy (rare), enuresis, eosinophilia, erythema multiforme, Fanconi-like syndrome (rare, in children), galactorrhea, hematoma formation, hemorrhage, hepatic failure, hepatotoxicity, hostility, hyperactivity, hyperammonemia, hyperammonemic encephalopathy (in patients with UCD), hyperglycinemia, hypersensitivity reactions (severe, with multiorgan dysfunction), hypofibrinogenemia, hyponatremia, hypothermia, inappropriate ADH secretion, intermittent porphyria, LDH increased, leukopenia, lupus, lymphocytosis, macrocytosis, menstrual irregularities, pancytopenia parkinsonism, parotid gland swelling, photosensitivity, platelet aggregation inhibited, polycystic ovary disease (rare), psychosis, seeing "spots before the eyes," Stevens-Johnson syndrome, suicidal behavior/ideation, thyroid function tests abnormal, toxic epidermal necrolysis (rare), urinary tract infection

Drug Interactions

Metabolism/Transport Effects Substrate of CYP2A6 (minor), CYP2B6 (minor), CYP2C19 (minor), CYP2C9 (minor), CYP2E1 (minor); **Note:** Assignment of Major/Minor substrate status based on clinically relevant drug interaction potential; **Inhibits** CYP2C9 (weak); **Induces** CYP2A6 (weak/moderate)

Avoid Concomitant Use

Avoid concomitant use of Valproic Acid and Derivatives with any of the following: Cosyntropin

Increased Effect/Toxicity

Valproic Acid and Derivatives may increase the levels/ effects of: Barbiturates; Ethosuximide; LamoTRIgine; LORazepam; Paliperidone; Primidone; RisperiDONE; Rufinamide; Sodium Oxybate; Temozolomide; Tricyclic Antidepressants; Vorinostat; Zidovudine

The levels/effects of Valproic Acid and Derivatives may be increased by: ChlorproMAZINE; Cosyntropin; Felbamate; GuanFACINE; Primidone; Salicylates; Topiramate

Decreased Effect

Valproic Acid and Derivatives may decrease the levels/ effects of: CarBAMazepine; Fosphenytoin-Phenytoin; OLANZapine; OXcarbazepine; Urea Cycle Disorder Agents

The levels/effects of Valproic Acid and Derivatives may be decreased by: Barbiturates; CarBAMazepine; Carbapenems; Ethosuximide; Fosphenytoin-Phenytoin; Methylfolate; Protease Inhibitors; Rifampin

Food Interactions Food may delay but does not affect the extent of absorption. Management: May administer with food if GI upset occurs.

Stability Hazardous agent; use appropriate precautions for handling and disposal (NIOSH, 2012).

Depakote® tablets and Depakene® solution: Store below 30°C (86°F)

Depakote® Sprinkles: Store below 25°C (77°F)

Depakote® ER tablets: Store at 25°C (77°F); excursions permitted to 15°C to 30°C (59°F to 86°F)

Depakene® capsules: Store at 15°C to 25°C (59°F to 77°F)

Depacon® injection: Store intact vials at 15°C to 30°C (59°F to 86°F). Stable for at least 24 hours at room temperature when diluted in D_5W, NS, or LR and stored in glass or polyvinyl chloride bags.

Stavzor™ capsules: Store at 25°C (77°F); excursions permitted to 15°C to 30°C (59°F to 86°F)

Mechanism of Action Causes increased availability of gamma-aminobutyric acid (GABA), an inhibitory neurotransmitter, to brain neurons or may enhance the action of GABA or mimic its action at postsynaptic receptor sites

Pharmacokinetics (Adult data unless noted)

Protein binding: 80% to 90% (concentration dependent); free fraction: ~10% at serum concentration at 40 mcg/mL and ~18.5% at 130 mcg/mL; decreased protein binding in neonates and patients with renal impairment or chronic hepatic disease

Distribution: Distributes into CSF at concentrations similar to unbound concentration in plasma (ie, ~10% of total plasma concentration)

V_d:

Total valproate: 11 L/1.73 m²

Free valproate: 92 L/1.73 m²

Metabolism: Extensively hepatic via glucuronide conjugation (30% to 50% of administered dose) and 40% via mitochondrial beta-oxidation; other oxidative metabolic pathways occur to a lesser extent. The relationship between dose and total valproate concentration is nonlinear; concentration does not increase proportionally with the dose, but increases to a lesser extent due to saturable plasma protein binding. The kinetics of unbound drug are linear.

Bioavailability: Oral: All products, except Depakote®-ER, are equivalent to I.V. **Depakote®-ER tablets are not equivalent to Depakote® delayed release tablets and are not interchangeable**; mean bioavailability of Depakote®-ER tablets is 89%, relative to Depakote® delayed release tablets. In pediatric patients 10-17 years of age, once-daily administration of Depakote®-ER produced valproate plasma concentration-time profiles similar to adults.

Half-life: Increased with liver disease

Newborns (exposed to VPA *in utero*): 30-60 hours

Neonates 1st week of life: 40-45 hours

Neonates <10 days: 10-67 hours

Infants and Children >2 months: 7-13 hours

Children and Adolescents 2-14 years: 9 hours (Range: 3.5-20 hours) (Cloyd, 1993)

Adults: 9-16 hours

Time to peak serum concentration:

Oral: Depakote ® tablet and sprinkle capsules: ~4 hours; Depakote® ER: 4-17 hours; Stavzor™: 2 hours

Rectal: 1-3 hours (Graves, 1987)

I.V.: End of the infusion

Elimination: Urine (30% to 50% as glucuronide conjugate, <3% as unchanged drug); faster clearance in children who receive other antiepileptic drugs and those who are younger; age and polytherapy explain 80% of interpatient variability in total clearance; children >10 years of age have pharmacokinetic parameters similar to adults

Dialysis: Hemodialysis reduces valproate concentrations by ~20%

Dosing: Neonatal Note: Due to the increased risk of valproic acid and derivatives-associated hepatotoxicity, valproic acid and derivatives are not preferred agents for use in neonates.

Refractory seizures: Limited data available: Oral: Loading dose: 20 mg/kg, followed by a maintenance dose of 5-10 mg/kg/dose every 12 hours; adjust dose according to serum concentrations; dosing based on a report of six neonates (GA: 30-41 weeks) that showed oral valproic acid effectively controlled seizure activity in five of six patients; however, therapy was discontinued in 50% of the patients due to hyperammonemia; frequent monitoring is recommended (Evans, 1998; Gal, 1988).

Refractory status epilepticus: Limited data available: I.V.: Loading dose: 20-40 mg/kg followed by a continuous I.V. infusion of 5 mg/kg/**hour** was used in five neonates; once patients were seizure-free for 12 hours and no longer had seizure activity on EEG, the infusion rate was decreased every 2 hours by 1 mg/kg/**hour** (Uberall, 2000).

Dosing: Usual

Infants, Children, and Adolescents: **Note:** Use of Depakote®-ER in pediatric patients <10 years of age is not recommended; do not confuse Depakote®-ER with Depakote®. **Erroneous substitution of Depakote® (delayed release tablets) for Depakote®-ER has resulted in toxicities; only Depakote®-ER is intended for once daily administration.**

Migraine prophylaxis:

Depakote®: Adolescents ≥16 years: Oral: 250 mg twice daily; adjust dose based on patient response; maximum daily dose: 1000 mg/**day**

Stavzor™: Children and Adolescents ≥12 years: Oral: 250 mg twice daily; adjust dose based on patient response; maximum daily dose: 1000 mg/**day**

Depakote® ER: Children and Adolescents ≥12 years: Oral: 500 mg once daily for 7 days, may increase to 1000 mg once daily; adjust dose based on patient response; usual dosage range 500-1000 mg/day; dose should be individualized; if smaller dosage adjustments are needed, use Depakote® delayed release tablets

Seizures disorders: Note: Due to the increased risk of valproic acid and derivatives-associated hepatotoxicity in patients <2 years, valproic acid and derivatives are not preferred agents in this population.

Oral:

General dosing (including complex partial seizures): Initial: 10-15 mg/kg/day in 1-3 divided doses; increase by 5-10 mg/kg/day at weekly intervals until seizures are controlled or side effects preclude further increases; daily doses >250 mg should be given in divided doses; maintenance: 30-60 mg/kg/day in 2-3 divided doses; Depakote® and Depakote® Sprinkle can be given twice daily; **Note:** Children receiving more than 1 anticonvulsant (ie, polytherapy) may require doses up to 100 mg/kg/day in 3-4 divided doses.

Simple and complex absence seizures: Initial: 15 mg/kg/day in 1-3 divided doses; increase by 5-10 mg/kg/day at weekly intervals until seizures are controlled or side effects preclude further increases; daily doses >250 mg should be given in divided doses; maintenance: 30-60 mg/kg/day in 2-3 divided doses; Depakote® and Depakote® Sprinkle can be given twice daily

Conversion to Depakote® ER from a stable dose of Depakote®: May require an increase in the total daily dose between 8% and 20% to maintain similar serum concentrations

Conversion to monotherapy from adjunctive therapy: The concomitant antiepileptic drug (AED) can be decreased by ~25% every 2 weeks; dosage reduction of the concomitant AED may begin when valproate or derivative therapy is initiated or 1-2 weeks following valproate or derivative initiation

Parenteral: I.V.: Total daily I.V. dose is equivalent to the total daily oral dose; however, I.V. dose should be divided with a frequency of every 6 hours; if I.V. form is administered 2-3 times/day, close monitoring of trough concentrations is recommended; switch patients to oral product as soon as clinically possible as I.V. use >14 days has not been studied.

Rectal: Dilute oral syrup 1:1 with water for use as a retention enema (Graves, 1987):

Loading dose: 17-20 mg/kg once

Maintenance: 10-15 mg/kg/dose every 8 hours

Status epilepticus; refractory: Limited data available; optimal dose not established.

I.V.:

Loading dose: Initial: 20-40 mg/kg; some experts recommend an additional 20 mg/kg after 10-15 minutes if needed (Brophy, 2012); there is limited experience with loading doses >40 mg/kg in infants.

In one retrospective study, an initial loading dose of 25 mg/kg was effective in stopping seizure activity within 20 minutes after the end of the infusion in all 18 patients treated for status epilepticus (Yu, 2003). A separate retrospective trial found a higher efficacy rate in pediatric patients who received an initial loading dose of 30-40 mg/kg (73.3%, n=15) compared to 20-30 mg/kg (46.2%, n=26) or >40 mg/kg (40%, n=10) (Uberall, 2000). In an open-label, randomized comparative trial, an initial loading dose of 30 mg/kg was administered (n=20; age range: 7 months to 10 years of age; mean age: 3 years); a repeat bolus of 10 mg/kg could be administered if seizures were not controlled within 10 minutes; mean required dose: 37.5 ± 4.4 mg/kg; median required dose: 40 mg/kg (Mehta, 2007). Further studies are needed.

Maintenance dose: I.V. infusion: 5 mg/kg/**hour** after the loading dose was used in pediatric continuous I.V. infusion studies (Mehta, 2007; Uberall, 2000); once patients were seizure-free for 6 hours, the infusion rate was decreased by 1 mg/kg/**hour** every 2 hours (Mehta, 2007). Further studies are needed.

Rectal: Dilute oral syrup 1:1 with water for use as a retention enema (Snead, 1985):

Loading dose: 15-20 mg/kg once

Maintenance: 10-15 mg/kg/dose every 8 hours

Adults:

Seizures: Note: Administer doses >250 mg/day in divided doses.

Oral:

Simple and complex absence seizure: Initial: 15 mg/kg/day; increase by 5-10 mg/kg/day at weekly intervals until therapeutic concentrations are achieved; maximum daily dose: 60 mg/kg/**day**

Complex partial seizure: Initial: 10-15 mg/kg/day; increase by 5-10 mg/kg/day at weekly intervals until therapeutic concentrations are achieved; maximum daily dose: 60 mg/kg/**day**

Note: Regular release and delayed release formulations are usually given in 2-4 divided doses per day; extended release formulation (Depakote® ER) is usually given once daily. In patients previously maintained on regular release valproic acid therapy (Depakene®) who convert to delayed release divalproex sodium tablets (Depakote®) or valproic acid capsules (Stavzor™), the same daily dose and frequency as the regular release should be used; once

therapy is stabilized, the frequency of Depakote® or Stavzor™ may be adjusted to 2-3 times daily.

Conversion to Depakote® ER from a stable dose of Depakote®: May require an increase in the total daily dose between 8% and 20% to maintain similar serum concentrations

Conversion to monotherapy from adjunctive therapy: The concomitant antiepileptic drug (AED) can be decreased by ~25% every 2 weeks; dosage reduction of the concomitant AED may begin when the valproic acid or derivative is initiated or 1-2 weeks following valproic acid or derivative initiation

I.V.: Total daily I.V. dose should be equivalent to the total daily dose of the oral valproic acid or derivative; administer dose with the same frequency as oral products; switch patient to oral products as soon as possible.

Status epilepticus:

Loading dose: I.V.: 20-40 mg/kg administered at 3 to ≤6 mg/kg/minute; after 10 minutes an additional 20 mg/kg dose may be given if clinically indicated (Brophy, 2012)

Maintenance dose: I.V. infusion: 1-4 mg/kg/hour; titrate dose as needed based upon patient response and evaluation of drug-drug interactions

Mania: Oral:

Depakote® tablet, Stavzor™: Initial: 750 mg/day in divided doses; adjust dose as rapidly as possible to desired clinical effect; maximum daily dose: 60 mg/kg/**day**

Depakote® ER: Initial: 25 mg/kg/day given once daily; adjust dose as rapidly as possible to desired clinical effect; maximum daily dose: 60 mg/kg/**day**

Migraine prophylaxis: Oral:

Depakote® tablet, Stavzor™: Initial: 250 mg twice daily; adjust dose based on patient response, maximum daily dose: 1000 mg/day

Depakote® ER: Initial: 500 mg once daily for 7 days, may increase to 1000 mg once daily; adjust dose based on patient response; usual dosage range 500-1000 mg/day; dose should be individualized; if smaller dosage adjustments are needed, use Depakote® delayed release tablets

Dosing adjustment in renal impairment: No dosage adjustment required; however, protein binding is reduced in patients with renal impairment; monitoring **only** total valproate serum concentrations may be misleading.

Dosing adjustment in hepatic impairment: Valproic acid and derivatives are contraindicated in patients with hepatic disease or significant hepatic dysfunction. Potentially fatal hepatotoxicity may occur with valproic acid or derivative use. Clearance is decreased in patients with liver impairment. Hepatic disease is also associated with decreased albumin concentrations and 2- to 2.6-fold increase in the unbound fraction of valproate. Free concentrations of valproate may be elevated while total concentrations appear normal; therefore, monitoring **only** total valproate concentrations may be misleading.

Administration

Oral: May administer with food to decrease adverse GI effects; do not administer with carbonated drinks.

Depakote® ER: Swallow whole; do not crush or chew.

Depakote® sprinkle capsules: May be swallowed whole or may mix contents of capsule with semisolid food (eg, applesauce, pudding, mashed potatoes) and swallow immediately; do not crush or chew sprinkle beads; do not store drug food mixture for later use.

Depakene® capsule, Stavzor™: Swallow whole; do not break, crush, or chew.

Parenteral: I.V.:

Manufacturer recommendations: Dilute dose with at least 50 mL (in adults) of D$_5$W, NS, or LR; infuse over 60 minutes; maximum infusion rate: 20 mg/minute; **Note:** Rapid infusions may be associated with an increase in adverse effects; infusions of ≤15 mg/kg administered over 5-10 minutes (1.5-3 mg/kg/minute); were generally well tolerated (Ramsay, 2003). In pediatric patients, an infusion rate of 1.5-3 mg/kg/minute has been recommended (Brophy, 2012).

Rapid I.V. loading doses:

Infants and Children: Dilute dose; clinical trials usually diluted 1:1 with NS or D$_5$W (Mehta, 2007; Uberall, 2000); administer at 1.5-3 mg/kg/minute (Brophy, 2012). Further studies are needed.

Note: Faster infusion rates have been used in studies. One retrospective pediatric study administered loading doses of 25 mg/kg at a rate of ~3 mg/kg/minute (Yu, 2003). However, a prospective study administered 30 mg/kg of the drug diluted 1:1 in NS over 2-5 minutes (Mehta, 2007). Another retrospective study administered loading doses at a slightly faster rate: 20-40 mg/kg diluted 1:1 with NS or D$_5$W administered over 1-5 minutes (Uberall, 2000).

Adults: The European Federation of Neurological Societies (EFNS) recommends maximum administration rates of 6 mg/kg/minute (Meierkord, 2006). **Note:** In two adult studies, the drug was administered undiluted at rates as high as 10 mg/kg/minute (Limdi, 2007) and 500 mg/minute (Limdi, 2005). Further studies are needed.

Rectal: Dilute oral solution or syrup 1:1 with an equal volume of water prior to administration (Graves, 1987)

Hazardous agent; use appropriate precautions for handling and disposal (NIOSH, 2012).

Monitoring Parameters Liver enzymes (prior to therapy and at frequent intervals, especially during the first 6 months), bilirubin, serum ammonia (with symptoms of lethargy, mental status change), CBC with platelets (prior to initiation and periodically during therapy), serum concentrations, PT/PTT (especially prior to surgery); signs and symptoms of suicidality (eg, anxiety, depression, behavior changes), motor and cognitive function

Reference Range Note: In general, trough concentrations should be used to assess adequacy of therapy; peak concentrations may also be drawn if clinically necessary (eg, concentration-related toxicity). Additional patient-specific factors must be taken into consideration when interpreting drug concentrations, including indication, age, clinical response, pregnancy status, adherence, comorbidities, adverse effects, and concomitant medications (Patsalos, 2008; Reed, 2006).

Seizure disorder:

Therapeutic: 50-100 mcg/mL (SI: 350-690 micromoles/L); the relationship between plasma concentration and therapeutic response is not well documented; some patients may require lower concentrations to achieve therapeutic effect, and others may require higher concentration, but have a higher risk of toxicity

Toxic: >100-150 mcg/mL (SI: >690-1040 micromoles/L); probability of thrombocytopenia increases with total valproate concentrations ≥110 mcg/mL (SI: ≥760 micromoles/L) in females or ≥135 mcg/mL (SI: ≥930 micromoles/L) in males

Seizure control may improve at concentrations >100 mcg/mL (SI: >690 micromoles/L), but toxicity may occur.

Mania: Therapeutic trough: 50-125 mcg/mL (SI: 350-860 micromoles/L); risk of toxicity increases at concentrations >125 mcg/mL (SI: 875 micromole/L)

Test Interactions May cause a false-positive result for urine ketones (valproate partially eliminated as a keto-metabolite in the urine); may alter thyroid function tests

Additional Information Acute intoxications: Naloxone may reverse the CNS depressant effects but may also block the action of other anticonvulsants; carnitine may reduce the ammonia concentration

Dosage Forms Considerations

Strengths of divalproex sodium and valproate sodium products are expressed in terms of valproic acid

Dosage Forms Excipient information presented when available (limited, particularly for generics); consult specific product labeling.

Capsule, Oral, as valproic acid:
Depakene: 250 mg
Generic: 250 mg

Capsule Delayed Release, Oral, as valproic acid:
Stavzor: 125 mg, 250 mg, 500 mg [contains fd&c yellow #6 (sunset yellow)]

Capsule Sprinkle, Oral, as divalproex sodium:
Depakote Sprinkles: 125 mg [contains brilliant blue fcf (fd&c blue #1)]
Generic: 125 mg

Solution, Intravenous, as valproate sodium:
Depacon: 100 mg/mL (5 mL)

Solution, Intravenous, as valproate sodium [preservative free]:
Generic: 100 mg/mL (5 mL); 500 mg/5 mL (5 mL)

Solution, Oral, as valproate sodium:
Generic: 250 mg/5 mL (473 mL)

Syrup, Oral, as valproate sodium:
Depakene: 250 mg/5 mL (480 mL)
Generic: 250 mg/5 mL (5 mL, 10 mL, 473 mL)

Tablet Delayed Release, Oral, as divalproex sodium:
Depakote: 125 mg [contains brilliant blue fcf (fd&c blue #1), fd&c red #40]
Depakote: 250 mg [contains fd&c yellow #6 (sunset yellow)]
Depakote: 500 mg [contains fd&c blue #2 (indigotine)]
Generic: 125 mg, 250 mg, 500 mg

Tablet Extended Release 24 Hour, Oral, as divalproex sodium:
Depakote ER: 250 mg, 500 mg
Generic: 250 mg, 500 mg

References

Brophy GM, Bell R, Claassen J, et al, "Guidelines for the Evaluation and Management of Status Epilepticus," *Neurocrit Care*, 2012, 17(1):3-23.

Cloyd JC, Fischer JH, Kriel RL, et al, "Valproic Acid Pharmacokinetics in Children. IV. Effects of Age and Antiepileptic Drugs on Protein Binding and Intrinsic Clearance," *Clin Pharmacol Ther*, 1993, 53(1):22-9.

Cloyd JC, Kriel RL, Fischer JH, et al, "Pharmacokinetics of Valproic Acid in Children: I. Multiple Antiepileptic Drug Therapy," *Neurology*, 1983, 33(2):185-91.

Dreifuss FE, Santilli N, Langer DH, et al, "Valproic Acid Hepatic Fatalities: A Retrospective Review," *Neurology*, 1987, 37(3):379-85.

Evans D and Levene M, "Neonatal Seizures," *Arch Dis Child Fetal Neonatal Ed*, 1998, 78(1):70-5.

Freeman JM, Vining EP, Cost S, et al, "Does Carnitine Administration Improve the Symptoms Attributed to Anticonvulsant Medications?: A Double-Blinded, Crossover Study," *Pediatrics*, 1994, 93(6 Pt 1):893-5.

Gal P, Oles KS, Gilman JT, et al, "Valproic Acid Efficacy, Toxicity, and Pharmacokinetics in Neonates With Intractable Seizures," *Neurology*, 1988, 38(3):467-71.

Go CY, Mackay MT, Weiss SK, et al, "Evidence-Based Guideline Update: Medical Treatment of Infantile Spasms. Report of the Guideline Development Subcommittee of the American Academy of Neurology and the Practice Committee of the Child Neurology Society," *Neurology*, 2012, 78(24):1974-80.

Glauser T, Ben-Menachem E, Bourgeois B, et al, "ILAE Treatment Guidelines: Evidence-Based Analysis of Antiepileptic Drug Efficacy and Effectiveness as Initial Monotherapy for Epileptic Seizures and Syndromes," *Epilepsia*, 2006, 47(7):1094-120.

Graves NM and Kriel RL, "Rectal Administration of Antiepileptic Drugs in Children," *Pediatr Neurol*, 1987, 3(6):321-6.

Hagg S and Spigset O, "Anticonvulsant Use During Lactation," *Drug Saf*, 2000, 22(6):425-40.

Harden CL, Meador KJ, Pennell PB, et al, "Practice Parameter Update: Management Issues for Women With Epilepsy-Focus on Pregnancy

▶

(an Evidence-Based Review): Teratogenesis and Perinatal Outcomes: Report of the Quality Standards Subcommittee and Therapeutics and Technology Assessment Subcommittee of the American Academy of Neurology and American Epilepsy Society," *Neurology*, 2009, 73(2):133-41.

Harden CL, Pennell PB, Koppel BS, et al, "Practice Parameter Update: Management Issues for Women With Epilepsy-Focus on Pregnancy (an Evidence-Based Review): Vitamin K, Folic Acid, Blood Levels, and Breastfeeding: Report of the Quality Standards Subcommittee and Therapeutics and Technology Assessment Subcommittee of the American Academy of Neurology and American Epilepsy Society," *Neurology*, 2009, 73(2):142-9.

Hilmas E and Lee CK, "Valproic Acid-Related Reye's-Like Syndrome," *The Journal of Pediatric Pharmacy Practice*, 2000, 5(3):149-55.

Limdi NA, Knowlton RK, Cofield SS, et al, "Safety of Rapid Intravenous Loading of Valproate," *Epilepsia*, 2007, 48(3):478-83.

Limdi NA, Shimpi AV, Faught E, et al, "Efficacy of Rapid IV Administration of Valproic Acid for Status Epilepticus," *Neurology*, 2005, 64 (2):353-5.

Mehta V, Singhi P, and Singhi S, "Intravenous Sodium Valproate Versus Diazepam Infusion for the Control of Refractory Status Epilepticus in Children: A Randomized Controlled Trial," *J Child Neurol*, 2007, 22 (10):1191-7.

Meierkord H, Boon P, Engelsen B, et al, "EFNS Guideline on the Management of Status Epilepticus," *Eur J Neurol*, 2006, 13(5):445-50.

Murphy JV, Groover RV and Hodge C, "Hepatotoxic Effects in a Child Receiving Valproate and Carnitine," *J Pediatr*, 1993, 123(2):318-20.

National Institute for Occupational Safety and Health (NIOSH), "NIOSH List of Antineoplastic and Other Hazardous Drugs in Healthcare Settings 2012." Available at http://www.cdc.gov/niosh/docs/2012-150/pdfs/2012-150.pdf. Accessed January 21, 2013.

Patsalos PN, Berry DJ, Bourgeois BF, et al, "Antiepileptic Drugs – Best Practice Guidelines for Therapeutic Drug Monitoring: A Position Paper by the Subcommission on Therapeutic Drug Monitoring, ILAE Commission on Therapeutic Strategies," *Epilepsia*, 2008, 49 (7):1239-76.

Ramsay RE, Cantrell D, Collins SD, et al, "Safety and Tolerance of Rapidly Infused Depacon. A Randomized Trial in Subjects With Epilepsy," *Epilepsy Res*, 2003, 52(3):189-201.

Raskind JY and El-Chaar GM, "The Role of Carnitine Supplementation During Valproic Acid Therapy," *Ann Pharmacother*, 2000, 34(5):630-8.

Reed RC and Dutta S, "Does It Really Matter When a Blood Sample for Valproic Acid Concentration Is Taken Following Once-Daily Administration of Divalproex-ER?" *Ther Drug Monit*, 2006, 28(3):413-8.

Snead OC 3rd and Miles MV, "Treatment of Status Epilepticus in Children With Rectal Sodium Valproate," *J Pediatr*, 1985, 106 (2):323-5.

Uberall MA, Trollmann R, Wunsiedler U, et al, "Intravenous Valproate in Pediatric Epilepsy Patients With Refractory Status Epilepticus," *Neurology*, 2000, 54(11):2188-9.

Yu KT, Mills S, Thompson N, et al, "Safety and Efficacy of Intravenous Valproate in Pediatric Status Epilepticus and Acute Repetitive Seizures," *Epilepsia*, 2003, 44(5):724-6.

Valsartan (val SAR tan)

Medication Safety Issues

Sound-alike/look-alike issues:

Valsartan may be confused with losartan, Valstar, Valturna

Diovan may be confused with Zyban

International issues:

Diovan [U.S., Canada, and multiple international markets] may be confused with Dianben, a brand name for metformin [Spain]

Brand Names: U.S. Diovan

Brand Names: Canada Apo-Valsartan; Ava-Valsartan; CO Valsartan; Diovan; Mylan-Valsartan; PMS-Valsartan; Ran-Valsartan; Sandoz-Valsartan; Teva-Valsartan

Therapeutic Category Angiotensin II Receptor Blocker; Antihypertensive Agent

Generic Availability (U.S.) No

Use Treatment of primary hypertension alone or in combination with other antihypertensive agents (FDA approved in ages 6-16 years and adults); reduction of cardiovascular mortality in clinically stable patients with left ventricular failure or left ventricular dysfunction postmyocardial infarction (FDA approved in adults); treatment of heart failure (NYHA Class II-IV) (FDA approved in adults)

Pregnancy Risk Factor D

Pregnancy Considerations [U.S. Boxed Warning]: Drugs that act on the renin-angiotensin system can cause injury and death to the developing fetus. Discontinue as soon as possible once pregnancy is detected. The use of drugs which act on the renin-angiotensin system are associated with oligohydramnios. Oligohydramnios, due to decreased fetal renal function, may lead to fetal lung hypoplasia and skeletal malformations. Use is also associated with anuria, hypotension, renal failure, skull hypoplasia, and death in the fetus/neonate. in The exposed fetus should be monitored for fetal growth, amniotic fluid volume, and organ formation. Infants exposed *in utero* should be monitored for hyperkalemia, hypotension, and oliguria (exchange transfusions or dialysis may be needed). These adverse events are generally associated with maternal use in the second and third trimesters.

Untreated chronic maternal hypertension is also associated with adverse events in the fetus, infant, and mother. The use of angiotensin II receptor blockers is not recommended to treat chronic uncomplicated hypertension in pregnant women and should generally be avoided in women of reproductive potential (ACOG, 2013).

Breast-Feeding Considerations It is not known if valsartan is found in breast milk. Due to the potential for serious adverse reactions in the nursing infant, the manufacturer recommends a decision be made whether to discontinue nursing or to discontinue the drug, taking into account the importance of treatment to the mother. The Canadian labeling contraindicates use in nursing women.

Contraindications Hypersensitivity to valsartan, any component, or other angiotensin II receptor blockers

Warnings Drugs that act on the renin-angiotensin system can cause injury and death to the developing fetus. Discontinue as soon as possible once pregnancy is detected **[U.S. Boxed Warning]**. Symptomatic hypotension may occur, especially in patients with an activated renin-angiotensin system (eg, volume- or salt-depleted patients receiving high doses of diuretic agents); use with caution in these patients; correct depletion before starting therapy or initiate therapy under close medical supervision. Use with caution in patients with heart failure or post-MI; symptomatic hypotension may occur. Concomitant use of an ACE inhibitor or renin inhibitor (eg, aliskiren) is associated with an increased risk of hypotension, hyperkalemia, and renal dysfunction. Concomitant use with aliskiren should be avoided in patients with GFR <60 mL/minute and is contraindicated in patients with diabetes mellitus (regardless of GFR).

Angioedema has been reported rarely with some angiotensin II receptor antagonists (ARBs) and may occur at any time during treatment (especially following first dose); it may involve the head and neck (potentially compromising airway) or the intestine (presenting with abdominal pain). Patients with idiopathic or hereditary angioedema or previous angioedema associated with ACE-inhibitor therapy may be at an increased risk. Prolonged frequent monitoring may be required, especially if tongue, glottis, or larynx are involved, as they are associated with airway obstruction. Patients with a history of airway surgery may have a higher risk of airway obstruction. Discontinue therapy immediately if angioedema occurs. Aggressive early management is critical. Intramuscular (I.M.) administration of epinephrine may be necessary. Do not readminister to patients who have had angioedema with ARBs.

Precautions Use with caution in hepatic impairment; clearance of valsartan is reduced. Use with caution in impaired renal function; use is associated with deterioration of renal function and/or increases in serum creatinine, particularly in patients with low renal blood flow (eg, renal artery stenosis, heart failure); deterioration may result in oliguria, acute renal failure, and progressive azotemia. Small increases in serum creatinine may occur following initiation; consider discontinuation in patients with progressive and/or significant deterioration in renal function. Not recommended for use in children with GFR <30 mL/minute/1.73 m^2; has not been studied. Hyperkalemia may occur; risk factors include renal dysfunction, diabetes mellitus, concomitant use of potassium-sparing diuretics, potassium supplements, and/or potassium-containing salts; use with caution in these patients and with these agents; monitor potassium closely.

In a hypertension clinical trial of 90 children <6 years, five severe adverse events occurred in the treatment group, including two deaths (causes were identified as viral gastroenteritis and pneumonia) and three cases of increased liver enzymes; all patients also had significant comorbidities (primarily renal or urinary abnormalities); a causal relationship to valsartan could not be established nor excluded; use not recommended in this age group per manufacturer labeling (Flynn, 2008).

Adverse Reactions

Cardiovascular: Hypotension, orthostatic hypotension, syncope

Central nervous system: Dizziness, fatigue, headache, orthostatic dizziness, vertigo

Endocrine & metabolic: Serum potassium increased, hyperkalemia

Gastrointestinal: Abdominal pain (including upper), diarrhea, nausea

Hematologic & oncologic: Neutropenia

Infection: Viral infection

Neuromuscular & skeletal: Arthralgia, back pain

Ophthalmic: Blurred vision

Otic: Vertigo

Renal: Increased blood urea nitrogen, increased serum creatinine, renal insufficiency

Respiratory: Cough

All indications: Rare but important or life-threatening: Alopecia, anaphylaxis, anemia, angioedema, anorexia, bullous dermatitis, decreased hematocrit, decreased hemoglobin, dyspepsia, flatulence, hepatitis (rare), hypersensitivity reaction, impotence, insomnia, liver function tests increased, microcytic anemia, myalgia, palpitation, paresthesia, photosensitivity, pruritus, renal failure, rhabdomyolysis, skin rash, taste disorder, thrombocytopenia (very rare), vasculitis, xerostomia

Drug Interactions

Metabolism/Transport Effects Substrate of SLCO1B1; **Inhibits** CYP2C9 (weak)

Avoid Concomitant Use There are no known interactions where it is recommended to avoid concomitant use.

Increased Effect/Toxicity

Valsartan may increase the levels/effects of: ACE Inhibitors; Amifostine; Antihypertensives; CycloSPORINE (Systemic); DULoxetine; Hydrochlorothiazide; Hypotensive Agents; Lithium; Nonsteroidal Anti-Inflammatory Agents; Obinutuzumab; Potassium-Sparing Diuretics; RiTUXimab; Sodium Phosphates

The levels/effects of Valsartan may be increased by: Alfuzosin; Aliskiren; Barbiturates; Brimonidine (Topical); Canagliflozin; Diazoxide; Eltrombopag; Eplerenone; Heparin; Heparin (Low Molecular Weight); Herbs (Hypotensive Properties); Hydrochlorothiazide; MAO Inhibitors; Pentoxifylline; Phosphodiesterase 5 Inhibitors; Potassium Salts; Prostacyclin Analogues; Tolvaptan; Trimethoprim

Decreased Effect

The levels/effects of Valsartan may be decreased by: Herbs (Hypertensive Properties); Methylphenidate; Nonsteroidal Anti-Inflammatory Agents; Yohimbine

Food Interactions Food decreases the peak plasma concentration and extent of absorption by 50% and 40%, respectively. Management: Administer consistently with regard to food.

Stability Store at 25°C (77°F); excursions permitted to 15°C to 30°C (59°F to 86°F). Protect from moisture; dispense in tightly closed container.

Mechanism of Action Valsartan produces direct antagonism of the angiotensin II (AT2) receptors, unlike the ACE inhibitors. It displaces angiotensin II from the AT1 receptor and produces its blood pressure-lowering effects by antagonizing AT1-induced vasoconstriction, aldosterone release, catecholamine release, arginine vasopressin release, water intake, and hypertrophic responses. This action results in more efficient blockade of the cardiovascular effects of angiotensin II and fewer side effects than the ACE inhibitors.

Pharmacodynamics

Antihypertensive effect:

Onset of action: 2 hours postdose

Maximum effect: Within 6 hours postdose; with chronic dosing, substantial hypotensive effects are seen within 2 weeks; maximum effect: After 4 weeks

Duration: 24 hours

Pharmacokinetics (Adult data unless noted)

Distribution: V_d: 17 L

Protein binding: 95%, primarily albumin

Metabolism: To inactive metabolite (valeryl 4-hydroxy valsartan) via unidentified enzyme(s)

Bioavailability:

Tablet: 25% (range: 10% to 35%)

Suspension: ~40% (~1.6 times more than tablet)

Half-life, elimination:

Pediatric patients:

1-5 years: ~4 hours (Blumer, 2009)

6-16 years: ~5 hours (Blumer, 2009)

Adults: ~6 hours

Time to peak serum concentration:

Pediatric patients 1-16 years: Oral suspension: 2 hours (Blumer, 2009)

Adults: Tablets: 2-4 hours

Elimination: Feces (83%) and urine (13%) primarily as unchanged drug; 20% of dose is recovered as metabolites

Clearance: Found to be similar per kg bodyweight in children vs adults receiving a single dose of the suspension (Blumer, 2009)

Dialysis: Not removed by hemodialysis

Dosing: Usual

Children and Adolescents: **Hypertension: Oral: Note:** Due to increased bioavailability of extemporaneously prepared oral suspension (not commercially available), patients may require a higher dose when converting from oral suspension to tablet dosage form.

Children 1-5 years, weighing ≥8 kg: Limited data available: Reported dosage range: 0.4-3.4 mg/kg/dose once daily; maximum daily dose dependent upon patient weight: <18 kg: 40 mg/**day**; ≥18 kg: 80 mg/**day**. Dosing based on a single multicenter, international, placebo-controlled, dose-finding, crossover trial of 90 children 1-5 years (mean age: 3.2 years; minimum patient weight: 8 kg) which randomized patients to receive low, medium, or high doses according to patient body weight. Patients <18 kg received low dose: 5 mg once daily; medium dose: 20 mg once daily; or high dose: 40 mg once daily. Patients ≥18 kg received low dose: 10 mg once daily; medium dose: 40 mg once daily; or high dose: 80 mg once daily. Results showed significant antihypertensive effects in all dose level groups; five severe adverse events were reported during treatment (Flynn, 2008).

Children and Adolescents 6-16 years: Initial: 1.3 mg/kg once daily; maximum initial daily dose: 40 mg/**day**; may titrate to effect up to a maximum dose of 2.7 mg/kg/dose once daily or maximum daily dose: 160 mg/**day**, whichever is lower; doses greater than this have not been studied

Adolescents ≥17 years: Initial: 80 mg or 160 mg once daily (in patients who are not volume depleted); dose may be increased to achieve desired effect; maximum daily dose: 320 mg/**day**; in adults, usual dosage range (JNC 7): 80-320 mg once daily

Adults:

Hypertension: Oral: Initial: 80 mg or 160 mg once daily (in patients who are not volume depleted); dose may be increased to achieve desired effect; maximum recommended dose: 320 mg once daily; usual dosage range (JNC 7): 80-320 mg once daily

Heart failure: Oral: Initial: 40 mg twice daily; titrate dose to 80-160 mg twice daily, as tolerated; maximum dose: 320 mg/day in divided doses

Left ventricular dysfunction after MI: Initial: 20 mg twice daily; titrate dose to target of 160 mg twice daily as tolerated; may initiate ≥12 hours following MI

Dosing adjustment in renal impairment:

Children ≥6 years and Adolescents:

CrCl ≥30 mL/minute: No dosage adjustment necessary.

CrCl <30 mL/minute or Dialysis: There are no dosage adjustments provided in manufacturer's labeling; has not been studied; use not recommended.

Adults:

CrCl ≥30 mL/minute: No dosage adjustment necessary.

CrCl <30 mL/minute: There are no dosage adjustments provided in manufacturer's labeling; safety and efficacy have not been established.

Dialysis: Not significantly removed.

Dosing adjustment in hepatic impairment: Children ≥6 years, Adolescents, and Adults:

Mild to moderate impairment: No dosage adjustment necessary; use caution in patients with liver disease. Patients with mild to moderate chronic disease have twice the exposure as healthy volunteers.

Severe impairment: There are no dosage adjustments provided in manufacturer's labeling; has not been studied.

Administration May be administered without regard to food

Monitoring Parameters Blood pressure, BUN, serum creatinine, renal function, baseline and periodic serum electrolytes

Dosage Forms Excipient information presented when available (limited, particularly for generics); consult specific product labeling.

Tablet, Oral:

Diovan: 40 mg [scored]

Diovan: 80 mg, 160 mg, 320 mg

Extemporaneous Preparations A 4 mg/mL oral suspension may be made from tablets, Ora-Plus®, and Ora-Sweet® SF. Add 80 mL of Ora-Plus® to an 8-ounce amber glass bottle containing eight valsartan 80 mg tablets. Shake well for ≥2 minutes. Allow the suspension to stand for a minimum of 1 hour, then shake for ≥1 minute. Add 80 mL of Ora-Sweet SF® to the bottle and shake for ≥10 seconds. Store in amber glass prescription bottles; label "shake well". Stable for 30 days at room temperature or 75 days refrigerated.

Diovan® prescribing information, Novartis Pharmaceuticals Corp, East Hanover, NJ, 2012.

References

American College of Obstetricians and Gynecologists (ACOG), "ACOG Practice Bulletin No. 125: Chronic Hypertension in Pregnancy," *Obstet Gynecol*, 2012, 119(2 Pt 1):396-407.

Blumer J, Batisky DL, Wells T, et al, "Pharmacokinetics of Valsartan in Pediatric and Adolescent Subjects With Hypertension," *J Clin Pharmacol*, 2009, 49(2):235-41.

Chobanian AV, Bakris GL, Black HR, et al, "The Seventh Report of the Joint National Committee on Prevention, Detection, Evaluation, and Treatment of High Blood Pressure: The JNC 7 Report," *JAMA*, 2003, 289(19):2560-71.

Conlin P, Moore T, Swartz S, et al, "Effect of Indomethacin on Blood Pressure Lowering by Captopril and Losartan in Hypertensive Patients," *Hypertension*, 2000, 36(3):461-5.

Flynn JT, Meyers KE, Neto JP, et al, "Efficacy and Safety of the Angiotensin Receptor Blocker Valsartan in Children With Hypertension Aged 1 to 5 Years," *Hypertension*, 2008, 52(2):222-8.

◆ **Valtrex** *see* ValACYclovir *on page 2097*

◆ **Valtrex® (Can)** *see* ValACYclovir *on page 2097*

◆ **Val-Vancomycin (Can)** *see* Vancomycin *on page 2110*

◆ **Vanceril** *see* Beclomethasone (Oral Inhalation) *on page 265*

◆ **Vancocin (Can)** *see* Vancomycin *on page 2110*

◆ **Vancocin HCl** *see* Vancomycin *on page 2110*

Vancomycin (van koe MYE sin)

Medication Safety Issues

Sound-alike/look-alike issues:

I.V. vancomycin may be confused with INVanz

Vancomycin may be confused with clindamycin, gentamicin, tobramycin, valACYclovir, vecuronium, Vibramycin

High alert medication:

The Institute for Safe Medication Practices (ISMP) includes this medication (intrathecal administration) among its list of drug classes which have a heightened risk of causing significant patient harm when used in error.

Related Information

Prevention of Infective Endocarditis *on page 2336*

Brand Names: U.S. First-Vancomycin 25; First-Vancomycin 50; Vancocin HCl

Brand Names: Canada PMS-Vancomycin; Sterile Vancomycin Hydrochloride, USP; Val-Vancomycin; Vancocin; Vancomycin Hydrochloride for Injection; Vancomycin Hydrochloride for Injection, USP

Therapeutic Category Antibiotic, Miscellaneous

Generic Availability (U.S.) Yes

Use

Parenteral: Treatment of patients with the following infections or conditions: Infections due to documented or suspected methicillin-resistant *S. aureus* or beta-lactam resistant coagulase negative *Staphylococcus*; serious or life-threatening infections (eg, endocarditis, meningitis, osteomyelitis) due to documented or suspected staphylococcal or streptococcal infections in patients who are allergic to penicillins and/or cephalosporins; empiric therapy of infections associated with central lines, VP shunts, hemodialysis shunts, vascular grafts, prosthetic heart valves (FDA approved in all ages)

Oral: Treatment of *C. difficile*-associated diarrhea and enterocolitis caused by *Staphylococcus aureus* (including methicillin-resistant strains) [FDA approved in pediatric patients (age not specified) and adults]

Pregnancy Risk Factor B (oral); C (injection)

Pregnancy Considerations Adverse events have not been observed in animal reproduction studies. Vancomycin crosses the placenta and can be detected in fetal serum, amniotic fluid, and cord blood (Bourget, 1991; Reyes, 1989). Adverse fetal effects, including sensorineural hearing loss or nephrotoxicity, have not been reported following maternal use during the second or third trimesters of pregnancy.

The pharmacokinetics of vancomycin may be altered during pregnancy and pregnant patients may need a higher dose of vancomycin. Maternal half-life is unchanged, but the volume of distribution and the total plasma clearance may be increased (Bourget, 1991). Individualization of therapy through serum concentration monitoring may be warranted. Vancomycin is recommended for the treatment of mild, moderate, or severe *Clostridium difficile* infections in pregnant women (Surawicz, 2013). Vancomycin is recommended as an alternative agent to prevent the transmission of group B streptococcal (GBS) disease from mothers to newborns (ACOG, 2011; CDC, 2010).

Breast-Feeding Considerations Vancomycin is excreted in human milk following I.V. administration. If given orally to the mother, the minimal systemic absorption of the dose would limit the amount available to pass into the milk. Vancomycin is recommended for the treatment of mild, moderate, or severe *Clostridium difficile* infections in breast-feeding women (Surawicz, 2013). Due to the potential for serious adverse reactions in the nursing infant, the manufacturer recommends a decision be made whether to discontinue nursing or to discontinue the drug, taking into account the importance of treatment to the mother. Non-dose-related effects could include modification of bowel flora.

Contraindications Hypersensitivity to vancomycin or any component

Premixed solutions: Hypersensitivity to corn or corn products

Warnings May cause nephrotoxicity with intravenous therapy, although limited data suggest direct causal relationship; usual risk factors include preexisting renal impairment, concomitant nephrotoxic medications, advanced age, and dehydration. Nephrotoxicity has also been reported following treatment with oral vancomycin (typically in patients >65 years of age). If multiple sequential (≥2) serum creatinine concentrations demonstrate an increase of 0.5 mg/dL or ≥50% increase from baseline (whichever is greater) in the absence of an alternative explanation, the patient should be identified as having vancomycin-induced nephrotoxicity (Rybak, 2009). Discontinue treatment if signs of nephrotoxicity occur; renal damage is usually reversible. Clinically significant serum concentrations have been reported in patients with inflammatory disorders of the intestinal mucosa who have taken oral vancomycin (multiple doses) for the treatment of *C. difficile*-associated diarrhea. Although use may be warranted, the risk for adverse reactions may be higher in this situation; consider monitoring serum trough concentrations, especially with renal insufficiency, severe colitis, concurrent rectal vancomycin administration, and/or concomitant I.V. aminoglycosides. The IDSA suggests that it is appropriate to obtain trough concentrations when a patient is receiving high doses (eg, ≥2 g/day in adults) for prolonged courses (Cohen, 2010). Accumulation may occur after multiple oral doses of vancomycin in patients with renal impairment; consider monitoring trough concentrations in this circumstance.

May cause neurotoxicity; usual risk factors include preexisting renal impairment, concomitant neuro-/nephrotoxic medications, advanced age, and dehydration. Ototoxicity, although rarely associated with monotherapy, is proportional to the amount of drug given and the duration of treatment. Tinnitus or vertigo may be indications of vestibular injury and impending bilateral irreversible damage. Discontinue treatment if signs of ototoxicity occur.

Neutropenia has been reported; risk increased with prolonged therapy (>1 week) or total doses exceeding 25 g in adults; prompt reversal of neutropenia is expected with discontinuation of therapy.

Oral vancomycin is not effective for systemic infections; parenteral vancomycin is not effective for the treatment of colitis due to *C. difficile* and enterocolitis due to *S. aureus*. **Note:** In adults, the Infectious Disease Society of America (IDSA) recommends the use of oral metronidazole for initial treatment of mild to moderate *C. difficile* infection

and the use of oral vancomycin for initial treatment of severe *C. difficile* infection (Cohen, 2010).

IInfusion-related reaction may occur. Rapid infusion or doses ≥15-20 mg/kg/hour associated with red neck or red man syndrome described as erythema multiforme-like reaction with intense pruritus, tachycardia, hypotension; rash involving face, neck, upper trunk, back, and upper arms; reaction usually dissipates in 30-60 minutes.

Intravenous use may result in fungal or bacterial super-infection, including *C. difficile*-associated diarrhea (CDAD) and pseudomembranous colitis; CDAD has been observed >2 months postantibiotic treatment.

Precautions Use with caution in patients with renal impairment or those receiving other nephrotoxic or ototoxic drugs; dosage modification required in patients with impaired renal function. Chemical peritonitis syndrome has been reported with intraperitoneal administration.

Adverse Reactions

Injection:
Cardiovascular: Hypotension accompanied by flushing
Central nervous system: Chills, drug fever
Dermatologic: Erythematous rash on face and upper body (red neck or red man syndrome)
Hematologic: Eosinophilia, reversible neutropenia
Local: Phlebitis
Rare but important or life-threatening: Drug rash with eosinophilia and systemic symptoms (DRESS), ototoxicity (rare; use of other ototoxic agents may increase risk), renal failure (limited data suggesting direct relationship), Stevens-Johnson syndrome, thrombocytopenia, vasculitis

Oral:
Cardiovascular: Peripheral edema
Central nervous system: Fatigue, fever, headache
Gastrointestinal: Abdominal pain, bad taste (with oral solution), diarrhea, flatulence, nausea, vomiting
Genitourinary: Urinary tract infection
Neuromuscular & skeletal: Back pain
Rare but important or life-threatening: Creatinine increased, interstitial nephritis, ototoxicity, renal failure, renal impairment, thrombocytopenia, vasculitis

Drug Interactions

Metabolism/Transport Effects None known.

Avoid Concomitant Use
Avoid concomitant use of Vancomycin with any of the following: BCG

Increased Effect/Toxicity
Vancomycin may increase the levels/effects of: Aminoglycosides; Colistimethate; Neuromuscular-Blocking Agents

The levels/effects of Vancomycin may be increased by: Nonsteroidal Anti-Inflammatory Agents

Decreased Effect
Vancomycin may decrease the levels/effects of: BCG; Sodium Picosulfate; Typhoid Vaccine

The levels/effects of Vancomycin may be decreased by: Bile Acid Sequestrants

Stability
Parenteral:
Powder for injection: Store intact vials at 20°C to 25°C (68°F to 77°F). After reconstitution, vials may be stored under refrigeration for 14 days. **Note:** Vials contain no bacteriostatic agent. Upon further dilution with NS or D₅W, may refrigerate and use within 96 hours.
Premixed solution (manufacturer premixed): Store at -20°C (-4°F); once thawed, solutions are stable for 72 hours at room temperature or for 30 days refrigerated. Do not refreeze.
Oral: Capsules: Stored at 15°C to 30°C (59°F to 86°F).

◀ **Mechanism of Action** Inhibits bacterial cell wall synthesis by blocking glycopeptide polymerization through binding tightly to D-alanyl-D-alanine portion of cell wall precursor

Pharmacodynamics Displays time-dependent antimicrobial killing; slowly bacteriocidal

Pharmacokinetics (Adult data unless noted)

Absorption:

Oral: Poor; may be enhanced with bowel inflammation

I.M.: Erratic

Intraperitoneal: Can result in 38% systemic absorption

Distribution: Wide and variable distribution in body tissues and fluids including pericardial, pleural, ascites, and synovial fluids; low concentration in CSF

V_d:

Neonate, term: 0.57-0.69 L/kg (de Hoog, 2004)

Neonates, receiving ECMO (mean age: ~39 weeks): Variable; 1.1 L/kg (range: 0.6-2.1 L/kg) (Amaker, 1996); others have reported lower values: 0.45 ± 0.18 L/kg (Buck, 1998)

Pediatric patients: Median: 0.57 L/kg (range: 0.26-1.05 L/kg) (Marsot, 2012)

Adult: 0.4-1 L/kg (Rybak, 2009)

Relative diffusion from blood into CSF: Distribution improved with inflamed meninges and typically exceeds usual MICs

Children:

CSF concentrations: 0.2-17.3 mcg/mL (de Hoog, 2004)

CSF:blood level ratio: Normal meninges: Nil; Inflamed meninges: 7.1% to 68% (de Hoog, 2004)

Adults:

Uninflamed meninges: 0-4 mcg/mL; serum concentration dependent (Rybak, 2009)

Inflamed meninges: 6-11 mcg/mL; serum concentration dependent (Rybak, 2009)

CSF:blood level ratio: Normal meninges: Nil; Inflamed meninges: 20% to 30%

Protein binding: 55%

Metabolism: <3%

Half-life, biphasic: Prolonged significantly with reduced renal function

Terminal:

Newborns: 6-10 hours

3 months to 4 years: 4 hours

>3 years: 2.2-3 hours

Adults: 5-8 hours

Elimination: Primarily via glomerular filtration; excreted as unchanged drug in the urine (80% to 90%); oral doses are excreted primarily in the feces; presence of malignancy in children is associated with an increase in vancomycin clearance

Clearance:

Neonates: 0.63-1.5 mL/minute/kg; dependent on GA and/or PMA (de Hoog, 2004)

Neonates, receiving ECMO: 0.78 mL/minute/kg (range: 0.49-1.07 mL/minute/kg) (Amaker, 1996)

Pediatric patients: Median: 1.1 mL/minute/kg (range: 0.33-1.87 mL/minute/kg) (Marsot, 2012)

Adults: 0.71-1.31 mL/minute/kg (de Hoog, 2004)

Dialysis: Poorly dialyzable by intermittent hemodialysis (0% to 5%); however, use of high-flux membranes and continuous renal replacement therapy (CRRT) increases vancomycin clearance, and generally requires replacement dosing

Dosing: Neonatal

General dosing, susceptible infection: Note: Consider single-dose administration with serum concentration monitoring rather than scheduled dosing in patients with urine output <1 mL/kg/hour or if serum creatinine significantly increases from baseline (eg, doubles). Consider prolongation of dosing interval when coadministered with ibuprofen or indomethacin or in neonates with history of

the following: Birth depression, birth hypoxia/asphyxia, or cyanotic congenital heart disease.

Initial dosage recommendation:

Renal function-based dosing (Capparelli, 2001; *Nelson's Pocket Book of Pediatric Antimicrobial Therapy,* 2012): I.V.:

PNA ≤60 days:

≤28 weeks GA:

S_{cr} <0.5 mg/dL: 15 mg/kg/dose every 12 hours

S_{cr} 0.5-0.7 mg/dL: 20 mg/kg/dose every 24 hours

S_{cr} 0.8-1 mg/dL: 15 mg/kg/dose every 24 hours

S_{cr} 1.1-1.4 mg/dL: 10 mg/kg/dose every 24 hours

S_{cr} >1.4 mg/dL: 15 mg/kg/dose every 48 hours

>28 weeks GA:

S_{cr} <0.7 mg/dL: 15 mg/kg/dose every 12 hours

S_{cr} 0.7-0.9 mg/dL: 20 mg/kg/dose every 24 hours

S_{cr} 1-1.2 mg/dL: 15 mg/kg/dose every 24 hours

S_{cr} 1.3-1.6 mg/dL: 10 mg/kg/dose every 24 hours

S_{cr} >1.6 mg/dL: 15 mg/kg/dose every 48 hours

PNA >60 days: 30-40 mg/kg/**day** divided every 6-8 hours

Weight-based dosing (*Red Book,* 2009): I.V.:

PNA <7 days:

<1200 g: 15 mg/kg/dose every 24 hours

1200-2000 g: 10-15 mg/kg/dose every 12-18 hours

>2000 g: 10-15 mg/kg/dose every 8-12 hours

PNA ≥7 days:

<1200 g: 15 mg/kg/dose every 24 hours

1200-2000 g: 10-15 mg/kg/dose every 8-12 hours

>2000 g: 10-15 mg/kg/dose every 6-8 hours

ECMO, initial dosing in full-term neonates: I.V.: 15-20 mg/kg/dose every 18-24 hours (Buck, 2003); closely monitor serum concentrations; more frequent dosing may be needed for some patients

CNS Infection:

Meningitis (Tunkel, 2004): **Note:** Maintain trough serum concentrations of 15-20 mcg/mL; for neonates <2 kg, consider use of smaller doses and longer intervals. I.V.:

PNA ≤7 days and ≥2 kg: 20-30 mg/kg/**day** divided every 8-12 hours

PNA >7days and ≥2 kg: 30-45 mg/kg/**day** divided every 6-8 hours

VP-shunt infection, ventriculitis: Limited data available: Intrathecal/intraventricular (**use a preservative-free preparation**): 5-10 mg/day (Tunkel, 2004)

Dosing adjustment in renal impairment: Monitor vancomycin serum concentrations and adjust accordingly.

Dosing: Usual Initial dosage recommendation: **Note:** Doses require adjustment in renal impairment. Consider single-dose administration with serum concentration monitoring rather than scheduled dosing in patients with urine output <1 mL/kg/hour or if serum creatinine significantly increases from baseline (eg, doubles):

Infants, Children, and Adolescents:

General dosing, susceptible infection:

Infants ≤2 months:

Weight-based dosing (*Red Book,* 2012): **Note:** Every 6 hour dosing recommended as initial dosage regimen if targeting trough serum concentrations >10 mcg/mL (Benner, 2009; Frymoyer, 2009) in patients with normal renal function. Close monitoring of serum concentrations and assurance of adequate hydration status is recommended.

Mild to moderate infection: I.V.: 40-45 mg/kg/**day** divided every 6-8 hours; dose and frequency should be individualized based on serum concentrations; usual maximum daily dose: 2000 mg/**day**

Severe infection: I.V.: 45-60 mg/kg/**day** divided every 6-8 hours; dose and frequency should be individualized based on serum concentrations; usual maximum daily dose: 4000 mg/**day**

Renal function-based dosing (Capparelli, 2001; *Nelson's Pocket Book of Pediatric Antimicrobial Therapy*, 2012):

>28 weeks GA:

S_{cr} <0.7 mg/dL: 15 mg/kg/dose every 12 hours

S_{cr} 0.7-0.9 mg/dL: 20 mg/kg/dose every 24 hours

S_{cr} 1-1.2 mg/dL: 15 mg/kg/dose every 24 hours

S_{cr} 1.3-1.6 mg/dL: 10 mg/kg/dose every 24 hours

S_{cr} >1.6 mg/dL: 15 mg/kg/dose every 48 hours

Infants >2 months, Children, and Adolescents (*Red Book*, 2012): **Note:** Every 6 hour dosing recommended as initial dosage regimen if targeting trough serum concentrations >10 mcg/mL (Benner, 2009; Frymoyer, 2009) in patients with normal renal function. Close monitoring of serum concentrations and assurance of adequate hydration status is recommended.

Mild to moderate infection: I.V.: 40-45 mg/kg/**day** divided every 6-8 hours; dose and frequency should be individualized based on serum concentrations; usual maximum daily dose: 2000 mg/**day**

Severe infection: I.V.: 45-60 mg/kg/**day** divided every 6-8 hours; dose and frequency should be individualized based on serum concentrations; usual maximum daily dose: 4000 mg/**day**

Bacteremia [S. aureus (methicillin-resistant)]: I.V.: 15 mg/kg/dose every 6 hours for 2-6 weeks depending on severity (Liu, 2011)

Bone and joint infection:

Osteomyelitis [*S. aureus* (methicillin-resistant)]: I.V.: 15 mg/kg/dose every 6 hours for a minimum of 4-6 weeks (Liu, 2011)

Septic arthritis [*S. aureus* (methicillin-resistant)]: I.V.: 15 mg/kg/dose every 6 hours for minimum of 3-4 weeks (Liu, 2011)

Endocarditis:

Treatment: I.V.: 40 mg/kg/**day** divided every 6-12 hours for 4-6 weeks; dosage should be adjusted to target peak serum concentrations of 30-45 mcg/mL and trough serum concentrations of 10-15 mcg/mL; may combine with gentamicin for 2-6 weeks based on organism, resistance pattern and type of valve. (Baddour, 2005; Ferrieri, 2002). **Note:** Recommended by the AHA as an alternative agent in β-lactam allergic patients.

S. aureus (methicillin-resistant):

AHA Guidelines: I.V.: 40 mg/kg/**day** divided every 6-12 hours for at least 6 weeks; dosage should be adjusted to target peak serum concentrations of 30-45 mcg/mL and trough serum concentrations of 10-15 mcg/mL; **Note:** For prosthetic valves, combination with rifampin for the entire duration of therapy and gentamicin for the first 2 weeks has been recommended (Baddour, 2005; Ferrieri, 2002).

IDSA Guidelines: I.V.: 60 mg/kg/**day** divided every 6 hours for at least 6 weeks (Liu, 2011)

Prophylaxis, GI or genitourinary procedures: I.V.: 20 mg/kg over 1 hour; complete infusion 30 minutes prior to the procedure (Wilson, 2007). **Note:** Recommended by the AHA as an alternative agent in β-lactam allergic patients. As of April 2007, routine prophylaxis for GI/GU procedures is no longer recommended by the AHA.

Enterocolitis (S. aureus): Oral: 40 mg/kg/**day** divided every 6-8 hours for 7-10 days; maximum daily dose: 2000 mg/**day**

Intra-abdominal infection, complicated (MRSA): I.V.: 40 mg/kg/**day** divided every 6-8 hours (Solomkin, 2010)

Peritonitis (CAPD) (Warady, 2012):

Prophylaxis:

Touch contamination of PD line (if known MRSA colonization): Intraperitoneal: 25 mg per liter

High-risk gastrointestinal procedures: **Note:** Use should be reserved for patients at high risk for

MRSA: I.V.: 10 mg/kg administered 60-90 minutes before procedure; maximum dose: 1000 mg

Treatment: Intraperitoneal:

Intermittent: Initial dose: 30 mg/kg in the long dwell; subsequent doses: 15 mg/kg/dose every 3-5 days during the long dwell; **Note:** Increased clearance may occur in patients with residual renal function; subsequent doses should be based on serum concentration obtained 2-4 days after the previous dose; redosing should occur when serum concentration <15 mg/mL.

Continuous: Loading dose: 1000 mg per liter of dialysate; maintenance dose: 25 mg per liter

Pneumonia:

Community-acquired pneumonia (CAP): Infants ≥3 months, Children, and Adolescents: I.V.: 40-60 mg/kg/**day** every 6-8 hours; dosing to achieve AUC/MIC >400 has been recommended for treating moderate to severe MRSA infections (Bradley, 2011)

Alternate regimen: *S. aureus* (methicillin-resistant): Infants, Children, and Adolescents: I.V.: 60 mg/kg/**day** divided every 6 hours for 7-21 days depending on severity (Liu, 2011)

Healthcare-associated pneumonia (HAP), *S. aureus* (methicillin-resistant): I.V.: 60 mg/kg/**day** divided every 6 hours for 7-21 days depending on severity (Liu, 2011)

Septic thrombosis of cavernous or dural venous sinus [S. aureus (methicillin-resistant)]: I.V.: 15 mg/kg/dose every 6 hours for 4-6 weeks (some experts combine with rifampin) (Lui, 2011)

Skin and skin structure infections, complicated: [MRSA or S. aureus (methicillin sensitive) in penicillin allergic patients]: I.V.: 40 mg/kg/**day** divided every 6 hours (Stevens, 2005)

Alternate regimen: *S. aureus* (methicillin-resistant): I.V.: 60 mg/kg/**day** divided every 6 hours for 7-14 days (Liu, 2011)

CNS infection:

Brain abscess, subdural empyema, spinal epidural abscess [*S. aureus* (methicillin-resistant)]: I.V.: 15 mg/kg/dose every 6 hours for 4-6 weeks (some experts combine with rifampin) (Lui, 2011)

Meningitis: I.V.: 15 mg/kg/dose every 6 hours; **Note:** Maintain trough serum concentrations of 15-20 mcg/mL (Tunkel, 2004)

S. aureus (methicillin-resistant): 15 mg/kg/dose every 6 hours for 2 weeks (some experts combine with rifampin) (Liu, 2011)

VP-shunt infection, ventriculitis: Limited data available: Intrathecal/intraventricular **(use a preservative-free preparation):** 5-20 mg/**day**; usual dose: 10 or 20 mg/**day** (Tunkel, 2004)

C. difficile-**associated diarrhea (CDAD):** Oral: 40 mg/kg/**day** divided every 6-8 hours for 7-10 days; maximum daily dose: 2000 mg/**day**; **Note:** Metronidazole is initial drug of choice (*Red Book*, 2012)

Adults:

Usual dosage range: Initial intravenous dosing should be based on actual body weight; subsequent dosing adjusted based on serum trough vancomycin concentrations.

I.V.: 2000-3000 mg/**day** (or 30-60 mg/kg/**day**) in divided doses every 8-12 hours (Rybak, 2009); **Note:** Dose requires adjustment in renal impairment.

Oral: 500-2000 mg/**day** in divided doses every 6 hours

Indication-specific dosing:

Catheter-related infections: Antibiotic lock technique (Mermel, 2009): 2 mg/mL ± 10 units heparin/mL **or** 2.5 mg/mL ± 2500 **or** 5000 units heparin/mL **or** 5 mg/mL ± 5000 units heparin/mL (preferred regimen); instill into catheter port with a volume sufficient to fill the catheter (2-5 mL). **Note:** May use SWI/NS or D_5W

as diluents. Do not mix with any other solutions. Dwell times generally should not exceed 48 hours before renewal of lock solution. Remove lock solution prior to catheter use, then replace.

C. difficile-associated diarrhea (CDAD): Oral:

Manufacturer recommendations: 125 mg 4 times daily for 10 days

IDSA guideline recommendations: Severe infection: 125 mg every 6 hours for 10-14 days; Severe, complicated infection: 500 mg every 6 hours with or without concurrent I.V. metronidazole. May consider vancomycin retention enema (in patients with complete ileus) (Cohen, 2010)

Complicated infections in seriously ill patients: I.V.: Loading dose: 25-30 mg/kg (based on actual body weight) may be used to rapidly achieve target concentration; then 15-20 mg/kg/dose every 8-12 hours (Rybak, 2009)

Endocarditis:

Treatment: I.V.: 1000 mg every 12 hours for 4-6 weeks; may combine with gentamicin for 2-6 weeks based on organism, resistance pattern and type of valve (Gould, 2012)

Prophylaxis (Wilson, 2007):

Dental, oral, or upper respiratory tract surgery: I.V.: 1000 mg 1 hour before surgery. **Note:** AHA guidelines now recommend prophylaxis only in patients undergoing invasive procedures and in whom underlying cardiac conditions may predispose to a higher risk of adverse outcomes should infection occur.

GI/GU procedure: I.V.: 1000 mg 1 hour prior to surgery; must be used in combination with gentamicin. **Note:** As of April 2007, routine prophylaxis for GI/GU procedures no longer recommended by the AHA.

Enterocolitis (S. aureus): Oral: 500-2000 mg/day in 3-4 divided doses for 7-10 days (usual dose: 125-500 mg every 6 hours)

Meningitis:

I.V.: 30-60 mg/kg/day in divided doses every 8-12 hours (Rybak, 2009) or 500-750 mg every 6 hours (with third generation cephalosporin for PCN-resistant Streptococcus pneumoniae)

Intrathecal, intraventricular: 5-20 mg/day

MRSA infections (Liu, 2011): I.V.: 15-20 mg/kg/dose every 8-12 hours; duration of therapy dependent upon site of infection and clinical response

Susceptible (MIC ≤1 mcg/mL) gram-positive infections: I.V.: 15-20 mg/kg/dose (usual: 750-1500 mg) every 8-12 hours. **Note:** If MIC ≥2 mcg/mL, alternative therapies are recommended (Rybak, 2009)

Dosing adjustment in renal impairment: Vancomycin levels should be monitored in patients with any renal impairment:

Infants, Children, and Adolescents: The following adjustments have been recommended (Aronoff, 2007): **Note:** Renally adjusted dose recommendations are based on doses of 10 mg/kg/dose every 6 hours or 15 mg/kg/dose every 8 hours:

GFR 30-50 mL/minute/1.73 m^2: 10 mg/kg/dose every 12 hours

GFR 10-29 mL/minute/1.73 m^2: 10 mg/kg/dose every 18-24 hours

GFR <10 mL/minute/1.73 m^2: 10 mg/kg/dose; redose based on serum concentrations

Intermittent hemodialysis: 10 mg/kg/dose; redose based on serum concentrations

Peritoneal dialysis (PD): 10 mg/kg/dose; redose based on serum concentrations

Continuous renal replacement therapy (CRRT): 10 mg/kg/dose every 12-24 hours; monitor serum concentrations

Adults: Some experts suggest:

CrCl >50 mL/minute: Start with 15-20 mg/kg/dose (usual: 750-1500 mg) every 8-12 hours

CrCl 20-49 mL/minute: Start with 15-20 mg/kg/dose (usual: 750-1500 mg) every 24 hours

CrCl <20 mL/minute: Will need longer intervals; determine by serum concentration monitoring

Note: In the critically ill patient with renal insufficiency, the initial loading dose (25-30 mg/kg) should not be reduced; however, subsequent dosage adjustments should be made based on renal function and trough serum concentrations.

Poorly dialyzable by intermittent hemodialysis (0% to 5%); however, use of high-flux membranes and continuous renal replacement therapy (CRRT) increases vancomycin clearance and generally requires replacement dosing.

Intermittent hemodialysis (IHD) (administer after hemodialysis on dialysis days): Following loading dose of 15-25 mg/kg, give either 500-1000 mg or 5-10 mg/kg after each dialysis session. (Heintz, 2009). **Note:** Dosing dependent on the assumption of 3 times/week, complete IHD sessions.

Redosing based on pre-HD serum concentrations:

<10 mg/L: Administer 1000 mg after HD

10-25 mg/L: Administer 500-750 mg after HD

>25 mg/L: Hold vancomycin

Redosing based on post-HD serum concentrations:

<10-15 mg/L: Administer 500-1000 mg

Peritoneal dialysis (PD):

Administration via PD fluid: 15-30 mg/L (15-30 mcg/mL) of PD fluid

Systemic: Loading dose of 1000 mg, followed by 500-1000 mg every 48-72 hours with close monitoring of levels

Continuous renal replacement therapy (CRRT) (Heintz, 2009; Trotman, 2005): Drug clearance is highly dependent on the method of renal replacement, filter type, and flow rate. Appropriate dosing requires close monitoring of pharmacologic response, signs of adverse reactions due to drug accumulation, as well as drug concentrations in relation to target trough (if appropriate). The following are general recommendations only (based on dialysate flow/ultrafiltration rates of 1-2 L/hour and minimal residual renal function) and should not supersede clinical judgment:

CVVH: Loading dose of 15-25 mg/kg, followed by either 1000 mg every 48 hours or 10-15 mg/kg every 24-48 hours

CVVHD: Loading dose of 15-25 mg/kg, followed by either 1000 mg every 24 hours or 10-15 mg/kg every 24 hours

CVVHDF: Loading dose of 15-25 mg/kg, followed by either 1000 mg every 24 hours or 7.5-10 mg/kg every 12 hours

Note: Consider redosing patients receiving CRRT for vancomycin serum concentrations <10-15 mg/L.

Dosage adjustment in hepatic impairment: Degrees of hepatic dysfunction do not affect the pharmacokinetics of vancomycin (Marti, 1996)

Oral: No adjustment provided in the manufacturer's labeling

Administration

Oral: Vancomycin powder for injection may be reconstituted and used for oral administration (Cohen, 2010). Reconstituted powder for injection (not premixed solution) may be administered orally by diluting in 30 mL of water; common flavoring syrups may be added to improve taste. The unflavored, diluted solution may also be administered via nasogastric tube. Also see Extemporaneous Preparations section.

Parenteral: Administer intermittent I.V. infusion over 60 minutes at a final concentration not to exceed 5 mg/mL;

if a maculopapular rash appears on face, neck, trunk, and upper extremities, slow the infusion rate to administer dose over 90-120 minutes and increase the dilution volume; the reaction usually dissipates in 30-60 minutes; administration of antihistamines just before the infusion may also prevent or minimize this reaction

Intrathecal/Intraventricular: Dilute in NS without preservatives to a final concentration between 2-5 mg/mL

Monitoring Parameters Periodic renal function tests (especially when targeting higher serum concentrations), urinalysis, serum vancomycin concentrations, WBC; audiogram (in patients who concurrently receive ototoxic chemotherapy); fluid status

Reference Range Measure trough serum concentrations to assess efficacy. Peak concentrations may be helpful in the setting of atypical pharmacokinetic profile. Trough serum concentration typically obtained at steady state (ie, prior to the fourth dose). Target trough serum concentration may vary depending on organism, MIC, source of infection, and/or other patient factors (Rybak, 2009).

15-20 mcg/mL: For organisms with an MIC = 1 mcg/mL or complicated infections (bacteremia, endocarditis, osteomyelitis, meningitis, and hospital-acquired pneumonia caused by *Staphylococcus* spp.) (Rybak, 2009)

10-15 mcg/mL: Current recommendation for all other infections with an organism with an MIC <1 mcg/mL

5-10 mcg/mL: Traditional recommendation; may be adequate to treat some infections based on site and MIC; however, this range is not recommended in the adult guidelines for vancomycin use due to resistance development potential

Note: Although AUC/MIC is the preferred method to determine clinical effectiveness, trough serum concentrations may be used as a surrogate marker and is recommended as the most accurate and practical method of vancomycin monitoring.

Additional Information "Red man syndrome," characterized by skin rash and hypotension, is not an allergic reaction but rather is associated with too rapid infusion of the drug. To alleviate or prevent the reaction, infuse vancomycin at a rate of ≥30 minutes for each 500 mg of drug being administered (eg, 1 g over ≥60 minutes); 1.5 g over ≥90 minutes. When treating pathogens with a vancomycin MIC ≥2 mcg/mL, alternative antibiotics should be considered.

Dosage Forms Excipient information presented when available (limited, particularly for generics); consult specific product labeling.

Capsule, Oral:
Vancocin HCl: 125 mg, 250 mg
Generic: 125 mg, 250 mg

Solution, Intravenous:
Generic: 500 mg/100 mL (100 mL); 750 mg/150 mL (150 mL); 1 g/200 mL (200 mL)

Solution, Oral:
First-Vancomycin 25: 25 mg/mL (150 mL, 300 mL) [contains fd&c red #40, fd&c yellow #10 (quinoline yellow), sodium benzoate; white grape flavor]

First-Vancomycin 50: 50 mg/mL (150 mL, 210 mL, 300 mL) [contains fd&c red #40, fd&c yellow #10 (quinoline yellow), sodium benzoate; white grape flavor]

Solution Reconstituted, Intravenous:
Generic: 500 mg (1 ea); 750 mg (1 ea); 1000 mg (1 ea); 5000 mg (1 ea); 10 g (1 ea)

Solution Reconstituted, Intravenous [preservative free]:
Generic: 1000 mg (1 ea); 5000 mg (1 ea); 10 g (1 ea)

Extemporaneous Preparations Note: A vancomycin (25 mg/mL or 50 mg/mL) suspension is commercially available as a compounding kit (First-Vancomycin).

Using a vial of vancomycin powder for injection (reconstituted to 50 mg/mL), add the appropriate volume for the dose to 30 mL of water and administer orally or via NG tube. For oral administration, common flavoring syrups may be added to improve taste.

Vancomycin Hydrochloride for Injection, USP (prescribing information), Schaumburg, II, APP Pharmaceuticals, LLC, 2011.

A vancomycin 25 mg/mL solution in Ora-Sweet® and water (1:1) may be prepared by reconstituting vancomycin for injection with sterile water, then dilute with a 1:1 mixture of Ora-Sweet® and distilled water to a final concentration of 25 mg/mL; transfer to amber prescription bottle. Stable for 75 days refrigerated or for 26 days at room temperature.

Ensom MH, Decarie D, and Lakhani A, "Stability of Vancomycin 25 mg/mL in Ora-Sweet and Water in Unit-Dose Cups and Plastic Bottles at 4°C and 25°C," Can J Hosp Pharm, 2010, 63(5):366-72.

References

Amaker RD, DiPiro JT, and Bhatia J, "Pharmacokinetics of Vancomycin in Critically Ill Infants Undergoing Extracorporeal Membrane Oxygenation," Antimicrob Agents Chemother, 1996, 40(5):1139-42.

American Academy of Pediatrics Committee on Infectious Diseases, "Treatment of Bacterial Meningitis," Pediatrics, 1988, 81(6):904-7.

American College of Obstetricians and Gynecologists Committee on Obstetric Practice, "ACOG Committee Opinion No. 485: Prevention of Early-Onset Group B Streptococcal Disease in Newborns," Obstet Gynecol, 2011, 117(4):1019-27.

American Thoracic Society and Infectious Diseases Society of America, "Guidelines for the Management of Adults With Hospital-Acquired, Ventilator-Associated, and Healthcare-Associated Pneumonia," Am J Respir Crit Care Med, 2005, 171(4):388-416.

Aronoff GR, Bennett WM, Berns JS, et al, Drug Prescribing in Renal Failure: Dosing Guidelines for Adults and Children, 5th ed. Philadelphia, PA: American College of Physicians; 2007, 154.

Baddour LM, Wilson WR, Bayer AS, et al, "Infective Endocarditis: Diagnosis, Antimicrobial Therapy, and Management of Complications: A Statement for Healthcare Professionals From the Committee on Rheumatic Fever, Endocarditis, and Kawasaki Disease, Council on Cardiovascular Disease in the Young, and the Councils on Clinical Cardiology, Stroke, and Cardiovascular Surgery and Anesthesia, American Heart Association: Endorsed by the Infectious Diseases Society of America," Circulation, 2005, 111(23):e394-434.

Benner KW, Worthington MA, Kimberlin DW, et al, "Correlation of Vancomycin Dosing to Serum Concentrations in Pediatric Patients: A Retrospective Database Review," J Pediatr Pharmacol Ther, 2009, 14:86-93.

Bourget P, Fernandez H, Delouis C, et al, "Transplacental Passage of Vancomycin During the Second Trimester of Pregnancy," Obstet Gynecol, 1991, 78(5 Pt 2):908-11.

Bradley JS, Byington CL, Shah SS, et al, "The Management of Community-Acquired Pneumonia in Infants and Children Older Than 3 Months of Age: Clinical Practice Guidelines by the Pediatric Infectious Diseases Society and the Infectious Diseases Society of America", Clin Infect Dis, 2011, 53(7):e25-76.

Buck ML, "Pharmacokinetic Changes During Extracorporeal Membrane Oxygenation: Implications for Drug Therapy of Neonates," Clin Pharmacokinet, 2003, 42(5):403-17.

Buck ML, "Vancomycin Pharmacokinetics in Neonates Receiving Extracorporeal Membrane oxygenation," Pharmacotherapy, 1998, 18(5):1082-6.

Capparelli EV, Lane JR, Romanowski GL, et al, "The Influences of Renal Function and Maturation on Vancomycin Elimination in Newborns and Infants," J Clin Pharmacol, 2001, 41(9):927-34.

Centers for Disease Control and Prevention (CDC), "Prevention of Perinatal Group B Streptococcal Disease—Revised Guidelines From CDC, 2010," MMWR Recomm Rep, 2010, 59(RR-10):1-36.

Chang D, "Influence of Malignancy on the Pharmacokinetics of Vancomycin in Infants and Children," Pediatr Infect Dis J, 1995, 14 (8):667-73.

Chang D, Liem L, and Malogolowkin M, "A Prospective Study of Vancomycin Pharmacokinetics and Dosage Requirements in Pediatric Cancer Patients," Pediatr Infect Dis J, 1994, 13(11):969-74.

Cohen SH, Gerding DN, Johnson S, et al, "Clinical Practice Guidelines for Clostridium difficile Infection in Adults: 2010 Update by the Society for Healthcare Epidemiology of America (SHEA) and the Infectious Diseases Society of America (IDSA)," Infect Control Hosp Epidemiol, 2010, 31(5):431-55.

de Hoog M, Mouton JW, and van den Anker JN, "Vancomycin: Pharmacokinetics and Administration Regimens in Neonates," Clin Pharmacokinet, 2004, 43(7):417-40.

Ferrieri P, Gewitz MH, Gerber MA, et al, "Unique Features of Infective Endocarditis in Childhood," Circulation, 2002, 105(17):2115-26.

Frymoyer A, Hersh AL, Benet LZ, et al, "Current Recommended Dosing of Vancomycin for Children With Invasive Methicillin-Resistant Staphylococcus aureus Infections Is Inadequate," Pediatr Infect Dis J, 2009, 28(5):398-402.

Gould FK, Denning DW, Elliott TS, et al, "Guidelines for the Diagnosis and Antibiotic Treatment of Endocarditis in Adults: A Report of the Working Party of the British Society for Antimicrobial Chemotherapy," *J Antimicrob Chemother*, 2012, 67(2):269-89.

Heintz BH, Matzke GR, Dager WE, "Antimicrobial Dosing Concepts and Recommendations for Critically Ill Adult Patients Receiving Continuous Renal Replacement Therapy or Intermittent Hemodialysis," *Pharmacotherapy*, 2009, 29(5):562-77.

Leonard MB, Koren G, Stevenson DK, et al, "Vancomycin Pharmacokinetics in Very Low Birth Weight Neonates," *Pediatr Infect Dis J*, 1989, 8(5):282-6.

Liu C, Bayer A, Cosgrove SE, et al, "Clinical Practice Guidelines by the Infectious Diseases Society of America for the Treatment of Methicillin-Resistant *Staphylococcus aureus* Infections in Adults and Children: Executive Summary," *Clin Infect Dis*, 2011, 52(3):285-92.

Marsot A, Boulamery A, Bruguerolle B, et al, "Vancomycin: A Review of Population Pharmacokinetic Analyses," *Clin Pharmacokinet*, 2012, 51 (1):1-13.

Martí R, Rosell M, Pou L, et al, "Influence of Biochemical Parameters of Liver Function on Vancomycin pharmacokinetics," *Pharmacol Toxicol*, 1996, 79(2):55-9.

Matzke GR, Zhanel GG, and Guay DRP, "Clinical Pharmacokinetics of Vancomycin," *Clin Pharmacokinet*, 1986, 11(4):257-82.

Mermel LA, Allon M, Bouza E, et al, "Clinical Practice Guidelines for the Diagnosis and Management of Intravascular Catheter-Related Infection: 2009 Update by the Infectious Diseases Society of America," *Clin Infect Dis*, 2009, 49(1):1-45.

Nelson's Pocket Book of Pediatric Antimicrobial Therapy, 19th ed, Bradley JS, Nelson JD, Kimberlin DK, et al, eds, Philadelphia, PA: Lippincott Williams & Wilkins, 2012.

Red Book: 2012 Report of the Committee on Infectious Diseases, "Antibacterial Drugs Dosage Tables," 29th ed, Pickering LK, ed, Elk Grove Village, IL: American Academy of Pediatrics, 2012, 808-16.

Reyes MP and Ostrea EM Jr, "Toxicity of Vancomycin Given During Pregnancy (Reply)," *Am J Obstet Gynecol*, 1990, 163(4 Pt 1):1376.

Rodvold KA, Everett JA, Pryka RD, and Kraus DM, "Pharmacokinetics and Administration Regimens of Vancomycin in Neonates, Infants and Children," *Clin Pharmacokinet*, 1997, 33(1):32-51.

Rybak MJ, Albrecht LM, Boike SC, et al, "Nephrotoxicity of Vancomycin, Alone and With an Aminoglycoside," *J Antimicrob Chemother*, 1990, 25(4):679-87.

Rybak M, Lomaestro B, Rotschafer JC, et al, "Therapeutic Monitoring of Vancomycin in Adult Patients: A Consensus Review of the American Society of Health-System Pharmacists, the Infectious Diseases Society of America, and the Society of Infectious Diseases Pharmacists," *Am J Health-Syst Pharm*, 2009, 66(1):82-98.

Solomkin JS, Mazuski JE, Bradley JS, et al, "Diagnosis and Management of Complicated Intra-abdominal Infection in Adults and Children: Guidelines by the Surgical Infection Society and the Infectious Diseases Society of America," *Clin Infect Dis*, 2010, 50(2):133-64.

Stevens DL, Bisno AL, Chambers HF, et al, "Practice Guidelines for the Diagnosis and Management of Skin and Soft-Tissue Infections," *Clin Infect Dis*, 2005, 41(10):1373-406.

Surawicz CM, Brandt LJ, Binion DG, et al. Guidelines for diagnosis, treatment, and prevention of *Clostridium difficile* infections. *Am J Gastroenterol*. 2013;108(4):478-498.

Trotman RL, Williamson JC, Shoemaker DM, et al, "Antibiotic Dosing in Critically Ill Adult Patients Receiving Continuous Renal Replacement Therapy," *Clin Infect Dis*, 2005, 41:1159-66.

Tunkel AR, Hartman BJ, Kaplan SL, et al, "Practice Guidelines for the Management of Bacterial Meningitis," *Clin Infect Dis*, 2004, 39 (9):1267-84.

Warady BA, Bakkaloglu S, Newland J, et al, "Consensus Guidelines for the Prevention and Treatment of Catheter-Related Infections and Peritonitis in Pediatric Patients Receiving Peritoneal Dialysis: 2012 Update," *Perit Dial Int*, 2012, (32 Suppl 2):S32-86.

Wilson W, Taubert KA, Gewitz M, et al, "Prevention of Infective Endocarditis: Guidelines From the American Heart Association: A Guideline From the American Heart Association Rheumatic Fever, Endocarditis, and Kawasaki Disease Committee, Council on Cardiovascular Disease in the Young, and the Council on Clinical Cardiology, Council on Cardiovascular Surgery and Anesthesia, and the Quality of Care and Outcomes Research Interdisciplinary Working Group," *Circulation*, 2007, 116(15):1736-54. Available at http://circ.-ahajournals.org/cgi/reprint/CIRCULATIONAHA.106.183095v1

◆ **Vancomycin Hydrochloride** see Vancomycin on page 2110

◆ **Vancomycin Hydrochloride for Injection (Can)** see Vancomycin on page 2110

◆ **Vancomycin Hydrochloride for Injection, USP (Can)** see Vancomycin on page 2110

◆ **Vandazole** see MetroNIDAZOLE (Topical) on page 1404

◆ **Vanos** see Fluocinonide on page 894

◆ **Vantas** see Histrelin on page 1016

◆ **Vantin** see Cefpodoxime on page 410

◆ **VAQTA** see Hepatitis A Vaccine on page 1005

◆ **VAR** see Varicella Virus Vaccine on page 2116

◆ **Varicella, Measles, Mumps, and Rubella Vaccine** see Measles, Mumps, Rubella, and Varicella Virus Vaccine on page 1310

Varicella Virus Vaccine

(var i SEL a VYE rus vak SEEN)

Medication Safety Issues

Sound-alike/look-alike issues:

Varicella virus vaccine has been given in error (instead of the indicated varicella immune globulin) to pregnant women exposed to varicella.

Other safety concerns:

Both varicella vaccine and zoster vaccine are live, attenuated strains of varicella-zoster virus. Their indications, dosing, and composition are distinct. Varicella is indicated in children to prevent chickenpox, while zoster vaccine is indicated in older individuals to prevent reactivation of the virus which causes shingles. Zoster vaccine is **not** a substitute for varicella vaccine and should not be used in children.

Related Information

Immunization Administration Recommendations on page 2368

Immunization Guidelines on page 2373

Brand Names: U.S. Varivax

Brand Names: Canada Varilrix; Varivax III

Therapeutic Category Vaccine

Generic Availability (U.S.) No

Use Immunization against varicella in individuals who do not have evidence of immunity (FDA approved in ages ≥12 months and adults).

The ACIP (CDC/ACIP [Marin, 2007]) recommends vaccination for all children, adolescents, and adults who do not have evidence of immunity. Vaccination is especially important for:

• Healthcare personnel
• Persons with close contact to those at high risk for severe disease
• Persons living or working in environments where transmission is likely (teachers, childcare workers, residents, and staff of institutional settings)
• Persons in environments where transmission has been reported
• Nonpregnant women of childbearing age
• Adolescents and adults in households with children
• International travelers

Postexposure prophylaxis: Vaccination within 3 days (possibly 5 days) after exposure to rash is effective in preventing illness or modifying severity of disease (CDC/ACIP [Marin, 2007]).

Pregnancy Considerations Varicella virus vaccine is contraindicated for use in pregnant females and pregnancy should be avoided for 3 months (per manufacturer labeling; 1 month per ACIP) following vaccination. Varicella disease during the 1st or 2nd trimesters may result in congenital varicella syndrome. The onset of maternal varicella infection from 5 days prior to 2 days after delivery may cause varicella infection in the newborn. All women should be assessed for immunity during a prenatal visit; those without evidence of immunity should be vaccinated upon completion or termination of pregnancy (CDC, 2007). Based on information collected from 1995-2013 using the manufacturer's pregnancy registry, of 820 women who received a varicella containing vaccine, there were no infants born with abnormalities consistent with congenital varicella syndrome. Any exposures to the vaccine during pregnancy or within 3 months prior to pregnancy should be reported to the manufacturer (Merck & Co, 877-888-4231) or to VAERS (800-822-7967) as suspected adverse reactions.

Breast-Feeding Considerations Following immunization, varicella virus was not detected in the milk samples of 12 breast-feeding women and none of the breast-fed infants seroconverted. Immunization should not be delayed due to breast-feeding (CDC, 2007). The manufacturer recommends that caution be exercised when administering varicella virus vaccine to nursing women. Breast-feeding infants should be vaccinated according to the recommended schedules (CDC, 2011).

Contraindications Hypersensitivity (severe allergy or anaphylactic) to any component of the vaccine, including gelatin; a history of anaphylactoid reaction to neomycin; immunosuppressed or immunodeficient individuals including individuals with leukemia, lymphomas, or other malignant neoplasms affecting the bone marrow or lymphatic systems; persons with AIDS or other clinical manifestations of HIV (per manufacturer labeling); those receiving immunosuppressive therapy (including immunosuppressive doses of corticosteroids); primary and acquired immunodeficiency states; active, untreated tuberculosis; current febrile illness (per manufacturer labeling); pregnancy

Warnings Immediate treatment (including epinephrine 1:1000) for anaphylactic and/or hypersensitivity reaction should be available during vaccine use. Salicylates should be avoided for 6 weeks after vaccination; varicella may increase the risk of Reye's syndrome. Varicella vaccine and antibody-containing products (eg, immune globulin, blood products) should not be administered simultaneously. Guidelines with suggested administration intervals are available (CDC/ACIP [Kroger, 2011]).

Vaccinated individuals should not have close association with susceptible high-risk individuals (newborns of mothers without evidence of immunity, all infants born <28 weeks gestation regardless of maternal immunity, pregnant women without evidence of immunity, immunocompromised persons) for 6 weeks following vaccination (per the manufacturer). However, the CDC notes that transmission of the virus is rare and recommends that vaccine recipients who develop a vaccine-related rash avoid contact with susceptible individuals at high risk for complications until the lesions are resolved (crusted over or fade away) or until no new lesions appear for 24 hours. According to the CDC guidelines, having a pregnant household member is not a contraindication to vaccination (CDC/ACIP [Marin, 2007]).

Although administration to persons with HIV is a contraindication per the manufacturer, guidelines for use are available. Children with HIV infection with age-specific CD4+ T-lymphocyte percentages ≥15% may receive live attenuated varicella vaccine. Vaccination may be considered for adolescents and adults with CD4+ T-lymphocyte counts ≥200 cells/µL (CDC/ACIP [Marin, 2007]). Syncope has been reported with use of injectable vaccines and may be accompanied by transient visual disturbances, weakness, or tonic-clonic movements. Procedures should be in place to avoid injuries from falling and to restore cerebral perfusion if syncope occurs (CDC, 57(17), 2008).

Products may contain albumin, gelatin, and/or neomycin. Use is contraindicated in patients with history of anaphylactic/anaphylactoid reactions to neomycin; contact dermatitis due to neomycin is not a contraindication to the vaccine.

Precautions Although fever is a contraindication per the manufacturer, current guidelines allow for administration to patients with mild acute illness (with or without low grade fever) (CDC/ACIP [Marin, 2007]). Vaccination may not

result in effective immunity in all patients. Response depends upon multiple factors (eg, type of vaccine, age of patient) and may be improved by administering the vaccine at the recommended dose, route, and interval. Vaccines may not be effective if administered during periods of altered immune competence (CDC/ACIP [Kroger, 2011]). Defer use in patients with a family history of congenital or hereditary immunodeficiency until immune competence in the vaccine recipient is demonstrated (CDC/ACIP [Marin, 2007]). Use of this vaccine is contraindicated in persons who are immunosuppressed or immunodeficient. In general, live vaccines should be administered ≥4 weeks prior to planned immunosuppression and avoided within 2 weeks of immunosuppression when feasible (IDSA [Rubin, 2014]).

Antipyretics have not been shown to prevent febrile seizures; antipyretics may be used to treat fever or discomfort following vaccination (CDC/ACIP [Kroger, 2011]). One study reported that routine prophylactic administration of acetaminophen to prevent fever prior to vaccination decreased the immune response of some vaccines; the clinical significance of this reduction in immune response has not been established (Prymula, 2009).

Use of this vaccine for specific medical and/or other indications (eg, immunocompromising conditions, hepatic or kidney disease, diabetes) is also addressed in the ACIP Recommended Immunization Schedule (CDC/ACIP [Akinsanya-Beysolow, 2014]; CDC/ACIP [Bridges, 2014]). Specific recommendations for use of this vaccine in immunocompromised patients with asplenia, cancer, HIV infection, cerebrospinal fluid leaks, cochlear implants, hematopoietic stem cell transplant (prior to or after), sickle cell disease, solid organ transplant (prior to or after), or those receiving immunosuppressive therapy for chronic conditions, as well as contacts of immunocompromised patients, are available from the IDSA (Rubin, 2014).

Adverse Reactions All serious adverse reactions must be reported to the U.S. Department of Health and Human Services (DHHS) Vaccine Adverse Event Reporting System (VAERS) 1-800-822-7967 or online at https://vaers.hhs.gov/esub/index. In Canada, adverse reactions may be reported to local provincial/territorial health agencies or to the Vaccine Safety Section at Public Health Agency of Canada (1-866-844-0018).

Central nervous system: Chills, disturbed sleep, fatigue, headache, irritability, malaise, nervousness

Dermatologic: Contact dermatitis, dermatitis, diaper rash, eczema, miliaria, pruritus, rash at injection site (varicella-like), urticaria, varicella-like rash, xeroderma

Gastrointestinal: Abdominal pain, constipation, decreased appetite, diarrhea, nausea, period of tooth development, vomiting

Genitourinary: Herpes labialis

Hematologic & oncologic: Lymphadenopathy

Hypersensitivity: Hypersensitivity reaction

Local: Injection site reaction

Neuromuscular & skeletal: Arthralgia, myalgia, neck stiffness

Otic: Otitis

Respiratory: Cough, respiratory tract disease (lower/upper)

Miscellaneous: Fever

Rare but important or life-threatening: Anaphylactic shock, anaphylaxis, aplastic anemia, aseptic meningitis, ataxia, Bell's palsy, cerebrovascular accident, encephalitis, erythema multiforme, febrile seizures, Guillain-Barre syndrome, hemiparesis (acute), hepatitis, herpes zoster, IgA vasculitis, necrotizing retinitis (immunocompromised patients), pneumonitis, seizure (nonfebrile), Stevens-Johnson syndrome, thrombocytopenia (including immune thrombocytopenia), transverse myelitis, varicella (disseminated or vaccine strain)

◄ **Drug Interactions**

Metabolism/Transport Effects None known.

Avoid Concomitant Use

Avoid concomitant use of Varicella Virus Vaccine with any of the following: Belimumab; Fingolimod; Immunosuppressants

Increased Effect/Toxicity

The levels/effects of Varicella Virus Vaccine may be increased by: 5-ASA Derivatives; Belimumab; Corticosteroids (Systemic); Dimethyl Fumarate; Fingolimod; Hydroxychloroquine; Immunosuppressants; Leflunomide; Mercaptopurine; Methotrexate; Salicylates; Smallpox Vaccine

Decreased Effect

Varicella Virus Vaccine may decrease the levels/effects of: Tuberculin Tests

The levels/effects of Varicella Virus Vaccine may be decreased by: Dimethyl Fumarate; Fingolimod; Immune Globulins; Immunosuppressants

Stability

Vaccine: Store intact vials in freezer at -50°C to -15°C (-58°F to 5°F); use of dry ice may subject vaccine to temperatures colder than -58°F (-50°C); may be stored at 2°C to 8°C (36°F to 46°F) for 72 hours; if not used within 72 hours, vaccine should be discarded; protect from light. Diluent: Store at 20°C to 25°C (68°F to 77°F) or in refrigerator.

Reconstituted vaccine: Discard after 30 minutes if not used; do not freeze reconstituted vaccine.

Mechanism of Action As a live, attenuated vaccine, varicella virus vaccine offers active immunity to disease caused by the varicella-zoster virus by inducing cell mediated and humoral immune responses

Pharmacodynamics

Onset of action: Seroconversion occurred in 97% of healthy children ~4 to 6 weeks following a one-dose regimen; using a two-dose regimen, the seroconversion rate was 99.9% 6 weeks after the second dose. In adolescents≥13 years of age and adults, the seroconversion rate was ~75% 4 weeks after the first dose and 99% 4 weeks after the second dose

Duration: Antibody titers detectable at 10 years postvaccination. Actual antibody titers vary by year and age group but are ~99% to 100% for children at 10 years and 100% for adolescents and adults at 6 years postvaccination. Exposure to wild-type varicella may boost antibody levels.

Dosing: Usual

Pediatric:

Primary immunization: Children ≥12 months:

CDC (ACIP) recommendations: SubQ: 0.5 mL per dose for a total of 2 doses administered as follows: 12 to 15 months of age and 4 to 6 years of age. The second dose may be administered earlier provided ≥3 months have elapsed after the first dose (CDC/ACIP [Marin, 2007]). If the second dose was administered ≥4 weeks after the first dose, it may be considered as valid (CDC/ACIP [Akinsanya-Beysolow, 2014]).

Manufacturer's labeling: SubQ: 0.5 mL per dose; a second dose may be administered ≥3 months later

Catch-up immunization: CDC (ACIP) recommendations (Akinsany-Beysolow, 2014): **Note:** Do not restart the series. If doses have been given, begin the below schedule at the applicable dose number. SubQ: 0.5 mL per dose for a total of 2 doses administered as follows: First dose given on the elected date

Second dose given at least 3 months after the first dose (if age <13 years) or at least 4 weeks after the first dose (if age ≥13 years)

Postexposure prophylaxis (healthy, previously unvaccinated individuals): Children (≥12 months) and Adolescents: SubQ: 0.5 mL administered ideally within 72 hours postexposure but may be used up to 120 hours (5 days) postexposure

Adult:

Primary immunization: All patients without evidence of immunity (CDC/ACIP [Bridges, 2014]):

Varicella vaccine-naïve: SubQ: 0.5 mL per dose, followed by a second dose at least 4 to 8 weeks later

Previously received 1 dose of varicella vaccine: SubQ: 0.5 mL as a single dose

Postexposure prophylaxis (healthy, previously unvaccinated individuals): SubQ: 0.5 mL administered ideally within 72 hours postexposure but may be used up to 120 hours (5 days) postexposure

Dosage adjustment in renal impairment: There are no dosage adjustments provided in manufacturer's labeling.

Dosage adjustment in hepatic impairment: There are no dosage adjustments provided in manufacturer's labeling.

Administration Reconstitute vaccine with 0.7 mL of the provided diluent. Gently agitate to mix thoroughly. Total volume of reconstituted vaccine will be ~0.5 mL. Inject subcutaneously into the outer aspect of the upper arm or anterolateral aspect of the thigh; **not for I.V. or I.M. administration**. Adolescents and adults should be vaccinated while seated or lying down. U.S. law requires that the date of administration, the vaccine manufacturer, lot number of vaccine, and the administering person's name, title, and address be entered into the patient's permanent medical record.

Monitoring Parameters Rash, fever; observe for syncope for 15 minutes following administration. If seizure-like activity associated with syncope occurs, maintain patient in supine or Trendelenburg position to re-establish adequate cerebral perfusion.

Additional Information Evidence of immunity to varicella includes any of the following (CDC/ACIP [Marin, 2007]):

Documentation of age-appropriate vaccination with varicella vaccine.

Laboratory evidence of immunity or laboratory confirmation of disease.

Birth in the United States prior to 1980 (except for health care personnel, pregnant women, and the immunocompromised).

Diagnosis or verification of varicella disease by health care provider.

Diagnosis or verification of herpes zoster by health care provider.

In order to maximize vaccination rates, the ACIP recommends simultaneous administration (ie, >1 vaccine on the same day at different anatomic sites) of all age-appropriate vaccines (live or inactivated) for which a person is eligible at a single visit, unless contraindications exist. If available, the use of combination vaccines is generally preferred over separate injections, taking into consideration provider assessment, patient preference, and potential adverse events. If separate vaccines being used, evaluate product information regarding same syringe compatibility of vaccines. Separate needles and syringes should be used for each injection. The ACIP prefers each dose of specific vaccine in a series come from the same manufacturer if possible (CDC/ACIP [Kroger, 2011]).

For additional information, please refer to the following website: http://www.cdc.gov/vaccines/vpd-vac/.

Dosage Forms Excipient information presented when available (limited, particularly for generics); consult specific product labeling.

Injectable, Subcutaneous [preservative free]:

Varivax: 1350 PFU/0.5 mL (1 ea)

References

AAP Steering Committee on Quality Improvement and Management, Subcommittee on Febrile Seizures American Academy of Pediatrics, "Febrile Seizures: Clinical Practice Guideline for the Long-Term Management of the Child With Simple Febrile Seizures," *Pediatrics,* 2008, 121(6):1281-6.

Akinsanya-Beysolow I, Advisory Committee on Immunization Practices (ACIP), ACIP Child/Adolescent Immunization Work Group, et al. Advisory committee on immunization practices recommended immunization schedule for adults aged 19 years or older - United States, 2014. *MMWR Morb Mortal Wkly Rep.* 2014; 63(5):108-109. Full schedule available at http://www.cdc.gov/vaccines/schedules/downloads/child/0-18yrs-child-combined-schedule.pdf

Bridges CB, Coyne-Beasley T, Advisory Committee on Immunization Practices (ACIP), ACIP Adult Immunization Work Group; Centers for Disease Control and Prevention (CDC). Advisory committee on immunization practices recommended immunization schedule for adults aged 19 years or older - United States, 2014. *MMWR Morb Mortal Wkly Rep.* 2014; 63(5):108-109. Available at: http://www.cdc.gov/vaccines/schedules/downloads/adult/adult-combined-schedule.pdf

Centers for Disease Control and Prevention (CDC), "Prevention of Varicella: Recommendations of the Advisory Committee on Immunization Practices (ACIP)," *MMWR Recomm Rep,* 2007, 56(RR-4):1-40. Available at http://www.cdc.gov/mmwr/preview/mmwrhtml/rr5604a1.htm

Centers for Disease Control and Prevention (CDC), "Recommendations of the Advisory Committee on Immunization Practices (ACIP): General Recommendations on Immunization," *MMWR Recomm Rep,* 2011, 60(2):1-61. Available at http://www.cdc.gov/mmwr/pdf/rr/rr6002.pdf

Centers for Disease Control and Prevention (CDC), "Syncope After Vaccination-United States, January 2005-July 2007," *MMWR Morb Mortal Wkly Rep,* 2008, 57(17):457-60.

Chaves SS, Gargiullo P, Zhang JX, et al, "Loss of Vaccine-Induced Immunity to Varicella Over Time," *N Engl J Med,* 2007, 356 (11):1121-9.

Kroger AT, Atkinson WL, Marcuse EK, Pickering LK. General recommendations on immunization - recommendations of the Advisory Committee on Immunization Practices (ACIP). *MMWR Recomm Rep.* 2011;60(RR-2):1-64.

Kuter BJ, Weibel RE, Guess HA, et al, "Oka/Merck Varicella Vaccine in Healthy Children: Final Report of a 2-Year Efficacy Study and 7-Year Follow-Up Studies," *Vaccine,* 1991, 9(9):643-7.

Marin M, Güris D, Chaves SS, Schmid S, Seward JF, Advisory Committee on Immunization Practices. Prevention of varicella: recommendations of the Advisory Committee on Immunization Practices (ACIP). *MMWR Recomm Rep.* 2007;56(RR-4):1-40. Available at http://www.cdc.gov/mmwr/preview/mmwrhtml/rr5604a1.htm

Prymula R, Siegrist CA, Chlibek R, et al, "Effect of Prophylactic Paracetamol Administration at Time of Vaccination on Febrile Reactions and Antibody Responses in Children: Two Open-Label, Randomised Controlled Trials," *Lancet,* 2009, 374(9698):1339-50.

Rubin LG, Levin MJ, Ljungman P, et al. 2013 IDSA clinical practice guideline for vaccination of the immunocompromised host. *Clin Infect Dis.* 2014;58(3):e44-e100.

◆ **Varicella Zoster** *see* Varicella-Zoster Immune Globulin (Human) *on page 2119*

Varicella-Zoster Immune Globulin (Human)

(var i SEL a- ZOS ter i MYUN GLOB yoo lin HYU man)

Medication Safety Issues
Sound-alike/look-alike issues:
Varicella virus vaccine has been given in error (instead of the indicated varicella immune globulin) to pregnant women exposed to varicella.

Related Information
Immunization Administration Recommendations *on page 2368*

Immunization Guidelines *on page 2373*

Brand Names: U.S. VariZIG

Brand Names: Canada VariZIG

Therapeutic Category Immune Globulin

Generic Availability (U.S.) No

Use Postexposure prophylaxis of varicella in high-risk individuals including: Immunocompromised children and adults; newborns of mothers with varicella shortly before or after delivery; premature infants, neonates, and infants <1 year of age; adults without evidence of immunity; pregnant women (FDA approved in all ages)

The Advisory Committee on Immunization Practices (ACIP) recommends varicella-zoster immune globulin (VZIG) for patients who are at high risk for severe varicella infection and complications, patients who were exposed to varicella or herpes zoster, and patients for whom varicella vaccine is contraindicated. The decision to use VZIG should take into consideration if the patient lacks evidence of immunity, if exposure is likely to result in an infection, and if the patient is at greater risk for varicella complications than the general population. The following are patient groups for whom VZIG is recommended (CDC, 2013):

- Immunocompromised patients without evidence of immunity, including those with neoplastic disease (eg, leukemia or lymphoma), primary or acquired immunodeficiency, and immunosuppressive therapy (including steroid therapy equivalent to prednisone ≥2 mg/kg or 20 mg/day)
- Newborn of mother who had onset of chickenpox within 5 days before delivery or within 48 hours after delivery
- Hospitalized premature infants (≥28 weeks gestation) who were exposed during the neonatal period and whose mother has no history of chickenpox
- Hospitalized premature infants (<28 weeks gestation or ≤1000 g) regardless of maternal history and who were exposed during the neonatal period
- Pregnant women without evidence of immunity who have been exposed

Pregnancy Risk Factor C

Pregnancy Considerations Animal reproduction studies have not been conducted. Endogenous immune globulins cross the placenta. Clinical use of other immunoglobulins suggest that there are no adverse effects on the fetus. Women who do not have evidence of immunity to varicella may be at increased risk of complications if infected during pregnancy. Varicella infection in the mother can also lead to intrauterine infection in the fetus. VZIG is primarily used to prevent maternal complications, not fetal infection (CDC, 2007).

Breast-Feeding Considerations It is not known if this preparation is excreted into breast milk; endogenous immune globulins can be found in breast milk (Agarwal, 2011). The manufacturer recommends that caution be used if administered to breast-feeding women.

Contraindications Hypersensitivity to VZIG, immune globulin, or any component; IgA deficiency with the presence of anti-IgA antibodies and a history of hypersensitivity

Warnings Varicella zoster immune globulin should be administered as soon as possible following exposure (within 96 hours, preferred) to reduce the severity of varicella. There is no evidence which shows therapy will reduce the incidence of chickenpox infection after exposure to varicella zoster virus or that it will effect established varicella zoster virus infections. According to CDC guidelines, healthy and immunocompromised patients [except bone marrow transplant (BMT) recipients] with positive history of varicella infection are considered immune. BMT patients who had varicella infection *prior to* transplant are **not** considered immune. BMT patients who develop varicella infection *after* transplant **are** considered immune. Patients receiving monthly treatments of high-dose intravenous immunoglobulins (IVIG) (≥400 mg/kg) are likely to be protected and probably do not require VZIG if the last dose of IVIG was given in the 3 weeks before exposure. Patients who are fully vaccinated, but later became immunocompromised, should be monitored closely; treatment with VZIG is not indicated, but other therapy may be needed if disease occurs (CDC, 2007).

Hypersensitivity and anaphylactic reactions can occur; immediate treatment (including epinephrine 1:1000) ▶

should be available. Reactions can occur in patients with IgA deficiency or hypersensitivity reactions to human globulin. Product of human plasma; may potentially contain infectious agents which could transmit disease. Screening of donors, as well as testing and/or inactivation or removal of certain viruses, reduces the risk. Infections thought to be transmitted by this product should be reported to the manufacturer (Cangene Corporation 800-768-2304).

Thrombotic events may occur during or following treatment with intravenous immune globulin products; those at risk include patients with multiple cardiovascular risk factors, history of atherosclerosis, advanced age, impaired cardiac output, coagulation disorders, prolonged periods of immobilization, and/or known hyperviscosity disorders; consider baseline assessment of blood viscosity in patients at risk for hyperviscosity (patients with cryoglobulins, fasting chylomicronemia/markedly high triglycerides, or monoclonal gammopathies). Contains polysorbate 80 (Tween 80) which may cause allergic reactions in susceptible individuals. In premature neonates, thrombocytopenia, ascites, pulmonary deterioration, and renal and hepatic failure have been reported after receiving parenteral products containing polysorbate 80 (Alade, 1986; CDC, 1984).

Precautions Use with caution in patients with a history of bleeding disorders (including thrombocytopenia) and/or patients on anticoagulant therapy; bleeding/hematoma may occur from I.M. administration.

Adverse Reactions
U.S. labeling:
Central nervous system: Chills, fatigue. headache
Dermatologic: Skin rash
Gastrointestinal: Nausea
Local: Pain at injection site
Rare but important or life-threatening: Deep vein thrombosis, hypersensitivity reaction, serum sickness, thrombosis

Canadian labeling:
Cardiovascular: Flushing
Central nervous system: Chills, dizziness, fatigue, headache, insomnia, pain
Dermatologic: Dermatitis, skin rash (including erythematous)
Gastrointestinal: Dysgeusia, nausea
Local: Injection site reaction (bruising, itching, pain, or tenderness), pain at injection site
Neuromuscular & skeletal: Myalgia, neck pain
Miscellaneous: Fever

Drug Interactions
Metabolism/Transport Effects None known.
Avoid Concomitant Use There are no known interactions where it is recommended to avoid concomitant use.
Increased Effect/Toxicity There are no known significant interactions involving an increase in effect.
Decreased Effect
Varicella-Zoster Immune Globulin (Human) may decrease the levels/effects of: Vaccines (Live)

Stability Store at 2°C to 8°C (36°F to 46°F); do not freeze. Reconstituted solution can be stored for up to 12 hours at 2°C to 8°C (36°F to 46°F) prior to use.

Mechanism of Action Antibodies obtained from pooled human plasma of individuals with high titers of varicella-zoster provide passive immunity.

Pharmacodynamics Duration: 3 weeks

Pharmacokinetics (Adult data unless noted)
Half-life: 26.2 ± 4.6 days
Time to peak serum concentration: Within 5 days

Dosing: Neonatal Postexposure prophylaxis, varicella:
I.M.: **Note:** Administration should begin as soon as possible and within 10 days after exposure (CDC, 2013). High-risk, susceptible patients who are re-exposed >3 weeks after a prior dose of VZIG should receive another full dose;

there is no evidence VZIG modifies established varicella-zoster infections. The minimum dose is 62.5 units.
≤2 kg: 62.5 units
2.1 to 10 kg: 125 units

Dosing: Usual Note: Administration should begin as soon as possible and within 10 days after exposure (CDC, 2013). In hematopoietic cell transplant (HCT) recipients who are exposed to varicella or zoster or a varicella zoster vaccine vaccinee who develops a varicella-like rash, administration should occur within 96 hours, ideally within 48 hours (Tomblyn, 2009). High-risk, susceptible patients who are re-exposed >3 weeks after a prior dose of VZIG should receive another full dose; there is no evidence VZIG modifies established varicella-zoster infections. The minimum dose is 62.5 units and the maximum dose is 625 units.

Pediatric: **Postexposure prophylaxis, varicella:** Infants, Children, and Adolescents: I.M.:
2.1 to 10 kg: 125 units
10.1 to 20 kg: 250 units
20.1 to 30 kg: 375 units
30.1 to 40 kg: 500 units
>40 kg: 625 units

Adult: **Postexposure prophylaxis, varicella:** Patient weight >40 kg: I.M.: 625 units; **Note:** Refer to pediatric dosing for weight based dosing in adults ≤40 kg.

Administration For I.M. administration only. Reconstitute with 1.25 mL of diluent; use only the provided diluent; inject diluent slowly and at an angle onto the inside glass wall of the vial. Gently invert vial and swirl to dissolve; do not shake. Final concentration: 100 units/mL.

Administer I.M. into deltoid muscle or anterolateral aspect of upper thigh; avoid gluteal region; may require ≥2 injections depending on patient size. Do not exceed 3 mL per injection site.

Monitoring Parameters Observe for adverse effects following administration; baseline assessment of blood viscosity in patients at risk for hyperviscosity; signs and symptoms of varicella infection for 28 days after VZIG administration (CDC, 2013).

Test Interactions May cause false-positive test for immunity to VZV for 3 months following administration. May cause a false-positive Coomb's test.

Additional Information In susceptible children and adults for whom the varicella vaccine is not contraindicated, live varicella virus vaccine can be given within 3-5 days after exposure to prevent or modify infection severity. There is no evidence VZIG modifies established varicella-zoster infections.

VZIG contains <40 mcg/mL of IgA

Dosage Forms Excipient information presented when available (limited, particularly for generics); consult specific product labeling.
Solution Reconstituted, Injection [preservative free]:
VariZIG: 125 units (1 ea) [contains polysorbate 80]

References
Agarwal S, Karmaus W, Davis S, et al, "Immune Markers in Breast Milk and Fetal and Maternal Body Fluids: A Systematic Review of Perinatal Concentrations," *J Hum Lact*, 2011, 27(2):171-86.

Alade SL, Brown RE, and Paquet A Jr, "Polysorbate 80 and E-Ferol Toxicity," *Pediatrics*, 1986, 77(4):593-7.

Centers for Disease Control and Prevention (CDC), "FDA Approval of an Extended Period for Administering VariZIG for Postexposure Prophylaxis of Varicella," *MMWR Morb Mortal Wkly Rep*, 2012, 61 (12):212.

Centers for Disease Control and Prevention (CDC), "Prevention of Varicella: Recommendations of the Advisory Committee on Immunization Practices (ACIP), *MMWR Recomm Rep*, 2007, 56(RR-4):1-40. Available at http://www.cdc.gov/mmwr/preview/mmwrhtml/rr5604a1.htm

Centers for Disease Control and Prevention (CDC), "Unusual Syndrome With Fatalities Among Premature Infants: Association With a New Intravenous Vitamin E Product," *MMWR Morb Mortal Wkly Rep*, 1984, 33(14):198-9.

Centers for Disease Control and Prevention (CDC), "Updated Recommendations for Use of VariZIG - United States, 2013," *MMWR Morb Mortal Wkly Rep*, 2013, 62(28):574-6.

Tomblyn M, Chiller T, Einsele H, et al. Guidelines for preventing infectious complications among hematopoietic cell transplantation recipients: a global perspective. *Biol Blood Marrow Transplant*. 2009;15(10):1143-1238.

◆ **Varicella-Zoster Virus (VZV) Vaccine (Varicella)** *see* Varicella Virus Vaccine *on page 2116*

◆ **Varilrix (Can)** *see* Varicella Virus Vaccine *on page 2116*

◆ **Varivax** *see* Varicella Virus Vaccine *on page 2116*

◆ **Varivax III (Can)** *see* Varicella Virus Vaccine *on page 2116*

◆ **VariZIG** *see* Varicella-Zoster Immune Globulin (Human) *on page 2119*

◆ **VasoClear [OTC]** *see* Naphazoline (Ophthalmic) *on page 1470*

◆ **VasoClear-A [OTC]** *see* Naphazoline (Ophthalmic) *on page 1470*

◆ **Vasocon® (Can)** *see* Naphazoline (Ophthalmic) *on page 1470*

Vasopressin (vay soe PRES in)

Medication Safety Issues
High alert medication:
The Institute for Safe Medication Practices (ISMP) includes this medication (I.V. or intraosseous administration) among its list of drugs which have a heightened risk of causing significant patient harm when used in error.

Administration issues:
Use care when prescribing and/or administering vasopressin solutions. Close attention should be given to concentration of solution, route of administration, dose, and rate of administration (units/minute, units/kg/minute, units/kg/hour).

Related Information
Adult ACLS Algorithms *on page 2198*
Management of Drug Extravasations *on page 2255*

Brand Names: U.S. Pitressin Synthetic

Brand Names: Canada Pressyn®; Pressyn® AR

Therapeutic Category Antidiuretic Hormone Analog; Hormone, Posterior Pituitary

Generic Availability (U.S.) Yes

Use Treatment of diabetes insipidus; prevention and treatment of postoperative abdominal distention; differential diagnosis of diabetes insipidus [FDA approved in pediatric patients (age not specified) and adults]. Has also been used as an adjunct in the treatment of acute massive hemorrhage of GI tract or esophageal varices; treatment of pulseless arrest, ventricular fibrillation or tachycardia, and asystole/pulseless electrical activity; vasodilatory/septic shock with hypotension unresponsive to fluid resuscitation or exogenous catecholamines; cardiac arrest secondary to anaphylaxis (unresponsive to epinephrine); and donor management of brain-dead patients (hormone replacement therapy).

Pregnancy Risk Factor C

Pregnancy Considerations Animal reproduction studies have not been conducted. Vasopressin and desmopressin have been used safely during pregnancy based on case reports.

Breast-Feeding Considerations Based on case reports, vasopressin and desmopressin have been used safely during nursing.

Contraindications Hypersensitivity to vasopressin or any component

Warnings I.V. infiltration may lead to severe vasoconstriction and localized tissue necrosis. May cause water intoxication; early signs include drowsiness, listlessness, and headache; these should be recognized to prevent coma and seizures.

Precautions Use with caution in patients with seizure disorders, migraine, asthma, vascular disease, renal disease, cardiac disease, goiter with cardiac complications, arteriosclerosis, chronic nephritis with nitrogen retention; an increased risk of cardiac arrest has been reported in adults receiving I.V. infusions at rates >0.05 units/minute

Adverse Reactions
Cardiovascular: Arrhythmia, asystole (>0.04 units/minute), blood pressure increased, cardiac output decreased (>0.04 units/minute), chest pain, MI, vasoconstriction (with higher doses), venous thrombosis

Central nervous system: Fever, pounding in head, vertigo

Dermatologic: Circumoral pallor, ischemic skin lesions, urticaria

Gastrointestinal: Abdominal cramps, flatulence, mesenteric ischemia, nausea, vomiting

Genitourinary: Uterine contraction

Neuromuscular & skeletal: Tremor

Respiratory: Bronchial constriction

Miscellaneous: Diaphoresis

Drug Interactions
Metabolism/Transport Effects None known.

Avoid Concomitant Use There are no known interactions where it is recommended to avoid concomitant use.

Increased Effect/Toxicity There are no known significant interactions involving an increase in effect.

Decreased Effect There are no known significant interactions involving a decrease in effect.

Food Interactions Ethanol may decrease the antidiuretic effect. Management: Avoid ethanol.

Mechanism of Action Increases cyclic adenosine monophosphate (cAMP) which increases water permeability at the renal tubule resulting in decreased urine volume and increased osmolality; causes peristalsis by directly stimulating the smooth muscle in the GI tract; direct vasoconstrictor without inotropic or chronotropic effects

Pharmacodynamics I.M., SubQ:
Onset of action: 1 hour
Duration: 2-8 hours

Pharmacokinetics (Adult data unless noted)
Destroyed by trypsin in GI tract, must be administered parenterally

Metabolism: Most of dose is rapidly metabolized in liver and kidney

Half-life: 10-35 minutes

Dosing: Neonatal I.V.: **Note:** Units of measure vary by indication and age (ie, milliunits/kg/**hour**, units/kg/**hour**, milliunits/kg/minute, units/kg/minute); extra precautions should be taken.

Vasodilatory shock with hypotension unresponsive to fluid resuscitation and exogenous catecholamines: Note: Limited information available; efficacy results variable; optimal dose and timing have not been clearly established: Continuous I.V. infusion: 0.17-10 milliunits/kg/minute (0.01-0.6 units/kg/**hour**) have been used; doses were initiated at the lower end of the range and titrated to effect in most studies. Dosing based on retrospective reviews and case reports that have shown increases in arterial blood pressure and urine output and also allowed for dosage reductions of additional vasopressors (Bidegain, 2010; Brierley, 2009; Choong, 2008; Ikegami, 2010; Meyer, 2008); further studies needed.

Dosing: Usual Note: Units of measure vary by indication and age (ie, milliunits/kg/**hour**, units/kg/**hour**, milliunits/kg/minute, units/kg/minute); extra precautions should be taken.

Diabetes insipidus:

I.M., SubQ: (Highly variable dosage; titrate dosage based upon serum and urine sodium and osmolality in addition to fluid balance and urine output)

Children: 2.5-10 units 2-4 times/day

Adults: 5-10 units 2-4 times/day as needed

Continuous I.V. infusion: Children and Adults: Initial: 0.5 milliunits/kg/**hour** (0.0005 units/kg/**hour**); double dosage as needed every 30 minutes to a maximum of 10 milliunits/kg/**hour** (0.01 units/kg/**hour**)

Donor management in brain-dead patients (hormone replacement therapy): Continuous I.V. infusion:

Infants, Children, and Adolescents: (Nakagawa/NATCO Guidelines, 2008): 0.5-1 milliunits/kg/**hour** (0.0005-0.001 units/kg/**hour**); titrate dose to maintain urine output at 3-4 mL/kg/**hour**. In one retrospective case-controlled study (n=34, age: 8.2 ± 6.2 years), the average dose was 41 milliunits/kg/**hour** (0.041 units/kg/**hour**) (Katz, 2000).

Adults: Initial: 1 unit bolus, followed by 0.5-4 units/**hour** (Rosendale, 2003; UNOS Critical Pathway, 2002)

GI hemorrhage: Continuous I.V. infusion (may also be infused directly into the superior mesenteric artery):

Children: Initial: 2-5 milliunits/kg/minute (0.002-0.005 units/kg/minute); titrate dose as needed; maximum dose: 10 milliunits/kg/minute (0.01 units/kg/minute) (Tuggle, 1988)

Alternative: Initial: 0.1 units/minute; increase by 0.05 units/minute to a maximum of:

<5 year: 0.2 units/minute

5-12 years: 0.3 units/minute

>12 years: 0.4 units/minute

If bleeding stops for 12 hours, then taper off over 24-48 hours.

Adults: Initial: 0.2-0.4 units/minute, then titrate dose as needed (maximum dose: 0.8 units/minute); if bleeding stops, continue at same dose for 12 hours, then taper off over 24-48 hours

Pulseless arrest, ventricular fibrillation, ventricular tachycardia:

Infants, Children, and Adolescents: I.V.: Limited data available: 0.4 units/kg after traditional resuscitation methods and at least two doses of epinephrine have been administered; **Note:** Due to insufficient evidence, no formal recommendations for or against the routine use of vasopressin during pediatric cardiac arrest are provided (Duncan, 2009; Mann, 2002; PALS, 2010).

Adults: I.V., I.O.: 40 units; may give one dose to replace first or second dose of epinephrine. I.V./I.O. drug administration is preferred, but if no access, may give endotracheally. ACLS guidelines do not recommend a specific endotracheal dose; however, may be given endotracheally using the same I.V. dose (ACLS, 2010; Wenzel, 1997).

Vasodilatory shock with hypotension unresponsive to fluid resuscitation and exogenous catecholamines: Continuous I.V. infusion:

Infants and Children: 0.17-8 milliunits/kg/minute (0.01-0.48 units/kg/**hour** has been used; efficacy results have varied; optimal dose and timing has not been established. Dosing based on retrospective reviews and case reports that have shown increases in arterial blood pressure and urine output and also allowed for dosage reductions of additional vasopressors (Brierley, 2009; Choong, 2008; Meyer, 2008). The only double-blind, placebo-controlled trial (n=65, age: 3-14 years) evaluated a dose of 0.5-2 milliunits/kg/minute (0.03-0.12 units/kg/**hour**) at multiple centers and found no significant difference in the time to reach hemodynamic stability and a trend toward increased mortality in the vasopressin group was noted. Based on these findings, the authors did not recommend

routine use of vasopressin; further evaluations of dosing regimens needed (Choong, 2009)

Adults: Initial: 0.01-0.04 units/minute; titrate to effect (doses >0.04 units/minute have been associated with increased risk of cardiovascular side effects); most case reports have used 0.04 units/minute continuous infusion as a fixed dose

Note: Abrupt discontinuation of infusion may result in hypotension; to discontinue gradually taper infusion

Dosing adjustment in hepatic impairment: Some patients with cirrhosis respond to much lower doses

Administration Parenteral:

I.V.: Continuous infusion: Dilute in NS or D$_5$W to a final concentration of 0.1-1 unit/mL. In one clinical trial with lower dosing (eg, 0.0005 units/kg/**hour**) in pediatric patients, a more diluted solution (eg, 20 units in 500 mL D$_5$W) was employed (Wise-Faberowski, 2004). Infusion through central line is strongly recommended.

I.M.: Administer without further dilution.

Endotracheal: Administer, then flush with 5-10 mL NS, followed by several manual ventilations.

Vesicant/Extravasation Risk Vesicant

Monitoring Parameters Fluid intake and output, urine specific gravity, urine and serum osmolality, serum and urine sodium; hemoglobin and hematocrit (GI bleeding)

Reference Range Vasopressin concentration:

Basal: <4 pg/mL

Water deprivation: 10 pg/mL

Shock: 100-1000 pg/mL (biphasic response)

Dosage Forms Excipient information presented when available (limited, particularly for generics); consult specific product labeling.

Solution, Injection:

Pitressin Synthetic: 20 units/mL (1 mL) [contains chlorobutanol (chlorobutol)]

Generic: 20 units/mL (0.5 mL, 1 mL, 10 mL)

References

Bidegain M, Greenberg R, Simmons C, et al, "Vasopressin for Refractory Hypotension in Extremely Low Birth Weight Infants," *J Pediatr,* 2010, 157(3):502-4.

Brierley J, Carcillo JA, Choong K, et al, "Clinical Practice Parameters for Hemodynamic Support of Pediatric and Neonatal Septic Shock: 2007 Update From the American College of Critical Care Medicine," *Crit Care Med,* 2009, 37(2):666-88.

Choong K and Kissoon N, "Vasopressin in Pediatric Shock and Cardiac Arrest," *Pediatr Crit Care Med,* 2008, 9(4):372-9.

Choong K, Bohn D, Fraser DD, et al, "Vasopressin in Pediatric Vasodilatory Shock: A Multicenter Randomized Controlled Trial," *Am J Respir Crit Care Med,* 2009, 180(7):632-9.

Duncan JM, Meaney P, Simpson P, et al, "Vasopressin for In-Hospital Pediatric Cardiac Arrest: Results From the American Heart Association National Registry of Cardiopulmonary Resuscitation," *Pediatr Crit Care Med,* 2009, 10(2):191-5.

Field JM, Hazinski MF, Sayre MR, et al, "Part 1: Executive Summary: 2010 American Heart Association Guidelines for Cardiopulmonary Resuscitation and Emergency Cardiovascular Care," *Circulation,* 2010, 122(18 Suppl 3):S640-56.

Hodges BM and Fraser G, "Vasopressin for Vasodilatory Shock," *Hosp Pharm,* 2002, 37(11):1149-57.

Ikegami H, Funato M, Tamai H, et al, "Low-Dose Vasopressin Infusion Therapy for Refractory Hypotension in ELBW Infants," *Pediatr Int,* 2010, 52(3):368-73.

Katz K, Lawler J, Wax J, et al, "Vasopressin Pressor Effects in Critically Ill Children During Evaluation for Brain Death and Organ Recovery," *Resuscitation,* 2000, 47(1):33-40.

Kleinman ME, Chameides L, Schexnayder SM, et al, "Part 14: Pediatric Advanced Life Support: 2010 American Heart Association Guidelines for Cardiopulmonary Resuscitation and Emergency Cardiovascular Care," *Circulation,* 2010, 122(18 Suppl 3):S876-908.

Koshman SL, Zed PJ, and Abu-Laban RB, "Vasopressin in Cardiac Arrest," *Ann Pharmacother,* 2005, 39(10):1687-92.

Liedel JL, et al, "The Successful Use of Vasopressin in Children With Hypotension," *Crit Care Med,* 2001, 29(12):A63.

Mann K, Berg RA, and Nadkarni V, "Beneficial Effects of Vasopressin in Prolonged Pediatric Cardiac Arrest: A Case Series," *Resuscitation,* 2002, 52(2): 149-56.

Meyer S, Gortner L, McGuire W, et al, "Vasopressin in Catecholamine-Refractory Shock in Children," *Anaesthesia,* 2008, 63(3):228-34.

Nakagawa TA, "Pediatric Donor Management Guidelines. NATCO, The Organization for Transplant Professionals," 2008, *UpToDate®*, Basow DS, ed, Waltham, MA: *UpToDate®*, 2011. Available at http://www.uptodate.com

Neumar RW, Otto CW, Link MS, et al, "Part 8: Adult Advanced Cardiovascular Life Support: 2010 American Heart Association Guidelines for Cardiopulmonary Resuscitation and Emergency Cardiovascular Care," *Circulation*, 2010, 122(18 Suppl 3):S729-67.

Rosendale JD, Kauffman HM, McBride MA, et al, "Aggressive Pharmacologic Donor Management Results in More Transplanted Organs," *Transplantation*, 2003, 75(4):482-7.

Rosenzweig EB, Starc TJ, Chen JM, et al, "Intravenous Arginine-Vasopressin in Children With Vasodilatory Shock After Cardiac Surgery," *Circulation*, 1999, 100(19 Suppl):II182-6.

Tuggle DW, Bennett KG, Scott J, et al, "Intravenous Vasopressin and Gastrointestinal Hemorrhage in Children," *J Pediatr Surg*, 1988, 23 (7):627-9.

UNOS, "Critical Pathway for Donation After Cardiac Death." Available at http://www.unos.org/docs/Critical_Pathway_DCD_Donor.pdf

Wenzel V, Lindner KH, Prengel AW, et al, "Endobronchial Vasopressin Improves Survival During Cardiopulmonary Resuscitation in Pigs," *Anesthesiology*, 1997, 86(6):1375-81.

Wise-Faberowski L, Soriano SG, Ferrari L, et al, "Perioperative Management of Diabetes Insipidus in Children," *J Neurosurg Anesthesiol*, 2004, 16(3):220-5.

◆ **Vasotec** *see* Enalapril *on page 744*

◆ **Vasotec I.V (Can)** *see* Enalaprilat *on page 747*

◆ **Vaxigrip (Can)** *see* Influenza Virus Vaccine (Inactivated) *on page 1103*

◆ **Vectical** *see* Calcitriol *on page 342*

Vecuronium (vek ue ROE nee um)

Medication Safety Issues
Sound-alike/look-alike issues:
Vecuronium may be confused with valproate sodium, vancomycin
Norcuron® may be confused with Narcan®
High alert medication:
The Institute for Safe Medication Practices (ISMP) includes this medication among its list of drugs which have a heightened risk of causing significant patient harm when used in error.
Other safety concerns:
United States Pharmacopeia (USP) 2006: The Interdisciplinary Safe Medication Use Expert Committee of the USP has recommended the following:
- Hospitals, clinics, and other practice sites should institute special safeguards in the storage, labeling, and use of these agents and should include these safeguards in staff orientation and competency training.
- Healthcare professionals should be on high alert (especially vigilant) whenever a neuromuscular-blocking agent (NMBA) is stocked, ordered, prepared, or administered.

Brand Names: Canada Norcuron®
Therapeutic Category Neuromuscular Blocker Agent, Nondepolarizing; Skeletal Muscle Relaxant, Paralytic
Generic Availability (U.S.) Yes
Use Adjunct to anesthesia, to facilitate endotracheal intubation, and provide skeletal muscle relaxation during surgery or mechanical ventilation (FDA approved in ages >7 weeks to 16 years and adults)
Pregnancy Risk Factor C
Pregnancy Considerations There are no adequate and well-controlled studies in pregnant women. Use in cesarean section has been reported. Umbilical venous concentrations were 11% of maternal. Use only if the potential benefit justifies the potential risk to the fetus.
Breast-Feeding Considerations It is not known if vecuronium is excreted in breast milk. The manufacturer recommends that caution be exercised when administering vecuronium to nursing women.
Contraindications Hypersensitivity to vecuronium or any component

Warnings Ventilation must be supported during neuromuscular blockade; vecuronium should only be administered by individuals who are experienced in the maintenance of an adequate airway and respiratory support **[U.S. Boxed Warning]**. Vecuronium does not alter consciousness; use in conjunction with adequate sedation or anesthesia. Severe allergic reactions have been reported with neuromuscular blocking agents including vecuronium; cross-sensitivity with other neuromuscular blocking agents may occur; use extreme caution in patients with previous anaphylactic reactions.

Commercially supplied diluent contains benzyl alcohol which may cause allergic reactions in susceptible individuals; large amounts of benzyl alcohol (≥99 mg/kg/day) have been associated with a potentially fatal toxicity ("gasping syndrome") in neonates; the "gasping syndrome" consists of metabolic acidosis, respiratory distress, gasping respirations, CNS dysfunction (including convulsions, intracranial hemorrhage), hypotension, and cardiovascular collapse; *in vitro* and animal studies have shown that benzoate, a metabolite of benzyl alcohol, displaces bilirubin from protein binding sites; avoid use of benzyl alcohol containing diluent in neonates; SWI may be used for reconstitution in neonates.

Precautions Use with caution in patients with hepatic impairment, neuromuscular disease, myasthenia gravis. Many clinical conditions may potentiate or antagonize neuromuscular blockade, see table.

Clinical Conditions Affecting Neuromuscular Blockade

Potentiation	Antagonism
Acidosis	Alkalosis
Acute intermittent porphyria	Demyelinating lesions
Electrolyte abnormalities	Diabetes mellitus
Hypermagnesemia	Hypercalcemia
Severe hypocalcemia	Peripheral neuropathies
Severe hypokalemia	
Severe hyponatremia	
Hepatic failure	
Neuromuscular diseases	
Renal failure	

Adverse Reactions Rare but important or life-threatening: Acute quadriplegic myopathy syndrome (prolonged use), Bradycardia, circulatory collapse, edema, flushing; hypersensitivity reaction (hypotension, tachycardia, erythema, rash, urticaria); itching, myositis ossificans (prolonged use), rash
Drug Interactions
Metabolism/Transport Effects None known.
Avoid Concomitant Use
Avoid concomitant use of Vecuronium with any of the following: QuiNINE
Increased Effect/Toxicity
Vecuronium may increase the levels/effects of: Cardiac Glycosides; Corticosteroids (Systemic); OnabotulinumtoxinA; RimabotulinumtoxinB

The levels/effects of Vecuronium may be increased by: AbobotulinumtoxinA; Aminoglycosides; Calcium Channel Blockers; Capreomycin; Clindamycin (Topical); Colistimethate; CycloSPORINE (Systemic); Dantrolene; Fosphenytoin-Phenytoin; Inhalational Anesthetics; Ketorolac (Nasal); Ketorolac (Systemic); Lincosamide Antibiotics; Lithium; Loop Diuretics; Magnesium Salts; Piperacillin; Polymyxin B; Procainamide; QuiNIDine; QuiNINE; Spironolactone; Tetracycline Derivatives; Vancomycin

Decreased Effect

The levels/effects of Vecuronium may be decreased by: Acetylcholinesterase Inhibitors; CarBAMazepine; Fosphenytoin-Phenytoin; Loop Diuretics

Stability Store intact vials at 20°C to 25°C (68°F to 77°F); protect from light. Stable for 5 days at room temperature or under refrigeration when reconstituted with bacteriostatic water; stable for 24 hours under refrigeration when reconstituted with preservative-free SWI or other compatible I.V. fluid (dextrose, NS, or LR) (avoid preservatives in neonates); do not mix with alkaline drugs

Mechanism of Action Blocks acetylcholine from binding to receptors on motor endplate inhibiting depolarization

Pharmacodynamics

Onset of action: Within 1-3 minutes

Duration (dose dependent): 30-40 minutes

Pharmacokinetics (Adult data unless noted)

Distribution: V_d:

Infants: 0.36 L/kg

Children: 0.2 L/kg

Adults: 0.27 L/kg

Protein binding: 60% to 80%

Half-life, distribution: Adults: 4 minutes

Half-life, elimination:

Infants: 65 minutes

Children: 41 minutes

Adults: 65-75 minutes

Elimination: Vecuronium bromide and its metabolite(s) appear to be excreted principally in feces via biliary elimination (50%); the drug and its metabolite(s) are also excreted in urine (25%); the rate of elimination is appreciably reduced with hepatic dysfunction but not with renal dysfunction

Dosing: Neonatal Paralysis/skeletal muscle relaxation: I.V.: 0.1 mg/kg/dose; maintenance: 0.03-0.15 mg/kg/dose every 1-2 hours as needed

Dosing: Usual Paralysis/skeletal muscle relaxation:

Infants >7 weeks to 1 year:

I.V.: 0.1 mg/kg/dose; repeat every hour as needed

Continuous I.V. infusion: 1-1.5 **mcg**/kg/minute (0.06-0.09 mg/kg/**hour**)

Children and Adolescents >1-16 years:

I.V.: 0.1 mg/kg/dose; repeat every hour as needed

Continuous I.V. infusion: 1.5-2.5 **mcg**/kg/minute (0.09-0.15 mg/kg/**hour**)

Adults:

I.V.: 0.1 mg/kg/dose; repeat every hour as needed

Continuous I.V. infusion: 0.8-1.7 **mcg**/kg/minute (0.05-0.1 mg/kg/**hour**)

Dosing adjustment in hepatic impairment: Dose reductions are necessary in patients with cirrhosis or cholestasis

Usual Infusion Concentrations: Neonatal I.V. infusion: 1 mg/mL

Usual Infusion Concentrations: Pediatric I.V. infusion: 0.1 mg/mL, 0.2 mg/mL, 1 mg/mL

Administration Parenteral: I.V.: Dilute vial to a maximum concentration of 2 mg/mL and administer by rapid direct injection; for continuous infusion, dilute to a maximum concentration of 1 mg/mL in D_5W, NS, or LR; use SWI instead of provided diluent (contains benzyl alcohol) in neonates

Monitoring Parameters Assisted ventilation status, heart rate, blood pressure, peripheral nerve stimulator measuring twitch response

Additional Information Produces minimal, if any, histamine release

Dosage Forms Excipient information presented when available (limited, particularly for generics); consult specific product labeling.

Solution Reconstituted, Intravenous, as bromide:

Generic: 10 mg (1 ea); 20 mg (1 ea)

Solution Reconstituted, Intravenous, as bromide [preservative free]:

Generic: 10 mg (1 ea); 20 mg (1 ea)

References

Kumar P, Denson SE, Mancuso TJ, et al, "Premedication for Nonemergency Endotracheal Intubation in the Neonate," *Pediatrics*, 2010, 125(3):608-15.

Martin LD, Bratton SL, and O'Rourke PP, "Clinical Uses and Controversies of Neuromuscular Blocking Agents in Infants and Children," *Crit Care Med*, 1999, 27(7):1358-68.

Phillips MS, "Standardizing I.V. Infusion Concentrations: National Survey Results," *Am J Health Syst Pharm*, 2011, 68(22):2176-82.

Velaglucerase Alfa (vel a GLOO ser ase AL fa)

Brand Names: U.S. Vpriv

Brand Names: Canada VPRIV

Therapeutic Category Enzyme, Glucocerebrosidase; Gaucher's Disease, Treatment Agent

Generic Availability (U.S.) No

Use Long-term enzyme replacement therapy (ERT) for patients with Type 1 Gaucher's disease (FDA approved in ages ≥4 years and adults)

Pregnancy Risk Factor B

Pregnancy Considerations Teratogenic effects were not observed in animal reproduction studies. Pregnancy may exacerbate existing type I Gaucher disease or result in new symptoms. Women with type I Gaucher disease have an increased risk of spontaneous abortion if disease is not well controlled. Adverse pregnancy outcomes, including hepatosplenomegaly and thrombocytopenia, may occur.

Breast-Feeding Considerations It is not known if velaglucerase alfa is excreted in breast milk. The manufacturer recommends that caution be used if administered to nursing women.

Contraindications Hypersensitivity to velaglucerase alfa or any component

Warnings Hypersensitivity reactions, including anaphylaxis, have been reported; appropriate medical support should be readily available. Hypersensitivity reactions including asthenia, dizziness, fatigue, fever, headache, hypo-/hypertension, and nausea were frequently reported (during clinical trials: ~52% in treatment-naïve, 22% previous enzyme replacement therapy); majority of reactions mild and occurred more frequently during the first 6 months of treatment and decreased with frequency over time. Management strategies are based on severity; more severe reactions may require symptomatic treatment, pretreatment with antihistamines, antipyretics and/or corticosteroids; and slowing the infusion rate. Treatment should be discontinued if anaphylaxis or other acute reactions occur.

Precautions Development of IgG antibodies has been reported; the clinical significance is unknown. Patients with an immune response to other enzyme replacement therapies who are switching to velaglucerase alfa should be monitored for antibody development. Pediatric patients (4-17 years) may experience a higher frequency) of some adverse effects than adults (>10% difference in incidence), including: Fever, rash, prolonged aPTT, and upper respiratory tract infection.

Adverse Reactions

Cardiovascular: Flushing, hypertension, hypotension, tachycardia

Central nervous system: Dizziness, fatigue, headache

Dermatologic: Skin rash (more common in children), urticaria

Gastrointestinal: Abdominal pain, nausea

Hematologic & oncologic: Prolonged partial thromboplastin time (more common in children)

Hypersensitivity: Hypersensitivity reaction (including one case of anaphylaxis)

Immunologic: Immunogenicity

Neuromuscular & skeletal: Arthralgia (knee), back pain, ostealgia

Respiratory: Upper respiratory tract infection (more common in children)

Miscellaneous: Fever (more common in children)

Drug Interactions

Metabolism/Transport Effects None known.

Avoid Concomitant Use There are no known interactions where it is recommended to avoid concomitant use.

Increased Effect/Toxicity There are no known significant interactions involving an increase in effect.

Decreased Effect There are no known significant interactions involving a decrease in effect.

Stability Store in refrigerator at 2°C to 8°C (36°F to 46°F); do not freeze; protect from light. Reconstituted or diluted solution stable for 24 hours at 2°C to 8°C (36°F to 46°F); do not use if opaque particles or solution discoloration seen; infusion should be completed within 24 hours of reconstitution of vial

Mechanism of Action Velaglucerase alfa, which contains the same amino acid sequence as endogenous glucocerebrosidase, catalyzes the hydrolysis of glucocerebroside to glucose and ceramide in the lysosome. In patients with type 1 Gaucher's disease, glucocerebrosidase deficiency results in accumulation of glucocerebroside in macrophages, thereby causing the associated signs and symptoms. Velaglucerase alfa is used to diminish hepatosplenomegaly and improve anemia, thrombocytopenia, and bone disease.

Pharmacokinetics (Adult data unless noted) Note: Values reported below based on combined pediatric patient (4-17 years) and adult data.

Distribution: V_{dss}: 0.08-0.11 L/kg

Half-life: 11-12 minutes

Dosing: Usual Note: Pretreatment with antihistamines and/or corticosteroids can be considered for prevention of subsequent infusion reactions in patients with hypersensitivity reactions requiring symptomatic treatment; during clinical studies, patients were not routinely premedicated prior to infusion.

Pediatric: **Gaucher's disease (type 1):** Children and Adolescents 4 to 17 years: I.V.: 60 units/kg every other week; adjust based upon disease activity; dosing range: 15 to 60 units/kg every other week. **Note:** When switching from imiglucerase to velaglucerase alfa, initiate velaglucerase alfa treatment 2 weeks after the last imiglucerase dose and at the same dose as stable imiglucerase therapy.

Adult: **Gaucher's disease (type 1):** I.V.: 60 units/kg administered every 2 weeks; adjust dose based upon disease activity (range: 15 to 60 units/kg evaluated in clinical trials). **Note:** When switching from imiglucerase to velaglucerase alfa in stable patients, initiate treatment 2 weeks after the last imiglucerase dose and at the same dose.

Dosing adjustment in renal impairment: There are no dosage adjustments provided in manufacturer's labeling.

Dosing adjustment in hepatic impairment: There are no dosage adjustments provided in manufacturer's labeling.

Administration Parenteral: For I.V. administration. Reconstitute the 400 unit vial with 4.3 mL of SWI which results in 100 units/mL concentration; further dilute in 100 mL NS; gently mix; do not shake; slight flocculation (white irregular-shaped particles) may occur and is acceptable for administration. Infuse over 60 minutes through an in-line low protein-binding 0.2 micron filter

Monitoring Parameters CBC, liver enzymes, IgG antibodies; MRI, CT, or US of liver and spleen; bone density studies; monitor antibodies in those patients who developed antibodies to other enzyme replacement therapies

Additional Information Gaucher Disease Registry: https://www.registrynxt.com/Gaucher/Pages/Home.aspx

Dosage Forms Excipient information presented when available (limited, particularly for generics); consult specific product labeling.

Solution Reconstituted, Intravenous [preservative free]:

Vpriv: 400 units (1 ea)

References

Baldellou A, Andria G, Campbell PE, et al. Paediatric non-neuronopathic Gaucher disease: recommendations for treatment and monitoring. *Eur J Pediatr.* 2004;163(2):67-75.

Charrow J, Andersson HC, Kaplan P, et al. Enzyme replacement therapy and monitoring for children with type 1 Gaucher disease: consensus recommendations. *J Pediatr.* 2004;144(1):112-120.

VPRIV (velaglucerase alfa) [prescribing information]. Cambridge, MA: Shire Human Genetic Therapies; November 2013.

◆ **Velban** *see* VinBLAStine *on page 2136*

◆ **Veletri** *see* Epoprostenol *on page 770*

◆ **Veltin™** *see* Clindamycin and Tretinoin *on page 503*

Venlafaxine (ven la FAX een)

Medication Safety Issues

Sound-alike/look-alike issues:

Effexor may be confused with Effexor XR

BEERS Criteria medication:

This drug may be potentially inappropriate for use in geriatric patients (Quality of evidence - moderate; Strength of recommendation - strong).

Related Information

Antidepressant Agents *on page 2219*

Oral Medications That Should Not Be Crushed or Altered *on page 2438*

Brand Names: U.S. Effexor XR

Brand Names: Canada Apo-Venlafaxine XR; CO Venlafaxine XR; Dom-Venlafaxine XR; Effexor XR; GD-Venlafaxine XR; Mylan-Venlafaxine XR; PMS-Venlafaxine XR; Ran-Venlafaxine XR; Riva-Venlafaxine XR; Sandoz-Venlafaxine XR; Teva-Venlafaxine XR; Venlafaxine XR

Therapeutic Category Antidepressant, Serotonin/Norepinephrine Reuptake Inhibitor

Generic Availability (U.S.) Yes

Use Treatment of major depressive disorder, generalized anxiety disorder, social anxiety disorder (social phobia), and panic disorder (all indications: FDA approved in adults); has also been used to treat ADHD and autism in children and obsessive-compulsive disorder and chronic fatigue syndrome in adults

Medication Guide Available Yes

Pregnancy Risk Factor C

Pregnancy Considerations Adverse events have been observed in some animal reproduction studies. Venlafaxine and its active metabolite ODV cross the human placenta. An increased risk of teratogenic effects following venlafaxine exposure during pregnancy has not been observed, based on available data. The risk of spontaneous abortion may be increased. Neonatal seizures and neonatal abstinence syndrome have been noted in case reports following maternal use of venlafaxine during pregnancy. Nonteratogenic effects in the newborn following SSRI/SNRI exposure late in the third trimester include respiratory distress, cyanosis, apnea, seizures, temperature instability, feeding difficulty, vomiting, hypoglycemia, hyper- or hypotonia, hyper-reflexia, jitteriness, irritability, constant crying, and tremor. Symptoms may be due to the toxicity of the SNRI or a discontinuation syndrome and may be consistent with serotonin syndrome associated with treatment. The long-term effects of *in utero* SNRI/SSRI exposure on infant development and behavior are not known.

Due to pregnancy-induced physiologic changes, some pharmacokinetic parameters of venlafaxine may be altered. Women should be monitored for decreased effi-cacy. The ACOG recommends that therapy with SSRIs or SNRIs during pregnancy be individualized; treatment of depression during pregnancy should incorporate the clin-ical expertise of the mental health clinician, obstetrician, primary healthcare provider, and pediatrician. According to the American Psychiatric Association (APA), the risks of medication treatment should be weighed against other treatment options and untreated depression. For women who discontinue antidepressant medications during preg-nancy and who may be at high risk for postpartum depres-sion, the medications can be restarted following delivery. Treatment algorithms have been developed by the ACOG and the APA for the management of depression in women prior to conception and during pregnancy.

Breast-Feeding Considerations Venlafaxine and ODV are found in breast milk and the serum of nursing infants. Adverse events have not been observed; however, it is recommended to monitor the infant for adverse events if the decision to breast-feed has been made. The long-term effects on neurobehavior have not been studied, thus one should prescribe venlafaxine to a mother who is breast-feeding only when the benefits outweigh the potential risks. The manufacturer does not recommend breast-feeding during therapy.

Contraindications Hypersensitivity to venlafaxine or any component; use of MAO inhibitors within 14 days (poten-tially fatal reactions may occur); do not initiate MAO inhibitor within 7 days of discontinuing venlafaxine

Warnings Clinical worsening of depression or suicidal ideation and behavior may occur in children and adults with major depressive disorder **[U.S. Boxed Warning]**. In clinical trials, antidepressants increased the risk of suicidal thinking and behavior (suicidality) in children, adolescents, and young adults (18-24 years of age) with major depres-sive disorder and other psychiatric disorders. This risk must be considered before prescribing antidepressants for any clinical use. Short-term studies did **not** show an increased risk of suicidality with antidepressant use in patients >24 years of age and showed a decreased risk in patients ≥65 years.

Patients of all ages who are treated with antidepressants for any indication require appropriate monitoring and close observation for clinical worsening of depression, suicidal-ity, and unusual changes in behavior, especially during the first few months after antidepressant initiation or when the dose is adjusted. Family members and caregivers should be instructed to closely observe the patient (ie, daily) and communicate condition with healthcare provider. Patients should also be monitored for associated behaviors (eg, anxiety, agitation, panic attacks, insomnia, irritability, hos-tility, aggressiveness, impulsivity, akathisia, hypomania, mania) which may increase the risk for worsening depres-sion or suicidality. Worsening depression or emergence of suicidality (or associated behaviors listed above) that is abrupt in onset, severe, or not part of the presenting symptoms, may require discontinuation or modification of drug therapy.

Avoid abrupt discontinuation; discontinuation symptoms (including agitation, dysphoria, anxiety, confusion, dizzi-ness, hypomania, nightmares, and other symptoms) may occur if therapy is abruptly discontinued or dose reduced; risk of discontinuation symptoms may be increased at higher doses and with longer duration of therapy; to discontinue therapy in patients receiving venlafaxine for >1 week, taper the dose to minimize risks of discontinua-tion symptoms; to discontinue therapy in patients receiving venlafaxine for ≥6 weeks, taper the dose gradually over at least 2 weeks; **Note:** Clinical trials of Effexor XR® tapered the daily dose slowly at 1 week intervals by increments of 75 mg; if intolerable symptoms occur following a decrease in dosage or upon discontinuation of therapy, consider

resuming the previous dose with a more gradual taper. To reduce risk of intentional overdose, write prescriptions for the smallest quantity consistent with good patient care.

Screen individuals for bipolar disorder prior to treatment (using antidepressants alone may induce manic episodes in patients with this condition). Venlafaxine may cause sustained increase in blood pressure (dose dependent; monitor blood pressure; dose reduction or discontinuation may be needed). Serotonin syndrome or other serious adverse reactions may occur when venlafaxine is used in combination with serotonergic drugs (eg, triptans) or drugs that impair the metabolism of serotonin (eg, MAO inhib-itors).

Precautions Use with caution; decrease the dose in patients with renal or hepatic impairment or concomitant diseases that may affect hepatic metabolism. Use with caution in patients with seizure disorders; seizures have been reported; discontinue if seizures occur. Use with caution in patients receiving diuretics or those who are volume-depleted; may cause hyponatremia or SIADH. May cause mydriasis; use with caution and closely monitor patients with increased IOP or those at risk of acute narrow-angle glaucoma. May cause anxiety, nervousness, and insomnia. In children treated for ADHD, an increase in hyperactivity (behavioral activation) was reported (Olvera, 1996). Use with caution in patients with a history of mania; may activate mania or hypomania. Use with caution in suicidal patients, children, or during breast-feeding in lactating women. Use with caution during late third trimes-ter of pregnancy; newborns may experience adverse effects or venlafaxine withdrawal symptoms; consider risks and benefits.

May cause anorexia and significant, dose-related weight loss; use with caution in patients where weight loss is undesirable; may adversely affect weight and height in children; monitor closely in pediatric patients; weight loss in pediatric patients was not limited to those with venlafax-ine-associated anorexia; reduction in growth rate, as assessed by height, was greater in children <12 years of age than in adolescents.

Use with caution in patients with diseases that may affect hemodynamic responses (eg, unstable cardiac disease, recent MI); dose-related increases in systolic and diastolic blood pressure have been documented; monitor blood pressure regularly, and if sustained increases noted, con-sider dose reduction or discontinuation. May cause abnor-mal bleeding (eg, ecchymosis); use with caution in patients with abnormal platelet function. A case of priapism has been reported in an adolescent patient (Samuel, 2000). May cause tachycardia; mean increases of 4 bpm and 8.5 bpm have been reported; use with caution in patients with underlying medical conditions (eg, recent MI, heart failure, hyperthyroidism) that may worsen with tachycardia, espe-cially at doses >200 mg/day in adults. In adult studies of depression, Effexor XR® was associated with an increase in QT_c interval of 4.7 msec from baseline (versus a 1.9 msec decrease for placebo); clinical significance of this effect is not known.

Adverse Reactions

Cardiovascular: Chest pain, edema, hypertension, ortho-static hypotension, tachycardia, vasodilation

Central nervous system: Abnormal dreams, abnormal thinking, agitation, amnesia, anxiety, chills, confusion, depression, depersonalization, dizziness, fever, head-ache, hypoesthesia, insomnia, migraine, nervousness, somnolence, vertigo, yawning

Dermatologic: Bruising, pruritus, rash

Endocrine & metabolic: Libido decreased

Gastrointestinal: Abdominal pain, anorexia, appetite increased, belching, constipation, diarrhea, dyspepsia, flatulence, nausea, taste perversion, weight gain/loss, xerostomia

Genitourinary: Abnormal ejaculation/orgasm, impotence, metrorrhagia, prostatic disorder, urinary frequency, urinary impairment, urinary retention, vaginitis

Neuromuscular & skeletal: Arthralgia, hypertonia, neck pain, paresthesia, tremor, trismus, twitching, weakness

Ocular: Abnormal or blurred vision, accommodation abnormal, mydriasis

Otic: Tinnitus

Renal: Albuminuria

Respiratory: Bronchitis, cough increased, dyspnea, pharyngitis, sinusitis

Miscellaneous: Diaphoresis, flu-like syndrome, infection, trauma

Rare but important or life-threatening: Agranulocytosis, anaphylaxis, anemia, aneurysm, angina pectoris, angioedema, anuria, aplastic anemia, appendicitis, arrhythmia (including atrial and ventricular tachycardia, fibrillation, and torsade de pointes), arteritis, asthma, ataxia, atelectasis, atrioventricular block, bacteremia, balance/coordination impaired, basophilia, bigeminy, biliary pain, bilirubinemia, bleeding time increased, bradycardia, bradykinesia, BUN increased, bundle branch block, carcinoma, cardiac arrest, cardiovascular disorder (mitral valve and circulatory disturbance), cataract, catatonia, cellulitis, cerebral ischemia, cholelithiasis, congestive heart failure, coronary artery disease, CPK increased, creatinine increased, crystalluria, cyanosis, deafness, DVT, dehydration, delusions, dementia, diabetes mellitus, dystonia, ECG abnormalities (including QT prolongation), embolus, eosinophilia, erythema multiforme, exfoliative dermatitis, extrapyramidal symptoms, extrasystoles, facial paralysis, fasciitis, fatty liver, gastrointestinal ulcer, glaucoma, glycosuria, granuloma, Guillain-Barré syndrome, hematemesis, hematoma, hemorrhage (eye, GI, mucocutaneous, rectal), hepatic necrosis, hepatic failure, hepatitis, homicidal ideation, hostility, hyperacusis, hypercalcinuria, hyperchlorhydria, hyper-/hypoglycemia, hyper-/hypokalemia, hyper-/hypophosphatemia, hyper-/hypothyroidism, hyperuricemia, hypocholesteremia, hyponatremia, hypoproteinemia, hypotension, interstitial lung disease (including eosinophilic pneumonia), intestinal obstruction, jaundice, kidney function abnormal, larynx edema, leukocytosis, leukoderma, leukopenia, liver enzymes increased, loss of consciousness, lymphadenopathy, lymphocytosis, maculopapular rash, menstrual abnormalities, MI, miliaria, moniliasis, multiple myeloma, myasthenia, myoclonus, myopathy, neck rigidity, neuroleptic malignant-like syndrome, neuropathy, neutropenia, osteoporosis, pancreatitis, pancytopenia, peripheral vascular disorder, pleurisy, pneumonia, pyelonephritis, pyuria, renal failure, rhabdomyolysis, rheumatoid arthritis, seizure, serotonin syndrome, SIADH, skin atrophy, Stevens-Johnson syndrome, suicidal ideation, suicide attempt, syncope, tendon rupture, thrombocythemia, thrombocytopenia, tongue edema, toxic* epidermal necrolysis, withdrawal syndrome

Drug Interactions

Metabolism/Transport Effects Substrate of CYP2C19 (minor), CYP2C9 (minor), CYP2D6 (major), CYP3A4 (major); **Note:** Assignment of Major/Minor substrate status based on clinically relevant drug interaction potential; **Inhibits** CYP2B6 (weak), CYP2D6 (weak), CYP3A4 (weak)

Avoid Concomitant Use

Avoid concomitant use of Venlafaxine with any of the following: Conivaptan; Fusidic Acid (Systemic); Iobenguane I 123; Linezolid; MAO Inhibitors; Methylene Blue; Pimozide; Urokinase

Increased Effect/Toxicity

Venlafaxine may increase the levels/effects of: Agents with Antiplatelet Properties; Alpha-/Beta-Agonists; Anticoagulants; Antipsychotics; Apixaban; ARIPiprazole; Aspirin; Collagenase (Systemic); Dabigatran Etexilate; Highest Risk QTc-Prolonging Agents; Ibritumomab; Lomitapide; Methylene Blue; Moderate Risk QTc-Prolonging Agents; NSAID (Nonselective); Pimozide; Rivaroxaban; Salicylates; Serotonin Modulators; Thrombolytic Agents; Tositumomab and Iodine I 131 Tositumomab; TraZODone; Urokinase; Vitamin K Antagonists

The levels/effects of Venlafaxine may be increased by: Abiraterone Acetate; Alcohol (Ethyl); Antiemetics (5HT3 Antagonists); Antipsychotics; Ceritinib; Conivaptan; CYP2D6 Inhibitors (Moderate); CYP2D6 Inhibitors (Strong); CYP3A4 Inhibitors (Moderate); CYP3A4 Inhibitors (Strong); Dasatinib; Fusidic Acid (Systemic); Glucosamine; Herbs (Anticoagulant/Antiplatelet Properties); Ibrutinib; Ivacaftor; Linezolid; Luliconazole; MAO Inhibitors; Metoclopramide; Mifepristone; Multivitamins/Fluoride (with ADE); Multivitamins/Minerals (with ADEK; Folate, Iron); Multivitamins/Minerals (with AE, No Iron); Nonsteroidal Anti-Inflammatory Agents; Omega-3 Fatty Acids; Pentosan Polysulfate Sodium; Pentoxifylline; Propafenone; Prostacyclin Analogues; Simeprevir; Stiripentol; Vitamin E; Voriconazole

Decreased Effect

Venlafaxine may decrease the levels/effects of: Alpha2-Agonists; Indinavir; Iobenguane I 123; Ioflupane I 123

The levels/effects of Venlafaxine may be decreased by: Bosentan; CYP3A4 Inducers (Strong); Dabrafenib; Deferasirox; Mitotane; Nonsteroidal Anti-Inflammatory Agents; Peginterferon Alfa-2b; Siltuximab; St Johns Wort; Tocilizumab

Stability Tablets and capsules: Store at controlled room temperature, 20°C to 25°C (68°F to 77°F); Effexor XR® 37.5 mg capsules: Protect from light and dispense in light resistant container

Mechanism of Action Venlafaxine and its active metabolite, O-desmethylvenlafaxine (ODV), are potent inhibitors of neuronal serotonin and norepinephrine reuptake and weak inhibitors of dopamine reuptake. Venlafaxine and ODV have no significant activity for muscarinic cholinergic, H_1-histaminergic, or alpha$_2$-adrenergic receptors. Venlafaxine and ODV do not possess MAO-inhibitory activity.

Pharmacokinetics (Adult data unless noted)

Absorption: Oral: ≥92%

Distribution: Distributes into breast milk; breast milk to plasma ratio: Venlafaxine: 2.8-4.8 (mean: 4.1); ODV: 2.8-3.8 (mean: 3.1) (Ilett, 1998)

Mean V_d (apparent): Adults:

Venlafaxine: 7.5 ± 3.7 L/kg

ODV: 5.7 ± 1.8 L/kg

Protein binding: Venlafaxine: 27%; ODV: 30%

Metabolism: Extensive in the liver, primarily via cytochrome P450 CYP2D6 to o-desmethylvenlafaxine (ODV; active metabolite); also metabolized to N-desmethylvenlafaxine, N,O-desmethylvenlafaxine, and other minor metabolites. **Note:** Clinically important differences between CYP2D6 poor and extensive metabolizers is not expected (sum of venlafaxine and ODV serum concentrations is similar in poor and extensive metabolizers; ODV is approximately equal in activity and potency to venlafaxine)

Bioavailability: Oral: 45%

Half-life:

Adults: Venlafaxine: 5 ± 2 hours; ODV: 11 ± 2 hours

Adults with cirrhosis: Venlafaxine: Half-life prolonged by ~30%; ODV: Half-life prolonged by ~60%

Adults with renal impairment (GFR: 10-70 mL/minute): Venlafaxine: Half-life prolonged by ~50%; ODV: Half-life prolonged by ~40%

Adults on dialysis: Venlafaxine: Half-life prolonged by ~180%; ODV: Half-life prolonged by 142%

Time to peak serum concentration:

Immediate release: Venlafaxine: 2 hours; ODV: 3 hours

Extended release: Venlafaxine: 5.5 hours; ODV: 9 hours

Elimination: ~87% of dose is excreted in urine within 48 hours; 5% as unchanged drug, 29% as unconjugated ODV, 26% as conjugated ODV, and 27% as other minor metabolites

Clearance:

Adults with cirrhosis: Venlafaxine: Clearance is decreased by ~50%; ODV: Clearance is decreased by ~30%

Adults with more severe cirrhosis: Venlafaxine: Clearance is decreased by ~90%

Adults with renal impairment (GFR: 10-70 mL/minute): Venlafaxine: Clearance is decreased by ~24%; ODV: Clearance unchanged versus normal subjects

Adults on dialysis: Venlafaxine: Clearance decreased by ~57%; ODV: Clearance decreased by ~56%

Dialysis: Not likely to significantly remove drug due to large volume of distribution

Dosing: Usual Oral:

Children and Adolescents: Note: Not FDA approved. Limited information is available.

ADHD: One open-label clinical trial and one case report are available; 16 children and adolescents (8-16 years of age; mean: 11.6 ± 2.3 years) were enrolled in a 5-week open trial of venlafaxine; doses were initiated at 12.5 mg/day for the first week; for children <40 kg, the daily dose was increased (if tolerated) by 12.5 mg each week to a maximum of 50 mg/day divided in 2 doses; for patients ≥40 kg, the daily dose was increased (if tolerated) by 25 mg each week to a maximum of 75 mg/day divided in 3 doses; mean dose: 60 mg/day (1.4 mg/kg/day) in 2-3 divided doses; 10 patients completed the study [2 were lost to follow-up; 5 discontinued therapy due to adverse effects (4 had an increase in hyperactivity; 1 had severe nausea)]; venlafaxine decreased behavioral symptoms (but not cognitive symptoms) in 7 of 16 subjects (44%) (Olvera, 1996). An initial dose of 37.5 mg given 3 times/day was used in an 11-year-old female with ADHD; the dose was slowly titrated to 100 mg given 3 times/day; after 6 weeks the patient showed moderate to marked improvement in symptoms, but developed hypertension; the dose was then decreased to 75 mg given 3 times/day with normalization of blood pressure (Pleak, 1995). Further studies are needed.

Autism: One retrospective report is available; 10 patients (3-21 years of age; mean 10.5 ± 5.6 years) with autism spectrum disorders (autism, Asperger's syndrome, and pervasive developmental disorders not otherwise specified) received initial doses of 12.5 mg/day administered once daily at breakfast; doses were gradually titrated based on clinical response and side effects; mean final dose: 24.4 mg/day; range: 6.25-50 mg/day; 6 of the 10 patients were sustained-treatment responders (Hollander, 2000). Further studies are needed.

Depression: Note: Due to the lack of demonstrated efficacy and concerns about an increased risk for suicidal behavior, venlafaxine should be reserved for pediatric patients with major depression who do not respond to fluoxetine or sertraline (Dopheide, 2006).

One double-blind, placebo-controlled, 6-week study is available; 33 children and adolescents (8-17 years of age) with major depression completed the trial (16 received venlafaxine; Note: One patient who did not complete the study, discontinued venlafaxine due to development of a manic episode requiring hospitalization and lithium therapy); immediate release venlafaxine was used; for children 8-12 years, doses were initiated at 12.5 mg once daily for 3 days, then

increased to 12.5 mg twice daily for 3 days, then increased to 12.5 mg given 3 times/day for the rest of the study; for adolescents 13-17 years, doses were initiated at 25 mg once daily for 3 days, then increased to 25 mg twice daily for 3 days, then increased to 25 mg given 3 times/day for the rest of the study; both venlafaxine and placebo patients improved over time; however, no significant difference in symptoms was noted between groups (ie, venlafaxine did not have a significant effect on symptoms or specific behaviors); the authors suggest this lack of efficacy may be due to the low doses used and short duration of treatment (Mandoki, 1997).

A large multicenter double-blind, placebo-controlled study of venlafaxine-ER in children and adolescents 7-17 years of age with major depression is ongoing; this study is using higher doses; initial: 37.5 mg/day for 1 week; with increases to 75 mg/day for weeks 2-8; results are not yet available (Weller, 2000). One report of two 16-year-old patients used higher doses of venlafaxine (final doses: 112.5 mg/day and 150 mg/day) in combination with lithium to successfully treat major depression (Walter, 1998). Further studies are needed.

Adults:

Immediate release: Depression: Initial: 75 mg/day in 2-3 divided doses; dose may be increased (if needed) by increments of up to 75 mg/day at intervals of ≥4 days as tolerated, up to 225 mg/day. Note: Doses >225 mg/day for outpatients (moderately depressed patients) were not more effective; more severely depressed patients may require 350 mg/day; maximum: 375 mg/day in 3 divided doses

Extended release:

Depression: Initial: Usual: 75 mg/day; may start with 37.5 mg/day for 4-7 days to allow patient to adjust to medication, then increase to 75 mg/day; dose may be increased (if needed) by increments of up to 75 mg/day at intervals of ≥4 days as tolerated, up to a maximum of 225 mg/day. Note: Although higher doses of the immediate release tablets have been used in more severely depressed inpatients (see above), experience with extended release capsule in doses >225 mg/day is very limited.

Generalized anxiety disorder and social anxiety disorder: 75 mg/day; may start with 37.5 mg/day for 4-7 days to allow patient to adjust to medication, then increase to 75 mg/day. Note: Although a dose-response relationship has not been clearly established, certain patients may benefit from doses >75 mg/day; dose may be increased (if needed) by increments of up to 75 mg/day at intervals of ≥4 days as tolerated, up to a maximum of 225 mg/day.

Panic disorder: Initial: 37.5 mg once daily for 7 days; may increase to 75 mg daily; dose may be increased further (if needed) by increments of up to75 mg/day at intervals of ≥7 days; maximum dose: 225 mg/day

Dosing adjustment in renal impairment: Adults: GFR 10-70 mL/minute: Decrease total daily dose by 25% to 50%

Dosing adjustment in patients on dialysis: Decrease total daily dose by 50%; withhold dose until completion of dialysis treatment; further individualization of dose may be needed

Dosing adjustment in hepatic impairment: Moderate hepatic impairment: Decrease total daily dose by 50%; further individualization of dose may be needed

Administration

Immediate release tablet: Administer with food

Extended release capsule: Administer with food once daily at about the same time each day; swallow whole with fluid; do not crush, chew, divide, or place in water; capsule may be opened and entire contents sprinkled on spoonful of applesauce; swallow drug/food mixture immediately. Do not store for future use; do not chew contents (ie, pellets) of capsule; follow drug/food mixture with water to ensure complete swallowing of pellets.

Monitoring Parameters Monitor blood pressure regularly, especially in patients with high baseline blood pressure; monitor renal and hepatic function (for possible dose reductions), heart rate, weight, height, serum cholesterol and sodium. Monitor patient periodically for symptom resolution; monitor for worsening depression, suicidality, and associated behaviors (especially at the beginning of therapy or when doses are increased or decreased)

Test Interactions May interfere with urine detection of phencyclidine and amphetamine (false-positives).

Additional Information Drug release from extended release capsules is not pH dependent (it is controlled by diffusion through the coating membrane on the spheroids); patients with depression who are receiving immediate release tablets may be switched to Effexor XR® using the nearest mg/day equivalent dose (dosing may require further individualization)

Long-term usefulness of venlafaxine should be periodically re-evaluated in patients receiving the drug for extended periods of time. Neonates born to women receiving venlafaxine, other SNRIs (serotonin and norepinephrine reuptake inhibitors), and SSRIs late during the third trimester may experience respiratory distress, apnea, cyanosis, temperature instability, vomiting, feeding difficulty, hypoglycemia, constant crying, irritability, hypotonia, hypertonia, hyper-reflexia, tremor, jitteriness, and seizures; these symptoms may be due to a direct toxic effect, withdrawal syndrome, or (in some cases) serotonin syndrome. Withdrawal symptoms occur in 30% of neonates exposed to SSRIs and SNRIs *in utero*; monitor newborns for at least 48 hours after birth; long-term effects of *in utero* exposure to SSRIs and SNRIs are unknown (Levinson-Castiel, 2006).

Dosage Forms Excipient information presented when available (limited, particularly for generics); consult specific product labeling.

Capsule Extended Release 24 Hour, Oral:
Effexor XR: 37.5 mg, 75 mg, 150 mg
Generic: 37.5 mg, 75 mg, 150 mg
Tablet, Oral:
Generic: 25 mg, 37.5 mg, 50 mg, 75 mg, 100 mg
Tablet Extended Release 24 Hour, Oral:
Generic: 37.5 mg, 75 mg, 150 mg, 225 mg

References
Dopheide JA, "Recognizing and Treating Depression in Children and Adolescents," *Am J Health Syst Pharm*, 2006, 63(3):233-43.
Emslie GJ, Yeung PP, and Knox NR, "Long-Term, Open-Label Venlafaxine Extended-Release Treatment in Children and Adolescents With Major Depressive Disorder," *CNS Spectr*, 2007, 12(3):223-33.
Hollander E, Kaplan A, Cartwright C, et al, "Venlafaxine in Children, Adolescents, and Young Adults With Autism Spectrum Disorders: An Open Retrospective Clinical Report," *J Child Neurol*, 2000, 15 (2):132-5.
Ilett KF, Hackett LP, Dusci LJ, et al, "Distribution and Excretion of Venlafaxine and O-Desmethylvenlafaxine in Human Milk," *Br J Clin Pharmacol*, 1998, 45(5):459-62.
Lessard E, Yessine MA, Hamelin BA, et al, "Diphenhydramine Alters the Disposition of Venlafaxine Through Inhibition of CYP2D6 Activity in Humans," *J Clin Psychopharmacol*, 2001, 21(2):175-84.
Levinson-Castiel R, Merlob P, Linder N, et al, "Neonatal Abstinence Syndrome After *in utero* Exposure to Selective Serotonin Reuptake Inhibitors in Term Infants," *Arch Pediatr Adolesc Med*, 2006, 160 (2):173-6.
Mandoki MW, Tapia MR, Tapia MA, et al, "Venlafaxine in the Treatment of Children and Adolescents With Major Depression," *Psychopharmacol Bull*, 1997, 33(1):149-54.
Olvera RL, Pliszka SR, Luh J, et al, "An Open Trial of Venlafaxine in the Treatment of Attention-Deficit/Hyperactivity Disorder in Children and Adolescents," *J Child Adolesc Psychopharmacol*, 1996, 6(4):241-50.
Pleak RR and Gormly LJ, "Effects of Venlafaxine Treatment for ADHD in a Child," *Am J Psychiatry*, 1995, 152(7):1099.
Samuel RZ, "Priapism Associated With Venlafaxine Use," *J Am Acad Child Adolesc Psychiatry*, 2000, 39(1):16-7.
Walter G, Lyndon B, and Kubb R, "Lithium Augmentation of Venlafaxine in Adolescent Major Depression," *Aust N Z J Psychiatry* 1998, 32 (3):457-9.
Weller EB, Weller RA, and Davis GP, "Use of Venlafaxine in Children and Adolescents: A Review of Current Literature," *Depress Anxiety*, 2000, 12(Suppl 1):85-9.

◆ **Venlafaxine XR (Can)** see Venlafaxine on page 2125
◆ **Venofer** see Iron Sucrose on page 1155
◆ **Ventolin Diskus (Can)** see Albuterol on page 84
◆ **Ventolin HFA** see Albuterol on page 84
◆ **Ventolin I.V. Infusion (Can)** see Albuterol on page 84
◆ **Ventolin Nebules P.F. (Can)** see Albuterol on page 84
◆ **VePesid** see Etoposide on page 815
◆ **Vepesid™ (Can)** see Etoposide on page 815
◆ **Veramyst** see Fluticasone (Nasal) on page 913

Verapamil (ver AP a mil)

Medication Safety Issues
Sound-alike/look-alike issues:
Calan may be confused with Colace, diltiazem
Covera-HS may be confused with Provera
Isoptin may be confused with Isopto Tears
Verelan may be confused with Voltaren

High alert medication:
The Institute for Safe Medication Practices (ISMP) includes this medication (I.V. formulation) among its list of drug classes which have a heightened risk of causing significant patient harm when used in error.

Administration issues:
Significant differences exist between oral and I.V. dosing. Use caution when converting from one route of administration to another.

International issues:
Dilacor [Brazil] may be confused with Dilacor XR brand name for diltiazem [U.S.]

Related Information
Medications for Which a Single Dose May Be Fatal When Ingested by a Toddler on page 2408
Oral Medications That Should Not Be Crushed or Altered on page 2438

Brand Names: U.S. Calan; Calan SR; Isoptin SR; Verelan; Verelan PM

Brand Names: Canada Apo-Verap; Apo-Verap SR; Covera; Covera-HS; Dom-Verapamil SR; Isoptin SR; Mylan-Verapamil; Mylan-Verapamil SR; Novo-Veramil; Novo-Veramil SR; Nu-Verap; Nu-Verap SR; PHL-Verapamil SR; PMS-Verapamil SR; PRO-Verapamil SR; Riva-Verapamil SR; Verapamil Hydrochloride Injection, USP; Verapamil SR; Verelan

Therapeutic Category Antianginal Agent; Antiarrhythmic Agent, Class IV; Antihypertensive Agent; Calcium Channel Blocker; Calcium Channel Blocker, Nondihydropyridine

Generic Availability (U.S.) Yes

Use
Oral: Treatment of hypertension (all oral products) (FDA approved in adults); angina pectoris (vasospastic, chronic stable, unstable) (Calan®, Covera-HS®) (FDA approved in adults); supraventricular tachyarrhythmia [PSVT (prophylaxis), atrial fibrillation/flutter (rate control)] (Calan®) (FDA approved in adults)
I.V.: Supraventricular tachyarrhythmia [PSVT; atrial fibrillation/flutter (rate control)] (FDA approved in all ages)

Pregnancy Risk Factor C

Pregnancy Considerations Adverse events were observed in some animal reproduction studies in doses which also caused maternal toxicity. Verapamil crosses the placenta. Use during pregnancy may cause adverse fetal effects (bradycardia, heart block, hypotension) (Tan, 2001). Verapamil may be used to control atrial fibrillation in pregnant women (Fuster, 2006). Women with hypertrophic cardiomyopathy who are controlled with verapamil prior to pregnancy may continue therapy, but increased fetal monitoring is recommended (Gersh, 2011). Verapamil is not the preferred treatment for paroxysmal supraventricular tachycardia (PSVT) in pregnant women (Blomström-Lundqvist, 2003). Untreated chronic maternal hypertension is associated with adverse events in the fetus, infant, and mother. If treatment for hypertension during pregnancy is needed, other agents are preferred (ACOG, 2013).

Breast-Feeding Considerations Verapamil is excreted into breast milk; the estimated exposure to the nursing infant is <1% of the maternal dose. Breast-feeding is not recommended by some manufacturers.

Contraindications Hypersensitivity to verapamil or any component; severe left ventricular dysfunction; hypotension or cardiogenic shock; sick sinus syndrome (except in patients with a functioning artificial ventricular pacemaker); second- or third-degree AV block (except in patients with a functioning artificial ventricular pacemaker); atrial flutter or fibrillation associated with an accessory bypass tract [Wolff-Parkinson-White (WPW) syndrome, Lown-Ganong-Levine syndrome]

I.V.: Additional contraindications include concurrent use of I.V. beta-blocking agents; ventricular tachycardia; severe congestive heart failure (unless secondary to supraventricular tachycardia that is treatable with verapamil)

Warnings Avoid I.V. use in neonates and young infants due to severe apnea, bradycardia, hypotensive reactions, cardiac arrest. I.V. use is discouraged in children due to hypotension and myocardial depression. Although effective in terminating SVT in older children, verapamil is not the drug of choice (due to adverse effects) and is not included in the current PALS tachyarrhythmia algorithm. Monitor ECG and blood pressure closely in patients receiving I.V. therapy; have I.V. calcium chloride available at bedside to treat hypotension. I.V. administration, hypertrophic cardiomyopathy, sick sinus syndrome, moderate to severe CHF, concomitant therapy with beta-blockers or digoxin can all increase the incidence of adverse effects.

Use caution when using verapamil together with agents with SA/AV nodal-blocking properties. Administration of I.V. verapamil and an I.V. beta-blocker within a few hours of each other may result in asystole and should be avoided; simultaneous administration is contraindicated. Use with other agents known to reduce SA node function and/or AV nodal conduction (eg, digoxin) or reduce sympathetic outflow (eg, clonidine) may increase the risk of serious bradycardia.

Precautions Use with caution in patients with hypertrophic cardiomyopathy (especially obstructive) or concomitant therapy with beta-blockers or digoxin (verapamil may significantly increase digoxin serum concentrations; adjust digoxin dose). Use caution in patients with hepatic or renal impairment (verapamil dosage reduction may be needed; monitor for signs of overdosage, including hypotension or PR prolongation on ECG). Verapamil may decrease neuromuscular transmission in patients with Duchenne's muscular dystrophy and may worsen myasthenia gravis (use with caution in these patients; verapamil dosage reduction may be needed). Use Covera-HS® with caution in patients with severe GI narrowing (table is nondeformable) and in patients with extremely short GI transit time (<7 hours) (dosage adjustment may be required; pharmacokinetic data are not available).

Adverse Reactions

Cardiovascular: AV block, bradycardia, CHF/pulmonary edema, flushing, hypotension, peripheral edema

Central nervous system: Dizziness, fatigue, headache, lethargy, pain, sleep disturbance

Dermatologic: Rash

Gastrointestinal: Constipation, diarrhea, dyspnea, gingival hyperplasia, nausea

Hepatic: Liver enzymes increased

Neuromuscular & skeletal: Myalgia, paresthesia

Respiratory: Dyspnea

Miscellaneous: Flu-like syndrome

Rare but important or life-threatening:

Oral: Abdominal discomfort, alopecia, angina, arthralgia, atrioventricular dissociation, blurred vision, bruising, cerebrovascular accident, chest pain, claudication, confusion, diaphoresis, ECG abnormal, equilibrium disorders, erythema multiforme, exanthema, extrapyramidal symptoms, galactorrhea/hyperprolactinemia, gastrointestinal distress, gynecomastia, hyperkeratosis, impotence, insomnia, macules, MI, muscle cramps, palpitation, psychosis, purpura (vasculitis), shakiness, somnolence, spotty menstruation, Stevens-Johnson syndrome, syncope, tinnitus, urination increased, urticaria, weakness, xerostomia

I.V.: Bronchi/laryngeal spasm, depression, diaphoresis, itching, muscle fatigue, respiratory failure, rotary nystagmus, seizure, sleepiness, urticaria, vertigo

Postmarketing and/or case reports: Asystole, eosinophilia, EPS, exfoliative dermatitis, GI obstruction, hair color change, paralytic ileus, Parkinsonian syndrome, pulseless electrical activity, shock, ventricular fibrillation

Drug Interactions

Metabolism/Transport Effects Substrate of CYP1A2 (minor), CYP2B6 (minor), CYP2C9 (minor), CYP2E1 (minor), CYP3A4 (major), P-glycoprotein; **Note:** Assignment of Major/Minor substrate status based on clinically relevant drug interaction potential; **Inhibits** CYP1A2 (weak), CYP2C9 (weak), CYP2D6 (weak), CYP3A4 (moderate), P-glycoprotein

Avoid Concomitant Use

Avoid concomitant use of Verapamil with any of the following: Bosutinib; Ceritinib; Conivaptan; Dantrolene; Disopyramide; Dofetilide; Fusidic Acid (Systemic); Ibrutinib; Ivabradine; Lomitapide; PAZOPanib; Pimozide; Silodosin; Simeprevir; Tolvaptan; Topotecan; Ulipristal; VinCRIStine (Liposomal)

Increased Effect/Toxicity

Verapamil may increase the levels/effects of: Afatinib; Alcohol (Ethyl); Aliskiren; Amifostine; Amiodarone; Antihypertensives; ARIPiprazole; AtorvaSTATin; Atosiban; Avanafil; Benzodiazepines (metabolized by oxidation); Beta-Blockers; Bosentan; Bosutinib; Bradycardia-Causing Agents; Brentuximab Vedotin; Budesonide (Systemic, Oral Inhalation); BusPIRone; Calcium Channel Blockers (Dihydropyridine); Cannabis; CarBAMazepine; Cardiac Glycosides; Ceritinib; Colchicine; Corticosteroids (Systemic); CycloSPORINE (Systemic); CYP3A4 Substrates; Dabigatran Etexilate; Disopyramide; Dofetilide; DOXOrubicin (Conventional); Dronabinol; Dronedarone; DULoxetine; Eletriptan; Eplerenone; Everolimus; FentaNYL; Fexofenadine; Fingolimod; Flecainide; Fosphenytoin; Halofantrine; Hypotensive Agents; Ibrutinib; Imatinib; Ivabradine; Ivacaftor; Lithium; Lomitapide; Lovastatin; Lurasidone; Magnesium Salts; Midodrine; Neuromuscular-Blocking Agents (Nondepolarizing); Nitroprusside; Obinutuzumab; OxyCODONE; PAZOPanib; P-glycoprotein/ABCB1 Substrates; Phenytoin; Pimecrolimus; Pimozide; Propafenone; Prucalopride; QuiNIDine; Ranolazine; Red Yeast Rice; Rifaximin; RisperiDONE; RiTUXimab; Rivaroxaban; Salicylates; Salmeterol; Saxagliptin; Silodosin; Simeprevir; Simvastatin; Tacrolimus (Systemic); Tacrolimus (Topical); Tetrahydrocannabinol; Tolvaptan; Topotecan; Ulipristal; Vilazodone; VinCRIStine (Liposomal); Zuclopenthixol

The levels/effects of Verapamil may be increased by: Alfuzosin; Alpha1-Blockers; Anilidopiperidine Opioids;

Antifungal Agents (Azole Derivatives, Systemic); AtorvaSTATin; Barbiturates; Brimonidine (Topical); Calcium Channel Blockers (Dihydropyridine); Cimetidine; CloNIDine; Conivaptan; CycloSPORINE (Systemic); CYP3A4 Inhibitors (Moderate); CYP3A4 Inhibitors (Strong); Dantrolene; Dasatinib; Diazoxide; Dronedarone; Fluconazole; Fusidic Acid (Systemic); Grapefruit Juice; Herbs (Hypotensive Properties); Ivabradine; Luliconazole; Macrolide Antibiotics; Magnesium Salts; MAO Inhibitors; Mifepristone; Pentoxifylline; P-glycoprotein/ABCB1 Inhibitors; Phosphodiesterase 5 Inhibitors; Prostacyclin Analogues; Protease Inhibitors; QuiNIDine; Regorafenib; Stiripentol; Telithromycin

Decreased Effect

Verapamil may decrease the levels/effects of: Clopidogrel; Ifosfamide

The levels/effects of Verapamil may be decreased by: Barbiturates; Bosentan; Calcium Salts; CarBAMazepine; CYP3A4 Inducers (Strong); Dabrafenib; Deferasirox; Efavirenz; Herbs (Hypertensive Properties); Methylphenidate; Mitotane; Nafcillin; P-glycoprotein/ABCB1 Inducers; Rifamycin Derivatives; Siltuximab; St Johns Wort; Tocilizumab; Yohimbine

Food Interactions

Ethanol: Verapamil may increase ethanol levels. Management: Monitor patients and caution about increased effects.

Food: Grapefruit juice may increase the serum concentration of verapamil. Management: Avoid grapefruit juice or use with caution and monitor for effects.

Stability

Injection: Store at controlled room temperature of 15°C to 30°C (59°F to 86°F); protect from light; use only clear solutions. Compatible in solutions of pH of 3-6, but may precipitate in solutions having a pH ≥6

Calan®: Store at 15°C to 25°C (59°F to 77°F); protect from light; dispense in tightly closed, light-resistant container.

Calan® SR: Store at 15°C to 25°C (59°F to 77°F); protect from light and moisture; dispense in tightly closed, light-resistant container.

Covera-HS®: Store at controlled room temperature of 20°C to 25°C (68°F to 77°F); dispense in tightly closed, light-resistant container.

Isoptin® SR: Store at 25°C (77°F); excursions permitted to 15°C to 30°C (59°F to 86°F); protect from light and moisture; dispense in tightly closed, light-resistant container.

Verelan®: Store at controlled room temperature of 20°C to 25°C (68°F to 77°F); avoid excessive heat; dispense in tightly closed, light-resistant container.

Verelan® PM: Store at 25°C (77°F); excursions permitted to 15°C to 30°C (59°F to 86°F); protect from moisture; dispense in tightly closed, light-resistant container.

Mechanism of Action

Inhibits calcium ion from entering the "slow channels" or select voltage-sensitive areas of vascular smooth muscle and myocardium during depolarization; produces relaxation of coronary vascular smooth muscle and coronary vasodilation; increases myocardial oxygen delivery in patients with vasospastic angina; slows automaticity and conduction of AV node.

Pharmacodynamics

Maximum effect:
Oral (nonsustained tablets): 2 hours
I.V.: 1-5 minutes
Duration:
Oral: 6-8 hours
I.V.: 10-20 minutes

Pharmacokinetics (Adult data unless noted)

Absorption: Well-absorbed
Distribution: V_d: 3.89 L/kg (Storstein, 1984)
Protein binding:
Neonates: ~60%

Adults: ~90%
Metabolism: Extensive first-pass effect, metabolized in the liver to several inactive dealkylated metabolites; major metabolite is norverapamil which possesses weak hemodynamic effects (20% that of verapamil)
Bioavailability: Oral: 20% to 30%
Half-life:
Infants: 4.4-6.9 hours
Adults (single dose): 2-8 hours, increased up to 12 hours with multiple dosing
Adults: Severe hepatic impairment: 14-16 hours
Elimination: 70% of dose excreted in urine as metabolites (3% to 4% as unchanged drug), and 16% in feces
Dialysis: Not removed by hemodialysis

Dosing: Usual

I.V.: **Note:** Although verapamil is effective in the treatment of SVT, it is not included in the PALS tachyarrhythmia algorithm due to its adverse effects (PALS, 2010).

Infants: **Should not be used in infants without expert consultation and is generally not recommended**; administer with continuous ECG monitoring, have I.V. calcium available at bedside: 0.1-0.2 mg/kg/dose (usual: 0.75-2 mg/dose) may repeat dose in 30 minutes if adequate response not achieved; **Note:** Optimal interval for subsequent doses is unknown and must be individualized for each specific patient.

Children 1-15 years: 0.1-0.3 mg/kg/dose; maximum dose: 5 mg/dose; may repeat dose in 30 minutes if adequate response not achieved; maximum for second dose: 10 mg/dose; **Note:** Optimal interval for subsequent doses is unknown and must be individualized for each specific patient.

Oral: Dose not well established:
Children: 4-8 mg/kg/day in 3 divided doses
or
1-5 years: 40-80 mg every 8 hours
>5 years: 80 mg every 6-8 hours
Note: A mean daily dose of ~5 mg/kg/day (range: 2.3-8.1 mg/kg/day) was used in 22 children 15 days to 17 years of age receiving chronic oral therapy for SVT (n=20) or hypertrophic cardiomyopathy (n=2) (Piovan, 1995).

Adults:
I.V. (ACLS 2010 guidelines): PSVT (narrow complex, unresponsive to vagal maneuvers and adenosine, in patients with preserved cardiac function): Initial: 2.5-5 mg; if no response in 15-30 minutes and no adverse effects seen, give 5-10 mg every 15-30 minutes to a maximum total dose of 20-30 mg

I.V.: Manufacturer's recommendations: 5-10 mg (0.075-0.15 mg/kg); may repeat 10 mg (0.15 mg/kg) 30 minutes after the initial dose if needed and if patient tolerated initial dose; **Note:** Optimal interval for subsequent doses is unknown and must be individualized for each specific patient.

Angina: Oral: **Note:** When switching from immediate release to extended/sustained release formulations, the total daily dose remains the same unless formulation strength does not allow for equal conversion.

Immediate release: Initial: 80-120 mg 3 times/day (small stature: 40 mg 3 times/day); usual dose range (Gibbons, 2003): 80-160 mg 3 times/day

Extended release: Covera-HS®: Initial: 180 mg once daily at bedtime; if inadequate response, may increase dose at weekly intervals to 240 mg once daily, then 360 mg once daily, then 480 mg once daily; maximum dose: 480 mg/day

Chronic atrial fibrillation (rate control), PSVT prophylaxis: Oral: Immediate release: 240-480 mg/day in 3-4 divided doses; usual dose range (European Heart Rhythm Association, 2006): 120-360 mg/day

Hypertension: Oral: **Note:** When switching from immediate release to extended/sustained release formulations, the total daily dose remains the same unless formulation strength does not allow for equal conversion.

Immediate release: 80 mg 3 times/day; usual dose range (JNC 7): 80-320 mg/day in 2 divided doses

Sustained release: Usual dose range (JNC 7): 120-480 mg/day in 1-2 divided doses; **Note:** There is no evidence of additional benefit with doses >360 mg/day.

Calan® SR, Isoptin® SR: Initial: 180 mg once daily in the morning (small stature: 120 mg/day); if inadequate response, may increase dose at weekly intervals to 240 mg once daily, then 180 mg twice daily (or 240 mg in the morning followed by 120 mg in the evening); maximum dose: 240 mg twice daily

Verelan®: Initial: 180 mg once daily in the morning (small stature: 120 mg/day); if inadequate response, may increase dose at weekly intervals to 240 mg once daily, then 360 mg once daily, then 480 mg once daily; maximum dose: 480 mg/day

Extended release: Usual dose range (JNC 7): 120-360 mg once daily (once daily dosing is recommended at bedtime)

Covera-HS®: Initial: 180 mg once daily at bedtime; if inadequate response, may increase dose at weekly intervals to 240 mg once daily, then 360 mg once daily, then 480 mg once daily; maximum dose: 480 mg/day

Verelan® PM: Initial: 200 mg once daily at bedtime (small stature: 100 mg once daily); if inadequate response, may increase dose at weekly intervals to 300 mg once daily, then 400 mg once daily; maximum dose: 400 mg/day

Dosing adjustment in renal impairment: Children and Adults: Use with caution and closely monitor ECG for PR prolongation, blood pressure, and other signs of overdose; dosage reduction may be needed. The manufacturer of Verelan® PM recommends an initial adult dose of 100 mg/day at bedtime. **Note:** A number of studies show no difference in verapamil (or norverapamil metabolite) disposition between chronic renal failure and control patients, suggesting that dosage adjustment is not required in renal impairment (Beyerlein, 1990; Hanyok, 1988; Mooy, 1985; Zachariah, 1991). However, a study in adults suggests reduced renal clearance of verapamil and its metabolite (norverapamil) with advanced renal failure (Storstein, 1984). Additionally, several clinical papers report adverse effects of verapamil in patients with chronic renal failure receiving recommended doses of verapamil (Pritza, 1991; Váquez, 1996). Thus, prudence dictates cautious use, close monitoring, and dosage adjustment if needed.

Dosing adjustment in hepatic impairment: Children and Adults: In patients with cirrhosis, reduce dose to 20% and 50% of normal dose for oral and intravenous administration, respectively; monitor blood pressure for hypotension and ECG for prolongation of PR interval (Somogyi, 1981). The manufacturer of Verelan PM® recommends an initial adult dose of 100 mg/day at bedtime. The manufacturers of Calan®, Calan® SR, Covera-HS®, Isoptin® SR, and Verelan® recommend giving 30% of the normal dose to patients with severe hepatic impairment.

Administration

Oral: Nonsustained-release tablets can be administered with or without food. Swallow extended and sustained released preparations whole, do not break, chew, or crush. Administer Calan® SR and Isoptin® SR with food on a once daily or twice daily schedule; administer Covera-HS® and Verelan® PM once daily at bedtime. Administer Verelan® (sustained release capsules) once daily in the morning; capsule may be opened and contents sprinkled on a spoonful of applesauce; swallow immediately, do not chew; do not store for future use;

follow with water to ensure complete swallowing of capsule pellets; do not divide capsule

Parenteral: I.V.: Infuse I.V. dose over 2-3 minutes; infuse I.V. over 3-4 minutes if blood pressure is in the lower range of normal: Maximum concentration: 2.5 mg/mL

Monitoring Parameters ECG, blood pressure, heart rate; hepatic enzymes with long-term use

Test Interactions May interfere with urine detection of methadone (false-positive).

Dosage Forms Excipient information presented when available (limited, particularly for generics); consult specific product labeling. [DSC] = Discontinued product

Capsule Extended Release 24 Hour, Oral, as hydrochloride:

Verelan: 120 mg [DSC]

Verelan: 120 mg [contains fd&c red #40, methylparaben, propylparaben]

Verelan: 180 mg [DSC]

Verelan: 180 mg [contains fd&c red #40, methylparaben, propylparaben]

Verelan: 240 mg [DSC]

Verelan: 240 mg [contains brilliant blue fcf (fd&c blue #1), fd&c red #40, methylparaben, propylparaben]

Verelan: 360 mg [DSC]

Verelan: 360 mg [contains brilliant blue fcf (fd&c blue #1), fd&c red #40, methylparaben, propylparaben]

Verelan PM: 100 mg [DSC]

Verelan PM: 100 mg [contains brilliant blue fcf (fd&c blue #1), fd&c red #40]

Verelan PM: 200 mg [DSC]

Verelan PM: 200 mg [contains brilliant blue fcf (fd&c blue #1), fd&c red #40]

Verelan PM: 300 mg [DSC]

Verelan PM: 300 mg [contains brilliant blue fcf (fd&c blue #1), fd&c red #40]

Generic: 100 mg, 120 mg, 180 mg, 200 mg, 240 mg, 300 mg, 360 mg

Solution, Intravenous, as hydrochloride:

Generic: 2.5 mg/mL (2 mL, 4 mL)

Tablet, Oral, as hydrochloride:

Calan: 80 mg, 120 mg [scored]

Generic: 40 mg, 80 mg, 120 mg

Tablet Extended Release, Oral, as hydrochloride:

Calan SR: 120 mg

Calan SR: 180 mg [scored]

Calan SR: 240 mg [scored; contains fd&c blue #2 aluminum lake, fd&c yellow #10 aluminum lake]

Isoptin SR: 120 mg

Isoptin SR: 180 mg [scored]

Isoptin SR: 240 mg [scored; contains fd&c blue #2 aluminum lake, fd&c yellow #10 aluminum lake]

Generic: 120 mg, 180 mg, 240 mg

Extemporaneous Preparations A 50 mg/mL oral suspension may be made with immediate release tablets and either a 1:1 mixture of Ora-Sweet and Ora-Plus or a 1:1 mixture of Ora-Sweet SF and Ora-Plus or cherry syrup. When using cherry syrup, dilute cherry syrup concentrate 1:4 with simple syrup, NF. Crush seventy-five verapamil hydrochloride 80 mg tablets in a mortar and reduce to a fine powder. Add small portions of chosen vehicle (40 mL total) and mix to a uniform paste; mix while adding the vehicle in incremental proportions to **almost** 120 mL; transfer to a calibrated bottle, rinse mortar with vehicle, and add quantity of vehicle sufficient to make 120 mL. Label "shake well", "refrigerate", and "protect from light". Stable for 60 days refrigerated (preferred) or at room temperature (Allen, 1996).

A 50 mg/mL oral suspension may be made with immediate release tablets, a 1:1 preparation of methylcellulose 1% and simple syrup, and purified water. Crush twenty 80 mg verapamil tablets in a mortar and reduce to a fine powder. Add 3 mL purified water USP and mix to a uniform paste;

mix while adding the vehicle incremental proportions to **almost** 32 mL; transfer to a calibrated bottle, rinse mortar with vehicle, and add quantity of vehicle sufficient to make 32 mL. Label "shake well" and "refrigerate". Stable for 91 days refrigerated (preferred) or at room temperature (Nahata, 1997).

Allen LV Jr and Erickson MA 3rd, "Stability of Labetalol Hydrochloride, Metoprolol Tartrate, Verapamil Hydrochloride, and Spironolactone With Hydrochlorothiazide in Extemporaneously Compounded Oral Liquids," *Am J Health Syst Pharm*, 1996, 53(19):304-9.

Nahata MC, "Stability of Verapamil in an Extemporaneous Liquid Dosage Form," *J Appl Ther Res*, 1997,1(3):271-3.

References

American College of Obstetricians and Gynecologists (ACOG), "ACOG Practice Bulletin No. 125: Chronic Hypertension in Pregnancy," *Obstet Gynecol*, 2012, 119(2 Pt 1):396-407.

Beyerlein C, Csaszar G, Hollmann M, et al, "Verapamil in Antihypertensive Treatment of Patients on Renal Replacement Therapy - Clinical Implications and Pharmacokinetics," *Eur J Clin Pharmacol*, 1990, 39 Suppl 1:S35-7.

Blomström-Lundqvist C, Scheinman MM, Aliot EM, et al, "ACC/AHA/ ESC Guidelines for the Management of Patients With Supraventricular Arrhythmias-Executive Summary: A Report of the American College of Cardiology/American Heart Association Task Force on Practice Guidelines and the European Society of Cardiology Committee for Practice Guidelines (Writing Committee to Develop Guidelines for the Management of Patients With Supraventricular Arrhythmias)," *Circulation*, 2003, 108(15):1871-909.

Chobanian AV, Bakris GL, Black HR, et al, "The Seventh Report of the Joint National Committee on Prevention, Detection, Evaluation, and Treatment of High Blood Pressure: The JNC 7 report," *JAMA*, 2003, 289(19):2560-72.

European Heart Rhythm Association; Heart Rhythm Society, Fuster V, et al, "ACC/AHA/ESC 2006 Guidelines for the Management of Patients With Atrial Fibrillation - Executive Summary: A Report of the American College of Cardiology/American Heart Association Task Force on Practice Guidelines and the European Society of Cardiology Committee for Practice Guidelines (Writing Committee to Revise the 2001 Guidelines for the Management of Patients With Atrial Fibrillation)," *J Am Coll Cardiol*, 2006, 48(4):854-906.

Field JM, Hazinski MF, Sayre MR, et al, "Part 1: Executive Summary: 2010 American Heart Association Guidelines for Cardiopulmonary Resuscitation and Emergency Cardiovascular Care," *Circulation*, 2010, 122(18 Suppl 3):S640-56.

Fuster V, Ryden LE, Cannom DS, et al, "ACC/AHA/ESC 2006 Guidelines for the Management of Patients With Atrial Fibrillation-Executive Summary. A Report of the American College of Cardiology/American Heart Association Task Force on Practice Guidelines and the European Society of Cardiology Committee for Practice Guidelines (Writing Committee to Revise the 2001 Guidelines for the Management of Patients With Atrial Fibrillation). Developed in Collaboration With the European Heart Rhythm Association and the Heart Rhythm Society," *J Am Coll Cardiol*, 2006, 48(4):854-906.

Gersh BJ, Maron BJ, Bonow RO, et al, "2011 ACCF/AHA Guideline for the Diagnosis and Treatment of Hypertrophic Cardiomyopathy: A Report of the American College of Cardiology Foundation/American Heart Association Task Force on Practice Guidelines," *Circulation*, 2011, 124(24):e783-831.

Gibbons RJ, Abrams J, Chatterjee K, et al, "ACC/AHA 2002 Guideline Update for the Management of Patients With Chronic Stable Angina - Summary Article: A Report of the American College of Cardiology/ American Heart Association Task Force on Practice Guidelines (Committee on the Management of Patients With Chronic Stable Angina)," *J Am Coll Cardiol*, 2003, 41(1):159-68.

Hanyok JJ, Chow MS, Kluger J, et al, "An Evaluation of the Pharmacokinetics, Pharmacodynamics, and Dialyzability of Verapamil in Chronic Hemodialysis Patients," *J Clin Pharmacol*, 1988, 28(9):831-6.

Kleinman ME, Chameides L, Schexnayder SM, et al, "Part 14: Pediatric Advanced Life Support: 2010 American Heart Association Guidelines for Cardiopulmonary Resuscitation and Emergency Cardiovascular Care," *Circulation*, 2010, 122(18 Suppl 3):S876-908.

Mooy J, Schols M, v Baak M, et al, "Pharmacokinetics of Verapamil in Patients With Renal Failure," *Eur J Clin Pharmacol*, 1985, 28(4):405-10.

Neumar RW, Otto CW, Link MS, et al, "Part 8: Adult Advanced Cardiovascular Life Support: 2010 American Heart Association Guidelines for Cardiopulmonary Resuscitation and Emergency Cardiovascular Care," *Circulation*, 2010, 122(18 Suppl 3):729-67.

Piovan D, Padrini R, Svalato Moreolo G, et al, "Verapamil and Norverapamil Plasma Levels in Infants and Children During Chronic Oral Treatment," *Ther Drug Monit*, 1995, 17(1):60-7.

Pritza DR, Bierman MH, and Hammeke MD, "Acute Toxic Effects of Sustained-Release Verapamil in Chronic Renal Failure," *Arch Intern Med*, 1991, 151(10):2081-4.

Sapire DW, O'Riordan AC, and Black IF, "Safety and Efficacy of Short- and Long-Term Verapamil Therapy in Children With Tachycardia," *Am J Cardiol*, 1981, 48(6):1091-7.

Shakibi JG, "Arrhythmias in Infants and Children," *Pediatrician*, 1981, 10(1-3):117-22.

Somogyi A, Albrecht M, Kliems G, et al, "Pharmacokinetics, Bioavailability and ECG Response of Verapamil in Patients With Liver Cirrhosis," *Br J Clin Pharmacol*, 1981, 12(1):51-60.

Storstein L, Larsen A, Midtbø K, et al, "Pharmacokinetics of Calcium Blockers in Patients With Renal Insufficiency and in Geriatric Patients," *Acta Med Scand Suppl*, 1984, 681:25-30.

Tan HL and Lie KI, "Treatment of Tachyarrhythmias During Pregnancy and Lactation," *Eur Heart J*, 2001, 22(6):458-64.

Váquez C, Huelmos A, Alegría E, et al, "Verapamil Deleterious Effects in Chronic Renal Failure," *Nephron*, 1996, 72(3):461-4.

Zachariah PK, Moyer TP, Theobald HM, et al, "The Pharmacokinetics of Racemic Verapamil in Patients With Impaired Renal Function," *J Clin Pharmacol*, 1991, 31(1):45-53.

◆ **Verapamil Hydrochloride** *see* Verapamil *on page 2129*

◆ **Verapamil Hydrochloride Injection, USP (Can)** *see* Verapamil *on page 2129*

◆ **Verapamil SR (Can)** *see* Verapamil *on page 2129*

◆ **Verelan** *see* Verapamil *on page 2129*

◆ **Verelan PM** *see* Verapamil *on page 2129*

◆ **Veripred 20** *see* PrednisoLONE (Systemic) *on page 1727*

◆ **Vermox** *see* Mebendazole *on page 1313*

◆ **Vermox® (Can)** *see* Mebendazole *on page 1313*

◆ **Versacloz** *see* CloZAPine *on page 527*

◆ **Versed** *see* Midazolam *on page 1411*

◆ **Versel® (Can)** *see* Selenium Sulfide *on page 1877*

◆ **Vertin-32 [OTC]** *see* Meclizine *on page 1317*

◆ **Vesanoid** *see* Tretinoin (Systemic) *on page 2068*

◆ **Vesanoid® (Can)** *see* Tretinoin (Systemic) *on page 2068*

◆ **Vfend** *see* Voriconazole *on page 2150*

◆ **VFEND (Can)** *see* Voriconazole *on page 2150*

◆ **Vfend IV** *see* Voriconazole *on page 2150*

◆ **Viagra** *see* Sildenafil *on page 1884*

◆ **Vibramycin** *see* Doxycycline *on page 721*

◆ **Vibra-Tabs (Can)** *see* Doxycycline *on page 721*

◆ **Vicks 44E [OTC]** *see* Guaifenesin and Dextromethorphan *on page 987*

◆ **Vicks DayQuil Mucus Control DM [OTC]** *see* Guaifenesin and Dextromethorphan *on page 987*

◆ **Vicks Nature Fusion Cough [OTC]** *see* Dextromethorphan *on page 636*

◆ **Vicks Nature Fusion Cough & Chest Congestion [OTC]** *see* Guaifenesin and Dextromethorphan *on page 987*

◆ **Vicks Pediatric Formula 44E [OTC]** *see* Guaifenesin and Dextromethorphan *on page 987*

◆ **Vicodin®** *see* Hydrocodone and Acetaminophen *on page 1027*

◆ **Vicodin ES®** *see* Hydrocodone and Acetaminophen *on page 1027*

◆ **Vicodin HP®** *see* Hydrocodone and Acetaminophen *on page 1027*

◆ **Videx** *see* Didanosine *on page 654*

◆ **Videx® (Can)** *see* Didanosine *on page 654*

◆ **Videx EC** *see* Didanosine *on page 654*

◆ **Videx® EC (Can)** *see* Didanosine *on page 654*

Vigabatrin (vye GA ba trin)

Medication Safety Issues

Sound-alike/look-alike issues:
Vigabatrin may be confused with Vibativ

Related Information

Safe Handling of Hazardous Drugs *on page 2419*

Brand Names: U.S. Sabril

Brand Names: Canada Sabril

Therapeutic Category Anticonvulsant, Miscellaneous; Infantile Spasms, Treatment

Generic Availability (U.S.) No

Use

Powder for oral solution: Monotherapy for treatment of infantile spasms in patients for whom the potential benefits outweigh the potential risk of vision loss (FDA approved in ages 1 month to 2 years); has also been used in children as adjunct therapy for refractory complex partial seizures

Tablet: Adjunct therapy for refractory complex partial seizures not controlled by usual treatments in patients for whom the potential benefits outweigh the potential risk of vision loss (FDA approved in adults)

Prescribing and Access Restrictions As a requirement of the REMS program, access to this medication is restricted. Vigabatrin is only available in the U.S. under a special restricted distribution program (SHARE). Under the SHARE program, only prescribers and pharmacies registered with the program are able to prescribe and distribute vigabatrin. Vigabatrin may only be dispensed to patients who are enrolled in and meet all conditions of SHARE. Contact the SHARE program at 1-888-45-SHARE.

Medication Guide Available Yes

Pregnancy Risk Factor C

Pregnancy Considerations Adverse events were observed in animal reproduction studies. Vigabatrin crosses the placenta in humans (Tran, 1998). Birth defects have been reported following use in pregnancy and include: cardiac defects, limb defects, male genital malformations, fetal anticonvulsant syndrome, renal and ear abnormalities. Time of exposure or maternal dosage was not reported and information is not available relating to the incidence or types of these outcomes in comparison to the general epilepsy population. Visual field examinations have been conducted following in utero exposure in a limited number of children tested at ≥6 years of age; no visual field loss was observed in 4 children and results were inconclusive in 2 others (Lawthorn, 2009; Sorri 2005). Use during pregnancy is contraindicated in Canadian product labeling.

Patients exposed to vigabatrin during pregnancy are encouraged to enroll in the North American Antiepileptic Drug (NAAED) Pregnancy Registry by calling 1-888-233-2334. Additional information is available at www.aedpregnancyregistry.org.

Breast-Feeding Considerations Small amounts of vigabatrin are found in human milk (≤4% of the weight-adjusted maternal dose based on 2 cases) (Tran, 1998). Due to the potential for serious adverse reactions in the nursing infants, the manufacturer recommends a decision be made whether to discontinue nursing or to discontinue the drug, taking into account the importance of the drug to the mother.

Use while breast-feeding is contraindicated in Canadian product labeling.

Contraindications Hypersensitivity to vigabatrin or any component

Warnings Hazardous agent; use appropriate precautions for handling and disposal (NIOSH, 2012). Vigabatrin causes permanent vision loss in a high percentage of patients, including infants, children, and adults. Vision loss is most frequently described as progressive, bilateral concentric visual field constriction; decreased visual acuity has also been reported. Neither type of vision loss is reliably prevented through periodic vision testing. There is no known exposure level of vigabatrin without risk of vision loss; however, risk has been shown to increase with total cumulative dose or duration of therapy **[U.S. Boxed Warning]**. The onset of vision loss is unpredictable, occurring within weeks of starting treatment or sooner, or at any time during treatment, even after months or years of therapy. It has also been reported to worsen despite discontinuation of therapy. Most information characterizing frequency and extent of vision loss is from adult data since vision loss assessment is difficult in infants and children. Vigabatrin causes permanent bilateral concentric visual field constriction in >30% of patients ranging in severity from mild to severe, including tunnel vision to within 10 degrees of visual fixation, and can result in disability. In some cases, vigabatrin can damage the central retina and decrease visual acuity. In infants and children, symptoms of vision loss are unlikely to be recognized by the parent or caregiver until loss is severe. Vision loss of milder severity, although potentially unrecognized by the parent or caregiver, may still adversely affect function. Vision should be assessed to the extent possible at baseline (no later than 4 weeks after initiation), at least every 3 months during therapy, and at 3-6 months after discontinuation. Once detected, vision loss is not reversible. Due to the risk of vision loss and because vigabatrin provides an observable symptomatic benefit when it is effective, the lowest dose and shortest exposure consistent with clinical objectives should be used. If the patient fails to show substantial clinical benefit within a short period of time after initiation of treatment (2-4 weeks for infantile spasms; ≤3 months in adults), vigabatrin therapy should be withdrawn. If in the clinical judgment of the prescriber, evidence of treatment failure becomes obvious earlier in the treatment course, vigabatrin should be discontinued at that time. The interaction of other types of irreversible vision damage with vision damage from vigabatrin has not been well-characterized, but is likely adverse. Vigabatrin should not be used with other drugs associated with serious adverse ophthalmic effects such as retinopathy or glaucoma unless the benefits clearly outweigh the risks. The possibility that vision loss from vigabatrin may be more common, more severe or have more severe functional consequences in infants and children than in adults cannot be excluded. In the U.S., vigabatrin is only available under a special restricted distribution program (SHARE) **[U.S. Boxed Warning]**. Under the SHARE program, only prescribers and pharmacies registered with the program are able to prescribe and distribute vigabatrin. Vigabatrin may only be dispensed to patients who are enrolled in and meet all conditions of SHARE.

Antiepileptic drugs (AEDs) increase the risk of suicidal behavior and ideation in patients receiving these medications for any indication. Pooled analyses of placebo-controlled trials involving 11 different AEDs (regardless of indication) showed a twofold increased risk of suicidal thoughts or behavior (estimated incidence rate: 0.43% in AED treated patients compared to 0.24% of patients receiving placebo); increased risk was observed as early as 1 week after initiation of AED and continued through duration of trials (most trials ≤24 weeks); risk did not vary significantly by age (age range: 5-100 years). Consider risks and benefits of AEDs before prescribing. Monitor all patients receiving an AED for emergence of suicidal thoughts or behavior, thoughts of self-harm, any unusual changes in behavior or mood, or the emergence or worsening of depressive symptoms; notify healthcare provider immediately if symptoms or concerning behavior occur.

Note: The FDA requires a Medication Guide for all anti-epileptic drugs informing patients of this risk.

Precautions Use with caution and reduce dose in patients with renal dysfunction. Anticonvulsants should not be discontinued abruptly because of the possibility of increasing seizure frequency; vigabatrin should be withdrawn gradually to minimize the potential of increased seizure frequency; to withdraw therapy in infants and children, decrease the dose by 25-50 mg/kg/day every 3-4 days; in adults decrease the dose by 1 g/day every week. Vigabatrin should not be used as monotherapy or first line therapy for complex partial seizures. Use with caution when initiating therapy, particularly in patients with myoclonic seizures, as an increase in seizure frequency or onset of new types of seizures may occur.

Dose-dependent, asymptomatic MRI abnormalities have been reported in infants treated with vigabatrin for infantile spasms; resolution of abnormalities generally occurs upon vigabatrin discontinuation; abnormalities resolved in a few infants, despite continued use; some infants displayed coincident motor abnormalities, but no causal relationship has been established; risk for long-term clinical sequelae has not been studied. Animal models have shown intramyelinic edema in the brain; current evidence suggests that this does not occur in humans; however, patients should be monitored for neurotoxicity. A relationship between MRI abnormalities in infants and animal model findings has not been established. In adult patients, peripheral neuropathy manifesting as numbness or tingling in the toes or feet, reduced distal lower limb vibration or position sensation, or progressive loss of reflexes, starting at the ankles, has been reported.

Anemia has been reported; in some cases with a significant reduction in hemoglobin (<8 g/dL) and/or hematocrit (<24%). Somnolence and fatigue can occur with use; higher incidence reported in infants compared to adults (infants: ≤45%; adults: ≤24%); patients must be cautioned about performing tasks which require mental alertness (eg, operating machinery or driving). May cause fever; higher incidence reported in infants than adults (≤30% vs 6%). May cause vomiting; higher incidence in infants (up to 20%). Peripheral edema independent of hypertension, heart failure, weight gain, or renal or hepatic dysfunction has been reported; in adults, an average weight gain of 3.5 kg has been associated with use. Vigabatrin has been reported to decrease AST and ALT activity in the plasma in up to 90% of patients, causing the enzymes to become undetectable in some patients; this may preclude use of AST and ALT as markers for hepatic injury. Infants may experience a higher frequency of other adverse effects than adults, including vomiting and upper respiratory tract infections.

Adverse Reactions

Cardiovascular: Edema, peripheral edema

Central nervous system: Abnormal behavior, abnormal thinking, aggression, anxiety, confusion, coordination impaired, depression, disturbance in attention, dizziness, fatigue, fever, headache, hypoesthesia, hypotonia, insomnia, irritability, lethargy, memory impairment, postictal state, sedation, seizure, sensory disturbance, somnolence, status epilepticus, vertigo

Dermatologic: Contusion, rash

Endocrine & metabolic: Dysmenorrhea, fluid retention

Gastrointestinal: Abdominal distention, abdominal pain, appetite decreased/increased, constipation, diarrhea, dyspepsia, hemorrhoidal symptoms, nausea, viral gastroenteritis, vomiting, weight gain

Genitourinary: Urinary tract infection

Neuromuscular & skeletal: Arthralgia, back pain, dysarthria, extremity pain, hyper-reflexia, hyporeflexia, joint swelling, muscle spasms, myalgia, paresthesia, shoulder pain, tremor, weakness

Ocular: Blurred vision, conjunctivitis, diplopia, eye strain, nystagmus, strabismus, visual field constriction

Otic: Otitis media, tinnitus

Respiratory: Bronchitis, cough, dyspnea, nasal congestion, pharyngitis, pharyngolaryngeal pain, pneumonia, sinus headache, sinusitis, upper respiratory tract infection

Miscellaneous: Candidiasis, croup, influenza, thirst, viral infection

Rare but important or life-threatening: Acute psychosis, angioedema, cholestasis, deafness, delayed puberty, delirium, encephalopathy, facial edema, gastrointestinal hemorrhage, hypomania, laryngoedema, malignant hyperthermia, multiorgan failure, optic neuritis, pruritus, psychotic disorder, pulmonary embolism, respiratory failure, Stevens-Johnson syndrome, toxic epidermal necrolysis

Drug Interactions

Metabolism/Transport Effects Induces CYP2C9 (weak/moderate)

Avoid Concomitant Use

Avoid concomitant use of Vigabatrin with any of the following: Azelastine (Nasal); Paraldehyde; Thalidomide

Increased Effect/Toxicity

Vigabatrin may increase the levels/effects of: Alcohol (Ethyl); Azelastine (Nasal); Buprenorphine; ClonazePAM; CNS Depressants; Hydrocodone; Methotrimeprazine; Metyrosine; Mirtazapine; Paraldehyde; Pramipexole; ROPINIRole; Rotigotine; Selective Serotonin Reuptake Inhibitors; Thalidomide; Zolpidem

The levels/effects of Vigabatrin may be increased by: Brimonidine (Topical); Cannabis; Doxylamine; Dronabinol; Droperidol; HydrOXYzine; Kava Kava; Magnesium Sulfate; Methotrimeprazine; Nabilone; Perampanel; Rufinamide; Sodium Oxybate; Tapentadol; Tetrahydrocannabinol

Decreased Effect

Vigabatrin may decrease the levels/effects of: Fosphenytoin; Phenytoin

The levels/effects of Vigabatrin may be decreased by: Ketorolac (Nasal); Ketorolac (Systemic); Mefloquine; Orlistat

Stability Hazardous agent; use appropriate precautions for handling and disposal (NIOSH, 2012). Store tablet and powder for oral solution at 20°C to 25°C (68°F to 77°F).

Mechanism of Action Irreversibly inhibits gamma-aminobutyric acid transaminase (GABA-T), increasing the levels of the inhibitory compound gamma amino butyric acid (GABA) within the brain. Duration of effect is dependent upon rate of GABA-T resynthesis.

Pharmacodynamics Note: A correlation between serum concentrations and efficacy has not been established.

Duration of action: Variable; dependent on rate of GABA-T resynthesis

Pharmacokinetics (Adult data unless noted)

Absorption: Rapid

Distribution: V_{dss}: 1.1 L/kg

Protein binding: Does not bind to plasma proteins

Metabolism: Minimal

Bioavailability: Oral: Tablet and oral solution are bioequivalent

Half-life: Infants: 5.7 hours; adults: 7.5 hours; prolonged in renal impairment

Time to peak serum concentration: Infants: 2.5 hours; children and adults: 1 hour

Elimination: Urine (80% as unchanged drug)

Clearance:
Infants: 2.4 ± 0.8 L/hour
Children: 5.7 ± 2.5 L/hour
Adults: 7 L/hour

Dialysis: Effect of dialysis has not been adequately studied; in case reports, hemodialysis decreased vigabatrin plasma concentrations by 40% to 60%

Dosing: Usual

Infants, Children, and Adolescents:

Infantile spasms: Infants and Children 1 month to 2 years of age: Oral: Initial: 50 mg/kg/day divided twice daily; may titrate upwards by 25-50 mg/kg/day increments every 3 days based on response and tolerability; maximum dose: 150 mg/kg/day divided twice daily; **Note:** To taper, decrease dose by 25-50 mg/kg/day every 3-4 days.

Refractory complex partial seizures; adjunctive treatment: Limited data available: Oral:

Children ≥10 kg and Adolescents <16 years: Initial: 40 mg/kg/day divided twice daily; maintenance dosages based on patient weight (Camposano, 2008; Coppola, 2004; Willmore, 2009):

10-15 kg: 500-1000 mg/day divided twice daily
16-30 kg: 1000-1500 mg/day divided twice daily
31-50 kg: 1500-3000 mg/day divided twice daily
>50 kg: 2000-3000 mg/day divided twice daily

Adolescents ≥16 years: Initial: 500 mg twice daily; increase daily dose by 500 mg increments at weekly intervals based on response and tolerability; recommended dose: 3000 mg/day divided twice daily; **Note:** To taper, decrease dose by 1000 mg/day on a weekly basis.

Adults: **Refractory complex partial seizures; adjunctive treatment:** Initial: 500 mg twice daily; increase daily dose by 500 mg increments at weekly intervals based on response and tolerability; recommended dose: 3000 mg/day divided twice daily; **Note:** To taper, decrease dose by 1000 mg/day on a weekly basis.

Dosing adjustment in renal impairment: Adults:

CrCl >50-80 mL/minute: Decrease dose by 25%
CrCl >30-50 mL/minute: Decrease dose by 50%
CrCl >10-30 mL/minute: Decrease dose by 75%

Dosing adjustment in hepatic impairment: There are no dosage adjustment provided in manufacturer's labeling; has not been studied; however, does not undergo appreciable hepatic metabolism.

Administration Hazardous agent; use appropriate precautions for handling and disposal (NIOSH, 2012). May be administered without regard to food.

Powder for oral solution: Dissolve each 500 mg powder packet in 10 mL (may use provided syringe to measure) of cold or room temperature water to make a 50 mg/mL solution; discard solution if it is not clear (or free of particles) and colorless. The appropriate dose aliquot should be administered immediately; may use provided oral syringe. Any remaining liquid should be discarded.

Monitoring Parameters Ophthalmologic examination by an ophthalmic professional with expertise in visual field interpretation and the ability to perform dilated indirect ophthalmoscopy of the retina at baseline (no later than 4 weeks after therapy initiation), periodically during therapy (every 3 months), and 3-6 months after discontinuation of therapy; assessment should include visual acuity and visual field whenever possible including mydriatic peripheral fundus examination and visual field perimetry. Observe patient for excessive sedation, especially when instituting or increasing therapy; frequency, duration, and severity of seizure episodes; hemoglobin and hematocrit; renal function; weight; signs and symptoms of suicidality (eg, anxiety, depression, behavior changes), neurotoxicity, peripheral neuropathy, and edema.

Reference Range A correlation between serum concentrations and efficacy has not been established.

Test Interactions Vigabatrin has been reported to decrease AST and ALT activity in the plasma in up to 90% of patients, causing the enzymes to become undetectable in some patients; this may preclude use of AST and ALT as markers for hepatic injury. Vigabatrin may increase amino acids in the urine leading to false-positive tests for rare genetic metabolic disorders

Additional Information Vigabatrin is not effective in absence or febrile seizures; exacerbation of certain seizure types or onset of new types of seizures have been seen after initiation of vigabatrin.

Dosage Forms Excipient information presented when available (limited, particularly for generics); consult specific product labeling.

Packet, Oral:
Sabril: 500 mg (50 ea)

Tablet, Oral:
Sabril: 500 mg [scored]

References

Bar-Oz B, Nulman I, Koren G, et al, "Anticonvulsants and Breast-Feeding: A Critical Review," *Paediatr Drugs*, 2000, 2(2):113-26.

Camposano SE, Major P, Halpern E, et al, "Vigabatrin in the Treatment of Childhood Epilepsy: A Retrospective Chart Review of Efficacy and Safety Profile," *Epilepsia*, 2008, 49(7):1186-91.

Challier JC, Rey E, Bintein T, et al, "Passage of S(+) and R(-) Gamma-Vinyl-GABA Across the Human Isolated Perfused Placenta," *Br J Clin Pharmacol*, 1992, 34(2):139-43.

Coppola G, "Treatment of Partial Seizures in Childhood: An Overview," *CNS Drugs*, 2004, 18(3):133-56.

Lawthom C, Smith PE, and Wild JM, "*In utero* Exposure to Vigabatrin: No Indication of Visual Field Loss," *Epilepsia*, 2009, 50(2):318-21.

Mackay MT, Weiss SK, Adams-Webber T, et al, "Practice Parameter: Medical Treatment of Infantile Spasms: Report of the American Academy of Neurology and the Child Neurology Society," *Neurology*, 2004, 62(10):1668-81.

National Institute for Occupational Safety and Health (NIOSH), "NIOSH List of Antineoplastic and Other Hazardous Drugs in Healthcare Settings 2012." Available at http://www.cdc.gov/niosh/docs/2012-150/pdfs/2012-150.pdf. Accessed January 21, 2013.

Pearl PL, Vezina LG, Saneto RP, et al, "Cerebral MRI Abnormalities Associated With Vigabatrin Therapy," *Epilepsia*, 2009, 50(2):184-94.

Sorri I, Herrgård E, Viinikainen K, et al, "Ophthalmologic and Neurologic Findings in Two Children Exposed to Vigabatrin *in utero*," *Epilepsy Res*, 2005, 65(1-2):117-20.

Tran A, O'Mahoney T, Rey E, et al, "Vigabatrin: Placental Transfer *in vivo* and Excretion Into Breast Milk of the Enantiomers," *Br J Clin Pharmacol*, 1998, 45(4):409-11.

Wheless JW, Carmant L, Bebin M, et al, "Magnetic Resonance Imaging Abnormalities Associated With Vigabatrin in Patients With Epilepsy," *Epilepsia*, 2009, 50(2):195-205.

Willmore LJ, Abelson MB, Ben-Menachem E, et al, "Vigabatrin: 2008 Update," *Epilepsia*, 2009, 50(2):163-73.

◆ **Vigamox** see Moxifloxacin (Ophthalmic) on page 1451

◆ **Vigamox® (Can)** see Moxifloxacin (Ophthalmic) on page 1451

◆ **Vimpat** see Lacosamide on page 1189

VinBLAStine (vin BLAS teen)

Medication Safety Issues

Sound-alike/look-alike issues:

VinBLAStine may be confused with vinCRIStine, vinorelbine

High alert medication:

The Institute for Safe Medication Practices (ISMP) includes this medication among its list of drug classes which have a heightened risk of causing significant patient harm when used in error.

Administration issues:

Must be dispensed in overwrap which bears the statement **"Do not remove covering until the moment of injection. Fatal if given intrathecally. For I.V. use only."** Syringes should be labeled: **"Fatal if given intrathecally. For I.V. use only."**

Related Information

Emetogenic Potential of Antineoplastic Agents in Children on page 2327

Management of Drug Extravasations on page 2255

Safe Handling of Hazardous Drugs on page 2419

Brand Names: Canada Vinblastine Sulphate Injection

Therapeutic Category Antineoplastic Agent, Antimicrotubular; Antineoplastic Agent, Mitotic Inhibitor; Antineoplastic Agent, Vinca Alkaloid

Generic Availability (U.S.) Yes

Use Palliative treatment of Hodgkin's disease; advanced testicular germinal-cell cancers; non-Hodgkin's lymphoma, histiocytosis X (Letterer-Siwe disease), choriocarcinoma, breast cancer, mycosis fungoides, and Kaposi's sarcoma [FDA approved in pediatrics (age not specified) and adults]. Has been used for the treatment of bladder cancer, melanoma, and nonsmall cell lung cancer (NSCLC)

Pregnancy Risk Factor D

Pregnancy Considerations Animal studies have demonstrated resorption and teratogenic effects. There are no adequate and well-controlled studies in pregnant women. Women of childbearing potential should avoid becoming pregnant during vinblastine treatment. Aspermia has been reported in males who have received treatment with vinblastine.

Breast-Feeding Considerations Due to the potential for serious adverse reactions in the nursing infant, breast-feeding is not recommended.

Contraindications Hypersensitivity to vinblastine or any component; severe granulocytopenia; presence of bacterial infection. **I.T. administration is contraindicated (may result in death).**

Warnings Hazardous agent; use appropriate precautions for handling and disposal (NIOSH, 2012); vinblastine can cause fetal toxicity when administered to pregnant women; for I.V. use only; **intrathecal administration may result in death [U.S. Boxed Warning].** Must be dispensed in overwrap which bears the statement: **"Do not remove covering until the moment of injection. Fatal if given intrathecally. For I.V. use only."** Vinblastine is a moderate vesicant; avoid extravasation **[U.S. Boxed Warning].** Assure proper needle or catheter placement prior to administration. Should be administered by individuals experienced in the administration of vinblastine.

Injection (solution) contains benzyl alcohol which may cause allergic reactions in susceptible individuals; large amounts of benzyl alcohol (≥99 mg/kg/day) have been associated with a potentially fatal toxicity ("gasping syndrome") in neonates; the "gasping syndrome" consists of metabolic acidosis, respiratory distress, gasping respirations, CNS dysfunction (including convulsions, intracranial hemorrhage), hypotension and cardiovascular collapse; avoid use of vinblastine products containing benzyl alcohol in neonates; *in vitro* and animal studies have shown that benzoate, a metabolite of benzyl alcohol, displaces bilirubin from protein binding sites

Precautions Use with caution in patients with ischemic heart disease. Acute shortness of breath and severe bronchospasm have been reported in association with concurrent administration of mitomycin; may occur within minutes to several hours following vinblastine administration or up to 14 days following a dose of mitomycin; use caution in patients with preexisting pulmonary disease. Leukopenia is common; granulocytopenia may be severe with higher doses; leukopenia may be more pronounced in cachectic patients and patients with skin ulceration. Thrombocytopenia and anemia may occur rarely. Dosage modification required in patients with impaired liver function or neurotoxicity (may rarely cause reversible disabling neurotoxicity); dosage should be reduced in patients with recent exposure to radiation therapy or chemotherapy.

Itraconazole and erythromycin may decrease the metabolism of vinblastine via CYP3A4 inhibition, and itraconazole may increase the effects of vinblastine via P-glycoprotein effects; severe myelosuppression and neurotoxicity may occur. Should be administered by individuals experienced in the administration of vinblastine **[U.S. Boxed Warning].**

Adverse Reactions

Common:
Cardiovascular: Hypertension
Central nervous system: Malaise
Dermatologic: Alopecia
Gastrointestinal: Constipation
Hematologic: Myelosuppression, leukopenia/granulocytopenia (nadir: 5-10 days; recovery: 7-14 days; dose-limiting toxicity)
Neuromuscular & skeletal: Bone pain, jaw pain, tumor pain

Less common:
Cardiovascular: Angina, cerebrovascular accident, coronary ischemia, ECG abnormalities, limb ischemia, MI, myocardial ischemia, Raynaud's phenomenon
Central nervous system: Depression, dizziness, headache, neurotoxicity (duration: >24 hours), seizure, vertigo
Dermatologic: Dermatitis, photosensitivity (rare), rash, skin blistering
Endocrine & metabolic: Aspermia, hyperuricemia, SIADH
Gastrointestinal: Abdominal pain, anorexia, diarrhea, gastrointestinal bleeding, hemorrhagic enterocolitis, ileus, metallic taste, nausea (mild), paralytic ileus, rectal bleeding, stomatitis, toxic megacolon, vomiting (mild)
Genitourinary: Urinary retention
Hematologic: Anemia, thrombocytopenia (recovery within a few days), thrombotic thrombocytopenic purpura
Local: Cellulitis (with extravasation), irritation, phlebitis (with extravasation), radiation recall
Neuromuscular & skeletal: Deep tendon reflex loss, myalgia, paresthesia, peripheral neuritis, weakness
Ocular: Nystagmus
Otic: Auditory damage, deafness, vestibular damage
Renal: Hemolytic uremic syndrome
Respiratory: Bronchospasm, dyspnea, pharyngitis

Drug Interactions

Metabolism/Transport Effects Substrate of CYP2D6 (minor), CYP3A4 (major), P-glycoprotein; **Note:** Assignment of Major/Minor substrate status based on clinically relevant drug interaction potential; **Inhibits** CYP2D6 (weak), CYP3A4 (weak); **Induces** P-glycoprotein

Avoid Concomitant Use
Avoid concomitant use of VinBLAStine with any of the following: BCG; CloZAPine; Conivaptan; Dabigatran Etexilate; Dipyrone; Fusidic Acid (Systemic); Natalizumab; Pimecrolimus; Pimozide; Sofosbuvir; Tacrolimus (Topical); Tofacitinib; Vaccines (Live); VinCRIStine (Liposomal)

Increased Effect/Toxicity
VinBLAStine may increase the levels/effects of: ARIPiprazole; CloZAPine; Dofetilide; Leflunomide; Lomitapide; MitoMYcin (Systemic); Natalizumab; Pimozide; Tofacitinib; Tolterodine; Vaccines (Live)

The levels/effects of VinBLAStine may be increased by: Ceritinib; Conivaptan; CYP3A4 Inhibitors (Moderate); CYP3A4 Inhibitors (Strong); Dasatinib; Denosumab; Dipyrone; Fusidic Acid (Systemic); Itraconazole; Ivacaftor; Lopinavir; Luliconazole; Macrolide Antibiotics; MAO Inhibitors; Mifepristone; P-glycoprotein/ABCB1 Inhibitors; Pimecrolimus; Posaconazole; Ritonavir; Roflumilast; Simeprevir; Stiripentol; Tacrolimus (Topical); Trastuzumab; Voriconazole

Decreased Effect
VinBLAStine may decrease the levels/effects of: Afatinib; BCG; Brentuximab Vedotin; Coccidioidin Skin Test; Dabigatran Etexilate; DOXOrubicin (Conventional); Linagliptin; P-glycoprotein/ABCB1 Substrates; Sipuleucel-T; Sofosbuvir; Vaccines (Inactivated); Vaccines (Live); VinCRIStine (Liposomal)

The levels/effects of VinBLAStine may be decreased by: Bosentan; CYP3A4 Inducers (Strong); Dabrafenib; ▸

Deferasirox; Echinacea; Mitotane; Peginterferon Alfa-2b; P-glycoprotein/ABCB1 Inducers; Siltuximab; St Johns Wort; Tocilizumab

Stability Hazardous agent; use appropriate precautions for handling and disposal (NIOSH, 2012). Store vials at 2°C to 8°C (36°F to 46°F); 1 mg/mL solution prepared with preserved NS injection is stable for 28 days when refrigerated and protected from light. **Note:** Vinblastine must be dispensed in overwrap which bears the statement "Do not remove covering until the moment of injection. Fatal if given intrathecally. For I.V. use only."

Mechanism of Action Vinblastine binds to tubulin and inhibits microtubule formation, therefore, arresting the cell at metaphase by disrupting the formation of the mitotic spindle; it is specific for the M and S phases. Vinblastine may also interfere with nucleic acid and protein synthesis by blocking glutamic acid utilization.

Pharmacokinetics (Adult data unless noted)
Distribution: Poor penetration into CSF; rapidly distributed into body tissues; V_{dss}: 27.3 L/kg
Protein binding: 99%
Metabolism: Extensive in the liver via CYP3A4 to an active metabolite
Half-life, terminal: 24.8 hours
Elimination: Biliary excretion (95%), urine (<1% as unchanged drug)

Dosing: Usual Vinblastine may be administered at intervals of every 7 days or greater and only after leukocyte count has returned to at least 4000/mm³; maintenance therapy should be titrated according to leukocyte count

I.V. (refer to individual protocols):
Children:
Hodgkin's disease: 2.5-6 mg/m²/day once every 1-2 weeks for 3-6 weeks; maximum weekly dose: 12.5 mg/m²
Histiocytosis X: 0.4 mg/kg once every 7-10 days
Germ cell tumor: 0.2 mg/kg on days 1 and 2 of cycle every 3 weeks times 4 cycles
Adults: 3.7-18.5 mg/m²/day every 7-10 days

Dosing adjustment in hepatic impairment: Children and Adults: Direct serum bilirubin concentration >3 mg/dL: Reduce dose 50%

Administration Hazardous agent; use appropriate precautions for handling and disposal (NIOSH, 2012).

Parenteral: **Do not administer intrathecally, death may occur**; do not administer I.M. or SubQ since the drug is very irritating; may be administered IVP directly into the vein or through a Y-site of a freely running I.V. over a 1-minute period at a concentration for administration of 1 mg/mL; I.V. continuous infusion: Prolonged administration times and/or increased administration volumes may run the risk of vein irritation and extravasation. Assure proper needle or catheter placement prior to administration.

Vesicant/Extravasation Risk Vesicant

Monitoring Parameters CBC with differential and platelet count, serum uric acid, hepatic function tests

Additional Information Myelosuppressive effects:
Nadir (days): 4-10
Recovery (days): 7-14

Dosage Forms Excipient information presented when available (limited, particularly for generics); consult specific product labeling.
Solution, Intravenous, as sulfate:
Generic: 1 mg/mL (10 mL)
Solution Reconstituted, Intravenous, as sulfate:
Generic: 10 mg (1 ea)

References

Balis FM, Holcenberg JS and Bleyer WA, "Clinical Pharmacokinetics of Commonly Used Anticancer Drugs," *Clin Pharmacokinet*, 1983, 8 (3):202-32.

Bashir H, Motl S, Metzger ML, et al, "Itraconazole-Enhanced Chemotherapy Toxicity in a Patient With Hodgkin Lymphoma," *J Pediatr Hematol Oncol*, 2006, 28(1):33-5.

Crom WR, Glynn-Barnhart AM, Rodman JH, et al, "Pharmacokinetics of Anticancer Drugs in Children," *Clin Pharmacokinet*, 1987, 12 (3):168-213.

Gadner H, Grois N, Arico M, et al, "A Randomized Trial of Treatment for Multisystem Langerhans' Cell Histiocytosis," *J Pediatr*, 2001, 138 (5):728-34.

National Institute for Occupational Safety and Health (NIOSH), "NIOSH List of Antineoplastic and Other Hazardous Drugs in Healthcare Settings 2012." Available at http://www.cdc.gov/niosh/docs/2012-150/pdfs/2012-150.pdf. Accessed January 21, 2013.

Tannock I, Ehrlichman C, Perrault D, et al, "Failure of 5-Day Vinblastine Infusion in the Treatment of Patients With Advanced Refractory Breast Cancer," *Cancer Treat Rep*, 1982, 66(9):1783-4.

Yap HY, Blumenschein GR, Keating MJ, et al, "Vinblastine Given as a Continuous 5-Day Infusion in the Treatment of Refractory Breast Cancer," *Cancer Treat Rep*, 1980, 64(2-3):279-83.

◆ **Vinblastine Sulfate** *see* VinBLAStine *on page 2136*

◆ **Vinblastine Sulphate Injection (Can)** *see* VinBLAStine *on page 2136*

◆ **Vincaleukoblastine** *see* VinBLAStine *on page 2136*

◆ **Vincasar PFS** *see* VinCRIStine *on page 2138*

VinCRIStine (vin KRIS teen)

Medication Safety Issues
Sound-alike/look-alike issues:
VinCRIStine may be confused with vinBLAStine, vinorelbine
VinCRIStine conventional may be confused with vinCRIStine liposomal
Oncovin may be confused with Ancobon

High alert medication:
This medication is in a class the Institute for Safe Medication Practices (ISMP) includes among its list of drug classes which have a heightened risk of causing significant patient harm when used in error.

BEERS Criteria medication:
This drug may be potentially inappropriate for use in geriatric patients (Quality of evidence - moderate; Strength of recommendation - strong).

Administration issues:
For I.V. use only. Fatal if administered by other routes. To prevent fatal inadvertent intrathecal injection, it is strongly recommended that vincristine doses be dispensed in a small minibag (25 to 50 mL of a compatible solution), and **NOT** a syringe (ISMP, 2014). Vincristine should **NOT** be prepared during the preparation of any intrathecal medications. After preparation, keep vincristine in a location **away** from the separate storage location recommended for intrathecal medications. Vincristine should **NOT** be delivered to the patient at the same time with any medications intended for central nervous system administration.

Related Information
Emetogenic Potential of Antineoplastic Agents in Children *on page 2327*
Management of Drug Extravasations *on page 2255*
Safe Handling of Hazardous Drugs *on page 2419*

Brand Names: U.S. Vincasar PFS

Brand Names: Canada Vincristine Sulfate Injection; Vincristine Sulfate Injection USP

Therapeutic Category Antineoplastic Agent, Antimicrotubular; Antineoplastic Agent, Mitotic Inhibitor; Antineoplastic Agent, Vinca Alkaloid

Generic Availability (U.S.) Yes

Use Treatment of acute lymphocytic leukemia (ALL), Hodgkin lymphoma, neuroblastoma, non-Hodgkin lymphomas, Wilms' tumor, and rhabdomyosarcoma [FDA approved in pediatrics (age not specified) and adults]; has also been used in the treatment of central nervous system tumors, chronic lymphocytic leukemia (CLL), Ewing's sarcoma, gestational trophoblastic tumors (high-risk), multiple myeloma, retinoblastoma, and small cell lung cancer

Pregnancy Risk Factor D

Pregnancy Considerations Animal reproduction studies have demonstrated teratogenicity and fetal loss. May cause fetal harm if administered during pregnancy. Women of childbearing potential should avoid becoming pregnant during treatment.

Breast-Feeding Considerations It is not known if vincristine is excreted in breast milk. Due to the potential for serious adverse reactions in the nursing infant, the decision to discontinue vincristine or to discontinue breast-feeding should take into account the benefits of treatment to the mother.

Contraindications Hypersensitivity to vincristine or any component; patients with demyelinating form of Charcot-Marie-Tooth syndrome

Warnings Hazardous agent; use appropriate precautions for handling and disposal (NIOSH, 2012); avoid eye contamination. **For I.V. administration only; intrathecal administration usually results in death [U.S. Boxed Warning].** To prevent administration errors, the World Health Organization recommends dispensing vincristine diluted in a minibag (WHO, 2007); **if not dispensed in a minibag, affix an auxiliary label stating "For intravenous use only - fatal if given by other routes" and also place in an overwrap labeled "Do not remove covering until moment of injection."** Vincristine should **NOT** be prepared during the preparation of any intrathecal medications. After preparation, keep vincristine in a location **away** from the separate storage location recommended for intrathecal medications. Vincristine should **NOT** be delivered to the patient at the same time with any medications intended for central nervous system administration.

Vincristine is a vesicant; avoid extravasation. Ensure proper catheter or needle position prior to (and during) infusion, individuals administering should be experienced in vincristine administration; discontinue administration immediately if extravasation occurs and initiate appropriate extravasation management, including local injection of hyaluronidase and moderate heat application to the affected area. Use a separate vein to complete administration **[U.S. Boxed Warning]**.

Precautions Should only be prescribed and administered by individuals experienced in the use of chemotherapeutic agents **[U.S. Boxed Warning]**. Use with caution in patients with impaired hepatic function or hepatobiliary dysfunction; may be associated with hepatic sinusoidal obstruction syndrome (SOS; formerly called veno-occlusive disease [VOD]), increased risk in children <3 years of age; monitor for signs or symptoms of hepatic SOS, including bilirubin >1.4 mg/dL, unexplained weight gain, ascites, hepatomegaly, or unexplained right upper quadrant pain (Arndt, 2004).

Use with caution in patients with preexisting neuromuscular disease and/or with concomitant neurotoxic agents; may cause neurotoxicity; typically follows a sequence with initial paresthesia and sensory impairment reported followed by neuritic pain and finally motor impairment; alterations in mental status such as depression, confusion, or insomnia may also occur; neurologic effects are dose-dependent and dose-limiting; effects may be additive with spinal cord irradiation; dosage adjustment may be required. Acute uric acid nephropathy has been reported after vincristine administration; monitor serum uric acid during induction. Acute shortness of breath and broncho-spasm have been reported following administration of a vinca alkaloids usually in combination with mitomycin-C; onset may be several minutes to hours after vincristine administration and up to 2 weeks after mitomycin-C; progressive dyspnea requiring treatment may develop;

permanently discontinue vincristine if pulmonary dysfunction occurs.

May cause constipation, paralytic ileus, intestinal necrosis, and/or perforation; constipation may present as upper colon impaction with an empty rectum (may require flat film of abdomen for diagnosis); generally responds to high enemas and laxatives; patients should be on a prophylactic bowel management regimen. May cause SIADH (rarely); reported more frequently in Asian patients although the exact mechanism has not been determined (Moore, 2009).

Potentially significant interactions may exist, requiring dose or frequency adjustment, additional monitoring, and/ or selection of alternative therapy. Consult drug interactions database for more detailed information.

Adverse Reactions

Cardiovascular: Edema, hyper-/hypotension, MI, myocardial ischemia

Central nervous system: Ataxia, coma, cranial nerve dysfunction (auditory damage, extraocular muscle impairment, laryngeal muscle impairment, paralysis, paresis, vestibular damage, vocal cord paralysis), dizziness, fever, headache, neurotoxicity (dose-related), neuropathic pain (common), seizure, vertigo

Dermatologic toxicity: Alopecia (common), rash

Endocrine & metabolic: Hyperuricemia, parotid pain, SIADH (rare)

Gastrointestinal: Abdominal cramps, abdominal pain, anorexia, constipation (common), diarrhea, intestinal necrosis, intestinal perforation, nausea, oral ulcers, paralytic ileus, vomiting, weight loss

Genitourinary: Bladder atony, dysuria, polyuria, urinary retention

Hematologic: Anemia (mild), leukopenia (mild), thrombocytopenia (mild), thrombotic thrombocytopenic purpura

Hepatic: Hepatic sinusoidal obstruction syndrome (SOS); veno-occlusive liver disease)

Local: Phlebitis, tissue irritation/necrosis (if infiltrated)

Neuromuscular & skeletal: Back pain, bone pain, deep tendon reflex loss, difficulty walking, foot drop, gait changes, jaw pain, limb pain, motor difficulties, muscle wasting, myalgia, paralysis, paresthesia, peripheral neuropathy (common), sensorimotor dysfunction, sensory loss

Ocular: Cortical blindness (transient), nystagmus, optic atrophy with blindness

Otic: Deafness

Renal: Acute uric acid nephropathy, hemolytic uremic syndrome

Respiratory: Bronchospasm, dyspnea, pharyngeal pain

Miscellaneous: Allergic reactions (rare), anaphylaxis (rare), hypersensitivity (rare)

Drug Interactions

Metabolism/Transport Effects Substrate of CYP3A4 (major), P-glycoprotein; **Note:** Assignment of Major/Minor substrate status based on clinically relevant drug interaction potential; **Inhibits** CYP3A4 (weak)

Avoid Concomitant Use

Avoid concomitant use of VinCRIStine with any of the following: BCG; Conivaptan; Fusidic Acid (Systemic); Natalizumab; Pimecrolimus; Pimozide; Tacrolimus (Topical); Tofacitinib; Vaccines (Live)

Increased Effect/Toxicity

VinCRIStine may increase the levels/effects of: ARIPiprazole; Dofetilide; Leflunomide; Lomitapide; MitoMYcin (Systemic); Natalizumab; Pimozide; Tofacitinib; Vaccines (Live); Vitamin K Antagonists

The levels/effects of VinCRIStine may be increased by: Ceritinib; Conivaptan; CYP3A4 Inhibitors (Moderate); CYP3A4 Inhibitors (Strong); Dasatinib; Denosumab; Fusidic Acid (Systemic); Itraconazole; Ivacaftor;

Lopinavir; Luliconazole; Macrolide Antibiotics; MAO Inhibitors; Mifepristone; NIFEdipine; P-glycoprotein/ABCB1 Inhibitors; Pimecrolimus; Posaconazole; Ritonavir; Roflumilast; Simeprevir; Stiripentol; Tacrolimus (Topical); Teniposide; Trastuzumab; Voriconazole

Decreased Effect

VinCRIStine may decrease the levels/effects of: BCG; Cardiac Glycosides; Coccidioidin Skin Test; Fosphenytoin; Phenytoin; Sipuleucel-T; Vaccines (Inactivated); Vaccines (Live); Vitamin K Antagonists

The levels/effects of VinCRIStine may be decreased by: Bosentan; CYP3A4 Inducers (Strong); Dabrafenib; Deferasirox; Echinacea; Fosphenytoin; Mitotane; P-glycoprotein/ABCB1 Inducers; Phenytoin; Siltuximab; St Johns Wort; Tocilizumab

Stability Hazardous agent; use appropriate precautions for handling and disposal (NIOSH, 2012).

Store intact vials at 2°C to 8°C (36°F to 46°F); protect from light; store vials upright. Solution further diluted in 25 to 50 mL of NS or D₅W (minibag) are stable for 7 days under refrigeration or 2 days at room temperature; in ambulatory infusion devices, solution is stable for 7 days at room temperature. **Note:** In order to prevent inadvertent intrathecal administration, the World Health Organization (WHO) and the Institute for Safe Medical Practices (ISMP) recommend dispensing vincristine in a minibag (rather than a syringe). Vincristine should **NOT** be prepared during the preparation of any intrathecal medication. After preparation, keep vincristine in a location away from the separate storage location recommended for intrathecal medications.

If dispensing vincristine in a syringe, affix an auxiliary label stating "For intravenous use only - fatal if given by other routes" to the syringe and the syringe must be packaged in the manufacturer-provided overwrap which bears the statement **"Do not remove covering until the moment of injection. For intravenous use only. Fatal if given intrathecally."**

Mechanism of Action Binds to tubulin and inhibits microtubule formation, therefore, arresting the cell at metaphase by disrupting the formation of the mitotic spindle; it is specific for the M and S phases. Vincristine may also interfere with nucleic acid and protein synthesis by blocking glutamic acid utilization.

Pharmacokinetics (Adult data unless noted) Note: In pediatric patients, significant intrapatient and interpatient variability has been reported (Gidding, 1999).

Distribution: Rapidly removed from bloodstream and tightly bound to tissues; poor penetration into the CSF

Metabolism: Extensive in the liver via CYP3A

Half-life, terminal: 85 hours (range: 19 to 155 hours)

Elimination: Primarily in feces (~80%); urine (10% to 20%; <1% as unchanged drug)

Clearance: In pediatric patients, correlation with diagnosis has been reported; clearance in patients with ALL and non-Hodgkin lymphoma higher than Wilms' tumor (Gidding, 1999):

Infants: Vincristine clearance is lower compared to children; more closely related to body weight than to body surface area (Crom, 1994)

Children and Adolescents 2 to 18 years: Reported means: 357 to 482 mL/minute/m²; some suggest faster clearance in children <10 years of age than in adolescents (Crom, 1994); however, more recent data does not support this finding nor a dosage reduction in adolescent patients (Frost, 2003; Gidding, 1999)

Dosing: Neonatal Note: Dosing and frequency may vary by protocol and/or treatment phase; refer to specific protocol. In pediatric patients, dosing may be based on either BSA (mg/m²) or weight (mg/kg); use extra precaution to verify dosing parameters during calculations.

Neuroblastoma (CE-CAdO regimen): I.V.:

Newborns: 0.035 mg/**kg** on day 1 every 21 days for 2 cycles (Rubie, 1998) or on days 1 and 5 for 2 cycles (Rubie, 2001)

Older neonates: 0.75 mg/m² to 1.05 mg/m² on days 1 and 5 every 21 days for 2 cycles (Rubie, 1998) or 0.05 mg/**kg** on days 1 and 5 for 2 cycles (Rubie, 2001)

Dosing: Usual Note: Doses may be capped at a maximum of 2 mg/dose. Dosing and frequency may vary by protocol and/or treatment phase; refer to specific protocol.

Pediatric: **Note:** In pediatric patients, dosing may be based on either BSA (mg/m²) or weight (mg/kg); use extra precaution to verify dosing parameters during calculations.

Malignancy, general dosing: Manufacturer's labeling: I.V.:

≤10 kg: 0.05 mg/**kg**/dose once weekly

>10 kg: 1.5 to 2 mg/m²/dose; frequency may vary based on protocol; maximum dose: 2 mg

Acute lymphocytic leukemia (ALL): I.V.: Children: 1.5 mg/m²/dose; maximum dose: 2 mg; reported frequency variable; both regimens studied in children ≤10 years:

Bostrom, 2003: Administer dose on the following days: Induction phase: Days 0, 7, 14, and 21; Consolidation phase: Days 0, 28, and 56; Delayed intensification phase: Days 0, 7, and 14; Maintenance phase: Days 0, 28, and 56

Avramis, 2003: Administer dose on the following days: Induction phase: Days 0, 7, 14, and 21; Consolidation phase: Days 0, 28, and 56; Interim maintenance phases: Days 0 and 28; Delayed intensification phase: Days 0, 7, and 14; Maintenance phase: Every 4 weeks

Burkitt lymphoma and B-cell ALL: I.V.: Children and Adolescents: 1.5 mg/m²/dose; maximum dose: 2 mg; reported frequency variable

Bowman, 1996: Administer dose on days 4 and 11 of initial phase cycle; initial phase is in combination with cyclophosphamide, doxorubicin, and CNS prophylaxis (alternates with secondary phase) for a total of 4 cycles of each phase

Reiter, 1999: Administer dose on day 1 of cycle AA in combination with dexamethasone, ifosfamide, methotrexate, cytarabine, etoposide, and CNS prophylaxis and of cycle BB in combination with dexamethasone, cyclophosphamide, methotrexate, doxorubicin, and CNS prophylaxis

Ewing sarcoma: Limited data available: I.V.: Children and Adolescents: Dose and frequency regimens variable:

Grier, 2003: 2 mg/m²/dose on day 1 of a 21 day cycle, administer either every cycle or during odd-numbered cycles; maximum dose: 2 mg

Kolb, 2003: 0.67 mg/m²/**day** as a continuous I.V. infusion on days 1, 2, and 3; total dose for cycle: 2 mg/m²/**cycle** (maximum dose/cycle: 2 mg) during cycles 1, 2, 3, and 6

Hodgkin lymphoma: I.V.: Children and Adolescents: BEACOPP regimen: 2 mg/m² on day 7 of a 21-day treatment cycle; maximum dose: 2 mg (Kelly, 2002)

Neuroblastoma: I.V.:

Infants: CE-CAdO regimen:

Body surface area-directed (Rubie, 1998):

<10 kg: 0.75 mg/m² to 1.05 mg/m² on days 1 and 5 every 21 days for 2 cycles; some infants may only receive on day 1. **Note:** This dosing equates to a 30% to 50% reduction in the dose used for patients ≥10 kg.

≥10 kg: 1.5 mg/m² on days 1 and 5 every 21 days for 2 cycles; maximum dose: 2 mg

Weight-based: 0.05 mg/**kg** on days 1 and 5 for 2 cycles (Rubie, 2001)

Children and Adolescents:

CE-CAdO regimen (Rubie, 1998):

<10 kg: 0.75 mg/m^2 to 1.05 mg/m^2 on days 1 and 5 every 21 days for 2 cycles

≥10 kg: 1.5 mg/m^2 on days 1 and 5 every 21 days for 2 cycles; maximum dose: 2 mg

CAV-P/VP regimen: 0.033 mg/**kg**/day as a continuous infusion days 1, 2, and 3 (total dose: 0.1 mg/**kg**), then 1.5 mg/m^2 bolus day 9 of courses 1, 2, 4, and 6; maximum dose: 2 mg/dose (Kushner, 1994)

Retinoblastoma: Limited data available: I.V.:

Infants and Children ≤36 months: 0.05 mg/**kg**/dose; maximum dose: 2 mg; reported frequency variable

Rodriguez-Galindo, 2003: Administer dose on day 1 every 21 days in combination with carboplatin for 8 cycles

Freidman, 2000: Administer dose day 0 every 28 days in combination with carboplatin and etoposide for 6 cycles

Children >36 months: 1.5 mg/m^2 on day 0 every 28 days in combination with carboplatin and etoposide for 6 cycles; maximum dose: 2 mg (Friedman, 2000)

Rhabdomyosarcoma: Infants, Children, and Adolescents (Crist, 2001):

VA regimen:

Infants: Initial: 0.75 mg/m^2/dose as a single dose during week 1; if tolerated, may increase to dose to 1.13 mg/m^2/dose as a single dose for week 2 and further increase to 1.5 mg/m^2/dose weekly for weeks 3 to 8, weeks 13 to 20, and weeks 25 to 32

Children and Adolescents: 1.5 mg/m^2/dose weekly (maximum dose: 2 mg/dose) for weeks 1 to 8, weeks 13 to 20, and weeks 25 to 32

VAC regimen:

Infants: 0.75 mg/m^2/dose weekly for weeks 0 to 12, week 16, and weeks 20 to 25; continuation therapy: Weeks 29 to 34 and weeks 38 to 43

Children and Adolescents: 1.5 mg/m^2/dose weekly (maximum dose: 2 mg/dose) for weeks 0 to 12, week 16, and weeks 20 to 25; continuation therapy: weeks 29 to 34 and weeks 38 to 43

Wilm's tumor: Dose and frequency regimens variable; regimens studies in infants, children, and adolescents

Pritchard, 1995:

Infants: 0.75 mg/m^2/dose weekly for 10 to 11 weeks then every 3 weeks for 15 additional weeks

Children and Adolescents: 1.5 mg/m^2/dose weekly for 10 to 11 weeks then every 3 weeks for 15 additional weeks

Green, 2007:

Infants and Children ≤30 kg: 0.05 mg/**kg**/dose (maximum dose: 2 mg) weeks 1, 2, 4, 5, 6, 7, 8, 10, and 11, followed by 0.067 mg/**kg**/dose (maximum dose: 2 mg) weeks 12, 13, 18, and 24

Children and Adolescents >30 kg: 1.5 mg/m^2/dose (maximum dose: 2 mg) weeks 1, 2, 4, 5, 6, 7, 8, 10, and 11, followed by 2 mg/m^2/dose (maximum dose: 2 mg) weeks 12, 13, 18, and 24

Adult:

General dosing: Manufacturer's labeling: 1.4 mg/m^2/dose; frequency may vary based on protocol; maximum dose: 2 mg/dose

ALL:

Hyper-CVAD regimen: 2 mg/dose days 4 and 11 during odd-numbered cycles (cycles 1, 3, 5, 7) of an 8-cycle phase, followed by maintenance treatment (if needed) of 2 mg monthly for 2 years (Kantarjian, 2004)

Larson (CALBG 8811) regimen: Induction phase: 2 mg/dose days 1, 8, 15, and 22 (4-week treatment cycle); Early intensification phase: 2 mg/dose days 15 and 22 (4-week treatment cycle, repeat once); Late intensification phase: 2 mg/dose days 1, 8, 15 (8-week treatment cycle); Maintenance phase: 2 mg/dose day 1 every 4 weeks until 24 months from diagnosis (Larson, 1995)

Central nervous system tumors: I.V.: PCV regimen: 1.4 mg/m^2/dose (maximum dose: 2 mg) on days 8 and 29 of a 6-week treatment cycle for a total of 6 cycles (van de Bent, 2006) **or** 1.4 mg/m^2/dose (no maximum dose) on days 8 and 29 of a 6-week treatment cycle for up to 4 cycles (Cairncross, 2006)

Hodgkin lymphoma:

BEACOPP regimen: 1.4 mg/m^2/dose (maximum dose: 2 mg) on day 8 of a 21-day treatment cycle (Diehl, 2003)

Stanford V regimen: 1.4 mg/m^2/dose (maximum dose: 2 mg) in weeks 2, 4, 6, 8, 10, and 12 (Horning, 2000; Horning, 2002)

Non-Hodgkin lymphoma:

Burkitt lymphoma:

CODOX-M/IVAC: Cycles 1 and 3 (CODOX-M): 1.5 mg/m^2 (no maximum dose) days 1 and 8 of cycle 1 and days 1, 8, and 15 of cycle 3 (Magrath, 1996) **or** 1.5 mg/m^2 (maximum dose: 2 mg) days 1 and 8 of cycles 1 and 3 (Mead, 2002; Mead, 2008); CODOX-M is in combination with cyclophosphamide, doxorubicin, methotrexate, and CNS prophylaxis and alternates with IVAC (etoposide, ifosfamide, and cytarabine) for a total of 4 cycles

Hyper-CVAD: 2 mg (flat dose) days 4 and 11 of courses 1, 3, 5, and 7 (in combination with cyclophosphamide, doxorubicin, and dexamethasone) and alternates with even courses 2, 4, 6, and 8 (methotrexate and cytarabine) (Thomas, 2006)

Follicular lymphoma: CVP regimen: 1.4 mg/m^2/dose (maximum dose: 2 mg) on day 1 of a 21-day treatment cycle for 8 cycles (Marcus, 2005)

Large B-cell lymphoma:

CHOP regimen: 1.4 mg/m^2/dose (maximum dose: 2 mg) on day 1 of a 21-day treatment cycle for 8 cycles (Coiffier, 2002)

EPOCH regimen: 0.4 mg/m^2/day continuous infusion for 4 days (over 96 hours) (total 1.6 mg/m^2/cycle; dose not usually capped) of a 21-day treatment cycle (Wilson, 2002)

Dosing adjustment for renal impairment: Adults: No dosage adjustment necessary (Kintzel, 1995)

Dosing adjustment for hepatic impairment: All patients: The manufacturer's labeling recommends the following adjustment: Serum bilirubin >3 mg/dL: Administer 50% of normal dose.

The following adjustments have also been recommended:

Floyd, 2006: Serum bilirubin 1.5 to 3 mg/dL or transaminases 2 to 3 times ULN or alkaline phosphatase increased: Administer 50% of dose.

Superfin, 2007:

Serum bilirubin 1.5-3 mg/dL: Administer 50% of dose.

Serum bilirubin >3 mg/dL: Avoid use.

Administration Hazardous agent; use appropriate precautions for handling and disposal (NIOSH, 2012). **Note: For I.V. administration only; fatal if given intrathecally;** vincristine should **NOT** be delivered to the patient with any medications intended for central nervous system administration. **Note:** In order to prevent inadvertent intrathecal administration, the World Health Organization (WHO) and the Institute for Safe Medical Practices (ISMP) recommend dispensing vincristine in a minibag (rather than a syringe). Vincristine should **NOT** be prepared during the preparation of any intrathecal medication. After preparation, keep vincristine in a location away from the separate storage location recommended for intrathecal medications. If dispensing vincristine in a syringe, affix an auxiliary label stating **"For intravenous use only - fatal if given by other routes"** to the syringe and the syringe must be packaged in the manufacturer-provided overwrap which bears the statement **"Do not remove covering until the moment of injection. For intravenous use only. Fatal if given intrathecally."**

Parenteral: For I.V. use only; avoid extravasation; may further dilute in NS or D_5W and administer as a short 5-10 minute infusion (preferred); may also be administered undiluted (1 mg/mL) slow I.V. push (over 1 minute) or as a 24-hour continuous I.V. infusion (depending on protocol)

Vincristine is a vesicant; ensure proper needle or catheter placement prior to and during infusion; avoid extravasation. If extravasation occurs, stop infusion immediately and disconnect (leave cannula/needle in place); gently aspirate extravasated solution (do **NOT** flush the line); initiate hyaluronidase antidote; apply dry warm compresses for 20 minutes 4 times a day for 1-2 days; elevate extremity. Hyaluronidase: If needle/cannula still in place, administer 1-6 mL hyaluronidase (150 units/mL) into the existing I.V. line; the usual dose is 1 mL hyaluronidase for each 1 mL of extravasated drug (Perez Fidalgo, 2012; Schulmeister, 2011). If needle/cannula has been removed, inject 1-6 mL (150 units/mL) subcutaneously in a clockwise manner using 1 mL for 1 mL of drug extravasated (Schulmeister, 2011) **or** administer 1 mL (150 units/mL) as 5 separate 0.2 mL injections (25-gauge needle) subcutaneously into the extravasation site (Polovich, 2009). Remaining portion of the vincristine dose should be infused through a separate vein.

Note: Do not administer to patients while they are receiving radiation therapy through ports that include the liver. If used in combination with L-asparaginase, administer vincristine 12-24 hours before L-asparaginase to minimize toxicity.

Vesicant/Extravasation Risk Vesicant

Monitoring Parameters Serum electrolytes (sodium), hepatic function tests, neurologic examination, CBC with differential, serum uric acid, monitor infusion site, monitor for constipation/ileus and for signs/symptoms of peripheral neuropathy

Additional Information Ten times the usual recommended dose of vincristine in children <13 years of age has been lethal; doses of 3 to 4 mg/m^2 can be expected to produce severe toxic manifestations. Treatment is supportive and symptomatic, including anticonvulsants, fluid restriction, and diuretics to prevent adverse effects from SIADH and enemas or cathartics to prevent ileus. Use of leucovorin calcium may be helpful in treating vincristine overdose. Leucovorin calcium 100 mg I.V. every 3 hours for 24 hours, then every 6 hours for at least 48 hours has been administered in case reports.

Dosage Forms Excipient information presented when available (limited, particularly for generics); consult specific product labeling.

Solution, Intravenous, as sulfate:
Vincasar PFS: 1 mg/mL (1 mL, 2 mL)
Solution, Intravenous, as sulfate [preservative free]:
Generic: 1 mg/mL (1 mL, 2 mL)

References

Arndt C, Hawkins D, Anderson JR, et al, "Age Is a Risk Factor for Chemotherapy-Induced Hepatopathy With Vincristine, Dactinomycin, and Cyclophosphamide," *J Clin Oncol*, 2004, 22(10):1894-901.

Aronoff GR, Bennett WM, Berns JS, et al, *Drug Prescribing in Renal Failure: Dosing Guidelines for Adults and Children*, 5th ed, Philadelphia, PA: American College of Physicians, 2007, 120, 174.

Avramis VI, Sencer S, Periclou AP, et, al, "A Randomized Comparison of Native Escherichia Coli Asparaginase and Polyethylene Glycol Conjugated Asparaginase for Treatment of Children With Newly Diagnosed Standard-Risk Acute Lymphoblastic Leukemia: A Children's Cancer Group Study," *Blood*, 2002, 99(6):1986-94.

Bostrom BC, Sensel MR, Sather HN, et al, "Dexamethasone Versus Prednisone and Daily Oral Versus Weekly Intravenous Mercaptopurine for Patients With Standard-Risk Acute Lymphoblastic Leukemia: A Report From the Children's Cancer Group," *Blood*, 2003, 101 (10):3809-17.

Bowman WP, Shuster JJ, Cook B, et al, "Improved Survival for Children With B-Cell Acute Lymphoblastic Leukemia and Stage IV Small Noncleaved-Cell Lymphoma: A Pediatric Oncology Group Study," *J Clin Oncol*, 1996, 14(4):1252-61.

Cairncross G, Berkey B, Shaw E, et al, "Phase III Trial of Chemotherapy Plus Radiotherapy Compared With Radiotherapy Alone for Pure and Mixed Anaplastic Oligodendroglioma: Intergroup Radiation Therapy Oncology Group Trial 9402," *J Clin Oncol*, 2006, 24(18):2707-14.

Crist WM, Anderson JR, Meza JL, et al, "Intergroup Rhabdomyosarcoma Study-IV: Results for Patients With Nonmetastatic Disease," *J Clin Oncol*, 2001, 19(12):3091-102.

Crom WR, deGraaf SS, Synold T, et al, "Pharmacokinetics of Vincristine in Children and Adolescents With Acute Lymphocytic Leukemia," *J Pediatr*, 1994, 125(4):642-9.

Diehl V, Franklin J, Pfreundschuh M, et al, "Standard and Increased-Dose BEACOPP Chemotherapy Compared With COPP-ABVD for Advanced Hodgkin's Disease," *N Engl J Med*, 2003, 348(24):2386-95.

Floyd JD, Nguyen DT, Lobins RL, et al, "Cardiotoxicity of Cancer Therapy," *J Clin Oncol*, 2005, 23(30):7685-96.

Floyd J, Mirza I, Sachs B, et al, "Hepatotoxicity of Chemotherapy," *Semin Oncol*, 2006, 33(1):50-67.

Friedman DL, Himelstein B, Shields CL, et al, "Chemoreduction and Local Ophthalmic Therapy for Intraocular Retinoblastoma," *J Clin Oncol*, 2000, 18(1):12-7.

Frost BM, Lönnerholm G, Koopmans P, et al, "Vincristine in Childhood Leukaemia: No Pharmacokinetic Rationale for Dose Reduction in Adolescents," *Acta Paediatr*, 2003, 92(5):551-7.

Granowetter L, Womer R, Devidas M, et al, "Dose-Intensified Compared With Standard Chemotherapy for Nonmetastatic Ewing Sarcoma Family of Tumors: A Children's Oncology Group Study," *J Clin Oncol*, 2009, 27(15):2536-41.

Green DM, Cotton CA, Malogolowkin M, et al, "Treatment of Wilms Tumor Relapsing After Initial Treatment With Vincristine and Actinomycin D: A Report From the National Wilms Tumor Study Group," *Pediatr Blood Cancer*, 2007, 48(5):493-9.

Grier HE, Krailo MD, Tarbell NJ, et al, "Addition of Ifosfamide and Etoposide to Standard Chemotherapy for Ewing's Sarcoma and Primitive Neuroectodermal Tumor of Bone," *N Engl J Med*, 2003, 348(8):694-701.

Horning SJ, Hoppe RT, Breslin S, et al, "Stanford V and Radiotherapy for Locally Extensive and Advanced Hodgkin's Disease: Mature Results of a Prospective Clinical Trial," *J Clin Oncol*, 2002, 20 (3):630-7.

Horning SJ, Williams J, Bartlett NL, et al, "Assessment of the Stanford V Regimen and Consolidative Radiotherapy for Bulky and Advanced Hodgkin's Disease: Eastern Cooperative Oncology Group Pilot Study E1492," *J Clin Oncol*, 2000, 18(5):972-80.

Jacobson JO, Polovich M, McNiff KK, et al, "American Society of Clinical Oncology/Oncology Nursing Society Chemotherapy Administration Safety Standards," *J Clin Oncol*, 2009, 27(32):5469-75.

Kantarjian H, Thomas D, O'Brien S, et al, "Long-Term Follow-Up Results of Hyperfractionated Cyclophosphamide, Vincristine, Doxorubicin, and Dexamethasone (Hyper-CVAD), A Dose-Intensive Regimen, in Adult Acute Lymphocytic Leukemia," *Cancer*, 2004, 101 (12):2788-801.

Kelly KM, Hutchinson RJ, Sposto R, et al, "Feasibility of Upfront Dose-Intensive Chemotherapy in Children With Advanced-Stage Hodgkin's Lymphoma: Preliminary Results From the Children's Cancer Group Study CCG-59704," *Ann Oncol*, 2002, 13(Suppl 1):107-11.

Kintzel PE and Dorr RT, "Anticancer Drug Renal Toxicity and Elimination: Dosing Guidelines for Altered Renal Function," *Cancer Treat Rev*, 1995, 21(1):33-64.

Kolb EA, Kushner BH, Gorlick R, et al, "Long-Term Event-Free Survival After Intensive Chemotherapy for Ewing's Family of Tumors in Children and Young Adults," *J Clin Oncol*, 2003, 21(18):3423-30.

Kushner BH, LaQuaglia MP, Bonilla MA, et al, "Highly Effective Induction Therapy for Stage 4 Neuroblastoma in Children Over 1 Year of Age," *J Clin Oncol*, 1994, 12(12):2607-13.

Larson RA, Dodge RK, Burns CP, et al, "A Five-Drug Remission Induction Regimen With Intensive Consolidation for Adults With Acute Lymphoblastic Leukemia: Cancer and Leukemia Group B Study 8811," *Blood*, 1995, 85(8):2025-37.

Legha SS, "Vincristine Neurotoxicity. Pathophysiology and Management," *Med Toxicol*, 1986, 1(6):421-7.

Magrath I, Adde M, Shad A, et al, "Adults and Children With Small Noncleaved-Cell Lymphoma Have a Similar Excellent Outcome When Treated With the Same Chemotherapy Regimen," *J Clin Oncol*, 1996, 14(3):925-34.

McCune JS and Lindley C, "Appropriateness of Maximum-Dose Guidelines for Vincristine," *Am J Health Syst Pharm*, 1997, 54(15):1755-8.

Mead GM, Barrans SL, Qian W, et al, "A Prospective Clinicopathologic Study of Dose-Modified CODOX-M/IVAC in Patients With Sporadic Burkitt Lymphoma Defined Using Cytogenetic and Immunophenotypic Criteria (MRC/NCRI LY10 Trial)," *Blood*, 2008, 112(6):2248-60.

Mead GM, Sydes MR, Walewski J, et al, "An International Evaluation of CODOX-M and CODOX-M Alternating With IVAC in Adult Burkitt's Lymphoma: Results of United Kingdom Lymphoma Group LY06 Study," *Ann Oncol*, 2002, 13(8):1264-74.

Moore A and Pinkerton R, "Vincristine: Can Its Therapeutic Index Be Enhanced?" *Pediatr Blood Cancer*, 2009, 53(7):1180-7.

Morgan C, Tillett T, Braybrooke J, et al, "Management of Uncommon Chemotherapy-Induced Emergencies," *Lancet Oncol*, 2011, 12 (8):806-14.

National Institute for Occupational Safety and Health (NIOSH), "NIOSH List of Antineoplastic and Other Hazardous Drugs in Healthcare Settings 2012." Available at http://www.cdc.gov/niosh/docs/2012-150/pdfs/2012-150.pdf. Accessed January 21, 2013.

Pérez Fidalgo JA, García Fabregat L, Cervantes A, et al, "Management of Chemotherapy Extravasation: ESMO-EONS Clinical Practice Guidelines," *Ann Oncol*, 2012, 23(Suppl 7):167-73.

Polovich M, Whitford JN, and Olsen M, *Chemotherapy and Biotherapy Guidelines and Recommendations for Practice*, 3rd ed, Pittsburgh, PA: Oncology Nursing Society, 2009.

Pritchard J, Imeson J, Barnes J, et al, "Results of the United Kingdom Children's Cancer Study Group First Wilms' Tumor Study," *J Clin Oncol*, 1995, 13(1):124-33.

Reiter A, Schrappe M, Tiemann M, et al, "Improved Treatment Results in Childhood B-Cell Neoplasms With Tailored Intensification of Therapy: A Report of the Berlin-Frankfurt-Münster Group Trial NHL-BFM 90," *Blood*, 1999, 94(10):3294-306.

Rodriguez-Galindo C, Wilson MW, Haik BG, et al, "Treatment of Intraocular Retinoblastoma With Vincristine and Carboplatin," *J Clin Oncol*, 2003, 21(10):2019-25.

Rubie H, Michon J, Plantaz D, et al, "Unresectable Localized Neuroblastoma: Improved Survival After Primary Chemotherapy Including Carboplatin-Etoposide. Neuroblastoma Study Group of the Societe Francaise d'Oncologie Pediatrique (SFOP)," *Br J Cancer*, 1998, 77 (12):2310-7.

Rubie H, Plantaz D, Coze C, et al, "Localised and Unresectable Neuroblastoma in Infants: Excellent Outcome With Primary Chemotherapy. Neuroblastoma Study Group, Société Française d'Oncologie Pédiatrique," *Med Pediatr Oncol*, 2001, 36(1):247-50.

Schulmeister L, "Extravasation Management: Clinical Update," *Semin Oncol Nurs*, 2011, 27(1):82-90.

Shields CL, Honavar SG, Meadows AT, et al, "Chemoreduction for Unilateral Retinoblastoma," *Arch Ophthalmol*, 2002, 120(12):1653-8.

Stefanou A and Dooley M, "Simple Method to Eliminate the Risk of Inadvertent Intrathecal Vincristine Administration," *J Clin Oncol*, 2003, 21(10):2044.

Superfin D, Iannucci AA, and Davies AM, "Commentary: Oncologic Drugs in Patients With Organ Dysfunction: A Summary," *Oncologist*, 2007, 12(9):1070-83.

Thomas DA, Faderi S, O'Brien S, et al, "Chemoimmunotherapy With Hyper-CVAD Plus Rituximab for the Treatment of Adult Burkitt and Burkitt-Type Lymphoma or Acute Lymphoblastic Leukemia," *Cancer*, 2006, 106(7):1569-80.

Wilson WH, Grossbard ML, Pittaluga S, et al, "Dose-Adjusted EPOCH Chemotherapy for Untreated Large B-Cell Lymphomas: A Pharmacodynamic Approach With High Efficacy," *Blood*, 2002, 99(8):2685-93.

Woods WG, O'Leary M, and Nesbit ME, "Life-Threatening Neuropathy and Hepatotoxicity in Infants During Induction Therapy for Acute Lymphoblastic Leukemia," *J Pediatr*, 1981, 98(4):642-5.

World Health Organization, "Vincristine (and Other Vinca Alkaloids) Should Only Be Given Intravenously Via a Minibag," July, 2007, Alert 115. Available at http://www.who.int/medicines/publications/druga-lerts/Alert_115_vincristine.pdf

◆ **Vincristine (Conventional)** *see* VinCRIStine *on page 2138*

◆ **Vincristine Sulfate** *see* VinCRIStine *on page 2138*

◆ **Vincristine Sulfate Injection (Can)** *see* VinCRIStine *on page 2138*

◆ **Vincristine Sulfate Injection USP (Can)** *see* VinCRIStine *on page 2138*

Vinorelbine (vi NOR el been)

Medication Safety Issues
Sound-alike/look-alike issues:
Vinorelbine may be confused with vinBLAStine, vinCRIStine

High alert medication:
This medication is in a class the Institute for Safe Medication Practices (ISMP) includes among its list of drug classes which have a heightened risk of causing significant patient harm when used in error.

Administration issues:
Vinorelbine is intended **for I.V. use only**: Inadvertent intrathecal administration of other vinca alkaloids has resulted in death. Syringes containing vinorelbine should be labeled **"For I.V. use only. Fatal if given intrathecally."** Vinorelbine should **NOT** be prepared during the preparation of any intrathecal medications. After preparation, keep vinorelbine in a location **away** from the separate storage location recommended for intrathecal medications.

Related Information
Emetogenic Potential of Antineoplastic Agents in Children *on page 2327*
Management of Drug Extravasations *on page 2255*
Safe Handling of Hazardous Drugs *on page 2419*

Brand Names: U.S. Navelbine

Brand Names: Canada Navelbine; Vinorelbine Injection, USP; Vinorelbine Tartrate for Injection

Therapeutic Category Antineoplastic Agent, Antimicrotubular; Antineoplastic Agent, Vinca Alkaloid

Generic Availability (U.S.) Yes

Use Treatment of nonsmall cell lung cancer (FDA approved in adults); has also been used for refractory/recurrent solid tumors, Hodgkin's lymphoma, and leukemias

Pregnancy Risk Factor D

Pregnancy Considerations Animal reproduction studies have demonstrated embryotoxicity, fetotoxicity, decreased fetal weight, and delayed ossification. May cause fetal harm if administered during pregnancy. Women of childbearing potential should avoid becoming pregnant during vinorelbine treatment.

Breast-Feeding Considerations It is not known if vinorelbine is excreted in breast milk. Due to the potential for serious adverse reactions in the nursing infant, breastfeeding should be discontinued during treatment.

Contraindications Hypersensitivity to vinorelbine or any component; pretreatment granulocyte counts <1000/mm^3

Documentation of allergic cross-reactivity for drugs in this class is limited; however, because of similarities in chemical structure and/or pharmacologic actions, the possibility of cross-sensitivity cannot be ruled out with certainty.

Warnings Hazardous agent; use appropriate precautions for handling and disposal (NIOSH, 2012); avoid eye contamination (exposure may cause severe irritation). Severe granulocytopenia may occur with treatment (may lead to infection); granulocyte counts should be ≥1000 cells/mm^3 prior to treatment initiation; dosage adjustment may be required based on blood counts; monitor blood counts prior to each dose **[U.S. Boxed Warning]**. Granulocytopenia is a dose-limiting toxicity; nadir is generally 7-10 days after administration and recovery occurs within the following 7-14 days. Monitor closely for infections and/or fever in patients with severe granulocytopenia. Use with extreme caution in patients with compromised marrow reserve due to prior chemotherapy or radiation therapy.

Fatal cases of interstitial pulmonary changes and ARDS have been reported with single-agent therapy (mean onset of symptoms: 1 week). Promptly evaluate changes in baseline pulmonary symptoms or any new-onset pulmonary symptoms (eg, dyspnea, cough, hypoxia). Acute shortness of breath and severe bronchospasm have been reported with vinca alkaloids, usually when used in combination with mitomycin. May cause severe constipation (grades 3-4), paralytic ileus, intestinal obstruction, necrosis, and/or perforation; some events were fatal.

For I.V. use only; intrathecal administration of other vinca alkaloids has resulted in death **[U.S. Boxed Warning]**. If dispensed in a syringe, should be labeled "for intravenous use only - fatal if given intrathecally". Vinorelbine should **NOT** be prepared during the preparation of any intrathecal medications. After preparation, keep vinorelbine in a location **away** from the separate storage location recommended for intrathecal medications.

Vinorelbine is a vesicant; ensure proper catheter or needle position prior to (and during) infusion. Avoid extravasation. Extravasation may cause local tissue necrosis and/or thrombophlebitis **[U.S. Boxed Warning]**.

Precautions May cause new-onset or worsening of pre-existing neuropathy; use with caution in patients with neuropathy; monitor for new or worsening signs/symptoms of neuropathy; dosage adjustment required. Vinorelbine elimination is predominantly hepatic; while there is no evidence that toxicity is enhanced in patients with elevated transaminases, use with caution in patients with severe hepatic injury or impairment; dosage modification required for elevated total bilirubin. May have radiosensitizing effects with prior or concurrent radiation therapy; radiation recall reactions may occur in patients who have received prior radiation therapy. Potentially significant interactions may exist, requiring dose or frequency adjustment, additional monitoring, and/or selection of alternative therapy. Consult drug interactions database for more detailed information. Should be administered under the supervision of an experienced cancer chemotherapy physician **[U.S. Boxed Warning]**.

Adverse Reactions

Cardiovascular: Chest pain

Central nervous system: Fatigue

Dermatologic: Alopecia, rash

Gastrointestinal: Constipation, diarrhea, nausea, paralytic ileus, vomiting

Hematologic: Anemia, granulocytopenia (nadir: 7-10 days; recovery 14-21 days), leukopenia, neutropenia, neutropenic fever/sepsis, thrombocytopenia

Hepatic: AST increased, total bilirubin increased

Local: Injection site pain, injection site reaction (includes erythema and vein discoloration), phlebitis

Neuromuscular & skeletal: Arthralgia, jaw pain, myalgia, peripheral neuropathy, loss of deep tendon reflexes, weakness

Otic: Ototoxicity

Respiratory: Dyspnea

Rare but important or life-threatening: Abdominal pain, allergic reactions, anaphylaxis, angioedema, back pain, DVT, dysphagia, esophagitis, flushing, gait instability, headache, hemolytic uremic syndrome, hemorrhagic cystitis, hyper-/hypotension, hyponatremia, intestinal necrosis, intestinal obstruction, intestinal perforation, interstitial pulmonary changes, local rash, local urticaria, MI (rare), mucositis, muscle weakness, myocardial ischemia, pancreatitis, paralytic ileus, pneumonia, pruritus, pulmonary edema, pulmonary embolus, radiation recall (dermatitis, esophagitis), skin blistering, syndrome of inappropriate ADH secretion, tachycardia, thromboembolic events, thrombotic thrombocytopenic purpura, tumor pain, urticaria, vasodilation

Drug Interactions

Metabolism/Transport Effects Substrate of CYP2D6 (minor), 3A4 (major); **Inhibits** CYP2D6 (weak), 3A4 (weak)

Avoid Concomitant Use

Avoid concomitant use of Vinorelbine with any of the following: BCG; CloZAPine; Conivaptan; Dipyrone; Fusidic Acid (Systemic); Natalizumab; Pimecrolimus; Pimozide; Tacrolimus (Topical); Tofacitinib; Vaccines (Live)

Increased Effect/Toxicity Previous or simultaneous use with mitomycin-C has resulted in acute shortness of breath and severe bronchospasm within minutes or several hours after Vinca alkaloid injection and may occur up to 2 weeks after the dose of mitomycin. CYP3A4 inhibitors may increase the levels/effects of vinorelbine; example inhibitors include azole antifungals, ciprofloxacin, clarithromycin, diclofenac, doxycycline, erythromycin, imatinib, isoniazid, nefazodone, nicardipine, propofol, protease inhibitors, quinidine, and verapamil. Incidence of granulocytopenia is significantly higher in cisplatin/vinorelbine combination therapy than with single-agent vinorelbine.

Decreased Effect CYP3A4 inducers may decrease the levels/effects of vinorelbine; example inducers include aminoglutethimide, carbamazepine, nafcillin, nevirapine, phenobarbital, phenytoin, and rifamycins.

Stability Store intact vials at 2°C to 8°C (36°F to 46°F); do not freeze. Protect from light. Intact vials are stable at 25°C (77°F) for up to 72 hours. Solutions diluted for infusion in polypropylene syringes or polyvinyl chloride bags are stable for 24 hours at 5°C to 30°C (41°F to 86°F). After preparation, keep vinorelbine in a location **away** from the separate storage location recommended for intrathecal medications.

Mechanism of Action Semisynthetic vinca alkaloid which binds to tubulin and inhibits microtubule formation, therefore, arresting the cell at metaphase by disrupting the formation of the mitotic spindle; it is specific for the M and S phases. Vinorelbine may also interfere with nucleic acid and protein synthesis by blocking glutamic acid utilization.

Pharmacokinetics (Adult data unless noted)

Distribution: Binds extensively to human platelets and lymphocytes (80% to 91%); V_d:

Children and Adolescents 2-17 years: 21.1 ± 12.2 L/kg (Johansen, 2006)

Adults: 25-40 L/kg

Protein binding: 80% to 91%

Metabolism: Extensively hepatic, via CYP3A4, to two metabolites, deacetylvinorelbine (active) and vinorelbine N-oxide

Half-life elimination: Triphasic:

Children and Adolescents 2-17 years: Terminal: 16.5 ± 9.7 hours (Johansen, 2006)

Adults: Terminal: 28-44 hours

Elimination: Feces (46%); urine (18%, 10% to 12% as unchanged drug)

Dosing: Usual

Infants, Children, and Adolescents:

Hodgkin's lymphoma; refractory or recurrent: Limited data available: I.V.: Children ≥10 years and Adolescents: 25 mg/m² once weekly on days 1 and 8 of a 21-day cycle in combination with gemcitabine (Cole, 2009)

Leukemias; acute (ALL, AML), refractory, or recurrent: Limited data available: I.V.:

Infants: 0.67 mg/**kg** once weekly on days 0, 7, 14 of a 14-day cycle in combination with topotecan, clofarabine, and thiotepa (TVTC regimen) (Steinherz, 2010)

Children and Adolescents: 20 mg/m² once weekly on days 0, 7, and 14 of a 14-day cycle in combination with topotecan, clofarabine, and thiotepa (TVTC regimen) (Shuka, 2014; Steinherz, 2010)

Solid tumors; refractory or recurrent: Limited data available: Children and Adolescents: I.V.:

Monotherapy: 30 mg/m^2 once weekly for weeks 1-6 of an 8-week cycle for 10 courses; may reduce dosage to 27 mg/m^2 for Grade 3 or 4 hematologic toxicity in patients who demonstrate objective response or who have had treatment delay beyond 63 days (week 9) from the previous course (Kuttesch, 2009)

Combination therapy: 25 mg/m^2 once weekly for 3 weeks on days 1, 8, and 15 of each 28-day cycle in combination with cyclophosphamide (Casanova, 2004; Minard-Colin, 2012)

Adults: **Nonsmall cell lung cancer (NSCLC):** I.V.: **Note:** Utilize patient's actual body weight (full weight) for calculation of body surface area- or weight-based dosing, particularly when the intent of therapy is curative; manage regimen-related toxicities in the same manner as for nonobese patients; if a dose reduction is utilized due to toxicity, consider resumption of full weight-based dosing with subsequent cycles, especially if cause of toxicity (eg, hepatic or renal impairment) is resolved (Griggs, 2012).

Monotherapy: 30 mg/m^2 every 7 days until disease progression or unacceptable toxicity

Combination therapy: 25-30 mg/m^2 every 7 days in combination with cisplatin

Dosing adjustment in hematological toxicity: Adults: **Note:** In patients with concurrent hematologic toxicity and hepatic impairment, administer the lower of the doses determined from the adjustment recommendations.

Granulocyte counts should be ≥1000 cells/mm^3 prior to the administration of vinorelbine. Adjustments in the dosage of vinorelbine should be based on granulocyte counts obtained on the day of treatment as follows:

Granulocytes ≥1500 cells/mm^3 on day of treatment: Administer 100% of starting dose

Granulocytes 1000-1499 cells/mm^3 on day of treatment: Administer 50% of starting dose

Granulocytes <1000 cells/mm^3 on day of treatment: Do not administer. Repeat granulocyte count in 1 week; if 3 consecutive doses are held because granulocyte count is <1000 cells/mm^3, discontinue vinorelbine.

For patients who, during treatment, have experienced fever and/or sepsis while granulocytopenic or had 2 consecutive weekly doses held due to granulocytopenia, subsequent doses of vinorelbine should be:

75% of starting dose for granulocytes ≥1500 cells/mm^3

37.5% of starting dose for granulocytes 1000-1499 cells/mm^3

Dosage adjustment for neurotoxicity: Adults: Neurotoxicity ≥grade 2: Discontinue treatment

Dosage adjustment for other adverse events: Adults: Severe adverse events: Reduce dose or discontinue treatment

Dosing adjustment in renal impairment: Adults:

Renal insufficiency: No dosage adjustment necessary

Hemodialysis: Initial: I.V.: Reduce dose to 20 mg/m^2/week; administer either after dialysis (on dialysis days) or on nondialysis days (Janus, 2010)

Dosing adjustment in hepatic impairment: All patients: **Note:** In patients with concurrent hematologic toxicity and hepatic impairment, administer the lower of the doses determined from the adjustment recommendations. Administer with caution in patients with hepatic insufficiency. In patients who develop hyperbilirubinemia during treatment with vinorelbine, the dose should be adjusted for total bilirubin as follows:

Serum bilirubin ≤2 mg/dL: Administer 100% of dose

Serum bilirubin 2.1-3 mg/dL: Administer 50% of dose (Ecklund, 2005; Floyd, 2006; Superfin, 2006)

Serum bilirubin >3 mg/dL: Administer 25% of dose (Ecklund, 2005; Floyd, 2006; Superfin, 2006)

Administration Hazardous agent; use appropriate precautions for handling and disposal (NIOSH, 2012).

For I.V. use only; FATAL IF GIVEN INTRATHECALLY. Administer as a direct intravenous push or rapid bolus, over 6-10 minutes (up to 30 minutes); in pediatric trials, vinorelbine typically administered over 6-10 minutes. Longer infusions may increase the risk of pain and phlebitis. Intravenous doses should be followed by at least 75-125 mL of saline or D$_5$W to reduce the incidence of phlebitis and inflammation.

Vesicant; avoid extravasation. Assure proper needle or catheter position prior to administration. If extravasation occurs, stop infusion immediately and disconnect (leave cannula/needle in place); gently aspirate extravasated solution (do **NOT** flush the line); initiate hyaluronidase antidote (See Management of Drug Extravasations for more details); apply dry warm compresses for 20 minutes 4 times a day for 1-2 days; elevate extremity (Pérez Fidalgo, 2012). Remaining portion of the vinorelbine dose should be infused through a separate vein.

Vesicant/Extravasation Risk Vesicant.

Monitoring Parameters CBC with differential and platelet count (prior to each dose, and after treatment), hepatic function tests; monitor for new-onset pulmonary symptoms (or worsening from baseline); monitor for neuropathy (new or worsening symptoms; monitor infusion site; monitor for signs symptoms of constipation/ileus

Dosage Forms Excipient information presented when available (limited, particularly for generics); consult specific product labeling.

Solution, Intravenous:

Navelbine: 10 mg/mL (1 mL); 50 mg/5 mL (5 mL)

Generic: 10 mg/mL (1 mL); 50 mg/5 mL (5 mL)

Solution, Intravenous [preservative free]:

Generic: 10 mg/mL (1 mL); 50 mg/5 mL (5 mL)

References

Casanova M, Ferrari A, Bisogno G, et al, "Vinorelbine and Low-Dose Cyclophosphamide in the Treatment of Pediatric Sarcomas: Pilot Study for the Upcoming European Rhabdomyosarcoma Protocol," *Cancer*, 2004, 101(7):1664-71.

Casanova M, Ferrari A, Spreafico F, et al, "Vinorelbine in Previously Treated Advanced Childhood Sarcomas: Evidence of Activity in Rhabdomyosarcoma," *Cancer*, 2002, 94(12):3263-8.

Cole PD, Schwartz CL, Drachtman RA, et al. Phase II study of weekly gemcitabine and vinorelbine for children with recuerent or refractory Hodgkin's Disease: a children's oncology group report. *J Clin Oncol*. 2009;27(9):1456-1461.

Ecklund JW, Trifilio S, and Mulcahy MF, "Chemotherapy Dosing in the Setting of Liver Dysfunction," *Oncology (Williston Park)*, 2005, 19 (8):1057-63.

Floyd J, Mirza I, Sachs B, Perry MC. Hepatotoxicity of chemotherapy. *Semin Oncol*. 2006;33(1):50-67.

Griggs JJ, Mangu PB, Anderson H, et al, "Appropriate Chemotherapy Dosing For Obese Adult Patients With Cancer: American Society of Clinical Oncology Clinical Practice Guideline," *J Clin Oncol*, 2012, 30 (13):1553-61.

Jacobson JO, Polovich M, McNiff KK, et al, "American Society of Clinical Oncology/ Oncology Nursing Society Chemotherapy Administration Safety Standards," *J Clin Oncol*, 2009, 27(32):5469-75.

Janus N, Thariat J, Boulanger H, et al, "Proposal for Dosage Adjustment and Timing of Chemotherapy in Hemodialyzed Patients," *Ann Oncol*, 2010, 21(7):1395-403.

Johansen J, Kuttesch J, Bleyer WA, et al. Phase I evaluation of oral and intravenous vinorelbine in pediatric cancer patients: a report from the children's oncology group. *Clin Cancer Res*. 2006;12(2):516-522.

Kuttesch JF, Krailo MD, Madden T, et al. Phase II evaluation of intravenous vinorelbine (Navelbine) in recurrent or refractory pediatric malignancies: a children's oncology group study. *Pediatr Blood Cancer*. 2009;53(4):590-593.

LeVeque D and Jehl F, "Clinical Pharmacokinetics of Vinorelbine," *Clin Pharmacokinet*, 1996, 31(3):184-97.

Minard-Colin V, Ichante JL, Nguyen L, et al. Phase II study of vinorelbine and continuous low doses cyclophosphamide in children and young adults with relapsed or refractory malignant solid tumour: good tolerance profile and efficacy in rhabdomyosarcoma – a report from the Société Française des Cancers et leucémies de l'Enfant et de l'adolescent (SFCE). *Eur J Cancer*. 2012;48:2409-2416.

National Institute for Occupational Safety and Health (NIOSH), "NIOSH List of Antineoplastic and Other Hazardous Drugs in Healthcare Settings 2012." Available at http://www.cdc.gov/niosh/docs/2012-150/pdfs/2012-150.pdf. Accessed January 21, 2013.

Navelbine (vinorelbine tartrate) [prescribing information]. Parsippany, NJ: Pierre Fabre Médicament; October 2007.

Pérez Fidalgo JA, García Fabregat L, Cervantes A, et al, "Management of Chemotherapy Extravasation: ESMO-EONS Clinical Practice Guidelines," *Ann Oncol*, 2012, 23(Suppl 7):167-73.

Polovich M, Whitford JN and Olsen M, *Chemotherapy and Biotherapy Guidelines and Recommendations for Practice*, 3rd ed, Pittsburgh, PA: Oncology Nursing Society, 2009.

Schulmeister L, "Extravasation Management: Clinical Update," *Semin Oncol Nurs*, 2011, 27(1):82-90.

Shukla N, Kobos R, Renaud T, et al. Phase II trial of clofarabine with topotecan, vinorelbine and thiotepa for pediatric patients with relapsed or refractory acute leukemia. *Pediatr Blood Cancer*. 2014;61:431-435.

Steinherz PG, Shukla N, Kobos R, et al. Remission re-induction chemotherapy with clofarabine, topotecan, thiotepa and vinorelbine for patients with relapsed or refractory leukemia. *Pediatr Blood Cancer*. 2010;54:687-693.

Superfin D, Iannucci AA, and Davies AM, "Commentary: Oncologic Drugs in Patients With Organ Dysfunction: A Summary," *Oncologist*, 2007, 12(9):1070-83.

◆ **Vinorelbine Injection, USP (Can)** *see* Vinorelbine *on page 2143*

◆ **Vinorelbine Tartrate** *see* Vinorelbine *on page 2143*

◆ **Vinorelbine Tartrate for Injection (Can)** *see* Vinorelbine *on page 2143*

◆ **Viokace** *see* Pancrelipase *on page 1591*

◆ **Viokase (Can)** *see* Pancrelipase *on page 1591*

◆ **Viosterol** *see* Ergocalciferol *on page 774*

◆ **Viracept** *see* Nelfinavir *on page 1479*

◆ **Viramune** *see* Nevirapine *on page 1487*

◆ **Viramune® (Can)** *see* Nevirapine *on page 1487*

◆ **Viramune XR** *see* Nevirapine *on page 1487*

◆ **Viramune XR® (Can)** *see* Nevirapine *on page 1487*

◆ **Virasal** *see* Salicylic Acid *on page 1860*

◆ **Virazole** *see* Ribavirin *on page 1818*

◆ **Viread** *see* Tenofovir *on page 1977*

◆ **Viroptic** *see* Trifluridine *on page 2084*

◆ **Viroptic® (Can)** *see* Trifluridine *on page 2084*

◆ **Virtussin A/C** *see* Guaifenesin and Codeine *on page 985*

◆ **Viscous Lidocaine** *see* Lidocaine (Topical) *on page 1242*

◆ **Visine-LR [OTC]** *see* Oxymetazoline (Ophthalmic) *on page 1578*

◆ **Visipaque** *see* Iodixanol *on page 1142*

◆ **Visipaque™ (Can)** *see* Iodixanol *on page 1142*

◆ **Vistaril** *see* HydrOXYzine *on page 1054*

◆ **Vistide** *see* Cidofovir *on page 466*

◆ **Vita-C [OTC]** *see* Ascorbic Acid *on page 206*

◆ **Vitamin C** *see* Ascorbic Acid *on page 206*

Vitamin A (VYE ta min aye)

Medication Safety Issues
Sound-alike/look-alike issues:
Aquasol® may be confused with Anusol®

Related Information
Multivitamin Product Table *on page 2227*

Brand Names: U.S. A-25 [OTC]; AFirm 1X [OTC]; AFirm 2X [OTC]; AFirm 3X [OTC]; Aquasol A; Gordons-Vite A [OTC]; Vitamin A Fish [OTC]

Therapeutic Category Nutritional Supplement; Vitamin, Fat Soluble

Generic Availability (U.S.) May be product dependent

Use Treatment of vitamin A deficiency (injection: FDA approved in all ages; oral: FDA approved in adults); has also been used for prevention of vitamin A deficiency, supplementation in infants and children ≤5 years with measles, and prevention of chronic lung disease in premature neonates

Pregnancy Risk Factor X

Pregnancy Considerations Adverse events have been observed in animal reproduction studies. In humans, the critical period of exposure is the first trimester of pregnancy. Excess vitamin A during pregnancy may cause craniofacial malformations, as well as CNS, heart, and thymus abnormalities. Maternal vitamin A deficiency also causes adverse effects in the fetus, and vitamin A requirements are increased in pregnant women (IOM, 2000). The manufacturer notes that the safety of doses >6000 units/day in pregnant women has not been established and doses greater than the RDA are contraindicated in pregnant women or those who may become pregnant. High doses are used in some areas of the world for supplementation where deficiency is a public health problem (eg, to prevent night blindness); however, single doses >25,000 units should be avoided within 60 days of conception. High-dose supplementation is otherwise not recommended as part of routine antenatal care (WHO, 2011c).

Breast-Feeding Considerations Vitamin A requirements are increased in breast-feeding women (IOM, 2000). High-dose supplementation (eg, doses higher than the RDA) is not recommended in otherwise healthy women who receive adequate nutrition (WHO, 2011b).

Contraindications Hypersensitivity to vitamin A or any component; hypervitaminosis A; pregnancy (dose exceeding RDA); intravenous administration of Aquasol A®

Warnings Patients receiving >25,000 units/day should be closely monitored for toxicity. Injection contains polysorbate 80 (Tween 80®) which may cause allergic reactions in susceptible individuals. In premature neonates, thrombocytopenia, ascites, pulmonary deterioration, and renal and hepatic failure have been reported after receiving parenteral products containing polysorbate 80 (Alade, 1986; CDC, 1984).

Adverse Reactions Miscellaneous: Allergic reactions (rare), anaphylactic shock (following I.V. administration)

Drug Interactions

Metabolism/Transport Effects None known.

Avoid Concomitant Use
Avoid concomitant use of Vitamin A with any of the following: Retinoic Acid Derivatives

Increased Effect/Toxicity
The levels/effects of Vitamin A may be increased by: Retinoic Acid Derivatives

Decreased Effect
The levels/effects of Vitamin A may be decreased by: Orlistat

Food Interactions Excessive ethanol intake depletes the liver of vitamin A and may enhance vitamin A toxicity (IOM, 2000)

Stability Injection: Store at 2°C to 8°C (36°F to 46°F); do not freeze. Protect from light.

Mechanism of Action Vitamin A is a fat soluble vitamin needed for visual adaptation to darkness, maintenance of epithelial cells, immune function and embryonic development.

Pharmacokinetics (Adult data unless noted)
Absorption: Vitamin A in dosages **not** exceeding physiologic replacement is well absorbed in the small intestine after oral administration; water miscible preparations are absorbed more rapidly than oil preparations; large oral doses, conditions of fat malabsorption, low protein intake, or hepatic or pancreatic disease reduce oral absorption

Distribution: Large amounts concentrate for storage in the liver

Metabolism: Converted in the small intestine to retinol and further metabolized in the liver; conjugated with glucuronide, undergoes enterohepatic circulation

Elimination: In feces via biliary elimination

Dosing: Neonatal 1 unit vitamin A = 0.3 mcg retinol

Adequate Intake (AI): 400 mcg (1330 units)

Chronic lung disease, prevention in ELBW: I.M.: 5000 units/dose 3 times weekly (ie, MWF) initiated within the first 96 hours of life and continued for 4 weeks was used in 405 neonates (mean GA: 26.8 weeks; mean birth weight: 770 g; range: 400-1000 g) (Tyson, 1999).

Dosing: Usual 1 unit vitamin A = 0.3 mcg retinol

Dietary Reference Intake for vitamin A (presented as retinol activity equivalent [RAE] (IOM, 2000): Oral:

Adequate Intake (AI) (IOM, 2000):

1-6 months: 400 mcg/day (1330 units/day)

6-12 months: 500 mcg/day (1670 units/day)

Recommended Daily Allowance (RDA) (IOM, 2000): Oral:

1-3 years: 300 mcg/day (1000 units/day)

4-8 years: 400 mcg/day (1330 units/day)

9-13 years: 600 mcg/day (2000 units/day)

>13 years and Adults: Female: 700 mcg/day (2330 units/day); Male: 900 mcg/day (3000 units/day)

Pregnant females:

14-18 years: 750 mcg/day (2500 units/day)

≥19 years: 770 mcg/day (2560 units/day)

Lactating females:

14-18 years: 1200 mcg/day (4000 units/day)

≥19 years: 1300 mcg/day (4330 units/day)

Measles infection, supplementation (WHO, 2004; WHO, 2010): Infants and Children: Oral:

Infants <6 months: 50,000 units daily for 2 days

Infants 6-11 months: 100,000 units daily for 2 days

Children ≥12 months to 5 years: 200,000 units daily for 2 days

Note: If severe malnutrition or ophthalmologic evidence of vitamin A deficiency is present, repeat a single dose 2-4 weeks after the second dose.

Vitamin A deficiency (varying recommendations available):

Prophylaxis for at-risk populations (eg, potential HIV infection, local prevalence of nightblindness >1% in ages 24-59 months or prevalence of serum retinol ≤0.7 mmol/L is ≥20% in ages 6-59 months) (WHO, 2008; WHO, 2010; WHO, 2011a; WHO, 2011b; WHO, 2011c; WHO, 2011d): Oral:

Infants <6 months: Not recommended

Infants 6-12 months: 100,000 units; administer as a single dose; repeat every 4-6 months, but do not readminister within 30 days of previous dose

Children and Adolescents: 200,000 units; administer as a single dose; repeat every 4-6 months, but do not readminister within 30 days of previous dose

Adults: 200,000 units/dose every 6 months

Pregnant women: Maximum 10,000 units once daily or 25,000 units once weekly. Administer for a minimum of 12 weeks during pregnancy or until delivery.

Postpartum women: 200,000 units at delivery or within 8 weeks of delivery

Treatment:

Infants:

I.M.: 7500-15,000 units once daily for 10 days followed by oral supplementation

Oral: 5000-10,000 units daily for 2 months following I.M. dosing

Children 1-8 years:

I.M.: 17,500-35,000 units once daily for 10 days followed by oral supplementation

Oral: 5000-10,000 units once daily for 2 months following I.M. dosing

Children >8 years and Adults:

I.M.: 100,000 units once daily for 3 days; then 50,000 units once daily for 14 days followed by oral supplementation

Oral: 10,000-20,000 units once daily for 2 months following I.M. dosing

Xerophthalmia (WHO, 1997; WHO, 2010): Oral:

Infants <6 months: 50,000 units administered as a single dose; repeat the next day and again after at least 2 weeks for a total of 3 doses

Infants 6-12 months: 100,000 units administered as a single dose; repeat the next day and again after at least 2 weeks for a total of 3 doses

Children and Adolescents: 200,000 units administered as a single dose; repeat the next day and again after at least 2 weeks for a total of 3 doses

Adults: 200,000 units once daily for 2 days; repeat with single dose in 2 weeks. **Note:** Females of reproductive age with night blindness or Bitot's spots should receive 5000-10,000 units daily or ≤25,000 units once weekly; if severe xerophthalmia, females of reproductive age may receive high dose (ie, 200,000 unit regimen) regardless of pregnancy status.

Malabsorption syndrome (prophylaxis): Children >8 years and Adults: Oral: 10,000-50,000 units/day of water miscible product

Administration

Oral: Administer with food or milk; for infants and children <24 months of age, capsules may be cut open and contents squeezed into the mouth

Parenteral: **For I.M. use only;** for neonatal patients, a 0.3 mL syringe and 29-gauge needle should be used for I.M. dose administration

Additional Information 1 USP vitamin A unit = 0.3 mcg of all-*trans* isomer of retinol; 1 RAE (retinol activity equivalent) = 1 mcg of all-*trans*-retinol = 12 mcg of dietary beta-carotene (IOM, 2000)

Dosage Forms Excipient information presented when available (limited, particularly for generics); consult specific product labeling.

Capsule, Oral:

A-25: 25,000 units

Vitamin A Fish: 7500 units

Generic: 10,000 units

Capsule, Oral [preservative free]:

A-25: 25,000 units [dye free]

Generic: 8000 units

Cream, External:

AFirm 1X: 0.15% (30 g) [fragrance free; contains benzyl alcohol, cetyl alcohol, disodium edta, methylparaben, peg-10 soya sterol, trolamine (triethanolamine)]

AFirm 2X: 0.3% (30 g) [fragrance free; contains benzyl alcohol, cetyl alcohol, disodium edta, methylparaben, peg-10 soya sterol, trolamine (triethanolamine)]

AFirm 3X: 0.6% (30 g) [fragrance free; contains benzyl alcohol, cetyl alcohol, disodium edta, methylparaben, peg-10 soya sterol, trolamine (triethanolamine)]

Gordons-Vite A: 100,000 units/g (75 g, 120 g, 480 g, 2400 g)

Lotion, External:

Gordons-Vite A: 100,000 units (120 mL, 4000 mL)

Solution, Intramuscular:

Aquasol A: 50,000 units/mL (2 mL) [contains chlorobutanol (chlorobutol)]

Tablet, Oral:

Generic: 10,000 units, 15,000 units, Vitamin A 10000 units and beta carotene 1000 units

References

Alade SL, Brown RE, and Paquet A Jr, "Polysorbate 80 and E-Ferol Toxicity," *Pediatrics*, 1986, 77(4):593-7.

Centers for Disease Control (CDC), "Unusual Syndrome With Fatalities Among Premature Infants: Association With a New Intravenous Vitamin E Product," *MMWR Morb Mortal Wkly Rep*, 1984, 33 (14):198-9.

Committee on Infectious Diseases, "Vitamin A in the Treatment of Measles," *Pediatrics*, 1993, 91(5):1014-5.

DeMaeyer EM, "The WHO Programme of Prevention and Control of Vitamin A Deficiency, Xerophthalmia, and Nutritional Blindness," *Nutr Health*, 1986, 4(2):105-12.

Hussey GD and Klein M, "A Randomized, Controlled Trial of Vitamin A in Children With Severe Measles," *N Engl J Med*, 1990, 323(3):160-4.

IOM (Institute of Medicine), *Dietary Reference Intakes for Vitamin A, Vitamin K, Arsenic, Boron, Chromium, Copper, Iodine, Iron, Manganese, Molybdenum, Nickel, Silicon, Vanadium, and Zinc*, Washington, DC: National Academy Press, 2000.

Tyson JE, Wright LL, Oh W, et al, "Vitamin A Supplementation for Extremely-Low-Birth-Weight Infants. National Institute of Child Health and Human Development Neonatal Research Network," *N Engl J Med*, 1999, 340(25):1962-8.

WHO Guideline, "Vitamin A Supplementation in Infants 1–5 Months of Age," Geneva: World Health Organization, 2011a. Available at http://www.who.int/nutrition/publications/micronutrients/guidelines/vas_infants_1-5/en/

WHO Guideline, "Vitamin A Supplementation in Postpartum Women," Geneva: World Health Organization, 2011b. Available at http://www.who.int/nutrition/publications/micronutrients/guidelines/vas_postpartum/en/

WHO Guideline, "Vitamin A Supplementation in Pregnant Women," Geneva: World Health Organization, 2011c. Available at http://www.who.int/nutrition/publications/micronutrients/guidelines/vas_pregnant/en/

WHO Guideline, "Vitamin A Supplementation in Infants 6-59 Months of Age," Geneva: World Health Organization, 2011d. Available at http://www.who.int/nutrition/publications/micronutrients/guidelines/vas_6to59_months/en/index.html

WHO Model Formulary, 2008. Available at http://apps.who.int/medicinedocs/en/m/abstract/Js16879e/

WHO Model Formulary for Children, 2010. Available at http://apps.who.int/medicinedocs/en/m/abstract/Js17151e/

WHO/UNICEF/IVACG Task Force, *Vitamin A Supplements. A Guide to Their Use in the Treatment and Prevention of Vitamin A Deficiency and Xerophthalmia*, 2nd ed. Geneva: World Health Organization, 1997. Available at http://www.who.int/nutrition/publications/micronutrients/vitamin_a_deficiency/9241545062/en/

◆ **Vitamin A Acid** *see* Tretinoin (Topical) *on page 2071*

◆ **Vitamin A Fish [OTC]** *see* Vitamin A *on page 2146*

◆ **Vitamin B₁** *see* Thiamine *on page 2009*

◆ **Vitamin B₂** *see* Riboflavin *on page 1821*

◆ **Vitamin B₃** *see* Niacin *on page 1491*

◆ **Vitamin B₆** *see* Pyridoxine *on page 1778*

◆ **Vitamin B₁₂** *see* Cyanocobalamin *on page 556*

◆ **Vitamin B₁₂ₐ** *see* Hydroxocobalamin *on page 1045*

◆ **Vitamin Bw** *see* Biotin *on page 292*

◆ **Vitamin D2** *see* Ergocalciferol *on page 774*

◆ **Vitamin D3 Super Strength [OTC]** *see* Cholecalciferol *on page 455*

Vitamin E (VYE ta min ee)

Medication Safety Issues
Sound-alike/look-alike issues:
Aquasol E may be confused with Anusol

Related Information
Multivitamin Product Table *on page 2227*

Brand Names: U.S. Alph-E [OTC]; Alph-E-Mixed 1000 [OTC]; Alph-E-Mixed [OTC]; Aquasol E [OTC]; Aquavit-E [OTC]; Aqueous Vitamin E [OTC]; E-400 [OTC]; E-400-Clear [OTC]; E-400-Mixed [OTC]; E-Max-1000 [OTC]; E-Pherol [OTC]; Formula E 400 [OTC]; Gordons-Vite E [OTC]; Natural Vitamin E [OTC]; Nutr-E-Sol [OTC]; Vita-Plus E [OTC]; Vitamin E Beauty [OTC]; Vitec [OTC]; Xtra-Care [OTC]

Therapeutic Category Nutritional Supplement; Vitamin, Fat Soluble; Vitamin, Topical

Generic Availability (U.S.) May be product dependent

Use Prevention and treatment of vitamin E deficiency

Pregnancy Considerations Vitamin E crosses the placenta. Maternal serum concentrations of α tocopherol increase with lipid concentrations as pregnancy progresses; however, placental transfer remains constant. Additional supplementation is not needed in pregnant women without deficiency (IOM, 2000).

Breast-Feeding Considerations Vitamin E is found in breast milk; concentrations decrease over time and are highest immediately postpartum. Breast milk concentrations may be affected by maternal intake; however, additional supplementation is not needed in nursing women (IOM, 2000).

Contraindications Hypersensitivity to vitamin E or any component

Warnings Necrotizing enterocolitis has been associated with oral administration of large dosages (eg, >200 units/day) of a hyperosmolar vitamin E preparation in low birth weight infants. May induce vitamin K deficiency (Corkins, 2010). Excessive intake of vitamin E may be associated with adverse effects including hemorrhagic effects; use caution when total daily intake from all sources exceeds the recommended age-based daily upper limit: 1-3 years: 200 mg; 4-8 years: 300 mg; 9-13 years: 600 mg; 14-18 years: 800 mg; ≥19 years: 1000 mg; monitor serum concentrations (IOM, 2000).

Aquasol E contains polysorbate 80 (Tween 80) which may cause allergic reactions in susceptible individuals. In premature neonates, thrombocytopenia, ascites, pulmonary deterioration, and renal and hepatic failure have been reported after receiving parenteral products containing polysorbate 80 (Alade, 1986; CDC, 1984).

Adverse Reactions
Central nervous system: Fatigue, headache

Dermatologic: Contact dermatitis with topical preparation, rash

Endocrine & metabolic: Creatinuria, gonadal dysfunction, hypercholesterolemia, hypertriglyceridemia, serum thyroxine decreased, serum triiodothyronine decreased

Gastrointestinal: Diarrhea, intestinal cramps, nausea, necrotizing enterocolitis (infants)

Neuromuscular & skeletal: CPK increased, weakness

Ocular: Blurred vision

Renal: Serum creatinine increased

Drug Interactions
Metabolism/Transport Effects None known.

Avoid Concomitant Use There are no known interactions where it is recommended to avoid concomitant use.

Increased Effect/Toxicity
Vitamin E may increase the levels/effects of: Agents with Antiplatelet Properties; Anticoagulants

The levels/effects of Vitamin E may be increased by: Tipranavir

Decreased Effect
Vitamin E may decrease the levels/effects of: CycloSPORINE (Systemic)

The levels/effects of Vitamin E may be decreased by: Orlistat

Stability Protect from light.

Mechanism of Action Prevents oxidation of vitamin A and C; protects polyunsaturated fatty acids in membranes from attack by free radicals and protects red blood cells against hemolysis

Pharmacokinetics (Adult data unless noted)
Absorption: Oral: Depends upon the presence of bile; absorption is reduced in conditions of malabsorption, in low birth weight premature infants, and as dosage increases; water miscible preparations are better absorbed than oil preparations

Metabolism: Hepatic to glucuronides

Elimination: Feces

Dosing: Neonatal
Adequate intake (AI): Oral: 4 mg/day; **Note:** Adequate intake represents α-tocopherol intake from dietary consumption.

Cholestasis, chronic; supplementation: Oral: 25 to 50 units/day; a water soluble formulation is preferred (Kleigman, 2011)

Deficiency, vitamin E: Oral:

Treatment: 25 to 50 units/day for 1 week, followed by adequate dietary intake (Kleigman, 2011)

Prevention: Aquasol E drops: 5 units/day

Cystic fibrosis supplementation: Oral: 40 to 50 units/day (Borowitz, 2002)

Dosing: Usual

Infants, Children, and Adolescents:

Adequate intake (AI): Oral: **Note:** Adequate intake represents α-tocopherol intake from dietary consumption

1 to 6 months: 4 mg/day

7 to 12 months: 5 mg/day

Recommended daily allowance (RDA): Oral: **Note:** Recommended daily allowance represents α-tocopherol intake from dietary consumption.

1 to 3 years: 6 mg/day

4 to 8 years: 7 mg/day

9 to 13 years: 11 mg/day

14 to 18 years: 15 mg/day

Cholestasis, chronic; supplementation: Oral:

Infants: 20 to 50 units/kg/day; in the trials, a water soluble formulation was used (Corkins, 2010; Sokol, 1993)

Biliary atresia, post-hepatoportoenterostomy (HPE): Initial: 100 units/day using AquaADEK (2 mL); titrate dose based upon serum concentrations in 25 units/kg/day increments up to 100 units/kg/day to target α-tocopherol serum concentration range: 3.8 to 20.3 mcg/mL, vitamin E:total serum lipids ratio of 0.6 mg/g; patients with a total bilirubin <2 mg/dL may require lower doses (Shneider, 2012)

Children: 1 unit/kg/day; a water soluble formulation is preferred (Kleigman, 2011)

Deficiency, vitamin E: Oral:

Treatment (associated with malabsorption): Children: 1 unit/kg/day; adjust dose based on serum concentrations; a water soluble formulation is preferred (Kleigman, 2011)

Prevention: Aquasol E:

Infants: 5 units/day

Children <4 years: 10 units/day

Children ≥4 years and Adolescents: 15 units/day

Cystic fibrosis supplementation (Borowitz, 2002): Oral:

1 to 12 months: 40 to 50 units/day

1 to 3 years: 80 to 150 units/day

4 to 8 years: 100 to 200 units/day

>8 years: 200 to 400 units/day

Superficial dermatologic irritation: Children and Adolescents: Topical: Apply a thin layer over affected area

Adults:

Recommended daily allowance (RDA): Oral: **Note:** Recommended daily allowance represents α-tocopherol intake from dietary consumption. 15 mg/day

Lactating female: 19 mg/day

Superficial dermatologic irritation: Topical: Apply a thin layer over affected area

Administration Oral: May administer with or without food. Swallow capsules whole; do not crush or chew.

Monitoring Parameters Plasma tocopherol concentrations

Reference Range Plasma tocopherol: 6-14 mcg/mL

Additional Information Vitamin E, also known as α-tocopherol, occurs as several different isomers: RRR-α-tocopherol (the only form of α-tocopherol that occurs naturally in foods) and the 2,S and 2,R sterioisomers that occur in fortified foods and supplements [also known as all racemic (all rac)-α-tocopherol]. Only the 2,R-stereoisomeric forms of α-tocopherol are biologically active, thus a higher amount of all racemic (all rac)-α-tocopherol is needed than the vitamin E found naturally in foods (based on milligram amount) (IOM, 2000).

In the past, the recommended daily allowance (RDA) for vitamin E had been expressed in units. The term units has been replaced by milligrams (mg) of α-tocopherol or may also be expressed as alpha tocopherol equivalents (ATE), which refer to the biologically active (R) stereoisomer content. While international units are no longer recognized, many fortified foods and supplements continue to use this term. USP units are now used by the pharmaceutical industry when labeling vitamin E supplements. Both IUs and USP units are based on the same equivalency. One unit of vitamin E=1 mg of all racemic (all-rac)-α-tocopheryl acetate (synthetic Vitamin E; also known as dl-α-tocopherol acetate) or 0.67 mg RRR-α-tocopherol (naturally occurring vitamin E; also known as d-α-tocopherol) (IOM, 2000).

Dosage Forms Excipient information presented when available (limited, particularly for generics); consult specific product labeling.

Capsule, Oral:

Alph-E: 400 units

Alph-E-Mixed: 200 units

Alph-E-Mixed 1000: 1000 units

Alph-E-Mixed: 400 units [corn free, milk free, sugar free, wheat free, yeast free]

Formula E 400: 400 units

Vita-Plus E: 400 units

Generic: 100 units, 200 units, 400 units, 1000 units

Capsule, Oral [preservative free]:

E-400: 400 units [corn free, gluten free, milk derivatives/products, no artificial color(s), no artificial flavor(s), sodium free, soy free, starch free, sugar free, yeast free]

E-400-Clear: 400 units [dye free]

E-400-Mixed: 400 units [dye free]

E-Max-1000: 1000 units [dye free]

Generic: 100 units, 400 units

Cream, External:

Gordons-Vite E: 1500 units/30 g (15 g, 75 g, 480 g, 2400 g)

Generic: 1000 units (112 g)

Liquid, External:

Generic: 920 units/mL (28.5 mL, 57 mL, 114 mL)

Liquid, Oral:

Nutr-E-Sol: 400 units/15 mL (473 mL) [color free, starch free, sugar free]

Lotion, External:

Vitec: (113 g)

Xtra-Care: (2 mL, 59 mL, 118 mL, 237 mL, 621 mL, 1000 mL, 3840 mL)

Oil, External:

Vitamin E Beauty: 24,000 units/52 mL (52 mL); 49,000 units/52 mL (52 mL)

Solution, Oral:

Aquasol E: 15 units/0.3 mL (12 mL, 30 mL) [contains polysorbate 80, propylene glycol, saccharin]

Aquavit-E: 15 units/0.3 mL (30 mL) [butterscotch flavor]

Aqueous Vitamin E: 15 units/0.3 mL (30 mL) [anise-butterscotch flavor]

Generic: 15 units/0.3 mL (12 mL)

Tablet, Oral:
E-Pherol: 400 units
Natural Vitamin E: 200 units, 400 units [animal products free, gelatin free, gluten free, kosher certified, lactose free, no artificial color(s), no artificial flavor(s), starch free, sugar free, yeast free]
Generic: 100 units, 200 units, 400 units

References

Alade SL, Brown RE, Paquet A. Polysorbate 80 and e-ferol toxicity. *Pediatrics.* 1986;77(4):593-597.

Borowitz D, Baker RD, Stallings V. Consensus report on nutrition for pediatric patients with cystic fibrosis. *J Pediatr Gastroenterol Nutr.* 2002;35(3):246-259.

Center for Disease Control and Prevention (CDC). Unusual syndrome with fatalities among premature infants: association with a new intravenous vitamin E product. *MMWR.* 1984;33(14):198-199.

Corkins MR, ed. *The A.S.P.E.N. pediatric nuitrition support core curriculum. The American Society for Parenteral and Enteral Nutrition.* Silver Spring, MD; 2010.

IOM (Institute of Medicine). *Dietary Reference Intakes for Vitamin C, Vitamin E, Selenium, and Carotenoids.* Washington, DC: National Academy Press; 2000.

Kliegman RM, Stanton BF, St. Gemell JW, et al, eds. *Nelson Textbook of Pediatrics.* 19th ed. Philadelphia, PA: Saunders Elsevier; 2011.

Office of Dietary Supplements, National Institutes of Health, "Dietary Supplement Fact Sheet: Vitamin E." Available at: http://ods.od.nih.gov/factsheets/vitamine/

Schneider BL, Magee JC, Bezerra JA, et.al. Efficacy of fat-soluble vitamin supplementation in infants with biliary atresia. *Pediatrics.* 2012;130:607-614.

Sokol RJ, Butler-Simon N, Conner C. Multicenter trial of d-alpha-tocopheryl polyethylene glycol 1000 succinate for treatment of vitamin E deficiency in children with chronic cholestasis. *Gastroenterology.* 1993;104(6):1727-1735.

◆ **Vitamin E Beauty [OTC]** *see* Vitamin E *on page 2148*

◆ **Vitamin G** *see* Riboflavin *on page 1821*

◆ **Vitamin H** *see* Biotin *on page 292*

◆ **Vitamin K** *see* Phytonadione *on page 1671*

◆ **Vitamin K₁** *see* Phytonadione *on page 1671*

◆ **Vita-Plus E [OTC]** *see* Vitamin E *on page 2148*

◆ **Vitec [OTC]** *see* Vitamin E *on page 2148*

◆ **Vitrase** *see* Hyaluronidase *on page 1020*

◆ **Vitrasert [DSC]** *see* Ganciclovir (Ophthalmic) *on page 957*

◆ **Vituz** *see* Hydrocodone and Chlorpheniramine *on page 1030*

◆ **Vi Vaccine** *see* Typhoid Vaccine *on page 2093*

◆ **Vivactil** *see* Protriptyline *on page 1767*

◆ **Viva-Drops® [OTC]** *see* Artificial Tears *on page 205*

◆ **Vivarin® [OTC]** *see* Caffeine *on page 338*

◆ **Vivelle-Dot** *see* Estradiol (Systemic) *on page 796*

◆ **Vivotif** *see* Typhoid Vaccine *on page 2093*

◆ **VLB** *see* VinBLAStine *on page 2136*

◆ **VM-26** *see* Teniposide *on page 1976*

◆ **Vogelxo** *see* Testosterone *on page 1986*

◆ **Vogelxo Pump** *see* Testosterone *on page 1986*

◆ **Voltaren** *see* Diclofenac (Systemic) *on page 645*

◆ **Voltaren** *see* Diclofenac (Topical) *on page 649*

◆ **Voltaren Emulgel (Can)** *see* Diclofenac (Topical) *on page 649*

◆ **Voltaren Ophtha (Can)** *see* Diclofenac (Ophthalmic) *on page 648*

◆ **Voltaren Rapide (Can)** *see* Diclofenac (Systemic) *on page 645*

◆ **Voltaren SR (Can)** *see* Diclofenac (Systemic) *on page 645*

◆ **Voltaren-XR** *see* Diclofenac (Systemic) *on page 645*

◆ **Volulyte (Can)** *see* Tetrastarch *on page 1998*

◆ **Voluven** *see* Tetrastarch *on page 1998*

◆ **von Willebrand Factor/Factor VIII Complex** *see* Antihemophilic Factor/von Willebrand Factor Complex (Human) *on page 177*

◆ **Voraxaze** *see* Glucarpidase *on page 972*

Voriconazole (vor i KOE na zole)

Medication Safety Issues
Sound-alike/look-alike issues:
Voriconazole may be confused with fluconazole, itraconazole, posaconazole

Brand Names: U.S. Vfend; Vfend IV

Brand Names: Canada VFEND

Therapeutic Category Antifungal Agent, Systemic; Antifungal Agent, Triazole

Generic Availability (U.S.) Yes

Use Treatment of invasive aspergillosis; treatment of candidemia in non-neutropenic patients, deep tissue *Candida* infections and esophageal candidiasis; treatment of serious fungal infections caused by *Scedosporium apiospermum* or *Fusarium* spp (including *Fusarium solanae*) (All indications: FDA approved in ages ≥12 years and adults)

Pregnancy Risk Factor D

Pregnancy Considerations Voriconazole can cause fetal harm when administered to a pregnant woman. Voriconazole was teratogenic and embryotoxic in animal studies, and lowered plasma estradiol in animal models. Women of childbearing potential should use effective contraception during treatment. Should be used in pregnant woman only if benefit to mother justifies potential risk to the fetus.

Breast-Feeding Considerations It is not known if voriconazole is excreted in breast milk. Due to the potential for serious adverse reactions in the nursing infant, the manufacturer recommends a decision be made whether to discontinue nursing or to discontinue the drug, taking into account the importance of treatment to the mother.

Contraindications Hypersensitivity to voriconazole or any component; coadministration with astemizole, barbiturates (long acting), carbamazepine, cisapride, efavirenz (≥400 mg/day in adults), ergot derivatives (ergotamine and dihydroergotamine), pimozide, quinidine, rifampin, rifabutin, ritonavir (≥800 mg/day in adults), sirolimus, St John's wort, terfenadine

Documentation of allergic cross-reactivity for imidazole antifungals is limited; however, because of similarities in chemical structure and/or pharmacologic actions, the possibility of cross-sensitivity cannot be ruled out with certainty.

Warnings Serious (and rarely fatal) hepatic toxicity, including hepatitis, cholestasis, and fulminant hepatic failure, has been reported with azole therapy, including voriconazole; usually reversible upon discontinuation of therapy; most serious incidences have occurred in patients with multiple critical underlying medical conditions; however, hepatic reactions have occurred in patients without risk factors. In adults, liver function test abnormalities may be associated with higher plasma drug concentrations and/or doses; in pediatric patients, this possible correlation has not been clearly observed (Driscoll, 2011; Neely, 2010; Soler-Palacín, 2012). Monitor liver function and bilirubin at baseline and periodically during therapy; if abnormal LFT's occur during therapy, additional close monitoring for more severe hepatic injury recommended; if develops, discontinuation of therapy should be considered. Use caution with preexisting hepatic impairment; in patients with mild to moderate hepatic impairment (Child-Pugh class A or B), dosage reduction required; voriconazole has not been studied in severe impairment of patients with chronic hepatitis B or C;

risk vs benefits should be considered and patients closely monitored.

Visual changes, such as blurred vision, photophobia, and changes in visual acuity and color perception, are commonly associated with treatment (reported incidence: ~19%); postmarketing cases of optic neuritis and papilledema (lasting >1 month) have also been reported. Patients should be warned to avoid tasks which depend on vision, including operating machinery or driving. Visual changes are reversible on discontinuation following brief exposure/ treatment regimens (≤28 days); reversibility following long-term administration has not been evaluated; patients on long-term therapy should be monitored.

QT interval prolongation has been associated with voriconazole use; rare cases of arrhythmia (including torsade de pointes), cardiac arrest, and sudden death have been reported, usually in seriously ill patients with comorbidities and/or risk factors (eg, prior cardiotoxic chemotherapy, cardiomyopathy, electrolyte imbalance, or concomitant QT_c-prolonging drugs). Use with caution in these patient populations; correct electrolyte abnormalities (eg, hypokalemia, hypomagnesemia, hypocalcemia) prior to initiating therapy.

Rare cases of malignancy (melanoma, squamous cell carcinoma) have been reported in patients (mostly immunocompromised) with prior onset of severe photosensitivity reactions and exposure to long-term voriconazole therapy. Other serious exfoliative cutaneous reactions, including Stevens-Johnson syndrome, have also been reported. Reports of a causal relationship to dose and/or serum concentration have been mixed; in pediatric patients, a dose- and/or concentration-dependent relationship has been reported by some (Bernard, 2012; Soler-Palacín, 2012); however, others have reported phototoxicities without any relation to dose and/or concentration (Frick 2010; Hansford 2012). In pediatric patients, an increased risk and earlier onset of photosensitivity reactions have been observed with concurrent methotrexate therapy (van Hasselt, 2013). Patients should avoid strong, direct exposure to sunlight; may cause photosensitivity, especially with long-term use. Discontinue use in patients who develop an exfoliative cutaneous reaction or a skin lesion consistent with squamous cell carcinoma or melanoma. Periodic total body skin examinations should be performed, particularly with prolonged use.

If used during pregnancy, the patient should be informed that voriconazole may cause fetal harm. Voriconazole tablets contain lactose; avoid use in patients with rare hereditary problems of galactose intolerance, Lapp lactase deficiency, or glucose-galactose malabsorption. Voriconazole oral suspension contains sucrose; avoid use in patients with rare hereditary problems of fructose intolerance, sucrose-isomaltase deficiency, or glucose-galactose malabsorption.

Voriconazole is metabolized by cytochrome P450 enzymes resulting in interactions with other drugs. Due to potential serious and/or life-threatening drug interactions, some drugs are contraindicated.

Voriconazole oral suspension contains sodium benzoate; benzoic acid (benzoate) is a metabolite of benzyl alcohol; large amounts of benzyl alcohol (≥99 mg/kg/day) have been associated with a potentially fatal toxicity ("gasping syndrome") in neonates; the "gasping syndrome" consists of metabolic acidosis, respiratory distress, gasping respirations, CNS dysfunction (including convulsions, intracranial hemorrhage), hypotension and cardiovascular collapse; use voriconazole oral suspension containing sodium benzoate with caution in neonates; *in vitro* and animal studies have shown that benzoate displaces bilirubin from protein binding sites

Precautions Use caution in patients with hypersensitivity to other azole antifungal agents since cross-reaction may occur but has not been established. Use with caution in patients with severe renal impairment; avoid administration of voriconazole injection if CrCl <50 mL/minute; the I.V. formulation contains sulfobutyl ether beta-cyclodextrin (SBECD) which may accumulate in renal insufficiency. Acute renal failure has been observed in severely ill patients; use with caution in patients receiving concomitant nephrotoxic medications. Do not infuse concomitantly with blood products or short-term concentrated electrolyte solutions, even if the two infusions are running in separate intravenous lines (or cannulas). Infusion-related anaphylactoid-type reactions (chest tightness, dyspnea, faintness, fever, flushing, nausea, pruritus, rash, sweating, and tachycardia) have been reported (uncommon); consider discontinuation of infusion if reaction is severe. Use with caution in patients (children and adults) at risk for acute pancreatitis (eg, recent chemotherapy or hematopoietic stem cell transplantation); postmarketing occurrences of pancreatitis in children have been reported; pancreatic function should be monitored. With long-term use, fluorosis (teeth mottling) and periostitis have been reported; if occurs, discontinue therapy.

In pediatric patients <12 years, bioequivalence between the oral tablet and suspension has not been determined; due to possible shortened gastric transit time in infants and children, absorption of tablets may be different than adults; it is recommended that infants and children <12 years only receive oral suspension formulation. Additionally, data suggests that children <12 years have approximately a 50% reduction in bioavailability than adults; in some pediatric patients, voriconazole therapy should be initiated with the parenteral formulation with conversion to oral therapy once significant clinical improvement has been observed [Karlsson, 2009; Vfend prescribing information (Europe Medicines Agency), 2013]; consider monitoring serum concentrations (Chen, 2012).

Adverse Reactions

Cardiovascular: Tachycardia

Central nervous system: Chills, hallucinations, headache

Dermatologic: Skin rash

Endocrine & metabolic: Hypokalemia

Gastrointestinal: Nausea, vomiting

Hepatic: Cholestatic jaundice, increased serum alkaline phosphatase, increased serum ALT, increased serum AST

Ophthalmic: Photophobia, visual disturbance

Renal: Increased serum creatinine

Miscellaneous: Fever

Rare but important or life-threatening: Acute renal failure, adrenocortical insufficiency, agranulocytosis, alopecia, anaphylactoid reaction, anemia (aplastic, hemolytic, macrocytic, megaloblastic, or microcytic), angioedema, anorexia, anuria, arthritis, ascites, ataxia, atrial arrhythmia, atrial fibrillation, atrioventricular block, bacterial infection, bigeminy, blighted ovum, bone marrow depression, bradycardia, brain disease, bundle branch block, cardiac arrest, cardiac failure, cardiomegaly, cardiomyopathy, cellulitis, cerebral edema, cerebral hemorrhage, cerebral ischemia, cerebrovascular accident, chest pain, cholecystitis, cholelithiasis, cholestasis, chromatopsia, color blindness, coma, confusion, convulsions, corneal opacity, cyanosis, deafness, deep vein thrombophlebitis, deep vein thrombosis, delirium, dementia, dental fluorosis, depersonalization, depression, diabetes insipidus, diarrhea, discoid lupus erythematosus, disseminated intravascular coagulation, drowsiness, duodenal ulcer (active), duodenitis, dyspnea, eczema, edema, encephalitis, endocarditis, eosinophilia, erythema multiforme, esophageal ulcer, exfoliative dermatitis, extrapyramidal reaction, extrasystoles, fixed drug eruption, fungal infection, gastric ulcer, gastrointestinal hemorrhage, glucose tolerance decreased, graft versus host disease, Guillain-Barre syndrome, hematemesis, hemorrhagic cystitis, hepatic coma, hepatic failure, hepatitis, hepatomegaly, herpes simplex infection, hydronephrosis, hyperbilirubinemia, hypercholesterolemia, hyper-/hypocalcemia, hyper-/hypoglycemia, hyper-/hypomagnesemia, hyper-/hyponatremia, hyper-/hypotension, hyper-/hypothyroidism, hyperkalemia, hypersensitivity reaction, hyperuricemia, hypophosphatemia, hypoxia, impotence, increased blood urea nitrogen, increased gamma-glutamyl transferase, increased lactate dehydrogenase, increased susceptibility to infection, intestinal perforation, intracranial hypertension, jaundice, leukopenia, lymphadenopathy, lymphangitis, maculopapular rash, malignant melanoma, melanosis, multi-organ failure, myasthenia, myocardial infarction, myopathy, nephritis, nephrosis, neuropathy, nocturnal amblyopia, nodal arrhythmia, nodule, nystagmus, oculogyric crisis, optic atrophy, optic neuritis, orthostatic hypotension, osteomalacia, osteonecrosis, osteoporosis, otitis externa, palpitations, pancreatitis, pancytopenia, papilledema, paresthesia, perforated duodenal ulcer, periosteal disease, peripheral edema, peritonitis, petechia, pleural effusion, pneumonia, prolonged bleeding time, prolonged QT interval on ECG, pruritus, pseudomembranous colitis, pseudoporphyria, psoriasis, psychosis, pulmonary edema, pulmonary embolism, purpura, rectal hemorrhage, renal insufficiency, renal tubular necrosis, respiratory distress syndrome, respiratory tract infection, retinal hemorrhage, retinitis, seizure, sepsis, skin discoloration, skin photosensitivity, splenomegaly, squamous cell carcinoma, Stevens-Johnson syndrome, subconjunctival hemorrhage, substernal pain, suicidal ideation, supraventricular extrasystole, supraventricular tachycardia, syncope, thrombocytopenia, thrombophlebitis, thrombotic thrombocytopenic purpura, tongue edema, tonic-clonic seizures, torsades de pointes, toxic epidermal necrolysis, uremia, urinary incontinence, urinary retention, urinary tract infection, urticaria, uterine hemorrhage, uveitis, vaginal hemorrhage, vasodilation, ventricular arrhythmia, ventricular fibrillation, ventricular tachycardia, visual field defect

Drug Interactions

Metabolism/Transport Effects Substrate of CYP2C19 (major), CYP2C9 (major), CYP3A4 (minor); **Note:** Assignment of Major/Minor substrate status based on clinically relevant drug interaction potential; **Inhibits** CYP2C19 (moderate), CYP2C9 (moderate), CYP3A4 (strong)

Avoid Concomitant Use

Avoid concomitant use of Voriconazole with any of the following: Ado-Trastuzumab Emtansine; Alfuzosin; Apixaban; Astemizole; Atazanavir; Avanafil; Axitinib; Barbiturates; Bosutinib; Cabozantinib; CarBAMazepine; Ceritinib; Cisapride; Conivaptan; Crizotinib; Darunavir; Dihydroergotamine; Dofetilide; Dronedarone; Eletriptan; Eplerenone; Ergoloid Mesylates; Ergonovine; Ergotamine; Everolimus; Fluconazole; Halofantrine; Highest Risk QTc-Prolonging Agents; Ibrutinib; Ivabradine; Lapatinib; Lomitapide; Lopinavir; Lovastatin; Lurasidone; Macitentan; Methylergonovine; Mifepristone; Nilotinib; Nisoldipine; Pimozide; QuiNIDine; Ranolazine; Red Yeast Rice; Regorafenib; Rifamycin Derivatives; Ritonavir; Rivaroxaban; Saccharomyces boulardii; Salmeterol; Silodosin; Simeprevir; Simvastatin; Sirolimus; St Johns Wort; Tamsulosin; Terfenadine; Ticagrelor; Tolvaptan; Toremifene; Ulipristal; Vemurafenib; VinCRIStine (Liposomal); Vorapaxar

Increased Effect/Toxicity

Voriconazole may increase the levels/effects of: Ado-Trastuzumab Emtansine; Alfentanil; Alfuzosin; Almotriptan; Alosetron; Antineoplastic Agents (Vinca Alkaloids); Apixaban; ARIPiprazole; Astemizole; AtorvaSTATin; Avanafil; Axitinib; Bedaquiline; Benzodiazepines (metabolized by oxidation); Boceprevir; Bortezomib; Bosentan; Bosutinib; Brentuximab Vedotin; Brinzolamide; Budesonide (Nasal); Budesonide (Systemic, Oral Inhalation); BusPIRone; Busulfan; Cabozantinib; Calcium Channel Blockers; Cannabis; Carvedilol; Ceritinib; Cilostazol; Cisapride; Cobicistat; Colchicine; Conivaptan; Contraceptives (Estrogens); Contraceptives (Progestins); Corticosteroids (Orally Inhaled); Corticosteroids (Systemic); Crizotinib; CycloSPORINE (Systemic); CYP2C19 Substrates; CYP2C9 Substrates; CYP3A4 Substrates; Diclofenac (Systemic); Diclofenac (Topical); Dienogest; Dihydroergotamine; DOCEtaxel; Dofetilide; DOXOrubicin (Conventional); Dronabinol; Dronedarone; Dutasteride; Efavirenz; Eletriptan; Elvitegravir; Enzalutamide; Eplerenone; Ergoloid Mesylates; Ergonovine; Ergotamine; Etravirine; Everolimus; FentaNYL; Fesoterodine; Fluticasone (Nasal); Fluticasone (Oral Inhalation); Fosamprenavir; Fosphenytoin; GuanFACINE; Halofantrine; Highest Risk QTc-Prolonging Agents; Ibrutinib; Ibuprofen; Imatinib; Ivabradine; Ivacaftor; Ixabepilone; Lacosamide; Lapatinib; Levomilnacipran; Lomitapide; Losartan; Lovastatin; Lurasidone; Macitentan; Macrolide Antibiotics; Maraviroc; Meloxicam; Methadone; Methylergonovine; Methyl-PREDNISolone; Moderate Risk QTc-Prolonging Agents; Nelfinavir; Nilotinib; Nisoldipine; Ospemifene; OxyCODONE; Paricalcitol; PAZOPanib; Phenytoin; Pimecrolimus; Pimozide; PONATinib; Proton Pump Inhibitors; QuiNIDine; Ranolazine; Red Yeast Rice; Regorafenib; Repaglinide; Reverse Transcriptase Inhibitors (Non-Nucleoside); Rifamycin Derivatives; Rilpivirine; Rivaroxaban; Ruxolitinib; Salmeterol; Saxagliptin; Sildenafil; Silodosin; Simeprevir; Simvastatin; Sirolimus; Solifenacin; Sulfonylureas; SUNItinib; Tacrolimus (Systemic); Tacrolimus (Topical); Tadalafil; Tamsulosin; Telaprevir; Terfenadine; Tetrahydrocannabinol; Ticagrelor; Tofacitinib; Tolterodine; Tolvaptan; Toremifene; Ulipristal; Vardenafil; Vemurafenib; Venlafaxine; Vilazodone; VinCRIStine (Liposomal); Vitamin K Antagonists; Vorapaxar; Zolpidem

The levels/effects of Voriconazole may be increased by: Atazanavir; Boceprevir; Chloramphenicol; Cobicistat; Contraceptives (Estrogens); Contraceptives (Progestins); CYP2C19 Inhibitors (Moderate); CYP2C19 Inhibitors (Strong); CYP2C9 Inhibitors (Moderate); CYP2C9 Inhibitors (Strong); Etravirine; Fluconazole; Fosamprenavir; Ivabradine; Luliconazole; Macrolide Antibiotics; Mifepristone; Proton Pump Inhibitors; QTc-Prolonging Agents (Indeterminate Risk and Risk Modifying); Telaprevir

Decreased Effect

Voriconazole may decrease the levels/effects of: Amphotericin B; Atazanavir; Clopidogrel; Ifosfamide; Prasugrel; Saccharomyces boulardii; Ticagrelor

The levels/effects of Voriconazole may be decreased by: Atazanavir; Barbiturates; CarBAMazepine; CYP2C19 Inducers (Strong); CYP2C9 Inducers (Strong); Dabrafenib; Darunavir; Didanosine; Efavirenz; Etravirine; Fosphenytoin; Lopinavir; Peginterferon Alfa-2b; Phenytoin; Reverse Transcriptase Inhibitors (Non-Nucleoside); Rifamycin Derivatives; Ritonavir; St Johns Wort; Sucralfate; Telaprevir

Food Interactions Food may decrease voriconazole absorption. Management: Oral voriconazole should be taken 1 hour before or 1 hour after a meal. Maintain adequate hydration unless instructed to restrict fluid intake.

Stability

Oral:

Tablets: Store at 15°C to 30°C (59°F to 86°F).

Powder for oral suspension: Store at 2°C to 8°C (36°F to 46°F) prior to reconstitution. Once reconstituted, oral suspension is stable for 14 days at 15°C to 30°C (59°F to 86°F); do not refrigerate or freeze reconstituted oral suspension.

Parenteral: Store intact vials at 15°C to 30°C (59°F to 86°F); reconstituted solution is stable for up to 24 hours at 2°C to 8°C (36°F to 46°F). Voriconazole is incompatible with TPN, blood products, sodium bicarbonate, and electrolyte supplement infusions.

Mechanism of Action Interferes with fungal cytochrome P450 activity (selectively inhibits 14-alpha-lanosterol demethylation), decreasing ergosterol synthesis (principal sterol in fungal cell membrane) and inhibiting fungal cell membrane formation.

Pharmacokinetics (Adult data unless noted) Note: Overall, in pediatric patients, voriconazole pharmacokinetics are complex. In adolescents >14 years and pediatric patients 12-14 years and weighing >50 kg, data suggests that pharmacokinetics are similar to adults (Friberg, 2012). In pediatric patients <12 years, the full pharmacokinetic profile for voriconazole is not completely defined and for patients <2 years, the data is sparse. In children 2 to <12 years, current data suggests voriconazole undergoes a high degree of variability in exposure with linear elimination at lower doses and nonlinear at higher doses; therefore, to achieve similar AUC as adults, higher mg/kg dosing is necessary in children (Friberg, 2012; Karlsson, 2009; Walsh, 2010).

Absorption: Oral: Rapid and complete

Distribution: Extensive tissue distribution; CSF concentration ~50% of plasma concentration (Walsh, 2008)

Children 2 to <12 years: Biphasic, V_d (central): 0.81 L/kg; V_d (peripheral): 2.2 L/kg (Karlsson, 2009)

Adults: V_d: 4.6 L/kg

Protein binding: 58%

Metabolism: Metabolized by cytochrome P450 enzymes CYP2C19, CYP2C9, and CYP3A4 to voriconazole N-oxide (minimal antifungal activity); CYP2C19 is significantly involved in metabolism of voriconazole; CYP2C19 exhibits genetic polymorphism (15% to 20% Asians may be poor metabolizers of voriconazole; 3% to 5% Caucasians and African Americans may be poor metabolizers). In children 2-12 years, metabolic clearance is faster than in adults (Walsh, 2010) and current data suggests that CYP2C19 genotype has no apparent effect on exposure (Driscoll, 2011).

Bioavailability: Oral:

Children 2 to <12 years: Reported range highly variable: ~45% to 64% (Friberg, 2012; Karlsson, 2009) and values as high as 80% have been reported (Neely, 2010)

Adults: 96%

Half-life: Variable, dose dependent

Time to peak serum concentration: Oral:

Children 2 to <12 years: Median: 1.1 hours (range: 0.73-8.03 hours) (Driscoll, 2011)

Adults: 1-2 hours

Elimination: Urine (as inactive metabolites; <2% as unchanged drug)

Dosing: Neonatal Fungal infection, severe; treatment: Limited data available (case series and reports); dosing regimens variable: I.V.: Usual reported dose: 12-20 mg/kg/day divided every 8-12 hours; doses up to 24 mg/kg/day have been used; dosing based on experience in 23 neonates of which the majority were premature (minimum GA: 24 weeks) (Celik, 2013; Doby, 2012; Turan, 2011); earlier data describes lower daily doses of 4-8 mg/kg/day divided every 12 hours (Celik, 2013; Frankenbusch, 2006; Kohli, 2008; Santos, 2007). In the rare instance in which conversion to oral therapy described, oral therapy was initiated at same I.V. dose. **Note:** Pharmacokinetic neonatal data is sparse; consider monitoring serum concentrations (trough); the frequency dependent upon several factors and some suggest more frequent monitoring in neonates (Chen, 2012); further studies are needed.

Dosing: Usual

Pediatric: **Note:** In pediatric patients <12 years, bioequivalence between the oral tablet and suspension has not been determined; due to possible shortened gastric transit time in infants and children, absorption of tablets may be different than adults; it is recommended that infants and children <12 years only receive oral suspension formulation [Vfend prescribing information (Europe Medicines Agency), 2013].

Infants and Children <2 years: **Fungal infection; treatment, including empiric therapy:** Limited data available (small case series, n=17 patients): I.V., Oral suspension: Initial: 9 mg/kg/dose every 12 hours followed by monitoring of serum trough concentrations typically initiated after 3 doses; adjust dose to achieve target value (>1 mcg/mL); median final dosage: 31.5 mg/kg/**day** (12-71 mg/kg/**day**) divided every 12 hours; dosing based on experience which showed lower initial regimens (7 mg/kg/dose every 12 hours) achieved therapeutic troughs in only 14% of infants and children <2 years (Bartenlink, 2013; Gerin, 2011)

Children 2 to <12 years: Limited data available:

General dosing, susceptible infection (*Red Book*, 2012):

I.V.:

Loading dose: 9 mg/kg/dose every 12 hours for 2 doses on day 1

Maintenance: 9 mg/kg/dose every 12 hours; maximum single dose: 350 mg

Oral: 9 mg/kg/dose every 12 hours; maximum single dose: 350 mg; **Note:** In most patients, oral therapy has not been recommended as initial therapy for treatment; it has been recommended to convert parenteral to oral therapy only after significant clinical improvement has been observed [Vfend prescribing information (Europe Medicines Agency), 2013]. Earlier data had suggested a fixed dose (200 mg twice daily) in children 2-12 years (Karlsson, 2009); however, additional trials have shown interpatient variability and low drug exposure in older or heavier children within this age range; weight-based dosing is now recommended (Driscoll, 2011; Frieberg, 2012); **Note:** Clinical trials have only used the oral suspension product in this population; due to difference in GI transit time and lack of data with the tablet dosage form in these patients, only the oral suspension is recommended [Vfend prescribing information (Europe Medicines Agency), 2013].

Aspergillosis, invasive, including disseminated and extrapulmonary infection; treatment: Duration of therapy should be a minimum of 6-12 weeks or throughout period of immunosuppression (Walsh, 2008):

I.V.: **Note:** Recent data suggest higher doses (mg/kg) are required; consider using a loading dose: 9 mg/kg/dose every 12 hours for 2 doses on day 1, followed by a maintenance dose: 8-9 mg/kg/dose every 12 hours; maximum dose: 350 mg. Monitoring of concentrations may be warranted (Driscoll, 2011; *Red Book*, 2012)

Non-HIV-exposed/-positive: 5-7 mg/kg/dose every 12 hours (Walsh, 2008); see Note regarding higher dose recommendations (Walsh, 2008)

HIV-exposed/-positive (CDC, 2009): See Note regarding higher dose recommendations.

Loading dose: 6-8 mg/kg/dose (maximum: 400 mg/dose) every 12 hours for 2 doses on day 1

Maintenance dose: 7 mg/kg/dose (maximum: 200 mg/dose) every 12 hours; change to oral administration when able; duration of therapy (I.V. and oral combined): ≥12 weeks but should be individualized

Oral suspension: May consider oral therapy once patient stable

Non-HIV-exposed/-positive: 9 mg/kg/dose every 12 hours (*Red Book*, 2012)

HIV-exposed/-positive (CDC, 2009): **Note:** Recent data suggest higher doses (mg/kg) are required (9 mg/kg every 12 hours) (*Red Book*, 2012)

Loading dose: 8 mg/kg/dose (maximum: 400 mg/dose) every 12 hours for 2 doses on day 1

Maintenance dose: 7 mg/kg/dose (maximum: 200 mg/dose) every 12 hours

Candidiasis or other serious fungal infection, treatment: I.V.: Loading dose: 9 mg/kg/dose every 12 hours for 2 doses on day 1, followed by a maintenance dose: 8-9 mg/kg/dose every 12 hours; maximum dose: 350 mg (Driscoll, 2011; *Red Book*, 2012)

Children ≥12 years and Adolescents:

Aspergillosis, invasive, including disseminated and extrapulmonary infection; treatment: Duration of therapy should be a minimum of 6-12 weeks or throughout period of immunosuppression (Walsh, 2008):

I.V.: Initial: Loading dose: 6 mg/kg every 12 hours for 2 doses; followed by maintenance dose of 4 mg/kg every 12 hours

Oral: Maintenance dose:

Manufacturer's labeling: Patient weight:
<40 kg: 100 mg every 12 hours; maximum daily dose: 300 mg/**day**
≥40 kg: 200 mg every 12 hours; maximum daily dose: 600 mg/**day**

IDSA recommendations (Walsh, 2008): May consider oral therapy in place of I.V. with dosing of 4 mg/kg (rounded up to convenient tablet dosage form) every 12 hours; however, I.V. administration is preferred in serious infections since comparative efficacy with the oral formulation has not been established.

Candidemia and other deep tissue *Candida* infections; non-neutropenic patient: Treatment should continue for a minimum of 14 days following resolution of symptoms or following last positive culture, whichever is longer.

I.V.: Initial: Loading dose 6 mg/kg every 12 hours for 2 doses; followed by maintenance dose of 3-4 mg/kg every 12 hours

Oral:

Manufacturer's labeling: Maintenance dose: Patient weight:
<40 kg: 100 mg every 12 hours; maximum daily dose: 300 mg/**day**
≥40 kg: 200 mg every 12 hours; maximum daily dose: 600 mg/**day**

IDSA recommendations (Pappas, 2009): Initial: Loading dose: 400 mg every 12 hours for 2 doses; followed by 200 mg every 12 hours

Candidiasis, esophageal: Treatment should continue for a minimum of 14 days, and for at least 7 days following resolution of symptoms: Oral: Patient weight:
<40 kg: 100 mg every 12 hours; maximum daily dose: 300 mg/**day**
≥40 kg: 200 mg every 12 hours; maximum daily dose: 600 mg/**day**

Endophthalmitis, fungal: I.V.: 6 mg/kg every 12 hours for 2 doses, then 3-4 mg/kg every 12 hours (Pappas, 2009)

Scedosporiosis, fusariosis:

I.V.: Initial: Loading dose: 6 mg/kg every 12 hours for 2 doses; followed by maintenance dose of 4 mg/kg every 12 hours

Oral: Maintenance dose: Patient weight:
<40 kg: 100 mg every 12 hours; maximum daily dose 300 mg/**day**
≥40 kg: 200 mg every 12 hours; maximum daily dose: 600 mg/**day**

Adult:

Candidemia and other deep tissue *Candida* infections: Treatment should continue for a minimum of 14 days following resolution of symptoms or following last positive culture, whichever is longer.

I.V.: Initial: Loading dose 6 mg/kg every 12 hours for 2 doses; followed by maintenance dose of 3-4 mg/kg every 12 hours

Oral: Manufacturer's labeling: Maintenance dose: Patient weight:
<40 kg: 100 mg every 12 hours; maximum: 300 mg/day
≥40 kg: 200 mg every 12 hours; maximum: 600 mg/day

Esophageal candidiasis: Oral: Treatment should continue for a minimum of 14 days, and for at least 7 days following resolution of symptoms: Patient weight:
<40 kg: 100 mg every 12 hours; maximum: 300 mg/day
≥40 kg: 200 mg every 12 hours; maximum: 600 mg/day

Scedosporiosis, fusariosis:

I.V.: Initial: Loading dose: 6 mg/kg every 12 hours for 2 doses; followed by maintenance dose of 4 mg/kg every 12 hours

Oral: Maintenance dose: Patient weight:
<40 kg: 100 mg every 12 hours; maximum 300 mg/day
≥40 kg: 200 mg every 12 hours; maximum: 600 mg/day

Dosage adjustment in patients unable to tolerate treatment: Children ≥12 years, Adolescents, and Adults:

I.V.: Dose may be reduced to 3 mg/kg every 12 hours

Oral: Patient weight:
<40 kg: Dose may be reduced in 50 mg decrements to a minimum 100 mg every 12 hours
≥40 kg: Dose may be reduced in 50 mg decrements to a minimum dosage of 200 mg every 12 hours

Dosage adjustment in patients receiving concomitant CYP450 enzyme inducers or substrates: Children ≥12 years, Adolescents, and Adults:

Efavirenz: Oral: Increase maintenance dose of voriconazole to 400 mg every 12 hours and reduce efavirenz dose to 300 mg once daily; upon discontinuation of voriconazole, return to the initial dose of efavirenz

Phenytoin:

I.V.: Increase voriconazole maintenance dosage to 5 mg/kg every 12 hours

Oral: Patient weight:
<40 kg: Increase voriconazole dose to 200 mg every 12 hours
≥40 kg: Increase voriconazole dose to 400 mg every 12 hours

Dosing adjustment in renal impairment: Children ≥12 years, Adolescents, and Adults:
Oral: No adjustment necessary
Parenteral: I.V.:
Mild (CrCl ≥50 mL/minute): No adjustment necessary
Moderate to severe (CrCl <50 mL/minute): Accumulation of the intravenous vehicle occurs. After initial I.V. loading dose, oral voriconazole should be administered, unless an assessment of the risk:benefit justifies the use of I.V. voriconazole. Monitor serum creatinine and change to oral voriconazole therapy when possible.
Dialysis: Poorly dialyzed; no supplemental dose or dosage adjustment necessary, including patients on intermittent hemodialysis, peritoneal dialysis, or continuous renal replacement therapy (eg, CVVHD)

Dosing adjustment in hepatic impairment: Children ≥12 years, Adolescents, and Adults:
Mild to moderate hepatic dysfunction (Child-Pugh Class A and B): Use standard loading dose regimen, then decrease maintenance dose by 50%
Severe hepatic impairment (Child-Pugh Class C): Not recommended for use unless benefit outweighs the risk; monitor closely for toxicity; not studied

Administration

Oral: Administer at least one hour before or one hour after a meal; shake suspension for approximately 10 seconds before use; do not mix suspension with other medications, flavoring agents, or other fluids. Maintain adequate hydration unless instructed to restrict fluid intake.
Parenteral: I.V.: **Do not administer I.V. push;** voriconazole must be administered by I.V. infusion over 1-2 hours at a rate not to exceed 3 mg/kg/hour; final concentration for administration should be 0.5-5 mg/mL. Do not infuse concomitantly into same line or cannula with other drug infusions, including TPN.

Monitoring Parameters Serum electrolytes, periodic renal function tests (particularly serum creatinine), hepatic function tests, and bilirubin; monitor visual activity, visual field, and color perception if treatment course continues >28 days; ECG in select patients; pancreatic function in patients at risk for acute pancreatitis; voriconazole trough levels in patients exhibiting signs of toxicity or not responding to treatment; total body skin examination yearly or more frequently if lesions occur

Reference Range Trough: 1-6 mcg/mL; some have suggested a higher minimum trough (2 mcg/mL) for disseminated infections or those in isolated sites (Chen, 2012)

Dosage Forms Excipient information presented when available (limited, particularly for generics); consult specific product labeling.
Solution Reconstituted, Intravenous:
Generic: 200 mg (1 ea)
Solution Reconstituted, Intravenous [preservative free]:
Vfend IV: 200 mg (1 ea) [latex free]
Vfend IV: 200 mg (1 ea)
Suspension Reconstituted, Oral:
Vfend: 40 mg/mL (75 mL) [contains sodium benzoate; orange flavor]
Generic: 40 mg/mL (75 mL)
Tablet, Oral:
Vfend: 50 mg, 200 mg
Generic: 50 mg, 200 mg

References

Bartelink IH, Wolfs T, Jonker M, et al, "Highly Variable Plasma Concentrations of Voriconazole in Pediatric Hematopoietic Stem Cell Transplantation Patients," *Antimicrob Agents Chemother*, 2013, 57 (1):235-40.

Bernhard S, Kernland Lang K, Ammann RA, et al, "Voriconazole-Induced Phototoxicity in Children," *Pediatr Infect Dis J*, 2012, 31 (7):769-71.

Celik IH, Demirel G, Oguz SS, et al, "Compassionate Use of Voriconazole in Newborn Infants Diagnosed With Severe Invasive Fungal Sepsis," *Eur Rev Med Pharmacol Sci*, 2013, 17(6):729-34.

Centers for Disease Control and Prevention (CDC), "Guidelines for the Prevention and Treatment of Opportunistic Infections Among HIV-Exposed and HIV-Infected Children," *MMWR Recomm Rep*, 2009, 58(RR-11):1-166. Available at http://aidsinfo.nih.gov/contentfiles/Pediatric_OI.pdf

Cesaro S, Strugo L, Alaggio R, et al, "Voriconazole for Invasive Aspergillosis in Oncohematological Patients: A Single-Center Pediatric Experience," *Support Care Cancer*, 2003, 11(11):722-7.

Chen J, Chan C, Colantonio D, et al, "Therapeutic Drug Monitoring of Voriconazole in Children," *Ther Drug Monit*, 2012, 34(1):77-84.

Cowen EW, Nguyen JC, Miller DD, et al, "Chronic Phototoxicity and Aggressive Squamous Cell Carcinoma of the Skin in Children and Adults During Treatment With Voriconazole," *J Am Acad Dermatol*, 2010, 62(1):31-7.

DHHS Panel on Opportunistic Infections (OI) in HIV-Infected Adults and Adolescents, "Guidelines for Prevention and Treatment of Opportunistic Infections in HIV-Infected Adults and Adolescents: Recommendations from the Centers for Disease Control and Prevention (CDC), the National Institutes of Health (NIH), and the HIV Medicine Association (HIVMA) of the Infectious Diseases Society of America (IDSA)," May 7, 2013. Available at http://aidsinfo.nih.gov/contentfiles/lvguidelines/adult_oi.pdf

Doby EH, Benjamin DK Jr, Blaschke AJ, et al, "Therapeutic Monitoring of Voriconazole in Children Less Than Three Years of Age: A Case Report and Summary of Voriconazole Concentrations for Ten Children," *Pediatr Infect Dis J*, 2012, 31(6):632-5.

Driscoll TA, Yu LC, Frangoul H, et al, "Comparison of Pharmacokinetics and Safety of Voriconazole Intravenous-to-Oral Switch in Immunocompromised Children and Healthy Adults," *Antimicrob Agents Chemother*, 2011, 55(12):5770-9.

Frankenbusch K, Eifinger F, Kribs A, et al, "Severe Primary Cutaneous Aspergillosis Refractory to Amphotericin B and the Successful Treatment With Systemic Voriconazole in Two Premature Infants With Extremely Low Birth Weight," *J Perinatol*, 2006, 26(8):511-4.

Friberg LE, Ravva P, Karlsson MO, et al, "Integrated Population Pharmacokinetic Analysis of Voriconazole in Children, Adolescents, and Adults," *Antimicrob Agents Chemother*, 2012, 56(6):3032-42.

Frick MA, Soler-Palacín P, Martín Nalda A, et al, "Photosensitivity in Immunocompromised Patients Receiving Long-Term Therapy With Oral Voriconazole," *Pediatr Infect Dis J*, 2010, 29(5):480-1.

Gerin M, Mahlaoui N, Elie C, et al, "Therapeutic Drug Monitoring of Voriconazole After Intravenous Administration in Infants and Children With Primary Immunodeficiency," *Ther Drug Monit*, 2011, 33(4):464-6.

Hansford JR, Cole C, Blyth CC, et al, "Idiosyncratic Nature of Voriconazole Photosensitivity in Children Undergoing Cancer Therapy," *J Antimicrob Chemother*, 2012, 67(7):1807-9.

Karlsson MO, Lutsar I, and Milligan PA, "Population Pharmacokinetic Analysis of Voriconazole Plasma Concentration Data From Pediatric Studies," *Antimicrob Agents Chemother*, 2009, 53(3):935-44.

Kohli V, Taneja V, Sachdev P, et al, "Voriconazole in Newborns," *Indian Pediatr*, 2008, 45(3):236-8.

McCarthy KL, Playford EG, Looke DF, et al, "Severe Photosensitivity Causing Multifocal Squamous Cell Carcinomas Secondary to Prolonged Voriconazole Therapy," *Clin Infect Dis*, 2007, 44(5):e55-6.

Miller DD, Cowen EW, Nguyen JC, et al, "Melanoma Associated With Long-Term Voriconazole Therapy: A New Manifestation of Chronic Photosensitivity," *Arch Dermatol*, 2010, 146(3):300-4.

Neely M, Rushing T, Kovacs A, et al, "Voriconazole Pharmacokinetics and Pharmacodynamics in Children," *Clin Infect Dis*, 2010, 50 (1):27-36.

Pappas PG, Kauffman CA, Andes D, et al, "Clinical Practice Guidelines for the Management of Candidiasis: 2009 Update by the Infectious Diseases Society of America," *Clin Infect Dis*, 2009, 48(5):503-35.

Red Book: 2012 Report of the Committee on Infectious Diseases, 29th ed, Pickering LK, ed, Elk Grove Village, IL: American Academy of Pediatrics, 2012.

Romero AJ, Pogamp PL, Nilsson LG, et al, "Effect of Voriconazole on the Pharmacokinetics of Cyclosporine in Renal Transplant Patients," *Clin Pharmacol Ther*, 2002, 71(4):226-34.

Santos RP, Sánchez PJ, Mejias A, et al, "Successful Medical Treatment of Cutaneous Aspergillosis in a Premature Infant Using Liposomal Amphotericin B, Voriconazole and Micafungin," *Pediatr Infect Dis J*, 2007, 26(4):364-6.

Scott LJ and Simpson D, "Voriconazole: A Review of its Use in the Management of Invasive Fungal Infections," *Drugs*, 2007, 67 (2):269-98.

Soler-Palacín P, Frick MA, Martín-Nalda A, et al, "Voriconazole Drug Monitoring in the Management of Invasive Fungal Infection in Immunocompromised Children: A Prospective Study," *J Antimicrob Chemother*, 2012, 67(3):700-6.

Steinbach WJ, "Antifungal Agents in Children," *Pediatr Clin North Am*, 2005, 52(3):895-915.

Turan O, Ergenekon E, Hirfanoğlu IM, et al, "Combination Antifungal Therapy With Voriconazole for Persistent Candidemia in Very Low Birth Weight Neonates," *Turk J Pediatr*, 2011, 53(1):19-26.

van Hasselt JG, van Eijkelenburg NK, Huitema AD, et al, "Severe Skin Toxicity in Pediatric Oncology Patients Treated With Voriconazole and Concomitant Methotrexate," *Antimicrob Agents Chemother*, 2013, 57 (6):2878-81.

Walsh TJ, Anaissie EJ, Denning DW, et al, "Treatment of Aspergillosis: Clinical Practice Guidelines of the Infectious Diseases Society of America," *Clin Infect Dis*, 2008, 46(3):327-60.

Walsh TJ, Driscoll T, Milligan PA, et al, "Pharmacokinetics, Safety, and Tolerability of Voriconazole in Immunocompromised Children," *Antimicrob Agents Chemother*, 2010, 54(10):4116-23.

Walsh TJ, Karlsson MO, Driscoll T, et al, "Pharmacokinetics and Safety of Intravenous Voriconazole in Children After Single- or Multiple-Dose Administration," *Antimicrob Agents Chemother*, 2004, 48(6):2166-72.

Walsh TJ, Lutsar I, Driscoll T, et al, "Voriconazole in the Treatment of Aspergillosis, Scedosporiosis and Other Invasive Fungal Infections in Children," *Pediatr Infect Dis J*, 2002, 21(3):240-8.

Walsh TJ, Pappas P, Winston DJ, et al, "Voriconazole Compared With Liposomal Amphotericin B for Empirical Antifungal Therapy in Patients With Neutropenia and Persistent Fever," *N Engl J Med*, 2002, 346(4):225-34.

◆ **VoSpire ER** *see* Albuterol *on page 84*

◆ **VP-16** *see* Etoposide *on page 815*

◆ **VP-16-213** *see* Etoposide *on page 815*

◆ **Vpriv** *see* Velaglucerase Alfa *on page 2124*

◆ **VPRIV (Can)** *see* Velaglucerase Alfa *on page 2124*

◆ **VSL #3® [OTC]** *see* Lactobacillus *on page 1191*

◆ **VSL #3®-DS** *see* Lactobacillus *on page 1191*

◆ **Vumon® (Can)** *see* Teniposide *on page 1976*

◆ **VWF/FVIII Concentrate** *see* Antihemophilic Factor/von Willebrand Factor Complex (Human) *on page 177*

◆ **VWF:RCo** *see* Antihemophilic Factor/von Willebrand Factor Complex (Human) *on page 177*

◆ **vWF:RCof** *see* Antihemophilic Factor/von Willebrand Factor Complex (Human) *on page 177*

◆ **VX-770** *see* Ivacaftor *on page 1169*

◆ **Vytorin** *see* Ezetimibe and Simvastatin *on page 829*

◆ **Vyvanse** *see* Lisdexamfetamine *on page 1260*

◆ **VZIG** *see* Varicella-Zoster Immune Globulin (Human) *on page 2119*

◆ **VZV Vaccine (Varicella)** *see* Varicella Virus Vaccine *on page 2116*

Warfarin (WAR far in)

Medication Safety Issues

Sound-alike/look-alike issues:

Coumadin® may be confused with Avandia®, Cardura®, Compazine, Kemadrin

Jantoven® may be confused with Janumet®, Januvia®

High alert medication:

The Institute for Safe Medication Practices (ISMP) includes this medication among its list of drugs which have a heightened risk of causing significant patient harm when used in error.

National Patient Safety Goals:

The Joint Commission on Accreditation of Healthcare Organizations requires healthcare organizations that provide anticoagulant therapy to have a process in place to reduce the risk of anticoagulant-associated patient harm. Patients receiving anticoagulants should receive individualized care through a defined process that includes standardized ordering, dispensing, administration, monitoring and education. This does not apply to routine short-term use of anticoagulants for prevention of venous thromboembolism when the expectation is that the patient's laboratory values will remain within or close to normal values (NPSG.03.05.01).

Brand Names: U.S. Coumadin; Jantoven

Brand Names: Canada Apo-Warfarin®; Coumadin®; Mylan-Warfarin; Novo-Warfarin; Taro-Warfarin

Therapeutic Category Anticoagulant

Generic Availability (U.S.) May be product dependent

Use Prophylaxis and treatment of venous thrombosis, pulmonary embolism, and thromboembolic disorders; prevention and treatment of thromboembolic complications in patients with prosthetic heart valves or atrial fibrillation; reduction of the risk of death, recurrent MI, and thromboembolic events such as systemic embolization or stroke after MI; has also been used for the prevention of recurrent arterial ischemic stroke and TIAs.

Medication Guide Available Yes

Pregnancy Risk Factor D (women with mechanical heart valves)/X (other indications)

Pregnancy Considerations Warfarin crosses the placenta; concentrations in the fetal plasma are similar to maternal values. Teratogenic effects have been reported following first trimester exposure and may include coumarin embryopathy (nasal hypoplasia and/or stippled epiphyses; limb hypoplasia may also be present). Adverse CNS events to the fetus have also been observed following exposure during any trimester and may include CNS abnormalities (including ventral midline dysplasia, dorsal midline dysplasia). Spontaneous abortion, fetal hemorrhage, and fetal death may also occur. Use is contraindicated during pregnancy (or in women of reproductive potential) except in women with mechanical heart valves who are at high risk for thromboembolism; use is also contraindicated in women with threatened abortion, eclampsia, or preeclampsia. Frequent pregnancy tests are recommended for women who are planning to become pregnant and adjusted-dose heparin or low molecular weight heparin (LMWH) should be substituted as soon as pregnancy is confirmed or adjusted-dose heparin or LMWH should be used instead of warfarin prior to conception.

In pregnant women with high-risk mechanical heart valves, the benefits of warfarin therapy should be discussed with the risks of available treatments; when possible avoid warfarin use during the first trimester and close to delivery. Adjusted-dose LMWH or adjusted-dose heparin may be used throughout pregnancy or until week 13 of gestation when therapy can be changed to warfarin. LMWH or heparin should be resumed close to delivery. In women who are at a very high risk for thromboembolism (older generation prothesis in mitral position or history of thromboembolism), warfarin can be used throughout pregnancy and replaced with LMWH or heparin near term; the use of low-dose aspirin is also recommended. Women who require long-term anticoagulation with warfarin and who are considering pregnancy, LMWH substitution should be done prior to conception when possible. When choosing therapy, fetal outcomes (ie, pregnancy loss, malformations), maternal outcomes (ie, VTE, hemorrhage), burden of therapy, and maternal preference should be considered (Bates, 2012).

Breast-Feeding Considerations Breast-feeding women may be treated with warfarin. Based on available data, warfarin does not pass into breast milk. Women who are breast-feeding should be carefully monitored to avoid excessive anticoagulation. According to the American College of Chest Physicians (ACCP), warfarin may be used in lactating women who wish to breast-feed their infants (Bates, 2012). Monitor nursing infants for bruising or bleeding (per manufacturer).

Contraindications Hypersensitivity to warfarin or any component; hemorrhagic tendencies or blood dyscrasias; recent or contemplated surgery of the CNS, eye, or traumatic surgery with large open wounds; active ulceration or overt bleeding of GI, GU, or respiratory tracts; CNS hemorrhage; cerebral aneurysms; dissecting aortic aneurysms; pericarditis and pericardial effusions; bacterial endocarditis; spinal puncture or other procedures with potential for uncontrollable bleeding; major regional or lumbar block anesthesia; neurosurgical procedures; malignant hypertension; pregnancy (except in women with mechanical heart valves who are at high risk for thromboembolism), threatened abortion, eclampsia, pre-eclampsia; inadequate laboratory facilities; unsupervised patients with conditions associated with a high potential for noncompliance

Warnings Hazardous agent; use appropriate precautions for handling and disposal. Serious and potentially fatal bleeding may occur **[U.S. Boxed Warning]**. Bleeding is more likely during initiation of treatment (within first month) and with higher doses. Risk factors for bleeding include high intensity anticoagulation (INR >4), age (≥65 years), highly variable INRs, history of GI bleeding, hypertension, cerebrovascular disease, serious heart disease, anemia, severe diabetes, malignancy, trauma, renal insufficiency, polycythemia vera, vasculitis, open wound, history of PUD, indwelling catheters, menstruating and postpartum women, drug-drug interactions, and long duration of therapy. Regular monitoring of INR is required **[U.S. Boxed Warning]**. Dosage must be individualized for each patient. Medications, dietary changes, and other factors affect INR levels achieved with warfarin therapy **[U.S. Boxed Warning]**. Patients must be instructed about preventative measures to minimize risk of bleeding and to report bleeding, accidents, or falls as well as any new or discontinued medications, herbal, or alternative products used, or significant changes in smoking or dietary habits **[U.S. Boxed Warning]**.

Necrosis and/or gangrene of the skin and other tissues may occur (rarely) due to early hypercoagulability; risk is increased in patients with protein C deficiency; tissue debridement or amputation may be required; permanent disability or death has been reported; discontinue warfarin if warfarin-associated necrosis occurs; consider heparin for anticoagulation.

Warfarin therapy may release atheromatous plaque emboli; symptoms depend on site of embolization, most commonly kidneys, pancreas, liver, and spleen. In some cases, emboli may lead to necrosis or death. "Purple toe" syndrome, due to cholesterol microembolization, has been rarely described with coumarin-type anticoagulants. Typically, this occurs after several weeks of therapy, and may present as a dark, purplish, mottled discoloration of the plantar and lateral surfaces. Other manifestations of cholesterol microembolization may include rash; livedo reticularis; gangrene; abrupt and intense pain in lower extremities; abdominal, flank, or back pain; hematuria; renal insufficiency; hypertension; cerebral ischemia; spinal cord infarction; or other symptoms of vascular compromise.

May cause hypersensitivity reactions, including anaphylaxis; use with caution in patients with anaphylactic

disorders. Concomitant use with vitamin K may decrease anticoagulant effect; monitor carefully. Concomitant use with ethacrynic acid, indomethacin, NSAIDs, phenylbutazone, or aspirin increases warfarin's anticoagulant effect and may cause severe GI irritation. Oral anticoagulant therapy is usually avoided in neonates due to a greater potential risk of bleeding (Monagle, 2001) and other problems (Monagle, 2008).

Precautions Do not switch brands once desired therapeutic response has been achieved. Use with caution in patients with acute infection or active tuberculosis (antibiotics and fever may alter the response to warfarin), prolonged dietary insufficiencies (vitamin K deficiency), diabetes mellitus, thyroid disease, moderate-to-severe renal or hepatic impairment, or heparin-induced thrombocytopenia with deep vein thrombosis (limb ischemia, necrosis, and gangrene have occurred when warfarin was started or continued after heparin was stopped; warfarin monotherapy is contraindicated in the initial treatment of active HIT; warfarin initially inhibits the synthesis of protein C, potentially accelerating the underlying active thrombotic process. Use with caution in patients with or at risk for hemorrhage, necrosis, or gangrene. Use care in the selection of patients appropriate for this treatment; ensure patient cooperation especially from the alcoholic, illicit drug user, demented, or psychotic patient. Safety and efficacy have not been established in pediatric patients; monitor closely; rare hair loss and tracheal calcification have been reported in children.

Periodic monitoring of INR (preferred) or prothrombin time is essential. A large number of factors (alone or in combination), including changes in diet, medications, and herbal remedies, may influence the patient's response to warfarin; monitor patients more closely when these factors change. Genetic variations in the CYP2C9 and vitamin K oxidoreductase (VKORC1) enzymes may also influence the patient's response to warfarin; presence of the CYP2C9*2 or *3 allele and/or polymorphism of the VKORC1 gene may increase the risk of bleeding. The *2 allele is reported to occur with a frequency of 4% to 11% in African-Americans and Caucasians, respectively, while the *3 allele frequencies are 2% to 7%, respectively. Other variant 2C9 alleles (eg, *5, *6, *9, and *11) are also associated with reduced metabolic activity and thus may increase risk of bleeding, but are much less common. Lower doses may be required in these patients; genetic testing may help determine appropriate dosing.

Adverse Reactions Bleeding is the major adverse effect of warfarin. Hemorrhage may occur at virtually any site. Risk is dependent on multiple variables, including the intensity of anticoagulation and patient susceptibility.

Cardiovascular: Vasculitis

Central nervous system: Signs/symptoms of bleeding (eg, dizziness, fatigue, fever, headache, lethargy, malaise, pain)

Dermatologic: Alopecia, bullous eruptions, dermatitis, rash, pruritus, urticaria

Gastrointestinal: Abdominal pain, diarrhea, flatulence, gastrointestinal bleeding, nausea, taste disturbance, vomiting

Genitourinary: Hematuria

Hematologic: Anemia, retroperitoneal hematoma, unrecognized bleeding sites (eg, colon cancer) may be uncovered by anticoagulation

Hepatic: Hepatitis (including cholestatic hepatitis), transaminases increased

Neuromuscular & skeletal: Osteoporosis (potential association with long-term use), paralysis, paresthesia, weakness

Respiratory: Respiratory tract bleeding, tracheobronchial calcification

Miscellaneous: Anaphylactic reaction, hypersensitivity/allergic reactions, skin necrosis, gangrene, "purple toes" syndrome

Drug Interactions

Metabolism/Transport Effects Substrate of CYP1A2 (minor), CYP2C19 (minor), CYP2C9 (major), CYP3A4 (minor); **Note:** Assignment of Major/Minor substrate status based on clinically relevant drug interaction potential; **Inhibits** CYP2C19 (weak), CYP2C9 (weak)

Avoid Concomitant Use

Avoid concomitant use of Warfarin with any of the following: Apixaban; Dabigatran Etexilate; Enzalutamide; Omacetaxine; Rivaroxaban; Streptokinase; Tamoxifen; Urokinase; Vorapaxar

Increased Effect/Toxicity

Warfarin may increase the levels/effects of: Anticoagulants; Collagenase (Systemic); Deferasirox; Ethotoin; Fosphenytoin; Ibritumomab; Omacetaxine; Phenytoin; Regorafenib; Rivaroxaban; Sulfonylureas; Tositumomab and Iodine I 131 Tositumomab

The levels/effects of Warfarin may be increased by: Acetaminophen; Agents with Antiplatelet Properties; Allopurinol; Amiodarone; Androgens; Antineoplastic Agents; Apixaban; Atazanavir; Bicalutamide; Boceprevir; Capecitabine; Cephalosporins; Ceritinib; Chloral Hydrate; Chloramphenicol; Cimetidine; Clopidogrel; Cloxacillin; Cobicistat; Corticosteroids (Systemic); Cranberry; CYP2C9 Inhibitors (Moderate); CYP2C9 Inhibitors (Strong); Dabigatran Etexilate; Dasatinib; Desvenlafaxine; Dexmethylphenidate; Disulfiram; Dronedarone; Econazole; Efavirenz; Erythromycin (Ophthalmic); Esomeprazole; Ethacrynic Acid; Ethotoin; Etoposide; Exenatide; Fenofibrate and Derivatives; Fenugreek; Fibric Acid Derivatives; Fluconazole; Fluorouracil (Systemic); Fluorouracil (Topical); Fosamprenavir; Fosphenytoin; Fusidic Acid (Systemic); Gefitinib; Ginkgo Biloba; Glucagon; Green Tea; Herbs (Anticoagulant/Antiplatelet Properties); HMG-CoA Reductase Inhibitors; Ibrutinib; Ifosfamide; Imatinib; Itraconazole; Ivermectin (Systemic); Ketoconazole (Systemic); Lansoprazole; Leflunomide; Levomilnacipran; Lomitapide; Macrolide Antibiotics; Methylphenidate; Metreleptin; MetroNIDAZOLE (Systemic); Miconazole (Oral); Miconazole (Topical); Mifepristone; Milnacipran; Mirtazapine; Multivitamins/Fluoride (with ADE); Multivitamins/Minerals (with ADEK, Iron); Multivitamins/Minerals (with AE, No Iron); Nelfinavir; Neomycin; Nonsteroidal Anti-Inflammatory Agents; NSAID (COX-2 Inhibitor); NSAID (Nonselective); Omega-3 Fatty Acids; Omeprazole; Orlistat; Penicillins; Pentosan Polysulfate Sodium; Pentoxifylline; Phenytoin; Posaconazole; Proguanil; Propafenone; Prostacyclin Analogues; QuiNIDine; QuiNINE; Quinolone Antibiotics; Ranitidine; RomiDEPsin; Salicylates; Saquinavir; Selective Serotonin Reuptake Inhibitors; Sitaxentan; SORAfenib; Streptokinase; Sugammadex; Sulfinpyrazone [Off Market]; Sulfonamide Derivatives; Sulfonylureas; Tamoxifen; Tegafur; Telaprevir; Tetracycline Derivatives; Thrombolytic Agents; Thyroid Products; Tibolone; Tigecycline; Tipranavir; Tolterodine; Toremifene; Torsemide; TraMADol; Tricyclic Antidepressants; Urokinase; Venlafaxine; Vitamin E; Vorapaxar; Voriconazole; Vorinostat; Zafirlukast; Zileuton

Decreased Effect

The levels/effects of Warfarin may be decreased by: Adalimumab; Alcohol (Ethyl); Aminoglutethimide;

Antineoplastic Agents; Antithyroid Agents; Aprepitant; AzaTHIOprine; Barbiturates; Bile Acid Sequestrants; Boceprevir; Bosentan; CarBAMazepine; Cloxacillin; Coenzyme Q-10; Contraceptives (Estrogens); Contraceptives (Progestins); CYP2C9 Inducers (Strong); Dabrafenib; Darunavir; Dicloxacillin; Efavirenz; Elvitegravir; Enzalutamide; Eslicarbazepine; Estrogen Derivatives; Floxacillin; Fosaprepitant; Ginseng (American); Glutethimide; Green Tea; Griseofulvin; Lopinavir; Mercaptopurine; Metreleptin; Multivitamins/Minerals (with ADEK, Folate, Iron); Nafcillin; Nelfinavir; Peginterferon Alfa-2b; Phytonadione; Progestins; Rifamycin Derivatives; Ritonavir; St Johns Wort; Sucralfate; Telaprevir; Teriflunomide; TraZODone

Food Interactions

Ethanol: Acute ethanol ingestion (binge drinking) decreases the metabolism of oral anticoagulants and increases PT/INR. Chronic daily ethanol use increases the metabolism of oral anticoagulants and decreases PT/INR. Management: Avoid ethanol.

Food: The anticoagulant effects of warfarin may be decreased if taken with foods rich in vitamin K. Vitamin E may increase warfarin effect. Cranberry juice may increase warfarin effect. Management: Maintain a consistent diet; consult prescriber before making changes in diet. Take warfarin at the same time each day.

Stability

Tablets: Store at controlled room temperature of 15°C to 30°C (59°F to 86°F). Protect from light. Dispense in tight, light-resistant container.

Injection: Store unopened vials in box at controlled room temperature of 15°C to 30°C (59°F to 86°F). Protect from light. After reconstitution, store at controlled room temperature and use within 4 hours after reconstitution. Do not refrigerate. Discard unused portion (does not contain preservative). Reconstituted solution is stable in D_5LR, $D_5^{1}/_2NS$, D_5NS, D_5W, $D_{10}W$; **variable stability (consult detailed reference)** in LR, NS.

Mechanism of Action Hepatic synthesis of coagulation factors II, VII, IX, and X, as well as proteins C and S, requires the presence of vitamin K. These clotting factors are biologically activated by the addition of carboxyl groups to key glutamic acid residues within the proteins' structure. In the process, "active" vitamin K is oxidatively converted to an "inactive" form, which is then subsequently reactivated by vitamin K epoxide reductase complex 1 (VKORC1). Warfarin competitively inhibits the subunit 1 of the multi-unit VKOR complex, thus depleting functional vitamin K reserves and hence reduces synthesis of active clotting factors.

Pharmacodynamics Anticoagulation effects:

Onset of action: 24-72 hours

Maximum effect: Within 5-7 days

Duration of action (single dose): 2-5 days

Pharmacokinetics (Adult data unless noted)

Absorption: Oral: Rapid

Distribution: Adults: V_d: 0.14 L/kg

Protein binding: 99%

Metabolism: Hepatic, primarily via CYP2C9; minor pathways include CYP2C19, 1A2, and 3A4

Genomic variants: Clearance of S-warfarin is reduced by ~37% in patients heterozygous for 2C9 (*1/*2 or *1/*3), and reduced by ~70% in patients homozygous for reduced function alleles (*2/*2, *2/*3, or *3/*3)

Half-life, elimination: Adults: 20-60 hours; mean: 40 hours; highly variable among individuals

Elimination: Urine (92%, primarily as metabolites; very little warfarin is excreted unchanged in the urine)

Dosing: Usual Note: Dosing must be individualized. **Note:** New product labeling identifies genetic factors which may increase patient sensitivity to warfarin. Specifically, genetic variations in the proteins CYP2C9 and VKORC1, responsible for warfarin's primary metabolism and pharmacodynamic activity, respectively, have been identified as predisposing factors associated with decreased dose requirement and increased bleeding risk. A genotyping test is available and may provide important guidance on initiation of anticoagulant therapy.

Oral:

Infants and Children: **To maintain an International Normalized Ratio (INR) between 2-3:**

Initial loading dose on day 1 (if baseline INR is 1-1.3): 0.2 mg/kg (maximum dose: 10 mg); use initial loading dose of 0.1 mg/kg if patient has liver dysfunction or has undergone a Fontan procedure (Streif, 1999)

Loading dose for days 2-4: doses are dependent upon patient's INR

if INR is 1.1-1.3, repeat the initial loading dose

if INR is 1.4-1.9, give 50% of the initial loading dose

if INR is 2-3, give 50% of the initial loading dose

if INR is 3.1-3.5, give 25% of the initial loading dose

if INR is >3.5, hold the drug until INR <3.5, then restart at 50% of previous dose

Maintenance dose guidelines for day 5 of therapy and beyond: Doses are dependent upon patient's INR

if INR is 1.1-1.4, increase dose by 20% of previous dose

if INR is 1.5-1.9, increase dose by 10% of previous dose

if INR is 2-3, do not change the dose

if INR is 3.1-3.5, decrease dose by 10% of previous dose

if INR is >3.5, hold the drug and check INR daily until INR <3.5, then restart at 20% less than the previous dose

Usual maintenance dose: ~0.1 mg/kg/day; range: 0.05-0.34 mg/kg/day; the dose in mg/kg/day is inversely related to age. In the largest pediatric study (n=319; Streif, 1999), infants <12 months of age required a mean dose of 0.33 mg/kg/day, but children 13-18 years required a mean dose of 0.09 mg/kg/day; a target INR of 2-3 was used for a majority of these patients (75% of warfarin courses). Overall, children required a mean dose of 0.16 mg/kg/day to achieve a target INR of 2-3. In another study (Andrew, 1994), to attain an INR of 1.3-1.8, infants <12 months (n=2) required 0.24 and 0.27 mg/kg/day, but children >1 year required a mean of 0.08 mg/kg/day (range: 0.03-0.17 mg/kg/day). Consistent anticoagulation may be difficult to maintain in children <5 years of age. Children receiving phenobarbital, carbamazepine, or enteral nutrition may require higher maintenance doses (Streif, 1999).

Adults: **Note:** Initial dosing must be individualized. Consider patient factors (hepatic function, cardiac function, age, nutritional status, concurrent therapy, risk of bleeding) in addition to prior dose response (if available) and the clinical situation. Initial dose: 2-5 mg daily for 2 days **or** 5-10 mg daily for 1-2 days (Ansell, 2008); then adjust dose according to results of INR; usual maintenance dose ranges from 2-10 mg daily; individual patients may require loading and maintenance doses outside these general guidelines.

Note: Lower starting doses may be required for patients with hepatic impairment, poor nutrition, CHF, elderly, high risk of bleeding, patients who are debilitated, or those with reduced function genomic variants of the catabolic enzymes CYP2C9 (*2 or *3 alleles) or VKORC1 (-1639 polymorphism); see table. Higher initial doses may be reasonable in selected patients (ie, receiving enzyme-inducing agents and with low risk of bleeding).

Range[1] of Expected Therapeutic Maintenance Dose Based on CYP2C9[2] and VKORC1[3] Genotypes

VKORC1	CYP2C9					
	*1/*1	*1/*2	*1/*3	*2/*2	*2/*3	*3/*3
GG	5-7 mg	5-7 mg	3-4 mg	3-4 mg	3-4 mg	0.5-2 mg
AG	5-7 mg	3-4 mg	3-4 mg	3-4 mg	0.5-2 mg	0.5-2 mg
AA	3-4 mg	3-4 mg	0.5-2 mg	0.5-2 mg	0.5-2 mg	0.5-2 mg

Note: Must also take into account other patient-related factors when determining initial dose (eg, age, body weight, concomitant medications, comorbidities)

[1]Ranges derived from multiple published clinical studies.

[2]Patients with CYP2C9 *1/*3, *2/*2, *2/*3, and *3/*3 alleles may take up to 4 weeks to achieve maximum INR with a given dose regimen.

[3]VKORC1 -1639G>A (rs 9923231) variant is used in this table; other VKORC1 variants may also be important determinants of dose.

I.V.: (For patients who cannot take oral form): I.V. dose is equal to oral dose

Dosing adjustment in renal disease: No adjustment required; however, patients with renal failure have an increased risk of bleeding complications. Monitor closely.

Dosing adjustment in hepatic disease: Monitor effect at usual doses; the response to oral anticoagulants may be markedly enhanced in obstructive jaundice (due to reduced vitamin K absorption) and also in hepatitis and cirrhosis (due to decreased production of vitamin K-dependent clotting factors); INR should be closely monitored

Administration

Oral: May administer on an empty or full stomach. Take at the same time each day.

Parenteral: For I.V. use only; do not administer I.M. Reconstitute 5 mg vial with 2.7 mL SWI to produce 2 mg/mL solution. Administer by slow I.V. injection over 1-2 minutes into peripheral vein

Monitoring Parameters INR (preferred) or prothrombin time; hemoglobin, hematocrit, signs and symptoms of bleeding; consider genotyping of CYP2C9 and VKORC1 prior to initiation of therapy, if available.

Reference Range The INR is now the standard test used to monitor warfarin anticoagulation; the desired INR is based upon indication; due to the lack of pediatric clinical trials assessing optimal INR ranges and clinical outcomes, the desired INR ranges for children are extrapolated from adult studies; the optimal therapeutic INR ranges may possibly be lower in children versus adults. Further pediatric studies are needed (Monagle, 2008). **Note:** If INR is not available, prothrombin time should be $1^{1}/_{2}$ to 2 times the control.

Targeted INR and Ranges for Children, Based on Indication[a,b,c]

Indication	Targeted INR	Targeted INR Range
Systemic venous thromboembolism[d]	2.5	2-3
Central venous line-related thrombosis, initial 3 months of therapy	2.5	2-3
Central venous line-related thrombosis after first 3 months of warfarin therapy (**Note:** This is a prophylactic dose)	1.7	1.5-1.9
Central venous line, long-term home TPN (prophylactic dose) (Not recommended routinely)		2-3
Primary prophylaxis following Fontan procedure	2.5	2-3
Primary prophylaxis for dilated cardiomyopathy	2.5	2-3
Primary prophylaxis for biological prosthetic heart valves in children	Follow adult guidelines in table below	
Primary prophylaxis for mechanical prosthetic heart valves in children	Follow adult guidelines in table below	
Kawasaki disease with giant coronary aneurysms	2.5	2-3
Cerebral sinovenous thrombosis **Note:** INR recommendations from 2004 Chest guidelines	2.5	2-3

[a]Information from Monagle, 2004 and Monagle, 2008.

[b]Children are defined in the Chest guidelines as patients aged 28 days to 16 years of age.

[c]See Monagle, 2008 for timing of initiation and adjunct antithrombotic and antiplatelet therapy.

[d]Anticoagulant therapy with UFH or LMWH is recommended for children with first episode of venous thromboembolism (central venous line and noncentral venous line related).

Adult Target INR Ranges Based Upon Indication

Indication	Targeted INR	Targeted INR Range
Cardiac		
Acute myocardial infarction (high risk)[a]	2.5	2-3[b,c]
Atrial fibrillation or atrial flutter	2.5	2-3
Valvular		
Bileaflet or Medtronic Hall tilting disk mechanical aortic valve in normal sinus rhythm and normal LA size	2.5	2-3
Bileaflet or tilting disk mechanical mitral valve	3	2.5-3.5
Caged ball or caged disk mechanical valve	3	2.5-3.5
Mechanical prosthetic valve with systemic embolism despite adequate anticoagulation	3 or 3.5[d]	2.5-3.5[d] or 3-4[d]
Mechanical valve and risk factors for thromboembolism (eg, AF, MI[e], LA enlargement, hypercoagulable state, low EF) or history of atherosclerotic vascular disease	3	2.5-3.5[f]
Bioprosthetic mitral valve	2.5	2-3[g]
Bioprosthetic mitral or aortic valve with prior history of systemic embolism	2.5	2-3[g]
Bioprosthetic mitral or aortic valve with evidence of LA thrombus at surgery	2.5	2-3[h]

Indication	Targeted INR	Targeted INR Range
Bioprosthetic mitral or aortic valve with risk factors for thromboembolism (eg, AF, hypercoagulable state or low EF)	2.5	2-3[i]
Prosthetic mitral valve thrombosis (resolved)	4	3.5-4.5[c]
Prosthetic aortic valve thrombosis (resolved)	3.5	3-4[c]
Rheumatic mitral valve disease and normal sinus rhythm (LA diameter >5.5 cm), AF, previous systemic embolism, or LA thrombus	2.5	2-3
Thromboembolism Treatment		
Venous thromboembolism	2.5	2-3[j,k]
Thromboprophylaxis		
Chronic thromboembolic pulmonary hypertension (CTPH)	2.5	2-3
Lupus inhibitor (no other risk factors)	2.5	2-3
Lupus inhibitor and recurrent thromboembolism	3	2.5-3.5
Major trauma patients with impaired mobility undergoing rehabilitation	2.5	2-3
Spinal cord injury (acute) undergoing rehabilitation	2.5	2-3
Total hip or knee replacement (elective) or hip fracture surgery	2.5	2-3[l]
Other Indications		
Cerebral venous sinus thrombosis	2.5	2-3[m]
Ischemic stroke due to AF	2.5	2-3

[a]High-risk includes large anterior MI, significant heart failure, intracardiac thrombus, atrial fibrillation, history of thromboembolism.

[b]Maintain anticoagulation for 3 months.

[c]Combine with aspirin 81 mg/day.

[d]Combine with aspirin 81 mg/day, if not previously receiving, **and/or** if previous target INR was 2.5, then new target INR should be 3 (2.5-3.5). If previous target INR was 3, then new target INR should be 3.5 (3-4).

[e]MI refers to anterior-apical ST-segment elevation myocardial infarction.

[f]Combine with aspirin 81 mg/day unless patient is at high risk of bleeding (eg, history of GI bleed, age >80 years).

[g]Maintain anticoagulation for 3 months after valve insertion, then switch to aspirin 81 mg/day if no other indications for warfarin exist or clinically reassess need for warfarin in patients with prior history of systemic embolism.

[h]Maintain anticoagulation with warfarin until thrombus resolution.

[i]If patient has history of atherosclerotic vascular disease, combine with aspirin 81 mg/day unless patient is at high risk of bleeding (eg, history of GI bleed, age >80 years).

[j]Treat for 3 months in patients with VTE due to transient reversible risk factor. Treat for a minimum of 3 months in patients with unprovoked VTE and evaluate for long-term therapy. Other risk groups (eg, cancer) may require >3 months of therapy.

[k]In patients with unprovoked VTE who prefer less frequent INR monitoring, low-intensity therapy (INR range: 1.5-1.9) with less frequent monitoring is recommended over stopping treatment.

[l]Continue for at least 10 days and up to 35 days after surgery.

[m]Continue for up to 12 months.

Warfarin levels are not used for monitoring degree of anticoagulation. They may be useful if a patient with unexplained coagulopathy is using the drug surreptitiously or if it is unclear whether clinical resistance is due to true drug resistance or lack of drug intake.

Normal prothrombin time (PT): 10.9-12.9 seconds. Healthy premature newborns have prolonged coagulation test screening results (eg, PT, aPTT, TT) which return to normal adult values at approximately 6 months of age. However, healthy premature newborns (ie, those not receiving antithrombotic agents), do not develop spontaneous

(continued)

hemorrhage or thrombotic complications because of a balance between procoagulants and inhibitors.

Additional Information Usual duration of therapy in children (Monagle, 2008):

DVT:

Idiopathic TE: ≥6 months

Recurrent idiopathic TE: Indefinite

Secondary thrombosis (with resolved risk factors): ≥3 months

Recurrent secondary TE: Anticoagulate until removal of precipitating factor (≥3 months)

Primary prophylaxis for Glenn or Bilateral Cavopulmonary Shunts (BCPS): Continue until ready for Fontan surgery

Post-Fontan surgery: Optimal duration not defined

Cardiomyopathy in children eligible for transplant: Until transplant

Primary pulmonary hypertension: Duration not listed

Biological prosthetic heart valves: Follow adult recommendations

Mechanical prosthetic heart valves: Follow adult recommendations

Ventricular assist device (VAD) placement: Until transplant or weaned from VAD

Kawasaki disease: Treatment depends on severity of coronary involvement

Cerebral sinovenous thrombosis (CSVT) in neonates: 6 weeks-3 months

CSVT in children: ≥3 months

Neonates with homozygous protein C deficiency: Long-term

Note: Overdoses of warfarin may be treated with vitamin K, to reverse warfarin's anticoagulation effect. Prospective genotyping is available and may provide important guidance on initiation of anticoagulant therapy. Commercial testing with PGxPredict™:WARFARIN is now available from PGxHealth™ (Division of Clinical Data, Inc, New Haven, CT). The test genotypes patients for presence of the CYP2C9*2 or *3 alleles and the VKORC1 -1639G>A polymorphism. The results of the test allow patients to be phenotyped as extensive, intermediate, or poor metabolizers (CYP2C9) and as low, intermediate, or high warfarin sensitivity (VKORC1). Ordering information is available at 888-592-7327 or warfarininfo@pgxhealth.com.

Dosage Forms Excipient information presented when available (limited, particularly for generics); consult specific product labeling. [DSC] = Discontinued product

Solution Reconstituted, Intravenous, as sodium:

Coumadin: 5 mg (1 ea [DSC])

Tablet, Oral, as sodium:

Coumadin: 1 mg [scored]

Coumadin: 2 mg [scored; contains fd&c blue #2 aluminum lake, fd&c red #40 aluminum lake]

Coumadin: 2.5 mg [scored; contains fd&c blue #1 aluminum lake, fd&c yellow #10 aluminum lake]

Coumadin: 3 mg [scored; contains fd&c blue #2 aluminum lake, fd&c red #40 aluminum lake, fd&c yellow #6 aluminum lake]

Coumadin: 4 mg [scored; contains fd&c blue #1 aluminum lake]

Coumadin: 5 mg [scored; contains fd&c yellow #6 aluminum lake]

Coumadin: 6 mg [scored; contains fd&c blue #1 aluminum lake, fd&c yellow #6 aluminum lake]

Coumadin: 7.5 mg [scored; contains fd&c yellow #10 aluminum lake, fd&c yellow #6 aluminum lake]

Coumadin: 10 mg [scored; dye free]

Jantoven: 1 mg [scored; contains fd&c red #40 aluminum lake]

Jantoven: 2 mg [scored; contains fd&c blue #2 aluminum lake, fd&c red #40 aluminum lake]

Jantoven: 2.5 mg [scored; contains fd&c blue #1 aluminum lake, fd&c yellow #10 aluminum lake]

Jantoven: 3 mg [scored]

Jantoven: 4 mg [scored; contains fd&c blue #1 aluminum lake]

Jantoven: 5 mg [scored; contains fd&c yellow #6 aluminum lake]

Jantoven: 6 mg [scored; contains fd&c blue #1 aluminum lake]

Jantoven: 7.5 mg [scored; contains fd&c yellow #10 aluminum lake, fd&c yellow #6 aluminum lake]

Jantoven: 10 mg [scored]

Generic: 1 mg, 2 mg, 2.5 mg, 3 mg, 4 mg, 5 mg, 6 mg, 7.5 mg, 10 mg

References

Andrew M, Marzinotto V, Brooker LA, et al, "Oral Anticoagulation Therapy in Pediatric Patients: A Prospective Study," *Thromb Haemost*, 1994, 71(3):265-9.

Ansell J, Hirsh J, Poller L, et al, "The Pharmacology and Management of the Vitamin K Antagonists: The Seventh ACCP Conference on Antithrombotic and Thrombolytic Therapy," *Chest*, 2004, 126(3 Suppl):204S-33S.

Arepally GM and Ortel TL, "Clinical Practice. Heparin-Induced Thrombocytopenia," *N Engl J Med*, 2006, 355(8):809-17

Bates SM, Greer IA, Middeldorp S, et al. "VTE, Thrombophilia, Antithrombotic Therapy, and Pregnancy: Antithrombotic Therapy and Prevention of Thrombosis, 9th ed: American College of Chest Physicians Evidence-Based Clinical Practice Guidelines," *Chest*, 2012, 141(2 Suppl):e691-736.

David M and Andrew M, "Venous Thromboembolic Complications in Children," *J Pediatr*, 1993, 123(3):337-46.

Fihn SD "Aiming for Safe Anticoagulation," *N Engl J Med*, 1995, 333 (1):54-5.

Hirsh J, Dalen JE, Anderson DR, et al, "Oral Anticoagulants. Mechanism of Action, Clinical Effectiveness, and Optimal Therapeutic Range," *Chest*, 2001, 119:8S-21S.

Monagle P, Chalmers E, Chan A, et al, "Antithrombotic Therapy in Neonates and Children: American College of Chest Physicians Evidence-Based Clinical Practice Guidelines (8th Edition)," *Chest*, 2008, 133(6 Suppl):887S-968S.

Monagle P, Chan A, Massicotte P, et al, "Antithrombotic Therapy in Children: The Seventh ACCP Conference on Antithrombotic and Thrombolytic Therapy," *Chest*, 2004, 126(3 Suppl):645S-87S.

Monagle P, Michelson AD, Bovill E, et al, "Antithrombotic Therapy in Children," *Chest*, 2001, 119:344S-70S.

Salem DN, O'Gara PT, Madias C, et al, "Valvular and Structural Heart Disease: American College of Chest Physicians Evidence-Based Clinical Practice Guidelines (8th Edition)," *Chest*, 2008, 133(6 Suppl):593S-629S.

Salem DN, Stein PD, Al-Ahmad A, et al, "Antithrombotic Therapy in Valvular Heart Disease - Native and Prosthetic: The Seventh ACCP Conference on Antithrombotic and Thrombolytic Therapy," *Chest*, 2004, 126(3 Suppl):457S-82S.

Streif W, Andrew M, Marzinotto V, et al, "Analysis of Warfarin Therapy in Pediatric Patients: A Prospective Cohort Study of 319 Patients," *Blood*, 1999, 94(9):3007-14.

Suvarna R, Pirmohamed M, and Henderson L, "Possible Interaction Between Warfarin and Cranberry Juice," *BMJ*, 2003, 327(7429):1454.

Wells PS, Holbrook AM, Crowther NR, et al, "Interactions of Warfarin With Drugs and Food," *Ann Intern Med*, 1994, 121(9):676-83.

◆ **Warfarin Sodium** *see* Warfarin *on page 2156*

◆ **4-Way Fast Acting [OTC]** *see* Phenylephrine (Nasal) *on page 1660*

◆ **4-Way Menthol [OTC]** *see* Phenylephrine (Nasal) *on page 1660*

◆ **4-Way Saline [OTC]** *see* Sodium Chloride *on page 1902*

◆ **Welchol** *see* Colesevelam *on page 539*

◆ **Wellbutrin** *see* BuPROPion *on page 327*

◆ **Wellbutrin XL** *see* BuPROPion *on page 327*

◆ **Wellbutrin SR** *see* BuPROPion *on page 327*

◆ **Westcort** *see* Hydrocortisone (Topical) *on page 1038*

◆ **Westcort® (Can)** *see* Hydrocortisone (Topical) *on page 1038*

◆ **Westhroid** *see* Thyroid, Desiccated *on page 2018*

◆ **Westhroid-P [DSC]** *see* Thyroid, Desiccated *on page 2018*

◆ **White Mineral Oil** *see* Mineral Oil *on page 1419*

◆ **Wilate®** *see* Antihemophilic Factor/von Willebrand Factor Complex (Human) *on page 177*

- Winpred (Can) see PredniSONE on page 1732
- WinRho SDF see Rho(D) Immune Globulin on page 1815
- WinRho® SDF (Can) see Rho(D) Immune Globulin on page 1815
- Woman's Laxative [OTC] (Can) see Bisacodyl on page 293
- Womens Laxative [OTC] see Bisacodyl on page 293
- Wound Wash Saline [OTC] see Sodium Chloride on page 1902
- WP Thyroid see Thyroid, Desiccated on page 2018
- WR-2721 see Amifostine on page 116
- WR-139007 see Dacarbazine on page 578
- WR-139013 see Chlorambucil on page 437
- WR-139021 see Carmustine on page 382
- Wycillin see Penicillin G Procaine on page 1634
- Wycillin® (Can) see Penicillin G Procaine on page 1634
- Wydase see Hyaluronidase on page 1020
- Xanax see ALPRAZolam on page 100
- Xanax® (Can) see ALPRAZolam on page 100
- Xanax TS™ (Can) see ALPRAZolam on page 100
- Xanax XR see ALPRAZolam on page 100
- Xartemis XR see Oxycodone and Acetaminophen on page 1573
- Xerclear see Acyclovir and Hydrocortisone on page 69
- Xerese™ see Acyclovir and Hydrocortisone on page 69
- Xifaxan see Rifaximin on page 1826
- Xilep see Rufinamide on page 1858
- Ximino™ see Minocycline on page 1420
- Xodol® 5/300 see Hydrocodone and Acetaminophen on page 1027
- Xodol® 7.5/300 see Hydrocodone and Acetaminophen on page 1027
- Xodol® 10/300 see Hydrocodone and Acetaminophen on page 1027
- Xolair see Omalizumab on page 1533
- Xolegel see Ketoconazole (Topical) on page 1179
- Xolido XP [OTC] see Lidocaine (Topical) on page 1242
- Xolox [DSC] see Oxycodone and Acetaminophen on page 1573
- Xopenex see Levalbuterol on page 1218
- Xopenex Concentrate see Levalbuterol on page 1218
- Xopenex HFA see Levalbuterol on page 1218
- Xpect [OTC] see GuaiFENesin on page 984
- X-Seb T Pearl [OTC] see Coal Tar on page 532
- X-Seb T Plus [OTC] see Coal Tar on page 532
- Xtra-Care [OTC] see Vitamin E on page 2148
- Xylocaine see Lidocaine (Systemic) on page 1239
- Xylocaine see Lidocaine (Topical) on page 1242
- Xylocaine (Cardiac) see Lidocaine (Systemic) on page 1239
- Xylocaine-MPF see Lidocaine (Systemic) on page 1239
- Xylocaine® MPF With Epinephrine see Lidocaine and Epinephrine on page 1245
- Xylocaine Viscous see Lidocaine (Topical) on page 1242
- Xylocaine® With Epinephrine see Lidocaine and Epinephrine on page 1245
- Xylocard® (Can) see Lidocaine (Systemic) on page 1239
- Xyntha see Antihemophilic Factor (Recombinant) on page 172
- Xyntha Solofuse see Antihemophilic Factor (Recombinant) on page 172
- Xyzal see Levocetirizine on page 1227

Yellow Fever Vaccine (YEL oh FEE ver vak SEEN)

Related Information
Immunization Administration Recommendations on page 2368

Immunization Guidelines on page 2373

Brand Names: U.S. YF-VAX

Brand Names: Canada YF-VAX

Therapeutic Category Vaccine

Generic Availability (U.S.) No

Use To provide active immunity to yellow fever virus to individuals who are either traveling to or living in endemic yellow fever areas (FDA approved in ages ≥9 months and adults)

The Advisory Committee on Immunization Practices (ACIP) recommends vaccination for: Persons traveling to or living in areas at risk for yellow fever transmission; persons traveling to countries which require vaccination for international travel; laboratory personnel who may be exposed to the yellow fever virus or concentrated preparations of the vaccine.

Although the vaccine is approved for use in children ≥9 months of age, the CDC recommends use in children as young as 6 months under unusual circumstances (eg, travel to an area where exposure is unavoidable). Children <6 months of age should **never** receive the vaccine.

Pregnancy Risk Factor C

Pregnancy Considerations Animal reproduction studies have not been conducted. Adverse events were not observed in the mother or fetus following vaccination during the third trimester of pregnancy in Nigerian women; however, maternal seroconversion was reduced. Inadvertent exposure early in the first trimester of pregnancy in Brazilian women did not show decreased maternal seroconversion; no major congenital abnormalities were noted. Cord blood from an infant whose mother was vaccinated during the first trimester tested positive for IgM antibodies; no adverse events were noted in the infant. Vaccine should be administered if travel to an endemic area is unavoidable and the infant should be monitored after birth. Tests to verify maternal immune response may be considered. If a pregnant woman is to be vaccinated only to satisfy an international requirement (as opposed to decreasing risk of infection), efforts should be made to obtain a waiver letter. Women should wait 4 weeks after receiving vaccine before conceiving (CDC, 2010).

Breast-Feeding Considerations Laboratory confirmed transmission of 17DD yellow fever vaccine virus via breast-feeding has been documented. Yellow fever vaccine was administered to a nursing mother 15 days postpartum. She was exclusively breast-feeding her newborn. Eight days after maternal vaccination, the infant developed a fever, was irritable, refused to nurse, then was hospitalized for seizures the next day. Yellow fever virus specific to the vaccine and IgM antibodies were detected in the newborn CSF. The child was discharged after 24 days in the hospital; growth and neurodevelopment were normal through 6 months of age. Breast-feeding is contraindicated by the manufacturer, particularly in infants <9 months of age. If travel to an endemic area cannot be avoided or postponed, women who are nursing should be vaccinated. Breast-feeding does not adversely affect immunization (CDC, 2010; WHO, 2013).

Contraindications Hypersensitivity to the vaccine, egg or chick embryo protein, or any component; children <6 months of age (per CDC guidelines) (<9 months of age per manufacturer); acute or febrile disease; breast-feeding; immunosuppressed individuals including those with blood dyscrasias, leukemia, lymphomas, thymic disease, or other malignant neoplasms affecting the bone marrow or lymphatic systems; concurrent immunosuppressive therapy (corticosteroids, alkylating drugs, antimetabolites) or radiation; transplant; family history of congenital or hereditary immunodeficiency; primary and acquired immunodeficiency states including patients with symptomatic HIV infection or CD4+ counts <200/mm^3 (or <15% of total lymphocytes in ages ≤6 years) (per CDC)

Warnings Not for use in patients who are immunosuppressed due to an increased risk of encephalitis with yellow fever vaccine administration; consider delaying travel or obtaining a waiver letter. Patients on low-dose or short-term corticosteroids are not considered immunosuppressed and may receive the vaccine. Use caution when administering the vaccine to patients with asymptomatic HIV infection with CD4+ counts 200-499/mm^3 (or 15 to 24% of total lymphocytes in children <6 years of age). Chicken embryos are used in the manufacture of this vaccine; use caution in patients with immediate-type hypersensitivity reactions to eggs; immediate treatment for anaphylactic reactions should be available during vaccine use.

Avoid use in infants <9 months and pregnant women unless travel to high-risk areas are unavoidable; use in infants <6 months of age is contraindicated due to risk of encephalitis. The decision to use in children between 6-9 months of age must weigh the risks of exposure to the virus with the theoretic risks of vaccine-associated encephalitis (*Red Book*, 2009). Advice regarding use of this vaccine can be obtained from the Division of Vector-Borne Infectious Diseases of the CDC. Syncope has been reported with use of injectable vaccines and may be accompanied by transient visual disturbances, weakness, or tonic-clonic movements. Procedures should be in place to avoid injuries from falling and to restore cerebral perfusion if syncope occurs. In general, household and close contacts of persons with altered immune competence may receive all age-appropriate vaccines.

Precautions Malnourished persons may have a decreased response to vaccination. Antipyretics have not been shown to prevent febrile seizures; antipyretics may be used to treat fever or discomfort following vaccination (CDC, 2011). One study reported that routine prophylactic administration of acetaminophen to prevent fever prior to vaccination decreased the immune response of some vaccines; the clinical significance of this reduction in immune response has not been established (Prymula, 2009). Transfusion-related transmission of yellow fever vaccine virus has been reported; wait 2 weeks after immunization with yellow fever vaccine to donate blood. Latex is used in stopper of the vial which may cause allergic reactions in susceptible individuals. May cause fever; reported incidence variable depending on the study, as low as <5% and as high as 10% to 30% has been reported.

Adverse Reactions All serious adverse reactions must be reported to the U.S. Department of Health and Human Services (DHHS) Vaccine Adverse Event Reporting System (VAERS) 1-800-822-7967 or online at https://vaers.hhs.gov/esub/index. In Canada, adverse reactions may be reported to local provincial/territorial health agencies or to the Vaccine Safety Section at Public Health Agency of Canada (1-866-844-0018).

Adverse reactions may be increased in patients <9 months or ≥60 years of age):

Central nervous system: Chills, fever, focal neurological defects, headache, malaise, seizure

Dermatologic: Rash, urticaria

Local: Injection site reactions (edema, erythema, hypersensitivity, mass, pain, pruritus, rash, warmth)

Neuromuscular & skeletal: Myalgia, weakness

Miscellaneous: Guillain-Barré syndrome (GBS), hypersensitivity (immediate), vaccine-associated neurotropic disease (rare), viscerotropic disease (rare; may be associated with multiorgan failure)

Vaccine-associated neurologic disease (YEL-AND) may manifest as meningoencephalitis (neurotropic disease), GBS, acute disseminated encephalomyelitis, and bulbar palsy. Vaccine-associated viscerotropic disease (YEL-AVD) mimics naturally-acquired yellow fever disease; risk may be increased in older patients and those with a history of thymus disease or thymectomy.

Drug Interactions

Metabolism/Transport Effects None known.

Avoid Concomitant Use

Avoid concomitant use of Yellow Fever Vaccine with any of the following: Belimumab; Fingolimod; Immunosuppressants

Increased Effect/Toxicity

The levels/effects of Yellow Fever Vaccine may be increased by: Belimumab; Corticosteroids (Systemic); Dimethyl Fumarate; Fingolimod; Hydroxychloroquine; Immunosuppressants; Leflunomide; Mercaptopurine; Methotrexate

Decreased Effect

Yellow Fever Vaccine may decrease the levels/effects of: Tuberculin Tests

The levels/effects of Yellow Fever Vaccine may be decreased by: Dimethyl Fumarate; Fingolimod; Immunosuppressants

Stability Store at 2°C to 8°C (35°F to 46°F); do not freeze. Must be used within 60 minutes of reconstitution; keep reconstituted suspension refrigerated until used.

Pharmacodynamics Onset of action: Seroconversion: 10-14 days

Dosing: Usual Children ≥6 months and Adults: SubQ: One dose (0.5 mL) ≥10 days before travel; Booster: Repeat same dosage every 10 years if at continued risk of exposure (CDC, 2010).

Administration Parenteral: Use entire contents of provided diluent to reconstitute vaccine. Gently swirl until a uniform suspension forms; swirl well before withdrawing dose. Avoid vigorous shaking to prevent foaming of suspension. Use within 60 minutes following reconstitution; keep suspension refrigerated until used. Administer by SubQ injection into the anterolateral aspect of the thigh or arm; **not for I.V. administration.** If inadvertently administered I.M., the dose does not need to be repeated. Use of expired vaccine is not considered a valid dose and should be repeated after 28 days. For booster doses, if the date of previous vaccination cannot be determined and the patient requires vaccination, the booster dose can be given. Adolescents and adults should be vaccinated while seated or lying down

Monitoring Parameters Observe for syncope for 15 minutes following administration. If seizure-like activity associated with syncope occurs, maintain patient in supine or Trendelenburg position to reestablish adequate cerebral perfusion.

Additional Information A desensitization procedure is available for persons with severe egg sensitivity. Consult manufacturer's labeling for details. Some countries require a valid International Certification of Vaccination or Prophylaxis (ICVP) showing receipt of vaccine. Certificate is valid beginning 10 days after and for 10 years following vaccination (booster doses received within 10 years are valid from the date of vaccination). The WHO requires revaccination every 10 years to maintain traveler's vaccination certificate. Current requirements and recommendations for immunization related to travel destination can be obtained from the CDC Travelers' Health Web site (www.cdc.gov/travel). All travelers to endemic areas should be advised of the risks of yellow fever disease and all available methods to prevent it. All travelers should take protective measures to avoid mosquito bites.

In order to maximize vaccination rates, the ACIP recommends simultaneous administration (ie, >1 vaccine on the same day at different anatomic sites) of all age-appropriate vaccines (live or inactivated) for which a person is eligible at a single visit, unless contraindications exist. If available, the use of combination vaccines is generally preferred over separate injections, taking into consideration provider assessment, patient preference, and potential adverse events. If separate vaccines being used, evaluate product information regarding same syringe compatibility of vaccines. Separate needles and syringes should be used for each injection. The ACIP prefers each dose of specific vaccine in a series come from the same manufacturer if possible (CDC, 2011).

The following CDC agencies may be contacted if serologic testing is needed or for advice when administering yellow fever vaccine to pregnant women, children <9 months, or patients with altered immune status:

Division of Vector-Borne Infectious Diseases: 970-221-6400

Division of Global Migration and Quarantine: 404-498-1600

Dosage Forms Excipient information presented when available (limited, particularly for generics); consult specific product labeling.

Injection, powder for reconstitution [17D-204 strain]:

YF-VAX®: ≥4.74 Log$_{10}$ plaque-forming units (PFU) per 0.5 mL dose [single-dose or 5-dose vial; produced in chicken embryos; contains gelatin; packaged with diluent; vial stopper contains latex]

References

AAP Steering Committee on Quality Improvement and Management, Subcommittee on Febrile Seizures American Academy of Pediatrics, "Febrile Seizures: Clinical Practice Guideline for the Long-Term Management of the Child With Simple Febrile Seizures," *Pediatrics*, 2008, 121(6):1281-6.

Centers for Disease Control and Prevention (CDC), "General Recommendations on Immunization. Recommendations of the Advisory Committee on Immunization Practices (ACIP)," *MMWR Recomm Rep*, 2006, 55(RR-15):1-48. Available at: http://www.cdc.gov/mmwr/preview/mmwrhtml/rr5515a1.htm.

Centers for Disease Control and Prevention, "Guidelines for Preventing Opportunistic Infections Among Hematopoietic Stem Cell Transplant Recipients. Recommendations of CDC, the Infectious Disease Society of America, and the American Society of Blood and Marrow Transplantation," *MMWR Recomm Rep*, 2004, 49(RR-10):89-90.

Centers for Disease Control and Prevention (CDC), "Syncope After Vaccination-United States, January 2005-July 2007," *MMWR Morb Mortal Wkly Rep*, 2008, 2;57(17):457-60.

Centers for Disease Control and Prevention, "Transfusion-Related Transmission of Yellow Fever Vaccine Virus – California, 2009," *MMWR Morb Mortal Wkly Rep*, 2010, 59(2):34-7.

National Center for Immunization and Respiratory Diseases, "General Recommendations on Immunization - Recommendations of the Advisory Committee on Immunization Practices (ACIP)," *MMWR Recomm Rep*, 2011, 60(2):1-64.

Prymula R, Siegrist CA, Chlibek R, et al, "Effect of Prophylactic Paracetamol Administration at Time of Vaccination on Febrile Reactions and Antibody Responses in Children: Two Open-Label, Randomised Controlled Trials," *Lancet*, 2009, 374(9698):1339-50.

Red Book: 2009 Report of the Committee on Infectious Diseases, "International Travel," 28th ed, Pickering LK, ed, Elk Grove Village, IL: American Academy of Pediatrics, 2009, 98-104.

Staples JE, Gershman M, Fischer M, et al, "Yellow Fever Vaccine: Recommendations of the Advisory Committee on Immunization Practices (ACIP)," *MMWR Recomm Rep*, 2010, 59(RR-7):1-27.

World Health Organization (WHO), "Meeting of the Strategic Advisory Group of Experts on Immunization, April 2013 – Conclusions and Recommendations," *Wkly Epidemiol Rec*, 2013, 88(20):201-6.

◆ **YF-VAX** *see* Yellow Fever Vaccine *on page 2162*

◆ **YM-08310** *see* Amifostine *on page 116*

◆ **Yodoxin** *see* Iodoquinol *on page 1144*

◆ **Z4942** *see* Ifosfamide *on page 1068*

◆ **Zaclir Cleansing** *see* Benzoyl Peroxide *on page 275*

◆ **Zaditor [OTC]** *see* Ketotifen (Ophthalmic) *on page 1185*

◆ **Zaditor® (Can)** *see* Ketotifen (Ophthalmic) *on page 1185*

Zafirlukast (za FIR loo kast)

Medication Safety Issues
Sound-alike/look-alike issues:
Accolate® may be confused with Accupril®, Accutane®, Aclovate®

Brand Names: U.S. Accolate

Brand Names: Canada Accolate®

Therapeutic Category Antiasthmatic; Leukotriene Receptor Antagonist

Generic Availability (U.S.) Yes

Use Prophylaxis and chronic treatment of asthma (FDA approved in ages ≥5 years and adults)

Pregnancy Risk Factor B

Pregnancy Considerations Adverse events were not observed in animal reproduction studies except with doses that were also maternally toxic. Based on limited data, an increased risk of teratogenic effects has not been observed with zafirlukast use in pregnancy (Bakhireva, 2007). Uncontrolled asthma is associated with adverse events on pregnancy (increased risk of perinatal mortality, pre-eclampsia, preterm birth, low birth weight infants). Zafirlukast may be considered for use in women who had a favorable response prior to becoming pregnant; however, initiating a leukotriene receptor antagonist during pregnancy is an alternative (but not preferred) treatment option for mild persistent asthma (NAEPP, 2005).

Breast-Feeding Considerations Zafirlukast is excreted into breast milk. In women receiving zafirlukast 40 mg twice daily, maternal serum concentrations were 225 ng/mL and breast milk concentrations were 50 ng/mL. Due to the potential for adverse reactions in the nursing infant, breast-feeding is not recommended by the manufacturer.

Contraindications Hypersensitivity to zafirlukast or any component; hepatic impairment (including hepatic cirrhosis)

Warnings Zafirlukast is not indicated for use in the reversal of bronchospasm in acute asthma attacks, including status asthmaticus. Therapy with zafirlukast can be continued during acute exacerbations of asthma. An increased proportion of zafirlukast patients (>55 years of age) reported infections as compared to placebo-treated patients; these infections were mostly mild or moderate in intensity, predominantly affected the respiratory tract, were dose-proportional to the total milligrams of zafirlukast exposure, and associated with coadministration of inhaled corticosteroids.

Serious hepatic adverse events (including hepatitis, hyperbilirubinemia, and hepatic failure) have been reported with use; female patients may be at greater risk. Periodic testing of liver function may be considered (early detection coupled with therapy discontinuation is generally believed to improve the likelihood of recovery). Advise patients to be alert for and to immediately report symptoms (eg, anorexia, right upper quadrant abdominal pain, nausea). If hepatic dysfunction is suspected (due to clinical signs/symptoms), discontinue use immediately and measure liver function tests (particularly ALT); resolution observed in most but not all cases upon discontinuation of therapy. Do not resume or restart if hepatic function studies indicate dysfunction.

Use in patients with hepatic impairment (including hepatic cirrhosis) is contraindicated.

In rare cases, patients may present with systemic eosinophilia, sometimes presenting with clinical features of vasculitis consistent with Churg-Strauss syndrome, a condition which is often treated with systemic corticosteroid therapy. Healthcare providers should be alert to eosinophilia, vasculitic rash, worsening pulmonary symptoms, cardiac complications, and/or neuropathy presenting in their patients. A causal association between zafirlukast and these underlying conditions has not been established.

Postmarketing reports of neuropsychiatric events including agitation, aggression, anxiousness, dream abnormalities, hallucinations, depression, insomnia, irritability, restlessness, suicidal thinking and behavior (including suicide) and tremor have been observed.

Precautions Use caution with concomitant warfarin therapy; use with warfarin results in a clinically significant increase in INR; closely monitor INR with concurrent use. An increased proportion of patients >55 years of age reported infections as compared to placebo-treated patients. These infections were mostly mild or moderate in intensity and predominantly affected the respiratory tract. Infections occurred equally in both sexes, were dose-proportional to total milligrams of zafirlukast exposure, and were associated with coadministration of inhaled corticosteroids.

Adverse Reactions

Central nervous system: Dizziness, fever, headache, pain
Gastrointestinal: Abdominal pain, diarrhea, dyspepsia, nausea, vomiting
Hepatic: ALT increased
Neuromuscular & skeletal: Back pain, myalgia, weakness
Miscellaneous: Infection
Rare but important or life-threatening: Agranulocytosis, angioedema, arthralgia, bleeding, bruising, depression, edema, eosinophilia (systemic), eosinophilic pneumonia, hepatic failure, hepatitis, hyperbilirubinemia, hypersensitivity reactions, insomnia, malaise, pruritus, rash, urticaria, vasculitis with clinical features of Churg-Strauss syndrome (rare)

Drug Interactions

Metabolism/Transport Effects Substrate of CYP2C9 (major); **Note:** Assignment of Major/Minor substrate status based on clinically relevant drug interaction potential; **Inhibits** CYP1A2 (weak), CYP2C19 (weak), CYP2C8 (weak), CYP2C9 (moderate), CYP2D6 (weak), CYP3A4 (weak)

Avoid Concomitant Use

Avoid concomitant use of Zafirlukast with any of the following: Pimozide

Increased Effect/Toxicity

Zafirlukast may increase the levels/effects of: ARIPiprazole; Bosentan; Cannabis; Carvedilol; CYP2C9 Substrates; Dofetilide; Dronabinol; Lomitapide; Pimozide; Tetrahydrocannabinol; Theophylline Derivatives; Vitamin K Antagonists

The levels/effects of Zafirlukast may be increased by: Ceritinib; CYP2C9 Inhibitors (Moderate); CYP2C9 Inhibitors (Strong); Mifepristone

Decreased Effect

The levels/effects of Zafirlukast may be decreased by: CYP2C9 Inducers (Strong); Dabrafenib; Erythromycin (Systemic); Peginterferon Alfa-2b; Theophylline Derivatives

Food Interactions Food decreases bioavailability of zafirlukast by 40%. Management: Take on an empty stomach 1 hour before or 2 hours after meals.

Stability Store tablets at 20°C to 25°C (68°F to 77°F); protect from light and moisture; dispense in original airtight container

Mechanism of Action Zafirlukast is a selectively and competitive leukotriene-receptor antagonist (LTRA) of leukotriene D4 and E4 (LTD4 and LTE4), components of slow-reacting substance of anaphylaxis (SRSA). Cysteinyl leukotriene production and receptor occupation have been correlated with the pathophysiology of asthma, including airway edema, smooth muscle constriction, and altered cellular activity associated with the inflammatory process, which contribute to the signs and symptoms of asthma.

Pharmacodynamics Asthma symptom improvement:
Maximum effect: 2-6 weeks
Duration: 12 hours

Pharmacokinetics (Adult data unless noted)
Absorption: Rapid
Bioavailability: Food decreases bioavailability by ~40%
Distribution: Extensively excreted into breast milk; breast milk to plasma ratio: 0.15
V_{dss}: ~70 L
Protein binding: ≥99%, predominantly albumin
Metabolism: Extensively metabolized by liver via cytochrome P450 isoenzyme CYP2C9 pathway
Half-life, elimination: ~10 hours (range: 8-16 hours)
Time to peak serum concentration:
Children: 2-2.5 hours
Adults: 3 hours
Elimination: Fecal (~90%) and urine (~10%)
Clearance:
Children 5-6 years: 9.2 L/hour
Children 7-11 years: 11.4 L/hour
Adults: 20 L/hour

Dosing: Usual Oral:
Children 5-11 years: 10 mg twice daily
Children ≥12 years and Adults: 20 mg twice daily

Dosing adjustment in renal impairment: Dosage adjustment is not necessary.

Dosing adjustment in hepatic impairment: Use is contraindicated.

Administration Oral: Administer at least 1 hour before or 2 hours after a meal

Monitoring Parameters Pulmonary function tests (FEV-1, PEF), improvement in asthma symptoms, periodic liver function tests

Reference Range Obtaining plasma concentrations not clinically indicated; plasma zafirlukast serum concentrations exceeding 5 ng/mL at 12-14 hours following oral doses have correlated with activity; mean trough serum levels at doses of 20 mg twice daily were 20 ng/mL

Dosage Forms Excipient information presented when available (limited, particularly for generics); consult specific product labeling.
Tablet, Oral:
Accolate: 10 mg, 20 mg
Generic: 10 mg, 20 mg

References

Bakhireva LN, Jones KL, Schatz M, et al, "Organization of Teratology Information Specialists Collaborative Research Group. Safety of Leukotriene Receptor Antagonists in Pregnancy," *J Allergy Clin Immunol*, 2007, 119(3):618-25.

"Guidelines for the Diagnosis and Management of Asthma. NAEPP Expert Panel Report 3," August 2007, www.nhlbi.nih.gov/guidelines/asthma/asthgdln.pdf.

"National Asthma Education and Prevention Program. Expert Panel Report: Guidelines for the Diagnosis and Management of Asthma Update on Selected Topics–2002," *J Allergy Clin Immunol*, 2002, 110 (5 Suppl):S141-219.

National Heart, Lung, and Blood Institute; National Asthma Education and Prevention Program Asthma and Pregnancy Working Group, "NAEPP Expert Panel Report. Managing Asthma During Pregnancy: Recommendations for Pharmacologic Treatment - 2004 Update," *J Allergy Clin Immunol*, 2005, 115(1):34-46.

◆ **Zamicet™** *see* Hydrocodone and Acetaminophen *on page 1027*

Zanamivir (za NA mi veer)

Medication Safety Issues

Sound-alike/look-alike issues:

Relenza® may be confused with Albenza®, Aplenzin™

Brand Names: U.S. Relenza Diskhaler

Brand Names: Canada Relenza®

Therapeutic Category Antiviral Agent; Neuraminidase Inhibitor

Generic Availability (U.S.) No

Use Treatment of influenza A or B infection in patients who have been symptomatic for no more than 2 days (FDA approved in children ≥7 years and adults); prophylaxis of influenza A or B infection (FDA approved in children ≥5 years and adults); has also been used for treatment of patients symptomatic for >2 days with severe illness (CDC, 2010)

The Advisory Committee on Immunization Practices (ACIP) recommends that antiviral **treatment** be considered for the following (see specific antiviral product monograph for appropriate patient selection):

- Persons with severe, complicated or progressive illness
- Hospitalized persons
- Persons at higher risk for influenza complications:
  - Children <2 years of age (highest risk in children <6 months of age)
  - Adults ≥65 years of age
  - Persons with chronic disorders of the pulmonary (including asthma) or cardiovascular systems (except hypertension)
  - Persons with chronic metabolic diseases (including diabetes mellitus), hepatic disease, renal dysfunction, hematologic disorders (including sickle cell disease), or immunosuppression (including immunosuppression caused by medications or HIV)
  - Persons with neurologic/neuromuscular conditions (including conditions such as spinal cord injuries, seizure disorders, cerebral palsy, stroke, mental retardation, moderate-to-severe developmental delay, or muscular dystrophy) which may compromise respiratory function, the handling of respiratory secretions, or that can increase the risk of aspiration
  - Pregnant or postpartum women (≤2 weeks after delivery)
  - Persons <19 years of age on long-term aspirin therapy
  - American Indians and Alaskan Natives
  - Persons who are morbidly obese (BMI ≥40)
  - Residents of nursing homes or other chronic care facilities
- Use may also be considered for previously healthy, nonhigh risk outpatients with confirmed or suspected influenza based on clinical judgment when treatment can be started within 48 hours of illness onset.

The ACIP recommends that **prophylaxis** be considered for the following (see specific antiviral product monograph for appropriate patient selection):

- Postexposure prophylaxis may be considered for family or close contacts of suspected or confirmed cases, who are at higher risk of influenza complications, and who have not been vaccinated against the circulating strain at the time of the exposure or if exposure occurred within 2 weeks of vaccination.
- Postexposure prophylaxis may be considered for unvaccinated healthcare workers who had occupational exposure without protective equipment.
- Pre-exposure prophylaxis should only be used for persons at very high risk of influenza complications and who cannot be otherwise protected at times of high risk for exposure. Prophylaxis should also be administered to all eligible residents of institutions that house patients at high risk when needed to control outbreaks.

Prescribing and Access Restrictions Zanamivir *aqueous solution* intended for nebulization or intravenous (I.V.) administration is **not** currently approved for use. Data on safety and efficacy via these routes of administration are limited. However, limited supplies of zanamivir aqueous solution may be made available through the Zanamivir Compassionate Use Program for qualifying patients for the treatment of serious influenza illness. For information, contact the GlaxoSmithKline Clinical Support Help Desk at 1-866-341-9160 or gskclinicalsupportHD@gsk.com.

Pregnancy Risk Factor C

Pregnancy Considerations Adverse events were not observed in animal reproduction studies. Influenza infection may be more severe in pregnant women. Untreated influenza infection is associated with an increased risk of adverse events to the fetus and an increased risk of complications or death to the mother. Oseltamivir and zanamivir are currently recommended for the treatment or prophylaxis of influenza in pregnant women and women up to 2 weeks postpartum. Oseltamivir and zanamivir are currently recommended as an adjunct to vaccination and should not be used as a substitute for vaccination in pregnant women (consult current CDC guidelines).

Breast-Feeding Considerations It is not known if zanamivir is found in human milk and the manufacturer recommends that caution be exercised when administering zanamivir to nursing women. According to the CDC, breast-feeding while taking zanamivir can be continued. The CDC recommends that women infected with the influenza virus follow general precautions (eg, frequent hand washing) to decrease viral transmission to the child. Mothers with influenza-like illnesses at delivery should consider avoiding close contact with the infant until they have received 48 hours of antiviral medication, fever has resolved, and cough and secretions can be controlled. These measures may help decrease (but not eliminate) the risk of transmitting influenza to the newborn. During this time, breast milk can be expressed and bottle-fed to the infant by another person who is well. Protective measures, such as wearing a face mask, changing into a clean gown or clothing, and strict hand hygiene should be continued by the mother for ≥7 days after the onset of symptoms or until symptom-free for 24 hours. Infant care should be performed by a noninfected person when possible (consult current CDC guidelines). Influenza may cause serious illness in postpartum women and prompt evaluation for febrile respiratory illnesses is recommended.

Contraindications Hypersensitivity to zanamivir, milk proteins, or any component

Warnings Bronchospasm, decreased lung function, and other serious adverse reactions, including those with fatal outcomes, have been reported in patients with and without airway disease; discontinue with bronchospasm or signs of decreased lung function. For a patient with an underlying airway disease where a medical decision has been made to use zanamivir, a fast-acting bronchodilator should be made available, and used prior to each dose. Not recommended for use in patients with underlying respiratory disease, such as asthma or COPD, due to lack of efficacy and risk of serious adverse effects. Rare occurrences of neuropsychiatric events (including confusion, delirium, hallucinations, and/or self-injury) have been reported from postmarketing surveillance; direct causation is difficult to establish (influenza infection may also be associated with behavioral and neurologic changes); pediatric patients with influenza may be at increased risk of seizures, confusion, or abnormal behavior early in their illness (monitor for abnormal behavior).

Relenza® inhalation powder should only be administered via inhalation using the provided Diskhaler® delivery device; the commercially available formulation is **not** intended to be solubilized or administered via any nebulizer/mechanical ventilator; inappropriate administration has resulted in death. Allergic-like reactions, including anaphylaxis, oropharyngeal edema, and serious skin rashes have been reported; powder for oral inhalation contains lactose; use contraindicated in patients allergic to milk proteins.

Precautions Use caution in renal or hepatic impairment; safety and efficacy have not been established. Zanamivir is not a substitute for annual influenza vaccination; indicated for children ≥5 years of age (for influenza prophylaxis) and children ≥7 years of age (for influenza treatment); children ages 5-6 years may have inadequate inhalation (via Diskhaler®) for the treatment of influenza. Effectiveness has not been established for prophylaxis of influenza in nursing home patients (per manufacturer). The CDC recommends zanamivir to be used to control institutional outbreaks of influenza when circulating strains are suspected of being resistant to oseltamivir (refer to current guidelines).

Antiviral treatment should begin within 48 hours of symptom onset; however, the CDC recommends that treatment may still be beneficial and should be started in hospitalized patients with severe, complicated, or progressive illness if >48 hours. Treatment should not be delayed while awaiting results of laboratory tests for influenza. Nonhospitalized persons who are not at high risk for developing severe or complicated illness and who have a mild disease are not likely to benefit if treatment is started >48 hours after symptom onset. Nonhospitalized persons who are already beginning to recover do not need treatment. Effectiveness has not been established in patients with significant underlying medical conditions. Patients must be instructed in the use of the delivery system. Safety and efficacy of repeated courses have not been established.

Adverse Reactions
Central nervous system: Dizziness, fatigue, fever/chills, headache, malaise
Dermatologic: Urticaria
Gastrointestinal: Abdominal pain, anorexia, appetite decreased, diarrhea, nausea, throat/tonsil discomfort/pain, vomiting
Neuromuscular & skeletal: Arthralgia, articular rheumatism, muscle pain, musculoskeletal pain
Respiratory: Bronchitis, cough, infection, nasal inflammation, nasal signs and symptoms, sinusitis
Miscellaneous: Viral infection
Rare but important or life-threatening: Allergic or allergic-like reaction (including oropharyngeal edema), arrhythmia, bronchospasm, consciousness altered, delusions, dyspnea, hallucinations, neuropsychiatric events (self-injury, confusion, delirium), nightmares, rash (including serious cutaneous reactions [eg, erythema multiforme, Stevens-Johnson syndrome, toxic epidermal necrolysis]), seizure, syncope

Drug Interactions
Metabolism/Transport Effects None known.
Avoid Concomitant Use There are no known interactions where it is recommended to avoid concomitant use.
Increased Effect/Toxicity There are no known significant interactions involving an increase in effect.
Decreased Effect
Zanamivir may decrease the levels/effects of: Influenza Virus Vaccine (Live/Attenuated)

Stability Store at 25°C (77°F); excursions permitted to 15°C to 30°C (59°F to 86°F). Do not puncture Rotadisk blister until taking a dose using the Diskhaler.

Mechanism of Action Zanamivir inhibits influenza virus neuraminidase enzymes, potentially altering virus particle aggregation and release.

Pharmacokinetics (Adult data unless noted)
Absorption: Systemic: 4% to 17%
Protein binding: <10%

Metabolism: None
Half-life: 2.5-5.1 hours; mild-to-moderate renal impairment: 4.7 hours; severe renal impairment: 18.5 hours
Time to peak serum concentration: 1-2 hours
Elimination: Urine (as unchanged drug); feces (unabsorbed drug)

Dosing: Usual Note: 10 mg dose is provided by 2 inhalations (one 5 mg blister per inhalation):
Pediatric:
Influenza virus A and B; treatment: Oral inhalation: Children ≥7 years and Adolescents: Two inhalations (10 mg) twice daily for 5 days; doses on first day should be separated by at least 2 hours; on subsequent days, doses should be spaced by ~12 hours. Begin within 2 days of signs or symptoms. Longer treatment may be considered for patients who remain severely ill after 5 days.
Influenza virus A and B; prophylaxis: Oral inhalation:
Manufacturer's labeling:
Household setting: Children ≥5 years and Adolescents: Two inhalations (10 mg) once daily for 10 days; begin within 36 hours following onset of signs or symptoms of index case
Community outbreak: Adolescents: Two inhalations (10 mg) once daily for 28 days; begin within 5 days of outbreak
Alternate dosing: Children ≥5 years and Adolescents:
Household setting: CDC Recommendation: Two inhalations (10 mg) once daily for 7 days after last known exposure (CDC, 2012)
Community outbreak: IDSA/PIDS recommendations: Two inhalations (10 mg) once daily; continue until influenza activity in community subsides or immunity obtained from immunization; up to 28 days has been well tolerated (Bradley, 2011; CDC, 2011)
Institutional outbreak: CDC recommendations: Two inhalations (10 mg) once daily; continue for ≥2 weeks and until ~7 days after identification of illness onset in the last patient. Zanamivir is to be used to control institutional outbreaks of influenza when circulating strains are suspected of being resistant to oseltamivir (CDC, 2012).
HIV-exposed/-positive: Two inhalations (10 mg) once daily for 10 days after last known exposure (DHHS [pediatric], 2013)
Adult: **Influenza virus A and B:**
Manufacturer's labeling: Oral inhalation:
Prophylaxis, household setting: Two inhalations (10 mg) once daily for 10 days. Begin within 36 hours following onset of signs or symptoms of index case.
Prophylaxis, community outbreak: Two inhalations (10 mg) once daily for 28 days. Begin within 5 days of outbreak.
Treatment: Two inhalations (10 mg total) twice daily for 5 days. Doses on first day should be separated by at least 2 hours; on subsequent days, doses should be spaced by ~12 hours. Begin within 2 days of signs or symptoms. Longer treatment may be considered for patients who remain severely ill after 5 days.
Alternate dosing: Oral inhalation:
Prophylaxis, household exposure: Two inhalations (10 mg) once daily for 7 days after last known exposure (CDC, 2012)
Prophylaxis, institutional outbreak: Two inhalations (10 mg) once daily; continue for ≥2 weeks and until ~7 days after identification of illness onset in the last patient. Zanamivir is to be used to control institutional outbreaks of influenza when circulating strains are suspected of being resistant to oseltamivir (CDC, 2012).
Prophylaxis, community outbreak (IDSA/PIDS, 2011): Two inhalations (10 mg) once daily; continue until influenza activity in community subsides or immunity

obtained from immunization; up to 28 days has been well tolerated (CDC, 2011)

Dosing adjustment in renal impairment: Children, Adolescents, and Adults: Adjustment not necessary following a 5-day course of treatment due to low systemic absorption; however, the potential for drug accumulation should be considered.

Administration Oral Inhalation: **Inhalation powder not for use via nebulizer:** Use a Diskhaler® delivery device (a special breath-activated plastic inhaler). The foil blister disk containing zanamivir inhalation powder should not be manipulated or solubilized. Load Relenza® Rotadisk® into the diskhaler; a blister that contains medication is pierced and the drug is dispersed into the air stream created when the patient inhales through the mouthpiece. Patients scheduled to take inhaled bronchodilators at the same time as zanamivir should be advised to use their bronchodilator before taking zanamivir.

Monitoring Parameters Monitor respiratory function, changes in behavior; if used for prophylaxis, signs/symptoms of influenza infection

Dosage Forms Excipient information presented when available (limited, particularly for generics); consult specific product labeling.
Aerosol Powder Breath Activated, Inhalation:
Relenza Diskhaler: 5 mg/blister (20 ea) [contains lactose]

References
American Academy of Pediatrics Committee on Infectious Diseases, "Antiviral Therapy and Prophylaxis for Influenza in Children," *Pediatrics*, 2007, 119(4):852-60.

Bradley JS, Byington CL, Shah SS, et al, "The Management of Community-Acquired Pneumonia in Infants and Children Older Than 3 Months of Age: Clinical Practice Guidelines by the Pediatric Infectious Diseases Society and the Infectious Diseases Society of America", *Clin Infect Dis*, 2011, 53(7):e25-76.

Centers for Disease Control and Prevention (CDC), "Antiviral Agents for the Treatment and Chemoprophylaxis of Influenza-Recommendations of the Advisory Committee on Immunization Practices (ACIP)," *MMWR Recomm Rep*, 2011, 60(1):1-24.

Centers for Disease Control and Prevention (CDC), "Influenza Antiviral Medications: Summary for Clinicians." Available at http://www.cdc.gov/flu/professionals/antivirals/summary-clinicians.htm. Last accessed: November 26, 2012.

DHHS. Guidelines for the prevention and treatment of opportunistic infections among HIV-exposed and HIV-infected children: recommendations from the National Institutes of Health, Centers for Disease Control and Prevention, the HIV Medicine Association of the Infectious Diseases Society of America, the Pediatric Infectious Diseases Society, and the American Academy of Pediatrics. November 6, 2013. Available at http://aidsinfo.nih.gov

Harper SA, Bradley JS, Englund JA, et al, "Seasonal Influenza in Adults and Children - Diagnosis, Treatment, Chemoprophylaxis, and Institutional Outbreak Management: Clinical Practice Guidelines of the Infectious Diseases Society of America," *Clin Infect Dis*, 2009, 48 (8):1003-32.

◆ **Zantac** see Ranitidine on page 1805

◆ **Zantac 75 [OTC]** see Ranitidine on page 1805

◆ **Zantac 75 (Can)** see Ranitidine on page 1805

◆ **Zantac 150 Maximum Strength [OTC]** see Ranitidine on page 1805

◆ **Zantac Maximum Strength Non-Prescription (Can)** see Ranitidine on page 1805

◆ **Zarontin** see Ethosuximide on page 809

◆ **Zarontin® (Can)** see Ethosuximide on page 809

◆ **Zaroxolyn** see Metolazone on page 1394

◆ **ZD9238** see Fulvestrant on page 946

◆ **ZDV** see Zidovudine on page 2168

◆ **ZDV, Abacavir, and Lamivudine** see Abacavir, Lamivudine, and Zidovudine on page 41

◆ **Zeasorb-AF [OTC]** see Miconazole (Topical) on page 1410

◆ **Zecuity** see SUMAtriptan on page 1958

◆ **Zegerid** see Omeprazole and Sodium Bicarbonate on page 1538

◆ **Zegerid OTC [OTC]** see Omeprazole and Sodium Bicarbonate on page 1538

◆ **Zeldox** see Ziprasidone on page 2178

◆ **Zemplar** see Paricalcitol on page 1606

◆ **Zemuron** see Rocuronium on page 1847

◆ **Zemuron® (Can)** see Rocuronium on page 1847

◆ **Zenatane** see ISOtretinoin on page 1161

◆ **Zenhale™ (Can)** see Mometasone and Formoterol on page 1436

◆ **Zenpep** see Pancrelipase on page 1591

◆ **Zenzedi** see Dextroamphetamine on page 629

◆ **Zephrex-D [OTC]** see Pseudoephedrine on page 1770

◆ **Zerit** see Stavudine on page 1932

◆ **Zerit® (Can)** see Stavudine on page 1932

◆ **Zestril** see Lisinopril on page 1262

◆ **Zetia** see Ezetimibe on page 827

◆ **Zetonna** see Ciclesonide (Nasal) on page 464

◆ **Ziagen** see Abacavir on page 36

◆ **Ziagen® (Can)** see Abacavir on page 36

◆ **Ziana®** see Clindamycin and Tretinoin on page 503

Zidovudine (zye DOE vyoo deen)

Medication Safety Issues
Sound-alike/look-alike issues:
Azidothymidine may be confused with azaTHIOprine, aztreonam
Retrovir® may be confused with acyclovir, ritonavir
Other safety concerns:
AZT is an error-prone abbreviation (mistaken as azathioprine, aztreonam)

Related Information
Adult and Adolescent HIV on page 2348
Pediatric HIV on page 2338
Perinatal HIV on page 2356
Safe Handling of Hazardous Drugs on page 2419
Brand Names: U.S. Retrovir
Brand Names: Canada Apo-Zidovudine®; AZT™; Novo-AZT; Retrovir®; Retrovir® (AZT™)
Therapeutic Category Antiretroviral Agent; HIV Agents (Anti-HIV Agents); Nucleoside Reverse Transcriptase Inhibitor (NRTI)
Generic Availability (U.S.) May be product dependent
Use Treatment of HIV infection in combination with other antiretroviral agents [Oral: FDA approved in ages ≥4 weeks and adults; Injection (short-term use): FDA approved in adults] (**Note:** HIV regimens consisting of three antiretroviral agents are strongly recommended); chemoprophylaxis to reduce perinatal HIV transmission [Oral, injection: FDA approved in ages 0 days to 6 weeks (postpartum therapy of HIV-1 exposed neonate) and adults (antepartum and intrapartum therapy of HIV-1 infected mother)]; has also been used as HIV postexposure prophylaxis (eg, chemoprophylaxis after occupational exposure to HIV)
Pregnancy Risk Factor C
Pregnancy Considerations Adverse events have been observed in some animal reproduction studies. Zidovudine has a high level of transfer across the human placenta and the placenta also metabolizes zidovudine to the active metabolite. No increased risk of overall birth defects has been observed following first trimester exposure according to data collected by the antiretroviral pregnancy registry. The pharmacokinetics of zidovudine are not significantly altered in pregnancy and dosing adjustment is not needed.

The DHHS Perinatal HIV Guidelines consider zidovudine in combination with lamivudine to be a preferred NRTI backbone for use in antiretroviral-naïve pregnant women. Zidovudine should be administered I.V. near delivery regardless of antepartum regimen or mode of delivery in women with HIV RNA >1000 copies/mL or unknown HIV RNA status.

Cases of lactic acidosis/hepatic steatosis syndrome related to mitochondrial toxicity have been reported in pregnant women with prolonged use of nucleoside analogues. It is not known if pregnancy itself potentiates this known side effect; however, women may be at increased risk of lactic acidosis and liver damage. In addition, these adverse events are similar to other rare but life-threatening syndromes which occur during pregnancy (eg HELLP syndrome). Hepatic enzymes and electrolytes should be monitored in women receiving nucleoside analogues and clinicians should watch for early signs of the syndrome. In addition, mitochondrial dysfunction may develop in infants following *in utero* exposure.

Regardless of CD4 count or HIV RNA copy number, all HIV-infected pregnant women should receive a combination antiretroviral (ARV) drug regimen. A combination of antepartum, intrapartum, and infant ARV prophylaxis is recommended. ARV therapy should be started as soon as possible in women with symptomatic infection. Although earlier initiation may be more effective in reducing the perinatal transmission of HIV, initiation may be delayed until after 12 weeks gestation in women who do not require immediate treatment after careful consideration of maternal conditions (eg, nausea and vomiting) and the potential risks of first trimester fetal exposure for specific agents. A scheduled cesarean delivery at 38 weeks gestation is recommended for all women with HIV RNA >1000 copies/mL or unknown concentrations near delivery in order to decrease transmission. If ARV therapy must be interrupted for <24 hours during the peripartum period, stop then restart all medications simultaneously in order to decrease the chance of developing resistance. Long-term follow-up is recommended for all infants exposed to ARV medications. In couples who want to conceive, the HIV-infected partner should attain maximum viral suppression prior to conception.

Health care providers are encouraged to enroll pregnant women exposed to antiretroviral medications in the Antiretroviral Pregnancy Registry (1-800-258-4263 or www.APRegistry.com). Health care providers caring for HIV-infected women and their infants may contact the National Perinatal HIV Hotline (888-448-8765) for clinical consultation (DHHS [perinatal], 2014).

Breast-Feeding Considerations Zidovudine is excreted into breast milk. Concentrations of zidovudine in breast milk are similar to those in the maternal serum. Maternal or infant antiretroviral therapy does not completely eliminate the risk of postnatal HIV transmission. In addition, multiclass-resistant virus has been detected in breast-feeding infants despite maternal therapy. Therefore, in the United States, where formula is accessible, affordable, safe, and sustainable, and the risk of infant mortality due to diarrhea and respiratory infections is low, complete avoidance of breast-feeding by HIV-infected women is recommended to decrease potential transmission of HIV (DHHS [perinatal], 2014).

Contraindications Life-threatening hypersensitivity to zidovudine or any component

Warnings Hazardous agent; use appropriate precautions for handling and disposal (NIOSH, 2012). Hematologic toxicity including neutropenia and severe anemia requiring transfusions may occur **[U.S. Boxed Warning]**; use with caution in patients with ANC <1000 cells/mm^3 or hemoglobin <9.5 g/dL; consider interruption of therapy for significant anemia (Hgb <7.5 g/dL or reduction >25% of baseline; neonates: Hgb <7 g/dL) or neutropenia (ANC <750 cells/mm^3 or reduction >50% from baseline; neonates ANC <500 cells/mm^3); use of erythropoietin or filgrastim may be necessary in some patients. Prolonged use of zidovudine may cause myositis and myopathy **[U.S. Boxed Warning]**.

Cases of lactic acidosis, severe hepatomegaly with steatosis, and death have been reported in patients receiving nucleoside analogues **[U.S. Boxed Warning]**; most of these cases have been in women; prolonged nucleoside use, obesity, and prior liver disease may be risk factors; use with extreme caution in patients with other risk factors for liver disease; discontinue therapy in patients who develop laboratory or clinical evidence of lactic acidosis or pronounced hepatotoxicity. Concomitant use of combination antiretroviral therapy with interferon alfa (with or without ribavirin) has resulted in hepatic decompensation (with some fatalities) in patients coinfected with HIV and HCV; monitor patients closely, especially for hepatic decompensation, neutropenia, and anemia; consider discontinuation of zidovudine if needed; consider dose reduction or discontinuation of interferon alfa, ribavirin, or both if clinical toxicities, including hepatic decompensation, worsen.

Syrup contains sodium benzoate; benzoic acid (benzoate) is a metabolite of benzyl alcohol; large amounts of benzyl alcohol (≥99 mg/kg/day) have been associated with a potentially fatal toxicity ("gasping syndrome") in neonates; the "gasping syndrome" consists of metabolic acidosis, respiratory distress, gasping respirations, CNS dysfunction (including convulsions, intracranial hemorrhage), hypotension and cardiovascular collapse; use syrup containing sodium benzoate with caution in neonates; *in vitro* and animal studies have shown that benzoate displaces bilirubin from protein binding sites.

Precautions Use with caution in patients with bone marrow compromise or in patients with impaired renal or hepatic function; reduce dosage or interrupt therapy in patients with anemia, granulocytopenia, or myopathy; reduce dosage in patients with severe renal or hepatic impairment. Fat redistribution and accumulation [ie, central obesity, peripheral wasting, facial wasting, breast enlargement, dorsocervical fat enlargement (buffalo hump), and cushingoid appearance] have been observed in patients receiving antiretroviral agents (causal relationship not established).

Immune reconstitution syndrome (an acute inflammatory response to residual or indolent opportunistic infections) may occur in HIV patients during initial treatment with combination antiretroviral agents; this syndrome may require further patient assessment and therapy. Autoimmune disorders (eg, Grave's disease, Guillain-Barré syndrome, and polymyositis) have been reported in patients experiencing immune reconstitution; time to onset is variable and may occur many months after antiretroviral treatment is initiated.

In perinatally HIV-exposed infants, the sensitivity of diagnostic virologic assays, particularly HIV RNA assays, may be affected by infant combination antiretroviral prophylactic therapy. Thus, a negative result of a diagnostic virologic assay should be repeated 2 to 4 weeks after cessation of neonatal combination antiretroviral prophylactic therapy (DHHS [pediatric], 2014).

Use of zidovudine with stavudine is not recommended due to antagonistic effects. Zidovudine should not be used concurrently with combination products that also contain zidovudine as a component (eg, Combivir or Trizivir).

Adverse Reactions

Cardiovascular: ECG abnormality (children), edema (children), heart failure (children), left ventricular dilation (children)

Central nervous system: Chills, fatigue, fever (children), headache, insomnia, irritability (children), malaise, nervousness (children)

Dermatologic: Rash (more common in children)

Gastrointestinal: Abdominal cramps, abdominal pain, anorexia, constipation (adults), diarrhea (children), dyspepsia, nausea (more common in adults), vomiting (more common in adults), weight loss (children)

Genitourinary: Hematuria (children)

Hematologic: Anemia (more common in neonates), granulocytopenia, macrocytosis (children), neutropenia (children), thrombocytopenia (children)

Hepatic: Hepatomegaly (children), transaminases increased

Neuromuscular & skeletal: Arthralgia, musculoskeletal pain, myalgia, neuropathy, weakness

Otic: Hearing loss

Respiratory: Cough (children)

Rare but important or life-threatening: Allergic reactions, amblyopia, anaphylaxis, angioedema, anxiety, aplastic anemia, back pain, body fat redistribution, cardiomyopathy, confusion, CPK increased, depression, diabetes, dizziness, dyslipidemias, dyspnea, gynecomastia, hearing loss, hemolytic anemia, hepatitis, hepatomegaly with steatosis, immune reconstitution syndrome, insulin resistance, jaundice, lactic acidosis, LDH increased, leukopenia, loss of mental acuity, lymphadenopathy, macular edema, mania, myopathy, myositis, oral mucosa pigmentation, pancreatitis, pancytopenia with marrow hypoplasia, paresthesia, photophobia, pruritus, pure red cell aplasia, rhabdomyolysis, seizure, skin/nail pigmentation changes (blue), Stevens-Johnson syndrome, syncope, taste perversion, toxic epidermal necrolysis, tremor, urticaria, vertigo

Drug Interactions

Metabolism/Transport Effects Substrate of CYP2A6 (minor), CYP2C19 (minor), CYP2C9 (minor), CYP3A4 (minor); **Note:** Assignment of Major/Minor substrate status based on clinically relevant drug interaction potential

Avoid Concomitant Use

Avoid concomitant use of Zidovudine with any of the following: CloZAPine; Dipyrone; Stavudine

Increased Effect/Toxicity

Zidovudine may increase the levels/effects of: CloZAPine; Ribavirin

The levels/effects of Zidovudine may be increased by: Acyclovir-Valacyclovir; Clarithromycin; Dipyrone; DOXOrubicin (Conventional); DOXOrubicin (Liposomal); Fluconazole; Ganciclovir-Valganciclovir; Interferons; Methadone; Probenecid; Raltegravir; Valproic Acid and Derivatives

Decreased Effect

Zidovudine may decrease the levels/effects of: Stavudine

The levels/effects of Zidovudine may be decreased by: Clarithromycin; DOXOrubicin (Conventional); DOXOrubicin (Liposomal); Protease Inhibitors; Rifamycin Derivatives

Stability

I.V.: Store intact vials at 15°C to 25°C (59°F to 77°F); protect from light. Diluted solution in D$_5$W to ≤4 mg/mL is physically and chemically stable for 24 hours at room temperature and 48 hours if refrigerated; to minimize the potential for microbial contamination, manufacturer recommends administering diluted I.V. solution within 8 hours if stored at room temperature and within 24 hours if refrigerated.

Oral: Tablets, capsules, syrup: Store at 15°C to 25°C (59°F to 77°F); protect capsules from moisture

Mechanism of Action Zidovudine is a thymidine analog which interferes with the HIV viral RNA-dependent DNA polymerase resulting in inhibition of viral replication; nucleoside reverse transcriptase inhibitor

Pharmacokinetics (Adult data unless noted) Note: In general, pharmacokinetic data for pediatric patients >3 months to 12 years of age are similar to data in adult patients.

Absorption: Oral: Well absorbed

Distribution: Significant penetration into the CSF

CSF/plasma ratio:

Infants 3 months to Children 12 years (n=38): Median: 0.68; range: 0.03 to 3.25

Adults (n=39): Median: 0.6; range: 0.04 to 2.62

V$_d$: 1.6 L/kg

Protein binding: 25% to 38%

Metabolism: Extensive first-pass effect; hepatic via glucuronidation to inactive metabolites

Bioavailability: Oral: Similar for tablets, capsules, and syrup

Neonates <14 days: 89%

Infants 14 days to 3 months: 61%

Infants 3 months to Children 12 years: 65%

Adults: 64% ± 10%

Half-life, terminal:

Premature neonate: 6.3 hours

Full-term neonates: 3.1 hours

Infants 14 days to 3 months: 1.9 hours

Infants 3 months to Children 12 years: 1.5 hours

Adults: 0.5 to 3 hours (mean: 1.1 hours)

Time to peak serum concentration: Within 30 to 90 minutes

Elimination: Urinary excretion (63% to 95%)

Oral: 72% to 74% of drug excreted in urine as metabolites and 14% to 18% as unchanged drug

I.V.: 45% to 60% excreted in urine as metabolites and 18% to 29% as unchanged drug

Dosing: Neonatal

HIV infection, treatment (DHHS [pediatric], 2014): Use in combination with other antiretroviral agents; standard neonatal doses may be excessive in premature neonates:

Oral:

GA <30 weeks: 2 mg/kg/dose every 12 hours; at 4 weeks of age, increase dose to 3 mg/kg/dose every 12 hours

GA ≥30 weeks and <35 weeks: 2 mg/kg/dose every 12 hours; at PNA 15 days, increase dose to 3 mg/kg/dose every 12 hours

GA ≥35 weeks: 4 mg/kg/dose every 12 hours

I.V.: **Use I.V. route only until oral therapy can be administered:**

GA <30 weeks: 1.5 mg/kg/dose every 12 hours; at 4 weeks of age, increase dose to 2.3 mg/kg/dose every 12 hours

GA ≥30 weeks and <35 weeks: 1.5 mg/kg/dose every 12 hours; at PNA 15 days, increase dose to 2.3 mg/kg/dose every 12 hours

GA ≥35 weeks: 3 mg/kg/dose every 12 hours

Perinatal transmission, prevention: Note: A 6-week course of zidovudine in the neonate is generally recommended for all HIV-exposed neonates to prevent perinatal transmission of HIV; a shorter 4-week course may be considered for neonates ≥35 weeks' gestation at birth if the mother received standard combination antiretroviral therapy during pregnancy, viral suppression was consistent, and maternal adherence is not a concern. In addition, the recommended regimen in the U.S. to prevent perinatal transmission of HIV also includes maternal antepartum oral zidovudine and maternal intrapartum I.V. zidovudine. Use of zidovudine in combination with nevirapine is recommended in the neonate in select situations (eg, infants born to HIV-infected mothers with no antepartum antiretroviral therapy prior to labor or during labor; or infants born to mothers with only intrapartum antiretroviral therapy) and may be considered in other situations (eg, infants born to mothers with suboptimal viral suppression at delivery; or infants born to mothers with known antiretroviral drug-resistant virus). **Note:** Zidovudine dosing should begin as soon as possible after birth (within 6 to 12 hours after delivery) and continue for the first 6 weeks of life. If neonate is diagnosed as HIV positive, discontinue prevention (prophylaxis) dosing and begin treatment regimen (see above). **Use I.V. route only until oral therapy can be administered** (DHHS [perinatal], 2014).

Premature neonates (DHHS [pediatric, perinatal], 2014): **Note:** Standard neonatal doses may be excessive in premature neonates.

Oral:

GA <30 weeks: 2 mg/kg/dose every 12 hours; at 4 weeks of age, increase dose to 3 mg/kg/dose every 12 hours

GA ≥30 weeks and <35 weeks: 2 mg/kg/dose every 12 hours; at PNA 15 days, increase dose to 3 mg/kg/dose every 12 hours

GA ≥35 weeks: 4 mg/kg/dose every 12 hours

I.V.: **Use I.V. route only until oral therapy can be administered**:

GA <30 weeks: 1.5 mg/kg/dose every 12 hours; at 4 weeks of age, increase dose to 2.3 mg/kg/dose every 12 hours

GA ≥30 weeks and <35 weeks: 1.5 mg/kg/dose every 12 hours; at PNA 15 days, increase dose to 2.3 mg/kg/dose every 12 hours

GA ≥35 weeks: 3 mg/kg/dose every 12 hours

Full-term neonates:

Oral:

Manufacturer's labeling: 2 mg/kg/dose every 6 hours

AIDS*info* recommendation: 4 mg/kg/dose every 12 hours (DHHS [pediatric, perinatal], 2014)

World Health Organization simplified dosing regimen: For use in low resource settings: **Note:** With the WHO regimen, neonates who weigh >3.75 kg at birth will receive a smaller zidovudine dose (compared with the mg/kg/dose method) and infants <3.75 kg will receive a larger zidovudine dose (WHO, 2010)

Birth weight ≤2.5 kg: 10 mg twice daily

Birth weight >2.5 kg: 15 mg twice daily

I.V.: **Use I.V. route only until oral therapy can be administered**:

Manufacturer's labeling: 1.5 mg/kg/dose every 6 hours

AIDS*info* recommendation: 3 mg/kg/dose every 12 hours (DHHS [pediatric, perinatal], 2014)

Dosage adjustment for hematologic toxicity: Consider interruption of therapy for significant anemia (Hgb <7.5 g/dL or >25% decrease from baseline; neonates: HgB <7 g/dL) and/or significant neutropenia (ANC <750 cells/mm^3 or >50% decrease from baseline; neonates ANC <500 cells/mm^3) until evidence of bone marrow recovery occurs; once bone marrow recovers, dose may be resumed using appropriate adjunctive therapy (eg, epoetin alfa)

Dosing: Usual

Pediatric:

HIV infection, treatment: Use in combination with other antiretroviral agents.

Infants 4 to <6 weeks and full-term at birth:

Oral:

Manufacturer's labeling: Patient weight 4 to <9 kg: 12 mg/kg/dose twice daily or 8 mg/kg/dose 3 times daily; **Note:** The 3-times-daily dosing is approved but rarely used in practice (DHHS [pediatric], 2014).

AIDS*info* recommendation: 4 mg/kg/dose every 12 hours (DHHS [pediatric], 2014)

I.V.: **Use I.V. route only until oral therapy can be administered**: 3 mg/kg/dose every 12 hours (DHHS [pediatric], 2014)

Infants ≥6 weeks, Children, and Adolescents: **Note:** Dosage may be calculated by body weight (in kg) or body surface area and should not exceed the recommended adult dose. Doses calculated by body weight may not be the same as those calculated by body surface area.

Oral: **Note:** The 3-times-daily dosing is approved but rarely used in practice (DHHS [pediatric], 2014).

BSA-directed dosing: 240 mg/m^2/dose every 12 hours (maximum single dose: 300 mg) or 160 mg/m^2/dose every 8 hours (maximum single dose: 200 mg)

Weight-directed dosing:

4 to <9 kg: 12 mg/kg/dose twice daily or 8 mg/kg/dose 3 times/day

≥9 to <30 kg: 9 mg/kg/dose twice daily or 6 mg/kg/dose 3 times/day

≥30 kg: 300 mg twice daily or 200 mg 3 times/day

I.V.: **Use I.V. route only until oral therapy can be administered**:

Infants >6 weeks and Children <12 years: 120 mg/m^2/dose every 6 hours or as a continuous I.V. infusion at 20 mg/m^2/hour (Briars, 2004)

Children ≥12 years and Adolescents: 1 mg/kg/dose every 4 hours

HIV postexposure prophylaxis: Children ≥12 years and Adolescents: Oral: 300 mg twice daily **or** 200 mg 3 times daily (with food) in combination with lamivudine or emtricitabine, with or without a protease inhibitor depending on risk; begin therapy within 2 hours of exposure if possible; continue for four weeks (CDC, 2005).

Perinatal transmission, prevention: Note: A 6-week course of zidovudine in the neonate is generally recommended for all HIV-exposed neonates to prevent perinatal transmission of HIV; a shorter 4-week course may be considered for infants ≥35 weeks' gestation at birth if the mother received standard combination antiretroviral therapy during pregnancy, viral suppression was consistent, and maternal adherence is not a concern. In addition, the recommended regimen in the U.S. to prevent perinatal transmission of HIV also includes maternal antepartum oral zidovudine and maternal intrapartum I.V. zidovudine. Use of zidovudine in combination with nevirapine is recommended in the neonate in select situations (eg, infants born to HIV-infected mothers with no antepartum antiretroviral therapy) prior to labor or during labor; or infants born to mothers with only intrapartum antiretroviral therapy) and may be considered in other situations (eg, infants born to mothers with suboptimal viral suppression at delivery; or infants born to mothers with known antiretroviral drug-resistant virus). **Note:** Zidovudine dosing should begin as soon as possible after birth (within 6 to 12 hours after delivery) and continue for the first 6 weeks of life. If neonate is diagnosed as HIV positive, discontinue prevention (prophylaxis) dosing and begin treatment regimen (see above). **Use I.V. route only until oral therapy can be administered** (DHHS [perinatal], 2014).

Infants <6 weeks and full-term at birth:

Oral:

Manufacturer's labeling: 2 mg/kg/dose every 6 hours

AIDS*info* recommendation: 4 mg/kg/dose every 12 hours (DHHS [perinatal], 2014)

I.V.: **Use I.V. route only until oral therapy can be administered:**
Manufacturer's labeling: 1.5 mg/kg/dose every 6 hours
AIDS*info* recommendation: 3 mg/kg/dose every 12 hours (DHHS [pediatric, perinatal], 2014)

Adult:

HIV infection, treatment:
Oral: 300 mg twice daily or 200 mg 3 times daily
I.V.: 1 mg/kg/dose administered every 4 hours around-the-clock (5 to 6 doses daily)

HIV postexposure prophylaxis: Oral: 300 mg twice daily **or** 200 mg 3 times daily (with food) in combination with lamivudine or emtricitabine. A third agent may be added for high risk exposures. Therapy should be started within 2 hours of exposure and continued for 4 weeks (CDC, 2005).

Perinatal transmission, prevention: Maternal dose: **Note:** Dose adjustment not required in pregnant women. Begin oral therapy with usual recommended doses based on current guidelines. Zidovudine should be administered by continuous I.V. infusion during labor and delivery regardless of antepartum regimen or mode of delivery in women with HIV RNA >1000 copies/mL or unknown HIV RNA status. If oral zidovudine was part of the antepartum regimen, discontinue during intrapartum I.V. infusion. Other antiretroviral agents should be continued orally. Zidovudine I.V. is not required in women receiving combination antiretroviral therapy who have HIV RNA ≤1000 copies/mL consistently in late pregnancy and/or near delivery and have no adherence or tolerance concerns (DHHS [perinatal], 2014).
During labor and delivery, administer zidovudine I.V.: 2 mg/kg as loading dose, followed by a continuous I.V. infusion of 1 mg/kg/hour until delivery. For scheduled cesarean delivery, begin I.V. zidovudine 3 hours before surgery.

Dosing adjustment in renal impairment:
Infants >6 weeks, Children, and Adolescents:
The following adjustments have been recommended (Aronoff, 2007): **Note:** Renally adjusted dose recommendations are based on oral doses of 160 mg/**m²**/dose every 8 hours and I.V. dose of 120 mg/**m²**/dose every 6 hours.
GFR ≥10 mL/minute/1.73 m²: No adjustment required
GFR <10 mL/minute/1.73 m²: Administer 50% of dose every 8 hours
Intermittent hemodialysis (IHD): Administer 50% of dose every 8 hours
Peritoneal dialysis (PD): Administer 50% of dose every 8 hours
Continuous renal replacement therapy (CRRT): No adjustment required

Adults:
End-stage renal disease patients (CrCl <15 mL/minute) maintained on hemodialysis or peritoneal dialysis:
Oral:
Manufacturer's labeling: 100 mg every 6 to 8 hours
AIDS*info* guidelines: 100 mg every 8 hours or 300 mg once daily (DHHS [adult], 2014)
I.V.: 1 mg/kg/dose every 6 to 8 hours
Continuous renal replacement therapy (CRRT): No adjustment needed (Aronoff, 2007)

Dosing adjustment in hepatic impairment: Specific recommendations currently unknown; dosage reduction may be required; use with caution; monitor for hematologic toxicities frequently.

Dosing adjustment for hematologic toxicity: Consider interruption of therapy for significant anemia (Hgb <7.5 g/dL or >25% decrease from baseline) and/or significant neutropenia (ANC <750 cells/mm³ or >50% decrease from baseline) until evidence of bone marrow recovery occurs; once bone marrow recovers, dose may

be resumed using appropriate adjunctive therapy (eg, epoetin alfa).

Administration Hazardous agent; use appropriate precautions for handling and disposal (NIOSH, 2012).
Oral: May be administered without regard to meals
Parenteral: Do not administer I.M.; do not administer I.V. push or by rapid infusion; infuse I.V. zidovudine over 1 hour at a final concentration not to exceed 4 mg/mL; I.V. dose may be infused over 30 minutes in neonates

Monitoring Parameters Note: Monitor CD4 percentage (if <5 years of age) or CD4 count (if ≥5 years of age) at least every 3 to 4 months (DHHS [pediatric], 2014)

Prior to initiation of therapy: Genotypic resistance testing, CD4 and viral load (every 3 to 4 months), CBC with differential, LFTs, BUN, creatinine, electrolytes, glucose, urinalysis (every 6 to 12 months), and assessment of readiness for adherence with medication regimen. At initiation and with any change in treatment regimen: CBC with differential, electrolytes, calcium, phosphate, glucose, LFTs, bilirubin, urinalysis (at initiation), BUN, creatinine, albumin, total protein, lipid panel (at initiation), CD4, and viral load. After 1 to 2 weeks of therapy: Signs of medication toxicity and adherence. After 2 to 4 weeks of therapy: CBC with differential, viral load, signs of medication toxicity and adherence; then every 3 to 4 months: CBC with differential, electrolytes, glucose, LFTs, bilirubin, BUN, creatinine, CD4, viral load, signs of medication toxicity, and adherence. Lipid panel and urinalysis every 6 to 12 months. CD4 monitoring frequency may be decreased to every 6 to 12 months in children who are adherent to therapy if the value is well above the threshold for opportunistic infections, viral suppression is sustained, and the clinical status is stable for more than 2 to 3 years (DHHS [pediatric], 2014). Monitor for growth and development, signs of HIV-specific physical conditions, HIV disease progression, opportunistic infections, hepatotoxicity, anemia, or lactic acidosis.

Additional Information Conversion from oral to I.V. dose: I.V. dose = ²/₃ of the oral dose. Zidovudine-associated reduction in Hgb may occur as early as 2 to 4 weeks after initiation of therapy; onset of neutropenia usually occurs after 6 to 8 weeks.

Dosage Forms Excipient information presented when available (limited, particularly for generics); consult specific product labeling.
Capsule, Oral:
Retrovir: 100 mg [contains soybean lecithin]
Generic: 100 mg
Solution, Intravenous [preservative free]:
Retrovir: 10 mg/mL (20 mL)
Syrup, Oral:
Retrovir: 50 mg/5 mL (240 mL) [contains sodium benzoate; strawberry flavor]
Generic: 50 mg/5 mL (240 mL)
Tablet, Oral:
Generic: 300 mg

References

Briars LA, Hilao JJ, and Kraus DM, "A Review of Pediatric Human Immunodeficiency Virus Infection," *Journal of Pharmacy Practice*, 2004, 17(6):407-31.
Center for Disease Prevention (CDC), "Updated U.S. Public Health Service Guidelines for the Management of Occupational Exposures to HIV and Recommendations for Postexposure Prophylaxis," *MMWR Recomm Rep*, 2005, 54(RR-9):1-17.
DHHS Panel on Antiretroviral Guidelines for Adults and Adolescents, "Guidelines for the Use of Antiretroviral Agents in HIV-Infected Adults and Adolescents," May 1, 2014. Available at http://www.aidsinfo.nih.gov
DHHS Panel on Antiretroviral Therapy and Medical Management of HIV-Infected Children, "Guidelines for the Use of Antiretroviral Agents in Pediatric HIV Infection," February 12, 2014. Available at http://aidsinfo.nih.gov
DHHS Panel on Treatment of HIV-Infected Pregnant Women and Prevention of Perinatal Transmission, "Recommendations for the Use of Antiretroviral Drugs in Pregnant HIV-1-Infected Women for

Maternal Health and Interventions to Reduce Perinatal HIV-1 Transmission in the United States," March 28, 2014. Available at http://aidsinfo.nih.gov

Mueller BU, Jacobsen F, Butler KM, et al, "Combination Treatment With Azidothymidine and Granulocyte Colony-Stimulating Factor in Children With Human Immunodeficiency Virus Infection," *J Pediatr*, 1992, 121(5 Pt 1):797-802.

National Institute for Occupational Safety and Health (NIOSH), "NIOSH List of Antineoplastic and Other Hazardous Drugs in Healthcare Settings 2012." Available at http://www.cdc.gov/niosh/docs/2012-150/pdfs/2012-150.pdf. Accessed January 21, 2013.

Volberding PA, Lagakos SW, Koch MA, et al, "Zidovudine in Asymptomatic Human Immunodeficiency Virus Infection. A Controlled Trial in Persons With Fewer Than 500 CD4-Positive Cells Per Cubic Millimeter. The AIDS Clinical Trials Group of the National Institute of Allergy and Infectious Diseases," *N Engl J Med*, 1990, 322(14):941-9.

World Health Organization, "Antiretroviral Drugs for Treating Pregnant Women and Preventing HIV Infection in Infants: Recommendations for a Public Health Approach," 2010. Available at http://www.who.int/hiv/pub/mtct/antiretroviral2010/en/index.html

◆ **Zidovudine, Abacavir, and Lamivudine** see Abacavir, Lamivudine, and Zidovudine on page 41

◆ **Zidovudine and Lamivudine** see Lamivudine and Zidovudine on page 1198

◆ **Zilactin [OTC]** see Benzyl Alcohol on page 278

◆ **Zilactin-B® (Can)** see Benzocaine on page 273

◆ **Zilactin Baby [OTC]** see Benzocaine on page 273

◆ **Zilactin Baby® (Can)** see Benzocaine on page 273

Zileuton (zye LOO ton)

Related Information
Oral Medications That Should Not Be Crushed or Altered on page 2438

Brand Names: U.S. Zyflo; Zyflo CR

Therapeutic Category 5-Lipoxygenase Inhibitor

Generic Availability (U.S.) No

Use For prophylaxis and chronic treatment of asthma (FDA approved in ages ≥12 years and adults); **NOT** indicated for the relief of acute bronchospasm; therapy may continue during asthma exacerbations

Pregnancy Risk Factor C

Pregnancy Considerations Adverse events were observed in animal reproduction studies. If a leukotriene modifier is needed during pregnancy, other agents are preferred (ACOG, 2008).

Breast-Feeding Considerations It is not known if zileuton is excreted into breast milk. Due to the potential tumorigenicity of zileuton in animal studies, the manufacturer does not recommend breast-feeding.

Contraindications Hypersensitivity to zileuton or any component, active liver disease, or transaminase elevations ≥3 times ULN

Warnings Zileuton is not appropriate or indicated for the reversal of bronchospasm in acute asthma attacks, including status asthmaticus; therapy may be continued during acute asthma exacerbations. Increased serum transaminase levels and bilirubin have been reported (incidence: 3.2%); females >65 years of age and patients with preexisting elevated transaminases may be at greater risk. Serum ALT test is the most sensitive indicator of zileuton-associated liver injury; hepatic changes may resolve with continued treatment (usually within 3 weeks), remain unchanged, or progress to clinically significant injury. Monitor hepatic function at initiation and monthly during first 3 months of therapy, then every 2-3 months for the remainder of first year of therapy, and then periodically thereafter. Discontinue therapy and follow transaminases until normal if signs or symptoms of hepatic dysfunction present (eg, right upper quadrant pain, nausea, fatigue, lethargy, pruritus, jaundice, or "flu-like" symptoms) or serum transaminases ≥5 times ULN. Due to the risk of hepatotoxicity, the manufacturer does not recommend use

of zileuton in children <12 years of age. Zileuton increases serum theophylline concentrations (approximately doubled); consider theophylline dosage adjustment and monitor levels closely. Concomitant administration with warfarin may result in increased prothrombin times; monitor prothrombin times and adjust warfarin dose accordingly. Concomitant administration with propranolol may result in increased propranolol AUC (approximately doubled); monitor patients closely, propranolol dosage adjustment may be necessary.

Precautions Use caution in females >65 years of age, patients with history of liver disease, and/or in those patients who consume substantial quantities of ethanol. Postmarketing reports of behavioral changes (eg, agitation, aggression, depression, insomnia, tremor) and sleep disorders have been noted; patients should be monitored accordingly and instructed to notify prescriber if neuropsychiatric changes occur.

Adverse Reactions
Cardiovascular: Chest pain

Central nervous system: Dizziness, fever, headache, insomnia, malaise, nervousness, pain, somnolence

Dermatologic: Pruritus, rash

Gastrointestinal: Abdominal pain, constipation, diarrhea, dyspepsia, flatulence, nausea, vomiting

Genitourinary: Urinary tract infection, vaginitis

Hematologic: Leukopenia

Hepatic: ALT increased, hepatotoxicity

Neuromuscular & skeletal: Arthralgia, hypertonia, myalgia, neck pain/rigidity

Ocular: Conjunctivitis

Respiratory: Pharyngolaryngeal pain, sinusitis, upper respiratory tract infection

Miscellaneous: Hypersensitivity reactions, lymphadenopathy

Rare but important or life-threatening: Behavior/mood changes, hepatitis, hyperbilirubinemia, jaundice, liver failure, suicidality, suicide

Drug Interactions
Metabolism/Transport Effects Substrate of CYP1A2 (minor), CYP2C9 (minor), CYP3A4 (minor); **Note:** Assignment of Major/Minor substrate status based on clinically relevant drug interaction potential; **Inhibits** CYP1A2 (weak)

Avoid Concomitant Use
Avoid concomitant use of Zileuton with any of the following: Pimozide

Increased Effect/Toxicity
Zileuton may increase the levels/effects of: Pimozide; Propranolol; Theophylline; Warfarin

Decreased Effect There are no known significant interactions involving a decrease in effect.

Food Interactions Zyflo CR®: Improved absorption when administered with food. Management: Administer with food.

Stability Store tablets at 20°C to 25°C (68°F to 77°F). Protect from light.

Mechanism of Action Specific 5-lipoxygenase inhibitor which inhibits leukotriene formation. Leukotrienes augment neutrophil and eosinophil migration, neutrophil and monocyte aggregation, leukocyte adhesion, increased capillary permeability, and smooth muscle contraction (which contribute to inflammation, edema, mucous secretion, and bronchoconstriction in the airway of the asthmatic.)

Pharmacokinetics (Adult data unless noted)
Absorption: Well-absorbed

Distribution: 1.2 L/kg

Protein binding: 93%, primarily albumin

Metabolism: Hepatic and gastrointestinal; zileuton and N-dehydroxylated metabolite can be metabolized by CYP1A2, 2C9, and 3A4

Half-life, elimination: ~3 hours

Time to peak serum concentration: Immediate release: 1.7 hours

Elimination: Urine (~95% primarily as metabolites); feces (~2%)

Dialysis: <0.5% removed by hemodialysis

Dosing: Usual Oral: Children, Adolescents ≥12 years, and Adults:

Immediate release: 600 mg 4 times/day

Extended release: 1200 mg twice daily

Dosing adjustment in renal impairment: No dosage adjustment necessary in renal impairment or with hemodialysis.

Dosing adjustment in hepatic impairment: Contraindicated with hepatic impairment.

Administration Extended release: Do not crush, cut, or chew tablet; administer within 1 hour after morning and evening meals.

Monitoring Parameters Hepatic transaminases (prior to initiation and during therapy), specifically monitor serum ALT (prior to initiation, once a month for the first 3 months, every 2-3 months for the remainder of the first year, and periodically thereafter for patients receiving long-term therapy). Monitor vital signs and lung sounds prior to and periodically during therapy.

Dosage Forms Excipient information presented when available (limited, particularly for generics); consult specific product labeling.

Tablet, Oral:

Zyflo: 600 mg [scored]

Tablet Extended Release 12 Hour, Oral:

Zyflo CR: 600 mg

References

ACOG Committee on Practice Bulletins-Obstetrics, "ACOG Practice Bulletin: Clinical Management Guidelines for Obstetrician-Gynecologists Number 90, February 2008: Asthma in Pregnancy," *Obstet Gynecol*, 2008, 111(2 Pt 1):457-64.

The American College of Obstetricians and Gynecologists (ACOG) and The American College of Allergy, Asthma and Immunology (ACAAI), "The Use of Newer Asthma and Allergy Medications During Pregnancy," *Ann Allergy Asthma Immunol*, 2000, 84(5):475-80

◆ **Zinacef** see Cefuroxime on page 422

◆ **Zinacef in Sterile Water** see Cefuroxime on page 422

◆ **Zinc** see Trace Elements on page 2059

◆ **Zinc 15 [OTC]** see Zinc Sulfate on page 2176

◆ **Zinc-220 [OTC]** see Zinc Sulfate on page 2176

Zinc Acetate (zink AS e tate)

Brand Names: U.S. Galzin

Therapeutic Category Trace Element

Generic Availability (U.S.) No

Use Maintenance treatment of Wilson's disease following initial chelation therapy (FDA approved in ages ≥10 years and adults)

Pregnancy Risk Factor A

Pregnancy Considerations The risk of fetal harm appears remote with use of zinc acetate during pregnancy. An increased risk of fetal abnormalities has not been observed in pregnant women receiving zinc acetate (regardless of trimester).

Breast-Feeding Considerations Women receiving zinc therapy should avoid nursing due to risks for zinc-induced copper deficiency in nursing infants.

Contraindications Hypersensitivity to zinc salts or any component

Precautions Not recommended for initial treatment of Wilson's disease in symptomatic patients; effects on copper are not immediate. May be used as maintenance therapy after patient has been stabilized on initial chelation therapy. Neurological deterioration may occur with initial therapy as copper stores are mobilized. Hepatic copper

levels should not be used to manage therapy as they do not differentiate between potentially toxic free copper and safely bound copper. May cause gastric irritation/upset, particularly with morning dose. Use with caution in hepatic or renal impairment; use has not been studied.

Adverse Reactions

Central nervous system: Neurologic deterioration (uncommon)

Endocrine & metabolic: Amylase increased, lipase increased

Gastrointestinal: Gastric irritation

Hepatic: Alkaline phosphatase increased, hepatic function decreased (rare)

Drug Interactions

Metabolism/Transport Effects None known.

Avoid Concomitant Use There are no known interactions where it is recommended to avoid concomitant use.

Increased Effect/Toxicity There are no known significant interactions involving an increase in effect.

Decreased Effect

Zinc Acetate may decrease the levels/effects of: Ceftibuten; Cephalexin; Deferiprone; Dolutegravir; Eltrombopag; Quinolone Antibiotics; Tetracycline Derivatives; Trientine

The levels/effects of Zinc Acetate may be decreased by: Trientine

Food Interactions Food and beverages other than water may interfere with zinc absorption. Management: Administer on empty stomach at least 1 hour before or 2-3 hours after meals and 1 hour away from beverages other than water. Can give 1 hour after breakfast if GI irritation occurs.

Stability Store at 25°C (77°F); excursions permitted to 15°C to 30°C (59°F to 86°F); protect from light.

Mechanism of Action Zinc induces production of the copper binding protein metallothionein in enterocytes. Copper binding within enterocytes results in an impairment of the intestinal absorption of dietary copper and reabsorption of endogenously secreted copper in saliva, bile, gastric acid. Following enterocyte desquamation, bound copper is eliminated in the feces.

Pharmacodynamics

Onset of action: Slow

Duration of action: Inhibition of copper uptake: ~11 days following cessation of therapy (Anderson, 1998)

Pharmacokinetics (Adult data unless noted)

Absorption: pH dependent (enhanced at pH ≤3); impaired by food (Anderson, 1998)

Elimination: Primarily in feces

Dosing: Usual Note: Dose expressed in mg **elemental** zinc

Children and Adolescents: **Wilson's disease:** Oral:

Manufacturer labeling: Children ≥10 years and Adolescents: 25 mg 3 times daily; may increase to 50 mg 3 times daily if inadequate response to lower dose

AASLD recommendations (Roberts, 2008): Note: Three times daily dosing recommended; doses must be administered at least twice daily to be effective:

Children >5 years and <50 kg: Limited data available: 25 mg 3 times daily

Children >50 kg and Adolescents: 50 mg 3 times daily

Adults: **Wilson's disease:** Oral:

Males and nonpregnant females: 50 mg 3 times daily

Pregnant females: 25 mg 3 times daily; may increase to 50 mg 3 times daily if inadequate response to lower dose

Administration Administer on empty stomach at least 1 hour before or 2-3 hours after meals, and 1 hour away from beverages other than water. Gastric irritation most commonly associated with morning dose; may administer 1 hour after breakfast if gastric irritation occurs. Swallow capsule whole; do not chew or open.

Monitoring Parameters Serum non-ceruloplasmin bound copper, 24-hour urinary copper excretion, 24-hour urinary zinc levels, LFTs, iron and/or other trace minerals, neurologic evaluation including speech, periodic ophthalmic exam

Reference Range Target ranges for patients with Wilson's disease on zinc acetate therapy:

24-hour urinary copper excretion: ≤75 mcg/24 hours (patients on chelation therapy will have increased urinary copper due to chelated copper)

Non-ceruloplasmin plasma copper (free copper): <20 mcg/dL

Dosage Forms Considerations

Strength of Galzin capsule is expressed as elemental zinc

Dosage Forms Excipient information presented when available (limited, particularly for generics); consult specific product labeling.

Capsule, Oral:

Galzin: 25 mg, 50 mg

References

Anderson LA, Hakojarvi SL, and Boudreaux SK, "Zinc Acetate Treatment in Wilson's Disease," *Ann Pharmacother*, 1998, 32(1):78-87.

Roberts EA and Schilsky ML, "Diagnosis and Treatment of Wilson Disease: An Update. American Association for Study of Liver Diseases (AASLD)," *Hepatology*, 2008, 47(6):2089-111.

Zinc Chloride (zink KLOR ide)

Therapeutic Category Trace Element

Generic Availability (U.S.) Yes

Use Prevention of zinc deficiency as an additive to parenteral nutrition (FDA approved in all ages)

Pregnancy Risk Factor C

Pregnancy Considerations Zinc crosses the placenta and can be measured in the cord blood and placenta. Fetal concentrations are regulated by the placenta (de Moraes, 2011).

Breast-Feeding Considerations

Zinc is found in breast milk; concentrations decrease over the first 6 months of lactation. Concentrations are generally not affected by dietary supplementation (IOM, 2000)

Contraindications Hypersensitivity to zinc salts or any component; peripheral undiluted administration

Warnings Do not administer undiluted by direct injection into a peripheral vein due to potential for phlebitis, tissue irritation, and potential increased renal loss of minerals from a bolus injection.

Precautions Administration of zinc in absence of copper may decrease plasma copper levels. The parenteral product contains aluminum; toxic aluminum concentrations may be seen with high doses, prolonged use, or renal dysfunction. Premature neonates are at higher risk due to immature renal function and aluminum intake from other parenteral sources. Parenteral aluminum exposure of >4-5 mcg/kg/day is associated with CNS and bone toxicity and tissue loading may occur at lower doses.

Adverse Reactions Rare but important or life-threatening: Hypotension, indigestion, jaundice, leukopenia, nausea, neutropenia, pulmonary edema, vomiting

Drug Interactions

Metabolism/Transport Effects None known.

Avoid Concomitant Use There are no known interactions where it is recommended to avoid concomitant use.

Increased Effect/Toxicity There are no known significant interactions involving an increase in effect.

Decreased Effect

Zinc Chloride may decrease the levels/effects of: Dolutegravir; Eltrombopag; Trientine

The levels/effects of Zinc Chloride may be decreased by: Trientine

Stability Store intact vial at 20°C to 25°C (68°F to 77°F).

Pharmacokinetics (Adult data unless noted)

Distribution: Storage sites are liver and skeletal muscle; serum levels do not adequately reflect whole-body zinc status

Protein binding: 55% bound to albumin; 40% bound to alpha 1-macroglobulin

Elimination: Primarily in feces (Anderson, 1998)

Dosing: Neonatal Parenteral nutrition, maintenance requirement: I.V.: **Note:** Dosage expressed in terms of **elemental** zinc:

ASPEN recommendations:

Premature neonates <3 kg: 400 mcg/kg/day (Mirtallo, 2004); higher doses have been suggested in premature neonates: 450-500 mcg/kg/day (Vanek, 2012)

Term neonates ≥3 kg: 50-250 mcg/kg/day (Mirtallo, 2004; Vanek, 2012)

Manufacturer's labeling:

Premature neonates <3 kg: 300 mcg/kg/day

Term neonates ≥3 kg: 100 mcg/kg/day

Dosing: Usual Note: Dosages may be presented in units of mcg or mg, use caution to ensure correct units. Clinical response may not occur for up to 6-8 weeks:

Infants, Children, and Adolescents: **Parenteral nutrition, maintenance requirement:** I.V.: **Note:** Dosage expressed in terms of **elemental** zinc; higher doses may be needed if impaired intestinal absorption or an excessive loss of zinc (eg, excessive, prolonged diarrhea, high-output intestinal fistula, burns)

ASPEN recommendations:

Age-directed dosing (Vanek, 2012):

Infants <3 months: 250 mcg/kg/day

Infants ≥3 months: 50 mcg/kg/day

Children: 50 mcg/kg/day; maximum daily dose: 5000 mcg/**day**

Weight-directed dosing (Mirtallo, 2004):

Infants <10 kg: 50-250 mcg/kg/day

Children 10-40 kg: 50-125 mcg/kg/day; maximum daily dose: 5000 mcg/**day**

Adolescents >40 kg: 2-5 mg/day

Manufacturer labeling: Infants >3 kg and Children ≤5 years: 100 mcg/kg/day

Adults: **Parenteral nutrition, maintenance requirement:** I.V.: **Note:** Dosage expressed in terms of **elemental** zinc:

Acute metabolic states: 4.5-6 mg/day

Metabolically stable: 2.5-4 mg/day

Replacement for small bowel fluid loss (metabolically stable): An additional 12.2 mg zinc/L of fluid lost or an additional 17.1 mg zinc per kg of stool or ileostomy output

Administration Dilute as component of daily parenteral nutrition or maintenance fluids; must be diluted in ≥100 mL; do not give undiluted by direct injection into a peripheral vein due to potential for phlebitis and tissue irritation and potential to increase renal losses of minerals from a bolus injection

Monitoring Parameters Patients on parenteral nutrition should have periodic serum copper and serum zinc levels; alkaline phosphatase, taste acuity, mental depression

Dosage Forms Considerations

Strength of zinc chloride injection is expressed as elemental zinc

Dosage Forms Excipient information presented when available (limited, particularly for generics); consult specific product labeling.

Solution, Intravenous:

Generic: 1 mg/mL (10 mL)

References

American Academy of Pediatrics Committee on Nutrition, "Zinc," *Pediatrics*, 1978, 62(3):408-12.

Anderson LA, Hakojarvi SL, and Boudreaux SK, "Zinc Acetate Treatment in Wilson's Disease," *Ann Pharmacother*, 1998, 32(1):78-87.

de Moraes ML, de Faria Barbosa R, Santo RE, et al, "Maternal-Fetal Distribution of Calcium, Iron, Copper, and Zinc in Pregnant Teenagers and Adults," *Biol Trace Elem Res*, 2011, 139(2):126-36.

◄ Department Health & Human Services, Food Drug Administration, "Aluminum in Large and Small Volume Parenterals Used in Total Parenteral Nutrition," *Federal Register*, 2000, 65(17):4103-11.

IOM (Institute of Medicine), *Dietary Reference Intakes for Vitamin A, Vitamin K, Arsenic, Boron, Chromium, Copper, Iodine, Iron, Manganese, Molybdenum, Nickel, Silicon, Vanadium, and Zinc*, Washington, DC: National Academy Press, 2000.

Mirtallo J, Canada T, Johnson D, et al, "Safe Practices for Parenteral Nutrition," *JPEN J Parenter Enteral Nutr*, 2004, 28(6):S39-70.

Vanek VW, Borum P, Buchman A, et al, "A.S.P.E.N. Position Paper: Recommendations for Changes in Commercially Available Parenteral Multivitamin and Multi-trace Element Products," *Nutr Clin Pract*, 2012, 27(4):440-91.

◆ **Zincofax® (Can)** *see* Zinc Oxide *on page 2176*

Zinc Oxide (zink OKS ide)

Brand Names: U.S. Ammens® Original Medicated [OTC]; Ammens® Shower Fresh [OTC]; Balmex® [OTC]; Boudreaux's® Butt Paste [OTC]; Critic-Aid Skin Care® [OTC]; Desitin® Creamy [OTC]; Desitin® [OTC]

Brand Names: Canada Zincofax®

Therapeutic Category Topical Skin Product

Generic Availability (U.S.) Yes: Ointment

Use Protective coating for mild skin irritations and abrasions; soothing and protective ointment to promote healing of chapped skin, diaper rash

Pregnancy Considerations Zinc oxide is not expected to be absorbed systemically following topical administration to healthy skin (Newman, 2009). Systemic absorption would be required in order for zinc oxide to cross the placenta and reach the fetus.

Contraindications Hypersensitivity to zinc oxide or any component

Adverse Reactions Local: Irritation, skin sensitivity

Drug Interactions

Metabolism/Transport Effects None known.

Avoid Concomitant Use There are no known interactions where it is recommended to avoid concomitant use.

Increased Effect/Toxicity There are no known significant interactions involving an increase in effect.

Decreased Effect There are no known significant interactions involving a decrease in effect.

Stability Avoid prolonged storage at temperatures >30°C

Mechanism of Action Mild astringent with weak antiseptic properties

Dosing: Neonatal Topical: Apply several times daily to affected area

Dosing: Usual Infants, Children, and Adults: Topical: Apply several times daily to affected area

Administration Topical: For external use only; do not use in the eyes

Dosage Forms Excipient information presented when available (limited, particularly for generics); consult specific product labeling.

Cream, topical:
Balmex®: 11.3% (60 g, 120 g, 480 g) [contains aloe, benzoic acid, soybean oil, and vitamin E]

Cream, topical [stick]:
Balmex®: 11.3% (56 g) [contains aloe, benzoic acid, soybean oil, and vitamin E]

Ointment, topical: 20% (30 g, 60 g, 454 g); 40% (120 g)
Desitin®: 40% (30 g, 60 g, 90 g, 120 g, 270 g, 480 g) [contains cod liver oil and lanolin]
Desitin® Creamy: 10% (60 g, 120 g)

Paste, topical:
Boudreaux's® Butt Paste: 16% (30 g, 60 g, 120 g, 480 g) [contains castor oil, boric acid, mineral oil, and Peruvian balsam]
Critic-Aid Skin Care®: 20% (71 g, 170 g)

Powder, topical:
Ammens® Original Medicated: 9.1% (312 g)
Ammens® Shower Fresh: 9.1% (312 g)

References
Adam R, "Skin Care of the Diaper Area," *Pediatr Dermatol*, 2008, 25 (4):427-33.

Newman MD, Stotland M, and Ellis JI, "The Safety of Nanosized Particles in Titanium Dioxide- and Zinc Oxide-Based Sunscreens," *J Am Acad Dermatol*, 2009, 61(4):685-92.

Visscher MO, "Update on the Use of Topical Agents in Neonates," *Newborn & Infant Nursing Reviews*, 2009, 9(1):33362-80.

Zinc Sulfate (zink SUL fate)

Medication Safety Issues
Sound-alike/look-alike issues:
ZnSO$_4$ is an error-prone abbreviation (mistaken as morphine sulfate)

Brand Names: U.S. Eye-Sed [OTC]; Orazinc [OTC]; Zinc 15 [OTC]; Zinc-220 [OTC]

Brand Names: Canada Anuzinc; Rivasol

Therapeutic Category Mineral, Oral; Mineral, Parenteral; Trace Element

Generic Availability (U.S.) Yes

Use
Oral: Dietary supplementation of zinc (OTC: FDA approved in adults); has also been used to help reduce the duration and severity of diarrhea in malnourished patients

Parenteral: Prevention of zinc deficiency as an additive to parenteral nutrition (FDA approved in all ages)

Pregnancy Risk Factor C

Pregnancy Considerations Zinc crosses the placenta and can be measured in the cord blood and placenta. Fetal concentrations are regulated by the placenta (de Moraes, 2011).

Breast-Feeding Considerations Zinc is found in breast milk; concentrations decrease over the first 6 months of lactation. Concentrations are generally not affected by dietary supplementation (IOM, 2000).

Contraindications Hypersensitivity to zinc salts or any component

Parenteral: Peripheral I.V. undiluted administration

Warnings Do not administer undiluted by direct injection into a peripheral vein due to potential for phlebitis, tissue irritation, and potential increased renal loss of minerals from a bolus injection; excessive intake in healthy persons may be deleterious as decreases in HDL (high-density lipoproteins) and impairment of immune system function have been reported

Precautions Administration of zinc in absence of copper may decrease plasma copper levels. The parenteral product contains aluminum; toxic aluminum concentrations may be seen with high doses, prolonged use, or renal dysfunction. Premature neonates are at higher risk due to immature renal function and aluminum intake from other parenteral sources. Parenteral aluminum exposure of >4-5 mcg/kg/day is associated with CNS and bone toxicity and tissue loading may occur at lower doses.

Adverse Reactions
Central nervous system: Dizziness, headache
Gastrointestinal: Abdominal cramps, diarrhea, nausea, vomiting

Drug Interactions

Metabolism/Transport Effects None known.

Avoid Concomitant Use There are no known interactions where it is recommended to avoid concomitant use.

Increased Effect/Toxicity There are no known significant interactions involving an increase in effect.

Decreased Effect
Zinc Sulfate may decrease the levels/effects of: Ceftibuten; Cephalexin; Deferiprone; Dolutegravir; Eltrombopag; Quinolone Antibiotics; Tetracycline Derivatives; Trientine

The levels/effects of Zinc Sulfate may be decreased by:
Trientine

Food Interactions Avoid foods high in calcium or phosphorus.

Stability
Oral:
Capsule: Store at 15°C to 30°C (59°F to 86°F).
Tablet (Orazinc®): Store at 13°C to 24°C (55°F to 76°F).
Parenteral: Store intact vial at 20°C to 25°C (68°F to 77°F); excursions permitted to 15°C to 30°C (59°F to 86°F).

Pharmacokinetics (Adult data unless noted)
Absorption: pH-dependent; enhanced at lower pH; (pH <3); impaired by food (Anderson, 1998)
Distribution: Storage sites are liver and skeletal muscle; serum levels do not adequately reflect whole-body zinc status
Protein binding: 55% bound to albumin; 40% bound to alpha 1-macroglobulin
Elimination: Primarily in feces (Anderson, 1998)

Dosing: Neonatal Note: Clinical response may not occur for up to 6-8 weeks.
Adequate intake (AI): Oral: 2 mg **elemental** zinc/day
Parenteral nutrition, maintenance requirement: I.V.:
Note: Dosage expressed in terms of **elemental** zinc:
ASPEN recommendations:
Premature neonates <3 kg: 400 mcg/kg/day (Mirtallo, 2004); higher doses have been suggested in premature neonates: 450-500 mcg/kg/day (Vanek, 2012)
Term neonates ≥3 kg: 50-250 mcg/kg/day (Mirtallo, 2004; Vanek, 2012)
Manufacturer's labeling:
Premature neonates <3 kg: 300 mcg/kg/day
Term neonates ≥3 kg: 100 mcg/kg/day

Dosing: Usual Note: Dosages may be presented in units of mcg or mg; use caution to ensure correct units. Clinical response may not occur for up to 6-8 weeks:
Infants, Children, and Adolescents:
Adequate intake (AI): Oral: Infants 1-6 months: 2 mg **elemental** zinc/day
Recommended daily allowance (RDA): Oral:
Infants 7-12 months and Children 1-3 years: 3 mg **elemental** zinc/day
Children 4-8 years: 5 mg **elemental** zinc/day
Children and Adolescents 9-13 years: 8 mg **elemental** zinc/day
Adolescents 14-18 years:
Female: 9 mg **elemental** zinc/day
Male: 11 mg **elemental** zinc/day
Zinc deficiency, treatment: Oral:
Infants and Children: 0.5-1 mg **elemental** zinc/kg/day in divided doses 1-3 times daily; higher doses may be needed if impaired intestinal absorption or an excessive loss of zinc (eg, excessive, prolonged diarrhea, high-output intestinal fistula, burns)
Adolescents: 25-50 mg **elemental** zinc (110-220 mg zinc sulfate) 3 times daily; higher doses may be needed if impaired intestinal absorption or an excessive loss of zinc (eg, excessive, prolonged diarrhea, high-output intestinal fistula, burns)
Parenteral nutrition, maintenance requirement: I.V.:
Note: Dosage expressed in terms of **elemental** zinc; higher doses may be needed if impaired intestinal absorption or an excessive loss of zinc (eg, excessive, prolonged diarrhea, high-output intestinal fistula, burns)
ASPEN recommendations:
Age-directed dosing (Vanek, 2012):
Infants <3 months: 250 mcg/kg/day
Infants ≥3 months: 50 mcg/kg/day
Children: 50 mcg/kg/day; maximum daily dose: 5000 mcg/**day**
Weight-directed dosing (Mirtallo, 2004):
Infants <10 kg: 50-250 mcg/kg/day

Children 10-40 kg: 50-125 mcg/kg/day; maximum daily dose: 5000 mcg/**day**
Adolescents >40 kg: 2-5 mg/day
Manufacturer labeling: Infants >3 kg and Children ≤5 years: 100 mcg/kg/day; maximum daily dose: 5000 mcg/**day**

Diarrhea, treatment; malnourished patient (WHO/UNICEF, 2004): Oral: **Note:** Dosage expressed in terms of **elemental** zinc; **Note:** Zinc should be started in conjunction with oral rehydration solutions at first sign of diarrhea:
Infants <6 months: 10 mg once daily for 10-14 days
Infants >6 months and Children: 20 mg once daily for 10-14 days
Adults:
Recommended daily allowance (RDA): Oral:
Female: 8 mg **elemental** zinc/day
Male: 11 mg **elemental** zinc/day
Zinc deficiency, treatment: Oral: 25-50 mg **elemental** zinc/dose (110-220 mg zinc sulfate) 3 times daily
Parenteral nutrition, maintenance requirement: I.V.:
Note: Dosage expressed in terms of **elemental** zinc:
Acute metabolic states: 4.5-6 mg/day
Metabolically stable: 2.5-4 mg/day
Replacement for small bowel fluid loss (metabolically stable): An additional 12.2 mg zinc/L of fluid lost, or an additional 17.1 mg zinc per kg of stool or ileostomy output

Administration
Oral: Administer with food if GI upset occurs
Parenteral: Dilute as component of daily parenteral nutrition or maintenance fluids; do not give undiluted by direct injection into a peripheral vein due to potential for phlebitis and tissue irritation and potential to increase renal losses of minerals from a bolus injection

Monitoring Parameters Patients on parenteral nutrition or chronic therapy should have periodic serum copper and serum zinc levels; alkaline phosphatase, taste acuity, mental depression

Dosage Forms Considerations
Strength of zinc sulfate injection is expressed as elemental zinc
Oral zinc sulfate is approximately 23% elemental zinc

Dosage Forms Excipient information presented when available (limited, particularly for generics); consult specific product labeling.
Capsule, Oral:
Orazinc: 220 mg
Zinc-220: 220 mg
Generic: 220 mg
Solution, Intravenous:
Generic: 1 mg/mL (10 mL); 5 mg/mL (5 mL)
Solution, Ophthalmic:
Eye-Sed: 0.217% (15 mL) [contains benzalkonium chloride, boric acid]
Tablet, Oral:
Orazinc: 110 mg
Zinc 15: 66 mg
Generic: 50 mg, 220 mg
Tablet, Oral [preservative free]:
Generic: 220 mg

References
American Academy of Pediatrics Committee on Nutrition, "Zinc," *Pediatrics*, 1978, 62(3):408-12.
Anderson LA, Hakojarvi SL, and Boudreaux SK, "Zinc Acetate Treatment in Wilson's Disease," *Ann Pharmacother*, 1998, 32(1):78-87.
Clinical Management of Acute Diarrhoea, Geneva, NY: World Health Organization/UNICEF, 2004. Available at http://www.unicef.org/nutrition/files/ENAcute_Diarrhoea_reprint.pdf. Accessed 2/13/2013.
de Moraes ML, de Faria Barbosa R, Santo RE, et al, "Maternal-Fetal Distribution of Calcium, Iron, Copper, and Zinc in Pregnant Teenagers and Adults," *Biol Trace Elem Res*, 2011, 139(2):126-36.
Department Health & Human Services, Food Drug Administration, "Aluminum in Large and Small Volume Parenterals Used in Total Parenteral Nutrition," *Federal Register*, 2000, 65(17):4103-11.

IOM (Institute of Medicine), *Dietary Reference Intakes for Vitamin A, Vitamin K, Arsenic, Boron, Chromium, Copper, Iodine, Iron, Manganese, Molybdenum, Nickel, Silicon, Vanadium, and Zinc*, Washington, DC: National Academy Press, 2001. Available at http://www.nal.usda.gov/fnic/DRI//DRI_Vitamin_A/vitamin_a_full_report.pdf

Mirtallo J, Canada T, Johnson D, et al, "Safe Practices for Parenteral Nutrition," *JPEN J Parenter Enteral Nutr*, 2004, 28(6):S39-70.

Vanek VW, Borum P, Buchman A, et al, "A.S.P.E.N. Position Paper: Recommendations for Changes in Commercially Available Parenteral Multivitamin and Multi-trace Element Products," *Nutr Clin Pract*, 2012, 27(4):440-91.

◆ **Zinc Undecylenate** *see* Undecylenic Acid and Derivatives *on page 2095*

◆ **Zinda-Letrozole (Can)** *see* Letrozole *on page 1211*

◆ **Zinecard** *see* Dexrazoxane *on page 626*

Ziprasidone (zi PRAS i done)

Medication Safety Issues
Sound-alike/look-alike issues:
Ziprasidone may be confused with TraZODone
BEERS Criteria medication:
This drug may be potentially inappropriate for use in geriatric patients (Quality of evidence - moderate; Strength of recommendation - strong).

Related Information
Oral Medications That Should Not Be Crushed or Altered *on page 2438*
Safe Handling of Hazardous Drugs *on page 2419*

Brand Names: U.S. Geodon
Brand Names: Canada Zeldox
Therapeutic Category Antipsychotic Agent, Atypical
Generic Availability (U.S.) May be product dependent
Use Due to its greater capacity to prolong the QT interval, ziprasidone is generally not considered to be a first-line agent.

Oral: Treatment of schizophrenia (FDA approved in adults); treatment as monotherapy of acute manic or mixed episodes associated with bipolar disorder with or without psychosis (FDA approved in adults); maintenance adjunctive therapy (to lithium or valproate) for bipolar I disorder (FDA approved in adults). **Note:** In June 2009, an FDA advisory panel advised that ziprasidone is effective in patients 10-17 years of age for the treatment of mixed and manic episodes of bipolar disorder, but did not conclude that it was safe due to large number of subjects lost to follow-up and ambiguity within QT$_c$ prolongation data. Has also been used in children and adolescents for treatment of Tourette's syndrome, tic disorders, irritability associated with autism, and pervasive development disorders not otherwise specified (PDD-NOS)

Injection: Acute agitation in patients with schizophrenia (FDA approved in adults)

Pregnancy Risk Factor C
Pregnancy Considerations Adverse events were observed in animal reproduction studies. Antipsychotic use during the third trimester of pregnancy has a risk for abnormal muscle movements (extrapyramidal symptoms [EPS]) and/or withdrawal symptoms in newborns following delivery. Symptoms in the newborn may include agitation, feeding disorder, hypertonia, hypotonia, respiratory distress, somnolence, and tremor; these effects may be self-limiting or require hospitalization. Ziprasidone may cause hyperprolactinemia, which may decrease reproductive function in both males and females.

The ACOG recommends that therapy during pregnancy be individualized; treatment with psychiatric medications during pregnancy should incorporate the clinical expertise of the mental health clinician, obstetrician, primary healthcare provider, and pediatrician. Safety data related to atypical antipsychotics during pregnancy is limited and routine use is not recommended. However, if a woman is inadvertently exposed to an atypical antipsychotic while pregnant, continuing therapy may be preferable to switching to a typical antipsychotic that the fetus has not yet been exposed to; consider risk:benefit (ACOG, 2008).

Healthcare providers are encouraged to enroll women 18-45 years of age exposed to ziprasidone during pregnancy in the Atypical Antipsychotics Pregnancy Registry (1-866-961-2388 or http://www.womensmentalhealth.org/pregnancyregistry).

Breast-Feeding Considerations It is not known if ziprasidone is excreted into breast milk. Breast-feeding is not recommended by the manufacturer.

Contraindications Hypersensitivity to ziprasidone or any component; known history or current prolonged QT interval; congenital long-QT syndrome; recent myocardial infarction; history of arrhythmias; uncompensated heart failure; concurrent use of other QT$_c$-prolonging agents, including arsenic trioxide, chlorpromazine, cisapride, class Ia antiarrhythmics (disopyramide, quinidine, procainamide), class III antiarrhythmics (amiodarone, dofetilide, ibutilide, sotalol), dolasetron, droperidol, gatifloxacin, halofantrine, levomethadyl, mefloquine, mesoridazine, moxifloxacin, pentamidine, pimozide, probucol, sparfloxacin, tacrolimus, and thioridazine

Warnings Hazardous agent; use appropriate precautions for handling and disposal (NIOSH, 2012). Ziprasidone is generally not considered to be a first-line agent; dose-related prolongation of the QT$_c$ may occur and may be associated with torsade de pointes and sudden death. Observed QT$_c$ prolongation with ziprasidone was greater than with other atypical antipsychotic agents (eg, risperidone, olanzapine, quetiapine), but less than with thioridazine. A prospective study followed 20 children (mean age: 13.2 years) for an average of 4.6 months and reported significant QT$_c$ prolongation at relatively low ziprasidone doses (mean daily dose: 30 mg ± 13 mg/day); the authors suggest the effect is not dose-dependent in children unlike adults and recommend reserving ziprasidone use as second- or third-line for patients at risk for QT$_c$ prolongation or when using doses >40 mg/day (Blair, 2005). Hypokalemia or hypomagnesemia may increase risk of torsade de pointe and/or sudden death; baseline electrolyte measurements are recommended. Use caution in patients with bradycardia. Discontinue in patients found to have persistent QT$_c$ intervals >500 msec. Patients with symptoms of dizziness, palpitations, or syncope should receive further cardiac evaluation.

May cause neuroleptic malignant syndrome; symptoms include hyperpyrexia, altered mental status, muscle rigidity, autonomic instability, acute renal failure, rhabdomyolysis, and increased CPK. May cause extrapyramidal reactions, including pseudoparkinsonism, acute dystonic reactions, akathisia, and tardive dyskinesia. Risk of these reactions is dose-dependent. To decrease risk of tardive dyskinesia: Use smallest dose and shortest duration possible; evaluate continued need periodically. Risk of dystonia is increased with the use of high potency and higher doses of conventional antipsychotics and in males and younger patients. May cause hyperglycemia, which may be severe and include potentially fatal ketoacidosis or hyperosmolar coma; use with caution and monitor glucose closely in patients with diabetes mellitus (or with risk factors such as family history or obesity); measure fasting blood glucose at the beginning of therapy and periodically during therapy in these patients; monitor for symptoms of hyperglycemia in all patients treated with ziprasidone; measure fasting blood glucose in patients who develop symptoms. May cause development of a dose-related rash and/or urticaria (5%) which may also involve systemic illness; discontinue if alternative cause cannot be identified. Leukopenia, neutropenia, and agranulocytosis (sometimes fatal) have been reported in clinical trials and postmarketing reports with antipsychotic use; presence of risk factors (eg, preexisting low WBC or history of drug-induced leuko-/neutropenia) should prompt periodic blood count assessment. Discontinue therapy at first signs of blood dyscrasias or if absolute neutrophil count <1000/mm^3.

An increased risk of death has been reported with the use of antipsychotics in elderly patients with dementia-related psychosis **[U.S. Boxed Warning]**; most deaths seemed to be cardiovascular (eg, sudden death, heart failure) or infectious (eg, pneumonia) in nature. An increased incidence of cerebrovascular adverse events (eg, transient ischemic attack, stroke), including fatalities, has been reported with the use of antipsychotics in elderly patients with dementia-related psychosis. Ziprasidone is not approved for the treatment of patients with dementia-related psychosis.

Pediatric psychiatric disorders are frequently serious mental disorders which present with variable symptoms that do not always match adult diagnostic criteria. Conduct a thorough diagnostic evaluation and carefully consider risks of psychotropic medication before initiation in pediatric patients. Medication therapy for pediatric patients with bipolar disorder is indicated as part of a total treatment program that frequently includes educational, psychological, and social interventions.

Precautions Use with caution in patients with seizure disorders (rare seizure reports); in suicidal patients, in patients with concomitant systemic illnesses or unstable heart disease or a recent history of MI (these patients not adequately studied); and in patients at risk of aspiration pneumonia (esophageal dysmotility and aspiration have been associated with antipsychotic agents). May cause orthostatic hypotension; use with caution in patients at risk for this effect or in those who would not tolerate transient hypotensive episodes (eg, cerebrovascular disease, cardiovascular disease, hypovolemia, or concurrent medication which predisposes to hypotension). Use with caution in patients with breast cancer or other prolactin-dependent tumors; ziprasidone increases prolactin concentrations; high concentrations of prolactin may reduce pituitary gonadotropin secretion; galactorrhea, amenorrhea, gynecomastia, impotence, decreased bone density may occur. Use with caution in children and adolescents; adverse effects due to increased prolactin concentrations have been observed; long-term effects on growth or sexual maturation have not been evaluated. May cause somnolence (dose-related), priapism (rarely), alteration of temperature regulation; use with caution in patients exposed to temperature extremes. Dyslipidemia has been reported with atypical antipsychotics; risk profile may differ between agents.

Use with caution in patients with hepatic disease or impairment. Use with caution during diarrheal illnesses; monitor electrolytes closely (K and Mg) (Blair, 2004). Use the intramuscular formulation with caution in patients with renal impairment due to cyclodextrin excipient, an excipient which may accumulate in renal insufficiency.

Adverse Reactions

Cardiovascular: Bradycardia, chest pain, facial edema, hypertension, orthostatic hypotension, tachycardia, vasodilation

Central nervous system: Agitation, akathisia, akinesia, amnesia, anxiety, ataxia, chills, confusion, coordination abnormal, delirium, dizziness, dystonia, extrapyramidal symptoms, fever, headache, hostility, hypothermia, insomnia, oculogyric crisis, personality disorder, psychosis, somnolence, speech disorder, vertigo

Dermatologic: Fungal dermatitis, photosensitivity reaction, rash

Endocrine & metabolic: Dysmenorrhea

Gastrointestinal: Abdominal pain, anorexia, buccoglossal syndrome, constipation, diarrhea, dyspepsia, dysphagia, nausea, rectal hemorrhage, salivation increased, tongue edema, vomiting, weight gain, xerostomia

Genitourinary: Priapism

Local: Injection site pain

Neuromuscular & skeletal: Abnormal gait, back pain, choreoathetosis, cogwheel rigidity, dysarthria, dyskinesia, hyper-/hypokinesia, hyper-/hypotonia, hypoesthesia, myalgia, neuropathy, paresthesia, tremor, twitching, weakness

Ocular: Diplopia, vision abnormal

Respiratory: Cough, dyspnea, infection, pharyngitis, rhinitis

Miscellaneous: Diaphoresis, flank pain, flu-like syndrome, furunculosis, withdrawal syndrome

Rare but important or life-threatening: Abnormal ejaculation, albuminuria, alkaline phosphatase increased, allergic reaction, alopecia, amenorrhea, anemia, angioedema, angina, anorgasmia, atrial fibrillation, AV block (first degree), basophilia, blepharitis, bruising, BUN increased, bundle branch block, cardiomegaly, cataract, cerebral infarction, cerebrovascular accident, cholestatic jaundice, circumoral paresthesia, conjunctivitis, contact dermatitis, CPK increased, creatinine (serum) increased, dehydration, depression, dry eyes, eczema, enuresis, eosinophilia, epistaxis, exfoliative dermatitis, facial droop, fatty liver, fecal impaction, galactorrhea, GGT increased, gingival bleeding, glycosuria, gout, gynecomastia, hematemesis, hemoptysis, hematuria, hepatitis, hepatomegaly, hyper-/hypochloremia, hyper-/hypocholesterolemia, hyper-/hypoglycemia, hyper-/hypokalemia, hyper-/hypothyroidism, hyperlipemia, hyperreflexia, hyperuricemia, hypocalcemia, hypomagnesemia, hyponatremia, hypoproteinemia, impotence, jaundice, keratitis, keratoconjunctivitis, ketosis, lactation (female), laryngismus, LDH increased, leukocytosis, leukopenia, leukoplakia (mouth), lymphadenopathy, lymphedema, lymphocytosis, maculopapular rash, mania/hypomania, melena, menorrhagia, metrorrhagia, monocytosis, myocarditis, myoclonus, myopathy, neuroleptic malignant syndrome, nocturia, nystagmus, ocular hemorrhage, oliguria, opisthotonos, paralysis, peripheral edema, phlebitis, photophobia, pneumonia, polycythemia, polyuria, pulmonary embolism, QT$_c$ prolongation >500 msec, respiratory alkalosis, seizure, serotonin syndrome, sexual dysfunction (male and female), syncope, tardive dyskinesia, tenosynovitis, thirst, thrombocytopenia, thrombocythemia, thrombophlebitis, thyroiditis, tinnitus, torsade de pointes, torticollis, transaminases increased, trismus, urinary incontinence, urinary retention, urticaria, uterine hemorrhage, vaginal hemorrhage, vesiculobullous rash, visual field defect

Drug Interactions

Metabolism/Transport Effects Substrate of CYP1A2 (minor), CYP3A4 (minor); **Note:** Assignment of Major/Minor substrate status based on clinically relevant drug interaction potential; **Inhibits** CYP2D6 (weak), CYP3A4 (weak)

Avoid Concomitant Use

Avoid concomitant use of Ziprasidone with any of the following: Amisulpride; Azelastine (Nasal); FLUoxetine; Highest Risk QTc-Prolonging Agents; Ivabradine; Metoclopramide; Mifepristone; Moderate Risk QTc-Prolonging Agents; Paraldehyde; Pimozide; Sulpiride; Thalidomide

Increased Effect/Toxicity

Ziprasidone may increase the levels/effects of: Alcohol (Ethyl); Amisulpride; Azelastine (Nasal); Buprenorphine; CNS Depressants; FLUoxetine; Highest Risk QTc-Prolonging Agents; Hydrocodone; Lomitapide; Methotrimeprazine; Methylphenidate; Metyrosine; Paraldehyde;

Pimozide; Selective Serotonin Reuptake Inhibitors; Serotonin Modulators; Sulpiride; Thalidomide; Zolpidem

The levels/effects of Ziprasidone may be increased by: Acetylcholinesterase Inhibitors (Central); Brimonidine (Topical); Cannabis; Doxylamine; Dronabinol; FLUoxetine; HydrOXYzine; Ivabradine; Kava Kava; Magnesium Sulfate; Methotrimeprazine; Methylphenidate; Metoclopramide; Metyrosine; Mifepristone; Moderate Risk QTc-Prolonging Agents; Nabilone; Perampanel; QTc-Prolonging Agents (Indeterminate Risk and Risk Modifying); Rufinamide; Serotonin Modulators; Sodium Oxybate; Tapentadol; Tetrahydrocannabinol

Decreased Effect

Ziprasidone may decrease the levels/effects of: Amphetamines; Anti-Parkinson's Agents (Dopamine Agonist); Quinagolide

The levels/effects of Ziprasidone may be decreased by: CarBAMazepine

Food Interactions Administration with food increases serum levels twofold. Management: Administer with food.

Stability Hazardous agent; use appropriate precautions for handling and disposal (NIOSH, 2012).

Oral: Store at controlled room temperature of 25°C (77°F); excursions permitted to 15°C to 30°C (59°F to 86°F).

Injection: Store at controlled room temperature of 25°C (77°F); excursions permitted to 15°C to 30°C (59°F to 86°F). Protect from light. Following reconstitution, injection may be stored at room temperature up to 24 hours or up to 7 days if refrigerated and protected from light.

Mechanism of Action Ziprasidone is a benzylisothiazolylpiperazine antipsychotic. The exact mechanism of action is unknown. However, *in vitro* radioligand studies show that ziprasidone has high affinity for D_2, D_3, $5-HT_{2A}$, $5-HT_{1A}$, $5-HT_{2C}$, $5-HT_{1D}$, and alpha$_1$-adrenergic; moderate affinity for histamine H_1 receptors; and no appreciable affinity for alpha$_2$-adrenergic receptors, beta-adrenergic, $5-HT_3$, $5-HT_4$, cholinergic, mu, sigma, or benzodiazepine receptors. Ziprasidone functions as an antagonist at the D_2, $5-HT_{2A}$, and $5-HT_{1D}$ receptors and as an agonist at the $5-HT_{1A}$ receptor. Ziprasidone moderately inhibits the reuptake of serotonin and norepinephrine.

Pharmacokinetics (Adult data unless noted)

Absorption: Well absorbed; presence of food increases by up to twofold

Distribution: Apparent V_d: 1.5 L/kg

Protein binding: 99%, primarily to albumin and alpha$_1$-acid glycoprotein

Metabolism: Extensively hepatic, primarily chemical and enzymatic reductions via glutathione and aldehyde oxidase, respectively; less than 1/3 of total metabolism via CYP3A4 and CYP1A2 (minor)

Bioavailability: I.M.: 100%, Oral: ~60% under fed conditions

Half-life:
I.M.: 2-5 hours
Oral:
Children: Mean: 3.3-4.1 hours (Sallee, 2006)
Adult: 7 hours

Time to peak serum concentration:
I.M.: ≤60 minutes
Oral:
Children: Mean: 5-5.5 hours (Sallee, 2006)
Adult: 6-8 hours

Elimination: Feces (66%) and urine (20%) as metabolites; little as unchanged drug (<1% urine, <4% feces)

Clearance:
Children: Mean: 11.5-13.1 mL/minute/kg (Sallee, 2006)
Adult: Mean: 7.5 mL/minute/kg

Dialysis: Not removed by hemodialysis

Dosing: Usual

Children and Adolescents:

Acute agitation (schizophrenia): Limited data available (Barzman, 2007; Khan, 2006; Staller, 2004): I.M.: Children 5-11 years: 10 mg
Adolescents ≥12 years: 10-20 mg; **Note:** One study (n=59; age range: 5-19 years) reported that 69% of 20 mg doses surpassed the desired calming therapeutic effect and caused varying degrees of sedation (4% of patients were unable to be aroused) (Barzman, 2007)

Autism and PDD-NOS irritability: Limited data available: Oral: Children ≥8 years and Adolescents: Reported final dose range: 20-160 mg/day divided twice daily
A prospective, open-labeled study of 12 patients (12-18 years) used the following individually titrated doses (Malone, 2007)
Patient weight ≤35 kg: Initial: 20 mg every other day given at bedtime for 2 doses; then increase dose in weekly increments based on clinical response and tolerability: Week 1: 10 mg twice daily (20 mg/day); Week 2: 20 mg twice daily (40 mg/day); Week 3: 40 mg twice daily (80 mg/day); Week 4: 80 mg twice daily (160 mg/day)
Patient weight >35 kg: Initial: 20 mg/day at bedtime for 3 doses; then increase dose in weekly increments based on clinical response and tolerability: Week 1: 20 mg twice daily (40 mg/day); Week 2: 40 mg twice daily (80 mg/day); Week 4: 80 mg twice daily (160 mg/day)
A case series of 12 patients (8-20 years) initiated therapy at 20 mg/day given at bedtime and then increased by 10-20 mg/week divided twice daily based on clinical response and tolerability; final ziprasidone dosage ranged between 20-120 mg/day (mean: ~60 mg/day) divided twice daily (McDougle, 2002)

Bipolar I disorder: Oral: Children and Adolescents 10-17 years: **Note:** In June 2009, an FDA advisory panel advised that ziprasidone is effective in patients 10-17 years of age for the treatment of mixed and manic episodes of bipolar disorder, but did not conclude that it was safe due to large number of subjects lost to follow-up and ambiguity within QT_c prolongation data; limited data available (DelBello, 2008; DelBello, 2008a; Elbe, 2008; Findling, 2008; Mechcatie, 2009)
Initial dose: 20 mg/day; titrate dose upwards as tolerated, using twice daily dosing over a 2-week period to the weight-based target range: 60-80 mg/day (≤45 kg) divided into twice daily doses or 120-160 mg/day (>45 kg) divided into twice daily doses.
Alternate dosing: An open-label, 8-week study of 21 patients [6-17 years (mean: 10.3 years)] with bipolar disorder and comorbid conditions (eg, ADHD, depression, conduct disorder) used the following weight-based dosing regimen (Biederman, 2007):
Initial dose: 1 mg/kg/day divided twice daily; increase to 1.5 mg/kg/day divided twice daily by Week 2 and increase to 2 mg/kg/day divided twice daily by Week 3 if tolerated; maximum dose: 160 mg/day; **Note:** Only 14 of the 21 patients completed the study; five dropped out due to lack of efficacy; two dropped out due to adverse reactions; patients experienced a high incidence of sedation (46%) and headaches (38%).

Tourette's syndrome, tic disorder: Limited data available: Oral: Children and Adolescents 7-16 years: Initial dose: 5 mg/day for 3 days then using twice daily dosing, titrate dose as tolerated up to 40 mg/day divided twice daily. Dosing is based on a double-blind, placebo-controlled pilot study (n=28), mean daily dose at the end of trial: 28.2 + 9.6 mg/day (Sallee, 2000).

Adults:

Acute agitation (schizophrenia): I.M.: 10 mg every 2 hours **or** 20 mg every 4 hours; maximum: 40 mg/day; oral therapy should replace I.M. administration as soon as possible. Use >3 days has not been studied.

Bipolar mania: Oral: Initial: 40 mg twice daily; adjustment: May increase to 60 or 80 mg twice daily on second day of treatment; average dose 40-80 mg twice daily

Schizophrenia: Oral: Initial: 20 mg twice daily; adjustment: Increases (if indicated) should be made no more frequently than every 2 days; ordinarily patients should be observed for improvement over several weeks before adjusting the dose. Maintenance: Range: 20-100 mg twice daily; however, dosages >80 mg twice daily are generally not recommended

Dosing adjustment in renal impairment: Adults:

Oral: No dosage adjustment is recommended

I.M.: Cyclodextrin, an excipient in the I.M. formulation, is cleared by renal filtration; use with caution

Ziprasidone is not removed by hemodialysis.

Dosing adjustment in hepatic impairment: No dosage adjustment is recommended; however, drug undergoes extensive hepatic metabolism and systemic exposure may be increased. Use with caution.

Administration Hazardous agent; use appropriate precautions for handling and disposal (NIOSH, 2012).

Oral: Administer with food.

Injection: Injection is for I.M. use only; do not administer I.V. Reconstitute with 1.2 mL SWI for final concentration 20 mg/mL

Monitoring Parameters Vital signs; serum potassium and magnesium; CBC with differential; fasting lipid profile and fasting blood glucose/Hb A_{1c} (prior to treatment, at 3 months, then annually); weight, BMI, waist circumference; personal/family history of diabetes; blood pressure; mental status, abnormal involuntary movement scale (AIMS), extrapyramidal symptoms. Weight should be assessed prior to treatment, at 4 weeks, 8 weeks, 12 weeks, and then at quarterly intervals. Consider titrating to a different antipsychotic agent for a weight gain ≥5% of the initial weight. Monitor patient periodically for symptom resolution. In children, baseline and periodic (eg, when initially reach steady state, with dose changes or addition of an interacting drug) ECG monitoring in children has been recommended by several pediatric clinicians (Blair, 2004; Blair, 2005; Elbe, 2008). Discontinue drug in patients found to have persistent QT_c intervals >500 msec.

Additional Information Long-term usefulness of ziprasidone should be periodically re-evaluated in patients receiving the drug for extended periods of time. A Phase III trial designed to evaluate ziprasidone in adolescents with schizophrenia was terminated early due to lack of efficacy; no safety concerns were noted.

Agitation and/or aggression after traumatic brain injury (TBI): A case series of 20 patients [ages: 9 months to 17 years (median: 8 years)] reported using age-based ziprasidone dosing during the immediate TBI recovery phase with a total duration of therapy range of 3-8 days. To discontinue, ziprasidone dose was tapered over ~2 days. Doses were initiated at a low dose and titrated up based on agitation level and Riker SAS score; however, minimal dosage adjustments were required during the study. The drug appeared to be safe and effective; further studies are needed (Scott, 2009). Initial dosing:

<2 years: 1.7 mg/kg/day divided 2-3 times/day (final dose: 1.8 mg/kg/day)

2-6 years: 0.9 mg/kg/day divided twice daily (final dose: 1.5 mg/kg/day)

7-12 years: 0.7 mg/kg/day divided twice daily (final dose: 1.5 mg/kg/day)

≥13 years: 0.6 mg/kg/day divided twice daily (final dose: 0.7 mg/kg/day)

Dosage Forms Excipient information presented when available (limited, particularly for generics); consult specific product labeling.

Capsule, Oral, as hydrochloride:

Geodon: 20 mg, 40 mg, 60 mg, 80 mg

Generic: 20 mg, 40 mg, 60 mg, 80 mg

Solution Reconstituted, Intramuscular, as mesylate [strength expressed as base]:

Geodon: 20 mg (1 ea)

Extemporaneous Preparations Hazardous agent: Use appropriate precautions for handling and disposal.

A 2.5 mg/mL oral solution may be made with the injection. Use 8 vials of the 20 mg injectable powder. Add 1.2 mL of distilled water to each vial to make a 20 mg/mL solution. Once dissolved, transfer 7.5 mL to a calibrated bottle and add quantity of vehicle (Ora-Sweet®) sufficient to make 60 mL. Label "shake well" and "refrigerate". Stable for 14 days at room temperature or 42 days refrigerated (preferred).

Green K and Parish RC, "Stability of Ziprasidone Mesylate in an Extemporaneously Compounded Oral Solution," *J Pediatr Pharmacol Ther,* 2010, 15:138-41.

References

ACOG Committee on Practice Bulletins-Obstetrics, "ACOG Practice Bulletin: Clinical Management Guidelines for Obstetrician-Gynecologists Number 92, April 2008 (Replaces Practice Bulletin Number 87, November 2007). Use of Psychiatric Medications During Pregnancy and Lactation," *Obstet Gynecol,* 2008, 111(4):1001-20.

Barzman DH, DelBello MP, Forrester JJ, et al, "A Retrospective Chart Review of Intramuscular Ziprasidone for Agitation in Children and Adolescents on Psychiatric Units: Prospective Studies Are Needed," *J Child Adolesc Psychopharmacol,* 2007, 17(4):503-9.

Biederman J, Mick E, Spencer T, et al, "A Prospective Open-Label Treatment Trial of Ziprasidone Monotherapy in Children and Adolescents With Bipolar Disorder," *Bipolar Disord,* 2007, 9(8):888-94.

Blair J, Scahill L, State M, et al, "Electrocardiographic Changes in Children and Adolescents Treated With Ziprasidone: A Prospective Study," *J Am Acad Child Adolesc Psychiatry,* 2005, 44(1):73-9.

Blair J, Taggart B, and Martin A, "Electrocardiographic Safety Profile and Monitoring Guidelines in Pediatric Psychopharmacology," *J Neural Transm,* 2004, 111(7):791-815.

DelBello MP, Findling RL, Wang PP, et al, "Efficacy and Safety of Ziprasidone in Pediatric Bipolar Disorder," Presented at the 161st Annual Meeting of the American Psychiatric Association (APA); May 3-8, 2008; Washington DC (poster).

DelBello MP, Versavel M, Ice K, et al, "Tolerability of Oral Ziprasidone in Children and Adolescents With Bipolar Mania, Schizophrenia, or Schizoaffective Disorder," *J Child Adolesc Psychopharmacol,* 2008a, 18(5):491-9.

Elbe D and Carandang CG, "Focus on Ziprasidone: A Review of Its Use in Child and Adolescent Psychiatry," *J Can Acad Child Adolesc Psychiatry,* 2008, 17(4):220-9.

Findling RL, DelBello MP, Wang PP, et al, "Long-Term Safety and Tolerability of Ziprasidone in Pediatric Bipolar Disorder," Presented at the 161st Annual Meeting of the American Psychiatric Association (APA); May 3-8, 2008; Washington DC (poster).

Juncos JL, Shea SA, Stover N, et al, "Safety and Efficacy of Ziprasidone in Tourette Syndrome," *Movement Disord,* 2002, 17(5):S340 (abstract).

Khan SS and Mican LM, "A Naturalistic Evaluation of Intramuscular Ziprasidone Versus Intramuscular Olanzapine for the Management of Acute Agitation and Aggression in Children and Adolescents," *J Child Adolesc Psychopharmacol,* 2006, 16(6):671-7.

Malone RP, Delaney MA, Hyman SB, et al, "Ziprasidone in Adolescents With Autism: An Open-Label Pilot Study," *J Child Adolesc Psychopharmacol,* 2007, 17(6):779-90.

McDougle CJ, Kem DL, and Posey DJ, "Case Series: Use of Ziprasidone for Maladaptive Symptoms in Youths With Autism," *J Am Acad Child Adolesc Psychiatry,* 2002, 41(8):921-7.

Mechcatie, E, "MD Consult: News: Mixed Votes on Ziprasidone's Safety and Efficacy for Pediatric Indications, " June 16, 2009. Date accessed: January 20, 2010.

National Institute for Occupational Safety and Health (NIOSH), "NIOSH List of Antineoplastic and Other Hazardous Drugs in Healthcare Settings 2012." Available at http://www.cdc.gov/niosh/docs/2012-150/pdfs/2012-150.pdf. Accessed January 21, 2013.

Sallee FR, Miceli JJ, Tensfeldt T, et al, "Single-Dose Pharmacokinetics and Safety of Ziprasidone in Children and Adolescents," *J Am Acad Child Adolesc Psychiatry,* 2006, 45(6):720-8.

Sallee FR, Kurlan R, Goetz CG, et al, "Ziprasidone Treatment of Children and Adolescents With Tourette's Syndrome: A Pilot Study," *J Am Acad Child Adolesc Psychiatry*, 2000, 39(3):292-9.

Scott LK, Green R, McCarthy PJ, et al, "Agitation and/or Aggression After Traumatic Brain Injury in the Pediatric Population Treated With Ziprasidone. Clinical Article," *J Neurosurg Pediatr*, 2009, 3(6):484-7.

Staller JA, "Intramuscular Ziprasidone in Youth: A Retrospective Chart Review," *J Child Adolesc Psychopharmacol*, 2004, 14(4):590-2.

◆ **Ziprasidone Hydrochloride** *see* Ziprasidone on page 2178

◆ **Ziprasidone Mesylate** *see* Ziprasidone on page 2178

◆ **Zipsor** *see* Diclofenac (Systemic) on page 645

◆ **Zirgan** *see* Ganciclovir (Ophthalmic) on page 957

◆ **Zithromax** *see* Azithromycin (Systemic) on page 247

◆ **Zithromax® (Can)** *see* Azithromycin (Systemic) on page 247

◆ **Zithromax® For Intravenous Injection (Can)** *see* Azithromycin (Systemic) on page 247

◆ **Zithromax TRI-PAK™** *see* Azithromycin (Systemic) on page 247

◆ **Zithromax Tri-Pak** *see* Azithromycin (Systemic) on page 247

◆ **Zithromax Z-PAK®** *see* Azithromycin (Systemic) on page 247

◆ **Zithromax Z-Pak** *see* Azithromycin (Systemic) on page 247

◆ **Zmax** *see* Azithromycin (Systemic) on page 247

◆ **Zmax SR™ (Can)** *see* Azithromycin (Systemic) on page 247

◆ **ZnSO₄ (error-prone abbreviation)** *see* Zinc Sulfate on page 2176

◆ **Zocor** *see* Simvastatin on page 1892

◆ **Zofran** *see* Ondansetron on page 1544

◆ **Zofran® (Can)** *see* Ondansetron on page 1544

◆ **Zofran ODT** *see* Ondansetron on page 1544

◆ **Zofran® ODT (Can)** *see* Ondansetron on page 1544

◆ **Zoloft** *see* Sertraline on page 1879

Zolpidem (zole PI dem)

Medication Safety Issues
Sound-alike/look-alike issues:
Ambien may be confused with Abilify, Ativan, Ambi 10
Sublinox may be confused with Suboxone
Zolpidem may be confused with lorazepam, zaleplon
BEERS Criteria medication:
This drug may be potentially inappropriate for use in geriatric patients (Quality of evidence - moderate; Strength of recommendation - strong).
International issues:
Ambien [U.S., Argentina, Israel] may be confused with Amyben brand name for amiodarone [Great Britain]

Related Information
Oral Medications That Should Not Be Crushed or Altered on page 2438

Brand Names: U.S. Ambien; Ambien CR; Edluar; Intermezzo; Zolpimist

Brand Names: Canada Sublinox

Therapeutic Category Hypnotic, Nonbenzodiazepine

Generic Availability (U.S.) May be product dependent

Use Oral:
Tablets:
Ambien: Short-term treatment of insomnia (with difficulty of sleep onset) (FDA approved in age ≥18 years and adults)
Ambien CR: Treatment of insomnia (with difficulty of sleep onset and/or sleep maintenance) (FDA approved in age ≥18 years and adults)

Sublingual:
Edluar: Short-term treatment of insomnia (with difficulty of sleep onset) (FDA approved in age ≥18 years and adults)
Intermezzo: "As needed" treatment of middle-of-the-night insomnia with ≥4 hours of sleep time remaining (FDA approved in age age ≥18 years and adults)
Oral spray: Zolpimist: Short-term treatment of insomnia (with difficulty of sleep onset) (FDA approved in age ≥18 years and adults)

Medication Guide Available Yes

Pregnancy Risk Factor C

Pregnancy Considerations Adverse events were observed in some animal reproduction studies. Zolpidem crosses the placenta (Juric, 2009). Severe neonatal respiratory depression has been reported when zolpidem was used at the end of pregnancy, especially when used concurrently with other CNS depressants. Children born of mothers taking sedative/hypnotics may be at risk for withdrawal; neonatal flaccidity has been reported in infants following maternal use of sedative/hypnotics during pregnancy. Additional adverse effects to the fetus/newborn have been noted in some studies (Wang, 2010; Wikner, 2011).

Breast-Feeding Considerations Zolpidem is excreted in breast milk. The manufacturer recommends that caution be exercised when administering zolpidem to nursing women.

Contraindications Hypersensitivity to zolpidem tartrate or any component

Warnings Evaluate patient carefully for medical or psychiatric causes of insomnia prior to initiation of drug treatment; failure of zolpidem to treat insomnia (after 7-10 days of therapy), a worsening of insomnia, or the emergence of behavioral changes or thinking abnormalities may indicate a medical or psychiatric illness requiring evaluation; these effects also have been reported with zolpidem use. Abnormal thinking and behavior changes may occur with sedative/hypnotic use, including decreased inhibition (eg, aggressiveness, extroversion that seems out of character); visual and auditory hallucinations, agitation, bizarre behavior, and depersonalization have been reported with zolpidem use. Hallucinations have been reported more frequently in children and adolescents receiving zolpidem for insomnia associated with ADHD than in adults (7.4% vs ≤1%). Worsening of depression, including suicide or suicidal ideation, may occur; use with caution in patients with depression; to reduce the risk of overdose, prescriptions should be written for the smallest quantity consistent with good patient care. Abrupt discontinuation after prolonged use may result in withdrawal symptoms and signs.

Hypersensitivity reactions, including anaphylaxis and angioedema, may occur; angioedema may involve the tongue, glottis, or larynx; occurrence of dyspnea, throat closing, or nausea and vomiting suggest anaphylaxis; angioedema of the throat, glottis, or larynx may result in potentially fatal airway obstruction; do not rechallenge patients who develop angioedema after receiving zolpidem. Hazardous sleep-related activities, such as sleep-driving (driving while not fully awake without any recollection of driving), preparing and eating food, and making phone calls while asleep have also been reported; increased risk of these type of events has been reported with greater than recommended zolpidem dosages as well as concomitant ethanol or CNS depressant use; amnesia may also occur; discontinue treatment in patients who report a sleep-driving episode. Effects of other sedative drugs or ethanol may be potentiated.

May cause CNS depression impairing physical and mental capabilities; patients should be cautioned about performing tasks which require mental alertness (eg, operating machinery or driving). Zolpidem should only be administered immediately prior to bedtime or after the patient has gone to bed but is having difficulty falling asleep and when the patient is able to stay in bed a full night (7-8 hours) before being active again; Intermezzo should only be administered if patient awakens in middle of night and has difficulty returning to sleep and has at least 4 hours left to stay in bed. Zolpidem may continue to affect alertness the next morning; risk is higher in patients who take extended release formulations and with higher dose. Caution patients about risk associated with next-morning alertness; patients may have diminished alertness even if they feel fully awake; use lowest effective dose. Women may be more sensitive to morning effects due to decreased elimination; pharmacokinetic studies involving zolpidem have shown a significant increase in maximum concentration and exposure in females compared to males at the same dose; dosage adjustment is recommended.

Some oral, immediate release tablet dosage forms may contain polysorbate 80 which may cause allergic reactions in susceptible individuals.

Precautions Use with caution in patients with sleep apnea, COPD, or respiratory compromise; myasthenia gravis; and concomitant illnesses which may affect zolpidem metabolism or hemodynamic response. Use with caution and decrease the dose in patients with hepatic impairment and in debilitated patients; monitor for impaired cognitive and/or motor function. Use with caution in patients with renal impairment or with a history of drug dependence.

The most common adverse effects observed in children include the following: Dizziness, headache, hallucinations, affect lability, enuresis, gastroenteritis, and anxiety (Blumer, 2009).

Potentially significant interactions may exist, requiring dose or frequency adjustment, additional monitoring, and/or selection of alternative therapy. Consult drug interactions database for more detailed information.

Adverse Reactions

Cardiovascular: Chest discomfort, increased blood pressure, palpitations

Central nervous system: Abnormal dreams, amnesia, anxiety, apathy, ataxia, burning sensation, confusion, depersonalization, depression, disinhibition, disorientation, dizziness, drowsiness, drugged feeling, eating disorder (binge eating), emotional lability, equilibrium disturbance, euphoria, fatigue, hallucination, headache, hypoesthesia, increased body temperature, insomnia, lack of concentration, lethargy, memory impairment, paresthesia, psychomotor retardation, sleep disorder, stress, vertigo

Dermatologic: Skin rash, urticaria, wrinkling of skin

Endocrine & metabolic: Hypermenorrhea

Gastrointestinal: Abdominal distress, abdominal tenderness, change in appetite, constipation, diarrhea, dyspepsia, flatulence, frequent bowel movements, gastroenteritis, gastroesophageal reflux disease, hiccups, nausea, vomiting, xerostomia

Genitourinary: Dysuria, urinary tract infection, vaginal dryness

Hypersensitivity: Hypersensitivity reaction

Neuromuscular & skeletal: Arthralgia, back pain, muscle cramps, muscle spasm, myalgia, neck pain, tremor, weakness

Ophthalmic: Accommodation disturbance, asthenopia, blurred vision, diplopia, eye redness, visual disturbance (including altered depth perception)

Otic: Labyrinthitis, tinnitus

Respiratory: Dry throat, flu-like symptoms, lower respiratory tract infection, pharyngitis, sinusitis, throat irritation, upper respiratory tract infection

Miscellaneous: Fever

Rare but important or life-threatening: Abnormal hepatic function tests, acute renal failure, aggressive behavior, anaphylaxis, anemia, angina pectoris, angioedema, anorexia, arteritis, arthritis, breast fibroadenosis, breast neoplasm, bronchitis, cardiac arrhythmia, cerebrovascular disease, circulatory shock, cognitive dysfunction, corneal ulcer, delusions, dementia, dermatitis, drug tolerance, dysarthria, dysphagia, edema, extrasystoles, glaucoma, hepatic insufficiency, hyperbilirubinemia, hyperglycemia, hyperlipidemia, hypertension, hypotension, hysteria, illusion, impotence, leukopenia, lymphadenopathy, migraine, myocardial infarction, neuralgia, neuritis, neuropathy, orthostatic hypotension, panic disorder, personality disorder, psychoneurosis, pulmonary edema, pulmonary embolism, pyelonephritis, respiratory depression, restless leg syndrome, rhinitis, scleritis, somnambulism, syncope, tachycardia, tenesmus, tetany, thrombosis, urinary incontinence, vaginitis, ventricular tachycardia

Drug Interactions

Metabolism/Transport Effects Substrate of CYP1A2 (minor), CYP2C19 (minor), CYP2C9 (minor), CYP2D6 (minor), CYP3A4 (major); **Note:** Assignment of Major/Minor substrate status based on clinically relevant drug interaction potential

Avoid Concomitant Use

Avoid concomitant use of Zolpidem with any of the following: Azelastine (Nasal); Conivaptan; Fusidic Acid (Systemic); Paraldehyde; Sodium Oxybate; Thalidomide

Increased Effect/Toxicity

Zolpidem may increase the levels/effects of: Alcohol (Ethyl); Azelastine (Nasal); Buprenorphine; CarBAMazepine; Hydrocodone; Methotrimeprazine; Metyrosine; Paraldehyde; Pramipexole; ROPINIRole; Rotigotine; Selective Serotonin Reuptake Inhibitors; Sodium Oxybate; Thalidomide

The levels/effects of Zolpidem may be increased by: Antifungal Agents (Azole Derivatives, Systemic); Brimonidine (Topical); Cannabis; Ceritinib; CNS Depressants; Conivaptan; CYP3A4 Inhibitors (Moderate); CYP3A4 Inhibitors (Strong); Dasatinib; Dronabinol; Droperidol; Fluconazole; FluvoxaMINE; Fusidic Acid (Systemic); Ivacaftor; Kava Kava; Luliconazole; Magnesium Sulfate; Methotrimeprazine; Mifepristone; Nabilone; Perampanel; Rufinamide; Simeprevir; Stiripentol; Tapentadol; Tetrahydrocannabinol

Decreased Effect

The levels/effects of Zolpidem may be decreased by: Bosentan; CarBAMazepine; CYP3A4 Inducers (Strong); Dabrafenib; Deferasirox; Flumazenil; Mitotane; Peginterferon Alfa-2b; Rifamycin Derivatives; Siltuximab; St Johns Wort; Telaprevir; Tocilizumab

Food Interactions Maximum plasma concentration and bioavailability are decreased with food; time to peak plasma concentration is increased; half-life remains unchanged. Grapefruit juice may decrease the metabolism of zolpidem. Management: Do not administer with (or immediately after) a meal. Avoid grapefruit juice.

Stability

Ambien®; Edluar™, Intermezzo®: Store at 20°C to 25°C (68°F to 77°F). Protect sublingual tablets from light and moisture.

Ambien CR®: Store at 15°C to 25°C (59°F to 77°F); limited excursions up to 30°C (86°F) are permissible.

Zolpimist®: Store container in upright position at 25°C (77°F). Do not freeze. Avoid prolonged exposure to temperatures >30°C (86°F).

Mechanism of Action Zolpidem, an imidazopyridine hypnotic that is structurally dissimilar to benzodiazepines, enhances the activity of the inhibitory neurotransmitter, γ-aminobutyric acid (GABA), via selective agonism at the benzodiazepine-1 (BZ_1) receptor; the result is increased chloride conductance, neuronal hyperpolarization, inhibition of the action potential, and a decrease in neuronal excitability leading to sedative and hypnotic effects. Because of its selectivity for the BZ_1 receptor site over the BZ_2 receptor site, zolpidem exhibits minimal anxiolytic, myorelaxant, and anticonvulsant properties (effects largely attributed to agonism at the BZ_2 receptor site).

Pharmacodynamics

Onset of action: Immediate release: 30 minutes

Duration: Immediate release: 6-8 hours

Pharmacokinetics (Adult data unless noted) Note:

C_{max} and AUC are increased by ~45% in female patients

Absorption: Oral:

Immediate release and sublingual: Rapid

Extended release: Biphasic absorption; rapid initial absorption (similar to immediate release product); then provides extended concentrations in the plasma beyond 3 hours postadministration

Distribution: V_d, apparent:

Children 2-6 years: 1.8 ± 0.8 L/kg (Blumer, 2008)

Children >6-12 years: 2.2 ± 1.7 L/kg (Blumer, 2008)

Adolescents: 1.2 ± 0.4 L/kg (Blumer, 2008)

Adults: 0.54 L/kg (Holm, 2004)

Protein binding: ~93%

Metabolism: Hepatic methylation and hydroxylation via CYP3A4 (~60%), CYP2C9 (~22%), CYP1A2 (~14%), CYP2D6 (~3%), and CYP2C19 (~3%) to three inactive metabolites

Bioavailability: 70% (Holm, 2004)

Half-life elimination:

Children 2-6 years: Tablet (immediate release): 1.8 hours (Blumer, 2008)

Children >6 years and Adolescents: Tablet (immediate release): 2.3 hours (Blumer, 2008)

Adults:

Spray (Zolpimist): ~3 hours (range: 1.7-8.4 hours)

Sublingual tablet (Edluar, Intermezzo): ~3 hours (range: 1.4-6.7 hours)

Tablet (immediate release, extended release): ~2.5 hours (range: 1.4-4.5 hours); Cirrhosis: 9.9 hours (range: 4.1-25.8 hours)

Time to peak serum concentration:

Children 2-6 years: Tablet (immediate release): 0.9 hours (Blumer, 2008)

Children >6-12 years: Tablet (immediate release): 1.1 hours (Blumer, 2008)

Adolescents: Tablet (immediate release): 1.3 hours (Blumer, 2008)

Adults:

Spray (Zolpimist): ~0.9 hours

Sublingual tablet:

Edluar: ~1.4 hours; with food: ~1.8 hours

Intermezzo: 0.6-1.3 hours; with food: ~3 hours

Tablet: Immediate release: 1.6 hours; with food: 2.2 hours; Extended release: 1.5 hours; with food: 4 hours

Elimination: Urine (48% to 67%, primarily as metabolites); feces (29% to 42%, primarily as metabolites)

Clearance, apparent:

Children and Adolescents (Blumer, 2008):

Children 2-6 years: 11.7 ± 7.9 mL/minute/kg

Children >6-12 years: 9.7 ± 10.3 mL/minute/kg

Adolescents: 4.8 ± 2 mL/minute/kg

Adults: Intermezzo: Males: 4 mL/minute/kg; Females: 2.7 mL/minute/kg

Dosing: Usual Note: The lowest effective dose should be used; higher doses may be more likely to impair next-morning activities.

Children and Adolescents ≤17 years: **Insomnia:** Oral: Limited data available; efficacy results variable and have **not** been demonstrated in randomized placebo-controlled trials. An open-label, dose escalation pharmacokinetic evaluation showed zolpidem was well-tolerated in pediatric patients 2-18 years of age and recommended a dose of 0.25 mg/kg at bedtime for evaluation in future efficacy trials (Blumer, 2008). A single case report

describes an 18-month-old infant who was effectively treated with zolpidem for primary insomnia (Bhat, 2008). However, zolpidem has **not** been shown to be effective in a randomized placebo-controlled trial (n=201) of children aged 6-17 years with ADHD-associated insomnia; zolpidem 0.25 mg/kg/dose (maximum dose: 10 mg) administered nightly did **not** decrease sleep latency; in addition, hallucinations occurred in 7.4% of patients (Blumer, 2009). A comparative, randomized controlled trial of zolpidem and haloperidol in pediatric burn patients (n=40, mean age: 9.4 ± 0.7 years) showed zolpidem dosed at 0.5 mg/kg nightly for one week (maximum dose: 20 mg) minimally increased Stage 3/4 sleep and REM but not total sleep time; the authors no longer use zolpidem to try to improve sleep in their pediatric burn patients (Armour, 2008).

Adolescents ≥18 years and Adults: **Insomnia:** Oral:

Immediate release tablet, spray: 5 mg (females) or 5-10 mg (males) immediately before bedtime; maximum dose: 10 mg

Extended release tablet: 6.25 mg (females) or 6.25-12.5 mg (males) immediately before bedtime; maximum dose: 12.5 mg

Sublingual tablet:

Edluar: 5 mg (females) or 5-10 mg (males) immediately before bedtime; maximum dose: 10 mg daily

Intermezzo: **Note:** Should be taken if patient awakens in middle of night, has difficulty returning to sleep, and has at least 4 hours left before waking.

Females: 1.75 mg once per night as needed; maximum dose: 1.75 mg/night

Males: 3.5 mg once per night as needed; maximum dose: 3.5 mg/night

Dosage adjustment with concomitant CNS depressants: Females and males: 1.75 mg once per night as needed; dose adjustment of concomitant CNS depressant(s) may be necessary

Dosing adjustment for renal impairment: Adults: There are no dosage adjustments provided in manufacturer's labeling; however, some zolpidem labeling recommends monitoring patients with renal impairment closely.

Dosing adjustment for hepatic impairment: Adults:

Immediate release tablet, spray: 5 mg immediately before bedtime

Extended release tablet: 6.25 mg immediately before bedtime

Sublingual tablet:

Edluar: 5 mg immediately before bedtime

Intermezzo: Females and males: 1.75 mg once per night as needed. **Note:** Take only if ≥4 hours left before waking.

Administration

All formulations (excluding Intermezzo): Administer immediately before bedtime due to rapid onset of action. For faster sleep onset, do not administer with (or immediately after) a meal.

Sublingual tablets (Edluar, Intermezzo): Examine blister-pack before use; do not use if blisters are broken, torn, or missing. Separate individual blisters at perforation; peel off top layer of paper; push tablet through foil. Place under the tongue and allow to disintegrate; do not swallow or administer with water. Intermezzo should be taken in bed if patient awakens in the middle of the night and has at least 4 hours left before waking.

Oral spray (Zolpimist): Spray directly into the mouth over the tongue. Prior to initial use, pump should be primed by spraying 5 times. If pump is not used for at least 14 days, reprime pump with 1 spray.

Extended release tablets (Ambien CR): Swallow whole; do not divide, crush, or chew.

Monitoring Parameters Daytime alertness; respiratory rate; behavior profile

Test Interactions Increased aminotransferase [ALT/AST], bilirubin (S); decreased RAI uptake

Controlled Substance C-IV

Dosage Forms Excipient information presented when available (limited, particularly for generics); consult specific product labeling.

Solution, Oral, as tartrate:
Zolpimist: 5 mg/actuation (7.7 mL) [contains benzoic acid, propylene glycol; cherry flavor]

Tablet, Oral, as tartrate:
Ambien: 5 mg [contains fd&c red #40, polysorbate 80]
Ambien: 10 mg
Generic: 5 mg, 10 mg

Tablet Extended Release, Oral, as tartrate:
Ambien CR: 6.25 mg
Ambien CR: 12.5 mg [contains fd&c blue #2 (indigotine)]
Generic: 6.25 mg, 12.5 mg

Tablet Sublingual, Sublingual, as tartrate:
Edluar: 5 mg, 10 mg [contains saccharin sodium]
Intermezzo: 1.75 mg, 3.5 mg

References

Armour A, Gottschlich MM, Khoury J, et al, "A Randomized, Controlled Prospective Trial of Zolpidem and Haloperidol for Use as Sleeping Agents in Pediatric Burn Patients," *J Burn Care Res*, 2008, 29 (1):238-47.

Bhat T, Pallikaleth SJ, and Shah N, "Primary Insomnia Treated With Zolpidem in an 18-Month Old Child," *Indian J Psychiatry*, 2008,50 (1):59-60.

Blumer JL, Findling RL, Shih WJ, et al, "Controlled Clinical Trial of Zolpidem for the Treatment of Insomnia Associated With Attention-Deficit/Hyperactivity Disorder in Children 6 to 17 Years of Age," *Pediatrics*, 2009, 123(5):e770-6.

Blumer JL, Reed MD, Steinberg F, et al, "Potential Pharmacokinetic Basis for Zolpidem Dosing in Children With Sleep Difficulties," *Clin Pharmacol Ther*, 2008, 83(4):551-8.

Holm KJ, Goa KL. Zolpidem: An update of its pharmacology, therapeutic efficacy and tolerability in the treatment of insomnia. *Drugs*. 2000;59(4):865-889.

Juric S, Newport DJ, Ritchie JC, et al, "Zolpidem (Ambien) in Pregnancy: Placental Passage and Outcome," *Arch Womens Ment Health*, 2009, 12(6):441-6.

Wang LH, Lin HC, Lin CC, et al, "Increased Risk of Adverse Pregnancy Outcomes in Women Receiving Zolpidem During Pregnancy," *Clin Pharmacol Ther*, 2010, 88(3):369-74.

Wikner BN and Källén B, "Are Hypnotic Benzodiazepine Receptor Agonists Teratogenic in Humans?" *J Clin Psychopharmacol*, 2011, 31(3):356-9.

◆ **Zolpidem Tartrate** see Zolpidem on page 2182

◆ **Zolpimist** see Zolpidem on page 2182

◆ **Zolvit® [DSC]** see Hydrocodone and Acetaminophen on page 1027

◆ **Zonalon** see Doxepin (Topical) on page 717

◆ **Zonalon (Can)** see Doxepin (Systemic) on page 715

◆ **Zonalon® (Can)** see Doxepin (Topical) on page 717

◆ **Zonegran** see Zonisamide on page 2185

Zonisamide (zoe NIS a mide)

Medication Safety Issues
Sound-alike/look-alike issues:
Zonegran® may be confused with SINEquan®
Zonisamide may be confused with lacosamide

Related Information
Safe Handling of Hazardous Drugs on page 2419

Brand Names: U.S. Zonegran

Therapeutic Category Anticonvulsant, Miscellaneous

Generic Availability (U.S.) Yes

Use Adjunctive treatment of partial seizures (FDA approved in ages >16 years and adults); has been used investigationally for the treatment of generalized epilepsies including, generalized tonic-clonic seizures, absence seizures, infantile spasms, myoclonic epilepsies, and Lennox-Gastaut syndrome (Leppik, 1999; Oommen, 1999)

Medication Guide Available Yes

Pregnancy Risk Factor C

Pregnancy Considerations Teratogenic effects were observed in animal reproduction studies; therefore, zonisamide is classified as pregnancy category C. Zonisamide crosses the placenta and can be detected in the newborn following delivery. Although adverse fetal events have been reported, the risk of teratogenic effects following maternal use of zonisamide in not clearly defined. Other agents may be preferred until additional data is available. Newborns should be monitored for transient metabolic acidosis after birth. Zonisamide clearance may increase in the second trimester of pregnancy, requiring dosage adjustment. Women of childbearing potential are advised to use effective contraception during therapy.

Patients exposed to zonisamide during pregnancy are encouraged to enroll themselves into the AED Pregnancy Registry by calling 1-888-233-2334. Additional information is available at http://www.aedpregnancyregistry.org.

Breast-Feeding Considerations Zonisamide is excreted into breast milk in concentrations similar to those in the maternal plasma and has been detected in the plasma of a nursing infant. According to the manufacturer, the decision to continue or discontinue breast-feeding during therapy should take into account the risk of exposure to the infant and the benefits of treatment to the mother.

Contraindications Hypersensitivity to zonisamide, sulfonamides, or any component

Warnings Hazardous agent; use appropriate precautions for handling and disposal (NIOSH, 2012). Zonisamide is a sulfonamide; although rare, severe, and life-threatening sulfonamide reactions may occur (eg, Stevens-Johnson syndrome, toxic epidermal necrolysis, aplastic anemia, agranulocytosis, other blood dyscrasias, and fulminant hepatic necrosis); discontinue zonisamide in patients with signs of hypersensitivity reaction or other serious reactions; consider discontinuation of zonisamide in any patient who develops a rash or monitor very closely; deaths due to serious rashes have been reported; rashes usually appear within 2-16 weeks of starting therapy.

Use may be associated with the development of hyperchloremic, non-anion gap, metabolic acidosis (generally dose-dependent); predisposing conditions or therapies include renal disease, severe respiratory disease, diarrhea, surgery, ketogenic diet, and other medications (such as acetazolamide or topiramate). Pediatric patients may also be at an increased risk and may have more severe metabolic acidosis. Serum bicarbonate should be monitored prior to initiation and during therapy; if metabolic acidosis occurs, consider decreasing the dose or discontinuing use with appropriate dose tapering. If use continues despite acidosis, alkali treatment should be considered. Untreated metabolic acidosis may increase the risk of developing nephrolithiasis, nephrocalcinosis, osteomalacia (or rickets in children), or osteoporosis; pediatric patients may also have decreased growth rates.

Oligohydrosis (decreased sweating) and hyperthermia have been reported in 40 pediatric patients; many cases occurred after exposure to elevated environmental temperatures; some cases resulted in heat stroke requiring hospitalization; pediatric patients may be at an increased risk; monitor patients, especially pediatric patients, for decreased sweating and hyperthermia, especially in warm or hot weather; use zonisamide with caution in patients receiving drugs that predispose to heat-related disorders (eg, anticholinergic agents, carbonic anhydrase inhibitors); safety and efficacy in pediatric patients <16 years of age has not been established.

Do not abruptly discontinue therapy; abrupt withdrawal may precipitate seizures; withdraw gradually to lessen chance for increased seizure frequency (unless a more rapid withdrawal is required due to safety concerns). CNS ▶

adverse effects may occur including fatigue or somnolence, psychiatric symptoms (eg, depression, psychosis), and cognitive symptoms [difficulty concentrating, speech or language problems (especially word-finding difficulties), and psychomotor slowing]; fatigue and somnolence usually occur within the first month of starting therapy, most commonly at higher doses (eg, in adults at doses of 300-500 mg/day). Patients should be cautioned about performing tasks which require mental alertness (eg, operating machinery or driving).

Antiepileptic drugs (AEDs) increase the risk of suicidal behavior and ideation in patients receiving these medications for any indication. Pooled analyses of placebo-controlled trials involving 11 different AEDs (regardless of indication) showed a twofold increased risk of suicidal thoughts or behavior (estimated incidence rate: 0.43% in AED treated patients compared to 0.24% of patients receiving placebo); increased risk was observed as early as 1 week after initiation of AED and continued through duration of trials (most trials ≤24 weeks); risk did not vary significantly by age (age range: 5–100 years). Consider risks and benefits of AEDs before prescribing. Monitor all patients receiving an AED for emergence of suicidal thoughts or behavior, thoughts of self-harm, any unusual changes in behavior or mood, or the emergence or worsening of depressive symptoms; notify healthcare provider immediately if symptoms or concerning behavior occur. **Note:** The FDA requires a Medication Guide for all antiepileptic drugs informing patients of this risk.

Precautions Use with caution in patients with renal or hepatic dysfunction; do not use in patients with GFR <50 mL/minute; zonisamide may cause kidney stones (ensure patients have adequate fluid intake); zonisamide may decrease GFR and increase serum creatinine and BUN; discontinue therapy in patients who develop acute renal failure or a persistent significant increase in serum creatinine or BUN. In children, agitation, anxiety, ataxia, and behavior disorders have been reported (Kimura, 1994).

Adverse Reactions

Central nervous system: Agitation/irritability, anxiety, ataxia, concentration decreased, confusion, depression, difficulty in verbal expression, dizziness fatigue, headache, hyperesthesia, incoordination, insomnia, memory impairment, mental slowing, nervousness, schizophrenic/schizophreniform behavior, seizure, somnolence, speech disorders, status epilepticus, tiredness, tremor

Dermatologic: Bruising, pruritus, rash

Gastrointestinal: Abdominal pain, anorexia, constipation, diarrhea, dyspepsia, diarrhea, dyspepsia, nausea, taste perversion, vomiting, weight loss, xerostomia

Neuromuscular & skeletal: Abnormal gait, paresthesia, weakness

Ocular: Amblyopia, diplopia, nystagmus

Otic: Tinnitus

Renal: Kidney stones

Respiratory: Cough increased, pharyngitis, rhinitis

Rare (but important or life threatening symptoms): Agranulocytosis, allergic reaction, alopecia, amenorrhea, aplastic anemia, apnea, arthritis, atrial fibrillation, bladder calculus, bradycardia, cerebrovascular accident, cholangitis, cholecystitis, cholestatic jaundice, colitis, deafness, duodenitis, encephalopathy, fecal incontinence, gingivitis, GI ulcer, glaucoma, heart failure, hematuria, hemoptysis, hirsutism, hyper-/hypotension, hyperthermia, hypoglycemia, hyponatremia, immunodeficiency, impotence, iritis, leukopenia, lupus erythematosus, lymphadenopathy, mastitis, menorrhagia, metabolic acidosis, neuropathy, oculogyric crisis, oligohidrosis (children), pancreatitis, photophobia, pulmonary embolus, rectal hemorrhage, Stevens-Johnson syndrome, stroke, suicidal behavior/ideation, syncope, thrombocytopenia,

thrombophlebitis, toxic epidermal necrolysis, urinary incontinence, ventricular extrasystoles

Drug Interactions

Metabolism/Transport Effects Substrate of CYP2C19 (minor), CYP3A4 (major); **Note:** Assignment of Major/Minor substrate status based on clinically relevant drug interaction potential

Avoid Concomitant Use

Avoid concomitant use of Zonisamide with any of the following: Azelastine (Nasal); Carbonic Anhydrase Inhibitors; Conivaptan; Fusidic Acid (Systemic); Paraldehyde; Thalidomide

Increased Effect/Toxicity

Zonisamide may increase the levels/effects of: Alcohol (Ethyl); Alpha-/Beta-Agonists (Indirect-Acting); Amphetamines; Anticonvulsants (Barbiturate); Anticonvulsants (Hydantoin); Azelastine (Nasal); Buprenorphine; Carbonic Anhydrase Inhibitors; CNS Depressants; Flecainide; Hydrocodone; Memantine; MetFORMIN; Methotrimeprazine; Metyrosine; Mirtazapine; Paraldehyde; Pramipexole; QuiNIDine; ROPINIRole; Rotigotine; Selective Serotonin Reuptake Inhibitors; Thalidomide; Zolpidem

The levels/effects of Zonisamide may be increased by: Brimonidine (Topical); Cannabis; Ceritinib; Conivaptan; CYP3A4 Inhibitors (Moderate); CYP3A4 Inhibitors (Strong); Dasatinib; Doxylamine; Dronabinol; Droperidol; Fusidic Acid (Systemic); HydrOXYzine; Ivacaftor; Kava Kava; Luliconazole; Magnesium Sulfate; Methotrimeprazine; Mifepristone; Nabilone; Perampanel; Rufinamide; Salicylates; Simeprevir; Sodium Oxybate; Stiripentol; Tapentadol; Tetrahydrocannabinol

Decreased Effect

Zonisamide may decrease the levels/effects of: Lithium; Methenamine

The levels/effects of Zonisamide may be decreased by: Bosentan; CYP3A4 Inducers (Strong); Dabrafenib; Deferasirox; Fosphenytoin; Ketorolac (Nasal); Ketorolac (Systemic); Mefloquine; Mitotane; Orlistat; PHENobarbital; Phenytoin; Siltuximab; St Johns Wort; Tocilizumab

Food Interactions Food delays time to maximum concentration, but does not affect bioavailability. Management: Administer without regard to meals.

Stability Hazardous agent; use appropriate precautions for handling and disposal (NIOSH, 2012). Store at controlled room temperature 25°C (77°C). Protect from moisture and light.

Mechanism of Action The exact mechanism of action is not known. May stabilize neuronal membranes and suppress neuronal hypersynchronization through action at sodium and calcium channels. Does not affect GABA activity.

Pharmacokinetics (Adult data unless noted)

Absorption: Oral: Rapid and complete

Distribution: V_d (apparent): 1.45 L/kg; highly concentrated in erythrocytes

Protein binding: 40%

Metabolism: Hepatic; undergoes acetylation to form N-acetyl zonisamide and reduction via cytochrome P450 isoenzyme CYP3A4 to 2-sulfamoylacetylphenol (SMAP); SMAP then undergoes conjugation with glucuronide

Half-life: ~63 hours (range: 50-68 hours)

Time to peak serum concentration: 2-6 hours

Elimination: Urine: 62% (35% as unchanged drug, 15% as N-acetyl zonisamide, 50% as SMAP glucuronide); feces (3%); **Note:** Of the dose recovered in Japanese patients, 28% is as unchanged drug, 52% is as N-acetyl zonisamide, and 19% is as SMAP glucuronide (Glauser, 2002)

Dosing: Usual Oral:

Infants and Children: In a review article of 20 Japanese pediatric studies, the following doses were recommended

(Glauser, 2002): Initial: 1-2 mg/kg/day given in two divided doses/day; increase dose in increments of 0.5-1 mg/kg/day every 2 weeks; usual dose: 5-8 mg/kg/day.

Higher initial and maximum doses have been recommended by others (Leppik, 1999; Oommen, 1999): Initial: 2-4 mg/kg/day given in two divided doses/day; titrate dose upwards if needed every 2 weeks; usual dose: 4-8 mg/kg/day; maximum dose: 12 mg/kg/day

Infantile spasms: Several studies used a faster titration of zonisamide to control infantile spasms. Suzuki treated 11 newly diagnosed infants (mean age: ~6 months) with zonisamide monotherapy starting at doses of 3-5 mg/kg/day given in 2 divided doses/day; doses were increased every 4th day until seizures were controlled or a maximum dose of 10 mg/kg/day was attained; 4 of 11 patients responded at doses of 4-5 mg/kg/day (Suzuki, 1997). Yanai treated 27 newly diagnosed infantile spasm patients with zonisamide add-on or monotherapy starting at doses of 2-4 mg/kg/day given in 2 divided doses/day; doses were increased by 2-5 mg/kg every 2-4 days until seizures were controlled or a maximum of 10-20 mg/kg/day was attained; 9 of 27 patients responded at a mean effective dose of 7.8 mg/kg/day (range: 5-12.5 mg/kg/day); non-responders received doses of 8-20 mg/kg/day (mean: 10.8 mg/kg/day) (Yania, 1999). Suzuki treated 54 newly diagnosed infants (11 of which were previously reported) with zonisamide monotherapy starting at doses of 3-4 mg/kg/day given in 2 divided doses; doses were increased every 4th day until seizures were controlled or a maximum dose of 10-13 mg/kg/day was attained; 11 of 54 infants responded at a mean effective dose of 7.2 mg/kg/day (range: 4-12 mg/kg/day); the majority of infants who responded did so at a dose of 4-8 mg/kg/day and within 1-2 weeks of starting therapy (Suzuki, 2001). Further studies are needed.

Adolescents >16 years and Adults: Initial: 100 mg once daily; dose may be increased to 200 mg/day after 2 weeks; further increases in dose should be made in increments of 100 mg/day and only after a minimum of 2 weeks between adjustments; usual effective dose: 100-600 mg/day. **Note:** There is no evidence of increased benefit with doses >400 mg/day. Steady-state serum concentrations fluctuate 27% with once daily dosing, and 14% with twice daily dosing; patients may benefit from divided doses given twice daily (Leppik, 1999)

Dosage adjustment in renal impairment: Slower dosage titration and more frequent monitoring are recommended. Do not use if GFR <50 mL/minute. Marked renal impairment (CrCl <20 mL/minute) was associated with a 35% increase in AUC.

Dosage adjustment in hepatic impairment: Slower titration and frequent monitoring are indicated.

Administration Hazardous agent; use appropriate precautions for handling and disposal (NIOSH, 2012). May be administered without regard to meals; swallow capsule whole; do not crush, chew, or break capsule.

Monitoring Parameters Seizure frequency, duration, and severity; symptoms of CNS adverse effects; skin rash; periodic BUN and serum creatinine; serum bicarbonate prior to initiation and periodically during therapy; serum electrolytes, including chloride, phosphorus, and calcium; alkaline phosphatase; serum albumin; symptoms of metabolic acidosis; monitor patients, especially pediatric patients, for decreased sweating and hyperthermia, especially in warm or hot weather; signs and symptoms of suicidality (eg, anxiety, depression, behavior changes)

Reference Range Monitoring of plasma concentrations may be useful; proposed therapeutic range: 10-20 mcg/mL; patients may benefit from higher concentrations

(ie, up to 30 mcg/mL), but concentrations >30 mcg/mL have been associated with adverse effects (Leppik, 1999; Oommen, 1999)

Dosage Forms Excipient information presented when available (limited, particularly for generics); consult specific product labeling.

Capsule, Oral:
  Zonegran: 25 mg, 100 mg
  Generic: 25 mg, 50 mg, 100 mg

Extemporaneous Preparations Hazardous agent; use appropriate precautions during preparation and disposal.

A 10 mg/mL suspension may be made using capsules and either simple syrup or methylcellulose 0.5%. Empty contents of ten 100 mg capsules into glass mortar. Reduce to a fine powder and add a small amount of Simple Syrup, NF and mix to a uniform paste; mix while adding the chosen vehicle in incremental proportions to **almost** 100 mL; transfer to an amber calibrated plastic bottle, rinse mortar with vehicle, and add quantity of vehicle sufficient to make 100 mL. Label "shake well" and "refrigerate". When using simple syrup vehicle, stable 28 days at room temperature or refrigerated (preferred). When using methylcellulose vehicle, stable 7 days at room temperature or 28 days refrigerated. **Note:** Although no visual evidence of microbial growth was observed, storage under refrigeration would be recommended to minimize microbial contamination.

Abobo CV, Wei B, and Liang D, "Stability of Zonisamide in Extemporaneously Compounded Oral Suspensions," *Am J Health Syst Pharm*, 2009, 66(12):1105-9.

References

Glauser TA and Pellock JM, "Zonisamide in Pediatric Epilepsy: Review of the Japanese Experience," *J Child Neurol*, 2002, 17(2):87-96.

Kawada K, Itoh S, Kusaka T, et al, "Pharmacokinetics of Zonisamide in Perinatal Period," *Brain Dev*, 2002, 24(2):95-7.

Kimura S, "Zonisamide-Induced Behavior Disorder in Two Children," *Epilepsia*, 1994, 35(2):403-5.

Leppik IE, "Zonisamide," *Epilepsia*, 1999, 40(Suppl 5):S23-9.

National Institute for Occupational Safety and Health (NIOSH), "NIOSH List of Antineoplastic and Other Hazardous Drugs in Healthcare Settings 2012." Available at http://www.cdc.gov/niosh/docs/2012-150/pdfs/2012-150.pdf. Accessed January 21, 2013.

Oommen KJ and Mathews S, "Zonisamide: A New Antiepileptic Drug," *Clin Neuropharmacol*, 1999, 22(4):192-200.

Suzuki Y, Nagai T, Ono J, et al, "Zonisamide Monotherapy in Newly Diagnosed Infantile Spasms," *Epilepsia*, 1997, 38(9):1035-8.

Suzuki Y, "Zonisamide in West Syndrome," *Brain Dev*, 2001, 23 (7):658-61.

Yanai S, Hanai T, and Narazaki O, "Treatment of Infantile Spasms With Zonisamide," *Brain Dev*, 1999, 21(3):157-61.

◆ **Zorbtive** *see* Somatropin *on page 1920*

◆ **Zortress** *see* Everolimus *on page 821*

◆ **Zorvolex** *see* Diclofenac (Systemic) *on page 645*

◆ **Zostrix® [OTC]** *see* Capsaicin *on page 367*

◆ **Zostrix® (Can)** *see* Capsaicin *on page 367*

◆ **Zostrix® Diabetic Foot Pain [OTC]** *see* Capsaicin *on page 367*

◆ **Zostrix®-HP [OTC]** *see* Capsaicin *on page 367*

◆ **Zostrix® H.P. (Can)** *see* Capsaicin *on page 367*

◆ **Zosyn** *see* Piperacillin and Tazobactam *on page 1679*

◆ **Zovirax** *see* Acyclovir (Systemic) *on page 63*

◆ **Zovirax** *see* Acyclovir (Topical) *on page 68*

◆ **Z-Pak** *see* Azithromycin (Systemic) *on page 247*

◆ **Zubsolv** *see* Buprenorphine and Naloxone *on page 324*

◆ **Zuplenz®** *see* Ondansetron *on page 1544*

◆ **Zuplenz** *see* Ondansetron *on page 1544*

◆ **Zyban** *see* BuPROPion *on page 327*

◆ **Zydone® [DSC]** *see* Hydrocodone and Acetaminophen *on page* 1027

◆ **Zyflo** *see* Zileuton *on page* 2173

◆ **Zyflo CR** *see* Zileuton *on page* 2173

◆ **Zyloprim** *see* Allopurinol *on page* 97

◆ **ZYM-Amlodipine (Can)** *see* AmLODIPine *on page* 135

◆ **Zymar (Can)** *see* Gatifloxacin *on page* 958

◆ **Zymaxid** *see* Gatifloxacin *on page* 958

◆ **ZYM-Carvedilol (Can)** *see* Carvedilol *on page* 385

◆ **ZYM-Cholestyramine-Light (Can)** *see* Cholestyramine Resin *on page* 457

◆ **ZYM-Cholestyramine-Regular (Can)** *see* Cholestyramine Resin *on page* 457

◆ **ZYM-Clonazepam (Can)** *see* ClonazePAM *on page* 514

◆ **ZYM-Cyclobenzaprine (Can)** *see* Cyclobenzaprine *on page* 558

◆ **ZYM-Fluconazole (Can)** *see* Fluconazole *on page* 877

◆ **ZYM-Fluoxetine (Can)** *see* FLUoxetine *on page* 901

◆ **ZYM-Ondansetron (Can)** *see* Ondansetron *on page* 1544

◆ **ZYM-Pravastatin (Can)** *see* Pravastatin *on page* 1720

◆ **ZYM-Simvastatin (Can)** *see* Simvastatin *on page* 1892

◆ **ZYM-Sotalol (Can)** *see* Sotalol *on page* 1925

◆ **ZYM-Topiramate (Can)** *see* Topiramate *on page* 2046

◆ **ZYM-Trazodone (Can)** *see* TraZODone *on page* 2065

◆ **Zyncof [OTC]** *see* Guaifenesin and Dextromethorphan *on page* 987

◆ **ZyPREXA** *see* OLANZapine *on page* 1525

◆ **Zyprexa (Can)** *see* OLANZapine *on page* 1525

◆ **Zyprexa Intramuscular (Can)** *see* OLANZapine *on page* 1525

◆ **ZyPREXA Relprevv** *see* OLANZapine *on page* 1525

◆ **Zyprexa Zydis** *see* OLANZapine *on page* 1525

◆ **ZyPREXA Zydis** *see* OLANZapine *on page* 1525

◆ **ZyrTEC Allergy [OTC]** *see* Cetirizine *on page* 431

◆ **ZyrTEC Allergy Childrens [OTC]** *see* Cetirizine *on page* 431

◆ **ZyrTEC Childrens Allergy [OTC]** *see* Cetirizine *on page* 431

◆ **ZyrTEC Childrens Hives Relief [OTC]** *see* Cetirizine *on page* 431

◆ **ZyrTEC Hives Relief [OTC]** *see* Cetirizine *on page* 431

◆ **ZyrTEC Itchy Eye [OTC]** *see* Ketotifen (Ophthalmic) *on page* 1185

◆ **Zytram XL (Can)** *see* TraMADol *on page* 2060

◆ **Zyvox** *see* Linezolid *on page* 1251

◆ **Zyvoxam (Can)** *see* Linezolid *on page* 1251

◆ **ZzzQuil [OTC]** *see* DiphenhydrAMINE (Systemic) *on page* 673

APPENDIX TABLE OF CONTENTS

Cardiology / Pulmonary
  Emergency Drip Calculations..2191
  Newborn Resuscitation Algorithm...2193
  Maternal Cardiac Arrest...2194
  Pediatric ALS (PALS) Algorithms...2195
  Adult ACLS Algorithms..2198
  Normal Pediatric Heart Rates...2201
  Normal Respiratory Rates..2203
  Measuring Pediatric Blood Pressure...2204
  Hypotension, Definitions by Age Group...2206
  Hypertension, Classification by Age Group 2207
  Blood Pressure in Premature Infants, Normal..2208
  Blood Pressure Measurements, Age-Specific Percentiles...2209
  New York Heart Association (NYHA) Classification of Functional Capacity of Patients With Diseases of the Heart,
    1994 Revisions..2217
  World Health Organization (WHO) Functional Classification of Pulmonary Hypertension...............2218
Comparative Drug Charts
  Antidepressant Agents...2219
  Corticosteroids Systemic Equivalencies...2222
  Inhaled Corticosteroids..2223
  Topical Corticosteroids...2224
  Immune Globulin Product Comparison...2226
  Multivitamin Product Table..2227
  Opioid Conversion Table...2242
Conversion Tables
  Apothecary/Metric Equivalents..2244
  Pounds/Kilograms Conversion...2245
  Temperature Conversion...2246
Cytochrome P450 Enzymes and Drug Metabolism
  Cytochrome P450 Enzymes: Substrates, Inhibitors, and Inducers...2247
Dermatology
  Management of Drug Extravasations..2255
  Burn Management..2265
Endocrinology
  Contraceptive Comparison Table...2266
Gastroenterology and Nutrition
  Enteral Nutrition Product Comparison..2274
  Fluid and Electrolyte Requirements in Children..2308
  H. pylori Treatment in Pediatric Patients..2311
  Pediatric Parenteral Nutrition..2312
Growth and Development
  Growth Charts...2317
  Ideal Body Weight Calculation..2323
  Body Surface Area of Children and Adults...2324
  Average Weights and Surface Areas...2325
  Physical Development..2326
Hematology / Oncology
  Emetogenic Potential of Antineoplastic Agents in Children..2327
  Tumor Lysis Syndrome...2329
  Total Blood Volume..2333
Hepatology
  Assessment of Liver Function...2334
Hotline Numbers
  Hotline and Important Phone Numbers...2335
Infectious Diseases / Immunology
  Prevention of Infective Endocarditis..2336
  Pediatric HIV..2338
  Adult and Adolescent HIV...2348
  Perinatal HIV..2356
  Immunization Administration Recommendations...2368
  Immunization Guidelines..2373
  Skin Tests for Delayed Hypersensitivity...2383
Laboratory
  Reference Values for Children...2385
  Acid/Base Assessment...2393
  Laboratory Calculations..2394
Neonatology
  Apgar Scoring System...2396

Nephrology
    Renal Function Estimation in Adult Patients...2397
    Renal Function Estimation in Pediatric Patients..2400
Neurology
    Preprocedure Sedatives in Children.. 2402
    Coma Scales..2404
    Serotonin Syndrome... 2405
Toxicology
    Acetaminophen Serum Level Nomogram.. 2407
    Medications for Which a Single Dose May Be Fatal When Ingested by a Toddler....................................... 2408
Miscellaneous
    Controlled Substances..2409
    Milliequivalent and Millimole Calculations and Conversions...2410
    Patient Information for Disposal of Unused Medications..2412
    Pediatric Medication Administration... 2413
    Safe Handling of Hazardous Drugs... 2419
    Carbohydrate Content of Medications..2428
    Oral Medications That Should Not Be Crushed or Altered..2438
    WHO Model Formulary for Children..2448

EMERGENCY DRIP CALCULATIONS

The availability of a limited number of standard concentrations for emergency medications (eg, vasopressors) within an institution is required by The Joint Commission (JCAHO, 2004). With standardized concentrations, the equation below can be used to calculate the rate of infusion (mL/hour) for a given dose (mcg/kg/minute):

$$\text{Rate (mL/hour)} = \frac{\text{dose (mcg/kg/minute) x weight (kg) x 60 minute/hour}}{\text{concentration (mcg/mL)}}$$

If a standardized concentration delivers the dose in too low of a volume (eg, <1 mL/hour) then a lower standardized concentration (ie, more dilute) is used. If a standardized concentration delivers the dose in too high of a volume (depending on patient's size and fluid status), a higher standardized concentration (ie, more concentrated) is used.

In 2011, the Institute for Safe Medication Practices (ISMP) and the Vermont Oxford Network (VON), a group of healthcare professionals working to improve neonatal care, collaborated along with U.S. neonatal intensive care units to identify and recommend standard concentrations for use in neonatal patients. The following table represents their recommendations for emergency medications. For a complete list of all their recommended standard concentrations, go to www.ismp.org/Tools/PediatricConcentrations.pdf

ISMP/VON Recommended Standardized Neonatal Concentrations for Emergency Medications

Drug	Concentration (mcg/mL)
Alprostadil	10
DOBUTamine	2000
DOPamine	1600
EPINEPHrine	10
Norepinephrine	16

Some centers use the following pediatric standardized concentrations according to patient weight (Campbell, 1994):

Standardized Concentrations by Patient Weight

Drug	Patient Weight (kg)	Concentration (mcg/mL)
DOPamine	2 to 3 4 to 8 9 to 15 >15	200 400 800 1600
EPINEPHrine, Isoproterenol, or Norepinephrine	2 to 3 4 to 8 ≥9	5 10 20

Other centers use the following standardized concentrations depending on both patient weight and dose (Hodding, 2010):

Drug	Standardized Concentrations (mcg/mL)			
DOBUTamine	800	1600	3200	6400
DOPamine	800	1600	3200	6400
EPINEPHrine	20	40	60	120
Norepinephrine	20	40	60	120
Isoproterenol	20	40	60	120

Some centers also limit the number of standardized concentrations to only two per emergency medication (Larsen, 2005)

Drug	Standardized Concentrations (mcg/mL)	
DOBUTamine	1000	4000
DOPamine	800	3200
EPINEPHrine	8	64
Norepinephrine	8	64
Isoproterenol	8	64

An example of how different standardized concentrations are used for different patient weights and doses is given below for dopamine. Each table lists the dopamine infusion rate in mL/hour for a specific patient weight (in kg) and dose (in mcg/kg/minute) for a specific standardized concentration. The first table is for dopamine **1600** mcg/mL and the second table for **800** mcg/mL.

DOPamine Infusion Rate (mL/hour) According to Patient Weight (kg) and Dose (mcg/kg/minute) Using Standardized Concentration of 1600 mcg/mL

Weight (kg)	Dose (mcg/kg/minute)				
	5	7.5	10	15	20
2	0.4*	0.6*	0.8*	1.1	1.5
3	0.6*	0.8*	1.1	1.7	2.3
4	0.8*	1.1	1.5	2.3	3.0
5	0.9*	1.4	1.9	2.8	3.8
7	1.3	2.0	2.6	3.9	5.3
10	1.9	2.8	3.8	5.6	7.5
12	2.3	3.4	4.5	6.8	9.0
14	2.6	3.9	5.3	7.9	10.5
16	3.0	4.5	6.0	9.0	12.0
18	3.4	5.1	6.8	10.1	13.5
20	3.8	5.6	7.5	11.3	15.0
25	4.7	7.0	9.4	14.1	18.8
30	5.6	8.4	11.3	16.9	22.5
35	6.6	9.8	13.1	19.7	26.3
40	7.5	11.3	15.0	22.5	30.0
45	8.4	12.7	16.9	25.3	33.8
50	9.4	14.1	18.8	28.1	37.5

*For rates <1 mL/hour, use 800 mcg/mL concentration

DOPamine Infusion Rate (mL/hour) According to Patient Weight (kg) and Dose (mcg/kg/minute) Using Standardized Concentration of 800 mcg/mL

Weight (kg)	Dose (mcg/kg/minute)				
	5	7.5	10	15	20
2	0.8	1.1	1.5	2.3	3.0
3	1.1	1.7	2.3	3.4	4.5
4	1.5	2.3	3.0	4.5	6.0
5	1.9	2.8	3.8	5.6	7.5

BACKGROUND INFORMATION
The Joint Commission (formerly called JCAHO) and the "Rule of Six"

In its 2004 National Patient Safety Goals (NPSG), The Joint Commission (TJC) required organizations to "standardize and limit the number of drug concentrations available in the organization" to meet patient safety goal # 3 ("Improve the safety of using high-alert medications"). High-alert medications are drugs that possess a great risk of causing significant injury to patients when they are used in error. Emergency medications (eg, vasopressors) qualify as high-alert drugs.

Historically, the "Rule of Six" was used to calculate patient-specific I.V. concentrations of emergency medication infusions, so that 1 mL/hour would deliver a set mcg/kg/minute dose.

TJC has determined that using the "Rule of Six" or other methods to individualize a concentration of a high-alert drug for a specific patient (ie, use of a nonstandardized concentration) is **not** in compliance with the requirement of the above NPSG goal. In addition, the "Rule of Six" is not recommended by the Institute for Safe Medication Practices (ISMP). Limiting and standardizing the number of drug concentrations (as opposed to using the "Rule of Six") is thought to be safer and less error prone.

REFERENCES
Campbell MM, Taeubel MA, Kraus DM. Updated bedside charts for calculating pediatric doses of emergency medications. *Am J Hosp Pharm*. 1994;51 (17):2147-2152.
Hodding JH, Executive Director, Pharmacy and Nutritional Services, Long Beach Memorial Medical Center and Miller Children's Hospital, Long Beach, CA, personal correspondence, April 2010.
Joint Commission on Accreditation of Healthcare Organizations (JCAHO). 2004 national patient safety goals, frequently asked questions: updated 8/30/04. August 30, 2004.
Joint Commission on Accreditation of Healthcare Organizations (JCAHO). Transition plan from 'rule of 6'. JCAHOnline, December 2004/January 2005.
Larsen GY, Parker HB, Cash J, O'Connell M, Grant MC. Standard drug concentrations and smart-pump technology reduce continuous-medication-infusion errors in pediatric patients. *Pediatrics*. 2005;116(1):e21-e25.

NEWBORN RESUSCITATION ALGORITHM

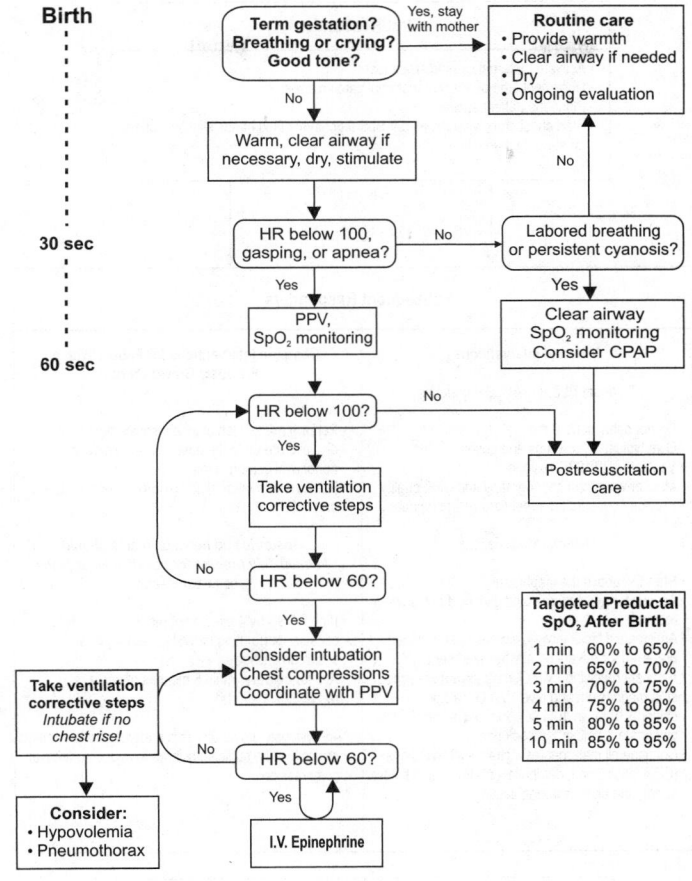

Epinephrine dose for neonatal resuscitation: I.V.: 0.01-0.03 mg/kg (0.1-0.3 mL/kg of **1:10,000** solution) every 3-5 minutes. **Note:** I.V. is the preferred neonatal route. While obtaining I.V. access, one may consider higher doses via E.T.: 0.05-0.1 mg/kg (0.5-1 mL/kg of **1:10,000** solution).

MATERNAL CARDIAC ARREST

First Responder

- Activate maternal cardiac arrest team
- Document time of onset of maternal cardiac arrest
- Place the patient supine
- Start chest compressions as per BLS algorithm; place hands slightly higher on sternum than usual

---

Subsequent Responders

Maternal Interventions

Treat per BLS and ACLS Algorithms

- Do not delay defibrillation
- Give typical ACLS drugs and doses
- Ventilate with 100% oxygen
- Monitor waveform capnography and CPR quality
- Provide post-cardiac arrest care as appropriate

Maternal Modifications

- Start I.V. above the diaphragm
- Assess for hypovolemia and give fluid bolus when required
- Anticipate difficult airway; experienced provider preferred for advanced airway placement
- If patient receiving I.V./I.O. magnesium prearrest, stop magnesium and give I.V./I.O. calcium chloride 10 mL in 10% solution, or calcium gluconate 30 mL in 10% solution
- Continue all maternal resuscitative interventions (CPR, positioning, defibrillation, drugs, and fluids) during and after cesarean section

Obstetric Interventions for Patient With an Obviously Gravid Uterus*

- Perform manual left uterine displacement (LUD) - displace uterus to the patient's left to relieve aortocaval compression
- Remove both internal and external fetal monitors if present

Obstetric and neonatal teams should immediately prepare for possible emergency cesarean section

- If no ROSC by 4 minutes of resuscitative efforts, consider performing immediate emergency cesarean section
- Aim for delivery within 5 minutes of onset of resuscitative efforts

*An obviously gravid uterus is a uterus that is deemed clinically to be sufficiently large to cause aortocaval compression

---

Search for and Treat Possible Contributing Factors (BEAU-CHOPS)

Bleeding/DIC
Embolism: Coronary/pulmonary/amniotic fluid embolism
Anesthetic complications
Uterine atony
Cardiac disease (MI/ischemia/aortic dissection/cardiomyopathy)
Hypertension/pre-eclampsia/eclampsia
Other: Differential diagnosis of standard ACLS guidelines
Placenta abruptio/previa
Sepsis

PEDIATRIC ALS (PALS) ALGORITHMS

Pediatric Bradycardia
With a Pulse and Poor Perfusion

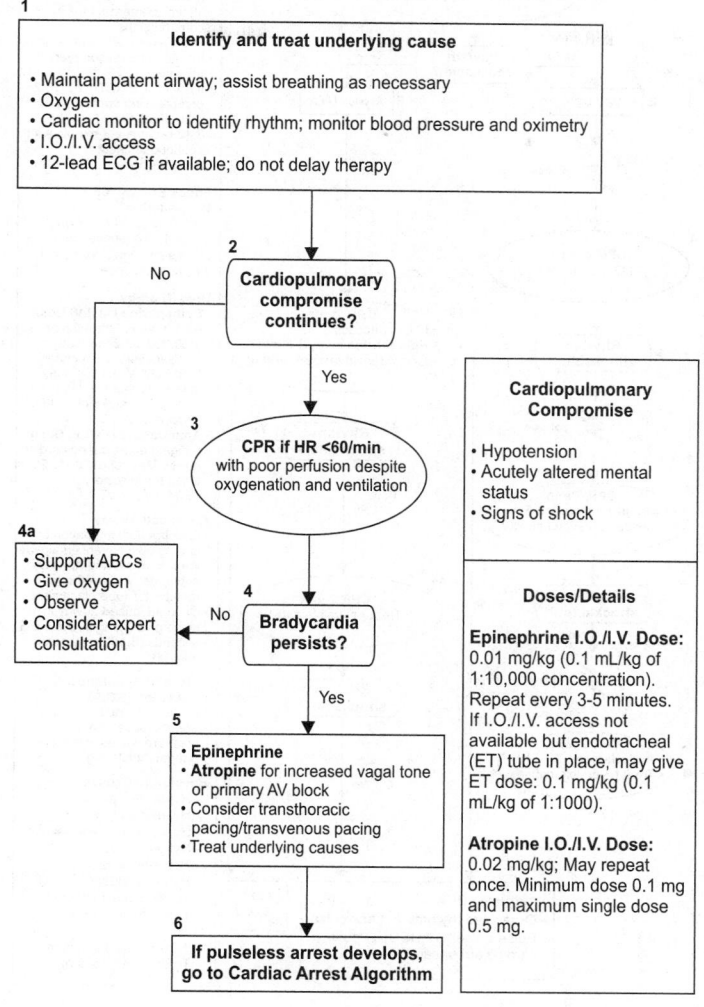

1

Identify and treat underlying cause

• Maintain patent airway; assist breathing as necessary
• Oxygen
• Cardiac monitor to identify rhythm; monitor blood pressure and oximetry
• I.O./I.V. access
• 12-lead ECG if available; do not delay therapy

2

No

Cardiopulmonary compromise continues?

Yes

3

CPR if HR <60/min with poor perfusion despite oxygenation and ventilation

4a

• Support ABCs
• Give oxygen
• Observe
• Consider expert consultation

4

No

Bradycardia persists?

Yes

5

• **Epinephrine**
• **Atropine** for increased vagal tone or primary AV block
• Consider transthoracic pacing/transvenous pacing
• Treat underlying causes

6

If pulseless arrest develops, go to Cardiac Arrest Algorithm

Cardiopulmonary Compromise

• Hypotension
• Acutely altered mental status
• Signs of shock

Doses/Details

Epinephrine I.O./I.V. Dose:
0.01 mg/kg (0.1 mL/kg of 1:10,000 concentration). Repeat every 3-5 minutes. If I.O./I.V. access not available but endotracheal (ET) tube in place, may give ET dose: 0.1 mg/kg (0.1 mL/kg of 1:1000).

Atropine I.O./I.V. Dose:
0.02 mg/kg; May repeat once. Minimum dose 0.1 mg and maximum single dose 0.5 mg.

Pediatric Cardiac Arrest

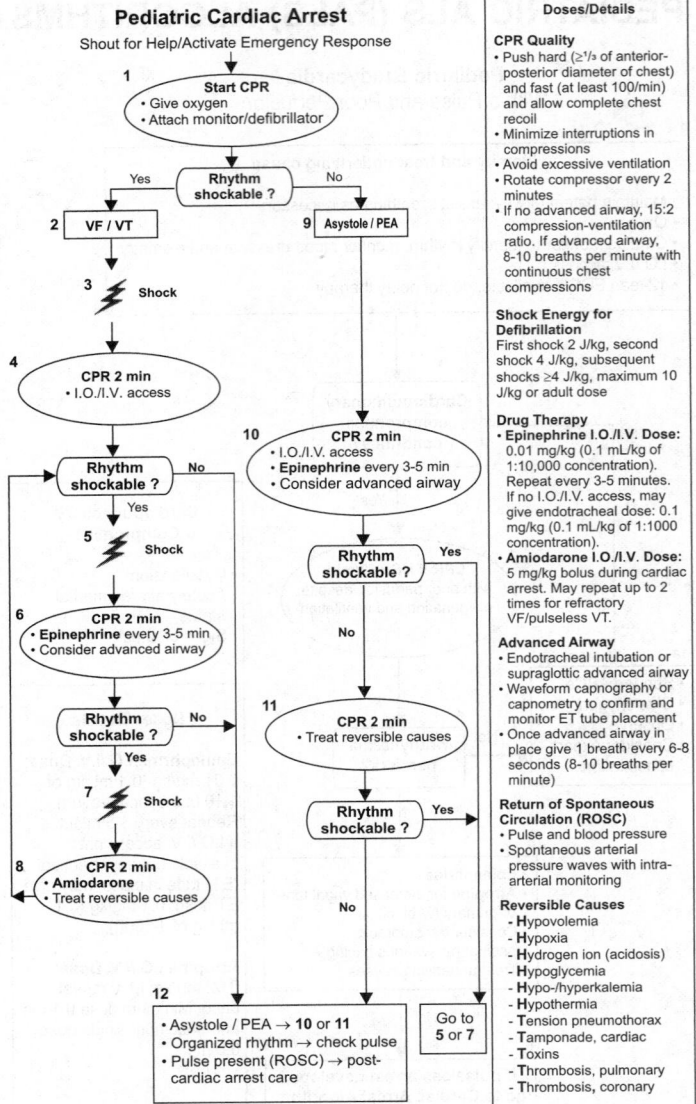

Shout for Help/Activate Emergency Response

1
Start CPR
• Give oxygen
• Attach monitor/defibrillator

Rhythm shockable ? — Yes / No

2 VF / VT

9 Asystole / PEA

3 Shock

4 CPR 2 min
• I.O./I.V. access

Rhythm shockable ? — No / Yes

5 Shock

6 CPR 2 min
• Epinephrine every 3-5 min
• Consider advanced airway

Rhythm shockable ? — No / Yes

7 Shock

8 CPR 2 min
• Amiodarone
• Treat reversible causes

10 CPR 2 min
• I.O./I.V. access
• Epinephrine every 3-5 min
• Consider advanced airway

Rhythm shockable ? — Yes / No

11 CPR 2 min
• Treat reversible causes

Rhythm shockable ? — Yes / No

12
• Asystole / PEA → **10** or **11**
• Organized rhythm → check pulse
• Pulse present (ROSC) → post-cardiac arrest care

Go to **5 or 7**

Doses/Details

CPR Quality
• Push hard (≥$^1/_3$ of anterior-posterior diameter of chest) and fast (at least 100/min) and allow complete chest recoil
• Minimize interruptions in compressions
• Avoid excessive ventilation
• Rotate compressor every 2 minutes
• If no advanced airway, 15:2 compression-ventilation ratio. If advanced airway, 8-10 breaths per minute with continuous chest compressions

Shock Energy for Defibrillation
First shock 2 J/kg, second shock 4 J/kg, subsequent shocks ≥4 J/kg, maximum 10 J/kg or adult dose

Drug Therapy
• **Epinephrine I.O./I.V. Dose:** 0.01 mg/kg (0.1 mL/kg of 1:10,000 concentration). Repeat every 3-5 minutes. If no I.O./I.V. access, may give endotracheal dose: 0.1 mg/kg (0.1 mL/kg of 1:1000 concentration).
• **Amiodarone I.O./I.V. Dose:** 5 mg/kg bolus during cardiac arrest. May repeat up to 2 times for refractory VF/pulseless VT.

Advanced Airway
• Endotracheal intubation or supraglottic advanced airway
• Waveform capnography or capnometry to confirm and monitor ET tube placement
• Once advanced airway in place give 1 breath every 6-8 seconds (8-10 breaths per minute)

Return of Spontaneous Circulation (ROSC)
• Pulse and blood pressure
• Spontaneous arterial pressure waves with intra-arterial monitoring

Reversible Causes
- **H**ypovolemia
- **H**ypoxia
- **H**ydrogen ion (acidosis)
- **H**ypoglycemia
- **H**ypo-/hyperkalemia
- **H**ypothermia
- **T**ension pneumothorax
- **T**amponade, cardiac
- **T**oxins
- **T**hrombosis, pulmonary
- **T**hrombosis, coronary

Pediatric Tachycardia
With a Pulse and Poor Perfusion

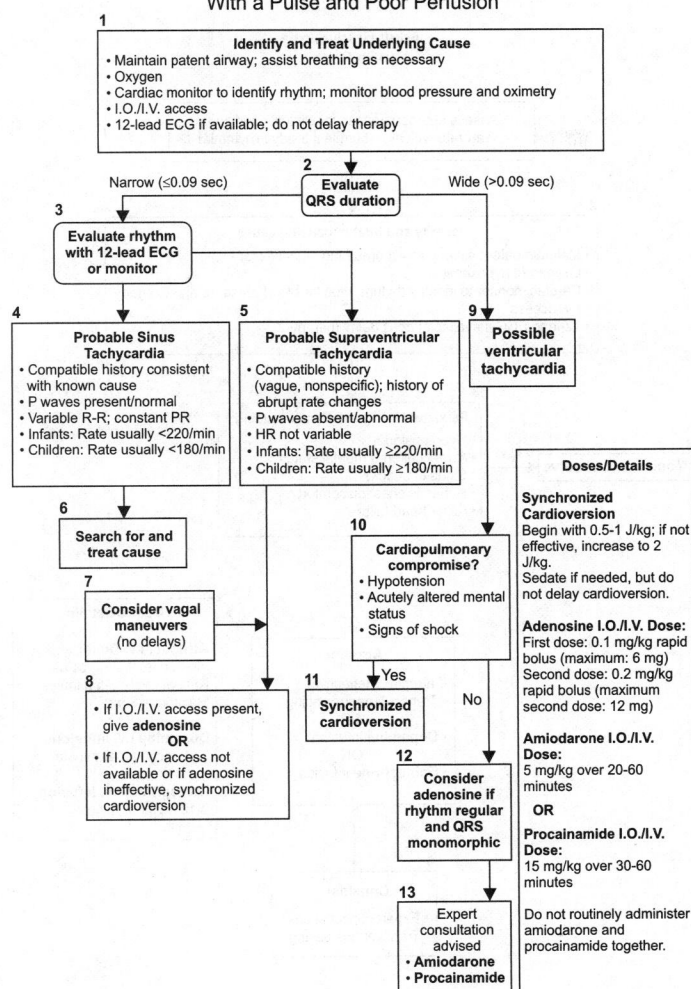

Reprinted with permission: 2010 American Heart Association guidelines for cardiopulmonary resuscitation and emergency cardiovascular care – Part 14: pediatric advanced life support. *Circulation*. 2010;122(Suppl 3):S876-S908. ©2010 American Heart Association, Inc.
See http://circ.ahajournals.org/cgi/content/full/122/18_suppl_3/S876.
All requests to use this information must come through the AHA.

ADULT ACLS ALGORITHMS

Adult Bradycardia
(With Pulse)

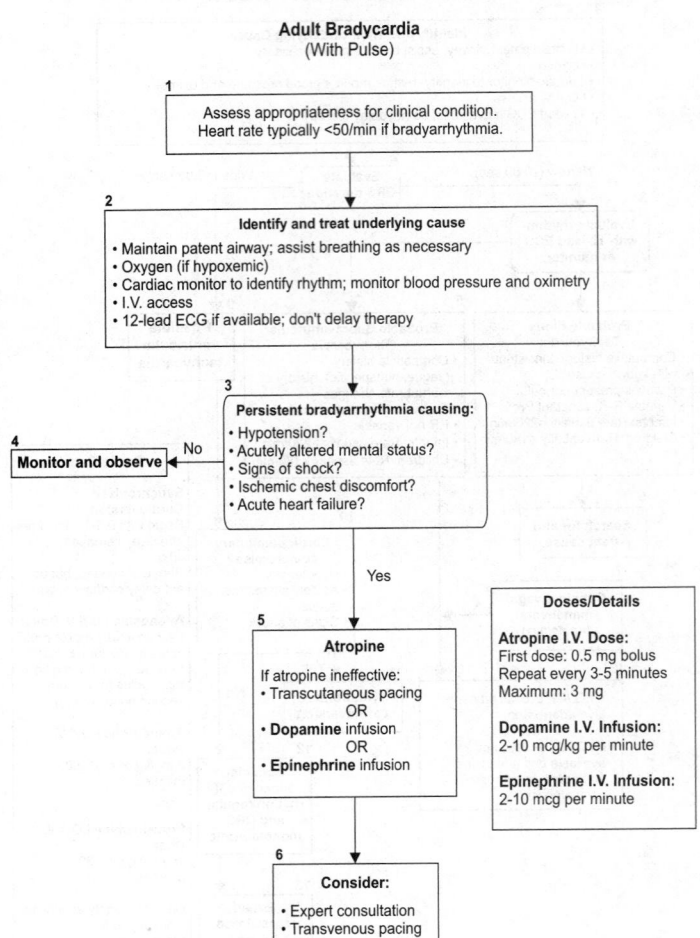

1

Assess appropriateness for clinical condition.
Heart rate typically <50/min if bradyarrhythmia.

2

Identify and treat underlying cause

- Maintain patent airway; assist breathing as necessary
- Oxygen (if hypoxemic)
- Cardiac monitor to identify rhythm; monitor blood pressure and oximetry
- I.V. access
- 12-lead ECG if available; don't delay therapy

3

Persistent bradyarrhythmia causing:

- Hypotension?
- Acutely altered mental status?
- Signs of shock?
- Ischemic chest discomfort?
- Acute heart failure?

No →

4

Monitor and observe

Yes

5

Atropine

If atropine ineffective:
- Transcutaneous pacing
  OR
- **Dopamine** infusion
  OR
- **Epinephrine** infusion

Doses/Details

Atropine I.V. Dose:
First dose: 0.5 mg bolus
Repeat every 3-5 minutes
Maximum: 3 mg

Dopamine I.V. Infusion:
2-10 mcg/kg per minute

Epinephrine I.V. Infusion:
2-10 mcg per minute

6

Consider:

- Expert consultation
- Transvenous pacing

Adult Cardiac Arrest

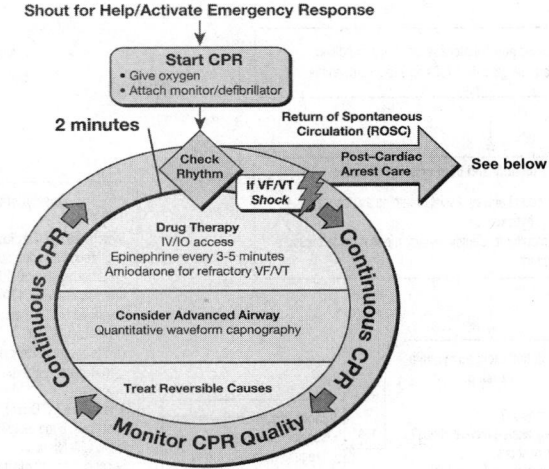

Shout for Help/Activate Emergency Response

Start CPR
• Give oxygen
• Attach monitor/defibrillator

2 minutes

Check Rhythm

If VF/VT Shock

Drug Therapy
IV/IO access
Epinephrine every 3-5 minutes
Amiodarone for refractory VF/VT

Consider Advanced Airway
Quantitative waveform capnography

Treat Reversible Causes

Monitor CPR Quality

Continuous CPR

Return of Spontaneous Circulation (ROSC)

Post–Cardiac Arrest Care

See below

© 2010 American Heart Association

CPR Quality

- Push hard (≥2 inches [5 cm]) and fast (≥100/min) and allow complete chest recoil
- Minimize interruptions in compressions
- Avoid excessive ventilation
- Rotate compressor every 2 minutes
- If no advanced airway, 30:2 compression-ventilation ratio
- Quantitative waveform capnography
  - If PETCO$_2$ <10 mm Hg, attempt to improve CPR quality
- Intra-arterial pressure
  - If relaxation phase (diastolic) pressure <20 mm Hg, attempt to improve CPR quality

Return of Spontaneous Circulation (ROSC)

- Pulse and blood pressure
- Abrupt sustained increase in PETCO$_2$ (typically ≥40 mm Hg)
- Spontaneous arterial pressure waves with intra-arterial monitoring

Shock Energy

- **Biphasic:** Manufacturer recommendation (120 to 200 J); if unknown, use maximum available. Second and subsequent doses should be equivalent, and higher doses may be considered.
- **Monophasic:** 360 J

Drug Therapy

- Epinephrine I.V./I.O. Dose: 1 mg every 3 to 5 minutes
- Vasopressin I.V./I.O. Dose: 40 units can replace first or second dose of epinephrine
- Amiodarone I.V./I.O. Dose: First dose: 300 mg bolus; Second dose: 150 mg

Advanced Airway

- Supraglottic advanced airway or endotracheal intubation
- Waveform capnography to confirm and monitor ET tube placement
- 8 to 10 breaths per minute with continuous chest compressions

Reversible Causes

- Hypovolemia; Hypoxia; Hydrogen ion (acidosis); Hypo-/hyperkalemia; Hypothermia
- Tension pneumothorax; Tamponade, cardiac; Toxins; Thrombosis, pulmonary; Thrombosis, coronary

Adult Tachycardia
(With Pulse)

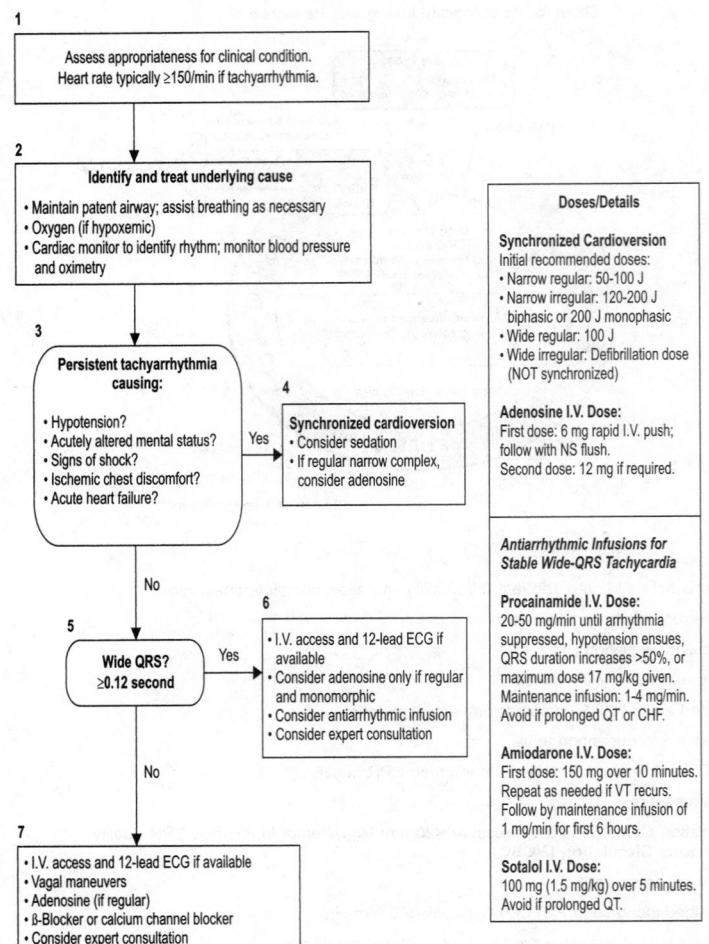

1

Assess appropriateness for clinical condition.
Heart rate typically ≥150/min if tachyarrhythmia.

2

Identify and treat underlying cause

- Maintain patent airway; assist breathing as necessary
- Oxygen (if hypoxemic)
- Cardiac monitor to identify rhythm; monitor blood pressure and oximetry

3

Persistent tachyarrhythmia causing:

- Hypotension?
- Acutely altered mental status?
- Signs of shock?
- Ischemic chest discomfort?
- Acute heart failure?

Yes →

4

Synchronized cardioversion
- Consider sedation
- If regular narrow complex, consider adenosine

No ↓

5

Wide QRS?
≥0.12 second

Yes →

6

- I.V. access and 12-lead ECG if available
- Consider adenosine only if regular and monomorphic
- Consider antiarrhythmic infusion
- Consider expert consultation

No ↓

7

- I.V. access and 12-lead ECG if available
- Vagal maneuvers
- Adenosine (if regular)
- ß-Blocker or calcium channel blocker
- Consider expert consultation

Doses/Details

Synchronized Cardioversion
Initial recommended doses:
- Narrow regular: 50-100 J
- Narrow irregular: 120-200 J biphasic or 200 J monophasic
- Wide regular: 100 J
- Wide irregular: Defibrillation dose (NOT synchronized)

Adenosine I.V. Dose:
First dose: 6 mg rapid I.V. push; follow with NS flush.
Second dose: 12 mg if required.

Antiarrhythmic Infusions for Stable Wide-QRS Tachycardia

Procainamide I.V. Dose:
20-50 mg/min until arrhythmia suppressed, hypotension ensues, QRS duration increases >50%, or maximum dose 17 mg/kg given. Maintenance infusion: 1-4 mg/min. Avoid if prolonged QT or CHF.

Amiodarone I.V. Dose:
First dose: 150 mg over 10 minutes. Repeat as needed if VT recurs. Follow by maintenance infusion of 1 mg/min for first 6 hours.

Sotalol I.V. Dose:
100 mg (1.5 mg/kg) over 5 minutes. Avoid if prolonged QT.

Note: Sotalol injection is no longer available.

Reprinted with permission: 2010 American Heart Association guidelines for cardiopulmonary resuscitation and emergency cardiovascular care − Part 8: adult advanced cardiovascular life support. *Circulation.* 2010;122(Suppl 3):S729-S767. ©2010 American Heart Association, Inc.

See http://circ.ahajournals.org/cgi/content/full/122/18_suppl_3/S729.

All requests to use this information must go through the AHA.

NORMAL PEDIATRIC HEART RATES

Age	Mean Heart Rate (beats/minute)	Heart Rate Range (2nd to 98th percentile)
<1 d	123	93 to 154
1 to 2 d	123	91 to 159
3 to 6 d	129	91 to 166
1 to 3 wk	148	107 to 182
1 to 2 mo	149	121 to 179
3 to 5 mo	141	106 to 186
6 to 11 mo	134	109 to 169
1 to 2 y	119	89 to 151
3 to 4 y	108	73 to 137
5 to 7 y	100	65 to 133
8 to 11 y	91	62 to 130
12 to 15 y	85	60 to 119

Adapted from: *The Harriet Lane Handbook.* 12th ed. Greene MG, ed. St Louis, MO: Mosby Yearbook; 1991.

Normal QRS Axes (in degrees)

Age	Mean	Range
1 wk to 1 mo	+110	+30 to +180
1 to 3 mo	+70	+10 to +125
3 mo to 3 y	+60	+10 to +110
>3 y	+60	+20 to +120
Adults	+50	−30 to +105

INTERVALS AND SEGMENTS
OF AN ECG CYCLE

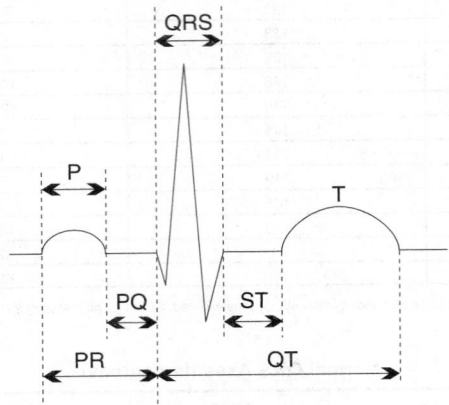

HEXAXIAL REFERENCE
SYSTEM

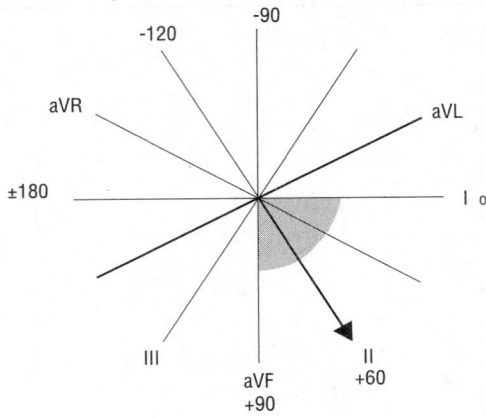

NORMAL RESPIRATORY RATES

Hour After Birth	Average Respiratory Rate	Range
1st hour	60 breaths/minute	20 to 100
2 to 6 hours	50 breaths/minute	20 to 80
>6 hours	30 to 40 breaths/minute	20 to 60

Age (years)	Mean RR (breaths/minute)
0 to 2	25 to 30
3 to 9	20 to 25
10 to 18	16 to 20

MEASURING PEDIATRIC BLOOD PRESSURE

Figure 1. Determination of Proper Cuff Size, Step 1

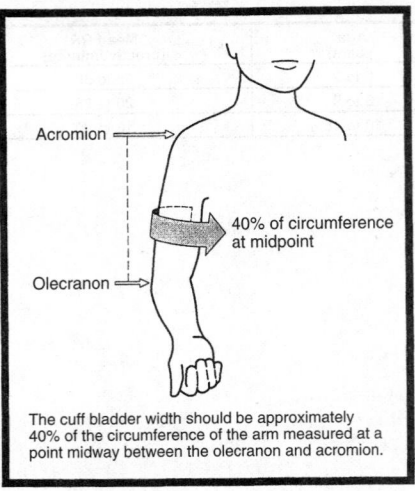

The cuff bladder width should be approximately 40% of the circumference of the arm measured at a point midway between the olecranon and acromion.

Figure 2. Determination of Proper Cuff Size, Step 2

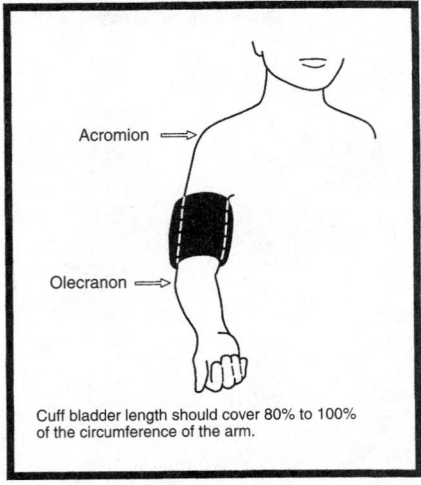

Cuff bladder length should cover 80% to 100% of the circumference of the arm.

Figure 3. Blood Pressure Measurement

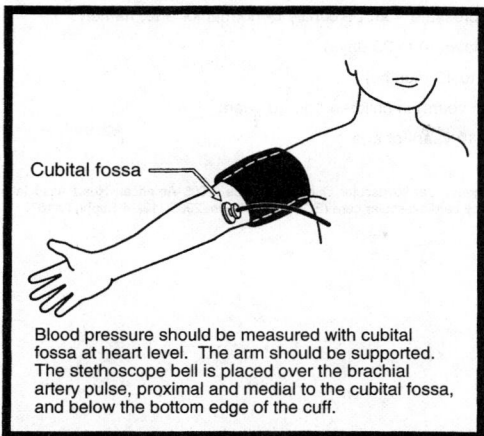

Cubital fossa

Blood pressure should be measured with cubital
fossa at heart level. The arm should be supported.
The stethoscope bell is placed over the brachial
artery pulse, proximal and medial to the cubital fossa,
and below the bottom edge of the cuff.

Used with permission: Perloff D, Grim C, Flack J, et al, "Human Blood Pressure
Determination by Sphygmomanometry," *Circulation*, 1993, 88:2460-7.

HYPOTENSION, DEFINITIONS BY AGE GROUP

Hypotension is a *systolic* blood pressure <5th percentile of normal for age, namely:

- <60 mm Hg in term neonates (0 to 28 days)
- <70 mm Hg in infants (1 to 12 months)
- <70 mm Hg + (2 x age in years) in children 1 to 10 years
- <90 mm Hg in children ≥10 years of age

REFERENCE

American Heart Association Emergency Cardiovascular Care Committee. 2005 American Heart Association (AHA) guidelines for cardiopulmonary resuscitation (CPR) and emergency cardiovascular care (ECC). *Circulation*. 2005;112(24 Suppl):IV-167.

HYPERTENSION, CLASSIFICATION BY AGE GROUP[1]

Age Group	Significant Hypertension (mm Hg)	Severe Hypertension (mm Hg)
Newborn (7 d)		
systolic BP	≥96	≥106
Newborn (8 to 30 d)		
systolic BP	≥104	≥110
Infant (<2 y)		
systolic BP	≥112	≥118
diastolic BP	≥74	≥82
Children (3 to 5 y)		
systolic BP	≥116	≥124
diastolic BP	≥76	≥84
Children (6 to 9 y)		
systolic BP	≥122	≥130
diastolic BP	≥78	≥86
Children (10 to 12 y)		
systolic BP	≥126	≥134
diastolic BP	≥82	≥90
Adolescents (13 to 15 y)		
systolic BP	≥136	≥144
diastolic BP	≥86	≥92
Adolescents (16 to 18 y)		
systolic BP	≥142	≥150
diastolic BP	≥92	≥98

Adapted from Horan MJ. *Pediatrics*. 1987;79:1-25.

[1]See also Blood Pressure Measurement, Age Specific Percentiles, and 90th and 95th Percentiles of Blood Pressure by Percentiles of Height

BLOOD PRESSURE IN PREMATURE INFANTS, NORMAL

(Birth weight 600 to 1750 g)[1]

Day	600 to 999 g		1000 to 1249 g	
	S (± 2SD)	D (± 2SD)	S (± 2SD)	D (± 2SD)
1	37.9 (17.4)	23.2 (10.3)	44 (22.8)	22.5 (13.5)
3	44.9 (15.7)	30.6 (12.3)	48 (15.4)	36.5 (9.6)
7	50 (14.8)	30.4 (12.4)	57 (14)	42.5 (16.5)
14	50.2 (14.8)	37.4 (12)	53 (30)	
28	61 (23.5)	45.8 (27.4)	57 (30)	

Day	1250 to 1499 g		1500 to 1750 g	
	S (± 2SD)	D (± 2SD)	S (± 2SD)	D (± 2SD)
1	48 (18)	27 (12.4)	47 (15.8)	26 (15.6)
3	59 (21.1)	40 (13.7)	51 (18.2)	35 (10)
7	68 (14.8)	40 (11.3)	66 (23)	41 (24)
14	64 (21.2)	36 (24.2)	76 (34.8)	42 (20.3)
28	69 (31.4)	44 (26.2)	73 (5.6)	50 (9.9)

[1]Blood pressure was obtained by the Dinamap method

S = systolic, D = diastolic, SD = standard deviation

Modified from Ingelfinger JR, Powers L, Epstein MF. Blood pressure norms in low-weight infants: birth through four weeks. *Pediatr Res.* 1983;17:319A.

BLOOD PRESSURE MEASUREMENTS, AGE-SPECIFIC PERCENTILES

Blood Pressure Measurements: Ages 0 to 12 Months, <u>BOYS</u>

Korotkoff phase IV (K4) used for diastolic BP. Reproduced with permission from Horan MJ. *Pediatrics*. 1987;79:11-25.

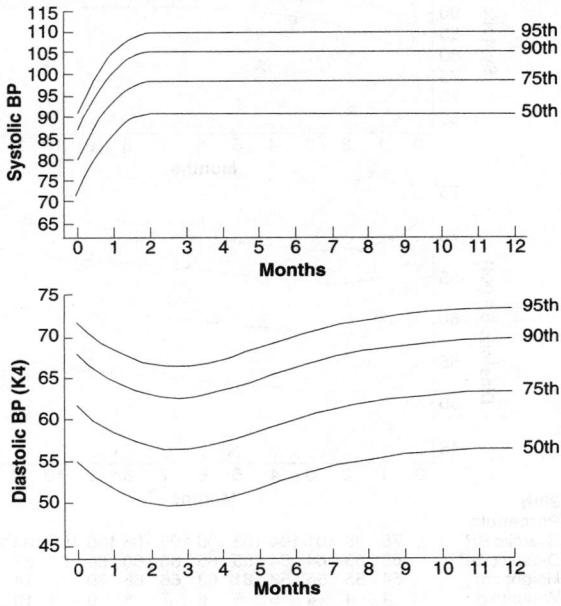

90th Percentile

Systolic BP	87	101	106	106	106	105	105	105	105	105	105	105	105
Diastolic BP	68	65	63	63	63	65	66	67	68	68	69	69	69
Height cm	51	59	63	66	68	70	72	73	74	76	77	78	80
Weight kg	4	4	5	5	6	7	8	9	9	10	10	11	11

Blood Pressure Measurements: Ages 0 to 12 Months, <u>GIRLS</u>

Korotkoff phase IV (K4) used for diastolic BP. Reproduced with permission from Horan MJ. *Pediatrics*. 1987;79:11-25.

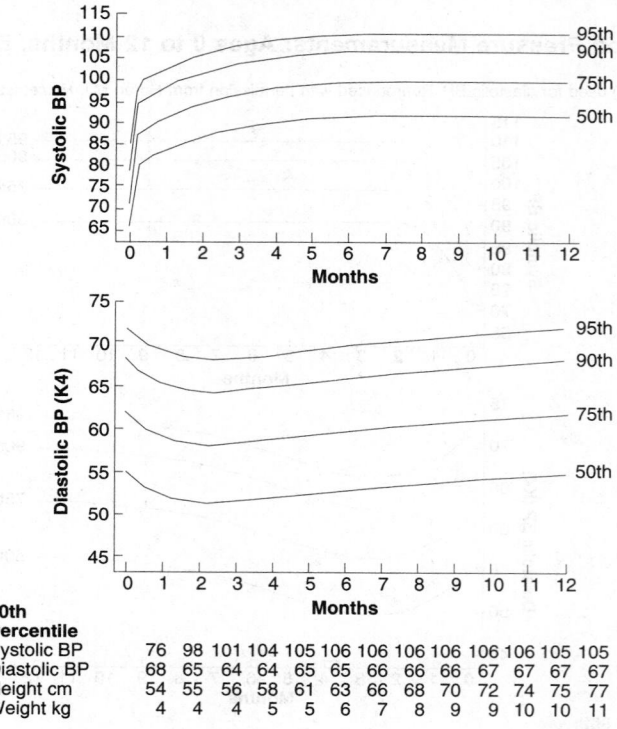

90th Percentile													
Systolic BP	76	98	101	104	105	106	106	106	106	106	106	105	105
Diastolic BP	68	65	64	64	65	65	66	66	66	67	67	67	67
Height cm	54	55	56	58	61	63	66	68	70	72	74	75	77
Weight kg	4	4	4	5	5	6	7	8	9	9	10	10	11

Blood Pressure Levels for <u>BOYS</u> by Age and Height Percentile

CARDIOLOGY / PULMONARY

Age (y)	BP Percentile[1]	Systolic BP (mm Hg) Height Percentile[3]							Diastolic BP (mm Hg)[2] Height Percentile[3]						
		5%	10%	25%	50%	75%	90%	95%	5%	10%	25%	50%	75%	90%	95%
1	50th	80	81	83	85	87	88	89	34	35	36	37	38	39	39
	90th	94	95	97	99	100	102	103	49	50	51	52	53	53	54
	95th	98	99	101	103	104	106	106	54	54	55	56	57	58	58
	99th	105	106	108	110	112	113	114	61	62	63	64	65	66	66
2	50th	84	85	87	88	90	92	92	39	40	41	42	43	44	44
	90th	97	99	100	102	104	105	106	54	55	56	57	58	58	59
	95th	101	102	104	106	108	109	110	59	59	60	61	62	63	63
	99th	109	110	111	113	115	117	117	66	67	68	69	70	71	71
3	50th	86	87	89	91	93	94	95	44	44	45	46	47	48	48
	90th	100	101	103	105	107	108	109	59	59	60	61	62	63	63
	95th	104	105	107	109	110	112	113	63	63	64	65	66	67	67
	99th	111	112	114	116	118	119	120	71	71	72	73	74	75	75
4	50th	88	89	91	93	95	96	97	47	48	49	50	51	51	52
	90th	102	103	105	107	109	110	111	62	63	64	65	66	66	67
	95th	106	107	109	111	112	114	115	66	67	68	69	70	71	71
	99th	113	114	116	118	120	121	122	74	75	76	77	78	78	79
5	50th	90	91	93	95	96	98	98	50	51	52	53	54	55	55
	90th	104	105	106	108	110	111	112	65	66	67	68	69	69	70
	95th	108	109	110	112	114	115	116	69	70	71	72	73	74	74
	99th	115	116	118	120	121	123	123	77	78	79	80	81	81	82
6	50th	91	92	94	96	98	99	100	53	53	54	55	56	57	57
	90th	105	106	108	110	111	113	113	68	68	69	70	71	72	72
	95th	109	110	112	114	115	117	117	72	72	73	74	75	76	76
	99th	116	117	119	121	123	124	125	80	80	81	82	83	84	84
7	50th	92	94	95	97	99	100	101	55	55	56	57	58	59	59
	90th	106	107	109	111	113	114	115	70	70	71	72	73	74	74
	95th	110	111	113	115	117	118	119	74	74	75	76	77	78	78
	99th	117	118	120	122	124	125	126	82	82	83	84	85	86	86
8	50th	94	95	97	99	100	102	102	56	57	58	59	60	60	61
	90th	107	109	110	112	114	115	116	71	72	72	73	74	75	76
	95th	111	112	114	116	118	119	120	75	76	77	78	79	79	80
	99th	119	120	122	123	125	127	127	83	84	85	86	87	87	88

Blood Pressure Levels for BOYS by Age and Height Percentile continued

Age (y)	BP Percentile[1]	Systolic BP (mm Hg)[2] Height Percentile[3]							Diastolic BP (mm Hg)[2] Height Percentile[3]						
		5%	10%	25%	50%	75%	90%	95%	5%	10%	25%	50%	75%	90%	95%
9	50th	95	96	98	100	102	103	104	57	58	59	60	61	61	62
	90th	109	110	112	114	115	117	118	72	73	74	75	76	76	77
	95th	113	114	116	118	119	121	121	76	77	78	79	80	81	81
	99th	120	121	123	125	127	128	129	84	85	86	87	88	88	89
10	50th	97	98	100	102	103	105	106	58	59	60	61	61	62	63
	90th	111	112	114	115	117	119	119	73	73	74	75	76	77	78
	95th	115	116	117	119	121	122	123	77	78	79	80	81	81	82
	99th	122	123	125	127	128	130	130	85	86	86	88	88	89	90
11	50th	99	100	102	104	105	107	107	59	59	60	61	62	63	63
	90th	113	114	115	117	119	120	121	74	74	75	76	77	78	78
	95th	117	118	119	121	123	124	125	78	78	79	80	81	82	82
	99th	124	125	127	129	130	132	132	86	86	87	88	89	90	90
12	50th	101	102	104	106	108	109	110	59	60	61	62	63	63	64
	90th	115	116	118	120	121	123	123	74	75	75	76	77	78	79
	95th	119	120	122	123	125	127	127	78	79	80	81	82	82	83
	99th	126	127	129	131	133	134	135	86	87	88	89	90	90	91
13	50th	104	105	106	108	110	111	112	60	60	61	62	63	64	64
	90th	117	118	120	122	124	125	126	75	75	76	77	78	79	79
	95th	121	122	124	126	128	129	130	79	79	80	81	82	83	83
	99th	128	130	131	133	135	136	137	87	87	88	89	90	91	91
14	50th	106	107	109	111	113	114	115	60	61	62	63	64	65	65
	90th	120	121	123	125	126	128	128	75	76	77	78	79	79	80
	95th	124	125	127	128	130	132	132	80	80	81	82	83	84	84
	99th	131	132	134	136	138	139	140	87	88	89	90	91	92	92
15	50th	109	110	112	113	115	117	117	61	62	63	64	65	66	66
	90th	122	124	125	127	129	130	131	76	77	78	79	80	80	81
	95th	126	127	129	131	133	134	135	81	81	82	83	84	85	85
	99th	134	135	136	138	140	142	142	88	89	90	91	92	93	93
16	50th	111	112	114	116	118	119	120	63	63	64	65	66	67	67
	90th	125	126	128	130	131	133	134	78	78	79	80	81	82	82
	95th	129	130	132	134	135	137	137	82	83	83	84	85	86	87
	99th	136	137	139	141	143	144	145	90	90	91	92	93	94	94

Blood Pressure Levels for BOYS by Age and Height Percentile *continued*

Age (y)	BP Percentile[1]	Systolic BP (mm Hg)							Diastolic BP (mm Hg)[2]						
		Height Percentile[3]													
		5%	10%	25%	50%	75%	90%	95%	5%	10%	25%	50%	75%	90%	95%
17	50th	114	115	116	118	120	121	122	65	66	66	67	68	69	70
	90th	127	128	130	132	134	135	136	80	80	81	82	83	84	84
	95th	131	132	134	136	138	139	140	84	85	86	87	87	88	89
	99th	139	140	141	143	145	146	147	92	93	93	94	95	96	97

[1]Blood pressure percentile determined by a single measurement

[2]Korotkoff phase V (K5) used for diastolic BP

[3]Height percentile determined by standard growth curves

Source: National High Blood Pressure Education Program Working Group on High Blood Pressure in Children and Adolescents. The fourth report on the diagnosis, evaluation, and treatment of high blood pressure in children and adolescents. *Pediatrics.* 2004;114(2 Suppl 4th report):555-576.

Blood Pressure Levels for GIRLS by Age and Height Percentile

Age (y)	BP Percentile[1]	Systolic BP (mm Hg)[2]							Diastolic BP (mm Hg)[2]						
		Height Percentile[3]							Height Percentile[3]						
		5%	10%	25%	50%	75%	90%	95%	5%	10%	25%	50%	75%	90%	95%
1	50th	83	84	85	86	88	89	90	38	39	39	40	41	41	42
	90th	97	97	98	100	101	102	103	52	53	53	54	55	55	56
	95th	100	101	102	104	105	106	107	56	57	57	58	59	59	60
	99th	108	108	109	111	112	113	114	64	64	65	65	66	67	67
2	50th	85	85	87	88	89	91	91	43	44	44	45	46	46	47
	90th	98	99	100	101	103	104	105	57	58	58	59	60	61	61
	95th	102	103	104	105	107	108	109	61	62	62	63	64	65	65
	99th	109	110	111	112	114	115	116	69	69	70	70	71	72	72
3	50th	86	87	88	89	91	92	93	47	48	48	49	50	50	51
	90th	100	100	102	103	104	106	106	61	62	62	63	64	64	65
	95th	104	104	105	107	108	109	110	65	66	66	67	68	68	69
	99th	111	111	113	114	115	116	117	73	73	74	74	75	76	76
4	50th	88	88	90	91	92	94	94	50	50	51	52	52	53	54
	90th	101	102	103	104	106	107	108	64	64	65	66	67	67	68
	95th	105	106	107	108	110	111	112	68	68	69	70	71	71	72
	99th	112	113	114	115	117	118	119	76	76	76	77	78	79	79
5	50th	89	90	91	93	94	95	96	52	52	53	54	55	55	56
	90th	103	103	105	106	107	109	109	66	66	67	68	69	69	70
	95th	107	107	108	110	111	112	113	70	70	71	72	73	73	74
	99th	114	114	116	117	118	120	120	78	78	79	79	80	81	81
6	50th	91	92	93	94	96	97	98	54	54	55	56	56	57	58
	90th	104	105	106	108	109	110	111	68	68	69	70	70	71	72
	95th	108	109	110	111	113	114	115	72	72	73	74	74	75	76
	99th	115	116	117	119	120	121	122	80	80	80	81	82	83	83
7	50th	93	93	95	96	97	99	99	55	56	56	57	58	58	59
	90th	106	107	108	109	111	112	113	69	70	70	71	72	72	73
	95th	110	111	112	113	115	116	116	73	74	74	75	76	76	77
	99th	117	118	119	120	122	123	124	81	81	82	82	83	84	84
8	50th	95	95	96	98	99	100	101	57	57	57	58	59	60	60
	90th	108	109	110	111	113	114	114	71	71	71	72	73	74	74
	95th	112	112	114	115	116	118	118	75	75	75	76	77	78	78
	99th	119	120	121	122	123	125	125	82	82	83	83	84	85	86

Blood Pressure Levels for GIRLS by Age and Height Percentile *continued*

Age (y)	BP Percentile[1]	Systolic BP (mm Hg)							Diastolic BP (mm Hg)[2]						
		Height Percentile[3]							Height Percentile[3]						
		5%	10%	25%	50%	75%	90%	95%	5%	10%	25%	50%	75%	90%	95%
9	50th	96	97	98	100	101	102	103	58	58	58	59	60	61	61
	90th	110	110	112	113	114	116	116	72	72	72	73	74	75	75
	95th	114	114	115	117	118	119	120	76	76	76	77	78	79	79
	99th	121	121	123	124	125	127	127	83	83	84	84	85	86	87
10	50th	98	99	100	102	103	104	105	59	59	59	60	61	62	62
	90th	112	112	114	115	116	118	118	73	73	73	74	75	76	76
	95th	116	116	117	119	120	121	122	77	77	77	78	79	80	80
	99th	123	123	125	126	127	129	129	84	84	85	86	86	87	88
11	50th	100	101	102	103	105	106	107	60	60	60	61	62	63	63
	90th	114	114	116	117	118	119	120	74	74	74	75	76	77	77
	95th	118	118	119	121	122	123	124	78	78	78	79	80	81	81
	99th	125	125	126	128	129	130	131	85	85	86	87	87	88	89
12	50th	102	103	104	105	107	108	109	61	61	61	62	63	64	64
	90th	116	116	117	119	120	121	122	75	75	75	76	77	78	78
	95th	119	120	121	123	124	125	126	79	79	79	80	81	82	82
	99th	127	127	128	130	131	132	133	86	86	87	88	88	89	90
13	50th	104	105	106	107	109	110	110	62	62	62	63	64	65	65
	90th	117	118	119	121	122	123	124	76	76	76	77	78	79	79
	95th	121	122	123	124	126	127	128	80	80	80	81	82	83	83
	99th	128	129	130	132	133	134	135	87	87	88	89	89	90	91
14	50th	106	106	107	109	110	111	112	63	63	63	64	65	66	66
	90th	119	120	121	122	124	125	125	77	77	77	78	79	80	80
	95th	123	123	125	126	127	129	129	81	81	81	82	83	84	84
	99th	130	131	132	133	135	136	136	88	88	89	90	90	91	92
15	50th	107	108	109	110	111	113	113	64	64	64	65	66	67	67
	90th	120	121	122	123	125	126	127	78	78	78	79	80	81	81
	95th	124	125	126	127	129	130	131	82	82	82	83	84	85	85
	99th	131	132	133	134	136	137	138	89	89	90	91	91	92	93
16	50th	108	108	110	111	112	114	114	64	64	65	66	66	67	68
	90th	121	122	123	124	126	127	128	78	78	79	80	81	81	82
	95th	125	126	127	128	130	131	132	82	82	83	84	85	85	86
	99th	132	133	134	135	137	138	139	90	90	90	91	92	93	93

Blood Pressure Levels for GIRLS by Age and Height Percentile *continued*

Age (y)	BP Percentile[1]	Systolic BP (mm Hg)							Diastolic BP (mm Hg)[2]						
		Height Percentile[3]							Height Percentile[3]						
		5%	10%	25%	50%	75%	90%	95%	5%	10%	25%	50%	75%	90%	95%
17	50th	108	109	110	111	113	114	115	64	65	65	66	67	67	68
	90th	122	122	123	125	126	127	128	78	79	79	80	81	81	82
	95th	125	126	127	129	130	131	132	82	83	83	84	85	85	86
	99th	133	133	134	136	137	138	139	90	90	91	91	92	93	93

[1]Blood pressure percentile determined by a single measurement

[2]Korotkoff phase V (K5) used for diastolic BP

[3]Height percentile determined by standard growth curves

Source: National High Blood Pressure Education Program Working Group on High Blood Pressure in Children and Adolescents. The fourth report on the diagnosis, evaluation, and treatment of high blood pressure in children and adolescents. *Pediatrics*. 2004;114(2 Suppl 4th report):555-576.

NEW YORK HEART ASSOCIATION (NYHA) CLASSIFICATION OF FUNCTIONAL CAPACITY OF PATIENTS WITH DISEASES OF THE HEART, 1994 REVISIONS

Class I

Patients with cardiac disease but without resulting limitation of physical activity. Ordinary physical activity does not cause undue fatigue, palpitation, dyspnea, or anginal pain.

Class II

Patients with cardiac disease resulting in slight limitation of physical activity. They are comfortable at rest. Ordinary physical activity results in fatigue, palpitation, dyspnea, or anginal pain.

Class III

Patients with cardiac disease resulting in marked limitation of physical activity. They are comfortable at rest. Less than ordinary activity causes fatigue, palpitation, dyspnea, or anginal pain.

Class IV

Patients with cardiac disease resulting in inability to carry on any physical activity without discomfort. Symptoms of heart failure or the anginal syndrome may be present even at rest. If any physical activity is undertaken, discomfort increases.

REFERENCE

The Criteria Committee of the New York Heart Association. *Nomenclature and Criteria for Diagnosis of Diseases of the Heart and Great Vessels*. 9th ed. Boston, MA: Little, Brown & Co; 1994;253-256.

WORLD HEALTH ORGANIZATION (WHO) FUNCTIONAL CLASSIFICATION OF PULMONARY HYPERTENSION

Class I

Patients with pulmonary hypertension but without resulting limitation of physical activity. Ordinary physical activity does not cause undue dyspnea or fatigue, chest pain, or near syncope.

Class II

Patients with pulmonary hypertension resulting in slight limitation of physical activity. They are comfortable at rest. Ordinary physical activity causes undue dyspnea or fatigue, chest pain, or near syncope.

Class III

Patients with pulmonary hypertension resulting in marked limitation of physical activity. They are comfortable at rest. Less than ordinary activity causes undue dyspnea or fatigue, chest pain, or near syncope.

Class IV

Patients with pulmonary hypertension with inability to carry out any physical activity without symptoms. These patients manifest signs of right heart failure. Dyspnea and/or fatigue may be present even at rest. Discomfort is increased by any physical activity.

REFERENCE

Widlitz A, Barst RJ. Pulmonary arterial hypertension in children. *Eur Respir J.* 2003;21(1):155-176.

ANTIDEPRESSANT AGENTS

Comparison of Usual Adult Dosage, Mechanism of Action, and Adverse Effects

Drug	Initial Adult Dose	Usual Adult Dosage (mg/d)	Dosage Forms	ACH	Drowsiness	Orthostatic Hypotension	Conduction Abnormalities	GI Distress	Weight Gain	Comments
						Adverse Effects				
Tricyclic Antidepressants and Related Compounds[1]										
Amitriptyline	25 to 75 mg qhs	100 to 300	T	4+	4+	3+	3+	1+	4+	Also used in chronic pain, migraine, and as a hypnotic; contraindicated with cisapride
Amoxapine	50 mg bid	100 to 400	T	2+	2+	2+	2+	0	2+	May cause extrapyramidal symptom (EPS)
ClomiPRAMINE[2] (Anafranil)	25 to 75 mg qhs	100 to 250	C	4+	4+	2+	3+	1+	4+	Only approved for OCD
Desipramine (Norpramin)	25 to 75 mg qhs	100 to 300	T	1+	2+	2+	2+	0	1+	Blood levels useful for therapeutic monitoring
Doxepin	25 to 75 mg qhs	100 to 300	C, L, T	3+	4+	2+	2+	0	4+	
Imipramine (Tofranil, Tofranil-PM)	25 to 75 mg qhs	100 to 300	T, C	3+	3+	4+	3+	1+	4+	Blood levels useful for therapeutic monitoring
Maprotiline	25 to 75 mg qhs	100 to 225	T	2+	3+	2+	2+	0	2+	
Nortriptyline (Pamelor)	25 to 50 mg qhs	50 to 150	C, L	2+	2+	1+	2+	0	1+	Blood levels useful for therapeutic monitoring
Protriptyline (Vivactil)	15 mg qAM	15 to 60	T	2+	1+	2+	3+	1+	1+	
Trimipramine (Surmontil)	25 to 75 mg qhs	100 to 300	C	4+	4+	3+	3+	0	4+	
Selective Serotonin Reuptake Inhibitors[3]										
Citalopram (Celexa)	20 mg qAM	20 to 60	T, L	0	0	0	0	3+[4]	1+	
Escitalopram (Lexapro)	10 mg qAM	10 to 20	T, L	0	0	0	0	3+	1+	S-enantiomer of citalopram
FLUoxetine (PROzac, PROzac Weekly, Sarafem, Selfemra)	10 to 20 mg qAM	20 to 80	C, CDR, L, T	0	0	0	0	3+[4]	1+	CYP2B6 and 2D6 inhibitor
FluvoxaMINE[2] (Luvox CR)	50 mg qhs	100 to 300	T, CXR	0	0	0	0	3+[4]	1+	Contraindicated with pimozide, thioridazine, mesoridazine, CYP1A2, 2B6, 2C19, and 3A4 inhibitors
PARoxetine (Paxil, Paxil CR, Pexeva)	10 to 20 mg qAM	20 to 50	T, CXR, L	1+	1+	0	0	3+[4]	2+	CYP2B6 and 2D6 inhibitor
Sertraline (Zoloft)	25 to 50 mg qAM	50 to 200	T, L	0	0	0	0	3+[4]	1+	CYP2B6 and 2C19 inhibitor
Vilazodone (Viibryd)	10 mg qAM	10 to 40	T	0	0	0	0	3+	0	CYP2C8, 2C19, and 2D6 inhibitor; also is a 5-HT$_{1A}$ partial agonist

Comparison of Usual Adult Dosage, Mechanism of Action, and Adverse Effects *continued*

Drug	Initial Adult Dose	Usual Adult Dosage (mg/d)	Dosage Forms	Adverse Effects						Comments
				ACH	Drowsiness	Orthostatic Hypotension	Conduction Abnormalities	GI Distress	Weight Gain	
Dopamine-Reuptake Blocking Compounds										
BuPROPion (Aplenzin, Buproban, Budeprion SR, Budeprion XL, Wellbutrin XL, Wellbutrin, Wellbutrin XL, SR, Zyban)	100 mg bid-tid IR[5]; 150 mg qAM-bid SR[6]	300 to 450	T, TSR, TXR	0	0	0	1+/0	1+	0	Contraindicated with seizures, bulimia, and anorexia; low incidence of sexual dysfunction. IR: A 6-h interval between doses preferred. SR: An 8-h interval between doses preferred. XL: Administer once daily
Serotonin/Norepinephrine Reuptake Inhibitors[7]										
Desvenlafaxine (Pristiq)	50 mg/d	50 to 100	TXR	0	1+	1+	0	3+[4]	0	Active metabolite of venlafaxine
DULoxetine (Cymbalta)	40 to 60 mg/d	40 to 60	CDR	1+	1+	0	1+	3+	0	Also indicated for GAD, management of pain associated with diabetic neuropathy, and management of fibromyalgia
Levomilnacipran (Fetzima)	20 mg/d	20 to 120	CXR	1+	0	2+	1+	2+	0	1S,2R-enantiomer of milnacipram
Milnacipran[8] (Savella)	12.5 mg/d	100 to 200	T	2+	1+	0	1+	3+	0	Only indicated for fibromyalgia
Venlafaxine (Effexor, Effexor XR)	25 mg bid-tid IR; 37.5 mg qd XR	75 to 375 IR; 75 to 225 XR	T, TXR, CXR	1+	1+	0	1+	3+[4]	0	High-dose may be useful to treat refractory depression; frequency of hypertension increases with dosage >225 mg/d
5-HT$_2$ Receptor Antagonist Properties										
Nefazodone	100 mg bid	300 to 600	T	1+	1+	2+	1+	1+	0	Contraindicated with carbamazepine, pimozide, astemizole, cisapride, and terfenadine; caution with triazolam and alprazolam; low incidence of sexual dysfunction
TraZODone (Oleptro)	50 mg tid IR; 150 mg qhs XR	150 to 600 IR; 150 to 375 XR	T, TXR	0	4+	3+	1+	1+	2+	
5-HT$_3$ Receptor Antagonist Properties										
Vortioxetine (Brintellix)	10 mg/d	5 to 20	T	0	0	0	0	3+	0	Also is a 5-HT$_{1A}$ agonist; moderate incidence of sexual dysfunction
Noradrenergic Antagonist										
Mirtazapine (Remeron, Remeron SolTab)	15 mg qhs	15 to 45	T, TOD	1+	3+	1+	1+	0	3+	Dose >15 mg/d less sedating, low incidence of sexual dysfunction

Comparison of Usual Adult Dosage, Mechanism of Action, and Adverse Effects *continued*

Drug	Initial Adult Dose	Usual Adult Dosage (mg/d)	Dosage Forms	ACH	Drowsiness	Orthostatic Hypotension	Conduction Abnormalities	GI Distress	Weight Gain	Comments
						Adverse Effects				
						Monoamine Oxidase Inhibitors				
Isocarboxazid (Marplan)	10 mg tid	10 to 30	T	2+	2+	2+	1+	1+	2+	Diet must be low in tyramine; contraindicated with sympathomimetics and other antidepressants
Phenelzine (Nardil)	15 mg tid	15 to 90	T	2+	2+	2+	0	1+	3+	
Tranylcypromine (Parnate)	10 mg bid	10 to 60	T	2+	1+	2+	1+	1+	2+	
Selegiline (EmSam)	6 mg/d	6 to 12	Transdermal	2+	1+	2+	0	1+	0	Low tyramine diet not required for 6 mg/d dosage

ACH = anticholinergic effects (dry mouth, blurred vision, urinary retention, constipation); 0 - 4+ = absent or rare - relatively common; T = tablet; TSR = tablet, sustained release; TXR = tablet, extended release; TOD = tablet, orally disintegrating; L = liquid; C = capsule; CDR = capsule, delayed release; CXR = capsule, extended release; IR = immediate release; SR = sustained release; XR = extended release

[1]**Important note:** A 1-week supply taken all at once in a patient receiving the maximum dose can be fatal.

[2]Not approved by FDA for depression; approved for OCD

[3]Flat dose response curve, headache, nausea, and sexual dysfunction are common side effects for SSRIs.

[4]Nausea is usually mild and transient.

[5]R: 100 mg bid; may be increased to 100 mg tid no sooner than 3 days after beginning therapy

[6]SR: 150 mg qAM; may be increased to 150 mg bid as early as day 4 of dosing. To minimize seizure risk, do not exceed SR 200 mg/dose.

[7]Do not use with sibutramine; relatively safe in overdose

[8]Milnacipran is only approved for fibromyalgia.

CORTICOSTEROIDS SYSTEMIC EQUIVALENCIES

Glucocorticoid	Approximate Equivalent Dose (mg)	Routes of Administration	Relative Anti-inflammatory Potency	Relative Mineralocorticoid Potency	Protein Binding (%)	Half-life Plasma (min)
Short-Acting						
Cortisone	25	P.O., I.M.	0.8	0.8	90	30
Hydrocortisone	20	I.M., I.V.	1	1	90	90
Intermediate-Acting						
MethylPREDNISolone[1]	4	P.O., I.M., I.V.	5	0	—	180
PrednisoLONE	5	P.O., I.M., I.V., intra-articular, intradermal, soft tissue injection	4	0.8	90 to 95	200
PredniSONE	5	P.O.	4	0.8	70	60
Triamcinolone[1]	4	I.M., intra-articular, intradermal, intrasynovial, soft tissue injection	5	0	—	300
Long-Acting						
Betamethasone	0.75	P.O., I.M., intra-articular, intradermal, intrasynovial, soft tissue injection	25	0	64	100 to 300
Dexamethasone	0.75	P.O., I.M., I.V., intra-articular, intradermal, soft tissue injection	25 to 30	0	—	100 to 300
Mineralocorticoids						
Fludrocortisone	—	P.O.	10	125	42	200

[1]May contain propylene glycol as an excipient in injectable forms

Asare K. Diagnosis and treatment of adrenal insufficiency in the critically ill patient. *Pharmacotherapy.* 2007;27(11):1512-1528.

INHALED CORTICOSTEROIDS

Estimated Comparative Daily Dosage

Children ≥12 Years of Age and Adults

Drug	Low Daily Dose	Medium Daily Dose	High Daily Dose
Beclomethasone aerosol solution inhalation	80 to 240 mcg	>240 to 480 mcg	>480 mcg
Budesonide aerosol powder breath-activated inhalation	180 to 600 mcg	>600 to 1200 mcg	>1200 mcg
Flunisolide aerosol solution inhalation	320 mcg	>320 to 640 mcg	>640 mcg
Fluticasone HFA	88 to 264 mcg	>264 to 440 mcg	>440 mcg
Fluticasone aerosol powder breath-activated inhalation	100 to 300 mcg	>300 to 500 mcg	>500 mcg
Mometasone aerosol powder breath-activated inhalation	200 mcg	400 mcg	>400 mcg

HFA = hydrofluoroalkane

Children <12 Years of Age

Drug	Low Daily Dose	Medium Daily Dose	High Daily Dose
Beclomethasone inhalation	0 to 4 years: NA 5 to 11 years: 80 to 160 mcg	0 to 4 years: NA 5 to 11 years: >160 to 320 mcg	0 to 4 years: NA 5 to 11 years: >320 mcg
Budesonide aerosol powder breath-activated inhalation	0 to 4 years: NA 5 to 11 years: 180 to 400 mcg	0 to 4 years: NA 5 to 11 years: >400 to 800 mcg	0 to 4 years: NA 5 to 11 years: >800 mcg
Budesonide nebulized	0 to 4 years: 0.25 to 0.5 mg 5 to 11 years: 0.5 mg	0 to 4 years: >0.5 to 1 mg 5 to 11 years: 1 mg	0 to 4 years: >1 mg 5 to 11 years: 2 mg
Flunisolide aerosol solution inhalation	0 to 4 years: NA 5 to 11 years: 160 mcg	0 to 4 years: NA 5 to 11 years: 320 mcg	0 to 4 years: NA 5 to 11 years: ≥640 mcg
Fluticasone HFA	0 to 4 years: 176 mcg 5 to 11 years: 88 to 176 mcg	0 to 11 years: >176 to 352 mcg	0 to 11 years: >352 mcg
Fluticasone aerosol powder breath-activated inhalation	0 to 4 years: NA 5 to 11 years: 100 to 200 mcg	0 to 4 years: NA 5 to 11 years: >200 to 400 mcg	0 to 4 years: NA 5 to 11 years: >400 mcg
Mometasone aerosol powder breath-activated inhalation	NA	NA	NA

HFA = hydrofluoroalkane, NA = not approved for use in this age group or no data available

REFERENCE

Expert Panel Report 3. Guidelines for the diagnosis and management of asthma. *Clinical Practice Guidelines*, National Institutes of Health, National Heart, Lung, and Blood Institute, NIH Publication No. 08-4051. Available at http://www.nhlbi.nih.gov/guidelines/asthma/asthgdln.htm

TOPICAL CORTICOSTEROIDS

GUIDELINES FOR SELECTION AND USE OF TOPICAL CORTICOSTEROIDS

The quantity prescribed and the frequency of refills should be monitored to reduce the risk of adrenal suppression. In general, short courses of high-potency agents are preferable to prolonged use of low potency. After control is achieved, control should be maintained with a low potency preparation.

1. Low-to-medium potency agents are usually effective for treating thin, acute, inflammatory skin lesions; whereas, high or super-potent agents are often required for treating chronic, hyperkeratotic, or lichenified lesions.

2. Since the stratum corneum is thin on the face and intertriginous areas, low-potency agents are preferred but a higher potency agent may be used for 2 weeks.

3. Because the palms and soles have a thick stratum corneum, high or super-potent agents are frequently required.

4. Low potency agents are preferred for infants and the elderly. Infants have a high body surface area to weight ratio; elderly patients have thin, fragile skin.

5. The vehicle in which the topical corticosteroid is formulated influences the absorption and potency of the drug. Ointment bases are preferred for thick, lichenified lesions; they enhance penetration of the drug. Creams are preferred for acute and subacute dermatoses; they may be used on moist skin areas or intertriginous areas. Solutions, gels, and sprays are preferred for the scalp or for areas where a nonoil-based vehicle is needed.

6. In general, super-potent agents should not be used for longer than 2 to 3 weeks unless the lesion is limited to a small body area. Medium-to-high potency agents usually cause only rare adverse effects when treatment is limited to 3 months or less, and use on the face and intertriginous areas are avoided. If long-term treatment is needed, intermittent vs continued treatment is recommended.

7. Most preparations are applied once or twice daily. More frequent application may be necessary for the palms or soles because the preparation is easily removed by normal activity and penetration is poor due to a thick stratum corneum. Every-other-day or weekend-only application may be effective for treating some chronic conditions.

Relative Potency of Selected Topical Corticosteroids

	Steroid	Dosage Form
Very High Potency		
0.05%	Betamethasone dipropionate, augmented	Cream, gel, lotion, ointment
0.05%	Clobetasol propionate	Cream, foam, gel, lotion, ointment, shampoo, spray
0.05%	Diflorasone diacetate	Ointment
0.05%	Halobetasol propionate	Cream, ointment
High Potency		
0.1%	Amcinonide	Cream, ointment, lotion
0.05%	Betamethasone dipropionate, augmented	Cream
0.05%	Betamethasone dipropionate	Cream, ointment
0.1%	Betamethasone valerate	Ointment
0.05%	Desoximetasone	Gel
0.25%	Desoximetasone	Cream, ointment
0.05%	Diflorasone diacetate	Cream, ointment
0.05%	Fluocinonide	Cream, ointment, gel
0.1%	Halcinonide	Cream, ointment
0.5%	Triamcinolone acetonide	Cream, spray
Intermediate Potency		
0.05%	Betamethasone dipropionate	Lotion
0.1%	Betamethasone valerate	Cream
0.1%	Clocortolone pivalate	Cream
0.05%	Desoximetasone	Cream
0.025%	Fluocinolone acetonide	Cream, ointment
0.05%	Flurandrenolide	Cream, ointment, lotion, tape
0.005%	Fluticasone propionate	Ointment
0.05%	Fluticasone propionate	Cream, lotion
0.1%	Hydrocortisone butyrate[1]	Ointment, solution
0.2%	Hydrocortisone valerate[1]	Cream, ointment
0.1%	Mometasone furoate[1]	Cream, ointment, lotion
0.1%	Prednicarbate	Cream, ointment
0.025%	Triamcinolone acetonide	Cream, ointment, lotion
0.1%	Triamcinolone acetonide	Cream, ointment, lotion

Relative Potency of Selected Topical Corticosteroids *(continued)*

	Steroid	Dosage Form
	Low Potency	
0.05%	Alclometasone dipropionate[1]	Cream, ointment
0.05%	Desonide	Cream, ointment
0.01%	Fluocinolone acetonide	Cream, solution
0.5%	Hydrocortisone[1]	Cream, ointment, lotion
0.5%	Hydrocortisone acetate[1]	Cream, ointment
1%	Hydrocortisone acetate[1]	Cream, ointment
1%	Hydrocortisone[1]	Cream, ointment, lotion, solution
2.5%	Hydrocortisone[1]	Cream, ointment, lotion

[1] Not fluorinated

IMMUNE GLOBULIN PRODUCT COMPARISON

Brand Name	Concentration	pH	Initial Rate		Max Rate		IgA Content (mcg/mL)	Osmolarity/ Osmolality (mOsmol/kg)	Comments
			I.V.	SubQ[1]	I.V.[2]	SubQ[1]			
Bivigam	10%	4 to 4.6	0.3 mL/kg/h	–	3.6 mL/kg/h	–	≤200	Not available	Contains polysorbate 80
Carimune NF[3]	3%	6.4 to 6.8	1 mL/kg/h		6 mL/kg/h		Trace[4]	192 to 498[5]	Contains sucrose
	12%		0.24 mL/kg/h		1.5 mL/kg/h			768 to 1074[5]	
Flebogamma DIF	5%	5 to 6	0.6 mL/kg/h		6 mL/kg/h		<50	240 to 370	
	10%		0.6 mL/kg/h		4.8 mL/kg/h		<100		
GamaSTAN S/D	15% to 18%	6.4 to 7.2	–	–	–	–	Not available	Not available	For I.M. use
Gammagard S/D	5%	6.4 to 7.2	0.5 mL/kg/h	–	4 mL/kg/h	–	≤1[6]	636	Contains polysorbate 80
	10%		0.5 mL/kg/h		8 mL/kg/h		≤2[6]	1250	
Gammagard Liquid	10%	4.6 to 5.1	0.5 mL/kg/h	<40 kg: 15 mL/h/site with a maximum of 8 sites; ≥40 kg: 20 mL/h/site with a maximum of 8 sites	5 mL/kg/h; 5.4 mL/kg/h (MMN only)	<40 kg: 20 mL/h/site with a maximum of 8 sites; maximum **total** rate: 160 mL/h; ≥40 kg: 30 mL/h/site with a maximum of 8 sites; maximum **total** rate: 240 mL/h	37	240 to 300	
Gammaked	10%	4 to 4.5	0.6 mL/kg/h; 1.2 mL/kg/h (CIDP only)	20 mL/h/site with a maximum of 8 sites	4.8 mL/kg/h	Not determined	46	258	
Gammaplex	5%	4.8 to 5	0.6 mL/kg/h	–	4.8 mL/kg/h	–	<10	420 to 500	Contains polysorbate 80
Gamunex-C	10%	4 to 4.5	0.6 mL/kg/h; 1.2 mL/kg/h (CIDP only)	20 mL/h/site with a maximum of 8 sites	4.8 mL/kg/h	Not determined	46	258	
Hizentra	20%	4.6 to 5.2	–	15 mL/h/site with a maximum of 4 sites	–	Up to 25 mL/h/site with a maximum of 4 sites; maximum **total** rate: 50 mL/h	≤50	380	Contains L-proline and polysorbate 80
Octagam	5%	5.1 to 6	0.6 mL/kg/h	–	4 mL/kg/h	–	≤200	310 to 380	Contains maltose
Privigen	10%	4.6 to 5	0.3 mL/kg/h	–	2.4 mL/kg/h (ITP); 4.8 mL/kg/h	–	≤25	240 to 440	Contains L-proline

CIDP = chronic inflammatory demyelinating polyneuropathy, ITP = immune (idiopathic) thrombocytopenic purpura, MMN = multifocal motor neuropathy

[1] Subcutaneous administration **only** for the treatment of primary humoral immunodeficiency (PI)

[2] Lower infusion rates should be used in patients at risk for renal dysfunction or thrombotic complications; see specific product information for details.

[3] Other concentrations may be prepared; see product information for additional details.

[4] Per product information; other sources list IgA content as 1000 to 2000 mcg/mL for 6% solution (Siegel J. Immune globulins: therapeutic, pharmaceutical, cost, and administration considerations. *Pharm Prac News.* 2013).

[5] Osmolarity depends on concentration and diluent used; see product information for details.

[6] Data presented is based on the maximum concentration that can be prepared. The 5% solution with IgA content <2.2 mcg/mL has been discontinued. The lower IgA product (ie, IgA <1 mcg/mL for the 5% prepared solution) is available by special request; contact manufacturer or see specific product information for details.

MULTIVITAMIN PRODUCT TABLE

Injectable Formulations

Product	A (units)	B$_1$ (mg)	B$_2$ (mg)	B$_6$ (mg)	B$_{12}$ (mcg)	C (mg)	D (units)	E (units)	K (mcg)	Additional Information
Solution										
Infuvite Adult (*per 10 mL*)	3300	6	3.6	6	5	200	200	10	150	Supplied as two 5 mL vials. Biotin 60 mcg, folic acid 600 mcg, niacinamide 40 mg, dexpanthenol 15 mg
Infuvite Pediatric (*per 5 mL*)	2300	1.2	1.4	1	1	80	400	7	200	Supplied as one 4 mL vial and one 1 mL vial. Biotin 20 mcg, folic acid 140 mcg, niacinamide 17 mg, dexpanthenol 5 mg
M.V.I.-12 (*per 10 mL*)	3300	6	3.6	6	5	200	200	10		Supplied as a single 2-chambered 10 mL vial. Biotin 60 mcg, folic acid 600 mcg, niacinamide 40 mg, dexpanthenol 15 mg
M.V.I. Adult (*per 10 mL*)	3300	6	3.6	6	5	200	200	10	150	Supplied as two 5 mL vials or a single 2-chambered 10 mL vial. Also available in a pharmacy bulk package (two 50 mL vials). Biotin 60 mcg, folic acid 600 mcg, niacinamide 40 mg, dexpanthenol 15 mg
Powder for Reconstitution										
M.V.I. Pediatric	2300	1.2	1.4	1	1	80	400	7	200	Biotin 20 mcg, folic acid 140 mcg, niacinamide 17 mg, dexpanthenol 5 mg, aluminum, polysorbate 80

Adult Formulations

Product	A (units)	B$_1$ (mg)	B$_2$ (mg)	B$_6$ (mg)	B$_{12}$ (mcg)	C (mg)	D (units)	E (units)	Additional Information
Caplet									
Glutofac-ZX	5000	20	20	25	2500	200	400	100	Biotin 200 mcg, Cr 200 mcg, Cu 2.5 mg, folic acid 2800 mcg, lutein 500 mcg, lycopene 500 mcg, Mg 100 mg, Mn 2.5 mg, niacinamide 100 mg, pantothenic acid 10 mg, Se 100 mcg, Zn 15 mg
Strovite Forte	4000	20	20	25	50	500	400	60	Biotin 0.15 mg, Cr 0.05 mg, Cu 3 mg, Fe (as ferrous fumarate) 10 mg, folic acid 1 mg, Mg 50 mg, Mo 20 mg, niacinamide 100 mg, pantothenic acid 25 mg, Se 50 mcg, Zn 15 mg; contains soy products
Strovite Plus	5000	20	20	25	50	500		30	Biotin 0.15 mg, Cr 0.1 mg, Cu 3 mg, Fe (as ferrous fumarate) 27 mg, folic acid 0.8 mg, Mg 50 mg, Mn 5 mg, niacinamide 100 mg, pantothenic acid 25 mg, Zn 22.5 mg; contains soy products
Capsule									
Ferrex 150 Forte Plus					25	60 mg ascorbic acid 0.8 mg threonic acid			Fe [elemental] 150 mg, folic acid 1 mg, succinic acid 50 mg
Foltrin					15	75			Fe [elemental] 110 mg, folic acid 0.5 mg, special liver-stomach concentrate 240 mg
Hemocyte Plus		10	6	5	15	200			Cu 0.8 mg, Fe [elemental] 106 mg, folic acid 1 mg, Mg 6.9 mg, Mn 1.3 mg, niacinamide 30 mg, pantothenic acid 10 mg, Zn 18.2 mg
Ocuvite Lutein [OTC]						60		30	Cu 2 mg, lutein 6 mg, Zn 15 mg
Tandem Plus		10	6	5	15	200			Cu 0.8 mg, Fe (as ferrous fumarate) 162 mg, Fe (as polysaccharide) 115.2 mg, folic acid 1 mg, Mn 1.3 mg, niacinamide 30 mg, pantothenic acid 10 mg, Zn 18.2 mg
Capsule, Softgel									
Ocuvite Adult 50+ [OTC]						150		30	Cu 1 mg, lutein 6 mg, omega-3 150 mg, Zn 9 mg; contains soy products
PreserVision Lutein [OTC]						226		200	Cu 0.8 mg, lutein 5 mg, Zn 34.8 mg; contains soy products
Gummy									
One A Day VitaCraves Gummies [OTC] (2 per serving)	4000			2	10	60	400	40	Biotin 150 mcg, choline 60 mcg, folic acid 400 mcg, inositol 40 mcg, iodine 80 mcg, pantothenic acid 10 mg, Zn 5 mg
One A Day VitaCraves Sour Gummies [OTC] (2 per serving)	4000			2	10	60	400	40	Biotin 150 mcg, choline 60 mcg, folic acid 400 mcg, inositol 40 mcg, iodine 80 mcg, pantothenic acid 10 mg, Zn 5 mg
One A Day VitaCraves Gummies Plus Immunity Support [OTC] (2 per serving)	4000			2	10	125	400	40	Biotin 150 mcg, folic acid 400 mcg, iodine 80 mcg, pantothenic acid 20 mg, Se 35 mcg, Zn 5 mg
Liquid									
Centamin [OTC] (per 15 mL)	1300	1.5	1.7	2	6	60	400	30	Biotin 300 mcg, Cr 25 mcg, Fe 9 mg, iodine 150 mcg, Mo 25 mcg, niacin 20 mg, pantothenic acid 10 mg, Zn 3 mg (237 mL)
Centrum [OTC] (per 15 mL)		1.5	1.7	2	6	60		30	Biotin 300 mcg, Cr 25 mcg, Fe 9 mg, iodine 150 mcg, Mn 2 mg, Mo 25 mcg, niacin 20 mg, pantothenic acid 10 mg, Zn 3 mg; contains alcohol 5.7%, sodium benzoate (236 mL)

Adult Formulations *continued*

Product	A (units)	B₁ (mg)	B₂ (mg)	B₆ (mg)	B₁₂ (mcg)	C (mg)	D (units)	E (units)	Additional Information
Drinkables Fruits and Vegetables [OTC] *(per 1 oz)*	1812	100 mcg	100 mcg	100 mcg	0.2	38	142	11	Biotin 30 mcg, Ca 10 mg, choline 1 mg, Cr 43 mcg, Fe 180 mcg, folic acid 142 mcg, inositol 1 mg, lutein 100 mcg, lycopene 100 mcg, Mg 3 mg, Mn 0.7 mg, niacin 1 mg, PABA 1 mg, pantothenic acid 4 mg, phosphorus 7 mg, potassium 35 mg, sodium 10 mg, Stevia extract 18 mg, vitamin K 28 mcg, proprietary blend 22 g (887 mL)
Drinkables Multi Vitamins [OTC] *(per 1 oz)*	5000	1.5	1.7	2	6	80	400	30	Biotin 300 mcg, choline 3 mg, Cr 120 mcg, folic acid 400 mcg, inositol 3 mg, lutein 250 mcg, lycopene 300 mcg, Mn 2 mg, niacin 20 mg, PABA 3 mg, pantothenic acid 10 mg, vitamin K 80 mcg, proprietary trace mineral blend 252 mg (444 mL, 976 mL)
Geriation [OTC] *(per 30 mL)*		5	2.5	1	1				Choline 100 mg, Fe 15 mg, iodine 100 mcg, Mg 2 mg, Mn 2 mg, niacinamide 50 mg, pantothenic acid 10 mg, Zn 2 mg (473 mL); contains alcohol 18%
Geritol Tonic [OTC] *(per 15 mL)*		2.5	2.5	0.5					Choline 50 mg, Fe 18 mg, methionine 25 mg, niacin 50 mg, pantothenic acid 2 mg (120 mL, 360 mL)
Multi-Delyn [OTC] *(per 5 mL)*	2250	0.8	1	0.9	4	54	360	13.5	Niacin 12 mg; alcohol free, sugar free (240 mL, 473 mL)
Soft Chews									
Viactiv [OTC]	2500	1.5	1.7	2	6	60	400	33	Biotin 30 mcg, Ca 200 mg, folic acid 400 mcg, niacin 15 mg, pantothenic acid 10 mg; sodium 10 mg; contains soy products
Viactiv With Calcium [OTC]							500		Ca 500 mg, sodium 10 mg, vitamin K 40 mcg; contains soy products
Tablet									
Androvite [OTC] *(per 6 tablets)*	25,000	50	50	100	125	1000	400	400	Betaine 100 mg, biotin 125 mcg, boron 3 mg, Cr 200 mcg, Cu 2 mg, Fe (as amino acid chelate) 18 mg, folic acid 400 mcg, hesperidin 35 mg, inositol 36 mg, iodine 150 mcg, Mg 500 mg, Mn 10 mg, niacinamide 50 mg, PABA 25 mg, pancreatin 4X 75 mg, pantothenic acid 100 mg, rutin 25 mg, Se 200 mcg, Zn 50 mg
Centrum [OTC]	3500	1.5	1.7	2	6	60	400	30	Biotin 30 mcg, boron 75 mcg, Ca 200 mg, chloride 72 mg, Cr 35 mcg, Cu 0.5 mg, Fe 18 mg, folic acid 400 mcg, iodine 150 mcg, Mg 50 mg, Mn 2.3 mg, Mo 45 mcg, niacin 20 mg, nickel 5 mcg, pantothenic acid 10 mg, phosphorus 20 mg, potassium 80 mg, Se 55 mcg, silicon 2 mg, tin 10 mcg, vanadium 10 mcg, vitamin K 25 mcg, Zn 11 mg; contains sodium benzoate
Centrum Cardio [OTC] *(per tablet; dose: 2 tablets daily)*	1750	0.75	0.85	2.5	100	30	200	15	Biotin 15 mcg, boron 16 mcg, Ca 54 mcg, chloride 29 mcg, Cr 60 mcg, Cr 0.35 mg, Fe 3 mg, folic acid 200 mcg, iodine 75 mcg, Mg 20 mg, Mn 1 mg, Mo 37.5 mcg, niacin 10 mg, nickel 2.5 mcg, pantothenic acid 5 mg, phosphorus 40 mg, phytosterols 400 mg, potassium 32 mg, Se 10 mcg, silicon 1 mg, tin 5 mcg, vanadium 5 mcg, vitamin K 12.5 mcg, Zn 3.75 mcg; contains sodium benzoate, soy products
Centrum Performance [OTC]	3500	4.5	5.1	6	18	120	400	60	Biotin 50 mcg, boron 60 mcg, chloride 72 mg, Ca 100 mg, Cr 120 mcg, Cu 0.9 mg, Fe 18 mg, folic acid 400 mcg, ginseng root 50 mg, iodine 150 mcg, Mg 40 mg, Mn 4 mg, Mo 75 mcg, niacin 40 mg, nickel 5 mcg, pantothenic acid 12 mg, phosphorus 48 mg, potassium 80 mg, Se 70 mcg, silicon 4 mg, tin 10 mcg, vanadium 10 mcg, vitamin K 25 mcg, Zn 11 mg; contains sodium benzoate
Centrum Silver [OTC]	2500	1.5	1.7	3	25	60	500	50	Biotin 30 mcg, boron 150 mcg, Ca 220 mg, chloride 72 mg, Cr 45 mcg, Cu 0.5 mg, folic acid 400 mcg, iodine 150 mcg, lutein 250 mcg, lycopene 300 mcg, Mg 50 mg, Mn 2.3 mg, Mo 45 mcg, niacin 20 mg, nickel 5 mcg, pantothenic acid 10 mg, phosphorus 20 mg, potassium 80 mg, Se 55 mcg, silicon 2 mg, vanadium 10 mcg, vitamin K 30 mcg, Zn 11 mg; contains sodium benzoate
Centrum Silver Ultra Men's [OTC]	3500	1.5	1.7	6	100	120	600	60	Biotin 30 mcg, boron 150 mcg, Ca 250 mcg, chloride 72 mg, Cr 60 mcg, Cu 0.7 mg, folic acid 300 mcg, iodine 150 mcg, lutein 300 mcg, lycopene 600 mcg, Mg 50 mg, Mn 4 mg, Mo 50 mcg, niacin 20 mg, nickel 5 mcg, pantothenic acid 10 mg, phosphorus 20 mg, potassium 80 mg, Se 100 mcg, silicon 2 mg, vanadium 10 mcg, vitamin K 60 mcg, Zn 15 mg; contains soy products

MULTIVITAMIN PRODUCT TABLE

Adult Formulations *continued*

Product	A (units)	B₁ (mg)	B₂ (mg)	B₆ (mg)	B₁₂ (mcg)	C (mg)	D (units)	E (units)	Additional Information
Centrum Silver Ultra Women's [OTC]	3500	1.1	1.1	5	50	100	800	35	Biotin 30 mcg, boron 150 mcg, Ca 500 mg, chloride 72 mg, Cr 50 mcg, Cu 0.5 mg, Fe (as ferrous fumarate) 8 mg, folic acid 400 mcg, iodine 150 mcg, lutein 300 mcg, Mg 50 mg, Mn 2.3 mg, Mo 50 mcg, nickel 5 mcg, pantothenic acid 5 mg, phosphorus 20 mg, potassium 80 mg, Se 55 mcg, silicon 2 mg, vanadium 10 mcg, vitamin K 50 mcg, Zn 15 mg; contains soy products
Centrum Ultra Men's [OTC]	3500	1.2	1.3	2	6	90	600	45	Biotin 40 mcg, boron 150 mcg, Ca 210 mg, chloride 72 mg, Cr 35 mcg, Cu 0.9 mg, Fe (as ferrous fumarate) 8 mg, folic acid 200 mcg, iodine 150 mcg, lycopene 600 mcg, Mg 100 mg, Mn 2.3 mg, Mo 50 mcg, niacin 16 mg, nickel 5 mcg, pantothenic acid 15 mg, phosphorus 20 mg, potassium 80 mg, Se 100 mcg, silicon 2 mg, tin 10 mcg, vanadium 10 mcg, vitamin K 60 mcg, Zn 11 mg; contains soy products
Centrum Ultra Women's [OTC]	3500	1.1	1.1	2	6	75	800	35	Biotin 40 mcg, boron 150 mcg, Ca 500 mg, chloride 72 mg, Cr 25 mcg, Cu 0.9 mg, Fe (as ferrous fumarate) 18 mg, folic acid 400 mcg, iodine 150 mcg, Mg 100 mg, Mn 1.8 mg, Mo 50 mcg, niacin 14 mg, nickel 5 mcg, pantothenic acid 15 mg, phosphorus 20 mg, potassium 80 mg, Se 55 mcg, silicon 2 mg, tin 10 mcg, vanadium 10 mcg, vitamin K 50 mcg, Zn 8 mg; contains soy products
DiatxZN		1.5	1.5	50	2 mg	60			Biotin 300 mcg, Cu 1.5 mg, folic acid 5 mg, niacinamide 20 mg, pantothenic acid 10 mg, Zn 25 mg; gluten free, sugar free
Freedavite [OTC]	5000	1.5	1.7	2	6	60	400	30	Biotin 30 mcg, Ca 20 mg, Cu 0.1 mg, Fe (as ferrous fumarate) 1.8 mg, folic acid 400 mcg, iodine 75 mcg, Mg 8 mg, Mn 0.625 mg, niacinamide 20 mg, pantothenic acid 10 mg, Se 35 mcg, Zn 1.5 mg
Geri-Freeda [OTC]	5000	15	15	15	15	150	400	15	Betaine 10 mcg, biotin 15 mcg, Ca 50 mg, choline 10 mg, Cr 60 mcg, Cu 0.5 mg, folic acid 400 mcg, hesperidin 10 mg, inositol 10 mg, iodine 150 mcg, L-lysine 25 mg, Mn 1 mg, niacinamide 50 mg, PABA 10 mg, pantothenic acid 15 mg, Se 35 mcg, Zn 7.5 mg
Gerital Complete [OTC]	6100	1.5	1.7	2	6.7	57	400	30	Biotin 44 mcg, Ca 148 mg, chloride 20 mg, Cr 12 mcg, Cu 1.8 mg, Fe 16 mg, folic acid 0.38 mg, iodine 120 mcg, Mg 86 mg, Mn 2.4 mg, Mo 1 mg, niacin 20 mg, pantothenic acid 13 mg, phosphorus 118 mg, potassium 36 mg, selenium 1 mg, vitamin K 24 mcg, Zn 13.5 mg
Gynovite Plus [OTC] (*per 6 tablets*)	5000	10	10	20	125	180	400	400	Betaine 100 mg, biotin 125 mcg, boron 3 mg, Ca 500 mg, Cr 200 mcg, Cu 2 mg, Fe (as amino acid chelate) 18 mg, folic acid 400 mcg, hesperidin 35 mg, inositol 50 mg, iodine 150 mcg, Mg 600 mg, Mn 10 mg, niacinamide 20 mg, PABA 25 mg, pancreatin 4X 93 mg, pantothenic acid 10 mg, rutin 25 mg, Se 200 mcg, Zn 15 mg
Hi-Kovite [OTC] (*per contents of 1 vitamin tablet plus 1 mineral tablet*)	5000	10	10	10	10	200	400	30	Bioflavonoids 10 mg, biotin 30 mcg, Ca 120 mg, Cu 0.5 mg, Fe (as ferrous fumarate) 9 mg, folic acid 400 mcg, inositol 10 mg, iodine 75 mcg, L-lysine 10 mg, Mg 60 mg, Mn 1 mg, niacinamide 100 mg, PABA 10 mg, pantothenic acid 10 mg, potassium 35 mg, Se 17.5 mcg, Zn 7.5 mg
Iberet-500		6	6	5	25	500			Iron 105 mg, niacin 30 mg, pantothenic acid 10 mg
ICaps AREDS Formula [OTC] (*per 2 tablets*)	28640					452		400	Cu 1.6 mg, Zn 69.6 mg
ICaps Lutein and Zeaxanthin Formula [OTC] (*per 2 tablets*)	6600					400		150	Cu 4 mg, lutein/zeaxanthin 4 mg, Mn 10 mg, Se 40 mg, Zn 60 mg
ICaps Multivitamin [OTC] (*per 4 tablets*)	5000	1.5	10	2	6	512	400	430	Biotin 30 mcg, Ca 333 mg, Cr 120 mcg, Cu 3.6 mg, folic acid 400 mcg, iodine 150 mcg, lutein 6.67 mg, lycopene 0.3 mg, Mg 100 mg, Mn 2 mg, Mo 75 mcg, niacin 10 mg, pantothenic acid 10 mg, phosphorus 140 mg, Se 40 mcg, vitamin K 25 mcg, zeaxanthin 3.3 mg, Zn 84.6 mg
Maxaron Forte					250 (methylcobalamin)	200			Fe (as ferrous fumarate) 70 mg, Fe (as iron glycinate sulfate) 80 mg, l-methylfolate 1.13 mg

Adult Formulations *continued*

Product	A (units)	B$_1$ (mg)	B$_2$ (mg)	B$_6$ (mg)	B$_{12}$ (mcg)	C (mg)	D (units)	E (units)	Additional Information
Monocaps [OTC]	5000	15	15	15	15	120	400	15	Biotin 15 mcg, Ca 50 mg, Cu 0.1 mg, Fe (as ferrous fumarate) 14 mg, folic acid 400 mcg, iodine 150 mcg, lecithin 10 mg, L-lysine 10 mg, Mg 30 mg, Mn 1 mg, niacinamide 40 mg, pantothenic acid 15 mg, Se 35 mcg, Zn 3.75 mg
Multilex [OTC]	10,000	10	5	1.7	3	100	400	5.5	Ca 10 mg, Cu 1 mg, Fe 15 mg, Mg 5 mg, Mn 1 mg, niacinamide 30 mg, potassium iodide 0.15 mg, Zn 1.5 mg
Multilex-T&M [OTC]	10,000	15	10	2	7.5	150	400	5.5	Ca 10 mg, Cu 1 mg, Fe 15 mg, Mg 5 mg, Mn 1 mg, niacinamide 100 mg, potassium iodide 0.15 mg, Zn 1.5 mg
Myadec [OTC]	5000	1.7	2	3	6	60	400	30	Biotin 30 mcg, boron 150 mcg, Ca 162 mg, chloride 36 mg, Cr 25 mcg, Cu 2 mg, Fe 18 mg, folic acid 400 mcg, iodine 150 mcg, Mg 100 mg, Mn 2.5 mg, Mo 25 mcg, niacin 20 mg, nickel 5 mcg, pantothenic acid 10 mg, phosphorus 125 mg, potassium 40 mg, Se 25 mcg, silicon 10 mg, vanadium 10 mcg, vitamin K 25 mcg, Zn 15 mg; contains soy products
NicAzel Forte				8					Azerizin 700 mg (proprietary blend of nicotinamide, azelaic acid, quercetin, and curcumin), Cu 2 mg, folic acid 500 mcg, Zn 12 mg; contains tartrazine
Ocuvite [OTC]	1000					200		60	Cu 2 mg, lutein 2 mg, Se 55 mcg, Zn 40 mg
One A Day Cholesterol Plus [OTC]	2500	1.5	1.7	2	6	60	400	30	Biotin 50 mcg, boron 150 mcg, Ca 100 mg, Cr 120 mcg, Cu 2 mg, folic acid 400 mcg, iodine 150 mcg, Mg 100 mg, Mn 2 mg, Mo 75 mcg, niacin 20 mg, pantothenic acid 10 mg, phytosterols 100 mg, potassium 99 mg, Se 70 mcg, Zn 15 mg; contains soy products
One A Day Energy [OTC]	3500	3	3.4	4	12	60	400	22.5	Biotin 300 mcg, boron 150 mcg, caffeine 90 mg, Ca 250 mg, Cr 100 mcg, Cu 2 mg, Fe 9 mg, folic acid 400 mcg, guarana seed powder 110 mg, iodine 150 mcg, Mg 40 mg, Mn 2 mg, Mo 25 mcg, niacin 40 mg, nickel 5 mcg, pantothenic acid 10 mg, potassium 99 mg, Se 45 mcg, silicon 5 mg, tin 10 mcg, vitamin K 25 mcg, Zn 15 mg; contains tartrazine
One A Day Essential [OTC]	3000	1.5	1.7	2	6	60	400	30	Ca 45 mg, folic acid 400 mcg, niacin 20 mg, pantothenic acid 10 mg; contains soy products
One A Day Maximum [OTC]	2500	1.5	1.7	2	6	60	400	30	Biotin 30 mcg, boron 150 mcg, Ca 162 mg, chloride 72 mg, Cr 65 mcg, Cu 2 mg, Fe 18 mg, folic acid 400 mcg, iodine 150 mcg, Mg 100 mg, Mn 3.5 mg, Mo 160 mcg, niacin 20 mg, nickel 5 mcg, pantothenic acid 10 mg, phosphorus 109 mg, potassium 80 mg, Se 20 mcg, silicon 2 mg, tin 10 mcg, vanadium 10 mcg, vitamin K 25 mcg, Zn 15 mg; contains soy products
One A Day Menopause Formula [OTC]	2500	3	3.4	8	12	60	800	33	Biotin 300 mcg, boron 1500 mcg, Ca 300 mg, Cr 120 mcg, Cu 1 mg, folic acid 400 mcg, iodine 150 mcg, Mg 50 mg, Mn 2 mg, Mo 37.5 mcg, niacin 20 mg, pantothenic acid 15 mg, Se 20 mcg, soybean extract 60 mg, Zn 15 mg; contains soy products
One A Day Men's 50+ Advantage [OTC]	2500	4.5	3.4	6	25	60	700	22.5	Biotin 30 mcg, Ca 120 mg, Cr 180 mcg, folic acid 400 mcg, ginko biloba extract 120 mg, iodine 150 mcg, lycopene 300 mcg, Mg 100 mg, Mn 4 mg, molybdenum 90 mcg, niacin 20 mg, pantothenic acid 15 mg, Se 110 mcg, vitamin K 20 mcg, Zn 22.5 mg
One A Day Men's Health Formula [OTC]	3500	1.2	1.7	3	18	60	700	22.5	Biotin 30 mcg, Ca 210 mg, Cr 120 mcg, Cu 2 mg, folic acid 400 mcg, lycopene 300 mcg, Mg 120 mg, Mn 2 mg, niacin 16 mg, pantothenic acid 5 mg, Se 110 mcg, vitamin K 20 mcg, Zn 15 mg
One A Day Men's Pro Edge [OTC]	3500	3	3.4	4	12	80	800	33	Biotin 300 mcg, Ca 200 mg, Cr 120 mcg, Cu 2 mg, folic acid 400 mcg, Mg 200 mg, Mn 2 mg, niacin 25 mg, pantothenic acid 15 mg, Se 70 mcg, vitamin K 20 mcg, Zn 15 mg; contains tartrazine
One A Day Teen Advantage for Her [OTC]	2500	2.3	2.6	3	9	120	800	30	Biotin 300 mcg, Ca 300 mg, Cr 120 mcg, Cu 2 mg, Fe 18 mg, folic acid 400 mcg, Mg 50 mg, Mn 2 mg, niacin 30 mg, pantothenic acid 10 mg, Se 20 mcg, vitamin K 25 mcg, Zn 15 mg
One A Day Teen Advantage for Him [OTC]	2500	3.75	4.25	5	15	120	400	30	Biotin 30 mcg, Ca 200 mg, Cr 120 mcg, Cu 2 mg, Fe 9 mg, folic acid 400 mcg, Mg 100 mg, Mn 2 mg, niacin 30 mg, pantothenic acid 10 mg, Se 20 mcg, vitamin K 25 mcg, Zn 15 mg
One A Day Women's [OTC]	2500	1.5	1.7	2	6	60	1000	22.5	Biotin 30 mcg, Ca 500 mg, Cr 120 mcg, Cu 2 mg, Fe 18 mg, folic acid 400 mcg, Mg 50 mg, Mn 2 mg, niacin 10 mg, pantothenic acid 5 mg, Se 20 mcg, vitamin K 25 mcg, Zn 15 mg; contains tartrazine

Adult Formulations *continued*

Product	A (units)	B₁ (mg)	B₂ (mg)	B₆ (mg)	B₁₂ (mcg)	C (mg)	D (units)	E (units)	Additional Information
One A Day Women's 50+ Advantage [OTC]	2500	4.5	3.4	6	25	60	1000	22.5	Biotin 30 mcg, Ca 500 mg, Cr 180 mcg, Cu 2 mg, folic acid 400 mcg, ginkgo biloba extract 120 mg, iodine 150 mcg, Mg 50 mg, Mn 4 mg, Mo 90 mcg, niacin 20 mg, pantothenic acid 15 mg, Se 20 mcg, vitamin K 20 mcg, Zn 22.5 mg; contains tartrazine
One A Day Women's Active Metabolism [OTC]	2500	2.4	2.7	3.2	9.5	60	800	22.5	Biotin 30 mcg, Ca 300 mg, caffeine 120 mg, Cr 120 mcg, Cu 2 mg, Fe 18 mg, folic acid 400 mcg, guarana seed 50 mg, Mg 50 mg, Mn 2 mg, niacin 10 mg, pantothenic acid 5 mg, Se 20 mcg, vitamin K 25 mcg, Zn 15 mg; contains soy products
One A Day Women's Active Mind & Body [OTC]	2500	2.4	2.7	3.2	9.5	60	800	30	Biotin 30 mcg, Ca 300 mg, Cr 120 mcg, Cu 2 mg, Fe 18 mg, folic acid 400 mcg, guarana blend 180 mg, Mg 50 mg, Mn 2 mg, niacin 10 mg, pantothenic acid 5 mg, Se 20 mcg, vitamin K 25 mcg, Zn 15 mg; contains tartrazine
Optivite P.M.T. [OTC] *(per 6 tablets)*	12,500	25	25	300	60	1500	100	100	Betaine 100 mg, bioflavonoids 250 mg, biotin 60 mcg, Ca 125 mg, choline 313 mg, Cr 100 mcg, Fe (as amino acid chelate) 15 mg, folic acid 200 mcg, inositol 24 mg, iodine 75 mcg, Mg 250 mg, Mn 10 mg, niacinamide 25 mg, PABA 25 mg, pancreatin 4X 93 mg, pantothenic acid 25 mg, potassium 48 mg, rutin 25 mg, Se 100 mcg, Zn 25 mg
PreserVision AREDS [OTC] *(per 2 tablets)*	14,320					226		200	Cu 0.8 mg, Zn 34.8 mg
Quintabs [OTC]	5000	30	30	30	30	300	400	50	Biotin 30 mcg, folic acid 400 mcg, niacinamide 100 mg, pantothenic acid 30 mg
Quintabs-M [OTC]	5000	30	30	30	30	300	400	50	Biotin 30 mcg, Ca 30 mg, Cu 0.2 mg, Fe (as ferrous fumarate) 10 mg, folic acid 400 mcg, iodine 150 mcg, Mg 15 mg, Mn 2 mg, niacinamide 100 mg, pantothenic acid 30 mg, Se 35 mcg, Zn 7.5 mg
Quintabs-M Iron-Free [OTC]	5000	30	30	30	30	300	400	50	Biotin 30 mcg, Ca 30 mg, Cu 0.2 mg, folic acid 400 mcg, iodine 150 mcg, Mg 15 mg, Mn 2 mg, niacinamide 100 mg, pantothenic acid 30 mg, Se 35 mcg, Zn 7.5 mg
Repliva 21/7					10	140 mg as ascorbic acid 60 mg as Ester-C supplement			Fe [elemental] 151 mg, folic acid 1 mg, succinic acid 150 mg
Theragran-M [OTC]	5000	3	3.4	6	12	90	400	60	Biotin 30 mcg, boron 150 mcg, Ca 40 mg, chloride 7.5 mg, Cr 50 mcg, Cu 2 mg, Fe 9 mg, folic acid 400 mcg, iodine 150 mcg, Mg 100 mg, Mn 2 mg, Mo 75 mcg, Ni 5 mcg, niacin 20 mg, pantothenic acid 10 mg, phosphorous 31 mg, potassium 7.5 mg, Se 70 mcg, silicon 2 mg, tin 10 mcg, vanadium 10 mcg, vitamin K 28 mcg, Zn 15 mg; contains soy products
Thera-M [OTC]	5000	3	3.4	6	12	90	400		Biotin 30 mcg, boron 150 mcg, Ca 40 mg, chloride 7.5 mg, Cr 50 mcg, Cu 2 mg, Fe (as ferrous fumarate) 9 mg, folic acid 400 mcg, iodine 150 mcg, Mg 100 mg, Mn 2 mg, Mo 75 mcg, Ni 5 mcg, niacinamide 20 mg, pantothenic acid 10 mg, phosphorous 31 mg, potassium 7.5 mg, Se 70 mcg, silicon 2 mg, tin 10 mcg, vanadium 10 mcg, vitamin K 28 mcg, Zn 15 mg; contains soy products
T-Vites [OTC]		25	25	25	30	100	400	200	Biotin 30 mcg, folic acid 400 mcg, Mg 100 mg, Mn 0.5 mg, niacinamide 150 mg, pantothenic acid 25 mg, potassium 35 mg, Zn 3.75 mg
Ultra Freeda A-Free [OTC] *(per 3 tablets)*		50	50	50	100	1000	400	200	Base (choline, inositol, PABA) 100 mg, bioflavonoids 100 mg, biotin 300 mcg, Ca 250 mg, Cr 200 mcg, Fe (as ferrous fumarate) 18 mg, folic acid 800 mcg, iodine 150 mcg, Mg 100 mg, Mn 10 mg, Mo 12.5 mcg, niacinamide and niacin 100 mg, pantothenic acid 100 mg, potassium 35 mg, Se 100 mcg, Zn 22.5 mg
Ultra Freeda Iron-Free [OTC] *(per 3 tablets)*	5000	50	50	50	100	1000	400	200	Base (choline, inositol) 100 mg, bioflavonoids 100 mg, biotin 300 mcg, Ca 250 mg, Cr 200 mcg, folic acid 800 mcg, iodine 150 mcg, Mg 100 mg, Mn 10 mg, Mo 12.5 mcg, niacinamide and niacin 100 mg, pantothenic acid 100 mg, potassium 35 mg, Se 100 mcg, Zn 22.5 mg

Adult Formulations *continued*

Product	A (units)	B_1 (mg)	B_2 (mg)	B_6 (mg)	B_{12} (mcg)	C (mg)	D (units)	E (units)	Additional Information
Ultra Freeda With Iron [OTC] *(per 3 tablets)*	5000	50	50	50	100	1000	400	200	Base (choline, inositol) 100 mg, bioflavonoids 100 mg, biotin 300 mcg, Ca 250 mg, Cr 200 mcg, Fe (as ferrous fumarate) 18 mg, folic acid 800 mcg, iodine 150 mcg, Mg 100 mg, Mn 10 mg, Mo 12.5 mcg, niacinamide and niacin 100 mg, pantothenic acid 100 mg, potassium 35 mg, Se 100 mcg, Zn 22.5 mg
Xtramins [OTC]	1000	5	2	5	10	50	100	10	Boron 1 mg, Ca 250 mg, Cr 40 mcg, Cu 500 mcg, Fe (as iron gluconate) 10 mg, folic acid 400 mcg, iodine 150 mcg, Mg 20 mg, Mn 2 mg, niacinamide 15 mg, PABA 5 mg, pantothenic acid 5 mg, potassium 45 mg, Se 30 mcg, Zn 10 mg; gluten free, sugar free
Yelets [OTC]	5000	10	10	10	10	100	400	30	Biotin 30 mcg, Ca 60 mg, Fe (as ferrous fumarate) 18 mg, folic acid 400 mcg, iodine 150 mcg, L-lysine 10 mg, Mg 20 mg, Mn 1 mg, niacinamide 25 mg, pantothenic acid 10 mg, Se 17.5 mcg, Zn 7.5 mg
Tablet, Chewable									
Centrum [OTC]	3500	1.5	1.7	2	6	60	400	30	Biotin 45 mcg, Ca 108 mg, Cr 20 mcg, Cu 2 mg, Fe 18 mg, folic acid 400 mcg, iodine 150 mcg, Mg 40 mg, Mn 1 mg, Mo 20 mg, niacin 20 mg, pantothenic acid 10 mg, phosphorus 50 mg, vitamin K 10 mcg, Zn 15 mg; contains sodium benzoate, soy products
Centrum Silver [OTC]	4000	2.2	2.7	7	25	75	400	70	Biotin 45 mcg, Ca 200 mg, Cr 100 mcg, Cu 2 mg, folic acid 400 mcg, iodine 100 mcg, lutein 250 mcg, Mg 50 mg, Mn 4.5 mg, Mo 25 mg, niacin 12 mg, nickel 5 mcg, pantothenic acid 10 mg, phosphorus 125 mg, Se 22.5 mcg, silicon 4 mg, tin 10 mcg, vanadium 10 mcg, Zn 15 mg; contains phenylalanine, sodium benzoate, soy products
Tablet, dissolving									
ProBarimin QT	5000	3	1.7	5	250	60	800	30	Biotin 300 mcg, Ca 120 mg, Cu 2 mg, Fe (as ferrous fumarate) 8 mg, folic acid 600 mcg, Mn 2 mg, molybdenum 75 mcg, niacinamide 20 mg, pantothenic acid 10 mg, Se 55 mcg, Zn 15 mg; sugar free
Wafers									
CalciFol				10	25		200		Boron 1 mg, Ca 1342 mg, folic acid 1.6 mg, magnesium 50 mg
Calcifolic-D				10	125		300		Boron 250 mcg, Ca 1342 mg, folic acid 1 mg, magnesium 50 mg
Combination Package									
Encora									
AM tablet				25		25	200		Ca 400 mg, folic acid 2 mg
PM tablet				12.5		25	600		Ca 600 mg, folic acid 0.5 mg
AM/PM gelatin capsule								50	Linoleic acid 10 mg, omega-3 fatty acids 650 mg including DHA and EPA 550 mg and ALA 100 mg

ALA = α-linolenic acid, Ca = calcium, Cr = chromium, Cu = copper, DHA = docosahexaenoic acid, EPA = eicosapentaenoic acid, Fe = iron, Mg = magnesium, Mn = manganese, Mo = molybdenum, Se = selenium, Zn = zinc

Pediatric Formulations

Product	A (units)	B_1 (mg)	B_2 (mg)	B_6 (mg)	B_{12} (mcg)	C (mg)	D (units)	E (units)	Additional Information
Capsule, softgel									
AquADEKs [OTC]	18,167 (92% as beta carotene)	1.5	1.7	1.9	12	75	800	150 units as d-alpha tocopherol and 80 mg as mixed tocopherols	Beta-carotene 10 mg, biotin 100 mcg, coenzyme Q_{10} 10 mg, folic acid 200 mcg, niacinamide 20 mg, pantothenic acid 12 mg, selenium 75 mcg, vitamin K 700 mcg, Zn 10 mg; dye free
SourceCF [OTC]	16000 (88% as beta carotene)	1.5	1.7	1.9	6	100	1000	200	Biotin 100 mcg, folic acid 200 mcg, niacinamide 20 mg, pantothenic acid 12 mg, vitamin K 800 mcg, Zn 15 mg; contains soy products
Drops									
AquADEKs [OTC] (per mL)	5751 (87% as beta carotene)	0.6	0.6	0.6		45	400	50 units as d-alpha tocopherol and 15 mg as mixed tocopherols	Beta-carotene 3 mg, biotin 15 mcg, enzyme Q_{10} 2 mg, niacinamide 6 mg, pantothenic acid 3 mg, selenium 10 mcg, vitamin K 400 mcg, Zn 5 mg; contains sodium benzoate; dye free (60 mL)
MyKidz Iron [OTC] (*per 2 mL*)	1500					35	400		Fe [elemental] 10 mg; alcohol free, sugar free, dye free
MyKidz Iron FL (*per 2 mL*)	1500					35	400		Fe [elemental] 10 mg, fluoride 0.25 mg; alcohol free, sugar free, dye free (118 mL)
Poly-Vi-Sol [OTC] (*per mL*)	1500	0.5	0.6	0.4	2	35	400	5	Niacin 8 mg; gluten free (50 mL)
Poly-Vi-Sol With Iron [OTC] (*per mL*)	1500	0.5	0.6	0.4		35	400	5	Fe [elemental] 10 mg, niacin 8 mg; gluten free (50 mL)
SourceCF [OTC] (*per mL*)	4627 (75% as beta carotene)	0.6	0.6	0.6	4	45	500	50	Biotin 15 mcg, niacinamide 6 mg, pantothenic acid 3 mg, vitamin K 400 mcg, Zn 5 mg; contains sodium benzoate (60 mL)
Tri-Vi-Sol [OTC] (*per mL*)	1500					35	400		Gluten free (50 mL)
Gummy									
Flintstones Gummies [OTC] (*per 2 gummies*)	2000			1	5	30	200	20	Biotin 75 mcg, choline 38 mcg, folic acid 200 mcg, inositol 20 mcg, iodine 40 mcg, pantothenic acid 5 mg, zinc 2.5 mg
Flintstones Gummies Plus Immunity Support [OTC] (*per 2 gummies*)	2000			1	5	125	200	20	Biotin 75 mcg, folic acid 200 mcg, inositol 20 mcg, iodine 40 mcg, pantothenic acid 5 mg, Zn 2.5 mg
Flintstones Gummies Plus Bone Building Support [OTC] (*per 2 gummies*)	1600			1	5	30	400	20	Biotin 75 mcg, Ca 100 mg, iodine 40 mcg, pantothenic acid 5 mg, Zn 2.5 mg
Flintstones Sour Gummies [OTC] (*per 2 gummies*)	2000			1	5	30	200	20	Biotin 75 mcg, choline 38 mcg, folic acid 200 mcg, inositol 20 mcg, iodine 40 mcg, pantothenic acid 5 mg, zinc 2.5 mg; contains tartrazine
One A Day Kids Jolly Rancher Gummies [OTC] (*per 2 gummies*)	2000			1	5	30	200	20	Biotin 75 mcg, choline 30 mcg, folic acid 200 mcg, inositol 20 mcg, iodine 40 mcg, pantothenic acid 5 mg, Zn 2.5 mg; contains tartrazine

Pediatric Formulations *continued*

Product	A (units)	B₁ (mg)	B₂ (mg)	B₆ (mg)	B₁₂ (mcg)	C (mg)	D (units)	E (units)	Additional Information
One A Day Kids Jolly Rancher Sour Gummies [OTC] (*per 2 gummies*)	2000			1	5	30	200	20	Biotin 75 mcg, choline 30 mcg, folic acid 200 mcg, inositol 20 mcg, iodine 40 mcg, pantothenic acid 5 mg, Zn 2.5 mg; contains tartrazine
One A Day Kids Scooby-Doo! Gummies [OTC] (*per 2 gummies*)	2000			1	5	30	200	20	Biotin 75 mcg, choline 30 mcg, folic acid 200 mcg, inositol 20 mcg, iodine 40 mcg, pantothenic acid 5 mg, zinc 2.5 mg
Tablet, Chewable									
ADEKs [OTC]	4000	1.2	1.3	1.5	12	60	400	150	Beta carotene 3 mg, biotin 50 mcg, folic acid 0.2 mg, niacinamide 10 mg, pantothenic acid 10 mg, vitamin K 150 mcg, Zn 7.5 mg
Centrum Kids [OTC]	3500	1.5	1.7	2	6	60	400	30	Biotin 45 mcg, Ca 108 mg, Cr 20 mcg, Cu 2 mg, Fe 18 mg, folic acid 400 mcg, iodine 150 mcg, Mg 40 mg, Mn 1 mg, Mo 20 mcg, niacin 20 mg, pantothenic acid 10 mg, phosphorus 50 mg, vitamin K 10 mcg, Zn 15 mg; contains phenylalanine, sodium benzoate, soy products
Flintstones Complete [OTC]	3000	1.5	1.7	2	6	60	400	30	Biotin 40 mcg, Ca 100 mg, choline 38 mg, Cu 2 mg, Fe 18 mg, folic acid 400 mcg, iodine 150 mcg, Mg 20 mg, niacin 15 mg, pantothenic acid 10 mg, phosphorus 100 mg, sodium 10 mg, Zn 12 mg; contains phenylalanine, soy products
Flintstones Plus Bone Building Support [OTC]	2500	1.05	1.2	1.05	4.5	60	400	15	Calcium 200 mg, folic acid 300 mcg, niacin 13.5 mg, sodium 10 mg; contains phenylalanine, soy products
Flintstones Plus Immunity Support [OTC]	2500	1.05	1.2	1.05	4.5	250	400	15	Folic acid 300 mcg, niacin 13.5 mg, sodium 25 mg
Flintstones Plus Iron [OTC]	2500	1.05	1.2	1.05	4.5	60	400	15	Fe 15 mg, folic acid 300 mcg, niacin 13.5 mg, sodium 10 mg; contains soy products
My First Flintstones [OTC]	1998	1.05	1.2	1.05	4.5	60	400	15	Folic acid 300 mcg, niacin 10 mg, sodium 10 mg; contains soy products
One A Day Kids Scooby-Doo! Complete [OTC]	3000	1.5	1.7	2	6	60	400	30	Biotin 40 mcg, Ca 100 mg, Cu 2 mg, Fe 18 mg, folic acid 400 mcg, iodine 150 mcg, Mg 20 mg, niacin 15 mg, pantothenic acid 10 mg, phosphorus 100 mg, sodium 10 mg, Zn 12 mg; contains phenylalanine; sugar free
Quflora	1200	1.2	1.3	1.5	4	60	400	15	Cu 1 mg, folic acid 100 mcg, l-methylfolate 108 mcg, Mg 15 mg, niacinamide 5 mg; grape flavor. Available in three fluoride strengths: 0.25 mg, 0.5 mg, 1 mg
SourceCF [OTC]	16000	1.5	1.7	1.9	6	100	1000	200	Biotin 100 mcg, folic acid 200 mcg, niacinamide 10 mg, pantothenic acid 12 mg, vitamin K 800 mcg, Zn 15 mg
Vitalets [OTC]	2500	0.75	0.85	1	3	40	200	15	Biotin 150 mcg, Ca 80 mg, Fe (as ferrous fumarate) 10 mg, folic acid 200 mcg, Mg 20 mg, Mn 0.1 mg, niacinamide 10 mg, pantothenic acid 5 mg, phosphorus 60 mg, Zn 0.8 mg

Ca = calcium, Cr = chromium, Cu = copper, Fe = iron, Mg = magnesium, Mn = manganese, Mo = molybdenum, Zn = zinc

Prenatal Formulations

Product	A (units)	B₁ (mg)	B₂ (mg)	B₆ (mg)	B₁₂ (mcg)	C (mg)	D (units)	E (units)	Additional Information
Caplet									
Néevo		3	3.4	2.6	0.5	80	400	30	Biotin 30 mcg, Ca 200 mg, Cu 2 mg, Fe (as polysaccharide iron complex) 29 mg, folic acid 0.4 mg, l-methylfolate 1.3 mg, Mg 40 mg, niacinamide 20 mg, pantothenic acid 7 mg, Zn 15 mg; contains sodium benzoate
Prenate chewable				10	125		300	30	Biotin 280 mcg, blueberry extract 25 mg, boron 250 mcg, Ca 500 mg, folate 1 mg (folic acid 400 mcg, Quatrefolic 600 mcg), Mg 50 mg
Select-OB [OTC]	1700	1.6	1.8	2.5	5	60	400	30	Fe (as polysaccharide iron complex) 29 mg, folic acid 1 mg, Mg 25 mg, niacinamide 15 mg, Zn 15 mg; gluten free
Vitafol-OB [OTC]	2700	1.6	1.8	2.5	12	70	400	30	Ca 100 mg, Cu 2 mg, Fe [elemental] 65 mg, folic acid 1 mg, Mg 25 mg, niacinamide 18 mg, Zn 25 mg; gluten free, sugar free
Vitafol-PN	1700	1.6	1.8	2.5	5	60	400	30	Ca 125 mg, Fe [elemental] 65 mg, folic acid 1 mg, Mg 25 mg, niacinamide 15 mg, Zn 15 mg
Capsule									
Concept OB		5	5	25	10	210		30	Biotin 300 mcg, Cu 0.8 mg, DHA 156 mg, EPA 39 mg, Fe (as ferrous fumarate) 130 mg, Fe (as polysaccharide iron complex) 92.4 mg, folic acid 1 mg, Mn 1.3 mg, niacin 20 mg, pantothenic acid 7 mg, Zn 18.2 mg
Nexa Plus				25		28	800	30	Biotin 250 mcg, Ca 160 mg, DHA 350 mg, docusate calcium 55 mg, Fe 29 mg, folic acid 1.25 mg; contains soy products
PrimaCare One				25		25	170	30	Ca 150 mg, Fe [elemental] 27 mg, folic acid 1 mg, linolenic acid 30 mg; 330 mg omega-3 fatty acids, including alpha-linolenic acid 30 mg; contains soy products
R-Natal OB		2	4	20	30	100	400	30	Cu 2 mg, DHA 320 mg, Fe (as carbonyl iron) 20 mg, folic acid 1 mg, Zn 30 mg; contains soy products
Vitafol Ultra		1.6	1.8	2.5	12	30	1000	20	Algal oil 415 mg, beta carotene 1100 units, Cu 2 mg, DHA 200 mg, Fe (as polysaccharide iron complex) 29 mg, folic acid 0.4 mg, l-methylfolate 0.6 mg, Mg 20 mg, niacinamide 15 mg, potassium iodide 150 mcg, Zn 25 mg; contains soy products
Capsule, Softgel									
CitraNatal Harmony				25			400	30	Algal oil 650 mg, Ca 104 mg, DHA 265 mg, docusate sodium 50 mg, Fe (as carbonyl iron) 29 mg, folic acid 1 mg
Concept DHA		2	3	25	12.5	25		15	Biotin 300 mcg, Cu 2 mg, Fe (as ferrous fumarate) 53.5 mg, Fe (as polysaccharide iron complex) 38 mg, folic acid 1 mg, Mg 5 mg, niacin 1.8 mg, pantothenic acid 5 mg, Zn 10 mg
Folcaps Care One			1.5	50		25	800	30	Alpha-linolenic acid 50 mg, biotin 300 mcg, Ca 100 mg, DHA 350 mg, EPA 150 mg, docusate sodium 50 mg, Fe 27 mg, folic acid 1 mg, iodine 150 mcg, Mg 50 mg, niacinamide 10 mg, Zn 5 mg; contains soy products
Natelle One				25		30		30	Ca 102 mg, DHA 250 mg, EPA not more than 0.625 mg, Fe (as ferrous fumarate) 28 mg, folic acid 1 mg; contains soy products
NeevoDHA				25	1	40	400	30	Ca 75 mg, DHA 250 mg, Fe (as ferrous fumarate) 27 mg, folic acid 400 mcg, l-methylfolate 1.13 mg; contains soy products
PreferaOB One				50	12	25		10	Biotin 30 mg, DHA 200 mg, Fe 28 mg (22 mg as polysaccharide complex and 6 mg as heme iron polypeptide), folic acid 1 mg, iodine 175 mcg, niacinamide 17 mg, pantothenic acid 10 mg, Zn 15 mg; contains soy products
Prenate DHA				26	13	90	220	10	Ca 145 mg, DHA 300 mg, Fe (as ferrous fumarate) 28 mg, folate 1 mg (folic acid 400 mcg, Quatrefolic 600 mcg), Mg 50 mg; contains soy products
Prenate Essential				26	13	90	220	10	Biotin 280 mcg, Ca 145 mg, DHA 300 mg, EPA 40 mg, Fe (as ferrous fumarate) 29 mg, folate 1 mg (folic acid 400 mcg, Quatrefolic 600 mcg), iodine 150 mcg, Mg 50 mg; contains soy products, tartrazine

Prenatal Formulations *continued*

Product	A (units)	B₁ (mg)	B₂ (mg)	B₆ (mg)	B₁₂ (mcg)	C (mg)	D (units)	E (units)	Additional Information
Prenate Mini				26	13	60	220	10	Biotin 280 mcg, blueberry extract (*vaccinium angustifolium*) 25 mg, Ca 100 mg, DHA 350 mg, Fe (as carbonyl iron) 29 mg, folate 1 mg (folic acid 400 mcg, Quatrefolic 600 mcg), iodine 150 mcg, Mg 25 mg; contains soy products
PreNexa Premier				25		28	800	30	Ca 160 mg, DHA 310 mg, docusate sodium 55 mg, Fe 27 mg, folic acid 1.25 mg; contains soy products
TriCare Prenatal DHA One		3	3.4	25	100	60	800	30	Biotin 300 mcg, Cu 2 mg, DHA 215 mg, docusate sodium 25 mg, EPA 45 mg, Fe (as ferrous fumarate) 27 mg, folic acid 1 mg, niacin 20 mg, Zn 10 mg
vitaMedMD One Rx		1.5	1.7	25	8	60	400	21	Biotin 300 mcg, DHA 200 mg, Fe 30 mg, folate 1 mg (folic acid 400 mcg, Quatrefolic 600 mcg), niacinamide 20 mg, pantothenic acid 10 mg, Zn 7.5 mg
vitaPearl		1.7	2	25	8	30	400	30	Biotin 300 mcg, DHA 200 mg, Fe 30 mg, folic acid 1.4 mg, niacinamide 20 mg, pantothenic acid 10 mg, potassium iodide 150 mcg, zinc 7.5 mg; gluten, lactose, and sugar free
Tablet									
A-Free Prenatal [OTC] (*per 3 tablets*)		6	6	3	6	100	400	30	Biotin 30 mcg, calcium 1000 mg, Cu 0.3 mg, Fe (as ferrous fumarate) 27 mg, folic acid 800 mcg, Mg 100 mg, Mn 0.3 mg, niacinamide 30 mg, pantothenic acid 15 mg, Zn 22.5 mg; natural base contains bioflavonoids and hesperidin 66 mg
B-Nexa				42					Calcium 124 mg, folic acid 1.22 mg, ginger root powder extract 100 mg
CitraNatal Rx		3	3.4	20		120	400	30	Fe 125 mg, Cu 2 mg, docusate sodium 50 mg, Fe (as carbonyl iron, ferrous gluconate) 27 mg, folic acid 1 mg, iodine 150 mcg, niacinamide 20 mg, Zn 25 mg
Femecal OB		1.5	1.6	50	12		400	10	Biotin 30 mcg, Cu 0.8 mg, Fe 28 mg (22 mg as polysaccharide iron complex and 6 mg as ferrous aspartate and iron glycinate), folic acid 1 mg, iodine 175 mcg, niacinamide 17 mg, pantothenic acid 10 mg, Se 65 mcg, Zn 15 mg
Focalgin-B				42					Ca 124.23 mg, folic acid 1.22 mg, ginger 100 mg
Foltabs Prenatal		3	3.4	20	8	120	400	30	Ca 125 mg, Cu 2 mg, docusate sodium 50 mg, Fe 27 mg, folic acid 1 mg, iodine 150 mcg, niacinamide 20 mg, Zn 25 mg
Gesticare		3	3	50	6	120	420	30	Ca 200 mg, choline 55 mg, Fe (as ferrous fumarate) 28 mg, folic acid 1 mg, iodine 150 mcg, niacinamide 20 mg, Zn 15 mg
KPN Prenatal [OTC] (*per 3 tablets*)	2000	6	6	3	6	100	400	30	Biotin 30 mcg, Ca 1000 mg, Cu 0.3 mg, Fe (as ferrous fumarate) 27 mg, folic acid 800 mcg, Mg 100 mg, Mn 0.3 mg, niacinamide 30 mg, pantothenic acid 15 mg, Zn 22.5 mg; natural base contains 66 mg bioflavonoids and hesperidin
Mini-Prenatal [OTC]	2000	2	3	3	10	100	400	15	Biotin 100 mcg, Ca 200 mg, Cu 2 mg, Fe (as ferrous fumarate) 27 mg, folic acid 800 mcg, Mg 60 mg, Mn 2 mg, niacinamide 20 mg, pantothenic acid 20 mg, Zn 15 mg
Multi-Nate 30	3000	1.8	4	25	12	120	400	30	Ca 200 mg, Cu 2 mg, Fe 29 mg, folic acid 1 mg, Mg 25 mg, niacin 20 mg, Zn 25 mg; contains soy products
PreferaOB		1.5	1.6	50	12		400	10	Biotin 30 mcg, Cu 0.8 mg, Fe 34 mg (28 mg as polysaccharide complex and 6 mg as heme iron polypeptide), folic acid 1 mg, iodine 250 mcg, niacin 17 mg, pantothenic acid 10 mg, Se 65 mg, Zn 4.5 mg
Prenaissance Next-B				42					Ca 124.23 mg, folic acid 1.22 mg, ginger 100 mg; contains tartrazine
Prenatabs FA	4000	3	3	3	8	120	400	30	Ca 200 mg, Fe (as ferrous fumarate) 29 mg, folic acid 1 mg, iodine 150 mcg, niacin 20 mg, Zn 15 mg
Prenatabs Rx	4000	3	3	3	8	120	400	30	Beta carotene 4000 units, biotin 30 mcg, Ca 200 mg, Cu 3 mg, Fe (as iron carbonyl) 29 mg, folic acid 1 mg, Mg 100 mg, niacinamide 20 mg, pantothenic acid 7 mg, potassium iodide 150 mcg, Zn 15 mg; contains soy products
Prenatal One Daily [OTC]	2000	2	3	3	10	100	400	15	Biotin 100 mcg, Ca 200 mg, Cu 2 mg, Fe (as ferrous fumarate) 27 mg, folic acid 800 mcg, Mg 60 mg, Mn 2 mg, niacinamide 20 mg, pantothenic acid 10 mg, Zn 15 mg
Prenatal Rx 1	4000	1.5	1.6	4	2.5	80	400	15	Biotin 30 mcg, Ca 200 mg, Cu 3 mg, Fe (as ferrous fumarate) 60 mg, folic acid 1 mg, Mg 100 mg, niacinamide 17 mg, pantothenic acid 7 mg, Zn 25 mg

Prenatal Formulations *continued*

Product	A (units)	B₁ (mg)	B₂ (mg)	B₆ (mg)	B₁₂ (mcg)	C (mg)	D (units)	E (units)	Additional Information
Prenatal With Beta Carotene [OTC]	1500	3	3	10	12	100	250	30	Biotin 30 mg, Ca 250 mg, Cu 2 mg, Fe 29 mg, folic acid 990 mcg, niacinamide 20 mg, pantothenic acid 20 mg, Zn 25 mg
Prenate Elite	2600	3	3.5	21	13	75	450	10	Biotin 330 mcg, Ca 100 mg, Cu 1.5 mg, Fe (as ferrous fumarate) 26 mg, folate 1 mg (folic acid 400 mcg, Quatrefolic 600 mcg), iodine 150 mcg, niacinamide 21 mg, pantothenic acid 6 mg, Zn 15 mg
Stuart Prenatal [OTC]	4000	1.8	1.7	2.6	8	120	400	30	Ca 200 mg, Fe 28 mg, folic acid 800 mcg, niacin 20 mg, Zn 25 mg
TriCare Prenatal		1.6	1.6	3.1	12	100	400	30	Ca 200 mg, Cu 2 mg, Fe (as ferrous fumarate) 27 mg, folic acid 1 mg, niacinamide 20 mg, Zn 10 mg
Vitafol-Nano				2.5	12		1000		Fe (as ferrous fumarate) 18 mg, folic acid 0.4 mg, l-methylfolate 0.6 mg, potassium iodide 150 mcg
VP-Heme OB		1.5	1.6	50	12		400	10	Biotin 30 mcg, Cu 0.8 mg, Fe 34 mg (28 mg as polysaccharide iron complex and 6 mg as heme iron polypeptide), folic acid 1 mg, niacinamide 17 mg, potassium iodide 250 mcg, selenium 65 mcg, Zn 4.5 mg
Tablet, Chewable									
NataChew [OTC]	1000	2	3	10	12	120	400	11	Fe (as ferrous fumarate) 29 mg, folic acid 1 mg, niacinamide 20 mg
PreCare				2		50	6 mcg	3.5	Ca 250 mg, Cu 2 mg, Fe (as ferrous fumarate) 40 mg, folic acid 1 mg, Mg 50 mg, Zn 15 mg
Select-OB	1700	1.6	1.8	2.5	5	60	400	30	Fe 29 mg, folic acid 1 mg, Mg 25 mg, niacin 15 mg, Zn 15 mg
Vinate Care				2		50	6 mcg	3.5	Ca 250 mg, Cu 2 mg, Fe (as ferrous fumarate) 40 mg, folic acid 1 mg, Mg 50 mg, Zn 15 mg
vitaMedMD RediChew Rx			1.7	2	8		400		Folate 1 mg (folic acid 400 mcg, Quatrefolic 600 mcg)
Combination Package									
CitraNatal 90 DHA (*tablet*)		3	3.4	20		120	400	30	Ca 159 mg, Cu 2 mg, docusate sodium 50 mg, Fe 90 mg (as carbonyl iron and ferrous gluconate), folic acid 1 mg, iodine 150 mcg, niacinamide 20 mg, Zn 25 mg. Packaged with *gelatin capsule* containing DHA 300 mg and EPA 0.75 mg
CitraNatal Assure		3	3.4	25		120	400	30	Ca 125 mg, Cu 2 mg, docusate sodium 50 mg, Fe (as carbonyl iron and ferrous gluconate) 35 mg, folic acid 1 mg, iodine 150 mcg, niacin 20 mg, Zn 25 mg. Packaged with *softgel capsule* containing DHA 300 mg
CitraNatal B-Calm				25		120	400	30	Ca 125 mg, Fe (as carbonyl iron) 20 mg, folic acid 1 mg. Packaged with two B₆ 25 mg tablets
CitraNatal DHA (*tablet*)		3	3.4	20		120	400	30	Ca 125 mg, Cu 2 mg, docusate sodium 50 mg, Fe 27 mg (as carbonyl iron and ferrous gluconate), folic acid 1 mg, iodine 150 mcg, niacinamide 20 mg, Zn 25 mg. Packaged with *gelatin capsule* containing DHA 250 mg
CitraNatal 90 DHA (*tablet*)		3	3.4	20		120	400	30	Ca 200 mg, Cu 2 mg, docusate sodium 50 mg, Fe 90 mg (as carbonyl iron), folic acid 1 mg, iodine 150 mcg, niacinamide 20 mg, Zn 25 mg. Packaged with *gelatin capsule* containing DHA 250 mg
Duet DHA Balanced (*tablet*)	2840	1.5	4	50	12	120	840	2	Ca 215 mg, Cu 2 mg, Fe 26 mg, folic acid 1 mg, iodine 210 mcg, Mg 25 mg, niacinamide 20 mg, Zn 25 mg. Packaged with purified omega-3 fatty acids 278 mg *softgel capsule*
Foltabs Prenatal Plus DHA		3	3.4	20		120	400	30	Ca 125 mg, Cu 2 mg, docusate sodium 50 mg, Fe 27 mg, folic acid 1 mg, iodine 150 mcg, niacinamide 20 mg, Zn 25 mg. Packaged with *gelatin capsule* containing DHA 250 mg
Gesticare DHA		3	3	50	8	120	410	30	Ca 200 mg, choline 55 mg, Fe (as ferrous fumarate) 27 mg, folic acid 1 mg, iodine 150 mcg, niacinamide 20 mg, Zn 15 mg. Packaged with *gelatin capsule* containing DHA 250 mg and EPA not more than 0.625 mg

Prenatal Formulations *continued*

Product	A (units)	B_1 (mg)	B_2 (mg)	B_6 (mg)	B_{12} (mcg)	C (mg)	D (units)	E (units)	Additional Information
One A Day Women's Prenatal [OTC] (*tablet*)	4000	1.7	2	2.5	8	60	400	30	Biotin 300 mcg, Ca 300 mg, Cu 2 mg, Fe 28 mg, folic acid 800 mcg, iodine 150 mcg, Mg 50 mg, niacin 20 mg, pantothenic acid 10 mg, Zn 15 mg. Packaged with omega-3 fatty acids 440 mg *liquid gel* containing 200 mg DHA and 240 mg eicosapentaenoic acid; contains soy products.
OptiNate (*tablet*)		3	3.4	20	12	120	400	10	Biotin 30 mcg, Ca 200 mg, Cu 2 mg, docusate sodium 50 mg, Fe [elemental] 90 mg, folate 1 mg, Mg 30 mg, niacinamide 20 mg, pantothenic acid 6 mg, Zn 15 mg; contains sodium benzoate. Packaged with *Omega-3 L-Vcaps capsule* containing DHA 250 mg.
Paire OB Plus DHA		1.5	1.6	50	12		400	10	Biotin 30 mcg, Cu 0.8 mg, Fe 28 mg, folic acid 1 mg, iodine 175 mcg, niacinamide 17 mg, pantothenic acid 10 mg, Se 65 mcg, Zn 15 mg. Packaged with *softgel capsule* containing DHA 200 mg
PreferaOB + DHA		1.5	1.6	50	12		400	10	Biotin 30 mcg, Cu 0.8 mg, Fe 34 mg (28 mg as polysaccharide complex and 6 mg as heme iron polypeptide), folic acid 1 mg, iodine 250 mcg, niacin 17 mg, pantothenic acid 10 mg, Se 65 mg, Zn 4.5 mg. Packaged with *softgel capsule* containing DHA 200 mg
Vitafol-OB+DHA (*caplet*)	2700	1.6	1.8	2.5	12	70	400	30	Ca 100 mg, Cu 2 mg, Fe [elemental] 65 mg, folic acid 1 mg, Mg 25 mg, niacinamide 18 mg, Zn 25 mg; gluten free, sugar free. Packaged with *gelatin capsule* containing DHA 250 mg
vitaMedMD Plus Rx		3	3.4	25	12	60	600	30	Biotin 300 mcg, calcium 150 mg, Cu 2 mg, Fe 30 mg (folic acid 400 mcg, Quatrefolic 600 mcg), iodine 150 mcg, niacinamide 20 mg, pantothenic acid 10 mg, Zn 15 mg. Packaged with *softgel capsule* containing DHA 300 mg
VitaPhil + DHA	2600	3	3.5	30	12	120	420	20	Biotin 30 mcg, Ca 8 mg, choline 60 mg, Cu 2 mg, Fe 26 mg, folic acid 1 mg, niacinamide 20 mg, Mg 50 mg, Se 50 mg, Zn 15 mg; contains soy products. Packaged with *softgel capsule* containing DHA 200 mg
VP-Heme OB + DHA (*tablet*)		1.5	1.6	50	12		400	10	Biotin 30 mcg, Ca 10 mg, Cu 0.8 mg, Fe 34 mg (28 mg as polysaccharide iron complex and 6 mg as heme iron polypeptide), folic acid 1 mg, niacinamide 17 mg, potassium iodide 250 mcg, selenium 65 mcg, Zn 4.5 mg. Packaged with *softgel capsule* containing omega-3 long chain fatty acids 203 mg

Ca = calcium, Cr = chromium, Cu = copper, DHA = doccosahexaenoic acid (from omega-3 fatty acids), Fe = iron, Mg = magnesium, Mn = manganese, Mo = molybdenum, Se = selenium, Zn = zinc

Vitamin B Complex Combinations

Product	B₁ (mg)	B₂ (mg)	B₆ (mg)	B₁₂ (mcg)	C (mg)	E (units)	Additional Information
Caplet							
Allbee with C [OTC]	15	10.2	5		300		Biotin 300 mcg, folic acid 400 mcg, niacinamide 50 mg, pantothenic acid 10 mg
Allbee C-800 [OTC]	15	17	25	12	800	45	Biotin 300 mcg, folic acid 400 mcg, niacinamide 100 mg, pantothenic acid 25 mg
Allbee C-800 + Iron [OTC]	15	17	25	12	800	45	Biotin 300 mcg, Fe 27 mg, folic acid 0.4 mg, niacinamide 100 mg, pantothenic acid 25 mg
Nephronex	1.5	1.7	10	10	60		Biotin 300 mcg, folic acid 1 mg, nicotinic acid 20 mg, pantothenic acid 10 mg
Capsule							
Metanx			35 (pyridoxal 5-phosphate)	2 mg (methylco-balamin)			L-methylfolate 3 mg, schizochytrium algae
Virt-Caps	1.5	1.7	10	6	100		Biotin 150 mcg, folic acid 1 mg, niacinamide 20 mg, pantothenic acid 5 mg
Elixir							
Eldertonic (per 15 mL)	0.5	0.6	0.7	2			Mg 0.7 mg, Mn 0.7 mg, niacin 7 mg, pantothenic acid 3 mg, Zn 5 mg [contains alcohol 13.5%]
Liquid							
Gevrabon [OTC] (per 30 mL)	5	2.5	1	1			Choline 10 mg, Fe 15 mg, iodine 100 mcg, Mn 2 mg, niacinamide 50 mg, pantothenic acid 10 mg, Zn 2 mg; alcohol, benzoic acid; sherry wine flavor (480 mL)
Nephronex (per 5 mL)	1.5	1.7	10	10	60		Biotin 300 mcg, folic acid 900 mcg, nicotinic acid 20 mg, pantothenic acid 10 mg
Softgel							
Nephrocaps	1.5	1.7	10	6	100		Biotin 150 mcg, folate 1 mg, niacinamide 20 mg, pantothenic acid 5 mg
Renal Caps	1.5	1.7	10	6	100		Biotin 150 mcg, folic acid 1 mg, niacinamide 20 mg, pantothenic acid 5 mg
Tablet							
Bee Zee [OTC]	15	10.2	10	6	600	45	Biotin 300 mcg, folic acid 400 mcg, niacinamide 100 mg, pantothenic acid 25 mg, Zn 22.5 mg
DexFol	1.5	1.5	50	1	60		Biotin 300 mcg, cobalamin 1 mg, folic acid 400 mcg, folacin 5 mg, niacinamide 20 mg, pantothenic acid 10 mg [dye, sugar, and lactose free]
Foltanx			35 (pyridoxal 5-phosphate)	2 mg (methylco-balamin)			L-methylfolate 3 mg
Foltx	25		25	2 mg			L-methylfolate 1.13 mg
Kobee [OTC]	10	10	10	10			Biotin 10 mcg, choline citrate 10 mg, folic acid 400 mcg, inositol 10 mg, niacinamide 50 mg, PABA 10 mg, pantothenic acid 10 mg
NephPlex Rx	1.5	1.7	10	6	60		Biotin 300 mcg, folic acid 1 mg, niacinamide 20 mg, pantothenic acid 10 mg, zinc 12.5 mg
Nephro-Vite [OTC]	1.5	1.7	10	6	60		Biotin 300 mcg, folic acid 0.8 mg, niacinamide 20 mg, pantothenic acid 10 mg
Nephro-Vite Rx	1.5	1.7	10	6	60		Biotin 300 mcg, folic acid 1 mg, niacinamide 20 mg, pantothenic acid 10 mg
Nephron FA	1.5	1.7	10	6	40		Biotin 300 mcg, docusate sodium 75 mg, ferrous fumarate 200 mg, folic acid 1 mg, niacinamide 20 mg, pantothenic acid 10 mg
Quin B Strong [OTC]	25	25	25	25			Biotin 25 mcg, folic acid 400 mcg, niacinamide 100 mg, pantothenic acid 25 mg (in a base containing 25 mg of choline citrate and inositol)
Quin B Strong with C and Zinc [OTC]	25	25	25	25	500		Biotin 25 mcg, folic acid 400 mcg, niacinamide 100 mg, pantothenic acid 25 mg, Zn 15 mg (in a base containing 25 mg of choline citrate and inositol)
Rena-Vite [OTC]	1.5	1.7	10	6	60		Biotin 300 mcg, folic acid 800 mcg, niacin 20 mg, pantothenic acid 10 mg

Vitamin B Complex Combinations *continued*

Product	B₁ (mg)	B₂ (mg)	B₆ (mg)	B₁₂ (mcg)	C (mg)	E (units)	Additional Information
Rena-Vite RX	1.5	1.7	10	6	60		Biotin 300 mcg, folate 1 mg, niacin 20 mg, pantothenic acid 10 mg
Stresstabs High Potency Advanced [OTC]	10	10	5	12	250	30	Biotin 45 mcg, Ca 70 mg, Cu 3 mg, folic acid 400 mcg, niacinamide 100 mg, pantothenic acid 20 mg, phosphorus 30 mg, Zn 23.9 mg
Stresstabs High Potency Energy [OTC]	10	10	5	5	300	30	Biotin 45 mcg, Ca 20 mg, Fe 4 mg, folic acid 400 mcg, niacinamide 100 mg, pantothenic acid 20 mg, phosphorus 15 mg
Stresstabs High Potency Weight [OTC]	10	10	5	12	300	30	Biotin 45 mcg, Ca 44 mg, chromium 200 mcg, EGCG 32 mg, folic acid 400 mcg, niacinamide 100 mg, pantothenic acid 20 mg, phosphorus 32 mg
Super Dec B 100 [OTC]	100	100	100	100			Biotin 100 mcg, folic acid 400 mcg, niacinamide 100 mg, pantothenic acid 100 mg (in a base containing 100 mg of choline citrate and inositol)
Superplex-T [OTC]	15	10	5	10	500		Niacinamide 100 mg, pantothenic acid 18.3 mg, sodium 70 mg
Super Quints 50 [OTC]	50	50	50	50			Biotin 50 mcg, folic acid 400 mcg, niacinamide 50 mg, pantothenic acid 50 mg (in a base containing 50 mg of choline citrate, glutaminic acid, glutamine, glycine, inositol, and lysine)
Surbex-T [OTC]	12.4	9	3.7	9	450		Niacinamide 90.7 mg, pantothenic acid 16.6 mg, sodium 65 mg
Z-Bec [OTC]	15	10.2	10	6	600	45	Biotin 300 mcg, folic acid 400 mcg, niacinamide 100 mg, pantothenic acid 25 mg, Zn 22.5 mg

Ca = calcium, Cu = copper, Fe = iron, Mg = magnesium, Mn = manganese, Se = selenium, Zn = zinc

OPIOID CONVERSION TABLE

This table serves as a general guide to opioid conversion. Utilization of a direct conversion without a detailed patient and medication assessment is not recommended and may result in over- or underdosing. Values are based on single-dose adult studies. Duration of action may be shorter in children due to faster elimination (in general) compared to adults. The pharmacokinetics of opioids in children and infants >6 months of age are similar to adults, but infants <6 months of age, especially those who are premature or physically compromised, may demonstrate decreased clearance and are at risk of apnea.

Drug	Onset (min)	Duration (h)	Equianalgesic I.M. Dose (mg)	Equianalgesic P.O. Dose[1] (mg)	Parenteral Oral Ratio
Alfentanil	I.V.: Immediate	<0.25 to 0.33	No data	—	—
Codeine[2]	I.M.: 10 to 30, P.O.: 30 to 60	4 to 6	100 to 130	200	1/2 to 2/3
FentaNYL	I.M.: 7 to 15, I.V.: Immediate	I.M.: 1 to 2, I.V.: 0.5 to 1	0.1	—	—
HYDROcodone	P.O.: 10 to 20	3 to 6	—	30 to 45	—
HYDROmorphone	P.O.: 15 to 30	4 to 5	1.5	7.5	1/5
Meperidine[3]	P.O., I.M., SubQ: 10 to 15, I.V.: ≤5	P.O., I.M., SubQ: 2 to 4, I.V.: 2 to 3	75	300	1/3 to 1/2
Methadone[4]	P.O.: 30 to 60, I.V.: 10 to 20	Acute: 4 to 6, Chronic: >8	Pediatrics: Acute: 10, Chronic: Not established[5]	Pediatrics: Acute: 20, Chronic: Not established[5] Adults[6]. See Guidelines for Conversion to Oral Methadone in Adults	
Morphine	P.O. (immediate release): 15 to 60, I.V.: ≤5	P.O. (immediate release), I.V., I.M., SubQ: 3 to 5, Extended release tablets: 8 to 12	10	30	1/6: ratio decreases to 1/1.5 to 2.5 upon chronic dosing
OxyCODONE	P.O. (immediate release): 15 to 30	P.O.: Immediate release: 4 to 5, Controlled release: 12	—	20	—
Pentazocine	P.O., I.M., SubQ: 15 to 30, I.V.: ≤2 to 3	I.V., I.M., SubQ: 2 to 3	30	50	1/3

Guidelines for Conversion to Oral Methadone in Adults[6]

Oral Morphine Dose or Equivalent (mg/day)	Oral Morphine:Oral Methadone (Conversion Ratio)
<90	4:1
90 to 300	8:1
>300	12:1

[1] Chronic administration may alter pharmacokinetics and change parenteral oral ratio.

[2] Codeine should not be used in infants <6 months of age due to slow metabolism, accumulation of morphine (major metabolite), and risk of apnea/death. In addition, 10% of the population cannot convert codeine to morphine and therefore will not experience analgesia. Conversely, ultra-rapid metabolizers may have an exaggerated opioid response.

[3] Not recommended for routine use due to potential accumulation of a neurotoxic metabolite

[4] Conversion to methadone requires close observation for delayed sedation which may occur 3 to 5 days postconversion. Dosing interval needs to be increased after the initial 1 to 2 days of treatment to avoid late sedation.

[5] A conversion factor for pediatric patients receiving chronic opioids has not been identified; doses lower than those listed for acute opioid administration would be recommended based on adult data. Some experts recommend against the use of an "equianalgesic" dosage of methadone (to prevent or treat opioid withdrawal) because calculated methadone doses may be unnecessarily high for this indication (Lugo, 2001).

[6] Conversion of higher doses may be guided by the following (consult a pain or palliative care specialist if unfamiliar with methadone prescribing): As the total daily dose of morphine increases, the equianalgesic dose ratio (methadone:morphine) changes in adults (American Pain Society, 2008). Total daily dose should be divided by 3 and administered every 8 hours. Methadone is significantly more potent with repetitive dosing. Begin methadone at lower doses and gradually titrate. Use these conversion guidelines only in adult patients; do not use in pediatric patients; applicability to pediatric patients is unknown and may be dangerous or potentially lethal.

REFERENCES

Friedrichsdorf SJ, Kang TI. The management of pain in children with life-limiting illnesses. *Pediatr Clin North Am.* 2007;54(5):645-672.

Lugo RA, MacLaren R, Cash J, Pribble CG, Vernon DD. Enteral methadone to expedite fentanyl discontinuation and prevent opioid abstinence syndrome in the PICU. *Pharmacotherapy.* 2001;21(12):1566-1573.

National Cancer Institute. Pain (PDQ). Available at http://www.cancer.gov/cancertopics/pdq/supportivecare/pain/HealthProfessional/page1. Accessed May 7, 2009.

National Comprehensive Cancer Network (NCCN). Clinical practice guidelines in oncology: adult cancer pain. Version 1, 2009. Available at http://www.nccn.org/professionals/physician_gls/PDF/pain.pdf

Patanwala AE, Duby J, Waters D, Erstad BL. Opioid conversions in acute care. *Ann Pharmacother.* 2007;41(2):255-266.

Principles of Analgesic Use in the Treatment of Acute Pain and Cancer Pain. 6th ed. Glenview, IL: American Pain Society; 2008.

APOTHECARY/METRIC EQUIVALENTS

Apothecary-Metric Exact Equivalents

1 gram (g)	=	15.43 grains (gr)		0.1 mg	=	1/600 gr
1 milliliter (mL)	=	16.23 minims		0.12 mg	=	1/500 gr
1 minim	=	0.06 mL		0.15 mg	=	1/400 gr
1 gr	=	64.8 milligrams (mg)		0.2 mg	=	1/300 gr
1 fluid ounce (fl oz)	=	29.57 mL		0.3 mg	=	1/200 gr
1 pint (pt)	=	473.2 mL		0.4 mg	=	1/150 gr
1 ounce (oz)	=	28.35 g		0.5 mg	=	1/120 gr
1 pound (lb)	=	453.6 g		0.6 mg	=	1/100 gr
1 killogram (kg)	=	2.2 lb		0.8 mg	=	1/80 gr
1 quart (qt)	=	946.4 mL		1 mg	=	1/65 gr

Apothecary-Metric Approximate Equivalents[1]

Liquids			**Solids**		
1 teaspoonful	=	5 mL	¼ grain	=	15 mg
1 tablespoonful	=	15 mL	½ grain	=	30 mg
			1 grain	=	60 mg
			1½ grain	=	100 mg
			5 grains	=	300 mg
			10 grains	=	600 mg

[1]Use exact equivalents for compounding and calculations requiring a high degree of accuracy.

POUNDS/KILOGRAMS CONVERSION

1 pound = 0.45359 kilograms
1 kilogram = 2.2 pounds

lb	=	kg		lb	=	kg		lb	=	kg
1		0.45		70		31.75		140		63.50
5		2.27		75		34.02		145		65.77
10		4.54		80		36.29		150		68.04
15		6.80		85		38.56		155		70.31
20		9.07		90		40.82		160		72.58
25		11.34		95		43.09		165		74.84
30		13.61		100		45.36		170		77.11
35		15.88		105		47.63		175		79.38
40		18.14		110		49.90		180		81.65
45		20.41		115		52.16		185		83.92
50		22.68		120		54.43		190		86.18
55		24.95		125		56.70		195		88.45
60		27.22		130		58.91		200		90.72
65		29.48		135		61.24				

TEMPERATURE CONVERSION

Celsius to Fahrenheit = (°C x 9/5) + 32 = °F
Fahrenheit to Celsius = (°F - 32) x 5/9 = °C

°C	=	°F		°C	=	°F		°C	=	°F
100.0		212.0		39.0		102.2		36.8		98.2
50.0		122.0		38.8		101.8		36.6		97.9
41.0		105.8		38.6		101.5		36.4		97.5
40.8		105.4		38.4		101.1		36.2		97.2
40.6		105.1		38.2		100.8		36.0		96.8
40.4		104.7		38.0		100.4		35.8		96.4
40.2		104.4		37.8		100.1		35.6		96.1
40.0		104.0		37.6		99.7		35.4		95.7
39.8		103.6		37.4		99.3		35.2		95.4
39.6		103.3		37.2		99.0		35.0		95.0
39.4		102.9		37.0		98.6		0		32.0
39.2		102.6								

CYTOCHROME P450 ENZYMES: SUBSTRATES, INHIBITORS, AND INDUCERS

INTRODUCTION

Most drugs are eliminated from the body, at least in part, by being chemically altered to less lipid-soluble products (ie, metabolized), and thus are more likely to be excreted via the kidneys or the bile. Phase I metabolism includes drug hydrolysis, oxidation, and reduction, and results in drugs that are more polar in their chemical structure, while Phase II metabolism involves the attachment of an additional molecule onto the drug (or partially metabolized drug) in order to create an inactive and/or more water soluble compound. Phase II processes include (primarily) glucuronidation, sulfation, glutathione conjugation, acetylation, and methylation.

Virtually any of the Phase I and II enzymes can be inhibited by some xenobiotic or drug. Some of the Phase I and II enzymes can be induced. Inhibition of the activity of metabolic enzymes will result in increased concentrations of the substrate (drug), whereas induction of the activity of metabolic enzymes will result in decreased concentrations of the substrate. The well-documented enzyme-inducing effects of phenobarbital may include a combination of Phase I and II enzymes. Phase II glucuronidation may be increased via induced UDP-glucuronosyltransferase (UGT) activity, whereas Phase I oxidation may be increased via induced cytochrome P450 (CYP) activity. However, for most drugs, the primary route of metabolism (and the primary focus of drug-drug interaction) is Phase I oxidation.

CYP enzymes may be responsible for the metabolism (at least partial metabolism) of approximately 75% of all drugs, with the CYP3A subfamily responsible for nearly half of this activity. Found throughout plant, animal, and bacterial species, CYP enzymes represent a superfamily of xenobiotic metabolizing proteins. There have been several hundred CYP enzymes identified in nature, each of which has been assigned to a family (1, 2, 3, etc), subfamily (A, B, C, etc), and given a specific enzyme number (1, 2, 3, etc) according to the similarity in amino acid sequence that it shares with other enzymes. Of these many enzymes, only a few are found in humans, and even fewer appear to be involved in the metabolism of xenobiotics (eg, drugs). The key human enzyme subfamilies include CYP1A, CYP2A, CYP2B, CYP2C, CYP2D, CYP2E, and CYP3A. However, the number of distinct isozymes (eg, CYP2C9) found to be functionally active in humans, as well as, the number of genetically variant forms of these isozymes (eg, CYP2C9*2) in individuals continues to expand.

CYP enzymes are found in the endoplasmic reticulum of cells in a variety of human tissues (eg, skin, kidneys, brain, lungs), but their predominant sites of concentration and activity are the liver and intestine. Though the abundance of CYP enzymes throughout the body is relatively equally distributed among the various subfamilies, the relative contribution to drug metabolism is (in decreasing order of magnitude) CYP3A4 (nearly 50%), CYP2D6 (nearly 25%), CYP2C8/9 (nearly 15%), then CYP1A2, CYP2C19, CYP2A6, and CYP2E1. Owing to their potential for numerous drug-drug interactions, those drugs that are identified in preclinical studies as substrates of CYP3A enzymes are often given a lower priority for continued research and development in favor of drugs that appear to be less affected by (or less likely to affect) this enzyme subfamily.

Each enzyme subfamily possesses unique selectivity toward potential substrates. For example, CYP1A2 preferentially binds medium-sized, planar, lipophilic molecules, while CYP2D6 preferentially binds molecules that possess a basic nitrogen atom. Some CYP subfamilies exhibit polymorphism (ie, genetic variation that results in a modified enzyme with small changes in amino acid sequences that may manifest differing catalytic properties). The best described polymorphisms involve CYP2C9, CYP2C19, and CYP2D6. Individuals possessing "wild type" genes exhibit normal functioning CYP capacity. Others, however, possess genetic variants that leave the person with a subnormal level of catalytic potential (so called "poor metabolizers"). Poor metabolizers would be more likely to experience toxicity from drugs metabolized by the affected enzymes (or less effects if the enzyme is responsible for converting a prodrug to it's active form as in the case of codeine). The percentage of people classified as poor metabolizers varies by enzyme and population group. As an example, approximately 7% of Caucasians and only about 1% of Asians appear to be CYP2D6 poor metabolizers.

CYP enzymes can be both inhibited and induced by other drugs, leading to increased or decreased serum concentrations (along with the associated effects), respectively. Induction occurs when a drug causes an increase in the amount of smooth endoplasmic reticulum, secondary to increasing the amount of the affected CYP enzymes in the tissues. This "revving up" of the CYP enzyme system may take several days to reach peak activity, and likewise, may take several days, even months, to return to normal following discontinuation of the inducing agent.

CYP inhibition occurs via several potential mechanisms. Most commonly, a CYP inhibitor competitively (and reversibly) binds to the active site on the enzyme, thus preventing the substrate from binding to the same site, and preventing the substrate from being metabolized. The affinity of an inhibitor for an enzyme may be expressed by an inhibition constant (Ki) or IC50 (defined as the concentration of the inhibitor required to cause 50% inhibition under a given set of conditions). In addition to reversible competition for an enzyme site, drugs may inhibit enzyme activity by binding to sites on the enzyme other than that to which the substrate would bind, and thereby cause a change in the functionality or physical structure of the enzyme. A drug may also bind to the enzyme in an irreversible (ie, "suicide") fashion. In such a case, it is not the concentration of drug at the enzyme site that is important (constantly binding and releasing), but the number of molecules available for binding (once bound, always bound).

Although an inhibitor or inducer may be known to affect a variety of CYP subfamilies, it may only inhibit one or two in a clinically important fashion. Likewise, although a substrate is known to be at least partially metabolized by a variety of CYP enzymes, only one or two enzymes may contribute significantly enough to its overall metabolism to warrant concern when used with potential inducers or inhibitors. Therefore, when attempting to predict the level of risk of using two drugs that may affect each other via altered CYP function, it is important to identify the relative effectiveness of the inhibiting/inducing drug on the CYP subfamilies that significantly contribute to the metabolism of the substrate. The contribution of a specific CYP pathway to substrate metabolism should be considered not only in light of other known CYP pathways, but also other nonoxidative pathways for substrate metabolism (eg, glucuronidation) and transporter proteins (eg, P-glycoprotein) that may affect the presentation of a substrate to a metabolic pathway.

◄ # HOW TO USE THIS TABLE

The following table provides a clinically relevant perspective on drugs that are affected by, or affect, cytochrome P450 (CYP) enzymes. Not all human, drug-metabolizing CYP enzymes are specifically (or separately) included in the table. Some enzymes have been excluded because they do not appear to significantly contribute to the metabolism of marketed drugs (eg, CYP2C18). In the case of CYP3A4, the industry routinely uses this single enzyme designation to represent all enzymes in the CYP3A subfamily. CYP3A7 is present in fetal livers. It is effectively absent from adult livers. CYP3A4 (adult) and CYP3A7 (fetal) appear to share similar properties in their respective hosts. The impact of CYP3A7 in fetal and neonatal drug interactions has not been investigated.

An enzyme that appears to play a clinically significant (major) role in a drug's metabolism is indicated by "S". A clinically significant designation is the result of a two-phase review. The first phase considered the contribution of each CYP enzyme to the overall metabolism of the drug. The enzyme pathway was considered potentially clinically relevant if it was responsible for at least 30% of the metabolism of the drug. If so, the drug was subjected to a second phase. The second phase considered the clinical relevance of a substrate's concentration being increased twofold, or decreased by one-half (such as might be observed if combined with an effective CYP inhibitor or inducer, respectively). If either of these changes was considered to present a clinically significant concern, the CYP pathway for the drug was designated "major." If neither change would appear to present a clinically significant concern, or if the CYP enzyme was responsible for a smaller portion of the overall metabolism (ie, <30%), then no association between the enzyme and the drug will appear in the table.

Enzymes that are strongly or moderately inhibited by a drug are indicated by "↓". Enzymes that are weakly inhibited are not identified in the table. The designations are the result of a review of published clinical reports, available Ki data, and assessments published by other experts in the field. As it pertains to Ki values set in a ratio with achievable serum drug concentrations ([I]) under normal dosing conditions, the following parameters were employed: [I]/Ki ≥1 = strong; [I]/Ki 0.1 to 1 = moderate; [I]/Ki <0.1 = weak.

Enzymes that appear to be effectively induced by a drug are indicated by "↑". This designation is the result of a review of published clinical reports and assessments published by experts in the field.

In general, clinically significant interactions are more likely to occur between substrates ("S") and either inhibitors or inducers of the same enzyme(s), which have been indicated by "↓" and "↑", respectively. However, these assessments possess a degree of subjectivity, at times based on limited indications regarding the significance of CYP effects of particular agents. An attempt has been made to balance a conservative, clinically-sensitive presentation of the data with a desire to avoid the numbing effect of a "beware of everything" approach. It is important to note that information related to CYP metabolism of drugs is expanding at a rapid pace, and thus, the contents of this table should only be considered to represent a "snapshot" of the information available at the time of publication.

SELECTED READINGS

Bjornsson TD, Callaghan JT, Einolf HJ, et al. The conduct of in vitro and in vivo drug-drug interaction studies: a PhRMA perspective. J Clin Pharmacol. 2003;43(5):443-469.
Drug-Drug Interactions. Rodrigues AD, ed. New York, NY: Marcel Dekker, Inc; 2002.
Metabolic Drug Interactions. Levy RH, Thummel KE, Trager WF, et al, eds. Philadelphia, PA: Lippincott Williams & Wilkins; 2000.
Michalets EL. Update: clinically significant cytochrome P-450 drug interactions. Pharmacotherapy. 1998;18(1):84-112.
Thummel KE, Wilkinson GR. In vitro and in vivo drug interactions involving human CYP3A. Annu Rev Pharmacol Toxicol. 1998;38:389-430.
Zhang Y, Benet LZ. The gut as a barrier to drug absorption: combined role of cytochrome P450 3A and P-Glycoprotein. Clin Pharmacokinet. 2001;40 (3):159-168.

SELECTED WEBSITES

http://www.imm.ki.se/CYPalleles
http://medicine.iupui.edu/flockhart
http://www.fda.gov/Drugs/DevelopmentApprovalProcess/DevelopmentResources/DrugInteractionsLabeling/ucm080499.htm

CYP: Substrates, Inhibitors, Inducers

S = substrate; ↓ = inhibitor; ↑ = inducer

Drug	1A2	2A6	2B6	2C8	2C9	2C19	2D6	2E1	3A4
Acenocoumarol	S				S				
Alfentanil									S
Alfuzosin									S
Alosetron	S								
ALPRAZolam									S
Ambrisentan						S			S
Aminophylline	S								
Amiodarone		↓		S	↓		↓		S, ↓
Amitriptyline							S		
AmLODIPine	↓								S
Amobarbital		↑							
Amoxapine							S		
Aprepitant									S, ↓

CYP: Substrates, Inhibitors, Inducers *(continued)*

Drug	1A2	2A6	2B6	2C8	2C9	2C19	2D6	2E1	3A4
ARIPiprazole							S		S
Armodafinil						↓			S, ↑
Atazanavir									S, ↓
Atomoxetine							S		
Atorvastatin									S
Benzphetamine									S
Betaxolol	S						S		
Bisoprolol									S
Bortezomib						S, ↓			S
Bosentan					S, ↑				S, ↑
Bromazepam									S
Bromocriptine									S
Budesonide									S
Buprenorphine									S
BuPROPion			S						
BusPIRone									S
Busulfan									S
Caffeine	S								↓
Captopril							S		
CarBAMazepine	↑		↑	↑	↑	↑			S, ↑
Carisoprodol						S			
Carvedilol					S		S		
Celecoxib				↓	S				
ChlordiazePOXIDE									S
Chloroquine							S, ↓		S
Chlorpheniramine							S		
ChlorproMAZINE							S, ↓		
Chlorzoxazone								S	
Ciclesonide									S
Cilostazol									S
Cimetidine	↓					↓	↓		↓
Cinacalcet							↓		
Ciprofloxacin	↓								
Cisapride									S
Citalopram						S			S
Clarithromycin									S, ↓
Clobazam						S			S
ClomiPRAMINE	S					S	S, ↓		
ClonazePAM									S
Clorazepate									S
Clotrimazole									↓
CloZAPine	S						↓		
Cocaine							↓		S
Codeine[1]							S		
Colchicine									S
Conivaptan									S, ↓
Cyclobenzaprine	S								
Cyclophosphamide[2]			S						S
CycloSPORINE									S, ↓
Dacarbazine	S							S	
Dantrolene									S
Dapsone					S				S

CYP: Substrates, Inhibitors, Inducers (continued)

Drug	1A2	2A6	2B6	2C8	2C9	2C19	2D6	2E1	3A4
Darifenacin							↓		S
Darunavir									S
Dasatinib									S
Delavirdine					↓	↓	↓		S, ↓
Desipramine		↓	↓				S, ↓		↓
Desogestrel						S			
Dexamethasone									S, ↑
Dexlansoprazole						S, ↓			S
Dexmedetomidine		S					↓		
Dextromethorphan							S		
Diazepam						S			S
Diclofenac	↓								
Dihydroergotamine									S
Diltiazem									S, ↓
DiphenhydrAMINE							↓		
Disopyramide									S
Disulfiram								↓	
DOCEtaxel									S
Doxepin							S		
DOXOrubicin			↓				S		S
Doxycycline									↓
DULoxetine	S						S, ↓		
Efavirenz[3]			S		↓	↓			S, ↓, ↑
Eletriptan									S
Enflurane								S	
Eplerenone									S
Ergoloid mesylates									S
Ergonovine									S
Ergotamine									S
Erlotinib									S
Erythromycin									S, ↓
Escitalopram						S			S
Esomeprazole						S, ↓			S
Estradiol	S								S
Estrogens, conjugated A/synthetic	S								S
Estrogens, conjugated equine	S								S
Estrogens, esterified	S								S
Estropipate	S								S
Eszopiclone									S
Ethinyl estradiol									S
Ethosuximide									S
Etoposide									S
Exemestane									S
Felbamate									S
Felodipine				↓					S
FentaNYL									S
Flecainide							S		
Fluconazole					↓	↓			↓
Flunisolide									S
FLUoxetine	↓				S	↓	S, ↓		
FluPHENAZine							S		
Flurazepam									S

CYP: Substrates, Inhibitors, Inducers *(continued)*

Drug	1A2	2A6	2B6	2C8	2C9	2C19	2D6	2E1	3A4
Flurbiprofen					↓				
Flutamide	S								S
Fluticasone									S
Fluvastatin					S, ↓				
FluvoxaMINE	S, ↓					↓	S		
Fosamprenavir (as amprenavir)									S, ↓
Fosaprepitant									S, ↓
Fosphenytoin (as phenytoin)			↑	↑	S, ↑	S, ↑			↑
Fospropofol	↓		S		S	↓			↓
Gefitinib									S
Gemfibrozil	↓			↓	↓	↓			
Glimepiride					S				
GlipiZIDE					S				
Guanabenz	S								
Haloperidol							S, ↓		S, ↓
Halothane								S	
Ibuprofen					↓				
Ifosfamide[4]		S				S			S
Imatinib							↓		S, ↓
Imipramine						S	S, ↓		S
Indinavir									S, ↓
Indomethacin					↓				
Irbesartan				↓	↓				
Irinotecan			S						S
Isoflurane								S	
Isoniazid		↓				↓	↓	S, ↓	
Isosorbide dinitrate									S
Isosorbide mononitrate									S
Isradipine									S
Itraconazole									S, ↓
Ixabepilone									S
Ketamine			S		S				S
Ketoconazole	↓	↓			↓	↓	↓		S, ↓
Lansoprazole						S, ↓			S
Lapatinib									S
Letrozole		↓							
Levonorgestrel									S
Lidocaine							S, ↓		S, ↓
Lomustine							S		
Lopinavir									S
Loratadine							↓		
Losartan				↓	S, ↓				S
Lovastatin									S
Maprotiline							S		
Maraviroc									S
MedroxyPROGESTERone									S
Mefenamic acid					↓				
Mefloquine									S
Mephobarbital						S			
Mestranol[5]					S				S
Methadone							↓		S
Methamphetamine							S		

CYP: Substrates, Inhibitors, Inducers *(continued)*

Drug	1A2	2A6	2B6	2C8	2C9	2C19	2D6	2E1	3A4
Methoxsalen	↓	↓							
Methsuximide						S			
Methylergonovine									S
MethylPREDNISolone									S
Metoprolol							S		
MetroNIDAZOLE									↓
Mexiletine	S, ↓						S		
Miconazole	↓	↓			↓	↓	↓	↓	S, ↓
Midazolam									S
Mirtazapine	S						S		S
Moclobemide						S	S		
Modafinil							↓		S
Montelukast					S				S
Nafcillin									↑
Nateglinide					S				S
Nebivolol							S		
Nefazodone							S		S, ↓
Nelfinavir						S			S, ↓
Nevirapine			↑						S, ↑
NiCARdipine					↓	↓	↓		S, ↓
NIFEdipine	↓								S
Nilotinib									S
Nilutamide						S			
NiMODipine									S
Nisoldipine									S
Norethindrone									S
Norfloxacin	↓								↓
Norgestrel									S
Nortriptyline							S		
Ofloxacin	↓								
OLANZapine	S								
Omeprazole					↓	S, ↓			S
Ondansetron									S
OXcarbazepine									↑
PACLitaxel				S	S				S
Pantoprazole						S, ↓			
Paricalcitol									S
PARoxetine			↓				S, ↓		
PAZOPanib									S
Pentamidine						S			
PENTobarbital		↑							↑
Perphenazine							S		
PHENobarbital	↑	↑	↑	↑	↑	S			↑
Phenytoin			↑	↑	S, ↑	S, ↑			↑
Pimozide	S								S
Pindolol							S		
Pioglitazone				S, ↓					
Piroxicam					↓				
Posaconazole									↓
Primaquine	↓								S
Primidone	↑		↑	↑	↑				↑
Procainamide							S		

CYP: Substrates, Inhibitors, Inducers *(continued)*

Drug	1A2	2A6	2B6	2C8	2C9	2C19	2D6	2E1	3A4
Progesterone						S			S
Promethazine			S				S		
Propafenone							S		
Propofol	↓		S		S	↓			↓
Propranolol	S						S		
Protriptyline							S		
Pyrimethamine					↓				
Quazepam						S			S
QUEtiapine									S
QuiNIDine							↓		S, ↓
QuiNINE				↓	↓		↓		S
RABEprazole				↓		S, ↓			S
Ramelteon	S								
Ranolazine							↓		S
Rasagiline	S								
Repaglinide				S					S
Rifabutin									S, ↑
Rifampin	↑	↑	↑	↑	↑	↑			↑
Rifapentine				↑	↑				↑
Riluzole	S								
RisperiDONE							S		
Ritonavir				↓			S, ↓		S, ↓
ROPINIRole	S								
Ropivacaine	S								
Rosiglitazone				S, ↓					
Salmeterol									S
Saquinavir									S, ↓
Secobarbital		↑			↑	↑			
Selegiline			S						
Sertraline			↓			S, ↓	S, ↓		↓
Sevoflurane								S	
Sibutramine									S
Sildenafil									S
Simvastatin									S
Sirolimus									S
Sitaxsentan					↓	↓			↓
Solifenacin									S
SORAfenib			↓	↓	↓				
Spiramycin									S
SUFentanil									S
SulfADIAZINE					S, ↓				
Sulfamethoxazole					S, ↓				
SUNItinib									S
Tacrine	S								
Tacrolimus									S
Tadalafil									S
Tamoxifen				↓	S		S		S
Tamsulosin							S		S
Telithromycin									S, ↓
Temsirolimus									S
Teniposide									S
Terbinafine							↓		

CYP: Substrates, Inhibitors, Inducers (continued)

Drug	1A2	2A6	2B6	2C8	2C9	2C19	2D6	2E1	3A4
Tetracycline									S, ↓
Theophylline	S							S	S
Thiabendazole	↓								
Thioridazine							S, ↓		
Thiotepa			↓						
Thiothixene	S								
TiaGABine									S
Ticlopidine						↓	↓		S
Timolol							S		
Tinidazole									S
Tipranavir									S
TiZANidine	S								
TOLBUTamide					S, ↓				
Tolterodine							S		S
Toremifene									S
Torsemide					S				
TraMADol[1]							S		S
Tranylcypromine	↓	↓				↓	↓		
TraZODone									S
Tretinoin				S					
Triazolam									S
Trifluoperazine	S								
Trimethoprim				↓	S, ↓				S
Trimipramine						S	S		S
Vardenafil									S
Venlafaxine							S		S
Verapamil									S, ↓
VinBLAStine									S
VinCRIStine									S
Vinorelbine									S
Voriconazole					S	S			↓
Warfarin					S, ↓				
Zafirlukast					S, ↓				
Zileuton	↓								
Zolpidem									S
Zonisamide									S
Zopiclone					S				S
Zuclopenthixol							S		

[1] This opioid analgesic is bioactivated *in vivo* via CYP2D6. Inhibiting this enzyme would decrease the effects of the analgesic. The active metabolite might also affect, or be affected by, CYP enzymes.

[2] Cyclophosphamide is bioactivated *in vivo* to acrolein via CYP2B6 and 3A4. Inhibiting these enzymes would decrease the effects of cyclophosphamide.

[3] Data have shown both induction (*in vivo*) and inhibition (*in vitro*) of CYP3A4.

[4] Ifosfamide is bioactivated *in vivo* to acrolein via CYP3A4. Inhibiting this enzyme would decrease the effects of ifosfamide.

[5] Mestranol is bioactivated *in vivo* to ethinyl estradiol via CYP2C8/9. See Ethinyl Estradiol for additional CYP information.

MANAGEMENT OF DRUG EXTRAVASATIONS

A potential complication of drug therapy is extravasation. A variety of symptoms, including erythema, ulceration, pain, tissue sloughing, and necrosis, are possible. A variety of drugs have been reported to cause tissue damage if extravasated.

DEFINITIONS

- **Extravasation:** Unintentional or inadvertent leakage (or instillation) of fluid out of a blood vessel into surrounding tissue

- **Irritant:** An agent that causes aching, tightness, and phlebitis with or without inflammation, but does not typically cause tissue necrosis. Irritants can cause necrosis if the extravasation is severe or left untreated.

- **Vesicant:** An agent that has the potential to cause blistering, severe tissue injury, or tissue necrosis when extravasated

- **Flare:** Local, nonpainful, possibly allergic reaction often accompanied by reddening along the vein

PREVENTING EXTRAVASATIONS

Although it is not possible to prevent all extravasations, a few precautions can minimize the risk to the patient. The vein used should be a large, intact vessel with good blood flow. Veins in the forearm (ie, basilic, cephalic, and median antebrachial) are usually good options for peripheral infusions. To minimize the risk of dislodging the catheter, avoid using veins in the hands, dorsum of the foot, and any joint space (eg, antecubital). It is important to remember to not administer chemotherapy distal to a recent venipuncture.

A frequently recommended precaution against drug extravasation is the use of a central venous catheter. Use of a central line has several advantages, including high patient satisfaction, reliable venous access, high flow rates, and rapid dilution of the drug. Many institutions encourage or require use of a vascular access device for administration of vesicant agents. Despite their benefit, central lines are not an absolute solution. Vascular access devices are subject to a number of complications. Misplacement/migration of the catheter or improper placement of the needle in accessing injection ports, and cuts, punctures, infections, or rupture of the catheter itself have all been reported.

Education of both the patient and practitioner is imperative. Educate the patient to immediately report any signs of pain, itching, tingling, burning, redness, swelling, or discomfort, all of which could be early signs of extravasation. Symptoms of extravasation which may appear later include blistering, ulceration, and necrosis. Ensure the healthcare team is informed of the risks and management strategies for both prevention and treatment of extravasations. Absence of blood return, resistance upon administration, or interruption of the I.V. flow should raise suspicion of potential extravasation.

INITIAL EXTRAVASATION MANAGEMENT

1. **Stop the infusion:** At the first suspicion of extravasation, the drug infusion and I.V. fluids should be stopped.

2. **Do NOT remove the catheter/needle:** The I.V. tubing should be disconnected, but the catheter/needle should be left in place to facilitate aspiration of fluid from the extravasation site and, if appropriate, administration of an antidote.

3. **Aspirate fluid:** To the extent possible, the extravasated drug solution should gently be removed from the subcutaneous tissues. It is important to avoid any friction or pressure to the area.

4. **Do NOT flush the line:** Flooding the infiltration site with saline or dextrose in an attempt to dilute the drug solution is not recommended.

5. **Remove the catheter/needle:** If an antidote is not going to be administered into the extravasation site, the catheter/ needle should be removed. If an antidote is to be injected into the area, it should be injected through the catheter to ensure delivery of the antidote to the extravasation site. When this has been accomplished, the catheter should then be removed.

6. **Elevate:** The affected extremity should be elevated.

7. **Monitor and document:** Mark the extravasation site (using a surgical felt pen, gently draw an outline on the skin of the extravasation area) and photograph if possible. Monitor and document the event and follow-up activities according to institutional policy.

Table 1. Vesicant Agents and Extravasation Management

Extravasated Medication	Preferred Antidote	Antidote Administration	Supportive Management	Comments
Amino Acids (4.25%)/parenteral nutrition	Hyaluronidase	Hyaluronidase: Intradermal or SubQ: Inject a total of 1 mL (15 units/mL) as five separate 0.2 mL injections (using a 25-gauge needle) into area of extravasation at the leading edge in a clockwise manner (MacCara, 1983; Zenk, 1981)	Apply dry cold compresses (Hurst, 2004)	
Aminophylline	Hyaluronidase	Hyaluronidase: Intradermal or SubQ: Inject a total of 1 mL (15 units/mL) as five separate 0.2 mL injections (using a 25-gauge needle) into area of extravasation at the leading edge in a clockwise manner (MacCara, 1983; Zenk, 1981)	Apply dry cold compresses (Hurst, 2004)	
Amsacrine	No known antidote	No known antidote	Apply dry warm compresses (Schulmeister, 2011)	Not commercially available in the U.S.
Bendamustine	Sodium Thiosulfate	May be managed in the same manner as mechlorethamine extravasation (Schulmeister, 2011): Sodium thiosulfate 1/6 M solution: Inject subcutaneously into extravasation area using 2 mL for each mg of mechlorethamine suspected to have extravasated (Pérez Fidalgo, 2012; Polovich, 2009)	Apply dry cold compresses for 20 minutes 4 times/day for 1 to 2 days (Pérez Fidalgo, 2012)	Irritant with vesicant-like properties (reports of both irritant and vesicant reactions)
Calcium Chloride (≥10%)	Hyaluronidase	Hyaluronidase: Intradermal or SubQ: Inject a total of 1 mL (15 units/mL) as five separate 0.2 mL injections (using a 25-gauge needle) into area of extravasation at the leading edge in a clockwise manner (MacCara, 1983; Zenk, 1981)	Apply dry cold compresses (Hurst, 2004)	
Calcium Gluconate	Hyaluronidase	Hyaluronidase: Intradermal or SubQ: Inject a total of 1 mL (15 units/mL) as five separate 0.2 mL injections (using a 25-gauge needle) into area of extravasation at the leading edge in a clockwise manner (MacCara, 1983; Zenk, 1981)	Apply dry cold compresses (Hurst, 2004)	
CISplatin (>0.4 mg/mL)	Sodium Thiosulfate	Sodium thiosulfate 1/6 M solution: Inject 2 mL into existing I.V. line for each 100 mg of cisplatin extravasated; then consider also injecting 1 mL as 0.1 mL subcutaneous injections (clockwise) around the area of extravasation; may repeat subcutaneous injections several times over the next 3 to 4 hours (Ener, 2004)	Information conflicts regarding use of warm or cold compresses	
Contrast Media	Hyaluronidase	Dimethyl sulfoxide (DMSO) may also be considered an option. Apply topically to a region covering twice the affected area every 8 hours for 7 days; begin within 10 minutes of extravasation; do not cover with a dressing (Pérez Fidalgo, 2012). Hyaluronidase: Intradermal or SubQ: Inject a total of 1 mL (15 units/mL) as five separate 0.2 mL injections (using a 25-gauge needle) into area of extravasation at the leading edge in a clockwise manner (MacCara, 1983; Zenk, 1981) The injection of a total of 5 mL (150 units/mL) as five separate 1 mL injections around the extravasation site has been also used successfully (Rowlett, 2012)	Apply dry cold compresses (Hurst, 2004)	
DACTINomycin	No known antidote	No known antidote	Apply dry cold compress for 20 minutes 4 times/day for 1 to 2 days (Pérez Fidalgo, 2012)	
Dantrolene	No known antidote	No known antidote	No recommendation	
DAUNOrubicin (Conventional)	Dexrazoxane or topical Dimethyl Sulfoxide (DMSO)	Adults: Dexrazoxane 1000 mg/m² (maximum dose: 2000 mg) I.V. (administer in a large vein remote from site of extravasation) over 1 to 2 hours days 1 and 2, then 500 mg/m² (maximum dose: 1000 mg) I.V. over 1 to 2 hours day 3; begin within 6 hours after extravasation (Mouridsen, 2007; Pérez Fidalgo, 2012). **Note:** Reduce dexrazoxane dose by 50% in patients with moderate to severe renal impairment (CrCl <40 mL/min). Pediatrics and Adults: DMSO: Apply topically to a region covering twice the affected area every 8 hours for 7 days; begin within 10 minutes of extravasation; do not cover with a dressing (Pérez Fidalgo, 2012)	Apply dry cold compress for 20 minutes 4 times/day for 1 to 2 days (Pérez Fidalgo, 2012). Withhold cooling for 15 minutes before and after dexrazoxane.	If using dexrazoxane, do not use DMSO. Administer dexrazoxane through a large vein remote from area of the extravasation.

Table 1. Vesicant Agents and Extravasation Management *continued*

Extravasated Medication	Preferred Antidote	Antidote Administration	Supportive Management	Comments
Dextrose (≥10%)	Hyaluronidase	Hyaluronidase: **Dextrose 10%:** Intradermal or SubQ: Inject a total of 1 mL (15 units/mL) as five separate 0.2 mL injections (using a 25-gauge needle) into area of extravasation at the leading edge in a clockwise manner (MacCara, 1983; Zenk, 1981) **Dextrose 50%:** Injection of a total of 1 mL (150 units/mL) as five separate 0.2 mL injections administered along the leading edge of erythema has been used successfully (Wiegand, 2010)	Apply dry cold compresses (Hurst, 2004)	
Diazepam	No known antidote	No known antidote	Apply dry cold compresses (Hurst, 2004)	
Digoxin	No known antidote	No known antidote	No recommendation	
DOCEtaxel	No known antidote	No known antidote	Information conflicts regarding use of warm or cold compresses	Irritant with vesicant-like properties (reports of both irritant and vesicant reactions)
DOPamine	Phentolamine	Phentolamine: Dilute 5 to 10 mg in 10 to 15 mL NS and administer into extravasation site as soon as possible after extravasation (Peberdy, 2010) *Alternatives to phentolamine (due to shortage):* Nitroglycerin topical 2% ointment (based on limited case reports in neonates/infants): Apply 4 mm/kg as a thin ribbon to the affected areas; may repeat after 8 hours if needed (Wong, 1992) **or** apply a 1-inch strip on the affected site (Denkler, 1989) Terbutaline (based on limited case reports): Infiltrate extravasation area using a solution of terbutaline 1 mg diluted to 10 mL in NS (large extravasation site; administration volume varied from 3 to 10 mL, **or** 1 mg diluted in 1 mL 0.9% NS (small/distal extravasation site; administration volume varied from 0.5 to 1 mL). (Stier, 1999)	Apply dry warm compresses (Hurst, 2004)	
DOXOrubicin (Conventional)	Dexrazoxane or topical DMSO	Adults: Dexrazoxane 1000 mg/m² (maximum dose: 2000 mg) I.V. (administer in a large vein remote from site of extravasation) over 1 to 2 hours days 1 and 2, then 500 mg/m² (maximum dose: 1000 mg) I.V. over 1 to 2 hours day 3; begin within 6 hours after extravasation (Mouridsen, 2007; Pérez Fidalgo, 2012). **Note:** Reduce dexrazoxane dose by 50% in patients with moderate to severe renal impairment (CrCl <40 mL/min). Pediatrics and Adults: DMSO: Apply topically to a region covering twice the affected area every 8 hours for 7 days; begin within 10 minutes of extravasation; do not cover with a dressing (Pérez Fidalgo, 2012)	Apply dry cold compress for 20 minutes 4 times/day for 1 to 2 days (Pérez Fidalgo, 2012). Withhold cooling for 15 minutes before and after dexrazoxane.	If using dexrazoxane, do not use DMSO. Administer dexrazoxane through a large vein remote from area of the extravasation.
EPINEPHrine	Phentolamine	Phentolamine: Dilute 5 to 10 mg in 10 to 15 mL NS and administer into extravasation site as soon as possible after extravasation (Peberdy, 2010) *Alternatives to phentolamine (due to shortage):* Nitroglycerin topical 2% ointment (based on limited case reports in neonates/infants): Apply 4 mm/kg as a thin ribbon to the affected areas; may repeat after 8 hours if needed (Wong, 1992) **or** apply a 1-inch strip on the affected site (Denkler, 1989) Terbutaline (based on limited case reports): Infiltrate extravasation area using a solution of terbutaline 1 mg diluted to 10 mL in NS (large extravasation site; administration volume varied from 3 to 10 mL) **or** 1 mg diluted in 1 mL NS (small/distal extravasation site; administration volume varied from 0.5 to 1 mL) (Stier, 1999)	Apply dry warm compresses (Hurst, 2004)	

Table 1. Vesicant Agents and Extravasation Management *continued*

Extravasated Medication	Preferred Antidote	Antidote Administration	Supportive Management	Comments
EPIrubicin	Dexrazoxane or topical DMSO	Adults: Dexrazoxane 1000 mg/m² (maximum dose: 2000 mg) I.V. (administer in a large vein remote from site of extravasation) over 1 to 2 hours days 1 and 2, then 500 mg/m² (maximum dose: 1000 mg) I.V. over 1 to 2 hours day 3; begin within 6 hours after extravasation (Mouridsen, 2007; Pérez Fidalgo, 2012). **Note:** Reduce dexrazoxane dose by 50% in patients with moderate to severe renal impairment (CrCl <40 mL/min). Pediatrics and Adults: DMSO: Apply topically to a region covering twice the affected area every 8 hours for 7 days; begin within 10 minutes of extravasation; do not cover with a dressing (Pérez Fidalgo, 2012)	Apply dry cold compress for 20 minutes 4 times/day for 1 to 2 days (Pérez Fidalgo, 2012). Withhold cooling for 15 minutes before and after dexrazoxane.	If using dexrazoxane, do not use DMSO. Administer dexrazoxane through a large vein remote from area of the extravasation.
Esmolol	No known antidote	No known antidote	No recommendation	
HydrOXYzine	No known antidote	No known antidote	No recommendation	**Note:** Labeled route of administration for parenteral hydroxyzine is by I.M. injection only; I.V. administration is contraindicated.
IDArubicin	Dexrazoxane or topical DMSO	Adults: Dexrazoxane 1000 mg/m² (maximum dose: 2000 mg) I.V. (administer in a large vein remote from site of extravasation) over 1 to 2 hours days 1 and 2, then 500 mg/m² (maximum dose: 1000 mg) I.V. over 1 to 2 hours day 3; begin within 6 hours after extravasation (Mouridsen, 2007; Pérez Fidalgo, 2012). **Note:** Reduce dexrazoxane dose by 50% in patients with moderate to severe renal impairment (CrCl <40 mL/min). Pediatrics and Adults: DMSO: Apply topically to a region covering twice the affected area every 8 hours for 7 days; begin within 10 minutes of extravasation; do not cover with a dressing (Pérez Fidalgo, 2012)	Apply dry cold compress for 20 minutes 4 times/day for 1 to 2 days (Pérez Fidalgo, 2012). Withhold cooling for 15 minutes before and after dexrazoxane.	If using dexrazoxane, do not use DMSO. Administer dexrazoxane through a large vein remote from area of the extravasation.
Mannitol (>5%)	Hyaluronidase	Hyaluronidase: SubQ: Administer multiple 0.5 to 1 mL injections of a 15 units/mL solution around the periphery of the extravasation (Kumar, 2003)	No recommendation	
Mechlorethamine	Sodium Thiosulfate	Sodium thiosulfate 1/6 M solution: Inject subcutaneously into extravasation area using 2 mL for each mg of mechlorethamine suspected to have extravasated (Pérez Fidalgo, 2012; Polovich, 2009)	Apply ice for 6 to 12 hours after sodium thiosulfate administration (Mustargen prescribing information, 2012; Polovich, 2009) **or** may apply dry cold compresses for 20 minutes 4 times/day for 1 to 2 days (Perez Fidalgo, 2012)	
MitoMYcin	Topical DMSO	DMSO: Apply topically to a region covering twice the affected area every 8 hours for 7 days; begin within 10 minutes of extravasation; do not cover with a dressing (Pérez Fidalgo, 2012)	Apply dry cold compress for 20 minutes 4 times/day for 1 to 2 days (Pérez Fidalgo, 2012)	
MitoXANtrone	Dexrazoxane or topical DMSO	Adults: Dexrazoxane 1000 mg/m² (maximum dose: 2000 mg) I.V. (administer in a large vein remote from site of extravasation) over 1 to 2 hours days 1 and 2, then 500 mg/m² (maximum dose: 1000 mg) I.V. over 1 to 2 hours day 3; begin within 6 hours after extravasation (Mouridsen, 2007; Pérez Fidalgo, 2012). **Note:** Reduce dexrazoxane dose by 50% in patients with moderate to severe renal impairment (CrCl <40 mL/min). Pediatrics and Adults: DMSO: Apply topically to a region covering twice the affected area every 8 hours for 7 days; begin within 10 minutes of extravasation; do not cover with a dressing (Pérez Fidalgo, 2012)	Apply dry cold compress for 20 minutes 4 times/day for 1 to 2 days (Pérez Fidalgo, 2012)	Irritant with vesicant-like properties (reports of both irritant and vesicant reactions). Administer dexrazoxane through a large vein remote from area of the extravasation.
Nafcillin	Hyaluronidase	Hyaluronidase: Intradermal or SubQ: Inject a total of 1 mL (15 units/mL) as five separate 0.2 mL Injections (using a 25-gauge needle) into area of extravasation at the leading edge in a clockwise manner (MacCara, 1983; Zenk, 1981)	Apply dry cold compresses (Hurst, 2004)	

Table 1. Vesicant Agents and Extravasation Management *continued*

Extravasated Medication	Preferred Antidote	Antidote Administration	Supportive Management	Comments
Norepinephrine	Phentolamine	Phentolamine: Dilute 5 to 10 mg in 10 to 15 mL NS and administer into extravasation site as soon as possible after extravasation (Peberdy, 2010) **or** dilute 5 to 10 mg in 10 mL NS and administer into extravasation area (within 12 hours of extravasation) (Phentolamine product information, 1999) *Alternatives to phentolamine (due to shortage):* Nitroglycerin topical 2% ointment (based on limited case reports in neonates/infants): Apply 4 mm/kg as a thin ribbon to the affected areas; may repeat after 8 hours if needed (Wong, 1992) **or** apply a 1-inch strip on the affected site (Denkler, 1989) Terbutaline (based on limited case reports): Infiltrate extravasation area using a solution of terbutaline 1 mg diluted to 10 mL in NS (large extravasation site; administration volume varied from 3 to 10 mL) **or** 1 mg diluted in 1 mL NS (small/distal extravasation site; administration volume varied from 0.5 to 1 mL) (Stier, 1999)	Apply dry warm compresses (Hurst, 2004)	
Oxaliplatin	No known antidote	No known antidote	Information conflicts regarding use of warm or cold compresses Cold compresses could potentially precipitate or exacerbate peripheral neuropathy (de Lemos, 2005)	Irritant with vesicant-like properties (reports of both irritant and vesicant reactions)
PACLitaxel	Hyaluronidase	Hyaluronidase: *If needle/cannula still in place:* Administer 1 to 6 mL (150 units/mL) into existing I.V. line; usual dose is 1 mL for each 1 mL of extravasated drug; if needle/cannula has been removed, inject subcutaneously in a clockwise manner around area of extravasation; may repeat several times over the next 3 to 4 hours (Ener, 2004)	Information conflicts regarding use of warm or cold compresses	Irritant with vesicant-like properties (reports of both irritant and vesicant reactions)
Pentamidine	No known antidote	No known antidote	Dry warm compresses (Reynolds, 2014)	Irritant with vesicant-like properties (reports of both irritant and vesicant reactions)
Phenylephrine	Phentolamine	Phentolamine: Dilute 5 to 10 mg in 10 to 15 mL NS and administer into extravasation site as soon as possible after extravasation (Peberdy, 2010) *Alternatives to phentolamine (due to shortage):* Nitroglycerin topical 2% ointment (based on limited case reports in neonates/infants): Apply 4 mm/kg as a thin ribbon to the affected areas; may repeat after 8 hours if needed (Wong, 1992) **or** apply a 1-inch strip on the affected site (Denkler, 1989) Terbutaline (based on limited case reports): Infiltrate extravasation area using a solution of terbutaline 1 mg diluted to 10 mL in NS (large extravasation site; administration volume varied from 3 to 10 mL) **or** 1 mg diluted in 1 mL NS (small/distal extravasation site; administration volume varied from 0.5 to 1 mL) (Stier, 1999)	Apply dry warm compresses (Hurst, 2004)	
Phenytoin	No antidote **or** Hyaluronidase	Conflicting information: Do not use antidotes (pediatrics) (Montgomery, 1999) Hyaluronidase: SubQ: Inject four separate 0.2 mL injections of 15 units/mL (using a 25-gauge needle) into area of extravasation (Sokol, 1998)	No recommendation	
Potassium Acetate (>0.1 mEq/mL)	Hyaluronidase	Hyaluronidase: Intradermal or SubQ: Inject a total of 1 mL (15 units/mL), as five separate 0.2 mL injections (using a 25-gauge needle) into area of extravasation at the leading edge in a clockwise manner (MacCara, 1983; Zenk, 1981)	Apply dry cold compresses (Hurst, 2004)	Reports of both irritant and vesicant reactions

Table 1. Vesicant Agents and Extravasation Management *continued*

Extravasated Medication	Preferred Antidote	Antidote Administration	Supportive Management	Comments
Potassium Chloride (>0.1 mEq/mL)	Hyaluronidase	Hyaluronidase: Intradermal or SubQ: Inject a total of 1 mL (15 units/mL) as five separate 0.2 mL injections (using a 25-gauge needle) into area of extravasation at the leading edge in a clockwise manner (MacCara, 1983; Zenk, 1981)	Apply dry cold compresses (Hurst, 2004)	Reports of both irritant and vesicant reactions
Promethazine	No known antidote	No known antidote	Apply dry cold compresses (Hurst, 2004)	**Note:** Preferred route of administration for promethazine is by deep intramuscular (I.M.) injection. If I.V. route is used, discontinue infusion immediately with onset of burning/pain; evaluate for inadvertent arterial injection or extravasation.
Sodium Bicarbonate (≥8.4%)	Hyaluronidase	Hyaluronidase: SubQ: Inject four to five separate 0.2 mL injections of 15 units/mL around area of extravasation (Hurst, 2004)	Apply dry cold compresses (Hurst, 2004)	
Sodium Chloride (>1%)	No known antidote	No known antidote	Apply dry warm compresses (Hastings-Tolsma, 1993)	
Streptozocin	No known antidote	No known antidote	No recommendation	Irritant with vesicant-like properties (reports of both irritant and vesicant reactions)
Trabectedin	No known antidote	No known antidote	No recommendation	Not commercially available in the U.S.
Tromethamine	No known antidote	No known antidote	No recommendation	
Vasopressin	Phentolamine	Phentolamine: Dilute 5 to 10 mg in 10 to 15 mL NS and administer into extravasation site as soon as possible after extravasation (Peberdy, 2010) *Alternatives to phentolamine (due to shortage):* Nitroglycerin topical 2% ointment (based on limited case reports in neonates/infants): Apply 4 mm/kg as a thin ribbon to the affected areas; may repeat after 8 hours if needed (Wong, 1992) **or** apply a 1-inch strip on the affected site (Denkler, 1989) Terbutaline (based on limited case reports): Infiltrate extravasation area using a solution of terbutaline 1 mg diluted to 10 mL in NS (large extravasation site; administration volume varied from 3 to 10 mL) **or** 1 mg diluted in 1 mL NS (small/distal extravasation site; administration volume varied from 0.5 to 1 mL) (Stier, 1999)	No recommendation	
VinBLAStine	Hyaluronidase	Hyaluronidase: *If needle/cannula still in place:* Administer 1 to 6 mL (150 units/mL) into existing I.V. line; usual dose is 1 mL for each 1 mL of extravasated drug (Pérez Fidalgo, 2012; Schulmeister, 2011) *If needle/cannula was removed:* Inject 1 to 6 mL (150 units/mL) subcutaneously in a clockwise manner using 1 mL for each 1 mL of drug extravasated (Schulmeister, 2011) or administer 1 mL (150 units/mL) as five separate 0.2 mL injections (using a 25-gauge needle) into the extravasation site (Polovich, 2009)	Apply dry warm compress for 20 minutes 4 times/day for 1 to 2 days (Pérez Fidalgo, 2012)	

Table 1. Vesicant Agents and Extravasation Management *continued*

Extravasated Medication	Preferred Antidote	Antidote Administration	Supportive Management	Comments
VinCRIStine	Hyaluronidase	**Hyaluronidase:** *If needle/cannula still in place:* Administer 1 to 6 mL (150 units/mL) into existing I.V. line; usual dose is 1 mL for each 1 mL of extravasated drug (Pérez Fidalgo, 2012; Schulmeister, 2011) *If needle/cannula was removed:* Inject 1 to 6 mL (150 units/mL) subcutaneously in a clockwise manner using 1 mL for each 1 mL of drug extravasated (Schulmeister, 2011) **or** administer 1 mL (150 units/mL) as five separate 0.2 mL injections (using a 25-gauge needle) into the extravasation site (Polovich, 2009)	Apply dry warm compress for 20 minutes 4 times/day for 1 to 2 days (Pérez Fidalgo, 2012)	
Vindesine	Hyaluronidase	**Hyaluronidase:** *If needle/cannula still in place:* Administer 1 to 6 mL (150 units/mL) into existing I.V. line; usual dose is 1 mL for each 1 mL of extravasated drug (Pérez Fidalgo, 2012; Schulmeister, 2011) *If needle/cannula was removed:* Inject 1 to 6 mL (150 units/mL) subcutaneously in a clockwise manner using 1 mL for each 1 mL of drug extravasated (Schulmeister, 2011) **or** administer 1 mL (150 units/mL) as five separate 0.2 mL injections (using a 25-gauge needle) into the extravasation site (Polovich, 2009)	Apply dry warm compress for 20 minutes 4 times/day for 1 to 2 days (Pérez Fidalgo, 2012)	Not commercially available in the U.S.
Vinorelbine	Hyaluronidase	**Hyaluronidase:** *If needle/cannula still in place:* Administer 1 to 6 mL (150 units/mL) into existing I.V. line; usual dose is 1 mL for each 1 mL of extravasated drug (Pérez Fidalgo, 2012; Schulmeister, 2011) *If needle/cannula was removed:* Inject 1 to 6 mL (150 units/mL) subcutaneously in a clockwise manner using 1 mL for each 1 mL of drug extravasated (Schulmeister, 2011) **or** administer 1 mL (150 units/mL) as five separate 0.2 mL injections (using a 25-gauge needle) into the extravasation site (Polovich, 2009)	Apply dry warm compress for 20 minutes 4 times/day for 1 to 2 days (Pérez Fidalgo, 2012)	

SUPPORTIVE MANAGEMENT

Compresses: Two issues for which there is less consensus are the application of warm or cold compresses and the use of various antidotes for extravasation management. A variety of recommendations exists for each of these concerns; however, there is no consensus concerning the proper approach.

Cold: Intermittent cooling of the area of extravasation results in vasoconstriction, potentially restricting the spread of the drug and decreasing the pain and inflammation in the area. Application of dry cold compresses for 20 minutes 4 times/day for 1 to 2 days is usually recommended as immediate treatment for most drug extravasations, including anthracycline, antibiotic (eg, mitomycin or dactinomycin), or alkylating agent extravasation (Pérez Fidalgo, 2012). Cold dry compresses may also be utilized in the management of nonvesicant extravasations.

Warm: Application of dry warm compresses results in a localized vasodilation and increased blood flow. Increased circulation is believed to facilitate removal of the drug from the area of extravasation. Application of dry warm compresses for 20 minutes 4 times/day for 1 to 2 days is generally recommended for extravasation of vinca alkaloid, taxane, and platinum derivatives (Pérez Fidalgo, 2012). Avoid moist heat. Most data are from animal studies with relatively few human case reports. Animal models indicate application of heat exacerbates the damage from anthracycline extravasations.

For some agents, such as oxaliplatin and taxanes, there are conflicting recommendations. Some reports recommend application of cold; others recommend warm.

Table 2: Antineoplastic Agents Associated With Irritation or Occasional Extravasation Reactions

Acyclovir (>7 mg/mL)	Fluorouracil
Arsenic Trioxide	Gemcitabine
Bendamustine[1]	Ibritumomab
Bleomycin	Ifosfamide
Bortezomib	Irinotecan
Busulfan	Ixabepilone
CARBOplatin	Melphalan
Carmustine	MitoXANtrone[1]
CISplatin (≤0.4 mg/mL)	Oxaliplatin[1]
Cladribine	PACLitaxel[1]
Cyclophosphamide	PACLitaxel (Protein Bound)
Dacarbazine	Pentamidine[1]
DAUNOrubicin Citrate (Liposomal)	Streptozocin[1]
DOCEtaxel[1]	Teniposide
DOXOrubicin (Liposomal)	Thiopental[1]
Etoposide	Thiotepa
Etoposide Phosphate	Topotecan

[1]Irritant with vesicant-like properties (there have been reports of both irritant and vesicant reactions)

The nurse administering the vesicant agent should monitor the patient and I.V. site frequently. Prior to drug administration, verify the patency of the I.V. line. The line should be flushed with 5 to 10 mL of a saline or dextrose solution (depending on compatibility) and the drug(s) infused through the side of a free-flowing I.V. line over 2 to 5 minutes. If an extravasation occurs, it is important to monitor the site closely at 24 hours, 1 week, 2 weeks, and as necessary for any signs and symptoms of extravasation.

EXTRAVASATION-SPECIFIC ANTIDOTES

Dexrazoxane: Dexrazoxane, a derivative of EDTA, is an intracellular chelating agent initially approved as a cardioprotective agent in patients receiving anthracycline therapy. It is believed that the cardioprotective effect of dexrazoxane is a result of chelating iron following intracellular hydrolysis. Dexrazoxane is not an effective chelator itself but is hydrolyzed intracellularly to an open-ring chelator form, which complexes with iron, other heavy metals, and doxorubicin complexes to inhibit the generation of free radicals. In the management of anthracycline-induced extravasation, dexrazoxane may act by reversibly inhibiting topoisomerase II, protecting tissue from anthracycline cytotoxicity, thereby decreasing tissue damage.

Dexrazoxane is administered as 3 I.V. infusions over 1 to 2 hours through a different venous access location: 1000 mg/m^2 within 6 hours, 1000 mg/m^2 after 24 hours, and 500 mg/m^2 after 48 hours of the actual extravasation up to a maximum total dose of 2000 mg on days 1 and 2 and 1000 mg on day 3, respectively (Mouridsen, 2007). Localized cooling was permitted (except within 15 minutes before and after dexrazoxane infusion). Prior to administering dexrazoxane, discontinue DMSO as studies suggest the single agent is more effective than when used in combination with DMSO. **Note:** Reduce dexrazoxane dose by 50% in patients with moderate to severe renal impairment (CrCl <40 mL/minute).

Dimethyl sulfoxide (DMSO): Case reports and small studies have suggested that DMSO is an effective treatment for certain chemotherapy extravasations (anthracyclines, mitomycin, and mitoxantrone). DMSO has free-radical scavenger properties, which increases removal of vesicant drugs from tissues to minimize tissue damage in extravasation management (Pérez Fidalgo, 2012). Common dosing is to apply topically by gently painting DMSO 50% solution onto an area twice the size of the extravasation with a saturated gauze pad or cotton swab every 8 hours for 7 days (Pérez Fidalgo, 2012). Allow the site to dry. Do not cover with a dressing, as severe blistering may result. During application, DMSO may cause local erythema. Clinical reports of DMSO use are difficult to interpret due to variations in DMSO concentration (50% to 99%); the product is only commercially available in the United States at a concentration of 50% (vol/vol) solution in water.

Hyaluronidase: Hyaluronidase is an enzyme that destroys hyaluronic acid, an essential component of connective tissue. This results in increased permeability of the tissue, facilitating diffusion and absorption of fluids. It is postulated that increasing the diffusion of extravasated fluids results in more rapid absorption, thereby limiting tissue damage. In individual case reports, hyaluronidase has been reported effective in preventing tissue damage from a wide variety of agents, including vinca alkaloids, epipodophyllotoxins, and taxanes. The ESMO/EONS guidelines suggest that 150 to 900 units may be administered subcutaneously around the area of chemotherapy extravasation (Pérez Fidalgo, 2012). Administration as 5 separate 0.2 mL (15 units/mL) SubQ or intradermal injections into the extravasation site has been reported (MacCara, 1983). A 24-gauge or smaller needle should be used. It is recommended to use a new syringe for each injection site. If needle/cannula still in place, administration of a 1 to 6 mL hyaluronidase (150 units/mL) has been reported in the management of plant alkaloid extravasation (Pérez Fidalgo, 2012; Schulmeister, 2011) and paclitaxel extravasation (Ener, 2004). Refer to Table 1 for vesicant-specific management.

Phentolamine: Phentolamine minimizes tissue injury due to extravasation of norepinephrine and other sympathomimetic vasoconstrictors. Inject 5 to 10 mg diluted in 10 to 15 mL normal saline and inject/infiltrate into the extravasation area; begin as soon as possible after extravasation but within 12 hours.

Sodium thiosulfate: Sodium thiosulfate (1/6 molar) has been recommended for treatment of mechlorethamine, concentrated cisplatin, and bendamustine extravasations. Sodium thiosulfate provides a substrate for alkylation by mechlorethamine, preventing the alkylation and subsequent destruction in subcutaneous tissue.

Preparation of a 1/6 molar solution of sodium thiosulfate:

- Dilute 4 mL of a sodium thiosulfate 10% solution into a syringe with 6 mL of sterile water for injection, resulting in 10 mL of 1/6 molar solution

  or

- Dilute 1.6 mL of a sodium thiosulfate 25% solution with 8.4 mL of sterile water for injection, resulting in 10 mL of 1/6 molar solution

Inject the 1/6 molar sodium thiosulfate solution either into the existing needle/cannula or subcutaneously around the edge of the extravasation site using a tuberculin syringe, using a new syringe for each injection site. The dose of sodium thiosulfate and route of administration depend on the amount of drug extravasated. Refer to Table 1 for vesicant-specific dosing.

Topical nitroglycerin or terbutaline (alternatives to phentolamine): Terbutaline and topical nitroglycerin have been used (case reports) as alternatives to phentolamine in the event of phentolamine supply shortages. Topical nitroglycerin (2% ointment) is reported to reverse the vasoconstriction at the extravasation site caused by infiltration of sympathomimetic vasoconstrictors; case reports for use in neonates/infants suggest resolution of ischemia (Denkler, 1989; Wong, 1992).

REFERENCES

Albanell J, Baselga J. Systemic therapy emergencies. *Semin Oncol.* 2000;27(3):347-361.

Bellin MF, Jakobsen JA, Tomassin I, et al. Contrast medium extravasation injury: guidelines for prevention and management. *Eur Radiol.* 2002;12 (11):2807-2812.

Bertelli G. Prevention and management of extravasation of cytotoxic drugs. *Drug Saf.* 1995;12(4):245-255.

Boyle DM, Engelking C. Vesicant extravasation: myths and realities. *Oncol Nurs Forum.* 1995;22(1):57-67.

de Lemos ML, Walisser S. Management of extravasation of oxaliplatin. *J Oncol Pharm Pract.* 2005;11(4):159-162.

de Lemos ML. Role of dimethylsulfoxide for mangement of chemotherapy extravasation. *J Oncol Pharm Practice.* 2004;10(4):197-200.

Denkler KA, Cohen BE. Reversal of dopamine extravasation injury with topical nitroglycerin ointment. *Plast Reconstr Surg.* 1989;84(5):811-813.

Doellman D, Hadaway L, Bowe-Geddes LA, et al. Infiltration and extravasation: update on prevention and management. *J Infus Nurs.* 2009;32 (4):203-211.

Dorr RT. Antidotes to vesicant chemotherapy extravasations. *Blood Rev.* 1990;4(1):41-60.

Dorr RT, Soble M, Alberts DS. Efficacy of sodium thiosulfate as a local antidote to mechlorethamine skin toxicity in the mouse. *Cancer Chemother Pharmacol.* 1988;22(4):299-302.

Ener RA, Meglathery SB, Styler M. Extravasation of systemic hemato-oncological therapies. *Ann Oncol.* 2004;15(6):858-862.

Hadaway L. Infiltration and extravasation. *Am J Nurs.* 2007;107(8):64-72.

Hastings-Tolsma MT, Yucha CB, Tompkins J, Robson L, Szeverenyi N. Effect of warm and cold applications on the resolution of I.V. infiltrations. *Res Nurs Health.* 1993;16(3):171-178.

Hurst S, McMillan M. Innovative solutions in critical care units: extravasation guidelines. *Dimens Crit Care Nurs.* 2004;23(3):125-128.

Kumar MM, Sprung J. The use of hyaluronidase to treat mannitol extravasation. *Anesth Analg.* 2003;97(4):1199-1200.

Kurul S, Saip P, Aydin T. Totally implantable venous-access ports: local problems and extravasation injury. *Lancet Oncol.* 2002;3(11):684-692.

Larson DL. Alterations in wound healing secondary to infusion injury. *Clin Plast Surg.* 1990;17(3):509-517.

Larson DL. Treatment of tissue extravasation by antitumor agents. *Cancer.* 1982;49(9):1796-1799.

Larson DL. What is the appropriate management of tissue extravasation by antitumor agents? *Plast Reconstr Surg.* 1985;75(3):397-405.

MacCara ME. Extravasation: a hazard of intravenous therapy. *Drug Intell Clin Pharm.* 1983;17(10):713-717.

Montgomery LA, Hanrahan K, Kottman K, Otto A, Barrett T, Hermiston B. Guideline for I.V. infiltrations in pediatric patients. *Pediatr Nurs.* 1999;25 (2):167-169, 173-180.

Mouridsen HT, Langer SW, Buter J, et al. Treatment of anthracycline extravasation with savene (dexrazoxane): results from two prospective clinical multicentre studies. *Ann Oncol.* 2007;18(3):546-550.

Mustargen product information, Lundbeck, 2012

Peberdy MA, Callaway CW, Neumar RW, et al. Part 9: post-cardiac arrest care: 2010 American Heart Association guidelines for cardiopulmonary resuscitation and emergency cardiovascular care. *Circulation.* 2010;122(18 Suppl 3):S768-S786.

Pérez Fidalgo JA, García Fabregat L, Cervantes A, et al. Management of chemotherapy extravasation: ESMO-EONS clinical practice guidelines. *Ann Oncol.* 2012;23(Suppl 7):vii167-173.

Perry MC. Extravasation. *The Chemotherapy Source Book.* 4th ed. Philadelphia, PA; 2008.

Phentolamine product information, Bedford Laboratories, 1999

Polovich M, Whitford JN, Olsen M. *Chemotherapy and Biotherapy Guidelines and Recommendations for Practice.* 3rd ed. Pittsburgh, PA: Oncology Nursing Society; 2009.

Reynolds PM, Maclaren R, Mueller SW, Fish DN, Kiser TH. Management of extravasation injuries: a focused evaluation of noncytotoxic medications [published online January 13, 2014]. *Pharmacotherapy.*

Rowlett J. Extravasation of contrast media managed with recombinant human hyaluronidase. *Am J Emerg Med.* 2012;30(9):2102.

Schrijvers DL. Extravasation: a dreaded complication of chemotherapy. *Ann Oncol.* 2003;14(Suppl 3):iii26-iii30.

Schulmeister L, Camp-Sorrell D. Chemotherapy extravasation from implanted ports. *Oncol Nurs Forum.* 2000;27(3):531-538.

Schulmeister L. Extravasation management: clinical update. *Semin Oncol Nurs.* 2011;27(1):82-90.

Schulmeister L. Preventing and managing vesicant chemotherapy extravasations. *J Support Oncol.* 2010;8(5):212-215.

Sokol DK, Dahlmann A, Dunn DW. Hyaluronidase treatment for intravenous phenytoin extravasation. *J Child Neurol.* 1998;13(5):246-247.

Stanford BL, Hardwicke F. A review of clinical experience with paclitaxel extravasations. *Support Care Cancer*. 2003;11(5):270-277.

Stier PA, Bogner MP, Webster K, Leikin JB, Burda A. Use of subcutaneous terbutaline to reverse peripheral ischemia. *Am J Emerg Med*. 1999;17(1):91-94.

Wang CL, Cohan RH, Ellis JH, Adusumilli S, Dunnick NR. Frequency, management, and outcome of extravasation of nonionic iodinated contrast medium in 69,657 intravenous injections. *Radiology*. 2007;243(1):80-87.

Wiegand R, Brown J. Hyaluronidase for the management of dextrose extravasation. *Am J Emerg Med*. 2010;28(2):257.

Wong AF, McCulloch LM, Sola A. Treatment of peripheral tissue ischemia with topical nitroglycerin ointment in neonates. *J Pediatr*. 1992;121(6):980-983.

Zenk KE. Management of intravenous extravasations. *Infusion*. 1981;5(4):77-79.

BURN MANAGEMENT

Modified Lund-Browder Burn Assessment Chart Estimation of Total Body Surface Area of Burn Involvement[1] (% by site and age)

Site[2]	0 to 1 years	1 to 4 years	5 to 9 years	10 to 14 years	15 years	Adult
Head	9.5	8.5	6.5	5.5	4.5	3.5
Neck	0.5	0.5	0.5	0.5	0.5	0.5
Trunk	13	13	13	13	13	13
Upper arm	2	2	2	2	2	2
Forearm	1.5	1.5	1.5	1.5	1.5	1.5
Hand	1.5	1.5	1.5	1.5	1.5	1.5
Perineum	1	1	1	1	1	1
Buttock (each)	2.5	2.5	2.5	2.5	2.5	2.5
Thigh	2.75	3.25	4	4.25	4.5	4.75
Leg	2.5	2.5	2.75	3	3.25	3.5
Foot	1.75	1.75	1.75	1.75	1.75	1.75

[1]Applies only to second- and third-degree burns.

[2]Percentage for each site is only for **a single extremity with** anterior **OR** posterior involvement. Percentage should be **doubled if both anterior and posterior** involvement of a single extremity.

The total body surface area of burn involvement is determined by the sum of the percentages of each site.

Adapted from: Coren CV. Burn injuries in children. *Pediatric Annals.* 1987;16(4):328-339.

Parkland Fluid Replacement Formula

A guideline for replacement of deficits and ongoing losses (**Note:** For infants, maintenance fluids may need to be added to this): Administer 4 mL/kg/% burn of Ringer's lactate (glucose may be added but beware of stress hyperglycemia) over the first 24 hours; half of this total is given over the first 8 hours **calculated from the time of injury**; the remaining half is given over the next 16 hours. The second 24-hour fluid requirements average 50% to 75% of first day's requirement. Concentrations and rates best determined by monitoring weight, serum electrolytes, urine output, NG losses, etc.

Colloid may be added after 18 to 24 hours (1 g/kg/day of albumin) to maintain serum albumin >2 g/100 mL.

Potassium is generally withheld for the first 48 hours due to the large amount of potassium that is released from damaged tissues. To manage serum electrolytes, monitor urine electrolytes twice weekly and replace calculated urine losses.

CONTRACEPTIVE COMPARISON TABLE

Combination Oral Contraceptive Categories and Regimens

Monophasic contraceptives: Constant dose of estrogen and progestin provided in the active pills per cycle

Biphasic and triphasic contraceptive: Dose of estrogen and progestin vary in the active pills. Decreases the total doses of hormones per cycle; however, may not be associated with a significant increase in safety or efficacy

21/7 regimen: Considered to be the "conventional" regimen; consists of 21 days of active tablets, followed by 7 days of inactive tablets; provides monthly withdrawal bleeding. Symptoms of hormone withdrawal may occur during the hormone-free (inactive) interval and include bloating, breast tenderness, headaches, pelvic pain, and swelling

24/4 regimen: Consists of 24 days of active tablets, followed by 4 days of inactive tablets. Decreases the hormone-free interval from 7 to 4 days to decrease the symptoms associated with hormone withdrawal; provides monthly withdrawal bleeding with decreased duration and lighter blood flow as compared to 21/7 regimens

24/2/2 and 21/2/5 regimens: Multiphasic contraceptive. Decreases the hormone-free interval from 7 to 0 to 2 days by providing a lower, noncontraceptive dose of ethinyl estradiol (0.01 mg) in place of some or all of the placebo tablets to decrease the symptoms associated with hormone withdrawal. Provides monthly withdrawal bleeding with decreased duration and lighter blood flow as compared to 21/7 regimens

84/7 regimen: Extended-cycle contraceptive. Consists of 84 days of active tablets, followed by 7 days of inactive tablets. Decreases withdrawal bleeding to 4 times/year

365-day regimen: Extended-cycle contraceptive. Consists of 365 days of active tablets; eliminates withdrawal bleeding

Ferrous fumarate may be provided in place of placebo tablets in some formulations to facilitate ease of administration; not for therapeutic purposes.

Levomefolate may be provided in place of placebo tablets in some formulations to reduce the risk of neural tube defects if pregnancy occurs during or shortly after use.

Combination Oral Contraceptive Formulations – Monophasic

Brand Name	Regimen (# of pills/pack)	Formulation Content			Additional Information
		Estrogen	Progestin	Other	
Gianvi Loryna Yaz	24/4 regimen (28)	Day 1 to 24: Ethinyl estradiol 0.02 mg	Day 1 to 24: Drospirenone 3 mg	Day 25 to 28: Inactive tablets	
Beyaz	24/4 regimen (28)	Day 1 to 24: Ethinyl estradiol 0.02 mg	Day 1 to 24: Drospirenone 3 mg	Day 1 to 28: Levomefolate calcium 0.451 mg	
Loestrin 24 Fe Lomedia 24 Fe	24/4 regimen (28)	Day 1 to 24: Ethinyl estradiol 0.02 mg	Day 1 to 24: Norethindrone acetate 1 mg	Day 25 to 28: Ferrous fumarate 75 mg	
Generess Fe	24/4 regimen (28)	Day 1 to 24: Ethinyl estradiol 0.025 mg	Day 1 to 24: Norethindrone 0.8 mg	Day 25 to 28: Ferrous fumarate 75 mg	Chewable tablet; efficacy in women with a BMI >35 kg/m² has not been evaluated
Gildess 1/20 Junel 1/20 Larin 1/20 Loestrin 21 1/20 Microgestin 1/20	21/7 regimen (21)	Day 1 to 21: Ethinyl estradiol 0.02 mg	Day 1 to 21: Norethindrone acetate 1 mg		
Aviane Lutera Orsythia Sronyx	21/7 regimen (28)	Day 1 to 21: Ethinyl estradiol 0.02 mg	Day 1 to 21: Levonorgestrel 0.1 mg	Day 22 to 28: Inactive tablets	
Gildess Fe 1/20 Junel Fe 1/20 Larin Fe 1/20 Loestrin Fe 1/20 Microgestin Fe 1/20	21/7 regimen (28)	Day 1 to 21: Ethinyl estradiol 0.02 mg	Day 1 to 21: Norethindrone acetate 1 mg	Day 22 to 28: Ferrous fumarate 75 mg	
Safyral	21/7 regimen (28)	Day 1 to 21: Ethinyl estradiol 0.03 mg	Day 1 to 21: Drospirenone 3 mg	Day 1 to 28: Levomefolate calcium 0.451 mg	
Levora Nordette 28 Portia 28	21/7 regimen (28)	Day 1 to 21: Ethinyl estradiol 0.03 mg	Day 1 to 21: Levonorgestrel 0.15 mg	Day 22 to 28: Inactive tablets	
Gildess 1.5/30 Junel 1.5/30 Larin 1.5/30 Loestrin 21 1.5/30 Microgestin 1.5/30	21/7 regimen (21)	Day 1 to 21: Ethinyl estradiol 0.03 mg	Day 1 to 21: Norethindrone acetate 1.5 mg		
Gildess Fe 1.5/30 Junel Fe 1.5/30 Larin Fe 1.5/30 Loestrin Fe 1.5/30 Microgestin Fe 1.5/30	21/7 regimen (28)	Day 1 to 21: Ethinyl estradiol 0.03 mg	Day 1 to 21: Norethindrone acetate 1.5 mg	Day 22 to 28: Ferrous fumarate 75 mg	
Cryselle 28 Low-Ogestrel Lo/Ovral-28	21/7 regimen (28)	Day 1 to 21: Ethinyl estradiol 0.03 mg	Day 1 to 21: Norgestrel 0.3 mg	Day 22 to 28: Inactive tablets	
Balziva Briellyn Ovcon 35 Philith Vyfemla Zenchent (28s)	21/7 regimen (28)	Day 1 to 21: Ethinyl estradiol 0.035 mg	Day 1 to 21: Norethindrone 0.4 mg	Day 22 to 28: Inactive tablets	

Combination Oral Contraceptive Formulations – Monophasic continued

Brand Name	Regimen (# of pills/pack)	Formulation Content			Additional Information
		Estrogen	Progestin	Other	
Femcon Fe Wymzya Fe Zenchent Fe	21/7 regimen (28)	Day 1 to 21: Ethinyl estradiol 0.035 mg	Day 1 to 21: Norethindrone 0.4 mg	Day 22 to 28: Ferrous fumarate 75 mg	Chewable tablets
Modicon Necon 0.5/35 Nortrel 0.5/35	21/7 regimen (28)	Day 1 to 21: Ethinyl estradiol 0.035 mg	Day 1 to 21: Norethindrone 0.5 mg	Day 22 to 28: Inactive tablets	
Necon 1/35 Norinyl 1+35 Nortrel 1/35 Ortho-Novum 1/35	21/7 regimen (28)	Day 1 to 21: Ethinyl estradiol 0.035 mg	Day 1 to 21: Norethindrone 1 mg	Day 22 to 28: Inactive tablets	
Nortrel 1/35	21/7 regimen (21)	Day 1 to 21: Ethinyl estradiol 0.035 mg	Day 1 to 21: Norethindrone 1 mg		
MonoNessa Ortho-Cyclen Sprintec	21/7 regimen (28)	Day 1 to 21: Ethinyl estradiol 0.035 mg	Day 1 to 21: Norgestimate 0.25 mg	Day 22 to 28: Inactive tablets	
Ovcon 50	21/7 regimen (28)	Day 1 to 21: Ethinyl estradiol 0.05 mg	Day 1 to 21: Norethindrone 1 mg	Day 22 to 28: Inactive tablets	
Ogestrel	21/7 regimen (28)	Day 1 to 21: Ethinyl estradiol 0.05 mg	Day 1 to 21: Norgestrel 0.5 mg	Day 22 to 28: Inactive tablets	
Necon 1/50 Norinyl 1+50	21/7 regimen (28)	Day 1 to 21: Mestranol 0.05 mg	Day 1 to 21: Norethindrone 1 mg	Day 22 to 28: Inactive tablets	

Combination Oral Contraceptive Formulations – Multiphasic

Brand Name	Regimen (# of pills/pack)	Formulation Content			Additional Information
		Estrogen	Progestin	Other	
Lo Loestrin Fe	24/2/2 regimen (28)	Day 1 to 24: Ethinyl estradiol 0.01 mg	Day 1 to 24: Norethindrone acetate 1 mg		Efficacy in women with a BMI >35 kg/m^2 has not been evaluated
		Day 25 to 26: Ethinyl estradiol 0.01 mg			
				Day 27 to 28: Ferrous fumarate 75 mg	
Azurette Kariva Mircette	21/2/5 regimen (28)	Day 1 to 21: Ethinyl estradiol 0.02 mg	Day 1 to 21: Desogestrel 0.15 mg		
				Day 22 to 23: Inactive tablets	
		Day 24 to 28: Ethinyl estradiol 0.01 mg			

Combination Oral Contraceptive Formulations – Biphasic

Brand Name	Regimen (# of pills/pack)	Formulation Content			Additional Information
		Estrogen	Progestin	Other	
Necon 10/11	21/7 regimen (28)	Day 1 to 10: Ethinyl estradiol 0.035 mg	Day 1 to 10: Norethindrone 0.5 mg		
		Day 11 to 21: Ethinyl estradiol 0.035 mg	Day 11 to 21: Norethindrone 1 mg		
				Day 22 to 28: Inactive tablets	

Combination Oral Contraceptive Formulations – Triphasic

Brand Name	Regimen (# of pills/pack)	Formulation Content			Additional Information
		Estrogen	Progestin	Other	
Estrostep Fe Tilia Fe Tri-Legest Fe	21/7 regimen (28)	Day 1 to 5: Ethinyl estradiol 0.02 mg Day 6 to 12: Ethinyl estradiol 0.03 mg Day 13 to 21: Ethinyl estradiol 0.035 mg	Day 1 to 5: Norethindrone acetate 1 mg Day 6 to 12: Norethindrone acetate 1 mg Day 13 to 21: Norethindrone acetate 1 mg		Escalating dose of estrogen; constant dose of progestin
Caziant Cyclessa Velivet	21/7 regimen (28)	Day 1 to 7: Ethinyl estradiol 0.025 mg Day 8 to 14: Ethinyl estradiol 0.025 mg Day 15 to 21: Ethinyl estradiol 0.025 mg	Day 1 to 7: Desogestrel 0.1 mg Day 8 to 14: Desogestrel 0.125 mg Day 15 to 21: Desogestrel 0.15 mg	Day 22 to 28: Inactive tablets	Constant dose of estrogen; escalating dose of progestin
Ortho Tri-Cyclen Lo	21/7 regimen (28)	Day 1 to 7: Ethinyl estradiol 0.025 mg Day 8 to 14: Ethinyl estradiol 0.025 mg Day 15 to 21: Ethinyl estradiol 0.025 mg	Day 1 to 7: Norgestimate 0.18 mg Day 8 to 14: Norgestimate 0.215 mg Day 15 to 21: Norgestimate 0.25 mg	Day 22 to 28: Inactive tablets	Constant dose of estrogen; escalating dose of progestin
Enpresse Trivora	21/7 regimen (28)	Day 1 to 6: Ethinyl estradiol 0.03 mg Day 7 to 11: Ethinyl estradiol 0.04 mg Day 12 to 21: Ethinyl estradiol 0.03 mg	Day 1 to 6: Levonorgestrel 0.05 mg Day 7 to 11: Levonorgestrel 0.075 mg Day 12 to 21: Levonorgestrel 0.125 mg	Day 22 to 28: Inactive tablets	Escalating doses of estrogen and progestin
Necon 7/7/7 Nortrel 7/7/7 Ortho-Novum 7/7/7	21/7 regimen (28)	Day 1 to 7: Ethinyl estradiol 0.035 mg Day 8 to 14: Ethinyl estradiol 0.035 mg Day 15 to 21: Ethinyl estradiol 0.035 mg	Day 1 to 7: Norethindrone 0.5 mg Day 8 to 14: Norethindrone 0.75 mg Day 15 to 21: Norethindrone 1 mg	Day 22 to 28: Inactive tablets	Constant dose of estrogen; escalating dose of progestin
Aranelle Leena Tri-Norinyl	21/7 regimen (28)	Day 1 to 7: Ethinyl estradiol 0.035 mg Day 8 to 16: Ethinyl estradiol 0.035 mg Day 17 to 21: Ethinyl estradiol 0.035 mg	Day 1 to 7: Norethindrone 0.5 mg Day 8 to 16: Norethindrone 1 mg Day 17 to 21: Norethindrone 0.5 mg	Day 22 to 28: inactive tablets	
Ortho Tri-Cyclen TriNessa Tri-Sprintec	21/7 regimen (28)	Day 1 to 7: Ethinyl estradiol 0.035 mg Day 8 to 14: Ethinyl estradiol 0.035 mg Day 15 to 21: Ethinyl estradiol 0.035 mg	Day 1 to 7: Norgestimate 0.18 mg Day 8 to 14: Norgestimate 0.215 mg Day 15 to 21: Norgestimate 0.25 mg	Day 22 to 28: Inactive tablets	Constant dose of estrogen; escalating dose of progestin

Combination Oral Contraceptive Formulations – Four-phase

Brand Name	Regimen (# of pills/pack)	Formulation Content			Additional Information
		Estrogen	Progestin	Other	
Natazia	26/2 regimen (28)	Day 1 to 2: Estradiol valerate 3 mg			Efficacy in women with BMI >30 kg/m^2 has not been evaluated; not recommended for women who are taking strong CYP3A4 inducers
		Day 3 to 7: Estradiol valerate 2 mg	Day 3 to 7: Dienogest 2 mg		
		Day 8 to 24: Estradiol valerate 2 mg	Day 8 to 24: Dienogest 3 mg		
		Day 25 to 26: Estradiol valerate 1 mg			
				Days 27 to 28: Inactive tablets	

Combination Oral Contraceptive Formulations – Extended cycle

Brand Name	Regimen (# of pills/pack)	Formulation Content			Additional Information
		Estrogen	Progestin	Other	
Amethyst Lybrel	365-day regimen (28)	Daily: Ethinyl estradiol 0.02 mg	Daily: Levonorgestrel 0.09 mg		No hormone-free interval; no withdrawal bleeding episodes; 365 days of active pills
Introvale Jolessa Seasonale Quasense	84/7 regimen (91)	Day 1 to 84: Ethinyl estradiol 0.03 mg	Day 1 to 84: Levonorgestrel 0.15 mg		Four withdrawal bleeding episodes/year
				Days 85 to 91: Inactive tablets	

Combination Oral Contraceptive Formulations – Extended cycle/multiphasic

Brand Name	Regimen (# of pills/pack)	Formulation Content			Additional Information
		Estrogen	Progestin	Other	
LoSeasonique	(91)	Day 1 to 84: Ethinyl estradiol 0.02 mg	Day 1 to 84: Levonorgestrel 0.1 mg		No hormone-free interval; four withdrawal bleeding episodes/year
		Day 85 to 91: Ethinyl estradiol 0.01 mg			
Amethia Camrese Seasonique	(91)	Day 1 to 84: Ethinyl estradiol 0.03 mg	Day 1 to 84: Levonorgestrel 0.15 mg		No hormone-free interval; four withdrawal bleeding episodes/year
		Day 85 to 91: Ethinyl estradiol 0.01 mg			

Progestin-Only Oral Contraceptives

Brand Name	Progestin	Additional Information
Camila Errin Heather Jolivette Nora-BE Nor-QD Ortho Micronor	Norethindrone 0.35 mg	No hormone-free interval
Next Choice	Levonorgestrel 0.75 mg	For emergency contraception
Plan B One Step	Levonorgestrel 1.5 mg	For emergency contraception

Additional Hormonal Contraceptive Products[1]

Brand Name	Route	Formulation Content			Additional Information
		Estrogen	Progestin	Other	
Depo-Provera Contraceptive	I.M.		Medroxyprogesterone 150 mg		Dosed every 3 months
depo-subQ provera 104	SubQ		Medroxyprogesterone 104 mg		Dosed every 3 months
ella	Oral			Ulipristal acetate 30 mg	Selective progesterone receptor modulator for emergency contraception
Implanon, Nexplanon	Subdermal		Etonogestrel 68 mg; 60 to 70 µg/day initially (week 5 to 6) and decreases to ~25 to 30 µg/ day at the end of the third year		Long-acting reversible contraception (up to 3 years)
Mirena	Intrauterine		Levonorgestrel 20 mcg/day		Long-acting reversible contraception (up to 5 years)
NuvaRing	Vaginal	Day 1 to 21: Ethinyl estradiol 0.015 mg	Day 1 to 21: Etonogestrel 0.12 mg		21/7 regimen
Ortho Evra Xulane	Transdermal	Day 1 to 21: Ethinyl estradiol 0.02 mcg	Day 1 to 21: Norelgestromin 0.15 mg		21/7 regimen
Skyla	Intrauterine		Levonorgestrel ~6 mcg/day		Long-acting reversible contraception (up to 3 years)

[1]Products presented in alphabetical order by brand name

Estrogens Used for Contraception

Ethinyl estradiol (EE)	• Low-dose combination hormonal contraceptives contain ≤35 mcg EE • Original combination oral contraceptive pills contained EE in doses ≤150 mcg; the highest dose currently available is EE 50 mcg and should not be used unless medically indicated • Decreasing doses of EE decrease the risk of VTE, MI; also associated with bleeding irregularities (amenorrhea, infrequent bleeding, prolonged or frequent bleeding, unscheduled bleeding, spotting) • Increased doses of EE are associated with bloating, breast tenderness, and nausea
Estradiol valerate (E2V)	• Metabolized to EE • ~3% of the dose is directly bioavailable as estradiol
Mestranol	• Original estrogen used in oral contraceptives • Metabolized to EE (large variability)

Progestins Used for Contraception

Desogestrel	• Structurally related to testosterone • Converted into etonogestrel
Dienogest	• Structurally related to testosterone • Antiandrogenic activity and is devoid of estrogenic, androgenic, glucocorticoid, and mineralocorticoid activities • Potential uses include hormone replacement therapy or endometriosis
Drospirenone	• Spironolactone analogue with antimineralocorticoid and antiandrogenic activity • When combined with ethinyl estradiol, used to treat premenstrual dysphoric disorder and acne
Ethynodiol diacetate	• Structurally related to testosterone
Etonogestrel	• Biologically active metabolite of desogestrel • Progestational activity with minimal intrinsic androgenicity
Levonorgestrel	• Structurally related to testosterone
Medroxyprogesterone acetate	• Structurally related to progesterone
Norelgestromin	• Biologically active metabolite of norgestimate
Norethindrone	• Structurally related to testosterone
Norethindrone acetate	• Structurally related to testosterone • Converted to norethindrone
Norgestimate	• Structurally related to testosterone • High progestational activity with minimal intrinsic androgenicity

CLINICAL PRACTICE GUIDELINES

Centers for Disease Control and Prevention (CDC). U.S. medical eligibility criteria for contraceptive use, 2010. *MMWR*. May 2010.

Centers for Disease Control and Prevention (CDC). U.S. medical eligibility criteria for contraceptive use, 2010, update. *MMWR*. July 2011.

Centers for Disease Control and Prevention (CDC). U.S. selected practice recommendations for contraceptive use, 2013. *MMWR*. June 2013.

Medicines and Healthcare Products Regulatory Agency (MHRA – United Kingdom). Combined oral contraceptives (the pill): when to start taking the pill, and missed pill advice. May 2011.

PATIENT INFORMATION

Food and Drug Administration (FDA) Office of Women's Health – Birth Control Poster

Food and Drug Administration (FDA) Office of Women's Health – Emergency Contraception (Emergency Birth Control) Fact Sheet

Food and Drug Administration (FDA) Office of Women's Health – Birth Control Methods Fact Sheet

REFERENCES

Burkman R, Bell C, Serfaty D. The evolution of combined oral contraception: improving the risk-to-benefit ratio. *Contraception*. 2011;84(1):19-34.

Centers for Disease Control and Prevention (CDC). Update to CDC's U.S. medical eligibility criteria for contraceptive use, 2010: revised recommendations for the use of contraceptive methods during the postpartum period. *MMWR Morb Mortal Wkly Rep*. 2011;60(26):878-883.

Centers for Disease Control and Prevention (CDC). U.S. medical eligibility criteria for contraceptive use, 2010. *MMWR Recomm Rep*. 2010;59(RR-4):1-86.

Choice of contraceptives. *Treat Guidel Med Lett*. 2010;8(100):89-96.

Cremer M, Phan-Weston S, Jacobs A. Recent innovations in oral contraception. *Semin Reprod Med*. 2010;28(2):140-146.

Goldzieher JW, Brody SA. Pharmacokinetics of ethinyl estradiol and mestranol. *Am J Obstet Gynecol*. 1990;163(6 Pt 2):2114-2119.

Grossman Barr N. Managing adverse effects of hormonal contraceptives. *Am Fam Physician*. 2010;82(12):1499-1506.

Practice Committee of American Society for Reproductive Medicine. Hormonal contraception: recent advances and controversies. *Fertil Steril*. 2008;90(5 Suppl):S103-S113.

Read CM. New regimens with combined oral contraceptive pills – moving away from traditional 21/7 cycles. *Eur J Contracept Reprod Health Care*. 2010;15(Suppl 2):S32-S41.

Sitruk-Ware R, Nath A. The use of newer progestins for contraception. *Contraception*. 2010;82(5):410-417.

ENTERAL NUTRITION PRODUCT COMPARISON

PREMATURE NEONATAL PRODUCTS

Premature Formula[1,2] – Initial Hospitalization

Indication: Premature infant formulas designed for rapidly growing LBW infants

	Preterm Human Milk	Enfamil Premature 20 Cal[3]	Enfamil Premature 24 Cal[3,4]	Enfamil Premature 30 Cal[3,5]	Similac Special Care 20 With Iron[6]	Similac Special Care 24 With Iron[4,6]	Similac Special Care 30 With Iron[6]	Gerber Good Start Premature 20	Gerber Good Start Premature 24[4]
Calories /100 mL	67	68	81	100	68	81	101	68	81
Protein g/100 mL	1.62	2	2.48 (2.8)[4]	3	2.03	2.43 (2.68)[4]	3.04	2	2.4 (2.9)[4]
Protein source	Preterm human milk	Nonfat milk and whey protein concentrate	Nonfat milk and whey protein concentrate	Nonfat milk and whey protein concentrate	Nonfat milk and whey protein concentrate	Nonfat milk and whey protein concentrate	Nonfat milk and whey protein concentrate	100% enzymatically hydrolyzed whey protein isolate (milk)	100% enzymatically hydrolyzed whey protein isolate (milk)
Carbohydrate g/100 mL	6.64	7.4	8.9 (8.5)[4]	11.2	6.97	8.4 (8.1)[4]	7.84	7.1	8.5 (7.9)[4]
Carbohydrate source	Lactose	Corn syrup solids and lactose	Corn syrup solids and lactose	Maltodextrin	Corn syrup solids and lactose (50:50)	Corn syrup solids and lactose	Corn syrup solids and lactose (50:50)	Lactose, maltodextrin (50:50)	Lactose, maltodextrin (50:50)
Fat g/100 mL	3.89	3.4	4.1	5.2	3.67	4.41	6.71	3.5	4.2
Fat source (essential fatty acid amounts are per 100 kcal)	Preterm human milk	40% MCT, soy, and high oleic vegetable oils (sunflower/safflower); DHA[7] (17 mg); ARA[7] (34 mg); linoleic acid (810 mg); linolenic acid (90 mg)	40% MCT, soy, and high oleic vegetable oils (sunflower/safflower); DHA[7] (17 mg); ARA[7] (34 mg); linoleic acid (810 mg); linolenic acid (90 mg)	40% MCT, soy, and high oleic vegetable oils (sunflower/safflower); DHA[7] (17 mg); ARA[7] (34 mg); linoleic acid (810 mg); linolenic acid (90 mg); soy lecithin	MCT, soy, and coconut oils (50:30:18) with DHA and ARA[7]	MCT, soy, and coconut oils (50:30:18) with DHA and ARA[7], soy lecithin	MCT, soy, and coconut oils (50:30:18) with DHA and ARA[7], soy lecithin	MCT, high oleic sunflower or safflower, soy oils, single cell DHA[7] (0.32%), ARA[7] (0.64%), linoleic acid (950 mg), linolenic acid (100 mg) (40:29:29:2)	MCT, high oleic sunflower or safflower, soy oils, single cell DHA[7] (0.32%), ARA[7] (0.64%), linoleic acid (950 mg), linolenic acid (100 mg) (40:29:29:2)
Osmolality mOsm/kg H_2O	290	240	300	320	235	280	325	229	275
Osmolarity mOsm/L		220	260	270	188	240	282	187	225
Sodium mEq/L (mg/L)	10.8 (248)	(390)	(470)	(590)	12.6 (291)	15.2 (349)	19 (436)	(370)	(450)
Potassium mEq/L (mg/L)	14.6 (570)	(660)	(800)	(1030)	22.3 (872)	26.8 (1047)	33.5 (1308)	(810)	(970)
Chloride mEq/L (mg/L)	15.6 (550)	(610)	(730)	(860)	15.5 (548)	18.6 657	23.2 (821)	(570)	(690)
Calcium mEq/L (mg/L)	12.4 (248)	(1120)	(1340)	(1670)	60.7 (1217)	72.9 (1461)	91.3 (1826)	(1110)	(1330)
Phosphorus mEq/L (mg/L)	(128)	(560)	(670)	(840)	(676)	(812)	(1014)	(570)	(690)
Iron mg/L	1	12.2 (3.4)[8]	14.6 (4.1)[8]	18.3	12.2 (2.5)[8]	14.6	18.3	12	15
% free water	90	90	88	85	90	89	85		

Premature Formula[1,2] – Initial Hospitalization continued

	Preterm Human Milk	Enfamil Premature 20 Cal[3]	Enfamil Premature 24 Cal[3,4]	Enfamil Premature 30 Cal[3,5]	Similac Special Care 20 With Iron[6]	Similac Special Care 24 With Iron[4,6]	Similac Special Care 30 With Iron[6]	Gerber Good Start Premature 20	Gerber Good Start Premature 24[4]
Manufacturer	Mothers	Mead Johnson	Mead Johnson	Mead Johnson	Abbott	Abbott	Abbott	Gerber	Gerber
Special information		Gluten-free	Gluten-free	Gluten-free	Kosher, Halal	Kosher, Halal	Kosher, Halal		

[1] Information based on manufacturer's literature as of 2013 and is subject to change

[2] To approximate values of 24-cal/oz formulation, multiply the values desired, found in the 20-cal/oz formula, by 1.2.

[3] Not recommended for use in patients >2.5 kg because may receive excessive fat soluble vitamin quantities with continued use

[4] Also available as high-protein formula; carbohydrate and protein amounts for the high-protein formulas are listed in parentheses

[5] Can use as a ready-to-feed formula, mix with Enfamil Premature 24 kcal/oz to make 25 to 29 kcal/oz, or mix with Enfamil Premature 24 kcal/oz high-protein to increase protein and kcal/oz

[6] Provides 2 mg of elemental iron per kg/day if providing 120 kcal/kg/day; not recommended for use in patients >3.6 kg

[7] DHA (docosahexaenoic acid) and ARA (arachidonic acid) are fatty acids found naturally in breast milk. DHA is provided via *Crypthecodinium cohnii* oil. ARA is provided via *Mortierella alphia* oil.

[8] Low-iron formulation in parentheses

Human Milk Fortifiers[1,2]

Indication: Add to human milk as a supplement for premature and low birth weight infants

	Enfamil Human Milk Fortifier	Enfamil Human Milk Fortifier Acidified Liquid[3]	Similac Human Milk Fortifier
Calories /packet	3.5	7.5/5 mL vial	3.5
Protein g/packet	0.28	0.55	0.25
Protein source	Milk protein isolate and whey protein hydrolysate	Wey protein isolate hydrolysate (milk)	Nonfat milk and whey protein concentrate
Carbohydrate g/packet	<0.1	<0.3	0.45
Carbohydrate source	Corn syrup solids	Pectin	Corn syrup solids
Fat g/packet	0.25	0.58	0.09
Fat source (essential fatty acid amounts are per 100 kcal)	MCT and soybean oils and soy lecithin (140 mg of linoleic acid and 17 mg of linolenic acid/4 packets)	MCT, vegetable oils (soy, high oleic sunflower oils), DHA[3,5] (24 mg), ARA[3,5] (38 mg), linoleic acid (730 mg), linolenic acid (60 mg)	MCT oil and soy lecithin
Osmolality mOsm/kg H_2O	Additional 35 when added to breast milk	Additional 36 when added to human milk	
Sodium mEq/packet (mg/packet)	(4)	(6.75)	0.16 (3.75)
Potassium mEq/packet (mg/packet)	(7.25)	(11.3)	0.4 (15.8)
Chloride mEq/packet (mg/packet)	(3.25)	(7)	0.27 (9.5)
Calcium mEq/packet (mg/packet)	(22.5)	(29)	1.46 (29.3)
Phosphorus mEq/packet (mg/packet)	(12.5)	(16)	0.54 (16.8)
Iron mg/packet	0.36	0.44	0.088
Manufacturer	Mead Johnson	Mead Johnson	Abbott
Special information	Gluten-free	Gluten-free	Kosher, Halal

[1]Information based on manufacturer's literature as of 2013 and is subject to change

[2]May be mixed with human milk or fed alternatively with human milk to low birth weight infants.

[3]Meets ADA and CDC feeding preparation guidelines. Contains 4 g of protein/100 kcal with human milk; pH of 4.3 by itself; pH of 4.7 with human milk. Four 5 mL vials contain 12 mg of DHA, 188 international units of vitamin D, and 1.76 mg of elemental iron. One 5 mL vial + 25 mL of human milk/100 kcal would provide 24 mg of DHA and 38 mg of ARA. One 5 mL vial + 50 mL of human milk increases caloric content by 2 kcal/oz. Two 5 mL vials + 25 mL of human milk increases caloric content by 4 kcal/oz.

[4]Not recommended for use in patients >3.6 kg

[5]DHA (docosahexaenoic acid) and ARA (arachidonic acid) are fatty acids found naturally in breast milk. DHA is provided via *Crypthecodinium cohnii* oil. ARA is provided via *Mortienella alphia* oil.

Premature Formula – Enhanced Caloric Preparations

Indications: Premature Neonates Who Need High Calorie Low Volume Feedings

Similac Special Care Liqui-Mix System[1]

	22 calorie/oz formula	26 calorie/oz formula	27 calorie/oz formula	27 calorie/oz formula	28 calorie/oz formula
Base formula to begin with	Similac Special Care 20 With Iron (SSC 20)	Similac Special Care 24 With Iron[2] (SSC 24)	Similac Special Care 20 With Iron (SSC 20)	Similac Special Care 24 With Iron[2] (SSC 24)	Similac Special Care 24 With Iron[2] (SSC 24)
Formula used to increase caloric content	Similac Special Care 24 With Iron[2] (SSC 24)	Similac Special Care 30 With Iron (SSC 30)	Similac Special Care 30 With Iron (SSC 30)	Similac Special Care 30 With Iron (SSC 30)	Similac Special Care 30 With Iron (SSC 30)
Mixing instructions	15 mL SSC 20 + 15 mL SSC 24	20 mL SSC 24 + 10 mL SSC 30	10 mL SSC 20 + 20 mL SSC 30	15 mL SSC 24 + 15 mL SSC 30	10 mL SSC 24 + 20 mL SSC 30
Ratio	1:1	2:1	1:2	1:1	1:2
Calories /100 mL	74	88	90	91	95
Protein g/100 mL	2.23 (2.35)[2]	2.64 (2.8)[2]	2.71	2.74 (2.86)[2]	2.84 (2.92)[2]
Protein source	Nonfat milk and whey protein concentrate	Nonfat milk and whey protein concentrate	Nonfat milk and whey protein concentrate	Nonfat milk and whey protein concentrate	Nonfat milk and whey protein concentrate
Carbohydrate g/100 mL	7.7 (7.5)[2]	8.2 (8)[2]	7.5	8.1 (8)[2]	8 (7.9)[2]
Carbohydrate source	Corn syrup solids and lactose (50:50)	Corn syrup solids and lactose (50:50)	Corn syrup solids and lactose (50:50)	Corn syrup solids and lactose (50:50)	Corn syrup solids and lactose (50:50)
Fat g/100 mL	4.04	5.17	5.69	5.56	5.94
Fat source (essential fatty acid amounts are per 100 kcal)	MCT, soy, and coconut oils (50:30:18) with DHA and ARA[3]; soy lecithin	MCT, soy, and coconut oils (50:30:18) with DHA and ARA[3]; soy lecithin	MCT, soy, and coconut oils (50:30:18) with DHA and ARA[3]; soy lecithin	MCT, soy, and coconut oils (50:30:18) with DHA and ARA[3]; soy lecithin	MCT, soy, and coconut oils (50:30:18) with DHA and ARA[3]; soy lecithin
Osmolality mOm/kg H_2O	258	295	295	305	310
Sodium mEq/L (mg/L)	13.9 (320)	16 (380)	16.9 (390)	17 (390)	18 (410)
Potassium mEq/L (mg/L)	24.5 (960)	29 (1130)	29.7 (1160)	30 (1180)	31 (1220)
Chloride mEq/L (mg/L)	17 (600)	20 (710)	20.6 (730)	21 (740)	22 (770)
Calcium mEq/L (mg/L)	(1340)	(1580)	(1620)	(1640)	(1700)
Phosphorus mEq/L (mg/L)	(740)	(880)	(900)	(910)	(950)
Iron mg/L	13	15.8	13.5	16.4	17
Manufacturer	Abbott	Abbott	Abbott	Abbott	Abbott

[1] Information based on manufacturer's literature as of 2011 and is subject to change

[2] Also available as high-protein formula; carbohydrate and protein amounts for the high-protein formula are listed in parentheses

[3] DHA (docosahexaenoic acid) and ARA (arachidonic acid) are fatty acids found naturally in breast milk. DHA is provided via *Crypthecodinium cohnii* oil. ARA is provided via *Mortierella alpha* oil.

Enfamil Mixing Instructions[1]

	26 calorie/oz formula	27 calorie/oz formula	28 calorie/oz formula
Base formula to begin with	Enfamil Premature High Protein 24 Cal (EPHP 24)	Enfamil Premature High Protein 24 Cal (EPHP 24)	Enfamil Premature High Protein 24 Cal (EPHP 24)
Formula used to increase caloric content	Enfamil Premium Infant Concentrate (EPIC)	Enfamil Premium Infant Concentrate (EPIC)	Enfamil Premium Infant Concentrate (EPIC)
Mixing instructions	60 mL EPHP 24 + 8 mL EPIC	60 mL EPHP 24 + 14 mL EPIC	60 mL EPHP 24 + 20 mL EPIC
Calories /100 mL	88	92	95
Protein g/100 mL	2.9	2.9	2.9
Protein source	Nonfat milk and whey protein concentrate	Nonfat milk and whey protein concentrate	Nonfat milk and whey protein concentrate
Carbohydrate g/100 mL	9.3	9.7	10.1
Carbohydrate source	Corn syrup soids, lactose, galactooligosaccharides[2,3], polydextrose	Corn syrup soids, lactose, galactooligosaccharides[2,3], polydextrose	Corn syrup soids, lactose, galactooligosaccharides[2,3], polydextrose
Fat g/100 mL	4.5	4.7	4.8
Fat source (essential fatty acid amounts are per 100 kcal)	MCT, soy, high oleic vegetable (sunflower/safflower), palm olein, and coconut oils; DHA[4] (14.9 mg); ARA[4] (30 mg); linoleic acid; linolenic acid; and soy lecithin	MCT, soy, high oleic vegetable (sunflower/safflower), palm olein, and coconut oils; DHA[4] (15.6 mg); ARA[4] (32 mg); linoleic acid; linolenic acid; and soy lecithin	MCT, soy, high oleic vegetable (sunflower/safflower), palm olein, and coconut oils; DHA[4] (16.2 mg); ARA[4] (33 mg); linoleic acid; linolenic acid; and soy lecithin
Sodium mEq/L (mg/L)	(460)	(450)	(440)
Potassium mEq/L (mg/L)	(880)	(920)	(960)
Chloride mEq/L (mg/L)	(750)	(750)	(760)
Calcium mEq/L (mg/L)	(1300)	(1290)	(1270)
Phosphorus mEq/L (mg/L)	(670)	(660)	(660)
Iron mg/L	15.8	16.4	17.1
Manufacturer	Mead Johnson	Mead Johnson	Mead Johnson

[1]Information based on manufacturer's literature as of 2011 and is subject to change

[2]Contains Bifidus BL, beneficial cultures like those found in breast milk to help support a healthy immune system

[3]Prebiotic

[4]DHA (docosahexaenoic acid) and ARA (arachidonic acid) are fatty acids which are found naturally in breast milk. DHA is provided via *Crypthecodinium cohnii* oil. ARA is provided via *Mortienella alphia* oil.

Premature Formula[1,2] – At Discharge

Indication: Premature infant formulas designed for rapidly growing LBW infants

	Enfamil EnfaCare[3]	Similac Expert Care Neosure	Gerber Good Start Nourish
Calories /100 mL	73	74	74
Protein g/100 mL	2.1	2.08	2.1
Protein source	Nonfat milk and whey protein concentrate	Nonfat milk and whey protein concentrate	100% enzymatically hydrolyzed whey protein isolate (milk)
Carbohydrate g/100 mL	7.7	7.51	7.8
Carbohydrate source	Powder: Corn syrup solids, lactose Liquid: Maltodextrin, lactose	Corn syrup solids, lactose	Lactose, maltodextrin (60:40)
Fat g/100 mL	3.9	4.09	3.9
Fat source (essential fatty acid amounts are per 100 kcal)	High oleic vegetable (sunflower/ safflower), soy, 20% MCT, and coconut oils; DHA[4] (17 mg); ARA[4] (34 mg); linoleic acid (860 to 950 mg)[5]; linolenic acid (90 to 95 mg)[6]	Soy, high oleic safflower, MCT, and coconut oils with DHA and ARA[4]; soy lecithin	High oleic sunflower or safflower, MCT, and soy oils; single cell DHA[4] (0.32%); ARA[4] (0.64%); linoleic acid (900 mg); linolenic acid (60 mg); soy lecithin
Osmolality mOsm/kg H_2O	250 (liquid) 310 (powder)	250	275
Osmolarity mOsm/L	220 (liquid) 280 (powder)	187	180
Sodium mEq/L (mg/L)	(260 – liquid) (280 – powder)	10.7 (245)	(260)
Potassium mEq/L (mg/L)	(780)	27 (1056)	(781)
Chloride mEq/L (mg/L)	(580)	15.7 (558)	(551)
Calcium mEq/L (mg/L)	(890)	39 (781)	(893)
Phosphorus mEq/L (mg/L)	(490)	(461)	(484)
Iron mg/L	13.3	13.4	13
% free water	89	89	
Manufacturer	Mead Johnson	Abbott	Gerber
Special information	Gluten-free	Kosher, Halal	

[1]Information based on manufacturer's literature as of 2013 and is subject to change

[2]To approximate values of 24-cal/oz formulation, multiply the values desired found in the 20-cal/oz formula by 1.2.

[3]Recommended minimum patient weight >1.8 kg

[4]DHA (docosahexaenoic acid) and ARA (arachidonic acid) are fatty acids found naturally in breast milk. DHA is provided via *Crypthecodinium cohnii* oil. ARA is provided via *Mortienella alphia* oil.

[5]Amount of linoleic acid varies depending on product and size: 860 mg in the powder, 900 mg in the 2 fl oz ready-to-feed, 950 mg in the 32 fl oz ready-to-feed

[6]Amount of linolenic acid varies depending on product and size: 90 mg in the 2 fl oz ready-to-feed, 95 mg in the 32 fl oz ready-to-feed and the powder

INFANT PRODUCTS

Infant Milk-Based Formulas[1,2]

Indications: Feeding normal term infants or sick infants without special nutritional requirements

	Human Milk	Enfamil Premium[3]	Similac Advance[4]	Similac Advance Organic[5]	Gerber Good Start Gentle	Gerber Good Start Protect[6]	Enfamil A.R.[7]	Similac Sensitive RS
Calories /100 mL	68	67	68	68	68	68	68	68
Protein g/100 mL	1	1.4	1.4	1.4	1.49	1.49	1.67	1.5
Protein source	Mature Term human milk	Nonfat milk, whey protein concentrate	Nonfat milk, whey protein concentrate	Organic nonfat milk	100% whey protein concentrate (milk)	100% whey protein concentrate (milk)	Nonfat milk	Milk protein isolate
Carbohydrate g/100 mL	7.2	7.5	7.2	7.1	7.85	7.58	7.5	7.2
Carbohydrate source	Lactose	Lactose, galactooligosac-charides[8,9], polydextrose	Lactose and galactooligosac-charides[8]	Organic maltodextrin, organic sugar, fructooligosacchar-ides[8]	Corn (30%) maltodextrin, lactose (70%), galactooligosac-charides[8] (4 g/L)	Lactose and corn maltodextrin	Rice starch, lactose, maltodextrin, galactooligosac-charides[8,9], polydextrose	Corn syrup, rice starch, sugar (50:30:20)
Fat g/100 mL	3.91	3.5	3.78	3.8	3.45	3.42	3.4	3.7
Fat source (essential fatty acid amounts are per 100 kcal)	Human milk, fat	Vegetable oil (palm olein, coconut, soy, and high oleic sunflower oils), DHA[10] (17 mg), ARA[10] (34 mg), linoleic acid (860 mg, 80 mg), soy lecithin	High oleic safflower, soy, and coconut oils (40:30:29) DHA: 0.15%[10] ARA: 0.40%[10]	Organic high oleic sunflower, organic soy, and organic coconut oils (40:30:29; DHA & ARA)[10]	Vegetable oil (palm, soy, coconut, and high oleic safflower or sunflower oils), DHA[10] (0.32%), ARA[10] (0.64%), linoleic acid (900 mg), linolenic acid (46:26:20:6:2), soy lecithin	Vegetable oil (palm, soy, coconut, and high oleic safflower or sunflower oils), DHA[10] (0.32%), ARA[10] (0.64%), linoleic acid (900 mg), linolenic acid (46:26:20:6:2), soy lecithin	Vegetable oils (palm olein, soy, coconut, and high oleic safflower oils), DHA[10] (17 mg), ARA[10] (34 mg), linoleic acid (860 mg), linolenic acid (85 mg)	High oleic safflower, soy, and coconut oils, DHA and ARA[10] (40:30:29)
Osmolality mOsm/kg H_2O	286	300	310	225	250	250	240 (liquid) 230 (powder)	270
Osmolarity mOsm/L	270	270	127	127	133	133	220 (liquid) 210 (powder)	240
Sodium mEq/L (mg/L)	7.7 (177)	(180)	7.1 (162)	7.1 (163)	(183)	(183)	(267)	(240)
Potassium mEq/L (mg/L)	13.6 (531)	(720)	18.2 (710)	18.1 (710)	(730)	(730)	(720)	(867)
Chloride mEq/L (mg/L)	11.9 (422)	(420)	12.4 (440)	12.4 (442)	(440)	(440)	(500)	(534)
Calcium mEq/L (mg/L)	16 (280)	27 (520)	26.3 (528)	26.3 (530)	(453)	(453)	(520)	(1301)
Phosphorus mEq/L (mg/L)	9 (143)	(287)	18.8 (284)	(285)	(257)	(257)	(354)	(867)
Iron mg/L	0.27	12	12.2	12.2	10.1	10.1	12	12.2
% free water	80 to 90	89	90	90	90	90	89	90
Manufacturer	Mothers	Mead Johnson	Abbott	Abbott	Gerber	Gerber	Mead Johnson	Abbott

Infant Milk-Based Formulas[1,2] *continued*

	Human Milk	Enfamil Premium[3]	Similac Advance[4]	Similac Advance Organic[5]	Gerber Good Start Gentle	Gerber Good Start Protect[6]	Enfamil A.R.[7]	Similac Sensitive RS
Special information							Gluten-free	
Special uses							Thickened with added rice starch for babies who spit up frequently	With added rich starch to help reduce spit-up; milk-based, lactose-free formula

[1] Information based on manufacturer's literature as of 2013 and is subject to change

[2] To approximate values for the content of a 24-, 27-, or 30-cal/oz formula (made by dilution of a powder-based formulation), multiply the value desired, found in the above 20-cal/oz formula, by the following factors: 1.2 (24-cal/oz), 1.35 (27-cal/oz), or 1.5 (30-cal/oz).

[3] Available as newborn and infant products. Newborn product is for birth to 3 months of age and provides 400 international units of vitamin D in 27 fl oz and is similar to breast milk 3 to 5 days after initiation of lactation. Infant product is for 0 to 12 months of age.

[4] Contains nucleotides and prebiotics for enhanced immune function.

[5] Certified USDA organic

[6] Contains Bifidus BL, beneficial cultures like those found in breast milk to help support a healthy immune system

[7] Viscosity in the bottle is 10 times routine formula, yet it flows freely through a standard nipple

[8] Prebiotic

[9] Polydextrose + galactooligosaccharides = Natural Defense Dual Prebiotics from Mead Johnson. They support the growth of healthy gut bacteria which help support immune function.

[10] DHA (docosahexaenoic acid) and ARA (arachidonic acid) are fatty acids which are found naturally in breast milk. DHA is provided via *Crypthecodinium cohnii* oil. ARA is provided via *Mortierella alphia* oil.

Infant Milk-Based Formulas − Reduced Lactose and Lactose Free[1,2]

Indications: Feeding normal term infants or sick infants without special nutritional requirements

	Enfamil Gentlease[3]	Similac Sensitive	Gerber Good Start Soothe[4]
Calories /100 mL	67	68	68
Protein g/100 mL	1.5	1.45	1.5
Protein source	Partially hydrolyzed nonfat milk and whey protein concentrate (soy)	Milk protein isolate	100% whey partially hydrolyzed
Carbohydrate g/100 mL	7.2	7.5	7.58
Carbohydrate source	Corn syrup solids	Corn maltodextrin, sugar, galactooligosaccaharides[5] (55:43:4)	Maltodextrin, lactose (70:30)
Fat g/100 mL	3.5	3.65	3.45
Fat source (essential fatty acid amounts are per 100 kcal)	Vegetable oil (palm olein, soy, coconut, and high oleic sunflower oils), DHA[6] (17 mg), ARA[6] (34 mg), linoleic acid (860 mg), linolenic acid (80 mg)	High oleic safflower, soy, and coconut oils (40:30:29) DHA: 0.15% ARA: 0.40%[6]	Vegetable oil (palm olein, soy, coconut, and high oleic safflower or sunflower oils), DHA[6] (0.32%), ARA[6] (0.64%), linoleic acid (900 mg), linolenic acid (85 mg)
Osmolality mOsm/kg H_2O	230 (powder) 220 (liquid)	200	132
Osmolarity mOsm/L	210 (powder) 200 (liquid)	135	195
Sodium mEq/L (mg/L)	(240)	8.8 (203)	(183)
Potassium mEq/L (mg/L)	(720)	18.5 (724)	(730)
Chloride mEq/L (mg/L)	(420)	12.4 (440)	(440)
Calcium mEq/L (mg/L)	(547)	28.3 (568)	(487)
Phosphorus mEq/L (mg/L)	(307)	21.6 (379)	(271)
Iron mg/L	12	12.2	10
% free water	89	90	90
Manufacturer	Mead Johnson	Abbott	Gerber
Special information	Gluten-free	Kosher, Halal	

[1]Information based on manufacturer's literature as of 2013 and is subject to change

[2]To approximate values for the content of a 24-, 27-, or 30-cal/oz formula (made by dilution of a powder-based formulation), multiply the value desired, found in the above 20-cal/oz formula, by the following factors: 1.2 (24-cal/oz), 1.35 (27-cal/oz), or 1.5 (30-cal/oz).

[3]Previous product Enfamil LactoFree LIPIL discontinued. Recommend using Enfamil Gentlease instead. Enfamil Gentlease contains 1/5 the lactose of regular milk-based formulas and is for infants who have shown transient intolerance to lactose and is marketed for fussiness/gas.

[4]30% lactose of regular milk-based formulas

[5]Prebiotic

[6]DHA (docosahexaenoic acid) and ARA (arachidonic acid) are fatty acids found naturally in breast milk. DHA is provided via *Crypthecodinium cohnii* oil. ARA is provided via *Mortienella alphia* oil.

Casein Hydrolysate Formulas[1,2]

Indication: For infants requiring low molecular weight peptides or amino acids

	Nutramigen[3]	Pregestimil[4]	Pregestimil 24	Similac Expert Care Alimentum
Calories /100 mL	67	68	81	68
Protein g/100 mL	1.87	1.89	2.3	1.86
Protein source	Casein hydrolysate, L-cystine, L-tyrosine, L-tryptophan, taurine	Casein hydrolysate (milk), L-cystine, L-tyrosine, L-tryptophan, taurine	Casein hydrolysate (milk), L-cystine, L-tyrosine, L-tryptophan, taurine	Casein hydrolysate, L-cystine, L-tyrosine, L-tryptophan
Carbohydrate g/100 mL	6.87	6.9	8.3	6.9
Carbohydrate source	Corn syrup solids and modified corn starch	Corn syrup solids and modified corn starch	Corn syrup solids and modified cornstarch	Corn maltodextrin and sugar (70:30)
Fat g/100 mL	3.54	3.78	4.5	3.75
Fat source (essential fatty acid amounts are per 100 kcal)	Vegetable oils (palm olein, soy, coconut, and high oleic sunflower oils), DHA[4] (17 mg), ARA[4] (34 mg), linoleic acid (940 mg), linolenic acid (80 to 85 mg)[5]	55% MCT, soy, and high oleic vegetable (sunflower/safflower) oils; DHA[4] (17 mg); ARA[4] (34 mg); linoleic acid (940 mg); linolenic acid (95 to 120 mg)[6]	55% MCT, soy, corn, and high oleic vegetable (sunflower/safflower) oils; DHA[4] (17 mg); ARA[4] (34 mg); linoleic acid (940 mg); linolenic acid (120 mg)	High oleic safflower, 33% medium chain triglycerides, and soy oils; DHA[4] (0.15%); ARA[4] (0.4%) (35:33:28:4); DATEM[7]
Osmolality mOsm/kg H_2O	260 to 320[8] (liquid) 300 (powder)	290 (liquid) 320 (powder)	340	370
Osmolarity mOsm/L	230 to 290[9] (liquid) 270 (powder)	260 (liquid) 280 (powder)	300	171
Sodium mEq/L (mg/L)	(313)	(313)	(373)	12.9 (298)
Potassium mEq/L (mg/L)	(734)	(733)	(872)	20.3 (798)
Chloride mEq/L (mg/L)	(574)	(574)	(682)	15.5 (541)
Calcium mEq/L (mg/L)	(627)	(627)	(743)	35.4 (710)
Phosphorus mEq/L (mg/L)	(347)	(347)	(412)	(507)
Iron mg/L	12	12	14.3	12.2
% free water	89	89	86	90
Manufacturer	Mead Johnson	Mead Johnson	Mead Johnson	Abbott
Special information	Lactose-free, gluten-free, galactose-free, sucrose-free	Lactose-free, gluten-free, galactose-free, sucrose-free	Lactose-free, gluten-free, galactose-free, sucrose-free	Ready-to-feed is corn-free
Special uses	Sensitivity to intact proteins found in milk and soy formulas, patients with colic, and patients with galactosemia	Fat malabsorption or sensitivity to intact proteins; may be used in cystic fibrosis, short bowel syndrome, intractable diarrhea, severe protein calorie malnutrition, and patients with galactosemia	Fat malabsorption or sensitivity to intact proteins; may be used in cystic fibrosis, short bowel syndrome, intractable diarrhea, severe protein calorie malnutrition, and patients with galactosemia	Severe food allergies, sensitivity (including colic) to intact proteins, protein maldigestion or fat malabsorption

[1]Information based on manufacturer's literature as of 2013 and is subject to change

[2]To approximate values for the content of a 24-, 27-, or 30-cal/oz formula (made by dilution of a powder-based formulation), multiply the value desired, found in the above 20-cal/oz formula, by the following factors: 1.2 (24-cal/oz), 1.35 (27-cal/oz), or 1.5 (30-cal/oz)

[3]Also available with EnfloraLGG, which is a probiotic to support the strength of the intestinal barrier and to support digestive health

[4]DHA (docosahexaenoic acid) and ARA (arachidonic acid) are fatty acids found naturally in breast milk. DHA is provided via *Crypthecodinium cohnii* oil. ARA is provided via *Mortienella alphia* oil.

[5]Amount of linolenic acid varies depending on product and size: 80 mg in the 8 fl oz concentrate and 2, 8, and 32 fl oz ready-to-feed; 85 mg in the 6 fl oz ready-to-feed and the 13 fl oz concentrate

[6]Amount of linolenic acid varies depending on product and size: 95 mg in the powder; 120 mg in the ready-to-feed

[7]Diacetyl tartaric acid esters of mono-diglycerides is an emulsifier derived from soy, palm, or canola oil.

[8]Osmolality varies depending on product and size: 260 mOsm/kg H_2O for the 13 fl oz concentrates and the 6 fl oz ready-to-feed; 270 mOsm/kg H_2O for the 8 and 32 fl oz ready-to-feed; 320 mOsm/kg H_2O for the 2 fl oz ready-to-feed

[9]Osmolarity varies depending on product and size: 230 mOsm/L for the 6 oz ready-to-feed and the 13 fl oz concentrate; 240 mOsm/L for the 8 and 32 fl oz ready-to-feeds; 290 mOsm/L for the 2 fl oz ready-to-feed

Infant Soy Formulas[1,2]

Indications: Lactase deficiency, milk intolerance, or galactosemia; not recommended for premature infants with birthweight <1.8 kg

	Enfamil ProSobee	Similac Soy Isomil	Gerber Good Start Soy
Calories /100 mL	68	67.6	67.6
Protein g/100 mL	1.67	1.66	1.69
Protein source	Soy protein isolate, L-methionine, taurine	Soy protein isolate, L-methionine	Enzymatically hydrolyzed soy protein isolate, L-methionine, taurine
Carbohydrate g/100 mL	7.1	7	7.51
Carbohydrate source	Corn syrup solids	Corn syrup solids, sugar, fructoolgiosaccharide[3] (78:19:3)	Corn maltodextrin sucrose (79:21)
Fat g/100 mL	3.5	3.69	3.45
Fat source (essential fatty acid amounts are per 100 kcal)	Vegetable oils (palm olein, soy, coconut, and high oleic sunflower oils), DHA[4] (17 mg), ARA[4] (34 mg), linoleic acid (860 mg), linolenic acid (80 to 85 mg)[5]	High oleic safflower, soy, and coconut oils (41:30:28); DHA[4] (0.15%), ARA[4] (0.4%)	Vegetable oils (palm olein, soy, coconut, and high oleic safflower or sunflower oils), DHA[4] (0.32%), ARA[4] (0.64%), linoleic acid (920 mg), linolenic acid (85 mg), soy lecithin
Osmolality mOsm/kg H2O	170 to 200[6]	200	180
Osmolarity mOsm/L	153 to 180[7]	155	156
Sodium mEq/L (mg/L)	(240)	12.9 (298)	(271)
Potassium mEq/L (mg/L)	(800)	18.7 (730)	(785)
Chloride mEq/L (mg/L)	(533)	11.8 (419)	(473)
Calcium mEq (mg/L)	(700)	35.4 (710)	(710)
Phosphorus mEq/L (mg/L)	(460)	32.9 (507)	(426)
Iron mg/L	12	12.2	12.1
% free water	89	90	90
Manufacturer	Mead Johnson	Abbott	Gerber
Special information	Gluten-free, lactose-free, galactose-free		Kosher, Halal

[1]Information based on manufacturer's literature as of 2013 and is subject to change

[2]To approximate values for the content of a 24-, 27-, or 30-cal/oz formula (made by dilution of a powder-based formulation), multiply the value desired, found in the above 20-cal/oz formula, by the following factors: 1.2 (24-cal/oz), 1.35 (27-cal/oz), or 1.5 (30-cal/oz).

[3]Prebiotic

[4]DHA (docosahexaenoic acid) and ARA (arachidonic acid) are fatty acids found naturally in breast milk. DHA is provided via *Crypthecodinium cohnii* oil. ARA is provided via *Mortienella alphia* oil.

[5]Amount of linolenic acid varies depending on product and size: 80 mg in the powder, 8 and 13 fl oz concentrates, and 2 and 8 fl oz ready-to-feed; 85 mg in the 6 and 32 fl oz ready-to-feed

[6]Osmolality varies depending on product and size: 170 mOsm/kg H2O for the 8 and 13 fl oz concentrates and the 6, 8, and 32 fl oz ready-to-feed; 180 mOsm/kg H2O for the powder; 190 mOsm/kg H2O for the 2 fl oz ready-to-feed

[7]Osmolarity varies depending on product and size: 153 mOsm/L for the 6 and 32 fl oz ready-to-feed; 155 mOsm/L for the 8 and 13 fl oz concentrates and the 8 fl oz ready-to-feed; 162 mOsm/L for the powder; 180 mOsm/L for the 2 fl oz ready-to-feed

Infant Elemental Enteral Formulas[1]

	EleCare DHA/ARA[2,3] (20 kcal/oz)	Neocate Infant DHA & ARA[2,3] (20 kcal/oz)	Neocate Nutra[4]	PurAmino
Calories/mL	0.68	0.67	4.7/g	0.68
Carbohydrate g/100 mL	7.2	7.8	67.4/100 g	6.9
Carbohydrate source	Corn syrup solids	Corn syrup solids		Corn syrup solids
Protein g/100 mL	2.09	2.1	8.2/100 g	1.87
Protein source	Free amino acids	Free L-amino acids	Free L-amino acids	Free L-amino acids
Fat g/100 mL	3.24	3	18.8/100 g	3.53
Fat source (essential fatty acid amounts are per 100 kcal)	High oleic safflower, MCT, and soy oils (39:33:28)	33% MCT (palm kernel/ coconut), high oleic sunflower, and soy oils; DHA and ARA[2]	4% MCT refined vegetable oils (fractionated coconut, high oleic sunflower, canola, and sunflower oils)	Vegetable oil (palm olein, coconut, soy, and high oleic sunflower oils), DHA and ARA[2], linoleic acid (860 mg)
Osmolality mOsm/kg	350 unflavored	375		350
Osmolarity mOsm/L	187			320
Sodium mEq/L (mg/L)	13.5 (304)	(250)	(38/100 g)	(313)
Potassium mEq/L (mg/L)	26.4 (1014)	(1033)	(<20/100 g)	(734)
Chloride mEq/L (mg/L)	11.5 (405)	(517)	(44/100 g)	(574)
Calcium mEq/L (mg/L)	39.2 (784)	(831)	(667/100 g)	(627)
Phosphorus mg/L	548	624	(340/100 g)	347
Iron mg/L	9.9	12.4	5.9/100 g	12
% Free water	90			89
Manufacturer	Abbott	Nutricia	Nutricia	Mead Johnson

[1]Information based on manufacturer's literature as of 2013 and is subject to change

[2]DHA (docosahexaenoic acid) and ARA (arachidonic acid) are fatty acids which are found naturally in breast milk. DHA is provided via *Crypthecodinium cohnii* oil. ARA is provided via *Mortienella alphia* oil.

[3]Indicated for 0 to 12 month olds

[4]First and only amino acid-based semi-solid medical food

OLDER INFANT/TODDLER PRODUCTS

Older Infant/Toddler Milk-Based Formulas[1]

	Enfagrow Premium Next Step[2]	Enfagrow Gentlease Next Step[3]	Similac Go & Grow Milk-Based formula	Gerber Graduates Gentle	Gerber Graduates Protect[4]
Calories /100 mL	67	67	65	68	68
Protein g/100 mL	1.73	1.73	1.95	1.47	1.47
Protein source	Nonfat milk	Partially hydrolyzed nonfat milk and whey protein concentrate solids (soy)	Nonfat milk, lactose	100% whey protein concentrate (milk)	100% whey protein concentrate (milk)
Carbohydrate g/100 mL	7	7	6.6	7.73	7.47
Carbohydrate source	Corn syrup solids, lactose, galactooligosaccharides[5], polydextrose[5]	Corn syrup solids, galactooligosaccharides[5], polydextrose[5]	Lactose, galactooligosaccharides[5]	Lactose, maltodextrin (70:30), and galactooligosaccharides[5] (4 g/L)	Lactose and maltodextrin (70:30)
Fat g/100 mL	3.54	3.5	3.5	3.4	3.4
Fat source	Vegetable oils (palm olein, soy, coconut, and high oleic sunflower oils), DHA[6] (17 mg), ARA[6] (34 mg), linoleic acid (860 mg), linolenic acid (85 mg)	Vegetable oils (palm olein, soy, coconut, and high oleic sunflower oils), DHA[6] (17 mg), ARA[6] (34 mg), linoleic acid (860 mg), linolenic acid (85 mg)	High oleic safflower, soy, and coconut oil; DHA and ARA[6]	Palm olein, soy, coconut, and high oleic safflower or sunflower oils; DHA[6] (0.32%); ARA[6] (0.64%); linoleic acid (900 mg); linolenic acid (85 mg); soy lecithin	Palm olein, soy, coconut, and high oleic safflower or sunflower oils; DHA[6] (0.32%); ARA[6] (0.64%); linoleic acid (900 mg); linolenic acid (85 mg); soy lecithin
Osmolality mOsm/kg H_2O	270	230	300	180	250
Osmolarity mOsm/L	240	210	135	148	148
Sodium mEq/L (mg/L)	(240)	(267)	(195)	(180)	(180)
Potassium mEq/L (mg/L)	(867)	(867)	(975)	(720)	(720)
Chloride mEq/L (mg/L)	(534)	(534)	(520)	(434)	(434)
Calcium mEq/L (mg/L)	(1301)	(1301)	(1268)	(1267)	(1267)
Phosphorus mEq/L (mg/L)	(867)	(867)	(845)	(707)	(707)
Iron mg/L	13.3	13.3	13.5	13.3	13.3
% free water	89	89	90	89	89
Manufacturer	Mead Johnson	Mead Johnson	Abbott	Gerber	Gerber
Special information	Gluten-free	Gluten-free	Gluten-free, Kosher, Halal		
Special uses	Infants and toddlers 9 to 36 months	Infants 9 to 36 months	Infants and toddlers 9 to 24 months; specifically formulated to help bridge nutritional gaps that can be associated with transition to table foods.	Infants 9 to 24 months	Infants 9 to 24 months

[1]Information based on manufacturer's literature as of 2013 and is subject to change

[2]Also available as Enfagrow Premium Older Toddler for 12 to 36 months in either vanilla or natural milk flavor. Contains polydextrose + galactooligosaccharides – Natural Defense Dual Prebiotics from Mead Johnson. They support the growth of healthy gut bacteria which help support immune function.

[3]Contains ⅛ the lactose of other milk-based infant/toddler formulas. Contains polydextrose + galactooligosaccharides – Natural Defense Dual Prebiotics from Mead Johnson. They support the growth of healthy gut bacteria which help support immune function.

[4]Contains Bifidus BL, beneficial cultures like those found in breast milk to help support a healthy immune system

[5]Prebiotic

[6]DHA (docosahexaenoic acid) and ARA (arachidonic acid) are fatty acids found naturally in breast milk. DHA is provided via *Crypthecodinium cohnii* oil. ARA is provided via *Mortierella alpina* oil.

Older Infant/Toddler Soy Formulas[1,2]

Indications: Lactase deficiency, milk intolerance, or galactosemia

	Enfagrow Soy Next Step[3]	Gerber Graduates Soy[4]	Similac Go & Grow Soy-Based formula[4]
Calories /100 mL	67	68	68
Protein g/100 mL	2.2	1.87	1.89
Protein source	Soy protein isolate, L-methionine, taurine	Enzymatically hydrolyzed soy protein isolate, L-methionine, taurine	Soy protein isolate, L-methionine, taurine
Carbohydrate g/100 mL	7.87	7.3	6.96
Carbohydrate source	Corn syrup solids	Corn maltodextrin, sucrose (79:21)	Corn syrup solids, sugar, fructooligosaccharides[5]
Fat g/100 mL	2.93	3.3	3.7
Fat source	Vegetable oils (palm olein, soy, coconut, and high oleic sunflower oils), DHA[6] (17 mg), ARA[6] (34 mg), linoleic acid (720 mg), linolenic acid (70 mg)	Vegetable oils (palm olein, soy, coconut, and high oleic sunflower oils), DHA[6], ARA[6] (46:26:20:6:2), linoleic acid (920 mg), soy lecithin	High oleic safflower, soy, and coconut oils; DHA[6]; ARA[6]
Osmolality mOsm/kg H_2O	230	180	200
Osmolarity mOsm/L	200	156	160
Sodium mEq/L (mg/L)	(240)	(269)	12.9 (298)
Potassium mEq/L (mg/L)	(800)	(774)	(811)
Chloride mEq/L (mg/L)	(534)	(474)	11.8 (419)
Calcium mEq/L (mg/L)	(1301)	(1267)	(1318)
Phosphorus mEq/L (mg/L)	56 (867)	(707)	(879)
Iron mg/L	13.3	13.3	13.5
% free water	88	89	90
Manufacturer	Mead Johnson	Gerber	Abbott
Special information	Gluten-free, lactose-free, galactose-free	Lactose-free	

[1]Information based on manufacturer's literature as of 2013 and is subject to change

[2] To approximate values for the content of a 24-, 27-, or 30-cal/oz formula (made by dilution of a powder-based formulation), multiply the value desired, found in the above 20-cal/oz formula, by the following factors: 1.2 (24-cal/oz), 1.35 (27-cal/oz), or 1.5 (30-cal/oz)

[3]Indicated for infants and toddlers ≥9 months

[4]Indicated for infants and toddlers 9 to 24 months

[5]Prebiotic

[6]DHA (docosahexaenoic acid) and ARA (arachidonic acid) are fatty acids which are found naturally in breast milk. DHA is provided via *Crypthecodinium cohnii* oil. ARA is provided via *Mortienella alphia* oil.

Soy Formula[1] – Special Indications

Indications: Dietary management of diarrhea in infants >6 months and toddlers

	Similac Expert Care for Diarrhea
Calories /100 mL	68
Protein g/100 mL	1.8
Protein source	Soy protein isolate, L-methionine
Carbohydrate g/100 mL	6.83
Carbohydrate source	Corn syrup solids and sugar (60:40)
Fat g/100 mL	3.69
Fat source	Soy and coconut oils (60:40)
Osmolality mOsm/kg H_2O	240
Osmolarity mOsm/L	163
Sodium mEq/L (mg/L)	12.9 (298)
Potassium mEq/L (mg/L)	18.7 (730)
Chloride mEq/L (mg/L)	11.8 (419)
Calcium mEq/L (mg/L)	35.4 (710)
Phosphorus mEq/L (mg/L)	(507)
Iron mg/L	12.2
% free water	90
Manufacturer	Abbott
Special information	Lactose-free, gluten-free, Kosher, Halal

[1]Information based on manufacturer's literature as of 2013 and is subject to change

PEDIATRIC PRODUCTS

Pediatric Enteral Formulas[1]

A selection of the commonly used enteral feedings for children 1 to 13 years of age

	PediaSure Enteral Formula[2]	PediaSure Enteral Formula With Fiber[2]	Peptamen Junior[3-6]	Compleat Pediatric[4,6]	Compleat Pediatric Reduced Calorie[4,8]
Calories/oz	30	30	30	30	18
Calories/mL	1	1	1	1	0.6
Carbohydrate g/100 mL	13.9	14.3	13.6	13.2	7.5
Carbohydrate source	Corn maltodextrin, sugar	Corn maltodextrin, sugar	Maltodextrin, sugar, corn starch, guar gum, sucralose	Corn syrup, green pea, green bean puree, peach and cranberry juice, maltodextrin	Corn syrup, green pea, green bean, and peach puree; tomato, carrot, and cranberry juice
Protein g/100 mL	3	3	3	3.76	3
Protein source	Milk protein concentrate	Milk protein concentrate	Enzymatically hydrolyzed whey protein (milk)	Chicken, sodium caseinate, and pea puree	Chicken, sodium caseinate, and pea puree
Fat g/100 mL	3.8	3.8	3.8	3.9	2
Fat source	High oleic safflower, soy, and MCT oils; soy lecithin	High oleic safflower, soy, and MCT oils; soy lecithin	MCT (coconut and/or palm kernel), soybean, and canola oils; lecithin	Canola and MCT (coconut and/or palm kernel) oils; hydroxylated soy lecithin	Canola and MCT (coconut and/or palm kernel) oils; hydroxylated soy lecithin
Osmolality mOsm/kg	335 vanilla	350 vanilla	260 unflavored 380 vanilla/chocolate 400 strawberry	380	300
Osmolarity mOsm/L	278	278	255		
Sodium mEq/L (mg/L)	17 (380)	17 (380)	20 (460)	33 (760)	33.5 (770)
Potassium mEq/L (mg/L)	33 (1308)	34 (1310)	33.8 (1320)	42 (1640)	45.1 (1760)
Chloride mEq/L (mg/L)	32 (1139)	32 (1140)	30.4 (1080)	15.7 (560)	15.7 (560)
Calcium mEq/L (mg/L)	53 (1055)	53 (1055)	(1120)	(1440)	(1440)
Phosphorus mEq/L (mg/L)	(844)	(844)	(840)	(1000)	(1050)
Iron (mg/L)	11	11	14	14	13
% Free water	84	85	85	82	87
Fiber (g/unit dose)		Dietary: 0.8 scFOS: 2		Dietary: 1.7[9]	Dietary: 1.7[9]
Manufacturer	Abbott	Abbott	Nestle	Nestle	Nestle

Pediatric Enteral Formulas[1] continued

	PediaSure Enteral Formula[2]	PediaSure Enteral Formula With Fiber[2]	Peptamen Junior[3-6]	Compleat Pediatric[4,6]	Compleat Pediatric Reduced Calorie[4,8]
Indication			For patients with impaired GI function, short bowel syndrome, cerebral palsy, cystic fibrosis, Crohn's, malabsorption, chronic diarrhea, delayed gastric emptying, growth failure, transitioning from parenteral nutrition		For patients with decreased caloric needs
Special information	Gluten-free, lactose-free, Kosher, Halal (not for galactosemia)		Gluten-free, lactose-free (not Kosher)	Blenderized tube feeding formula containing real food; equivalent to 2 servings of fruits/vegetables for patients 1 to 4 years of age; equivalent to 1.6 servings of fruits/vegetables for patients >4 years of age; lactose-free, gluten-free (not for galactosemia)	Equivalent to 3 servings of fruits/vegetables for patients 1 to 4 years of age; equivalent to 2 servings of fruits/vegetables for patients >4 years of age

[1]Information based on manufacturer's literature as of 2013 and is subject to change

[2]Prebiotic Nutraflora scFOS (short chain fructooligosaccharides) provides fuel for beneficial bacteria in the digestive tract that help to support a healthy immune system.

[3]Also available with Prebio (3.6 g/L) prebiotic formulation

[4]Contains CalciLock blend of essential nutrients to help support healthy bone development

[5]Closed system with SpikeRight PLUS port, the first available proximal-end enteral connector system designed to be incompatible with I.V. equipment

[6]Meets or exceed 100% DRIs for protein and 25 key vitamins and minerals in 1000 mL for patients 1 to 8 years of age and in 1500 mL for patients 9 to 13 years of age

[7]1.7 oz dry packet mixed with 220 mL of water produces 250 mL of formula.

[8]Meets or exceed 100% DRIs for protein and 25 key vitamins and minerals in 1000 mL for patients 1 to 8 years of age and in 1200 mL for patients 9 to 13 years of age

[9]Nutrisource fiber is a soluble fiber (6.8 g/L), PHGG

Pediatric Enteral Formulas[1] (continued)

A selection of the commonly used enteral feedings for children 1 to 13 years of age

	Peptamen Junior with Fiber[2-4]	Nutren Junior[2,3,5]	Nutren Junior with Fiber[2-5]	Pediasure Peptide 1.0 Cal[3,6]
Calories/oz	30	30	30	30
Calories/mL	1	1	1	1
Carbohydrate g/100 mL	13.6	11	11	13.4
Carbohydrate source	Maltodextrin, sugar, corn starch, pea fiber, fructooligosaccharide[6,8], inulin	Maltodextrin, sugar	Maltodextrin, sugar, pea fiber, fructooligosaccharide[7], inulin	Corn maltodextrin
Protein g/100 mL	3	3	3	3
Protein source	Enzymatically hydrolyzed whey protein (milk)	Milk protein concentrate, 50% whey protein concentrate	Milk protein concentrate, 50% whey protein concentrate	Whey protein hydrolysate, hydrolyzed sodium caseinate
Fat g/100 mL	3.8	5	5	4.05
Fat source	MCT (coconut and/or palm kernel), soybean, and canola oils; soy lecithin	Soybean, canola, and MCT (coconut and/or palm kernel) oils; soy lecithin	Soybean, canola, and MCT (coconut and/or palm kernel) oils; soy lecithin	Structured lipid (interesterified canola and MCTs), MCTs, canola oils, soy lecithin
Osmolality mOsm/kg	390 vanilla	350 vanilla	350 vanilla	390 vanilla, strawberry 250 unflavored
Osmolarity mOsm/L	255	256	256	
Sodium mEq/L (mg/L)	20 (460)	20 (460)	20 (460)	31.2 (717)
Potassium mEq/L (mg/L)	33.8 (1320)	33.8 (1320)	33.8 (1320)	34.6 (1350)
Chloride mEq/L (mg/L)	30.4 (1080)	30.4 (1080)	30.4 (1080)	28.5 (1010)
Calcium mEq/L (mg/L)	(1120)	(1200)	(1200)	(1060)
Phosphorus mEq/L (mg/L)	(840)	(840)	(840)	(844)
Iron (mg/L)	14	14	14	14
% Free water	84	85	85	84.5
Fiber (g/unit dose)	Dietary 1.85 Soluble: 0.9 Insoluble: 0.95		Dietary 1.5 Soluble: 0.55 Insoluble: 0.95	Dietary: 0.7 scFOS: 0.7
Manufacturer	Nestle	Nestle	Nestle	Abbott
Special information	(not Kosher)	Gluten-free, lactose-free, Kosher	Gluten-free, lactose-free, Kosher	Gluten-free, lactose-free, Kosher

[1]Information based on manufacturer's literature as of 2013 and is subject to change
[2]Contains CalciLock blend of essential nutrients to help support healthy bone development
[3]Meets or exceed 100% DRIs for protein and 25 key vitamins and minerals in 1000 mL for patients 1 to 8 years of age and in 1500 mL for patients 9 to 13 years of age
[4]Contains Prebio, a soluble fiber (3.6 g/L) to help promote the growth of beneficial bacteria and 3.8 g/L insoluble fiber to help support normal bowel function
[5]Closed system with SpikeRight PLUS port, the first available proximal-end enteral connector system designed to be incompatible with I.V. equipment
[6]Prebiotic Nutraflora scFOS (short chain fructooligosaccharides) provides fuel for beneficial bacteria in the digestive tract that help to support a healthy immune system.
[7]Meets or exceed 100% DRIs for protein and 25 key vitamins and minerals in 667 mL (1000 kcal) for patients 1 to 8 years of age and in 1000 mL (1500 kcal) for patients 9 to 13 years of age
[8]Prebiotic
[9]Lipid blend provides 720 mg/L of EPA and DHA to help modulate pro-inflammatory mediators

Pediatric Elemental Enteral Formulas[1]

	EleCare Jr (30 kcal/oz)	Neocate Junior[2,3] (30 kcal/oz)	Vivonex Pediatric[4-7]
Calories/mL	1.01	1	0.8
Carbohydrate g/100 mL	10.7	10.4	13
Carbohydrate source	Corn syrup solids	Corn syrup solids	Maltodextrin, modified cornstarch
Protein g/100 mL	3.1	3.3	2.4
Protein source	Free amino acids	Free L-amino acids	100% free L-amino acids
Fat g/100 mL	4.91	5	2.3
Fat source (essential fatty acid amounts are per 100 kcal)	High oleic safflower, MCT, and soy oils (39:33:28)	35% MCT, refined vegetable oils (palm kernel and/or coconut, canola, and high oleic safflower oils)	MCT (coconut and/or palm kernel) and soybean oils
Osmolality mOm/kg	590 unflavored/vanilla	550 unflavored 630 tropical 650 chocolate/vanilla[3]	360
Osmolarity mOsm/L	280		
Sodium mEq/L (mg/L)	20 (459)	(500)	17 (400)
Potassium mEq/L (mg/L)	39 (1526)	(1370)	31 (1200)
Chloride mEq/L (mg/L)	17 (608)	(762)	28 (1000)
Calcium mEq/L (mg/L)	58.7 (1174)	(1180)	(1120)
Phosphorus mg/L	822	799	(840)
Iron mg/L	14.9	16	10
% free water	84		89
Manufacturer	Abbott	Nutricia	Nestle

[1]Information based on manufacturer's literature as of 2013 and is subject to change

[2]Indicated for 1- to 10-year-olds

[3]Also available in product containing prebiotics

[4]For patients with severe impaired GI function, transitioning from parenteral nutrition, severe short bowel syndrome, malabsorption syndrome, Crohn's, intestinal failure, status post-GI trauma/surgery, or burns; not for children <1 year of age; gluten-free, lactose-free, Kosher

[5]Contains CalciLock blend of essential nutrients to help support healthy bone development

[6]Meets or exceeds 100% DRIs for protein and 25 key vitamins and minerals in 1000 mL for patients 1 to 8 years of age and in 1500 mL for patients 9 to 13 years of age

[7]1.7 oz dry packet mixed with 220 mL of water produces 250 mL of formula

Pediatric High Caloric Density Enteral Formulas[1]

	Pediasure 1.5 Cal[2]	Pediasure 1.5 Cal With Fiber[2]	Peptamen Junior 1.5[2,4]	Pediasure Peptide 1.5 Cal[3,7]
Calories/mL	1.5	1.5	1.5	1.5
Carbohydrate g/100 mL	16	16.5	18	20.1
Carbohydrate source	Corn maltodextrin	Corn maltodextrin	Maltodextrin, cornstarch, fructooligosaccharide[3,5], inulin, guar gum	Corn maltodextrin
Protein g/100 mL	5.9	5.9	4.5	4.51
Protein source	Milk protein concentrate	Milk protein concentrate	Enzymatically, hydrolyzed whey protein (milk)	Whey protein hydrolysate, hydrolyzed sodium caseinate
Fat g/100 mL	6.8	6.8	6.8	6
Fat source	High oleic safflower, soy, and MCT oils; soy lecithin; DHA (from cohnii oil)	High oleic safflower, soy, and MCT oils; soy lecithin; DHA (from cohnii oil)	60% MCT (coconut and/or palm kernel), soybean, and canola oils; soy lecithin[6]	Structured lipid (interesterified canola and MCTs), MCTs, canola oils, soy lecithin
Osmolality mOsm/kg	370 vanilla	390 vanilla	450 unflavored	450 vanilla
Osmolarity mOsm/L	278	278	385	
Sodium mEq/L (mg/L)	16.5 (380)	16.5 (380)	30 (692)	46.7 (1075)
Potassium mEq/L (mg/L)	42 (1650)	42 (1650)	50.8 (1980)	51.9 (2025)
Chloride mEq/L (mg/L)	32 (1140)	32 (1140)	45.6 (1620)	42.8 (1520)
Calcium mEq/L (mg/L)	74 (1480)	74 (1480)	(1650)	(1580)
Phosphorus mEq/L (mg/L)	(1055)	(1055)	(1352)	(1265)
Iron (mg/L)	11	11	21	21
% free water	78.1	78.1	77	76.8
Fiber (g/unit dose)	Dietary: 3 scFOS: 1.5[3]	Dietary: 3 scFOS: 1.5[3]	Soluble: 1.34	Dietary: 1.1 scFOS: 1.1[3]
Manufacturer	Abbott	Abbott	Nestle	Abbott
Special uses/ information	For patients 1 to 13 years of age Gluten-free, lactose-free, Kosher, Halal	For patients 1 to 13 years of age Gluten-free, lactose-free, Kosher, Halal	For patients who need volume/fluid restriction with impaired GI function, short bowel syndrome, cerebral palsy, cystic fibrosis, Crohn's, malabsorption, chronic diarrhea, growth failure, transitioning from parenteral nutrition, critical illness/trauma, transplant	

[1] Information based on manufacturer's literature as of 2013 and is subject to change

[2] Meets or exceeds 100% DRIs for protein and 25 key vitamins and minerals in 1000 mL for patients 1 to 8 years of age and in 1500 mL for patients 9 to 13 years of age

[3] Prebiotic Nutraflora scFOS (short chain fructooligosaccharides) provides fuel for beneficial bacteria in the digestive tract that helps to support a healthy immune system.

[4] Contains CalciLock blend of essential nutrients to help support healthy bone development

[5] Prebiotic

[6] Lipid blend provides 720 mg/L of EPA and DHA to help modulate pro-inflammatory mediators

[7] Meets or exceeds 100% DRIs for protein and 25 key vitamins and minerals in 667 mL (1000 kcal) for patients 1 to 8 years of age and in 1000 mL (1500 kcal) for patients 9 to 13 years of age

Pediatric Nutritionally Complete Drinks[1]

A selection of the commonly used supplemental drinks

	Boost Kid Essentials[2,3]	Boost Kid Essentials 1.5[2,4]	Boost Kid Essentials 1.5 with Fiber[2,4]	Resource Breeze	Carnation Breakfast Essentials (ready-to-drink)	Carnation Breakfast Essentials[5] (powder)	PediaSure	PediaSure with Fiber	PediaSure SideKicks	PediaSure Sidekicks Clear	EO28 Splash
Calories/oz	30	45	45	30	24	24	30	30	18.9	17.6	30
Calories/mL	1	1.5	1.5	1.06	0.8	0.8	1	1	0.63	0.6	1
Carbohydrate g/100 mL	13.4	16.4	16.4	22.8	10.3	3.9	13.9	13.9	8.9	12	14.6
Carbohydrate source	Maltodextrin, sugar	Maltodextrin, sugar	Maltodextrin, sugar	Sugar, corn syrup, maltodextrin	Sugar, maltodextrin, sucralose	Sugar, maltodextrin, lactose	Sucrose and corn maltodextrin	Sucrose and corn maltodextrin	Sugar	Corn maltodextrin, sugar	Maltodextrin and sugar
Protein g/100 mL	2.8	4.2	4.2	3.8	3.5	13	3	3	3	3	2.5
Protein source	Sodium and calcium caseinates, whey protein concentrate	Sodium and calcium caseinates, whey protein concentrate	Sodium and calcium caseinates, whey protein concentrate	Whey protein isolate (milk)	Calcium caseinate	Nonfat milk	Milk protein concentrate, whey protein concentrate, soy protein isolate	Milk protein concentrate and soy protein isolate	Milk protein concentrate, soy protein isolate, whey protein concentrate	Whey protein isolate	Free L-amino acids
Fat g/100 mL	3.8	7.6	7.6		1.5	0.5 g/serving	3.8	3.8	2.1		3.5
Fat source	High oleic sunflower, soybean, MCT (coconut and/or palm kernel), and soy oils; soy lecithin	MCT, soy, and sunflower oils, soy lecithin	Soybean, high oleic sunflower, MCT (coconut and/or palm kernel), soy, and sunflower oils; soy lecithin		Corn oil	Trace butterfat	High oleic safflower oil, canola oil	High oleic safflower oil, canola oil	Soy oil, soy lecithin		Fractionated coconut, canola, and high oleic sunflower oils
Osmolality mOsm/kg	550 vanilla 600 chocolate 570 strawberry	390 vanilla	405 vanilla	750 orange	480 classic French vanilla 490 chocolate splash		480 vanilla, strawberry, banana, berry 540 chocolate	480 vanilla	420 vanilla	325 tropical fruit, wild berry	820 grape, tropical fruit, and orange-pineapple
Osmolarity mOsm/L							278	278	278	278	
Sodium mEq/L (mg/L)	23.7 (546)	30.1 (693)	30.1 (693)	14.8 (338)	23.6 (545)	8.3/serving (190/serving)	17 (380)	17 (380)	17 (380)	(175)	(200)
Potassium mEq/L (mg/L)	29 (1134)	33.3 (1302)	33.3 (1302)	0.4 (21.1)	25.8 (1000)	18 (700)	33 (1308)	33 (1308)	41.5 (1646)	(150)	(930)
Chloride mEq/L (mg/L)	15.4 (546)	21 (748)	21 (748)				32 (1139)	32 (1139)	32 (1139)		(350)
Calcium mEq/L (mg/L)	(1260)	(1470)	(1470)		(1515)	(500)	53 (1055)	53 (1055)	53 (1055)	(175)	(620)

Pediatric Nutritionally Complete Drinks[1] continued

	Boost Kid Essentials[2,3]	Boost Kid Essentials 1.5[2,4]	Boost Kid Essentials 1.5 with Fiber[2,4]	Resource Breeze	Carnation Breakfast Essentials (ready-to-drink)	Carnation Breakfast Essentials[5] (powder)	PediaSure	PediaSure with Fiber	PediaSure SideKicks	PediaSure SideKicks Clear	EO28 Splash
Phosphorus mEq/L (mg/L)	(882)	(1260)	(1260)	(633)	(1515)	(500)	(844)	(844)	(844)	(750)	(620)
Iron (mg/L)	13.9	13.9	13.9	11.4	13.6		11	11	11	9	7.7
% Free water	84	72	71	83	86		84	84	89.5	90	80
Fiber (g/unit dose)			Dietary: 2.1 Insoluble: 0.5			Dietary: <1/ serving	Dietary: 1 scFOS: 1[6]	Dietary: 3 scFOS: 1.8[6]	Dietary: 3 scFOS: 2.4[6]		
Indication	1 to 13 years old	1 to 13 years old	1 to 13 years old			Reduced calorie	1 to 13 years old	1 to 13 years old	All the nutrition of Pediasure with less calories and less fat than Pediasure	For supplemental use in 1- to 3-year-olds only; no more than 1 serving per day	>1 year old; nutritionally complete, ready-to-drink amino acid-based
Manufacturer	Nestle	Nestle	Nestle	Nestle	Nestle	Nestle	Abbott	Abbott	Abbott	Abbott	Nutricia
Special information	Gluten-free, lactose-free, Kosher	Gluten-free, lactose-free, Kosher		Fruit-flavored, clear liquid; gluten-free, lactose-free, Kosher, Halal (all flavors)	Available in sugar-free form; Kosher; cholesterol-restricted	Available in sugar-free form; Kosher; cholesterol-restricted	Gluten-free, lactose-free, Kosher, contains DHA (from tuna oil) of 32 mg per 8 fl oz			Suitable for clear liquid diet and fat-restricted diet	

[1]Information based on manufacturer's literature as of 2013 and is subject to change

[2]Contains CalciLock blend of essential nutrients to help support healthy bone development

[3]Meets or exceed 100% DRIs for protein and 25 key vitamins and minerals in 1000 mL for patients 1 to 8 years of age and in 1500 mL for patients 9 to 13 years of age

[4]Meets or exceed 100% DRIs for protein and 25 key vitamins and minerals in 750 mL for patients 1 to 8 years of age and in 1000 mL for patients 9 to 13 years of age

[5]One envelope (6 level tablespoons) added to 8 oz of fat-free milk; mix with soy or lactose-reduced milk for decreased lactose content

[6]Prebiotic Nutraflora scFOS (short chain fructooligosaccharides) provides fuel for beneficial bacteria in the digestive tract that help to support a healthy immune system.

ADOLESCENT/ADULT PRODUCTS

Adolescent and Adult Enteral Formulas[1]

	Osmolite 1 Cal	Jevity	Nutren 1[2]	Ensure	Boost[3]
Calories/mL	1.06	1.06	1	1.05	1
Carbohydrate g/100 mL	14.4	15.5	12.8	16.9	17.1
Carbohydrate source	Corn maltodextrin, corn syrup solids	Corn maltodextrin, corn syrup solids, soy fiber	Maltodextrin, sugar	Sugar, corn maltodextrin	Corn syrup solids, sugar
Protein g/100 mL	4.43	4.43	4	3.8	4.2
Protein source	Sodium and calcium caseinate, soy protein isolate	Sodium and calcium caseinates, soy protein isolate	Calcium-potassium caseinate (milk)	Milk protein concentrate and soy protein concentrate	Milk protein concentrate, soy protein isolate
Fat g/100 mL	3.47	3.47	3.8	2.5	1.7
Fat source	Canola, corn, and MCT oils, and soy lecithin	Canola, corn, and MCT oils, and soy lecithin	Canola, MCT (coconut and/or palm kernel), and corn oils; soy lecithin	Soy, canola, and corn oils, soy lecithin	Vegetable oils (canola, high oleic sunflower, and corn); soy lecithin
Osmolality mOsm/kg H₂O	300 unflavored	300 unflavored	370 vanilla	620 strawberry, vanilla, butter pecan 640 creamy milk chocolate, rich dark chocolate	625 vanilla, chocolate, or strawberry
Osmolarity mOsm/L	374	370	370	329	
Sodium mEq/L (mg/L)	40.4 (930)	40.4 (930)	38 (880)	36.7 (844)	27.1 (625)
Potassium mEq/L (mg/L)	40.2 (1570)	40.2 (1570)	31.7 (1240)	40 (1561)	49.2 (1917)
Chloride mEq/L (mg/L)	40.7 (1440)	37 (1310)	33.8 (1200)	33.3 (1181)	31.7 (1133)
Calcium mEq/L (mg/L)	(760)	(910)	(668)	(1266)	(1250)
Phosphorus mEq/L (mg/L)	(760)	(760)	(668)	(1055)	(1250)
Iron (mg/L)	14	14	12	19	18.8
% free water	84	84	85	83	85
Fiber (g/unit dose)		Dietary: 1.4/100 mL	Also available with fiber[4]		
Manufacturer	Abbott	Abbott	Nestle	Abbott	Nestle
Special uses	Low residue, isotonic formula	Isotonic formula with fiber	Normal protein/normal calorie requirements	Supplement; for interim sole-source feeding	Nutritionally complete drink
Special information		Gluten-free, lactose-free, Kosher	Gluten-free, lactose-free, Kosher		Gluten-free, lactose-free, Kosher (not for galactosemia)

[1]Information based on manufacturer's literature as of 2013 and is subject to change

[2]Also available with fiber with Prebio (prebiotics)

[3]Contains CalciLock blend of essential nutrients to help support healthy bone development

[4]Prebio is a fiber blend to help promote healthy microbiota and contains 3.5 g of dietary fiber with 1.3 g of soluble fiber and 2.2 g of insoluble fiber.

Adolescent and Adult Elemental Enteral Formulas With Modified Protein[1]

	Peptamen	Peptamen 1.5[2]	Tolerex[3] (powder)	Vivonex Plus[4] (powder)	Vivonex RFT[2]	Vivonex T.E.N.[5] (powder)	Vital 1.0 Cal[6]	Vital 1.5 Cal[6]
Calories/mL	1	1.5	1	1	1	1	1	1.5
Carbohydrate g/100 mL	12.8	18.4	22.6	18.8	17.6	20.4	13	18.7
Carbohydrate source	Maltodextrin, cornstarch, guar gum	Maltodextrin, cornstarch, guar gum	Maltodextrin, modified corn starch	Maltodextrin (corn), modified cornstarch	Maltodextrin, modified corn starch	Maltodextrin (corn), modified cornstarch	Maltodextrin, sugar, scFOS[5], sucralose	Maltodextrin, sugar, scFOS[5], sucralose
Protein g/100 mL	4	6.8	2.1	4.5	5	3.8	4	6.75
Protein source	Enzymatically hydrolyzed whey (milk)	Enzymatically hydrolyzed whey (milk)	Free L-amino acids	Free L-amino acids (30% from branched chain amino acids)	Free L-amino acids (29% from branched chain amino acids)	Free L-amino acids	Whey protein hydrolysate, partially hydrolyzed sodium caseinate	Whey protein hydrolysate, partially hydrolyzed sodium caseinate
Fat g/100 mL	3.9	5.6	0.2	0.66	1.2	0.26	3.8	5.71
Fat source	70% MCT (coconut and/or palm kernel) and soybean oils; soy lecithin	70% MCT (coconut and/or palm kernel) and soybean oils; soy lecithin	Safflower oil	Soybean oil	Soybean oil	Safflower oil	Structured lipid (interesterified canola oil and MCT), canola oil, and MCT	Structured lipid (interesterified canola oil and MCT), canola oil, and MCT
Osmolality mOsm/kg	270 unflavored 380 vanilla	550 unflavored, vanilla	550 unflavored	650	630 unflavored	630 unflavored	390 vanilla	610 vanilla
Osmolarity mOsm/L							340	544
Sodium mEq/L (mg/L)	24.3 (560)	44.3 (1020)	22 (500)	26 (605)	30.4 (700)	26 (610)	(1055)	(1500)
Potassium mEq/L (mg/L)	38.5 (1500)	48 (1860)	30 (1167)	25 (969)	31 (1200)	23 (928)	(1400)	(2000)
Chloride mEq/L (mg/L)	28.2 (1000)	49 (1740)	26 (935)	26 (933)	23 (800)	24 (841)	(1055)	(1500)
Calcium mEq/L (mg/L)	(800)	(1000)	(550)	(550)	(668)	(500)	(705)	(1000)
Phosphorus mg/L	(700)	(1000)	(551)	(550)	(668)	(500)	(705)	(1000)
Fiber g/unit dose							Dietary: 1 scFOS: 1[6]	Dietary: 1 scFOS: 1[6]
Iron mg/L	18	27	10	10	12	9	13	18
% Free water	85	77	84	83	85	83	84.2	76.4
Manufacturer	Nestle	Nestle	Nestle	Nestle	Nestle	Nestle	Abbott	Abbott

Adolescent and Adult Elemental Enteral Formulas With Modified Protein[1] *continued*

	Peptamen	Peptamen 1.5[2]	Tolerex[3] (powder)	Vivonex Plus[4] (powder)	Vivonex RFT[2]	Vivonex T.E.N.[5] (powder)	Vital 1.0 Cal[6]	Vital 1.5 Cal[6]
Indication	For patients with impaired GI function related to: Malabsorption, pancreatitis, short bowel syndrome, chronic diarrhea, cystic fibrosis, delayed gastric emptying, cerebral palsy, Crohn's disease/IBD, malabsorption related to cancer treatment, malnutrition, and Celiac disease with malabsorption; also for early enteral feeding and transition from or dual feeding with parenteral nutrition	For patients with impaired GI function related to: Malabsorption, pancreatitis, short bowel syndrome, chronic diarrhea, cystic fibrosis, delayed gastric emptying, cerebral palsy, Crohn's disease/IBD, malabsorption related to cancer treatment; also for early enteral feeding, transition from parenteral nutrition, shortened feeding schedules, elevated protein requirements, and fluid/volume restrictions	For patients with severely impaired GI function related to: Severe protein and fat malabsorption and specialized nutrient needs	Provides nutrition to patients with severely impaired GI function, severe protein and fat malabsorption, extensive bowel resection, malabsorption syndrome, select trauma/surgery, intestinal failure, chylothorax, and pancreatitis; also for parenteral nutrition alternative, dual feeding with parenteral nutrition, transitional feeding, early postoperative feeding, and trophic feeding	Provides nutrition to patients with severely impaired GI function, severe protein and fat malabsorption, extensive bowel resection, malabsorption syndrome, select trauma/surgery, intestinal failure, chylothorax, and pancreatitis; also for parenteral nutrition alternative, dual feeding with parenteral nutrition, transitional feeding, early postoperative feeding, and trophic feeding	Provides nutrition to patients with severely impaired GI function, severe protein and fat malabsorption, extensive bowel resection, malabsorption syndrome, select trauma/surgery, intestinal failure, chylothorax, and pancreatitis; also for parenteral nutrition alternative, dual feeding with parenteral nutrition, transitional feeding, early postoperative feeding, and trophic feeding	Peptide-based elemental formula for malabsorption, maldigestion, or impaired GI function or for symptoms of GI intolerance	Peptide-based elemental formula for malabsorption, maldigestion, or impaired GI function or for symptoms of GI intolerance
Special information	Gluten-free, lactose-free, low residue (not for galactosemia)	Gluten-free, lactose-free, low residue (not for galactosemia)	100% free amino acids with only 2% of calories from fat Gluten-free, lactose-free, Kosher (not for galactosemia)	Gluten-free, lactose-free, low residue, Kosher	Gluten-free, lactose-free, low residue, Kosher (not for galactosemia)	Gluten-free, lactose-free, low-residue, Kosher	Gluten-free, lactose-free, low-residue	Gluten-free, lactose-free, low-residue

[1]Information based on manufacturer's literature as of 2013 and is subject to change

[2]Closed system with SpikeRight PLUS port, the first available proximal-end enteral connector system designed to be incompatible with I.V. equipment

[3]2.82 oz dry packet mixed with 255 mL of water produces 300 mL of formula

[4]2.8 oz dry packet mixed with 250 mL of water produces 300 mL of formula; not for children 0 to 3 years of age

[5]2.84 oz dry packet mixed with 250 mL of water produces 300 mL of formula

[6]Prebiotic Nutraflora scFOS (short chain fructooligosaccharides) provide fuel for beneficial bacteria in the digestive tract that help to support a healthy immune system

Adolescent and Adult High Caloric Density Enteral Formulas[1]

	Ensure Plus	Osmolite 1.2 Cal	Osmolite 1.5 Cal	Nutren 1.5[2]	Nutren 2[2]	Jevity 1.2 Cal	Jevity 1.5 Cal	Isosource 1.5 Cal[2]	Hi-Cal
Calories/mL	1.5	1.2	1.5	1.5	2	1.2	1.5	1.5	2
Carbohydrate g/100 mL	21.5	15.8	20.4	16.8	19.6	16.9	21.6	16.8	21.6
Carbohydrate source	Corn, maltodextrin, sugar, scFOS[3]	Corn, maltodextrin	Corn, maltodextrin	Maltodextrin	Corn syrup solids, maltodextrin, sugar	Corn, maltodextrin, corn syrup solids, fructooligosaccharides, soy fiber, and oat fiber	Corn, maltodextrin, corn syrup solids, fructooligosaccharides, soy fiber, and oat fiber	Maltodextrin, sugar, soy fiber, and partially hydrolyzed guar gum	Corn syrup solids, sugar, corn maltodextrin
Protein g/100 mL	5.5	5.55	6.27	6	8	5.6	6.4	6.8	8.4
Protein source	Milk protein, caseinate, soy protein concentrate, whey protein concentrate	Sodium and calcium caseinates	Sodium and calcium caseinates, soy protein isolate	Calcium-potassium caseinate (milk)	Calcium-potassium caseinate (milk)	Sodium and calcium caseinates, soy protein isolate	Sodium and calcium caseinates, soy protein isolate	Sodium and calcium caseinates (milk)	Sodium and calcium caseinates
Fat g/100 mL	4.6	3.93	4.91	6.8	10.4	3.9	5	6.5	8.9
Fat source	Canola, and corn oils; soy lecithin	High oleic safflower, canola, and MCT oils; soy lecithin	High oleic safflower, canola, and MCT oils; soy lecithin	50% MCT (coconut and/or palm kernel), canola, and corn oils; soy lecithin	75% MCT (coconut and/or palm kernel), canola, and corn oils; soy lecithin	Canola, corn, and MCT oils; soy lecithin	Canola, corn, and MCT oils; soy lecithin	Canola, MCT (coconut and/or palm kernel), and soy oils; hydroxylated soy lecithin	Corn oil and soy lecithin
Osmolality mOsm/kg	680 vanilla, strawberry, butter pecan, milk chocolate	360 unflavored	525 unflavored	430 unflavored 510 vanilla	745 vanilla	450 unflavored	525 unflavored	650 unflavored 585 vanilla	705 vanilla
Osmolarity mOsm/L		465	512			465	518		
Sodium mEqL (mg/L)	40.5 (928)	58.3 (1340)	60.9 (1400)	50.4 (1160)	56.5 (1300)	58.7 (1350)	60.9 (1400)	56.5 (1300)	63 (1456)
Potassium mEqL (mg/L)	45 (1772)	46.4 (1810)	46 (1800)	48.2 (1880)	49.2 (1920)	47.3 (1850)	55.1 (2150)	55 (2140)	62 (2447)
Chloride mEqL (mg/L)	32 (1139)	43.5 (1540)	48 (1700)	49 (1740)	52.8 (1876)	42.4 (1500)	38.4 (1360)	45 (1610)	40.5 (1435)
Calcium mEqL (mg/L)	(1266)	(1200)	(1000)	(1000)	(1340)	(1200)	(1200)	(1072)	(844)
Phosphorus mEqL (mg/L)	(1266)	(1200)	(1000)	(1000)	(1340)	(1200)	(1200)	(1020)	(844)
Iron (mg/L)	19	18	18	18	24	18	18	19	15.2
% free water	75.9	82	76.2	76	70	80.7	76	78	70

Adolescent and Adult High Caloric Density Enteral Formulas[1] continued

	Ensure Plus	Osmolite 1.2 Cal	Osmolite 1.5 Cal	Nutren 1.5[2]	Nutren 2[2]	Jevity 1.2 Cal	Jevity 1.5 Cal	Isosource 1.5 Cal[2]	Hi-Cal
Fiber (g/unit dose)	Dietary: 3 scFOS: 3[3]					Dietary: 1.8 scFOS: 8[3]	Dietary: 2.2 scFOS: 1[3]	Dietary: 2/can[4] Soluble: 1.1/can Insoluble: 0.9/can	
Manufacturer	Abbott	Abbott	Abbott	Nestle	Nestle	Abbott	Abbott	Nestle	Abbott
Special uses/ information	For those with fluid restrictions or require volume-limited feedings; supplement; for interim sole-source feeding	Increased calories, increased protein, decreased residue	Increased calories, increased protein, decreased residue	Increased calories Gluten-free, lactose-free, Kosher	Calorically dense Gluten-free, lactose-free, Kosher	Increased protein with fiber Gluten-free, lactose-free, Kosher, Halal	Increased protein with fiber Gluten-free, lactose-free, Kosher, Halal	High calorie, high nitrogen formula with fiber Gluten-free, lactose-free, Kosher	Increased calories fortified with vitamins and minerals

[1]Information based on manufacturer's literature as of 2013 and is subject to change

[2]Closed system with SpikeRight PLUS port, the first available proximal-end enteral connector system designed to be incompatible with I.V. equipment

[3]Prebiotic Nutraflora scFOS (short chain fructooligosaccharides) provides fuel for beneficial bacteria in the digestive tract that helps to support a healthy immune system.

[4]NUTRISOURCE FIBER (soy)

SPECIALTY PRODUCTS

Casein Hydrolysate Formulas[1,2]

Indication: For infants predisposed to or being treated for hypocalcemia due to hyperphosphatemia whose renal or cardiovascular functions would benefit from lowered mineral concentrations

	Similac PM 60/40
Calories /100 mL	68
Protein g/100 mL	1.5
Protein source	Whey protein caseinate, sodium caseinate
Carbohydrate g/100 mL	6.9
Carbohydrate source	Lactose
Fat g/100 mL	3.79
Fat source	High oleic safflower, soy, coconut oils (41:30:29)
Osmolality mOsm/kg H_2O	280
Osmolarity mOsm/L	124
Sodium mEq/L (mg/L)	7.1 (162)
Potassium mEq/L (mg/L)	13.8 (541)
Chloride mEq/L (mg/L)	11.3 (399)
Calcium mEq/L (mg/L)	18.9 (379)
Phosphorus mEq/L (mg/L)	(189)
Iron mg/L	4.7
% free water	90
Manufacturer	Abbott
Special information	Gluten-free, Kosher, Halal
Special uses	Renal and cardiovascular disease

[1]Information based on manufacturer's literature as of 2013 and is subject to change

Nutrition for the Ketogenic Diet[1]

Indications: Dietary management of intractable epilepsy, pyruvate dehydrogenase deficiency, glucose transport type-1 deficiency

	KetoCal 3:1[2,3]	KetoCal 4:1[2,4]	KetoCal 4:1 LQ[2,5]
Calories /mL	1	1.44	1.5
Protein g/100 mL	2.2	3	3.1
Protein source	Milk protein, L-cystine, L-tryptophan, taurine	Dry whole milk, L-isoleucine, L-tryptophan, taurine	Sodium caseinate (milk), L-cystine, L-tryptophan, whey protein concentrate (milk)
Carbohydrate g/100 mL	1	0.6	1.73
Carbohydrate source	Lactose	Corn syrup solids	Soy fiber, cornstartch, inulin
Fat g/100 mL	9.7	14.4	14.8
Fat source (essential fatty acid amounts are per 100 kcal)	Refined vegetable oil (palm and soy oils)	Hydrogenated soybean oil, refined soybean oil, soy lecithin	Refined vegetable oil (high oleic sunflower, soy, and palm oils), soy lecithin, DHA[6] (37 mg), ARA[6] (37 mg), linoleic acid (2152 mg), linolenic acid (209 mg)
Osmolality mOsm/kg H_2O	180	197	260 vanilla 280 unflavored
Sodium mEq/L (mg/L)	(411)	(600)	(1030)
Potassium mEq/L (mg/L)	(1290)	(2160)	(1650)
Chloride mEq/L (mg/L)	(629)	(1000)	(1550)
Calcium mEq/L (mg/L)	(1090)	(1600)	(884)
Phosphorus mEq/L (mg/L)	(730)	(1300)	(884)
Iron mg/L	16	22	15
% free water			77.8
Manufacturer	Nutricia	Nutricia	Nutricia
Special information		Recommend reconstitution ratio of 4 mL of water for each 1 g of powder	

[1]Information based on manufacturer's literature as of 2013 and is subject to change

[2]Ratio represents fats to carbohydrates plus protein

[3]For patients up to 8 years of age; powder formulation to initiate the ketogenic diet

[4]For patients >1 year of age; powder formulation

[5]For patients ≤13 years of age; ready-to-use formulation

[6]DHA (docosahexaenoic acid) and ARA (arachidonic acid) are fatty acids which are found naturally in breast milk. DHA is provided via *Crypthecodinium cohnii* oil. ARA is provided via *Mortienella alphia* oil.

Low Long Chain Fatty Acids Formulas[1]

	Portagen	Enfaport
Calories /100 mL	100	100
Protein g/100 mL	3.5	3.6
Protein source	Sodium caseinate	Calcium and sodium caseinates (milk)
Carbohydrate g/100 mL	11.5	10.3
Carbohydrate source	75% corn syrup solids and 25% sugar	Corn syrup solids
Fat g/100 mL	4.8	5.5
Fat source (essential fatty acid amounts are per 100 kcal)	87% MCT, 13% corn oils, soy lecithin	84% MCT and 13% soy oils, 3% DHA[2] (17 mg), ARA[2] (34 mg), linoleic acid (350 mg), linolenic acid (50 mg), soy lecithin
Osmolality mOsm/kg	350	280
Osmolarity mOsm/L	300	240
Sodium mEq/L (mg/L)	(552)	(300)
Potassium mEq/L (mg/L)	(1250)	(1170)
Chloride mEq/L (mg/L)	(865)	(880)
Calcium mEq/L (mg/L)	(938)	(950)
Phosphorus mEq/L (mg/L)	(708)	(530)
Iron mg/L	18.8	18.3
% free water	87	84
Manufacturer	Mead Johnson	Mead Johnson
Indication	For children and adults with defects in the intraluminal hydrolysis of fats (decreased bile salts, decreased pancreatic lipase); defective mucosal fat absorption (decreased mucosal permeability, decreased absorptive surface); and/or defective lymphatic transport of fat (ie, intestinal lymphatic obstruction); if used long-term, not nutritionally complete and will require supplementation of essential fatty acids and ultra trace minerals	Iron-fortified, milk-based infant formula with 84% of fat as MCT for infants with chylothorax or LCHAD deficiency (long chain 3-hydroxyacyl CoA dehydrogenase − inherited disorder of fat oxidation)
Special information	Gluten-free, lactose-free	Gluten-free, lactose-free, sucrose-free

[1]Information based on manufacturer's literature as of 2013 and is subject to change

[2]DHA (docosahexaenoic acid) and ARA (arachidonic acid) are fatty acids which are found naturally in breast milk. DHA is provided via *Crypthecodinium cohnii* oil. ARA is provided via *Mortienella alphia* oil.

NUTRITIONAL MODULARS

Nutritional Modulars – Carbohydrate and Protein Supplements[1]

	Polycose Powder	ProMod Liquid Protein[2,3]	Benecalorie (liquid)	Beneprotein (powder)	Liquid Protein Fortifier	Resource Benefiber	Duocal
Indication	Carbohydrate additive for use as a caloric supplement which is readily mixable in most foods, enteral formulas or beverages without appreciably altering their taste	Protein supplement which mixes readily in enteral formulas, most foods, or beverages without appreciably altering their taste; indicated for wounds, protein-energy malnutrition, involuntary weight loss, pre- and postsurgery anorexia, stress, trauma, cancer, burns	Calorie and protein supplement which mixes well into most foods and beverages	Protein supplement; 100% high quality whey proteins; mixes instantly in a variety of foods/beverages without compromising taste or texture	Protein supplement for preterm infants; peptides and amino acids for easy digestion and absorption; for use with breast milk or infant formula	For dietary management of occasional constipation; mixes instantly in a variety of foods/beverages without compromising taste or texture	To increase calories by adding to food and beverages; contains no protein; neutral flavor
Calories	3.8/g[4]	3.3/mL	7.5/mL[5]	3.6/g[6]	0.67/mL	4/g[7]	4.9/g[8]
Protein (g)		0.33/mL	0.16/mL	0.86/g	0.17/mL		
Protein source		Hydrolyzed beef collagen	Calcium caseinate (milk)	Whey protein isolate (milk)	Casein hydrolysate (milk)		
Carbohydrate (g)	0.94/g	0.47/mL				1/g	0.73/g
Carbohydrate source	Glucose polymers derived from controlled hydrolysis of cornstarch	Glycerin	Sucralose			Partially hydrolyzed guar gum	Hydrolyzed corn starch
Fat (g)			0.75/mL				0.22/g
Fat source			High oleic sunflower oil	Soy lecithin			Corn/coconut oil and MCT oils (fractionated coconut, palm kernel)
Osmolality mOsm/kg					1 mL contributes 12 for 100 mL feeding		1 scoop = 5 g; for 1:3 dilution; 310; 0.93 mOsm/g powder
Osmolarity mOsmL	247[9]	59.9					
Sodium mEq/L (mg/L)	<0.057/g (<1.3/g)	(<0.0018/mL)		2.1/g (0.09/g)		3.76/g (0.175/g)	<0.2/g
Potassium mEq/L (mg/L)	<0.003/g (<0.1/g)	(<0.0007/mL)		4.3/g (0.11/g)		3.76/g (0.1/g)	<0.05/g
Chloride mEq/L (mg/L)	<0.063/g (<2.23/g)						<0.2/g
Calcium mEq/L (mg/L)	<0.015/g (<0.3/g)	(0.002)		(2.9/g)			<0.05/g
Phosphorus mEq/L (mg/L)	(<0.15/g)	(<0.003/mL)					<0.05/g

Nutritional Modulars – Carbohydrate and Protein Supplements[1] continued

	Polycose Powder	ProMod Liquid Protein[2,3]	Benecalorie (liquid)	Beneprotein (powder)	Liquid Protein Fortifier	Resource Benefiber	Duocal
Manufacturer	Abbott	Abbott	Nestle	Nestle	Abbott	Nestle	Nutricia
Special information		Powder displacement is 0.63 mL/g. Gluten-free, Kosher	Gluten-free, lactose-free, cholesterol-free, Kosher	Gluten-free, lactose-free, Kosher	The first and only commercially sterile, extensively hydrolyzed liquid protein designed for preterm infant feedings. Eliminates the need for powder mixing and meets ADA and CDC recommendations to reduce risk of contamination		Milk protein-free

[1]These products are not complete formulations and should not be used as a sole source of nutrition; information based on manufacturer's literature as of 2013 and is subject to change

[2]Comes in fruit punch flavor

[3]Promod Powder is no longer commercially available.

[4]1 teaspoon (2 g) = 8 calories, 1 tablespoon (6 g) = 23 calories, ¼ cup (24 g) = 91 calories.

[5]Serving is a 1.5 fl oz package

[6]1 scoop = 7 g packet = 1.5 tablespoons

[7]1 tbsp = 4 g packet, usually mix with 2 to 4 fl oz. This provides 3 g of soluble dietary fiber.

[8]42 cal/tablespoon

[9]Approximate osmotic contribution to solution mixed into is 1.6 mOsm/g with a low renal solute load of 0.13 mOsm/g

Nutritional Modulars – Fat Supplement[1]

	Vegetable Oil[2]	Microlipid	MCT Oil[3]	Whole Milk
Indications	Inexpensive fat source for calories and essential fatty acids	50% fat emulsion for use as a source of calories or essential fatty acids; it mixes easily and stays in emulsion	Fat supplement for use in patients who cannot efficiently digest and absorb long-chain fats	For children >1 year of age
Calories	8.3/mL	4.5/mL	7.7/mL	157/8 oz
Protein (g)	—	—	—	8.2/8 oz
Protein source	—	—	—	82% casein, 18% whey
Carbohydrate (g)	—	—	—	11.5/8 oz
Carbohydrate source	—	—	—	Lactose
Fat (g)	0.93/mL	0.5/mL	0.93/mL	8.2/8 oz
Fat source	Corn, soybean, sunflower or safflower oils[5]	Safflower oil[4], polyglycerol esters, soy lecithin	Modified coconut/palm kernel oils	Butter fat
Osmolality mOsm/kg	—	62	—	285
Sodium mEq/L (mg/L)	—	—	—	5.3/8 oz (120/8 oz)
Potassium mEq/L (mg/L)	—	—	—	9.6/8 oz (377/8 oz)
Calcium mEq/L (mg/L)	—	—	—	14.9/8 oz (295/8 oz)
Phosphorus mEq/L (mg/L)	—	—	—	(230/8 oz)
Iron mg/L	—	—	—	Trace
% free water	—	45	—	91
Manufacturer		Nestle	Nestle	
Special information		Can administer 15 mL via syringe through the feeding tube and flush afterwards with 30 mL water Gluten-free, lactose-free, Kosher	Recommended initial volume is 15 mL administrated gradually. Recommended max volume over 24 hrs is 100 mL as indicated, given in divided doses not to exceed 15 to 20 mL. Can administer 15 mL via syringe through the feeding tube and flush afterwards with 30 mL water. For oral consumption, may mix with juice, milk, sauces, salad dressings, or other foods. Gluten-free, lactose-free, Kosher	

[1]These products are not complete formulations and should not be used as a sole source of nutrition; information based on manufacturer's literature as of 2013 and is subject to change

[2]1 tablespoon = 14 g

[3]Does not contain essential fatty acids

[4]Rich source of polyunsaturated fat

[5]% of linoleic from fat: Soybean oil 51%, corn oil 58%, sunflower oil 65%, safflower oil 77%

ELECTROLYTE REPLACEMENT

Oral Electrolyte Maintenance Solution[1]

	Pedialyte[2]	Pedialyte Freezer Pop[3]	Enfamil Enfalyte[4,5]
Indications	Replace fluids and electrolytes lost during diarrhea and vomiting to prevent dehydration in infants/children	Replace fluids and electrolytes lost during diarrhea and vomiting to prevent dehydration in infants/children	Oral electrolyte maintenance solution using rice syrup solids as carbohydrate source to help replace electrolytes and water one might lose from vomiting and diarrhea; for infants and children
Calories	0.1/mL	0.1/mL	0.126/mL
Protein (g)			
Protein source			
Carbohydrate (g)	25	25	30
Carbohydrate source	Dextrose	Dextrose	Rice syrup solids
Fat (g)			
Fat source			
Osmolality mOsm/kg	250 unflavored 270 flavored	270 flavored	160
Osmolarity mOsm/L			168
Sodium mEq/L (mg/L)	45	45	50 (1150)
Potassium mEq/L (mg/L)	20	20	25 (980)
Chloride mEq/L (mg/L)	35	35	45 (160)
Calcium mEq/L (mg/L)			
Phosphorus mEq/L (mg/L)			
Iron mg/L			
Manufacturer	Abbott	Abbott	Mead Johnson
Special information	Kosher, Halal (only certain flavors)		

[1]These products are not complete formulations and should not be used as a sole source of nutrition; information based on manufacturer's literature as of 2013 and is subject to change

[2]Unflavored but available as grape, fruit, bubblegum, strawberry, and apple

[3]Each freezer pop is 2.1 fl oz. Grape, cherry, orange, and blue raspberry are not Kosher.

[4]Cherry

[5]Contains citrate 34 mEq/L

FLUID AND ELECTROLYTE REQUIREMENTS IN CHILDREN

Maintenance Fluids (Two methods)

Surface area method (most commonly used in children >10 kg): 1500 to 2000 mL/m^2/day

Body weight method[A]

Weight	Daily Fluids (Holliday-Segar Method)	Hourly Rate (Holliday-Segar Estimate)
<10 kg	100 mL/kg/day	4 mL/kg/hour
11 to 20 kg	1000 mL + 50 mL/kg (for each kg >10)	40 mL/hour + 2 mL/kg/hour (for each kg >10)
>20 kg	1500 mL + 20 mL/kg (for each kg >20)	60 mL/hour + 1 mL/kg/hour (for each kg >20)

[A]Should not be used in patients <14 days; generally overestimates needs.

Maintenance Electrolytes (See specific monographs for more detailed information)

Sodium: 3 to 4 mEq/kg/day
Potassium: 2 to 3 mEq/kg/day

Alterations of Maintenance Fluid Requirements

Fever	Increase maintenance fluids by 5 mL/kg/day for each degree of temperature above 38°C
Hyperventilation	Increase maintenance fluids by 10 to 60 mL/100 kcal BEE (basal energy expenditure)
Sweating	Increase maintenance fluids by 10 to 25 mL/100 kcal BEE (basal energy expenditure)
Hyperthyroidism	Variable increase in maintenance fluids: 25% to 50%
Renal disease	Monitor and analyze output; adjust therapy accordingly
Renal failure	Maintenance fluids are equal to insensible losses (300 mL/m^2) + urine replacement (mL for mL)
Diarrhea	Increase maintenance fluids on a mL/mL loss basis

Dehydration Fluid Therapy

Goals of therapy:

* Restore circulatory volume to prevent shock (10% to 15% dehydration)

* Restore combined intracellular and extracellular deficits of water and electrolytes within 24 hours for isotonic or hyponatremic dehydration. For hypertonic dehydration restore over 48 hours.

* Maintain adequate water and electrolytes

* Resolve homeostatic distortions (eg, acidosis)

* Replace ongoing losses

Analysis of the Severity of Dehydration by Physical Signs

Clinical Sign	Mild	Moderate	Severe
Degree of dehydration Infant Child/Adult	 <5% <3%	 5% to 10% 3% to 6%	 >10% >6%
Skin turgor	Normal	Decreased	Markedly decreased
Mucous membranes	Thirsty	Dry	Parched
Skin color	Normal	Pale	Mottled
Urine output	Decreased	Oliguria	Anuria
Blood pressure	Normal	Normal, ↓	↓↓
Heart rate	Normal, ↑	↑	↑↑
Capillary refill	Normal	Delayed (>1.5 seconds)	Very delayed (>3 seconds)
Fontanelle (<7 mo)	Flat	Sunken	Very sunken
CNS	Consolable	Irritable/lethargic	Limp, depressed consciousness

Adapted from *Nelson's Textbook of Pediatrics*. 19th ed. Saunders; 2011 and *Current Pediatric Diagnosis & Treatment*. 20th ed. McGraw Hill; 2011.

Classification of Dehydration (based upon the serum sodium concentration)

Isotonic	130 to 150 mEq/L
Hypotonic	<130 mEq/L
Hypertonic	>150 mEq/L

Water deficit may also be calculated (in isotonic dehydration):

$$\text{Water deficit (mL)} = \frac{\% \text{ dehydration} \times \text{wt (kg)} \times 1000 \text{ g/kg}}{100}$$

Fluid Replacement

Rehydration begins with a fluid bolus if adequate perfusion is not present. Fluid boluses of 20 mL/kg (maximum single dose: 1000 mL) using crystalloids (eg, normal saline or lactated Ringers) are administered over 20 to 60 minutes or as rapidly as possible if necessary; repeat doses until circulation is improved [eg, warm skin, decreased heart rate (towards normal), improved capillary refill time, urine output restored]. Once perfusion has been restored then fluid replacement (maintenance plus deficit) is continued over the next 24 hours (isotonic/hypotonic dehydration) or 48 hours (hypertonic dehydration).

For 24 hour replacement, half the deficit fluid is given in the first 8 hours and the second half is given over the last 16 hours. Although $D_5\frac{1}{4}NS$ provides the estimated sodium requirement for most patients when used as a maintenance fluid, there is a risk of developing iatrogenic hyponatremia. To prevent hyponatremia, many clinicians use $\frac{1}{2}NS$ instead. Some clinicians have suggested NS should be used for maintenance fluids.

For hypernatremic dehydration the total deficit volume plus the maintenance volume for 48 hours should be combined and the total administered over 48 hours. This is done to prevent osmotic fluid shifts which could lead to cerebral edema and possibly seizures. The fluid used for replacement should be hypotonic (eg, $D_5\frac{1}{4}NS$) to ensure sodium is not corrected by more than 10 mEq/L/day.

Example of Fluid Replacement (assume 10 kg infant with 10% isotonic dehydration)

	Water	Sodium (mEq)	Potassium (mEq)
Maintenance	1000 mL	40	20
Deficit[A]	1000 mL	80	80
Total	2000 mL	120	100

[A]Reduce this total by any fluid boluses given initially.

First 8 hours:	Replace $\frac{1}{3}$ maintenance water	=	330 mL
	Replace $\frac{1}{2}$ deficit water	=	500 mL
	Total		830 mL/8 h = 103 mL/h

Replace $\frac{1}{2}$ of Na^+ & K^+ = 60 mEq sodium/803 mL; 50 mEq potassium/803 mL (It is suggested that the maximum initial potassium concentration used is 40 mEq/L and is **not** started until urine output has been established.)

The actual order would appear as: $D_5\frac{1}{2}NS$ at 103 mL/hour for 8 hours; add 40 mEq/L KCl after patient voids.

Second 16 hours:	Replace $\frac{2}{3}$ maintenance water	=	670 mL
	Replace $\frac{1}{2}$ deficit water	=	500 mL
	Total		1260 mL/16 h = 79 mL/h

Replace remainder of sodium and potassium.

The actual order would appear as: $D_5\frac{1}{2}NS$ with KCl 40 mEq/L at 79 mL/hour for 16 hours.

Analysis of Ongoing Losses

Electrolyte Composition of Biological Fluids (mEq/L)

Fluid Type	Sodium	Potassium	HCO_3^-
Gastric	20 to 80	5 to 20	0
Small intestine	100 to 140	5 to 15	40
Diarrheal stool	10 to 90	10 to 80	40
Ileostomy	45 to 135	3 to 15	40

CURRENT Diagnosis and Treatment Pediatrics, 20th ed, McGraw-Hill, 2011.

Because of the wide range of normal values, specific analyses are suggested in individual cases.

Oral Rehydration

Due to the high worldwide incidence of dehydration from infantile diarrhea, effective, inexpensive oral rehydration solutions have been developed. In the U.S., a typical effective solution for rehydration contains 45 to 75 mEq/L sodium, 20 to 25 mEq/L potassium, 30 to 34 mEq/L bicarbonate or its equivalent, and sufficient chloride to provide electroneutrality. Two percent to 3% glucose helps facilitate electrolyte and water absorption in the intestine and provides short-term calories. Oral replacement fluids should be administered frequently in small quantities (5 to 15 mL) to provide 50 mL/kg over 4 hours in mild dehydration and 100 mL/kg over 6 hours for moderate dehydration. Oral rehydration should **not** be used if any of the following exists: Altered level of consciousness, respiratory distress, acute surgical abdomen, >10% volume depletion in infants, hemodynamic instability, severe hyponatremia (Na <120 mEq/L) or severe hypernatremia (Na >160 mEq/L). Clear liquids such as broth, juice, tea, and soda are not appropriate for fluid replacement due to high osmolarity and limited electrolytes and should be avoided. The following table describes the electrolyte/sugar content of commonly used oral rehydration solutions.

Composition of Frequently Used Oral Electrolyte Replacement Solutions

Solutions	Carbohydrate (g/L)	Na$^+$ (mEq/L)	K$^+$ (mEq/L)	Cl$^-$ (mEq/L)	Base^A (mEq/L)
WHO solution, modified	13.5	75	20	65	30
Pedialyte	25	45	20	35	30
Enfalyte	30	50	25	45	34
Oralyte	25	45	20	35	30

^{A}Actual or potential bicarbonate (eg, acetate, citrate, or lactate)

Adapted from Centers for Disease Control and Prevention (CDC). Managing acute gastroenteritis among children: oral rehydration, maintenance, and nutritional therapy. *MMWR*. 2003;52(RR-16):1-16 and manufacturer's labeling.

REFERENCES

Centers for Disease Control and Prevention (CDC). Managing acute gastroenteritis among children: oral rehydration, maintenance, and nutritional therapy. *MMWR Recomm R*. 2003;52(RR-16):1-16.

Ford DM. Fluid, electrolyte, & acid-base disorders & therapy. *CURRENT Diagnosis and Treatment Pediatrics*. 20th ed. Hay WW, Levin MJ, Sondheimer JM, et al, eds. New York: McGraw-Hill; 2011;1299-1307.

Greenbaum LA. Deficit therapy. *Nelson Textbook of Pediatrics*. 19th ed. Kliegman RM, Stanton BF, St. Geme JW, et al, eds. Philadelphia, PA: Saunders; 2011;245-249.

Meyers RS. Pediatric fluid and electrolyte therapy. *J Pediatr Pharmacol Ther*. 2009;14(4):204-211.

H. PYLORI TREATMENT IN PEDIATRIC PATIENTS

Medication Regimen	Dosages	Duration of Therapy
	First-Line Therapy (Option 1)	
Omeprazole[1]	0.5 mg/kg/dose twice daily maximum dose: 20 mg twice daily	7 to 14 days
plus		
Amoxicillin	25 mg/kg/dose twice daily maximum dose: 1000 mg twice daily	7 to 14 days
plus		
Clarithromycin	7.5 mg/kg/dose twice daily maximum dose: 500 mg twice daily	7 to 14 days
	First-Line Therapy (Option 2)	
Omeprazole[1]	0.5 mg/kg/dose daily maximum dose: 20 mg twice daily	7 to 14 days
plus		
Amoxicillin	25 mg/kg/dose twice daily maximum dose: 1000 mg twice daily	7 to 14 days
plus		
MetroNIDAZOLE	10 mg/kg/dose twice daily maximum dose: 500 mg twice daily	7 to 14 days
	First-Line Therapy (Option 3)	
Omeprazole[1]	0.5 mg/kg/dose daily maximum dose: 20 mg twice daily	7 to 14 days
plus		
Clarithromycin	7.5 mg/kg/dose twice daily maximum dose: 500 mg twice daily	7 to 14 days
plus		
MetroNIDAZOLE	10 mg/kg/dose twice daily maximum dose: 500 mg twice daily	7 to 14 days
	Second-Line Therapy	
Bismuth Subsalicylate	262 mg 4 times/day	7 to 14 days
plus		
Omeprazole[1]	0.5 mg/kg/dose twice daily maximum dose: 20 mg twice daily	7 to 14 days
plus		
MetroNIDAZOLE	10 mg/kg/dose twice daily maximum dose: 500 mg twice daily	7 to 14 days
plus		
Amoxicillin or Tetracycline[2] or Clarithromycin	Amoxicillin: 25 mg/kg/dose twice daily maximum dose: 1000 mg twice daily **or** Tetracycline: 25 mg/kg/dose twice daily maximum dose: 1000 mg twice daily **or** Clarithromycin: 7.5 mg/kg/dose twice daily maximum dose: 500 mg twice daily	7 to 14 days

[1]Comparable doses of other proton pump inhibitors may be considered.

[2]Should only be used in children ≥12 years

REFERENCE

Gold BD, Colletti RB, Abbott M, et al. *Helicobacter pylori* infection in children: recommendations for diagnosis and treatment. *J Pediatr Gastroenterol Nutr.* 2000;31(5):490-497.

PEDIATRIC PARENTERAL NUTRITION

The following information is intended as a brief overview of the use of PN in infants and children.

Goal: The therapeutic goal of PN in infants and children is both to maintain nutrition status and to achieve balanced somatic growth; in premature infants, the goal is to mimic intrauterine growth.

General Indications for Use: PN is the provision of required nutrients by the intravenous route to replenish, optimize, or maintain nutritional status.

Specific Indications

PN of **all** required nutrients (total parenteral nutrition) is indicated in patients for whom it is expected that it would be impossible or dangerous to enterally administer nutrition. PN in combination with enteral nutrition is indicated in patients who are expected to be unable to meet their nutritional needs by the enteral route alone within 5 days. Peripheral PN is indicated only for partial nutritional supplementation or as bridge therapy for patients awaiting central venous access.

1. Patients with an inability to absorb nutrients via the gastrointestinal tract, which may include the following: Severe diarrhea, short bowel syndrome, developmental anomalies of the GI tract, inflammatory bowel disease, cystic fibrosis, or anatomic or functional loss of GI integrity

2. Severe malnutrition

3. Severe catabolic states, such as burns, trauma, or sepsis

4. Patients undergoing high dose chemotherapy, radiation, and bone marrow transplantation

5. Patients whose clinical condition may necessitate complete bowel rest (eg, necrotizing enterocolitis, pancreatitis, GI fistulas, or recent GI surgery)

6. Intensive care low-birth-weight infants

7. Neonatal asphyxia

8. Meconium ileus

9. Respiratory distress syndrome (RDS)

Nutritional Assessment

Nutritional screening may be done on admission by staff nurses or dietitian to identify patients who are malnourished or at risk of malnutrition. Patients identified through the screening process as being at risk should receive a complete nutritional assessment which may include anthropometric measurements, diet history, laboratory values, and physical exam. As many as 44% of hospitalized pediatric patients are malnourished and require nutritional therapy. The type of nutritional support indicated depends on the underlying disease, the degree of gastrointestinal function, and the severity of malnutrition. Acutely malnourished patients have an increased risk for serious infection, postoperative complications, and death. Indicators of acute protein-calorie malnutrition include low weight for height, low serum albumin, lymphopenia, decreased body fat folds, and decreased arm muscle area.

Nutritional Requirements

Energy requirements vary based on age. The following table provides an estimate for caloric and protein requirements at various ages for normal subjects.

Daily Caloric and Protein Requirements for Pediatric Patients

Age	kcal/kg/day	Protein g/kg/day
Preterm neonate	90 to 120	3 to 4
Term infant <1 year	85 to 105	2 to 3
1 to 7 years	75 to 90	1.5 to 3
7 to 10 years	50 to 75	1.5 to 3
11 to 12 years	50 to 75	0.8 to 2.5
>12 to 18 years	30 to 50	0.8 to 2.5

Patients who are severely malnourished or markedly catabolic may require higher levels to achieve catch-up growth or meet increased requirements. Patients who are well-nourished and/or inactive may require less.

During parenteral nutrition, 10% to 16% of calories should be in the form of amino acids to achieve optimal benefit (approximately 3 to 4 g/kg/day in preterm infants, 2 to 3 g/kg/day in infants, 1.5 to 3 g/kg/day in children (1 to 10 years), and 0.8 to 2.5 g/kg/day in adolescents). Exceptions include patients with renal or hepatic failure (where less protein is indicated), or in the treatment of severe trauma, head injury, or sepsis (where more protein may be indicated).

PN ORDERING

Fluid Intake

The patient should be given a total volume of fluid reasonable for his/her age and cardiovascular status. It is generally safe to start with the fluid maintenance level of 1500 mL/m^2/day in children >10 kg or use the Holliday-Segar weight-based method in children >2 weeks (see Fluid and Electrolyte Requirements in Children). The fluid requirements in preterm infants are extremely variable due to much greater insensible water losses from radiant warmers and bili-lights. While the standard fluid maintenance of 100 mL/kg/day may be sufficient for term infants, intakes of up to 150 mL/kg/day may be necessary in the very low birth weight infants. Be sure to consider significant fluid intake from medications or other I.V. fluids and enteral diets in planning the fluids available for PN.

Amino Acids

Amino acids may be described as either a "standard" mixture of essential and nonessential amino acids or "specialized" mixtures. Specialized mixtures are intended for use in patients whose physiologic or metabolic needs may not be met with the "standard" amino acid compositions. Examples of specialized solutions include:

TrophAmine, Aminosyn PF, PremaSol	Indicated for use in premature infants and young children due to addition of taurine, L-glutamic acid, L-aspartic acid, increased amounts of histidine, and reduction in amounts of methionine, alanine, phenylalanine, and glycine. Supplementation with a cysteine[1] additive has been recommended.
HepatAmine	Indicated for treatment in patients with hepatic encephalopathy due to cirrhosis or hepatitis or in patients with liver disease who are intolerant of standard amino acid solutions. Contains higher percentage of branched-chain amino acids and a lower percentage of aromatic amino acids than standard mixtures.
NephrAmine, Aminosyn RF	Indicated for use in patients with compromised renal function who are intolerant of standard amino acid solutions. Contains a mixture of essential amino acids and histidine.

[1]Supplementation is usually provided as a fixed ratio to the amino acid solution: 40 mg of cysteine per gram of amino acid; duration of supplementation is usually for the first year of life, but practice varies widely.

Protein provides 4 kcal per gram.

Amino acid calculations:

% amino acid	=	amino acid (g)/100mL
Grams of protein	=	grams of nitrogen x 6.25
% amino acid desired	=	$\dfrac{\text{(g amino acid/kg) x weight (kg) x 100}}{\text{total PN fluid volume (mL)}}$

Dextrose

For central PN, dextrose is usually begun with a 10% to 12.5% solution or a solution providing dextrose at no more than 5 mg/kg/minute (in neonates and premature infants). The concentration is advanced, if tolerated, by 2.5% to 5% per day (2 to 2.5 mg/kg/minute increments in neonates and premature infants) to the desired caloric density, usually 20% to 25% dextrose. Fluid restricted patients often need 30% to 35% dextrose to meet their energy needs. For peripheral PN, 5% to 12.5% dextrose is utilized.

Dextrose provides 3.4 kcal per gram.

Dextrose calculations:

% Dextrose = dextrose (g)/100 mL		
Dextrose infusion rate (mg/kg/minute)	=	$\dfrac{\text{rate (mL/h) x% dextrose x 0.166}}{\text{weight (kg)}}$
% Dextrose desired[1]	=	$\dfrac{\text{desired rate (mg/kg/min) x weight (kg)}}{\text{0.166 x rate (mL/h)}}$

[1]Do not use dextrose concentrations <5% due to hypotonicity.

Fat Emulsion (FE)

There are three roles for intravenous fat in parenteral nutrition:

1. To provide nonprotein calories
2. To provide essential fatty acids and a "balanced" calorie source
3. To provide calories in catabolic patients with limited ability to excrete CO_2

The FE dosage is increased as tolerated daily (see General Guidelines for Initiation and Advancement for PN following). The maximum fat intake is 3.5 g/kg/day and no more than 60% of the total daily caloric intake. It is administered as a continuous infusion over 24 hours or at a rate no greater than 0.15 to 0.17 g/kg/hour via a Y-connector with the dextrose-amino acid I.V. line. In patients receiving cyclic PN, the FE should be administered over the duration of the PN infusion. The triglyceride concentration should be checked on initiation and then weekly. Triglyceride concentrations should be maintained at <200 mg/dL in neonates, <350 mg/dL in renal patients, and <250 mg/dL in other patients. FE should be used cautiously in neonates with hyperbilirubinemia due to displacement of bilirubin from albumin by the free fatty acids. An increase in free bilirubin may increase the risk of kernicterus. Significant displacement occurs when the free fatty acid to serum albumin molar ratio (FFA/SA) >6. For example, infants with a total bilirubin >8 to 10 mg/dL (assuming an albumin concentration of 2.5 to 3 g/dL) should not receive more parenteral FE than required to meet the essential fatty acid requirement of 0.5 to 1 g/kg/day.

Note: Avoid use of 10% FE in preterm infants because a greater accumulation of plasma lipids occurs due to the greater phospholipid load of the 10% concentration.

Fat emulsion 10% provides 1.1 kcal/mL or 11 kcal/g

Fat emulsion 20% provides 2 kcal/mL or 10 kcal/g

Fat emulsion calculations:

20% FE = 20 g fat/100 mL = 2 kcal/mL

$$\text{Desired 20\% FE (mL)} = \frac{(\% \text{ total kcal as fat}) \times (\text{total kcal})}{2 \text{ kcal/mL}}$$

or as an alternative

$$\text{Desired 20\% FE (mL)} = \text{FE (g/kg)} \times \text{weight (kg)} \times 5 \text{ mL/g}$$

General Guidelines for Initiation and Advancement of PN[1]

Age	Initiation and Advancement[2]	Protein (g/kg/day)	Dextrose	Fat (g/kg/day)
	Initial	1.5 to 3	5 to 7 mg/kg/min	1 to 2
Premature infant	Daily increase	1	1 to 2.5 mg/kg/min or 1% to 2.5% increments	0.5 to 1
	Goal	3 to 4	8 to 12 mg/kg/min (max: 14 to 18 mg/kg/min)	3 to 3.5
	Initial	1 to 3	6 to 9 mg/kg/min	1 to 2
Term infant <1 y	Daily increase	1	1 to 2 mg/kg/min or 2.5% to 5% increments	0.5 to 1
	Goal	2 to 3	12 mg/kg/min (max: 14 to 18 mg/kg/min)	3
	Initial	1 to 2	10%	1 to 2
Children 1 to 10 y	Daily increase	1	1 to 2 mg/kg/min or 5% increments	0.5 to 1
	Goal	1.5 to 3	8 to 10 mg/kg/min	2 to 3
	Initial	0.8 to 1.5	3.5 mg/kg/min or 10%	1
>10 y	Daily increase	1	1 to 2 mg/kg/min or 5% increments	1
	Goal	0.8 to 2.5	5 to 6 mg/kg/min	1 to 2.5

[1]Rate of advancement may be limited by metabolic tolerance (eg, hyperglycemia, azotemia, hypertriglyceridemia)

[2]Timely intervention in premature infants is essential with initiation of dextrose as soon as possible after birth, amino acids within the first 12 hours, and fat emulsion within 24 to 48 hours of life.

ELECTROLYTES AND MINERALS

Guideline for Daily Electrolyte and Mineral Requirements

	Preterm Neonates (mEq/kg)	Infants/Children (mEq/kg)	Adolescents/Children >50 kg
Sodium	2 to 5[1]	2 to 5	1 to 2 mEq/kg
Potassium	2 to 4	2 to 4	1 to 2 mEq/kg
Calcium gluconate[2]	2 to 4[3]	0.5 to 4	10 to 20 mEq/day
Magnesium	0.3 to 0.5	0.3 to 0.5	10 to 30 mEq/day
Phosphate[2]	1 to 2 mmol/kg[3]	0.5 to 2 mmol/kg	10 to 40 mmol/day

[1]Premature infants lose sodium in urine due to the immature resorptive function of kidney and diuretic use. Hyponatremia may lead to poor tissue growth and adverse developmental outcomes. Sodium content in PN may be adjusted to a maximum of 154 mEq/L (NS) to achieve normal sodium serum levels.

[2]Calcium-phosphate stability in parenteral nutrition solutions is dependent upon the pH of the solution, temperature, and relative concentration of each ion. The pH of the solution is primarily dependent upon the amino acid concentration. The higher the percentage amino acids the lower the pH, the more soluble the calcium and phosphate. Individual commercially available amino acid solutions vary significantly with respect to pH lowering potential and consequent calcium phosphate compatibility. See the pharmacist for specific calcium phosphate stability information.

[3]A 1.7:1 calcium to phosphate ratio in PN allows for the highest absolute retention of both minerals and simulates the *in utero* accretion of calcium and phosphate.

VITAMINS AND TRACE ELEMENTS

Vitamins

A pediatric parenteral multivitamin product is indicated for children <11 years of age and <40 kg. Children >40 kg or >11 years of age may receive adult multivitamin formulations.

Dosage:

Pediatric MVI[1]:
  Neonates: 2 mL/kg/day; maximum 5 mL/day
  Infants and Children ≤11 years: 5 mL/day
  Children >40 kg or >11 years and Adults: Use adult formulation[2] 10 mL/day

Trace Element Daily Requirements[1]

	Preterm Neonates <3 kg (mcg/kg/day)	Term Neonates 3 to 10 kg (mcg/kg/day)	Children 10 to 40 kg (mcg/kg/day)	Adolescents >40 kg (per day)
Chromium[2]	0.05 to 0.2	0.2	0.14 to 0.2	5 to 15 mcg
Copper[3]	20	20	5 to 20	200 to 500 mcg
Manganese[4]	1	1	1	40 to 100 mcg
Selenium[2,5]	1.5 to 2	2	1 to 2	40 to 60 mcg
Zinc	400	50 to 250	50 to 125	2 to 5 mg

[1]Recommended intakes of trace elements cannot be achieved through the use of a single pediatric trace element product. Only through the use of individualized trace element products can recommended intakes be achieved.

[2]Reduce dose in patients with renal dysfunction.

[3]Reduce dose by 50% in patients with impaired biliary excretion or cholestatic liver disease.

[4]Omit in patient with impaired biliary excretion or cholestatic liver disease.

[5]Indicated for use in long-term parenteral nutrition patients.

These are recommended daily trace element requirements. Additional supplementation may be indicated in clinical conditions resulting in excessive losses. For example, additional zinc may be needed in situations of excessive gastrointestinal losses.

DEVELOPING THE PN GOAL REGIMEN

The purpose of this example is to illustrate the thought process in determining what dextrose and amino acid solution and fat emulsion intake would provide the desired daily fluid calorie and protein goals. The following example utilizes the method of calculating calories from protein, dextrose, and fat. However, some clinicians do not include protein calories since protein is used as a building block for adequate growth and development, rather than a calorie source.

1. Calculate the fluid, protein, and caloric goals. Example:

    Weight = 10 kg

    Fluids = 100 mL/kg/day = 1000 mL

    Calories = 100 kcal/kg/day = 1000 kcal

    Protein = 2.5 g/kg/day = 25 g

2. If fat emulsion (FE) comprises 30% to 35% of the total daily calories, using the above example: 30% of 1000 kcal = 300 kcal.
    300 kcal ÷ 2 kcal/mL (20% FE) = 150 mL

3. Calculate percent amino acid solution to achieve goal protein intake. Example:
    [25 g (total protein) ÷ 850 mL (total fluid)] x 100 = 2.9%

4. Determine the calories from protein. Example:
    25 g x 4 kcal/g = 100 kcal

5. To determine the goal dextrose concentration calculate the total daily calories remaining. Example:

1000 kcal	(total daily calories)
-100 kcal	(daily calories from protein)
-300 kcal	(daily calories from fats)
600 kcal	(total daily calories remaining)

6. Determine the concentration of dextrose to achieve the total daily calories remaining. Example:
    600 kcal ÷ 3.4 kcal/g x [100 ÷ 850 mL[1]] = 21%
    [1]Total daily fluids desired minus that from fats.

7. Calculate the goal dextrose infusion rate (DIR) in mg/kg/minute. Example:
    (850 mL ÷ 24 hours) x 21% x 0.166 ÷ 10kg = 12.3 mg/kg/minute
    This patient's goal regimen would be: Dextrose 21%, amino acid 2.9%, 850 mL/day plus fat emulsion 20% 150 mL/day.

Suggested PN Monitoring Guidelines

Parameter	Suggested Frequency	
	Initial/Hospitalized	Follow-up/Outpatient
Growth		
Weight	Daily	Daily to every visit
Height/length	Weekly	Weekly to every visit
Body composition (triceps skinfold, bone age)	Initially	Monthly to annually
Metabolic (Serum[1])		
Electrolytes	Daily to twice weekly	Weekly to every visit
Magnesium	Daily to weekly	Weekly to every visit
Phosphorus	Daily to weekly	Weekly to every visit
BUN/creatinine	Weekly	Weekly to every visit
Acid-base status	Until stable	As indicated
Prealbumin	Weekly	Weekly to every visit
Glucose	Daily to weekly	Weekly to every visit
Triglyceride	Weekly	Weekly to every visit
Liver function tests	Weekly	Weekly to every visit
Complete blood count/differential	Weekly	Weekly to every visit
Platelets, PT/PTT	Weekly	As indicated
Iron indices	As indicated	Biannually to annually
Trace elements	As indicated	Annually
Carnitine	As indicated	As indicated
Folate/vitamin B_{12}	As indicated	As indicated
Ammonia	As indicated	As indicated
Bilirubin, direct	Weekly	As indicated
Clinical Calculations		
Fluid balance	Daily	As indicated
Projected vs actual intake	Daily	Weekly to every visit
Calorie/protein intake	Daily	As indicated

Frequency depends on clinical condition

[1]For metabolically unstable patients, need to check more frequently

Adapted from: Guidelines for the use of parenteral and enteral nutrition in adult and pediatric patients. ASPEN board of directors and the clinical guidelines task force. *JPEN J Parenter Enteral Nutr.* 2002;26(1 Suppl):1-138SA.

Pharmacologic considerations of mixing medications with PN solutions include:

- Adsorption — bag, bottle, tubing, filter
- Blood levels
- Site of injection/administration
- Flush
- Amino acid-dextrose concentrations
- pH factors
- Temperature
- Additives in solution
- Heparin dose

REFERENCES

ASPEN Board of Directors and The Clinical Guidelines Task Force. Guidelines for the use of parenteral and enteral nutrition in adult and pediatric patients. *JPEN J Parenter Enteral Nutr.* 2002;26(1 Suppl):1-138SA.

Carney LN, Nepa A, Cohen SS, et al. Parenteral and enteral nutrition support: determining the best way to feed. *The A.S.P.E.N Pediatric Nutrition Support Core Curriculum.* Corkins MR, Balint J, Bobo E, et al, eds. Silver Spring, MD: American Society of Parenteral and Enteral Nutrition. 2010;433-447.

Mirtallo J, Canada T, Johnson D, et al. Safe practices for parenteral nutrition. *JPEN J Parenter Enteral Nutr.* 2004;28(6):S39-S70.

GROWTH CHARTS

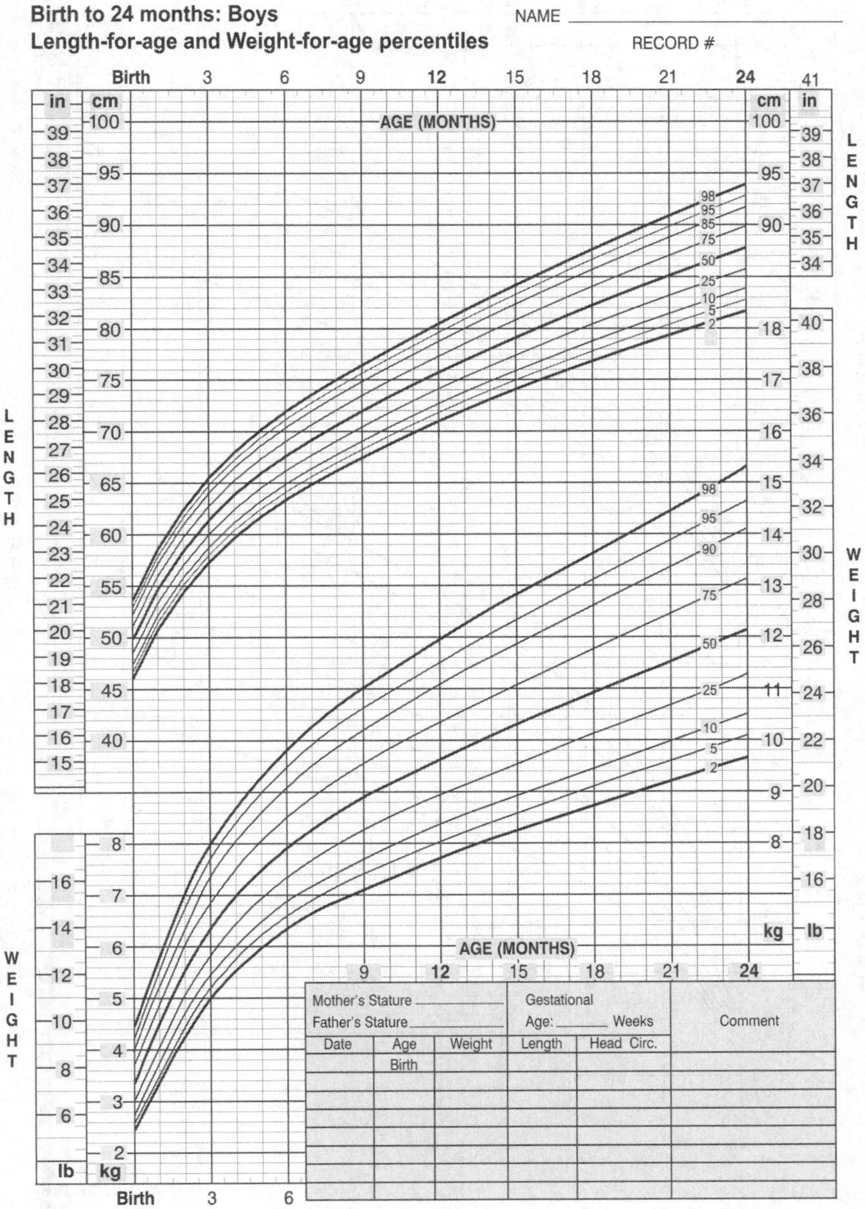
Birth to 24 months: Boys
Length-for-age and Weight-for-age percentiles
NAME
RECORD #
Birth
3
6
9
12
15
18
21
24
AGE (MONTHS)
in
cm
LENGTH
WEIGHT
98
95
85
75
50
25
10
5
2
98
95
90
75
50
25
10
5
2
kg
lb
Mother's Stature
Father's Stature
Gestational
Age:
Weeks
Comment
Date
Age
Weight
Length
Head Circ.
Birth

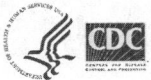

Published by the Centers for Disease Control and Prevention, November 1, 2009
SOURCE: WHO Child Growth Standards (http://www.who.int/childgrowth/en)

Birth to 24 months: Girls
Length-for-age and Weight-for-age percentiles

NAME _____

RECORD # _____

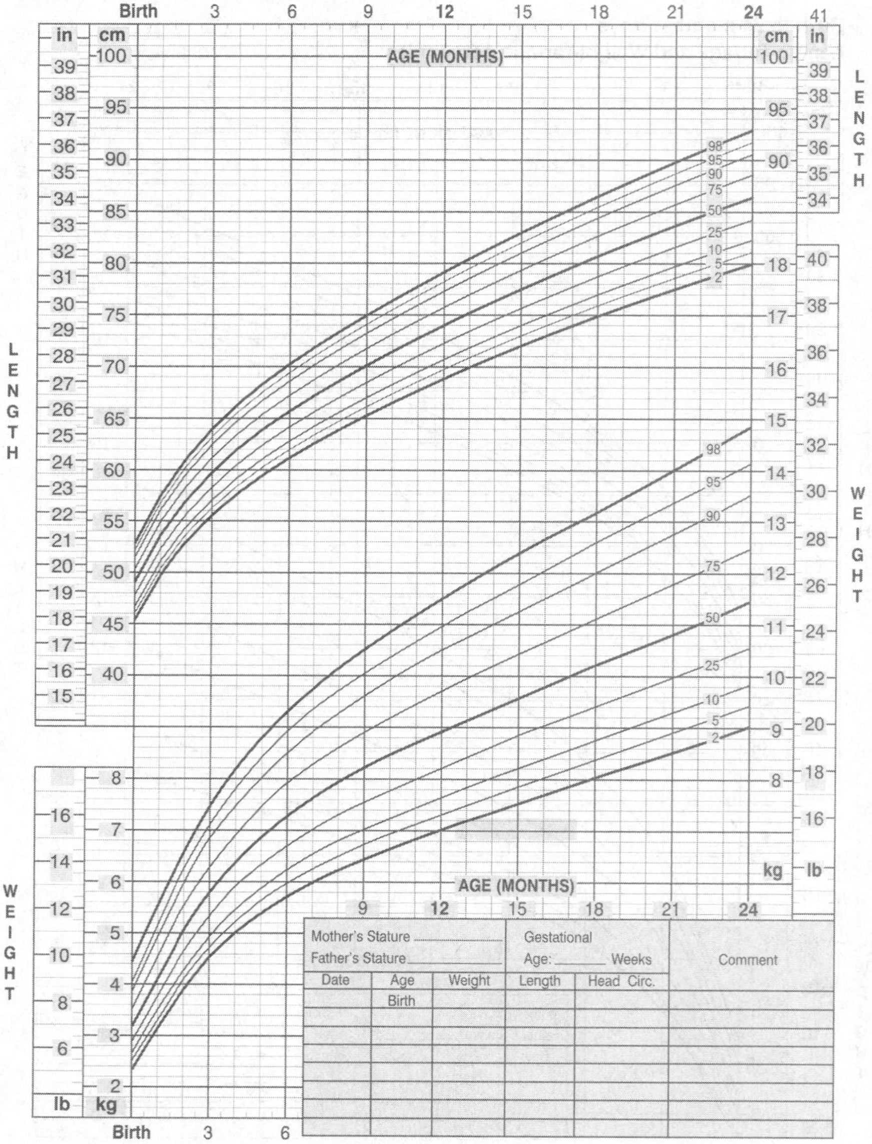

Birth 3 6 9 12 15 18 21 24 41

AGE (MONTHS)

in | cm

L
E
N
G
T
H

W
E
I
G
H
T

Mother's Stature _____
Father's Stature _____

Date	Age	Weight	Length	Head Circ.	Comment
Birth					

Gestational Age: _____ Weeks

Published by the Centers for Disease Control and Prevention, November 1, 2009
SOURCE: WHO Child Growth Standards (http://www.who.int/childgrowth/en)

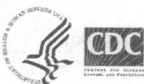

2318

2 to 20 years: Boys
Stature-for-age and Weight-for-age percentiles

NAME _____

RECORD # _____

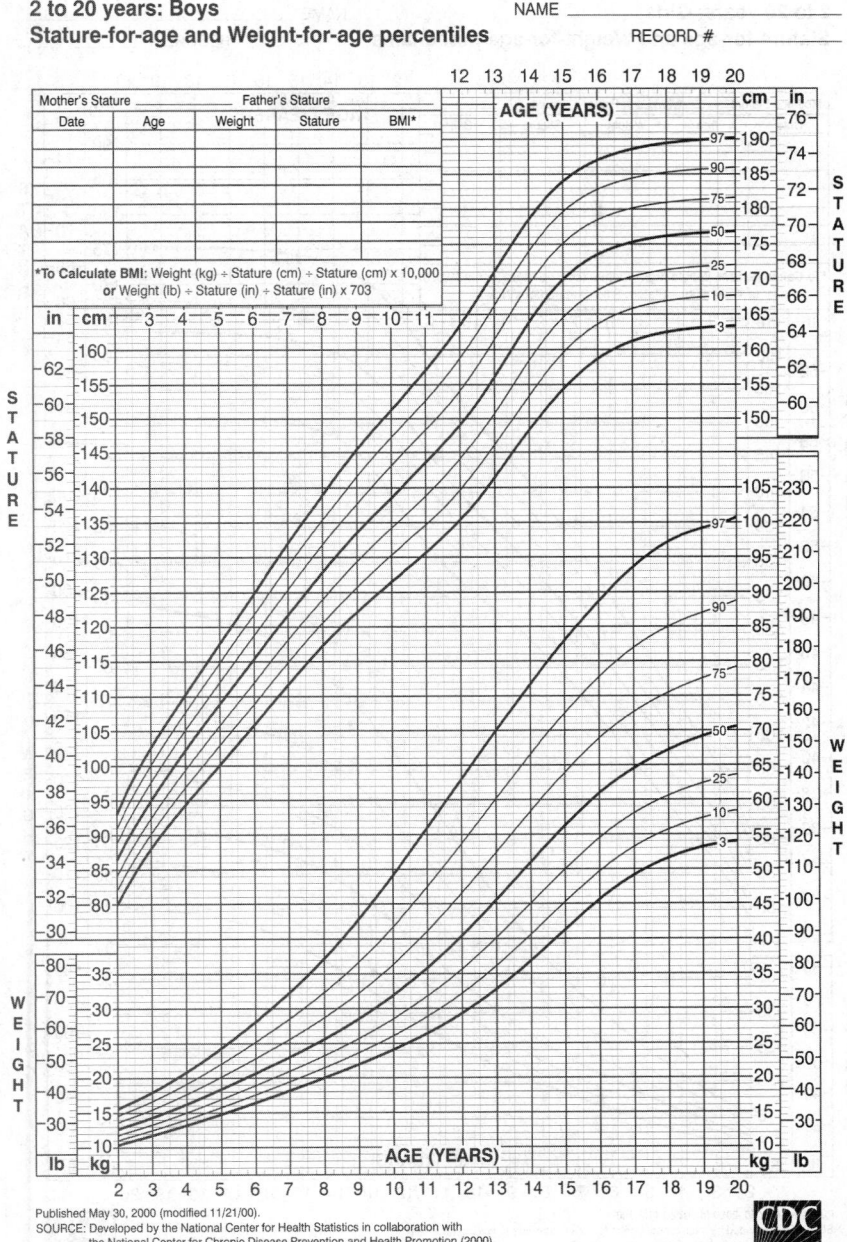

*To Calculate BMI: Weight (kg) ÷ Stature (cm) ÷ Stature (cm) x 10,000
or Weight (lb) ÷ Stature (in) ÷ Stature (in) x 703

Published May 30, 2000 (modified 11/21/00).
SOURCE: Developed by the National Center for Health Statistics in collaboration with
the National Center for Chronic Disease Prevention and Health Promotion (2000).
http://www.cdc.gov/growthcharts

CDC

SAFER · HEALTHIER · PEOPLE™

2 to 20 years: Girls
Stature-for-age and Weight-for-age percentiles

NAME _____

RECORD # _____

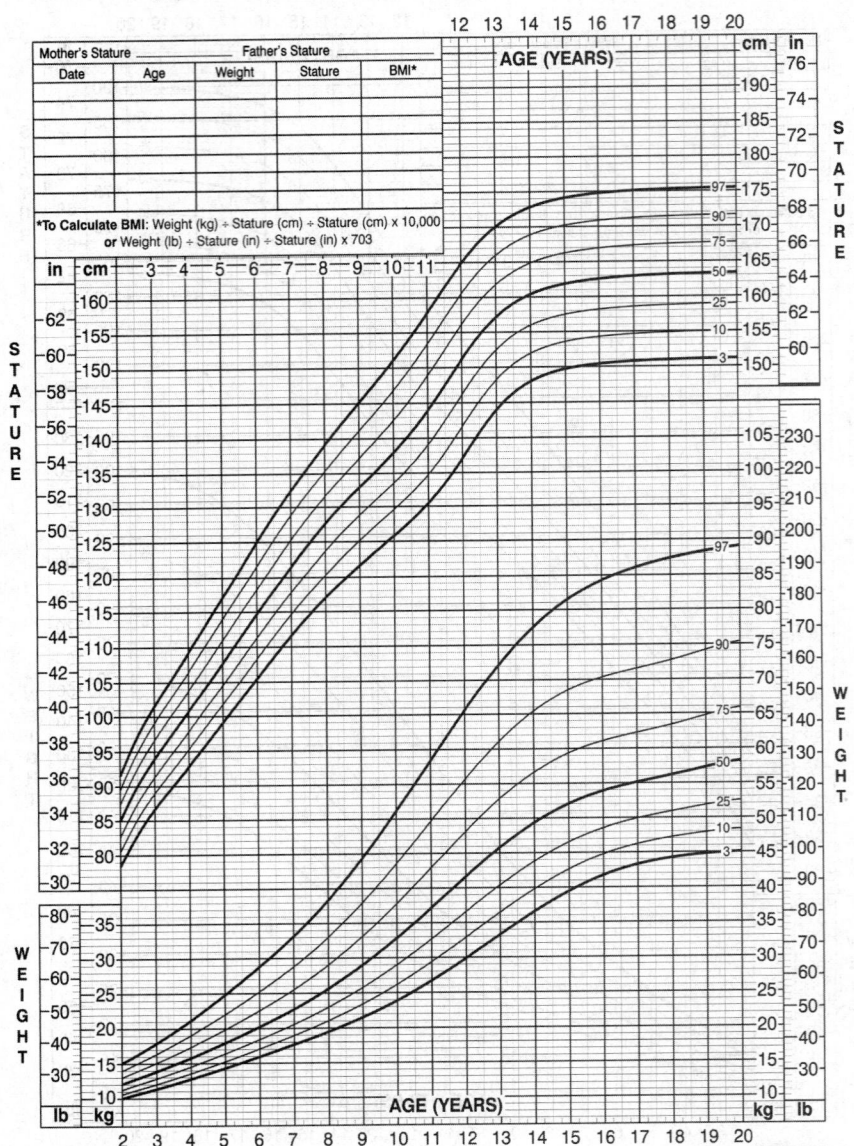

Mother's Stature		Father's Stature		
Date	Age	Weight	Stature	BMI*

*To Calculate BMI: Weight (kg) ÷ Stature (cm) ÷ Stature (cm) x 10,000
or Weight (lb) ÷ Stature (in) ÷ Stature (in) x 703

AGE (YEARS)

STATURE

WEIGHT

Published May 30, 2000 (modified 11/21/00).
SOURCE: Developed by the National Center for Health Statistics in collaboration with
the National Center for Chronic Disease Prevention and Health Promotion (2000).
http://www.cdc.gov/growthcharts

CDC
SAFER · HEALTHIER · PEOPLE™

2320

Birth to 24 months: Boys
Head circumference-for-age and
Weight-for-length percentiles

NAME _____

RECORD # _____

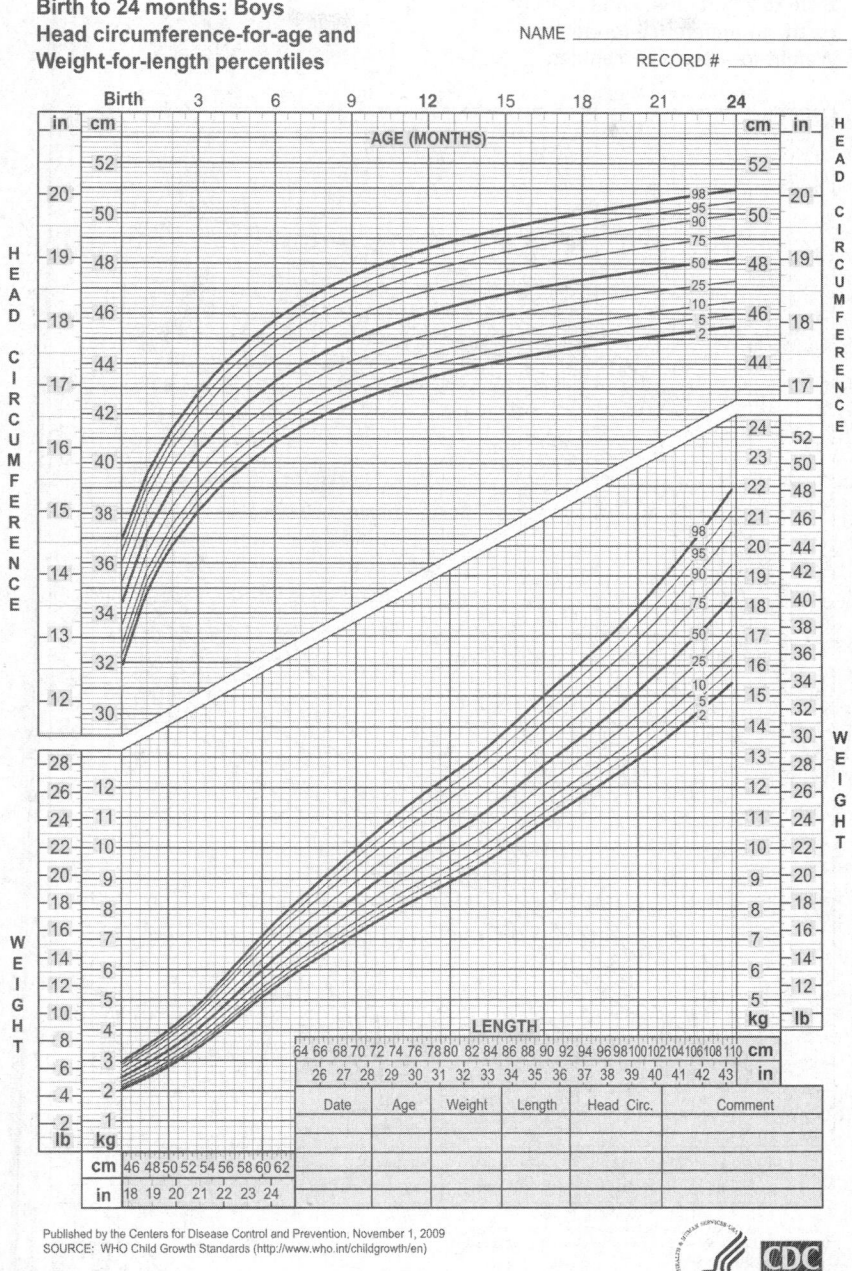

Date	Age	Weight	Length	Head Circ.	Comment

Published by the Centers for Disease Control and Prevention, November 1, 2009
SOURCE: WHO Child Growth Standards (http://www.who.int/childgrowth/en)

CDC

Birth to 24 months: Girls
Head circumference-for-age and
Weight-for-length percentiles

NAME _____

RECORD # _____

Birth to 24 months: Girls — Head circumference-for-age and Weight-for-length percentiles growth chart.

LENGTH

| | cm | 64 66 68 70 72 74 76 78 80 82 84 86 88 90 92 94 96 98 100 102 104 106 108 110 |
| | in | 26 27 28 29 30 31 32 33 34 35 36 37 38 39 40 41 42 43 |

Date	Age	Weight	Length	Head Circ.	Comment

| cm | 46 48 50 52 54 56 58 60 62 |
| in | 18 19 20 21 22 23 24 |

Published by the Centers for Disease Control and Prevention, November 1, 2009
SOURCE: WHO Child Growth Standards (http://www.who.int/childgrowth/en)

2322

IDEAL BODY WEIGHT CALCULATION

Adults (18 years and older)

        IBW (male) = 50 + (2.3 x height in inches over 5 feet)

        IBW (female) = 45.5 + (2.3 x height in inches over 5 feet)

        IBW is in kg.

Children

    a. 1 to 18 years (Traub and Johnson, 1980)

$$IBW = \frac{(height^2 \times 1.65)}{1000}$$

        IBW is in kg.

        Height is in cm.

    b. 5 feet and taller (Traub and Johnson, 1980)

        IBW (male) = 39 + (2.27 x height in inches over 5 feet)

        IBW (female) = 42.2 + (2.27 x height in inches over 5 feet)

        IBW is in kg.

    c. 1 to 17 years (Traub and Kichen, 1983)

        $IBW = 2.396e^{0.01863 \; (height)}$

        IBW is in kg.

        Height is in cm.

REFERENCES

Traub SL, Johnson CE. Comparison of methods of estimating creatinine clearance in children. *Am J Hosp Pharm*. 1980;37(2):195-201.

Traub SL, Kichen L. Estimating ideal body mass in children. *Am J Hosp Pharm*. 1983;40(1):107-110.

BODY SURFACE AREA OF CHILDREN AND ADULTS

Calculating Body Surface Area in Children

In a child of average size, find weight and corresponding surface area on the boxed scale to the left or use the nomogram to the right. Lay a straightedge on the correct height and weight points for the child, then read the intersecting point on the surface area scale. (**Note:** 2.2 lb = 1 kg)

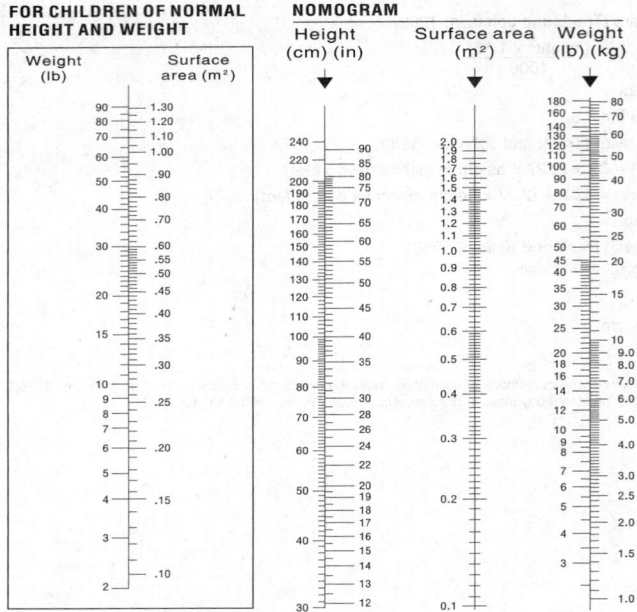

BODY SURFACE AREA FORMULA
(Adult and Pediatric)

$$BSA\ (m^2) = \sqrt{\frac{Ht\ (in)\ x\ Wt\ (lb)}{3131}} \quad \text{or, in metric: } BSA\ (m^2) = \sqrt{\frac{Ht\ (cm)\ x\ Wt\ (kg)}{3600}}$$

References

Lam TK and Leung DT, "More on Simplified Calculation of Body Surface Area," *N Engl J Med*, 1988, 318(17):1130 (Letter).

Mosteller RD, "Simplified Calculation of Body Surface Area", *N Engl J Med*, 1987, 317(17):1098 (Letter).

AVERAGE WEIGHTS AND SURFACE AREAS

Average Height, Weight, and Surface Area by Age and Gender

Age	Girls			Boys		
	Height (cm)	Weight (kg)	BSA (m²)	Height (cm)	Weight (kg)	BSA (m²)
Birth	49.5	3.4	0.22	50	3.6	0.22
3 mo	59	5.6	0.3	61	6	0.32
6 mo	65	7.2	0.36	67	7.9	0.38
9 mo	70	8.3	0.4	72	9.3	0.43
12 mo	74.5	9.5	0.44	75.5	10.3	0.46
15 mo	77	10.3	0.47	79	11.1	0.49
18 mo	80	11	0.49	82	11.7	0.52
21 mo	83	11.6	0.52	85	12.2	0.54
2 y	86	12	0.54	87.5	12.6	0.55
2.5 y	91	13	0.57	92	13.5	0.59
3 y	94.5	13.8	0.6	96	14.3	0.62
3.5 y	97	15	0.64	98	15	0.64
4 y	101	16	0.67	102	16	0.67
4.5 y	104	17	0.7	105	17	0.7
5 y	107.5	18	0.73	109	18.5	0.75
6 y	115	20	0.80	115	21	0.82
7 y	121.5	23	0.88	122	23	0.88
8 y	127.5	25.5	0.95	127.5	26	0.96
9 y	133	29	1.04	133.5	28.5	1.03
10 y	138	33	1.12	138.5	32	1.1
11 y	144	37	1.22	143.5	36	1.2
12 y	151	41.5	1.32	149	40.5	1.29
13 y	157	46	1.42	156	45.5	1.4
14 y	160.5	49.5	1.49	163.5	51	1.52
15 y	162	52	1.53	170	56	1.63
16 y	162.5	54	1.56	173.5	61	1.71
17 y	163	55	1.58	175	64.5	1.77
Adult[1]	163.5	58	1.62	177	83.5	2.03

Data extracted from the CDC growth charts based on the 50th percentile height and weight for a given age[2]

Body surface area calculation[3]: Square root of [(Ht x Wt) / 3600]

[1]McDowell MA, Fryar CD, Hirsch R, Ogden CL. Anthropometric reference data for children and adults: U.S. population, 1999-2002. *Adv Data.* 2005; (361):1-5.

[2]Centers for Disease Control and Prevention (CDC). 2000 CDC growth charts: United States. Available at http://www.cdc.gov/growthcharts. Accessed November 16, 2007.

[3]Mosteller RD. Simplified calculation of body-surface area *N Engl J Med.* 1987;317(17):1098.

PHYSICAL DEVELOPMENT

Weight gain first 6 weeks
20 g/day

Birth weight
regained by day 14
doubles by age 4 mo
triples by age 12 mo
quadruples by age 2 y

Teeth
1st tooth 6 to 18 mo
teeth = age (mo) − 6 (until 30 mo)

Head circumference
35 cm at birth
44 cm by 6 mo
47 cm by 1 y
1 cm/mo for 1st y
0.25 cm/mo 2nd y

Length
increases 50% by age 1 y
doubles by age 4 y
triples by age 13 y

Tanner Stages of Sexual Development

Stage	Characteristics	Age at Onset (mean ± SD)
Genital stages: Male		
1	Prepubertal	
2	Scrotum and testes enlarge; skin of scrotum reddens and rugations appear	11.4 ± 1.1 y
3	Penis lengthens; testes enlarge further	12.9 ± 1 y
4	Penis growth continues in length and width; glans develops adult form	13.8 ± 1 y
5	Development completed; adult appearance	14.9 ± 1.1 y
Breast development: Female		
1	Prepubertal	
2	Breast buds appear; areolae enlarge	11.2 ± 1.1 y
3	Elevation of breast contour; areolae enlarge	12.2 ± 1.1 y
4	Areolae and papilla form a secondary mound on breast	13.1 ± 1.2 y
5	Adult form	15.3 ± 1.7 y
Menarche		
Pubic hair: Both sexes		13.5 ± 1 y
1	Prepubertal, no coarse hair	
2	Longer, silky hair appears at base of penis or along labia	F: 11.7 ± 1.2 y M: 12 ± 1 y
3	Hair coarse, kinky, spreads over pubic bone	F: 12.4 ± 1.1 y M: 13.9 ± 1 y
4	Hair of adult quality but not spread to junction of medial thigh with perineum	F: 13 ± 1 y M: 14.4 ± 1.1 y
5	Spread to medial thigh	F: 14.4 ± 1.1 y M: 15.2 ± 1.1 y
6	"Male escutcheon"	Variable if occurs
Maximum growth rate		
Male at 14.1 ± 0.9 y		
Female at 12.1 ± 0.9 y		

EMETOGENIC POTENTIAL OF ANTINEOPLASTIC AGENTS IN CHILDREN

Note: Unless otherwise specified, emetogenic potential listed is for single agent treatment. For multi-agent regimens, if not otherwise specified, emetogenic potential is based on the component with the higher emetic potential.

Highly Emetogenic Chemotherapy (Frequency of Emesis: >90%)

Altretamine
CARBOplatin
Carmustine >250 mg/m^2
CISplatin
Cyclophosphamide >1000 mg/m^2
Cytarabine 3000 mg/m^2
Dacarbazine
DACTINomycin
Mechlorethamine
Methotrexate ≥12 g/m^2
Procarbazine (oral)
Streptozocin

Thiotepa ≥300 mg/m^2
Multi-agent regimens:
    Cyclophosphamide + Anthracycline (doxorubicin or epirubicin)
    Cyclophosphamide + Etoposide
    Cytarabine 150 to 200 mg/m^2 + Daunorubicin
    Cytarabine 300 mg/m^2 + Etoposide
    Cytarabine 300 mg/m^2 + Teniposide
    Doxorubicin + Ifosfamide
    Doxorubicin + Methotrexate 5 g/m^2
    Etoposide + Ifosfamide

Moderately Emetogenic Chemotherapy (Frequency of Emesis: 30% to 90%)

Aldesleukin >12 to 15 million units/m^2
Amifostine >300 mg/m^2
Arsenic trioxide
AzaCITIDine
Bendamustine
Busulfan (I.V.)
Carmustine ≤250 mg/m^2
Clofarabine
Cyclophosphamide ≤1000 mg/m^2 (I.V.)
Cyclophosphamide (oral)
Cytarabine >200 mg/m^2 to <3000 mg/m^2
DAUNOrubicin
DOXOrubicin
EPIrubicin

Etoposide (oral)
IDArubicin
Ifosfamide
Imatinib
Intrathecal treatment (methotrexate and/or cytarabine ± hydrocortisone)
Irinotecan
Lomustine
Melphalan >50 mg/m^2
Methotrexate ≥250 **mg**/m^2 to <12 **g**/m^2
Mitotane
Oxaliplatin ≥75 mg/m^2
Temozolomide (I.V.)
Temozolomide (oral)

Low Emetogenic Chemotherapy (Frequency of Emesis: 10% to 30%)

Aldesleukin ≤12 million units/m^2
Amifostine ≤300 mg/m^2
Bexarotene (oral)
Busulfan (oral)
Capecitabine
Cytarabine ≤200 mg/m^2
DOCEtaxel
DOXOrubicin (liposomal)
Etoposide (I.V.)
Everolimus
Fludarabine (oral)
Fluorouracil
Gemcitabine

Ixabepilone
Methotrexate >50 to <250 mg/m^2
MitoMYcin
MitoXANtrone
Nilotinib
PACLitaxel
PACLitaxel (protein bound)
PEMEtrexed
Teniposide
Thiotepa <300 mg/m^2
Topotecan
Tretinoin
Vorinostat

Minimal Emetogenic Chemotherapy (Frequency of Emesis: <10%)

Alemtuzumab
Asparaginase
Bevacizumab
Bleomycin
Bortezomib
Cetuximab
Chlorambucil
Cladribine
Dasatinib
Decitabine
Denileukin diftitox
Dexrazoxane
Erlotinib
Fludarabine (I.V.)
Gefitinib
Gemtuzumab ozogamicin
Hydroxyurea
Interferon alfa
Lapatinib
Lenalidomide

Melphalan (oral, low dose)
Mercaptopurine (oral)
Methotrexate ≤50 mg/m^2
Methotrexate (oral)
Nelarabine
Panitumumab
Pegaspargase
Peginterferon alfa
Pentostatin
RiTUXimab
SORAfenib
SUNItinib
Temsirolimus
Thalidomide
Thioguanine (oral)
Trastuzumab
Valrubicin
VinBLAStine
VinCRIStine
Vinorelbine (I.V.)

REFERENCES

Basch E, Prestrud AA, Hesketh PJ, et al. Antiemetics: American Society of Clinical Oncology clinical practice guideline update. *J Clin Oncol*. 2011;29 (31):4189-4198.

Dupuis LL, Boodhan S, Sung L, et al. Guideline for the classification of the acute emetogenic potential of antineoplastic medication in pediatric cancer patients. *Pediatr Blood Cancer*. 2011;57(2):191-198.

Multinational Association of Supportive Care in Cancer. MASCC/ESMO antiemetic guideline 2011. http://www.mascc.org/assets/documents/MASCC_-Guidelines_English_2011.pdf. Accessed April 2011.

National Comprehensive Cancer Network (NCCN). NCCN clinical practice guidelines in oncology: antiemesis. 2013. http://www.nccn.org/professionals/physician_gls/PDF/antiemesis.pdf

TUMOR LYSIS SYNDROME

INTRODUCTION

Tumor lysis syndrome (TLS) is a potentially life-threatening disorder that is characterized as an acute metabolic disturbance resulting from the rapid destruction of tumor cells. Cellular destruction releases intracellular constituents (nucleic acids, anions, cations, peptides) that overwhelm the body's normal mechanisms for their utilization, excretion, and elimination. Signs and symptoms of TLS often develop within 72 hours of beginning cytotoxic chemotherapy in patients with newly diagnosed acute leukemias (acute lymphoblastic leukemia [ALL] and acute myeloid leukemia [AML]) or lymphoproliferative malignancies (Burkitt's and non-Burkitt's lymphomas). Moreover, TLS can occur spontaneously in malignant diseases with vigorous cell turnover. Although most commonly reported in patients with hematologic and lymphoid malignancies, TLS has also been reported with solid tumors such as breast cancer, colon cancer, melanoma, ovarian cancer, prostate cancer, small cell lung cancer, and testicular cancer. Acute TLS attributed to administration of a corticosteroid, imatinib, rituximab, sorafenib, and zoledronic acid in patients with treatment-sensitive tumors have been reported in the medical literature. Additional treatment and diagnostic procedures attributed to causing tumor lysis syndrome include total body irradiation, splenic irradiation, staging laparotomy, laparoscopic splenectomy preceded by splenic artery embolization, and radiofrequency interstitial thermal ablation of metastatic hepatic lesions. Metabolic abnormalities associated with acute TLS include hyperphosphatemia, hyperkalemia, hyperuricemia, azotemia, hypocalcemia, and metabolic acidosis. Cardiac arrhythmias, seizures, and major organ failure can occur in severe cases of TLS. Hyperkalemia, hyperuricemia, and hypocalcemia can produce cardiac arrhythmias, tetany, and sudden death. Acute renal failure can occur due to precipitation of uric acid and calcium phosphate in the renal tubules.

PREDISPOSING FACTORS

1. Bulky disease (>10 cm); leukemia with high white blood cell count (>25,000/mm^3) or rapidly increasing peripheral blast count

2. Acute myeloid leukemia with history of chronic myelomonocytic leukemia

3. Marked sensitivity of the tumor to a particular treatment modality

4. Renal impairment, including preexisting volume depletion

5. Elevated pretreatment lactic dehydrogenase serum concentrations (>2 times ULN)

6. Elevated pretreatment uric acid serum concentrations (>7.5 mg/dL) independent of renal impairment

CLINICAL FEATURES AND TREATMENT

Classification and Risk Stratification

TLS can be described as either laboratory (LTLS) or clinical (CTLS) type. LTLS is the presence of 2 or more abnormal lab values or a 25% change in lab values within 3 days before or 7 days after chemotherapy. Laboratory values to monitor include uric acid, potassium, phosphorus, and calcium. CTLS is defined as LTLS with at least one clinical manifestation such as renal insufficiency, seizures, cardiac arrhythmias, or sudden death.

Certain patients have greater risk for developing LTLS and/or CTLS and should be treated more aggressively to prevent its occurrence. Risk stratification guides what type of prophylaxis and management therapies should be used for which patients. Patients classified as high risk should have aggressive prophylactic treatment with hydration and rasburicase while being monitored closely in an ICU or similarly monitored setting. Intermediate risk patients should receive prophylactic treatment with hydration and allopurinol; if hyperuricemia does develop in these patients, consider rasburicase. Initial management of pediatric patients at intermediate risk may include rasburicase. Patients at low risk for developing TLS require no prophylactic therapy but should be monitored closely and treated as necessary.

Risk Stratification

Type of Cancer	High Risk	Intermediate Risk	Low Risk
Non-Hodgkin's lymphoma (NHL)	Burkitt's, Burkitt's-ALL (B-ALL), lymphoblastic lymphoma	Diffuse large B-cell lymphoma (DLBCL)	Indolent NHL
Acute lymphoblastic leukemia (ALL)	WBC ≥100,000 cells/mm^3	WBC 50,000 to 100,000 cells/mm^3	WBC ≤50,000 cells/mm^3
Acute myeloid leukemia (AML)	WBC ≥50,000 cells/mm^3; monoblastic; rapidly increasing peripheral blast count	WBC 10,000 to 50,000 cells/mm^3	WBC ≤10,000 cells/mm^3
Chronic lymphocytic leukemia (CLL)		WBC 10,000 to 100,000 cells/mm^3; treatment with fludarabine	WBC ≤10,000 cells/mm^3
Other hematologic malignancies (chronic myeloid leukemia [CML], multiple myeloma) and solid tumors		Rapid proliferation with expected rapid response to therapy	Remainder of patients

Monitoring

High risk patients should have laboratory and clinical parameters (serum uric acid, phosphate, calcium, creatinine, LDH, and fluid input and output) monitored 4 to 6 hours after initiating chemotherapy. For all patients treated with rasburicase, monitor serum uric acid 4 hours after administration, then every 6 to 8 hours thereafter until resolution of TLS occurs. Frequent assessment of serum chemistries and fluid balance is necessary to avert pathophysiologic adverse events and guide the duration of rasburicase therapy. Electrolyte and fluid abnormalities must be addressed at the time that they are identified. However, rasburicase is administered no more frequently than once daily to achieve uric acid control for a duration of 5 to 7 doses (has also been administered as a single dose schedule with repeat doses, if needed, based on serum uric acid level).

Intermediate risk patients should be monitored throughout and for at least 24 hours after completion of chemotherapy. If rasburicase is not used, laboratory parameters should be monitored 8 hours after initiation of chemotherapy and regularly thereafter according to the patient's clinical condition and institutional practice.

Low risk patients should be monitored as determined by the institution and patient factors. If TLS has not occurred within 2 days, development is very unlikely.

General Principles

Prevention and early management of TLS are aimed at decreasing the risk of morbidity and mortality from cardiac arrhythmias, seizures, and organ failure. In patients with high or intermediate risk, vigorous hydration is the cornerstone of the initial management for acute or potential TLS. Patients should be hydrated with 2 to 3 L/m^2/day (200 mL/kg/day if ≤10 kg) intravenous fluid (Children: D$_5$W$^1/_4$NS; Adults: Not specified) to maintain urine output of 80 to 100 mL/m^2/hour (4 to 6 mL/kg/hour if ≤10 kg), with diuretic use if necessary (avoid or minimize diuretic use in patients with hypovolemia or obstructive uropathy). Due to the tendency for calcium phosphate nephrocalcinosis and the potential for metabolic alkalosis, urinary alkalinization with sodium bicarbonate is no longer universally recommended for the treatment and prevention of TLS (Coiffier, 2008).

Allopurinol should be administered to intermediate risk patients to decrease endogenous uric acid production and reduce associated urinary obstruction; dose reductions may be required for renal dysfunction (Coiffier, 2008). In adult or pediatric patients, give 150 to 300 mg/m^2/day (or 10 mg/kg/day in pediatric patients) divided every 8 hours (maximum 800 mg/day) orally or 200 to 400 mg/m^2/day I.V. (in 1 to 3 divided doses; maximum 600 mg/day). The time to maximum effect of allopurinol is 27 hours. While allopurinol decreases uric acid production, it is ineffective in reducing markedly elevated uric acid concentrations which may allow renotubular crystal formation and obstruction despite its administration. In addition, allopurinol impedes the clearance of purine analogues such as mercaptopurine and azathioprine.

Rasburicase is administered to rapidly reduce uric acid concentrations; significant reduction in plasma uric acid concentrations is measurable four hours following drug administration. Rasburicase, which is a recombinant form of urate oxidase produced in *Saccharomyces cerevisiae*, catalyzes the degradation of uric acid to allantoin which is more soluble and readily excreted by the kidneys. Rasburicase is reserved for patients at high risk for TLS (or considered in intermediate risk pediatric patients), patients with elevated uric acid concentrations, or patients with signs of moderate to severe renal impairment or other major organ dysfunction. The major risks associated with administration of rasburicase include anaphylaxis, hypersensitivity reactions, methemoglobinemia, and hemolysis. Rasburicase is contraindicated in patients with glucose-6-phosphate dehydrogenase deficiency due to an increased risk of hemolysis. An additional concern with rasburicase administration is the development of neutralizing antibodies. This phenomenon was observed in 64% of 28 normal, healthy volunteers studied; the effect of neutralizing antibodies on the efficacy of this product with repeated usage is unknown. Rasburicase appears to be less immunogenic in patients with hematologic or lymphoid malignancies receiving chemotherapy. One study reported detection of neutralizing antibodies in 2% of 184 patients with hematologic or lymphoid malignancies treated with rasburicase before and throughout chemotherapy (Cortes, 2010).

Rasburicase is approved for use in pediatric and adult patients, with the labeled dose of 0.2 mg/kg/dose daily for up to five days. Due to the costs and risks of therapy plus the immediate and measurable effects of rasburicase, some centers administer a single dose which is repeated daily as warranted by plasma uric acid concentrations. The following doses (based on risk for TLS) and duration of treatment based on plasma uric acid concentrations have been recommended for children: 0.2 mg/kg once daily (duration based on plasma uric acid concentrations) for high risk patients, 0.15 mg/kg once daily (duration based on plasma uric acid concentrations) for intermediate risk, and 0.05 to 0.1 mg/kg once daily (duration based on clinical judgment) if used for low-risk patients (Coiffier, 2008). Weight- and risk-based dosing as detailed above has been reported in adults. Fixed-dose rasburicase, ranging from 3 to 7.5 mg as a single dose (Hutcherson, 2006; McDonnell, 2006; Reeves, 2008; Trifilio, 2006) with doses (1.5 to 6 mg) repeated if needed (based on serum uric acid concentrations) has also been reported in adults. The optimal timing of rasburicase administration (with respect to chemotherapy administration) is not specified in the manufacter's labeling. In some studies, chemotherapy was administered 4 to 24 hours after the first rasburicase dose (Cortes, 2010; Kikuchi, 2009; Vadhan-Raj, 2012); however, rasburicase generally may be administered irrespective of chemotherapy timing.

Upon rasburicase administration, serum uric acid levels generally decrease within 4 hours. In order to allow for appropriate therapeutic effect and to accurately assess the need for a repeat dose, repeat uric acid levels should be drawn no earlier than 4 hours post-rasburicase dose. Rasburicase will degrade uric acid *in vitro* when the blood sample is stored at room temperature. Consequently, to prevent artifactually depressed uric acid concentrations, plasma samples must be collected in prechilled tubes, then immediately placed in an ice water bath until centrifuged at 4°C. Plasma must be analyzed within four hours of collection.

Clinical features and treatment for specific metabolic disorders are discussed in the following sections.

Hyperuricemia

Cytolysis during TLS releases purine and pyrimidine nucleotides into the bloodstream and extracellular tissues. Oxidation of the purines hypoxanthine and xanthine yields uric acid, which can precipitate in the renal tubules and cause oliguric renal failure. A high concentration of uric acid and an acidic urine pH promote uric acid crystallization and renotubular precipitation. Maintenance of urine flow is utilized to reduce purine precipitation and preserve renal function. Allopurinol blocks the endogenous production of uric acid by inhibiting the enzyme xanthine oxidase, which oxidizes hypoxanthine and xanthine to uric acid. Allopurinol is used prophylactically during the early management of TLS in intermediate risk patients. Rasburicase decreases existing uric acid concentrations by conversion of this molecule to the inactive and soluble metabolite allantoin, which is readily excreted by the kidneys. Rasburicase should be used prophylactically in high risk patients or in patients with preexisting hyperuricemia or acute renal impairment.

Hyperkalemia

Potassium is primarily an intracellular ion that is released during massive cellular breakdown. Increasing concentrations of serum potassium can be dangerous, leading to cardiac arrhythmias or sudden death, especially in the presence of hypocalcemia (see following discussion). Standard treatments to remove potassium from the blood stream and extracellular fluids should be initiated as warranted by the patient's serum potassium concentration and electrocardiographic abnormalities. Other sources of potassium intake (including nutritional sources, medications, and intravenous solutions) should be eliminated in patients at risk for or with TLS. Pharmaceutical measures routinely used to manage hyperkalemia in patients with TLS include volume expansion with forced diuresis, administration of insulin with glucose, and the cation exchange product sodium polystyrene sulfonate. Sodium bicarbonate can be administered I.V. push to induce influx of potassium into cells. Textbook algorithms for management of hyperkalemia include instructions for administration of calcium as a cardioprotective measure; however, this is **not** a standard intervention in the setting of TLS. Calcium gluconate administration must be done judiciously in the patient with TLS as it can precipitate as calcium phosphate in highly perfused tissues. Monitor patient ECG and cardiac rhythm closely for arrhythmias.

Hyperphosphatemia

The release of intracellular inorganic phosphate following massive cellular breakdown sets into motion several important clinical features. Serum phosphate concentrations will quickly exceed the threshold for normal renal excretion, with phosphate excretion becoming limited by the glomerular filtration rate. Any azotemia that develops during therapy will hinder phosphate excretion. Treatment includes the use of phosphate binders such as aluminum hydroxide, sevelamer, calcium carbonate (avoid use in patients with hypercalcemia and limit use to pediatric patients), or lanthanum carbonate (avoid use in pediatric patients). In severe cases of hyperphosphatemia, hemodialysis or hemofiltration may be necessary.

Hypocalcemia

High phosphate concentrations will also cause reciprocal hypocalcemia. Although generally asymptomatic, hypocalcemia may cause neuromuscular irritation, tetany, and cardiac dysrhythmias. Symptomatic patients may receive calcium gluconate intravenously (slowly, with ECG monitoring) to increase serum calcium concentrations. Unfortunately, despite hypocalcemia, the solubility product of calcium and phosphate may be exceeded in acute TLS due to high concentrations of phosphate, resulting in tissue calcification and organ failure. For this reason, calcium gluconate should be administered cautiously and only if necessary.

Hemodialysis/Hemofiltration

Due to the unpredictability of TLS, renal replacement therapy may be needed and can be lifesaving. Hemodialysis or hemofiltration may be used to control and maintain fluid volume and/or to remove uric acid, phosphate, and potassium from serum. Intermittent hemodialysis, continuous arteriovenous hemodialysis, or continuous veno-venous hemodiafiltration should be considered as warranted by the severity of serum chemistry abnormalities, major organ dysfunction, and the patient's response to pharmaceutical treatments.

Leukoreduction/Plasmapheresis

Leukoreduction, which utilizes plasmapheresis and hydroxyurea to rapidly decrease the peripheral white blood cell count, is performed in some cases of acute myeloid leukemia. The primary goal of leukoreduction is to reduce the risk of complications from serum hyperviscosity syndrome consequent to a very high white blood cell count. However, leukoreduction can indirectly reduce the risk of TLS as removal of circulating blasts diminishes the primary source of cells undergoing lysis in patients with acute myeloid leukemia. Plasmapheresis is used infrequently and very cautiously in patients with acute promyelocytic leukemia due to the inherent disease-related risks of coagulopathy, hemorrhage, and hypotension in this population. Plasmapheresis is rarely used for leukoreduction in patients with lymphocytic or lymphoblastic leukemias as these patients are at lower risk for hyperviscosity syndrome despite a high white blood cell count. This is because lymphocytes do not have the same 'sticky' quality as myeloid cells. Hydroxyurea can be used without plasmapheresis to achieve leukoreduction.

REFERENCES

Abu-Alfa AK, Younes A. Tumor lysis syndrome and acute kidney injury: evaluation, prevention, and management. *Am J Kidney Dis.* 2010;55(5 Suppl 3): S1-S13.

Al-Kali A, Farooq S, Tfayli A. Tumor lysis syndrome after starting treatment with gleevec in a patient with chronic myelogenous leukemia. *J Clin Pharm Ther.* 2009;34(5):607-610.

Arnold TM, Reuter JP, Delman BS, Shanholtz CB. Use of single-dose rasburicase in an obese female. *Ann Pharmacother.* 2004;38(9):1428-1431.

Barry BD, Kell MR, Redmond HP. Tumor lysis syndrome following endoscopic radiofrequency interstitial thermal ablation of colorectal liver metastases. *Surg Endosc.* 2002;16(7):1109.

Cairo MS, Bishop M. Tumor lysis syndrome: new therapeutic strategies and classification. *Br J Haematol.* 2004;127(1):3-11.

Cairo MS, Coiffier B, Reiter A, Younes A; TLS Expert Panel. Recommendations for the evaluation of risk and prophylaxis of tumour lysis syndrome (TLS) in adults and children with malignant diseases: an expert TLS panel consensus. *Br J Haematol.* 2010;149(4):578-586.

Chen SW, Hwang WS, Tsao CJ, Liu HS, Huang GC. Hydroxyurea and splenic irradiation-induced tumour lysis syndrome: a case report and review of the literature. *J Clin Pharm Ther.* 2005;30(6):623-625.

Coiffier B, Altman A, Pui CH, Younes A, Cairo MS. Guidelines for the management of pediatric and adult tumor lysis syndrome: an evidence-based review. *J Clin Oncol.* 2008;26(16):2767-2778.

Coiffier B, Mounier N, Bologna S, et al. Efficacy and safety of rasburicase (recombinant urate oxidase) for the prevention and treatment of hyperuricemia during induction chemotherapy of aggressive non-hodgkin's lymphoma: results of the GRAAL1 (Groupe d'Etude Des Lymphomes De l'Adulte trial on rasburicase activity in adult lymphoma) study. *J Clin Oncol.* 2003;21(23):4402-4406.

Cortes J, Moore JO, Maziarz RT, et al. Control of plasma uria acid in adults at risk for tumor lysis syndrome: efficacy and safety of rasburicase alone and rasburicase followed by allopurinol compared with allopurinol alone – results of a multicenter phase III study. *J Clin Oncol.* 2010;28(27):4207-4213.

Duzova A, Cetin M, Gümrük F, Yetgin S. Acute tumour lysis syndrome following a single-dose corticosteroid in children with acute lymphoblastic leukaemia. *Eur J Haematol.* 2001;66(6):404-407.

Gemici C. Tumour lysis syndrome in solid tumours. *Clin Oncol (R Coll Radiol).* 2006;18(10):773-780.

Habib GS, Saliba WR. Tumor lysis syndrome after hydrocortisone treatment in metastatic melanoma: a case report and review of the literature. *Am J Med Sci.* 2002;323(3):155-157.

Huang WS, Yang CH. Sorafenib induced tumor lysis syndrome in an advanced hepatocellular carcinoma patient. *World J Gastroenterol.* 2009;15 (35):4464-4466.

Hutcherson DA, Gammon DC, Bhatt MS, Faneuf M. Reduced-dose rasburicase in the treatment of adults with hyperuricemia associated with malignancy. *Pharmacotherapy*. 2006;26(2):242-247.

Jabr FI. Acute tumor lysis syndrome induced by rituximab in diffuse large B-cell lymphoma. *Int J Hematol*. 2005;82(4):312-314.

Kikuchi A, Kigasawa H, Tsurusawa M, et al. A study of rasburicase for the management of hyperuricemia in pediatric patients with newly diagnosed hematologic malignancies at high risk for tumor lysis syndrome. *Int J Hematol*. 2009;90(4):492-500.

Kurt M, Onal IK, Elkiran T, Altun B, Altundag K, Gullu I. Acute tumor lysis syndrome triggered by zoledronic acid in patient with metastatic lung adenocarcinoma. *Med Oncol*. 2005;22(2):203-206.

Lee MH, Cheng KI, Jang RC, Hsu JH, Dai ZK, Wu JR. Tumour lysis syndrome developing during an operation. *Anaesthesia*. 2007;62(1):85-87.

Lee AC, Li CH, So KT, Chan R. Treatment of impending tumor lysis with single-dose rasburicase. *Ann Pharmacother*. 2003;37(11):1614-1617.

Leibowitz AB, Adamsky C, Gabrilove J, Labow DM. Intraoperative acute tumor lysis syndrome during laparoscopic splenectomy preceded by splenic artery embolization. *Surg Laparosc Endosc Percutan Tech*. 2007;17(3):210-211.

Lerza R, Botta M, Barsotti B, et al. Dexamethazone-induced acute tumor lysis syndrome in a T-cell malignant lymphoma. *Leuk Lymphoma*. 2002;43(5):1129-1132.

Linck D, Basara N, Tran V, et al. Peracute onset of severe tumor lysis syndrome immediately after 4 Gy fractionated TBI as part of reduced intensity preparative regimen in a patient with T-ALL with high tumor burden. *Bone Marrow Transplant*. 2003;31(10):935-937.

Liu CY, Sims-McCallum RP, Schiffer CA. A single dose of rasburicase is sufficient for the treatment of hyperuricemia in patients receiving chemotherapy. *Leuk Res*. 2005;29(4):463-465.

Mato AR, Riccio BE, Qin L, et al. A predictive model for the detection of tumor lysis syndrome during AML induction therapy. *Leuk Lymphoma*. 2006;47(5):877-883.

McDonnell AM, Lenz KL, Frei-Lahr DA, Hayslip J, Hall PD. Single-dose rasburicase 6 mg in the management of tumor lysis syndrome in adults. *Pharmacotherapy*. 2006;26(6):806-812.

National Comprehensive Cancer Network (NCCN). Practice guidelines in oncology: acute myeloid leukemia, version 1.2011. http://www.nccn.org/professionals/physician_gls/PDF/aml.pdf

Oztop I, Demirkan B, Yaren A, et al. Rapid tumor lysis syndrome in a patient with metastatic colon cancer as a complication of treatment with 5-fluorouracil/leucoverin and irinotecan. *Tumori*. 2004;90(5):514-516.

Reeves DJ, Bestul DJ. Evaluation of a single fixed dose of rasburicase 7.5 mg for the treatment of hyperuricemia in adults with cancer. *Pharmacother*. 2008;28(6):685-690.

Riccio B, Mato A, Olson EM, Berns JS, Luger S. Spontaneous tumor lysis syndrome in acute myeloid leukemia: two cases and a review of the literature. *Cancer Biol Ther*. 2006;5(12):1614-1617.

Rostom AY, El-Hussainy G, Kandil A, Allam A. Tumor lysis syndrome following hemi-body irradiation for metastatic breast cancer. *Ann Oncol*. 2000;11(10):1349-1351.

Sorscher SM. Tumor lysis syndrome following docetaxel therapy for extensive metastatic prostate cancer. *Cancer Chemother Pharmacol*. 2004;54(2):191-192.

Theodorou D, Lagoudianakis E, Pattas M, et al. Pretreatment tumor lysis syndrome associated with bulky retroperitoneal tumors. Recognition is the mainstay of therapy. *Tumori*. 2006;92(6):540-541.

Trifilio S, Gordon L, Singhal S, et al. Reduced-dose rasburicase (recombinant xanthine oxidase) in adult cancer patients with hyperuricemia. *Bone Marrow Transplant*. 2006;37(11):997-1001.

Vadhan-Raj S, Fayad LE, Fanale MA, et al. A randomized trial of a single-dose rasburicase versus five-daily doses in patients at risk for tumor lysis syndrome. *Ann Oncol*. 2012;23(6):1640-1645.

Yahata T, Nishikawa N, Aoki Y, Tanaka K. Tumor lysis syndrome associated with weekly paclitaxel treatment in a case with ovarian cancer. *Gynecol Oncol*. 2006;103(2):752-754.

Zigrossi P, Brustia M, Bobbio F, Campanini M. Flare and tumor lysis syndrome with atypical features after letrozole therapy in advanced breast cancer. A case report. *Ann Ital Med Int*. 2001;16(2):112-117.

TOTAL BLOOD VOLUME

Age	Example Weight (kg) [age]	Approximate Total Blood Volume (mL/kg)[1]	Estimated Total Blood Volume (mL)
Premature infant	1.5	89 to 105	134 to 158
Term newborn	3.4	78 to 86	265 to 292
1 to 12 months	7.6 [6 months]	73 to 78	555 to 593
1 to 3 years	12.4 [2 years]	74 to 82	918 to 1017
4 to 6 years	18.2 [5 years]	80 to 86	1456 to 1565
7 to 18 years	45.5 [13 years]	83 to 90	3777 to 4095
Adults	70.0	68 to 88	4760 to 6160

[1]Approximate total blood volume information compiled from: *Nathan and Oski's Hematology of Infancy and Childhood*. 5th ed. Nathan DG, Orkin SH, eds. Philadelphia, PA: WB Saunders; 1998.

ASSESSMENT OF LIVER FUNCTION

Child-Pugh Score

Component	Score Given for Observed Findings		
	1	2	3
Encephalopathy grade[1]	None	1 to 2	3 to 4
Ascites	None	Mild or controlled by diuretics	Moderate or refractory despite diuretics
Albumin (g/dL)	>3.5	2.8 to 3.5	<2.8
Total bilirubin (mg/dL)	<2 (<34 micromoles/L)	2 to 3 (34 to 50 micromoles/L)	>3 (>50 micromoles/L)
or			
Modified total bilirubin[2]	<4	4 to 7	>7
Prothrombin time (seconds prolonged)	<4	4 to 6	>6
or			
INR	<1.7	1.7 to 2.3	>2.3

[1]**Encephalopathy Grades**
Grade 0: Normal consciousness, personality, neurological examination, electroencephalogram
Grade 1: Restless, sleep disturbed, irritable/agitated, tremor, impaired handwriting, 5 cps waves
Grade 2: Lethargic, time-disoriented, inappropriate, asterixis, ataxia, slow triphasic waves
Grade 3: Somnolent, stuporous, place-disoriented, hyperactive reflexes, rigidity, slower waves
Grade 4: Unrousable coma, no personality/behavior, decerebrate, slow 2 to 3 cps delta activity

Alternative Encephalopathy Grades
Grade 1: Mild confusion, anxiety, restlessness, fine tremor, slowed coordination
Grade 2: Drowsiness, disorientation, asterixis
Grade 3: Somnolent but rousable, marked confusion, incomprehensible speech, incontinent, hyperventilation
Grade 4: Coma, decerebrate posturing, flaccidity

[2]Modified total bilirubin used to score patients who have Gilbert's syndrome or who are taking indinavir.

CHILD-PUGH CLASSIFICATION

Class A (mild hepatic impairment): Score 5 to 6
Class B (moderate hepatic impairment): Score 7 to 9
Class C (severe hepatic impairment): Score 10 to 15

REFERENCES

Centers for Disease Control and Prevention (CDC). Report of the NIH panel to define principles of therapy of HIV infection and guidelines for the use of antiretroviral agents in HIV-infected adults and adolescents. March 2004. Available at http://www.aidsinfo.nih.gov

U.S. Department of Health and Human Services Food and Drug Administration. Guidance for industry, pharmacokinetics in patients with impaired hepatic function: study design, data analysis, and impact on dosing and labeling. May 2003. Available at http://www.fda.gov/OHRMS/DOCKETS/98fr/99D-5047-GDL00002.pdf

HOTLINE AND IMPORTANT PHONE NUMBERS

AIDS Hotline (National)	800-232-4636
American Association of Poison Control Centers (AAPCC)	800-222-1222
American College of Clinical Pharmacy (ACCP)	913-492-3311
American Dental Association (ADA)	312-440-2500
American Medical Association (AMA)	800-621-8335
American Pharmacists Association (APhA)	202-628-4410
American Society of Health-System Pharmacists	866-279-0681
Animal Poison Control Center (24-hours)	888-426-4435
Canadian Pharmacists Association	613-523-7877
Center for Disease Control	1-800-CDC-INFO
FDA (Rare Diseases/Orphan Drugs)	301-796-8660
National Cancer Institute	1-800-4-CANCER
Asthma and Allergy Foundation of America	1-800-7-ASTHMA
Epilepsy Foundation	800-332-1000
National Council on Patient Information & Education	301-340-3940
National Institute of Health	301-496-4000
National Capital Poison Center	202-362-3867
Emergency	800-222-1222
Pediatric Pharmacy Advocacy Group (PPAG) Membership Information	901-380-3617
National Pesticide Information Center	800-858-7378
Rocky Mountain Poison Control Information	800-222-1222

PREVENTION OF INFECTIVE ENDOCARDITIS

Recommendations by the American Heart Association
(*Circulation*, 2007;116(15):1736-1754.)

The recommendations were formulated by a writing group under the auspices of the American Heart Association (AHA), and included representation from the Infectious Diseases Society of America (IDSA), the American Academy of Pediatrics (AAP), and the American Dental Association (ADA). Additionally, input was received from both national and international experts on infective endocarditis (IE). These guidelines are based on expert interpretation and review of scientific literature from 1950 through 2006. The consensus statement was subsequently reviewed by outside experts not affiliated with the writing group and by the Science Advisory and Coordinating Committee of the American Heart Association. These guidelines are meant to aid practitioners but are not intended as the standard of care or as a substitute for clinical judgment.

In a major departure from the former recommendations, the current guidelines have been greatly simplified to place a much greater emphasis on a very limited number of underlying cardiac conditions (see Table 1). These specific conditions have been associated with the highest risk of adverse outcomes due to IE. Patients should receive IE prophylaxis only if they are undergoing certain invasive procedures (see Table 2) and have at least one of the underlying cardiovascular conditions specified below.

Common situations for which routine prophylaxis was previously, but no longer recommended, include mitral valve prolapse, general dental cleanings and local anesthetic administration (noninfected tissue), and bronchoscopy (see Table 2).

Table 1. Cardiac Conditions Associated With the Highest Risk of Adverse Outcome From Endocarditis

Prophylaxis With Dental Procedures Is Recommended
Previous infective endocarditis
Prosthetic cardiac valves
Congenital heart disease (CHD)
Unrepaired cyanotic CHD, including palliative shunts and conduits
Completely repaired congenital heart defect with prosthetic material or device, whether placed by surgery or by catheter intervention, during the first 6 months after the procedure[1]
Repaired CHD with residual defects at the site or adjacent to the site of a prosthetic patch or prosthetic device (which inhibit endothelialization)
Cardiac transplantation recipients who develop cardiac valvulopathy

[1]Prophylaxis is recommended because endothelialization of prosthetic material occurs within 6 months after the procedure.

Table 2. Guidance for Use of Prophylactic Antibiotic Therapy Based on Procedure or Condition[1]

Location of Procedure	Prophylaxis Recommended	Prophylaxis NOT Recommended
Dental	All invasive manipulations of the gingival or periapical region or perforation of oral mucosa (includes biopsies, suture removal, placement of orthodontic bands)	Anesthetic injections through noninfected tissue, radiographs, placement/adjustment/removal prosthodontics/orthodontic appliances or brackets, shedding of deciduous teeth, trauma-induced bleeding from lips, gums, or oral mucosa
Respiratory tract	Biopsy/incision of respiratory mucosa (eg, tonsillectomy/adenoidectomy); drainage of abscess or empyema[2]	Bronchoscopy (unless incision of mucosa required)
Gastrointestinal (GI) or genitourinary (GU) tract	Established GI/GU infection or prevention of infectious sequelae[3]; elective cystoscopy or other urinary tract procedure with established enterococci infection/colonization[3,4]	Routine diagnostic procedures, including esophagogastroduodenoscopy or colonoscopy in the absence of active infection; vaginal delivery and hysterectomy
Skin, skin structure, or musculoskeletal	Any surgical procedure involving infected tissue	Procedures conducted in noninfected tissue; tattoos and ear/body piercing

[1]Patients should receive prophylactic antibiotic therapy if they meet the criteria for a specified procedure/condition in this table and they have a high-risk cardiovascular condition listed in the preceding text.

[2]If infection is known or suspected to be caused by *Staphylococcus aureus*, consider antistaphylococcal penicillin or cephalosporin, or vancomycin in beta-lactam-sensitive patients.

[3]Consider alternate agents with activity against enterococci (ampicillin, penicillin, piperacillin); vancomycin (for beta-lactam-sensitive patients)

[4]Eradication of enterococci from the urinary tract should be considered.

Table 3. Prophylactic Regimens for Dental Procedures

Situation	Agent	Regimen to Be Given 30 to 60 Minutes Before Procedure	
		Adults	Children[1]
Standard general prophylaxis	Amoxicillin	2000 mg P.O.	50 mg/kg P.O.
Unable to take oral medications	Ampicillin **or**	2000 mg I.M./I.V.	50 mg/kg I.M./I.V.
	CeFAZolin or cefTRIAXone	1000 mg I.M./I.V.	50 mg/kg I.M./I.V.
Allergic to penicillin	Clindamycin **or**	600 mg P.O.	20 mg/kg P.O.
	Cephalexin[2] or other dose-equivalent first/second generation cephalosporin[2] **or**	2000 mg P.O	50 mg/kg P.O.
	Azithromycin or clarithromycin	500 mg P.O.	15 mg/kg P.O.
Allergic to penicillin and unable to take oral medications	Clindamycin **or**	600 mg I.M./I.V.	20 mg/kg I.M./I.V.
	CeFAZolin[2] or cefTRIAXone[2]	1000 mg I.M./I.V.	50 mg/kg I.M./I.V.

[1]Total children's dose should not exceed adult dose.

[2]Cephalosporins should not be used in individuals with immediate-type hypersensitivity reaction (urticaria, angioedema, or anaphylaxis) to penicillins.

Gastrointestinal/Genitourinary/Respiratory Procedures and Surgery Involving Skin, Skin Structure, or Musculoskeletal Tissue

In general, antibiotic prophylaxis solely to prevent IE is **not** recommended in patients undergoing GI/GU procedures or surgery involving skin, skin structure, or musculoskeletal tissue, unless infection is present at the site where the procedure is to occur. For patients with conditions listed in Table 1 undergoing an invasive respiratory tract procedure to treat an established infection (eg, drainage of an abscess or empyema) and the infection is known or suspected to be caused by *Staphlococcus aureus* (*S. aureus*), an antistaphlococcal penicillin or cephalosporin is recommended. In those patients with infections of the GI or GU tract undergoing GI/GU procedures, it may be reasonable to administer an agent with activity against enterococci (eg, ampicillin, penicillin, piperacillin); amoxicillin or ampicillin is preferred. In patients with a condition listed in Table 1 undergoing surgery involving infected skin, skin structure, or musculoskeletal tissue, it is reasonable that the regimen contain an agent with activity against staphylococci and beta-hemolytic streptococci (eg, antistaphlococcal penicillin or cephalosporin). In any case, vancomycin (or clindamycin in the setting of infected skin, skin structure, or musculoskeletal tissue) may be administered to patients unable to tolerate a beta-lactam (eg, ampicillin). Vancomycin should be administered with any infection known or suspected to be caused by a methicillin-resistant *S. aureus*.

Table 4. Vancomycin Dosing

	Dosage for Adults	Dosage for Children
Vancomyin	1000 mg I.V. infused **slowly over 1 hour**; complete infusion within 30 minutes before procedure	20 mg/kg (maximum: 1000 mg) I.V. infused **slowly over 1 hour**; complete infusion within 30 minutes before procedure

If infection is caused by a known or suspected strain of resistant enterococcus, consult with an infectious diseases expert.

REFERENCE

Wilson W, Taubert KA, Gewitz M, et al. Prevention of infective endocarditis. Guidelines from the American Heart Association. A guideline from the American Heart Association Rheumatic Fever, Endocarditis, and Kawasaki Disease Committee, Council on Cardiovascular Disease in the Young, and the Council on Clinical Cardiology, Council on Cardiovascular Surgery and Anesthesia, and the Quality of Care and Outcomes Research Interdisciplinary Working Group. *Circulation*. 2007;116(15):1736-1754.

PEDIATRIC HIV

Selected information from: The Panel on Antiretroviral Therapy and Medical Management of HIV-Infected Children. Guidelines for the use of antiretroviral agents in pediatric HIV infection. February 12, 2014. Available at http://aidsinfo.nih.gov/contentfiles/PediatricGuidelines.pdf

1994 Revised Human Immunodeficiency Virus (HIV) Pediatric Classification System: Immune Categories Based on Age-Specific CD4 T cell and Percentage[1]

Immune Category	<12 mo		1 to 5 y		6 to 12 y	
	No./mm^3	%	No./mm^3	%	No./mm^3	%
Category 1 no suppression	≥1500	≥25	≥1000	≥25	≥500	≥25
Category 2 moderate suppression	750 to 1499	15 to 24	500 to 999	15 to 24	200 to 499	15 to 24
Category 3 severe suppression	<750	<15	<500	<15	<200	<15

[1]Modified from: Centers of Disease Control and Prevention (CDC). 1994 revised classification system for human immunodeficiency virus infection in children less than 13 years of age. *MMWR*. 1994;43(RR-12):1-10.

1994 REVISED HIV PEDIATRIC (<13 YEARS OF AGE) CLASSIFICATION SYSTEM: CLINICAL CATEGORIES

Category N: Not Symptomatic

Children who have no signs or symptoms considered to be the result of HIV infection or who have only **one** of the conditions listed in category A

Category A: Mildly Symptomatic

Children with **two** or more of the following conditions, but none of the conditions listed in categories B and C:

- Lymphadenopathy (≥0.5 cm at more than two sites; bilateral = one site)
- Hepatomegaly
- Splenomegaly
- Dermatitis
- Parotitis
- Recurrent or persistent upper respiratory infection, sinusitis, or otitis media

Category B: Moderately Symptomatic

Children who have symptomatic conditions attributed to HIV infection, other than those listed for category A or category C. Examples of conditions in clinical category B include, but are not limited to the following:

- Anemia (<8 g/dL), neutropenia (<1000/mm^3), or thrombocytopenia (<100,000/mm^3) persisting ≥30 days
- Bacterial meningitis, pneumonia, or sepsis (single episode)
- Candidiasis, oropharyngeal (ie, thrush) persisting for >2 months in children aged >6 months
- Cardiomyopathy
- Cytomegalovirus infection with onset before age 1 month
- Diarrhea, recurrent or chronic
- Hepatitis
- Herpes simplex virus (HSV) stomatitis, recurrent (ie, more than two episodes within 1 year)
- HSV bronchitis, pneumonitis, or esophagitis with onset before age 1 month
- Herpes zoster (ie, shingles) involving at least two distinct episodes or more than one dermatome
- Leiomyosarcoma
- Lymphoid interstitial pneumonia (LIP) or pulmonary lymphoid hyperplasia complex
- Nephropathy
- Nocardiosis
- Fever lasting >1 month
- Toxoplasmosis with onset before age 1 month
- Varicella, disseminated (ie, complicated chickenpox)

Category C: Severely Symptomatic

Children who have any condition listed in the 1987 surveillance case definition for acquired immunodeficiency syndrome (below), with the exception of LIP (which is a category B condition).

- Serious bacterial infections, multiple or recurrent (ie, any combination of at least two culture confirmed infections within a 2-year period), of the following types: Septicemia, pneumonia, meningitis, bone or joint infection, or abscess of an internal organ or body cavity (excluding otitis media, superficial skin or mucosal abscesses, and indwelling catheter-related infections)

- Candidiasis, esophageal or pulmonary (bronchi, trachea, lungs)

- Coccidioidomycosis, disseminated (at site other than or in addition to lungs or cervical or hilar lymph nodes)

- Cryptococcosis, extrapulmonary

- Cryptosporidiosis or isosporiasis with diarrhea persisting >1 month

- Cytomegalovirus disease with onset of symptoms at age >1 month (at site other than liver, spleen, or lymph nodes)

- Encephalopathy (at least one of the following progressive findings present for at least 2 months in the absence of a concurrent illness other than HIV infection that could explain the findings):

  – Failure to attain or loss of developmental milestones or loss of intellectual ability, verified by standard developmental scale or neuropsychological tests;

  – Impaired brain growth or acquired microcephaly demonstrated by head circumference measurements or brain atrophy demonstrated by CT or MRI (serial imaging is required for children <2 years of age);

  – Acquired symmetric motor deficit manifested by two or more of the following: Paresis, pathologic reflexes, ataxia, or gait disturbance

- HSV infection causing a mucocutaneous ulcer that persist for >1 month; or bronchitis, pneumonitis, or esophagitis for any duration affecting a child >1 month of age

- Histoplasmosis, disseminated (at site other than or in addition to lungs or cervical or hilar lymph nodes)

- Kaposi's sarcoma

- Lymphoma, primary, in brain

- Lymphoma, small, noncleaved cell (Burkitt's), or immunoblastic or large cell lymphoma of B-cell or unknown immunologic phenotype

- Mycobacterium tuberculosis, disseminated or extrapulmonary

- Mycobacterium, other species or unidentified species, disseminated (at site other than or in addition to lungs, skin, or cervical or hilar lymph nodes)

- *Mycobacterium avium* complex or *Mycobacterium kansasii*, disseminated (at site other than or in addition to lungs, skin, or cervical lymph nodes)

- *Pneumocystis jiroveci* pneumonia

- Progressive multifocal leukoencephalopathy

- Salmonella (nontyphoid) septicemia, recurrent

- Toxoplasmosis of the brain with onset at >1 month of age

- Wasting syndrome in the absence of a concurrent illness other than HIV infection that could explain the following findings:

  – Persistent weight loss >10% of baseline; **OR**

  – Downward crossing of at least two of the following percentile lines on the weight-for-age chart (eg, 95th, 75th, 50th, 25th, 5th) in a child ≥1 year of age; **OR**

  – <5th percentile on weight-for-height chart on two consecutive measurements, ≥30 days apart **PLUS**

    - Chronic diarrhea (ie, ≥two loose stools per day for >30 days); **OR**

    - Documented fever (for ≥30 days, intermittent or constant)

REFERENCE

Centers for Disease Control and Prevention (CDC). 1994 revised classification system for human immunodeficiency virus infection in children less than 13 years of age. *MMWR*. 1994;43(RR-12):1-10.

INDICATIONS FOR INITIATION OF ANTIRETROVIRAL THERAPY IN HIV-INFECTED CHILDREN

This table provides general guidance rather than absolute recommendations for an individual patient. Factors to be considered in decisions about initiation of therapy include the risk of disease progression as determined by CD4 percentage or count and plasma HIV RNA copy number, the potential benefits and risks of therapy, and the ability of the caregiver to adhere to administration of the therapeutic regimen. Issues associated with adherence should be fully assessed, discussed, and addressed with the caregiver and child, if age-appropriate, before the decision to initiate therapy is made.

Patients/caregivers may choose to postpone therapy, and on a case-by-case basis, providers may elect to defer therapy based on clinical and/or psychosocial factors. Children in whom antiretroviral therapy is deferred need close follow-up. Factors to consider in deciding when to initiate therapy in children in whom treatment was deferred include: Increasing HIV RNA levels (such as HIV RNA levels approaching 100,000 copies/mL); CD4 cell count or percentage values approaching the age-related threshold for treatment; development of clinical symptoms; and the ability of caregiver and child to adhere to the prescribed regimen.

Age/Criteria	Recommendation
<12 months	
• Regardless of clinical symptoms, immune status, or viral load	Treat
1 to <3 years	
• AIDS or significant HIV-related symptoms[a]	Treat
• CD4 cell count <1000 cells/mm^3 or CD4 percentage <25%[b]	Treat
• Asymptomatic or mild symptoms[c] **and** CD4 cell count ≥1000 cells/mm^3 or CD4 percentage ≥25%	Consider treatment
3 to <5 years	
• AIDS or significant HIV-related symptoms[a]	Treat
• CD4 cell count <750 cells/mm^3 or CD4 percentage <25%[b]	Treat
• Asymptomatic or mild symptoms[c] **and** CD4 cell count ≥750 cells/mm^3 or CD4 percentage ≥25%	Consider treatment
≥5 years	
• AIDS or significant HIV-related symptoms[a]	Treat
• CD4 cell count ≤500 cells/mm^{3b}	Treat[d]
• Asymptomatic or mild symptoms[c] **and** CD4 cell count >500 cells/mm^3	Consider treatment
All ages	
• HIV RNA levels >100,000 copies/mL[e]	Treat

[a]CDC clinical category C and B (except for the following category B condition: Single episode of serious bacterial infection)

[b]Laboratory data should be confirmed with a second test to meet the treatment criteria before initiation of antiretroviral therapy

[c]CDC clinical category A or N or the following category B condition: Single episode of serious bacterial infection

[d]The guidelines recommend treatment for patients in this group when CD4 cell count is ≤500 cells/mm^3; rating of evidence is strongest for treatment when CD4 cell count is <350 cells/mm^3

[e]To avoid overinterpretation of temporary blips in viral load (eg, which can occur during intercurrent illnesses), plasma HIV RNA level >100,000 copies/mL should be confirmed by a second level before initiating antiretroviral therapy.

ANTIRETROVIRAL REGIMENS RECOMMENDED FOR INITIAL THERAPY FOR HIV INFECTION IN CHILDREN

A combination antiretroviral regimen in treatment-naïve children generally contains 1 NNRTI plus a 2-NRTI backbone or 1 PI (generally with low-dose ritonavir boosting) plus a 2-NRTI backbone. Regimens should be individualized based on advantages and disadvantages of each combination.

Preferred Regimen

Children ≥14 days and <3 years of age[1]	2 NRTIs **plus** lopinavir/ritonavir
Children ≥3 years to <6 years of age	2 NRTIs **plus** efavirenz[2] 2 NRTIs **plus** lopinavir/ritonavir
Children ≥6 years of age	2 NRTIs **plus** atazanavir **plus** low-dose ritonavir 2 NRTIs **plus** efavirenz[2] 2 NRTIs **plus** lopinavir/ritonavir

Alternative Regimens

Children >14 days of age	2 NRTIs **plus** nevirapine[3]
Children ≥3 years to <12 years of age	2 NRTIs **plus** twice-daily darunavir **plus** low-dose ritonavir
Children ≥12 years of age	2 NRTIs **plus** once-daily darunavir **plus** low-dose ritonavir[4]

Regimens for Use in Special Circumstances

Children ≥6 months of age[5]	2 NRTIs **plus** fosamprenavir **plus** low-dose ritonavir
Children ≥2 years of age	2 NRTIs **plus** nelfinavir 2 NRTIs **plus** raltegravir
Children ≥12 years of age	2 NRTIs **plus** dolutegravir
Treatment-naïve adolescents ≥13 years of age and weighing >39 kg	2 NRTIs **plus** atazanavir unboosted

Preferred 2-NRTI Backbone Options for Use in Combination With Additional Drugs

Children of any age	Zidovudine **plus** (lamiVUDine **or** emtricitabine)
Children ≥3 months of age	Abacavir **plus** (lamiVUDine **or** emtricitabine) Zidovudine **plus** (lamiVUDine **or** emtricitabine)
Adolescents at Tanner stage 4 or 5	Abacavir **plus** (lamiVUDine **or** emtricitabine) Tenofovir **plus** (lamiVUDine **or** emtricitabine) Zidovudine **plus** (lamiVUDine **or** emtricitabine)

Alternative 2-NRTI Backbone Options for Use in Combination With Additional Drugs

Children ≥2 weeks of age	Didanosine **plus** (lamiVUDine **or** emtricitabine) Zidovudine **plus** didanosine
Children ≥3 months of age	Zidovudine **plus** abacavir
Children at Tanner stage 3 and Adolescents	Tenofovir **plus** (lamiVUDine **or** emtricitabine)

2-NRTI Backbone Options for Use in Special Circumstances

	Stavudine **plus** (lamiVUDine **or** emtricitabine) Tenofovir **plus** (lamiVUDine **or** emtricitabine) (prepubertal children ≥2 years of age and adolescents, Tanner stage 1 or 2)

NRTI = nucleoside analogue reverse transcriptase inhibitor, NNRTI = non-nucleoside analogue reverse transcriptase inhibitor, PI = protease inhibitor

[1]Lopinavir/ritonavir should not be administered to neonates before a postmenstrual age (first day of the mother's last menstrual period to birth plus the time elapsed after birth) of 42 weeks and a postnatal age of at least 14 days.

[2]Efavirenz should only be used in children ≥3 months of age with weight ≥3.5 kg but is not recommended as initial therapy in children ≥3 months to 3 years of age. Unless adequate contraception can be assured, efavirenz-based therapy is not recommended for adolescent females who are sexually active and may become pregnant.

[3]Nevirapine should not be used in postpubertal girls with CD4 count >250/mm^3, unless the benefit clearly outweighs the risk. Nevirapine is FDA approved for treatment of infants ≥15 days of age.

[4]Darunavir once daily should not be used if resistance-associated substitutions are present (V11I, V32I, L33F, I47V, I50V, I54L, I54M, T74P, L76V, I84V, and L89V).

[5]Fosamprenavir with low-dose ritonavir should only be administered to infants born at ≥38 weeks GA who have attained a PNA of 28 days and to infants born before 38 weeks GA who have reached a PMA of 42 weeks.

Antiretroviral Regimens or Components Not Recommended for Initial Treatment of HIV Infection in Children

Regimen or Antiretroviral Component	Rationale for Being Not Recommended
Unboosted atazanavir-containing regimens in children <13 years of age and/or <39 kg	Reduced exposure
Darunavir-based regimens once-daily in children ≥3 years to <12 years of age	Insufficient data to recommend
Unboosted darunavir	Use without ritonavir has not been studied
Dual (full-dose) PI regimens	Insufficient data to recommend
Dual NRTI combination of abacavir **plus** didanosine	Insufficient data to recommend
Dual NRTI combination of abacavir **plus** tenofovir	Insufficient data to recommend
Dual NRTI combination of stavudine **plus** didanosine	Significant toxicities
Dual NRTI combination of tenofovir **plus** didanosine	Increase in concentrations; high rate of virologic failure
Efavirenz-based regimens for children <3 years of age	Appropriate dose not determined
Enfuvirtide (T-20)-containing regimens	Insufficient data to recommend; injectable preparation
Etravirine-based regimens	Insufficient data to recommend
Elvitegravir-based regimens	Insufficient data to recommend
Fosamprenavir without ritonavir boosting	Reduced exposure; medication burden
Indinavir-based regimens	Renal toxicities
Once-daily lopinavir/ritonavir	Reduced drug exposure
Maraviroc-based regimens	Insufficient data to recommend
Nelfinavir-containing regimens for children <2 years of age	Appropriate dose not determined
Regimens containing only NRTIs	Inferior virologic efficacy
Regimens containing three drug classes	Insufficient data to recommend
Full-dose ritonavir or use of ritonavir as the sole PI	GI intolerance; metabolic toxicity
Regimens containing three NRTIs and an NNRTI	Insufficient data to recommend
Rilpivirine-based regimens	Insufficient data to recommend
Saquinavir-based regimens	Limited dosing and outcome data burden
Tenofovir-containing regimens in children <2 years of age	Potential bone toxicity; appropriate dose has yet to be determined
Tipranavir-based regimens	Increased dose of ritonavir for boosting; reported cases of intracranial hemorrhage

NNRTI = non-nucleoside analogue reverse transcriptase inhibitor, NRTI = nucleoside analogue reverse transcriptase inhibitor, PI = protease inhibitor

Antiretroviral Regimens or Components That Should Never Be Recommended for Treatment of HIV Infection in Children

	Rationale	Exception
Antiretroviral Regimens Never Recommended for Children		
One antiretroviral drug alone (monotherapy)	• Rapid development of resistance	HIV-exposed infants (with negative viral testing) during 6-week period of prophylaxis to prevent perinatal transmission
	• Inferior antiretroviral activity compared to combination with ≥3 antiretroviral drugs	LamiVUDine or emtricitabine interim "bridging regimen" in special circumstances of children with treatment failure associated with drug resistance and persistent nonadherence
Two NRTIs alone	• Rapid development of resistance	Not recommended for initial therapy; for patients currently on this treatment, some clinicians may opt to continue if virologic goals are achieved
	• Inferior antiretroviral activity compared to combination with ≥3 antiretroviral drugs	
Tenofovir **plus** abacavir **plus** lamiVUDine **or** emtricitabine as triple NRTI regimen	High rate of early virologic failure when this triple NRTI regimen used as initial therapy in treatment-naïve adults	No exception
Tenofovir **plus** didanosine **plus** lamiVUDine **or** emtricitabine as triple NRTI regimen	High rate of early virologic failure when this triple NRTI regimen used as initial therapy in treatment-naïve adults	No exception
Antiretroviral Components Never Recommended as Part of Antiretroviral Regimen for Children		
Atazanavir **plus** indinavir	Potential additive hyperbilirubinemia	No exception
Dual NNRTI combinations	Enhanced toxicity	No exception
Dual NRTI combinations:		
LamiVUDine **plus** emtricitabine	Similar resistance profile and no additive benefit	No exception
Stavudine **plus** zidovudine	Antagonistic effect on HIV	No exception
Efavirenz in 1st trimester of pregnancy or in sexually active adolescent girls of childbearing potential when reliable contraception cannot be ensured	Potential for teratogenicity	When no other antiretroviral option is available and potential benefits outweigh risks
Nevirapine in adolescent girls with CD4$^+$ T-cell count >250 cells/mm^3 or adolescent boys with CD4$^+$ T-cell count >400 cells/mm^3	Increased incidence of symptomatic (including serious and potentially fatal) hepatic events in these patient groups	Only if benefit clearly outweighs the risk
Unboosted saquinavir, darunavir, or tipranavir	• Poor oral bioavailability	No exception
	• Inferior virologic activity compared to other protease inhibitors	

NNRTI = non-nucleoside analogue reverse transcriptase inhibitor, NRTI = nucleoside analogue reverse transcriptase inhibitor

DEFINITIONS OF TREATMENT FAILURE IN HIV-INFECTED CHILDREN

Virologic Failure[1]

- **Incomplete viral response to therapy:**

    Incomplete virologic response to therapy is defined for all children as a plasma HIV RNA >200 copies/mL after 6 months of therapy, or repeated HIV RNA above the level of quantification using the most sensitive assay after 12 months of therapy.

    Occassionally, infants with higher plasma HIV RNA levels at initiation of therapy may take longer to reach undetectable viral load. HIV-infected adults with HIV RNA detectable above the level of quantification but <200 copies/mL after 6 months of continuous antiretroviral therapy often ultimately achieve virologic suppression without regimen change.

- **Viral rebound:**
    Viral rebound is defined as repeated detection of plasma HIV RNA above the level of quantification after a child had achieved virologic suppression in response to therapy. Isolated episodes of plasma HIV RNA detection above the level of quantification but <500 copies/mL, followed by return to viral suppression (often called "blips"), are common and not generally reflective of virologic failure. However, repeated or persistent viremia (especially if >500 copies/mL) after having achieved virologic suppression usually represents viral rebound.

Immunologic Failure[2]

- **Incomplete immunologic response to therapy:** Failure to maintain or achieve a CD4 cell count or percentage that is at least above the age-specific range for severe immunodeficiency. Some experts define as a failure by a child <5 years old with severe immune suppression (CD4 percentage <15%) to increase CD4 percentage by ≥5 percentage points or a failure by a child ≥5 years old with severe immune suppression (CD4 <200 cells/mm^3), to increase absolute CD4 values by ≥50 cells/mm^3 above baseline within the first year of therapy.

- **Immunologic decline:** Sustained decline of 5 percentage points in CD4 percentage below pretherapy baseline in any age, or decline to below pretherapy baseline in CD4 absolute cell count in children who are ≥5 years old.[3]

Clinical Failure

- **Progressive neurodevelopmental deterioration:** Two or more of the following on repeated assessments:
  - Impairment in brain growth
  - Decline of cognitive function documented by psychometric testing
  - Clinical motor dysfunction
- **Growth failure:** Persistent decline in weight-growth velocity despite adequate nutritional support and without other explanation
- **Severe or recurrent infection or illness:** Recurrence or persistence of AIDS-defining conditions or other serious infections

[1]**Virologic suppression** is defined as having plasma HIV RNA below the level of quantification using the most sensitive assay (<20 to 75 copies/mL). Older assays with lower limits of 200 or 400 copies/mL are not recommended.
[2]At least two measurements (taken 1 week apart) should be performed before considering a change in therapy.
[3]Declines that represent a change to a more advanced category of immunosuppression compared to baseline (eg, from CD4 percentage of 28% to 23%, or from CD4 count of 250 cells/mm³ to 150 cells/mm³) or to more severe immunosuppression in those already suppressed at baseline (eg, from CD4 percentage of 14% to 9%, or from CD4 count of 150 cells/mm³ to 100 cells/mm³) are of particular concern.

Assessment of Causes of Virologic Antiretroviral Treatment Failure

Assessment	Assessment Method	Intervention

Nonadherence	1. Interview child and caretaker
	• 24-hour or 7-day recall
	• Description of:
	  – WHO gives medication
	  – WHAT is given (names, doses)
	  – WHERE medications are kept, administered
	  – WHEN they are taken/given
	  – HOW medications make child feel
	• Conduct open-ended discussion of experiences taking/giving medications and barriers/challenges
		Identify or re-engage family members to support/supervise adherence.
		
		Establish fixed daily times and routines for medication administration.
		
		Avoid confusion with drug names by explaining that drug therapies have generic names, trade names, and many agents are coformulated under a third or fourth name.
		
		Explore opportunities for facility or home-based DOT.

	2. Review pharmacy records • Assess timeliness of refills	
	3. Observe medication administration • Observe dosing/administration in clinic • Home-based observation by visiting health professional • Hospital admission for trial of therapy – Observe administration/tolerance monitor treatment response	Simplify medication regimen if feasible. Substitute new agents if single ARV is poorly tolerated. Consider gastric tube placement to facilitate adherence. Consider DOT Utilization of tools to simplify administration (pill boxes, reminders including alarms, integrated medication packaging for AM or PM dosing, others). Relaxation techniques.

	4. Psychosocial assessment
	• Comprehensive family-focused assessment of factors likely to impact on adherence with particular attention toward recent changes:
	  – Status of caregiver, financial stability, housing, child/caretaker relationships
	  – School and achievement
	  – Substance abuse (child, caretaker, family members)
	  – Mental health and behavior
	  – Child/youth and caretaker beliefs toward antiretroviral therapy
	  – Disclosure status (to child and others)
	  – Peer pressure
		Address competing needs through appropriate social services.
		
		Address and treat concomitant mental illness and behavioral disorders. Initiate disclosure discussions with family/child.
		
		Consider need for child protection services and alternate care settings when necessary.

Pharmacokinetics and Dosing Issues	1. Recalculate doses for individual medications using weight or body surface area. 2. Identify concomitant medications including prescription, over-the-counter, and recreational substances; assess for drug-drug interactions. 3. Consider drug levels for specific antiretroviral drugs	Adjust drug doses. Discontinue or substitute competing medications. Reinforce applicable food restrictions.
Antiretroviral Resistance Testing	1. Perform genotypic and phenotypic resistance assays 2. Perform tropism assay, as appropriate.	If no resistance detected to current drugs, focus on improving adherence. If resistance to current regimen detected, optimize adherence and evaluate potential for new regimen.

Options for Regimens With at Least Two Fully Active Agents With Goal of Virologic Suppression in Patients With Failed Antiretroviral Therapy and Evidence of Viral Resistance[1]

Prior Regimen	Recommended Change (in order of relative preference)[1]
2 NRTIs + NNRTI	• 2 NRTIs + PI
	• 2 NRTIs + integrase inhibitor
2 NRTIs + PI	• 2 NRTIs + NNRTI
	• 2 NRTIs + different ritonavir-boosted PI
	• 2 NRTIs + integrase inhibitor
	• NRTI(s) + integrase inhibitor + (NNRTI or different ritonavir-boosted PI)
3 NRTIs	• 2 NRTIs + (NNRTI or PI)
	• 2 NRTIs + integrase inhibitor
	• Integrase inhibitor + 2 other active agents [chosen from NNRTI, PI, NRTI(s)]
Failed regimen(s) that included NRTI(s), NNRTI(s), and PI(s)	• 1 NRTI + ritonavir-boosted PI
	• NRTI(s) + ritonavir-boosted PI + integrase inhibitor [consider adding enfuvirtide and/or maraviroc[2] if additional active drug(s) are needed]
	• NRTI(s) + ritonavir-boosted darunavir, lopinavir, or saquinavir + etravirine [consider adding one or more of maraviroc[2], enfuvirtide, or integrase inhibitor if additional active drug(s) are needed]
	• >1 NRTI + 2 ritonavir-boosted PIs (lopinavir/ritonavir + saquinavir or lopinavir/ritonavir + atazanavir) [consider adding enfuvirtide or an integrase inhibitor if additional active drug(s) are needed]

[1]Antiretroviral therapy regimens should be chosen based on treatment history and drug-resistance testing to optimize antiretroviral drug effectiveness in the subsequent regimen. This is particularly important in selecting NRTI components of an NNRTI-based regimen where drug resistance may occur rapidly to the NNRTI if the virus is not sufficiently sensitive to the NRTIs. Regimens should contain at least two, but preferably three, fully active drugs for durable, potent virologic suppression. Please see individual drug monographs for information about drug interactions and dose adjustment when designing a regimen for children with multiclass drug resistance. Collaboration with a pediatric HIV specialist is especially important when choosing regimens for children with multiclass drug resistance. Regimens in this table are listed in relative order of preference and are provided as examples, but this list in not exhaustive.

[2]No current Food and Drug Administration (FDA)-approved pediatric indication for maraviroc

ROLE OF THERAPEUTIC DRUG MONITORING IN MANAGEMENT OF PEDIATRIC HIV INFECTION[1]

Evaluation of antiretroviral drug plasma concentrations is not routinely required in the management of pediatric HIV but should be considered in children receiving combination antiretroviral therapy in the following scenarios:

- Use of antiretroviral drugs with limited pharmacokinetic data and therapeutic experience in children (eg, for use of efavirenz in children <3 years of age and darunavir with once-daily dosing in children <12 years of age)
- Significant drug-drug interactions and food-drug interactions
- Unexpected suboptimal treatment response (eg, lack of virologic suppression with history of medical adherence and lack of resistance mutations)
- Suspected suboptimal absorption of the drug
- Suspected dose-dependent toxicity

Evaluation of the genetic G516T polymorphism of drug metabolizing enzyme cytochrome P450 (CYP450) 2B6 in combination with the evaluation of plasma efavirenz concentrations is recommended for children <3 years of age receiving efavirenz due to significant association of this polymorphism with efavirenz concentrations.

[1]See table in the Adult and Adolescent HIV on page 2348 appendix piece for "Suggested Minimum Target Trough Concentrations" of antiretroviral drugs

ANTIRETROVIRAL DRUG RESISTANCE TESTING

- Antiretroviral drug resistance testing is recommended at the times of HIV diagnosis, before initiation of therapy, in all treatment-naïve patients. Genotypic resistance testing is preferred for this purpose.
- Antiretroviral drug resistance testing is recommended prior to changing therapy for treatment failure.
- Resistance testing in the setting of virological failure should be obtained while the patient is still on the failing regimen, or within 4 weeks of discontinuation of the regimen.
- Phenotypic resistance testing should be used (usually in addition to genotypic resistance testing) for patients with known or suspected complex drug resistance mutation patterns, which generally arise after virologic failure of successive antiretroviral therapy regimens.
- The absence of detectable resistance to a drug does not ensure that its use will be successful, especially if it shares cross-resistance with drugs previously used. In addition, current resistance assays are not sensitive enough to fully exclude the presence of resistant virus. Thus, the history of past antiretroviral use and previous resistance test results must be reviewed when making decisions regarding the choice of new agents for patients with virologic failure.

- Viral Coreceptor (tropism) assays should be used whenever the use of a CCR5 antagonist is being considered. Tropism assays should also be considered for patients who demonstrate virologic failure while receiving therapy that contains a CCR5 antagonist.

- Consultation with a pediatric HIV specialist is recommended for interpretation of resistance assays when considering initiating or changing an antiretroviral regimen in a pediatric patient.

STRATEGIES TO IMPROVE ADHERENCE TO ANTIRETROVIRAL MEDICATION REGIMENS IN CHILDREN

Initial Intervention Strategies

- Establish trust and identify mutually acceptable goals for care with patient and caregiver.

- Obtain explicit agreement on need for treatment and adherence with patient and caregiver.

- Identify depression, low self-esteem, substance abuse, or other mental health issues for the child/adolescent and/or caregiver that may decrease adherence. Treat prior to starting therapy, if possible.

- Identify family, friends, health team members, or others who can help with adherence support.

- Educate patient and family about the critical role of adherence in therapy outcome.

- Specify the adherence target: ≥95% of prescribed doses.

- Educate patient and family about the relationship between partial adherence and resistance.

- Educate patient and family about resistance and constraint of later choices of antiretroviral drug; explain that while a failure of adherence may be temporary, the effects on treatment choice may be permanent.

- Develop a treatment plan that the patient and family understand and to which they feel committed.

- Establish readiness to take medication by practice sessions or other means.

- For patient education and to assess tolerability of medications chosen, consider a brief period of hospitalization at start of therapy in selected circumstances.

Medication Strategies

- Choose the simplest regimen possible, reducing dosing frequency and number of pills.

- Choose a regimen with dosing requirements that best conform to daily and weekly routines and variations in patient and family activities.

- Choose the most palatable medicine possible (pharmacists may be able to add syrups or flavoring agents to increase palatability).

- Choose drugs with the fewest side effects; provide anticipatory guidance for management of side effects.

- Simplify food requirements for medication administration.

- Prescribe drugs carefully to avoid adverse drug-drug interactions.

- Assess pill swallowing capacity and offer pill-swallowing training.

Follow-up Intervention Strategies

- Monitor adherence at each visit, as well as in between visits by telephone or letter as needed.

- Provide ongoing support, encouragement, and understanding of the difficulties of the demands of attaining 95% adherence with medication doses.

- Use patient education aids including pictures, calendars, and stickers.

- Encourage use of pillboxes, reminders, alarms, pagers, and timers.

- Provide follow-up clinic visits, telephone calls, and SMS text messages to support and assess adherence.

- Provide access to support groups, peer groups, or one-on-one counseling for caregivers and patients especially for those with known depression or drug use issues, which are known to decrease adherence.

- Provide pharmacist-based adherence support, such as medication education counseling, blister packs, refill reminders, automatic refills, and home delivery of medications.

- Consider directly observed therapy (DOT) at home, in the clinic, or in select circumstances, during a brief inpatient hospitalization.

- Consider gastrostomy tube use in selected circumstances.

Modifying Antiretroviral Regimens in Children With Sustained Virologic Suppression on Antiretroviral Therapy

For children who have sustained virologic suppression on their current regimen, changing to a new antiretroviral regimen with improved pill burden or tolerance should be considered in order to facilitate continued adherence and increase safety.

Examples of Changes in Antiretroviral Regimen Components That Are Made for Reasons of Simplification, Convenience, and Safety Profile in Children Who Have Sustained Virologic Suppression on Their Current Regimen

Antiretroviral Drug(s)	Current Age	Body Size Attained	Potential Antiretroviral Regimen Change	Comment
Zidovudine or didanosine (or stavudine)	≥1 year	N/A	Abacavir	Once-daily dosing; less long-term mitochondrial toxicity
Abacavir twice daily	≥1 year	Any	Abacavir once daily	
Lopinavir/ritonavir	≥1 year	≥3 kg	Raltegravir	Better palatability; less adverse lipid effect
Lopinavir/ritonavir twice daily	≥3 years	N/A	Efavirenz	Once-daily dosing; better palatability; less adverse lipid effect
Lopinavir/ritonavir twice daily	≥6 years	15 kg	Ritonavir-boosted atazanavir	Once-daily dosing; lower pill burden; less adverse lipid effect
Zidovudine or didanosine	Adolescence	Pubertal maturity (Tanner stage IV or V)	Tenofovir or abacavir	Once-daily dosing; less long-term mitochondrial toxicity; coformulation with other ARVs can further reduce pill burden
Lopinavir/ritonavir twice daily	≥12 years	40 kg	Ritonavir-boosted darunavir	Once-daily dosing possible; lower pill burden
Any	Adolescence	Pubertal maturity (Tanner stage IV or V)	Co-formulated: • Tenofovir/emtricitabine/efavirenz (Atripla) • Elvitegravir/cobicistat/emtricitabine/tenofovir (Stribild) • Emtricitabine/rilpivirine/tenofovir (Complera)	Once-daily dosing; single pill; alignment with adult regimens

ADULT AND ADOLESCENT HIV

Selected information from the Panel on Antiretroviral Guidelines for Adults and Adolescents. Guidelines for the use of antiretroviral agents in HIV-1-infected adults and adolescents. Department of Health and Human Services. May 1, 2014. Available at http://www.aidsinfo.nih.gov/ContentFiles/AdultandAdolescentGL.pdf

Goals of HIV Therapy and Strategies to Achieve Them

Goals of Therapy

- Maximal and durable suppression of viral load
- Restoration and/or preservation of immunologic function
- Improvement of quality of life
- Reduction of HIV-related morbidity and mortality
- Prevention of HIV transmission

Strategies to Achieve Goals of Therapy

- Rational sequencing of drugs
- Preservation of future treatment options
- Selection of appropriate combination therapy
- Maximize adherence to the antiretroviral regimen
- Optimize initial regimen with use of pretreatment genotypic drug resistance testing
- Optimize antiretroviral regimen with use of therapeutic drug monitoring in selected clinical settings

Recommendations on the Indications and Frequency of Viral Load and CD4 Count Monitoring[1]

Clinical Scenario	Viral Load Monitoring	CD4 Count Monitoring
Before initiating ART	At entry into care. If ART initiation is deferred, repeat viral load before initiating ART. In patients not initiating ART, repeat testing is optional	At entry into care. If ART is deferred, repeat CD4 count every 3 to 6 months[2]
After initiating ART	Preferably within 2 to 4 weeks (and no later than 8 weeks) after initiation of ART; thereafter, repeat every 4 to 8 weeks until viral load is suppressed	3 months after initiation of ART
After modifying ART because of drug toxicities or for regimen simplification in a patient with viral suppression	4 to 8 weeks after modification of ART to confirm effectiveness of new regimen	Monitor according to prior CD4 count and duration on ART, as outlined below
After modifying ART because of virologic failure	Preferably within 2 to 4 weeks (but no later than 8 weeks) after modification; thereafter, repeat every 4 to 8 weeks until viral load is suppressed. If viral suppression is not possible, repeat viral load every 3 months or more frequently if indicated	Every 3 to 6 months
During the first 2 years of ART	Every 3 to 4 months	Every 3 to 6 months[1]
After 2 years of ART (viral load consistently suppressed, CD4 consistently 300 to 500 cells/mm³)	Can extend to every 6 months for patients with consistent viral suppression for ≥2 years	Every 12 months
After 2 years of ART (viral load consistently suppressed, CD4 consistently >500 cells/mm³)	Can extend to every 6 months for patients with consistent viral suppression for ≥2 years	Optional
While on ART with detectable viremia (viral load repeatedly >200 copies/mL)	Every 3 months or more frequently if clinical indicated	Every 3 to 6 months
Change in clinical status (eg, new HIV clinical symptom or initiation of interferon, chronic systemic corticosteroids, or antineoplastic therapy	Every 3 months	Perform CD4 count and repeat ad clinically indicated[3]

ART = antiretroviral therapy

[1]Monitoring of lymphocyte subsets other than CD4 (eg, CD8, CD19) has not proven clinically useful, adds to costs, and is not routinely recommended

[2]Some experts may repeat CD4 count every 3 months in patients with low baseline CD4 count (<200 to 300 cells/mm³) before ART but every 6 months in those who initiated ART at higher CD4 cell count (eg, >300 cells/mm³)

[3]The following are examples of clinically indicated scenarios: Changes in a patient's clinical status that may decrease CD4 count and thus prompt initiation of prophylaxis for opportunistic infections, such as new HIV-associated symptoms, or initiation of treatment with medications which are known to reduce CD4 cell count

Initiating Antiretroviral Therapy in Treatment-Naïve HIV-1-Infected Patient[1,2]

Clinical Condition	Recommendations
• HIV-infected patient	Antiretroviral therapy is recommended for all HIV-infected individuals[3]
• Patients who are at risk of transmitting HIV to sexual partners	Antiretroviral therapy is recommended for HIV-infected individuals for prevention of transmission of HIV
• AIDS-defining illness, including HIV-associated dementia • Pregnant women[4] • Acute opportunistic infections • Lower CD4 counts (<200 cells/mm³) • Patients with HIV-associated nephropathy • Acute/recent infection • Patients coinfected with hepatitis B virus (HBV) • Patients coinfected with hepatitis C virus (HCV) • Rapidly declining CD4 counts (>100 cells/mm³ decrease per year) • Higher viral loads (>100,000 copies/mL)	Antiretroviral therapy is strongly recommended regardless of CD4 count; these conditions favor more rapid initiation of therapy

[1]Patients initiating antiretroviral therapy should be willing and able to commit to lifelong treatment, and should understand the benefits and risks of therapy and the importance of adherence.

[2]Patients may choose to postpone therapy, and providers, on a case-by-case basis, may elect to defer therapy based on clinical and/or psychosocial factors.

[3]The strength of this recommendation varies on the basis of pretreatment CD4 cell count:
  • CD4 count <350 cells/mm³: Strong recommendation with evidence from randomized controlled trials
  • CD4 count 350 to 500 cells/mm³: Strong recommendation with evidence from well-designed nonrandomized trials or observational cohort studies with long-term clinical outcomes
  • CD4 count >500 cells/mm³: Moderate recommendation; expert opinion

[4]Combination antiretroviral therapy is recommended for all HIV-infected pregnant women to prevent maternal-to-child transmission, even if the mother does not require antiretroviral therapy for her own health. Following delivery, considerations regarding continuation of the maternal antiretroviral regimen for therapeutic indications are the same as for other nonpregnant individuals. For more detailed discussion, please refer to: Recommendations for use of antiretroviral drugs in pregnant HIV-1-infected women for maternal health and interventions to reduce perinatal HIV transmission in the United States. Available at http://www.aidsinfo.nih.gov/guidelines/

Conditions in Which Deferral of Therapy Might Be Considered

Some patients and their clinicians may decide to defer therapy for a period of time based on clinical or personal circumstances. The degree to which these factors might support deferral of therapy depends on the CD4 count and viral load. Although deferring therapy for the reasons listed below may be reasonable for patients with high CD4 counts (eg, >500 cells/mm³), deferral for patients with much lower CD4 counts (eg, <200 cells/mm³) should be considered only in rare situations and should be undertaken with close clinical follow-up. A brief delay in initiating therapy may be considered to allow a patient more time to prepare for lifelong treatment. Deferral may be considered in the following conditions:

• When there are significant barriers to adherence.

• Presence of comorbidities that complicate or prohibit antiretroviral therapy.
  Examples include:

  – Patients requiring surgery that might result in an extended interruption of antiretroviral therapy.

  – Patients taking medications that have clinically significant drug interactions with antiretroviral agents and for whom alternative therapy is not available.

  – Patients with a poor prognosis due to a concomitant medical condition who would not be expected to derive survival or quality-of-life benefits from antiretroviral therapy.

• Elite HIV controllers or long-term nonprogressors (**Note:** Antiretroviral therapy is recommended for nonprogressors who have consistently detectable viremia (HIV >200 to 1000 copies/mL) and elite controllers who exhibit evidence of disease progression (as defined by declining CD4 counts or development of HIV-related complications).

Antiretroviral Regimens Recommended for Treatment-Naïve Patients

Patients who are naïve to antiretroviral therapy should be started on one of the following types of combination regimens:

- **NNRTI + 2 NRTIs; or**
- **PI (generally boosted with ritonavir) + 2 NRTIs; or**
- **INSTI + 2 NRTIs**

Selection of a regimen should be individualized based on virologic efficacy, toxicity, pill burden, dosing frequency, drug-drug interaction potential, resistance testing results, and comorbid conditions. The regimens in each category are listed in alphabetical order.

For more detailed recommendations on antiretroviral choices and dosing in HIV-infected pregnant women, please refer to: Recommendations for use of antiretroviral drugs in pregnant HIV-1-infected women for maternal health and interventions to reduce perinatal HIV transmission in the United States. Available at http://www.aidsinfo.nih.gov/guidelines

Recommended Initial ART Regimen Options for All Patients, Regardless of Pre-ART Viral Load or CD4 Cell Count

NNRTI-based Regimen • EFV/TDF/FTC[1]
PI-based Regimens • ATV/r + TDF/FTC[1] • DRV/r + TDF/FTC[1]
INSTI-based Regimen • DTG + ABC/3TC[1] – **only** for patients who are HLA-B*5701 negative • DTG + TDF/FTC[1] • EVG/COBI/TDF/FTC – **only** for patients with pretreatment estimated CrCl ≥70 mL/min • RAL + TDF/FTC[1]
In addition to the regimens listed above, the following regimens are also recommended but only for patients with pre-ART plasma HIV RNA <100,000 copies/mL
NNRTI-based Regimen • EFV + ABC/3TC[1] – **only** for patients who are HLA-B*5701 negative • RPV/TDF/FTC[1] – **only** for patients with CD4 cell count >200 cells/mm^3
PI-based Regimens • ATV/r + ABC/3TC[1] – **only** for patients who are HLA-B*5701 negative
Alternative Initial ART Regimen Options (Regimens that are effective and tolerable but have potential disadvantages when compared with the recommended regimen listed above or have less data from randomized clinical trials. An alternative regimen may be the preferred regimen for some patients.)
PI-based Regimens (in alphabetical order) • DRV/r + ABC/3TC[1] – **only** for patients who are HLA-B*5701 negative • LPV/r (once[2] or twice daily) + ABC/3TC[1] – **only** for patients who are HLA-B*5701 negative • LPV/r (once[2] or twice daily) + TDF/FTC[1]
INSTI-based Regimen • RAL + ABC/3TC[1] – **only** for patients who are HLA-B*5701 negative

3TC = lamiVUDine, ABC = abacavir, ART = antiretroviral therapy, ATV = atazanavir, COBI = cobicistat, ddI = didanosine, DRV = darunavir, DTG = dolutegravir, EFV = efavirenz, EVG = elvitegravir, FPV = fosamprenavir, FTC = emtricitabine, INSTI = integrase strand transfer inhibitor, LPV = lopinavir, MVC = maraviroc, NNRTI = nonnucleoside reverse transcriptase inhibitor, NRTI = nucleos(t)ide reverse transcriptase inhibitor, NVP = nevirapine, PI = protease inhibitor, r = low-dose ritonavir, RAL = raltegravir, RPV = rilpivirine, TDF = tenofovir, ZDV = zidovudine

The following combinations in the recommended list above are available as fixed-dose combination formulations: ABC/3TC, EFV/TDF/FTC, EVG/COBI/TDF/FTC, LPV/r, RPV/TDF/FTC, and TDF/FTC

[1]3TC may substitute for FTC or vice versa.

[2]Once daily LPV/r is not recommended for pregnant patients.

Antiretroviral Components Not Recommended as Initial Therapy

Antiretroviral Drugs or Components (in alphabetical order)	Reasons for Not Recommending as Initial Therapy
Abacavir/lamivudine/zidovudine (coformulated) as triple-NRTI combination regimen	• Inferior virologic efficacy
Abacavir + lamiVUDine + zidovudine + tenofovir as quadruple NRTI combination	• Inferior virologic efficacy
Atazanavir (unboosted)	• Less potent than ritonavir-boosted atazanavir
Darunavir (unboosted)	• Usage without ritonavir has not been studied
Delavirdine	• Inferior virologic efficacy • Inconvenient dosing (3 times/day)
Didanosine + lamiVUDine (or emtricitabine)	• Inferior virologic efficacy • Limited clinical trial experience in treatment-naïve patients • Didanosine toxicity, such as pancreatitis and peripheral neuropathy
Didanosine + tenofovir	• High rate of early virologic failure • Rapid selection of resistant mutations • Potential for immunologic nonresponse/CD4$^+$ decline • Increased didanosine drug exposure and toxicities
Enfuvirtide	• No clinical trial experience in treatment-naïve patients • Requires twice daily subcutaneous injections
Etravirine	• Insufficient data in treatment-naïve patients
Fosamprenavir (unboosted or ritonavir-boosted)	• Virologic failure with unboosted fosamprenavir-based regimen may select mutations that confer resistance to darunavir • Less clinical trial data for ritonavir-boosted fosamprenavir than for other ritonavir-boosted protease inhibitors
Indinavir (unboosted)	• Inconvenient dosing (3 times/day with meal restrictions) • Fluid requirement • Indinavir toxicities, such as nephrolithiasis and crystalluria
Indinavir (ritonavir-boosted)	• Fluid requirement • Indinavir toxicities, such as nephrolithiasis and crystalluria
Maraviroc	• Requires testing for CCR5 tropism before initiation of therapy • No virologic benefit when compared with other recommended regimens • Requires twice-daily dosing
Nelfinavir	• Inferior virologic efficacy • Diarrhea
Nevirapine	• Associated with serious and potentially fatal toxicity (hepatic events and severe rash, including Stevens-Johnson syndrome and toxic epidermal necrolysis) • When compared with efavirenz, nevirapine did not meet noninferiority criteria
Ritonavir as sole PI	• High pill burden • Gastrointestinal intolerance • Metabolic toxicity
Saquinavir (unboosted)	• Inadequate bioavailability • Inferior virologic efficacy
Saquinavir (ritonavir-boosted)	• High pill burden • Can cause QT and PR prolongation; requires pretreatment and follow-up ECG
Stavudine + lamiVUDine	• Significant toxicities including lipoatrophy, peripheral neuropathy, and hyperlactatemia, including symptomatic and life-threatening lactic acidosis, hepatic steatosis, and pancreatitis
Tipranavir (ritonavir-boosted)	• Inferior virologic efficacy • Higher rate of adverse events than other ritonavir-boosted protease inhibitors • Higher dose of ritonavir required for boosting than with other protease inhibitors
Zidovudine + lamiVUDine	• Greater toxicities (including bone marrow suppression; GI toxicities; mitochondrial toxicities, such as lipoatrophy, lactic acidosis, and hepatic steatosis; skeletal muscle myopathy; and cardiomyopathy) compared to recommended NRTIs

Antiretroviral Regimens or Components That Should Not Be Offered at Any Time

	Rationale	Exception
Antiretroviral Regimens Not Recommended		
Monotherapy with NRTI	• Rapid development of resistance • Inferior antiretroviral activity when compared to combination with three or more antiretrovirals	• No exception
Dual-NRTI regimens	• Rapid development of resistance • Inferior antiretroviral activity when compared to combination with three or more antiretrovirals	• No exception
Triple-NRTI regimens except for abacavir/zidovudine/lamivudine or possibly tenofovir + zidovudine/ lamivudine	• High rate of early virologic nonresponse seen when triple NRTI combinations including ABC/TDF/3TC or TDF/ddl/ 3TC were used as initial regimen in treatment-naive patients • Other triple-NRTI regimens have not been evaluated	• Abacavir/zidovudine/lamivudine; and possibly tenofovir + zidovudine/ lamivudine in selected patients where other combinations are not desirable
Antiretroviral Components Not Recommended as Part of Antiretroviral Regimen		
Atazanavir + indinavir	Potential additive hyperbilirubinemia	• No exception
Didanosine + stavudine	• High incidence of toxicities – peripheral neuropathy, pancreatitis, and hyperlactatemia • Reports of serious, even fatal, cases of lactic acidosis with hepatic steatosis with or without pancreatitis in pregnant women	• No exception
Didanosine + tenofovir	• Increased didanosine concentrations and serious didanosine-associated toxicities • Potential for immunologic nonresponse and/or CD4 cell count decline • High rate of virologic failure • Rapid selection of resistance mutations at failure	• Clinicians caring for patients who are clinically stable on regimens containing tenofovir + didanosine should consider altering the NRTIs to avoid this combination
2-NNRTI combination	• When EFV combined with NVP, higher incidence of clinical adverse events seen when compared to either EFV- or NVP-based regimen • Both EFV and NVP may induce metabolism and may lead to reductions in etravirine (ETR) exposure; thus, should not be used in combination	• No exception
Efavirenz in first trimester of pregnancy or in women with significant childbearing potential	• Teratogenic in nonhuman primates	• When no other antiretroviral options are available and potential benefits outweigh the risks
Emtricitabine + lamiVUDine	• Similar resistance profile • No potential benefit	• No exception
Etravirine + unboosted PI	• Etravirine may induce metabolism of these PIs, appropriate doses not yet established.	• No exception
Etravirine + ritonavir-boosted atazanavir or fosamprenavir	• Etravirine may alter the concentrations of these PIs, appropriate doses not yet established.	• No exception
Etravirine + ritonavir-boosted tipranavir	• Etravirine concentration may be significantly reduced by RTV-boosted tipranavir	• No exception
Nevirapine in treament-naïve women with CD4 >250 or men with CD4 >400	• High incidence of symptomatic hepatotoxicity	• If no other antiretroviral option available, if used, patients should be closely monitored
Stavudine + zidovudine	• Antagonistic effect on HIV-1	• No exception
Unboosted darunavir, saquinavir, or tipranavir	• Inadequate bioavailability	• No exception

Recommendations for Using Drug-Resistance Assays

Clinical Setting/Recommendation	Rationale
Drug-Resistance Assay Recommended	
In acute HIV infection: Drug resistance testing is recommended, regardless of whether treatment will be initiated immediately or deferred. A genotypic assay is generally preferred.	If treatment is to be initiated, drug resistance testing will determine whether drug-resistant virus was transmitted and will help in the design of initial or changed (if therapy was initiated prior to test results) regimens.
	Genotypic testing is preferable to phenotypic testing because of lower cost, faster turnaround time, and greater sensitivity for detecting mixtures of wild-type and resistant virus.
If treatment is deferred, repeat resistance testing should be considered at the time ART is initiated. A genotypic assay is generally preferred.	If treatment is deferred, testing still should be performed because of the greater likelihood that transmitted resistance-associated mutations will be detected earlier in the course of HIV infection; results of testing may be important when treatment is eventually initiated. Repeat testing at the time ART is initiated should be considered because of the possibility that the patient may have acquired drug-resistant virus.
In treatment-naïve patients with chronic HIV infection: Drug resistance testing is recommended at the time of entry into HIV care, regardless of whether therapy is initiated immediately or deferred. A genotypic assay is generally preferred.	Transmitted HIV with baseline resistance to at least one drug may be seen in 6% to 16% of patients. Suboptimal virologic responses may be seen in patients with baseline resistant mutations. Some drug resistance mutations can remain detectable for years in untreated chronically infected patients.
If therapy is deferred, repeat resistance testing should be considered at the time ART is initiated. A genotypic assay is generally preferred.	Repeat testing prior to initiation of ART should be considered because that the patient may have acquired a drug-resistant virus.
	Genotypic testing is preferred for the reasons noted previously.
If an INSTI is considered for an ART-naïve patient and transmitted INSTI resistance is a concern, providers may wish to supplement standard resistance testing with a specific INSTI genotypic resistance assay	Standard genotypic drug-resistance assays test only for mutations in the RT and PR genes.
If use of a CCR5 antagonist is being considered, a coreceptor tropism assay should be performed.	A phenotypic tropism assay is preferred to determine HIV-1 coreceptor usage.
	A genotypic tropism assay should be considered as an alternative test to predict HIV-1 coreceptor usage.
In patients with virologic failure: Drug resistance testing is recommended in persons on combination antiretroviral therapy with HIV RNA levels >1000 copies/mL. In persons with HIV RNA levels >500 but <1000 copies/mL, testing may be unsuccessful but should still be considered.	Testing can help determine the role of resistance in drug failure and maximize the clinician's ability to select active drugs for the new regimen. Drug resistance testing should be performed while the patient is taking prescribed antiretroviral drugs or, if not possible, within 4 weeks after discontinuing therapy.
A genotypic assay is generally preferred in those experiencing virologic failure on their first or second regimens.	Genotypic testing is generally preferred for the reasons noted previously.
In patients failing INSTI-based regimens, genotypic testing for INSTI resistance should be performed to determine whether to include drugs from this class in subsequent regimens.	Standard genotypic drug-resistance assays test only for mutations in the RT and PR genes.
If use of a CCR5 antagonist is being considered, a coreceptor tropism assay should be performed.	A phenotypic tropism assay is preferred to determine HIV-1 coreceptor usage.
	A genotypic tropism assay should be considered as an alternative test to predict HIV-1 coreceptor usage.
Addition of phenotypic assay to genotypic assay is generally preferred for those with known or suspected complex drug resistance patterns, particularly to protease inhibitors.	Phenotypic testing can provide useful additional information for those with complex drug resistance mutation patterns, particularly to protease inhibitors.
In patients with suboptimal suppression of viral load: Drug resistance testing is recommended in persons with suboptimal suppression of viral load after initiation of antiretroviral therapy.	Testing can help determine the role of resistance and thus assist in identifying the number of active drugs available for a new regimen.
In HIV-infected pregnant women: Genotypic resistance testing is recommended for all pregnant women prior to initiation of therapy and for those entering pregnancy with detectable HIV RNA levels while on therapy.	The goals of antiretroviral therapy in HIV-infected pregnant women are to achieve maximal viral suppression for treatment of maternal HIV infection as well as for prevention of perinatal HIV transmission. Genotypic resistance testing will assist the clinician in selecting the optimal regimen for the patient.
Drug-Resistance Assay Not Usually Recommended	
After therapy discontinued: Drug resistance testing is not usually recommended after discontinuation (>4 weeks) of antiretroviral drugs.	Drug-resistance mutations may become minor species in the absence of selective drug pressure, and available assays may not detect minor drug-resistant species. If testing is performed in this setting, the detection of drug resistance may be of value, but its absence does not rule out the presence of minor drug-resistant species.
In patients with low HIV RNA levels: Drug resistance testing is not usually recommended in persons with a plasma viral load <500 copies/mL.	Resistance assays cannot be consistently performed because of low HIV RNA levels

Therapeutic Drug Monitoring

As with other notable drug classes (eg, antibiotics, anticonvulsants), the goal of therapeutic drug monitoring (TDM) is to maximize therapeutic efficacy and minimize drug-related toxicities. The utility of TDM in the setting of antiretroviral drug therapy is supported by data showing considerable interpatient variability with respect to drug concentrations among patients taking similar doses, as well as data demonstrating concentration/effect and concentration/toxicity correlations. The optimal plasma concentrations of many antiretroviral drugs have yet to be determined (eg, NRTIs). Those drugs for which target trough levels are defined are shown below.

Suggested Minimum Target Trough Concentrations

Drug	Concentration (ng/mL)
Suggested minimum target trough concentrations in patients with HIV-1 susceptible to the antiretroviral drug	
Fosamprenavir	400 (concentration assayed as amprenavir)
Atazanavir	150
Indinavir	100
Lopinavir	1000
Nelfinavir[1]	800
Saquinavir	100 to 250
Efavirenz	1000
Nevirapine	3000
Suggested minimum target trough concentrations for treatment-experienced patients who have resistant HIV-1 strains	
Maraviroc	>50
Tipranavir	20,500
Median (Range) Trough Concentrations From Clinical Trials	
Darunavir (600 mg twice daily)	3,300 (1,255 to 7,368)
Etravirine	275 (81 to 2,980)
Raltegravir	72 (29 to 118)

[1]Measurable active M8 metabolite.

Identifying, Diagnosing, and Managing Acute and Recent HIV-1 Infection

1. **Suspecting acute HIV infection:** Signs or symptoms of acute HIV infection with recent (within 2 to 6 weeks) high HIV risk exposure[1]

    • Signs/symptoms/laboratory findings may include but are not limited to one or more of the following: Fever, lymphadenopathy, skin rash, myalgia/arthralgia, headache, diarrhea, oral ulcers, leucopenia, thrombocytopenia, transaminase elevation

    • High-risk exposures include sexual contact with a person infected with HIV or at risk for HIV, sharing of injection drug use paraphernalia, or contact of potentially infectious blood with mucous membranes or breaks in skin[1]

2. **Differential diagnosis:** Includes but is not limited to viral illnesses, such as EBV- and non-EBV (eg, CMV)-related infectious mononucleosis syndromes, influenza, viral hepatitis, streptococcal infection, syphilis

3. **Evaluation/diagnosis of acute HIV infection:**

    • Acute infection is defined as detectable HIV RNA or p24 antigen [the antigen used in currently available HIV antigen/antibody (Ag/Ab) combination assays], in serum or plasma in the setting of a negative or indeterminate HIV antibody test result.

       – A reactive HIV antibody test or Ag/Ab test must be followed by supplemental confirmatory testing.

       – A negative or indeterminate HIV antibody test in a person with a positive Ag/Ab test or in whom acute HIV infection is suspected requires assessment of plasma HIV RNA[2] to assess for acute HIV infection.

       – A positive plasma HIV RNA test in the setting of a negative or indeterminate antibody result is consistent with acute HIV infection.

    • Patients presumptively diagnosed with acute HIV infection should have serologic testing repeated over the next 3 to 6 months to document seroconversion.

4. **Considerations for antiretroviral therapy during early HIV infection:**
    *   All pregnant women with early HIV infection should start on a combination ARV regimen as soon as possible because of the high risk of mother-to-child transmission of HIV
    *   Treatment for early HIV infection should be offered to all nonpregnant people
    *   The risks of antiretroviral therapy during early infection are consistent with those for initiating antiretroviral therapy in chronically infected asymptomatic patients with high CD4 counts
    *   If therapy is initiated, the goal should be for sustained plasma virologic suppression
    *   Enrollment in clinical trial should be considered

[1]In some settings, behaviors conducive to acquisition of HIV infection might not be ascertained or might not be perceived as "high-risk" by the healthcare provider or the patient or both. Thus, symptoms and signs consistent with acute retroviral syndrome should motivate consideration of this diagnosis, even in the absence of reported high-risk behaviors.

[2]Plasma HIV RNA can be measured by a variety of quantitative assays, including branched DNA (bDNA) and reverse transcriptase-polymerase chain reaction (RT-PCR)-based assays, as well as by a qualitative transcription-mediated amplification (APTIMA, GenProbe).

Associated Signs and Symptoms of Acute Retroviral Syndrome and Percentage of Expected Frequency

*   Fever (96%)
*   Lymphadenopathy (74%)
*   Pharyngitis (70%)
*   Rash (70%)
    *   Erythematous maculopapular with lesions on face and trunk and sometimes extremities, including palms and soles
    *   Mucocutaneous ulceration involving mouth, esophagus, or genitals
*   Myalgia or arthralgia (54%)
*   Diarrhea (32%)
*   Headache (32%)
*   Nausea and vomiting (27%)
*   Hepatosplenomegaly (14%)
*   Weight loss (13%)
*   Thrush (12%)
*   Neurologic symptoms (12%)
    *   Meningoencephalitis or aseptic meningitis
    *   Peripheral neuropathy or radiculopathy
    *   Facial palsy
    *   Guillain-Barré syndrome
    *   Brachial neuritis
    *   Cognitive impairment or psychosis

REFERENCE
Niu MT, Stein DS, Schnittman SM. Primary human immunodeficiency virus type 1 infection: review of pathogenesis and early treatment intervention in humans and animal retrovirus infections. *J Infect Dis.* 1993;168(6):1490-1501.

PERINATAL HIV

Overview and Rationale of Perinatal Antiretroviral Therapy

Antiretroviral agents are used during pregnancy for two reasons: 1) To treat maternal human immunodeficiency virus (HIV) infection and 2) To reduce the risk of perinatal HIV transmission. The pivotal clinical trial that demonstrated the benefits of antiretroviral prophylaxis to decrease the risk of perinatal HIV transmission was the Pediatric AIDS Clinical Trials Group (PACTG) 076 (Connor, 1994). In this randomized, double-blind, placebo-controlled trial, zidovudine monotherapy was administered in three phases: 1) Antepartum (to the pregnant woman), 2) Intrapartum (during labor to the pregnant woman) and 3) Postpartum (to the newborn infant for 6 weeks). A relative reduction of 67.5% in the risk of perinatal HIV transmission was observed in this study; the mother to infant HIV transmission rate decreased from 25.5% in the placebo group to 8.3% in the zidovudine group.

Many studies have been conducted and much has been learned since publication of that pivotal study. Currently, antiretroviral monotherapy is **not** considered to be appropriate for the treatment of HIV infection. Maternal use of combination highly active antiretroviral therapy (ie, HAART) is considered to be the standard of care, both for the treatment of maternal HIV infection and to reduce the risk of perinatal HIV transmission. Optimal reduction of the risk of perinatal HIV transmission still includes a three-phase approach with appropriate antiretroviral medications administered 1) Antepartum (to the pregnant woman), 2) Intrapartum (during labor to the pregnant woman) and 3) Postpartum (to the newborn infant). The antepartum HAART regimen should contain at least three antiretroviral agents (see below) and include one or more nucleoside reverse transcriptase inhibitor (NRTI) drugs with a high placental transfer rate (eg, zidovudine, lamivudine, emtricitabine, tenofovir, abacavir). Intrapartum zidovudine is recommended for HIV-infected pregnant women with HIV RNA >1000 copies/mL (or unknown HIV RNA) near delivery, regardless of their antiretroviral regimen or mode of delivery. A 6-week course of zidovudine is generally recommended for all newborns born to women who are HIV positive; however, a 4-week course of zidovudine may be considered in the infant when the mother has received standard combination antiretroviral therapy during pregnancy with consistent viral suppression and there are no concerns related to maternal adherence (see Table 3). A two-drug postpartum regimen, consisting of a 6-week course of zidovudine plus a three-dose course of nevirapine, is recommended for newborns whose mothers have not received antepartum antiretroviral therapy (see Table 4). Use of combination antiretroviral prophylaxis may be considered on a case-by-case basis in newborns in special circumstances who are at higher risk of HIV perinatal transmission (eg, infants born to HIV-infected mothers with no antiretroviral therapy prior to labor or during labor; infants born to mothers with only intrapartum antiretroviral therapy; infants born to mothers with suboptimal viral suppression at delivery; or infants born to mothers with known antiretroviral drug-resistant virus). Today, with the use of antepartum HAART therapy, prenatal HIV counseling and testing, antiretroviral prophylaxis, scheduled cesarean delivery, and avoidance of breastfeeding, the perinatal transmission rate of HIV infection has decreased to <2% in the United States and Europe.

Note: In 2013, a case of "functional cure" was reported in an HIV-positive newborn who received a three-drug combination antiretroviral regimen in therapeutic doses from 30 hours until 18 months of age. Medication was discontinued by the infant's mother at that time. Blood samples at 23 through 30 months of age demonstrated an undetectable viral load and were negative for HIV-antibodies (Persaud, 2013). In the absence of antiretroviral medications, the infant was free of detectable HIV for more than 2 years. However, recently the child (who is almost 4 years of age) was found to have a detectable viral load (>10,000 copies/mL), a decreased CD4 count, and HIV antibodies. The child was restarted on antiretroviral therapy. This case indicates that early three-drug antiretroviral treatment provided a sustained HIV remission after discontinuation of medication; however, it did not completely eliminate the reservoir of HIV-infected cells. Further studies are needed to assess the reasons why administration of a three-drug combination antiretroviral treatment regimen to an HIV-positive newborn caused a sustained remission in the absence of antiretroviral medications and what could be done to increase this period of remission (NIAID, 2014). Note that discontinuation of antiretroviral medication in HIV-positive individuals is not recommended in the *AIDSinfo* guidelines.

Specific recommendations for the use of antiretroviral drugs during pregnancy are updated regularly by the Department of Health and Human Services Panel on Treatment of HIV-Infected Pregnant Women and Prevention of Perinatal Transmission. The latest guidelines are available at http://AIDSinfo.nih.gov. Health care professionals are encouraged to contact the antiretroviral pregnancy registry to monitor outcomes of pregnant women exposed to antiretroviral medications (800-258-4263 or www.APRegistry.com).

The 2014 Panel recommendations include the following (information is summarized here for the reader):

General Principles

Note: Combined antepartum, intrapartum and infant antiretroviral prophylaxis is recommended for the prevention of perinatal HIV.

Preconception:

- Discussion of childbearing intentions with all women of childbearing age should be conducted on an ongoing basis throughout the course of their care.

- Effective and appropriate contraception should be selected to avoid unintended pregnancy.

- Preconception counseling concerning safer sexual practices (and elimination of alcohol, illicit drug use, and smoking) should be conducted.

- All HIV-infected women who wish to become pregnant should be receiving a maximally suppressive antiretroviral regimen.

- Evaluation or selection of antiretroviral therapy should consider efficacy for maternal treatment, hepatitis B virus disease status, the potential for teratogenicity if pregnancy should occur, and possible adverse outcomes for mother and fetus.

- Peri-contraception administration of antiretroviral pre-exposure prophylaxis (PrEP) for HIV-uninfected partners may offer an additional tool to reduce the risk of sexual transmission. The utility of PrEP of the uninfected partner when the infected partner is receiving ART and has a suppressed viral load has not been studied.

- For both concordant and discordant couples, the HIV-infected partner should attain maximum viral suppression before attempting conception. Refer to Perinatal Guidelines for additional information about reproductive options for HIV-concordant and serodiscordant couples.

Antepartum:

- Known risks and benefits of antiretroviral therapy during pregnancy should be discussed with all HIV-infected women.

- Combined antepartum, intrapartum, and infant antiretroviral prophylaxis is recommended because antiretroviral drugs reduce perinatal transmission by several mechanisms, including lowering maternal antepartum viral load and providing infant pre- and post-exposure prophylaxis.

- Assessment of HIV disease status and recommendations about initial antiretroviral therapy or changes to current regimen should be included in initial evaluation of pregnant women infected with HIV. The National Perinatal HIV Hotline (888-448-8765) provides free clinical consultation on all aspects of perinatal HIV care.

- All HIV-infected pregnant women should receive a combination antepartum antiretroviral drug regimen containing at least three agents regardless of plasma HIV RNA copy number or CD4 count.

- In general, the same antiretroviral regimens as recommended for treatment of nonpregnant adults should be used in pregnant women, unless there are known adverse effects for women, fetuses, or infants that outweigh benefits.

- Multiple factors must be considered when choosing a regimen for a pregnant woman, including comorbidities, convenience, adverse effects, drug interactions, resistance testing results, pharmacokinetics, and experience with use in pregnancy.

- Pharmacokinetic changes in pregnancy may lead to lower plasma concentrations of drugs and necessitate increased dosages, more frequent dosing, or ritonavir boosting, especially of protease inhibitors.

- For antiretroviral-naïve pregnant women, a combination regimen including two NRTIs and either a protease inhibitor (PI) with low-dose ritonavir or a non-nucleoside reverse transcriptase inhibitor (NNRTI) is preferred. Some clinicians prefer a ritonavir-boosted PI regimen because clinically significant resistance to PIs is less common than resistance to NNRTIs in antiretroviral-naïve individuals. In addition, the preferred NNRTI is efavirenz which has a potential risk for teratogenicity and should be avoided during the first 8 weeks of pregnancy. **Note:** A possible small increased risk of preterm birth in pregnant women receiving PI-based combination antiretroviral therapy exists; however, due to the clear benefits of such regimens, PIs should not be withheld for fear of altering pregnancy outcome.

- A combination antepartum antiretroviral regimen is more effective than a single-drug regimen to reduce perinatal HIV transmission. Combination antiretroviral regimens are recommended both for women who require HIV treatment for their own health and for prevention of perinatal transmission in pregnant HIV-infected women who do not yet require HIV therapy.

- Resistance studies should be conducted prior to starting/modifying therapy if HIV RNA is detectable (eg, >500 to 1000 copies/mL). If HIV is diagnosed late in pregnancy, antiretroviral therapy or prophylaxis should be initiated promptly without waiting for results of resistance testing.

- Optimal adherence to antiretroviral medications is a key part of the strategy to avoid failure and reduce the development of resistance.

- Coordination of services among prenatal care providers, primary care and HIV specialty care providers, mental health and drug abuse treatment services, and public assistance programs, is essential to ensure that HIV-infected women adhere to their antiretroviral drug regimens.

- Additional specific medication issues:

  - At least one NRTI drug with high placental transfer (eg, zidovudine, lamivudine, emtricitabine, tenofovir, abacavir) should be included in the regimen.

  - Preferred two-NRTI combinations include abacavir plus lamivudine, tenofovir plus emtricitabine (or lamivudine), and zidovudine plus lamivudine.

  - Efavirenz: Due to the risk of teratogenicity, pregnancy should be avoided in women receiving efavirenz and treatment with efavirenz should be avoided during the first 8 weeks of pregnancy (the primary period of fetal organogenesis) whenever possible. Because the risk of neural tube defects is restricted to the first 5 to 6 weeks of pregnancy and pregnancy is rarely recognized before 4 to 6 weeks of pregnancy, and unnecessary antiretroviral drug changes during pregnancy may be associated with loss of viral control and increased risk of perinatal transmission, efavirenz may be continued in pregnant women receiving an efavirenz-based regimen who present for antenatal care in the first trimester, provided there is virologic suppression on the regimen.

  - Nevirapine use as initial therapy in pregnant women with a CD4 cell count >250 cells/mm^3 should generally be avoided and should only be used if the benefit clearly outweighs the risk of increased hepatic toxicity. Nevirapine can be continued in pregnant women who are virologically suppressed and tolerating therapy regardless of CD4 count. **Note:** Women with CD4 counts >250 cells/mm^3 are at increased risk for rash-associated nevirapine-related hepatotoxicity including severe, life-threatening and potentially fatal hepatic events. Elevated transaminase levels at baseline may also increase the risk of nevirapine toxicity.

- Lopinavir/ritonavir and ritonavir-boosted atazanavir are the preferred protease inhibitors for antiretroviral-naïve pregnant women. Alternative protease inhibitors include ritonavir-boosted darunavir and ritonavir-boosted saquinavir.

- Protease inhibitors may require dosing adjustments during pregnancy.

- Glucose screening with a standard, 1-hour, 50 g glucose loading test at 24 to 28 weeks of gestation should be performed in HIV-infected pregnant women taking antiretroviral drug regimens. Some experts recommend earlier glucose screening in women receiving protease inhibitor-based regimens initiated before pregnancy, similar to recommendations for women with high-risk factors for glucose intolerance.

- Combination of stavudine and didanosine is not recommended during pregnancy; stavudine and didanosine in combination may cause lactic acidosis, hepatic failure, and maternal/neonatal mortality with prolonged use during pregnancy.

- NRTIs may be associated with lactic acidosis; monitor.

- Mitochondrial dysfunction should be considered in uninfected children with perinatal exposure to antiretroviral medications who present with severe clinical findings of unknown etiology, particularly neurologic findings.

- Long-term clinical follow-up for any child with *in utero* exposure to antiretroviral medications is recommended.

Intrapartum:

- Scheduled cesarean delivery at 38 weeks is recommended for women with suboptimal viral suppression near delivery (eg, HIV RNA >1000 copies/mL) or with unknown HIV RNA near the time of delivery.

- A rapid HIV antibody test should be performed in women with unknown HIV status who present in labor. If positive, a confirmatory HIV test should be sent as soon as possible and maternal intravenous (I.V.) zidovudine and infant combination antiretroviral drug prophylaxis should be initiated without waiting for test results. If the HIV test is positive, infant antiretroviral drugs should be continued for 6 weeks; if the maternal HIV test is negative, the infant antiretroviral drugs should be stopped.

- HIV-infected pregnant women with HIV RNA >1000 copies/mL (or unknown HIV RNA) near delivery should receive intrapartum I.V. zidovudine, regardless of their antepartum HAART regimen or mode of delivery. In situations in which I.V. administration is not possible, oral administration can be considered.

- I.V. zidovudine is not required for HIV-infected women receiving antiretroviral regimens who have HIV RNA ≤1000 copies/mL consistently during late pregnancy and near delivery and no concerns regarding adherence to the regimen.

- Pregnant women with HIV RNA >1000 copies/mL and documented zidovudine resistance who are not currently taking zidovudine for their own health should receive I.V. zidovudine during labor, in addition to their established regimens, except in women with documented histories of hypersensitivity.

- HIV-infected pregnant women in labor who have not received antepartum antiretroviral drugs should receive I.V. zidovudine.

- Women who are receiving an antepartum combination antiretroviral treatment regimen should continue their regimen on schedule as much as possible during labor and prior to scheduled cesarean delivery. Women with HIV RNA >1000 copies/mL who are receiving oral fixed-dose combination regimens that include zidovudine should have zidovudine administered I.V. during labor while other antiretroviral components are continued orally.

- Nevirapine use as a single dose is not recommended for women in the U.S. who are receiving standard antiretroviral prophylaxis regimens or for women who have **not** received antepartum antiretroviral drugs.

- If antepartum antiretroviral drugs were **not** administered, intrapartum therapy (I.V. zidovudine administered to the mother) and infant combination antiretroviral prophylaxis for 6 weeks is recommended.

Postpartum:

- Postnatal infant prophylaxis with a 6-week course of zidovudine is generally recommended for all infants born to HIV-infected women. However, a 4-week neonatal chemoprophylaxis regimen can be considered when the mother has received standard combined antiretroviral therapy during pregnancy with consistent viral suppression and there are no concerns related to maternal adherence.

- Zidovudine, at gestation age-appropriate doses, should be initiated as close to the time of birth as possible, preferably within 6 to 12 hours of delivery

- If antepartum or intrapartum antiretroviral drugs were not administered, or suboptimal viral suppression or antiretroviral drug resistance is known, most experts recommend postnatal infant prophylaxis with nevirapine (3 doses administered in the first week of life – at birth, 48 hours later, and 96 hours after the second dose) in combination with a 6-week course of zidovudine.

- Breast-feeding is not recommended for HIV-infected women in the United States, including those receiving antiretroviral therapy.

- The decision to continue maternal antiretroviral therapy after delivery should be based on current recommendations for initiation of antiretroviral therapy, current and nadir CD4 counts and trajectory, HIV RNA levels, adherence issues, clinical symptoms/disease stage, presence of other indications for antiretroviral therapy, whether the woman has an HIV-uninfected sexual partner, and patient preference.

- Arrangements for new or continued supportive services should be made prior to hospital discharge for women continuing antiretroviral therapy postpartum.

- Contraceptive counseling should be included in the prenatal period, as well as immediately postpartum, as a critical aspect of postpartum care.

Special Situations

HIV/hepatitis B virus coinfection:

- Screening for hepatitis B virus (HBV) with hepatitis B surface antigen (HBsAg), hepatitis B core antibody (anti-HBc), and hepatitis B surface antibody (anti-HBs) is recommended for all pregnant women not already screened during current pregnancy.
- All pregnant women who screen negative for HBV should receive the HBV vaccine series.
- Women with chronic HBV should also be screened for hepatitis A virus (HAV) because they are at increased risk of complications from coinfection with other viral hepatitis infections.
- Women with chronic HBV infection who are negative for hepatitis A immunoglobulin G should receive the HAV vaccine series.
- All pregnant women with chronic hepatitis B virus (HBV) infection and HIV coinfection should receive a combination antiretroviral regimen, including a dual NRTI backbone with two drugs active against both HIV and HBV. Tenofovir plus lamiVUDine or emtricitabine is the preferred backbone.
- Consultation with an expert is strongly recommended for pregnant women coinfected with HIV/HBV.
- Interferon alfa and pegylated interferon alfa are not recommended during pregnancy.
- Pregnant women with HBV and HIV coinfection receiving antiretroviral medications should be monitored for liver toxicity.
- If antiretroviral drugs are discontinued postpartum in women coinfected with HIV/HBV, liver function tests should be monitored frequently for potential exacerbation of HBV infection.
- Infants born to hepatitis B infected women should receive hepatitis B immune globulin (HBIG) and initiate the three-dose hepatitis B vaccination series within 12 hours of birth.

HIV/hepatitis C virus coinfection:

- Screening for hepatitis C is recommended for all HIV-infected women not already screened during current pregnancy.
- Women with chronic hepatitis C virus (HCV) infection should also be screened for hepatitis A virus (HAV) because they are at increased risk of complications from coinfection with other viral hepatitis infections.
- Women with chronic HBC infection who are negative for hepatitis A immunoglobulin G should receive the HAV vaccine series
- Consultation with an expert is strongly recommended for pregnant women coinfected with HIV/HCV.
- Interferon alfa and pegylated interferon alfa are not recommended during pregnancy.
- Recommendations for antiretroviral drug use during pregnancy are the same for women who have chronic HCV infection as for those without HIV/HCV coinfection.
- Pregnant women with HCV and HIV coinfection and receiving antiretroviral medications should be monitored for liver toxicity.
- Decisions concerning mode of delivery should be based on standard obstetric and HIV-related indications alone.
- Infants born to women coinfected with HCV and HIV should be evaluated for both HIV and HCV infection. For evaluation of HCV, HCV RNA virologic testing can be performed after 2 months of age and HCV antibody testing should be conducted after 18 months of age.

The following recommendations in Table 1 are for pregnant HIV-infected women who have never received antiretroviral therapy previously (antiretroviral-naïve) and are predicated on lack of evidence of resistance to regimen components. See Table 2 for more information on specific drugs in pregnancy. Within each drug class, regimens are listed alphabetically and the order does not indicate a ranking of preference. It is recommended that women who become pregnant while on a stable antiretroviral regimen with viral suppression remain on that same regimen.

A combination antiretroviral regimen in treatment-naïve pregnant women generally contains one PI (with low-dose ritonavir boosting) plus a 2-NRTI backbone or an NNRTI plus a 2-NRTI backbone. Regimens should be individualized based on advantages and disadvantages of each combination.

Table 1. What to Start: Initial Combination Regimens for Antiretroviral-Naïve HIV-Infected Pregnant Women

Drug	Comments
PREFERRED REGIMENS	
Regimens with clinical trial data in adults demonstrating optimal efficacy and durability with acceptable toxicity and ease of use. Pharmacokinetic data available in pregnancy and no evidence to date of teratogenic effects or established adverse outcomes for mother, fetus, or newborn. To minimize the risk of resistance, a PI regimen is preferred for women who may stop antiretroviral therapy during the postpartum period.	
Preferred Two-NRTI Backbone	
Abacavir plus lamivudine	Available as fixed-drug combination (Epzicom); can be administered once daily. Potential hypersensitivity reaction; abacavir should not be used in patients who test positive for HLA-B*5701.
Tenofovir plus emtricitabine or lamivudine	Tenofovir/emtricitabine available as fixed-drug combination (Truvada). Either tenofovir/ emtricitabine or tenofovir plus lamivudine can be administered once daily. Tenofovir has potential renal toxicity, thus tenofovir-based dual NRTI combinations should be used with caution in patients with renal insufficiency.
Zidovudine plus lamivudine	Available as fixed-drug combination (Combivir). NRTI combination with most experience for use in pregnancy but has disadvantages of requirement for twice-daily administration and increased potential for hematologic toxicity.
PI Regimens	
Atazanavir/ritonavir **plus** a preferred two-NRTI backbone	Once-daily administration
Lopinavir/ritonavir **plus** a preferred two-NRTI backbone	Twice-daily administration. Once-daily lopinavir/ritonavir is not recommended for use in pregnant women.
NNRTI Regimen	
Efavirenz **plus** a preferred two-NRTI backbone **Note:** May be initiated after the first 8 weeks of pregnancy	Concern because of birth defects seen in primate study; risk in humans is unclear (see Table 2). Postpartum contraception must be ensured. Preferred regimen in women requiring co-administration of drugs with significant interactions with PIs.
ALTERNATIVE REGIMENS	
Regimens with clinical trial data demonstrating efficacy in adults but one or more of the following apply: Experience in pregnancy is limited, data are lacking or incomplete on teratogenicity, or regimen is associated with dosing, formulation, toxicity, or interaction issues.	
PI Regimens	
Darunavir/ritonavir **plus** a preferred two-NRTI backbone	Less experience with use in pregnancy than atazanavir/ritonavir and lopinavir/ritonavir
Saquinavir/ritonavir **plus** a preferred two-NRTI backbone	Baseline ECG is recommended before initiation of saquinavir/ritonavir because of potential PR and QT prolongation; contraindicated with preexisting cardiac conduction system disease. Large pill burden.
NNRTI Regimen	
Nevirapine **plus** a preferred two-NRTI backbone	Nevirapine should be used with caution when initiating antiretroviral therapy in women with CD4 T-lymphocyte (CD4) cell count >250 cells/mm^3. Use nevirapine and abacavir together with caution; both can cause hypersensitivity reactions within the first few weeks after initiation.
Integrase Inhibitor Regimen	
Raltegravir plus a preferred two-NRTI backbone	Limited data on raltegravir use in pregnancy but may be considered when drug interactions with PI regimens are a concern.
INSUFFICIENT DATA IN PREGNANCY TO RECOMMEND ROUTINE USE IN ANTIRETROVIRAL-NAIVE WOMEN	
Drugs that are approved for use in adults but lack adequate pregnancy-specific pharmacokinetic or safety data	
Dolutegravir	No data on use in pregnancy
Elvitegravir/cobicistat/emtricitabine/ tenofovir (Stribild)	No data on use of elvitegravir/cobicistat component in pregnancy
Fosamprenavir/ritonavir	Limited data on use in pregnancy
Maraviroc	Requires tropism testing before use; few case reports of use in pregnancy
Rilpivirine	Rilpivirine not recommended with pretreatment HIV RNA >100,000 copies/mL or CD4 cell count <200 cells/mm^3. Do not use with proton pump inhibitor. Limited data on use in pregnancy.
NOT RECOMMENDED	
Drugs whose use is not recommended because of toxicity, lower rate of viral suppression, or because not recommended in antiretroviral-naïve populations	
Abacavir/lamivudine/zidovudine	Generally not recommended due to inferior virology efficacy
Stavudine	Not recommended due to toxicity
Didanosine	Not recommended due to toxicity

Table 1. What to Start: Initial Combination Regimens for Antiretroviral-Naïve HIV-Infected Pregnant Women *(continued)*

Drug	Comments
Indinavir/ritonavir	Concerns of kidney stones, hyperbilirubinemia
Nelfinavir	Lower rate of viral suppression with nelfinavir compared to lopinavir/ritonavir or efavirenz in adult trials
Ritonavir	Ritonavir as a single PI is not recommended because of inferior efficacy and increased toxicity
Etravirine	Not recommended in antiretroviral-naïve populations
Enfuvirtide	Not recommended in antiretroviral-naïve populations
Tipranavir	Not recommended in antiretroviral-naïve populations

NNRTI = non-nucleoside analogue reverse transcriptase inhibitor, NRTI = nucleoside analogue reverse transcriptase inhibitor, PI = protease inhibitor

Table 2. Antiretroviral Drug Use in Pregnant HIV-Infected Women: Pharmacokinetic and Toxicity Data in Human Pregnancy and Recommendations for Use in Pregnancy[a]

Drug	Pharmacokinetic and Dosing Considerations in Pregnancy	Recommendations for Use in Pregnancy
NRTIs		NRTIs are recommended for use as part of combinations regimens, usually including 2 NRTIs with either an NNRTI or one or more PIs. Use of single or dual NRTIs alone is not recommended for treatment of HIV infection.
Abacavir	Pharmacokinetics not significantly altered in pregnancy. No change in dose indicated during pregnancy.	High placental transfer to fetus[b]
		No evidence of human teratogenicity (can rule out 2-fold increase in overall birth defects)
		Hypersensitivity reactions occur in ~5% to 8% of nonpregnant individuals; a much smaller percentage are fatal and are usually associated with rechallenge. Rate in pregnancy is unknown. Testing for HLA-B*5701 allele identifies patients at risk of reactions and should be done and documented as negative before starting abacavir. Patients should be educated regarding symptoms of hypersensitivity reaction.
Didanosine	Pharmacokinetics not significantly altered in pregnancy. No change in dose indicated during pregnancy.	Low to moderate placental transfer to fetus[b]
		In the APR, an increased rate of birth defects with didanosine compared to general population was noted after both first-trimester and later exposure. No specific pattern of defects was noted and clinical relevance is uncertain.
		Didanosine should not be used with stavudine; lactic acidosis, sometimes fatal, has been reported in pregnant women receiving didanosine and stavudine together.
Emtricitabine	Pharmacokinetics not significantly altered in pregnancy. No change in dose indicated during pregnancy.	High placental transfer to fetus[b]
		No evidence of human teratogenicity (can rule out 2-fold increase in overall birth defects)
		If hepatitis B coinfected, it is possible that a hepatitis B flare may occur if emtricitabine is discontinued postpartum.
LamiVUDine	Pharmacokinetics not significantly altered in pregnancy. No change in dose indicated during pregnancy.	High placental transfer to fetus[b]
		No evidence of human teratogenicity (can rule out 1.5-fold increase in overall birth defects)
		If hepatitis B coinfected, it is possible that a hepatitis B flare may occur if LamiVUDine is discontinued postpartum.
Stavudine	Pharmacokinetics not significantly altered in pregnancy. No change in dose indicated during pregnancy.	High placental transfer to fetus[b]
		No evidence of human teratogenicity (can rule out 2-fold increase in overall birth defects)
		Stavudine should not be used with didanosine; lactic acidosis, sometimes fatal, has been reported in pregnant women receiving didanosine and stavudine together. Do not use stavudine with zidovudine due to antagonism.
Tenofovir	AUC lower in third trimester than postpartum but trough levels adequate. No change in dose indicated during pregnancy.	High placental transfer to fetus[b]
		No evidence of human teratogenicity (can rule out 2-fold increase in overall birth defects). Studies in monkeys show decreased fetal growth and reduction in fetal bone porosity within 2 months of starting maternal therapy. Human studies demonstrate no effect on intrauterine growth, but one study demonstrated lower length and head circumference with exposure.
		Tenofovir should be used in combination with LamiVUDine or emtricitabine in women with chronic hepatitis B infection. If hepatitis B coinfected, it is possible that a hepatitis B flare may occur if tenofovir is discontinued postpartum.
		Monitor renal function due to potential for renal toxicity.
Zidovudine	Pharmacokinetics not significantly altered in pregnancy. No change in dose indicated during pregnancy.	High placental transfer to fetus[b]
		No evidence of human teratogenicity (can rule out 1.5-fold increase in overall birth defects).

Table 2. Antiretroviral Drug Use in Pregnant HIV-Infected Women: Pharmacokinetic and Toxicity Data in Human Pregnancy and Recommendations for Use in Pregnancy[a] *continued*

Drug	Pharmacokinetics and Dosing Considerations in Pregnancy	Recommendations for Use in Pregnancy
NNRTIs		NNRTIs are recommended for use in combination regimens with 2 NRTI drugs.
		Hypersensitivity reactions, including hepatic toxicity and rash, more common in women; unclear if increased in pregnancy
Efavirenz	AUC decreased during third trimester, compared with postpartum, but nearly all third-trimester participants exceeded target exposure.	Moderate placental transfer to fetus[b]
		Potential fetal safety concern: FDA Pregnancy Class D. Cynomolgus monkeys receiving efavirenz during the first trimester at a dose resulting in plasma concentrations comparable to systemic human therapeutic exposure had 3 of 20 infants with significant CNS or other malformations.
	No change in dose indicated during pregnancy	In humans, there is no increase in overall birth defects with first-trimester efavirenz exposure. However, in humans with first-trimester exposure, there have been 6 retrospective case reports and 1 prospective case report of CNS defects and 1 prospective case report of anophthalmia with facial clefts. The relative risk with first-trimester exposure is unclear.
		Nonpregnant women of childbearing potential should undergo pregnancy testing before efavirenz initiation and counseling about potential risk to the fetus and desirability of avoiding pregnancy while on efavirenz-containing regimens. Alternate antiretroviral regimens that do not include efavirenz should be strongly considered in women who are planning to become pregnant or who are sexually active and not using effective contraception, assuming these alternative regimens are acceptable to the provider and are not thought to compromise the health of the woman.
		Because the risk of neural tube defects is restricted to the first 5 to 6 weeks of pregnancy and pregnancy is rarely recognized before 4 to 6 weeks of pregnancy, and unnecessary antiretroviral drug changes during pregnancy may be associated with loss of viral control and increased risk of perinatal transmission, efavirenz may be continued in pregnant women receiving an efavirenz-based regimen who present for antenatal care in the first trimester, provided there is virologic suppression on the regimen.
Etravirine	Limited pharmacokinetic data in pregnancy (n=4) suggests no differences from nonpregnant adults. Insufficient data to make dosing recommendation during pregnancy.	Moderate placental transfer (data from one mother-infant pair)[b]
		Insufficient data to assess for teratogenicity in humans. No evidence of teratogenicity in rats or rabbits.
Nevirapine	Pharmacokinetics not significantly altered in pregnancy. No change in dose indicated during pregnancy.	High placental transfer to fetus[b]
		No evidence of human teratogenicity (can rule out 1.5-fold increase in overall birth defects and 2-fold increase in risk of birth defects in more common classes, cardiovascular and genitourinary)
		Increased risk of symptomatic, often rash-associated, and potentially fatal liver toxicity among women with CD4 counts ≥250/mm³ when first initiating therapy; pregnancy does not appear to increase risk
		Nevirapine should be initiated in pregnant women with CD4 counts ≥250/mm³ only if benefit clearly outweighs risk because of potential increased risk of life-threatening hepatotoxicity in women with high CD4 cell counts. Elevated transaminase levels at baseline may increase the risk of nevirapine toxicity.
		Women who become pregnant while taking nevirapine-containing regimens and are tolerating them well can continue therapy, regardless of CD4 count.
Rilpivirine	No pharmacokinetic studies in human pregnancy; no dosing recommendations can be made	Unknown placental transfer to fetus in humans
	Insufficient data to make dosing recommendation during pregnancy	No evidence of teratogenicity in rats or rabbits. Insufficient data to assess for teratogenicity in humans.

Table 2. Antiretroviral Drug Use in Pregnant HIV-Infected Women:
Pharmacokinetic and Toxicity Data in Human Pregnancy and Recommendations for Use in Pregnancy[a] *continued*

Drug	Pharmacokinetics and Dosing Considerations in Pregnancy	Recommendations for Use in Pregnancy
Protease Inhibitors		PIs are recommended for use in combination regimens with 2 NRTI drugs. Hyperglycemia, new onset or exacerbation of diabetes mellitus, and diabetic ketoacidosis reported with PI use; unclear if pregnancy increases risk. Conflicting data regarding preterm delivery in women receiving PIs.
Atazanavir **Note:** Must be combined with low-dose ritonavir boosting in pregnancy	Atazanavir concentrations are reduced during pregnancy; also reduced when given concomitantly with tenofovir or H$_2$-receptor antagonist. Use of unboosted atazanavir is **not** recommended during pregnancy. Use of an increased dose (400 mg atazanavir plus 100 mg ritonavir once daily with food) during the second and third trimester results in plasma concentrations equivalent to those in nonpregnant adults on standard dosing. Although some experts recommend increased atazanavir dosing in all women during the second and third trimesters, the package insert recommends increased atazanavir dosing only for antiretroviral-experienced pregnant women in the second and third trimesters also receiving either tenofovir or H^2-receptor antagonist.	Low placental transfer to fetus[b] No evidence of human teratogenicity (can rule out 2-fold increase in overall birth defects) Must be given as low-dose ritonavir-boosted regimen in pregnancy Effect of *in utero* atazanavir exposure on infant's indirect bilirubin levels is unclear. Nonpathologic elevations of neonatal hyperbilirubinemia have been observed in some but not all clinical trials to date.
Darunavir **Note:** Must be combined with low-dose ritonavir boosting	Exposure is decreased in pregnancy. Once-daily dosing is **not** recommended during pregnancy. Twice-daily dosing is recommended for all pregnant women. Increased twice-daily darunavir dose (darunavir 800 mg plus ritonavir 100 mg with food) in pregnancy is being investigated.	Low placental transfer to fetus[b] Insufficient data to assess for teratogenicity in humans. No evidence of teratogenicity in mice, rats, or rabbits. Must be given as low-dose ritonavir-boosted regimen
Fosamprenavir **Note:** Must be combined with low-dose ritonavir boosting in pregnancy	With ritonavir boosting, AUC is reduced during third trimester. However, exposure is greater during the third trimester with boosting than in nonpregnant adults without boosting and trough concentrations achieved during the third trimester were adequate for patients without PI resistance mutations. Use of unboosted fosamprenavir is **not** recommended during pregnancy. No change in standard boosted dose is indicated.	Low placental transfer to fetus[b] Insufficient data to assess for teratogenicity in humans. Increased fetal loss in rabbits but no increase in defects in rats and rabbits. Must be given as low-dose ritonavir-boosted regimen in pregnancy
Indinavir **Note:** Must be combined with low-dose ritonavir boosting in pregnancy	Indinavir exposure markedly reduced when administered without ritonavir boosting during pregnancy. Indinavir exposure low with indinavir 400 mg plus ritonavir 100 mg dosing during pregnancy; no pharmacokinetic data available on alternative boosted dosing regimens in pregnancy. Use of unboosted indinavir is **not** recommended during pregnancy.	Minimal placental transfer to fetus[b] No evidence of human teratogenicity (can rule out 2-fold increase in overall birth defects) Must be given as low-dose ritonavir-boosted regimen in pregnancy Theoretical concern regarding increased indirect bilirubin levels, which may exacerbate physiologic hyperbilirubinemia in neonates. Minimal placental passage mitigates this concern.

2364

Table 2. Antiretroviral Drug Use in Pregnant HIV-Infected Women: Pharmacokinetic and Toxicity Data in Human Pregnancy and Recommendations for Use in Pregnancy[a] *continued*

Drug	Pharmacokinetics and Dosing Considerations in Pregnancy	Recommendations for Use in Pregnancy
Lopinavir/ ritonavir	Pharmacokinetic studies suggest increased dose (lopinavir 600 mg plus ritonavir 150 mg twice daily without regard to meals) should be used in second and third trimesters, especially in PI-experienced patients. If standard dosing is used, monitor virologic response and lopinavir drug concentrations, if available. No data to address if drug concentrations are adequate with once-daily dosing in pregnancy. Once-daily dosing **is not** recommended during pregnancy. Some experts recommend increased dose of lopinavir 600 mg plus ritonavir 150 mg twice daily without regard to meals in second and third trimesters.	Low placental transfer to fetus[b] No evidence of human teratogenicity (can rule out 2-fold increase in overall birth defects) Oral solution contains 42% alcohol and 15% propylene glycol and is not recommended for use in pregnancy. Once-daily lopinavir/ritonavir dosing is not recommended during pregnancy.
Nelfinavir	Lower nelfinavir exposure in third trimester than postpartum in women receiving nelfinavir 1250 mg twice daily; however, generally adequate drug concentrations are achieved during pregnancy, although concentrations are variable in late pregnancy. Nelfinavir dosing of 750 mg 3 times daily with food is not recommended during pregnancy. No change in standard dose (1250 mg twice daily with food) is indicated.	Minimal to low placental transfer to fetus[b] No evidence of human teratogenicity (can rule out 1.5-fold increase in overall birth defects and 2-fold increase in risk of birth defects in more common classes, cardiovascular and genitourinary)
Ritonavir	Lower concentrations during pregnancy compared with postpartum but no dosage adjustment necessary when used as booster Use only as low-dose booster with other protease inhibitors	Low placental transfer to fetus[b] No evidence of human teratogenicity (can rule out 2-fold increase in overall birth defects) Oral solution contains 43% alcohol and is not recommended for use in pregnancy.
Saquinavir	Based on limited data, saquinavir exposure may be reduced in pregnancy but not sufficient to warrant a dose change. No change in dose indicated during pregnancy	Minimal placental transfer to fetus[b] Insufficient data to assess for teratogenicity in humans. No evidence of teratogenicity in rats or rabbits. Must be given as low-dose ritonavir-boosted regimen Baseline ECG recommended before starting therapy because PR and/or QT interval prolongations have been observed. Contraindicated in patients with preexisting cardiac conduction system disease.
Tipranavir	Limited pharmacokinetic data in human pregnancy. Insufficient data to make dosing recommendation.	Moderate placental transfer to fetus reported in one patient[b] Insufficient data to assess for teratogenicity in humans. No evidence of teratogenicity in rats or rabbits. Must be given as low-dose ritonavir-boosted regimen.
Entry Inhibitors		
Enfuvirtide	No pharmacokinetic data in human pregnancy. Insufficient data to make dosing recommendation.	Minimal to low placental transfer to fetus[b] No data on human teratogenicity
Maraviroc	Limited pharmacokinetic data in human pregnancy. Insufficient data to make dosing recommendation.	Minimal to low placental transfer to fetus[b] No data on human teratogenicity

Table 2. Antiretroviral Drug Use in Pregnant HIV-Infected Women:
Pharmacokinetic and Toxicity Data in Human Pregnancy and Recommendations for Use in Pregnancy[a] *continued*

Drug	Pharmacokinetics and Dosing Considerations in Pregnancy	Recommendations for Use in Pregnancy
Integrase Inhibitors		
Dolutegravir	No pharmacokinetic data in human pregnancy. Insufficient data to make dosing recommendation.	Unknown placental transfer to fetus. Insufficient data to assess for teratogenicity in humans. No evidence of teratogenicity in mice, rats, or rabbits.
Elvitegravir plus cobicistat	No pharmacokinetic data in human pregnancy. Insufficient data to make dosing recommendation.	No data on placental transfer of elvitegravir plus cobicistat are available. Insufficient data to assess for teratogenicity in humans. No evidence of teratogenicity in rats or rabbits.
Raltegravir	Limited data suggest pharmacokinetics not significantly altered in pregnancy. No change in dose indicated during pregnancy.	High placental transfer to fetus[b]. Insufficient data to assess for teratogenicity in humans. Increased skeletal variants in rats; no increase in defects in rabbits. Case report of markedly elevated liver transaminases with use in late pregnancy. Severe, potentially life-threatening, and fatal skin and hypersensitivity reactions have been reported in nonpregnant adults. Chewable tables contain phenylalanine.

APR = antiretroviral pregnancy registry

[a]Individual antiretroviral drug dosages may need to be adjusted in renal or hepatic insufficiency (for details, see individual drug monographs).

[b]Placental transfer categories: Mean or median cord blood to maternal delivery plasma drug ratio: High: >0.6; Moderate: 0.3 to 0.6; Low: 0.1 to 0.3; Minimal: <0.1

Table 3. Intrapartum Maternal and Neonatal Zidovudine Dosing for Prevention of Perinatal Transmission of HIV

Drug	Dosing	Duration
Maternal Intrapartum		
Zidovudine	2 mg/kg I.V. over 1 hour followed by continuous infusion of 1 mg/kg/h	Onset of labor until delivery of infant
Neonatal		
Zidovudine (≥35 weeks gestational age at birth)	4 mg/kg/dose P.O. twice daily, started as soon as possible after birth (preferably within 6 to 12 hours after delivery); or, if unable to tolerate oral agents, 3 mg/kg/dose I.V. beginning within 6 to 12 hours of delivery, then every 12 hours	Birth through 4 to 6 weeks[1]
Zidovudine (≥30 weeks to <35 weeks gestational age at birth)	2 mg/kg/dose P.O. (1.5 mg/kg/dose if given I.V.) started as soon as possible after birth (preferably within 6 to 12 hours after delivery), then every 12 hours; advance to 3 mg/kg/dose P.O. (or 2.3 mg/kg/dose if given I.V.) every 12 hours at 15 days of age	Birth through 6 weeks
Zidovudine (<30 weeks gestational age at birth)	2 mg/kg/dose P.O. (1.5 mg/kg/dose if given I.V.) started as soon as possible after birth (preferably within 6 to 12 hours after delivery), then every 12 hours; advance to 3 mg/kg/dose P.O. (or 2.3 mg/kg/dose if given I.V.) every 12 hours after 4 weeks of age	Birth through 6 weeks

[1]All HIV-exposed infants should receive postpartum antiretroviral drugs to reduce perinatal transmission of HIV. A 6-week course of neonatal zidovudine is generally recommended. A 4-week neonatal zidovudine chemoprophylaxis regimen may be considered when the mother has received standard antiretroviral therapy during pregnancy with consistent viral suppression and there are no concerns related to maternal adherence.

Table 4. Additional Antiretroviral Prophylaxis Agents for HIV-Exposed Infants of Women Who Received No Antepartum Antiretroviral Prophylaxis (Initiate as Soon as Possible After Delivery)[1]

Drug	Dosing	Duration
Neonatal Two-drug regimen: Zidovudine + Nevirapine		
Zidovudine	Use dosing from table above	Birth through 6 weeks
Nevirapine	Birth weight 1.5 to 2 kg: 8 mg/dose P.O. Birth weight >2 kg: 12 mg/dose P.O.	**Three** doses in the first week of life: • First dose within 48 hours of birth (birth to 48 hours) • Second dose 48 hours after first • Third dose 96 hours after second

[1]The Panel recommends 6 weeks of zidovudine plus 3 doses of nevirapine in the first week of life for infants whose mothers have not received antepartum antiretroviral agents and for infants whose mothers have not received antepartum or intrapartum antiretroviral agents. Most experts feel the potential benefit of combining zidovudine infant prophylaxis with additional antiretroviral drugs may exceed the risk of multiple drug exposure in the following cases: Infants born to HIV-infected mothers with no antiretroviral therapy prior to labor or during labor; infants born to mothers with only intrapartum antiretroviral therapy (ie, no antepartum antiretroviral therapy); infants born to mothers with suboptimal viral suppression at delivery (especially if delivery was vaginal); or infants born to mothers with known antiretroviral drug-resistant virus. However, risk of HIV transmission depends on a number of maternal and infant factors, including viral load, mode of delivery, and gestational age at delivery. Data from the NICHD-HPTN 040/PACTG 1043 study supports the use of the zidovudine plus nevirapine two-drug regimen in newborns whose mothers have not received antepartum antiretroviral therapy. In all other scenarios, decisions about the use of combination antiretroviral prophylaxis in infants should be made in consultation with a pediatric HIV specialist before delivery, if possible, and should be accompanied by a discussion with the mothers about potential risks and benefits of this approach.

REFERENCES

Connor EM, Sperling RS, Gelber R, et al. Reduction of maternal-infant transmission of human immunodeficiency virus type 1 with zidovudine treatment. Pediatric AIDS clinical trials group protocol 076 study group. *N Engl J Med.* 1994;331(18):1173-1180.

National Institute of Allergy and Infectious Disease (NIAID). "Mississippi baby" now has detectable HIV, researchers find. July 10, 2014. Available at http://www.niaid.nih.gov/news/newsreleases/2014/Pages/MississippiBabyHIV.aspx

Panel on Treatment of HIV-Infected Pregnancy Women and Prevention of Perinatal Transmission. Recommendations for use of antiretroviral drugs in pregnant HIV-infected women for maternal health and interventions to reduce perinatal HIV transmission in the United States. March 28, 2014. Available at http://aidsinfo.nih.gov/contentfiles/PerinatalGL.pdf

Persaud D, Gay H, Ziemniak C, et al. Absence of detectable HIV-1 viremia after treatment cessation in an infant. *N Engl J Med.* 2013;369(19): 1828-1835.

IMMUNIZATION ADMINISTRATION RECOMMENDATIONS

The following tables are taken from the General Recommendations on Immunization, 2011:

- Guidelines for Spacing of Live and Inactivated Antigens
- Guidelines for Administering Antibody-Containing Products and Vaccines
- Recommended Intervals Between Administration of Antibody-Containing Products and Measles- or Varicella-Containing Vaccine, by Product and Indication for Vaccination
- Vaccination of persons with Primary and Secondary Immunodeficiencies
- Needle length and Injection Site of I.M. injections

Guidelines for Spacing of Live and Inactivated Antigens

Antigen Combination	Recommended Minimum Interval Between Doses
Two or more inactivated[1]	May be administered simultaneously or at any interval between doses
Inactivated and live	May be administered simultaneously or at any interval between doses
Two or more live injectable[2]	28 days minimum interval, if not administered simultaneously

[1]Certain experts suggest a 28-day interval between tetanus toxoid, reduced diphtheria toxoid, and reduced acellular pertussis (Tdap) vaccine and tetravalent meningococcal conjugate vaccine if they are not administered simultaneously.

[2]Live oral vaccines (eg, Ty21a typhoid vaccine and rotavirus vaccine) may be administered simultaneously or at any interval before or after inactivated or live injectable vaccines.

Adapted from American Academy of Pediatrics. Pertussis. Pickering LK, Baker CJ, Kimberlin DW, et al, eds. *Red Book*: 2009 Report of the Committee on Infectious Diseases. 28th ed. Elk Grove Village, IL: American Academy of Pediatrics; 2009;22.

Guidelines for Administering Antibody-Containing Products[1] and Vaccines

Simultaneous Administration (during the same office visit)

Products Administered	Recommended Minimum Interval Between Doses
Antibody-containing products and inactivated antigen	Can be administered simultaneously at different anatomic sites or at any time interval between doses.
Antibody-containing products and live antigen	Should **not** be administered simultaneously.[2] If simultaneous administration of measles-containing vaccine or varicella vaccine is unavoidable, administer at different sites and revaccinate or test for seroconversion after the recommended interval.

Nonsimultaneous Administration

Products Administered		Recommended Minimum Interval Between Doses
Administered first	Administered second	
Antibody-containing products	Inactivated antigen	No interval necessary
Inactivated antigen	Antibody-containing products	No interval necessary
Antibody-containing products	Live antigen	Dose-related[2,3]
Live antigen	Antibody-containing products	2 weeks[2]

[1]Blood products containing substantial amounts of immune globulin include intramuscular and intravenous immune globulin, specific hyperimmune globulin (eg, hepatitis B immune globulin, tetanus immune globulin, varicella zoster immune globulin, and rabies immune globulin), whole blood, packed red blood cells, plasma, and platelet products.

[2]Yellow fever vaccine, rotavirus vaccine, oral Ty21a typhoid vaccine, live-attenuated influenza vaccine, and zoster vaccine are exceptions to these recommendations. These live-attenuated vaccines can be administered at any time before, after, or simultaneously with an antibody-containing product.

[3]The duration of interference of antibody-containing products with the immune response to the measles component of measles-containing vaccine, and possibly varicella vaccine, is dose-related.

Recommended Intervals Between Administration of Antibody-Containing Products and Measles- or Varicella-Containing Vaccine, by Product and Indication for Vaccination

Product/Indication	Dose (mg IgG/kg) and Route[1]	Recommended Interval Before Measles- or Varicella-Containing Vaccine[2] Administration (mo)
Tetanus IG	I.M.: 250 units (10 mg IgG/kg)	3
Hepatitis A IG		
Contact prophylaxis	I.M.: 0.02 mL/kg (3.3 mg IgG/kg)	3
International travel	I.M.: 0.06 mL/kg (10 mg IgG/kg)	3
Hepatitis B IG	I.M.: 0.06 mL/kg (10 mg IgG/kg)	3
Rabies IG	I.M.: 20 int. units/kg (22 mg IgG/kg)	4

Recommended Intervals Between Administration of Antibody-Containing Products and Measles- or Varicella-Containing Vaccine, by Product and Indication for Vaccination (continued)

Product/Indication	Dose (mg IgG/kg) and Route[1]	Recommended Interval Before Measles- or Varicella-Containing Vaccine[2] Administration (mo)
Varicella IG	I.M.: 125 units/10 kg (60 to 200 mg IgG/kg) (maximum: 625 units)	5
Measles prophylaxis IG		
Standard (ie, nonimmunocompromised) contact	I.M.: 0.25 mL/kg (40 mg IgG/kg)	5
Immunocompromised contact	I.M.: 0.50 mL/kg (80 mg IgG/kg)	6
Blood transfusion		
Red blood cells (RBCs), washed	I.V.: 10 mL/kg (negligible IgG/kg)	None
RBCs, adenine-saline added	I.V.: 10 mL/kg (10 mg IgG/kg)	3
Packed RBCs (hematocrit 65%)[3]	I.V.: 10 mL/kg (60 mg IgG/kg)	6
Whole blood cells (hematocrit 35% to 50%)[3]	I.V.: 10 mL/kg (80 to 100 mg IgG/kg)	6
Plasma/platelet products	I.V.: 10 mL/kg (160 mg IgG/kg)	7
Cytomegalovirus intravenous immune globulin (IGIV)	150 mg/kg maximum	6
IGIV		
Replacement therapy for immune deficiencies[4]	I.V.: 300 to 400 mg/kg[4]	8
Immune thrombocytopenic purpura treatment	I.V.: 400 mg/kg	8
Postexposure varicella prophylaxis[5]	I.V.: 400 mg/kg	8
Immune thrombocytopenic purpura treatment	I.V.: 1000 mg/kg	10
Kawasaki disease	I.V.: 2 g/kg	11
Monoclonal antibody to respiratory syncytial virus F protein (Synagis [Medimmune])[6]	I.M.: 15 mg/kg	None

HIV = human immunodeficiency virus, IG = immune globulin, IgG = immune globulin G, IGIV = intravenous immune globulin, mg IgG/kg = milligrams of immune globulin G per kilogram of body weight, I.M. = intramuscular, I.V. = intravenous, RBCs = red blood cells

[1]This table is not intended for determining the correct indications and dosages for using antibody-containing products. Unvaccinated persons might not be fully protected against measles during the entire recommended interval, and additional doses of IG or measles vaccine might be indicated after measles exposure. Concentrations of measles antibody in an IG preparation can vary by manufacturer's lot. Rates of antibody clearance after receipt of an IG preparation also might vary. Recommended intervals are extrapolated from an estimated half-life of 30 days for passively acquired antibody and an observed interference with the immune response to measles vaccine for 5 months after a dose of 80 mg IgG/kg.

[2]Does not include zoster vaccine. Zoster vaccine may be given with antibody-containing blood products.

[3]Assumes a serum IgG concentration of 16 mg/mL

[4]Measles and varicella vaccinations are recommended for children with asymptomatic or mildly symptomatic HIV infection but are contraindicated for persons with severe immunosuppression from HIV or any other immunosuppressive disorder.

[5]The investigational product VariZIG, similar to licensed varicella-zoster IG (VZIG), is a purified human IG preparation made from plasma containing high levels of anti-varicella antibodies (IgG). The interval between VariZIG and varicella vaccine (Var or MMRV) is 5 months.

[6]Contains antibody only to respiratory syncytial virus

Vaccination of Persons With Primary and Secondary Immunodeficiencies

Category	Specific Immunodeficiency	Contraindicated Vaccines[1]	Risk-Specific Recommended Vaccines[1]	Effectiveness and Comments
Primary				
B-lymphocyte (humoral)	Severe antibody deficiencies (eg, X-linked agammaglobulinemia and common variable immunodeficiency)	Oral poliovirus (OPV)[2] Smallpox Live-attenuated influenza vaccine (LAIV) BCG Ty21a (live oral typhoid) Yellow fever	Pneumococcal Consider measles and varicella vaccination	The effectiveness of any vaccine is uncertain if it depends only on the humoral response (eg, PPSV or MPSV4) IGIV interferes with the immune response to measles vaccine and possibly varicella vaccine
	Less severe antibody deficiencies (eg, selective IgA deficiency and IgG subclass deficiency)	OPV[2] BCG Yellow Fever Other live-vaccines appear to be safe	Pneumococcal	All vaccines likely effective; immune response may be attenuated
T-lymphocyte (cell-mediated and humoral)	Complete defects (eg, severe combined immunodeficiency [SCID] disease, complete DiGeorge syndrome)	All live vaccines[3,4,5]	Pneumococcal	Vaccines might be ineffective
	Partial defects (eg, most patients with DiGeorge syndrome, Wiskott-Aldrich syndrome, ataxia-telangiectasia)	All live vaccines[3,4,5]	Pneumococcal Meningococcal Hib (if not administered in infancy)	Effectiveness of any vaccine depends on degree of immune suppression
Complement	Persistent complement, properdin, or factor B deficiency	None	Pneumococcal Meningococcal	All routine vaccines likely effective
Phagocytic function	Chronic granulomatous disease, leukocyte adhesion defect, and myeloperoxidase deficiency	Live bacterial vaccines[3]	Pneumococcal[6]	All inactivated vaccines safe and likely effective; live viral vaccines likely safe and effective
Secondary				
	HIV/AIDS	OPV[2] Smallpox BCG LAIV Withhold MMR and varicella in severely immunocompromised persons Yellow fever vaccine might have a contraindication or a precaution depending on clinical parameters of immune function[9]	Pneumococcal Consider Hib (if not administered in infancy) and meningococcal vaccination.	MMR, varicella, rotavirus, and all inactivated vaccines, including inactivated influenza, might be effective.[7]
	Malignant neoplasm, transplantation, immunosuppressive or radiation therapy	Live viral and bacterial, depending on immune status[3,4]	Pneumococcal	Effectiveness of any vaccine depends on degree of immune suppression

Vaccination of Persons With Primary and Secondary Immunodeficiencies *continued*

Category	Specific Immunodeficiency	Contraindicated Vaccines[1]	Risk-Specific Recommended Vaccines[1]	Effectiveness and Comments
	Asplenia	None	Pneumococcal Meningococcal Hib (if not administered in infancy)	All routine vaccines likely effective
	Chronic renal disease	LAIV	Pneumococcal Hepatitis B[8]	All routine vaccines likely effective

AIDS = acquired immunodeficiency syndrome; BCG = bacille Calmette-Guerin; Hib = *Haemophilus influenzae* type b; HIV = human immunodeficiency virus; IG = immunoglobulin; IGIV = immune globulin intravenous; LAIV = live, attenuated influenza vaccine; MMR = measles, mumps, and rubella; MPSV4 = quadrivalent meningococcal polysaccharide vaccine; OPV = oral poliovirus vaccine (live); PPSV = pneumococcal polysaccharide vaccine; TIV = trivalent inactivated influenza vaccine

[1]Other vaccines that are universally or routinely recommended should be administered if not contraindicated.

[2]OPV is no longer available in the United States.

[3]Live bacterial vaccines: BCG and oral Ty21a *Salmonella typhi* vaccine

[4]Live viral vaccines: MMR, MMRV, OPV, LAIV, yellow fever, zoster, rotavirus, varicella, and vaccinia (smallpox). Smallpox vaccine is not recommended for children or the general public.

[5]Regarding T-lymphocyte immunodeficiency as a contraindication for rotavirus vaccine, data exist only for severe combined immunodeficiency.

[6]Pneumococcal vaccine is not indicated for children with chronic granulomatous disease beyond age-based universal recommendations for PCV. Children with chronic granulomatous disease are not at increased risk for pneumococcal disease.

[7]HIV-infected children should receive IG after exposure to measles and may receive varicella and measles vaccine if CD4[+] lymphocyte count is ≥15%.

[8]Indicated based on the risk from dialysis-based bloodborne transmission

[9]Symptomatic HIV infection or CD4[+] T-lymphocyte count of <200/mm[3] or <15% of total lymphocytes for children aged <6 years is a contraindication to yellow fever vaccine administration. Asymptomatic HIV infection with CD4[+] T-lymphocyte count of 200 to 499/mm[3] for persons aged ≥6 years or 15% to 24% of total lymphocytes for children aged <6 years is a precaution for yellow fever vaccine administration. Details of yellow fever vaccine recommendations are available from the CDC. (CDC. Yellow fever vaccine: recommendations of the Advisory Committee on Immunization Practices [ACIP]. *MMWR Recomm Rep.* 2010;59[No. RR-7].)

Adapted from American Academy of Pediatrics. Passive immunization. Pickering LK, Baker CJ, Kimberlin DW, et al, eds. *Red Book:* 2009 Report of the Committee on Infectious Diseases. 28th ed. Elk Grove Village, IL: American Academy of Pediatrics; 2009:74-75.

Needle Length and Injection Site of I.M. for Children Aged ≤18 years (by age) and Adults Aged ≥19 years (by sex and weight)

Age Group	Needle Length	Injection Site
Children (birth to 18 y)		
Neonates[1]	5/8" (16 mm)[2]	Anterolateral thigh
Infant 1 to 12 mo	1" (25 mm)	Anterolateral thigh
Toddler 1 to 2 y	1" to 1¼" (25 to 32 mm)	Anterolateral thigh[3]
	5/8"[2] to 1" (16 to 25 mm)	Deltoid muscle of the arm
Children 3 to 18 y	5/8"[2] to 1" (16 to 25 mm)	Deltoid muscle of the arm[3]
	1" to 1¼" (25 to 32 mm)	Anterolateral thigh
Adults ≥19 y		
Men and women <60 kg (130 lb)	1" (25 mm)[4]	Deltoid muscle of the arm
Men and women 60 to 70 kg (130 to 152 lb)	1" (25 mm)	
Men 70 to 118 kg (152 to 260 lb)	1" to 1½" (25 to 38 mm)	
Women 70 to 90 kg (152 to 200 lb)		
Men >118 kg (260 lb)	1½" (38 mm)	
Women >90 kg (200 lb)		

I.M. = intramuscular

[1] First 28 days of life

[2] If skin is stretched tightly and subcutaneous tissues are not bunched

[3] Preferred site

[4] Some experts recommend a 5/8" needle for men and women who weigh <60 kg.

Adapted from Poland GA, Borrud A, Jacobsen RM, et al. Determination of deltoid fat pad thickness: implications for needle length in adult immunization. *JAMA.* 1997;277:1709-1711.

RECOMMENDATIONS FOR TRAVELERS

The Centers for Disease Control and Prevention (CDC) also provides guidance to assist travelers and their health care providers in deciding the vaccines, medications, and other measures necessary to prevent illness and injury during international travel. Available at http://wwwnc.cdc.gov/travel

REFERENCE

Centers for Disease Control and Prevention (CDC). Recommendations of the Advisory Committee on Immunization Practices (ACIP): general recommendations on immunization. *MMWR Recomm Rep.* 2011;60(2):1-61.

IMMUNIZATION GUIDELINES

Vaccine	Birth	1 mo	2 mos	4 mos	6 mos	9 mos	12 mos	15 mos	18 mos	19–23 mos	2–3 yrs	4–6 yrs	7–10 yrs	11–12 yrs	13–15 yrs	16–18 yrs
Hepatitis B[1] (HepB)	1st dose	2nd dose			3rd dose											
Rotavirus[2] (RV) RV-1 (2-dose series); RV-5 (3-dose series)			1st dose	2nd dose	see footnote 2											
Diphtheria, tetanus & acellular pertussis[3] (DTaP: <7 yrs)			1st dose	2nd dose	3rd dose			4th dose				5th dose				
Tetanus & diphtheria & acellular pertussis[4] (Tdap: ≥ 7 yrs)														(Tdap)		
Haemophilus influenzae type b[5] (Hib)			1st dose	2nd dose	see footnote 5		3rd or 4th dose, see footnote 5									
Pneumococcal conjugate[6] (PCV13)			1st dose	2nd dose	3rd dose		4th dose									
Pneumococcal polysaccharide[6] (PPSV23)																
Inactivated poliovirus[7] (IPV) (<18 years)			1st dose	2nd dose			3rd dose					4th dose				
Influenza[8] (IIV;LAIV) 2 doses for some: see footnote 8						Annual vaccination (IIV only)						Annual vaccination (IIV or LAIV)				
Measles, mumps, rubella[9] (MMR)							1st dose					2nd dose				
Varicella[10] (VAR)							1st dose					2nd dose				
Hepatitis A[11] (Hep A)							2 dose series see footnote 11									
Human papillomavirus[12] (HPV2: females only; HPV4: males and females)														(3 dose series)		
Meningococcal[13] (Hib-MenCY ≥ 6 wks; MenACWY-D ≥ 9 mos; MenACWY-CRM ≥ 2 mos.)					see footnote 13									1st dose		booster

Recommended Immunization Schedule for Persons 0 to 18 Years of Age — United States, 2014[a]

- Range of recommended ages for all children.
- Range of recommended ages for catch-up immunization.
- Range of recommended ages for certain high-risk groups.
- Range of recommended ages during which catch-up is encouraged and for certain high-risk groups.
- Not routinely recommended.

NOTE: The recommendations in the tables must be read along with the following footnotes.

[a] This schedule includes recommendations in effect as of January 1, 2014. Any dose not administered at the recommended age should be administered at a subsequent visit, when indicated and feasible. The use of a combination vaccine generally is preferred over separate injections of its equivalent component vaccines. Vaccination providers should consult the relevant Advisory Committee on Immunization Practices (ACIP) statement for detailed recommendations, available online at http://www.cdc.gov/vaccines/hcp/acip-recs/index. html. Clinically significant adverse events that follow vaccination should be reported to the Vaccine Adverse Event Reporting System (VAERS) online (http://www.vaers.hhs.gov) or by telephone (800-822-7967).Suspected cases of vaccine-preventable diseases should be reported to the state or local health department. Additional information, including precautions and contraindications for vaccination, is available from CDC online (http://www.cdc.gov/vaccines/recs/vac-admin/contraindications.htm) or by telephone (800-CDC-INFO [800-232-4636]). This schedule is approved by the Advisory Committee on Immunization Practices (http://www.cdc.gov/vaccines/acip), the American Academy of Pediatrics (http://www.aap.org), the American Academy of Family Physicians (http://www.aafp.org), and the American College of Obstetricians and Gynecologists (http://www.acog.org).

This schedule includes recommendations in effect as of January 1, 2014. Any dose not administered at the recommended age should be administered at a subsequent visit, when indicated and feasible. The use of a combination vaccine generally is preferred over separate injections of its equivalent component vaccines. Vaccination providers should consult the relevant Advisory Committee on Immunization Practices (ACIP) statement for detailed recommendations, available at **http://www.cdc.gov/vaccines/hcp/acip-recs/index.html**. Clinically significant adverse events that follow vaccination should be reported to the Vaccine Adverse Event Reporting System (VAERS), available at http://vaers.hhs.gov/index or by telephone at **(800) 822-7967**. Also see the footnotes after the following "Catch-up Immunization Schedule" for more specific information about the vaccines.

Catch-up Immunization Schedule for Persons 4 Months to 18 Years of Age Who Start Late or Who Are >1 Month Behind − United States, 2014

This table provides catch-up schedules and minimum intervals between doses for children whose vaccinations have been delayed. A vaccine series does not need to be restarted, regardless of the time that has elapsed between doses. Use the section appropriate for the child's age. Always use this table in conjunction with the previous "Recommended immunization schedule for persons aged 0 through 18 years" and the footnotes that follow.

Vaccine	Minimum Age for Dose 1	Minimum Interval Between Doses			
		Dose 1 to Dose 2	Dose 2 to Dose 3	Dose 3 to Dose 4	Dose 4 to Dose 5
Catch-up Schedule for Persons 4 Months to 6 Years of Age					
Hepatitis B[1]	Birth	**4 weeks**	**8 weeks** and ≥16 weeks after first dose; minimum age for final dose is 24 weeks		
Rotavirus[2]	6 weeks	**4 weeks**	**4 weeks**[2]		
Diphtheria, tetanus, and acellular pertussis[3]	6 weeks	**4 weeks**	**4 weeks**	**6 months**	**6 months**[3]
Haemophilus influenzae type b[5]	6 weeks	**4 weeks** if first dose administered at <12 months of age **8 weeks** (as final dose) if first dose administered at 12 to 14 months of age **No further doses needed** if first dose administered at ≥15 months of age	**4 weeks**[5] if currently <12 months of age and first dose administered at <7 months of age **8 weeks** and 12 to 59 months of age (as final dose)[5] if currently <12 months of age and first dose administered between 7 to 11 months of age (regardless of Hib vaccine [PRP-T or PRP-OMP] used for first dose); **or** if currently 12 to 59 months of age and first dose administered at <12 months of age; **or** first 2 doses were PRP-OMP and administered at <12 months of age **No further doses needed** if previous dose administered at ≥15 months of age	**8 weeks** (as final dose) This dose only necessary for children 12 to 59 months of age who received 3 (PRP-T) doses before 12 months of age and started primary series before 7 months of age	
Pneumococcal[6]	6 weeks	**4 weeks** if first dose administered at <12 months of age **8 weeks** (as final dose for healthy children) if first dose administered at ≥12 months of age **No further doses needed** for healthy children if first dose administered at ≥24 months of age	**4 weeks** if currently <12 months of age **8 weeks** (as final dose for healthy children) if currently ≥12 months of age **No further doses needed** for healthy children if previous dose administered at ≥24 months of age	**8 weeks** (as final dose) This dose only necessary for children 12 to 59 months of age who received 3 doses before 12 months of age or for children at high risk who received 3 doses at any age	
Inactivated poliovirus[7]	6 weeks	**4 weeks**[7]	**4 weeks**[7]	**6 months**[7] minimum 4 years of age for final dose	
Meningococcal[13]	6 weeks	**8 weeks**[13]	See footnote 13	See footnote 13	
Measles, mumps, rubella[9]	12 months	**4 weeks**			
Varicella[10]	12 months	**3 months**			
Hepatitis A[11]	12 months	**6 months**			
Catch-up Schedule for Persons 7 to 18 Years of Age					
Tetanus, diphtheria; tetanus, diphtheria, and acellular pertussis[4]	7 years[4]	**4 weeks**	**4 weeks** if first dose of DTaP/DT administered at <12 months of age **6 months** if first dose of DTaP/DT administered at ≥12 months of age and then no further doses needed for catch-up	**6 months** if first dose of DTaP/DT administered at <12 months of age	
Human papillomavirus[12]	9 years	Routine dosing intervals are recommended[12]			
Hepatitis A[11]	12 months	**6 months**			
Hepatitis B[1]	Birth	**4 weeks**	**8 weeks** (and ≥16 weeks after first dose)		
Inactivated poliovirus[7]	6 weeks	**4 weeks**	**4 weeks**[7]	**6 months**[7]	
Meningococcal[13]	6 weeks	**8 weeks**[13]			

Vaccine	Minimum Age for Dose 1	Minimum Interval Between Doses				
		Dose 1 to Dose 2	Dose 2 to Dose 3	Dose 3 to Dose 4	Dose 4 to Dose 5	
Measles, mumps, rubella[9]	12 months	**4 weeks**				
Varicella[10]	12 months	**3 months** if person is <13 years of age **4 weeks** if person is ≥13 years of age				

Footnotes to Recommended Immunization Schedule for Persons 0 to 18 Years of Age and the Catch-up Immunization Schedule

Note: For further guidance on the use of the vaccines mentioned below, see http://www.cdc.gov/vaccines/hcp/acip-recs/index.html. For vaccine recommendations for persons ≥19 years of age, see the adult immunization schedule.

[1]**Hepatitis B vaccine (HepB)** *(Minimum age: Birth)*
Routine vaccination:
  At birth:

- Administer monovalent HepB vaccine to all newborns before hospital discharge.

- For infants born to hepatitis B surface antigen (HB$_s$Ag)-positive mothers, administer HepB vaccine and 0.5 mL of hepatitis B immune globulin (HBIG) within 12 hours of birth. These infants should be tested for HB$_s$Ag and antibody to HB$_s$Ag (anti-HBs) 1 to 2 months after completion of the HepB series at 9 to 18 months of age (preferably at the next well-child visit).

- If the mother's HB$_s$Ag status is unknown, within 12 hours of birth, administer HepB vaccine to all infants regardless of birth weight. For infants weighing <2000 grams, administer HBIG in addition to HepB vaccine within 12 hours of birth. Determine the mother's HB$_s$Ag status as soon as possible and, if she is HB$_s$Ag-positive, also administer HBIG for infants weighing ≥2000 grams as soon as possible but no later than 7 days of age.

  Doses following the birth dose:

- The second dose should be administered at 1 or 2 months of age. Monovalent HepB vaccine should be used for doses administered before 6 weeks of age.

- Infants who did not receive a birth dose should receive 3 doses of a HepB-containing vaccine on a schedule of 0, 1 to 2 months, and 6 months of age starting as soon as feasible. See the previous "Catch-up Immunization Schedule".

- Administer the second dose 1 to 2 months after the first dose (minimum interval of 4 weeks); administer the third dose at least 8 weeks after the second dose **and** at least 16 weeks after the **first** dose. The final (third of fourth) dose in the HepB vaccine series should be administered **no earlier than 24 weeks of age**.

- Administration of a total of 4 doses of HepB vaccine is permitted when a combination vaccine containing HepB is administered after the birth dose.

  Catch-up vaccination:

- Unvaccinated persons should complete a 3-dose series.

- A 2-dose series (doses separated by at least 4 months) of adult formulation Recombivax HB is licensed for use in children 11 to 15 years of age.

- For other catch-up guidance, see the previous "Catch-up Immunization Schedule".

[2]**Rotavirus vaccine (RV)** *(Minimum age: 6 weeks for both RV-1 [Rotarix] and RV-5 [RotaTeq])*
Routine vaccination:

- Administer a series of RV vaccine to all infants as follows:

    – If Rotarix is used, administer a 2-dose series at 2 and 4 months of age.

    – If RotaTeq is used, administer a 3-dose series at ages 2, 4, and 6 months of age.

    – If any dose in the series was RotaTeq or vaccine product is unknown for any dose in the series, a total of 3 doses of RV vaccine should be administered.

  Catch-up vaccination:

- The maximum age for the first dose in the series is 14 weeks, 6 days; vaccination should not be initiated for infants ≥15 weeks, 0 days of age.

- The maximum age for the final dose in the series is 8 months, 0 days.

- For other catch-up guidance, see the previous "Catch-up Immunization Schedule".

[3]**Diphtheria and tetanus toxoids and acellular pertussis vaccine (DTaP)** *(Minimum age: 6 weeks; exception: DTaP-IPV [Kinrix]: 4 years)*
Routine vaccination:

- Administer a 5-dose series of DTaP vaccine at 2, 4, 6, and 15 to 18 months of age, and at 4 to 6 years of age. The fourth dose may be administered as early as 12 months of age, provided at least 6 months have elapsed since the third dose.

  Catch-up vaccination:

- The fifth dose of DTaP vaccine is not necessary if the fourth dose was administered at ≥4 years of age.

- For other catch-up guidance, see the previous "Catch-up Immunization Schedule".

⁴Tetanus and diphtheria toxoids and acellular pertussis vaccine (Tdap) *(Minimum age: 10 years for Adacel and Boostrix)*
Routine vaccination:

- Administer 1 dose of Tdap vaccine to all adolescents 11 to 12 years of age.

- Tdap can be administered regardless of the interval since the last tetanus and diphtheria toxoid-containing vaccine.

- Administer 1 dose of Tdap vaccine to pregnant adolescents during each pregnancy (preferred during 27 to 36 weeks gestation), regardless of time since prior Td or Tdap vaccination.

Catch-up vaccination:

- Persons ≥7 years of age who are not fully immunized with DTaP vaccine series should receive Tdap vaccine as 1 (preferably the first) dose in the catch-up series; if additional doses are needed, use Td vaccine. For children 7 to 10 years of age who receive a dose of Tdap as part of the catch-up series, an adolescent Tdap vaccine dose at 11 to 12 years of age should **not** be administered. Td should be administered instead 10 years after the Tdap dose.

- Persons 11 to 18 years of age who have not received Tdap vaccine should receive a dose, followed by tetanus and diphtheria toxoids (Td) booster doses every 10 years thereafter.

- Inadvertent doses of DTaP vaccine:

    – If administered inadvertently to a child 7 to 10 years of age, may count as part of the catch-up series. This dose can count as the adolescent Tdap dose or the child can later receive a Tdap booster dose at 11 to 12 years of age.

    – If administered inadvertently to an adolescent 11 to 18 years of age, the dose should be counted as the adolescent Tdap booster.

- For other catch-up guidance, see the previous "Catch-up Immunization Schedule".

⁵*Haemophilus influenzae* type b conjugate vaccine (Hib) *(Minimum age: 6 weeks for PRP-T [ActHIB, DTaP-IPV/Hib (Pentacel), and Hib-MenCY (MenHibrix)], PRP-OMP [PedvaxHIB or COMVAX], 12 months for PRP-T [Hiberix])*
Routine vaccination:

- Administer a 2- or 3-dose Hib vaccine primary series and a booster dose (dose 3 or 4 depending on vaccine used in primary series) at 12 to 15 months of age to complete a full Hib vaccine series.

- The primary series with ActHIB, MenHibrix, or Pentacel consists of 3 doses and should be administered at 2, 4, and 6 months of age. The primary series with PedvaxHib or COMVAX consists of 2 doses and should be administered at 2 and 4 months of age; a dose at 6 months of age is not indicated.

- One booster dose (dose 3 or 4 depending on vaccine used in primary series) of any Hib vaccine should be administered at 12 to 15 months of age. An exception is Hiberix vaccine. Hiberix should only be used for the booster (final) dose in children 12 months to 4 years of age who have received at least 1 prior dose of Hib-containing vaccine.

- For recommendations on the use of MenHibrix in patients at increased risk for meningococcal disease, please refer to the meningococcal vaccine footnotes and also to *MMWR*, 2013, 62(RR02);1-22, available at http://www.cdc.gov/mmwr/pdf/rr/rr6202.pdf.

Catch-up vaccination:

- If dose 1 was administered at 12 to 14 months of age, administer a second (final) dose at least 8 weeks after dose 1, regardless of Hib vaccine used in the primary series.

- If the first 2 doses were PRP-OMP (PedvaxHIB or COMVAX) and were administered at ≤11 months of age, the third (and final) dose should be administered at 12 to 15 months of age and at least 8 weeks after the second dose.

- If the first dose was administered at 7 to 11 months of age, administer the second dose at least 4 weeks later and a third (and final) dose at 12 to 15 months of age or 8 weeks after the second dose, whichever is later, regardless of Hib vaccine used for the first dose.

- If the first dose is administered at <12 months of age and the second dose is given between 12 to 14 months of age, a third (and final) dose should be given 8 weeks later.

- For unvaccinated children ≥15 months of age, administer only 1 dose.

- For other catch-up guidance, see the previous "Catch-up Immunization Schedule". For catch-up guidance related to MenHibrix, please see the meningococcal vaccine footnotes and also *MMWR*, 2013, 62(RR02);1-22, available at http://www.cdc.gov/mmwr/pdf/rr/rr6202.pdf.

Vaccination of persons with high-risk conditions:

- Children 12 to 59 months of age who are at increased risk for Hib disease, including chemotherapy recipients and whose with anatomic or functional asplenia (including sickle cell disease), human immunodeficiency virus (HIV) infection, immunoglobulin deficiency, or early component complement deficiency, who have received either no doses or only 1 dose of Hib vaccine before 12 months of age, should receive 2 additional doses of Hib vaccine 8 weeks apart; children who received ≥2 doses of Hib vaccine before 12 months of age should receive 1 additional dose.

- For patients <5 years of age undergoing chemotherapy or radiation treatment who received a Hib vaccine dose(s) within 14 days of starting therapy or during therapy, repeat the dose(s) at least 3 months following therapy completion.

- Recipients of hematopoietic stem cell transplant (HSCT) should be revaccinated with a 3-dose regimen of Hib vaccine starting 6 to 12 months after successful transplant, regardless of vaccination history; doses should be administered at elast 4 weeks apart.

- A single dose of any Hib-containing vaccine should be administered to unimmunized* children and adolescents ≥15 months of age undergoing an elective splenectomy; if possible, vaccine should be administered at least 14 days before the procedure.

- Hib vaccine is not routinely recommended for patients ≥5 years of age. However, 1 dose of Hib vaccine should be administered to unimmunized* persons ≥5 years of age who have anatomic or functional asplenia (including sickle cell disease) and unvaccinated persons 5 to 18 years of age with human immunodeficiency virus (HIV) infection.

*Patients who have not received a primary series and booster dose or at least 1 dose of Hib vaccine after 14 months of age are considered unimmunized.

[6]Pneumococcal vaccines *(Minimum age: 6 weeks for PCV13, 2 years for PPSV23)*

Routine vaccination with PCV13:

- Administer a 4-dose series of PCV13 vaccine at 2, 4, 6, and 12 to 15 months of age.

- For children 14 to 59 months of age who have received an age-appropriate series of 7-valent PCV (PCV7), administer a single supplemental dose of 13-valent PCV (PCV13).

Catch-up vaccination with PCV13:

- Administer 1 dose of PCV13 to all healthy children 24 to 59 months of age who are not completely vaccinated for their age.

- For other catch-up guidance, see the previous "Catch-up Immunization Schedule".

Vaccination of persons with high-risk conditions with PCV13 and PPSV23:

- All recommended PCV13 doses should be administered prior to PPSV23 vaccination if possible.

- For children 2 to 5 years of age with any of the following conditions: Chronic heart disease (particularly cyanotic congenital heart disease and cardiac failure); chronic lung disease (including asthma if treated with high-dose oral corticosteroid therapy); diabetes mellitus; cerebrospinal fluid leak; cochlear implant; sickle cell disease and other hemoglobuinopathies; anatomic or functional asplenia; HIV infection; chronic renal failure; nephrotic syndrome; diseases associated with treatment with immunosuppressive drugs or radiation therapy, including malignant neoplasms, leukemias, lymphomas, and Hodgkin disease; solid organ transplantation; or congenital immunodeficiency:

  1. Administer 1 dose of PCV13 if 3 doses of PCV (PCV7 and/or PCV13) were received previously.

  2. Administer 2 doses of PCV13 at least 8 weeks apart if fewer than 3 doses of PCV (PCV7 and/or PCV13) were received previously.

  3. Administer 1 supplemental dose of PCV13 if 4 doses of PCV7 or other age-appropriate complete PCV7 series was received previously.

  4. The minimum interval between doses of PCV (PCV7 or PCV13) is 8 weeks.

  5. For children with no history of PPSV23 vaccination, administer PPSV23 at least 8 weeks after the most recent dose of PCV13.

- For children 6 to 18 years of age who have cerebrospinal fluid leak; cochlear implant; sickle cell disease and other hemoglobinopathies; anatomic or functional asplenia; congenital or acquired immunodeficiencies; HIV infection; chronic renal failure; nephrotic syndrome; diseases associated with treatment with immunosuppressive drugs or radiation therapy, including malignant neoplasms, leukemias, lymphomas, and Hodgkin disease; generalized malignancy; solid organ transplantation; or multiple myeloma:

  1. If neither PCV13 nor PPSV23 has been received previously, administer 1 dose of PCV13 now and 1 dose of PPSV23 at least 8 weeks later.

  2. If PCV13 has been received previously but PPSV23 has not, administer 1 dose of PPSV23 at least 8 weeks after the most recent dose of PCV13.

  3. If PPSV23 has been received but PCV13 has not, administer 1 dose of PCV13 at least 8 weeks after the most recent dose of PPSV23.

- For children 6 to 18 years of age with chronic heart disease (particularly cyanotic congenital heart disease and cardiac failure), chronic lung disease (including asthma if treated with high-dose oral corticosteroid therapy), diabetes mellitus, alcoholism, or chronic liver disease, who have not received PPSV23, administer 1 dose of PPSV23. If PCV13 has been received previously, then PPSV23 should be administered at least 8 weeks after any prior PCV13 dose.

- A single revaccination with PPSV23 should be administered 5 years after the first dose to children with sickle cell disease or other hemoglobinopathies; anatomic or functional asplenia; congenital or acquired immunodeficiencies; HIV infection; chronic renal failure; nephrotic syndrome; diseases associated with treatment with immunosuppressive drugs or radiation therapy, including malignant neoplasms, leukemias, lymphomas, and Hodgkin disease; generalized malignancy; solid organ transplantation; or multiple myeloma.

[7]Inactivated poliovirus vaccine (IPV) *(Minimum age: 6 weeks)*

Routine vaccination:

- Administer a 4-dose series of IPV at 2, 4, and 6 to 18 months of age and at 4 to 6 years of age. The final dose in the series should be administered on or after the fourth birthday and at least 6 months after the previous dose.

Catch-up vaccination:

- In the first 6 months of life, minimum age and minimum intervals are only recommended if the person is at risk for imminent exposure to circulating poliovirus (ie, travel to a polio-endemic region or during an outbreak).

- If ≥4 doses are administered before 4 years of age, an additional dose should be administered at 4 to 6 years of age and at least 6 months after the previous dose.

- A fourth dose is not necessary if the third dose was administered at ≥4 years of age and at least 6 months after the previous dose.

- If both OPV and IPV were administered as part of a series, a total of 4 doses should be administered, regardless of the child's current age. IPV is not routinely recommended for U.S. residents ≥18 years of age.

- For other catch-up guidance, see the previous "Catch-up Immunization Schedule".

[8]**Influenza vaccines** (*Minimum age: 6 months for inactivated influenza vaccine [IIV]; 2 years for live, attenuated influenza vaccine [LAIV]*)
Routine vaccination:

- Administer influenza vaccine annually to all children beginning at 6 months of age. For most healthy, nonpregnant persons 2 to 49 years of age, either LAIV or IIV may be used. However, LAIV should **not** be administered to some persons, including 1) those with asthma, 2) children 2 to 4 years of age who had wheezing in the past 12 months, or 3) those who have any other underlying medical conditions that predispose them to influenza complications. For all other contraindications to use of LAIV, see *MMWR*, 2013, 62(No. RR-7);1-43, available at http://www.cdc.gov/mmwr/pdf/rr/rr6207.pdf.

For children 6 months to 8 years of age:

- For the 2013 to 2014 season, administer 2 doses (separated by at least 4 weeks) to children who are receiving influenza vaccine for the first time. Some children in this age group who have been vaccinated previously will also need 2 doses. For additional guidance, follow dosing guidelines in the 2013 to 2014 ACIP influenza vaccine recommendations. See *MMWR*, 2013, 62(No. RR-7);1-43, available at http://www.cdc.gov/mmwr/pdf/rr/rr6207.pdf.

- For the 2014 to 2015 season, follow dosing guidelines in the 2014 ACIP influenza vaccine recommendations.

For persons ≥9 years of age:

- Administer 1 dose.

[9]**Measles, mumps, and rubella vaccine (MMR)** (*Minimum age: 12 months for routine vaccination*)
Routine vaccination:

- Administer a 2-dose series of MMR vaccine at 12 to 15 months of age and 4 to 6 years of age. The second dose may be administered before 4 years of age, provided at least 4 weeks have elapsed since the first dose.

- Administer 1 dose of MMR vaccine to infants 6 to 11 months of age before departure from the United States for international travel. These children should be revaccinated with 2 doses of MMR vaccine, the first at 12 to 15 months of age (12 months if the child remains in an area where disease risk is high) and the second dose at least 4 weeks later.

- Administer 2 doses of MMR vaccine to children ≥12 months of age before departure from the United States for international travel. The first dose should be administered at ≥12 months of age and the second dose at least 4 weeks later.

Catch-up vaccination:

- Ensure that all school-aged children and adolescents have had 2 doses of MMR vaccine; the minimum interval between the 2 doses is 4 weeks.

- For other catch-up guidance, see the previous "Catch-up Immunization Schedule".

[10]**Varicella vaccine (VAR)** (*Minimum age: 12 months*)
Routine vaccination:

- Administer a 2-dose series of VAR vaccine at 12 to 15 months of age and 4 to 6 years of age. The second dose may be administered before 4 years of age, provided at least 3 months have elapsed since the first dose. If the second dose was administered at least 4 weeks after the first dose, it can be accepted as valid.

Catch-up vaccination:

- Ensure that all persons 7 to 18 years of age without evidence of immunity (see *MMWR*, 2007, 56[No. RR-4], available at http://www.cdc.gov/mmwr/pdf/rr/rr5604.pdf) have 2 doses of varicella vaccine. For children 7 to 12 years of age, the recommended minimum interval between doses is 3 months (if the second dose was administered at least 4 weeks after the first dose, it can be accepted as valid); for persons ≥13 years of age, the minimum interval between doses is 4 weeks.

- For other catch-up guidance, see the previous "Catch-up Immunization Schedule".

[11]**Hepatitis A vaccine (HepA)** (*Minimum age: 12 months*)
Routine vaccination:

- Initiate the 2-dose HepA vaccine series at 12 to 23 months of age; separate the 2 doses by 6 to 18 months.

- Children who have received 1 dose of HepA vaccine before 24 months of age should receive a second dose 6 to 18 months after the first dose.

- For any person ≥2 years of age who has not already received the HepA vaccine series, 2 doses of HepA vaccine separated by 6 to 18 months may be administered if immunity against hepatitis A virus infection is desired.

Catch-up vaccination:

- The minimum interval between the 2 doses is 6 months.

- For other catch-up guidance, see the previous "Catch-up Immunization Schedule".

Special populations:

- Administer 2 doses of HepA vaccine at least 6 months apart to previously unvaccinated persons who live in areas where vaccination programs target older children or who are at increased risk for infection. This includes persons traveling to or working in countries that have high or intermediate endemicity of infection; men having sex with men; users of injection and noninjection illicit drugs; persons who work with HAV-infected primates or with HAV in a research laboratory; persons with clotting-factor disorders; persons with chronic liver disease; and persons who anticipate close, personal contact (eg, household or regular babysitting) with an international adoptee during the first 60 days after arrival in the United States from a country with high or intermediate endemicity. The first dose should be administered as soon as the adoption is planned, ideally ≥2 weeks before the arrival of the adoptee.

[12]**Human papillomavirus vaccines (HPV)** *(Minimum age: 9 years for HPV2 [Cervarix] and HPV4 [Gardasil])*

Routine vaccination:

- Administer a 3-dose series of HPV vaccine on a schedule of 0, 1 to 2, and 6 months to all adolescents 11 to 12 years of age. Either HPV4 or HPV2 may be used for females and only HPV4 may be used for males.

- The vaccine series can be started beginning at 9 years of age.

- Administer the second dose 1 to 2 months after the first dose (minimum interval of 4 weeks) and administer the third dose 24 weeks after the first dose and 16 weeks after the second dose (minimum interval of 12 weeks).

Catch-up vaccination:

- Administer the vaccine series to females (either HPV2 or HPV4) and males (HPV4) at 13 to 18 years of age if not previously vaccinated.

- Use recommended routine dosing intervals (see above) for vaccine series catch-up.

- For other catch-up guidance, see the previous "Catch-up Immunization Schedule".

[13]**Meningococcal conjugate vaccines (MCV)** *(Minimum age: 6 weeks for Hib-MenCY [MenHibrix], 9 months for MenACWY-D [Menactra], 2 months for MenACWY-CRM [Menveo])*

Routine vaccination:

- Administer a single dose of Menactra or Menveo vaccine at 11 to 12 years of age with a booster dose at 16 years of age.

- Adolescents 11 to 18 years of age with human immunodeficiency virus (HIV) infection should receive a 2-dose primary series of Menactra or Menveo with at least 8 weeks between doses.

- For children 2 months to 18 years of age with high-risk conditions, see below.

Catch-up vaccination:

- Administer Menactra or Menveo vaccine at 13 to 18 years of age if not previously vaccinated.

- If the first dose is administered at 13 to 15 years of age, a booster dose should be administered at 16 to 18 years of age with a minimum interval of at least 8 weeks between doses.

- If the first dose is administered at ≥16 years of age, a booster dose is not needed.

- For other catch-up guidance, see the previous "Catch-up Immunization Schedule".

Vaccination of persons with high-risk conditions and other persons at increased risk of disease:

- Children with anatomic or functional asplenia (including sickle cell disease):

  1. For children <19 months of age, administer a 4-dose infant series of MenHibrix or Menveo at 2, 4, 6, and 12 to 15 months of age.

  2. For children 19 to 23 months of age who have not completed a series of MenHibrix or Menveo, administer 2 primary doses of Menveo at least 3 months apart.

  3. For children ≥24 months of age who have not received a complete series of MenHibrix, Menveo, or Menactra, administer 2 primary doses of either Menactra or Menveo at least 2 months apart. If Menactra is administered to a child with asplenia (including sickle cell disease), do not administer Menactra until 2 years of age and at least 4 weeks after the completion of all PCV13 doses.

- Children with persistent complement component deficiency:

  1. For children <19 months of age, administer a 4-dose infant series of either MenHibrix or Menveo at 2, 4, 6, and 12 to 15 months of age.

  2. For children 7 to 23 months of age who have not initiated vaccination, two options exist depending on age and vaccine brand:

     a. For children who initiate vaccination with Menveo at 7 to 23 months of age, a 2-dose series should be administered with the second dose after 12 months of age and at least 3 months after the first dose.

     b. For children who initiate vaccination with Menactra at 9 to 23 months of age, a 2-dose series of Menactra should be administered at least 3 months apart.

     c. For children ≥24 months of age who have not received a complete series of MenHibrix, Menveo, or Menactra, administer 2 primary doses of either Menactra or Menveo at least 2 months apart.

- For children who travel to or reside in countries in which meningoccoal disease is hyperendemic or epidemic, including countries in the African meningitis belt or the Hajj, administer an age-appropriate formulation and series of Menactra or Menveo for protection against serogroups A and W meningococcal disease. Prior receipt of MenHibrix is not sufficient for children traveling to the meningitis belt or the Hajj because it does not contain serogroups A or W.

- For children at risk during a community outbreak attributable to a vaccine serogroup, administer or complete an age- and formulation-appropriate series of MenHibrix, Menactra, or Menveo.

- For booster doses among persons with high-risk conditions, refer to *MMWR*, 2013, 62(RR02);1-22, available at http://www.cdc.gov/mmwr/preview/mmwrhtml/rr6202a1.htm.

Catch-up recommendations for persons with high-risk conditions:

1. If MenHibrix is administered to achieve protection against meningococcal disease, a complete age-appropriate series of MenHibrix should be administered.

2. If the first dose of MenHibrix is given at or after 12 months of age, a total of 2 doses should be given at least 8 weeks apart to ensure protection against serogroups C and Y meningococcal disease.

3. For children who initiate vaccination with Menveo at 7 to 9 months of age, a 2-dose series should be administered with the second dose after 12 months of age and at least 3 months after the first dose.

4. For other catch-up recommendations for these persons, refer to *MMWR*, 2013, 62(RR02);1-22, available at http://www.cdc.gov/mmwr/preview/mmwrhtml/rr6202a1.htm.

For complete information on the use of meningococcal vaccines, including guidance related to vaccination of persons at increased risk of infection, see *MMWR*, 2013, 62(RR02);1-22, available athttp://www.cdc.gov/mmwr/preview/mmwrhtml/rr6202a1.htm

This schedule is approved by the Advisory Committee on Immunization Practices (**http://www.cdc.gov/vaccines/acip/index.-html**), the American Academy of Pediatrics (**http://www.aap.org**), the American Academy of Family Physicians (**http://www.aafp.org**), and the American College of Obstetricians and Gynecologists (**http://www.acog.org**).

REFERENCE

Centers for Disease Control and Prevention (CDC). Advisory Committee on Immunization Practices (ACIP) recommended immunization schedules for persons aged 0 through 18 years and adults aged 19 years and older – United States, 2014. Available at http://www.cdc.gov/vaccines/schedules/hcp/child-adolescent.html

VACCINE INJURY TABLE

The Vaccine Injury Table makes it easier for some people to get compensation. The table lists and explains injuries/conditions that are presumed to be caused by vaccines. It also lists time periods in which the first symptom of these injuries/conditions must occur after receiving the vaccine. If the first symptom of these injuries/conditions occurs within the listed time period, it is presumed that the vaccine was the cause of the injury or condition, unless another cause is found. For example, if the patient received the tetanus vaccines and had a severe allergic reaction (anaphylaxis) within 4 hours after receiving the vaccine, then it is presumed that the tetanus vaccine caused the injury if no other cause is found.

If the injury/condition is not on the table or if the injury/condition did not occur within the time period on the table, it must be proven that the vaccine caused the injury/condition. Such proof must be based on medical records or opinion, which may include expert witness testimony.

Vaccine Injury Table[1]

Vaccine		Illness, Disability, Injury, or Condition Covered	Time Period for First Symptom or Manifestation of Onset or of Significant Aggravation After Vaccine Administration
Vaccines containing tetanus toxoid (eg, DTaP, DTP, DT, Td, TT)	A.	Anaphylaxis or anaphylactic shock	4 hours
	B.	Brachial neuritis	2 to 28 days
	C.	Any acute complication or sequela (including death) of an illness, disability, injury, or condition referred to above which illness, disability, injury, or condition arose within the time period prescribed	Not applicable
Vaccines containing whole cell pertussis bacteria, extracted or partial cell pertussis bacteria, or specific pertussis antigen(s) (eg, DTP, DTaP, P, DTP-Hib)	A.	Anaphylaxis or anaphylactic shock	4 hours
	B.	Encephalopathy (or encephalitis)	72 hours
	C.	Any acute complication or sequela (including death) of an illness, disability, injury, or condition referred to above which illness, disability, injury, or condition arose within the time period prescribed	Not applicable
Measles, mumps, and rubella vaccine or any of its components (eg, MMR, MR, M, R)	A.	Anaphylaxis or anaphylactic shock	4 hours
	B.	Encephalopathy (or encephalitis)	5 to 15 days
	C.	Any acute complication or sequela (including death) of an illness, disability, injury, or condition referred to above which illness, disability, injury, or condition arose within the time period prescribed	Not applicable
Vaccines containing rubella virus (eg, MMR, MR, R)	A.	Chronic arthritis	7 to 42 days
	B.	Any acute complication or sequela (including death) of an illness, disability, injury, or condition referred to above which illness, disability, injury, or condition arose within the time period prescribed	Not applicable
Vaccines containing measles virus (eg, MMR, MR, M)	A.	Thrombocytopenic purpura	7 to 30 days
	B.	Vaccine-strain measles viral infection in an immunodeficient recipient	6 months
	C.	Any acute complication or sequela (including death) of an illness, disability, injury, or condition referred to above which illness, disability, injury, or condition arose within the time period prescribed	Not applicable
Vaccines containing polio live virus (OPV)	A.	Paralytic polio	
		• In a nonimmunodeficient recipient	30 days
		• In an immunodeficient recipient	6 months
		• In a vaccine-associated community case	Not applicable
	B.	Vaccine-strain polio viral infection	
		• In a nonimmunodeficient recipient	30 days
		• In an immunodeficient recipient	6 months
		• In a vaccine-associated community case	Not applicable
	C.	Any acute complication or sequela (including death) of an illness, disability, injury, or condition referred to above which illness, disability, injury, or condition arose within the time period prescribed	Not applicable
Vaccines containing polio inactivated (eg, IPV)	A.	Anaphylaxis or anaphylactic shock	4 hours
	B.	Any acute complication or sequela (including death) of an illness, disability, injury, or condition referred to above which illness, disability, injury, or condition arose within the time period prescribed	Not applicable
Hepatitis B vaccines	A.	Anaphylaxis or anaphylactic shock	4 hours
	B.	Any acute complication or sequela (including death) of an illness, disability, injury, or condition referred to above which illness, disability, injury, or condition arose within the time period prescribed	Not applicable
Hemophilus influenzae type b polysaccharide conjugate vaccines		No condition specified	Not applicable
Varicella vaccine		No condition specified	Not applicable

Vaccine Injury Table[1] *(continued)*

Vaccine	Illness, Disability, Injury, or Condition Covered	Time Period for First Symptom or Manifestation of Onset or of Significant Aggravation After Vaccine Administration
Rotavirus vaccine	No condition specified	Not applicable
Pneumococcal conjugate vaccines	No condition specified	Not applicable
Hepatitis A vaccines	No condition specified	Not applicable
Trivalent influenza vaccines	No condition specified	Not applicable
Meningococcal vaccines	No condition specified	Not applicable
Human papillomavirus (HPV) vaccines	No condition specified	Not applicable
Any new vaccine recommended by the Centers for Disease Control and Prevention for routine administration to children, after publication by the secretary of a notice of coverage*	No condition specified	Not applicable

*Now includes all vaccines against seasonal influenza (except trivalent influenza vaccines, which are already covered), effective November 12, 2013

[1]Effective date: July 22, 2011; available at http://www.hrsa.gov/vaccinecompensation/vaccinetable.html

SKIN TESTS FOR DELAYED HYPERSENSITIVITY

Skin tests for delayed hypersensitivity are used diagnostically to assess previous infection (ie, PPD, histoplasmin, and coccidioidin) or used to evaluate cellular immune function by testing for anergy (ie, mumps, *Candida*, tetanus toxoid, trichophyton, PPD). Anergy, a defect in cell-mediated immunity, is characterized by a depressed response or lack of response to skin testing with injected antigens. Anergy has been associated with congenital and acquired immunodeficiencies and malnutrition.

Candida 1:100

Dose = 0.1 mL intradermally (30% of children younger than 18 months of age and 50% older than 18 months of age respond)

Can be used as a control antigen

Histoplasmin 1:100

Dose = 0.1 mL intradermally (yeast derived)

Mumps 40 cfu per mL

Dose = 0.1 mL intradermally (contraindicated in patients allergic to eggs, egg products, or thimerosal)

Purified Protein Derivatives 5 TU (PPD[1] Mantoux Tuberculin)

Screening for tuberculosis:

Children who have no risk factors but who reside in high-prevalence regions: skin test at 4 to 6 years and 11 to 16 years of age

Children exposed to HIV-infected individuals, homeless, residents of nursing homes, institutionalized adolescents, users of illicit drugs, incarcerated adolescents and migrant farm workers: skin test every 2 to 3 years

Children at high risk (children infected with HIV, incarcerated adolescents): annual skin testing

Dose = 0.1 mL intradermally

Definition of positive Mantoux skin test (regardless of previous BCG administration):

Reaction ≥5 mm for high-risk group (children in close contact with known or suspected infectious cases of tuberculosis; children suspected to have disease based on clinical and/or roentgenographic evidence; and children with underlying host factors (immunosuppressive conditions, receiving immunosuppressive therapy, and HIV infection).

Reaction ≥10 mm for children <4 years; those with medical diseases who are at increased risk for dissemination or for those at increased risk because of environmental exposure.

Reaction ≥15 mm for children ≥4 years of age including those with no risk factors.

[1]PPD 1 TU (first strength) is only used in individuals suspected of being highly sensitive. PPD 250 TU (second strength) is used only for individuals who fail to respond to a previous injection of 5 TU, or anergic patients in whom TB is suspected.

Tetanus Toxoid 1:5

Dose = 0.1 mL intradermally (29% of children younger than 2 years of age and 78% older than 2 years of age respond if they have received 3 immunizing doses)

Can be used as a control antigen.

Tine Test

Indication: survey and screen for exposure to tuberculosis (grasp forearm firmly; stretch the skin of the volar surface tightly; apply the tines to the selected site; press for at least one second so that a circular halo impression is left on the skin)

General Information

1. Intradermal skin tests should be injected in the flexor surface of the forearm.

2. A pale wheal 6 to 10 mm in diameter should form over the needle tip as soon as the injection is administered. If no bleb forms, the injection must be repeated.

3. Space skin tests at least 2 inches apart to prevent reactions from overlapping.

4. Read skin tests for diameter of induration and presence of erythema at 24, 48, and 72 hours. Reactions occurring before 24 hours are indicative of an immediate rather than a delayed hypersensitivity reaction.

5. False-negative results may occur in patients with malnutrition, viral infections, febrile illnesses, immunodeficiency disorders, severe disseminated infections, uremia, patients who have received immunosuppressive therapy (steroids, antineoplastic agents), patients who have received a recent live attenuated virus vaccine (MMR, measles).

6. False-positive results may occur in patients sensitive to ingredients in the skin test solution such as thimerosal; cross-sensitivity between similar antigens; or with improper interpretation of skin test.

7. Side effects are pain, blisters, extensive erythema and necrosis at the injection site.
   Emergency equipment and epinephrine should be readily available to treat severe allergic reactions that may occur.

Recommended Interpretation of Skin Test Reactions

Reaction	Local Reaction	
	After Intradermal Injections of Antigens	**After Dinitrochlorobenzene**
1+	Erythema >10 mm and/or induration >1 to 5 mm	Erythema and/or induration covering <1/2 area of dosing site
2+	Induration 6 to 10 mm	Induration covering >1/2 area of dose site
3+	Induration 11 to 20 mm	Vesiculation and induration at dose site or spontaneous flare at days 7 to 14 at the site
4+	Induration >20 mm	Bulla or ulceration at dose site or spontaneous flare at days 7 to 14 at the site

REFERENCES

American Academy of Pediatrics Committee on Infectious Diseases. Screening for tuberculosis in infants and children. *Pediatrics*. 1994;93(1):131-134.

American Academy of Pediatrics Committee on Infectious Diseases. Update on tuberculosis skin testing of children. *Pediatrics*. 1996;97(2):282-284.

REFERENCE VALUES FOR CHILDREN

	Normal Values	
	Age	**Serum Concentration**
CHEMISTRY		
	Premature 1 day	1.8 to 3 g/dL
	Full-term <6 days	2.5 to 3.4 g/dL
Albumin	8 days to 1 year	1.9 to 4.9 g/dL
	1 to 3 years	3.4 to 4.2 g/dL
	4 to 19 years	3.5 to 5.6 g/dL
Ammonia	All ages	19 to 60 mcg/dL
Amylase	1 to 19 years	30 to 100 units/L
Bilirubin, total	*See nomogram for age-specific neonatal values*	
	1 month to Adult	<1 mg/dL
	Cord blood	9 to 11.5 mg/dL
	Newborn 3 to 24 hours	9 to 10.6 mg/dL
	Newborn 24 to 48 hours	7 to 12 mg/dL
Calcium, total	4 to 7 days	9 to 10.9 mg/dL
	Child	8.8 to 10.8 mg/dL
	Adolescent to Adult	8.4 to 10.2 mg/dL
	Cord blood	5 to 6 mg/dL
Calcium, ionized, whole blood	Newborn 3 to 24 hours	4.3 to 5.1 mg/dL
	Newborn 24 to 48 hours	4 to 4.7 mg/dL
	≥2 days	4.8 to 4.92 mg/dL (2.24 to 2.46 mEq/L)
	Newborn	27 to 40 mm Hg
	Infant	27 to 41 mm Hg
Carbon dioxide (PCO_2)	Child to Adult:	
	Male	35 to 48 mm Hg
	Female	32 to 45 mm Hg
Chloride		95 to 105 mEq/L
Cholesterol	*See following tables for age- and gender-specific values*	
Creatinine	0 to 4 years	0.03 to 0.5 mg/dL
	4 to 7 years	0.03 to 0.59 mg/dL
	7 to 10 years	0.22 to 0.59 mg/dL
	10 to 14 years	0.31 to 0.88 mg/dL
(IDMS) Enzymatic	>14 years	0.5 to 1.06 mg/dL
	Cord blood	45 to 96 mg/dL
	Premature	20 to 60 mg/dL
	Neonate	30 to 60 mg/dL
Glucose	Newborn 1 day	40 to 60 mg/dL
	>1 day	50 to 90 mg/dL
	Child	60 to 100 mg/dL
	Adult	70 to 105 mg/dL
Iron	All ages	22 to 184 mcg/dL
Iron binding capacity, total	Infant	100 to 400 mcg/dL
	≥1 year to Adult	250 to 400 mcg/dL
	1 to 12 months	10 to 21 mg/dL
Lactic acid, lactate	1 to 7 years	7 to 14 mg/dL
	7 to 15 years	5 to 8 mg/dL
Lead, whole blood	Child	<10 mcg/dL
	Toxic	≥70 mcg/dL
Lipase	1 to 18 years	145 to 216 units/L
Magnesium		1.5 to 2.5 mEq/L
Osmolality, serum	Child to Adult	275 to 295 mOsm/kg

		Normal Values	
CHEMISTRY	**Age**	**Serum Concentration**
	Newborn 0 to 5 days	4.8 to 8.2 mg/dL
	1 to 3 years	3.8 to 6.5 mg/dL
Phosphorus	4 to 11 years	3.7 to 5.6 mg/dL
	12 to 15 years	2.9 to 5.4 mg/dL
	16 to 19 years	2.7 to 4.7 mg/dL
	Newborn	4.5 to 7.2 mEq/L
	2 days to 3 months	4 to 6.2 mEq/L
Potassium, plasma	3 months to 1 year	3.7 to 5.6 mEq/L
	1 to 16 years	3.5 to 5 mEq/L
	Premature neonate	4.3 to 7.6 g/dL
	Newborn	4.6 to 7.4 g/dL
Protein, total	1 to 7 years	6.1 to 7.9 g/dL
	8 to 12 years	6.4 to 8.1 g/dL
	13 to 19 years	6.6 to 8.2 g/dL
Sodium		136 to 145 mEq/L
Triglycerides	*See following tables for age- and gender-specific values*	
	Cord blood	21 to 40 mg/dL
	Premature (1 week)	3 to 25 mg/dL
Urea nitrogen, blood	Newborn	3 to 12 mg/dL
	Infant to Child	5 to 18 mg/dL
	Adolescent to Adult	7 to 18 mg/dL
	1 to 3 years	1.8 to 5 mg/dL
	4 to 6 years	2.2 to 4.7 mg/dL
	7 to 9 years	2 to 5 mg/dL
	10 to 11 years:	
	Male	2.3 to 5.4 mg/dL
	Female	3 to 4.7 mg/dL
Uric acid	12 to 13 years: Male	2.7 to 6.7 mg/dL
	14 to 15 years: Male	2.4 to 7.8 mg/dL
	12 to 15 years: Female	3 to 5.8 mg/dL
	16 to 19 years:	
	Male	4 to 8.6 mg/dL
	Female	3 to 5.9 mg/dL
ENZYMES		
	≤7 days	6 to 40 units/L
	8 to 30 days:	
	Male	10 to 40 units/L
Alanine aminotransferase (ALT) (SGPT)	Female	8 to 32 units/L
	1 to 12 months	12 to 45 units/L
	1 to 19 years	5 to 45 units/L
	1 to 9 years	145 to 420 units/L
	10 to 11 years	140 to 560 units/L
	12 to 13 years:	
	Male	200 to 495 units/L
	Female	105 to 420 units/L
Alkaline phosphatase (ALKP)	14 to 15 years:	
	Male	130 to 525 units/L
	Female	70 to 230 units/L
	16 to 19 years:	
	Male	65 to 260 units/L
	Female	50 to 130 units/L

ENZYMES

<u>Normal Values</u>

	Age	Serum Concentration
	Newborn ≤7 days:	
	Male	30 to 100 units/L
	Female	24 to 95 units/L
	8 to 30 days	22 to 71 units/L
	1 to 12 months	22 to 63 units/L
Aspartate aminotransferase (AST) (SGOT)	1 to 3 years	20 to 60 units/L
	3 to 9 years	15 to 50 units/L
	10 to 15 years	10 to 40 units/L
	16 to 19 years:	
	Male	15 to 45 units/L
	Female	5 to 30 units/L
	Cord blood	70 to 380 units/L
	Newborn 5 to 8 hours	214 to 1175 units/L
Creatine kinase (CK)	Newborn 24 to 33 hours	130 to 1200 units/L
	Newborn 72 to 100 hours	87 to 725 units/L
	Adult	5 to 130 units/L
	<1 year	170 to 580 units/L
Lactate dehydrogenase (LDH)	1 to 9 years	150 to 500 units/L
	10 to 19 years	120 to 330 units/L

Blood Gases

	Arterial	Capillary	Venous
pH	7.35 to 7.45	7.35 to 7.45	7.32 to 7.42
pCO_2 (mm Hg)	35 to 45	35 to 45	38 to 52
pO_2 (mm Hg)	70 to 100	60 to 80	24 to 48
HCO_3 (mEq/L)	19 to 25	19 to 25	19 to 25
TCO_2 (mEq/L)	19 to 29	19 to 29	23 to 33
O_2 saturation (%)	90 to 95	90 to 95	40 to 70
Base excess (mEq/L)	-5 to +5	-5 to +5	-5 to +5

Hyperbilirubinemia Assessment in the Newborn Infant

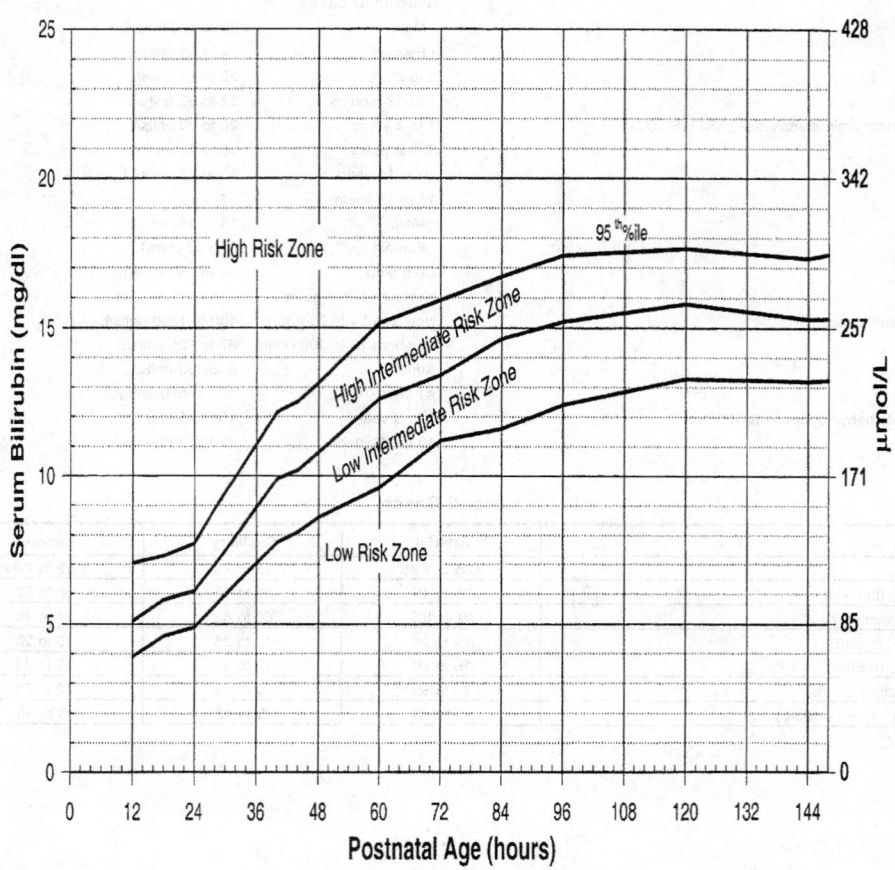

Nomogram for designation of risk in 2840 well newborns at ≥36 weeks gestational age with birth weight of ≥2000 g or ≥35 weeks gestational age and birth weight of ≥2500 g based on the hour-specific serum bilirubin values. The serum bilirubin level was obtained before discharge and the zone in which the value fell predicted the likelihood of a subsequent bilirubin level exceeding the 95th percentile (high-risk zone).

Classification of Serum Lipid Concentrations[1]

Classification	Total Cholesterol[2] (mg/dL)		LDL-C[2] (mg/dL)		HDL-C[2] (mg/dL)			Apolipoprotein A-1	Triglycerides[3] (mg/dL)			Apolipoprotein B
	Children and Adolescents	Young Adults	Children and Adolescents	Young Adults	Children and Adolescents	Young Adults		Children and Adolescents	Children 0 to 9 years	Children ≥10 years and Adolescents <19 years	Young Adults	Children and Adolescents
Low					<40	<40		<115				
Borderline low						40 to 44						
Acceptable/ optimal	<170	<190	<110	<120	>45	>45		>120	<75	<90	<115	<90
Borderline high	170 to 199	190 to 224	120 to 159	130 to 159	40 to 45			115 to 120	75 to 99	90 to 129	115 to 149	90 to 109
High	≥200	≥225	≥130	≥160					≥100	≥130	≥150	≥110

[1]Adapted from: Expert panel on integrated guidelines for cardiovascular health and risk reduction in children and adolescents: summary report. *Pediatrics.* 2011;128(Suppl 5):S213-S256.

[2]To convert cholesterol results to SI units, divide value by 38.6.

[3]To convert triglyceride results to SI units, divide value by 88.6.

Serum Lipid Concentrations by Age and Gender

	Males (mg/dL)			Females (mg/dL)		
	5 to 9 years	10 to 14 years	15 to 19 years	5 to 9 years	10 to 14 years	15 to 19 years
Total Cholesterol						
50th percentile	153	161	152	164	159	157
75th percentile	168	173	168	177	171	176
90th percentile	183	191	183	189	191	198
95th percentile	186	201	191	197	205	208
Triglycerides						
50th percentile	48	58	68	57	68	64
75th percentile	58	74	88	74	85	85
90th percentile	70	94	125	103	104	112
95th percentile	85	111	143	120	120	126
LDL-C						
50th percentile	90	94	93	98	94	93
75th percentile	103	109	109	115	110	110
90th percentile	117	123	123	125	126	129
95th percentile	129	133	130	140	136	137
HDL						
5th percentile	38	37	30	36	37	35
10th percentile	43	40	34	38	40	38
25th percentile	49	46	39	48	45	43
50th percentile	55	55	46	52	52	51

Adapted from: American Academy of Pediatrics Committee on Nutrition. Lipid screening and cardiovascular health in childhood. *Pediatrics.* 2008;122:(1) 198-208.

Thyroid Function Tests

	Age	Normal Range
T_4 (thyroxine) serum concentrations	1 to 7 days	10.1 to 20.9 mcg/dL
	8 to 14 days	9.8 to 16.6 mcg/dL
	1 month to 1 year	5.5 to 16 mcg/dL
	>1 year	4 to 12 mcg/dL
Free Thyroxine Index (FTI)	1 to 3 days	9.3 to 26.6
	1 to 4 weeks	7.6 to 20.8
	1 to 4 months	7.4 to 17.9
	4 to 12 months	5.1 to 14.5
	1 to 6 years	5.7 to 13.3
	>6 years	4.8 to 14
T_3 serum concentration	Newborn	100 to 470 ng/dL
	1 to 5 years	100 to 260 ng/dL
	5 to 10 years	90 to 240 ng/dL
	10 years to Adult	70 to 210 ng/dL
T_3 uptake		35% to 45%
TSH serum concentration	Cord sample	3 to 22 micro international units/mL
	1 to 3 days	<40 micro international units/mL
	3 to 7 days	<25 micro international units/mL
	>7 days	≤10 micro international units/mL

Hematology Values

Age	Hgb (g/dL)	Hct (%)	RBC (mill/mm³)	RDW	MCV (fL)	MCH (pg/cell)	MCHC (%)	PLTS (x 10³/mm³)
≤30 days	15 to 24	44 to 70			99 to 115	33 to 39		84 to 478*
1 to 23 months	10.5 to 14	32 to 42			72 to 88	24 to 30		
2 to 9 years	11.5 to 14.5	33 to 43			76 to 90	25 to 31		
10 to 17 years (male)	12.5 to 16.1	36 to 47	4 to 5.5	12% to 15%	78 to 95	26 to 32	32 to 36	150 to 450
10 to 17 years (female)	12 to 15	35 to 45			78 to 95	26 to 32		
≥18 years (male)	13.5 to 18	42 to 52			78 to 100	27 to 31		
≥18 years (female)	12.5 to 16	37 to 47			78 to 100	27 to 31		

*Value for ages 0 to 7 days, for ages >7 days similar to range for all patient ages

WBC and Diff

Age	WBC (x 10³/mm³)	Segs	Bands	Lymphs	Monos	Eosinophils	Basophils	Myelocytes
≤30 days	9.1 to 34							
1 to 23 months	6 to 14							
2 to 9 years	4 to 12	54% to 62%	3% to 5%	25% to 33%	3% to 7%	1% to 3%	≤0.75%	0%
10 to 17 years	4 to 10.5							
≥18 years	4 to 10.5							

Segs = segmented neutrophils, bands = band neutrophils, lymphs = lymphocytes, monos = monocytes

Erythrocyte Sedimentation Rates and Reticulocyte Counts

Sedimentation rate, Westergren	Child	0 to 20 mm/hour
	Adult male	0 to 15 mm/hour
	Adult female	0 to 20 mm/hour
Sedimentation rate, Wintrobe	Child	0 to 13 mm/hour
	Adult male	0 to 10 mm/hour
	Adult female	0 to 15 mm/hour
Reticulocyte count: Neonatal and infant data based on capillary specimen	1 day	0.4% to 0.6%
	7 days	<0.1% to 1.3%
	1 to 4 weeks	<1% to 1.2%
	5 to 6 weeks	<0.1% to 2.4%
	7 to 8 weeks	0.1% to 2.9%
	9 to 10 weeks	<0.1% to 2.6%
	11 to 12 weeks	0.1% to 1.3%
Reticulocyte count: Whole blood specimen	Adult	0.5% to 1.5%

Cerebrospinal Fluid Values, Normal

		% PMNs
Cell count:		
Preterm mean	9 (0 to 25.4 WBC/mm^3)	57%
Term mean	8.2 (0 to 22.4 WBC/mm^3)	61%
>1 month	0.7	0
Glucose:		
Preterm	24 to 63 mg/dL	mean 50 mg/dL
Term	34 to 119 mg/dL	mean 52 mg/dL
Child	40 to 80 mg/dL	
CSF glucose/blood glucose:		
Preterm	55% to 105%	
Term	44% to 128%	
Child	50%	
Lactic acid dehydrogenase	5 to 30 units/mL	mean 20 units/mL
Myelin basic protein	<4 ng/mL	
Pressure: Initial LP (mm H$_2$O):		
Newborn	80 to 110 (<110)	
Infant/Child	<200 (lateral recumbent position)	
Respiratory movements	5 to 10	
Protein:		
Preterm	65 to 150 mg/dL	mean 115 mg/dL
Term	20 to 170 mg/dL	mean 90 mg/dL
Child:		
Ventricular	5 to 15 mg/dL	
Cisternal	5 to 25 mg/dL	
Lumbar	5 to 40 mg/dL	

ACID/BASE ASSESSMENT

Henderson-Hasselbalch Equation

$pH = 6.1 + \log ([HCO_3^-] / (0.03) [PaCO_2])$

Normal arterial blood pH: 7.4 (normal range: 7.35 to 7.45)

Where:

$[HCO_3^-]$ = Serum bicarbonate concentration

$PaCO_2$ = Arterial carbon dioxide partial pressure

Alveolar Gas Equation

P_iO_2 = F_iO_2 x (total atmospheric pressure – vapor pressure of H_2O at 37°C)

  = F_iO_2 x (760 mm Hg – 47 mm Hg)

PAO_2 = $P_iO_2 – (PaCO_2 / R)$

Alveolar-arterial oxygen (A-a) gradient = $PAO_2 – PaO_2$

or

A-a gradient = $[(F_iO_2 \times 713) – (PaCO_2/0.8)] – PaO_2$

A-a gradient normal ranges:

Children	15 to 20 mm Hg
Adults	20 to 25 mm Hg

where:

P_iO_2 = Oxygen partial pressure of inspired gas (mm Hg) (150 mm Hg in room air at sea level)

F_iO_2 = Fractional pressure of oxygen in inspired gas (0.21 in room air)

PAO_2 = Alveolar oxygen partial pressure

PaO_2 = Arterial oxygen partial pressure

$PaCO_2$ = Arterial carbon dioxide partial pressure

R = Respiratory exchange quotient (typically 0.8, increases with high carbohydrate diet, decreases with high fat diet)

Acid-Base Disorders

Acute metabolic acidosis:
$PaCO_2$ expected = 1.5 ($[HCO_3^-]$) + 8 ± 2 **or**
Expected decrease in $PaCO_2$ = 1.3 (1-1.5) x decrease in $[HCO_3^-]$

Acute metabolic alkalosis:
Expected increase in $PaCO_2$ = 0.6 (0.5-1) x increase in $[HCO_3^-]$

Acute respiratory acidosis (<6 h duration):
For every $PaCO_2$ increase of 10 mm Hg, $[HCO_3^-]$ increases by 1 mEq/L

Chronic respiratory acidosis (>6 h duration):
For every $PaCO_2$ increase of 10 mm Hg, $[HCO_3^-]$ increases by 4 mEq/L

Acute respiratory alkalosis (<6 h duration):
For every $PaCO_2$ decrease of 10 mm Hg, $[HCO_3^-]$ decreases by 2 mEq/L

Chronic respiratory alkalosis (>6 h duration):
For every $PaCO_2$ decrease of 10 mm Hg, $[HCO_3^-]$ increases by 5 mEq/L

LABORATORY CALCULATIONS

ANION GAP

Definition: The difference in concentration between unmeasured cation and anion equivalents in serum.

Anion gap = $Na^+ - (Cl^- + HCO_3^-)$
(The normal anion gap is 10 to 14 mEq/L)

Differential Diagnosis of Increased Anion Gap Acidosis

Organic anions
Lactate (sepsis, hypovolemia, seizures, large tumor burden)
Pyruvate
Uremia
Ketoacidosis (beta-hydroxybutyrate and acetoacetate)
Amino acids and their metabolites
Other organic acids (eg, formate from methanol, glycolate from ethylene glycol)

Inorganic anions
Hyperphosphatemia
Sulfates
Nitrates

Medications and toxins
Penicillins and cephalosporins
Salicylates (including aspirin)
Cyanide
Carbon monoxide

Differential Diagnosis of Decreased Anion Gap

Organic cations
Hypergammaglobulinemia

Inorganic cations
Hyperkalemia
Hypercalcemia
Hypermagnesemia

Medications and toxins
Lithium

Hypoalbuminemia

OSMOLALITY

Definition: The summed concentrations of all osmotically active solute particles

Predicted serum osmolality =

$$mOsm/L = (2 \times serum\ Na^{++}) + \frac{serum\ glucose}{18} + \frac{BUN}{2.8}$$

The normal range of serum osmolality is 285 to 295 mOsm/L.

Calculated Osm

Note: Osm is a term used to reconcile osmolality and osmolarity

Osmol gap = measured Osm – calculated Osm

0 to +10: Normal
>10: Abnormal
<0: Probable lab or calculation error

Differential Diagnosis of Increased Osmol Gap
(increased by >10 mOsm/L)
Ethanol
Ethylene glycol
Glycerol
Iodine (questionable)
Isopropanol (acetone)
Mannitol
Methanol
Sorbitol

CORRECTED SODIUM FOR HYPERGLYCEMIA

Corrected Na^+ = serum Na^+ + [1.5 x (glucose − 150 divided by 100)]

Note: Do not correct for glucose <150.

CORRECTED TOTAL SERUM CALCIUM FOR ALBUMIN LEVEL

[(Normal albumin − patient's albumin) x 0.8] + patient's measured total calcium

BICARBONATE DEFICIT

HCO_3^- deficit = (0.4 x wt in kg) x (HCO_3^- desired − HCO_3^- measured)

Note: In clinical practice, the calculated quantity may differ markedly from the actual amount of bicarbonate needed or that which may be safely administered.

APGAR SCORING SYSTEM

	Score		
Sign	0	1	2
Heart rate	Absent	Under 100 beats per minute	Over 100 beats per minute
Respiratory effort	Absent	Slow (irregular)	Good crying
Muscle tone	Limp	Some flexion of extremities	Active motion
Reflex irritability	No response	Grimace	Cough or sneeze
Color	Blue, pale	Pink body, blue extremities	All pink

From Apgar V. A proposal for a new method of evaluation of the newborn infant. *Anesth Analg.* 1953;32:260.

FETAL HEART RATE MONITORING

Normal Heart Rates

Fetal heart rate (FHR) 120 to 160 bpm. Isolated accelerations are normal and considered reassuring. Mild (100 to 120 bpm) and transient bradycardias may be normal. Normal fetal heart rate tracings show beat-to-beat variability of 5 to 10 bpm (poor beat-to-beat variability suggests fetal hypoxia).

Abnormal Heart Rates

Bradycardia (FHR <120 bpm): Potential causes include fetal distress, drugs, congenital heart block (associated with maternal SLE, congenital cardiac defects).

Tachycardia (FHR >160 bpm): Potential causes include maternal fever, chorioamnionitis, drugs, fetal dysrhythmias, eg, SVT (with or without fetal CHF).

Decreased Beat-to-Beat Variability

Results from fetal CNS depression. Potential causes include fetal hypoxia, fetal sleep, fetal immaturity, and maternal narcotic/sedative administration.

Fetal Heart Rate Decelerations

Type 1 (early decelerations)

- Seen most commonly in late labor
- Mirror uterine contractions in time of onset, duration, and resolution
- Uniform shape
- Usually associated with good beat-to-beat variability
- Heart rate may dip to 60 to 80 bpm
- Associated with fetal head compression (increases vagal tone)
- Considered benign, and not representative of fetal hypoxia

Type 2 (late decelerations)

- Deceleration 10 to 30 seconds after onset of uterine contraction
- Heart rate fails to return to baseline after contraction is completed
- Asymmetrical shape (longer deceleration, shorter acceleration)
- Late decelerations of 10 to 20 bpm may be significant
- Probably associated with fetal CNS and myocardial depression

Type 3 (variable decelerations)

- Heart rate variations do not correlate with uterine contractions
- Variable shape and duration
- Occur occasionally in many normal labors
- Concerning if severe (HR <60 bpm), prolonged (duration >60 seconds), associated with poor beat-to-beat variability, or combined with late decelerations
- Associated with cord compression (including nuchal cord)

REFERENCE

Manual of Neonatal Care, Joint Program in Neonatology. 3rd ed. Cloherty JP, Stark AR, eds. Boston, MA: Little, Brown; 1991.

RENAL FUNCTION ESTIMATION IN ADULT PATIENTS

Evaluation of a patient's renal function often includes the use of equations to estimate glomerular filtration rate (GFR) (eg, estimated GFR [eGFR] creatinine clearance [CrCl]) using an endogenous filtration marker (eg, serum creatinine) and other patient variables. For example, the Cockcroft-Gault equation estimates renal function by calculating CrCl and is typically used to steer medication dosing. Equations which calculate eGFR are primarily used to categorize chronic kidney disease (CKD) staging and monitor progression. The rate of creatinine clearance does not always accurately represent GFR; creatinine may be cleared by other renal mechanisms in addition to glomerular filtration and serum creatinine concentrations may be affected by nonrenal factors (eg, age, gender, race, body habitus, illness, diet). In addition, these equations were developed based on studies in limited populations and may either over- or underestimate the renal function of a specific patient.

Nevertheless, most clinicians estimate renal function using CrCl as an indicator of actual renal function for the purpose of adjusting medication doses. For medications that require dose adjustment for renal impairment, utilization of eGFR (ie, Modification of Diet in Renal Disease [MDRD]) may overestimate renal function by up to 40% which may result in supra-therapeutic medication doses (Hermsen, 2009). These equations should only be used in the clinical context of patient-specific factors noted during the physical exam/work-up. The 2012 National Kidney Foundation (NKF)-Kidney Disease Improving Global Outcomes (KDIGO) CKD guidelines state that drug dosing should be based on an e-GFR which is **not** adjusted for body surface area (BSA) (ie, reported in units of mL/minute/1.73 m^2) since the effect of eGFR adjusted for BSA compared to eGFR without adjustments for BSA has not been extensively studied. **Decisions regarding drug therapy and doses must be based on clinical judgment.**

RENAL FUNCTION ESTIMATION EQUATIONS

Commonly used equations to estimate renal function utilizing the endogenous filtration marker serum creatinine include the Cockcroft-Gault, Jelliffe, four-variable Modification of Diet in Renal Disease (MDRD), six-variable MDRD (aka, MDRD extended), and Chronic Kidney Disease Epidemiology Collaboration (CKD-EPI). All of these equations, except for the CKD-EPI, were originally developed using a serum creatinine assay measured by the alkaline picrate-based (Jaffe) method. Many substances, including proteins, can interfere with the accuracy of this assay and overestimate serum creatinine concentration. The NKF and The National Kidney Disease Education Program (NDKEP) advocated for a universal creatinine assay, in order to ensure an accurate estimate of renal function in patients. As a result, a more specific enzymatic assay with an isotope dilution mass spectrometry (IDMS)-traceable international standard was developed. Compared to the older methods, IDMS-traceable assays may report lower serum creatinine values and may, therefore, overestimate renal function when used in the original equations not re-expressed for use with a standardized serum creatinine assay (eg, Cockcroft-Gault, Jelliffe, original MDRD). Updated four-variable MDRD and six-variable MDRD equations based on serum creatinine measured by the IDMS-traceable method has been proposed for adults (Levey, 2006); the Cockcroft-Gault and Jelliffe equations have not been re-expressed and may overestimate renal function when used with a serum creatinine measured by the IDMS-traceable method. However, at this point, all laboratories should be using creatinine methods calibrated to be IDMS traceable.

The CKD-EPI creatinine equation, published in 2009, uses the same four variables as the four-variable MDRD (serum creatinine, age, sex, and race), but allows for more precision when estimating higher GFR values (eg, eGFR >60 mL/minute/1.73 m^2) as compared to the MDRD equation. The NKDEP has not made a recommendation on the general implementation of the CKD-EPI equation but does suggest that laboratories which report numeric values for eGFR >60 mL/minute/1.73 m^2 should consider the use of CKD-EPI. The NKD-KDIGO 2012 CKD guidelines recommend that clinicians use a creatinine-derived equation for the evaluation and management of CKD and specifically recommend that clinical laboratories use the 2009 CKD-EPI equation when reporting eGFR in adults.

The following factors may contribute to an inaccurate estimation of renal function (Stevens, 2006):

- Increased creatinine generation (may underestimate renal function):
    - Black or African American patients
    - Muscular body habitus
    - Ingestion of cooked meats
- Decreased creatinine generation (may overestimate renal function):
    - Increased age
    - Female patients
    - Hispanic patients
    - Asian patients
    - Amputees
    - Malnutrition, inflammation, or deconditioning (eg, cancer, severe cardiovascular disease, hospitalized patients)
    - Neuromuscular disease
    - Vegetarian diet
- Rapidly changing serum creatinine (either up or down): In patients with rapidly rising serum creatinines (ie, increasing by >0.5 to 0.7 mg/dL/day), it is best to assume that the patient's renal function is severely impaired

Use extreme caution when estimating renal function in the following patient populations:

- Low body weight (actual body weight <ideal body weight)

- Liver transplant
- Elderly (>90 years of age)
- Dehydration
- Recent kidney transplantation (serum creatinine values may decrease rapidly and can lead to renal function under-estimation; conversely, delayed graft function may be present)

Note: In most situations, the use of the patient's ideal body weight (IBW) is recommended for estimating renal function, except when the patient's actual body weight (ABW) is less than ideal. Use of actual body weight (ABW) in obese patients (and possibly patients with ascites) may significantly overestimate renal function. Some clinicians prefer to use an adjusted body weight in such cases [eg, IBW + 0.4 (ABW - IBW)]; the adjustment factor may vary based on practitioner and/or institutional preference.

IDMS-traceable methods

Method 1: MDRD equation[1]:

$$eGFR = 175 \times (Creatinine)^{-1.154} \times (Age)^{-0.203} \times (Gender) \times (Race)$$
where:
  eGFR = estimated GFR; calculated in mL/minute/1.73 m^2
  Creatinine is input in mg/dL
  Age is input in years
  Gender: Females: Gender = 0.742; Males: Gender = 1
  Race: Black: Race = 1.212; White or other: Race = 1

Method 2: MDRD Extended equation:

$$eGFR = 161.5 \times (Creatinine)^{-0.999} \times (Age)^{-0.176} \times (SUN)^{-0.170} \times (Albumin)^{0.318} \times (Gender) \times (Race)$$
where:
  eGFR = estimated GFR; calculated in mL/minute/1.73 m^2
  Creatinine is input in mg/dL
  Age is input in years
  SUN = Serum Urea Nitrogen; input in mg/dL
  Albumin = Serum Albumin; input in g/dL
  Gender: Females: Gender = 0.762; Males: Gender = 1
  Race: Black: Race = 1.18; White or other: Race = 1

Method 3: CKD-EPI equation[2]:

$$eGFR = 141 \times (Creatinine/k)^{Exp} \times (0.993)^{Age} \times (Gender) \times (Race)$$
where:
  eGFR = estimated GFR; calculated in mL/minute/1.73 m^2
  (Creatinine/k):
    Creatinine is input in mg/dL
    k: Females: k = 0.7; Males: k = 0.9
    Exp:
      When (Creatinine/k) is ≤1: Females: Exp = -0.329; Males: Exp = -0.411
      When (Creatinine/k) is >1: Exp = -1.209
  Age is input in years
  Gender: Females: Gender = 1.018; Males: Gender = 1
  Race: Black: Race = 1.159; White or other: Race = 1

Alkaline picrate-based (Jaffe) methods

Note: These equations have not been updated for use with serum creatinine methods traceable to IDMS. Use with IDMS-traceable serum creatinine methods may overestimate renal function; use with caution.

Method 1: MDRD equation:

$$eGFR = 186 \times (Creatinine)^{-1.154} \times (Age)^{-0.203} \times (Gender) \times (Race)$$
where:
  eGFR = estimated GFR; calculated in mL/minute/1.73 m^2
  Creatinine is input in mg/dL
  Age is input in years
  Gender: Females: Gender = 0.742; Males: Gender = 1
  Race: Black: Race = 1.212; White or other: Race = 1

Method 2: MDRD Extended equation:

$$eGFR = 170 \times (Creatinine)^{-0.999} \times (Age)^{-0.176} \times (SUN)^{-0.170} \times (Albumin)^{0.318} \times (Gender) \times (Race)$$
where:
  eGFR = estimated GFR; calculated in mL/minute/1.73 m^2
  Creatinine is input in mg/dL
  Age is input in years
  SUN = Serum Urea Nitrogen; input in mg/dL
  Albumin = Serum Albumin; input in g/dL
  Gender: Females: Gender = 0.762; Males: Gender = 1
  Race: Black: Race = 1.18; White or other: Race = 1

Method 3: Cockroft-Gault equation[3]

Males: CrCl = [(140 - Age) X Weight] / (72 X Creatinine)
Females: CrCl = {[(140 - Age) X Weight] / (72 X Creatinine)} X 0.85
where:
CrCl = creatinine clearance; calculated in mL/minute
Age is input in years
Weight is input in kg
Creatinine is input in mg/dL

Method 4: Jelliffe equation

Males: CrCl = {98 - [0.8 X (Age - 20)]} / (Creatinine)
Females: CrCl = Use above equation, then multiply result by 0.9
where:
CrCl = creatinine clearance; calculated in mL/minute/1.73 m^2
Age is input in years
Creatinine is input in mg/dL

FOOTNOTES
[1]Preferred equation for CKD staging National Kidney Disease Education Program
[2]Recommended equation for the reporting of eGFR by the NKD-KDIGO guidelines
[3]Equation typically used for adjusting medication doses

REFERENCES
Cockcroft DW, Gault MH. Prediction of creatinine clearance from serum creatinine. *Nephron*. 1976;16(1):31-41.

Dowling TC, Matzke GR, Murphy JE, Burckart GJ. Evaluation of renal drug dosing: prescribing information and clinical pharmacist approaches. *Pharmacotherapy*. 2010;30(8):776-786.

Hermsen ED, Maiefski M, Florescu MC, Qiu F, Rupp ME. Comparison of the modification of diet in renal disease and Cockcroft-Gault equations for dosing antimicrobials. *Pharmacotherapy*. 2009;29(6):649-655.

Jelliffe RW. Letter: creatinine clearance: bedside estimate. *Ann Intern Med*. 1973;79(4):604-605.

Kidney disease: improving global outcomes (KDIGO) CKD work group. KDIGO 2012 clinical practice guidelines for the evaluation and management of chronic kidney disease. *Kidney Inter*. 2013;3:1-150. http://www.kdigo.org/clinical_practice_guidelines/pdf/CKD/KDIGO_2012_CKD_GL.pdf

Levey AS, Bosch JP, Lewis JB, Greene T, Rogers N, Roth D. A more accurate method to estimate glomerular filtration rate from serum creatinine: a new prediction equation. Modification of diet in renal disease study group. *Ann Intern Med*. 1999;16;130(6):461–470.

Levey AS, Coresh J, Greene T, et al. Using standardized serum creatinine values in the modification of diet in renal disease study equation for estimating glomerular filtration rate. *Ann Intern Med*. 2006;145(4):247-254.

Levey AS, Stevens LA, Schmid CH, et al. A new equation to estimate glomerular filtration rate. *Ann Intern Med*. 2009;150(9):604-612.

National Kidney Disease Education Program. GFR calculators. http://www.nkdep.nih.gov/professionals/gfr_calculators. Accessed April 24, 2013.

Stevens LA, Coresh J, Greene T, Levey AS. Assessing kidney function – measured and estimated glomerular filtration rate. *N Engl J Med*. 2006;354(23):2473-2483.

RENAL FUNCTION ESTIMATION IN PEDIATRIC PATIENTS

Evaluation of a patient's renal function often includes the use of equations to estimate glomerular filtration rate (GFR) (eg, estimated GFR [eGFR] creatinine clearance [CrCl]) using an endogenous filtration marker (eg, serum creatinine) and other patient variables. For example, the Schwartz equation estimates renal function by calculating eGFR and is typically used to steer medication dosing or categorize chronic kidney disease (CKD) staging and monitor progression. The rate of creatinine clearance does not always accurately represent GFR; creatinine may be cleared by other renal mechanisms in addition to glomerular filtration and serum creatinine concentrations may be affected by nonrenal factors (eg, age, gender, race, body habitus, illness, diet). In addition, these equations were developed based on studies in limited populations and may either over- or underestimate the renal function of a specific patient.

Nevertheless, most clinicians use an eGFR or CrCl as an indicator of renal function in pediatric patients for the purposes of adjusting medication doses. These equations should be used in the clinical context of patient-specific factors noted during the physical exam/work-up. **Decisions regarding drug therapy and doses must be made on clinical judgment.**

RENAL FUNCTION ESTIMATION EQUATIONS

Commonly used equations to estimate renal function utilizing the endogenous filtration marker serum creatinine include the Schwartz and Traub-Johnson equations. Both equations were originally developed using a serum creatinine assay measured by the alkaline picrate-based (Jaffe) method. Many substances, including proteins, can interfere with the accuracy of this assay and overestimate serum creatinine concentration. The National Kidney Foundation and The National Kidney Disease Education Program advocated for a universal creatinine assay, in order to ensure an accurate estimate of GFR in patients. As a result, a more specific enzymatic assay with an isotope dilution mass spectrometry (IDMS)-traceable international standard was developed. Compared to the older methods, IDMS-traceable assays may report lower serum creatinine values and may, therefore, overestimate renal function when used in the original equations. An updated Schwartz equation (eg, Bedside Schwartz) based on serum creatinine measured by the IDMS-traceable method has been proposed for pediatrics (Schwartz, 2009); the Traub-Johnson equation has not been re-expressed. The original Schwartz and Traub-Johnson equations may overestimate renal function when used with a serum creatinine measured by the IDMS-traceable method. However, at this point, all laboratories should be using creatinine methods calibrated to be IDMS traceable.

The following factors may contribute to an inaccurate estimation of renal function (Stevens, 2006):

- Increased creatinine generation (may underestimate renal function):
  - Black or African American patients
  - Muscular body habitus
  - Ingestion of cooked meats
- Decreased creatinine generation (may overestimate renal function):
  - Increased age
  - Female patients
  - Asian patients
  - Amputees
  - Malnutrition, inflammation, or deconditioning (eg, cancer, severe cardiovascular disease, hospitalized patients)
  - Neuromuscular disease
  - Vegetarian diet
- Rapidly changing serum creatinine (either up or down):
  - In patients with rapidly rising serum creatinines (ie, increasing by >0.5 to 0.7 mg/dL/day), it is best to assume that the patient's renal function is severely impaired

Use extreme caution when estimating renal function in the following patient populations:

- Low body weight (actual body weight <ideal body weight)
- Liver transplant
- Prematurity (especially very low birth weight)
- Dehydration
- Recent kidney transplantation (serum creatinine values may decrease rapidly and can lead to renal function under-estimation; conversely, delayed graft function may be present)

IDMS-traceable method: Bedside Schwartz[1]

Note: This equation is for use in ages 1 to 16 years.

eGFR = (0.413 X Height) / Creatinine

where:

eGFR = estimated GFR; calculated in mL/minute/1.73 m^2

Height (length) is input in cm

Creatinine = Sr_{Cr} input in mg/dL

Alkaline picrate-based (Jaffe) methods

Note: These equations have not been updated for use with serum creatinine methods traceable to IDMS. Use with IDMS-traceable serum creatinine methods may overestimate renal function; use with caution.

Method 1: Schwartz equation

Note: This equation may not provide an accurate estimation of creatinine clearance for infants <6 months of age or for patients with severe starvation or muscle wasting.

eGFR = (k X Height) / Creatinine

where:

eGFR = estimated GFR; calculated in mL/minute/1.73 m^2

Height (length) is input in cm

k = constant of proportionality that is age-specific

<1 year preterm: 0.33

<1 year full-term: 0.45

1 to 12 years: 0.55

>12 years female: 0.55

>12 years male: 0.7

Creatinine is input in mg/dL

Method 2: Traub-Johnson equation

Note: This equation is for use in ages 1 to 18 years.

CrCl = (0.48 X Height) / Creatinine

where:

CrCl = estimated creatinine clearance; calculated in mL/minute/1.73 m^2

Height (length) is input in cm

Creatinine = Sr_{Cr} input in mg/dL

FOOTNOTES

[1]National Kidney Disease Education Program preferred equation

REFERENCES

Dowling TC, Matzke GR, Murphy JE, Burckart GJ. Evaluation of renal drug dosing: prescribing information and clinical pharmacist approaches. *Pharmacotherapy.* 2010;30(8):776-786.

Myers GL, Miller WG, Coresh J, et al. Recommendations for improving serum creatinine measurement: a report from the laboratory working group of the National Kidney Disease Education Program. *Clin Chem.* 2006;52(1):5-18.

National Kidney Disease Education Program. GFR calculators. http://www.nkdep.nih.gov/professionals/gfr_calculators. Accessed April 24, 2013.

Pottel H, Mottaghy FM, Zaman Z, Martens F. On the relationship between glomerular filtration rate and serum creatinine in children. *Pediatr Nephrol.* 2010;25(5):927-934.

Schwartz GJ, Brion LP, Spitzer A. The use of plasma creatinine concentration for estimating glomerular filtration rate in infants, children, and adolescents. *Pediatr Clin North Am.* 1987;34(3):571-590.

Schwartz GJ, Haycock GB, Edelmann CM Jr, Spitzer A. A simple estimate of glomerular filtration rate in children derived from body length and plasma creatinine. *Pediatrics.* 1976;58(2):259-263.

Schwartz GJ, Muñoz A, Schneider MF, et al. New equations to estimate GFR in children with CKD. *J Am Soc Nephrol.* 2009;20(3):629-637.

Staples A, LeBlond R, Watkins S, Wong C, Brandt J. Validation of the revised Schwartz estimating equation in a predominantly non-CKD population. *Pediatr Nephrol.* 2010;25(11):2321-2326.

Stevens LA, Coresh J, Greene T, Levey AS. Assessing kidney function − measured and estimated glomerular filtration rate. *N Engl J Med.* 2006;354 (23):2473-2483.

Traub SL, Johnson CE. Comparison of methods of estimating creatinine clearance in children. *Am J Hosp Pharm.* 1980;37(2):195-201.

PREPROCEDURE SEDATIVES IN CHILDREN

PURPOSE

The following table is a guide to aid the clinician in the selection of the most appropriate sedative to sedate a child for a procedure. One must also consider:

- Not all patients require sedation. It is dependent on the procedure and age of the child.

- When sedation is desired, one must consider the time of onset, the duration of action, and the route of administration.

- Each of the following drugs is well absorbed when given by the suggested routes and doses.

- Each drug was assigned an "intensity" based upon the class of drug, dose, and route. However, it should be noted that any drug can produce a deeper level of sedation.

- Practitioners performing a specific level of sedation must be prepared to manage the patient who slips into the next deeper level of sedation (eg, when performing moderate sedation, be prepared to manage deep sedation). This may occur regardless of which sedation drug is used.

- Those drugs classified as producing deep sedation require more frequent monitoring postprocedure.

- For painful procedures, an analgesic agent needs to be administered.

LEVELS OF SEDATION

- Minimal sedation (formerly anxiolysis): A medically controlled state in which patients respond appropriately to verbal commands; cognitive and coordination function may be impaired, but cardiovascular and ventilatory function are not affected.

- Moderate sedation (formerly conscious sedation): A medically controlled drug-induced depression of consciousness during which patients respond purposefully to verbal commands either alone or accompanied by light tactile stimulation. No interventions are required to maintain a patent airway, and spontaneous ventilation is adequate. Cardiovascular function is usually maintained.

- Deep sedation: A medically controlled state of depressed consciousness associated with partial or complete loss of protective airway reflexes. Patients cannot be easily aroused, but respond purposefully after repeated verbal or painful stimulation. Cardiovascular function is usually maintained.

- General anesthesia (Note: This level of sedation is reserved for patients in an operating room setting): A medically controlled state of loss of consciousness during which patients are not arousable, even with painful stimulation. Ventilatory function is usually impaired; patients require assistance with maintaining a patent airway; positive-pressure ventilation may be required. Cardiovascular function may be impaired.

Sedatives Used to Produce Moderate Sedation

Drug	Route	Dose (mg/kg)	Onset (min)	Duration (h)	Comments
Chloral hydrate	P.O./P.R.	25 to 100	10 to 20	4 to 8	Maximum single dose: Infants: 1 g; Children: 2 g
Diazepam (Valium)	P.O.	0.2 to 0.3; 45 to 60 min prior	Rapid	15 to 30 min	Maximum oral dose: 10 mg
	I.V.	0.05 to 0.1 over 3 to 5 min	1 to 3	15 to 30 min	Maximum total dose: 0.25 mg/kg
FentaNYL	Intranasal (using parenteral formulation)	1 to 2 mcg/kg	5 to 10	Related to blood level	Maximum total intranasal dose: 3 mcg/kg
	I.M.	1 to 3 mcg/kg	7 to 8	1 to 2	
	I.V.	1 to 3 mcg/kg	Immediate	30 to 60 min	
LORazepam (Ativan)	P.O.	0.05	60	8 to 12	
	I.M.	0.05	30 to 60	8 to 12	
	I.V.	0.01 to 0.05 over 5 to 10 min	15 to 30	8 to 12	
Meperidine (Demerol)	P.O.	2 to 4; 30 to 90 min prior	10 to 15	2 to 4	
	I.M.	0.5 to 1; 30 to 90 min prior	10 to 15	2 to 4	Maximum dose: 150 mg/dose
	I.V.	0.5 to 1; 30 to 90 min prior	5	2 to 3	

Sedatives Used to Produce Moderate Sedation (continued)

Drug	Route	Dose (mg/kg)	Onset (min)	Duration (h)	Comments
Midazolam (Versed)	P.O.	0.25 to 0.5	10 to 20	1 to 1.5	Maximum oral dose: 20 mg; patients <6 y may need doses as high as 1 mg/kg
	I.M.	0.1 to 0.15; 30 to 60 min prior	5	2	Maximum total dose: 10 mg
	I.V.	**6 mo to 5 y:** 0.05 to 0.1; **6 to 12 y:** 0.025 to 0.05; **>12 y to Adult:** 2.5 to 5 mg (total dose); over 10 to 20 min	1 to 5	23 to 30 min	Maximum concentration: 1 mg/mL; Maximum I.M./I.V. dose: 6 mo to 5 y: 6 mg 6 y to Adult: 10 mg
	P.R.	0.25 to 0.5	10 to 30	1 to 1.5	Dilute injection in 5 mL NS; administer rectally
	Intranasal	0.2 to 0.3	5	30 to 60 min	
Morphine	I.V.	0.05 to 0.1	Within 20 min	3 to 5	

Note: See individual drug monographs for further information.

Sedatives Used to Produce Deep Sedation

Drug	Route	Dose (mg/kg)	Onset (min)	Duration (h)	Comments
Methohexital (Brevital)	I.M.	5 to 10	2 to 10	1 to 1.5	Maximum concentration for I.M./I.V.: 50 mg/mL; maximum I.M./I.V. dose: 200 mg. Greater incidence of adverse effects with I.V. use.
	I.V.	0.5 to 2	1	7 to 10 min	
	P.R.	20 to 35	5 to 15	1 to 1.5	Rectal given as a 10% solution in sterile water; maximum dose rectal: 500 mg
PENTobarbital	P.O./I.M./P.R.	1.5 to 6	I.M.: 10 to 15 P.O./P.R.: 15 to 60	I.M.: 1 to 2 P.O./P.R.: 1 to 4	Maximum dose: 100 mg
	I.V.	1 to 2	3 to 5	15 to 45 min	

Note: See individual drug monographs for further information.

Sedatives Used to Produce Dissociative Anesthesia (Monitor as if Deep Sedation)

Drug	Route	Dose (mg/kg)	Onset (min)	Duration	Comments
Ketamine	P.O.	6 to 10; 30 min prior	30 to 45		May use injectable product orally diluted in a beverage of the patient's choice
	I.M.	3 to 7	3 to 4	12 to 25	
	I.V.	0.5 to 2	Within 30 seconds	5 to 10	

Note: See individual drug monographs for further information.

REFERENCES

American Academy of Pediatrics, American Academy of Pediatric Dentistry, Coté CJ, Wilson S, Work Group on Sedation. Guidelines for monitoring and management of pediatric patients during and after sedation for diagnostic and therapeutic procedures: an update. *Pediatrics.* 2006;118(6):2587-2602.

Cramton RE, Gruchala NE. Managing procedural pain in pediatric patients. *Curr Opin Pediatr.* 2012;24(4):530-538.

Elman DS, Denson JS. Preanesthetic sedation of children with intramuscular methohexital sodium. *Anesth Analg.* 1965;44(5):494-498.

Hegenbarth MA, American Academy of Pediatrics Committee on Drugs. Preparing for pediatric emergencies: drugs to consider. *Pediatrics.* 2008;121 (2):433-443.

Krauss B, Green SM. Procedural sedation and analgesia in children. *Lancet.* 2006;367(9512):766-780.

Miller JR, Grayson M, Stoelting VK. Sedation with intramuscular methohexital sodium for office and clinic ophthalmic procedures in children. *Am J Ophthalmol.* 1966;62(1):38-43.

Zeltzer LK, Altman A, Cohen D, LeBaron S, Munuksela EL, Schechter NL. American Academy of Pediatrics Report of the Subcommittee on the Management of Pain Associated with Procedures in Children with Cancer. *Pediatrics.* 1990;86(5 Pt 2):826-831.

COMA SCALES

Glasgow Coma Scale

Activity	Best Response	Score
Eye opening	Spontaneous	4
	Responds to voice	3
	Responds to pain	2
	No response	1
Verbal response	Oriented and appropriate	5
	Confused / disoriented conversation	4
	Inappropriate words	3
	Nonspecific sounds (incomprehensible)	2
	No response	1
Motor response	Follows commands	6
	Localizes pain	5
	Withdraws to pain	4
	Abnormal flexion (decorticate posturing)	3
	Abnormal extension (decerebrate posturing)	2
	No response	1

Modified Coma Scale for Infants

Activity	Best Response	Score
Eye opening	Spontaneous	4
	Responds to voice	3
	Responds to pain	2
	No response	1
Verbal response	Coos, babbles	5
	Irritable	4
	Cries to pain	3
	Moans to pain	2
	No response	1
Motor response	Normal spontaneous movements	6
	Withdraws to touch	5
	Withdraws to pain	4
	Abnormal flexion (decorticate posturing)	3
	Abnormal extension (decerebrate posturing)	2
	No response	1

Interpretation of Coma Scale Scores Maximum Score: 15; Minimum Score: 3 (low score indicates greater severity of coma)

Range of Score	Interpretation
3 to 8	Coma. Severe brain injury. Immediate action needed. Notify ICU staff STAT. Will require intubation regardless of respiratory status.
9 to 12	Lethargic. Needs close observation in special care unit. Frequent neuro checks. Notify ICU staff.
13 to 14	Needs observation
15	Normal

REFERENCES

James HE. Neurologic evaluation and support in the child with an acute brain insult. *Pediatr Ann.* 1986;15(1):16-22.

Jennett B, Teasdale G. Aspects of coma after severe head injury. *Lancet.* 1977;1(8017): 878-881.

SEROTONIN SYNDROME

Manifestations of Severe Serotonin Syndrome and Related Clinical Conditions

Condition	Medication History	Time Needed for Condition to Develop	Vital Signs	Pupils	Mucosa	Skin	Bowel Sounds	Neuromuscular Tone	Reflexes	Mental Status
Serotonin syndrome	Proserotonergic drug	<12 hours	Hypertension, tachycardia, tachypnea, hyperthermia (>41.1°C)	Mydriasis	Sialorrhea	Diaphoresis	Hyperactive	Increased, predominantly in lower extremities	Hyper-reflexia, clonus (unless masked by increased muscle tone)	Agitation, coma
Anticholinergic "toxidrome"	Anticholinergic agent	<12 hours	Hypertension (mild), tachycardia, tachypnea, hyperthermia (typically ≤38.8°C)	Mydriasis	Dry	Erythema, hot and dry to touch	Decreased or absent	Normal	Normal	Agitated delirium
Neuroleptic malignant syndrome	Dopamine antagonist	1 to 3 days	Hypertension, tachycardia, tachypnea, hyperthermia (>41.1°C)	Normal	Sialorrhea	Pallor, diaphoresis	Normal or decreased	"Lead-pipe" rigidity present in all muscle groups	Bradyreflexia	Stupor, alert mutism, coma
Malignant hyperthermia	Inhalational anesthesia	30 minutes to 24 hours after administration of inhalational anesthesia or succinylcholine	Hypertension, tachycardia, tachypnea, hyperthermia (can be as high as 46°C)	Normal	Normal	Mottled appearance, diaphoresis	Decreased	Rigor mortis-like rigidity	Hyporeflexia	Agitation

Reprinted with permission: Boyer EW, Shannon M. The serotonin syndrome. *N Engl J Med.* 2005;352(11):1112-1120. Copyright © 2005 Massachusetts Medical Society. All rights reserved.

Management of Serotonin Syndrome

1. Remove precipitating drugs
   a. Serotonergic agents (eg, antidepressants; especially SSRI and MAO Inhibitors)
   b. Be mindful of half-life elimination and active metabolites
2. Supportive care
   a. Intravenous fluids
   b. Correct vital signs
3. Control agitation
   a. Benzodiazepines (diazepam)
   b. Avoid physical restraints
4. 5-HT$_{2A}$ antagonists
   a. Cyproheptadine: 12 to 32 mg/day (may be crushed and administered via nasogastric tube)
   b. ChlorproMAZINE: I.M.: 50 to 100 mg (monitor vitals)
5. Control autonomic instability
   a. Norepinephrine **or**
   b. Phenylephrine **or**
   c. EPINEPHrine
   d. Nitroprusside or esmolol for hypertension and tachycardia
6. Control hyperthermia
   a. Benzodiazepines
   b. Neuromuscular paralysis with vecuronium (**Note:** Avoid succinylcholine)
   c. Intubation
   d. Do not use antipyretic agents
7. Other
   a. Do not use propranolol, bromocriptine, and dantrolene

ACETAMINOPHEN SERUM LEVEL NOMOGRAM

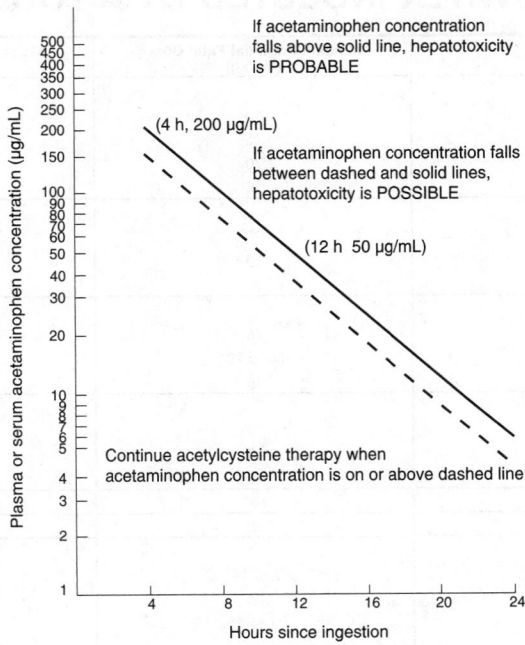

If acetaminophen concentration falls above solid line, hepatotoxicity is PROBABLE

(4 h, 200 µg/mL)

If acetaminophen concentration falls between dashed and solid lines, hepatotoxicity is POSSIBLE

(12 h 50 µg/mL)

Continue acetylcysteine therapy when acetaminophen concentration is on or above dashed line

Plasma or serum acetaminophen concentration (µg/mL)

Hours since ingestion

Nomogram relating plasma or serum acetaminophen concentration and probability of hepatotoxicity at varying intervals following ingestion of a single toxic dose of acetaminophen. Modified from Rumack BH, Matthew H, "Acetaminophen Poisoning and Toxicity", Pediatrics, 1975, 55:871-6,
© American Academy of Pediatrics, 1975, and from Rumack BH, et al, "Acetaminophen Overdose", Arch Intern Med, 1981, 141:380-5,
© American Medical Association.

MEDICATIONS FOR WHICH A SINGLE DOSE MAY BE FATAL WHEN INGESTED BY A TODDLER

Medication[1]	Minimal Potential Fatal Dose (mg/kg)	Maximal Dose Unit Available (mg)
Antiarrhythmics		
Disopyramide	15	150
Flecainide	25	150
Procainamide	70	1000
QuiNIDine	15	324
Antimalarials		
Chloroquine	20	500
Hydroxychloroquine	20	200
QuiNINE	80	650
Antipsychotics		
ChlorproMAZINE	25	200
Loxapine	30 to 70	50
Thioridazine	15	200
Calcium channel blockers		
Diltiazem	15	360
NIFEdipine	15	90
Verapamil	15	360
Camphor	100	1 g/5 mL
Methyl salicylate	200	1.4 g/mL
Narcotics		
Codeine	7 to 14	60
HYDROcodone	1.5	60 mg/5 mL
Methadone	1 to 2	40
Morphine		200
Oral hypoglycemics		
ChlorproPAMIDE	5	25
Glibenclamide	0.1	2.5
GlipiZIDE	0.1	5
Podophyllin 25%	15 to 20	1.25 g/5 mL
Theophylline	8.4	500
Tricyclic antidepressants		
Amitriptyline	15	100
Desipramine	15	150
Imipramine	15	75

[1]Assumptions: Toddler would weigh 10 kg; the lowest described or estimated fatal dose (adjusted for body weight) was used; the toddler is healthy, with normal drug metabolism.

Adapted from Bar-Oz B, Levichek Z, Koren G. Medications that can be fatal for a toddler with one tablet or teaspoonful: a 2004 update. *Paediatr Drugs.* 2004;6(2):123-126.

CONTROLLED SUBSTANCES

Note: These are federal classifications. Your individual state may place a substance into a more restricted category. When this occurs, the more restricted category applies. Consult your state law.

Schedule I = C-I

The drugs and other substances in this schedule have no legal medical uses except research. They have a **high** potential for abuse. They include opiates, opium derivatives, and hallucinogens.

Schedule II = C-II

The drugs and other substances in this schedule have legal medical uses and a **high** abuse potential which may lead to severe dependence. They include former "Class A" narcotics, amphetamines, barbiturates, and other drugs.

Schedule III = C-III

The drugs and other substances in this schedule have legal medical uses and a **lesser** degree of abuse potential which may lead to **moderate** dependence. They include former "Class B" narcotics and other drugs.

Schedule IV = C-IV

The drugs and other substances in this schedule have legal medical uses and **low** abuse potential which may lead to **moderate** dependence. They include barbiturates, benzodiazepines, propoxyphenes, and other drugs.

Schedule V = C-V

The drugs and other substances in this schedule have legal medical uses and **low** abuse potential which may lead to **moderate** dependence. They include narcotic cough preparations, diarrhea preparations, and other drugs.

MILLIEQUIVALENT AND MILLIMOLE CALCULATIONS AND CONVERSIONS

DEFINITIONS AND CALCULATIONS

Definitions

mole	=	gram molecular weight of a substance (aka molar weight)
millimole (mM)	=	milligram molecular weight of a substance (a millimole is 1/1000 of a mole)
equivalent weight	=	gram weight of a substance which will combine with or replace 1 gram (1 mole) of hydrogen; an equivalent weight can be determined by dividing the molar weight of a substance by its ionic valence
milliequivalent (mEq)	=	milligram weight of a substance which will combine with or replace 1 milligram (1 millimole) of hydrogen (a milliequivalent is 1/1000 of an equivalent)

Calculations

moles	=	$\dfrac{\text{weight of a substance (grams)}}{\text{molecular weight of that substance (grams)}}$
millimoles	=	$\dfrac{\text{weight of a substance (milligrams)}}{\text{molecular weight of that substance (milligrams)}}$
equivalents	=	moles x valence of ion
milliequivalents	=	millimoles x valence of ion
moles	=	$\dfrac{\text{equivalents}}{\text{valence of ion}}$
millimoles	=	$\dfrac{\text{milliequivalents}}{\text{valence of ion}}$
millimoles	=	moles x 1000
milliequivalents	=	equivalents x 1000

Note: Use of equivalents and milliequivalents is valid only for those substances which have fixed ionic valences (eg, sodium, potassium, calcium, chlorine, magnesium, bromine, etc). For substances with variable ionic valences (eg, phosphorous), a reliable equivalent value cannot be determined. In these instances, one should calculate millimoles (which are fixed and reliable) rather than milliequivalents.

MILLIEQUIVALENT CONVERSIONS

To convert mg/100 mL to mEq/L the following formula may be used:

$$\frac{(\text{mg/100 mL}) \times 10 \times \text{valence}}{\text{atomic weight}} \quad = \quad \text{mEq/L}$$

To convert mEq/L to mg/100 mL the following formula may be used:

$$\frac{(\text{mEq/L}) \times \text{atomic weight}}{10 \times \text{valence}} \quad = \quad \text{mg/100 mL}$$

To convert mEq/L to volume of percent of a gas the following formula may be used:

$$\frac{(\text{mEq/L}) \times 22.4}{10} \quad = \quad \text{volume percent}$$

Valences and Atomic Weights of Selected Ions

Substance	Electrolyte	Valence	Molecular Wt
Calcium	Ca^{++}	2	40
Chloride	Cl^-	1	35.5
Magnesium	Mg^{++}	2	24
Phosphate	HPO_4^{--} (80%)	1.8	96[1]
pH = 7.4	$H_2PO_4^-$ (20%)	1.8	96[1]
Potassium	K^+	1	39
Sodium	Na^+	1	23
Sulfate	SO_4^{--}	2	96[1]

[1]The molecular weight of phosphorus only is 31, and sulfur only is 32.

Approximate Milliequivalents — Weights of Selected Ions

Salt	mEq/g Salt	mg Salt/mEq
Calcium carbonate [$CaCO_3$]	20	50
Calcium chloride [$CaCl_2 \cdot 2H_2O$]	14	74
Calcium gluceptate [$Ca(C_7H_{13}O_8)_2$]	4	245
Calcium gluconate [$Ca(C_6H_{11}O_7)_2 \cdot H_2O$]	5	224
Calcium lactate [$Ca(C_3H_5O_3)_2 \cdot 5H_2O$]	7	154
Magnesium gluconate [$Mg(C_6H_{11}O_7)_2 \cdot H_2O$]	5	216
Magnesium oxide [MgO]	50	20
Magnesium sulfate [$MgSO_4$]	17	60
Magnesium sulfate [$MgSO_4 \cdot 7H_2O$]	8	123
Potassium acetate [$K(C_2H_3O_2)$]	10	98
Potassium chloride [KCl]	13	75
Potassium citrate [$K_3(C_6H_5O_7) \cdot H_2O$]	9	108
Potassium iodide [KI]	6	166
Sodium acetate [$Na(C_2H_3O_2)$]	12	82
Sodium acetate [$Na(C_2H_3O_2) \cdot 3H_2O$]	7	136
Sodium bicarbonate [$NaHCO_3$]	12	84
Sodium chloride [$NaCl$]	17	58
Sodium citrate [$Na_3(C_6H_5O_7) \cdot 2H_2O$]	10	98
Sodium iodine [NaI]	7	150
Sodium lactate [$Na(C_3H_5O_3)$]	9	112
Zinc sulfate [$ZnSO_4 \cdot 7H_2O$]	7	144

PATIENT INFORMATION FOR DISPOSAL OF UNUSED MEDICATIONS

Federal guidelines and the Food and Drug Administration (FDA) recommend that disposal of most unused medications should NOT be accomplished by flushing them down the toilet or drain unless specifically stated in the drug label prescribing information. (See "Disposal of Unused Medications Not Specified to be Flushed" below.)

However, certain drugs can potentially harm an individual for whom it is not intended, even in a single dose, depending on the size of the individual and strength of the medication. Accidental (or intentional) ingestion of one of these drugs by an unintended individual (eg, child or pet) can cause hypotension, somnolence, respiratory depression, or other severe adverse events that could lead to coma or death. For this reason, certain unused medications **should** be disposed of by flushing them down a toilet or sink.

Disposal by flushing of these medications is not believed to pose a risk to human health or the environment. Trace amounts of medicine in the water system have been noted, mainly from the body's normal elimination through urine or feces, but there has been no evidence of these small amounts being harmful. Disposal by flushing of these select, few medications contributes a small fraction to the amount of medicine in the water system. The FDA believes that the benefit of avoiding a potentially life-threatening overdose by accidental ingestion outweighs the potential risk to the environment by flushing these medications.

Medications Recommended for Disposal by Flushing Down the Toilet

Medication	Active Ingredient
Abstral, sublingual tablet	FentaNYL citrate
Actiq, oral transmucosal lozenge	FentaNYL citrate
AVINza, capsule (extended release)	Morphine sulfate
Butrans, transdermal patch	Buprenorphine
Daytrana, transdermal patch	Methylphenidate
Demerol, tablet[1]	Meperidine hydrochloride
Demerol, oral solution[1]	Meperidine hydrochloride
Diastat/Diastat AcuDial, rectal gel	Diazepam
Dilaudid, tablet[1]	HYDROmorphone hydrochloride
Dilaudid, oral liquid[1]	HYDROmorphone hydrochloride
Dolophine, tablet (as hydrochloride)[1]	Methadone hydrochloride
Duragesic, patch (extended release)[1]	FentaNYL
Embeda, capsule (extended release)	Morphine sulfate and naltrexone hydrochloride
Fentora, tablet (buccal)	FentaNYL citrate
Kadian, capsule (extended release)	Morphine sulfate
Methadone hydrochloride (oral solution)[1]	Methadone hydrochloride
Methadose, tablet[1]	Methadone hydrochloride
Morphine sulfate, tablet (immediate release)[1]	Morphine sulfate
Morphine sulfate, oral solution[1]	Morphine sulfate
MS Contin, tablet (extended release)[1]	Morphine sulfate
Onsolis, soluble film (buccal)	FentaNYL citrate
Opana, tablet (immediate release)	Oxymorphone hydrochloride
Opana ER, tablet (extended release)	Oxymorphone hydrochloride
Oramorph SR, tablet (sustained release)	Morphine sulfate
OxyCONTIN, tablet (extended release)[1]	OxyCODONE hydrochloride
Percocet, tablet[1]	Oxycodone hydrochloride and acetaminophen
Percodan, tablet[1]	Oxycodone hydrochloride and aspirin
Xyrem, oral solution	Sodium oxybate
Zohydro ER, capsule (extended release)	Hydrocodone bitartrate
Zubsolv, tablet	Buprenorphine and naloxone

[1]Medications available in generic formulations

DISPOSAL OF UNUSED MEDICATIONS NOT SPECIFIED TO BE FLUSHED

The majority of medications should be disposed of without flushing them down a toilet or drain. These medications should be removed from the original container, mixed with an unappealing substance (eg, coffee grounds, cat litter), sealed in a plastic bag or other closable container, and disposed of in the household trash.

Another option for disposal of unused medications is through drug take-back programs. For information on availability of drug take-back programs in your area, contact city or county trash and recycling service.

For more information on unused medication disposal, see specific drug product labeling information or call the FDA at (888) INFO-FDA (1-888-463-6332).

REFERENCE

U.S. Food and Drug Administration (FDA). Disposal by flushing of certain unused medicines: what you should know. Available at: http://www.fda.gov/Drugs/ResourcesForYou/Consumers/BuyingUsingMedicineSafely/EnsuringSafeUseofMedicine/SafeDisposalofMedicines/ucm186187.htm Accessed October 20, 2009.

PEDIATRIC MEDICATION ADMINISTRATION

Adapted from *Giving Your Child Medicine – Ways to Ensure Your Child Receives the Correct Dose of Medicine,* patient booklet, Lexi-Comp, Inc, 2002.

GENERAL ADVICE

Administering medicine to a sick child can be extremely challenging for parents and caregivers. Dosages are calculated by taking the child's age and/or weight into consideration. Infants and young children require very small doses of medicines, thus making accurate measurement very important.

Special measuring devices are available to accurately and easily provide the prescribed dosage. Measuring out a dose with common household utensils can lead to unacceptable inaccuracies. Improper measurement can also cause increased side effects, and over- or under-dosing.

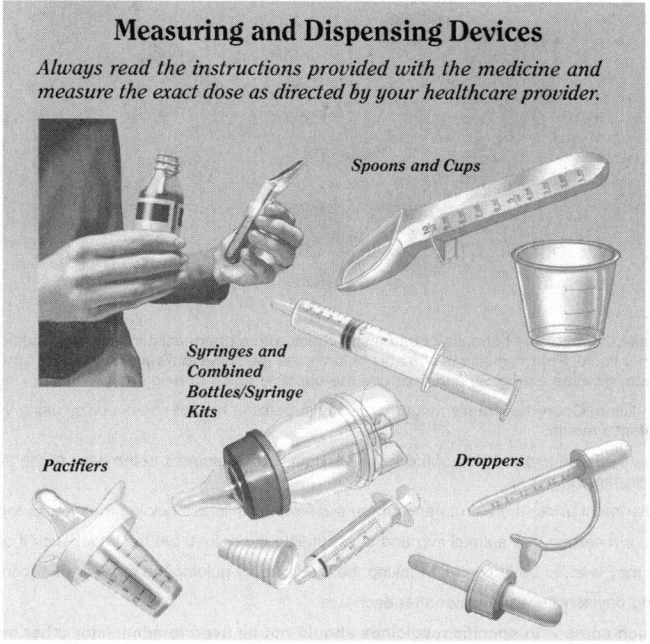

Measuring and Dispensing Devices

Always read the instructions provided with the medicine and measure the exact dose as directed by your healthcare provider.

Spoons and Cups

Syringes and Combined Bottles/Syringe Kits

Pacifiers

Droppers

LIQUIDS

Use either an oral syringe, a medicine dropper, a medicine spoon, or a medicine cup (only for older children) when giving your child oral liquids. You can purchase any of these at a local pharmacy if not provided with your child's medicine. There are specialized pacifiers and bottles designed as medicine delivery aids for children <2 years of age.

- If the medicine can be given on an empty stomach, give right before a feeding.

- Hold an infant in the normal feeding position, or put in a highchair or car seat.

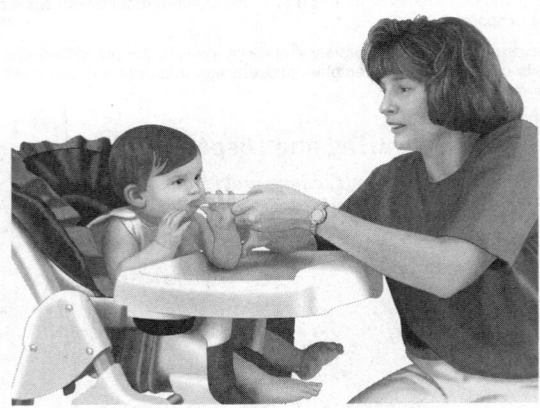

If the child refuses to take the medicine because of bad taste, check with a pharmacist to see if the medicine can be mixed with fruit juice, milk, or another liquid. Pharmacists may be able to flavor the medicine to disguise the taste. You may use a popsicle to partially numb the mouth, give the medicine, and then use the popsicle again to help improve taste.

- Prepare the medicine. Open the infant's mouth by gently squeezing his/her cheeks or by using your finger to pull out a corner of the infant's mouth.

- Slowly squirt the medicine into the side of the infant's mouth. Do not squirt it to the back of the throat because this can cause choking or gagging.

- Gently stroke the infant under the chin to encourage swallowing while still holding the cheeks together.

- Alternatively, pour medicine into a small cup and dip your little finger in it. Let the infant suck it off your finger.

- Young children may want to be in control of taking the medicine by guiding the dropper or spoon into their mouth.

- Rinse measuring device with warm water after each use.

Droppers or cups which come with specific medicines should not be used to administer other medicine.

EYE DROPS AND OINTMENTS

- Wash your hands before and after use.
- Hold container between hands to bring eye drops or ointment to room temperature before using.
- Clean child's eye of secretions and old medicine if necessary.
- Gently wipe the eye with a damp gauze or cotton pad.
- Tilt child's head back and to the side of the affected eye.
- Do not touch the container tip to eye, lid, or other skin.

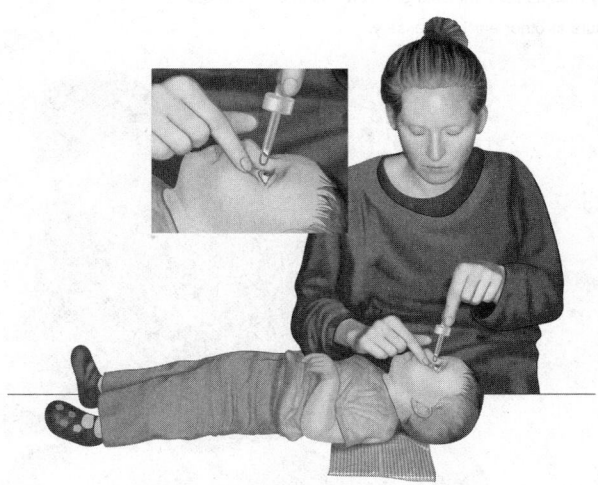

Drops

- If the drops are a suspension, shake the bottle well.
- Gently press the skin under the lower eyelid and pull the lower eyelid away from the eye slightly until you can see a small pouch.
- Insert 1 drop. Wait 1 minute between drops if more than one eye medicine is prescribed.
- After using medicine, ask the child to keep eyes closed. Apply light pressure to the inside corner of the eye.
- Do this for 3 to 5 minutes. This keeps the medicine in the eye.

Ointment

- If you are using an ointment, gently pull down the lower lid and squeeze in the prescribed amount.
- Release the lower eyelid and instruct the child to keep eyes closed for 1 to 2 minutes. This will put the medicine in contact with the eye.

EAR DROPS

- Wash your hands before and after use.
- Warm the medicine by holding the bottle between your hands.
- If the drops are a suspension, shake the bottle well.
- For children <3 years of age, pull the outer ear outward and downward.
- For children ≥3 years of age, pull the outer ear outward and upward.
- Instill prescribed number of drops in affected ear without touching dropper to ear.
- Have child stay on side for 2 minutes or insert cotton plug into ear.
- Repeat procedure in other ear if necessary.

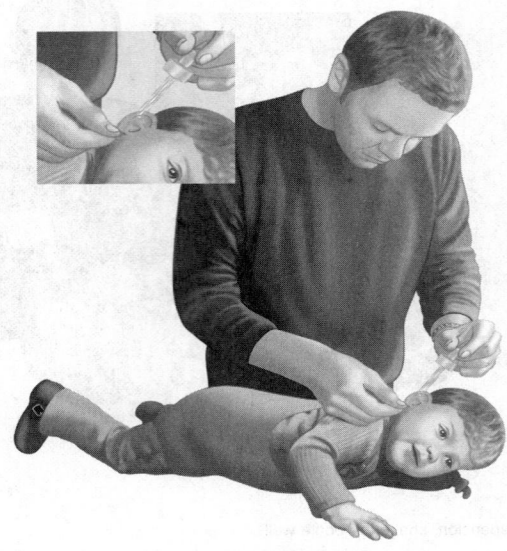

TOPICAL CREAMS AND OINTMENTS

If no specific directions have been given, follow these general guidelines:

- For use on skin only. Keep out of mouth, nose, and eyes (may burn).
- Wash your hands before and after use.
- Clean affected area and dry well before use.
- Apply a thin layer of medicine to the affected skin and rub in gently. Some medicines can be poured or squeezed onto a gauze pad, cotton swab, or cotton ball to apply.
- Do not put coverings (bandages, dressings) over the area unless told to do so by a healthcare provider.

NOSE DROPS

- Wash your hands before and after use.
- Warm the medicine by holding the bottle between your hands.
- If the drops are a suspension, shake the bottle well.
- Try to clear mucus out of nose. For infants and small children, you can use a nasal aspirator (bulb syringe) or gently twirl a moist cotton swab inside each nostril.
  Do not reach too far into the nostril with the swab or bulb syringe.
  For older children, have the child blow nose.
- Infants can be cradled in your arms in a lying position with head tilted back slightly.

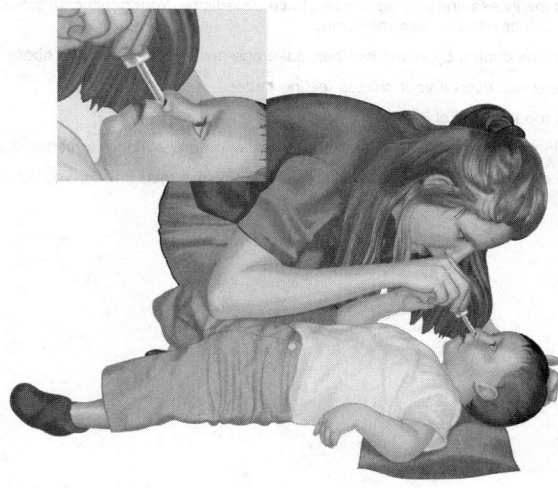

- Young children should lie on their back with a small pillow between their shoulders.
- Have them tilt head back over top of pillow. Older children can sit up with the head tilted back.
- Tell older children they may be able to taste the medicine.
- Draw the correct amount of medicine into the dropper, insert the dropper slightly into the nostril, and squeeze the medicine in without touching dropper to the nose.
- Repeat procedure in other nostril if necessary.
- Keep the child's head tilted back for 2 minutes.
- If child coughs, sit him/her upright.

RECTAL SUPPOSITORIES

- Wash your hands before and after use.
- If appropriate, store suppository in refrigerator or run it under cold water with the wrapper still on to make it firm enough to place in rectum. Ask pharmacist if you are able to safely store medicine in a refrigerator.
- Infants should be facedown across your knees. An older child can lie on his/her side with knees drawn to chest.
- Remove the wrapper.
- Moisten suppository with water or place a small amount of petroleum jelly on the tip.
- Consider use of a disposable glove.
- Gently insert the smooth, rounded end of the suppository into the rectum and up beyond the sphincter (1/2 to 1 inch beyond the sphincter). Use your pinky finger for children <3 years of age and your index finger for those ≥3 years.
- If the suppository is inserted far enough, it should stay in place. If it comes out, reinsert it slightly farther than before.
- Hold the buttocks together for a couple of minutes to prevent the child from expelling the suppository.
- Have child remain in the same position for about 20 minutes, if possible. If not, have him/her sit or lie down without going to the bathroom.

> **If in doubt...**
>
> Speak to your healthcare provider or your pharmacist about any concerns you have regarding the medicine prescribed for your child.
>
> **IF YOUR CHILD HAS A REACTION TO ANY MEDICINE, GET HELP IMMEDIATELY.**

DO'S AND DON'TS

DO wash your child's hands immediately if medicine gets on them.

DO use distractions such as toys, songs, stories, or rhymes to keep your child busy while trying to give medicine.

DO get another adult to help hold the infant while you give the medicine, or use a car seat to hold the infant or child still.

DO try a different form of the medicine. A child might prefer a chewable tablet or a form that can be sprinkled on food.

DO teach your child about the illness and why he/she has to take medicine. Your healthcare provider or librarian may have books about children who are sick or need to take medicine.

DO help your child gain some control by letting him/her make age-appropriate decisions about care.

DO use prescription as directed, even if your child is feeling better.

DO store medicine out of the reach of children and pets.

DO NOT measure medicine for an infant with a medicine cup (use an oral syringe, a medicine dropper, or a medicine spoon).

DO NOT use a teaspoon or tablespoon from your silverware to measure medicine for your child.

SAFE HANDLING OF HAZARDOUS DRUGS

Early concerns regarding the identification and exposure risk of hazardous drugs in healthcare setting were primarily focused on antineoplastic medications, but now have expanded to numerous other agents (eg, antivirals, hormones, bioengineered medications). The criteria for a hazardous drug include one or more of the following characteristics:

- Carcinogenic
- Teratogenic (or other developmental toxicity)
- Causing reproductive toxicity
- Organotoxic at low doses
- Genotoxic
- New agents with structural or toxicity profiles similar to existing hazardous agents

Agencies have developed definitions, created lists, and generated guidelines to minimize risk of exposure to products considered hazardous. The Environmental Protection Agency (EPA), National Institute for Occupational Safety and Health (NIOSH), and American Society of Health-System Pharmacists (ASHP) have created definitions of hazardous agents (table 1) which may be useful. Based on their definitions, these agencies developed lists of agents which are identified as hazardous drugs or should be handled as hazardous (table 2).

Table 1. Criteria for Defining Hazardous Agents

EPA	NIOSH	ASHP
Meets one of the following criteria:	Carcinogenic	Genotoxic
Ignitability: Create fire (under certain conditions) or are spontaneously combustible and have a flash point <60°C (140°F)	Teratogenic or other developmental toxicity	Carcinogenic
Corrosivity: Acids or bases (pH ≤2 or ≥12.5) capable of corroding metal containers	Causing reproductive toxicity Organotoxic at low doses	Teratogenic or impairs fertility
Reactivity: Unstable under "normal" conditions; may cause explosions, toxic fumes, gases, or vapors if heated, compressed, or mixed with water	Genotoxic New drugs with structural and toxicity profiles similar to existing hazardous agents	Causes serious organ or other toxic manifestation at low doses
Toxicity: Harmful or fatal if ingested or absorbed; may leach from the waste and pollute ground water when disposed of on land		
OR		
Appears on one of the following lists:		
F: Wastes (nonspecific) from common or industrial manufacturing processes from nonspecific sources		
K: Specific (source) wastes from specific industries (eg, petroleum or pesticides)		
P (acutely toxic) or U (toxic): Wastes (unused form) from certain discarded commercial chemical products		

NIOSH updated its list of antineoplastic and hazardous drugs in 2012. Medications with special handling precautions in the product labeling and medications with hazardous characteristics or with structural/toxicity profiles similar to agents on the NIOSH list are also listed in Table 2.

Table 2. Drugs Listed as or Considered Hazardous

	NIOSH List[1]	EPA List[2,3]	Product Labeling[4]	Structure or Toxicity Profile Similar to Existing Hazardous Agents	Radiopharmaceutical	Not on NIOSH List, but Meets NIOSH Criteria
Abiraterone				X		X
Acitretin	X					
Ado-Trastuzumab Emtansine			X			X
Afatinib				X		X
Aldesleukin	X					
Alefacept	X					
Alitretinoin	X					
Altretamine	X		X			
Ambrisentan	X		X			
Amsacrine	X		X			
Anastrozole	X					
Arsenic Trioxide	X	P-listed	X			
Asparaginase	X					
Axitinib				X		X
AzaCITIDine	X		X			
AzaTHIOprine	X		X			
BCG Vaccine	X		X			

Table 2. Drugs Listed as or Considered Hazardous *(continued)*

	NIOSH List[1]	EPA List[2,3]	Product Labeling[4]	Structure or Toxicity Profile Similar to Existing Hazardous Agents	Radiopharmaceutical	Not on NIOSH List, but Meets NIOSH Criteria
Bendamustine	X		X			
Bevacizumab						X
Bexarotene	X					
Bicalutamide	X					
Bleomycin	X		X			
Bortezomib	X		X			
Bosentan	X					
Bosutinib			X	X		X
Brentuximab Vedotin			X			X
Buserelin				X		X
Busulfan	X		X			
Cabazitaxel			X	X		X
Cabergoline	X					
Cabozantinib				X		X
Capecitabine	X		X			
CarBAMazepine	X					
Carbon 14 Urea			X		X	
CARBOplatin	X		X			
Carfilzomib				X		X
Carmustine	X		X			
Ceritinib				X		X
Cetrorelix	X					
Chlorambucil	X	U-listed	X			
Chloramphenicol	X					
Choriogonadotropin Alfa	X					
Chromic Phosphate P 32			X		X	
Cidofovir	X		X			
CISplatin	X		X			
Cladribine	X		X			
Clofarabine	X		X			
ClonazePAM	X					
Colchicine	X					
Crizotinib				X		X
Cyclophosphamide	X	U-listed	X			
CycloSPORINE	X					
Cyproterone				X		X
Cytarabine	X		X			
Cytarabine (Liposomal)	X		X			
Dabrafenib				X		X
Dacarbazine	X		X			
DACTINomycin	X		X			
Dasatinib	X		X			
DAUNOrubicin	X	U-listed	X			
DAUNOrubicin (Liposomal)	X	U-listed	X			
Decitabine	X		X			
Degarelix	X		X			
Denileukin	X					
Dexrazoxane			X			X
Dichlorodifluoromethane		U-listed				
Diethylstilbestrol	X	U-listed				
Dihydroergotamine				X		X
Dinoprostone	X					
Divalproex	X					
DOCEtaxel	X		X			
DOXOrubicin	X		X			
DOXOrubicin (Liposomal)	X		X			
Dronedarone	X					
Dutasteride	X		X			
Entecavir	X					

Table 2. Drugs Listed as or Considered Hazardous *(continued)*

	NIOSH List[1]	EPA List[2,3]	Product Labeling[4]	Structure or Toxicity Profile Similar to Existing Hazardous Agents	Radiopharmaceutical	Not on NIOSH List, but Meets NIOSH Criteria
Enzalutamide				X		X
EPINEPHrine (does not include epinephrine salts)		P-listed				
EPIrubicin	X		X			
Ergoloid Mesylates				X		X
Ergonovine/ Methylergonovine	X					
Ergotamine				X		X
Eribulin				X		X
Erlotinib				X		X
Estradiol	X					
Estramustine	X					
Estrogen-Progestin Combinations	X					
Estrogens (Conjugated)	X					
Estrogens (Esterified)	X					
Estrone	X					
Estropipate	X					
Etoposide	X		X			
Etoposide Phosphate	X		X			
Everolimus	X		X			
Exemestane	X					
Finasteride	X		X			
Florbetapir F18			X		X	
Floxuridine	X		X			
Fluconazole						X
Fludarabine	X		X			
Fludeoxyglucose F 18			X		X	
Fluorouracil	X		X			
Fluoxymesterone	X					
Flutamide	X					
Formaldehyde		U-listed				
Fulvestrant	X					
Gallium Citrate Ga-67			X		X	
Ganciclovir	X		X			
Ganirelix	X					
Gefitinib				X		X
Gemcitabine	X					
Gemtuzumab Ozogamicin	X		X			
Gonadotropin, Chorionic	X					
Goserelin	X					
Hexachlorophene		U-listed				
Histrelin				X		X
Hydroxyurea	X		X			
Ibritumomab			X		X	
Ibrutinib				X		X
IDArubicin	X		X			
Ifosfamide	X		X			
Imatinib	X		X			
Indium 111 Capromab Pendetide			X		X	
Indium 111 Oxyquinoline			X		X	
Indium In-111 Pentetreotide			X		X	
Iobenguane I 123			X		X	
Iodinated I 131 Albumin			X		X	
Iodine I-125 Human Serum Albumin			X		X	
Iodine I-125 Iothalamate			X		X	
Ioflupane I 123			X		X	
Irinotecan	X		X			
Isotretinoin				X		X

Table 2. Drugs Listed as or Considered Hazardous (continued)

	NIOSH List[1]	EPA List[2,3]	Product Labeling[4]	Structure or Toxicity Profile Similar to Existing Hazardous Agents	Radiopharmaceutical	Not on NIOSH List, but Meets NIOSH Criteria
Ixabepilone	X		X			
Lapatinib				X		X
Leflunomide	X					
Lenalidomide	X		X			
Letrozole	X					
Leuprolide	X					
Lindane		U-listed				
Liraglutide						X
Lomustine	X		X			
Macitentan				X		X
Mechlorethamine	X		X			
MedroxyPROGESTERone	X					
Megestrol	X					
Melphalan	X	U-listed	X			
Menotropins	X					
Mercaptopurine	X		X			
Mercury		U-listed				
Methotrexate	X		X			
Methoxsalen						X
MethylTESTOSTERone	X					
Mifepristone	X					
Misoprostol				X		X
MitoMYcin	X	U-listed	X			
Mitotane	X		X			
MitoXANtrone	X		X			
Mycophenolate	X		X			
Nafarelin	X					
Nelarabine	X		X			
Nicotine		P-listed				
Nilotinib	X					
Nilutamide	X					
Nitrogen 13 Ammonia			X		X	
Nitroglycerin (doses in "finished form" are excluded)		P-listed				
Omacetaxine			X	X		X
Ospemifene				X		X
Oxaliplatin	X		X			
OXcarbazepine	X					
Oxytocin	X					
PACLitaxel	X		X			
PACLitaxel (Protein Bound)	X		X			
Palifermin	X					
Pamidronate				X		X
Paraldehyde		U-listed				
PARoxetine	X					
PAZOPanib	X					
Pegaspargase	X					
PEMEtrexed	X		X			
Pentamidine	X					
Pentetate Calcium Trisodium	X					
Pentetate Indium Disodium In 111			X		X	
Pentostatin	X		X			
Pertuzumab				X		X
Phenacetin		U-listed				
Phenol		U-listed				
Phenoxybenzamine	X					
Physostigmine		P-listed				
Pimecrolimus				X		X

Table 2. Drugs Listed as or Considered Hazardous *(continued)*

	NIOSH List[1]	EPA List[2,3]	Product Labeling[4]	Structure or Toxicity Profile Similar to Existing Hazardous Agents	Radiopharmaceutical	Not on NIOSH List, but Meets NIOSH Criteria
Pipobroman	X					
Plerixafor	X					
Podofilox	X					
Podophyllum Resin	X					
Pomalidomide			X	X		X
PONATinib				X		X
Porfimer			X			X
PRALAtrexate	X		X			
Procarbazine	X		X			
Progesterone	X					
Progestins	X					
Radium Ra 223 Dichloride			X		X	
Raloxifene	X					
Raltitrexed			X	X		X
Ramucirumab						X
Rasagiline	X					
Regorafenib				X		X
Reserpine		U-listed				
Resorcinol		U-listed				
Ribavirin	X					
RisperiDONE	X					
RomiDEPsin	X		X			
Rubidium-82 Chloride			X		X	
Ruxolitinib				X		X
Saccharin		U-listed				
Samarium Sm 153 Lexidronam			X		X	
Selenium Sulfide		U-listed				
Sirolimus	X					
Sodium Fluoride F18			X		X	
Sodium Iodide I[123]			X		X	
Sodium Iodide I[131]			X		X	
SORAfenib	X					
Streptozocin	X	U-listed	X			
Strontium-89			X		X	
Sunitinib	X					
Tacrolimus	X					
Tamoxifen	X					
Technetium Tc 99m Bicisate			X		X	
Technetium Tc 99m Diethylene Triamine Penta-Acetic Acid			X		X	
Technetium Tc 99m Disofenin			X		X	
Technetium Tc 99m Exametazime			X		X	
Technetium Tc 99m Gluceptate			X		X	
Technetium Tc 99m-Labeled Red Blood Cells			X		X	
Technetium Tc 99m Mebrofenin			X		X	
Technetium Tc 99m Oxidronate			X		X	
Technetium Tc 99m Pyrophosphate			X		X	
Technetium Tc 99m Succimer			X		X	
Technetium Tc 99m Sulfur Colloid			X		X	
Technetium Tc 99m Tetrofosmin			X		X	
Technetium Tc 99m Tilmanocept			X		X	

Table 2. Drugs Listed as or Considered Hazardous (continued)

	NIOSH List[1]	EPA List[2,3]	Product Labeling[4]	Structure or Toxicity Profile Similar to Existing Hazardous Agents	Radiopharmaceutical	Not on NIOSH List, but Meets NIOSH Criteria
Tegafur and Uracil			X	X		X
Telavancin	X					
Temozolomide	X		X			
Temsirolimus	X		X			
Teniposide	X		X			
Teriflunamide				X		X
Tesamorelin						X
Testolactone	X					
Testosterone	X					
Tetracycline	X					
Thalidomide	X		X			
Thioguanine	X		X			
Thiotepa	X		X			
Topiramate				X		X
Topotecan	X		X			
Toremifene	X					
Tositumomab			X		X	
Trabectedin	X					X
Trametinib				X		X
Trastuzumab				X		X
Tretinoin	X					
Trichloromonofluoromethane		U-listed				
Trifluridine	X					
Triptorelin	X					
Ulipristal				X		X
Uracil Mustard	X	U-listed				
ValGANciclovir	X		X			
Valproic Acid	X					
Valrubicin	X		X			
Vandetanib			X	X		X
Vemurafenib			X	X		X
Vidarabine	X					
Vigabatrin	X					
VinBLAStine	X		X			
VinCRIStine	X		X			
VinCRIStine (Liposomal)	X		X			
Vindesine			X	X		X
Vinorelbine	X		X			
Vismodegib				X		X
Vorinostat	X		X			
Warfarin		<0.3%: U-listed; >0.3%: P-listed				X
Zidovudine	X					
Ziprasidone	X					
Zoledronic Acid	X					
Zonisamide	X					

[1]National Institute for Occupational Safety and Health (NIOSH). NIOSH list of antineoplastic and other hazardous drugs in health care settings, 2012. http://www.cdc.gov/niosh/docs/2012-150/pdfs/2012-150.pdf. Accessed July 10, 2012.

[2]Healthcare Environmental Resource Center (HERC). Pharmaceutical wastes in healthcare facilities. http://www.hercenter.org/hazmat/pharma.cfm#listed. Accessed September 15, 2010.

[3]Healthcare Environmental Resource Center (HERC). Hazardous waste determination. http://www.hercenter.org/hazmat/hazdeterm.cfm. Accessed September 15, 2010.

[4]Product labeling indicates precautions for safe handling and disposal should be followed.

Hazardous drugs must be stored, transported, prepared, administered, and disposed of under conditions that protect the healthcare worker from either acute or chronic/low level exposure. Institutional policies or guidelines to minimize occupational exposure to hazardous drugs should include a focus on the following areas:

- Development and maintenance of a facility-specific hazardous drugs list

  - Working definition/criteria of a hazardous drug

  - Volumes, formulations, and frequency of hazardous drugs handled: Injection, oral (liquid, solid), topical

  - Oral dosage forms and administration (uncoated tablets or alteration of forms by crushing or preparation of oral solutions may result in exposure; coated tablets or capsules administered intact may pose a lower exposure risk)

Each institution or facility must create its own policy or guideline, including a facility-specific list of drugs deemed hazardous. According to the Joint Commission standards, organizations should minimize risks associated with handling hazardous medications. Orientation and routine training related to safe handling of hazardous drugs is recommended. Until proven otherwise, most institutions consider investigational drugs to be hazardous and to be handled accordingly, particularly if the mechanism of action suggests a potential for concern. Hazardous drug procedures must include all possible routes of administration.

Additional information regarding development and implementation of an institutional policy/guideline, areas at risk, personnel at risk, risk management, spill management, personnel training, and surveillance may be found at:

ASHP Guidelines on Handling Hazardous Drugs:
  http://www.ashp.org/DocLibrary/BestPractices/PrepGdlHazDrugs.aspx
Environmental Protection Agency Recommendations:
  http://hercenter.org/hazmat/hazdeterm.cfm
  http://hercenter.org/hazmat/pharma.cfm
NIOSH List of Antineoplastic and Other Hazardous Drugs in Healthcare Settings:
  http://www.cdc.gov/niosh/docs/2012-150/pdfs/2012-150.pdf
U.S. Nuclear Regulatory Commission (radiopharmaceuticals, such as ibritumomab or tositumomab):
  http://www.nrc.gov/materials/miau/med-use.html

- Identification of personnel and locations in the facility at risk for occupational exposure to hazardous drugs

  - Pharmacy

    - Receiving storage and inventory

    - Dose preparation and dispensing

    - Drug waste disposal

  - Nursing Unit

    - Drug administration

    - Drug waste disposal

    - Patient waste disposal

  - Other areas

    - Laboratory

    - Operating/procedure rooms

    - Veterinary department

    - Facility shipping/receiving

    - Environmental/laundry services

    - Maintenance services

While the greatest risk of occupational exposure to hazardous drugs occurs during preparation and administration of these agents, it is important to recognize that a risk of exposure can occur throughout the facility from the moment of delivery through the disposal of product and contaminated human waste. Drug preparation and administration may occur in nontraditional areas of the institution including the operating room and in veterinary facilities. Procedures should address the importance of proper labeling and packaging and separation of hazardous vs nonhazardous inventories throughout the facility. Drug containers should be examined upon their arrival at the pharmacy. Containers that show signs of damage should be handled carefully and may require quarantine and decontamination before being placed in stock. Give consideration to routinely quarantining and decontaminating all hazardous drug containers as part of the inspection process before placing in stock.

- Mechanisms/routes of occupational exposure

  - Inhalation of dust or aerosolized droplets (most common)

  - Absorption through skin (most common)

  - Ingestion from contaminated food/drink

  - Accidental injection during preparation/administration/disposal

- Potential adverse effects of hazardous exposure
  - Skin disorders
  - Reproductive effects (eg, spontaneous abortion, stillbirth, congenital malformation)
  - Leukemia and other cancers
- Risk management
  - Use and maintenance of equipment designed to minimize exposure during handling
    - Buffer/Ante transition area
    - Biological safety cabinets, isolators
    - Closed system drug-transfer devices
    - Personal protective equipment
    - Deactivation, decontamination, and cleaning procedures

Barrier protection through the use of ventilation controls and personal protective equipment is the current standard to minimize exposure when handling hazardous drugs. NIOSH and ASHP recommend the use of Class II biological safety cabinets (type B2 preferred), but other options include the totally enclosed Class III biological safety cabinets, appropriate isolators, and robotic systems. Self-contained or closed system devices have been recommended to minimize workplace contamination by preventing escape of drug or vapor out of the device. Devices available include PhaSeal, ONGARD, TEVADAPTOR, Equashield, and CLAVE systems; other systems may also be commercially available. Gloves, gowns, respiratory protection, hair and shoe covers, and eye protection represent the core of personal protective equipment. Guidelines for choice of gowns and gloving, and the circumstances to employ this protection are published by ASHP, NIOSH, and in USP 797.

Procedures for safe handling should be followed with oral dosage forms of antineoplastics (Goodin, 20110). Appropriate personal protective equipment should be worn, automatic counting machines should not be utilized, compounding should be performed in a biologic safety cabinet, separate equipment (eg, counting trays) should be used, disposable equipment should be used if possible, cytotoxic waste should be disposed of, and non-disposable equipment used for preparation should be appropriately decontaminated.

  - Hazardous drug spill management
    - Size and location
    - Spill kit use
    - Worker contamination

Procedures for handling spills throughout a facility are well described by ASHP and NIOSH. Institutional procedures should focus on location and size of the spill, how to handle a spill when a spill kit is not available, and how to respond to a worker contamination (emergent treatment, follow-up care).

  - Personnel training in the handling of hazardous drugs
    - Prior to handling hazardous drugs
    - Periodic and ongoing testing

Personnel throughout a facility must have training in the handling of hazardous drugs that are relevant to their job description. Pharmacy personnel who compound and dispense hazardous drugs must be fully trained in the storing, preparation, dispensing, and disposal of these agents. Such training should include didactic, as well as demonstrating hands-on technique, and such validation should be repeated on a regular schedule. Special training may be necessary for hazardous drugs administered by routes outside of traditional administration routes and when administered in settings outside of traditional settings (eg, at home).

  - Environmental and medical surveillance
    - Components of a comprehensive medical surveillance program
    - Reproductive and health questionnaires (at time of hire and periodically)
    - Drug handling history (to estimate current and prior exposure)
    - Baseline clinical evaluation plan (including related medical history, physical exam, lab work)
    - Follow-up plan (for those with health changes suggestive of toxicity or acute exposure)
    - Potential use of environmental sampling techniques
    - Use of common marker hazardous drugs for assay purposes

The goal of medical surveillance is to minimize adverse effects on the health of workers exposed to hazardous drugs. NIOSH recommends that medical surveillance be employed by the facility, and may include the basic observation of employee symptom complaints or monitoring for changes in health status as part of routine checkups. Some programs follow the employee more closely and procedures may include periodic lab studies (eg, blood counts), physical exam, detailed medical history and occupational exposure history, and/or biologic studies. Environmental sampling to look for surface contamination in hazardous drug preparation and administration areas may be considered, particularly in institutions with high volumes. Certain hazardous drugs serve as markers which allow for assay for measurable contamination, and can alert the facility for proper follow-up.

- Work practices regarding reproductive risks to healthcare workers
  - Alternative duty options

Since hazardous drugs are associated with reproductive risks, policies and guidelines should address healthcare workers whom are pregnant, attempting to conceive or father a child, and whom are breast-feeding. Workers of reproductive capability should acknowledge in writing that they understand the risk of handling hazardous drugs and be given the opportunity for reassignment or alternate work duty.

REFERENCES

American Society of Hospital Pharmacists. ASHP guidelines on handling hazardous drugs. 2006;63(12):1172-1193.

Baker ES, Connor TH. Monitoring occupational exposure to cancer chemotherapy drugs. *Am J Health Syst Pharm.* 1996;53(22):2713-2723.

Bos RP, Sessink PJ. Biomonitoring of occupational exposures to cytostatic anticancer drugs. *Rev Environ Health.* 1997;12(1):43-58.

Connor TH, Anderson RW, Sessink PJ, Broadfield L, Power LA. Surface contamination with antineoplastic agents in six cancer treatment centers in Canada and the United States. *Am J Health Syst Pharm.* 1999;56(14):1427-1432.

Connor TH, McDiarmid MA. Preventing occupational exposures to antineoplastic drugs in health care settings. *CA Cancer J Clin.* 2006;56(6):354-365.

Connor TH, DeBord DG, Pretty JR, et al. Evaluation of antineoplastic drug exposure of health care workers at three university-based US cancer centers. *J Occup Environ Med.* 2010;52(10):1019-1027.

Connor TH. Permeability of nitrile rubber, latex, polyurethane, and neoprene gloves to 18 antineoplastic drugs. *Am J Health Syst Pharm.* 1999;56(23):2450-2453.

Connor TH, Sessink PJ, Harrison BR, et al. Surface contamination of chemotherapy drug vials and evaluation of new vial-cleaning techniques: results of three studies. *Am J Health Syst Pharm.* 2005;62(5):475-484.

Goodin S, Griffith N, Chen B, et al. Safe handling of oral chemotherapeutic agents in clinical practice: recommendations from an international pharmacy panel. *J Oncol Pract.* 2011;7(1):7-12.

Healthcare Environmental Resource Center (HERC). Hazardous waste determination. http://www.hercenter.org/hazmat/hazdeterm.cfm. Accessed September 15, 2010.

Healthcare Environmental Resource Center (HERC). Pharmaceutical wastes in healthcare facilities. http://www.hercenter.org/hazmat/pharma.cfm#listed. Accessed September 15, 2010.

Lawson CC, Rocheleau CM, Whelan EA, et al. Occupational exposures among nurses and risk of spontaneous abortion. *Am J Obstet Gynecol.* 2012;206(4):327.

McDiarmid MA, Oliver MS, Roth TS, Rogers B, Escalante C. Chromosome 5 and 7 abnormalities in oncology personnel handling anticancer drugs. *J Occup Environ Med.* 2010;52(10):1028-1034.

National Institute for Occupational Safety and Health (NIOSH). Medical surveillance for healthcare workers exposed to hazardous drugs. 2012. http://www.cdc.gov/niosh/docs/wp-solutions/2013-103/. Accessed January 22, 2013.

National Institute for Occupational Safety and Health (NIOSH). NIOSH list of antineoplastic and other hazardous drugs in health care settings, 2010. http://www.cdc.gov/niosh/docs/2010-167/pdfs/2010-167.pdf. Accessed September 15, 2010.

National Institute for Occupational Safety and Health (NIOSH). NIOSH list of antineoplastic and other hazardous drugs in healthcare settings 2012. http://www.cdc.gov/niosh/docs/2012-150/pdfs/2012-150.pdf. Accessed July 11, 2012.

National Institute for Occupational Safety and Health (NIOSH). Preventing occupational exposure to antineoplastic and other hazardous drugs in health care settings. http://www.cdc.gov/niosh/docs/2004-165/2004-165d.html#o. Accessed October 1, 2007.

Polovich M. *Safe Handling of Hazardous Drugs.* 2nd ed. Pittsburgh, PA: Oncology Nursing Society; 2011.

Sessink PJ, Bos RP. Drugs hazardous to healthcare workers. Evaluation of methods for monitoring occupational exposure to cytostatic drugs. *Drug Saf.* 1999;20(4):347-359.

Sessink PJ, Anzion RB, Van den Broek PH, Bos RP. Detection of contamination with antineoplastic agents in a hospital pharmacy department. *Pharm Weekbl Sci.* 1992;14(1):16-22.

Sessink PJ, Boer KA, Scheefhals AP, Anzion RB, Bos RP. Occupational exposure to antineoplastic agents at several departments in a hospital. Environmental contamination and excretion of cyclophosphamide and ifosfamide in urine of exposed workers. *Int Arch Occup Environ Health.* 1992;64(2):105-112.

Sorsa M, Anderson D. Monitoring of occupational exposure to cytostatic anticancer agents. *Mutat Res.* 1996;355(1-2):253-261.

CARBOHYDRATE CONTENT OF MEDICATIONS[1]

Description (Brand Name)	Dosage Unit	Grams Carbohydrate per Dosage Unit
Acetaminophen extra strength caplets (Tylenol)	500 mg	<0.125
Acetaminophen chewable tablets (Tylenol Meltaways)	80 mg	<0.56
Acetaminophen suspension (Children's Tylenol)	160 mg/5 mL	<5
Acetaminophen regular strength caplets (Tylenol)	325 mg	<0.075
Acetaminophen extra strength liquid (Tylenol)	1000 mg/30 mL	<5.7
Acetaminophen elixir with codeine (Tylenol With Codeine) *0.35 g ethyl alcohol/5 mL	120 mg/5 mL	3
Acetaminophen with codeine tablets (Tylenol With Codeine)	All strengths	0.05
Acyclovir suspension (Zovirax) *1.75 g sorbitol	200 mg/5 mL	0
Acyclovir tablets (Zovirax)	400 mg	0.02
Acyclovir capsules (Zovirax)	200 mg	0.21
Alendronate tablets (Fosamax)	70 mg	<0.12
Alendronate solution (Fosamax)	70 mg/5 mL	0
ALPRAZolam solution (Alprazolam Intensol)	1 mg/mL	0
Aluminum hydroxide, magnesium hydroxide, and simethicone (Maalox Advanced Regular Strength)	5 mL	0.903
Aluminum hydroxide, magnesium hydroxide, and simethicone (Maalox Advanced Maximum Strength)	5 mL	0.93
Aminocaproic acid syrup (Amicar)	250 mg/mL	0.26
Amoxicillin suspension (Amoxil)	200 mg/5 mL	1.688/5 mL
Amoxicillin suspension (Amoxil)	400 mg/5 mL	1.877/5 mL
Amoxicillin tablets (Amoxil)	500 mg	0.142
Amoxicillin tablets (Amoxil)	875 mg	0.248
Amoxicillin oral suspension (Amoxil)	125 mg/5 mL	1.7
Amoxicillin oral suspension (Amoxil)	250 mg/5 mL	1.85
Amoxicillin chewable tablets (Amoxil)	125 mg	0.05
Amoxicillin chewable tablets (Amoxil)	250 mg	0.34
Amoxicillin capsules (Amoxil)	250 mg	0
Amoxicillin capsules (Amoxil)	500 mg	0
Amoxicillin and clavulanate potassium oral suspension (Augmentin)	125 mg/5 mL	0.52
Amoxicillin and clavulanate potassium oral suspension (Augmentin)	200 mg/5 mL	0.06
Amoxicillin and clavulanate potassium oral suspension (Augmentin)	250 mg/5 mL	0.6
Amoxicillin and clavulanate potassium oral suspension (Augmentin)	400 mg/5 mL	0.06
Amoxicillin and clavulanate potassium chewable tablets (Augmentin)	200 mg	0.206
Amoxicillin and clavulanate potassium chewable tablets (Augmentin)	400 mg	0.36
Amoxicillin and clavulanate potassium tablets (Augmentin)	250 mg	0.02
Amoxicillin and clavulanate potassium tablets (Augmentin)	500 mg	0.02
Amoxicillin and clavulanate potassium tablets (Augmentin)	875 mg	0.03
Amoxicillin and clavulanate potassium suspension (Augmentin)	600 mg/5mL	0.049
Amoxicillin and clavulanate potassium extended release tablets (Augmentin XR)	1000 mg	0.018
Ampicillin oral suspension (Omnipen)	125 mg/5 mL	4
Ampicillin oral suspension (Omnipen)	250 mg/5 mL	4
ARIPiprazole tablets (Abilify)	10 mg	0.062
ARIPiprazole tablets (Abilify)	15 mg	0.057
ARIPiprazole tablets (Abilify)	20 mg	0.124
ARIPiprazole tablets (Abilify)	30 mg	0.187
ARIPiprazole solution (Abilify)	1 mg/mL	.6/mL
AtoMOXetine capsules (Strattera)	10 mg	0.18 to 0.22
AtoMOXetine capsules (Strattera)	18 mg	0.18 to 0.22
AtoMOXetine capsules (Strattera)	25 mg	0.18 to 0.22

(continued)

Description (Brand Name)	Dosage Unit	Grams Carbohydrate per Dosage Unit
AtoMOXetine capsules (Strattera)	40 mg	0.18 to 0.22
AtoMOXetine capsules (Strattera)	60 mg	0.18 to 0.22
Azithromycin oral suspension (Zithromax)	100 mg/5 mL	3.86
Azithromycin oral suspension (Zithromax)	200 mg/5 mL	3.87
Azithromycin tablets (Zithromax)	250 mg	0.036
Azithromycin tablets (Zithromax)	500 mg	0.071
Calcium and vitamin D caplet (Citracal Maximum)	Caplet	0
Calcium and vitamin D chewable tablets (Caltrate 600+D)	Chewable tablets	1.9
Calcium and vitamin D tablets (Caltrate 600+D)	Tablets	0.25
Calcium and vitamin D tablets (Caltrate 600+Soy)	Tablets	0.25
Calcium and vitamin D tablets (Citracal Petites, Citracal Regular)	Tablets	0
Calcium carbonate capsules (Calci-Mix)	1250 mg	0
Calcium carbonate tablets (Caltrate 600)	1500 mg	0.25
Calcium carbonate tablets	640 mg	0.05
Calcium carbonate suspension	1250 mg/5 mL	1.75
Calcium carbonate, iron, vitamin D tablets (Caltrate 600 + Iron and Vitamin D)	1500 mg	0.25
Calcium carbonate gelcap (Liqui-Cal)	600 mg	0.16
Calcium carbonate tablets (Mylanta Children's Chewables)	400 mg	0.93
Calcium carbonate suspension (Mylanta Children's Suspension)	400 mg/5 mL	1.5
Calcium carbonate tablets (Tums Regular)	500 mg	0.75
Calcium carbonate tablets (Tums 500)	1250 mg	1.9
Calcium carbonate extra strength tablets (Tums E-X)	750 mg	1.1
Calcium carbonate ultra tablets (Tums Ultra)	1000 mg	1.5
Calcium carbonate sugar free extra strength tablets (Tums Extra Strength Sugar Free)	750 mg	0.5
Calcium citrate capsules (Citracal)	2,376 mg	0
Calcium citrate (Citracal)	950 mg	0
CarBAMazepine extended release caplets (Carbatrol)	100 mg	<0.04
CarBAMazepine extended release caplets (Carbatrol)	200 mg	0.08 whole, <0.02 without shell
CarBAMazepine extended release caplets (Carbatrol)	300 mg	0.121 whole, <0.03 without shell
CarBAMazepine tablets (Equetro)	100 mg	<0.04
CarBAMazepine tablets (Equetro)	200 mg	0.08
CarBAMazepine tablets (Equetro)	300 mg	0.121
CarBAMazepine extended release tablets (TEGretol-XR)	100 mg	0.028
CarBAMazepine extended release tablets (TEGretol-XR)	200 mg	0.055
CarBAMazepine extended release tablets (TEGretol-XR)	400 mg	Unknown
CarBAMazepine suspension (TEGretol)	100 mg/5 mL	3.35
CarBAMazepine chewable tablets (TEGretol)	100 mg	0.28
CarBAMazepine tablets (TEGretol)	200 mg	0.06
Carnitine solution (Carnitor)	1 g/10 mL	0.48
Cefaclor oral suspension (Ceclor)	125 mg/5 mL	2.95
Cefaclor oral suspension (Ceclor)	187 mg/5 mL	2.83
Cefaclor oral suspension (Ceclor)	250 mg/5 mL	2.83
Cefaclor oral suspension (Ceclor)	375 mg/5 mL	2.6
Cefaclor pulvules (Ceclor)	250 mg	0.04
Cefaclor pulvules (Ceclor)	500 mg	0.07
Cefadroxil oral suspension (Duricef)	250 mg/5 mL	3
Cefadroxil capsules (Duricef)	500 mg	0.13
Cefadroxil film-coated tablets (Duricef)	1 g	0.13
Cefdinir suspension (Omnicef)	125 mg/5 mL	2.87/5 mL
Cefdinir suspension (Omnicef)	250 mg/5 mL	2.7/5 mL
Cefdinir capsules (Omnicef)	300 mg	0
Cefixime oral suspension (Suprax)	100 mg/5 mL	2.7
Cefixime tablets (Suprax)	200 mg	0.06
Cefpodoxime proxetil oral suspension (Vantin)	50 mg/5 mL	3
Cefpodoxime proxetil oral suspension (Vantin)	100 mg/5 mL	3.05

(continued)

Description (Brand Name)	Dosage Unit	Grams Carbohydrate per Dosage Unit
Cefpodoxime proxetil tablets (Vantin)	100 mg	0.04
Cefpodoxime proxetil tablets (Vantin)	200 mg	0.08
Cefprozil oral suspension (Cefzil)	125 mg/5 mL	2
Cefprozil oral suspension (Cefzil)	250 mg/5 mL	1.9
Cefprozil tablets (Cefzil)	250 mg	0.02
Cefprozil tablets (Cefzil)	500 mg	0.03
Cefuroxime axetil suspension (Ceftin)	125 mg/5 mL	3.062
Cefuroxime axetil suspension (Ceftin)	250 mg/5 mL	2.289
Cefuroxime axetil tablets (Ceftin)	125 mg	0
Cefuroxime axetil tablets (Ceftin)	250 mg	0
Cefuroxime axetil tablets (Ceftin)	500 mg	0
Cephalexin oral suspension (Keflex)	125 mg/5 mL	3.13
Cephalexin oral suspension (Keflex)	250 mg/5 mL	3.03
Cephalexin pulvules (Keflex)	250 mg	0.13
Cephalexin pulvules (Keflex)	500 mg	0.13
Cetirizine syrup (ZyrTEC)	5 mg/5 mL	2.025
Cetirizine tablets (ZyrTEC)	5 mg	0.08
Cetirizine tablets (ZyrTEC)	10 mg	0.16
Chlorothiazide suspension (Diuril) *0.025 ethyl alcohol/5 mL	250 mg/5 mL	2
Chlorpheniramine maleate and phenylephrine hydrochloride liquid (Triaminic Cold and Allergy)	1 mg chlorpheniramine maleate and 2.5 mg phenylephrine hydrochloride/5 mL	8.13/5 mL
Cholecalciferol oral solution (D-Vi-Sol)	400 units/mL	0.630
Cimetidine tablets (Tagamet)	200 mg	0.01
Ciprofloxacin tablets (Cipro)	250 mg	0.04
Ciprofloxacin tablets (Cipro)	500 mg	0.07
Ciprofloxacin tablets (Cipro)	750 mg	0.11
Ciprofloxacin oral suspension (Cipro)	250 mg/5 mL	1.4
Ciprofloxacin oral suspension (Cipro)	500 mg/5 mL	1.3
Citalopram solution (CeleXA)	10 mg/5 mL	2.5
Citalopram tablets (CeleXA)	10 mg	0.239
Citalopram tablets (CeleXA)	20 mg	0.229
Citric acid, sodium citrate, and potassium citrate solution (Cytra-3)	5 mL	1.5
Clarithromycin suspension (Biaxin)	125 mg/5 mL	3
Clarithromycin suspension (Biaxin)	250 mg/5 mL	2.3
Clarithromycin tablets (Biaxin)	250 mg	0.07
Clarithromycin tablets (Biaxin)	500 mg	0
Clindamycin solution (Cleocin)	75 mg/5 mL	1.89
Clobazam tablets (Onfi)	10 mg	0.1
Clobazam tablets (Onfi)	20 mg	0.21
Clobazam suspension (Onfi)	2.5 mg/mL	0.19
ClonazePAM orally disintegrating tablets	All strengths	0.0075
ClonazePAM tablets (KlonoPIN)	0.5 mg	0.14
ClonazePAM tablets (KlonoPIN)	1 mg	0.14
ClonazePAM tablets (KlonoPIN)	2 mg	0.14
CloNIDine tablets (Catapres)	0.1 mg	0.12
CloNIDine tablets (Catapres)	0.2 mg	0.11
CloNIDine tablets (Catapres)	0.3 mg	0.16
Clorazepate tablets (Tranxene)	3.75 mg	0
CycloSPORINE capsules (Gengraf)	25 mg	0.019
CycloSPORINE capsules (Gengraf)	100 mg	0.077
CycloSPORINE capsules (Neoral)	25 mg	0.01
CycloSPORINE capsules (Neoral)	100 mg	0.04
CycloSPORINE oral suspension (Neoral)	100 mg/mL	0
CycloSPORINE oral suspension (SandIMMUNE) *0.12 ethyl alcohol/mL	100 mg/mL	0
CycloSPORINE capsules (SandIMMUNE)	25 mg	0
CycloSPORINE capsules (SandIMMUNE)	50 mg	0.01

(continued)

Description (Brand Name)	Dosage Unit	Grams Carbohydrate per Dosage Unit
CycloSPORINE capsules (SandIMMUNE)	100 mg	0
Dantrolene caplets (JHP Pharmaceuticals)	50 mg	0.245
Desloratadine orally disintegrating tablets (Clarinex)	5 mg	0.03
Desloratadine tablets (Clarinex)	5 mg	0.107
Dexamethasone oral solution	0.5 mg/5 mL	1.7
Dexamethasone oral concentrate solution (Intensol) *0.3 ethyl alcohol/mL	1 mg/mL	0
Dexmethylphenidate capsules (Focalin XR)	All strengths	0.25
Dextroamphetamine and amphetamine extended release caplets (Adderall XR)	5 mg	0.038
Dextroamphetamine and amphetamine extended release caplets (Adderall XR)	10 mg	0.076
Dextroamphetamine and amphetamine extended release caplets (Adderall XR)	15 mg	0.113
Dextroamphetamine and amphetamine extended release caplets (Adderall XR)	20 mg	0.151
Dextroamphetamine and amphetamine extended release caplets (Adderall XR)	25 mg	0.188
Dextroamphetamine and amphetamine extended release caplets (Adderall XR)	30 mg	0.226
Dextromethorphan guaifenesin syrup (Robitussin DM)	10 mg/5 mL	2.24 g sorbitol/5 mL
Diazepam solution (Diazepam Intensol)	5 mg/mL	0
Diazepam oral solution	5 mg/5 mL	1
Diazepam tablets (Valium)	2 mg	0.167
Diazepam tablets (Valium)	5 mg	0.164
Diazepam tablets (Valium)	10 mg	0.159
Digoxin pediatric elixir (Lanoxin) *0.1 ethyl alcohol/mL	0.05 mg/mL	0.3
Digoxin tablets (Lanoxin)	0.25 mg	0.10
Digoxin tablets (Lanoxin)	0.125 mg	0.09
DimenhyDRINATE chewable tablets (Dramamine)	50 mg	<0.5
DiphenhydrAMINE elixir (Benadryl)	5 mL	1.5
Divalproex tablet	125 mg	0.025
Docusate sodium sorbitol glycerin capsules (Correctol Extra Gentle Stool Softener)	100 mg	0.13
Docusate sodium liquigels (Surfak)	240 mg	0.37
Docusate sodium syrup	20 mg/5 mL	1.4
Erythromycin powder suspension (EryPed)	200 mg/5mL	0.606/mL
Erythromycin powder suspension (EryPed)	400 mg/5mL	0.604/mL
Erythromycin base tablets (Ery-Tab)	333 mg	0
Erythromycin base tablets (Ery-Tab)	500 mg	0
Erythromycin ethylsuccinate granules (E.E.S.)	200 mg/5 mL	1.5
Erythromycin ethylsuccinate filmtabs (E.E.S.)	400 mg	0.2
Erythromycin ethyl + sulfisoxazole acetyl suspension (Pediazole)	200 mg erythromycin and 600 mg sulfisoxazole/5 mL	1.9
Ethosuximide syrup (Zarontin)	250 mg/5 mL	3.63
Ethosuximide capsules (Zarontin)	250 mg	0.13
Esomeprazole delayed release caplets (NexIUM)	20 mg	<0.024
Esomeprazole delayed release caplets (NexIUM)	40 mg	<0.047
Esomeprazole packets (NexIUM)	All strengths	<3
Ezogabine (Potiga)	All strengths	Negligible*
Famotidine tablets (Pepcid AC)	10 mg	Negligible
Famotidine oral suspension (Pepcid)	40 mg/5 mL	1.19
Famotidine tablets (Pepcid)	20 mg	0.09
Famotidine tablets (Pepcid)	40 mg	0.08
Famotidine, calcium carbonate, and magnesium hydroxide cherry-flavored chewable tablets (Pepcid Complete)	10 mg	<0.662
Famotidine, calcium carbonate, and magnesium hydroxide mint-flavored chewable tablets (Pepcid Complete)	10 mg	<0.76
Felbamate solution (Felbatol)	600 mg/5 mL	1.5
Felbamate tablets (Felbatol)	400 mg	0.13

(continued)

Description (Brand Name)	Dosage Unit	Grams Carbohydrate per Dosage Unit
Felbamate tablets (Felbatol)	600 mg	0.19
Ferrous fumarate (Ferro-Sequels)	Capsules	0.5
Ferrous sulfate drops (Fer-In-Sol)	75 mg/1 mL	0.61
Ferrous sulfate syrup (Fer-In-Sol)	90 mg/5 mL	6.25
Fexofenadine tablets (Allegra)	30 mg	.103
Fexofenadine tablets (Allegra)	60 mg	.206
Fexofenadine tablets (Allegra)	180 mg	.618
Fluconazole tablets (Diflucan)	150 mg	0.132
Fluconazole tablets (Diflucan)	200 mg	0.175
Fluconazole tablets (Teva Pharmaceuticals)	50 mg	0.04
Fluconazole tablets (Teva Pharmaceuticals)	100 mg	0.08
Fluconazole tablets (Teva Pharmaceuticals)	150 mg	0.122
Fluconazole tablets (Teva Pharmaceuticals)	200 mg	0.163
Fluconazole oral suspension (Teva Pharmaceuticals)	10 mg/mL	0.52/mL
Fluconazole oral suspension (Teva Pharmaceuticals)	40 mg/mL	0.5/mL
Fluconazole tablets (Greenstone Pharmaceuticals)	50 mg	0.044
Fluconazole tablets (Greenstone Pharmaceuticals)	100 mg	0.088
Fluconazole tablets (Greenstone Pharmaceuticals)	150 mg	0.132
Fluconazole oral suspension (Greenstone Pharmaceuticals)	10 mg/mL	0.578/mL
Fluconazole oral suspension (Greenstone Pharmaceuticals)	40 mg/mL	0.548/mL
Fluconazole tablets (Greenstone Pharmaceuticals)	200 mg	0.175
Fluconazole oral suspension (Diflucan)	10 mg/mL	0.578
Fluconazole oral suspension (Diflucan)	40 mg/mL	0.548
Fluconazole tablets (Diflucan)	50 mg and 100 mg	0
FLUoxetine capsules (PROzac)	40 mg	0.22
FLUoxetine liquid (Greenstone)	4 mg/5 mL	0.8
FLUoxetine capsules (PROzac)	10 mg	0.22
FLUoxetine capsules (PROzac)	20 mg	0.21
Fluticasone intranasal suspension (Flonase)	50 mcg	0
Furosemide tablets (Lasix)	20 mg	0.06
Furosemide tablets (Lasix)	40 mg	0.11
Furosemide tablets (Lasix)	80 mg	0.22
Furosemide elixir (Lasix)	10 mg/mL	0.8
Gabapentin tablets (Neurontin)	600 mg	0.049
Gabapentin tablets (Neurontin)	800 mg	0.066
Gabapentin solution (Neurontin)	250 mg/5 mL	Unknown
Gabapentin tablets (Neurontin)	100 mg	0.03
Gabapentin tablets (Neurontin)	300 mg	0.07
Gabapentin tablets (Neurontin)	400 mg	0.1
Glycopyrrolate tablets (Robinul)	1 mg	0.1
Glycopyrrolate tablets (Robinul)	2 mg	0.18
Glycerin suppositories	82.5% glycerin/1.35 g	1.11
Granisetron tablets	1 mg	0.098
Guanfacine extended release tablets (Intuniv)	1 mg	0.024
Guanfacine extended release tablets (Intuniv)	2 mg	0.047
Guanfacine extended release tablets (Intuniv)	3 mg	0.04
Guanfacine extended release tablets (Intuniv)	4 mg	0.053
Hydrocodone and acetaminophen tablets (Vicodin)	5 mg/500 mg	0.038
HydrOXYzine syrup (Atarax)	10 mg/5 mL	5.88
HydrOXYzine tablets (Atarax)	10 mg	0.04
HydrOXYzine tablets (Atarax)	25 mg	0.05
HydrOXYzine tablets (Atarax)	50 mg	0.07
HydrOXYzine tablets (Atarax)	100 mg	0.1
HydrOXYzine suspension (Vistaril)	25 mg/5 mL	5.83
HydrOXYzine capsules (Vistaril)	25 mg	0.03
HydrOXYzine capsules (Vistaril)	50 mg	0.07
HydrOXYzine capsules (Vistaril)	100 mg	0.11

(continued)

Description (Brand Name)	Dosage Unit	Grams Carbohydrate per Dosage Unit
Hyoscyamine Sublingual tablets (Ethex pharmaceuticals)	0.125 mg	<0.0001
Hyoscyamine tablets (Ethex pharmaceuticals)	0.125 mg	<0.0001
Ibuprofen tablets (Advil)	200 mg	0.23
Ibuprofen tablets (Motrin Junior)	100 mg	<0.56
Ibuprofen drops (Motrin Infants)	50 mg/1.25 mL	<0.525/1.25 mL
Ibuprofen drops dye free (Motrin Infants')	50 mg/1.25 mL	<0.525/1.25 mL
Ibuprofen suspension (Motrin Children's)	100 mg/5 mL	<2.15
Ibuprofen dye free suspension (Motrin Children's)	100 mg/5 mL	<2.15
Ibuprofen chewable tablets (Motrin)	100 mg	<0.56
Insulin oral inhalation (Exubera)	1 mg	Unknown
Insulin oral inhalation (Exubera)	3 mg	Unknown
Iron, vitamins A, D, E, C drops (Vi-Daylin + Iron Drops)	20 mg/mL	0.75
Iron, vitamins A, D, E, C liquid (Vi-Daylin Liquid With Iron)	10 mg/5 mL	5
Iron, vitamins A, D, E, C, folic acid chewable tablets (Vi-Daylin Chewable With Iron)	12 mg	0.43
Iron, vitamins A, D, E, C, folic acid chewable tablets (Vi-Daylin Chewable With Iron)	0.3 mg	0.43
Iron, vitamin B, vitamin D drops (Poly-Vi-Sol With Iron)	10 mg/mL	0.85
Ketotifen oral syrup (Zaditen)	1 mg/5 mL	4
Lacosamide tablets (Vimpat)	All strengths	0
Lactase oral caplet (Lactaid)	Original	0.33
Lactobacillus capsules (Culturelle)	Capsules	<0.00001
Lactobacillus capsules (iFlora)	Capsules	0.41
Lactobacillus chewable tablets (Lactinex)	500 mg	0.377
Lactobacillus granules (Culturelle)	Granules	<0.0001
Lactobacillus granules (Lactinex)	1 g/packet	0.438
Lactobacillus oral packet (Culturelle)	Packet	<0.00001
LamoTRIgine chewable/dispersible tablets (LaMICtal)	2 mg	0.006
LamoTRIgine chewable/dispersible tablets (LaMICtal)	5 mg	0.015
LamoTRIgine chewable/dispersible tablets (LaMICtal)	25 mg	0.01
LamoTRIgine orally disintegrating tablets (LaMICtal ODT)	25 mg	0.07
LamoTRIgine orally disintegrating tablets (LaMICtal ODT)	50 mg	0.139
LamoTRIgine orally disintegrating tablets (LaMICtal ODT)	100 mg	0.278
LamoTRIgine orally disintegrating tablets (LaMICtal ODT)	200 mg	0.557
LamoTRIgine tablets (LaMICtal)	25 mg	0.03
LamoTRIgine tablets (LaMICtal)	100 mg	0.11
LamoTRIgine tablets (LaMICtal)	150 mg	0.16
LamoTRIgine tablets (LaMICtal)	200 mg	0.14
Lansoprazole delayed release capsules (Prevacid)	15 mg	0.124
Lansoprazole delayed release capsules (Prevacid)	30 mg	0.248
Lansoprazole delayed release orally disintegrating tablets (Prevacid)	15 mg	0.169
Lansoprazole delayed release orally disintegrating tablets (Prevacid)	30 mg	0.338
Leucovorin tablets (Barr Pharmaceuticals)	5 mg	0.11 to 0.15
LevETIRAcetam tablets (Keppra)	250 mg	0
LevETIRAcetam tablets (Keppra)	500 mg	0
LevETIRAcetam tablets (Keppra)	750 mg	0
LevETIRAcetam oral solution (Keppra)	100 mg/mL	0.5/mL
LevOCARNitine solution (Carnitor SF)	100 mg/mL	0
Levothyroxine tablets (Levoxyl)	All strengths	0
Levothyroxine tablets (Sandoz generic)	All strengths	0.123
Levothyroxine tablets (Synthroid)	All strengths	0.126
Lisinopril tablets (Prinivil)	5 mg	0.04
Lisinopril tablets (Prinivil)	10 mg	0.08
Lisinopril tablets (Prinivil)	20 mg	0.08
Loperamide (Imodium A-D) *0.26 ethyl alcohol/5 mL	1 mg/5 mL	4.13
Loracarbef oral suspension (Lorabid)	100 mg/5 mL	3.15

(continued)

Description (Brand Name)	Dosage Unit	Grams Carbohydrate per Dosage Unit
Loracarbef oral suspension (Lorabid)	200 mg/5 mL	3.03
Loracarbef pulvules (Lorabid)	200 mg	0.22
Loracarbef pulvules (Lorabid)	400 mg	0.11
Loratadine orally disintegrating tablets (Alavert)	10 mg	0.2
Loratadine orally disintegrating tablets (Claritin RediTabs 24 Hour Allergy)	10 mg	0.007
Loratadine oral syrup	5 mg/5 mL	8
Loratadine tablets (Alavert)	10 mg	0.08
LORazepam solution (Lorazepam Intensol)	2 mg/mL	0
Magaldrate, simethicone suspension (Riopan Plus)	5 mL	0.37
Magnesium Hydroxide (Milk of Magnesia)	Mint (400 mg/5mL)	0
Magnesium hydroxide in purified water and mineral oil	300 mg/5 mL	0
Magnesium hydroxide (Phillips' MOM Mint)	40 mEq elem mg/15 mL	0
Magnesium hydroxide, aluminum hydroxide, simethicone (Mylanta)	Tablets – regular strength	0.49
Magnesium hydroxide, aluminum hydroxide, simethicone (Mylanta)	Tablets – double strength	0.83
Magnesium hydroxide, aluminum hydroxide, simethicone (different flavors available) (Mylanta)	Liquid – regular strength, 5 mL	0.67
Magnesium hydroxide, aluminum hydroxide, simethicone (Mylanta)	Liquid – double strength, 5 mL	0.67
Meclizine tablets (Dramamine II)	25 mg	<0.25
Mesalamine capsules (Pentasa)	250 mg	0.23
Methadone (Methadone Intensol)	10 mg/mL	0
Methylphenidate extended release tablets (Concerta)	18 mg	0.007
Methylphenidate extended release tablets (Concerta)	27 mg	0.005
Methylphenidate extended release tablets (Concerta)	36 mg	0.015
Methylphenidate extended release tablets (Concerta)	54 mg	0.008
Methylphenidate tablets (Ritalin)	5 mg	0.087
Methylphenidate tablets (Ritalin)	10 mg	0.124
Methylphenidate tablets (Ritalin)	20 mg	0.155
Methylphenidate extended release caplets (Ritalin LA)	All strengths	0.25
Methylphenidate sustained release tablets (Ritalin-SR)	20 mg	0.092
Metoclopramide syrup (Reglan)	5 mg/5 mL	1.75
Metoclopramide tablets (Reglan)	5 mg	0.11
Metoclopramide tablets (Reglan)	10 mg	0.1
Modafinil tablets (Provigil)	All strengths	0.1
Mometasone intranasal suspension (Nasonex)	50 mcg/spray	Negligible
Montelukast chewable tablets (Singulair)	4 mg	0.161
Montelukast chewable tablets (Singulair)	5 mg	0.201
Montelukast tablets (Singulair)	10 mg	0.089
Montelukast granules (Singulair)	4 mg	0.484
Multiple vitamin and mineral supplement (Bugs Bunny Complete)	Chewable tablets (sugar free)	0.37
Multiple vitamin and mineral supplement (Bugs Bunny Plus Iron)	Chewable tablets	0.47
Multiple vitamin and mineral supplement (Bugs Bunny With Extra C)	Chewable tablets	0.32
Multiple vitamin and mineral supplement (Centrum Advanced Formula Liquid)	15 mL	6.25
Multiple vitamin and mineral supplement (Centrum Advanced Formula tablets)	Tablets	0.25
Multiple vitamin and mineral supplement (Flintstones Plus Extra C)	Chewable tablets	<0.6
Multiple vitamin and mineral supplement (Flintstones Plus Iron)	Chewable tablets	0.65
Multiple vitamin and mineral supplement (Flintstones Plus Calcium)	Chewable tablets	0.11
Multiple vitamin and mineral supplement (Flintstones Original)	Chewable tablets	0.70
Multiple vitamin and mineral supplement (Flintstones Complete)	Chewable tablets (sugar free)	0.37
Multiple vitamin and mineral supplement (Unicap)	Tablets	0.25
Multiple vitamin and mineral supplement (Unicap)	Capsules	0.25
NIFEdipine capsules (Procardia)	10 mg	0.10
NIFEdipine capsules (Procardia)	20 mg	0.12

(continued)

Description (Brand Name)	Dosage Unit	Grams Carbohydrate per Dosage Unit
Nitrofurantoin oral suspension (Furadantin)	25 mg/5 mL	0.7
Nystatin oral suspension	100,000 units/mL	0.61
Nystatin oral suspension (Mycostatin)	100,000 units/mL	0.60
Nystatin tablets (Mycostatin)	500,000 units	0.11
Omeprazole capsules (PriLOSEC)	10 mg	<0.179
Omeprazole capsules (PriLOSEC)	20 mg	<0.179
Omeprazole capsules (PriLOSEC)	30 mg	<0.202
Omeprazole and sodium bicarbonate powder for suspension (Zegerid)	All strengths	4
Ondansetron tablets (Zofran)	4 mg	0.082
Ondansetron tablets (Zofran)	8 mg	0.176
Ondansetron oral solution (Zofran)	4 mg/ 5 mL	53%
Ondansetron orally disintegrating tablets (Zofran)	4 mg	Unknown
Ondansetron orally disintegrating tablets	8 mg	Unknown
Ora-Plus oral liquid	Liquid	0
Ora-Sweet oral syrup	Syrup	0.8/mL
Oseltamivir capsules (Tamiflu)	30 mg	0.017
Oseltamivir capsules (Tamiflu)	45 mg	0.025
Oseltamivir capsules (Tamiflu)	75 mg	0.042
OXcarbazepine tablets (Trileptal)	150 mg	0.01
OXcarbazepine tablets (Trileptal)	300 mg	0.017
OXcarbazepine tablets (Trileptal)	600 mg	0.031
OXcarbazepine suspension (Trileptal)	300 mg/5 mL	0.305/mL
Oxymetazoline nasal spray	0.05%	0
PARoxetine oral suspension (Paxil)	10 mg/5mL	2/5 mL
PARoxetine tablets (Paxil)	10 mg	0.003
PARoxetine tablets (Paxil)	20 mg	0.006
PARoxetine tablets (Paxil)	30 mg	0.009
PARoxetine tablets (Paxil)	40 mg	0.012
PARoxetine tablets (Paxil CR)	12.5 mg	0.109
Penicillin suspension (Stada Pharmaceuticals)	125 mg/5 mL	2.645/5 mL
Penicillin suspension (Stada Pharmaceuticals)	250 mg/ 5 mL	2.645/5 mL
Penicillin V potassium oral suspension	125 mg/5 mL	2.53
Penicillin V potassium oral suspension	250 mg/5 mL	3.28
Penicillin V potassium tablets	250 mg	0.09
Penicillin V potassium tablets	500 mg	0
PHENobarbital elixir *0.71 g ethyl alcohol/5 mL	20 mg/5 mL	3.4
PHENobarbital tablets	15 mg	0.06
PHENobarbital tablets	30 mg	0.07
PHENobarbital tablets	60 mg	0.1
Phenylephrine (Neo-Synephrine Pediatric Formula Nasal Drops)	0.125%	0
Phenytoin suspension (Dilantin)	125 mg/5 mL	1.39
Phenytoin infatabs (Dilantin)	50 mg	0.48
Phenytoin kapseal (Dilantin)	30 mg	0.15
Phenytoin kapseal (Dilantin)	100 mg	0.11
Polycarbophil (Konsyl Fiber)	625 mg	0.5/tsp
Polyethylene Glycol 3350 powder (MiraLAX)	17 g	0
Potassium chloride 10% *0.25 ethyl alcohol/5 mL	6.67 mEq/5 mL	0.25
Potassium citrate and citric acid oral solution (Cytra-K)	5 mL	1 (brown bottle) 0.5 (white bottle)
Potassium citrate and citric acid powder for oral solution (Cytra-K)	Packet	0.063
Potassium citrate and sodium citrate (Polycitra)	–	0.442/mL
Potassium phosphate and sodium phosphate packet (Phos-NaK)	Packet	0.23
PrednisoLONE solution (Orapred)	15 mg/5 mL	1.86/5 mL
PrednisoLONE syrup (Prelone)	5 mg/5 mL	2.01
PrednisoLONE syrup (Prelone)	15 mg/5 mL	3.55

Description (Brand Name)	Dosage Unit	Grams Carbohydrate per Dosage Unit
PrednisoLONE oral solution (Pediapred)	5 mg/5 mL	1.53
PredniSONE solution (PredniSONE Intensol)	5 mg/mL	0
PredniSONE oral solution *0.25 ethyl alcohol/5 mL	5 mg/5 mL	1.8
Primidone oral suspension (Mysoline)	250 mg/5 mL	0
Primidone tablets (Mysoline)	50 mg	0.03
Primidone tablets (Mysoline)	250 mg	0.03
Psyllium powder (Konsyl Easy Mix)	All strengths	0.5/tsp
QUEtiapine tablets (SEROquel)	25 mg	0.037
QUEtiapine tablets (SEROquel)	50 mg	0.047
QUEtiapine tablets (SEROquel)	100 mg	0.095
QUEtiapine tablets (SEROquel)	200 mg	0.19
QUEtiapine tablets (SEROquel)	300 mg	0.285
QUEtiapine tablets (SEROquel)	400 mg	0.38
Ranitidine syrup (Zantac)	150 mg/10 mL	1
Ranitidine tablets (Zantac)	All strengths	0
RisperiDONE orally disintegrating tablets (RisperDAL M-Tab)	0.25 mg	0.02
RisperiDONE orally disintegrating tablets (RisperDAL M-Tab)	0.5 mg	0.039
RisperiDONE orally disintegrating tablets (RisperDAL M-Tab)	1 mg	0.044
RisperiDONE orally disintegrating tablets (RisperDAL M-Tab)	2 mg	0.044
RisperiDONE orally disintegrating tablets (RisperDAL M-Tab)	3 mg	0.066
RisperiDONE orally disintegrating tablets (RisperDAL M-Tab)	4 mg	0.088
RisperiDONE solution (RisperDAL)	1 mg/mL	0
RisperiDONE tablets (RisperDAL)	1 mg	0.177
RisperiDONE tablets (RisperDAL)	4 mg	0.352
Rufinamide suspension (Banzel)	40 mg/mL	0.25
Rufinamide tablets (Banzel)	100 mg	0.077
Rufinamide tablets (Banzel)	200 mg	0.153
Rufinamide tablets (Banzel)	400 mg	0.306
Saccharomyces boulardii caplets (Florastor)	250 mg	0.505
Saccharomyces boulardii powder (Florastor Kids)	250 mg/packet	0.505
Salmeterol oral inhalation (Serevent Diskus)	50 mcg	0
Senna children's syrup (Senokot Children's)	5 mL	3.3
Senna syrup (Senokot)	5 mL	3.8
Senna granules (Senokot)	Teaspoonful	2
Senna tablets (Senokot)	Tablets	0.03
Senna tablets (Senokot-S)	Tablets	0.05
Senna tablets (SenokotXTRA)	Tablets	0.08
Simethicone drops (Mylicon)	40 mg/0.6 mL	<0.071
Sodium citrate and citric acid solution (Bicitra)	1 mEq/mL	.230/mL
Sodium citrate and citric acid solution (Cytra-2)	5 mL	0.8 (brown bottle) 1.5 (white bottle)
Sodium divalproex sprinkle capsules (Depakote)	125 mg	0
Sodium divalproex tablets (Depakote)	125 mg	0.03
Sodium divalproex tablets (Depakote)	250 mg	0.05
Sodium divalproex tablets (Depakote)	500 mg	0.1
Sodium fluoride (Luride Drops) (peach flavor)	0.5 mg/mL (fluoride ion)	0.7
Sodium phosphate enema (mono- and dibasic) (Fleets)	Enema	0
Tegaserod tablets (Zelnorm)	2 mg	Unknown
Tegaserod tablets (Zelnorm)	6 mg	0.038
Theophylline elixir (Elixophyllin) *0.86 ethyl alcohol/5 mL	26.67 mg/5 mL	0.31
TiaGABine tablets (Gabitril)	4 mg	0.05
TiaGABine tablets (Gabitril)	12 mg	0.14
TiaGABine tablets (Gabitril)	16 mg	0.19
TiaGABine tablets (Gabitril)	20 mg	0.23
Topiramate caplets (Topamax)	15 mg	0.05
Topiramate caplets (Topamax)	25 mg	0.083
Topiramate tablets (Topamax)	25 mg	0.04

(continued)

Description (Brand Name)	Dosage Unit	Grams Carbohydrate per Dosage Unit
Topiramate tablets (Topamax)	50 mg	0.083
Topiramate tablets (Topamax)	100 mg	0.17
Topiramate tablets (Topamax)	200 mg	0.09
Triamcinolone intranasal suspension (Nasacort AQ)	55 mcg/spray	0.14/inhalation
Trimethoprim (TMP) and sulfamethoxazole (SMX) suspension (Hi-Tech Pharmacal)	40 mg TMP/200 mg SMX/5 mL	3.16/5 mL
Trimethoprim (TMP) and sulfamethoxazole (SMX) grape suspension (Septra)	40 mg TMP/200 mg SMX/5 mL	2.35
Trimethoprim (TMP) and sulfamethoxazole (SMX) tablets (Septra)	80 mg TMP/400 mg SMX	0
Trimethoprim (TMP) and sulfamethoxazole (SMX) double strength tablets (Septra)	160 mg TMP/800 mg SMX	0
Triprolidine pseudoephedrine syrup (Actifed)	1.25 mg/5 mL 30 mg/5 mL	5
Valacyclovir caplets (Valtrex)	All strengths	0
Valproic acid syrup (Depakene)	250 mg/5 mL	4.5
Valproic acid capsules (Depakene)	250 mg	0
Vigabatrin tablets (Sabril)	500 mg	0.014
Vigabatrin powder for oral solution (Sabril)	500 mg/packet	0
Vitamin D drops (Drisdol)	8000 units/mL	0
Vitamin E drops (Aquasol E)	15 units/0.3 mL	0.06
Xylometazoline (Otrivin Pediatric Nasal Drops)	0.05%	0
Zidovudine syrup (Retrovir)	50 mg/5 mL	2.15
Zidovudine tablets (Retrovir)	300 mg	0.02
Zidovudine capsules (Retrovir)	100 mg	0.09
Zonisamide capsules (Zonegran)	25 mg	0
Zonisamide capsules (Zonegran)	50 mg	0
Zonisamide capsules (Zonegran)	100 mg	0

[1]The nature of information is subject to change; while great care has been taken to ensure the accuracy of the information, the reader is advised to also refer to manufacturers for product-specific data.

*Contact manufacturer for additional information

REFERENCES

Feldstein TJ. Carbohydrate and alcohol content of 200 oral liquid medications for use in patients receiving ketogenic diets. *Pediatrics.* 1996;97(4):506-511.

Ketomeds. A source of information for carbohydrate content of medications. 7-14-11. Available at http://www.ketomeds.com/KetoMeds.pdf

McGhee B, Katyal N. Avoid unnecessary drug-related carbohydrates for patients consuming the ketogenic diet. *J Am Diet Assoc.* 2001;101(1):87-101.

ORAL MEDICATIONS THAT SHOULD NOT BE CRUSHED OR ALTERED

There are a variety of reasons for crushing tablets or capsule contents prior to administering to the patient. Patients may have nasogastric tubes which do not permit the administration of tablets or capsules, an oral solution for a particular medication may not be available from the manufacturer or readily prepared by pharmacy, patients may have difficulty swallowing capsules or tablets, or mixing of powdered medication with food or drink may make the drug more palatable.

Generally, medications which should not be crushed fall into one of the following categories:

- **Extended Release Products:** The formulation of some tablets is specialized as to allow the medication within it to be slowly released into the body. This may be accomplished by centering the drug within the core of the tablet, with a subsequent shedding of multiple layers around the core. Wax melts in the GI tract, releasing drug contained within the wax matrix (eg, OxyCONTIN). Capsules may contain beads which have multiple layers which are slowly dissolved with time.

  Common Abbreviations for Extended Release Products

CD	Controlled dose
CR	Controlled release
CRT	Controlled release tablet
LA	Long-acting
SR	Sustained release
TR	Timed release
TD	Time delay
SA	Sustained action
XL	Extended release
XR	Extended release

- **Medications Which Are Irritating to the Stomach:** Tablets which are irritating to the stomach may be enteric-coated which delays release of the drug until the time when it reaches the small intestine. Enteric-coated aspirin is an example of this.

- **Foul-Tasting Medication:** Some drugs are quite unpleasant to taste so the manufacturer coats the tablet in a sugar coating to increase its palatability. By crushing the tablet, this sugar coating is lost and the patient tastes the unpleasant tasting medication.

- **Sublingual Medication:** Medication intended for use under the tongue should not be crushed. While it appears to be obvious, it is not always easy to determine if a medication is to be used sublingually. Sublingual medications should indicate on the package that they are intended for sublingual use.

- **Effervescent Tablets:** These are tablets which, when dropped into a liquid, quickly dissolve to yield a solution. Many effervescent tablets, when crushed, lose their ability to quickly dissolve.

- **Potentially Hazardous Substances:** Certain drugs, including antineoplastic agents, hormonal agents, some antivirals, some bioengineered agents, and other miscellaneous drugs, are considered potentially hazardous when used in humans based on their characteristics. Examples of these characteristics include carcinogenicity, teratogenicity, reproductive toxicity, organ toxicity at low doses, genotoxicity, or new drugs with structural and toxicity profiles similar to existing hazardous drugs. Exposure to these substances can result in adverse effects and should be avoided. Crushing or breaking a tablet or opening a capsule of a potentially hazardous substance may increase the risk of exposure to the substance through skin contact, inhalation, or accidental ingestion. The extent of exposure, potency, and toxicity of the hazardous substance determines the health risk. Institutions have policies and procedures to follow when handling any potentially hazardous substance. **Note:** All potentially hazardous substances may not be represented in this table. Refer to institution-specific guidelines for precautions to observe when handling hazardous substances.

RECOMMENDATIONS

1. It is not advisable to crush certain medications.

2. Consult individual monographs prior to crushing capsule or tablet.

3. If crushing a tablet or capsule is contraindicated, consult with your pharmacist to determine whether an oral solution exists or can be compounded.

Drug Product	Dosage Form	Dosage Reasons/Comments
Accutane	Capsule	Mucous membrane irritant; teratogenic potential
Aciphex	Tablet	Extended release
Aciphex Sprinkle	Capsule	Slow release. Capsule may be opened and contents sprinkled on soft food (eg, applesauce, fruit- or vegetable-based baby food, yogurt) or emptied into a small amount of liquid (eg, infant formula, apple juice, pediatric electrolyte solution). Granules should not be chewed or crushed.
Actiq	Lozenge	Slow release. This lollipop delivery system requires the patient to dissolve it slowly.
Actoplus Met XR	Tablet	Variable release
Actonel	Tablet	Irritant. Chewed, crushed, or sucked tablets may cause oropharyngeal irritation.
Adalat CC	Tablet	Extended release
Adderall XR	Capsule	Extended release[1]
Adenovirus (Types 4, 7) Vaccine	Tablet	Teratogenic potential; enteric-coated; do not disrupt tablet to avoid releasing live adenovirus in upper respiratory tract
Advicor	Tablet	Variable release
Afeditab CR	Tablet	Extended release
Afinitor	Tablet	Mucous membrane irritant; teratogenic potential; hazardous substance[11]
Aggrenox	Capsule	Extended release. Capsule may be opened; contents include an aspirin tablet that may be chewed and dipyridamole pellets that may be sprinkled on applesauce.
Alavert Allergy and Sinus D-12	Tablet	Extended release
Allegra-D	Tablet	Extended release
ALPRAZolam ER	Tablet	Extended release
Altoprev	Tablet	Extended release
Ambien CR	Tablet	Extended release
Amitiza	Capsule	Manufacturer recommended
Amnesteem	Capsule	Mucous membrane irritant; teratogenic potential
Ampyra	Tablet	Extended release
Amrix	Capsule	Extended release
Aplenzin	Tablet	Extended release
Apriso	Capsule	Extended release[1]; maintain pH at ≤6
Aptivus	Capsule	Taste. Oil emulsion within spheres
Aricept 23 mg	Tablet	Film-coated; chewing or crushing may increase rate of absorption
Arava	Tablet	Teratogenic potential; hazardous substance[11]
Arthrotec	Tablet	Delayed release; enteric-coated
Asacol	Tablet	Slow release
Aspirin enteric-coated	Capsule, tablet	Delayed release; enteric-coated
Astagraf XL	Capsule	Extended release
Atelvia	Tablet	Extended release; tablet coating is an important part of the delayed release
Augmentin XR	Tablet	Extended release[2, 8]
AVINza	Capsule	Slow release[1] (not pudding)
Avodart	Capsule	Capsule should not be handled by pregnant women due to teratogenic potential[10]; hazardous substance[11]
Azulfidine EN-tabs	Tablet	Delayed release
Bayer Aspirin EC	Caplet	Enteric-coated
Bayer Aspirin, Low Adult 81 mg	Tablet	Enteric-coated
Bayer Aspirin, Regular Strength 325 mg	Caplet	Enteric-coated
Biaxin XL	Tablet	Extended release
Biltricide	Tablet	Taste[8]

(continued)

Drug Product	Dosage Form	Dosage Reasons/Comments
Bisac-Evac	Tablet	Enteric-coated[3]
Bisacodyl	Tablet	Enteric-coated[3]
Boniva	Tablet	Irritant. Chewed, crushed, or sucked tablets may cause oropharyngeal irritation.
Bosulif	Tablet	Hazardous substance[11]
Budeprion SR	Tablet	Extended release
Buproban	Tablet	Extended release
BuPROPion SR	Tablet	Extended release
Calan SR	Tablet	Extended release[8]
Campral	Tablet	Delayed release; enteric-coated
Caprelsa	Tablet	Teratogenic potential; hazardous substance[11]
Carbatrol	Capsule	Extended release[1]
Cardene SR	Capsule	Extended release
Cardizem	Tablet	Not described as slow release but releases drug over 3 hours.
Cardizem CD	Capsule	Extended release
Cardizem LA	Tablet	Extended release
Cardura XL	Tablet	Extended release
Cartia XT	Capsule	Extended release
Casodex	Tablet	Teratogenic potential; hazardous substance[11]
CeeNU	Capsule	Teratogenic potential; hazardous substance[11]
Cefaclor extended release	Tablet	Extended release
Ceftin	Tablet	Taste[2]. Use suspension for children.
Cefuroxime	Tablet	Taste[2]. Use suspension for children.
CellCept	Capsule, tablet	Teratogenic potential; hazardous substance[9,11]
Charcoal Plus DS	Tablet	Enteric-coated
Chlor-Trimeton 12-Hour	Tablet	Extended release[2]
Cipro XR	Tablet	Extended release[2]
Claravis	Capsule	Mucous membrane irritant; teratogenic potential
Claritin-D 12-Hour	Tablet	Extended release[2]
Claritin-D 24-Hour	Tablet	Extended release[2]
Colace	Capsule	Taste[5]
Colestid	Tablet	Slow release
Cometriq	Capsule	Teratogenic potential; hazardous substance[11]
Commit	Lozenge	Integrity compromised by chewing or crushing
Concerta	Tablet	Extended release
ConZip	Capsule	Variable release; tablet disruption may cause overdose
Coreg CR	Capsule	Extended release[1]; may add contents to chilled applesauce
Cotazym-S	Capsule	Enteric-coated[1]
Covera-HS	Tablet	Extended release
Creon	Capsule	Extended release[1]; enteric-coated contents
Crixivan	Capsule	Taste. Capsule may be opened and mixed with fruit puree (eg, banana).
Cyclophosphamide	Capsule, tablet	Hazardous substance[11]; manufacturer recommendation
Cymbalta	Capsule	Enteric-coated[1]; may add contents to apple juice or applesauce but not chocolate
Depakene	Capsule	Slow release; mucous membrane irritant[2]; hazardous substance[11]
Depakote	Tablet	Delayed release; hazardous substance[11]
Depakote ER	Tablet	Extended release; hazardous substance[11]
Depakote Sprinkles	Capsule	Extended release[1]
Detrol LA	Capsule	Extended release
Dexedrine	Capsule	Extended release

(continued)

Drug Product	Dosage Form	Dosage Reasons/Comments
Dexilant	Capsule	Delayed release[1]
Diamox Sequels	Capsule	Extended release
Dibenzyline	Capsule	Hazardous substance[11]
Diclegis	Tablet	Delayed release; manufacturer recommendation
Dilacor XR	Capsule	Extended release
Dilatrate-SR	Capsule	Extended release
Dilt-CD	Capsule	Extended release
Dilt-XR	Capsule	Extended release
Diltia XT	Capsule	Extended release
Ditropan XL	Tablet	Extended release
Divalproex ER	Tablet	Extended release
Donnatal Extentab	Tablet	Extended release[2]
Doxidan	Tablet	Enteric-coated[3]
Drisdol	Capsule	Liquid filled[4]
Droxia	Capsule	May be opened; wear gloves to handle; hazardous substance[11]
Duavee	Tablet	Manufacturer recommendation; hazardous substance[11]
Dulcolax	Capsule	Liquid-filled
Dulcolax	Tablet	Enteric-coated[3]
EC-Naprosyn	Tablet	Delayed release; enteric-coated
Ecotrin Adult Low Strength	Tablet	Enteric-coated
Ecotrin Maximum Strength	Tablet	Enteric-coated
Ecotrin Regular Strength	Tablet	Enteric-coated
E.E.S.	Tablet	Enteric-coated[2]
Effer-K	Tablet	Effervescent tablet[6]
Effervescent Potassium	Tablet	Effervescent tablet[6]
Effexor XR	Capsule	Extended release
Embeda	Capsule	Extended release[1]; do not give via NG tube
E-Mycin	Tablet	Enteric-coated
Enablex	Tablet	Slow release
Entocort EC	Capsule	Extended release; enteric-coated[1]
Epanova	Capsule	Manufacturer recommendation
Equetro	Capsule	Extended release[1]
Ergomar	Tablet	Sublingual form[7]
Erivedge	Capsule	Teratogenic potential[11]
Eryc	Capsule	Enteric-coated
Ery-Tab	Tablet	Delayed release; enteric-coated
Erythromycin Stearate	Tablet	Enteric-coated
Erythromycin Base	Tablet	Enteric-coated
Erythromycin Delayed-Release	Capsule	Enteric-coated pellets[1]
Etoposide	Capsule	Hazardous substance[11]
Evista	Tablet	Taste; teratogenic potential[10]; hazardous substance[11]
Exalgo	Tablet	Extended release; breaking, chewing, crushing, or dissolving before ingestion or injecting increases the risk of overdose
Exjade	Tablet	Do not chew or swallow whole; do not give as tablets meant to be given as a liquid
Fareston	Tablet	Teratogenic potential; hazardous substance[11]
Feldene	Capsule	Mucous membrane irritant
Fentanyl	Lozenge	Slow release; lollipop delivery system requires the patient to slowly dissolve in mouth
Fentora	Tablet	Buccal tablet; swallowing whole or crushing may reduce effectiveness
Feosol	Tablet	Enteric-coated[2]

(continued)

Drug Product	Dosage Form	Dosage Reasons/Comments
Fergon	Tablet	Enteric-coated
Ferro-Sequels	Tablet	Slow release
Flagyl ER	Tablet	Extended release
Fleet Laxative	Tablet	Enteric-coated[3]
Flomax	Capsule	Slow release
Focalin XR	Capsule	Extended release[1]
Forfivo XL	Capsule	Extended release
Fortamet	Tablet	Extended release
Fosamax	Tablet	Mucous membrane irritant
Fosamax Plus D	Tablet	Mucous membrane irritant
Fulyzaq	Tablet	Delayed release
Gengraf	Capsule	Teratogenic potential; hazardous substance[11]
Geodon	Capsule	Hazardous substance[11]
Gleevec	Tablet	Taste[8]. May be dissolved in water or apple juice; hazardous substance[11]
GlipiZIDE XL	Tablet	Extended release
Glucophage XR	Tablet	Extended release
Glucotrol XL	Tablet	Extended release
Glumetza	Tablet	Extended release
Gralise	Tablet	Extended release
Halfprin	Tablet	Enteric-coated
Hetlioz	Capsule	Manufacturer recommendation
Hexalen	Capsule	Teratogenic potential; hazardous substance[11]
Horizant	Tablet	Extended release
Hycamtin	Capsule	Teratogenic potential; hazardous substance[11]
Hydrea	Capsule	Can be opened and mixed with water; wear gloves to handle; hazardous substance[11]
Iclusig	Tablet	Teratogenic potential; hazardous substance[11]
Imbruvica	Capsule	Teratogenic potential; hazardous substance[11]
Imdur	Tablet	Extended release[8]
Inderal LA	Capsule	Extended release
Indomethacin SR	Capsule	Slow release[1,2]
Inlyta	Tablet	Teratogenic potential; hazardous substance[11]
InnoPran XL	Capsule	Extended release
Intelence	Tablet	Tablet should be swallowed whole and not crushed; tablet may be dispersed in water
Intermezzo	Tablet	Sublingual form[7]
Intuniv	Tablet	Extended release
Invega	Tablet	Extended release
IsoDitrate	Tablet	Extended release
Isoptin SR	Tablet	Extended release[8]
Isosorbide Dinitrate Sublingual	Tablet	Sublingual form[7]
ISOtretinoin	Capsule	Mucous membrane irritant
Jalyn	Capsule	Capsule should not be handled by pregnant women due to teratogenic potential[10]; hazardous substance[9,11]
Janumet XR	Tablet	Extended release
Juxtapid	Capsule	Manufacturer recommendation
Kadian	Capsule	Extended release[1]. Do not give via NG tubes; may add contents to applesauce without crushing.
Kaletra	Tablet	Film-coated; pregnant women or women who may become pregnant should not handle crushed or broken tablets; active ingredients surrounded by wax matrix to prevent healthcare exposure
Kapidex	Capsule	Delayed release[1]

(continued)

Drug Product	Dosage Form	Dosage Reasons/Comments
Kapvay	Tablet	Extended release
Kazano	Tablet	Not scored; manufacturer recommended
K-Dur	Tablet	Slow release
Keppra	Tablet	Taste[2]
Keppra XR	Tablet	Extended release[2]
Ketek	Tablet	Slow release
Khedezia	Tablet	Extended release
Klor-Con	Tablet	Extended release[2]
Klor-Con M	Tablet	Slow release[2]; some strengths are scored; to make liquid, place tablet in 120 mL of water; disperse 2 minutes; stir
K-Lyte/Cl	Tablet	Effervescent tablet[6]
Kombiglyze XR	Tablet	Extended release; tablet matrix may remain in stool
K-Tab	Tablet	Extended release[2]
LaMICtal XR	Tablet	Extended release
Lescol XL	Tablet	Extended release
Letairis	Tablet	Film-coated; slow release; hazardous substance[11]
Leukeran	Tablet	Teratogenic potential; hazardous substance[11]
Levbid	Tablet	Extended release[8]
Lialda	Tablet	Delayed release, enteric-coated
Lithobid	Tablet	Extended release
Lovaza	Capsule	Contents of capsule may erode walls of styrofoam or plastic materials
Luvox CR	Capsule	Extended release
Lysodren	Tablet	Hazardous substance[11]
Mag-Tab SR	Tablet	Extended release
Matulane	Capsule	Teratogenic potential; hazardous substance[11]
Maxiphen DM	Tablet	Slow release[8]
Mestinon ER	Tablet	Extended release[2]
Metadate CD	Capsule	Extended release[1]
Metadate ER	Tablet	Extended release
Metoprolol ER	Tablet	Extended release
MicroK Extencaps	Capsule	Extended release[1,2]
Minocin	Capsule	Slow release
Mirapex ER	Tablet	Extended release
Morphine sulfate extended-release	Tablet	Extended release
Motrin	Tablet	Taste[5]
Moxatag	Tablet	Extended release
MS Contin	Tablet	Extended release[2]
Mucinex	Tablet	Slow release
Mucinex DM	Tablet	Slow release[2]
Multaq	Tablet	Hazardous substance[11]
Myfortic	Tablet	Delayed release; teratogenic potential; hazardous substance[11]
Myrbetriq	Tablet	Extended release
Namenda XR	Capsule	Extended release[1]
Naprelan	Tablet	Extended release
Neoral	Capsule	Teratogenic potential; hazardous substance[11]
NexIUM	Capsule	Delayed release[1]
Niaspan	Tablet	Extended release
Nicotinic Acid	Capsule, Tablet	Slow release[8]
Nifediac CC	Tablet	Extended release
Nifedical XL	Tablet	Extended release

(continued)

Drug Product	Dosage Form	Dosage Reasons/Comments
NIFEdipine ER	Tablet	Extended release
Nitrostat	Tablet	Sublingual route[7]
Norpace CR	Capsule	Extended release; form within a special capsule
Norvir	Tablet	Crushing tablets has resulted in decreased bioavailability of drug[2]
Noxafil	Tablet	Delayed release
Nucynta ER	Tablet	Extended release; tablet disruption may cause a potentially fatal overdose
Oleptro	Tablet	Extended release[8]
Omtryg	Capsule	Manufacturer recommendation
Onglyza	Tablet	Film-coated
Opana ER	Tablet	Extended release; tablet disruption may cause a potentially fatal overdose
Opsumit	Tablet	Teratogenic potential; hazardous substance[11]
Oracea	Capsule	Delayed release
Oramorph SR	Tablet	Extended release[2]
Oravig	Tablet	Buccal tablet
Orphenadrine citrate ER	Tablet	Extended release
Otezla	Tablet	Manufacturer recommendation
Oxtellar XR	Tablet	Extended release
OxyCONTIN	Tablet	Extended release; surrounded by wax matrix; tablet disruption may cause a potentially fatal overdose
Oxymorphone ER	Tablet	Extended release
Pancrease MT	Capsule	Enteric-coated[1]
Pancreaze	Capsule	Slow-release[1]; enteric-coated contents
Pancrelipase	Capsule	Slow-release[1]; enteric-coated contents
Paxil CR	Tablet	Extended release
Pentasa	Capsule	Slow release[1]
Pertzye	Capsule	Slow-release[1]; enteric-coated contents
Plendil	Tablet	Extended release
Pomalyst	Capsule	Teratogenic potential; hazardous substance[11]; healthcare workers should avoid contact with capsule contents/body fluids
Pradaxa	Capsule	Bioavailability increases by 75% when the pellets are taken without the capsule shell
Prevacid	Capsule	Delayed release[1]
Prevacid	Suspension	Slow release. Contains enteric-coated granules. Not for use in NG tubes; mix with water only
Prevacid SoluTab	Tablet	Orally disintegrating. Do not swallow; dissolve in water only and dispense via dosing syringe or NG tube.
PriLOSEC	Capsule	Delayed release
PriLOSEC OTC	Tablet	Delayed release
Pristiq	Tablet	Extended release
Procardia XL	Tablet	Extended release
Procysbi	Capsule	Delayed release[1]
Propecia	Tablet	Women who are, or may become, pregnant should not handle crushed or broken tablets due to teratogenic potential[10]; hazardous substance[11]
Proscar	Tablet	Women who are, or may become, pregnant should not handle crushed or broken tablets due to teratogenic potential[10]; hazardous substance[11]
Protonix	Tablet	Slow release
PROzac Weekly	Capsule	Enteric-coated
Purinethol	Tablet	Teratogenic potential[10]; hazardous substance[11]
Pytest	Capsule	Hazardous substance[11]
Qudexy XR	Capsule	Extended release
QuiNIDine ER	Tablet	Extended release[8]; enteric-coated

(continued)

Drug Product	Dosage Form	Dosage Reasons/Comments
Ranexa	Tablet	Slow release
Rapamune	Tablet	Hazardous substance[11]; pharmacokinetic NanoCrystal technology may be affected[2]
Rayos	Tablet	Delayed release; release is dependent upon intact coating
Razadyne ER	Capsule	Extended release
Renagel	Tablet	Expands in liquid if broken/crushed.
Renvela	Tablet	Enteric-coated[2]; expands in liquid if broken or crushed
Requip XL	Tablet	Extended release
Rescriptor	Tablet	If unable to swallow, may dissolve 100 mg tablets in water and drink; 200 mg tablets must be swallowed whole
Revlimid	Capsule	Teratogenic potential; hazardous substance[11]; healthcare workers should avoid contact with capsule contents/body fluids
RisperDAL M-Tab	Tablet	Orally disintegrating. Do not chew or break tablet; after dissolving under tongue, tablet may be swallowed
Ritalin LA	Capsule	Extended release[1]
Ritalin-SR	Tablet	Extended release
Rythmol SR	Capsule	Extended release
Ryzolt	Tablet	Extended release; tablet disruption may cause overdose
SandIMMUNE	Capsule	Teratogenic potential; hazardous substance[11]
Saphris	Tablet	Sublingual form[7]
Sensipar	Tablet	Tablets are not scored and cutting may cause inaccurate dosage
SEROquel XR	Tablet	Extended release
Sinemet CR	Tablet	Extended release[8]
Slo-Niacin	Tablet	Slow release[8]
Slow-Mag	Tablet	Delayed release
Solodyn	Tablet	Extended release
Somnote	Capsule	Liquid filled
Soriatane	Capsule	Teratogenic potential; hazardous substance[11]
Sprycel	Tablet	Film-coated. Active ingredients are surrounded by a wax matrix to prevent healthcare exposure. Women who are, or may become pregnant, should not handle crushed or broken tablets; teratogenic potential; hazardous substance[11]
Stavzor	Capsule	Delayed release; hazardous substance[11]
Stivarga	Tablet	Manufacturer recommendation; teratogenic potential; hazardous substance[11]
Strattera	Capsule	Capsule contents can cause ocular irritation.
Sudafed 12-Hour	Capsule	Extended release[2]
Sudafed 24-Hour	Capsule	Extended release[2]
Sulfazine EC	Tablet	Delayed release, enteric-coated
Sular	Tablet	Extended release
Sustiva	Tablet	Tablets should not be broken (capsules should be used if dosage adjustment needed)
Symax Duotab	Tablet	Controlled release
Symax SR	Tablet	Extended release
Syprine	Capsule	Potential risk of contact dermatitis
Tabloid	Tablet	Teratogenic potential; hazardous substance[11]
Tafinlar	Capsule	Teratogenic potential; hazardous substance[11]
Tamoxifen	Tablet	Teratogenic potential; hazardous substance[11]
Targretin	Capsule	Manufacturer recommended; teratogenic potential; hazardous substance[11]
Tasigna	Capsule	Hazardous substance[11]; altering capsule may lead to high blood levels, increasing the risk of toxicity
Taztia XT	Capsule	Extended release[1]
Tecfidera	Capsule	Manufacturer recommendation; delayed release; irritant
TEGretol-XR	Tablet	Extended release[2]

(continued)

Drug Product	Dosage Form	Dosage Reasons/Comments
Temodar	Capsule	Teratogenic potential; hazardous substance[11]. **Note:** If capsules are accidentally opened or damaged, rigorous precautions should be taken to avoid inhalation or contact of contents with the skin or mucous membranes.
Tessalon Perles	Capsule	Swallow whole; pharmacologic action may cause choking if chewed or opened and swallowed.
Tetracycline	Capsule	Hazardous substance[11]
Thalomid	Capsule	Teratogenic potential; hazardous substance[11]
Theo-24	Capsule	Extended release[1]; contains beads that dissolve through GI tract
Theochron	Tablet	Extended release
Theophylline ER	Tablet	Extended release
Tiazac	Capsule	Extended release[1]
Topamax	Capsule	Taste[1]
Topamax	Tablet	Taste
Toprol XL	Tablet	Extended release[8]
Toviaz	Tablet	Extended release
Tracleer	Tablet	Teratogenic potential; hazardous substance[10,11]; women who are or may be pregnant should not handle crushed or broken tablets
TRENtal	Tablet	Extended release
Treximet	Tablet	Unique formulation enhances rapid drug absorption
TriLipix	Capsule	Extended release
Trokendi XR	Capsule	Extended release
Tylenol Arthritis Pain	Caplet	Controlled release
Tylenol 8 Hour	Caplet	Extended release
Uceris	Tablet	Extended release; coating on tablet designed to break down at pH of ≥7
Ultram ER	Tablet	Extended release. Tablet disruption my cause a potentially fatal overdose.
Ultresa	Capsule	Delayed release; enteric-coated contents
Ultrase	Capsule	Enteric-coated[1]
Ultrase MT	Capsule	Enteric-coated[1]
Uniphyl	Tablet	Slow release
Urocit-K	Tablet	Wax-coated; prevents upper GI release
Uroxatral	Tablet	Extended release
Valcyte	Tablet	Irritant potential[2]; teratogenic potential; hazardous substance[11]
Vascepa	Capsule	Manufacturer recommendation
Verapamil SR	Tablet	Extended release[8]
Verelan	Capsule	Sustained release[1]
Verelan PM	Capsule	Extended release[1]
Vesanoid	Capsule	Teratogenic potential; hazardous substance[11]
VESIcare	Tablet	Enteric-coated
Videx EC	Capsule	Delayed release
Vimovo	Tablet	Delayed release
Viokace	Tablet	Mucous membrane irritant
Viramune XR	Tablet	Extended release[2]
Voltaren-XR	Tablet	Extended release
VoSpire ER	Tablet	Extended release
Votrient	Tablet	Crushing significantly increases AUC and T_{max}; hazardous substance[11]; crushed or broken tablets may cause dangerous skin problems
Wellbutrin	Tablet	Film-coated
Wellbutrin SR	Tablet	Extended release
Wellbutrin XL	Tablet	Extended release

(continued)

Drug Product	Dosage Form	Dosage Reasons/Comments
Xalkori	Capsule	Teratogenic potential; hazardous substance[11]
Xanax XR	Tablet	Extended release
Xeloda	Tablet	Teratogenic potential; hazardous substance[11].
Xtandi	Capsule	Teratogenic potential; hazardous substance[11]
Zegerid OTC	Capsule	Delayed release[2]
Zelboraf	Tablet	Teratogenic potential; hazardous substance[11]
Zenpep	Capsule	Delayed release[1]; enteric-coated contents
Zohydro ER	Capsule	Extended release; capsule disruption may cause a potentially fatal overdose
Zolinza	Capsule	Irritant; avoid contact with skin or mucous membranes; use gloves to handle; teratogenic potential; hazardous substance[11]
Zomig-ZMT	Tablet	Oral-disintegrating form[7]
Zortress	Tablet	Mucous membrane irritant; teratogenic potential; hazardous substance[11]
Zyban	Tablet	Slow release
Zyflo CR	Tablet	Extended release
ZyrTEC-D Allergy & Congestion	Tablet	Extended release
Zytiga	Tablet	Teratogenic potential; hazardous substance[11]; women who are or may be pregnant should wear gloves if handling tablets

[1]Capsule may be opened and the contents taken without crushing or chewing; soft food, such as applesauce or pudding, may facilitate administration; contents may generally be administered via nasogastric tube using an appropriate fluid, provided entire contents are washed down the tube.

[2]Liquid dosage forms of the product are available; however, dose, frequency of administration, and manufacturers may differ from that of the solid dosage form.

[3]Antacids and/or milk may prematurely dissolve the coating of the tablet.

[4]Capsule may be opened and the liquid contents removed for administration.

[5]The taste of this product in a liquid form would likely be unacceptable to the patient; administration via nasogastric tube should be acceptable.

[6]Effervescent tablets must be dissolved in the amount of diluent recommended by the manufacturer.

[7]Tablets are made to disintegrate under (or on) the tongue.

[8]Tablet is scored and may be broken in half without affecting release characteristics.

[9]Skin contact may enhance tumor production; avoid direct contact.

[10]Prescribing information recommends that women who are, or may become, pregnant should not handle medication, especially if crushed or broken; avoid direct contact.

[11]Potentially hazardous or hazardous substance; refer to institution-specific guidelines for precautions to observe when handling this substance.

REFERENCES

Mitchell JF. Oral dosage forms that should not be crushed. Available at http://www.ismp.org/tools/DoNotCrush.pdf. Accessed November 11, 2011.

National Institute for Occupational Safety and Health (NIOSH). NIOSH list of antineoplastic and other hazardous drugs in healthcare settings 2012. Available at http://www.cdc.gov/niosh/docs/2012-150/pdfs/2012-150.pdf. Accessed July 11, 2012.

WHO MODEL FORMULARY FOR CHILDREN

The World Health Organization (WHO) has developed a Model List of Essential Medicines for children (EMLc) in response to a 2007 resolution recognizing the need for further research and development of pediatric medicines. The following drugs are included in the WHO model formulary, which is based on the EMLc and intended for children up to 12 years of age. Medications not included on this list may be available to or recommended in children, but they are not considered essential by WHO.

Abacavir
Acetaminophen
Acetic Acid
Acetylcysteine
Acetylsalicylic Acid
Acyclovir
Albendazole
Albuterol
Allopurinol
Amikacin
Amitriptyline
Amodiaquine
Amoxicillin
Amoxicillin and Clavulanic Acid
Amphotericin B
Ampicillin
Antitetanus Immunoglubulin (Human)
Antivenom Immunoglobulin
Artemether
Artemether and Lumefantrine
Artesunate
Ascorbic Acid
Asparaginase
Atazanavir
Atropine
AzaTHIOprine
Azithromycin
Barium Sulfate
BCG Vaccine
Benzathine Benzylpenicillin
Benznidazole
Benzoyl Peroxide
Benzyl Benzoate
Benzylpenicillin
Betamethasone
Bleomycin
Budesonide
Bupivacaine
Caffeine Citrate
Calamine Lotion
Calcium Folinate
Calcium Gluconate
Capreomycin
CarBAMazepine
CARBOplatin
Cefalexin
CeFAZolin
Cefotaxime
CefTAZidime
CefTRIAXone
Charcoal, Activated
Chlorambucil
Chloramphenicol
Chlorhexidine
Chlorine Base Compound
Chloroquine
Chloroxylenol
Chlorphenamine
ChlorproMAZINE
Cholera Vaccine
Ciclosporin
Ciprofloxacin
Clindamycin
Clofazimine
Cloxacillin

Coal Tar
Colecalciferol
Cyclizine
Cyclophosphamide
CycloSERINE
Cytarabine
Dacarbazine
DACTINomycin
Dapsone
DAUNOrubicin
Deferoxamine
Dexamethasone
Diazepam
Didanosine
Diethylcarbamazine
Digoxin
Diloxanide
Dimercaprol
Diphtheria Antitoxin
Diphtheria Vaccine
Docusate Sodium
DOPamine
DOXOrubicin
Doxycycline
Efavirenz
Eflornithine
Emtricitabine
Enalapril
EPINEPHrine
Erythromycin
Ethambutol
Ethanol
Ethionamide
Ethosuximide
Etoposide
Factor IX Complex (Coagulation Factors, II, VII, IX, X)
   Concentrate
Factor VIII Concentrate
Ferrous Salt
Fluconazole
Flucytosine
Fludrocortisone
Fluorescein
Fluorouracil
FLUoxetine
Folic Acid
Furosemide
Gentamicin
Glucose
Glucose With Sodium Chloride
Glutaral
Griseofulvin
Haemophilus Influenzae Type B Vaccine
Haloperidol
Halothane
Heparin Sodium
Hepatitis A Vaccine
Hepatitis B Vaccine
Human Normal Immunoglubulin
Hydrochlorothiazide
Hydrocortisone
Hydroxocobalamin
Hyoscine Hydrobromide
Ibuprofen
Imipenem and Cilastatin

Influenza Vaccine
Insulin Injection (Soluble)
Intermediate-Acting Insulin
Intraperitoneal Dialysis Solution (of Appropriate Composition)
Iodine
Isoniazid
Ivermectin (Systemic)
Japanese Encephalitis Vaccine
Kanamycin
Ketamine
Lamivudine
Lamivudine, Nevirapine, and Stavudine
Lamivudine, Nevirapine, and Zidovudine
Lamivudine and Zidovudine
Levamisole
Levothyroxine
Lidocaine
Lidocaine and Epinephrine
Lopinavir and Ritonavir
Lorazepam
Lugol's Solution
Mannitol
Measles Vaccine
Mebendazole
Mefloquine
Melarsoprol
Meningococcal Meningitis Vaccine
Mercaptopurine
MetFORMIN
Methotrexate
Methylrosanilinium Chloride (Gentian Violet)
Metoflopramide
MetroNIDAZOLE
Miconazole
Midazolam
Morphine
Mumps Vaccine
Naloxone
Neostigmine
Nevirapine
Niclosamide
Nifurtimox
Nitrofurantoin
Nitrous Oxide
Nystatin
Ofloxacin
Omeprazole
Ondansetron
Oral Rehydration Salts
Oxamniquine
Oxygen
P-Aminosalicylic Acid
Pancreatic Enzymes
Paromomycin
Penicillamine
Pentamidine
Permethrin
Pertussis Vaccine
PHENobarbital
Phenoxymethylpenicillin
Phenytoin
Phytomenadione
Pneumococcal Vaccine
Podophyllum Resin
Poliomyelitis Vaccine
Polyvidone Iodine
Potassium Chloride
Potassium Iodide
Potassium Permanganate

Praziquantel
PrednisoLONE
Primaquine
Procaine Benzylpenicillin
Procarbazine
Proguanil
Propranolol
Propylthiouracil
Prostaglandin E
Protamine Sulfate
Pyrantel
Pyrazinamide
Pyridostigmine
Pyridoxine
Pyrimethamine
QuiNINE
Rabies Immunoglobulin
Rabies Vaccine
Ranitidine
Retinol
Ribavirin
Riboflavin
Rifampicin
Ritonavir
Rotavirus Vaccine
Rubella Vaccine
Salicylic Acid
Saquinavir
Selenium Sulfide
Senna
Silver Sulfadiazine
Sodium Calcium Edetate
Sodium Chloride
Sodium Fluoride
Sodium Hydrogen Carbonate
Sodium Lactate, Compound Solution
Sodium Stibogluconate or Meglumine Antimoniate
Spironolactone
Stavudine
Streptomycin
SulfADIAZINE
Sulfadoxine and Pyrimethamine
Sulfamethoxazole and Trimethoprim
Suramin Sodium
Surfactant
Suxamethonium
Tetanus Vaccine
Tetracaine
Tetracycline
Thiamine
Thiopental
Triclabendazole
Trimethoprim
Tropicamide
Tuberculin, Purified Protein Derivative
Typhoid Vaccine
Urea
Valproic Acid (Sodium Valproate)
Vancomycin
Varicella Vaccine
Vecuronium
VinBLAStine
VinCRIStine
Warfarin
Water for Injection
Xylometazoline
Yellow Fever Vaccine
Zidovudine
Zinc Sulfate

THERAPEUTIC CATEGORY & KEY WORD INDEX

Acne Products

Adapalene 73
Adapalene and Benzoyl Peroxide 74
Azelaic Acid 244
Benzoyl Peroxide 275
Clindamycin and Benzoyl Peroxide 502
Clindamycin and Tretinoin 503
Clindamycin (Topical) 500
ISOtretinoin 1161
Sulfacetamide (Topical) 1944
Tazarotene 1971
Tetracycline 1996
Tretinoin (Topical) 2071

Adjuvant Therapy, Penicillin Level Prolongation

Probenecid 1739

Adrenal Corticosteroid

Alclometasone 87
Beclomethasone (Oral Inhalation) 265
Budesonide and Formoterol 314
Budesonide (Nasal) 313
Budesonide (Systemic, Oral Inhalation) 308
Ciclesonide (Oral Inhalation) 461
Clobetasol 506
Corticotropin 545
Cortisone 548
Cosyntropin 549
Dexamethasone (Systemic) 615
Fludrocortisone 887
Fluocinolone (Otic) 892
Fluocinolone (Topical) 892
Fluocinonide 894
Fluorometholone 897
Fluticasone and Salmeterol 916
Fluticasone (Oral Inhalation) 910
Halobetasol 997
Hydrocortisone (Systemic) 1034
MethylPREDNISolone 1386
Mometasone and Formoterol 1436
Prednicarbate 1725
PrednisoLONE (Systemic) 1727
PredniSONE 1732
Triamcinolone (Systemic) 2072

Adrenergic Agonist Agent

Albuterol 84
Budesonide and Formoterol 314
CloNIDine 516
Dexmedetomidine 621
DOBUTamine 696
DOPamine 708
EPHEDrine (Systemic) 759
EPINEPHrine (Systemic, Oral Inhalation) 761
Fluticasone and Salmeterol 916
Formoterol 929
Isoproterenol 1160
Levalbuterol 1218
Metaproterenol 1352
Mometasone and Formoterol 1436
Norepinephrine 1510
Phenylephrine (Nasal) 1660
Phenylephrine (Ophthalmic) 1661
Phenylephrine (Systemic) 1658
Phenylephrine (Topical) 1662
Pirbuterol 1683
Pseudoephedrine 1770
Salmeterol 1862
Terbutaline 1984

Adrenergic Agonist Agent, Ophthalmic

Cyclopentolate and Phenylephrine 560
Dipivefrin 692
Naphazoline (Ophthalmic) 1470

Oxymetazoline (Ophthalmic) 1578
Phenylephrine (Ophthalmic) 1661

Alcohol Free

Acetaminophen and Codeine 53
Benzocaine 273
Cetirizine 431
Chlorpheniramine 448
Cholecalciferol 455
Citric Acid, Sodium Citrate, and Potassium
  Citrate 487
Dextromethorphan 636
DiphenhydrAMINE (Systemic) 673
Docusate 701
Ferrous Sulfate 868
GuaiFENesin 984
Ibuprofen 1059
Loratadine 1278
LORazepam 1280
Phenylephrine (Systemic) 1658
Polysaccharide-Iron Complex 1701
PrednisoLONE (Systemic) 1727
Pseudoephedrine 1770
Salicylic Acid 1860
Simethicone 1891
Sodium Chloride 1902
Sodium Citrate and Citric Acid 1906
Sorbitol 1924
Trimethoprim 2087

Alkalinizing Agent, Oral

Citric Acid, Sodium Citrate, and Potassium
  Citrate 487
Potassium Citrate and Citric Acid 1710
Sodium Bicarbonate 1901
Sodium Citrate and Citric Acid 1906

Alkalinizing Agent, Parenteral

Sodium Acetate 1899
Sodium Bicarbonate 1901
Tromethamine 2091

Alpha$_2$-Adrenergic Agonist

GuanFACINE 989

Alpha-Adrenergic Agonist

CloNIDine 516
Dexmedetomidine 621
Norepinephrine 1510
Phenylephrine (Nasal) 1660
Phenylephrine (Ophthalmic) 1661
Phenylephrine (Systemic) 1658
Phenylephrine (Topical) 1662

Alpha-Adrenergic Agonist, Ophthalmic

Brimonidine (Ophthalmic) 303

Alpha-Adrenergic Blocking Agent, Intranasal

Dihydroergotamine 665

Alpha-Adrenergic Blocking Agent, Oral

Doxazosin 712
Ergotamine 776
Ergotamine and Caffeine 777
Phenoxybenzamine 1655
Prazosin 1724
Terazosin 1981

Alpha-Adrenergic Blocking Agent, Parenteral

Dihydroergotamine 665
Phentolamine 1656

Alpha-Adrenergic Inhibitors, Central

Methyldopa 1376

Alpha-/Beta-Adrenergic Blocker

Labetalol 1186

Amebicide
Chloroquine 444
Iodoquinol 1144
MetroNIDAZOLE (Systemic) 1399
Paromomycin 1608
Tinidazole 2029

5-Aminosalicylic Acid Derivative
Balsalazide 261
Mesalamine 1347
Olsalazine 1532
SulfaSALAzine 1954

Ammonium Detoxicant
Lactulose 1193
Neomycin 1482
Sodium Benzoate 1900
Sodium Phenylacetate and Sodium Benzoate 1911
Sodium Phenylbutyrate 1912

Amphetamine
Dextroamphetamine 629
Dextroamphetamine and Amphetamine 632
Lisdexamfetamine 1260
Methamphetamine 1359

Analgesic, Narcotic
Acetaminophen and Codeine 53
Alfentanil 93
Belladonna and Opium 269
Buprenorphine 320
Buprenorphine and Naloxone 324
Codeine 534
FentaNYL 853
Hydrocodone and Acetaminophen 1027
HYDROmorphone 1041
Meperidine 1337
Methadone 1355
Morphine (Liposomal) 1449
Morphine (Systemic) 1440
Nalbuphine 1464
Opium Tincture 1548
OxyCODONE 1569
Oxycodone and Acetaminophen 1573
Oxycodone and Aspirin 1575
Paregoric 1605
Pentazocine 1639
Remifentanil 1811
SUFentanil 1942

Analgesic, Non-narcotic
Acetaminophen 47
Aspirin 212
Choline Magnesium Trisalicylate 459
Diclofenac (Ophthalmic) 648
Diclofenac (Systemic) 645
Diclofenac (Topical) 649
Etodolac 812
Flurbiprofen (Systemic) 908
Ibuprofen 1059
Indomethacin 1096
Ketorolac (Systemic) 1180
Meloxicam 1325
Naproxen 1470
Oxaprozin 1562
Piroxicam 1683
Sulindac 1957
Tolmetin 2042

Analgesic, Non-narcotic (Epidural)
CloNIDine 516

Analgesic, Nonopioid
Sucrose 1941

Analgesic, Opioid
TraMADol 2060

Analgesic, Topical
Benzocaine 273
Benzyl Alcohol 278
Capsaicin 367
Cocaine 533
Dibucaine 645
Lidocaine and Prilocaine 1246
Lidocaine and Tetracaine 1248
Lidocaine (Topical) 1242
Tetracaine (Topical) 1995

Analgesic, Urinary
Phenazopyridine 1651

Androgen
Danazol 582
Fluoxymesterone 906
Oxandrolone 1560
Testosterone 1986

Angiogenesis Inhibitor
Thalidomide 2000

Angiotensin II Receptor Blocker
Candesartan 363
Irbesartan 1147
Losartan 1283
Olmesartan 1530
Valsartan 2108

Angiotensin-Converting Enzyme (ACE) Inhibitor
Benazepril 270
Captopril 368
Enalapril 744
Enalaprilat 747
Fosinopril 938
Lisinopril 1262
Quinapril 1788

Anorexiant
Dextroamphetamine 629
Dextroamphetamine and Amphetamine 632
Methamphetamine 1359

Antacid
Aluminum Hydroxide 110
Aluminum Hydroxide and Magnesium Hydroxide 111
Calcium Carbonate 346
Magnesium Hydroxide 1294
Sodium Bicarbonate 1901

Anthelmintic
Albendazole 80
Ivermectin (Systemic) 1170
Mebendazole 1313
Praziquantel 1723
Pyrantel Pamoate 1774

Antiallergic, Ophthalmic
Azelastine (Ophthalmic) 247
Epinastine 761
Ketotifen (Ophthalmic) 1185
Nedocromil 1474

Antianginal Agent
AmLODIPine 135
Atenolol 222
Diltiazem 667
Metoprolol 1396
Nadolol 1460
NiCARdipine 1493
NIFEdipine 1497
Nitroglycerin 1504
Propranolol 1759
Verapamil 2129

Antianxiety Agent
ALPRAZolam 100

BusPIRone 332
Diazepam 640
Doxepin (Systemic) 715
HydrOXYzine 1054
LORazepam 1280

Antiarrhythmic Agent, Class I-A
Disopyramide 694
Procainamide 1740
QuiNIDine 1791

Antiarrhythmic Agent, Class I-B
Lidocaine (Systemic) 1239
Mexiletine 1406
Phenytoin 1663

Antiarrhythmic Agent, Class I-C
Flecainide 874

Antiarrhythmic Agent, Class II
Esmolol 791
Metoprolol 1396
Nadolol 1460
Propranolol 1759
Sotalol 1925

Antiarrhythmic Agent, Class III
Amiodarone 127
Sotalol 1925

Antiarrhythmic Agent, Class IV
Verapamil 2129

Antiarrhythmic Agent, Miscellaneous
Adenosine 76
Digoxin 658

Antiasthmatic
Albuterol 84
Aminophylline 124
Atropine 234
Beclomethasone (Oral Inhalation) 265
Budesonide and Formoterol 314
Budesonide (Systemic, Oral Inhalation) 308
Ciclesonide (Oral Inhalation) 461
Cromolyn (Systemic, Oral Inhalation) 551
EPINEPHrine (Systemic, Oral Inhalation) 761
Fluticasone and Salmeterol 916
Fluticasone (Oral Inhalation) 910
Formoterol 929
Hydrocortisone (Systemic) 1034
Ipratropium (Oral Inhalation) 1144
Isoproterenol 1160
Levalbuterol 1218
Metaproterenol 1352
MethylPREDNISolone 1386
Mometasone (Oral Inhalation) 1432
Montelukast 1438
Pirbuterol 1683
PrednisoLONE (Systemic) 1727
PredniSONE 1732
Salmeterol 1862
Terbutaline 1984
Theophylline 2005
Triamcinolone (Systemic) 2072
Zafirlukast 2164

Antibacterial, Otic
Hydrogen Peroxide 1040
Neomycin, Polymyxin B, and Hydrocortisone 1485

Antibacterial, Topical
Chlorhexidine Gluconate 441
Gentian Violet 968
Hexachlorophene 1016
Hydrogen Peroxide 1040
Potassium Iodide and Iodine 1713

Antibiotic, Aminoglycoside
Amikacin 118
Gentamicin (Ophthalmic) 966
Gentamicin (Systemic) 962
Gentamicin (Topical) 967
Neomycin 1482
Streptomycin 1935
Tobramycin (Ophthalmic) 2039
Tobramycin (Systemic, Oral Inhalation) 2034

Antibiotic, Anaerobic
Clindamycin (Systemic) 495
Clindamycin (Topical) 500
MetroNIDAZOLE (Systemic) 1399

Antibiotic, Beta-lactam and Beta-lactamase Combination
Amoxicillin and Clavulanate 144
Ampicillin and Sulbactam 162
Ticarcillin and Clavulanate Potassium 2022

Antibiotic, Beta-lactam and Beta-lactamase Inhibitor Combination
Piperacillin and Tazobactam 1679

Antibiotic, Carbapenem
Ertapenem 778
Imipenem and Cilastatin 1077
Meropenem 1345

Antibiotic, Cephalosporin (First Generation)
Cefadroxil 392
CeFAZolin 393
Cephalexin 429

Antibiotic, Cephalosporin (Second Generation)
Cefaclor 391
CefoTEtan 407
CefOXitin 408
Cefprozil 412
Cefuroxime 422

Antibiotic, Cephalosporin (Third Generation)
Cefdinir 395
Cefditoren 397
Cefixime 401
Cefotaxime 404
Cefpodoxime 410
CefTAZidime 413
Ceftibuten 416
CefTRIAXone 417

Antibiotic, Cephalosporin (Fourth Generation)
Cefepime 398

Antibiotic/Corticosteroid, Otic
Ciprofloxacin and Dexamethasone 477
Ciprofloxacin and Hydrocortisone 477

Antibiotic, Cyclic Lipopeptide
DAPTOmycin 589

Antibiotic, Fluoroquinolone
Besifloxacin 281
Moxifloxacin (Ophthalmic) 1451

Antibiotic, Glycylcycline
Tigecycline 2025

Antibiotic, Macrolide
Azithromycin (Systemic) 247
Clarithromycin 490
Erythromycin and Sulfisoxazole 785
Erythromycin (Ophthalmic) 784
Erythromycin (Systemic) 780
Erythromycin (Topical) 785

Antibiotic, Miscellaneous
Aztreonam 254

Bacitracin 256
Capreomycin 365
Chloramphenicol 439
Clindamycin and Tretinoin 503
Clindamycin (Systemic) 495
Clindamycin (Topical) 500
Colistimethate 541
CycloSERINE 563
Methenamine 1361
Nitrofurantoin 1502
Pentamidine 1637
Polymyxin B 1699
Rifabutin 1822
Rifampin 1824
Rifaximin 1826
Tinidazole 2029
Trimethoprim 2087
Vancomycin 2110

Antibiotic, Ophthalmic
Azithromycin (Ophthalmic) 253
Bacitracin and Polymyxin B 257
Bacitracin, Neomycin, and Polymyxin B 258
Bacitracin, Neomycin, Polymyxin B, and
    Hydrocortisone 258
Besifloxacin 281
Ciprofloxacin (Ophthalmic) 475
Erythromycin (Ophthalmic) 784
Gatifloxacin 958
Gentamicin (Ophthalmic) 966
Levofloxacin (Ophthalmic) 1233
Moxifloxacin (Ophthalmic) 1451
Neomycin, Polymyxin B, and Dexamethasone 1484
Neomycin, Polymyxin B, and Hydrocortisone 1485
Ofloxacin (Ophthalmic) 1523
Polymyxin B 1699
Prednisolone and Gentamicin 1731
Sulfacetamide (Ophthalmic) 1943
Tetracycline 1996
Tobramycin (Ophthalmic) 2039
Trimethoprim and Polymyxin B 2089

Antibiotic, Oral Rinse
Chlorhexidine Gluconate 441
Hydrogen Peroxide 1040

Antibiotic, Otic
Bacitracin, Neomycin, Polymyxin B, and
    Hydrocortisone 258
Ciprofloxacin (Otic) 476
Neomycin, Polymyxin B, and Hydrocortisone 1485
Ofloxacin (Otic) 1524

Antibiotic, Oxazolidinone
Linezolid 1251

Antibiotic, Penicillin
Amoxicillin 140
Amoxicillin and Clavulanate 144
Ampicillin 159
Ampicillin and Sulbactam 162
Penicillin V Potassium 1635
Penicillin G Benzathine 1629
Penicillin G (Parenteral/Aqueous) 1631
Penicillin G Procaine 1634

Antibiotic, Penicillin (Antipseudomonal)
Piperacillin and Tazobactam 1679
Ticarcillin and Clavulanate Potassium 2022

Antibiotic, Penicillin (Antistaphylococcal)
Dicloxacillin 652
Nafcillin 1462
Oxacillin 1555

Antibiotic, Quinolone
Ciprofloxacin (Otic) 476

Ciprofloxacin (Systemic) 471
Gatifloxacin 958
Levofloxacin (Ophthalmic) 1233
Levofloxacin (Systemic) 1228
Ofloxacin (Ophthalmic) 1523
Ofloxacin (Otic) 1524
Ofloxacin (Systemic) 1521

Antibiotic, Streptogramin
Quinupristin and Dalfopristin 1796

Antibiotic, Sulfonamide Derivative
Erythromycin and Sulfisoxazole 785
Sulfacetamide (Ophthalmic) 1943
Sulfacetamide (Topical) 1944
SulfADIAZINE 1945
Sulfamethoxazole and Trimethoprim 1948

Antibiotic, Sulfone
Dapsone (Systemic) 586

Antibiotic, Tetracycline Derivative
Demeclocycline 607
Doxycycline 721
Minocycline 1420
Tetracycline 1996

Antibiotic, Topical
Bacitracin 256
Bacitracin and Polymyxin B 257
Bacitracin, Neomycin, and Polymyxin B 258
Bacitracin, Neomycin, Polymyxin B, and
    Hydrocortisone 258
Erythromycin (Topical) 785
Gentamicin (Topical) 967
Mafenide 1290
MetroNIDAZOLE (Topical) 1404
Mupirocin 1452
Neomycin 1482
Neomycin and Polymyxin B 1483
Neomycin, Polymyxin B, and Hydrocortisone 1485
Silver Sulfadiazine 1890
Tetracycline 1996

Antibiotic, Urinary Irrigation
Neomycin and Polymyxin B 1483
Polymyxin B 1699

Anticholinergic Agent
Atropine 234
Benztropine 276
Dicyclomine 652
Glycopyrrolate 977
Hyoscyamine 1056
Hyoscyamine, Atropine, Scopolamine, and
    Phenobarbital 1058
Ipratropium (Nasal) 1146
Ipratropium (Oral Inhalation) 1144
Propantheline 1754
Scopolamine (Systemic) 1872
Tolterodine 2045
Trihexyphenidyl 2085

Anticholinergic Agent, Ophthalmic
Atropine 234
Cyclopentolate 560
Cyclopentolate and Phenylephrine 560
Homatropine 1018
Scopolamine (Ophthalmic) 1874

Anticholinergic Agent, Transdermal
Scopolamine (Systemic) 1872

Anticoagulant
Enoxaparin 752
Heparin 1001

Protein C Concentrate (Human) 1766
Warfarin 2156

Anticoagulant, Thrombin Inhibitor
Argatroban 192

Anticonvulsant
Magnesium Sulfate 1297

Anticonvulsant, Barbiturate
Amobarbital 138
PENTobarbital 1641
PHENobarbital 1651
Primidone 1737

Anticonvulsant, Benzodiazepine
CloBAZam 504
ClonazePAM 514
Clorazepate 524
Diazepam 640
LORazepam 1280
Midazolam 1411

Anticonvulsant, Hydantoin
Fosphenytoin 941
Phenytoin 1663

Anticonvulsant, Miscellaneous
AcetaZOLAMIDE 56
CarBAMazepine 372
Felbamate 848
Gabapentin 950
Lacosamide 1189
LamoTRIgine 1199
LevETIRAcetam 1219
OXcarbazepine 1564
TiaGABine 2020
Topiramate 2046
Valproic Acid and Derivatives 2102
Vigabatrin 2134
Zonisamide 2185

Anticonvulsant, Succinimide
Ethosuximide 809
Methsuximide 1375

Anticonvulsant, Triazole Derivative
Rufinamide 1858

Anticystine Agent
Cysteamine (Systemic) 571

Antidepressant, Dopamine-Reuptake Inhibitor
BuPROPion 327

Antidepressant, Miscellaneous
Lithium 1266

Antidepressant, Selective Serotonin Reuptake Inhibitor (SSRI)
Citalopram 484
Escitalopram 788
FLUoxetine 901
FluvoxaMINE 922
PARoxetine 1609
Sertraline 1879

Antidepressant, Serotonin/Norepinephrine Reuptake Inhibitor
Venlafaxine 2125

Antidepressant, Serotonin Reuptake Inhibitor/Antagonist
Nefazodone 1474
TraZODone 2065

Antidepressant, Tricyclic (Secondary Amine)
Desipramine 608
Nortriptyline 1512
Protriptyline 1767

Antidepressant, Tricyclic (Tertiary Amine)
Amitriptyline 133
ClomiPRAMINE 510
Doxepin (Systemic) 715
Imipramine 1080

Antidiabetic Agent, Alpha-glucosidase Inhibitor
Acarbose 46

Antidiabetic Agent, Biguanide
MetFORMIN 1353

Antidiabetic Agent, Dopamine Agonist
Bromocriptine 304

Antidiabetic Agent, Insulin
Insulin NPH 1130

Antidiabetic Agent, Oral
Acarbose 46
Bromocriptine 304
GlipiZIDE 968
GlyBURIDE 974
MetFORMIN 1353
Rosiglitazone 1850

Antidiabetic Agent, Parenteral
Insulin Aspart 1114
Insulin Aspart Protamine and Insulin Aspart 1117
Insulin Detemir 1119
Insulin Glargine 1121
Insulin Lispro 1125
Insulin Lispro Protamine and Insulin Lispro 1128
Insulin NPH and Insulin Regular 1132
Insulin Regular 1134

Antidiabetic Agent, Sulfonylurea
GlipiZIDE 968
GlyBURIDE 974

Antidiabetic Agent, Thiazolidinedione
Rosiglitazone 1850

Antidiarrheal
Attapulgite 238
Bismuth 294
Charcoal, Activated 432
Diphenoxylate and Atropine 678
Lactobacillus 1191
Loperamide 1270
Octreotide 1518
Opium Tincture 1548
Paregoric 1605

Antidiuretic Hormone Analog
Vasopressin 2121

Antidote
Aluminum Hydroxide 110
Carglumic Acid 381
Dexrazoxane 626
Glucarpidase 972
Insulin Regular 1134
Mesna 1350
Octreotide 1518
Sodium Nitrite and Sodium Thiosulfate 1909

Antidote, Acetaminophen
Acetylcysteine 60

Antidote, Adsorbent
Charcoal, Activated 432

Antidote, Aluminum Toxicity
Deferoxamine 604

Antidote, Anticholinergic Agent
Physostigmine 1670

Antidote, Anticholinesterase
Pralidoxime 1719

Antidote, Arsenic Toxicity
Dimercaprol 672

Antidote, Benzodiazepine
Flumazenil 888

Antidote, Cisplatin
Amifostine 116

Antidote, Copper Toxicity
PenicillAMINE 1627

Antidote, Cyanide
Amyl Nitrite 165
Hydroxocobalamin 1045
Methylene Blue 1377
Sodium Thiosulfate 1919

Antidote, Cyclophosphamide-induced Hemorrhagic Cystitis
Mesna 1350

Antidote, Cycloserine Toxicity
Pyridoxine 1778

Antidote, Digoxin
Digoxin Immune Fab 663

Antidote, Drug-induced Dystonic Reactions
Benztropine 276
DiphenhydrAMINE (Systemic) 673
Trihexyphenidyl 2085

Antidote, Drug-induced Methemoglobinemia
Methylene Blue 1377

Antidote, Ethylene Glycol Toxicity
Alcohol (Ethyl) 88
Fomepizole 927

Antidote, Extravasation
Hyaluronidase 1020
Phentolamine 1656
Sodium Thiosulfate 1919

Antidote for Narcotic Agonists
Naloxone 1466

Antidote, Gold Toxicity
Dimercaprol 672

Antidote, Heparin
Protamine 1764

Antidote, Hydrazine Toxicity
Pyridoxine 1778

Antidote, Hydrofluoric Acid
Calcium Gluconate 354

Antidote, Hypercalcemia
Calcitonin 340
Etidronate 810
Pamidronate 1587

Antidote, Hyperkalemia
Sodium Polystyrene Sulfonate 1917

Antidote, Hypersensitivity Reactions
DiphenhydrAMINE (Systemic) 673
EPINEPHrine (Systemic, Oral Inhalation) 761

Antidote, Ifosfamide-induced Hemorrhagic Cystitis
Mesna 1350

Antidote, Insulin
Dextrose 637

Antidote, Iron Toxicity
Deferoxamine 604

Antidote, Lead Toxicity
Dimercaprol 672
Edetate CALCIUM Disodium 729
PenicillAMINE 1627
Succimer 1937

Antidote, Malignant Hyperthermia
Dantrolene 583

Antidote, Mercury Toxicity
Dimercaprol 672

Antidote, Methanol Toxicity
Alcohol (Ethyl) 88
Fomepizole 927

Antidote, Methotrexate
Leucovorin Calcium 1213

Antidote, Mushroom Toxicity
Pyridoxine 1778

Antidote, Neuromuscular Blocking Agent
Edrophonium 730
Neostigmine 1486
Pyridostigmine 1776

Antidote, Oral Hypoglycemic
Dextrose 637

Antidote, Organophosphate Poisoning
Atropine 234
Pralidoxime 1719

Anti-ectoparasitic Agent
Ivermectin (Systemic) 1170

Antiemetic
Aprepitant 190
ChlorproMAZINE 450
Dexamethasone (Systemic) 615
DimenhyDRINATE 670
Dolasetron 703
Dronabinol 725
Droperidol 725
Fosaprepitant 934
Granisetron 980
HydrOXYzine 1054
LORazepam 1280
Meclizine 1317
Metoclopramide 1391
Nabilone 1459
Ondansetron 1544
Palonosetron 1586
Perphenazine 1648
Prochlorperazine 1745
Promethazine 1748
Trimethobenzamide 2086

Antifibrinolytic Agent
Tranexamic Acid 2063

Antiflatulent
Charcoal, Activated 432
Simethicone 1891

Antifungal Agent
Pentamidine 1637

Antifungal Agent, Echinocandin
Caspofungin 388
Micafungin 1407

Antifungal Agent, Oral Nonabsorbed
Clotrimazole (Oral) 526

Antifungal Agent, Systemic
Amphotericin B (Conventional) 147
Amphotericin B (Lipid Complex) 152
Amphotericin B (Liposomal) 155

Caspofungin 388
Fluconazole 877
Flucytosine 882
Griseofulvin 982
Itraconazole 1166
Ketoconazole (Systemic) 1177
Micafungin 1407
Posaconazole 1703
Voriconazole 2150

Antifungal Agent, Topical
Amphotericin B (Conventional) 147
Ciclopirox 465
Clotrimazole (Topical) 527
Econazole 728
Gentian Violet 968
Ketoconazole (Topical) 1179
Miconazole (Topical) 1410
Nystatin (Topical) 1517
Terbinafine (Topical) 1984
Tolnaftate 2044
Undecylenic Acid and Derivatives 2095

Antifungal Agent, Triazole
Posaconazole 1703
Voriconazole 2150

Antifungal Agent, Vaginal
Clotrimazole (Topical) 527
Miconazole (Topical) 1410
Nystatin (Topical) 1517

Antigout Agent
Allopurinol 97
Colchicine 537
Probenecid 1739

Antihemophilic Agent
Antihemophilic Factor (Human) 170
Antihemophilic Factor (Recombinant) 172
Antihemophilic Factor/von Willebrand Factor Complex
    (Human) 177
Anti-inhibitor Coagulant Complex (Human) 180
Desmopressin 612
Factor IX Complex (Human) [(Factors II, IX, X)] ... 833
Factor IX (Human) 835
Factor IX (Recombinant) 838
Factor VIIa (Recombinant) 831
Tranexamic Acid 2063

Antihemorrhagics
Octreotide 1518

Antihistamine
Carbinoxamine 377
Cetirizine 431
Chlorpheniramine 448
Clemastine 494
Cyproheptadine 569
Desloratadine 611
DimenhyDRINATE 670
DiphenhydrAMINE (Systemic) 673
DiphenhydrAMINE (Topical) 677
Fexofenadine 870
Hydrocodone and Chlorpheniramine 1030
HydrOXYzine 1054
Levocetirizine 1227
Loratadine 1278
Meclizine 1317

Antihistamine/Decongestant Combination
Brompheniramine and Pseudoephedrine 306
Loratadine and Pseudoephedrine 1279
Promethazine and Phenylephrine 1752
Promethazine, Phenylephrine, and Codeine 1752
Triprolidine and Pseudoephedrine 2090

Antihistamine, Nasal
Azelastine (Nasal) 245

Antihypertensive Agent
AMILoride 121
AmLODIPine 135
Atenolol 222
Benazepril 270
Bumetanide 316
Candesartan 363
Captopril 368
Carvedilol 385
Chlorothiazide 446
CloNIDine 516
Diltiazem 667
Doxazosin 712
Esmolol 791
Ethacrynic Acid 806
Felodipine 850
Fosinopril 938
Furosemide 948
HydrALAZINE 1022
Hydrochlorothiazide 1023
Irbesartan 1147
Isradipine 1164
Labetalol 1186
Lisinopril 1262
Losartan 1283
Methyldopa 1376
Metolazone 1394
Metoprolol 1396
Nadolol 1460
NiCARdipine 1493
NIFEdipine 1497
Nitroglycerin 1504
Nitroprusside 1507
Olmesartan 1530
Phenoxybenzamine 1655
Phentolamine 1656
Prazosin 1724
Propranolol 1759
Quinapril 1788
Spironolactone 1930
Terazosin 1981
Timolol (Systemic) 2026
Torsemide 2057
Triamterene 2079
Valsartan 2108
Verapamil 2129

Antihypertensive Agent, Combination
Hydrochlorothiazide and Spironolactone 1025

Antihypoglycemic Agent
Diazoxide 643
Glucagon 970

Anti-infective Agent, Topical
Alcohol (Ethyl) 88

Anti-inflammatory Agent
Alclometasone 87
Aspirin 212
Balsalazide 261
Beclomethasone (Oral Inhalation) 265
Budesonide and Formoterol 314
Budesonide (Nasal) 313
Budesonide (Systemic, Oral Inhalation) 308
Choline Magnesium Trisalicylate 459
Ciclesonide (Oral Inhalation) 461
Clobetasol 506
Colchicine 537
Cortisone 548
Dexamethasone (Systemic) 615
Diclofenac (Ophthalmic) 648

Diclofenac (Systemic) 645
Diclofenac (Topical) 649
Etodolac 812
Fluocinolone (Otic) 892
Fluocinolone (Topical) 892
Fluocinonide 894
Flurbiprofen (Systemic) 908
Fluticasone and Salmeterol 916
Fluticasone (Oral Inhalation) 910
Halobetasol 997
Hydrocortisone (Systemic) 1034
Hydrocortisone (Topical) 1038
Ibuprofen 1059
Indomethacin 1096
Ketorolac (Ophthalmic) 1184
Ketorolac (Systemic) 1180
Meloxicam 1325
Mesalamine 1347
MethylPREDNISolone 1386
Mometasone and Formoterol 1436
Mometasone (Nasal) 1433
Mometasone (Oral Inhalation) 1432
Mometasone (Topical) 1435
Naproxen 1470
Olsalazine 1532
Oxaprozin 1562
Piroxicam 1683
Prednicarbate 1725
PrednisoLONE (Systemic) 1727
PredniSONE 1732
SulfaSALAzine 1954
Sulindac 1957
Triamcinolone (Nasal) 2076
Triamcinolone (Systemic) 2072

Anti-inflammatory Agent, Ophthalmic
Dexamethasone (Ophthalmic) 619
Fluorometholone 897
Flurbiprofen (Ophthalmic) 910
PrednisoLONE (Ophthalmic) 1730
Triamcinolone (Ophthalmic) 2077

Anti-inflammatory Agent, Rectal
Hydrocortisone (Topical) 1038
Mesalamine 1347

Anti-inflammatory Agent, Topical
Triamcinolone (Topical) 2078

Antilipemic Agent
AtorvaSTATin 227
Ezetimibe 827
Ezetimibe and Simvastatin 829
Fluvastatin 920
Lovastatin 1286
Niacin 1491
Pravastatin 1720
Simvastatin 1892

Antilipemic Agent, Bile Acid Sequestrant
Cholestyramine Resin 457
Colesevelam 539
Colestipol 540

Antilipemic Agent, HMG-CoA Reductase Inhibitor
Rosuvastatin 1853

Antimalarial Agent
Artemether and Lumefantrine 203
Atovaquone and Proguanil 231
Chloroquine 444
Hydroxychloroquine 1048
Mefloquine 1321
Primaquine 1735
Pyrimethamine 1780
QuiNIDine 1791

QuiNINE 1794
Sulfadoxine and Pyrimethamine 1947

Antimanic Agent
Lithium 1266

Antimigraine Agent
Almotriptan 99
Amitriptyline 133
Dihydroergotamine 665
Ergotamine 776
Ergotamine and Caffeine 777
Metoprolol 1396
Nadolol 1460
Papaverine 1599
Propranolol 1759
Rizatriptan 1845
SUMAtriptan 1958
Timolol (Systemic) 2026

Antineoplastic Agent, Alkylating Agent
Busulfan 333
CARBOplatin 379
Carmustine 382
Chlorambucil 437
CISplatin 481
Cyclophosphamide 561
Ifosfamide 1068
Lomustine 1268
Mechlorethamine (Systemic) 1315
Melphalan 1328
Oxaliplatin 1557
Temozolomide 1972
Thiotepa 2014

Antineoplastic Agent, Alkylating Agent (Nitrogen Mustard)
Chlorambucil 437
Cyclophosphamide 561
Mechlorethamine (Systemic) 1315
Melphalan 1328

Antineoplastic Agent, Alkylating Agent (Nitrosourea)
Carmustine 382
Lomustine 1268

Antineoplastic Agent, Anthracenedione
MitoXANtrone 1427

Antineoplastic Agent, Anthracycline
DAUNOrubicin (Conventional) 599
DOXOrubicin (Conventional) 718
IDArubicin 1067

Antineoplastic Agent, Antibiotic
Bleomycin 295
DACTINomycin 580
DAUNOrubicin (Conventional) 599
DOXOrubicin (Conventional) 718
MitoXANtrone 1427

Antineoplastic Agent, Anti-CD20
RiTUXimab 1841

Antineoplastic Agent, Antimetabolite
Clofarabine 508
Cytarabine (Conventional) 573
Fludarabine 885
Fluorouracil (Systemic) 897
Fluorouracil (Topical) 900
Mercaptopurine 1342
Methotrexate 1367
Nelarabine 1477
Pentostatin 1644
Thioguanine 2010

Antineoplastic Agent, Antimetabolite (Purine Analog)
Cladribine 488
Fludarabine 885

Pentostatin 1644
Thioguanine 2010

Antineoplastic Agent, Antimetabolite (Purine Antagonist)
Clofarabine 508
Fludarabine 885
Pentostatin 1644

Antineoplastic Agent, Antimetabolite (Pyrimidine Antagonist)
Gemcitabine 959

Antineoplastic Agent, Antimicrotubular
DOCEtaxel 697
PACLitaxel 1579
VinBLAStine 2136
VinCRIStine 2138
Vinorelbine 2143

Antineoplastic Agent, Aromatase Inhibitor
Letrozole 1211

Antineoplastic Agent, BCR-ABL Tyrosine Kinase Inhibitor
Imatinib 1072

Antineoplastic Agent, Biologic Response Modulator
Aldesleukin 90
Interferon Alfa-2b 1138
Peginterferon Alfa-2b 1621

Antineoplastic Agent, Camptothecin
Irinotecan 1149
Topotecan 2053

Antineoplastic Agent, Enzyme
Asparaginase (E. coli) 208
Asparaginase (Erwinia) 211
Pegaspargase 1615

Antineoplastic Agent, Estrogen Receptor Antagonist
Fulvestrant 946
Tamoxifen 1968

Antineoplastic Agent, Hormone (Gonadotropin Hormone-Releasing Analog)
Leuprolide 1215

Antineoplastic Agent, Miscellaneous
Aldesleukin 90
Arsenic Trioxide 201
Asparaginase (E. coli) 208
Asparaginase (Erwinia) 211
Dacarbazine 578
Hydroxyurea 1051
Megestrol 1324
Mitotane 1425
Pegaspargase 1615
Procarbazine 1743
Tretinoin (Systemic) 2068

Antineoplastic Agent, Mitotic Inhibitor
Etoposide 815
VinBLAStine 2136
VinCRIStine 2138

Antineoplastic Agent, Monoclonal Antibody
Bevacizumab 288
RiTUXimab 1841

Antineoplastic Agent, mTOR Kinase Inhibitor
Everolimus 821

Antineoplastic Agent, Platinum Analog
CARBOplatin 379
CISplatin 481

Antineoplastic Agent, Podophyllotoxin Derivative
Teniposide 1976

Antineoplastic Agent, Purine
Mercaptopurine 1342

Antineoplastic Agent, Retinoic Acid Derivatives
ISOtretinoin 1161
Tretinoin (Systemic) 2068

Antineoplastic Agent, Taxane Derivative
DOCEtaxel 697
PACLitaxel 1579

Antineoplastic Agent, Topoisomerase I Inhibitor
Irinotecan 1149

Antineoplastic Agent, Topoisomerase II Inhibitor
DAUNOrubicin (Conventional) 599
DOXOrubicin (Conventional) 718
IDArubicin 1067
MitoXANtrone 1427
Teniposide 1976

Antineoplastic Agent, Topoisomerase Inhibitor
Etoposide 815
Topotecan 2053

Antineoplastic Agent, Tyrosine Kinase Inhibitor
Imatinib 1072

Antineoplastic Agent, Vascular Endothelial Growth Factor (VEGF) Inhibitor
Bevacizumab 288

Antineoplastic Agent, Vinca Alkaloid
VinBLAStine 2136
VinCRIStine 2138
Vinorelbine 2143

Antiparasitic Agent, Topical
Benzyl Alcohol 278
Ivermectin (Topical) 1172
Lindane 1250
Malathion 1300
Permethrin 1647
Spinosad 1930

Anti-Parkinson's Agent
Benztropine 276
Trihexyphenidyl 2085

Anti-Parkinson's Agent (Dopamine Agonist)
Amantadine 112

Antiplatelet Agent
Anagrelide 166
Aspirin 212
Clopidogrel 521
Dipyridamole 693

Antiprotozoal
Atovaquone 229
MetroNIDAZOLE (Systemic) 1399
Nitazoxanide 1500
Pentamidine 1637

Antiprotozoal, Nitroimidazole
Tinidazole 2029

Antipruritic, Topical
Lidocaine and Prilocaine 1246

Antipsoriatic Agent, Topical
Coal Tar 532

Antipsychotic Agent
CloZAPine 527

Antipsychotic Agent, Atypical
ARIPiprazole 196
CloZAPine 527
OLANZapine 1525
Paliperidone 1581
QUEtiapine 1783
RisperiDONE 1831
Ziprasidone 2178

Antipsychotic Agent, Benzisoxazole
Paliperidone 1581
RisperiDONE 1831

Antipsychotic Agent, Typical
Pimozide 1677

Antipsychotic Agent, Typical, Butyrophenone
Haloperidol 998

Antipsychotic Agent, Typical, Phenothiazine
ChlorproMAZINE 450
Perphenazine 1648
Prochlorperazine 1745
Thioridazine 2012
Thiothixene 2015
Trifluoperazine 2082

Antipyretic
Acetaminophen 47
Aspirin 212
Choline Magnesium Trisalicylate 459
Ibuprofen 1059
Indomethacin 1096
Ketorolac (Systemic) 1180
Naproxen 1470

Antiretroviral Agent
Abacavir 36
Abacavir and Lamivudine 39
Abacavir, Lamivudine, and Zidovudine 41
Atazanavir 218
Darunavir 595
Didanosine 654
Efavirenz 731
Efavirenz, Emtricitabine, and Tenofovir 735
Emtricitabine 738
Emtricitabine and Tenofovir 741
Enfuvirtide 750
Etravirine 819
Fosamprenavir 931
Indinavir 1093
LamiVUDine 1194
Lamivudine and Zidovudine 1198
Lopinavir and Ritonavir 1272
Maraviroc 1304
Nelfinavir 1479
Nevirapine 1487
Ritonavir 1837
Saquinavir 1867
Stavudine 1932
Tenofovir 1977
Zidovudine 2168

Antiretroviral Agent, Reverse Transcriptase Inhibitor (Nucleotide)
Adefovir 75

Antiretroviral, CCR5 Antagonist (Anti-HIV)
Maraviroc 1304

Antiretroviral, Integrase Inhibitor (Anti-HIV)
Dolutegravir 705
Raltegravir 1802

Antirheumatic, Disease Modifying
Abatacept 44
Adalimumab 70
Anakinra 168
Etanercept 803
Hydroxychloroquine 1048
InFLIXimab 1099
Methotrexate 1367
Tocilizumab 2040

Antirheumatic Miscellaneous
Cyclophosphamide 561
RiTUXimab 1841

Antiseborrheic Agent, Topical
Coal Tar 532
Selenium Sulfide 1877
Sulfur and Salicylic Acid 1956

Antisecretory Agent
Octreotide 1518

Antispasmodic Agent, Gastrointestinal
Atropine 234
Dicyclomine 652
Glycopyrrolate 977
Hyoscyamine 1056
Hyoscyamine, Atropine, Scopolamine, and Phenobarbital 1058
Propantheline 1754

Antispasmodic Agent, Urinary
Belladonna and Opium 269
Oxybutynin 1568
Propantheline 1754

Antithyroid Agent
Methimazole 1362
Potassium Iodide 1711
Potassium Iodide and Iodine 1713
Propylthiouracil 1762

Antitubercular Agent
Capreomycin 365
CycloSERINE 563
Ethambutol 807
Ethionamide 808
Isoniazid 1158
Pyrazinamide 1775
Rifabutin 1822
Rifampin 1824
Streptomycin 1935

Antitussive
Codeine 534
Dextromethorphan 636
Guaifenesin and Codeine 985
Guaifenesin and Dextromethorphan 987
Hydrocodone and Acetaminophen 1027
Hydrocodone and Chlorpheniramine 1030
Hydrocodone and Homatropine 1032
HYDROmorphone 1041
Promethazine and Codeine 1750
Promethazine, Phenylephrine, and Codeine 1752

Antivenin
Antivenin (Latrodectus mactans) 185
Centruroides Immune F(ab')₂ (Equine) 428
Crotalidae Polyvalent Immune Fab (Ovine) 553

Antiviral Agent
Amantadine 112
Dolutegravir 705
Entecavir 757
Raltegravir 1802
Tipranavir 2031
ValGANciclovir 2099
Zanamivir 2166

Antiviral Agent, Adamantane
Amantadine 112

Antiviral Agent, Inhalation Therapy
Ribavirin 1818

Antiviral Agent, Ophthalmic
Trifluridine 2084

Antiviral Agent, Oral
Acyclovir (Systemic) 63
Famciclovir 842
Oseltamivir 1551
Rimantadine 1830
ValACYclovir 2097

Antiviral Agent, Parenteral
Acyclovir (Systemic) 63
Cidofovir 466
Foscarnet 936
Ganciclovir (Systemic) 955

Antiviral Agent, Topical
Acyclovir and Hydrocortisone 69
Acyclovir (Topical) 68
Penciclovir 1627

Barbiturate
Amobarbital 138
Methohexital 1365
PENTobarbital 1641
PHENobarbital 1651
Primidone 1737
Secobarbital 1875

Benzodiazepine
ALPRAZolam 100
ClonazePAM 514
Clorazepate 524
Diazepam 640
Flurazepam 907
LORazepam 1280
Midazolam 1411
Triazolam 2080

Beta₁ & Beta₂-Adrenergic Agonist Agent
Isoproterenol 1160

Beta₂-Adrenergic Agonist
Albuterol 84
Budesonide and Formoterol 314
Fluticasone and Salmeterol 916
Formoterol 929
Levalbuterol 1218
Metaproterenol 1352
Mometasone and Formoterol 1436
Pirbuterol 1683
Salmeterol 1862
Terbutaline 1984

Beta-Adrenergic Blocker
Atenolol 222
Esmolol 791
Metoprolol 1396
Nadolol 1460
Propranolol 1759
Sotalol 1925
Timolol (Ophthalmic) 2028
Timolol (Systemic) 2026

Beta-Adrenergic Blocker, Nonselective With Alpha-Blocking Activity
Carvedilol 385

Beta-Adrenergic Blocker, Ophthalmic
Levobunolol 1223
Timolol (Ophthalmic) 2028

Bile Acid
Chenodiol 434

Biological Response Modulator
Aldesleukin 90
Interferon Alfa-2b 1138
Oprelvekin 1549
Peginterferon Alfa-2b 1621

Biotinidase Deficiency, Treatment Agent
Biotin 292

Bisphosphonate Derivative
Etidronate 810
Pamidronate 1587

Blood Product Derivative
Albumin 82
Antihemophilic Factor (Human) 170
Antihemophilic Factor/von Willebrand Factor Complex (Human) 177
Anti-inhibitor Coagulant Complex (Human) 180
C1 Inhibitor (Human) 337
Factor IX Complex (Human) [(Factors II, IX, X)] 833
Factor IX (Human) 835
Immune Globulin 1084
Protein C Concentrate (Human) 1766

Blood Viscosity Reducer Agent
Pentoxifylline 1646

Bronchodilator
Albuterol 84
Aminophylline 124
Atropine 234
Budesonide and Formoterol 314
EPINEPHrine (Systemic, Oral Inhalation) 761
Fluticasone and Salmeterol 916
Formoterol 929
Ipratropium (Oral Inhalation) 1144
Isoproterenol 1160
Levalbuterol 1218
Metaproterenol 1352
Mometasone and Formoterol 1436
Pirbuterol 1683
Salmeterol 1862
Terbutaline 1984
Theophylline 2005

Calcium Channel Blocker
AmLODIPine 135
Diltiazem 667
Felodipine 850
Isradipine 1164
NiCARdipine 1493
NIFEdipine 1497
Verapamil 2129

Calcium Channel Blocker, Dihydropyridine
AmLODIPine 135
Felodipine 850
Isradipine 1164
NiCARdipine 1493
NIFEdipine 1497

Calcium Channel Blocker, Nondihydropyridine
Diltiazem 667
Verapamil 2129

Calcium Salt
Calcium Acetate 344
Calcium Carbonate 346
Calcium Chloride 349
Calcium Citrate 351
Calcium Glubionate 353
Calcium Gluconate 354
Calcium Lactate 358
Calcium Phosphate (Tribasic) 359

Caloric Agent
Fat Emulsion (Plant Based) 846
Medium Chain Triglycerides 1318

Carbonic Anhydrase Inhibitor
AcetaZOLAMIDE 56

Carbonic Anhydrase Inhibitor, Ophthalmic
Dorzolamide 710

Cardiac Glycoside
Digoxin 658

Cardioprotective Agent
Dexrazoxane 626

CCR5 Antagonist
Maraviroc 1304

Central Nervous System Stimulant
Caffeine 338
Dexmethylphenidate 623
Dextroamphetamine 629
Dextroamphetamine and Amphetamine 632
Doxapram 711
Lisdexamfetamine 1260
Methamphetamine 1359
Methylphenidate 1379
Modafinil 1429

Chelating Agent
Dexrazoxane 626

Chelating Agent, Oral
Deferasirox 601
PenicillAMINE 1627
Succimer 1937

Chelating Agent, Parenteral
Deferoxamine 604
Dimercaprol 672
Edetate CALCIUM Disodium 729

Chemoprotectant Agent
Dexrazoxane 626
Mesna 1350

Cholesterol Absorption Inhibitor
Ezetimibe 827
Ezetimibe and Simvastatin 829

Cholinergic Agent
Bethanechol 288
Edrophonium 730
Neostigmine 1486
Physostigmine 1670
Pilocarpine (Ophthalmic) 1675
Pilocarpine (Systemic) 1674
Pyridostigmine 1776

Cholinergic Agent, Ophthalmic
Acetylcholine 59
Physostigmine 1670
Pilocarpine (Ophthalmic) 1675

Colony-Stimulating Factor
Darbepoetin Alfa 592
Epoetin Alfa 766
Filgrastim 872
Sargramostim 1870

Contraceptive, Oral
Norethindrone 1511

Contraceptive, Progestin Only
MedroxyPROGESTERone 1318
Norethindrone 1511

Controlled Substance II
Alfentanil 93
Amobarbital 138
Belladonna and Opium 269
Cocaine 533
Codeine 534
Dexmethylphenidate 623
Dextroamphetamine 629
Dextroamphetamine and Amphetamine 632

FentaNYL 853
HYDROmorphone 1041
Lisdexamfetamine 1260
Meperidine 1337
Methadone 1355
Methamphetamine 1359
Methylphenidate 1379
Morphine (Liposomal) 1449
Morphine (Systemic) 1440
Nabilone 1459
Opium Tincture 1548
OxyCODONE 1569
Oxycodone and Acetaminophen 1573
Oxycodone and Aspirin 1575
PENTobarbital 1641
Remifentanil 1811
Secobarbital 1875
SUFentanil 1942

Controlled Substance III
Acetaminophen and Codeine 53
Buprenorphine 320
Buprenorphine and Naloxone 324
Dronabinol 725
Fluoxymesterone 906
Guaifenesin and Codeine 985
Hydrocodone and Acetaminophen 1027
Ketamine 1175
Paregoric 1605
Testosterone 1986

Controlled Substance IV
ALPRAZolam 100
Chloral Hydrate 436
CloBAZam 504
ClonazePAM 514
Clorazepate 524
Diazepam 640
Flurazepam 907
LORazepam 1280
Methohexital 1365
Midazolam 1411
Modafinil 1429
Pentazocine 1639
PHENobarbital 1651
Triazolam 2080
Zolpidem 2182

Controlled Substance V
Acetaminophen and Codeine 53
Diphenoxylate and Atropine 678
Guaifenesin and Codeine 985
Lacosamide 1189
Promethazine and Codeine 1750
Promethazine, Phenylephrine, and Codeine 1752

Corticosteroid, Inhalant (Oral)
Beclomethasone (Oral Inhalation) 265
Budesonide and Formoterol 314
Budesonide (Systemic, Oral Inhalation) 308
Ciclesonide (Oral Inhalation) 461
Fluticasone and Salmeterol 916
Fluticasone (Oral Inhalation) 910
Mometasone and Formoterol 1436
Mometasone (Oral Inhalation) 1432

Corticosteroid, Intranasal
Beclomethasone (Nasal) 267
Budesonide (Nasal) 313
Ciclesonide (Nasal) 464
Flunisolide (Nasal) 890
Fluticasone (Nasal) 913
Mometasone (Nasal) 1433
Triamcinolone (Nasal) 2076

Corticosteroid, Ophthalmic
Bacitracin, Neomycin, Polymyxin B, and
  Hydrocortisone 258
Dexamethasone (Ophthalmic) 619
Fluocinolone (Ophthalmic) 891
Fluorometholone 897
Neomycin, Polymyxin B, and Dexamethasone 1484
Neomycin, Polymyxin B, and Hydrocortisone 1485
Prednisolone and Gentamicin 1731
PrednisoLONE (Ophthalmic) 1730
Triamcinolone (Ophthalmic) 2077

Corticosteroid, Otic
Bacitracin, Neomycin, Polymyxin B, and
  Hydrocortisone 258
Neomycin, Polymyxin B, and Hydrocortisone 1485

Corticosteroid, Rectal
Hydrocortisone (Topical) 1038

Corticosteroid, Systemic
Betamethasone (Systemic) 282
Cortisone 548
Dexamethasone (Systemic) 615
Fludrocortisone 887
Hydrocortisone (Systemic) 1034
MethylPREDNISolone 1386
PrednisoLONE (Systemic) 1727
PredniSONE 1732
Triamcinolone (Systemic) 2072

Corticosteroid, Topical
Acyclovir and Hydrocortisone 69
Alclometasone 87
Bacitracin, Neomycin, Polymyxin B, and
  Hydrocortisone 258
Betamethasone (Topical) 285
Clobetasol 506
Fluocinolone (Topical) 892
Fluocinonide 894
Fluticasone (Topical) 915
Halobetasol 997
Hydrocortisone (Topical) 1038
Mometasone (Topical) 1435
Neomycin, Polymyxin B, and Hydrocortisone 1485
Prednicarbate 1725
Triamcinolone (Topical) 2078

Cough Preparation
Codeine 534
Dextromethorphan 636
Guaifenesin and Codeine 985
Guaifenesin and Dextromethorphan 987
Hydrocodone and Acetaminophen 1027
Hydrocodone and Chlorpheniramine 1030
Hydrocodone and Homatropine 1032
Promethazine and Codeine 1750
Promethazine, Phenylephrine, and Codeine 1752

**Cystic Fibrosis Transmembrane Conductance Regulator
Potentiator**
Ivacaftor 1169

Cytoprotective Agent
Amifostine 116

Decongestant
Pseudoephedrine 1770

Decongestant/Analgesic
Pseudoephedrine and Ibuprofen 1772

Decongestant, Nasal
EPINEPHrine (Nasal) 765
Naphazoline (Nasal) 1469
Oxymetazoline (Nasal) 1577

Diagnostic Agent
Benzylpenicilloyl Polylysine 279

Diagnostic Agent, Adrenocortical Insufficiency
Cosyntropin 549

**Diagnostic Agent, Gastrinoma (Zollinger-Ellison
Syndrome)**
Secretin 1876

Diagnostic Agent, Growth Hormone Function
Arginine 195

Diagnostic Agent, Hypothalamic-Pituitary ACTH Function
Metyrapone 1405

Diagnostic Agent, Myasthenia Gravis
Edrophonium 730
Neostigmine 1486

Diagnostic Agent, Pancreatic Exocrine Insufficiency
Secretin 1876

Diagnostic Agent, Pheochromocytoma
Phentolamine 1656

Diuretic
Caffeine 338

Diuretic, Carbonic Anhydrase Inhibitor
AcetaZOLAMIDE 56

Diuretic, Combination
Hydrochlorothiazide and Spironolactone 1025

Diuretic, Loop
Bumetanide 316
Ethacrynic Acid 806
Furosemide 948
Torsemide 2057

Diuretic, Miscellaneous
Metolazone 1394

Diuretic, Osmotic
Mannitol 1301

Diuretic, Potassium Sparing
AMILoride 121
Spironolactone 1930
Triamterene 2079

Diuretic, Thiazide
Chlorothiazide 446
Chlorthalidone 453
Hydrochlorothiazide 1023

Dopamine Agonist
Fenoldopam 852

Drug-induced Neuritis, Treatment Agent
Pyridoxine 1778

Dye Free
Acetaminophen 47
Aluminum Hydroxide and Magnesium Hydroxide 111
Benzocaine 273
Brompheniramine and Pseudoephedrine 306
Calcium Carbonate 346
Calcium Citrate 351
Calcium Gluconate 354
Calcium Lactate 358
Cetirizine 431
Cholecalciferol 455
Copper 544
Cysteine 572
Dextromethorphan 636
DiphenhydrAMINE (Systemic) 673
Erythromycin (Systemic) 780
Ferrous Sulfate 868
Fexofenadine 870

Fluoride 894
Folic Acid 925
GuaiFENesin 984
Guaifenesin and Dextromethorphan 987
Ibuprofen 1059
Loratadine 1278
LORazepam 1280
Methadone 1355
Metoclopramide 1391
Nystatin (Oral) 1516
Phenylephrine (Systemic) 1658
Polysaccharide-Iron Complex 1701
Potassium Gluconate 1711
PrednisoLONE (Systemic) 1727
Psyllium 1773
Salicylic Acid 1860
Sodium Citrate and Citric Acid 1906
Stavudine 1932
Trimethoprim 2087
Vitamin A 2146
Vitamin E 2148
Warfarin 2156

Electrolyte Supplement, Oral
Calcium Carbonate 346
Calcium Citrate 351
Calcium Glubionate 353
Calcium Gluconate 354
Calcium Lactate 358
Calcium Phosphate (Tribasic) 359
Magnesium L-aspartate Hydrochloride 1295
Magnesium Chloride 1291
Magnesium Gluconate 1293
Magnesium Oxide 1296
Magnesium Sulfate 1297
Potassium Bicarbonate 1707
Potassium Bicarbonate and Potassium
  Chloride 1707
Potassium Chloride 1708
Potassium Gluconate 1711
Potassium Phosphate and Sodium Phosphate 1718
Sodium Bicarbonate 1901
Sodium Chloride 1902
Sodium Phosphates 1913

Electrolyte Supplement, Parenteral
Calcium Acetate 344
Calcium Chloride 349
Calcium Gluconate 354
Magnesium Chloride 1291
Magnesium Sulfate 1297
Potassium Acetate 1705
Potassium Chloride 1708
Potassium Phosphate 1715
Sodium Acetate 1899
Sodium Bicarbonate 1901
Sodium Chloride 1902
Sodium Glycerophosphate Pentahydrate 1907
Sodium Phosphates 1913

Endothelin Receptor Antagonist
Bosentan 298

Enzyme
Alglucosidase Alfa 95
Galsulfase 953
Glucarpidase 972
Laronidase 1210
Protein C Concentrate (Human) 1766
Rasburicase 1808

Enzyme, α-galactosidase A
Agalsidase Beta 79

Enzyme, Glucocerebrosidase
Imiglucerase 1076
Velaglucerase Alfa 2124

Enzyme, Inhalant
Dornase Alfa 709

Enzyme, Pancreatic
Pancrelipase 1591

Ergot Alkaloid
Ergotamine 776
Ergotamine and Caffeine 777

Ergot Alkaloid and Derivative
Dihydroergotamine 665

Ergot Derivative
Bromocriptine 304

Erythropoiesis Stimulating Protein
Darbepoetin Alfa 592

Estrogen Derivative
Estradiol (Systemic) 796
Estrogens (Conjugated/Equine, Systemic) 799
Estrogens (Conjugated/Equine, Topical) 801

Estrogen Derivative, Vaginal
Estrogens (Conjugated/Equine, Topical) 801

Expectorant
GuaiFENesin 984
Guaifenesin and Codeine 985
Guaifenesin and Dextromethorphan 987
Potassium Iodide 1711

Fabry's Disease, Treatment Agent
Agalsidase Beta 79

Fat Occlusion (Central Venous Catheter), Treatment Agent
Alcohol (Ethyl) 88

Fluid Replacement, Enteral
Dextrose 637

Fluid Replacement, Parenteral
Dextrose 637

Folic Acid Derivative
Leucovorin Calcium 1213

Fusion Inhibitor
Enfuvirtide 750

Gallstone Dissolution Agent
Ursodiol 2095

Gastric Acid Secretion Inhibitor
Esomeprazole 793
Lansoprazole 1206
Omeprazole 1535
Pantoprazole 1595
RABEprazole 1797

Gastrointestinal Agent, Gastric or Duodenal Ulcer Treatment
Aluminum Hydroxide 110
Aluminum Hydroxide and Magnesium Hydroxide 111
Bismuth 294
Cimetidine 469
Esomeprazole 793
Famotidine 843
Lansoprazole 1206
Nizatidine 1508
Omeprazole 1535
Pantoprazole 1595
RABEprazole 1797
Ranitidine 1805
Sucralfate 1940

Gastrointestinal Agent, Gastric Ulcer Treatment
Misoprostol 1423

Gastrointestinal Agent, Miscellaneous
Adalimumab 70
InFLIXimab 1099

Gastrointestinal Agent, Prokinetic
Cisapride 478
Metoclopramide 1391

Gaucher's Disease, Treatment Agent
Imiglucerase 1076
Velaglucerase Alfa 2124

General Anesthetic
Alfentanil 93
Amobarbital 138
Etomidate 814
FentaNYL 853
Ketamine 1175
Methohexital 1365
PENTobarbital 1641
Propofol 1755
Remifentanil 1811
SUFentanil 1942

Genitourinary Irrigant
Neomycin and Polymyxin B 1483

Glaucoma, Treatment Agent
Brimonidine (Ophthalmic) 303

Glucocorticoid
Alclometasone 87
Beclomethasone (Oral Inhalation) 265
Budesonide and Formoterol 314
Budesonide (Nasal) 313
Budesonide (Systemic, Oral Inhalation) 308
Ciclesonide (Oral Inhalation) 461
Clobetasol 506
Cortisone 548
Dexamethasone (Systemic) 615
Fludrocortisone 887
Fluocinolone (Topical) 892
Fluocinonide 894
Fluorometholone 897
Fluticasone and Salmeterol 916
Fluticasone (Oral Inhalation) 910
Halobetasol 997
Hydrocortisone (Systemic) 1034
Hydrocortisone (Topical) 1038
MethylPREDNISolone 1386
Mometasone and Formoterol 1436
Mometasone (Nasal) 1433
Mometasone (Oral Inhalation) 1432
Mometasone (Topical) 1435
Prednicarbate 1725
PrednisoLONE (Systemic) 1727
PredniSONE 1732
Triamcinolone (Nasal) 2076
Triamcinolone (Systemic) 2072
Triamcinolone (Topical) 2078

Gold Compound
Auranofin 239
Gold Sodium Thiomalate 979

Gonadotropin
Chorionic Gonadotropin (Human) 460

Gonadotropin Releasing Hormone Agonist
Histrelin 1016

Growth Factor
Epoetin Alfa 766

Growth Hormone
Mecasermin 1313
Somatropin 1920

Hematopoietic Agent
Darbepoetin Alfa 592
Epoetin Alfa 766
Filgrastim 872
Pegfilgrastim 1616
Sargramostim 1870

Hemorrhoidal Treatment Agent
Phenylephrine (Topical) 1662

Hemostatic Agent
Aminocaproic Acid 122
Desmopressin 612
Thrombin (Topical) 2017
Tranexamic Acid 2063

Histamine H$_1$ Antagonist, Ophthalmic
Ketotifen (Ophthalmic) 1185

Histamine H$_2$ Antagonist
Cimetidine 469
Famotidine 843
Nizatidine 1508
Ranitidine 1805

HIV Agents (Anti-HIV Agents)
Abacavir 36
Abacavir and Lamivudine 39
Abacavir, Lamivudine, and Zidovudine 41
Atazanavir 218
Darunavir 595
Didanosine 654
Dolutegravir 705
Efavirenz 731
Efavirenz, Emtricitabine, and Tenofovir 735
Emtricitabine 738
Emtricitabine and Tenofovir 741
Enfuvirtide 750
Etravirine 819
Fosamprenavir 931
Indinavir 1093
LamiVUDine 1194
Lamivudine and Zidovudine 1198
Lopinavir and Ritonavir 1272
Maraviroc 1304
Nelfinavir 1479
Nevirapine 1487
Raltegravir 1802
Ritonavir 1837
Saquinavir 1867
Stavudine 1932
Tenofovir 1977
Tipranavir 2031
Zidovudine 2168

HMG-CoA Reductase Inhibitor
AtorvaSTATin 227
Ezetimibe and Simvastatin 829
Fluvastatin 920
Lovastatin 1286
Pravastatin 1720
Simvastatin 1892

Homocystinuria, Treatment Agent
Betaine 281

Hormone, Posterior Pituitary
Desmopressin 612
Vasopressin 2121

5-HT$_3$ Receptor Antagonist
Granisetron 980

Ondansetron 1544
Palonosetron 1586

Hyperammonemia Agent
Lactulose 1193
Neomycin 1482
Sodium Benzoate 1900
Sodium Phenylacetate and Sodium Benzoate 1911
Sodium Phenylbutyrate 1912

Hyperglycemic Agent
Dextrose 637

Hyperkalemia, Adjunctive Treatment Agent
Dextrose 637
Insulin Regular 1134

Hyperthermia, Treatment
Dantrolene 583

Hypnotic
Amobarbital 138
Chloral Hydrate 436
Diazepam 640
Flurazepam 907
LORazepam 1280
Midazolam 1411
PENTobarbital 1641
PHENobarbital 1651
Secobarbital 1875
Triazolam 2080

Hypnotic, Nonbenzodiazepine
Zolpidem 2182

Hypoglycemic Agent, Oral
GlipiZIDE 968
GlyBURIDE 974
MetFORMIN 1353

Immune Globulin
Botulism Immune Globulin (Intravenous-Human) 301
Cytomegalovirus Immune Globulin (Intravenous-Human) 576
Hepatitis B Immune Globulin (Human) 1008
Immune Globulin 1084
Rabies Immune Globulin (Human) 1800
Rh₀(D) Immune Globulin 1815
Tetanus Immune Globulin (Human) 1991
Varicella-Zoster Immune Globulin (Human) 2119

Immunomodulating Agent, Topical
Pimecrolimus 1675

Immunomodulator, Systemic
Interferon Alfa-2b 1138
Peginterferon Alfa-2b 1621

Immunosuppressant Agent
Antithymocyte Globulin (Equine) 182
Antithymocyte Globulin (Rabbit) 184
AzaTHIOprine 241
Cyclophosphamide 561
CycloSPORINE (Ophthalmic) 569
CycloSPORINE (Systemic) 564
Everolimus 821
InFLIXimab 1099
Mycophenolate 1453
RiTUXimab 1841
Sirolimus 1895
Tacrolimus (Systemic) 1963
Thalidomide 2000

Infantile Spasms, Treatment
Corticotropin 545
Valproic Acid and Derivatives 2102
Vigabatrin 2134

Inhalation, Miscellaneous
Cromolyn (Nasal) 553
Cromolyn (Systemic, Oral Inhalation) 551

Insulin, Combination
Insulin Aspart Protamine and Insulin Aspart 1117
Insulin Lispro Protamine and Insulin Lispro 1128
Insulin NPH and Insulin Regular 1132

Insulin, Intermediate-Acting
Insulin Detemir 1119
Insulin NPH 1130

Insulin, Long-Acting
Insulin Glargine 1121

Insulin, Rapid-Acting
Insulin Aspart 1114
Insulin Glulisine 1123
Insulin Lispro 1125

Insulin, Short-Acting
Insulin Regular 1134

Integrase Inhibitor
Dolutegravir 705
Raltegravir 1802

Interferon
Interferon Alfa-2b 1138
Peginterferon Alfa-2a 1617
Peginterferon Alfa-2b 1621

Interleukin-1 Receptor Antagonist
Anakinra 168
Canakinumab 361
Rilonacept 1828

Interleukin-6 Receptor Antagonist
Tocilizumab 2040

Intravenous Nutritional Therapy
Dextrose 637
Fat Emulsion (Plant Based) 846

Iron Salt
Ferrous Fumarate 865
Ferrous Gluconate 866
Ferrous Sulfate 868
Polysaccharide-Iron Complex 1701

Iron Salt, Parenteral
Ferric Gluconate 864
Iron Dextran Complex 1153
Iron Sucrose 1155

Keratolytic Agent
Podophyllum Resin 1693
Salicylic Acid 1860
Tazarotene 1971

Laxative, Bowel Evacuant
Polyethylene Glycol-Electrolyte Solution 1697

Laxative, Bulk-Producing
Psyllium 1773

Laxative, Hyperosmolar
Sorbitol 1924

Laxative, Lubricant
Mineral Oil 1419

Laxative, Miscellaneous
Lactulose 1193

Laxative, Osmotic
Glycerin 976
Magnesium Citrate 1292
Magnesium Hydroxide 1294
Magnesium Oxide 1296
Polyethylene Glycol 3350 1696

Polyethylene Glycol-Electrolyte Solution 1697
Sorbitol 1924

Laxative, Saline
Sodium Phosphates 1913

Laxative, Stimulant
Bisacodyl 293
Castor Oil 390
Docusate and Senna 702
Senna 1877

Laxative, Surfactant
Docusate 701
Docusate and Senna 702

Leprostatic Agent
Dapsone (Systemic) 586

Leukotriene Receptor Antagonist
Montelukast 1438
Zafirlukast 2164

5-Lipoxygenase Inhibitor
Zileuton 2173

Local Anesthetic, Injectable
Bupivacaine 318
Chloroprocaine 442
Lidocaine and Epinephrine 1245
Lidocaine (Systemic) 1239
Mepivacaine 1341
Ropivacaine 1849
Tetracaine (Systemic) 1994

Local Anesthetic, Ophthalmic
Lidocaine (Ophthalmic) 1241
Proparacaine 1755
Tetracaine (Ophthalmic) 1995

Local Anesthetic, Oral
Benzocaine 273
Dyclonine 727

Local Anesthetic, Topical
Benzocaine 273
Cocaine 533
Dibucaine 645
Lidocaine and Prilocaine 1246
Lidocaine and Tetracaine 1248
Lidocaine (Topical) 1242
Tetracaine (Topical) 1995

Local Anesthetic, Transdermal
Lidocaine (Topical) 1242

Local Anesthetic, Urinary
Phenazopyridine 1651

Low Molecular Weight Heparin (LMWH)
Enoxaparin 752

Lubricant, Ocular
Ocular Lubricant 1521
Sodium Chloride 1902

Lung Surfactant
Beractant 280
Calfactant 360
Lucinactant 1289
Poractant Alfa 1702

Luteinizing Hormone-Releasing Hormone Analog
Leuprolide 1215

Magnesium Salt
Magnesium L-aspartate Hydrochloride 1295
Magnesium Chloride 1291
Magnesium Citrate 1292
Magnesium Gluconate 1293

Magnesium Oxide 1296
Magnesium Sulfate 1297

Metabolic Alkalosis Agent
Ammonium Chloride 138
Arginine 195
Carglumic Acid 381

Mineralocorticoid
Fludrocortisone 887

Mineral, Oral
Ferrous Fumarate 865
Ferrous Gluconate 866
Ferrous Sulfate 868
Fluoride 894
Zinc Sulfate 2176

Mineral, Oral Topical
Fluoride 894

Mineral, Parenteral
Ferric Gluconate 864
Iron Dextran Complex 1153
Iron Sucrose 1155
Trace Elements 2059
Zinc Sulfate 2176

Monoclonal Antibody
Adalimumab 70
Basiliximab 263
Canakinumab 361
InFLIXimab 1099
Palivizumab 1584
RiTUXimab 1841
Tocilizumab 2040

Monoclonal Antibody, Anti-Asthmatic
Omalizumab 1533

mTOR Kinase Inhibitor
Sirolimus 1895

Mucolytic Agent
Acetylcysteine 60
Dornase Alfa 709

Mucopolysaccharidosis I (MPS I) Disease, Treatment Agent
Laronidase 1210

Muscle Contracture, Treatment
OnabotulinumtoxinA 1541
RimabotulinumtoxinB 1829

Nasal Agent, Vasoconstrictor
Naphazoline (Nasal) 1469
Oxymetazoline (Nasal) 1577
Phenylephrine (Nasal) 1660

Neuraminidase Inhibitor
Oseltamivir 1551
Zanamivir 2166

Neurolytic
Alcohol (Ethyl) 88

Neuromuscular Blocker Agent, Depolarizing
Succinylcholine 1938

Neuromuscular Blocker Agent, Nondepolarizing
Atracurium 232
Cisatracurium 479
Pancuronium 1593
Rocuronium 1847
Vecuronium 2123

Nitrate
Nitroglycerin 1504

Non-nucleoside Reverse Transcriptase Inhibitor (NNRTI)
Efavirenz 731
Efavirenz, Emtricitabine, and Tenofovir 735
Etravirine 819
Nevirapine 1487

Nonsteroidal Anti-inflammatory Drug (NSAID), COX-2 Selective
Celecoxib 425

Nonsteroidal Anti-inflammatory Drug (NSAID), Ophthalmic
Diclofenac (Ophthalmic) 648
Flurbiprofen (Ophthalmic) 910
Ketorolac (Ophthalmic) 1184

Nonsteroidal Anti-inflammatory Drug (NSAID), Oral
Aspirin 212
Choline Magnesium Trisalicylate 459
Diclofenac (Systemic) 645
Etodolac 812
Flurbiprofen (Systemic) 908
Ibuprofen 1059
Indomethacin 1096
Ketorolac (Systemic) 1180
Meloxicam 1325
Naproxen 1470
Oxaprozin 1562
Piroxicam 1683
Sulindac 1957
Tolmetin 2042

Nonsteroidal Anti-inflammatory Drug (NSAID), Parenteral
Ibuprofen 1059
Indomethacin 1096
Ketorolac (Systemic) 1180

Norepinephrine Reuptake Inhibitor, Selective
AtoMOXetine 224

Nucleoside Analog Reverse Transcriptase Inhibitor (NRTI)
Abacavir and Lamivudine 39
Abacavir, Lamivudine, and Zidovudine 41

Nucleoside Reverse Transcriptase Inhibitor (NRTI)
Abacavir 36
Didanosine 654
Efavirenz, Emtricitabine, and Tenofovir 735
Emtricitabine 738
Emtricitabine and Tenofovir 741
LamiVUDine 1194
Lamivudine and Zidovudine 1198
Stavudine 1932
Zidovudine 2168

Nucleotide Reverse Transcriptase Inhibitor (NRTI)
Efavirenz, Emtricitabine, and Tenofovir 735
Emtricitabine and Tenofovir 741
Tenofovir 1977

Nutritional Supplement
Ascorbic Acid 206
Biotin 292
Cholecalciferol 455
Cyanocobalamin 556
Cysteine 572
Ergocalciferol 774
Folic Acid 925
Hydroxocobalamin 1045
LevOCARNitine 1224
Medium Chain Triglycerides 1318
Niacin 1491
Phytonadione 1671
Pyridoxine 1778
Riboflavin 1821
Thiamine 2009
Vitamin A 2146
Vitamin E 2148

Ophthalmic Agent
Besifloxacin 281

Ophthalmic Agent, Miotic
Acetylcholine 59
Pilocarpine (Ophthalmic) 1675

Ophthalmic Agent, Miscellaneous
Artificial Tears 205
Ocular Lubricant 1521
Silver Nitrate 1889

Ophthalmic Agent, Mydriatic
Atropine 234
Cyclopentolate 560
Cyclopentolate and Phenylephrine 560
Homatropine 1018
Phenylephrine (Ophthalmic) 1661
Scopolamine (Ophthalmic) 1874
Tropicamide 2092

Ophthalmic Agent, Toxin
OnabotulinumtoxinA 1541

Ophthalmic Agent, Vasoconstrictor
Dipivefrin 692
Naphazoline (Ophthalmic) 1470

Opioid Partial Agonist
Buprenorphine 320
Buprenorphine and Naloxone 324
Nalbuphine 1464
Pentazocine 1639

Otic Agent, Analgesic
Antipyrine and Benzocaine 181

Otic Agent, Anti-infective
Acetic Acid 58

Otic Agent, Cerumenolytic
Antipyrine and Benzocaine 181
Carbamide Peroxide 377

Ovulation Stimulator
Chorionic Gonadotropin (Human) 460

Pancreatic Enzyme
Pancrelipase 1591

Pediculocide
Benzyl Alcohol 278
Ivermectin (Topical) 1172
Lindane 1250
Malathion 1300
Permethrin 1647
Spinosad 1930

Phenothiazine Derivative
ChlorproMAZINE 450
Perphenazine 1648
Prochlorperazine 1745
Promethazine 1748
Promethazine and Codeine 1750
Thioridazine 2012
Thiothixene 2015
Trifluoperazine 2082

Phosphate Binder
Sevelamer 1882

Phosphate Salt
Potassium Phosphate 1715
Potassium Phosphate and Sodium Phosphate 1718

Phosphodiesterase Enzyme Inhibitor
Anagrelide 166
Milrinone 1417

Phosphodiesterase Type-5 (PDE5) Inhibitor
Sildenafil 1884

Phosphodiestrerase-3 Enzyme Inhibitor
Anagrelide 166

Plasma Volume Expander
Albumin 82
Dextran 628
Hetastarch 1014

Plasma Volume Expander, Colloid
Tetrastarch 1998

Polyclonal Antibody
Antithymocyte Globulin (Equine) 182

Potassium Salt
Potassium Phosphate 1715
Potassium Phosphate and Sodium Phosphate 1718

Preservative Free
Abatacept 44
Acetaminophen 47
AcetaZOLAMIDE 56
Acetylcysteine 60
Adalimumab 70
Adenosine 76
Albumin 82
Albuterol 84
Alcohol (Ethyl) 88
Aldesleukin 90
Alfentanil 93
Alglucosidase Alfa 95
Allopurinol 97
Amifostine 116
Amikacin 118
Ampicillin 159
Anakinra 168
Antihemophilic Factor (Recombinant) 172
Anti-inhibitor Coagulant Complex (Human) 180
Artificial Tears 205
Ascorbic Acid 206
Atracurium 232
Atropine 234
AzaTHIOprine 241
Azithromycin (Systemic) 247
Aztreonam 254
Bacitracin 256
Baclofen 259
Basiliximab 263
Bevacizumab 288
Bleomycin 295
Botulism Immune Globulin (Intravenous-Human) 301
Bupivacaine 318
C1 Inhibitor (Human) 337
Caffeine 338
Calcium Carbonate 346
Calcium Chloride 349
Calcium Citrate 351
Calcium Gluconate 354
Calcium Lactate 358
Canakinumab 361
CARBOplatin 379
CeFAZolin 393
CefOXitin 408
CefTAZidime 413
Centruroides Immune F(ab')₂ (Equine) 428
Chloroprocaine 442
Cholecalciferol 455
Cidofovir 466
Ciprofloxacin (Otic) 476
Ciprofloxacin (Systemic) 471
Cisatracurium 479
CISplatin 481
Cladribine 488
Clofarabine 508
CloNIDine 516

Copper 544
Cosyntropin 549
Cromolyn (Systemic, Oral Inhalation) 551
Cyanocobalamin 556
CycloSPORINE (Ophthalmic) 569
Cysteine 572
Cytarabine (Conventional) 573
Cytomegalovirus Immune Globulin (Intravenous-Human) 576
Dacarbazine 578
DAPTOmycin 589
Darbepoetin Alfa 592
DAUNOrubicin (Conventional) 599
Dexamethasone (Ophthalmic) 619
Dexamethasone (Systemic) 615
Dexmedetomidine 621
Digoxin Immune Fab 663
Diltiazem 667
DiphenhydrAMINE (Systemic) 673
Diphtheria and Tetanus Toxoids 679
Diphtheria and Tetanus Toxoids, Acellular Pertussis, and Poliovirus Vaccine 682
Diphtheria and Tetanus Toxoids, and Acellular Pertussis Vaccine 686
Diphtheria, Tetanus Toxoids, Acellular Pertussis, Hepatitis B (Recombinant), and Poliovirus (Inactivated) Vaccine 690
DOBUTamine 696
DOXOrubicin (Conventional) 718
Doxycycline 721
Enoxaparin 752
EPHEDrine (Systemic) 759
EPINEPHrine (Systemic, Oral Inhalation) 761
Epoetin Alfa 766
Esmolol 791
Etanercept 803
Etomidate 814
Factor VIIa (Recombinant) 831
Famotidine 843
FentaNYL 853
Ferrous Gluconate 866
Ferrous Sulfate 868
Filgrastim 872
Fluconazole 877
Fludarabine 885
Folic Acid 925
Fomepizole 927
Furosemide 948
Gemcitabine 959
Glucarpidase 972
Granisetron 980
Haemophilus b Conjugate and Hepatitis B Vaccine 993
Haemophilus b Conjugate Vaccine 994
Haloperidol 998
Heparin 1001
Hepatitis A Vaccine 1005
Hepatitis B Immune Globulin (Human) 1008
Hepatitis B Vaccine (Recombinant) 1009
Hyaluronidase 1020
Hydrocortisone (Systemic) 1034
HYDROmorphone 1041
Ibuprofen 1059
IDArubicin 1067
Immune Globulin 1084
InFLIXimab 1099
Influenza Virus Vaccine (Inactivated) 1103
Influenza Virus Vaccine (Live/Attenuated) 1109
Iodixanol 1142
Ipratropium (Oral Inhalation) 1144
Irinotecan 1149
Iron Sucrose 1155
Ketorolac (Ophthalmic) 1184

Leucovorin Calcium 1213
Leuprolide 1215
Levalbuterol 1218
LevOCARNitine 1224
Levofloxacin (Systemic) 1228
Levothyroxine 1234
Lidocaine and Epinephrine 1245
Lidocaine (Ophthalmic) 1241
Lidocaine (Systemic) 1239
Lidocaine (Topical) 1242
Magnesium L-aspartate Hydrochloride 1295
Magnesium Gluconate 1293
Magnesium Oxide 1296
Measles, Mumps, and Rubella Virus Vaccine 1307
Measles, Mumps, Rubella, and Varicella Virus
   Vaccine 1310
Meningococcal (Groups A / C / Y and W-135)
   Diphtheria Conjugate Vaccine 1330
Mepivacaine 1341
Methotrexate 1367
MethylPREDNISolone 1386
Metoclopramide 1391
MetroNIDAZOLE (Systemic) 1399
Midazolam 1411
Milrinone 1417
Morphine (Systemic) 1440
Nafcillin 1462
Naloxone 1466
Niacin 1491
Norepinephrine 1510
Nystatin (Oral) 1516
Ocular Lubricant 1521
OnabotulinumtoxinA 1541
Ondansetron 1544
Oprelvekin 1549
Oxacillin 1555
Oxaliplatin 1557
PACLitaxel 1579
Palivizumab 1584
Pamidronate 1587
Papillomavirus (Types 6, 11, 16, 18) Vaccine (Human,
   Recombinant) 1600
Papillomavirus (Types 16, 18) Vaccine (Human,
   Recombinant) 1603
Pegaspargase 1615
Pegfilgrastim 1616
Peginterferon Alfa-2a 1617
Peginterferon Alfa-2b 1621
Penicillin G (Parenteral/Aqueous) 1631
Phenylephrine (Ophthalmic) 1661
Phytonadione 1671
Polymyxin B 1699
Poractant Alfa 1702
Potassium Gluconate 1711
Propofol 1755
Protamine 1764
Protein C Concentrate (Human) 1766
Psyllium 1773
Pyridoxine 1778
Rabies Immune Globulin (Human) 1800
Rabies Vaccine 1801
Ranitidine 1805
Remifentanil 1811
Rh$_o$(D) Immune Globulin 1815
Riboflavin 1821
Rilonacept 1828
RimabotulinumtoxinB 1829
RiTUXimab 1841
Rocuronium 1847
Ropivacaine 1849
Rotavirus Vaccine 1855
Sodium Chloride 1902
Sodium Phosphates 1913

Sodium Thiosulfate 1919
Somatropin 1920
Sucrose 1941
SUFentanil 1942
SUMAtriptan 1958
Tetracaine (Systemic) 1994
Thiamine 2009
Thrombin (Topical) 2017
Timolol (Ophthalmic) 2028
Tobramycin (Systemic, Oral Inhalation) 2034
Tocilizumab 2040
Topotecan 2053
Trace Elements 2059
Valproic Acid and Derivatives 2102
Vancomycin 2110
Varicella Virus Vaccine 2116
Varicella-Zoster Immune Globulin (Human) 2119
Vecuronium 2123
Velaglucerase Alfa 2124
VinCRIStine 2138
Vitamin A 2146
Vitamin E 2148
Zidovudine 2168
Zinc Sulfate 2176

Progestin
Hydroxyprogesterone Caproate 1049
MedroxyPROGESTERone 1318
Megestrol 1324
Norethindrone 1511

Prostaglandin
Alprostadil 103
Epoprostenol 770
Misoprostol 1423

Protease Inhibitor
Atazanavir 218
Darunavir 595
Fosamprenavir 931
Indinavir 1093
Lopinavir and Ritonavir 1272
Nelfinavir 1479
Ritonavir 1837
Saquinavir 1867
Tipranavir 2031

Protectant, Topical
Aluminum Hydroxide 110

Proton Pump Inhibitor
Esomeprazole 793
Lansoprazole 1206
Omeprazole 1535
Omeprazole and Sodium Bicarbonate 1538
Pantoprazole 1595
RABEprazole 1797

Radiological/Contrast Media, Nonionic
Iodixanol 1142

Recombinant Human Erythropoietin
Epoetin Alfa 766

Respiratory Stimulant
Aminophylline 124
Caffeine 338
Doxapram 711
Theophylline 2005

Retinoic Acid Derivative
Clindamycin and Tretinoin 503
ISOtretinoin 1161
Tretinoin (Systemic) 2068
Tretinoin (Topical) 2071

Rickets, Treatment Agent
Calcitriol 342

Salicylate
Aspirin 212
Choline Magnesium Trisalicylate 459

Scabicidal Agent
Crotamiton 555
Lindane 1250
Malathion 1300
Permethrin 1647

Sedative
Amobarbital 138
Chloral Hydrate 436
Clorazepate 524
Dexmedetomidine 621
Diazepam 640
DiphenhydrAMINE (Systemic) 673
Flurazepam 907
HydrOXYzine 1054
LORazepam 1280
Methohexital 1365
Midazolam 1411
Pentazocine 1639
PENTobarbital 1641
PHENobarbital 1651
Promethazine 1748
Secobarbital 1875
Triazolam 2080

Selective 5-HT$_3$ Receptor Antagonist
Dolasetron 703

Serotonin 5-HT$_{1D}$ Receptor Agonist
Almotriptan 99
Rizatriptan 1845

Shampoos
Lindane 1250
Selenium Sulfide 1877

Skeletal Muscle Relaxant, Miscellaneous
QuiNINE 1794

Skeletal Muscle Relaxant, Nonparalytic
Baclofen 259
Chlorzoxazone 454
Cyclobenzaprine 558
Dantrolene 583
Methocarbamol 1364

Skeletal Muscle Relaxant, Paralytic
Atracurium 232
Cisatracurium 479
Pancuronium 1593
Rocuronium 1847
Succinylcholine 1938
Vecuronium 2123

Smoking Cessation Aid
BuPROPion 327

Soap
Hexachlorophene 1016

Sodium Salt
Potassium Phosphate and Sodium Phosphate 1718
Sodium Acetate 1899
Sodium Bicarbonate 1901
Sodium Chloride 1902
Sodium Phosphates 1913

Somatostatin Analog
Octreotide 1518

Stool Softener
Docusate 701
Docusate and Senna 702

Substance P/Neurokinin 1 Receptor Antagonist
Aprepitant 190
Fosaprepitant 934

Substituted Benzimidazole
Omeprazole and Sodium Bicarbonate 1538

Sucrase Deficiency, Treatment Agent
Sacrosidase 1859

Sugar Free
Acetaminophen 47
Aluminum Hydroxide and Magnesium Hydroxide 111
Arginine 195
Ascorbic Acid 206
Aspirin 212
Benzocaine 273
Bismuth 294
Brompheniramine and Pseudoephedrine 306
Calcium Carbonate 346
Cetirizine 431
Chlorpheniramine 448
Cholecalciferol 455
Cholestyramine Resin 457
Citric Acid, Sodium Citrate, and Potassium
   Citrate 487
Colesevelam 539
Dextromethorphan 636
DiphenhydrAMINE (Systemic) 673
Docusate 701
Docusate and Senna 702
Ferrous Gluconate 866
Fluoride 894
Folic Acid 925
GuaiFENesin 984
Guaifenesin and Codeine 985
Guaifenesin and Dextromethorphan 987
Immune Globulin 1084
LevOCARNitine 1224
Loratadine 1278
LORazepam 1280
Magnesium L-aspartate Hydrochloride 1295
Magnesium Chloride 1291
Magnesium Hydroxide 1294
Methadone 1355
Niacin 1491
Phenylephrine (Systemic) 1658
Polysaccharide-Iron Complex 1701
Potassium Chloride 1708
Potassium Citrate and Citric Acid 1710
Potassium Gluconate 1711
Potassium Phosphate and Sodium Phosphate 1718
PrednisoLONE (Systemic) 1727
Pseudoephedrine 1770
Psyllium 1773
Pyrantel Pamoate 1774
Pyridoxine 1778
Ranitidine 1805
Sodium Citrate and Citric Acid 1906
Sodium Phosphates 1913
Sorbitol 1924
Tamoxifen 1968
Vitamin E 2148

Sympathomimetic
Albuterol 84
DOBUTamine 696
DOPamine 708
EPHEDrine (Systemic) 759
EPINEPHrine (Systemic, Oral Inhalation) 761
Formoterol 929

Isoproterenol 1160
Levalbuterol 1218
Metaproterenol 1352
Norepinephrine 1510
Phenylephrine (Nasal) 1660
Phenylephrine (Ophthalmic) 1661
Phenylephrine (Systemic) 1658
Phenylephrine (Topical) 1662
Pirbuterol 1683
Pseudoephedrine 1770
Terbutaline 1984
Triprolidine and Pseudoephedrine 2090

Theophylline Derivative
Aminophylline 124
Theophylline 2005

Thrombolytic Agent
Alteplase 104

Thrombopoietic Growth Factor
Oprelvekin 1549

Thrombotic Occlusion (Central Venous Catheter), Treatment Agent
Alteplase 104

Thyroid Product
Levothyroxine 1234
Liothyronine 1256
Liotrix 1258
Thyroid, Desiccated 2018

Tocolytic Agent
Terbutaline 1984

Topical Skin Product
Acetic Acid 58
Adapalene and Benzoyl Peroxide 74
Aluminum Acetate 110
Benzoyl Peroxide 275
Benzyl Alcohol 278
Calamine 340
Capsaicin 367
Clindamycin and Benzoyl Peroxide 502
Iodine 1141
Lactic Acid and Ammonium Hydroxide 1191
Silver Nitrate 1889
Sulfacetamide (Topical) 1944
Zinc Oxide 2176

Topical Skin Product, Acne
Adapalene and Benzoyl Peroxide 74

Trace Element
Zinc Acetate 2174
Zinc Chloride 2175
Zinc Sulfate 2176

Trace Element, Multiple, Neonatal
Trace Elements 2059

Trace Element, Parenteral
Copper 544
Trace Elements 2059

Transient Receptor Potential Vanilloid 1 (TRPV1) Agonist
Capsaicin 367

Tumor Necrosis Factor (TNF) Blocking Agent
Adalimumab 70
Etanercept 803
InFLIXimab 1099
Thalidomide 2000

Tyrosinemia Type 1, Treatment Agent
Nitisinone 1501

Urea Cycle Disorder (UCD) Treatment Agent
Arginine 195

Carglumic Acid 381
Sodium Benzoate 1900
Sodium Phenylacetate and Sodium Benzoate 1911
Sodium Phenylbutyrate 1912

Uric Acid Lowering Agent
Allopurinol 97
Probenecid 1739
Rasburicase 1808

Uricosuric Agent
Probenecid 1739

Urinary Acidifying Agent
Ammonium Chloride 138
Ascorbic Acid 206

Urinary Tract Product
Cysteamine (Systemic) 571

Vaccine
Diphtheria and Tetanus Toxoids 679
Diphtheria and Tetanus Toxoids, Acellular Pertussis, and Poliovirus Vaccine 682
Diphtheria and Tetanus Toxoids, Acellular Pertussis, Poliovirus and Haemophilus b Conjugate Vaccine 684
Diphtheria and Tetanus Toxoids, and Acellular Pertussis Vaccine 686
Diphtheria, Tetanus Toxoids, Acellular Pertussis, Hepatitis B (Recombinant), and Poliovirus (Inactivated) Vaccine 690
Haemophilus b Conjugate and Hepatitis B Vaccine 993
Haemophilus b Conjugate Vaccine 994
Hepatitis A Vaccine 1005
Hepatitis B Vaccine (Recombinant) 1009
Influenza Virus Vaccine (Inactivated) 1103
Influenza Virus Vaccine (Live/Attenuated) 1109
Meningococcal Polysaccharide Vaccine (Groups A / C / Y and W-135) 1336
Papillomavirus (Types 6, 11, 16, 18) Vaccine (Human, Recombinant) 1600
Pneumococcal Polysaccharide Vaccine (Polyvalent) 1691
Rabies Vaccine 1801
Tetanus Toxoid (Adsorbed) 1993
Typhoid Vaccine 2093
Varicella Virus Vaccine 2116
Yellow Fever Vaccine 2162

Vaccine, Inactivated Bacteria
Meningococcal (Groups A / C / Y and W-135) Diphtheria Conjugate Vaccine 1330
Meningococcal Polysaccharide (Groups C and Y) and Haemophilus b Tetanus Toxoid Conjugate Vaccine 1334
Poliovirus Vaccine (Inactivated) 1694

Vaccine, Inactivated (Bacterial)
Pneumococcal Conjugate Vaccine (13-Valent) 1688

Vaccine, Inactivated (Viral)
Papillomavirus (Types 16, 18) Vaccine (Human, Recombinant) 1603

Vaccine, Inactivated Virus
Influenza Virus Vaccine (Inactivated) 1103
Japanese Encephalitis Virus Vaccine (Inactivated) 1173

Vaccine, Live/Attenuated
Influenza Virus Vaccine (Live/Attenuated) 1109

Vaccine, Live Virus
Measles, Mumps, and Rubella Virus Vaccine 1307

Measles, Mumps, Rubella, and Varicella Virus
Vaccine 1310
Rotavirus Vaccine 1855

Vaccine, Recombinant
Influenza Virus Vaccine (Recombinant) 1112

Vascular Endothelial Growth Factor (VEGF) Inhibitor
Bevacizumab 288

Vasoconstrictor, Nasal
Oxymetazoline (Nasal) 1577

Vasoconstrictor, Ophthalmic
Oxymetazoline (Ophthalmic) 1578

Vasodilator
Diazoxide 643
Doxazosin 712
HydrALAZINE 1022
Nitroglycerin 1504
Nitroprusside 1507
Papaverine 1599
Phenoxybenzamine 1655
Phentolamine 1656
Prazosin 1724
Terazosin 1981

Vasodilator, Coronary
Amyl Nitrite 165
Dipyridamole 693
Nitroglycerin 1504

Vasopressin Analog, Synthetic
Desmopressin 612

Vitamin D Analog
Calcitriol 342
Cholecalciferol 455
Ergocalciferol 774
Paricalcitol 1606

Vitamin A Derivative
ISOtretinoin 1161

Vitamin, Fat Soluble
Calcitriol 342
Cholecalciferol 455
Ergocalciferol 774
Paricalcitol 1606
Phytonadione 1671
Vitamin A 2146
Vitamin E 2148

Vitamin, Topical
Tretinoin (Topical) 2071
Vitamin E 2148

Vitamin, Water Soluble
Ascorbic Acid 206
Biotin 292
Cyanocobalamin 556
Folic Acid 925
Hydroxocobalamin 1045
Niacin 1491
Pyridoxine 1778
Riboflavin 1821
Thiamine 2009

NOTES

NOTES

NOTES

NOTES

NOTES

NOTES

NOTES

NOTES

NOTES

NOTES

NOTES